ABPI DATA SHEET COMPENDIUM

1991–92

With The Code of Practice for the Pharmaceutical Industry

Compiled by Gillian Walker

Datapharm Publications Limited
12 Whitehall, London SW1A 2DY

THIS COMPENDIUM CAN BE USED UNTIL JANUARY 1993 WHEN IT WILL BE SUPERSEDED BY THE 1993–94 EDITION.

Responsibility for Data Sheets

The data sheets in this Compendium are prepared independently by each participating company and each proof is checked and the text confirmed as correct by the participant concerned. Neither Datapharm Publications Limited nor The Association of the British Pharmaceutical Industry (ABPI) give any guarantee whatsoever as to the accuracy of the information contained in the data sheets and accept no liability whatsoever in respect of any loss, damage or expense arising from any such information or for any error or omission in the data sheets and in particular (but without prejudice to the generality of the foregoing) shall not be liable for any consequential damages or expenses or any loss of profit or any liability to third parties incurred by anyone relying on the information contained in the data sheets appearing in this Compendium.

Published by Datapharm Publications Limited

Compiled by Gillian Walker
Produced by David Massam

ISBN 0 907102 06 9
ISSN 0306-9133

Printed and bound in Great Britain
by William Clowes Limited, Beccles and London

THE COMPENDIUM

Data sheets are supplied to practitioners in order to comply with the requirements of the Medicines Act 1968.

They are prepared by the individual companies concerned and, in consequence, vary somewhat in style. However, all follow the requirements laid down by 'The Medicines (Data Sheet) Regulations 1972'.

Participation in the Compendium is open to all companies supplying medicinal products intended for use under medical supervision.

Data sheets are intended for members of the medical and pharmaceutical professions and are written with them in mind. Any member of the public who reads them should bear in mind the need to take professional advice before making any decision affecting his or her own medication.

DATE OF PREPARATION

The data sheets included in this Compendium were finalised during the second quarter of 1991 and the Compendium itself was published in October 1991.

REVISED DATA SHEETS

Individual participating companies may issue loose leaf data sheets which supersede those included in this Compendium.

It is advisable to retain any such revised data sheets which are received and to indicate that fact on the corresponding data sheets in the Compendium.

LEGAL CATEGORY

The following abbreviations are used under the heading 'Legal category' in data sheets in the Compendium.

- GSL A preparation which is included in the General Sale List.
- P A pharmacy sale medicine which can be sold only from a retail pharmacy.
- POM A prescription only medicine.
- CD A preparation controlled by the Misuse of Drugs Act 1971 and Regulations. The CD is followed by (Sch 1), (Sch 2), (Sch 3), (Sch 4) or (Sch 5) depending on the schedule to the Misuse of Drugs Regulations 1985, as amended, in which the preparation is included.

Doctors are reminded that certain of the particulars must be in their own handwriting on prescriptions for preparations coming within Schedule 2 and Schedule 3 (except phenobarbitone) to the Misuse of Drugs Regulations 1985, as amended.

SYMBOLS AND ABBREVIATIONS

An asterisk (*) by the name of a product indicates that the name is a trade mark. The company symbols which appear in certain participants' sections are also trade marks.

An inverted triangle (▼) by the name of a product indicates that that product is newly introduced and there are special requirements as to the reporting of adverse reactions (see page xvi).

OP in the 'Package quantities' section of a data sheet indicates that the pack is an 'original pack'.

FURTHER INFORMATION

The regulations which relate to data sheets restrict the scope of the material which may be given under the heading 'Further information' and require insertion of the word 'Nil' in any data sheet where there is no entry under that heading. Companies are, of course, none the less always willing to provide additional information on their products upon request.

Enquiries should be directed to the companies concerned. Addresses and telephone numbers are provided in the Directory of Participants at the end of the Compendium.

Contents

Code of Practice for the Pharmaceutical Industry

First Revision of the Seventh Edition (January 1991)

For many years members of The Association of the British Pharmaceutical Industry have voluntarily agreed to observe the principles set out in a *Code of Practice for the Pharmaceutical Industry*; a Code which regulates the standards of conduct to be followed in the marketing of medicines intended for use under medical supervision.

The Code was first published in 1958 and has been regularly revised to take account of changes in marketing practices. A first revision of the seventh edition was introduced in 1991, publication following consultation with the British Medical Association and the Department of Health. The Code embodies the basic principles and procedures which the pharmaceutical industry believes to be essential for the conduct of its marketing activities and for the maintenance of standards which are in the interests alike of the public, the medical and allied professions and the industry.

On occasion, the criticism has been made that members of the medical profession were not aware of the provisions of the Code and, consequently, that the Code had been less effective than might otherwise have been the case. To ensure that these provisions become better known, the Code is reproduced in its entirety below.

Those who feel that the promotion of a medical speciality product has fallen below the standards which are required by the Code may write, if they so wish, to the Secretary, Code of Practice Committee, The Association of the British Pharmaceutical Industry, 12 Whitehall, London SW1A 2DY, and ask that the matter be investigated.

INTRODUCTION

a This Code of Practice for the Pharmaceutical Industry has been drawn up after consultation with the British Medical Association and the Department of Health.

b The Code owes its origin to the determination of the Association of the British Pharmaceutical Industry to secure the acceptance and adoption of high standards of conduct in the marketing of medical products designed for use under medical supervision.

c Medical products usually owe their existence to research carried out by their manufacturers or to the development by them of results of academic research. Before a medical product is placed on the market the manufacturer will have accumulated considerable toxicological, pharmacological and clinical evidence and will have met all the statutory requirements for the testing, manufacture and marketing of that product. Comprehensive legislation has been introduced to safeguard the public by ensuring that all products meet standards of quality, efficacy and safety which are acceptable in the state of present knowledge and experience.

d It is necessary, however, for the manufacturer, operating as he does in a keenly competitive industry and serving professions for which freedom of choice is essential, to draw attention to the existence and nature of a particular product; for example, by appropriate promotional measures and the dissemination of further knowledge and experience gained in widespread use.

e While it is possible to legislate satisfactorily for the testing, manufacture and control of medical products, the Association believes that appropriate standards of marketing conduct cannot be defined by the same means. For this reason, members of the Association have concurred in the promulgation of the Code of Practice and submitted to its restraints.

f The Code emphasises the importance in the public interest of providing the medical and allied professions with accurate, fair and objective information on medical products so that rational prescribing decisions can be made. Moreover, the Code accepts the principle that such information should be presented in a form and by ways and means which conform not only to legal requirements but also to ethical standards and canons of good taste.

The industry recognises its obligations to provide information about medical products to the pharmaceutical profession and the principles set out in this Code, therefore, apply equally to communications addressed to that profession. However, there may be instances where compliance with every provision of the Code would be inappropriate; for example, in connection with promotional material the purpose of which is to convey information of a commercial nature to pharmacists or pharmaceutical distributors.

g The Code, therefore, represents an act of self-discipline. Acceptance and observance of its provisions are a condition of membership of the Association of the British Pharmaceutical Industry. Member companies also acknowledge that the Code itself is to be applied in the spirit, as well as in the letter.

Pharmaceutical companies outside the Association are invited to accept and observe the Code because it is considered that high ethical standards should be followed throughout the whole industry if it is to maintain the confidence of all the interests which it serves.

h The Code is administered by a Committee established by the Board of Management of the Association. The Committee, with an independent legally qualified Chairman from outside the industry, consists of three independent members who are medically qualified persons not engaged in the industry, and fourteen members who are drawn from the senior management of member companies, including at least five medical directors or medically qualified persons of equivalent status.

The Chairman has general authority to obtain expert assistance in any field, and has an original and a casting vote.

i The Committee meets regularly to deal with complaints, to secure compliance with the Code, and to make such recommendations as it deems fit for the amendment of the provisions of the Code.

j An outstanding feature has been the success of voluntary compliance with the provisions of the Code and acceptance of the rulings of the Committee. It has not been found necessary to apply sanctions to secure compliance because members of the Association are anxious to ensure that their marketing activities conform to the highest standard.

k It is important, therefore, that the Code should accurately reflect that standard and for this reason it is kept under constant review by the Board of Management and amended from time to time where necessary to clarify it and bring it up to date. Notes for the guidance of member companies are issued periodically to keep them informed of the rulings and recommendations of the Committee and of any alterations to the Code.

l This edition of the Code supersedes all previous issues and is the seventh edition since the Code was established in 1958. It embodies the basic principles and provisions which the pharmaceutical industry believes are essential for the conduct of its marketing activities and for the maintenance of standards which are in the interests alike of the public, the medical and allied professions and the industry.

PROVISIONS OF THE CODE

The supplementary text, which appears in italics, is intended to give guidance as to the interpretation of the Code.

1 Definition of certain terms

1.1 The term 'promotion' means those informational and marketing activities, undertaken by a pharmaceutical company or with its authority, the purpose of which is to induce the prescribing, supply or administration of its medical products.

It includes the activities of representatives and all other aspects of sales promotion in whatever form, such as journal and direct mail advertising; participation in exhibitions; the use of audio-cassettes, films, records, tapes and video recordings; the use of viewdata systems and data storage devices such as memory discs accessed and reproduced on television apparatus, visual display units and the like; the provision of samples, gifts and hospitality.

The term 'promotion' does not extend to:

(i) Replies made in response to enquiries from particular doctors or to replies in response to a specific communication, whether of enquiry or comment, including letters published in a medical journal.

(ii) Announcements of pack changes, adverse reaction warnings or recall of products provided they contain no product claims.

(iii) 'Trade advertisements' as defined in the Medicines (Advertising of Medicinal Products) Regulations 1975, i.e. catalogues, price lists or other documents issued with a view to wholesale dealing but not containing any reference to product usage other than a therapeutic classification.

By 'wholesale dealing' is meant the sale of a product to a person who, during the course of his business or professional practice, buys it for the purpose of selling it or administering it or causing it to be administered to one or more human beings.

1.2 The term 'medical product' means any unbranded or branded pharmaceutical product intended for use in humans which is promoted to the medical profession rather than directly to the lay public.

1.3 The term 'medical profession', 'practice of medicine', 'practitioner' and 'doctor' should be interpreted to extend to the dental profession and be construed accordingly.

1.4 The term 'medical representative' means a representative whose duties comprise or include calling upon members of the medical profession.

2 Methods of promotion

Methods of promotion must never be such as to bring discredit upon, or reduce confidence in, the pharmaceutical industry.

The issue of rubber stamps to doctors for use as aids to prescription writing is one of the methods of promotion barred by this Clause.

3 Grant of product licence

A medical product must not be promoted prior to the grant of the product licence authorising its sale or supply.

This prohibition does not apply to any product which is exempt from the need to be the subject of a product licence.

4 Nature and availability of information

4.1 Upon reasonable request, the company concerned shall promptly provide members of the medical profession with accurate and relevant information about the medical products which the company markets.

4.2 Information about medical products should accurately reflect current knowledge or responsible opinion.

4.3 Information about medical products must be accurate, balanced and must not mislead either directly or by implication.

Claims for superior potency per unit weight are meaningless and best avoided unless they can be linked with some practical advantage, e.g. reduction in side-effects or cost of effective dosage.

4.4 Information must be capable of substantiation, such substantiation being provided without delay at the request of members of the medical profession.

The application of Clauses 4 and 5 of the Code is not limited to information or claims of a medical or scientific nature. It includes, inter alia, information or claims relating to pricing and market share.

Thus, for example, any claim relating to market share of a product must be substantiated without delay to members of the medical profession upon request.

5 Claims and comparisons

5.1 Claims for a medical product must be based on an up-to-date evaluation of all the evidence and must reflect this evidence accurately and clearly.

5.2 Exaggerated or all-embracing claims must not be made and superlatives must not be used. Claims should not imply that a medical product, or an active ingredient, has some special merit, quality or property unless this can be substantiated.

5.3 Any statement about side-effects should be specific and based on data submitted with the licence application or notified to the licensing authority, or on published data to which references are given. It should not be stated that a product has no side-effects, toxic hazards or risks of addiction. The word 'safe' must not be used without qualification.

5.4 The word 'new' should not be used to describe any product or presentation which has been generally available, or any therapeutic indication which has been generally promoted, for more than twelve months in the United Kingdom.

5.5 Comparisons of products must be factual, fair, and capable of substantiation. In presenting a comparison, care must be taken to ensure that it does not mislead by distortion, by undue emphasis, or in any other way.

'Hanging' comparatives, which merely claim that a product is 'better' or 'stronger', etc, must not be used.

5.6 Brand names of products of other companies must not be used unless the prior consent of the proprietors has been obtained.

6 Disparaging references

6.1 The products or services of other companies should not be disparaged either directly or by implication.

Substantiated comparative claims inviting fair comparisons with a group of products or with other products in the same field are permissible, provided that such claims are not presented in a way which is likely to mislead, whether by distortion, undue emphasis or otherwise.

6.2 The clinical and scientific opinions of members of the medical and allied professions should not be disparaged either directly or by implication.

7 Printed promotional material

7.1 The Medicines Act 1968 requires a pharmaceutical company to provide a practitioner with a data sheet before promoting a product directly to him. The content of such data sheets is determined by Regulations made under the Medicines Act.

Data Sheets for many prescription products are published in the ABPI Data Sheet Compendium which is issued at regular intervals. Copies of the Compendium are supplied to members of the medical and pharmaceutical professions.

7.2 All other printed material (including journal advertising) which is issued for promotional purposes by the product licence holder or with his authority must include certain information specified in this Code.

The requirements of Clause 7.3 or 7.4, as appropriate, must be complied with in any advertising directed towards the medical profession even if it is of a general nature, e.g. prestige advertisements listing a company's products.

An advertisement which would not otherwise conform with the Code should not be regarded as doing so by reason only of the fact that the content of the data sheet is reproduced as part of the advertisement or because a data sheet is sent with the advertisement.

7.3(i) Except for 'abbreviated advertisements', as defined in Clause 7.4, the following information must be given clearly and concisely on printed promotional material:

a The number of the relevant product licence and the name and address of the holder of the licence, or the business name and address of the part of his business responsible for the sale of the product.

b A quantitative list of the active ingredients, using approved names where such exist, or other non-proprietary names; alternatively, the non-proprietary name of the product if it is the subject of an accepted monograph.

Attention is drawn to the fact that the Medicines (Advertising to Medical and Dental Practitioners) Regulations 1978 (SI 1978 No. 1020) impose additional requirements which relate to the position and type size of this information.

c At least one authorised indication for use consistent with the data sheet.

d A succinct statement of the information in the data sheet relating to the dosage and method of use relevant to the indications quoted in the advertisement and, where not otherwise obvious, the route of administration.

e A succinct statement of the side-effects, precautions and contra-indications relevant to the indications in the advertisement, giving, in an abbreviated form, the substance of the relevant information in the data sheet.

f Any warning issued by the Medicines Commission, a committee appointed under Section 4 of the Medicines Act 1968 or the licensing authority, which is required to be included in advertisements.

g The cost of a product, except in the case of advertisements in journals which have an appreciable proportion of their circulation outside the United Kingdom.

The cost of a product is the cost (excluding value added tax) of either a specified package of the product, or a specified quantity or recommended daily dose, calculated by reference to any specified package of the product.

Attention is drawn to the fact that the Medicines (Advertising to Medical and Dental Practitioners) Regulations 1978 (SI 1978 No. 1020) impose a specific requirement to that proportion of the circulation of a journal which has to be outside the United Kingdom in order to qualify for the exception to this requirement.

7.3(ii) The information required by Clause 7.3 (i) (d), (e) and (f) must be printed in such type and in such a position that its relationship to the claims and indications is readily appreciated by the reader.

7.4(i) The requirements of Clause 7.3 do not apply in the case of an 'abbreviated advertisement'. An 'abbreviated advertisement' is one, the text of which contains in relation to the product no more than:

a The brand name of the product.

b The approved names of the active ingredients, where such names exist, or other non-proprietary names; alternatively, the non-proprietary name of the product if it is the subject of an accepted monograph.

Attention is drawn to the fact that the Medicines (Advertising to Medical and Dental Practitioners) Regulations 1978 (SI 1978 No. 1020), impose additional requirements which relate to the position and type of this information.

c The name and address of the product licence holder, or the business name and address of the part of his business responsible for the sale of the product.

d One indication for use, or more than one indication provided that these are related, consistent with the data sheet.

e A concise statement, consistent with the data sheet, giving the reason why the product is recommended for such indication or indications.

f A form of words which indicates clearly that further information is available on request to the licence holder or is to be found in the data sheet relating to the product.

7.4(ii) An 'abbreviated advertisement' must always contain the information required by Clause 7.4(i) (a), (b), (c) and (f). The information required by Clause

7.4(i) (d) and (e) is optional. An 'abbreviated advertisement' must not include any illustration which is likely to convey any information about the product or imply claims which are additional to those provided in accordance with Clause 7.4(i) (a) to (e) inclusive.

7.4(iii) An 'abbreviated advertisement' directed towards a doctor is permissible only when it constitutes an advertisement appearing in a publication sent or delivered wholly or mainly to doctors. A loose insert included in such a publication cannot be an 'abbreviated advertisement'. A promotional mailing or representative leave-piece cannot be an 'abbreviated advertisement' and an 'abbreviated advertisement' cannot appear as part of another promotional item, such as in a brochure consisting of a full advertisement for another of a company's products.

Attention is drawn to the fact that the Medicines (Advertising to Medical and Dental Practitioners) Regulations 1978 (SI 1978 No. 1020) impose additional requirements which relate to the maximum permitted size of an 'abbreviated advertisement'.

7.4(iv) An 'abbreviated advertisement' is not permissible where the Medicines Commission, a committee appointed under Section 4 of the Medicines Act 1968 or the licensing authority, has required a warning to be included in any advertisement relating to the medical product, and the licensing authority has issued a direction that 'abbreviated advertisements' should not be issued.

7.5 Promotional material, such as mailings and journal advertisements, must not be designed to disguise its real nature.

Doctors rightly resent receiving promotional material in the guise of personal communications, as when advertisements are enclosed in a plain envelope or are addressed in real or facsimile handwriting on letters or postcards.

Envelopes should not be used for the dispatch of promotional material if they bear words implying that the contents are non-promotional, e.g. that the contents provide information relating to safety.

It is advisable to use first class mail only for important communications of a non-promotional nature such as notifications of warnings or cautions or the withdrawal or recall of a product.

Advertisements in journals should not be designed so as to resemble editorial matter.

7.6 Promotional material should conform, both in text and illustration, to canons of good taste and should recognise the professional standing of the recipients.

Representations of the nude female form (even in silhouette) or partly clothed figures should not be used in promotional material in such a way as to arouse a visual or emotional response in order to attract attention to the text.

Displays of part of the naked body which are necessary to illustrate pictorially the message of the text are permissible provided that they conform to the dictates of decency and good taste.

7.7 Doctors' names or photographs must not be used in a prominent manner in promotional material or in any other way that is contrary to the ethical code of the medical profession.

7.8 Promotional material should not imitate the devices, copy, slogans or general layout adopted by other companies in a way that is likely to mislead or confuse.

7.9 Where appropriate, for example, in technical and other informative material, the date of printing or the last review should be stated.

7.10 (i) Extremes of format, size or cost of printed material should be avoided.

7.10 (ii) No advertisement included in a journal may consist of more than two consecutive pages.

7.10 (iii) No advertisement taking the form of a loose insert in a journal may consist of more than a single sheet of a size no larger than the page size of the journal itself, printed on one or both sides.

Large size mailings which cannot be put through letter boxes are a source of irritation to doctors and should be avoided as far as possible.

7.11 Postcards, other exposed mailings, envelopes or wrappers should not carry matter which might be regarded as advertising to the lay public or which could be considered unsuitable for public view.

Postcards and other exposed mailings should not contain copy or illustrations which ought not to be read or seen by lay persons.

7.12 'Telemessages' and 'Telex' must not be used for promotional purposes.

7.13 In a two page journal advertisement only one page need include the information required by Clause 7.3 of the Code provided that the other page (except where it faces the page on which the information is printed) includes a reference, on an outer edge, in at least 8 point type, indicating where that information appears. Where the two pages of the advertisement are not facing, neither must be false or misleading when read in isolation.

Where an advertisement consists of a double-sided insert in a journal, neither side must be false or misleading when read in isolation.

By 'two page journal advertisement' is meant an advertisement on two pages in a journal where the pages follow on without interruption. Where the pages do not follow on without interruption, each individual page is regarded as a separate advertisement.

Promotional material on two consecutive right-hand pages in a journal cannot, for example, be a single advertisement.

7.14 In a multi-page advertisement other than a press advertisement, the information required by Clause 7.3 of the Code must appear on one or more continuous pages and, where such an advertisement consists of more than four pages, the advertisement must include a clear indication as to where this information may be found.

8 References to official bodies

Promotional material should not include any reference to the Medicines Commission, a committee appointed under Section 4 of the Medicines Act 1968 or the licensing authority, unless this is specifically required by the licensing authority.

9 References to the National Health Service

9.1 Where reference is made to the prescribing of a product under the National Health Service, the phrase 'freely prescribable' or similar phrases suggesting a lack of restriction or restraint must not be used.

This Clause was inserted in the first edition of the Code in deference to the wishes of the then Ministry of Health. 'Freely' in this context means 'without restriction or restraint'.

Although NHS doctors are free to prescribe whatever medicines they consider necessary for the treatment of a patient, they are nevertheless required to exercise due economy.

9.2 Reproductions of official documents, such as prescription form FP 10, should not be used for promotional purposes unless the agreement of the appropriate Government department has been received.

The term 'reproduction' includes any depiction which simulates or might be taken to simulate the document in question.

10 Artwork, graphs, illustrations, etc.

10.1 Illustrations must not mislead as to the nature of the claims or comparisons being made, nor as to the purposes for which the product is used; nor should illustrations detract from warnings or contra-indications.

10.2 Artwork and graphs must conform to the letter and the spirit of the Code. Graphs and tables should be presented in such a way as to give a clear, fair, balanced view of the matters with which they deal, and should only be included if they are strictly relevant to the claims or comparisons being made.

10.3 Graphs and tables must not be used in any way which might mislead; for example, by their incompleteness or by the use of suppressed zeros or unusual scales.

11 Reprints, abstracts and quotations

11.1 Reprints of articles by members of the medical profession must not be included in mailings but may be supplied to individual doctors on request. It is permissible to include in promotional material reasonably brief abstracts of, or quotations from, articles by members of the medical profession and to include in such material reference to doctors' names in a bibliography of published works. In no case, however, should doctors' names be used in a prominent manner in promotional material.

11.2 Quotations from medical literature, or from personal communications received from doctors, must accurately reflect the meaning of the author and the significance of the study.

11.3 Quotations relating to medical products taken from public broadcasts (e.g. radio and television) and from private occasions, such as medical conferences or symposia, may not be used without the written permission of the speaker.

11.4 The utmost care must be taken to avoid ascribing claims or views relating to medical products to authors when such claims or views no longer represent, or may not represent, the current views of the authors concerned.

12 Distribution of printed promotional material

12.1 Promotional material should only be sent or distributed to those categories of persons whose need for, or interest in, the particular information can reasonably be assumed.

12.2 Any information designed to encourage the use of medical products in clinics, industrial concerns, clubs or schools must be addressed to the medical adviser or medical officer or to medical auxiliary staff.

12.3 Restraint should be exercised on the frequency of distribution and on the volume of promotional material distributed.

The style of mailings is relevant to their acceptability to doctors and criticism of their frequency is most likely to arise where their informational content is limited or where they appear to be elaborate and expensive. A higher frequency rate will be accepted for mailings on 'new' products than for others.

12.4 Mailing lists must be kept up-to-date. Requests from doctors to be removed from promotional mailing lists must be complied with promptly and no name may be restored except at the doctor's request or with his permission.

13 Audio-visual material

The expression 'audio-visual material' is to be interpreted as including material which consists either of sound only or of projected moving or still pictures only. It includes sound recordings, cinematograph films, tape-slide presentations, video-recordings and sound or television broadcasting. It does not include information reproduced on television apparatus, visual display units and the like which comes within the scope of Clause 14.

13.1 Audio-visual material must comply with all relevant requirements of the Code, with the exception of Clause 7.3.

13.2 When audio-visual material is used to promote a product, the information required by Clause 7.3 (i) of the Code must be provided either by way of a document made available to all persons to whom the material is played or shown, or to whom it is sent, or, except in the case of material which consists of sound only, by way of inclusion as part of the audio-visual material.

13.3 Where the information required by Clause 7.3 (i) is provided as part of the audio-visual material, it must appear visually in or with the advertisement and be of sufficient clarity and duration that it can be read easily.

The information provided in accordance with Clause 13.3 must not be separate from the advertisement itself but must appear as part of it or immediately before or after it.

13.4 Audio-visual promotional material is subject to the certification requirements of Clause 15.

14 Material reproduced on television apparatus, visual display units and the like

14 (i) Promotional material which is made available to hospitals, doctors, pharmacists etc., by systems which enable the material to be accessed and reproduced on to television apparatus, visual display units and the like, must comply with all relevant requirements of the Code, with the exception of Clauses 7.3 and 7.14.

Such material includes viewdata systems, memory discs and the like, but not video-tapes, which come within the scope of Clause 13.

14 (ii) The obligatory information required by Clause 7.3(i)(a) to (f) must be available through the system conveying the promotional material and instructions for accessing that information must be displayed with the promotional material

14 (iii) Promotional material made available in this way is subject to the certification requirements of Clause 15.

Copies of promotional information made available in this way must be made in permanent form and retained for not less than three years.

15 Certification of printed promotional material

15.1 No promotional material shall be issued unless the final text and layout have been certified by two persons on behalf of the company in the manner provided by this Clause. One of the two persons shall be a doctor. The other shall be a pharmacist or some other appropriately qualified person or a senior official of the company. The doctor, pharmacist or other qualified person must be a senior employee of the company or an appropriately qualified person whose services are retained for that purpose.

15.2 The names of those nominated, together with their qualifications, shall be notified in advance to the licensing authority. The names and qualifications of designated alternative signatories must also be given. Changes in the names of nominees must be promptly notified.

15.3 The certificate shall certify that the signatories have examined the material in its final form and that in their belief it is in accordance with the requirements of the relevant advertising regulations and this Code of Practice, is consistent with the product licence and the data sheet, and is a fair and truthful presentation of the facts about the product.

15.4 Companies shall preserve all certificates, together with the material in the form certified, for not less than three years and produce them upon request from the licensing authority or the Association at the instance of the Code of Practice Committee.

15.5 The foregoing procedure shall apply, with the necessary variations, to audio-visual material prepared by or on behalf of companies in accordance with Clause 13, to promotional material provided by or with the authority of companies for reproduction on television apparatus, visual display units and the like in accordance with Clause 14 and to briefing material for representatives prepared in accordance with Clause 17.12.

16 Suspension of advertisements or practices

In the event of the Code of Practice Committee requiring a company either:

(i) to suspend the use of an advertisement pending its decision on a complaint by the licensing authority relevant to the safe or proper use of the product, in accordance with paragraph 8 of the 'Constitution and Procedure for the Code of Practice Committee', or,

(ii) to suspend a practice or the use of an advertisement in accordance with paragraph 13 of the 'Constitution and Procedure for the Code of Practice Committee',

the company shall comply forthwith.

17 Medical representatives

17.1 Medical representatives must be adequately trained and possess sufficient medical and technical knowledge to present information on the company's products in an accurate and responsible manner.

17.2 Medical representatives should at all times maintain a high standard of ethical conduct in the discharge of their duties.

17.3 The requirements of the Code which aim at accuracy, fairness, balance, and good taste apply to oral representations as well as printed material.

17.4 Unfair or misleading comparisons or comparisons implying a therapeutic advantage which is not in fact justified must be avoided by medical representatives.

17.5 Claims made for products by medical representatives must be limited to the indications permitted by the product licence.

17.6 Medical representatives must not employ any inducement or subterfuge to gain an interview. No payment of a fee should be made for the grant of an interview.

The practice of gaining or extending an interview on the pretext of carrying out a survey is to be avoided. This does not preclude the use of medical representatives to obtain bona fide survey information, but it is essential that the survey should be devised and conducted so as to leave no doubt in the doctor's mind that the survey will produce medically useful information.

17.7 Medical representatives must ensure that the frequency, timing and duration of calls on doctors, or on hospitals, together with the manner in which they are made, do not cause inconvenience. The wishes of an individual doctor, or the arrangements in force at any particular establishment, must be observed by medical representatives.

The number of calls made on a medical practitioner and the intervals between successive visits are relevant to the determination of frequency.

Companies should arrange that intervals between visits do not cause inconvenience to practitioners and the number of calls made by a medical representative each year should not normally exceed, on average, three visits to each doctor.

Averages are to be calculated separately for general practitioners and other members of the medical profession to whom visits are made.

The calculation should exclude:

(i) Attendance by a medical representative at a scientific meeting or an audio-visual presentation given to a group of doctors.

(ii) A visit which is requested by a doctor or a call which is made in order to respond to a specific enquiry.

(iii) A visit to follow up a report of an adverse reaction.

A medical representative should not stay in a surgery in which another medical representative is already waiting, except with the doctor's or receptionist's approval.

Medical representatives must always endeavour to treat the doctor's time with the utmost respect and give him no cause to believe that his time might have been wasted. If, for any unavoidable reasons, an appointment with a doctor cannot be kept, the longest possible notice must be given.

Calls on hospital medical staff should generally be limited to matters likely to be of specific interest to them. The majority are specialists and medical representatives should ensure that their specialised interests are borne in mind. It is preferable for most hospital staff to be seen only after making a prior appointment, at which time subjects for discussion should be identified.

17.8 Medical representatives must take adequate precautions to ensure the security of medical products in their possession.

17.9 Medical representatives must not use the telephone to promote products to the medical profession unless prior arrangement has been made with individual doctors.

17.10 Medical representatives should be paid on the basis of a fixed basic salary, and any addition proportional to sales of prescription medicines should not constitute an undue proportion of their remuneration.

17.11 When discussion about a product is initiated by a medical representative, he should place before the doctor for reference either a data sheet in respect of that product or another document with the same content. If, however, the doctor asks a question about a different product, then the medical representative will not be required to produce such data in respect of that other product.

17.12 Companies must prepare detailed briefing material for medical representatives on the technical aspects of any product which the medical representative is to promote. A copy of such material must be made available to the licensing authority on request. Briefing material must comply with the relevant requirements of the Code and, in particular, is subject to the certification requirements of Clause 15.

17.13 Medical representatives should not make a claim for a product based on the regulatory treatment of that product, or of competing products, or based on any warnings issued in relation to other products, unless in accordance with a specific requirement. However, a medical representative may refer to such matters in answer to a specific question.

17.14 A company may only employ as medical representatives persons who have passed the examination established by the Association except that:

17.14(i) Persons with an acceptable professional qualification, e.g. in pharmacy, medicine or nursing, who were employed as medical representatives at any time before 1 October 1984 are exempt from this requirement.

17.14(ii) Persons who were employed as medical representatives on 1 October 1979 are exempt from this requirement.

17.14(iii) Trainee medical representatives may be employed for a period of up to two years from the date of commencing training as a medical representative.

18 Samples

18.1 Samples intended for treatment should be provided to a doctor only in response to a signed request.

A company may make available to a doctor a pre-printed request form or card; such a form or card may bear no more than the doctor's name, the company's name and address and an identifying reference, together with guidance as to the further information which the doctor himself must add. This limitation as to the provision of information on a pre-printed request form or card does not apply, however, in the case of a product controlled under the Misuse of Drugs Act 1971.

If such a pre-printed form or card is presented by a representative, then the doctor himself must complete the form by inserting the requisite information.

Wherever practicable, an individual sample should not represent more than four days' treatment for a single patient.

18.2 A signed request is not required when samples are provided to assist doctors in the recognition or identification of a product, or to demonstrate the use of a particular apparatus or equipment. Only the minimum quantity necessary for this purpose should be supplied.

18.3 No samples should be mailed to doctors except in response to a request. Samples which are sent by post must be packed so as to be reasonably secure against the package being opened by young children.

18.4 Where samples of products restricted by law to supply on prescription are distributed by a representative, the sample must be handed direct to the doctor or given to a person authorised to receive the sample on his behalf. A similar practice must be adopted for products which it would be unsafe to use except under medical supervision.

18.5 Samples of products restricted by law to supply on prescription, which are made available to representatives for distribution, should be strictly limited in quantity and an adequate system of accountability should be established.

18.6 Distribution of samples in hospitals should comply with individual hospital regulations, if any.

19 Gifts and inducements

19.1 Subject to Clause 19.2 no gift or financial inducement shall be offered or given to members of the medical profession for purposes of sales promotion.

Schemes designed to test the extent to which mailings are opened and read and which involve a reward, e.g. a reward for the return of a voucher included in the mailing, are unacceptable if the gift is one which would not come within Clause 19.2.

19.2 Gifts in the form of articles designed as promotional aids, whether related to a particular product or of general utility, may be distributed to members of the medical and allied professions provided the gift is inexpensive and relevant to the practice of medicine or pharmacy.

Amongst other items, nail brushes, book matches and pens have been held to be reasonable gifts. Gifts of table mats have been held to be in contravention of the Code as being irrelevant to the practice of medicine or pharmacy.

19.3 The requirements of Clause 7.3 or Clause 7.4 do not apply if a promotional aid of the type mentioned in Clause 19.2 bears no more than one or more of the following particulars:

(i) The name of the product.

(ii) The name of the product licence holder or the name of that part of his business responsible for the sale of the product.

(iii) The address of the product licence holder or the address of the part of his business responsible for the sale of the product.

(iv) An indication that the product name is a trade mark.

If a promotional aid consists of a note pad in which the individual pages bear advertising material, there is no need for the individual pages to comply with Clause 7 provided that the information required by the Clause is given elsewhere in the pad; for example, on the cover.

20 Hospitality

Entertainment or other hospitality offered to members of the medical and allied professions for purposes of sales promotion should always be secondary to the main purpose of the meeting. It should not extend beyond members of the professions. The level of hospitality should be appropriate and not out of proportion to the occasion; its cost should not exceed that level which the recipients might normally adopt when paying for themselves.

Medical and group meetings are desirable and are to be encouraged. Both the British Medical Association and the Association share the opinion that such meetings should only take place if the advertising content is supported by a clear educational content. If hospitality is offered at meetings attendance should be restricted to members of the medical and allied professions.

It follows, therefore, that invitations to such medical and group meetings should not be extended to wives or husbands unless they themselves are practising members of the medical or allied professions.

When organising a meeting at which hospitality will be offered, a factor to be taken into account is the impression which will be created in the minds of the recipients or those who hear about it. Hospitality which becomes little more than pure entertainment has limited value in terms of the provision of information and promotion; such hospitality can only be regarded, therefore, as irrelevant and wasteful.

21 Marketing research

Marketing research is the collection and analysis of information and must be unbiased and non-promotional. The use to which the statistics or information is put may be promotional. The two phases should be kept distinct.

21.1 Methods used for marketing research must never be such as to bring discredit upon, or to reduce confidence in, the pharmaceutical industry. The following provisions apply whether the research is carried out directly by the company concerned or by an organisation acting on the company's behalf.

21.2 The following information must be made available to the informant at first approach:

(i) The nature of the survey.

(ii) The name and address of the organisation carrying out the work.

(iii) The identity of the interviewer.

(iv) The nature and length of the interview.

The requirement in Clause 21.2(ii) does not mean that the organisation is also obliged to reveal the identity of its client. This must depend upon the contract between the client and the organisation.

21.3 Questions intended to solicit disparaging references to competing products or companies must be avoided.

21.4 Any written or oral statement given or made to an informant in order to obtain co-operation must be both factually correct and honoured.

21.5 Any incentives offered to the informants should be kept to a minimum and be commensurate with the work involved.

21.6 Marketing research must not in any circumstances be used as a disguised form of sales promotion and the research *per se* must not have as a direct objective the influencing of the opinions of the informant.

21.7 The identity of an informant must be treated as being confidential, unless he has specifically agreed otherwise.

In the absence of this agreement it follows that the information provided (as distinct from the overall results of the research) must not be used as the basis upon which a subsequent approach is made to that informant for the purpose of sales promotion.

21.8 Precautions should be taken to ensure that no embarrassment results for informants following on from an interview, or from any subsequent communication concerning the research project.

22 Relations with the general public

22.1 Medicines which cannot legally be sold or supplied to the public otherwise than in accordance with a prescription, or which are legally limited to promotion for sale or supply only on prescription, must not be advertised to the general public.

22.2 Information about medicines which is made available to the general public either directly or indirectly must be factual and presented in a balanced way so as to avoid the risks of raising unfounded hopes of successful treatment or of misleading with respect to the safety of the product.

Statements must not be made for the purpose of encouraging members of the public to ask their doctors to prescribe a product.

22.3 Requests from individual members of the public for information or advice on personal medical matters must always be refused and the enquirer recommended to consult his or her own doctor.

The provision of information about medicines to members of the public who request it is not precluded by the requirements of Clause 22.3, provided that the requirements of Clauses 22.1 and 22.2 are complied with.

22.4 The introduction of a new medicine should not be made known to the general public until all reasonable steps have been taken to inform the medical profession of its availability.

23 Operative date

This First Revision of the Seventh Edition of the Code shall take effect on 1 January 1991.

Post-marketing Surveillance Guidelines

INTRODUCTION

These guidelines are intended for company sponsored post marketing surveillance studies, whether carried out by a company directly, or indirectly through an agency or other intermediary. They have been formulated and approved by: The Association of the British Pharmaceutical Industry; the British Medical Association; the Committee on Safety of Medicines and the Royal College of General Practitioners.

Any departure from these guidelines, which gives cause for concern that a PMS study appears to be promotional in intent, may be submitted to the Code of Practice Committee of the ABPI for adjudication as a possible breach of that Code.

GUIDELINES

1 These guidelines are intended for post-marketing surveillance (PMS) observational cohort studies sponsored by pharmaceutical companies.

2 Post-marketing surveillance involves the collection of clinical data, primarily on drug safety, on marketed medicines used in everyday clinical practice.

3 PMS studies will normally entail the use of the product in accordance with the Summary of Product Characteristics (Data Sheet). However, information collected about marketed medicines used at the discretion of clinicians outside the terms of the Product Licence should not be excluded from the analysis of the results of a PMS study, but should be separately reported.

4 The following features are essential in the design of company sponsored PMS. There should be a valid medical reason for undertaking the study. The design and methods used must permit the achievement of the stated scientific and medical objectives. The study must not be designed for, or conducted as a promotional exercise.

5 Before the start of such a PMS study, a document must be drawn up explaining the aims and objectives of the study, the methods to be used and the record keeping which is to be maintained.

6 The plans of all PMS studies by pharmaceutical companies will be filed in a register held by the Medicines Division of the DoH. The ABPI will hold a voluntary register.

7 It is useful to distinguish between prospective and retrospective PMS studies. In 'prospective' studies the patient is recruited from the day the qualifying prescription is written and clinical experience is monitored from that time onwards. In 'retrospective' studies, the patient is identified at some point after the medicine has been prescribed. The clinical record will be studied from the date of the qualifying prescription. Studies on these patients can be continued thereafter by further monitoring, either on or off the treatment.

8 In prospective studies patients should be identified for inclusion in the study only *after* the decision to prescribe a particular medicine has been taken. The clinical justification for prescribing the particular medicine for each individual patient must be recorded at the outset by the prescribing doctor in the study documents for that patient.

9 The Committee on Safety of Medicines (CSM) has indicated the type of drugs on which PMS will normally be expected. Detailed proposals regarding such studies should be produced when a product licence application is originally submitted to the Licensing Authority. Any subsequent proposed variation in the study plan should be reviewed prior to implementation with the Adverse Drug Reactions Unit of the CSM Secretariat.

10 Any PMS study which gives cause for concern because it appears to be a sales promotion may also be reported to the Code of Practice Committee of the ABPI for adjudication regarding a possible breach of the Code of Practice.

11 The medicines used in company sponsored PMS studies shall be prescribed and supplied to patients by prescription in the normal way, eg. in NHS practice by an FP10 form written by the GP or by the usual hospital methods.

12 The company must not indicate that a study has been 'approved' or 'requested' by the CSM in any literature or communication which is not confidential to the CSM and/or DoH.

13 Responsibility for the design, conduct and analysis of the study shall be vested in a company Medical Department under the supervision of a Medical Practitioner registered in the UK, and whose name will be recorded in the documents.

14 Company representatives should not be involved in such a way that the study can be seen as a promotional exercise.

15 Interim and final reports should be made available without undue delay to participating doctors and lodged with the CSM. A final report should be made available for publication.

16 Doctors must be reminded of their commitment to notify adverse drug reactions to the CSM. Any reporting requirements of adverse drug reactions imposed by the CSM or Medicines Division, DoH, or the industry must be observed. Participating companies should ensure that doctors taking part in sponsored PMS studies notify the company's Medical Department immediately of any serious suspected adverse drug reaction which occurs during the course of the study.

17 Normal standards of professional confidentiality must be exercised.

REMUNERATION

18 No inducement to undertake a study shall be offered to, requested by, or given to a doctor participating in a company sponsored PMS study.

19 Subject to compatibility with NHS guidance and terms of service, reasonable payment may be offered to the doctor as a recompense for completing record forms and expenses incurred in the work involved in a company sponsored PMS study. Appropriate fees have been agreed between ABPI and BMA.

The reporting of adverse reactions

Suspected adverse reactions to any therapeutic agents should be reported. These agents include drugs, vaccines, blood products, X-ray contrast media, dental or surgical materials, intra-uterine contraceptive devices, absorbable sutures, contact lens fluids.

Newer drugs marked ▼

Doctors are asked to report any adverse or unexpected event, however minor, which could conceivably be attributed to the drug. Reports should be made despite uncertainty in the doctor's mind about a causal relationship, irrespective of whether the reaction is well recognised, and even if other drugs have been given concurrently.

Established drugs

Doctors are asked to report any suspected adverse drug reaction which was potentially dangerous, incapacitating or lethal. These should be reported even though the toxic effect is well recognised. Examples include anaphylaxis, blood dyscrasias, endocrine disturbances, effects on fertility, haemorrhage from any site, renal impairment, jaundice, ophthalmic disorders, severe CNS effects, severe skin reactions, reactions in pregnant women, and any drug interactions. For established drugs doctors are asked not to report well known, relatively minor side effects such as dry mouth with tricyclic antidepressants, constipation with opiates, or nausea with digoxin.

Special problems

(i) Delayed drug effects Doctors are reminded that some reactions (e.g., the development of cancers, chloroquine retinopathy and retroperitoneal fibrosis) may become manifest months or years after drug exposure. Please report any suspicion of such an association.

(ii) Drugs in the elderly Doctors are asked to be particularly alert to the possibility of adverse reactions when drugs are given to the elderly.

(iii) Congenital abnormalities When an infant is born with a congenital abnormality or there is a malformed aborted fetus, doctors are asked to consider the possibility that this might be an adverse reaction to a drug and to report all drugs (including self-medication) taken by the mother during pregnancy.

(iv) Adverse reactions to vaccines Doctors are asked to report all suspected reactions to both new and established vaccines. The balance between risks and benefits from vaccines is liable to change and needs to be kept under continuous review.

Special postage-paid forms ('yellow cards') are provided for reports. Some of these are included at the back of the Compendium and supplies can also be obtained from the Committee on Safety of Medicines at Market Towers, 1 Nine Elms Lane, London SW8 5NQ, telephone 071-720 2188.

The above statement and the symbols marking certain products have been included in the Compendium at the request of the Medicines Division of the Department of Health.

The individual companies concerned would find it helpful to be informed by practitioners of any adverse reactions to their products which are reported.

Abbott Laboratories Limited
Queenborough
Kent ME11 5EL

CORDILOX*

Presentation
Cordilox tablets 40 mg: Yellow, biconvex, film-coated Verapamil Hydrochloride Tablets BP imprinted with 'Cordilox' and '40' on one face and on the other containing 40 mg Verapamil Hydrochloride BP per tablet.

Cordilox tablets 80 mg: Yellow, biconvex, film-coated Verapamil Hydrochloride Tablets BP imprinted with 'Cordilox' and '80' on one face and on the other containing 80 mg Verapamil Hydrochloride BP per tablet.

Cordilox tablets 120: Yellow, biconvex, film-coated Verapamil Hydrochloride Tablets BP imprinted with 'Cordilox' and '120' on one face and on the other containing 120 mg Verapamil Hydrochloride BP per tablet.

Cordilox 160: Yellow, biconvex, film-coated Verapamil Hydrochloride Tablets BP imprinted with 'Cordilox' and '160' on one face and on the other containing 160 mg Verapamil Hydrochloride BP per tablet.

Cordilox IV: Colourless glass 2 ml ampoules with break-line containing 5 mg Verapamil Hydrochloride BP per ampoule.

Uses
Cordilox tablets:
(1) The treatment of mild to moderate hypertension and renal hypertension, used alone or in conjunction with other antihypertensive therapy.
(2) The treatment and prophylaxis of angina pectoris, and variant angina.
(3) The treatment and prophylaxis of paroxysmal supraventricular tachycardia and atrial flutter/fibrillation (verapamil should not be used when atrial flutter/fibrillation complicates Wolff-Parkinson-White syndrome, see 'Precautions').

Cordilox IV: The treatment of supraventricular arrhythmias.

Mode of Action: Cordilox is a calcium channel blocker which inhibits the inward movement of calcium in smooth muscle cells of the systemic and coronary arteries and in the cells of cardiac muscle and the intracardiac conduction system.

Cordilox lowers peripheral vascular resistance with little or no reflex tachycardia. Its efficacy in reducing both raised systolic and diastolic blood pressure is thought to be primarily due to this mode of action.

The decrease in systemic and coronary vascular resistance and the sparing effect on intracellular oxygen consumption appear to explain the anti-anginal properties of the product.

Because of its effect on the movement of calcium in the intracardiac conduction system, it reduces automaticity, decreases conduction velocity and increases the refractory period.

Dosage and administration
Hypertension (oral administration)

Adults: The usual dosage is 160 mg twice a day. However, a minority of patients may be successfully controlled on 120 mg b.d. while others may require up to 480 mg daily given in divided doses. A further reduction in blood pressure may be obtained by combining Cordilox with other antihypertensive agents, e.g. thiazide diuretics. For concomitant administration of beta-blockers, see 'Precautions'.

Children: Up to 10 mg/kg/day orally in divided doses according to the severity of disease.

Angina (oral administration)

Adults: The usual dosage is 120 mg three times a day. 80 mg t.d.s. can be completely satisfactory in some patients with angina of effort. Less than 120 mg t.d.s. is not likely to be effective in angina at rest and variant angina.

Children: No data available.

Supraventricular arrhythmias
Non-acute (oral administration)

Adults: 40–120 mg t.d.s. according to the severity of the condition.

Children: Up to 2 years: ½ 40 mg tablet 2–3 times a day. 2 years and above: 1–3 40 mg tablets 2–3 times a day according to age.

Acute (IV injection)

Adults: For the treatment of tachyarrhythmias, 5–10 mg (1–2 ampoules) should be injected intravenously over a period of 30 seconds with continuous observation of the patient and, preferably, with simultaneous ECG monitoring.

In cases of paroxysmal tachyarrhythmias a further 5 mg may, if necessary, be injected 5–10 minutes after the first injection with the same precautions being observed.

Higher doses are not usually necessary.

Children:	Newborn:	0.75–1 mg (0.3–0.4 ml)
	Infants:	0.75–2 mg (0.3–0.8 ml)
	1–5 years:	2–3 mg (0.8–1.2 ml)
	6–15 years:	2.5–5 mg (1.0–2.0 ml).

In many cases smaller doses than those mentioned above are sufficient. The injection should be stopped at the onset of the desired effect.

For concomitant administration with beta-blockers see 'Precautions'.

Elderly: No special dosage recommendations except in those patients with impaired liver function or cardiac conduction disturbances (see 'Precautions').

Contra-indications, warnings, etc
Contra-indications: Hypotension, marked bradycardia (less than 50 beats/minute), second and third degree atrioventricular block, sick sinus syndrome, uncompensated heart failure. Combination with beta-blockers is contra-indicated in patients with poor ventricular function.

Precautions: Cordilox may affect impulse conduction and should be used with caution in patients with first degree atrioventricular block. The effects of Cordilox and beta-blockers or other drugs with a cardio-depressive action may be additive both with respect to conduction and contraction, therefore care must be exercised when these are administered concurrently or closely together. This is especially true when either drug is administered intravenously.

Patients with atrial fibrillation/flutter and an accessory pathway (e.g. W-P-W syndrome) may rarely develop increased conduction across the anomalous pathway and ventricular tachycardia may be precipitated.

If there are signs of tachycardia-induced heart failure (energetic exhaustion of the myocardium) digitalisation is necessary before intravenous administration of Cordilox.

Cordilox may have an additive effect with other antihypertensive drugs. Thus, in many cases, with

Cordilox, a reduction in the dose of the other antihypertensive drug may be possible.

There is a possibility of an interaction between verapamil and quinidine, causing hypotension, when Cordilox is administered by the intravenous route.

Verapamil hydrochloride has been shown to increase the serum concentration of digoxin and caution should be exercised with regard to digitalis toxicity.

Cordilox may affect left ventricular contractility as a result of its mode of action. This effect is small and normally not important but cardiac failure may be precipitated or aggravated if it exists. In cases of poor ventricular function therefore, Cordilox should only be given after appropriate therapy for cardiac failure such as digitalis, etc.

Caution should be observed in the acute phase of myocardial infarction.

In patients with impaired liver function, particular attention should be paid to the dosage because of reduced drug metabolism.

Long term verapamil therapy may give rise to potentiation of neuromuscular blocking agents during anaesthesia.

Use in pregnancy and lactation: Verapamil is excreted in breast milk at concentrations approximately equal to 0.5 to 1.0 times that coexisting in maternal plasma. However, the amount ingested in such circumstances is less than 1% of the recommended therapeutic oral infant dose, assuming normal suckling rates. Animal studies have not shown any teratogenic effect. Cordilox should not be given during pregnancy unless, in the clinician's judgement, it is essential for the welfare of the patients. The possibility that Cordilox can cause relaxation of the uterine muscle should be considered at term.

Side-effects:
Oral administration: Cordilox is generally well tolerated. Constipation is not uncommon, flushing is observed occasionally, headaches rarely. Nausea and vomiting have seldom been reported and allergic reactions even more rarely. On very rare occasions a reversible impairment of liver function characterised by an increase in transaminases and/or alkaline phosphatase, may occur during verapamil treatment and is most probably a hypersensitivity reaction.

Parenteral administration: Cordilox is well tolerated and does not exert a bronchoconstrictor effect.

Due to its mode of action, undesired effects on atrioventricular conduction and blood pressure are possible. This applies particularly to patients with atrioventricular block and/or considerably impaired myocardial function. On rare occasions the intravenous administration of Cordilox may lead to an undesired blocking of conduction and, in extreme cases, to asystole. The asystole is usually of short duration and normally sinus rhythm returns spontaneously after a few seconds. However, if on rare occasions asystole persists, treatment should be carried out as described below.

Intravenous administration of Cordilox may lead to a slight transient fall in blood pressure due to a reduction in peripheral resistance. Rarely this may result in severe hypotension.

Treatment of acute cardiovascular side-effects: If acute complications occur after intravenous injection of Cordilox (asystole, atrioventricular block or ventricular fibrillation) the usual emergency measures should be applied, e.g. cardiac massage, mechanical ventilation, the intravenous injection of adrenaline, and the intravenous injection of 10–20 ml of calcium gluconate 10% solution. Hypotension following intravenous injection of Cordilox may, if necessary, be controlled without difficulty by the use of vasoconstrictor substances.

Overdosage
Oral administration: Usual emergency measures for acute cardiovascular side-effects should be followed as above. In the case of second and third degree AV block, atropine, isoprenaline or a temporary pace-maker may be necessary. If myocardial insufficiency occurs, dopamine, dobutamine, cardiac glycosides or calcium gluconate (10–20 ml of a 10% solution) may be required. Appropriate positioning of the patient and vasoconstrictor drugs may be indicated in the case of hypotension.

Parenteral administration: See 'Treatment of acute cardiovascular side-effects'.

Pharmaceutical precautions Cordilox IV is incompatible with alkaline solutions (e.g. Sodium Bicarbonate Intravenous Infusion BP) as this may lead to a precipitation of the verapamil base.

Legal category POM.

Package quantities

Cordilox 40 mg:	Containers of 100 tablets
Cordilox 80 mg:	Containers of 100 tablets
Cordilox 120:	Containers of 100 and 500 tablets
Cordilox 160:	Blister packs of 56 tablets
Cordilox IV:	Containers of 5 × 2 ml ampoules.

Further information
Metabolisable carbohydrate:

Cordilox 40 mg:	3.2 mg/tablet
Cordilox 80 mg:	6.4 mg/tablet
Cordilox 120:	9.6 mg/tablet
Cordilox 160:	12.8 mg/tablet
Cordilox IV:	Nil.
Cordilox IV:	Sodium content: 0.30 mmol/ ampoule (0.15 mmol/ml).

Product licence numbers

Cordilox 40 mg:	0037/0098
Cordilox 80 mg:	0037/0085
Cordilox 120:	0037/0084
Cordilox 160:	0037/0131
Cordilox IV:	0037/5903

DOPAMINE HYDROCHLORIDE IN 5% DEXTROSE INJECTION

Presentation Dopamine hydrochloride in 5% dextrose solution is a sterile, nonpyrogenic solution for administration by intravenous infusion. It is presented in 250 ml flexible containers of 400 mg (1600 mcg/ml) and 800 mg (3200 mcg/ml) Dopamine Hydrochloride USP in 5% dextrose injection.

It is intended for use as a single-dose injection.

Uses Dopamine administered intravenously is a positive myocardial inotropic agent, which also may increase mesenteric and renal blood flow plus urinary output.

Dopamine hydrochloride in 5% dextrose is indicated in patients with poor perfusion, low cardiac output, impending renal failure and for the correction of haemodynamic imbalances present in shock due to myocardial infarction, trauma, endotoxic septicaemia, open heart surgery, renal failure and chronic cardiac decompensation as in refractory congestive failure.

Dosage and administration Where appropriate, the circulating blood volume must be restored with a suitable plasma expander or whole blood, prior to administration of dopamine hydrochloride.

Begin infusion of dopamine hydrochloride solution at doses of 2.5 mcg/kg/min in patients who are likely to respond to modest increments of heart force and renal perfusion.

In more seriously ill patients, begin infusion of dopamine hydrochloride at doses of 5 mcg/kg/min and increase gradually using 5 to 10 mcg/kg/min increments up to a rate of 20 to 50 mcg/kg/min as needed. If doses in excess of 50 mcg/kg/min are required, it is advisable to check urine output frequently. Should urinary flow begin to decrease in the absence of hypotension, reduction of dopamine dosage should be considered. It has been found that more than 50% of patients have been satisfactorily maintained on doses less than 20 mcg/kg/min.

In patients who do not respond to these doses, additional increments of dopamine may be given in an effort to achieve adequate blood pressure, urine flow and perfusion generally.

Treatment of all patients requires constant evaluation of therapy in terms of blood volume, augmentation of cardiac contractility, and distribution of peripheral perfusion and urinary output.

Dosage of dopamine should be adjusted according to the patient's response, with particular attention to diminution of established urine flow rate, increasing tachycardia or development of new dysrhythmias as indications for decreasing or temporarily suspending the dosage.

Contra-indications, warnings, etc
Contra-indications: Dopamine hydrochloride should not be used in patients with phaeochromocytoma. Dextrose solutions without electrolytes should not be administered simultaneously with blood through the same infusion set because of the possibility that pseudoagglutination of red cells may occur.

Warnings: Dopamine should not be administered in the presence of uncorrected tachyarrhythmias or ventricular fibrillation.

Patients who have been treated with monoamine oxidase (MAO) inhibitors prior to administration of dopamine should receive substantially reduced dosage of the latter. The starting dose in such patients should be reduced to at least one-tenth (1/10) of the usual dose.

Excess administration of potassium-free solutions may result in significant hypokalaemia.

The intravenous administration of these solutions can cause fluid and/or solute overloading resulting in dilution of serum electrolyte concentrations, overhydration, congested states or pulmonary oedema.

Precautions: Hypovolaemia should be corrected where necessary prior to treatment with dopamine.

If a disproportionate rise in diastolic pressure (i.e. a marked decrease in pulse pressure) is observed, the infusion rate should be decreased and the patients observed carefully for further evidence of predominant vasoconstriction activity, unless such an effect is desired.

Patients with a history of peripheral vascular disease should be closely monitored for any changes in colour or temperature of the skin of the extremities. If a change of skin colour or temperature occurs and is thought to be the result of compromised circulation to the extremities, the benefits of continued dopamine infusion should be weighed against the risk of possible necrosis. These changes may be reversed by decreasing the rate or discontinuing the infusion.

Dopamine hydrochloride in 5% dextrose injection should be infused into a large vein whenever possible to prevent the possibility of infiltration of perivascular tissue adjacent to the infusion site. Extravasation may cause necrosis and sloughing of the surrounding tissue. Ischaemia can be reversed by infiltration of the affected area with 10–15 ml of saline containing 5 to 10 mg phentolamine mesylate. A syringe with a fine hypodermic needle should be used to liberally infiltrate the ischaemic area as soon as extravasation is noted.

Dopamine should be used with extreme caution in patients inhaling cyclopropane or halogenated hydrocarbon anaesthetics due to the arterial arrhythmogenic potential.

Dextrose solutions should be used with caution in patients with known subclinical or overt diabetes mellitus.

Adverse reactions: The most frequently reported adverse reactions to dopamine have been ectopic beats, tachycardia, nausea, vomiting, anginal pain, palpitations, dyspnoea, headache, hypotension and vasoconstriction.

Very rarely reported reactions include aberrant conduction, bradycardia, piloerection, widened QRS complex, azotaemia and elevated blood pressure.

Usage in pregnancy: Animal studies have shown no evidence of teratogenic effects with dopamine. The drug may be used in pregnant women when, in the judgment of the physician, the expected benefits outweigh the potential risk to the foetus.

Usage in children: Safety and effectiveness in children have not been established.

Overdosage: Accidental overdosage as evidenced by excessive blood pressure elevation can be controlled by dose reduction or discontinuing the administration for a short period until the patient's condition stabilises.

If these measures fail, an infusion of phentolamine mesylate should be considered.

Pharmaceutical precautions Do not add sodium bicarbonate or other alkaline substances, since dopamine is inactivated in alkaline solution.

Do not administer unless solution is clear and seal is intact. Discard unused portion.

Additive medications should not be delivered via this solution.

Recommended storage: Room temperature (25°C). Store away from heat. Protect from freezing.

Legal category POM.

Package quantities 250 ml flexible containers containing:

Dopamine hydrochloride 400 mg in 5% dextrose injection.

Dopamine hydrochloride 800 mg in 5% dextrose injection.

Further information Nil.

Product licence numbers 400 mg 0037/0146
800 mg 0037/0147

ENDURON*

Presentation Each square, pink tablet engraved with a bisect line on one face and the a logo on the other, contains 5 mg methyclothiazide, an oral diuretic.

Uses Enduron is a thiazide diuretic agent which exerts its diuretic and saluric effects through the inhibition of the renal tubular reabsorption of electrolytes. The excretion of sodium and chloride is greatly enhanced whilst potassium excretion is increased but to a variable degree.

Indications:

1. Treatment of mild to moderate hypertension.
2. As an adjunct to other antihypertensive drugs in the treatment of resistant hypertension.
3. Treatment and control of oedema associated with congestive heart failure, nephrotic syndrome, hepatic cirrhosis, pre-menstrual tension and steroid administration.

Dosage and administration The usual adult oral dose is 2.5–5 mg daily. This may be increased to 10 mg once daily, if necessary, but doses larger than 10 mg have little additional therapeutic effect. Enduron is not recommended for use in children.

Elderly: No special dosage recommendations except in those patients with renal or hepatic disease (see 'Contra-indications'). Borderline renal or hepatic insufficiency may be unpredictably aggravated by thiazides. See also warnings.

Contra-indications, warnings, etc
Contra-indications: Known sensitivity to thiazide derivatives. It should not be administered in the presence of severe renal or hepatic disease, Addison's disease, hypercalcaemia and concurrent lithium therapy.

Warnings:

1. Diabetes may be precipitated or aggravated.
2. Gout may be precipitated or aggravated.
3. Renal function should be monitored.
4. Patients on corticosteroids, or with impending hepatic coma, cirrhotic oedema or ascites may require potassium supplements, and should be carefully evaluated clinically.
5. Pancreatitis may be precipitated.
6. Particular caution is needed in the case of elderly patients because of their likely susceptibility to electrolyte imbalance.

Use in pregnancy and lactation: Diuretics are best avoided for the management of oedema in pregnancy or hypertension in pregnancy as their use may be associated with hypovolaemia, increased blood viscosity and reduced placental perfusion. There is inadequate evidence of safety in human pregnancy and some workers have described foetal bone marrow depression and thrombocytopaenia. Foetal and neonatal jaundice have also been reported.

As diuretics pass into breast milk they should be avoided in mothers who wish to breast feed.

Precautions and side-effects: Enduron is a benzothiadiazine derivative, and the physician should be alert for the side-effects inherent in this type of medication. If potassium depletion occurs, potassium or a potassium sparing drug should be given. Myocardial sensitivity to digitalis is increased in the presence of reduced potassium and signs of digitalis intoxication may be produced by formerly tolerated doses of digitalis. Hypokalaemia can cause an increase in arrhythmias. Hypochloraemic alkalosis is a possibility with any potent benzothiadiazine. Dilutional hyponatremia may occur in oedematous patients in hot weather; appropriate therapy is water restriction, rather than administration of salt, except in rare instances when the hyponatremia is life threatening. Elevation of the blood urea nitrogen, serum uric acid, blood sugar have occurred with the use of thiazide drugs. In common with other thiazides impotence may occur. Blood dyscrasias including thrombocytopenia with purpura, agranulocytosis and aplastic anaemia have also been reported but are rare.

Overdosage: Symptoms: Electrolyte imbalance; dehydration; hypotension; signs of hypokalaemia; dizziness; muscular weakness and gastro-intestinal disturbances may occur.

Treatment: Employ general supportive measures. Blood pressure and fluid/electrolyte balance should be monitored. Replacement of fluids and electrolytes may be indicated. For recent ingestion gastric lavage or emesis should be considered.

Pharmaceutical precautions Nil.

Legal category POM.

Package quantities Enduron is supplied in containers of 100 tablets.

Further information Metabolisable carbohydrate content: Approx. 0.18 g per tablet.

Product licence number 0037/5028.

ENFLURANE

Presentation Enflurane is an inhalation anaesthetic with a pleasant ethereal odour. No additives or stabilisers are present.

Uses Enflurane may be used for induction and maintenance of general anaesthesia. Adequate data are not available yet to establish its full place in obstetric anaesthesia other than in caesarean section. High concentrations of enflurane may produce marked uterine relaxation.

Enflurane may be used for outpatient and dental anaesthesia in view of the rapidity of action and recovery, with stability of the cardiovascular system. Enflurane can be used in children.

Actions: Induction and recovery are rapid. It does not stimulate excessive salivation, tracheobronchial secretions or cause bronchial constriction. Pharyngeal and laryngeal reflexes are diminished quickly. The level of anaesthesia changes rapidly with enflurane. Tachypnoea does not usually occur. Spontaneous respiration becomes depressed as the depth of anaesthesia increases.

Enflurane provokes a 'sigh' response reminiscent of that seen with diethyl ether.

During induction there is a decrease in blood pressure followed by a return to near normal levels, which may or may not be associated with surgical stimulation.

Blood pressure tends to fall in direct relation to the depth of anaesthesia but cardiac rate and rhythm remain stable. Enflurane appears to 'sensitise' the myocardium to adrenaline in man to a lesser extent than halothane. Available data indicate that subcutaneous injections of adrenaline may be safely administered to humans in concentrations of 1:100,000 or less at a dose of 10 ml in any given 10 minute period and not more than 30 ml/hour. All the usual precautions in the use of vasoconstrictor substances must be observed.

Good muscular relaxation is obtained with enflurane, but should greater relaxation be necessary minimal doses of an intravenous muscle relaxant may be used with measures to ensure adequate ventilation.

All commonly used intravenous muscle relaxants are compatible with enflurane.

Note: Enflurane potentiates the effect of the non-depolarising muscle relaxants which should therefore be used in reduced dosage. Neostigmine does not reverse the direct effect of enflurane.

Enflurane produces little post-operative analgesia.

Metabolism of enflurane in the human body proceeds at a low rate; inorganic fluoride is formed but serum levels in healthy individuals have not been shown to rise to significant levels.

Dosage and administration Vaporisers calibrated specifically for enflurane should be used so that the concentration being delivered is known.

The inspired concentration required to achieve clinical anaesthesia depends upon the age of the patient and to a minimal extent on body temperature. The MAC value is higher in children and decreases with advancing age, falling from an average in oxygen of 2.4% in the newborn and 2.5% at puberty, to 1.9% in young adults, and 1.7% at middle age. As with other agents, lesser concentrations of enflurane are normally required to maintain surgical anaesthesia in elderly patients. MAC values increase with increasing body temperature.

Premedication: Drugs used for premedication should be selected for each individual patient. The use of anticholinergic drugs is a matter of choice.

Induction: To avoid excitement a short-acting barbiturate or other intravenous induction agent should be administered, followed by inhalation of the enflurane mixture. Enflurane and oxygen alone or oxygen-nitrous oxide mixtures may be used.

It is recommended that enflurane induction be initiated at a concentration of 0.4% and gradually increased by 0.5% increments after every few breaths until surgical anaesthesia is achieved.

The maximum inspired concentration during induction should be no more than 4.5%. High inspired concentrations should be lowered as rapidly as possible to maintenance levels to prevent overdosage, and the blood pressure carefully observed.

Maintenance: In conjunction with nitrous oxide, surgical levels of anaesthesia may be maintained with a 0.5%–3% concentration of enflurane. A 3% concentration should not be exceeded for maintenance during spontaneous respiration. With controlled respiration techniques, during prolonged operations, single or supplementary doses of muscle relaxants may be used if required, bearing in mind the possibility of some slight potentiation. Ventilation to maintain the carbon dioxide tension in arterial blood in the the 4.7–6.0 kPa (35–45 mmHg) range is preferred to hyper- or hypoventilation, in order to minimise the possibility of CNS excitation.

Blood pressure levels during maintenance depend on enflurane concentration in the absence of other complicating factors. Excessive decreases (unless related to hypovolaemia) may be due to depth of anaesthesia and in such instances should be corrected by reducing the inspired enflurane concentration.

Elderly: As with other agents, lesser concentrations of enflurane are normally required to maintain surgical anaesthesia in elderly patients.

Contra-indications, warnings, etc

Contra-indications: Known sensitivity to enflurane and in patients with known or suspected genetic susceptability to malignant hyperthermia.

Precautions: Enflurane should be used with caution in patients who, by virtue of medical or drug history, may be considered more susceptible to cerebral stimulation produced by this drug. Increasing depth of anaesthesia with enflurane may produce changes in the electroencephalogram characterised by high voltage, fast frequency waves progressing through spike-dome complexes alternating with periods of electrical silence to frank seizure activity patterns. The latter may or may not be associated with motor movement. Motor activity, when encountered, generally consists of twitching or 'jerks' of various muscle groups; it is self-limiting and can be terminated by lowering the anaesthetic concentration. This electroencephalographic pattern associated with deep anaesthesia may be exacerbated by hyperventilation producing low arterial carbon dioxide tension. The pattern serves as a warning that depth of anaesthesia is excessive. Cerebral blood flow and metabolism studies in normal volunteers during seizure patterns show no evidence of cerebral hypoxia, and recovery appears to be uncomplicated.

In susceptible individuals, enflurane anaesthesia may trigger a skeletal muscle hypermetabolic state and the clinical syndrome known as malignant hyperthermia. The syndrome includes non-specific features such as muscle rigidity, tachycardia, tachypnoea, cyanosis, arrhythmias and unstable blood pressure.

Treatment includes discontinuing enflurane anaesthesia, administration of dantrolene sodium and supportive therapy. Renal failure may appear later and urine flow should be sustained if possible.

Since levels of anaesthesia may be altered easily and rapidly, only vaporisers which deliver a predictable output with reasonable accuracy should be used. Hypotension and respiratory exchange can serve as a guide to anaesthetic depth. With deep levels of anaesthesia, more marked hypotension and respiratory depression are encountered.

The action of non-depolarising relaxants is augmented by enflurane, so less than the usual amounts of those drugs should be used.

Overdosage or unduly rapid absorption of adrenaline administered topically or by subcutaneous or submucosal injection during enflurane anaesthesia may give rise to cardiac arrhythmias (see 'Actions' section). Care must be taken to avoid intravenous injection.

Bromsulphthalein (BSP) retention is mildly raised post-operatively in some cases. There is some elevation of blood glucose and white blood cell count intra-operatively.

Use in pregnancy: Reproduction studies have been performed in rats and rabbits. Following single and multiple maternal administrations, no evidence of teratogenicity due to enflurane was found in the developing foetuses in these species. The relevance of these studies to the human is not known. Since there is no adequate experience in pregnant women who have received the drug, safety in pregnancy has not been established.

It is not known whether enflurane is excreted in breast milk and caution should therefore be exercised when enflurane is administered to a nursing mother.

Adverse reactions:

1. Motor activity exemplified by movement of various muscle groups and seizures may be encountered with deep levels of enflurane anaesthesia, particularly with hyperventilation.
2. Hypotension, respiratory depression and arrhythmias have been reported.
3. Elevation of the white blood cell count has been observed. It has not been determined whether this is related to enflurane or to surgical stress.
4. A mild increase in serum glucose concentration has been observed in some normal and diabetic patients, as with other anaesthetic agents. There seems to be no contra-indication to the use of the agent in these patients for whom rapid recovery is advantageous.
5. Hepatic enzyme changes occur less frequently and to a lesser degree after multiple enflurane anaesthetics when compared with multiple exposures to halothane. While jaundice and significant hepatic enzyme increases occasionally occur after halothane anaesthesia, this is extremely rare after the administration of enflurane in the absence of complicating factors such as blood transfusion or concomitant administration of hepatotoxic drugs.
6. Increased serum inorganic fluoride levels have been found during and immediately after enflurane anaesthesia due to biodegradation of the agent. These levels normally remain well below the postulated threshold for nephrotoxicity and, after reaching a peak within eight hours of the end of the anaesthetic, rapidly return to preoperative values.

Although there is no evidence that enflurane anaesthesia adversely affects the normal or diseased kidney it may be prudent to avoid its use in cases of chronic renal failure.

Side-effects: Nausea, vomiting, hiccups or shivering may occur occasionally.

Pharmaceutical precautions Store away from heat. Keep well closed.

Legal category P.

Package quantities Enflurane is supplied in bottles of 250 ml.

Further information Nil.

Product licence number 0037/0053.

ERYTHROCIN* 250
ERYTHROCIN* 500

Presentation Erythrocin 250 and Erythrocin 500 are white, film-coated tablets containing respectively 250 mg and 500 mg of erythromycin as Erythromycin Stearate BP. They are Erythromycin Stearate Tablets BP.

Uses For the prophylaxis and treatment of infections caused by erythromycin-sensitive organisms.

Clinical indications:

1. Upper respiratory tract infections.
2. Lower respiratory tract infections.
3. Skin and soft tissue infections.
4. Bone infections.
5. Sexually transmitted diseases.
6. Oral/dental infections.
7. Eye infections.
8. Gastro-intestinal infections.
9. Prophylaxis.

Erythromycin has also proved to be of value in endocarditis and septicaemia but in these conditions initial administration of erythromycin lactobionate by the intravenous route is advised.

Microbiological indications: Erythromycin has been shown to be active in vitro against the following organisms: Staphylococci, Streptococci, *Haemophilus influenzae*, L-forms, *Mycoplasma pneumoniae*, *Legionella pneumophila*, *Branhamella catarrhalis*, *Bordetella pertussis*, *Corynebacterium diphtheriae* (as an adjunct to antitoxin), Neisseria, *Treponema pallidum*, *Chlamydia trachomatis*, Clostridia, *Ureaplasma urealytica*, Campylobacter.

Dosage and administration

Adults and children over 8 years: For mild to moderate infections 1–2 g daily in divided doses. For severe infections this may be increased to 4 g daily in divided doses. Tablets should be taken before or with meals.

Elderly: No special dosage recommendations.

Children under 8 years: Erythroped suspension is recommended.

Period of dosing with regard to indication

Upper respiratory tract infections	5–10 days.
Lower respiratory tract infections	7–14 days or until signs and symptoms indicate a cure. Legionnaires' disease may require prolonged treatment. Initially administration of erythromycin lactobionate by the intravenous route is recommended.

Skin and soft tissue infections	5–10 days. Acne may require prolonged treatment.
Sexually transmitted diseases	
NGU and syphilis	10–21 days. Some conditions may require prolonged treatment.
Oral/dental infections	At least 5 days.
Eye infections	
Chlamydial inclusion conjunctivitis	3 weeks.
Gastro-intestinal infections	
Campylobacter	Minimum 5 days.

Contra-indications, warnings, etc
Contra-indications: Known sensitivity to erythromycin.

Precautions: Erythromycin is excreted principally by the liver, so caution should be exercised in administering the antibiotic to patients with impaired hepatic function or concomitantly receiving potentially hepatotoxic agents.

The administration of erythromycin has been infrequently associated with the occurrence of reversible cholestatic jaundice.

The use of erythromycin in patients who are receiving digoxin, warfarin, carbamazepine and high doses of theophylline may result in the potentiation of their effects due to reduction in the rates of excretion.

Use in pregnancy: There is no evidence of hazard from erythromycin in human pregnancy. It has been in wide use for many years without apparent ill consequence. Animal studies have shown no hazard.

Side-effects: Occasional side-effects such as nausea, abdominal discomfort, vomiting and diarrhoea may be experienced. Reversible hearing loss associated with doses of erythromycin usually greater than 4 g per day has been reported. Allergic reactions are rare and mild, although anaphylaxis has occurred extremely rarely. There are no reports implicating erythromycin products with abnormal tooth development and only rare reports of damage to the blood, kidneys, liver or central nervous system.

Overdosage: Symptoms: Hearing loss, severe nausea, vomiting and diarrhoea.

Treatment: Gastric lavage, general supportive measures.

Pharmaceutical precautions Keep bottle tightly closed. Protect from light. Store below 25°C.

Legal category POM.

Package quantities Erythrocin 250: Containers of 100, 500 and 1000 tablets.

Erythrocin 500: Containers of 100 and 500 tablets and blister packs of 10, 15 and 56 tablets.

Further information Erythrocin 250 and 500 contain no dyes. They contain respectively 0.07 g and 0.15 g Maize Starch BP.

Product licence number
Erythrocin 250 0037/5079R
Erythrocin 500 0037/5044R

ERYTHROCIN IV LACTOBIONATE IN THE ABBOTT ADD-VANTAGE DRUG DELIVERY SYSTEM

Presentation This is a sterile lyophilised presentation of erythromycin as erythromycin lactobionate in the Abbott ADD-Vantage glass vial. The vial is designed specifically for use with Abbott ADD-Vantage flexible container (PVC bag) containing Sodium Chloride Intravenous Infusion BP (0.9% w/v).

The following strength is available: 1.0 g erythromycin for dilution to 250 ml.

Erythrocin IV lactobionate is not suitable for intramuscular use.

The product is intended for intravenous infusion.

Uses
Clinical indications: Erythromycin lactobionate is indicated in severe and immunocomprised cases of infections caused by sensitive organisms where high blood levels are required at the earliest opportunity or when the oral route is comprised.

1. Upper respiratory tract infections.
2. Lower respiratory tract infections.
3. Skin and soft tissue infections.
4. Gastro-intestinal and biliary infections.
5. Prophylaxis: Peri-operative secondary infection prophylaxis, severe trauma and burns secondary infection prophylaxis, endocarditis prophylaxis (dental procedures).
6. Endocarditis.
7. Septicaemia.
8. Oral/dental infections.

Microbiological indications: Erythromycin has been shown to be active in vitro against the following organisms: Staphylococci, Streptococci, *Haemophilus influenzae*, L-forms, *Mycoplasma pneumoniae*, *Legionella pneumophila*, *Branhamella catarrhalis*, *Bordetella pertussis*, *Corynebacterium diphtheriae* (as an adjunct to antitoxin), Neisseria, *Treponema pallidum*, *Chlamydia trachomatis*, Clostridia, *Ureaplasma urealytica*, Campylobacter.

Dosage and administration
Recommended dosage

Adults, children and neonates: Severe and immunocompromised infections, 50 mg/kg/day (equivalent to 4 g per day for adults).

Mild to moderate infections (oral route compromised) 25 mg/kg/day.

Elderly: No special dosage recommendations.

Recommended administration: When reconstituted the erythromycin concentration is 4 mg/ml. Intermittent administration is recommended, with infusion over 20 to 60 minutes. The interval between infusions should not be more than 6 hours. Alternatively, continuous administration may be employed. However, the infusion should be completed within 8 hours of preparation to ensure potency.

Preparation of solution for administration

To assemble vial and flexible diluent container:

To open: Peel overwrap from the corner and remove container: (Use aseptic technique).

1. Remove the protective covers from the top of the vial and the vial port on the diluent container.
2. Screw the vial into the vial port until it is firmly seated and will go no further.
3. Label appropriately.

To reconstitute the drug:

1. Squeeze the bottom of the diluent container gently to inflate the portion of the container surrounding the end of the drug vial.
2. With the other hand, push the drug vial down into the container, telescoping the walls of the container. Grasp the inner cap of the vial through the walls of the container.
3. With a rocking motion, pull the inner cap from the drug vial.
4. Mix container contents thoroughly and use within the specified time.

Reconstituted product should be used within 8 hours and checked for freedom from gel formation and particulate matter prior to use.

Contra-indications, warnings, etc
Contra-indications: Known sensitivity to erythromycin. Intravenous saline solution may be contra-indicated in patients with impaired renal or cardiac function.

Precautions: Extravasation should be avoided. Erythromycin is excreted principally by the liver, so caution should be exercised in administering the antibiotic to patients with impaired hepatic function or concomitantly receiving potentially hepatotoxic agents.

The administration of erythromycin has been infrequently associated with the occurrence of reversible cholestatic jaundice.

The use of erythromycin in patients who are receiving digoxin, warfarin, carbamazepine and high doses of theophylline may result in the potentiation of their effects due to reduction in the rates of excretion.

Caution must be exercised in the administration of parenteral fluids, especially those containing sodium ions, to patients receiving corticosteroids or corticotrophin.

Use in pregnancy: There is no evidence of hazard from erythromycin in human pregnancy and it has been in wide use for many years without apparent ill consequence. Animal studies have shown no hazard.

Side-effects: Occasional side-effects such as nausea, abdominal discomfort, vomiting and diarrhoea may be experienced. Reversible hearing loss associated with doses of erythromycin usually greater than 4 g per day has been reported. Allergic reactions are rare and mild, although anaphylaxis has occurred extremely rarely. There are no reports implicating erythromycin products with abnormal tooth development and only rare reports of damage to the blood, kidneys, liver or central nervous system.

Compatibility with other IV additives has not been established.

Overdosage: Symptoms: Hearing loss, severe nausea, vomiting and diarrhoea.

Treatment: General supportive measures.

Pharmaceutical precautions Erythrocin IV Lactobionate vial: None.

ADD-Vantage flexible container: Protect from freezing. Store at room temperature.

Legal category POM.

Package quantities Carton containing one 1.0 g vial and one 250 ml bag.

Further information Nil.

Product licence numbers
Abbott ADD-Vantage system:

1.0 g vial:	0037/0168
250 ml bag (saline):	0037/0169

ERYTHROMID*
ERYTHROMID DS*

Presentation Erythromid and Erythromid DS are orange-coloured, enteric-coated, film-coated tablets containing respectively 250 mg and 500 mg of Erythromycin BP. They are Erythromycin Tablets BP.

Uses For the prophylaxis and treatment of infections caused by erythromycin-sensitive organisms.

Clinical indications:

1. Upper respiratory tract infections.
2. Lower respiratory tract infections.
3. Skin and soft tissue infections.
4. Bone infections.
5. Sexually transmitted diseases.
6. Oral/dental infections.
7. Eye infections.
8. Gastro-intestinal infections.
9. Prophylaxis.

Erythromycin has also proved to be of value in endocarditis and septicaemia, but in these conditions initial administration of erythromycin lactobionate by the intravenous route is advised.

Microbiological indications: Erythromycin has been shown to be active in vitro against the following organisms: Staphylococci, Streptococci, *Haemophilus influenzae*, L-forms, *Mycoplasma pneumoniae*, *Legionella pneumophila*, *Branhamella catarrhalis*, *Bordetella pertussis*, *Corynebacterium diphtheriae* (as an adjunct to antitoxin), Neisseria, *Treponema pallidum*, *Chlamydia trachomatis*, Clostridia, *Ureaplasma urealytica*, Campylobacter.

Dosage and administration
Adults and children over 8 years: For mild to moderate infections 1–2 g daily in divided doses. For severe infections this may be increased to 4 g daily in divided doses. Tablets should be taken before or with meals.

Elderly: No special dosage recommendations.

Children under 8 years: Erythroped suspension is recommended.

Period of dosing with regard to indication

Upper respiratory tract infections	5–10 days.
Lower respiratory tract infections	7–14 days or until signs and symptoms indicate a cure. Legionnaires' disease may require prolonged treatment. Initially administration of erythromycin lactobionate by the intravenous route is recommended.
Skin and soft tissue infections	5–10 days. Acne may require prolonged treatment.
Sexually transmitted diseases	
NGU and syphilis	10–21 days. Some conditions may require prolonged treatment.
Oral/dental infections	At least 5 days.
Eye infections	
Chlamydial inclusion conjunctivitis	3 weeks.
Gastro-intestinal infections	
Campylobacter	Minimum 5 days.

Contra-indications, warnings, etc
Contra-indications: Known sensitivity to erythromycin.

Precautions: Erythromycin is excreted principally by the liver, so caution should be exercised in administering the antibiotic to patients with impaired hepatic function or concomitantly receiving potentially hepatotoxic agents.

The administration of erythromycin has been infrequently associated with the occurrence of reversible cholestatic jaundice.

The use of erythromycin in patients who are receiving digoxin, warfarin, carbamazepine and high doses of theophylline may result in the potentiation of their effects due to reduction in the rates of excretion.

Use in pregnancy: There is no evidence of hazard from erythromycin in human pregnancy. It has been in wide use for many years without apparent ill consequence. Animal studies have shown no hazard.

Side-effects: Occasional side-effects such as nausea, abdominal discomfort, vomiting and diarrhoea may be experienced. Reversible hearing loss associated with doses of erythromycin usually greater than 4 g per day has been reported. Allergic reactions are rare and mild, although anaphylaxis has occurred extremely rarely. There are no reports implicating erythromycin products with abnormal tooth development and only rare reports of damage to the blood, kidneys, liver or central nervous system.

Overdosage: Symptoms: Hearing loss, severe nausea, vomiting and diarrhoea.

Treatment: Gastric lavage, general supportive measures.

Pharmaceutical precautions Keep bottle tightly closed. Protect from light. Store below 25°C.

Legal category POM.

Package quantities Erythromid: Containers of 50, 100, 500 and 1000 tablets.

Erythromid DS: Containers of 25, 100 and 500 tablets.

Further information Erythromid and Erythromid DS each contain two azo dyes (not tartrazine), E110 and E124. No metabolisable carbohydrate is present.

Product licence numbers
Erythromid 0037/5019R
Erythromid DS 0037/0121

ERYTHROMYCIN LACTOBIONATE

Presentation A sterile, white, lyophilised presentation of 1.0 g of erythromycin as erythromycin lactobionate in a vial.

When reconstituted with 20 ml Water for Injections BP provides 22 ml of solution. Deliberate overage ensures that each 20 ml of this solution contains 1.0 g of erythromycin as erythromycin lactobionate.

The solution must be further diluted prior to intravenous administration (see dosage and administration).

Erythromycin Lactobionate is not suitable for intramuscular use.

Uses

Clinical indications: Erythromycin lactobionate is indicated in severe and immunocompromised cases of infections caused by sensitive organisms where high blood levels are required at the earliest opportunity or when the oral route is compromised.

1. Upper respiratory tract infections.
2. Lower respiratory tract infections.
3. Skin and soft tissue infections.
4. Gastro-intestinal and biliary infections.
5. Prophylaxis: Peri-operative secondary infection prophylaxis, severe trauma and burns secondary infection prophylaxis, endocarditis prophylaxis (dental procedures).
6. Endocarditis.
7. Septicaemia.
8. Oral/dental infections.

Microbiological indications: Erythromycin has been shown to be active in vitro against the following organisms: Staphylococci, Streptococci, *Haemophilus influenzae*, L-forms, *Mycoplasma pneumoniae*, *Legionella pneumophila*, *Branhamella catarrhalis*, *Bordetella pertussis*, Corynebacterium diphtheriae (as an adjunct to antitoxin), Neisseria, *Treponema pallidum*, *Chlamydia trachomatis*, Clostridia, *Ureaplasma urealytica*, Campylobacter.

Dosage and administration

Recommended dosage

Adults, children and neonates: Severe and immunocompromised infections, 50 mg/kg/day, preferably by continuous infusion (equivalent to 4 g per day for adults).

Mild to moderate infections (oral route compromised) 25 mg/kg/day.

Elderly: No special dosage recommendations.

Recommended administration: Continuous intravenous infusion with an erythromycin concentration of 1 mg/ml (0.1% solution) is recommended.

If required, solution strengths up to 5 mg/ml (0.5% solution) may be used, but should not be exceeded. Higher concentrations may result in pain along the vein.

Bolus injection is not recommended.

However, if it is decided to administer the daily dose as 4 doses once every 6 hours, then the erythromycin concentration should not exceed 5 mg/ml and the time of each infusion should be between 20 and 60 minutes.

Preparation of solution for intravenous administration

Step 1: Inject 20 ml of Water for Injections BP into the vial and shake to dissolve contents. Do not use saline or other diluents. This will give 22 ml of solution.

20 ml of this solution will contain 1.0 g erythromycin (50 mg erythromycin/ml).

Use within 24 hours of preparation. Keep in a refrigerator between 2°C and 8°C.

This solution must be further diluted before administration, see Step 2.

Step 2: Solutions for administration are prepared with Sodium Chloride Intravenous Infusion BP 0.9% w/v (see also below).

Dose required	*Volume from Step 1*	*Volume of sterile 0.9% saline*	*Total volume*	*Erythromycin concentration*
1.0 g 500 mg	20 ml 10 ml	1000 ml 500 ml	1020 ml 510 ml	1.0 mg/ml
1.0 g 500 mg	20 ml 10 ml	500 ml 250 ml	520 ml 260 ml	1.9 mg/ml
1.0 g 500 mg	20 ml 10 ml	200 ml 100 ml	220 ml 110 ml	4.6 mg/ml

If, for clinical reasons, 0.9% saline is not suitable, then neutralised Glucose Intravenous Infusion BP 5% w/v may be used. Neutralised glucose solution is prepared by the addition of 5 ml of sterile 8.4% w/v sodium bicarbonate solution to each litre of Glucose Intravenous Injection BP 5% w/v.

It is necessary to buffer the glucose solution in this way because the stability of Erythromycin Lactobionate is adversely affected below pH 5.5.

To ensure potency, all solutions for administration should be used within 8 hours of preparation.

Contra-indications, warnings, etc

Contra-indications: Known sensitivity to erythromycin.

Precautions: Erythromycin is excreted principally by the liver, so caution should be exercised in administering the antibiotic to patients with impaired hepatic function or concomitantly receiving potentially hepatotoxic agents.

The administration of erythromycin has been infrequently associated with the occurrence of reversible cholestatic jaundice.

The use of erythromycin in patients who are receiving digoxin, warfarin, carbamazepine and high doses of theophylline may result in the potentiation of their effects due to reduction in the rates of excretion.

Use in pregnancy: There is no evidence of hazard from erythromycin in human pregnancy. It has been in wide use for many years without apparent ill consequence. Animal studies have shown no hazard.

Side-effects: Occasional side-effects such as nausea, abdominal discomfort, vomiting and diarrhoea may be experienced. Reversible hearing loss associated with doses of erythromycin usually greater than 4 g per day has been reported. Allergic reactions are rare and mild, although anaphylaxis has occurred extremely rarely. There are no reports implicating erythromycin products with abnormal tooth development and only rare reports of damage to the blood, kidneys, liver or central nervous system.

Overdosage: Symptoms: Hearing loss, severe nausea, vomiting and diarrhoea.

Treatment: General supportive measures.

Pharmaceutical precautions The powder is stable at room temperature.

Legal category POM.

Package quantities 1 g vials of Erythromycin Lactobionate.

Further information Contains no sodium. Compatibility with other IV additives has not been established.

Product licence number 0037/0092.

ERYTHROPED* A
ERYTHROPED* A SACHET

Presentation

Erythroped A: Oval, yellow film coated tablet. Each tablet contains 500 mg erythromycin as erythromycin ethylsuccinate.

Erythroped A sachet: Each sachet contains 1.0 g of erythromycin as erythromycin ethylsuccinate in the form of free-flowing, orange-bramble flavoured, orange coloured granules. The granules give a palatable fine suspension, free from aggregates, when dispersed in approximately 100 ml of tap water in a cup or glass.

Uses For the prophylaxis and treatment of infections caused by erythromycin sensitive organisms.

Clinical indications:
1. Upper respiratory tract infections
2. Lower respiratory tract infections
3. Skin and soft tissue infections
4. Bone infections
5. Sexually transmitted diseases
6. Oral/dental infections
7. Eye infections
8. Gastro-intestinal infections
9. Prophylaxis.

Erythromycin has also proved to be of value in endocarditis and septicaemia, but in these conditions initial administration of erythromycin lactobionate by the intravenous route is advised.

Microbiological indications: Erythromycin has been shown to be active in vitro against the following organisms: Staphylococci, Streptococci, *Haemophilus influenzae*, L-forms, *Mycoplasma pneumoniae*, *Legionella pneumophila*, *Branhamella catarrhalis*, *Bordetella pertussis*, *Corynebacterium diphtheriae* (as an adjunct to antitoxin), Neisseria, *Treponema pallidum*, *Chlamydia trachomatis*, Clostridia, *Ureaplasma urealytica*, Campylobacter.

Dosage and administration
Adults and children over 8 years: For mild to moderate infections 2 g daily in divided doses. Up to 4 g daily in severe infections.

Elderly: No special dosage recommendations.

Children: Not recommended for children under 8 years as unit doses are too large. Erythroped PI and Erythroped are available for infants and younger children.

Period of dosing with regard to indication
Upper respiratory tract infections: 5–10 days
Lower respiratory tract infections: 7–14 days or until signs and symptoms indicate a cure. Legionnaires' disease may require prolonged treatment. Initially administration of erythromycin lactobionate by the intravenous route is recommended.
Skin and soft tissue infections: 5–10 days. Acne may require prolonged treatment.
Sexually transmitted diseases – NGU and syphilis: 10–21 days. Some conditions may require prolonged treatment.
Oral/dental infections. At least 5 days.
Eye infections – Chlamydial inclusion conjunctivitis: 3 weeks.
Gastro-intestinal infections – Campylobacter: Minimum 5 days.

Contra-indications, warnings, etc
Contra-indications: Known sensitivity to erythromycin.

Precautions: Erythromycin is excreted principally by the liver, so caution should be exercised in administering the antibiotic to patients with impaired hepatic function or concomitantly receiving potentially hepatotoxic agents.

The administration of erythromycin has been infrequently associated with the occurrence of reversible cholestatic jaundice.

The use of erythromycin in patients who are receiving digoxin, warfarin, carbamazepine and high doses of theophylline may result in the potentiation of their effects due to reduction in the rates of excretion.

Use in pregnancy: There is no evidence of hazard from erythromycin in human pregnancy. It has been in wide use for many years without apparent ill consequence. Animal studies have shown no hazard.

Side-effects: Occasional side-effects such as nausea, abdominal discomfort, vomiting and diarrhoea may be experienced. Reversible hearing loss associated with doses of erythromycin usually greater than 4 g per day has been reported. Allergic reactions are rare and mild, although anaphylaxis has occurred extremely rarely. There are no reports implicating erythromycin products with abnormal tooth development and only rare reports of damage to the blood, kidneys, liver or central nervous system.

Overdosage: Symptoms: Hearing loss, severe nausea, vomiting and diarrhoea.
Treatment: Gastric lavage, general supportive measures.

Pharmaceutical precautions Store below 30°C.

Legal category POM.

Package quantities Erythroped A: Blister packs of 28 tablets OP.
Erythroped A sachets: Cartons of 14 sachets.

Further information Dyes: Tablets contain E104 (non-azo). Sachets contain E110 (azo).
Sugar content: Tablets – sugar free. Sachets – 7.2 g sucrose per sachet.

Product licence numbers
Erythroped A tablets 0037/0137
Erythroped A sachets 0037/0141

ERYTHROPED* PI and ERYTHROPED* PI SACHET ERYTHROPED* and ERYTHROPED* SACHET ERYTHROPED* FORTE and ERYTHROPED* FORTE SACHET

Presentation *Suspensions:* Erythromycin as erythromycin ethylsuccinate in the form of granules which, when reconstituted, make a banana flavour suspension. It is available in three strengths:
1. Erythroped PI which contains 125 mg erythromycin per 5 ml or per sachet.
2. Erythroped, containing 250 mg erythromycin per 5 ml or per sachet.
3. Erythroped Forte, containing 500 mg erythromycin per 5 ml or per sachet.

Uses For the prophylaxis and treatment of infections caused by erythromycin sensitive organisms.

Clinical indications:
1. Upper respiratory tract infections
2. Lower respiratory tract infections
3. Skin and soft tissue infections
4. Bone infections
5. Sexually transmitted diseases
6. Oral/dental infections
7. Eye infections
8. Gastro-intestinal infections
9. Prophylaxis.

Erythromycin has also proved to be of value in endocarditis and septicaemia but in these conditions initial administration of erythromycin lactobionate by the intravenous route is advised.

Microbiological indications: Erythromycin has been shown to be active in vitro against the following organisms: Staphylococci, Streptococci, *Haemophilus influenzae*, L-forms, *Mycoplasma pneumoniae*, *Legionella pneumophila*, *Branhamella catarrhalis*, *Bordetella pertussis*, *Corynebacterium diphtheriae* (as an adjunct to antitoxin), Neisseria, *Treponema pallidum*, *Chlamydia trachomatis*, Clostridia, *Ureaplasma urealytica*, Campylobacter.

Dosage and administration
Adults and children over 8 years: For mild to moderate infections 2 g daily in divided doses. Up to 4 g daily in severe infections.

Elderly: No special dosage recommendations.

Children: Aged 2–8 years: for mild to moderate infections 1 g daily in divided doses.
Infants and babies up to 2 years: for mild to moderate infections 500 mg daily in divided doses.
For severe infections doses may be doubled.

Period of dosing with regard to indication
Upper respiratory tract infections: 5–10 days
Lower respiratory tract infections: 7–14 days or until

signs and symptoms indicate a cure. Legionnaires' disease may require prolonged treatment. Initially administration of erythromycin lactobionate by the intravenous route is recommended.

Skin and soft tissue infections: 5–10 days. Acne may require prolonged treatment.

Sexually transmitted disease – NGU and syphilis: 10–21 days. Some conditions may require prolonged treatment.

Oral/dental infections: At least 5 days.

Eye infections – Chlamydial inclusion conjunctivitis: 3 weeks.

Gastro-intestinal infections – Campylobacter: Minimum 5 days.

Contra-indications, warnings, etc
Contra-indications: Known sensitivity to erythromycin.

Precautions: Erythromycin is excreted principally by the liver, so caution should be exercised in administering the antibiotic to patients with impaired hepatic function or concomitantly receiving potentially hepatotoxic agents.

The administration of erythromycin has been infrequently associated with the occurrence of reversible cholestatic jaundice.

The use of erythromycin in patients who are receiving digoxin, warfarin, carbamazepine and high doses of theophylline may result in the potentiation of their effects due to reduction in the rates of excretion.

Use in pregnancy: There is no evidence of hazard from erythromycin in human pregnancy. It has been in wide use for many years without apparent ill consequence. Animal studies have shown no hazard.

Side-effects: Occasional side-effects such as nausea, abdominal discomfort, vomiting and diarrhoea may be experienced. Reversible hearing loss associated with doses of erythromycin usually greater than 4 g per day has been reported. Allergic reactions are rare and mild, although anaphylaxis has occurred extremely rarely. There are no reports implicating erythromycin products with abnormal tooth development and only rare reports of damage to the blood, kidneys, liver or central nervous system.

Overdosage: Symptoms: Hearing loss, severe nausea, vomiting and diarrhoea. Treatment: Gastric lavage, general supportive measures.

Pharmaceutical precautions Erythroped suspensions should be stored in a cool place and the container kept tightly closed. The suspensions should be used within 14 days of dispensing. Shake well before using.

Legal category POM.

Package quantities 140 ml bottles and containers of 28 single dose sachets OP.

Further information Contains dye E104 (non-azo).

Sugar content: Erythroped PI – 3.4 g/5 ml, 0.7 g per sachet; Erythroped – 3.2 g/5 ml, 1.5 g per sachet; Erythroped Forte – 2.9 g/5 ml, 2.9 g per sachet.

Product licence numbers

Erythroped PI	125 mg/5 ml	0037/0149
	125 mg/sachet	0037/0156
Erythroped	250 mg/5 ml	0037/0150
	250 mg/sachet	0037/0157
Erythroped Forte	500 mg/5 ml	0037/0151
	500 mg/sachet	0037/0158

ERYTHROPED* SUGAR FREE

Presentation Sachets containing 250 mg erythromycin as erythromycin ethylsuccinate in disaccharide- and dye-free granules. When dispersed in a little water, immediately before taking, the entire contents of one sachet provide a unit dose in the form of a cherry flavour suspension sweetened with mannitol.

Uses For the prophylaxis and treatment of infections caused by erythromycin sensitive organisms.

Clinical indications:
1. Upper respiratory tract infections.
2. Lower respiratory tract infections.
3. Skin and soft tissue infections.
4. Bone infections.
5. Sexually transmitted diseases.
6. Oral/dental infections.
7. Eye infections.
8. Gastro-intestinal infections.
9. Prophylaxis.

Erythromycin has also proved to be of value in endocarditis and septicaemia but in these conditions initial administration of erythromycin lactobionate by the intravenous route is advised.

Microbiological indications: Erythromycin has been shown to be active in vitro against the following organisms: Staphylococci, Streptococci, *Haemophilus influenzae*, L-forms, *Mycoplasma pneumoniae*, *Legionella pneumophila*, *Branhamella catarrhalis*, *Bordetella pertussis*, *Corynebacterium diphtheriae* (as an adjunct to antitoxin), Neisseria, *Treponema pallidum*, *Chlamydia trachomatis*, Clostridia, *Ureaplasma urealytica*, Campylobacter.

Dosage and administration
Adults and children over 8 years: For mild to moderate infections 2 g daily in divided doses. Up to 4 g daily in severe infections.

Elderly: No special dosage recommendations.

Children: Aged 2–8 years: For mild to moderate infections 1 g daily in divided doses.

Infants and babies up to 2 years: For mild to moderate infections 500 mg daily in divided doses.

For severe infections doses may be doubled.

Period of dosing with regard to indication

Upper respiratory tract infections	5–10 days.
Lower respiratory tract infections	7–14 days or until signs and symptoms indicate a cure. Legionnaires' disease may require prolonged treatment. Initially administration of erythromycin lactobionate by the intravenous route is recommended.
Skin and soft tissue infections	5–10 days. Acne may require prolonged treatment.
Sexually transmitted diseases	
NGU and syphilis	10–21 days. Some conditions may require prolonged treatment.
Oral/dental infections	At least 5 days.
Eye infections	
Chlamydial inclusion conjunctivitis	3 weeks.
Gastro-intestinal infections	
Campylobacter	Minimum 5 days.

Contra-indications, warnings, etc
Contra-indications: Known sensitivity to erythromycin.

Precautions: Erythromycin is excreted principally by the liver, so caution should be exercised in administering the antibiotic to patients with impaired hepatic function or concomitantly receiving potentially hepatotoxic agents.

The administration of erythromycin has been infrequently associated with the occurrence of reversible cholestatic jaundice.

The use of erythromycin in patients who are receiving digoxin, warfarin, carbamazepine and high doses of theophylline may result in the potentiation of their effects due to reduction in the rates of excretion.

Use in pregnancy: There is no evidence of hazard from erythromycin in human pregnancy. It has been in wide use for many years without apparent ill consequence. Animal studies have shown no hazard.

Side-effects: Occasional side-effects such as nausea,

abdominal discomfort, vomiting and diarrhoea may be experienced. Reversible hearing loss associated with doses of erythromycin usually greater than 4 g per day has been reported. Allergic reactions are rare and mild, although anaphylaxis has occurred extremely rarely. There are no reports implicating erythromycin products with abnormal tooth development and only rare reports of damage to the blood, kidneys, liver or central nervous system.

Overdosage: Symptoms: Hearing loss, severe nausea, vomiting and diarrhoea.

Treatment: Gastric lavage, general supportive measures.

Pharmaceutical precautions Store below 30°C.

Legal category POM.

Package quantities Cartons of 20 sachets.

Further information Nil.

Product licence number 0037/0135.

FERROGRAD*

Presentation Each red Filmtab* (film-coated tablet Abbott) contains Dried Ferrous Sulphate BP 325 mg (equivalent to 105 mg elemental iron) in a controlled release form (Gradumet*).

Uses For the prevention and treatment of iron-deficiency anaemia.

The Gradumet device allows controlled release of ferrous sulphate over a number of hours and reduces gastro-intestinal intolerance. The device consists of an inert plastic matrix, honeycombed by thousands of narrow passages which contain ferrous sulphate together with a water soluble channelling agent. As the tablet passes down the gastro-intestinal tract the iron is leached out. The spent matrix is finally excreted in the stools.

Dosage and administration

Recommended adult oral dosage: One tablet a day before food. As gastro intestinal intolerance is not a problem with Ferrograd, it should be given on an empty stomach when iron is most effectively absorbed.

Children: Not recommended for children under 12 years of age.

Elderly: The controlled release tablet and its inert plastic matrix may cause a safety hazard in some elderly or other patients suffering from delayed intestinal transit.

Contra-indications, warnings, etc

Contra-indications: Intestinal diverticula or any intestinal obstruction.

Precautions: Iron interacts with tetracyclines, magnesium trisilicate, trientine and zinc salts and absorption of all of these agents may be impaired. Ferrograd tablets should be kept out of children's reach. The controlled release tablet and its inert plastic matrix may cause a safety hazard in some elderly or other patients suffering from delayed intestinal transit.

Pregnancy: Ferrograd Folic is indicated for the prevention and treatment of iron deficiency anaemia of pregnancy and for prophylaxis of megaloblastic anaemia of pregnancy.

Side-effects: Side-effects reported are similar to those associated with conventional oral iron preparations, ie. nausea, vomiting, abdominal pain or discomfort, diarrhoea and/or constipation, but the incidence of side-effects is less owing to the controlled release of nature of the formulation.

Overdosage: Symptoms: Initial symptoms of iron overdosage include nausea, vomiting, diarrhoea, abdominal pain, haematemesis, rectal bleeding, lethargy and circulatory collapse. Hyperglycaemia and metabolic acidosis may also occur. The controlled release characteristic may delay excessive absorption of iron, and thus allow more time for counter measures to be implemented. However, initial symptoms of overdosage may be absent due to the controlled release formulation. Therefore, if overdosage is suspected, treatment should be implemented immediately. In severe cases, after a latent phase, relapse may occur after 24–48 hours, manifested by hypotension, coma and hepatocellular necrosis and renal failure.

Treatment: The following steps are recommended to minimise or prevent further absorption of the medication:

Children

1. Administer an emetic such as syrup of ipec.
2. Emesis should be followed by gastric lavage with desferrioxamine solution (2 g/l). This should then be followed by the instillation of desferrioxamine 5 g in 50–100 ml water, to be retained in the stomach. Inducing diarrhoea in children may be dangerous and should not be undertaken in young children. Keep the patient under constant surveillance to detect possible aspiration of vomitus – maintain suction apparatus and standby emergency oxygen in case of need.
3. Unleached tablets are radio-opaque. Therefore, an abdominal x-ray should be taken to determine the number of tablets retained in the stomach following emesis and gastric lavage.
4. Severe poisoning: in the presence of shock and/or coma with high serum iron levels (serum iron >90 μmol/l) immediate supportive measures plus i.v infusion of desferrioxamine should be instituted. Desferrioxamine 15 mg/kg body weight should be administered every hour by slow i.v infusion to a maximum 80 mg/kg/24 hours. Warning: hypotension may occur if the infusion rate is too rapid.
5. Less severe poisoning: i.m desferrioxamine 1 g 4–6 hourly is recommended.
6. Serum iron levels should be monitored throughout.

Adults

1. Administer an emetic.
2. Gastric lavage may be necessary to remove drug already released into the stomach. This should be undertaken using desferrioxamine solution (2 g/l). Desferrioxamine 5 g in 50–100 ml water should be introduced into the stomach following gastric emptying. Keep the patient under constant surveillance to detect possible aspiration of vomitus; maintain suction apparatus and standby emergency oxygen in case of need.
3. Unleached tablets are radio-opaque. Therefore, an abdominal x-ray of the patient should be taken to determine the number of tablets retained in the stomach following emesis and gastric lavage. The risk/benefit ratio of x-raying pregnant women must be carefully weighed but should be avoided if possible.
4. A drink of mannitol or sorbitol should be given to induce small bowel emptying.
5. Severe poisoning: in the presence of shock and/or coma with high serum iron levels (>142 μmol/l) immediate supportive measures plus i.v infusion of desferrioxamine should be instituted. The recommended dose of desferrioxamine is 5 mg/kg/h by slow i.v infusion up to a maximum of 80 mg/kg/24 hours. Warning: hypotension may occur if the infusion rate is too rapid.
6. Less severe poisoning: i.m desferrioxamine 50 mg/kg up to a maximum dose of 4 g should be given.
7. Serum iron levels should be monitored throughout.

Pharmaceutical precautions Nil.

Legal category P.

Package quantities Ferrograd is supplied in 5 carton packs, each containing 30 (3 × 10) tablets (OP).

Further information Nil.

Product licence number 0037/5000R.

FERROGRAD* C

Presentation Each two-layered, red Filmtab* (film-coated tablet Abbott) contains Dried Ferrous Sulphate BP 325 mg (equivalent to 105 mg elemental iron) in a controlled release form (Gradumet*) and 500 mg vitamin C, as sodium ascorbate.

Uses For the prevention and treatment of iron-deficiency anaemia. Ferrograd C combines the advantages of ferrous sulphate in the Gradumet matrix with a large dose of vitamin C further to enhance absorption and is indicated in iron-deficiency anaemia, especially when poor absorption is a problem, and to promote haemopoiesis in patients where an underlying vitamin C deficiency limits optimal haemoglobin formation. In patients whose haemoglobin has returned to normal, Ferrograd C may be of particular value in replenishing the depleted stores of iron.

The Gradumet device allows controlled release of ferrous sulphate over a number of hours and reduces gastro-intestinal intolerance. The device consists of an inert plastic matrix, honeycombed by thousands of narrow passages which contain ferrous sulphate together with a water-soluble channelling agent. As the tablet passes down the gastro-intestinal tract the iron is leached out. The spent matrix is finally excreted in the stools.

Dosage and administration
Recommended adult oral dosage: One tablet a day before food.

Children: Not recommended for children under 12 years of age.

Elderly: The controlled release tablet and its inert plastic matrix may cause a safety hazard in some elderly or other patients suffering from delayed intestinal transit.

Contra-indications, warnings, etc
Contra indications: Intestinal diverticula or any intestinal obstruction.

Warning: The administration of therapeutic doses of ascorbic acid may interfere with the Clinistix test for glucosuria giving a false negative result.

Precautions: Iron interacts with tetracyclines, magnesium trisilicate, trientine and zinc salts and absorption of all of these agents may be impaired. Ferrograd C tablets should be kept out of children's reach. The controlled release tablet and its inert plastic matrix may cause a safety hazard in some elderly or other patients suffering from delayed intestinal transit.

Side-effects: Side-effects reported are similar to those associated with conventional oral iron preparations, ie. nausea, vomiting, abdominal pain or discomfort, diarrhoea and/or constipation, but the incidence of side-effects is less owing to the controlled release nature of the formulation.

Overdosage: Symptoms: initial symptoms of iron overdosage include nausea, vomiting, diarrhoea, abdominal pain, haematemesis, rectal bleeding, lethargy and circulatory collapse. Hyperglycaemia and metabolic acidosis may also occur. The controlled release characteristic may delay excessive absorption of iron, and thus allow more time for counter measures to be implemented. However, initial symptoms of overdosage may be absent due to the controlled release formulation. Therefore, if overdosage is suspected, treatment should be implemented immediately. In severe cases, after a latent phase, relapse may occur after 24–48 hours, manifested by hypotension, coma and hepatocellular necrosis and renal failure. Vitamin C overdosage may cause acidosis and haemolytic anaemia in predisposed individuals (glucose – 6 – phosphate dehydrogenase deficiency). Renal failure may occur in massive vitamin C overdosage.

Treatment: The following steps are recommended to minimise or prevent further absorption of the medication:

Children

1. Administer an emetic such as syrup of ipec.
2. Emesis should be followed by gastric lavage with desferrioxamine solution (2 g/l). This should then be followed by the instillation of desferrioxamine 5 g in 50–100 ml water, to be retained in the stomach. Inducing diarrhoea in children may be dangerous and should not be undertaken in young children. Keep the patient under constant surveillance to detect possible aspiration of vomitus – maintain suction apparatus and standby emergency oxygen in case of need.
3. Unleached tablets are radio-opaque. Therefore, an abdominal x-ray should be taken to determine the number of tablets retained in the stomach following emesis and gastric lavage.
4. Severe poisoning: in the presence of shock and/or coma with high serum iron levels (serum iron >90 μmol/l) immediate supportive measures plus i.v. infusion of desferrioxamine should be instituted. Desferrioxamine 15 mg/kg body weight should be administered every hour by slow i.v infusion to a maximum 80 mg/kg/24 hours. Warning: hypotension may occur if the infusion rate is too rapid.
5. Less severe poisoning: i.m desferrioxamine 1 g 4–6 hourly is recommended.
6. Serum iron levels should be monitored throughout.

Adults

1. Administer an emetic.
2. Gastric lavage may be necessary to remove drug already released into the stomach. This should be undertaken using desferrioxamine solution (2 g/l). Desferrioxamine 5 g in 50–100 ml water should be introduced into the stomach following gastric emptying. Keep the patients under constant surveillance to detect possible aspiration of vomitus; maintain suction apparatus and standby emergency oxygen in case of need.
3. Unleached tablets are radio-opaque. Therefore, an abdominal x-ray of the patient should be taken to determine the number of tablets retained in the stomach following emesis and gastric lavage. The risk/benefit ratio of x-raying pregnant women must be carefully weighed but should be avoided if possible.
4. A drink of mannitol or sorbitol should be given to induce small bowel emptying.
5. Severe poisoning: in the presence of shock and/or coma with high serum iron levels (>142 μmol/l) immediate supportive measures plus i.v infusion of desferrioxamine should be instituted. The recommended dose of desferrioxamine is 5 mg/kg/h by slow i.v infusion up to a maximum of 80 mg/kg/24 hours. Warning: hypotension may occur if the infusion rate is too rapid.
6. Less severe poisoning: i.m desferrioxamine 50 mg/kg up to a maximum dose of 4 g should be given.
7. Serum iron levels should be monitored throughout.

Pharmaceutical precautions Nil.

Legal category P.

Package quantities Ferrograd C is supplied in 5 carton packs, each containing 30 (3 × 10) tablets (OP).

Further information Nil.

Product licence number 0037/5001R.

FERROGRAD* FOLIC

Presentation A two-layered (red and yellow), round, bi-convex Filmtab* (film-coated tablet Abbott). Each tablet contains Dried Ferrous Sulphate BP 325 mg (equivalent to 105 mg elemental iron) in a controlled release form (red half – Gradumet*) and 350 micrograms Folic Acid BP (yellow half).

Uses Ferrograd Folic is indicated:

1. For the prevention and treatment of iron-deficiency anaemia of pregnancy.
2. For the prophylaxis of megaloblastic anaemia of pregnancy.

Folic acid requirements in pregnancy can be met with supplements of between 300 and 400 micrograms daily. Without such supplements folate deficiency may develop leading to megaloblastic anaemia with attendant obstetric risks. Doses over 400 micrograms may mask undiagnosed primary B_{12} deficiency. In the extremely unlikely event of this condition occurring in a pregnant woman, the safe prophylactic dose is considered to be 350 micrograms.

The Gradumet device allows controlled release of ferrous sulphate over a number of hours, and reduces gastro-intestinal intolerance. The device consists of an inert plastic matrix, honeycombed by thousands of narrow passages which contain the ferrous sulphate together with water-soluble channelling agent. As the tablet passes down the gastro-intestinal tract the iron is leached out. The spent matrix is finally excreted in the stools.

Dosage and administration
Recommended adult oral dosage: One tablet daily before food throughout pregnancy and during the first month of the puerperium.

Children: Not recommended for children under 12 years of age.

Elderly: The controlled release tablet and its inert plastic matrix may cause a safety hazard in some elderly or other patients suffering from delayed intestinal transit.

Contra-indications, warnings, etc
Contra-indications: Megaloblastic anaemia due to primary vitamin B_{12} deficiency. Intestinal or any intestinal obstruction.

Precautions: Iron interacts with tetracyclines, magnesium trisilicate, trientine and zinc salts and absorption of all of these agents may be impaired. Ferrograd Folic tablets should be kept out of children's reach. The controlled release tablet and its inert plastic matrix may cause a safety hazard in some elderly or other patients suffering from delayed intestinal transit.

Side-effects: Side-effects reported are similar to those associated with conventional oral iron preparations, ie. nausea, vomiting, abdominal pain or discomfort, diarrhoea and/or constipation, but the incidence of side-effects is less owing to the controlled release nature of the formulation.

Overdosage: Symptoms: initial symptoms of iron overdosage include nausea, vomiting, diarrhoea, abdominal pain, haematemesis, rectal bleeding, lethargy and circulatory collapse. Hyperglycaemia and metabolic acidosis may also occur. The controlled release characteristic may delay excessive absorption of iron, and thus allow more time for counter measures to be implemented. However, initial symptoms of overdosage may be absent due to the controlled release formulation. Therefore, if overdosage is suspected, treatment should be implemented immediately. In severe cases, after a latent phase, relapse may occur after 24–48 hours, manifested by hypotension, coma and hepatocellular necrosis and renal failure.

Treatment: The following steps are recommended to minimise or prevent further absorption of the medication:

Children

1. Administer an emetic such as syrup of ipec.
2. Emesis should be followed by gastric lavage with desferrioxamine solution (2 g/l). This should then be followed by the instillation of desferrioxamine 5 g in 50–100 ml water, to be retained in the stomach. Inducing diarrhoea in children may be dangerous and should not be undertaken in young children. Keep the patient under constant surveillance to detect possible aspiration of vomitus – maintain suction apparatus and standby emergency oxygen in case of need.
3. Unleached tablets are radio-opaque. Therefore, an abdominal x-ray should be taken to determine the number of tablets retained in the stomach following emesis and gastric lavage.
4. Severe poisoning: in the presence of shock and/or coma with high serum iron levels (serum iron >90 μmol/l) immediate supportive measures plus i.v infusion of desferrioxamine should be instituted. Desferrioxamine 15 mg/kg body weight should be administered every hour by slow i.v infusion to a maximum 80 mg/kg/24 hours. Warning: hypotension may occur if the infusion rate is too rapid.
5. Less severe poisoning: i.m desferrioxamine 1 g 4–6 hourly is recommended.
6. Serum iron levels should be monitored throughout.

Adults

1. Administer an emetic.
2. Gastric lavage may be necessary to remove drug already released into the stomach. This should be undertaken using desferrioxamine solution (2 g/l). Desferrioxamine 5 g in 50–100 ml water should be introduced into the stomach following gastric emptying. Keep the patients under constant surveillance to detect possible aspiration of vomitus; maintain suction apparatus and standby emergency oxygen in case of need.
3. Unleached tablets are radio-opaque. Therefore, an abdominal x-ray of the patient should be taken to determine the number of tablets retained in the stomach following emesis and gastric lavage. The risk/benefit ratio of x-raying pregnant women must be carefully weighed but should be avoided if possible.
4. A drink of mannitol or sorbitol should be given to induce small bowel emptying.
5. Severe poisoning: in the presence of shock and/or coma with high serum iron levels (> 142 μmol/l) immediate supportive measures plus i.v infusion of desferrioxamine should be instituted. The recommended dose of desferrioxamine is 5 mg/kg/h by slow i.v infusion up to a maximum of 80 mg/kg/24 hours. Warning: hypotension may occur if the infusion rate is too rapid.
6. Less severe poisoning: i.m desferrioxamine 50 mg/kg up to a maximum dose of 4 g should be given.
7. Serum iron levels should be monitored throughout.

Pharmaceutical precautions Nil.

Legal category P.

Package quantities Ferrograd Folic is supplied in 5 carton packs, each containing 30 (3 × 10) tablets (OP).

Further information Nil.

Product licence number 0037/5002R.

HARMOGEN*

Presentation Peach-coloured, flat, elongated, scored tablets marked LV. Each tablet contains 1.5 mg Estropipate USP (piperazine oestrone sulphate), equivalent to 0.93 mg oestrone.

Uses Oestrogen replacement therapy for the relief of oestrogen deficiency symptoms during or after the menopause and following oophorectomy, e.g. vasomotor symptoms, senile atrophic vaginitis, vulvitis and urethral syndrome, postmenopausal osteoporosis, depression, irritability and sleep disturbances.

Dosage and administration
Adults: 1.5–4.5 mg daily, taken as a single or divided oral dose. It may be necessary to divide the dose if gastro-intestinal irritation becomes a problem.

Clinical studies indicate that two Harmogen tablets daily is a satisfactory starting dose. For maintenance, the lowest effective dose should be used for a period of 3–4 weeks followed by a rest period of 5–7 days. Unless the patient has undergone hysterectomy Harmogen should be given cyclically and accompanied by the administration of a progestogen. Withdrawal bleeding may occur towards the end of the rest period.

Elderly: As for adults.

Children: Not recommended.

Contra-indications, warnings, etc
Contra-indications: Oestrogen dependent carcinomas; history of thromboembolic disease; disorders of carbohydrate or lipid metabolism; undiagnosed bleeding from the genital tract; pregnancy; hepatic and renal disease; porphyria; history of herpes gestationis.

Precautions: The occurrence of abnormal, irregular bleeding at the commencement of, or during, therapy should be thoroughly investigated. Possible causes include incorrect dosage, fibroids or carcinoma.

Oestrogens may cause fluid retention, therefore caution should be exercised in patients with epilepsy, hypertension, migraine or cardiac disease.

Use with caution in patients with the combined factors of obesity, hypertension and smoking.

Prolonged exposure to unopposed oestrogens may increase the risk of the development of endometrial carcinoma.

Adverse effects of oestrogen therapy on blood pressure and gall bladder function have been reported.

In the unlikely event of the use of Harmogen in breast-feeding women, it should be remembered that oestrogens are excreted in the breast milk and inhibit milk flow.

Side-effects: The incidence of side-effects with Harmogen is low. Nausea is the most frequently reported side-effect; less common side-effects include fluid retention, breast swelling and tenderness, anorexia, vomiting, headaches, changes in liver function and breakthrough bleeding. Rare reactions include allergies, jaundice and changes in glucose metabolism and in libido. Oestrogens may precipitate porphyria cutanea tarda.

Overdosage: Overdosage is unlikely to cause serious problems. However, gastric lavage or emesis may be used when considered appropriate.

Pharmaceutical precautions Nil.

Legal category POM.

Package quantities Harmogen is supplied in containers of 100 tablets.

Further information Metabolisable carbohydrate content: Approx. 0.2 g per tablet.

The amount of piperazine in Harmogen is not sufficient to exert a pharmacological action, but its addition ensures solubility, stability and uniform potency.

Product licence number 0037/5064.

HYTRIN*

Presentation Hytrin (terazosin as terazosin hydrochloride) is presented as round flat bevelled tablets embossed with logo and triangular facets on one face and plain on the other. Hytrin tablets are available as follows: 1 mg white tablet; 2 mg yellow tablet; 5 mg tan tablet; 10 mg blue tablet.

Uses Orally administered Hytrin is indicated in the treatment of mild to moderate hypertension. It may be used in combination with thiazide diuretics and/or other antihypertensive drugs or as sole therapy where other agents are inappropriate or ineffective. The hypotensive effect is most pronounced on the diastolic pressure. Although the exact mechanism of the hypotensive action of terazosin is not established, the relaxation of peripheral blood vessels appears to be produced mainly by competitive antagonism of post-synaptic alpha$_1$-adrenoceptors. Hytrin usually produces an initial gradual decrease in blood pressure followed by a sustained antihypertensive action.

Hytrin has been administered to date without apparent interaction with the following types of drugs:

(a) analgesics/anti-inflammatories (e.g. paracetamol, aspirin, indomethacin, ibuprofen, phenylbutazone, dextropropoxyphene, tolmetin);

(b) cardiac glycosides (e.g. digoxin);

(c) hypoglycaemics (e.g. chlorpropamide, insulin, tolazamide, tolbutamide);

(d) antiarrhythmics (e.g. procainamide);

(e) anxiolytics/sedatives (e.g. clorazepate, chlordiazepoxide, diazepam, flurazepam);

(f) drugs used in the treatment of gout (e.g. allopurinol, probenecid);

(g) antibacterials (e.g. ampicillin, erythromycin, penicillin, tetracycline, trimethoprim and sulphamethoxazole);

(h) hormones/steroids (e.g. oestrogen supplements).

Long term administration of Hytrin has produced no pattern of clinically significant changes in the following laboratory parameters: glucose, uric acid, creatinine, urea, liver function tests, electrolytes, haematology.

Kinetics: The plasma concentration of the parent drug is at a maximum at about 1 hour post administration and then declines with a half-life of approximately 12 hours. Food has little or no effect on bioavailability. The drug is highly bound to plasma proteins.

Dosage and administration The dose of Hytrin should be adjusted according to the patient's blood pressure response. The following is a guide to its administration.

Guide to administration in adults

Initial dose: 1 mg before bedtime is the starting dose for all patients and should not be exceeded. Compliance with this initial dosage recommendation should be strictly observed to minimise the potential for acute first-dose hypotensive episodes.

Subsequent doses: The single daily dosage may be increased by approximately doubling the dosage at weekly intervals to achieve the desired blood pressure response.

The usual maintenance dose is 2 to 10 mg once daily. Doses over 20 mg rarely improve efficacy and doses over 40 mg have not been studied.

Use with thiazide diuretics and other antihypertensive agents: When adding a thiazide diuretic or another antihypertensive agent to a patient's regimen the dose of Hytrin should be reduced and retitration carried out if necessary. Caution should be observed when Hytrin is administered with thiazides or other antihypertensive agents as hypotension may develop.

Use in renal insufficiency: Pharmacokinetic studies indicate that patients with impaired renal function need no alteration in recommended dosage.

Use in children: Safety and efficacy in children has not been established.

Use in the elderly: Pharmacokinetic studies in the elderly indicate that no alteration in dosage recommendation is required.

Use in pregnancy: Although no teratogenic effects were seen in animal testing, the safety of Hytrin use during pregnancy or during lactation has not yet been established. Hytrin should not be used therefore in pregnancy unless the potential benefit outweighs the risk.

Contra-indications, warnings, etc

Contra-indications: Known sensitivity to alpha-adrenoceptor antagonists.

Warnings: Hytrin in common with other alpha-antagonists may cause syncope. In patients in clinical studies, the incidence of syncopal episodes was approximately one percent. In most cases this was believed to be due to an excessive postural hypotensive effect although occasionally the syncopal episode has been preceded by a bout of tachycardia with heart rates of 120 to 160 beats per minute.

Syncopal episodes have occurred within 30 to 90 minutes of the initial dose of the drug. Syncope has occasionally occurred in association with rapid dosage increases.

If syncope occurs the patient should be placed in a recumbent position and supportive treatment applied as necessary. This adverse effect is self-limiting and in most cases does not recur after the initial period of therapy or during subsequent dose titration.

Clinical trials to date have excluded patients having a history or diagnosis of orthostatic hypotension; fainting spells, blackouts; myocardial infarction; cerebrovascular accidents; transient ischemic attacks; angina pectoris; gastro-intestinal ulceration; alcoholism or other causes of liver disease; grade III or IV hypertensive retinopathy or insulin-dependent diabetes.

Carcinogenicity: Hytrin has been shown to produce tumours in male rats when administered at a high dose over a long period of time. No such occurrences were seen in a similar study in mice. The relevance of these findings with respect to the clinical use of the drug in man is unknown.

Precautions: Dizziness, lightheadedness or drowsiness may occur with the initial dose or in association with missed doses and subsequent reinitiation of Hytrin therapy. Patients should be cautioned about these possible adverse effects and the circumstances in which they may occur and advised to avoid driving or hazardous tasks for approximately the first 12 hours after the initial dose or when the dose is increased.

Dizziness, lightheadedness or fainting may occur when standing up quickly from a lying or sitting position. Patients should be advised of this possibility and instructed to lie down if these symptoms appear and then to sit for a few minutes before standing to prevent their recurrence.

Side-effects: Side-effects associated with the use of Hytrin have generally been mild to moderate in intensity. The most commonly reported side-effects in patients receiving up to 40 mg terazosin every day are dizziness, lack of energy and peripheral oedema. In most instances these side-effects have disappeared with continuing therapy or have been tolerated with no decrease in the dose of the drug.

Additional adverse reactions reported in clinical trials but not clearly associated with the use of terazosin included the following: headache; oedema; tachycardia; palpitations; vasodilations; constipation; diarrhoea; dry mouth; dyspepsia; flatulence; upset stomach; nausea; vomiting; weight gain; stiffness; swelling or weakness in joints; myalgia; depression; insomnia; decreased libido; nervousness; somnolence; paraesthesia; epistaxis; flu symptoms; pharyngitis; rhinitis; dyspnoea; cold symptoms; nasal congestion; increased cough; sinusitis; sweating; abnormal vision; amblyopia; conjunctivitis; eye disorder; tinnitus; impotence and urinary frequency.

Treatment of overdosage: Should administration of Hytrin lead to acute hypotension, cardiovascular support is of first importance. Restoration of blood pressure and normalisation of heart rate may be accomplished by keeping the patient in a supine position. If this measure is inadequate, shock should first be treated with volume expanders and if necessary, vasopressors could then be used. Renal function should be monitored and general supportive measures applied as required. Dialysis may not be of benefit since laboratory data indicate that terazosin is highly protein bound.

Pharmaceutical precautions Nil.

Legal category POM.

Package quantities
Starter Pack – blister pack containing 7 × 1 mg tablets and 21 × 2 mg tablets (OP).
2 mg tablet – blister packs containing 28 tablets (OP).
5 mg tablet – blister packs containing 28 tablets (OP).
10 mg tablet – blister packs containing 28 tablets (OP).

Further information Nil.

Product licence numbers
1 mg tablet 0037/0159
2 mg tablet 0037/0160
5 mg tablet 0037/0161
10 mg tablet 0037/0162

ISOFLURANE

Presentation Isoflurane is an inhalation anaesthetic with a mildly pungent ethereal odour. No additive or stabiliser is present.

Uses Inhalation anaesthesia.

Actions: Induction and particularly recovery are rapid. Although slight pungency may limit the rate of induction, excessive salivation and tracheobronchial secretions are not stimulated. Pharyngeal and laryngeal reflexes are diminished quickly. Levels of anaesthesia change rapidly with Isoflurane. Heart rhythm remains stable. Spontaneous respiration becomes depressed as depth of anaesthesia increases and should be closely monitored.

During induction there is a decrease in blood pressure which returns towards normal with surgical stimulation.

Blood pressure tends to fall during maintenance in direct relation to depth of anaesthesia, but cardiac rhythm remains stable. With controlled respiration and normal $PaCO_2$, cardiac output tends to be maintained despite increasing depth of anaesthesia, primarily through a rise in heart rate. With spontaneous respiration, the resulting hypercapnia may increase heart rate and cardiac output above awake levels.

Cerebral blood flow remains unchanged during light Isoflurane anaesthesia but tends to rise at deeper levels. Increases in cerebrospinal fluid pressure may be prevented or reversed by hyperventilating the patient before or during anaesthesia.

Electroencephalographic changes and convulsions are extremely rare with Isoflurane.

Isoflurane appears to sensitise the myocardium to adrenaline to an even lesser extent than enflurane. Limited data suggest that subcutaneous infiltration of up to 50 ml of 1:200,000 solution adrenaline does not induce ventricular arrhythmias in patients anaesthetised with Isoflurane.

Muscular relaxation may be adequate for some intra-abdominal operations at normal levels of anaesthesia, but should greater relaxation be required small doses of intravenous muscle relaxants may be used. All commonly used muscle relaxants are markedly potentiated by Isoflurane, the effect being most profound with non-depolarising agents. Neostigmine reverses the effects of non-depolarising muscle relaxants but has no effect on the relaxant properties of Isoflurane itself. All commonly used muscle relaxants are compatible with Isoflurane.

Isoflurane may be used for the induction and maintenance of general anaesthesia. Adequate data are not available to establish its place in pregnancy or obstetrics anaesthesia other than for caesarian section.

Relatively little metabolism of Isoflurane occurs in the human body. In the post-operative period only 0.17% of the isoflurane taken up can be recovered as urinary metabolites. Peak serum inorganic fluoride values usually average less than 5 micromol/litre and occur about four hours after anaesthesia, returning to normal levels within 24 hours. No signs of renal injury have been reported after Isoflurane administration.

Dosage and administration Vaporisers specially calibrated for Isoflurane should be used so that the concentration of anaesthetic delivered can be accurately controlled.

MAC values for Isoflurane vary with age. The table below indicates average MAC values for different age groups:

Age	*Average MAC value in oxygen*
0–1 month	1.6%
1–6 months	1.87%
6–12 months	1.8%
1–5 years	1.6%
mid-twenties	1.28%
mid-forties	1.15%
mid-sixties	1.05%

Premedication: Drugs used for premedication should be selected for the individual patient, bearing in mind the respiratory depressant effect of Isoflurane. The use of anticholinergic drugs is a matter of choice but may be advisable for inhalation induction in paediatrics.

Induction: A short-acting barbiturate or other intravenous induction agent is usually administered followed by inhalation of the Isoflurane mixture. Alternatively, Isoflurane with oxygen or with an oxygen/nitrous oxide mixture may be used.

It is recommended that induction with Isoflurane be initiated at a concentration of 0.5%. Concentrations of 1.5 to 3.0% usually produce surgical anaesthesia in 7 to 10 minutes.

Maintenance: Surgical levels of anaesthesia may be maintained with 1.0–2.5% Isoflurane in oxygen/nitrous oxide mixtures. An additional 0.5–1.0% Isoflurane may be required when given with oxygen alone.

For caesarian section, 0.5–0.75% Isoflurane in a mixture of oxygen/nitrous oxide is suitable to maintain anaesthesia for this procedure.

Arterial pressure levels during maintenance tend to be inversely related to alveolar Isoflurane concentrations in the absence of other complicating factors. Excessive falls in blood pressure may be due to depth of anaesthesia and, in these circumstances, should be corrected by reducing the inspired Isoflurane concentration.

Elderly: As with other agents, lesser concentrations of Isoflurane are normally required to maintain surgical anaesthesia in elderly patients. See above for MAC values.

Contra-indications, warnings, etc

Contra-indications: Known sensitivity to Isoflurane, or history of malignant hyperpyrexia following its administration should be considered contra-indications.

Precautions: Since levels of anaesthesia may be altered quickly and easily with Isoflurane, only vaporisers which deliver a predictable output with reasonable accuracy, or techniques during which inspired or expired concentrations can be monitored, should be used. The degree of hypotension and respiratory depression may provide some indication of anaesthetic depth.

Clinical experience with Isoflurane to date has not shown evidence of liver toxicity, even after prolonged administration. However, experience with repeated exposure to Isoflurane is limited and it is not yet possible to determine the effects of this on liver function.

As with other halogenated agents, Isoflurane must be used with caution in patients with increased intracranial pressure. In such cases hyperventilation may be necessary.

The action of non-depolarising relaxants is markedly potentiated with Isoflurane.

Use in pregnancy: Reproduction studies have been carried out on animals after repeated exposure to anaesthetic concentrations of Isoflurane. Studies with the rat demonstrated no effect on fertility, pregnancy or delivery or on the viability of the offspring. No evidence of teratogenicity was revealed. Comparable experiments in rabbits produced similar negative results. The relevance of these studies to the human is not known. Safety in pregnancy has not been established. Blood losses comparable with those found following anaesthesia with other inhalation agents have been observed with Isoflurane in patients undergoing induced abortion. Adequate data have not been developed to establish the safety of Isoflurane in obstetric anaesthesia, other than for caesarian section.

Adverse reactions

1. Arrhythmias have been occasionally reported.
2. Elevation of the white blood cell count has been observed, even in the absence of surgical stress.
3. Minimally raised levels of serum inorganic fluoride occur during and after Isoflurane anaesthesia, due to biodegradation of the agent. It is unlikely that the low levels of serum inorganic fluoride observed (mean 4.4 micromol/l in one study) could cause renal toxicity, as these are well below the proposed threshold levels for kidney toxicity.

Side-effects: As with other halogenated anaesthetics, hypotension and respiratory depression have been observed. Close monitoring of blood pressure and respiration is recommended. Supportive measures may be necessary to correct hypotension and respiratory depression resulting from excessively deep levels of anaesthesia. Undesirable effects during recovery (shivering, nausea and vomiting) are minor in nature and comparable in incidence with those found with other anaesthetics.

Pharmaceutical precautions Store away from heat. Keep container well closed.

Legal category P.

Package quantities Isoflurane is supplied in bottles of 100 ml.

Further information Nil.

Product licence number 0037/0115.

NORMETIC*

Presentation Flat, pale peach, bisected tablets with bevelled edges, 8.5 mm diameter and marked Normetic, containing Amiloride Hydrochloride BP equivalent to 5 mg anhydrous amiloride hydrochloride and 50 mg Hydrochlorothiazide BP.

Uses Antihypertensive and diuretic with potassium conserving properties. Indicated in the care of patients with hypertension, congestive heart failure, or hepatic cirrhosis with ascites, or where potassium depletion may occur. The amiloride hydrochloride in Normetic reduces the possibility of excessive potassium loss during prolonged and vigorous diuresis. Normetic is recommended in those conditions where potassium balance is particularly important, for example in patients with congestive heart failure receiving digitalis.

In hepatic cirrhosis and ascites, Normetic is likely to provide satisfactory diuresis with diminished potassium loss, thus lessening the risk of metabolic alkalosis.

Dosage and administration The rate of weight loss and the level of serum electrolytes should determine the dosage. The ideal target for weight loss after initiation of diuresis being in the range of 0.5–1.0 kg per day.

Hypertension: Usually 1 or 2 tablets once a day or in divided doses, which may be increased up to a maximum of 4 tablets per day.

Normetic may be used alone or in conjunction with other antihypertensive drugs. Since Normetic enhances the action of such agents, the antihypertensive dosage regimen may have to be altered to obviate any hypotensive reaction.

Hepatic cirrhosis with ascites: Starting with 1 tablet per day, dosage may be increased if required until there is effective diuresis provided the dose does not exceed 4 tablets per day. Ideally, a gradual weight loss is preferred in cirrhotic patients to minimise the occurrence of untoward reactions associated with diuretic therapy (your attention is drawn to the precautions section). Maintenance doses are sometimes less than the dosage necessary to initiate diuresis; consequently, the patient's weight should be stabilised before attempting to reduce dosage.

Congestive heart failure: The starting dose is 1 or 2 tablets per day, which may be altered if necessary to a maximum of 4 tablets per day. Serum potassium levels and diuretic response will establish the optimal dosage. On the establishment of initial diuresis, maintenance therapy is possible with a dosage reduction, or by the use of intermittent therapy.

Paediatric dosage: Normetic is not recommended for use in children since the safety of amiloride hydrochloride in this age group has not been established.

Use in the elderly: The dosage should be carefully adjusted according to renal function and clinical response. Where patients require reduced dosage, tablets may be halved by breaking along the bisect line.

Dosage in pregnancy: See 'Contra-indications, warnings, etc'.

Contra-indications, warnings, etc

Contra-indications: Hyperkalaemia (serum potassium over 5.5 mmol/litre); hypercalcaemia (serum calcium [total] over 2.6 mmol/litre; other potassium-conserving diuretics and potassium supplements; acute renal failure; severe progressive renal disease; diabetic nephropathy; hepatic failure; Addisons disease; anuria; patients with blood urea over 10 mmol/litre or serum creatinine over 130 micromol/litre in whom serum electrolyte and blood urea levels cannot be monitored with satisfaction and frequency; a known sensitivity to amiloride hydrochloride or hydrochlorothiazide.

The risk of lithium toxicity with patients combined on lithium and diuretics is very high and lithium should not be administered concurrently with Normetic.

In renal impairment, use of a potassium conserving agent may result in rapid development of hyperkalaemia.

Precautions: Diabetes Mellitus: Hyperkalaemia has been widely reported in diabetic patients on amiloride hydrochloride, mainly associated with chronic renal disease or pre-renal azotaemia. Renal function status should be established before prescribing Normetic to known or suspected diabetics. The taking of Normetic should be stopped prior to giving a glucose-tolerance test. Restabilising the insulin requirements of diabetic patients may be necessary. Latent diabetes mellitus may become manifest during thiazide therapy.

Metabolic or respiratory acidosis: severely ill patients likely to experience respiratory or metabolic acidosis on induction of potassium-conserving therapy, should be treated with caution. Categories such as decompensated diabetics or cardiopulmonary cases should be assessed for shifts in acid-base balance which may alter the balance of extracellular-intracellular potassium, and the development of acidosis may be associated with a marked rise in serum potassium.

Blood urea increases and electrolyte imbalance: Very infrequently, amiloride hydrochloride and hydrochlorothiazide, as combined in Normetic, fail to overcome any chloride deficit. Normal salt intake will, in the main, prevent any problem in this area.

Hyperkalaemia (serum potassium level over 5.5 mmol/litre): It has been noted that hyperkalaemia may be present in patients receiving amiloride hydrochloride either alone or in combination with other diuretics, especially in such categories as diabetics; the aged; congestive heart failure cases with known renal involvement; patients suffering from hepatic cirrhosis, or those subjected to vigorous diuretic therapy or the seriously ill. Careful observation of such categories of patients for manifestation of hyperkalaemia, using clinical, laboratory and ECG evidence should be undertaken as hyperkalaemia is not always accompanied by an abnormal ECG. In any development of hyperkalaemia, Normetic therapy should be stopped forthwith and, should it be desirable, reduction of serum potassium levels to normal values should be actively instituted. Reversible increases in blood urea have been reported in association with vigorous diuresis, notably in cases of hepatic cirrhosis with ascites and metabolic alkalosis or resistant oedema. In these cases, serum electrolyte and blood urea levels should be carefully monitored. Caution is advised in the use of Normetic with patients suffering renal impairment (see 'Contra-indications'). Care should be observed to avoid cumulative or toxic effects due to a reduced excretion of its components. Azotaemia may be precipitated or increased by hydrochlorothiazide. Normetic should be discontinued if increased azotaemia and oliguria occur during treatment.

Effects in cirrhotic patients: Patients with hepatic cirrhosis and ascites are more likely to experience adverse reactions during oral diuretic therapy owing to the fact that these patients are intolerant of acute shifts in electrolyte balance and because they may be subject to pre-existing hypokalaemia due to associated aldosteronism. Hepatic encephalopathy is characterised by coma, confusion and tremors has been reported with patients receiving amiloride hydrochloride and subjects receiving Normetic with no liver complications should be assessed for these conditions. A tenuous relationship between amiloride hydrochloride and a deepening of jaundice in cirrhotic patients has been postulated.

Additional precautions: Thiazides may produce sensitivity reactions in patients with or without a record of allergy or bronchial asthma. The action of other antihypertensive agents is potentiated by hydrochlorothiazide and a reduced dosage may be necessary at the introduction of Normetic. Reports indicate that there exists a possibility that thiazides may activate or exacerbate systemic lupus erythematosus.

Hydrochlorothiazide may reduce arterial responsiveness to noradrenaline, but not to such a degree as to prevent the effectiveness of noradrenaline in therapeutic usage. Thiazides may enhance the responsiveness to tubocurarine. In post-sympathectomy patients, the antihypertensive action of thiazides may be enhanced. Should orthostatic hypotension occur, it may be potentiated by narcotics, barbiturates and alcohol.

In some patients receiving thiazides, gout may be precipitated or hyperuricaemia may occur.

Acute pancreatitis associated with the use of hydrochlorothiazide has been reported.

Prolonged thiazide therapy has provoked isolated reports of pathological changes in the parathyroid glands accompanied by hypophosphataemia and hypercalcaemia. Serum BPI levels may be reduced by thiazide administration although not characterised by thyroid disturbance. The common complications of hyperparathyroidism have not been recorded. To establish parathyroid function, first discontinue thiazide administration.

As with any recently introduced preparations, patients should be monitored for possible signs of blood dyscrasias, liver dysfunction and idiosyncratic reactions.

Pregnancy and lactation warning: Owing to the limited clinical experience, the use of Normetic is not recommended during pregnancy and, as thiazides are found in breast milk, the patient should be instructed to stop nursing if continuation of the drug is thought to be essential. In general, as thiazides do cross the placental barrier and can be found in cord blood, the overall benefits of Normetic should be assessed against any potential harm to the foetus where pregnancy is present or suspected. Such problems noted have been thrombocytopaenia, foetal bone marrow depression, neonatal or foetal jaundice with the possibility of other side-effects associated with adult treatment. Diuretics are best avoided for the management of oedema of pregnancy or hypertension in pregnancy as their use may be associated with hypovolaemia, increased blood viscosity and reduced placental perfusion.

Side-effects: Related to diuresis: Orthostatic hypotension, muscle cramps, susceptibility to fatigue, weakness, dizziness, vertigo, salivary gland inflammation, transient blurred vision, paraesthesia, thirst, dry mouth.

Gastro-intestinal: Constipation and diarrhoea, pain, cramps, gastric irritation, abdominal fullness, vomiting, nausea, anorexia.

Additional side-effects: Side-effects associated with thiazide therapy are hyperuricaemia, glycosuria, hyperglycaemia, yellow vision, jaundice (intrahepatic cholestatic jaundice), restlessness, headache. Fever, necrotising angiitis (vasculitis, cutaneous vasculitis), photosensitivity, urticaria, rash, purpura, haemolytic anaemia, aplastic anaemia, agranulocytosis, leucopenia, thrombocytopenia, impotence, respiratory distress including pneumonitis and anaphylactic reactions have also been reported.

There have been a few reports of gastro-intestinal bleeding in subjects with a background of gastro-intestinal disease receiving amiloride hydrochloride alone; a causal relationship to amiloride, however, has not been established. Rare reversible abnormalities, possibly relating to Amiloride Hydrochloride, have been noted in liver function tests.

In the case of moderate or severe side-effects, the dosage of Normetic should be reduced or withdrawn altogether.

Treatment of overdosage: There is no specific antidote. Dehydration, electrolyte imbalance and hepatic coma are treated by the established procedures. If ingestion is recent, gastric lavage should be performed or emesis induced. Treatment is symptomatic and supportive. If hyperkalaemia occurs, prompt measures should be taken to lower the serum potassium levels. For respiratory impairment, oxygen or artificial respiration should be administered.

Pharmaceutical precautions Keep container tightly closed; store in a cool place, protected from light.

Legal category POM.

Package quantities Containers of 100 and 500 tablets.

Further information Oral potassium supplements must not be given with Normetic.

Onset of diuretic action begins within two to four hours after administration of Normetic, and reaches a peak at about the fourth hour; there is detectable activity for about 24 hours.

Product licence number 0037/0148.

SELSUN* SUSPENSION

Presentation Selsun suspension is presented as a viscous yellow suspension of Selenium Sulphide BP 2.5%.

Uses
Indications: For the treatment of simple dandruff and seborrhoeic dermatitis of the scalp.

Main pharmacological action: Selenium sulphide appears to have a cytostatic effect on cells of the epidermis and follicular epithelium, thus reducing corneocyte production. Selsun acts as an antiseborrhoeic agent which effectively controls itching and scaling dandruff. It has activity against certain dermatophytes including *Pityrosporum orbiculare* the organism causing pityriasis versicolor (tinea versicolor).

Dosage and administration
Adults and the elderly: A liberal application should be made twice a week for the first two weeks and then once a week for the next two weeks to control condition. After this initial course of treatment Selsun should not be used more often than necessary.

Children aged 5–14 years: Treatment as for adults.

Children under 5 years: Not recommended.

Contra-indications, warnings, etc
Contra-indications: Do not allow contact with broken skin.

Precautions: Very few cases of hypersensitivity reactions have been reported.

Selsun should be very thoroughly rinsed from the hair before dyeing, tinting or waving the hair. It should not be applied for a period of two days before or after any of these procedures. Contact with eyes should be avoided.

Use in pregnancy: It is not known whether Selsun can cause foetal harm when applied to the body surfaces of a pregnant woman or can affect reproductive capacity. Its effect on the milk of a lactating woman is unknown. As with all medications, avoid during the first 3 months of pregnancy.

Side-effects: Increased falling out of hair may occur with active treatment of any scalp condition. Oiliness of the hair may increase following the use of Selsun.

Overdosage

Topical application: None known.

Ingestion: Symptoms: Nausea and vomiting. Treatment: Vomiting should be provoked or gastric lavage undertaken. General supportive measures are required. A purgative may be administered to hasten elimination.

Pharmaceutical precautions Store in a cool place.

Legal category P.

Package quantities Selsun suspension is available in bottles of 50, 100 and 150 ml.

Further information Nil.

Product licence number 0037/5010R.

**Trade Mark*

Alcon Laboratories (U.K.) Limited

Imperial Way
Watford
Hertfordshire, WD2 4YR

BALANCED SALT SOLUTION ALCON BSS*

Presentation A sterile physiological balanced salt solution which is isotonic to the tissues of the eye. It is a lint free solution containing essential ions for normal cell metabolism. Each ml contains Sodium Chloride PhEur 0.64%, Potassium Chloride PhEur 0.075%, Calcium Chloride PhEur 0.048%, Magnesium Chloride Hexahydrate PhEur 0.03%, Sodium Acetate PhEur 0.39%, Sodium Citrate PhEur 0.17% and Water for Injection PhEur.

Uses As a physiologic irrigating solution.

Dosage and administration Sufficient to produce the required irrigation.

Administration:

15 ml and 30 ml Steri-Unit Drop-Tainer dispensers: The adaptor plug is designed to accept an ophthalmic irrigating needle. Intra-ocular tissue may be irrigated by attaching the needle to the Steri-Unit Drop-Tainer Bottle as follows:

1. Aseptically remove the Drop-Tainer by peeling off the paper backing.
2. Snap on surgical irrigator needle. Push well to ensure it is firmly in place.
3. Test patency of the assembly.

Squeeze out several drops before inserting into the anterior chamber. The needle should be removed from the chamber prior to releasing pressure to prevent suction.

250 ml and 500 ml bottles:

Note: Use an administration set with an air inlet in the plastic spike since the bottle does not contain a separate airway tube. Follow directions of the particular administration set to be used. Flip-off plastic cap from the aluminium seal and insert spike aseptically into the bottle through the centre target area of the rubber stopper. Allow the fluid to flow and remove air from the tubing before irrigation begins.

250 ml and 500 ml Viaflex containers: Following the directions of the particular administration set to be used, insert the spike of the administration set into the inlet port, break the membrane, allow the fluid to flow and remove air from the tubing before irrigation.

Contra-indications, warnings, etc

Contra-indications: There are no specific contra-indications for this product. When the corneal endothelium is abnormal, irrigation or any trauma may result in bullous keratopathy.

Not for intravenous infusion.

Pharmaceutical precautions This solution contains no preservative and should not be re-used.

Store in a cool place. Do not freeze.

15 and 30 ml presentations: If the blister or paper backing is damaged or broken, sterility of the enclosed bottle cannot be assured. Open under aseptic conditions only.

250 ml and 500 ml bottles: Do not use unless product is clear and vacuum is present.

Legal category P.

Package quantities 15 ml and 30 ml Steri-Unit Drop-Tainer dispensers; 250 ml and 500 ml glass infusion bottles and Viaflex containers.

Further information The enclosed Steri-Unit Drop-Tainers are sterile and may be safely handled by the surgeon.

Product licence numbers

15 ml and 30 ml Steri-Unit-Drop-Tainer 0649/0007
250 ml and 500 ml glass infusion bottle and Viaflex container 0649/0099

BETOPTIC*

Presentation A clear colourless to light yellow sterile solution containing 0.56% w/v betaxolol hydrochloride (equivalent to 0.5% w/v betaxolol base) and preserved with Benzalkonium Chloride PhEur 0.01% w/v.

Uses Betoptic is indicated for the reduction of elevated intra-ocular pressure in patients with ocular hypertension and chronic open-angle glaucoma.

Dosage and administration The usual dose is one drop of Betoptic instilled in the affected eye(s) twice daily. In some patients, the intra-ocular pressure lowering response to Betoptic may require a few weeks to stabilise and therefore clinical follow up should include a determination of the intra-ocular pressure during the first month of usage. Because of diurnal variations in intra-ocular pressure in individual patients, satisfactory response to twice a day therapy is best determined by measuring intra-ocular pressure at different times during the day.

If necessary concomitant therapy with pilocarpine, other miotics, adrenaline or systemically administered carbonic anhydrase inhibitors can be instituted.

Transfer from other agents: When only a single anti-glaucoma agent is being used, continue the agent and add one drop of Betoptic in the affected eye(s) twice a day. On the following day discontinue the previous agent completely and continue with Betoptic.

When several anti-glaucoma agents are being used, the patient should be assessed on an individual basis. Adjustment should involve one agent at a time at intervals of not less than one week. The physician may be able to discontinue some or all of the other anti-glaucoma agents.

Usage in children: Clinical studies to establish the safety and efficacy in children have not been performed and therefore Betoptic is currently not recommended for use in children.

Prescribing in the elderly: There are no special precautions to be followed.

Contra-indications, warnings, etc

Contra-indications: Betoptic is contra-indicated in patients with sinus bradycardia greater than a first degree block, cardiogenic shock or a history of overt cardiac failure and in patients with hypersensitivity to any component.

Warnings and precautions: Patients who are receiving a beta-adrenergic blocking agent orally and Betoptic should be observed for potential additive effect either on intraocular pressure or the known systemic effects of beta-blockade. While Betoptic has demonstrated a low potential for systemic effects, it should be used with caution in patients with diabetes (especially labile diabetes) or in patients suspected of developing thyrotoxicosis. Consideration should be given to the gradual withdrawal of beta-adrenergic blocking agents prior to general anaesthesia because of the reduced ability of the heart to respond to beta-adrenergically mediated sympathetic reflex stimuli.

Although cardioselective beta-blockers have less effect on lung function than non-selective beta-blockers caution should be exercised in the treatment of glaucoma patients with obstructive pulmonary disease. There have been reports of asthmatic attacks and pulmonary distress during Betoptic treatment in such patients. In individual cases the risk to benefit for each patient should be considered. An increase in airway resistance can be relieved by inhaled beta$_2$-mimetics.

In patients with angle-closure glaucoma, the immediate treatment objective is to re-open the angle by constriction of the pupil with a miotic agent. Betaxolol has no effect on the pupil; therefore, Betoptic should be used with a miotic to reduce elevated intra-ocular pressure in angle-closure glaucoma.

This product contains benzalkonium chloride and is not recommended for use when soft contact lenses are being worn.

Drug interactions: Although Betoptic used alone has little or no effect on pupil size, mydriasis resulting from concomitant therapy with Betoptic and adrenaline has been reported occasionally.

Close observation of the patient is recommended when a beta blocker is administered to patients receiving catecholamine-depleting drugs such as reserpine, because of possible additive effects and the production of hypotension and/or bradycardia. Caution should be exercised in patients using concomitant adrenergic psychotropic drugs.

Adverse reactions: Although Betoptic is generally well tolerated, discomfort of short duration may be experienced by some patients upon instillation and occasional tearing has been reported. Rare instances of decreased corneal sensitivity, erythema, itching, corneal punctate staining, keratitis, anisocoria and photophobia have been reported.

Systemic reactions following topical administration of Betoptic (eg: insomnia and depressive neurosis) have only rarely been reported.

Use in pregnancy: Although animal studies have not demonstrated any specific hazard there are no adequate and well-controlled studies in pregnant women. Because animal studies are not always predictive of human response this drug should be used during pregnancy only if clearly indicated.

Use by nursing mothers: It is not known whether Betoptic is excreted in human milk, caution should therefore be exercised when Betoptic is administered to nursing mothers.

Treatment of overdosage: A topical overdose of Betoptic may be flushed from the eye(s) with warm tap water.

Pharmaceutical precautions Keep the container tightly closed. Store at room temperature. Discard contents one month after opening.

Legal category POM.

Package quantities 5 ml containers.

Further information Betaxolol hydrochloride is a cardioselective (beta-1-adrenergic) receptor blocking agent, which is devoid of intrinsic sympathomimetic action and does not have significant membrane-stabilising activity. In controlled clinical studies ophthalmic betaxolol has shown minimal effect on pulmonary and cardiovascular parameters. Betoptic has been used successfully in glaucoma patients who have undergone laser trabeculoplasty and in aphakic patients.

Product licence number 0649/0097.

ISOPTO* ALKALINE

Presentation Isopto Alkaline is a sterile clear, colourless solution containing hydroxypropylmethylcellulose (Hypromellose) 1.0%, preserved with benzalkonium chloride 0.01%.

Uses Isopto Alkaline is used topically to provide tear-like lubrication for the symptomatic relief of dry eyes and eye irritation associated with deficient tear production. (Usually in cases of rheumatoic arthritis, keratoconjunctivitis sicca and xerophthalmia.) It may also be used as an ocular lubricant for artificial eyes.

Dosage and administration It is suitable for use both by adults and children. The dose depends upon the desired amount of lubrication, the usual dosage being one or two drops to be instilled into the eyes three times daily, or as needed.

Contra-indications, warnings, etc
Contra-indications: Isopto Alkaline is contra-indicated in those persons who have shown hypersensitivity to any component of the product. This product contains benzalkonium chloride and should not be used when soft contact lenses are worn.

Warnings: Isopto Alkaline may cause transient blurring of vision and mild stinging on instillation. Do not drive or operate hazardous machinery unless vision is clear. If irritation persists or worsens, or headache, eye pain, vision changes or continued redness occur, discontinue use and consult a physician. To preserve sterility do not allow the dropper to touch the eye or any other surface.

Use in pregnancy: There is insufficient evidence as to safety in pregnancy and this product should, therefore, only be used in pregnancy if it is considered essential by the physician.

Pharmaceutical precautions The eyedrops should be stored in a cool place. Discard one month after opening.

Legal category P.

Package quantities 10 ml containers.

Further information Isopto Alkaline eye-drops are contained in an unbreakable semi-rigid plastic dropper bottle with a screw-on cap.

Product licence number 0649/5900.

ISOPTO* ATROPINE 1.0%

Presentation Isopto Atropine is a clear, colourless, sterile solution containing atropine sulphate 1.0% and hydroxypropylmethylcellulose (Hypromellose) 0.5% and preserved with benzalkonium chloride 0.01%.

Uses Atropine is a powerful and long-acting anticholinergic agent used for producing cycloplegia and mydriasis. It is indicated for cycloplegic refraction, particularly in the determination of refraction in children below the age of six and in children with convergent strabismus. It is also indicated for the treatment of iritis and uveitis to immobilise the ciliary muscle and iris and to prevent or breakdown adhesions.

Dosage and administration *Adults and the Elderly:* For refraction, instil one drop into each eye twice daily for one or two days before examination. For uveitis, instil one or two drops into the eye(s) four times daily, or as required. Atropine should be used with particular caution in the elderly who are prone to systemic adverse effects and to the precipitation and exacerbation of glaucoma.

Usage in children: For refraction, instil one drop twice daily for one to three days before examination and one hour before examination. For uveitis, instil one drop up to three times daily. Do not use during the first three months of life due to possible association between the cycloplegia produced and the development of amblyopia. Safety and efficacy for use in children has not been established therefore use with extreme caution.

Contra-indications, warnings, etc
Contra-indications: Contra-indicated in persons with glaucoma or a tendency toward glaucoma, e.g., narrow anterior chamber angle, and in those persons showing

hypersensitivity to any component of this preparation. This product contains benzalkonium chloride and should not be used when soft contact lenses are worn.

Warnings: For topical use only – not for injection. The effects of anti-muscarinic agents may be enhanced by the concomitant administration of other drugs with anti-muscarinic properties such as amantadine, some anti-histamines, butyrophenones, phenothiazines and tri-cyclic anti-depressants. Extreme caution is advised for use in childen and individuals susceptible to belladonna alkaloids because of the increased risk of systemic toxicity.

Isopto Alkaline may cause blurred vision and sensitivity to light. Patients should be warned not to drive or engage in other hazardous activities unless vision is clear. Complete recovery from the effects of atropine eyedrops may take up to seven days. Parents should be warned of the oral toxicity of this preparation for children and advised to wash their hands after use.

Precautions: To reduce systemic absorption the lacrimal sac should be compressed at the medial canthus by digital pressure for at least one minute after instillation of the drops.

Adverse reactions: Local: Increased intraocular pressure, transient stinging, and sensitivity to light secondary to pupillary dilation. Prolonged administration may lead to local irritation, hyperaemia, oedema and conjunctivitis.

Systemic: Systemic anti-cholinergic toxicity is manifested by dryness in the mouth, flushing, dryness of the skin, bradycardia followed by tachycardia with palpitations and arrythmias, urinary urgency, difficulty and retention, reduction in the tone and motility of the gastrointestinal tract leading to constipation. Vomiting, giddiness and staggering may occur, a rash may be present in children and abdominal distension in infants. Toxic doses cause rapid respiration, hyperpyrexia and CNS stimulation or depression marked by restlessness, confusion, hallucinations and occasionally convulsions. In severe toxicity coma may lead to circulatory and respiratory failure and death.

Overdosage: Systemic toxicity may occur following topical use, particularly in children. It is manifested by flushing and dryness of the skin (a rash may be present in children), blurred vision, a rapid and irregular pulse, fever, abdominal distention in infants, convulsions and hallucinations and the loss of neuro-muscular co-ordination. Treatment is supportive (there is no evidence that physostigmine is superior to supportive management). In infants and small children the body surface must be kept moist. If accidentally ingested, induce emesis or perform gastric lavage.

Use in pregnancy: There is insufficient evidence as to drug safety in pregnancy and lactation. This product should not be used during pregnancy unless it is considered essential by a physician.

Pharmaceutical precautions Isopto Atropine should be stored in a cool place away from direct sunlight. Keep the container tightly closed. The contents should be discarded one month after opening.

Legal category POM.

Package quantities 5 ml containers.

Further information Isopto Atropine eye drops are contained in an unbreakable semi-rigid, plastic dropper bottle with screw-on cap.

Product licence number 0649/5901.

ISOPTO CARBACHOL 3%

Presentation Isopto Carbachol is a clear colourless sterile solution, containing 3% Carbachol and 1% hydroxypropyl methylcellulose (hypromellose), and preserved with benzalkonium chloride 0.005%.

Uses A directly acting miotic used for the treatment of glaucoma. May be used topically to control intraocular pressure in patients who become refractory to pilocarpine alone or who are unable to tolerate pilocarpine.

Dosage and administration Instil one or two drops up to four times daily. The frequency of instillation is determined by the severity of the glaucoma and the response to treatment. For adult use only, the safety and efficacy of use in children has not been established.

Contra-indications, warnings, etc
Contra-indications: In conditions where pupillary constriction is undesirable, e.g. acute iritis, anterior uveitis and some forms of secondary glaucoma. Contra-indicated in those persons showing hypersensitivity to any component of this preparation. This product contains benzalkonium chloride and should not be used when soft contact lenses are worn.

Warnings: For topical use only. Not for injection. Although systemic reactions rarely occur in the treatment of chronic simple glaucoma with the usual doses used, in the treatment of acute closed-angle glaucoma the possibility of systemic reactions must be considered because of the higher doses given. Caution is particularly advised with patients with acute heart failure, bronchial asthma, peptic ulceration, hypertension, urinary tract obstruction and Parkinson's disease. Carbachol penetrates the intact cornea poorly. To reduce the risk of systemic toxicity, use carbachol with caution in the presence of a corneal abrasion or damage to the epithelial barrier of the conjunctiva or cornea caused by topical anaesthesia or tonometry. Retinal detachments have been caused in susceptible individuals and those with pre-existing retinal disease, therefore, fundus examination is advised in all patients prior to the initiation of therapy.

Isopto Carbachol causes difficulty with dark adaptation, therefore, caution is necessary with night driving and when hazardous tasks are undertaken in poor illumination. May cause acccommodation spasm. Patients should be advised not to drive or use machinary if vision is not clear.

Adverse reactions: Local: Burning, itching, smarting, blurring, ciliary spasm, conjunctival vascular congestion, induced myopia, sensitisation of the lids and conjunctiva, reduced visual acuity in poor illumination, lens changes with chronic use, increased pupillary block, retinal detachments and vitreous haemorrhages. CNS: Browache and headache (especially in younger patients who have recently started therapy). Systemic: Systemic reactions following ocular use are rare but they may include hypertension, tachycardia, bronchial spasm, pulmonary oedema, salivation, sweating, nausea, vomiting, diarrhoea and lacrimation.

Overdosage: If accidentally ingested induce emesis or perform gastric lavage. Observe for signs of toxicity (salivation, lacrimation, sweating, nausea, vomiting and diarrhoea). If these occur, therapy with anti-cholinergic agents, such as atropine, may be necessary.

Use in pregnancy: Safety for use in pregnancy and lactation has not been established, therefore, use only when clearly indicated.

Pharmaceutical precautions Isopto Carbachol eye drops should be stored in a cool place away from direct sunlight. Keep the container tightly closed. Contents should be discarded one month after opening.

Legal category POM.

Package quantities 10 ml containers.

Further information Isopto Carbachol eye drops are contained in an unbreakable semi-rigid plastic dropper bottle with screw-on cap.

Product licence number 0649/5902.

ISOPTO* CARPINE 0.5%, 1.0%, 2.0%, 3.0%, 4.0%

Presentation Isopto Carpine is a clear, colourless, sterile solution available in five strengths; containing 0.5,

1, 2, 3 or 4% pilocarpine hydrochloride and 0.5% hydroxypropyl methylcellulose (hypromellose), and preserved with benzalkonium chloride 0.01%.

Uses Isopto Carpine is a directly-acting miotic used for the treatment of glaucoma. For topical instillation into the eye it is indicated for chronic simple glaucoma, patients may be maintained on pilocarpine as long as intraocular pressure is controlled and there is no deterioration in the visual fields. Also indicated for acute (closed angle glaucoma), pilocarpine may be used alone or in conjunction with other agents to decrease intraocular pressure prior to surgical treatment and for miosis to counter the effects of cycloplegic and mydriatic eye drops.

Dosage and administration One or two drops up to four times daily or as prescribed. The frequency of instillation and concentration of drops used are determined by the severity of the glaucoma and the response to treatment.

Usage in children: At the discretion of the physician. Safety and efficacy of use in children has not been established.

Contra-indications, warnings, etc
Contra-indications: Contraindicated in conditions where pupillary constriction is undesirable, e.g. acute iritis, anterior uveitis and some forms of secondary glaucoma. Hypersensitivity to any components of the preparation. Patients wearing soft contact lenses should not use this preparation.

Warnings: For topical use only. Not for injection. Although systemic reactions rarely occur in the treatment of chronic simple glaucoma with the usual doses used, in the treatment of acute closed-angle glaucoma the possibility of systemic reactions must be considered because of the higher doses given. Caution is particularly advised with patients with acute heart failure, bronchial asthma, peptic ulceration, hypertension, urinary tract obstruction and Parkinson's disease. As with all miotics rare cases of retinal detachment have been reported when used in certain susceptible individuals and those with pre-existing retinal disease, therefore fundus examination is advised in all patients prior to the initiation of therapy. The miosis usually causes difficulty with dark adaptation, therefore, caution is necessary with night driving and when hazardous tasks are undertaken in poor illumination. May cause accommodation spasm. Patients should be advised not to drive or use machinery if vision is not clear.

Adverse reactions: Local: Burning, itching, smarting, blurring, ciliary spasm, conjunctival vascular congestion, induced myopia, sensitisation of the lids and conjunctiva, reduced visual acuity in poor illumination, lens changes with chronic use, increased pupillary block, retinal detachments and vitreous haemorrhages.

CNS: Browache and headache (especially in younger patients who have recently started therapy).

Systemic: Systemic reactions following ocular use are rare but they may include hypertension, tachycardia, bronchial spasm, pulmonary oedema, salivation, sweating, nausea, vomiting, diarrhoea and lacrimation.

Overdosage: If accidentally ingested, induce emesis or perform gastric lavage. Observe for signs of toxicity (salivation, lacrimation, sweating, nausea, vomiting and diarrhoea). If these occur, therapy with anti-cholinergic agents, such as atropine, may be necessary.

Use in pregnancy: Safety for use in pregnancy and lactation has not been established, therefore, use only when clearly indicated.

Pharmaceutical precautions Isopto Carpine should be stored in a cool place away from direct sunlight. Keep the container tightly closed. The contents should be discarded one month after opening.

Legal category POM.

Package quantities 10 ml containers.

Further information Isopto Carpine eye drops are contained in an unbreakable semi-rigid, plastic dropper bottle with screw-on cap.

Product licence numbers
0.5% 0649/5903
1.0% 0649/5904
2.0% 0649/5905
3.0% 0649/5906
4.0% 0649/5907

ISOPTO* FRIN 0.12%

Presentation Isopto Frin is a clear, colourless sterile solution, containing Phenylephrine Hydrochloride BP 0.12% and Hydroxypropylmethylcellulose (Hypromellose) USP 0.5%, and preserved with Benzethonium Chloride USP 0.01%.

Uses For the temporary relief of redness of the eye due to minor eye irritations.

Dosage and administration One or two drops instilled topically into the eye up to four times a day. Isopto Frin is suitable for use by both adults and children.

Contra-indications, warnings, etc
Contra-indications: Not to be used by contact lens wearers except under medical supervision.

Interactions: Phenylephrine may interfere with the actions of antihypertensive agents while monoamine oxidase inhibitors and tricyclic antidepressants can exacerbate the systemic effects of phenylephrine.

Effects on ability to drive and to use machines: As with other eyedrops blurring of vision may occur immediately after instillation. Patients should be advised not to drive until any effects on vision have cleared.

Warnings and precautions: Patients being treated for high blood pressure or depression should consult their doctor before using these drops. If eye pain, changes in vision, continued redness of the eye are experienced or if the condition worsens or persists for more than 24 hours, patients should consult their doctor. Isopto Frin should not be used in patients with any eye disease or who have had eye surgery except under the advice and supervision of a doctor. Continued use of this product may increase redness of the eye. Care should be exercised in its use in small children, pressure should be put on the inner canthus of the eye for a few minutes after instillation to decrease systemic absorption through the conjunctiva. Use with caution on an inflamed eye, as hyperaemia greatly increases the rate of systemic absorption through the conjunctiva. Slight dilation of the pupil may occur in some patients. For this reason it should be used with care where narrow angle glaucoma may be present since its use may precipitate angle closure or in those with a shallow anterior chamber.

Pregnancy Warning: This product should only be used during pregnancy if considered essential by the physician.

Treatment of overdose: An overdose from a 0.12% solution of phenylephrine hydrochloride is extremely unlikely. Symptoms would however be those of acute hypertension. In such an event a quick acting adrenergic blocking agent such as 5 to 10 mg phentolamine mesylate, followed by a β-blocking agent such as 2.5 to 5 mg propranolol should be given.

Pharmaceutical precautions Isopto Frin eye drops should be stored in a cool place away from direct sunlight. Keep the container tightly closed. Contents should be discarded one month after opening. If the solution changes colour or becomes cloudy, do not use.

Legal category P.

Package quantities 10 ml containers.

Further information Isopto Frin eye drops are contained in an unbreakable semi-rigid plastic dropper bottle with screw-on cap.

Product licence number 0649/5911.

ISOPTO* PLAIN

Presentation Isopto Plain is a sterile, clear, colourless solution containing hydroxypropyl methylcellulose (hypromellose) 0.5%, and preserved with benzalkonium chloride 0.01%.

Uses Isopto Plain is used topically to provide tear-like lubrication for the symptomatic relief of dry eyes and eye irritation associated with deficient tear production. (Usually in cases of rheumatoid arthritis, keratoconjunctivitis, sicca and xerophthalmia.) Also used as an ocular lubricant for artificial eyes.

Dosage and administration It is suitable for use both by adults and children. The dose depends on the need for lubrication. Usually one to two drops to each eye three times daily or as prescribed.

Contra-indications, warnings, etc
Contra-indications: In those persons showing hypersensitivity to any component of the product. This product contains benzalkonium chloride and should not be used when soft contact lenses are worn.
Warnings: If irritation persists or worsens, or headache, eye pain, vision changes or continued redness occur, discontinue use and consult a physician. To preserve sterility do not allow the dropper to touch the eye or any other surface. This product may cause transient blurring of vision and mild stinging on instillation. Do not drive or operate hazardous machinery unless vision is clear.

Use in pregnancy: There is insufficient evidence as to safety in pregnancy and this product should, therefore, only be used in pregnancy if it is considered essential by the physician.

Pharmaceutical precautions The eye-drops should be stored in a cool place (8° to 25°C). Keep the container tightly closed. Keep out of reach of children. Discard contents one month after opening.

Legal category P.

Package quantities 10 ml containers.

Further information Isopto Plain eye-drops are contained in an unbreakable semi-rigid plastic dropper bottle with a screw-on cap.

Product licence number 0649/5920.

MAXIDEX*

Presentation Dexamethasone 0.1% in a vehicle containing 0.5% hydroxypropyl methylcellulose (hypromellose). A sterile, isotonic, ophthalmic suspension, preserved with benzalkonium chloride 0.01%.

Uses Indicated for treatment of steroid responsive inflammatory conditions of the conjunctiva, cornea and anterior segment of the eye, such as: anterior uveitis, iritis, cyclitis, allergic and vernal conjunctivitis, herpes zoster keratitis, superficial punctate keratitis and non specific superficial keratitis. Also indicated for the treatment of corneal injury from chemical, radiation or thermal burns or following penetration by foreign bodies. Indicated for post-operative use to reduce inflammatory reactions and suppress graft reaction.

Dosage and administration The frequency of instillation of drops and the duration of treatment will vary depending upon the severity of the underlying condition and the response to treatment. Severe inflammations require one or two drops instilled into the eye every thirty to sixty minutes until a satisfactory response occurs. Subconjunctival or systemic steroid therapy should be considered if there is no response. When a favourable response has been observed reduce the dosage towards one drop every four hours.

Contra-indications, warnings, etc
Contra-indications: Contra-indicated in herpes simplex and other viral diseases of the cornea and conjunctiva, fungal disease, ocular tuberculosis, untreated purulent infections and hypersensitivity to any component of the preparation. This product should not be used when soft lenses are being worn.

Warnings: Topical corticosteroids should never be given for an undiagnosed red eye as inappropriate use is potentially blinding. Because of the risk of "steroid glaucoma" and cataract formation the intraocular pressure and the lens must be checked frequently during use of this preparation. To avoid the risk of enhancement of herpetic corneal disease, frequent slit-lamp examination is essential. Topical steroids may mask or enhance the activity of acute purulent eye infections. In such cases antibiotic therapy is mandatory. Persistent corneal ulceration following long-term topical steroid use may be due to fungal invasion. Topical corticosteroids are not effective in mustard gas keratitis or Skogren's keratoconjunctivitis. Patient should be warned not to drive or use hazardous machinery if vision is not clear.

Precautions: This product may cause transient stinging on instillation or sensitivity to bright light.

Adverse reactions: Topical steroid use may result in increased intraocular pressure leading to optic nerve damage, reduced visual acuity and visual field defects. Intensive or prolonged use of topical corticosteroids may lead to the formation of posterior subcapsular cataracts. In those diseases causing thinning of the cornea or sclera, perforation of the globe may occur. Viral and fungal infections may be exacerbated by steroids. Transient stinging or burning may occur on instillation of the drops. Systemic side effects may occur with extensive use.

Use in pregnancy: There is inadequate evidence of safety in human pregnancy. Topical administration of corticosteroids to pregnant animals can cause abnormalities of foetal development including cleft palate and intra-uterine growth retardation. There may therefore be a very small risk of such effects in the human pregnancy.

Treatment of overdose: Long-term intensive topical use may lead to systemic effects. Oral ingestion of the contents of one bottle (up to 10 mls) is unlikely to lead to any serious adverse effects.

Pharmaceutical precautions Maxidex should be stored in a cool place away from direct sunlight. Keep the container tightly closed. The contents should be discarded one month after opening. Shake well before using.

Legal category POM.

Package quantities 5 ml and 10 ml containers.

Further information Maxidex eye drops are contained in an unbreakable semi-rigid, plastic dropper bottle with a screw-on cap, containing 5 ml or 10 ml of the preparation. Maxidex is a highly penetrating form of dexamethasone, a 0.1% microfine suspension especially formulated to provide maximum corneal absorption.

Product licence number 0649/5914.

MAXITROL* EYE DROPS
MAXITROL* EYE-OINTMENT

Presentation *Drops:* Dexamethasone BP 0.1%, Polymyxin B Sulphate USP 6,000 units/ml and Neomycin Sulphate equivalent to Neomycin 3.5 mg/ml in a vehicle containing 0.5% hydroxypropyl methylcellulose (hypromellose). A sterile, isotonic, ophthalmic suspension, preserved with benzalkonium chloride 0.004%.

Ointment: Dexamethasone BP 0.1%, Polymyxin B Sulphate USP 6,000 units/g and Neomycin Sulphate equivalent to Neomycin 3.5 mg/g in an ointment base, preserved with methylparaben 0.05% and propylparaben 0.01%.

Uses For the short-term treatment of steroid responsive conditions of the eye when prophylactic antibiotic treatment is also required, after excluding the presence of fungal and viral disease.

Dosage and administration *Maxitrol Suspension:*

One or two drops applied to each affected eye up to six times daily or more frequently if required. (Severe infections may require one or two drops every fifteen to twenty minutes initially reducing the frequency of instillation gradually as the infection is controlled.)

Maxitrol Ointment: Apply a small amount into the conjunctival sac(s) up to three or four times daily or, may be used adjunctively with drops at bedtime.

Not more than 20 ml or 8 g should be prescribed initially and the prescription should not be refilled without further evaluation as outlined in the section on warnings.

Contra-indications, warnings, etc
Contra-indications: Hypersensitivity to neomycin or to any component of the preparation. (Cross-sensitivity with other aminoglycoside antibiotics may occur.) Herpes simplex and other viral diseases of the cornea and conjunctiva, fungal disease, ocular tuberculosis, untreated purulent infections. This product contains benzalkonium chloride and should not be used when soft contact lenses are worn.

Warnings: Not for injection. In severe infections topical use should be supplemented with appropriate systemic treatment. Prolonged use should be avoided as it may lead to skin sensitisation and the emergence of resistant organisms.

Neomycin may cause irreversible partial or total deafness when given systemically or when applied topically to open wounds or damaged skin. This effect is dose-related and is enhanced by renal or hepatic impairment. Although this effect has not been reported following topical ocular use the possibility should be considered when high dose topical treatment is given to small children or infants.

Topical corticosteroids should never be given for an undiagnosed red eye as inappropriate use is potentially blinding. Because of the risk of "steroid glaucoma" and cataract formation the intraocular pressure and the lens must be checked frequently during use of this preparation. To avoid the risk of enhancement of herpetic corneal disease, frequent slit-lamp examination is essential. Topical steroids may mask or enhance the activity of acute purulent eye infections. In such cases antibiotic therapy is mandatory. Persistent corneal ulceration for long-term topical steroid use may be due to fungal invasion. Topical corticosteroids are not effective in mustard gas keratitis or Sjorgen's keratoconjunctivitis.

These products may cause transient blurring of vision on instillation. Patients should be warned not to drive or operate hazardous machinery unless vision is clear.

Adverse reactions: Hypersensitivity reactions, usually of the delayed type, occur frequently with local treatment with neomycin. Irritation, burning, stinging, itching and dermatitis may occur. Topical steroid use may result in increased intraocular pressure leading to optic nerve disease, reduced visual acuity and visual field defects. Intensive or prolonged use of topical corticosteroids may lead to formation of posterior subcapsular cataracts. In those diseases causing thinning of the cornea or sclera, perforation of the globe may occur. Viral and fungal infections may be exacerbated by steroids. Systemic side effects may occur with extensive use.

Treatment of overdosage: Long-term intensive topical use may lead to systemic effects. Oral ingestion of the contents of one bottle (up to 10 mls) is unlikely to lead to any serious adverse effects.

Use in pregnancy: Safety for use in pregnancy and lactation has not been established. Topical administration of corticosteroids to pregnant animals can cause abnormalities of foetal development including cleft palate and intra-uterine growth with retardation. There may therefore be a very small risk of such effects in human pregnancy. Use only when it is considered essential by the physician.

Pharmaceutical precautions Maxitrol eye-drops and eye-ointment should be stored in a cool place away from direct sunlight. Keep the container tightly closed. Contents should be discarded one month after opening. Drops should be well shaken before use.

Legal category POM.

Package quantities Drops 5 ml container. Ointment 3.5 g.

Further information Drops: Maxitrol eye-drops are contained in an unbreakable semi-rigid, plastic dropper bottle with screw-on cap.

Ointment: Maxitrol eye-ointment is contained in a tube with a screw-on cap.

Product licence numbers

Maxitrol Eye-Drops	0649/5915
Maxitrol Eye-Ointment	0649/5916

MYDRIACYL 0.5% w/v and 1.0% w/v

Presentation Mydriacyl is a sterile, clear, colourless solution containing Tropicamide 0.5% w/v or 1.0% w/v, packed in 5 ml Droptainers, and preserved with benzalkonium chloride 0.01%.

Uses Tropicamide is a short acting anti-cholinergic agent used as a mydriatic and cycloplegic. It is indicated for topical use for diagnostic purposes for fundoscopy and cycloplegic refraction. It may also be used in pre- and post-operative states where a short acting mydriasis is required.

Dosage and administration For fundoscopy: One or two drops of 0.5% solution instilled into the eyes 15 to 20 minutes prior to examination. For cycloplegic refraction: One or two drops of 1% solution repeated after 5 minutes. If the patient is not seen within 20 to 30 minutes an additional drop may be instilled to prolong the effect.

Use in children: Tropicamide has been reported to be inadequate for cycloplegia in children. A more powerful cycloplegic agent, such as atropine, may be required.

Contra-indications, warnings, etc
Contra-indications: Contra-indicated in glaucoma or a tendency towards glaucoma (e.g. narrow anterior chamber angle). Hypersensitivity to any component of the preparation. This preparation contains benzalkonium chloride and should not be used where soft contact lenses are worn.

Warnings: For topical uses only – not for injection. Because of the risk of precipitating angle-closure glaucoma in the elderly and others prone to raised intraocular pressure, an estimate of the depth of the angle of the anterior chamber should be made before use. Extreme caution is advised for use in children and individuals susceptible to belladonna alkaloids because of the increased risk of systemic toxicity. Parents should be warned of the oral toxicity of this preparation for children and advised to wash their hands after use. Use with caution in an inflamed eye as the hyperaemia greatly increases the rate of systemic absorption through the conjunctiva. The effect of anti-muscarinic agents may be enhanced by the concomitant administration of other drugs with anti-muscarinic properties such as amantadine, some anti-histamines, butyrophenones, phenothiazines and tricyclic anti-depressants. This product may cause blurred vision and sensitivity to light. Patients should be warned not to drive or engage in other hazardous activities unless vision is clear. Complete recovery from the effects of tropicamide eyedrops may take up to six hours.

Precautions: To reduce systemic absorption the lacrimal sac should be compressed at the medial canthus by digital pressure for at least one minute after instillation of the drops.

Adverse reactions: Local: Increased intraocular pressure, transient stinging and sensitivity to light secondary to pupillary dilation. Prolonged administration may lead to local irritation, hyperaemia, oedema and conjunctivitis. Systemic: Systemic anti-cholinergic toxicity is manifested by dryness of the mouth, flushing, dryness of the skin, bradycardia followed by tachycardia with palpitations and arrythmias, urinary urgency, difficulty and retention, reduction in the tone and mobility of the gastrointestinal tract leading to constipation. Vomiting, giddiness and staggering may occur, a rash may be present in children and abdominal distention in infants. Psychotic reactions, behavioural disturbances and cardio-respiratory collapse may occur in children.

Use in pregnancy: There is insufficient evidence as to drug safety in pregnancy and lactation. This product should be used during pregnancy only when considered essential by a physician.

Treatment of overdosage: Systemic toxicity may occur following topical use, particularly in children. It is manifested by flushing and dryness of the skin (a rash may be present in children), blurred vision, a rapid and irregular pulse, fever, abdominal distention in infants, convulsions and hallucinations and the loss of neuromuscular co-ordination. Treatment is supportive (there is no evidence that physostigmine is superior to supportive management). In infants and small children the body surface must be kept moist. If accidentally ingested, induce emesis or perform gastric lavage.

Pharmaceutical precautions Mydriacyl eye drops should be stored in a cool place, away from direct sunlight, but do not refrigerate. Keep the container tightly closed. Discard one month after opening.

Legal category POM.

Package quantities 5 ml containers.

Further information Mydriacyl eye drops are contained in a semi-rigid plastic dropper bottle with a screw-on-cap.

Product licence numbers
0.5% 0649/5917
1% 0649/5918

TEARS Naturale*

Presentation Tears Naturale is a clear, colourless sterile solution, presented in a 15 ml Drop-Tainer Dispenser, and contains the Duasorb water soluble polymeric system Dextran 70 0.1% and Hydroxypropyl Methylcellulose (Hypromellose) USP 0.3%, and preserved with Benzalkonium Chloride PhEur 0.01% and Disodium Edetate PhEur 0.05%.

Uses A soothing solution for use as an artificial tear and lubricant in the relief of dry eye syndromes associated with deficient tear secretion or deficient mucous.

Dosage and administration Instill 1 or 2 drops into the eye(s), as frequently as to relieve eye irritation symptoms.

Contra-indications, warnings, etc
Contra-indications: This product contains benzalkonium chloride, and should not be used when soft contact lenses are being worn.

Precautions: If irritation persists, discontinue use.

Pharmaceutical precautions To avoid contaminating the solution, do not let the dropper tip touch any surface. Keep the container tightly closed. Discard the contents 1 month after opening.

Legal category P.

Package quantities 15 ml.

Further information Tears Naturale eye-drops are contained in an unbreakable semi-rigid plastic dropper bottle with a screw-on cap.

Product licence number 0649/0031.

TOBRALEX*

Presentation A sterile, clear, colourless to very pale yellow ophthalmic solution containing Tobramycin BP 0.3% w/v, preserved with 0.01% Benzalkonium Chloride PhEur.

Uses Tobralex (tobramycin) Sterile Ophthalmic Solution is a bactericidal topical antibiotic indicated in the treatment of external bacterial conditions of the eye and its appendages. The spectrum of activity covers a wide range of Gram-positive organisms and many Gram-negative organisms.

A significant bacterial population resistant to tobramycin has not yet been reported. However, there is the possibility that bacterial resistance may develop following prolonged use.

Dosage and administration Adults and children: In mild to moderate cases, instil one or two drops into the affected eye every four hours. For severe infections, instil two drops into the eye hourly until there is an improvement and then reduce treatment, prior to discontinuation.

Contra-indications, warnings, etc
Contra-indications: Persons with known sensitivity to tobramycin or gentamicin.

Warnings: Sensitivity may occur in some patients. If so, discontinue use. Transient irritation may occur with some susceptible patients.

Tobralex ophthalmic solution is not for injection. This product contains benzalkonium chloride and should not be used when soft contact lenses are being worn.

Precautions: As with other antibiotics, prolonged use may result in the overgrowth of non-susceptible organisms, including fungi. If super-infection occurs, appropriate therapy should be initiated.

Use in pregnancy: Reproduction studies in animals at doses up to thirty-three times the normal human systemic dose have revealed no evidence of impaired fertility or harm to the foetus due to tobramycin. There are, however, no adequate and well-controlled studies in pregnant women. Because animal studies are not always predictive of human response, this drug should be used during pregnancy only if clearly needed.

Nursing mothers: Because of the potential for adverse reactions in nursing infants from Tobralex, a decision should be made whether to discontinue nursing the infant or discontinue the drug, taking into account the importance of the drug to the mother.

Adverse reactions: The most frequent adverse reactions to Tobralex Ophthalmic Solution are localized ocular toxicity and hypersensitivity, including lid itching and swelling, and conjunctival erythema. These reactions occur in less than 3% of patients treated with Tobralex. Similar reactions may occur with the topical use of other aminoglycoside antibiotics. Other adverse reactions have not been reported from Tobralex therapy, however, if topical ocular tobramycin is administered concomitantly with systemic aminoglycoside antibiotics, care should be taken to monitor the total serum concentration.

Overdosage: Clinically apparent signs and symptoms of an overdose of Tobralex Ophthalmic Solution (punctate keratitis, erythema, increased lacrimation, oedema and lid itching) may be similar to adverse reaction effects seen in some patients.

Pharmaceutical precautions Store at 8°C to 25°C. Do not freeze. Keep the container tightly closed. Discard contents one month after opening.

Sterile until opened.

Legal category POM.

Package quantities 5 ml.

Further information Tobralex eye drops are contained in an unbreakable semi-rigid plastic dropper bottle with screw-on cap.

Product licence number 0649/0044.

**Trade Mark*

Allen & Hanburys Limited
Stockley Park West
Uxbridge, Middlesex UB11 1BT

ALLEN & HANBURYS

BECLOFORTE* INHALER

Presentation Becloforte Inhaler is a metered-dose aerosol which delivers 250 micrograms Beclomethasone Dipropionate BP (as the trichlorofluoromethane solvate) per actuation into the mouthpiece of a specially designed actuator.

Becloforte Inhaler can be used as the sole inhalation device or as part of Becloforte-VM Inhalation System. This is designed to facilitate and improve the use of high doses of inhaled corticosteroids delivered from a metered-dose aerosol. It consists of a Becloforte Inhaler which is used in conjunction with a large (750 ml) spacer device – the Volumatic*, from which the active drug is inhaled.

Uses Beclomethasone Dipropionate BP given by inhalation has a potent glucocorticoid anti-inflammatory action within the lungs without the side effects observed when steroids are administered systemically.

Becloforte Inhaler is indicated for those asthmatic patients who have been shown to require high doses (greater than 800 micrograms to 1,000 micrograms daily) of Beclomethasone Dipropionate BP to control their symptoms. It may also be indicated for those patients whose asthma is no longer controlled by maximum maintenance doses of bronchodilators and Becotide* Inhalers.

Some patients with severe asthma require oral corticosteroid therapy in addition to Becotide Inhalers for the adequate control of their symptoms. Many of these patients may, on transfer to Becloforte Inhaler, be able to reduce significantly or eliminate their requirement for additional oral corticosteroids.

Some patients find difficulty in co-ordinating the firing of the inhaler with the early stages of the inspiratory cycle and therefore fail to maximise the potential benefit offered by treatment. By removing the need to synchronise these two operations Becloforte-VM may prove helpful for some patients since they can fire the inhaler and then breathe in.

Dosage and administration
Adults: Two inhalations (500 micrograms) twice daily, or one inhalation (250 micrograms) four times daily, is the recommended maintenance dosage. If necessary, dosage may be increased to two inhalations (500 micrograms) three or four times daily, according to response.

Children: Becloforte Inhaler is not indicated for use in children.

Contra-indications, warnings, etc
Contra-indications: Hypersensitivity to Becloforte Inhaler is a contra-indication; and special care is necessary in patients with active or quiescent pulmonary tuberculosis.

Pregnancy: There is inadequate evidence of safety in human pregnancy. Administration of corticosteroids to pregnant animals can cause abnormalities of fetal development, including cleft palate and intra-uterine growth retardation. There may therefore be a very small risk of such effects in the human fetus. It should be noted, however, that the fetal changes in animals occur after relatively high systemic exposure. Because beclomethasone dipropionate is delivered directly to the lungs by the inhaled route it avoids the high level of exposure that occurs when corticosteroids are given by systemic routes.

The use of beclomethasone dipropionate in pregnancy requires that the possible benefits of the drug be weighed against the possible hazards. It should be noted that the drug has been in widespread use for many years without apparent ill consequence.

Lactation: No specific studies examining the transference of beclomethasone dipropionate into the milk of lactating animals have been performed. It is reasonable to assume that beclomethasone dipropionate is secreted in milk but at the dosages used for direct inhalation there is low potential for significant levels in breast milk. The use of beclomethasone dipropionate in mothers breast feeding their babies requires that the therapeutic benefits of the drug be weighed against the potential hazards to the mother and baby.

When using the Becloforte Inhaler alone, the patient's inhaler technique should be checked to make sure that aerosol actuation is synchronised with inspiration of breath for optimum dispersal of drug within the lungs.

Patients should also be made aware of the prophylactic nature of therapy with Becloforte Inhaler and that it should be taken regularly even when they are asymptomatic.

Patients being treated with Becotide Inhaler may be transferred directly to treatment with Becloforte Inhaler.

In the majority of patients no significant adrenal suppression occurs until doses of 1,500 micrograms per day are exceeded. Some patients receiving 2,000 micrograms of Becloforte per day may show a degree of adrenocortical suppression although short-term adrenal reserve remains intact. In such patients the risks of developing adrenal suppression should be balanced against the therapeutic advantages and precautions should be taken to provide systemic steroid cover in situations of prolonged stress.

Patients being treated with oral corticosteroids should be in a stable state before having Becloforte Inhaler added to their current therapy. Gradual withdrawal of the systemic steroid may be attempted after a week or two. Patients who have been treated with systemic steroids for long periods of time or at a high dose may have adrenocortical suppression. With these patients adrenocortical function should be monitored regularly and their dose of systemic steroid reduced cautiously.

Patients recently transferred from oral steroids to Becloforte Inhaler together with those still receiving oral steroids should carry a warning card indicating that they may need to start or increase the dosage of oral steroids in times of stress, e.g. surgery, chest infections or worsening asthmatic attacks but that this can be reduced again after the stress has been resolved. A small supply of oral steroids can be given to them for emergency use.

Replacement of systemic steroid treatment with Becloforte Inhaler sometimes unmasks allergies such as rhinitis or eczema previously controlled by the systemic drug. These allergies should be symptomatically treated with antihistamine and/or topical preparations.

Treatment with Becloforte Inhaler should not be stopped abruptly.

Side-effects: Candidiasis of the mouth and throat occurs in some patients but the incidence is no greater than that with Becotide Inhaler. Patients with high blood levels of Candida precipitins, indicating a previous infection, are more likely to develop this complication. Some patients may find it helpful to rinse their mouth thoroughly with water after using the Inhaler. Symptomatic candidiasis can be treated with topical anti-fungal therapy whilst still continuing with Becloforte Inhaler.

In some patients, beclomethasone dipropionate may

cause hoarseness or throat irritation. It may be helpful to rinse the mouth out with water after inhalation.

As with other inhalation therapy, the potential for paradoxical bronchospasm should be kept in mind. If it occurs, treatment should be discontinued immediately and alternative therapy instituted.

Overdosage: If Becloforte Inhaler is used excessively over a long period, this could lead to adrenal suppression. In such cases, the patient should be transferred to oral corticosteroid therapy and when the condition has stabilised, be returned to the inhaled therapy at the recommended dose. To guard against the unexpected event of adrenal suppression regular tests of adrenal function are advised.

Pharmaceutical precautions Becloforte Inhaler should be stored at a temperature below 30°C.

As with most inhaled medications in aerosol canisters, the therapeutic effect of this medication may decrease when the canister is cold.

Protect from frost and direct sunlight.

The canister should not be punctured, broken or burnt even if it is apparently empty.

Legal category POM.

Package quantities Each canister of Becloforte Inhaler provides 200 inhalations. It is available as a standard metered-dose aerosol or as Becloforte-VM when two aerosols are packed together with a large volume (750 ml) spacer device.

Further information Nil.

Product licence number 0045/0125

BECODISKS*

Presentation Each Becodisk comprises eight, regularly spaced, double-foil blisters each containing a mixture of microfine beclomethasone dipropionate, 100 micrograms, 200 micrograms or 400 micrograms and larger particle lactose. Each dosage strength is identified in the centre of the disk as 'Becodisk 100 mcg', 'Becodisk 200 mcg' or 'Becodisk 400 mcg'.

Becodisks are intended only for use in a specific drug delivery device known as the Becotide Diskhaler*. The contents of each blister are deposited into the beige Diskhaler device when pierced with an integral needle. The contents are then available to the patient to inhale by breath operation which allows the drug to be fully available even at low inspiratory flow rates.

Becodisks, therefore, provide reliable drug delivery for many patients, but a rather larger unit dose relative to Becotide 50 or Becotide 100 Inhaler is necessary for the same therapeutic effect.

Uses Beclomethasone Dipropionate BP given by inhalation has a potent glucocorticoid anti-inflammatory action within the lungs but does not cause adverse systemic glucocorticoid effects at therapeutic doses. Becodisks, therefore, are indicated for a wide range of patients with bronchial asthma. These patients include: those whose asthma is poorly controlled by bronchodilators alone; those who are inadequately controlled by sodium cromoglycate in addition to bronchodilators; those with severe asthma who are dependent on systemic corticosteroids, or adrenocorticotrophic hormone (ACTH) or its synthetic equivalent.

Becodisks are particularly important for managing severe asthma in children because good control can be achieved without retardation of growth.

Dosage and administration Becodisks are for inhalation use only, using a Becotide Diskhaler. For optimum results Becodisks should be used regularly.

Adults: The contents of one 400 micrograms blister or two 200 microgram blisters twice daily is the usual maintenance dose. Alternatively, 200 micrograms may be administered three or four times daily.

Children: 100 micrograms two, three or four times a day according to the response. Alternatively, 200 micrograms twice daily may be administered.

Contra-indications, warnings, etc
Contra-indications: Hypersensitivity to Becodisks is a contra-indication; and special care is necessary in patients with active or quiescent pulmonary tuberculosis.

Precautions: Patients should be instructed in the proper use of the Diskhaler to ensure that the drug reaches the target areas within the lungs. They should also be made aware that Becodisks have to be used regularly for optimum benefit.

In the majority of patients no significant adrenal suppression occurs until doses of 1,500 micrograms per day are exceeded. Reduction of plasma cortisol levels has been reported in some patients who received 2,000 micrograms per day of inhaled beclomethasone dipropionate.

Pregnancy: There is inadequate evidence of safety in human pregnancy. Administration of corticosteroids to pregnant animals can cause abnormalities of fetal development including cleft palate and intra-uterine growth retardation. There may therefore be a very small risk of such effects in the human fetus. It should be noted, however, that the fetal changes in animals occur after relatively high systemic exposure. Because beclomethasone dipropionate is delivered directly to the lungs by the inhaled route it avoids the high level of exposure that occurs when corticosteroids are given by systemic routes.

The use of beclomethasone dipropionate in pregnancy requires that the possible benefits of the drug be weighed against the possible hazards. It should be noted that the drug has been in widespread use for many years without apparent ill consequence.

Lactation: No specific studies examining the transference of beclomethasone dipropionate into the milk of lactating animals have been performed. It is reasonable to assume that beclomethasone dipropionate is secreted in milk but, at the dosages used for direct inhalation, there is low potential for significant levels in breast milk.

The use of beclomethasone dipropionate in mothers breast feeding their babies requires that the therapeutic benefits of the drug be weighed against the potential hazards to the mother and baby.

Patients inadequately controlled by bronchodilator therapy: The use of Becodisks in patients who have never taken oral corticosteroids or taken only occasional courses of oral corticosteroids is straightforward. An improvement in respiratory function is normally obvious within a week. The few patients who do not respond during this period usually have excessive mucus in their bronchi so that the drug is unable to penetrate to its site of action. In such cases a short course of systemic steroid in relatively high dosage should be given to control secretion of mucus and other inflammatory changes in the lungs. Continuation of treatment with Becodisks usually maintains the improvement achieved, the oral steroid being gradually withdrawn. Exacerbation of asthma caused by infection is usually controlled by appropriate antibiotic treatment, by increasing the dose of Becodisks and, if necessary, by giving systemic corticosteroid.

Patients being treated with oral corticosteroids: The transfer of steroid-dependent patients to Becodisks and their subsequent management needs special care mainly because recovery from impaired adrenocortical function, caused by prolonged systemic steroid therapy, is slow. The patient should be in a reasonably stable state before being given Becodisks in addition to his usual maintenance dose of systemic steroid. After about a week, gradual withdrawal of the systemic steroid is started by reducing the daily dose by one milligram prednisolone, or its equivalent at not less than weekly intervals. Patients treated with systemic steroids for long periods of time or who have received high doses may have adrenocortical suppression. With these patients adrenocortical function should be monitored regularly and their dose of systemic steroid reduced cautiously. Transferred patients whose adrenocortical function is impaired should carry a warning card indicating that they need supplementary systemic steroid during periods of stress, e.g., surgery, chest infection or worsening asthma attacks. Consideration should be given to supplying such patients with oral steroids to use in an emergency. The dose of Becodisks should be increased at this time and then reduced to the maintenance level after the systemic steroid has been discontinued.

Replacement of systemic steroid treatment with Becodisks sometimes unmasks allergies such as allergic rhinitis or eczema previously controlled by the systemic drug. These allergies should be symptomatically treated with antihistamine and/or topical preparations.

Side-effects: Candidiasis of the mouth and throat (thrush) occurs in some patients. Patients with high blood levels of Candida precipitins, indicating a previous infection, are more likely to develop this complication. Some patients may find it helpful to rinse their mouth thoroughly with water after using Becodisks. Symptomatic candidiasis can be treated with topical antifungal therapy whilst still continuing with the treatment.

In some patients inhaled beclomethasone dipropionate may cause hoarseness or throat irritation. It may be helpful to rinse the mouth out with water immediately after inhalation.

As with other inhalation therapy, the potential for paradoxical bronchospasm should be kept in mind. If it occurs, the preparation should be discontinued immediately and alternative therapy instituted.

Overdosage: The acute toxicity of beclomethasone dipropionate is low. The only harmful effect that follows inhalation of large amounts of the drug over a short time period is suppression of hypothalamic-pituitary-adrenal (HPA) function. No special emergency action need be taken. Treatment with Becodisks should be continued at the recommended dose to control the asthma; HPA function recovers in a day or two.

If Becodisks are used excessively over a long period this could lead to adrenal suppression. In such a case, the patient should be transferred to oral corticosteroid therapy, and when the condition has stabilised, be returned to inhaled therapy at the recommended dose.

To guard against the unexpected event of adrenal suppression, regular tests of adrenal function are advised. Oral steroids should then be slowly withdrawn, as for steroid-dependent patients.

Pharmaceutical precautions Whilst the Becodisks provide a good protection to the blister contents from the effect of the atmosphere, they should not be exposed to extremes of temperature and should be stored below 30°C. A Becodisk may be kept in the Diskhaler at all times but a blister should only be pierced immediately prior to use. Failure to observe this instruction may affect the operation of the Diskhaler.

Legal category POM.

Package quantities Becodisks 100 micrograms and 200 micrograms are supplied in cartons of 14 (OP), together with a Diskhaler device. Becodisks 400 micrograms are supplied in cartons of 7 (OP), together with a Diskhaler device.

Further information Nil.

Product licence number
Becodisks 100 micrograms 0045/0136
Becodisks 200 micrograms 0045/0137
Becodisks 400 micrograms 0045/0142

BECONASE* AQUEOUS NASAL SPRAY

Presentation Beconase Aqueous Nasal Spray is a presentation of an aqueous suspension of microfine Beclomethasone Dipropionate BP delivered by a metering, atomising pump. Each 100 mg spray delivered by the nasal applicator contains 50 micrograms Beclomethasone Dipropionate BP.

Uses Beconase Aqueous Nasal Spray is indicated for the prophylaxis and treatment of perennial and seasonal allergic rhinitis including hay fever, and vasomotor rhinitis. Beclomethasone Dipropionate BP has a potent anti-inflammatory effect within the respiratory tract at doses which are not systemically active.

Dosage and administration Beconase Aqueous Nasal Spray is for administration by the intranasal route only.

Adults and children: The recommended dosage is two sprays into each nostril twice daily. For some patients, a dosage regimen of a single spray into each nostril three or four times daily may be preferred. Total daily administration should not normally exceed eight sprays.

For full therapeutic benefit, regular usage is essential. The co-operation of the patient should be sought to comply with the regular dosage schedule and it should be explained that maximum relief may not be obtained within the first few doses.

For children under six years old, there are insufficient clinical data to recommend use.

Contra-indications, warnings, etc
Contra-indications: Beconase Aqueous Nasal Spray is contra-indicated in patients with a history of hypersensitivity to any of its components.

Precautions: Infections of the nasal passages and paranasal sinuses should be appropriately treated but do not constitute a specific contra-indication to treatment with Beconase Aqueous Nasal Spray.

Care must be taken while transferring patients from systemic steroid treatment to Beconase Aqueous Nasal Spray if there is any reason to suppose that their adrenal function is impaired.

Although Beconase Aqueous Nasal Spray will control seasonal allergic rhinitis in most cases, an abnormally heavy challenge of summer allergens may in certain instances necessitate appropriate additional therapy particularly to control eye symptoms.

Pregnancy: There is inadequate evidence of safety in human pregnancy. Administration of corticosteroids to pregnant animals can cause abnormalities of fetal development, including cleft palate and intra-uterine growth retardation. There may therefore be a very small risk of such effects in the human fetus. It should be noted, however, that the fetal changes in animals occur after relatively high systemic exposure; direct intranasal application ensures minimal systemic exposure.

The use of beclomethasone dipropionate in pregnancy requires that the possible benefits of the drug be weighed against the possible hazards. It should be noted that the drug has been in widespread use for many years without apparent ill consequence.

Lactation: No specific studies examining the transference of beclomethasone dipropionate into the milk of lactating animals have been performed. It is reasonable to assume that beclomethasone dipropionate is secreted in milk but at the dosages used for direct inhalation, there is low potential for significant levels in breast milk. The use of beclomethasone dipropionate in mothers breast feeding their babies requires that the therapeutic benefits of the drug be weighed against the potential hazards to the mother and baby.

Side-effects: No major side effects attributable to the use of recommended doses of Beconase Aqueous Nasal Spray have been reported.

As with other nasal sprays, dryness and irritation of the nose and throat, unpleasant taste and smell and epistaxis have been reported rarely.

Overdosage: The only harmful effect that follows inhalation of large amounts of the drug over a short time period is suppression of hypothalamic-pituitary-adrenal (HPA) function. No special emergency action need be taken. Treatment with Beconase Aqueous Nasal Spray should be continued at the recommended dose. HPA function recovers in a day or two.

Pharmaceutical precautions Beconase Aqueous Nasal Spray should be protected from light and stored below 30°C. Do not refrigerate.

Legal category POM.

Package quantities Beconase Aqueous Nasal Spray is supplied in an amber glass bottle fitted with a metering, atomising pump and nasal applicator. Each bottle provides approximately 200 metered sprays in recommended use.

Further information Beconase Aqueous Nasal Spray is an alternative intranasal presentation of Beclomethasone Dipropionate BP to Beconase Nasal Spray and is available for those who may prefer an aqueous product.

Product licence number 0045/0127

BECONASE* NASAL SPRAY

Presentation Beconase Nasal Spray is a metered-dose aerosol which delivers 50 micrograms Beclomethasone Dipropionate BP (as the trichlorofluoromethane solvate) per actuation into a specially designed nasal applicator.

Uses Beconase is indicated for the prophylaxis and treatment of perennial and seasonal allergic rhinitis including hay fever, and vasomotor rhinitis. Beclomethasone Dipropionate BP has a potent anti-inflammatory effect within the respiratory tract at doses which are not systemically active.

Beconase Aqueous Nasal Spray is available for those who may prefer an aqueous presentation.

Dosage and administration Beconase is for administration by the intranasal route only. The recommended dosage is two applications into each nostril twice daily (400 micrograms/day).

For some patients, a dosage regimen of a single application into each nostril three or four times daily may be preferred. Total daily administration should not normally exceed 8 puffs.

For full therapeutic benefit regular usage is essential. The co-operation of the patient should be sought to comply with the regular dosage schedule and it should be explained that maximum relief may not be obtained within the first few applications.

For children under six years old, there are insufficient clinical data to recommend use.

Contra-indications, warnings, etc
Contra-indications: Beconase Nasal Spray is contra-indicated in patients with a history of hypersensitivity to any of its components.

Precautions: Infections of the nasal passages and paranasal sinuses should be appropriately treated but do not constitute a specific contra-indication to treatment with Beconase.

Care must be taken while transferring patients from systemic steroid treatment to Beconase if there is any reason to suppose that their adrenal function is impaired.

Although Beconase Nasal Spray will control seasonal allergic rhinitis in most cases, an abnormally heavy challenge of summer allergens may in certain instances necessitate appropriate additional therapy particularly to control eye symptoms.

Pregnancy: There is inadequate evidence of safety in human pregnancy. Administration of corticosteroids to pregnant animals can cause abnormalities of fetal development, including cleft palate and intra-uterine growth retardation. There may therefore be a very small risk of such effects in the human fetus. It should be noted, however, that the fetal changes in animals occur after relatively high systemic exposure; direct intranasal application ensures minimal systemic exposure.

Lactation: No specific studies examining the transference of beclomethasone dipropionate into the milk of lactating animals have been performed. It is reasonable to assume that beclomethasone dipropionate is secreted in milk but, at the dosages used for direct inhalation, there is low potential for significant levels in breast milk. The use of beclomethasone dipropionate in mothers breast feeding their babies requires that the therapeutic benefits of the drug be weighed against the potential hazards to the mother and baby.

Side-effects: Extremely rare cases of nasal septal perforation have been reported following the use of intranasal aerosol corticosteroids.

Occasionally, sneezing attacks have followed immediately after the use of an aerosol.

As with other nasal sprays, dryness and irritation of the nose and throat, unpleasant taste and smell and epistaxis have been reported rarely.

Overdosage: The only harmful effect that follows inhalation of large amounts of the drug over a short time period is suppression of hypothalamic-pituitary-adrenal (HPA) function. No special emergency action need be taken. Treatment with Beconase Nasal Spray should be continued at the recommended dose. HPA function recovers in a day or two.

Pharmaceutical precautions Beconase Nasal Spray should be stored at a temperature below 30°C.

As with most inhaled medications in aerosol canisters, the therapeutic effect of this medication may decrease when the canister is cold.

Protect from frost and direct sunlight.

The canister should not be punctured, broken or burnt even if it is apparently empty.

Legal category POM.

Package quantities Beconase Nasal Spray is a metered-dose aerosol with a specially designed nasal applicator. Each canister provides 200 sprays.

Further information When Beconase is administered as two applications into each nostril the first puff should be directed at the upper and the second at the lower part of the nasal cavity.

Product licence number 0045/0093R

BECOTIDE* 50 INHALER
BECOTIDE* 100 INHALER
BECOTIDE* 200 INHALER

Presentation Becotide 50 Inhaler is a metered-dose aerosol which delivers 50 micrograms Beclomethasone Dipropionate BP (as the trichlorofluoromethane solvate) per actuation into the mouthpiece of a specially designed actuator.

Becotide 100 Inhaler is a metered-dose aerosol which delivers 100 micrograms Beclomethasone Dipropionate BP per actuation into the mouthpiece of a specially designed actuator.

Becotide 200 Inhaler is a metered-dose aerosol which delivers 200 micrograms Beclomethasone Dipropionate BP per actuation into the mouthpiece of a specially designed actuator.

Uses Beclomethasone Dipropionate BP given by inhalation has a potent glucocorticoid anti-inflammatory action within the lungs but does not cause adverse systemic glucocorticoid effects at therapeutic doses. Becotide 50 Inhaler, Becotide 100 Inhaler and Becotide 200 Inhaler therefore are indicated for a wide range of patients with bronchial asthma.

These patients include: those whose asthma is becoming worse and the relief provided by bronchodilators is less effective; those who are inadequately controlled by sodium cromoglycate in addition to bronchodilators; those with severe asthma who are dependent on systemic corticosteroids, or adrenocorticotrophic hormone (ACTH) or its synthetic equivalent.

Becotide 50 Inhaler or Becotide 100 Inhaler are particularly important for managing severe asthma in children because good control can be achieved without retardation of growth.

Becotide 200 is unsuitable for administration to children.

Dosage and administration
Adults: 200 micrograms twice a day. Alternatively, the total daily dose may be administered as three or four

divided doses. In more severe cases dosage may be started at 600 to 800 micrograms per day and subsequently reduced when the patient begins to respond.

Children: 50 to 100 micrograms should be given two, three or four times daily, according to the response. Alternatively, 100 micrograms or 200 micrograms twice daily may be administered.

Contra-indications, warnings, etc
Contra-indications: Hypersensitivity to any Becotide Inhaler is a contra-indication; and special care is necessary in patients with active or quiescent pulmonary tuberculosis.

Precautions: Patients should be instructed on the proper use of the inhaler to ensure that the drug reaches the target areas within the lungs. They should also be made aware that Becotide Inhaler has to be used regularly for optimum benefit. Patients should be made aware of the prophylactic nature of therapy with Becotide Inhaler and that it should be taken regularly, even when they are asymptomatic.

In the majority of patients no significant adrenal suppression occurs until doses of 1,500 micrograms per day are exceeded.

Reduction of plasma cortisol levels has been reported in some patients who have received 2,000 micrograms per day of inhaled beclomethasone dipropionate.

Pregnancy: There is inadequate evidence of safety in human pregnancy. Administration of corticosteroids to pregnant animals can cause abnormalities of fetal development, including cleft palate and intra-uterine growth retardation. There may, therefore, be a very small risk of such effects in the human fetus. It should be noted, however, that the fetal changes in animals occur after relatively high systemic exposure. Because beclomethasone dipropionate is delivered directly to the lungs by the inhaled route it avoids the high level of exposure that occurs when corticosteroids are given by systemic routes.

The use of beclomethasone dipropionate in pregnancy requires that the possible benefits of the drug be weighed against the possible hazards. It should be noted that the drug has been in widespread use for many years without apparent ill consequence.

Lactation: No specific studies examining the transference of beclomethasone dipropionate into the milk of lactating animals have been performed. It is reasonable to assume that beclomethasone dipropionate is secreted in milk but at the dosages used for direct inhalation, there is low potential for significant levels in breast milk. The use of beclomethasone dipropionate in mothers breast feeding their babies requires that the therapeutic benefits of the drug be weighed against the potential hazards to the mother and baby.

Patients inadequately controlled by bronchodilator therapy: The use of Becotide Inhaler in patients who have never taken steroids or taken only occasional courses of steroids is straightforward. An improvement in respiratory function is normally obvious within a week. The few patients who do not respond during this period usually have excessive mucus in their bronchi so that the drug is unable to penetrate to its site of action. In such cases, a short course of systemic steroid in relatively high dosage should be given to control secretion of mucus and other inflammatory changes in the lungs. Continuation of treatment with Becotide Inhaler usually maintains the improvement achieved, the oral steroid being gradually withdrawn. Exacerbation of asthma caused by infection is usually controlled by appropriate antibiotic treatment, by increasing the dose of Becotide Inhaler and if necessary by giving a systemic steroid.

Patients being treated with oral corticosteroids: The patient should be in a reasonably stable state before being given Becotide Inhaler in addition to his usual maintenance dose of systemic steroid. After about a week, gradual withdrawal of the systemic steroid is started by reducing the daily dose by one milligram prednisolone, or its equivalent, at not less than weekly intervals. Patients treated with systemic steroids for long periods of time or who have received high doses may have adrenocortical suppression. With these patients, adrenocortical function should be monitored regularly and their dose of systemic steroid reduced cautiously. Transferred patients whose adrenocortical function is impaired should carry a warning card indicating that they need supplementary systemic steroids during periods of stress, e.g., surgery, chest infection or worsening asthma attacks. Consideration should be given to supplying such patients with oral steroids to use in an emergency. The dose of Becotide Inhaler should be increased at this time and then reduced to the maintenance level after the systemic steroid has been discontinued.

Replacement of systemic steroid treatment with Becotide Inhaler sometimes unmasks allergies such as allergic rhinitis or eczema previously controlled by the systemic drug. These allergies should be symptomatically treated with antihistamine and/or topical preparations.

Side-effects: Candidiasis of the mouth and throat (thrush) occurs in some patients, the incidence of which is increased with doses greater than 400 micrograms beclomethasone dipropionate per day. Patients with high blood levels of Candida precipitins, indicating a previous infection, are most likely to develop this complication. Some patients may find it helpful to rinse their mouth thoroughly with water after using the Inhaler. Symptomatic candidiasis can be treated with topical antifungal therapy whilst still continuing with the Becotide Inhaler.

In some patients, inhaled beclomethasone dipropionate may cause hoarseness or throat irritation. It may be helpful to rinse the mouth out with water immediately after inhalation.

As with other inhalation therapy, the potential for paradoxical bronchospasm should be kept in mind. If it occurs, the preparation should be discontinued immediately and alternative therapy instituted.

Overdosage: The acute toxicity of beclomethasone dipropionate is low. The only harmful effect that follows inhalation of large amounts of the drug over a short time period is suppression of hypothalamic-pituitary-adrenal (HPA) function. No special emergency action need be taken. Treatment with Becotide Inhalers should be continued at the recommended dose to control the asthma; HPA function recovers in a day or two.

If Becotide Inhalers are used excessively over a long period, this could lead to adrenal suppression. In such a case, the patient should be transferred to oral corticosteroid therapy and when the condition has stabilised, be returned to the inhaled therapy at the recommended dose. To guard against the unexpected event of adrenal suppression regular tests of adrenal function are advised.

Oral steroids should then be slowly withdrawn, as for steroid dependent patients.

Pharmaceutical precautions Becotide Inhalers should be stored at a temperature below 30°C.

As with most inhaled medications in aerosol canisters, the therapeutic effect of this medication may decrease when the canister is cold.

Protect from frost and direct sunlight.

The canister should not be punctured, broken or burnt even if it is apparently empty.

Legal category POM.

Package quantities Becotide Inhalers are metered-dose aerosols with a specially designed actuator.

Becotide 50 Inhaler, Becotide 100 Inhaler and Becotide 200 Inhaler are available in canisters providing 200 inhalations.

Further information Nil.

Product licence numbers

Becotide 50 Inhaler	0045/0089R
Becotide 100 Inhaler	0045/0131
Becotide 200 Inhaler	0045/0152

BECOTIDE* ROTACAPS*

Presentation Becotide Rotacaps capsules, an alternative inhalation form of beclomethasone dipropionate to Becotide Inhaler, are especially valuable for treating patients who are unable to use pressurised inhalers effectively or who might use them incorrectly.

Becotide Rotacaps contain a mixture of microfine beclomethasone dipropionate and large particle lactose in hard gelatin capsules. Each Rotacap contains 100 micrograms (buff/colourless), 200 micrograms (brown/colourless) or 400 micrograms (dark brown/colourless) of beclomethasone dipropionate and is marked Becotide 100, Becotide 200 or Becotide 400, respectively.

The contents of a Rotacap are inhaled using a specially developed device called a Rotahaler* inhaler which separates the capsule into halves that rotate and release the drug when the patient inhales. This breath actuation is very sensitive so the drug is fully available even at the lowest inspiratory flow rates. The Rotahaler is therefore a more reliable drug delivery system for many patients but a rather larger unit dose relative to Becotide Inhaler is necessary for the same therapeutic effect.

Uses Beclomethasone dipropionate given by inhalation has a potent glucocorticoid anti-inflammatory action within the lungs but does not cause adverse systemic glucocorticoid effects at therapeutic doses. Becotide Rotacaps therefore are indicated for a wide range of patients with bronchial asthma. These patients include: those whose asthma is becoming worse and the relief provided by bronchodilators is less effective; those who are inadequately controlled by sodium cromoglycate in addition to bronchodilators; those with severe asthma who are dependent on systemic corticosteroids, or adrenocorticotrophic hormone (ACTH) or its synthetic equivalent.

Becotide Rotacaps are particularly important for managing severe asthma in children because good control can be achieved without retardation of growth.

Dosage and administration Becotide Rotacaps are for inhalation use only, using a Becotide Rotahaler. For optimum results, Becotide Rotacaps should be used regularly.

Adults: One 400 micrograms Rotacap or two 200 microgram Rotacaps twice a day is the usual maintenance dose. Alternatively, one 200 micrograms Rotacap may be given three or four times daily.

Children: One 100 micrograms Rotacap two, three or four times a day, according to the response. Alternatively, 200 micrograms twice a day may be administered.

Contra-indications, warnings, etc

Contra-indications: Hypersensitivity to Becotide is a contra-indication. Special care is necessary in patients with active or quiescent pulmonary tuberculosis.

Precautions: Patients should be instructed in the proper use of the Rotahaler to ensure that the drug reaches the target areas within the lungs. Patients should be made aware of the prophylactic nature of therapy with inhaled beclomethasone dipropionate and that it should be taken regularly, even when they are asymptomatic.

In the majority of patients no significant adrenal suppression occurs until doses of 1,500 micrograms per day are exceeded.

Reduction of plasma cortisol levels has been reported in some patients who received 2,000 micrograms per day of inhaled beclomethasone dipropionate.

Pregnancy: There is inadequate evidence of safety in human pregnancy. Administration of corticosteroids to pregnant animals can cause abnormalities of fetal development including cleft palate and intra-uterine growth retardation. There may therefore be a very small risk of such effects in the human fetus. It should be noted, however, that the fetal changes in animals occur after relatively high systemic exposure. Because beclomethasone dipropionate is delivered directly to the lungs by the inhaled route it avoids the high level of exposure that occurs when corticosteroids are given by systemic routes.

The use of beclomethasone dipropionate in pregnancy requires that the possible benefits of the drug be weighed against the possible hazards. It should be noted that the drug has been in widespread use for many years without apparent ill consequence.

Lactation: No specific studies examining the transference of beclomethasone dipropionate into the milk of lactating animals have been performed. It is reasonable to assume that beclomethasone dipropionate is secreted in milk but, at the dosages used for direct inhalation, there is low potential for significant levels in breast milk. The use of beclomethasone dipropionate in mothers breast feeding their babies requires that the therapeutic benefits of the drug be weighed against the potential hazards to the mother and baby.

Patients inadequately controlled by bronchodilator therapy: The use of Becotide Rotacaps in patients who have never taken steroids or taken only occasional courses of steroids is straightforward. An improvement in respiratory function is normally obvious within a week. The few patients who do not respond during this period usually have excessive mucus in their bronchi so that the drug is unable to penetrate to its site of action. In such cases, a short course of systemic steroid in relatively high dosage should be given to control secretion of mucus and other inflammatory changes in the lungs. Continuation of treatment with inhaled beclomethasone dipropionate usually maintains the improvement achieved, the oral steroid being gradually withdrawn. Exacerbation of asthma caused by infection is usually controlled by appropriate antibiotic treatment, by increasing the dose of inhaled beclomethasone dipropionate and if necessary by giving systemic steroid.

Patients being treated with oral corticosteroids: The transfer of steroid-dependent patients to Becotide Rotacaps and their subsequent management needs special care mainly because recovery from impaired adrenocortical function, caused by prolonged systemic steroid therapy, is slow. The patient should be in a reasonably stable state before being given Becotide Rotacaps in addition to his usual maintenance dose of systemic steroid. After about a week, gradual withdrawal of the systemic steroid is started by reducing the daily dose by one milligram prednisolone, or its equivalent, at not less than weekly intervals. Patients treated with systemic steroids for long periods of time or who have received high doses may have adrenocortical suppression. With these patients, adrenocortical function should be monitored regularly and their dose of systemic steroid reduced cautiously. Transferred patients whose adrenocortical function is impaired should carry a warning card indicating that they need supplementary systemic steroid during periods of stress, e.g., surgery, chest infection or worsening asthma attacks. Consideration should be given to supplying such patients with oral steroids to use in an emergency. The dose of Becotide Rotacaps, should be increased at this time and then reduced to the maintenance level after the systemic steroid has been discontinued.

Replacement of systemic steroid treatment with Becotide Rotacaps sometimes unmasks allergies such as allergic rhinitis or eczema previously controlled by the systemic drug. These allergies should be symptomatically treated with antihistamine and/or topical preparations.

Side-effects: Candidiasis of the mouth and throat (thrush) occurs in some patients treated with beclomethasone dipropionate. Patients with high blood levels of *Candida precipitins*, indicating a previous infection, are more likely to develop this complication. Some patients may find it helpful to rinse their mouth thoroughly with water after using the Rotahaler. Symptomatic candidiasis can be treated with topical anti-fungal therapy whilst still continuing with the treatment.

In some patients inhaled beclomethasone dipropionate may cause hoarseness or throat irritation. It may be helpful to rinse the mouth out with water immediately after inhalation.

As with other inhalation therapy, the potential for paradoxical bronchospasm should be kept in mind. If it occurs, the preparation should be discontinued immediately and alternative therapy instituted.

Overdosage: The acute toxicity of beclomethasone

dipropionate is low. The only harmful effect that follows inhalation of large amounts of the drug over the short time period is suppression of hypothalamic-pituitary-adrenal (HPA) function. No special emergency action need be taken. Treatment with Becotide Rotacaps should be continued at the recommended dose to control the asthma; HPA function recovers in a day or two.

If Becotide Rotacaps are used excessively over a long period this could lead to adrenal suppression. In such a case, the patient should be transferred to oral corticosteroid therapy, and when the condition has stabilised, be returned to inhaled therapy at the recommended dose. To guard against the unexpected event of adrenal suppression, regular tests of adrenal function are advised. Oral steroids should then be slowly withdrawn, as for steroid-dependent patients.

Pharmaceutical precautions To keep the Rotacaps in good condition it is important that they are stored in a dry place below 30°C where they will not be exposed to extremes of temperature. A convenient supply may be carried in the special container for the Rotahaler. The Rotacaps should be inserted into the Rotahaler immediately prior to use to avoid softening. Failure to observe this instruction may affect the delivery of the drug.

Legal category POM.

Package quantities Becotide Rotacaps 100 micrograms, 200 micrograms and 400 micrograms are supplied in containers of 112 (OP).

Further information Nil.

Product licence numbers

Becotide Rotacaps 100 micrograms	0045/0119
Becotide Rotacaps 200 micrograms	0045/0120
Becotide Rotacaps 400 micrograms	0045/0141

BECOTIDE* SUSPENSION FOR NEBULISATION

Presentation Becotide Suspension for Nebulisation is an aqueous suspension of Beclomethasone Dipropionate BP adjusted with a buffer to about pH 4.5 and preserved with benzalkonium chloride 0.01% w/v. The concentration of beclomethasone dipropionate is 50 micrograms per ml of suspension.

Uses Becotide Suspension for Nebulisation is indicated for the management of infants and children whose asthma is inadequately controlled by bronchodilators and/or sodium cromoglycate, thus necessitating additional treatment with steroids, and who are unable to use a pressurised inhaler (e.g., Becotide Inhaler) effectively or unable to inhale the drug in powder form (e.g., Becotide Rotacaps Capsules).

Becotide Suspension for Nebulisation is not a substitute for injectable or oral corticosteroids in emergency situations.

Dosage and administration Becotide Suspension for Nebulisation should be administered as an aerosol produced by a nebuliser with an adequate flow rate and using a suitable mouthpiece to enable delivery of the drug.

The exact dose delivered to the patient varies slightly depending on the equipment used (e.g., driving source, nebuliser chamber).

For optimum results, Becotide Suspension for Nebulisation should be used according to a regular daily schedule.

Infants: (Up to one year) 1 ml (50 micrograms) administered two, three or four times daily is the usual maintenance dose.

Children: (One to 12 years) 2 ml (100 micrograms) administered two, three or four times daily is the usual maintenance dose.

Becotide Suspension for Nebulisation should be used with a respirator or nebuliser only under the close supervision of a physician. Patients receiving treatment with Becotide Suspension for Nebulisation must be warned that if their clinical condition deteriorates they should not increase the dose or the frequency of administration but should seek medical advice.

To aid administration of small volumes of the suspension it may be diluted immediately before use with up to an equal volume of normal saline.

Adults: Because of the large volumes which would be necessary, Becotide Suspension for Nebulisation is not suitable for administering high doses of beclomethasone dipropionate.

Contra-indications, warnings, etc
Contra-indications: Hypersensitivity to Becotide Suspension for Nebulisation is a contra-indication; and special care is necessary in patients with active or quiescent pulmonary tuberculosis.

Precautions: Becotide Suspension for Nebulisation is not a substitute for injectable or oral corticosteroids if these are indicated, and it should not be injected or administered orally. It is advisable to administer the suspension via a mouthpiece to avoid the possibility of atrophic changes of facial skin which may occur with prolonged use with a face-mask. Patients and/or parents should be made aware that Becotide Suspension for Nebulisation has to be used regularly for optimum benefit.

Non-isotonic solutions, or those which are not of neutral pH or which contain benzalkonium chloride, may rarely cause paradoxical bronchospasm in some patients.

In the majority of patients no significant adrenal suppression occurs until doses of 1,500 micrograms per day are exceeded. Reduction of plasma cortisol levels has been reported in some patients who received 2,000 micrograms per day of inhaled beclomethasone dipropionate.

Pregnancy: There is inadequate evidence of safety in human pregnancy. Administration of corticosteroids to pregnant animals can cause abnormalities of fetal development including cleft palate and intra-uterine growth retardation. There may therefore be a very small risk of such effects in the human fetus. It should be noted, however, that the fetal changes in animals occur after relatively high systemic exposure. Because beclomethasone dipropionate is delivered directly to the lungs by the inhaled route it avoids the high level of exposure that occurs when corticosteroids are given by systemic routes.

The use of beclomethasone dipropionate in pregnancy requires that the possible benefits of the drug be weighed against the possible hazards. It should be noted that the drug has been in widespread use for many years without apparent ill consequence.

Lactation: No specific studies examining the transference of beclomethasone dipropionate into the milk of lactating animals have been performed. It is reasonable to assume that beclomethasone dipropionate is secreted in milk but, at the dosages used for direct inhalation, there is low potential for significant levels in breast milk. The use of beclomethasone dipropionate in mothers breast feeding their babies requires that the therapeutic benefits of the drug be weighed against the potential hazards to the mother and baby.

Patients inadequately controlled by bronchodilator therapy: The use of Becotide Suspension for Nebulisation in patients who have never taken steroids or taken only occasional courses of steroids is normally straightforward. An improvement in respiratory function is obvious within a week. The few patients who do not respond during this period usually have excessive mucus in their bronchi so that the drug is unable to penetrate to its site of action. In such cases, a short course of systemic steroid in relatively high dosage should be given to control secretion of mucus and other inflammatory changes in the lungs. Continuation of treatment with inhaled beclomethasone dipropionate usually maintains the improvement achieved, the oral steroid being gradually withdrawn. Exacerbation of asthma caused by infection is usually controlled by appropriate antibiotic treatment, by increasing the dose of Becotide Suspension for Nebulisation and, if necessary, by giving systemic steroid.

Patients being treated with oral corticosteroids: The transfer to Becotide Suspension for Nebulisation of steroid-dependent patients unable to use an aerosol or Rotahaler and their subsequent management needs special care mainly because recovery from impaired adrenocortical function, caused by prolonged systemic steroid therapy, is slow. Initially, patients should be given Becotide Suspension for Nebulisation in addition to their usual maintenance dose of systemic steroid. After about a week, gradual withdrawal of the systemic steroid is started by reducing the daily dose by one milligram of prednisolone, or its equivalent, at not less than weekly intervals. Patients treated with systemic steroids for long periods of time or who have received high doses may have adrenocortical suppression. With these patients, adrenocortical function should be monitored regularly and the dose of systemic steroid reduced cautiously. Transferred patients whose adrenocortical function is impaired should carry a warning card indicating that they need supplementary systemic steroid during periods of stress, e.g., surgery, chest infection or worsening asthma attacks. Consideration should be given to supplying such patients with oral steroids to use in an emergency. The dose of Becotide Suspension for Nebulisation should be increased at this time and then reduced to the maintenance level after the systemic steroid has been discontinued.

Replacement of systemic steroid treatment with Becotide Suspension for Nebulisation may unmask allergies such as allergic rhinitis or eczema previously controlled by the systemic drug. These allergies should be symptomatically treated with antihistamine and/or topical preparations.

Side-effects: Administration of Becotide Suspension for Nebulisation has been associated with occasional reports of paradoxical bronchospasm. If it occurs, the preparation should be discontinued immediately and alternative therapy instituted.

Candidiasis of the mouth and throat (thrush) is known to occur in some patients treated with beclomethasone dipropionate. Patients with high blood levels of Candida precipitins, indicating a previous infection, are the most likely to develop this complication. Some patients may find it helpful to rinse their mouth thoroughly with water after using the nebuliser. The condition usually responds to topical antifungal therapy without discontinuing treatment with Becotide Suspension for Nebulisation.

In some patients inhaled beclomethasone dipropionate may cause hoarseness or throat irritation. It may be helpful to rinse the mouth out with water immediately after inhalation.

Overdosage: If Becotide Suspension for Nebulisation is used excessively over a long period this could lead to adrenal suppression. In such a case, the patient should be transferred to oral corticosteroid therapy and when the condition has stabilised, be returned to the inhaled therapy at the recommended dose. To guard against the unexpected event of adrenal suppression, regular tests of adrenal function are advised.

Oral steroids should then be withdrawn slowly, as for steroid-dependent patients.

Pharmaceutical precautions Becotide Suspension for Nebulisation should be stored between 2 and 30°C and protected from light.

The suspension may be diluted immediately before use with up to an equal volume of normal saline.

The suspension should not be mixed with other agents.

Once the bottle has been opened the contents should be discarded after one month. Any unused suspension in the chamber of the nebuliser should be discarded.

Legal category POM.

Package quantities Becotide Suspension for Nebulisation is supplied in screw-capped amber glass bottles of 10 ml.

Further information As many nebulisers operate on a continuous flow basis, it is likely that nebulised drug will be released in the local environment. Becotide Suspension for Nebulisation should therefore be administered in a well ventilated room, particularly in hospitals when several patients may be using nebulisers at the same time.

Product licence number 0045/0126

EUDEMINE* TABLETS 50 mg
EUDEMINE* INJECTION

Presentation Eudemine Tablets 50 mg are white, sugar-coated tablets each containing Diazoxide BP 50 mg. Identification code AH/8D.

Eudemine Injection. Ampoules of 20 ml containing Diazoxide BP 300 mg in an aqueous, colourless solution with sodium hydroxide at pH 11.6.

Uses Diazoxide is a benzothiadiazine analogue which has two main therapeutic actions. It is used orally and intravenously in the treatment of intractable hypoglycaemia and intravenously for the acute treatment of severe hypertension associated with renal disease.

Diazoxide also causes salt and water retention.

Hypoglycaemia: Eudemine administered orally is indicated for the treatment of intractable hypoglycaemia with severe symptoms from a variety of causes including: idiopathic hypoglycaemia in infancy, leucine-sensitive or unclassified; functional islet-cell tumours both malignant and benign if inoperable; extra-pancreatic neoplasms producing hypoglycaemia; glycogen storage disease; hypoglycaemia of unknown origin.

Hypertensive emergencies: Eudemine Injection is used particularly for the emergency treatment of acute hypertensive crises, especially those occurring in association with acute hypertensive encephalopathy, congestive heart failure, acute glomerular nephritis, eclampsia or pre-eclampsia.

Severe hypertension: It is also indicated for the control of severe hypertension associated with renal disease.

In hypertensive patients requiring such diagnostic procedures as renal biopsy, arteriography or cardiac catheterisation, Eudemine Injection may be given to facilitate the procedure and reduce the danger of haemorrhage due to hypertension. Eudemine Injection is only indicated in patients who have failed to respond to other hypotensive agents.

Dosage and administration

Hypoglycaemia: In hypoglycaemia the dosage schedule of Eudemine Tablets is determined according to the clinical needs and the response of the individual patient. For both adults and children a starting oral dose of 5 mg/kg body weight divided into 2 or 3 equal doses per 24 hours will establish the patient's response and thereafter the dose can be increased until the symptoms and blood glucose level respond satisfactorily. Regular determinations of the blood glucose in the initial days of treatment are essential. In children with leucine-sensitive hypoglycaemia, a dosage range of 15 to 20 mg/kg/day is suggested.

In adults with benign or malignant islet-cell tumours producing large quantities of insulin, high dosages of up to 1,000 mg per day have been used.

Hypertensive emergencies and severe hypertension: In the treatment of hypertension, Eudemine Injection is administered by the intravenous route only and it should never be given intramuscularly or subcutaneously.

Adults: A full dose of 300 mg in 20 ml will be required by most patients. However, an adequate fall in blood pressure in some patients may be obtained with as little as 150 mg. Patients must be recumbent during the injection which must be rapid and not exceed 30 seconds.

Children: On the rare occasions that Eudemine Injection is indicated for hypertension in children the dosage should be based on a level of 5 mg per kg body weight by injection.

A response occurs within five minutes and usually

persists for at least four hours. One injection is often effective, but further injections may be required, particularly in hypertensive crises or in accelerating disease refractory to other hypotensive agents. Up to four ampoules of 300 mg may be given in 24 hours. An initial dose of 600 mg is recommended only in life-threatening situations. Once the blood pressure is controlled by Eudemine Injection, treatment with anti-hypertensive agents designed for maintenance therapy can be initiated. It appears that if hypertensive patients treated with Eudemine Injection are allowed an unrestricted sodium intake then the subsequent response to oral hypotensive agents will be improved.

Contra-indications, warnings, etc
Contra-indications: In the treatment of hypoglycaemia, Eudemine is contra-indicated in all cases which are amenable to surgery or other specific therapy.

There are no absolute contra-indications to Eudemine for the control of hypertension but it should be used with discretion. Agents which can be given by infusion, such as hydralazine or labetalol, should have been shown to be ineffective before a bolus injection of diazoxide is given.

Hypersensitivity to any component of the preparation or to other thiazides.

Precautions: Each of the two main therapeutic actions of Eudemine tend to be unwanted effects when the product is used for the alternative main indication. Thus in the treatment of hypoglycaemia it is necessary that the blood pressure be monitored regularly, whilst in the treatment of hypertension, therapy with Eudemine necessitates regular monitoring of the blood glucose levels.

Eudemine Injection should be used with care in patients who have impaired cerebral or cardiac circulation i.e. in patients in whom abrupt reduction in blood pressure might be detrimental. Prolonged hypotension should be avoided so as not to aggravate pre-existing renal failure.

In either indication, retention of sodium and water is likely to necessitate therapy with an oral diuretic such as frusemide or ethacrynic acid. The dosage of either of the diuretics mentioned may be up to 1 g daily. It must be appreciated that if diuretics are employed then both the hypotensive and the hyperglycaemic activities of diazoxide will be potentiated and it is likely that the dosage of diazoxide will require adjustment downwards. In patients with severe renal failure it is desirable to maintain with diuretic therapy, urinary volumes in excess of 1 litre daily. Hypokalaemia should be avoided by adequate potassium replacement.

Whenever Eudemine is given over a prolonged period regular haematological examinations are indicated to exclude changes in white blood cell and platelet counts. Also in children, there should be regular assessment of growth, bone and psychological maturation.

With Eudemine Injection the high alkalinity of the solution necessitates that great care is taken to ensure that the injection is given directly into a vein without leakage into surrounding tissues.

The very rapid, almost complete protein binding of diazoxide requires cautious dosage to be used in patients whose plasma proteins may be lower than normal.

Pregnancy: Eudemine Tablets are only to be used in pregnant women when the indicated condition is deemed to put the mother's life at risk.

Side-effects: In the treatment of hypertension the hyperglycaemia induced by diazoxide is generally inevitable. Each injection of diazoxide usually means a transient rise in blood sugar of about 10%. Fortunately, the hyperglycaemia in hypertensive patients can be readily controlled with tolbutamide, or exceptionally with insulin. A hypotensive effect in normotensive patients is of minor importance and rarely requires any specific therapy. An oral diuretic may be indicated to control sodium and water retention.

With Eudemine Injection reflex tachycardia is not uncommon in the first few minutes after injection and is more frequent in digitalised patients. Orthostatic hypotension is unlikely but it may occur in those recently treated with adrenergic blocking agents. When it is used during labour for the treatment of toxaemia, the smooth muscle relaxant effect can cause delay in the second stage. This should be counteracted with oxytocic agents.

With oral therapy nausea is common in the first two or three weeks and may require relief with an antinauseant. Prolonged therapy has given rise to reports of hypertrichosis lanuginosa, anorexia and hyperuricaemia.

Extra-pyramidal side effects have been reported with oral diazoxide. It was found that extra-pyramidal effects such as Parkinsonian tremor, cogwheel rigidity and oculogyric crises could be easily suppressed by intravenous injection of an anti-Parkinsonian drug such as procyclidine and that they could be prevented by maintenance therapy with such a drug given orally.

Prolonged oral therapy of Eudemine during pregnancy has been reported to cause alopecia in the newborn.

Other adverse effects of Eudemine which have been reported are hyperosmolar non-ketotic coma, cardiomegaly, leucopenia and thrombocytopenia.

Drugs potentiated by diazoxide therapy include: oral diuretics, antihypertensive agents and anticoagulants.

Overdosage: Excessive dosage of Eudemine can result in hyperglycaemia which will respond to insulin and/or to hypotension which will necessitate maintenance of blood volume with intravenous fluids.

Pharmaceutical precautions *Tablets:* Store below 30°C.

Injection: It is particularly important that Eudemine Injection is protected from light.

Eudemine Injection should never be mixed with other drugs and it should not be diluted. Store below 25°C.

Legal category POM.

Package quantities Eudemine Tablets 50 mg are packed in containers of 100 (OP).

Eudemine Injection is in ampoules individually boxed in packs of five.

Further information Nil.

Product licence numbers

Eudemine Tablets 50 mg	0045/5081R
Eudemine Injection	0045/0084

FENTAZIN* TABLETS

Presentation
Fentazin Tablets 2 mg each contain Perphenazine BP 2 mg. Identification code is AH/1C.

Fentazin Tablets 4 mg each contain Perphenazine BP 4 mg. Identification code is AH/2C.

Both are white, sugar-coated tablets.

Uses Fentazin is a potent tranquilliser and anti-emetic of the phenothiazine group. It is indicated in the following: as an adjunct to the short-term management of anxiety, severe psychomotor agitation, excitement, violent or dangerously impulsive behaviour; schizophrenia, treatment of symptoms and prevention of relapse, other psychoses, especially paranoid, mania and hypomania; nausea and vomiting. Because of the hazard of severe extra-pyramidal reactions, Fentazin is not indicated for the treatment of agitation and restlessness in the elderly.

Dosage and administration
Adults: Fentazin Tablets are administered orally in a usual dosage of 4 mg perphenazine three times daily. As there may be great variability of individual response and dosage requirement, the dose may have to be adjusted upwards or downwards according to the patient response. The total daily dose should not exceed 24 mg.

Treatment should be started and dosage increased under close supervision. Treatment should be reviewed at intervals so as to avoid indiscriminate or unduly prolonged use.

Elderly: One quarter or one half the recommended

starting dose for adults may be sufficient for therapeutic response in the elderly.

Children: Fentazin should not be given to children under the age of fourteen years.

Contra-indications, warnings, etc

Contra-indications: Fentazin should not be administered to patients with leucopenia or in association with drugs liable to cause bone-marrow depression or to patients in comatose states.

Precautions: The possibility of suicide in depressed patients remains during treatment and until significant remission occurs. Fentazin should be used with caution in patients with liver disease; cardiac arrhythmias; congestive cardiac failure; coronary artery disease; severe respiratory disease; renal failure; epilepsy, conditions predisposing to epilepsy (e.g., alcohol withdrawal or brain damage); Parkinson's disease; patients who have shown hypersensitivity to other phenothiazines; personal or family history of narrow-angle glaucoma; hypothyroidism; myasthenia gravis; phaeochromocytoma; prostatic hypertrophy. Since temperature regulation may be impaired, care should be taken in extremely hot weather, and in cold weather, especially in the elderly and frail because of risk of hypothermia.

Pregnancy: The safety of perphenazine in pregnancy has not yet been established.

Drug interactions: Fentazin can increase the central nervous system depression produced by other CNS-depressant drugs including alcohol, hypnotics, sedatives or strong analgesics. It may antagonise the action of adrenaline and other sympathomimetic agents and reverses the blood pressure-lowering effects of adrenergic-blocking agents such as guanethidine and clonidine. It may impair the metabolism of tricyclic antidepressants, the anti-parkinson effects of levodopa and the effects of anti-convulsants.

Undesirable anticholinergic effects can be enhanced by anti-parkinson or other anticholinergic drugs. Phenothiazines may enhance the cardiac-depressant effects of quinidine, the effect of diazoxide and of neuromuscular blocking agents and the absorption of corticosteroids and digoxin.

Fentazin may affect the control of diabetes and the action of anticoagulants. The possibility of interactions with lithium should be borne in mind.

Fentazin should not be taken with tea or coffee as absorption may be impaired by the formation of insoluble precipitates. Antacids can also impair its absorption.

Side-effects: Not all the following side effects have been reported with this specific drug; however, pharmacological similarities with other phenothiazine derivatives require that each be considered. Many of these side-effects may be prevented by a reduction in dosage.

Drowsiness, sedation, dry mouth and nasal stuffiness may occur, particularly with high dosage and at the start of treatment. Dose-related postural hypotension may occur, particularly in the elderly. Other dose-related anticholinergic-type side effects including blurring of vision, tachycardia, constipation and urinary hesitancy or retention. Adynamic ileus rarely occurs with phenothiazine therapy, but is of particular concern in psychiatric patients who may fail to seek treatment of the condition.

Perphenazine may impair alertness, especially at the start of treatment. These effects may be potentiated by alcohol. Patients should be warned of the risks of sedation and advised not to drive or operate machinery during treatment, until their susceptibility is known.

Extra-pyramidal reactions may occur even at low dosage. Acute dystonias may occur early in treatment. Parkinsonian rigidity, tremor, akathisia tend to appear less rapidly. Oculogyric crises have been reported. Anti-parkinson agents should not be prescribed routinely, because of the possible risks of aggravating anticholinergic side effects of perphenazine, of precipitating toxic-confusional states or of impairing its therapeutic efficacy. They should only be given as required.

Tardive dyskinesia is a syndrome of irregularly repetitive involuntary movements which may occur during administration or after withdrawal of perphenazine and other neuroleptic drugs. It is characterised by abnormal writhing movements or protrusions of the tongue with lip-smacking, puckering or chewing movements and facial grimaces. Choreoathetoid movements of the extremities or repetitive movements of the neck or trunk may accompany the orofacial dyskinesia or can occur alone. The syndrome is common among patients treated with moderate to high doses of antipsychotic drugs for prolonged periods of time and may prove irreversible, particularly in patients over the age of 50. It is unlikely to occur in the short term when low or moderate doses are used as recommended, but since its occurrence may be related to duration of treatment as well as daily dose, perphenazine should be given in the minimal effective dose for the minimum possible time, unless it is established that long-term administration for the treatment of schizophrenia is required. The potential seriousness and unpredictability of tardive dyskinesia and the fact that it has occasionally been reported to occur when neuroleptic antipsychotic drugs have been prescribed for relatively short periods in low dosage means that the prescribing of such agents requires especially careful assessment of risks versus benefit. Tardive dyskinesia can be precipitated or aggravated by anti-parkinson drugs. Short-lived dyskinesias may occur after abrupt drug withdrawal.

In schizophrenia, the response to antipsychotic drug treatment may be delayed. If drugs are withdrawn, recurrence of symptoms may not become apparent for several weeks or months. Perphenazine may also cause abnormalities of cerebrospinal fluid proteins.

Perphenazine, even in low dosage in susceptible (especially non-psychotic) individuals, may cause unpleasant subjective feelings of being mentally dulled or slowed down, nausea, dizziness, headache or paradoxical effects of excitement, agitation or insomnia. Confusional states or epileptic fits can occur. The elderly are more susceptible to the sedative and hypotensive effects.

The effects of phenothiazines on the heart are dose-related. ECG changes with prolongation of the QT interval and T-wave changes have been reported commonly in patients treated with moderate to high dosage; they are reversible on reducing the dose. In a very small number of cases, they have been reported to precede serious arrhythmias, including ventricular tachycardia and fibrillation, which have also occurred after overdosage.

Hormonal effects of antipsychotic neuroleptic drugs include hyperprolactinaemia, which may cause galactorrhoea, gynaecomastia and oligo or amenorrhoea. Sexual function, including erection and ejaculation is sometimes impaired by perphenazine. Weight gain may occur. Oedema has been reported with phenothiazine medication. Perphenazine administration may also result in false-positive pregnancy tests.

Agranulocytosis has been reported very rarely, most commonly in the first three months of treatment, but occasionally later. Blood counts should be performed if the patient develops signs of a persistent infection. Transient leucopenia can also occur. The occurrence of antinuclear antibodies has been reported with phenothiazines. Systemic lupus erythematosus has very rarely occurred.

Raised serum cholesterol and rarely hyperglycaemia have been reported in association with phenothiazines.

Perphenazine rarely causes increased susceptibility to sunburn and patients should be warned to avoid excessive exposure. Skin rashes have occurred rarely. Fine deposits in the cornea and lens and pigmented retinopathy have been reported after long-term therapy.

Perphenazine may impair body temperature-regulation and cases of severe hypothermia or hyperpyrexia have been reported, usually in association with moderate or high dosage of phenothiazines. The elderly or hypothyroid patient may be particularly susceptible to hypothermia. The hazard of hyperthermia may be increased by especially hot or humid weather or by drugs, such as anti-parkinson agents, which impair sweating.

Perphenazine can very rarely cause obstructive jaundice associated with stasis in biliary canaliculi. It has been thought to be a hypersensitivity reaction. Transient abnormalities of liver function tests may occur in the absence of jaundice.

Withdrawal: Acute withdrawal symptoms including nausea, vomiting and insomnia, have very rarely been described after abrupt cessation of high doses of phenothiazines. Gradual withdrawal is advisable.

Overdosage: Gastric lavage is recommended. Emetics are likely to be of little value because of the potent anti-emetic activity of the drug. Hypotension is not usually a problem, especially if the patient is passing urine satisfactorily. Severe hypotension may require fluid infusion therapy. If a vasopressor is needed, norepinephrine may be used. Central nervous system depression is best treated conservatively; analeptics should not be used. Rewarming measures should not be employed unless the body temperature falls below 30°C. Convulsions may be controlled with standard methods, but the use of barbiturates should be avoided. Cardiac monitoring for at least 48 hours is recommended.

Pharmaceutical precautions Store below 30°C.

Legal category POM.

Package quantities Fentazin Tablets 2 mg and 4 mg are issued in cartons each containing 100 tablets (OP) in 10 foil strips of 10 (5 × 2) tablets.

Further information Perphenazine is a phenothiazine with piperazine side chain. Its pharmacological profile of activity includes moderate sedative and hypotensive properties and a fairly pronounced tendency to cause extra-pyramidal reactions.

Product licence numbers

Fentazin Tablets 2 mg	0045/5082R
Fentazin Tablets 4 mg	0045/5083R

PIRITON* TABLETS
PIRITON SYRUP
PIRITON INJECTION

Presentation Piriton is a potent antihistamine (Chlorpheniramine Maleate BP) presented as tablets, sustained-action tablets, syrup and injection.

Piriton Tablets: Round, biconvex, cream tablets each containing Chlorpheniramine Maleate BP 4 mg. Identification engraved Piriton AH.

Piriton Syrup: Each 10 ml of Piriton Syrup contains Chlorpheniramine Maleate BP 4 mg. It is colourless.

Piriton Injection: Each 1 ml of Piriton Injection contains Chlorpheniramine Maleate BP 10 mg. It is colourless.

Uses The oral preparations of Piriton are indicated for symptomatic control of all allergic conditions responsive to antihistamines, including hay fever, vasomotor rhinitis, urticaria, angioneurotic oedema, food allergy, drug and serum reactions, insect bites.

Piriton Injection is indicated for acute urticaria, control of allergic reactions to insect bites and stings, angioneurotic oedema, drug and serum reactions, desensitisation reactions, hay fever, vasomotor rhinitis, severe pruritus of non-specific origin.

Dosage and administration

Piriton Tablets

Adults: 1 tablet four to six-hourly (daily max: 24 mg).

Children (aged 6–12 years): ½ tablet four to six-hourly (daily max: 12 mg).

Elderly: As in adults but such patients are prone to confusional psychosis and other neurological anticholinergic effects.

Piriton Syrup

Adults: Two 5 ml spoonfuls four to six-hourly (daily max: 24 mg i.e., 60 ml).

Children between 6–12 years: one 5 ml spoonful four to six-hourly (daily max: 12 mg i.e., 30 ml).

Children between 2–5 years: 2.5 ml four to six-hourly (daily max: 6 mg i.e., 15 ml).

Children between 1–2 years: 2.5 ml twice daily. Not recommended in children below 1 year.

Elderly: As in adults but such patients are prone to confusional psychosis and other neurological anticholinergic effects.

When Piriton Syrup is dispensed to meet prescriptions involving doses of 2.5 ml it should be diluted with an equal quantity of unpreserved Syrup BP. The resultant mixture should be used within fourteen days.

Piriton Injection

The injection may be subcutaneous, intramuscular or intravenous. The latter is recommended when a rapid effect is desired as in anaphylactic reactions. For the intravenous route Piriton should be diluted in the syringe with 5 to 10 ml of blood and then injected slowly over a period of one minute. Any drowsiness, giddiness or hypotension which may follow is usually transitory.

The usual dose of Piriton Injection for adults is 10 to 20 mg, but not more than 40 mg should be given per 24 hours.

In the event of a blood transfusion reaction a dose of 10 to 20 mg of Piriton should be given by the subcutaneous route. This can be repeated to a total of 40 mg per 24 hours or oral forms of Piriton may be given until the symptoms subside. Though Piriton may be helpful in the prevention of delayed reactions to penicillin and other drugs it cannot be relied on to prevent anaphylactic reactions in patients known to be allergic to a particular drug. Piriton Injection 10 mg should be injected separately by the intramuscular route immediately prior to injection of any other drug.

In the event of an anaphylactic reaction Piriton Injection 10 to 20 mg may be given by slow intravenous injection in addition to the emergency therapy of adrenaline, corticoids, oxygen and supportive therapy.

Contra-indications, warnings, etc

Contra-indications: Piriton is contra-indicated in patients who are hypersensitive to antihistamines and those that have had monoamine oxidase inhibitor therapy within the previous fourteen days.

Precautions: Chlorpheniramine may have an additive effect when used concurrently with hypnotics and anxiolytics causing potentiation of drowsiness. A similar additive effect will result from concurrent usage of alcohol with chlorpheniramine. Monoamine oxidase inhibitor therapy intensifies the anticholinergic effects of chlorpheniramine. Chlorpheniramine inhibits phenytoin metabolism and can lead to phenytoin toxicity.

The anticholinergic properties of chlorpheniramine may cause drowsiness, dizziness, blurred vision and psychomotor impairment, which can seriously hamper the patients' ability to drive and use machinery.

Pregnancy: Safety for the use of Piriton during pregnancy has not been established. Piriton should only be used during pregnancy when clearly needed and when potential benefit outweighs the potential unknown risks to the fetus. Use during the third trimester may result in reactions in the newborn or premature neonates.

Small amounts of antihistamines are excreted in breast milk. Use by nursing mothers is not recommended because of the risks of adverse effects in the infant. Antihistamines may inhibit lactation.

Side-effects: Sedation varying from slight drowsiness to deep sleep. Inability to concentrate, lassitude, blurred vision, gastro-intestinal disturbances such as nausea, vomiting and diarrhoea may occasionally occur. Urinary retention, headaches, dryness of the mouth. Dizziness, palpitation, tachycardia, arrhythmias, hypotension, tightness of the chest, abdominal pain, dyspepsia, anorexia, hepatitis including jaundice, thickening of bronchial secretions, haemolytic anaemia and other blood dyscrasias infrequently occur.

Allergic reactions including exfoliative dermatitis, photosensitivity and skin reactions. Urticaria, twitching, muscular weakness and inco-ordination. Tinnitus, depression, irritability and nightmares infrequently occur.

Paradoxical excitation in children and confusional psychosis in the elderly can occur.

The effects of alcohol may be increased. In common

with other drugs having anticholinergic effects, chlorpheniramine should be used with caution in epilepsy, prostatic hypertrophy, glaucoma, hepatic disease, bronchitis, bronchiectasis, thyrotoxicosis, raised intra-ocular pressure, severe hypertension or cardiovascular disease and bronchial asthma. Children and the elderly are more likely to experience the neurological anticholinergic effects.

Overdosage: The estimated lethal dose of Piriton is 25 to 50 mg/kg body weight. Symptoms and signs include sedation, paradoxical stimulation of CNS, toxic psychosis, seizures, apnoea, convulsions, anticholinergic effects, dystonic reactions and cardiovascular collapse including arrhythmias. Treatment includes gastric lavage or emesis using syrup of ipecacuanha. Following these measures activated charcoal and cathartics may be administered to minimise absorption.

If overdosage is by the oral route other symptomatic and supportive measures should be provided with special attention to cardiac, respiratory, renal and hepatic functions and fluid and electrolyte balance.

Treat hypotension and arrhythmias vigorously. CNS convulsions may be treated with i.v. diazepam or phenytoin. Haemoperfusion may be used in severe cases.

Pharmaceutical precautions
Storage: Piriton Tablets should be stored below 30°C. Piriton Injection should be stored below 25°C and protected from light. Piriton Syrup should be stored at a temperature not exceeding 25°C and protected from light.

Dilution: If it is necessary to dilute Piriton Syrup then the suitable diluent is unpreserved Syrup BP. The resulting mixture will keep for fourteen days at room temperature.

Legal category
Tablets P.
Syrup P.
Injection POM.

Package quantities
Piriton Tablets are supplied in containers of 100.
Piriton Syrup is supplied in bottles of 150 ml (OP).
Piriton Injection is supplied in boxes of 5 ampoules.

Further information No Piriton preparation contains tartrazine.

Product licence numbers

Piriton Tablets	0045/5077R
Piriton Syrup	0045/5019R
Piriton Injection	0045/5056R

SEREVENT* DISKHALER▼

Presentation The active ingredient is presented in a disk comprising 4 regularly spaced double foil blisters each delivering a mixture of 50 micrograms salmeterol as the hydroxynaphthoate (xinafoate) and lactose.

Uses *Indications:* Long-term regular treatment of reversible airways obstruction in asthma (including patients with nocturnal asthma and exercise-induced asthma) and chronic bronchitis.

Mode of action: Serevent is a new class of selective $beta_2$-adrenoceptor agonist and, at therapeutic dosage, it has little or no measurable cardiovascular effect.

Salmeterol has been shown to produce long-lasting bronchodilatation of up to at least 12 hours in subjects with reversible airways obstruction. Regular dosing will produce sustained improvement in lung function, so reducing symptoms of airways obstruction and symptoms of nocturnal asthma. In the majority of patients it will remove the need for additional symptomatic bronchodilator medication.

In vitro tests have shown salmeterol to be a potent and long-lasting inhibitor of the release, from human lung, of mast cell derived mediators, such as histamine, leukotrienes and prostaglandin D_2. In man, salmeterol inhibits the early and late phase response to inhaled allergen and after single dosing attenuates bronchial hyper-responsiveness indicating anti-inflammatory as well as bronchodilator activity.

Dosage and administration Serevent Diskhaler is for inhalation use only.

Adults: One blister (50 micrograms of salmeterol) twice daily.
In patients with more severe airways obstruction up to two blisters (2 × 50 micrograms of salmeterol) twice daily.

There are insufficient clinical data in children at present to recommend the use of Serevent.

There is no need to adjust the dose in the elderly.

In patients with impaired renal function there is no need to adjust the dose.

In order to gain full therapeutic benefit, regular usage of Serevent is recommended in the treatment of reversible airways obstruction. The onset of the bronchodilator effect of salmeterol usually occurs in approximately 5 to 10 minutes. The full benefits will be apparent after the first or second dose of the drug. The bronchodilator effects of salmeterol usually last for 12 hours, this is particularly useful in the treatment of nocturnal asthma symptoms and in the management of exercise-induced asthma.

As there may be adverse effects associated with excessive dosing, the dosage or frequency of administration should only be increased on medical advice.

Contra-indications, warnings, etc
Contra-indications: Hypersensitivity to any ingredient of the preparation.

Precautions: With commencement of Serevent therapy the requirement for symptomatic bronchodilator therapy is usually reduced such that the majority of patients do not need any additional symptomatic bronchodilator. If symptoms persist patients should take a short-acting inhaled beta-agonist (e.g., salbutamol) for relief but, this need is usually an indication that control of their airways obstruction is sub-optimal and further treatment should be considered. This may involve increasing the dose of Serevent and/or commencing or increasing the dose of prophylactic treatment such as inhaled corticosteroids.

Inhaled Serevent is designed for twice daily regular dosing and, as such, should be seen as complementary to other prophylactic agents such as inhaled corticosteroids. Patients treated with inhaled steroid or other prophylactic treatments should continue with these at the same dosage when Serevent is introduced.

In most patients, requirement for additional bronchodilator will be significantly reduced. If patients develop increasing consumption of a short-acting beta-agonist (e.g., salbutamol) over a short period of time then medical attention should be sought. Acute exacerbations of asthma should be treated in the normal way with nebulised and/or parenteral bronchodilators and parenteral corticosteroids.

Potentially serious hypokalaemia may result from $beta_2$-agonist therapy. Particular caution is advised in acute severe asthma as this effect may be potentiated by concomitant treatment with xanthine derivatives, steroids, diuretics and by hypoxia. It is recommended that serum potassium levels are monitored in such situations.

Salmeterol should be administered with caution in patients suffering from thyrotoxicosis.

Pregnancy: In animal studies, some effects on the fetus, typical for a $beta_2$-agonist, occurred at exposure levels substantially higher than those that occur with therapeutic use. Extensive experience with other $beta_2$-agonists has provided no evidence that such effects are relevant for women receiving clinical doses.

As yet, experience of the use of salmeterol during pregnancy is limited. As with any medicine, use during pregnancy should be considered only if the expected benefit to the mother is greater than any risk to the fetus.

Lactation: Plasma levels of salmeterol after inhaled therapeutic doses are negligible and, therefore, levels in milk should be correspondingly low. Nevertheless, as there is no experience of the use of salmeterol in nursing mothers its use in such circumstances should only be considered if the expected benefit to the mother is greater than any possible risk to the infant. Studies in lactating animals support the view that salmeterol is likely to be secreted in only very small amounts into breast milk.

Side effects: Tremor has been rarely reported. This tends to be transient, dose related and reduces with regular therapy. In clinical trials, headache and subjective palpitations were also rarely reported but the incidence was not significantly different from placebo.

Potentially serious hypokalaemia may result from $beta_2$-agonist therapy. As with other inhalation therapy, the potential for paradoxical bronchospasm, should be kept in mind. If it occurs, the preparation should be discontinued immediately and alternative therapy instituted.

Drug interactions: Non-selective beta-blocking drugs, such as propranolol, should never be prescribed in asthma, and cardioselective beta-blocking drugs should only be used with caution in asthmatics.

Overdosage: The symptoms and signs of salmeterol overdosage are tremor, headache and tachycardia. The preferred antidote for overdosage with Serevent is a cardioselective beta-blocking agent. Cardioselective beta-blocking drugs should be used with caution in patients with a history of bronchospasm.

Pharmaceutical precautions Whilst Serevent Diskhaler provides good protection to the blister contents from the effect of the atmosphere, the product should not be exposed to extremes of temperature and should be stored below 25°C.

A disk may be kept in the Diskhaler device at all times but a blister should only be pierced immediately prior to use. Failure to observe this instruction will affect operation of the Serevent Diskhaler.

Legal category POM.

Package quantities Serevent Diskhaler is supplied as a carton containing 14 × 4 blisters (14 disks), together with a Diskhaler Inhaler.

Further information Nil.

Product licence number 0045/0158

SEREVENT* INHALER▾

Presentation Pressurised metered-dose inhaler delivering 25 micrograms salmeterol as the hydroxynaphthoate (xinafoate) with each actuation. Each canister provides 120 actuations.

Uses *Indications:* Long-term regular treatment of reversible airways obstruction in asthma (including patients with nocturnal asthma and exercise-induced asthma) and chronic bronchitis.

Mode of action: Serevent is a new class of selective $beta_2$-adrenoceptor agonist and, at therapeutic dosage, it has little or no measurable cardiovascular effect.

Salmeterol has been shown to produce long-lasting bronchodilatation of up to at least 12 hours in subjects with reversible airways obstruction. Regular dosing will produce sustained improvement in lung function, so reducing symptoms of airways obstruction and symptoms of nocturnal asthma. In the majority of patients it will remove the need for additional symptomatic bronchodilator medication.

In vitro tests have shown salmeterol to be a potent and long-lasting inhibitor of the release, from human lung, of mast cell derived mediators, such as histamine, leukotrienes and prostaglandin D_2. In man, salmeterol inhibits the early and late phase response to inhaled allergen and after single dosing attenuates bronchial hyper-responsiveness indicating anti-inflammatory as well as bronchodilator activity.

Dosage and administration Serevent is administered by the inhaled route only.

Adults: Two inhalations (2 × 25 micrograms of salmeterol) twice daily. In patients with more severe airways obstruction, four inhalations (4 × 25 micrograms of salmeterol) twice daily.

There are insufficient clinical data in children at present to recommend the use of Serevent.

There is no need to adjust the dose in the elderly.

In patients with impaired renal function there is no need to adjust the dose.

In order to gain full therapeutic benefit, regular usage of Serevent is recommended in the treatment of reversible airways obstruction. The onset of the bronchodilator effect of salmeterol usually occurs in approximately 5 to 10 minutes. The full benefits will be apparent after the first or second dose of the drug. The bronchodilator effects of salmeterol usually last for 12 hours, this is particularly useful in the treatment of nocturnal asthma symptoms and in the management of exercise-induced asthma.

As there may be adverse effects associated with excessive dosing, the dosage or frequency of administration should only be increased on medical advice.

In patients who find co-ordination of a pressurised metered-dose inhaler difficult a Volumatic* spacer may be used with Serevent Inhaler.

Contra-indications, warnings, etc
Contra-indications: Hypersensitivity to any ingredient of the preparation.

Precautions: With commencement of Serevent therapy the requirement for symptomatic bronchodilator therapy is usually reduced such that the majority of patients do not need any additional symptomatic bronchodilator. If symptoms persist patients should take a short-acting inhaled beta-agonist (e.g., salbutamol) for relief but, this need is usually an indication that control of their airways obstruction is sub-optimal and further treatment should be considered. This may involve increasing the dose of Serevent and/or commencing or increasing the dose of prophylactic treatment such as inhaled corticosteroids.

Inhaled Serevent is designed for twice daily regular dosing and, as such, should be seen as complementary to other prophylactic agents such as inhaled corticosteroids. Patients treated with inhaled steroid or other prophylactic treatments should continue with these at the same dosage when Serevent is introduced.

In most patients, requirement for additional bronchodilator will be significantly reduced. If patients develop increasing consumption of a short-acting beta-agonist (e.g., salbutamol) over a short period of time then medical attention should be sought. Acute exacerbations of asthma should be treated in the normal way with nebulised and/or parenteral bronchodilators and parenteral corticosteroids.

Potentially serious hypokalaemia may result from $beta_2$-agonist therapy. Particular caution is advised in acute severe asthma as this effect may be potentiated by concomitant treatment with xanthine derivatives, steroids, diuretics and by hypoxia. It is recommended that serum potassium levels are monitored in such situations.

Salmeterol should be administered with caution in patients suffering from thyrotoxicosis.

Pregnancy: In animal studies, some effects on the fetus, typical for a $beta_2$-agonist, occurred at exposure levels substantially higher than those that occur with therapeutic use. Extensive experience with other $beta_2$-agonists has provided no evidence that such effects are relevant for women receiving clinical doses.

As yet, experience of the use of salmeterol during pregnancy is limited. As with any medicine, use during pregnancy should be considered only if the expected benefit to the mother is greater than any risk to the fetus.

Lactation: Plasma levels of salmeterol after inhaled therapeutic doses are negligible and, therefore, levels in milk should be correspondingly low. Nevertheless, as there is no experience of the use of salmeterol in nursing mothers its use in such circumstances should only be considered if the expected benefit to the mother is greater than any possible risk to the infant. Studies in lactating animals support the view that salmeterol is likely to be secreted in only very small amounts into breast milk.

Side effects: Tremor has been rarely reported. This tends to be transient, dose related and reduces with regular therapy. In clinical trials, headache and subjective palpitations were also rarely reported but the incidence was not significantly different from placebo.

Potentially serious hypokalaemia may result from beta$_2$-agonist therapy. As with other inhalation therapy, the potential for paradoxical bronchospasm, should be kept in mind. If it occurs, the preparation should be discontinued immediately and alternative therapy instituted.

Drug interactions: Non-selective beta-blocking drugs, such as propranolol, should never be prescribed in asthma, and cardioselective beta-blocking drugs should only be used with caution in asthmatics.

Overdosage: The symptoms and signs of salmeterol overdosage are tremor, headache and tachycardia. The preferred antidote for overdosage with Serevent Inhaler is a cardioselective beta-blocking agent. Cardioselective beta-blocking drugs should be used with caution in patients with a history of bronchospasm.

Pharmaceutical precautions Serevent Inhaler should be stored below 30°C, protected from frost and direct sunlight. The canister should not be broken, punctured or burnt, even when apparently empty.

As with most inhaled medications in pressurised metered-dose inhalers, the therapeutic effect of this medication may decrease when the canister is cold.

Legal category POM.

Package quantities Serevent Inhaler is a metered-dose aerosol with a specially designed actuator. Each canister provides 120 actuations.

Further information Nil.

Product licence number 0045/0157

TRIPTAFEN* TRIPTAFEN*-M

Presentation Triptafen are sugar-coated pink tablets, coded AH/1D, each containing Amitriptyline Hydrochloride BP 25 mg and Perphenazine BP 2 mg.

Triptafen-M are sugar-coated, light salmon pink tablets, coded AH/2D, each containing Amitriptyline Hydrochloride BP 10 mg and Perphenazine BP 2 mg.

Uses Amitriptyline hydrochloride is a tricyclic compound with antidepressive activity. Perphenazine is a piperazine derivative of phenothiazine which has potent tranquillising activity.

Triptafen and Triptafen-M are indicated for the treatment of mild to moderate depression associated with anxiety.

Dosage and administration Triptafen preparations are administered orally.

Adults: Triptafen: 1 tablet three times daily with a further tablet at night if necessary.

Triptafen-M: 1 tablet three times daily with a further tablet at night if necessary.

Failure to respond within four weeks is an indication to review treatment. In all cases treatment should not continue beyond three months without reassessment.

Children: Triptafen preparations are not suitable for administration to children under fourteen years of age.

Contra-indications, warnings, etc
Contra-indications: Glaucoma; urinary retention; congestive heart failure; coronary artery disease; epilepsy; severely impaired liver function; concurrent administration of other antidepressive drugs, particularly monoamine oxidase inhibitors (MAOIs). No Triptafen preparation should be given to patients with leucopenia or in association with drugs liable to cause bone-marrow depression.

Precautions: Triptafen or Triptafen-M should not be given in conjunction with MAOIs and, because of the persistent action of the latter, an interval of at least fourteen days should be allowed to elapse between withdrawal of an MAOI and the introduction of a Triptafen preparation.

Persistent oral dyskinesia has been reported occasionally, particularly in elderly female patients, after long-term treatment with potent phenothiazine drugs including perphenazine. Consequently, Triptafen preparations should be prescribed with regular patient reassessments.

Pregnancy: Unless there are compelling reasons, these preparations should not be used during pregnancy, especially during the first and last trimesters. There is inadequate evidence of safety of these preparations in human pregnancy, although they have been in wide use for many years without apparent ill-effect. There is evidence of harmful effects in pregnancy in animals when given in exceptionally high doses.

Side-effects: Amitriptyline may give rise to dryness of the mouth, drowsiness and occasionally tachycardia and blurred vision. Perphenazine may cause mild drowsiness and a slight fall in blood pressure and in addition tremor and extra-pyramidal side effects have been reported. Idiosyncratic side-effects, such as pruritus, nausea, diarrhoea and indigestion may occur.

Overdosage: Gastric lavage should be performed as soon as possible. If convulsions occur or threaten they should be controlled with standard methods, but barbiturates should be avoided. In severe cases haemodialysis may be performed if practicable. It is recommended that patients who have taken an overdose of Triptafen should be observed for at least 48 hours even if symptoms are not severe.

Pharmaceutical precautions
Storage: No special storage conditions are necessary for either of the Triptafen preparations.

Legal category POM.

Package quantities Triptafen Tablets and Triptafen-M Tablets are issued in cartons containing 100 tablets (OP) in foil strips of 10.

Further information Nil.

Product licence numbers

Triptafen Tablets	0045/0128
Triptafen-M Tablets	0045/0129

VENTIDE* INHALER

Presentation Ventide Inhaler is a metered-dose aerosol which delivers 100 micrograms Salbutamol BP and 50 micrograms Beclomethasone Dipropionate BP (as the trichlorofluoromethane solvate) per actuation, into the mouthpiece of a specially designed actuator.

Uses This association of Salbutamol BP with Beclomethasone Dipropionate BP is specially provided for those patients who require regular doses of both drugs for treatment of their obstructive airways disease. Ventide Inhaler is not intended for use as a first-line treatment but is for use once the need for inhaled corticosteroid therapy has been established.

Dosage and administration
Adults: Two inhalations (200 micrograms salbutamol and 100 micrograms beclomethasone dipropionate) three or four times a day.

Children: One or two inhalations (100 micrograms to 200 micrograms salbutamol and 50 micrograms to 100 micrograms beclomethasone dipropionate) two, three or four times a day.

Contra-indications, warnings, etc
Contra-indications: Although intravenous salbutamol and occasionally salbutamol tablets are used in the management of premature labour uncomplicated by conditions such as placenta praevia, ante-partum haemorrhage or toxaemia of pregnancy, Ventide Inhaler is not appropriate for managing premature labour. Ventide Inhaler should not be used for threatened abortion during the first or second trimesters of pregnancy.

Ventide Inhaler is contra-indicated in patients with a history of hypersensitivity to any of its components.

Precautions: Patients should be instructed in the proper use of the inhaler to ensure that the drugs reach the target areas within the lungs. Patients should be made aware than Ventide Inhaler should be used regularly for optimum benefit. However, patients should be regularly reassessed so that their continuing need for corticosteroid therapy can also be reviewed.

Ventide Inhaler is not for use in acute attacks but for routine long-term management so some patients will require a separate Ventolin* Inhaler for relief of acute bronchospasm. However, should the effect of the additional Ventolin Inhaler or the relief provided by the Ventide Inhaler last for less than four hours, patients should be advised that this may indicate that their asthma is worsening and to seek medical advice in case treatment with inhaled corticosteroids needs to be increased or treatment with systemic corticosteroids needs to be started or increased.

In the majority of patients no significant adrenal suppression occurs until doses of 1,500 micrograms of beclomethasone dipropionate per day are exceeded. Reduction of plasma cortisol levels has been reported in some patients who received 2,000 micrograms per day of inhaled beclomethasone dipropionate.

For those patients who are steroid-dependent it is advisable to commence therapy with beclomethasone dipropionate as the separate aerosol, Becotide Inhaler. Instructions regarding the introduction of Becotide Inhaler as full or part replacement for systemic steroids are given in the Data Sheet for Becotide Inhaler.

Patients who have been weaned in the previous few months from long-term systemic corticosteroids need special consideration until the hypothalamic-pituitary-adrenal system has recovered sufficiently to enable the patient to cope with emergencies such as trauma, surgery or infections. Such patients should carry a warning card indicating that they need supplementary systemic steroid during periods of stress, until their adrenocortical function has become normal. These patients should also be given a supply of oral steroid to use in emergency when their airways obstruction worsens.

Special care is necessary in patients with active or quiescent pulmonary tuberculosis.

Salbutamol should be administered cautiously to patients suffering from thyrotoxicosis.

Salbutamol and non-selective beta-blocking drugs such as propranolol, should not normally be prescribed together.

Potentially serious hypokalaemia may result from $beta_2$-agonist therapy. Particular caution is advised in acute severe asthma as this effect may be potentiated by concomitant treatment with xanthine derivatives, steroids, diuretics and by hypoxia. It is recommended that serum potassium levels are monitored in such situations.

Pregnancy: Administration of drugs during pregnancy should only be considered if the expected benefit to the mother is greater than any possible risk to the fetus. Salbutamol has been in widespread use for many years in human beings without apparent ill consequence; this includes its well established use in the management of premature labour. However, as with the majority of drugs, there is little published evidence of its safety in the early stages of human pregnancy, but in animal studies there was evidence of some harmful effects on the fetus at very high dose levels.

There is inadequate evidence of safety of beclomethasone dipropionate in human pregnancy. Administration of corticosteroids to pregnant animals can cause abnormalities of fetal development including cleft palate and intra-uterine growth retardation. There may, therefore, be a very small risk of such effects on the human fetus. It should be noted however, that the fetal changes in animals occur after relatively high systemic exposure. Because beclomethasone dipropionate is delivered directly to the lungs by the inhaled route it avoids the high level of exposure that occurs when corticosteroids are given by systemic routes.

The use of salbutamol and beclomethasone dipropionate (or Ventide) in pregnancy requires that the possible benefit of the drugs be weighed against the possible hazards.

Lactation: No specific studies examining the transference of beclomethasone dipropionate into the milk of lactating animals have been performed. It is reasonable to assume that beclomethasone dipropionate is secreted in milk but at the dosages used for direct inhalation, there is low potential for significant levels in breast milk. As salbutamol is probably also secreted in breast milk the use of Ventide in nursing mothers should be restricted to situations where it is felt that the expected benefit to the mother is likely to outweigh any potential risk to the neonate.

Side-effects:
Salbutamol: Mild tremor and headache have been rarely reported. They usually disappear with continued treatment.

There have been very rare reports of transient muscle cramps.

Hypersensitivity reactions including angioedema and urticaria, bronchospasm, hypotension and collapse have been reported very rarely.

Potentially serious hypokalaemia may result from $beta_2$-agonist therapy.

Beclomethasone Dipropionate: Candidiasis of the mouth and throat (thrush) occurs in some patients inhaling beclomethasone dipropionate. Patients with high blood levels of Candida precipitins, indicating a previous infection, are most likely to develop this complication. Such patients may find it helpful to rinse their mouth with water after using the inhaler. The condition usually responds to topical antifungal therapy without discontinuing treatment with Ventide Inhaler.

In some patients inhaled beclomethasone dipropionate may cause hoarseness or throat irritation. It may be helpful to rinse the mouth out with water immediately after inhalation.

As with other inhalation therapy, the potential for paradoxical bronchospasm should be kept in mind. If it occurs, the preparation should be discontinued immediately and alternative therapy instituted.

Overdosage: The preferred antidote for overdosage with Ventide Inhaler is a cardio-selective, beta-blocking agent, to counteract the salbutamol component, but beta-blocking drugs should be used with caution in patients with a history of bronchospasm. The acute toxicity of beclomethasone dipropionate is low. The only harmful effect that follows inhalation of large amounts of the drug over a short time period is suppression of hypothalamic-pituitary-adrenal (HPA) function. No special emergency action need be taken. Treatment with Ventide Inhaler should be continued at the recommended dose to control the asthma; HPA function recovers in a day or two.

In the unlikely event of grossly excessive intake of beclomethasone dipropionate for weeks or months a degree of adrenocortical atrophy could occur in addition to suppression of HPA function. The patient should be treated as steroid-dependent and transferred to a suitable maintenance dose of a systemic steroid such as prednisolone. Once the patient's condition is stabilised the reintroduction of inhaled corticosteroids should be considered.

Pharmaceutical precautions *Storage:* Ventide Inhaler should be stored below 30°C, protected from direct sunlight, heat and from frost.

As with most inhaled medications in aerosol canisters, the therapeutic effect of this medication may decrease when the canister is cold.

The canister should not be punctured, broken or burnt even if it is apparently empty.

Legal category POM.

Package quantities Ventide Inhaler is a metered-dose aerosol with a specially designed actuator. Each canister provides 200 inhalations.

Further information Products containing salbutamol do not cause difficulty in micturition because, unlike sympathomimetic drugs such as ephedrine, salbutamol does not stimulate alpha-adrenoreceptors. Salbutamol products are not contra-indicated in patients under treatment with monoamine oxidase inhibitors (MAOIs).

Product licence number 0045/0122

VENTIDE* ROTACAPS*

Presentation Ventide Rotacaps, an alternative inhalation form of the combination of salbutamol and beclomethasone dipropionate to Ventide Inhaler, are especially valuable for treating patients who are unable to use pressurised inhalers effectively or who might use them incorrectly.

Ventide Rotacaps contain a mixture of microfine salbutamol sulphate, microfine beclomethasone dipropionate and larger particle lactose in grey/colourless hard gelatin cartridges. Each light grey Rotacap contains 200 micrograms salbutamol (as sulphate) plus 100 micrograms beclomethasone dipropionate, and each dark grey Rotacap contains 400 micrograms salbutamol (as sulphate) plus 200 micrograms beclomethasone dipropionate. The Rotacaps are marked 'Ventide paed' or 'Ventide' respectively. The contents of a Rotacap are inhaled using a specially developed device called a Rotahaler which separates the cartridge into halves that rotate and release the drugs when the patient inhales. This breath actuation is very sensitive and so the drugs are fully available even at low inspiratory flow rates. The Rotahaler is therefore a more reliable drug delivery system for many patients but a rather larger unit dose of the drugs relative to Ventide Inhaler is necessary for the same therapeutic effect.

Uses This association of Salbutamol BP with Beclomethasone Dipropionate BP is specially provided for those patients who require regular doses of both drugs for treatment of their obstructive airways disease. Ventide Rotacaps are not intended for use as a first-line treatment but are for use once the need for inhaled corticosteroid therapy has been established.

Dosage and administration Ventide Rotacaps are for inhalation use only, using a Ventide Rotahaler.

Adults: One Ventide Rotacap containing 400 micrograms salbutamol (as sulphate) and 200 micrograms beclomethasone dipropionate three or four times a day.

Children: One Ventide Paediatric Rotacap containing 200 micrograms salbutamol (as sulphate) and 100 micrograms beclomethasone dipropionate two, three or four times a day.

Contra-indications, warnings, etc
Contra-indications: Although intravenous salbutamol and occasionally salbutamol tablets are used in the management of premature labour, uncomplicated by conditions such as placenta praevia, ante-partum haemorrhage or toxaemia of pregnancy, Ventide Rotacaps are not appropriate for managing premature labour. Ventide Rotacaps should not be used for threatened abortion during the first or second trimesters of pregnancy.

Ventide Rotacaps are contra-indicated in patients with a history of hypersensitivity to any of their components.

Precautions: Patients should be instructed in the proper use of the Rotahaler to ensure that the drugs reach the target areas within the lungs. Patients should be made aware that Ventide Rotacaps should be used regularly for optimum benefit. However, patients should be regularly reassessed so that their continuing need for corticosteroid therapy can also be reviewed.

Ventide Rotacaps are not intended for use in acute attacks but are indicated for routine long-term management, so some patients will require a separate bronchodilator for inhalation for relief of acute bronchospasm. However, should the effect of the additional inhaled bronchodilator or the relief provided by the Ventide Rotacaps last for less than four hours, patients should be advised that this may indicate that their asthma is worsening and to seek medical advice in case treatment with inhaled corticosteroids needs to be increased or treatment with systemic corticosteroids needs to be started or increased.

In the majority of patients no significant adrenal suppression occurs until doses of 1,500 micrograms of beclomethasone dipropionate per day are exceeded. Reduction of plasma cortisol levels has been reported in some patients who received 2,000 micrograms per day of inhaled beclomethasone dipropionate.

For those patients who are steroid-dependent it is advisable to commence therapy with beclomethasone dipropionate as the separate Rotacaps, Becotide Rotacaps. Instructions regarding the introduction of Becotide Rotacaps as full or part replacement for systemic steroids are given in the Data Sheet for Becotide Rotacaps.

Patients who have been weaned in the previous few months from long-term systemic corticosteroids need special consideration until the hypothalamic-pituitary-adrenal system has recovered sufficiently to enable the patient to cope with emergencies such as trauma, surgery or infections. Such patients should carry a warning card indicating that they need supplementary systemic steroid during periods of stress, until their adrenocortical function has become normal. These patients should also be given a supply of oral steroid to use in emergency when their airways obstruction worsens.

Special care is necessary in patients with active or quiescent pulmonary tuberculosis.

Salbutamol should be administered cautiously to patients suffering from thyrotoxicosis.

Salbutamol and non-selective beta-blocking drugs, such as propranolol, should not normally be prescribed together.

Potentially serious hypokalaemia may result from $beta_2$-agonist therapy. Particular caution is advised in acute severe asthma as this effect may be potentiated by concomitant treatment with xanthine derivatives, steroids, diuretics and by hypoxia. It is recommended that serum potassium levels are monitored in such situations.

Pregnancy: Administration of drugs during pregnancy should only be considered if the expected benefit to the mother is greater than any possible risk to the fetus. Salbutamol has been in widespread use for many years in human beings without apparent ill consequence; this includes its well established use in the management of premature labour. However, as with the majority of drugs, there is little published evidence of its safety in the early stages of human pregnancy, but in animal studies there was evidence of some harmful effects on the fetus at very high dose levels.

There is inadequate evidence of safety of beclomethasone dipropionate in human pregnancy. Administration of corticosteroids to pregnant animals can cause abnormalities of fetal development including cleft palate and intra-uterine growth retardation. There may, therefore, be a very small risk of such effects on the human fetus. It should be noted however, that the fetal changes in animals occur after relatively high systemic exposure. Because beclomethasone dipropionate is delivered directly to the lungs by the inhaled route it avoids the high level of exposure that occurs when corticosteroids are given by systemic routes.

The use of salbutamol and beclomethasone dipropionate (or Ventide) in pregnancy requires that the possible benefit of the drugs be weighed against the possible hazards.

Lactation: No specific studies examining the transference of beclomethasone dipropionate into the milk of lactating animals have been performed. It is reasonable to assume that beclomethasone dipropionate is secreted in milk but at the dosages used for direct inhalation, there is low potential for significant levels in breast milk. As salbutamol is probably also secreted in breast milk the use of Ventide in nursing mothers should be restricted to situations where it is felt that the expected benefit to the mother is likely to outweight any potential risk to the neonate.

Side-effects:
Salbutamol: Mild tremor and headache have been rarely reported. They usually disappear with continued treatment.

There have been very rare reports of transient muscle cramps.

Hypersensitivity reactions including angioedema and urticaria, bronchospasm, hypotension and collapse have been reported very rarely.

Potentially serious hypokalaemia may result from beta$_2$-agonist therapy.

Beclomethasone Dipropionate: Candidiasis of the mouth and throat (thrush) occurs in some patients inhaling beclomethasone dipropionate. Patients with high blood levels of Candida precipitins, indicating a previous infection, are most likely to develop this complication. Such patients may find it helpful to rinse their mouth with water after using the Rotahaler. The condition usually responds to topical antifungal therapy without discontinuing treatment with Ventide Rotacaps.

In some patients inhaled beclomethasone dipropionate may cause hoarseness or throat irritation. It may be helpful to rinse the mouth out with water immediately after inhalation.

As with other inhalation therapy, the potential for paradoxical bronchospasm should be kept in mind. If it occurs, the preparation should be discontinued immediately and alternative therapy instituted.

Overdosage: The preferred antidote for overdosage with Ventide Rotacaps is a cardio-selective, beta-blocking agent, to counteract the salbutamol component, but beta-blocking drugs should be used with caution in patients with a history of bronchospasm.

The acute toxicity of beclomethasone dipropionate is low. The only harmful effect that follows inhalation of large amounts of beclomethasone dipropionate over a short time period is suppression of hypothalamic-pituitary-adrenal (HPA) function and no special emergency action need be taken for this. Treatment with Ventide Rotacaps should be continued at the recommended dose to control the asthma; HPA function recovers in a day or two.

In the unlikely event of grossly excessive intake of beclomethasone dipropionate for weeks or months a degree of adrenocortical atrophy could occur in addition to suppression of HPA function. The patient should be treated as steroid-dependent and transferred to a suitable maintenance dose of a systemic steroid such as prednisolone. Once the patient's condition is stabilised the re-introduction of inhaled corticosteroids should be considered.

Pharmaceutical precautions *Storage:* To keep the Rotacaps in good condition it is important that they are stored in a dry place below 30°C, where they will not be exposed to extremes of temperature. A convenient supply may be carried in the special container for the Rotahaler. The Rotacaps should only be inserted into the Rotahaler immediately prior to use. Failure to observe this instruction may affect the operation of the Rotahaler.

Legal category POM.

Package quantities Ventide Rotacaps and Ventide Paediatric Rotacaps are supplied in containers of 112 (OP).

Further information Products containing salbutamol do not cause difficulty in micturition because, unlike sympathomimetic drugs such as ephedrine, salbutamol does not stimulate alpha-adrenoreceptors. Salbutamol products are not contra-indicated in patients under treatment with monoamine oxidase inhibitors (MAOIs).

Product licence numbers

Ventide Rotacaps	0045/0138
Ventide Paediatric Rotacaps	0045/0139

VENTODISKS*

Presentation Each Ventodisk comprises eight regularly spaced double foil blisters each containing a mixture of microfine salbutamol (as sulphate), 200 micrograms or 400 micrograms, and larger particle lactose. Each dosage strength is identified in the centre of the disk as 'Ventodisk 200 mcg' (light blue) or 'Ventodisk 400 mcg' (dark blue).

Ventodisks are intended only for use in a specific drug delivery device known as the Ventolin Diskhaler. The contents of each blister are deposited into the blue Diskhaler device when pierced with an integral needle. The contents are then available to the patients to inhale by breath operation which allows the drug to be fully available even at low inspiratory flow rates.

Ventodisks therefore provide reliable drug delivery for many patients, but a rather larger unit dose relative to Ventolin Inhaler is necessary for the same therapeutic effect.

Uses Salbutamol BP is a beta-adrenergic stimulant which has a highly selective action on bronchial beta$_2$-adrenoceptors and little or no effect on cardiac beta$_1$-receptors at therapeutic doses.

Salbutamol is also highly active in preventing antigen-induced release of histamine and slow reacting substance of anaphylaxis, SRS (A), from mast cells in human lung sensitised with IgE antibody. Such Type 1 hypersensitivity reactions are generally considered to be the primary triggers of the allergic asthma syndrome.

Ventodisks are therefore indicated both for the treatment and prophylaxis of bronchial asthma and also for the treatment of other conditions, such as bronchitis and emphysema, with associated reversible airways obstruction. Inhaled salbutamol has a long duration of action and is ideally suited for routine maintenance therapy and prophylaxis in chronic asthma, both to relieve persistent bronchospasm and to suppress the allergic response within the lungs. Regular use is also indicated for the treatment of persistent bronchospasm as in chronic bronchitis.

Salbutamol acts rapidly and Ventodisks may be used when necessary to relieve attacks of acute dyspnoea. They may also be used before exertion to prevent exercise-induced bronchospasm or before exposure to a known unavoidable allergen challenge.

The effective dose of salbutamol from Ventodisks is only one tenth of the usual oral dose and so the skeletal muscle tremor sometimes associated with oral therapy occurs rarely.

The selective action of salbutamol on the bronchi and its lack of effect on the cardiovascular system make Ventodisks suitable for treating patients with coexisting heart disease or hypertension.

Dosage and administration Ventodisks are for inhalation use only, using a Ventolin Diskhaler.

Adults: For the relief of acute bronchospasm and for managing intermittent episodes of asthma, 200 micrograms or 400 micrograms may be administered as a single dose.

The recommended dose for chronic maintenance or prophylactic therapy is 400 micrograms three or four times a day.

To prevent exercise-induced bronchospasm, 400 micrograms should be taken before exertion.

Children: 200 micrograms is the recommended dose for relief of acute bronchospasm, in the management of episodic asthma or before exercise. 200 micrograms should be administered three or four times a day for routine maintenance or prophylactic therapy.

For optimum results, in most patients, Ventodisks should be used regularly.

The bronchodilator effect of each administration of inhaled salbutamol lasts for at least four hours, except in patients whose asthma is becoming worse. Such patients should be warned not to increase their usage of Ventodisks but should seek medical advice in case treatment with an inhaled and/or systemic glucocorticosteroid is indicated.

Contra-indications, warnings, etc
Contra-indications: Although intravenous salbutamol and occasionally salbutamol tablets are used in the

management of premature labour uncomplicated by conditions such as placenta praevia, ante-partum haemorrhage, or toxaemia of pregnancy, inhaled salbutamol preparations are not appropriate for managing premature labour. Salbutamol presentations should not be used for threatened abortion during the first and second trimesters of pregnancy.

Ventodisks are contra-indicated in patients with a history of hypersensitivity to any of their components.

Precautions: In the event of a previously effective dose of inhaled salbutamol failing to give relief lasting at least three hours, the patient should be advised to seek medical advice in order that any necessary additional treatment may be instituted.

Salbutamol should be administered cautiously to patients suffering from thyrotoxicosis.

Salbutamol and non-selective beta-blocking drugs such as propranolol, should not usually be prescribed together.

Potentially serious hypokalaemia may result from $beta_2$-agonist therapy. Particular caution is advised in acute severe asthma as this effect may be potentiated by concomitant treatment with xanthine derivatives, steroids, diuretics and by hypoxia. It is recommended that serum potassium levels are monitored in such situations.

Pregnancy: Administration of the drug during pregnancy should only be considered if the expected benefit to the mother is greater than any possible risk to the fetus.

Salbutamol has been in widespread use for many years in human beings without apparent ill consequence; this includes its well established use in the management of premature labour. However, as with the majority of drugs, there is little published evidence of its safety in the early stages of human pregnancy, but in animal studies there was evidence of some harmful effects on the fetus at very high dose levels.

Lactation: As salbutamol is probably secreted in breast milk its use in nursing mothers requires careful consideration. It is not known whether salbutamol has a harmful effect on the neonate and so its use should be restricted to situations where it is felt that the expected benefit to the mother is likely to outweigh any potential risk to the neonate.

Side-effects: Mild tremor and headache have been rarely reported. They usually disappear with continued treatment.

There have been very rare reports of transient muscle cramps.

Hypersensitivity reactions including angioedema and urticaria, bronchospasm, hypotension and collapse have been reported very rarely.

Potentially serious hypokalaemia may result from $beta_2$-agonist therapy.

As with other inhalation therapy, the potential for paradoxical bronchospasm should be kept in mind. If it occurs, the preparation should be discontinued immediately and alternative therapy instituted.

Overdosage: The preferred antidote for overdosage with salbutamol is a cardioselective beta-blocking agent but beta-blocking drugs should be used with caution in patients with a history of bronchospasm.

Pharmaceutical precautions Whilst Ventodisks provide a good protection to the blister contents from the effect of the atmosphere they should not be exposed to extremes of temperature and should be stored below 30°C. A Ventodisk may be kept in the Diskhaler at all times but a blister should only be pierced immediately prior to use. Failure to observe this instruction may affect the operation of the Diskhaler.

Legal category POM.

Package quantities Ventodisks 200 micrograms and 400 micrograms are supplied in cartons of 14 (OP), together with a Diskhaler device.

Further information Salbutamol does not cause difficulty in micturition because, unlike sympathomimetic drugs such as ephedrine, it does not stimulate alpha-adrenoceptors. Salbutamol is not contra-indicated in patients under treatment with monoamine oxidase inhibitors (MAOIs).

Product licence numbers

Ventodisks 200 micrograms	0045/0134
Ventodisks 400 micrograms	0045/0135

VENTOLIN* INHALER

Presentation Metered-dose aerosol delivering 100 micrograms Salbutamol BP per actuation, with a specially designed actuator.

Uses Salbutamol BP is a beta-adrenergic stimulant which has a highly selective action on the receptors in bronchial muscle and, in therapeutic dosage, little or no action on the cardiac receptors.

Salbutamol is also highly active in preventing antigen-induced release of histamine and slow-reacting substance of anaphylaxis, SRS(A), from mast cells in human lung sensitised with IgE antibody. Such Type 1 hypersensitivity reactions are generally considered to be the primary triggers of the allergic asthma syndrome. Ventolin Inhaler is therefore indicated both for the treatment and prophylaxis of bronchial asthma, and also for the treatment of other conditions, such as bronchitis and emphysema, with associated reversible airways obstruction. Because Ventolin is long-acting, it is ideally suited for routine maintenance therapy in chronic asthma and chronic bronchitis. The inhaler drug-delivery system, using salbutamol in microgram dosage, avoids the skeletal muscle tremor sometimes associated with oral therapy.

Ventolin Inhaler acts rapidly and may be used when necessary to relieve attacks of acute dyspnoea. Doses may be taken prophylactically before exertion or to prevent exercise-induced asthma.

Because of its selective action on the bronchi and its lack of effects on the cardiovascular system, Ventolin Inhaler is suitable for treating bronchospasm in patients with co-existing heart disease or hypertension.

Dosage and administration *Adults:* For the relief of acute bronchospasm and for managing intermittent episodes of asthma, one or two inhalations may be administered as a single dose. The recommended dose for chronic maintenance or prophylactic therapy is two inhalations three or four times a day.

To prevent exercise-induced bronchospasm, two inhalations should be taken before exertion.

Children: One inhalation is the recommended dose for the relief of acute bronchospasm, in the management of episodic asthma or before exercise. One inhalation should be administered three or four times a day for routine maintenance or prophylactic therapy. These doses may be increased to two inhalations if necessary.

For optimum results, in most patients, Ventolin Inhaler should be used regularly. The bronchodilator effect of each administration of inhaled Ventolin lasts for at least four hours, except in patients whose asthma is becoming worse. Such patients should be warned not to increase their usage of Inhaler, but should seek medical advice in case treatment with an inhaled and/or systemic glucocorticosteroid is indicated.

Contra-indications, warnings, etc

Contra-indications: Although intravenous salbutamol and occasionally salbutamol tablets are used in the management of premature labour uncomplicated by conditions such as placenta praevia, ante-partum haemorrhage or toxaemia of pregnancy, inhaled salbutamol preparations are not appropriate for managing premature labour. Salbutamol presentations should not be used for threatened abortion during the first or second trimesters of pregnancy.

Ventolin Inhaler is contra-indicated in patients with a history of hypersensitivity to any of its components.

Precautions: In the event of a previously effective dose of Ventolin Inhaler failing to give relief for at least three hours, the patient should be advised to seek medical advice in order that any necessary additional steps may be taken. Salbutamol should be administered cautiously to patients suffering from thyrotoxicosis.

Salbutamol and non-selective beta-blockers such as propranolol should not usually be prescribed together.

Potentially serious hypokalaemia may result from beta$_2$-agonist therapy. Particular caution is advised in acute severe asthma as this effect may be potentiated by concomitant treatment with xanthine derivatives, steroids, diuretics and by hypoxia. It is recommended that serum potassium levels are monitored in such situations.

Pregnancy: Administration of the drug during pregnancy should only be considered if the expected benefit to the mother is greater than any possible risk to the fetus.

Salbutamol has been in widespread use for many years in human beings without apparent ill consequence; this includes its well established use in the management of premature labour. However, as with the majority of drugs, there is little published evidence of its safety in the early stages of human pregnancy, but in animal studies there was evidence of some harmful effects on the fetus at very high dose levels.

Lactation: As salbutamol is probably secreted in breast milk its use in nursing mothers requires careful consideration. It is not known whether salbutamol has a harmful effect on the neonate and so its use should be restricted to situations where it is felt that the expected benefit to the mother is likely to outweigh any potential risk to the neonate.

Side-effects: Mild tremor and headache have been rarely reported. They usually disappear with continued treatment.

There have been very rare reports of transient muscle cramps.

Hypersensitivity reactions including angioedema and urticaria, bronchospasm, hypotension and collapse have been reported very rarely.

Potentially serious hypokalaemia may result from beta$_2$-agonist therapy.

As with other inhalation therapy, the potential for paradoxical bronchospasm should be kept in mind. If it occurs, the preparation should be discontinued immediately and alternative therapy instituted.

Overdosage: The preferred antidote for overdosage with Ventolin Inhaler is a cardioselective beta-blocking agent, but beta-blocking drugs should be used with caution in patients with a history of bronchospasm.

Pharmaceutical precautions Ventolin Inhaler should be stored below 30°C protected from direct sunlight, heat and from frost. The canister should not be broken, punctured or burnt, even when apparently empty.

As with most inhaled medications in aerosol canisters, the therapeutic effect of this medication may decrease when the canister is cold.

Legal category POM.

Package quantities Ventolin Inhaler is a metered-dose aerosol with a specially designed actuator. Each canister provides 200 inhalations.

Further information Ventolin does not cause difficulty in micturition because, unlike sympathomimetic drugs such as ephedrine, it does not stimulate alpha-adrenoceptors. Ventolin is not contra-indicated in patients under treatment with monoamine oxidase inhibitors (MAOIs).

Product licence number 0045/5022R

VENTOLIN* NEBULES* 2.5 mg and 5.0 mg

Presentation Ventolin Nebules 2.5 mg are a plastic ampoule presentation containing a sterile, aqueous, colourless to pale yellow solution of Salbutamol BP as the sulphate in normal saline. The concentration, which is expressed in terms of Salbutamol BP is 0.1% (1 mg Salbutamol BP as the sulphate in 1 ml). Each Nebule contains 2.5 ml of solution equivalent to 2.5 mg salbutamol. The solution is adjusted to pH 4.0.

Ventolin Nebules 5.0 mg are a plastic ampoule presentation containing a sterile, aqueous, colourless to pale yellow solution of Salbutamol BP as the sulphate in normal saline. The concentration, which is expressed in terms of Salbutamol BP is 0.2% (2 mg Salbutamol BP as the sulphate in 1 ml). Each Nebule contains 2.5 ml of solution equivalent to 5.0 mg salbutamol. The solution is adjusted to pH 4.0.

Uses Ventolin Nebules are indicated for use in the routine management of chronic bronchospasm unresponsive to conventional therapy and in the treatment of acute severe asthma.

Dosage and administration

Adults and children: An appropriate starting dose of salbutamol by wet aerosol is 2.5 mg. This may be increased to 5 mg. However, in domiciliary practice the benefits of increasing the dose of nebulised salbutamol should be weighed against the risk that a deterioration in the patient's underlying condition may be masked. In such circumstances, a medical assessment should be considered since alternative therapy may be indicated. Treatment may be repeated up to four times daily by means of a nebuliser.

Delivery of the aerosol may be by face mask or 'T' piece.

Ventolin Nebules are intended to be used undiluted. However, if prolonged delivery time is desirable (more than 10 minutes) dilution with normal saline for injection may be required.

Clinical efficacy of nebulised salbutamol in infants under 18 months is uncertain. As transient hypoxaemia may occur, supplemental oxygen therapy should be considered.

Contra-indications, warnings, etc

Contra-indications: Although intravenous salbutamol and occasionally salbutamol tablets are used in the management of premature labour uncomplicated by conditions such as placenta praevia, ante-partum haemorrhage or toxaemia of pregnancy, inhaled salbutamol preparations are not appropriate for managing premature labour. Salbutamol presentations should not be used for threatened abortion during the first or second trimesters of pregnancy.

Ventolin Nebules are contra-indicated in patients with a history of hypersensitivity to any of their components.

Precautions: Ventolin Nebules should be used with care in patients known to have received large doses of other sympathomimetic drugs. They should be administered cautiously to patients suffering from thyrotoxicosis.

Ventolin Nebules are to be used with a nebuliser, only under the direction of a physician. The solution should not be injected or administered orally.

Patients receiving treatment at home with Ventolin Nebules must be warned that if either the usual relief is diminished or the usual duration of action reduced, they should not increase the dose or its frequency of administration, but should seek medical advice.

Solutions which are not of neutral pH may rarely cause paradoxical bronchospasm in some patients.

Salbutamol and non-selective beta-blocking drugs such as propranolol, should not usually be prescribed together.

Potentially serious hypokalaemia may result from beta$_2$-agonist therapy. Particular caution is advised in acute severe asthma as this effect may be potentiated by concomitant treatment with xanthine derivatives, steroids, diuretics and by hypoxia. It is recommended that serum potassium levels are monitored in such situations.

Pregnancy: Administration of the drug during pregnancy should only be considered if the expected benefit to the mother is greater than any possible risk to the fetus.

Salbutamol has been in widespread use for many years in human beings without apparent ill consequence; this includes its well established use in the management of premature labour. However, as with the majority of drugs, there is little published evidence of its safety in the early stages of human pregnancy, but in animal studies there was evidence of some harmful effects on the fetus at very high dose levels.

Lactation: As salbutamol is probably secreted in breast milk its use in nursing mothers requires careful consideration. It is not known whether salbutamol has a harmful effect on the neonate and so its use should be restricted to situations where it is felt that the expected benefit to the mother is likely to outweigh any potential risk to the neonate.

Side-effects: A small increase in heart rate may occur in patients who inhale large doses of Ventolin. This is not usually accompanied by any changes in the electrocardiogram.

Other side effects which occur with very high doses of Ventolin by inhalation are peripheral vasodilatation and fine tremor of skeletal muscle.

Headaches have been rarely reported. They usually disappear with continued treatment.

There have been very rare reports of transient muscle cramps.

Hypersensitivity reactions including angioedema and urticaria, bronchospasm, hypotension and collapse have been reported very rarely.

Potentially serious hypokalaemia may result from beta$_2$-agonist therapy.

As with other inhalation therapy, the potential for paradoxical bronchospasm should be kept in mind. If it occurs, the preparation should be discontinued immediately and alternative therapy instituted.

Overdosage: The preferred antidote to overdosage with Ventolin Nebules is a cardio-selective beta-blocking agent, but beta-blocking drugs should be used with caution in patients with a history of bronchospasm.

Pharmaceutical precautions
Storage: Ventolin Nebules should be stored at a temperature below 25°C and protected from light.

Dilution: Ventolin Nebules may be diluted with Sodium Chloride Injection BP (normal saline). Solutions in nebulisers should be replaced daily.

Legal category POM.

Package quantities Ventolin Nebules 2.5 mg and 5.0 mg are each available in boxes containing 20 Nebules in strips of 10.

Further information Ventolin does not cause difficulty in micturition because, unlike sympathomimetic drugs such as ephedrine, it does not stimulate alpha-adrenoceptors. Ventolin is not contra-indicated in patients under treatment with monoamine oxidase inhibitors (MAOIs).

Ventolin Nebules are suitable for treating bronchospasm in patients with co-existing heart disease or hypertension.

Ventolin Nebules are a sterile, preservative-free presentation.

Product licence numbers

Ventolin Nebules 2.5 mg	0045/0123
Ventolin Nebules 5.0 mg	0045/0133

VENTOLIN* PARENTERAL PREPARATIONS
VENTOLIN* INJECTION 500 micrograms (0.5 mg) in 1 ml (500 micrograms/ml)
VENTOLIN* INJECTION 250 micrograms (0.25 mg) in 5 ml (50 micrograms/ml)
VENTOLIN* SOLUTION FOR INTRAVENOUS INFUSION 5 mg in 5 ml (1 mg/ml)

Presentation Ventolin Injection 500 micrograms (0.5 mg) in 1 ml (500 micrograms/ml) is presented as ampoules of 1 ml each containing 500 micrograms salbutamol as Salbutamol Sulphate BP, in a sterile isotonic solution adjusted to pH 3.5 with sulphuric acid.

Ventolin Injection 250 micrograms (0.25 mg) in 5 ml (50 micrograms/ml) is presented as ampoules of 5 ml each containing 250 micrograms salbutamol as Salbutamol Sulphate BP, in a sterile isotonic solution adjusted to pH 3.5 with sulphuric acid.

Ventolin Solution for Intravenous Infusion 5 mg in 5 ml (1 mg/ml) is presented as ampoules of 5 ml each containing 5 mg salbutamol as Salbutamol Sulphate BP, in a sterile isotonic solution adjusted to pH 3.5 with sulphuric acid.

The ampoules are of clear, neutral glass and the solution is colourless or faintly straw-coloured.

Uses Salbutamol BP is a beta-adrenergic stimulant that has a selective action on the beta$_2$-adrenoceptors in the bronchi and uterus and much less action on the beta$_1$-adrenoceptors in the heart.

Ventolin Parenteral Preparations are indicated for two distinct clinical situations:

1. For the relief of severe bronchospasm associated with asthma or bronchitis and for the treatment of status asthmaticus.
2. For the management of premature labour uncomplicated by conditions such as placenta praevia, antepartum haemorrhage or toxaemia of pregnancy, in the last trimester of pregnancy.

Dosage and administration
1. In severe bronchospasm and status asthmaticus

Adults
Subcutaneous route: 500 micrograms (8 micrograms/kg body weight) and repeated every four hours as required.

Intramuscular route: 500 micrograms (8 micrograms/kg body weight) and repeated every four hours as required.

Intravenous route: 250 micrograms (4 micrograms/kg body weight) injected slowly. If necessary the dose may be repeated. Ventolin Injection 250 micrograms in 5 ml (50 micrograms/ml) is a suitably dilute preparation for slow intravenous injection but if Ventolin Injection 500 micrograms in 1 ml (500 micrograms/ml) is used the injection may be facilitated by dilution with Water for Injections BP.

Infusion: In status asthmaticus, infusion rates of 3 to 20 micrograms per minute are generally adequate, but in patients with respiratory failure, higher dosage has been used with success. A starting dose of 5 micrograms per minute is recommended with appropriate adjustment in dosage according to patient response.

A suitable solution for infusion may be prepared by diluting 5 ml of Ventolin Solution for Intravenous Infusion in 500 ml of an infusion solution such as Sodium Chloride and Dextrose Injection BP to provide a salbutamol dose of 10 micrograms/ml of solution.

Children
At present there is insufficient evidence to recommend a dosage regimen for routine use in children.

2. In the management of premature labour

For this indication Ventolin Solution for Intravenous Infusion is recommended using a solution prepared as in 1. above.

Infusion rates of 10 to 45 micrograms per minute are generally adequate to control uterine contractions, but greater or lesser infusion rates may be required according to the strength and frequency of contractions. A starting rate of 10 micrograms per minute is recommended, increasing the rate at 10-minute intervals until there is evidence of patient response shown by diminution in strength, frequency or duration of contractions.

Thereafter, the infusion rate may be increased slowly until contractions cease. The maternal pulse rate should be monitored and the infusion rate adjusted to avoid excessive maternal heart rates (above 140 beats per minute). Once uterine contractions have ceased the infusion rate should be maintained at the same level for one hour and then reduced by 50% decrements at six-hourly intervals. Treatment may be continued orally with Ventolin Tablets 4 mg given three or four times daily.

As an alternative procedure or to counteract inadvertent overdosage with oxytocic drugs Ventolin Injection may be administered as a single injection by the intravenous or intramuscular routes. The usual recommended dose is 100 to 250 micrograms of salbutamol. The dose may be repeated according to the response of the patient.

Note. The contents of the ampoules of Ventolin Solution for Intravenous Infusion must not be injected undiluted. The concentration should be reduced by 50% before administration.

Ventolin parenteral preparations should not be administered in the same syringe or infusion as any other medication.

Contra-indications, warnings, etc

Contra-indications: Although intravenous salbutamol and occasionally salbutamol tablets are used in the management of premature labour uncomplicated by conditions such as placenta praevia, ante-partum haemorrhage or toxaemia of pregnancy, salbutamol preparations should not be used for threatened abortion during the first or second trimesters of pregnancy. Ventolin Parenteral Preparations are contra-indicated in patients with a history of hypersensitivity to any of their components.

Precautions: Salbutamol and non-selective beta-blocking drugs, such as propranolol, should not usually be prescribed together.

The use of Ventolin Parenteral Preparations in the treatment of severe bronchospasm or status asthmaticus does not obviate the requirement for glucocorticoid steroid therapy as appropriate. When practicable, administration of oxygen concurrently with parenteral Ventolin is recommended, particularly when it is given by intravenous infusion to hypoxic patients. In common with other beta-adrenoceptor agonists, salbutamol can induce reversible metabolic changes such as hypokalaemia and increased blood glucose levels. The diabetic patient may be unable to compensate for the increase in blood glucose and the development of ketoacidosis has been reported. Concurrent administration of corticosteroids can exaggerate this effect. Therefore, diabetic patients and those concurrently receiving corticosteroids should be monitored frequently during intravenous infusion of Ventolin so that remedial steps (e.g., an increase in insulin dosage) can be taken to counter any metabolic change occurring. For these patients it may be preferable to dilute Ventolin Solution for Intravenous Infusion in Sodium Chloride Injection BP rather than Sodium Chloride and Dextrose Injection BP.

Potentially serious hypokalaemia may result from $beta_2$-agonist therapy. Particular caution is advised in acute severe asthma as this effect may be potentiated by concomitant treatment with xanthine derivatives, steroids, diuretics and by hypoxia. It is recommended that serum potassium levels are monitored in such situations.

Salbutamol should be administered cautiously to patients suffering from thyrotoxicosis. In patients being treated to inhibit uterine contractions in premature labour by intravenous infusion of salbutamol, increases in maternal heart rate of the order of 20 to 50 beats per minute usually accompany the infusion. The maternal pulse rate should be monitored and not normally allowed to exceed a steady rate of 140 beats per minute. Maternal blood pressure may fall slightly during the infusion; the effect being greater on diastolic than on systolic pressure. Falls in diastolic pressure are usually within the range of 10 to 20 mmHg. The effect of infusion on fetal heart rate is less marked, but increases of up to 20 beats per minute may occur. In the treatment of premature labour before Ventolin Parenteral Preparations are given to any patient with known heart disease, an adequate assessment of the patient's cardiovascular status should be made by a physician experienced in cardiology.

Pregnancy: Administration of the drug during pregnancy should only be considered if the expected benefit to the mother is greater than any possible risk to the fetus.

Salbutamol has been in widespread use for many years in human beings without apparent ill consequence; this includes its well established use in the management of premature labour. However, as with the majority of drugs, there is little published evidence of its safety in the early stages of human pregnancy, but in animal studies there was evidence of some harmful effects on the fetus at very high dose levels.

Lactation: As salbutamol is probably secreted in breast milk its use in nursing mothers requires careful consideration. It is not known whether salbutamol has a harmful effect on the neonate and so its use should be restricted to situations where it is felt that the expected benefit to the mother is likely to outweigh any potential risk to the neonate.

Side-effects: Intramuscular use of the undiluted injection may produce slight pain or stinging. Enhancement of physiological tremor may occur with Ventolin. This effect is caused by a direct action on skeletal muscle and is common to all beta-adrenergic stimulants.

Ventolin Parenteral Preparations may dilate some peripheral arterioles leading to a small reduction in arterial pressure and a compensatory increase in cardiac rate. Increases in heart rate are more likely to occur in patients with normal heart rates and these increases are dose-dependent. In patients with pre-existing sinus tachycardia, especially those in status asthmaticus, the heart rate tends to fall as the condition of the patient improves.

There have been very rare reports of transient muscle cramps.

Hypersensitivity reactions including angioedema, urticaria, bronchospasm, hypotension and collapse have been reported rarely.

In the management of premature labour, intravenous infusion of Ventolin has occasionally been associated with nausea, vomiting and headaches.

Potentially serious hypokalaemia may result from $beta_2$-agonist therapy.

Overdosage: The preferred antidote for overdosage with Ventolin is a cardio-selective beta-blocking agent. Beta-blocking drugs should be used with caution in patients with a history of bronchospasm.

Pharmaceutical precautions Ventolin Parenteral Preparations may be diluted with Water for Injections BP, Sodium Chloride Injection BP, Sodium Chloride and Dextrose Injection BP or Dextrose Injection BP. These are the only recommended diluents.

Ventolin Parenteral Preparations should not be administered in the same syringe or infusion as any other medication.

The contents of the ampoule of Ventolin Solution for Intravenous Infusion must not be injected in the undiluted form; the concentration should be reduced by at least 50% before administration.

Storage: Ventolin Parenteral Preparations should be protected from light and stored at a temperature below 30°C.

All unused admixtures of Ventolin Parenteral Preparations with infusion fluids should be discarded twenty-four hours after preparation.

Legal category POM.

Package quantities Ventolin Injection 500 micrograms (0.5 mg) in 1 ml (500 micrograms/ml) is available in boxes of 5 ampoules.

Ventolin Injection 250 micrograms (0.25 mg) in 5 ml (50 micrograms/ml) is available in boxes of 10 ampoules.

Ventolin Solution for Intravenous Infusion 5 mg in 5 ml (1 mg/ml) is available in boxes of 10 ampoules.

Further information Ventolin does not cause difficulty in micturition because, unlike sympathomimetic drugs such as ephedrine, it does not stimulate alpha-adrenoceptors. Ventolin is not contra-indicated in patients under treatment with monoamine oxidase inhibitors (MAOIs).

Product licence numbers

Ventolin Injection 500 micrograms (0.5 mg) in 1 ml (500 micrograms/ml) 0045/0102R

Ventolin Injection 250 micrograms (0.25 mg) in 5 ml (50 micrograms/ml) 0045/0108R
Ventolin Solution for Intravenous Infusion 5 mg in 5 ml (1 mg/ml) 0045/0103R

VENTOLIN* RESPIRATOR SOLUTION

Presentation Ventolin Respirator Solution is an aqueous, colourless solution of Salbutamol Sulphate BP adjusted to pH 3.5 and preserved with benzalkonium chloride 0.01% w/v. The concentration, which is expressed in terms of Salbutamol BP, is 0.5% or 5 mg per ml of solution.

Uses Ventolin Respirator Solution is indicated for the treatment of severe acute asthma (status asthmaticus) and other forms of bronchospasm.

Dosage and administration
1. By intermittent administration: Adults: Ventolin Respirator Solution 0.5 to 1.0 ml (2.5 to 5.0 mg of salbutamol) should be diluted to a final volume of 2.0 to 4.0 ml with normal saline for injection. The resulting solution is inhaled from a suitably driven nebuliser until aerosol generation ceases. Using a correctly matched nebuliser and driving source this should take about ten minutes.

Ventolin Respirator Solution may be used undiluted for intermittent administration. For this, 2.0 ml of Ventolin Respirator Solution (10.0 mg salbutamol) is placed in the nebuliser and the patient allowed to inhale the nebulised solution until bronchodilatation is achieved. This usually takes three to five minutes.

Some adult patients may require higher doses of salbutamol up to 10 mg, in which case nebulisation of the undiluted solution may continue until aerosol generation ceases.

Children: The same mode of administration for intermittent administration is also applicable to children. The usual dosage for children under the age of twelve years is 0.5 ml (2.5 mg salbutamol) diluted to 2.0 to 4.0 ml with normal saline. Some children may however require higher doses of salbutamol up to 5.0 mg.

Intermittent treatment may be repeated four times daily.

2. By continuous administration: Ventolin Respirator Solution is diluted with normal saline for injection to contain 50 to 100 micrograms of salbutamol per ml (1 to 2 ml solution made up to 100 ml with diluent). The diluted solution is administered as an aerosol by a suitably driven nebuliser. The usual rate of administration is 1 to 2 mg per hour.

Delivery of the aerosol may be by facemask, 'T' piece or via an endotracheal tube. Intermittent positive pressure ventilation may be used but is rarely necessary. When there is a risk of anoxia through hypoventilation, oxygen should be added to the inspired air.

Clinical efficacy of nebulised salbutamol in infants under 18 months is uncertain. As transient hypoxaemia may occur, supplemental oxygen therapy should be considered.

Contra-indications, warnings, etc
Contra-indications: Although intravenous salbutamol and occasionally salbutamol tablets are used in the management of premature labour uncomplicated by conditions such as placenta praevia, ante-partum haemorrhage, or toxaemia of pregnancy, inhaled salbutamol preparations are not appropriate for managing premature labour. Salbutamol preparations should not be used for threatened abortion during the first or second trimesters of pregnancy.

Ventolin Respirator Solution is contra-indicated in patients with a history of hypersensitivity to any of its components.

Precautions: Ventolin Respirator Solution should be used with care in patients known to have received large doses of other sympathomimetic drugs.

It should be administered cautiously to patients suffering from thyrotoxicosis.

Ventolin Respirator Solution is to be used with a respirator or nebuliser only, under the direction of a physician. It is not to be injected or administered orally.

Patients receiving treatment at home with Ventolin Respirator Solution must be warned that if either the usual relief is diminished or the usual duration of action reduced, they should not increase the dose or its frequency of administration, but should seek medical advice.

Salbutamol and non-selective beta-blocking drugs such as propranolol, should not usually be prescribed together.

Non-isotonic solutions, or those which are not of neutral pH, or which contain benzalkonium chloride, may rarely cause paradoxical bronchospasm in some patients.

Potentially serious hypokalaemia may result from $beta_2$-agonist therapy. Particular caution is advised in acute severe asthma as this effect may be potentiated by concomitant treatment with xanthine derivatives, steroids, diuretics and by hypoxia. It is recommended that serum potassium levels are monitored in such situations.

Pregnancy: Administration of the drug during pregnancy should only be considered if the expected benefit to the mother is greater than any possible risk to the fetus.

Salbutamol has been in widespread use for many years in human beings without apparent ill consequence; this includes its well established use in the management of premature labour. However, as with the majority of drugs, there is little published evidence of its safety in the early stages of human pregnancy, but in animal studies there was evidence of some harmful effects on the fetus at very high dose levels.

Lactation: As salbutamol is probably secreted in breast milk its use in nursing mothers requires careful consideration. It is not known whether salbutamol has a harmful effect on the neonate and so its use should be restricted to situations where it is felt that the expected benefit to the mother is likely to outweigh any potential risk to the neonate.

Side-effects: A small increase in heart rate may occur in patients who inhale large doses of Ventolin. This is not usually accompanied by any changes in the electrocardiogram. Other side effects which may occur with very high doses of Ventolin by inhalation are peripheral vasodilatation and fine tremor of skeletal muscle.

Headaches have been rarely reported. They usually disappear with continued treatment.

There have been rare reports of transient muscle cramps.

Hypersensitivity reactions including angioedema and urticaria, bronchospasm, hypotension and collapse have been reported very rarely.

Potentially serious hypokalaemia may result from $beta_2$-agonist therapy.

As with other inhalation therapy, the potential for paradoxical bronchospasm should be kept in mind. If it occurs, the preparation should be discontinued immediately and alternative therapy instituted.

Overdosage: During continuous administration of Ventolin Respirator Solution any signs of overdosage can usually be counteracted by withdrawal of the drug.

The preferred antidote for overdosage with Ventolin Respirator Solution is a cardioselective beta-blocking agent, but beta-blocking drugs should be used with caution in patients with a history of bronchospasm.

Pharmaceutical precautions *Storage:* Ventolin Respirator Solution should be stored at a temperature below 25°C and protected from light. Once the bottle has been opened the contents should be discarded after one month.

Dilution: Ventolin Respirator Solution may be diluted with Sodium Chloride Injection BP (normal saline).

Solutions in nebulisers should be replaced daily.

Legal category POM.

Package quantities Ventolin Respirator Solution is supplied in screw-capped bottles of 20 ml.

Further information Ventolin does not cause difficulty

in micturition because, unlike sympathomimetic drugs such as ephedrine, it does not stimulate alpha-adrenoceptors. Ventolin is not contra-indicated in patients under treatment with monoamine oxidase inhibitors (MAOIs).

Ventolin Respirator Solution is suitable for treating bronchospasm in patients with co-existing heart disease or hypertension.

Product licence number 0045/5023R

VENTOLIN* ROTACAPS*

Presentation Ventolin Rotacaps, an alternative inhalation form of salbutamol to Ventolin Inhaler, are especially valuable for treating patients who are unable to use pressurised inhalers effectively or who might use them unwisely.

Ventolin Rotacaps contain a mixture of microfine salbutamol sulphate and larger particle lactose in blue/colourless hard gelatin cartridges. Each Rotacap contains 200 micrograms (light blue) or 400 micrograms (dark blue) of salbutamol (as sulphate) and is marked Ventolin 200 or Ventolin 400. The contents of a Rotacap are inhaled using a specially developed device called a Rotahaler* which separates the cartridge into halves that rotate and release the drug when the patient inhales. This breath actuation is very sensitive and so the drug is fully available even at the lowest inspiratory flow rates. The Rotahaler is, therefore, a more reliable drug delivery system for many patients, but a rather larger unit dose relative to Ventolin Inhaler is necessary for the same therapeutic effect.

Uses Salbutamol BP is a beta-adrenergic stimulant which has a highly selective action on bronchial beta-adrenoceptors and little or no effect on cardiac beta-receptors at therapeutic doses.

Salbutamol is also highly active in preventing antigen-induced release of histamine and slow-reacting substance of anaphylaxis, SRS(A), from mast cells in human lung sensitised with IgE antibody. Such Type I hypersensitivity reactions are generally considered to be the primary triggers of the allergic asthma syndrome.

Ventolin Rotacaps are therefore indicated both for the treatment and prevention of bronchial asthma, and also for the treatment of other conditions, such as bronchitis and emphysema, with associated reversible airway obstruction. Inhaled salbutamol has a long duration of action and Ventolin Rotacaps are ideally suited for routine maintenance therapy and prophylaxis in chronic asthma, both to relieve persistent bronchospasm and to suppress the allergic response within the lungs. Their regular use is also indicated for controlling persistent bronchospasm in chronic bronchitis.

Ventolin Rotacaps act rapidly and may be used when necessary to relieve attacks of acute dyspnoea. Rotacaps may also be used before exertion to prevent exercise-induced asthma or before exposure to a known unavoidable allergen challenge.

The effective dose of salbutamol from Rotacaps is only one tenth of the usual oral dose and so the skeletal muscle tremor sometimes associated with oral therapy occurs rarely.

The selective action of salbutamol on the bronchi and its lack of effects on the cardiovascular system make Ventolin Rotacaps suitable for treating patients with co-existing heart disease or hypertension.

Dosage and administration Ventolin Rotacaps are for inhalation use only, using a Ventolin Rotahaler.

Adults: For the relief of acute bronchospasm and for managing intermittent episodes of asthma, 200 micrograms or 400 micrograms may be administered as a single dose.

The recommended dose for chronic maintenance or prophylactic therapy is 400 micrograms three or four times a day.

To prevent exercise-induced bronchospasm, 400 micrograms should be taken before exertion.

Children: 200 micrograms is the recommended dose for the relief of acute bronchospasm, in the management of episodic asthma or before exercise.

200 micrograms should be administered three or four times a day for routine maintenance or prophylactic therapy.

For optimum results, in most patients Ventolin Rotacaps should be used regularly.

The bronchodilator effect of each administration of inhaled Ventolin lasts for at least four hours, except in patients whose asthma is becoming worse. Such patients should be warned not to increase their usage of Rotacaps but should seek medical advice in case treatment with an inhaled and/or systemic glucocorticosteroid is indicated.

Contra-indications, warnings, etc

Contra-indications: Although intravenous salbutamol and occasionally salbutamol tablets are used in the management of premature labour uncomplicated by conditions such as placenta praevia, ante-partum haemorrhage or toxaemia of pregnancy, inhaled salbutamol preparations are not appropriate for managing premature labour. Salbutamol presentations should not be used for threatened abortion during the first or second trimester of pregnancy. Ventolin Rotacaps are contra-indicated in patients with a history of hypersensitivity to any of their components.

Precautions: In the event of a previously effective dose of inhaled Ventolin failing to give relief lasting at least three hours, the patient should be advised to seek medical advice in order that any necessary additional steps may be taken. Salbutamol should be administered cautiously to patients suffering from thyrotoxicosis.

Salbutamol and non-selective beta-blocking drugs such as propranolol, should not usually be prescribed together.

Potentially serious hypokalaemia may result from $beta_2$-agonist therapy. Particular caution is advised in acute severe asthma as this effect may be potentiated by concomitant treatment with xanthine derivatives, steroids, diuretics and by hypoxia. It is recommended that serum potassium levels are monitored in such situations.

Pregnancy: Administration of the drug during pregnancy should only be considered if the expected benefit to the mother is greater than any possible risk to the fetus.

Salbutamol has been in widespread use for many years in human beings without apparent ill consequence; this includes its well established use in the management of premature labour. However, as with the majority of drugs, there is little published evidence of its safety in the early stages of human pregnancy, but in animal studies there was evidence of some harmful effects on the fetus at very high dose levels.

Lactation: As salbutamol is probably secreted in breast milk its use in nursing mothers requires careful consideration. It is not known whether salbutamol has a harmful effect on the neonate and so its use should be restricted to situations where it is felt that the expected benefit to the mother is likely to outweigh any potential risk to the neonate.

Side-effects: Mild tremor and headache have been rarely reported. They usually disappear with continued treatment.

There have been very rare reports of transient muscle cramps.

Hypersensitivity reactions including angioedema and urticaria, bronchospasm, hypotension and collapse have been reported very rarely.

Potentially serious hypokalaemia may result from $beta_2$-agonist therapy.

As with other inhalation therapy, the potential for paradoxical bronchospasm should be kept in mind. If it occurs, the preparation should be discontinued immediately and alternative therapy instituted.

Overdosage: The preferred antidote for overdosage with salbutamol is a cardioselective beta-blocking agent, but beta-blocking drugs should be used with caution in patients with a history of bronchospasm.

Pharmaceutical precautions To keep the Rotacaps

in good condition it is important that they are stored in a dry place below 30°C where they will not be exposed to extremes of temperature. A convenient supply may be carried in the special container for the Rotahaler. The Rotacaps should only be inserted in the Rotahaler immediately prior to use. Failure to observe this instruction may affect the operation of the Rotahaler.

Legal category POM.

Package quantities Ventolin Rotacaps 200 micrograms and 400 micrograms are supplied in containers of 112 (OP).

Further information Ventolin does not cause difficulty in micturition because, unlike sympathomimetic drugs such as ephedrine, it does not stimulate alpha-adrenoceptors. Ventolin is not contra-indicated in patients under treatment with monoamine oxidase inhibitors (MAOIs).

Product licence numbers

Ventolin Rotacaps 200 micrograms	0045/0116
Ventolin Rotacaps 400 micrograms	0045/0117

VENTOLIN* CR TABLETS

Presentation Ventolin CR Tablets 8 mg: White hexagonal controlled-release tablets each containing 8 mg salbutamol as Salbutamol Sulphate BP. Printed 8 on one side.

Ventolin CR Tablets 4 mg: White hexagonal controlled-release tablets each containing 4 mg salbutamol as Salbutamol Sulphate BP. Printed 4 on one side.

The tablet consists of an outer semi-permeable membrane and an inner core containing salbutamol sulphate. There is a hole in the outer coat which allows osmotically controlled release of the drug.

Uses Salbutamol BP is a beta-adrenergic stimulant which has a highly selective action on $beta_2$-receptors in bronchial smooth muscle and, in therapeutic dosage, little or no action on the cardiac $beta_1$-receptors.

Ventolin CR Tablets are indicated for the treatment of reversible airways obstruction of all types including bronchial asthma, chronic asthma, chronic bronchitis and emphysema.

Dosage and administration Ventolin CR Tablets must be swallowed whole with a glass of water and not chewed or crushed.

Adults: The recommended dose is one 8 mg tablet twice daily.

Elderly: There is no need to adjust the dose in the elderly.

Children: In children aged 3 to 12 years, the recommended dose is one 4 mg tablet twice daily.

Contra-indications, warnings, etc

Contra-indications: Although intravenous salbutamol and occasionally salbutamol tablets are used in the management of premature labour uncomplicated by conditions such as placenta praevia, ante-partum haemorrhage or toxaemia of pregnancy, presentations containing salbutamol should not be used for threatened abortion during the first or second trimester of pregnancy.

Ventolin CR Tablets are contra-indicated in patients with a history of hypersensitivity to any of their components.

Precautions: Salbutamol should be administered cautiously to patients suffering from thyrotoxicosis.

Salbutamol and non-selective beta-blocking drugs, such as propranolol, should not usually be prescribed together.

Potentially serious hypokalaemia may result from $beta_2$-agonist therapy. Particular caution is advised in acute severe asthma as this effect may be potentiated by concomitant treatment with xanthine derivatives, steroids, diuretics and by hypoxia. It is recommended that serum potassium levels are monitored in such situations.

Pregnancy: Administration of the drug during pregnancy should only be considered if the expected benefit to the mother is greater than any possible risk to the fetus.

Salbutamol has been in widespread use for many years in human beings without apparent ill consequence; this includes its well established use in the management of premature labour. However, as with the majority of drugs, there is little published evidence of its safety in the early stages of human pregnancy, but in animal studies there was evidence of some harmful effects on the fetus at very high dose levels.

Lactation: As salbutamol is probably secreted in breast milk its use in nursing mothers requires careful consideration. It is not known whether salbutamol has a harmful effect on the neonate and so its use should be restricted to situations where it is felt that the expected benefit to the mother is likely to outweigh any potential risk to the neonate.

Side-effects: Ventolin CR Tablets may cause a fine tremor of skeletal muscle in some patients; usually the hands are most obviously affected. This effect is common to all beta-adrenergic stimulants. The incidence of tremor with this preparation is similar to that seen with standard salbutamol tablets. A few patients experience feelings of tension; this is also due to the effects on skeletal muscle and not to direct CNS stimulation. In patients who are usually sensitive to beta-adrenergic stimulants, peripheral vasodilatation and a compensatory small increase in heart rate may occur. Occasionally, headaches have been reported.

There have been very rare reports of transient muscle cramps.

Hypersensitivity reactions including angioedema and urticaria, bronchospasm, hypotension and collapse have been reported very rarely.

Potentially serious hypokalaemia may result from $beta_2$-agonist therapy.

Overdosage: The preferred antidote for overdosage with salbutamol is a cardioselective beta-blocking agent, but beta-blocking drugs should be used with caution in patients with a history of bronchospasm.

Pharmaceutical precautions *Storage:* Ventolin CR Tablets should be stored at a temperature not exceeding 30°C.

Ventolin CR Tablets should not be removed from their foil pack until required for administration.

Legal category POM.

Package quantities Ventolin CR Tablets are supplied in double-foil blisters of 14 in cartons of 56.

Further information Ventolin CR does not cause difficulty in micturition because, unlike sympathomimetic drugs such as ephedrine, it does not stimulate alpha-adrenoceptors.

Ventolin CR is not contra-indicated in patients under treatment with monoamine oxidase inhibitors (MAOI's).

Product licence numbers

Ventolin CR Tablets 4 mg	0045/0143
Ventolin CR Tablets 8 mg	0045/0144

VENTOLIN* TABLETS 2 mg and 4 mg VENTOLIN* SYRUP

Presentation

Ventolin Tablets 2 mg: Pink tablets each containing salbutamol 2 mg as Salbutamol Sulphate BP. Engraved with the code $\frac{AH}{1K}$ on one side.

Ventolin Tablets 4 mg: Pink tablets each containing salbutamol 4 mg as Salbutamol Sulphate BP. Engraved with the code $\frac{AH}{2K}$ on one side.

Ventolin Syrup: Salbutamol 2 mg as Salbutamol Sulphate BP in each 5 ml of a fruit-flavoured, sugar-free syrup, which is devoid of artificial colouring agents.

Uses Salbutamol BP is a beta-adrenergic stimulant which has a highly selective action on the receptors in bronchial muscle and, in therapeutic dosage, little or no action on the cardiac receptors.

Ventolin Tablets 2 mg and 4 mg, and Syrup are indicated for the relief of bronchospasm in bronchial asthma of all types, chronic bronchitis and emphysema.

Ventolin Syrup is suitable oral therapy for children or those adults who prefer liquid medicines.

Because of their selective action on the bronchi and their lack of effects on the cardiovascular system, Ventolin oral preparations are suitable for treating bronchospasm in patients with co-existing heart disease or hypertension.

The selective action of salbutamol on the B_2-adrenoceptor has led to the use of parenteral Ventolin, usually as a continuous intravenous infusion, for the management of premature labour uncomplicated by conditions such as placenta praevia, ante-partum haemorrhage or toxaemia of pregnancy during the third trimester of pregnancy. Once the uterine contractions have ceased and the infusion of Ventolin has been gradually withdrawn, maintenance therapy can be effected with Ventolin Tablets.

Dosage and administration *Ventolin Tablets 2 mg and 4 mg and Syrup: Adults:* The usual effective dose is 4 mg (one tablet 4 mg or 10 ml of syrup) three or four times per day. If adequate bronchodilatation is not obtained each single dose may be gradually increased to as much as 8 mg.

However, it has been established that some patients obtain adequate relief with 2 mg three or four times daily. In elderly patients or in those known to be unusually sensitive to beta-adrenergic stimulant drugs, it is advisable to initiate treatment with 2 mg three or four times per day.

Children: The following doses should be administered three or four times daily:

2–6 years: 1 to 2 mg as 2.5 to 5 ml syrup or half to one tablet 2 mg.

6–12 years: 2 mg as 5 ml Syrup or 1 tablet 2 mg.

Over 12 years: 2 to 4 mg as 5 to 10 ml Syrup or 1 tablet 2 mg or 1 tablet 4 mg.

The drug is well tolerated by children so that, if necessary, these doses may be cautiously increased.

In the management of premature labour, after uterine contractions have been controlled by intravenous infusion of Ventolin and the infusion has been withdrawn, maintenance therapy can be continued with oral Ventolin. The usual dosage is 4 mg three or four times daily.

Contra-indications, warnings, etc
Contra-indications: Although intravenous salbutamol and occasionally salbutamol tablets are used in the management of premature labour, uncomplicated by conditions such as placenta praevia, ante-partum haemorrhage or toxaemia of pregnancy, salbutamol presentations should not be used for threatened abortion during the first or second trimester of pregnancy.

Ventolin oral preparations are contra-indicated in patients with a history of hypersensitivity to any of their components.

Precautions: Salbutamol oral preparations and non-selective beta-blocking drugs, such as propranolol, should not usually be prescribed together.

Salbutamol should be administered cautiously to patients suffering from thyrotoxicosis.

Potentially serious hypokalaemia may result from $beta_2$-agonist therapy. Particular caution is advised in acute severe asthma as this effect may be potentiated by concomitant treatment with xanthine derivatives, steroids, diuretics and by hypoxia. It is recommended that serum potassium levels are monitored in such situations.

Pregnancy: Administration of the drug during pregnancy should only be considered if the expected benefit to the mother is greater than any possible risk to the fetus.

Salbutamol has been in widespread use for many years in human beings without apparent ill consequence; this includes its well established use in the management of premature labour. However, as with the majority of drugs, there is little published evidence of its safety in the early stages of human pregnancy, but in animal studies there was evidence of some harmful effects on the fetus at very high dose levels.

Lactation: As salbutamol is probably secreted in breast milk its use in nursing mothers requires careful consideration. It is not known whether salbutamol has a harmful effect on the neonate and so its use should be restricted to situations where it is felt that the expected benefit to the mother is likely to outweigh any potential risk to the neonate.

Side-effects: Ventolin oral preparations may cause fine tremor of skeletal muscle which occurs in some patients, usually the hands are most obviously affected. This effect is dose related and is common to all beta-adrenergic stimulants. A few patients feel tense; this is also due to the effects on skeletal muscle and not to direct CNS stimulation. With doses of Ventolin higher than those recommended or in patients who are unusually sensitive to beta-adrenergic stimulants, peripheral vasodilatation and a compensatory small increase in heart rate may occur. Occasionally headaches have been reported.

There have been very rare reports of transient muscle cramps. Hypersensitivity reactions including angioedema, urticaria, bronchospasm, hypotension and collapse have been reported very rarely.

Potentially serious hypokalaemia may result from $beta_2$-agonist therapy.

Overdosage: The preferred antidote for overdosage with Ventolin is a cardio-selective beta-blocking agent, but beta-blocking drugs should be used with caution in patients with a history of bronchospasm.

Pharmaceutical precautions *Storage:* Ventolin Tablets 2 mg and 4 mg and Ventolin Syrup should be stored at a temperature not exceeding 30°C. Ventolin Syrup should be protected from light. Ventolin Tablets should be stored in a dry place and the cap replaced securely after use.

Dilution: Ventolin Syrup does not contain sugars. It may be diluted with Purified Water BP. The resulting mixture should be protected from light and used within 28 days. A 50% v/v dilution of Ventolin Syrup has been shown to be adequately preserved against microbial contamination. However, to avoid the possibility of introducing excessive microbial contamination, the Purified Water used for dilution should be recently prepared or alternatively it should be boiled and cooled immediately before use. Dilution of Ventolin Syrup with Syrup BP or Sorbitol solution is not recommended as this may result in precipitation of the cellulose thickening agent. Admixture of Ventolin Syrup with other liquid preparations is not recommended.

Legal category POM.

Package quantities Ventolin Tablets 2 mg are supplied in containers of 100 (OP) and 500.

Ventolin Tablets 4 mg are supplied in containers of 100 (OP) and 500.

Ventolin Syrup is supplied in bottles of 150 ml (OP) and 2 litres.

Further information The Syrup preparation does not contain sugars, so it is unlikely to predispose to dental caries with long-term use.

Ventolin does not cause difficulty in micturition because, unlike sympathomimetic drugs such as ephedrine, it does not stimulate alpha-adrenoceptors.

Ventolin is not contra-indicated in patients under treatment with monoamine oxidase inhibitors (MAOIs).

Product licence numbers

Ventolin Tablets 2 mg	0045/5079R
Ventolin Tablets 4 mg	0045/0088R
Ventolin Syrup	0045/5024R

ZIRTEK* TABLETS

Presentation Zirtek is available as white oblong film-coated tablets, each containing 10 mg cetirizine dihydrochloride. Each tablet is scored and bears the code Y/Y. The tablets are supplied in blister packs.

Uses Cetirizine is a potent antihistamine with a low potential for drowsiness at pharmacologically active doses and with additional anti-allergic properties. It is a selective H_1-antagonist with negligible effects on other receptors and so is virtually free from anti-cholinergic and anti-serotonin effects. Cetirizine inhibits the histamine-mediated 'early' phase of the allergic reaction and also reduces the migration of inflammatory cells and the release of mediators associated with the 'late' allergic response.

Zirtek is indicated for the treatment of perennial rhinitis, seasonal allergic rhinitis (hay fever) and chronic idiopathic urticaria.

Dosage and administration
Adults and children over 12: one 10 mg tablet daily.

At present there are insufficient clinical data to recommend the use of cetirizine in children under the age of 12.

At present there are no data to suggest that the dose need be reduced in elderly patients. In patients with renal insufficiency dosage should be reduced to half a tablet daily.

Contra-indications, warnings, etc
Contra-indications: Zirtek tablets are contra-indicated in patients with a history of hypersensitivity to any of their constituents.

Zirtek is contra-indicated in lactating women since the active ingredient, cetirizine, is excreted in breast milk.

Precautions: Studies in healthy volunteers at 20 and 25 mg/day have not revealed effects on alertness or reaction time, however patients are advised not to exceed the recommended dose if driving or operating machinery.

Pregnancy: No adverse effects have been reported from animal studies. There has been little or no use of Zirtek in pregnancy. As with other drugs the use of Zirtek in pregnancy should be avoided.

Drug interactions: To date, there are no known interactions with other drugs. Studies with diazepam and cimetidine have revealed no evidence of interactions. As with other antihistamines it is advisable to avoid excessive alcohol consumption.

Side-effects: In objective tests of psychomotor function, the incidence of sedation with cetirizine was similar to that of placebo.

There have been occasional reports of mild and transient side effects such as headache, dizziness, drowsiness, agitation, dry mouth and gastro-intestinal discomfort. If desired the dose may be taken as 5 mg in the morning and 5 mg in the evening.

Overdosage: Drowsiness can be a symptom of overdosage, occurring from administration of 50 mg of Zirtek as a single dose. In the case of massive overdosage, gastric lavage should be performed together with the usual supportive measures. To date, there is no specific antidote.

Pharmaceutical precautions Store below 30°C.

Legal category POM.

Package quantities Zirtek tablets are supplied in cartons each containing 30 tablets in blister packs of 10.

Further information Peak blood levels of the order of 0.3 micrograms/ml are reached between thirty and sixty minutes after administration of a 10 mg dose of cetirizine. Its plasma half-life is approximately 11 hours. Absorption is very consistent from one subject to the next. Its renal clearance is 30 ml/minute and the excretion half-life is approximately nine hours. Cetirizine is strongly bound to plasma proteins.

Product licence number 5221/0001.
Product licence holder: UCB S.A., Pharmaceutical Sector, B-1050 Brussels, Belgium.

Distributor Allen & Hanburys Limited, Uxbridge, Middlesex UB11 1BT

**Trade Mark*

Allergan Ltd
Crown Centre
Coronation Road
Cressex Industrial Estate
High Wycombe
Buckinghamshire HP12 3SH

BETAGAN*

Presentation Clear, colourless to light yellow, sterile ophthalmic solution containing levobunolol hydrochloride 0.5% (w/v). Also contains Liquifilm* (Polyvinyl Alcohol USP) 1.4% (w/v), Benzalkonium Chloride PhEur 0.004% (w/v), Disodium Edetate PhEur 0.0127% (w/v), with Sodium Metabisulphite BP, Sodium Phosphate Dibasic USP, Potassium Phosphate Monobasic USP, Sodium Chloride PhEur and Purified Water PhEur.

Uses Betagan is indicated for the reduction of intraocular pressure in chronic open-angle glaucoma and ocular hypertension.

Dosage and administration The usual adult dose is one drop instilled in the affected eye(s) once or twice daily.

In common with other topical ophthalmic beta-adrenergic blocking agents, full clinical response may take several weeks to occur. Intraocular pressure should therefore be measured approximately four weeks after starting treatment. Because of diurnal variations in intraocular pressure, satisfactory response is best determined by measuring the intraocular pressure at different times during the day.

Use in the elderly: The recommended dosage is suitable for use in the elderly.

Use in children: Betagan is not currently recommended for use in children.

Concomitant administration: If the patient's intraocular pressure is not satisfactory on this regimen, concomitant therapy with dipivefrin or adrenaline, and/or pilocarpine and other miotics, and/or systemically administered carbonic anhydrase inhibitors can be instituted.

Contra-indications, warnings, etc
Contra-indications: Bronchial asthma; history of bronchial asthma; chronic obstructive pulmonary disease; sinus bradycardia; second and third degree atrioventricular block; cardiac failure; cardiogenic shock; hypersensitivity to any component.

Warnings: As with other topically applied ophthalmic drugs, Betagan may be absorbed systemically and adverse reactions typical of oral beta-adrenoceptor blocking agents may occur.

Respiratory and cardiac reactions have been reported including, rarely, death due to bronchospasm or associated with cardiac failure.

Congestive heart failure should be adequately controlled before commencing therapy with Betagan. In patients with a history of cardiac disease pulse rates should be monitored.

Diabetic control should be monitored during Betagan therapy in patients with labile diabetes.

Betagan has little or no effect on pupil size and if administered in angle-closure glaucoma, for reduction of intraocular pressure, must only be given in combination with a miotic.

Betagan contains benzalkonium chloride and should not be used in patients continuing to wear soft (hydrophilic) contact lenses.

Use in pregnancy: Betagan has not been studied in human pregnancy. It is recommended that Betagan be avoided in pregnancy.

Use during lactation: If treatment with Betagan during lactation is considered necessary for the benefit of the mother, consideration should be given to the cessation of breast feeding.

Interactions: Use with caution in patients receiving oral beta-adrenergic blocking agents, because of the potential for additive effects on systemic blockade.

Side-effects:

Ocular: Transient burning and stinging on instillation; blepharoconjunctivitis and iridocyclitis have been reported occasionally. The pharmacological and physical properties of levobunolol indicate a potential for post-instillation reduction in corneal sensitivity: this potential has not been confirmed in clinical studies with Betagan.

Cardiovascular: Bradycardia and hypotension have been reported occasionally.

Respiratory: There have been reports of dyspnoea and asthma.

CNS: Headache, transient ataxia and dizziness, and lethargy have been reported occasionally.

Dermatological: Urticaria and pruritis have been rarely reported.

Overdosage: There are no data available on human overdosage with Betagan, which is unlikely to occur via the ocular route. Should accidental ocular overdosage occur, flush the eye(s) with water or normal saline. If accidentally ingested, systemic symptoms may result.

The symptoms associated with systemic overdosage are most likely to be bradycardia, hypotension, bronchospasm and cardiac failure. Therapy for overdosage of a beta-adrenergic blocking agent should be instituted, such as intravenous administration of atropine sulphate 0.25 to 2 mg to induce vagal blockade. Conventional therapy for hypotension, bronchospasm, heart block and cardiac failure may be necessary.

Pharmaceutical precautions Betagan should be stored at room temperature, protected from light. Discard any unused contents 28 days after opening the bottle.

Legal category POM.

Package quantities Betagan is supplied in plastic dropper bottles containing 5 ml of 0.5% w/v solution.

Further information In controlled clinical studies of approximately two years' duration, intraocular pressure was well controlled in approximately 80% of subjects treated with Betagan 0.5% b.i.d. No significant effect on pupil size, tear production or corneal sensitivity was observed.

In a 3 month study, one drop once-a-day of Betagan 0.5% controlled intraocular pressure in 72% of subjects.

The onset of action is detected within one hour of instillation, with maximum effect seen between 2 and 6 hours. A significant decrease in intraocular pressure can be maintained for up to 24 hours following a single dose.

Diminished response after prolonged therapy has been reported in some patients.

Betagan reduces intraocular pressure with little or no effect on pupil size or accommodation, so the blurred vision and night blindness associated with miotics would not be expected and have not been reported with use of Betagan. This is particularly important in cataract patients with central lens opacities who experience decreased visual acuity with pupillary constriction on miotic therapy.

Product licence number 0426/0060.

EPIFRIN* 1%

Presentation Clear, colourless to very slightly straw coloured, sterile, aqueous ophthalmic solution containing 1.0% (w/v) Adrenaline BP, present as the hydrochloride. Also contains Benzalkonium Chloride PhEur 0.004% (w/v), Disodium Edetate PhEur 0.00127% (w/v) with Sodium Metabisulphite BP and Purified Water PhEur.

Uses For the treatment of primary open angle glaucoma. It may be used in conjunction with miotic or carbonic anhydrase inhibitor therapy.

Dosage and administration The usual dosage is one drop in the affected eye(s) once or twice daily. The dosage should be adjusted to meet the needs of the individual patient.

Contra-indications, warnings, etc
Contra-indications: Epifrin should not be used in the presence of a narrow angle between the iris and cornea as pupillary dilation may precipitate angle closure.

Topical adrenaline has been shown occasionally to cause macular oedema in aphakic eyes and thus the use of adrenaline-containing eyedrops in aphakic patients is not recommended.

Use in pregnancy: The safety of intensive or protracted use of adrenaline therapy during pregnancy has not been substantiated.

Precautions: Systemic effects of topical adrenaline therapy may exacerbate the clinical condition of patients with thyrotoxicosis, hypertension or cardiovascular disease, including tachycardia.

This product contains benzalkonium chloride and should not be used by patients continuing to wear soft (hydrophilic) contact lenses.

Side-effects:

Ocular: Ocular discomfort, irritation and red eye have been reported. As with other adrenaline preparations adrenochrome deposits in the conjunctiva and cornea have been reported occasionally following prolonged therapy.

CNS: Headache has been reported rarely.

Skin: Rare reports of local skin reactions.

Pharmaceutical precautions Protect from light and excessive heat. If the solution discolours or a precipitate forms it should be discarded. Discard any unused contents 28 days after opening the bottle.

Legal category P.

Package quantities Epifrin 1% is available in a 10 ml plastic dropper bottle.

Further information Adrenaline appears to exert its therapeutic effect by decreasing aqueous production and enhancing outflow facility. Unlike cholinergic agents, adrenaline has little or no effect on pupil size or accommodation, so the blurred vision and night blindness associated with miotics do not occur with Epifrin. This is particularly important in cataract patients with central lens opacities who experience decreased visual acuity with pupillary constriction on miotic therapy.

Product licence number 0426/0018R.

FML*

Presentation White, microfine, sterile ophthalmic suspension of Fluorometholone USP 0.1% (w/v). Contains Liquifilm* (Polyvinyl Alcohol USP) 1.4% (w/v), Disodium Edetate PhEur 0.127% (w/v), Benzalkonium Chloride PhEur 0.004% (w/v), with Polysorbate 80 BP, Sodium Phosphate PhEur, Sodium Chloride PhEur and Purified Water PhEur.

Uses Topical ophthalmic suspension for steroid responsive inflammation of the palpebral and bulbar conjunctiva, cornea and anterior segment of the globe.

Dosage and administration 1 to 2 drops instilled into the conjunctival sac two to four times daily. During the initial 24 to 48 hours the dosage may be safely increased to 2 drops every hour. Care should be taken not to discontinue therapy prematurely.

Contra-indications, warnings, etc
Contra-indications: Acute superficial herpes simplex (dendritic) keratitis, vaccinia, varicella and most other viral diseases of the conjunctiva and cornea. Ocular tuberculosis. Fungal diseases of the eye. Hypersensitivity to any of the constituents of the medication.

Warnings: Steroid medication in the treatment of herpes simplex keratitis (involving the stroma) requires great caution: frequent slit-lamp microscopy is mandatory. Prolonged use may result in glaucoma, damage to the optic nerve, defects in visual acuity and fields of vision, posterior subcapsular cataract formation, or may aid in the establishment of secondary ocular infections from fungi or viruses liberated from ocular tissue.

In those diseases causing thinning of the cornea or sclera, perforation has been known to occur with use of topical steroids.

Safety and effectiveness have not been demonstrated in children of the age group two years or below.

This preparation contains benzalkonium chloride and should not be used by patients continuing to wear soft (hydrophilic) contact lenses.

Use in pregnancy: There is inadequate evidence of safety in human pregnancy. Administration of corticosteroids to pregnant animals can cause abnormalities of foetal development including cleft palate and intra-uterine growth retardation. There may therefore be a very small risk of such effects in the human foetus.

Precautions: As fungal infections of the cornea are particularly prone to develop coincidentally with long-term local steroid applications, fungus invasion must be suspected in any persistent corneal ulceration where a steroid has been used or is in use.

Intraocular pressure should be checked frequently.

Side-effects: Glaucoma with optic nerve damage, visual acuity or field defects, posterior subcapsular cataract formation, secondary ocular infection from pathogens liberated from ocular tissues, perforation of the globe.

Local side-effects of steroid therapy, i.e. skin atrophy, striae and telangiectasia, are especially likely to affect facial skin.

Pharmaceutical precautions Protect from freezing. Discard any unused contents 28 days after opening the bottle.

Legal category POM.

Package quantities Supplied in plastic dropper bottles containing 5 ml and 10 ml.

Further information Nil.

Product licence number 0426/0028.

FML-NEO*

Presentation White, microfine, sterile ophthalmic suspension of Fluorometholone USP 0.1% (w/v) and Neomycin Sulphate PhEur 0.5% (w/v) (equivalent to 0.35% neomycin base). Also contains Liquifilm* (Polyvinyl Alcohol USP) 1.4% (w/v), Disodium Edetate PhEur 0.127% (w/v), Benzalkonium Chloride PhEur 0.004% (w/v), with Polysorbate 80 BP, Sodium Phosphate PhEur, Sodium Chloride PhEur, Sodium Thiosulphate BP and Purified Water PhEur.

Uses FML-Neo is indicated for use in the following situations:

1. In the treatment of infectious conjunctivitis due to organisms sensitive to neomycin;

2. For the treatment of corneal and anterior segment inflammatory disorders which may be threatened with, or complicated by, organisms sensitive to neomycin;

3. Prophylactically following removal of foreign bodies, as well as before and after surgery, where the possibility exists of infection with susceptible organisms.

Dosage and administration One to two drops in the conjunctival sac two to four times daily. During the initial 24 to 48 hours, the dosage may be safely increased to one drop every hour. Care should be taken not to discontinue treatment prematurely.

Contra-indications, warnings, etc
Contra-indications: Acute untreated purulent ocular infections. Acute superficial herpes simplex (dendritic) keratitis, vaccinia, varicella and most other viral diseases of the conjunctiva and cornea. Ocular tuberculosis. Fungal diseases of the eye. Hypersensitivity to any of the constituents of the medication.

Warnings: In diseases due to micro-organisms resistant to neomycin, infection may be masked, enhanced or activated by the steroid. Prolonged use may result in overgrowth of nonsusceptible organisms.

If sensitivity or other untoward reactions occur, discontinue the medication.

As fungal infections of the cornea have been reported coincidentally with long-term steroid applications, fungal invasion may be suspected in any persistent corneal ulceration where a steroid has been used, or is in use, over a prolonged period of time.

Use of steroid medication in the presence of stromal herpes simplex requires great caution; frequent slit lamp microscopy is required.

This preparation contains benzalkonium chloride and should not be used by patients continuing to wear soft (hydrophilic) contact lenses.

Use in pregnancy: There is inadequate evidence of safety in human pregnancy. Administration of corticosteroids to pregnant animals can cause abnormalities of foetal development including cleft palate and intra-uterine growth retardation. There may therefore be a very small risk of such effects in the human foetus.

Precautions: Patients with a history of herpes simplex keratitis should be treated with caution.

Use of topical steroids may increase intraocular pressure. Eye drops containing corticosteroids should not be used for more than one week except under strict ophthalmic supervision with regular determination of intraocular pressure.

Articles in current medical literature indicate an increase in the prevalence of persons sensitive to neomycin. The possibility of such a reaction should be borne in mind.

Side-effects: In those diseases causing thinning of the cornea, perforation has been known to have occurred with the use of topical steroids.

Acute purulent untreated infections of the eye may be masked, enhanced or activated by the presence of steroid medication. Secondary ocular infection may occur from pathogens liberated from ocular tissues.

Reports in the literature indicate that posterior subcapsular lenticular opacities have occurred after heavy or protracted use of topical ophthalmic corticosteroids.

Local side effects of steroid therapy, i.e. skin atrophy, striae and telangiectasia, are especially likely to affect facial skin.

Pharmaceutical precautions Shake well before using. Do not freeze. Discard any unused contents 28 days after opening the bottle.

Legal category POM.

Package quantities Available in plastic dropper bottles containing 5 ml.

Further information Nil.

Product licence number 0426/0043.

KERECID* OPHTHALMIC SOLUTION

Presentation A clear, colourless and odourless aqueous ophthalmic solution of Idoxuridine PhEur 0.1% (w/v). Also contains Liquifilm* (Polyvinyl Alcohol USP) 1.4% (w/v), Disodium Edetate PhEur 0.0127% (w/v), Benzalkonium Chloride PhEur 0.004% (w/v), with Sodium Chloride PhEur and Purified Water PhEur.

Uses Kerecid is an antiviral agent for the treatment of keratitis caused by the herpes simplex virus and other DNA viruses sensitive to idoxuridine.

Dosage and administration Adults and children.

For optimal results, the infected tissues should be kept 'saturated' with Kerecid. One of the following schedules is recommended:

1. Instil one drop in the infected eye(s) every hour during the day. At night, the dosage may be reduced to one drop every other hour.

2. Instil one drop every minute for 5 minutes. This schedule should be repeated every 4 hours – night and day.

To minimise recurrences, continue treatment for five to seven days after healing appears to be complete, that is, after complete loss of corneal staining with fluorescein. Treatment should not usually be continued for more than 21 days.

Observe patients frequently during treatment. Improvement in dendritic keratitis and other superficial infections is generally seen within a week, but may occasionally occur much earlier. Some strains of herpes simplex virus appear resistant to the action of idoxuridine. If superficial infections show no sign of improvement after seven to eight days, alternative treatment is indicated. A faint dendritic pattern in the deeper epithelial layers that neither stains nor produces symptoms may persist for two to four weeks. This does not indicate failure of treatment or a need for continued therapy.

Antibiotics may be used to control secondary infections; and atropine preparations may be given if needed. Do not, however, mix Kerecid with these adjuvant medications.

Contra-indications, warnings, etc
Contra-indications: Hypersensitivity to the active ingredient or other components of this medication. Do not administer boric acid during treatment as it may cause irritation in the presence of Kerecid.

Warnings: Kerecid contains benzalkonium chloride and should not be used by patients continuing to wear soft (hydrophilic) contact lenses.

Use in pregnancy: In common with other antiviral agents, idoxuridine is potentially mutagenic. There is some evidence from animal studies that idoxuridine may be embryotoxic, but there is no clinical evidence of any hazard to the foetus in human use arising from over 20 years clinical experience. Kerecid should not be administered in pregnancy, especially during the first trimester, and should be administered to women of childbearing potential only if adequate contraceptive precautions are taken.

Precautions: Caution is required with concomitant use of topical corticosteroids which may encourage the spread of viral infection. They should not be used in the presence of active corneal ulceration, but may be considered when the stromal disease seriously affects vision, or when oedema or uveitis is present. Kerecid should be continued for several days after corticosteroid treatment has been completed.

Adverse reactions: Transient irritation and pain on administration may occur; itching, inflammation, oedema and, rarely, allergic reactions and occlusion of the lachrymal punctum have been reported.

Overdosage: Excessive use may damage the corneal epithelium. Toxic effects are unlikely to follow ingestion.

Pharmaceutical precautions Store at controlled room temperature (15–30°C) and protect from light. The contents are sterile until the pack is opened; discard any unused contents 28 days after opening.

Legal category POM.

Package quantities Polythene bottle with integral dropper, containing 15 ml.

Further information Nil.

Product licence number 0426/0019R

LACRI-LUBE*

Presentation Off-white, smooth, preservative-free, sterile ophthalmic ointment containing white petrolatum, mineral oil and non-ionic lanolin derivatives.

Uses Useful as adjunctive therapy to lubricate and protect the eye in conditions such as exposure keratitis, decreased corneal sensitivity, recurrent corneal erosions, keratitis sicca, and also in ophthalmic surgery and non-ophthalmic surgery.

Dosage and administration For topical administration. Pull lower lid down to form a pocket and apply a small amount as required. There is no variation of dosage for age.

Contra-indications, warnings, etc No known contra-indications.

Pharmaceutical precautions Store away from heat. To avoid contamination during use, do not touch tip to any surface.

Legal category P.

Package quantities Lacri-Lube is available in 3.5 g and 5 g ophthalmic ointment tubes.

Further information Dry eye symptoms commonly persist at night – Lacri-Lube has been specifically formulated to lubricate and protect the dry eye during sleep.

Lacri-Lube can provide prophylactic ocular care during general surgical procedures as an adjunct to taping of the eyelids.

Product licence number 0426/0041.

LIQUIFILM* TEARS

Presentation Clear, colourless to slightly straw-coloured, sterile, aqueous ophthalmic solution containing Liquifilm* (Polyvinyl Alcohol USP) 1.4% (w/v). Also contains Disodium Edetate PhEur 0.015% (w/v), Benzalkonium Chloride PhEur 0.005% (w/v) with Sodium Chloride PhEur, Sodium Phosphate PhEur, and Purified Water PhEur.

Uses Liquifilm Tears is an ocular lubricant for the relief of dry eye and dry eye symptoms.

Dosage and administration For all ages. One or two drops administered topically to the affected eye(s) as required.

Contra-indications, warnings, etc
Contra-indications: Sensitivity to any of the components. Not for use with soft (hydrophilic) contact lenses because of the presence of benzalkonium chloride as a preservative.

Warnings: If irritation increases or persists, discontinue use.

Pharmaceutical precautions Store at room temperature. Discard any unused contents 28 days after opening the bottle.

Legal category P.

Package quantities Liquifilm Tears is available in plastic dropper bottles containing 15 ml.

Further information Liquifilm Tears (polyvinyl alcohol) lowers the surface tension at the surface of the corneal epithelium, providing a lubricant layer which enhances patient comfort. Liquifilm Tears can help to restore normal tear film tonicity and to act as a wetting agent for lipid-, aqueous- and mucin-deficient eyes.

Product licence number 0426/0009R.

PRED FORTE*

Presentation White, microfine, sterile ophthalmic suspension containing Prednisolone Acetate USP 1.0% (w/v). Also contains Benzalkonium Chloride PhEur 0.006% (w/v) and Disodium Edetate PhEur 0.0127% (w/v), with Hydroxypropylmethylcellulose PhEur, Polysorbate 80 BP, Boric Acid BP, Sodium Citrate PhEur, Sodium Chloride PhEur and Purified Water PhEur.

Uses For short-term treatment of steroid-responsive inflammatory conditions of the eye, after excluding the presence of viral, fungal and bacterial pathogens.

Dosage and administration One to two drops instilled into the conjunctival sac two to four times daily. During the initial 24–48 hours the dosage may be safely increased to 2 drops every hour. Care should be taken not to discontinue therapy prematurely.

Contra-indications, warnings, etc
Contra-indications: Acute untreated purulent ocular infections. Acute superficial herpes simplex (dendritic) keratitis, vaccinia, varicella and most other viral diseases of the cornea and conjunctiva. Fungal diseases of the eye. Ocular tuberculosis. Sensitivity to any component of the formulation.

Warnings: Acute purulent infections of the eye may be masked or enhanced by the use of topical steroids. Pred Forte contains no antimicrobial agent. If infection is present, appropriate measures must be taken to counteract the infective organisms.

Fungal infections of the cornea have been reported coincidentally with long-term steroid application, and fungal invasion may be suspected in any persistent corneal ulceration where a steroid has been used, or is in use.

Various ocular diseases and long-term use of topical corticosteroids have been known to cause corneal or scleral thinning. Use of topical corticosteroids in the presence of thin corneal or scleral tissue may lead to perforation.

Pred Forte contains benzalkonium chloride as a preservative and should not be used in patients continuing to wear soft (hydrophilic) contact lenses.

Use in pregnancy: There is inadequate evidence of safety in human pregnancy. Administration of corticosteroids to pregnant animals can cause abnormalities of foetal development including cleft palate and intra-uterine growth retardation. There may therefore be a very small risk of such effects in the human foetus.

Precautions: Patients with a history of herpes simplex keratitis should be treated with caution. Use of steroid medication in the presence of stromal herpes simplex requires caution and should be followed by frequent, mandatory, slit lamp microscopy.

Use of topical corticosteroids may cause an increase in intraocular pressure in certain individuals. This may result in damage to the optic nerve with resultant defects in visual fields. It is advisable that intraocular pressure be checked frequently during treatment with Pred Forte.

Side-effects:

Ocular: Increased intraocular pressure; secondary ocular infections from fungi or viruses liberated from ocular tissues; perforation of the globe when used in conditions where there is a thinning of the cornea or sclera.

Posterior subcapsular cataract formation has been reported after heavy or protracted use of topical ophthalmic corticosteroids.

Systemic: Extensive topical use of corticosteroids may lead to systemic side effects.

Overdosage: There is no clinical experience of overdosage. Acute overdosage is unlikely to occur via the ophthalmic route.

Pharmaceutical precautions Protect from freezing. Shake the bottle well before use. Discard any unused contents 28 days after opening the bottle.

Legal category POM.

Package quantities Plastic dropper bottle containing 5 ml or 10 ml.

Further information Ocular steroid preparations may be differentiated by the basic potency of the steroid and by the chemical derivative used in the formulation. Alternative chemical forms of the same steroid can give rise to marked differences in steroid concentrations in aqueous humour. Pred Forte contains prednisolone, a relatively mild steroid, which, due to the presence of the acetate group, has been shown to possess excellent corneal penetrative properties.

Product licence number 0426/0051.

PROPINE*

Presentation Sterile ophthalmic solution containing Dipivefrin Hydrochloride USP 0.1% (w/v). Also contains Benzalkonium Chloride PhEur 0.005% (w/v), Disodium Edetate PhEur 0.015% (w/v), with Sodium Chloride PhEur and Purified Water PhEur.

Uses Propine is indicated for the reduction of intraocular pressure in chronic open angle glaucoma or ocular hypertensive patients with anterior chamber open angles.

Dosage and administration The usual dosage is one drop in the affected eye(s) every 12 hours.

Contra-indications, warnings, etc
Contra-indications: Patients suffering from closed angle glaucoma.

Use in pregnancy: The safety of the intensive or protracted use of dipivefrin during pregnancy has not been substantiated.

Precautions: Dipivefrin should be used with caution in patients with narrow angles since dilation of the pupil may trigger an attack of angle closure glaucoma.

Macular oedema is a rare occurrence with adrenaline use in aphakic patients. Prompt reversal generally follows discontinuance of the drug. Macular oedema with dipivefrin does present as a possibility in the aphakic patient.

This product contains benzalkonium chloride and should not be used by patients continuing to wear soft (hydrophilic) contact lenses.

Side-effects:

Cardiovascular: Tachycardia, arrhythmias and hypertension have been reported with ocular administration of adrenaline, and may occur rarely with Propine therapy.

Ocular: The most frequently reported side effects are conjunctival injection, and burning and stinging on instillation.

Rebound vasodilation, mydriasis and allergic reactions, including blepharoconjunctivitis, have been reported occasionally.

Adrenochrome deposits in the conjunctiva and cornea have been associated rarely with use of dipivefrin.

Follicular conjunctivitis has been reported during long term therapy with Propine. The condition is reversible upon discontinuance of the drug.

Pharmaceutical precautions Store at room temperature. Discard any unused contents 28 days after opening the bottle.

Legal category POM.

Package quantities Plastic dropper bottles containing 5 ml or 10 ml.

Further information The active ingredient in Propine, dipivefrin HCl, is a prodrug of adrenaline. Its lipophilic nature facilitates penetration into the anterior chamber where it is hydrolysed to the active substance. Propine is a more efficient way of delivering adrenaline with fewer side effects than associated with conventional therapy. Unlike cholinergic agents, dipivefrin has little or no effect on pupil size or accommodation, so the blurred vision and night blindness associated with miotics do not occur with Propine.

Product licence number 0426/0040.

**Trade Mark*

Alpha Therapeutic UK Limited
Howlett Way
Fison Way Industrial Estate
Thetford
Norfolk IP24 1HZ

ALBUTEIN* 5%

Presentation Albutein 5% is Albumin Solution BP 5% and each 100 ml of solution contains 5 g of human serum albumin. It is a clear, almost colourless to amber sterile aqueous solution for single dose intravenous administration.

Uses Albumin is a highly soluble globular protein (MW 66,500) which is important in regulating the osmotic pressure of plasma. Albutein 5% solution supplies the oncotic equivalent of approximately its own volume of normal human plasma and will increase the circulating plasma volume by an amount equal to the volume infused. The degree and duration of volume expansion depend upon the initial blood volume. The effect of infused albumin persists longer in patients with diminished blood volume than in individuals with normal blood volume. Albumin is also a transport protein and binds naturally occurring, therapeutic and toxic materials in the circulation. The binding properties of albumin may in special circumstances provide an indication for its clinical use. For such purposes, however, Albutein 20% or Albutein 25% should be used.

Albutein 5% is indicated:
(i) For the treatment of hypovolaemic shock.
(ii) In conditions in which there is severe hypoalbuminaemia. However unless the pathologic condition responsible for the hypoalbuminaemia can be corrected, administration of albumin can afford only symptomatic or supportive relief.
(iii) For the treatment of burns.
(iv) As an adjunct in cardiopulmonary bypass procedures.

In those conditions in which the colloid requirement is high and there is less need for fluid, albumin should be administered as the 20% or 25% solutions.

Dosage and administration Albutein 5% is intended for intravenous administration. The total dosage will vary with the individual.

Adults: An initial infusion of 500 ml is suggested. This may be repeated in 15–30 minutes if the initial dose is inadequate. Additional amounts should be administered as clinically indicated.

The rate of administration should be 1–2 ml per minute in patients with slightly low or normal blood volume. In patients with shock and/or greatly reduced blood volume, Albutein 5% may be administered as rapidly as necessary.

Children: Dosage will vary with clinical state and body weight. A dose of one-quarter to one-half of the adult dose may be administered or dosage may be calculated on the basis of 3–5 ml per kilogram of body weight. The rate of administration should be calculated on one-quarter of the adult rate.

Contra-indications, warnings, etc Albutein 5% is contra-indicated in patients with severe anaemia or cardiac failure in the presence of normal or increased intravascular volume and in patients with a history of allergic reactions to albumin products.

Albutein 5% should be administered with caution to patients with low cardiac reserve. Additional fluids may be required for patients with marked dehydration. Rapid infusion may cause vascular overload with resultant pulmonary oedema. Patients should be closely monitored for signs of increased venous pressure. A rapid rise in blood pressure following infusion necessitates careful observation of injured or postoperative patients to detect and treat severed blood vessels that may not have bled at a lower pressure.

Do not use for control of haemorrhage due to deficiencies or defects in the clotting mechanism. The product is not intended for use in dialysis patients or in premature infants.

Albumin naturally binds a variety of therapeutic and toxic materials and thus administration of Albutein 5% may modify the pre-existing distribution of certain substances.

Adverse reactions are rare. However allergic or pyrogenic reactions, characterised primarily by fever and chills, nausea, vomiting, tachycardia and hypotension have been reported.

If such reactions occur the infusion should be discontinued and appropriate therapy (e.g. antihistamine) or specific support treatment should be given.

Reproduction studies have not been conducted with albumin. Human albumin should be given to a pregnant woman only if clearly needed.

Administration of large quantities of albumin may require supplementation with red cell concentrates to help overcome any resulting relative anaemia.

Pharmaceutical precautions Do not use if the solution appears turbid or contains a deposit. Since the solution does not contain a preservative it should be used within 3 hours of penetration of the container. Discard any unused portion.

Do not administer protein hydrolysates or alcohol via the same administration set used for Albutein 5%.

Albutein 5% should be stored between 2° and 25°C protected from light.

Legal category POM.

Package quantities Albutein 5% is supplied in:
250 ml glass vials containing 12.5 g albumin.
500 ml glass vials containing 25.0 g albumin.

Further information Albutein 5% is prepared from plasma obtained from carefully selected and rigorously screened donors. The final product is heated at 60°C for 10 hours. However as with all blood products the risk of viral transmission with this product cannot be absolutely excluded. Nevertheless there are no known cases of viral transmission resulting from the administration of Albutein 5%.

Product licence number 4447/0007.

ALBUTEIN* 20%

Presentation Albutein 20% is Albumin Solution BP 20% and each 100 ml of solution contains 20 g of human serum albumin. It is a clear, almost colourless to amber sterile aqueous solution for single dose intravenous administration.

Uses Albumin is a highly soluble globular protein (MW 66,500) which is important in regulating the osmotic pressure of plasma. Albutein 20% solution supplies the oncotic equivalent of approximately 4 times its own volume of normal human plasma. It will increase the circulating plasma volume by an amount approximately 2.5 times the volume infused within 15 minutes, if the recipient is adequately hydrated. The degree and duration of volume expansion depend upon the initial blood volume. The effect of infused albumin persists longer in patients with diminished blood volume than in individuals with normal blood volume. Albumin is also a transport protein and binds naturally occurring, therapeutic and toxic materials in the circulation. The binding properties of albumin may in special circumstances provide an indication for its clinical use.

Albutein 20% is indicated:

(i) For the treatment of hypovolaemic shock.

(ii) In conditions in which there is severe hypoalbuminaemia. However unless the pathologic condition responsible for the hypoalbuminaemia can be corrected, administration of albumin can afford only symptomatic or supportive relief.

(iii) For the treatment of burns.

(iv) As an adjunct in cardiopulmonary bypass procedures.

(v) In conjunction with exchange transfusion in the treatment of neonatal hyperbilirubinaemia.

Dosage and administration Albutein 20% is intended for intravenous administration. The total dosage will vary with the individual.

Adults: An initial infusion of 100 ml is suggested for Albutein 20%. This may be repeated in 15–30 minutes if the initial dose is inadequate. Additional amounts should be administered as clinically indicated.

The rate of administration should be 1 ml per minute in patients with slightly low or normal blood volume. In patients with shock and/or greatly reduced blood volume, Albutein 20% may be administered as rapidly as necessary.

Children: Dosage will vary with clinical state and body weight. Dosage may be calculated on the basis of 1 ml per kilogram body weight for Albutein 20%.

The rate of administration should be calculated on one-quarter to one-half of the adult rate.

Contra-indications, warnings, etc Albutein 20% is contra-indicated in patients with severe anaemia or cardiac failure in the presence of normal or increased intravascular volume and in patients with a history of allergic reactions to albumin products.

Albutein 20% should be administered with caution to patients with low cardiac reserve. Additional fluids may be required for patients with marked dehydration. Rapid infusion may cause vascular overload with resultant pulmonary oedema. Patients should be closely monitored for signs of increased venous pressure. A rapid rise in blood pressure following infusion necessitates careful observation of injured or postoperative patients to detect and treat severed blood vessels that may not have bled at a lower pressure.

Do not use for control of haemorrhage due to deficiencies or defects in the clotting mechanism. The product is not intended for use in dialysis patients or in premature infants.

Albumin naturally binds a variety of therapeutic and toxic materials and thus administration of Albutein 20% may modify the pre-existing distribution of certain substances.

Adverse reactions are rare. However allergic or pyrogenic reactions, characterised primarily by fever and chills, nausea, vomiting, tachycardia and hypotension have been reported.

If such reactions occur the infusion should be discontinued and appropriate therapy (e.g. antihistamine) or specific support treatment should be given.

Reproduction studies have not been conducted with albumin. Human albumin should be given to a pregnant woman only if clearly needed.

Administration of large quantities of albumin may require supplementation with red cell concentrates to help overcome any resulting relative anaemia.

Pharmaceutical precautions Do not use if the solution appears turbid or contains a deposit. Since the solution does not contain a preservative it should be used within 3 hours of penetration of the container. Discard any unused portion.

Do not administer protein hydrolysates or alcohol via the same administration set used for Albutein 20%.

Albutein 20% should be stored between 2° and 25°C protected from light.

Legal category POM.

Package quantities Albutein 20% is supplied in:
50 ml glass vials containing 10 g of albumin.
100 ml glass vials containing 20 g of albumin.

Further information Albutein 20% is prepared from plasma obtained from carefully selected and rigorously screened donors. The final product is heated at 60°C for 10 hours. However as with all blood products the risk of viral transmission with this product cannot be absolutely excluded. Nevertheless there are no known cases of viral transmission resulting from the administration of Albutein 20%.

Product licence number 4447/0008.

ALBUTEIN* 25%

Presentation Albutein 25% is Albumin Solution BP 25% and each 100 ml of solution contains 25 g of human serum albumin. It is a clear, almost colourless to amber sterile aqueous solution for single dose intravenous administration.

Uses Albumin is a highly soluble globular protein (MW 66,500) which is important in regulating the osmotic pressure of plasma. Albutein 25% solution supplies the oncotic equivalent of approximately 5 times its own volume of normal human plasma. It will increase the circulating plasma volume by an amount approximately 3.5 times the volume infused within 15 minutes, if the recipient is adequately hydrated. The degree and duration of volume expansion depend upon the initial blood volume. The effect of infused albumin persists longer in patients with diminished blood volume than in individuals with normal blood volume. Albumin is also a transport protein and binds naturally occurring, therapeutic and toxic materials in the circulation. The binding properties of albumin may in special circumstances provide an indication for its clinical use.

Albutein 25% is indicated:

(i) For the treatment of hypovolaemic shock.

(ii) In conditions in which there is severe hypoalbuminaemia. However unless the pathologic condition responsible for the hypoalbuminaemia can be corrected, administration of albumin can afford only symptomatic or supportive relief.

(iii) For the treatment of burns.

(iv) As an adjunct in cardiopulmonary bypass procedures.

(v) In conjunction with exchange transfusion in the treatment of neonatal hyperbilirubinaemia.

Dosage and administration Albutein 25% is intended for intravenous administration. The total dosage will vary with the individual.

Adults: An initial infusion of 100 ml is suggested for Albutein 25%. This may be repeated in 15–30 minutes if the initial dose is inadequate. Additional amounts should be administered as clinically indicated.

The rate of administration should be 1 ml per minute in patients with slightly low or normal blood volume. In patients with shock and/or greatly reduced blood volume, Albutein 25% may be administered as rapidly as necessary.

Children: Dosage will vary with clinical state and body weight. Dosage may be calculated on the basis of 1 ml per kilogram body weight for Albutein 25%.

The rate of administration should be calculated on one-quarter to one-half of the adult rate.

Contra-indications, warnings, etc Albutein 25% is

contra-indicated in patients with severe anaemia or cardiac failure in the presence of normal or increased intravascular volume and in patients with a history of allergic reactions to albumin products.

Albutein 25% should be administered with caution to patients with low cardiac reserve. Additional fluids may be required for patients with marked dehydration. Rapid infusion may cause vascular overload with resultant pulmonary oedema. Patients should be closely monitored for signs of increased venous pressure. A rapid rise in blood pressure following infusion necessitates careful observation of injured or postoperative patients to detect and treat severed blood vessels that may not have bled at a lower pressure.

Do not use for control of haemorrhage due to deficiencies or defects in the clotting mechanism. The product is not intended for use in dialysis patients or in premature infants.

Albumin naturally binds a variety of therapeutic and toxic materials and thus administration of Albutein 25% may modify the pre-existing distribution of certain substances.

Adverse reactions are rare. However allergic or pyrogenic reactions, characterised primarily by fever and chills, nausea, vomiting, tachycardia and hypotension have been reported.

If such reactions occur the infusion should be discontinued and appropriate therapy (e.g. antihistamine) or specific support treatment should be given.

Reproduction studies have not been conducted with albumin. Human albumin should be given to a pregnant woman only if clearly needed.

Administration of large quantities of albumin may require supplementation with red cell concentrates to help overcome any resulting relative anaemia.

Pharmaceutical precautions Do not use if the solution appears turbid or contains a deposit. Since the solution does not contain a preservative it should be used within 3 hours of penetration of the container. Discard any unused portion.

Do not administer protein hydrolysates or alcohol via the same administration set used for Albutein 25%.

Albutein 25% should be stored between 2° and 25°C protected from light.

Legal category POM.

Package quantities Albutein 25% is supplied in:
20 ml glass vials containing 5 g of albumin.
50 ml glass vials containing 12.5 g of albumin.
100 ml glass vials containing 25 g of albumin.

Further information Albutein 25% is prepared from plasma obtained from carefully selected and rigorously screened donors. The final product is heated at 60°C for 10 hours. However as with all blood products the risk of viral transmission with this product cannot be absolutely excluded. Nevertheless there are no known cases of viral transmission resulting from the administration of Albutein 25%.

Product licence number 4447/0009.

FLUOSOL* ▼

Presentation Fluosol (20% Intravascular Perfluorochemical Emulsion) is a stable, white emulsion of perfluorodecalin (Perflunafene, INN) and perfluorotri-n-propylamine (Perfluamine INN) in Water for Injection. The formulation is a sterile, non-pyrogenic fluid intended for intravascular administration.

Fluosol consists of three separate parts which must be mixed prior to use: (1) the Fluosol emulsion; (2) Solution 1; and (3) Solution 2. The additive solutions serve to adjust pH, ionic strength and osmotic pressure in the final 20% emulsion, and must be added separately and sequentially prior to administration. The Fluosol emulsion is supplied as a 400 ml volume in a 500 ml flexible plastic container. Solutions 1 and 2 are supplied in glass vials, 30 ml and 70 ml, respectively, as sterile, non-pyrogenic aqueous solutions.

The quantitative composition of each of the constituents is shown below:

Fluosol Emulsion		*g/100 ml*
Perfluorodecalin (Perflunafene)		17.5
Perfluorotri-n-propylamine (Perfluamine)		7.5
Poloxamer 188		3.4
Glycerin (Glycerol)		1.0
Egg Yolk Phospholipid		0.5
Potassium Oleate		0.04
Water for Injection		qs
Solution 1	*%w/v*	*g/30 ml*
Sodium Bicarbonate	3.5	1.05
Potassium Chloride	0.56	0.168
Water for Injection	qs	qs

The pH of Solution 1 is adjusted with carbon dioxide gas.

Solution 2	*%w/v*	*g/70 ml*
Sodium Chloride	4.29	3.004
Dextrose (Glucose)	1.29	0.901
Magnesium Chloride hexahydrate	0.305	0.214
Calcium Chloride dihydrate	0.254	0.178
Water for Injection	qs	qs

When the Fluosol emulsion and the two solutions are mixed for administration the resultant composition is as follows:

Composition of Fluosol when prepared for administration

Ingredient	*g/100 ml*
Perfluorodecalin (Perflunafene)	14.0
Perfluorotri-n-propylamine (Perfluamine)	6.0
Poloxamer 188	2.72
Glycerin (Glycerol)	0.80
Sodium Chloride	0.60
Egg Yolk Phospholipid	0.40
Sodium Bicarbonate	0.21
Dextrose (Glucose)	0.18
Magnesium Chloride hexahydrate	0.043
Calcium Chloride dihydrate	0.036
Potassium Chloride	0.034
Potassium Oleate	0.032
Water for Injection	qs

The concentration of electrolytes in the final 20% emulsion when prepared for administration is as follows:

Electrolyte	*mEq/litre*	*mmol/litre*
Sodium (Na^+)	127.6	127.6
Potassium (K^+)	5.5	5.5
Calcium (Ca^{++})	4.8	2.4
Magnesium (Mg^{++})	4.2	2.1
Chloride (Cl^-)	116.2	116.2
Bicarbonate (HCO_3^-)	25.0	25.0

Fluosol has an osmolarity of approximately 410 mosmol/litre and contains emulsified perfluorochemical particles with a mean particle diameter of less than 270 nm as determined by laser light scattering spectrophotometry. The content of particles greater than 400 nm is less than 10%. The pH of the emulsion when prepared for administration is approximately 7.3. The fluoride ion content is less than 2 ppm.

Uses *Action:* Fluosol functions as an acellular oxygen transport emulsion and is intended for use as a hypoxia modifying agent. Prior to use the perfluorochemical emulsion is mixed with the salt Solutions 1 and 2, oxygenated and warmed to 37°C. The Fluosol perfluorochemical emulsion particles are the active constituent. They absorb, transport and release the physiologically important gases oxygen and carbon dioxide. The solubilities of these gases at 37°C and at a partial pressure of oxygen (pO_2) of 760 mmHg, are 7 volumes % and 66 volumes % respectively. The dissociation curves for both gases are linear. The amount of gas dissolved in Fluosol is a direct function of the partial pressure of that gas. The oxygen transport properties of Fluosol are due to loading of oxygen at a high partial pressure during oxygenation in the bag and unloading to tissues at a low partial pressure. Similarly carbon dioxide is loaded at high partial pressure in the tissues and unloaded at low partial pressure in the lungs.

Fluosol is intended for use during Percutaneous Transluminal Coronary Angioplasty (PTCA). When the emulsion is oxygenated and injected transluminally through a coronary angioplasty balloon catheter it will deliver oxygen to the myocardium distal to the point of balloon inflation. The small particle size and elasticity of the perfluorochemical emulsion particles, together with the lower viscosity of Fluosol relative to blood, render the product especially suitable for this task.

Indications: Fluosol is indicated for use during percutaneous transluminal coronary angioplasty to reduce or prevent intraprocedural myocardial ischaemia. The use of Fluosol during the procedure preserves ventricular wall motion and global ejection fraction. These actions of Fluosol enable balloon inflation times to be selected by the clinician more appropriately in accordance with the characteristics of the stenotic lesions being treated and the needs of the individual patients.

Dosage and administration Oxygenated Fluosol should be administered only via intracoronary perfusion during balloon angioplasty by means of an angiographic power injector.

Administration: The Fluosol emulsion must be thawed and mixed with Solutions 1 and 2 prior to administration. The thawed and reconstituted emulsion must be oxygenated to 600 mmHg partial pressure of oxygen prior to use. The oxygenation procedure should be carried out with "Carbogen" (95% O_2/5% CO_2). Do not oxygenate the emulsion with 100% O_2 as this will adversely affect the pH of the emulsion. Refer to the 'Directions for Use' which are packaged with the Oxygenation Kit.

Fluosol emulsion should be thawed in a water bath at not warmer than 70°C or at room temperature. For full details see 'Pharmaceutical precautions' and Package Insert. After mixing and oxygenation are complete, the prepared product should be filled into an angiographic power injector and maintained at 37°C by means of a warming jacket on the injector. The oxygenated Fluosol is administered via the angiographic power injector through the central lumen of the angioplasty balloon catheter with or without the guidewire in place. (See also *Dosage* below).

Strict asepsis should be maintained during thawing, addition and mixing of additive solutions, oxygenation, and filling of the power injector. Carry out each operation inside a controlled aseptic environment using a laminar air flow cabinet or other suitable system.

Fluosol must be oxygenated and warmed to 37°C prior to administration.

Dosage: Fluosol should not be administered more than once in six months. Prior to administration it is advisable to give a 0.5 ml intravenous test dose, especially in patients with a known hypersensitivity to angiographic contrast media.

The 0.5 ml test dose should be withdrawn from the container of Fluosol prepared for administration and injected into a peripheral vein. The 0.5 ml test dose may be performed with or without prior oxygenation of the Fluosol. The patient should be observed for 10 minutes after receiving the test dose and if no untoward event occurs, the intracoronary administration may proceed.

Adverse reactions to the 0.5 ml intravenous test dose are rare. If the patient experiences an adverse reaction after receiving the test dose, Fluosol should not be administered; in this case the patient should be treated by an alternative procedure, such as angioplasty without distal perfusion or coronary artery bypass graft surgery. Intravenous chlorpheniramine and/or hydrocortisone may be given to treat reactions to the test dose.

Oxygenated Fluosol should be injected at a rate of approximately 60 ml/minute at 37°C during the period of balloon inflation depending on the size of the distal vessel bed.

It may be helpful to initiate oxygenated Fluosol perfusion shortly before balloon inflation and to continue momentarily after balloon deflation. Balloon inflation time should be limited by the patient's tolerance and by the physician's judgement of clinical status and desired therapeutic result. An angiographic power injector reservoir, filled with 260 ml of oxygenated Fluosol, will allow more than 4 minutes of perfusion time at a flow rate of 60 ml/minute. Perfusion rates above 120 ml/minute and total intracoronary perfusion volumes above 500 ml have not been studied.

The selection of an angioplasty balloon catheter and guidewire can affect the perfusion of oxygenated Fluosol. Fluosol is compatible with a range of coronary angioplasty catheters, however, for specific information please contact Alpha Therapeutic UK Limited.

Contra-indications, warnings, etc

Contra-indications: Intracoronary perfusion of Fluosol during PTCA is contra-indicated in patients with a functionally critical secondary stenosis in the dilated and perfused vessel distal to the treated lesion. Fluosol should not be administered to patients with a known sensitivity to any of its constituents.

Warnings: Oxygenated Fluosol must be warmed to approximately 37°C prior to administration. Intracoronary infusion of ambient temperature emulsion has been associated with ventricular fibrillation requiring cardioversion.

Any coronary angioplasty procedure carries some degree of risk of coronary arterial dissection with occlusion, coronary artery spasm and vasospastic angina; myocardial infarction, distal intraluminal thrombus, arrhythmia, tachycardia, bradycardia, and ventricular fibrillation requiring cardioversion. Supportive treatment and personnel must be available to handle these procedural complications.

Precautions: Perfusion with oxygenated Fluosol should be performed only with lumened catheters and guidewire systems which permit pressure monitoring and/or contrast agent delivery. Prior to initiating oxygenated Fluosol perfusion, the operator must verify proper positioning of the balloon catheter.

During percutaneous transluminal coronary angioplasty the patient should be continuously monitored for signs of hypoxia. Electrocardiographic monitoring should be performed.

If the position of the balloon catheter occludes side branches which will not receive perfusion from oxygenated Fluosol, ischaemic ST segment changes, angina, and creatine kinase elevation may result. The operator should be aware of potential complications of coronary angioplasty which may occur in spite of oxygenated Fluosol perfusion. A characteristic electrocardiographic pattern of ST segment elevation, reaching a plateau at 30–40 seconds of balloon inflation with an amplitude of 1.2 mm, has been observed in many patients receiving distal perfusion with oxygenated Fluosol. This phenomenon is thought to be a mechanical artifact of the perfusion and is not an indicator of ischaemia. It has also been observed in experimental animals in which oxygenated Fluosol was administered to coronary arteries without ischaemia. It invariably decreased with return-to-normal ST patterns upon balloon deflation and reperfusion by blood. The pattern of the ST changes seen in these patients was distinctly different from ischaemic ST elevations in control patients which continue to rise after balloon inflation.

The perfluorochemicals in Fluosol are taken up by the reticuloendothelial system, primarily in the liver, spleen and bone marrow. No metabolism of the perfluorochemicals has been observed; the molecules are excreted intact via the lungs. In view of this, asplenic patients or patients with compromised liver or lung function may display altered distribution or prolonged half-life of perfluorochemical emulsion particles.

Adverse reactions: Adverse reactions occurring during oxygenated Fluosol perfusion in angioplasty may be difficult to separate from complications attributable to the procedure itself. Some levels of hypoxia, evidenced by angina and ST segment elevation, may occur. A transient increase in pulmonary artery wedge pressure above baseline levels was observed in some patients receiving multiple balloon inflations with Fluosol perfusion. Wedge pressure returned to near baseline levels within 3–5 minutes after the procedure.

Clinical studies have shown that transient liver enzyme elevations have occurred in some patients. These have not been found to be clinically significant.

Potential adverse reactions, occurring in less than 0.4% of patients, may include mild pruritus, bradycardia, chest discomfort following procedure, dyspnoea, hypotension, increased respiratory rate and coughing.

In clinical trials 1.2% of patients reacted to a 0.5 ml intravenous test dose of Fluosol. If the patient experiences an adverse reaction (mild generalised pruritus, mild chills, nausea, vomiting, urticaria, or mild back pain) after receiving the test dose, Fluosol should not be administered; in this case the patient should be treated by an alternative procedure, such as angioplasty without distal perfusion or coronary artery bypass graft surgery. Intravenous chlorpheniramine and/or hydrocortisone may be given to treat reactions to the intravenous test dose.

Drug interactions: Administration of Fluosol may prolong the action of lipid soluble anaesthetics. In animal studies the hepatotoxic effects of carbon tetrachloride were enhanced by the prior or post administration of perfluorochemicals.

Drug/laboratory test interactions: Centrifuged samples of blood containing Fluosol may contain a packed layer of perfluorochemicals at the bottom of the tube. Packed red blood cells will be above the layer of perfluorochemicals and plasma will be at the top. The volume % of perfluorochemicals in the sample is defined as the fluorocrit.

At high concentrations in blood (well above those expected in angioplasty perfusion), Fluosol may cause an upward displacement of the standard curve in some radioimmunoassays. Additionally, at high concentrations in blood, Fluosol may interfere with some spectrophotometric tests due to turbidity.

Use during pregnancy and lactation: Reproduction studies have been performed in rats at approximately three times the human dose and have revealed no evidence of impaired fertility or harm to the foetus due to Fluosol. There are, however, no adequate and well controlled studies in pregnant women. Because animal reproduction studies are not always predictive of human response, this drug should be used during pregnancy only if clearly needed.

Perfluorodecalin has been found in human breast milk. One day after peripheral intravenous infusion of 20 ml/kg of Fluosol when the fluorocrit was 0.5%, a sample of breast milk was obtained. Perfluorodecalin was detected in the breast milk at a level of 0.58 mg/ml; no perfluorotri-n-propylamine was detected. It is recommended that after administration of Fluosol nursing mothers should not breast feed the baby, even though the perfluorochemicals will not be absorbed orally.

Pharmaceutical precautions The 400 ml container of Fluosol emulsion must be stored in the frozen state between −5 and −30°C. Do not use any container in which there is evidence that the emulsion has thawed during transit.

Solutions 1 and 2 may be stored at room temperature not exceeding 30°C. *Do not freeze Solutions 1 and 2.*

Do not thaw the emulsion in a microwave oven. This may cause uneven warming and localized overheating. Thaw the frozen emulsion in a water bath or warming cabinet not warmer than 70°C or at room temperature.

Additives other than Solution 1, Solution 2 and Carbogen gas must not be made to the container of Fluosol emulsion. Fluosol is for single dose use only; any unused contents must be discarded and should not be stored or re-sterilised for later use.

Filters should not be used when Fluosol is administered as this may disturb the emulsion.

Do not administer the contents of any container in which there appears to be a separation of the emulsion or any container of emulsion which may have thawed during storage.

Parenteral drug products should be inspected visually for particulate matter and discolouration prior to administration.

For further information on the correct administration of Fluosol please refer to the Package Insert contained within the Oxygenation Kit.

It is recommended that a temperature of approximately 37°C is used to thaw the Fluosol emulsion. This will take approximately 25 minutes. Once thawed the emulsion may be kept for up to seven days at 2–8°C.

If a more rapid thaw is required the emulsion may be thawed at up to 70°C without affecting the seven days refrigerated shelf life. However caution should be exercised if higher thaw temperatures are implemented since Fluosol must only be infused at a temperature of approximately 37°C.

In addition provided the emulsion (1) has been *thawed at 40°C or less and* (2) has been stored at 2–8°C for no more than two days *and* (3) Solutions 1 and 2 have not been incorporated the Fluosol emulsion may be re-frozen. Once re-thawed it must be stored at 2–8°C and used within 2 days.

Strict aseptic technique must be employed during addition of Solutions 1 and 2. Once the solutions have been added the Fluosol emulsion may be kept for 24 hours at 2–8°C. However, once the Fluosol emulsion has been oxygenated it must be administered at 37°C within 8 hours. For full details contact Alpha Therapeutic UK Ltd.

Legal category POM.

Package quantities Fluosol consists of three components which must be mixed before administration.

The components included are:
Fluosol Emulsion, 400 ml in a flexible plastic bag.
Solution 1, 30 ml in a glass vial.
Solution 2, 70 ml in a glass vial.

The additive solutions are supplied in a separate kit which includes accessories for effecting oxygenation. The Oxygenation Kit includes the following accessories:
Solution 1 (30 ml partial fill in 50 ml vial)
Solution 2 (70 ml partial fill in 100 ml vial)
Gas Cartridge: 95 ml cartridge containing 95% Oxygen/5% Carbon Dioxide
Piercing Device
Sterile Filter: 0.2 micron membrane filter
One 18 Gauge needle
Protective plastic bag

Further information The Product Licence holder can be consulted for full information on the use of this product.

Product licence number 4447/0015.

PLASMATEIN* 5%

Presentation Plasmatein 5% is Plasma Protein Solution BP 5% and each 100 ml of solution contains 5 g protein of which at least 85% is albumin. It is a clear, pale yellow, sterile aqueous solution intended for single dose intravenous administration.

Uses Plasmatein 5% is a stabilised isotonic solution of protein of which at least 85% is albumin and the remainder is heat stable alpha- and beta-globulins. As such Plasmatein 5% behaves clinically in a similar way to albumin and can be used to regulate the osmotic pressure of plasma. It is osmotically equivalent to an equal volume of plasma. The intravenous administration of Plasmatein 5% results therefore in expansion of intravascular volume by providing and holding fluid in the vascular space.

Plasmatein 5% is indicated:
(i) For the treatment of hypovolaemic shock.
(ii) In conditions in which there is severe hypoproteinaemia. However unless the pathologic condition responsible for the hypoproteinaemia can be corrected, administration of Plasmatein 5% can afford only symptomatic or supportive relief.
(iii) For the treatment of burns.

(iv) As an adjunct in haemodialysis.

Dosage and administration Plasmatein 5% is intended for intravenous administration. The total dosage will vary with the clinical condition and size of the individual.

Adults: An initial infusion of 500 ml is suggested. Additional amounts may be administered as clinically indicated.

The rate of administration should not normally be greater than 10 ml per minute.

Children: Dosage will vary with clinical condition and body weight. A dose of one-quarter to one-half of the adult dose may be administered or dosage may be calculated on the basis of 3–5 ml per kilogram of body weight.

The rate of administration should be calculated on one-quarter of the adult rate.

Contra-indications, warnings, etc Plasmatein 5% is contra-indicated in patients on cardiopulmonary bypass; in patients with severe anaemia or cardiac failure in the presence of normal or increased intravascular volume; in patients with a history of allergic reactions to albumin products.

Plasmatein 5% may produce hypotension if infused rapidly (greater than 10 ml/minute). Blood pressure should be monitored during use and infusion slowed or discontinued if sudden hypotension occurs. Rapid infusion may cause vascular overload with resultant pulmonary oedema. Patients should be closely monitored for signs of increased venous pressure. Plasmatein 5% should be administered with caution to patients with low cardiac reserve. Additional fluids may be necessary for patients with marked dehydration. A rapid rise in blood pressure following infusion necessitates careful observation of injured or postoperative patients to detect and treat severed blood vessels that may not have bled at a lower pressure.

Do not use for control of haemorrhage due to deficiencies or defects in the clotting mechanism.

Albumin naturally binds a variety of therapeutic and toxic materials and thus administration of Plasmatein 5% may modify the pre-existing distribution of certain substances.

Adverse reactions are rare. However Plasmatein 5% administration may result in hypotension, particularly following rapid infusion. Allergic or pyrogenic reactions, characterised primarily by fever and chills, rash, nausea, vomiting, tachycardia and hypotension have also been reported.

If such reactions occur the infusion should be discontinued and appropriate therapy (e.g. antihistamine) or specific support treatment should be given.

Reproduction studies have not been conducted with plasma protein solution. Plasmatein 5% should be given to a pregnant woman only if clearly needed.

Administration of large quantities of plasma protein solution may require supplementation with red cell concentrates to help overcome any resulting relative anaemia.

Pharmaceutical precautions Do not use if the solution appears turbid or contains a deposit which does not readily disappear on shaking. Since the solution does not contain a preservative it should be used within 3 hours of penetration of the container. Discard any unused portion.

Do not administer protein hydrolysates or alcohol via the same administration set used for Plasmatein 5%.

Legal category POM.

Package quantities Plasmatein 5% is supplied in:
250 ml glass vials containing 12.5 g plasma protein.
500 ml glass vials containing 25.0 g plasma protein.

Further information Plasmatein 5% is prepared from plasma obtained from carefully selected and rigorously screened donors. However as with all blood products the risk of viral transmission with this product cannot be absolutely excluded. Nevertheless there are no known cases of viral transmission resulting from the administration of Plasmatein 5%.

Product licence number 4447/0010.

PROFILATE*-SD

Presentation Profilate-SD is a preparation of Dried Factor VIII Fraction BP. It is a stable, highly purified, freeze-dried concentrate of Factor VIII (Antihaemophilic Factor, Antihaemophilic Globulin) which has been treated during manufacture with an organic solvent, Tri-(n-butyl) phosphate (TNBP) and a detergent, Polysorbate 80 in order to inactivate certain viruses known to be transmissible by human blood.

Profilate-SD is a sterile preparation intended for intravenous administration. Each vial is a single dose container having the Factor VIII activity expressed on the label in International Units (IU). One International Unit approximates to the activity of one ml of fresh pooled human plasma. The specific activity of the product is at least 3.0 IU of Factor VIII per milligram of protein. Profilate-SD, when reconstituted contains not more than 2 units of heparin per ml and not more than 20 milligrams of fibrinogen per ml.

Uses For the prevention and control of bleeding in patients with moderate or severe Factor VIII deficiency due to classical haemophilia A or acquired Factor VIII deficiency.

Dosage and administration

Dosage: The dose of Profilate-SD to be administered must be adjusted according to the needs of the patient. The patient's plasma level of Factor VIII should be determined and monitored during treatment. The formula below provides a guide to dosage calculations:

Bodyweight in kg × 0.5 × Desired increase in Factor VIII (*as a percentage*) = Number of Factor VIII units required

Example:
50 kg × 0.5 IU/kg × 30% = 750 IU Profilate-SD

Mild to moderate haemorrhages may usually be treated with a single administration sufficient to raise the plasma Factor VIII level to 20–30 percent. In the event of more serious haemorrhage the patient's plasma Factor VIII level should be raised to 30–50 percent, infusions are generally required at twice daily intervals over several days.

Surgery in patients with Factor VIII deficiency requires that the Factor VIII level be raised to 50–80 percent with the level maintained at or above 30 percent for approximately two weeks post-operatively. For dental extractions, the Factor VIII level should be raised to 50 percent immediately prior to the procedure; further Factor VIII may be given if bleeding recurs.

In patients with severe Factor VIII deficiency who experience frequent haemorrhages, Profilate-SD should be administered prophylactically on a daily or every other day schedule so as to raise the Factor VIII level to approximately 15 percent.

Reconstitution: Use only the diluent provided. Use aseptic technique.

1. Warm diluent and concentrate bottles to at least room temperature (but not above 37°C).
2. Remove plastic flip-off caps from the diluent and concentrate vials.
3. Swab the exposed rubber surfaces with alcohol. Do not leave excess cleaning agent in indentation on the stoppers.
4. Remove covering from one end of a double-ended needle to expose the short needle. Insert this exposed short needle through the depression in the centre of the stopper in the vial of diluent.
5. Remove plastic cap from the upper end of the double-ended needle now seated in the stopper of the diluent vial. Hold concentrate vial in one hand, invert the vial of diluent in the other hand and push the exposed end of the needle through the depression in the centre

of the stopper, making certain that the diluent is always above the vial of concentrate. There should be enough vacuum in the vial to draw in all the diluent.
6. Disconnect the two vials by removing the needle from the concentrate vial stopper. Swirl the concentrate vial until all concentrate is dissolved. Reconstitution normally requires less than five minutes. When the reconstitution procedure is strictly followed a few small particles may occasionally remain. The microaggregate filter will retain particles and the labelled potency will not be reduced.

Administration: Profilate-SD is intended for intravenous administration only and should be used within 3 hours of reconstitution.

By syringe: Use aseptic technique.

1. Peel cover from microaggregate filter package and securely install the syringe into the exposed luer inlet of the filter using a slight clockwise twisting motion.
2. Remove filter from packaging. Remove protective sleeve from the spike end of the filter using clockwise twisting motion.
3. Pull back plunger to aspirate sufficient air into the syringe to allow reconstituted product to be withdrawn as described in the next step.
4. Insert the spike end of the filter into the reconstituted concentrate vial. Inject air and aspirate the reconstituted product from the vial into the syringe.
5. Remove and discard the filter from the syringe. Attach syringe to an infusion set, expel air from syringe and infusion set. Perform venepuncture and administer slowly.
6. If the patient is to receive more than one vial of concentrate, the infusion set will allow this to be performed with a single venepuncture.
7. Discard all administration equipment after use.

By administration set: Use aseptic technique.

1. Close clamp on the administration set.
2. With vial upright, insert piercing pin straight through stopper centre. Do not twist or angle.
3. Immediately invert vial to automatically establish proper fluid level in drip chamber (half full).
4. Attach infusion set, open clamp and allow solution to expel air from tubing and needle, then close clamp.
5. Perform venepuncture and adjust flow, not to exceed 10 ml/minute.
6. Discard all administration equipment after use.

Contra-indications, warnings, etc

Contra-indications: There are no known contra-indications to the use of Profilate-SD.

Warnings: This product is prepared from pooled units of human plasma derived from screened donors. Each unit has been individually tested and found nonreactive for hepatitis B surface antigen and antibody to Human Immunodeficiency Virus (HIV). The plasma used in the preparation of this product has been tested for alanine aminotransferase (ALT) levels in an effort to reduce the risk of transmission of non-A, non-B hepatitis. Each unit used in the manufacture of this product has been found to have an ALT level less than 2 times the upper limit of normal for the test. Incubation in an organic solvent/ detergent mixture during the manufacturing process is designed to reduce the risk of transmitting viral infection. The effectiveness of this processing step has been demonstrated by *in vitro* inactivation studies using live viruses added to Profilate-SD.

However, testing methods presently available are not sensitive enough to detect all units of potentially infectious plasma and no treatment method has yet been shown to be totally effective in eliminating viral infectivity from coagulation factor products. Despite all precautions taken by the manufacturer it cannot be assumed that this product is totally free of HIV or hepatitis virus. As with all drugs the risks associated with use must be weighed against the benefits of therapy.

Since animal reproduction studies have not been conducted with Profilate-SD, it should only be given to pregnant women if clearly indicated.

Precautions: Profilate-SD should not be administered at a rate exceeding 10 ml/minute. Rapid administration may result in vasomotor reactions.

Some haemophiliacs develop inhibitors to Factor VIII. In these patients the response to Profilate-SD may be much less than would otherwise be expected and larger doses are often required. The management of patients with inhibitors requires careful monitoring, especially if surgical procedures are indicated.

Nursing personnel and others who administer this material should exercise appropriate caution in handling because of the risk of exposure to viral infection such as hepatitis.

Discard any unused contents. Discard administration equipment after single use. Do not resterilize components. Do not use any vials which on reconstitution appear to totally lack vacuum.

Adverse reactions: Occasionally, mild reactions occur following the administration of Factor VIII concentrates. These may include allergic reactions, urticaria, fever, chills, nausea, vomiting, headache, somnolence or lethargy. If a reaction is noted and the patient requires additional Profilate-SD, product from a different lot should be administered.

Massive doses of Factor VIII concentrate have rarely resulted in acute haemolytic anaemia, increased bleeding tendency or hyperfibrinogenaemia. Profilate-SD contains blood group isoagglutinins and when large and/or frequent doses are required in patients of blood group A, B or AB, the patient should be monitored for signs of intravascular haemolysis and falling haematocrit. Should this condition occur, the administration of serologically compatible type O red blood cells or the administration of Dried Factor VIII Fraction BP produced from group specific plasma should be considered.

Pharmaceutical precautions Profilate-SD should be protected from light and stored at temperatures between 2° and 8°C. Do not freeze. Profilate-SD may be stored at room temperature not to exceed 30°C for up to three months.

Legal category POM.

Package quantities Profilate-SD is supplied in cartons containing ten vials of freeze dried concentrate. The potency is stated on each vial label. Accessory packs containing either 10 ml or 25 ml vials of diluent are provided with each carton of concentrate.

Further information The organic solvent detergent treatment process has been shown to provide a high level of virus kill without compromising protein structure and function. The susceptibility of human pathogenic viruses such as human immunodeficiency virus (HIV), hepatitis B virus, non-A, non-B hepatitis virus and marker viruses such as Sindbis Virus and Vesicular Stomatitis Virus to inactivation by organic solvent detergent treatment has been discussed in the literature. *In vitro* inactivation studies sponsored by Alpha Therapeutic Corporation to evaluate the organic solvent detergent treatment step used in the manufacture of Profilate-SD show inactivation of greater than 10 logs of HIV as well as 6.8 logs of Vesicular Stomatitis Virus (VSV) and 6.4 logs of Sindbis Virus.

Product licence number 4447/0005.

SOYACAL*

Presentation A sterile milky white emulsion of soybean oil in Water for Injection suitable for intravenous administration and containing:

	Soyacal 10%	*Soyacal 20%*
Purified soybean oil	10.0 g	20.0 g
Purified egg yolk phospholipids	1.2 g	1.2 g
Glycerol	2.21 g	2.21 g
Sodium hydroxide	to pH7	to pH7
Water for injection	to 100.0 ml	to 100.0 ml

Uses Soybean oil is a refined natural product consisting of a mixture of neutral triglycerides of mainly unsaturated fatty acids. The major component fatty acids are linoleic (49%–60%), oleic (21%–26%), palmitic (9%–13%), linolenic (6%–9%) and stearic (3%–5%).

Soyacal is a concentrated source of energy available as either 10% or 20% emulsions which will supply 1,100 kcal (4.6MJ) and 2,000 kcal (8.4MJ) per litre respectively.

Soyacal 10% and 20% have osmolarities of approximately 280 and 315 mosm per litre respectively and contain emulsified fat particles averaging approximately 0.33 microns in diameter, similar to naturally occurring chylomicrons.

Soyacal has been designed as part of a balanced intravenous feeding regimen in patients unable to receive sufficient nutrients enterally.

Indications:

(1) As a source of calories and essential fatty acids for patients requiring parenteral nutrition for extended periods of time.

(2) As a source of essential fatty acids when a deficiency occurs.

Dosage and administration Patients receiving Soyacal should be monitored for their capacity to eliminate the infused fat from the circulation. Lipaemia must clear between infusions.

Soyacal may be administered by slow intravenous infusion as part of a supplemental or total parenteral nutrition (TPN) regimen via a peripheral vein or by central venous catheter.

Patients receiving TPN should be monitored for electrolyte and fluid imbalances prior to initiating TPN and regularly throughout feeding. The appropriate alterations in fluid and electrolyte should be made as necessary.

Adults: The initial infusion rate in adults should be 1.0 ml per minute for Soyacal 10% and 0.5 ml per minute for Soyacal 20% for the first 15 to 30 minutes of infusion. If no untoward reactions occur, the infusion rate can be increased so that 500 ml of Soyacal 10% or 250 ml of Soyacal 20% will be infused over a period of 4–6 hours. No more than 500 ml of Soyacal 10% or 250 ml of Soyacal 20% should be infused on the first day of therapy. If the patient has no untoward reactions the dose may be increased on the following day. The daily dosage should not normally exceed 2.5 g (equivalent to 25 ml of Soyacal 10% or 12.5 ml of Soyacal 20%) fat per kg body weight. Intravenous fat emulsion should make up no more than 60% of the total caloric input of the patient. Carbohydrate and a source of amino acids should comprise the remaining 40% or more of the caloric input.

Children: Dosage is governed by the maturity and birth weight of the infant. In all cases the infant's ability to eliminate infused fat from the circulation should be checked daily. If lipaemia is present re-testing should be carried out after an interval of four hours.

(1) Infants: The initial infusion rate in paediatric patients should be 0.1 ml per minute for Soyacal 10% or 0.05 ml per minute for Soyacal 20% for the first 10 to 15 minutes. If no untoward reactions occur, the rate can be increased to permit infusion of 1 g fat per kg of body weight in four hours. The dosage should not exceed 4 g fat (equivalent to 40 ml of Soyacal 10% or 20 ml of Soyacal 20%) per kg of body weight in any 24 hour period. Intravenous fat emulsion should make up no more than 60% of the total caloric input of the patient. Carbohydrate and a source of amino acids should comprise the remaining 40% or more of the caloric input.

(2) Low birth weight/premature infants: The maximum fat removal capacity of pre-term infants has been estimated at 0.3 g fat/kg/hour. A commencing dosage of 0.5 g fat (equivalent to 5 ml of Soyacal 10% or 2.5 ml of Soyacal 20%) per kg of body weight in 24 hours is recommended. In the absence of measurement of serum triglycerides the dosage should not exceed 2 g fat (equivalent to 20 ml of Soyacal 10% or 10 ml of Soyacal 20%) per kg of body weight in 24 hours.

Fatty acid deficiency: When Soyacal is administered to correct fatty acid deficiency 8–10% of the caloric input should be supplied by the fat emulsion in order to provide adequate linoleic acid to correct the deficiency.

Contra-indications, warnings, etc

Contra-indications: Soyacal is contra-indicated in patients with acute circulatory shock and in patients with a disturbance of normal fat metabolism such as pathologic hyperlipaemia, lipoid nephrosis and acute pancreatitis if accompanied by hyperlipaemia.

Warnings: Premature and small for gestational age infants have poor clearance of intravenous fat emulsion and increased fatty acid plasma levels following fat emulsion infusion. Intravenous fat overload has caused intravascular fat accumulation in the lungs and displacement of bilirubin from circulatory plasma albumin. Serious consideration must be given to administration of less than the maximum recommended doses in these patients.

The presence of Soyacal in blood samples may interfere with certain laboratory measurements.

Precautions: When Soyacal is administered the patient's capacity to eliminate the infused fat from the circulation must be monitored. The lipaemia must clear between infusions. Avoid overdosage absolutely.

Too rapid administration of Soyacal can cause fluid and/or fat overloading. This can result in dilution of serum electrolyte concentrations, overhydration, pulmonary oedema, impaired pulmonary diffusion capacity or metabolic acidosis. Caution should be exercised in administering Soyacal to patients with severe liver damage, pulmonary disease, anaemia or blood coagulation disorders or when there is a danger of fat embolism.

Consideration should be given to performing liver function tests during long term therapy and to performing platelet counts in neonatal patients receiving parenteral nutrition.

Overdosage: In the event of fat overdose during therapy, stop the infusion until visual inspection of the plasma, determination of triglyceride concentrations, or measurement of plasma light-scattering activity by nephelometry indicates that the lipid has cleared. Institute appropriate corrective measures and re-evaluate the patient periodically.

Side-effects: Rare adverse reactions occurring soon after infusion include fever, chills, headache and other poorly defined complaints such as nausea, fatigue and allergic-type reactions.

Delayed adverse reactions which have been reported infrequently in patients receiving intravenous nutrition include cholestasis, thrombocytopaenia, transient increase in liver function tests, altered platelet counts and hepatomegaly.

Pregnancy: Reproduction studies have been performed in rats and rabbits at doses up to 3–6 times the adult human dose and have revealed no evidence of impaired fertility or teratogenicity. However, no adequate studies in pregnant women have been carried out. Therefore Soyacal should be used during pregnancy only if clearly needed.

Pharmaceutical precautions Store below 25°C and protect from light. Do not freeze. Do not use any leaking vials. Do not administer any bottle in which there appears to be separation of the emulsion.

Soyacal is supplied in single dose containers. Unused contents must be discarded.

Antibiotics and other drugs must not be added to the Soyacal emulsion container.

Admixtures may be incompatible. See 'Further information' below.

Lipid containing fluids have a propensity to extract phthalates from certain plasticised PVC. Although the amount is very small and no adverse clinical effects have been reported from administration of such small amounts of phthalate it may be advisable to consider use of non-phthalate containers and infusion sets for Soyacal administration.

Legal category POM.

Package quantities Soyacal is available in concentrations of 10% and 20%. Bottles containing 50 ml, 100 ml, 250 ml and 500 ml are available.

Further information Soyacal can be infused concurrently into the same vein as carbohydrate-amino acid solutions by means of a Y-connector located near the infusion site; the flow rate of each fluid should be controlled separately by an infusion pump.

Soyacal can be mixed with other solutions in a single container (e.g. a 3 litre bag). Studies have shown that mixtures of Soyacal with amino acid injections (5.2% to 10% with or without electrolytes) and dextrose injection (10% to 70%) are stable for short periods of time. Such mixing must follow defined formulae and mixing techniques. Detailed information on compatible admixtures and mixing techniques is available on request.

Product licence numbers

Soyacal 10%	4447/0012
Soyacal 20%	4447/0013

VENOGLOBULIN*

Presentation Venoglobulin is a sterile white crystalline freeze-dried preparation of highly purified human normal immunoglobulin contained in glass vials. It is supplied with a diluent vial containing sterile Water for Injections BP. When reconstituted as directed Venoglobulin contains Immunoglobulin G (Human) 50 mg/ml, Albumin (Human) 10 mg/ml, D-Mannitol 20 mg/ml and Sodium Chloride 5 mg/ml and has a pH of 6.8. The purity of the IgG portion of the presentation is typically more than 99%. Trace amounts of IgA and IgM may be present. The product is suitable for intravenous administration. It is available in vials containing 0.5 g, 2.5 g or 5.0 g immunoglobulin per vial.

Uses

Pharmacological actions: Venoglobulin is a high purity human immunoglobulin class G (IgG) preparation which contains antibodies against the wide spectrum of antigens to which the plasma donor population has been exposed. The distribution of IgG subclasses in the preparation corresponds to that found in normal plasma.

Venoglobulin retains the biological functions of endogenous gammaglobulin and has very low anticomplementary activity. The precise mode of action in idiopathic thrombocytopenic purpura has yet to be elucidated.

Indications:

1. Replacement therapy for congenital agammaglobulinaemia and hypogammaglobulinaemia.

For hypogammaglobulinaemic patients who require an immediate and substantial increase in serum immunoglobulin levels or who have limited muscle mass or who have bleeding tendencies and for whom intramuscular injections are contra-indicated.

For maintenance treatment of patients with primary immunodeficiency syndromes who are unable to produce sufficient amounts of IgG antibodies e.g. common variable immunodeficiency, X-linked agammaglobulinaemia, severe combined immunodeficiency and Wiskott–Aldrich syndrome.

2. Treatment of idiopathic thrombocytopenic purpura.

Dosage and administration

Dosage:

Immunodeficiency Syndromes: The usual dosage of Venoglobulin in immunodeficiency syndromes is 200 mg/kg bodyweight usually administered once a month by intravenous infusion. If the clinical response is inadequate or the level of serum IgG achieved is felt to be insufficient the dose may be increased to 300–400 mg/kg bodyweight or the infusion may be repeated more frequently than once a month.

Idiopathic thrombocytopenic purpura: The usual treatment regimen is 400 mg/kg bodyweight daily for 5 days. Maintenance doses of 400 mg/kg bodyweight may be given every few weeks as required to maintain the platelet count.

Reconstitution: Use aseptic technique. For full details, see Package Insert.

1. Remove the plastic flip-off caps from the diluent and Venoglobulin vials.
2. Swab the exposed rubber surfaces with alcohol. Do not leave excess cleaning agents on stoppers.
3. Remove the protective plastic cap from one end of the double ended transfer needle. Insert the exposed end of the needle through the stopper into the vial of sterile Water for Injections BP.
4. Remove the plastic cap from the other end of the transfer needle, invert the vial of diluent and push the exposed end of the needle through the stopper into the vial of Venoglobulin. The vacuum will draw the diluent into the vial.
5. Swirl the container gently to effect dissolution. *Do not shake the solution.* Avoid foaming. Venoglobulin normally dissolves in a few minutes but in exceptional cases it may require up to 20 minutes. *Use only if the solution is free of turbidity and undissolved particles.*

Administration: Venoglobulin should be infused at a rate of 0.01–0.02 ml per kg bodyweight per minute for the first thirty minutes. If the patient does not experience any discomfort the rate may be increased up to 0.04 ml per kg per minute and if tolerated subsequent infusions to the same patient may be at the higher rate. If adverse effects occur the rate should be reduced or the infusion interrupted until the symptoms subside. The infusion may then be resumed at a rate which is tolerated by the patient.

Contra-indications, warnings, etc

Contra-indications: Venoglobulin is contra-indicated in individuals with a history of anaphylactic or severe systemic response to intramuscular or intravenous immune globulin preparations.

As with all blood products containing IgA, Venoglobulin is contra-indicated in patients with selective IgA deficiency who possess antibody to IgA.

Warnings: Patients with agamma- or extreme hypogammaglobulinaemia who have never before received immunoglobulin therapy or whose time from last treatment is greater than 8 weeks may be at risk of developing inflammatory reactions on infusion of Venoglobulin. Such reactions are rare and appear to be related to the rate of infusion. They are manifested by a rise in temperature, chills, nausea and vomiting. Vital signs should be monitored continuously and the patient should be carefully observed throughout the infusion. The rate of administration specified in *Dosage and administration* should be closely followed, at least until the physician has had sufficient experience with a given patient. Adrenaline should be available for treatment of any acute anaphylactoid reaction.

Animal reproduction studies have not been conducted with Venoglobulin. It is also not known whether Venoglobulin can cause foetal harm when administered to pregnant women or can affect reproduction capacity. Venoglobulin should, therefore, be given to a pregnant woman only if clearly needed.

This product is prepared from pooled units of human plasma which have been individually tested and found non-reactive for hepatitis B surface antigen and antibody to human immunodeficiency virus (HIV). The plasma used in the preparation of this product has been screened for alanine aminotransferase (ALT) in order to reduce the risk of transmission of non-A, non-B hepatitis. Each unit used in manufacture has been found to have an ALT level of less than twice the upper limit of normal for the test. Other screening procedures are used to eliminate high risk plasma donors. Furthermore, in-vitro inactivation studies indicate that the manufacturing process is capable of removing significant quantities of HIV virus. However, despite all precautions taken by the manufacturer the risk of transmission of infection, in particular non-A, non-B hepatitis, by intravenous immunoglobulin preparations cannot be entirely excluded.

Adverse reactions: Clinical investigations have confirmed that Venoglobulin is well tolerated and not likely to produce side effects when infused at the recommended rates. However, the first infusion of immunoglobulin particularly in previously untreated agamma- and hypogammaglobulinaemic patients or patients who have previously received another immunoglobulin preparation may lead to systemic side effects. Some of the effects may occur as a result of a reaction between the antibodies administered and free antigens in the blood and tissues of the patient.

Adverse reactions may include flushing of the face, tightness of the chest, chills, fever, dizziness, nausea, mild back pain and hypotension.

Overdosage: Overdosage with Venoglobulin has not been reported but is unlikely to have any harmful effects.

Pharmaceutical precautions Venoglobulin should be stored below 30°C and should be protected from light. Do not use after expiry date printed on the label.

Venoglobulin should be reconstituted only with the diluent provided. Do not mix with any other drugs or intravenous fluids. Administer via a separate intravenous line.

Venoglobulin should be infused within 3 hours of reconstitution. Discard any unused solution. If large volumes are to be administered it may be advisable to warm the solution to near body temperature prior to infusion.

Legal category POM.

Package quantities
0.5 g vial supplied with 10 ml sterile Water for Injections BP and transfer needle.
2.5 g vial supplied with 50 ml sterile Water for Injections BP and transfer needle.
5.0 g vial supplied with 100 ml sterile Water for Injections BP and transfer needle.

Product licence number 4447/0014

**Trade Mark*

Approved Prescription Services Limited
Water Street
Towngate, Wyke
West Yorkshire BD12 9AF

APSIFEN*
APSIFEN*-F

Presentation Apsifen is available in two presentations:
Apsifen: Round, biconvex, pink sugar-coated tablets, marked 'APS' or plain on one side and coded 200 0521 or 400 0525 for the 200 and 400 mg strengths respectively.
Apsifen-F: Round, biconvex, pink, film-coated tablets marked 'APS' on one side and plain on the other side.

Both presentations contain the same active ingredient, Ibuprofen BP, and both are available in two strengths, 200 mg and 400 mg. They comply with the monograph for Ibuprofen Tablets BP.

Apsifen-F is also available in a 600 mg strength; this tablet is pink, capsule-shaped, biconvex, film-coated and marked 'APS' or plain on one side and 600 0531 on the other side.

Apsifen contains sucrose, colours E110, E127 and E211. Apsifen-F contains colours E127, E464 and E171.

Uses Ibuprofen is a non-steroidal anti-inflammatory agent with analgesic and anti-pyretic activity. Its principal effects are to relieve pain and stiffness and to reduce swelling.

Apsifen and Apsifen-F may therefore be used in the management of:
(a) Rheumatoid Arthritis including Still's disease;
(b) Osteoarthrosis and seronegative (non rheumatoid) arthropothies;
(c) Ankylosing Spondylitis.

Like other similar agents, ibuprofen has also been used in non-articular rheumatic conditions and in soft-tissue injuries, and for the relief of mild to moderate pain such as dysmenorrhoea, dental and post-operative pain.

Dosage and administration (Oral)
Adults: Initially 1200 mg per day in divided doses. In severe conditions up to 1800 mg per day may be given until the acute phase of the condition has been brought under control. Some patients may be maintained on doses in the range 600–1200 mg per day. Under no circumstances should the dose of ibuprofen exceed 2400 mg in any 24 hours.

Children: 20 mg/kg of body weight given daily in divided doses. The tablets are not suitable for children weighing less than 20 kg and no more than two 200 mg tablets should be given in 24 hours to those weighing less than 30 kg.

The Elderly: A separate dosage schedule is not recommended because ibuprofen is well tolerated and overdosage is not usually dangerous, but see precaution (d) below.

Contra-indications, warnings, etc
Contra-indications: Ibuprofen should not be used in patients with:
(a) active peptic ulceration;
(b) a history of severe peptic ulceration.

Precautions: Special care must be taken when using ibuprofen in the following situations:
(a) In patients with asthma;
(b) In allergic patients or in patients who have developed bronchospasm with other non-steroidal anti-inflammatory agents;
(c) Pregnancy: As with other agents the use of ibuprofen during pregnancy should be avoided if possible;
(d) In elderly patients, in whom increased tissue levels may result from the normal processes of ageing with an attendant increase in the risk of adverse reactions (which are more likely to be masked by concurrent therapy or disease in the elderly).

Adverse Reactions: As with other non-steroidal anti-inflammatory agents, the most common unwanted effects with ibuprofen include dyspepsia, gastro-intestinal intolerance and bleeding. Other unwanted effects include a variety of skin rashes and, less commonly, thrombocytopenia. A few cases of toxic amblyopia which recovered on withdrawal of treatment have been reported. Signs of intolerance or unwanted effects are indications for stopping treatment.

Overdosage: There is no specific antidote to ibuprofen. Management usually includes gastric lavage associated with special care of plasma electrolytes and any other appropriate symptomatic relief.

Pharmaceutical precautions Apsifen and Apsifen-F Tablets should be stored at room temperature in a dry place and protected from light.

Legal category POM.

Package quantities
Apsifen and Apsifen-F 200 mg: polypropylene tubes of 100 and 500 tablets.
Apsifen and Apsifen-F 400 mg: polypropylene tubes of 100 and 250 tablets.
Apsifen-F 600 mg: polypropylene tubes of 100 tablets.

Further information Nil.

Product licence numbers
Apsifen Tablets 200 mg 0289/0029
Apsifen Tablets 400 mg 0289/0037
Apsifen-F Tablets 200 mg 0289/0062
Apsifen-F Tablets 400 mg 0289/0063
Apsifen-F Tablets 600 mg 0289/0069

APSIN* VK

Presentation Apsin VK is available in two presentations, tablets and granules for syrup.

Apsin VK Tablets are white, round, biconvex, film-coated, scored on one side and marked 'APS' on the other side. The tablets are also marked with the strength (250) and code number (2102) on the scored side. They contain the equivalent of 250 mg penicillin V (as the potassium salt) per tablet and comply with the monograph for Phenoxymethylpenicillin Tablets BP.

Apsin VK Syrups are prepared by adding water to the granules to produce an orange coloured and flavoured clear syrup. Each 5 ml syrup contains the equivalent of 125 mg or 250 mg penicillin V (as the potassium salt). The products comply with the specification for Phenoxymethylpenicillin Oral Solution BP. The syrups contain sucrose and colours E110 and E124.

Uses Phenoxymethylpenicillin is a bactericidal agent active against penicillin-sensitive Gram-positive bacteria.

Apsin VK may therefore be used in the management of infections due to penicillin-sensitive organisms, in particular streptococci and staphylococci.

As with other similar agents phenoxymethylpenicillin has occasionally been used prophylactically, when appropriate before and after surgery or dental treatment in patients at risk from bacterial endocarditis owing to congenital or acquired cardiac valvular disease – eg. rheumatic heart disease.

Dosage and administration (Oral).
Adults: 250 mg every 4 hours, or for prophylaxis 125 mg every 12 hours.

Children: aged 6 to 12 years, 250 mg every six hours; aged 1 to 5 years, 125 mg every six hours.

Infants: under 12 months old should receive 62.5 mg every six hours.

The Elderly: Phenoxymethylpenicillin is erratically absorbed from the gastro-intestinal tract, and this phenomenon is likely be exaggerated in the elderly, so the efficacy of treatment may be less predictable in these patients. A separate dosage schedule is not recommended.

It is recommended that doses are taken 30 minutes before food.

In patients with beta-haemolytic streptococcal infection, it is usual to continue treatment at the full dosage for 10 days in order to minimise the occurrence of secondary complications such as acute nephritis and rheumatic fever.

Contra-indications, warnings, etc
Contra-indications: Phenoxymethylpenicillin should not be used in patients with:
(a) chronic or deep-seated infections such as subacute bacterial endocarditis, meningitis or syphilis.
(b) hypersensitivity to penicillins.

Precautions: Special care must be taken when using phenoxymethylpenicillin in patients with a history of allergy, as they are more likely to develop hypersensitivity reactions. For this reason, penicillin should not be used for trivial infections.

Adverse Reactions: Occasionally patients suffer from transient diarrhoea. Hypersensitivity reactions such as urticaria are less common and usually milder than those associated with penicillins given by injection. However, as with all penicillins, anaphylaxis can occur in susceptible hypersensitive individuals and is an acute emergency. Normally, sensitivity reactions may be controlled with antihistamines or, if these fail, with systemic corticosteroids or pressor amines such as adrenaline.

Overdosage: There are no serious sequelae reported, and management should be symptomatic.

Pharmaceutical precautions
Storage: Apsin VK Tablets and granules for Syrup should be stored below 20°C in a dry place, not in a refrigerator. The tablets should be dispensed in airtight containers.

Apsin VK Syrups, when reconstituted, should be used within seven days. They will retain potency for this period if stored below 15°C.

Dilution: Apsin VK Syrups can be diluted with Syrup BP if required. Such dilutions must be freshly prepared.

Legal category POM.

Package quantities
Apsin VK Tablets: polypropylene tubes of 100, 500 and 1000 tablets.

Apsin VK Syrups: granules to produce 100 ml of Syrup when reconstituted with 60 ml water for 250 mg/5 ml Syrup or 65 ml water for 125 mg/5 ml Syrup.

Further information Nil.

Product licence numbers

Apsin VK Tablets 250 mg	0289/5130
Apsin VK Syrup 125 mg/5 ml	0289/5278
Apsin VK Syrup 250 mg/5 ml	0289/5279

APSOLOL*

Presentation
1. Pink, film-coated, Propranolol Tablets BP 10 mg embossed BERK 1Z1 or 1Z1, with breakline on reverse.
2. Pink, film-coated, Propranolol Tablets BP 40 mg embossed BERK 2Z1 or 2Z1, with breakline on reverse.
3. Pink, film-coated, Propranolol Tablets BP 80 mg embossed BERK 3Z1 or 3Z1, with breakline on reverse.
4. Pink, film-coated, Propranolol Tablets BP 160 mg embossed BERK 4Z1 or 4Z1, quadrisected with double breakline on reverse.

Uses Apsolol is a competitive blocker of adrenergic β-receptor sites. It is used in the treatment of hypertension, angina pectoris, cardiac dysrhythmias, anxiety tachycardia, essential tremor and for the long term prevention of sudden cardiac death in patients who have shown evidence of dysrhythmias during the acute phase of myocardial infarction. It may also be used as a prophylactic in migraine, and as adjunctive therapy in thyrotoxicosis.

Dosage and administration Dosage requires individual adjustment. A heart rate of 55/min or less is an indication that dosage should be increased no further.

Adults: Hypertension: Initially, 80 mg twice daily, increased where necessary at weekly intervals. The usual maintenance dosage is 160–320 mg daily. Lower doses may be effective when a diuretic or other antihypertensive drug is given concurrently.

Angina pectoris: Initially, 40 mg twice or thrice daily increased by the same amount at weekly intervals until control is achieved, or the maximum daily dose of 480 mg is reached.

Prophylaxis against recurrence of myocardial infarction: For long term prevention of sudden cardiac death in patients who have survived the acute phase of myocardial infarction, clinical study has shown that treatment should be commenced four to six days after the infarction at a dose of 40 mg four times daily which should then be maintained. As the overriding principle is to maintain adequate β-blockade the dose may need to be varied for some patients.

Anxiety, migraine, essential tremor: 40 mg twice or thrice daily, increased at weekly intervals if needed to a daily total of 160 mg.

Dysthythmias, anxiety tachycardia, hypertrophic obstructive cardiomyopathy, thyrotoxicosis: 10–40 mg three or four times daily.

Children: Dysrhythmias, thyrotoxicosis: The minimum effective dosage, based on 0.25–0.5 mg/kg bodyweight, three or four times daily.

Migraine: Children under the age of 12 may be given 20 mg two or three times daily. Older children may be given adult dosage.

Elderly: No specific dosage recommendations. However, the optimum dose should be determined individually according to clinical response. In patients with impaired hepatic function a reduced dosage should be considered initially.

Contra-indications, warnings, etc
Contra-indications: Propranolol is contra-indicated in patients with second or third degree heart block; bronchial asthma or a history of small airways disease particularly if associated with bronchospasm; metabolic acidosis or after prolonged fasting.

Precautions: Apsolol should be used with great caution in patients with heart failure, unless that is due to thyrotoxicosis alone. Concomitant therapy with digitalis and diuretics is usually desirable in heart failure.

Particular care should be taken in the elderly where hepatic clearance may be reduced thus requiring an appropriate reduction in dosage.

Apsolol should be withdrawn 24 hours before elective surgery, as it may interfere with response to stress. If this cannot be done, 1–2 mg atropine should be given intravenously before anaesthesia commences and anaesthetics such as ether, chloroform, cyclopropane and trichloroethylene, which may cause myocardial depression, should not be used.

Warnings and adverse reactions: Treatment with beta-blocking agents must not be stopped suddenly. If it is necessary to withdraw Apsolol, this should be done gradually, or another beta-blocker should be substituted.

Bradycardia and hypotension are usually a sign of overdosage, but may rarely be due to intolerance of the drug. In the latter case Apsolol should be withdrawn and, if necesary, the patient should be treated as for overdosage. Heart block and congestive heart failure have been reported due to propranolol.

Dry eyes and skin rash have been reported during treatment with β-adrenergic blocking agents. If these symptoms are not attributable to some other cause, Apsolol should be withdrawn.

Apsolol may cause or precipitate Raynaud's phenomenon, intermittent claudication or peripheral arterial insufficiency. Bronchospasm may occur, particularly in patients with a history of asthma or hay fever.

There have been rare reports of blood dyscrasias during treatment with propranolol.

Minor side-effects include cold extremities, nausea, vomiting, diarrhoea, fatigue or insomnia. These are usually transient and are less common if the drug is introduced gradually.

Use in pregnancy: Although there is no evidence that propranolol is teratogenic, Apsolol should not be used in pregnancy unless it is considered essential.

Treatment of overdosage: The clinical features can include bradycardia, severe hypotension, bronchospasm, hypoglycaemia, delirium and unconsciousness. Initially isoprenaline should be infused, and if marked bradycardia is present atropine should be given intravenously (0.6–3 mg; 50 microgram/kg in children): if the response is limited, glucagon therapy must be instituted (50–150 microgram/kg intravenously over one minute followed by 1–5 mg/hour infused). Bronchospasm may be treated by nebulized salbutamol or intravenous aminophylline or salbutamol.

Pharmaceutical precautions Protect from light.

Legal category POM.

Package quantities
Apsolol 10, 40 and 80 mg: polypropylene tubes of 500 and 1000 tablets

Apsolol 160 mg: polypropylene tubes of 100 tablets

Further information Nil.

Product licence numbers

Apsolol Tablets	10 mg	0152/0150
Apsolol Tablets	40 mg	0152/0151
Apsolol Tablets	80 mg	0152/0152
Apsolol Tablets	160 mg	0152/0153

Product licence holder: Berk Pharmaceuticals Ltd.

APSOLOX*

Presentation Apsolox is presented as round, biconvex, film-coated tablets marked 'APS' on one side, while the strength and code number are marked on the other side. The tablets contain Oxprenolol Hydrochloride BP and comply with the monograph for Oxprenolol Tablets BP. Four strengths are available:

Apsolox 20 mg (of Oxprenolol Hydrochloride BP) marked '20/0220' and coloured white.
Apsolox 40 mg (of Oxprenolol Hydrochloride BP) marked '40/0221' and coloured white.
Apsolox 80 mg (of Oxprenolol Hydrochloride BP) marked '80/0222' and coloured yellow.
Apsolox 160 mg (of Oxprenolol Hydrochloride BP) marked '160/0223' and coloured orange.

All strengths of tablets contain sucrose; in addition the 20 mg and 40 mg strengths contain colour E171; the 80 mg strength colours E464, E171 and E102 and the 160 mg strength contains colours E464, E171 and E110.

Uses Oxprenolol is a beta adrenergic receptor blocking agent. As with propranolol its principal effects are on the cardiovascular system. However, oxprenolol is dissimilar in having partial agonist activity (sometimes termed intrinsic sympathomimetic activity).

Apsolox may therefore be used in the management of:

(a) Angina Pectoris
(b) Hypertension
(c) Some forms of Cardiac Dysrhythmias
(d) Anxiety-induced Tachycardia
(e) Hypertrophic Obstructive Cardiomyopathy

Beta adrenergic blocking agents, including oxprenolol, are also used as an adjunct to the management of Thyrotoxicosis and Cardiac Dysrhythmias associated with anaesthesia.

Dosage and administration (Oral)
Adults: Angina Pectoris: The usual dose range is 120–480 mg per day in divided doses to suit the patient's requirements.

Adults: Hypertension: The usual initial dose is 80 mg twice daily and may be increased at weekly intervals as necessary. Most patients will be managed with a dose in the range 160–320 mg per day. It is usual to add a suitable diuretic to the management of most hypertensives who require the higher doses of a beta-blocker.

Adults: Dysrhythmias, Anxiety-induced Tachycardia, Hypertrophic Obstructive Cardiomyopathy and Thyrotoxicosis: Initially 20–40 mg three times per day. This dose may be increased up to 480 mg per day (in divided doses) to achieve the desired effect.

Children: Occasionally beta-blockers have been given to children for the management of dysrhythmias. There is no accepted dosage scheme, but it has been found useful to start with a dose based on 1 mg/kg body weight per day.

The Elderly: Older patients tend to be more susceptible to the effects of beta blockade, so reduced dosages should be used initially. The presence of minor complaints such as cold extremities should be considered as a reason for using alternative treatment regimes if available. Patients already stabilised on beta blockade may require reduced dosage with increasing age.

Contra-indications, warnings, etc
Contra-indications: Oxprenolol should not be used:

(a) In patients with 2nd or 3rd degree heart-block.
(b) In patients with a history of bronchospasm (Asthma).
(c) In patients with marked bradycardia (less than 55 b/minute).
(d) In patients with cardiogenic shock or uncontrolled heart failure.
(e) In patients receiving verapamil or other calcium antagonists. Several days should be allowed for complete elimination of one agent before administering the other.

Precautions: Special care must be taken when using beta-blockers such as oxprenolol in the following situations:

(a) *Cardiac Failure:* If there is evidence of cardiac failure this must be controlled before initiating and during treatment with oxprenolol.
(b) *Pulse Rate:* If the pulse rate falls below 50 b/min, treatment should be withdrawn temporarily and resumed at a lower dose.
(c) *Metabolic Disorders:* In patients with metabolic disorders including alcoholism and diabetic acidosis, great care should be taken in the administration of oxprenolol. Treatment with beta-blockers is liable to mask symptoms and deepen the underlying abnormality in hypoglycaemia and other disorders of carbohydrate metabolism. In patients with labile or insulin-dependent diabetes in whom it is proposed to initiate beta-blocker treatment, it may prove necessary to adjust the dosage of the antidiabetic therapy.
(d) *High Doses:* When high doses of a beta-blocker such as oxprenolol are used, excessive reduction in blood pressure or pulse rate may occur, particularly when used in conjunction with other hypotensive agents such as neurone blocking agents, vasodilators, reserpine or diuretics.
(e) *Pregnancy:* Many beta-blockers such as oxprenolol

have been known to cause bradycardia in the foetus, and this may persist after birth. As with all treatment during pregnancy, labour and lactation, extra care should be taken, and as far as possible treatment should be avoided during these periods, to protect the foetus or the suckling new-born child.

(f) *Other Anti-arrhythmic Agents:* Care should be exercised during co-administration or sequential administration, because serious interactions have been reported between some beta-blocking agents and other antiarrhythmics/cardiac depressants besides verapamil.

(g) *Anaesthesia:* Should treatment with oxprenolol be continued over the period of anaesthesia, then atropine (1–2 mg intravenously) should be included in the pre-medication and special care taken to avoid anaesthetics with negative inotropic activity or that encourage vagal dominance, such as ether, cyclopropane, halothane and trichloroethylene. Similarly, some muscle relaxants – for example suxamethonium – may also increase bradycardia. Otherwise withdrawal should be gradual and completed 24 hours before anaesthesia.

(h) *Renal Failure:* An increased interval between doses may be required to avoid accumulation of oxprenolol.

(i) *Elderly Patients:* See the entry under *Dosage and administration.*

Adverse Reactions: Like other beta-blockers, oxprenolol is well tolerated in normal use. In general untoward effects are minor and include dizziness, headache, insomnia, drowsiness, excitability, gastrointestinal disturbances and rarely bradycardia. Like other beta-blockers, oxprenolol may precipitate bronchospasm, heart failure, or be associated with cold extremities, skin rashes and/or dry eyes. The occurrence of any of these latter symptoms is a reason for discontinuing treatment. (See next paragraph about stopping treatment).

Cessation of Treatment: Withdrawal should be gradual, as several beta-blockers, including oxprenolol, have been associated with a significant increase in symptoms of angina or increase in blood pressure following abrupt withdrawal. If clonidine is co-prescribed, then clonidine should not be withdrawn until several days after Apsolox withdrawal has been completed. (Please refer to prescribing information on clonidine for further information).

Overdosage: Excessive bradycardia and hypotension may be treated with atropine 1–2 mg intravenously and, if necessary, this may be followed by a beta receptor stimulant such as isoprenaline hydrochloride 25 micrograms intravenously. Where cardiogenic shock has supervened, glucagon 5–10 mg intravenously has been reported to be useful. Bronchospasm may be countered by appropriate $beta_2$ receptor stimulants such as salbutamol, either by inhalation or 4 micrograms/kg body weight by slow intravenous injection.

Pharmaceutical precautions Apsolox Tablets should be stored at room temperature in a dry place. The 80 mg and 160 mg strengths should be protected from light.

Legal category POM.

Package quantities
Apsolox 20 and 160 mg: polypropylene tubes of 100 tablets.

Apsolox 40 and 80 mg: polypropylene tubes of 100 and 500 tablets.

Further information Hypertension is a condition which can benefit from the use of both a beta-blocking agent as contained in Apsolox and a thiazide diuretic such as bendrofluazide. This is because their separate pharmacological actions are complementary in hypertension and may allow adequate treatment with smaller doses of each than would be required if either were to be used alone.

The time-to-peak plasma level in fasted healthy young human volunteers following a single dose of Apsolox is approximately 1½–2 hours, and the excretion half-life of oxprenolol in plasma is about 1½ hours. However, as with most other beta-blocking agents the onset of biological activity is delayed and the duration is prolonged relative to the plasma concentration. The decay half-life of the biological effect following a single-dose in normal volunteers has been reported to be 13 hours for oxprenolol, the measure of 'effect' being the reduction in exercise-induced double product (maximum heart rate × systolic blood pressure).†

Product licence numbers

Apsolox Tablets	20 mg	0289/0050
Apsolox Tablets	40 mg	0289/0051
Apsolox Tablets	80 mg	0289/0052
Apsolox Tablets	160 mg	0289/0053

†Vukovich R. A. et al. *Br. J. Clin. Pharmacol.* 1979; 7 Supp 2: 167S–172S.

APSTIL* TABLETS

Presentation Apstil is presented as pink, biconvex, film-coated tablets marked APS on one side with the strength and a code number on the reverse. The tablets contain Stilboestrol BP and comply with the monograph for Stilboestrol Tablets BP.

There are two strengths available: Apstil 1 mg Tablets marked 1/1313; and Apstil 5 mg Tablets marked 5/1314. The tablets also contain lactose and colours E171, E127, E110 and E132.

Uses Stilboestrol is a synthetic non-steroidal oestrogen hormone. It has been in use for many years. However, it has carcinogenic potential, so its use is now only justified in the management of malignant disease.

It may be used to suppress androgenic hormonal activity in the management of androgen-dependent carcinomas such as carcinoma of the prostate in males and some post-menopausal carcinomas such as breast cancer in females.

Apstil Tablets may therefore be used in:
a. Carcinoma of the prostate;
b. Metastatic post-menopausal carcinoma of the breast.

Dosage and administration
Adults:
Management of prostatic carcinoma 1–3 mg daily.
Management of post-menopausal breast carcinoma 10–20 mg daily.

Children: Not suitable.

The elderly: As the conditions for which Apstil is indicated primarily occur in the elderly, the recommended dosage remains unchanged.

Contra-indications, warnings, etc
Contra-indications: Stilboestrol is contra-indicated in:

a. pregnancy – it is not suitable for pre-menopausal women;
b. children;
c. any oestrogen-dependent neoplasms especially of the genital tract;
d. pre-menopausal carcinoma of the breast;
e. endometrial hyperplasia;
f. uterine fibromyomata (fibroids);

or where there is:

g. undiagnosed vaginal bleeding;
h. a history of herpes gestationis;
i. porphyria;
j. moderate to severe hypertension;
k. severe or active liver disease;
l. a history of thrombo-embolism or conditions predisposing to it such as sickle cell anaemia, untreated polycythaemia and pulmonary hypertension;
m. hyperlipoproteinaemia;
n. any cardiovascular or cerebrovascular disorder.

Warnings: The use of any oestrogens predisposes a patient to develop endometrial neoplasia. This is in addition to the known risk of inducing malignant disease with stilboestrol.

Stilboestrol may exacerbate or precipitate cardiac failure and increase the risks of attacks of epilepsy or migraine in patients with a history of these conditions. It is very important that stilboestrol is not used in the groups of patients noted under contra-indications above.

Precautions: Care should be taken when administering Stilboestrol preparations to patients with:

a. cardiac failure;
b. hypertension;
c. diabetes;
d. epilepsy;
e. migraine;
f. depression;
g. contact lenses;
h. cholelithiasis;
i. a history of or with cholestatic jaundice from any cause e.g., jaundice of pregnancy or following the use of oral contraceptives;
j. any evidence of renal dysfunction.

During treatment with Apstil the blood pressure should be monitored at regular intervals and if hypertension develops treatment should be stopped. In addition, if surgery is contemplated or signs or symptoms of thrombosis develop treatment should also be discontinued. This is because of the significant increase in risk of deep vein thrombosis in the presence of high oestrogen activity.

In patients who suffer from diabetes, glucose tolerance may be lowered, and the need for insulin or other antidiabetic drugs may be increased.

In thyroid disease or investigations of thyroid function, thyroid hormone binding globulin may be increased leading to increased circulating total thyroid hormone, which may lead to difficulty in interpreting thyroid function tests.

Pregnancy: Apstil is NOT indicated for pre-menopausal women.

Children: Apstil is NOT suitable for children.

Adverse Reactions: As high doses of stilboestrol in early pregnancy have caused vaginal carcinoma in female offspring 16–20 years later, it should not be used in premenopausal women.

As with other oestrogens the following hormonal disturbances may occur – fluid retention, headache, nausea and vomiting, weight gain, hypertension, breast discomfort, chloasma, skin rashes, erythema nodosum, cholelithiasis and cholestatic jaundice. Venous thrombosis, thromboembolism and possibly cerebral and coronary thrombosis are also risks.

In women, Stilboestrol may cause an increase in the size of uterine fibromyomata, endometrial proliferation and/or an aggravation or recurrence of endometriosis and an excessive production of cervical mucous. The risk of endometrial neoplasia is increased significantly.

In both sexes the use of Stilboestrol may cause tenderness, pain, enlargement and secretion of milk like fluid from the breast. It also may aggravate corneal discomfort in patients with contact lenses and be associated with fluctuating moods (both elation and depression) and headaches including an increase in incidence of migraine.

The general metabolic effects of Stilboestrol include sodium and water retention, reduced glucose tolerance and changes in body weight (usually increases).

In men there will be some feminization, e.g. gynaecomastia and testicular atrophy, and impotence.

Other effects may be withdrawal bleeding in women and an increased incidence of cholelithiasis. In the event of prolonged usage there is an increased risk of endometrial carcinoma.

Overdosage: There is no specific antidote to stilboestrol. The commonest symptoms of overdosage are nausea and vomiting. Management may include gastric lavage associated with special care of plasma electrolytes and any other appropriate symptomatic relief. Should the overdose (abuse) be in female children, an oestrogen-withdrawal bleed may be induced.

Pharmaceutical precautions Apstil Tablets should be stored in a dry place below 25°C and protected from light.

Legal category POM.

Package quantities
Apstil Tablets 1 mg: Blister packs of 56.
Apstil Tablets 5 mg: Blister packs of 28.

Further information Apstil should not be used in children or young adults because it has carcinogenic potential.

In prostatic carcinoma and metastatic post-menopausal breast carcinoma, stilboestrol causes temporary disease regression in approximately 80% and 30% of patients respectively.

Product licence numbers
Apstil Tablets 1 mg 0289/5188
Apstil Tablets 5 mg 0289/5189

ASMAVEN*

Presentation
Asmaven Tablets are pink, round, flat-faced with bevelled edges, marked 'APS' or plain on one side, while the strength and code number are marked on the other side. The tablets contain Salbutamol BP as the sulphate and comply with the monograph for Salbutamol Tablets BP. Two strengths are available:
Asmaven 2 mg (of Salbutamol BP) marked '2/1507'.
Asmaven 4 mg (of Salbutamol BP) marked '4/1508'.

Both strengths of tablets contain lactose and colours E127 and E131.

Asmaven Inhaler (not available in the UK at the time of writing) is a metered-dose metal aerosol canister mounted in a specially-designed blue plastic actuator with white plastic cap. It delivers 100 micrograms of Salbutamol BP to the patient per actuation and contains sufficient for at least 200 metered inhalations. The whole is enclosed in a carton with an instruction leaflet for the patient. Asmaven Inhaler complies with the monograph for Salbutamol Aerosol Inhalation BPC.

Uses *Tablets and Inhaler:* Salbutamol is a beta-adrenergic stimulant which has a selective action on the beta-adrenergic receptors in bronchial muscle and, in therapeutic dosage, little or no action on the cardiac beta-adrenergic receptors. In view of the selective action on the bronchi, salbutamol preparations are suitable for treating bronchospasm in patients with co-existing heart disease or hypertension.

Salbutamol is also active, when used locally in human lung sensitised with IgE antibody, in preventing antigen-induced release of histamine and slow reacting substance of anaphylaxis, SRS(A), from mast cells. Such Type I hypersensitivity reactions are generally considered to be the primary triggers of the allergic asthma syndrome.

The inhaler delivers a much smaller dose than the tablets. The small dose is effective because it is delivered locally to the tissues responsible for bronhco-constriction, but it minimises the unwanted systemic effects such as the skeletal muscle tremor sometimes associated with the higher systemic doses arising from tablet usage. The increased therapeutic ratio when salbutamol is used locally makes the inhaler suitable for use in those patients also receiving beta-blocking agents. The inhaler also has the advantage of a rapid local onset of action and a relatively prolonged duration of effect.

Asmaven preparations (tablets or inhaler) may therefore be used in the management of:

(a) Bronchial Asthma
(b) Other conditions with associated reversible airways obstruction such as Bronchitis and Emphysema

} including patients with co-existing heart disease or hypertension.

The Asmaven Inhaler is particularly suitable for:

(a) Relieving attacks of Acute Dyspnoea
(b) Routine maintenance therapy in Chronic Asthma
(c) Routine maintenance therapy in Chronic Bronchitis
(d) Prophylaxis before exertion to prevent exercise-induced Asthma

} including patients also receiving beta-blocking agents.

Tablets in Premature Labour: Asmaven Tablets may be used following the administration of salbutamol as a continuous intravenous infusion for the management of premature labour during the third trimester of pregnancy. Once the uterine contractions have ceased and the infusion has been withdrawn, maintenance therapy may be continued with Asmaven Tablets.

Dosage and administration (Oral)
Asmaven Tablets.

Adults: The usual effective dose is 4 mg three or four times per day. If adequate bronchodilation is not obtained, each single dose may be gradually increased to as much as 8 mg. However, it has been established that some patients obtain adequate relief with 2 mg three or four times daily.

Children: The following doses should be administered three or four times daily:
2–6 years: ½ to 1 of the 2 mg tablets.
6–12 years: 1 of the 2 mg tablets.
Over 12 years: 1–2 of the 2 mg tablets or 1 of the 4 mg tablets.

Salbutamol is well tolerated by children so that, if necessary, these doses may be cautiously increased.

The Elderly: In elderly patients or in those known to be unusually sensitive to beta-adrenergic stimulants, it is advisable to initiate treatment with 2 mg three or four times per day.

Premature Labour: In the management of premature labour, after uterine contractions have been controlled by intravenous salbutamol and the infusion has been withdrawn, maintenance therapy may be continued with Asmaven Tablets. The usual dosage is 4 mg three or four times daily.

Asmaven Inhaler
Adults: Acute Bronchospasm and intermittent episodes of Asthma: One or two inhalations as a single dose.

Adults: Chronic Maintenance or Prophylactic Therapy: Two inhalations three or four times a day.

Adults: Prevention of Exercise-induced Bronchospasm: Two inhalations before exertion.

Children: Acute Bronchospasm, Episodic Asthma, or before exercise: One inhalation.

Children: Routine Maintenance or Prophylactic Therapy: One inhalation three or four times a day.

These doses may be increased to two inhalations if necessary.

Duration of effect: The bronchodilator effect of each administration of inhaled salbutamol lasts at least four hours except in patients whose asthma is worsening. Such patients should be warned not to increase their usage of inhaler but to seek medical advice in case treatment with a glucocorticoid is indicated.

Contra-indications, warnings, etc
Contra-indications: Care should be taken when administering salbutamol preparations to patients suffering from diabetes mellitus, serious cardiovascular disorders or hypertension.
Pregnancy: Although intravenous salbutamol and salbutamol tablets are used in the management of premature labour, these preparations should not be used for threatened abortion during the first or second trimester of pregnancy.

Beta-blocking Agents: Salbutamol tablets should not usually be prescribed for patients under treatment with beta-blocking agents, but note that the inhaler may be prescribed for such patients.

Precautions: Thyrotoxicosis: Care should be taken when administering salbutamol preparations to patients suffering from thyrotoxicosis.

Hypokalaemia: Potentially serious hypokalaemia may result from $beta_2$ agonist therapy. Particular caution is advised in severe asthma as this effect may be potentiated by concomitant treatment with xanthine derivatives, steroids, diuretics and by hypoxia. It is recommended that serum potassium levels are monitored in such situations.

Pregnancy: As with other agents the use of salbutamol during pregnancy should be avoided if possible (except for the management of premature labour).

Duration of Inhaler Action: Patients using salbutamol inhaler should be warned to seek medical advice if a previously effective dose fails to continue relief for at least three hours; treatment with a glucocorticoid may then be indicated.

Adverse Reactions: Potentially serious hypokalaemia may result from $beta_2$ agonist therapy. The only other side-effect of significance with salbutamol tablets is a fine tremor of skeletal muscle which occurs in some patients; usually the hands are most obviously affected. This effect is dose related and is common to all beta-adrenergic stimulants. A few patients feel tense; this is also due to the effects on skeletal muscle and not to direct CNS stimulation. With doses of salbutamol higher than those recommended or in patients who are unusually sensitive to beta-adrenergic stimulants peripheral vasodilation and a compensatory small increase in heart rate may occur. Occasionally headaches have been reported.

No important adverse reactions have been reported following therapy with salbutamol inhaler. This is presumably due to the small size of the effective dose and the correspondingly increased therapeutic ratio.

Overdosage: The preferred antidote for overdosage with salbutamol is a cardioselective beta-blocking agent, but such agents should be used with caution in patients with a history of bronchospasm.

Pharmaceutical precautions
Asmaven Tablets should be stored below 25°C and protected from light.

Asmaven Inhaler should be stored in a cool place, protected from frost, direct heat and sunlight. The canister should not be broken, punctured or burnt even when apparently empty.

Legal category POM.

Package quantities
Asmaven Tablets 2 mg: Polypropylene tubes of 500 tablets.
Asmaven Tablets 4 mg: Polypropylene tubes of 100 and 500 tablets.
Asmaven Inhaler: One aerosol canister mounted in a plastic actuator and enclosed in a carton with an instruction leaflet. The inhaler is not available in the U.K at the time of writing.

Further information Unlike sympathomimetic agents such as ephedrine, salbutamol does not stimulate alpha-adrenoceptors and, therefore, does not cause difficulty in micturition. Therefore salbutamol is not contra-indicated in patients under treatment with monoamine oxidase inhibitors (MAOIs).

Product licence numbers

Asmaven Tablets 2 mg	0289/0064
Asmaven Tablets 4 mg	0289/0065
Asmaven Inhaler	0289/0068

CALABREN*

Presentation Calabren is presented as white biconvex tablets marked 'APS' or plain on one side and with the strength and code number on the other side. They contain Glibenclamide BP and comply with the monograph for Glibenclamide Tablets BP. Two strengths are available:

2.5 mg – round tablets coded 3103;
5 mg – elongated tablets coded 3104 with a break-line.
Both strengths of tablets contain lactose.

Uses Glibenclamide is an oral hypoglycaemic agent. Calabren may therefore be used in the management of non-insulin-dependent diabetes mellitus in patients who have responded poorly to dietary measures alone.

Dosage and administration Oral.
Adults: Previously untreated Diabetes Mellitus: Treatment should be started with 5 mg daily, taken during or immediately following breakfast or the first main meal of the day. It is wise to start at a lower dose of 2.5 mg daily if the patient is elderly or debilitated – see 'Contra-indications, warnings, etc.' If control of diabetic symptoms remains inadequate, the daily dose may be increased not more frequently than weekly in steps of 2.5 mg (usual) or 5 mg (maximum) daily to a maximum dose not exceeding 15 mg daily. This is normally given as a single dose during or immediately after breakfast or the first main meal of the day. However, care should be taken to apportion the diet with the daily activity schedule and the final dosage schedule for each individual patient.

Adults: Changing from other oral sulphonyl-urea hypoglycaemic agents: These changes may be made without any formal break in treatment. Where the patient is already well controlled, Calabren treatment should commence with one 5 mg dose daily, adjusted weekly in increments not exceeding 5 mg to a maximum of 15 mg daily – see above. Where control has not been adequate on previous therapy, Calabren treatment may be started on the approximately equivalent dose provided this does not exceed 10 mg daily. It may then be raised at weekly intervals to a maximum dose of 15 mg daily.

5 mg of Glibenclamide BP is approximately equivalent to:

Tolbutamide	1 g
Glymidine	1 g
Acetohexamide	500 mg
Tolazamide	250 mg
Chlorpropamide	250 mg
Glibonuride	25 mg
Glipizide	5 mg

Adults: Changing from biguanides such as metformin: Calabren treatment should be started at a dose of 2.5 mg daily and the biguanide then withdrawn. To achieve control the dose of Calabren should be adjusted at weekly intervals in increments of 2.5 mg daily but not exceeding the maximum dose of 15 mg daily.

Adults: Combination Therapy with biguanides: Where control of diabetic symptoms has not been achieved with a single oral hypoglycaemic agent such as glibenclamide at the maximum dosage of 15 mg daily, control may often be achieved by adding a biguanide derivative to the regime.

Adults: Changing from an insulin regime: A few patients with very low daily insulin requirements may remain controlled if transferred to glibenclamide and should be treated as new patients. Tablets should always be taken with or immediately after the first main meal of the day, and the insulin dose should be reduced further with each increased dose level of glibenclamide.

Children: Juvenile-onset diabetes mellitus is normally insulin-dependent, and consequently glibenclamide is not suitable for use in children.

The elderly: The initial dose in elderly or debilitated patients should be 2.5 mg daily.

Contra-indications, warnings, etc
Contra-indications: Glibenclamide should not be used:
(a) in patients suffering from or with a history of diabetic keto-acidosis.
(b) in patients with serious impairment of function in the kidneys, liver or adrenal glands.
(c) in patients undergoing surgery.
(d) in pregnant patients, for whom insulin treatment is normally preferred.

Warning: The hypoglycaemic effect of glibenclamide may be ENHANCED (occasionally dramatically) by:
(a) coumarin anticoagulants.
(b) monoamine oxidase inhibitors.
(c) beta-adrenergic blocking agents.
(d) sulphonamides.
(e) phenylbutazone.
(f) chloramphenicol
(g) cyclophosphamide
(h) salicylates e.g., aspirin.

Conversely the hypoglycaemic effect of glibenclamide may be DIMINISHED by:
(a) sympathomimetic agents e.g., adrenalin.
(b) steroids including oral contraceptives.
(c) thiazide diuretics.

Precautions: Special care must be taken when using glibenclamide in the following situations:
(a) *Elderly or Debilitated Patients:* These patients are more likely to suffer from hypoglycaemia – see treatment of overdosage.
(b) *Pregnancy and Lactation:* There is no adequate information on the use of glibenclamide in human pregnancy. It is normal practice to manage diabetes in pregnant patients with insulin, although there appear to be no specific reasons to stop a pre-existing regime which includes glibenclamide. There is no evidence of teratogenicity in animal experiments. However, as with other sulphonylurea hypoglycaemic agents, it is wise to assume that glibenclamide is present in human breast milk. Consequently, its use is best avoided where the patient expresses a desire to breast-feed.

Adverse Reactions: Like other oral hypoglycaemic agents, glibenclamide is well tolerated in normal use. Untoward effects are usually mild and rarely require treatment to be discontinued. Among these mild effects are gastro-intestinal symptoms (anorexia, diarrhoea and nausea) and allergic-type skin reactions. Leucopenia and thrombocytopenia have been reported, and are reversible on stopping treatment. Transient changes in liver enzymes and function tests have been reported during glibenclamide treatment, although a definite relationship to treatment has yet to be established. As with all other oral hypoglycaemic agents, an over-response to treatment may occur, especially in relation to unexpected heavy exercise. These hypoglycaemic attacks are not usually prolonged and should be managed as for overdosage.

Overdosage: Conscious Patients with early signs of hypoglycaemia – faintness, nausea, cold-sweats and/or palpitation – may be treated with glucose water or 3–4 lumps of sugar (sucrose) with water. This treatment may be repeated as necessary and, if symptoms continue to recur at intervals, may be supplemented with half a pint of milk after successful management of the current recurrence of symptoms.

Overdosage: Comatose Patients should receive glucose administered as a continuous intravenous infusion, because a bolus injection may lead to a more severe and prolonged rebound hypoglycaemia. An alternative approach is to administer 1 mg of glucagon as a subcutaneous or intramuscular injection. The objective of both treatments is to achieve rapid recovery of consciousness, when further 'feeding' should be instituted, as above.

Pharmaceutical precautions Calabren Tablets should be stored below 25°C.

Legal category POM.

Package quantities
Calabren 2.5 mg: polypropylene tubes of 100 tablets.
Calabren 5 mg: polypropylene tubes of 100 and 500 tablets.

Further information Nil.

Product licence numbers

Calabren Tablets 2.5 mg	0289/0047
Calabren Tablets 5 mg	0289/0048

**Trade Mark*

Armour Pharmaceutical Company Limited
St. Leonards House
St. Leonards Road
Eastbourne
East Sussex BN21 3YG

ALBUMINAR*-5

Presentation Albuminar-5 is a sterile aqueous solution of Human Albumin 5% obtained from large pools of adult human venous plasma. Each 100 ml of Albuminar-5 contains 5 g of human albumin which is osmotically equivalent to normal human plasma.

The product conforms to the monograph for Human Albumin Solution PhEur.

Indications Albuminar-5 is indicated in: The emergency treatment of shock and in other conditions where the restoration of blood volume is urgent.

Serious burns to prevent haemoconcentration and to combat fluid and sodium losses.

Clinical situations associated with low plasma protein (Hypoproteinaemia) with or without oedema, provided that sodium restriction is not imperative.

Therapeutic Plasma Exchange as a replacement fluid for apheresed plasma.

Dosage and administration (a) *Administration*: Albuminar-5 is for intravenous infusion.

Albuminar-5 may be given intravenously without further dilution; 5% solution is approximately isotonic and isosmotic with citrated plasma.

When albumin solution is administered to patients with normal blood volume, particular attention should be given to the rate of infusion so that the plasma volume is not expanded too rapidly.

(b) *Standard dose: Urgent restoration of blood volume:* In the emergency treatment of shock, the amount of albumin and duration of therapy must be based on the responsiveness of the patient as indicated by blood pressure, central venous pressure, degree of pulmonary congestion and haematocrit. The initial dose may be followed by additional albumin within 15–30 minutes if the response is deemed inadequate. If there has been considerable loss of blood, transfusion with whole blood is indicated, or if there is continued loss of protein, blood or plasma it may also be desirable to give whole blood and/or other blood fractions.

Burns: Albuminar-5 may be used to prevent marked haemoconcentration and to maintain appropriate electrolyte balance. An optimal regimen involving the use of albumin, crystalloids and water has not been established. Suggested therapy in the treatment of burns includes administration of large volumes of crystalloid solution during the first 24 hours to maintain an adequate plasma volume, even when albumin is infused. Continuation of therapy beyond 24 hours usually requires more albumin and less crystalloid solution. Duration of treatment varies depending on the extent of protein loss through renal excretion, denuded areas of skin and decreased albumin synthesis. Attempts to raise the albumin level above 40 g/litre may only result in an increased rate of catabolism.

Conditions associated with hypoproteinaemia: In these conditions, 1,000 to 1,500 ml of Albuminar-5 may be required to reduce oedema and to bring serum protein values to normal. Since such patients usually have approximately normal blood volume, doses of more than 500 ml of Albuminar-5 should not be given faster than 500 ml in 30–45 minutes to avoid circulatory embarrassment. If slower administration is desired, e.g. in patients with hypertension or cardiac insufficiency, 1,000 ml of Albuminar-5 may be administered by continuous drip at a rate of 100 ml of this solution per hour. Unless the pathological condition responsible for the hypoproteinaemia can be corrected, albumin in any form can afford only symptomatic or supportive relief. The 5% solution should not be administered in situations where sodium restriction is imperative.

Therapeutic plasma exchange: In plasma exchange procedures the volume of plasma removed may be replaced with an equivalent volume of Albuminar-5.

(c) *Children:* The amount of albumin given and the duration of therapy must be determined by the child's condition, response and other parameters, as stated under '*Standard Dose*'. However, when treating children, their body weight should also be taken into account.

Use in pregnancy: There is some experience of albumin being used in the treatment of pre-eclampsia and eclampsia. However, there is very little experience of the use of albumin in the early stages of pregnancy. There is no evidence either in human pregnancy or in animal work that administration of albumin is free from hazard.

Pharmacology: Action: Albuminar-5 is active osmotically and is therefore important in regulating the volume of circulating blood. When the circulating blood volume has been depleted, the haemodilution following albumin administration persists for many hours. In individuals with normal blood volumes, it usually lasts only a few hours.

Contra-indications, warnings, etc *Contra-indications:* Albuminar-5 may be contra-indicated in patients with severe anaemia or cardiac failure.

Precautions: If dehydration is present additional fluids must accompany or follow the administration of Albuminar-5.

The rise in blood pressure which may follow rapid administration of albumin necessitates careful observation of the injured patient to detect bleeding points, which failed to bleed at the lower blood pressure; otherwise new haemorrhage and shock may occur.

Albuminar-5 should be administered with caution to patients with low cardiac reserve or with no albumin deficiency, because a rapid increase in plasma volume may cause circulatory embarrassment or pulmonary oedema. In cases of hypertension or cardiac insufficiency, a slower rate of administration is desirable, at a rate of 5 g of albumin (100 ml) per hour. A careful watch must be kept for the possible development of pulmonary oedema. Should pulmonary oedema occur, the infusion must be stopped immediately.

Warnings and adverse effects: Do not use if the solution is turbid or contains a deposit. Since the solution contains no preservative, it should be used within 3 hours after entering the vial.

The incidence of adverse reactions to Human Albumin Solution 5% is low, although nausea, vomiting, increased salivation and febrile reactions may occasionally occur.

Toxicity and treatment of overdosage: Administration of large quantities of albumin should be supplemented with red cell concentrates or replaced by whole blood to combat the relative anaemia which would follow such use. If circulatory embarrassment or pulmonary oedema should develop, the infusion must be stopped immediately and specific treatment given.

Pharmaceutical precautions
(a) *Presentation and Composition:* Albuminar-5 is a sterile, clear, brownish, slightly viscous aqueous solution of human serum albumin. It is stabilised with 0.004 M sodium acetyltryptophanate and 0.004 M sodium caprylate and the pH of the solution is adjusted with sodium bicarbonate or acetic acid. The solution contains approximately 145 mmol/l of sodium and not more than 200 micrograms/l of aluminium. The solution contains no preservative.

(b) *Storage:* Albuminar-5 should be stored at a temperature between 2° and 25°C. Freezing will not harm the solution, but might damage the container and allow contamination of the contents.

Protect solution from light.

When stored as directed Albuminar-5 has a shelf-life of 3 years.

Legal category POM.

Package quantities
Albuminar-5 is supplied as a 5% solution in:
250 ml glass vials containing 12.5 grams of albumin
500 ml glass vials containing 25.0 grams of albumin
1,000 ml glass vials containing 50.0 grams of albumin.

Further information Albuminar-5 is prepared from blood that was non-reactive for hepatitis B surface antigen (HBsAg) when tested with licensed reagents. The likelihood of the presence of viable hepatitis viruses has been further minimised by pasteurising the product at 60°C for 10 hours. Such treatment has been shown to be effective in this respect even when prepared from plasma known to be infective and albumin so prepared, unlike whole blood or plasma, is considered free of the danger of homologous serum hepatitis. All units of source plasma are tested for antibody to the human immunodeficiency virus (HIV) and found to be negative. Albuminar-5 may be given in conjunction with other parenteral fluids, such as whole blood, plasma, saline, dextrose, or sodium lactate. It is convenient to use, since no cross-matching is required and the absence of cellular elements removes the danger of sensitisation with repeated infusions.

Albuminar-5 contains none of the recognised components of the clotting mechanism of normal blood or plasma. It does not interfere with the normal clotting of blood.

Product licence number 0231/0056.

ALBUMINAR-20

Presentation Albuminar-20 is a sterile aqueous solution of Human Albumin 20% obtained from large pools of adult human venous plasma. Each 100 ml of Albuminar-20 contains 20 g of human serum albumin which is osmotically equivalent to 400 ml of normal human plasma.

The product conforms to the monograph for Human Albumin Solution Ph Eur.

Indications Albuminar-20 is indicated in: The emergency treatment of shock and in other conditions where the restoration of blood volume is urgent.

Serious burns to prevent haemoconcentration and to combat fluid and sodium losses.

Clinical situations associated with low plasma protein (hypoproteinaemia) with or without oedema.

As an adjunct to exchange transfusion for the treatment of hyperbilirubinaemia in haemolytic disease of the newborn.

In priming heart lung machines for cardiopulmonary by-pass surgery.

Dosage and administration
(a) *Administration:* Albuminar-20 is for intravenous infusion.

Albuminar-20 may be given intravenously without dilution or it may be diluted with normal saline or 5% dextrose before administration, 250 ml per litre gives a solution which is approximately isotonic and isosmotic with citrated plasma.

When undiluted albumin solution is administered to patients with normal blood volume, particular attention should be given to the rate of infusion so that the plasma volume is not expanded too rapidly.

(b) *Standard dose: Urgent restoration of blood volume:* In these conditions effectiveness of Albuminar-20 depends on its ability to draw tissue fluid into the blood stream, when such fluid is available. Therefore, if dehydration is present, other fluids must be administered by any available route, either with albumin or following it. In the emergency treatment of shock, the amount of albumin and duration of therapy must be based on the responsiveness of the patient as indicated by blood pressure, central venous pressure, degree of pulmonary congestion and haematocrit. The initial dose may be followed by additional albumin within 15–30 minutes if the response is deemed inadequate. If there has been considerable loss of blood, transfusion with whole blood is indicated, or if there is continued loss of protein, blood or plasma it may also be desirable to give whole blood and/or other blood fractions.

Burns: Albuminar-20 may be used in conjunction with normal saline or dextrose to prevent marked haemoconcentration and to maintain appropriate electrolyte balance. An optimal regimen involving the use of albumin, crystalloids and water has not been established. Suggested therapy in the treatment of burns includes administration of large volumes of crystalloid solution during the first 24 hours to maintain an adequate plasma volume, even when albumin is infused. Continuation of therapy beyond 24 hours usually requires more albumin and less crystalloid solution. Duration of treatment varies depending on the extent of protein loss through renal excretion, denuded areas of skin and decreased albumin synthesis. Attempts to raise the albumin level above 40 g/litre may only result in an increased rate of catabolism.

Conditions associated with hypoproteinaemia: In these conditions, 200 to 300 ml of Albuminar-20 may be required to reduce oedema and to bring serum protein values to normal. Since such patients usually have approximately normal blood volume, doses of more than 100 ml of Albuminar-20 should not be given faster than 100 ml in 30–45 minutes to avoid circulatory embarrassment. If slower administration is desired, e.g. in patients with hypertension or cardiac insufficiency, 250 ml of Albuminar-20 may be mixed with 250 ml of 10% dextrose solution and administered by continuous drip at a rate of 100 ml of this dextrose solution per hour. Unless the pathological condition responsible for the hypoproteinaemia can be corrected, albumin in any form can afford only symptomatic or supportive relief.

Hyperbilirubinaemia in haemolytic disease of the newborn: In neonates, with serum bilirubin levels above 20 mg per 100 ml severe cerebral damage can develop due to kernicterus. In hypoalbuminaemia the reserve binding capacity for bilirubin is decreased and consequently bilirubin toxicity increases and with it the risk of cerebral damage. The risk of cerebral damage can be reduced by correction of the bilirubin binding capacity with Albuminar-20.

If immediate protection of the patient is required an intravenous injection of 1.0–1.5 g/kg albumin (5–7 ml Albuminar-20/kg bodyweight) can be given. Following this injection the exchange transfusion procedure should be instituted within 6 hours.

If albumin is intended for increasing the removal of bilirubin during exchange transfusion, it is suggested that 1.5–2.5 g albumin (7–12 ml Albuminar-20) is added to each 100 ml donor blood during exchange transfusion.

In Priming Heart Lung Machines for Cardiopulmonary By-Pass Surgery: Pre-operative dilution of the blood by use of a pump prime consisting of only albumin and crystalloid has been shown to be well tolerated during clinical studies. An albumin concentration of 5 g per cent has been widely used. A commonly employed programme is an albumin and crystalloid pump prime adjusted so as to achieve a haematocrit reading of 20 per cent and a plasma albumin level of 2.5 g/100 ml in the patient.

(c) *Children*: The amount of albumin given and the duration of therapy must be determined by the child's condition, response and other parameters, as stated under *'Standard Dose'*. However, when treating children, their body weight should also be taken into account.

Use in pregnancy: There is some experience of albumin being used in the treatment of pre-eclampsia and eclampsia. However, there is very little experience of the use of albumin in the early stages of pregnancy. There is no evidence either in human pregnancy or in animal work that administration of albumin is free from hazard.

Pharmacology: Action: Albuminar-20 is active osmotically and is therefore important in regulating the volume of circulating blood. When injected intravenously, 50 ml of Albuminar-20 draws approximately 3 volumes of additional fluid into the circulation within 15 minutes, except in the presence of marked dehydration. This extra fluid reduces haematocrit and blood viscosity. The degree of volume expansion is dependent on the initial blood volume. When circulating blood volume has been depleted, the haemodilution following albumin administration persists for many hours. In individuals with normal blood volume, it usually lasts only a few hours.

Contra-indications, warnings, etc
Contra-indications: Albuminar-20 may be contra-indicated in patients with severe anaemia or cardiac failure.

Precautions: If dehydration is present additional fluids must accompany or follow the administration of Albuminar-20.

The rise in blood pressure which may follow rapid administration of albumin necessitates careful observation of the injured patient to detect bleeding points, which failed to bleed at the lower blood pressure; otherwise new haemorrhage and shock may occur.

Albuminar-20 should be administered with caution to patients with low cardiac reserve or with no albumin deficiency, because a rapid increase in plasma volume may cause circulatory embarrassment or pulmonary oedema. In cases of hypertension or cardiac insufficiency, a slower rate of administration is desirable: 250 ml of Albuminar-20 may be mixed with 250 ml of 10% dextrose solution and administered at a rate of 10 g of albumin (100 ml) per hour. A careful watch must be kept for the possible development of pulmonary oedema. Should pulmonary oedema occur, the infusion must be stopped immediately.

Warnings and adverse effects: Do not use if the solution is turbid or contains a deposit. Since the solution contains no preservative, it should be used within 3 hours after entering the vial.

The incidence of adverse reactions to Human Albumin Solution 20% is low, although nausea, vomiting, increased salivation and febrile reactions may occasionally occur.

Toxicity and treatment of overdosage: Administration of large quantities of albumin should be supplemented with red cell concentrates or replaced by whole blood to combat the relative anaemia which would follow such use.

If circulatory embarrassment or pulmonary oedema should develop, the infusion must be stopped immediately and specific treatment given.

Pharmaceutical precautions
(a) *Presentation and composition:* Albuminar-20 is a sterile, clear, brownish, slightly viscous aqueous solution of human albumin. It is stabilised with 0.016 M sodium acetyltryptophanate and 0.016 M sodium caprylate and the pH of the solution is adjusted with sodium bicarbonate or acetic acid. The solution contains approximately 124 mmol/l of sodium and not more than 200 micrograms/l of aluminium. The solution contains no preservative.

(b) *Storage:* Albuminar-20 should be stored at a temperature between 2° and 25°C. Freezing will not harm the solution, but might damage the container and allow contamination of the contents. Protect solution from light.

When stored as directed, Albuminar-20 has a shelf-life of 3 years.

Legal category POM.

Package quantities Albuminar-20 is supplied as a 20% solution in:
50 ml vials containing 10.0 grams of albumin;
100 ml vials containing 20.0 grams of albumin.

Further information Albuminar-20 is prepared from blood that was non-reactive for hepatitis B surface antigen (HBsAg) when tested with licensed reagents. The likelihood of the presence of viable hepatitis viruses has been further minimised by pasteurising the product at 60°C for 10 hours. Such treatment has been shown to be effective in this respect even when prepared from plasma known to be infective and albumin so prepared, unlike whole blood or plasma, is considered free of the danger of homologous serum hepatitis. All units of source plasma are tested for antibody to the human immunodeficiency virus (HIV) and found to be negative.

Albuminar-20 may be given in conjunction with other parenteral fluids, such as whole blood, plasma, saline, dextrose, or sodium lactate. It is convenient to use, since no cross-matching is required and the absence of cellular elements removes the danger of sensitisation with repeated infusions.

Albuminar-20 contains none of the recognised components of the clotting mechanism of normal blood or plasma. It does not interfere with the normal clotting of blood.

Product licence number 0231/0057

ALBUMINAR-25

Presentation Albuminar-25 is a sterile aqueous solution of Human Albumin 25% obtained from large pools of adult human venous plasma. Each 100 ml of Albuminar-25 contains 25 g of human serum albumin which is osmotically equivalent to 500 ml of normal human plasma.

The product conforms to the monograph for Human Albumin Solution Ph Eur.

Indications Albuminar-25 is indicated in: The emergency treatment of shock and in other conditions where the restoration of blood volume is urgent.

Serious burns to prevent haemoconcentration and to combat fluid and sodium losses.

Clinical situations associated with low plasma protein (hypoproteinaemia) with or without oedema.

As an adjunct to exchange transfusion for the treatment of hyperbilirubinaemia in haemolytic disease of the newborn.

In priming heart-lung machines for cardiopulmonary by-pass surgery.

Dosage and administration
(a) *Administration:* Albuminar-25 is for intravenous infusion.

Albuminar-25 may be given intravenously without dilution or it may be diluted with normal saline or 5% dextrose before administration; 200 ml per litre gives a solution which is approximately isotonic and isosmotic with citrated plasma.

When undiluted albumin solution is administered to patients with normal blood volume, particular attention should be given to the rate of infusion so that it is slow enough to prevent too rapid expansion of plasma volume.

(b) *Standard dose: Urgent restoration of blood volume:* In these conditions effectiveness of Albuminar-25 depends on its ability to draw tissue fluid into the blood stream, when such fluid is available. Therefore, if dehydration is present, other fluids must be administered by any available route, either with albumin or following it. In the emergency treatment of shock, the amount of albumin and duration of therapy must be based on the responsiveness of the patient as indicated by blood pressure, central venous pressure, degree of pulmonary congestion and haematocrit. The initial dose may be followed by additional albumin within 15–30 minutes if the response is deemed inadequate. If there has been considerable loss of blood, transfusion with whole blood is indicated, or if there is continued loss of protein, blood or plasma it may also be desirable to give whole blood and/or other blood fractions.

Burns: Albuminar-25 may be used in conjunction with normal saline or dextrose to prevent marked haemoconcentration and to maintain appropriate electrolyte balance. An optimal regimen involving the use of albumin, crystalloids and water has not been established. Suggested therapy in the treatment of burns includes administration of large volumes of crystalloid solution during the first 24 hours to maintain an adequate plasma volume, even when albumin is infused. Continuation of therapy beyond 24 hours usually requires more albumin and less crystalloid solution. Duration of treatment varies depending on the extent of protein loss through renal excretion, denuded areas of skin and decreased albumin synthesis. Attempts to raise the albumin level above 40 g/litre may only result in an increased rate of catabolism.

Conditions associated with hypoproteinaemia: In these conditions, 200 to 300 ml of Albuminar-25 may be required to reduce oedema and to bring serum protein values to normal. Since such patients usually have approximately normal blood volume, doses of more than 100 ml of Albuminar-25 should not be given faster than 100 ml in 30–45 minutes to avoid circulatory embarrassment. If slower administration is desired, e.g. in patients with hypertension or cardiac insufficiency, 200 ml of Albuminar-25 may be mixed with 300 ml of 10% dextrose solution and administered by continuous drip at a rate of 100 ml of this dextrose solution per hour. Unless the pathological condition responsible for the hypoproteinaemia can be corrected, albumin in any form can afford only symptomatic or supportive relief.

Hyperbilirubinaemia in haemolytic disease of the newborn: In neonates with serum bilirubin levels above 20 mg per 100 ml severe cerebral damage can develop due to kernicterus. In hypoalbuminaemia the reserve binding capacity for bilirubin is decreased and consequently bilirubin toxicity increases and with it the risk of cerebral damage. The risk of cerebral damage can be reduced by correction of the bilirubin binding capacity with Albuminar-25.

If immediate protection of the patient is required an intravenous injection of 1.0–1.5 g/kg albumin (4–6 ml Albuminar-25/kg bodyweight) can be given. Following this injection the exchange transfusion procedure should be instituted within 6 hours.

If albumin is intended for increasing the removal of bilirubin during exchange transfusion, it is suggested that 1.5–2.5 g albumin (6–10 ml Albuminar-25) is added to each 100 ml donor blood during exchange transfusion.

In Priming Heart Lung Machines for Cardiopulmonary By-Pass Surgery: Pre-operative dilution of the blood by use of a pump prime consisting of only albumin and crystalloid has been shown to be well tolerated during clinical studies. An albumin concentration of 5 g per cent has been widely used. A commonly employed programme is an albumin and crystalloid pump prime adjusted so as to achieve a haematocrit reading of 20 per cent and a plasma albumin level of 2.5 g/100 ml in the patient.

(c) *Children*: The amount of albumin given and the duration of therapy must be determined by the child's condition, response and other parameters, as stated under *'Standard Dose'*. However, when treating children, their body weight should also be taken into account.

Use in pregnancy: There is some experience of albumin being used in the treatment of pre-eclampsia and eclampsia. However, there is very little experience of the use of albumin in the early stages of pregnancy. There is no evidence either in human pregnancy or in animal work that administration of albumin is free from hazard.

Pharmacology: Action: Albuminar-25 is active osmotically and is therefore important in regulating the volume of circulating blood. When injected intravenously, 50 ml of Albuminar-25 draws approximately 175 ml of additional fluid into the circulation within 15 minutes, except in the presence of marked dehydration. This extra fluid reduces haematocrit and blood viscosity. The degree of volume expansion is dependent on the initial blood volume. When circulating blood volume has been depleted, the haemodilution following albumin administration persists for many hours. In individuals with normal blood volume, it usually lasts only a few hours.

Contra-indications, warnings, etc

Contra-indications: Albuminar-25 may be contra-indicated in patients with severe anaemia or cardiac failure.

Precautions: If dehydration is present additional fluids must accompany or follow the administration of Albuminar-25.

The rise in blood pressure which may follow rapid administration of albumin necessitates careful observation of the injured patient to detect bleeding points, which failed to bleed at the lower blood pressure; otherwise new haemorrhage and shock may occur.

Albuminar-25 should be administered with caution to patients with low cardiac reserve or with no albumin deficiency, because a rapid increase in plasma volume may cause circulatory embarrassment or pulmonary oedema. In cases of hypertension or cardiac insufficiency, a slower rate of administration is desirable: 200 ml of Albuminar-25 may be mixed with 300 ml of 10% dextrose solution and administered at a rate of 10 g of albumin (100 ml) per hour. A careful watch must be kept for the possible development of pulmonary oedema. Should pulmonary oedema occur, the infusion must be stopped immediately.

Warnings and adverse effects: Do not use if the solution is turbid or contains a deposit. Since the solution contains no preservative, it should be used within 3 hours after entering the vial.

The incidence of untoward reactions to Human Albumin Solution 25% is low, although nausea, vomiting, increased salivation and febrile reactions may occasionally occur.

Toxicity and treatment of overdosage: Administration of large quantities of albumin should be supplemented with red cell concentrates or replaced by whole blood to combat the relative anaemia which would follow such use.

If circulatory embarrassment or pulmonary oedema should develop, the infusion must be stopped immediately and specific treatment given.

Pharmaceutical precautions

(a) *Presentation and composition:* Albuminar-25 is a sterile, clear, brownish, slightly viscous aqueous solution of human albumin. It is stabilised with 0.02 M sodium acetyltryptophanate and 0.02 M sodium caprylate and the pH of the solution is adjusted with sodium bicarbonate or acetic acid. The solution contains approximately 145 mmol/l of sodium and not more than 200 micrograms/l of aluminium. The solution contains no preservative.

(b) *Storage:* Albuminar-25 should be stored at a temperature between 2° and 25°C. Freezing will not harm the solution, but might damage the container and allow contamination of the contents. Protect solution from light.

When stored as directed, Albuminar-25 has a shelf-life of 3 years.

Legal category POM.

Package quantities Albuminar-25 is supplied as a 25% solution in:

50 ml vials containing 12.5 grams of albumin;
100 ml vials containing 25.0 grams of albumin.

Further information Albuminar-25 is prepared from blood that was non-reactive for hepatitis B surface antigen (HBsAg) when tested with licensed reagents. The likelihood of the presence of viable hepatitis viruses has been further minimised by pasteurising the product at 60°C for 10 hours. Such treatment has been shown to be effective in this respect even when prepared from plasma known to be infective and albumin so prepared, unlike whole blood or plasma, is considered free of the danger of homologous serum hepatitis. All units of source plasma are tested for antibody to the human immunodeficiency virus (HIV) and found to be negative.

Albuminar-25 may be given in conjunction with other parenteral fluids, such as whole blood, plasma, saline, dextrose, or sodium lactate. It is convenient to use, since no cross-matching is required and the absence of cellular elements removes the danger of sensitisation with repeated infusions.

Albuminar-25 contains none of the recognised components of the clotting mechanism of normal blood or plasma. It does not interfere with the normal clotting of blood.

Product licence number 0231/0045.

MONOCLATE-P* ▼

Presentation Freeze-Dried Human Coagulation Factor VIII, Monoclate-P, Factor VIII: C Pasteurised is a sterile, stable, lyophilised concentrate of Factor VIII: C with reduced amounts of Factor VIII: R and purified of extraneous plasma-derived protein by use of affinity chromatography. A murine monoclonal antibody to Factor VIII: R is used as an affinity ligand to first isolate the Factor VIII Complex. Factor VIII: C is then dissociated from VIII: R, recovered, formulated and provided as a sterile lyophilised powder.

The concentrate as formulated contains Human Albumin Solution as a stabiliser, resulting in a concentrate with a specific activity between 5 and 10 units/mg of total protein. In the absence of this added Human Albumin Solution stabiliser, specific activity has been determined to exceed 3,000 units/mg of protein. Monoclate-P has been prepared from pooled human plasma and is intended for use in therapy of classical haemophilia (Haemophilia A).

This concentrate has been pasteurised by heating at 60°C for 10 hours in aqueous solution form during its manufacture in order to further reduce the risk of viral transmission. The product conforms to the monograph for Freeze Dried Human Coagulation Factor VIII BP PhEur.

Uses Freeze-Dried Human Coagulation Factor VIII, Monoclate-P, Factor VIII: C Pasteurised is indicated for treatment of classical haemophilia (Haemophilia A). Affected individuals frequently require therapy following minor accidents. Surgery, when required in such individuals, must be preceded by temporary correction of the clotting abnormality. Presurgical correction of severe AHF deficiency can be accomplished with a small volume of Monoclate-P.

Monoclate-P is not effective in controlling the bleeding of patients with von Willebrand's disease.

Dosage and administration Freeze-Dried Human Coagulation Factor VIII, Monoclate-P, Factor VIII: C Pasteurised is for intravenous administration only. As a general rule one unit of AHF activity per kg will increase the circulating AHF level by 2%. The following formula provides a guide for dosage calculations:

$$\text{Number of AHF IU Required} = \frac{\text{Body weight}}{\text{(in kg)}} \times \frac{\text{desired Factor VIII}}{\text{increase (\% normal)}} \times 0.5$$

Although dosage must be individualised according to the needs of the patient (weight, severity of haemorrhage, presence of inhibitors), the following general dosages are suggested.

Mild haemorrhages: Minor haemorrhagic episodes will generally subside with a single infusion if a level of 30% of normal or more is attained.

Moderate haemorrhage and minor surgery: For more serious haemorrhages and minor surgical procedures, the patient's Factor VIII level should be raised to 30–50% of normal, which usually requires an initial dose of 15–25 IU per kg. If further therapy is required a maintenance dose is 10–15 IU per kg every 8–12 hours.

Severe haemorrhage: In haemorrhages near vital organs (neck, throat, subperitoneal) it may be desirable to raise the Factor VIII level to 80–100% of normal which can be achieved with an initial dose of 40–50 IU per kg and a maintenance dose of 20–25 IU per kg every 8–12 hours.

Major surgery: For surgical procedures a dose of AHF sufficient to achieve a level 80–100% of normal should be given an hour prior to surgery. A second dose, half the size of the priming dose, should be given five hours after the first dose. Factor VIII levels should be maintained at a daily minimum of at least 30% of normal for a period of 10–14 days postoperatively. Close laboratory control to maintain AHF plasma levels deemed appropriate to maintain haemostasis is recommended.

Reconstitution and administration: Specific instructions for reconstitution and administration are included on the package insert and patient instruction leaflet.

Monoclate-P is for intravenous injection only. Plastic disposable syringes are recommended with Monoclate-P solution. The ground glass surfaces of all-glass syringes tend to stick with solutions of this type.

A winged infusion needle with microbore tubing is supplied with each pack. Use of other winged needles without microbore tubing, although compatible with the concentrate, will result in a larger retention of solution within the infusion set.

Contra-indications, warnings, etc
Contra-indications: None known.

Warnings: Monoclate-P is prepared from pooled units of human plasma which may contain the causative agents of hepatitis B, nonA nonB hepatitis, acquired immune deficiency syndrome (AIDS) and other viral diseases. Each unit of plasma used in the production of Monoclate-P has been tested and found nonreactive for hepatitis B surface antigen (HB_sAg) and negative for antibody to human immunodeficiency virus (Anti-HIV) by FDA approved tests, and has been shown to have ALT levels not exceeding two times the upper limit of normal. Additional screening procedures used to eliminate high risk plasma donors, and the purification techniques and pasteurisation step used in the manufacturing process, are all designed to reduce the risk of transmitting viral infection. However, testing methods presently available are not sensitive enough to detect all units of potentially infectious plasma, and treatment methods have not been shown to be totally effective in eliminating any of the aforementioned viral diseases from this concentrate. Accordingly, the benefits and risks of treatment with this concentrate should be carefully assessed prior to use.

Individuals who have not received multiple infusions of blood or plasma products are likely to develop signs and/or symptoms of some viral infections, especially nonA nonB hepatitis as shown by recent data, when treated with coagulant factor concentrates. A group of such patients treated with an earlier form of the concentrate which had not undergone liquid pasteurisation (Antihaemophilic Factor (Human), Monoclate, Factor VIII: C, Heat-Treated) did not demonstrate signs or symptoms of nonA nonB hepatitis over observation periods ranging from six to 23 months.

Precautions: Patients should be informed of the early signs of hypersensitivity reactions including hives, generalised urticaria, tightness of the chest, wheezing, hypotension and anaphylaxis, and should be advised to discontinue use of the concentrate and contact their physician if these symptoms occur.

Adverse reactions: Products of this type are known to cause allergic reactions, mild chills, nausea or stinging at the infusion site.

Pharmaceutical precautions Monoclate-P should not be mixed with other drugs before injection.

Storage: When stored at refrigerator temperature, 2°–8°C (36°–46°F), Monoclate-P, is stable for the period indicated by the expiration date on its label. Within this period, Monoclate-P may be stored at room temperature not to exceed 30°C (85°F), for up to six months. Avoid freezing which may damage container for the diluent.

Legal category POM.

Package quantities Monoclate-P is supplied in a single dose vial. IU activity is stated on the label of each vial. A patient user kit is supplied with each containing sterile Water for Injections, sterile 10 ml plastic syringe, sterile vented filter spike, sterile winged infusion set, sterile double ended transfer needle, sterile plaster dressing, disposable alcohol swabs and plastic disposal bag.

Further information Upon reconstitution, a clear, colourless solution is obtained, containing 50 to 150 times as much Factor VIII: C as does an equal volume of plasma.

Each vial contains the labelled amount of antihaemophilic factor (AHF) activity as expressed in terms of International Units of antihaemophilic activity. One unit of antihaemophilic activity is equivalent to that quantity of AHF present in one ml of normal human plasma. When reconstituted as recommended, the resulting solution contains approximately 300 to 450 millimoles of sodium ions per litre and has 2–3 times the tonicity of saline. It contains approximately 2–3 millimoles of calcium per litre, contributed as calcium chloride, approximately 1–2% Human Albumin Solution, 0.8% mannitol, and 1.2 mM histidine. The pH is adjusted with hydrochloric acid and/or sodium hydroxide. Monoclate-P also contains trace amounts (less than 50 ng per 100 AHF activity units) of mouse protein.

Clinical evaluation of Monoclate-P for its half-life characteristics in haemophilic patients showed it to be comparable to other commercially available Freeze-Dried Human Coagulation Factor VIII materials.

The mean half-life obtained from six patients was 17.5 hours with a mean recovery of 1.9 IU/dl rise/IU/kg.

The pasteurisation process used in the manufacture of this concentrate has demonstrated in vitro inactivation of 10.5 logs of Human Immunodeficiency Virus (HIV). Evidence of the capability of the purification and preparative steps used in the production of Monoclate-P, to reduce viral bioburden, was obtained in studies involving the addition of known quantities of virus to cryoprecipitate. These studies were conducted using an earlier form of the concentrate which had not undergone liquid pasteurisation (Antihaemophilic Factor (Human), Monoclate, Factor VIII: C, Heat-Treated). These studies provide evidence that the combined effects of the manufacturing steps, which purify the Factor VIII: C and prepare the concentrate in a final sterile container as a lyophilised powder, contribute viral reduction capabilities of approximately 5–6 logs. In a separate study, aluminium hydroxide treatment followed by antibody affinity chromatography reduced vaccinia virus infectivity by 4.81 logs. These studies indicate that the purification and preparative steps of the manufacturing process are capable of providing a non-specific, viral reduction independent of the pasteurisation process

Product licence numbers

250 IU/vial	0231/0090
500 IU/vial	0231/0091
1,000 IU/vial	0231/0092
Diluent	0231/0093, 0094, 0095

**Trade Mark*

Astra Pharmaceuticals Limited
Home Park Estate
Kings Langley
Herts WD4 8DH

ASTRA

BETALOC* TABLETS 50 mg and 100 mg

Presentation White tablets containing either 50 mg (coded A/BB) or 100 mg (coded A/ME) metoprolol tartrate.

Inactive ingredients: Lactose, microcrystalline cellulose, sodium starch glycolate, colloidal silicon, polyvidone.

Uses In the management of hypertension and angina pectoris. Cardiac arrhythmias, especially supraventricular tachyarrhythmias.

Adjunct to the treatment of hyperthyroidism.

Early intervention with Betaloc in acute myocardial infarction reduces infarct size and the incidence of ventricular fibrillation. Pain relief may also decrease the need for opiate analgesics.

Betaloc has been shown to reduce mortality when administered to patients with acute myocardial infarction.

Prophylaxis of migraine.

Dosage and administration The dose must always be adjusted to the individual requirements of the patient. The following are guide lines:

Hypertension: Total daily dosage Betaloc 100–400 mg to be given as a single or twice daily dose.

The starting dose is 100 mg per day. This may be increased by 100 mg per day at weekly intervals.

If full control is not achieved using a single daily dose, a b.d. regimen should be initiated. Combination therapy with a diuretic or other anti-hypertensive agent may also be considered.

Angina: Usually Betaloc 50–100 mg twice or three times daily.

Cardiac arrhythmias: Betaloc 50 mg b.i.d. or t.i.d. should usually control the condition. If necessary the dose can be increased up to 300 mg per day in divided doses.

Following the treatment of an acute arrhythmia with Betaloc injection, continuation therapy with Betaloc tablets should be initiated 4–6 hours later. The initial oral dose should not exceed 50 mg t.i.d.

Hyperthyroidism: Betaloc 50 mg four times a day. The dose should be reduced as the euthyroid state is achieved.

Myocardial infarction: Early intervention – to achieve optimal benefits from intravenous Betaloc, suitable patients should present within 12 hours of the onset of chest pain. Therapy should commence with 5 mg i.v. every 2 minutes to a maximum of 15 mg total as determined by blood pressure and heart rate. The second or third dose should not be given if the systolic blood pressure is <90 mmHg, the heart rate is <40 beats/min and the P-Q time is >0.26 seconds, or if there is any aggravation of dyspnoea or cold sweating. Orally, therapy should commence 15 minutes after the last injection with 50 mg every 6 hours for 48 hours. Patients who fail to tolerate the full intravenous dose should be given half the suggested oral dose.

Maintenance – The usual maintenance dose is 200 mg daily, given in divided doses.

Migraine prophylaxis: Betaloc 100–200 mg daily given in divided doses.

Elderly: There are no special dosage requirements in otherwise healthy elderly patients.

Significant hepatic dysfunction: A reduction in dosage may be necessary.

Contra-indications, warnings, etc

Contra-indications: AV block. Uncontrolled heart failure. Severe bradycardia. Sick-sinus syndrome. Cardiogenic shock. Severe peripheral arterial disease. Known hypersensitivity to Betaloc or other β-blockers.

Betaloc is also contra-indicated when myocardial infarction is complicated by significant bradycardia, first degree heart block, systolic hypotension (<100 mmHg) and/or severe heart failure.

Warnings: Betaloc may aggravate bradycardia, symptoms of peripheral arterial circulatory disorders and anaphylactic shock.

Abrupt interruption of β-blockers is to be avoided. When possible, Betaloc should be withdrawn gradually over a period of 10 days, in diminishing doses to 25 mg daily for the last 6 days. During its withdrawal patients should be kept under close surveillance, especially those with known ischaemic heart disease.

Betaloc may be administered when heart failure has been controlled. Digitalisation and/or diuretic therapy should also be considered for patients with a history of heart failure, or patients known to have a poor cardiac reserve.

Although cardioselective beta-blockers may have less effect on lung function than non-selective beta-blockers, as with all beta-blockers these should be avoided in patients with reversible obstructive airways disease unless there are compelling clinical reasons for their use. When administration is necessary, use of a $beta_2$-bronchodilator (e.g. terbutaline) may be advisable in some patients.

In labile and insulin-dependent diabetes it may be necessary to adjust the hypoglycaemic therapy.

In patients with a phaeochromocytoma, an alpha-blocker should be given concomitantly.

In the presence of liver cirrhosis the bioavailability of Betaloc may be increased.

The administration of adrenaline to patients undergoing beta-blockade can result in an increase in blood pressure and bradycardia, although this is less likely to occur with β_1-selective drugs.

Betaloc therapy must be reported to the anaesthetist prior to general anaesthesia. If withdrawal of Betaloc is considered desirable, this should if possible be completed at least 48 hours before general anaesthesia. However, in some patients it may be desirable to employ a β-blocker as premedication. By shielding the heart against the effects of stress the β-blocker may prevent excessive sympathetic stimulation provoking cardiac arrhythmias or acute coronary insufficiency. If a β-blocker is given for this purpose, an anaesthetic with little negative inotropic activity should be selected to minimise the risk of myocardial depression.

Pregnancy: Betaloc should not be used in pregnancy or nursing mothers unless the physician considers that the benefit outweighs the possible hazard to the foetus/infant. As with all beta-blockers Betaloc may cause side-effects e.g. bradycardia, hypoglycaemia in the foetus, and in the newborn and breastfed infant. Betaloc has, however, been used in pregnancy associated hypertension under close supervision, after 20 weeks gestation. Although Betaloc crosses the placental barrier and is present in cord blood, no evidence of foetal abnormalities has been reported.

Lactation: The amount of Betaloc ingested via breast milk should not produce significant β-blocking effects in the neonate if the mother is treated with normal therapeutic doses.

Interactions: The effects of Betaloc and other antihypertensive drugs on blood pressure are usually additive, and care should be taken to avoid hypotension. However, combinations of antihypertensive drugs may often be used with benefit to improve control of hypertension.

Betaloc can reduce myocardial contractility and impair intracardiac conduction. Care should be exercised when drugs with similar activity, e.g. antiarrhythmic agents, general anaesthetics, are given concurrently. Like all other β-blockers, Betaloc should not be given in combination with verapamil since this may cause bradycardia, hypotension and asystole. Care should also be exercised when β-blockers are given in combination with sympathetic ganglion blocking agents, other β-blockers (i.e. eye drops) or MAO inhibitors. If combination treatment with clonidine is to be discontinued, metoprolol should be withdrawn several days before clonidine.

As β-blockers may affect the peripheral circulation, care shoud be exercised when drugs with similar activity e.g. ergotamine are given concurrently.

Betaloc will antagonise the β_1-effects of sympathomimetic agents but should have little influence on the bronchodilator effects of β_2-agonists at normal therapeutic doses. Enzyme inducing agents (e.g. rifampicin) may reduce plasma concentrations of Betaloc, whereas enzyme inhibitors (e.g. cimetidine) may increase plasma concentrations. Betaloc may impair the elimination of lignocaine.

Indomethacin may reduce the antihypertensive effect of β-blockers.

Side-effects: These are usually mild and infrequent. The most common appear to be lassitude, GI disturbances (nausea, vomiting or abdominal pain) and disturbances of sleep pattern. In many cases these effects have been transient or have disappeared after a reduction in dosage.

Effects related to the CNS which have been reported occasionally are dizziness and headache and rarely paraesthesia, muscle cramps, depression and decreased mental alertness. There have also been isolated reports of personality disorders.

Cardiovascular effects which have been reported occasionally are bradycardia, postural hypotension and rarely, heart failure, palpitations, cardiac arrhythmias, Raynauds phenomenon, peripheral oedema and precordial pain. There have also been isolated reports of cardiac conduction abnormalities, and gangrene in patients with pre-existing severe peripheral circulatory disorders.

Common gastro-intestinal disturbances have been described above but rarely diarrhoea or constipation also occur and there have been isolated cases of dry mouth and abnormal liver function.

Skin rashes (urticaria, psoriasiform, dystrophic skin lesions) and positive anti-nuclear antibodies (not associated with SLE) occur rarely. Isolated cases of photosensitivity, increased sweating and alopecia have been reported. Respiratory effects include occasional reports of dyspnoea on exertion and rare reports of bronchospasm and isolated cases of rhinitis.

Isolated cases of weight gain, thrombocytopenia, disturbances of vision, conjunctivitis, tinnitus and dry or irritated eyes have also been reported.

The reported incidence of skin rashes and/or dry eyes is small and in most cases the symptoms have cleared when treatment was withdrawn. Discontinuation of the drug should be considered if any such reaction is not otherwise explicable.

Overdosage: Poisoning due to an overdose of Betaloc may lead to severe hypotension, sinus bradycardia, atrioventricular block, heart failure, cardiogenic shock, cardiac arrest, bronchospasm, impairment of consciousness, coma, nausea, vomiting, cyanosis, hypoglycaemia and, occasionally, hyperkalaemia. The first manifestations usually appear 20 minutes to 2 hours after drug ingestion.

Treatment should include close monitoring of cardiovascular, respiratory and renal function, and blood glucose and electrolytes. Further absorption may be prevented by induction of vomiting, gastric lavage or administration of activated-charcoal if ingestion is recent. Cardiovascular complications should be treated symptomatically, which may require the use of sympathomimetic agents (e.g. noradrenaline, metaraminol), atropine or inotropic agents (e.g. dopamine, dobutamine). Temporary pacing may be required for AV block. Glucagon can reverse the effects of excessive β-blockade, given in a dose of 1–10 mg intravenously. Intravenous β_2-stimulants e.g. terbutaline may be required to relieve bronchospasm.

Betaloc cannot be effectively removed by haemodialysis.

Pharmaceutical precautions Protect from light, heat and moisture.

Legal category POM.

Package quantities

Tablets 50 mg:	Calendar packs of 56
Tablets 50 mg, 100 mg:	Blister pack of 100.
	Securitainers of 500.

Further information Betaloc is well absorbed after oral administration, peak plasma concentrations occurring 1.5–2 hours after dosing. The bioavailability of a single dose is approximately 50%, increasing to approximately 70% during repeated administration. The bioavailability also increases if metoprolol is given with food.

Elimination is mainly by hepatic metabolism and the average elimination half-life is 3.5 hours (range 1 to 9 hours). Rates of metabolism vary between individuals, with poor metabolisers (approximately 10%) showing higher plasma concentrations and slower elimination than extensive metabolisers. Within individuals, however, plasma concentrations are stable and reproducible.

Because of variation in rates of metabolism, the dose of Betaloc should always be adjusted to the individual requirements of the patient. As the therapeutic response, adverse effects and relative cardioselectivity are related to plasma concentration, poor metabolisers may require lower than normal doses. Dosage adjustment is not routinely required in the elderly or in patients with renal failure, but dosage may need to be reduced in patients with significant hepatic dysfunction when Betaloc elmination may be impaired.

Product licence numbers

Betaloc Tablets 50 mg	0017/0073R
Betaloc Tablets 100 mg	0017/0074R.

BETALOC* I.V. INJECTION

Presentation
Ampoules: Each ampoule of 5 ml contains 5 mg metoprolol tartrate.

Inactive ingredients: Sodium chloride, water for injection.

Uses Control of tachyarrhythmias, especially supraventricular tachyarrhythmias.

Early intervention with Betaloc in acute myocardial infarction reduces infarct size and the incidence of ventricular fibrillation. Pain relief may also decrease the need for opiate analgesics.

Betaloc has been shown to reduce mortality when administered to patients with acute myocardial infarction.

Dosage and administration *Control of tachyarrhythmias:* Initially up to 5 mg injected i.v. at a rate of 1–2 mg per minute. The injection can be repeated at 5 minute intervals until a satisfactory response has been obtained. A total dose of 10–15 mg generally proves sufficient.

Because of the risk of a pronounced drop of blood pressure, the i.v. administration of Betaloc to patients with a systolic blood pressure below 100 mm Hg should only be given with special care.

During anaesthesia: 2–4 mg injected slowly i.v. at induction is usually sufficient to prevent the development of arrhythmias during anaesthesia. The same dosage can also be used to control arrhythmias developing during anaesthesia. Further injections of 2 mg may be given as required to a maximum overall dose of 10 mg.

Myocardial infarction: Early intervention. To achieve optimal benefits from intravenous Betaloc, suitable patients should present within 12 hours of the onset of chest pain. Therapy should commence with 5 mg i.v. every 2 minutes to a maximum of 15 mg total as determined by blood pressure and heart rate. The second or third dose should not be given if the systolic blood pressure is <90 mg Hg, the heart rate is <40 beats/min and the P-Q time is >0.26 seconds, or if there is any aggravation of dyspnoea or cold sweating. Orally, therapy should commence 15 minutes after the injection with 50 mg every 6 hours for 48 hours. Patients who fail to tolerate the full intravenous dose should be given half the suggested oral dose.

Elderly: There are no special dosage requirements in otherwise healthy elderly patients.

Significant hepatic dysfunction: A reduction in dosage may be necessary.

Contra-indications, warnings, etc

Contra-indications: AV Block. Uncontrolled heart failure. Severe bradycardia. Sick sinus syndrome. Cardiogenic shock. Severe peripheral arterial disease. Known hypersensitivity to Betaloc or other β-blockers.

Betaloc i.v. is also contra-indicated when myocardial infarction is complicated by significant bradycardia, first degree heart block, systolic hypotension (<100 mm Hg) and/or severe heart failure.

Warnings: Betaloc i.v. may aggravate bradycardia, symptoms of peripheral arterial circulatory disorders and anaphylactic shock.

Betaloc i.v. may be administered when heart failure has been controlled. Digitalisation and/or diuretics should also be considered for patients with a history of heart failure, or patients known to have a poor cardiac reserve.

Although cardioselective beta-blockers may have less effect on lung function than non-selective beta-blockers, as with all beta-blockers these should be avoided in patients with reversible obstructive airways disease unless there are compelling clinical reasons for their use. When administration is necessary, use of a beta$_2$-bronchodilator (e.g. terbutaline) may be advisable in some patients.

In labile and insulin-dependent diabetes it may be necessary to adjust the hypoglycaemic therapy.

In patients with a phaeochromocytoma, an alpha-blocker should be given concomitantly.

The administration of adrenaline to patients undergoing beta-blockade can result in an increase in blood pressure and bradycardia although this is less likely to occur with β_1-selective drugs.

Betaloc i.v. therapy must be reported to the anaesthetist prior to general anaesthesia. However, in some patients it may be desirable to employ a β-blocker as premedication. By shielding the heart against the effects of stress the β-blocker may prevent excessive sympathetic stimulation provoking cardiac arrhythmias or acute coronary insufficiency. If a β-blocker is given for this purpose, an anaesthetic with little negative inotropic activity should be selected to minimise the risk of myocardial depression.

Pregnancy: Betaloc i.v. should not be used in pregnancy or nursing mothers unless the physician considers that the benefit outweighs the possible hazard to the foetus/infant. As with all beta-blockers metoprolol may cause side-effects e.g. bradycardia, hypoglycaemia in the foetus, and in the newborn and breastfed infant. Metoprolol has, however, been used in pregnancy associated hypertension under close supervision, after 20 weeks gestation. Although Betaloc i.v. crosses the placental barrier and is present in cord blood, no evidence of foetal abnormalities has been reported.

Lactation: The amount of Betaloc i.v. ingested via breast milk should not produce significant β-blocking effects in the neonate if the mother is treated with normal therapeutic doses.

Interactions: The effects of Betaloc i.v. and other antihypertensive drugs on blood pressure are usually additive, and care should be taken to avoid hypotension.

Betaloc i.v. can reduce myocardial contractility and impair intracardiac conduction. Care should be exercised when drugs with similar activity, e.g. antiarrhythmic agents, general anaesthetics, are given concurrently. Like all other β-blockers, Betaloc i.v. should not be given in combination with verapamil since this may cause bradycardia, hypotension and asystole. Care should also be exercised when β-blockers are given in combination with sympathetic ganglion blocking agents, other β-blockers (i.e. eye drops) or MAO inhibitors.

As β-blockers may affect the peripheral circulation, care should be exercised when drugs with similar activity e.g. ergotamine are given concurrently.

Betaloc i.v. will antagonise the β_1-effects of sympathomimetic agents but should have little influence on the broncohodilator effects of β_2-agonists at normal therapeutic doses. Enzyme inducing agents (e.g. rifampicin) may reduce plasma concentrations of Betaloc, whereas enzyme inhibitors (e.g. cimetidine) may increase plasma concentrations. Betaloc i.v. may impair the elimination of lignocaine.

Side-effects: As in the case of other β-blockers, a marked fall in blood pressure may sometimes occur following intravenous injection of Betaloc. Other side effects are usually mild and infrequent. The most common appear to be lassitude, GI disturbances (nausea, vomiting or abdominal pain) and disturbances of sleep pattern. In many cases these effects have been transient or have disappeared after a reduction in dosage.

Effects related to the CNS which have been reported occasionally are dizziness and headache and rarely paraesthesia, muscle cramps, depression and decreased mental alertness. There have also been isolated reports of personality disorders.

Cardiovascular effects which have been reported occasionally are bradycardia, postural hypotension and rarely, heart failure, palpitations, cardiac arrhythmias, Raynauds phenomenon, peripheral oedema and precordial pain. There have also been isolated reports of cardiac conduction abnormalities, and gangrene in patients with pre-existing severe peripheral circulatory disorders.

Common gastro-intestinal disturbances have been described above but rarely diarrhoea or constipation also occur and there have been isolated cases of dry mouth and abnormal liver function.

Skin rashes (urticuria, psoriasiform, dystrophic skin lesions) and positive anti-nuclear antibodies (not associated with SLE) occur rarely. Isolated cases of photosensitivity, increased sweating and alopecia have been reported. Respiratory effects include occasional reports of dyspnoea on exertion and rare reports of bronchospasm and isolated cases of rhinitis.

Isolated cases of weight gain, thrombocytopenia, disturbances of vision, conjunctivitis, tinnitus and dry or irritated eyes have also been reported.

The reported incidence of skin rashes and/or dry eyes is small and in most cases the symptoms have cleared when treatment was withdrawn. Discontinuation of the drug should be considered if any such reaction is not otherwise explicable.

Overdosage: Poisoning due to an overdose of Betaloc i.v. may lead to severe hypotension, sinus bradycardia, atrioventricular block, heart failure, cardiogenic shock, cardiac arrest, bronchospasm, impairment of consciousness, coma, nausea, vomiting, cyanosis, hypoglycaemia and, occasionally, hyperkalaemia. The first manifestations usually appear 20 minutes to 2 hours after drug ingestion.

Treatment should include close monitoring of cardiovascular, respiratory and renal function, and blood glucose and electrolytes. Cardiovascular complications should be treated symptomatically, which may require the use of sympathomimetic agents (e.g. noradrenaline, metaraminol), atropine or inotropic agents (e.g. dopamine, dobutamine). Temporary pacing may be required for AV block. Glucagon can reverse the effects of excessive β-blockade, given in a dose of 1–10 mg intravenously. Intravenous β_2-stimulants e.g. terbutaline may be required to relieve bronchospasm.

Betaloc i.v. cannot be effectively removed by haemodialysis.

Pharmaceutical precautions Protect from light.

Legal category POM.

Package quantities 4 × 5 ml ampoules.

Further information Betaloc is a cardioselective β_1-receptor blocker exhibiting no intrinsic sympathomimetic activity. Elimination is mainly by hepatic metabolism and the average elimination half-life is 3.5 hours (range 1 to 9 hours). Rates of metabolism vary between individuals, with poor metabolisers (approximately 10%) showing higher plasma concentrations and slower elimination than extensive metabolisers. Within individuals, however, plasma concentrations are stable and reproducible.

Product licence number 0017/0072.

BETALOC*-SA

Presentation White tablets (coded A/MD) containing 200 mg metoprolol tartrate as Durules (sustained release tablets).

Inactive ingredients: Aluminium silicate, paraffin special, magnesium stearate, ethylcellulose, hydroxypropyl methylcellulose, polyethylene glycol, titanium dioxide.

Uses In the management of angina pectoris and hypertension.

Prophylaxis of migraine.

Dosage and administration *Angina pectoris and hypertension:* One tablet daily, in the morning. In rare cases two tablets may be indicated.

Migraine Prophylaxis: One tablet daily, in the morning.

Betaloc SA tablets should be swallowed whole and not broken or chewed.

Elderly: There are no special dosage requirements in otherwise healthy elderly patients.

Significant hepatic dysfunction: A reduction in dosage may be necessary.

Contra-indications, warnings, etc

Contra-indications: AV block. Uncontrolled heart failure. Severe bradycardia. Sick-sinus syndrome. Cardiogenic shock. Severe peripheral arterial disease. Known hypersensitivity to Betaloc SA or other β-blockers.

Warnings: Betaloc SA may aggravate bradycardia, symptoms of peripheral arterial circulatory disorders and anaphylactic shock.

Abrupt interruption of β-blockers is to be avoided. When possible, Betaloc SA should be withdrawn gradually over a period of 10 days. During its withdrawal patients should be kept under close surveillance, especially those with known ischaemic heart disease.

Betaloc SA may be administered when heart failure has been controlled. Digitalisation and/or diuretic therapy should also be considered for patients with a history of heart failure, or patients known to have a poor cardiac reserve.

Although cardioselective beta-blockers may have less effect on lung function than non-selective beta-blockers, as with all beta-blockers these should be avoided in patients with reversible obstructive airways disease unless there are compelling clinical reasons for their use. When administration is necessary, use of a $beta_2$-bronchodilator (e.g. terbutaline) may be advisable in some patients.

In labile and insulin-dependent diabetes it may be necessary to adjust the hypoglycaemic therapy.

In patients with phaeochromocytoma, an alpha-blocker should be given concomitantly.

In the presence of liver cirrhosis the bioavailability of Betaloc SA may be increased.

The administration of adrenaline to patients undergoing beta-blockade can result in an increase in blood pressure and bradycardia although this is less likely to occur with β_1-selective drugs.

Betaloc SA therapy must be reported to the anaesthetist prior to general anaesthesia. If withdrawal of metoprolol is considered desirable, this should if possible be completed at least 48 hours before general anaesthesia. However, in some patients it may be desirable to employ a β-blocker as premedication. By shielding the heart against the effects of stress the β-blocker may prevent excessive sympathetic stimulation provoking cardiac arrhythmias or acute coronary insufficiency. If a β-blocker is given for this purpose, an anaesthetic with little negative inotropic activity should be selected to minimise the risk of myocardial depression.

Pregnancy: Betaloc SA should not be used in pregnancy or nursing mothers unless the physician considers that the benefit outweighs the possible hazards to the foetus/infant. As with all beta-blockers metoprolol may cause side-effects e.g. bradycardia, hypoglycaemia in the foetus, and in the newborn and breastfed infant. Metoprolol has, however, been used in pregnancy associated hypertension under close supervision, after 20 weeks gestation. Although Betaloc SA crosses the placental barrier and is present in cord blood, no evidence of foetal abnormalities has been reported.

Lactation: The amount of metoprolol ingested via breast milk should not produce significant β-blocking effects in the neonate if the mother is treated with normal therapeutic doses.

Interactions: The effects of Betaloc SA and other antihypertensive drugs on blood pressure are usually additive, and care should be taken to avoid hypotension. However, combinations of antihypertensive drugs may often be used with benefit to improve control of hypertension.

Betaloc SA can reduce myocardial contractility and impair intracardiac conduction. Care should be exercised when drugs with similar activity, e.g. antiarrhythmic agents, general anaesthetics, are given concurrently. Like all other β-blockers, Betaloc SA should not be given in combination with verapamil since this may cause bradycardia, hypotension and asystole. Care should also be exercised when β-blockers are given in combination with sympathetic ganglion blocking agents, other β-blockers (i.e. eye drops) or MAO inhibitors. If combination treatment with clonidine is to be discontinued, Betaloc SA should be withdrawn several days before clonidine.

As β-blockers may affect the peripheral circulation, care should be exercised when drugs with similar activity e.g. ergotamine are given concurrently.

Betaloc SA will antagonise the β_1-effects of sympathomimetic agents but should have little influence on the bronchodilator effects of β_2-agonists at normal therapeutic doses. Enzyme inducing agents (e.g. rifampicin) may reduce plasma concentrations of Betaloc SA, whereas enzyme inhibitors (e.g. cimetidine) may increase plasma concentrations. Betaloc SA may impair the elimination of lignocaine.

Indomethacin may reduce the antihypertensive effect of β-blockers.

Side-effects: These are usually mild and infrequent. The most common appear to be lassitude, GI disturbances (nausea, vomiting or abdominal pain) and disturbances of sleep pattern. In many cases these effects have been transient or have disappeared after a reduction in dosage.

Effects related to the CNS which have been reported occasionally are dizziness and headache and rarely paraesthesia, muscle cramps, depression and decreased mental alertness. There have also been isolated reports of personality disorders.

Cardiovascular effects which have been reported occasionally are bradycardia, postural hypotension and rarely, heart failure, palpitations, cardiac arrhythmias, Raynauds phenomenon, peripheral oedema and precordial pain. There have also been isolated reports of cardiac conduction abnormalities, and gangrene in patients with pre-existing severe peripheral circulatory disorders.

Common gastro-intestinal disturbances have been

described above but rarely diarrhoea or constipation also occur and there have been isolated cases of dry mouth and abnormal liver function.

Skin rashes (urticaria, psoriasiform, dystrophic skin lesions) and positive anti-nuclear antibodies (not associated with SLE) occur rarely. Isolated cases of photosensitivity, increased sweating and alopecia have been reported. Respiratory effects include occasional reports of dyspnoea on exertion and rare reports of bronchospasm and isolated cases of rhinitis.

Isolated cases of weight gain, thrombocytopenia, disturbances of vision, conjunctivitis, tinnitus and dry or irritated eyes have also been reported.

The reported incidence of skin rashes and/or dry eyes is small and in most cases the symptoms have cleared when treatment was withdrawn. Discontinuation of the drug should be considered if any such reaction is not otherwise explicable.

Overdosage: Poisoning due to an overdose of Betaloc SA may lead to severe hypotension, sinus bradycardia, atrioventricular block, heart failure, cardiogenic shock, cardiac arrest, bronchospasm, impairment of consciousness, coma, nausea, vomiting, cyanosis, hypoglycaemia and, occasionally, hyperkalaemia. The first manifestations usually appear 20 minutes to 2 hours after drug ingestion.

Treatment should include close monitoring of cardiovascular, respiratory and renal function, and blood glucose and electrolytes. Further absorption may be prevented by induction of vomiting, gastric lavage or administration of activated-charcoal if ingestion is recent. Cardiovascular complications should be treated symptomatically, which may require the use of sympathomimetic agents (e.g. noradrenaline, metaraminol), atropine or inotropic agents (e.g. dopamine, dobutamine). Temporary pacing may be required for AV block. Glucagon can reverse the effects of excessive β-blockade, given in a dose of 1–10 mg intravenously. Intravenous β_2-stimulants e.g. terbutaline may be required to relieve bronchospasm.

Metoprolol cannot be effectively removed by haemodialysis.

Pharmaceutical precautions Protect from light, heat and moisture.

Legal category POM.

Package quantities Calendar pack of 28 tablets. Securitainers of 300 tablets.

Further information Administration of Betaloc SA results in a controlled release of active substance which means that the peak plasma levels are reduced. Compared to Betaloc tablets the absorption phase is prolonged and the duration of effect is extended. The substance is completely absorbed and the maximal beta-blocking effect is reached after about four hours.

These factors may lead to a more convenient dosage and an improved degree of $beta_1$-selectivity.

The effect on the pulse and blood pressure remain pronounced 24 hours after administration.

Elimination is mainly by hepatic metabolism and the average elimination half-life is 3.5 hours (range 1 to 9 hours). Rates of metabolism vary between individuals, with poor metabolisers (approximately 10%) showing higher plasma concentrations and slower elimination than extensive metabolisers. Within individuals, however, plasma concentrations are stable and reproducible.

Product licence number 0017/0093.

BRICANYL* INHALER
BRICANYL* SPACER INHALER

Presentation *Bricanyl Inhaler:* Metered dose aerosol delivering 0.25 mg terbutaline sulphate per actuation.

Bricanyl Spacer Inhaler: Metered dose aerosol with extended mouthpiece delivering 0.25 mg terbutaline sulphate per actuation.

Bricanyl Refill Canister: Canister containing 400 doses of terbutaline sulphate 0.25 mg. For use with the Nebuhaler or as a refill for Bricanyl Spacer Inhaler.

Inactive ingredients: All the above contain sorbitan trioleate and chlorofluorocarbons 11, 12 and 114.

Nebuhaler: 750 ml plastic cone with a one-way valve. For use in conjunction with Bricanyl refill canister.

Both the Bricanyl Spacer Inhaler and the Nebuhaler are recommended to enable patients with difficulty coordinating conventional aerosols to derive greater therapeutic benefit. A package insert is provided giving simple operating instructions.

Uses A selective $beta_2$-adrenergic agonist recommended for prophylactic treatment and relief of an acute attack of allergic, intrinsic and exercise induced asthma, chronic bronchitis, emphysema and other bronchopulmonary disorders on which bronchospasm is a complicating factor.

Dosage and administration
Bricanyl Inhaler: Adults and children: Prophylaxis and relief of acute attack: One or two inhalations as required, with a short interval between each inhalation at 6 hourly intervals. Not more than 8 inhalations should be necessary in any 24 hours, but medical advice should be sought and treatment reviewed if condition fails to improve.

Bricanyl Spacer Inhaler: Adults and children: Prophylaxis and relief of acute attack: One or two inhalations as required, with a short interval between each inhalation at 6 hourly intervals. Not more than 8 inhalations should be necessary in any 24 hours, but medical advice should be sought and treatment reviewed if condition fails to improve.

Nebuhaler: Adults and children: The dose must always be adjusted to patient response and severity of the bronchospasm. Patients must be instructed to actuate the aerosol and breathe in slowly and deeply through the mouthpiece. Ideally two inspirations per actuation are required to empty the Nebuhaler.

Prophylaxis and relief of acute attack: One or two inhalations as required, with a short interval between each inhalation at 6 hourly intervals. Not more than 8 inhalations should be necessary in any 24 hours, but medical advice should be sought and treatment reviewed if condition fails to improve.

Bricanyl via the Nebuhaler may also be used in conditions such as severe bronchospasm and severe acute asthma which are normally managed by administration of nebulised bronchodilators.

For hospital use in acute asthma: Adults: The initial dose should be 2 mg (8 actuations); this may be repeated up to a total dose of 8 mg in one hour. Thereafter a dose of up to 4 mg may be given four times daily.

A similar dose range may be used for domiciliary use, but patients should be warned that if either the usual relief or duration of action is diminished, they should seek medical advice immediately.

Children over 5 years: Dosage must be individualised but clinical studies have shown that when used for the management of acute asthma in children, the following dosages given over a 15 minute period have been as effective as equal doses administered by nebuliser.

Children under 25 Kg	1.25–2.5 mg (5–10 puffs)
Children over 25 Kg	2.5–5.0 mg (10–20 puffs)

Elderly: Dosage as for adults. Because of the difficulty experienced by many elderly patients in coordinating inhalation with actuation, Bricanyl Spacer inhaler or use via the Nebuhaler will provide a more certain delivery of drug.

Contra-indications, warnings, etc
Contra-indications: Bricanyl preparations are contra-indicated in patients with a history of sensitivity to any of their constituents.

Precautions: Care should be taken with patients suffering from myocardial insufficiency or thyrotoxicosis. Due to the hyperglycaemic effects of β_2-stimulants, additional blood glucose controls are initially recommended when Bricanyl therapy is commenced in diabetic patients. If treatment becomes less effective or shorter acting the patients general condition should be reviewed.

Potentially serious hypokalaemia may result from beta$_2$-agonist therapy. Particular caution is advised in severe asthma as this effect may be potentiated by concomitant treatment with xanthine derivatives, steroids, diuretics and by hypoxia. It is recommended that serum potassium levels are monitored in such situations.

Interactions with other medicaments: Non-selective β-blocking agents such as propranolol may partially or totally inhibit the effect of β-stimulants. Therefore Bricanyl and non-selective β-blockers should not normally be administered concurrently. Bricanyl should be used with caution in patients receiving other sympathomimetics.

Pregnancy and lactation: Although no teratogenic effects have been observed in animals or in patients Bricanyl should only be administered with caution during the first trimester of pregnancy. Terbutaline is secreted via breast milk, but influence on the infant is unlikely at therapeutic doses.

Side-effects: The frequency of side effects is low at recommended doses. Side effects which have been recorded such as tremor, tonic cramp and palpitations are all characteristic of sympathomimetic amines. A few patients feel tense; this is also due to the effects on skeletal muscle and not to direct CNS stimulation. Whenever these side effects have occurred the majority have usually been spontaneously reversible within the first week of treatment.

Potentially serious hypokalaemia may result from beta$_2$-agonist therapy.

Overdose

(i) *Possible symptoms and signs:* Headache, anxiety, tremor, tonic cramp, palpitations, arrhythmia. A fall in blood pressure sometimes occurs. Laboratory findings: hypokalaemia, hyperglycaemia and lactoacidosis sometimes occur.

(ii) *Treatment: Mild and moderate cases:* Reduce the dose.

Severe cases: Determination of acid-base balance, blood sugar and electrolytes. Monitoring of heart rate and rhythm and blood pressure. Metabolic changes should be corrected. A cardioselective β-blocker (e.g. metoprolol) is recommended for the treatment of arrhythmias causing a haemodynamic deterioration. The β-blocker should be used with care because of the possibility of inducing bronchoconstriction. If the β$_2$-mediated reduction in peripheral vascular resistance significantly contributes to the fall in blood pressure, a volume expander should be given.

Pharmaceutical precautions Store at temperatures not exceeding 25°C.

Legal category POM.

Package quantities Bricanyl Inhaler: Aerosol containing 400 metered doses.

Bricanyl Spacer Inhaler: Aerosol containing 400 metered doses complete with extended mouthpiece.

Bricanyl Refill Canister: Canister containing 400 doses:

Nebuhaler: 750 ml plastic cone with a one-way valve.

Further information Bricanyl is also available as Respirator Solution, Tablets, Syrup, Injection and Expectorant.

Product licence number 0017/0061R.

BRICANYL* TABLETS
BRICANYL* SYRUP

Presentation

Bricanyl Tablets 5 mg: Off-white tablet, scored on one side, symbol "5" on the reverse containing Terbutaline Sulphate BP.

Inactive ingredients: Lactose, maize starch, providone, microcrystalline cellulose, magnesium stearate.

Bricanyl Syrup: A clear colourless raspberry-flavoured aqueous syrup containing 0.3 mg Terbutaline Sulphate BP per ml.

Inactive ingredients: Bricanyl Syrup is sorbitol based and contains in addition edetic acid and sodium benzoate.

Uses Terbutaline is a selective β$_2$-adrenergic agonist recommended for use in the following indications:

Prophylactic treatment and relief of an acute attack of allergic, intrinsic and exercise-induced asthma; chronic bronchitis; emphysema; other bronchopulmonary disorders in which bronchospasm is a complicating factor; for the management of uncomplicated premature labour.

Dosage and administration

(1) *Use in bronchospasm*

Adults:

Tablets: During the first 1–2 weeks 2.5 mg (½ tablet) 3 times in a 24 hour period is recommended. The dose may then be increased to 5 mg (1 tablet) 3 times in 24 hours to achieve adequate bronchodilation.

Syrup: 2 to 3 × 5 ml spoonfuls 3 times in 24 hours.

Elderly: Dosage as for adults.

Children:

Tablets: 7–15 years 2.5 mg (½ tablet) 2 or 3 times in 24 hours.

Syrup: The following dosage is recommended – 0.075 mg (0.25 ml)/kg body weight 3 times in a 24 hour period.

e.g. 3–7 years: ½–1 × 5 ml, 3 times in 24 hours.
7–15 years: 1–2 × 5 ml, 3 times in 24 hours.

(2) *Use in the management of premature labour:* After uterine contractions have been controlled by intravenous infusion of Bricanyl Injection, maintenance therapy can be continued with subcutaneous injections (0.25 mg, 4 times in a 24 hour period for 3 days) after which oral treatment (5 mg, 3 times in a 24-hour period) is commenced. Oral treatment should be continued until the end of the 36th week of pregnancy.

Contra-indications, warnings, etc

Contra-indications: Bricanyl oral preparations are contra-indicated in patients with a history of hypersensitivity to any of their constituents.

Although Bricanyl Injection and Tablets are used in the management of uncomplicated premature labour, their use in the following conditions is contra-indicated: Any condition of the mother or foetus in which prolongation of the pregnancy is hazardous, e.g. severe toxaemia, ante-partum haemorrhage, intra-uterine infection, ablatio placentae, threatened abortion during the first and second trimesters, or cord compression.

Precautions: Care should be taken with patients suffering from myocardial insufficiency or thyrotoxicosis. Due to the hyperglycaemic effects of β$_2$-stimulants, additional blood glucose controls are initially recommended when Bricanyl therapy is commenced in diabetic patients. If treatment becomes less effective or shorter acting the patients general condition should be reviewed.

Potentially serious hypokalaemia may result from beta$_2$-agonist therapy. Particular caution is advised in severe asthma as this effect may be potentiated by concomitant treatment with xanthine derivatives, steroids, diuretics and by hypoxia. It is recommended that serum potassium levels are monitored in such situations.

Interactions with other medicaments: Non selective β-blocking agents such as propranolol may partially or totally inhibit the effect of β-stimulants. Therefore Bricanyl oral preparations and non-selective β-blockers should not normally be administered concurrently. Bricanyl should be used with caution in patients receiving other sympathomimetics.

Use in pregnancy and lactation: Although no teratogenic effects have been observed in animals or in patients, Bricanyl should only be administered with caution during the first trimester of pregnancy.

Terbutaline is secreted via breast milk, but influence on the infant is unlikely at therapeutic doses.

Side-effects: The frequency of side-effects is low at the recommended doses. Side-effects which have been recorded such as tremor, tonic cramp and palpitations are all characteristic of sympathomimetic amines. A few patients feel tense; this is also due to the effects on skeletal muscle and not to direct CNS stimulation. Whenever these side-effects have occurred the majority have usually been spontaneously reversible within the first week of treatment.

Potentially serious hypokalaemia may result from beta$_2$-agonist therapy.

Overdosage

Possible symptoms and signs: Headache, anxiety, tremor, tonic cramp, palpitations, arrhythmia. A fall in blood pressure sometimes occurs. Laboratory findings: hypokalaemia, hyperglycaemia and lactoacidosis sometimes occur.

Treatment: (a) *Mild and moderate cases:* Reduce the dose. Then increase the dose more slowly if the bronchodilator effect is insufficient.

(b) *Severe cases:* Gastric lavage, activated charcoal. Determination of acid-base balance, blood sugar and electrolytes. Monitoring of heart rate and rhythm and blood pressure. Metabolic changes should be corrected. A cardioselective β-blocker (e.g. metoprolol) is recommended for the treatment of arrhythmias causing a haemodynamic deterioration. The β-blocker should be used with care because of the possibility of inducing bronchoconstriction. If the β_2-mediated reduction in peripheral vascular resistance significantly contributes to the fall in blood pressure, a volume expander should be given.

Pharmaceutical precautions Store at room temperature. The recommended diluent for Bricanyl Syrup is water.

Legal category POM.

Package quantities
Bricanyl Tablets: Securitainers of 100 and 500 tablets.
Bricanyl Syrup: Bottles of 300 ml and 1 litre.

Further information Bricanyl Tablets and Syrup exert a prolonged bronchodilation, in clinical trials demonstrated for up to 8 hours. Maximum plasma concentration is reached 1–4 hours after dosing.

Bricanyl oral preparations contain no colouring agents and are sugar-free.

A suitable regime for providing eight-hourly oral administration is: on rising, in the mid-afternoon, on retiring.

Product licence numbers
Bricanyl Tablets 0017/0047R
Bricanyl Syrup 0017/0058R.

BRICANYL* INJECTION

Presentation Clear aqueous solution for injection containing 0.5 mg terbutaline sulphate per ml and sodium chloride.

Bricanyl injection is available in 1 ml and 5 ml ampoules. Bricanyl injection in 1 ml ampoules is intended for subcutaneous, intramuscular or intravenous injection. Bricanyl injection in 5 ml ampoules is intended for infusion after dilution with infusion solutions.

Uses

1. *For bronchodilatation.* A selective β_2 adrenergic stimulant recommended for the relief of allergic and intrinsic asthma, chronic bronchitis, emphysema and other broncho-pulmonary disorders in which bronchospasm is a complicating factor.

2. *For the management of uncomplicated premature labour.*

Dosage and administration

1. *For bronchodilatation.* When a rapid therapeutic response is required, Bricanyl can be administered by any of the three standard parenteral routes: subcutaneous, intramuscular, or i.v. bolus. The preferred routes will usually be subcutaneous or intramuscular. When given as an i.v. bolus the injection must be made slowly noting patient response.

Adults: 0.5 ml–1 ml (0.25–0.5 mg) up to four times a day.

Children: 2–15 years. 0.01 mg/kg body weight to a maximum of 0.3 mg total.

Age	*Average weight*		*mg terbutaline*	*ml volume*
	kg	*(lb)*		
<3	10	(22)	0.1	0.2
3	15	(33)	0.15	0.3
6	20	(44)	0.2	0.4
8	25	(55)	0.25	0.5
10+	30+	(66+)	0.3	0.6

By infusion: 3 to 5 ml (1.5–2.5 mg) in 500 ml dextrose, saline or dextrose/saline solution given by continuous intravenous infusion at a rate of 10–20 drops (0.5–1 ml) per minute for 8 to 10 hours. A corresponding reduction in dosage should be made for children.

Elderly: Dosages as for adults.

2. *For management of premature labour.* The dose must be individually titrated with reference to suppression of contractions, increase in pulse rate and changes in blood pressure, which are limiting factors.

These parameters should be carefully monitored during treatment. A maternal heart rate of more than 135 beats/min should be avoided. 10 microgram/min i.v. should be infused during the first hour. This can be increased by 5 microgram/min at 10 min intervals until the contractions stop. The highest dose should be 25 microgram/min. During the next seven hours, the dose should be decreased in 30 minute periods by 5 microgram/min to the lowest maintenance dose that produces continued suppression of the contractions. After this initial treatment, subcutaneous injections (0.25 mg) should be given four times a day for three days. During this period, oral treatment should be started (5 mg three times a day). The oral treatment should be continued until the end of the 36th week of pregnancy. Suggestion for dilution: 5 mg (2×5 ml ampoules) in 1,000 ml of dextrose solution (40 drops contain approximately 10 microgram).

Contra-indications, warnings, etc

1. *Contra-indications:* Bricanyl preparations are contra-indicated in patients with a history of sensitivity to any of their constituents.

Although Bricanyl injection and tablets are used in the management of uncomplicated premature labour, their use in the following conditions is contra-indicated: Any condition of the mother or foetus in which prolongation of the pregnancy is hazardous e.g. severe toxaemia, ante-partum haemorrhage, intra-uterine infection, ablatio placentae, threatened abortion during the first and second trimesters or cord compression.

Precautions: Care should be taken with patients suffering from myocardial insufficiency or thyrotoxicosis. Due to the hyperglycaemic effects of beta-2 stimulants, additional blood glucose measurements are initially recommended when Bricanyl therapy is commenced in diabetic patients. If treatment becomes less effective or shorter-acting, the patient's general condition should be reviewed.

Potentially serious hypokalaemia may result from beta$_2$-agonist therapy. Particular caution is advised in severe asthma as this effect may be potentiated by concomitant treatment with xanthine derivatives, steroids, diuretics and by hypoxia. It is recommended that serum potassium levels are monitored in such situations.

In premature labour in a patient with known or suspected cardiac disease a physician experienced in cardiology should assess the suitability of treatment before i.v. infusion with Bricanyl.

Warnings: In treatment of premature labour, hyperglycaemia and ketoacidosis have been found in pregnant women with diabetes after treatment with β_2-stimulants. It may therefore be necessary to adjust the insulin dose when β_2-stimulants are used in the treatment.

During infusion treatment in pregnant women with β_2-

stimulants in combination with corticosteroids a rare complication with a pathological picture resembling pulmonary oedema, has been reported.

Increased tendency to uterine bleeding has been reported in connection with Caesarean section. However, this can be effectively stopped by propranolol 1–2 mg injected intravenously.

Interactions with other medicaments: Non-selective beta-blocking agents such as propranolol may partially or totally inhibit the effect of beta-stimulants. Therefore Bricanyl and non-selective beta-blockers should not normally be administered concurrently. Bricanyl should be used with caution in patients receiving other sympathomimetics.

Pregnancy and lactation: Although no teratogenic effects have been observed in animals or in patients, Bricanyl should only be administered with caution during the first trimester of pregnancy.

Terbutaline is secreted via breast milk, but effect on the infant is unlikely at therapeutic doses.

Side-effects: When used as a bronchodilator the frequency of side-effects is low. Side-effects which have been recorded such as tremor, tonic cramp and palpitations are all characteristics of sympathomimetic amines. A few patients feel tense; this is also due to the effects on skeletal muscle and not to direct CNS stimulation. Whenever these side-effects have occurred the majority have usually been spontaneously reversible within the first week of treatment.

Potentially serious hypokalaemia may result from beta$_2$-agonist therapy.

Overdosage: Possible symptoms and signs: Headache, anxiety, tremor, tonic cramp, palpitations, arrhythmia. A fall in blood pressure sometimes occurs. Laboratory findings: hypokalaemia, hyperglycaemia and lactic acidosis sometimes occur.

Treatment: Mild and moderate cases: Reduce the dose. Severe cases: Determination of acid-base balance, blood sugar and electrolytes. Monitoring of heart rate and rhythm and blood pressure. Metabolic changes should be corrected. A cardioselective beta-blocker (e.g. metroprolol) is recommended for the treatment of arrhythmias causing haemodynamic deterioration. The beta-blocker should be used with care because of the possibility of inducing bronchoconstriction. If the beta$_2$-mediated reduction in peripheral vascular resistance significantly contributes to the fall in blood pressure, a volume expander should be given.

Pharmaceutical precautions No special storage conditions are necessary. The recommended diluent is water for injection, or sterile saline or dextrose.

Legal category POM.

Package quantities Packs of 5 × 1 ml ampoules and 10 × 5 ml ampoules.

Further information Nil.

Product licence number 0017/0048R.

BRICANYL* EXPECTORANT

Presentation A clear aqueous raspberry/menthol flavoured solution containing:

Terbutaline Sulphate BP	0.3 mg/ml
Guaiphenesin	13.3 mg/ml

Inactive ingredients: Sorbitol, glycerol, citric acid, sodium hydroxide, sodium benzoate, disodium edetate, saccharin sodium, flavour raspberry, flavour lemon limette, menthol natural, ethanol, water.

Uses Terbutaline is a selective β_2-adrenergic agonist recommended for use in the following indications: Prophylactic treatment and relief of an acute attack of allergic, intrinsic and exercise-induced asthma; chronic bronchitis; emphysema; other bronchopulmonary disorders in which brochospasm is a complicating factor.

Dosage and administration
Adults: 2–3 × 5 ml spoonfuls 3 times in 24 hours.
Elderly: Dosage as for adults.
Children: Not recommended for children.

Contra-indications, warnings, etc
Contra-indications: Bricanyl oral preparations are contra-indicated in patients with a history of hypersensitivity to any of their constituents.

Precautions: Care should be taken with patients suffering from myocardial insufficiency or thyrotoxicosis. Due to the hyperglycaemic effects of β_2-stimulants, additional blood glucose controls are initially recommended when Bricanyl therapy is commenced in diabetic patients. If treatment becomes less effective or shorter acting the patients' general condition should be reviewed.

Potentially serious hypokalaemia may result from beta$_2$-agonist therapy. Particular caution is advised in severe asthma as this effect may be potentiated by concomitant treatment with xanthine derivatives, steroids, diuretics and by hypoxia. It is recommended that serum potassium levels are monitored in such situations.

Interactions with other medicaments: Non selective β-blocking agents such as propranolol may partially or totally inhibit the effect of β-stimulants. Therefore, Bricanyl oral preparations and non-selective β-blockers should not normally be administered concurrently. Bricanyl should be used with caution in patients receiving other sympathomimetics.

Use in pregnancy and lactation: Although no teratogenic effects have been observed in animals or in patients, Bricanyl should only be administered with caution during the first trimester of pregnancy.

Terbutaline is secreted via breast milk, but influence on the infant is unlikely at therapeutic doses.

Side-effects: The frequency of side-effects is low at the recommended doses. Side-effects which have been recorded such as tremor, tonic cramp and palpitations are all characteristic of sympathomimetic amines. A few patients feel tense; this is also due to the effects of skeletal muscle and not to direct CNS stimulation. Whenever these side-effects have occurred the majority have usually been spontaneously reversible within the first week of treatment.

Potentially serious hypokalaemia may result from beta$_2$-agonist therapy.

Overdosage

Possible symptoms and signs: Headache, anxiety, tremor, tonic cramp, palpitations, arrhythmia. A fall in blood pressure sometimes occurs.

Laboratory findings: hypokalaemia, hyperglycaemia and lactic acidosis sometimes occur.

Treatment: (a) *Mild and moderate cases:* Reduce the dose. Then increase the dose more slowly if the broncholytic effect is insufficient.

(b) *Severe cases:* Gastric lavage, activated charcoal. Determination of acid-base balance, blood sugar and electrolytes. Monitoring of heart rate and rhythm and blood pressure. Metabolic changes should be corrected. A cardioselective β-blocker (e.g. metoprolol) is recommended for the treatment of arrhythmias causing a haemodynamic deterioration. The β-blocker should be used with care because of the possibility of inducing bronchoconstriction. If the β_2-mediated reduction in peripheral vascular resistance significantly contributes to the fall in blood pressure, a volume expander should be given.

Pharmaceutical precautions Store at room temperature. The recommended diluent for Bricanyl Expectorant is water.

Legal category POM.

Package quantities Bottles of 300 ml.

Further information Bricanyl Expectorant exerts a prolonged bronchodilation, in clinical trials demonstrated for up to 8 hours. Maximum plasma concentration is reached 1–4 hours after dosing.

Bricanyl Expectorant contains no colouring agents and is sugar-free.

A suitable regime for providing eight-hourly oral

administration is: on rising; in the mid-afternoon; on retiring.

Product licence numbers
Bricanyl Expectorant Syrup 0017/0068R.

BRICANYL* RESPIRATOR SOLUTION

Presentation A clear aqueous solution for nebulisation.

Single dose unit ampoules, Respules, containing 5 mg terbutaline sulphate in 2 ml. Multidose bottles containing 100 mg in 10 ml. These solutions also contain sodium chloride and sodium edetate. Multidose bottles also contain chlorobutanol.

Uses For the relief of severe bronchospasm.

Dosage and administration In most patients the use of terbutaline sulphate, based on the doses below, given 2–4 times daily will be sufficient to relieve bronchospasm. In acute severe asthma additional doses may be necessary.

Bricanyl Respules:
Adults: 1 or 2 Respules (5 or 10 mg)
Children: (>25 kg) 1 Respule (5 mg)
Children: (<25 kg) use multidose bottles.

Multidose bottles:
Adults: 0.5 to 1 ml (5 to 10 mg) diluted to required nebuliser volume with sterile physiological saline.

Children: 0.2 to 0.5 mls (2 to 5 mg), see table, diluted to required nebuliser volume with sterile physiological saline.

Table illustrating ml undiluted solution from multidose bottle required for administration to children.

Age	*Average weight kg*	*Average weight lb*	*mg terbutaline*	*ml undiluted solution*
<3	10	22	2.0	0.2
3	15	33	3.0	0.3
6	20	44	4.0	0.4
8+	25+	55+	5.0	0.5

Elderly: Dosage as for adults.

Contra-indications, warnings, etc No contra-indications are known.

Precautions: Care should be taken with patients suffering from myocardial insufficiency or thyrotoxicosis.

Potentially serious hypokalaemia may result from $beta_2$-agonist therapy. Particular caution is advised in severe asthma as this effect may be potentiated by concomitant treatment with xanthine derivatives, steroids, diuretics and by hypoxia. It is recommended that serum potassium levels are monitored in such situations.

Pregnancy: Although no teratogenic effects have been observed in animal experiments, caution is recommended during the first trimester of pregnancy.

Lactation: Terbutaline is excreted in breast milk, but influence on the infant is unlikely at therapeutic doses.

Side-effects: The frequency of side-effects is low and those which have been recorded, e.g. tremor and palpitations, are all characteristic of sympathomimetic amines. Whenever these have occurred, the majority have been spontaneously reversible within the first week of treatment.

Potentially serious hypokalaemia may result from $beta_2$-agonist therapy.

Overdose: In the event of a large overdose the most significant symptom would be a reflex tachycardia. Other symptoms may include tremor, restlessness, nausea, vomiting and headache. Hypokalaemia metabolic acidosis and hyperglycaemia may occur. Treatment should be symptomatic. Hypokalaemia should be corrected. If tachycardia or ventricular arrhythmias requiring therapy occur, treatment with a beta-blocker given i.v. may be considered. A selective beta-blocker such as metoprolol is preferable.

Pharmaceutical precautions Store at room temperature away from light. Single dose plastic units (Respules) in an opened foil envelope must be used within 3 months. Bricanyl Respules will not normally require dilution at recommended doses.

Bricanyl Respirator Solution in multidose bottles contains preservative and must be diluted before use with sterile physiological saline. Solution in nebulisers should be replaced daily.

Legal category POM.

Package quantities Single dose units (Respules): Packs of 20 × 2 ml. (Strips of 5 units wrapped in a foil envelope).
Multidose bottles: 10 ml bottle.

Further information Nil.

Product licence numbers
Single dose units Respules 0017/0228
Multidose bottles 0017/0078

BRICANYL* SA

Presentation White tablet with engraving $\frac{A}{BD}$ containing 7.5 mg terbutaline sulphate in a sustained-release formulation.

Inactive ingredients: Polyvinyl chloride, colloidal silicon dioxide, tartaric acid, ethyl cellulose, stearyl alcohol.

Uses For relief of bronchospasm in bronchial asthma and in chronic bronchitis, emphysema and other pulmonary disorders in which bronchospasm is a complicating factor.

Dosage and administration
Adults: 1 tablet morning and evening. The tablet may not be divided or chewed, but must be swallowed whole together with liquid.

Elderly: Dosage as for adults.

Contra-indications, warnings, etc
Contra-indications: Bricanyl oral preparations are contra-indicated in patients with a history of hypersensitivity to any of their constituents.

Precautions: Care should be taken with patients suffering from myocardial insufficiency or thyrotoxicosis. Due to the hyperglycaemic effects of β_2-stimulants, additional blood glucose controls are initially recommended when Bricanyl therapy is commenced in diabetic patients. If treatment becomes less effective or shorter acting the patients' general condition should be reviewed.

Potentially serious hypokalaemia may result from $beta_2$-agonist therapy. Particular caution is advised in severe asthma as this effect may be potentiated by concomitant treatment with xanthine derivatives, steroids, diuretics and by hypoxia. It is recommended that serum potassium levels are monitored in such situations.

Interactions with other medicaments: Non-selective β-blocking agents such as propranolol may partially or totally inhibit the effect of β-stimulants. Therefore, Bricanyl oral preparations and non-selective β-blockers should not normally be administered concurrently. Bricanyl should be used with caution in patients receiving other sympathomimetics.

Use in pregnancy and lactation: Although no teratogenic effects have been observed in animals or in patients, terbutaline should only be administered with caution during the first trimester of pregnancy.

Terbutaline is secreted via breast milk, but influence on the infant is unlikely at therapeutic doses.

Side-effects: The frequency of side-effects is low at the recommended doses. Side-effects which have been recorded such as tremor, tonic cramp and palpitations are all characteristic of sympathomimetic amines. A few patients feel tense; this is also due to the effects of skeletal muscle and not to direct CNS stimulation.

Whenever these side-effects have occurred the majority have usually been spontaneously reversible within the first week of treatment.

Potentially serious hypokalaemia may result from beta$_2$-agonist therapy.

Overdosage

Possible symptoms and signs: Headache, anxiety, tremor, tonic cramp, palpitations, arrhythmia. A fall in blood pressure sometimes occurs.

Laboratory findings: hypokalaemia, hyperglycaemia and lactacidosis sometimes occur.

Treatment: (a) *Mild and moderate cases:* Reduce the dose. Then increase the dose more slowly if the bronchodilator effect is insufficient.

(b) *Severe cases:* Gastric lavage, activated charcoal. Determination of acid-base balance, blood sugar and electrolytes. Monitoring of heart rate and rhythm and blood pressure. Metabolic changes should be corrected. A cardioselective β-blocker (e.g. metoprolol) is recommended for the treatment of arrhythmias causing a haemodynamic deterioration. The β-blocker should be used with care because of the possibility of inducing bronchoconstriction. If the β_2-mediated reduction in peripheral vascular resistance significantly contributes to the fall in blood pressure, a volume expander should be given.

Pharmaceutical precautions No special storage conditions are necessary.

Legal category POM.

Package quantities Glass bottles containing 60 tablets.

Further information The inactive components in Bricanyl SA form a matrix which is insoluble in the digestive juices. The empty matrix may sometimes pass through the digestive system unchanged and be excreted.

Product licence number 0017/0110.

BRICANYL* TURBOHALER

Presentation Breath-actuated metered dose powder inhaler delivering 0.5 mg terbulatine sulphate per actuation. Each inhaler contains 100 doses. Bricanyl Turbohaler is free from propellants, lubricants, preservatives, carrier substances or other additives.

Uses For the relief of bronchospasm in bronchial asthma and in chronic bronchitis, emphysema and other pulmonary disorders in which bronchospasm is a complicating factor.

Dosage and administration

Adults and children: One inhalation (0.5 mg) as required. Not more than 4 inhalations should be necessary in any 24 hour period.

Elderly: Dosage as for adults.

Contra-indications, warnings, etc No contra-indications are known.

Precautions: Care should be used in patients suffering from myocardial insufficiency or thyrotoxicosis.

Patients should be warned that if either the usual relief or duration of action is diminished they should seek medical advice immediately.

Potentially serious hypokalaemia may result from beta$_2$-agonist therapy. Particular caution is advised in severe asthma as this effect may be potentiated by concomitant treatment with xanthine derivatives, steroids, diuretics and by hypoxia. It is recommended that serum potassium levels are monitored in such situations.

Use in pregnancy and lactation: Although no teratogenic effects have been observed in animals or in patients, terbutaline should only be administered with caution during the first trimester of pregnancy.

Terbutaline is secreted via breast milk, but influence on the infant is unlikely at therapeutic doses.

Non-selective beta-blocking agents may partly or totally inhibit the effect of beta-stimulants. Patients should be warned that if either the usual relief or duration of action is diminished they should seek medical advice immediately.

Side-effects: The frequency of side-effects is low. Those which have been recorded e.g. tremor, tonic cramp and palpitations are all characteristic of sympathomimetic amines. Whenever these have occurred, the majority have been spontaneously reversible within the first week of treatment.

Potentially serious hypokalaemia may result from beta$_2$-agonist therapy.

Overdose: Possible symptoms and signs of overdose include headache, anxiety, tremor, tonic cramp, palpitations and arrhythmia. A fall in blood pressure, hypokalaemia, hyperglycaemia and metabolic acidosis may also occur.

Treatment of overdose: Treatment should be symptomatic. Hypokalaemia should be corrected. If tachycardia or ventricular arrhythimas requiring therapy occur, treatment with a beta-blocker given i.v. may be considered. A selective beta-blocker such as metoprolol is preferred.

Pharmaceutical precautions Protect from moisture. Store at room temperature.

Legal category POM.

Package quantities Powder inhaler containing 100 doses.

Further information Bricanyl Turbohaler is breath-actuated and therefore there is no need to co-ordinate the release of the dose and the inhalation. Treatment with Bricanyl Turbohaler is effective even at low inspiratory flow rates, like those present during an acute asthmatic attack.

Product licence number 0017/0241.

CITANEST*

Presentation A sterile clear aqueous solution of prilocaine hydrochloride 0.5%, 1.0%. Each ml contains prilocaine hydrochloride 5 mg; 10 mg respectively. In addition all Citanest presentations contain sodium chloride to produce an isotonic solution.

Inactive ingredients: Sodium hydroxide. The multidose vials contain methylparahydroxybenzoate.

Uses Citanest is a local anaesthetic solution for use in infiltration anaesthesia, intravenous regional anaesthesia and nerve blocks.

Dosage and administration The dose is adjusted according to the response of the patient and the site of administration. The lowest concentration and smallest dose producing the required effect should be given. The maximum dose for healthy adults should not exceed 400 mg.

Children and elderly or debilitated patients require smaller doses, commensurate with age and physical status.

Contra-indications, warnings, etc Known hypersensitivity to anaesthetics of the amide type. Citanest should be avoided in patients with anaemia or congenital or acquired methaemoglobinaemia.

Precautions In common with other local anaesthetics, Citanest should be used cautiously in patients with epilepsy, impaired cardiac conduction, impaired respiratory function, and in patients with liver or kidney damage, if the dose or site of administration is likely to result in high blood levels.

Facilities for resuscitation should be available when local anaesthetics are administered.

The effect of local anaesthetics may be reduced if an injection is made into an inflamed or infected area.

Use in pregnancy: Although there is no evidence from animal studies of harm to the foetus, as with all drugs, Citanest should not be given during early pregnancy unless the benefits are considered to outweigh the risks.

Side-effects: In common with other local anaesthetics, adverse reactions to Citanest are rare and are usually the result of excessively high blood concentrations due to inadvertent intravascular injection, excessive dosage, rapid absorption or occasionally to hypersensitivity, idiosyncracy or diminished tolerance on the part of the patient. In such circumstances systemic effects occur involving the central nervous system and/or the cardiovascular system.

CNS reactions are excitatory and/or depressant, and may be characterised by nervousness, dizziness, blurred vision and tremors, followed by drowsiness, convulsions, unconsciousness and possibly respiratory arrest. The excitatory reactions may be very brief or may not occur at all, in which case the first manifestations of toxicity may be drowsiness, merging into unconsciousness and respiratory arrest. Cardiovascular reactions are depressant, and may be characterised by hypotension, myocardial depression, bradycardia and possibly cardiac arrest.

Allergic reactions are extremely rare. They may be characterised by cutaneous lesions, urticaria, oedema or anaphylactoid reactions. Detection of sensitivity by skin testing is of doubtful value.

Hypotension may occur as a physiological response to central nerve blocks.

Clinically significant levels of methaemoglobin may occur with cyanosis when doses of prilocaine exceed 600 mg. Methaemoglobinaemia may be treated by the intravenous administration of a 1% solution of methylene blue in a dose of 1 mg/kg.

Pharmaceutical precautions Store at room temperature.

Legal category POM.

Package quantities
Single dose vial: 0.5%: Packs of 5 × 50 ml.
Multidose vials: 0.5%, 1.0%: Packs of 5 × 20 ml and packs of 5 × 50 ml.

Further information Citanest 0.5% SDV (single dose vial) is preservative free and should therefore be used on one occasion only.

Product licence numbers

0.5% (multi-dose vial)	0017/5047R
1.0% (multi-dose vial)	0017/5048R
0.5% (single-dose vial)	0017/0208

CITANEST* 2% SOLUTION

Presentation A sterile clear aqueous solution of Prilocaine Hydrochloride BP 20.0 mg/ml.

Inactive ingredients: Sodium chloride to produce an isotonic solution. No preservative is added.

Uses Infiltration anaesthesia, epidurals, nerve blocks, analgesia.

Dosage and administration The dose is adjusted according to the response of the patient and the site of administration.

The smallest dose to produce the required effect should be given.

The maximum dose for healthy adults should not exceed 400 mg.

Children and elderly or debilitated patients require smaller doses, commensurate with age and physical status.

Contra-indications, warnings, etc
Contra-indications: Known hypersensitivity to anaesthetics of the amide type.

Use in patients with anaemia or congenital or acquired methaemoglobinaemia.

Precautions and warnings Use cautiously in patients with epilepsy, impaired cardiac conduction, impaired respiratory function, and in patients with liver or kidney damage, if the dose or site of administration is likely to result in high blood levels. Facilities for resuscitation should be available when local anaesthetics are administered.

The effect of local anaesthetics may be reduced if an injection is made into an inflamed or infected area.

Use in pregnancy: Although there is no evidence from animal studies of harm to the foetus, as with all drugs Citanest should not be given during early pregnancy unless the benefits are considered to outweigh the risks.

Adverse reactions: In common with other local anaesthetics, adverse reactions to Citanest are rare and are usually the result of excessively high blood concentrations due to inadvertent intravascular injection, excessive dosage, rapid absorption or occasionally to hypersensitivity, idiosyncracy or diminished tolerance on the part of the patient. In such circumstances systemic effects occur involving the central nervous system and/or the cardiovascular system.

CNS reactions are excitatory and/or depressant, and may be characterised by nervousness, dizziness, blurred vision and tremors, followed by drowsiness, convulsions, unconsciousness and possibly respiratory arrest. The excitatory reactions may be very brief or may not occur at all, in which case the first manifestations of toxicity may be drowsiness, merging into unconsciousness and respiratory arrest. Cardiovascular reactions are depressant, and may be characterised by hypotension, myocardial depression, bradycardia and possibly cardiac arrest.

Allergic reactions are extremely rare. They may be characterised by cutaneous lesions, urticaria, oedema or anaphylactoid reactions. Detection of sensitivity by skin testing is of doubtful value.

Hypotension may occur as a physiological response to central nerve blocks.

Clinically significant levels of methaemoglobin may occur with cyanosis when doses of prilocaine exceed 600 mg. Methaemoglobinaemia may be treated by the intravenous administration of a 1% solution of methylene blue in a dose of 1 mg/kg.

Pharmaceutical precautions Store at room temperature.

Legal category POM.

Package quantities Packs of 5 × 10 ml single dose vials.

Further information Nil.

Product licence number 0017/0090.

CITANEST* 3% WITH OCTAPRESSIN*

Presentation Sterile clear aqueous solution for dental anaesthesia; prilocaine hydrochloride 30 mg/ml, felypressin 0.03 i.u. per ml. In addition Citanest 3% with Octapressin cartridges contain sodium chloride to produce an isotonic solution.

Uses Local anaesthetic solution with vasoconstrictor for dental infiltration anaesthesia where there is no necessity for profound ischaemia in the area injected. For all dental nerve-block techniques.

Dosage and administration 1–2 ml should be sufficient for the majority of procedures. The addition of Octapressin decreases the rate of absorption of the injected solution. For this reason the recommended maximum dosage for Citanest with Octapressin is higher than that recommended for a plain solution, but total dosage of Citanest should not exceed 600 mg in a healthy adult of body weight 70 kg. The total dose should not exceed 20 ml. In aged and debilitated patients the dose must be reduced. In children the maximum dose is considerably less and should be calculated in relation to body weight.

Contra-indications, warnings, etc In known cases of ischaemic heart disease not more than four cartridges should be used at one sitting.

Known sensitivity to local anaesthetics of the amide type.

Adverse reactions: The type of toxic reaction is unpredictable and depends on dosage, route of administration and state of the patient. The reactions are primarily of two types, and typified by stimulation and depression of the cerebral cortex and medulla respectively. Slow onset – stimulation leading to nervousness, dizziness, blurred vision, nausea, tremors, convulsions and respiratory arrest. Rapid onset – depression leading to respiratory arrest, cardiovascular collapse and cardiac arrest. Symptoms occur rapidly and with little warning.

Precautions: Adequate resuscitation equipment must be available whenever local or general anaesthesia is administered. Though clinical tolerance is remarkably good, overdosage or accidental intravenous injection may give rise to toxic reactions. Care should be observed in patients suffering from epilepsy.

Pharmaceutical precautions Store at room temperature.

Legal category POM.

Package quantities Glass cartridges of 2.2 ml standard, and 2.2 ml self-aspirating, in boxes of 100.

Further information Citanest 3% with Octapressin solution is free of preservative.

Product licence number 0017/5003.

CITANEST* 4%

Presentation Sterile clear aqueous solution. Each ml contains prilocaine hydrochloride 40 mg.

Inactive ingredients: Sodium chloride to produce an isotonic solution and sodium hydroxide.

Uses Local anaesthetic solution without vasoconstrictor for dental infiltration anaesthesia where there is no necessity for profound ischaemia in the area injected. For all dental nerve-block techniques. For all dental injections where a vasoconstrictor is contra-indicated.

Dosage and administration 1–2 ml. In a healthy adult of a normal body weight (70 kg) the maximum dose should not exceed 400 mg. In aged and debilitated patients the dose must be reduced, and in children the maximum dose should be calculated in relation to body weight, i.e. 3 mg per lb or 6 mg per kg.

Contra-indications, warnings, etc
Contra-indications: Known hypersensitivity to anaesthetics of the amide type.

Side-effects: Systemic effects due to the use of Citanest in dental practice are practically unknown due to the small dosages employed.

Citanest should be avoided in patients with anaemia or congenital or acquired methaemoglobinaemia.

Precautions: In common with other local anaesthetics, Citanest should be used cautiously in patients with epilepsy, impaired cardiac conduction, impaired respiratory function and in patients with liver or kidney damage, if the dose or site of administration is likely to result in high blood levels.

Though clinical tolerance is remarkably good, overdosage or accidental intravenous injection may give rise to toxic reactions. These are best avoided by aspiration before making an injection, in order to avoid accidental intravascular injection.

Warnings: Facilities for resuscitation should be available when local anaesthetics are administered.

The effect of local anaesthetics may be reduced if an injection is made into an inflamed or infected area.

The type of toxic reaction is unpredictable, and depends on dosage, route of administration and state of patient. Reactions are primarily of two types typified by stimulation and depression of the cerebral cortex and medulla respectively. Slow onset – stimulation leading to nervousness, dizziness, blurred vision, nausea, tremors, convulsions and respiratory arrest. Rapid onset – depression leading to respiratory arrest, cardiovascular collapse and cardiac arrest. Symptoms occur rapidly and with little warning.

Pharmaceutical precautions Store at room temperature.

Legal category POM.

Package quantities Glass cartridges of 2.2 ml standard cartridges in boxes of 100.

Further information Citanest 4% solution is free of preservative.

Product licence number 0017/5050R.

CO-BETALOC*

Presentation White scored tablets (coded A/MH) containing 100 mg metoprolol tartrate and 12.5 mg hydrochlorothiazide.

Inactive ingredients: Lactose, microcrystalline cellulose, sodium starch glycolate, polyvinylpyrrolidone, colloidal silica, magnesium stearate.

Uses In the management of mild or moderate hypertension. Co-Betaloc may be suitable for use when satisfactory control of arterial blood pressure cannot be obtained with either a diuretic or a beta-adrenoreceptor blocking drug used alone.

Dosage and administration The dose will depend on patient response. Usually 1–3 tablets per day as a single or divided dose.

Elderly: There are no special dosage requirements in otherwise healthy elderly patients.

Significant hepatic dysfunction: A reduction in dosage may be necessary.

Contra-indications, warnings, etc
Contra-indications: AV block. Uncontrolled heart failure. Severe bradycardia. Sick-sinus syndrome. Cardiogenic shock. Severe peripheral arterial disease. Known hypersensitivity to Betaloc or other β-blockers.

Severe kidney and liver failure. Therapy resistant hypokalaemia and hyponatraemia. Hypercalcaemia, symptomatic hyperuricaemia. Anuria. Known hypersensitivity to hydrochlorothiazide or other sulphonamide derivatives.

An anti-diuretic effect has been reported following concomitant treatment with diuretics and lithium. As with all products which contain diuretics, Co-Betaloc is contra-indicated during lithium therapy.

Warnings: Metoprolol may aggravate bradycardia, symptoms of peripheral arterial circulatory disorders and anaphylactic shock.

Abrupt interruption of β-blockers is to be avoided. When possible, Co-Betaloc should be withdrawn gradually over a period of 10 days. During its withdrawal patients should be kept under close surveillance, especially those with known ischaemic heart disease.

Co-Betaloc may be administered when heart failure has been controlled. Digitalisation and/or additional diuretic therapy should also be considered for patients with a history of heart failure, or patients known to have a poor cardiac reserve.

Although cardioselective beta-blockers may have less effect on lung function than non-selective beta-blockers, as with all beta-blockers these should be avoided in patients with reversible obstructive airways disease unless there are compelling clinical reasons for their use. When administration is necessary, use of a $beta_2$-bronchodilator (e.g. terbutaline) may be advisable in some patients.

In labile and insulin-dependent diabetes it may be necessary to adjust the hypoglycaemic therapy.

In patients with a phaeochromocytoma, an alpha-blocker should be given concomitantly.

In the presence of liver cirrhosis the bioavailability of metoprolol may be increased.

The administration of adrenaline to patients undergoing beta-blockade can result in an increase in blood pressure and bradycardia although this is less likely to occur with β_1-selective drugs.

Co-Betaloc therapy must be reported to the anaesthetist prior to general anaesthesia. If withdrawal of metoprolol is considered desirable, this should if possible be completed at least 48 hours before general anaesthesia.

Co-Betaloc does not interfere with potassium balance. However, at higher doses of hydrochlorothiazide disturbances in the electrolyte and water balance may be experienced. Hyperuricaemia may occur or frank gout may be precipitated in certain patients receiving higher doses of thiazide therapy. Latent diabetes may become manifest during thiazide therapy.

Diuretics in higher doses may precipitate azotemia in patients with renal disease. Cumulative effects of hydrochlorothiazide may develop in patients with impaired renal function. If renal impairment becomes evident metoprolol/hydrochlorothiazide therapy should be discontinued.

Pregnancy: Co-Betaloc should not be used in pregnancy or nursing mothers unless the physician considers that the benefit outweighs the possible hazard to the foetus/infant. As with all beta-blockers metoprolol may cause side-effects e.g. bradycardia, hypoglycaemia in the foetus, and in the newborn and breastfed infant. Metoprolol has, however, been used in pregnancy associated hypertension under close supervision, after 20 weeks gestation. Although the drug crosses the placental barrier and is present in cord blood, no evidence of foetal abnormalities has been reported.

Hydrochlorothiazide can reduce the plasma volume as well as the uteroplacental blood circulation.

Lactation: The amount of metoprolol ingested via breast milk should not produce significant β-blocking effects in the neonate if the mother is treated with normal therapeutic doses.

As hydrochlorothiazide passes into breast milk, consideration should be given to withdrawal of Co-Betaloc, replacement by metoprolol in monotherapy or breast-feeding stopped.

Interactions: The effects of Co-Betaloc and other antihypertensive drugs on blood pressure are usually additive, and care should be taken to avoid hypotension. However, combinations of antihypertensive drugs may often be used with benefit to improve control of hypertension.

Metoprolol can reduce myocardial contractility and impair intracardiac conduction. Care should be exercised when drugs with similar activity, e.g. antiarrhythmic agents, general anaesthetics, are given concurrently. Like all other β-blockers, metoprolol should not be given in combination with verapamil since this may cause bradycardia, hypotension and asystole. Care should also be exercised when β-blockers are given in combination with sympathetic ganglion blocking agents, other β-blockers (i.e. eye drops) or MAO inhibitors. If combination treatment with clonidine is to be discontinued, metoprolol should be withdrawn several days before clonidine.

As β-blockers may affect the peripheral circulation, care should be exercised when drugs with similar activity e.g. ergotamine are given concurrently.

Metoprolol will antagonise the β_1-effects of sympathomimetic agents but should have little influence on the bronchodilator effects of β_2-agonists at normal therapeutic doses. Enzyme inducing agents (e.g. rifampicin) may reduce plasma concentrations of metoprolol, whereas enzyme inhibitors (e.g. cimetidine) may increase plasma concentrations. Metoprolol may impair the elimination of lignocaine.

Indomethacin may reduce the antihypertensive effect of β-blockers.

In general reported interactions have occurred with doses of hydrochlorothiazide higher than those used in this combination. Insulin requirements in diabetic patients may be altered and lithium renal clearance is reduced, increasing the risk of lithium toxicity. Responsiveness to turbocurarine may be increased and arterial responsiveness to noradrenaline may be decreased, but not enough to preclude effectiveness of the pressor agent for therapeutic use. Hypokalaemia may develop during concomitant use of steroids or ACTH, and may sensitise or exaggerate the response of the heart to toxic effects of digitalis.

Side-effects: Side effects to metoprolol are usually mild and infrequent. The most common appear to be lassitude, GI disturbances (nausea, vomiting or abdominal pain) and disturbances of sleep pattern. In many cases these effects have been transient or have disappeared after a reduction in dosage.

Effects related to the CNS which have been reported occasionally are dizziness and headache and rarely paraesthesia, muscle cramps, depression and decreased mental alterness. There have also been isolated reports of personality disorders.

Cardiovascular effects which have been reported occasionally are bradycardia, postural hypotension and rarely, heart failure, palpitations, cardiac arrhythmias, Raynauds phenomenon, peripheral oedema and precordial pain. There have also been isolated reports of cardiac conduction abnormalities, and gangrene in patients with pre-existing severe peripheral circulatory disorders.

Common gastro-intestinal disturbances have been described above but rarely diarrhoea or constipation also occur and there have been isolated cases of dry mouth and abnormal liver function.

Skin rashes (urticaria, psoriasiform, dystrophic skin lesions) and positive anti-nuclear antibodies (not associated with SLE) occur rarely. Isolated cases of photosensitivity, increased sweating and alopecia have been reported. Respiratory effects include occasional reports of dyspnoea on exertion and rare reports of bronchospasm and isolated cases of rhinitis.

Isolated cases of weight gain, thrombocytopenia, disturbances of vision, conjunctivitis, tinnitus and dry or irritated eyes have also been reported.

The reported incidence of skin rashes and/or dry eyes is small and in most cases the symptoms have cleared when treatment was withdrawn. Discontinuation of the drug should be considered if any such reaction is not otherwise explicable.

Hydrochlorothiazide is generally well tolerated at the dose used (12.5 mg) in the combination. However the familiar side-effects of thiazide diuretics may be expected e.g. gastro-intestinal disturbances, metabolic and electrolyte changes, disturbances in sleep patterns, skin rashes and effects relating to the CNS.

Overdosage: Poisoning due to an overdose of Co-Betaloc may lead to severe hypotension, sinus bradycardia, atrioventricular block, heart failure, cardiogenic shock, cardiac arrest, bronchospasm, impairment of consciousness, coma, nausea, vomiting, cyanosis, hypoglycaemia and, occasionally, hyperkalaemia. The first manifestations usually appear 20 minutes to 2 hours after drug ingestion.

The most prominent feature of poisoning due to hydrochlorothiazide is acute loss of fluid and electrolytes. The following symptoms may also be observed: dizziness, sedation/impairment of consciousness, hypotension and muscle cramps.

Treatment should include close monitoring of cardiovascular, respiratory and renal function, and blood glucose and electrolytes. Further absorportion may be prevented by induction of vomiting, gastric lavage or administration of activated-charcoal if ingestion is recent. Cardiovascular complications should be treated symptomatically, which may require the use of sympathomimetic agents (e.g. noradrenaline, metaraminol), atropine or inotropic agents (e.g. dopamine, dobutamine). Temporary pacing may be required for AV block. Glucagon can reverse the effects of excessive β-blockade, given a dose of 1–10 mg intravenously. Intravenous β_2-stimulants e.g. terbutaline may be required to relieve bronchospasm.

Intravenous volume and electrolyte-replacement may be necessary.

Metoprolol cannot be effectively removed by haemodialysis.

Pharmaceutical precautions Store in a cool dry place.

Legal category POM.

Package quantities Calendar packs of 28 tablets. Securitainers of 300 tablets.

Further information Metoprolol is well absorbed after oral administration, peak plasma concentrations occurring 1.5–2 hours after dosing. The bioavailability of a single dose is approximately 50%, increasing to approximately 70% during repeated administration. The bioavailability also increases if metoprolol is given with food.

Elimination is mainly by hepatic metabolism and the average elimination half-life is 3.5 hours (range 1 to 9 hours). Rates of metabolism vary between individuals, with poor metabolisers (approximately 10%) showing higher plasma concentrations and slower elimination than extensive metabolisers. Within individuals, however, plasma concentrations are stable and reproducible.

Because of variation in rates of metabolism, the dose of metoprolol should always be adjusted to the individual requirements of the patient. As the therapeutic response, adverse effects and relative cardioselectivity are related to plasma concentration, poor metabolisers may require lower than normal doses. Dosage adjustment is not routinely required in the elderly or in patients with renal failure, but dosage may need to be reduced in patients with significant hepatic dysfunction when metoprolol elimination may be impaired.

Product licence number 0017/0092.

CO-BETALOC* SA

Presentation Yellow, biconvex, film coated tablets engraved $\frac{A}{MC}$

Each tablet contains metoprolol tartrate 200 mg embedded in a white tablet layer, from which release takes place slowly, and hydrochlorothiazide 25 mg, in a yellow layer, which is rapidly released.

Inactive ingredients: Aluminium silicate, paraffin special, ethyl cellulose, magnesium stearate, lactose, microcrystalline cellulose, maize starch, polyvinylpyrrolidone, riboflavin, sodium stearyl fumerate, hydroxypropylmethylcellulose, polyethylene glycol, iron oxide yellow, titanium dioxide.

Uses In the management of mild or moderate hypertension. Co-Betaloc SA may be suitable for use when satisfactory control of arterial blood pressure cannot be obtained with either a diuretic or a beta-adrenoreceptor blocking drug used alone.

Dosage and administration The dose will depend on patient response. Usually 1 tablet daily, taken whole and swallowed with water.

Elderly: There are no special dosage requirements in otherwise healthy elderly patients.

Significant hepatic dysfunction: A reduction in dosage may be necessary.

Contra-indications, warnings, etc

Contra-indications: AV block. Uncontrolled heart failure. Severe bradycardia. Sick sinus syndrome. Cardiogenic shock. Severe peripheral arterial disease. Known hypersensitivity to metoprolol or other β-blockers.

Severe kidney and liver failure. Therapy resistant hypokalaemia and hyponatraemia. Hypercalcaemia, symptomatic hyperuricaemia. Anuria. Known hypersensitivity to hydrochlorothiazide or other sulphonamide derivatives.

An anti-diuretic effect has been reported following concomitant treatment with diuretics and lithium. As with all products which contain diuretics, Co-Betaloc SA is contra-indicated during lithium therapy.

Warnings: Metoprolol may aggravate bradycardia, symptoms of peripheral arterial circulatory disorders and anaphylactic shock.

Abrupt interruption of Co-Betaloc SA is to be avoided. When possible, the drug should be withdrawn gradually over a period of 10 days using Co-Betaloc to help reduce the dose. During withdrawal from treatment patients should be kept under close surveillance, especially those with known ischaemic heart disease.

Co-Betaloc SA may be administered when heart failure has been controlled. Digitalisation and/or diuretic therapy should also be considered for patients with a history of heart failure, or patients known to have a poor cardiac reserve.

Although cardioselective beta-blockers may have less effect on lung function than non-selective beta-blockers, as with all beta-blockers these should be avoided in patients with reversible obstructive airways disease unless there are compelling clinical reasons for their use. When administration is necessary, use of a $beta_2$-bronchodilator (e.g. terbutaline) may be advisable in some patients.

In labile and insulin dependent diabetes, it may be necessary to adjust the hypoglycaemic therapy.

In patients with phaeochromocytoma, an alpha-blocker should be given concomitantly.

The bioavailability of metoprolol may be increased in the presence of liver cirrhosis.

The administration of adrenaline to patients undergoing beta-blockade can result in an increase in blood pressure and bradycardia although this is less likely to occur with β_1-selective drugs.

Metoprolol therapy must be reported to the anaesthetist prior to general anaesthesia. If it is desirable to withdraw metoprolol in patients who are to undergo anaesthesia the withdrawal should if possible be completed at least 48 hours before anaesthesia.

Co-Betaloc SA does not interfere with potassium balance. However, at higher doses of hydrochlorothiazide disturbances in the electrolyte and water balance may be experienced. Hyperuricaemia may occur or frank gout may be precipitated in certain patients receiving higher doses of thiazide therapy. Latent diabetes may become manifest during thiazide therapy.

Diuretics in higher doses may precipitate azotemia in patients with renal disease. Cumulative effects of hydrochlorothiazide may develop in patients with impaired renal function. If renal impairment becomes evident metoprolol/hydrochlorothiazide therapy should be discontinued.

Pregnancy: Co-Betaloc SA should not be used in pregnancy or nursing mothers unless the physician considers that the benefit outweighs the possible hazard to the foetus/infant. As with all beta-blockers metoprolol may cause side-effects e.g. bradycardia, hypoglycaemia in the foetus, and in the newborn and breastfed infant. Metoprolol has, however, been used in pregnancy associated hypertension under close supervision, after 20 weeks gestation. Although metoprolol crosses the placental barrier and is present in cord blood, no evidence of foetal abnormalities has been reported.

Hydrochlorothiazide can reduce the plasma volume as well as the uteroplacental blood circulation.

Lactation: The amount of metoprolol ingested via breast milk should not produce significant β-blocking effects in the neonate if the mother is treated with normal therapeutic doses.

As hydrochlorothiazide passes into breast milk, consideration should be given to withdrawal of Co-Betaloc SA, replacement by metoprolol in monotherapy or breast-feeding stopped.

Interactions: The effects of metoprolol and other anti-hypertensive drugs on blood pressure are usually additive, and care should be taken to avoid hypotension. However, combinations of antihypertensive drugs may often be used with benefit to improve control of hypertension.

Metoprolol can reduce myocardial contractility and impair intracardiac conduction. Care should be exercised when drugs with similar activity, e.g. antiarrhythmic agents, general anaesthetics, are given concurently. Like all other β-blockers, metoprolol should not be given in combination with verapamil since this may cause bradycardia, hypotension and asystole. Care should also be exercised when β-blockers are given in combination with sympathetic ganglion blocking agents, other β-blockers (i.e. eye drops) or MAO inhibitors. If combination treatment with clonidine is to be discontinued, metoprolol should be withdrawn several days before clonidine.

As β-blockers may affect the peripheral circulation, care should be exercised when drugs with similar activity e.g. ergotamine are given concurrently.

Metoprolol will antagonise the β_1-effects of sympathomimetic agents but should have little influence on the bronchodilator effects of β_2-agonists at normal therapeutic doses. Enzyme inducing agents (e.g. rifampicin) may reduce plasma concentrations of metoprolol, whereas enzyme inhibitors (e.g. cimetidine) may increse plasma concentrations. Metoprolol may impair the elimination of lignocaine.

Indomethacin may reduce the antihypertensive effect of β-blockers.

In general reported interactions have occurred with doses of hydrochlorothiazide higher than those used in this combination. Insulin requirements in diabetic patients may be altered and lithium renal clearance is reduced, increasing the risk of lithium toxicity. Responsiveness to tubocurarine may be increased and arterial responsiveness to noradrenaline may be decreased, but not enough to preclude effectiveness of the pressor agent for therapeutic use. Hypokalaemia may develop during concomitant use of steroids or ACTH, and may sensitize or exaggerate the response of the heart to toxic effects of digitalis.

Side-effects: Side-effects to metoprolol are usually mild and infrequent. The most common appear to be lassitude, GI disturbances (nausea, vomiting or abdominal pain) and disturbances of sleep pattern. In many cases these effects have been transient or have disappeared after a reduction in dosage.

Effects related to the CNS which have been reported occasionally are dizziness and headache and rarely paraesthesia, muscle cramps, depression and decreased mental alertness. There have also been isolated reports of personality disorders.

Cardiovascular effects which have been reported occasionally are bradycardia, postural hypotension and rarely, heart failure, palpitations, cardiac arrhythmias, Raynauds phenomenon, peripheral oedema and precordial pain. There have also been isolated reports of cardiac conduction abnormalities, and gangrene in patients with pre-existing severe peripheral circulatory disorders.

Common gastro-intestinal disturbances have been described above but rarely diarrhoea or constipation also occur and there have been isolated cases of dry mouth and abnormal liver function.

Skin rashes (urticaria, psoriasiform, dystrophic skin lesions) and positive anti-nuclear antibodies (not associated with SLE) occur rarely. Isolated cases of photosensitivity, increased sweating and alopecia have been reported. Respiratory effects include occasional reports of bronchospasm and isolated cases of rhinitis.

Isolated cases of weight gain, thrombocytopenia, disturbances of vision, conjunctivitis, tinnitus and dry or irritated eyes have also been reported.

The reported incidence of skin rashes and/or dry eyes is small and in most cases the symptoms have cleared when treatment was withdrawn. Discontinuation of the drug should be considered if any such reaction is not otherwise explicable.

Hydrochlorothiazide is generally well tolerated at the dose used (25 mg) in the combination. However the familiar side-effects of thiazide diuretics may be expected e.g. gastro-intestinal disturbances, metabolic and electrolyte changes, disturbances in sleep pattern, skin rashes and effects relating to the CNS.

Overdosage: Poisoning due to an overdose of metoprolol may lead to severe hypotension, sinus bradycardia, atrioventricular block, heart failure, cardiogenic shock, cardiac arrest, bronchospasm, impairment of consciousness, coma, nausea, vomiting, cyanosis, hypoglycaemia and, occasionally, hyperkalaemia. The first manifestations usually appear 20 minutes to 2 hours after drug ingestion.

The most prominent feature of poisoning due to hydrochlorothiazide is acute loss of fluid and electrolytes. The following symptoms may also be observed: dizziness, sedation/impairment of consciousness, hypotension and muscle cramps.

Treatment should include close monitoring of cardiovascular, respiratory and renal function, and blood glucose and electrolytes. Further absorption may be prevented by induction of vomiting, gastric lavage or administration of activated-charcoal if ingestion is recent. Cardiovascular complications should be treated symptomatically, which may require the use of sympathomimetic agents (e.g. noradrenaline, metaraminol), atropine or inotropic agents (e.g. dopamine, dobutamine). Temporary pacing may be required for AV block. Glucagon can reverse the effects of excessive β-blockade, given in a dose of 1–10 mg intravenously. Intravenous β_2-stimulants e.g. terbutaline may be required to relieve bronchospasm.

Intravenous volume and elctrolyte-replacement may be necessary.

Metoprolol cannot be effectively removed by haemodialysis.

Pharmaceutical precautions Store in a cool dry place.

Legal category POM.

Package quantities Calendar packs of 28 tablets.

Further information Metoprolol is well absorbed after oral administration, peak plasma concentrations occurring 1.5–2 hours after dosing. The bioavailability of a single dose is approximately 50%, increasing to approximately 70% during repeated administration. The bioavailability also increases if metoprolol is given with food.

Elimination is mainly by hepatic metabolism and the average elimination half-life is 3.5 hours (range 1 to 9 hours). Rates of metabolism vary between individuals, with poor metabolisers (approximately 10%) showing higher plasma concentrations and slower elimination than extensive metabolisers. Within individuals, however, plasma concentrations are stable and reproducible.

Because of variation in rates of metabolism, the dose of metoprolol should always be adjusted to the individual requirements of the patient. As the therapeutic response, adverse effects and relative cardioselectivity are related to plasma concentrations, poor metabolisers may require lower than normal doses. Dosage adjustment is not routinely required in the elderly or in patients with renal failure, but dosage may need to be reduced in patients with significant hepatic dysfunction when metoprolol elimination may be impaired.

Product licence number 0017/0202.

DIRYTHMIN-SA*

Presentation White, film-coated sustained release tablets (Durules), engraved $_{D}A_{R}$ on one side containing 150 mg disopyramide base as the phosphate.

Inactive ingredients: Paraffin, polyvinyl acetate, carboxypolymethylene, magnesium stearate, ethanol 95%, hydroxypropylmethyl-cellulose, polyethylene glycol 6000, titanium dioxide.

Uses Dirythmin-SA is a Class I antiarrhythmic drug, indicated for treatment of a wide range of supraventricular and ventricular arrhythmias including:

- Atrial or ventricular ectopic beats.
- Paroxysmal atrial or ventricular tachycardia.
- Arrhythmias associated with myocardial infarction.
- Wolff-Parkinson-White syndrome.
- Maintenance of sinus rhythm following electroconversion.

Dirythmin-SA can be used in both digitilised and non-digitalised patients.

Dosage and administration The dosage should be adjusted dependant on the patient response and tolerance. The normal adult dosage is 2 tablets 12 hourly

(600 mg daily). Dosage should not normally exceed 750 mg daily.

In patients with moderate renal insufficiency (creatinine clearance>40 ml/min) or hepatic insufficiency, dosage should be limited to 1 Dirythmin-SA tablet b.d. In patients with creatinine clearance<40 ml/min standard capsules are advised.

Dirythmin-SA tablets should be swallowed whole.

Patients treated with conventional disopyramide capsules q.i.d. can be transferred to the equivalent dosage of Dirythmin-SA e.g. 150 mg disopyramide q.i.d. is equivalent to 2 × 150 mg Dirythmin-SA tablets b.d.

Elderly: The renal function of the patient must be considered in relation to the dose as above.

Children: The safety and efficacy of Dirythmin-SA in children has not been established.

Contra-indications, warnings, etc

Contra-indications: Dirythmin is contra-indicated in patients with second or third degree AV block, if no pacemaker is present, cardiogenic shock and hypersensitivity to disopyramide phosphate. Patients with heart failure or who are susceptible to heart failure should be fully digitalised before Dirythmin therapy in order to ensure its mild negative inotropic effect does not contribute to any cardiac insufficiency.

Dirythmin-SA should not be administered to patients with hypotension.

Warnings and precautions: In view of the serious nature of many of the conditions being treated, it is suggested that Dirythmin injection should only be used when facilities exist for cardiac monitoring or defibrillation should the need arise.

Dirythmin should only be used with caution in patients with atrial flutter or atrial tachycardia with block, as conversion of partial AV block to a 1:1 response may occur.

Prior digitalisation is recommended in such patients.

Dirythmin may be given to patients with glaucoma if it appears that the potential benefits of therapy outweigh the risks of treatment. Careful monitoring and aggressive therapy of the glaucoma should be undertaken. Administration of Dirythmin to patients who have or may develop urinary retention is possible, but appropriate corrective methods (e.g. catheterisation or transurethral resection) should be taken. The potential benefits of Dirythmin should be weighed against the disadvantages of treatment in such patients.

Dirythmin possesses anticholinergic properties. Caution should be observed in patients with benign prostatic hypertrophy, myasthenia gravis and in patients receiving other anticholinergic drugs.

Dirythmin should be used with caution in the presence of digitalis intoxication.

Care should be taken when prescribing Dirythmin for patients with sick-sinus syndrome or bundle branch block. The effect of Dirythmin in these conditions is uncertain at present.

Hepatic impairment causes an increase in the plasma half-life of Dirythmin. Dosage should be reduced for such patients. If treatment is warranted, patients should be closely monitored.

Disopyramide is eliminated predominantly by glomerular filtration. The dose administered to patients with significant renal impairment may consequently require adjustment. Antiarrhythmic drugs may be ineffective in patients with hypokalaemia. Dirythmin should be used with caution in patients receiving concurrent therapy with diuretics which are likely to result in hypokalaemia. Significant potassium deficits should be corrected before initiating Dirythmin therapy.

Dirythmin should not be given with other negative inotropic drugs, including other Class 1 antiarrhythmic agents and/or beta receptor antagonists unless life-threatening arrhythmias demonstrably unresponsive to single-drug therapy are present. Patients receiving more than one antiarrhythmic agent must be carefully monitored.

Use in pregnancy and lactation: The safety of Dirythmin in pregnancy has not been established. Animal teratology and reproduction studies have demonstrated no adverse effects. The benefits of Dirythmin therapy must be weighed against the possible hazards to the mother and foetus. Dirythmin has been reported to stimulate contractions of the pregnant uterus. However, it is not known whether the use of Dirythmin during labour has any effect on either the foetus or the course of labour and delivery.

Whether Dirythmin is excreted in human milk is unknown. Animal studies have shown a higher concentration of metabolites in milk than in plasma. Therefore, if use of the drug is considered essential, an alternative method of infant feeding should be instituted.

Side-effects: Severe hypotension following Dirythmin administration has been observed primarily in patients with primary cardiomyopathy or inadequately compensated congestive heart failure. If hypotension develops, Dirythmin should be discontinued promptly (unless the hypotension is due to cardiac arrhythmia) and subsequently may be restarted at a lower dose without an initial loading dose. Such patients should be closely monitored.

If first degree heart block develops in a patient receiving Dirythmin the dosage should be reduced. If first degree AV block persists, unless it is controlled by a ventricular pacemaker, the risks of continuing treatment must be weighed against the benefits.

Development of second or third degree AV block or unifascicular, bifascicular or trifascicular block requires discontinuation of therapy, unless the ventricular rate is adequately controlled by a temporary or implanted ventricular pacemaker.

There have been reports of ventricular tachycardia, ventricular fibrillation, or torsade de pointes in patients receiving disopyramide. These have usually but not always, been associated with significant widening of the QRS complex or a prolonged Q-T interval. Dirythmin should therefore be discontinued if there is significant (greater than 25%) QRS widening or Q-T prolongation.

Treatment of overdosage: The stomach should be emptied by aspiration and lavage. Supportive or symptomatic treatment should be instigated.

Pharmaceutical precautions Store in a cool, dry place.

Legal category POM.

Package quantities Amber glass bottles of 100 tablets.

Further information Nil.

Product licence number 0017/0100.

EMLA* CREAM 5%

Presentation White cream. Each gram contains lignocaine base 25 mg and prilocaine base 25 mg in a eutectic mixture as an oil water emulsion containing carboxypolymethylene and sodium hydroxide.

Uses Local anaesthetic for topical use to produce anaesthesia of the skin.

For topical use on the genital mucosa to facilitate the removal of warts in adults.

Dosage and administration
Adults (including elderly) and children >1 year:

Surface	*Procedure*	*Application*
Skin (apply a thick layer of cream under an occlusive dressing)	Minor dermatological procedures e.g. needle insertion and surgical treatment of localised lesions	Approximately 2 g Emla applied for a minimum of 60 minutes, maximum 5 hours
	Dermal procedures on larger areas e.g. split skin grafting	Approximately 1.5–3 g/10 cm² Emla applied for a minimum of 2 hours, maximum 5 hours
Genital mucosa (Adults) (no occlusive dressing required)	Surgical treatment of localised lesions	Apply up to 10 g Emla for 5–10 minutes. Commence procedure immediately thereafter

Analgesic efficacy may decline if the skin application time is more than 5 hours. Procedures on intact skin should begin soon after the occlusive dressing is removed.

On the genital mucosa analgesic efficacy declines after 10–15 minutes and therefore the procedure should be commenced immediately.

Not recommended in infants.

Contra-indications, warnings, etc
Contra-indications: Known hypersensitivity to anaesthetics of the amide type.

Precautions: Until further clinical experience is available, Emla Cream should not be applied to wounds, mucous membranes or in areas of atopic dermatitis.

Emla Cream should not be applied to genital mucosa in children.

Emla causes corneal irritation and should not be applied to or near the eyes. Emla, like other local anaesthetics may be ototoxic and should not be instilled in the middle ear nor should it be used for procedures which might allow penetration into the middle ear.

Although the systemic availability of prilocaine by percutaneous absorption of Emla is low, caution should be exercised in patients with anaemia, congenital or acquired methaemoglobinaemia or patients on concomitant therapy known to produce such conditions.

Pregnancy and lactation: Lidocaine and prilocaine cross the placental barrier. However, both drugs have been in widespread clinical use for many years and a large number of women of childbearing age have been exposed to them. No specific effects on the reproductive process have been reported.

Lidocaine and prilocaine are excreted in breast milk in small amounts.

Adverse events: Transient paleness, redness and oedema have been reported.

Prilocaine has been known to cause methaemoglobinaemia when given parenterally.

In rare cases local anaesthetics have been associated with allergic reactions including anaphylactic shock.

Interactions: Methaemoglobinaemia may be accentuated in patients already taking drugs known to induce the condition, e.g. sulphonamides.

The risk of additional systemic toxicity should be considered when large doses of Emla are applied to patients already using other local anaesthetics or structurally related drugs e.g. tocainide.

Overdosage: Overdosage with Emla is unlikely but signs of systemic toxicity will be similar in nature to those observed after administration of other local anaesthetics.

Pharmaceutical precautions Store at room temperature.

Legal category POM.

Package quantities 'Pre-medication pack' containing 10 × 5 g tubes Emla and 25 occlusive dressings. 5 g tube Emla without dressings. 30 g tube Emla.

Further information Nil.

Product licence number 0017/0213.

FOSCAVIR* ▼

Presentation Solution for intravenoius infusion containing foscarnet 24 mg/ml.

1 ml contains 24 mg (80 μmol) foscarnet trisodium hexahydrate for injection, hydrochloric acid for injection q.s. and water for injection q.s. The solution is sterile, clear and isotonic with a pH of 7.4.

Uses Therapeutic conditions: Foscavir is indicated for the treatment of cytomegalovirus (CMV) retinitis in patients with AIDS in whom ganciclovir is contra-indicated or inappropriate.

Treatment with Foscavir has produced stabilization of retinal lesions in approximately 80% of cases treated. However, as CMV is usually a latent infection, relapses are likely in the majority of patients with persistent immunodeficiency once treatment is discontinued. In such cases, further courses of Foscavir may be given.

Foscavir is not recommended for the treatment of CMV infections other than retinitis, or for use in non-AIDS patients. Foscavir is not recommended for use in patients undergoing haemodialysis as dosage guidelines have not been established.

Dosage and administration
Method of administration: Foscavir must be administered intravenously either by a central venous line, or after dilution, by peripheral vein. Dilution with dextrose 5% to a concentration of 12 mg/ml or less is recommended for administration by peripheral vein. No other dilution fluids may be used, and the dilution should be performed under aseptic conditions immediately prior to administration.

Adults: Foscavir treatment is started with an intravenous infusion of 20 mg/kg body weight over a period of 30 minutes, followed by a continuous intravenous infusion at a rate determined by renal function as measured by serum creatinine (see below).

S-Creatinine	*Foscavir dose mg/kg/24 hrs.*
<110	200
111–130	199–129
131–150	129–115
151–170	115–100
171–190	100–86
191–210	86–72
211–230	72–43
231–250	43–21
>250	Not recommmended

The recommended dose rates are intended to provide a plasma foscarnet concentration of 150 mg/l (500 μmol/l): the concentration of foscarnet producing 50% inhibition of CMV isolates (ID_{50}) is 80 mg/l (270 μmol/l).

A treatment period of 2–3 weeks is recommended, depending on the clinical response.

There is some evidence that renal toxicity can be minimised by adequate hydration of the patient e.g. intravenous saline 2.5 litres/day.

Elderly: As for adults.

Children: There is no experience of the use of Foscavir in children.

Renal or hepatic insufficiency: The dose rate should be reduced in patients with renal insufficiency, according to the serum creatinine level, as described in the table above. Dose adjustment is not required in patients with hepatic insufficiency.

Contra-indications, warnings, etc
Contra-indications: Hypersensitivity to Foscavir, pregnancy and lactation.

Precautions and warnings: Serum creatinine should be measured every second day in all patients during treatment and all patients should be adequately hydrated. Impairment of renal function, sometimes associated with flank pain, has been observed in approximately 45% of patients treated with Foscavir. Some patients have required haemodialysis for acute renal failure. The maximum increase in serum creatinine was usually reached a few days after end of treatment. Serum creatinine usually normalised within 8–10 weeks of discontinuing treatment in the patients studied, suggesting that the renal impairment can be of a reversible nature. Extreme caution is advised when Foscavir is used in combination with other potentially nephrotoxic drugs such as intravenous pentamidine because of the risk of additive toxicity. Care should also be taken when administering Foscavir to patients with pre-existing renal impairment.

Serum calcium should be measured every second day during administration of Foscavir. Increases and decreases in serum calcium have been observed. Symptomatic hypocalcaemia (paraesthesia, cramp, positive Trousseau's sign) necessitating calcium administration has occurred in some patients. Particular caution is advised in patients with decreased calcium levels before treatment, and those receiving other drugs known to influence serum calcium levels such as intravenous pentamidine.

Hypoglycaemia has been observed rarely although the relationship to Foscavir is uncertain.

Epileptic seizures have occurred during treatment with Foscavir. In most cases there were other possible explanations, but an association with Foscavir, hypocalcaemia or hypoglycaemia cannot be excluded.

Decreases in haemoglobin concentration have been observed during treatment. There have been no significant changes in white blood cell or platelet counts.

Administration of undiluted Foscavir 24 mg/ml solution has been associated with thrombophlebitis when given by peripheral vein.

Headache, nausea/vomiting, fatigue and rash can occur during treatment.

Use during pregnancy and lactation: Foscavir is contraindicated in pregnancy. Breast feeding should be discontinued before starting Foscavir treatment.

Interactions: Foscavir can impair renal function and additive toxicity may occur when used in combination with other nephrotoxic drugs.

Foscavir can cause hypocalcaemia, particularly in combination with intravenous pentamidine.

The elimination of foscarnet may be impaired by drugs which inhibit renal tubular secretion.

There is no evidence of an interaction or increased myelotoxicity when Foscavir is used in combination with Zidovudine (AZT).

Overdose: Inadvertent administration of 12 g Foscavir during a 30 minute infusion in one patient was associated with paraesthesia. In another, administration of 10 g Foscavir during a 2 hour infusion was not associated with any symptoms. Epileptic seizures coinciding with high plasma concentrations of foscarnet have been reported in one patient.

Haemodialysis increases foscarnet elimination and may be of benefit in severe overdosage.

Special warnings: Use on one patient during one treatment only. Discard unused contents.

Effects on ability to drive and use machines: None known. Foscarnet has no sedative effect.

Pharmaceutical precautions
Incompatibilities: Foscavir may be diluted with dextrose 5% for infusion into a peripheral vein. No other drug or infusion fluid should be mixed with Foscavir, either in the infusion vessel or the infusion line.

Special precautions for storage: Store between 8°C and 25°C. Do not refrigerate. Foscavir contains no preservative and once the sterility seal of a bottle has been broken the solution should be used within 24 hours. Use immediately following dilution.

Package quantities: 250 ml and 500 ml glass bottles.

Further information Nil.

Product licence number 0017/0248

HEMINEVRIN* 0.8% INFUSION

Presentation Colourless aqueous solution containing Chlormethiazole Edisylate 8 mg/ml BP.

Inactive ingredients: Dextrose anhydrous, sodium hydroxide.

Uses Heminevrin is a short acting hypnotic and sedative with anticonvulsant effects used for the treatment of: Pre-eclamptic toxaemia, eclampsia, status epilepticus, acute alcohol withdrawal symptoms where oral administration is not practicable; as a sedative during regional anaesthesia.

Dosage and administration When Heminevrin is given by i.v. infusion, the dosage should always be controlled by the desired effect and the patient's response. Exact recommendations on dosage cannot be given because of individual patient variation and the presence or absence of other CNS depressant drugs such as diazepam, paraldehyde or alcohol. The doses given below therefore are guides only and due account must be taken of the patient's age (i.e. children and the very elderly), the general condition and any previous medication.

In general, the infusion should be given as a loading dose to produce the required effect, followed by a maintenance dose. As is the case with intravenous anaesthetics, Heminevrin's brief action is due to redistribution of the drug and not to rapid elimination. Thus stopping the drug, will allow rapid reversal of its sedative effect initially but after large and prolonged dosage, recovery may be considerably delayed. The patient should be closely and constantly observed.

Pre-eclamptic toxaemia: Heminevrin is used to sedate the patient and raise the threshold for eclamptic convulsions.

It is indicated in moderate or severe pre-eclamptic toxaemia under the following circumstances: rapid progression of the disease, symptoms and signs associated with impending eclampsia, when labour is to be induced, during labour and post-partum (a) for up to 12 hours in patients with adequate urine output or (b) until recovery diuresis in patients with poor urinary output.

During labour most patients will require an average of 0.5 to 0.75 ml/min of Heminevrin 0.8%. As the majority of patients are delivered within 24 hours, prolonged infusion is not necessary. Heminevrin has no analgesic properties and pain relief must be given as necessary. After delivery the intravenous infusion is maintained at 0.5 ml/min for 12 hours. Thereafter oral therapy is continued.

Eclampsia: Heminevrin is used to control eclamptic fits or to prevent their recurrence. It is used in conjunction with antihypertensive drugs. If seizures are occurring, Heminevrin 0.8% should be started at an infusion rate of 5–10 ml/min until the fits stop. Once this is achieved the infusion rate is decreased to 0.5–1 ml/min, though this may be varied to suit the individual patient, who should be well sedated but communicative.

If the patient is not having a fit at the start of treatment then Heminevrin is given at 3–5 ml/min until deep sedation occurs. Once the desired level of sedation is achieved this is maintained with an infusion rate of 0..5 to 1.0 ml/min, though this may be varied to suit the individual patient.

The patient should be lying on one side and adequate oxygenation assured. Loss of the airway, pulmonary aspiration of gastric contents, ventilatory failure and circulatory collapse may occur unless the patient is constantly monitored by experienced staff with oxygen and resuscitation equipment available.

Status epilepticus: Adults: 5–15 ml/min should be infused intravenously up to a total of 40–100 ml of Heminevrin 0.8%. This will usually stop convulsions. Thereafter the infusion rate will depend on the patient's response but in most cases 0/.5–1 ml/min will be required. The patient should be nursed in the lateral position, to avoid airway obstruction, and turned every 2 hours. The sedation must be maintained until the epileptic convulsions do not recur if the infusion is slowed or stopped. If a prolonged infusion is necessary, fluid and electrolyte balance must be checked.

Children: An initial infusion rate of 0.01 ml/kg/min (0.08 mg/kg/min). If seizures continue the dose is increased every 2 to 4 hours until seizures are abolished or drowsiness occurs. When seizures have ceased for 2 days the rate of infusion may be gradually reduced every 4 to 6 hours. If seizures recur the dose should be increased to the previous level at which they were controlled.

Acute alcohol withdrawal symptoms; including delirium tremens: Most patients can be treated with oral Heminevrin but in severe cases an i.v. infusion will give rapid control. The dosing principles mentioned previously, that is, a loading dose for a short period of time followed by maintenance infusion should be used. The initial drip rate should be set in the range of 3 to 7.5 ml/min until shallow sleep is induced from which the patient can easily be awakened. Thereafter, the drip rate should be reduced to a maintenance level, usually 0.5 to 1.0 ml/min, to achieve the lowest possible rate to maintain shallow sleep and adequate spontaneous breathing.

The patients should be nursed on their side to prevent airway obstruction and turned every 2 hours.

For those patients who urgently require deep sedation, an alternative is to give intravenously 40–100 ml of the 0.8% solution over a period of 3–5 minutes. Such treatment should only be given under direct medical supervision. Thereafter maintenance therapy can be established as indicated above.

Because there is a risk of producing unconsciousness with too high a rate of infusion, special attention should be paid to 'Precautions' regarding intravenous administration.

Intravenous administration is usually carried out over a period of 6 to 12 hours during which time usually 500 to 1000 ml of the 0.8% infusion is given. The level of consciousness and the effect of therapy on symptoms should be checked by interrupting the drip flow at intervals. The level of consciousness should lighten rapidly on stopping the drip flow but the longer the administration lasts, the longer the recovery will take. It is desirable to limit the period of intravenous use and to transfer the patient to oral therapy as soon as possible. During prolonged intravenous administation careful attention should be paid to fluid balance and nutrition.

Sedative during regional anaesthesia: Pre-medication with atropine or similar antisialogogue will help to prevent nasal congestion and upper airway mucus secretion that otherwise may occur with chlormethiazole. As judged by unresponsiveness to sound and loss of eyelash reflex, unconsciousness should be induced by a fast running intravenous infusion (approx. 25 ml/min) for 1–2 minutes. Thereafter, maintenance must be judged on the patient's reaction but the dose required is of the order of 1–4 ml/min.

If being used as an intravenous sedative in association with regional block anaesthesia e.g. spinal or epidural, the block must be fully effective before surgery begins. Chlormethiazole has no analgesic properties and the patient will respond to painful stimuli by moving.

If the regional block does not fully relieve the pain of operation it is better to give an i.v. opioid analgesic or convert to a volatile inhalation anaesthetic rather than try to increase the dosage of chlormethiazole.

At the end of an operation, stopping the chlormethiazole allows the patient to awaken usually in 1–5 minutes.

Elderly: Caution is advised as there may be delayed elimination of chlormethiazole.

Contra-indications, warnings, etc

Contra-indications: Known sensitivity to chlormethiazole. Acute pulmonary insufficiency.

Precautions and warnings: Heminevrin should be used cautiously in patients with chronic pulmonary insufficiency because there is a risk of respiratory depression.

Heminevrin may potentiate or be potentiated by centrally acting depressant drugs, including alcohol and benzodiazepines. Fatal cardiorespiratory collapse has been reported when chlormethiazole was combined with other CNS depressant drugs. When used concomitantly, dosage shold be appropriately reduced.

The patient should be kept under close and constant observation by a nurse during the period of continuous infusion. With too high a rate of infusion the sleep induced with Heminevrin can pass unnoticed into deep unconsciousness with the consequent risk of mechanical airway obstruction. With overdosage there is always the possibility of causing centrally induced respiratory depression and circulatory collapse.

Because of the possible danger of mechanical airway obstruction occurring in deep sedation during Heminevrin therapy, the patient's airway may be maintained where necessary by the use of an oral airway tube. In addition, facilities for intubation and resuscitation equipment should always be close at hand.

Hypoxia resulting from, for example, respiratory insufficiency, can manifest itself as an acute confusional state. Recognition and specific treatment of the cause is essential in such patients and other sedative/hypnotics should be avoided.

Moderate liver disorders associated with alcoholism do not preclude the use of chlormethiazole, but delayed elimination of the drug may require reduced dosage. Great caution should be observed in patients with gross liver damage and decreased liver function, particularly as sedation can mask the onset of liver coma.

Caution should be observed in patients with chronic renal disease.

A combination of chlormethiazole and diazoxide should be avoided as an adverse neonatal reaction suspected to be due to the maternal administration of this combination has been reported.

There is evidence to indicate that the metabolism of chlormethiazole is inhibited by cimetidine, thus the co-administration of these drugs may lead to increased blood/plasma levels of chlormethiazole.

Nasopharyngeal/bronchial secretions may be increased at a time when the heavily sedated patient may be unable to cough or maintain the airway.

There has been a report of thrombophlebitis, fever and headache in young children during prolonged Heminevrin infusion. This may have been due to interaction with plastic i.v. infusion sets and silastic i.v. cannulae. For administration in small children a motor driven glass syringe should be used in preference to a drip set. A teflon intravenous cannula should be used which can be connected to the syringe by a polythene extension tube. If an infusion set is used it should be changed at least every 24 hours.

As Heminevrin is sorbed by PVC giving sets, there may be some loss in concentration before the drug reaches the patient. Dosage must therefore be adjusted to the patient's response and not given on a fixed milligram basis.

When i.v. Heminevrin is given for longer than 24 hours, there is a possibility of electrolyte imbalance due to the water load involved with the glucose vehicle. Electrolytes such as Na, K, Ca and Cl can be added to the infusion bottle to produce physiological concentrations. They will not affect the stability of chlormethiazole over a 24 hour period. Other drugs however, must not be added.

Pregnancy and lactation: Do not use in pregnancy, especially during the first trimester, unless there are compelling reasons. There is no evidence of safety in human pregnancy nor is there evidence from animal studies that it is entirely free from hazard.

Chlormethiazole is excreted into breast milk. The effects of even small quantities of sedative/hypnotic and anticonvulsant drugs on the infant brain is not established.

Adverse effects: The most common side-effect appears to be a tingling sensation in the nose and sneezing occurring immediately after the start of the intravenous infusion. Conjunctival irritation has also been noted in some cases. Occasionally these symptoms may be severe and may be associated with severe headache. In rare cases anaphylactic reactions have occurred.

Intravenous administration of Heminevrin solution may be followed by moderate tachycardia and a slight but temporary decrease in blood pressure, which is less pronounced the slower the infusion is given. Rapid infusion may cause apnoea and hypotension. Care is needed in patients in whom these events may cause cerebral or cardiac complications e.g. elderly. Thrombophlebitis may occur at the site of injection with intravenous infusion. Neither heparin nor cortisone has been shown to be helpful in preventing such reactions.

Overdosage: Overdosage can produce unconsciousness with deep coma accompanied by respiratory and cardiovascular depression similar to that seen with barbiturate overdosage. Treatment consists of securing the airway, giving oxygen (with assisted or controlled ventilation if necessary) and supporting the circulation.

Legal category POM.

Pharmaceutical Precautions Store between 5°C–8°C.

Package quantities Bottles of 500 ml.

Further information Nil.

Product licence number 0017/5007R.

HEMINEVRIN* CAPSULES
HEMINEVRIN* SYRUP

Presentation *Capsules:* Greyish-brown gelatine capsules containing chlormethiazole (base) 192 mg.

Inactive ingredients: Miglyol 812.

Syrup: Clear, colourless, aqueous solution containing chlormethiazole edisylate 50 mg/ml.

Inactive ingredients: Ethanol, sorbital 70%, cineol, methanol, sodium hydroxide.

Uses Neuropharmacological studies in animals show that Heminevrin possesses sedative/hypnotic and anticonvulsant properties. Whilst the mode of action is uncertain, the anticonvulsant effect may involve direct or indirect actions on GABA-systems in the CNS. The sedative/hypnotic properties involve actions on both catecholaminergic and gabaergic systems.

Indications: Heminevrin is indicated in the management of restlessness and agitation in the elderly, in the short term treatment of severe insomnia in the elderly and in the control of symptoms arising from acute withdrawal from alcohol where close hospital supervision is also provided.

Dosage and administration Doses of capsules and syrup are not strictly equivalent: one capsule contains 192 mg chlormethiazole base; 5 ml of syrup contains the equivalent of 157 mg base.

Management of restlessness and agitation in the elderly: One capsule or 5 ml syrup three times daily.

Management of restlessness and agitation in the elderly: One capsule or 5 ml syrup three times daily.

Severe insomnia in the elderly: 1–2 capsules or 5–10 ml of the syrup before going to bed. The lower dose should be tried first. As with all psychotropic drugs, treatment should be kept to a minimum, reviewed regularly and discontinued as sooon as possible.

Alcohol withdrawal states: Heminevrin is not a specific 'cure' for alcoholism. Alcohol withdrawal should be treated in hospital or, in exceptional circumstances, on an outpatient basis by specialist units when the daily dosage of Heminevrin must be monitored closely by community health staff. The dosage should be adjusted to patient response. The patient should be sedated but rousable. A suggested regimen is:

Initial dose: 2 to 4 capsules, if necessary repeated after some hours.

Day 1, first 24 hours: 9 to 12 capsules, divided into 3 or 4 doses.

Day 2: 6 to 8 capsules, divided into 3 or 4 doses.

Day 3: 4 to 6 capsules, divided into 3 or 4 doses.

Days 4 to 6: A gradual reduction in dosage until final dose.

Administration for more than nine (9) days is not recommended. 5 ml of Heminevrin syrup can be substituted for each capsule administered, if desired.

Heminevrin is not recommended for use in children.

Contra-indications, warnings, etc
Contra-indications: Known sensitivity to chlormethiazole. Acute pulmonary insufficiency.

Precautions: Heminevrin should be used cautiously in patients with chronic pulmonary insufficiency. Heminevrin may potentiate or be potentiated by centrally acting depressant drugs including alcohol and benzodiazepines. Fatal cardiorespiratory collapse has been reported when chlormethiazole was combined with other CNS depressant drugs. When used concomitantly dosage should be appropriately reduced.

Hypoxia, resulting from, for example, cardiac and/or respiratory insufficiency, can manifest itself as an acute confusional state. Recognition and specific treatment of the cause is essential in such patients and in such cases sedative/hypnotics should be avoided.

Moderate liver disorders associated with alcoholism do not preclude the use of chlormethiazole, though an associated increase in systemic availability or oral doses and delayed elimination of the drug may require reduced dosage. Great caution should be observed in patients with gross liver damage and decreased liver function, particularly as sedation can mask the onset of liver coma.

Caution should be observed in patients with chronic renal disease.

Caution must be exercised in prescribing for individuals known to be addiction prone or for those whose histories suggest they may increase the dose on their own initiative since chlormethiazole is not free from the risk of producing psychological and/or physical dependence. After prolonged administrration of high doses, physical dependence has been reported with withdrawal symptoms such as convulsions, tremors, and organic psychosis. These reports have mainly been associated with indiscriminate prescribing to outpatient alcoholics and Heminevrin should not be prescribed to patients who continue to abuse alcohol.

As with all centrally acting depressant drugs, the driving of vehicles and the operating of machinery are to be avoided when under treatment.

A combination of chlormethiazole and diazoxide should be avoided as an adverse neonatal reaction suspected to be due to the maternal administration of this combination has been reported.

The combination of propranolol and chlormethiazole produced profound bradycardia in one patient possibly due to increased bioavailability of propranolol.

There is evidence to indicate that the metabolism of chlormethiazole is inhibited by cimetidine, thus the co-administration of these drugs may lead to increased blood/plasma levels of chlormethiazole.

Elderly: Caution is advised as there may be increased bioavailability and delayed elimination of chlormethiazole.

Children: Oral Heminevrin is not recommended for use in children.

Pregnancy: Do not use in pregnancy especially during the first and last trimesters, unless there are compelling reasons. There is no evidence of safety in human pregnancy, nor is there evidence from animal studies that it is entirely free from hazard.

Lactation: Chlormethiazole is excreted into the breast milk. The effect of even small quantities of sedative/hypnotic and anticonvulsant drugs on the infant brain is not established.

Chlormethiazole should only be used in nursing mothers where the physician considers that the benefit outweighs the possible hazard to the infant.

Alcoholism: Alcohol combined with chlormethiazole particularly in alcoholics with cirrhosis can lead to fatal respiratory depression even with short term use. It should not therefore be prescribed for alcoholics who continue to drink alcoholic beverages.

Adverse effects: The most common side-effect is nasal congestion and irritation, which may occur 15 to 20 minutes after drug ingestion. Conjunctival irritation has also been noted in some cases and, occasionally, these symptoms may be severe and may be associated with severe headache. Gastrointestinal disturbances have been reported.

In rare cases anaphylactic reactions have occurred.

When Heminevrin has been given at higher than recommended doses for other than recommended indications over prolonged periods of time, physical dependence, tolerance and withdrawal reactions have been reported.

Great caution is required in prescribing Heminevrin for patients with a history of chronic alcoholism, drug abuse or marked personality disorder.

When used as a night-time hypnotic, hangover effects in the elderly are uncommon due to the short half-life but may occur.

Excessive sedation may occur, especially with higher doses or when given to the elderly for daytime sedation. Paradoxical excitement or confusion may occur rarely.

Overdose: The main symptoms to be expected with overdose of Heminevrin are: coma, respiratory depression, hypotension and hypothermia.

Hypothermia is thought to be due to a direct central effect as well as a result of lying unconscious for several hours. In addition, patients have increased secretion in the upper airways, which in one series was associated with a high incidence of pneumonia. The effects of overdosage are not usually severe in patients with no evidence of alcoholic liver disease, but they may be exacerbated when chlormethiazole is taken in combination with alcohol and/or CNS depressant drugs, particularly those that are metabolised by the liver. There is no specific antidote to chlormethiazole. Treatment of overdosage should therefore be carried out on a symptomatic basis, applying similar principles to those used in the treatment of barbiturate overdosage.

Further information Heminevrin has a short half life and therefore a low incidence of daytime sedation when prescribed as an hypnotic.

In the elderly, the safety and efficacy of Heminevrin has been established in controlled studies of up to three months duration. However, as with all psychotropic drugs, treatment should be kept to a minimum, reviewed regularly and discontinued as soon as possible.

Pharmaceutical precautions Heminevrin Syrup should be stored in a cool place.

Legal category POM.

Package quantities
Capsules: Bottles of 60.

Syrup: Bottles of 300 ml.

Product licence numbers
Capsules 0017/5009R
Syrup 0017/0063R

HEWLETTS* CREAM

Presentation White scented cream containing zinc oxide, 80 mg/g, hydrous wool fat 40 mg/g, oleic acid, arachis oil, soft white paraffin, oil of rose.

Uses Topical ointment for nursing hygiene and care of skin and chapped and sore hands.

Dosage and administration Applied as required.

Contra-indications, warnings, etc
Contra-indication: Not to be administered to large areas of broken skin.

Warnings: Use sparingly and if healing does not occur within a few days a physician should be consulted.

Pharmaceutical precautions Store at room temperature.

Legal category GSL.

Package quantities 35 g tubes. 400 g jars.

Further information Nil.

Product licence number 0017/5010R.

IMDUR*

Presentation Yellow oval biconvex film coated tablet, scored both sides and coded A/ID. Each tablet contains 60 mg isosorbide mononitrate in a sustained release formulation based on Durules*.

Uses Prophylactic treatment of angina pectoris.

Dosage and administration
Adults: One tablet once daily given in the morning. The dose may be increased to two tablets daily, both tablets given in the morning. If headache occurs the dose may initially be reduced to half a tablet daily.

Imdur tablets should not be chewed or crushed and should be swallowed with half a glass of fluid.

Children: The safety and efficacy of Imdur in children has not been established.

Elderly: No evidence of a need for routine dosage adjustment in the elderly has been found, but special care may be needed in those with increased susceptibility to hypotension or marked hepatic or renal insufficiency.

Contra-indications, warnings, etc Severe cerebrovascular insufficiency or hypotension are relative contra-indications to the use of Imdur.

Precautions: Imdur is not indicated for relief of acute angina attacks; in the event of an acute attack, sublingual or buccal glyceryl trinitrate tablets should be used. The safety and efficacy of Imdur during pregnancy or lactation has not been established.

Side-effects: Headache may occur when treatment is initiated but usually disappears after 1–2 weeks of treatment. Hypotension with symptoms such as dizziness and nausea has occasionally been reported. These symptoms generally disappear during long term treatment.

Overdose: Treatment should be symptomatic. The main symptom is likely to be hypotension.

Pharmaceutical precautions Nil.

Legal category POM.

Package quantities Amber glass bottles of 100 tablets. Calendar packs of 28 tablets.

Further information Isosorbide mononitrate is an active metabolite of isosorbide dinitrate and exerts qualitatively similar effects. Isosorbide mononitrate is completely absorbed and not metabolised during the first passage through the liver. This reduces the fluctuations in plasma levels and leads to predictable and reliable clinical effects.

Administration of Imdur results in a controlled release of active substance leading to reduced peak plasma levels. Compared to ordinary tablets the absorption phase is prolonged and the duration of effect is extended.

With Imdur 60 mg or 120 mg once daily no development of tolerance with respect to antianginal effects has been detected.

Product licence number 0017/0226.

JECTOFER*

Presentation Dark brown liquid for intramuscular injection; Iron Sorbitol Citric Acid Complex BP (50 mg elemental iron per ml). Jectofer also contains sodium chloride.

Uses For the treatment of iron-deficiency anaemia and the rapid replenishment of iron stores.

Dosage and administration The recommended single dose of Jectofer is 1.5 mg per kg body weight by intramuscular injection to a maximum of 100 mg per injection. A series of daily injections of this single dose should be given to restore haemoglobin levels to normal and replenish iron stores based on the following table.

Hb gm/100 ml	5.0	6.0	7.0	8.0	9.0	10.0	11.0
Hb%	33	40	46	53	60	66	73
No. of injections	24	22	20	17	14	12	10

In elderly or debilitated patients who have a low tolerance threshold to intramuscular iron the injections should be given on alternate days. Not recommended in children under 3 kg (7 lb) body weight.

Elderly: Dosage as for adults.

Contra-indications, warnings, etc
Contra-indications: Severe liver damage, acute kidney infection, untreated urinary tract infection.

Side-effects: A few cases have been reported of serious reactions of a cardiovascular type with cardiac arrhythmia.

Precautions and warnings: Jectofer should not be used to treat anaemias other than iron deficiency anaemia. Care should be taken when treating patients with iron-shortage diseases or haemoglobinopathies. The importance of using the correct recommended dose in relation to body weight is emphasised, especially in patients who are already markedly underweight. Jectofer should not be given intravenously. Oral iron should be discontinued 24 hours before Jectofer is administered.

Pharmaceutical precautions Store at room temperature, do not refrigerate.

Legal category POM.

Package quantities 10 × 2 ml ampoules for intramuscular use.

Further information Nil.

Product licence number 0017/5011R.

KINIDIN DURULES*

Presentation Film-coated white oval tablets, each containing 250 mg quinidine bisulphate (equivalent to 200 mg Quinidine Sulphate BP) in a sustained action form.

Inactive ingredients: Hydroxypropyl methylcellulose, polyethylene glycol, paraffin special, polyvinyl chloride, polyvinyl acetate, magnesium stearate, colour E171.

Uses Maintenance of sinus rhythm following cardioversion of atrial fibrillation. Suppression of supraventricular and ventricular tachyarrhythmias.

Dosage and administration An initial test dose of one tablet should be given to detect hypersensitivity. Dosage is adjusted according to individual patient requirements.

The usual dose is 2 to 5 tablets morning and evening. Tablets should be swallowed whole with water.

Contra-indications, warnings, etc
Contra-indications: Kinidin Durules are contra-indicated in patients with known hypersensitivity to quinidine, a history of quinidine induced thrombocytopenia or complete heart block.

Quinidine should be used with extreme caution in patients with incomplete atrio-ventricular block uncompensated cardiac failure, digitalis toxicity, myocarditis, severe myocardial damage, or myasthenia gravis.

Precautions: Hypokalaemia should be corrected prior to treatment with Kinidin.

Use in pregnancy and lactation: The use of Kinidin Durules is contra-indicated in pregnancy.

Quinidine is excreted in breast milk but is unlikely to cause effects at therapeutic doses.

Drug interactions: In digitalised patients quinidine may increase the concentration of digitalis in plasma by up to 100%.

Quinidine may enhance the effects of antihypertensive agents and vasodilators, oral anticoagulants, and non-depolarising skeletal muscle relaxants.

Drugs with enzyme-inducing effects may enhance the metabolism of quinidine, and thus reduce its effects.

Cimetidine decreases the clearance of quinidine thus increasing the plasma levels.

Side-effects: Quinidine may cause gastro-intestinal irritation with nausea, vomiting and diarrhoea.

Signs of cinchonism with tinnitus, blurred vision, headache and dizziness may occur but are usually associated with overdosage.

Hypersensitivity reactions are rare. Symptoms include urticaria, fever, and thrombocytopenia. Granulomatous hepatitis with raised liver enzymes, reversible on stopping therapy has also been reported.

Heart block and serious disturbances of rhythm such as extrasystoles, venticular tachycardia and ventricular fibrillation can occur. Occasional cases of photosensitivity have been reported.

Overdosage: Poisoning due to an overdose of Kinidin Durules may lead to widening of the QRS complex and prolongation of the QT interval, atrioventricular block, sinoatrial block or arrest, asystole, paroxysmal ventricular tachycardia, flutter or fibrillation, myocardial depression, severe hypotension and cardiac arrest. Cinchonism, nausea, vomiting, drowsiness and sometimes convulsions also occur. Metabolic acidosis and hypokalaemia may complicate severe poisoning.

Treatment should include close monitoring of cardiovascular, respiratory and renal function, electrolytes and continuous ECG monitoring. Further absorption may be prevented by induction of vomiting or gastric lavage, or administration of activated charcoal if ingestion is recent. Cardiovascular complications should be treated symptomatically, which may require the use of sympathomimetic agents (e.g. noradrenaline, metaraminol) or inotropic agents (e.g. dopamine, dobutamine). Temporary pacing may be required for AV block. Glucagon may be used to treat hypotension and intravenous sodium bicarbonate to correct acidosis and intravenous diazepam for convulsions.

Quinidine and its metabolites cannot be removed effectively by peritoneal or haemodialysis or charcoal column haemoperfusion, but repeated oral administration of activated charcoal may enhance elimination. Forced acid diuresis is not recommended.

As Kinidin Durules is a sustained release preparation, treatment of overdosage may be required for an extended period.

Pharmaceutical precautions Store in a cool dry place.

Legal category POM.

Package quantities Securitainers of 100 and 250.

Further information The therapeutic plasma concentration is 2 to 4 microgram per ml (6 to 12 micromoles per litre) when determined using method of Cramer and Isaksson, Scand. *J. Clin. Lab. Invest*, 1963, **15**, 553.

Product licence number 0017/5015R.

LIGNOSTAB*, LIGNOSTAB A

Presentation Lignostab is a sterile clear aqueous solution of Lignocaine Hydrochloride 2%.

Lignostab A is a sterile clear aqueous solution of Lignocaine Hydrochloride 2% with Adrenaline 1:80,000.

All are supplied in glass cartridges designed for use with dental-type syringes. Each cartridge contains 2.0 ml of solution.

Inactive ingredients: Lignostab solutions all contain sodium chloride. Lignostab A also contains disodium edetate and sodium metabisulphite.

Uses Local anaesthetic solution for use mainly in dental procedures.

Lignostab A contains adrenaline. The effect of this vasoconstrictor is to prolong the local anaesthesia by delaying the diffusion of the anaesthetic into the surrounding tissues.

Dosage and administration The dosage is adjusted according to the response of the patient and the site of administration. The lowest concentration and smallest dose producing the required effect should be given. The maximum single dose of lignocaine hydrochloride is 200 mg when given alone or 500 mg when given with a vasoconstrictor.

Children and elderly or debilitated patients require smaller doses, commensurate with age and physical status.

Contra-indications, warnings, etc
Contra-indications: Known hypersensitivity to anaesthetics of the amide type or the other constituents.

The use of a vasoconstrictor is contra-indicated for anaesthesia of fingers, toes, tip of nose, ears and penis.

Intravenous use.

Precautions: As for other local anaesthetics, use cautiously in patients with epilepsy, impaired cardiac conduction, impaired respiratory function, and in patients with impaired hepatic function, if the dose or site of administration is likely to result in high blood levels.

Facilities for resusicitation should be available when local anaesthetics are administered.

The effect of local anaesthetics may be reduced if an injection is made into an inflamed or infected area.

Solutions containing a vasoconstrictor should be used with caution in patients with hypertension, cardiac disease, cerebrovascular insufficiency, thyrotoxicosis, in patients taking tricyclic antidepressants, MAOI's, or receiving potent general anaesthetic agents.

Solutions containing adrenaline should be used where possible so as to prolong anaesthesia and reduce systemic absorption. This is particularly important in highly vascular areas.

Use on one patient during one treatment only. Discard unused contents.

Use in pregnancy: Although this product crosses the placenta, the low doses used in dental anaesthesia would not be expected to give rise to signs of toxicity in the foetus.

Side-effects: In common with other local anaesthetics, adverse reactions are rare and are usually the result of excessively high blood concentrations due to inadvertent intravascular injection, excessive dosage, rapid absorption or occasionally to hypersensitivity, idiosyncracy or diminished tolerance on the part of the patient. In such circumstances systemic effects occur involving the central nervous system and/or the cardiovascular system.

CNS reactions are excitatory and/or depressant, and may be characterised by nervousness, dizziness, blurred vision and tremors, followed by drowsiness, convulsions, unconsciousness and possibly respiratory arrest. The excitatory reactions may be very brief or may not occur at all, in which case the first manifestations of toxicity may be drowsiness, merging into unconsciousness and respiratory arrest.

Cardiovascular reactions are depressant, and may be characterised by hypotension, myocardial depression, bradycardia and possibly cardiac arrest.

Allergic reactions are extremely rare. They may be characterised by cutaneous lesions, urticaria, oedema or anaphylactoid reactions. Detection of sensitivity by skin testing is of doubtful value.

Hypotension may occur as a physiological response to central nerve blocks.

Symptoms and treatment of overdosage: The injection of excessive amounts of Lignostab A may, due to the vasoconstrictor, cause ischaemia. This can be followed by a reactive hyperaemia resulting in post extraction bleeding. Respiratory failure may need assisted ventilation. The circulation can be maintained with electrolyte or plasma infusions. Should convulsions develop these can be controlled with diazepam or a short acting barbiturate.

In cases of overdosage with adrenaline or noradrenaline containing solutions, intravenous phentolamine may be required to control blood pressure, with the addition of a beta-blocker in cases of adrenaline overdosage.

Pharmaceutical precautions Store at 2°–25°C. Protect from light.

Legal category: POM.

Package quantities: Boxes of 500 cartridges.

Product licence numbers

Lignostab	0017/0256
Lignostab A	0017/0257

LOSEC* ▼

Presentation Losec capsules 20 mg: hard gelatine capsules with an opaque pink body, marked 20 and an opaque reddish-brown cap marked A/OM in black ink. Each capsule contains omeprazole 20 mg as enteric-coated granules.

Uses Healing of erosive reflux oesophagitis. Symptom relief is rapid, and the majority of patients are healed after 4 weeks.

Treatment of patients with benign peptic ulcers unresponsive to an adequate dose and duration of conventional therapy including those complicating NSAID therapy.

Zollinger-Ellision syndrome.

Dosage and administration For erosive reflux oesophagitis the recommended dosage is 20 mg Losec once daily, given for 4 weeks. For those patients not fully healed after the initial course, healing usually occurs during a further 4 weeks' treatment.

Losec has also been used in a dose of 40 mg once daily in patients with reflux oesophagitis refractory to other therapy. Healing usually occurred within 8 weeks.

For duodenal ulcer the usual dose is 20 mg Losec once daily for 4 weeks. For gastric ulcer the usual dose is 20 mg Losec once daily for 8 weeks. In severe cases, the dose may be increased to 40 mg Losec once daily.

Long-term maintenance treatment with Losec is not recommended.

Zollinger-Ellison syndrome: The recommended initial dosage is 60 mg Losec once daily. The dosage should be adjusted individually and treatment continued as long as clinically indicated. More than 90% of patients with severe disease and inadequate response to other therapies have been effectively controlled on doses of 20–120 mg daily. With doses above 80 mg daily, the dose should be divided and given twice daily.

Elderly: Dose adjustment is not required in the elderly.

Children: There is no experience of the use of Losec in children.

Impaired renal or hepatic function: Dose adjustment is not required in patients with impaired renal or hepatic function. Patients with severe liver disease should not require more than 20 mg Losec daily.

Contra-indications, warnings, etc There are no known contra-indications to the use of Losec. When gastric ulcer is suspected, the possibility of malignancy should be excluded before treatment with Losec is instituted, as treatment may alleviate symptoms and delay diagnosis.

Use in pregnancy and lactation: There is no evidence on the safety of Losec in human pregnancy. Animal studies have revealed no teratogenic effect, but reproduction studies have revealed reduced litter weights. Avoid in pregnancy unless there is no safer alternative.

There is no information available on the passage of Losec into milk or its effects on the neonate. Breast feeding should therefore be discontinued if the use of Losec is considered essential.

Adverse reactions: Losec is well tolerated. Nausea, headache, diarrhoea, constipation and flatulence have been reported but are rare. Skin rashes have occurred in a few patients. These events have usually been mild and transient and there has been no consistent relationship with treatment.

Interactions: Losec can delay the elimination of diazepam, phenytoin and warfarin. Monitoring of patients receiving warfarin or phenytoin is recommended and a reduction of warfarin or phenytoin dose may be necessary when omeprazole is added to treatment. There is no evidence of an interaction with theophylline, propranolol or antacids.

Overdosage: There is no information available on the effects of overdosage in man. However, Losec is very specific in action and no particular problems are anticipated. Symptomatic and supportive therapy should be given as appropriate. Single oral doses of up to 160 mg have been given without adverse effects.

Animal toxicology: Gastric ECL-cell hyperplasia and carcinoids, localised to the oxyntic mucosa, have been observed in life-long studies in rats. These changes have been related to sustained hypergastrinaemia. No treatment related mucosal changes have been observed in patients treated continuously for periods up to 4 years.

Pharmaceutical precautions Use within one month of opening. Replace cap firmly after use. Dispense in original containers.

Legal category POM.

Package quantities Bottles of 5 or 28 capsules.

Further information Losec is a specific inhibitor of the gastric proton pump (H^+, K^+ ATPase) in the parietal cell. There is produces dose-dependent inhibition of acid secretion by binding to the enzyme, and effectively reduces gastric acid secretion.

Oral dosing with 20 mg Losec once daily produces inhibition of gastric acid secretion within 1–2 hours of the first dose. The maximum effect is achieved within 4 days of starting treatment after which the degree of acid inhibition remains constant. The mean decrease in pentagastrin-stimulated peak acid output twenty-four hours after dosing with Losec is about 70%. The inhibition of acid secretion is directly related to the area under the plasma concentration-time curve (AUC) but not to the plasma concentration at any given time.

Product licence number 0017/0238.

MARCAIN*
MARCAIN* WITH ADRENALINE

Presentation Clear, colourless, aqueous, sterile solution 0.25%, 0.5% anhydrous bupivacaine HCl with and without adrenaline and 0.75% anhydrous bupivacaine HCl without adrenaline.

0.25% Marcain – 10 ml ampoule containing bupivacaine hydrochloride BP 2.64 mg/ml.

0.25% Marcain with adrenaline – 10 ml ampoule containing bupivacaine hydrochloride BP 2.64 mg/ml with adrenaline 1 in 200,000.

0.5% Marcain – 10 ml ampoule containing bupivacaine hydrochloride BP 5.28 mg/ml.

0.5% Marcain with adrenaline – 10 ml ampoule containing bupivacaine hydrochloride BP 5.28 mg/ml with adrenaline 1 in 200,000.

0.75% Marcain – 10 ml ampoule containing bupivacaine hydrochloride BP 7.92 mg/ml.

Inactive ingredients: All the above solutions contain sodium chloride to produce isotonic solutions. Those containing adrenaline also contain sodium metabisulphite.

Uses Marcain 0.25% and 0.5% solutions are used for the production of local anaesthesia by percutaneous infiltration, peripheral nerve block(s) and central neural block (caudal or epidural), that is, for specialist use in situations where prolonged anaesthesia is required. Because sensory nerve block is more marked than motor block, Marcain is especially useful in the relief of pain, e.g. during labour.

A list of indications and the suggested dose and strength of solution appropriate for each are shown in the following table.

Marcain 0.75% solution produces a more prolonged motor block than 0.25% or 0.5% solutions and is, therefore, recommended for epidural anaesthesia for surgical purposes. Epidural anaesthesia is usually maintained for 3 to 4 hours.

Dosage and administration The utmost care should be taken to prevent an accidental intravascular injection, always including careful aspiration. For epidural anaesthesia, a test dose of 3–5 ml of bupivacaine containing adrenaline should be administered, since an intravascular injection of adrenaline will be quickly recognised by an increase in heart rate. Verbal contact and repeated measurement of heart rate should be maintained throughout a period of 5 minutes following the test dose. Aspiration should be repeated prior to administration of the total dose. The main dose should be injected slowly, *25–50 mg/min*, in incremental doses under constant contact with the patient. If mild toxic symptoms occur, the injection should be stopped immediately.

The dosage varies and depends upon the area to be anaesthetised, the vascularity of the tissues, the number of neuronal segments to be blocked, individual tolerance and the technique of anaesthesia used. The lowest dosage needed to provide effective anaesthesia should be administered. For most indications, the duration of anaesthesia with Marcain solutions is such that a single dose is sufficient.

The maximum dosage must be determined by evaluating the size and physical status of the patient and considering the usual rate of systemic absorption from a particular injection site. Experience to date indicates a single dose of up to 150 mg bupivacaine hydrochloride. Doses of up to 50 mg 2-hourly may subsequently be used. The dosages in the following table are recommended as a guide for use in the average adult. For young, elderly or debilitated patients, these doses should be reduced.

Contra-indications, warnings, etc Bupivacaine hydrochloride solutions are contra-indicated in patients with a known hypersensitivity to local anaesthetic agents of the amide type or to other components of the injectable formulation.

Solutions of bupivacaine hydrochloride are contra-indicated for intravenous regional anaesthesia (Bier's-block).

Solutions containing adrenaline are contra-indicated in patients with thyrotoxicosis or severe heart disease, particularly when tachycardia is present.

Solutions of bupivacaine hydrochloride with adrenaline should not be used in connection with anaesthesia in areas of the body supplied by end arteries or otherwise having a compromised blood supply such as digits, nose, external ear, penis, etc.

0.75% solution is contra-indicated for epidural use in obstetrics.

Epidural anaesthesia, regardless of the local anaesthetic used, has its own contra-indications which include: Active disease of the central nervous system such as meningitis, poliomyelitis, intracranial haemorrhage, subacute combined degeneration of the cord due to pernicious anaemia and cerebral and spinal tumours. Tuberculosis of the spine. Pyogenic infection of the skin at or adjacent to the site of lumbar puncture. Cardiogenic or hypovolaemic shock. Coagulation disorders or ongoing anticoagulation treatment.

Precautions: There have been reports of cardiac arrest with difficult resuscitation or death during use of bupivacaine for epidural anaesthesia in obstetrical patients. In most cases, this has followed use of the 0.75% concentration. Resuscitation has been difficult or impossible despite apparently adequate preparation and appropriate management. Cardiac arrest has occurred after convulsions resulting from systemic toxicity, presumably following unintentional intravascular injection. The 0.75% concentration should be reserved for surgical procedures where a high degree of muscle relaxation and prolonged effect are necessary.

Type of block	*% Conc*	*Each dose*		*Motor block†*
		ml	*mg*	
Local infiltration	0.25	up to 60	up to 150	—
Lumbar epidural				
Surgical operations	0.50	10 to 20	50 to 100	Moderate to complete
	0.75	10 to 20	75 to 150	Complete
Analgesia in labour	0.50	6 to 12	30 to 60	Moderate to complete
	0.25	6 to 12	15 to 30	Minimal
Caudal epidural				
Surgical operations	0.50	15 to 30	75 to 150	Moderate to complete
Children (aged up to 10 yrs):				
Up to lower thoracic (T10)	0.25	0.3 to 0.4 ml/kg	0.75 to 1 mg/kg	
Up to mid-thoracic (T6)	0.25	0.4 to 0.6 ml/kg	1.0 to 1.5 mg/kg	
If total amount greater than 20 ml reduce concentration to 0.2%.				
Analgesia in labour	0.50	10 to 20	50 to 100	Moderate to complete
	0.25	10 to 20	25 to 50	Moderate
Peripheral nerves	0.50	up to 30	up to 150	Moderate to complete
	0.25	up to 60	up to 150	Slight to moderate
Sympathetic blocks	0.25	20 to 50	50 to 125	—

† With continuous (intermittent) techniques, repeat doses increase the degree of motor block. The first repeat dose of 0.5% may produce complete motor block for intra-abdominal surgery.

Epidural blockade and large nerve plexus blocks should only be employed by those with the necessary training and experience.

Adequate resuscitation equipment should be available whenever local or general anaesthesia is administered. Overdosage or accidental intravenous injection may give rise to toxic reactions.

Injection of repeated doses of bupivacaine hydrochloride may cause significant increases in blood levels with each repeated dose due to slow accumulation of the drug. Tolerance varies with the status of the patient. Debilitated, elderly or acutely ill patients should be given reduced doses commensurate with their physical status.

Only in rare cases have amide local anaesthetics been associated with allergic reactions (in most severe instances anaphylactic shock).

Patients allergic to ester-type local anaesthetic drugs (procaine, tetracaine, benzocaine, etc.) have not shown cross-sensitivity to agents of the amide type such as bupivacaine.

Local anaesthetics should be used with caution for epidural anaesthesia in patients with impaired cardiovascular function since they may be less able to compensate for functional changes associated with the prolongation of A-V conduction produced by these drugs.

Since bupivacaine is metabolised in the liver, it should be used cautiously in patients with liver disease or with reduced liver blood flow.

Epidural anaesthesia with any local anaesthetic can cause hypotension and bradycardia which should be anticipated and appropriate precautions taken. These may include pre-loading the circulation with crystalloid or colloid solution. If hypotension develops it should be treated with a vasopressor such as ephedrine 10–15 mg intravenously. Severe hypotension may result from hypovolaemia due to haemorrhage or dehydration, or aorto-caval occlusion in patients with massive ascites, large abdominal tumours or late pregnancy. Marked hypotension should be avoided in patients with cardiac decompensation.

Patients with hypovolaemia due to any cause can develop sudden and severe hypotension during epidural anaesthesia.

Epidural anaesthesia can cause intercostal paralysis and patients with pleural effusions may suffer respiratory embarrassment. Septicaemia can increase the risk of intraspinal abscess formation in the postoperative period.

Paracervical block may have a greater adverse effect on the foetus than other nerve blocks used in obstetrics. Due to the systemic toxicity of bupivacaine special care should be taken when using bupivacaine for paracervical block.

Small doses of local anaesthetics injected into the head and neck, including retrobulbar, dental and stellate ganglion blocks, may produce systemic toxicity due to inadvertent intra-arterial injection.

Clinicians who perform retrobulbar blocks should be aware that there have been reports of respiratory arrest following local anaesthetic injection. Prior to retrobulbar block, necessary equipment, drugs and personnel should be immediately available as with all other regional procedures.

Solutions containing adrenaline should be used with caution in patients with hypertension, arteriosclerotic heart disease, cerebrovascular insufficiency or diabetes.

Drug interactions: Bupivacaine should be used with care in patients receiving anti-arrhythmic drugs with local anaesthetic activity, e.g. lignocaine, since their toxic effects may be additive.

Solutions containing adrenaline should be used with caution in those patients receiving drugs known to produce blood pressure alterations, i.e. MAO inhibitors, tricyclic antidepressants, phenothiazines, etc., as severe and sustained hypotension or hypertension may occur.

Serious cardiac arrhythmias may occur if preparations containing a vasconstrictor drug are employed in patients during or following the administration of chloroform, halothane, cyclopropane, trichlorethylene or other related agents.

Pregnancy and lactation: Bupivacaine enters the mother's milk, but in such small quantities that there is no risk of affecting the child at therapeutic dose levels.

There is no evidence of untoward effects in human pregnancy. In large doses there is evidence of decreased pup surivival in rats and an embryological effect in rabbits if Marcain is administered in pregnancy. Marcain should not therefore be given in early pregnancy unless the benefits are considered to outweigh the risks.

Side-effects: Serious systemic adverse reactions are rare, but may occur in connection with overdosage or unintentional intravascular injection.

Bupivacaine causes systemic toxicity similar to that observed with other local anaesthetic agents. It is caused by high plasma concentrations as a result of excessive dosage, rapid absorption or, most commonly, inadvertent intravascular injection. Pronounced acidosis or hypoxia may increase the risk and severity of toxic reactions. Such reactions involve the central nervous system and the cardiovascular system. CNS reactions are characterised by numbness of the tongue, lightheadedness, dizziness, blurred vision and muscle twitch, followed by drowsiness, convulsions, unconsciousness and possibly respiratory arrest.

Cardiovascular reactions are related to depression of

the conduction system of the heart and myocardium leading to decreased cardiac output, heart block, hypotension, bradycardia and sometimes ventricular arrhythmias, including ventricular tachycardia, ventricular fibrillation and cardiac arrest. Usually these will be preceded or accompanied by major CNS toxicity, i.e. convulsions, but in rare cases cardiac arrest has occurred without prodromal CNS effects.

Epidural anaesthesia itself can cause adverse reactions regardless of the local anaesthetic agent used. These include hypotension and bradycardia due to sympathetic blockade and/or vasovagal fainting.

In severe cases cardiac arrest may occur.

Accidental sub-arachnoid injection can lead to very high spinal anaesthesia possibly with apnoea and severe hypotension.

Neurological damage is a rare but well recognised consequence of regional and particularly epidural and spinal anaesthesia. It may be due to several causes, e.g. direct injury to the spinal cord or spinal nerves, anterior spinal artery syndrome, injection of an irritant substance, or an injection of a non-sterile solution. These may result in localised areas of paraesthesia or anaesthesia, motor weakness, loss of sphincter control and paraplegia. Occasionallly these are permanent.

Treatment of side-effects: Treatment of a patient with systemic toxicity consists of arresting convulsions and ensuring adequate ventilation with oxygen, if necessary by assisted or controlled ventilation (respiration). If convulsions occur they must be treated promptly by intravenous injection of thiopentone 100 to 200 mg or diazepam 5 to 10 mg. Alternatively succinyl choline 50 mg–100 mg i.v. may be used providing the clinician is capable of performing endotracheal intubation and managing a fully paralysed patient.

Once convulsions have been controlled and adequate ventilation of the lungs ensured, no other treatment is generally required. If hypotension is present, however, a vasopressor, preferably one with inotropic activity, e.g. ephedrine 15 to 30 mg, should be given intravenously.

Cardiac arrest due to bupivacaine can be resistant to electrical defibrillation and resuscitation must be continued energetically for a prolonged period.

High or total spinal blockade causing respiratory paralysis and hypotension during epidural anaesthesia should be treated by ensuring and maintaining a patent airway and giving oxygen by assisted or controlled ventilation.

Hypotension should be treated by the use of vasopressors, e.g. ephedrine 10–15 mg intravenously and repeated until the desired level of arterial pressure is reached. Intravenous fluids, both electrolytes and colloids, given rapidly can also reverse hypotension.

Pharmaceutical precautions No special requirements.

Legal category POM.

Package quantities 0.25% Marcain 10 × 10 ml Steripack sterile wrapped ampoules.

0.25% Marcain with adrenaline 10 × 10 ml Steripack sterile wrapped ampoules.

0.5% Marcain 10 × 10 ml Steripack sterile wrapped ampoules.

0.5% Marcain with adrenaline 10 × 10 ml Steripack sterile wrapped ampoules.

0.75% Marcain 10 × 10 ml Steripack sterile wrapped ampoules.

Further information: Nil

Product licence numbers

0.25% plain	0017/0116
0.25% with adrenaline	0017/0118
0.5% plain	0017/0117
0.5% with adrenaline	0017/0119
0.75% plain	0017/0133

MARCAIN* HEAVY

Presentation Clear, colourless solution containing bupivacaine hydrochloride 5 mg per ml and glucose 80 mg per ml. The specific gravity of the solution is 1.026 at 20°C.

Inactive ingredients: Sodium hydroxide and water.

Uses Spinal anaesthesia for surgery (urological and lower limb surgery lasting 2–3 hours, abdominal surgery lasting 45–60 minutes). Bupivacaine is a long acting local anaesthetic agent of the amide type. Marcain Heavy has rapid onset of action and long duration. The duration of analgesia in the T_{10}–T_{12} segments is 2–3 hours.

Marcain Heavy produces a moderate muscular relaxation of the lower extremities lasting 2–2.5 hours. The motor blockade of the abdominal muscles makes the solution suitable for performance of abdominal surgery lasting 45–60 minutes. The duration of motor blockade does not exceed the duration of analgesia. The cardiovascular effects of Marcain Heavy are similar or less than those seen with other spinal agents. Bupivacaine 5 mg/ml with glucose 80 mg/ml is exceptionally well tolerated by all tissues with which it comes in contact.

Dosage and administration The dose should be regarded as a guide for use in the average adult.

Spinal anaesthesia for surgery: 2–4 ml (10–20 mg bupivacaine hydrochloride).

The spread of anaesthesia obtained with Marcain Heavy depends on several factors, the most important being the volume of solution introduced and the position of the patient.

When injected in the L_3–L_4 intervertebral space with the patient in the sitting position, 3 ml of Marcain Heavy spreads to the T_7–T_{10} segments. With the patient receiving the injection in the horizontal position and then turned supine, the blockade spreads to T_4–T_7 spinal segments. It should be understood that the level of spinal anaesthesia achieved with any local anaesthetic can be unpredictable in a given patient.

If the patient is in the lateral position the blockade spreads to T_4. The effects of injections of Marcain Heavy exceeding 4 ml have not yet been studied and such volumes can therefore not be recommended.

Contra-indications, warnings, etc Known hypersensitivity to local anaesthetics of the amide type.

Spinal anaesthesia, regardless of the local anaesthetic used, has its own contra-indications which include:

Active disease of the central nervous system such as meningitis, poliomyelitis, intracranial haemorrhage, subacute combined degeneration of the cord due to pernicious anaemia and cerebral and spinal tumours.

Tuberculosis of the spine.

Pyogenic infection of the skin at or adjacent to the site of lumbar puncture.

Cardiogenic or hypovolaemic shock.

Coagulation disorders or ongoing anticoagulation treatment.

Precautions: Spinal anaesthesia should only be undertaken by clinicians with the necessary knowledge and experience. Resuscitative equipment and drugs should be immediately available and the anaesthetist should remain in constant attendance. Spinal anaesthesia with any local anaesthetic can cause hypotension and bradycardia which should be anticipated and appropriate precautions taken. These may include pre-loading the circulation with crystalloid or colloid solution. If hypotension develops it should be treated with a vasopressor such as ephedrine 10–15 mg intravenously. Severe hypotension may result from hypovolaemia due to haemorrhage or dehydration, or aorto-caval occlusion in patients with massive ascites, large abdominal tumours of late pregnancy. Marked hypotension should be avoided in patients with cardiac decompensation.

Patients with hypovolaemia due to any cause can develop sudden and severe hypotension during spinal anaesthesia.

Spinal anaesthesia can cause intercostal paralysis and patients with pleural effusions may suffer respiratory embarrassment. Septicaemia can increase the risk of intraspinal abscess formation in the postoperative period.

Pregnancy and lactation: Bupivacaine enters the mother's milk but in such small quantities that there is generally no risk of affecting the child at therapeutic dose levels.

There is no evidence of untoward effects in human pregnancy. In large doses there is evidence of decreased pup survival in rats and an embryological effect in rabbits if Marcain is administered in pregnancy. Marcain should not therefore be given in early pregnancy unless the benefits are considered to outweigh the risks.

Drug interactions: Bupivacaine should be used with care in patients receiving antiarrhythmic drugs with local anaesthetic activity, as their toxic effects may be additive.

Side-effects: The safety of Marcain Heavy is comparable to that of other local anaesthetics used for spinal anaesthesia.

In rare cases bupivacaine has been associated with allergic reactions and anaphylactic shock.

Spinal anaesthesia itself can cause adverse reactions regardless of the local anaesthetic agent used. These include hypotension and bradycardia due to sympathetic blockade and/or vasovagal fainting.

In severe cases cardiac arrest can occur.

High spinal anaesthesia may result in paralysis of all respiratory muscles.

Postoperatively a post lumbar puncture headache can occur.

Neurological damage is a rare but well recognised consequence of regional and particularly spinal anaesthesia. It may be due to several causes, e.g. direct injury to the spinal cord or spinal nerves, anterior spinal artery syndrome, injection of an irritant substance, or an injection of a non-sterile solution. These may result in localisd areas of paraesthesia or anaesthesia, motor weakness, loss of sphincter control and paraplegia. Occasionally these are permanent. Neurological complications of this type have been reported after the use of all local anaesthetics used for spinal anaesthesia.

Systemic toxicity: Rarely associated with spinal anaesthesia but might occur after accidental intravascular injection. Systemic adverse reactions are characterized by numbness of the tongue, lightheadedness, dizziness and tremors, followed by convulsions and cardiovascular disorders.

Treatment of side-effects: High or total spinal blockade causing respiratory paralysis should be treated by ensuring and maintaining a patent airway and giving oxygen by assisted or controlled ventilation.

Hypotension should be treated by the use of vasopressors, e.g. ephedrine 10–15 mg intravenously and repeated until the desired level of arterial pressure is reached. Intravenous fluids, both electrolytes and colloids, given rapidly can also reverse hypotension.

Treatment of systemic toxicity: No treatment is required for milder symptoms of systemic toxicity but if convulsions occur then it is important to ensure adequate oxygenation and to arrest the convulsions if they last more than 15–30 seconds. Oxygen should be given by face mask and the respiration assisted or controlled if necessary. Convulsions can be arrested by injection of thiopentone 100–150 mg intravenously or with diazepam 5–10 mg intravenously. Alternatively, succinyl choline 50–100 mg intravenously may be given but only if the clinician has the ability to perform endotracheal intubation and to manage a totally paralysed patient.

Pharmaceutical precautions The solution must not be stored in contact with metals, e.g. needles or metal parts of syringes, as dissolved metal ions may cause swelling at the site of the injection.

The solution should be used immediately after opening of the ampoule. Any remaining solution should be discarded.

Legal category POM.

Package quantities Sterile wrapped ampoules 4 × 4 ml.

Product licence number 0017/0139.

PENSACAINE* 2% WITH ADRENALINE 1:80,000

Presentation Sterile, clear aqueous solution. Each ml contains lignocaine hydrochloride anhydrous 20 mg/ml equivalent to Lignocaine Hydrochloride BP 21.4 mg/ml and Adrenaline Tartrate EP 22.7 micrograms equivalent to adrenaline 12.5 micrograms.

Inactive ingredients: Sodium chloride to produce an isotonic solution, sodium metabisulphite, sodium hydroxide and hydrochloric acid.

Uses Pensacaine 2% with adrenaline is a local anaesthetic solution for use in dental infiltration anaesthesia and all dental nerve-block techniques.

Dosage and administration Infiltration – usual dose is 1 ml. Nerve block – usual dose is 1.5 to 2 ml.

The recommended maximum dose for lignocaine hydrochloride when given with adrenaline is 500 mg.

Children and elderly or debilitated patients require smaller doses.

Contra-indications, warnings, etc Known hypersensitivity to local anaesthetics of the amide type.

The use of a vasoconstrictor is contra-indicated for anaesthesia of fingers, toes, tip of nose, ears and penis.

Pensacaine with adrenaline should not be given intravenously.

Precautions: In common with other local anaesthetics, Pensacaine with adrenaline should be used cautiously in patients with epilepsy, impaired cardiac conduction, imparied respiratory function, and in patients with impaired hepatic function if the dose or site of administration is likely to result in high blood levels.

Facilities for resuscitation should be available when local anaesthetics are administered.

The effect of local anaesthetics may be reduced if an injection is made into an inflamed or infected area. Solutions containing adrenaline should be used with caution in patients with hypertension, cardiac disease, cerebrovascular insufficiency or thyrotoxicosis.

Solutions containing adrenaline should be used where possible so as to prolong anaesthesia and reduce systemic absorption. This is particularly important in highly vascular areas.

Use on one patient during one treatment only.

Use in pregnancy and lactation: Although there is no evidence from animal studies of harm to the foetus, as with all drugs, lignocaine should not be given in early pregnancy unless the benefits are considered to outweigh the risks.

Adverse reactions: In common with other local anaesthetics, adverse reactions to Pensacaine with adrenaline are extremely rare in dental practice and are usually the result of excessively high blood concentrations due to inadvertent intravascular injection, excessive dosage, rapid absorption or occasionally to hypersensitivity, idiosyncracy or diminished tolerance on the part of the patient. In such circumstances systemic effects occur involving the central nervous system and/or the cardiovascular system.

CNS reactions are excitatory and/or depressant, and may be characterized by nervousness, dizziness, blurred vision and tremors, followed by drowsiness, convulsions, unconsciousness and possibly respiratory arrest. The excitatory reactions may be very brief or may not occur at all, in which case the first manifestations of toxicity may be drowsiness, merging into unconsciousness and respiratory arrest.

Cardiovascular reactions are depressant, and may be characterized by hypotension, myocardial depression, bradycardia and possibly cardiac arrest.

Allergic reactions are extremely rare. They may be characterized by cutaneous lesions, urticaria, oedema or anaphylactoid reactions. Detection of sensitivity by skin testing is of doubtful value.

Pharmaceutical precautions Store below 15°C.

Legal category POM.

Package quantities Glass cartridges of 2 ml standard and 2 ml self-aspirating, in boxes of 100.

Further information Dental cartridges of Pensacaine 2% with adrenaline 1:80,000 do not contain an antimicrobial agent.

Product licence number 0017/5027R.

PROCAINAMIDE DURULES*

Presentation Slightly yellow, circular, convex tablets containing 500 mg procainamide hydrochloride.

Uses Supraventricular tachyarrhythmias (atrial premature beats, paroxysmal atrial tachycardia, atrial flutter, atrial fibrillation, AV junctional tachycardia and premature beats).

Ventricular arrhythmias (ectopic beats, premature beats, and tachycardia).

Digitalis induced arrhythmias.

Dystrophia myotonia; myotonia congenita (Thomsen).

Dosage and administration Ideally the dosage should be adjusted to maintain a serum concentration between 4–8 micrograms per ml, usually 2–3 tablets three times a day (3–4.5 g daily).

Guidelines: Anti-arrhythmic prophylaxis after acute myocardial infarction, initially 3–4 Durules followed by 2–3 Durules thrice daily as maintenance. During transition from lignocaine therapy, treatment with Procainamide Durules should be initiated two hours prior to discontinuation of infusion of lignocaine. It may occasionally be necessary to divide the daily dose into 4 doses per day.

The Durules should be swallowed whole, not broken or chewed.

Elderly: Lower doses will be required if renal insufficiency or heart failure are present.

Children: Not recommended in children under 12.

Contra-indications, warnings, etc
Contra-indications: Procainamide hypersensitivity. Second or third degree AV block and bifascicular block with AV block type 1 if the patient does not have a pacemaker. Bronchial asthma, myasthenia gravis and SLE are relative contraindications.

Precautions: In patients with renal insufficiency or heart failure, accumulation of procainamide may occur; caution should therefore be observed and the dose adjusted if necessary. Accumulation leads to an impairment of hepatic and/or renal function.

Side-effects: Procainamide is generally well tolerated, but anorexia, nausea and vomiting and diarrhoea may occur. Occasional cases of flushing, skin rash, pruritus, depression, vertigo, psychosis with hallucinations, shivering, fever, joint and muscle pain, 'bitter taste' and muscle weakness have been reported. A possible lupus erythematosus-like syndrome may occur during treatment. Serological tests for ANF should therefore be made before commencement of treatment and regularly thereafter. The blood should also be examined for LE-type cells at the same time. If the ANF titre rises or LE cells appear, then cessation of treatment should be considered. Usually these increases are noted before overt clinical symptoms are detectable. The syndrome is usually completely reversible. Serious side-effects in the form of leucopenia and agranulocytosis may occur during long-term treatment.

Overdosage: Poisoning due to an overdose of Procainamide Durules may lead to widening of the QRS complex, atrioventricular block, sinoatrial block or arrest, asystole, myocardial depression, severe hypotension and cardiac arrest. Paroxysmal ventricular and supra-ventricular tachyarrhythmias are less frequent. Nausea, vomiting, oliguria and CNS symptoms such as confusion, hallucinations or convulsions can also occur.

Treatment should include close monitoring of cardiovascular, respiratory and renal function, electrolytes and continuous ECG monitoring. Further absorption may be prevented by induction of vomiting or gastric lavage, or administration of activated charcoal if ingestion is recent. Cardiovascular complications should be treated symptomatically, which may require the use of sympathomimetic agents (e.g. noradrenaline, metaraminol), or inotropic agents (e.g. dopamine, dobutamine). Temporary pacing may be required for AV block. Glucagon may be used to treat hypotension, intravenous sodium bicarbonate to correct acidosis and intravenous diazepam for convulsions.

Procainamide and its active metabolite (N-acetyl procainamide) can be removed by haemodialysis, or charcoal column haemoperfusion and repeated oral administration of activated charcoal may enhance elimination.

As Procainamide Durules is a sustained release preparation, treatment of overdosage may be required for an extended period.

Pharmaceutical precautions Procainamide Durules may be stored at room temperature.

Legal category POM.

Package quantities 500 mg tablets in bottles of 100.

Further information Procainamide Durules are a sustained release formulation which enable therapeutic blood levels of procainamide to be conveniently attained and maintained.

Product licence number 0017/0071.

PLENDIL* ▼

Presentation Circular biconvex film coated extended release tablets containing either 5 mg felodipine coded A/FM or 10 mg felodipine coded A/FE.

Uses In the management of hypertension. Plendil is effective in all grades of hypertension.

Dosage and administration
Adults including elderly: The dose should be adjusted to the individual requirements of the patient. The recommended starting dose is 5 mg once daily. Doses higher than 20 mg daily are not usually needed.

The tablets should be taken in the morning, swallowed with water and must not be divided, crushed or chewed.

Children: The safety and efficacy of Plendil in children has not been established.

Plendil can be used in combination with β-blockers or diuretics. The effects on blood pressure are likely to be additive and combination therapy will usually enhance the antihypertensive effect. Care should be taken to avoid hypotension.

In patients with severely impaired liver function the dose of felodipine should be low. The pharmacokinetics are not significantly affected in patients with impaired renal function.

Contra-indications, warnings, etc
Contra-indications: Plendil should not be used in women of child bearing potential.

Hypersensitivity to felodipine.

Pregnancy and lactation: In a study on fertility and general reproductive performance in rats, prolongation of parturition resulting in difficult labour and increased foetal deaths and early postnatal deaths was observed in the medium and high dose groups. Reproduction studies in rabbits have shown a dose-related reversible enlargement of the mammary glands of parent animals and dose-related digital abnormalities in the foetuses.

It is not known whether Plendil is excreted in breast milk, or whether it has harmful effects on the new born.

Precautions: As with other vasodilators, Plendil may in rare cases precipitate significant hypotension with tachycardia which in susceptible individuals may result in myocardial ischaemia.

Interactions: Enzyme inhibitors such as cimetidine, impairs the elimination of Plendil, and Plendil dosage may need to be reduced when drugs are given concomitantly. Conversely powerful enzyme inducing agents such as some anticonvulsants (phenytoin, carbamazepine, phenobarbitone) can increase Plendil elimination, and higher than normal Plendil doses may be required in patients taking the drugs.

No dosage adjustment is required when Plendil is given concomitantly with digoxin.

Side-effects: As with other calcium antagonists, flushing, headache, palpitations, dizziness and fatigue may occur. These reactions are usually transient and are most likely to occur at the start of treatment or after an increase in dosage.

As with other calcium antagonists ankle swelling, resulting from precapillary vasodilation may occur. The degree of ankle swelling is dose related.

Skin reactions such as rash and pruritis have been reported.

In patients with gingivitis/periodontitis mild gingival enlargement has been reported with Plendil, as with other calcium antagonists. The enlargement can be avoided or reversed by careful dental hygiene.

Overdose: Overdosage may cause excessive peripheral vasodilatation with marked hypotension which may sometimes be accompanied by bradycardia. Severe hypotension should be treated symptomatically, with the patient placed supine and the legs elevated. Bradycardia, if present, should be treated with atropine 0.5–1 mg i.v. If this is not sufficient, plasma volume should be increased by infusion of e.g. glucose, saline or dextran. Sympathomimetic drugs with predominant effect on the $\alpha 1$ adrenoceptor may be given e.g. metaraminol or phenylephrine.

Pharmaceutical precautions Store at room temperature.

Legal category POM.

Package quantities Calendar pack of 28 tablets.

Further information Plendil is a calcium antagonist and lowers arterial blood pressure by decreasing vascular resistance. In general a reduction in blood pressure is evident 2 hours after the first oral dose and at steady state lasts for at least 24 hours after dose.

Plendil exhibits a high degree of selectivity for smooth muscles in the arterioles and in therapeutic doses has no direct effect on cardiac contractility. Felodipine does not affect venous smooth muscle and adrenergic vasomotor control.

Electrophysiological studies have shown that felodipine has no direct effect of conduction in the specialised conducting system of the heart and no effect of the AV nodal refractoriness.

Plendil produces a slight and transient increase in heart rate, which can be counteracted by combined administration with beta-blockers.

Plendil possesses a mild natriuretic/diuretic effect and does not produce general fluid retention, nor affect daily potassium excretion. Plendil is well tolerated in patients with angina pectoris and congestive heart failure.

Although Plendil is approximately 99% protein bound it does not appear to affect the unbound fraction of other extensively bound drugs such as warfarin.

Product licence numbers
Plendil 5 mg 0017/0301
Plendil 10 mg 0017/0302

PULMICORT*

Presentation Pulmicort Inhaler is a metered dose aerosol delivering 200 micrograms budesonide per actuation via a standard or Spacer adapter. Pulmicort L.S. inhaler is a metered dose aerosol delivering 50 micrograms budesonide per actuation via a standard or L.S. Spacer adapter.

Inactive ingredients: Sorbitan trioleate and chlorofluorocarbons 11, 12 and 114.

Uses Pulmicort Inhaler and Pulmicort LS Inhaler contain the potent, non-halogenated corticosteroid budesonide. Inhaled budesonide possesses a local anti-inflammatory action in the lungs without giving rise to systemic corticosteroid effects.

Pulmicort is recommended in patients with bronchial asthma.

The specially designed Spacer adapter permits the aerosol propellants to evaporate and the particle velocity to decrease, resulting in reduced drug deposition in the oral cavity. In addition the Spacer adapter diminishes the need for co-ordination between aerosol actuation and inhalation, making this inhaler suitable for patients who have difficulty using conventional inhalers.

Dosage and administration *Adults:* 200 micrograms twice daily, in the morning and in the evening. During periods of severe asthma the daily dosage can be increased to up to 1600 micrograms.

In patients well controlled the daily dose may be reduced below 400 micrograms, but should not go below 200 micrograms.

Children: 50 to 400 micrograms to be given twice daily. During periods of severe asthma the daily dosage can be increased up to 800 micrograms.

Elderly: Dosage as for adults.

Contra-indications, warnings, etc No specific contra-indications are known, but special care is needed in patients with lung tuberculosis, fungal and viral infections in the airways.

Precautions *Pregnancy and breast feeding:* In pregnant animals, administration of budesonide causes abnormalities of foetal development. The relevance of this finding to man has not been established. Administration during pregnancy should be avoided unless there are compelling reasons. As yet there is no information regarding the passage of budesonide into breast milk.

Patients not dependent on steroids: Treatment with the recommended doses of Pulmicort usually gives a therapeutic benefit within 7 days. However, certain patients may have an excessive collection of mucous secretion in the bronchi, which reduces penetration of the active substance into the airways. In these cases a short course of oral corticosteroids (usually 1 to 2 weeks) should be given in addition to the aerosol. After the course of the oral drug the inhaler alone should be sufficient therapy. Exacerbations of asthma caused by bacterial infections are usually controlled by appropriate antibiotic treatment and possibly increasing the Pulmicort dosage or if necessary, by giving systemic steroids.

Steroid dependent patients: Transfer of patients dependent upon oral steroids to treatment with Pulmicort demands special care mainly due to the slow restitution of the disturbed hypothalamic-pituitary function caused by extended treatment with oral corticosteroids. When the Pulmicort treatment is initiated the patient should be in a relatively stable phase. Pulmicort is then given in combination with the previously used oral steroid dose for about 10 days.

After this period of time the reduction of the oral corticoid dose can be started with a dose reduction corresponding to about 1 mg prednisolone per day every week. The oral dose is thus reduced to the lowest level which in combination with Pulmicort gives a stable respiratory capacity.

In many cases it may eventually be possible to withdraw completely the oral steroid with Pulmicort treatment, but other cases may have to be maintained on a low oral steroid dosage.

Some patients may experience uneasiness during the withdrawal period due to a decreased steroid effect. The physician may have to explain the reason for the Pulmicort treatment in order to encourage the patient to continue. The length of time needed for the body to regain its natural production of corticosteroid in sufficient amounts is often extensive. Thus during physically stressing situations such as severe infections, trauma and surgical operations it will be necessary to give the patient an additional oral steroid dose. Acute exacerbations, accompanied by increased mucous viscosity and mucous plugging, require complementary treatment with a short course of oral corticosteroids.

During transfer from oral therapy to Pulmicort a generally lower systemic steroid action will be experienced which may result in the appearance of allergic or arthritic symptoms such as rhinitis, eczema and muscle and joint pain. Specific treatment should be initiated for these conditions.

Side effects: Occasional cases of mild irritation in the throat and hoarseness have been reported. Due to drug deposition in the oral cavity candidiasis of the mouth and throat occurs in some patients. However, the incidence should be less with the Spacer adapter or Nebuhaler as these reduce oral deposition. Advising the patient to rinse the mouth with water after each dosing occasion is also recommended. In most cases this condition responds to topical anti-fungal therapy without discontinuing treatment with Pulmicort.

Overdosage: The only harmful effect that follows inhalation of large amounts of the drug over a short period is suppression of hypothalamic-pituitary adrenal (HPA) function. No special emergency action needs to be taken. Treatment with Pulmicort inhaler should be continued at the recommended dose to control the asthma.

Pharmaceutical precautions To be stored at room temperature.

Legal category POM.

Package quantities Pulmicort Inhaler (200 micrograms/puff). Aerosol canister containing 200 metered doses complete with standard and Spacer delivery systems.

Pulmicort L.S. Inhaler (50 micrograms/puff). Aerosol canister containing 200 metered doses complete with standard and Spacer delivery systems.

Pulmicort (200 micrograms/puff) and Pulmicort L.S. (50 micrograms/puff) refill canisters are available.

Further information Pulmicort and Pulmicort L.S. may also be administered via the Nebuhaler.

Product licence numbers
Pulmicort Inhaler (200 micrograms/puff) 0017/0128
Pulmicort L.S. Inhaler (50 micrograms/puff) 0017/0113

PULMICORT* RESPULES

Presentation A white to off-white suspension for nebulisation. Respules (2 ml single dose unit ampoules), containing 0.25 mg/ml or 0.5 mg/ml budesonide.

Inactive ingredients: Sodium chloride, polysorbate 80, citric acid, sodium citrate and disodium edetate.

Uses Pulmicort Respules contain the potent non-halogenated corticosteroid, budesonide for use in bronchial asthma in patients where use of a pressurised inhaler or dry powder formulation is unsatisfactory or inappropriate.

Dosage and administration
Dosage schedules: Pulmicort Respules should be administered from suitable nebulisers. The dose delivered to the patient varies depending on the nebulising equipment used. The nebulisation time and the dose delivered is dependent on flow rate, volume of nebuliser chamber and volume fill. A suitable volume fill for most nebulisers is 2–4 ml. The dosage of Pulmicort Respules should be adjusted to the need of the individual. When treatment is started, during periods of severe asthma and while reducing or discontinuing oral glucocorticosteroids the recommended dose of Pulmicort Respules is:

Adults (including elderly): Usually 1–2 mg twice daily. In very severe cases the dosage may be further increased.

Children 12 years and older: Dosage as for adults.

Children 3 months to 12 years: 0./5–1 mg twice daily.

The maintenance dose should be the lowest dose which keeps the patient symptom-free.

Recommended doses are:

Adults (including elderly and children 12 years and older): 0.5–1 mg twice daily.

Children (3 months–12 years): 0.25–0.5 mg twice daily.

Recommended dosage table

	Pulmicort Respule Presentation	
Dose (mg)	*0.25 mg/ml Volume (ml)*	*0.5 mg/ml*
0.25	1	—
0.5	2	1
0.75	3	—
1.0	4	2
1.5	6	3
2.0	8	4

Where an increased therapeutic effect is desired, especially in those patients without major mucus secretion in the airways, an increased dose of Pulmicort is recommended rather than combined treatment with oral corticosteroids because of the lower risk of systemic effects.

Contra-indications, warnings, etc
Contra-indications: Hypersensitivity to any of the constituents.

Special warnings and precautions: Special care is needed in patients with pulmonary tuberculosis and viral infections in the airways.

Non-steroid dependent patients: A therapeutic effect is usually reached within 10 days. In patients with excessive mucus secretion in the bronchi a short (about 2 weeks) additional oral corticosteroid regimen can be given initially. After the course of the oral drug Pulmicort Respules alone should be sufficient therapy.

Steroid dependent patients: When transfer from oral corticosteroid to treatment with Pulmicort is initiated the patient should be in a relatively stable phase. Pulmicort is then given in combination with the previously used oral steroid dose for about 10 days.

After that the oral dose should be gradually reduced (by for example 2.5 mg prednisolone or the equivalent each month) to the lowest possible level. In many cases, it is possible to completely substitute Pulmicort for the oral corticosteroid.

During transfer from oral therapy to Pulmicort a generally lower systemic corticosteroid action will be experienced which may result in the appearance of allergic or arthritic symptoms such as rhinitis, eczema and muscle and joint pain. Specific treatment should be initiated for these conditions.

Acute exacerbations of asthma may need additional treatment with a short course of oral corticosteroid.

The nebuliser chamber should be cleaned after every administration. Wash the nebuliser chamber and mouthpiece or face-mask in hot water using a mild detergent. Rinse well and dry by connecting the nebuliser chamber to the compressor or air inlet.

Pulmicort does not affect the ability to drive and use machines.

Pulmicort Respules can be mixed with 0.9% saline and with solutions of terbutaline, salbutamol, sodium chromoglycate or ipratropium bromide.

Side-effects: Mild irritation in the throat, coughing and hoarseness. Candida infection in the oropharynx has been reported. To minimize oropharyngeal thrush the mouth should be rinsed with water after administration. In rare cases inhaled drugs may provoke bronchoconstriction in hyperreactive patients. Facial skin irritation has occurred in a few cases when a nebuliser with face mask has been used. To prevent irritation facial skin should be washed after use of the face mask. Coughing can usually be prevented by inhaling a beta-2-agonist (e.g. terbutaline) 5–10 minutes before inhalation of Pulmicort Respules.

Use in pregnancy and lactation: In pregnant animals administration of budesonide causes abnormalities of foetal development. The relevance of this finding to man has not been established. Administration during pregnancy should be avoided unless there are compelling reasons. As yet there is no information regarding the passage of budesonide into breast milk.

Overdosage: Pulmicort Respules contains 0.1 mg/ml disodium edetate which has been shown to cause bronchoconstriction at levels above 1.2 mg/ml. Acute overdosage with Pulmicort should not present a clinical problem.

Pharmaceutical precautions Store below 30°C. Use within 3 months of opening the foil envelope. Protect opened ampoule from light. Use within 12 hours of opening.

Legal category POM.

Further information Nil.

Product licence numbers

Pulmicort Respules 0.25 mg/ml	0017/0309
Pulmicort Respules 0.5 mg/ml	0017/0310

PULMICORT* TURBOHALER

Presentation Pulmicort Turbohaler 200 is a breath-actuated metered dose powder inhaler delivering 200 micrograms budesonide per actuation. Pulmicort Turbohaler 400 is a breath-actuated metered dose powder inhaler delivering 400 micrograms budesonide per actuation. Pulmicort Turbohaler 200 and Pulmicort Turbohaler 400 are free from propellants, lubricants, preservatives, carrier substances or other additives.

Uses Pulmicort Turbohaler 200 and Pulmicort Turbohaler 400 contain the potent, non-halogenated corticosteroid budesonide. Clinical studies have shown inhaled budesonide to possess a local anti-inflammatory action in the lungs without giving rise to systemic corticosteroid effects. Investigations with Pulmicort have documented good therapeutic results in bronchial asthma, whilst being well tolerated during prolonged treatment.

Pulmicort is, therefore, recommended in patients with bronchial asthma who have not previously been well controlled on bronchodilators and/or anti-allergic agents.

Dosage and administration The dosage of Pulmicort Turbohaler 200 and Pulmicort Turbohaler 400 should be individualised. When starting treatment, during periods of severe asthma and while reducing or discontinuing oral glucocorticosteroids the dosage in adults should be 200–1600 micrograms daily in divided doses. In less severe cases 200–800 micrograms daily may be used; during periods of severe asthma the daily dosage can be increased to up to 1600 micrograms.

Children: 200–800 micrograms daily in divided doses. During periods of severe asthma the daily dose can be increased up to 800 micrograms.

Elderly: Dosage as for adults.

The maintenance dose should be individualised and should be the lowest possible. Administration twice daily (morning and evening) is usually sufficient.

In patients where an increased therapeutic effect is desired, an increased dose of Pulmicort is recommended because of the lower risk of systemic effects as compared with a combined treatment with oral glucocorticosteroids.

The patient should rinse the mouth with water after each administration.

Contra-indications, warnings, etc No specific contra-indications are known, but special care is needed in patients with lung tuberculosis, fungal and viral infections in the airways.

Precautions: Non-steroid dependent patients: A therapeutic effect is usually reached within 10 days. In patients with excessive mucus secretion in the bronchi a short (about 2 weeks) additional oral corticosteroid regimen can be given initially.

Steroid dependent patients: When transferral from oral steroids to Pulmicort Turbohaler is started, the patient should be in a relatively stable phase. A high dose of Pulmicort Turbohaler is given in combination with the previously used oral steroid for about 10 days. After that the oral dose should be gradually reduced (by for example 2.5 mg prednisolone or the equivalent each month) to the lowest possible level. In many cases, it is possible to completely substitute Pulmicort for the oral steroid.

Note: During transfer from oral therapy to Pulmicort a generally lower systemic steroid action will be experienced which may result in the appearance of allergic or arthritic symptoms such as rhinitis, eczema and muscle and joint pain. Specific treatment should be initiated for these conditions.

Acute exacerbations of asthma may need additional treatment with a short course of oral corticosteroid.

Pregnancy and breast feeding: In pregnant animals, administration of budesonide causes abnormalities of foetal development. The relevance of this finding to man has not been established. Administration during pregnancy should be avoided unless there are compelling reasons. If treatment with glucocorticosteroids during pregnancy is unavoidable, inhaled glucocorticosteroids should be preferred because of their lower systemic effect compared with equipotent anti-asthmatic doses of oral glucocorticosteroids. There is no information regarding the passage of budesonide into breast milk.

Side-effects: Mild irritation in the throat and hoarseness. Candida infection in the oropharynx has been reported. Advising the patient to rinse the mouth with water after each administration is recommended. In most cases this condition responds to topical anti-fungal therapy without discontinuing treatment with Pulmicort.

Rare cases of cataract after prolonged use of corticosteroid aerosols have been reported.

Overdosage: The only harmful effect that follows inhalation of large amounts of the drug over a short period is suppression of hypothalamic-pituitary-adrenal (HPA) function. No special emergency action needs to be taken. Treatment with Pulmicort Turbohaler should be continued at the recommended dose to control the asthma.

Pharmaceutical precautions Store at room temperature.

Legal category POM.

Package quantities Pulmicort Turbohaler 200: containing 100 or 200 doses.

Pulmicort Turbohaler 400: containing 50, 100 or 200 doses.

Further information Pulmicort Turbohaler is breath-actuated and therefore there is no need to co-ordinate the release of the dose and the inhalation.
Treatment with Pulmicort Turbohaler is effective even at low inspiratory flow rates.

Product licence numbers

Pulmicort Turbohaler 200	0017/0272
Pulmicort Turbohaler 400	0017/0271

RHINOCORT*

Presentation Rhinocort is a metered-dose aerosol for nasal application delivering 50 micrograms budesonide per actuation. Rhinocort aerosol contains sorbitan trioleate and chlorofluorocarbons 11, 12 and 114.

Uses Seasonal and perennial, allergic rhinitis and vasomotor rhinitis.

Dosage and administration Two applications into each nostril morning and evening. (Total dose 400 micrograms). When good effect has been achieved the dosage may be reduced to one application into each nostril morning and evening.

Contra-indications, warnings, etc No specific contra-indications are known, but special care is needed in fungal and viral infections in the airways, and in patients with lung tuberculosis.

Precautions: Pregnancy and breast feeding: In pregnant animals, administration of budesonide causes abnormalities of foetal developments. The relevance of this to man has not been established. Administration during pregnancy should be avoided unless there are compelling reasons. As yet there is no information regarding the passage of budesonide into breast milk.

The patient should be informed that the full effect of Rhinocort is not achieved until after a few days. Concomitant treatment with an antihistamine may sometimes be necessary to counteract potential eye symptoms caused by the allergy. In continuous long-term treatment with Rhinocort the nasal mucosa should be inspected regularly, at least once a year. Until greater experience has been achieved continuous long-term treatment of children is not recommended.

Side-effects: Occasionally, sneezing attacks may follow immediately after the use of the aerosol. Slight haemorrhagic secretions may occur.

Pharmaceutical precautions *Storage:* Store at room temperature.

Legal category POM.

Package quantities Rhinocort Nasal Aerosol is an aerosol cannister containing 7 g suspension corresponding to 200 doses.

Further information In pharmacological investigations and investigations in human beings budesonide (a non-halogenated corticosteroid) has shown a favourable relationship between anti-inflammatory effects and systemic effects due to the fact that budesonide is inactivated very rapidly in the liver after systemic absorption. With the recommended dosage of Rhinocort, an effective corticosteroid treatment of the nasal mucous membrane is attained with very little risk of systemic side-effects. The duration of action of Rhinocort is such that application morning and evening is sufficient.

Product licence number 0017/0204.

RHINOCORT* AQUA

Presentation Rhinocort Aqua is a metered pump spray for nasal application delivering 100 micrograms budesonide per dose. Rhinocort Aqua also contains disodium edetate, potassium sorbate, glucose, cellulose carboxymethylcellulose sodium, polysorbate 80, hydrochloric acid and water.

Uses Season and perennial allergic rhinitis and vasomotor rhinitis.

Dosage and administration
Adults: The recommended dose is 400 mcg. Rhinocort Aqua may be given once daily (two applications into each nostril in the morning). When good effect has been achieved the dosage may be reduced to one application into each nostril.

Rhinocort Aqua may also be given twice daily (one application into each nostril morning and evening).

Elderly: Dosage as for adults.

Children: There are insufficient data to recommend the use of Rhinocort Aqua in children. However it is unlikely that the risk/benefit ratio in children is different from that in adults.

Contra-indications, warnings, etc
Contra-indication: Hypersensitivity to any of the ingredients.

Precautions and warnings: Special care is needed in patients with fungal and viral infections in the airways, and in patients with lung tuberculosis.

The patient should be informed that full effect of Rhinocort is not achieved until after a few days treatment. Treatment of seasonal rhinitis should, if possible, start before exposure to the allergens. Concomitant treatment may sometimes be necessary to counteract eye symptoms caused by the allergy. In continuous long-term treatment, the nasal mucosa should be inspected regularly e.g. every 6 months.

Until greater experience has been achieved, continuous long-term treatment of children is not recommended.

Rhinocort Aqua does not affect the ability to drive and operate machinery.

Pregnancy and lactation: Administation during pregnancy should be avoided unless there are compelling reasons. In pregnant animals administration of budesonide causes abnormalities of foetal development. The relevance of this to man has not been established. There is no information available regarding the passage of budesonide into breast milk.

Side-effects: Occasionally sneezing may follow immediately after the use of the spray. Slight haemorrhagic secretion may occur.

Overdose: Acute overdose with Rhinocort should not present a clinical problem.

Pharmaceutical precautions Store below 30°C. Use within 2 months of starting treatment.

Legal category POM.

Package quantities Rhinocort Aqua is a nasal spray containing 100 × 100 microgram doses budesonide INN.

Further information In pharmacological investigations and investigations in human beings budesonide (a non-halogenated corticosteroid) has shown a favourable relationship between anti-inflammatory effects and systemic effects due to the fact that budesonide is inactivated very rapidly in the liver after systemic absorption. With the recommended dosage of Rhinocort Aqua an effective corticosteroid treatment of the nasal mucous membrane is attained with very little risk of systemic side effects.

Product licence number 0017/0304.

ROXIAM* ▼

Presentation
Composition: 150 mg remoxipride hydrochloride monohydrate (equivalent to 131.2 mg remoxipride base).

300 mg remoxipride hydrochloride monohydrate (equivalent to 262.4 mg remoxipride base).

Roxiam also contains microcrystalline cellulose, carboxy methylcellulose sodium, ethyl cellulose, triethyl citrate, indigotine (E132), erythrosine (E127) and titanium oxide (E1710).

Pharmaceutical form: Opaque blue hard gelatin extended release capsules imprinted as follows: 150 mg capsule – RMX 150c and Astra logo.
300 mg – RMX 300c and Astra logo.

Uses Roxiam is indicated for the treatment of acute and chronic schizophrenic psychoses, and other psychoses where delusions, hallucinations, and thought disorder are prominent symptoms except those due to depressive illness.

Dosage and administration
Dosage
Adults: An initial dose of 300 mg once daily is recommended. This dose can be adjusted up or down according to the individual response. Most patients respond to a dose of 150–450 mg once daily. In individual cases the daily dose may be increased up to 600 mg.

For maintenance treatment 150–300 mg once daily is recommended for the majority of patients.

Capsules should be swallowed whole and not opened or chewed because of the bitter taste of their contents.

Elderly: A starting daily dose of 150 mg is recommended which can be individually adjusted within the same dose range as above. Experience is limited. Use with caution until further experience is gained.

Children: Not recommended.

Renal or hepatic insufficiency: In cases of severe renal insufficiency (creatinine clearance <25 ml/min) or severe hepatic insufficiency a starting dose of 150 mg/day is recommended which can be adjusted individually.

Moderate impairment of renal or hepatic function does not warrant dose reduction.

Contra-indications, warnings, etc
Contra-indications: No absolute contra-indications are known.

Undesirable effects: Roxiam is generally well tolerated and in many instances it has been difficult to differentiate adverse effects from symptoms of the underlying disease.

Undesirable effects which have been reported include:

Central nervous system: tiredness, drowsiness, insomnia, concentration difficulties, restlessness, anxiety, agitation and aggressiveness. These are usually mild and transient. Nausea, headache, dizziness and changes in body weight can also occur.

Extrapyramidal system: akathisia, hypokinesia, rigidity, tremor, acute dystonia and dyskinesia. The incidence and severity are less than with haloperidol, and fewer patients require drug withdrawal or treatment.

Autonomic system: blurred vision, dry mouth, salivation, constipation and micturition disorders. Clinically significant hypotension and orthostatic reactions are rare.

Endocrine system: menstrual disorders. The incidence of gynaecomastia and galactorrhoea is low.

Liver: increase of liver transaminases. The incidence is similar to that with haloperidol, and the changes usually small and transient.

Skin: skin rash and urticaria.

Special precautions for use: Despite the limited potential of Roxiam to induce extrapyramidal symptoms, caution is advised in patients with Parkinson's disease.

Neuroleptics are known to affect the seizure threshold. Although animal data and studies in humans do not indicate any such risk with Roxiam caution is recommended in treating patients with unstable epilepsy.

In women with existing breast cancer or a history of this disease possible risks should be weighed against benefits of therapy when considering treatment with hyperprolactinemia-inducing drugs, including Roxiam.

Use during pregnancy and lactation: Until clinical experience has been gained use with caution during pregnancy and in women of childbearing potential unless adequate contraceptive precautions are taken. Animal studies have shown that remoxipride penetrates the placental barrier but there is no evidence of teratogenic effects.

Remoxipride enters breast milk; the amount ingested by the infant would be less than 3% of the dose given to the mother. It is recommended that breast feeding should be avoided, but benefits may outweigh potential hazards for the child.

Interactions: There are no pharmacokinetic interactions between remoxipride and biperiden (anticholinergic), warfarin (anticoagulant), diazepam (sedative) or ethanol.

Remoxipride is partly metabolised by debrisoquine hydroxylase and it causes induction of liver microsomal enzymes in animals. Pharmacokinetic interactions with other drugs being metabolised by these enzymes cannot be excluded.

Overdose: Experience is limited. Sedation and extrapyramidal symptoms have been reported. In cases of severe intoxication, intensive care unit procedures are recommended. Parenteral antiparkinson medication should be given to counteract extrapyramidal symptoms. Benzodiazepines may be of value for controlling agitation or excitation related to akathisia.

Specal warnings: Roxiam like neuroleptics in general, may sometimes paradoxically aggravate symptoms of excitation, agitation and aggressiveness. Dose reduction or drug withdrawal may be necessary.

Neuroleptics may cause tardive dyskinesia (TD). Until further experience has been gained with Roxiam in long term treatment it is not possible to exclude TD as a potential risk.

Unexplained hyperthermia in patients on treatment with neuroleptics could be an indicator of the neuroleptic malignant syndrome. In this event, all neuroleptic drugs, including Roxiam, should be withheld until the origin of the fever has been determined.

Effects on ability to drive and use machines: Roxiam has a low potential for causing drowsiness and does not generally impair co-ordination or motor performance. However, patients should be advised not to drive or operate machinery until their individual susceptibility is known.

Pharmaceutical precautions
Incompatibilities: Not applicable.

Shelf life: The shelf life of Roxiam is 2 years.

Special precautions for storage: Store at room temperature.

Legal category POM.

Package quantities Blister packs of 28 capsules. Bottles of 100 capsules.

Further information Nil.

Product licence numbers
Roxiam 150 0017/0281
Roxiam 300 0017/0282.

THEO-DUR*

Presentation A slow release tablet containing Theophylline BP (anhydrous), designed to give therapeutic blood levels over 8–12 hours.
200 mg tablet: Off white mottled flat elliptical scored tablet.
300 mg tablet: Off-white mottled bi-convex oblong scored tablet.

Uses As a bronchodilator in the symptomatic or prophylactic treatment of bronchospasm associated with chronic obstructive airways disease including asthma and chronic bronchitis.

Dosage and administration
Standard dosing
Adults: the usual maintenance dose is one 300 mg tablet 12 hourly.

Children: <35 kg body weight: 100 mg (half a 200 mg tablet) 12 hourly. >35 kg body weight: 200 mg 12 hourly.

Elderly and patients with liver disease: Plasma half life of theophylline may be prolonged and individual dosing should be adopted (see below).

Theophylline clearance is increased in cigarette smokers and such patients may require increased doses of Theo-Dur to achieve a therapeutic effect.

Individual dosing: If sufficient therapeutic effect is not achieved or if side-effects occur, the dose of Theo-Dur may be increased or decreased by 100 mg (half a 200 mg tablet) or 150 mg (half a 300 mg tablet)stages. If doses higher than the usual maintenance doses are to be given, it is recommended that the patient's serum theophylline level is determined and the dose adjusted to maintain this level between 10–20 microgram/ml (55–110 micromols/l). The following procedure is recommended.

Adults: 150 mg (half a 300 mg tablet) 12 hourly for 4–7 days then 300 mg 12 hourly for 7–10 days.

Children: <35 kg body weight: 100 mg (half a 200 mg tablet) 12 hourly for 7–14 days. >35 kg body weight: 100 mg (half a 200 mg tablet) 12 hourly for 4–7 days then 200 mg 12 hourly for 7–10 days.

Blood for theophylline assay should be taken 3–8 hours after a dose when there has been no dosage adjustment for at least 4 days and no doses have been missed for 48 hours. The dose of Theo-Dur may be adjusted as follows:

Peak serum theophylline level	*Dosage adjustment*
<7.9 microgram/ml	Increase dose by 50%.*
8–9.9 microgram/ml	Increase dose by 20%* to the nearest 50 mg.
10–13.9 microgram/ml	If the patient's symptoms persist, increase the dose by 10% to the nearest 50 mg.

14–19.9 microgram/ml	Do not adjust the dose unless side-effects occur in which case a 10% decrease, to the nearest 50 mg may be necessary.
20–24.9 microgram/ml	Decrease dose by 10% to the nearest 50 mg.
25–29.9 microgram/ml	Miss next dose and decrease maintenance dose by 25%.*
>30 microgram/ml	Miss next two doses and decrease maintenance dose by 50%*.

* With patients falling into these categories it is advisable to re-check the serum theophylline concentration 3–5 days after dosage adjustment.

Nocturnal asthma: For the control of symptoms of nocturnal asthma the appropriately individualised dosage of Theo-Dur should be administered once daily at approximately 8 p.m.

Note:

1. The tablet must not be crushed or chewed but swallowed whole or as a half.
2. Any previous theophylline or aminophylline therapy should be discontinued.
3. If a patient has not previously been treated with theophylline or aminophylline, it is advisable to give half the maintenance dose of Theo-Dur (100 mg or 150mg) for the first 4–7 days of treatment. This procedure should reduce the incidence of side-effects.

It is not possible to ensure bioequivalence between different sustained release theophylline products. It should therefore be emphasised that patients once titrated to an effective dose should not be changed from Theo-dur tablets to other sustained release preparations or vice versa without retitration and clinical assessment.

After an effective therapeutic regime is attained, it is important that practitioners, pharmacists and patients are aware of the possible dangers of inefficacy or toxicity if an alternative sustained release theophylline preparation is substituted. This may be a particular hazard because the products are available without prescription. Likewise there may be a hazard if the doctor prescribes "generically" or if the preparation used in hospital is unknown by the general practitioner.

Contra-indications, warnings, etc
Contra-indications: None known.

Precautions: Theophylline should be given with caution to patients with congestive heart failure, liver disease or viral infections, and in the elderly. Plasma half-life of theophylline is prolonged in most of these patients, and the drug may accumulate to toxic concentrations.

Use in pregnancy and lactation: Caution is recommended during pregnancy and lactation. When theophylline is prescribed to pregnant and nursing women, the risk-benefit of the treatment must be taken into account.

Theophylline crosses the placenta, but no influence on foetal development or reproductive capacity has been established. Theophylline should not be used routinely in nursing women even though only very small amounts of theophylline are excreted into breast milk.

Premature children with low birthweight have an extremely prolonged theophylline half-life, which may lead to high theophylline plasma levels causing insomnia, agitation and/or anxiety. Full capacity to eliminate theophylline is not reached until the age of 6–12 months. Caution should be used when theophylline is given to infants who cannot complain of minor adverse reactions.

Side-effects: Side-effects of theophylline depend to a great extent on serum concentration and are frequent only at theophylline concentration exceeding 20 micrograms/ml. The Theo-Dur slow-release formulation reduces fluctuation in serum levels of theophylline, thereby reducing the incidence of side-effects.

The most common side-effects are gastro-intestinal disturbances (nausea, vomiting and anorexia) which, in most cases, disappear on reducing the dose. Monitoring of the serum concentration of theophylline is recommended.

The CNS stimulating effect of theophylline can cause restlessness, irritability, anxiety and insomnia in some patients. Cardiovascular effects such as palpitations and tachycardia may appear.

Severe side-effects (cramps, convulsions and supraventricular tachycardia) may appear at very high serum concentration, in which case the medication should be discontinued.

Drug interactions: The plasma theophylline concentration may increase in patients receiving cimetidine, quinolone derivatives such as ciprofloxacin or macrolide antibiotics such as erythromycin and troleandomycin, concurrently with theophylline preparations. Increase in the theophylline plasma concentration is also seen with oestrogen, allopurinol and propranolol. The serum concentration may be reduced during concurrent therapy with phenobarbital, phenytoin and rifampicin as these drugs may increase theophylline clearance. Theophylline has been shown to decrease the plasma concentration of lithium.

Concurrent administration of ketamine with theophylline may reduce the threshold value for inducing convulsions.

Xanthines may potentiate hypokalaemia resulting from beta$_2$-agonist therapy, steroids, diuretics and hypoxia. Particular caution is advised in severe asthma. It is recommended that serum potassium levels are monitored in such situations.

Treatment of overdosage: Gastric lavage and symptomatic treatment to maintain fluid and electrolyte balance. Give oxygen as necessary. Monitor serum theophylline levels. Oral activated charcoal may reduce serum theophylline concentration. In severe cases charcoal haemoperfusion may be required. Tablets in the intestine may continue to release theophylline for several hours.

Possible signs and symptoms of overdosage are insomnia, anorexia, agitation, anxiety, nausea, vomiting, convulsions, hypotension, palpitations, tachycadia and cardiac arrhythmias. Serious toxicity is not always preceded by less severe adverse effects.

Pharmaceutical precautions Nil.

Legal category P.

Package quantities 100 tablets.

Further information Theophylline clearance is decreased in patients with hepatic cirrhosis, congestive heart failure, acute pulmonary oedema, acute febrile illness, concomitant administration of erythromycin, cimetidine or influenza vaccine; in these circumstances, patients may require a reduced dose of Theo-Dur to avoid the occurrence of side-effects.

If a patient taking an oral theophylline preparation develops acute asthma, intravenous aminophylline should not be administered unless the serum theophylline level is known.

In patients with congestive heart failure associated with chronic obstructive airways disease, theophylline treatment may be of additional benefit because of its cardiac stimulant effect.

Product licence numbers
200 mg 0017/0098.
300 mg 0017/0099.

TONOCARD*

Presentation Yellow, biconvex, film coated tablets containing tocainide hydrochloride, either 400 mg (coded A/TT).

Inactive ingredients: Methyl cellulose, magnesium stearate, hydroxypropylmethylcellulose, polyethylene glycol, titanium dioxide, iron oxide yellow and paraffin powder.

Injection vials of 15 ml, each 1 ml of clear aqueous sterile solution for injection contains 50 mg tocainide hydrochloride.

Uses For the treatment of patients with life-threatening symptomatic ventricular tachyarrhythmias associated with severely compromised left ventricular function who do not respond to other therapy or for whom other therapy is contra-indicated.

Dosage and administration *Acute Treatment:* 500–750 mg by infusion or by slow intravenous injection given over 15–30 minutes, followed immediately by 600–800 mg orally.

Maintenance treatment: 8 hours after acute treatment, commence maintenance therapy with 1200 mg daily, divided into two or three oral doses.

Chronic ventricular tachyarrhythmias: 1200 mg daily, divided into two or three oral doses.

The oral daily dosage of Tonocard may be increased to 1800–2400 mg in divided doses, if necessary.

Not to be administered to children.

Elderly: Dosage reduction may be necessary if renal disease is present.

In patients with severe renal insufficiency (creatinine clearance <30 ml/min) the dose should be reduced to 800 mg/day (400 mg every 12 hours). If treatment is indicated in patients with total renal insufficiency or severe hepatic insufficiency the initial dose should be reduced to 600 mg daily.

Contra-indications, warnings, etc *Contra-indications:* Known hypersensitivity to amide drugs. Second or third degree AV block, in the absence of a pacemaker.

Precautions: Tonocard therapy should only be instituted when facilities are available for regular monitoring of blood counts.

Agranulocytosis, bone marrow depression, leucopenia, neutropenia, aplastic hypoplastic anaemia and thrombocytopenia have been reported in patients receiving Tonocard; the incidence of neutropenia may be as high as 1 in 300. Fatalities have occurred. Patients should be instructed to promptly report the development of bruising or bleeding and any signs of infection such as fever, sore throat or chills. Since most of these events have been noted during the first 12 weeks of therapy, it is recommended that blood counts be performed weekly during this period, and monthly thereafter. If any of these haematological disorders are identified, specialist advice should be sought with a view to discontinuing Tonocard therapy and substituting other appropriate treatment.

Pulmonary fibrosis, interstitial pneumonitis and fibrosing alveolitis have been reported in patients receiving Tonocard and fatalities have occurred. The cases are usually characterised by bilateral infiltrates on X-ray, frequently associated with dyspnoea and cough. Fever may or may not be present. The condition may be confused with pulmonary oedema or pneumonia. Patients should be instructed to promptly report the development of any pulmonary symptoms such as exertional dyspnoea, cough or wheezing. Chest X-rays are advisable at that time. If any of these pulmonary disorders is confirmed, specialist advice should be sought with a view to discontinuing Tonocard therapy and substituting other appropriate treatment.

Like other drugs, Tonocard should be used with caution in patients with severe hepatic or renal disease and in the elderly because of the potential risk of accumulation. Caution is also advised in patients with uncompensated heart failure and in patients receiving other antiarrhythmic agents.

Like other antiarrhythmic drugs, Tonocard may aggravate arrhythmias in some patients.

Hypokalaemia reduces the antiarrhythmic effects of tocainide and should be corrected, if possible, before the initiation of treatment.

Use in pregnancy: Reproduction studies in animals have shown maternal and foetal toxicity. The safety of Tonocard in human pregnancy has not been tested and the potential benefit should be weighed against possible hazard.

It is not known whether tocainide is excreted in breast milk.

Side-effects: Reported side effects are mainly neurological or gastro-intestinal. CNS symptoms are usually dose-related and may include tremor, dizziness, lightheadedness, paraesthesia, visual hallucinations and convulsions. Gastro-intestinal symptoms include nausea and vomiting. Abnormal liver function tests, hepatitis and jaundice have been reported. Fever and skin reactions have also been reported. The skin reactions include rash, Steven Johnson syndrome and exfoliative dermatitis. Bradycardia and hypotension may occur after i.v. injection. Positive ANF titres, clinical manifestation of lupus erythematous syndrome and fibrosing alveolitis have been reported during Tonocard therapy. Agranulocytosis, aplastic anaemia and thrombocytopenia have occurred (see 'Precautions'). Pulmonary fibrosis has been reported (see 'Precautions').

Interactions: Caution should be exercised in the use of multiple drug therapy. Specific interaction studies with digoxin and metoprolol have been conducted. No clinically significant interaction was seen with digoxin, but tocainide and metoprolol had additive effects, increasing pulmonary wedge pressure and reducing cardiac index.

Tocainide has been use clinically with digitalis and other antiarrhythmic agents (lignocaine, quinidine, disopyramide, procainamide) as well as beta-blocking agents, without evidence of untoward effects. However, concurrent use of tocainide and lignocaine may lead to potentiation of CNS effects.

Overdosage: Poisoning due to an overdose of Tonocard may lead to CNS excitation with paraesthesia, muscle twitching and convulsions, atrioventricular block, sinoatrial block or arrest, asystole, myocardial depression, severe hypotension and cardiac arrest.

Treatment should include close mointoring of cardiovascular and respiratory function and electrolytes. Further absorption may be prevented by induction of vomiting, gastric lavage or administration of activated charcoal if ingestion is recent. If convulsions occur, maintenance of a patent airway is mandatory and assisted or controlled ventilation with oxygen may be required. Convulsions may be controlled with intravenous diazepam or a short-acting barbiturate.

Cardiovascular complications should be treated symptomatically, which may require the use of sympathomimetic agents (e.g. noradrenaline, metaraminol), or inotropic agents (e.g. dopamine, dobutamine). Temporary pacing may be required for AV block and intravenous sodium bicarbonate to correct acidosis.

Tocainide can be removed by haemodialysis and probably also by charcoal column haemoperfusion.

Due to the relatively long half-life of tocainide, treatment of overdosage may be required for an extended period.

Pharmaceutical precautions Recommended diluents for i.v. injection (50 mg/ml) are sodium chloride injection or 5% dextrose injection.

Legal category POM.

Package quantities *Tablets:* 400 mg, bottle of 100 tablets.

Injection: Packs of 5 × 15 ml injection vials 50 mg/ml.

Further information Tonocard is a primary amine analogue of lignocaine, with a high oral bioavailability. Its electrophysiological properties are similar to lignocaine and, as such, Tonocard has been shown to be effective in the treatment of ventricular arrhythmias. In therapeutic plasma concentration, no clinically significant adverse haemodynamic changes have been reported, even in patients with acute myocardial infarction or those pre-treated with beta-blockers.

Product licence numbers

400 mg tablets	0017/0106
50 mg/ml I.V. Injection	0017/0108

XYLOCAINE*

Presentation A sterile clear aqueous solution of Lignocaine Hydrochloride BP. Each ml contains:

0.5% solution: Lidocaine hydrochloride PhEur 5.35 mg equivalent to lidocaine hydrochloride anhydrous 5 mg.

1.0% solution: Lidocaine hydrochloride PhEur 10.7 mg equivalent to lidocaine hydrochloride anhydrous 10 mg.
1.5% solution: Lidocaine hydrochloride PhEur 16 mg equivalent to lidocaine hydrochloride anhydrous 15 mg.
2% solution: Lidocaine hydrochloride PhEur 21.4 mg equivalent to lidocaine hydrochloride anhydrous 20 mg.

All the above contain sodium chloride to produce isotonic solutions.

Uses Xylocaine is a local anaesthetic solution for use in infiltration anaesthesia, intravenous regional anaesthesia and nerve blocks.

Dosage and administration The dosage is adjusted according to the response of the patient and site of administration. The lowest concentration and smallest dose producing the required effect should be given. The maximum dose for healthy adults should not exceed 200 mg.

Children and elderly or debilitated patients require smaller doses, commensurate with age and physical status.

Contra-indications, warnings, etc Known hypersensitivity to anaesthetics of the amide type.

Precautions: In common with other local anaesthetics, Xylocaine should be used cautiously in patients with epilepsy, impaired cardiac conduction, bradycardia, impaired respiratory function, and in patients with impaired hepatic function, if the dose or site of administration is likely to result in high blood levels.

Facilities for resuscitation should be available when local anaesthetics are administered.

The effect of local anaesthetics may be reduced if an injection is made into an inflamed or infected area.

Use in pregnancy: Although there is no evidence from animal studies of harm to the foetus, as with all drugs, Xylocaine should not be given during early pregnancy unless the benefits are considered to outweigh the risks.

Side-effects: In common with other local anaesthetics, adverse reactions to Xylocaine are rare and are usually the result of excessively high blood concentrations due to inadvertent intravascular injection, excessive dosage, rapid absorption or occasionally to hypersensitivity, idiosyncracy or diminished tolerance on the part of the patient. In such circumstances systemic effects occur involving the central nervous system and/or the cardiovascular system.

CNS reactions are excitatory and/or depressant, and may be characterized by nervousness, dizziness, blurred vision and tremors, followed by drowsiness, convulsions, unconsciousness and possibly respiratory arrest. The excitatory reactions may be very brief or may not occur at all, in which case the first manifestations of toxicity may be drowsiness, merging into unconsciousness and respiratory arrest. Cardiovascular reactions are depressant, and may be characterized by hypotension, myocardial depression, bradycardia and possibly cardiac arrest.

Allergic reactions are extremely rare. They may be characterized by cutaneous lesions, urticaria, oedema or anaphylactoid reactions. Detection of sensitivity by skin testing is of doubtful value.

Hypotension may occur as a physiological response to central nerve blocks.

Interactions: Cimetidine can impair the metabolism of lidocaine absorbed into the circulation. Elimination will be delayed and the risk of adverse reactions increased.

Pharmaceutical precautions Store at room temperature.

Legal category POM.

Package quantities
Vials:
0.5% solution – 20 ml. Packs of 5 vials.
1.0% solution – 20 ml. Packs of 5 vials.
2.0% solution – 20 ml. Packs of 5 vials.
Ampoules:
1.5% solution – 25 ml.

Further information Multidose vials of Xylocaine contain methylparahydroxybenzoate PhEur 1 mg/ml.

Product licence numbers
Vials
0.5% 0017/5031R
1.0% 0017/5032R
2.0% 0017/5034R
Ampoules
1.5% 0017/5033R

XYLOCAINE* WITH ADRENALINE 1:200,000

Presentation A sterile clear aqueous solution of Lignocaine Hydrochloride BP. Each ml contains:

0.5% solution: Lignocaine hydrochloride anhydrous 5 mg equivalent to Lignocaine Hydrochloride BP 5.35 mg, Adrenaline Tartrate PhEur 10 micrograms equivalent to adrenaline 5 micrograms.
1% solution: Lignocaine hydrochloride anhydrous 10 mg equivalent to Lignocaine Hydrochloride BP 10.70 mg, Adrenaline Tartrate PhEur 10 micrograms equivalent to adrenaline 5 micrograms.
2% solution: Lignocaine hydrochloride anhydrous 20 mg equivalent to Lignocaine Hydrochloride BP 21.40 mg, Adrenaline Tartrate PhEur 10 micrograms equivalent to adrenaline 5 micrograms.

Inactive ingredients: Sodium chloride, sodium metabisulphite, methyl parahydroxybensoate.

Uses Xylocaine with Adrenaline is a local anaesthetic solution for use in infiltration anaesthesia and nerve blocks.

Dosage and administration The dosage is adjusted according to the response of the patient and the site of administration. The lowest concentration and smallest dose producing the required effect should be given. The maximum single dose of Xylocaine when given with adrenaline is 500 mg.

Children and elderly or debilitated patients require smaller doses, commensurate with age and physical status.

Contra-indications, warnings, etc Known hypersensitivity to anaesthetics of the amide type.

The use of a vasoconstrictor is contra-indicated for anaesthesia of fingers, toes, tip of nose, ears and penis.

Xylocaine with adrenaline should not be given intravenously.

Precautions: In common with other local anaesthetics, Xylocaine with adrenaline should be used cautiously in patients with epilepsy, impaired cardiac conduction, impaired respiratory function, and in patients with impaired hepatic function, if the dose or site of administration is likely to result in high blood levels.

Facilities for resuscitation should be available when local anaesthetics are administered.

The effect of local anaesthetics may be reduced if an injection is made into an inflamed or infected area.

Solutions containing adrenaline should be used with caution in patients with hypertension, cardiac disease, cerebrovascular insufficiency, thyrotoxicosis, in patients taking tricyclic antidepressants, MAOI's, or receiving potent general anaesthetic agents.

Solutions containing adrenaline should be used where possible so as to prolong anaesthesia and reduce systemic absorption. This is particularly important in highly vascular areas.

Use in pregnancy: Although there is no evidence from animal studies of harm to the foetus, as with all drugs, Xylocaine should not be given during early pregnancy unless the benefits are considered to outweigh the risks.

Side-effects: In common with other local anaesthetics,

adverse reactions to Xylocaine with adrenaline are rare and are usually the result of excessively high blood concentrations due to inadvertent intravascular injection, excessive dosage, rapid absorption or occasionally to hypersensitivity, idiosyncracy or diminished tolerance on the part of the patient. In such circumstances systemic effects occur involving the central nervous system and/or the cardiovascular system.

CNS reactions are excitatory and/or depressant, and may be characterized by nervousness, dizziness, blurred vision and tremors, followed by drowsiness, convulsions, unconsciousness and possibly respiratory arrest. The excitatory reactions may be very brief or may not occur at all, in which case the first manifestations of toxicity may be drowsiness, merging into unconsciousness and respiratory arrest.

Cardiovascular reactions are depressant, and may be characterized by hypotension, myocardial depression, bradycardia and posssibly cardiac arrest.

Allergic reactions are extremely rare. They may be characterized by cutaneous lesions, urticaria, oedema or anaphylactoid reactions. Detection of sensitivity by skin testing is of doubtful value.

Hypotension may occur as a physiological response to central nerve blocks.

Pharmaceutical precautions Store at room temperature.

Legal category POM.

Package quantities
0.5% with adrenaline 20 ml. Packs of 5 vials
1.0% with adrenaline 20 ml. Packs of 5 vials
2.0% with adrenaline 20 ml. Packs of 5 vials

Further information Multidose vial preparations of Xylocaine with adrenaline 1 : 200,000 contain methylhydroxybenzoate 1 mg/ml.

Product licence numbers
Vials
0.5% 0017/5028R
1.0% 0017/5029R
2.0% 0017/5030R

XYLOCAINE* 2% WITH ADRENALINE 1 : 80,000

Presentation Sterile, clear aqueous solution. Each ml contains Lignocaine Hydrochloride Anhydrous BP 20 mg/ml equivalent to Lignocaine Hydrochloride BP 21.4 mg/ml and Adrenaline Tartrate EP 22.7 micrograms equivalent to adrenaline 12.5 micrograms.

Inactive ingredients: Sodium chloride to produce an isotonic solution, sodium metabisulphite, sodium hydroxide and hydrochloric acid.

Uses Xylocaine 2% with adrenaline is a local anaesthetic solution for use in dental infiltration anaesthesia and all dental nerve-block techniques.

Dosage and administration Infiltration – usual dose is 1 ml. Nerve block – usual dose is 1.5 to 2 ml.

The recommended maximum dose for Xylocaine when given with adrenaline is 500 mg.

Children and elderly or debilitated patients require smaller doses.

Contra-indications, warnings, etc Known hypersensitivity to anaesthetics of the amide type.

The use of a vasoconstrictor is contra-indicated for anaesthesia of fingers, toes, tip of nose, ears and penis.

Xylocaine with adrenaline should not be given intravenously.

Precautions: In common with other local anaesthetics, Xylocaine with adrenaline should be used cautiously in patients with epilepsy, impaired cardiac conduction, impaired respiratory function, and in patients with impaired hepatic function if the dose or site of administration is likely to result in high blood levels.

Facilities for resuscitation should be available when local anaesthetics are administered.

The effect of local anaesthetics may be reduced if an injection is made into an inflamed or infected area. Solutions containing adrenaline should be used with caution in patients with hypertension, cardiac disease, cerebrovascular insufficiency, thyrotoxicosis.

Solutions containing adrenaline should be used where possible so as to prolong anaesthesia and reduce systemic absorption. This is particularly important in highly vascular areas.

Use on one patient during one treatment only.

Use in pregnancy and lactation: Although there is no evidence from animal studies of harm to the foetus, as with all drugs lignocaine should not be given in early pregnancy unless the benefits are considered to outweigh the risks.

Adverse reactions: In common with other local anaesthetics, adverse reactions to Xylocaine with adrenaline are extremely rare in dental practice and are usually the result of excessively high blood concentrations due to inadvertent intravascular injection, excessive dosage, rapid absorption or occasionally to hypersensitivity, idiosyncracy or diminished tolerance on the part of the patient. In such circumstances systemic effects occur involving the central nervous system and/or the cardiovascular system.

CNS reactions are excitatory and/or depressant, and may be characterised by nervousness, dizziness, blurred vision and tremors, followed by drowsiness, convulsions, unconsciousness and possibly respiratory arrest. The excitatory reactions may be very brief or may not occur at all, in which case the first manifestations of toxicity may be drowsiness, merging into unconsciousness and respiratory arrest.

Cardiovascular reactions are depressant, and may be characterized by hypotension, myocardial depression, bradycardia and possibly cardiac arrest.

Allergic reactions are extremely rare. They may be characterized by cutaneous lesions, urticaria, oedema or anaphylactoid reactions. Detection of sensitivity by skin testing is of doubtful value.

Pharmaceutical precautions Store in a cool place.

Legal category POM.

Package quantities Glass cartridges of 2 ml standard and 2 ml self-aspirating, in boxes of 100.

Further information Dental cartridges of Xylocaine 2% with adrenaline 1 : 80,000 do not contain an antimicrobial agent.

Product licence number 0017/5027R.

XYLOCAINE* ANTISEPTIC GEL

Presentation Clear sterile viscous gel. Each millilitre contains Lignocaine Hydrochloride BP 21.4 mg (equivalent to 20 mg lignocaine hydrochloride anhydrous), Chlorhexidine Gluconate Solution BPC 0.0025 ml in a water-miscible base.

Inactive ingredients: Hydroxypropylmethyl cellulose, sodium hydroxide.

Uses Anaesthetic gel for anaesthesia of the urethra and topical application on mucous membrane wherever an anaesthetic/antiseptic effect is required.

Dosage and administration *Men:* 10 ml injected initially, followed by 3–5 ml.

Women: 3–5 ml injected into the urethra.

Contra-indications, warnings, etc Known hypersensitivity to anaesthetics of the amide type.

Warning: Care should be taken to avoid instillation of excessive amounts of Xylocaine antiseptic gel into the rectum. This is of particular importance in infants and children. Systemic absorption of lignocaine may occur from the rectum and large doses may result in CNS side effects. On rare occasions convulsions have occurred in children.

Pharmaceutical precautions Store in a cool place.

Legal category P.

Package quantities 20 g tubes and 20 g Accordion* Syringes.

Further information The use of an Accordion syringe pack eliminates the necessity to attach a separate nozzle prior to catheterisation.

Product licence numbers

Tubes	0017/0244
Accordion Syringe	0017/5035

XYLOCAINE* GEL

Presentation A topical anaesthetic for urological procedures and lubrication of endotracheal tubes. 1 g Xylocaine Gel contains:

Active constituent: Lidocaine hydrochloride monohydrate for injection EP corresponding to lidocaine hydrochloride 20 mg.

Inactive constituents: Hydroxypropyl methylcellulose EP, sodium hydroxide qs, hydrochloric acid qs, water, purified EP q.s.

Uses

Action: Xylocaine Gel 2% provides prompt and profound anaesthesia of mucous membranes and lubrication which reduces friction. Its water miscible base, characterised by high viscosity and low surface tension, brings the anaesthetic into intimate and prolonged contact with the tissue for effective anaesthesia of long duration (approx. 20–30 min).

Anaesthesia usually occurs rapidly (within 5 minutes depending upon area of application).

The active ingredient of Xylocaine Gel 2% is lidocaine, which stabilises the neuronal membrane and prevents the initiation and conduction of nerve impulses, thereby affecting local anaesthetic action. Lidocaine is absorbed following application to mucous membranes. The absorption occurs most rapidly after intratracheal administration. Blood concentrations of lidocaine after instillation in urethra of doses up to 800 mg are of low range and below toxic levels. The metabolism of lidocaine takes place in the liver and metabolites and unchanged drug are excreted by the kidney.

Indications: Surface anaesthesia and lubrication:

- The male and female urethra during cystoscopy, catheterisation, exploration by sound and other endourethral operations.
- Nasal and pharyngial cavities in endoscopic procedures such as gastroscopy and bronchoscopy.
- During proctoscopy and rectoscopy.
- Intubation.

Symptomatic treatment of pain in connection with cystitis and urethritis.

Dosage and administration As with any local anaesthetic, reactions and complications are best averted by employing the minimal effective dosage. Debilitated, elderly patients and children should be given doses commensurate with their age and physical condition.

Urethral anaesthesia: Surface anaesthesia of the male adult urethra: For adequate analgesia in males 20 ml (= 400 mg lidocaine hydrochloride) jelly is required. The jelly is instilled slowly until almost half the syringe (10 ml = 200 mg lidocaine hydrochloride) is emptied. A penile clamp is then applied for several minutes at the corona; then the rest of the jelly is instilled.

When anaesthesia is especially important, e.g. during sounding or cystoscopy, a larger quantity of jelly, for example 30–40 ml, may be instilled in 3–4 portions and allowed to work for 10–12 minutes before insertion of the instrument.

Surface anaesthesia of the female adult urethra: Instil 5–10 ml in small portions to fill the whole urethra. In order to obtain adequate anaesthesia, several minutes should be allowed prior to performing urological procedures.

Endoscopy: Instillation of 10–20 ml is recommended for adequate analgesia and a small amount should be applied on the instrument for lubrication.

Lubrication for endotracheal intubation: About 5 ml applied on the surface of the tube just prior to insertion. Care should be taken to avoid introducing the product into the lumen of the tube.

Contra-indications, warnings, etc

Contra-indications: Known history of hypersensitivity to local anaesthetics of the amide type or other components of the gel.

Precautions: Absorption from wound surfaces and mucous membranes is relatively high, especially in the bronchial tree. Xylocaine Gel should be used with caution in patients with traumatised mucosa and/or sepsis in the region of the proposed application.

If the dose or site of administration is likely to result in high blood levels, lidocaine, in common with other local anaesthetics, should be used cautiously in patients with epilepsy, impaired cardiac condition, bradycardia, impaired hepatic function and in severe shock.

The use of oral topical anaesthetic agents may interfere with swallowing and thus enhance the danger of aspiration. This is particularly important in children because of their frequency of eating. Numbness of the tongue or buccal mucosa may increase the danger of biting trauma.

When used for endotracheal tube lubrication care should be taken to avoid introduction of the jelly into the lumen of the tube. The jelly may dry on the inner surface leaving residue which tend to clump with flexion, narrowing the lumen. There have been rare reports in which this residue has caused the lumen to occlude.

Care should be taken to avoid instillation of excessive amounts of Xylocaine Gel into the rectum. This is of particular importance in infants and children. Systemic absorption of lidocaine may occur from the rectum, and large doses may result in CNS side-effects. On rare occasions convulsions have occurred in children.

Pregnancy: Although there is no evidence from animal studies of harm to the foetus, as with all drugs, Xylocaine should not be given during early pregnancy unless the benefits outweight the risks.

Lactation: Lidocaine enters the mother's milk, but in such small quantities that there is generally no risk of affecting the child at therapeutic dose levels.

Side-effects: In extremely rare cases local anaesthetic preparations have been associated with allergic reactions (in the most severe instances anaphylactic shock).

Systemic adverse reactions are rare and may result from high plasma levels due to excessive dosage, rapid absorption or may result from hypersensitivity, idiosyncracy or diminished tolerance on the part of the patient. Such reactions involve the central nervous system and/or the cardiovascular system.

CNS reactions are excitatory and/or depressant and may be characterised by nervousness, dizziness, convulsions, unconsciousness and, possibly, respiratory arrest. The excitatory reactions may be very brief or may not occur at all, in which case the first manifestations of toxicity may be drowsiness, merging into unconsciousness and respiratory arrest.

Cardiovascular reactions are depressant and may be characterised by hypotension, myocardial depression, bradycardia and possibly cardiac arrest.

Interaction: Lidocaine should be used with caution in patients receiving antiarrhythmic drugs, such as tocainide, since the toxic effects are additive.

Overdosage: Treatment of a patient with toxic manifestations consists of ensuring adequate ventilation and arresting convulsions. Ventilation should be maintained with oxygen by assisted or controlled respiration as required. If convulsions occur, they should be treated rapidly by intravenous administration of succinylcholine 50–100 mg and/or 5–15 mg diazepam. As succinylcholine will arrest respiration it should only be used if the clinician has the ability to perform endotracheal intubation and to manage a totally paralysed patient. Thiopentone may also be used to abort convulsions in dosage

100–200 mg. If ventricular fibrillation or cardiac arrest occurs effective cardiovascular resuscitation must be instituted. Adrenaline in repeated doses and sodium bicarbonate should be given as rapidly as possible.

Pharmaceutical precautions Xylocaine Accordion Gel is sterile and is meant for single use only.

Legal category P.

Package quantities Packs of 10 × 20 g Accordion Syringes. 20 g tubes.

Further information Nil.

Product licence numbers

Tubes	0017/0242
Accordion Syringe	0017/5037R.

XYLOCAINE* OINTMENT 5%

Presentation A water-soluble topical anaesthetic ointment.

1 g Xylocaine Ointment contains: Lignocaine 50 mg, propylene glycol, polyethylene glycols, water purif. q.s.

Uses

Action: Xylocaine Ointment contains lignocaine which is dissolved in a vehicle consisting of carbowaxes and propylene glycol. Lignocaine penetrates the tissues and exerts a topical anaesthetic effect. The onset of action is 3–5 minutes on mucous membrane. It is ineffective when applied to intact skin. Propylene glycol in the ointment base has an antibacterial effect against many pathogenic microrganisms. The carbowax base melts readily at body temperature and spreads evenly. The ointment is easily removed with water.

Lignocaine stabilises the neuronal membrane and prevents the initiation and conduction of nerve impulses effecting local anaesthetic action. Lignocaine is absorbed following the application to mucous membranes. The absorption occurs most rapidly after intratracheal administration. The metabolism of lignocaine takes place in the liver and metabolites and unchanged drug are excreted by the kidney.

Indications: Temporary relief of pain associated with minor burns and abrasions of the skin, e.g. sunburn, herpes zoster and labialis, pruritus, sore nipples, insect bites.

Anaesthesia of mucous membranes, e.g. various anal conditions such as haemorrhoids and fissures.

For the alleviation of pain during examination and instrumentation, e.g. proctoscopy, sigmoidoscopy, cystocopy, endotracheal intubation.

Dentistry: Surface anaesthesia of the gums prior to injection, before deep scaling and in conjunction with the fitting of new dentures.

Dosage and administration As with any local anaesthetic, reactions and complications are best averted by employing the minimal effective dosage. Debilitated, elderly patients and children should be given dosage commensurate with their age and physical condition.

The ointment should be applied in a thin layer for adequate control of symptoms. A sterile gauze pad is suggested for application to broken and burned tissue.

Apply to tube prior to endotracheal intubation.

In dentistry, apply to previously dried oral mucosa, allow at least 3-5 minutes for anaesthesia to become effective. When inserting new dentures, apply to all denture surfaces contacting mucosa.

For tender nipples, apply on a small piece of gauze; the ointment must be washed away before next feeding.

Not more than 35 g of the ointment should be administered in any 24 hour period.

Contra-indications, warnings, etc

Contra-indications: Known history of hypersensitivity to local anaesthetics of the amide type or to other components of the ointment.

Precautions: Absorption from wound surfaces and mucous membranes is relatively high, especially in the bronchial tree. This should be taken into special consideration when the ointment is used in children for treatment of large areas.

Xylocaine ointment should be used with caution in patients with traumatized mucosa and/or sepsis in the region at the proposed application.

If the dose or site of administration is likely to result in high blood levels, lignocaine, in common with other local anaesthetics should be used cautiously in patients with epilepsy, impaired cardiac condition, bradycardia, impaired hepatic function and in severe shock.

The use of oral topical anaesthetic agents may interfere with swallowing and thus enhance the danger of aspiration. This is particularly important in children because of their frequency of eating. Numbness of the tongue or buccal mucosa may increase the danger of biting trauma.

When used for endotracheal tube lubrication care should be taken to avoid introduction of the ointment into the lumen of the tube. The ointment may dry on the inner surface leaving residue which tend to clump with flexion, narrowing the lumen. There have been rare reports in which this residue has caused the lumen to occlude.

Pregnancy: There is no or inadequate evidence of safety of the drug in human pregnancy but it has been in wide use for many years without apparent ill consequence, animal studies have shown no hazard. If drug therapy is need in pregnancy, thus drug can be used if there is no safer alternative.

Lactation: Lignocaine enters the mother's milk, but in such small quantities that there is generally no risk of affecting the child at therapeutic dose levels.

Side-effects: In extremely rare cases local anaesthetic preparations have been associated with allergic reactions (in the most severe instances anaphylactic shock).

Systemic adverse reactions are rare and may result from high plasma levels due to excessive dosage, rapid absorption or may result from hypersensitivity, idiosyncracy or diminished tolerance on the part of the patient. Such reactions involve the central nervous system and/or the cardiovascular system.

CNS reactions are excitatory and/or depressant, and may be characterised by nervousness, dizziness, convulsions, unconsciousness and possible respiratory arrest. The excitatory reactions may be very brief or may not occur at all, in which case the first manifestations of toxicity may be drowsiness, merging into unconsciousness and respiratory arrest.

Cardiovascular reactions are depressant, and may be characterised by hypotension, myocardial depression, bradycardia and possibly cardiac arrest.

Interaction: Lignocaine should be used with caution in patients receiving antiarrhythmic drugs, such as tocainide, since the toxic effects are additive.

Overdosage: Treatment of a patient with toxic manifestations consists of ensuring adequate ventilation and arresting convulsions. Ventilation should be maintained with oxygen by assisted or controlled respiration as required. If convulsions occur, they should be treated rapidly by intravenous administration of succinylcholine 50–100 mg and/or 5–15 mg diazepam. As succinylcholine will arrest respiration it should only be used if the clinician has the ability to perform endotracheal intubation and to manage a totally paralysed patient. Thiopentone may also be used to abort convulsions in doage 100–200 mg. If ventricular fibrillation or cardiac arrest occurs, effective cardiovascular resuscitation must be instituted. Adrenaline in repeated doses and sodium bicarbonate should be given as rapidly as possible.

Pharmaceutical precautions Store at room temperature.

Legal category P.

Package quantities 15 g tubes.

Further information Nil.

Product licence number 0017/5038R.

XYLOCAINE* SPRAY

Presentation Topical anaesthetic aerosol containing lignocaine 10.378% w/w.

Inactive ingredients: Cetyl pyridiniumchloride, polyethylene glycol, trichloro- and dichlorofluoromethane, alcohol, menthol, cineole.

Uses For the prevention of pain associated with the following procedures:

Otorhinolaryngology: Puncture of the maxillary sinus and minor surgical procedures in the nasal cavity, pharynx and epipharynx.

Paracentesis.

Obstetrics: During the final stages of delivery and before episiotomy and perineal suturing as supplementary pain control.

Introduction of instruments and catheters into the respiratory and digestive tract: Provides surface anaesthesia for the otopharyngeal and tracheal areas to reduce reflex activity, attentuate haemodynamic response and to facilitate insertion of the tube or the passage of instruments during endotracheal intubation, laryngoscopy, bronchoscopy and oesophagoscopy.

Dental practice: Before injections, dental impressions, X-ray photography, removal of calculus, seating or adjustment of dentures.

Dosage and administration As with any local anaesthetic, reactions and complications are best averted by employing the minimal effective dosage. Debilitated or elderly patients and children should be given doses commensurate with their age and physical condition.

Each activation of the metered dose valve delivers 10 mg lignocaine base. It is unnecessary to dry the site prior to application. No more than 20 spray applications should be used in any adult to produce the desired anaesthetic effect.

The number of sprays depend on the extent of the area to be anaesthetised.

Dental practice: 1–5 applications to the mucous membranes.

Otorhinolaryngology: 3 applications for puncture of the maxillary sinus.

During delivery: Up to 20 applications (200 mg lignocaine base).

Introduction of instruments and catheters into the respiratory and digestive tract: Up to 20 applications (200 mg lignocaine base) for procedures in pharynx, larynx, and trachea.

Contra-indications, warnings, etc

Contra-indications: Known history of hypersensitivity to local anaesthetics of the amide type or to other components of the spray solution.

Precautions: Absorption from wound surfaces and mucous membranes is relatively high, especially in the bronchial tree. Xylocaine Spray should be used with caution in patients with traumatised mucosa and/or sepsis in the region of the proposed application.

If the dose or site of administration is likely to result in high blood levels, lignocaine, in common with other local anaesthetics, should be used with caution in patients with epilepsy, impaired cardiac conduction, bradycardia, impaired hepatic function and in severe shock.

The oropharyngeal use of topical anaesthetic agents may interfere with swallowing and thus enhance the danger of aspiration. This is particularly important in children because of their frequency of eating. Numbness of the tongue or buccal mucosa may increase the danger of biting trauma.

Avoid contact with the eyes.

Use in pregnancy and lactation: There is no or inadequate evidence of safety of the drug in human pregnancy but it has been in wide use for many years without apparent ill consequence, animal studies having shown no hazard. If drug therapy is needed in pregnancy, this drug can be used if there is no safer alternative.

Lignocaine enters the mother's milk, but in such small quantities that there is generally no risk of the child being affected at therapeutic dose levels.

Side-effects: In extremely rare cases local anaesthetic preparations have been associated with allergic reactions (in the most severe instances anaphylactic shock).

Systemic adverse reactions are extremely rare and may result from high plasma levels due to excessive dosage or rapid absorption or from hypersensitivity, idiosyncracy or reduced tolerance on the part of the patient. Such reactions involve the central nervous system and/or the cardiovascular system.

CNS reactions are excitatory and/or depressant and may be characterised by nervousness, dizziness, convulsions, unconsciousness and possible respiratory arrest. The excitatory reactions may be very brief or may not occur at all, in which case the first manifestations of toxicity may be drowsiness, merging into unconsciousness and respiratory arrest.

Cardiovascular reactions are depressant and may be characterised by hypotension, myocardial depression, bradycardia and possibly cardiac arrest.

Interaction: Lignocaine should be used with caution in patients receiving antiarrhythmic drugs, such as tocainide, since the toxic effects are additive.

Overdosage: The treatment of a patient with toxic manifestations consists of ensuring adequate ventilation and arresting convulsions. Ventilation should be maintained with oxygen by assisted or controlled respiration as required. If convulsions occur, they should be treated rapidly by the intravenous administration of succinylcholine 50–100 mg and/or 5–15 mg diazepam. As succinylcholine will arrest respiration, it should only be used if the clinician has the ability to perform endotracheal intubation and to manage a totally paralysed patient. Thiopentone may also be used to abort convulsions in the dosage 100–200 mg. If ventricular fibrillation or cardiac arrest occurs, effective cardiovascular resuscitation must be instituted. Adrenaline in repeated doses and sodium bicarbonate should be given as rapidly as possible.

Pharmaceutical precautions Each depression of the metered valve delivers 10 mg lignocaine base. The contents of the spray bottle are sufficient to provide approximately 800 sprays. A metal spray nozzle is included in the package. If sterilisation of the nozzle is desired, the entire nozzle is autoclavable. Do not remove the white cap from the nozzle.

Store in a cool place. Keep away from excessive heat.

Legal category P.

Package quantities 80 g spray bottles (approx. 800 spray doses) with a metering valve complete with adjustable spray nozzle which can be steam sterilised at 115°C or 121°C.

Further information Nil.

Product licence number 0017/5039R.

XYLOCAINE* 4% TOPICAL

Presentation Topical anaesthetic for use on mucous membranes.

1 ml Xylocaine 4% Topical Solution contains lignocaine hydrochloride monohydrate for injection corresponding to lignocaine hydrochloride 40 mg, methylparahydroxybenzoate for injection, sodium hydroxide, water for injection q.s. to 1 ml, anhydrous and methylhydroxybenzoate.

Uses

Action: The active agent of Xylocaine Topical Solution is lignocaine, which provides prompt and profound anaesthesia of accessible mucous membranes. Anaesthesia usually occurs rapidly (within 1–5 minutes depending upon area of application) and persists for approximately 15–30 minutes.

Lignocaine stabilises the neuronal membrane and prevents the initiation of nerve impulses, thereby affecting local anaesthetic action. Lignocaine may be absorbed following topical administration. Its rate of absorption and percentage of dose absorbed depend upon concentration and total dose administered, the specific site of application and duration of exposure. In general, the rate of absorption of local anaesthetic agents following topical application occurs most rapidly after intratracheal administration. The metabolism of lignocaine takes place in the liver and metabolities and unchanged drug are excreted by the kidney. The elimination half-life of lignocaine is approximately 1.6 hours.

Indications: Anaesthesia of mucous membranes of the oropharyngeal, tracheal and bronchial areas e.g. in bronchoscopy, bronchography, larygoscopy, oesophagoscopy and endotracheal intubation.

Biopsy in the mouth and throat: puncture of the maxillary sinus or polypectomy. Tonsillectomy: resection of nasal turbinates; in dentistry.

Dosage and administration As with any local anaesthetic, reactions and complications are best averted by employing the minimal effective dosage. Debilitated, elderly patients and children should be given dosage commensurate with their age and physical condition.

The suggested dosage for adults is 1–7.5 ml Xylocaine Topical Solution (=40–300 mg lignocaine HCl). For children, smaller amounts and a weaker concentration should be administered depending on their age and weight. Doses exceeding 7.5 ml (=300 mg lignocaine) may result in plasma levels which have been associated with toxic manifestations.

Biopsy: 3–4 ml may be sprayed on the area or the solution may be applied for a few minutes with a swab. Adrenaline may be added to this solution in order to produce vasoconstriction (add 1–2 drops, 0.05 ml, 1:1,000 solution to 5 ml Xylocaine 4% solution.

Puncture of maxillary sinus or polypectomy: A swab soaked in the solution may be applied for two to three minutes. The addition of adrenaline is advised in these procedures, made up on the lines indicated above.

The Xylocaine Topical Solution may be applied from a swab, which should be discarded after use. Surface anaesthesia may also be achieved by instillation into a cavity or on to a surface. When spraying, the solution should be transferred from the original container to an atomiser.

Contra-indications, warnings, etc
Contra-indications: Known history of hypersensitivity to local anaesthetics of the amide type or other components of the solution.

Precautions: Absorption from wound surfaces and mucous membranes is relatively high, especially in the bronchial tree. Xylocaine Topical Solution should therefore be used with caution in patients with traumatized mucosa and/or sepsis in the region of the proposed application.

If the dose or site of administration is likely to result in high blood levels, lignocaine, in common with other local anaesthetics, should be used with caution in patients with epilepsy, impaired cardiac conduction, bradycardia, impaired hepatic function and in severe shock.

The use of oral topical anaesthetic agents may interfere with swallowing and thus enhance the danger of aspiration. This is particularly important in children because of their frequency of eating.

Numbness of the tongue or buccal mucosa may increase the danger of biting trauma.

Use in pregnancy and lactation: There is no or inadequate evidence of safety of the drug in human pregnancy but it has been in wide use for many years without apparent ill consequence, animal studies have shown no hazard. If drug therapy is needed in pregnancy, this drug can be used if there is no safer alternative.

Lignocaine enters the mother's milk, but in such small quantities that there is generally no risk of affecting the child at therapeutic dose levels.

Adverse reactions: In extremely rare cases amide-type local anaesthetic preparations have been associated with allergic reactions (in the most severe instances anaphylactic shock).

Systemic adverse reactions are rare and may result from high plasma levels due to excessive dosage, rapid absorption or may result from hypersensitivity, idiosyncracy or diminished tolerance on the part of the patient. Such reactions are systemic in nature and involve the central nervous system and/or the cardiovascular system.

CNS reactions are excitatory and/or depressant and may be characterised by nervousness, dizziness, blurred vision and tremors followed by drowsiness, convulsions, unconsciousness and, possibly, respiratory arrest. The excitatory reactions may be very brief or may not occur at all, in which case the first manifestations of toxicity may be drowsiness, merging into unconsciousness and respiratory arrest.

Cardiovascular reactions are depressant and may be characterised by hypotension, myocardial depression, bradycardia and, possibly, cardiac arrest.

Interactions: Lignocaine should be used with caution in patients receiving antiarrhythmic drugs, such as tocainide, since the toxic effects are additive.

Overdosage: Treatment of a patient with toxic manifestations consists of ensuring adequate ventilation and arresting convulsions. Ventilation should be maintained with oxygen by assisted or controlled respiration as required. If convulsions occur, they must be treated rapidly by intravenous administration of succinylcholine 50–100 mg and/or 5–15 mg diazepam. As succinycholine will arrest respiration, it should only be used if the clinician has the ability to perform endotracheal intubation and to manage a totally paralysed patient. Thiopentone may also be used to abort convulsions in dosage 100–200 mg. Adrenaline in repeated doses and sodium bicarbonate should be given as rapidly as possible.

Pharmaceutical precautions Store at room temperature.

Legal category P.

Package quantities Bottles of 30 ml.

Further information Nil.

Product licence number 0017/5040R.

XYLOCARD*

Presentation *Xylocard 100 mg intravenous bolus injection:* Clear aqueous sterile solution in pre-loaded 5 ml syringe: lignocaine hydrochloride anhydrous 20 mg/ml, equivalent to 21.2 mg Lignocaine Hydrochloride Monohydrate for Injection USP.

Xylocard 1 g and 2 g for addition to intravenous infusion: Sterile aqueous solution in pre-loaded 5 ml or 10 ml syringe: lignocaine hydrochloride anhydrous 200 mg/ml, equivalent to 212 mg Lignocaine Hydrochloride for Injection USP.

Inactive ingredients: Water for injection, sodium hydroxide for pH adjustment.

Uses Prevention of ventricular tachyarrhythmias in patients with suspected or proven acute myocardial infarction. Treatment of ventricular tachyarrhythmias associated with acute myocardial infarction. Ventricular extrasystoles and ventricular tachycardia. As antiarrhythmic cover in cases of ventricular fibrillation being DC converted.

Dosage and administration
Adults:
Xylocard 100 mg I.V. bolus injection: 1 mg/kg body weight. Normal doses 50–100 mg (2.5–5 ml) as initial treatment to be injected slowly over a period of two minutes. When necessary injection can be repeated once or twice at 5–10 minute intervals. Effect can be observed within two minutes and usually persists for 15–20 minute intervals. Not more than 200–300–mg should be administered during one hour.

Xylocard 1 g and 2 g for addition to I.V. Infusion: A concentration of 0.2% lignocaine infusion may be recommended for most cases. This is achieved by adding 1 × Xylocard 1 g syringe (or half × Xylocard 2 g syringe) to 500 ml infusion solution. Normal dose 2–4 mg/min. Based on a concentration of 0.2% this is equivalent to an infusion rate of 1–2 ml/min.

Children: The safety and efficacy of lignocaine in children has not been established.

Elderly: In patients with cardiac failure, total plasma clearance will be reduced and lower dosages may be required.

Contra-indications, warnings, etc Lignocaine is contra-indicated in patients with a known history of hypersensitivity.

Atrioventricular block is an absolute or relative contra-indication, according to severity.

Other serious conduction disturbances, and cardiac decompensation not dependent on treatable tachyarrhythmias, are also contra-indications.

Precautions: In bradycardia complicated by ventricular tachyarrhythmias, Xylocard may need to be combined with atropine or atropine-like drugs or pacemaker therapy.

Patients with severe liver damage should be given lower doses and the effect carefully monitored. Manifest renal insufficiency calls for special care in infusion therapy.

Use with caution in combination with other antiarrhythmic or myocardial depressant drugs as the impairment of cardiac conduction and left ventricular function may be additive. Lignocaine may rarely aggravate or induce ventricular arrhythmias.

Hypokalaemia reduces the antiarrhythmic effects of lignocaine and should be corrected, if possible, before initiation of treatment.

Pregnancy and lactation: It is not known whether lignocaine is excreted in breast milk.

Side-effects: Dizziness, paraesthesia or drowsiness often occur when intravenous injections of Xylocard are given too rapidly. These mild side-effects are transient and do not require special therapeutic measures.

Central nervous side-effects: Drowsiness, persistent dizziness, paraesthesia, tinnitus, disorientation, blurred vision, tremor, convulsions, loss of consciousness and respiratory depression.

Cardiovascular side-effects: Hypotension and bradycardia, which may lead to cardiac arrest.

With the recommended dosage, central nervous and cardiovascular side-effects are rare.

Overdosage: Poisoning due to an overdose of lignocaine may lead to CNS excitation with paraesthesia, muscle twitching and convulsions, atrioventricular block, sinoatrial block or arrest, asystole, myocardial depression, severe hypotension and cardiac arrest.

Treatment should include close monitoring of cardiovascular and respiratory function and electrolytes. If convulsions occur, maintenance of a patent airway is mandatory and assisted or controlled ventilation with oxygen may be required. Convulsions may be controlled with intravenous diazepam or a short-acting barbiturate.

Cardiovascular complications should be treated symptomatically, which may require the use of sympathomimetic agents (e.g. noradrenaline, metaraminol), or inotropic agents (e.g. dopamine, dobutamine). Temporary pacing may be required for AV block.

Lignocaine is usually eliminated rapidly from the body, but elimination may be delayed in severe hypotension, cardiac failure or cardiogenic shock.

Interactions: Propranolol and cimetidine can impair the metabolism or lignocaine. Elimination will be delayed, the duration of action prolonged and the risk of adverse reactions increased.

Pharmaceutical precautions Store in a cool place.

The contents of the Xylocard 1 g and 2 g syringes are for dilution in infusion fluid only. Under no circumstances are they to be administered undiluted.

Legal category POM.

Package quantities *Xylocard 100 mg 5 ml (20 mg/ml):* Pre-loaded syringe for immediate use. Box of 10.

Xylocard 1 g (5 ml) and Xylocard 2 g (10 ml) both 200 mg/ml: Pre-loaded syringe for addition to infusion bottles and bags. Box of 10.

Further information All Xylocard syringes are free of bacteriostat and preservatives.

Product licence numbers

Xylocard 100 mg I.V. bolus	0017/5018R
Xylocard 1 g for I.V. infusion	0017/0064R
Xylocard 2 g for I.V. infusion	0017/0064R

XYLOPROCT* OINTMENT

Presentation White water-miscible cream. Each gram contains: Lignocaine 50 mg, Hydrocortisone Acetate BP 2.75 mg.

Inactive ingredients: Zinc Oxide BP 180 mg, aluminium acetate 35 mg, polyethylene glycol, stearyl alcohol, cetanol, carbowax.

Uses For the relief of symptoms such as anal and perianal pruritis, pain and inflammation associated with haemorrhoids, anal fissure, fistulas, proctitis. Pruritis vulva.

Dosage and administration To be applied several times a day according to the severity of the condition.

Contra-indications, warnings, etc
Contra-indications: Known hypersensitivity to local anaesthetics of the amide type or any of the other ingredients.

Precautions and warnings: Xyloproct is intended for use for limited periods and when the presence of infection has been excluded.

When using the special applicator, care should be taken to avoid instillation of excessive amounts of Xyloproct ointment into the rectum. This is of particular importance in infants and children. Systemic absorption of lignocaine may occur from the rectum and large doses may result in CNS side effects. On rare occasions convulsions have occurred in children. Xyloproct suppositories should be used in preference to ointment for treatment of proctitis or internal haemorrhoids.

Local reactions such as dermatitis have been reported with the use of Xyloproct ointment.

Use in pregnancy: Do not use in pregnancy unless considered essential by the physician.

Pharmaceutical precautions Store in a cool place.

Legal category POM.

Package quantities *Tubes:* 30 g ointment complete with applicator.

Further information Nil.

Product licence number 0017/5023R.

XYLOPROCT* SUPPOSITORIES

Presentation White cone-shaped suppositories. Each suppository contains: Xylocaine (lignocaine) 60 mg, hydrocortisone Acetate BP 5 mg, Zinc Oxide BP 400 mg, Aluminium acetate 50 mg.

Inactive ingredients: Hard fat BP.

Uses For the treatment of symptoms associated with haemorrhoids and other disorders of the anal canal such as proctitis, anal fissure.

Dosage and administration Remove protective foil. Use 1 suppository at night before retiring and repeat the treatment after each bowel action.

Contra-indications, warnings, etc
Contra-indications: Known hypersensitivity to local anaesthetics of the amide type or any of the other ingredients.

Precautions: Xyloproct is intended for use for limited

periods and when the presence of peri-anal thrush has been excluded.

Xyloproct suppositories should be used in preference to ointment for the treatment of proctitis or internal haemorrhoids. Local reactions such as dermatitis have been reported with the use of Xyloproct ointment.

Use in pregnancy: Do not use in pregnancy unless considered essential by the physician.

Pharmaceutical precautions Store in a cool place.

Legal category POM.

Package quantities Packs containing 10 separate foil-protected suppositories.

Further information Nil.

Product licence number 0017/5024R.

XYLOTOX* 2% E.80

Presentation Sterile clear aqueous solution: lignocaine hydrochloride 24.7 mg equivalent to lignocaine base 20 mg/ml. Adrenaline BP 1:80,000. In addition Xylotox 2% E80 contains sodium chloride, calcium chloride, potassium chloride and sodium metabisulphite.

Uses Local anaesthetic solution with vasoconstrictor for dental infiltration anaesthesia where a vasoconstrictor is indicated. For all dental nerve-block techniques.

Dosage and administration *Infiltration:* 1 ml. *Nerve block:* 1.5 to 2 ml. *Extensive surgery:* 3 to 10 ml. Adult maximum dose 500 mg.

In children the maximum dose is considerably less and should be calculated in relation to the body weight.

Contra-indications, warnings, etc Patients with thyrotoxicosis and cardiac disease, particularly with arrhythmia or hypertension. Known hypersensitivity to local anaesthetics of the amide type.

Side-effects: The type of toxic reaction is unpredictable and depends on dosage, route of administration and state of patient, the reactions are primarily of two types, typified by stimulation and depression of the cerebral cortex and medulla respectively. Slow onset – stimulation leading to nervousness, dizziness, blurred vision, nausea, tremor convulsions and respiratory arrest. Rapid onset – depression leading primarily to respiratory arrest, cardiovascular collapse and cardiac arrest. Symptoms occur rapidly and with little warning.

Precautions: Adequate resuscitation equipment must be available whenever local or general anaesthesia is administered. Though clinical tolerance is remarkably good, overdosage or accidental intravenous injection may give rise to toxic reactions. These are best avoided by aspiration before making an injection in order to avoid accidental intravascular injection.

Care should be observed in patients taking tricyclic anti-depressants.

Pharmaceutical precautions Store in a cool place.

Legal category POM.

Package quantities Glass cartridges of 2.2 ml and 1.8 ml in boxes of 100.

Further information Nil.

Product licence number 0017/0141.

**Trade Mark*

Bayer UK Limited
Pharmaceutical Business Group
Bayer House
Strawberry Hill
Newbury, Berkshire, RG13 1JA

ADALAT*
ADALAT* 5

Presentation *Adalat capsules:* Orange, soft gelatin ovoid capsules containing a yellow viscous fluid. Each capsule is overprinted with 'ADALAT' and the Bayer cross and contains 10 mg nifedipine.

Adalat 5 capsules: Orange, soft gelatin ovoid capsules containing a yellow viscous fluid. Each capsule is overprinted with 'ADALAT 5' and the Bayer cross and contains 5 mg nifedipine.

Uses
Mode of action: As a specific and potent calcium antagonist, the main action of Adalat is to relax arterial smooth muscle both in the coronary and peripheral circulation.

In angina pectoris, Adalat capsules relax peripheral arteries so reducing the load on the left ventricle. Additionally, Adalat dilates submaximally both clear and pre-stenotic, stenotic and post-stenotic coronary arteries, thus protecting the heart against coronary artery spasm and improving perfusion to the ischaemic myocardium.

Adalat capsules reduce the frequency of painful attacks and ischaemic ECG changes, irrespective of the relative contribution from coronary artery spasm or atherosclerosis.

Adalat causes a reduction in blood pressure such that the percentage lowering is directly related to its initial height. In normotensive individuals, Adalat has little or no effect on blood pressure.

Indications: For the treatment and prophylaxis of angina pectoris, and the treatment of Raynaud's phenomenon and all grades of hypertension.

Dosage and administration For oral administration, the capsules should be taken with a little fluid during or after food. The recommended dose is one 10 mg capsule three times daily with subsequent titration of dosage according to response. The dosage may be adjusted within the range 5 mg three times daily to 20 mg three times daily.

If an immediate anti-anginal effect is required, the capsule should be bitten open and the liquid contents held in the mouth.

Adalat 5 capsules permit titration of initial dosage in the elderly and those patients on concomitant medication. The recommended dose is one Adalat 5 capsule three times daily.

Patients with hepatic dysfunction should commence therapy at 5 mg three times daily with careful monitoring. Patients with renal impairment should not require adjustment of dosage.

There are no recommendations for use in children.

Treatment may be continued indefinitely.

Contra-indications, warnings, etc
Contra-indications: Adalat should not be administered to patients with known hypersensitivity to nifedipine, to women capable of child-bearing or to nursing mothers. Adalat should not be used in cardiogenic shock.

Warnings and precautions: Adalat may be used in combination with beta-blocking drugs and other anti-hypertensive agents but the possibility of an additive effect resulting in postural hypotension should be borne in mind. Adalat will not prevent possible rebound effects after cessation of other antihypertensive therapy.

Adalat should be used with caution in patients whose cardiac reserve is poor.

Caution should be exercised in patients with severe hypotension.

Ischaemic pain has been reported in a small proportion of patients within 30 to 60 minutes of the introduction of Adalat therapy. Although a 'steal' effect has not been demonstrated, patients experiencing this effect should discontinue Adalat.

The use of Adalat in diabetic patients may require adjustment of their control.

The antihypertensive effect of Adalat may be potentiated by simultaneous administration of cimetidine. When used in combination with nifedipine, serum quinidine levels have been shown to be suppressed regardless of dosage of quinidine.

Side-effects: Most side-effects are consequences of the vasodilator effects of nifedipine and include headache, dizziness and flushing. Gravitational oedema, not associated with heart failure or weight gain, has also been reported.

Other less commonly reported side-effects include, rash, nausea, lethargy and increased frequency of micturition.

There are reports of gingival hyperplasia which may regress on withdrawal of therapy.

Rare cases of hypersensitivity-type jaundice have been reported.

Overdosage: Reports of overdosage are limited and symptoms are not necessarily dose-related. Severe hypotension, bradycardia and unconsciousness have been observed.

Gastric lavage and charcoal instillation have been employed. Intravenous calcium gluconate or calcium chloride appear most helpful, with intravenous atropine for bradycardia. Metaraminol has been beneficially combined with calcium salts in the experimental situation.

Pharmaceutical precautions The capsules should be protected from strong light and stored in the manufacturer's original container.

Legal category POM.

Package quantities Adalat and Adalat 5 capsules are available in foil strips of 10 in packs of 100. Hospital packs containing 500 Adalat 10 mg capsules are also available.

Further information Adalat has no therapeutic anti-arrhythmic effect. Since Adalat does not cause a rise in intraocular pressure, it can be used in patients with glaucoma.

Adalat can be used in patients with obstructive airways disease with coexisting hypertension or angina pectoris. Long term metabolic disturbances have not been observed.

Product licence numbers

Adalat	0010/0021
Adalat 5	0010/0079

ADALAT* RETARD
ADALAT* RETARD 10

Presentation *Adalat retard:* Pink-grey lacquered tablets each containing 20 mg nifedipine, one side marked 1U, and the reverse side with the Bayer cross. *Adalat retard 10:* Pink-grey lacquered tablets each containing 10 mg nifedipine, one side marked A10 and the reverse side with the Bayer cross.

Uses
Mode of action: Nifedipine is a specific and potent calcium antagonist. In hypertension, the main action of Adalat retard is to cause peripheral vasodilatation and thus reduce peripheral resistance.

Adalat retard administered twice daily provides 24 hour control of raised blood pressure. Adalat retard causes reduction in blood pressure such that the percentage lowering is directly related to its initial height. In normotensive individuals, Adalat retard has little or no effect on blood pressure.

Indications: For the treatment of all grades of hypertension and the prophylaxis of angina pectoris.

Dosage and administration The recommended dose of Adalat retard is one tablet (20 mg) twice daily swallowed with a little fluid during or after food, with subsequent titration of dosage according to response. The dosage may be adjusted within the range 10 mg twice daily to 40 mg twice daily.

Adalat retard 10 permits titration of initial dosage. The recommended dose is one Adalat retard 10 tablet (10 mg) twice daily.

Patients with hepatic dysfunction should commence therapy at 10 mg twice daily with careful monitoring. Patients with renal impairment should not require adjustment of dosage.

There are no recommendations for use in children.

Treatment may be continued indefinitely.

Contra-indications, warnings, etc
Contra-indications: Adalat retard should not be administered to patients with known hypersensitivity to nifedipine, to women capable of child-bearing or to nursing mothers. Adalat retard should not be used in cardiogenic shock.

Warnings and precautions: Adalat retard may be used in combination with beta-blocking drugs and other antihypertensive agents but the possibility of an additive effect resulting in postural hypotension should be borne in mind. Adalat retard will not prevent possible rebound effects after cessation of other antihypertensive therapy.

Adalat retard should be used with caution in patients whose cardiac reserve is poor.

Caution should be exercised in patients with severe hypotension.

Ischaemic pain has been reported in a small proportion of patients within one to four hours of the introduction of Adalat retard therapy. Although a 'steal' effect has not been demonstrated, patients experiencing this effect should discontinue Adalat retard.

The use of Adalat retard in diabetic patients may require adjustment of their control.

The antihypertensive effect of Adalat retard may be potentiated by simultaneous administration of cimetidine. When used in combination with nifedipine, serum quinidine levels have been shown to be suppressed regardless of dosage of quinidine.

Side-effects: Most side-effects are consequences of the vasodilator effects of nifedipine and include headache, dizziness and flushing. Gravitational oedema, not associated with heart failure or weight gain, has also been reported.

Other less commonly reported side-effects include rash, nausea, lethargy and increased frequency of micturition.

There are reports of gingival hyperplasia which may regress on withdrawal of therapy.

Rare cases of hypersensitivity-type jaundice have been reported.

Overdosage: Reports of overdosage are limited and symptoms are not necessarily dose-related. Severe hypotension, bradycardia and unconsciousness have been observed.

Gastric lavage and charcoal instillation have been employed. Intravenous calcium gluconate or calcium chloride appear most helpful, with intravenous atropine for bradycardia. Metaraminol has been beneficially combined with calcium salts in the experimental situation.

Pharmaceutical precautions The tablets should be protected from strong light and stored in the manufacturer's original container.

Legal category POM.

Package quantities Adalat retard tablets: strips of 10 in packs of 100.

Adalat retard 10 tablets: strips of 14 in packs of 56.

Further information Adalat retard has no therapeutic antiarrhythmic effect. Since Adalat retard does not cause a rise in intraocular pressure, it can be used in patients with glaucoma.

Adalat retard can be used in patients with obstructive airways disease with coexisting hypertension or angina pectoris. Long term metabolic disturbances have not been observed.

Product licence numbers

Adalat retard	0010/0078
Adalat retard 10	0010/0151

ALRHEUMAT*

Presentation Opaque 'off-white' hard gelatin capsules each containing 50 mg ketoprofen.

Uses Alrheumat is recommended for the management of the rheumatic diseases: rheumatoid arthritis, osteoarthrosis, ankylosing spondylitis, sero-negative (non-rheumatoid) arthropathies, non-articular rheumatism and soft tissue rheumatism.

Alrheumat is also recommended for the treatment of dysmenorrhoea and as an analgesic for the symptomatic relief of muscular aches and pains (including backache), dental pain and post-operative pain.

Dosage and administration Alrheumat capsules are administered orally and should be taken with food.

Rheumatic diseases: Dosage is usually 1 capsule (50 mg) three times daily. This dosage may be increased to 1 capsule four times daily or decreased to 1 capsule twice daily depending on body weight and clinical condition of the patient and the severity of the disease.

Dysmenorrhoea: One capsule (50 mg) up to three times a day. Treatment is normally required for 3 to 4 days from the onset of menstruation or symptoms of dysmenorrhoea.

Analgesia: One capsule (50 mg) up to three times daily. Prolonged use is not recommended for minor conditions such as the relief of mild to moderate pain.

Children: Paediatric dosage has not been established.

Contra-indications, warnings, etc
Contra-indications: Alrheumat should not be given to patients known to be sensitive to aspirin or other non-steroidal anti-inflammatory agents which are prostaglandin inhibitors. In such patients, and in those with a history of bronchial asthma or allergic disease, severe bronchospasm may be precipitated.

Alrheumat should not be given to patients with active peptic ulceration.

Precautions: Patients with a history of peptic ulcer or chronic dyspepsia should be carefully monitored. Care should also be taken in patients with a history of impaired hepatic function. Alrheumat, in common with other propionic acid derivatives, exhibits moderate plasma protein binding. Patients receiving anticoagulants, hydantoins and protein-bound sulphonamides must therefore be closely monitored. The required dose of these drugs may well be beneficially reduced if taken concurrently with Alrheumat.

In patients with renal, cardiac or hepatic impairment, caution is required since the use of NSAIDs may result in deterioration of renal function. The dose should be kept as low as possible and renal function monitored.

Use in pregnancy and lactation: No embryotoxic or teratogenic effects have been reported, but, on principle, caution should be exercised when prescribing during pregnancy and lactation.

Side-effects: Occasional gastro-intestinal disturbances occur and in some such cases a reduction in dosage has been helpful. In common with most other anti-inflammatory agents, there have been very rare reports of gastro-intestinal haemorrhage. Skin rashes have been rare.

Non-steroidal anti-inflammatory agents have been reported to cause nephrotoxicity in various forms, and their use can lead to interstitial nephritis, nephrotic syndrome and renal failure.

Pharmaceutical precautions Nil.

Legal category POM.

Package quantities Alrheumat capsules are available in blister strips of 10 packed in boxes of 100 and 500 capsules.

Further information Nil.

Product licence number 0010/0025R

BAYCARON*

Presentation A white scored tablet 7 mm × 2 mm, one side scored L/1 and the reverse side with the Bayer cross, containing 25 mg mefruside.

Uses Baycaron is a diuretic agent and is intended for the treatment of hypertension and oedema.

Dosage and administration Baycaron is best taken with a little fluid after meals.

Hypertension: 25 mg to 50 mg initially for 10 to 14 days, then maintenance dose of 25 mg each morning. Alternate day dosage may also be used.

Oedema: 25 mg to 50 mg every morning increasing if necessary to 75 mg to 100 mg to obtain the desired response. For long-term therapy intermittent dosage is preferable e.g. 25 mg to 50 mg every second or third day.

Daily doses in excess of 100 mg do not usually increase diuresis further.

Paediatric dosage has not been established.

Contra-indications, warnings, etc
Contra-indications: Severe renal failure, hepatic coma, Addisons disease, severe hypercalcaemia.

Warnings and precautions: It is often necessary to give extra potassium during treatment with diuretics and potassium supplements may be necessary during long-term treatment with Baycaron, especially in patients with impaired liver function or in those also receiving digoxin and other cardiac glycosides.

Particular care is necessary in the elderly because of their susceptibility to electrolyte imbalance.

Although there is no short-term alteration of carbohydrate metabolism in normal subjects on a 50 mg daily dose, the glucose tolerance curve may be prolonged in some diabetics. After Baycaron administration serum uric acid may be raised and therefore it should be used with caution in potential cases of gout.

Baycaron is not suitable for the treatment of acute conditions of fluid excess such as pulmonary and cerebral oedema and glaucoma.

Baycaron should not be administered concurrently with lithium carbonate. Patients with known sulphonamide sensitivity may show allergic reactions to Baycaron. Care should be exercised when prescribed with non-steroidal anti-inflammatory drugs. It is always advisable to monitor renal function. Thiazide and thiazide-like diuretics have been implicated in blood dyscrasias and pancreatitis.

Pregnancy warning: Baycaron has not been shown to produce teratogenic effects, either after administration to animals, or when used to treat toxaemia of pregnancy. However, the benefits should be carefully weighed against possible risks in the first trimester of pregnancy.

Diuretics are best avoided for the management of oedema of pregnancy or hypertension in pregnancy as their use may be associated with hypovolaemia, increased blood viscosity and reduced placental perfusion.

There is inadequate evidence of safety in human pregnancy and some workers have described foetal bone marrow depression and thrombocytopenia. Foetal and neonatal jaundice have also been described.

Lactation warning: As diuretics pass into breast milk they should be avoided in mothers who wish to breast feed.

Side-effects: Baycaron is very well tolerated. Occasionally, with daily doses of up to 100 mg, dyspepsia and nausea are encountered initially, but usually subside on continued treatment. There are no reports of postural hypotension nor of any impairment of micturition or bowel habit. Due to its profile of diuretic action, Baycaron does not precipitate acute retention of urine in, for example, cases of prostatic hypertrophy. Impotence is rarely associated with mefruside.

Overdosage: There is no special antidote and general supportive measures should be offered together with monitoring of blood pressure, fluid and electrolyte balance, correcting when necessary.

Pharmaceutical precautions There are no special precautions or requirements regarding the storage of Baycaron.

Legal category POM.

Package quantities Bottles of 150 tablets.

Further information
Hypertension: Baycaron, with its powerful natriuretic effect is particularly suited to the treatment of hypertension, especially in the long term. Baycaron may be administered alone or in combination with other anti-hypertensive agents.

Oedema: By virtue of its prolonged and smooth natriuretic action, Baycaron is suitable for the long-term treatment of oedematous conditions, for example: oedema of cardiac, hepatic, or renal origin, and premenstrual tension. Its profile of action leads to minimum patient inconvenience. Diuresis begins two to four hours following oral administration and is maximal between six and twelve hours after administration.

Product licence number 0010/5903R.

BAYOLIN*

Presentation A white cream. Each 100 g cream contains heparinoid 'Bayer' 5,000 HDBu., glycol salicylate 10 g, benzyl nicotinate 2.5 g.

Uses Bayolin is a rubefacient used to provide symptomatic relief of muscular pain and stiffness including backache, sciatica, lumbago, fibrositis and rheumatic pain.

Dosage and administration *Adults, and children over the age of 12 years:* Topical application two or three times daily, the cream being massaged gently into the affected area until absorbed.

Children under 12 years of age: Not recommended.

Contra-indications, warnings, etc
Contra-indications: None.

Warnings and precautions: Some reddening and warming of the skin is to be expected, but in rare cases an allergic reaction may occur. Always apply to a small test area before application. Do not use near eyes or mucous membranes. Bayolin should be applied to unbroken skin only. Do not apply immediately after a hot bath. Bayolin is very well tolerated but should not be used on children under 12 years of age or sensitive body areas. It is advisable for the hands to be washed after application.

Side-effects: Occasionally a skin reaction to the nicotinic acid component of Bayolin may be seen.

Use in pregnancy: As with all medicines, Bayolin should be used with caution during pregnancy.

Overdosage/Accidental oral ingestion: In the event of Bayolin being taken orally, treat symptomatically.

Pharmaceutical precautions There are no special requirements for storage or other precautions to be taken.

Legal category P.

Package quantities Bayolin Cream is available in 35 g tubes.

Further information Nil.

Product licence number 0010/5907.

BETA-ADALAT*

Presentation Beta-Adalat is presented as reddish brown capsules bearing the name Beta-Adalat with the Bayer cross. Each capsule contains nifedipine retard 20 mg, and atenolol 50 mg.

Uses Management of hypertension and of angina pectoris where therapy with either a calcium channel blocker or a beta-blocker proves inadequate.

Mode of action: Atenolol effects a marked negative inotropic and chronotropic effect thereby reducing cardiac output, myocardial oxygen demand and blood pressure, particularly during exercise. Nifedipine is a powerful coronary and peripheral vasodilator which increases myocardial oxygen supply and reduces blood pressure (afterload) and peripheral resistance. Concomitant use of $beta_1$-blockade, therefore, ameliorates the reflex sympathetic response to nifedipine monotherapy by blocking the rise in heart rate, while atenolol's tendency to increase peripheral resistance is balanced by the vasodilation and increased sympathetic tone induced by the calcium antagonist. Consequently, greater antihypertensive or antianginal efficacy is achieved by the concomitant use of nifedipine and atenolol than either drug alone.

Dosage and administration
Adults: Hypertension: One capsule daily. If necessary, the dosage may be increased to one capsule dosed twice daily. Patients can be transferred to the combination from other antihypertensive treatments with the exception of clonidine (see 'Precautions' below).

Angina: One capsule dosed twice daily. Where additional efficacy is necessary, prophylactic nitrate therapy or additional nifedipine may be of benefit.

Children: There is no paediatric experience with Beta-Adalat and, therefore, this preparation should not be used in children.

Elderly: Dosage should not exceed one capsule daily in hypertension or one capsule twice daily in angina.

Contra-indications, warnings, etc
Contra-indications: Beta-Adalat must not be administered to women capable of childbearing or to nursing mothers.

Beta-Adalat must not be used in the presence of second or third degree heart block.

Beta-Adalat must not be used in patients with cardiogenic shock or evidence of overt heart failure.

Beta-Adalat must not be used in conjunction with other drugs with a cardio-depressant action e.g. verapamil, as conduction disturbances may ensue.

Precautions
Cardiac: Particular care should be taken with patients with conduction defects or whose cardiac reserve is poor. However, in patients already treated with a beta-adrenoceptor antagonist, and/or where signs of cardiac failure have been controlled, Beta-Adalat may be substituted with care if necessary.

Care should be taken in prescribing a beta-adrenoceptor blocking drug with Class 1 antidysrhythmic agents such as disopyramide.

One of the pharmacological actions of beta-adrenoceptor blocking drugs is to reduce heart rate. In the rare instances where symptoms may be attributable to the slow heart rate at a dose of one capsule daily, the drug should be discontinued.

Cessation of therapy with a beta-adrenoceptor blocking drug in patients with ischaemic heart disease should be gradual.

Caution should be exercised when transferring patients from clonidine to beta-adrenoceptor blocking drugs. If beta-adrenoceptor drugs are given concurrently, clonidine should not be discontinued until several days after withdrawal of the beta-adrenoceptor blocking drug.

Obstructive airways disease: Although cardioselective ($beta_1$) beta-blockers may have less effect on lung function than non-selective beta-blockers, as with all beta-blockers these should be avoided in patients with reversible obstructive airways disease unless there are compelling clinical reasons for their use. Where such reasons exist, Beta-Adalat may be used with caution. Occasionally some increase in airways resistance may occur in asthmatic patients, however, and this may usually be reversed by standard doses of bronchodilators such as salbutamol or isoprenaline.

Renal impairment: In patients with marked renal impairment (i.e. creatinine clearance below 15 ml/min/1.73 m^2, serum creatinine greater than 600 micromol/litre) the use of the combination is considered inappropriate.

Hepatic impairment: Care should be taken in patients with marked hepatic impairment. Although no dosage adjustment is suggested from the systemic availability of the monocomponents in patients with cirrhosis, hypertensive patients with clinically significant liver disease have not been studied.

Anaesthesia: It is not advisable to withdraw beta-adrenoceptor blocking drugs prior to surgery in the majority of patients. However, care should be taken when using anaesthetic agents such as ether, cyclopropane and trichloroethylene. Vagal dominance, if it occurs, may be corrected with atropine (1–2 mg intravenously).

Diabetes: The use of nifedipine in diabetic patients may require adjustment of their control.

Beta-Adalat modifies the tachycardia of hypoglycaemia.

Interactions: The antihypertensive effect of nifedipine can be potentiated by simultaneous administration of cimetidine. When used in combination with nifedipine, serum quinidine levels may be suppressed regardless of dosage of quinidine.

Side-effects: Side-effects which have been reported during treatment with the combination include headache, flushing, fatigue, dizziness and oedema. Side-effects of nifedipine such as flushing and headache may occur at the beginning of the treatment. They are, however, mostly slight and diminish with continuous use. Rare cases of hypersensitivity-type jaundice have been reported with nifedipine. There are reports of gingival hyperplasia with nifedipine which may regress on withdrawal of therapy.

There have been reports of skin rashes and/or dry eyes associated with the use of beta-adrenoceptor blocking drugs. The reported incidence is small. Discontinuance of the drug should be considered if any such reaction is not otherwise explicable.

Overdosage: Excessive bradycardia can be countered with atropine 1–2 mg intravenously. If necessary, this may be followed by a bolus dose of glucagon 10 mg intravenously. If required, this may be repeated or followed by an intravenous infusion of glucagon 1–10 mg/hour depending on response. If no response to glucagon occurs or if glucagon is unavailable, a beta-adrenoceptor stimulant such as prenalterol 5 mg intravenously, followed if necessary by an intravenous infusion of 5 mg/hour or dobutamine 2.5 to 10 microgram/kg/minute by intravenous infusion may be given.

There is a possibility of hypotension occurring following the use of beta-adrenoceptor agonists but this will be reduced by more selective agents, prenalterol and dobutamine. In severe cases, cardiac pacing with appropriate cardiorespiratory support may be necessary.

Intravenous calcium gluconate combined with metaraminol may be beneficial for hypotension induced by nifedipine.

Pharmaceutical precautions Beta-Adalat capsules should be stored at room temperature, protected from light and moisture.

Legal category POM.

Package quantities Calendar packs of 28 capsules.

Further information When the combined antihypertensive effect of a beta-adrenoceptor antagonist and calcium antagonist is required, Beta-Adalat is a convenient and acceptable therapy. The combination of atenolol and nifedipine retard, given once daily, provides control of raised blood pressure over a 24 hour period and may be expected to improve patient compliance. Given twice daily the combination provides control of angina.

Product licence number 0010/0155.

CANESTEN* GYNAECOLOGICAL PRODUCTS

Presentation
Vaginal Tablets: White convex tablets, measuring 25 mm × 6.5 mm × 10 mm containing Clotrimazole BP.

100 mg tablet marked 'BAYER' on one side and 'AD' on the other.

200 mg tablet marked 'BAYER' on one side and 'F9' on the other.

500 mg tablet (Canesten 1) marked 'BAYER' on one side and 'MU' on the other.

2% Vaginal Cream: A white cream containing 2.0% Clotrimazole BP.

10% Vaginal Cream (Canesten 10% VC): A white cream containing 10.0% Clotrimazole BP.

Duopak: A combination pack comprising 6 Canesten vaginal tablets (each containing 100 mg Clotrimazole BP) plus a 20 g tube of Canesten cream (containing 1.0% Clotrimazole BP).

Uses Clotrimazole is a broad spectrum antifungal. It also exhibits activity against *Trichomonas*, staphylococci, streptococci and *Bacteroides*. It has no effect on lactobacilli.

Vaginal Tablets: The vaginal tablets are indicated for the treatment of candidal vaginitis and mixed vaginal infections where *Trichomonas* is present or suspected. Canesten is not recommended as sole treatment for pure trichomoniasis, except in cases where systemic therapy is contra-indicated.

2% Vaginal Cream: As for vaginal tablets.

10% Vaginal Cream: As for vaginal tablets.

Duopak: Vaginal tablets for candidal vaginitis; cream for associated vulvitis and to treat the sexual partner to prevent re-infection.

Dosage and administration
Adults: Vaginal Tablets 100 mg. Two vaginal tablets should be inserted daily, preferably at night, for three consecutive days. Alternatively, one vaginal tablet daily for six days may be inserted, preferably at night.

Vaginal Tablets 200 mg. One vaginal tablet should be inserted daily, preferably at night, for three consecutive days.

Vaginal Tablets 500 mg (Canesten 1). The single tablet should be inserted preferably at night.

2% Vaginal Cream: Insert one filled applicator, (5 g), intravaginally twice daily for three consecutive days, or once daily for six consecutive days, preferably at night.

10% Vaginal Cream (Canesten 10% VC): Insert the contents of the pre-filled applicator, (5 g), intravaginally, preferably at night.

Duopak: Two vaginal tablets should be inserted daily, preferably at night, for three consecutive days. Alternatively, one vaginal tablet daily for six days may be inserted, preferably at night. The cream should be applied night and morning to the vulva and surrounding area and/or to the partner's penis to prevent re-infection.

Using the applicator provided, each vaginal tablet or dose of vaginal cream should be inserted as deeply as is comfortable into the vagina. This is best achieved when lying back with the legs bent up.

Children: As the above products are used with an applicator paediatric usage is not recommended.

Contra-indications, warnings, etc
Contra-indications: Hypersensitivity to clotrimazole.

Side-effects: Rarely patients may experience local mild burning or irritation immediately after applying cream or inserting the vaginal tablets. Very rarely, the patient may find this irritation intolerable and stop treatment. Hypersensitivity reactions may occur.

Use in pregnancy: In animal studies clotrimazole has not been associated with teratogenic effects but following oral administration of high doses to rats there was evidence of foetotoxicity. The relevance of this effect to topical application in humans is not known. However, clotrimazole has been used in pregnant patients for over a decade without attributable adverse effects. It is therefore recommended that clotrimazole should be used in pregnancy only when considered necessary by the clinician. If used during pregnancy extra care should be taken when using the applicator to prevent the possibility of mechanical trauma.

Accidental oral ingestion: In the event, routine measures such as gastric lavage should be performed as soon as possible after ingestion.

Pharmaceutical precautions Do not store Canesten 10% Vaginal Cream above 25°C. No special storage precautions are necessary for other presentations.

Legal category POM.

Package quantities
Vaginal Tablets: 6 × 100 mg vaginal tablets packed in a blister strip. 3 × 200 mg vaginal tablets packed in a blister strip. 1 × 500 mg vaginal tablet (Canesten 1) packed in foil.

An applicator and a patient instruction leaflet are included.

Vaginal Cream 2%: 1 × 35 g tube of cream, together with 6 disposable applicators and a patient instruction leaflet.

Vaginal Cream 10% (Canesten 10% VC): A single pre-filled disposable applicator containing 5 g of Canesten 10% vaginal cream together with a patient instruction leaflet.

Duopak: 6 × 100 mg vaginal tablets packed in a blister strip plus a 20 g tube of 1% clotrimazole cream. An applicator for the vaginal tablets and patient instruction leaflet are included.

Further information Nil.

Product licence numbers

Vaginal Tablets 100 mg	0010/0015
Vaginal Tablets 200 mg	0010/0072
Vaginal Tablet 500 mg (Canesten 1)	0010/0083
2% Vaginal Cream	0010/0077
10% Vaginal Cream (Canesten 10% VC)	0010/0136
Duopak: Cream 1%	0010/0016
Vaginal Tablets 100 mg	0010/0015

CANESTEN* TOPICAL PRODUCTS

Presentation
Cream: A white cream containing 1.0% Clotrimazole BP.

Atomiser spray: A clear spray containing 1.0% Clotrimazole BP in 30% isopropanol. The spray is produced by an atomiser and contains no propellant.

Solution: A clear solution containing 1.0% Clotrimazole BP in polyethylene glycol 400.

Powder: A white powder containing 1.0% Clotrimazole BP.

Uses Clotrimazole is a broad spectrum antifungal. It also exhibits activity against *Trichomonas*, staphylococci, streptococci and *Bacteroides*.

Clotrimazole is recommended for the treatment of skin infections due to dermatophytes (e.g. *Trichophyton* species), yeasts (e.g. *Candida* species), moulds and other fungi. These include ringworm (tinea) infections, athlete's foot, paronychia, pityriasis versicolor, erythrasma and intertrigo.

Cream: The cream may also be used for the treatment of fungal nappy rash, candidal vulvitis and candidal balanitis.

Atomiser Spray: The spray is recommended in particular for infections covering large and/or hairy areas.

Solution: The solution is particularly suitable for use on hairy skin and in fungal infections of the outer and middle ear (otitis externa and otomycoses).

Powder: The powder is to be used as an adjunct to treatment with cream or atomiser spray and as a prophylactic against re-infection, particularly in infections such as athlete's foot. The powder should be applied to the lesions simultaneously and dusted inside articles of clothing in contact with infected areas.

Dosage and administration
Cream: Canesten cream should be thinly and evenly applied to the affected area two to three times daily and rubbed in gently.

Treatment should be continued for at least one month for dermatophyte infections, or for at least two weeks for *Candida* infections.

If the feet are infected, they should be thoroughly washed and dried, especially between the toes, before applying the cream.

Atomiser Spray: Canesten atomiser spray should be applied to the affected area two to three times daily. Treatment should be continued for at least one month for dermatophyte infections, or for at least two weeks for Candida infections and pityriasis versicolor infections.

Solution: Canesten solution should be thinly and evenly applied to the affected area two to three times daily. To prevent relapse treatment should be continued for at least two weeks after the disappearance of all signs of infection.

Powder: Sprinkle onto the affected areas two to three times daily after using the cream or atomiser spray. The powder may also be dusted inside articles of clothing and footwear which are in contact with the infected area.

Contra-indications, warnings, etc
Contra-indications: Hypersensitivity to clotrimazole or, (in the case of the atomiser spray), propylene glycol.

Warnings and precautions: Canesten atomiser spray should not be used near a naked flame, should not be allowed to come into contact with the eyes, ears or mucous membranes and should not be inhaled.

Side-effects: Rarely patients may experience local mild burning or irritation immediately after applying the cream, solution or atomiser spray. Very rarely, the patient may find this irritation intolerable and stop treatment. Hypersensitivity reactions may occur.

Use in pregnancy: In animal studies clotrimazole has not been associated with teratogenic effects but following oral administration of high doses to rats there was evidence of foetotoxicity. The relevance of this effect to topical application in humans is not known. However, clotrimazole has been used in pregnant patients for over a decade without attributable adverse effects. It is therefore recommended that clotrimazole should be used in pregnancy only when considered necessary by the clinician.

Accidental oral ingestion: In the event, routine measures such as gastric lavage should be performed as soon as possible after ingestion.

Pharmaceutical precautions No special storage precautions are necessary.

Legal category P.

Package quantities
Cream: Tubes containing 20 g or 50 g.
Atomiser Spray: Bottles containing 40 ml.
Solution: Dropper bottles containing 20 ml.
Powder: Packs containing 30 g.

Further information Nil.

Product licence numbers

Cream	0010/0016
Atomiser Spray	0010/0060
Solution	0010/0082
Powder	0010/0067

CANESTEN*HC

Presentation A white cream containing 1.0% Clotrimazole BP and 1.0% Hydrocortisone PhEur.

Uses Clotrimazole is a broad spectrum antifungal. It also exhibits activity against *Trichomonas*, staphylococci and *Bacteroides*. It has no effect on lactobacilli.

Hydrocortisone has a vasoconstrictive effect, thus reducing inflammation and oedema and also has an antipruritic effect.

Canesten HC is indicated for the treatment of the following skin infections where co-existing symptoms of inflammation, e.g. itching, require rapid relief:

1. All dermatomycoses due to dermatophytes, (e.g. Trichophyton species), moulds and other fungi.
2. All dermatomycoses due to yeasts (Candida species).
3. Skin diseases showing secondary infection with these fungi.
4. The treatment of nappy rash where infection due to *Candida albicans* is present. Candidal vulvitis, candidal balanitis and candidal intertrigo.

Dosage and administration Canesten HC should be thinly and evenly applied to the affected area twice daily and rubbed in gently.

Contra-indications, warnings, etc
Contra-indications: Hypersensitivity to any of the ingredients.

Warnings and precautions: As with all corticosteroids, long term continuous therapy to extensive areas of skin should be avoided, particularly in infants and children. In infants the napkin may act as an occlusive dressing and increase absorption.

Treatment should be for a maximum of 7 days.

Side-effects: Rarely patients may experience local mild burning or irritation immediately after applying the cream. Very rarely the patient may find this irritation intolerable and stop treatment. Hypersensitivity reactions may occur.

Use in pregnancy: Topical administration of corticosteroids to pregnant animals can cause abnormalities of foetal development. The relevance of this to humans has not been established.

In animal studies clotrimazole has not been associated with teratogenic effects but following oral administration of high doses to rats there was evidence of foetotoxicity. The relevance of this effect to topical application in humans is not known. However, clotrimazole has been used in pregnant patients for over a decade without attributable adverse effects.

It is therefore recommended that Canesten HC should

be used in pregnancy only when considered necessary by the clinician.

Accidental oral ingestion: In the event, routine measures such as gastric lavage should be performed as soon as possible after ingestion.

Pharmaceutical precautions Store in a cool place.

Legal category POM.

Package quantities Tubes containing 30 g.

Further information Nil.

Product licence number 0010/0120.

CIPROXIN*

Presentation
Infusion: Clear, almost colourless to pale yellow solution containing 254 mg ciprofloxacin lactate (equivalent to 200 mg ciprofloxacin) in 100 ml solution.

Tablets: White, scored, film-coated tablets, marked on one side with the Bayer cross, and with 'CIP 250' on the reverse side, each tablet containing 291.5 mg ciprofloxacin hydrochloride monohydrate (equivalent to 250 mg ciprofloxacin).

Uses Ciprofloxacin is a synthetic, 4-quinolone derivative with bactericidal activity against a wide range of Gram-negative and Gram-positive organisms.

Ciprofloxacin is indicated for the treatment of single infections or mixed infections caused by two or more susceptible organisms. It may be used for infections caused by organisms resistant to other antibiotics, including aminoglycosides, penicillins and cephalosporins.

The extensive tissue penetration of ciprofloxacin combined with its enhanced antibacterial activity (including anti-pseudomonal activity), enables ciprofloxacin to be used alone (pending sensitivity results) or in combination with an aminoglycoside or with beta-lactam antibiotics, for instance when severe neutropenia is present, or with an antibiotic active against anaerobes where the presence of these organisms is suspected.

Microbiology: In-vitro studies have shown that the antibacterial action of ciprofloxacin results from the inhibition of bacterial DNA gyrase. This mode of action differs from that of penicillins, cephalosporins, aminoglycosides and tetracyclines and, therefore, organisms resistant to these antibiotics are generally sensitive to ciprofloxacin.

Ciprofloxacin is active *in vitro* against the following Gram-negative and Gram-positive organisms: *Citrobacter* spp., *Edwardsiella tarda, Enterobacter* spp., *Escherichia coli, Hafnia alvei, Klebsiella* spp., *Morganella morganii, Proteus* spp. (indole positive and indole negative), *Providencia* spp., *Salmonella* spp., *Serratia* spp., *Shigella* spp., *Yersinia* spp., *Aeromonas* spp., *Campylobacter coli, Campylobacter jejuni, Plesiomonas shigelloides, Pseudomonas aeruginosa, Vibrio* spp., *Haemophilus* spp., *Branhamella catarrhalis, Pasteurella multocida, Moraxella* spp., *Neisseria* spp., *Legionella* spp., *Brucella melitensis, Staphylococcus* spp., *Streptococcus agalactiae, Listeria monocytogenes, Corynebacterium* spp.

Ciprofloxacin is less active against the following organisms. Sensitivity testing should be performed before treatment is commenced: *Acinetobacter* spp., *Alcaligenes* spp., *Flavobacterium* spp., non-*aeruginosa Pseudomonas* spp., *Gardnerella vaginalis, Chlamydia* spp., *Mycoplasma* spp., *Mycobacterium tuberculosis, Mycobacterium fortuitum, Enterococcus faecalis, Streptococcus pneumoniae, Streptococcus pyogenes, viridans* streptococci.

Anaerobes vary in their susceptibility from being moderately sensitive to resistant. In particular, the *Bacteroides fragilis* group and *Clostridium difficile* are resistant.

In addition, the following organisms are resistant to ciprofloxacin: *Ureaplasma urealyticum, Nocardia asteroides, Enterococcus faecium.*

Ciprofloxacin is not active against *Treponema pallidum.*

In-vitro studies have shown that additive activity often results when ciprofloxacin is used concomitantly with other antibacterial agents. Synergism is observed occasionally but antagonism is rarely seen.

Indications: Ciprofloxacin is indicated for the treatment of the following infections caused by sensitive bacteria:

Severe systemic infection: e.g. septicaemia, bacteraemia, peritonitis, infections in immunosuppressed patients with haematological or solid tumours and in patients in intensive care units with specific problems such as infected burns.

Respiratory tract infections: e.g. lobar and bronchopneumonia, acute and chronic bronchitis, acute exacerbation of cystic fibrosis, bronchiectasis, empyema. Ciprofloxacin is not recommended as first line therapy for the treatment of pneumococcal pneumonia. Ciprofloxacin may be used for treating Gram-negative pneumonia.

Ear, nose and throat infections: e.g. otitis media, sinusitis and mastoiditis, especially if due to Gram-negative bacteria (including *Pseudomonas spp.*). Ciprofloxacin is not recommended for the treatment of acute tonsillitis.

Urinary tract infections: e.g. uncomplicated and complicated urethritis, cystitis, pyelonephritis, prostatitis, epididymitis.

Skin and soft tissue infections: e.g. infected ulcers, wound infections, abscesses, cellulitis, otitis externa, erysipelas, infected burns.

Gastro-intestinal infections: e.g. enteric fever, infective diarrhoea.

Eye infections: e.g. bacterial conjunctivitis.

Infections of the biliary tract: e.g. cholangitis, cholecystitis, empyema of the gall bladder.

Intra-abdominal infections: e.g. peritonitis, intra-abdominal abscesses.

Bone and joint infections: e.g. osteomyelitis, septic arthritis.

Pelvic infections: e.g. salpingitis, endometritis, pelvic inflammatory disease.

Gonorrhoea: including urethral, rectal and pharyngeal gonorrhoea caused by beta-lactamase producing organisms or organisms moderately sensitive to penicillin.

Dosage and administration General dosage recommendations: the dosage of ciprofloxacin is determined by the severity and type of infection, the sensitivity of the causative organism(s) and the age, weight and renal function of the patient.

Adults
Ciproxin Infusion: Ciproxin Infusion in 50 ml (100 mg) and 100 ml (200 mg) infusion bottles may be infused directly and should be administered by short-term infusion over periods of 30–60 minutes. The dosage range for adults is 100–200 mg twice daily.

In gonorrhoea, a single dose of 100 mg.

Infections of the lower and upper urinary tract, 100 mg twice daily.

For both upper and lower respiratory tract infections, 200 mg twice daily.

Cystic fibrosis: In adults with pseudomonal infections of the lower respiratory tract, the normal dose is 200 mg twice daily. As the pharmacokinetics of ciprofloxacin remain unchanged in patients with cystic fibrosis, the low body weight of these patients should be taken into consideration when determining dosage.

In the majority of other infections, 200 mg twice daily should be administered.

Ciproxin Tablets: Ciproxin Tablets should be swallowed whole with an adequate amount of liquid. The dosage range for adults is 250–750 mg twice daily.

In gonorrhoea, a single dose of 250 mg.

Infections of the lower and upper urinary tract (depending on severity), 250–500 mg twice daily.

In respiratory tract infections, 250–750 mg twice daily for both upper and lower respiratory tract infections, depending on severity. Although ciprofloxacin is not recommended as first line treatment for pneumococcal pneumonia, where it is considered to be appropriate, a dosage of 750 mg twice daily should be used.

Cystic fibrosis: In adults with pseudomonal infections of the lower respiratory tract, the normal dose is 750 mg twice daily. As the pharmacokinetics of ciprofloxacin remain unchanged in patients with cystic fibrosis, the low body weight of these patients should be taken into consideration when determining dosage.

In the majority of other infections, 500–750 mg twice daily should be administered. In severe infections, particularly due to *Pseudomonas*, staphylococci and streptococci, the higher dosage of 750 mg twice daily should be used.

Impaired renal function: Dosage adjustments are not usually required, except in patients with severe renal impairment (serum creatinine >265 micromole/l or creatinine clearance <20 ml/minute). If adjustment is necessary, this may be achieved by reducing the total daily dose by half, although monitoring of drug serum levels provides the most reliable basis for dose adjustment.

Elderly: Although higher ciprofloxacin serum levels are found in the elderly, no adjustment of dosage is necessary.

Adolescents and children: As with other drugs in its class, ciprofloxacin has been shown to cause arthropathy in weight-bearing joints of immature animals. Although the relevance of this to man is unknown, its use in children and growing adolescents is not recommended. However, where the benefit of using ciprofloxacin is considered to outweigh this potential risk, the dosage should be 5–10 mg/kg/day (intravenous) or 7.5–15 mg/kg/day (oral) depending upon the severity of infection, administered in two divided doses.

Duration of treatment: The duration of treatment depends upon the severity of infection, clinical response and bacteriological findings. For acute infections the usual treatment period is 5 to 7 days with Ciproxin Infusion or 5 to 10 days with Ciproxin Tablets. Generally, treatment should be continued for at least 3 days after the signs and symptoms of the infection have disappeared.

Initial intravenous administration may be followed by treatment with oral ciprofloxacin.

Contra-indications, warnings, etc

Contra-indications: Ciprofloxacin is contra-indicated in patients who have shown hypersensitivity to ciprofloxacin or other quinolones.

Ciprofloxacin is also contra-indicated in children and growing adolescents except where the benefits of treatment exceed the risks.

Warnings and precautions: Ciprofloxacin should be used with caution in epileptics and patients with a history of CNS disorders and only if the benefits of treatment are considered to outweigh the risk of possible CNS side-effects.

Ciprofloxacin could result in an impairment of the patient's ability to drive or operate machinery, particularly in conjunction with alcohol.

Crystalluria related to the use of ciprofloxacin has been reported. Patients receiving ciprofloxacin should be well hydrated and excessive alkalinity of the urine should be avoided.

Patients with latent or actual defects in glucose-6-phosphate dehydrogenase activity are prone to haemolytic reactions with quinolones, and so ciprofloxacin should be used with caution.

Drug interactions: Ciproxin Tablets should not be administered within 4 hours of medications containing magnesium, aluminium or iron salts as interference with absorption may occur. When appropriate, patients should be advised not to self-medicate with antacids or iron-containing preparations during therapy with Ciproxin.

Increased plasma levels of theophylline have been observed following concurrent administration with ciprofloxacin. It is recommended that the dose of theophylline should be reduced and plasma levels of theophylline monitored. Where monitoring of plasma levels is not possible, the use of ciprofloxacin should be avoided in patients receiving theophylline.

Prolongation of bleeding time has been reported during concomitant administration of ciprofloxacin and anticoagulants.

Animal data have shown that high doses of quinolones in combination with some non-steroidal anti-inflammatory drugs (e.g. fenbufen, but not acetylsalicylic acid) can lead to convulsions. However, this has not been reported in patients receiving ciprofloxacin.

Transient increases in serum creatinine have been seen following concomitant administration of ciprofloxacin and cyclosporin. Therefore, monitoring of serum creatinine levels is advisable.

Use in pregnancy and lactation: Reproduction studies performed in mice, rats and rabbits using parenteral and oral administration did not reveal any evidence of teratogenicity, impairment of fertility or impairment of peri-/post-natal development. However, as with other quinolones, ciprofloxacin has been shown to cause arthropathy in immature animals and therefore its use during pregnancy is not recommended. Studies have indicated that ciprofloxacin is secreted in breast milk. Administration to nursing mothers is thus not recommended.

Side-effects: Ciprofloxacin is generally well tolerated. The most frequently reported adverse reactions are: nausea, diarrhoea, vomiting, dyspepsia, abdominal pain, headache, restlessness, rash, dizziness and pruritus.

The following adverse reactions have been observed:

Gastro-intestinal disturbances, e.g. nausea, diarrhoea, vomiting, dyspepsia, abdominal pain, anorexia, flatulence, dysphagia.

CNS disturbances, e.g. headache, restlessness, dizziness, tremor, convulsions, confusion, hallucinations, somnolence.

Hypersensitivity/skin, e.g. rash, pruritus, urticaria, photosensitivity, systemic reactions including anaphylaxis.

Hepatic disturbances, e.g. transient increases in liver enzymes or serum bilirubin (particularly in patients with previous liver damage), hepatitis, jaundice and major liver disorders including hepatic necrosis.

Renal disturbances, e.g. transient increases in blood urea or serum creatinine, renal failure, crystalluria, nephritis.

Musculoskeletal disturbances, e.g. arthralgia, myalgia.

Effects on haematological parameters, e.g. eosinophilia, leukopenia, thrombocytopenia, thrombocytosis, altered prothrombin levels.

Special sense disturbances, e.g. blurred vision.

Other adverse events reported include vasculitis, pseudomembranous colitis, Stevens-Johnson syndrome, tachycardia.

In addition with Ciproxin Infusion, local irritation including pain at the site of injection has been reported, accompanied in a small number of patients by phlebitis or thrombophlebitis.

Overdosage: No information on overdosage is available. Routine measures such as gastric lavage should be performed as soon as possible after ingestion of Ciproxin Tablets.

Serum levels of ciprofloxacin are reduced by dialysis.

Pharmaceutical precautions Ciproxin Infusion is compatible with sodium chloride 0.9% solution, Ringer's Solution, glucose 5% and 10% solutions, glucose/saline and fructose 10% solution.

Ciproxin Infusion is incompatible with injection solutions (e.g. penicillins, heparin solutions) which are chemically or physically unstable at its pH of 3.9–4.5.

Unless compatibility is proven, the infusion should always be administered separately.

Since Ciproxin Infusion is light-sensitive, the bottles should always be stored in the cardboard outer container. No special precautions are required during the normal 30–60 minute infusion period.

No special storage precautions are necessary for Ciproxin Tablets.

Legal category POM.

Package quantities Ciproxin Infusion, bottles of 50 or 100 ml.

Ciproxin Tablets, blister strips of 10 in packs of 10, 20 and 100 tablets.

Further information Ciproxin Infusion contains 0.9% w/v sodium chloride, equivalent to approximately 154 mmol sodium per litre.

Product licence numbers
Ciproxin Infusion 0010/0150
Ciproxin Tablets 0010/0146

DTIC-DOME*

Presentation *Active ingredient:* 5-(3,3-dimethyl-1-triazeno) imidazole-4-carboxamide prepared as the citrate salt (dacarbazine).

100 mg and 200 mg vials of sterile dacarbazine.

DTIC-Dome is a colourless to ivory-coloured solid to be reconstituted with Water for Injections BP.

Uses *Actions:* Although the exact mechanism of action of dacarbazine is unknown, three hypotheses have been proposed:

1. Inhibition of DNA synthesis by acting as a purine analogue.
2. Action as an alkylating agent.
3. Interaction with sulphydryl groups.

The volume of distribution of dacarbazine exceeds body water content, suggesting localisation in some body tissues. Dacarbazine is only slightly (approximately 5%) protein bound. Its plasma half-life after intravenous administration is approximately 35 minutes. In animal studies, approximately 46% of radiolabelled dose was recovered from the urine after 6 hours. Of this 46%, almost half, was unchanged dacarbazine and a similar quantity was amino-imidazole carboxamide, a metabolite. Dacarbazine is subject to renal tubular secretion rather than glomerular filtration.

Indications: Metastatic malignant melanoma.
Sarcoma.
Hodgkin's disease.

In addition, dacarbazine has been shown, when used in combination with other cytotoxic agents, to be of value in treatment of other malignant diseases including: carcinoma of colon, ovary, breast, lung, testicular teratoma, and solid tumours in children.

Dosage and administration *Standard dose:* The following dosage schedules are recommended:

1. 2.0–4.5 mg/kg/day for 10 days, which may be repeated at 4 week intervals.
2. 250 mg/m^2/day for 5 days, which may be repeated at 3 week intervals.
3. A further alternative is to administer the total schedule dose on the first day.

Other schedules may be used at the discretion of the prescribing physician.

Children: The dosage for children is calculated on a mg/kg or mg/m^2 basis as per the standard dosage.

Administration: DTIC-Dome 100 mg and 200 mg vials are reconstituted with 9.9 ml and 19.7 ml, respectively, of Water for Injections BP. The resulting solution contains an equivalent of 10 mg/ml of dacarbazine. After the solution has been prepared, the calculated dose is drawn into a syringe and injected intravenously. Injection may be completed in one or two minutes.

If desired, the reconstituted solution may be further diluted with 125–250 ml of Dextrose Injection BP 5% or Sodium Chloride Injection BP 0.9% and administered by intravenous infusion over a period of 15 to 30 minutes.

Contra-indications, warnings, etc DTIC-Dome is contra-indicated in patients who have demonstrated a hypersensitivity to it in the past.

This product should not normally be administered to patients who are pregnant or to mothers who are breast feeding.

Studies have demonstrated this agent to have a carcinogenic and teratogenic effect when used on animals.

DTIC-Dome should be administered preferably to patients who are hospitalised and who can be observed carefully and frequently during and after therapy, with particular reference to the haemopoietic system.

Care must be taken to avoid extravasation of the drug subcutaneously during intravenous administration as this may result in tissue damage and severe pain.

Users should avoid contact of DTIC-Dome with the skin and eyes when reconstituting or administering.

It is recommended that DTIC-Dome be administered under the supervision of a physician experienced in the use of cancer chemotherapeutic agents. Since facilities for necessary laboratory studies must be available, hospitalisation is recommended.

Haemopoietic depression is the most common toxic side-effect of dacarbazine and involves primarily the leucocytes and platelets, although mild anaemia may sometimes occur. Leucopenia and thrombocytopenia may be severe enough to cause death. The possible bone marrow depression requires careful monitoring of white blood cell, red blood cell and platelet levels. Haemopoietic toxicity may warrant temporary suspension or cessation of dacarbazine therapy.

Symptoms of anorexia, nausea and vomiting are the most frequently noticed side-effects. Over 90% of patients are affected with the first few doses. The vomiting lasts for 1–12 hours and may be completely but unpredictably palliated by prochlorperazine. Rarely, dacarbazine causes diarrhoea. Some helpful suggestions include restricting the patient's oral intake of fluids and food for 4–6 hours prior to treatment. The rapid toleration of these symptoms suggests a central nervous system mechanism, and usually these symptoms subside after the first 1 or 2 days.

Infrequently, some patients have experienced an influenza-like syndrome of fever to 39°C, myalgias and malaise. This syndrome occurs usually after large single doses and approximately 7 days after treatment with dacarbazine and lasts 7–21 days, and may recur with successive treatments.

Alopecia has been noted as has facial flushing and facial paraesthesia.

Hepatic toxicity, accompanied by hepatic vein thrombosis and hepatocellular necrosis resulting in death, has been reported. The incidence of such reactions has been low; approximately 0.01% of patients treated. This toxicity has been observed mostly when dacarbazine has been administered concomitantly with other anti-neoplastic drugs; however, it has also been reported in some patients treated with dacarbazine alone.

Anaphylaxis can occur very rarely following administration of dacarbazine.

Erythematous and urticarial rashes have been observed infrequently after administration of dacarbazine.

Rarely photosensitivity reactions may occur.

Pharmaceutical precautions Store in a refrigerator between 2° and 8°C.

Dacarbazine, like all triazenes is sensitive to exposure to light and the reconstituted solution should be protected from light.

After reconstitution in the vial the solution may be stored, suitably protected from light, at 4°C for 72 hours or at normal room temperature for up to 8 hours.

If the reconstituted solution is further diluted in 5% Dextrose Injection BP or Sodium Chloride Injection BP 0.9% the resulting solution may be stored at 4°C for up to 24 hours.

Legal category POM.

Package quantities Vials containing 100 mg and 200 mg DTIC-Dome as sterile dacarbazine.

Further information When reconstituted, the injection contains dacarbazine 10 mg/ml in a solution containing citric acid and mannitol at pH 3.0–4.0.

Product licence numbers
100 mg 0010/0127
200 mg 0010/0128

FABAHISTIN*

Presentation Orange coloured sugar-coated tablets measuring approximately 8.5 mm × 5.5 mm, each tablet containing 50 mg mebhydrolin base.

Uses Fabahistin is an antihistamine recommended for the treatment of hay fever, urticaria, rhinitis and all other allergic disorders.

Dosage and administration Oral administration as follows:

Adults: 1 or 2 × 50 mg tablets three times a day.

Children: Over 10 years: 1 or 2 × 50 mg tablets three times a day.

Contra-indications, warnings, etc
Contra-indications: None known.

Precautions: The substance may cause drowsiness. If affected, do not drive or operate machinery. Avoid alcoholic drink.

No embryotoxic or teratogenic effects have been reported, but, on principle, caution should be exercised when prescribing any medication during pregnancy and lactation.

Side-effects: Very rarely cases of granulocytopenia or agranulocytosis associated with the use of mebhydrolin have been reported.

Overdosage: No symptoms have been reported in a patient receiving 140 × 50 mg tablets.

Pharmaceutical precautions There are no special requirements for storage.

Legal category POM.

Package quantities Strip packs of 100 tablets.

Further information Nil.

Product licence number 0010/5913.

MIGRAVESS*

Presentation Round, flat, white tablets, 22 mm diameter engraved with a breakline and a letter 'm' in each half of the tablet.

Each dry tablet contains:

Metoclopramide monohydrochloride	5 mg
Aspirin BP	325 mg
Sodium Bicarbonate PhEur	1180 mg
Citric Acid PhEur	850 mg

Uses Migravess is an analgesic and anti-emetic recommended for the rapid symptomatic relief of headache and nausea associated with migraine.

Dosage and administration *Adults:* Two tablets dissolved in water to be taken at the first symptoms of a migraine attack. If the attack persists the dose may be repeated up to a maximum of three doses (six tablets) per day.

Young adults (12–15 years): Half the adult dose.

Migravess must be dissolved completely in half a glass of water before taking.

Contra-indications, warnings, etc
Contra-indications: Migravess is contra-indicated in children under 12 years of age, in patients hypersensitive to aspirin or salicylates and in patients with haemostatic abnormalities or active peptic ulceration.

Use in pregnancy: Studies in several animal species have demonstrated no teratogenic effects with metoclopramide. Aspirin may prolong labour and contribute to maternal and neonatal bleeding. Therefore Migravess should only be used when there are compelling reasons. It is not advised during the first trimester and is best avoided at term. Migravess is not recommended during lactation because metoclopramide is excreted in breast milk.

Warnings and precautions: Aspirin may induce bronchospasm and asthma attacks in susceptible individuals or may induce gastro-intestinal haemorrhage.

Care should be taken in patients on other centrally acting drugs e.g. for epilepsy.

If vomiting persists the patient, especially if under 20 years of age, should be reassessed in order to avoid masking an underlying disorder e.g. cerebral irritation.

Side-effects: Various extra-pyramidal reactions to metoclopramide have been reported, particularly in the young and the elderly. The incidence may be increased if daily doses in excess of those recommended are administered. The reactions reported include spasm of facial, extra ocular or cervical muscles. There may be a generalised increase in muscle tone. Any side-effects normally disappear within 24 hours of withdrawal of the drug. Should treatment be required an anti-Parkinson drug of the anticholinergic type may be used to counteract these reactions.

In common with most anti-emetic drugs, metoclopramide may cause drowsiness but this is less common than with antihistamines. Other reported effects are lethargy, dizziness, insomnia, diarrhoea and flatulence.

Raised serum prolactin levels have been observed during metoclopramide administration. Metoclopramide may induce an acute hypertensive response in patients with phaeochromocytoma.

Interactions: Metoclopramide may result in altered absorption of other oral medication e.g. decrease in digoxin absorption and increase in the absorption of paracetamol and various antibiotics. The effects of sympathomimetic drugs and tricyclic antidepressants may be affected.

Aspirin may enhance the effect of anticoagulants and may inhibit the action of uricosuric agents. Migravess should not be administered concomitantly with atropine, any anticholinergic drug or concurrent with the administration of phenothiazines or butyrophenones.

Overdosage: If overdosage occurs treat with gastric lavage and supportive therapy. Atropine 2 mg intramuscularly should be given for dystonic reactions in adults.

Forced alkaline diuresis may be used. Restoration of the acid-base balance may be necessary.

Pharmaceutical precautions Store at room temperature in a dry place and do not remove tablets from the foil until required.

Legal category POM.

Package quantities Migravess is available in cartons of 30 tablets (15 strips of 2 tablets). The tablets are packed in moisture proof aluminium foil laminate.

Further information Each tablet contains 14 mEq Na^+. Migravess presents aspirin and metoclopramide in effervescent form intended to hasten gastric emptying and therefore absorption, with freedom from the side-effects often associated with ergotamine containing preparations.

Product licence number 0010/0109.

MIGRAVESS* FORTE

Presentation Round, flat, white tablets, 22 mm diameter engraved with a breakline and a letter 'f' in each half of the tablet.

Each dry tablet contains:

Metoclopramide monohydrochloride	5 mg
Aspirin BP	450 mg
Sodium Bicarbonate PhEur	1230 mg
Citric Acid PhEur	850 mg

Uses Migravess Forte is an analgesic and anti-emetic recommended for the rapid symptomatic relief of headache and nausea associated with severe migraine.

Dosage and administration *Adults:* Two tablets dissolved in water to be taken at the first symptoms of a migraine attack. If the attack persists the dose may be repeated up to a maximum of three doses (six tablets) per day.

Young adults (12–15 years): Half the adult dose.

Migravess Forte must be dissolved completely in half a glass of water before taking.

Contra-indications, warnings, etc

Contra-indications: Migravess Forte is contra-indicated in children under 12 years of age, in patients hypersensitive to aspirin or salicylates and in patients with haemostatic abnormalities or active peptic ulceration.

Use in pregnancy: Studies in several animal species have demonstrated no teratogenic effects with metoclopramide. Aspirin may prolong labour and contribute to maternal and neonatal bleeding. Therefore Migravess Forte should only be used when there are compelling reasons. It is not advised during the first trimester and is best avoided at term. Migravess Forte is not recommended during lactation because metoclopramide is excreted in breast milk.

Warnings and precautions: Aspirin may induce bronchospasm and asthma attacks in susceptible individuals or may induce gastro-intestinal haemorrhage.

Care should be taken in patients on other centrally acting drugs e.g. for epilepsy.

If vomiting persists the patient, especially if under 20 years of age, should be reassessed in order to avoid masking an underlying disorder e.g. cerebral irritation.

Side-effects: Various extra-pyramidal reactions to metoclopramide have been reported, particularly in the young and the elderly. The incidence may be increased if daily doses in excess of those recommended are administered. The reactions reported include spasm of facial, extra ocular or cervical muscles. There may be a generalised increase in muscle tone. Any side-effects normally disappear within 24 hours of withdrawal of the drug. Should treatment be required an anti-Parkinson drug of the anticholinergic type may be used to counteract these reactions.

In common with most anti-emetic drugs, metoclopramide may cause drowsiness but this is less common than with antihistamines. Other reported effects are lethargy, dizziness, insomnia, diarrhoea and flatulence.

Raised serum prolactin levels have been observed during metoclopramide administration. Metoclopramide may induce an acute hypertensive response in patients with phaeochromocytoma.

Interactions: Metoclopramide may result in altered absorption of other oral medication e.g. decrease in digoxin absorption and increase in the absorption of paracetamol and various antibiotics. The effects of sympathomimetic drugs and tricyclic antidepressants may be affected.

Aspirin may enhance the effect of anticoagulants and may inhibit the action of uricosuric agents. Migravess Forte should not be administered concomitantly with atropine, any anticholinergic drug or concurrent with the administration of phenothiazines or butyrophenones.

Overdosage: If overdosage occurs treat with gastric lavage and supportive therapy. Atropine 2 mg intramuscularly should be given for dystonic reactions in adults.

Forced alkaline diuresis may be used. Restoration of the acid-base balance may be necessary.

Pharmaceutical precautions Store at room temperature in a dry place and do not remove tablets from the foil until required.

Legal category POM.

Package quantities Migravess Forte is available in cartons of 30 tablets (15 strips of 2 tablets). The tablets are packed in moisture proof aluminium foil laminate.

Further information Each tablet contains 14.6 mEq Na^+. Migravess Forte presents aspirin and metoclopramide in effervescent form intended to hasten gastric emptying and therefore absorption, with freedom from the side-effects often associated with ergotamine containing preparations.

Product licence number 0010/0108.

NIMOTOP*

Presentation

Nimotop tablets: White to pale yellow film-coated tablets marked with the Bayer cross on one side with the letters SK on the reverse. Each tablet contains 30 mg nimodipine.

Nimotop solution: Vials for intravenous infusion, each containing 10 mg nimodipine in 50 ml (0.02%), or bottles for intravenous infusion each containing 50 mg nimodipine in 250 ml (0.02%) of sterile aqueous alcoholic solvent.

Mode of action: Nimodipine is a calcium channel blocker of the dihydropyridine group with preferential activity on cerebral vessels. Nimodipine increases cerebral perfusion, particularly in poorly perfused areas, by arterial dilatation, an effect which is proportionately greater in smaller than in larger vessels.

Indications: Nimotop tablets are recommended for the prevention of ischaemic neurological deficits following subarachnoid haemorrhage.

Nimotop solution is recommended for the treatment of neurological deficits following subarachnoid haemorrhage.

Dosage and administration

Prophylactic administration: The recommended dose is two tablets at 4-hourly intervals (total daily dose 360 mg), to be taken with water. Prophylactic administration should commence within four days of onset of subarachnoid haemorrhage and should be continued for 21 days.

In the event of surgical intervention, administration of Nimotop tablets should be continued (dose as above) to complete the 21 day treatment period.

Therapeutic administration: For the first two hours of treatment 1 mg of nimodipine i.e. 5 ml Nimotop solution (about 15 μg/kg bw/h), should be infused each hour. The dose should be increased after 2 hours to 2 mg nimodipine i.e. 10 ml Nimotop solution per hour (about 30 μg/kg bw/h), providing no severe decrease in blood pressure is observed.

Patients of bodyweight less than 70 kg or with unstable blood pressure should be started on a dose of 0.5 mg nimodipine per hour (2.5 ml of Nimotop solution), or less if necessary.

Therapeutic administration should commence as soon as cerebral ischaemia occurs, and should continue for at least 5 days up to a maximum of 14 days.

In the event of surgical intervention during treatment, administration of Nimotop solution should be continued (dose as above) for at least 5 days.

If cerebral ischaemia occurs during prophylactic administration, tablet treatment may be continued to complete the 21-day treatment period or substituted by Nimotop solution (dosage as above). Nimotop solution may be used with or without pre-treatment with Nimotop tablets. Nimotop solution and tablets should not be used concomitantly.

Nimotop solution should be administered only via a by-pass into a running drip (40 ml/h) of either sodium chloride 0.9%, glucose 5% solution or Ringer's solution using an infusion pump via a central catheter. Nimotop solution must not be added to an infusion bag or bottle.

Nimotop solution may be used during anaesthesia or surgical procedures.

Special precautions: Nimotop solution reacts with polyvinylchloride (PVC). Polyethylene or polypropylene are the recommended plastic materials to be used during nimodipine infusion.

Polyethylene tubes are supplied with Nimotop solution 50 ml vials but not with Nimotop solution 250 ml bottles. The recommendations on materials to be used during nimodipine infusion must be strictly adhered to, with only polyethylene or polypropylene tubes being suitable. (See also Pharmaceutical Precautions).

Contra-indications, warnings, etc

Contra-indications: None known.

Warnings: Nimotop tablets and solution should be used

with care when cerebral oedema or severely raised intracranial pressure are present.

Nimotop tablets should not be administered concomitantly with Nimotop solution.

Nimodipine may potentiate the hypotensive effect of anti-hypertensives. Concomitant administration of other calcium channel blockers (e.g. nifedipine, diltiazem, verapamil), or beta-blockers should be avoided. Where such co-administration is unavoidable, careful dose titration of nimodipine should be undertaken with possible reduction or discontinuation of the anti-hypertensive agent.

Patients with known renal disease and/or receiving nephrotoxic drugs, should have renal function monitored closely during intravenous treatment with Nimotop solution.

Use in pregnancy: No reproductive toxicology studies following parenteral administration are available. Reproductive toxicology studies in animals after oral administration showed no teratogenic effect. Nimotop tablets and solution should be used with caution in pregnant women and only when the benefit of treatment is considered to outweigh the risk.

Side-effects
Nimotop solution and tablets: The following have been reported: decrease in blood pressure, slight increase or decrease in heart rate, flushing, headache, gastro-intestinal disorders, nausea and feeling of warmth.

Nimotop solution: A transient rise in liver enzymes may occur during intravenous administration; this usually reverts to normal on completion of treatment. The infusion contains 20% ethanol and 17% polyethylene glycol-400; this should be taken into account during treatment.

Overdosage
Nimotop Tablets: If overdosage occurs, gastric lavage should be carried out and activated charcoal administered. If blood pressure is low, a vasopressor should be administered.

Nimotop Solution: If overdosage occurs, treatment should be discontinued immediately. If there is a large drop in blood pressure an intravenous injection of dopamine or noradrenaline may be indicated.

Pharmaceutical precautions Nimotop tablets should be stored in the manufacturer's original container in a dry place at a temperature not exceeding 25°C.

Nimotop solution is light sensitive and therefore should be stored only in the manufacturer's light-protective container within the cardboard carton at a temperature not exceeding 25°C. The solution when in the syringe or infusion pump must be protected from direct sunlight during administration, but it is stable in diffuse daylight and artificial light for up to 10 hours.

The solution should not be allowed to come into contact with PVC. The only plastic materials suitable for use are polyethylene or polypropylene. Nimotop solution is compatible with glass infusion bottles and infusion packs made of polyethylene (e.g. Polyfusor, Boots).

Nimotop solution 50 ml vials should be infused using a glass or rigid plastic (polyethylene or polypropylene) syringe and giving set (Gillette Sabre syringe; BD plastipak syringe; Monoject disposable syringe, Sherwood Medical Ltd; Combidyn tubes, Braun; Nitrocassette giving set, Imed Ltd.). Nimotop solution is incompatible with infusion bags and any giving sets made of PVC (e.g. Viaflex, Travenol; Steriflex, Boots).

Nimotop solution 250 ml bottles are for single use and the rubber stopper should be pierced only once. One 250 ml bottle is sufficient for 24 hours administration at the maximum recommended dose with a safety margin of 1 hour. A single bottle should not be used for longer than 25 hours regardless of whether all the solution has been used.

The bottle should be protected from direct sunlight at all times. If appropriate, infusion pumps and tubing should be protected with opaque covering, or black, brown, yellow or red infusion lines (Braun) can be used. If a peristaltic pump is used for administration, the infusion line supplied should be used. If a volumetric pump, e.g. Imed, is used then Nitrocassette cartridges that are polyethylene lined should be used.

Legal category POM.

Package quantities Nimotop tablets: Each pack contains 100 × 30 mg tablets in foil strips of 10.

Nimotop solution: 50 ml vials: Each pack contains 5 × 50 ml (0.02% solution) vials and 5 polyethylene infusion lines.

250 ml bottles: Each pack contains 1 × 250 ml (0.02% solution) bottle.

Further information Pharmacokinetic studies have shown the area under the curve to be similar following oral or intravenous administration of Nimotop at the recommended doses.

Product licence numbers

Nimotop tablets	0010/0137
Nimotop solution	0010/0138

NYSTAFORM*-HC OINTMENT
NYSTAFORM*-HC CREAM

Presentation *Nystaform-HC ointment: Active ingredients:* Nystatin BP 100,000 Units/g; Chlorhexidine acetate BP 1.0% w/w; Hydrocortisone PhEur 1.0% w/w.

Form and appearance: Nystaform-HC ointment is a yellow ointment containing the active ingredients in a water-repellent base.

Nystaform-HC cream: Active ingredients: Nystatin BP 100,000 Units/g; Chlorhexidine hydrochloride BP 1.0% w/w; Hydrocortisone PhEur 0.5% w/w.

Form and appearance: Nystaform-HC cream is a light yellow cream containing the active ingredients in a water miscible base.

Uses *Actions:* Nystatin is a fungistatic and fungicidal antibiotic primarily effective against *Candida albicans*. Chlorhexidine has activity against a wide range of bacteria. Hydrocortisone exercises a vasoconstrictive effect, thus reducing inflammation and oedema and also has an antipruritic effect.

Indications: Nystaform-HC preparations are indicated in infected dermatoses where fungal (particularly monilial) and/or bacterial infection is present. The choice of cream or ointment presentations will depend upon the severity, physical characteristics and site of the condition, and upon the physician's preference.

Dosage and administration For topical application only. Apply to infected areas 2–3 times daily. Treatment should be for a maximum period of 7 days. This dosage is recommended for both children and adults.

Contra-indications, warnings, etc
Contra-indications: Tuberculous lesions of the skin. Known sensitivity to any of the ingredients.

Precautions: For external use only. Keep out of eyes. In infants, long term continuous topical steroid therapy should be avoided. Adrenal suppression can occur even without occlusion. As with other topical corticosteroids, systemic absorption may occur when extensive areas are treated, particularly under occlusion.

Topical administration of corticosteroids to pregnant animals can cause abnormalities of foetal development. The relevance of this finding to humans has not been established. However, topical steroids should not be used extensively in the first trimester of pregnancy, i.e. in large amounts or for prolonged periods. However, the unproven theoretical teratogenic hazard must be placed in perspective against the need to maintain the health of the patient.

Overdosage: Not applicable.

Main side-effects/adverse reactions: None reported.

Pharmaceutical precautions *Storage:* Store in a cool place.

Legal category POM.

Package quantities Nystaform-HC cream 15 g and 30 g tubes. Nystaform-HC ointment 30 g tubes.

Further information If sensitivity occurs, or if new infection appears, discontinue use and institute appropriate therapy.

The micronisation and microdispersion of the hydrocortisone in Nystaform-HC preparations ensure that the dispersal of this active ingredient over the affected area is as uniform as possible.

The water miscible base of Nystaform-HC cream is particularly easy to apply to inflamed and tender skin. It is pleasant to use and does not leave the skin feeling greasy. The water repellent base of Nystaform-HC ointment spreads easily and helps to protect against urine when used in the nappy rash area.

Product licence numbers
Nystaform-HC ointment 0010/0124
Nystaform-HC cream 0010/0123

NYSTAFORM* OINTMENT NYSTAFORM* CREAM

Presentation *Nystaform ointment: Active ingredients:* Nystatin BP 100,000 Units/g; Chlorhexidine acetate BP 1.0% w/w.

Form and appearance: Nystaform ointment is a yellow ointment containing the active ingredients in a water-repellent base.

Nystaform cream: Active ingredients: Nystatin BP 100,000 Units/g; Chlorhexidine hydrochloride BP 1.0% w/w.

Form and appearance: Nystaform cream is a light yellow cream containing the active ingredients in a water miscible base.

Uses *Actions:* Nystatin is a fungistatic and fungicidal antibiotic primarily effective against *Candida albicans*. Chlorhexidine has activity against a wide range of bacteria.

Indications: For the treatment of infected skin conditions where fungal (particularly monilial) and/or bacterial infections are present.

Dosage and administration For topical application only. Apply to infected area 2–3 times daily. Continue application for one week after lesions have healed.

This dosage is recommended for both children and adults.

The patient should be advised that if the condition is not better within seven days, to return to the surgery for a further consultation. In any event the duration of this treatment should not normally exceed fourteen days.

Contra-indications, warnings, etc
Contra-indications: Known sensitivity to any of the ingredients.

Precautions: For external use only. Keep out of eyes.

Overdosage: Not applicable.

Main side-effects/adverse reactions: None reported.

Pharmaceutical precautions *Storage:* Store in a cool place.

Legal category POM.

Package quantities 30 g tubes.

Further information If sensitivity occurs, or if new infection appears, discontinue use and institute appropriate therapy.

The water miscible base of Nystaform cream is particularly easy to apply to inflamed and tender skin. It is pleasant to use and does not leave the skin feeling greasy. The water repellent base of Nystaform ointment spreads easily and helps to protect against urine when used in the nappy rash area.

Product licence numbers
Nystaform ointment 0010/0122
Nystaform cream 0010/0121

SECUROPEN*

Presentation Vials containing 0.5 g, 1.0 g, 2.0 g azlocillin as azlocillin sodium. Infusion vials containing 5.0 g azlocillin as azlocillin sodium.

Securopen infusion sets containing 3 × 5.0 g azlocillin, 3 × 50 ml Water for Injections BP, 3 transfer needles and 3 hanging bags.

Uses Azlocillin is a broad spectrum antibiotic with especially significant anti-pseudomonal activity. In addition to *Pseudomonas* strains the spectrum of activity of azlocillin includes the following Gram-negative and Gram-positive pathogens: *Escherichia coli, Klebsiella-Enterobacter-Serratia* group, *Proteus* (indole-positive and indole-negative), *Providencia, Citrobacter, Salmonella* and *Shigella,* enterococci, staphylococci (penicillin sensitive), *Haemophilus influenzae*, gonococci, meningococci, pneumococci, streptococci and *Corynebacterium*. The spectrum also includes the anaerobic organisms *Clostridia* and *Bacteroides* species, including *Bacteroides fragilis*.

Azlocillin is indicated for the treatment of systemic and/or local infections due to sensitive organisms, especially infections of the respiratory and urinary tracts and for septicaemia.

Azlocillin may be administered concomitantly with an aminoglycoside or with beta-lactamase stable isoxazolyl-penicillin, since there is evidence of synergy with these compounds.

Dosage and administration
Adult Dosage:
Patients with normal renal function: Life-threatening infections 5.0 g every 8 hours. In non life-threatening and urinary tract infections 2.0 g every 8 hours.

Children's Dosage:

Age	*Bodyweight (kg)*	*Daily dose (mg/kg-bodyweight)*	*(g)*
6–14 yrs	20–40	3 × 75	3 × 1.5–3.0
2–6 yrs	13–20	3 × 75	3 × 1.0–1.5
1–2 yrs	10–13	3 × 75	3 × 0.75–1.0
Infants 7 days–1 year	3–10	3 × 100	3 × 0.3–1.0
Neonates up to 7 days	3	2 × 100	2 × 0.3
Premature babies	2.5	2 × 50	2 × 0.125
	2.0	2 × 50	2 × 0.100
	1.5	2 × 50	2 × 0.075

Patients with impaired renal function: i.e. with serum creatinine above 177 micromol/l (2 mg/dl) or with creatinine clearance less than 30 ml/minute, the unit dose should be as above but at 12 hourly intervals.

In patients presenting with severe impairment of both renal and hepatic functions, a further reduction of the dose may be necessary.

Patients on haemodialysis: Azlocillin is dialysable. On non-dialysing days, patients should receive the recommended unit dose of azlocillin twice daily. Before each dialysis an additional unit dose should be given to compensate for the amount of azlocillin removed by dialysis.

Duration of Treatment: The duration of treatment depends upon the severity of the infection and also the clinical and bacteriological course of the disease. In principle, treatment should be maintained for at least 3 days after fever or clinical symptoms have disappeared. This on average requires 7–10 days therapy.

Administration: Azlocillin is administered intravenously as a 10% solution in Water for Injections. For doses of

2.0 g or less it is administered as a bolus injection and for higher doses it should be infused over 20–30 minutes.

Supplementary drugs should be injected through the drip tubing and not introduced into the bag or bottle containing azlocillin. In patients already receiving intravenous infusion therapy with other drugs, azlocillin should be infused during the intervening periods or as a parallel infusion. In order to achieve higher initial concentrations in the serum and tissues, up to half of the appropriate dose of azlocillin may be injected slowly through the tubing of the existing infusion.

Combination therapy: aminoglycosides, injectable tetracycline derivatives, ciprofloxacin, and metronidazole have proved to be incompatible with azlocillin and must therefore be administered separately. Before administering rarely used solutions or drugs, the compatibility of the individual components must be ascertained; precipitation, cloudiness or discolouration indicate possible incompatibility.

Contra-indications, warnings, etc
Contra-indications: A history of allergy to other penicillins and cephalosporins. Azlocillin is inactivated by beta-lactamases (penicillinases).

Use in pregnancy: Animal studies have shown no evidence of teratogenic or embryotoxic effects of azlocillin. However, as with all drugs, it should be administered with caution during the early months of pregnancy and its use requires that the anticipated benefits outweigh the possible risks.

Side-effects: Side-effects are uncommon and typical of other injectable penicillins. These may include: local irritation including pain at the site of injection; gastro-intestinal disturbances e.g. nausea, diarrhoea, vomiting, and occasionally pseudomembranous colitis; hypersensitivity reactions e.g. skin rashes, pruritus. Anaphylactic reactions may also occur.

Since very high serum levels of penicillins may induce seizures, dose adjustment is necessary in patients with severely impaired renal function.

Abnormal clinico-chemical and blood values, may be seen during therapy.

During treatment with high doses of azlocillin a prolongation of bleeding time may occur as a result of a dose-dependent disturbance of thrombocyte function.

Interactions: The duration of neuromuscular blockade due to vecuronium may be prolonged if azlocillin is administered at the end of the operation.

Patients being treated with azlocillin and concomitant heparin or other anticoagulants need more frequent control of coagulation parameters.

Overdosage: Overdosage should be treated by standard monitoring and supportive measures. Serum levels of azlocillin may be reduced by dialysis.

Pharmaceutical precautions *Storage:* Azlocillin should not be stored in temperatures exceeding 25°C. The expiry date is printed on the packaging.

Dilution and compatibility: Azlocillin should be freshly prepared immediately before administration by shaking the powder with a suitable volume of Water for Injections until completely dissolved to make a 10% solution – that is, 0.5 g in 5 ml, 1.0 g in 10 ml, 2.0 g in 20 ml and 5.0 g in 50 ml. If azlocillin has to be prepared in advance of administration, it may be kept as the 10% solution for 6 hours without loss of efficacy. Any unused solution should be discarded. Azlocillin is compatible and stable in the common infusion fluids provided that the solutions are freshly prepared as above. These include 5% and 10% glucose solutions, fructose 5%, Ringer's solution and sodium chloride 0.9%. Compatibility with rarely used solutions must be ascertained prior to administration; possible incompatibility is indicated by precipitation, cloudiness or discolouration.

Legal category POM.

Package quantities 0.5 g, 1.0 g, 2.0 g vials packed in boxes of 5.
5.0 g vial packed singly.
Infusion pack of 3 × 5.0 g with diluent, transfer needles and hanging bags.

Further information
Sodium content:
Each 5.0 g vial contains 10.84 mEq sodium (249.1 mg)
Each 2.0 g vial contains 4.33 mEq sodium (99.6 mg)
Each 1.0 g vial contains 2.17 mEq sodium (49.8 mg)
Each 0.5 g vial contains 1.08 mEq sodium (24.9 mg)
Displacement value 0.74 ml/g

Product licence numbers
Securopen 0010/0075
Water for Injections BP 0010/0095

TRASYLOL*

Presentation Colourless glass vials containing a solution of aprotinin for injection, each 50 ml vial containing 70 mg aprotinin (=500,000 Kallikrein Inactivator Units, KIU=277.8 European Pharmacopoeia Units, E.P. units) in 0.9% sodium chloride solution.

Uses
Mode of action: Trasylol is a protease inhibitor which contributes to the re-establishment of haemostasis by inactivating free plasmin, thus supplementing the natural plasmin inhibitors, like alpha-2-antiplasmin, which are depleted in the hyperplasminaemic state. Trasylol also inhibits the fibrinolytic activity of the plasmin-streptokinase complex formed following thrombolytic therapy with streptokinase.

Trasylol is indicated for the treatment of life-threatening haemorrhage due to hyperplasminaemia. Such haemorrhage has occasionally been observed during the mobilisation and dissection of malignant tumours, in acute promyelocytic leukaemia, and following thrombolytic therapy.

Dosage and administration Initially 500,000 KIU (277.8 E.P. units) to 1,000,000 KIU (555.6 E.P. units) should be given by slow intravenous injection or infusion (maximum rate 5 ml/min). If necessary, this should be followed by 200,000 KIU (111.1 E.P. units) hourly until bleeding stops.

The dose for children should be calculated in proportion to the adult dose on the basis of body weight. There is no specific dosage recommendation for the use of Trasylol in the elderly.

Contra-indications, warnings, etc
Contra-indications: Known hypersensitivity to aprotinin.

Side-effects: Trasylol is generally well tolerated but may occasionally cause local thrombophlebitis.

Hypersensitivity or pseudoallergic reactions can occur, not only after repeated courses of treatment but also with first administration. The symptoms range from skin eruptions, tachycardia, pallor or cyanosis, dyspnoea and nausea, to anaphylactic shock.

Trasylol should be administered slowly (maximum 5 ml/min) intravenously to the supine patient. If a hypersensitivity reaction occurs during the injection, administration should be stopped immediately and the usual therapeutic measures instituted, e.g. adrenaline, antihistamines and intravenous corticosteroids. Intravenous fluids, bronchodilators, and respiratory support may also be needed.

Use in pregnancy: No evidence of teratogenic or embryotoxic effects has been seen in animals. Experience in human pregnancy and lactation is limited and inadequate to assess safety. Since the recommended indication is life-threatening Trasylol may be used during pregnancy and lactation when the benefit of treatment is considered to outweigh the risk.

Overdosage: There is no special antidote or other action to be taken.

Pharmaceutical precautions Any unused solution should be discarded immediately. Trasylol vials are stable at room temperature. However if the contents are cloudy, the product must not be used. Do not use the contents of the vials after the expiry date shown on the label.

Trasylol has been shown to be incompatible with corticosteroids, heparin, nutrient solutions containing amino acids or fat emulsions, and tetracyclines. Administration of Trasylol in mixed infusions (particularly with beta-lactam antibiotics) should be avoided. Trasylol is compatible with electrolyte and sugar solutions.

Legal category POM.

Package quantities Trasylol is supplied as single 50 ml vials each containing 500,000 KIU (277.8 EP units).

Further information Nil.

Product licence number 0010/5900.

YOMESAN*

Presentation Yellowish tablets measuring 13 mm × 4 mm, each tablet containing 500 mg niclosamide BP. One side marked FE, the reverse side with the Bayer cross. The tablets are flavoured with vanilla.

Uses An anthelmintic for treatment of tapeworm infections:

Taenia saginata	(beef tapeworm)
Taenia solium	(pork tapeworm)
Diphyllobothrium latum	(fish tapeworm)
Hymenolepis nana	(dwarf tapeworm)

It has no effect in cysticercosis and echinococcosis due to cestode larvae (cysticerci) lodging in extra intestinal tissues.

Dosage and administration *Taenia saginata, Taenia solium, Diphyllobothrium latum.*

Adults and children over 6 years:	4 tablets
Children 2 to 6 years:	2 tablets
Children under 2 years:	1 tablet

In *Taenia solium* the tablets should be taken as a single dose after a light breakfast but in the case of *Taenia saginata* and *Diphyllobothrium latum* the dose may be divided, half being taken after breakfast and the remainder one hour later.

An aperient should be administered two hours later and in the case of *Taenia solium* a drastic purge should be given.

Infection due to *Hymenolepsis nana* should be treated for 7 days:

First day:

Adults and children over 6 years:	4 tablets
Children from 2 to 6 years:	2 tablets
Children under 2 years:	1 tablet

The subsequent 6 days:

Adults and children over 6 years:	2 tablets
Children from 2 to 6 years:	1 tablet
Children under 2 years:	½ tablet

It is important that the tablets are chewed thoroughly before washing down with water. In the case of small children the tablets should be ground up before administration.

Contra-indications, warnings, etc

Contra-indications: Hypersensitivity to niclosamide.

Side-effects: Very rarely the drug may cause mild transient GI disturbances (such as nausea, retching and abdominal pain), light headedness and pruritus.

Overdosage: Yomesan is not absorbed and no cases of overdosage have occurred. In the event of overdose a fast acting laxative and enema may be given. Vomiting should not be induced.

Use in Pregnancy: In common with most drugs it is wise to avoid treatment in the first trimester of pregnancy. Healthy children have been born to women treated with Yomesan in the first trimester of pregnancy.

Experimental studies in rats showed no embryotoxic or teratogenic effects.

Warning: In infections with *Taenia solium* there is always a danger of cysticercosis. A drastic purge is therefore recommended after treatment to eject the lower segment of the tapeworm containing mature eggs.

The hands should be thoroughly scrubbed after defaecation not only on the treatment day but for several days afterwards to avoid reinfection.

The consumption of alcohol during treatment must be avoided.

In the event of constipation it is imperative to restore regular bowel movements before Yomesan treatment.

Pharmaceutical precautions The tablets are light sensitive and should only be stored in the original foil.

Legal category P.

Package quantities Packs of 4 tablets of 0.5 g.

Further information Unless the tapeworm is expelled by a drastic purgative, residual parts of it may be eliminated with the stools during the next two or three days. Thereafter, neither tapeworm segments nor ova should be present in the stools. In re-infection with *Taenia saginata* and *Taenia solium* new tapeworm segments or ova should only appear after three months.

In infections with *Hymenolepis nana* the follow-up period is only 14 days as surviving scolices regenerate very rapidly to sexually mature tapeworms and accordingly, after approx. 10 days, ova are eliminated with the stools.

Product licence number 0010/5910R.

**Trade Mark*

Beecham Research
Welwyn Garden City
Hertfordshire AL7 1EY

BEECHAM RESEARCH

AMPICLOX* INJECTION

Presentation *Ampiclox Injection:* Vials containing 250 mg ampicillin as Ampicillin Sodium BP with 250 mg cloxacillin as Cloxacillin Sodium BP.

Uses Ampiclox is indicated for the immediate treatment of severe infections before the infecting organism is identified, and for mixed staphylococcal and Gram-negative infections.

Typical indications include: Bronchopneumonia, post-influenzal pneumonia and other severe respiratory infections. Post-operative chest and wound infections. Septic abortion and infections during the puerperium. Septicaemia. Infections in patients receiving immunosuppressive drugs. Prophylaxis in major surgery.

Dosage and administration *Adult dosage (including elderly patients): Intramuscular/Intravenous:* 1–2 vials four to six hourly.

Children's dosage: Up to 2 years: ¼ adult dose.†
2–10 years: ½ adult dose.

Administration: Intramuscular: Dissolve vial contents in 1.5 ml Water for Injections BP.

Intravenous: Dissolve vial contents in 10 ml Water for Injections BP and administer slowly (three to four minutes). Ampiclox may also be added to infusion fluids or injected, suitably diluted, into the drip tube over a period of three to four minutes.

Dosage may be further increased where necessary.

Contra-indications, warnings, etc
Contra-indications: Penicillin hypersensitivity; ocular administration.

Use in pregnancy and lactation: Animal studies have shown no teratogenic effects. The product has been in clinical use since 1968 and the limited number of reported cases of use in human pregnancy have shown no evidence of untoward effect. The use of Ampiclox in pregnancy should be reserved for cases considered essential by the clinician. During lactation, trace quantities of penicillins can be detected in breast milk.

Side-effects: Side-effects, as with other penicillins, are uncommon and mainly of a mild and transitory nature. Gastro-intestinal upsets (e.g. nausea, diarrhoea) and skin rashes have been reported infrequently. An urticarial rash suggests penicillin hypersensitivity; an erythematous rash may arise in patients receiving ampicillin who have glandular fever. If a skin rash occurs, treatment should be discontinued.

Overdosage: Problems of overdosage with Ampiclox are unlikely to occur; if encountered they may be treated symptomatically.

Pharmaceutical precautions Ampiclox should be stored in a cool, dry place.

Ampiclox solutions for injection should be used immediately.

Ampiclox may be added to most intravenous fluids (e.g. Water for Injections, sodium chloride 0.9%, glucose 5%, sodium chloride 0.18% with glucose 4%). In intravenous solutions containing glucose or other carbohydrates, Ampiclox should be infused within one hour of preparation. Intravenous solutions of Ampiclox in Water for Injections or sodium chloride 0.9% should be infused within 24 hours of preparation. Full particulars are given in the package enclosure leaflet. Preparation of Ampiclox infusion solutions must be carried out under appropriate aseptic conditions if these extended storage periods are required.

Ampiclox should not be mixed with blood products or other proteinaceous fluids (e.g. protein hydrolysates) or with intravenous lipid emulsions.

If Ampiclox is prescribed concurrently with an aminoglycoside the antibiotics should not be mixed in the syringe, intravenous fluid container or giving set because loss of activity of the aminoglycoside and possibly precipitation can occur under these conditions.

Legal category POM.

Package quantities *Ampiclox Injection:* Boxes of 10, with instructions for use.

Further information Nil.

Product licence number 0038/5003R.

† Ampiclox Neonatal (regd) is recommended for the treatment of infections in neonates and premature babies.

AMPICLOX* NEONATAL SUSPENSION

Presentation *Ampiclox Neonatal Suspension:* Bottles containing powder for the preparation of 10 ml suspension. When reconstituted each 0.6 ml dose contains 60 mg ampicillin as Ampicillin Trihydrate BP with 30 mg cloxacillin as Cloxacillin Sodium BP. A pipette to measure the 0.6 ml dose is provided.

Ampiclox Neonatal Suspension also contains inactive ingredients to make the medicine acceptable. Amongst these is sodium benzoate.

Ampiclox Neonatal Suspension is sugar-free and free from artificial colourings.

Uses Ampiclox Neonatal is indicated for the prophylaxis or treatment of infections in premature babies or neonates, particularly:

Suspected or confirmed infections.

Babies born of mothers with infected liquor or whose membranes ruptured more than 48 hours before delivery.

Babies requiring certain surgical procedures carrying risk of infection such as exchange transfusions.

Babies born with respiratory distress necessitating endotracheal procedures, when subsequent infection is a possible hazard.

Babies following difficult delivery, when inhalation of much liquor, mucus or meconium has occurred.

Dosage and administration *Dosage: Oral:* 0.6 ml suspension (90 mg) every four hours.

Contra-indications, warnings, etc
Contra-indications: Penicillin-hypersensitivity; ocular administration.

Precautions: Caution should be observed when administering Ampiclox Neonatal to babies whose mothers are hypersensitive to penicillin.

Side-effects: Side-effects, as with other penicillins, are uncommon and mainly of a mild and transitory nature. Gastro-intestinal upsets (e.g. nausea, diarrhoea) and skin rashes have been reported infrequently. An urticarial rash suggests penicillin hypersensitivity; an erythematous rash may arise in patients receiving ampicillin who have glandular fever. If a skin rash occurs, treatment should be discontinued.

Overdosage: Problems of overdosage with Ampiclox Neonatal are unlikely to occur; if encountered they may be treated symptomatically.

Pharmaceutical precautions Ampiclox Neonatal should be stored in a cool, dry place.

Once dispensed, Ampiclox Neonatal Suspension remains stable for five days if kept in a cool place.

Legal category POM.

Package quantities *Ampiclox Neonatal Suspension:* Original Pack of 10 ml with pipette and Patient Information Leaflet.

Further information Ampiclox Neonatal Suspension is sugar-free to minimise the risk of diarrhoea in the newborn.

If tube feeding is necessary the suspension can easily be passed down a Ryle's tube.

Product licence number 0038/5009R.

AUGMENTIN* TABLETS AUGMENTIN* DISPERSIBLE TABLETS AUGMENTIN* JUNIOR SUSPENSION AUGMENTIN* PAEDIATRIC SUSPENSION

Approved name: Co-amoxiclav

Presentation

Augmentin tablets: White oval film-coated tablets engraved 'Augmentin' on one side. Each tablet provides 250 mg amoxycillin with 125 mg clavulanic acid.

Augmentin Dispersible tablets: White round tablets engraved 'Augmentin'. Each tablet provides 250 mg amoxycillin with 125 mg clavulanic acid.

Augmentin Junior suspension: Bottles of powder for the preparation of 100 ml suspension. When reconstituted each 5 ml provides 125 mg amoxycillin with 62 mg clavulanic acid.

Augmentin Paediatric suspension: Bottles of powder for the preparation of 100 ml suspension. When reconstituted each 5 ml provides 125 mg amoxycillin with 31 mg clavulanic acid.

In all the above presentations the amoxycillin is present as amoxycillin trihydrate and the clavulanic acid is present as potassium clavulanate.

Augmentin oral presentations also contain inactive ingredients to make the medicine acceptable. Children's presentations: Amongst these ingredients are aspartame and lactose in Augmentin Junior and Paediatric suspensions.

Augmentin presentations do not contain sucrose, tartrazine or any other azo dyes and Augmentin Suspensions do not contain preservatives.

Uses Augmentin is an antibiotic agent with a notably broad spectrum of activity against the commonly occurring bacterial pathogens in general practice and hospital. The β-lactamase inhibitory action of clavulanate extends the spectrum of amoxycillin to embrace a wider range of organisms, including many resistant to other β-lactam antibiotics.

Augmentin oral preparations are indicated for short-term treatment of bacterial infections at the following sites:

Upper Respiratory Tract Infections (including ENT) e.g. tonsillitis, sinusitis, otitis media.

Lower Respiratory Tract Infections e.g. acute and chronic bronchitis, lobar and bronchopneumonia.

Genito-urinary Tract Infections e.g. cystitis, urethritis, pyelonephritis.

Skin and Soft Tissue Infections.

Bone and joint infections e.g. osteomyelitis.

Other infections e.g. septic abortion, puerperal sepsis, intra-abdominal sepsis.

Augmentin is bactericidal to a wide range of organisms including:

Gram-positive

Aerobes: *Streptococcus faecalis, Streptococcus pneumoniae, Streptococcus pyogenes, Streptococcus viridans, Staphylococcus aureus,* Corynebacterium species, *Bacillus anthracis, Listeria monocytogenes.*

Anaerobes: Clostridium species, Peptococcus species, Peptostreptococcus.

Gram-negative

Aerobes: *Haemophilus influenzae, Escherichia coli, Proteus mirabilis, Proteus vulgaris,* Klebsiella species, Salmonella species, Shigella species, *Bordetella pertussis,* Brucella species, *Neisseria gonorrhoeae, Neisseria meningitidis, Vibrio cholerae, Pasteurella multocida.*

Anaerobes: Bacteroides spp. including *B. fragilis.*

Dosage and administration

Usual dosages for the treatment of infection

Adults and children over 12 years	1 Augmentin tablet or Dispersible tablet three times a day. In severe infections this may be increased to two tablets three times a day. Therapy can be started parenterally and continued with an oral preparation.
Children 6–12 years	5 ml Augmentin Junior Suspension three times a day. In severe infections this may be increased to 10 ml three times a day.
Children 2–6 years	5 ml Augmentin Paediatric Suspension three times a day. In severe infections this may be increased to 10 ml three times a day.
Children 9 months–2 years	5 ml half-strength Augmentin Paediatric Suspension three times a day.
Children 3–9 months	2.5 ml half-strength Augmentin Paediatric Suspension three times a day.
Children 0–3 months	No suitable presentation is currently available for this age group.

Dosage in renal impairment
Adults

Mild impairment (Creatinine clearance >30 ml/min)	Moderate impairment (Creatinine clearance 10–30 ml/min)	Severe impairment (Creatinine clearance <10 ml/min)
No change in dosage.	1–2 tablets 12 hourly.	Not more than 1 tablet 12 hourly.

Children: Similar reductions in dosage should be made for children.

Each 375 mg tablet of Augmentin contains 0.63 mmol of potassium.

Administration

Oral: Tablets, dispersible tablets or suspensions. The absorption of Augmentin is unaffected by food. Dispersible tablets should be stirred into a little water before taking.

Treatment should not be extended beyond 14 days without review.

Contra-indications, warnings, etc

Contra-indication: Penicillin hypersensitivity.

Use in pregnancy and lactation: Animal studies with orally and parenterally administered Augmentin have shown no teratogenic effects. The product has been used orally in human pregnancy in a limited number of cases, with no untoward effect; however, use of Augmentin tablets in pregnancy is not recommended unless considered essential by the physician.

During lactation, trace quantities of penicillins can be detected in breast milk.

Precautions: Changes in liver function tests have been observed in some patients receiving Augmentin. The clinical significance of these changes is uncertain but Augmentin should be used with care in patients with evidence of severe hepatic dysfunction.

In patients with moderate or severe renal impairment Augmentin dosage should be adjusted as recommended in the 'Dosage' section.

Side-effects: Side-effects, as with amoxycillin, are uncommon and mainly of a mild and transitory nature.

Diarrhoea, pseudomembranous colitis, indigestion, nausea, vomiting and candidiasis have been reported. Nausea, although uncommon, is more often associated with higher oral dosages. If gastro-intestinal side-effects occur with oral therapy they may be reduced by taking Augmentin at the start of meals. Hepatitis and cholestatic jaundice have been reported.

Urticarial and erythematous rashes sometimes occur. Rarely erythema multiforme and Stevens-Johnson Syndrome have been reported. Erythematous rashes have been associated with glandular fever in patients receiving amoxycillin. Treatment should be discontinued if one of these types of rash appears. In common with other β-lactam antibiotics angioedema and anaphylaxis have been reported.

Overdosage: Problems of overdosage with Augmentin are unlikely to occur; if encountered they may be treated symptomatically. Augmentin may be removed from the circulation by haemodialysis.

Pharmaceutical precautions Augmentin preparations should be stored in a dry place.

Bottles of Augmentin tablets should be kept tightly closed and the tablets dispensed in moisture-proof containers.

Once dispensed, Augmentin Junior and Paediatric suspensions remain stable for 7 days if kept in a refrigerator (but not frozen).

For administration to children up to 2 years, Augmentin Paediatric suspension should be diluted to half-strength, using water.

Legal category POM

Package quantities *Augmentin tablets:* Original Pack of 21 with Patient Information Leaflet; also bottles of 30, 100 and 500.

Augmentin Dispersible tablets: Original Pack of 21 with Patient Information Leaflet.

Augmentin Junior suspension: Original Pack of 100 ml.

Augmentin Paediatric suspension: Original Pack of 100 ml.

Further information Augmentin is a novel concept in antibiotic therapy.

Resistance to many antibiotics is caused by bacterial enzymes which destroy the antibiotic before it can act on the pathogen. The clavulanate in Augmentin anticipates this defence mechanism by blocking the β-lactamase enzymes, thus rendering the organisms sensitive to amoxycillin's rapid bactericidal effect at concentrations readily attainable in the body. Clavulanate by itself has little antibacterial activity; however, in association with amoxycillin as Augmentin it produces a novel antibiotic agent of broad spectrum with wide application in hospital and general practice.

The pharmacokinetics of the two components of Augmentin are closely matched. Peak serum levels of both occur about 1 hour after oral administration. Both clavulanate and amoxycillin have low levels of serum binding; about 70% remains free in the serum.

Doubling the dosage of Augmentin approximately doubles the serum levels achieved.

Augmentin Junior and Paediatric Suspensions contain aspartame.

Augmentin is also available as Augmentin Intravenous for the short-term treatment of bacterial infections and for prophylaxis against infection which may be associated with major surgical procedures. Augmentin Intravenous is described in a separate data sheet.

Product licence numbers

Augmentin Tablets	0038/0270
Augmentin Dispersible Tablets	0038/0272
Augmentin Junior Suspension	0038/0274
Augmentin Paediatric Suspension	0038/0298

AUGMENTIN* INTRAVENOUS

Approved name: Co-amoxiclav

Presentation Augmentin Intravenous: Vials of sterile powder providing 500 mg amoxycillin with 100 mg clavulanic acid (600 mg Augmentin) or 1 g amoxycillin with 200 mg clavulanic acid (1.2 g Augmentin). For reconstruction as an intravenous injection or infusion.

The amoxycillin is present as amoxycillin sodium and the clavulanic acid is present as potassium clavulanate.

Uses Augmentin is an antibiotic agent with a notably broad spectrum of activity against the commonly occurring bacterial pathogens in general practice and hospital. The β-lactamase inhibitory action of clavulanate extends the spectrum of amoxycillin to embrace a wider range of organisms, including many resistant to other β-lactam antibiotics.

Augmentin Intravenous is indicated for short-term treatment of bacterial infections at the following sites:

Upper respiratory tract infections (including ENT) e.g. tonsillitis, sinusitis, otitis media.

Lower respiratory tract infections e.g. acute and chronic bronchitis, lobar and bronchopneumonia.

Genito-urinary tract infections e.g. cystitis, urethritis, pyelonephritis, female genital infections.

Skin and soft tissue infections.

Bone and joint infections e.g. osteomyelitis.

Other infections e.g. septic abortion, puerperal sepsis, intra-abdominal sepsis, septicaemia, peritonitis, post-surgical infections.

Augmentin Intravenous is also indicated for prophylaxis against infection which may be associated with major surgical procedures such as gastro-intestinal, pelvic, head and neck, cardiac, renal, joint replacement and biliary tract.

Augmentin is bactericidal to a wide range of organisms including:

Gram-positive

Aerobes: *Streptococcus faecalis, Streptococcus pneumoniae, Streptococcus pyogenes, Streptococcus viridans, Staphylococcus aureus,* Corynebacterium species, *Bacillus anthracis, Listeria monocytogenes.*

Anaerobes: Clostridium species, Peptococcus species, Peptostreptococcus.

Gram-negative

Aerobes: *Haemophilus influenzae, Escherichia coli, Proteus mirabilis, Proteus vulgaris,* Klebsiella species, Salmonella species, Shigella species, *Bordetella pertussis,* Brucella species, *Neisseria gonorrhoeae, Neisseria meningitidis, Vibrio cholerae, Pasteurella multocida.*

Anaerobes: Bacteroides species including *B. fragilis.*

Dosage and administration

Dosages for the treatment of infection

Adults and children over 12 years	Usually 1.2 g 8 hourly. In more serious infections, increase frequency to 6 hourly intervals.
Children 3 months–12 years	Usually 30 mg/kg† Augmentin 8 hourly. In more serious infections, increase frequency to 6 hourly intervals.
Children 0–3 months	30 mg/kg† Augmentin every 12 hours in premature infants and in full term infants during the perinatal period, increasing to 8 hours thereafter.

† Each 30 mg Augmentin provides 5 mg clavulanic acid with 25 mg amoxycillin.

Dosage for surgical prophylaxis: Surgical prophylaxis with Augmentin should aim to protect the patient for the period of risk of infection. Accordingly, procedures lasting for less than 1 hour are covered in adults by 1.2 g Augmentin IV given at induction of anaesthesia. Longer operations require subsequent doses of 1.2 g Augmentin IV (up to 4 doses in 24 hours), and this regime can be continued for several days if the procedure has significantly increased the risk of infection.

Clear clinical signs of infection at operation will require a normal course of intravenous or oral Augmentin therapy post-operatively.

Dosage in renal impairment
Adults

Mild impairment (Creatinine clearance >30 ml/min)	Moderate impairment (Creatinine clearance 10–30 ml/min)	Severe impairment (Creatinine clearance <10 ml/min)
No change in dosage.	1.2 g IV stat. followed by 600 mg IV 12 hourly.	1.2 g IV stat. followed by 600 mg IV 24 hourly. Dialysis decreases serum concentrations of Augmentin and an additional 600 mg IV dose may need to be given during dialysis and at the end of dialysis.

Children: Similar reductions in dosage should be made for children.

Each 1.2 g vial of Augmentin contains 1.0 mmol of potassium and 3.1 mmol of sodium (approx).

Administration: Augmentin Intravenous may be administered either by intravenous injection or by intermittent infusion. It is not suitable for intramuscular administration.

600 mg vial: To reconstitute dissolve in 10 ml Water for Injections BP. (Final volume 10.5 ml.)

1.2 g vial: To reconstitute dissolve in 20 ml Water for Injections BP. (Final volume 20.9 ml.)

Augmentin Intravenous should be given by slow intravenous injection over a period of 3–4 minutes and used within 20 minutes of reconstitution. It may be injected directly into a vein or via a drip tube.

Alternatively, Augmentin Intravenous may be infused in Water for Injections BP or Sodium Chloride Intravenous Injection BP (0.9% w/v). Add, without delay, 600 mg reconstituted solution to 50 ml infusion fluid or 1.2 g reconstituted solution to 100 ml infusion fluid (e.g. using a minibag or in-line burette). Infuse over 30–40 minutes and complete within 4 hours of reconstitution. For other appropriate infusion fluids: see package enclosure leaflet.

Any residual antibiotic solutions should be discarded.

Augmentin Intravenous is less stable in infusions containing glucose, dextran or bicarbonate. Reconstituted solution should, therefore, not be added to such infusions but may be injected into the drip tubing over a period of 3–4 minutes.

Augmentin Intravenous should not be mixed with blood products, other proteinaceous fluids such as protein hydrolysates or with intravenous lipid emulsions.

If Augmentin is prescribed concurrently with an aminoglycoside the antibiotics should not be mixed in the syringe, intravenous fluid container or giving set because loss of activity of the aminoglycoside can occur under these conditions.

Treatment should not be extended beyond 14 days without review.

Contra-indications, warnings, etc
Contra-indication: Penicillin hypersensitivity.

Use in pregnancy and lactation: Animal studies with orally and parenterally administered Augmentin have shown no teratogenic effects. The product has been used orally in human pregnancy in a limited number of cases with no untoward effect; however, use of Augmentin in pregnancy is not recommended unless considered essential by the physician.

There is no experience with Augmentin IV in human pregnancy; therefore its use in pregnancy cannot be recommended.

During lactation, trace quantities of penicillins can be detected in breast milk.

Precautions: Changes in liver function tests have been observed in some patients receiving Augmentin. The clinical significance of these changes is uncertain but Augmentin should be used with care in patients with evidence of severe hepatic dysfunction.

In patients with moderate or severe renal impairment Augmentin dosage should be adjusted as recommended in the 'Dosage' section.

Side-effects: Side-effects, as with amoxycillin, are uncommon and mainly of a mild and transitory nature.

Diarrhoea, pseudomembranous colitis, indigestion, nausea, vomiting and candidiasis have been reported. Nausea, although uncommon, is more often associated with higher oral dosages. Hepatitis and cholestatic jaundice have been reported. Phlebitis at the site of injection has also been reported.

Urticarial and erythematous rashes sometimes occur. Rarely erythema multiforme and Stevens-Johnson Syndrome have been reported. Erythematous rashes have been associated with glandular fever in patients receiving amoxycillin. Treatment should be discontinued if one of these types of rash appears. In common with other β-lactam antibiotics angioedema and anaphylaxis have been reported.

Overdosage: Problems of overdosage with Augmentin are unlikely to occur; if encountered they may be treated symptomatically. Augmentin may be removed from the circulation by haemodialysis.

Pharmaceutical precautions Augmentin preparations should be stored in a dry place. Augmentin vials should be stored below 25°C.

For Augmentin Intravenous, particulars of stability in solution and compatibilities are given under 'Administration' and in the package enclosure leaflet.

Legal category POM

Package quantities *Augmentin Intravenous:* 600 mg: Pack of 10. 1.2 g: Pack of 5. Each pack contains instructions for use.

Further information Augmentin is a novel concept in antibiotic therapy.

Resistance to many antibiotics is caused by bacterial enzymes which destroy the antibiotic before it can act on the pathogen. The clavulanate in Augmentin anticipates this defence mechanism by blocking the β-lactamase enzymes, thus rendering the organisms sensitive to amoxycillin's rapid bactericidal effect at concentrations readily attainable in the body.

Clavulanate by itself has little antibacterial activity; however, in association with amoxycillin as Augmentin it produces a novel antibiotic agent of broad spectrum with wide application in hospital and general practice.

The pharmacokinetics of the two components of Augmentin are closely matched. Both clavulanate and amoxycillin have low levels of serum binding; about 70% remains free in the serum.

Doubling the dosage of Augmentin approximately doubles the serum levels achieved.

Augmentin is also available as Tablets, Dispersible Tablets, Junior Suspension and Paediatric Suspension for the short term treatment of bacterial infections. Augmentin oral presentations are described in a separate Data Sheet.

Product licence numbers

Augmentin Intravenous 600 mg	0038/0320
Augmentin Intravenous 1.2 g	0038/0320

BACTROBAN* OINTMENT

Presentation *Bactroban Ointment:* A sterile presentation of mupirocin 2% w/w in a white, translucent, water-soluble, polyethylene glycol base.

Uses
Action: Bactroban is a topical antibacterial agent, active against those organisms responsible for the majority of skin infections, e.g. *Staphylococcus aureus*, including methicillin-resistant strains, other staphylococci, streptococci. It is also active against Gram-negative organisms such as *Escherichia coli* and *Haemophilus influenzae.*

Indications: Bacterial skin infections, e.g. impetigo, folliculitis, furunculosis.

Dosage and administration
Adults and children: Bactroban Ointment should be applied to the affected area up to three times a day, for up to 10 days. The area may be covered with a dressing or occluded if desired.

Contra-indications, warnings, etc
Contra-indications: Hypersensitivity to Bactroban or other ointments containing polyethylene glycols.

This Bactroban ointment formulation is not suitable for ophthalmic or intra-nasal use.

Use in pregnancy: Studies in experimental animals have shown mupirocin to be without teratogenic effects. However, there is inadequate evidence of safety to recommend the use of Bactroban during pregnancy.

Precautions: When Bactroban Ointment is used on the face, care should be taken to avoid the eyes.

Polyethylene glycol can be absorbed from open wounds and damaged skin and is excreted by the kidneys. In common with other polyethylene glycol based ointments, Bactroban Ointment should be used with caution if there is evidence of moderate or severe renal impairment.

Adverse reactions and side-effects: During clinical studies some minor adverse effects, localised to the area of application, were seen such as burning, stinging and itching.

Pharmaceutical precautions Bactroban Ointment may be stored at room temperature (below 25°C).

The ointment is supplied sterile; any remaining at the end of treatment should be discarded.

Legal category POM.

Package quantities *Bactroban Ointment:* Original Pack of 15 g (sealed tube in a carton).

Further information Bactroban is a novel antibiotic, both in chemical structure and mode of action; available only for topical application.

The active ingredient of Bactroban was previously described as pseudomonic acid in the published literature.

Bactroban Ointment is water soluble and does not stain the skin or clothing; it is easily removed by washing.

Product licence number 0038/0319.

BACTROBAN* NASAL

Presentation Bactroban Nasal Ointment: Calcium mupirocin equivalent to 2% w/w mupirocin in a white soft paraffin based ointment containing a glycerin ester.

Uses
Action: Bactroban is a topical antibacterial agent, active against those organisms responsible for the majority of skin infections, e.g. *Staphylococcus aureus*, including methicillin-resistant strains, other staphylococci, streptococci. It is also active against Gram-negative organisms such as *Escherichia coli* and *Haemophilus influenzae*.

Indication: The elimination of nasal carriage of staphylococci, including methicillin resistant *Staphylococcus aureus* (MRSA).

Dosage and administration
Adults and children: Bactroban Nasal Ointment should be applied to the anterior nares two to three times a day, as follows:

A small amount of the ointment (about the size of a match-head) should be placed on a cotton bud or on the little finger and applied to the anterior part of the inside of each nostril. The nostrils are closed by pressing the sides of the nose together; this will spread the ointment throughout the nares. A cotton bud should be used instead of the little finger for application in particular to infants or patients who are very ill.

Nasal carriage should normally clear within 5–7 days of treatment.

Contra-indications, warnings, etc
Contra-indications: Hypersensitivity to any of the constituents of Bactroban Nasal Ointment.

Use in pregnancy: Studies on experimental animals have shown mupirocin to be without teratogenic effects. However, there is inadequate evidence of safety to recommend the use of Bactroban Nasal Ointment during pregnancy.

Precautions: As with all topical preparations care should be taken to avoid the eyes.

Side-effects: During clinical studies some minor adverse effects were noted, such as a transient stinging sensation localised to the area of application.

Pharmaceutical precautions Bactroban Nasal Ointment may be stored at room temperature (below 25°C).

Any ointment remaining at the end of treatment should be discarded.

Legal category POM.

Package quantities *Bactroban Nasal Ointment:* Original Pack of 3 g (tube in a sealed carton) with instructions for use.

Further information Bactroban is a novel antibiotic, both in chemical structure and mode of action; available only for topical application.

To enhance the spreading properties of Bactroban Nasal Ointment, the preparation incorporates a glycerin ester as a lanolin substitute. This is based on synthetic triglycerides of naturally occurring fatty acids and has a low potential for sensitisation.

For the treatment of bacterial skin infections Bactroban Ointment should be used. See separate Bactroban Data Sheet for details.

The active ingredient of Bactroban was previously described as pseudomonic acid in the published literature.

Product licence number 0038/0347.

CELBENIN* INJECTION

Presentation *Celbenin Injection* (Methicillin Injection BP 1973): Vials containing 1 g Methicillin Sodium BP 1973.

Uses Celbenin is indicated for the treatment of infections suspected or confirmed to be caused by β-lactamase-producing staphylococci.

Typical indications include: Respiratory tract infections. Skin and soft tissue infections. Osteomyelitis and septic arthritis. Staphylococcal urinary tract infections. Enteritis. Endocarditis. Meningitis. Septicaemia.

Dosage and administration *Usual adult dosage (including elderly patients):*

Intramuscular: 1 g four to six hourly.
Intravenous: 1 g four to six hourly.

All recommended dosages are a guide only. In severe infections systemic dosages may be increased.

Intra-articular: 500 mg to 1 g once daily.
Intrapleural: 500 mg to 1 g once daily.
Subconjunctival: Up to 500 mg once daily.
By nebuliser: 500 mg four times a day.

Usual children's dosage: 2–10 years: $\frac{1}{2}$ adult dose.
Under 2 years: $\frac{1}{4}$ adult dose.

Administration: Intramuscular: Add 1.5 ml Water for Injections BP to 1 g vial contents.

Intravenous: Dissolve 1 g in 20 ml Water for Injections BP and give by slow injection (three to four minutes). Celbenin may also be added to infusion fluids or injected, suitably diluted, into the drip tube over a period of three to four minutes. Infusion bottles containing Celbenin should be changed every five hours.

Celbenin may be administered by other routes in conjunction with systemic therapy.

Intra-articular: Dissolve 1 g in 5 ml Water for Injections BP or 0.5% lignocaine hydrochloride solution.

Intrapleural: Dissolve 1 g in 10 ml Water for Injections BP.

Subconjunctival: Dissolve up to 500 mg in 0.5–0.75 ml of sterile water.

Nebuliser Solution: Dissolve 500 mg in 5 ml sterile water and administer by a suitable nebuliser.

Contra-indications, warnings, etc
Contra-indications: Penicillin hypersensitivity.

Use in pregnancy and lactation: Celbenin has been in clinical use since 1960 with no evidence of untoward effect in pregnancy. There are, however, inadequate animal and clinical data to recommend its use in pregnancy. During lactation, trace quantities of penicillins can be detected in breast milk.

Side-effects: Side-effects, as with other penicillins, are uncommon and mainly of a mild and transitory nature. Gastro-intestinal upsets (e.g. nausea, diarrhoea) and skin rashes have been reported infrequently. If a skin rash occurs, treatment should be discontinued.

Overdosage: Problems of overdosage with Celbenin are unlikely to occur; if encountered they may be treated symptomatically.

Pharmaceutical precautions Celbenin should be kept in a cool, dry place.

Solutions for IM or direct IV injection should normally be administered within 30 minutes of preparation. However, aqueous solutions of Celbenin Injection retain their activity for up to 5 hours at room temperature (25°C) and for up to 72 hours in a refrigerator (5°C).

Celbenin may be added to most intravenous fluids (e.g. Water for Injections, sodium chloride 0.9%, glucose 5%, sodium chloride 0.18% with glucose 4%). Intravenous solutions of Celbenin for infusion should be used within 4–6 hours of preparation. Full particulars are given in the package enclosure leaflet.

Reconstitution of Celbenin injections and preparation of Celbenin infusion solutions must be carried out under appropriate aseptic conditions if the extended storage periods are required.

Celbenin should not be mixed with blood products or other proteinaceous fluids (e.g. protein hydrolysates) or with intravenous lipid emulsions.

Legal category POM.

Package quantities Celbenin vials are supplied in boxes of 10. Each pack contains instructions for use.

Further information Nil.

Product licence number 0038/5024R.

EMINASE* ▼

Presentation Eminase is presented as a white to off-white sterile, freeze-dried solid in vials containing 30 Units of anistreplase.

Its chemical name is p-anisoylated (human) lys-plasminogen-streptokinase activator complex (APSAC). The approved name is anistreplase.

The potency of Eminase is measured using a reference standard which is specific for Eminase and is not comparable with units used for other thrombolytic agents.

Eminase includes the following inactive ingredients as solubilisers and stabilisers: aminocaproic acid, human albumin, lysine hydrochloride, mannitol, p-amidinophenyl-p'-anisate hydrochloride.

Uses
Indication: Eminase is indicated in the treatment of acute myocardial infarction to establish reperfusion, to preserve left ventricular function, to limit infarct size and to reduce mortality.

Clinical studies have shown that Eminase significantly reduces 30 day and 1 year mortality, limits infarct size and preserves left ventricular function.

Action: Eminase is a thrombolytic enzyme complex in which the catalytic centre of the activator complex is temporarily masked by an anisoyl group.

Eminase binds to fibrin strongly: this assists both its initial uptake and retention within the thrombus.

After intravenous injection, deacylation proceeds immediately with formation of the enzymatically active lys-plasminogen-streptokinase activator complex. Deacylation of Eminase proceeds in a controlled and sustained manner, resulting in a long plasma half-life which allows progressive clot uptake. This ensures sustained activation which may be useful in facilitating a low rate of early reocclusion.

The generation of lys-plasminogen-streptokinase activator complex within the thrombus converts fibrin-bound plasminogen to plasmin. The plasmin then dissolves the fibrin of the thrombus. The enzymatic efficiency of lys-plasminogen-streptokinase activator complex is enhanced by clot fibrin, ensuring efficient thrombolysis.

Dosage and administration
Dosage
Adults: Eminase is given as a single 30 Unit dose as a 4 to 5 minute intravenous injection.

Elderly: As above. See 'Precautions'.

Thrombolytic therapy should be administered as soon as possible after the onset of symptoms and preferably within 6 hours. The ease of administration of Eminase should facilitate early treatment of the patient with acute myocardial infarction, for whom time is critical.

Preparation: Eminase should be reconstituted by dissolving the contents of a 30 Unit vial in 5 ml Water for Injections BP. (5 ml Sodium Chloride Injection BP (0.9% w/v) is a suitable alternative.) To avoid foaming, the diluent should be directed against the wall of the vial and the powder dissolved by gently swirling. AVOID SHAKING. Eminase dissolves immediately to give a clear or slightly turbid, colourless to pale yellow solution.

NO OTHER MEDICATION SHOULD BE ADDED TO THE VIAL OR SYRINGE CONTAINING EMINASE.

Administration: Eminase should be given by slow intravenous injection over 4 to 5 minutes.

The reconstituted solution should be administered as soon as possible. If unused after 30 minutes the solution must be discarded.

Discoloured solutions should not be used.

RECONSTITUTED SOLUTION MUST NOT BE ADMINISTERED BY INTRAMUSCULAR INJECTION OR ADDED TO INFUSION FLUIDS.

Anticoagulation: The use of anticoagulants or antiplatelet drugs following administration of Eminase has not been shown to be of unequivocal benefit. In clinical studies a majority of patients treated with Eminase received heparin therapy 4 to 6 hours after Eminase during their hospital stay, followed by oral anticoagulation as appropriate.

Following Eminase, there is a decrease in plasma fibrinogen and plasminogen concentrations and an increase in fibrin degradation products. Values have generally returned to normal within 24 to 48 hours of therapy.

Contra-indications, warnings, etc
Contra-indications: Since all thrombolytic therapies increase the risk of bleeding, Eminase is contra-indicated in the following situations:
- After surgery or major trauma within the previous 10 days.
- Recent neurosurgical procedure (previous 2 months).
- Recent traumatic cardio-pulmonary resuscitation.
- In patients with active gastro-intestinal bleeding or other internal bleeding (within the previous 6 months), e.g. active peptic ulcer.
- History of cerebrovascular accident.
- In patients with known bleeding diathesis.
- In patients with severe, uncontrolled hypertension.
- In patients with known intracranial neoplasm, or aneurysm.
- in women with heavy vaginal bleeding.

Precautions: The most common complication associated with Eminase therapy is bleeding.

Patients with any condition in which bleeding constitutes a significant hazard, or which would be particularly difficult to manage because of its location, should be monitored carefully. The risks of Eminase therapy may be increased in such patients and should be weighed against the anticipated benefits.

Venepuncture and other invasive procedures should be kept to a minimum in order to reduce the risk of bleeding. In patients undergoing cardiac catheterisation the sheath should not be removed until 24 hours after dosing.

Patients with evidence of intramural ventricular thrombus or thrombus within abdominal aneurysms should be treated with caution as there is a risk of dissolution of clot with subsequent embolisation. This risk should be considered against the benefits of Eminase therapy.

Accelerated idioventricular rhythm may be associated with reperfusion of the coronary artery. Other arrhythmias (such as sinus bradycardia, ventricular tachycardia and ventricular fibrillation) may occur. These are not different from those often seen in the course of acute myocardial infarction and should be managed with standard measures.

Experience is limited in patients over 70 years of age and the benefits of Eminase should be balanced against risk in this group.

Because of the increased likelihood of resistance due to anti-streptokinase antibody, Eminase may not be effective if administered more than 5 days after prior Eminase or streptokinase therapy, particularly between 5 days and 12 months. Furthermore, increased anti-streptokinase antibody levels after Eminase or streptokinase may also increase the risk of allergic reactions following readministration.

Rapid injection of Eminase has been followed, in some patients, by a precipitate but transient fall in blood pressure. Eminase should be given by slow intravenous injection over 4 to 5 minutes.

Use in pregnancy and lactation: There is no evidence as to the drug safety in human pregnancy nor is there evidence from animal work that it is free from hazard. Avoid in pregnancy unless there is no safer alternative.

There is no information regarding the use of Eminase in lactating mothers.

Drug interactions: The interaction of Eminase and other drugs has not been formally studied.

Side-effects

Early reactions: Flushing, bradycardia and transient hypotension (usually within the first hour) as well as fever and nausea/vomiting (usually within 6 to 24 hours) have been reported but such reactions are generally not severe.

Allergic reactions including bronchoconstriction and anaphylaxis have been reported but are uncommon and usually reversible. A purpuric rash has occasionally been reported. All cases recovered spontaneously without sequelae.

Other reactions: The most common complication associated with thrombolytic therapy is bleeding, most frequently from arterial and venous puncture sites. Haemoptysis, haematuria, haematemesis and melaena have been reported occasionally. Cerebrovascular accidents have been reported but the incidence is low and there has usually been a predisposing factor.

Careful patient selection with due regard to risk factors and contra-indications can reduce the likelihood of haemorrhage.

Treatment of reactions: Local bleeding can be controlled with pressure. In cases of severe uncontrolled bleeding, if the haematocrit has fallen significantly transfusion with packed cells or whole blood may be necessary. Cryoprecipitate or purified clotting factor concentrates may also be used to correct the haemostatic deficiency. Tranexamic acid (10 mg/kg body weight given by slow intravenous injection) or aprotinin (see manufacturer's literature) will competitively inhibit the fibrinolytic action of Eminase.

Mild to moderate allergic reactions may be treated, if required, with an antihistamine. Severe anaphylactic reactions should be treated with adrenaline, corticosteroids and antihistamines as appropriate. Corticosteroids may be given prophylactically, if desired.

Treatment of overdosage: see under 'Treatment of reactions'.

Pharmaceutical precautions

Stability and storage: Eminase must be stored at 2–8°C (not frozen) and must not be used after the expiry date printed on the pack and vial. The IV Injection Pack, which includes Water for Injections, must not be frozen. Eminase vials must not be stored at room temperature. If a vial of Eminase is removed from the refrigerator in anticipation of being used, but is then not used, the vial can be returned to the refrigerator provided the material has not been reconstituted and is returned within 2 to 3 hours.

Reconstituted solution should be administered as soon as possible. If unused after 30 minutes the solution must be discarded.

Compatibility: No other medication should be added to the vial or syringe containing Eminase.

Legal category POM.

Package quantities

Vials of Eminase 30 Units, boxed singly.
Vials of Eminase 30 Units, boxed in packs of 5.
IV Injection Pack: 1 vial Eminase 30 Units, a 5 ml ampoule of Water for Injections BP, a 5 ml disposable syringe and needle.
Each pack contains instructions for use.

Further information Eminase belongs to a new class of thrombolytic agents designed for use in the treatment of acute myocardial infarction. Eminase can be given as a single, slow intravenous injection, over 4 to 5 minutes, unlike other thrombolytic agents which require intravenous infusions of various degrees of complexity. The ease of administration of Eminase facilitates early treatment of the patient with acute myocardial infarction, for whom time is critical.

The fibrinolytic mean half-life of Eminase is 94 minutes (range of 70 to 120 minutes).

At the recommended dose of 30 Units injected intravenously in patients with acute myocardial infarction of less than 6 hours duration, patency of coronary arteries has occurred in 70–80% of patients.

The incidence of early reocclusion with Eminase is low and is less than 10% in reported studies.

Clinical studies have shown that reperfusion with Eminase preserves myocardial function and improves patient survival.

Randomised controlled studies have demonstrated that treatment with Eminase reduces mortality for at least 1 year when administered within 6 hours after the onset of symptoms of acute myocardial infarction.

It is recommended that antiarrhythmic therapy for bradycardia and/or ventricular irritability be available when infusions of Eminase are administered as would normally be required in the early phase of acute myocardial infarction.

Product licence numbers

Eminase 30 Unit vial	0038/0353
Water for Injections BP	0038/0118

FLOXAPEN* CAPSULES
FLOXAPEN* SYRUPS
FLOXAPEN* INJECTION

Presentation *Floxapen Capsules* (Flucloxacillin Capsules BP): Black and caramel capsules overprinted Floxapen, containing 250 mg or 500 mg flucloxacillin as Flucloxacillin Sodium BP.

Floxapen Vials for Injection (Flucloxacillin Injection BP): Each vial contains 250 mg, 500 mg or 1 g flucloxacillin as Flucloxacillin Sodium BP.

Floxapen Syrups (Flucloxacillin Oral Suspension BP): Bottles containing powder for the preparation of 100 ml suspension. When reconstituted each 5 ml contains

125 mg or 250 mg flucloxacillin, as Flucloxacillin Magnesium BP.

Unidose sachets of powder for the preparation of a single dose of suspension. Each sachet contains 125 mg flucloxacillin as Flucloxacillin Magnesium BP.

Floxapen oral presentations also contain inactive ingredients to make the medicine acceptable. Children's presentations: amongst these ingredients are sodium benzoate and sucrose in Floxapen Syrup and Sachets.

Uses Floxapen is indicated for the treatment of infections due to Gram-positive organisms, including infections caused by β-lactamase-producing staphylococci. Typical indications include:

Skin and soft tissue infections: Boils. Abscesses. Carbuncles. Infected skin conditions, e.g. ulcer, eczema, and acne. Furunculosis. Cellulitis. Infected wounds. Infected burns. Protection for skin grafts. Otitis media and externa. Impetigo.

Respiratory tract infections: Pneumonia. Lung abscess. Empyema. Sinusitis. Pharyngitis. Tonsillitis. Quinsy.

Other infections caused by Floxapen-sensitive organisms: Osteomyelitis. Enteritis. Endocarditis. Urinary tract infection. Meningitis. Septicaemia.

Floxapen is also indicated for use as a prophylactic agent during major surgical procedures where appropriate; for example, cardiothoracic and orthopaedic surgery.

Dosage and administration

Usual adult dosage (including elderly patients)

Oral – 250 mg four times a day.
Intramuscular – 250 mg four times a day.
Intravenous – 250 mg – 1 g four times a day.

The above systemic dosages may be doubled where necessary; oral doses should be administered ½–1 hour before meals.

Osteomyelitis, endocarditis – Up to 8 g daily, in divided doses six to eight hourly.

Surgical prophylaxis – 1 to 2 g IV at induction of anaesthesia followed by 500 mg six hourly IV, IM, or orally for up to 72 hours.

Floxapen may be administered by other routes in conjunction with systemic therapy.

Intrapleural – 250 mg once daily.
By nebuliser – 125–250 mg four times a day.
Intra-articular – 250–500 mg once daily.

Usual children's dosage

2–10 years: ½ adult dose.
Under 2 years: ¼ adult dose.

Abnormal renal function: In common with other penicillins, Floxapen usage in patients with renal impairment does not usually require dosage reduction. However, in the presence of severe renal failure (creatinine clearance < 10 ml/min) a reduction in dose or an extension of dose interval should be considered.

Floxapen is not significantly removed by dialysis and hence no supplementary dosages need to be administered either during, or at the end of the dialysis period.

Administration

Intramuscular: Add 1.5 ml Water for Injections BP to 250 mg vial contents or 2 ml Water for Injections BP to 500 mg vial contents.

Intravenous: Dissolve 250–500 mg in 5–10 ml Water for Injections BP or 1 g in 15–20 ml Water for Injections BP. Administer by slow intravenous injection (three to four minutes). Floxapen may also be added to infusion fluids or injected, suitably diluted, into the drip tube over a period of three to four minutes.

Intrapleural: Dissolve 250 mg in 5–10 ml Water for Injections BP.

Intra-articular: Dissolve 250–500 mg in up to 5 ml Water for Injections BP or 0.5% lignocaine hydrochloride solution.

Nebuliser solution: Dissolve 125–250 mg of the vial contents in 3 ml sterile water.

Contra-indications, warnings, etc

Contra-indications: Penicillin hypersensitivity; ocular administration.

Use in pregnancy and lactation: Animal studies with Floxapen have shown no teratogenic effects. The product has been in clinical use since 1970 and the limited number of reported cases of use in human pregnancy have shown no evidence of untoward effect. The use of Floxapen in pregnancy should be reserved for cases considered essential by the clinician. During lactation, trace quantities of penicillins can be detected in breast milk.

Side-effects: Side-effects, as with other penicillins, are uncommon and mainly of a mild and transitory nature. Gastro-intestinal upsets (e.g. nausea, diarrhoea) and skin rashes have been reported. If a skin rash occurs, treatment should be discontinued. Hepatitis and cholestatic jaundice have been reported rarely. Pseudomembranous colitis has been reported rarely and has usually been associated with use of Floxapen in combination with other antibiotics.

Overdosage: Problems of overdosage with Floxapen are unlikely to occur; if encountered they may be treated symptomatically.

Pharmaceutical precautions Floxapen Capsules in Original Packs and Floxapen Syrups (bottles and sachets) should be stored in a dry place. Floxapen Capsules in reclosable containers and Floxapen Vials for Injection should be stored in a cool, dry place.

Once dispensed, Floxapen Syrups (bottles) remain stable for fourteen days when kept in a cool place. If a dilution of the reconstituted syrup is required, Syrup BP should be used.

Solutions for IM or direct IV injection should normally be administered within 30 minutes of preparation. However, aqueous solutions of Floxapen Injection retain their activity for up to 24 hours at room temperature (25°C) and up to 72 hours in a refrigerator (5°C).

Floxapen may be added to most intravenous fluids (e.g. Water for Injections, sodium chloride 0.9%, glucose 5%, sodium chloride 0.18% with glucose 4%). Intravenous solutions of Floxapen for infusion, stored up to 25°C, should be used within 24 hours of preparation. Full particulars are given in the package enclosure leaflet.

Reconstitution of Floxapen injections and preparation of Floxapen infusion solutions must be carried out under appropriate aseptic conditions if the extended storage periods are required.

Floxapen should not be mixed with blood products or other proteinaceous fluids (e.g. protein hydrolysates) or with intravenous lipid emulsions.

If Floxapen is prescribed concurrently with an aminoglycoside, the two antibiotics should not be mixed in the syringe, intravenous fluid container or giving set; precipitation may occur.

Legal category POM.

Package quantities

Floxapen Capsules 250 mg: Original Pack of 28 with Patient Information Leaflet; also containers of 20, 100 and 500.
Floxapen Capsules 500 mg: Original Pack of 28 with Patient Information Leaflet; also containers of 100.
Floxapen Vials 250 mg or 500 mg: boxes of 10 with instructions for use.
Floxapen Vials 1 g: boxes of 5 with instructions for use.
Floxapen Syrup 125 mg/5 ml: Original Pack of 100 ml with Patient Information Leaflet.
Floxapen Syrup 250 mg/5 ml: Original Pack of 100 ml with Patient Information Leaflet.
Floxapen Syrup 125 mg Unidose Sachets: boxes of 20 (hospital only). Each sachet contains instructions for preparation.

Further information Floxapen syrups are now formulated using the magnesium salt of flucloxacillin, in preference to the sodium salt, in order to provide two palatable strengths of suspension.

Following oral administration Floxapen gives blood levels comparable to those achieved by intramuscular injection.

Product licence numbers

Floxapen Capsules 250 mg	0038/5055R
Floxapen Capsules 500 mg	0038/5056R
Floxapen Vials for Injection 250 mg	0038/5051R
Floxapen Vials for Injection 500 mg	0038/5052R
Floxapen Vials for Injection 1 g	0038/5053R
Floxapen Syrup 125 mg/5 ml	0038/0309
Floxapen Syrup 250 mg/5 ml	0038/0310
Floxapen Syrup 125 mg Unidose Sachet	0038/0311

MAGNAPEN* CAPSULES
MAGNAPEN* SYRUP
MAGNAPEN* INJECTION

Approved name: Co-fluampicil

Presentation *Magnapen Capsules:* Black and turquoise capsules overprinted 'Magnapen', containing 250 mg ampicillin as Ampicillin Trihydrate BP with 250 mg flucloxacillin as Flucloxacillin Sodium BP.

Magnapen Syrup: Bottles containing powder for the preparation of 100 ml suspension. When reconstituted each 5 ml contains 125 mg ampicillin as Ampicillin Trihydrate BP with 125 mg flucloxacillin as Flucloxacillin Magnesium BP.

Magnapen Vials for Injection: 500 mg Vial: containing 250 mg ampicillin as Ampicillin Sodium BP with 250 mg flucloxacillin as Flucloxacillin Sodium BP.

1 g Vial: containing 500 mg ampicillin as Ampicillin Sodium BP with 500 mg flucloxacillin as Flucloxacillin Sodium BP.

Magnapen oral presentations also contain inactive ingredients to make the medicine acceptable. Children's presentation: amongst these ingredients are disodium edetate, sodium benzoate and sucrose in Magnapen Syrup.

Uses Magnapen is indicated for the treatment of severe infections where the causative organism is unknown, and for mixed infections involving β-lactamase-producing staphylococci. Typical indications include:

In general practice: Chest infections, ENT infections, skin and soft tissue infections, and infections in patients whose underlying pathology places them at special risk.

In hospital (prior to laboratory results being available): Severe respiratory tract infections. Post-operative chest and wound infections. Septic abortion; puerperal fever. Septicaemia. Prophylaxis in major surgery. Infections in patients receiving immuno-suppressive therapy.

The spectrum of activity of Magnapen also makes it suitable for the treatment of many mixed infections, particularly those where β-lactamase-producing staphylococci are suspected or confirmed.

Dosage and administration
Usual adult dosage (including elderly patients):
Oral: 1 capsule or 10 ml syrup four times a day.
Intramuscular/Intravenous: 500 mg four times a day.

Usual children's dosage:
Oral: Under 10 years: 5 ml syrup four times a day.†
Intramuscular/Intravenous: Under 2 years: $\frac{1}{4}$ adult dose.† 2–10 years: $\frac{1}{2}$ adult dose.

The above dosages for adults and children may be doubled where necessary.

Oral doses should be administered $\frac{1}{2}$–1 hour before meals.

Administration: Intramuscular: 500 mg Vial: add 1.5 ml Water for Injections BP to vial contents. 1 g Vial: add 2 ml Water for Injections BP to vial contents.

Intravenous: Dissolve 500 mg in 10 ml Water for Injections BP, or 1 g in 20 ml Water for Injections BP. Administer by slow intravenous injection (3–4 minutes). Magnapen Injection may be added to infusion fluids or injected, suitably diluted into the drip tube over a period of 3–4 minutes.

† Ampiclox Neonatal is recommended for the treatment of infections in neonates and premature babies.

Contra-indications, warnings, etc
Contra-indications: Penicillin hypersensitivity; ocular administration.

Use in pregnancy and lactation: Animal studies have shown no teratogenic effects. The product has been in clinical use since 1971 and the limited number of reported cases of use in human pregnancy have shown no evidence of untoward effect. The use of Magnapen in pregnancy should be reserved for cases considered essential by the clinician. During lactation, trace quantities of penicillins can be detected in breast milk.

Side-effects: Side-effects, as with other penicillins, are uncommon and mainly of a mild and transitory nature. Gastro-intestinal upsets (e.g. nausea, diarrhoea) and skin rashes have been reported. An urticarial rash suggests penicillin hypersensitivity; an erythematous rash may arise in patients receiving ampicillin who have glandular fever. If a skin rash occurs, treatment should be discontinued. Hepatitis and cholestatic jaundice have been reported rarely. Pseudomembranous colitis has been reported rarely.

Overdosage: Problems of overdosage with Magnapen are unlikely to occur; if encountered they may be treated symptomatically.

Pharmaceutical precautions Magnapen Capsules and Magnapen Vials for Injection should be stored in a cool, dry place. Magnapen Syrup should be stored in a dry place.

Once dispensed, Magnapen Syrup remains stable for 14 days when kept in a cool place. If a dilution of the reconstituted suspension is required, Syrup BP should be used.

Magnapen solutions for injection should be used immediately.

Magnapen may be added to most intravenous fluids (e.g. Water for Injections, sodium chloride 0.9%, glucose 5%, sodium chloride 0.18% with glucose 4%). In intravenous solutions containing glucose or other carbohydrates, Magnapen should be infused within two hours of preparation. Intravenous solutions of Magnapen in Water for Injections or sodium chloride 0.9% should be infused within 24 hours of preparation. Full particulars are given in the package enclosure leaflet. Preparation of Magnapen infusion solutions must be carried out under appropriate aseptic conditions if these extended storage periods are required.

Magnapen should not be mixed with blood products, other proteinaceous fluids (e.g. protein hydrolysates) or with intravenous lipid emulsions.

If Magnapen is prescribed concurrently with an aminoglycoside the antibiotics should not be mixed in the syringe, intravenous fluid container or giving set because loss of activity of the aminoglycoside and possibly precipitation can occur under these conditions.

Legal category POM.

Package quantities *Magnapen Capsules:* Containers of 20 and 100.
Magnapen Syrup: Original Pack of 100 ml with Patient Information Leaflet.
Magnapen Injections: Boxes of 10 vials with instructions for use.

Further information Infections encountered in medical practice can be of mixed bacteriology, often including β-lactamase-producing strains. Magnapen provides a broad spectrum of activity, which should be considered when dealing with such infections.

Magnapen Syrup is now formulated using the magnesium salt of flucloxacillin in preference to the sodium salt, in order to provide a more palatable suspension with extended stability.

Product licence numbers

Magnapen Capsules	0038/0090R
Magnapen Syrup	0038/0324

Magnapen Vials 500 mg	0038/0089R
Magnapen Vials 1 g	0038/0089R

MAXOLON* TABLETS
MAXOLON* SYRUP
MAXOLON* PAEDIATRIC LIQUID
MAXOLON* INJECTION

Presentation *Maxolon Tablets:* (Metoclopramide Tablets BP): Small, white, scored tablets, engraved 'Maxolon'. Each tablet contains 10 mg Metoclopramide Hydrochloride BP.

Maxolon Syrup: Clear colourless, lemon/lime flavoured oral solution. Each 5 ml dose contains 5 mg Metoclopramide Hydrochloride BP.

Maxolon Paediatric Liquid: Clear, colourless, lemon/lime flavoured oral solution, in a bottle with a 1 ml pipette. Each 1 ml contains 1 mg Metoclopramide Hydrochloride BP.

Maxolon Ampoules (Metoclopramide Injection BP): Clear, colourless aqueous solution. Each 2 ml ampoule contains 10 mg Metoclopramide Hydrochloride BP.

Maxolon presentations also contain inactive ingredients to make the medicine acceptable. Children's presentations: amongst these ingredients is parabens in Maxolon Syrup and Maxolon Paediatric Liquid. Maxolon Injection contains sodium chloride (isotonic agent) and sodium metabisulphite (antioxidant).

Maxolon Syrup and Maxolon Paediatric Liquid do not contain sugar, tartrazine or any other azo dyes.

Uses *Adults (20 years and over)*
Digestive disorders: Maxolon restores normal co-ordination and tone to the upper digestive tract.

Maxolon relieves the symptoms of gastro-duodenal dysfunction including: Dyspepsia; heartburn; flatulence; sickness; regurgitation of bile; pain.

These symptoms may be associated with such conditions as: Peptic ulcer. Reflux oesophagitis. Gastritis. Duodenitis. Hiatus hernia. Cholelithiasis and post-cholecystectomy dyspepsia.

Nausea and vomiting: Maxolon is indicated for the treatment of the nausea and vomiting associated with: Gastro-intestinal disorders. Cyclical vomiting. Intolerance to cytotoxic drugs. Congestive heart failure. Deep X-ray or cobalt therapy. Post-anaesthetic vomiting.

Migraine: Maxolon relieves symptoms of nausea and vomiting, and overcomes gastric stasis associated with attacks of migraine. This improvement in gastric emptying assists the absorption of concurrently administered oral anti-migraine therapy (e.g. paracetamol) which may otherwise be impaired in such patients.

Post-operative conditions: Post-operative gastric hypotonia. Post-vagotomy syndrome. Maxolon promotes normal gastric emptying and restores motility in vagotomised patients, and where post-operative symptoms suggest gastro-duodenal dysfunction.

Diagnostic procedures: Radiology. Duodenal intubation. Maxolon speeds up the passage of a barium meal by decreasing gastric emptying time, co-ordinating peristalsis and dilating the duodenal bulb. Maxolon also facilitates duodenal intubation procedures.

Young adults and children: The use of Maxolon in patients under 20 years should be restricted to the following: Severe intractable vomiting of known cause; vomiting associated with radiotherapy and intolerance to cytotoxic drugs; as an aid to gastro-intestinal intubation; as part of the premedication before surgical procedures.

Dosage and administration The dosage recommendations given below should be strictly adhered to if side-effects of the dystonic type are to be avoided. It should be noted that total daily dosage of Maxolon, especially for children and young adults, should not normally exceed 0.5 mg/kg body weight.

In patients with clinically significant degrees of renal or hepatic impairment, therapy should be at reduced dosage. Metoclopramide is metabolised in the liver and the predominant route of elimination of metoclopramide and its metabolites is via the kidney.

Medical indications
Oral

Adults 20 years and over: 10 mg three times daily.
For patients of less than 60 kg see below.

Elderly patients: As for adults. To avoid adverse reactions adhere strictly to dosage recommendations and where prolonged therapy is considered necessary, patients should be regularly reviewed.

Young adults and children: Maxolon should only be used after careful examination to avoid masking an underlying disorder, e.g. cerebral irritation. In the treatment of this group attention should be given primarily to body weight and treatment should commence at the lower dosage where stated.

Young adults:	
15–19 years	60 kg and over: 10 mg three times daily
	30–59 kg: 5 mg three times daily
Children:	
9–14 years	30 kg and over: 5 mg three times daily
5–9 years	20–29 kg: 2½ mg three times daily
3–5 years	15–19 kg: 2 mg two to three times daily
1–3 years	10–14 kg: 1 mg two to three times daily
Under 1 year	Up to 10 kg: 1 mg twice daily

Tablets should not be used in children under the age of 15. A liquid presentation should be used in the younger age groups; more accurate dosage is facilitated by the use of the Paediatric Liquid.

IM or IV: Maxolon may be administered, at the dosages stated above, either intramuscularly or by slow intravenous injection (1–2 minutes).

Diagnostic indications: A single dose of Maxolon may be given 5–10 minutes before the examination. Subject to body weight considerations (see above), the following dosages are recommended:

Adults:	20 years and over	10–20 mg
Young adults:	15–19 years	10 mg
Children:	9–14 years	5 mg
	5–9 years	2½ mg
	3–5 years	2 mg
	Under 3 years	1 mg

Contra-indications, warnings, etc
Use in pregnancy and lactation: Animal tests in several mammalian species and clinical experience have not indicated a teratogenic effect. Nevertheless, Maxolon should only be used when there are compelling reasons and is not advised during the first trimester.

During lactation, metoclopramide is found in breast milk.

Precautions: If vomiting persists the patient should be re-assessed to exclude the possibility of an underlying disorder, e.g. cerebral irritation.

Care should be exercised in patients being treated with other centrally active drugs e.g. in epilepsy.

Since extra-pyramidal symptoms may occur with both Maxolon and neuroleptics, such as the phenothiazines, particular care should be exercised in the event of these drugs being prescribed concurrently.

Following operations such as pyloroplasty or gut anastomosis Maxolon therapy should be withheld for three or four days as vigorous muscular contractions may not help healing.

Metoclopramide may induce an acute hypertensive response in patients with phaeochromocytoma.

Drug interactions: The action of Maxolon on the gastro-intestinal tract is antagonised by anticholinergics.

The absorption of any concurrently administered oral medication may be modified by the effect of Maxolon on gastric motility.

Side-effects: Various extra-pyramidal reactions to Maxolon, usually of the dystonic type, have been reported. The incidence of dystonic reactions, particularly in children and young adults, is increased if daily dosages higher than 0.5 mg per kg body weight are administered. Dystonic reactions include: spasm of the facial muscles, trismus, rhythmic protrusion of the tongue, a bulbar type of speech, spasm of extra-ocular muscles including oculogyric crises, unnatural positioning of the head and shoulders and opisthotonos. There may be a generalised increase in muscle tone. The majority of reactions occur within 36 hours of starting treatment and the effects usually disappear within 24 hours of withdrawal of the drug. Should treatment of a dystonic reaction be required an anticholinergic anti-Parkinsonian drug, or a benzodiazepine may be used.

Tardive dyskinesia has been reported during prolonged treatment in a small number of mainly elderly patients. Patients on prolonged treatment should be regularly reviewed.

Rarely, drowsiness, restlessness and diarrhoea have been reported in patients receiving metoclopramide therapy. Depression has been reported extremely rarely.

Raised serum prolactin levels have been observed during metoclopramide therapy: this effect is similar to that noted with many other compounds.

Overdosage: Overdosage should be treated by gastric lavage with appropriate supportive measures. For treatment of a dystonic reaction see above.

Pharmaceutical precautions Maxolon Syrup must be protected from light and should be dispensed into amber glass containers. It may be diluted with Purified Water BP to half strength but should not be stored diluted for more than one month.

Once dispensed Maxolon Paediatric Liquid should be used within 14 days.

If ampoules are removed from their carton, they should be stored away from light. If inadvertent exposure occurs, ampoules showing discoloration must be discarded.

Compatibility: If the standard formulation of Maxolon is used for the treatment of nausea and vomiting associated with cytotoxic drugs, the cytotoxic agent should be administered as a separate infusion (see Further Information).

Legal category POM.

Package quantities *Maxolon Tablets:* Original Packs of 21 and 84 with Patient Information Leaflet; also containers of 100 and 500.
Maxolon Syrup: Original Pack of 200 ml with Patient Information Leaflet; also bottle of 1 litre.
Maxolon Paediatric Liquid: Original Pack of 15 ml with 1 ml pipette and Patient Information Leaflet.
Maxolon Ampoules: Boxes of 12 with instructions for use.

Further information The action of Maxolon is closely associated with parasympathetic nervous control of the upper gastro-intestinal tract, where it has the effect of encouraging normal peristaltic action. This provides for a fundamental approach to the control of those conditions where disturbed gastro-intestinal motility is a common underlying factor.

Maxolon Syrup and Maxolon Paediatric Liquid are now tartrazine and sugar-free formulations.

A separate parenteral formulation is available as Maxolon 'High Dose' (100 mg/20 ml) for the IV treatment of nausea and vomiting associated with cytotoxic drugs; it is specially formulated to be compatible in solution with cisplatin. This is the subject of a separate Data Sheet available from the Company.

Product licence numbers

Maxolon Tablets	0038/5041
Maxolon Syrup	0038/5040
Maxolon Paediatric Liquid	0038/0095
Maxolon Ampoules	0038/0098

MAXOLON* 'HIGH DOSE'

Presentation *Maxolon 'High Dose' Ampoules:* Clear, colourless aqueous solution. Each 20 ml ampoule contains 100 mg Metoclopramide Hydrochloride BP.

Maxolon 'High Dose' also contains sodium chloride (isotonic agent).

Uses Maxolon 'High Dose' is indicated for the treatment of nausea and vomiting associated with intolerance to cytotoxic drugs.

Dosage and administration Maxolon 'High Dose' is administered by IV infusion, suitably diluted (see below). The recommended method of administration is by continuous infusion which allows steady serum levels of metoclopramide to be maintained.

Continuous infusion (recommended method): Maxolon 'High Dose' is given by IV infusion as a loading dose followed by a continuous infusion to maintain a metoclopramide serum concentration of 0.85–1.0 microgram per ml. The loading dose should be given before starting cytotoxic chemotherapy.

	Maxolon 'High Dose'	*Volume of diluent*	*IV infusion time*
Loading dose	2–4 mg/kg body weight	50–100 ml	15–30 minutes
Maintenance dose	3–5 mg/kg body weight	500 ml	8–12 hours

Total dosage in any 24-hour period should not normally exceed 10 mg/kg body weight.

Where cisplatin is to be used the loading dose of Maxolon 'High Dose' should be at least 3 mg/kg body weight and the maintenance dose at least 4 mg/kg body weight.

Intermittent infusion (alternative regimen): Maxolon 'High Dose' can be given by intermittent IV infusion suitably diluted. The initial dose should be given before starting cytotoxic chemotherapy.

	Maxolon 'High Dose'	*Volume of diluent*	*IV infusion time*
Initial dose	Up to 2 mg/kg body weight	At least 50 ml	At least 15 minutes
Repeat doses at 2 hourly intervals	Up to 2 mg/kg body weight	At least 50 ml	At least 15 minutes

Total dosage in any 24 hour period should not normally exceed 10 mg/kg body weight.

Abnormal renal or liver function: In patients with clinically significant degrees of renal or hepatic impairment, therapy should be at reduced dosage. Metoclopramide is metabolised in the liver and the predominant route of elimination of metoclopramide and its metabolites is via the kidney.

Compatibility with cytotoxic agents: Maxolon 'High Dose' is compatible with a number of cytotoxic drugs. However it should not be mixed in solution with therapeutic agents other than those stated.

Maxolon 'High Dose' is compatible with cisplatin, cyclophosphamide and doxorubicin hydrochloride and is stable over the concentration ranges listed below for 24 hours at room temperature when protected from light.

40–200 ml cisplatin (1 mg/ml) per 100 mg/20 ml Maxolon 'High Dose' in 1 litre of sodium chloride 0.9%.

Up to 40 mg doxorubicin hydrochloride (powder) per 100 mg/20 ml of Maxolon 'High Dose'.

Up to 4 g cyclophosphamide (1g/50 ml) per 100 mg/20 ml of Maxolon 'High Dose'.

Compatibility with morphine/diamorphine: Maxolon 'High Dose' is compatible with morphine hydrochloride and diamorphine hydrochloride and is stable over the concentration ranges listed below for 48 hours at room temperature under normal fluorescent lighting.

Up to 100 mg of morphine hydrochloride per 100 mg/20 ml of Maxolon 'High Dose'.

Up to 50 mg of diamorphine hydrochloride per 100 mg/20 ml of Maxolon 'High Dose'.

Maxolon 'High Dose' 100 mg/20 ml also remains stable for 48 hours at room temperature with 100 mg of morphine hydrochloride, or 50 mg diamorphine hydrochloride, when diluted 1 in 10 with sodium chloride 0.9%.

Stability in intravenous fluids: Ideally, intravenous solutions should be prepared at the time of infusion. However, Maxolon 'High Dose' has been shown to be stable for at least 48 hours at room temperature in the following solutions when administered in a PVC infusion bag (e.g. Viaflex* Travenol):

Sodium Chloride Intravenous Infusion BP (0.9% w/v)
Glucose Intravenous Infusion BP (5% w/v)
Sodium Chloride and Glucose Intravenous Infusion BP (sodium chloride 0.18% w/v; glucose 4% w/v)
Compound Sodium Lactate Intravenous Infusion BP (Ringer-Lactate Solution; Hartmann's Solution).

Note: Preparation must be under appropriate aseptic conditions if the above extended storage periods are required. The high dose ampoule presentation is not suitable for multidose use.

Contra-indications, warnings, etc
Use in pregnancy and lactation: Animal tests in several mammalian species and clinical experience have not indicated a teratogenic effect. Nevertheless, Maxolon should only be used when there are compelling reasons and is not advised during the first trimester.

During lactation, metoclopramide is found in breast milk.

Precautions: Care should be exercised in patients being treated with other centrally active drugs e.g. in epilepsy.

Since extrapyramidal symptoms may occur with both Maxolon and neuroleptics such as the phenothiazines, particular care should be exercised in the event of these drugs being prescribed concurrently.

Following operations such as pyloroplasty or gut anastomosis Maxolon therapy should be withheld for three or four days as vigorous muscular contractions may not help healing.

Metoclopramide may induce an acute hypertensive response in patients with phaeochromocytoma.

Drug interactions: The action of Maxolon on the gastro-intestinal tract is antagonised by anticholinergics.

The absorption of any concurrently administered oral medication may be modified by the effect of Maxolon on gastric motility.

Side-effects: When given at high dose in association with cancer chemotherapy, Maxolon has been found to be well tolerated with few adverse effects.

Various extrapyramidal reactions to Maxolon, usually of the dystonic type, have been reported. Studies of Maxolon given in doses up to 10 mg/kg body weight/day by IV infusion report an incidence of extrapyramidal reactions of less than 10%. The incidence of such reactions may be incresed in the younger patient.

Reactions to Maxolon have included: Spasm of the facial muscles, trismus, rhythmic protrusion of the tongue, a bulbar type of speech, spasm of extra-ocular muscles including oculogyric crises, unnatural positioning of the head and shoulders and opisthotonos. There may be a generalised increase in muscle tone. The majority of reactions occur within 36 hours of starting treatment and the effects usually disappear within 24 hours of withdrawal of the drug. Should treatment of a dystonic reaction be required an anticholinergic anti-Parkinsonian drug, or a benzodiazepine may be used.

Mild drowsiness and diarrhoea have been noted. Depression has been reported extremely rarely.

Raised serum prolactin levels have been observed during metoclopramide therapy: this effect is similar to that noted with many other compounds.

Pharmaceutical precautions If ampoules are removed from their carton they should be stored away from light. If inadvertent exposure occurs, ampoules showing discoloration must be discarded.

Legal category POM.

Package quantities 'High Dose' Ampoules: Boxes of 10 with instructions for use.

Further information Maxolon 'High Dose' is specifically for use in the management of cytotoxic intolerance. It is specially formulated to ensure compatibility in solution with cisplatin. The 20 ml ampoule provides ease of administration.

A number of published studies have indicated that other agents, e.g. dexamethasone, may be given in conjunction with Maxolon 'High Dose'.

Maxolon exerts a three-fold anti-emetic action: By inhibiting central dopamine receptors Maxolon raises the threshold of the chemoreceptor trigger zone, and reduces the reaction of the adjacent vomiting centre to centrally-acting emetics. Maxolon decreases the sensitivity of the visceral afferent nerves to the vomiting centre, reducing the effect of locally-acting emetics and irritant substances. In the upper gastro-intestinal tract Maxolon promotes normal gastric emptying and it may thus abolish gastric stasis which is part of the vomiting reflex.

Maxolon 'High Dose' is not intended for use in the wider range of indications for which Maxolon at standard dose is indicated. The separate Maxolon and Maxolon SR Data Sheets should be consulted for such uses.

Product licence number Maxolon 'High Dose' Ampoules for Injection: 0038/0300.

MAXOLON* SR

Presentation Maxolon SR capsules: Colourless, transparent capsules overprinted 'Maxolon SR 15'. Each capsule contains 15 mg Metoclopramide Hydrochloride BP in white sustained-release microgranules.

Maxolon SR also contains inactive ingredients to make the medicine acceptable.

Maxolon SR does not contain tartrazine or any other azo dyes.

Uses
Digestive disorders: Maxolon SR restores normal co-ordination and tone to the upper digestive tract. Maxolon SR relieves symptoms of gastro-duodenal dysfunction including: dyspepsia, heartburn, flatulence, sickness, pain, regurgitation of bile. These symptoms may be associated with such conditions as: reflux oesophagitis, hiatus hernia, gastritis, duodenitis, peptic ulcer, cholelithiasis and post-cholecystectomy dyspepsia.

Nausea and vomiting: Maxolon SR is indicated for the treatment of the nausea and vomiting associated with gastro-intestinal disorders and intolerance to cytotoxic drugs.

Dosage and administration Oral. In adults 20 years and over: 1 capsule (15 mg) twice daily, swallowed whole. Total daily dosage of Maxolon SR should not normally exceed 0.5 mg/kg body weight.

Elderly patients: As for other adults. To avoid adverse reactions adhere strictly to dosage recommendations and where prolonged therapy is considered necessary, patients should be regularly reviewed.

The interval between doses may need to be extended in patients with clinically significant degrees of renal or hepatic impairment. Metoclopramide is metabolised in the liver and the predominant route of elimination of metoclopramide and its metabolites is via the kidney.

Children and young adults: A presentation of Maxolon SR suitable for patients under 20 years of age is not available. Presentations suitable for patients of low body weight are described on the separate Maxolon Data Sheet.

Contra-indications, warnings, etc
Contra-indications: Maxolon SR is contra-indicated in patients under 20 years since the dose level cannot be reduced.

Use in pregnancy and lactation: Animal tests in several mammalian species and clinical experience with metoclopramide have not indicated a teratogenic effect.

Nevertheless Maxolon SR should only be used when there are compelling reasons and is not advised during the first trimester. During lactation, metoclopramide is found in breast milk.

Precautions: If vomiting persists the patient should be re-assessed to exclude the possibility of an underlying disorder, e.g. cerebral irritation.

Care should be exercised in patients being treated with other centrally active drugs e.g. in epilepsy.

Since extra-pyramidal symptoms may occur with both metoclopramide and neuroleptics, such as the phenothiazines, particular care should be exercised in the event of these drugs being prescribed concurrently.

Special care should be taken in cases of severe renal insufficiency (see also under dosage and administration).

Following operations such as pyloroplasty or gut anastomosis metoclopramide therapy should be withheld for three or four days as vigorous muscular contractions may not help healing.

Metoclopramide may induce an acute hypertensive response in patients with phaeochromocytoma.

Drug interactions: The action of metoclopramide on the gastro-intestinal tract is antagonised by anticholinergics.

The absorption of any concurrently administered oral medication may be modified by the effect of metoclopramide on gastric motility.

Side-effects: Various extra-pyramidal reactions to metoclopramide, usually of the dystonic type have been reported. The incidence of these reactions may be increased if daily dosages higher than 0.5 mg/kg body weight are administered. Dystonic reactions include: spasm of the facial muscles, trismus, rhythmic protrusion of the tongue, a bulbar type of speech, spasm of extraocular muscles including oculogyric crises, unnatural positioning of the head and shoulders and opisthotonos. There may be a generalised increase in muscle tone. The majority of reactions occur within 36 hours of starting treatment and the effects usually disappear within 24 hours of withdrawal of the drug. Should treatment of a dystonic reaction be required, an anticholinergic anti-Parkinsonian drug, or a benzodiazepine may be used.

Tardive dyskinesia has been reported during prolonged treatment in a small number of mainly elderly patients. Patients on prolonged treatment should be regularly reviewed.

Rarely, drowsiness, restlessness and diarrhoea have been reported in patients receiving metoclopramide therapy. Depression has been reported extremely rarely.

Raised serum prolactin levels have been observed during metoclopramide therapy: this effect is similar to that noted with many other compounds.

Overdosage: Overdosage should be treated by gastric lavage with appropriate supportive measures. For treatment of a dystonic reaction see above.

Pharmaceutical precautions Protect from direct light.

Legal category POM.

Package quantities *Maxolon SR Capsules:* Original Pack of 56 with Patient Information Leaflet.

Further information The action of metoclopramide is closely associated with parasympathetic nervous control of the upper gastro-intestinal tract, where it has the effect of encouraging normal peristaltic action. This provides for a fundamental approach to the control of those conditions where disturbed gastro-intestinal motility is a common underlying factor.

The use of Maxolon in a wider range of indications, and information on suitable presentations and dosages of Maxolon for patients under 20 years, are described on the separate Maxolon Data Sheet.

Product licence number 0038/0340.

ORBENIN* CAPSULES ORBENIN* INJECTION

Presentation *Orbenin Capsules* (Cloxacillin Capsules BP): Orange and black capsules overprinted 'Orbenin', containing 250 mg or 500 mg cloxacillin as Cloxacillin Sodium BP.

Orbenin Vials for Injection (Cloxacillin Injection BP): Each vial contains 250 mg or 500 mg cloxacillin as Cloxacillin Sodium BP.

Orbenin oral presentations also contain inactive ingredients to make the medicine acceptable.

Uses Orbenin is indicated for the treatment of infections caused by Gram-positive organisms, including infections caused by β-lactamase-producing staphylococci.

Typical indications include:

Skin and soft tissue infections: Boils. Abscesses. Carbuncles. Furunculosis. Cellulitis. Infected wounds. Infected burns. Protection for skin grafts. Otitis media and externa.

Infected skin conditions, e.g. ulcer, eczema and acne.

Respiratory tract infections: Pneumonia. Lung abscess. Empyema. Sinusitis. Pharyngitis. Tonsillitis. Quinsy.

Other infections caused by Orbenin-sensitive organisms: Osteomyelitis. Enteritis. Endocarditis. Urinary tract infection. Meningitis. Septicaemia.

Dosage and administration *Usual adult dosage (including elderly patients):*
Oral: 500 mg four times a day.
Intramuscular: 250 mg four to six hourly.
Intravenous: 500 mg four to six hourly.

Systemic dosages may be doubled where necessary: oral dosages should be administered ½–1 hour before meals.
Intrapleural: 500 mg once daily.
Intra-articular: 500 mg once daily.
By nebuliser: 125–250 mg four times a day.

Usual children's dosage:
2–10 years: ½ adult dose.

Administration: Intramuscular: Add 1.5 ml Water for Injections BP to 250 mg vial contents or 2 ml Water for Injections BP to 500 mg vial contents.
Intravenous: Dissolve 500 mg in 10 ml Water for Injections BP. Administer by slow intravenous injection (three to four minutes). Orbenin may also be added to infusion fluids or injected, suitably diluted, into the drip tube over a period of three to four minutes.

Orbenin may be administered by other routes in conjunction with systemic therapy.
Intrapleural: Dissolve 500 mg in 5–10 ml Water for Injections BP.
Intra-articular: Dissolve 500 mg in up to 5 ml Water for Injections BP or 0.5% lignocaine hydrochloride solution.

Nebuliser Solution: Dissolve 125–250 mg of the vial contents in 3 ml sterile water and administer by a suitable nebuliser.

Contra-indications, warnings, etc
Contra-indications: Penicillin hypersensitivity; ocular administration.

Use in pregnancy and lactation: Animal studies with Orbenin have shown no teratogenic effects. The product has been in clinical use since 1962 and the limited number of reported cases of use in human pregnancy have shown no evidence of untoward effect. The use of Orbenin in pregnancy should be reserved for cases considered essential by the clinician. During lactation, trace quantities of penicillins can be detected in breast milk.

Side-effects: Side-effects, as with other penicillins, are uncommon and mainly of a mild and transitory nature. Gastro-intestinal upsets (e.g. nausea, diarrhoea) and skin rashes have been reported infrequently. If a skin rash occurs, treatment should be discontinued.

Overdosage: Problems of overdosage with Orbenin are unlikely to occur; if encountered they may be treated symptomatically.

Pharmaceutical precautions Orbenin should be stored in a cool, dry place.

Solutions for IM or direct IV injection should normally be administered within 30 minutes of preparation. However, aqueous solutions of Orbenin Injection retain their activity for up to 24 hours at room temperature (25°C) and up to 72 hours in a refrigerator (5°C).

Orbenin may be added to most intravenous fluids (e.g. Water for Injections, sodium chloride 0.9%, glucose 5%, sodium chloride 0.18% with glucose 4%). Intravenous solutions of Orbenin for infusion, stored up to 25°C, should be used within 24 hours of preparation. Full particulars are given in the package enclosure leaflet.

Reconstitution of Orbenin injections and preparation of Orbenin infusion solutions must be carried out under appropriate aseptic conditions if the extended storage periods are required.

Orbenin should not be mixed with blood products or other proteinaceous fluids (e.g. protein hydrolysates) or with intravenous lipid emulsions.

If Orbenin is prescribed concurrently with an aminoglycoside, the two antibiotics should not be mixed in the syringe, intravenous fluid container or giving set; precipitation may occur.

Legal category POM.

Package quantities *Orbenin Capsules 250 mg or 500 mg:* Containers of 100.
Orbenin Vials 250 mg or 500 mg: Boxes of 10 with instructions for use.

Further information Nil.

Product licence numbers

Orbenin Capsules 250 mg	0038/5028R
Orbenin Capsules 500 mg	0038/5029R
Orbenin Vials for Injection 250 mg	0038/5025R
Orbenin Vials for Injection 500 mg	0038/5026R

PENBRITIN* CAPSULES
PENBRITIN* SYRUPS
PENBRITIN* PAEDIATRIC SUSPENSION
PENBRITIN* INJECTION

Presentation *Penbritin Capsules* (Ampicillin Capsules BP): black and red capsules overprinted 'Penbritin', containing 250 mg or 500 mg ampicillin as Ampicillin Trihydrate BP.

Penbritin Syrups (Ampicillin Oral Suspension BP): Bottles containing powder for the preparation of 100 ml pale cream-coloured suspension. When reconstituted each 5 ml contains 125 mg or 250 mg ampicillin as Ampicillin Trihydrate BP.

Penbritin Paediatric Suspension: Bottles containing powder for the preparation of 25 ml pink-coloured suspension. When reconstituted each 1.25 ml contains 125 mg ampicillin as Ampicillin Trihydrate BP. A pipette to measure the 1.25 ml dose is provided.

Penbritin Vials for Injection (Ampicillin Sodium BP for Injection): Each vial contains 250 mg or 500 mg ampicillin as Ampicillin Sodium BP.

Penbritin oral presentations also contain inactive ingredients to make the medicine acceptable. Children's presentations: amongst these ingredients are sodium benzoate and sucrose in Penbritin Syrups and Penbritin Paediatric Suspension: the latter also includes amaranth.

Uses Penbritin is a broad-spectrum penicillin, indicated for the treatment of a wide range of bacterial infections caused by ampicillin-sensitive organisms.

Typical indications include: Ear, nose and throat infections. Bronchitis. Pneumonia. Urinary tract infections. Gonorrhoea. Gynaecological infections. Septicaemia. Peritonitis. Endocarditis. Meningitis. Enteric fever. Gastro-intestinal infections.

Extraperitoneal application of Penbritin to wounds can be used to prevent infection following abdominal surgery.

Dosage and administration *Usual adult dosage* (including elderly patients) – oral, except where stated:

Ear, nose and throat infections: 250 mg four times a day.
Bronchitis: Routine therapy: 250 mg four times a day.
High-dosage therapy: 1 g four times a day.
Pneumonia: 500 mg four times a day.
Urinary tract infections: 500 mg three times a day.
Gonorrhoea: 2 g orally with 1 g probenecid as a single dose. Repeated doses are recommended for the treatment of females.
Gastro-intestinal infections: 500–750 mg three to four times daily.
Enteric: Acute: 1–2 g four times a day for two weeks.
Carriers: 1–2 g four times a day for four to twelve weeks.
Septicaemia, endocarditis, osteomyelitis: 500 mg four to six times a day IM or IV for one to six weeks.
Peritonitis, intra-abdominal sepsis: 500 mg four times a day IM or IV.
Meningitis: Adult dosage: 2 g six-hourly IV.
Children's dosage: 150 mg/kg daily IV in divided doses.

Usual children's dosage (under 10 years): ½ adult routine dosage.

All recommended dosages are a guide only. In severe infections the above dosages may be increased, or Penbritin given by injection. Oral doses of Penbritin should be taken half to one hour before meals.

Administration:
Intramuscular: Add 1.5 ml Water for Injections BP to 250 mg or 500 mg vial contents.
Intravenous: Dissolve 250 mg in 5 ml or 500 mg in 10 ml Water for Injections BP. Administer by slow injection (three to four minutes). Penbritin may also be added to infusion fluids or injected, suitably diluted, into the drip tube over a period of three to four minutes.

Penbritin may also be administered by other routes in conjunction with systemic therapy.
Intraperitoneal: 500 mg daily in up to 10 ml Water for Injections BP.
Intrapleural: 500 mg daily in 5–10 ml Water for Injections BP.
Intra-articular: 500 mg daily, in up to 5 ml Water for Injections BP or sterile 0.5% procaine hydrochloride solution.
Local use in abdominal surgery: 1 g sterile powder sprinkled into the wound extraperitoneally or into muscle layers to prevent wound infection post-operatively.

Contra-indications, warnings, etc
Contra-indications: Penicillin hypersensitivity.

Use in pregnancy and lactation: Animal studies with Penbritin have shown no teratogenic effects. The product has been in extensive clinical use since 1961 and its use in human pregnancy has been well documented in clinical studies. When antibiotic therapy is required during pregnancy, Penbritin may be considered appropriate.

During lactation, trace quantities of penicillins can be detected in breast milk.

Side-effects: Side-effects, as with other penicillins, are uncommon and mainly of a mild and transitory nature. Gastro-intestinal upsets (e.g., nausea, diarrhoea) and skin rashes have been reported infrequently. An urticarial rash suggests penicillin hypersensitivity; an erythematous rash may arise in patients receiving ampicillin who have glandular fever. If a skin rash occurs, treatment should be discontinued.

Overdosage: Problems of overdosage with Penbritin are unlikely to occur; if encountered they may be treated symptomatically.

Pharmaceutical precautions Penbritin should be stored in a cool dry place.

Once dispensed, Penbritin Syrups and Paediatric Suspension remain stable for seven days if kept in a cool place. If a dilution of the reconstituted syrup is required, Syrup BP should be used.

Penbritin solutions for injection should be used immediately.

Penbritin may be added to most intravenous fluids (e.g. Water for Injections, sodium chloride 0.9%, glucose 5%, sodium chloride 0.18% with glucose 4%). In intravenous solutions containing glucose or other carbohydrates, Penbritin should be infused within one hour of preparation. Intravenous solutions of Penbritin in Water for Injections or sodium chloride 0.9% should be infused within 24 hours of preparation. Full particulars are given in the package enclosure leaflet. Preparation of Penbritin infusion solutions must be carried out under approriate aseptic conditions if these extended storage periods are required.

Penbritin should not be mixed with blood products or other proteinaceous fluids (e.g. protein hydrolysates) or with intravenous lipid emulsions.

If Penbritin is prescribed concurrently with an aminoglycoside the antibiotics should not be mixed in the syringe, intravenous fluid container or giving set because loss of activity of the aminoglycoside can occur under these conditions.

Legal category POM.

Package quantities *Penbritin Capsules 250 mg:* Original Pack of 28 with Patient Information Leaflet; also containers of 100 and 500.
Penbritin Capsules 500 mg: Original Pack of 28 with Patient Information Leaflet; also containers of 100.
Penbritin Vials for Injection 250 mg, 500 mg: Boxes of 10 with instructions for use.
Penbritin Syrups: Original Packs of 100 ml.
Penbritin Paediatric Suspension: Original Pack of 25 ml with pipette and Patient Information Leaflet.

Further information Nil.

Product licence numbers

Penbritin Capsules 250 mg	0038/5074R
Penbritin Capsules 500 mg	0038/5075R
Penbritin Vials for Injection 250 mg	0038/5060R
Penbritin Vials for Injection 500 mg	0038/5061R
Penbritin Syrup 125 mg/5 ml	0038/0265
Penbritin Syrup 250 mg/5 ml	0038/0266
Penbritin Paediatric Suspension	0038/5066R

PYOPEN* INJECTION

Presentation *Pyopen 1 g Vial:* Vials containing 1 g carbenicillin as Carbenicillin Sodium BP.

Pyopen 5 g Vial: Vials containing 5 g carbenicillin as Carbenicillin Sodium BP.

Uses Pyopen is indicated primarily for the treatment of infections caused by sensitive Pseudomonas and Proteus species.

At recommended dosages, Pyopen is also effective against a wide range of other Gram-negative and Gram-positive bacteria, including: Escherichia coli, Haemophilus influenzae, Bacteroides fragilis and other anaerobes, Clostridium spp., Staphylococcus aureus (penicillin sensitive), Streptococcus spp.

Typical indications include: General Systemic Infections, Respiratory Tract Infections, Septicaemia, Urinary Tract Infections, Post-surgical Infections, Intra-abdominal sepsis, Endocarditis, Meningitis, Infected Burns, Infected Wounds.

In life-threatening infections, consideration should be given to the synergistic effects of Pyopen and a parenteral aminoglycoside; they should be given separately, at recommended dosages.

Dosage and administration *Dosage:* See table below.
Preparation
1 gram vial: Intramuscular: Add 2 ml Water for Injections BP to the contents of the vial and shake vigorously.
Intravenous: Add 5 ml Water for Injections BP to the contents of the vial and shake vigorously. Dilute to 20 ml.

5 gram vial (50 ml): Intravenous injection: Add at least 20 ml Water for Injections BP to the contents of the 5 g vial and shake vigorously.

Intravenous infusion: Add 20 ml Water for Injections BP to the contents of the 5 g vial, shake vigorously and add to a suitable volume of infusion fluid (approximately 100–150 ml).

Water for Injections BP is the preferred diluent for intravenous infusion of Pyopen as it will minimise the possibility of phlebitis. Alternatively, the antibiotic may be infused in a sterile solution of glucose of 5% or lower concentration. (The use of 0.9% sodium chloride solution as diluent will add to the sodium load of Pyopen and is, therefore, not usually recommended).

Heat is generated when Pyopen is dissolved; some warming of the contents of the vial may consequently be experienced.

N.B. Pyopen vials are not suitable for multi-dose use.

Administration: Intramuscular: Pyopen should be given every six hours.

Intravenous: Pyopen should be given every four to six hours by slow injection (three to four minutes) or by rapid infusion over 30–40 minutes (i.e. at a rate of approximately 50 drips per minute). Infusion over longer periods may result in sub-therapeutic serum concentrations.

Higher and more prolonged serum concentrations may be achieved with concurrent oral administration of probenecid (1 g three times a day in adults); however, caution should be exercised in the administration of probenecid to patients with impaired renal function.

Pyopen may be administered by other routes in conjunction with systemic therapy.

Intra-articular: Add 2–4 ml Water for Injections BP or 0.5% lignocaine hydrochloride solution to the contents of a 1 g vial. 500 mg to 1 g once daily is a suitable dosage.

Dosage of Pyopen

Infection	*Organism*	
	Pseudomonas	*Proteus spp.*
Adult (incl. elderly patients)		
Respiratory tract infections Chronic urinary tract infections Infected wounds and burns	5 g IV four to six-hourly	2 g IM six-hourly
Systemic infections Septicaemia, endocarditis, meningitis	5 g IV four-hourly	5 g IV six-hourly
Acute uncomplicated urinary tract infections	2 g IM six-hourly	1–2 g IM six-hourly
Children (daily dosage per kg body weight: to be administered in divided doses 4–8 hourly)		
Respiratory tract infections Chronic urinary tract infections Infected wounds and burns	250–400 mg per kg per day IV	100 mg per kg per day IM
Systemic infections Septicaemia, endocarditis, meningitis	400 mg per kg per day IV	250 mg per kg per day IV
Acute uncomplicated urinary tract infections	100 mg per kg per day IM	50–100 mg per kg per day IM

Intrapleural: Add 5 ml Water for Injections BP to the contents of a 1 g vial. Dilute to 10 ml. This dosage is normally given once daily.

Nebuliser Solution: Dissolve 250–500 mg Pyopen powder in 3–5 ml of water and administer four times daily by a suitable nebuliser.

Subconjunctival: A 25% solution (125 mg in 0.5 ml Lignocaine and Adrenaline Injection BP) is recommended.

Local irrigation: A 0.2% solution of Pyopen should be used.

Contra-indications, warnings, etc
Contra-indication: Penicillin hypersensitivity.

Use in pregnancy and lactation: Animal studies with Pyopen have shown no teratogenic effects. The product has been in clinical use since 1967 and the limited number of reported cases of use in human pregnancy have shown no evidence of untoward effect. The use of Pyopen in pregnancy should be reserved for cases considered essential by the clinician. Trace quantities of penicillins can be detected in the milk of lactating mothers. Breast feeding should therefore be discontinued during therapy.

Precautions: Except in cases of renal impairment, recommended dosages should never be reduced. Administration at less than full dosage may permit the multiplication of resistant strains, especially of Pseudomonas. Where renal function is impaired, Pyopen dosage may be reduced. However, monitoring is advisable in these cases to ensure that adequate serum antibiotic concentrations are achieved. Monitoring of sodium intake is also recommended. In treating patients on sodium restriction it should be noted that each 1 g vial of Pyopen contains 5.4 mmol sodium (approx. 124 mg), and each 5 g vial contains 27.1 mmol sodium. Potassium levels should be monitored and supplementation with potassium provided in appropriate cases.

When Pyopen is used with an aminoglycoside the usual dosage should be adopted; concurrent therapy is not an opportunity to secure dosage reduction unless indicated for other reasons – for instance renal failure.

Side-effects: Side-effects, as with other penicillins, are uncommon and mainly of a mild and transitory nature. Gastro-intestinal upsets (e.g. nausea, diarrhoea) and skin rashes have been reported infrequently. If a skin rash occurs, treatment should be discontinued.

If pain at the intramuscular injection site is troublesome, the vial contents may be dissolved in 0.5% lignocaine hydrochloride solution.

In rare cases, spontaneous skin and mucous membrane haemorrhages due to interference with normal clotting mechanisms have been reported.

Overdosage: Pyopen may be removed from the circulation by haemodialysis.

Pharmaceutical precautions *Stability and storage:* Pyopen is unstable to heat and is very hygroscopic. The vials of dry powder should be stored in a refrigerator at 5°C.

Solutions for IM or direct IV injection should normally be administered within 30 minutes of preparation. However, aqueous solutions of Pyopen Injection retain their activity for up to 24 hours at room temperature (25°C) and for up to 72 hours in a refrigerator (5°C).

Pyopen may be added to most intravenous fluids (e.g. Water for Injections, glucose 5%, sodium chloride 0.18% with glucose 4%). Intravenous solutions of Pyopen for infusion, stored up to 25°C, should be used within 24 hours of preparation. Full particulars are given in the package enclosure leaflet.

Reconstitution of Pyopen injections and preparation of Pyopen infusion solutions must be carried out under appropriate aseptic conditions if these extended storage periods are required.

Pyopen should not be mixed with blood products or other proteinaceous fluids (e.g. protein hydrolysates) or with intravenous lipid emulsions.

If Pyopen is prescribed concurrently with an aminoglycoside the antibiotics should not be mixed in the syringe, intravenous fluid container or giving set because loss of activity of the aminoglycoside can occur under these conditions.

Legal category POM.

Package quantities
Pyopen 1 g Vials: Cartons of 10.
Pyopen 5 g Vials: Cartons of 6 (50 ml vials).
Each pack contains instructions for use.

Further information Pyopen continues to be effective in patients with lowered host defences.

Product licence numbers

Pyopen 1 g Vials	0038/5035R
Pyopen 5 g Vials	0038/5037R

TALPEN*

Presentation *Talpen Tablets:* White film coated tablets, engraved Talpen on one side. Each tablet contains 250 mg of the ampicillin ester, talampicillin hydrochloride.

Talpen Syrup: Bottles containing powder for the preparation of 100 ml suspension. When reconstituted each 5 ml contains talampicillin napsylate (167 mg) equivalent to 125 mg talampicillin hydrochloride.

Talpen presentations also contain inactive ingredients to make the medicine acceptable. Children's presentation: amongst these ingredients are disodium edetate, lactose, monosodium glutamate, sodium benzoate, sodium methylhydroxybenzoate and sucrose in Talpen Syrup.

Uses Following oral administration, Talpen is particularly well absorbed and rapidly hydrolysed to give high blood levels of ampicillin. Talpen is indicated for the oral treatment of a wide range of bacterial infections caused by ampicillin-sensitive organisms, for example:

Gram-positive: Penicillin sensitive *Staph. aureus, Strep. pyogenes, Strep. faecalis, Strep. viridans, Strep. pneumoniae, Clostridium species, Bacillus anthracis, Corynebacterium diphtheriae.*

Gram-negative: Neisseria gonorrhoeae, Neisseria meningitidis, Escherichia coli, Haemophilus influenzae, Bordetella pertussis, Salmonella typhi, Salmonella paratyphi, Salmonellae (other), *Shigella* species, *Brucella* species, *Proteus mirabilis.*

Typical indications include: Acute and chronic bronchitis; Pneumonia; Ear, nose and throat infections; Gynaecological infections; Urinary tract infections; Skin and soft tissue infections; Gonorrhoea.

Dosage and administration *Usual adult oral dosage (including elderly patients):* †One Talpen tablet or 10 ml Talpen Syrup, three times a day.

Gonorrhoea: 1.5–2 g talampicillin hydrochloride as a single dose, is recommended.

Usual children's oral dosage: (2–10 years) †5 ml Talpen Syrup, three times a day. (Under two years) the equivalent of 3–7 mg talampicillin hydrochloride per kilogram body weight, three times a day.

Total ampicillin availability following oral administration of Talpen is unaffected by food.

Contra-indications, warnings, etc
Contra-indication: Penicillin hypersensitivity.

Use in pregnancy and lactation: Animal studies have shown no teratogenic effects. The product has been in clinical use since 1975 and the limited number of reported cases of use in human pregnancy have shown no evidence of untoward effect. The use of Talpen in pregnancy should be reserved for cases considered essential by the clinician. During lactation, trace quantities of penicillins can be detected in breast milk.

Precaution: Talpen is not recommended for patients with severe renal or hepatic impairment.

Side-effects: Side-effects, as with other penicillins, are

† *Dosage may be doubled in severe infections.*

uncommon and mainly of a mild and transitory nature. Gastro-intestinal upsets (e.g. nausea, diarrhoea) and skin rashes have been reported infrequently. An urticarial rash suggests penicillin hypersensitivity; an erythematous rash may arise in patients who have glandular fever. If a skin rash occurs, treatment should be discontinued.

Controlled clinical trials have shown that the incidence of diarrhoea as a side-effect is significantly lower following the administration of Talpen than following oral ampicillin.

Overdosage: Problems of overdosage with Talpen are unlikely to occur; if encountered they may be treated symptomatically.

Pharmaceutical precautions Talpen should be stored in tightly closed containers and kept in a cool dry place. Once dispensed, Talpen Syrup remains stable for seven days if kept in a cool place. If a dilution of the reconstituted syrup is required, Syrup BP should be used.

Legal category POM.

Package quantities
Talpen Tablets: Bottles of 100 and 500.
Talpen Syrup: Original Pack of 100 ml.

Further information Following oral administration of 250 mg Talpen, ampicillin peak serum concentrations are twice those obtained from 250 mg ampicillin capsules and are usually achieved in half the time. This excellent absorption is further reflected in urinary recovery studies.

Each 250 mg of talampicillin hydrochloride is chemically equivalent to 169 mg of ampicillin.

Product licence numbers

Talpen Tablets	0038/0209
Talpen Syrup	0038/0243

TICAR*

Presentation *Ticar 1 g vial:* Vials containing 1 g ticarcillin as ticarcillin sodium.

Ticar 5 g vial: Vials containing 5 g ticarcillin as ticarcillin sodium.

Ticar infusion: Infusion bottles containing 5 g ticarcillin as ticarcillin sodium.

Uses Ticar is an injectable broad-spectrum penicillin indicated for the treatment of severe infections including mixed infections, particularly those involving Pseudomonas, Proteus and other Gram-negative organisms. Sensitive organisms include:

Streptococcus species
Staphylococcus aureus (penicillin sensitive)
Clostridium species
Bacteroides species and other anaerobes
Pseudomonas species
Proteus species
E. coli
Haemophilus influenzae

Typical indications include:

General Systemic Infections
Respiratory Tract Infections
Septicaemia
Urinary Tract Infections
Peritonitis, intra-abdominal sepsis
Endocarditis
Infected burns
Infected wounds
Post-surgical infections

Ticar acts synergistically with aminoglycosides against Pseudomonas and other organisms. When Ticar is prescribed concurrently with an aminoglycoside the two products should be administered separately, at recommended dosages.

Dosage and administration *Dosage: Adults (including elderly patients):* The usual recommended daily dosage is 15–20 g administered in divided doses, usually at 4–8 hourly intervals.

For the treatment of acute uncomplicated urinary tract infections the usual recommended daily dosage is 3–4 g in divided doses, usually at 4–8 hourly intervals.

Children: The usual recommended dosage for children is 200–300 mg/kg/day in divided doses, usually at 4–8 hourly intervals.

For acute uncomplicated urinary tract infections the recommended dosage is 50–100 mg/kg/day in divided doses, usually at 4–8 hourly intervals.

Abnormal Renal Function: If renal function is impaired as indicated by urea or creatinine levels monitoring of antibiotic serum levels is advised and a reduction in dosage may need to be considered. In renal failure an appropriate adult dose would be 2 g every 8–12 hours. In such cases the serum half life may be as long as 13 hours compared with 70 minutes in normal subjects. (Corresponding reductions in dosage should be considered for children.)

Haemodialysis removes Ticar from the blood stream therefore a supplementary 2 g dose is recommended midway through the dialysis period.

Peritoneal dialysis removes Ticar at a slower rate than haemodialysis therefore a dosage of 2 g 8 hourly is recommended.

Preparation: 1 gram vial: Intramuscular – Add 2 ml Water for Injections BP and shake vigorously.

Intravenous – Add 5 ml Water for Injections BP and shake vigorously. Dilute to 20 ml.

5 gram vial: Intravenous injection: Add 20 ml Water for Injections BP and shake vigorously.

Intravenous infusion: Add 20 ml Water for Injections BP shake vigorously and add to a suitable volume of infusion fluid (approximately 100–150 ml).

Water for Injections BP is the preferred diluent for intravenous infusion of Ticar as it will minimise the possibility of phlebitis. Alternatively, the antibiotic may be infused in a sterile glucose solution of 5% or lower concentration. (The use of 0.9% sodium chloride solution as diluent will add to the sodium load of ticarcillin and is, therefore, not usually recommended).

Infusion pack: See detailed instructions on Transfer Needle leaflet and Package Enclosure leaflet.

Reconstituted solutions of Ticar are normally a pale straw colour.

Heat is generated when Ticar dissolves. Ticar vials may therefore become warm during preparation of solutions for injection.

Ticar vials are not suitable for multi-dose use.

Administration: When administered intravenously Ticar should be given by slow injection (three to four minutes) or by infusion over e.g. 30–40 minutes (i.e. at a rate of approximately 50 drops per minute). Infusion over long periods may result in subtherapeutic concentrations.

Higher and more prolonged serum concentrations may be achieved with concurrent oral administration of probenecid (1 g three times a day in adults); however, caution should be exercised in the administration of probenecid to patients with impaired renal function.

Contra-indications, warnings, etc
Contra-indication: Penicillin hypersensitivity.

Use in pregnancy and lactation: Animal studies with Ticar have shown no teratogenic effects. The product has been in clinical use since 1979 and the limited number of reported cases of use in human pregnancy have shown no evidence of untoward effect. The use of Ticar in pregnancy should be reserved for cases considered essential by the clinician. Trace quantities of penicillins can be detected in the milk of lactating mothers. Breast feeding should therefore be discontinued during therapy.

Precautions: Use of Ticar at less than recommended dosages may permit multiplication of resistant strains of bacteria especially of Pseudomonas. For patients with abnormal renal function see 'Dosage and Administration'. The sodium intake should be monitored in patients with renal impairment. In treating patients on sodium restriction it should be noted that each 1 g vial of Ticar contains 5.3 mmol of sodium (approx.) and each 5 g vial contains 26.7 mmol of sodium (approx.). Potassium levels should be monitored and supplementation with potassium provided in appropriate cases.

Side-effects: Side-effects, as with other penicillins, are uncommon and mainly of a mild and transitory nature. Gastro-intestinal upsets (e.g. nausea, diarrhoea) and skin rashes have been reported infrequently. If a skin rash occurs, treatment should be discontinued. Hypokalaemia and eosinophilia have been reported rarely.

If pain at the intramuscular injection site is troublesome the vial contents may be dissolved in 0.5% lignocaine hydrochloride solution.

In rare cases spontaneous skin and mucous membrane haemorrhages due to interference with normal clotting mechanisms have been reported.

Overdosage: There is an increased risk of bleeding if ticarcillin is given in excess doses. Ticar may be removed from the circulation by haemodialysis.

Pharmaceutical precautions *Stability and storage:* Vials of Ticar powder should be stored in a refrigerator (2–8°C).

Solutions for IM and direct IV injection should normally be administered within 30 minutes of preparation. However, aqueous solutions of Ticar retain their activity for up to 24 hours at room temperature (25°C) and for up to 72 hours in a refrigerator (5°C).

Ticar may be added to most intravenous fluids (e.g. Water for Injections, glucose 5%, sodium chloride 0.18% with glucose 4%). Intravenous solutions of Ticar for infusion, stored up to 25°C, should be used within 24 hours of preparation. Full particulars are given in the package enclosure leaflet.

Reconstitution of Ticar injections and preparation of Ticar infusion solutions must be carried out under appropriate aseptic conditions if these extended storage periods are required.

Compatibility: Ticar is compatible with intravenous solutions in general use except:

Proteinaceous fluids (e.g. protein hydrolysates)
Blood and plasma
Intravenous lipids

If Ticar is prescribed concurrently with an aminoglycoside the antibiotics should not be mixed in the syringe or giving set because loss of activity of the aminoglycoside can occur under these conditions.

Legal category POM.

Package quantities *Ticar 1 g vials:* Cartons of 10. *Ticar 5 g vials:* Cartons of 4.
Ticar infusion: 5 g infusion bottle with diluent and transfer needle, in packs of 4.

Each pack contains instructions for use.

Further information Ticar has proved to be particularly valuable in the treatment of patients with lowered host defences.

Synergy has been observed between Ticar and aminoglycosides, such as gentamicin, tobramycin and amikacin, against Pseudomonas and other organisms. When Ticar is used with an aminoglycoside the usual recommended dosages of both products should be used. Concurrent therapy is not an opportunity to secure dosage reduction unless indicated for other reasons – for example renal failure. (See manufacturers' literature for details of aminoglycoside prescribing information.)

As with other penicillins, Ticar is eliminated by glomerular filtration and tubular secretion. It is not highly bound to serum protein (approximately 45%) and is excreted unchanged in high concentrations in the urine.

Ticar can be detected in tissues and interstitial fluid following parenteral administration. Penetration into the cerebrospinal fluid, bile and pleural fluid has been demonstrated.

Product licence numbers

1 g vial	0038/0084
5 g vial	0038/0084
5 g infusion	0038/0084
Water for Injections BP	0038/0118

TIMENTIN*

Presentation Timentin presentations are for reconstitution as intravenous infusions.

Timentin 3.2 g: Vials of sterile powder providing 200 mg clavulanic acid with 3.0 g ticarcillin.

Timentin 1.6 g: Vials of sterile powder providing 100 mg clavulanic acid with 1.5 g ticarcillin.

The clavulanic acid is present as potassium clavulanate and the ticarcillin as ticarcillin sodium.

Uses Timentin is an injectable antibiotic agent with a broad spectrum of bactericidal activity against a wide range of Gram-positive and Gram-negative, aerobic and anaerobic bacteria. The presence of clavulanate in the formulation extends the spectrum of activity of ticarcillin to include many β-lactamase producing bacteria normally resistant to ticarcillin and other β-lactam antibiotics.

Timentin is indicated for the treatment of infections in which susceptible organisms have been detected or are suspected.

Typical indications include: Severe infections in hospitalised patients and proven or suspected infections in patients with impaired or suppressed host defences including: Septicaemia; bacteraemia; peritonitis; intra-abdominal sepsis; post-surgical infections; bone and joint infections; skin and soft tissue infections; respiratory tract infections; serious or complicated renal infections (e.g. pyelonephritis); ear, nose and throat infections.

Timentin acts synergistically with aminoglycosides against a number of organisms including Pseudomonas. Timentin prescribed concurrently with an aminoglycoside, may therefore be preferred in the treatment of life threatening infections, particularly in patients with impaired host defences. In such instances the two products should be administered separately, at recommended dosages.

Timentin is bactericidal to a wide range of organisms in vitro including: Gram-positive: Aerobes – Staphylococcus species including *Staph aureus* and *Staph epidermidis*, Streptococcus species including *Strep faecalis*. Anaerobes – Peptococcus species, Peptostreptococcus species, Clostridium species, Eubacterium species.

Gram-negative: Aerobes – *Escherichia coli*, Haemophilus species including *H influenzae*, *Branhamella catarrhalis*, Klebsiella species including *K pneumoniae*, Enterobacter species, Proteus species including indole positive strains, *Providencia stuartii*, Pseudomonas species, including *Ps aeruginosa*, Serratia species including *S marcescens*, Citrobacter species, Acinetobacter species. *Yersinia enterocolitica*. Anaerobes – Bacteroides species including *B fragilis*, Fusobacterium species, Veillonella species.

Dosage and administration
Dosage
Adults (including elderly patients): The usual dosage is 3.2 g Timentin given 6–8 hourly. The maximum recommended dosage is 3.2 g 4 hourly.

Dosage in renal impairment

Mild impairment (Creatinine clearance >30 ml/min)	Moderate impairment (Creatinine clearance 10–30 ml/min)	Severe impairment (Creatinine clearance <10 ml/min)
3.2 g 8 hourly	1.6 g 8 hourly	1.6 g 12 hourly

NOTE: 3.2 g Timentin contains approximately 1 mmol of potassium and 16 mmol of sodium.

Children: The usual dosage for children is 80 mg Timentin/kg bodyweight given every 6–8 hours.

For premature infants and full term infants during the perinatal period, the dosage is 80 mg Timentin/kg bodyweight every 12 hours, increasing to every 8 hours thereafter.

Children with renal impairment – Similar reductions in dosage should be made for children as for adults.

Administration: Timentin is for administration by intermittent IV infusion. Timentin should be infused preferably in Water for Injections BP or Glucose Intravenous Infusion BP (5% or less).

Reconstitution: Vials – The sterile powder should be dissolved in approximately 10 ml (1.6 g/3.2 g vial) prior to dilution into the infusion container (e.g. mini-bag) or in-line burette.

The following approximate infusion volumes are suggested:

	Water for Injections BP	*Glucose Intravenous Infusion BP (5% w/v)*
3.2 g	100 ml	100–150 ml
1.6 g	50 ml	100 ml

Detailed instructions are given in the package enclosure leaflet.

Each dose of Timentin should be infused intravenously over a period of 30–40 minutes; avoid continuous infusion over long periods as this may result in subtherapeutic concentrations.

800 mg Timentin has a displacement value of 0.55 ml.

Heat is generated when Timentin dissolves. Reconstituted solutions are normally a pale straw colour.

Timentin presentations are not for multi-dose use or for direct IV or IM injection. Any residual antibiotic solution should be discarded if less than the fully made up vial is used.

Particulars of stability in solution and compatibilities are given under 'Pharmaceutical Precautions' and in the package enclosure leaflet.

Contra-indications, warnings, etc

Contra-indication: Penicillin hypersensitivity.

Use in pregnancy and lactation: Animal studies with Timentin have shown no teratogenic effects. There is no experience of Timentin in human pregnancy; therefore its use in pregnancy cannot be recommended. Trace quantities of penicillins can be detected in the milk of lactating mothers. Breast feeding should therefore be discontinued during therapy.

Precautions: Changes in liver function tests have been observed in some patients receiving Timentin. The clinical significance of these changes is uncertain but Timentin should be used with care in patients with evidence of severe hepatic dysfunction.

For patients with abnormal renal function see 'Dosage and Administration'. The sodium intake should be monitored in patients with renal impairment. In treating patients on sodium restriction it should be noted that each gram of ticarcillin sodium contains 5.3 mmol of sodium (approx.). Potassium levels should be monitored and supplementation with potassium provided in appropriate cases.

In rare cases bleeding manifestations have been reported following high dosages of ticarcillin. If bleeding manifestations appear with Timentin, treatment should be discontinued and appropriate therapy instituted unless, in the opinion of the physician, no alternative is available.

Side-effects: Side-effects (gastro-intestinal upsets, rash) are uncommon and typical of other injectable penicillins. If a skin rash occurs, treatment should be discontinued. Hepatitis and cholestatic jaundice have been reported. Hypokalaemia and eosinophilia have been reported rarely.

Overdosage: There is an increased risk of bleeding if ticarcillin is given in excess doses. Timentin may be removed from the circulation by haemodialysis.

Pharmaceutical precautions Stability and storage: Timentin should be stored in a dry place below 25°C.

Ideally intravenous solutions should be prepared at the time of administration. However, Timentin has been shown to be stable in Water for Injections BP and Glucose Intravenous Infusion BP (5% w/v) at recommended dilutions for the following periods:

Intravenous infusions	*Stability period (hours)*	
	5°C	*25°C*
Water for Injections BP	72	24
Glucose Intravenous Infusion BP (5% w/v)	72	12

The infusion must be prepared under appropriate aseptic conditions if these extended storage periods are required.

Details of the stability of Timentin in other fluids are given in the package enclosure leaflet.

Compatibilities: Timentin is compatible with intravenous solutions in general use except: Proteinaceous fluids (e.g. protein hydrolysates); blood and plasma; intravenous lipids.

If Timentin is prescribed concurrently with an aminoglycoside the antibiotics should not be mixed in the syringe, intravenous fluid container or giving set because loss of activity of the aminoglycoside can occur under these conditions.

Legal category POM.

Package quantities

Timentin 3.2 g vial: Pack of 4
1.6 g vial: Pack of 4

Each pack contains instructions for use.

Further information Resistance to many antibiotics is caused by bacterial enzymes which destroy the antibiotic before it can act on the pathogen. The clavulanate in Timentin anticipates this defence mechanism by blocking the β-lactamase enzymes, thus rendering the organisms sensitive to ticarcillin's rapid bactericidal effect at concentrations readily attainable in the body.

Clavulanate, by itself, has little antibacterial effect; however, in association with ticarcillin, as Timentin it produces an antibiotic agent with a breadth of spectrum suitable for empiric use in a wide range of infections treated parenterally in hospital.

The pharmacokinetics of the two components are closely matched and both components are well distributed in body fluids and tissues. Both clavulanate and ticarcillin have low levels of serum binding; about 20% and 45% respectively.

As with other penicillins the major route of elimination for ticarcillin is via the kidney; clavulanate is also excreted by this route.

Product licence numbers

3.2 g 0038/0329
1.6 g 0038/0329

**Trade Mark*

Bencard
Welwyn Garden City Hertfordshire AL7 1EY

AMOXIL* CAPSULES AMOXIL* DISPERSIBLE TABLETS AMOXIL* SYRUPS SF AMOXIL* SACHETS SF AMOXIL* PAEDIATRIC SUSPENSION AMOXIL* INJECTION

Presentation *Amoxil Capsules:* (Amoxycillin Capsules BP) Maroon and gold capsules overprinted 'Amoxil 250', each providing 250 mg amoxycillin.

Maroon and gold capsules overprinted 'Amoxil 500', each providing 500 mg amoxycillin.

Amoxil Dispersible Tablets: Flat, white circular tablets, engraved 'Amoxil 500', each providing 500 mg amoxycillin.

Amoxil Syrups SF: (Amoxycillin Oral Suspension BP). Citrus flavoured sucrose free syrups providing 125 mg or 250 mg amoxycillin per 5 ml in a sorbitol base. Presented as powder in bottles for preparing 100 ml.

Amoxil Sachets SF: Sucrose-free sachets providing 750 mg or 3 g amoxycillin in a sorbitol base, for reconstitution in water. Each sachet carries instructions for preparation.

Amoxil Paediatric Suspension. Citrus flavoured suspension, providing 125 mg amoxycillin per 1.25 ml (measured by the pipette supplied). Presented as powder in bottles for preparing 20 ml. Each pack contains a Users Guide.

Amoxil Vials for Injection: Each vial provides 250 mg, 500 mg or 1 g amoxycillin. Presented as powder for reconstitution. Each pack contains instructions for use.

The amoxycillin content per dose unit is present as the trihydrate in Amoxil oral preparations and as the sodium salt in Amoxil injections. Each 1 g vial of Amoxil contains approximately 3.2 mmol of sodium.

All Amoxil oral presentations also contain inactive ingredients to make the medicine acceptable. Children's presentations: amongst these ingredients are disodium edetate, sodium benzoate and sorbitol in Amoxil Syrups SF; sorbitol in Amoxil Sachets SF; sodium benzoate and sucrose in Amoxil Paediatric Suspension. Amoxil Dispersible Tablets contain lactose.

Amoxil Syrups SF, Sachets SF and Dispersible Tablets are sucrose-free. All Amoxil presentations are free from tartrazine and other azo dyes.

Uses *Treatment of Infection:* Amoxil is a broad spectrum antibiotic indicated for the treatment of commonly-occurring bacterial infections such as:

Upper Respiratory Tract Infections
Otitis media
Acute and Chronic Bronchitis
Chronic Bronchial Sepsis
Lobar and Bronchopneumonia
Cystitis, Urethritis, Pyelonephritis
Bacteriuria in pregnancy
Gynaecological infections including puerperal sepsis and septic abortion
Gonorrhoea
Peritonitis
Intra-abdominal sepsis
Septicaemia
Bacterial endocarditis
Typhoid and Paratyphoid fever
Skin and Soft Tissue Infections
Osteomyelitis
Dental abscess (as an adjunct to surgical management)

In children with urinary tract infection the need for investigation should be considered.

Prophylaxis of endocarditis: Amoxil may be used for the prevention of bacteraemia, associated with procedures such as dental extraction, in patients at risk of developing bacterial endocarditis.

The wide range of organisms sensitive to the bactericidal action of Amoxil include:

Gram-positive	*Gram-negative*
Streptococcus faecalis	Haemophilus influenzae
Streptococcus pneumoniae	Escherichia coli
Streptococcus pyogenes	Proteus mirabilis
Streptococcus viridans	Salmonella species
Staphylococcus aureus (penicillin-sensitive)	Shigella species
	Bordetella pertussis
Clostridium species	Brucella species
Corynebacterium species	Neisseria gonorrhoeae
Bacillus anthracis	Neisseria meningitidis
Listeria monocytogenes	Vibrio cholerae
	Pasteurella septica

Dosage and administration *Treatment of Infection:*

Adult dosage (including elderly patients):

Oral:

Standard adult dosage: 250 mg three times daily, increasing to 500 mg three times daily for more severe infections.

High dosage therapy (maximum recommended oral dosage 6 g daily in divided doses): A dosage of 3 g twice daily is recommended in appropriate cases for the treatment of severe or recurrent purulent infection of the respiratory tract.

Short course therapy: Simple acute urinary tract infection: two 3 g doses with 10–12 hours between the doses. Dental abscess: two 3 g doses with 8 hours between the doses. Gonorrhoea: single 3 g dose.

Injectable:

500 mg IM eight hourly (or more frequently if necessary) in moderate infections. (This dose may be given by slow IV injection if more convenient.)

1 g IV six hourly in severe infections.

Children's dosage (up to 10 years of age): Oral: Standard children's dosage: 125 mg three times daily, increasing to 250 mg three times daily for more severe infections.

Amoxil Paediatric Suspension is recommended for children under six months of age.

In severe or recurrent acute otitis media, especially where compliance may be a problem, 750 mg twice a day for two days may be used as an alternative course of treatment in children aged 3 to 10 years. The use of Amoxil 750 mg Sachets SF is recommended.

Injectable: 50–100 mg/kg body weight a day, in divided doses.

Parenteral therapy is indicated if the oral route is considered impracticable or unsuitable, and particularly for the urgent treatment of severe infection.

In renal impairment the excretion of the antibiotic will be delayed and depending on the degree of impairment it may be necessary to reduce the total daily dosage.

Prophylaxis of endocarditis: see table on next page.

Administration: Oral: Using capsules, dispersible tablets, syrups, sachets or paediatric suspension.

Prophylaxis of Endocarditis:

Condition		*Adults' Dosage (including elderly)*	*Children's Dosage*	*Notes*
Dental Procedures: Prophylaxis for patients undergoing extraction, scaling or surgery involving gingival tissues, and who have not received a penicillin in the previous month. (N.B. Patients with prosthetic heart valves should be referred to hospital – see below.)	Patient not having general anaesthetic.	3 g Amoxil orally, 1 hour before procedure. A second dose may be given 6 hours later, if considered necessary.	Under 10: Half adult dose. Under 5: Quarter adult dose	*Note 1.* If prophylaxis with Amoxil is given twice within one month, emergence of resistant streptococci is unlikely to be a problem. Alternative antibiotics are recommended if more frequent prophylaxis is required, or if the patient has received a course of treatment with a penicillin during the previous month. *Note 2.* To minimise pain on injection, Amoxil should be dissolved in sterile 1% lignocaine solution (see 'Administration').
	Patient having general anaesthetic: if oral antibiotics considered to be appropriate.	Initially 3 g Amoxil orally 4 hours prior to anaesthesia, followed by 3 g orally (or 1 g IM if oral dose not tolerated) 6 hours after the initial dose.	The use of Amoxil 500 mg Dispersible Tablets or 750 mg Sachets SF is recommended.	
	Patient having general anaesthetic: if oral antibiotics not appropriate.	1 g Amoxil IM immediately before induction; with 500 mg orally, 6 hours later.	Under 10: Half adult dose.	
Dental Procedures: Patients for whom referral to hospital is recommended: (a) patients to be given a general anaesthetic who have been given a penicillin in the previous month. (b) patients to be given a general anaesthetic who have a prosthetic heart valve. (c) patients who have had one or more attacks of endocarditis.		Initially: 1 g Amoxil IM with 120 mg gentamicin IM, immediately prior to anaesthesia (if given) or 15 minutes prior to dental procedure. Followed by (6 hours later): 500 mg Amoxil orally.	Under 10: The doses of Amoxil should be half the adult dose; the dose of gentamicin should be 2 mg/kg.	See Note 2. *Note 3.* Amoxil and gentamicin should not be mixed in the same syringe. *Note 4.* Please consult the appropriate data sheet for full prescribing information on gentamicin.
Genito-urinary Surgery or Instrumentation: Prophylaxis for patients who have no urinary tract infection and who are to have genito-urinary surgery or instrumentation under general anaesthesia. *Obstetric and Gynaecological Procedures* / *Gastro-intestinal Procedures* }	Routine prophylaxis is recommended only for patients with prosthetic heart valves.	Initially: 1 g Amoxil IM with 120 mg gentamicin IM, immediately before induction. Followed by (6 hours later): 500 mg Amoxil orally or IM according to clinical condition.	Under 10: The doses of Amoxil should be half the adult dose; the dose of gentamicin should be 2 mg/kg.	See Notes 2, 3 and 4 above.
Surgery or Instrumentation of the Upper Respiratory Tract	Patients other than those with prosthetic heart valves.	1 g Amoxil IM immediately before induction; 500 mg Amoxil IM 6 hours later.	Under 10: Half adult dose.	See Note 2 above. *Note 5.* The second dose of Amoxil may be administered orally as Amoxil Syrup SF.
	Patients with prosthetic heart valves.	Initially: 1 g Amoxil IM with 120 mg gentamicin IM, immediately before induction; followed by (6 hours later) 500 mg Amoxil IM.	Under 10: The dose of Amoxil should be half the adult dose; the gentamicin dose should be 2 mg/kg.	See Notes 2, 3, 4 and 5 above.

Intravenous: Dissolve 250 mg in 5.0 ml Water for Injections BP. (Final volume=5.2 ml.)

Dissolve 500 mg in 10 ml Water for Injections BP. (Final volume=10.4 ml.)

Dissolve 1 g in 20 ml Water for Injections BP. (Final volume=20.8 ml.)

Amoxil injection, suitably diluted, may be injected directly into a vein or the infusion line over a period of 3–4 minutes.

Intravenous Infusion: Solutions may be prepared as described for intravenous injections and then added to an intravenous solution in a minibag or in-line burette and administered over a period of ½–1 hour. Alternatively, using a suitable reconstitution device, the appropriate volume of intravenous fluid may be transferred from the infusion bag into the vial and then drawn back into the bag after dissolution.

Intramuscular: 250 mg: Add 1.5 ml Water for Injections BP† and shake vigorously. (Final volume=1.7 ml.)

500 mg: Add 2.5 ml Water for Injections BP† and shake vigorously. (Final volume=2.9 ml.)

1 g: Add 2.5 ml of 1% sterile lignocaine hydrochloride solution and shake vigorously. (Final volume=3.3 ml.)

†If pain is experienced on intramuscular injection, a sterile 1% solution of lignocaine hydrochloride or 0.5% solution of procaine hydrochloride may be used in place of Water for Injections.

A transient pink colouration or slight opalescence may appear during reconstitution. Reconstituted solutions are normally a pale straw colour.

Contra-indications, warnings, etc Amoxil is a penicillin and should not be given to penicillin-hypersensitive patients.

Use in pregnancy and lactation: Animal studies with Amoxil have shown no teratogenic effects. The product has been in extensive clinical use since 1972 and its suitability in human pregnancy has been well documented in clinical studies. When antibiotic therapy is required during pregnancy, Amoxil may be considered appropriate. During lactation, trace quantities of Amoxil can be detected in breast milk.

Side-effects: Side-effects, as with other penicillins, are uncommon and mainly of a mild and transitory nature; they may include diarrhoea, indigestion, or occasionally rash, either urticarial or erythematous. An urticarial rash suggests penicillin hypersensitivity and the erythematous type rash may arise if Amoxil is administered to patients with glandular fever. In either case treatment should be discontinued. In common with other beta-lactam antibiotics angioedema and anaphylaxis have been reported.

Amoxil SF formulations contain sorbitol (see Further Information).

Overdosage: Gross overdosage will produce very high urinary concentrations, more so after parenteral administration. Problems are unlikely if adequate fluid intake and urinary output are maintained; however, crystalluria is a possibility. More specific measures may be necessary in patients with impaired renal function: the antibiotic is removed by haemodialysis.

Pharmaceutical precautions Prior to use, oral presentations of Amoxil should be stored in a dry place. Store Amoxil Sachets SF in a dry place at 25°C or below. Amoxil injections should be stored in a cool, dry place.

Once dispensed, Amoxil Syrups SF and Amoxil Paediatric Suspension should be used within the periods stated on the labels and any remaining should be discarded. If dilution of the reconstituted SF product is required, water should be used. Amoxil Paediatric Suspension may be diluted with water or Syrup BP.

When prepared for intramuscular or direct intravenous injection, Amoxil should be administered immediately after reconstitution. The stability of Amoxil in various infusion fluids is dependent upon the concentration and temperature: stability times are given in the package enclosure leaflet.

Amoxil should not be mixed with blood products, other proteinaceous fluids such as protein hydrolysates, or with intravenous lipid emulsions.

If Amoxil is prescribed concurrently with an aminoglycoside the antibiotics should not be mixed in the syringe, intravenous fluid container or giving set because loss of activity of the aminoglycoside can occur under these conditions.

Legal category POM.

Package quantities *Amoxil Capsules:* 250 mg Original Pack of 21 with Patient Information Leaflet; also container of 500. 500 mg Original Pack of 21 with Patient Information Leaflet; also container of 100.

Amoxil Dispersible Tablets: 500 mg: Original Pack of 21 with Patient Information Leaflet.

Amoxil Syrups SF: 125 mg and 250 mg per 5 ml: Original Pack of 100 ml with Patient Information Leaflet.

Amoxil 750 mg Sachet SF: Original Pack of 4. Each sachet carries instructions for preparation and each pack contains a Patient Information Leaflet.

Amoxil 3 g Sachet SF: Original Packs of 2 and 14. Each sachet carries instructions for preparation and each pack contains a Patient Information Leaflet.

Amoxil Paediatric Suspension: 125 mg per 1.25 ml: Original Pack of 20 ml with pipette and Patient Information Leaflet.

Amoxil Vials for Injection: 250 mg, 500 mg and 1 g: packs of 10, 10 and 5 respectively. Each pack carries instructions for use.

Further information Amoxil is well absorbed by the oral and parenteral routes. Oral administration, usually at convenient t.d.s. dosage, produces high serum levels independent of the time at which food is taken. Amoxil gives good penetration into bronchial secretions and high urinary concentrations of unchanged antibiotic. It is rapidly bactericidal and possesses the safety profile of a penicillin.

Sucrose content (approx.): Amoxil Paediatric Suspension (125 mg) 0.6 g per 1.25 ml.

Sorbitol content (approx.): Amoxil Syrup SF (125 mg) 0.75 g per 5 ml; Amoxil Syrup SF (250 mg) 0.57 g per 5 ml; Amoxil Sachet SF (750 mg) 1.1 g; Amoxil Sachet SF (3 g) 4.2 g.

Product licence numbers

Amoxil Capsules 250 mg	0038/0103
Amoxil Capsules 500 mg	0038/0105
Amoxil Dispersible Tablets 500 mg	0038/0277
Amoxil Syrup SF 125 mg per 5 ml	0038/0326
Amoxil Syrup SF 250 mg per 5 ml	0038/0327
Amoxil 750 mg Sachet SF	0038/0332
Amoxil 3 g Sachet SF	0038/0334
Amoxil Paediatric Suspension 125 mg per 1.25 ml	0038/0107
Amoxil Vials for Injection 250 mg	0038/0221
Amoxil Vials for Injection 500 mg	0038/0222
Amoxil Vials for Injection 1 g	0038/0225

ASERBINE* CREAM
ASERBINE* SOLUTION

Presentation *Aserbine Cream:* White cream in a tube.

Aserbine Solution: Clear colourless liquid in a polythene bottle.

Aserbine is prepared from:

	Aserbine cream %	*Aserbine solution %*
Propylene glycol	1.7	40.0
Malic acid	0.36	2.25
Benzoic acid	0.024	0.15
Salicylic acid	0.006	0.0375

Aserbine Cream is a water-in-oil emulsion containing the following inactive ingredients: white soft paraffin emulsified with sorbitan sesquiolate and cholesterol, parabens (preservative), allantoin and magnesium sulphate. Aserbine Solution (aqueous) contains oil of rose dissolved in ethanol.

Uses *Principal action:* Aserbine is a desloughing and cleansing agent which does not affect living tissue and has antibacterial properties to guard against wound infection.

Indications:

1. Whenever the presence of slough delays healing:
   Chronic skin ulcers:
   Venous (varicose) ulcers and other benign chronic ulcers; trophic ulcers including pressure sores.
   Burns.
   Traumatic injuries:
   Crushed limb injuries; multiple lesions.
   Surgical procedures where slough may be a problem:
   Preparation for skin grafting; mastectomies; amputations; post-surgical incisions.
2. Cleansing:
   Wounds and abrasions where coagulum, debris, dirt and grit, etc. are a problem.

Administration Aserbine is suitable for both adults and children and should be applied topically.

For desloughing: Aserbine Cream should be applied liberally to the wound surface and before each new application the wound should be washed with Aserbine Solution so that the loose slough and cream from the previous application are removed.

Dressing the wound twice daily has been found to produce the best results; however, more frequent dressings may be made if necessary.

Aserbine Solution may also be applied as a wet dressing which should be kept constantly moist.

For cleansing: Both Aserbine Cream and Solution have proved of value as cleansing agents in casualty work for the removal of coagulum, debris, dirt, grit, etc. from wounds and abrasions.

Contra-indications, warnings, etc
Contra-indications: None.

Warning: For external use only.

Use in pregnancy and lactation: There is no documented experience of its use in human pregnancy or lactation. As with all medicines, careful consideration should be given before the use of Aserbine during the first trimester.

Precautions: Care should be taken to avoid contact with the eyes because of Aserbine's low pH.

Overdosage: Not applicable.

Side-effects: Mild pyrexia, partially due to the absorption of protein products of slough breakdown from the wound, has been reported in severely burned patients. Irritation of the hypersensitive skin surrounding the wound may occur in a few patients. In these cases, Aserbine should be kept away from the growing epithelium at the periphery of the wound.

Occasionally a mild urticarial rash has been seen a small distance around the treated area. The discomfort was slight and readily controlled by antihistamines.

Drug interactions: No specific information available.

Pharmaceutical precautions Prolonged contact of Aserbine Solution with metallic surfaces is inadvisable.

Legal category P.

Package quantities *Aserbine Cream:* Original Pack of 100 g (tube). *Aserbine Solution:* 500 ml bottle.

Further information The acid pH of Aserbine Cream and Solution is such that, when applied to a wound, it causes maximum differential swelling between the living protein of healthy tissues and the dead protein of slough, leading to the separation of the dead tissue (desloughing). The wound surface is cleared from the presence of slough and debris without affecting the living tissue so that uninterrupted normal healing can proceed. Aserbine also has antibacterial properties which guard against wound infection.

Dressings with Aserbine Cream are non-adherent, odourless and do not stain the skin, clothing, etc.

Product licence numbers

Aserbine Cream	0038/5089
Aserbine Solution	0038/5090

DORALESE* TILTAB* TABLETS

Presentation Pale yellow, biconvex triangular, film-coated Tiltab tablets, with a small projection on each side. Each tablet contains 20 mg indoramin.

Uses Doralese is an alpha adrenoceptor antagonist that increases urinary flow rate by acting selectively and competitively on postsynaptic alpha$_1$-receptors.

It is indicated in the management of urinary outflow obstruction due to benign prostatic hypertrophy, particularly in patients in whom surgery is contra-indicated or delayed.

Dosage and administration
Adults only: 20 mg twice a day. If necessary the dosage may be increased, in increments of 20 mg at two-weekly intervals, to a maximum of 100 mg a day in divided doses.

Elderly: Since clearance of Doralese may be reduced, 20 mg at night may be adequate.

Contra-indications, warnings, etc
Contra-indications: Do not use in patients in established cardiac failure or those under treatment with an MAO inhibitor.

Precautions: If drowsiness occurs, patients should be warned not to drive or operate machinery and to avoid CNS depressants including alcohol.

Use with caution in patients with hepatic or renal insufficiency, Parkinson's disease which could be exacerbated, epilepsy, and those with a history of depression. Incipient cardiac failure should be controlled before treatment with Doralese.

At higher dosages indoramin is used in the management of hypertension. Concomitant use of Doralese with thiazide diuretics, beta-blockers or other antihypertensive drugs may enhance their hypotensive action. Titration of dosage of the latter may therefore be needed. Alcohol can increase both the rate and extent of absorption of indoramin, but no untoward effects have been reported at recommended doses.

Adverse reactions: Drowsiness or sedation can occur on starting treatment with Doralese, and also if the dosage is increased too rapidly. This usually responds to a reduction in dosage. Less commonly dry mouth, nasal congestion, weight gain, dizziness, retrograde ejaculation and depression may occur.

Overdosage: Experience of overdosage with indoramin is limited but symptoms have included deep sedation, coma, hypotension and convulsions. Animal work suggests that hypothermia may also occur. Suggested treatment includes gastric lavage, assisted ventilation if necessary, circulatory support and control of hypotension, intravenous diazepam for convulsions and slow rewarming if hypothermia occurs.

Pharmaceutical precautions Store below 25°C.

Legal category POM.

Package quantities Opaque blister packs (OP) of 60 (4 × 15).

Further information Postural hypotension has not been shown to be a significant problem. Reflex tachycardia has not been observed in clinical trials with doses of up to 100 mg.

Inactive ingredients include lactose.

Product licence number 0002/0168.

NACTON*
NACTON FORTE*

Presentation *Nacton (2 mg):* White-coloured, scored tablets engraved 'NACTON 2'.

Nacton Forte (4 mg): Orange-coloured, scored tablets engraved 'NACTON 4'.

Active ingredients: Nacton: Each tablet contains 2 mg of Poldine Methylsulphate BP.

Nacton Forte: Each tablet contains 4 mg of Poldine Methylsulphate BP.

Nacton presentations also contain inactive ingredients to make the medicine acceptable.

Uses *Principal action:* Poldine methylsulphate is a proven anticholinergic compound which at therapeutic doses acts mainly on the parietal or oxyntic cells of the stomach, causing gastric acid production to be reduced by over 50%.

Indications: Peptic ulcer; recurrent dyspepsia associated with hyperacidity; whenever acidity causes pain.

Dosage and administration
Standard Adult dosage: 1 tablet of Nacton Forte (4 mg) four times a day (the last at bedtime). This will give effective and continuous pain relief without side-effects in the majority of patients.

If necessary (e.g. in elderly patients), optimum dosage may be determined by adjusting to individual requirements. For example, initially 1 tablet of Nacton (2 mg) four times a day (the last at bedtime) followed by review after four days.

Tailored dosage: a tailored dosage schedule may be applied as follows: starting at one tablet of Nacton (2 mg) four times a day (the last at bedtime), increase by half a Nacton tablet (1 mg) per dose every four days. Continue until the first signs of any discomfort appear (e.g., dry mouth, blurred vision or hesitancy of micturition); then reduce each dose by half a Nacton tablet (1 mg). This should generally be the optimum therapeutic dose.

If treatment is suspended for more than a week and later resumed, the therapeutic dose should again be built up gradually. If the previous therapeutic dose was greater than 4 mg taken four times a day, the patient may resume treatment, building up from a starting dose of 4 mg four times a day.

Contra-indications, warnings, etc
Precautions: For patients in whom tachycardia, difficulty in micturition or increase in ocular tension might give rise to particular anxiety, Nacton and Nacton Forte should only be used under close supervision.

Use in pregnancy: There is no evidence that Nacton or Nacton Forte have teratogenic effects. However, treatment is not advised during the first trimester of pregnancy.

Side-effects. There should be no side-effects at therapeutic doses.

Overdosage: Mild overdosage: Signs of mild overdosage are, in order of frequency, dry mouth, blurred vision, hesitancy of micturition or tachycardia. They will usually disappear if one or two doses are omitted before resuming treatment at a lower dosage level.

Gross overdosage: Gastric aspiration and lavage should be performed immediately. A short-acting barbiturate such as thiopentone sodium may be given cautiously for the stage of excitement.

Pharmaceutical precautions Store in a dry place.

Legal category POM.

Package quantities *Nacton (2 mg):* Original Pack of 112 tablets.
Nacton Forte (4 mg): Original Pack of 112 tablets.

Further information Nacton and Nacton Forte provide an environment for ulcer healing by halving gastric acid production. Reduction of gastric acid secretion can be maintained over several years without development of tolerance to the dosage used. Pain is controlled even at night as each dose of Nacton or Nacton Forte is effective for 8–9 hours. Nacton and Nacton Forte permit patients a liberal diet and a return to normal working life.

Product licence numbers
Nacton 0038/5077
Nacton Forte 0038/5078

NORVAL*

Presentation *Norval tablets:* Orange film coated tablets engraved 'Norval' on one side and '30' on the other. Each tablet contains 30 mg Mianserin Hydrochloride BP.

Also available, orange film coated tablets containing 10 mg and 20 mg Mianserin Hydrochloride BP. Each tablet is engraved 'Norval' on one side and '10' or '20' respectively on the reverse.

Norval tablets also contain inactive ingredients to make the medicine acceptable.

Uses Symptoms of depressive illness.

Dosage and administration *For oral administration:* The tablets should be swallowed whole without chewing.

Adults: Treatment should normally be initiated, for the first few days, at 30–40 mg a day as a single bedtime dose, or in divided doses. The effective maintenance dosage will normally lie between 30 mg and 90 mg a day as indicated in the table, though higher levels may be required in some patients.

Degree of depression	*Usual daily dosage*
Mild to moderate	30–60 mg nocte or in divided doses.
Moderate to severe	60–90 mg nocte or in divided doses. If higher levels are required these should be given in divided doses.

Divided daily dosages up to 200 mg are well tolerated.

It is often advantageous to maintain antidepressant treatment for several months after initial clinical improvement has occurred.

Elderly: Not more than 30 mg a day initially. This starting dose should be increased with caution under close supervision. A lower maintenance dosage than is usual may be sufficient to produce a satisfactory clinical response.

Children: Not recommended.

Contra-indications, warnings, etc
Contra-indications: Use is contra-indicated in mania, severe liver disease and during breast feeding. (Breast feeding should be discontinued if antidepressant therapy is considered essential.)

Use in pregnancy: Do not use during pregnancy unless there are compelling reasons. There is no evidence of safety in human pregnancy. Animal studies have not shown hazard.

Precautions: Care should always be taken in patients with recent myocardial infarction or heart block. However, serious cardiotoxic effects appear to be rare at therapeutic dosage, even in patients with pre-existing cardiac disease, recent myocardial infarction or cardiac insufficiency.

The elderly are less liable to experience adverse reactions such as agitation, confusion and postural hypotension with Norval than with tricyclics or bridged tricyclics, but all antidepressant therapy should be used with caution in this group of patients.

Patients posing a high suicide risk always require close initial supervision.

Avoid, if possible, in patients with epilepsy.

When treating patients with diabetes, hepatic or renal insufficiency, normal precautions should be exercised and the dosages of any concurrent therapy kept under review.

Patients with narrow angle glaucoma or symptoms suggestive of prostatic hypertrophy, should also be monitored even though anticholinergic side-effects are not anticipated with Norval therapy.

There are indications that Norval, like other antidepressants, may precipitate hypomania in susceptible subjects with bipolar affective illness.

Norval may potentiate the central nervous depressant action of alcohol.

If surgery is necessary during Norval therapy, the anaesthetist should be informed of the treatment being given.

Drug interactions: Norval should not be given concurrently with, or within two weeks of cessation of therapy with, monoamine oxidase inhibitors.

Clinical experience has shown that Norval does not interact with the antihypertensives bethanidine, clonidine, hydralazine, guanethidine and propranolol. Nevertheless, the monitoring of blood pressure is recommended for those patients receiving concurrent antihypertensive therapy.

Phenytoin plasma levels should be monitored in patients treated concurrently with Norval.

Concurrent anticoagulant therapy of the coumarin-type (e.g. warfarin) is also permissible, but close additional monitoring should be undertaken.

Interactions have not been reported between Norval and sympathomimetic agents and are unlikely.

Warnings and adverse effects: As improvement may not occur during the first 2–4 weeks of treatment, patients should be closely monitored during this period. It may be advisable to maintain treatment for several months after initial clinical improvement has occurred.

The most commonly occurring side-effect is drowsiness, particularly during the first few days of therapy. Patients should be warned of the possible hazard in driving or operating machinery. Any drowsiness may be potentiated by alcohol.

Bone marrow depression, usually presenting as granulocytopenia or agranulocytosis, has been reported during treatment with Norval. These reactions have occurred most commonly after 4–6 weeks of treatment and were generally reversible on stopping treatment. A full blood count is recommended every four weeks during the first three months of treatment. In addition, monitoring of the patient's clinical condition should continue and if a patient develops fever, sore throat, stomatitis or other signs of infection, treatment should be stopped and a full blood count obtained. These adverse reactions have been observed in all age groups but appear to be more common in the elderly.

Jaundice, usually mild, hypomania and convulsions have also been reported at therapeutic dosage and under such circumstances treatment should be withdrawn.

Additional adverse effects that may occur include breast disorders (gynaecomastia, nipple tenderness and non-puerperal lactation), altered liver enzyme levels, dizziness, postural hypotension, polyarthropathy, skin rash, sweating and tremor.

Psychotic manifestations including mania and paranoid delusions may be exacerbated during antidepressant therapy.

The following adverse effects although not reported with Norval can occur with tricyclics and bridged tricyclics: interference with sexual function; withdrawal symptoms in adults; withdrawal symptoms (e.g. neuromuscular irritability) in neonates whose mothers received tricyclic or bridged tricyclic antidepressants during pregnancy.

Overdosage: Symptoms of overdosage are normally confined to prolonged sedation. Cardiac arrhythmias, severe hypotension, convulsions and respiratory depression are unlikely to occur. There is no specific antidote. Treatment is by gastric lavage with appropriate supportive therapy.

Pharmaceutical precautions Protect tablets from light.

Legal category POM.

Package quantities Norval 30 mg tablets: Original Pack of 28. Norval 10 mg tablets: Original Pack of 84. Norval 20 mg tablets: Original Pack of 28.

Further information Norval is an antidepressant with a distinctive tetracyclic structure which confers important benefits over the tricyclic compounds. Norval has also been shown to possess anxiolytic properties comparable with diazepam.

Antidepressant activity is at least equal to that of amitriptyline and imipramine, but Norval may be preferred for its absence of troublesome anticholinergic side-effects; this may be of special importance when treating depressed patients who may be at concurrent risk from conditions such as glaucoma, urinary retention and prostatic hypertrophy. There is also substantial evidence that anticholinergic effects such as dry mouth can be a psychosomatic feature of depressive illness; such symptoms have been shown to be alleviated with Norval therapy. Clinical experience has confirmed that Norval is significantly less toxic than either amitriptyline or imipramine and that cardiac problems are unlikely. Norval appears to be particularly effective in improving 'pessimistic thought' and 'suicidal ideation'. Moreover, its relatively high safety margin is of considerable importance in view of the high number of suicides attributed to tricyclic overdosage.

Product licence numbers

Norval 10 mg	0038/0230R
Norval 20 mg	0038/0247R
Norval 30 mg	0038/0248R

NULACIN*

Presentation Off-white coloured tablets embossed with the product name 'NULACIN'. Each tablet contains:

Whole milk combined with dextrins and maltose.

Magnesium trisilicate	230 mg
Heavy magnesium oxide	130 mg
Calcium carbonate	130 mg
Heavy magnesium carbonate	30 mg
Peppermint oil q.s.	

Calorific content per tablet: 11 calories.

Nulacin tablets also contain lactose and gluten.

Uses *Principal action:* The balanced combination of antacids and milk protein in Nulacin causes rapid and continuous neutralisation of excess gastric acid so that the gastric acidity is maintained at pH 3–4.

The milk fat in Nulacin helps to inhibit the formation of excess gastric juice.

Indications: Dyspepsia. Reflux oesophagitis. Hiatus hernia. Symptoms of peptic ulcer. Whenever gastric hyperacidity causes pain.

Dosage and administration (including elderly patients): One tablet repeated as required between meals and at bedtime, up to eight tablets per day.

For continuous therapeutic effect the tablet should be allowed to disperse slowly in the mouth, placed between cheek and gum. For quicker relief the tablet should be chewed and swallowed.

Contra-indications, warnings, etc
Contra-indication: As Nulacin contains gluten, it is contra-indicated in coeliac disease.

Use in pregnancy and lactation: As with all medicines, careful consideration should be given before the administration of Nulacin during the first trimester. Excessive usage of Nulacin should be avoided during pregnancy and lactation, when there may be a higher dietary intake of calcium.

Precautions: Caution is advised in patients with renal impairment.

Drug interactions: Antacids may reduce the absorption of a variety of agents (e.g. tetracyclines, phenytoin, iron, chloroquine, penicillamine, trientine) and such possibilities should be considered for Nulacin.

Side-effects: Nulacin may occasionally have a laxative effect.

Overdosage: Overdosage has not been reported. However, there is a theoretical risk of hypercalcaemia and, as with other antacids, of alkalosis, particularly in patients with renal impairment.

Pharmaceutical precautions Store in a cool dry place. Replace container cap after use.

Legal category GSL.

Package quantities 25 tablets.

Further information Nulacin contains effective doses of antacids to give rapid relief from gastric pain. Nulacin disperses slowly in the mouth to give continuous relief which is independent of the rate of stomach emptying. Nulacin is presented in convenient tablets which have a very acceptable malt and mint flavour.

Product licence number 0038/5079.

PARAMAX*

Presentation *Paramax Tablets:* White, round scored tablets, engraved 'Paramax' on one side.

Paramax Sachets: Sachets containing effervescent powder.

Each tablet or sachet contains 500 mg Paracetamol BP with 5 mg Metoclopramide Hydrochloride BP.

Paramax presentations also contain inactive ingredients to make the medicine acceptable.

Paramax presentations do not contain sucrose, tartrazine or any other azo dyes.

Uses *Indications:* Paramax is indicated for the symptomatic treatment of migraine.

Action: Paracetamol relieves pain. More rapid absorption is promoted by the action of metoclopramide which also relieves gastric stasis and overcomes nausea and vomiting.

Dosage and administration For oral administration only.

Paramax should be taken at the first warning of an attack. If symptoms persist, further doses may be taken at four-hourly intervals. Total dosage in any 24-hour period should not exceed the quantity stated.

The dosage recommendations given below should be strictly adhered to if side-effects of the dystonic type are to be avoided. It should be noted that total daily dosage of metoclopramide, especially for adolescents and young adults, should not normally exceed 0.5 mg/kg body weight.

Usual Recommended Dosage (Tablets or Sachets)

	Initial dose at first warning of attack	*Maximum dosage in any 24-hour period*
Adults (including elderly patients)	2	6
Young Adults (15–19 years)		
60 kg and over	2	5
30–59 kg	1	3
Adolescents (12–14 years)		
30 kg and over	1	3

Young adults and adolescents: Paramax should only be used after careful examination to avoid masking an underlying disorder, e.g. cerebral irritation. In the treatment of this group attention should be given primarily to bodyweight.

Children: A presentation of Paramax suitable for the treatment of children under 12 years of age is not available.

Paramax Sachets: Empty a sachet into about ¼ of a glass of water and stir before taking.

Contra-indications, warnings, etc
Use in pregnancy and lactation: There is no evidence that metoclopramide or paracetamol by themselves have teratogenic effects. Nevertheless, Paramax should only be used when there are compelling reasons and is not advised during the first trimester.

During lactation, metoclopramide and paracetamol may be found in breast milk.

Precautions: If vomiting persists the patient should be re-assessed to exclude the possibility of an underlying disorder, e.g. cerebral irritation.

Care should be exercised in patients being treated with other centrally active drugs e.g. in epilepsy.

Care should be exercised in the event of Paramax being prescribed concurrently with a phenothiazine since extra-pyramidal symptoms may occur with both products. The action of metoclopramide on the gastro-intestinal tract is antagonised by anticholinergics.

Metoclopramide may induce an acute hypertensive response in patients with phaeochromocytoma.

Side-effects: Various extra-pyramidal reactions to metoclopramide, usually of the dystonic type, have been reported. The incidence of these reactions may be increased if the metoclopramide dosage exceeds 0.5 mg/kg body weight/day. Reactions include: spasm of the facial muscles, trismus, rhythmic protrusion of the tongue, a bulbar type of speech, spasm of extra-ocular muscles, including oculogyric crises, unnatural positioning of the head and shoulders and opisthotonos. There may be a generalised increase in muscle tone. The majority of reactions occur within 36 hours of starting treatment and the effects usually disappear within 24 hours of withdrawal of the drug. Should treatment of a dystonic reaction be required, a benzodiazepine or an anticholinergic anti-Parkinsonian drug may be used.

Rarely, drowsiness, restlessness and diarrhoea have been reported in patients receiving metoclopramide therapy.

Raised serum prolactin levels have been observed during metoclopramide therapy; this effect is similar to that noted with many other compounds.

Overdosage: As with other paracetamol-containing products, an overdose of Paramax can be toxic to the liver. Overdosage should be treated by gastric lavage with appropriate supportive measures. Intravenous N-acetylcysteine or oral methionine if administered within 10 hours of paracetamol overdosage appears to exert a protective effect on the liver.

Pharmaceutical precautions Protect tablets from light. Store sachets in a dry place.

Legal category POM.

Package quantities *Paramax tablets:* Original Pack of 42 with Patient Information Leaflet.
Paramax sachets: Original Pack of 42. Each sachet carries instructions for preparation and each pack contains a Patient Information Leaflet.

Further information An acute attack of migraine is frequently characterised by impaired absorption of analgesics even when abdominal symptoms are absent. The beneficial effect of Paramax on delayed gastric emptying, nausea and vomiting contrasts with the gastric stasis which may occur following administration of phenothiazine or antihistamine antiemetics.

Product licence numbers
Paramax Tablets 0038/0256
Paramax Sachets 0038/0257

PARENTROVITE* IVHP
PARENTROVITE* IMHP

Presentation Paired amber glass ampoules for injectable administration; available in two different presentations. Intravenous High Potency (IVHP) and Intramuscular High Potency (IMHP).

Ingredients: See table overleaf.

Uses *Principal action:* Parentrovite IVHP and IMHP contain very high concentrations of the water-soluble vitamins B and C to correct disturbed carbohydrate metabolism.

Indications: Parentrovite is indicated only for the treatment of confirmed or imminent acute Wernicke's encephalopathy and Korsakoff's psychosis.

Parenteral therapy should be considered only when oral intake is impossible or inadequate.

Dosage and administration
Dosage in adults (including the elderly): 2 to 4 pairs Intravenous High Potency ampoules, repeated 4 to 8 hourly for up to 2 days as indicated clinically, followed by 1 pair Intravenous High Potency or Intramuscular High Potency ampoules daily for 5 to 7 days.

Children: Not recommended for use in children and adolescents.

Administration: For parenteral administration only.

The contents of each pair of ampoules (i.e. No. 1 and No. 2) should be mixed together in a single syringe immediately prior to administration. The intravenous and intramuscular presentations are not interchangeable. As a result of its high volume and lack of local anaesthetic, the intravenous presentation may cause unnecessary pain if administered intramuscularly. The presence of the anaesthetic in the intramuscular presentation makes it unsuitable for intravenous administration.

Intravenous Parentrovite: The contents of each pair of ampoules are to be mixed in the syringe immediately before use.

Very slow infusion should preferably be used, over a period of 10 minutes; dilution may be made with normal saline. When given by infusion with other drugs, Parentrovite should be injected slowly into the infusion tubing; slow administration should be ensured, i.e. 4–5 minutes.

When injecting directly into the vein, Parentrovite should be given slowly (4–5 minutes).

Intramuscular Parentrovite: The contents of each pair of ampoules are to be mixed in the syringe before injecting slowly into the lateral muscles of the thigh or into the gluteal region at one or more sites.

Contra-indications, warnings, etc
Contra-indications: Sensitivity to any of the vitamins present.

Use in pregnancy and lactation: It is important during pregnancy not to exceed the recommended dose. As with all medicines, careful consideration should be given before the administration of Parentrovite during the first trimester. Vitamins are excreted in breast milk.

Warnings and Precautions: Parentrovite may be used in patients being treated for Parkinson's disease with a levodopa preparation which includes a dopadecarboxylase inhibitor (e.g. carbidopa, benserazide) but should not be used with levodopa alone as pyridoxine may act as an antagonist.

Side-effects: On occasions, injections of Parentrovite have given rise to urticaria, angioedema or anaphylactic reactions. These reactions are more likely to occur with the intravenous high potency preparation. Flushing of the face has been reported occasionally. Treatment of anaphylaxis – On first appearance of any signs or symptoms of an allergic reaction, the administration should be stopped immediately. Treatment should include laying the patient flat with feet raised, and intramuscular administration of 0.5–1.0 ml Adrenaline Injection BP (adrenaline 1 in 1,000), repeated every ten minutes until improvement occurs. Antihistamines such as chlorpheniramine by slow intravenous injection are a useful adjunctive measure. Supportive treatment of hypotension with intravenous fluids, and of bronchospasm using bronchodilators, may be helpful. Intravenous steroids are of value, but their onset of action may be delayed for several hours.

Overdosage: Effects of overdosage are rare. It has been reported, however, that following administration of very large doses (for example over 10 pairs IVHP daily for three or more days) a state of excitement can result which is characterised by rapid mental activity. This subsides within 24 hours of stopping treatment, and there is often amnesia for the episode.

Pharmaceutical precautions Store below 15°C but do not freeze.

Legal category POM.

Package quantities
IV High Potency: 3 pairs, 12 pairs.
IM High Potency: 3 pairs, 12 pairs.
Each pack contains instructions for use.

Further Information Vitamins of the B complex play an integral part as co-enzymes in the intracellular metabolism of carbohydrates. The efficient functioning of this metabolism is essential for normal health. Similarly, ascorbic acid plays an important part in the biochemical reactions of cells and tissues and is normally present in the highest concentrations in those parts of the brain which are the most active metabolically.

Lack of the water-soluble vitamins results in impairment of normal intracellular metabolism. In some cases, such as an alcoholic who develops Wernicke's encephalopathy, lack of immediate treatment can result in permanent brain damage or even death.

The very high concentrations of the water-soluble vitamins contained in Parentrovite, rapidly replenish depleted cellular stores and speed the return of normal metabolism.

	Intravenous		*Intramuscular*	
	High potency (IVHP)		*High potency (IMHP)*	
Active ingredients of Parentrovite	*No. 1 (mg)*	*No. 2 (mg)*	*No. 1 (mg)*	*No. 2 (mg)*
Thiamine Hydrochloride (vitamin B_1)	250		250	
Riboflavine (vitamin B_2)	4		4	
Pyridoxine Hydrochloride (vitamin B_6)	50		50	
Nicotinamide		160		160
Ascorbic Acid (vitamin C)		500		500
Anhydrous Glucose		1,000		
*Benzyl Alcohol**			140	
				†
Volume per ampoule	5 ml	5 ml	5 ml	2 ml

* *To give 2% in the mixed ampoules* † *Contains 0.2% Chlorocresol*

Parentrovite presentations are aqueous solutions and contain sodium bicarbonate (buffer) and sodium metabisulphite (antioxidant).

Product licence numbers
IV High Potency: 0038/5095
IM High Potency: 0038/5097

PREGNAVITE FORTE* F

Presentation Lilac, sugar coated tablets, overprinted (FPF) in white.

Active ingredients

	Each tablet contains	*Hence daily dose (1 tab. three times a day) provides*
Dried ferrous sulphate	84 mg (equiv. to 25.2 mg Fe)	252 mg (equiv. to 75.6 mg Fe)
Calcium phosphate	160 mg	480 mg
Vitamin A	1,333 units	4,000 units
Vitamin D_2	133 units	400 units
Thiamine hydrochloride (vitamin B_1)	0.5 mg	1.5 mg
Riboflavine (vitamin B_2)	0.5 mg	1.5 mg
Pyridoxine hydrochloride (vitamin B_6)	0.33 mg	1.0 mg
Nicotinamide	5.0 mg	15 mg
Folic acid	0.12 mg	0.36 mg
Ascorbic acid (vitamin C)	13.3 mg	40 mg

Pregnavite Forte 'F' also contains inactive ingredients to make the medicine acceptable.

Uses To reduce the risk of spina bifida, or anencephaly, in babies born to women who have previously given birth to one or more babies (or aborted a foetus) with a neural tube defect.

Dosage and administration For oral administration only.

Adults: 1 tablet three times daily, during or after meals.

This dosage should be started not less than 28 days prior to conception and continue uninterrupted at least until the date of the second missed period.

Children: Pregnavite Forte F is not suitable for children.

Contra-indications, warnings, etc
Contra-indication: Pernicious anaemia. Sensitivity to any of the vitamins present.

Side-effects: These are rare but are occasionally encountered as mild gastro-intestinal upsets.

Precautions: Pregnavite Forte F may be used in patients being treated for Parkinson's disease with a levodopa preparation which includes a dopa-decarboxylase inhibitor (e.g. carbidopa, benserazide) but should not be used with levodopa alone as pyridoxine may act as an antagonist.

Use in pregnancy: Excessive vitamin A taken in pregnancy has been reported to be potentially dangerous. The recommended daily dose of Pregnavite Forte F has a vitamin content within the advised maximum daily intake in pregnancy and does not present a hazard. This should however be considered in the context of total dietary vitamin A.

Overdosage: In the event of overdosage, the patient should be referred to hospital, where desferrioxamine may be administered, if required, to reduce plasma iron levels. For full details please refer to the desferrioxamine data sheet.

Prolonged ingestion of massive doses of vitamins A and D can lead to hypervitaminosis states. Symptoms include dry, rough skin, painful joint swellings, anorexia and vomiting, but these disappear when treatment is discontinued.

Pharmaceutical precautions Store in a cool dry place.

Legal category P.

Package quantities *Tablets:* Original Pack of 84 with Patient Information Leaflet.

Further information NHS prescriptions on FP 10 must be endorsed 'S3B' by the prescriber ('S2B' in Scotland/N.Ireland).

Product licence number 0038/0339.

RELIFEX* TABLETS
RELIFEX* SUSPENSION

Presentation
Relifex Tablets: Red, film coated tablets marked 'Relifex' on one side and '500' on the other. Each tablet contains 500 mg nabumetone.

Relifex Suspension: A white to off-white suspension. Each 5 ml contains 500 mg nabumetone.

Relifex presentations also contain inactive ingredients to make the medicine acceptable. Amongst these are sodium benzoate (as a preservative) and sorbitol in Relifex Suspension.

Relifex presentations do not contain tartrazine or any other azo dyes.

Uses
Action: Nabumetone is a non-acidic non-steroidal anti-inflammatory agent which is a relatively weak inhibitor of prostaglandin synthesis. However, following absorption from the gastro-intestinal tract it is rapidly metabolised in the liver to the principal active metabolite, 6-methoxy-2-naphthylacetic acid, a potent inhibitor of prostaglandin synthesis.

Indications: Osteoarthritis and rheumatoid arthritis requiring anti-inflammatory and analgesic treatment.

Dosage and administration For oral administration. The tablets should be swallowed whole without chewing.

Adults: The recommended daily dose is two tablets or 10 ml suspension (1 g) taken as a single dose at bedtime.

For severe or persistent symptoms, or during acute exacerbations, an additional one or two tablets or 5–10 ml suspension (500 mg–1 g) may be given as a morning dose.

Use in the elderly: In common with many drugs, blood levels may be higher in elderly patients. The recommended daily dose of 1 g should not be exceeded in this age group and in some cases 500 mg may give satisfactory relief.

Use in children: There are no clinical data to recommend use of Relifex in children.

Contra-indications, warnings, etc
Contra-indications: Active peptic ulceration. Severe hepatic impairment (e.g. cirrhosis). Hypersensitivity to the drug.

Use in pregnancy and lactation: Studies in experimental animals have shown no teratogenic potential. As is common with other compounds administered to animals at doses high enough to be maternally toxic, indications of embryotoxicity were noted (studies in the rabbit, 300 mg/kg dose). High doses in rats (320 mg/kg) delayed parturition; this effect is considered to be due to inhibition of prostaglandin synthesis. The active metabolite of nabumetone has been found in the milk of lactating animals.

Safety in human pregnancy has not been established. Relifex is not recommended during pregnancy or in mothers who are breast feeding.

Precautions: Patients with established aspirin hypersensitivity may react similarly to nabumetone.

Patients with a history of peptic ulceration should be regularly reviewed for recurrence of symptoms.

Drug interactions: As the major circulating metabolite of Relifex is highly protein bound, patients receiving concurrent treatment with oral anti-coagulants, hydantoin anticonvulsants or sulphonylurea hypoglycaemics should be monitored for signs of overdosage of these drugs. Dosages should be adjusted if necessary.

Aluminium hydroxide gel, paracetamol and aspirin have not affected the bioavailability of Relifex in volunteer subjects.

Use in patients with impaired renal function: Urine is the major excretion route for the metabolites of Relifex. In patients with impaired renal function (creatinine clearance less than 30 ml/minute), dosage reduction should be considered. It is consistent with good clinical practice that patients with known renal impairment should be monitored regularly during therapy.

Liver function: Fluctuations in some parameters of liver function, particularly alkaline phosphatase, are frequently observed in patients with chronic inflammatory disorders; there is no evidence that Relifex accentuates these changes.

Side-effects: Side-effects include diarrhoea, dyspepsia, nausea, constipation, abdominal pain, flatulence, headache, dizziness, pruritus, rash and sedation. In clinical trials, increases in dose above 1 g did not lead to an increase in the incidence of side-effects.

Treatment of overdosage: There is no specific antidote. Treatment is with gastric lavage followed by activated charcoal using up to 60 g orally in divided doses, with appropriate supportive therapy.

Pharmaceutical precautions The tablets should be kept in their original pack, which protects them from light.

Legal category POM.

Package quantities
Relifex Tablets: Original Pack of 56 tablets in a square plastic bottle, with Patient Information Leaflet.

Relifex Suspension: Original Pack of 300 ml, with plastic measure (5/10 ml) and Patient Information Leaflet.

Further information Patients have been maintained on Relifex for more than three years with continuing clinical benefit.

Relifex Suspension is sucrose free (sorbitol content: approx. 1.25 g/5 ml).

Product licence numbers

Relifex Tablets	0038/0301
Relifex Suspension	0038/0352

RIDAURA* TILTAB* TABLETS

Presentation Pale yellow, film-coated, square Tiltab tablets, each containing 3 mg auranofin.

Uses Ridaura is an orally active gold preparation. Ridaura is indicated in the management of adults with active progressive rheumatoid arthritis only when non-steroidal anti-inflammatory drugs have been found to be inadequate alone to control the disease, i.e. when second-line therapy is required. In patients with adult rheumatoid arthritis, Ridaura has been shown to reduce disease activity reflected by synovitis, associated symptoms and appropriate laboratory parameters. Gold cannot reverse structural damage to joints caused by previous disease.

Ridaura does not produce an immediate response and therapeutic effects may be seen after 3–6 months of treatment.

Dosage and administration
Adults only: The usual starting dose is 6 mg daily as one 3 mg tablet twice a day in the morning and the evening. If this is well tolerated a single daily dose may be given as two 3 mg tablets with breakfast or the evening meal.

Treatment should be continued for a minimum of 3 to 6 months to assess response as Ridaura is a slow-acting drug. If response is inadequate after 6 months, an increase to 9 mg (one tablet 3 times a day) may be tolerated. If response remains inadequate after a 3-month trial of 9 mg daily, Ridaura therapy should be discontinued. Safety at dosages exceeding 9 mg daily has not been studied.

Absorption of gold from Ridaura tablets is rapid but incomplete (see *Further information*). Although mean blood gold levels are proportional to dose, no correlation between blood gold levels and safety or efficacy has been established. Dosage adjustments should therefore depend on monitoring clinical response and adverse events rather than on monitoring blood gold concentrations.

Anti-inflammatory drugs and analgesics may be prescribed as necessary with Ridaura.

Elderly: Dosage as above. As with all drugs, extra caution should be undertaken with administration to the elderly.

Contra-indications, warnings, etc
Contra-indications: Although not necessarily reported in association with Ridaura, do not use in patients with a history of any of the following gold-induced disorders: necrotizing enterocolitis, pulmonary fibrosis, exfoliative dermatitis, bone marrow aplasia or other severe blood dyscrasias. Use should also be avoided in progressive renal disease or severe active hepatic disease and in systemic lupus erythematosus. Ridaura should not be used in pregnancy (see *Use in pregnancy and lactation*).

Precautions: Use with caution in patients with any degree of renal impairment or hepatic dysfunction, inflammatory bowel disease, rash or history of bone marrow depression.

Close monitoring is essential. Full blood count with differential and platelet counts, which should be plotted, and tests for urinary protein must be performed prior to Ridaura therapy and at least monthly thereafter. Patients with gastro-intestinal symptoms, with rash or pruritus which may precede rash, or with stomatitis or a metallic taste which may precede stomatitis, should also be closely monitored (see *Adverse reactions*) as such symptoms may indicate a need for modification of dosage or withdrawal.

Prior to initiating treatment patients must be advised of the potential side effects associated with Ridaura. They should be warned to report promptly any unusual symptoms or signs during treatment such as pruritus, rash, metallic taste, sore throat or tongue, mouth ulceration, easy bruising, purpura, epistaxis, bleeding gums, menorrhagia or diarrhoea.

Gold has been shown to be carcinogenic in rodents although there was no evidence of carcinogenicity in 7-year dog studies.

Use in pregnancy and lactation: Gold is teratogenic in some animal species. Ridaura should not be used in pregnancy. Women of child-bearing potential should not be treated with Ridaura without full consideration of the benefits of treatment against the potential risk of teratogenicity. Women of child-bearing potential should practice effective contraception during treatment and for at least six months after; patients should be fully informed of the teratogenic risk, and termination of any pregnancy occurring during treatment should be considered in view of the possibility of foetal malformation. If women are to be treated post-partum with Ridaura, breast-feeding should be avoided.

Adverse reactions: Adverse reactions can occur throughout treatment with Ridaura, although the highest incidence can be expected during the first six months of treatment.

The most common reaction to Ridaura is diarrhoea or loose stools. Nausea may be present, and abdominal pain or other gastro-intestinal symptoms have been reported alone or in association. These usually resolve if dosage is temporarily reduced, e.g. from 6 mg to 3 mg a day, but if it is necessary to stop treatment, it can sometimes be started again at a lower dosage without further problem. About one patient in twenty will be unable to tolerate Ridaura because of diarrhoea. Ulcerative enterocolitis has been very rarely reported, as with all gold-containing drugs. Therefore, patients with gastro-intestinal symptoms should be carefully monitored for the appearance of gastro-intestinal bleeding and treatment stopped if this occurs.

Rashes, sometimes with pruritus, stomatitis and oral mucous membrane reactions, alopecia, conjunctivitis and taste disturbances including a metallic taste may occur but are usually not persistent and only occasionally require withdrawal of treatment. If, however, rash is persistent, especially if accompanied by pruritus, treatment should be stopped. Exfoliative dermatitis has been reported with other gold-containing drugs.

Blood dyscrasias, including leucopenia, granulocytopenia and thrombocytopenia can occur separately or in combination at any time during treatment. Agranulocytosis and aplastic anaemia have been reported very rarely. Ridaura should be withdrawn if the platelet count falls below 100,000/cu mm or signs and symptoms suggestive of thrombocytopenia occur. Transient decreases in haemoglobin or haematocrit early in treatment have been reported but were of no clinical significance.

Gold can produce the nephrotic syndrome or less severe glomerular disease with proteinuria and haematuria which are usually mild and transient. If, however, persistent or clinically significant proteinuria develops, treatment with Ridaura should be stopped promptly. Treatment may be restarted under close supervision after the proteinuria has cleared only in patients who experienced minimal proteinuria. Minor transient changes in renal function may also occur.

Pulmonary fibrosis may rarely occur. Attention should be paid to unexplained breathlessness and dry cough and chest X-ray is recommended at least annually.

Minor transient changes in liver function have been noted.

Overdosage: Ridaura overdosage experience is limited. One patient who took 27 mg Ridaura daily for 10 days developed an encephalopathy and peripheral neuropathy. Ridaura was discontinued and the patient eventually recovered.

In case of acute overdosage, immediate induction of vomiting or gastric lavage and appropriate supportive therapy are recommended.

Chelating agents (such as BAL) have been used with injectable gold and may be considered for Ridaura overdosage, although there has been no specific experience with Ridaura.

Pharmaceutical precautions No special storage precautions are necessary.

Legal category POM.

Package quantities Containers (OP) of 60 tablets.

Further information Rheumatologists may provide their patients with an information leaflet and a patient management card on which the results of laboratory tests carried out by both specialist and general practitioner can be recorded. This is helpful in the detection of adverse effects at an early stage.

About 20–30% of the gold in a dose of Ridaura is absorbed and although there is considerable variation in absorption this variability is less than that seen with parenteral gold. Steady-state blood concentrations are achieved 8–12 weeks after the start of treatment with Ridaura and are on average 5–10 times less than those following parenteral gold and do not correlate with clinical response or adverse events. About 70% of gold administered in Ridaura appears in the faeces during the first week following a single dose, and at 6 months after dosing less than 1% of the administered dose is retained in the body, in contrast to around 30% of a dose of gold given parenterally.

In contrast to injectable gold, which does not become cell-associated, 40% of the gold in the blood of Ridaura-treated patients is associated with blood cells. The metabolism of Ridaura is not fully understood, although it is clear from both animal studies and in vitro studies with human blood that both the sulphur and phosphorus ligands of Ridaura are rapidly dissociated from the gold.

Clinical studies have shown that patients may be safely transferred to Ridaura from injectable gold salt therapy without the need for overlap or a washout period.

Inactive ingredients include lactose.

Product licence number 0002/0082.

TEMOPEN* ▼

Presentation Vials containing 500 mg and 1 g of temocillin as temocillin sodium. Presented as an off-white/pale yellow sterile solid for reconstitution.

Uses

Action: Temopen is a bactericidal injectable penicillin which is active against most strains of Enterobacteriaceae (including *E. coli, Klebsiella* and *Proteus* species). Other sensitive organisms include *Haemophilus influenzae.* It is stable in the presence of the β-lactamase produced by many Gram-negative organisms and is, therefore, active against many strains of β-lactamase-producing Gram-negative aerobes which are resistant to a number of other antibiotics.

Temocillin is not generally active against *Pseudomonas* species, Gram-positive cocci or anaerobic organisms.

Indications: Temopen is indicated for the treatment of septicaemia, urinary tract infection and lower respiratory tract infection in which susceptible Gram-negative bacilli are suspected or confirmed.

In mixed infections where Gram-positive or anaerobic bacteria are also liable to be implicated, co-administration of flucloxacillin and metronidazole may be considered.

Dosage and administration

Adults (including the elderly): The usual dosage is 1–2 g every 12 hours. In the treatment of acute, uncomplicated urinary tract infections 1 g daily may be used, given as a single dose or in divided dosage.

Temopen may be administered by intravenous or intramuscular injection. High and prolonged serum concentrations are maintained, with an elimination half-life of 4 to 5 hours. The main route of excretion is via the kidney. Approximately 75% of a 1 g dose of Temopen is excreted unchanged in the urine within the first 24 hours.

Children: Insufficient data are available to recommend an appropriate dosage regime.

Dosage in patients with impaired renal or hepatic function (adults): No adjustment to the normal dosage is recommended for patients with a mild degree of renal impairment (creatinine clearance >30 ml/min). In more severe cases adjustment of the interval between doses is recommended (rather than a reduced dosage) as indicated below:

Degree of renal impairment	*Creatinine clearance (ml/min)*	*Recommended interval between doses*
Moderate	30–10	24 hours
Severe (not requiring dialysis)	<10	48 hours

Temopen is removed by haemodialysis. In patients receiving dialysis a further dose of Temopen should be given at the end of each period of dialysis.

Limited experience in patients with impaired hepatic function has not indicated a need for a reduction in dosage.

Preparation and administration: Temopen may be administered by intramuscular or intravenous injection, or by intermittent intravenous infusion. Temopen presentations are not intended for multi-dose use; any part-used antibiotic solution should be discarded. Solutions are normally a pale yellow colour.

Intravenous injection:

Dose	*Recommended volume of Water for Injections BP to be added for dissolution*	*Final volume*
500 mg	10 ml	10.4 ml
1–2 g	20 ml	—

Temopen solutions should be administered by slow injection into the vein or an infusion line over a period of 3–4 minutes.

Intravenous infusion: Solutions should be prepared as described for intravenous injection and then added to an intravenous infusion solution in a mini bag or in-line burette and administered over a period of 30–40 minutes. Alternatively, using a suitable reconstitution device, the appropriate volume of intravenous fluid may be transferred from the infusion bag into the vial and then drawn back into the bag after dissolution.

Intramuscular injection:

Vial strength	*Recommended volume of Water for Injections BP to be added for dissolution*	*Final volume*
500 mg	1.5 ml	1.9 ml
1 g	2.0 ml	2.7 ml

After addition of water to the vial, shake vigorously.

If pain is experienced at the site of injection, a sterile solution of lignocaine hydrochloride 0.5–1% may be used in place of Water for Injections.

Contra-indications, warnings, etc
Contra-indication: Penicillin hypersensitivity.

Use in pregnancy and lactation: Animal studies with Temopen have shown no teratogenic effect. There is no experience of Temopen in human pregnancy: therefore its use in pregnancy cannot be recommended. Trace quantities of penicillins can be detected in the milk of lactating mothers. Breast feeding should therefore be discontinued during therapy.

Precautions: In patients with moderate or severe renal impairment, the interval between doses should be increased (see dosage section).

Limited experience in patients with impaired hepatic function has not indicated a need for a reduction in dosage.

Side-effects: These are uncommon and typical of the injectable penicillins: they may include diarrhoea; pain at the site of IM injection; occasionally rash, either urticarial or erythematous. If a skin rash occurs treatment should be discontinued.

Overdosage: There have been no reported cases of overdosage. Dosages of up to 8 g daily have been administered to volunteers without untoward effects. Temopen may be removed from the circulation by haemodialysis.

Pharmaceutical precautions Vials of Temopen powder should be stored in a dry place, below 20°C. Temopen presentations are not intended for multi-dose use, and any part-used antibiotic solutions should be discarded.

Temopen solutions for direct injection or IV infusion should normally be administered within 30 minutes of preparation. However, they may be kept for up to 24 hours in a refrigerator (2–8°C). Refrigerated solutions should be restored to ambient temperature before use.

Full details of the stability of aseptically prepared Temopen infusions in standard IV fluids are available to Centralised Intravenous Additive Services on request.

Temopen is compatible with commonly used aqueous intravenous fluids including Water for Injections BP, Sodium Chloride (0.9% w/v) Intravenous Infusion BP, Glucose (5% w/v) Intravenous Infusion BP. Other appropriate infusion fluids are listed in the package enclosure leaflet.

Temopen may be mixed with cloxacillin or flucloxacillin in the same intravenous injection or infusion. Temopen is compatible with intravenous infusion solutions of metronidazole.

If Temopen is prescribed concurrently with an aminoglycoside the antibiotics should not be mixed in the syringe, intravenous fluid container or giving set because loss of activity of the aminoglycoside can occur under these conditions.

Temopen solutions should not be mixed with blood products or other proteinaceous fluids (e.g. protein hydrolysates) or with intravenous lipid emulsions.

Legal category POM.

Package quantities Temopen vials: 500 mg pack of 5; 1 g pack of 5.

Each pack contains instructions for use.

Further information Temopen offers selective parenteral treatment for appropriate Gram-negative systemic infections, with minimal disturbance of the normal intestinal flora. Each 1 g of Temopen contains approximately 5 mmol of sodium.

Temopen is not a significant inducer of β-lactamase production.

Product licence numbers

500 mg vial	38/0349
1 g vial	38/0350

**Trade Mark*

Berk Pharmaceuticals Limited
Towngate
Wyke
Bradford
West Yorkshire BD12 9AF

ALMODAN*

Presentation

Almodan Capsules: Yellow/brown capsules containing 250 mg and 500 mg amoxycillin as amoxycillin sodium and overprinted 'BERK 1R1' or '1R1' and 'BERK 2R1' or '2R1'. Other ingredients include sunset yellow (E110) and erythrosine (E127).

Almodan Syrup: Powder which when reconstituted with 59 ml of water makes 100 ml of syrup. It is available in two strengths providing 125 mg or 250 mg amoxycillin per 5 ml. Other ingredients include sucrose, sunset yellow (E110).

Almodan Injection: Clear glass vials containing 250 mg and 500 mg amoxycillin as amoxycillin sodium presented as powder for reconstitution.

Uses Treatment of infection: Amoxycillin is a broad spectrum antibiotic indicated for the treatment of commonly occurring bacterial infections such as: Upper respiratory infections; otitis media; acute and chronic bronchitis; lobar and bronchopneumonia; cystitis, urethritis, pyelonephritis; bacteriuria in pregnancy; gynaecological infections including puerperal sepsis and septic abortion; gonorrhoea; peritonitis; intra-abdominal sepsis; septicaemia; bacterial endocarditis; typhoid and paratyphoid fever; skin and soft tissue infections; osteomyelitis.

In children with urinary tract infection the need for investigation should be considered.

Prophylaxis of endocarditis: Amoxycillin may be used for the prevention of bacteraemia, associated with procedures such as dental extraction, in patients at risk of developing bacterial endocarditis.

The wide range of organisms sensitive to amoxycillin's bactericidal action include:

Gram-positive	*Gram-negative*
Streptococcus faecalis	*Haemophilus influenzae*
Streptococcus pneumoniae	*Escherichia coli*
Streptococcus pyogenes	*Proteus mirabilis*
Streptococcus viridans	Salmonella species
Staphylococcus aureus (penicillin-sensitive)	Shigella species
	Bordatella pertussis
Clostridium species	Brucella species
Corynebacterium species	*Neisseria gonorrhoeae*
Bacillus anthracis	*Neisseria meningitidis*
Listeria monocytogenes	*Vibrio cholerae*
	Pastuerella septica

Dosage and administration

DOSAGE

Adults (including elderly)

Oral: 250 mg three times daily, increasing to 500 mg three times daily for more severe infections.

High dose therapy: (Maximum recommended oral dosage 6 g daily in divided doses.) A dosage of 3 g twice daily is recommended in appropriate cases for the treatment of severe or recurrent purulent infection of the respiratory tract.

Short course therapy: Simple acute urinary tract infection: two 3 g doses with 10–12 hours between doses.

Gonorrhoea; Single 3 g dose.

Injectable: 500 mg intramuscularly eight hourly (or more frequently if necessary) in moderate infections.

1000 mg intravenously six hourly in severe infections.

Children (up to 10 years of age)

Oral: 125 mg three times daily, increasing to 250 mg three times daily for more severe infections.

Injectable: 50–100 mg/kg body weight/day in divided doses.

Parenteral therapy is indicated if the oral route is considered impracticable or unsuitable, and particularly for the urgent treatment of severe infection.

In renal impairment the excretion of the antibiotic will be delayed and depending on the degree of impairment it may be necessary to reduce the total daily dosage.

Prophylaxis of endocarditis

Dental procedures: Prophylaxis for patients undergoing extraction, scaling or surgery involving gingival tissues and who have not received a penicillin in the previous month (NB: Patients with prosthetic heart valves should be referred to hospital). If the patient has received a penicillin within the previous month prophylaxis with an alternative antibiotic should be considered.

Patients having no general anaesthetic: Adults (including elderly): 3 g Almodan orally, 1 hour before procedure. A second dose may be given 6 hours later if considered necessary.

Children: Under 10: Half adult dose
Under 5: Quarter adult dose.

Patients having general anaesthetic: If oral antibiotics considered appropriate: Adults (including elderly): Initially 3 g Almodan orally 4 hours prior to anaesthesia followed by 3 g orally (or 1 g IM if oral dose is not tolerated) 6 hours after initial dose.

Children: Under 10: Half adult dose
Under 5: Quarter adult dose.

If oral antibiotics not appropriate: Adults (including elderly): 1 g Almodan IM immediately before induction; with 500 mg orally six hours later.

Children: Under 10: Half adult dose.

Patients for whom referral to hospital is recommended: Patients to be given a general anaesthetic who have been given a penicillin in the previous month, patients to be given a general anaesthetic who have a prosthetic heart valve and patients who have had one or more attacks of endocarditis.

Adults (including elderly): Initially 1 g Almodan IM with 120 mg gentamicin IM immediately prior to anaesthesia (if given) or 15 minutes prior to dental procedure. Followed, 6 hours later by 500 mg Almodan, orally.

Children: Under 10: Half adult dose Almodan with 2 mg/kg gentamicin.

Almodan and gentamicin *should not* be mixed in the same syringe.

Genito-urinary surgery or instrumentation: Prophylaxis for patients who have no urinary tract infection and who are to have genito-urinary surgery or instrumentation under general anaesthesia.

Obstetric and gynaecological procedures/gastro-intestinal procedures: Routine prophylaxis is recommended only for patients with prosthetic heart valves.

Adults (including elderly): Initially 1 g Almodan IM with 120 mg gentamicin IM, immediately before induction, followed, 6 hours later, by 500 mg Almodan orally or IM according to clinical condition.

Children, under 10: Half adult dose Almodan with gentamicin 2 mg/kg.

Surgery or instrumentation of the upper respiratory tract: Patients other than those with prosthetic heart valves.

Adults (including elderly): 1 g Almodan IM immediately before induction; 500 mg Almodan IM or orally as syrup 6 hours later.

Children, under 10: Half the adult dose.

Patients with prosthetic heart valves: Adults (including elderly): Initially 1 g Almodan IM with 120 mg gentamicin IM, immediately before induction, followed, 6 hours later, by 500 mg Almodan IM or orally, as syrup.

Children, under 10: Half adult dose Almodan with gentamicin 2 mg/kg.

Almodan and gentamicin *should not* be mixed in the same syringe.

ADMINISTRATION

Oral: Using capsules or syrup.

Almodan Syrup is taken orally after reconstitution as follows:

Almodan Syrup 125 mg/5 ml: Add 59 ml of water to the powder and shake vigorously. This will make 100 ml of suspension, each 5 ml containing 125 mg of amoxycillin.

Almodan Syrup 250 mg/5 ml: Add 59 ml of water to the powder and shake vigorously. This will make 100 ml of suspension, each 5 ml containing 250 mg amoxycillin.

Intramuscular:

250 mg – add 1.5 ml Water for Injections BP and shake vigorously.

500 mg – add 2.5 ml Water for Injections BP and shake vigorously.

A transient pink colouration or slight opalescence may appear during reconstitution. Reconstituted solutions are normally a pale straw colour.

If pain is experienced on intramuscular injection, a sterile 1% solution of lignocaine hydrochloride or 0.5% solution of procaine hydrochloride may be used in place of water for injections.

Intravenous:

Dissolve 250 mg in 5.0 ml Water for Injections BP.

Dissolve 500 mg in 10 ml Water for Injections BP.

Amoxycillin injection, suitably diluted, may be injected directly into a vein or drip tube taking 3–4 minutes.

Contra-indications, warnings, etc Amoxycillin is a penicillin and should not be given to penicillin-hypersensitive patients.

Side-effects: Side-effects, as with other penicillins, are usually of a mild and transitory nature; they may include diarrhoea, indigestion, or occasionally rash, either urticarial or erythematous. An urticarial rash suggests penicillin hypersensitivity and the erythematous type rash may arise if amoxycillin is administered to patients with glandular fever. In either case, treatment should be discontinued. Since Almodan is a penicillin, problems of overdosage are unlikely to be encountered.

Pharmaceutical precautions Store in a cool dry place.

Syrup: Keep tightly closed. Use within 7 days after reconstitution. Shake well before use.

Injection: Administer immediately after reconstitution. Do not mix with blood products, other proteinaceous fluids such as protein hydrolysates or with intravenous lipid emulsions.

Legal category POM.

Package quantities
Capsules: Securitainers of 100 and 500
Syrup: 100 ml bottle
Injection: Packs of 10.

Further information Amoxycillin is well absorbed. Oral administration, usually at convenient tds dosage produces high serum levels independent of the time at which food is taken. Amoxycillin gives good penetration into bronchial secretions and high urinary concentrations of unchanged antibiotic. It is rapidly bactericidal and possesses the safety of the penicillins.

Product licence numbers

Almodan Capsules 250 mg	0152/0234
Almodan Capsules 500 mg	0152/0235
Almodan Syrup 125 mg/5 ml	0152/0236
Almodan Syrup 250 mg/5 ml	0152/0237
Almodan Injection 250 mg	0152/0231
Almodan Injection 500 mg	0152/0232

ANTIPRESSAN*

Presentation Orange, biconvex, film-coated tablets containing atenolol 50 mg (engraved BERK 1U1 or 1U1) and 100 mg (engraved BERK 2U1 or 2U1). Other ingredients include lactose and sunset yellow (E110).

Uses For the management of hypertension, angina pectoris, cardiac dysrhythmias and for use in the acute phase following myocardial infarction.

Dosage and administration

Adults:

Hypertension: While some patients will respond to a single oral daily dose of 50 mg, the usual dosage is 100 mg daily as a single dose. A period of approximately two weeks should be allowed for the full effect of atenolol to be realised.

Angina: The usual oral dose is 100 mg once daily or 50 mg given twice daily.

Dysrhythmias: Initial treatment is with atenolol given by the intravenous route commencing with atenolol 2.5 mg IV, administered at a rate of 1 mg/minute. This may be repeated at 5 minute intervals until a response is observed (to a maximum of 10 mg atenolol). If atenolol is given by infusion 0.15 mg/kg body-weight may be administered over a 20 minute period and may be repeated every 12 hours.

Following control of the dysrhythmia with IV atenolol, maintenance dosage is with oral atenolol 50 to 100 mg daily as a single dose.

Myocardial infarction: For suitable patients presenting within 12 hours of onset of chest pain, atenolol 5 mg should be given immediately by slow intravenous injection at a rate of 1 mg/minute. This should be followed 15 minutes later, provided no untoward effects were noted from the IV dose, by 50 mg atenolol orally. Twelve hours post-intravenous dose, a further 50 mg atenolol should be given orally and, thereafter, 100 mg daily as a single oral dose for up to 10 days.

Children: Atenolol is not recommended for use in children since appropriate data have not been generated.

Elderly patients: Dosage requirements may be reduced in elderly patients; particularly in those patients with impaired renal function.

Contra-indications, warnings, etc

Contra-indications: Atenolol must not be administered to patients with second or third degree heart block.

Precautions: Special care should be exercised in patients with poor cardiac reserve.

Reduction of heart rate is one of the pharmacological actions of atenolol. In the rare instances when symptoms may be attributable to the slow heart rate, the dose should be reduced.

Atenolol should be used with caution in patients with chronic obstructive airways disease. In asthmatic patients atenolol may precipitate an increase in airways resistance but this can usually be reversed with bronchodilators, e.g. salbutamol or isoprenaline.

In changing patients from clonidine to atenolol, care should be exercised. If the two agents are taken concurrently, clonidine should be continued for several days after withdrawal of atenolol.

In patients with ischaemic heart disease, atenolol should not be withdrawn abruptly.

Caution should be exercised with the concurrent administration of atenolol and antidysrhythmic agents, e.g. disopyramide. Similarly, the concurrent administration of atenolol and verapamil to patients with impaired ventricular function requires caution, while this combination should not be given to patients with abnormal conduction status.

Renal failure: Atenolol is excreted via the kidneys. Dosage adjustment should therefore be considered in patients with severe impairment of renal function. As a guide, for patients with a serum creatinine of 300–600 μmol/litre, the atenolol oral dose should be 50 mg daily or 100 mg once every two days. For patients with a serum creatinine of >600 μmol/litre the oral dose of atenolol should be 50 mg on alternate days or 100 mg once every four days.

Patients on haemodialysis should be given 50 mg atenolol orally following each dialysis. Because of the possibility of marked falls in blood pressure, this should be carried out under hospital supervision.

Anaesthesia: If it is decided to withdraw atenolol from patients prior to surgery, 48 hours should be allowed between the last dose of atenolol and anaesthesia. If atenolol is continued, vagal dominance may occur with anaesthetic agents such as trichloroethylene, ether or cyclopropane. If this occurs it may be corrected with atropine (1–2 mg IV).

Pregnancy: The use of atenolol in women who are pregnant, may become pregnant or who are nursing newborn infants should be made following risk/benefit considerations.

Side-effects: Side effects, as with other beta blocking agents, include bradycardia, coldness in the extremities, muscular fatigue and, rarely, sleep disturbances.

There have been reports of skin rashes and/or dry eyes associated with the use of beta blocking agents. The reported incidence is small and in most cases the symptoms have cleared when treatment was withdrawn. Discontinuance of the drug should be considered if any such reaction is not otherwise explicable. Cessation of beta blocker therapy should be gradual.

Overdosage: The most likely initial effect is excessive bradycardia which should respond to 1–2 mg atropine given intravenously. This may be followed if necessary by isoprenaline 25 micrograms initially or orciprenaline 0.5 mg given by slow IV injection.

Pharmaceutical precautions The tablets should be protected from light and moisture.

Legal category POM.

Package quantities Atenolol Tablets 50 mg and 100 mg: Packs of 100 tablets in securitainers. Calendar packs of 28 tablets.

Further information Nil.

Product licence numbers
Tablets 50 mg 0152/0238
Tablets 100 mg 0152/0239

ARBRALENE*

Presentation
50 mg tablets: White, round biconvex tablet containing 50 mg metoprolol tartrate, engraved BERK 4A5 or 4A5 on one side with a breakline on the reverse.

100 mg tablets: White, round biconvex tablet containing 100 mg metoprolol tartrate, engraved BERK 4A6 or 4A6 on one side with a breakline on the reverse.

Uses Management of hypertension and angina pectoris. Cardiac arrhythmias, especially supraventricular tachyarrhythmias. As an adjunct to the treatment of thyrotoxicosis. In early intervention in acute myocardial infarction to reduce infarct size and incidence of ventricular fibrillation. Pain relief may also decrease the need for opiate analgesics.

Metoprolol has been shown to reduce mortality when administered to patients with acute myocardial infarction.

Prophylaxis of migraine.

Dosage and administration
Hypertension: Initial dose is 100 mg per day. This may then be increased by 100 mg per day at weekly intervals depending upon response. If control is not achieved using a single daily dose then twice daily dosing should be initiated. Combination therapy with a diuretic or other hypotensive agent may also be considered.

Angina: 50 to 100 mg two or three times daily.

Cardiac arrhythmias: 50 mg two or three times daily should control the condition but if necessary this can be increased to 300 mg per day in divided doses.

Following the treatment of acute arrhythmia with a metoprolol injection, continuation therapy with Arbralene tablets, should be initiated 4 to 6 hours later at an initial dose not exceeding 50 mg three times daily.

Thyrotoxicosis: 50 mg four times daily.

Myocardial infarction: Early intervention. For optimal benefits suitable patients should present within 12 hours of the onset of chest pain. Therapy should commence with a 5 mg iv metoprolol injection every 2 minutes to a maximum of 15 mg total as determined by blood pressure and heart rate. Oral therapy should commence 15 minutes after the injection with 50 mg every 6 hours for 48 hours. Patients who fail to tolerate the full intravenous dose should be given half the suggested oral dose.

The usual maintenance dose is 200 mg daily.

Migraine prophylaxis: 100 to 200 mg daily administered in divided doses.

Elderly: There is no evidence to suggest that dosage requirements are different in the elderly.

Contra-indications, warnings, etc
Contra-indications: Atrioventricular block, digitalis refractory heart failure, severe bradycardia and cardiogenic shock.

Precautions: As for other beta-blockers, discontinuation of treatment should be gradual, i.e. over a period of 7 to 10 days, as abrupt interruption of the medication, particularly in patients with ischaemic heart disease, may lead to an acute deterioration in the patient's condition.

Metoprolol has been used in a significant number of asthmatic patients. Although it is a selective beta-blocker it is prudent to exercise particular care in the treatment of patients with chronic obstructive pulmonary disease. Use of a $beta_2$-bronchodilator, e.g. Terbutane, may become necessary in some patients, or current therapy may require adjustment.

In labile and insulin dependent diabetes it may be necessary to adjust the dosage of the hypoglycaemic therapy.

Metoprolol therapy must be reported to the anaesthetist prior to general anaesthetic. If it is desirable to withdraw metoprolol in patients who are to undergo anaesthesia, if possible withdrawal should be completed at least 48 hours before anaesthesia. However, for some patients undergoing elective surgery it may be desirable to employ a beta-blocker as premedication. By shielding the heart against the effects of stress, metoprolol may prevent excessive sympathetic stimulation which is liable to provoke such cardiac disturbance as arrhythmias or acute coronary insufficiency. In a patient under beta-blockade an anaesthetic with as little negative inotropic activity as possible should be selected.

Digitalis and/or diuretics should be considered for patients with a previous history of heart failure or in patients known to have a poor cardiac reserve.

Like all beta-blockers, metoprolol should not be given in combination with verapamil since this may cause bradycardia, hypotension and asystole.

Side-effects: Gastro-intestinal upsets, sleep disturbances and lassitude may occasionally occur. In most cases these effects have been transient or have disappeared after a reduction in dosage. There have been reports of skin rashes and/or dry eyes associated with the use of beta-adrenoceptor blocking drugs. The reported incidence is small and in most cases the symptoms have cleared on withdrawal of treatment. Discontinuation of the drug should be considered if any such reaction is not otherwise explicable.

Use in pregnancy and lactation: Metoprolol should not be used unless the physician considers that the benefit outweighs the possible hazard to the foetus or infant. As with all beta-blockers, metoprolol may cause side-effects, e.g. bradycardia in the foetus and in the newborn and breast fed infant. Although the drug crosses the placental barrier and is present in cord blood, no evidence of foetal abnormalities has been reported.

The amount of metoprolol ingested via breast milk appears to be negligible in terms of its beta-blocking effects if dosing is within the normal therapeutic range.

Overdosage: Overdosage may lead to marked hypotension and bradycardia. Such effects can be counteracted by using atropine sulphate 0.25 to 2.0 mg. If a satisfactory response is not achieved, agents such as dopamine or dobutamine can be administered. Glucagon in a dose of 1 to 10 mg can also be administered.

Pharmaceutical precautions Store in a cool, dry place. Protect from light.

Legal category POM.

Package quantities Containers of 100 and 500 tablets. Blister packs of 30 and 60 tablets.

Further information Nil.

Product licence numbers

Tablets 50 mg	0152/0269
Tablets 100 mg	0152/0270

BERKAPRINE*

Presentation Each tablet contains 50 mg Azathioprine BP. The tablets are yellow and marked BERK 1D2 or 1D2 on one side with a breakline on the reverse. Other ingredients include lactose.

Uses Azathioprine facilitates the survival and function of organ transplants.

Azathioprine has a significant therapeutic effect in a proportion of patients suffering from chronic active hepatitis, severe rheumatoid arthritis, systemic lupus erythematosus (SLE), idiopathic thrombocytopenic purpura, acquired haemolytic anaemia, severe cases of specified dermatological diseases (pemphigus vulgaris, dermatomyositis, polyarteritis nodosa, pyoderma gangrenosa) when these conditions are: (a) refractory to corticosteroids, or (b) when corticosteroids are contra-indicated, or (c) controlled by corticosteroids in dosages which are producing severe side-effects. In patients with such side-effects, the aim of azathioprine medication is to reduce the required maintenance dose of steroids.

In pemphigus and rheumatoid arthritis azathioprine has been shown to have significant therapeutic activity when used without corticosteroids.

The risks associated with azathioprine therapy should be considered against the severity of the patient's condition and the expected clinical effect.

The use of azathioprine in other indications must be regarded as experimental.

Dosage and administration

Adults: Transplantation: A loading dose of up to 5 mg/kg is usually given. The dosage during the first three months after transplantation is usually 1–4 mg/kg body weight per day (median 2.4 mg/kg body-weight per day). 1–2.5 mg/kg body-weight per day may be given intravenously as a maintenance dose, but only if oral therapy is impracticable. Cessation of azathioprine therapy, even after a period of years, carries a high risk of rejection within a few weeks.

Other conditions: For the treatment of the conditions listed under 'Uses', except for chronic active hepatitis, the dosage is usually between 2 and 2.5 mg/kg body weight per day. For the treatment of chronic active hepatitis the dosage is usually between 1 and 1.5 mg/kg body-weight per day.

The dosage of azathioprine and the duration of treatment may vary according to the condition, its severity and the clinical response obtained. A therapeutic response may not be evident for a few days or even weeks after initiation of therapy. If no discernible improvement occurs in the patient's condition within three months, consideration should be given to the withdrawal of the drug. Treatment is otherwise undertaken on long-term basis unless the patient exhibits evidence of intolerance to the drug.

Children: As for adults.

Elderly: It is advisable to monitor for developing leucopenia or thrombocytopenia particularly in cases of renal or hepatic insufficiency.

Contra-indications, warnings, etc

Contra-indications: Azathioprine hypersensitivity will generally be a contra-indication to continued use.

Precautions: There are potential hazards in the use of this preparation. Therefore, it should not be prescribed unless the patient can be adequately monitored for toxic effects throughout the duration of the therapy.

During the first eight weeks of therapy with azathioprine complete blood counts, including platelet counts, must be performed at least weekly (and more frequently when higher dosages are used or in the presence of disturbed renal or hepatic function), and with decreasing frequency thereafter.

Azathioprine may be given long-term unless the patient cannot tolerate the preparation. Withdrawal of an effective dose in certain instances, e.g. SLE with nephritis, may result in a serious relapse of the condition. In other instances, such as rheumatoid arthritis and certain haematological conditions, treatment may be withdrawn after a suitable interval without any ill-effect. Withdrawal should always be a gradual process performed under close supervision.

In the presence of severe renal or hepatic impairment careful monitoring is initially required, since the dosage of azathioprine may have to be reduced.

Severe secondary infections, often with uncommon organisms, are a hazard of immunosuppressive therapy. These are seen more frequently in transplant recipients than in patients being treated for other indications.

Azathioprine is potentially mutagenic and has been shown to cause chromosome damage in man. The clinical significance of these findings is unclear since the damage is apparently reversible on withdrawal.

Azathioprine has no detectable inhibitory effect on either male or female fertility. The depression of fertility accompanying chronic uraemia is generally reversed after transplantation and its accompanying azathioprine treatment.

An increased number of malignant tumours especially lymphoreticular and epithelial has been observed in transplant recipients. The skin tumours that have occurred in transplant patients have been primarily on sun-exposed skin. Patients should be cautioned against undue sun exposure, and the skin should be examined at regular intervals. There is, however, as yet no conclusive evidence of an increased incidence to tumours in other treated subjects. In such patients the risk may be indistinguishable from that accompanying some of the diseases under treatment.

The few cases reported show a different pattern from that seen in transplantation: tumour occurrence is much less common, has an increased latency, is seen mainly after prolonged continuous therapy, is less exclusively lymphoreticular and tends to occur in those patients also treated with alkylating agents. Use with caution in hyperplenism.

Concomitant allopurinol therapy: When azathioprine and allopurinol are given concomitantly only one quarter of the usual dosage of azathioprine should be given since allopurinol has an inhibitory effect on its metabolism.

Concomitant use of cytotoxics: Azathioprine should be used with caution in patients receiving, or who have recently received, other bone marrow suppressive agents.

Concomitant use of muscle relaxants: There is clinical evidence that azathioprine antagonises the effect of non-depolarising muscle relaxants such as curare, d-tubocurarine and pancuronium. Experimental data confirm that azathioprine reverses the neuromuscular blockage caused by d-tubocurarine, and show that azathioprine potentiates the neuromuscular blockage caused by succinylcholine.

Side-effects, adverse effects: The principal side-effect of azathioprine is a dose-related, generally reversible, depression of bone marrow function expressed as leucopenia, thrombocytopenia and rarely anaemia.

An additional form of haematological toxicity in patients receiving azathioprine is megaloblastic erythropoiesis and macrocytosis.

Haematological toxicity is most frequently noted at the outset of therapy but reports of the late occurrence of leucopenia and anaemia confirm the wisdom of continuing haematological surveillance of patients even on stable long-term treatment.

The report incidence of gastro-intestinal intolerance to oral administration of azathioprine is variable. It is manifested largely as nausea and anorexia with occasional vomiting. In some instances it seems to be a dose-related phenomenon and after a brief interruption administration may often be successfully reinstituted, at a lower dose. Doses should, when possible, be taken with food. Other more serious gastro-intestinal complications of therapy have been recorded. Pancreatitis is seen most commonly in transplant recipients and has also been reported in patients with granulomatous bowel disease treated with azathioprine.

Gastro-duodenal ulcer, intestinal haemorrhage and intestinal necrosis and perforation are complications seen only after transplantation and it appears likely that they are due to concomitant steroid therapy.

Azathioprine may occasionally cause cholestatic, dose-related reversible hepatotoxicity. In such cases withdrawal is advisable. A variety of possibly allergic manifestations has been reported. Drug fever, skin rash, myalgia and arthralgia are well documented though uncommon complications. There are also single case reports of possible azathioprine-related effects including acute renal insufficiency, haemolytic anaemia, acute restrictive lung disease and unexplained meningitis reactions.

Use in pregnancy and lactation: The potential teratogenicity of azathioprine should be borne in mind. Although it has been shown to be teratogenic in laboratory animals clinical evidence suggests that the risk is not appreciable in man. There is no doubt that azathioprine and its metabolites cross the placenta. A temporary impairment of immune function has been noted following exposure '*in utero*' to azathioprine combined with prednisone. The long-term consequences of these properties of azathioprine are unknown, but many children exposed '*in utero*' have now completed the first decade of life without reported problems.

It has not been possible to detect azathioprine or its metabolites in the breast milk of treated patients.

Treatment of overdosage: The most likely side-effect of overdosage is bone marrow depression, which may not reach its maximum until 9–14 days later. A single large dose of azathioprine is less likely to have a toxic effect than a chronic minor overdosage on prescription. Although the effects of overdosage may be delayed it is not uncommon for improvement to commence after day 12 provided that the patient has not had high doses during the intervening period. If overdosage occurs the blood picture and hepatic function in particular should be monitored. Azathioprine is known to be dialysable and dialysis may be used in severe cases.

Pharmaceutical precautions Store below 25°C. Protect from light. Keep dry.

Legal category POM.

Package quantities Securitainers of 100 tablets.

Further information Nil.

Product licence number 0152/0210.

BERKATENS* TABLETS

Presentation Yellow biconvex film-coated tablets containing Verapamil Hydrochloride BP 40 mg (engraved BERK 1T1 or $\frac{40}{0234}$), 80 mg (engraved BERK 2T1 or $\frac{80}{0235}$), 120 mg (engraved BERK 3T1 or $\frac{120}{0241}$) and 160 mg (engraved BERK 4T1 or $\frac{160}{0238}$). Other ingredients include lactose.

Uses Berkatens is indicated for the treatment and prophylaxis of angina pectoris. It may be used in the treatment and prophylaxis of supraventricular tachycardia, atrial fibrillation and atrial flutter; (Verapamil should not be used when atrial flutter/fibrillation complicates Wolff-Parkinson-White syndrome). Berkatens may also be used in the management of mild to moderate hypertension and renal hypertension.

Dosage and administration
Angina

Adults: The usual dosage is 120 mg three times daily. 80 mg three times daily may be satisfactory in some patients with angina of effort.

Supraventricular Tachycardias

Adults: 40–120 mg three times daily according to the severity of the condition. *Children:* 2 years and above: 1–3 40 mg tablets 2–3 times daily.

Hypertension

Adults: The usual dosage is 80–160 mg three times daily. *Children:* Up to 10 mg/kg/day, in divided doses according to the severity of condition.

Elderly: No specific dosage recommendations except in those patients with impaired liver function or cardiac conduction disturbances when a reduction in dose should be considered.

Contra-indications, warnings, etc
Contra-indications: Hypotension associated with cardiogenic shock, marked bradycardia, uncompensated heart failure, second or third degree atrioventricular block and sick sinus syndrome.

Precautions: Caution should be observed in the acute phase of myocardial infarction.

Care must be taken when verapamil and beta blockers are administered concurrently or closely together as their effects may be additive both with respect to conduction and contraction.

Verapamil may affect impulse conduction and should be used with caution in patients with first degree atrioventricular block. Patients with atrial fibrillation/flutter and an accessory pathway (e.g. Wolff-Parkinson-White syndrome) may rarely develop increased conduction across the anomalous pathway and ventricular tachycardia may be precipitated.

Verapamil may affect left ventricular contractility as a result of its mode of action. Although this effect is small and normally not important, cardiac failure may be precipitated or aggravated if it exists. Thus in patients with poor ventricular function verapamil should only be given after appropriate therapy for cardiac failure such as digitalis, etc.

Verapamil has been shown to increase the serum concentration of digoxin and caution should be exercised with regard to digitalis toxicity.

In patients with impaired liver function, particular attention should be paid to the dosage because of reduced drug metabolism.

Use in pregnancy: Although there is no published evidence that verapamil has any teratogenic effect, it should not be given during the first trimester of pregnancy, unless, in the clinician's judgement, it is essential for the welfare of the patient.

Side-effects: Berkatens is generally well-tolerated. Constipation may occur, flushing is observed occasionally, headaches rarely. Nausea, vomiting and allergic reactions have seldom been reported.

Treatment of overdosage: Usual emergency measures for acute cardiovascular side-effects should be applied, e.g.: in the case of second and third degree AV block: atropine, isoprenaline and, if required, pace-maker therapy; in the case of signs of myocardial insufficiency: dopamine, dobutamine, cardiac glycosides or calcium gluconate (10–20 ml of a 10% solution); in the case of hypotension: appropriate positioning of patient, dopamine, dobutamine, noradrenaline.

Pharmaceutical precautions Nil.

Legal category POM.

Package quantities
40 mg tablets: Securitainers of 100.
80 mg tablets: Securitainers of 100.
120 mg tablets: Securitainers of 100.
160 mg tablets: Securitainers of 100.

Further information Nil.

Product licence numbers

40 mg tablets	0152/0198
80 mg tablets	0152/0199
120 mg tablets	0152/0200
160 mg tablets	0152/0217

BERKMYCEN*

Presentation Yellow film-coated Oxytetracycline Tablets BP 250 mg engraved BERK 1C5 or 1C5 on one side. Other ingredients include lactose, tartrazine (E102).

Uses Antibiotic.

Infections caused by oxytetracycline-sensitive organisms. These include acute and chronic bronchitis, pneumonia, urinary tract infections, brucellosis, pertussis, rickettsial fevers and psittacosis.

Dosage and administration *Adults:* 250 mg every six hours. In severe infections dosage may be increased to 250 mg every three hours after an initial loading dose of 1 g.

Elderly: Usual adult dose. Caution should be observed as subclinical renal insufficiency may lead to drug accumulation.

Contra-indications, warnings, etc 'Berkmycen' should only be given to patients with renal dysfunction or failure if its use is considered essential.

Milk, or antacids containing aluminium, magnesium or calcium, interfere with the absorption of oxytetracycline. If gastric irritation occurs the tablets should be taken with food. As with all tetracyclines, 'Berkmycen' should be used with caution in patients with hepatic or renal dysfunction.

Bulging fontanelles in infants and benign intracranial hypertension in adults has been reported. Treatment should cease if evidence of raised intracranial pressure develops.

Like all tetracyclines, 'Berkmycen' may produce gastro-intestinal irritations, giving rise to nausea, abdominal discomfort and diarrhoea. Intestinal overgrowth of resistant organisms (*Candida albicans* in particular) may occur. Drug fever and allergic skin rashes may occur rarely.

Use in pregnancy: Berkmycen should not be used in late pregnancy or given to children during the period of tooth development, unless it is essential to use a tetracycline because of resistance to other antibiotics.

Treatment of overdosage: Serious symptoms are unlikely. Gastric lavage might be beneficial in the first hours after ingestion followed by conservative management. Milk will reduce absorption.

Pharmaceutical precautions Store in a cool place.

Legal category POM.

Package quantities Containers of 1000 and 5000.

Further information 'Berkmycen' oxytetracycline is an antimicrobial agent active against most pathogenic bacteria, both Gram-positive and Gram-negative, except for the majority of strains of *Proteus vulgaris* and *Pseudomonas aeruginosa.* Salmonella species and *Mycobacterium tuberculosis* show resistance, as do the yeasts and fungi, but 'Berkmycen' is effective against Actinomyces, *Entamoeba histolytica, Trichomonas vaginalis*, treponemata and some rickettsias and viruses.

Product licence number 0152/0094.

BERKOLOL*

Presentation
1. Pink, film-coated, Propranolol Tablets BP 10 mg embossed BERK 1Z1 or 1Z1, with breakline on reverse.
2. Pink, film-coated, Propranolol Tablets BP 40 mg embossed BERK 2Z1 or 2Z1, with breakline on reverse.
3. Pink, film-coated, Propranolol Tablets BP 80 mg embossed BERK 3Z1 or 3Z1, with breakline on reverse.
4. Pink, film-coated, Propranolol Tablets BP 160 mg embossed BERK 4Z1 or 4Z1, quadrisected with double breakline on reverse.

Other ingredients include lactose, erythrosine (E127).

Uses Berkolol is a competitive blocker of adrenergic β-receptor sites. It is used in the treatment of hypertension, angina pectoris, cardiac dysrhythmias, anxiety tachycardia, essential tremor and for the long term prevention of sudden cardiac death in patients who have shown evidence of dysrhythmias during the acute phase of myocardial infarction. It may also be used as a prophylactic in migraine, and as adjunctive therapy in thyrotoxicosis.

Dosage and administration Dosage requires individual adjustment. A heart rate of 55/min or less is an indication that dosage should be increased no further.

Adults: Hypertension: Initially, 80 mg twice daily, increased where necessary at weekly intervals. The usual maintenance dosage is 160–320 mg daily. Lower doses may be effective when a diuretic or other antihypertensive drug is given concurrently.

Angina pectoris: Initially, 40 mg twice or thrice daily increased by the same amount at weekly intervals until control is achieved, or the maximum daily dose of 480 mg is reached.

Prophylaxis against recurrence of myocardial infarction: For long term prevention of sudden cardiac death in patients who have survived the acute phase of myocardial infarction, clinical study has shown that treatment should be commenced four to six days after the infarction at a dose of 40 mg four times daily which should then be maintained. As the overriding principle is to maintain adequate β-blockade the dose may need to be varied for some patients.

Anxiety, migraine, essential tremor: 40 mg twice or thrice daily, increased at weekly intervals if needed to a daily total of 160 mg.

Dysrhythmias, anxiety tachycardia, hypertrophic obstructive cardiomyopathy, thyrotoxicosis: 10–40 mg three or four times daily.

Children: Dysrhythmias, thyrotoxicosis: The minimum effective dosage, based on 0.25–0.5 mg/kg body weight, three or four times daily.

Migraine: Children under the age of 12 may be given 20 mg two or three times daily. Older children may be given adult dosage.

Elderly: No specific dosage recommendations. However, the optimum dose should be determined individually according to clinical response. In patients with impaired hepatic function a reduced dosage shoud be considered initially.

Contra-indications, warnings, etc
Contra-indications: Propanolol is contra-indicated in patients with second or third degree heart block; bronchial asthma or a history of small airways disease particularly if associated with bronchospasm; metabolic acidosis or after prolonged fasting.

Precautions: Berkolol should be used with great caution in patients with heart failure, unless that is due to thyrotoxicosis alone. Concomitant therapy with digitalis and diuretics is usually desirable in heart failure.

Particular care should be taken in the elderly where hepatic clearance may be reduced thus requiring an appropriate reduction in dosage.

Berkolol should be withdrawn 24 hours before elective surgery, as it may interfere with response to stress. If this cannot be done, 1–2 mg atropine should be given intravenously before anaesthesia commences and anaesthetics such as ether, chloroform, cyclopropane and trichloroethylene, which may cause myocardial depression, should not be used.

Warnings and adverse reactions: Treatment with beta-blocking agents must not be stopped suddenly. If it is necessary to withdraw Berkolol, this should be done gradually, or another beta-blocker should be substituted.

Bradycardia and hypotension are usually a sign of overdosage, but may rarely be due to intolerance of the drug. In the latter case Berkolol should be withdrawn and, if necessary, the patient should be treated as for overdosage. Heart block and congestive heart failure have been reported due to propranolol.

Dry eyes and skin rash have been reported during treatment with β-adrenergic blocking agents. If these symptoms are not attributable to some other cause, Berkolol should be withdrawn.

Berkolol may cause or precipitate Raynaud's phenomenon, intermittent claudication or peripheral arterial insufficiency. Bronchospasm may occur, particularly in patients with a history of asthma or hay fever.

There have been rare reports of blood dyscrasias during treatment with propranolol.

Minor side-effects include cold extremities, nausea, vomiting, diarrhoea, fatigue or insomnia. These are usually transient and are less common if the drug is introduced gradually.

Use in pregnancy: Although there is no evidence that propranolol is teratogenic, Berkolol should not be used in pregnancy unless it is considered essential.

Treatment of overdosage: The clinical features can include bradycardia, severe hypotension, bronchospasm, hypoglycaemia, delirium and unconsciousness. Initially isoprenaline should be infused, and if marked bradycardia is present atropine should be given intravenously (0.6–3 mg; 50 microgram/kg in children): if the response is limited, glucagon therapy must be instituted (50–150 microgram/kg intravenously over one minute followed by 1–5 mg/hour infused). Bronchospasm may be treated by nebulized salbutamol or intravenous aminophylline or salbutamol.

Pharmaceutical precautions Protect from light.

Legal category POM.

Package quantities

Tablets 10 mg:	containers of 100 and 500
Tablets 40 mg:	containers of 100 and 1,000
Tablets 80 mg:	containers of 100 and 500
Tablets 160 mg:	containers of 100

Further information Nil.

Product licence numbers

Tablets 10 mg	0152/0150
Tablets 40 mg	0152/0151
Tablets 80 mg	0152/0152
Tablets 160 mg	0152/0153.

BERKOZIDE*

Presentation Plain white Bendrofluazide Tablets BP 2.5 mg and 5 mg. The 2.5 mg tablets are marked 1G5 on one side. The 5 mg tablets are marked 2G5 on one side with a breakline on the reverse. Other ingredients include lactose.

Uses Diuretic. Oedema, cardiac failure, inhibition of lactation, hypertension.

Dosage and administration In cardiac failure, 5–10 mg daily or on alternate days, a usual maintenance dosage being 5–10 mg on three days per week. For premenstrual oedema, 'Berkozide' may be given 5 mg daily for three to four days before menstruation. For inhibition of lactation 5 mg in the morning and 5 mg at noon for five days is usually adequate. In hypertension the dosage should be 2.5–5 mg daily. Bendrofluazide potentiates other antihypertensive agents, the dosage of which should be reduced and then adjusted as necessary.

Berkozide is not recommended for children.

Elderly: No special recommendations except in patients with renal or hepatic impairment (see below).

Contra-indications, warnings, etc 'Berkozide' is contra-indicated in severe renal insufficiency and hypercalcaemia and should be used with caution in patients with renal or hepatic disorders. It may precipitate hepatic coma in advanced cirrhosis.

Thiazide diuretics may induce water and electrolyte disturbances particularly in the elderly or when dosage is high or prolonged. Plasma electrolytes should be checked at regular intervals during therapy.

Potassium supplements should be given (preferably on non-diuretic days) when the dosage of 'Berkozide' is high or when diet is inadequate. It may be necessary to reduce the dosage of digitalis if this is given concurrently.

Toxic effects such as nausea, allergy, skin rashes or blood dyscrasias are rare. Hypokalaemia may develop with long use of 'Berkozide', but this risk is reduced by administration on alternate days. Like other thiazides, bendrofluazide may provoke hyperglycaemia and glycosuria in diabetic patients and may precipitate latent diabetes mellitus. It may also precipitate acute attacks of gout.

Use in lactation: Breast feeding should be avoided since thiazide diuretics are secreted in mother's milk.

Treatment of overdosage: Replace fluids with saline while monitoring plasma sodium and potassium. Potassium replacement may be required.

Pharmaceutical precautions No special precautions.

Legal category POM.

Package quantities *Tablets 2.5 mg:* Containers of 100 and 1,000.

Tablets 5 mg: Containers of 100 and 1,000.

Further information Bendrofluazide is an oral diuretic of the thiazide group which inhibits proximal tubular resorption of sodium chloride.

Product licence numbers

Tablets 2.5 mg	0152/5081R
Tablets 5 mg	0152/5084R

CALABREN*

Presentation Calabren is presented as white biconvex tablets marked 'APS' or plain on one side and with the strength and code number on the other side. They contain Glibenclamide BP and comply with the monograph for Glibenclamide Tablets BP. Two strengths are available: 2.5 mg – round tablets coded 3103; 5 mg – elongated tablets coded 3104 with a break-line. Both strengths of tablets contain lactose.

Uses Glibenclamide is an oral hypoglycaemic agent. Calabren may therefore be used in the management of non-insulin-dependent diabetes mellitus in patients who have responded poorly to dietary measures alone.

Dosage and administration Oral.
Adults: Previously untreated Diabetes Mellitus: Treatment should be started with 5 mg daily, taken during or immediately following breakfast or the first main meal of the day. It is wise to start at a lower dose of 2.5 mg daily if the patient is elderly or debilitated – see 'contra-indications, warnings, etc.' If control of diabetic symptoms remains inadequate, the daily dose may be increased not more frequently than weekly in steps of 2.5 mg (usual) or 5 mg (maximum) daily to a maximum dose not exceeding 15 mg daily. This is normally given as a single dose during or immediately after breakfast or the first main meal of the day. However, care should be taken to apportion the diet with the daily activity schedule and the final dosage schedule for each individual patient.

Adults: Changing from other oral sulphonyl-urea hypoglycaemic agents: These changes may be made without any formal break in treatment. Where the patient is already well controlled, treatment should commence with one 5 mg dose daily, adjusted weekly in increments not exceeding 5 mg to a maximum of 15 mg daily – see above. Where control has not been adequate on previous therapy, treatment may be started on the approximately equivalent dose provided this does not exceed 10 mg daily. It may then be raised at weekly intervals to a maximum of 15 mg daily.

5 mg of Glibenclamide BP is approximately equivalent to:

Tolbutamide	1 g
Glymidine	1 g
Acetohexamide	500 mg
Tolazamide	250 mg
Chlorpropamide	250 mg
Glibonuride	25 mg
Glipizide	5 mg

Adults: Changing from biguanides such as metformin: Calabren treatment should be started at a dose of 2.5 mg daily and the biguanide then withdrawn. To achieve control the dose of Calabren should be adjusted at weekly intervals in increments of 2.5 mg daily but not exceeding the maximum dose of 15 mg daily.

Adults: Combination therapy with biguanides: Where control of diabetic symptoms has not been achieved with a single oral hypoglycaemic agent such as glibenclamide at the maximum dosage of 15 mg daily, control may often be achieved by adding a biguanide derivative to the regime.

Adults: Changing from an insulin regime: A few patients with very low daily insulin requirements may remain controlled if transferred to glibenclamide and should be treated as new patients. Tablets should always be taken with or immediately after the first main meal of the day, and the insulin dose should be reduced further with each increased dose level of glibenclamide.

Children: Juvenile-onset diabetes mellitus is normally insulin-dependent, and consequently glibenclamide is not suitable for use in children.

The elderly: The initial dose in elderly or debilitated patients should be 2.5 mg daily.

Contra-indications, warnings, etc
Contra-indications: Glibenclamide should not be used:
(a) in patients suffering from or with a history of diabetic keto-acidosis.
(b) in patients with serious impairment of function in the kidneys, liver or adrenal glands.
(c) in patients undergoing surgery.
(d) in pregnant patients, for whom insulin treatment is normally preferred.

Warning: The hypoglycaemic effect of glibenclamide may be ENHANCED (occasionally dramatically) by:
(a) coumarin anticoagulants.
(b) monoamine oxidase inhibitors.
(c) beta-adrenergic blocking agents.
(d) sulphonamides.
(e) phenylbutazone.
(f) chloramphenicol.
(g) cyclophosphamide.
(h) salicylates e.g., aspirin.

Conversely the hypoglycaemic effect of glibenclamide may be DIMINISHED by:
(a) sympathomimetic agents e.g., adrenalin.
(b) steroids including oral contraceptives.
(c) thiazide diuretics.

Precautions: Special care must be taken when using glibenclamide in the following situations:
(a) *Elderly or debilitated patients:* These patients are more likely to suffer from hypoglycaemia – see treatment of overdosage.
(b) *Pregnancy and lactation:* There is no adequate information on the use of glibenclamide in human pregnancy. It is normal practice to manage diabetes in pregnant patients with insulin, although there appear to be no specific reasons to stop a pre-existing regime which includes glibenclamide. There is no evidence of teratogenicity in animal experiments. However, as with other sulphonylurea hypoglycaemic agents, it is wise to assume that glibenclamide is present in human breast milk. Consequently, its use is best avoided where the patient expresses a desire to breast-feed.

Adverse reactions: Like other oral hypoglycaemic agents, glibenclamide is well tolerated in normal use. Untoward effects are usually mild and rarely require treatment to be discontinued. Among these mild effects are gastrointestinal symptoms (anorexia, diarrhoea and nausea) and allergic-type skin reactions. Leucopenia and thrombocytopenia have been reported, and are reversible on stopping treatment. Transient changes in liver enzymes and function tests have been reported during glibenclamide treatment, although a definite relationship to treatment has yet to be established. As with all other oral hypoglycaemic agents, an over-response to treatment may occur, especially in relation to unexpected heavy exercise. These hypoglycaemic attacks are not usually prolonged and should be managed as for overdosage.

Overdosage: Conscious patients: with early signs of hypoglycaemia – faintness, nausea, cold-sweats and/or palpitation – may be treated with glucose water or 3–4 lumps of sugar (sucrose) with water. This treatment may be repeated as necessary and, if symptoms continue to recur at intervals, may be supplemented with half a pint of milk after successful management of the current recurrence of symptoms.

Overdosage: Comatose patients should receive glucose administered as a continuous intravenous infusion, because a bolus injection may lead to a more severe and prolonged rebound hypoglycaemia. An alternative approach is to administer 1 mg of glucagon as a subcutaneous or intramuscular injection. The objective of both treatments is to achieve rapid recovery of consciousness, when further 'feeding' should be instituted, as above.

Pharmaceutical precautions Tablets should be stored below 25°C.

Legal category POM.

Package quantities
Calabren 2.5 mg: polypropylene tubes of 100 tablets.
Calabren 5 mg: polypropylene tubes of 100 and 500 tablets.

Further information Nil.

Product licence numbers

Calabren Tablets 2.5 mg	0289/0047.
Calabren Tablets 5 mg	0289/0048

Product Licence holder: Approved Prescription Services Ltd.

CAPLENAL*

Presentation
100 mg tablets: white biconvex tablets containing 100 mg of Allopurinol BP, engraved BERK 1K1 or 1K1 on one side with a break-line on the reverse.
300 mg tablets: white biconvex tablets containing 300 mg of Allopurinol BP, engraved BERK 2K1 or 2K1 on one side with a break-line on the reverse.
Other ingredients include lactose.

Uses *Gout:* Primary hyperuricaemia.

Secondary hyperuricaemia: Prophylaxis of uric acid and calcium oxalate stones.

Dosage and administration *Adults:* The initial dose is 100–200 mg. The maintenance dose is 200–600 mg/daily. Maximum single dose 300 mg. It has rarely been found necessary to exceed 900 mg per day. The dose should be adjusted by monitoring serum uric acid and/or urinary uric acid levels at appropriate intervals until the desired effect is attained, which may take one to three weeks.

Children: 10–20 mg/kg body-weight/day. Use in children is mainly indicated in malignant conditions, especially leukaemia and certain enzyme disorders, for example Lesch-Nyhan syndrome.

Elderly: No specific dosage recommendations except in

those patients with impaired renal function when a dose reduction should be considered (see below).

Initiation of therapy: In the early stages of treatment with allopurinol, as with the uricosuric agents, an acute attack of gouty arthritis may be precipitated. Therefore it is advisable to give a prophylactic dose of a suitable anti-inflammatory agent or colchicine (0.5 mg three times a day) for at least one month.

Use with uricosurics: As allopurinol does not interfere with the action of uricosuric agents, they may be given concurrently. When changing from uricosuric therapy to allopurinol 1–3 weeks overlap of treatments is recommended to ensure a continuous hypouricaemic effect.

Use in neoplasia: When giving allopurinol to prevent uric acid nephropathy in neoplastic conditions, it is advisable to start treatment with allopurinol before cytotoxic therapy.

Dose recommendations in impaired renal function: Since allopurinol and its metabolites are excreted via the kidney, impairment of renal function may lead to retention of the drug and its metabolites with consequent prolongation of action. Thus, the amount and frequency of the dosage may require reduction as indicated by monitoring serum uric acid levels. The following schedule is provided for guidance in adults.

If creatinine clearance exceeds 20 ml/minute – give standard dose.

If creatinine clearance is between 10 and 20 ml/minute – give 100–200 mg/day.

If creatinine clearance is between 2 and 10 ml/minute – give 100 mg/day or at longer intervals.

Dose recommendations in renal dialysis: Allopurinol and its metabolites are removed by renal dialysis. If frequent dialysis is required an alternative schedule of 300–400 mg allopurinol after each dialysis with none in the interim should be considered.

Contra-indications, warnings, etc
Contra-indications: Acute gout. Known intolerance of allopurinol.

Precautions: Treatment should not be started during or immediately after an acute attack of gout. When 6-mercaptopurine or azathioprine is given concurrently with allopurinol, only one quarter of the usual dose of those drugs should be given because inhibition of xanthine oxidase will prolong their activity. There is no unequivocal evidence that allopurinol potentiates the activity of other cytotoxic drugs. If allopurinol is given concomitantly with chlorpropamide when renal function is poor, there may be an increased risk of prolonged hypoglycaemia activity.

The dosage of allopurinol should be reduced in patients with renal or hepatic diseases.

Particular care should be taken in the elderly where renal function may be reduced thus leading to a retention of the drug and its metabolites with the consequent prolongation of action.

Warnings and adverse reactions: Adverse reactions in association with allopurinol are usually rare and mostly of a minor nature. The incidence is higher in the presence of renal and/or hepatic disorders. The possible potentiation of anticoagulant action should be borne in mind when a patient on anticoagulants is given allopurinol.

Skin reactions are the most common reactions and may occur at any time during treatment. They may be pruritic, maculopapular, sometimes scaly or purpuric and rarely exfoliative. Allopurinol should be withdrawn immediately should such reactions occur. After recovery from mild reactions allopurinol may, if desired, be reintroduced at a low dose (e.g. 50 mg/day) which may be gradually increased. If the rash recurs, allopurinol should be permanently withdrawn.

Exfoliative skin reactions associated with other signs of hypersensitivity including fever, lymphadenopathy, arthralgia and eosinophilia occur rarely. If they do occur, it may be at any time during treatment. Allopurinol should then be withdrawn immediately and permanently. Corticosteroids may be beneficial in overcoming such reactions. Patients manifesting generalised hypersensitivity reactions usually have pre-existing renal and/or hepatic disorders.

Nausea and vomiting have been reported. This reaction is not a significant problem and can be avoided by taking allopurinol after meals.

There have been occasional reports of transient reduction in the numbers of circulating formed elements in the blood, usually in association with pre-existing renal and/or hepatic disorders. The clinical significance has yet to be demonstrated.

Exacerbation of acute gouty attacks may occur in the early stages of hypouricaemic therapy. In those conditions where the body's miscible urate pool is greatly increased (e.g. malignant diseases and its treatment: Lesch-Nyhan syndrome), the rise in xanthine concentration resulting from the action of allopurinol may lead to tissue deposition of xanthine. Adequate hydration will reduce the risk of xanthine deposition in the kidney and fluid intake should ensure adequate urinary output. Xanthine crystals have been seen in muscle tissue of patients receiving allopurinol but this appears to have no clinical significance.

The following complaints have been reported occasionally, but do not appear to have a clear cause and effect relationship with allopurinol: fever, general malaise, headache, vertigo, somnolence, taste perversion, hepatic necrosis, granulomatous hepatitis, abnormal liver function tests, hyperlipaemia, visual disorder, cataracts, macular changes, neuropathy, impotence, diabetes mellitus, furunculosis, alopecia, hypertension, haematuria, oedema.

Use in pregnancy: There is no evidence that allopurinol taken orally causes foetal abnormalities. However, as with all drugs, due caution should be exercised in pregnancy.

Treatment of overdosage: No reports of overdosage or acute intoxication with Caplenal are available.

Pharmaceutical precautions No special precautions.

Legal category POM.

Package quantities
100 mg tablets: containers of 100 and 500 tablets
300 mg tablets: containers of 100 tablets

Further information Nil.

Product licence numbers
Tablets 100 mg 0152/0154
Tablets 300 mg 0152/0176

CO-PROXAMOL

Presentation White, film-coated, oval shaped tablets, marked 2E2 on one side, containing Dextropropoxyphene Hydrochloride BP 32.5 mg and Paracetamol BP 325 mg.

Uses Analgesic for the relief of mild to moderate pain.

Dosage and administration
Adults: Two tablets, three or four times daily.

The elderly: As for adults but reduce dosage if renal or hepatic function is impaired.

Children: Not recommended for children.

Contra-indications, warnings, etc
Contra-indications: Hypersensitivity to dextropropoxyphene or paracetamol.

Precautions: Co-proxamol should be administered with caution to patients with severe renal or hepatic impairment as delayed elimination, or elevated serum levels may result.

Isolated reports suggest that dextropropoxyphene may inhibit the metabolism of some concurrently administered drugs. Patients receiving anticonvulsants, antidepressants or warfarin-like drugs should be monitored during therapy.

Warnings: Dextropropoxyphene is an analgesic with CNS depressant properties and should be used with caution in patients who are receiving other CNS depressants drugs as an additive affect may occur. Patients should be warned to avoid alcohol.

As with other drugs which affect the CNS, care should be taken when prescribing for patients with personality or other psychological disorders. Tolerance, psychological and physical dependence may rarely occur.

Overdosage of paracetamol may damage the liver due to the accumulation of intermediate metabolites which cause hepatic necrosis.

Dextropropoxyphene may impair the mental and physical reactions required for the performance of potentially hazardous tasks, such as driving and the operating of machines, to varying extents depending on dosage and individual susceptibility.

Side-effects: Dizziness, sedation, nausea and vomiting are possible side effects and seem to be more prominent in ambulatory than in non-ambulatory patients. Some of these effects may be alleviated if the patient lies down. Other reported side effects include constipation, abdominal pain, skin rashes, lightheadedness, headache, weakness, euphoria, dysphoria and minor visual disturbances.

Use in pregnancy: Safety for use in pregnancy has not been established.

Treatment of overdosage: The chronic ingestion of dextropropoxyphene in doses exceeding 720 mg as base (equivalent to 780 mg as hydrochloride) per day has caused toxic psychoses and convulsions. Symptoms of acute toxicity may be rapid in onset with the danger of respiratory arrest. Other recognised manifestations include respiratory depression, coma, circulatory collapse, pulmonary oedema, convulsions and cardiac arrhythmias.

Deterioration may be rapid, with fatal outcome. Paracetamol overdosage is associated with nausea and vomiting and frequently with abdominal pain.

Subsequent evidence of liver dysfunction may be apparent after 24 hours and if severe may lead to irreversible hepatic necrosis and death.

Firstly, adequate respiratory exchange should be re-established through provision of a patent airway and institution of assisted or controlled ventilation. The narcotic antagonist naloxone is a specific antidote against the respiratory depression produced by dextropropoxyphene. An initial dose of 0.4–2 mg should be administered intravenously with simultaneous efforts at respiratory resuscitation. If the desired degree of improvement is not obtained, the dose should be repeated at two to three minute intervals. Subsequent doses of naloxone may be necessary for up to 24 hours due to the slow elimination of dextropropoxyphene. Naloxone may also be administered by infusion. The rate of infusion should be such as to maximise the reversal of CNS depression.

In addition to the use of a narcotic antagonist, the patient may require careful titration with an anticonvulsant to control seizures. Analeptic drugs (for example, caffeine or amphetamine) should not be used because of their tendency to precipitate convulsions.

Early assessment of the severity of paracetamol poisoning by measurement of plasma paracetamol levels is essential if treatment, which should be instituted within 10 hours of ingestion, is to be effective. Present evidence suggests that cysteamine, methionine or N-acetylcysteine given within this period are effective in greatly reducing the toxic effects of paracetamol.

Oxygen, intravenous fluids, vasopressors and other supportive measures should be employed as indicated.

Gastric lavage may be helpful. Activated charcoal can absorb a significant amount of ingested dextropropoxyphene.

Pharmaceutical precautions Store in a cool, dry place.

Legal category CD (Sch 5), POM.

Package quantities Blister packs of 100 (10 strips of 10 tablets).

Further information Nil.

Product licence number 0152/0255.

DIAZEPAM

Presentation White Diazepam Tablets BP 2 mg, marked 'BERK 2' or '2', with single breakline. Other ingredients include lactose.

Yellow Diazepam Tablets BP 5 mg, marked 'BERK 5' or '5', with single breakline. Other ingredients include lactose, sunset yellow (E110).

Blue Diazepam Tablets BP 10 mg, marked 'BERK 10' or '10', with single breakline. Other ingredients include lactose.

Uses Diazepam is indicated for the short-term relief only (2–4 weeks) of anxiety that is severe, disabling or subjecting the individual to unacceptable distress, occurring alone or in association in insomnia or short-term psychosomatic, organic or psychotic illness.

The use of benzodiazepines to treat short-term 'mild' anxiety is considered to be inappropriate and unsuitable.

The short-term treatment of insomnia only when it is severe, disabling, or subjecting the individual to extreme distress.

Muscle spasm.

Premedication.

Dosage and administration The lowest dose which can control the symptoms should be used. Long-term chronic use is not recommended; treatment should not normally continue beyond 4 weeks. Treatment with benzodiazepines should always be withdrawn gradually. Patients who have been receiving treatment for a long time may require longer periods during which the doses are reduced.

Anxiety states: Severe anxiety states: 15–30 mg daily in divided doses.

Children: 1–5 mg daily in divided doses.

Insomnia associated with anxiety: 5–30 mg before retiring. Treatment should, if possible, be intermittent.

Conditions associated with muscle spasm: Spastic children with minimal brain damage: 2–40 mg daily in divided doses.

Cerebral palsy of adults, particularly associated with athetoid movements: 2–60 mg daily in divided doses.

Upper motor neuronic spasticity: 5–60 mg daily in divided doses.

Muscle spasm of varied aetiology, fibrositis, cervical spondylosis: 2–15 mg daily in divided doses.

Premedication for dental operation: One 5 mg tablet the night before the appointment, 5 mg on waking and 5 mg two hours before the appointment.

Elderly or diabetic patients: Doses should be half those recommended for ordinary adults.

Contra-indications, warnings, etc Benzodiazepines should not be used for phobic or obsessional states.

They should not be used alone to treat depression or anxiety associated with depression. Suicide may be precipitated in such patients.

They should not be used for the treatment of chronic psychosis.

Amnesia may occur.

In cases of loss or bereavement psychological adjustment may be inhibited by benzodiazepines.

Disinhibiting effects may be manifested in various ways. Suicide may be precipitated in patients who are depressed and aggressive behaviour toward self and others may be precipitated. Extreme caution should therefore be used in prescribing benzodiazepines in patients with personality disorders.

Withdrawal from benzodiazepines may be associated with physiological and psychological symptoms of withdrawal including depression. Withdrawal symptoms may occur following normal therapeutic doses given for short periods of time.

An underlying cause of insomnia should be sought before deciding upon the use of benzodiazepines for symptomatic relief.

Benzodiazepines are also contra-indicated in patients with known sensitivity to benzodiazepines, acute pulmonary insufficiency and acute narrow angle glaucoma.

Use in pregnancy: Not to be taken during pregnancy, especially in the first and third trimesters, unless there are compelling reasons.

Precautions: Chronic pulmonary insufficiency.

In chronic renal or hepatic disease.

In labour. High single doses or repeated low doses have been reported to produce hypotonia, poor sucking and hypothermia in the neonate and irregularities in the foetal heart.

Avoid, if possible, in lactation.

The concurrent use of other CNS depressant drugs should be avoided.

Adverse effects: Common adverse effects include drowsiness, sedation, unsteadiness and ataxia.

Performance and alertness may be impaired during the first week of administration. Patients should be warned of the possible hazard when driving or operating machinery. These effects may be potentiated by alcohol.

The elderly and the debilitated are particularly liable to experience these symptoms, together with confusion, especially if organic brain symptoms are present.

Rebound insomnia has been reported following abrupt cessation of treatment.

Abnormal psychological reactions to benzodiazepines have been reported. Rare behavioural adverse effects include paradoxical aggressive outbursts, excitement, confusion and the uncovering of depression and suicidal tendencies.

Other rare adverse effects including hypotension, gastrointestinal and visual disturbances, skin rashes, urinary retention, headache, vertigo, changes in libido, blood dyscrasias and jaundice have also been reported.

Treatment of overdosage: Ataxia is usually the most serious symptom. Gastric lavage may be carried out, followed by observation. Very occasionally a respirator may be required but diazepam generally causes few problems in overdosage. In children behavioural changes are likely.

Pharmaceutical precautions Store in a cool, dry place, protected from light.

Legal category CD (Sch 4), POM.

Package quantities Tablets 2 mg: Containers of 50, 250, 1000 and 5000
Tablets 5 mg: Containers of 50, 100, 200, 1000 and 5000
Tablets 10 mg: Containers of 500.

Further information Nil.

Product licence numbers
Tablets 2 mg 0152/0058R
Tablets 5 mg 0152/0059R
Tablets 10 mg 0152/0158.

DOMICAL*

Presentation Round film-coated bi-convex Amitriptyline Tablets BP marked 'D': 10 mg tablets are blue, 25 mg are orange and 50 mg are red-brown. Other ingredients include lactose; 25 mg tablet contains sunset yellow (E110).

Uses Amitriptyline is an antidepressant of the tricyclic group.

It is indicated for symptoms of a depressive illness especially when sedation is required.

Dosage and administration *Adults:* Initially 75 mg/day in divided doses or as a single dose at night, increasing to 200 mg/day according to clinical response. Maintenance dose is 50–100 mg at night.

Elderly or adolescent patients: 10–50 mg daily initially (see 'Precautions').

Children: Domical is not recommended for children under 12 years of age.

Contra-indications, warnings, etc
Contra indications: History of myocardial infarction, arrhythmias, particularly heart block of any degree, congestive cardiac failure, coronary artery insufficiency.

Receipt of monoamine oxidase inhibitors within the last two weeks.

Mania. Severe liver disease. Hypersensitivity to any tricyclic antidepressant. Breast feeding.

Precautions: The elderly or debilitated are particularly liable to experience toxic effects, especially agitation, confusion and postural hypotension. The initial dose should be increased with great caution under close supervision. Half the normal maintenance dose may be sufficient to produce a satisfactory clinical response.

All patients with severe depression should be closely supervised, particularly during the early stages of therapy when partial response may increase the risk of suicide.

Domical should be used with great caution in patients with a history of narrow angle glaucoma, urinary retention, epilepsy or recent convulsions, hepatic insufficiency, hyperthyroidism, cardiovascular disorders or blood dyscrasias, or symptoms suggestive of prostatic hypertrophy.

Tricyclic antidepressants potentiate the central nervous depressant action of alcohol.

Anaesthetics given during tri/tetracyclic antidepressant therapy may increase the risk of arrhythmias and hypotension. If surgery is necessary, the anaesthetist should be informed that a patient is being so treated.

Drug interactions: In patients who have been treated previously with monoamine oxidase inhibitors, at least two weeks should elapse before treatment with Domical is started, with great caution, commencing with low dosage and slow increments.

Amitriptyline may decrease the antihypertensive effect of guanethidine, debrisoquine, bethanidine and possibly clonidine. It is advisable to review all antihypertensive therapy during treatment with tricyclic antidepressants.

Amitriptyline should not be given with sympathomimetic agents such as ephedrine, isoprenaline, noradrenaline, phenylephrine and phenylpropanolamine, or with ethchlorvynol.

The antidepressant action of Domical may be decreased by barbiturates and increased by methylphenidate.

The dose of thyroid hormone medication may need to be reduced if amitriptyline is given concurrently.

Warnings and adverse reactions: As improvement may not occur during the first month of therapy, patients should be closely monitored during this period.

Cardiac arrhythmias and severe hypotension are likely to occur with high dosage or in deliberate overdosage. They may also occur in patients with pre-existing heart disease taking normal dosage.

Confusion may occur at high doses or in elderly patients, requiring reduction of dosage.

Drowsiness is not uncommon in the early stages of treatment, and patients should be warned not to drive or operate machinery until it has been established that their alertness is not impaired.

The following adverse effects, although not necessarily all reported with amitriptyline, have occurred with tricyclic antidepressants:

Atropine-like side-effects including dry mouth, disturbances of accommodation, tachycardia, constipation and hesitancy of micturition are common early in treatment, but usually lessen.

Other common adverse effects include nausea, sweating, postural hypotension, dizziness, tremor and rashes. Interference with sexual function may occur.

Serious adverse effects are rare. These include bone marrow depression, agranulocytosis, cholestatic jaundice, hypomania, convulsions and peripheral neuropathy.

Withdrawal symptoms which may occur on abrupt cessation of therapy include insomnia, irritability and excessive perspiration. There have also been reports of withdrawal symptoms in neonates whose mothers received tricyclic antidepressants during the third trimester of pregnancy.

Psychotic manifestations, including mania and paranoid delusions may be exacerbated during treatment with tricyclic antidepressants.

Use in pregnancy: Safety in pregnancy and lactation has not been established. Do not use during pregnancy nor in nursing mothers unless there are compelling reasons.

Treatment of overdosage: The major symptoms are likely to be coma and respiratory depression. Primary therapy must be aimed at correction of hypoxia, acidosis and electrolyte imbalance. Gastric lavage should be performed and the ECG monitored. If convulsions occur they may be treated with diazepam. Serious dysrhythmias are rare and DC conversion may be preferable to anticholinesterase agents, which can exacerbate convulsions.

Pharmaceutical precautions No special precautions.

Legal category POM.

Package quantities *Tablets 10 mg:* Containers of 500.
Tablets 25 mg: Containers of 500.
Tablets 50 mg: Containers of 100.

Further information Nil.

Product licence numbers
Tablets 10 mg 0152/0065R
Tablets 25 mg 0152/0066R
Tablets 50 mg 0152/0114R

DOPAMET*

Presentation Yellow film-coated Methyldopa Tablets BP. 125 mg (marked 'BERK 1C3' or '1C3'). 250 mg (marked 'BERK 2C3' or '2C3'). 500 mg (marked 'BERK 3C3' or '3C3'). Other ingredients include tartrazine (E102).

Uses Hypertension.

Dosage and administration *Adults:* 250 mg twice a day for two days, increased at intervals of not less than two days by an additional 250–500 mg daily until satisfactory control is achieved. This normally follows within 12–24 hours of reaching the effective dose for the individual patient, which is generally in the range of 500–2,000 mg daily. It is seldom necessary to exceed 3,000 mg daily and, because methyldopa is largely excreted by the kidneys, patients with impaired renal function may respond to comparatively low doses.

The requirement of Dopamet may be reduced by giving a thiazide diuretic concurrently: downward adjustments of dosage should likewise be made at intervals of not less than 48 hours.

In the few cases where tolerance develops, effective control can frequently be restored by increasing the dosage of Dopamet or by adding a diuretic to the regimen.

When patients are on other hypotensive agents and it is desired to change them over to Dopamet, drug interactions must be carefully watched for.

Reserpine and other Rauwolfia alkaloids, hydralazine and mebutamate when used alone or in any combination should be discontinued before treatment with Dopamet is started.

Ganglion blocking agents and adrenergic blocking agents used alone or in combination should be withdrawn cautiously and progressively. During the first week of transfer the dosage of blocking agent should be reduced by a half and Dopamet added at a dosage of 250 mg twice a day. The blocking agent is then reduced still further and the dosage of Dopamet adjusted upwards by 250–500 mg stages at two- to seven-day intervals to maintain optimal control of the blood pressure.

Monoamine oxidase inhibitors should be discontinued before treatment with Dopamet commences. It should then be used cautiously in case of delayed excretion of the monoamine oxidase inhibitors.

Elderly: The initial dose should not exceed 250 mg daily. This should be increased slowly as required but not to exceed a maximum daily dose of 2 g.

Contra-indications, warnings, etc
Contra-indications: Dopamet should not be given in cases of active liver disease, such as acute hepatitis and active cirrhosis, and in patients known to be sensitive to methyldopa.

Dopamet is not recommended where phaeochromocytoma is suspected, since methyldopa fluoresces at the same wavelengths as catecholamines in urine samples; spuriously high concentrations of urinary catecholamines may be reported and this will interfere in the diagnosis of phaeochromocytoma.

Dopamet should not be used with reserpine, other Rauwolfia alkaloids, hydralazine, mebutamate and monoamine oxidase inhibitors.

Precautions and warnings: When methyldopa is used with other antihypertensive agents, potentiation of antihypertensive action may occur. The progress of patients should be carefully followed to detect side reactions or manifestations of drug idiosyncrasy. Patients may require reduced doses of anaesthetics when on methyldopa. If hypotension does occur during anaesthesia, it can usually be controlled by vasopressors.

Use in pregnancy and lactation: Methyldopa crosses the placental barrier and appears in cord blood. Although no obvious teratogenic effects have been reported the possibility of foetal injury cannot be excluded and the drug should only be used in women who are or may become pregnant, if there are no safer alternatives and if the degree of hypertension carries risk for the mother or child.

Methyldopa is excreted in breast milk and should not be used by nursing mothers.

Side-effects: Sedation is the most frequent side-effect and may occur even at the starting dose level. It usually wears off after an effective maintenance dosage has been established. Depression may occur and corrective treatment with tricyclic antidepressants may antagonise the therapeutic effect of Dopamet.

Other minor side-effects are headache and feeling of weakness but again these wear off with time.

Symptoms of cerebrovascular insufficiency associated with effective lowering of blood pressure may also occur, including dizziness, light-headedness and faintness. If such symptoms occur, dosage should be reduced. Symptoms due to postural hypotension are fewer and less severe with Dopamet than with other hypotensive agents and exercise hypotension rarely occurs. If such symptoms do occur, the dose of Dopamet should be reduced.

Occasionally bradycardia, nasal stuffiness, mild dryness of the mouth and gastro-intestinal symptoms – including distension, constipation, flatus and diarrhoea – may occur. These are generally relieved by reducing the dosage.

Vomiting, pancreatitis and sore or black tongue have been reported.

Weight gain and oedema occur infrequently and are usually relieved by administering a thiazide diuretic. If oedema becomes progressive or other signs of heart failure appear after the addition of a thiazide diuretic, Dopamet should be discontinued.

Gynaecomastia, breast enlargement, lactation, disorders of sexual function, skin rash, mild arthralgia, myalgia, parasthesias, Parkinsonism, Bells palsy and psychic disturbances – including nightmares and reversible mild psychosis – have been reported.

A rise in blood urea has been found in some cases. Rarely, urine from patients receiving Dopamet may darken on exposure to air simply because of the chemical breakdown of methyldopa or its metabolites. Cases of acquired haemolytic anaemia have occurred in association with methyldopa. A condition resembling systemic lupus erythematosus has been reported. Should clinical symptoms suggest the possibility of anaemia, appropriate tests should be undertaken. If haemolysis is found to be present Dopamet should be discontinued. In addition some patients on continued therapy with methyldopa develop a positive direct Coombs test, but this rarely develops in the first six months of therapy and if it has not developed within 12 months it is not likely to do so. Prior knowledge of a positive Coombs reaction will aid in evaluation of cross-matching for transfusion. If a patient with a positive Coombs reaction shows an incompatible minor cross-match, an indirect Coombs test should be performed. If this is negative, transfusion with blood otherwise compatible in the major cross-match may be carried out. If positive, the advisability of transfusion should be determined by a haematologist.

A reversible thrombocytopenia has occurred on rare occasions and reversible reduction of the white blood cell count has been seen with a primary effect on the granulocytes. The granulocyte count, however, returns promptly to normal when the drug is discontinued. Rare cases of clinical agranulocytosis have been reported.

On rare occasions fever occurs, usually within the first three weeks of administering methyldopa, in some cases accompanied by eosinophilia or abnormalities in one or more liver function measurements. Jaundice with or without fever may also occur, usually within the first two to three months of therapy. In some patients the findings are consistent with cholestasis. Rare cases of fatal hepatic necrosis have been reported.

It is advisable to take a total and differential white blood cell count and to perform liver function tests at intervals during the first 6–12 weeks of treatment, or if the patient develops an unexplained fever. Should fever, abnormality in liver function or jaundice occur, therapy should be withdrawn. Dialysis may remove methyldopa. Hypertension may, therefore, recur after this procedure.

Rarely involuntary choreoathetotic movements have been observed during therapy with methyldopa in patients with severe bilateral cerebrovascular disease. Should these movements occur, therapy should be discontinued.

When a thiazide diuretic is added to the dosage regimen, an excessive drop in blood pressure may occur so that the dosage of Dopamet may be reduced by half when a thiazide is used additionally. Careful observation of changes in blood pressure must be made. If Dopamet is added to the regimen of a patient taking a thiazide diuretic then the initial dosage should be limited to 375 mg per day for the first two days and the dosage increased gradually at intervals of not less than two days until adequate control of the blood pressure is obtained.

Methyldopa may increase the neurotoxic potential of lithium without increasing plasma concentrations. Methyldopa may induce extra pyramidal side effects in patients receiving drugs for Parkinsonism.

Treatment of overdosage: Gastric lavage may be helpful if carried out within a reasonable time after ingestion and can be assisted by dialysis if the overdosage has been substantial. Other treatment should by symptomatic, with general support provided to maintain cardiac output, blood volume, electrolyte balance and urinary output. Administration of sympathomimetic agents may be indicated.

Pharmaceutical precautions Store in a cool dry place and protect from light.

Legal category POM.

Package quantities *Tablets 125 mg:* Containers of 250.

Tablets 250 mg: Containers of 250, 1,000 and 2,500.

Tablets 500 mg: Containers of 250 and 500.

Further information 'Dopamet' is an effective hypotensive agent which possesses significant advantages over the ganglion blocking and postganglion blocking agents, controlling high blood pressure throughout the day and night after a basic regimen particular to the patient has been established. It usually reduces supine as well as standing blood pressure and produces little or no postural or exertional hypotension. Normal or elevated plasma renin activity may decrease in the course of methyldopa therapy.

Product licence numbers
Tablets 125 mg 0152/0093
Tablets 250 mg 0152/5021R
Tablets 500 mg 0152/0080

DRYPTAL* TABLETS 40 mg

Presentation White Frusemide Tablets BP 40 mg marked 'BERK 2B2' or '2B2', single break line. Other ingredients include lactose.

Uses Diuretic. Oedema of cardiac, hepatic or renal origin. Pulmonary oedema. Toxaemia of pregnancy. Mild or moderate hypertension.

Dosage and administration The usual initial dosage is 1 tablet daily, thereafter adjusted to the minimum effective dose which may range from ½ tablet (20 mg) on alternate days to 3 tablets (120 mg) daily.

Children: From 1 to 3 mg/kg body weight.

Elderly: In the elderly elimination of frusemide is generally slower, dosage should therefore be titrated until the required response is achieved.

Contra-indications, warnings, etc Dryptal is contra-indicated in the presence of electrolyte deficiency, hepatic cirrhosis or digitalis intoxication and should be used with great caution in advanced renal failure. Patients with prostatic hypertrophy or impairment of micturition have an increased risk of developing acute retention. Cephaloridine nephrotoxicity may be increased by concomitant administration of potent diuretics such as frusemide.

During prolonged use and at high dosage a close check should be kept upon plasma electrolytes.

Dryptal may potentiate the action of cardiac glycosides and of hypotensive agents, the dosage of which may need to be reduced. Dryptal may also precipitate diabetes, or necessitate increased dosage of insulin.

Serum uric acid levels tend to rise during treatment with Dryptal and an acute attack of gout may occasionally be precipitated.

Elderly patients may be particularly susceptible to disturbances of water and electrolyte balance and micturition disorders during therapy with frusemide and particular caution should be exercised.

Other reported side-effects include nausea, gastric upset and malaise. The incidence of allergic reactions such as skin rashes is very low but when these occur treatment should be withdrawn. Bone marrow depression has been reported as a rare complication and necessitates withdrawal of treatment.

Use in pregnancy: Only when it is essential should Dryptal be given in the first trimester of pregnancy or to nursing mothers.

Treatment of overdosage: Correct dehydration and electrolyte depletion. Reversible deafness may occur.

Pharmaceutical precautions Store in a cool dry place protected from light.

Legal category POM.

Package quantities Containers of 50, 250 and 1,000.

Further information Nil.

Product licence number 0152/0083.

DRYPTAL* TABLETS 500 mg

Presentation Yellow, flat, bevel-edged Frusemide Tablets BP 500 mg engraved Berk 3B2 or 3B2 on one side and with a double breakline on the other. Other ingredients include lactose, sunset yellow (E110).

Uses Diuretic for the management of oliguria due to acute or chronic renal insufficiency with a GFR below 20 ml/minute.

Dosage and administration *Adults:* In patients with chronic renal insufficiency an initial daily dose of 250 mg (½ tablet) is employed. If a satisfactory diuresis is not produced then the dose may be increased in steps of 250 mg at four to six hourly intervals up to a maximum dose of 2,000 mg (4 tablets) as a single dose.

In cases of acute renal failure which have been initially controlled using Dryptal injection, oral therapy may be substituted for parenteral therapy regarding one 500 mg tablet as approximately equal to 250 mg of injection. Appropriate dosage adjustments may then be made according to the observed clinical response.

Elderly: In the elderly elimination of frusemide is generally slower, dosage should therefore be titrated until the required response is achieved.

Contra-indications, warnings, etc During treatment with high-dosage forms of Dryptal, fluid balance should be carefully controlled. In the case of patients with shock, steps should be taken to normalise blood pressure and circulating blood volume before commencing therapy. Regular checks of plasma electrolytes, particularly sodium, potassium, chloride and bicarbonate should be carried out, and electrolyte replacement therapy instituted if necessary.

Contra-indications: Dryptal tablets 500 mg are contra-indicated in renal failure as a result of poisoning by nephrotoxic or hepatotoxic agents and in renal failure associated with hepatic coma.

Warnings: The dosage of concurrently administered cardiac glycosides or antihypertensive agents may require adjustment.

Cephaloridine nephrotoxicity may be increased by concomitant administration of potent diuretics such as frusemide.

Latent diabetes may become manifest or the insulin requirements of diabetic patients may increase.

Precautions: Elderly patients may be particularly susceptible to disturbances of water and electrolyte balance and micturition disorders during therapy with frusemide and particular caution should be exercised.

Use in pregnancy: The safety of high dosage frusemide in pregnancy has not been established and Dryptal tablets 500 mg should be used with caution, weighing potential benefit to the patient against possible hazard to the foetus.

Treatment of overdosage: Correct dehydration and electrolyte depletion. Reversible deafness may occur.

Side-effects: Dryptal tablets 500 mg are generally well tolerated. Side-effects of a minor nature such as nausea, malaise or gastric upset may occur but are not usually severe enough to cause withdrawal of treatment. The incidence of allergic reactions such as skin rashes is very low but when these occur treatment should be withdrawn. In common with other sulphonamide-based diuretics hyperuricaemia may occur and, in rare cases, clinical gout may be precipitated. Bone marrow depression has been reported as a rare complication and necessitates withdrawal of treatment.

Pharmaceutical precautions Store in a cool dry place protected from light.

Legal category POM.

Package quantities Containers of 100.

Further information Nil.

Product licence number 0152/0145.

DRYPTAL* INJECTION 250 mg/25 ml

Presentation Dryptal 250 mg ampoules contain 250 mg Frusemide BP in 25 ml aqueous solution with sodium hydroxide.

Uses Dryptal 250 mg is a diuretic preparation for the management of oliguria due to acute or chronic renal insufficiency with a GFR below 20 ml/minute.

Dosage and administration *Adults:* Dryptal 250 mg should be administered by intravenous injection at a rate not exceeding 4 mg/minute.

The recommended initial dose is one 25 ml ampoule (250 mg) diluted in approximately 225 ml Sodium Chloride Injection BP or Ringer's Solution for Injection administered over one hour. This gives an approximate drip rate of 80 drops/minute, ensuring that the infusion is at the level of 4 mg/minute.

If a satisfactory increase in urine output, such as 40–50 ml/hour, is not attained within the next hour a second infusion of two 25 ml ampoules (500 mg) in an appropriate infusion fluid should be given, the total volume of the infusion being governed by the patient's state of hydration. If a satisfactory output is still not achieved within one hour of the end of the second infusion, a third infusion consisting of four 25 ml ampoules (1,000 mg) can be given. The rate of infusion should not exceed 4 mg/minute.

If the third infusion using the maximum intravenous dose of 1,000 mg over four hours is not effective, then dialysis will probably be required.

In oliguric or anuric patients with significant fluid overload, it may not be practicable to administer high-dose Dryptal injection by the method suggested above. Under these circumstances, the use of a constant-rate infusion pump (e.g. Sage pump) with micrometer screw-gauge adjustment may be considered for direct administration of the injection into the vein. The rate of administration should not exceed 4 mg/minute.

If the Dryptal infusion produces a satisfactory response of 40–50 ml/hour, then the effective dose (up to 1,000 mg) can be repeated every 24 hours. Alternatively, maintenance therapy can be continued with oral Dryptal 500 mg tablets when one 500 mg tablet may be regarded as being approximately equal to one 250 mg ampoule. Appropriate dosage adjustments may then be made according to the observed clinical response.

Elderly: In the elderly elimination of frusemide is generally slower, dosage should therefore be titrated until the required response is achieved.

Contra-indications, warnings, etc During treatment with high-dosage forms of Dryptal, fluid balance should be carefully controlled. In the particular case of patients with shock, steps should be taken to correct the blood pressure and circulating blood volume before commencing therapy. Regular checks of plasma electolytes, particularly sodium, potassium, chloride and bicarbonate, should be carried out, and electrolyte replacement therapy instituted accordingly.

Intravenous injections of Dryptal **must** be given slowly.

Infusion rates in excess of 4 mg/minute are associated with an increased risk of ototoxicity, usually reversible hearing loss.

Contra-indications: Dryptal injection 250 mg is contra-indicated in renal failure as a result of poisoning by nephrotoxic or hepatotoxic agents and in renal failure associated with hepatic coma.

Warnings: The dosage of concurrently administered cardiac glycosides or antihypertensive agents may require adjustment.

Cephaloridine nephrotoxicity may be increased by concomitant administration of potent diuretics such as frusemide.

Latent diabetes may become manifest or the insulin requirements of diabetic patients may increase.

Precautions: Elderly patients may be particularly susceptible to disturbances of water and electrolyte balance and micturition disorders during therapy with frusemide and particular caution should be exercised.

Use in pregnancy: The safety of high dosage frusemide in pregnancy has not been established and Dryptal injection 250 mg should be used with caution depending on the severity of the condition. As Dryptal may inhibit lactation it should be used with caution in nursing mothers.

Treatment of overdosage: Correct dehydration and electrolyte depletion. Reversible deafness may occur.

Side-effects: Dryptal injection 250 mg is generally well tolerated. Side-effects of a minor nature such as nausea, malaise or gastric upset may occur but are not usually severe enough to cause withdrawal of treatment.

The incidence of allergic reactions such as skin rashes is very low but when these occur treatment should be withdrawn.

In common with other sulphonamide-based diuretics

hyperuricaemia may occur and, in rare cases, clinical gout may be precipitated.

Bone marrow depression has been reported as a rare complication and necessitates withdrawal of treatment.

Pharmaceutical precautions Dryptal ampoules 250 mg should be stored in a cool place protected from light. Frusemide may precipitate in solutions of low pH and therefore dextrose solutions are not suitable infusion fluids for Dryptal injection 250 mg. The injection solution should not be mixed with other drugs in the infusion bottle.

Opened ampoules should be used immediately and any remainder of either the ampoule content or the prepared infusion solution should be discarded.

Legal category POM.

Package quantities Dryptal ampoules 250 mg are available in packs of 10 × 25 ml.

Further information Diuresis should commence within a few minutes and last for approximately two hours. A diuretic effect is seen during the infusion and its duration is related to the infusion time.

Product licence number 0152/0149.

EMBLON*

Presentation White tablets containing tamoxifen 10 mg (engraved BERK 1T7 or 1T7) and 20 mg (engraved BERK 2T7 or 2T7) as the citrate. Other ingredients include lactose.

Uses Emblon when used at the recommended dosage is an oestrogen antagonist. It does not have androgenic properties.

It is used for the treatment of breast cancer as an alternative to androgens or oestrogens. It produces fewer serious side-effects, consequently it may be more acceptable to the patient.

Emblon is also used to stimulate ovulation in the treatment of anovulatory infertility.

Dosage and administration
Adults (including elderly)

1. *Breast cancer:* Initial dose 10 mg twice daily. If a response is not observed within one month the dose should be increased to 20 mg twice daily.

2. *Infertility:* It is most important to exclude any possibility of pregnancy before any course of treatment is commenced.

In women who are menstruating regularly, the usual dose is 10 mg twice daily on day 2, 3, 4 and 5 of the menstrual cycle. Basal temperature measurement or assessment of pre-ovulatory cervical mucus should be made and if these indicate that this initial course has not been successful, the dose may be increased in subsequent cycles to 20 mg twice daily and then to 40 mg twice daily, on the same cycle days.

In women who are not menstruating regularly, the initial course of 10 mg twice daily may begin on any day. If the outcome of this initial course is negative then a further course with increased dosage as above may start 45 days later.

If the patient responds with menstruation, the next course of treatment should be commenced on the second day of the following cycle.

Contra-indications, warnings, etc
Contra-indications: Emblon must not be given during pregnancy. Pre-menopausal patients must undergo a careful examination to exclude any possibility of pregnancy before treatment with Emblon for breast cancer or infertility.

Precautions: Suppression of menstruation has been observed in a proportion of pre-menopausal patients receiving tamoxifen for the treatment of breast cancer. Reversible cystic ovarian swelling has occasionally been observed when such women have been treated with tamoxifen 40 mg twice daily for short periods.

Hypercalcaemia has been reported in a small number of patients with bony metastases when treated with tamoxifen. In such cases therapy should be stopped and the patient may be treated by rehydration, corticosteroids and if necessary mithramycin. There have been reports of serious potentiation of coumarin-type anticoagulants (Warfarin) by tamoxifen. Patients taking coumarin-type anticoagulants require close monitoring on the introduction or withdrawal of tamoxifen.

Side-effects: Side-effects from long term treatment are mainly associated with the anti-oestrogenic action of the drug such as hot flushes, vaginal bleeding and pruritus vulvae. Other side-effects which may occur are gastro-intestinal upsets, tumour pain, light headedness, dizziness, rashes and occasionally fluid retention.

These side-effects may be controlled by reduction of dosage without loss of control of the disease but if they are not, then it may be necessary to stop treatment.

Transient falls in platelet count, to levels between 80,000–90,000, but occasionally lower, have been reported in patients taking tamoxifen for breast cancer. These have not been associated with a haemorrhagic tendency and the platelet counts have recovered notwithstanding continuing treatment.

Emblon should be used with caution in patients with factors predisposing them to thromboembolism. A small number of endometrial hyperplasia, endometrial polyps and endometrial carcinomas have been reported in association with tamoxifen treatment. A definitive relationship to tamoxifen therapy has not been established.

A number of cases of visual disturbance including corneal changes, cataracts and retinopathy have been described in patients receiving Tamoxifen therapy.

Use in pregnancy: Emblon must not be given during pregnancy.

Treatment of overdosage: Theoretically, overdosage would be expected to enhance the anti-oestrogenic effect and consequently the side-effects described above. Animal studies would indicate that very high doses may produce oestrogenic effects.

Corneal and macular changes, resulting in blurred vision have been described when a small number of cases have been treated continuously with 12–16 times the recommended starting dose for over 17 months.

No specific antidote is known and treatment of overdosage should be aimed at alleviating symptoms.

Pharmaceutical precautions Emblon Tablets should be protected from heat and light.

Legal category POM.

Package quantities
10 mg tablets: Securitainers of 30 and 100 tablets. Blister packs of 30 and 250 tablets.
20 mg tablets: Securitainers of 30 and 100 tablets. Blister packs of 30 and 250 tablets.

Further information Nil.

Product licence numbers
10 mg tablets: 0152/0191
20 mg tablets: 0152/0240.

ERYCEN*

Presentation Plain orange film enteric coated erythromycin. Tablets BP 250 mg and 500 mg (Erythromycin base). Other ingredients include Ponceau 4R (E124), sunset yellow (E110)

Uses Infections caused by erythromycin-sensitive organisms especially Gram-positive pyogenic cocci and some Gram-negative bacteria, notably Haemophilus and Neisseria groups.

Dosage and administration *Adults:* Usual oral dose 250 mg every four to six hours. This may be increased to 4 g or more per day in unusually severe infections.

Elderly: No special dosage recommendations.

Contra-indications, warnings, etc Known sensitivity to erythromycin. Do not use in conjunction with other anti-infectives, except when specifically warranted. Erythromycin should not be administered concurrently with the anticoagulant warfarin unless essential to patient care as the effects of this drug may be potentiated by erythromycin resulting in dangerous haemorrhagic states.

Precautions: Caution should be exercised in administering erythromycin to patients with impaired hepatic function, since the antibiotic is excreted principally by the liver.

Side-effects are rare and usually mild. Nausea, vomiting, diarrhoea and pruritus have occurred. Allergic reactions are rare and mild, although anaphylaxis has occurred. Treatment should not usually be continued for longer than ten days. The rare possibility of superinfection caused by overgrowth of non-susceptible bacteria or fungi should be borne in mind during prolonged or repeated therapy, especially when other antibacterial agents are simultaneously employed.

Use in pregnancy: There is no evidence of hazard from erythromycin in human pregnancy.

Treatment of overdosage: It is unlikely that serious symptoms will occur; observation and conservative management are indicated.

Pharmaceutical precautions Store below 30°C and protect from light. Keep container tightly closed.

Package quantities Tablets 250 mg: Containers of 100 and 500.
Tablets 500 mg: Containers of 100 and 500.

Legal category POM.

Further information Erythromycin is bacteristatic and bactericidal, depending on the tissue concentration. Its anti-microbial spectrum is similar to that of penicillin G but it shows increased activity against some Gram-negative bacteria.

Product licence numbers
Tablets 250 mg 0152/0132
Tablets 500 mg 0152/0203

IMBRILON*

Presentation Opaque yellow Indomethacin Capsules BP 25 mg (marked 'BERK 1J3 25' or '1J3 25') and 50 mg (marked 'BERK 2J3 50' or '2J3 50'). Other ingredients include lactose, tartrazine (E102).

Cream-coloured Indomethacin Suppositories BP 100 mg. The base is polyethylene glycol.

Uses Non-steroidal analgesic and anti-inflammatory agent. Indicated in active rheumatoid arthritis, osteoarthritis, ankylosing spondylitis and acute gout. Also may be indicated in severe acute periarticular disorders such as bursitis, tendinitis, synovitis, tenosynovitis and capsulitis.

Dosage and administration Indomethacin Capsules should always be given with food, milk or an antacid to lessen the chance of gastro-intestinal disturbance.

Imbrilon Suppositories should be given singly, one night and morning.

Adults: 50–100 mg daily.

Children: Paediatric dosage not established.

Elderly: Elderly patients appear to be more susceptible to side-effects and dosage should be carefully monitored.

Contra-indications, warnings, etc
Contra-indications: Active peptic ulcer, a history of recurrent gastrointestinal lesions, sensitivity to indomethacin. Bronchospasm may be precipitated in bronchial asthma or in patients with a previous history of bronchospasm. Whilst there is little evidence to support total cross-sensitivity, indomethacin should be avoided in patients with a history of bronchospasm or allergic reactions induced by aspirin or other non-steroidal anti-inflammatory drugs.

Precautions and drug interactions: Indomethacin should be used with caution in patients with hepatic or renal dysfunction. Hepatitis and jaundice have been reported rarely. Patients should be warned not to drive or operate machinery, if they become dizzy.

In common with other anti-inflammatory analgesic antipyretic agents, indomethacin may mask the signs and symptoms of infectious disease and this should be borne in mind in order to avoid delay in starting treatment for infection.

Indomethacin should be used with caution in patients with an existing, albeit controlled, infection.

Particular care should be taken with older patients who are more susceptible to side-effects from indomethacin.

Use in pregnancy: It is not known if indomethacin is safe to use in children or in pregnancy or during lactation and it should not be given to such patients.

Treatment of overdosage: Gastric lavage should be given if indomethacin is considered still to be part of the stomach contents.

Otherwise supportive therapy is required and a watch should be kept for gastro-intestinal bleeding for several days.

Warnings and adverse effects: It must be expected that about 20% of patients will complain of side-effects, but starting treatment at a low dosage and increasing it gradually until symptomatic relief is obtained will minimise their incidence.

The most common side-effects are headache, dizziness and dyspepsia. If headache persists, even after dosage reduction, indomethacin should be withdrawn.

Other CNS side-effects which may occur include mental confusion, depression, convulsions, coma, depersonalisation and tinnitus. These are often transient and disappear with time or on reduction of dosage.

Indomethacin may aggravate psychiatric disorders, epilepsy and Parkinsonism.

Gastro-intestinal disorders which occur most frequently are nausea, anorexia, vomiting, epigastric distress, abdominal pain and diarrhoea. Giving indomethacin with food, milk or antacids lowers the incidence of these side-effects. Ulceration of the oesophagus, stomach or duodenum may also occur, accompanied by haemorrhage and perforation (a few fatalities have been reported). Gastro-intestinal bleeding without obvious ulceration may also occur. If this happens indomethacin treatment should be discontinued.

Blood dyscrasias, particularly thrombocytopenia, have been reported.

Blurred vision and orbital and peri-orbital pain are seen infrequently. Corneal deposits and retinal disturbances have been reported in some patients with rheumatoid arthritis on prolonged therapy with indomethacin, and ophthalmic examinations are desirable in patients given prolonged treatment.

Oedema and increased blood pressure also sometimes occur, as does haematuria.

Hypersensitivity reactions include pruritus, urticaria, angiitis, erythema nodosum. Skin rash and hair loss may also occur.

Acute respiratory distress including sudden dyspnoea and asthma, have been reported on rare occasions. Bronchospasm may be precipitated in patients suffering from, or with a previous history of bronchial asthma or allergic disease.

Pharmaceutical precautions Store in a cool place and protect from light.

Legal category POM.

Package quantities *Capsules 25 mg:* Containers of 500.

Capsules 50 mg: Containers of 100.

Suppositories 100 mg: Containers of 30.

Further information Nil.

Product licence numbers

Capsules 25 mg	0152/0072
Capsules 50 mg	0152/0074
Suppositories 100 mg	0152/0127.

LACTULOSE SOLUTION BP

Presentation A colourless to pale yellow solution containing 3.5 g/5 ml lactulose with 0.2 g/5 ml lactose and 0.47 g/5 ml galactose.

Uses
Mode of action: Lactulose solution provides a natural substrate for the saccharolytic bacterial flora in the colon. Lactulose is not affected by disaccharidases in the small intestine and passes unchanged with water into the colon where saccharolytic bacteria break down the lactulose to the monosaccharides galactose and fructose. These increase the osmotic pressure of the colonic contents and more water is drawn into the bowel with consequent increase in faecal bulk and stimulation of peristalsis.

The monosaccharides are then metabolised further to acetic and lactic acids with a subsequent lowering of the colonic pH and in hepatic encephalopathy the effectiveness of lactulose solution may be associated with this change which discourages the activity of ammonia producing organisms, resulting in a decrease in the relative concentration of free ammonia, effectively lowering blood ammonia concentration by reduced absorption.

Indications: Constipation. Hepatic encephalopathy (portal systemic encephalopathy): hepatic coma.

Dosage and administration
Constipation: Initially:

Adults 15 ml twice daily
Children 5–10 years 10 ml twice daily
Children under 5 years 5 ml twice daily
Babies 2.5 ml twice daily

Eventually the dosage should be adjusted to the needs of the individual.

Hepatic encephalopathy: 30–50 ml three times a day initially. The dose should be adjusted subsequently to produce two or three soft stools each day.

Elderly: Lactulose is a suitable laxative for the elderly. There is no evidence that the elderly require adjustment of dosages.

Contra-indications, warnings, etc
Contra-indications: Gastro-intestinal obstruction, galactosaemia.

Precautions: Diabetes mellitus, lactose intolerance.

Use in pregnancy: Lactulose solution like all laxatives should be used with caution during the first trimester of pregnancy.

Side-effects: Side-effects occur rarely. Mild nausea which generally subsides after the initial stage of treatment has been reported with lactulose solution.

High doses may provoke nausea, vomiting, flatulence or abdominal pain.

Pharmaceutical precautions Store below 20°C. Do not freeze. Dilution is not recommended.

Legal category P.

Package quantities 1 litre bottles.

Further information Due to the mode of action of lactulose solution it may take two to three days before the full benefit of treatment is obtained.

Product licence number 0152/0266.

LADROPEN*

Presentation Opaque orange/brown capsules containing 250 mg and 500 mg flucloxacillin as Flucloxacillin Sodium BP and overprinted 'BERK 1A8' or '1A8' and 'BERK 2A8' or '2A8' in white respectively.

Uses Treatment of infections caused by Gram-positive organisms including those caused by penicillin-resistant staphylococci.

Dosage and administration *Adults:* Oral: 250 mg four times daily. Capsules should be taken one hour before meals. This dosage may be doubled where necessary.

Elderly: No specific dosage recommendations, however, in those patients with severe renal impairment (creatinine clearance <10 mls/minute) a reduction in dose or extension of dose interval should be considered.

Contra-indications, warnings, etc
Contra-indications: Hypersensitivity to penicillin.

Warnings: Some patients may experience gastro-intestinal symptoms but these effects usually resolve rapidly when treatment is stopped. Urticarial or erythematous rashes occasionally occur. Treatment should be discontinued if either type of rash is observed.

Precautions: Patients with a known history of allergy are more likely to develop a hypersensitivity reaction.

Use in pregnancy: Safety in pregnancy has not been established.

Pharmaceutical precautions Flucloxacillin capsules should be stored in a cool, dry place.

Legal category POM.

Package quantities Capsules 250 mg: packs of 100 and 500 capsules.
Capsules 500 mg: packs of 100 capsules.

Further information Nil.

Product licence numbers

Capsules 250 mg	0152/0184.
Capsules 500 mg	0152/0185

LIDIFEN*

Presentation Lidifen is available in two presentations: Round, biconvex, pink sugar-coated tablets, marked 'APS' or plain on one side and coded 200 0521 or 400 0525 for the 200 and 400 mg strengths respectively.

Lidifen is also available in a 600 mg strength; this tablet is pink, capsule-shaped, biconvex, film-coated and marked 'APS' or plain on one side and 600 0531 on the other side.

Both presentations contain the same active ingredient, Ibuprofen BP, and comply with the monograph for Ibuprofen Tablets BP.

The 200 mg & 400 mg tablets contain sucrose, colours E110, E127 and E211. The 600 mg contains colours E127, E464 and E171.

Uses Ibuprofen is a non-steroidal anti-inflammatory agent with analgesic and anti-pyretic activity. Its principal effects are to relieve pain and stiffness and to reduce swelling.

Lidifen tablets may therefore be used in the management of:
(a) Rheumatoid Arthritis including Still's disease;
(b) Osteoarthrosis and seronegative (non rheumatoid) arthropothies;
(c) Ankylosing Spondylitis.

Like other similar agents, ibuprofen has been used in non-articular rheumatic conditions and in soft-tissue injuries, and for the relief of mild to moderate pain such as dysmenorrhoea, dental and post-operative pain.

Dosage and administration Oral.
Adult: Initially 1200 mg per day in divided doses. In severe conditions up to 1800 mg per day may be given until the acute phase of the condition has been brought under control. Some patients may be maintained on doses in the range 600–1200 mg per day. Under no circumstances should the dose of ibuprofen exceed 24,00 mg in any 24 hours.

Children: 20 mg/kg of body weight given daily in divided doses. The tablets are not suitable for children weighing less than 20 kg and no more than two 200 mg tablets should be given in 24 hours to those weighing less than 30 kg.

The elderly: A separate dosage schedule is not recommended because ibuprofen is well tolerated and overdosage is not usually dangerous, but see precaution (d) below.

Contra-indications, warnings, etc
Contra-indications: Ibuprofen should not be used in patients with:
(a) active peptic ulceration;
(b) a history of severe peptic ulceration.

Precautions: Special care must be taken when using ibuprofen in the following situations:
(a) In patients with asthma;
(b) In allergic patients or in patients who have developed bronchospasm with other non-steroidal anti-inflammatory agents;
(c) Pregnancy: As with other agents the use of ibuprofen during pregnancy should be avoided if possible;
(d) In elderly patients, in whom increased tissue levels may result from the normal processes of ageing with an attendant increase in the risk of adverse reactions (which are more likely to be masked by concurrent therapy or disease in the elderly).

Adverse reactions: As with other non-steroidal anti-inflammatory agents, the most common unwanted effects with ibuprofen include dyspepsia, gastro-intestinal intolerance and bleeding. Other unwanted effects include a variety of skin rashes and, less commonly, thrombocytopenia. A few cases of toxic amblyopia which recovered on withdrawal of treatment have been reported. Signs of intolerance or unwanted effects are indications for stopping treatment.

Overdosage: There is no specific antidote to ibuprofen. Management usually includes gastric lavage associated with special care of plasma electrolytes and any other appropriate symptomatic relief.

Pharmaceutical precautions Lidifen Tablets should be stored at room temperature in a dry place and protected from light.

Legal category POM.

Package quantities
Lidifen 200 mg: polypropylene tubes of 100 and 500 tablets.
Lidifen 400 mg: polypropylene tubes of 100 and 250 tablets.
Lidifen 600 mg: polypropylene tubes of 100 tablets.

Further information Nil.

Product licence numbers

Lidifen Tablets 200 mg	0289/0029
Lidifen Tablets 400 mg	0289/0037
Lidifen Tablets 600 mg	0289/0069

Product licence holder: Approved Prescription Services Ltd.

NITRAZEPAM TABLETS BP

Presentation White, round, flat, bevel-edged Nitrazepam Tablets BP, marked BERK 1N4 or 1N4, with single breakline on reverse, each containing 5 mg Nitrazepam BP. Other ingredients include lactose.

Uses Hypnotic of the benzodiazepine group, indicated for the short-term treatment of insomnia only when it is severe, disabling or subjecting the individual to extreme distress.

At therapeutic doses Nitrazepam induces sleep lasting some six to eight hours, from which the sleeper may be readily roused if necessary.

Dosage and administration The lowest effective dose should be used. Treatment should not be continued beyond 4 weeks and should, where possible, be intermittent. Long-term chronic use is not recommended. Treatment with benzodiazepines should always be withdrawn gradually. Patients who have been receiving treatment for a long time may require longer periods during which the doses are reduced.

Adults Usually 5 mg before retiring. This may be increased to 10 mg when necessary or to 20 mg in hospitalised patients.

Elderly Dose should not exceed half the recommended adult dose.

Children: Nitrazepam is not recommended for the routine treatment of children but 2.5 mg may be given when necessary to children aged one to six years and 5 mg to children aged seven or older.

Contra-indications, warnings, etc An underlying cause for insomnia should be sought before deciding upon the use of benzodiazepines for symptomatic relief.

Benzodiazepines should not be used for phobic or obsessional states.

They should not be used alone to treat depression or anxiety associated with depression. Suicide may be precipitated in such patients.

They should not be used for the treatment of chronic psychosis.

Amnesia may occur.

In cases of loss or bereavement psychological adjustment may be inhibited by benzodiazepines.

Disinhibiting effects may be manifested in various ways. Suicide may be precipitated in patients who are depressed and aggressive behaviour toward self and others may be precipitated. Extreme caution should therefore be used in prescribing benzodiazepines in patients with personality disorders.

Withdrawal from benzodiazepines may be associated with physiological and psychological symptoms of withdrawal including depression. Withdrawal symptoms may occur following normal therapeutic doses given for short periods of time.

Benzodiazepines are also contra-indicated in patients with known sensitivity to benzodiazepines and in acute pulmonary insufficiency.

Use in pregnancy: There is no information on the absolute safety of nitrazepam in human pregnancy. Do not use during pregancy, especially during the first and third trimesters, unless there are compelling reasons.

Precautions: Nitrazepam should only be used with great caution in patients with impairment of renal or hepatic function, or who are elderly or debilitated. Particular consideration should be given to respiratory function.

Concomitant administration with CNS depressants (including alcohol), general anaesthetics, narcotic analgesics, monoamine oxidase inhibitors and anti-depressants may result in an accentuation of their effects.

Patients should be warned of the possibility of drowsiness occurring, particularly in the first few days of therapy, and advised to moderate their use of alcohol. They should also be warned not to drive or operate machinery if Nitrazepam affects their alertness.

Adverse effects: Side-effects are few at the recommended dosage, although fatigue, drowsiness, ataxia or light-headedness, which are dose related, are occasionally noted. Confusion may occur in the elderly, especially if organic brain damage is present.

Treatment of overdosage: Drowsiness and ataxia will be the predominant initial symptoms and the patient may be unconscious for up to 36 hours. Gastric lavage may be useful but Nitrazepam causes few serious problems in overdosage. In children, behavioural changes are likely.

Pharmaceutical precautions Store in a cool place. Protect from light.

Legal category CD (Sch 4), POM.

Package quantities Containers of 50 and 500 tablets.

Further information Nil.

Product licence number 0152/0130.

PRIMPERAN*

Presentation *Tablets:* White tablet marked 'PRIMPERAN' or '1P5' with single break line on reverse. Each tablet contains 10 mg Metoclopramide Hydrochloride BP. Other ingredients include lactose.

Syrup: Each 5 ml of lime-coloured syrup contains 5 mg Metoclopramide Hydrochloride BP. Other ingredients include parabens and sunset yellow (E110).

Ampoules: Colourless solution for injection containing 10 mg Metoclopramide Hydrochloride BP in 2 ml with sodium metabisulphite and sodium chloride.

Uses *Adults (20 years and over):*
For the relief of upper gastro-intestinal symptoms: including heartburn, nausea, vomiting in flatulent dyspepsia, gastritis and duodenitis associated with gastro-intestinal disorders including peptic ulcers, and sequelae of gastrectomy.

As an anti-emetic agent: for the treatment of nausea and vomiting accompanying the following conditions:

- intolerance to cytotoxics.
- malignant disease.
- post-anaesthetic vomiting.
- post-operative gastric hypotonia.
- post vagotomy syndrome.
- migraine

and during deep X-ray and cobalt treatment.

In diagnosis: radiological investigation to facilitate duodenal intubation procedures; to facilitate barium meal examination.

For barium meal procedures:
(a) Where barium-meal studies are held up by spasm of the duodenal cap making examination for the presence of the ulcer difficult;
(b) To facilitate examination of the hypotonic stomach with delayed emptying, gastric stasis and pyloric channel syndrome.

Young adults and children: The use of Primperan in patients under 20 years should be restricted to the following: Severe intractable vomiting of known cause; vomiting associated with radiotherapy and intolerance to cytotoxic drugs; as an aid to gastro-intestinal intubation; as part of the pre-medication before surgical procedures.

Dosage and administration The daily dose level of Primperan is based upon 0.5 mg/kg body weight, in divided doses, which in normal circumstances should not be exceeded.

In patients with clinically significant degrees of renal or hepatic impairment, therapy should be initiated at a reduced dosage. The prominent route of elimination is via the kidney.

General therapeutic dosage:

Oral: (tablets and syrup).

Adults (20 years and over): 10 mg three times daily. For patients of less than 60 kg see below.

Elderly patients: As for adults.

Young adults and children: Primperan should only be used following careful examination to avoid masking an underlying disorder, e.g. cerebral irritation. The stated dosage recommendations should be strictly adhered to if side effects are to be avoided.

In treatment of this group attention should be given particularly to body weight and treatment should commence at a lower dose where stated.

Young adults:		
15–20 years	60 kg and over	10 mg three times daily
	30–59 kg	5 mg three times daily
Children:		
9–14 years	30 kg and over	5 mg three times daily
5–9 years	20–29 kg	2.5 mg three times daily
3–5 years	15–19 kg	2 mg two to three times daily
1–3 years	10–14 kg	1 mg two to three times daily
Under 1 year	Up to 10 kg	1 mg twice daily

The syrup presentation facilitates accurate dosage and tablets should not be used in children under the age of 15 years.

Intramuscular or intravenous administration: The dosages stated above are applicable to parenteral administration of Primperan.

Diagnostic dosage: (barium meal examination and small bowel intubation)

Primperan may be given 5–10 minutes before examination as a single dose subject to body-weight considerations (see Table).

The following doses are recommended:

Adults (20 years and over):	10–20 mg
Young adults (15–20 years):	10 mg
Children 9–14 years:	5 mg
5–9 years:	2.5 mg
3–5 years:	2 mg
Under 3 years:	1 mg

Contra-indications, warnings, etc
Contra-indications: There are no absolute contra-indications to the use of Primperan.

Warnings: The recommended dosage should not be exceeded, particularly in children, young adults and other patients of low body-weight, who may be more liable to dystonic reactions.

If vomiting persists the patient should be reassessed to exclude the possibility of an underlying disorder, e.g. cerebral irritation.

Since atropine effecively blocks the action of Primperan, the concomitant administration of this and other anticholinergic drugs should be avoided.

Precautions: As both Primperan and phenothiazines may cause benign transient dystonia, care should be exercised in the event of both drugs being prescribed concurrently.

Reduced renal clearance of metoclopramide may be observed in patients with impaired kidney function and dosage may therefore need adjustment. Particular caution should therefore be taken when treating the elderly.

Pregnancy: Primperan is not recommended during pregnancy, although animal tests in several mammalian species have revealed no teratogenic effect.

Side-effects: A low incidence of side-effects has been associated with the use of Primperan with absence of serious toxicity and excellent tolerance by oral and parenteral routes. Although rare, drowsiness and dystonic reactions have been reported. These are reversible, usually disappearing within 24 hours of stopping treatment.

Symptoms which can occur include spasm of facial, extra-ocular or cervical muscles which may be constant or rhythmic. There may also be a generalised increase in muscle tone. Anti-Parkinsonian drugs of the anticholinergic type may be used to counteract these reactions.

Tardive dyskinesia has been reported during prolonged treatment in a small number of mainly elderly patients. Patients on prolonged treatment should be regularly reviewed.

Metoclopramide may induce an acute hypertensive response in patients with phaeochromocytoma.

Treatment of overdosage: Gastric lavage and intensive supportive therapy should be initiated. Dystonic symptoms are likely and may be treated in severe cases with atropine, benztropine or other anticholinergic agents. Generalised convulsions may appear in infants.

Pharmaceutical precautions No known incompatibilities.

Diluent for Syrup: Purified water BP.

Protect from light. Store in a cool place.

Legal category POM.

Package quantities *Tablets:* Containers of 100 and 500.

Syrup: Bottles of 100 ml.

Ampoules: Boxes of 10 × 2 ml.

Further information Primperan has the unique action of normalising the hypomotile stomach and small intestine and also possesses powerful antiemetic effects.

Product licence numbers
Tablets 0152/5001R
Syrup 0152/5002R
Ampoules 0152/5003R

SALBUTAMOL SPRAY

Presentation Metered dose aerosol inhaler, delivering 100 micrograms of Salbutamol BP per actuation.

Uses Salbutamol inhaler is a beta-adrenergic stimulant which has a highly selective action on the receptors in bronchial muscle and, in therapeutic doses, little or no action on the cardiac receptors. Salbutamol is also highly active in preventing antigen-induced release of histamine and slow-reacting substance of anaphylaxis, SRS(A), from mast cells in human lung sensitised with IgE antibody. Such Type 1 hypersensitivity reactions are generally considered to be primary triggers of allergic asthma syndrome.

Salbutamol is therefore indicated both for the treatment and prophylaxis of bronchial asthma and also for the treatment of other conditions, such as bronchitis and emphysema, with associated reversible airways obstruction. Since salbutamol is long acting, it is ideally suited for routine maintenance therapy in chronic asthma and chronic bronchitis. The inhaler drug delivery system, using salbutamol in microgram dosage, avoids the skeletal muscle tremor sometimes associated with oral therapy. Salbutamol acts rapidly and may be used when necessary to relieve attacks of acute dyspnoea. Doses may be taken prophylactically before exertion or to prevent exercise-induced asthma.

As a result of its selective action on the bronchi and its lack of effects on the cardiovascular system, salbutamol is suitable for treating bronchospasm in patients with co-existing heart disease or hypertension, including those taking beta-blocking drugs which often impair respiratory function.

Dosage and administration
Adults: For the relief of acute bronchospasm and relieving intermittent episodes of asthma, one or two inhalations may be administered as a single dose. The recommended dose for chronic maintenance or prophylactic therapy is two inhalations three or four times a day. To prevent exercise-induced bronchospasm, two inhalations should be taken before exertion.

Children: One inhalation is the recommended dose for the relief of acute bronchospasm, in the management of episodic asthma or before exercise. One inhalation should be administered three or four times a day for routine maintenance or prophylactic therapy. These dosages may be increased to two inhalations, if necessary. For optimum results, in most patients, Salbutamol must be used regularly.

The bronchodilator effect of each administration of salbutamol lasts for at least four hours, except in patients whose asthma is becoming worse. Each patient should be warned not to increase their usage of inhaler, but should seek medical advice in case treatment with an inhaled and/or systemic glucocorticosteroid is indicated.

Contra-indications, warnings, etc
Contra-indications: Although intravenous salbutamol and occasionally salbutamol tablets are used in the management of uncomplicated premature labour, salbutamol presentations should not be used for threatened abortion during the first or second trimesters of pregnancy. Salbutamol is contra-indicated in patients with a history of hypersensitivity to any of its components.

Potentially serious hypokalaemia may result from $beta_2$ agonist therapy. Particular caution is advised in severe asthma as this effect may be potentiated by concomitant treatment with xanthine derivatives, steroids, diuretics and by hypoxia. It is recommended that serum potassium levels are monitored in such situations.

Precautions: In the event of a previously effective dose of salbutamol failing to give relief for at least three hours, the patient should be advised to seek medical advice in order that any necessary additional steps be taken.

Salbutamol should be administered cautiously to patients suffering from thyrotoxicosis.

Pregnancy: As with other drugs, the use of salbutamol should be avoided in the first and second trimesters of pregnancy.

Overdosage: The preferred antidote for overdosage with salbutamol is a cardioselective beta-blocking agent, but beta-blocking agents should be used with caution in patients with a history of bronchospasm.

Pharmaceutical precautions Salbutamol should be stored in a cool place, protected from frost and direct sunlight. The canister should not be broken, punctured or burnt, even when apparently empty.

Legal category POM.

Package quantities Salbutamol Spray is a metered dose aerosol. Each canister provides 200 inhalations.

Further information Unlike sympathomimetic agents such as ephedrine, salbutamol does not stimulate alpha-adrenoceptors and therefore does not cause difficulty in micturition. Thus, salbutamol is not contra-indicated in patients undergoing treatment with monoamine oxidase inhibitors (MAOIs).

Product licence number 0152/0281

SALBUTAMOL TABLETS

Presentation Salbutamol Tablets are pink, round, flat-faced with bevelled edges marked 'APS' or plain on one side, while the strength and code number are marked on the other side. The tablets contain Salbutamol BP as the sulphate and comply with the monograph for Salbutamol Tablets BP. Two strengths are available: Salbutamol 2 mg marked '2/1507', Salbutamol 4 mg marked '4/1508'.

Both strengths of tablets contain lactose and colours E127 and E131.

Uses Salbutamol is a beta-adrenergic stimulant which has a selective action on the beta-adrenergic receptors in bronchial muscle and, in therapeutic dosage, little or no action on the cardiac beta-adrenergic receptors. In view of the selective action on the bronchi, salbutamol preparations are suitable for treating bronchospasm in patients with co-existing heart disease or hypertension.

Salbutamol is also active, when used locally in human lung sensitised with IgE antibody, in preventing antigen-induced release of histamine and slow reacting substance of anaphylaxis, SRS(A), from mast cells. Such Type I hypersensitivity reactions are generally considered to be the primary triggers of the allergic asthma syndrome.

Salbutamol Tablets may therefore be used in the management of:
(a) Bronchial asthma.
(b) Other conditions with associated reversible airways obstruction such as bronchitis and emphysema (including patients with co-existing heart disease of hypertension).

Tablets in premature labour: Salbutamol Tablets may be used following the administration of salbutamol as a continuous intravenous infusion for the management of premature labour during the third trimester of pregnancy. Once the uterine concentrations have ceased and the infusion has been withdrawn, maintenance therapy may be continued with Salbutamol Tablets.

Dosage and administration Oral.

Adults: The usual effective dose is 4 mg three or four times per day. If adequate bronchodilation is not obtained, each single dose may be gradually increased to as much as 8 mg. However, it has been established that some patients obtain adequate relief with 2 mg three or four times daily.

Children: The following doses should be administered three or four times daily:
2–6 years: ¼ to 1 of the 2 mg tablets.
6–12 years: 1 of the 2 mg tablets.
Over 12 years: 1–2 of the 2 mg tablets or 1 of the 4 mg tablets.

Salbutamol is well tolerated by children so that, if necessary, these doses may be cautiously increased.

Elderly: In elderly patients or in those known to be unusually sensitive to beta-adrenergic stimulants, it is advisable to initiate treatment with 2 mg three or four times per day.

Premature labour: In the management of premature labour, after uterine contractions have been controlled by intravenous salbutamol and the infusion has been withdrawn, maintenance therapy may be continued with Salbutamol Tablets. The usual dosage is 4 mg three or four times daily.

Contra-indications, warnings, etc
Contra-indications: Care should be taken when administering salbutamol preparations to patients suffering from diabetes mellitus, serious cardiovascular disorders or hypertension.

Pregnancy: Although intravenous salbutamol and salbutamol tablets are used in the management of premature labour, these preparations should not be used for threatened abortion during the first or second trimester of pregnancy.

Beta-blocking agents: Salbutamol tablets should not usually be prescribed for patients under treatment with beta-blocking agents, but note that the inhaler may be prescribed for such patients.

Precautions: Thyrotoxicosis: Care should be taken when administering salbutamol preparation to patients suffering from thyrotoxicosis.

Hypokalaemia: Potentially serious hypokalaemia may result from $beta_2$ agonist therapy. Particular caution is advised in severe asthma as this effect may be potentiated by concomitant treatment with xanthine derivatives, steroids, diuretics and by hyponia. It is recommended that serum potassium levels are monitored in such situations.

Pregnancy: As with other agents the use of salbutamol during pregnancy should be avoided if possible (except for the management of premature labour).

Adverse reactions: Potentially serious hypokalaemia may result from $beta_2$ agonist therapy.

The only other side-effect of significance with salbutamol tablets is a fine tremor of skeletal muscle which occurs in some patients; usually the hands are most obviously affected. The effect is dose related and is common to all beta-adrenergic stimulants. A few patients feel tense; this is also due to the effects on skeletal muscle and not to direct CNS stimulation. With doses of salbutamol higher than those recommended or in patients who are usually sensitive to beta-adrenergic stimulants peripheral vasodilation and a compensatory small increase in heart rate may occur. Occasionally headaches have been reported.

No important adverse reactions have been reported following therapy with salbutamol inhaler. This is presumably due to the small size of the effective dose and the correspondingly increased therapeutic ratio.

Overdosage: The preferred antidote for overdosage with salbutamol is a cardioselective beta-blocking agent, but such agents should be used with caution in patients with a history of bronchospasm.

Pharmaceutical precautions Salbutamol Tablets should be stored below 25°C and protected from light.

Legal category POM.

Package quantities
Salbutamol Tablets 2 mg: Polypropylene tubes of 500 tablets.
Salbutamol Tablets 4 mg: Polypropylene tubes of 100 and 500 tablets.

Further information Unlike sympathomimetic agents such as ephedrine, salbutamol does not stimulate alpha-adrenoceptors and, therefore, does not cause difficulty in micturition. Therefore salbutamol is not contra-indicated in patients under treatment with monoamine oxidase inhibitors (MAOIs).

Product licence numbers

Salbutamol Tablets 2 mg	0289/0064
Salbutamol Tablets 4 mg	0289/0065

Product licence holder: Approved Prescription Services Ltd.

SPIROLONE*

Presentation Spirolone is presented as buff coloured, biconvex, film coated tablets marked 'APS' or plain on one side with a code number and strength on the reverse.

The tablets contain Spironolactone BP and comply with the monograph for Spironolactone Tablets BP.

There are two strengths available: Spirolone 25 mg tablets marked 25/0705; and Spirolone 100 mg tablets marked 100/0706. The tablets also contain lactose and the colours E171, E464 and E172.

Uses Spirolone is indicated for use in cirrhosis with ascites and oedema, malignant ascites, nephrotic syndrome, congestive cardiac failure, diagnosis and treatment of primary hyperaldosteronism.

Dosage and administration Oral. The tablets should be administered with fluid.

Adults: An initial dose of 100 mg/day increasing if necessary to 200 mg or possibily up to 400 mg daily. When oedema is controlled, the maintenance dose is determined on an individual basis, usually 75–200 mg/day.

Use of spironolactone in the treatment of nephrotic syndrome is only advised when glucocorticoids alone are insufficiently effective.

For treatment of cirrhosis with ascites and oedema the dosage is based on the urinary Na+/K+ ratio. If the ratio is greater than 1.0 a dosage of 100 mg daily is recommended and if less than 1.0 a daily dosage of 200–400 mg.

Diagnosis and treatment of primary hyperaldosteronism: Spironolactone may be used to provide presumptive evidence of primary aldosteronism while patients are on normal diets.

Long test: Administer 400 mg spironolactone per day for 3–4 weeks. If hypokalaemia and hypertension are corrected then consider a presumptive diagnosis of primary hyperaldosteronism.

Short test: Administer 400 mg spironolactone per day for 4 days. If serum potassium increases during treatment and drops on cessation of treatment then consider a presumptive diagnosis of primary aldosteronism.

On confirmation of hyperaldosteronism, spironolactone may be administered in preparation for surgery at a dosage of 100–400 mg daily. If surgery is unsuitable then spironolactone may be used for long term maintenance therapy at the lowest possible effective dosage.

Children: Initially 1.5–3 mg/kg body weight in divided doses, then adjust according to the patient's response and tolerance of one drug. If necessary the tablets may be crushed and taken with food or drink.

The elderly: Start with a low dose and increase as necessary to achieve maximum benefit.

Contra-indications, warnings, etc
Contra-indications: Spironolactone is contra-indicated in patients with: Renal failure, acute renal insufficiency; hyperkalaemia; and also during pregnancy and lactation.

Precautions: Spironolactone should not be administered with other potassium conserving diuretics as hyperkalaemia may be induced. Also, except in initial cases of potassium depletion, potassium supplements should be avoided unless considered essential, when serum electrolytes should be monitored.

Spironolactone may potentiate the effects of other

diuretics so their dosage may need to be reduced (by about 50%) and then adjusted as necessary.

Carbenoxolone may cause sodium retention and thus decrease the effectiveness of spironolactone. Conversely spironolactone inhibits the ulcer healing effect of carbenoxolone.

Spironolactone reduced the vascular responsiveness to noradrenaline. Caution should be exercised when patients being treated with Spironolactone are subject to local or general anaesthesia.

Aspirin and indomethacin antagonise the diuretic effect of spironolactone.

Patients should be advised not to drive or use dangerous machines if affected by drowsiness, dizziness or mental confusion.

Pregnancy: Administration of spironolactone during pregnancy and lactation should be avoided as it crosses the placental barrier and one of its metabolites has been found in breast milk.

Adverse reactions: Dosage related gynaecomastia and breast tenderness may occur rarely which is usually reversible on cessation of treatment.

Other fairly common minor adverse reactions include nausea, vomiting, abdominal pain, diarrhoea or constipation, drowsiness, ataxia, drug fever, skin rashes, hair loss, contact dermatitis, eosinophilia, agranulocytosis, facial pigmentation, menstrual irregularities, impotence and mild androgenic effects.

Overdosage: Acute overdosage symptoms may include drowsiness, mental confusion, nausea, vomiting, dizziness or diarrhoea.

Symptoms of hyperkalaemia may occur and these include cardiac irregularities, paraesthesia, weakness, flaccid paralysis or muscle spasm.

There is no specific antidote.

Overdose should be treated by withdrawal of spironolactone and instigation of general supportive measures which should include maintaining the fluid balance together with an adequate supply of electrolytes (not potassium).

Emergency treatment of hyperkalaemia is by the administration of glucose and insulin together, possibly as continuous infusions to acutely lower plasma potassium. Thiazide diuretics to enhance renal loss of body potassium or oral ion exchange resins to retain potassium in the gastro-intestinal tract may be used as adjunctive treatment or used alone when urgent reduction of plasma potassium is not required.

Pharmaceutical precautions Spirolone tablets should be stored below 25°C and protected from light.

Legal category POM.

Package quantities Spirolone 25 mg: Polypropylene tubes of 500 tablets.
Spirolone 100 mg: Polypropylene tubes of 100 tablets.

Further information Periodic estimation of serum electrolytes is recommended especially for elderly patients and those with renal impairment.

Long term treatment of rats with high doses of spironolactone has been shown to produce tumours. Although the clinical significance of this is uncertain, long term use of spironolactone in young patients requires careful consideration of benefits and potential hazards.

Product licence numbers
Spirolone 25 mg Tablets 0289/0071
Spirolone 100 mg Tablets 0289/0072

Product licence holder: Approved Prescription Services Ltd.

TEMAZEPAM

Presentation Green, soft gelatin capsules containing temazepam 10 mg or 20 mg in a dark green gel. The 10 mg capsules are marked 10 and the 20 mg capsules 20 in white.

Uses Temazepam is indicated for the short-term treatment of insomnia when it is severe, disabling or subjecting the individual to extreme distress.

It is also indicated for pre-medication before minor surgical and investigatory procedures, particularly for out-patients.

Dosage and administration The lowest dose which can control the symptoms should be used. Long-term chronic use is not recommended; treatment should not normally continue beyond 4 weeks. Treatment with benzodiazepines should always be withdrawn gradually. Patients who have been receiving treatment for a long time may require longer periods during which the doses are reduced.

Insomnia

Adults: 10 to 30 mg orally half an hour before retiring. This dose will prove satisfactory for most patients but may be increased to 40 or 60 mg for those patients who do not respond to the lower dose. Treatment should, if possible, be intermittent.

Elderly: The elderly may respond to lower doses and half the normal adult dose or less may be sufficient.

Children: Not recommended.

Pre-medication (adults only): 20 to 40 mg from half to one hour before the surgical or investigatory procedures are undertaken.

Contra-indications, warnings, etc Benzodiazepines should not be used for phobic or obsessional states.

They should not be used alone to treat depression or anxiety associated with depression. Suicide may be precipitated in such patients.

They should not be used for the treatment of chronic psychosis.

Amnesia may occur.

In cases of loss or bereavement psychological adjustment may be inhibited by benzodiazepines.

Disinhibiting effects may be manifested in various ways. Suicide may be precipitated in patients who are depressed and aggressive behaviour toward self and others may be precipitated. Extreme caution should therefore be used in prescribing benzodiazepines in patients with personality disorders.

Withdrawal from benzodiazepines may be associated with physiological and psychological symptoms of withdrawal including depression. Withdrawal symptoms may occur following normal therapeutic doses given for short periods of time.

An underlying cause for insomnia should be sought before deciding upon the use of benzodiazepines for symptomatic relief.

Temazepam is also contra-indicated in known sensitivity to benzodiazepines and in acute pulmonary insufficiency.

Use in pregnancy: There is no information on the absolute safety of temazepam in human pregnancy. Do not use in pregnancy, especially during the first and third trimesters, unless there are compelling reasons.

Precautions:

1. When used for the treatment of insomnia, daytime drowsiness is unlikely to occur; however, patients should be cautioned against driving or operating machinery until it is clearly established that hangover effects are not a problem whilst taking temazepam.

Such effects are more liable to occur on higher doses of temazepam and in patients new to hypnotic therapy or in the elderly.

2. Patients should be advised not to consume alcohol whilst taking temazepam. The effects of other CNS depressants such as general anaesthetics, antidepressant drugs and monoamine oxidase inhibitors will be accentuated.

3. Prolonged or excessive use of benzodiazepines may lead to dependence, particularly when high dosages are used or when given over longer periods.

The likelihood of psychological dependence is greater in patients with a history of alcoholism, drug abuse or those with personality disorders. Regular monitoring of such patients is essential.

4. Withdrawal symptoms such as sweating, depression,

nervousness, irritability, diarrhoea and rebound insomnia have been reported following sudden discontinuation, particularly of prolonged or excessive treatment. In such cases treatment should be withdrawn gradually.

5. Temazepam capsules should be given with caution to patients with chronic pulmonary insufficiency or renal or hepatic dysfunction. They should also be avoided if possible during lactation.

Side-effects: Temazepam has a short half-life and its effects are generally restricted to within a few hours after ingestion. Drowsiness, dizziness and blurring of vision rarely occur. Such effects are more common in the elderly and are potentiated by alcohol.

Other rare adverse effects including hypotension, gastrointestinal upsets, transient skin rashes, urinary retention, headache, changes in libido, blood dyscrasias and jaundice have been reported.

Overdosage: Overdosage is rarely life threatening. Treatment should be generally supportive and symptomatic. In spite of the drug's rapid absorption and short half-life, gastric lavage may be useful if performed soon after ingestion.

Pharmaceutical precautions Store in a cool, dry place. Dispense, if necessary, into well closed glass or plastic containers.

Legal category CD (Sch 4), POM.

Package quantities
10 mg – containers of 250 and 500 capsules.
20 mg – containers of 250 and 100 capsules.

Further information Temazepam is a benzodiazepine with a short half-life of approximately 8 hours and is rapidly absorbed from the gelatin capsule formulation. It is mainly metabolised to a pharmacologically inactive glucuronide.

These factors provide prompt induction of sleep with a low incidence of hangover effects.

The lack of accumulation and the short action of this benzodiazepine offers advantage in the treatment of those patients where daytime alertness is desirable.

Product licence numbers
Capsules 10 mg 0152/0215.
Capsules 20 mg 0152/0216.

TETRACHEL*

Presentation *Tablets:* Orange film-coated Tetracycline Tablets BP 250 mg engraved BERK 3C7 or 3C7. Other ingredients include lactose, sunset yellow (E110).

Capsules: Orange Tetracycline Capsules BP 250 mg. Other ingredients include lactose, sunset yellow (E110).

Uses Infections caused by organisms sensitive to tetracycline. These include pneumonia, acute and chronic bronchitis, urinary tract infections, stagnant loop syndrome, severe acne vulgaris, rickettsial fevers, chlamydial infections, cholera, brucellosis, amoebic dysentery, gonorrhoea and syphilis.

Dosage and administration *Adults:* 1–2 tablets or capsules every six hours.

Elderly: One tablet or capsule every six hours.

Children: Not recommended.

Contra-indications, warnings, etc Tetrachel is contra-indicated in patients with renal impairment, hypersensitivity to tetracyclines, in children under the age of 12, and in lactation and throughout pregnancy.

Precautions and warnings: Tetracyclines should only be administered with great caution to patients with hepatic insufficiency. Careful monitoring of dosage by serum levels is necessary.

Tetracyclines should only be used with great caution in conjunction with other potentially hepatotoxic drugs.

Tetrachel should not be used in conjunction with penicillins.

Prolonged use of an anti-infective agent may result in the development of superinfection due to micro-organisms resistant to the anti-infective. Cross-resistance between tetracyclines may develop in micro-organisms, and cross-sensitisation in patients.

Bulging fontanelles in infants and benign intracranial hypertension in adults has been reported. Treatment should cease if evidence of raised intracranial pressure develops.

Other side-effects may include nausea, vomiting or diarrhoea and skin photosensitivity. If symptoms of glossitis, stomatitis, vaginitis or pruritus ani due to candidal overgrowth occur, dosing with Tetrachel should be discontinued. Resistant staphylococci may occasionally give rise to enterocolitis. Skin rashes and allergic reactions are rare. Tetracyclines are absorbed to some extent by developing bones and teeth and may produce staining and enamel hyperplasia.

Use in pregnancy and lactation: Tetracycline is contra-indicated during pregnancy, breast feeding and in children up to the age of 12 years, and should not be administered unless considered essential by the physician, and for as short a treatment period as feasible. Repeated courses should be avoided. The effect appears to be related to total dosage given and not only to duration of treatment.

Use in the elderly: Reduced renal clearance of tetracycline may be observed in elderly patients and multiple drug therapy in such patients may compete for drug binding sites. It may be necessary to adjust dosage to compensate for these factors.

Drug interactions: Administration of Tetrachel with milk products, antacids, zinc salts, magnesium, calcium or iron preparations may impair absorption of tetracycline.

Tetracyclines may prolong the action of coumarin anticoagulants, and may themselves delay coagulation.

There have been reports that the reliability of oral contraceptives may be reduced when Tetrachel is administered concomitantly. Extra precautions against conceiving are therefore advised in any cycle in which tetracycline is given.

Treatment of overdosage: Serious symptoms are unlikely. Gastric lavage might be beneficial in the first hours after ingestion followed by conservative management. Milk will reduce absorption.

Pharmaceutical precautions Store in a cool place.

Legal category POM.

Package quantities *Tablets:* Packs of 100 and 1,000.
Capsules: Containers of 100 and 500.

Further information Nil.

Product licence numbers
Tablets 0152/0095
Capsules 0152/5005

TRIMOPAN*

Presentation
Trimopan 200 mg tablet: White, circular, biconvex tablets, marked 'Berk 3H7' or '3H7' on one side with a single breakline on the reverse. Each tablet contains 200 mg Trimethoprim BP. Other ingredients include lactose.

Trimopan 100 mg tablets: White, circular, biconvex tablets marked 'Berk 2H7' or '2H7' on one side with a single break-line on the reverse. Each tablet contains 100 mg Trimethoprim BP. Other ingredients include lactose.

Trimopan suspension: White suspension containing 50 mg Trimethoprim BP in each 5 ml. Other ingredients include parabens.

Uses Trimopan has potent antimicrobial activity due to its selective inhibition of bacterial dihydrofolate reductase. It is effective *in-vitro* against most Gram-positive and Gram-negative aerobic organisms, including *Haemophilus influenzae. Streptococcus pneumoniae, Klebsiella pneumoniae, Staphylococcus aureus, E. coli, Enterobacter, Proteus* and *Streptococcus faecalis.*

Exceptions include anaerobic bacteria. *Mycobacterium tuberculosis, Neisseria gonorrhoeae, Pseudomonas aeruginosa* and *Treponema pallidum*.

Indications: Treatment of susceptible infections caused by trimethoprim-sensitive organisms including urinary tract and respiratory tract infections.

Prophylaxis of recurrent urinary tract infections.

Dosage and administration
Adults and children over 12 years of age: Treatment of urinary tract infections and all other susceptible infections: 200 mg twice daily.

Long-term prophylaxis of recurrent urinary tract infections: 100 mg at night.

Children 4 months to 12 years of age: Treatment of urinary tract infections and all other susceptible infections is based on a dosage of 6 mg/kg body-weight daily subdivided into two equal doses. Suggested regimens are:

4 months–2 years	25 mg twice daily
2–6 years	50 mg twice daily
6–12 years	100 mg twice daily

Long-term prophylaxis of recurrent urinary tract infections is based on 2.5 mg/kg body-weight daily given as a single dose at night. Suggested regimens are:

4 months–2 years	25 mg at night
2–8 years	50 mg at night
8–12 years	100 mg at night

Dosage recommendations for treatment in renal impairment: Trimethoprim serum levels should be monitored from Day 2 onwards in severe renal failure and from Day 4 onwards in mild to moderate failure to provide guidance as to the appropriate dosage reduction.

Renal function	*Initial dose* (Day 1)	*Continuation* (Day 2 onwards)
Mild renal failure (Creatinine clearance above 25 ml/min)	200 mg Twice daily	200 mg Twice daily
Mild to moderate renal failure (Creatinine clearance 10–25 ml/min)	200 mg Twice daily	100 mg Twice daily
Severe renal failure or anuria/severe uraemia (Creatinine clearance below 10 ml/min)	200 mg Twice daily	50–100 mg Twice daily

Dialysis patients: Trimethoprim is removed by dialysis. It should not however be administered to dialysis patients unless plasma concentrations can be estimated regularly.

Elderly: No special dosage recommendations.

Contra-indications, warnings, etc *Contra-indications:* Severe hepatic insufficiency. Severe renal insufficiency, unless blood trimethoprim concentrations can be monitored regularly.

Megaloblastic anaemia and other blood dyscrasias.

Trimethoprim should not be administered to pregnant women, premature infants or children under 4 months of age.

Precautions: In patients with marked impairment of renal function, care should be taken to avoid accumulation and resulting adverse haematological effects. Regular haematological tests should be undertaken in patients receiving long-term treatment and those predisposed to folate deficiency. Particular care should be exercised in the haematological monitoring of children on long-term therapy. The usual caution in prescribing any drug for women of childbearing age should be exercised with trimethoprim. Trimethoprim is excreted in breast milk but is not contra-indicated for short term use in lactating mothers.

Side-effects: Nausea, vomiting, gastrointestinal disturbance, headache, skin rashes and pruritus have been reported but are rare.

Isolated cases of megaloblastic anaemia during prolonged therapy with trimethoprim with doses higher than those recommended have been reported but these are reversible with discontinuation of therapy and administration of calcium folinate.

Use in pregnancy: Trimethoprim should not be administered to pregnant women.

Treatment of overdosage: Symptomatic treatment, gastric lavage and forced diuresis can be used. Depression of haematopoiesis by trimethoprim can be counteracted by intramuscular administration of calcium folinate.

Pharmaceutical precautions Trimopan suspension is sugar-free and may be diluted with water or Sorbitol Solution BP. The suspension should be discarded after completion of course of treatment. Protect from light.

Legal category POM.

Package quantities

200 mg tablets:	Containers of 100 tablets Cartons of 70 tablets consisting of 5 calendar foils of 14 tablets each
100 mg tablets:	Containers of 100 tablets.
10 mg/ml suspension:	Bottles of 100 ml.

Further information Nil.

Product licence numbers

200 mg tablets	0152/0162
100 mg tablets	0152/0156
10 mg/ml suspension	0152/0160.

VIDOPEN*

Presentation Red and pink Ampicillin Capsules BP 250 mg marked VIDOPEN 250 or 250 and 500 mg marked VIDOPEN 500 or 500. Other ingredients include erythrosine (E127).

Pink powder for Syrup 125 mg/5 ml (Ampicillin Mixture BPC), or Syrup Forte 250 mg/5 ml (strong Ampicillin Mixture BPC), wild cherry flavoured and containing ampicillin trihydrate equivalent to the stated quantities of ampicillin. Other ingredients include sucrose, amaranth (E123).

Each vial of Vidopen Injection contains 250 mg or 500 mg Ampicillin BP.

Uses Ampicillin is a broad-spectrum antibiotic active against Shigella, *Escherichia coli, Proteus mirabilis, Haemophilus influenzae, Bordetella pertussis* and other Gram-negative bacteria. *Actinomyces muris ratti* and other Actinomycetes, as well as penicillin-sensitive Gram-positive pathogens. Vidopen is therefore indicated in a wide range of infections, particularly those of the respiratory, urinary and digestive tracts where there may be multiple pathogens.

Vidopen is not effective against organisms resistant to penicillin, since it is inactivated by penicillinase.

Dosage and administration Vidopen should be taken half an hour before meals.

Adults (including elderly):

ENT infections: 250 mg four times daily.

Bronchitis: 250 mg four times daily, or up to 1 g four times daily in acute exacerbations.

Pneumonia: 500 mg four times daily.

Urinary tract infections: 500 mg three times daily.

Gastro-intestinal infections: 500–750 mg three or four times daily.

Children: Over 20 kg bodyweight: Adult dosage.

Under 20 kg bodyweight:

Moderately severe infections: 100 mg/kg/day in divided doses every six or eight hours.

Severe infections: 200 mg/kg/day in divided doses every six hours.

All recommended dosages are a guide only. In severe infections the above dosages may be increased.

Parenteral therapy is indicated, particularly for the urgent treatment of severe infection.

Vidopen Injection 250 mg: Intramuscular: add 1.5 ml water for injection to 250 mg vial contents.

Intravenous: dissolve 250 mg in 5 ml Water for

Injections BP. Administer by slow injection (3–4 minutes).

Vidopen Injection 500 mg: Intramuscular: add 1.5 ml of water for injection to 500 mg vial contents.

Intravenous: dissolve 500 mg in 2×5 ml Water for Injections BP. Administer by slow injection (3–4 minutes).

Vidopen Injection should be administered immediately after reconstitution. It should not be mixed with blood products or other proteinaceous fluids (e.g., protein hydrolysates).

Contra-indications, warnings, etc Known sensitivity to penicillin or the cephalosporins is a contra-indication. Patients should be questioned on this before Vidopen is prescribed.

Side-effects are rare and usually of a mild, transitory nature. Two types of rash have been observed: an urticarial rash which is usually indicative of true penicillin hypersensitivity and an erythematous rash which is generally specific to ampicillin. The incidence of this erythematous rash is particularly high in patients with infectious mononucleosis. If a rash is reported it is advisable to discontinue treatment.

Gastro-intestinal symptoms may occur but usually resolve rapidly when treatment is stopped. If they persist they may indicate overgrowth of resistant organisms, requiring specific treatment.

Ampicillin is inactivated by penicillinase and should therefore not be used to treat infections which have survived treatment with penicillin.

Use in pregnancy: Safety in pregnancy has not been established.

Treatment of overdosage: Serious symptoms are unlikely. Observation.

Pharmaceutical precautions Store in a cool dry place.

The suspension, when made up, should be stored in a cool place and used within seven days. It may be diluted with Syrup BP.

Legal category POM.

Package quantities *Capsules 250 mg:* Containers of 250 and 1,000.

Capsules 500 mg: Containers of 100 and 500.

Syrup: Bottles of 100 ml.

Syrup Forte: Bottles of 100 ml.

Injection 250 mg: Packs of 10.

Injection 500 mg: Packs of 10.

Further information Nil.

Product licence numbers

Capsules 250 mg	0152/0118
Capsules 500 mg	0152/0119
Syrup 125 mg/5 ml	0152/0120
Syrup Forte 250 mg/5 ml	0152/0121
Injection 250 mg	0152/0249
Injection 500 mg	0152/0250

**Trade Mark*

Bioglan Laboratories Limited
1 The Cam Centre
Wilbury Way
Hitchin, Herts SG4 0TW

BIOGLAN

BARITOP* 100

Presentation A white, smooth, pleasant-tasting suspension containing Barium Sulphate EP 100% w/v, with carbon dioxide as an effervescent agent.

Uses Baritop 100 is designed for double-contrast radiography and used as an X-ray contrast medium for the gastro-intestinal tract. It may be used undiluted or diluted with water for examination by oral administration, or by enema, in accordance with the area to be examined and the examination methods.

Dosage and administration Recommended doses vary according to the parts to be examined and examination methods. The following provides a guide on the use of Baritop 100 for an adult:

Area	*Method of administration*	*Barium sulphate concentration (% w/v)*	*Dosage (ml)*
Oesophagus	Oral	50–100	10–150
Stomach and duodenum	Oral	30–100	10–300
Small intestine	Oral	30–100	100–300
Colon	Enema	20–100	200–2000

Contra-indications, warnings, etc
Contra-indications: Barium meal examination
(a) Patients with suspected perforation or with haemorrhage in digestive organs.

Contra-indications: Barium enema examination
(a) Patients with suspected perforation or with haemorrhage of intestinal organs.
(b) Patients with extreme exhaustion (prostration).

Warnings: Use extreme caution in the following:
Barium meal examinations:
(a) Patients with fistulae in digestive organs, or who show symptoms of fistulae.
(b) Patients with strictures or symptoms of obstruction.
(c) Patients suffering from extreme exhaustion.

Barium enema examinations:
(a) Patients with fistulae in digestive organs, or symptoms of fistulae.
(b) Patients who have disease of intestinal organs, which could lead to perforation; appendicitis, diverticulitis, ulcerative colitis, invagination tumour, parasitism, etc.

Side effects: Constipation, transient diarrhoea, abdominal pain, anal pain, bleeding, etc.

Cautions: Water and laxatives should be given to patients to prevent constipation. Keep out of the reach of children.

Pharmaceutical precautions Store in a warm place.

Legal category P.

Package quantities Sealed cans containing 300 ml, with ring-pull opening.

Further information Baritop 100 possesses excellent adherence properties to the mucosal surface, higher barium content and low viscosity with uniform dispersibility to allow X-ray examination of the barium distended tract to be made with better contrast using the double-contrast method.

Product licence number 0041/0024.

BARITOP* PLUS

Presentation Fine white granules of barium sulphate for suspension with water.

Uses X-ray contrast medium for radiography of the gastro-intestinal tract.

Dosage and administration Use Baritop Plus suspension prepared with the required amount of water, for examination by oral administration or by enema, utilising the appropriate examination method.

The table below provides a guide on the use of Baritop Plus.

Contra-indications, warnings, etc Suspected perforation of the gastro-intestinal tract, and caution should be exercised if there is a possibility of obstruction of the lower small bowel.

Side-effects: Side-effects may be experienced in some patients after examination. Constipation, transient diarrhoea, abdominal pain, anal pain, bleeding, etc.

Cautions: Caution after examination. Water and laxatives should be given to patients to prevent constipation. Keep out of the reach of children.

Pharmaceutical precautions Store in a dry place.

Legal category P.

Package quantities Supplied in sachets containing 200 g of barium sulphate powder.

Further information Nil.

Product licence number 0041/0025.

BENZAGEL* 5
BENZAGEL* 10

Presentation Benzagel 5 is a white gel containing 5% w/w micronised benzoyl peroxide.

Benzagel 10 is a white gel containing 10% w/w micronised benzoyl peroxide.

Uses Benzagel is indicated as an aid in the treatment of

Area	*Method of administration*	*Barium sulphate concentration (% w/v)*	*Dosage (ml)*	*Guide to prepare suspension (each 200 g of Baritop Plus)* Concentration	Water	Total volume
Oesophagus	Oral	50–200	10–150	140% w/v	85 ml	135 ml
Stomach and duodenum	Oral	30–200	10–300	150% w/v	75 ml	125 ml
Small bowel	Oral	30–150	100–300	200% w/v	45 ml	95 ml
Colon	Enema	20–130	200–2000			

acne, providing drying, desquamative and antiseptic activity.

Dosage and administration *Adults and children:* Commence treatment with Benzagel 5. Wash the affected areas with soap and water, dry and apply Benzagel once or twice daily.

The therapeutic response to benzoyl peroxide differs in individual patients and, in order to provide a satisfactory drying and desquamative action, it may be necessary to increase the strength to Benzagel 10.

Contra-indications, warnings, etc
Contra-indications: Patients with a known sensitivity to benzoyl peroxide.

Warnings: For external use only. To avoid irritation, take care to keep the product away from the mouth, eyes and other mucous membranes.

Precautions: The product should be applied with caution to sensitive areas, such as the neck and shoulders. Avoid contact with clothing and fabric.

Side-effects: In normal use a mild burning sensation will probably be felt on first application, and a moderate reddening and peeling of the skin will occur within a few days. During the first few weeks of treatment, a sudden increase in peeling will occur in most patients. This is not harmful and will subside within a day or two if the treatment is temporarily discontinued.

Pharmaceutical precautions Store in a cool place.

Legal category P.

Package quantities Benzagel 5 and Benzagel 10 are supplied in plastic tubes, each containing 40 g.

Further information The formulation of Benzagel contains micronised benzoyl peroxide which ensures a uniform dispersion of the active ingredient throughout the gel. Skin penetration is provided by the gel base, which dries to an invisible film.

Ingredients: Benzoyl Peroxide, Industrial Methylated Spirit 96 DMI, Carbopol 940, Sodium Hydroxide, Dioctyl Sodium Sulphosuccinate, Methyl Salicylate BP, Lemon Balm P14010, Purified Water BP.

Product licence numbers

Benzagel 5	3384/0005
Benzagel 10	3384/0006

BIOGLAN* EFFERVESCENT GRANULES

Presentation Fine white granules containing per dose of 3 g, Tartaric Acid EP 1.05 g, Sodium Bicarbonate EP 1.05 g, Dimethylpolysiloxane EP 0.15 g.

Uses Supplementary gas producing agent for double-contrast radiography of the stomach.

Dosage and administration One vial (3 g) granules should be placed at the back of the tongue and washed down immediately with either a small amount of water (10 ml) or barium suspension at the beginning of the double-contrast examination.

Contra-indications, warnings, etc Nil.

Pharmaceutical precautions Store in a cool, dry place.

Legal category P.

Package quantities Supplied in vials containing 3 g. 10 vials per tray, five trays per carton (50 doses per carton).

Further information Nil.

Product licence number 0603/0025.

BIORPHEN*

Presentation A colourless, aniseed flavoured solution for oral application, each 5 ml containing 25 mg of orphenadrine hydrochloride.

Uses Biorphen is an anticholinergic preparation for the treatment of the Parkinsonian syndrome. It is indicated for all forms of Parkinsonism, including the drug-induced neuroleptic syndrome.

Dosage and administration
Adults: Treatment is usually started at 150 mg daily, in divided doses. Optimum dosage is usually in the range of 150–300 mg daily in divided doses, and is achieved by raising the dose by 25–50 mg every two or three days.

Biorphen is suitable for drug-induced Parkinsonism, especially where mood elevation is required.

Contra-indications, warnings, etc
Contra-indications: Biorphen is contra-indicated in patients with glaucoma, prostatic hypertrophy and tardive dyskinesia.

Precautions and warnings: Caution must be observed in pregnancy, and obstructive disease in the gastro-intestinal or genito-urinary tracts. Due care should be taken with Biorphen therapy in patients with concomitant hypertension, cardiac, liver or kidney dysfunction.

Side effects: A transient feeling of numbness of the mouth and tongue, leading to subsequent dryness of the mouth. Disturbances of vision or micturition may also occur but may be resolved by adjustment to lower doses. Less commonly, tachycardia, hypersensitivity, nervousness, insomnia and euphoria may be experienced.

Overdosage: Give gastric lavage, emetic and high enema for severe anticholinergic intoxication. Cholinergic agents such as carbachol may be useful, together with non-specific general treatment.

Pharmaceutical precautions Store at room temperature, protect from light.

Legal category POM.

Package quantities Bottles of 200 ml and 1 litre, each containing 25 mg Orphenadrine Hydrochloride BP in 5 ml of sucrose-free base.

Further information Nil.

Product licence number 0041/0028.

BROFLEX*

Presentation A pink-coloured, blackcurrant flavoured syrup, each 5 ml containing 5 mg of benzhexol hydrochloride.

Uses Benzhexol is a parasympatholytic drug used in the treatment of Parkinsonian syndrome. It is indicated for post-encephalitic, arteriosclerotic and idiopathic Parkinsonism as well as drug-induced Parkinsonism, the neuroleptic syndrome caused by drugs such as reserpine and the phenothiazines acting on the central nervous system. Benzhexol antagonises some of the actions of acetylcholine, although it is less active than atropine.

Benzhexol increases mobility and decreases rigidity in patients with the Parkinsonian syndrome. The frequency of oculogyric crises are diminished; tremor and excessive salivation are also reduced.

Benzhexol is also useful in relieving the associated depression and mental inertia characteristic of Parkinsonism.

Dosage and administration Suitable for adults only.

Treatment is usually begun with a low dose of 1 mg per day, and gradually increased over a period of several days by 1 mg or 2 mg at a time. Similarly, if the dose of Broflex is to be decreased, this too should be done gradually. Elderly patients tend to respond to lower doses of the drug, whilst post-encephalitic patients generally tolerate the drug well and require higher doses.

Dosage ranges are as follows:

Parkinsonism: Usual treatment is within the dosage

range of 6–10 mg per day although, in cases of post-encephalitic Parkinsonism, the total daily dose may be as high as 15–20 mg.

Drug-induced Parkinsonism: The dose required for this category is usually between 5 mg and 15 mg per day.

The above doses are total daily doses and should be given as divided doses three or four times a day, either before or after food, depending on the response of the patient. In patients experiencing dryness of the mouth, Broflex should be taken before meals. If nausea occurs, the patient is advised to take Broflex after meals.

If patients already undergoing treatment with parasympathetic inhibitors, Broflex should be substituted as part of the therapy.

Contra-indications, warnings, etc
Precautions and warnings: Broflex therapy should be carefully monitored for allergic or other untoward reactions. This monitoring should be a continual process as therapy is long term. Incipient glaucoma can be precipitated by Broflex and caution should be used in patients with glaucoma. Caution must be observed in patients with obstructive disease in either the gastrointestinal or genito-urinary tract, and in elderly males with prostatic hypertrophy. Due care should be taken with Broflex therapy in patients with concomitant hypertension, cardiac, liver or kidney dysfunction.

Patients with arteriosclerosis or past history of other drug idiosyncrasy may display reactions of mental agitation and confusion, or nausea and vomiting. These patients should be started on the smaller dose, with gradual increases until an effective dose is reached. This titration of dosage may assist in minimising dose-related side-effects.

Side-effects: Giddiness, dryness of the mouth, nausea and vomiting, and blurred vision occur initially in a third to a half of all patients, but these effects diminish as therapy continues. Dosage reduction is advised if these effects continue.

Overdose: Give gastric lavage, emetic and high enema. Atropine antagonists may be useful. Usual general treatment, cold compresses and forced fluid intake are mandatory.

Pharmaceutical precautions Store at room temperature, protect from light. Syrup BP may be used as a diluent. Diluted syrups are stable for fourteen days.

Legal category POM.

Package quantities Bottles of 200 ml containing 5 mg benzhexol hydrochloride in 5 ml of syrup base.

Further information Nil.

Product licence number 0041/0029.

CITRAMAG*

Presentation A sachet containing a white, effervescent powder which produces 17.7 g magnesium citrate in aqueous solution, equivalent in alkalinity to 5 g magnesium oxide.

Uses For preparation of the patient for all radiological examinations requiring a completely evacuated bowel. May also be used for colorectal surgery.

Dosage and administration A high fluid, low-residue diet is begun on the day before the examination. Before 6.00 pm on the day before the examination, the aqueous solution of magnesium citrate is prepared and the solution is taken orally at 8.00 pm. On the day of the examination, no food should be consumed until after the examination, but plain water may be drunk.

Contra-indications, warnings, etc
Contra-indications: There are no contra-indications.

Precautions and warnings: For particular patients, chiefly those who are in renal failure, it may be necessary to modify the instructions supplied to the patient with Citramag, as explained below.

When any doubts exist about the suitability of the routine instructions, the advice of the treating physician should be obtained. It should be noted that fruit juice, which has a high content of potassium, should be avoided in conditions in which hyperkalaemia can occur, such as Addison's disease, selective hypoaldosteronism, and treatment with spironolactones, triamterene or amiloride.

Similarly, the risk of toxic hypermagnesaemia indicates the need for caution in the administration of magnesium citrate to patients in renal failure. The dosage of magnesium citrate solution may be reduced for very ill or very thin, elderly patients who may tolerate vigorous purgation poorly.

Pharmaceutical precautions Store in a cool, dry place – below 25°C.

Legal category P.

Package quantities Sachet containing 29.5 g of powder.

Further information Nil.

Product licence number 0041/0030.

HYDROCAL* CREAM

Presentation Hydrocal is a pale pink cream containing Hydrocortisone Acetate BP 1% w/w, in an emollient base containing Calamine BP.

Uses Hydrocal is indicated for the relief of the inflammatory manifestations of corticosteroid-responsive dermatoses including seborrhoeic dermatitis, eczema including atopic infantile discoid and stasis eczema, photodermatitis, primary irritant and allergic dermatitis, insect bite reactions and napkin rash or urinary dermatitis.

Dosage and administration
Adults, elderly: Apply three or four times daily.
Children, infants: A small quantity should be applied to the affected area two or three times daily.

Contra-indications, warnings, etc
Contra-indications: Tuberculosis, fungal, bacterial and viral infections; known hypersensitivity to Hydrocal or any of its ingredients.

Precautions: Extreme caution is required in dermatoses of infancy. In infants and children, long-term continuous topical therapy should be avoided where possible, as adrenal suppression can occur even without occlusion. In infants, the napkin may act as an occlusive dressing and increase absorption. Treatment should therefore be limited, if possible, to a maximum of seven days. Avoid use close to the eye.

Appropriate antimicrobial therapy should be used whenever treating inflammatory lesions which have become infected. Any spread of infection requires withdrawal of topical corticosteroid therapy, and administration of systemic antimicrobial agents.

As with all corticosteroids, prolonged application to the face is undesirable.

Pregnancy and lactation: There is inadequate evidence of safety in human pregnancy. Topical administration of corticosteroids to pregnant animals can cause abnormalities of foetal development. There may therefore be a very small risk of such effects in the human foetus.

Side-effects: Preparations containing hydrocortisone are usually well tolerated, but if signs of hypersensitivity appear, application should stop immediately.

Local atrophic changes may occur where skin folds are involved, or in sites such as the nappy area in small children, where constant moist conditions favour the absorption of hydrocortisone. Sufficient systemic absorption may also occur in such sites to produce the features of hypercorticism and suppression of the HPA axis after prolonged treatment. This effect is more likely to occur in infants and children, and if occlusive dressings are used.

Pharmaceutical precautions Store below 25°C.

Legal category POM.

Package quantities Hydrocal Cream is supplied in tubes containing 25 g.

Further information Ingredients: Hydrocortisone acetate BP, Calamine BP, emulsifying wax, oleyl alcohol, light mineral oil, Phenonip, Polysorbate 20, Bronopol BP, and Purified Water PhEur.

Product licence number 0041/0001.

ISOTRATE* 20

Presentation Isotrate 20 tablets are white, round biconvex uncoated tablets imprinted 'Bioglan ISMN 20' one face and plain on the reverse. Each tablet contains isosorbide mononitrate 20 mg.

Uses Isotrate is indicated for the prophylaxis of angina pectoris.

Isotrate is not indicated in the management of acute attacks of angina pectoris.

Mode of action: Isosorbide-5-mononitrate is an active metabolite of isosorbide dinitrate and from an oral dose exerts qualitatively similar effects. However, unlike the dinitrate which is subject to extensive 'first pass' hepatic metabolism, it has virtually complete systemic availability from an oral dose. Isosorbide mononitrate thus achieves predictable and sustained blood levels. Onset of pharmacological effects occur within 20 minutes of an oral dose and are maintained for more than 8 hours. Isosorbide-5-mononitrate is mainly eliminated via metabolism in the liver. The inactive metabolites are mainly excreted via the kidneys.

Dosage and administration
Adults: Usually one tablet twice or three times daily. Patients already accustomed to prophylactic nitrate therapy (for example with isosorbide dinitrate) may normally be transferred directly to a therapeutic dose of Isotrate. For patients not receiving prophylactic nitrate therapy, it is recommended that the initial dose should be one Isotrate tablet daily. Maintenance dose in individual patients will be between 20 mg and 120 mg daily.

Elderly patients: As for Adults, but particular care is required because of susceptibility to hypotension.

The tablets should be swallowed whole with a little fluid.

Children: Safety and efficacy in children has not been established.

Contra-indications, warnings, etc
Contra-indications: A known sensitivity to the drug or to isosorbide dinitrate, acute myocardial infarction with low filling pressures, acute circulatory failure (shock), severe hypotension or cerebral trauma, marked anaemia or hypovolaemia.

Precautions and warnings: Side-effects include hypotension, headache, dizziness and nausea. Usually, these respond to temporary reduction in dose on continued therapy.

Nitrates may give rise to symptoms of collapse after the first dose in patients with labile circulation. These symptoms can largely be avoided if the treatment is started with a low dose.

Isosorbide mononitrate should be used with caution in patients who are predisposed to closed angle glaucoma.

Headache may occur at the onset of treatment but will usually subside after a few days; if the headache persists dosage should be temporarily decreased.

Isosorbide mononitrate should be used with caution in patients suffering from hypothyroidism, hypothermia, malnutrition, severe liver or renal disease.

Pregnancy and lactation: As with other drugs, nitrates should not be administered to pregnant women and nursing mothers unless essential.

Overdosage: Overdosage should be treated symptomatically. The main symptom is likely to be hypotension and this may be treated by elevation of the legs to promote venous return.

Pharmaceutical precautions Store at room temperature. Protect from moisture.

Legal category P.

Package quantities Isotrate is blister packed in cartons of 60 tablets.

Further information Isosorbide mononitrate is the British Approved Name for Isosorbide-5-mononitrate.

Product licence number 0041/0006.

NOVARUCA*

Presentation A clear orange, water-miscible gel containing activated glutaraldehyde 10% w/w.

Uses For the topical treatment of viral warts including plantar warts, with the exception of warts on the face and those in the anal and perineal regions.

Dosage and administration To be applied to the wart twice daily. Cover with an adhesive dressing if required. Pare down any hard skin if it develops around the wart. If required, protect the surrounding skin with a thin film of petroleum jelly before application.

Contra-indications, warnings, etc
Contra-indications: The product should not be used on warts on the face, mucosa or perineum. Do not apply to broken skin.

Warnings: Keep away from the eyes. For external use only.

Other effects: Glutaraldehyde will stain the outer layers of the skin brown, thus indicating that treatment has been effected.

Pharmaceutical precautions Store in a cool place at a temperature below 25°C.

Legal category P.

Package quantity Tubes containing 15 g.

Further information Nil.

Product licence number 0041/0015

PRAGMATAR* CREAM

Presentation Pragmatar Cream is a pale, buff-coloured, oil-in-water cream containing 4% w/w cetyl alcohol-coal tar distillate, 3% w/w precipitated sulphur, and 3% w/w salicylic acid.

Uses Pragmatar has mild antipruritic, antiseptic, and keratolytic properties. It is indicated in the treatment of dandruff, other seborrhoeic conditions, and common scaly skin disorders.

Dosage and administration
Adults and children: For mild dandruff, apply the cream once a week when the hair is washed. For more severe cases, treat the entire scalp daily at bedtime, applying lightly but thoroughly with the fingertips. The cream can be washed out the next morning or when convenient. For other indicated subacute or chronic skin disorders, apply daily in small quantities to affected areas only.

For use in infants, the cream may be diluted by mixing with a few drops of water in the palm of the hand.

Contra-indications, warnings, etc
Contra-indication: Do not use in patients who are sensitive to sulphur, or in the presence of acute local infection.

Caution: Use with care near the eyes, mucous membranes, or on acutely inflamed areas. If any cream should accidentally enter the eye, flush with normal saline solution.

Adverse reactions: No side-effects are to be expected if

the cream is used according to directions. Excessive use, however, may cause erythema and irritation.

Overdosage: If ingestion occurs, gastro-intestinal disturbances may follow. Treatment consists of rinsing out the mouth together with symptomatic measures if necessary. Even with massive ingestion, salicylate poisoning seems unlikely.

Pharmaceutical precautions Store in a cool place.

Legal Category P.

Package quantities Tubes containing 25 g and 100 g.

Further information Any queries should be addressed to the Medical Information Department of the Product Licence Holder: Smith Kline & French Laboratories Ltd.

Ingredients: Cetyl alcohol-coal tar distillate, Precipitated Sulphur BP, Salicylic Acid BP, Sodium Carboxymethyl cellulose 7MF, Glycerol PhEur, Sodium Lauryl Sulphate BP, Cetyl Alcohol, light Liquid Paraffin BP, Perfume Bouquet 3522, Purified Water PhEur.

Product licence number 0002/5044.

Product licence holder: Smith Kline & French Laboratories Ltd, Welwyn Garden City.

VIRUDOX*

Presentation A clear, colourless solution containing Idoxuridine BP 5% in dimethyl sulphoxide.

Uses
Action: Idoxuridine exerts its antiviral activity by blocking the uptake of thymidine into viral DNA. It inhibits the replication of DNA-viruses, including adenovirus, cytomegalovirus, herpes simplex and vaccinia. Dimethyl sulphoxide aids the penetration of idoxuridine into the deeper layers of the epidermis where the virus is replicating.

Indications: Cutaneous herpes simplex and herpes zoster (shingles).

Dosage and administration
Adults (including the elderly): Virudox should be painted on the lesions and erythematous bases four times daily for four days. Treatment should be initiated upon diagnosis of the condition, preferably within two to three days of the rash appearing.

Treatment may be less successful if not started within seven days of onset of symptoms.

Children (under 12 years of age): Not recommended.

Contra-indications, warnings, etc
Contra-indications: Use in pregnancy. Known hypersensitivity to idoxuridine or dimethyl sulphoxide.

Use in pregnancy and lactation: Animal studies have shown idoxuridine to be teratogenic and therefore its use in pregnancy or patients at risk of becoming pregnant is contra-indicated.

The taste of breast milk may be made unpleasant if treatment is administered during lactation.

Side-effects: Transient stinging on application and a distinctive taste during the course of treatment are frequently experienced. Skin reactions have been reported.

Warnings: Accidental contact with the eye causes stinging and should be treated by washing out with water. Excessive usage may lead to maceration of the skin. Use inside the mouth is not advised.

Overdosage: There are no clinical reports of overdosage. Supportive measures should be instituted.

Pharmaceutical precautions Virudox should be stored in its original container at room temperature. Do not refrigerate as the contents of the bottle may solidify. In this case, the bottle should be warmed gently until the contents become liquid.

Legal category POM.

Package quantities Bottle containing 5 ml with brush.

Further information Virudox can damage synthetic materials and some printed cotton fabrics. Contact between Virudox and these materials should therefore be avoided.

Ingredients: Idoxuridine BP, Dimethyl Sulphoxide.

Product licence number 0041/0007.

**Trade Mark*

Boehringer Ingelheim Limited
Ellesfield Avenue
Bracknell
Berkshire RG12 4YS

ALUPENT*

Presentation *Alupent Tablets:* White/off white compressed tablets, scored and impressed with the letters 'At' on one side and with the Company symbol on the reverse. Each tablet contains orciprenaline sulphate 20 mg.

Alupent Syrup: Clear, colourless syrup with vanilla-like flavour. Each 5 ml contains orciprenaline sulphate 10 mg.

Alupent Metered Aerosol: 15 ml vial (300 metered doses) available as complete unit with mouthpiece or as refill vial only. Each metered dose contains orciprenaline sulphate 750 micrograms (670 micrograms available to the patient).

Uses *Action:* Alupent is a sympathomimetic amine with bronchodilator properties.

Indications: Alupent is indicated for the relief of bronchospasm, as in asthma, bronchitis and emphysema.

Alupent tablets and syrup are suggested for maintenance therapy.

Alupent metered aerosol is indicated for the relief of acute attacks.

Dosage and administration *Orally*

	Tablets 20 mg	*Syrup 10 mg in 5 ml*
Adults	1 four times daily	2 × 5 ml four times daily
Children 3–12 years	½ four times daily to 1 three times daily	1 × 5 ml four times daily to 2 × 5 ml three times daily
Children 1–3 years	Syrup recommended	½ × 5 ml four times daily to 1 × 5 ml four times daily
Children 0–1 year	Syrup recommended	½ × 5 ml three times daily to 1 × 5 ml three times daily

By inhalation

Metered Aerosol 750 micrograms per puff (670 micrograms available to the patient):

Adults: 1 or 2 puffs. Not to be repeated within 30 minutes. No more than 12 puffs in 24 hours.

Children 6–12 years: 1 or 2 puffs. Not to be repeated within 30 minutes. No more than 4 doses in 24 hours.

Children under 6 years: 1 puff. Not to be repeated within 30 minutes. No more than 4 puffs in 24 hours.

Diluents: Alupent Syrup may be diluted with either Syrup BP or Sorbitol Solution BP.

No specific information on the use of this product in the elderly is available. Clinical trials have included patients over 65 years and no adverse reactions specific to this age group have been reported.

Contra-indications, warnings, etc
Contra- indications: Thyrotoxicosis.

Precautions: Caution should be observed should it be necessary to administer Alupent to patients with myocardial insufficiency, angina, cardiac dysrhythmias, hypertension or hypertrophic subvalvular aortic stenosis. In view of the possible interaction between sympathomimetic amines and monoamine oxidase inhibitors, care should be exercised if it is proposed to administer an MAO inhibitor concurrently with Alupent. Caution should be observed with the use of Alupent if a patient is already receiving other sympathomimetic agents as cardiovascular effects may be additive.

Patients must be instructed in the correct use of a metered aerosol, and warned not to exceed the prescribed dose. Patients should also be warned to seek medical advice if a reduced response becomes apparent.

Although Alupent has been in wide general use for many years, there is no definite evidence of ill-consequence during human pregnancy. Only in doses much higher than the equivalent maximum therapeutic dose in man were effects on foetal development seen in animals. Alupent treatment may result in the prolongation of pregnancy and inhibition of labour. Medicines should not be used in pregnancy, especially the first trimester, unless the expected benefit is thought to outweigh any possible risk to the foetus.

Beta-adrenergic blocking agents may antagonise Alupent and reduce its bronchodilator effect if administered concurrently.

Side-effects: Transitory sympathomimetic side-effects, such as tremor, palpitation, tachycardia and headache, have occasionally been reported, as have nausea and abdominal discomfort.

Overdosage: No fatal doses have been reported but the following single dose should be considered toxic – 200 mg orally.

Overdosage may be manifest by tachycardia, palpitation, increase in systolic blood pressure, decrease in diastolic blood pressure, tremor and anxiety. It is suggested that the patient should be treated symptomatically, but care should be taken if beta-adrenergic blocking drugs are used in patients liable to bronchospasm.

Pharmaceutical precautions Alupent preparations should be protected from heat, light and air. Aerosol vials should not be incinerated or opened even when apparently empty.

Legal category POM.

Package quantities *Tablets:* Pack of 112 (OP).

Syrup: Packs of 300 ml (OP) and 2 litres.

Metered Aerosol: 15 ml vial (300 metered doses) (OP) complete with mouthpiece. 15 ml refill vial.

Further information Nil.

Product licence numbers

Alupent Tablets	0015/0046
Alupent Syrup	0015/0001
Alupent Metered Aerosol	0015/5002

ATROVENT*

Presentation *Metered dose inhaler:* 10 ml vial (200 metered doses) available as complete unit with mouthpiece. Each metered dose contains ipratropium bromide 20 micrograms of which 18 micrograms is available to the patient.

Uses *Action:* Atrovent is an anticholinergic bronchodilator.

Indications: Atrovent metered dose inhaler is indicated in the treatment of chronic reversible airways obstruction, particularly in chronic bronchitis.

Dosage and administration *Adults:* Usually 1 or 2 puffs three or four times daily, although some patients may need up to 4 puffs at a time to obtain maximum benefit during early treatment.

Children: 6–12 years: usually 1 or 2 puffs three times daily. Under 6 years: usually 1 puff three times daily.

In order to ensure that the inhaler is used correctly, administration should be supervised by an adult.

No specific information on the use of this product in the elderly is available. Clinical trials have included patients over 65 years and no adverse reactions specific to this age group have been reported.

Contra-indications, warnings, etc
Contra-indications: Known hypersensitivity to atropine.

Precautions: The patient should be warned to seek medical advice should a reduced response become apparent.

Patients must be instructed in the correct use of a metered dose inhaler and warned against the accidental release of the contents into the eye. Generally, caution is advocated in the use of anticholinergic agents in patients with glaucoma or prostatic hypertrophy. However, specific studies with Atrovent in patients with glaucoma showed that inhaling cumulative doses of 160 micrograms had no effect on the eye.

Atrovent has been in general use for several years and there is no definite evidence of ill-consequence during pregnancy; animal studies have shown no hazard. Nevertheless, medicines should not be used in pregnancy, especially during the first trimester, unless the expected benefit is thought to outweigh any possible risk to the foetus.

Side-effects: Anticholinergic side-effects are unlikely to occur at therapeutic doses although dry mouth has occasionally been reported. Urinary retention and constipation have only rarely been reported with Atrovent. There is no evidence that in the therapeutic dose range Atrovent has any adverse effect on bronchial secretion.

Overdosage: Inhaled doses of 5 mg produce an increase in heart rate and palpitation. Single doses of ipratropium bromide 30 mg by mouth caused anticholinergic side-effects but these were not severe and did not require specific reversal.

Pharmaceutical precautions Protect from heat including the sun. The vials should not be punctured or incinerated even when apparently empty. Protect from frost.

Legal category POM.

Package quantities 10 ml vial (200 metered doses) (OP) complete with mouthpiece.

Further information There is evidence that the concurrent administration of Atrovent and sympathomimetic drugs produces a greater relief of bronchospasm than either drug given alone.

Atrovent has been shown to produce effective bronchodilatation in patients receiving beta-adrenergic blocking agents.

Patients should be informed when starting treatment that the onset of action of Atrovent is slower than that of inhaled sympathomimetic bronchodilators.

Atrovent is also available as Atrovent Forte (40 micrograms per puff) and as a nebuliser solution (250 micrograms per ml).

Product licence number Atrovent metered dose inhaler 0015/0043

ATROVENT* FORTE METERED DOSE INHALER

Presentation Metered dose inhaler 10 ml (200 metered doses) available as complete unit with mouthpiece. Each metered dose contains ipratropium bromide 40 micrograms of which 36 micrograms is available to the patient.

Uses *Action:* Atrovent is an anticholinergic bronchodilator.

Indications: Atrovent is indicated in the treatment of chronic reversible airways obstruction, particularly in chronic bronchitis.

Dosage and administration
Adults: Usually 1 puff three or four times daily, although some patients may need 2 puffs at a time to obtain maximum benefit during early treatment.
Children: 6–12 years – usually 1 puff three times daily.

In order to ensure that the inhaler is used correctly, administration should be supervised by an adult.

No specific information on the use of this product in the elderly is available. Clinical trials with Atrovent MDI have included patients over 65 years and no adverse reactions specific to this age group have been reported.

Contra-indications, warnings, etc
Contra-indications: Known hypersensitivity to atropine.

Precautions: The patient should be warned to seek medical advice should a reduced response become apparent.

Patients must be instructed in the correct use of a metered dose inhaler and warned against accidental release of the contents into the eye. Generally, caution is advocated in the use of anticholinergic agents in patients with glaucoma or prostatic hypertrophy. However, specific studies with Atrovent in patients with glaucoma showed that inhaling cumulative doses of 160 micrograms had no effect on the eye.

Atrovent has been in general use for several years and there is no definite evidence of ill-consequence during pregnancy; animal studies have shown no hazard. Nevertheless, medicines should not be used in pregnancy, especially during the first trimester, unless the expected benefit is thought to outweigh any possible risk to the foetus.

Side-effects: Anticholinergic side-effects are unlikely to occur at therapeutic doses, although dry mouth has occasionally been reported. Urinary retention and constipation have only rarely been reported with Atrovent. There is no evidence that in the therapeutic dose range Atrovent has any adverse effect on bronchial secretion.

Overdosage: Inhaled doses of 5 mg produce an increase in heart rate and palpitation. Single doses of ipratropium bromide 30 mg by mouth caused anticholinergic side-effects but these were not severe and did not require specific reversal.

Pharmaceutical precautions Protect from heat including the sun. The vials should not be punctured or incinerated even when apparently empty.

Legal category POM

Package quantities 10 ml vial (200 metered doses) (OP) complete with mouthpiece.

Further information There is evidence that the concurrent administration of Atrovent and sympathomimetic drugs produces a greater relief of bronchospasm than either drug given alone.

Atrovent has been shown to produce effective bronchodilatation in patients receiving beta-adrenergic blocking agents.

Patients should be informed when starting treatment that the onset of action of Atrovent is slower than that of inhaled sympathomimetic bronchodilators.

Atrovent is also available as a metered dose inhaler providing 20 micrograms per metered dose and as a nebuliser solution (250 micrograms per ml).

Product licence number 0015/0107.

ATROVENT NEBULISER SOLUTION

Presentation Plastic vial containing an isotonic, preservative-free solution of ipratropium bromide 0.025% (250 micrograms/ml) for administration by inhalation. Two types of vial are available:

A vial containing 500 micrograms ipratropium bromide, i.e. 2 ml solution.

A vial containing 250 micrograms ipratropium bromide, i.e. 1 ml solution.

Uses
Action: Ipratropium bromide is an anticholinergic bronchodilator.

Indications: Atrovent Nebuliser Solution is indicated in the treatment of reversible airways obstruction.

Dosage and administration Atrovent Nebuliser Solution may be administered from an intermittent positive pressure ventilator or from suitable nebulisers.

The recommended dose is:

Adults: 0.4–2.0 ml solution (100–500 micrograms) up to 4 times daily.

Children: (3–14 years) 0.4–2.0 ml solution (100–500 micrograms) up to 3 times daily.

The dose of nebuliser solution may need to be diluted in order to obtain a final volume suitable for the particular nebuliser being used; if dilution is necessary use only sterile sodium chloride 0.9% solution.

There is no specific information on the use of isotonic Atrovent Nebuliser Solution in the elderly. Clinical trials with the previously available hypotonic formulation included patients over 65 years and no adverse reactions specific to this age group were reported.

Contra-indications, warnings, etc
Contra-indications: Known hypersensitivity to atropine.

Precautions: Administration of Atrovent nebuliser solution has been associated with occasional reports of paradoxical bronchospasm during early treatment. Use of the nebuliser solution should always be initiated in hospital and be subject to close medical supervision during the first week of treatment. The patient should be advised to seek medical advice should a reduced response become apparent.

Patients must be instructed in the correct administration of Atrovent nebuliser solution and warned not to allow the solution or mist to enter the eyes. Generally, caution is advocated in the use of anticholinergic agents in patients with glaucoma or prostatic hypertrophy. However, specific studies with Atrovent metered dose inhaler in patients with glaucoma showed that inhaling cumulative doses of 160 micrograms had no effect on the eye.

Atrovent has been in general use for several years and there is no definite evidence of ill-consequence during pregnancy; animal studies have shown no hazard. Nevertheless, medicines should not be used in pregnancy, especially during the first trimester, unless the expected benefit is thought to outweigh any possible risk to the foetus.

Side-effects: Anticholinergic side-effects are unlikely at therapeutic doses, but some patients may complain of a dry mouth. Urinary retention and constipation have only rarely been reported with Atrovent.

There is no evidence that in the therapeutic dose range Atrovent has any adverse effect on bronchial secretion.

Overdosage: Inhaled doses of 5 mg produce an increase in heart rate and palpitation but single doses of 2 mg have been given to adults and 1 mg to children without causing side-effects. Single doses of ipratropium bromide 30 mg by mouth cause anticholinergic side-effects but these are not severe and do not require specific reversal.

Pharmaceutical precautions Store at room temperature. Protect from heat and light. This product contains no preservative. A fresh vial should be used for each dose and the vial shold be opened immediately before administration. Any solution left in the vial should be discarded.

Legal category POM

Package quantities Pack of 10.

Further information There is evidence that the concurrent administration of Atrovent and sympathomimetic drugs produces a greater relief of bronchospasm than either drug given alone.

Atrovent has been shown to produce effective bronchodilatation in patients receiving β-blocking agents. Atrovent is also available as a metered dose inhaler.

Product licence number 0015/0108.

BEROTEC*

Presentation Pressurised metered inhaler: 10 ml vial (200 metered doses) available as complete unit with mouthpiece. Each metered dose contains fenoterol hydrobromide 200 micrograms (180 micrograms available to the patient).

Uses *Action:* Berotec is a highly potent, rapidly acting, selective beta$_2$ – adrenergic stimulant with a duration of action of 6–8 hours. The degree of selectivity coupled with administration by inhalation allows maximal bronchodilator effect with minimal side-effects.

Indications: For the treatment of reversible airways obstruction as in bronchial asthma, bronchitis and emphysema.

Dosage and administration By inhalation.

As Berotec has a longer duration of action than other bronchodilators a dosage of 1 or 2 puffs three times daily is usually sufficient to control bronchospasm in adults. If necessary this may be increased up to 2 puffs every four hours. Children (6–12 years) will normally require 1 puff three times daily but this may be increased up to 1 puff every four hours if necessary. It is recommended that administration of Berotec to children should be supervised by a responsible adult.

No specific information on the use of this product in the elderly is available. Clinical trials have included patients over 65 years and no adverse reactions specific to this age group have been reported.

Contra-indications, warnings, etc
Contra-indications: There are no absolute contra-indications to the use of Berotec.

Precautions: Caution should be observed should it be necessary to administer Berotec to patients with thyrotoxicosis, myocardial insufficiency, angina, cardiac dysrhythmias, hypertension or hypertrophic subvalvular aortic stenosis.

In view of the possible interaction between sympathomimetic amines and monoamine oxidase inhibitors or tricyclic anti-depressants, care should be exercised if it is proposed to administer these compounds concurrently with Berotec.

Berotec should be used with caution in patients already receiving other sympathomimetic agents as cardiovascular effects may be additive.

Potentially serious hypokalaemia may result from beta$_2$-agonist therapy. Particular caution is advised in severe asthma as this effect may be potentiated by concomitant treatment with xanthine derivatives, steroids, diuretics and by hypoxia. It is recommended that serum potassium levels are monitored in such situations.

Patients must be instructed in the correct use of a metered inhaler and warned not to exceed the prescribed dose. Patients should also be warned to seek medical advice should a reduced response become apparent.

Although Berotec has been in wide general use for several years, there is no definite evidence of ill consequence during human pregnancy. Animal studies have shown no hazard.

Beta-adrenergic agents have been shown to prolong pregnancy and inhibit labour although the amount in the prescribed dose of Berotec is probably insufficient to do so.

Medicines should not be used in pregnancy, especially in the first trimester, unless the expected benefit is thought to outweigh any possible risk to the foetus.

Beta-adrenergic blocking agents may antagonise Berotec and reduce its bronchodilator effect if administered concurrently.

Side-effects: Potentially serious hypokalaemia may result from beta$_2$-agonist therapy. Transient sympathomimetic side-effects, such as palpitation, tachycardia, headache and tremor may occur, as with other beta-adrenergic agonists, but are uncommon with administration by inhaler.

Overdosage: Accidental overdosage may give rise to tachycardia, palpitation and tremor. It is suggested that the patient should be treated symptomatically.

Should the administration of a beta-adrenergic blocking agent be considered necessary to counteract the effects of overdosage, its use in a patient liable to bronchospasm should be carefully monitored.

Pharmaceutical precautions Protect from heat, including the sun.

The inhaler vial should not be incinerated or opened even when empty.

Legal category POM.

Package quantities 10 ml vial (200 metered doses) (OP) complete with mouthpiece.

Further information There is evidence to suggest that Berotec may reduce the allergic response of tissues. Animal studies have shown that Berotec also produces an increase in the frequency of movement of the respiratory epithelial cilia and in the rate of mucus transport.

Long-term use has shown Berotec to be free from significant adverse effects, particularly with respect to the blood gases and general biochemistry. Tolerance is not a feature of long-term use.

Product licence number 0015/0034.

BEROTEC* NEBULISER SOLUTION

Presentation An aqueous hypotonic solution of fenoterol hydrobromide 0.5% (5 mg/ml) for administration by inhalation containing 0.05 mg/ml sodium metabisulphite and 0.5 mg/ml disodium edetate. The pH is approximately 3.2.

Uses *Action:* Berotec is a highly potent, rapidly acting, selective $beta_2$-adrenoceptor stimulant with a long duration of action. The degree of selectivity coupled with administration by inhalation allows maximal bronchodilator effect with minimal side-effects.

Indications: For the treatment of reversible airways obstruction as in bronchial asthma, bronchitis and emphysema.

Dosage and administration Berotec nebuliser solution may be administered from an intermittent positive pressure ventilator or from suitable nebulisers.

The recommended dose per inhalation ranges from 0.5–2.5 mg and this can be achieved by nebulising 0.1 to 0.5 ml solution. These volumes may be measured using the integral dropper (20 drops are approximately equivalent to 1 ml) and diluted with sterile sodium chloride 0.9% solution for ease of administration. Dilution should be carried out just before inhalation.

Adults: 0.5 mg–2.5 mg up to four times daily. Single doses of 5.0 mg have been safely used.

Children: (6–14 years) up to 1.0 mg up to three times daily.

The final volume depends on the type of nebuliser to be used and the administration time acceptable. 2 ml is a suitable final volume for most nebulisers such as the Bird micro-nebuliser, Bennett twin-jet, Acorn/OEM and Turrett No. 51. However, if a total volume of 2 ml is not suitable for the particular nebuliser to be used, the dilution should be adjusted to give the volume recommended by the manufacturer of the nebuliser.

No specific information on the use of this product in the elderly is available. Clinical trials have included patients over 65 years and no adverse reactions specific to this age group have been reported.

Contra-indications, warnings, etc
Contra-indications: There are no absolute contra-indications to the use of Berotec.

Precautions: The administration of nebuliser solutions which are hypotonic or of low pH or containing preservatives has been associated with cases of paradoxical bronchoconstriction.

Caution should be observed should it be necessary to administer Berotec to patients with thyrotoxicosis, myocardial insufficiency, angina, cardiac dysrhythmias, hypertension or hypertrophic subvalvular aortic stenosis.

In view of the possible interaction between sympathomimetic amines and monoamine oxidase inhibitors or tricyclic anti-depressants, care should be exercised if it is proposed to administer these compounds concurrently with Berotec.

Berotec should be used with caution in patients already receiving other sympathomimetic agents as cardiovascular effects may be additive.

Potentially serious hypokalaemia may result from $beta_2$-agonist therapy. Particular caution is advised in severe asthma as this effect may be potentiated by concomitant treatment with xanthine derivatives, steroids, diuretics and by hypoxia. It is recommended that serum potassium levels are monitored in such situations.

If relief is not obtained after correct use of the nebuliser solution the dose should not be exceeded and the patient should contact the doctor for advice.

Although Berotec has been in wide general use for several years, there is no definite evidence of ill-consequence during human pregnancy; animal studies have shown no hazard.

Beta-adrenergic agents have been shown to prolong pregnancy and inhibit labour although the amount in the prescribed dose of Berotec is probably insufficient to do so.

Medicines should not be used in pregnancy, especially during the first trimester, unless the expected benefit is thought to outweigh any possible risk to the foetus.

Beta-adrenergic blocking agents may antagonise Berotec and reduce its bronchodilator effect if administered concurrently.

Side-effects: Potentially serious hypokalaemia may result from $beta_2$-agonist therapy. As with other beta-adrenergic agonists transient sympathomimetic side-effects such as tremor, palpitation, tachycardia and headache may occur, but are uncommon with administration by inhalation.

Overdosage: Accidental overdosage may give rise to tachycardia, palpitation and tremor. It is suggested that the patient should be treated symptomatically.

Should the administration of a beta-adrenergic blocking agent be considered necessary to counteract the effects of overdose, its use in a patient liable to bronchospasm should be carefully monitored.

Pharmaceutical precautions Protect from light and heat.

Legal category POM.

Package quantities 20 ml amber glass bottle with integral dropper.

Further information There is evidence to suggest that Berotec may reduce the allergic response of tissues. Animal studies have shown that Berotec also produces an increase in the frequency of movement of the respiratory epithelial cilia and in the rate of mucus transport.

Long-term use has shown Berotec to be free from significant adverse effects, particularly with respect to the blood gases and general biochemistry.

Product licence number 0015/0082.

BUSCOPAN*

Presentation *Buscopan Tablets:* White, sugar-coated tablets, marked 'Buscopan' on one side. Each tablet contains hyoscine-N-butylbromide 10 mg.

Buscopan Ampoules: Ampoules for intramuscular or intravenous injection, each containing hyoscine-N-butylbromide 20 mg in 1 ml.

Uses *Action:* Buscopan is an antispasmodic agent, which relaxes smooth muscle of the organs of the abdominal and pelvic cavities. It is believed to act predominantly on the intramural parasympathetic ganglia of these organs.

Indications: Buscopan tablets are indicated in spasm of the gastro-intestinal or genito-urinary tracts and in spasmodic dysmenorrhoea.

Buscopan ampoules are indicated in acute spasm, as in renal or biliary colic; in radiology for differential diagnosis of obstruction and to reduce spasm and pain in pyelography, and in other diagnostic procedures where spasm may be a problem, e.g. gastro-duodenal endoscopy.

Dosage and administration *Adults: Orally:* 2 tablets four times daily. In spasmodic dysmenorrhoea, treatment should commence two days before the expected onset of the period and continue for three days after menstruation has begun.

By injection: 1 ampoule intramuscularly or intravenously repeated after half-an-hour if necessary. When used in endoscopy this dose may need to be repeated more frequently.

Children 6–12 years: Orally: 1 tablet three times daily.

Diluent: Buscopan injection solution may be diluted with dextrose or with sodium chloride 0.9% injection solutions. It is also miscible and compatible with most of the commonly used aqueous radiological contrast media such as sodium diatrizoate.

No specific information on the use of this product in the elderly is available. Clinical trials have included patients over 65 years and no adverse reactions specific to this age group have been reported.

Contra-indications, warnings, etc
Contra-indications: Because of a possible mydriatic effect, Buscopan should not be administered to patients with glaucoma.

Precautions: Although Buscopan has been in wide general use for many years, there is no definite evidence of ill-consequence during human pregnancy; animal studies have shown no hazard. Nevertheless, medicines should not be used in pregnancy, especially the first trimester, unless the expected benefit is thought to outweigh any possible risk to the foetus.

Side-effects: Dryness of the mouth, temporary loss of accommodation and tachycardia have very occasionally been reported.

Overdosage: Oral doses of up to 1090 mg produced only tiredness. Other features which may be encountered are dry mouth, loss of accommodation, tachycardia, orthostatic hypotension and Cheyne-Stokes respiration.

Gastric lavage should be employed where appropriate. Parasympathetic agents, e.g. pilocarpine or neostigmine, should be used as necessary.

Pharmaceutical precautions Buscopan tablets and ampoules should be protected from light and heat.

Legal category POM.

Package quantities *Tablets:* Packs of 56 (OP) and 560 (OP).

Ampoules: Packs of 10.

Further information Nil.

Product licence numbers
Buscopan Tablets 0015/0047
Buscopan Ampoules 0015/5005

CATAPRES*

Presentation *Catapres Tablets 100 micrograms:* White compressed tablets impressed with the motif C/Ɔ on one side and with the Company symbol on the reverse. Each tablet contains clonidine hydrochloride 100 micrograms.

Catapres Tablets 300 micrograms: White, compressed tablets impressed with the motif 03C/Ɔ30 and with the Company symbol on the reverse. Each tablet contains clonidine hydrochloride 300 micrograms.

Catapres PL Perlongets: red/yellow gelatin capsules imprinted with the notation Catapres PL, 11P and the Company symbol. Each Perlonget contains 5 mini-tablets constituting 250 micrograms clonidine hydrochloride in sustained release form.

Catapres Ampoules: Ampoules for injection. Each ampoule contains clonidine hydrochloride 150 micrograms in 1 ml.

Uses *Action:* Catapres is an antihypertensive agent with both central and peripheral sites of action. With long-term treatment Catapres reduces the responsiveness of peripheral vessels to vasoconstrictor and vasodilator substances and to sympathetic nerve stimulation. Early in treatment, however, blood pressure reduction is associated with a central reduction of sympathetic outflow and increased vagal tone.

Clinically there may be reduced venous return and slight bradycardia resulting in reduced cardiac output. Although initially peripheral resistance may be unchanged it tends to be reduced as treatment continues. There is no interference with myocardial contractility. Studies have shown that cardiovascular reflexes, as shown by the lack of postural hypotension and exercise hypotension, are preserved.

Indications: Catapres is indicated for the treatment of all grades of essential and secondary hypertension, hypertension during pregnancy and hypertensive crises.

Catapres PL is indicated for all degrees of hypertension excluding hypertensive crises.

Dosage and administration *Catapres Tablets:* Oral treatment should commence with 50–100 micrograms three times daily.

This dose should be increased gradually every second or third day until control is achieved. Most patients will be controlled on divided daily doses of 0.30–1.2 mg. However, some patients may require higher doses, e.g. 1.8 mg or more.

Catapres PL Perlongets: most patients will be satisfactorily controlled on one Perlonget daily (usually given in the evening). This dosage can be increased if necessary up to 2 or 3 Perlongets daily (one in the morning and one or two at night).

Catapres may be added to an existing antihypertensive regimen where blood pressure control has not been satisfactorily achieved. If side-effects with existing therapy are troublesome the concomitant use of Catapres may allow a lower dose of the established regimen to be employed. Patients changing treatment should have their existing therapy reduced gradually whilst Catapres is added to their regimen.

Catapres Ampoules: In hypertensive crises 1 or 2 Catapres ampoules should be given by slow intravenous injection.

An effect is usually seen within 10 minutes and reaches a maximum about 30 minutes to 1 hour after administration. The duration of effect depends upon the severity of the condition and is commonly of the order of 3–7 hours. Up to 5 ampoules may be given in 24 hours to achieve and maintain the desired blood pressure.

Patients undergoing anaesthesia should continue their Catapres treatment before, during and after anaesthesia, using oral or intravenous administration according to individual circumstances.

Diluent: Catapres injection solution is compatible with 0.9% sodium chloride solution and with 5% dextrose solution.

No specific information on the use of this product in the elderly is available. Clinical trials have included patients over 65 years and no adverse reactions specific to this age group have been reported.

Contra-indications, warnings, etc
Contra-indications: There are no known absolute contra-indications to the use of Catapres.

Precautions: This product may cause drowsiness. Patients who are affected should not drive or operate machinery. Sedation due to the drug may be increased by the concomitant use of other central nervous system depressants.

Sudden withdrawal of Catapres, particularly in those patients receiving high doses, may result in rebound hypertension. Termination of long-term therapy with Catapres for any reason should therefore be performed gradually. With Catapres PL this may be achieved by progressively increasing the interval between doses. If a hypertensive episode should nevertheless occur, reintroduction of oral or intravenous Catapres should reverse any such effect. If the use of Catapres is not practical then an alpha-adrenergic blocking drug, such as phentolamine, should be used.

If Catapres is being given concurrently with a β-blocker, Catapres should not be discontinued until several days after the withdrawal of the β-blocker.

Patients with a known history of depression should be carefully supervised while under long-term treatment with Catapres as there have been occasional reports of further depressive episodes during oral treatment in such patients.

Caution should be exercised in patients with Raynaud's disease or other occlusive peripheral vascular disease. As with all drugs used in hypertension, Catapres should be used with caution in patients with cerebrovascular, coronary or renal insufficiency.

Concomitant use of diuretics or other antihypertensive agents will usually result in an increased antihypertensive effect.

Concomitant administration of tricyclic antidepressants may reduce the antihypertensive effect of Catapres.

Alpha-adrenergic blocking drugs antagonise the acute effects of Catapres.

Although clonidine has been in wide general use for many years, there is no definite evidence of hazard during human pregnancy. In animal studies involving doses higher than the equivalent maximum therapeutic dose in man, effects on foetal development were seen only in one species. Foetal malformations did not occur. Medicines should not be used in pregnancy, especially the first trimester, unless the expected benefit is thought to outweigh any possible risk to the foetus.

Catapres should only be given to breast-feeding women if considered essential by the physician. There is as yet insufficient experience to enable Catapres to be recommended for children.

Intravenous injection of Catapres should be given slowly to avoid a possible transient pressor effect. This is particularly important in patients already under treatment with other antihypertensive agents such as guanethidine or reserpine.

Side-effects: Initially, sedation or dry mouth are encountered in a few patients. These effects usually subside as treatment continues. Other drug-related side-effects which have been mentioned in the literature include dizziness, headache, nocturnal unrest, nausea, euphoria, rash, constipation, impotence (rarely) and agitation on withdrawal of long-term therapy.

There are occasional reports of fluid retention during initial stages of oral treatment. This is usually transitory and can be corrected by the addition of a diuretic.

Facial pallor has been noted following injection.

A single case of toxic hepatitis has been reported, but the authors commented that the role of Catapres in hepatotoxicity in this patient remains questionable.

Acute administration in animals or in man has occasionally induced a transient elevation of blood sugar. This is believed to be due to the initial pharmacological effect of alpha-adrenergic stimulation. Investigators agree that this has no clinical significance. The inclusion of diabetic patients in many Catapres investigations has confirmed its suitability as an antihypertensive agent for such patients.

Overdosage: Accidental overdosage may cause hypotension, bradycardia, sedation and coma. Transient hypertension may be seen if the total dose is over 10 mg.

Gastric lavage should be performed where appropriate. In most cases all that is required are general supportive measures. Forced diuresis has been employed. Where bradycardia is severe atropine will increase the heart rate. If hypotension is giving rise to concern the administration of an alpha-adrenergic blocking drug such as phentolamine may help.

Pharmaceutical precautions Catapres tablets and ampoules should be protected from light and heat.

Legal category POM.

Package quantities *Tablets 100 micrograms:* Pack of 84 (OP).

Tablets 300 micrograms: Pack of 84 (OP).

Perlongets 250 micrograms: Calendar pack of 56 (OP).

Ampoules 150 micrograms in 1 ml: Pack of 5.

Further information No adverse reaction has been reported with the concurrent administration of digoxin, aminophylline, anticonvulsants or antiarrhythmic preparations. Monitoring of haematological and hepatic status in large numbers of patients has revealed no drug-related adverse effects. Renal blood flow and glomerular filtration rates are maintained and there is no deterioration in renal function. There is evidence that plasma renin levels are reduced. Catapres does not affect the estimation of VMA levels.

Clonidine hydrochloride is also available as Dixarit 25 micrograms tablets for the prophylactic management of migraine, recurrent vascular headache and menopausal flushing.

Product licence numbers

Catapres Tablets 100 micrograms	0015/5009
Catapres Tablets 300 micrograms	0015/5041
Catapres PL Perlongets 250 micrograms	0015/0072
Catapres Ampoules 150 micrograms in 1 ml	0015/5008

CELEVAC*

Presentation Pink tablets containing 500 mg Methylcellulose 450 BP.

Uses *Action:* Methylcellulose is a hydrophilic colloid which absorbs water to swell to a soft gel of uniform consistency.

Indications:

1. In the control of colostomy, ileostomy and diarrhoea.
2. In the management of diverticular disease.
3. In the management of simple constipation.
4. As an aid to appetite control and as an aid in the management of obesity.

Dosage and administration

1. *Colostomy and ileostomy control and for diarrhoea:* 3–6 tablets twice daily with the minimum of liquid. Liquids should be avoided for 30 minutes before and after each dose. Dosage should be adjusted to give stools the required consistency.

2. *Diverticular disease:* 3–6 tablets twice daily, adjusted according to the degree of constipation, diarrhoea or spastic pain.

3. *Simple constipation:* 3–6 tablets twice daily, to be taken with at least 300 ml of liquid. The dose may be reduced as normal bowel function is restored.

4. *Appetite control and obesity:* 3 tablets, with at least 300 ml of warm liquid, half an hour before each meal, and between meals when hunger pangs are severe.

No specific information on the use of this product in the elderly is available. Clinical trials have included patients over 65 years and no adverse reactions specific to this age group have been reported.

Contra-indications, warnings, etc Celevac should not be used in cases where the physician believes there is a pathological cause for the diarrhoea which would render the condition unsuitable for symptomatic medical treatment, e.g. infective bowel disease and imminent or threatened bowel obstruction. Bowel obstruction is a rare complication of treatment with any bulk-forming hydrophilic colloid.

Although Celevac has been in wide general use for many years there is no evidence of ill-consequence during human pregnancy.

Medicines should not be used in pregnancy, especially

the first trimester, unless the expected benefit is thought to outweigh any possible risk to the foetus.

Overdosage: Methylcellulose is not absorbed. The features to be expected would be abdominal distension which may be followed by intestinal obstruction.

Gastric lavage should be employed where appropriate. The patient should be observed and fluids given. If obstruction develops, appropriate measures such as rectal washout must be taken.

Pharmaceutical precautions Protect from heat and moisture.

Legal category GSL.

Package quantities Tablet pack of 112 (OP).

Further information Methylcellulose is a hydrophilic colloid which bonds loosely with H_2O and with H_2S, thus acting as a bulking agent and a deodorising agent. In diverticular disease its use has been associated with a fall in intracolonic pressures as well as relief of symptoms.

Product licence number 1416/5003.

CONOTRANE*

Presentation A white cream containing 0.1% w/w benzalkonium chloride and 22% w/w Dimethicone 350 BP.

Uses
Action: Conotrane combines the water repellent properties of dimethicone with the antiseptic activity of benzalkonium chloride.

Indications: Conotrane is used for protection of the skin from moisture, irritants, chafing and contamination with bacteria or yeasts; as in the prevention and treatment of napkin rash, in the prevention of pressure sores, and in the management of incontinence.

Dosage and administration The cream should be applied to the affected area several times a day as necessary or after every napkin change.

Contra-indications, warnings, etc
Contra-indications: Known hypersensitivity to benzalkonium chloride.

Side-effects: Local hypersensitivity to benzalkonium chloride is rare.

Pharmaceutical precautions Store in a cool place.

Legal category GSL.

Package quantities 50 g tube; 500 g jar.

Further information Nil.

Product licence number 0015/0113.

DEXA-RHINASPRAY*

Presentation Dexa-Rhinaspray metered nasal spray, complete with nasal applicator. Each 9 g vial contains about 125 metered doses. One metered dose contains: tramazoline hydrochloride 120 micrograms, dexamethasone-21 isonicotinate 20 micrograms, neomycin sulphate 100 micrograms.

Uses
Action: Tramazoline hydrochloride is a sympathomimetic substance with local vasoconstrictor activity. It has a quick-acting, long-lasting decongestant effect on the nasal mucosa.

Dexamethasone-21 isonicotinate is a corticosteroid with marked anti-inflammatory and anti-allergic properties. Neomycin sulphate is locally active against a wide range of both Gram-positive and Gram-negative bacteria.

Indication: Treatment of allergic rhinitis.

Dosage and administration
Adults: 1 metered dose can be applied into each nostril up to six times in 24 hours, although 2 or 3 applications a day are usually sufficient.

Children: 5–12 years – 1 metered dose into each nostril up to twice daily.

Children: under 5 years – not recommended.

No specific information on the use of this product in the elderly is available. Clinical trials have included patients over 65 years and no adverse reactions specific to this age group have been reported.

Contra-indications, warnings, etc
Contra-indications: Its use is contra-indicated in patients hypersensitive to neomycin or tramazoline and in infants.

Precautions: Prolonged use may result in the development of superinfection due to organisms resistant to neomycin. Care should be used to avoid contact with the eyes as conjunctival irritation may occur.

Although Dexa-Rhinaspray has been in general use for many years, there is no evidence of ill-consequence during human pregnancy; animal studies have shown no hazard. Nevertheless, medicines should not be used in pregnancy, especially the first trimester, unless the expected benefit is thought to outweigh the risk to the foetus.

Side-effects: A slight burning sensation in the nose, with sneezing, has been reported when using tramazoline hydrochloride alone.

Overdosage: There have been no reports of overdosage with Dexa-Rhinaspray, but absorption of tramazoline may produce pallor, sweating, tachycardia and anxiety. These should be treated symptomatically.

Pharmaceutical precautions Protect from extremes of temperature. The vials should not be punctured or incinerated even when apparently empty.

Legal category POM.

Package quantities 9 g vial (125 doses) (OP) complete with nasal applicator.

Further information Neomycin sulphate is rarely used systemically. Local use therefore does not prejudice the patient's response to later systemic antibiotic treatment.

Product licence number 0015/5010

DIXARIT*

Presentation Blue, bi-convex, sugar-coated tablets, One side plain, the obverse marked with DIXARIT. Each tablet contains clonidine hydrochloride 25 micrograms.

Uses *Action:* Treatment with Dixarit diminishes the responsiveness of peripheral vessels to constrictor and dilator stimuli, thereby preventing the vascular changes associated with migraine. The same direct action on peripheral vessels moderates the vascular changes associated with menopausal flushing.

Indications:

1. The prophylactic management of migraine or recurrent vascular headache.

2. The management of vasomotor conditions commonly associated with the menopause and characterised by flushing.

Dosage and administration *Adults:* Initially 2 tablets twice daily. If after two weeks there has been no remission, increase to 3 tablets twice daily.

Children: Not generally recommended for administration to children under 12 years.

The duration of treatment depends upon the severity of the condition.

No specific information on the use of this product in the elderly is available. Clinical trials have included patients over 65 years and no adverse reactions specific to this age group have been reported.

Contra-indications, warnings, etc
Contra-indications: There are no known absolute contra-indications to the use of Dixarit.

Precautions: Dixarit may be unsuitable for patients who

have co-existing or a previous history of depressive illness, since further depressive episodes have occasionally been reported in such patients.

Although clonidine has been in wide general use for many years there is no definite hazard during human pregnancy.

In animal studies involving doses higher than the equivalent maximum therapeutic dose in man, effects on foetal development were only seen in one species. Foetal malformations did not occur.

Medicines should not be used in pregnancy, especially the first trimester unless the expected benefit is thought to outweigh any possible risk to the foetus.

Using higher doses than those recommended above, clonidine is an effective antihypertensive agent. Caution should therefore be observed where antihypertensive agents are being used as potentiation of hypotensive effect may occur. Provided the recommended Dixarit dosage regimen is followed, no difficulty with hypotension should arise during the routine management of patients with either migraine or menopausal flushing.

Clonidine is available for the management of hypertension as Catapres Tablets (100 micrograms and 300 micrograms), Perlongets (250 micrograms) and Ampoules (150 micrograms in 1 ml). Where Catapres is already being used Dixarit therapy is obviously illogical.

Side-effects: Initially there may be sedation or dry mouth in some patients. Dizziness, nausea and nocturnal unrest have been reported, and occasionally rashes have been attributed to Dixarit.

In the management of hypertension a single case of toxic hepatitis has been reported with clonidine. However, the role of clonidine in hepatotoxicity in this patient remains questionable. Monitoring of haematological, renal and hepatic status in large numbers of patients has revealed no drug-related adverse effects.

Overdosage: Accidental overdosage may cause hypotension, bradycardia, sedation and coma. Transient hypertension may be seen if the total dose is over 10 mg.

Gastric lavage should be performed where appropriate. In most cases all that is required are general supportive measures. Forced diuresis has been employed. Where bradycardia is severe atropine will increase the heart rate. If hypotension is giving rise to concern the administration of an alpha-adrenergic blocking drug such as phentolamine may help.

Pharmaceutical precautions Protect from heat, moisture and light.

Legal category POM.

Package quantities Pack of 112 (OP).

Further information There is no information which suggests that Dixarit will interact with any other preparation used routinely in the management of either migraine or menopausal flushing.

Product licence number 0015/5014.

DUOVENT*

Presentation Pressurised metered dose inhaler: 10 ml vial (200 metered doses) available as complete unit with mouthpiece. Each metered dose contains fenoterol hydrobromide 100 micrograms (90 micrograms available to the patient) and ipratropium bromide 40 micrograms (36 micrograms available to the patient).

Uses *Action:* Fenoterol hydrobromide is a highly potent, rapidly acting selective beta$_2$-adrenoceptor stimulant. The degree of selectivity coupled with administration by inhalation allows maximal bronchodilator effect with minimal side-effects.

Ipratropium bromide is an anticholinergic drug with bronchodilator properties.

There is evidence that the concurrent administration of ipratropium bromide and a sympathomimetic drug produces a greater relief of bronchospasm than either drug given alone.

Indications: For the treatment of reversible airways obstruction as in bronchial asthma, bronchitis and emphysema.

Dosage and administration *Adults:* 1 or 2 puffs three or four times daily.

Children over 6 years: 1 puff three times daily. It is recommended that administration of Duovent to children be supervised by an adult.

No specific information on the use of this product in the elderly is available. Clinical trials have included patients over 65 years and no adverse reactions specific to this age group have been reported.

Contra-indications, warnings, etc
Contra-indications: Known sensitivity to atropine.

Precautions: Caution should be observed should it be necessary to administer Duovent to patients with thyrotoxicosis, myocardial insufficiency, angina, cardiac dysrhythmias, hypertension or hypertrophic subvalvular aortic stenosis. In view of the possible interaction between sympathomimetic amines and monoamine oxidase inhibitors or tricyclic anti-depressants, care should be exercised if it is proposed to administer these compounds concurrently with Duovent. Duovent should be used with caution in patients already receiving other sympathomimetic agents as cardiovascular effects may be additive.

Potentially serious hypokalaemia may result from beta$_2$ agonist therapy. Particular caution is advised in severe asthma as this effect may be potentiated by concomitant treatment with xanthine derivatives, steroids, diuretics and by hypoxia. It is recommended that serum potassium levels are monitored in such situations.

Generally, caution is advocated in the use of anticholinergic agents in patients with glaucoma and prostatic hypertrophy. However, specific studies with ipratropium bromide in patients with glaucoma showed that inhaling cumulative doses of 160 micrograms had no effect on the eye. Urinary retention and constipation have only rarely been reported.

Patients must be instructed in the correct use of a metered dose inhaler and warned against the accidental release of the contents into the eye. If relief is not obtained after correct use of the inhaler, the dose should not be exceeded and the patient should contact the doctor for advice.

Although both fenoterol hydrobromide and ipratropium bromide have been in general use for several years, there is no definite evidence of ill-consequence during human pregnancy; animal studies have shown no hazard. Beta-adrenergic agents have been shown to prolong pregnancy and inhibit labour although the amount in the prescribed dose of Duovent is probably insufficient to do so.

Medicines should not be used in pregnancy, especially the first trimester, unless the expected benefit is thought to outweigh any possible risk to the foetus.

Beta-adrenergic blocking agents may antagonise fenoterol hydrobromide and reduce its bronchodilator effect if administered concurrently.

Side-effects: Potentially serious hypokalaemia may result from beta$_2$ agonist therapy. Transient sympathomimetic side-effects, such as palpitation, tachycardia, headache and tremor may occur, as with other beta-adrenergic agonists, but are uncommon with administration by inhaler.

Anticholinergic side-effects are unlikely to occur at therapeutic doses but some patients may complain of a dry mouth. There is no evidence that in the therapeutic dose range Duovent has any adverse effect on bronchial secretion.

Overdosage: Accidental overdosage may give rise to tachycardia, palpitation and tremor. It is suggested that the patient should be treated symptomatically. Should the administration of a beta-adrenergic blocking agent be considered necessary to counteract the effects of over-dosage, its use in a patient liable to bronchospasm should be carefully monitored.

Very high doses (30 mg) of ipratropium bromide by mouth have been reported to cause anticholinergic side-effects but these were not severe and did not require specific reversal.

Pharmaceutical precautions Protect from heat, including the sun. The canister should not be incinerated or opened even when apparently empty.

Legal category POM.

Package quantities 10 ml vial (200 metered doses) (OP) complete with mouthpiece.

Further information There is evidence to suggest that fenoterol may reduce the allergic response of tissues. Animal studies have shown that fenoterol also produces an increase in the frequency of movement of the respiratory epithelial cilia and in the rate of mucus transport.

Long-term use has shown fenoterol and ipratropium to be free from significant adverse effects.

Product licence number 0015/0091.

HERPID*

Presentation A clear, colourless solution containing Idoxuridine BP 5% in dimethyl sulphoxide, of spectroscopic quality.

Uses *Action:* The antiviral agent idoxuridine arrests replication of DNA viruses, e.g. varicella/zoster; herpesvirus hominis; vaccinia. The idoxuridine is dissolved in dimethyl sulphoxide which penetrates the skin and carries the antiviral agent to the deeper levels of the epidermis where the virus is replicating.

Indications: Cutaneous herpes simplex and herpes zoster (shingles).

Dosage and administration Herpid should be painted on the lesions and their erythematous bases 4 times daily for four days. Treatment should start as soon as the condition has been diagnosed, ideally within two to three days after the rash appears. Good results are less likely if treatment is not started within seven days.

No specific information on the use of this product in the elderly is available. Clinical trials have included patients over 65 years and no adverse reactions specific to this age group have been reported.

Contra-indications, warnings, etc
Contra-indications: Animal studies have shown idoxuridine to be teratogenic. Consequently, Herpid should not be prescribed for women who are pregnant or at risk of becoming pregnant. In a small number of cases of women who used Herpid inadvertently in early pregnancy and who were followed to term, the infant was normal in each case.

Known hypersensitivity to either idoxuridine or dimethyl sulphoxide.

Dermographia.

Side-effects: Patients often experience stinging when applying Herpid and a distinctive taste during a course of treatment; both effects are transient.

Skin reactions have occasionally been reported.

Over-usage of the solution may lead to maceration of the skin.

Warning: Herpid in the eye causes stinging: treat by washing out with water.

Overdosage: There is no clinical experience of overdosage. Standard supportive measures should be adopted.

Pharmaceutical precautions Herpid should be stored in its box at room temperature. Do not refrigerate as the contents of the bottle may solidify. If crystals do form, allow to redissolve before use.

Legal category POM.

Package quantities 5 ml bottle, with brush (OP).

Further information Herpid can damage some synthetic materials (e.g. artificial silk and Terylene) and printed cotton fabrics. Contact between Herpid and these materials should therefore be avoided.

The use of Herpid in children with malignant disease might be justified but, although not a contra-indication, its use in children under the age of 12 years is not recommended.

Product licence number 1416/0001.

OXIVENT*▾

Presentation Pressurised metered inhaler: 10 ml vial (200 metered doses) available as a complete unit with mouthpiece. Each metered dose delivers 100 micrograms oxitropium bromide per puff.

Uses *Action:* Oxitropium is an anticholinergic bronchodilator

Indications: For the management of airways obstruction in patients suffering from chronic stable asthma and chronic obstructive pulmonary disease.

Dosage and administration *Adults:* Two puffs two or three times daily

Children: Oxivent has not been evaluated in children

Elderly patients: There are no special dosage requirements for the elderly.

All patients should be instructed in the correct use of a metered dose inhaler.

It should be noted that the time to peak bronchodilatation following the use of Oxivent is slow in comparison with the sympathomimetic bronchodilators.

Contra-indications, warnings, etc *Contra-indications:* Known hypersensitivity to atropine or ipratropium bromide.

Precautions: Patients should be warned to seek medical advice should a reduced response become apparent.

Symptoms of aerosol-induced bronchospasm including wheeze, cough and chest tightness, have been reported following the use of Oxivent. If patients report respiratory symptoms associated with use of the inhaler, treatment should be discontinued.

Accidental release into the eye should be avoided, although inhalation of doses of oxitropium up to 800 micrograms have been shown to have no effect on pupil diameter, intra-ocular pressure or accommodation.

Caution is advocated in patients with glaucoma or prostatic hypertrophy.

Use in pregnancy and lactation: The safety of this product for use in human pregnancy has not been established. Animal studies have shown reproductive toxicity with high doses of oxitropium. Oxivent should not be used during pregnancy, particularly the first trimester, unless the expected benefit is thought to outweigh any risk to the foetus. There is no information on the excretion of oxitropium bromide in breast milk.

Side-effects: Systemic anticholinergic side-effects such as blurring of vision or hesitancy of micturition are rare but may be important in the elderly. Local irritation of the throat and nose may occur and there are occasional reports of nausea. Dry mouth is reported by some patients.

Overdosage: Inhalation of doses up to 1200 micrograms (12 puffs) had no effect on systolic or diastolic blood pressure and doses up to 2000 micrograms (20 puffs) did not affect heart rate. There is no experience of higher doses. Expected symptoms would include disturbance of vision, urinary retention, reduction in salivation and increased heart rate. At very high doses symptoms resembling atropine poisoning are likely to occur. However, oxitropium bromide is poorly absorbed from the gastrointestinal tract.

Pharmaceutical precautions Protect from heat, including the sun. The vials should not be punctured or incinerated even when apparently empty.

Legal category POM

Package quantities 10 ml vial containing 200 doses, complete with mouthpiece.

Further information Oxivent at normal dose levels

has no effect on sputum production, sputum viscosity or mucociliary clearance.

In clinical studies Oxivent has been administered in conjunction with beta-agonists, xanthines, steroids and sodium cromoglycate with no evidence of adverse interaction. There is evidence that the administration of Oxivent with a beta-agonist produces greater bronchodilation than either drug used alone.

Product licence number 0015/0142.

PAVACOL-D*

Presentation Dark brown, sugar-free, tartrazine-free cough mixture. Each 5 ml contains Pholcodine BP 5 mg, together with balsam of tolu, oil of clove, tincture of ginger, oil of aniseed, tincture of capsicum, oil of peppermint, alcohol and chloroform.

Uses *Action:* Pholcodine exerts an inhibitory action on the cough centre, and has been found to be as effective as heroin as a cough suppressant. It is not a drug of addiction, and does not cause constipation.

Indications: For the symptomatic treatment of dry troublesome coughs.

Dosage and administration *Adults:* One or two 5 ml spoonfuls as required.

The dose may be increased to three 5 ml spoonfuls if necessary. No more than four doses should be taken in 24 hours.

Children: from 6 to 12 years: One 5 ml spoonful four or five times daily.

From 3 to 5 years: One 5 ml spoonful three times daily.

From 1 to 2 years: Half a 5 ml spoonful three or four times daily.

Pavacol-D may be diluted with Sorbitol Solution BPC. When diluted an in-use shelf-life of 14 days is recommended.

No specific information on the use of this product in the elderly is available. Clinical trials have included patients over 65 years and no adverse reactions specific to this age group have been reported.

Contra-indications, warnings, etc *Contra-indications:* Hypersensitivity to any of the ingredients, or liver disease.

Warnings: Nausea, drowsiness and constipation occur occasionally after pholcodine.

Cough suppressants may cause sputum retention and this may be harmful in patients with chronic bronchitis and bronchiectasis. Patients should be warned to consult the doctor if symptoms persist for more than 5 days.

Pregnancy: Although Pavacol-D has been in general use for many years, there is no evidence of ill-consequence during human pregnancy.

Medicines should not be used in pregnancy, especially the first trimester, unless the expected benefit is thought to outweigh any possible risk to the foetus.

Interactions: Alcohol or other CNS depressants may lead to greater drowsiness and sedation.

Overdosage: Symptoms of overdosage include nausea, drowsiness, restlessness, excitement, ataxia and respiratory depression. Treatment consists of emptying the stomach by aspiration and lavage. In case of severe poisoning the specific narcotic antagonist, naloxone may be used. Otherwise, treatment is supportive and symptomatic

Pharmaceutical precautions Store in a cool place and protect from light.

Legal category P.

Package quantities Bottles of 300 ml (OP).

Further information A sugar-free, tartrazine-free mixture suitable for both diabetic and non-diabetic patients.

Product licence number 1416/5039.

PERSANTIN*

Presentation Persantin tablets 25 mg: orange sugar-coated tablets, marked 'Persantin 25' on one side, containing dipyridamole 25 mg.

Persantin tablets 100 mg: white sugar-coated tablets, marked 'Persantin 100' on one side, containing dipyridamole 100 mg.

Uses
Action: Dipyridamole has an antithrombotic action based on its ability to modify various aspects of platelet function, such as platelet aggregation, adhesion and survival, which have been shown to be factors associated with the initiation of thrombus formation.

Indications: An adjunct to oral anticoagulation for prophylaxis of thromboembolism associated with prosthetic heart valves.

Dosage and administration
Adults: 300–600 mg daily in three or four doses.

Children: The normal total oral daily dose is 5 mg/kg in divided doses.

Persantin should usually be taken before meals.

Contra-indications, warnings, etc
Contra-indications: There are no absolute contra-indications to the administration of Persantin.

Precautions: Persantin is a potent vasodilator and should therefore be used with caution in patients with rapidly worsening angina, subvalvular aortic stenosis or haemodynamic instability associated with a recently sustained myocardial infarction.

There is inadequate evidence of safety in human pregnancy but Persantin has been used for many years without apparent ill-consequence. Animal studies have shown no hazards. Medicines should not be used in pregnancy, especially the first trimester, unless the expected benefit is thought to outweigh any possible risk to the foetus.

The concurrent administration of antacids may reduce the efficacy of Persantin.

It is possible that Persantin may enhance the effects of oral anticoagulants.

Persantin should be used with caution in patients with coagulation disorders.

Side-effects: If these occur it is usually during the early part of treatment and they are often dose-related. The vasodilating properties of Persantin may occasionally produce a vascular headache which normally disappears with dosage reduction. Dizziness, faintness, dyspepsia, mild diarrhoea and rash have also been reported occasionally.

Overdosage: Overdosage may lead to headache, gastrointestinal symptoms and hypotension. Coronary vasodilatation may cause chest pain in patients with ischaemic heart disease.

General supportive measures should be employed. Coronary vasodilatation may be reversed by administering aminophylline by slow IV injection, whilst monitoring the ECG.

Pharmaceutical precautions Protect from heat, light and moisture.

Legal category POM.

Package quantities Packs of 84 (OP), 100 and 1000 tablets.

Further information There is evidence that the effects of aspirin and dipyridamole on platelet behaviour are synergistic.

Product licence number
Persantin tablets 25 mg 0015/0052
Persantin tablets 100 mg 0015/5016

PERSANTIN* AMPOULES

Presentation Amber glass ampoules containing a yellow solution for intravenous injection. Each ampoule contains dipyridamole 10 mg in 2 ml.

Uses
Action: Dipyridamole is a powerful coronary vasodilator and produces a marked increase in coronary blood flow.

Indications: As an alternative to exercise stress in thallium-201 myocardial imaging, particularly in patients unable to exercise or in those for whom exercise may be contra-indicated.

Dosage and administration 0.56 mg/kg injected intravenously over 4 minutes. The injection of thallium-201 should be given from 1–2 minutes after completion of the dipyridamole injection.

The half-life of an intravenous bolus injection of dipyridamole is approximately 30 minutes and therefore repeat imaging to assess redistribution can be performed after 240 minutes.

Contra-indications, warnings, etc
Contra-indications: Patients with a known hypersensitivity to dipyridamole.

Subvalvular aortic stenosis, aortic disease, hypotension associated with a recently sustained myocardial infarction, significant valvular disease, or uncompensated congestive heart failure. Patients with known cardiac conduction defects or dysrhythmias.

Precautions: The product should be administered with care in unstable angina.

As with exercise-induced stress, the use of Persantin ampoules as an adjunct to thallium imaging may occasionally precipitate cardiac arrhythmia in patients with severe heart disease. Dipyridamole-thallium scanning should be performed with continual monitoring of the patient's ECG.

Concurrent administration of a vasodilator may cause a severe hypotensive effect.

There is inadequate evidence of safety in human pregnancy, but dipyridamole has been used for many years without apparent ill-consequence.

Side-effects: Some patients may experience chest pain or a worsening of their angina symptoms. These may be reversed, if necessary, with intravenous aminophylline.

Transient headache, dizziness, faintness, facial flushing and nausea are common side effects. A bitter taste has sometimes been experienced after intravenous injection.

Pharmaceutical precautions Protect from heat, light and moisture.

Legal category POM.

Package quantities Ampoules: Packs of 5.

Further information Persantin is also available as tablets (100 mg and 25 mg) for use as a platelet modifying drug.

Product licence number 0015/0119.

RINATEC*

Presentation Metered dose inhaler 10 ml (200 metered doses) available as complete unit with nasal applicator. Each metered dose contains ipratropium bromide 20 micrograms.

Uses
Action: Ipratropium bromide is an anticholinergic drug which acts as an antagonist against the muscarinic receptors of the mucoserous glands. Stimulation of these glands with the concomitant production of watery rhinorrhoea is thus prevented.

Indications: The treatment and management of watery rhinorrhoea associated with perennial rhinitis.

Dosage and administration
Adults: 1 or 2 puffs to the affected nostril(s), up to a maximum of 4 times a day while symptoms persist. In many patients symptoms of rhinorrhoea will be satisfactorily controlled at lower dose levels. Patients should adjust the dose according to the severity of their symptoms.
Children: The use of Rinatec has not been evaluated in children, therefore it is not recommended for use in patients below the age of 12 years.

Contra-indications, warnings, etc
Contra-indications: Known hypersensitivity to atropine or ipratropium bromide.

Precautions and warnings: Anticholinergic agents should only be used with caution in patients with glaucoma or prostate hypertrophy.

The patient should be adequately instructed in the correct use of the device and warned against accidental release into the eye. Release into the eye may result in pupillary dilatation. Generally, caution is advocated in the use of anticholinergic agents in patients with glaucoma or prostatic hypertrophy. However specific studies with Atrovent in patients with glaucoma showed that inhaling cumulative doses of 0.16 mg had no effect on the eye. If pupillary dilation associated with pain does occur, the patient should immediately contact the doctor for advice.

Excessive use or need for greater use may indicate a failure in control and response. The patient's condition should be reviewed.

The product should be used during pregnancy only if considered essential by the physician. Animal studies do not suggest a teratogenic effect and experience to date does not indicate a hazard during human pregnancy.

Side-effects: Treatment may result in dryness of the nasal mucosa. Symptoms of burning, bleeding, itching, stuffiness, crusting, sneezing and irritation have also been reported.

Overdosage: Accidental overdosage during intranasal use is unlikely and the resultant systemic effects are not likely to be significant. Single doses of ipratropium bromide 30 mg administered orally have caused anticholinergic side-effects but these were not severe and did not require specific reversal.

Pharmaceutical precautions Protect from heat including the sun. The vials should not be punctured or incinerated even when apparently empty.

Legal category POM.

Package quantities 10 ml vial (200 metered doses) (OP) complete with nasal applicator.

Further information Nil.

Product licence number 1416/0022.

TRANXENE*

Presentation Tranxene Capsules 15 mg: Pink/grey hard gelatin capsules imprinted with the notation 15 mg and the Company symbol. Each capsule contains dipotassium clorazepate 15 mg.

Tranxene Capsules 7.5 mg: Maroon/grey hard gelatin capsules imprinted with the product name, 7.5 mg and the Company symbol. Each capsule contains dipotassium clorazepate 7.5 mg.

Uses
Action: Tranxene is a tranquilliser exhibiting many characteristics of the benzodiazepine group of preparations. Particular features which distinguish Tranxene from other members of this group are the rapid appearance in the blood of the anxiolytic compound nordiazepam, the maintenance of satisfactory therapeutic effect in most patients with once daily administration, and little sedation.

Indications: For the short-term relief (2–4 weeks) only of anxiety that is severe, disabling or subjecting the individual to unacceptable distress, occurring alone or in association with insomnia or short-term psychosomatic, organic or psychotic illness.

The use of benzodiazepines to treat short-term 'mild' anxiety is considered to be inappropriate and unsuitable.

Dosage and administration Adults only, not generally recommended for children under 16 years. Tranxene 15 mg: one capsule daily, usually administered at night. Tranxene 7.5 mg: one capsule up to three times daily.

Half the normal dose may be sufficient for a therapeutic response in the elderly.

The lowest dose which can control symptoms should be used. It should not be continued beyond 4 weeks.

Long-term chronic use is not recommended.

Treatment should always be tapered off gradually.

Patients who have taken benzodiazepines for a long time may require a longer period during which doses are reduced.

Contra-indications, warnings, etc
Contra-indications: Known hypersensitivity to benzodiazepines; acute pulmonary insufficiency.

Precautions: Tranxene is not recommended for acute primary depressive states, chronic major psychoses, phobic or obsessional states. It should not be used alone for the treatment of depression or anxiety associated with depression. The action of Tranxene may potentiate other preparations with central nervous system depressant effects such as barbiturates, narcotics, phenothiazines and alcohol.

Although sedation has not proved to be a problem with Tranxene, in accordance with general principles patients should be advised that their ability to drive or to operate dangerous machinery may be impaired.

Amnesia may occur. In cases of loss or bereavement psychological adjustment may be inhibited by benzodiazepines.

There is no evidence as to drug safety in human pregnancy nor is there evidence from animal work that it is free from hazard. Do not use during pregnancy, especially during the first and last trimesters, unless there are compelling reasons.

Tranxene and its metabolites are excreted in human milk in minimal quantities and therefore use during lactation should be avoided if possible. In labour, high single doses or low repeated doses of benzodiazepines have been reported to produce irregularities of the foetal heart and hypotonia, and poor suckling and hypothermia in the neonate. Caution should be exercised in patients suffering from chronic pulmonary insufficiency, or chronic renal or hepatic disease.

Side-effects: Side-effects, which have been reported only rarely, include dizziness, gastro-intestinal upset, nervousness, blurred vision, dry mouth, headache, skin rashes and jaundice. Drowsiness has occasionally been reported but does not constitute a major problem.

Hypotension, urinary retention, changes in libido and blood dyscrasias have also been reported for benzodiazepines in general.

Abnormal psychological reactions to benzodiazepines have been reported. Disinhibiting effects may be manifested in various ways. Suicide may be precipitated in patients who are depressed and aggressive behaviour towards self and others may be precipitated. Extreme caution should therefore be used in prescribing benzodiazepines in patients with personality disorders.

Withdrawal from benzodiazepines may be associated with physiological and psychological symptoms including depression, nervousness, rebound insomnia, irritability, sweating and diarrhoea. Withdrawal symptoms occur with benzodiazepines following normal therapeutic doses given for short periods of time, but particularly on sudden discontinuation of the benzodiazepine, in patients with a history of drug abuse or alcoholism or in patients with marked personality disorders. In such patients treatment should be monitored closely and routine prescriptions avoided, with gradual drug withdrawal when appropriate.

Overdosage: An overdose of 900 mg has been reported, causing drowsiness, ataxia, respiratory depression and coma. If vomiting has not occurred spontaneously, it should be induced. Gastric lavage is recommended. General supportive therapy is indicated and specific measures to counteract central nervous system depressant effects may be necessary. Prolonged administration of doses as high as 120 mg daily has not given rise to organ toxicity. Abrupt withdrawal of excessive doses of benzodiazepines has been reported as occasionally producing confusion, toxic psychosis, convulsion or a condition resembling delirium tremens.

Pharmaceutical precautions Tranxene capsules should be protected from heat, light and moisture.

Legal category POM.

Package quantities Packs of 100 and 20 in aluminium foil strips.

Further information In common with other benzodiazepines, Tranxene has a central muscle-relaxant effect, and synergism with peripherally acting muscle relaxants is a theoretical possibility.

Product licence numbers

Tranxene capsules 15 mg	0015/0057.
Tranxene capsules 7.5 mg	0015/0045,

VILLESCON* LIQUID

Presentation Red, raspberry-flavoured liquid. Each 5 ml contains:

Prolintane hydrochloride	2.5 mg
Thiamine hydrochloride	1.67 mg
Riboflavine-5-phosphate sodium	1.36 mg
Pyridoxine hydrochloride	0.5 mg
Nicotinamide	5.0 mg

Uses *Action:* The principal ingredient of Villescon, prolintane hydrochloride, is a sympathomimetic amine with two main actions. It stimulates appetite and has a mild central action which produces an increased feeling of well-being in debilitated patients.

Indications: Villescon is indicated as a tonic after illness, surgery or labour, for apathy and anorexia in elderly patients, for institutional neuroses and for anorexia and lassitude following radiotherapy.

Dosage and administration *Adults:* 2×5 ml twice daily.

Children 5–12 years: ½×5 ml twice daily to 2×5 ml twice daily.

The normal course of treatment is 1–2 weeks.

It is recommended that the second daily dose be taken before four o'clock in the afternoon.

Diluent: Villescon Liquid may be diluted with purified water.

No specific information on the use of this product in the elderly is available. Clinical trials have included patients over 65 years and no adverse reactions specific to this age group have been reported.

Contra-indications, warnings, etc
Contra-indications: Thyrotoxicosis, epilepsy.

Precautions: Although no interaction between Villescon and MAO inhibitors has ever been demonstrated, the theoretical possibility of such an interaction should be borne in mind if these preparations are co-prescribed. It should be noted that even in very small quantities pyridoxine hydrochloride (vitamin B_6) inhibits the activity of levodopa.

There exists a proportion of patients whose ill-defined symptoms reflect a basic inadequacy of personality. Such patients are liable to misuse any drug with central activity, and it is advised that in these cases the recurrent prescription of Villescon should be avoided.

Although Villescon liquid has been in wide general use for many years, there is no definite evidence of ill-consequence during human pregnancy; animal studies have shown no hazard. Nevertheless, medicines should not be used in pregnancy, especially the first trimester, unless the expected benefit is thought to outweigh any possible risk to the foetus.

Side-effects: Tachycardia, nausea and colicky abdominal pains have been reported. Sleeplessness may be caused if Villescon is taken late in the day.

Overdosage: Accidental overdosage has been reported only rarely and may give rise to restlessness, insomnia, tachycardia and increase of blood pressure. An overdose of 300 mg prolintane has been reported in a young female who made a full recovery. Treatment should include gastric lavage and general supportive measures.

Sedation may be required to treat restlessness and insomnia.

Pharmaceutical precautions Villescon preparations should be protected from heat, light and moisture.

Legal category POM.

Package quantities Bottles of 150 ml (OP).

Further information Nil.

Product licence number 0015/0054.

VILLESCON* TABLETS

Presentation Orange, sugar-coated tablets, with the Company symbol on one side. Each tablet contains:

Prolintane hydrochloride	10.0 mg
Thiamine mononitrate	5.0 mg
Riboflavine	3.0 mg
Pyridoxine hydrochloride	1.5 mg
Nicotinamide	15.0 mg
Ascorbic acid	50.0 mg

Uses *Action:* The principal ingredient of Villescon, prolintane hydrochloride, is a sympathomimetic amine with two main actions. It stimulates appetite and has a mild central action which produces an increased feeling of well-being in debilitated patients.

Indications: Villescon is indicated as a tonic after illness, surgery or labour, for apathy and anorexia in elderly patients, for institutional neuroses and for anorexia and lassitude following radiotherapy.

Dosage and administration *Adults:* 1 tablet twice daily.

Children over 8 years: 1 tablet after breakfast.

The normal course of treatment is 1–2 weeks. It is recommended that the second daily dose be taken before four o'clock in the afternoon.

No specific information on the use of this product in the elderly is available. Clinical trials have included patients over 65 years and no adverse reactions specific to this age group have been reported.

Contra-indications, warnings, etc
Contra-indications: Thyrotoxicosis, epilepsy.

Precautions: Although no interaction between Villescon and MAO inhibitors has ever been demonstrated, the theoretical possibility of such an interaction should be borne in mind if these preparations are co-prescribed. It should be noted that even in very small quantities pyridoxine hydrochloride (vitamin B_6) inhibits the activity of levodopa.

There exists a proportion of patients whose ill-defined symptoms reflect a basic inadequacy of personality. Such patients are liable to misuse any drug with central activity, and it is advised that in these cases the recurrent prescription of Villescon should be avoided.

Although Villescon tablets have been in wide general use for many years there is no definite evidence of ill-consequence during human pregnancy; animal studies have shown no hazard. Medicines should not be used in pregnancy, especially the first trimester, unless the expected benefit is thought to outweigh any possible risk to the foetus.

Side-effects: Tachycardia, nausea and colicky abdominal pains have been reported. Sleeplessness may be caused if Villescon is taken late in the day.

Overdosage: Accidental overdosage has been reported only rarely and may give rise to restlessness, insomnia, tachycardia and increase of blood pressure. An overdose of 300 mg prolintane has been reported in a young female who made a full recovery. Treatment should include gastric lavage and general supportive measures. Sedation may be required to treat restlessness and insomnia.

Pharmaceutical precautions Villescon preparations should be protected from heat, light and moisture.

Legal category POM.

Package quantities Pack of 100.

Further information Nil.

Product licence number 0015/0055.

**Trade Mark*

Boehringer Ingelheim Hospital Division

A Division of Boehringer Ingelheim Limited
Ellesfield Avenue
Bracknell
Berkshire RG12 4YS

HOSPITAL DIVISION

ACTILYSE*

Presentation Dry powder for reconstitution.

Vials containing 50 mg (equivalent to 29 million IU) Actilyse (alteplase INN, recombinant human tissue-type plasminogen activator).

Vials containing 20 mg (equivalent to 11.6 million IU) Actilyse (alteplase INN, recombinant human tissue-type plasminogen activator).

The specific activity of Actilyse is 580,000 IU/mg.

Uses

Properties: Actilyse is a glycoprotein which activates the conversion of plasminogen to plasmin directly. When administered intravenously, Actilyse remains relatively inactive in the circulatory system until it binds to fibrin, for which it has a high affinity. Activation of Actilyse by fibrin binding causes a local conversion of plasminogen to plasmin, thus inducing thrombolysis of the fibrin clot. Systemic activity on components of the blood coagulation system is not marked, although an increased bleeding tendency may be seen (particularly at arterial puncture or venepuncture sites).

Actilyse has low antigenic potential.

Pharmacokinetics: Actilyse is cleared rapidly from the circulating blood and catabolised principally by the liver. The level of Actilyse in plasma falls to 50% of the initial level within 5 minutes of administration of an intravenous bolus, to approximately 20% after 10 minutes and to less than 10% after 20 minutes. Modest reductions of the levels of fibrinogen and other components of the coagulation system occur when Actilyse is administered at the recommended dosage.

Indications: Fibrinolytic therapy of acute thrombotic coronary artery occlusion.

Dosage and administration Under aseptic conditions the contents of a 50 mg injection vial of Actilyse dry substance should be dissolved in 50 ml Water for Injections, or a 20 mg vial dissolved in 20 ml Water for Injections. The contents of the reconstituted solution may be further diluted up to 1:5 with sterile Sodium Chloride Intravenous Infusion BP 0.9% w/v. Water for Injections or carbohydrate infusion solutions, (e.g. dextrose) must not be used for dilution of Actilyse.

Treatment should be initiated within 6 hours of the onset of chest pain.

A total dose of 100 mg Actilyse (equivalent to 58 million IU) should be given intravenously over 3 hours as follows:

10% of the total dose as an i.v. bolus over 1–2 minutes
50% of the total dose as an infusion over 1 hour
40% of the total dose as an infusion over the subsequent 2 hours

Patients weighing less than 67 kg should receive a total dose of 1.5 mg/kg (870,000 IU/kg) according to above schedule.

Contra-indications, warnings, etc

Contra-indications: Actilyse should not be used in cases of: History of cerebrovascular disease and uncontrolled hypertension, in view of the risks of cerebral haemorrhage.

Known bleeding diathesis.

Within 10 days of severe internal bleeding, major surgery or trauma, or puncture of major non-compressible blood vessels.

Active peptic ulceration.

Other known contra-indications to fibrinolytic therapy, e.g. acute pancreatitis, bacterial endocarditis.

Severe liver disease including hepatic failure, cirrhosis, portal hypertension (oesophageal varices) and active hepatitis.

Prolonged or traumatic resuscitation.

Precautions: Systemic disorders – Actilyse should be administered with caution to patients with diabetes mellitus and those with severe renal failure, as the arginine in the formulation (1.7 g per 50 mg vial and 0.7 g per 20 mg vial) might give rise to impaired glucose tolerance, and in renal failure might lead to hyperkalaemia.

There is no experience with the use of Actilyse in children.

Proliferative diabetic retinopathy.

Bleeding – during Actilyse infusion and in the immediate post-infusion period, special attention should be paid to potential bleeding sites. Intramuscular injections, venepuncture, and arterial puncture should be avoided during this period if possible; should arterial puncture be necessary it is preferable to use an upper limb vessel and check the site frequently for evidence of bleeding. Non-essential manipulation of the patient should be avoided during the Actilyse therapy.

Accelerated idioventricular rhythm may be associated with reperfusion of the coronary artery. Other arrhythmias (such as sinus bradycardia, ventricular tachycardia and ventricular fibrillation) may occur. These are not different from those often seen in the course of acute myocardial infarction and should be managed with standard antiarrhythmic measures.

Pregnancy: There is very little experience in the use of Actilyse during pregnancy. Actilyse does not cross the placental barrier in rats. In animal studies involving doses higher than the equivalent maximum therapeutic dose in man, no foetal malformations occurred. However, as for all medicines, Actilyse should not be used during pregnancy unless the expected benefit is thought to outweigh any possible risk to the foetus. There is a possibility of placental separation, particularly when Actilyse is administered during the third trimester.

Side-effects: Side effects reported in association with Actilyse therapy are generally minor.

Any bleeding which may occur is generally limited to the site of injection. In such cases it is not necessary to discontinue treatment with Actilyse. Should serious bleeding occur, fibrinolytic therapy with Actilyse should be discontinued. Intracerebral haemorrhage has occurred in approximately 0.5% of patients treated with 100 mg Actilyse. In view of the short half-life and modest systemic fibrinolytic effect, specific replacement of coagulation factors is not normally required.

Nausea and/or vomiting may occur and should be treated symptomatically.

Drug interactions: Prior or concomitant administration of anticoagulants may increase the risk of bleeding. Heparin has been commonly administered in association with Actilyse.

Overdosage: There is no experience of the effects of large overdoses of Actilyse, but one might expect depletion of fibrinogen and other blood coagulation components with consequent risk of bleeding. Actilyse infusion should be terminated. If serious bleeding complications occur, fresh frozen plasma or fresh whole blood should be infused; if necessary synthetic antifibrinolytic agents may be administered.

Pharmaceutical precautions Store below 25°C.

The reconstituted solution may be stored for up to 24 hours at 2–8°C, and up to 8 hours at temperatures below 25°C. Actilyse vials should be kept in the original carton until preparation.

Legal category POM.

Package quantities There are 3 types of pack available:

Pack containing 2 × 50 mg Actilyse (equivalent to 2 × 29 million IU) and 2 × 50 ml Water for Injections (PL 0015/0127) with 2 sterile transfer devices + 2 hanging bags.

Pack containing 1 × 50 mg Actilyse (equivalent to 29 million IU) and 1 × 50 ml Water for Injections (PL 0015/0127) with a sterile transfer device.

Pack containing 1 × 20 mg Actilyse (equivalent to 11.6 million IU) and 1 × 20 ml Water for Injections (PL 0015/0127) with a sterile transfer device.

Further information It is recommended that anti-arrhythmic therapy for bradycardia and/or ventricular irritability be available when infusions of Actilyse are administered, as would normally be required in the early phase treatment of acute myocardial infarction.

Product licence number 0015/0120.

MEXITIL*

Presentation *Mexitil Capsules 200 mg:* Red/red hard gelatin capsules imprinted with the notation 200 mg and the Company symbol. Each capsule contains mexiletine hydrochloride 200 mg.

Mexitil Capsules 50 mg: Red/purple hard gelatin capsules imprinted with the notation 50 mg and the Company symbol. Each capsule contains mexiletine hydrochloride 50 mg.

Mexitil Ampoules: Ampoules for intravenous injection. Each ampoule contains mexiletine hydrochloride 250 mg in 10 ml.

Uses *Action:* Mexitil is an anti-arrhythmic agent which depresses the maximum rate of depolarisation with little or no modification of resting potentials or the duration of action potentials.

Indications: For the treatment of existing or anticipated ventricular arrhythmias and ectopic beats such as those found after myocardial infarction and in ischaemic heart disease. IV mexiletine has been used successfully in the treatment of ventricular arrhythmias induced by digitalis or other drugs; mexiletine has also been proven to be of some benefit in idiopathic and other arrhythmic states. Mexiletine is often effective in patients with good left ventricular function, in suppressing ventricular arrhythmias refractory to other treatment. Mexiletine is not of proven value in arrhythmias in pre-excitation syndromes.

Dosage and administration

1. *Intravenous Mexitil:*

(a) *Loading dose:* IV injection of 4–10 ml (100–250 mg) Mexitil given at a suggested rate of 1 ml per minute (25 mg per minute).
Then
add 500 mg (2 ampoules) Mexitil to 500 ml of a suitable infusion solution (see 'Pharmaceutical Precautions'). Administer the first 250 ml by IV infusion over 1 hour (4 ml per minute).
Then
administer the second 250 ml by IV infusion over 2 hours (2 ml per minute).

(b) *Maintenance dose:* Add 250 mg (1 ampoule) Mexitil to 500 ml of a suitable infusion solution (see 'Pharmaceutical Precautions'). Administer by IV infusion at a suggested rate of 1 ml per minute (0.5 mg per minute), according to patient response. Continue for as long as required or until oral maintenance therapy is commenced.

2. *Oral Mexitil*

(a) *Loading dose:* Give 400 mg Mexitil.

(b) *Maintenance dose:* Give 200–250 mg Mexitil three to four times daily commencing 2 hours after the loading dose. The usual daily dose is between 600–800 mg in divided doses.

Note: Mexitil is absorbed in the upper part of the small intestine. In acute myocardial infarction and particularly when opiates have been given, *rate* of absorption *but not bioavailability* may be delayed and therefore a larger loading dose e.g. 600 mg may be preferable.

3. *Alternative loading dose regimes*

(a) *Combination IV Mexitil and Oral Mexitil loading dose:* IV injection of 8 ml (200 mg) Mexitil given at a suggested rate of 1 ml per minute. On completion of injection or infusion give 400 mg Mexitil orally.
Maintenance dose.
As in 2b.

(b) *Combination IV Lignocaine and Oral Mexitil loading dose:* Give IV lignocaine according to manufacturer's instructions.
On completion of injection give 400 mg Mexitil orally.
Maintenance dose.
As in 2b.

4. *Change over from IV to Oral Mexitil maintenance:* On discontinuing the IV infusion commence the maintenance dose. Give 200–250 mg Mexitil orally three or four times a day.

Notes:

1. The loading dose regime is designed to compensate for the rapid phase of tissue distribution which occurs especially with IV loading.

2. Side-effects are more likely to be encountered during the initial tissue loading phase in which case the rate of infusion should be reduced.

3. If the optimum therapeutic effect is not achieved the rate of infusion or oral dosage may be increased, side-effects permitting.

4. Gastric emptying time may be delayed in patients with myocardial infarction and/or to whom opiates have been given and thus it may be necessary to titrate the dose against therapeutic effects and side-effects.

5. The 50 mg capsule is available in order that a more precise dose titration may be undertaken should this be required. Smaller increments will also reduce the incidence of side-effects.

6. When mexiletine therapy is commenced, patients should be monitored closely (ECG and blood pressure, routine laboratory tests) particularly in the following situations:

Sinus node dysfunction, conduction defect, bradycardia, hypotension or cardiac, renal or hepatic failure. There may be potentiation of tremor in patients with Parkinsonism.

The duration of treatment required in any patient is of necessity variable, and although no precise guide can be given, withdrawal of treatment may be attempted after a suitable period free of arrhythmia. Gradual withdrawal, i.e. over 1–2 weeks, is preferable as arrhythmias which have been satisfactorily controlled may recur.

No specific information on the use of this product in the elderly is available. Clinical trials have included patients over 65 years and no adverse reactions specific to this age group have been reported.

Contra-indications, warnings, etc Hypersensitivity to mexiletine, cardiogenic shock and high degree A-V block unless a pacemaker is *in situ*.

Interactions with other medicaments and other forms of interaction:

(i) Drugs which delay the rate of absorption (narcotic analgesics, some antacids) may reduce peak plasma concentration of mexiletine.

(ii) Drugs which induce the hepatic mixed function oxidase system (e.g. rifampicin, phenytoin and phenobarbitone) can influence the metabolism and hence lower plasma levels of mexiletine.

(iii) Drugs which acidify or alkalinise urine will enhance or reduce (respectively) the rate of drug elimination.

(iv) No interactions have been observed with warfarin, diazepam or nitrazepam.

(v) Mexitil may be used concurrently with the cardiovascular drugs digoxin, amiodarone, quinidine and beta-adrenergic blocking agents. Concomitant IV therapy with other local anaesthetic-type agents such as lignocaine or procainamide is not recommended. However no problems have been encountered when oral mexiletine has been given in conjunction with these drugs.

Side-effects: Side-effects are mainly related to blood concentration and may therefore be seen during the initial phases of both IV and oral treatment when fluctuation may occur before the blood and tissue concentrations reach equilibrium. Reducing the rate of injection or infusion or delaying the next oral dose allows the blood concentration to fall and usually reduces side-effects. Generally side-effects are of four types:

Gastro-intestinal – nausea, vomiting, indigestion, constipation, diarrhoea, dry mouth, unpleasant taste, hiccoughs.

Central nervous system – light-headedness, drowsiness, confusion, dizziness, unco-ordination, diplopia, blurred vision, nystagmus, dysarthria, ataxia, tremor, paraesthesiae, convulsion, psychiatric disorders, insomnia. Animal studies using toxic doses have shown that benzodiazepines (diazepam) reduce the CNS effects.

Cardiovascular – hypotension, sinus bradycardia, atrial fibrillation, palpitation, conduction defects, exacerbation of arrhythmias and torsade de pointes.

When hypotension has occurred this has tended to be in patients with severe illness who have already been given a variety of anti-arrhythmic or other preparations and, if associated with bradycardia, may be reduced by the use of atropine.

Haematological – rash, jaundice, arthralgia, fever, thrombocytopenia and appearance of positive but symptomless antinuclear factor titres.

Although Mexitil has been in general use for several years, there is no definite evidence of safety during human pregnancy. Mexiletine freely crosses the placenta; however, animal studies have shown no hazard.

As with all medicines, mexiletine should not be used in pregnancy, especially the first trimester, unless the expected benefit is thought to outweigh any possible risk to the foetus.

Mexiletine is secreted in breast milk (at concentrations on average slightly higher than maternal blood), but has not been detected in the plasma of the suckling infant. Nevertheless caution should be exercised, particularly when nursing a premature infant.

Myocardial infarction results in prolonged absorption half-life of mexiletine. Plasma elimination half-life may be prolonged in moderate to severe hepatic disease, and in patients with creatinine clearance of less than 10 ml/min.

Overdosage: The minimum fatal dose is unknown but 4.40 g proved fatal in a healthy young adult.

The clinical features include nausea, vomiting, drowsiness, confusion, ataxia and convulsions. Blurred vision and paraesthesiae have also been reported. Hypotension, sinus bradycardia, atrial fibrillation and cardiac arrest are more specific effects.

Gastric lavage should be performed where appropriate and the patient should be transferred to an intensive/coronary care unit for possible cardiopulmonary support. Arrhythmias should be treated as appropriate and diazepam may be useful to control convulsions.

Acidification of the urine enhances the rate of drug elimination and so may be useful.

Pharmaceutical precautions Mexitil solution for injection is known to be compatible with the following infusion solutions: sodium chloride 0.9%; sodium chloride 0.9% with potassium chloride 0.3% or 0.6%; dextrose 5%; sodium bicarbonate 1.4%; sodium lactate (M/6).

Legal category POM.

Package quantities

Capsules 200 mg: pack of 100.
Capsules 50 mg: pack of 100.
Ampoules 250 mg in 10 ml: pack of 5.

Further information Mexitil has been used successfully within a few hours of myocardial infarction.

Mexitil is also available as Mexitil PL Perlongets, each containing 360 mg mexiletine hydrochloride in sustained release form.

Product licence numbers

Mexitil Capsules 200 mg	0015/0064
Mexitil Capsules 50 mg	0015/0062
Mexitil Ampoules 250 mg in 10 ml	0015/0065

MEXITIL* PL PERLONGETS*

Presentation Mexitil PL Perlongets: Turquoise/scarlet hard gelatin capsules. Each Perlonget contains 5 mini-tablets constituting 360 mg mexiletine hydrochloride in sustained release form.

Uses

Action: Mexitil is an anti-arrhythmic agent which depresses the maximum rate of depolarisation with little or no modification of resting potentials or the duration of action potentials.

Indications: For the treatment of existing or anticipated ventricular arrhythmias and ectopic beats such as those found after myocardial infarction and in ischaemic heart disease. Mexiletine has also been proven to be of some benefit in idiopathic and other arrhythmic states. Mexiletine is often effective in patients with good left ventricular function, in suppressing ventricular arrhythmias refractory to other treatment. Mexiletine is not of proven value in arrhythmias in pre-excitation syndromes.

Dosage and administration One Mexitil PL capsule twice daily (twelve hourly) will maintain therapeutic blood levels of mexiletine. If this regimen is used initially in new patients, therapeutic blood levels of mexiletine will be achieved after about 36 hours. If a more rapid effect is required, one of the following loading doses may be used:

(a) Two Mexitil PL capsules. This will give therapeutic blood levels of mexiletine within 6 hours.
(b) One Mexitil PL capsule together with 250 mg Mexitil as conventional capsules. This will give therapeutic blood levels of mexiletine within 2½ hours.
(c) Intravenous loading dose. See Mexitil capsules and injection data sheet for details. This will give therapeutic blood levels of mexiletine within 5 minutes.

Notes: Gastric emptying time may be delayed in patients with myocardial infarction and/or to whom opiates have been given and thus it may be necessary to titrate the dose against therapeutic effects and side-effects.

When mexiletine therapy is commenced, patients should be monitored closely (ECG and blood pressure, routine laboratory tests) particularly in the following situations:

Sinus node dysfunction, conduction defect, bradycardia, hypotension or cardiac, renal or hepatic failure. There may be potentiation of tremor in patients with Parkinsonism.

The duration of treatment required in any patient is of necessity variable, and although no precise guide can be given, withdrawal of treatment may be attempted after a suitable period free of arrhythmia. Gradual withdrawal, i.e. over 1–2 weeks, is preferable as arrhythmias which have been satisfactorily controlled may recur.

No specific information on the use of this product in the elderly is available. Clinical trials have included patients over 65 years and no adverse reactions specific to this age group have been reported.

Contra-indications, warnings, etc Hypersensitivity to mexiletine, cardiogenic shock and high degree A-V block unless a pacemaker is *in situ*.

Interactions with other medicaments and other forms of interaction:

(i) Drugs which delay the rate of absorption (narcotic analgesics, some antacids) may reduce peak plasma concentration of mexiletine.

(ii) Drugs which induce the hepatic mixed function oxidase system (e.g. rifampicin, phenytoin and phenobarbitone) can influence the metabolism and hence lower plasma levels of mexiletine.

(iii) Drugs which acidify or alkalinise urine will enhance or reduce (respectively) the rate of drug elimination.

(iv) No interactions have been observed with warfarin, diazepam or nitrazepam.

(v) Mexitil may be used concurrently with the cardiovascular drugs digoxin, amiodarone, quinidine and beta-adrenergic blocking agents. Concomitant IV therapy with other local anaesthetic-type agents such as lignocaine or procainamide is not recommended. However no problems have been encountered when oral mexiletine has been given in conjunction with these drugs.

Side-effects: Side-effects are mainly related to blood concentration and may therefore be seen during the initial phases of both i.v. and oral treatment when fluctuation may occur before the blood and tissue concentrations reach equilibrium. Reducing the rate of injection of infusion or delaying the next oral dose allows the blood concentration to fall and usually reduces side-effects. Generally side-effects are of four types:

Gastro-intestinal – nausea, vomiting, indigestion, constipation, diarrhoea, dry mouth, unpleasant taste, hiccoughs.

Central nervous system – light-headedness, drowsiness, confusion, dizziness, unco-ordination, diplopia, blurred vision, nystagmus, dysarthria, ataxia, tremor, paraesthesiae, convulsion, psychiatric disorders, insomnia. Animal studies using toxic doses have shown that benzodiazepines (diazepam) reduce the CNS effects.

Cardiovascular – hypotension, sinus bradycardia, atrial fibrillation, palpitation, conduction defects, exacerbation of arrhythmias and torsade de pointes.

When hypotension has occurred this has tended to be in patients with severe illness who have already been given a variety of anti-arrhythmic or other preparations and, if associated with bradycardia, may be reduced by the use of atropine.

Haematological – rash, jaundice, arthralgia, fever, thrombocytopenia and appearance of positive but symptomless antinuclear factor titres.

Although Mexitil has been in general use for several years, there is no definite evidence of safety during human pregnancy. Mexiletine freely crosses the placenta; however, animal studies have shown no hazard.

As with all medicines, mexiletine should not be used in pregnancy, especially the first trimester, unless the expected benefit is thought to outweigh any possible risk to the foetus.

Mexiletine is secreted in breast milk (at concentrations on average slightly higher than maternal blood), but has not been detected in the plasma of the suckling infant. Nevertheless caution should be exercised, particularly when nursing a premature infant.

Myocardial infarction results in prolonged absorption half-life of mexiletine. Plasma elimination half-life may be prolonged in moderate to severe hepatic disease, and in patients with creatinine clearance of less than 10 ml/min.

Overdosage: The minimum fatal dose is unknown but 4.40 g proved fatal in a healthy young adult.

The clinical features include: nausea, vomiting, drowsiness, confusion, ataxia and convulsions. Blurred vision and paraesthesiae have also been reported. Hypotension, sinus bradycardia, atrial fibrillation and cardiac arrest are more specific effects.

Gastric lavage should be performed where appropriate and the patient should be transferred to an intensive/coronary care unit for possible cardio-pulmonary support. Arrhythmias should be treated as appropriate and diazepam may be useful to control convulsions.

Acidification of the urine enhances the rate of drug elimination and so may be useful.

Legal category POM.

Package quantities 56 capsules in blister strips.

Further information Mexitil has been used successfully within a few hours of myocardial infarction.

Mexitil is also available as capsules containing 50 mg or 200 mg mexiletine hydrochloride, and as ampoules for intravenous administration containing 250 mg mexiletine hydrochloride in 10 ml.

Product licence number Mexitil PL Perlongets 0015/0084

MYDRILATE*

Presentation Isotonic, sterile, aqueous solutions of Cyclopentolate Hydrochloride BP 0.5% and 1.0% w/v buffered to pH5 and containing 0.01% w/v benzalkonium chloride.

Uses Cyclopentolate is an anti-muscarinic agent used topically in the eye as a mydriatic and cycloplegic. The effects are similar to those of atropine but with a more rapid onset and shorter duration of action. It is indicated for:

(i) Diagnostic purposes for fundoscopy and cycloplegic refraction.

(ii) Dilating the pupil in inflammatory conditions of the iris and uveal tract.

Dosage and administration

Adults (and the elderly)

(i) For refraction: instil one drop of 0.5% solution repeated after 15 minutes if necessary. NB: Maximum effect is reached after 30–60 minutes.

(ii) For uveitis: instil one or two drops of 0.5% solution up to four times daily or as required.

NB: For both indications deeply pigmented eyes may require use of a 1% solution.

Children

(i) For refraction: 6–16 years: one drop of 1% solution instilled into the eye approximately 40 minutes before examination.

Under 6 years: one or two drops of 1% solution instilled into the eye approximately 40 minutes before examination.

(ii) For uveitis: at the discretion of the physician.

Do not use during the first three months of life due to possible association between the cycloplegia produced and development of amblyopia and also the increased risks of systemic toxicity in neonates.

Cycloplegia following administration is quick in onset and short-lived. Maximal cycloplegia is achieved within 15–45 minutes of instillation, and lasts on average about 20 minutes. Recovery normally takes place in about four hours, but very occasionally some effect persists for up to 24 hours.

Mydriasis is produced very rapidly and an average pupil diameter of 7 mm is usually reached 15–30 minutes after instillation of 1 drop of 0.5% solution. Complete recovery from the mydriatic effect generally occurs spontaneously in not more than 20 hours.

No specific information on the use of this product in the elderly is available. Clinical trials have included patients over 65 years and no adverse reactions specific to this age group have been reported.

Contra-indications, warnings, etc Mydrilate is contra-indicated in: Glaucoma or a tendency towards glaucoma (e.g. narrow anterior chamber angle); hypersensitivity to cyclopentolate hydrochloride or benzalkonium chloride. This preparation contains benzalkonium chloride and should not be used whilst soft contact lenses are being worn.

Precautions: The effects of anti-muscarinic agents may be enhanced by the concomitant administration of other drugs with anti-muscarinic properties such as amantadine, some anti-histamines, butyrophenones, phenothiazines and tricyclic anti-depressants.

May cause blurred vision and sensitivity to light. Patients should be warned not to drive or engage in other hazardous activities unless vision is clear. Complete recovery from the effects of cyclopentolate eyedrops may take up to one day.

Side-effects: Local: Increased intraocular pressure, transient stinging, and sensitivity to light secondary to pupillary dilation. Prolonged administration may lead to local irritation, hyperaemia, oedema and conjunctivitis.

Systemic anti-cholinergic toxicity is manifested by dryness of the mouth, flushing, dryness of the skin, bradycardia followed by tachycardia with palpitations and arrhythmias, urinary urgency, difficulty and retention, reduction in the tone and motility of the gastro-intestinal tract leading to constipation.

Vomiting with giddiness and staggering may occur, a rash may be present in children and abdominal distention in infants. Psychotic reactions, behavioural disturbances and cardio-respiratory collapse may occur in children.

There is insufficient evidence as to drug safety in pregnancy and lactation. This product should not be used during pregnancy unless it is considered essential by a physician.

Because of the risk of precipitating angle-closure glaucoma in the elderly and others prone to raised intraocular pressure, an estimate of the depth of the angle of the anterior chamber should be made before use.

Extreme caution is advised for use in children and individuals susceptible to belladonna alkaloids because of the increased risk of systemic toxicity. Parents should be warned of the oral toxicity of this preparation for children, and advised to wash their hands after use.

Use with caution in an inflamed eye as the hyperaemia greatly increases the rate of systemic absorption through the conjunctiva.

To reduce systemic absorption the lacrimal sac should be compressed at the medial canthus by digital pressure for at least one minute after instillation of the drops.

Overdosage: Systemic toxicity may occur following topical use, particularly in children. It is manifested by flushing and dryness of the skin, (a rash may be present in children), blurred vision, a rapid and irregular pulse, fever, abdominal distention in infants, convulsions and hallucinations and the loss of neuro-muscular co-ordination.

Treatment is supportive (there is no evidence that physostigmine is superior to supportive management). In infants and small children the body surface must be kept moist. If accidentally ingested, induce emesis or perform gastric lavage.

Pharmaceutical precautions Store below 15°C, protect from light. Do not dilute or dispense from any container other than the original bottle. Discard one month after opening.

Legal category POM.

Package quantities 5 ml dropper bottles of 0.5% and 1.0% solutions.

Further information Mydrilate is non-irritant and sensitivity reactions are uncommon. The onset of cycloplegia is at least as fast as that obtained by any other preparation used for the purpose. In the normal eye it has little or no effect on intra-ocular tension.

Product licence numbers
Mydrilate 0.5% 1416/5030
Mydrilate 1.0% 1416/5031

ORAMORPH* CONCENTRATED ORAL SOLUTION

Presentation A clear, colourless solution of Morphine Sulphate BP 20 mg/ml.

Uses Oramorph Concentrated Oral Solution is indicated for the relief of severe pain.

Dosage and administration
Adults: Usual dose 10–20 mg (0.5–1.0 ml) every 4 hrs.

Children under 1 year: Not recommended.
1–5 years: Maximum dose 5 mg (0.25 ml) every 4 hrs.
6–12 years: Maximum dose 5–10 mg (0.25–0.5 ml) every 4 hrs.

Dosage can be increased under medical supervision according to the severity of the pain and the patient's previous history of analgesic requirements. Reductions in dosage may be appropriate in the elderly.

When patients are transferred from other morphine preparations to Oramorph Concentrated Oral Solution, dosage titration may be appropriate.

A calibrated dropper is supplied with this dosage form for accurate and convenient dose adjustment. The required dose may be added to a soft drink immediately prior to administration.

Morphine Sulphate BP is readily absorbed from the gastro-intestinal tract following oral administration. However, when Oramorph Concentrated Oral liquid is used in place of parenteral morphine, a 50% to 100% increase in dosage is usually required in order to achieve the same level of analgesia.

Contra-indications, warnings, etc Respiratory depression, obstructive airways disease, known morphine sensitivity, acute hepatic disease, acute alcoholism, head injuries, coma, convulsive disorders and where the intracranial pressure is raised. Concurrent administration of monoamine oxidase inhibitors or within two weeks of discontinuation of their use.

Precautions: Nausea and vomiting may be troublesome. Phenothiazine antiemetics may be given with morphine, but it should be noted that morphine potentiates the effects of tranquillizers, anaesthetics, hypnotics, sedatives and alcohol.

Care should be exercised if morphine sulphate is given in the first 24 hours post-operatively, in hyperthyroidism, and where there is reduced respiratory reserve, such as kyphoscoliosis, emphysema and severe obesity. Morphine sulphate should not be given if paralytic ileus is likely to occur. If constipation occurs, this may be treated with appropriate laxatives.

It is wise to reduce dosage in chronic hepatic and renal disease, myxoedema, adrenocortical insufficiency, prostatic hypertrophy or shock. Tolerance and dependence may occur.

Although morphine sulphate has been in general use for many years, there is inadequate evidence of safety in human pregnancy and lactation. Morphine is known to cross the placenta and is excreted in breast milk, and may thus cause respiratory depression in the new born infant.

Medicines should not be used in pregnancy, especially the first trimester, unless the expected benefit outweighs any possible risk to the foetus.

Patients should be warned not to drive or operate dangerous machinery after taking Oramorph.

Overdosage: Signs of morphine toxicity and overdosage: These are likely to consist of pin-point pupils, respiratory depression and hypotension. Circulatory failure and deepening coma may occur in more severe cases.

Treatment of morphine overdosage: Administer naloxone 0.4 mg intravenously. Repeat at 2–3 minute intervals as necessary, or by an infusion of 2 mg in 500 ml of normal saline or 5% dextrose (4 micrograms/ml). Empty the stomach. A 0.02% aqueous solution of potassium permanganate may be used for lavage. Assist respiration if necessary. Maintain fluid and electrolyte levels.

Pharmaceutical precautions Store at room temperature. Protect from light.

Legal category CD (Sch 2), POM.

Package quantities Bottles of 30 ml and 120 ml with calibrated dropper.

Further information Nil.

Product licence number 0015/0125.

ORAMORPH* ORAL SOLUTION

Presentation A clear, colourless solution of Morphine Sulphate BP 10 mg/5 ml.

Uses Oramorph Oral Solution is indicated for the relief of severe pain.

Dosage and administration
Adults: Usual dose 10–20 mg (5–10 ml) every 4 hrs.

Children under 1 year: Not recommended.
1–5 years: maximum dose 5 mg (2.5 ml) every 4 hrs.
6–12 years: maximum dose 5–10 mg (2.5–5 ml) every 4 hrs.

Dosage can be increased under medical supervision according to the severity of the pain and the patient's previous history of analgesic requirements. Reductions in dosage may be appropriate in the elderly.

Morphine Sulphate BP is readily absorbed from the gastro-intestinal tract following oral administration. However, when Oramorph Oral Solution is used in place of parenteral morphine, a 50% to 100% increase in dosage is usually required in order to achieve the same level of analgesia.

Contra-indications, warnings, etc Respiratory depression, obstructive airways disease, known morphine sensitivity, acute hepatic disease, acute alcoholism, head injuries, coma, convulsive disorders and where the intracranial pressure is raised. Concurrent administration of monoamine oxidase inhibitors or within two weeks of discontinuation of their use.

Precautions: Nausea and vomiting may be troublesome. Phenothiazine antiemetics may be given with morphine, but it should be noted that morphine potentiates the effects of tranquillizers, anaesthetics, hypnotics, sedatives and alcohol.

Care should be exercised if morphine sulphate is given in the first 24 hours post-operatively, in hyperthyroidism, and where there is reduced respiratory reserve, such as kyphoscoliosis, emphysema and severe obesity. Morphine sulphate should not be given if paralytic ileus is likely to occur. If constipation occurs, this may be treated with appropriate laxatives.

It is wise to reduce dosage in chronic hepatic and renal disease, myxoedema, adrenocortical insufficiency, prostatic hypertrophy or shock. Tolerance and dependence may occur.

Although morphine sulphate has been in general use for many years, there is inadequate evidence of safety in human pregnancy and lactation. Morphine is known to cross the placenta and is excreted in breast milk, and may thus cause respiratory depression in the new born infant.

Medicines should not be used in pregnancy, especially the first trimester, unless the expected benefit outweighs any possible risk to the foetus.

Patients should be warned not to drive or operate dangerous machinery after taking Oramorph.

Overdosage: Signs of morphine toxicity and overdosage: These are likely to consist of pin-point pupils, respiratory depression and hypotension. Circulatory failure and deepening coma may occur in more severe cases.

Treatment of morphine overdosage: Administer 400 micrograms naloxone intravenously. Repeat at 2–3 minute intervals as necessary, or by an infusion of 2 mg in 500 ml of normal saline or 5% dextrose (4 micrograms/ml). Empty the stomach. A 0.02% aqueous solution of potassium permanganate may be used for lavage. Assist respiration if necessary. Maintain fluid and electrolyte levels.

Pharmaceutical precautions Store at room temperature. Protect from light.

Legal category CD(Sch 5), POM.

Package quantities Bottles of 100 ml, 250 ml and 500 ml.

Further information Oramorph Oral Solution has been formulated to have a bland flavour to make it acceptable to the patient regardless of taste perception.

Product licence number 0015/0122.

WARFARIN

Presentation Compressed tablets containing Warfarin Sodium BP, impressed with the letters $\frac{\text{WBP}}{\text{W}}$ one side and coloured according to strength; 1 mg–brown; 3 mg–blue, 5 mg–pink.

Uses *Action:* Oral anticoagulant.

Indications: For prophylaxis against venous thrombosis and pulmonary embolism, and for use in the treatment of these conditions to prevent their extension. For the prophylaxis of systemic embolisation in patients with rheumatic heart disease and atrial fibrillation.

Dosage and administration Effective blood levels are rapidly reached by administering an *initial loading dose* usually of the order of 0.45–0.50 mg/kg for adults.

Maintenance dosage is started when the peak effect of the initial dosage is passed, usually after 48 hours. Its size depends on the prothrombin time or other appropriate coagulation tests. The single daily maintenance requirement is usually between 5 mg and 12 mg, but can vary between 2 mg and 30 mg.

The maintenance dose is omitted if the prothrombin time is excessively prolonged. Once the maintenance dose is stabilised in the therapeutic range it is rarely necessary to alter it.

Use in elderly patients: The elderly are generally more sensitive to the effects of warfarin and often require a smaller dose on a weight for weight basis than younger patients.

Contra-indications, warnings, etc
Contra-indications: Animal studies have shown warfarin to be teratogenic and there have been reports of foetal death associated with its administration during human pregnancy. Warfarin should not be prescribed for pregnant women.

Warfarin should not be given to patients within three days of surgery.

The use in patients known to be hypersensitive to warfarin is contra-indicated.

Warnings: When warfarin therapy is first introduced, patients should be told what to do if bleeding occurs.

Warfarin should be given with caution to patients with impaired liver or kidney function or in severe hypertension.

Warfarin should be given with caution to patients where there is a risk of serious haemorrhage such as haemorrhagic blood dyscrasias, haemophilia, ulcerative disorders, threatened abortion, subacute bacterial endocarditis, in the presence of extensive surgical wounds and after recent surgery to the eye and central nervous system.

Prothrombin times should be determined at least twice weekly for the first two weeks and subsequently at longer intervals (every two to three weeks).

Overdose: Overdosage may be manifest by haematuria or spontaneous bruising. This should be treated with vitamin K_1 (5–10 mg) intravenously. Significant correction occurs within four hours. Haemorrhage or severe overdose should be treated with an infusion of fresh frozen plasma (or whole blood if the former is not available). Intravenous vitamin K_1 (5–10 mg) may be used to supplement specific therapy with factor concentrations or before minor procedures such as dental extractions. The administration of vitamin K_1 may make the patient resistant to anticoagulation for some days. For this reason, fresh frozen plasma should be administered to those patients with prosthetic heart valves.

Many factors *potentiate* the effect of warfarin:

1. Warfarin in the circulation is firmly bound to plasma protein and will have an increased effect if displaced by other drugs such as diuretics, oral anti-diabetic agents, anti-inflammatory agents and amiodarone.
2. Certain drugs, for example D-thyroxine, potentiate the effects of warfarin by increasing its affinity for the hepatic receptor site.
3. Alcohol may inhibit liver enzymes, leading to a reduced dosage requirement of warfarin.
4. Other drugs which may potentiate the effect of warfarin include anabolic steroids, cimetidine, aspirin, clofibrate, sulphinpyrazone, chloral hydrate, some aminoglycoside antibiotics, chloramphenicol, erythromycin, disulfiram and paracetamol.
5. Renal damage may reduce the rate of excretion of warfarin and thus decrease the dose requirement.
6. Acute illness, weight loss and a decreased intake of vitamin K will exaggerate the response.

Other factors may *decrease* the effect of warfarin:

1. Warfarin is metabolised in the liver by microsomal enzymes. These enzymes are induced by drugs such as barbiturates and phenytoin leading to rapid metabolism of warfarin and necessitating an increased dose.
2. Oestrogens and oral contraceptives increase the concentration of vitamin K-dependent factors. Increased doses of warfarin may therefore be required.
3. Cholestyramine may absorb warfarin and thus reduce its effect.
4. Weight gain, gastro-intestinal upset and increased intake of vitamin K will necessitate an increase in maintenance dosage of warfarin.
5. Carbamazepine, glutethimide, phenazone, griseofulvin and rifampicin also diminish the effect of warfarin.

Pharmaceutical precautions Protect from heat, light and moisture.

Legal category POM.

Package quantities 1 mg, 3 mg and 5 mg tablets in containers of 100 and 500.

Further information Nil.

Product licence numbers

Tablets 1 mg	1416/5060
Tablets 3 mg	1416/5061
Tablets 5 mg	1416/5062

**Trade Mark*

Boehringer Mannheim UK (Pharmaceuticals) Limited
Simpson Parkway
Kirkton Campus
Livingston, West Lothian
EH54 7BH

BEZALIP*

Presentation Bezalip is available as white, film coated tablets each containing 200 mg bezafibrate. The tablets are marked BM on one face and G6 on the reverse. Lactose is present in the formulation.

Uses Bezalip is indicated for use in hyperlipidaemias of Type IIa, IIb, III, IV and V (Fredrickson Classification) which are illustrated below:

Type	*Major Lipid Elevation*
IIa	Cholesterol
IIb	Cholesterol and Triglycerides
III	Cholesterol and Triglycerides
IV	Triglycerides
V	Triglycerides (possibly cholesterol)

Bezalip is therefore indicated for use only in patients with a fully defined and diagnosed abnormality where diet alone is insufficient to correct the condition and in whom the long-term risks associated with the condition warrant treatment.

The rationale for the use of Bezalip to control abnormal elevations of serum lipids and lipoproteins is to reduce or prevent the long term adverse effects which have been shown by many major epidemiological studies to be positively and strongly correlated with such dyslipidaemias. The possible beneficial and adverse long-term consequences of some drugs used in the hyperlipidaemias are still the subject of scientific discussion, however, and there is currently no clinical evidence to demonstrate that Bezalip is effective in the prevention of heart disease.

Dosage and administration The recommended dosage of Bezalip is three tablets daily, equivalent to 600 mg bezafibrate. The tablets may be taken with or after food. Maintenance dosage may occasionally be reduced to two tablets daily, particularly in the treatment of hypertriglyceridaemia.

The initial response to therapy is normally rapidly apparent although a progressive response over a number of weeks may occur. The patient's response to Bezalip should be monitored at intervals. Treatment should be terminated if an adequate response has not been achieved within 4 to 6 months.

Contra-indications, warnings, etc Bezalip is contra-indicated in patients with severe liver dysfunction or primary biliary cirrhosis, and in those with severe renal disorders (serum creatinine values above 6 mg/100 ml). As bezafibrate is normally highly protein bound it should not be given to patients with the nephrotic syndrome. Although the drug substance has not been shown, in animal studies, to have any adverse effects on the foetus, it is recommended that Bezalip should not be administered either to pregnant women or to those who are breast-feeding. Bezalip is contra-indicated in patients hypersensitive to bezafibrate.

The chronic administration of the highest dose of bezafibrate to rats was associated with hepatic tumour formation in females. This dose was in the order of 30–40 times the human dose. No such adverse effect was apparent at reduced intake levels approximating more closely to the lipid-lowering dosage in humans.

Care is required in administering Bezalip to patients receiving anti-coagulant therapy. The dose of anti-coagulant should be reduced by 50 per cent initially and then titrated to the patient's needs. The dosage of Bezalip may need to be reduced in patients with mild to moderate renal dysfunction (contra-indicated in severe cases). At serum creatinine levels of 1.5 to 2.5 mg per 100 ml the dose of Bezalip should be reduced to two tablets daily, while one tablet daily is recommended when serum creatinine is in the range 2.6 to 6 mg per 100 ml.

Adverse effects in clinical use are rarely seen. Most commonly these effects are gastro-intestinal in nature, such as feelings of fullness of the stomach. This side effect is frequently transitory and does not normally require cessation of treatment. Other adverse effects may include a myositis-like syndrome and rarely disorders of potency and general hypersensitivity. The incidence of all these potential effects is low, and there is no evidence that administration is associated with an increased frequency of gallstones.

No serious clinical or biochemical effects are likely to occur in cases of acute overdosage and treatment in such cases, where necessary, should be symptomatic.

Pharmaceutical precautions Bezalip tablets require no special storage conditions. It is recommended, however, that they be stored in a cool, dry place in accordance with normal pharmaceutical practice.

Legal category POM.

Package quantities Packs of 100 tablets.

Further information The risks associated with hyperlipidaemia may be increased in a super-additive manner by the presence of other factors such as hypertension, obesity, smoking, genetic predisposition and diabetes. This increased risk of long term adverse effects should be taken into consideration when evaluating whether hyperlipidaemia in any particular patient warrants treatment with Bezalip.

Product licence number 0075/0036.

BEZALIP MONO*

Presentation Bezalip Mono is a white, round, film-coated tablet with a white core and is imprinted BM/D9. Each tablet contains 400 mg bezafibrate. Lactose is present in the formulation.

Uses Bezalip Mono is indicated for use in hyperlipidaemia of Type IIa, IIb, III, IV and V (Fredrickson Classification) which are illustrated below:

Type	*Major Lipid Elevation*
IIa	Cholesterol
IIb	Cholesterol and Triglycerides
III	Cholesterol and Triglycerides
IV	Triglycerides
V	Triglycerides (possibly cholesterol)

Bezalip Mono is indicated for use only in patients with a fully defined and diagnosed abnormality where diet alone is insufficient to correct the condition and in whom long-term risks associated with the condition warrant treatment.

The rationale for use of Bezalip Mono to control

abnormal elevations of serum lipids and lipoproteins is to reduce or prevent the long term adverse effects which have been shown by many major epidemiological studies to be positively and strongly correlated with such dyslipidaemias. The possible beneficial and adverse long term consequences of some drugs used in the hyperlipidaemias are still the subject of scientific discussion, however, and there is currently no clinical evidence to demonstrate that Bezalip Mono is effective in the prevention of heart disease.

Dosage and administration The dosage of Bezalip Mono is one tablet daily, equivalent to 400 mg bezafibrate. The tablets should be taken with or after the evening meal and should be swallowed whole without chewing.

The initial response to therapy is normally rapidly apparent although a progressive response over a number of weeks may occur. The patient's response should be monitored at intervals. Treatment should be terminated if an adequate response has not been achieved within 4 to 6 months.

Contra-indications, warnings, etc Bezalip Mono is contra-indicated in patients with severe liver dysfunction and in those with severe renal disorders (serum creatinine values above 530 μ moles/l). As bezafibrate is normally highly protein-bound it should not be given to patients with the nephrotic syndrome. Although the drug substance has not been shown, in animal studies, to have any adverse effects on the foetus, it is recommended that Bezalip Mono should not be administered either to pregnant women or to those who are breast-feeding. Bezalip Mono is contra-indicated in patients hypersensitive to bezafibrate.

The chronic administration of the highest dose of bezafibrate to rats was associated with hepatic tumour formation in females. This dose was in the order of 30–40 times the human dose. No such adverse effect was apparent at reduced intake levels approximating more closely to the lipid-lowering dosage in humans.

Care is required in administering Bezalip Mono to patients receiving anti-coagulant therapy. The dose of anti-coagulant should be reduced initially by 50 per cent and then titrated to the patient's needs. In patients with moderate renal impairment (serum creatinine 220 to 530 μ moles/l) Bezalip Mono should not be employed. Such patients may be treated with conventional Bezalip tablets (200 mg bezafibrate) using a much reduced dosage.

Adverse effects in clinical use are rarely seen. Most commonly these effects are gastro-intestinal in nature, such as feelings of fullness of the stomach. This side effect is frequently transitory and does not normally require cessation of treatment. Other adverse effects may include a myositis-like syndrome and rarely disorders of potency and general hypersensitivity. The incidence of all these potential effects is low, and there is no evidence that administration is associated with an increased frequency of gallstones.

No serious clinical or biochemical effects are likely to occur in cases of acute overdosage and treatment in such cases, where necessary, should be symptomatic.

Pharmaceutical precautions Bezalip Mono requires no special storage conditions. It is recommended, however, that the tablets be stored in a cool, dry place in accordance with normal pharmaceutical practice.

Legal category POM.

Package quantities Calendar packs of 28 tablets (OP).

Further information The risks associated with hyperlipidaemia may be increased in a super-additive manner by the presence of other factors such as hypertension, obesity, smoking, genetic predisposition and diabetes. This increased risk of long-term adverse effects should be taken into consideration when evaluating whether hyperlipidaemia in any patient warrants treatment with Bezalip Mono.

Product licence number 0075/0051.

CANTIL*

Presentation Cantil Tablets are yellow, circular, biconvex and bear a score line. Each tablet contains mepenzolate bromide 25 mg. Also present in the formulation are sucrose and the colouring agent E102.

Uses

Pharmacology: Cantil contains a synthetic anticholinergic agent, mepenzolate bromide, which exerts its actions preferentially on the smooth muscle of the lower gastro-intestinal tract.

Indications: Relief of spasm or hypermotility of the lower gastro-intestinal tract in conditions such as irritable colon syndrome, spastic and mucous colitis, spastic constipation, acute or chronic non-specific diarrhoeas, diverticulitis and ulcerative colitis.

Dosage and administration Adults and older children: 1 or 2 Cantil Tablets. Children aged 6 to 12 years: Not recommended. Elderly: As adults with caution.

Contra-indications, warnings, etc Cantil is contra-indicated in patients with glaucoma, those who are pregnant or breast-feeding and in those who are hypersensitive to mepenzolate bromide and other anticholinergics. Potential cardiac effects also warrant avoidance in patients with tachycardia, unstable angina pectoris or other serious cardiac dysfunction. As mepenzolate bromide slows gastro-intestinal motility it should not be employed in patients with hiatus hernia and gastric reflux, or in those with obstructive disease conditions, paralytic ileus or toxic megacolon. Cantil is also contra-indicated in patients with hepatic dysfunction or moderate to severe renal dysfunction. The use of the product is also inappropriate in severe cases of ulcerative colitis, in obstructive uropathy and in patients with myasthenia gravis.

Whilst no specific interactions with other drugs are known, it is possible that mepenzolate bromide may modify the bioavailability of other substances, due to its effect on gastro-intestinal motility, and that it may interact with drugs which act on the autonomic nervous system. There also may be a risk of an additive anticholinergic action with a range of other drugs such as tricyclic antidepressants, benzodiazepines, antihistamines and those used for control of psychoses and Parkinson's syndrome.

As Cantil exerts its action mainly on the lower gastro-intestinal tract, unwanted effects of treatment are generally mild and transient. Most commonly these present as dryness of the mouth and blurring of vision. Other potential adverse effects are those typical of anticholinergic agents and may include heartburn, constipation, dysphagia, nausea and vomiting, altered taste perception, feelings of fullness in the abdomen, impotence, urinary retention or hesitancy and impairment of visual accommodation. Other effects may include tachycardia or palpitations, dermal flushing, dizziness, weakness and CNS effects such as nervousness and insomnia. Suppression of lactation may occur, although Cantil is contra-indicated in patients who are breast-feeding. As anticholinergic agents may decrease sweating, fever associated with a dry skin may be seen, and there is the possibility of heat prostration in a high temperature environment. As with all drugs, allergic reactions also may occur. These effects may occur particularly in patients with impaired metabolism or excretion, such as in hypothyroid and elderly patients, or in those with predisposing conditions such as coronary heart disease, congestive heart failure, cardiac arrhythmias, hypertension, asthma, hyperthyroidism, renal or hepatic impairment and generally debilitated patients. Use of Cantil is contra-indicated in a number of such categories and in the others it should be employed with caution.

In the event of overdosage the apparent signs and symptoms may include all those typical of anticholinergic drugs such as dilated pupils and blurred vision; raised temperature with flushed, hot, dry skin; urinary retention or hesitancy; dry mouth, dysphagia and vomiting; muscular weakness or paralysis; CNS effects may include drowsiness, stupor, agitation, tremor, mental confusion or excitation and hallucinations, whilst cardiovascular actions may be evident as tachycardia and circulatory collapse with associated tachypnoea.

The treatment of overdosage is as for atropine and other anticholinergic drugs. Empty the stomach by aspiration and lavage to remove any unabsorbed drug substance. Administer a saline purgative to promote peristalsis (using, for example, 30 grams sodium sulphate in 250 ml warmed water). A short-acting sedative or hypnotic, such as i.v. diazepam, may be given with caution if excitation occurs. Peripheral symptoms may be treated with i.m. or s.c. injection of neostigmine methylsulphate 5 mg at suitable intervals. Assisted respiration may be necessary as may catheterisation if urine is retained. Fluids should be given freely.

Pharmaceutical precautions Cantil tablets require no special storage conditions. It is recommended, however, that they be stored in a cool, dry place in accordance with normal pharmceutical practice.

Legal category POM.

Package quantities Cantil Tablets are available in packs of 50 tablets.

Further information Relief from the pain and discomfort of intestinal spasm typically is apparent within 10 to 20 minutes and generally lasts for approximately 4 hours. Due to the relatively specific action on the large intestine, especially the colon, Cantil has a low incidence of systemic anticholinergic effects.

Product licence number 0075/5002R.

CORO-NITRO* SPRAY

Presentation A metered dose aerosol providing 0.4 mg glyceryl trinitrate per dose. Each aerosol contains 200 doses for buccal administration.

Uses Treatment and prophylaxis of angina pectoris.

Dosage and administration The normal dosage is one or two doses (0.4 to 0.8 mg glyceryl trinitrate) as required for relief of anginal pain or for short term prophylaxis before physical or emotional stress or other factors known to precipitate anginal attacks. Occasionally up to 3 doses (1.2 mg glyceryl trinitrate) may be needed at a single time in severe cases. In no circumstances should this be exceeded.

Coro-Nitro Spray is for buccal administration and patients must be warned not to inhale the spray. During use the aerosol should be held upright, close to the mouth. Pressure on the spray head will release a single dose of 0.4 mg glyceryl trinitrate. The spray should be directed into the mouth, preferably onto or under the tongue. Patients should be encouraged to practise using Coro-Nitro Spray, by test-firing into the air, when they first receive the product.

Coro-Nitro Spray is not recommended for children.

Contra-indications, warnings, etc Coro-Nitro Spray is contra-indicated in hypotensive disorders, including shock, in cases of significant cerebral trauma, and in patients hypersensitive to glyceryl trinitrate.

Use of Coro-Nitro Spray during pregnancy is not contra-indicated but is at the sole discretion of the prescribing doctor.

Adverse effects are similar to those normally seen with glyceryl trinitrate and may include headache, facial flushing, dizziness and nausea. Hypotensive effects may occur, especially when the patient has been consuming alcohol or is taking other hypotensive medication.

Excessive dosage may promote severe headache, facial flushing, hypotension and fainting and, rarely, cyanosis and methaemoglobinaemia. In some cases the effect of overdose will closely resemble shock. Recovery normally occurs spontaneously. The patient should lie in a supine position with the legs elevated to promote venous return. Symptomatic treatment may be needed if there is severe circulatory or respiratory collapse. Methaemoglobinaemia will respond to methylene blue infusion.

Note that if sprayed directly on to a naked flame the spray may briefly flare or sputter. Patients, especially those who smoke, should be warned not to use Coro-Nitro Spray near to a naked flame.

Pharmaceutical precautions Coro-Nitro Spray should not be stored in direct sunlight or near direct sources of heat. The aerosol container must not be punctured, broken or burnt, even if it appears to be empty.

Legal category P.

Package quantities Each Coro-Nitro Spray will deliver 200 metered doses of 0.4 mg glyceryl trinitrate (OP).

Further information Coro-Nitro Spray is extremely stable and has a shelf life in excess of 3 years.

Coro-Nitro Spray may be employed together with other anti-anginal agents when necessary, including those used for long term prophylaxis such as isosorbide mononitrate and betablockers.

Product licence number 0075/0052.

GASTROCOTE*

Presentation Gastrocote is presented as white, uncoated tablets which are engraved on one side with the name Gastrocote. Each tablet contains:

Alginic Acid BP	200 mg
Dried Aluminium Hydroxide Gel BP	80 mg
Magnesium Trisilicate BP	40 mg
Sodium Bicarbonate BP	70 mg

Uses Gastrocote acts to reduce the incidence of gastric reflux and thus of associated discomfort and pain. Gastrocote is indicated in heartburn, including heartburn of pregnancy, reflux oesophagitis, particularly where associated with hiatus hernia, and in all cases of epigastric distress associated with gastric reflux or regurgitation.

Dosage and administration *Adults and older children only:* 1 or 2 tablets to be chewed four times a day, that is, after main meals and at bedtime. Not to be given to children under 6 years.

Important: The tablets must be well chewed before swallowing.

Contra-indications, warnings, etc Care should be exercised in treating diabetic patients as the tablets each contain approximately 1 g of sucrose. Each tablet also contains 21 mg (0.91 mEq) of sodium which may be important for patients on a low sodium diet. There are no specific contra-indications to the use of Gastrocote and overdosage is virtually free of hazard although gastric bloating may occur.

Pharmaceutical precautions Gastrocote should be stored in a cool dry place.

Legal category P.

Package quantities Gastrocote tablets are supplied in containers of 100 tablets.

Further information When Gastrocote tablets are chewed sodium alginate is formed as a foam with the antacid constituents entrained. The foam coats the oesophagus with a demulcent, antacid layer when swallowed and then forms a viscous, colloidal foam gel floating on the stomach contents. This mild barrier physically impedes reflux. In the event of reflux being forced the demulcent alginate-antacid foam moves into the lower oesophagus before the stomach contents thus protecting the mucosa from further proteolytic attack and allowing healing to occur.

Product licence number 0075/0024.

GASTROCOTE* LIQUID

Presentation Gastrocote Liquid is a peach coloured suspension with an odour and taste reminiscent of butterscotch/mint. Each 5 ml contains:

Sodium Alginate BP	220 mg
Magnesium Trisilicate BP	40 mg
Dried Aluminium Hydroxide BP	80 mg
Sodium Bicarbonate BP	70 mg

The formulation also contains a hydroxybenzoate preservative and colouring agent E110.

Uses Gastrocote Liquid acts to reduce the incidence of gastric reflux and thus of associated discomfort and pain. It is indicated for use in heartburn, including heartburn of pregnancy, reflux oesophagitis, especially where associated with hiatus hernia, and in all cases of epigastric distress associated with gastric reflux or regurgitation.

Dosage and administration *Adults and older children only:* 5 to 15 ml (1 to 3 × 5 ml spoonfuls) to be taken four times daily, that is, after main meals and at bedtime. The container should be well shaken before each dose.

Contra-indications, warnings, etc There are no specific contra-indications to the use of Gastrocote Liquid.

Each 5 ml contains 42 mg sodium (1.8 mEq) which may be important for patients on a restricted salt intake.

No special dosage reduction is necessary in elderly patients although Gastrocote Liquid is not recommended for use in very young children and infants.

Acute overdosage is virtually free of hazard as Gastrocote Liquid is effective due to local physical actions rather than to a systemic pharmacological mechanism. Gastric bloating may be anticipated and, if necessary, should be treated symptomatically.

Pharmaceutical precautions It is recommended that Gastrocote Liquid be stored in a cool place. Gastrocote Liquid should be dispensed in the original pack and once opened should be used within one month.

Legal category P.

Package quantities Gastrocote Liquid is available in packs of 500 ml (OP).

Further information Gastrocote Liquid forms a low density foam gel raft in the stomach. The antacid constituents remain entrained in the foam gel raft and do not influence gastric pH. The foam gel raft floats on the gastric contents and physically impedes gastro-oesophageal reflux. In the event of reflux being forced the alginate-antacid foam enters the oesophagus first, thus coating the mucosa, providing demulcent, antacid protection and allowing healing to occur.

Product licence number 0075/0055.

ISMO*

Presentation Ismo tablets are white, circular, uncoated and contain isosorbide mononitrate.

The presentations available, which all contain lactose, are:

Ismo 10: 10 mg isosorbide mononitrate. Each tablet is marked Ismo on one face and 10 on the reverse.

Ismo 20: 20 mg isosorbide mononitrate. Each tablet is marked with a score line and BMB3 on both faces.

Ismo 40: 40 mg isosorbide mononitrate. Each tablet is marked Ismo on one face and 40 on the reverse.

The Ismo Starter Pack contains both Ismo 10 and Ismo 20 tablets for initiation of therapy in new patients.

Uses Ismo products are indicated for use in the treatment and prophylaxis of angina pectoris and as adjunctive therapy in congestive heart failure which does not respond adequately to cardiac glycosides and/or diuretics.

Dosage and administration The recommended dosage is from 20 to 120 mg isosorbide mononitrate daily in divided doses. The majority of patients will require a dosage in the range of 40 to 60 mg daily in divided doses. The tablets should be swallowed whole without chewing.

For patients who have not previously received prophylactic nitrate therapy it is recommended that the Ismo Starter Pack be employed. This provides an initial dosage of 10 mg isosorbide mononitrate (1 tablet) daily for 2 days followed by a dosage of 20 mg daily (1 tablet morning and evening) for a further 3 days. Subsequently the daily dosage may be increased to the normal prophylactic level using the Ismo 20 tablets also included in the Starter Pack. Patients already accustomed to chronic nitrate therapy normally may be transferred directly to a therapeutic dose of Ismo. For those previously treated with isosorbide dinitrate in conventional form the dosage of Ismo should be the same initially. Ismo is effectively twice as potent as sustained release forms of isosorbide dinitrate and patients transferred from such treatment initially should receive Ismo at half the previous dosage.

Contra-indications, warnings, etc Ismo tablets are contra-indicated in patients with a known hypersensitivity to isosorbide mononitrate or isosorbide dinitrate.

No dosage adjustment is necessary in the elderly, or in those with renal or hepatic impairment.

A number of nitrate-related adverse effects may occur during treatment including headache and feelings of dizziness. The incidence of such effects is normally highest at the commencement of treatment and tends to decline with time. The Ismo Starter Pack is provided to assist in minimising such effects initially. In highly sensitive patients hypotension may occur, especially after a high dose. Other reactions, similar to those associated with isosorbide dinitrate, may occur occasionally. In the event of overdosage the main sign is liable to be hypotension which should be treated by laying the patient in a supine position with the legs elevated to promote venous return.

Pharmaceutical precautions No special storage or handling precautions apply although it is recommended that Ismo products be kept in a cool, dry place in accordance with good pharmaceutical practice.

Legal category P.

Package quantities Ismo Starter Pack: 8 tablets of Ismo 10 in a calenderised blister strip and 56 tablets of Ismo 20 also in blister strips (OP).

Ismo 10: Packs of 100 tablets.
Ismo 20: Packs of 100 tablets.
Ismo 40: Packs of 100 tablets.

Further information Ismo provides long term nitrate treatment of angina pectoris and heart failure in a form with complete biological availability due to lack of any significant hepatic first-pass metabolism. This provides consistently uniform blood levels of drug substance and a predictable clinical response. The onset of activity occurs within 20 minutes and, depending on dosage, is maintained for up to 10 hours.

Product licence numbers 0075/0044, 0075/0045, 0075/0056.

ISMO* RETARD

Presentation Circular, white, sugar coated tablets containing 40 mg isosorbide mononitrate in a sustained release form. Lactose is present in the formulation.

Uses Ismo Retard is indicated for the prophylaxis of angina pectoris.

Dosage and administration Ismo Retard has been developed to provide a convenient, once daily dosage form of isosorbide mononitrate. It is designed to achieve therapeutic blood concentrations within 30 minutes which persist up to 17 hours. A nitrate free interval of up to 7 hours makes the development of anti-anginal tolerance during chronic therapy unlikely.

The tablets should be swallowed whole without chewing.

Adults: One tablet daily, to be taken in the morning.

Elderly: There is no evidence to suggest an adjustment of dose is necessary. However, caution may be required in elderly patients who are known to be susceptible to the effects of hypotensive medication.

Children: The safety and effficacy of Ismo Retard in children has not been established.

Contra-indications, warnings, etc Ismo Retard is contra-indicated in patients with a known hypersensitivity to isosorbide mononitrate or isosorbide dinitrate.

Ismo Retard is not indicated for relief of acute anginal attacks. In the event of an acute attack, sublingual or buccal glyceryl trinitrate tablets or spray should be used.

Patients who have not previously received nitrates may be started with a low dose, which should be increased gradually, before introducing Ismo Retard.

Caution is required in patients with increased susceptibility to hypotension and in patients with marked hepatic or renal insufficiency, closed angle glaucoma, marked anaemia and hypothyroidism.

There is inadequate evidence of safety of the drug in human pregnancy although nitrates have been in wide use for many years without ill consequence, animal studies having shown no adverse effects on the foetus. Nevertheless it is not advisable to use this drug during pregnancy and lactation.

A number of nitrate-related adverse effects may occur during treatment, including headache and feelings of dizziness. Other reactions, such as those associated with isosorbide dinitrate (e.g. flushing, postural hypotension, skin reactions) may occur occasionally.

Some of the effects of alcohol and the action of hypotensive agents may be potentiated by isosorbide mononitrate.

In the event of overdosage with Ismo Retard the main sign is likely to be hypotension. The stomach should be aspirated to remove any remaining tablets. The patient should be placed in a supine position with the legs elevated to promote venous return. Any other treatment should be symptomatic.

Pharmaceutical precautions No special handling or storage precautions apply. As with all medicines, however, it is recommended that Ismo Retard be stored in a cool, dry place.

Legal category P.

Package quantities Packs of 28 tablets (OP).

Further information Nil.

Product licence number 0075/0057.

LORON*▾

Presentation Loron capsules are white, size 0, hard gelatin capsules each containing 400 mg sodium clodronate for oral administration. Each capsule is marked BM B7.

Uses

Indication: Loron capsules are indicated for the maintenance of clinically acceptable serum calcium levels in patients with hypercalcaemia of malignancy initially treated with an intravenous infusion of sodium clodronate.

Properties: Sodium clodronate is a diphosphonate which has a high affinity to bone. It is mainly the portion of the dose adsorbed to bone which is pharmacologically active. The pharmacological effect of sodium clodronate is to suppress osteoclast-mediated bone resorption as judged by bone histology and decreases in serum calcium, urine calcium and urinary excretion of hydroxyproline, without adversely affecting mineralisation.

Dosage and administration

Adults: The recommended dose is 4 capsules (1600 mg sodium clodronate) daily. If necessary the dosage may be increased but should not exceed a maximum of 8 capsules (3200 mg sodium clodronate) daily. The capsules may be taken as a single dose or in two equally divided doses if necessary to improve gastro-intestinal tolerance. Loron capsules should be swallowed with a little fluid, but not milk, at least one hour before or one hour after food. The duration of treatment with Loron capsules should not exceed 6 months.

Elderly: No special dosage recommendations.

Children: Safety and efficacy in children has not been established.

Use in renal impairment: The effect of sodium clodronate in patients with moderate to severe renal impairment (serum creatinine greater than 440 micromol/l) has not been systematically examined in clinical trials. Since sodium clodronate is excreted unchanged by the kidney its use is contra-indicated in these patients. In patients with normal renal function or mild renal impairment (serum creatinine less than 440 micromol/l) serum creatinine should be monitored during therapy.

Contra-indications, warnings, etc

Contra-indications: Hypersensitivity to sodium clodronate. Acute, severe inflammatory conditions of the gastro-intestinal tract. Pregnancy and lactation. Moderate to severe renal failure (serum creatinine greater than 440 ml micromol/l). Concomitant use of other diphosphonates.

Precautions and warnings: No information is available on the potential carcinogenicity of sodium clodronate. The use of sodium clodronate should be restricted to 6 months as long-term toxicological data are not available.

It is recommended that appropriate monitoring of renal function with serum creatinine be carried out during treatment. Serum calcium and phosphate should be monitored periodically. Monitoring of liver enzymes and white cell counts is advised (see side effects).

Use in pregnancy and lactation: There are insufficient data either from animal studies or from experience in humans of the effects of sodium clodronate on the embryo and foetus. No studies have been conducted on excretion in breast milk. Consequently, sodium clodronate is contra-indicated in pregnancy and lactation.

Side effects: Patients may experience a mild gastro-intestinal upset, usually in the form of nausea or mild diarrhoea. The symptoms may respond to the use of a twice daily dosage regime, rather than a single dose. It is not normally required to withdraw therapy or to provide medication to control these effects. Asymptomatic hypocalcaemia has been noted rarely. A reversible elevation of serum parathyroid hormone may occur. In a small proportion of patients a mild, reversible increase in serum lactate dehydrogenase and a modest transient leucopenia have been reported although these may have been associated with concurrent chemotherapy. Allergic skin reactions have been observed in rare cases.

Interactions: No other diphosphonate drugs should be given with Loron capsules. There is no evidence from clinical experience that sodium clodronate interacts with other medication such as steroids, diuretics, NSAIDs, calcitonin or chemotherapeutic agents. Calcium rich foods, mineral supplements and antacids may impair absorption.

Overdosage: There is no experience of acute overdosage in humans. The development of hypocalcaemia is possible for up to 2 or 3 days following the overdosage. Serum calcium should be monitored and oral or parenteral calcium supplementation may be required. Acute overdosage may be associated with gastro-intestinal symptoms such as nausea and vomiting. Treatment should be symptomatic.

Pharmaceutical precautions No special handling or storage precautions apply. It is recommended however, that the capsules be stored in a cool, dry place in accordance with normal pharmaceutical practice.

Legal category POM.

Package quantities Original packs of 120 capsules.

Further information Sodium clodronate has been reported to improve bone pain in open and placebo controlled studies in patients with neoplastic bone disease from breast cancer, prostatic carcinoma or multiple myeloma.

Product licence numbers 0075/0063.

LORON* FOR INFUSION▾

Presentation Loron for Infusion is presented as a clear, colourless, sterile liquid containing 300 mg sodium clodronate per 10 ml ampoule, for use by intravenous infusion after dilution.

Uses
Indication: Loron for Infusion is indicated for the normalisation of serum calcium levels in hypercalcaemia of malignancy in conjunction with full rehydration of patients as appropriate.

Properties: Sodium clodronate is a diphosphonate which has a high affinity for bone. It is mainly the portion of a dose adsorbed to bone which is pharmacologically active. The pharmacological effect of sodium clodronate is to suppress osteoclast-mediated bone resorption, as judged by bone histology and decreases in serum calcium, urine calcium and urinary excretion of hydroxyproline, without adversely affecting mineralisation.

Dosage and administration Loron for Infusion is a concentrated presentation which must be diluted before use. The only recommended diluent is 0.9% w/v sodium chloride intravenous infusion. A single ampoule of Loron for Infusion (300 mg sodium clodronate) should be added aseptically to 500 ml of sodium chloride intravenous infusion (0.9%). No other drugs or nutrients may be added. The diluted infusion solution should be administered by slow intravenous infusion over a period of not less than 2 hours. Slow infusion is important for safety. It is recommended that oral or intravenous fluids be administered to establish or maintain full hydration.

Adults: The recommended dosage is 300 mg sodium clodronate/day. The duration of treatment with Loron for Infusion depends on patient response but should not exceed 10 days. In most cases an elevated serum calcium level can be lowered to within the normal range after treatment for 3 to 5 successive days. Normocalcaemia may be maintained thereafter with oral administration of Loron capsules. If hypercalcaemia recurs, the intravenous infusion may be reintroduced.

Elderly: No special dosage recommendations.

Children: Safety and efficacy in children has not been established.

Use in renal impairment: The effect of sodium clodronate in patients with moderate to severe renal impairment (serum creatinine greater than 440 micromol/l) has not been systematically examined in clinical trials. Since sodium clodronate is excreted unchanged by the kidney its use is contra-indicated in these patients. In patients with normal renal function or mild renal impairment (serum creatinine less than 440 micromol/l) serum creatinine should be monitored during therapy.

Contra-indications, warnings, etc
Contra-indications: Hypersensitivity to sodium clodronate. Pregnancy and lactation. Moderate to severe renal failure (serum creatinine greater than 440 micromol/l). Concomitant use of other diphosphonates.

Precautions and warnings: Intravenous infusion of sodium clondronate may be associated with a transient proteinuria immediately after infusion even when the correct dosage and administration recommendations are followed (see side effects). Hypercalcaemia may promote or worsen renal dysfunction and the use of sodium clodronate has normally been demonstrated to improve renal function as the serum calcium concentration is lowered. Nevertheless, care is required with the intravenous route of administration and the recommended dosage must not be exceeded.

It is recommended that appropriate monitoring of renal function with serum creatinine be carried out during treatment with Loron for Infusion. Serum calcium and phosphate should also be monitored periodically. Monitoring of liver enzymes and white cell counts is advised (see side effects).

Use in pregnancy and lactation: There are insufficient data either from animal studies or from experience in humans of the effects of sodium clodronate on the embryo and foetus. No studies have been conducted on excretion in breast milk. Consequently, sodium clodronate is contra-indicated in pregnancy and lactation.

Side-effects: Asymptomatic hypocalcaemia has been noted rarely. A reversible elevation of serum parathyroid hormone may occur. In a small proportion of patients a mild reversible increase in serum lactate dehydrogenase and a modest transient leucopenia have been reported although these may have been associated with concurrent or previous chemotherapy. Transient proteinuria has been reported immediately after intravenous infusion (see precautions and warnings). The clinical significance is uncertain. However chronic proteinuria following infusion has not been observed. Allergic skin reactions have been reported in rare cases.

Interactions: No other diphosphonate drugs should be given with Loron for Infusion. There is no evidence from clinical experience that sodium clodronate interacts with other medication such as steroids, diuretics, NSAIDs, calcitonin or chemotherapeutic agents.

Overdosage: There is no experience of acute overdosage in humans. An overdose by intravenous infusion, or injection of undiluted infusion concentrate, could provoke renal damage and renal function should be monitored. The development of hypocalcaemia is possible for up to 2 or 3 days after the overdose. Serum calcium should be monitored and oral or parenteral calcium supplementation may be required.

Pharmaceutical precautions No special storage conditions are required. Loron for Infusion must be diluted with the recommended solution before use. The prepared dilution should be administered over a period of not less than 2 hours and the infusion should be completed within 12 hours of preparation of the dilution.

Legal category POM.

Package quantities The ampoules are supplied in packs of 5.

Further information Sodium clodronate has been reported to improve bone pain in open and placebo controlled studies in patients with neoplastic bone disease from breast cancer, prostatic carcinoma or multiple myeloma.

Product licence numbers 0075/0064.

PALFIUM*

Presentation Palfium products contain Dextromoramide Tartrate BP, and the dose and strength are expressed as dextromoramide base. The presentations available cover the oral, parenteral and rectal routes of administration:

Palfium tablets, 5 mg: white, scored tablets for oral use (Dextromoramide Tablets BP, 5 mg).

Palfium tablets, 10 mg: peach, scored tablets for oral use (Dextromoramide Tablets BP, 10 mg).

Palfium injection, 5 mg and 10 mg per 1.0 ml of solution: a clear, colourless, aqueous solution for parenteral administration (Dextromoramide Tartrate Injection BP, 5 mg or 10 mg per 1 ml).

Palfium suppositories, 10 mg: light cream coloured suppositories for rectal administration.

Lactose is present in Palfium tablets and suppositories. Palfium tablets 10 mg contain colouring agent E 110 whilst sodium chloride is present to ensure isotonicity in both parenteral products.

Uses Palfium is a potent analgesic for relief of the severe pain of inoperable carcinoma and for the relief of other forms of severe and intractable pain.

Dosage and administration *Adult dosage: First dose:* Not more than 5 mg by mouth or by subcutaneous or intramuscular injection, or 10 mg rectally.

Subsequent doses: The size of subsequent doses depends upon the needs of the patient, that is, upon the severity of the pain. In cases of severe pain 10 mg

Palfium may be required, repeated as necessary in order to maintain analgesia. The dose required may also be influenced by the patient's body weight. Regardless of body weight, however, not more than 20 mg should be given as a single dose and usually not more than 15 mg by injection. The dose frequency and the total daily dosage may vary significantly and should be titrated according to the needs of the individual patient.

In postoperative pain the initial dose of Palfium in the immediate postoperative period should be restricted, for example, to 2.5 mg, as the patient may still be under the influence of circulating anaesthetic agents and pre-medications. For subsequent postoperative care, 5 mg three or four times daily as required is usually sufficient.

Administration: Palfium is as effective orally as by injection. The oral route of administration thus is to be preferred. Palfium tablets should be given before food, if possible. Palfium is also fully effective rectally and a 10 mg dose may be administered by suppository, particularly at night. When oral administration is impracticable Palfium injection may be administered by the intramuscular or subcutaneous route. Administration by the intravenous route is not recommended in normal practice.

Child dosage: A paediatric dosage regime has not yet been established. Should the need arise to administer Palfium to a child, the initial dosage should be not more than 0.08 mg per kg of body weight.

Contra-indications, warnings, etc Palfium is contra-indicated in patients with respiratory depression or obstructive airways disease, and in female patients during child-birth. It is also contra-indicated in patients receiving monoamine oxidase inhibitors and two to three weeks should be allowed to elapse before Palfium is administered to patients who have been treated with these agents.

The use of Palfium in pregnant patients is not recommended, although there is no evidence from animal studies to suggest that it is potentially harmful. In cases where the rate of metabolism of dextromoramide may be reduced, such as in the elderly and in patients with hypothyroidism or chronic hepatic insufficiency, it may be advisable to employ a reduced dosage regime.

Palfium may give rise to dizziness and sweating, especially in the ambulant patient. These effects may be minimised by advising the patient to rest, preferably supine, for a short period after administration of the first few doses. Nausea and vomiting may be troublesome but tend to occur only rarely. As with other potent analgesics tolerance and addiction may occur with continued use of Palfium. Concurrent administration of CNS depressants, including alcohol, must be carefully considered as such agents may enhance the central effects of Palfium and consequently the risk of respiratory depression.

Respiratory depression is unlikely to occur when Palfium is employed on its own in a normal therapeutic dosage. In the event of oral overdosage empty the stomach by aspiration and lavage using, for example, a 0.02% aqueous solution of potassium permanganate. If consciousness is impaired and respiration depressed suitable antagonists should be administered. Levallorphan tartrate 1.0 mg intravenously initially, followed by 1 or 2 doses of 0.5 mg may be used. Alternatively, nalorphine or naloxone may be administered using the appropriate dosage.

The circulation should be maintained with intravenous infusion of plasma or suitable electrolyte solutions and assisted respiration may be necessary until spontaneous breathing is restored.

Pharmaceutical precautions Palfium ampoules and tablets require no special precautions. As with all medicines, however, it is preferable that they be stored in a cool, dry place. Palfium suppositories must be stored in a cool location well away from radiators and other sources of heat.

Legal category CD (Sch 2) POM.

Package quantities Palfium tablets 5 mg and 10 mg, blister packs of 60.

Palfium injection, 5 mg and 10 mg per ml, packs of 10 1.1 ml ampoules.

Palfium suppositories, packs of 10.

Further information Palfium is as effective when given by mouth as when injected. The analgesic effect is rapid by all routes of administration (typically 20–30 minutes).

Palfium provides pain relief normally without clouding consciousness or mental activity, and does not cause constipation. It may be advantageous in some cases to provide simultaneous administration of a sedative, hypnotic or tranquilliser, such as chlorpromazine, with Palfium. A cautious approach should be made to establish the most satisfactory dosage regime. In most cases only half the normal dose of the ancillary drug will be required.

Product licence numbers

Palfium Tablets 5 mg	0075/5015R.
Palfium Tablets 10 mg	0075/0035R.
Palfium Injection 5 mg	0075/5012R.
Palfium Injection 10 mg	0075/5013R.
Palfium Suppositories	0075/5014R.

PIPTALIN*

Presentation Piptalin elixir is an orange-flavoured and orange coloured suspension. Each 5 ml of elixir contains pipenzolate bromide 4 mg and simethicone (activated dimethicone) 40 mg. The formulation also contains sodium benzoate as a preservative and colouring agent E110.

Uses

Pharmacology: Piptalin contains a synthetic anticholinergic agent, pipenzolate bromide, which provides both an antisecretory activity and an effect on smooth muscle spasm or hypermotility.

Indications: Piptalin is indicated for the alleviation of the discomfort and pain associated with spasm, hypermotility and gaseous distention in functional and organic digestive disorders. Piptalin is also indicated for functional abdominal pain in the school child and for flatulent dyspepsia, aerophagia, cardiospasm and pylorospasm.

Dosage and administration

Infants up to 10 kg body weight: 2.5 ml orally, 15 minutes before feeding, up to a maximum of four doses in each 24 hour period.

Young children: 10–20 kg body weight: 2.5–5.0 ml three or four times daily.

Older children: 20–40 kg body weight: 5.0 ml three or four times daily.

Adults: 10 ml three or four times daily.

Elderly: As adults with caution.

Piptalin elixir should be taken approximately 15 minutes before meals; if necessary it may be diluted with water.

Contra-indications, warnings, etc Piptalin is contra-indicated in pregnancy, lactation, and in those who are hypersensitive to pipenzolate bromide and other anticholinergics. Piptalin should be used with caution in patients with glaucoma and in those at a risk of urinary retention such as those with obstructive uropathy e.g. prostatic hypertrophy. Potential cardiac effects also warrant avoidance in patients with tachycardia, unstable angina pectoris or other serious cardiac dysfunction. As pipenzolate bromide slows gastro-intestinal motility it should not be employed in patients with obstructive disease conditions, pyloric stenosis, paralytic ileus or toxic megacolon. Piptalin is also contra-indicated in patients with hepatic dysfunction or moderate to severe renal dysfunction. The use of the product is also inappropriate in severe cases of ulcerative colitis and in patients with myasthenia gravis.

Whilst no specific interactions with other drugs are known it is possible that pipenzolate bromide may modify the bioavailability of other substances, due to its effect on gastro-intestinal motility, and that it may interact with drugs which act on the autonomic nervous system. There also may be a risk of an additive anticholinergic action with a range of other drugs such as tricyclic antidepressants, benzodiazepines, antihistamines and in those used for control of psychoses and Parkinson's syndrome.

As Piptalin exerts its action mainly on the gastro-intestinal tract, unwanted effects of treatment are generally mild and transient. Most commonly these present as dryness of the mouth. Other potential adverse effects are those typical of anticholinergic agents and may include constipation, dysphagia, nausea and vomiting, altered taste perception, feelings of fullness in the abdomen, impotence, urinary retention or hesitancy and impairment of visual accommodation.

Other effects may include tachycardia or palpitations, dermal flushing, dizziness, weakness and CNS effects such as nervousness and insomnia. Suppression of lactation may occur, although Piptalin is contra-indicated in patients who are breast-feeding. As anticholinergic agents may decrease sweating, fever associated with a dry skin may be seen, and there is the possibility of heat prostration in a high temperature environment. As with all drugs, allergic reactions may occur. Such effects may occur particularly in patients with impaired metabolism or excretion, such as in hypothyroid and elderly patients, or in those with predisposing conditions such as coronary heart disease, congestive heart failure, cardiac arrhythmias, hypertension, asthma, hyperthyroidism, renal or hepatic impairment and in generally debilitated patients.

Use of Piptalin is contra-indicated in a number of these categories and in the others it should be employed with caution.

In the event of overdosage the apparent signs and symptoms may include all those typical of anticholinergic drugs such as dilated pupils and blurred vision; raised temperature with flushed, hot, dry skin; urinary retention or hesitancy; dry mouth, dysphagia and vomiting; muscular weakness or paralysis; CNS effects may include drowsiness, stupor, agitation, tremor, mental confusion or excitation and hallucinations, whilst cardiovascular actions may be evident as tachycardia and circulatory collapse with associated tachypnoea.

Treatment of overdosage is as for atropine and other anticholinergic drugs. Empty the stomach by aspiration and lavage to remove any unabsorbed drug substance. Administer a saline purgative to promote peristalsis (using, for example, 30 g sodium sulphate in 250 ml warmed water). A short acting sedative or hypnotic, such as i.v. diazepam may be given with caution if excitation occurs. Peripheral symptoms may be treated with i.m. or s.c. injection of neostigmine methylsulphate 5 mg at suitable intervals. Assisted respiration may be necessary as may catheterisation if urine is retained. Fluid should be given freely.

Pharmaceutical precautions Piptalin Elixir should be shaken thoroughly before use. It may be diluted with water or syrup and is incompatible with alkaline solutions.

Legal category POM.

Package quantities Piptalin elixir is available in bottles of 100 ml and 500 ml.

Further information Relief from discomfort and pain due to spasm and flatulence usually occurs within 10 to 20 minutes and the duration of antispasmodic action is normally approximately four hours.

Piptalin combines the antispasmodic activity of pipenzolate bromide with the deflatulant effects of simethicone. The former relieves spasm and reduces hypermotility and gastric secretion while simethicone assists in elimination of entrapped gas and in prevention of the formation of mucous-occluded gas pockets in the gastro-intestinal tract.

Product licence number 0075/5017.

RECORMON*▼

Presentation Recormon contains epoetin beta (a recombinant human erythropoietin (rhEPO)) as a freeze-dried powder. Provided with each vial is an ampoule containing Water for Injections for reconstitution of the powder.

The presentations available are:
Recormon 1000: 1000 international units (IU) epoetin beta (corresponding to 8.3 micrograms erythropoietin) with 1 ml Water for Injections.
Recormon 2000: 2000 international units (IU) epoetin beta (corresponding to 16.6 micrograms erythropoietin) with 2 ml Water for Injections.
Recormon 5000: 5000 international units (IU) epoetin beta (corresponding to 41.5 micrograms erythropoietin) with 5 ml Water for Injections.

Uses Recormon is indicated for use in the correction of erythropoietin deficiency in dialysis patients with renal anaemia.

Dosage and administration There are two stages in the treatment with Recormon.

Adults:
(1) Correction of renally induced anaemia. The initial dosage for the first 4 weeks of treatment is 40 IU per kg of body weight three times per week, although this dosage may be increased after 1 month to 80 IU per kg of body weight if the initial haemoglobin response is less than 1 g per 100 ml per month. If necessary further increases of 20 IU per kg of body weight, at monthly intervals, may be made in order to achieve a haemoglobin between 10 to 12 g per 100 ml (haematocrit 30 to 35%). The maximum dosage should not exceed 240 IU per kg body weight three times a week.
(2) Maintenance therapy. To maintain a haemoglobin in the range 10 to 12 g per 100 ml (haematocrit 30 to 35%), the previous correction dose should be reduced by half initially. Subsequent doses are dependent upon the patient's response. As a general guideline, a dose of 30 IU per kg of body weight three times per week after dialysis may be considered as a typical maintenance dose.

Elderly: As for adults.

Children: A dosage regime has not yet been established.

Administration: For administration the freeze-dried powder must be dissolved using the contents of the ampoule of Water for Injections, also supplied, for each vial. The dissolved substance should be administered over approximately 2 minutes using the intravenous route, for example, in haemodialysis patients via the arteriovenous fistula on completion of the dialysis.

Whilst treatment with Recormon is normally a life-long therapy, it may be interrupted or terminated, if necessary, at any time at the discretion of the physician.

Contra-indications, warnings, etc
Contra-indications: There are no specific contra-indications.

Pregnancy and lactation: As experience in human pregnancy is inadequate and only limited animal teratogenicity studies have been conducted. Recormon is not recommended for use during pregnancy. Similarly there is little experience of the use of Recormon in patients who are breast feeding.

Precautions: Recormon should be used with caution in the presence of hypertension which is untreated, inadequately treated or difficult to control, in epilepsy, in patients with a raised platelet count (thrombocytosis), chronic hepatic failure, malignant conditions or known hypersensitivity to the product.

Deficiencies of folic acid and vitamin B_{12} should be excluded as they reduce the effectiveness of Recormon. In many cases, the increase in haemoglobin is accompanied by reduced serum ferritin values. Iron therapy, eg 200 to 300 mg/day orally or iron dextran intravenously twice weekly during the last hour of haemodialysis, is recommended for all patients with serum ferritin values below 100 micrograms per litre. Severe aluminium toxicity may delay the effectiveness of Recormon.

Interactions: There is no evidence from clinical usage so far to indicate that Recormon interacts with any other drug therapy.

Adverse events: Particularly at the commencement of treatment patients may experience flu-like symptoms such as headache, aching joints and feelings of weakness, dizziness and lassitude.

The most frequent adverse effect during treatment with Recormon is a dose-dependent increase in blood pressure or a worsening of existing hypertension. These increases in blood pressure may be treated with appropriate medication. Monitoring of blood pressure is recommended between dialysis sessions and especially at the commencement of therapy. In patients with normal or low blood pressure there have been isolated cases of hypertensive crisis with encephalopathy-like symptoms (headache and confusional state) and generalized tonic/clonic seizures requiring immediate medical attention. Particular attention should be paid to sudden stabbing migraine-like headaches as a possible warning sign.

There may be a moderate dose-dependent increase in the platelet count, within the normal range, during treatment with Recormon, the effect regressing as treatment continues. Development of thrombocytosis is extremely rare. It is recommended that the platelet count is monitored regularly during the first 8 weeks of therapy.

Due to the increase in haematocrit and haemoglobin during therapy the viscosity of the blood increases. An increase in the dose of heparin during haemodialysis frequently may be necessary, therefore, as occlusion of the dialysis system is possible if heparinisation is not optimised.

Shunt thromboses may also occur, especially in patients with a tendency to hypotension or who have had previous arteriovenous fistula complications, for example, as a result of stenosis, aneurysms, etc. Early shunt revision or prophylaxis against thrombosis is recommended.

As hyperkalaemia has been observed in isolated cases, it is recommended that serum potassium is monitored especially in the early phase of treatment. During clinical trials there were isolated reports of increases in serum creatinine, urea and phosphate levels, acne-like symptoms, myocardial infarction and one single anaphylactoid reaction.

Overdosage: No serious adverse effects are likely to occur in cases of acute overdosage. If necessary, treatment in such cases should be symptomatic.

Pharmaceutical precautions Recormon must be stored at a temperature of +2°C to +8°C, that is, in a refrigerator. Once reconstituted, any material which is not used immediately should be discarded as the sterility of the solution cannot be guaranteed thereafter. It is important, to avoid incompatibility or loss of activity,

— to avoid the use of glass; use only plastic materials for administration of the solution

— not to use any solvent other than that supplied

— not to mix the solvent with other drugs or infusion solutions.

Legal category POM.

Package quantities *Recormon 1000:* packs containing 10 vials of freeze-dried epoetin beta and 10 ampoules (1 ml) of Water for Injections.

Recormon 2000: packs containing 10 vials of freeze-dried epoetin beta and 10 ampoules (2 ml) of Water for Injections.

Recormon 5000: packs containing 5 vials of freeze-dried epoetin beta and 5 ampoules (5 ml) of Water for Injections.

Further information In the induction of increased erythropoiesis the target haemoglobin level in an individual patient is a matter for clinical judgement. On present evidence the typical target haemoglobin is 10–12 g per 100 ml.

Product licence numbers

Recormon	0075/0065
Water for Injections	0075/0066

SPIROCTAN*

Presentation Spiroctan products contain Spironolactone BP and are available as three dosage forms:

Spiroctan 25: Light-blue coated tablets marked BM B2 and containing 25 mg Spironolactone BP. Lactose, sucrose and the colouring agents E102 and E132 also are present.

Spiroctan 50: Green coated tablets marked BM A8 and containing 50 mg Spironolactone BP. Lactose, sucrose and the colouring agents E104, E110 and E132 also are present.

Spiroctan 100: Light-green hard gelatin capsules marked BM A7 and containing 100 mg Spironolactone BP. The capsule shells contain colouring agents E104 and E132 and lactose is present in the formulation.

Uses
Pharmacology: Spiroctan promotes diuresis by competitive inhibition of aldosterone, a sodium-retaining, potassium-excreting hormone. It acts on the distal portion of the renal tubule and may be used in conjunction with more proximally acting diuretics.

Indications for use: Spiroctan is recommended for the treatment of congestive cardiac failure, cirrhosis with ascites and oedema, malignant ascites, nephrotic syndrome and also for diagnosis and treatment of primary hyperaldosteronism.

Dosage and administration
Adults: Adequate maintenance dosage is usually between 50 and 200 mg daily, depending on the patient's response. This may be increased to 300 to 400 mg daily when necessary. An initial dosage of up to 600 mg daily may be employed in appropriate cases.

Elderly: In elderly patients caution is advised. It is suggested that treatment should begin at the lowest dose, increasing gradually up to the normal adult dose, until the desired response is achieved.

Children: The daily dosage for children is based on an intake of 1.5 to 3.0 mg per Kg body weight, as shown in the following guidelines.

Age 1 to 3 years (up to approximately 15 kg): One tablet Spiroctan 25 every other day.

Age 4 to 7 years (up to approximately 23 kg): One tablet Spiroctan 25 each day.

Age 8 to 12 years (up to approximately 37 kg): One tablet Spiroctan 25 twice daily.

Spiroctan tablets and capsules should be taken with fluid. When the daily dosage does not exceed 200 mg it may normally be taken as a single dose. For children who cannot swallow solid dose forms the tablets may be crushed and taken with food or drink.

Contra-indications, warnings, etc
Contra-indications: Spiroctan is contra-indicated in cases of renal failure, acute renal insufficiency, where hyperkalaemia or hyponatraemia is present, and in patients hypersensitive to spironolactone.

Pregnancy and lactation: Use of Spiroctan during pregnancy should be avoided. Animal teratogenicity studies have shown evidence of feminisation of the male foetus. As metabolites of spironolactone may be excreted in breast milk, the use of Spiroctan in patients who are breast feeding is not recommended.

Interactions: Potassium supplements should not be administered with Spiroctan except initially in cases of hypokalaemia and the use of Spiroctan with other potassium-sparing diuretics or ACE inhibitors should be avoided.

The effect of carbenoxolone may be decreased. Acetylsalicylic acid, indomethacin and other inhibitors of prostaglandin synthesis may reduce the inhibitory effect of Spiroctan on aldosterone.

The action of other diuretics may be potentiated. The initial dose should be half that normally administered and the dosage should be adjusted to the patient's needs. Spiroctan may enhance the effect of antihypertensive agents.

Precautions: Although the dose of Spiroctan does not generally need to be reduced in hepatic dysfunction such patients should be carefully monitored as hepatic coma may be precipitated in susceptible subjects.

Periodic estimation of serum electrolytes is recommended.

Adverse effects: These are infrequent and usually mild. They include drowsiness, mental confusion (especially in conjunction with alcohol), lethargy, ataxia and gastrointestinal effects. Drivers of vehicles or operators of dangerous machinery should be warned of the effects on alertness. Hyperkalaemia and hyponatraemia may occur but these effects are rare during long term therapy. There may be reversible increases in BUN. Gynaecomastia may occur rarely but is normally reversible on cessation of dosage. Very occasionally alterations in voice pitch occur and these may not be reversible. This risk should be carefully considered in patients for whom voice control is important, for example, in actors. Occasional reports of skin rashes, menstrual disorders, impotence, breast enlargement and nipple sensitivity have been made.

Carcinogenicity: Spironolactone has been shown to produce tumours in rats when administered at high doses over a long period of time. The significance of these findings with respect to clinical use is not certain. However, the long-term use of spironolactone in young patients requires careful consideration of the benefits and the potential hazard involved.

Overdosage: Toxic effects in overdosage are due to hyperkalaemia. Clinical symptoms include irregular pulse, lassitude and muscular weakness and it may be difficult clinically to differentiate from hypokalaemia. Treatment is by cessation of therapy, administration of potassium-excreting diuretics, use of ion-exchange resins, etc.

Pharmaceutical precautions No special storage precautions are necessary. As with all medicines, however, it is recommended that Spiroctan be stored in a cool, dry place.

Legal category POM.

Package quantities Spiroctan 25 Packs of 100 tablets. Spiroctan 50 Packs of 100 tablets. Spiroctan 100 Blister packs of 28 capsules.

Further information Spiroctan may be administered in combination with more proximally acting diuretics to increase diuresis and to prevent excessive potassium loss.

No metabolic changes occur with Spiroctan in incipient or overt diabetes.

Product licence numbers

Spiroctan 25	0075/0037.
Spiroctan 50	0075/0038.
Spiroctan 100	0075/0039.

SPIROCTAN-M* INJECTION

Presentation A clear, yellow, aqueous solution containing 200 mg potassium canrenoate in each 10 ml ampoule. The formulation also contains sodium carbonate and sodium chloride.

Uses Spiroctan-M Injection is indicated for use in patients with oedema associated with secondary aldosteronism in cases such as ascites, oedema associated with liver disease and oedema associated with chronic, decompensated heart disease.

Spiroctan-M Injection also is indicated for use in the diagnosis and treatment of primary hyperaldosteronism.

Use of Spiroctan-M Injection is recommended only when treatment with other diuretic agents is inadequate and when oral aldosterone antagonists cannot be administered.

Dosage and administration *Adult patients only:* The dosage of Spiroctan-M Injection should be adjusted to the needs and response of the individual patient. Depending upon the severity of the aldosterone excess, 1 to 2 ampoules (200 to 400 mg potassium canrenoate) should be administered daily, increasing to 4 ampoules (800 mg potassium canrenoate) daily in exceptional cases.

Administration is by the intravenous route, either by slow intravenous injection or by infusion following dilution in a suitable vehicle. In order to avoid irritation or pain at the site of injection, undiluted Spiroctan-M Injection should be administered slowly, 2 to 3 minutes per ampoule, and preferably not into a thin vein.

Contra-indications, warnings, etc Spiroctan-M Injection is contra-indicated in cases of hyperkalaemia, hyponatraemia and in renal patients where the serum creatinine is greater than 2 mg per 100 ml or the creatinine clearance is less than 30 ml per minute. Its use is not recommended in children nor in pregnant or breast-feeding patients.

It is possible that hyperkalaemia may be provoked if Spiroctan-M Injection is administered with amiloride, triamterene or ACE-inhibitors. Potentiation may occur with antihypertensive drugs and the action of carbenoxolone may be antagonised. Drugs such as aspirin and indomethacin may reduce the effectiveness of Spiroctan-M Injection. For long term therapy the electrolyte balance should be monitored regularly.

Adverse effects may include irritation or pain at the site of injection if undiluted Spiroctan-M Injection is not administered slowly. A transient confusion syndrome has been observed during therapy with high doses (1000 mg daily or more). Nausea and vomiting also may occur after a high dose and may be controlled by suitable anti-emetic medication. Hyperkalaemia may occur occasionally, especially in patients with renal dysfunction, and a reversible increase in BUN may occur even when kidney function is normal. It is theoretically possible that in chronic therapy there may be anti-androgenic effects, that is, nipple sensitivity, gynaecomastia in men and mastodynia in women. In rare cases there may be irreversible changes in voice pitch. Normally, however, treatment is of short duration and may be continued, if appropriate, using oral spironolactone capsules or tablets. The potency ratio of 0.7 should be considered in converting from Spiroctan-M Injection to oral spironolactone (spironolactone ÷ 0.7 = potassium canrenoate).

In long term studies of potassium canrenoate administered to rats for 2 years by the oral route myelocytic leukaemia and other neoplastic changes were observed. Use of Spiroctan-M Injection thus should be limited to as short a time as possible and the necessity for its use should be monitored continuously. Use in young patients particularly requires careful consideration of the benefits and potential hazards involved.

In overdosage, effects noted may include nausea, vomiting, transient confusion and possibly hyperkalaemia. Treatment is by cessation of therapy, anti-emetic medication and use of a potassium-eliminating drug if hyperkalaemia is present.

Pharmaceutical precautions Spiroctan-M Injection should be stored away from light. For slow intravenous infusion Spiroctan-M Injection may be diluted with 250 ml of either dextrose solution 5% or sodium chloride solution 0.9%. No other drugs or nutrients may be added. Use the diluted preparation within 12 hours and check visually for the absence of precipitation before use.

Legal category POM.

Package quantities The ampoules are supplied in packs of 5.

Further information Diuresis normally commences within the first 24 hours although long latent periods have been reported in refractory cases. Spiroctan-M Injection does not adversely affect glucose metabolism or the management of diabetes mellitus.

Product licence number 0075/0040.

SUSTAMYCIN*

Presentation Sustamycin is presented as light blue/dark blue hard gelatin capsules. Each capsule contains

250 mg Tetracycline Hydrochloride BP in a sustained release formulation. The colouring agents E 127 and E 131 are present in the capsule shells.

Uses Sustamycin is a sustained-action tetracycline formulation with an enhanced biological availability of tetracycline which allows for reduction of dose and of dose frequency. Sustamycin is indicated for use in chronic bronchitis, acute exacerbation of chronic bronchitis, severe acne, lymphogranuloma venereum, chancroid, non-specific urethritis, granuloma inguinale, chlamydial infections (psittacosis, trachoma and inclusion conjunctivitis), mycoplasma (respiratory and genital), Rickettsial infection (Q fever, typhus, Rocky Mountain spotted fever) and brucellosis. Sustamycin is also indicated as second or third line therapy in gonorrhoea and syphilis and in other infections due to sensitive organisms after bacteriological confirmation of sensitivity.

Dosage and administration Adults and children over 12 years only: usual dose is two capsules initially followed by one capsule every 12 hours. In more severe infections dosage may be increased at the discretion of the physician, for example, to two capsules twice daily for short periods. In mild infections one capsule daily may be sufficient.

Brucellosis: 4 capsules/day for 3 weeks.
Chlamydial infections: 4 capsules/day for 1 week.
Lymphogranuloma venereum: 4 capsules/day for 2 weeks.
Non-specific urethritis: 4 capsules/day for 10 to 21 days.
Severe acne: 4 capsules/day for 2–3 weeks followed by 1 capsule daily for 3 to 4 months.
Gonorrhoea: 3 capsules initially followed by 4 capsules/day to a maximum dose of 18 capsules (4.5 g) in total.
Syphilis: 60 to 80 capsules (15–20 g) over a period of 10–15 days.

Sustamycin should be taken in divided doses, preferably one hour before or two hours after main meals, and swallowed with a drink of water.

Contra-indications, warnings, etc Sustamycin is contra-indicated in patients with known hypersensitivity to tetracyclines and in cases of renal insufficiency. If tetracycline is administered to young children (under 12 years) or to pregnant or breast feeding women, it is selectively taken up in developing bones and teeth and dental staining and enamel hypoplasia may occur. Sustamycin should not be used in such patients unless the potential benefits justify the risks. As with all tetracyclines the concomitant intake of antacids, mineral supplements (calcium, magnesium and iron) and milk may diminish absorption from Sustamycin capsules. Tetracycline has also been reported to prolong the action of coumarin anticoagulants in some patients and a reduced coumarin dosage may be required. Patients using oral contraceptives may require additional contraceptive precautions. Serum lithium levels may be raised in patients on lithium therapy. Tetracyclines have been reported to reduce the effectiveness of concurrently administered penicillin.

The gastro-intestinal adverse effects common to the tetracyclines (i.e. nausea, vomiting and diarrhoea) occur only rarely due to the sustained release nature of Sustamycin. Hypersensitivity and photosensitivity reactions may be seen occasionally. Appropriate measures including discontinuation of therapy should be taken in the event of overgrowth of a non-susceptible organism (e.g. candidial overgrowth such as glossitis, stomatitis, vaginitis, pruritus ani or superinfections including fulminant staphylococcal enteritis). Other unwanted effects seen during tetracycline therapy may include hepatotoxicity and pancreatitis, haemolytic anaemia, eosinophilia, neutropenia and thrombocytopenia. Benign intracranial hypertension in adults and bulging fontanelles in infants have been reported as rare adverse effects of tetracyclines in general. Treatment should be withdrawn if there is evidence of raised intracranial pressure.

Caution is required when administering tetracyclines to elderly patients, those with hepatic dysfunction or receiving concurrent hepatotoxic medication, or to those with myasthenia gravis.

Treatment of overdosage is as for tetracyclines in general and depends on symptoms. Within the first few hours empty the stomach by aspiration and lavage and/or administer milk or antacids to reduce absorption. Gastro-intestinal effects may include nausea, vomiting and diarrhoea. More serious effects are unlikely, although in rare cases there may be allergic reactions or anaphylactic shock.

Pharmaceutical precautions Store in well closed containers at a temperature below 30°C.

Legal category POM.

Package quantities Sustamycin is available in containers of 50 capsules.

Further information Sustamycin contains tetracycline hydrochloride in a sustained release form facilitating twice daily dosage which leads to increased patient compliance compared with the four times daily dosage regimen of conventional tetracycline. The formulation enables tetracycline to be absorbed throughout the gastro-intestinal tract, not just in the stomach. This enhanced absorption allows a reduction in total tetracycline dosage while maintaining full clinical efficacy.

Product licence number 0075/0017.

**Trade Mark*

Boots Pharmaceuticals
1 Thane Road West
Nottingham NG2 3AA

BOOTS PHARMACEUTICALS

APRINOX*

Presentation Aprinox is Bendrofluazide BP, a diuretic of the thiazide group. Aprinox is available as white tablets in two strengths, 2.5 mg and 5 mg.

Inactive ingredients: Lactose.

Uses Aprinox is indicated in all cases where the reduction of fluid retention by diuresis is required i.e. oedema of cardiac, renal or hepatic origin; premenstrual, iatrogenic and all other types of oedema.

Aprinox will produce a moderate but useful prolonged fall of blood pressure in hypertensive patients and often gives adequate control when used alone; if necessary, Aprinox can be administered concurrently with other antihypertensive agents, allowing a reduction in the dosage of the latter.

Aprinox may also be used to effectively suppress lactation.

Dosage and administration *Diuretic:* Initially 5 to 10 mg once daily or on alternate days. Maintenance: 5 to 10 mg once or twice weekly. The dose should be taken early in the morning so as to complete diuresis by bedtime.

Antihypertensive: 2.5 to 5 mg once daily. When Aprinox is used concurrently with other antihypertensive agents the dose of the latter should be halved.

A suggested dosage for suppression of lactation is 5 mg in the morning and 5 mg at midday for about five days.

Children: Dosage in children may be up to 400 micrograms/kg bodyweight daily initially, reducing to 50–100 micrograms/kg bodyweight daily for maintenance.

Elderly: The dosage of thiazide diuretics may need to be reduced in the elderly, particularly when renal function is impaired because of the possibility of electrolyte imbalance.

Contra-indications, warnings, etc Aprinox is contra-indicated in severe renal failure and in patients with a known hypersensitivity to thiazides. It should be used with caution in patients with Addison's Disease, hypercalcaemia and hepatic or renal impairment. Renal function should be continuously monitored during thiazide therapy.

All the thiazide diuretics can produce a degree of electrolyte imbalance, especially in patients with renal or hepatic impairment or when dosage is high or prolonged. Serum electrolytes should be checked for abnormalities, particularly hypokalaemia, and the latter corrected by the addition of a potassium supplement to the regimen.

Note: Aprinox does not contain a potassium supplement.

Thiazide diuretics may raise the serum uric acid levels with consequent exacerbation of gout in susceptible subjects.

Thiazide derivatives sometimes lower carbohydrate tolerance and the insulin dosage of the diabetic patient may require adjustment. Care is necessary when bendrofluazide is administered to those with a known predisposition to diabetes.

Rarely blood dyscrasias, including agranulocytosis, aplastic anaemia, thrombocytopaenia and leucopaenia, and pancreatitis have been reported with long term therapy. Skin rashes and impotence have occasionally been reported.

Use in pregnancy and lactation: Diuretics are best avoided for the management of oedema of pregnancy or hypertension in pregnancy as their use may be associated with hypokalaemia, increased blood viscosity and reduced placental perfusion.

There is inadequate evidence of safety in human pregnancy and some workers have described foetal bone marrow depression and thrombocytopaenia. Foetal and neonatal jaundice have also been described.

As diuretics pass into breast milk, they should be avoided in mothers who wish to breast feed.

Drug interactions: Sensitivity to digitalis glycosides may be increased by the hypokalaemic effect of concurrent bendrofluazide. Patients should be observed for signs of digitalis intoxication, in particular arrhythmias, and if these appear, the dosage of digitalis glycosides should be temporarily reduced and a potassium supplement given to restore stability.

Serum lithium concentrations may be increased by concurrent use of thiazide diuretics.

Non-steroidal anti-inflammatory agents may blunt the diuretic and anti-hypertensive effects of thiazide diuretics.

ACTH, corticosteroids, acetazolamide and carbenoxolone may exacerbate the hypokalaemia associated with thiazide use. Thiazide diuretics may enhance the neuromuscular blocking effects of the non-depolarising muscle relaxants e.g. tubocurarine.

Interference with laboratory tests: Like all thiazides, bendrofluazide may interfere with a number of laboratory tests, including estimation of serum protein-bound iodine and tests of parathyroid function.

Treatment of overdosage: Monitor blood pressure, fluid and electrolyte balance and correct if necessary. Treatment is symptomatic and supportive; there is no specific antidote.

Pharmaceutical precautions Recommended storage conditions: 5°C to 20°C.

Legal category POM.

Package quantities Bottles of 100 and 500 tablets.

Further information A single dose of Aprinox will induce a diuresis extending over 12 to 18 hours.

Product licence numbers
Aprinox 2.5 mg 0014/5117
Aprinox 5 mg 0014/5118

ASILONE*

Presentation
Suspension: White suspension containing in each 5 ml, activated dimethicone 135 mg and the equivalent of Dried Aluminium Hydroxide BP 420 mg and Light Magnesium Oxide BP 70 mg. Inactive ingredients: potassium sorbate; methyl and propyl hydroxy-benzoate.

Uses
Asilone Suspension: Antiflatulent and antacid; for the relief of dyspeptic symptoms of functional or organic origin, including flatulence and associated abdominal distension; heartburn, including heartburn of pregnancy during the last two trimesters, hiatus hernia and oesophagitis; symptomatic management of gastritis and peptic ulceration.

Dosage and administration
Adults (including elderly):

Suspension: One or two 5 ml spoonfuls before meals and at bedtime.

Children: The suspension formulation is not recommended for children under 12 years.

Contra-indications, warnings, etc
Contra-indications: Antacid preparations should not be administered in severe debilitation or renal impairment.

Warnings: Antacids may interfere with the absorption of tetracyclines, rifampicin, warfarin and digoxin if given concomitantly.

Aluminium salts may cause constipation and magnesium salts diarrhoea. However, such bowel disturbances are rare with Asilone.

Asilone is not recommended in flatulent abdominal distension possibly related to intestinal obstruction.

Pregnancy: Antacid preparations are not recommended during the first trimester of pregnancy.

Overdosage: No cases of overdosage have been reported with Asilone. The components of Asilone are not expected to cause specific local or systemic toxicity even in acute overdosage in healthy individuals. No specific treatment; symptomatic management only if indicated.

Pharmaceutical precautions Do not freeze.

Legal category GSL.

Package quantities Suspension: Bottles of 100 ml, 300 ml and 500 ml.

Further information The sodium content of Asilone Suspension is low. Asilone is, therefore, particularly suited to the management of gastro-oesophageal conditions where a low sodium intake is indicated.

Asilone Suspension: typical sodium content 0·032 to 0·097 mmol per 10 ml.

Product licence numbers
Suspension 0327/0057

Product licence holder: Crookes Healthcare Ltd., Distributed by The Boots Co. P.L.C.

BRUFEN*

Presentation Brufen is available as sugar-coated tablets containing either 200 mg or 400 mg (Brufen 400) of Ibuprofen BP and film-coated tablets each containing 600 mg (Brufen 600) of Ibuprofen BP.

The tablets are light-magenta in colour and bear a black overprint as follows: 200 mg tablets – 'Brufen'; 400 mg tablets – 'Brufen 400'; 600 mg tablets – 'Brufen 600'.

For children, and for adults who have difficulty in swallowing tablets, Brufen is presented as Brufen Syrup, an orange flavoured liquid containing 100 mg of Ibuprofen BP in each 5 ml.

Brufen Granules are available as unit dose sachets each containing 600 mg of Ibuprofen BP in an effervescent, orange flavoured formulation. This product is not suitable for children under 12 years of age for whom Brufen Syrup is recommended.

Inactive ingredients: Brufen (200 mg) – Sodium benzoate; sucrose. Brufen 400 – Sodium benzoate; sucrose, Brufen granules – sucrose. Brufen Syrup – sucrose; methyl hydroxybenzoate; propyl hydroxybenzoate; sodium benzoate; sunset yellow.

Uses Brufen is indicated for its analgesic and anti-inflammatory effect in the treatment of rheumatoid arthritis (including juvenile rheumatoid arthritis or Still's disease), ankylosing spondylitis, osteoarthritis and other non-rheumatoid (seronegative) arthropathies.

In the treatment of non-articular rheumatic conditions, Brufen is indicated in periarticular conditions such as frozen shoulder (capsulitis), bursitis, tendinitis, tenosynovitis and low-back pain; Brufen can also be used in soft-tissue injuries such as sprains and strains.

Brufen is indicated for its analgesic effect in the relief of mild to moderate pain such as dysmenorrhoea, dental and post-operative pain and for symptomatic relief of headache including migraine headache.

Dosage and administration
Adult: The recommended dosage of Brufen is 1200–1800 mg daily in divided doses. Some patients can be maintained on 600–1200 mg daily. In severe or acute conditions it can be advantageous to increase the dosage until the acute phase is brought under control, provided that the total daily dosage does not exceed 2400 mg in divided doses.

Children: The daily dosage of Brufen is 20 mg/kg of body-weight in divided doses. This can be achieved as follows using the syrup:
1–2 years: One 2.5 ml spoonful (50 mg) three to four times a day.
3–7 years: One 5 ml spoonful (100 mg) three to four times a day.
8–12 years: Two 5 ml spoonfuls (200 mg) three to four times a day.

Not recommended for children weighing less than 7 kg.

In juvenile rheumatoid arthritis up to 40 mg/kg of body weight daily in divided doses may be taken.

Elderly: No special dosage modifications are required for elderly patients, unless renal or hepatic function is impaired, in which case dosage should be assessed individually.

Contra-indications, warnings, etc Brufen should not be given to patients with a history of or active peptic ulceration. Bronchospasm may be precipitated in patients suffering from, or with a previous history of, bronchial asthma. Brufen should not be given to patients in whom aspirin and other nonsteroidal anti-inflammatory drugs induce the symptoms of asthma, rhinitis or urticaria.

Nonsteroidal anti-inflammatory drugs have been reported to cause nephrotoxicity in various forms; interstitial nephritis, nephrotic syndrome and renal failure. In patients with renal, cardiac or hepatic impairment, caution is required since the use of Nonsteroidal anti-inflammatory drugs may result in deterioration of renal function. The dose should be kept as low as possible and renal function should be monitored in these patients.

Adverse effects reported include: Dyspepsia, gastro-intestinal intolerance and bleeding, and skin rashes of various types. Less frequently, thrombocytopenia has occurred.

Each Brufen Granules sachet contains 197 mg (approximately 9 mEq) sodium. This should be considered in patients whose overall intake of sodium must be markedly restricted.

Use in pregnancy and lactation: Whilst no teratogenic effects have been demonstrated in animal experiments, the use of Brufen during pregnancy should, if possible, be avoided. In the limited studies so far available, ibuprofen appears in the breast milk in very low concentration and is unlikely to affect the breast-fed infant adversely.

Drug interactions: In therapeutic doses, no evidence of clinically significant interactions with other commonly used drugs has so far been observed. However, as with other nonsteroidal anti-inflammatory agents, caution should be exercised in patients receiving oral anticoagulants and thiazide diuretics.

Interference with laboratory tests: There is no evidence so far that ibuprofen interferes with standard laboratory tests.

Treatment of overdosage: Gastric lavage and, if necessary, correction of serum electrolytes. There is no specific antidote to ibuprofen.

Pharmaceutical precautions Brufen 600 (600 mg tablets), Brufen Granules and Brufen Syrup should be stored below 25°C. Brufen Syrup should be protected from light.

Legal category POM.

Package quantities
Brufen 600 Tablets: pack of 100
Brufen 400 Tablets: pack of 100, pack of 250
Brufen Tablets 200 mg: pack of 100, pack of 500

Brufen Granules: Box of 20 sachets.
Brufen Syrup: Bottle of 200 ml.

Further information Taken on an empty stomach, peak serum levels of ibuprofen occur 45 minutes after ingestion whereas, taken after a meal, the peak is delayed up to 90 minutes. Since most people can take Brufen on an empty stomach without gastric discomfort, the initial dose of the day will be more rapidly effective if taken before food. This is particularly valuable in providing relief of the morning stiffness associated with arthritis.

Product licence numbers

Brufen 600 Tablets	0014/0264
Brufen 400 Tablets	0014/0158
Brufen Tablets 200 mg	0014/5132
Brufen Granules	0014/0378
Brufen Syrup	0014/0217

CHYMODIACTIN 4000 UNITS

Warning Chymodiactin should only be used in a hospital setting by clinicians experienced in the diagnosis and management of all spinal disorders and who have received specialised training in chemonucleolysis.

The proper selection of patients for the appropriate use of Chymodiatin in chemonucleolysis requires precise diagnosis in order to eliminate conditions other than herniated lumbar discs which may produce similar signs and symptoms of nerve root compression.

Chymodiactin should be used only in facilities where supporting personnel as well as clinicians are qualified and equipped to diagnose and manage all potential complications in the use of Chymodiactin, including anaphylaxis.

Presentation Chymodiactin is a sterile lyophilised powder of the proteolytic enzyme Chymopapain. The product is available in 2 ml vials exhibiting 4000 picoKatals activity (=4,000 Smith BAPNA assay units) of chymopapain with 1·4 mg sodium L-cysteinate hydrochloride as activator.

The proteolytic enzyme chymopapain is derived from the crude latex of Carica papaya and is purified by column chromatography which eliminates inactive protein components.

Definition of unit: The unit of chymopapain activity is the picoKatal. It forms under the conditions of the assay, 1 picomole of p-nitroaniline per second from DL-benzoylarginine-p-nitroanilide (BAPNA) substrate at pH 6·0 and 37°C.

The unit often employed in some European countries is the CTE unit. This unit of the enzymatic activity is defined as that amount of enzyme which produces, from acid denatured haemoglobin at pH 4·0 in one minute under the conditions of the test, an hydrolysate with an optical density at 275 nanometres equal to that of a tyrosine solution containing 1·0 microgram tyrosine/ml.

While the two units of activity are measured differently comparative experimental data has shown that the enzymatic activity of Chymodiactin vials was essentially identical whether haemoglobin or BAPNA methods are employed.

Uses Chymodiactin injection is indicated for the treatment of patients with clinically confirmed herniated lumbar intervertebral discs whose symptoms and signs have not responded to an adequate period or periods of conservative therapy.

Dosage and administration The lumbar intervertebral disc should be treated with a single injection of Chymodiactin on one occasion directly into the nucleus pulposus (see under 'Procedure').

Vials of Chymodiactin Injection 4000 picoKatals are reconstituted with 2 ml Water for Injections BP, the resulting solution containing 2000 picoKatals chymopapain per ml.

Recommended dosage is 2000–4000 picoKatals (1–2 ml) per disc preferably 3000 picoKatals (1·5 ml) per disc. The maximum dose in a single patient with multiple disc herniation is 8000 picoKatals (4 ml).

Children: Safety and effectiveness of Chymodiactin has not been studied in paediatric patients. Therefore its use is not recommended in children.

Elderly: There is insufficient evidence to recommend use in patients over 60 years.

Contra-indications, warnings, etc

Contra-indications: Chymodiactin is contra-indicated in patients with a known sensitivity to chymopapain, papaya or other papaya derivatives. Other contra-indications are severe spondylolisthesis; progressing paralysis or other increasing neurological dysfunction, and in patients with evidence of spinal cord tumour or a cauda equina lesion.

Chymopapain is a foreign protein and, as such, its injection has a potential for generating an immunological response. Therefore, patients who have previously received an injection of chymopapain should not be re-injected with Chymodiactin.

Patients with congestive cardiac failure, coronary artery disease and respiratory failure should be excluded from chymopapain therapy because of the cardiovascular risk in shock should an anaphylactic reaction occur. Additionally, patients on beta adrenoceptor blocking drug therapy should be excluded due to the blocking effects on rescue adrenaline administered and because such agents significantly potentiate the liberation of chemical mediators of anaphylaxis.

Chymodiactin is contra-indicated in patients in whom a pre-operative sensitivity screening test is performed and found to be positive.

Warnings and precautions:

1. Anaphylactic reactions have been observed in approximately 0·5% of patients after injection with Chymodiactin and may be life-threatening if not treated promptly. At least one open intravenous line must always be in place for such an occurrence. The reaction can be immediate or delayed for up to one hour after injection. A reaction may commence with almost immediate hypotension and/or bronchospasm, the former being more common. Subsequently laryngeal oedema, cardiac arrhythmia/arrest, coma and death may ensue. Speed in diagnosis and treatment is critical since the clinical signs, severity of progression and duration of an anaphylactic reaction are highly unpredictable. Other signs of allergic response must be watched for, e.g. erythema, pilomotor erection, rash, pruritis urticaria, conjunctivitis, vasomotor rhinitis, angioedema and various gastrointestinal disturbances, which may herald the imminent onset of a major reaction.

Post marketing surveillance data from the United States indicates that females are more likely to develop anaphylactic reactions than males. The rates being 0·9% and 0·3% respectively. There was a statistically significant difference in the frequency of anaphylaxis dependent on whether local or general anaesthesia was used for the procedure, rates of 0·4% and 0·6% being noted respectively.

2. Acute transverse myelitis/acute transverse myelopathy has been reported in association with the injection of chymopapain at a rate of about 1 in 18,000 patients. Although cause and effect relationship to the injection of chymopapain itself has not been established, the reported rate is significantly higher than the incidence reported in the medical literature. These patients are characterised clinically by the delayed (2–3 weeks) onset of paraplegia or paraparesis without prior signs or symptoms. Patients receiving injections at more than one disc space appear to be at increased risk.

Paraplegia, cerebral haemorrhage and other serious neurological complications have been reported soon after chymopapain injection in a small number of patients. Causal relationships to the drug when properly injected have not been established. Needle trauma and/or introduction of chymopapain and contrast media into the spinal fluid may be causal in some of these cases. Less severe neurological reactions have included sacral burning, leg pain, hypalgaesia, leg weakness, bilateral cramp, pain in the opposite leg and paresthesiae.

3. The drug is extremely toxic when injected intrathecally in animals. Therefore, great caution must be

exercised in ensuring that Chymodiactin is not introduced into the dural canal either directly or by leakage.

4. Several deaths have been reported in association with Chymodiactin injection. These have been related to complications secondary to anaphylaxis, to staphylococcal meningitis with disc abscess or of unknown aetiology. The mortality rate associated with Chymodiactin is estimated at 1 in 4,500 patients (0·02%).

5. Discitis, both bacterial and aseptic, has been reported in several patients.

6. Less severe, but more frequent, adverse reactions include back pain/stiffness/soreness in approximately 50% of treated patients and/or back spasm in approximately 30%. Less frequent adverse reactions occurring in less than 1% of patients studied include rash, itching, urticaria, nausea, paralytic ileus, urinary retention, headache and dizziness.

7. Certain radio-opaque contrast media are neurotoxic. It has been suggested that the toxicity of these materials may be enhanced by the co-administration of Chymodiactin. Intrathecal administration of Chymodiactin results in capillary disruption and bleeding which may again potentiate the neurotoxicity of contrast agents.

Consequently, it is recommended that discography is not performed as part of the chemonucleolysis procedure unless the operating surgeon determines that the risks of discography are outweighed by the benefits in a particular clinical situation.

8. *Pregnancy and lactation:* As adequate studies have not been performed in either pregnant or lactating women, Chymodiactin is not recommended for use in these patient groups.

Procedure

1. *Pre-Treatment* Because of the possibility of anaphylaxis during chemonucleolysis with Chymodiactin, a careful history should be conducted to determine if the patient has multiple allergies, especially a known allergy to papaya or papaya derivatives.

Pre-dose sensitivity testing to detect patients likely to be hypersensitive to Chymodiactin is recommended prior to Chymodiactin chemonucleolysis. Skin and serum testing methods are available.

The following pre-treatment may reduce the incidence, or decrease the severity, of the anaphylactic reaction.

(a) H_1 antagonist – e.g. chlorpheniramine – 4 mg orally, 6 hourly for 24 hours prior to chemonucleolysis to block H_1 effects.

(b) H_2 antagonists – e.g. cimetidine – 4–5 mg/kg bodyweight orally 2 hours prior to chemonucleolysis to block H_2 effects.

(c) Hydration should be ensured throughout the procedure. A secure, wide-bore venous access must be established pre-operatively and maintained for at least one hour after injection of the enzyme, to facilitate emergency intervention if required.

(d) Corticosteroid – e.g. hydrocortisone – orally or intravenously immediately prior to injection may stabilise membranes, decrease permeability and mediator release. Doses from 500–1,000 mg have been recommended.

(a), (b) and (c) are recommended and (d) is optional.

2. *Anaesthesia* The choice of anaesthesia for a specific patient should be made by the attending surgeon and anaesthetist. However, **it is recommended that supplemented local anaesthesia be used for chemonucleolysis whenever possible.**

Local anaesthesia: The use of supplemented local anaesthesia in preference to general anaesthesia provides an awake patient, more likely to be alert to pain, particularly if the needle impinges on nerve tissue. In addition, it is likely that a patient under local anaesthetic will not tolerate an excessive number of attempts to place the needle. Local anaesthesia is also associated with a lower frequency of anaphylaxis than general anaesthesia (0·4% v 0·6% respectively).

General anaesthesia: The advantages of general anaesthesia are thought to be ease of airway management if anaphylaxis should develop; more precise patient positioning for injection; less patient discomfort. The disadvantage of general anaesthesia is a higher rate of anaphylaxis (0·6%).

If halothane anaesthesia is used, it should be noted that if adrenaline is required for treatment of an anaphylactic reaction there is a potential arrhythmogenic interaction of the two drugs.

3. *Needle placement:* Needle placement for the intradiscal administration of Chymodiactin should be made by clinicians experienced in needle placement. Needle placement should be via the lateral approach to avoid puncture of the dura mater. Serious neurological toxicity has been reported using a posterior transdural approach. Therefore, this latter method should not be used.

Great care must be taken to ensure that the dura is not penetrated and that chymopapain or contrast agents (if used) do not enter the subarachnoid space. If there is any question regarding needle tip location within the nucleus of the disc, or if the contrast agent extravasates into the subarachnoid space, the procedure should be abandoned and chymopapain should not be injected.

Prior to injection of Chymodiactin, visualisation of the needle tip position in the disc must be confirmed using x-ray image intensifier for both the anteroposterior and lateral view.

As an additional aid in needle tip visualisation, surgeons performing chemonucleolysis may wish to consider the injection of saline or water into the nucleus pulposus (saline or water acceptance test). The use of this procedure does not supplant careful evaluation of high quality anteroposterior and lateral x-ray views of the disc.

Discography is not recommended at the time of the Chymodiactin injection unless the attending surgeon considers the risks to be outweighed by the benefits in the particular clinical situation. If, however, discography is considered to be essential, it should be performed using non-ionic water soluble contrast media, and at least 15 minutes should elapse after the administration of the radio-opaque contrast medium to allow for diffusion and absorption of the medium before injection of Chymodiactin through the same needle after removal of the obturator.

A volume of less than 0·5 ml of the contrast medium is ordinarily sufficient in determining the location of the needle tip.

If high quality x-ray equipment including an image intensifier is not available to perform chemonucleolysis the procedure should not be carried out. If there is any question about satisfactory needle placement or if needle placement is difficult, requiring repeated attempts, the procedure should be abandoned.

4. *Injection:* (a) For 3 minutes prior to Chymodiactin injection, 100% oxygen (O_2) may be administered to the patient by the anaesthetist to maximise oxygenation in case of anaphylaxis.

(b) Based on the increased frequency of neurological adverse reactions in patients with two or more disc level injections, **chemonucleolysis should be limited to one disc producing the patient's symptoms unless definitive signs, symptoms and diagnostic procedure indicate that more than one disc is at fault.**

Treatment of anaphylaxis: Clinical judgement, speed of therapy and choice of agents all enter into the treatment of anaphylaxis. It must be emphasised that adrenaline is the definitive therapeutic agent in the immediate treatment of the condition. Beta-blocker therapy may antagonise the action of adrenaline, and halothane, if used for general anaesthesia, and adrenaline, have an arrhythmogenic potential interaction when used together.

The recommended treatment for severe anaphylactoid reaction includes the immediate administration of a vasopressor such as 0·5–1·0 ml of 1:1,000 adrenaline, generally by the intramuscular route. Aminophylline and corticosteroids may be administered intravenously to relieve bronchospasm.

The severe manifestations of anaphylaxis include a sudden fall in blood pressure due to generalised vasodilation and increased capillary permeability, angio-oedema (including laryngeal oedema), and bronchospasm. Milder signs and symptoms include rhinitis, pruritis, urticaria, vomiting, diarrhoea and abdominal pain. The fall in cardiac output which accompanies a reduced venous return may cause secondary myocardial and tissue hypoxia, with cardiac arrhythmias and a metabolic acidosis completing a vicious circle in severe cases.

Immediate therapy of acute reaction: (a) The keystone of effective treatment is adrenaline: as soon as the reaction is recognised 500–1000 microgram (0·5 to 1·0 ml of 1:1,000 solution) should be injected intramuscularly (not subcutaneously).

(b) Intramuscular injections of adrenaline should be repeated every 15 minutes until improvement occurs.

(c) A slow intravenous injection of 20 mg of the H_1 antagonist chlorpheniramine should be given immediately after intramuscular adrenaline and repeated over the subsequent 24 to 48 hours to prevent relapse.

Intravenous corticosteroids (200 mg hydrocortisone hemisuccinate) have little place in the immediate management. Their beneficial effects are delayed for several hours. In severely ill patients, however, early administration may help prevent deterioration after the primary treatment has been given. Most patients respond to the combination of intramuscular adrenaline and an intravenous H_1-antagonist.

Continuation of therapy: Continuing deterioration with circulatory collapse, bronchospasm or laryngeal oedema requires further treatment. Circulatory collapse requires volume replacement by intravenous fluids monitored, if possible, by a central venous pressure line. If electrolyte solutions are used large volumes may be necessary because in severe anaphylactic shock the plasma loss may constitute 20–40% of the plasma volume. Colloid solutions such as plasma protein fraction or dextran are theoretically preferable but may themselves release histamine, though in severe anaphylaxis intracellular stores of histamine are likely to have been depleted. Bronchospasm, refractory to intramuscular adrenaline requires treatment with intravenous aminophylline, a nebulised beta-agonist (such as salbutamol or terbutaline), oxygen, and (if necessary) assisted ventilation. Respiratory obstruction due to laryngeal oedema may require emergency tracheostomy.

Effective treatment of anaphylactic shock clearly depends on the severity of the clinical conditions and the circumstances under which it occurs.

Pharmaceutical precautions Although Chymodiactin lyophilised powder is stable at room temperature (25°C) for periods of time up to 18 months without loss of potency, this product should be stored under refrigeration (2–8°C) prior to use.

The drug should be used within 2 hours of its reconstitution. A vial should be used for only one patient and unused drug discarded and not stored for future use.

Since inactivation of the enzyme will occur with some bacteriostatic agents in common use, diluents containing such agents should not be used.

Legal category POM.

Package quantities Cartons containing 1 vial of Chymodiactin injection 4000 picoKatals together with a package insert.

Further information Chymodiactin has previously been shown to dissolve the nucleus pulposus of dogs and rabbits at doses as low as 50 units/disc and 100 units/disc respectively. Doses of 3,000 units/disc cause thinning of only the inner portion of the annulus in rabbits but do not penetrate the entire structure, while doses as high as 24,000 units/disc in dogs resulted in no apparent significant change in the peripheral portion of the annulus. In vitro studies demonstrated that chymopapain solubilized the glycosaminoglycan protein complex of human nucleus pulposus, but did not attack the collagen of this structure.

When chymopapain was injected into dogs and rabbits, doses up to 100 times greater than that required to remove the nucleus pulposus were well tolerated when injected intravenously, intradiscally and epidurally. The drug is extremely toxic when injected intrathecally, the approximate LD_{50} is 15 units/kg in rabbits and 150 units/kg in dogs and 200 units/kg in baboons. Therefore, great caution must be exercised in assuring that Chymodiactin is not injected intrathecally into the dural canal in the human.

In experiments in baboons, the serial injection into the spinal fluid of contrast agents (Renografin, Conray or Amipaque) followed by Chymodiactin 15 minutes later produced serious neurotoxicity, including weakness, paralysis and death in doses that were harmless or only slightly toxic when administered as single agents. This information supports the clinical observation that the documented entry of contrast agent and presumed entry of chymopapain into the spinal fluid can produce serious neurotoxicity including paraplegia and cerebral haemorrhage.

Product licence number 0014/0397

CORTISTAB* TABLETS

Presentation Cortistab Tablets are white Cortisone Tablets BP, containing either 5 mg or 25 mg of Cortisone Acetate BP.

Inactive ingredients: Lactose.

Uses Cortisone Acetate has both glucocorticoid and mineralocorticoid properties. Cortistab Tablets are indicated in replacement therapy, such as Addison's disease, primary or secondary adrenal insufficiency or congenital adrenal hyperplasia.

Dosage and administration As with other corticosteroids, the dosage of Cortistab Tablets should be adjusted to the severity, prognosis and anticipated duration of the disease, and the response of the individual patient.

In replacement therapy the normal daily requirement is:

Adults: 12.5–50 mg.

Children: 5–25 mg in divided doses.

Elderly: Steroids should be used cautiously in the elderly, since adverse effects are enhanced in old age.

In patients requiring replacement therapy, the daily dose should be given when practicable, in two doses. The first dose in the morning should be larger than the second dose in the evening, simulating the normal diurnal rhythm of cortisol secretion.

After prolonged costicosteroid treatment, the function of the patient's own adrenal cortices is often suppressed. To allow normal adrenal function to be restored, Cortistab dosage should be reduced gradually, e.g. by 5 to 12.5 mg every few days.

Contra-indications, warnings, etc Caution is necessary when prescribing corticosteroids in the following conditions.

(a) Previous history of tuberculosis or characteristic appearance on chest X-ray. The emergence of active tuberculosis can, however, be prevented by the prophylactic use of antituberculous therapy.

(b) Diabetes mellitus (or a family history of diabetes).

(c) Osteoporosis (post menopausal females are particularly at risk).

(d) Hypertension.

(e) History of severe affective disorders (especially previous history of steroid psychosis).

(f) Glaucoma (or a family history of glaucoma).

(g) Previous steroid myopathy.

(h) Peptic ulceration.

(i) Epilepsy.

(j) Vaccination with live vaccines.

Precautions: During treatment, the patient should be observed for psychotic reactions, muscular weakness, electrocardiographic changes, hypertension and untoward hormonal effects.

Corticosteroids may mask some signs of infection and new infections may appear during the use. There may be decreased resistance and inability to localize infection when corticosteroids are used.

Killed vaccines or toxoids may be given though their effects may be attenuated.

Side-effects: The following side effects may be associated with the long term systemic use of corticosteroids.

Gastro-intestinal: Dyspepsia, peptic ulceration with perforation and haemorrhage, abdominal distension, oesophageal ulceration, oesophageal candidiasis, acute pancreatitis.

Musculoskeletal: Proximal myopathy, osteoporosis, vertebral and long bone fractures, avascular osteonecrosis, tendon rupture.

Fluid and electrolyte disturbance: Sodium and water retention, hypertension, hypokalemic alkalosis.

Dermatological: Impaired healing, skin atrophy, bruising, striae, acne.

Endocrine/metabolic: Suppression of the hypothalamo-pituitary adrenal axis, growth suppression in childhood and adolescence, menstrual irregularity and amenorrhoea. Cushingoid facies, hirsutism, weight gain, impaired carbohydrate tolerance with increased requirement for antidiabetic therapy, negative nitrogen balance.

Neuropsychiatric: Euphoria, psychological dependence, depression, insomnia. Intracranial hypertension in children. Aggravation of schizophrenia.

Ophthalmic: Increased intra-occular pressure, glaucoma, papilloedema, cataracts, corneal or scleral thinning, exacerbation of ophthalmic viral disease.

General: Opportunistic infection, recurrence of dormant tuberculosis, leucocytosis, hypersensitivity, thromboembolism, increased appetite, nausea, malaise.

Withdrawal symptoms: Fever, myalgia, arthralgia, adrenal insufficiency.

Use in pregnancy and lactation: There is inadequate evidence of safety in human pregnancy and there may be a very small risk of cleft palate and intra-uterine growth retardation in the fetus; there is evidence of harmful effects on pregnancy in animals.

In lactation, continuous therapy with high doses could possibly affect the child's adrenal function, monitor carefully.

Use in children: Corticosteroids cause growth retardation in infancy, childhood and adolescence. Treatment should be limited to the minimum dosage for the shortest possible time. In order to minimise suppression of the hypothalamo-pituitary adrenal axis and growth retardation, treatment should be administered where possible as a single dose on alternate days.

Use in the elderly: Treatment of elderly patients, particularly if long term, should be planned bearing in mind the more serious consequences of the common side effects of corticosteroids in old age, especially osteoporosis, diabetes, hypertension, susceptibility to infection and thinning of the skin.

Treatment of overdosage: Treatment is symptomatic but is unlikely to be required.

Warning: Cortisone itself is inactive and must be converted in the liver to its active metabolite hydrocortisone. In some liver disorders therefore, the bioavailability of Cortistab Tablets may be less reliable.

Drug interactions
Modification of other drug effects

Anticoagulants: The effectiveness of anticoagulants may be increased or decreased with concurrent corticosteroid therapy.

Salicylates: Serum levels of salicylates may increase considerably if corticosteroid therapy is withdrawn, possibly causing intoxication. Since both salicylates and corticosteroids are ulcerogenic, it is possible that there will be an increased rate of gastrointestinal ulceration.

Hypoglycaemic agents: The actions of hypoglycaemic drugs will be antagonized by the hyperglycaemic actions of cortisone.

Amphotericin: Since both amphotericin and corticosteroids have potassium-depleting effects, signs of hypokalaemia should be looked for during their concurrent use.

Methotrexate: There is a small amount of evidence that use of corticosteroids and methotrexate simultaneously, may cause increased methotrexate toxicity and possibly death, although this combination of drugs has been used very successfully.

Antagonistic/potentiating effects of other drugs

Barbiturates: The therapeutic effects of cortisone may be reduced by certain barbiturates (particularly when given in high doses).

Phenytoin: The therapeutic effects of cortisone may be reduced by concurrent use of phenytoin.

Rifampicin: The effects of cortisone may be reduced by concurrent use of rifampicin.

The concurrent usage of cortisone with antacids, cimetidine or theophylline appears to have no effect on the therapeutic use of either drug.

Pharmaceutical precautions Protect from light.

Legal category POM.

Package quantities Bottle of 100 tablets.

Further information Nil.

Product licence numbers
Cortistab 5 mg tablets 0014/5044
Cortistab 25 mg tablets 0014/5045

DELTASTAB* INJECTION

Presentation Deltastab Injection is a sterile suspension of 25 mg per ml of Prednisolone Acetate BP 1963.

Inactive ingredients: Benzyl alcohol; Tween 80; sodium chloride; sodium carboxymethylcellulose.

Uses Deltastab Injection is intended primarily for the local treatment by intra-articular or peri-articular injection of rheumatic and other inflammatory conditions. Indications include rheumatoid arthritis and osteoarthrosis when few joints are involved, and in traumatic arthritis, except when associated with fractures into the joint. In addition to articular use, Deltastab Injection injected into inflamed tendon sheaths and bursae will provide symptomatic treatment.

Deltastab Injection is suitable for parenteral administration by the intramuscular route in conditions requiring systemic corticosteroids.

Dosage and administration For articular use, 5 to 25 mg depending upon the size of the joint; the injections may be repeated when relapse occurs. Not more than three joints should be treated in any one day.

For parenteral use by intramuscular injection, the dosage of Deltastab Injection will depend upon the clinical circumstances and the judgement of the physician.

Suggested dosage: 25 to 100 mg once or twice weekly.

Elderly: Steroids should be used cautiously in the elderly, since adverse effects are enhanced by old age.

Contra-indications, warnings, etc Intra-articular and peri-articular injections of Deltastab Injection are contra-indicated when the joint or surrounding tissues are infected. The presence of infection also precludes injection into tendon sheaths and bursae. Deltastab Injection must not be injected directly into tendons, nor should it be injected into the spinal joints or any other than true diarthrodial joints.

Contra-indicated in patients with peptic ulcer, active tuberculosis, acute psychosis and acute bacterial or viral infection.

Precautions: It should be borne in mind that joints and tissues injected with corticosteroids have an increased susceptibility to infection and full aseptic precautions should be observed when making local injections of Deltastab.

Patients currently receiving steroid therapy or who have received such treatment within the previous year may require special control measures when involved in anaesthesia, surgical procedures and similar stress situations. Cessation of corticosteroid therapy may be followed by acute rebound exacerbation of disease, acute adrenocortical insufficiency and polyarthritis. Withdrawal of therapy should, therefore, be gradual and related to the period of use. Concurrent administration of barbiturates, phenylbutazone or phenytoin may increase corticosteroid levels. If anticoagulants are being given with corticosteroids, it is usually necessary to adjust the dosage of the former. The use of corticosteroids in the presence of disorders or drugs (e.g. hypoglycaemics) which impinge upon the effects of corticosteroids can result in inbalance of control.

Pregnancy and lactation: The systemic administration of corticosteroids to pregnant animals can lead to foetal abnormalities. The relevance of these findings to humans has not been fully established, though caution should be exercised when giving corticosteroids to patients suspected of being pregnant especially in the first trimester. Prednisone and prednisolone have been detected in breast milk at concentrations considered unlikely to be clinically significant.

Side-effects: With intra-articular and other local injections, the principal side-effect encountered is a temporary local exacerbation with increased pain and swelling. Normally, this subsides after a few hours. Particularly after high or prolonged local administration corticosteroids can be absorbed in amounts sufficient to produce systemic effects.

Note: When being given by intramuscular injection, the precautions, side-effects, contra-indications and withdrawal symptoms associated with the systemic use of corticosteroids become relevant to Deltastab Injection.

Treatment of overdosage: Treatment is symptomatic, but is unlikely to be required.

Pharmaceutical precautions Store between 15°C to 20°C. Protect from light. Shake well before use.

Legal category POM.

Package quantities 6 ampoules of 1 ml.

Further information Nil.

Product licence number 0014/5137.

DIMERCAPROL INJECTION

Presentation Dimercaprol Injection BP (B.A.L. Injection) is a sterile solution of dimercaprol in arachis oil containing 10% V/V benzyl benzoate. It is presented in 2 ml ampoules, and each ml of the injection contains 50 mg of Dimercaprol BP.

Inactive ingredients: Arachis oil; benzyl benzoate.

Uses Dimercaprol Injection is indicated in the treatment of acute poisoning by certain heavy metals – arsenic, mercury, gold, bismuth, antimony and possibly thallium. Although dimercaprol has not been successful in the treatment of lead poisoning when used alone, there is evidence that, used in conjunction with sodium calcium edetate, it can be used successfully in the treatment of lead poisoning, particularly in children.

Dosage and administration By intramuscular injection:

Adults: 400 to 800 mg, in divided doses, on the first day.
200 to 400 mg, in divided doses, on second and third days.
100 to 200 mg, in divided doses, on subsequent days.

Within the above dose range, individual dosage should be calculated on a body-weight basis, and will depend upon the severity of symptoms and the causative agent. As a general guide, single doses should not exceed 3 mg/kg; however, in severe acute poisoning, single doses up to 5 mg/kg may be required initially.

Children: Dimercaprol Injection is well tolerated by children and dosage should be calculated on the basis of body-weight, using the same unit dose per kilogram of body-weight as for an adult under similar clinical circumstances.

Precautions: The use of Dimercaprol Injection does not eliminate the need for the general treatment of poisoning due to the particular heavy metal. Any abnormal reaction (e.g. pyrexia) occurring after the initial injection of dimercaprol should be assessed before continuing treatment.

Elderly: There is no specific data on the use of dimercaprol in the elderly but since it is eliminated via the kidney, it should be used with caution in this age group.

Contra-indications, warnings, etc Dimercaprol Injection is contra-indicated in poisoning by iron and cadmium.

Dimercaprol Injection is contra-indicated in the presence of extensive hepatic insufficiency or damage.

Dimercaprol Injection should be used with caution in the hypertensive patient.

Side-effects are relatively frequent, but, at the therapeutic dosage usually employed, are seldom severe enough to warrant cessation of treatment and are almost invariably reversible. There is some evidence to indicate that 30–60 mg of ephedrine sulphate, by mouth, given half an hour before each injection of dimercaprol, will reduce these reactions. Also, a minimum interval of four hours between doses appears to reduce side-effects.

Dimercaprol Injection may cause the following side-effects particularly at the higher dosage levels:

Elevation of blood pressure accompanied by tachycardia; nausea and possibly vomiting; a burning sensation of the lips, mouth, throat and eyes; salivation and lachrymation; conjunctivitis; rhinorrhoea; muscle pain and spasm; abdominal pain; headache; tingling of the hands and other extremities; a feeling of constriction in the chest and throat; sweating of the forehead and hands.

Local pain may occur at the site of injection, and gluteal abscess has occasionally been encountered.

A side-effect apparently peculiar to children is a fever which develops after the second or third injection, and persists until treatment with dimercaprol is terminated.

Dimercaprol Injection may not be effective in cases of concomitant renal failure, e.g. in arsine poisoning and some cases of arsenic poisoning.

Pregnancy and lactation: Dimercaprol Injection has been used in Wilsons Disease with successful full-term pregnancies, but since there is no other experience of its use in pregnancy, it should be prescribed with caution. There is no information on the use of this product in lactation.

Pharmaceutical precautions Dimercaprol Injection may become cloudy in cold weather; if this occurs, warm slightly before use.

Protect from light.

Legal category POM.

Package quantities 12 ampoules of 2 ml.

Further information Nil.

Product licence number 0014/5509.

FROBEN*

Presentation Light yellow, sugar-coated tablets containing either 50 mg or 100 mg of Flurbiprofen BP. The 50 mg tablets are overprinted 'F50' in black; the 100 mg tablets are overprinted 'F100', in black.

White wax suppositories containing 100 mg of Flurbiprofen BP.

Inactive ingredients: Tablets – lactose; sucrose; sunset yellow; sodium benzoate; glucose.

Uses Froben is a nonsteroidal anti-inflammatory agent which has significant anti-inflammatory, analgesic and antipyretic properties and is indicated in the treatment of rheumatoid disease, osteoarthritis, ankylosing spondylitis. The tablets are also indicated in the relief of mild to moderate pain.

Dosage and administration The recommended daily dose is 150–200 mg in divided doses.

In patients with severe symptoms or disease of recent origin, or during acute exacerbations, the total daily dosage may be increased to 300 mg in divided doses.

Froben Suppositories are recommended for patients in whom rectal administration is preferable.

Although Froben is generally well tolerated in the

elderly, some patients, especially with impaired renal function, may eliminate nonsteroidal anti-inflammatory drugs more slowly than normal. In these cases Froben should be used with caution and dosage should be assessed individually.

Froben is not indicated for use in children.

Contra-indications, warnings, etc As with other nonsteroidal anti-inflammatory drugs Froben should be avoided in patients with peptic ulceration, gastrointestinal haemorrhage and ulcerative colitis.

Froben Suppositories are contra-indicated in patients with inflammatory diseases of the rectum and peri-anal area.

Fluid retention and oedema have been reported in common with other nonsteroidal anti-inflammatory agents. Froben should be used with caution in patients with a history of cardiac decompensation and hypertension.

Froben should not be given to patients with a history of asthma or to patients who have experienced bronchospasm, anaphylactic reactions, angioedema or other hypersensitivity type reactions from use of aspirin or other nonsteroidal anti-inflammatory drugs.

As it has been shown that Froben may prolong bleeding time, it should be used with caution in patients with a potential for abnormal bleeding.

Side-effects: Dyspepsia, nausea, vomiting, gastrointestinal haemorrhage, diarrhoea and ulcers of the mouth have been reported. Exacerbation of peptic ulceration and perforation have been reported.

Urticaria, angioedema and rashes of varying descriptions have been reported.

Very rarely cholestatic jaundice has been reported, which is reversible on withdrawal of the drug.

Thrombocytopenia has been reported. It is usually reversible on withdrawal of the drug.

Very rarely aplastic anaemia and agranulocytosis have been reported in association with the use of Froben but causality has not been established.

Nonsteroidal anti-inflammatory drugs have been reported to cause nephrotoxicity in various forms; interstitial nephritis, nephrotic syndrome and renal failure. In patients with renal, cardiac or hepatic impairment, caution is required since the use of nonsteroidal anti-inflammatory drugs may result in deterioration of renal function. The dose should be kept as low as possible and renal function should be monitored in these patients.

Occasional symptoms due to local irritation with the suppositories may occur, e.g. diarrhoea and pruritus.

Use in pregnancy and lactation: The safety of Froben during pregnancy or lactation has not been established. Pre-clinical studies have not revealed any teratogenic effects but parturition was delayed and prolonged.

Drug interactions: Special clinical studies have shown that the diuretic response to frusemide can occasionally be reduced by Froben. Similarly, interference with the action of anticoagulants has occasionally been reported.

Other studies have failed to show any interaction between Froben and digoxin, tolbutamide or antacids.

Interference with laboratory tests: There is no evidence so far that flurbiprofen interferes with standard laboratory tests.

Treatment of overdosage: Gastric lavage and, if necessary, correction of serum electrolytes. There is no specific antidote to flurbiprofen.

Pharmaceutical precautions Suppositories: Store in a cool, dry place between 2° and 25°C.

Legal category POM.

Package quantities
50 mg Tablets: Packs of 100 and 500 (strips of 10).
100 mg Tablets: Packs of 100 (strips of 10).
100 mg Suppositories: Packs of 12 (strips of 6).

Further information Froben is a potent inhibitor of prostaglandin synthetase which most probably explains its pharmacological effects.

Product licence numbers
Froben 50 mg Tablets 0014/0167
Froben 100 mg Tablets 0014/0168
Froben 100 mg Suppositories 0014/0252

FROBEN SR*

Presentation A hard gelatin capsule with a yellow opaque cap and a transparent yellow body containing white to off-white beads, printed 'FSR' in black. Each capsule contains 200 mg Flurbiprofen BP in sustained release form.

Uses Froben SR is a nonsteroidal anti-inflammatory agent which has significant analgesic and anti-inflammatory properties and is indicated in the treatment of osteoarthritis, rheumatoid disease and ankylosing spondylitis.

Dosage and administration The recommended daily dose is one 200 mg capsule, taken preferably in the evening, after food.

Froben SR Capsules are not recommended for children under 12 years.

Although flurbiprofen is generally well tolerated in the elderly, some patients, especially with impaired renal function, may eliminate nonsteroidal anti-inflammatory drugs more slowly than normal. In these cases, Froben SR should be used with caution.

Contra-indications, warnings, etc As with other nonsteroidal anti-inflammatory drugs Froben SR should be avoided in patients with peptic ulceration, gastrointestinal haemorrhage and ulcerative colitis.

Fluid retention and oedema have been reported with flurbiprofen, in common with other nonsteroidal anti-inflammatory agents. Froben SR should be used with caution in patients with a history of cardiac decompensation and hypertension.

Froben SR should not be given to patients with a history of asthma or to patients who have experienced bronchospasm, anaphylactic reactions, angioedema or other hypersensitivity type reactions from use of aspirin or other nonsteroidal anti-inflammatory drugs.

As it has been shown that flurbiprofen may prolong bleeding time, it should be used with caution in patients with a potential for abnormal bleeding.

Side-effects: Dyspepsia, nausea, vomiting, gastrointestinal haemorrhage, diarrhoea and ulcers of the mouth have been recorded with flurbiprofen. Occasionally peptic ulceration and perforation have also been reported.

Urticaria, angioedema and rashes of varying description have been reported. Photosensitivity has not been a problem.

Very rarely cholestatic jaundice has been reported. It is reversible on withdrawal of the drug.

Thrombocytopenia has been reported. It is usually reversible on withdrawal of the drug.

Very rarely aplastic anaemia and agranulocytosis have been reported in association with the use of flurbiprofen.

Nonsteroidal anti-inflammatory drugs have been reported to cause nephrotoxicity in various forms; interstitial nephritis, nephrotic syndrome and renal failure. In patients with renal, cardiac or hepatic impairment, caution is required since the use of nonsteroidal anti-inflammatory drugs may result in deterioration of renal function. The dose should be kept as low as possible and renal function should be monitored in these patients.

Use in pregnancy and lactation: The safety of flurbiprofen during pregnancy or lactation has not been established. Pre-clinical studies have not revealed any teratogenic effects but parturition was delayed and prolonged.

Drug interactions: Special clinical studies have shown that the diuretic response to frusemide can occasionally be reduced by flurbiprofen. Similarly, interference with the action of anticoagulants has occasionally been reported.

Other studies have failed to show any interaction between flurbiprofen and digoxin, tolbutamide or antacids.

Interference with laboratory tests: There is no evidence so far that flurbiprofen interferes with standard laboratory tests.

Treatment of overdosage: Gastric lavage and, if necessary, correction of serum electrolytes. There is no specific antidote to flurbiprofen.

Pharmaceutical precautions No special storage requirements are necessary.

Legal category POM.

Package quantities Pack of 30 capsules.

Further information Froben SR is a potent inhibitor of prostaglandin synthetase which most probably explains its pharmacological effects.

Taken once a day, preferably in the evening, Froben SR is particularly suitable for those patients where compliance may be a problem and for better control of morning stiffness.

Product licence number 0014/0327.

GASTROZEPIN*

Presentation Gastrozepin is pirenzepine dihydrochloride, available as white tablets each containing the equivalent of 50 mg of anhydrous substance. The tablets are scored on one face and impressed with 'G' on one side of the score and '50' on the other. The obverse is impressed with the symbol .

Inactive ingredients: Lactose.

Uses Gastrozepin is indicated in the treatment of gastric and duodenal ulcers.

Dosage and administration In most patients Gastrozepin should be given in a dosage of 100 mg daily as one tablet each morning and one at night. Freedom from discomfort is usually achieved with Gastrozepin after a few days but treatment should be continued for a total of 4–6 weeks to allow the condition to be completely healed.

In patients with severe symptoms, the total daily dosage may be increased to 150 mg, one tablet to be taken three times a day.

In patients requiring longer term therapy, Gastrozepin may be given continuously for up to three months.

The tablets are best taken half an hour or more before meals with a little liquid.

Elderly: There is no evidence to suggest that the dosage should be reduced in the elderly, provided normal renal function is maintained. The dosage may however need to be modified in patients with renal impairment, particularly those with end stage renal failure. Dosage modifications should take place by prolongation of the dosage interval.

Contra-indications, warnings, etc At doses sufficient to produce ulcer healing, pirenzepine does not cross the blood/brain barrier in significant amounts and so central pharmacological effects are likely to be minimal.

Contra-indicated in patients with known hypersensitivity to pirenzepine.

Pirenzepine should be avoided in patients with prostate enlargement, organic pyloric stenosis, paralytic ileus, closed angle glaucoma or those with a shallow anterior chamber.

No clinically significant interactions with pirenzepine have been reported, although anticholinergic side-effects may be enhanced when given together with other drugs with anticholinergic properties e.g. atropine, antihistamines, butyrophenones, phenothiazines and tricyclic antidepressants.

Pharmacological interaction between sympathomimetics or monoamine oxidase inhibitors and pirenzepine is a theoretical possibility.

Pregnancy and lactation: In animal studies pirenzepine had no teratogenic effects in the species tested, even at high dosages. The use of Gastrozepin is not recommended during pregnancy.

Pirenzepine appears in the milk of lactating mothers in minimal amounts after therapeutic doses but is not likely to adversely affect the infant.

Side Effects: Few side effects are associated with Gastrozepin. Occasionally dry mouth and accommodation difficulties may occur but these are transitory and rarely sufficiently severe to warrant discontinuation of therapy.

Interference with laboratory tests: There is no evidence so far that pirenzepine interferes with standard laboratory tests.

Treatment of Overdosage: There is no specific antidote to pirenzepine. The treatment of overdosage is entirely symptomatic.

Pharmaceutical precautions Recommended storage conditions: in a cool dry place.

Legal category POM.

Package quantities Gastrozepin tablets 50 mg – pack of 60.

Further information In animal studies pirenzepine has been shown to differentiate between muscarinic receptors in different tissues with preferential binding to receptors in the gastric mucosa. This property probably explains the selectivity of clinical activity throughout the normal therapeutic dose range, producing gastric antisecretory effects leading to ulcer healing without marked effects at other peripheral muscarinic receptor sites.

In addition to a reduction in acid secretion, pirenzepine also reduces the secretion of pepsinogen/pepsin.

Pirenzepine has a mean half-life of approximately 12 hours and therefore provides a continuous therapeutic activity from a twice daily dosage.

Product licence number 0014/0260

HYDRENOX*

Presentation Hydrenox Tablets are Hydroflumethiazide Tablets BP. They are white and each contains 50 mg of Hydroflumethiazide BP, a diuretic of the thiazide group.

Inactive ingredients: Lactose.

Uses Hydrenox is indicated in all cases where the reduction of fluid retention by diuresis is required, i.e. oedema of cardiac, renal or hepatic origin; premenstrual, iatrogenic and all other types of oedema. Hydrenox is also indicated in the treatment of hypertension, either used alone or in combination with other antihypertensive agents.

Dosage and administration *Diuretic:* 50 to 200 mg daily, depending upon the severity of the oedema, as a single dose in the morning. The daily dose should be given early enough to complete diuresis by bedtime. Doses of 25 to 50 mg on alternate days are usually adequate for maintenance therapy.

Antihypertensive: 25 to 50 mg daily; when given as an adjunct to other antihypertensive agents, the dose of the latter should be halved.

Children: Dosage in children will be at the discretion of the physician; 1 mg per kg of body-weight has been suggested as suitable for most cases.

Elderly: The dosage of thiazide diuretics may need to be reduced in the elderly, particularly when renal function is impaired because of the possibility of electrolyte imbalance.

Contra-indications, warnings, etc Hydrenox is contra-indicated in severe renal failure and in patients with a known hypersensitivity to thiazides. It should be used with caution in patients with Addison's Disease, hypercalcaemia and hepatic or renal impairment. Renal function should be continuously monitored during thiazide therapy.

All thiazide diuretics can produce a degree of electrolyte imbalance, especially in patients with renal or hepatic impairment or when dosage is high or prolonged. Serum electrolyte levels should be checked for abnormalities, particularly hypokalaemia, which should be corrected by the addition of potassium supplement to the regimen.

Note: Hydrenox does not contain a potassium supplement. Thiazide diuretics may raise serum acid levels with consequent exacerbation of gout in susceptible patients.

Thiazide diuretics sometimes lower carbohydrate tolerance and the insulin dosage of the diabetic patient may require adjustment. Care is necessary when hydroflumethiazide is given to those with a known pre-disposition to diabetes.

Rarely blood dyscrasias, including agranulocytosis, aplastic anaemia, thrombocytopaenia and leucopaenia and pancreatitis have been reported with long term thiazide therapy. Skin rashes and impotence have occasionally been reported.

Pregnancy and lactation: Diuretics are best avoided for the management of oedema of pregnancy or hypertension in pregnancy as their use may be associated with hypovolaemia, increased blood viscosity and reduced placental perfusion.

There is inadequate evidence of safety in human pregnancy and some workers have described foetal bone marrow depression and thrombocytopaenia. Foetal and neonatal jaundice have also been described.

As diuretics pass into breast milk, they should be avoided in mothers who wish to breast feed.

Drug interactions: Sensitivity to digitalis glycosides may be increased by the hypokalaemic effect of concurrent hydroflumethiazide. Patients should be observed for signs of digitalis intoxication, in particular arrhythmias, and if these appear, the dosage of digitalis glycosides should be reduced and a potassium supplement added to restore stability.

Serum lithium concentrations may be increased by concurrent use of thiazide diuretics.

Non-steroidal anti-inflammatory agents may blunt the diuretic and anti-hypertensive effects of thiazide diuretics.

ACTH, corticosteroids, acetazolamide and carbenoxolone may exacerbate the hypokalaemia associated with thiazide use. Thiazide diuretics may enhance the neuromuscular blocking effects of the non-depolarising muscle relaxants, e.g. tubocurarine.

Interference with laboratory tests: Like all thiazides, hydroflumethiazide may interfere with a number of laboratory tests, including estimation of serum protein-bound iodine and tests of parathyroid function.

Treatment of overdosage: Monitor blood pressure, fluid and electrolyte balance and correct if necessary. Treatment is symptomatic and supportive; there is no specific antidote.

Pharmaceutical precautions Recommended storage conditions, 5° to 20°C.

Legal category POM.

Package quantities Bottle of 100, bottle of 500.

Further information Nil.

Product licence number 0014/5119.

HYDROCORTISTAB* INJECTION

Presentation Hydrocortistab Injection is Hydrocortisone Acetate Injection BP, containing 25 mg of Hydrocortisone Acetate BP per ml.

Inactive ingredients: Benzyl alcohol; Tween 80; sodium chloride; sodium carboxymethylcellulose.

Uses Hydrocortistab Injection is indicated for the local treatment, by intra-articular or peri-articular injection of arthritic conditions such as rheumatoid arthritis and osteoarthritis when few joints are involved. It is also suitable for the symptomatic treatment, by the local injection, of certain non-articular inflammatory conditions such as inflamed tendon-sheaths and bursae.

Hydrocortistab Injection is not suitable for the production of systemic effects.

Dosage and administration By intra-articular or peri-articular injection.

Adults: 5–50 mg daily depending on the size of the joint.

Children: 5–30 mg daily in divided doses.

Not more than three joints should be treated in one day.

Elderly: Steroids should be used cautiously in the elderly, since adverse effects are enhanced in old age.

The injection may be repeated at intervals of about 3 weeks.

Caution is necessary when prescribing corticosteroids in the following conditions:

(a) Previous history of tuberculosis or characteristic appearance on chest X-ray. The emergence of active tuberculosis can, however, be prevented by the prophylactic use of antituberculous therapy.
(b) Diabetes mellitus (or a family history of diabetes).
(c) Osteoporosis (post menopausal females are particularly at risk).
(d) Hypertension.
(e) History of severe affective disorders (especially previous history of steroid psychosis).
(f) Glaucoma (or a family history of glaucoma).
(g) Previous steroid myopathy.
(h) Peptic ulceration.
(i) Epilepsy.
(j) Vaccination with live vaccines.

Contra-indications, warnings, etc As with all corticosteroids, the administration of Hydrocortistab Injection is contra-indicated when the affected site is infected. It should not be injected directly into tendons, nor should it be injected into spinal or any other than true diarthrodial joints.

Since joints and tissues injected with corticosteroids have an increased susceptibility to infection, local injections of Hydrocortistab should be carried out with full aseptic precautions.

Side-effects: The principal side-effect encountered with local injections of corticosteroids is a temporary local exacerbation, with increased pain and swelling. This usually subsides after a few hours. In certain circumstances, particularly after high or prolonged local dosage, corticosteroids can be absorbed in amounts sufficient to produce systemic effects.

The following side effects may be associated with the long term systemic use of corticosteroids.

Gastro-intestinal: Dyspepsia, peptic ulceration with perforation and haemorrhage, abdominal distension, oesophageal ulceration, oesophageal candidiasis, acute pancreatitis.

Musculoskeletal: Proximal myopathy, osteoporosis, vertebral and long bone fractures, avascular osteonecrosis, tendon rupture.

Fluid and electrolyte disturbance: Sodium and water retention, hypertension, hypokalemic alkalosis.

Dermatological: impaired healing, skin atrophy, bruising, striae, telangiectasia, acne.

Endocrine/metabolic: Suppression of the hypothalamo-pituitary adrenal axis, growth suppression in childhood and adolescence, menstrual irregularity and amenorrhoea. Cushingoid facies, hirsutism, weight gain, impaired carbohydrate tolerance with increased requirement for antidiabetic therapy, negative nitrogen balance.

Neuropsychiatric: Euphoria, psychological dependence, depression, insomnia. Intracranial hypertension in children. Aggravation of schizophrenia.

Ophthalmic: Increased intra-ocular pressure, glaucoma, papilloedema, cataracts, corneal or scleral thinning, exacerbation of ophthalmic viral disease.

General: Opportunistic infection, recurrence of dormant tuberculosis, leucocytosis, hypersensitivity, thromboembolism, increased appetite, nausea, malaise.

Withdrawal symptoms: Fever, myalgia, arthralgia, adrenal insufficiency.

Use in pregnancy and lactation: There is inadequate evidence of safety in human pregnancy and there may be a very small risk of cleft palate and intra-uterine growth retardation in the fetus; there is evidence of harmful effects on pregnancy in animals.

In lactation, continuous therapy with high doses could possibly affect the child's adrenal function, monitor carefully.

Use in children: Corticosteroids cause growth retardation in infancy, childhood and adolescence. Treatment should be limited to the minimum dosage for the shortest possible term. In order to minimise suppression of the hypothalamo-pituitary adrenal axis and growth retardation, treatment should be administered where possible as a single dose on alternate days.

Use in the elderly: Treatment of elderly patients, particularly if long term, should be planned bearing in mind the more serious consequences of the common side effects of corticosteroids in old age, especially osteoporosis, diabetes, hypertension, susceptibility to infection and thinning of the skin.

Warning: Withdrawal from glucocorticoid therapy, particularly if treatment has been long term may cause a variety of potentially serious symptoms. These effects, whilst only temporary, are due to drug-induced suppression of the hypothalamic-pituitary-adrenocortical axis and may be avoided by very gradual withdrawal from corticosteroid therapy.

Drug interactions

Modification of other drug effects

Anticoagulants: The effectiveness of anticoagulants may be increased or decreased with concurrent corticosteroid therapy.

Salicylates: Serum levels of salicylates may increase considerably if corticosteroid therapy is withdrawn, possibly causing intoxication. Since both salicylates and corticosteroids are ulcerogenic, it is possible that there will be an increased rate of gastrointestinal ulceration.

Hypoglycaemic agents: The actions of hypoglycaemic drugs will be antagonized by the hyperglycaemic actions of hydrocortisone acetate.

Amphotericin: Since both amphotericin and corticosteroids have potassium-depleting effects, signs of hypokalaemia should be looked for during their concurrent use.

Methotrexate: There is a small amount of evidence that use of corticosteroids and methotrexate simultaneously, may cause increased methotrexate toxicity and possibly death, although this combination of drugs has been used very successfully.

Antagonistic/potentiating effects of other drugs

Barbiturates: The therapeutic effects of hydrocortisone acetate may be reduced by certain barbiturates (particularly when given in high doses).

Phenytoin: The therapeutic effects of hydrocortisone acetate may be reduced by concurrent use of phenytoin.

Rifampicin: The effects of hydrocortisone acetate may be reduced by concurrent use of rifampicin.

The concurrent usage of hydrocortisone acetate with antacids, cimetidine or theophylline appears to have no effect on the therapeutic use of either drug.

Treatment of overdosage: Treatment is symptomatic but is unlikely to be required.

Pharmaceutical precautions Store between 15°C to 20°C; protect from light.

Legal category POM.

Package quantities 6 ampoules of 1 ml.

Further information Nil.

Product licence number 0014/5510.

HYDROCORTISTAB TABLETS

Presentation Hydrocortistab Tablets are Hydrocortisone Tablets BP, containing 20 mg of Hydrocortisone BP and are white in colour.

Inactive ingredients: Lactose.

Uses Hydrocortistab Tablets are indicated for replacement therapy in primary and secondary adrenal insufficiency, Addison's disease and congenital adrenal hyperplasia. Hydrocortistab tablets are also indicated as acute emergency treatment in severe bronchial asthma, drug hypersensitivity reactions, serum sickness, angioneurotic oedema and anaphylaxis.

Dosage and administration In replacement therapy the normal daily requirement is: Adults 20–30 mg. Children 10–30 mg. in divided doses.

In acute emergency 60–80 mg every 4–6 hours for 24 hours then gradually reducing the dose over several days.

Elderly: Steroids should be used cautiously in the elderly, since adverse effects are enhanced in old age.

Contra-indications, warnings, etc *Caution* is necessary when prescribing corticosteroids in the following conditions:

(a) Previous history of tuberculosis or characteristic appearance on chest X-ray. The emergence of active tuberculosis can, however, be prevented by the prophylactic use of antituberculous therapy.

(b) Diabetes mellitus (or a family history of diabetes).

(c) Osteoporosis (post menopausal females are particularly at risk).

(d) Hypertension.

(e) History of severe affective disorders (especially previous history of steroid psychosis).

(f) Glaucoma (or a family history of glaucoma).

(g) Previous steroid myopathy.

(h) Peptic ulceration.

(i) Epilepsy.

Side-effects: The following side-effects may be associated with the long term systemic use of corticosteroids.

Gastro-intestinal: Dyspepsia, peptic ulceration with perforation and haemorrhage, abdominal distension, oesophageal ulceration, oesophageal candidiasis, acute pancreatitis.

Musculoskeletal: Proximal myopathy, osteoporosis, vertebral and long bone fractures, avascular osteonecrosis, tendon rupture.

Fluid and electrolyte disturbance: Sodium and water retention, hypertension, hypokalaemic alkalosis.

Dermatological: Impaired healing, skin atrophy, bruising, striae, telangiectasia, acne.

Endocrine/metabolic: Suppression of the hypothalamo-pituitary adrenal axis, growth suppression in childhood and adolescence, menstrual irregularity and amenorrhoea. Cushingoid facies, hirsutism, weight gain, impaired carbohydrate tolerance with increased requirement for antidiabetic therapy, negative nitrogen balance.

Neuropsychiatric: Euphoria, psychological dependence, depression, insomnia. Intracranial hypertension in children. Aggravation of schizophrenia.

Ophthalmic: Increased intra-ocular pressure, glaucoma, papilloedema, cataracts, corneal or scleral thinning, exacerbation of ophthalmic viral disease.

General: Opportunistic infection, recurrence of dormant tuberculosis, leucocytosis, hypersensitivity, thromboembolism, increased appetite, nausea, malaise.

Withdrawal symptoms: Fever, myalgia, arthralgia, adrenal insufficiency.

Use in pregnancy: There is inadequate evidence of safety in human pregnancy and there may be a very small risk of cleft palate and intra-uterine growth retardation in the fetus; there is evidence of harmful effects on pregnancy in animals.

Use in children: Corticosteroids cause growth retardation in infancy, childhood and adolescence. Treatment should be limited to the minimum dosage for the shortest possible time. In order to minimise suppression of the hypothalamo-pituitary adrenal axis and growth retardation, treatment should be administered where possible as a single dose on alternate days.

Use in the elderly: Treatment of elderly patients, particularly if long term, should be planned bearing in mind the more serious consequences of the common side effects of corticosteroids in old age, especially osteoporosis, diabetes, hypertension, susceptibility to infection and thinning of the skin.

Special warning: Withdrawal from glucocorticoid therapy, particularly if treatment has been long term may cause a variety of potentially serious symptoms. These effects, whilst only temporary, are due to drug-induced suppression of the hypothalamic-pituitary-adrenocortical axis and may be avoided by very gradual withdrawal from corticosteroid therapy.

Treatment of overdosage: Treatment is symptomatic but is unlikely to be required.

Pharmaceutical precautions Store in a cool dry place.

Legal category POM.

Package quantities Hydrocortistab tablets 20 mg: bottle of 100.

Product licence number 0014/5383.

JUNIFEN*▼

Presentation Junifen is presented as an orange flavoured liquid containing 100 mg of ibuprofen in each 5 ml.

Inactive ingredients: Sucrose, sodium benzoate, methyl hydroxybenzoate, propyl hydroxybenzoate and sunset yellow.

Uses Junifen is indicated for the reduction of fever and the relief of mild to moderate pain in children older than one year.

Dosage and administration *Children:* The daily dosage of Junifen is 20 mg per kg of body-weight in divided doses. This can be achieved as follows:

1–2 years: One 2.5 ml spoonful three to four times a day
3–7 years: One 5 ml spoonful three to four times a day
8–12 years: Two 5 ml spoonfuls three to four times a day

A spoon with two ends is provided; one to measure 2.5 ml and the other 5 ml.

Not recommended for children under the age of 1 year or for children weighing less than 7 kg. For short term use only.

Contra-indications, warnings, etc Junifen should not be given to patients with a history of or active peptic ulceration. Bronchospasm may be precipitated in patients suffering from, or with a previous history of, bronchial asthma. Junifen should not be given to patients in whom aspirin and other non-steroidal anti-inflammatory drugs induce the symptoms of asthma, rhinitis or urticaria.

Adverse effects reported include: dyspepsia, gastrointestinal intolerance and bleeding, and skin rashes of various types. Less frequently, thrombocytopaenia has occurred.

Nonsteroidal anti-inflammatory drugs have been reported to cause nephrotoxicity in various forms; interstitial nephritis, nephrotic syndrome and renal failure. In patients with renal, cardiac or hepatic impairment, caution is required since the use of nonsteroidal anti-inflammatory drugs may result in deterioration of renal function. The dose should be kept as low as possible and renal function should be monitored in these patients.

Use in pregnancy and lactation: Whilst no teratogenic effects have been demonstrated in animal experiments, the use of Junifen during pregnancy should, if possible, be avoided. In the limited studies so far available, ibuprofen appears in the breast milk in very low concentrations and is unlikely to affect the breast-fed infant adversely.

Drug interactions: In therapeutic doses, no evidence of clinically significant interactions with other commonly used drugs has so far been observed. However, as with other non-steroidal anti-inflammatory agents, caution should be exercised in patients receiving oral anticoagulants and thiazide diuretics.

Interference with laboratory tests: There is no evidence so far that ibuprofen interferes with standard labatory tests.

Treatment of overdose: Gastric lavage and, if necessary, correction of serum electrolytes. There is no specific antidote to ibuprofen.

Pharmaceutical precautions Junifen should be stored below 25°C and protected from light.

Legal category POM.

Package quantities Bottle of 150 ml (with special dispensing spoon).

Product licence number 0014/0390.

KAODENE*

Presentation Kaodene is an aqueous suspension containing Codeine Phosphate BP 10 mg and Light Kaolin BP 3 g in each 10 ml. It is an off-white liquid with the odour and flavour of aniseed.

Inactive ingredients: methylhydroxybenzoate; propylhydroxybenzoate.

Uses Kaodene is indicated for the symptomatic relief of simple diarrhoea. It cannot be used as a substitute for rehydration therapy.

Dosage and administration *Adults and Children over 12 years:* 20 ml three or four times daily.

Children from 5 to 12 years: 10 ml three or four times daily.

Kaodene is not recommended for children under 5 years.

Contra-indications, warnings, etc Kaodene is contra-indicated in patients with pseudomembranous colitis and diverticular disease and must be used with caution in patients with ulcerative colitis and hepatic dysfunction.

Codeine phosphate is a narcotic analgesic and, given in large doses, may induce tolerance and psychological and physical dependence. At the recommended dosage, however, it is unlikely that such effects would be encountered with Kaodene.

Large doses of codeine may cause drowsiness and CNS depression, but this should not be a problem with the recommended doses of Kaodene.

The long term administration of Kaodene, particularly in the elderly, is not recommended.

Pregnancy and lactation: Whilst there is no adequate evidence of safety in human pregnancy, codeine has been widely used without apparent ill-effect for many years and studies in animals have not demonstrated any hazard. Codeine passes into breast milk in very small amounts which are probably insignificant.

Drug interactions: Kaodene may interfere with the absorption of some drugs from the gastro-intestinal tract.

Interference with laboratory tests: Administration of Kaodene may interfere with laboratory estimations of serum amylase and certain liver function tests.

Treatment of overdosage: Gastric lavage and symptomatic treatment as for codeine phosphate is recommended. Naloxone may be used to counteract CNS depression.

Pharmaceutical precautions *Recommended storage conditions:* 5°–20°C.

Legal category CD (Sch 5), P.

Package quantities Bottle of 250 ml.

Further information Nil.

Product licence number 0014/0233.

MUSTINE HYDROCHLORIDE FOR INJECTION BP

Presentation Synonyms: Nitrogen mustard; Mechlorethamine Hydrochloride USP; mustargen hydrochloride;

chlorethazine hydrochloride; Chlormethine Hydrochloride INN; 'HN$_2$'.

Mustine hydrochloride is di (2-chloroethyl) methylamine hydrochloride. It is a white or almost white hygroscopic, vesicant, crystalline powder or mass and is very soluble in water.

Mustine hydrochloride is supplied in sterile vials each containing 10 mg of the powder. The injection is prepared by dissolving this in Sodium Chloride Injection BP 0.9% w/v or Water for Injections BP.

Uses Mustine hydrocloride BP is a powerful cytotoxic agent used in the treatment of several neoplastic conditions. It is an alkylating agent and also possesses immunosuppressant properties.

The principal use of mustine hydrochloride is as part of combination treatment for Hodgkin's disease. It is sometimes used in non-Hodgkins lymphomas and carcinoma of bronchus, ovary and breast. It may be applied locally for the treatment of mycosis fungoides.

Dosage and administration *Route of administration:* Intravenous.

Recommended dose and dosage schedule: Single doses of 0.4 mg per kg bodyweight or a course of 4 daily doses of 0.1 mg per kg given by intravenous injection. The term 'bodyweight' is defined, in this case, as the actual bodyweight at the time of treatment except in cases where the weight has been artificially increased by oedema, ascites, or other fluid collections. The weight of the body before the increase is used in such cases.

UNDER NO CIRMCUMSTANCES SHOULD MUSTINE BE GIVEN INTRAMUSCULARLY

A repeat course of mustine therapy should not be undertaken for at least 6 weeks or until the bone marrow has recovered its haemopoietic activity.

Preparation of intravenous injection: A fresh solution is prepared by dissolving 10 mg of mustine hydrochloride in 10 ml of Sodium Chloride Injection BP 0.9% w/v, or Water for Injections BP. The best method of administration is to set up an intravenous drip of Sodium Chloride Injection BP 0.9% w/v or Dextrose Injection BP 5% w/v; the required dose of mustine prepared as above, is then injected into the tubing. This avoids the hazards of extravasation during injection. The drip rate should be fast at approximately 60 drops per minute and the injection of mustine should be carried out over 2 minutes. The drip rate should then be reduced to 20 drops per minute.

Alternatively the concentrated solution of mustine hydrochloride is freshly prepared as above and transferred aseptically to 500 ml of sterile Sodium Chloride Injection BP 0.9% w/v.

Topical use: Mycosis fungoides may be treated by topical application of a dilute solution of mustine hydrochloride. Various strengths of mustine hydrochloride have been used but 20 mg in 100 ml of 0.9% w/v Sodium Chloride Injection BP or Water for Injections BP is frequently recommended.

This solution is applied to the affected cutaneous area using a gauze pad. The person applying the solution should wear polyvinylchloride gloves to give protection.

Elderly: Elderly patients with generalised vascular disease may be more prone to local vascular and extravascular toxicity.

Contra-indications, warnings, etc Mustine should not be given during pregnancy or during lactation to mothers who are breastfeeding. The drug possesses foetotoxic and teratogenic potential.

Mustine should not be used in patients with severe leucopenia, thrombocytopenia or anaemia and in co-existent or suspected granuloma.

Precautions and warnings

1. *Extravasation:* Extravasation during injection should be avoided as this may cause severe tissue necrosis. Infusion should be stopped immediately if local pain is experienced. Where doubt occurs as to whether significant leakage has occurred, the infusion should be discontinued and the cannula resited in another vein. If extravasation does occur during injection the involved area should be infiltrated with isotonic sodium thiosulphate injection followed by the application of an ice compress intermittently for six to twelve hours. Management of extravasation must be carried out quickly because of mustine's rapid local toxic effects.

2. *Handling*

(a) Trained personnel should reconstitute the drug.

(b) This should be performed in a designated area, which has good general and local ventilation.

(c) The work surface should be covered with disposable plastic-backed absorbent paper.

(d) Protective gloves should be worn – polyvinylchloride gloves give adequate protection whereas rubber and polyethylene gloves have been shown to be ineffective.

(e) Mustine hydrochloride is a potent vesicant and local irritant to skin and mucous membranes. It can cause severe damage to eyes and the vapour irritates the respiratory tract. Precautions should be taken to prevent accidental contact with skin, eyes and clothing. Avoid ingestion and inhalation.

First aid measures:

(i) Eyes – Immediately irrigate with large amounts of water or 2% solution of sodium bicarbonate for at least 10 minutes and obtain urgent medical attention. The person concerned should then be seen by an ophthalmologist.

(ii) Skin – Wash away immediately with large amounts of water or, if at hand, sodium carbonate solution or an isotonic solution of sodium thiosulphate.

(iii) If accidentally ingested, wash out the mouth thoroughly with water and give water to drink.

(iv) If inhaled – remove to fresh air.

Urgent medical attention should be sought after any of these occurrences.

(f) Mustine hydrochloride should not be handled by pregnant staff.

(g) Adequate care and precautions should be taken in the disposal of items (syringes, needles, etc.) used to reconstitute cytotoxic drugs.

(h) After treatment with mustine all apparatus, including PVC gloves should be washed thoroughly. A 2.5% solution of sodium carbonate is particularly suitable for the lavage or the use of the following solution:

Decontamination solution: Distilled water 3 litres; Caustic soda solution SG 1.50–1 litre; Industrial Methylated Spirit (IMS) 66 OP–4.5 litres. This solution should be prepared at least 24 hours before use and placed under work bench near ventilation exhaust. Decontamination procedure – bottles (including caps), equipment, etc., must be dismantled as far as possible and immersed in the Decontamination solution for at least 48 hours. The solution should then be decanted to the sluice and bottles, equipment, etc. washed three times with clean water prior to disposal. Note: Bottles, equipment, etc. may be temporarily stored awaiting decontamination on a suitable tray which is then placed inside a plastic bag and securely tied.

(i) Use Luèr-lock fittings on all syringes and sets. Large bore needles are recommended to minimise pressure and the possible formation of aerosols. The latter may also be reduced by the use of a venting needle.

3. *Side-effects:* Intravenous use: Nausea, emesis, fever and/or leucopenia are the most common side-effects. Nausea and vomiting often occur during the eight hours following injection and appropriate sedation and anti-emetics should be prescribed 10–30 minutes before mustine is injected. Transient anorexia and occasional diarrhoea may occur and peptic ulcers have been reported.

Neurological disturbances including lightheadedness, headache, drowsiness, tinnitus and deafness may occur. Skin rashes and alopecia may occur.

Severe bone marrow depression may follow mustine therapy, with lymphocytopenia, granulocytopenia and occasionally agranulocytosis. It may lead to severe anaemia and thrombocytopenia. Peripheral blood counts should be checked prior to each treatment. Leucocytes and platelet counts in peripheral blood start to fall about one week after treatment with a nadir between 14 and 18 days. During the same period there is a fall in haemoglobin level. Both leucocyte and platelet counts return to normal before the end of the fourth week. Vein irritation leading to discolouration may occur, even in the absence of extravasation. Thrombophlebitis and venous thrombosis are potential complications to mustine therapy.

In non-pregnant women, delayed menstruation or temporary amenorrhoea may follow the treatment. In males a reduction of active spermatogenesis has been reported. Hyperuricaemia may develop in patients with large tumour masses.

Prolonged use of alkylating agents, particularly when combined with extensive radiation, is associated with a marked increase in the incidence of acute non-lymphocytic leukaemia.

Topical use: When mustine is applied topically, patients may develop a contact dermatitis, but systemic side-effects have not been reported.

4. *Treatment of overdose:* Sodium thiosulphate will neutralise an injection of mustine hydrochloride BUT ONLY IF GIVEN IMMEDIATELY AFTERWARDS. Each 10 mg mustine requires 640 mg sodium thiosulphate given as an isotonic solution. This is equivalent to approximately 1.5 ml of a 50% injection of sodium thiosulphate diluted with 20 ml 0.9% sodium chloride injection or approximately 21 ml of 3% sodium thiosulphate injection.

Interference with biochemical laboratory tests: Nil.

Pharmaceutical precautions Store at 2° to 15°C.

Stability of reconstituted solution: Whenever possible mustine injection should be reconstituted immediately before use. A recent study of the stability of mustine hydrochloride (1 mg/ml) in Sodium Chloride 0.9% Injection or Water for Injections, using an HPLC assay, specific for mustine, has suggested that to minimise accumulation of degradation products of mustine, reconstituted solutions should be used within 4 hours when stored at room temperature or 6 hours at 4°C. Solutions stored at −20°C in syringes degraded by about 5% in 4 weeks.

Incompatibilities: A 0.2% solution of mustine hydrochloride in water has a pH of 3 to 5 and it is recommended that mustine injection is administered in 0.9% sodium chloride or 5% dextrose since it is rapidly unstable in alkaline solutions.

Legal category POM.

Package quantities Pack of 10 vials.

Further information Following intravenous injection or infusion, mustine hydrochloride is rapidly converted to an ethyleneimmonium ion which alkylates and cross links guanine bases in the deoxyribonucleic acid of the chromosomes thus arresting cell division. Although its cytotoxic and growth-inhibitory action affects all cells, it has a special affinity for rapidly multiplying cells, including certain neoplastic growths, bone marrow and lymphatic tissues. The aim of treatment is, therefore to build up maximal concentrations in the neoplastic tissues and permit minimal amounts to reach the normal tissues.

Mustine usually disappears from the blood within approximately 10 minutes. Less than 0.1% of the drug is excreted unchanged in the urine.

Product licence number 0014/5512.

NIVEMYCIN* TABLETS AND ELIXIR

Presentation Nivemycin Tablets are Neomycin Tablets BP each containing 350000 units (approximately 500 mg) of Neomycin Sulphate BP.

Nivemycin Elixir is Neomycin Elixir BP. Each 1 ml contains 12,500 units (approximately 20 mg) of Neomycin Sulphate BP.

Inactive ingredients: Elixir – Benzoic acid; disodium edetate; alcohol; sunset yellow.

Uses Nivemycin is indicated for pre-operative sterilisation of the bowel and may also be useful in the treatment of impending hepatic coma, including portal systemic encephalopathy.

Dosage and administration Pre-operative sterilisation of the bowel:

Adults: 2 tablets every hour for 4 hours, then 2 tablets every 4 hours for 2 or 3 days before the operation.

Children over 12 years: 2 tablets every 4 hours for 2 or 3 days before the operation.

Children from 6 to 12 years: ½ to 1 tablet every 4 hours for 2 or 3 days before the operation.

In hepatic coma, the adult dose is 4 – 12 grams per day in divided doses for a period of 5 –7 days whilst for children, 50–100 mg/kg per day in divided doses appears to be appropriate. Chronic hepatic insufficiency may require up to 4 grams per day over an indefinite period.

Children up to 1 year: 2.5 to 10 ml every 4 hours for 2 or 3 days before the operation.

Children from 1 year to 5 years: 10 to 20 ml every 4 hours for two to three days before the operation.

Elderly: Elderly patients who are prescribed long-term Nivemycin should have a regular assessment made of renal function and hearing.

Contra-indications, warnings, etc Nivemycin should not be given when intestinal obstruction is present. Nivemycin should not be given to patients with hypersensitivity to aminoglycosides.

Caution: The absorption of Neomycin is poor from the alimentary tract, with about 97% of an orally administered dose being excreted unchanged in the faeces. Impaired gastro-intestinal motility however may increase absorption of the drug and it is therefore possible, as with other broad spectrum antibiotics, that prolonged therapy could result in ototoxicity and nephrotoxicity, particularly in patients with a degree of renal failure. When used as an adjunct in the management of hepatic coma, care should be taken that administration is of the minimal period necessary, since prolonged exposure to the drug may result in malabsorption. Neomycin should be used with caution in patients with neuromuscular disorders and parkinsonism.

There is almost complete cross-resistance between Neomycin, Kanamycin, Paromomycin and Framycetin. Cross-resistance with Gentamycin has also been reported.

Since prolonged therapy may result in the overgrowth of non-sensitive organisms, treatment should not be continued longer than necessary to prevent super-infection.

Nivemycin may impair absorption of other drugs including phenoxymethyl-penicillin and digoxin. The efficacy of oral contraceptives may be reduced. Care should be taken when considering the use of Nivemycin concurrently with drugs with a potential to cause nephrotoxic, ototoxic or neuromuscular activity.

Pregnancy and lactation: Whilst no reports linking the use of Neomycin to congenital defects have been located, the fact that this drug, together with other aminoglycosides, may have harmful effects on the foetus following oral absorption during pregnancy and the fact that small amounts of the drug are absorbed when given orally, the use of Nivemycin in pregnancy is recommended only when the benefits outweigh the potential risks.

Side-effects: Nausea, vomiting, diarrhoea, increased salivation, stomatitis, nephrotoxicity, ototoxicity, rise in serum levels of hepatic enzymes and bilirubin, blood dyscrasias, haemolytic anaemia, confusion, paraesthesia, disorientation, nystagmas, hypersensitivity reactions including dermatitis, pruritus, drug fever and anaphylaxis.

Treatment of overdosage: Monitor renal and auditory function. If these are impaired, dialysis is indicated.

Pharmaceutical precautions Nivemycin Tablets: Store below 30°C. Protect from light.
Nivemycin Elixir: Store in a cool place. Protect from light.

Legal category POM.

Package quantities Nivemycin Tablets: Bottle of 100. Nivemycin Elixir: 100 ml bottle.

Further information Nil.

Product licence numbers
Nivemycin Tablets 0014/5069.
Nivemycin Elixir 0014/5742.

PROTHIADEN*

Presentation Prothiaden is Dothiepin Hydrochloride BP an antidepressant of the tricyclic group. It is available as sugar-coated tablets, each containing 75 mg of Dothiepin Hydrochloride BP and as hard gelatin capsules, each containing 25 mg of Dothiepin Hydrochloride BP. The tablets are red in colour and bear the overprint 'P75' in white. The capsules are red/brown with the overprint 'P25' in white.

Inactive ingredients: Tablets – Sucrose; glucose; sunset yellow; Ponceau 4R; sodium benzoate. *Capsules* – Ponceau 4R.

Uses Prothiaden is indicated in the treatment of symptoms of depressive illness especially where an anti-anxiety effect is required.

Dosage and administration
Adults: Initially 75 mg/day in divided doses or as a single dose at night, increasing to 150 mg/day. In certain circumstances, e.g. in hospital use, dosages up to 225 mg daily have been used. Suggested regimens: 25 or 50 mg three times daily or, alternatively, 75 or 150 mg as a single dose at night. Should the regimen of 150 mg as a single night-time dose be adopted, it is better to give a smaller dose for the first few days.

Elderly: 50–75 mg daily initially. As with any antidepressant, the initial dose should be increased with caution under close supervision. Half the normal adult dose may be sufficient to produce a satisfactory clinical response.

Children: Not recommended.

Contra-indications, warnings, etc
Contra-indications: Recent myocardial infarction. Any degree of heart block or other cardiac arrhythmias. Mania. Severe liver disease.

Pregnancy and lactation: There is no evidence as to the drug safety in human pregnancy nor is there evidence from animal work that it is free from hazard.

Only use during pregnancy, especially during the first and last trimesters, if there are compelling reasons.

When administered during lactation the results from a study in two patients indicated that dothiepin is not actively secreted into the breast milk. Assuming a daily milk intake of 150 ml/kg/day (2½ oz/lb) on a weight-basis (mg/kg) the baby would ingest 1/650 of the adult dose (mg/kg) of the drug. Other factors to be taken into account include the range of maternal blood levels, the presence of metabolites and the lowered drug metabolising capacity of babies which may result in elevated serum levels of unchanged drug.

Precautions: The elderly are particularly liable to experience adverse reactions to antidepressants, especially agitation, confusion and postural hypotension. Patients posing a high suicidal risk require close supervision. Prothiaden should be given with caution to epileptic patients and to those with cardiovascular disorders.

Avoid if possible in patients with narrow angle glaucoma, symptoms suggestive of prostatic hypertrophy and a history of epilepsy.

Tricyclic antidepressants potentiate the central nervous depressant action of alcohol.

Anaesthetics given during tri/tetracyclic antidepressant therapy may increase the risk of arrythymias and hypotension. If surgery is necessary, the anaesthetist should be informed that a patient is being so treated.

Drug interactions: Prothiaden should not be given concurrently with an MAO Inhibitor nor within fourteen days of ceasing such treatment.

Prothiaden may alter the pharmacological effect of some concurrently administered drugs including CNS depressants such as alcohol and narcotic analgesics; the effect of these will be potentiated as will be the effects of adrenaline and noradrenaline (some local anaesthetics contain these sympathomimetics). The hypotensive activity of certain antihypertensive agents (e.g. bethanidine, debrisoquine, guanethidine) may be reduced by Prothiaden.

It would be advisable to review all antihypertensive therapy during treatment with tricyclic antidepressants.

Barbiturates may decrease and methyl phenidate may increase the serum concentration of dothiepin and thus affect its antidepressant action.

Warning: It may be two to four weeks from the start of treatment before there is an improvement in the patient's depression; the subject should be monitored closely during this period. The anxiolytic effect may be observed within a few days of commencing treatment. Initially, Prothiaden may impair alertness; patients likely to drive vehicles or operate machinery should be warned of this possibility.

Adverse effects: The following adverse effects, although not necessarily all reported with Prothiaden have occurred with other tricyclic antidepressants. Atropine-like side-effects including dry mouth, disturbances of accommodation, tachycardia, constipation and hesitancy of micturition are common early in treatment, but usually lessen.

Other adverse effects include drowsiness, sweating, postural hypotension, tremor and skin rashes. Interference with sexual function may occur. Serious adverse effects are rare. These include depression of the bone marrow, agranulocytosis, cholestatic jaundice, hypomania and convulsions. Psychotic manifestations, including mania and paranoid delusions may be exacerbated during treatment with tricyclic antidepressants. Withdrawal symptoms may occur on abrupt cessation of tricyclic therapy and include insomnia, irritability and excessive perspiration. Similar symptoms in neonates whose mothers received tricyclic antidepressants during the third trimester have also been reported, although this has not been observed following treatment with Prothiaden.

Cardiac arrhythmias and severe hypotension are likely to occur with high dosage or in deliberate overdosage. They may also occur in patients with pre-existing heart disease taking normal dosage.

Treatment of Overdosage: Gastric lavage; when the patient is unconscious or the cough reflex depressed the lungs should be protected by a cuffed endotracheal tube. Repeated gastric/intestinal aspiration or repeated administration of activated charcoal may remove drug and metabolites excreted into the gut via the bile. Continuous ECG monitoring is advisable. Abnormalities of cardiac rhythm and epileptic convulsions may occur and should be treated accordingly. Forced diuresis is *not* recommended. Bedrest is advisable, even after recovery.

Interference with laboratory tests: There is no evidence so far that dothiepin interferes with standard laboratory tests.

Pharmaceutical precautions Recommended storage conditions: 5°C to 20°C.

Legal category POM.

Package quantities
Prothiaden Tablets: 75 mg: Calender Pack of 28; Bottle of 500.

Prothiaden Capsules: 25 mg: Bottle of 100, Bottle of 600.

Further information It has been found that, in certain cases of depression, the daily dose of Prothiaden given as a single night-time dose is more effective and even better tolerated than the conventional divided day-time dosage. There is evidence that this single bed-time dose improves the sleep pattern of the depressed patient.

Product licence numbers
Prothiaden Capsules 0014/5941
Prothiaden Tablets 0014/0209

STABILLIN* V-K ELIXIRS AND TABLETS

Presentation Stabillin V-K Elixirs '62.5', '125' and '250' are preparations of dry granules which, when reconstituted with the specified volume of water, provide elixirs (Phenoxymethylpenicillin Elixir BPC) containing respectively the phenoxymethylpenicillin potassium equivalent to 62.5, 125 and 250 mg of phenoxymethylpenicillin in each 5 ml.

Stabillin V-K Tablets are Phenoxymethylpenicillin Tablets BP 250 mg.

Inactive ingredients: Elixir – Sucrose; 125 and 250 mg/5 ml only – Ponceau 4R; sunset yellow.

Uses Stabillin V-K preparations are indicated in the treatment of infections due to penicillin-sensitive organisms and to prevent the recurrence of rheumatic fever.

Dosage and administration Phenoxymethylpenicillin should be taken 30 minutes before food.

Adults: 0.5 to 2 g daily in divided doses at 6 hour intervals.

Children 6 to 12 years: 250 mg every 6 hours.

Children 1 to 5 years: 125 mg every 6 hours.

Children up to 1 year: 62.5 mg every 6 hours.

Elderly: As for adults except where there is renal impairment (see below).

As a prophylactic: 250 mg twice daily for adults; 125 mg twice daily for children.

Dosage in renal impairment: In patients with severe renal impairment, the dosage interval for all groups should be extended to 12 hours.

Contra-indications, warnings, etc Stabillin V-K is contra-indicated in patients with a known sensitivity to penicillin and should be given with caution to those with a history of allergy.

Sensitised patients will demonstrate cross-sensitivity to all other penicillins and may show hypersensitivity to the chemically related cephalosporins.

Since Penicillin V has a high therapeutic index, toxic blood levels are unlikely to occur after oral administration. Treatment is therefore likely to be symptomatic and supportive.

Pregnancy and lactation: Although Penicillin V is generally considered to be suitable for use during pregnancy, it is advisable to use the drug with caution, particularly during the first trimester. Phenyoxymethylpenicillin is secreted in the milk and should be used with caution in nursing mothers as it may cause an allergic reaction in the offspring.

Side-effects: Penicillin V is generally well tolerated but may occasionally cause transient nausea, diarrhoea, heartburn and pruritis ani. Occasionally, hypersensitivity reactions may occur with rash, urticaria, fever and angioneurotic oedema. Rarely, true anaphylaxis may occur.

Treatment of overdosage: Treatment is symptomatic, but is unlikely to be required.

Pharmaceutical precautions Stabillin V-K Elixir and the reconstituted Elixir should be stored in a cool place; the latter should be used within one week of preparation.

Legal category POM.

Package quantities
Stabillin V-K Elixirs: Bottle of granules to make 100 ml.
Stabillin V-K Tablets: Bottle of 500.

Further information Nil.

Product licence numbers
Stabillin V-K Elixir '62.5': 0014/5341
Stabillin V-K Elixir '125': 0014/5342
Stabillin V-K Elixir '250': 0014/5343
Stabillin V-K Tablets: 0014/5082

**Trade Mark*

B. Braun Medical Ltd
13/14, Farmbrough Close, Aylesbury Vale Industrial Park, Aylesbury, Bucks HP20 1DQ

AMINOPLASMAL* L5, L10

Presentation Colourless or faintly yellow-coloured sterile solutions for intravenous infusion, containing pure crystalline amino acids in the physiologically available L-form with added electrolytes. The product is supplied in two strengths and contains the following ingredients in each 1000 ml.

	L5	*L10*
Amino acids (g/l)		
L-Isoleucine	2.55	5.10
L-Leucine	4.45	8.90
L-Lysine HCl	3.50	7.00
L-Methionine	1.90	3.80
L-Phenylalanine	2.55	5.10
L-Threonine	2.05	4.10
L-Tryptophan	0.90	1.80
L-Valine	2.40	4.80
L-Arginine	4.60	9.20
L-Histidine	2.60	5.20
Aminoacetic Acid	3.95	7.90
L-Alanine	6.85	13.70
L-Proline	4.45	8.90
L-Aspartic Acid	0.65	1.30
L-Asparagine H_2O	1.86	3.72
L-Cysteine HCl H_2O	0.36	0.73
L-Glutamic Acid	2.30	4.60
L-Ornithine HCl	1.60	3.20
L-Serine	1.20	2.40
L-Tyrosine	0.30	0.30
N-Acetyl-L-Tyrosine	0.43	1.23
Electrolytes mmol/l (mEq/l)		
Sodium	48	48
Potassium	25	25
Magnesium	2.5	2.5
Acetate	59	59
Chloride	31	62
$H_2PO_4^-$	9	9
L-Malate^{2-}	7.5	7.5
α-Amino nitrogen (g/l)	5.78	11.56
Total nitrogen (g/l)	8.03	16.06
Caloric value: (kJ/l)	850	1700
(kcal/l)	200	400

Uses Aminoplasmal L is a physiologically balanced amino acid intravenous infusion which also provides in its electrolyte content maintenance requirements of sodium, potassium and magnesium.

Aminoplasmal L can be used in the following conditions:

Parenteral nutrition: Prophylaxis and therapy of protein deficiency resulting from increased protein losses and/or increased protein requirements.

Surgery: In pre- and post-operative or post-traumatic conditions.

After resections in the gastrointestinal area.

Internal medicine:
e.g. Malabsorptive states.
Inflammatory diseases of the G.I. tract.
Persisting diarrhoea and vomiting.

Nephrology: Renal insufficiency with only slightly raised residual nitrogen values after dialysis treatment.

Dosage and administration According to amino acid, electrolyte and fluid requirements, unless otherwise prescribed:

Adults (including the elderly): 20 to 30 ml Aminoplasmal L-5 per kg body weight per day or 10 to 20 ml Aminoplasmal L-10 per kg body weight per day.

Flow rate: Up to 60 drops per minute (180 ml per hour) Aminoplasmal L-5 or up to 40 drops per minute (120 ml per hour) Aminoplasmal L-10.

Children: 3rd to 5th year: 30 ml (1.5 g amino acid) Aminoplasmal L-5 per kg body weight per day or 15 ml (1.5 g amino acid) Aminoplasmal L-10 per kg body weight per day.

6th to 14th year: 20 ml (1.0 g amino acid) Aminoplasmal L-5 per kg body weight per day or 10 ml (1.0 g amino acid) Aminoplasmal L-10 per kg body weight per day.

Flow rate: Up to 2 ml (0.1 g amino acid) Aminoplasmal L-5 per kg body weight per hour or up to 1 ml (0.1 g amino acid) Aminoplasmal L-10 per kg body weight per hour.

Use in pregnancy and lactation: Aminoplasmal L can be given during pregnancy and lactation.

Contra-indications, warnings, etc

Contra-indications: Aminoplasmal L should not be administered in the following conditions: Advanced liver disease; disturbances of amino acid metabolism; congestive cardiac failure; renal failure with pathological blood nitrogen values; acidosis; overhydration; hyperkalaemia.

Warnings: Amino acid mixtures may precipitate acute folate deficiency and folic acid should be given daily.

Precautions: In order to ensure optimum metabolic utilisation of the amino acids administered, therapy should be adequately supported by an energy supply of 35 kcal (145 kJ) per gram of amino acids.

Fluid balance, serum-electrolytes, blood glucose level and acid base state should be regularly checked.

Side-effects: Providing the contra-indications are observed, side-effects are not to be anticipated.

Overdosage: Overdosage or a too rapid infusion may manifest in the form of nausea, shivering, vomiting and increased renal amino acid losses. In such cases the infusion should be interrupted and eventually continued at a reduced infusion rate.

Pharmaceutical precautions Do not store above 25°C.

It is not recommended that any additives should be incorporated into Aminoplasmal L solutions. They should, in preference, be given in the carbohydrate solution. However, if admixture with Aminoplasmal L is essential then the compatibility of the additive should be checked before administration.

Legal category POM.

Package quantities 500 ml and 1000 ml glass bottles.

Further information Nil.

Product licence numbers

Aminoplasmal L5	4296/0002
Aminoplasmal L10	4296/0003

AMINOPLASMAL* PED

Presentation Colourless or faintly yellow-coloured sterile solution for intravenous infusion, containing pure crystalline amino acids in the physiologically available L-form with added electrolytes. Each 1000 ml has the following composition:

Amino acids (g/l)	
L-Isoleucine	1.40
L-Leucine	2.50
L-Lysine Acetate	4.50
L-Methionine	0.80
L-Phenylalanine	1.90
L-Threonine	3.00
L-Tryptophan	0.60
L-Valine	1.60
L-Arginine	2.20
L-Histidine	3.00
Aminoacetic Acid	4.90
L-Alanine	5.80
L-Proline	2.70
L-Aspartic Acid	1.90
L-Asparagine H_2O	0.91
L-Cysteine HCl H_2O	1.46
L-Glutamic Acid	9.80
L-Ornithine HCl	1.14
L-Serine	1.00
L-Tyrosine	0.30
N-Acetyl-L-Tyrosine	0.86
Electrolytes mmol/l (mEq/l)	
Sodium	50
Potassium	25
Magnesium	2.5 (5.0)
Acetate	27
Chloride	15
Total amino acids (g/l)	50
α-Amino nitrogen (g/l)	5.7
Total nitrogen (g/l)	7.4
Caloric value: (kJ/l)	850
(kcal/l)	200

Uses Aminoplasmal Ped is a physiologically balanced paediatric amino acid intravenous infusion which also provides in its electrolyte content maintenance requirements of sodium, potassium and magnesium.

Aminoplasmal Ped can be used for prophylaxis and treatment of protein deficiency in paediatrics when oral food intake is either contra-indicated or impossible as in cases like:

Premature birth.
Small-for-date syndromes.
Gastro-intestinal diseases and malformations.
Peri-operatively in paediatric surgery.
Intensive care following burns and severe injuries.

Dosage and administration *Premature and newborn infants:* Unless otherwise prescribed 20–50 ml corresponding to 1–2.5 g amino acids per kg body weight per day. When administered during the first days of life, dosage should be restricted to 1 g amino acids per kg body weight per day and gradually increased to the above stated standard rate.

Babies: 40–60 ml corresponding to 2–3 g amino acids per kg body weight per day.

Flow rate: The flow rate should be adjusted so that the intended amount of solution to be administered is infused within 10–24 hours (preferably with an infusion pump).

Contra-indications, warnings, etc
Contra-indications: Aminoplasmal Ped should not be administered in the following conditions: Disturbances of protein metabolism; renal insufficiency; advanced liver disease; manifest cardiac insufficiency.

Warnings: Possible hyperhydration, hypotonic dehydration, hyperkalaemia, hyponatraemia as well as acidosis have to be treated prior to commencing the infusion.

Amino acid mixtures may precipitate acute folate deficiency and folic acid should be given daily.

Precautions: In order to ensure optimum metabolic utilisation of the amino acids administered, therapy with Aminoplasmal Ped should be adequately supported by an energy supply of 35 kcal (145 kJ) per gram of amino acids.

Fluid balance, serum-electrolytes, blood glucose level and acid base state should be regularly checked.

Side-effects: Providing the contra-indications are observed, side-effects are not to be anticipated.

Overdosage: Overdosage or a too rapid infusion may manifest in the form of nausea, shivering, vomiting and increased renal amino acid losses. In such cases the infusion should be interrupted and eventually continued at a reduced infusion rate.

Pharmaceutical precautions Do not store above 25°C.

It is not recommended that any additives should be incorporated into Aminoplasmal Ped solution. They should, in preference, be given in the carbohydrate solution. However, if admixture with Aminoplasmal Ped is essential then the compatibility of the additive should be checked before administration.

Legal category POM.

Package quantities 100 ml and 250 ml glass bottles in packs of 10 bottles.

Further information Nil.

Product licence number 4296/0004.

LIPOFUNDIN* MCT/LCT 10% AND 20% ▼

Presentation A sterile, pyrogen-free, white oil-in-water emulsion containing:

	10%	*20%*
Soya Oil BP	50 g	100 g
Medium-chain Triglycerides DAB	50 g	100 g
Egg Lecithin	12 g	12 g
Glycerol PhEur	25 g	25 g
Water for Injections PhEur to	1000 ml	1000 ml
Megajoules/l (approx)	4.43 (1058 kcal)	8.00 (1908 kcal)
Milliosmols/l (approx)	345	380
pH 6.5–8.5		

Uses Lipofundin MCT/LCT is indicated as a source of calories and essential fatty acids for patients requiring parenteral nutrition.

Dosage and administration
Adults: Lipofundin MCT/LCT can provide up to 60% of the daily non-protein calories at an average dose of 1–2 g of fat per kg body weight per day.

Only 500 ml of Lipofundin MCT/LCT 10% or 250 ml of Lipofundin MCT/LCT 20% should be infused into adults on the first day of therapy. If the patient shows no untoward reactions, the dose can be increased on the following day.

Duration of treatment should be limited to up to 10 days.

Flow rate (for 70 kg patient): The infusion rate during the first 15 minutes should not exceed 0.5–1.0 ml per kg body weight per hour of Lipofundin MCT/LCT 10% or 0.25–0.5 ml per kg body weight per hour of Lipofundin MCT/LCT 20%. If no adverse effects are observed during this initial infusion, the rate can be increased to 2 ml per kg body weight per hour for Lipofundin MCT/LCT 10% or 1 ml per kg body weight per hour for Lipofundin MCT/LCT 20%.

Since the lipaemia must clear between daily infusions, the patient's capacity to eliminate the infused fat from the circulation must be monitored and the dosage/flow rate adjusted accordingly.

Children: No data are available on the use of Lipofundin MCT/LCT in children.

The elderly: Experience of the use of Lipofundin MCT/LCT in the elderly is limited, although there is no evidence to suggest that dosage should be different from that recommended for other adult patients. Nevertheless, metabolic rates and patterns can vary in the elderly, so careful monitoring of this particular group of patients is always prudent.

Route of administration: Lipofundin MCT/LCT should be administered by intravenous infusion as part of a total parenteral nutrition regimen via a peripheral vein or central venous catheter.

Lipofundin MCT/LCT can be infused into the same central or peripheral vein as the carbohydrate and amino acid solutions by means of a short y-connector near the infusion site. This allows for mixing of the solutions immediately before entering the vein. Flow rates for each solution should be controlled separately by infusion pumps, if these are used.

Use in pregnancy: The safety of Lipofundin MCT/LCT during pregnancy and lactation has not been assessed, but its use during these periods is not considered to constitute a hazard. Nevertheless, medicines should not be used in pregnancy, especially during the first trimester, unless the expected benefit is thought to outweigh any possible risk to the foetus.

Contra-indications, warnings, etc
Contra-indications: The administration of Lipofundin MCT/LCT is contra-indicated in patients demonstrating disturbances in normal fat metabolism such as pathologic hyperlipaemia, lipoid nephrosis, or acute pancreatitis if accompanied by hyperlipaemia. It is further contra-indicated in patients with ketoacidosis or hypoxia, in thromboembolism and in acute shock states.

Warnings: Caution should be exercised in administering intravenous fat emulsions in patients with metabolic acidosis, severe liver damage, pulmonary disease, sepsis, diseases of the reticuloendothelial system, anaemia or blood coagulation disorders or when there is danger of fat embolism.

The too rapid infusion of fat emulsions can cause fluid and/or fat overloading resulting in dilution of serum electrolyte concentrations, overhydration, congested states, pulmonary oedema, impaired pulmonary diffusion capacity.

A too rapid infusion of Lipofundin MCT/LCT can also cause hyperketonaemia and/or metabolic acidosis, especially when carbohydrates are not administered simultaneously.

Precautions: Administration of Lipofundin MCT/LCT should be accompanied by simultaneous carbohydrate infusions making up to 40% (at least) of the total calorie intake. When Lipofundin MCT/LCT is administered, the patient's capacity to eliminate the infused fat from the circulation must be monitored. The lipaemia must clear between daily infusions.

Especially where fat emulsions are administered for extended periods of time, the patient's haemogram, blood coagulation, liver function and platelet count should be closely monitored.

Overdosage: In the event of fat overload during therapy, stop the infusion of Lipofundin MCT/LCT, until visual inspection of the plasma, determination of triglyceride concentrations, or measurement of plasma light-scattering activity by nephelometry indicate the lipid has cleared. Re-evaluate the patient and institute appropriate corrective measures.

Adverse reactions: Adverse reactions directly related to fat emulsions in general are of two types:

Immediate (acute) reactions: dyspnea, cyanosis, allergic reactions, hyperlipaemia, hypercoagulability, nausea, vomiting, headache, flushing, hyperthermia, sweating, chills, sleepiness, chest and back pain.

Delayed reactions: hepatomegaly, jaundice due to central lobular cholestasis, splenomegaly, thrombocytopenia, leucopenia, transient increases in liver function tests, and overloading syndrome. The deposition of a brown pigmentation in the reticuloendothelial system, the so-called 'intravenous fat pigment', has also been reported. The cause and the significance of this phenomenon are unknown.

Pharmaceutical precautions Lipofundin MCT/LCT should be stored below 25°C and not be allowed to freeze.

As a general rule, fat emulsions should not be mixed with electrolytes, drugs or any other additives in the infusion bottle. Lipofundin MCT/LCT may be used with nutrient mixing bag systems only if such resultant mixtures are compatible and stable. Any nutrient mixture prepared using Lipofundin MCT/LCT should be examined for compatibility and stability prior to administration. Attention should be paid especially to emulsion stability (visual and/or microscopic examination) and absence of deposits.

Legal category POM.

Package quantities 100 ml, 250 ml and 500 ml glass bottles in packs of 10 bottles.

Further information Medium-chain triglycerides are a mixture of neutral triglycerides of mainly caprylic (about 60%) and capric acid (about 40%).

Medium-chain triglycerides are cleared from the blood-stream at a faster rate and are oxidised more completely for energy production than long chain triglycerides. Therefore, they serve as a preferential energy source for the body.

Product licence numbers
Lipofundin MCT/LCT 10% 4296/0016
Lipofundin MCT/LCT 20% 4296/0019

LIPOFUNDIN* S 10% AND 20%

Presentation A sterile, pyrogen-free, white oil-in-water emulsion containing:

	10%	*20%*
Soybean Oil USP	100 g	200 g
Soybean Lecithin	7.5 g	15 g
Glycerol PhEur	25 g	25 g
Water for Injections PhEur to	1000 ml	1000 ml
Megajoules/l (approx)	4.47 (1068 kcal)	8.52 (2035 kcal)
Milliosmols/l (approx)	340	380

pH 6.5–8.5

Uses Lipofundin S is indicated as a source of calories for patients requiring parenteral nutrition. Where such nutrition is required for extended periods of time (more than 5 days), it is also indicated as a source of essential fatty acids to prevent the clinical manifestations of essential fatty acid deficiency (EFAD).

Dosage and administration
Adults including the elderly: Lipofundin S can provide up to 50% of the daily non-protein calories at an average dose of 1–2 g of fat per kg body weight per day, corresponding to 10–20 ml of Lipofundin S 10% or 5–10 ml of Lipofundin S 20% per kg body weight per day. Not more than 500 ml of Lipofundin S 10% or 250 ml of Lipofundin S 20% should be infused into adults on the first day of therapy. The dosage on subsequent days may be gradually increased as appropriate.

Flow rate (for 70 kg patient): For the first 15 minutes the infusion rate should not exceed 10–20 drops per minute or 0.5–1.0 ml per kg body weight per hour of Lipofundin S 10%, or 5–10 drops per minute or 0.25–0.5 ml per kg body weight per hour of Lipofundin S 20%. If no adverse effects are observed during this initial infusion, the rate can gradually be increased to 2.0 ml per kg body weight per hour for Lipofundin S 10% or 1.0 ml per kg body weight per hour for Lipofundin S 20%.

In patients with lower body weight the flow rate should be reduced accordingly.

Children: The usual dose is 1–2 g of fat per kg body weight per day, corresponding to 10–20 ml of Lipofundin S 10% or 5–10 ml of Lipofundin S 20% per kg body weight per day. The initial dose should be 0.5 g of fat per kg body weight per day. The intake on subsequent days may be gradually increased to the required dosage in relation to the patient's ability to eliminate fat.

Route of administration: Lipofundin S should be administered by intravenous infusion as part of a total parenteral nutrition regimen via a peripheral vein or central venous catheter.

Lipofundin S can be infused into the same central or peripheral vein as the carbohydrate and amino acid solutions by means of a short y-connector near the infusion site. This allows for mixing of the solutions immediately before entering the vein. Flow rates for each solution should be controlled separately by infusion pumps, if these are used.

Use in pregnancy: Animal reproduction studies have not been conducted with Lipofundin S. It is also not known whether Lipofundin S can cause fetal harm when administered to a pregnant woman or can affect reproduction capacity.

Contra-indications, warnings, etc
Contra-indications: The administration of Lipofundin S is contra-indicated in patients demonstrating disturbances in normal fat metabolism such as pathologic hyperlipaemia, lipoid nephrosis or acute pancreatitis if accompanied by hyperlipaemia. It is further contra-indicated in patients with advanced liver disease, patients with ketoacidosis or hypoxia, in thrombo-embolism and in acute shock states.

Warnings: Caution should be exercised in administering intravenous fat emulsions to patients with metabolic acidosis, pulmonary disease, sepsis, diseases of the reticuloendothelial system, anaemia or blood coagulation disorders, or when there is danger of fat embolism.

The too rapid infusion of fat emulsions can cause fluid and/or fat overloading resulting in dilution of serum electrolyte concentrations, overhydration, congested states, pulmonary oedema, impaired pulmonary diffusion capacity.

Precautions: It is important to monitor the patient's ability to eliminate the infused fat from the circulation. Especially if infusion of Lipofundin S is considered in patients with renal insufficiency, uncompensated diabetes mellitus, certain forms of liver insufficiency, metabolic disorders and sepsis, fat elimination should be checked daily. The lipaemia must clear between daily infusions.

Especially where fat emulsions are administered for extended periods of time, the patient's haemogram, blood coagulation, liver function and platelet count should be closely monitored.

Where shock, metabolic acidosis or severe dehydration is present, the condition should be corrected before the commencement of intravenous feeding.

Infusion of amino acid/carbohydrate solutions should accompany that of Lipofundin S to avoid hyperketonaemia and/or metabolic acidosis.

Overdosage: In the event of fat overload during therapy, stop the infusion of Lipofundin S, until visual inspection of the plasma, determination of triglyceride concentration, or measurement of plasma light-scattering activity by nephelometry indicate the lipid has cleared. Re-evaluate the patient and institute appropriate corrective measures.

Adverse reactions: Adverse reactions directly related to fat emulsions may be immediate or delayed:

Immediate reactions include dyspnea, cyanosis, allergic reactions, hyperlipaemia, hypercoagulability, nausea, vomiting, headache, flushing, hyperthermia, sweating, chills, sleepiness, chest and back pain.

Delayed reactions include hepatomegaly, jaundice due to central lobular cholestasis, splenomegaly, thrombocytopenia, leucopenia, transient increases in liver function tests, and overloading syndrome. Deposition of a brown pigmentation in the reticuloendothelial system, the so-called 'intravenous fat pigment', has also been reported. The cause and the significance of this phenomenon are unknown.

Pharmaceutical precautions Lipofundin S should be stored below 25°C and not be allowed to freeze.

As a general rule, fat emulsions should not be mixed with electrolytes, drugs or any other additives in the infusion bottle.

Lipofundin S may be used with nutrient bag systems only if such resultant mixtures are compatible and stable.

Legal category POM.

Package quantities 100 ml, 250 ml and 500 ml glass bottles in packs of 10 bottles.

Further information Nil.

Product licence numbers
Lipofundin S 10% 4296/0017
Lipofundin S 20% 4296/0018

8.4% w/v and 4.2% w/v SODIUM BICARBONATE INTRAVENOUS INFUSION BP

Presentation Clear, colourless, sterile, non-pyrogenic 8.4% w/v or 4.2% w/v solutions of Sodium Bicarbonate PhEur for intravenous infusion. The pH range for the solution is 7.0–8.5. Each 1000 ml of solution contains:

	8.4% w/v	4.2% w/v
Sodium Bicarbonate PhEur	84.0 g	42.0 g
Disodium Edetate · 2 H_2O PhEur	0.1 g	0.1 g
Water for Injections PhEur	to 1000 ml	to 1000 ml
Electrolytes:	mmol/l	mmol/l
Sodium	1000	500
Bicarbonate	1000	500
Milliosmols/l:	2000	1000

Uses Severe metabolic acidosis; lactic acidosis; rapid urine alkalinisation (for example in 'sulphonamide nephrosis', salicylate and barbiturate intoxication); as temporary therapy in case of imminent hyperkalaemia.

Dosage and administration
Adults (including the elderly) and children: A blind buffer therapy is to be performed only in life-threatening situations. The quantity of Sodium Bicarbonate Intravenous Infusion BP to be infused is determined by the blood gas values and is calculated according to the following formula:

$$\text{ml } 8.4\% \text{ w/v} = \text{negative base excess} \times \text{kg body weight} \times 0.3$$

$$\text{ml } 4.2\% \text{ w/v} = \text{negative base excess} \times \text{kg body weight} \times 0.3 \times 2$$

(The factor 0.3 corresponds to the proportion of the extracellular fluid in relation to total body fluid).

Correction of metabolic acidosis should not be effected too rapidly. It is advisable to start administering only half of the calculated dose and make continuation of the therapy conditional on further blood gas analysis.

Drop rate:
8.4%: 20–40 drops per minute, corresponding to 60–120 ml per hour
4.2%: up to 40 drops per minute, corresponding to 120 ml per hour.

Route of administration: 8.4% w/v and 4.2% w/v Sodium Bicarbonate Intravenous Infusion BP have osmolarities of about 2000 and 1000 mOsm/l respectively and must be given strictly I.V. When infused undiluted it should be administered only via a central venous catheter, preferably inserted into the vena cava.

Use during pregnancy and lactation: No adverse effects are anticipated if sodium bicarbonate infusion is given during pregnancy or when lactating. However, administration should be avoided during eclampsia.

Contra-indications, warnings, etc
Contra-indications: Sodium bicarbonate intravenous infusion is contra-indicated in cases of respiratory and metabolic alkalosis, hypoventilation, hypernatraemia, and in situations where supply of sodium is contra-indicated such as cardiac insufficiency, oedema, hypertension, eclampsia, renal impairment.

Warnings: Sodium Bicarbonate Intravenous Infusion BP must be administered strictly intravenously since paravenous administration may lead to tissue necrosis.

Special attention is to be paid to possible hypokalaemia.

If supply of sodium is contra-indicated but renal

function unimpaired, alkalinisation should preferably be performed with THAM solution.

Overdosage: Overdosage results in metabolic alkalosis, possibly followed by hypokalaemia or hypocalcaemic tetany.

In the unlikely event of overdosage with sodium bicarbonate intravenous infusion the infusion should be discontinued. To control the symptoms of alkalosis the patient should rebreathe expired air or, if more severe, administration of 0.9% sodium chloride intravenous infusion may be useful. In case of hypokalaemia potassium chloride may be indicated. If the patient develops tetany which cannot be controlled by rebreathing, administration of calcium gluconate may be necessary.

Pharmaceutical precautions 8.4% w/v and 4.2% w/v Sodium Bicarbonate Intravenous Infusion BP should not be stored below room temperature. A shelf life of two years is predicted when stored at temperatures up to 25°C. The container should be examined visually before use; possible crystallisation can be reversed by gently warming up the solution. As an additional protective measure against crystals being inadvertently infused with the solution, it is recommended to use an administration set fitted with an integral fluid filter.

No other medication or substance should be added to this solution unless known to be compatible.

Sodium bicarbonate infusions must not be administered simultaneously with solutions containing calcium, magnesium or phosphate.

Legal category POM.

Package quantities *8.4%:* 100 ml and 250 ml Type 1 (PhEur) glass bottles with an air inlet set or Sterifix Mini-Spike (100 ml pack only), in packs of 10 bottles.
4.2%: 500 ml Type 1 (PhEur) glass bottles with air inlet set in packs of 10 bottles.

Further information Sodium bicarbonate exerts a major pharmacological effect in the buffer system of the extracellular compartment.

The alkalinising effect sets in rapidly and the administration of sodium bicarbonate infusions requires unimpaired pulmonary ventilation as the buffer action involves enhanced liberation of carbon dioxide.

Product licence numbers
8.4% 4296/0005
4.2% 4296/0023

0.9% w/v SODIUM CHLORIDE INTRAVENOUS INFUSION BP

Presentation Clear, colourless, sterile solution of Sodium Chloride PhEur 0.9% w/v in Water for Injections PhEur packaged in pure polyethylene ampoules (Mini-Plasco*).

Uses 0.9% w/v Sodium Chloride Intravenous Infusion BP is used as a dissolvent and carrier solution for injectable drugs.

Dosage and administration
Adults (including the elderly) and children: As required, by intravenous or subcutaneous injection.

Contra-indications, warnings, etc
Contra-indications: None known.

Warnings and precautions: If to be administered subcutaneously, be aware that any additions to the isotonic normal saline solution could render it hypertonic and thus cause pain to the injection site.

Pharmaceutical precautions Do not store above 25°C.

0.9% w/v Sodium Chloride Intravenous Infusion BP is compatible with a wide range of medicaments. In case of doubt the compatibility of medicaments to this solution should be checked before use. Do not use unless the solution is clear and the ampoule undamaged.

Legal category POM.

Package quantities 5 ml, 10 ml and 20 ml polyethylene ampoules (Mini-Plasco) in packs of 20 ampoules.

Further information Nil.

Product licence number 4296/0021.

STRONG POTASSIUM CHLORIDE SOLUTION BP 1973

Presentation Clear, colourless, sterile concentrated solution for injection of Potassium Chloride PhEur 15% w/v in Water for Injections PhEur packaged in pure polyethylene ampoules (Mini-Plasco*).

Uses Strong Potassium Chloride Solution BP 1973 is indicated in the treatment of hypokalaemia and potassium deficiency in alkalotic conditions.

Dosage and administration
Adults (including the elderly) and children: Strong Potassium Chloride Solution BP 1973 must be given only diluted as additive to large volume intravenous fluids. 10 ml are diluted with not less than 500 ml of 0.9% Sodium Chloride Intravenous Infusion BP or other suitable diluent, and mixed well before use. Unless otherwise directed the dosage depends on the values obtained from the serum ionogram and the acid-base state. A potassium deficiency is calculated according to the following formula:

$$\text{mmol potassium} = \text{kg bw} \times 0.2 \times 2 \times (4.5 - \text{actual serum potassium (mmol)}).$$

(The extracellular volume is calculated from the body weight in kg × 0.2.)

Normally the calculated amount of Strong Potassium Chloride Solution BP 1973 required as a supplement is administered via not less than 500 ml of a vehicle solution. In case of a fluid deficit higher volumes of a vehicle solution may be given.

The maximum dosage is 20 mmol potassium per hour. It is recommended not to exceed 2–3 mmol potassium per kg body weight in 24 hours.

Contra-indications, warnings, etc
Contra-indications: Strong Potassium Chloride Solution BP 1973 is contra-indicated in hyperkalaemia, hyperchloraemia or where there is impaired renal function.

Warnings and precautions: Strong Potassium Chloride Solution BP 1973 must not be injected undiluted.

Overdosage: Hyperkalaemia after excessive parenteral administration is considered minimal if the serum concentration does not exceed 6.5 mmol/l, moderate between 6.5 and 8 mmol/l and severe above 8 mmol/l.

Symptoms of hyperkalaemia include cardiac arrhythmias, heart block, and cardiac arrest. Cardiac arrhythmias or a serum concentration above 6.5 mmol/l require immediate attention and may be treated by intravenous injection over 1 to 5 minutes of 10 to 20 ml of 10% Calcium Gluconate Injection BP with ECG monitoring. Serum concentrations may be reduced by infusion of 300 to 500 ml per hour of 10% to 25% glucose solutions, containing up to 10 units of insulin for each 20 g of glucose, or by the infusion of sodium bicarbonate solution.

Pharmaceutical precautions Do not store above 25°C. The compatibility of the large volume IV fluid intended for dilution should be checked before use. Do not use unless the solution is clear and the ampoule undamaged.

Legal category POM.

Package quantities 10 ml polyethylene ampoules (Mini-Plasco) in packs of 20 ampoules.

Further information Potassium is retained by spironolactone as well as triamterene. If administered concurrently with either of these two substances, severe hyperkalaemia may develop. Hyperkalaemia induced by either spironolactone or triamterene in conjunction with potassium chloride becomes particularly manifest in patients with impaired renal function. Hence all patients who are administered potassium chloride concurrently with spironolactone and/or triamterene, require close monitoring in order to diagnose a potential hyperkalaemic condition as early as possible. In case of already existing renal insufficiency neither spironolactone nor triamterene should be administered in combination with potassium chloride. Digitalis toxicity is enhanced in hypokalaemia.

Product licence number 4296/0020.

WATER FOR INJECTIONS BP

Presentation Clear, colourless, sterile preparation of Water for Injections PhEur packaged in pure polyethylene ampoules (Mini-Plasco*).

Uses Water for Injections BP is used as a dissolvent and diluent for injectable medicines.

Dosage and administration
Adults (including the elderly) and children: As required, by intravenous injection.

Contra-indications, warnings, etc None known.

Pharmaceutical precautions Do not store above 25°C. Do not use unless the solution is clear and the ampoule undamaged.

Legal category POM.

Package quantities 5 ml, 10 ml and 20 ml polyethylene ampoules (Mini-Plasco) in packs of 20 ampoules.

Further information Nil.

Product licence number 4296/0022.

**Trade Mark*

Bridge Pharmaceuticals
Welwyn Garden City
Hertfordshire AL7 1EY

DYSPAMET* CHEWTAB* TABLETS DYSPAMET* SUSPENSION

Presentation White, square, chewable tablets with a surface design consisting of a raised portion towards one side of the tablet and a curved depression over the rest of the surface. Each tablet contains 200 mg cimetidine.

A white vanilla-flavoured suspension. Each 5 ml dose contains 200 mg cimetidine.

Uses Cimetidine is a histamine H_2-receptor antagonist which rapidly inhibits both basal and stimulated gastric secretion of acid and reduces pepsin output.

Dyspamet is indicated in the treatment of duodenal and benign gastric ulceration, recurrent and stomal ulceration, oesophageal reflux disease and other conditions where reduction of gastric acid by cimetidine has been shown to be beneficial: persistent dyspeptic symptoms with or without ulceration, particularly meal-related upper abdominal pain; the prophylaxis of gastrointestinal haemorrhage from stress ulceration in seriously ill patients; before general anaesthesia in patients thought to be at risk of acid aspiration (Mendelson's) syndrome, particularly obstetric patients during labour; to reduce malabsorption and fluid loss in the short bowel syndrome; and in pancreatic insufficiency to reduce degradation of enzyme supplements. Dyspamet is also recommended in the management of the Zollinger-Ellison syndrome.

Dosage and administration Dyspamet Tablets should be chewed thoroughly before swallowing.

The total daily dose should not normally exceed 2.4 g. Dosage should be reduced in patients with impaired renal function (see *Precautions*).

Adults: Oral: The usual dosage is 400 mg twice a day with breakfast and at bedtime. For patients with duodenal or benign gastric ulceration, a single daily dose of 800 mg at bedtime is recommended. Other effective regimens are 200 mg three times a day with meals and 400 mg at bedtime (1.0 g/day) and, if inadequate, 400 mg four times a day (1.6 g) also with meals and at bedtime.

Symptomatic relief is usually rapid. Treatment should be given initially for at least four weeks (six weeks in benign gastric ulcer). Most ulcers will have healed by that stage, but those which have not will usually do so after a further course of treatment.

Treatment may be continued for longer periods in those patients who may benefit from reduction of gastric secretion and the dosage may be reduced as appropriate to 400 mg at bedtime or 400 mg in the morning and at bedtime.

In patients with benign peptic ulcer disease, relapse may be prevented by continued treatment, usually with 400 mg at bedtime; 400 mg in the morning and at bedtime has also been used.

In oesophageal reflux disease, 400 mg four times a day, with meals and at bedtime, for four to eight weeks is recommended to heal oesophagitis and relieve associated symptoms.

In patients with very high gastric acid secretion (e.g. Zollinger–Ellison syndrome) it may be necessary to increase the dose to 400 mg four times a day, or in occasional cases further.

Antacids can be made available to all patients until symptoms disappear.

In the prophylaxis of haemorrhage from stress ulceration in seriously ill patients, doses of 200–400 mg can be given every four to six hours.

In patients thought to be at risk of acid aspiration syndrome a dose of 400 mg can be given 90–120 minutes before induction of general anaesthesia or, in obstetric practice, at the start of labour. While such a risk persists, a dose of up to 400 mg may be repeated at four-hourly intervals as required up to the usual daily maximum of 2.4 g. The usual precautions to avoid acid aspiration should be taken.

In the short bowel syndrome, e.g. following substantial resection for Crohn's disease, the usual dosage range (see above) can be used according to individual response.

To reduce degradation of pancreatic enzyme supplements, 800–1600 mg a day may be given according to response in four divided doses, one to one and a half hours before meals.

Elderly: The normal adult dosage may be used unless renal function is markedly impaired (see *Precautions* and *Adverse reactions*).

Children: Experience in children is less than that in adults. In children more than one year old, cimetidine 25–30 mg/kg body weight per day in divided doses may be administered.

The use of cimetidine in infants under one year old is not fully evaluated; 20 mg/kg body weight per day in divided doses has been used.

Contra-indications, warnings, etc

Contra-indication: Hypersensitivity to cimetidine.

Precautions: Dosage should be reduced in patients with impaired renal function according to creatinine clearance. The following dosages are suggested: creatinine clearance of 0–15 ml per minute, 200 mg twice a day; 15–30 ml per minute, 200 mg three times a day; 30–50 ml per minute, 200 mg four times a day; over 50 ml per minute, normal dosage. Cimetidine is removed by haemodialysis, but not to any significant extent by peritoneal dialysis.

Cimetidine can prolong the elimination of drugs metabolised by oxidation in the liver. Although pharmacological interactions with a number of drugs, e.g. diazepam, propranolol, have been demonstrated, only those with oral anticoagulants, phenytoin, theophylline and intravenous lignocaine appear, to date, to be of clinical significance. Close monitoring of patients on Dyspamet receiving oral anticoagulants or phenytoin is recommended and a reduction in the dosage of these drugs may be necessary.

Clinical trials with cimetidine of over six years' continuous treatment and more than thirteen years' widespread use have not revealed unexpected adverse reactions related to long-term therapy. The safety of prolonged use is not, however, fully established and care should be taken to observe periodically patients given prolonged treatment.

Cimetidine treatment can mask the symptoms and allow transient healing of gastric cancer. The potential delay in diagnosis should particularly be borne in mind in patients of middle age and over with new or recently changed dyspeptic symptoms.

In patients on drug treatment or with illnesses that could cause falls in blood cell count, the possibility that H_2-receptor antagonism could potentiate this effect should be borne in mind.

Use in pregnancy and lactation: Although tests in animals and clinical evidence have not revealed any hazards from the administration of cimetidine during pregnancy or lactation, both animal and human studies have shown that it does cross the placental barrier and is excreted in milk. As with most drugs, the use of Dyspamet should be avoided during pregnancy and lactation unless essential.

Adverse reactions: More than 35 million patients have been treated with cimetidine worldwide and adverse reactions have been infrequent. Diarrhoea, dizziness or rash, usually mild and transient, and tiredness have been reported. Gynaecomastia has been reported and is almost always reversible on discontinuing treatment. Biochemical or biopsy evidence of reversible liver damage has been reported occasionally. Reversible confusional states have occurred, usually in elderly or already very ill patients, e.g. those with renal failure. There have been very rare reports of interstitial nephritis, acute pancreatitis, thrombocytopenia, agranulocytosis (see *Precautions*), headache, myalgia, arthralgia, sinus bradycardia, tachycardia and heart block, all reversible on withdrawal of treatment, and aplastic anaemia. Alopecia has been reported but no causal relationship has been established. Reversible impotence has also been very rarely reported but no causal relationship has been established at usual therapeutic doses. Isolated increases of plasma creatinine have been of no clinical significance.

Overdosage: Acute overdosage of up to 20 grams cimetidine has been reported several times with no significant ill effects. Induction of vomiting and/or gastric lavage may be employed together with symptomatic and supportive therapy.

Pharmaceutical precautions Store tablets in a dry place. Store suspension at a temperature not exceeding 25°C. Dilution of the suspension is not recommended.

Legal category POM.

Package quantities Chewable tablets, 200 mg, in opaque blister packs (OP) of 120 (20 × 6). Suspension in white plastic bottles (OP) of 600 ml.

Further information Inactive ingredients in the tablets include aspartame together with 900 mg lactose and 790 mg sorbitol per tablet, and in the suspension butyl paraben and propyl paraben together with 2.79 g sorbitol per 5 ml.

Product licence numbers

Dyspamet Chewtab Tablets	0002/0148.
Dyspamet Suspension	0002/0161.

DYTAC* CAPSULES

Presentation Opaque, maroon-coloured capsules, double-marked SKF, each containing 50 mg triamterene as a yellow, granular powder.

Uses Triamterene is a potassium-conserving diuretic, thought to act by directly inhibiting the exchange of sodium for potassium and hydrogen in the distal renal tubule.

Dytac is recommended for the control of oedema in cardiac failure, cirrhosis of the liver or the nephrotic syndrome, and in that associated with corticosteroid treatment. When Dytac is used as an adjuvant to potassium-depleting diuretics, such loss may be inhibited and diuresis enhanced.

Dosage and administration *Adults only:* When given alone, the usual dosage range is from 3 to a maximum of 5 Dytac capsules a day. The optimal daily dosage is 4 capsules, given in divided doses after breakfast and lunch. After the first week, treatment should preferably be given on alternate days to ensure satisfactory maintenance diuresis without an increase in blood urea levels. When given with another diuretic, lower dosages of both should be used initially.

Elderly: A lower dosage may be sufficient. The normally occurring reduction in glomerular filtration with age should be borne in mind.

Contra-indications, warnings, etc

Contra-indications: Do not give Dytac to patients with hyperkalaemia, progressive renal failure increasing hepatic dysfunction, Addison's disease, or known hypersensitivity to the drug. Potassium supplements, or other potassium-conserving drugs, including ACE inhibitors, should not be given routinely with Dytac.

Precautions: Use Dytac with caution in patients with hepatic or renal insufficiency; in those predisposed to gout since Dytac has been shown in rare instances to elevate uric acid levels; with hypotensive agents since an additive effect may result; and in diabetic nephropathy, due to increased risk of hyperkalaemia.

Folate antagonists combined with triamterene are inadvisable in patients with hepatic cirrhosis because of the increased theoretical risk of folate deficiency.

It is advisable to monitor blood urea, serum potassium levels and electrolytes periodically. This is important in the elderly, those with renal impairment and those receiving concomitant treatment with NSAIDs (see *Adverse reactions*).

Triamterene reduces the excretion of lithium and may thus precipitate intoxication.

Caution should be exercised if Dytac is used in conjunction with hypotensive agents. When Dytac is given with another diuretic, a lower dosage of both agents should be given initially.

Use in pregnancy and lactation: There is no clinical evidence to suggest any associated hazard to the foetus; however triamterene has been found to cross the placenta in humans. Nevertheless, drugs should be avoided in pregnancy unless essential, especially during the first trimester. Triamterene may appear in the breast milk and, if the drug is essential, the patient should stop breastfeeding. Folate antagonists combined with triamterene are inadvisable during pregnancy because of the increased theoretical risk of folate deficiency.

Adverse reactions: Nausea, vomiting, diarrhoea, weakness, headache, dry mouth, minor decreases in blood pressure, and rash have been reported. Photosensitivity is very rare. Anaphylaxis is a remote possibility.

Hyperkalaemia and/or hyponatraemia have been observed in some patients, and hypokalaemia has been described rarely in cirrhotic patients. Metabolic acidosis occasionally occurs. Electrolyte imbalance may also indicate excessive dosage or be secondary to the condition under treatment.

In common with most diuretics, Dytac may reduce glomerular filtration rate and cause a temporary increase in blood urea and creatinine levels; again this may also indicate excessive dosage or be secondary to the condition under treatment.

Renal failure, reversible on stopping treatment, has been reported very rarely and has been due to acute interstitial nephritis or an interaction between triamterene and some NSAIDs.

Triamterene has been found in renal stones both alone and in association with other usual calculus components. There is no evidence that stone formation is increased in patients taking triamterene-containing drugs.

Rare cases of thrombocytopenic purpura and megaloblastic anaemia have been reported.

Jaundice and abnormalities of serum levels of liver enzymes have also been reported.

Overdosage: Symptoms of electrolyte imbalance, especially hyperkalaemia, are likely. Symptoms include nausea, vomiting, weakness, lassitude, muscular weakness, hypotension and cardiac arrhythmias. Treatment consists of gastric lavage with careful monitoring of electrolytes and fluid balance. Cardiac rhythm should be monitored and appropriate measures taken to correct hyperkalaemia as necessary. There is no specific antidote. Renal dialysis may be of some benefit in cases of severe overdosage.

Pharmaceutical precautions Store in a dry place.

Legal category POM.

Package quantities Opaque blister packs (OP) of 30 (2 × 15) capsules.

Further information Triamterene may cause a blue fluorescence of the urine under certain light conditions.

Triamterene interferes with bioassay of folic acid.

Inactive ingredients include lactose.

Product licence number 0002/5014R.

DYTIDE* CAPSULES

Presentation Clear, colourless capsules with opaque, maroon caps, double-marked SKF, each containing 50 mg triamterene and 25 mg benzthiazide as a yellow, granular powder.

Uses Dytide is a potassium-conserving diuretic preparation for the control of oedema in cardiac failure, cirrhosis of the liver or the nephrotic syndrome, and in that associated with corticosteroid treatment.

Dosage and administration *Adults only:* The optimal dosage is 3 Dytide capsules a day, 2 being taken after breakfast and 1 after lunch. After the first week, treatment should preferably be given on alternate days, to ensure satisfactory maintenance diuresis without an increase in blood urea levels. Maintenance dosage may be reduced to 1 or 2 capsules every other day, taken after breakfast or after breakfast and lunch.

Elderly: A lower dosage may be sufficient. The normally occurring reduction in glomerular filtration with age should be borne in mind.

Contra-indications, warnings, etc

Contra-indications: Do not give Dytide to patients with hyperkalaemia, progressive renal failure, increasing hepatic dysfunction, hypercalcaemia, diabetic ketoacidosis, Addison's disease or known hypersensitivity to either constituent of the product. Potassium supplements, or other potassium-conserving drugs, including ACE inhibitors, should not be given routinely with Dytide.

Precautions: Use Dytide with caution in patients with hepatic or renal insufficiency; in those predisposed to gout since both components can elevate uric acid levels; with hypotensive agents, since an additive effect may result. Folate antagonists combined with triamterene are inadvisable in patients with hepatic crirrhosis because of the increased theoretical risk of folate deficiency. Since thiazide diuretics can provoke hyperglycaemia and glycosuria, diabetic patients should be treated with care, as should patients with diabetic nephropathy due to an increased risk of hyperkalaemia; the dosage of any concomitant sulphonylurea may need increasing. Pancreatitis may be aggravated.

It is advisable to monitor blood urea, serum potassium levels and electrolytes periodically. This is important in the elderly, those with renal impairment and those receiving concomitant treatment with NSAIDs (see *Adverse reactions*).

Triamterene and thiazides reduce excretion of lithium and may thus precipitate intoxication. There may be increased responsiveness to tubocurarine. Cholestyramine may delay or reduce the absorption of many drugs including diuretics.

Caution should be exercised if Dytide is used in conjunction with hypotensive agents. Also use with caution in conjunction with corticosteroids since an additive effect may result in excess potassium loss; with cardiac glycosides and antiarrhythmic drugs whose toxic potential is enhanced by hypokalaemia which may result from diuretic treatment; and with carbenoxolone which may antagonise the diuretic action of Dytide.

Use in pregnancy and lactation: Animal studies have not suggested foetal abnormalities. Nevertheless, both triamterene and thiazides have been shown to pass through the placenta in humans and also to pass into breast milk. In rare instances, thrombocytopenia, pancreatitis or hypoglycaemia have been reported in newborn infants of mothers treated with thiazides. Dytide is best avoided in pregnancy unless used for a pre-existing illness and then only after assessing risk versus benefit. It should also not be used in breastfeeding mothers. Folate antagonists combined with triamterene are inadvisable during pregnancy because of the increased theoretical risk of folate deficiency.

Adverse reactions: Nausea, vomiting, diarrhoea, muscle cramps, weakness, dizziness, headache, dry mouth, thirst, decreases in blood pressure, and rash have been reported. Photosensitivity is very rare. Anaphylaxis is a remote possibility.

Minor serum electrolyte changes have been observed infrequently, and marked fluctuations in serum potassium levels are uncommon. Metabolic acidosis occasionally occurs. Hyperglycaemia, increased uric acid levels which sometimes lead to gout, and hypercalcaemia that does not lead to tertiary hyperparathyroidism may also occur. Electrolyte imbalance may also indicate excessive dosage or be secondary to the condition under treatment.

In common with most diuretics, Dytide may reduce glomerular filtration rate and cause a temporary increase in blood urea and creatinine levels; again this may also indicate excessive dosage or be secondary to the condition under treatment. It can also cause increases in plasma lipid levels.

Renal failure, reversible on stopping treatment, has been reported very rarely and has been due to acute interstitial nephritis or an interaction between triamterene and some NSAIDs.

Triamterene has been found in renal stones both alone and in association with other usual calculus components. There is no evidence that stone formation is increased in patients taking triamterene-containing drugs.

Rare cases of thrombocytopenic purpura and megaloblastic anaemia have been reported with triamterene; thiazides alone have caused jaundice, acute pancreatitis and, rarely, blood dyscrasias including agranulocytosis, thrombocytopenia and leucopenia. Very rare cases of SLE have been reported associated with combined triamterene and hydrochlorothiazide.

Overdosage: Symptoms of electrolyte imbalance, especially hyperkalaemia, are likely. Symptoms include nausea, vomiting, weakness, lassitude, muscular weakness, hypotension and cardiac arrhythmias. Treatment consists of gastric lavage with careful monitoring of electrolytes and fluid balance. Cardiac rhythm should be monitored and appropriate measures taken to correct hyperkalaemia as necessary. There is no specific antidote. Renal dialysis may be of some benefit in cases of severe overdosage.

Pharmaceutical precautions Store in a dry place.

Legal category POM.

Package quantities Opaque blister packs (OP) of 30 (2 × 15) capsules.

Further information Triamterene may cause a blue fluorescence of the urine under certain light conditions.

Dytide interferes with some laboratory tests of thyroid and parathyroid functions, and bioassay of folic acid.

Inactive ingredients include lactose.

Product licence number 0002/5015R.

**Trade Mark*

Bristol-Myers Pharmaceuticals
Bristol-Myers Squibb House
Staines Road
Hounslow TW3 3JA

ALPHA KERI* BATH OIL

Presentation Alpha Keri Bath Oil is a clear colourless water dispersible anti-pruritic bath additive.

The product contains the following active ingredients: mineral oil (91.7%) and lanolin oil (3.0%).

Other ingredients: Oxybenzone, perfume, polyethylene dilaurate.

Uses Alpha Keri effectively deposits a thin uniform emulsified film of oil over the skin, and thus retards evaporation of moisture, helps to relieve itching, lubricates and softens the skin.

Alpha Keri is valuable as an aid in the management of dry pruritic skin, especially in senile pruritus, ichthyosis and other dermatoses where dermal hydration is an important part of the therapy (as in the prevention of decubitus ulcer).

Alpha Keri Bath Oil is particularly suitable for infant bathing. The preparation also overcomes the problem of cleansing the skin in conditions where the use of soaps, soap substitutes and colloid or oat-meal baths prove irritating.

Dosage and administration Alpha Keri should always be either added to water or rubbed onto wet skin.

Because of its inherent cleansing properties soap should not be used with Alpha Keri.

Bath: Add 10–20 ml to the bath water. Soak for 10–20 minutes.

Sponge bath: Add 10–20 ml to a basin of warm water. Apply over entire body with a sponge or flannel.

Infant bath: Add 5 ml to bath water.

Skin cleansing: Rub a small amount onto wet skin, rinse and pat dry.

Shower: Pour a small amount onto a wet sponge or flannel and rub onto wet skin, rinse and pat dry.

Contra-indications, warnings, etc As Alpha Keri deposits a film of oil over the skin, special care should be taken to guard against slipping, especially in the bath or shower.

Alpha Keri contains lanolin oil and is therefore contra-indicated in those patients allergic to this ingredient.

Pharmaceutical precautions Store at room temperature.

Legal category P.

Package quantities Alpha Keri Bath Oil is available in bottles containing 240 ml and 480 ml (original packs).

Further information Nil.

Product licence number 0125/0141.

AMIKIN*

Presentation *Amikin Injection:* Each vial contains in 2 ml, amikacin sulphate equivalent to amikacin activity 500 mg (500,000 international units).

Amikin Paediatric Injection: Each vial contains in 2 ml, amikacin sulphate equivalent to amikacin activity 100 mg (100,000 international units).

The product contains no preservatives.

Other ingredients: Sodium bisulphite, sodium citrate, sulphuric acid, water.

Uses AMIKIN is a semi-synthetic, aminoglycoside antibiotic which is active against a broad spectrum of Gram-negative organisms, including pseudomonas and some Gram-positive organisms.

Sensitive Gram-negative organisms include; Pseudomonas spp., *Escherichia coli,* indole-positive and indole-negative Proteus spp., Klebsiella-Enterobacter-Serratia spp., *Citrobacter freundii,* Salmonella, Shigella, Acinetobacter and Providencia spp.

Many strains of these Gram-negative organisms resistant to gentamicin and tobramycin show sensitivity to Amikin *in vitro.*

The principal Gram-positive organism sensitive to Amikin is *Staphylococcus aureus,* including methicillin-resistant strains. Amikin has some activity against other Gram-positive organisms including *Streptococcus pyogenes, Diplococcus pneumoniae,* and certain strains of enterococci.

Amikin is indicated in the short-term treatment of serious infections due to susceptible strains of Gram-negative bacteria, including Pseudomonas species. Although Amikin is not the drug of choice for infections due to staphylococci, at times it may be indicated for the treatment of known or suspected staphylococcal disease. These situations include: the initiation of therapy for severe infections when the organisms suspected are either Gram-negative or staphylococci, patients allergic to other antibiotics, and mixed staphylococcal/Gram-negative infections.

Therapy with Amikin may be instituted prior to obtaining the results of sensitivity testing.

Surgical procedures should be performed where indicated.

Dosage and administration At the recommended dosage level, uncomplicated infections due to sensitive organisms should respond to therapy within 24 to 48 hours.

If clinical response does not occur within three to five days, consideration should be given to alternative therapy.

Intramuscular or intravenous administration: For most infections the intramuscular route is preferred, but in life-threatening infections, or in patients in whom intramuscular injection is not feasible, the intravenous route, either slow bolus (two to three minutes) or infusion (0.25% over 30 minutes) may be used.

If required, suitable diluents for intravenous use are: normal saline, 5% glucose in water, lactated Ringer's injection and lactated Ringer's injection with 5% glucose. Once the product has been diluted the solution must be used as soon as possible and NOT STORED.

Adults and Children: 15 mg/kg/day in two equally divided doses (equivalent to 500 mg b.i.d. in adults):

Use of the 100 mg/2 ml strength is recommended for children for the accurate measurement of the appropriate dose.

Neonates and Premature Infants: An initial loading dose of 10 mg/kg followed by 15 mg/kg/day in two equally divided doses.

Sufficient extensive clinical use has not been achieved to enable firm dosage guidelines to be given in premature infants.

Elderly: Amikacin is excreted by the renal route, renal function should be assessed whenever possible and dosage adjusted as described under impaired renal function.

Life-threatening infections and/or those caused by pseudomonas: The adult dose may be increased to 500 mg every eight hours but should neither exceed 1.5 g/day nor be administered for a period longer than 10 days. A maximum total adult dose of 15 g should not be exceeded.

Urinary tract infections: (other than pseudomonal infections): 7.5 mg/kg/day in two equally divided doses (equivalent to 250 mg b.i.d. in adults). As the activity of amikacin is enhanced by increasing the pH, a urinary alkalinising agent may be administered concurrently.

Impaired renal function: In patients with impaired renal function, the daily dose should be reduced and/or the intervals between doses increased to avoid accumulation of the drug. A suggested method for estimating dosage in patients with known or suspected diminished renal function is to multiply the serum creatinine concentration (in mg/100 ml) by 9 and to use the resulting figure as the interval in hours between doses.

Serum Creatinine Concentration (mg/100 ml)		*Interval between Amikin doses of 7.5 mg/kg/IM (hours)*
1.5	X9=	13.5
2.0		18
2.5		22.5
3.0		27
3.5		31.5
4.0		36
4.5		40.5
5.0		45
5.5		49.5
6.0		54

As renal function may alter appreciably during therapy, the serum creatinine should be checked frequently and the dosage regimen modified as necessary.

Intraperitoneal use: Following exploration for established peritonitis, or after peritoneal contamination due to faecal spill during surgery, Amikin may be used as an irrigant after recovery from anaesthesia in concentrations of 0.25% (2.5 mg/ml). It may also be instilled into the wound at closure. If instillation is desired in adults, a single dose of 500 mg is diluted in 20 ml of sterile distilled water and may be instilled through a polyethylene catheter sutured into the wound at closure. If possible, instillation should be postponed until the patient has fully recovered from the effects of anaesthesia and muscle-relaxing drugs.

Other routes of administration: Amikin in concentrations of 0.25% (2.5 mg/ml) may be used satisfactorily as an irrigating solution in abscess cavities, the pleural space, the peritoneum and the cerebral ventricles.

Contra-indications, warnings, etc Patients should be well hydrated during Amikin therapy.

In patients with impaired renal function or diminished glomerular filtration, Amikin should be used cautiously. In such patients, renal function should be assessed by the usual methods prior to therapy and periodically during therapy. Daily doses should be reduced and/or the interval between doses lengthened in accordance with serum creatinine concentrations to avoid accumulation of abnormally high blood levels and to minimise the risk of ototoxicity.

If therapy is expected to last seven days or more in patients with renal impairment, or 10 days in other patients, a pre-treatment audiogram should be obtained and repeated during therapy. Amikin therapy should be stopped if tinnitus or subjective hearing loss develops, or if follow-up audiograms show significant loss of high-frequency response.

As with other aminoglycosides, ototoxicity and/or nephrotoxicity can result from the use of Amikin; precautions on dosage and adequate hydration should be observed.

If signs of renal irritation appear (such as albumin, casts, red or white blood cells), hydration should be increased and a reduction in dosage may be desirable. These findings usually disappear when treatment is completed. However, if azotaemia or a progressive decrease in urine output occurs, treatment should be stopped.

The use of Amikin in patients with a history of allergy to aminoglycosides or in patients who may have subclinical renal or eighth nerve damage induced by prior administration of nephrotoxic and/or ototoxic agents such as streptomycin, dihydrostreptomycin, gentamicin, tobramycin, kanamycin, bekanamycin, neomycin, polymyxin B, colistin, cephaloridine, or viomycin should be considered with caution, as toxicity may be additive. In these patients Amikin should be used only if, in the opinion of the physician, therapeutic advantages outweigh the potential risks.

The risk of ototoxicity is increased when Amikin is used in conjunction with rapidly acting diuretic drugs, particularly when the diuretic is administered intravenously. Such agents include frusemide and ethacrynic acid. Irreversible deafness may result.

The intraperitoneal use of Amikin is not recommended in young children or in patients under the influence of anaesthetics or muscle-relaxing drugs (including ether, halothane, d-tubocurarine, succinylcholine and decamethonium) as neuromuscular blockade and consequent respiratory depression may occur.

Pregnancy: The safety of Amikin in pregnancy has not yet been established.

Side-effects: When the recommended precautions and dosages are followed the incidence of toxic reactions, such as tinnitus, vertigo, and partial reversible or irreversible deafness, skin rash, drug fever, headache, paraesthesia, nausea and vomiting is low. Urinary signs of renal irritation (albumin, casts, and red or white cells), azotaemia and oliguria have been reported.

Overdosage: In the event of overdosage or toxic reaction, peritoneal dialysis or haemodialysis will aid in the removal of amikacin from the blood.

Pharmaceutical precautions At times, Amikin may be indicated as concurrent therapy with other antibacterial agents in mixed or superinfections. In such instances, Amikin should not be physically mixed with other antibacterial agents in syringes, infusion bottles or any other equipment. Each agent should be administered separately.

Amikin, as supplied, is stable at 25°C. The solution may darken from colourless to a pale yellow but this does not indicate a loss in potency.

Legal category POM.

Package quantities *Amikin Injection:* 2 ml vials packed in cartons of 5.

Amikin Paediatric Injection: 2 ml vials packed in cartons of 5.

Further information Amikin is rapidly absorbed after intramuscular injection. Peak serum levels of approximately 11 mg/l and 23 mg/l are reached one hour after i.m. doses of 250 mg and 500 mg respectively. Levels 10 hours after injection are of the order of 0.3 mg/l and 2.1 mg/l respectively.

Twenty per cent or less is bound to serum protein and serum concentrations remain in the bactericidal range for sensitive organisms for 10 to 12 hours.

Amikin diffuses readily through extracellular fluids and is excreted in the urine unchanged, primarily by glomerular filtration. Half-life in individuals with normal renal functions is two to three hours.

Following intramuscular administration of a 250 mg dose, about 65% is excreted in six hours and 91% within 24 hours. The urinary concentrations average 563 mg/l in the first six hours and 163 mg/l over 6 to 12 hours. Mean urine concentrations after a 500 mg i.m. dose average 832 mg/l in the first six hours.

Single doses of 500 mg administered to normal adults as an intravenous infusion over a period of 30 minutes produce a mean peak serum concentration of 38 mg/l at the end of the infusion. Repeated infusions do not produce drug accumulation.

Amikin has been found in cerebrospinal fluid, pleural fluid, amniotic fluid and in the peritoneal cavity following parenteral administration.

Product licence numbers

Paediatric Injection 100 mg/2 ml	0125/0090
Injection 500 mg/2 ml	0125/0092

ANGETTES 75*

Presentation White circular orange-flavoured tablets, each tablet containing Aspirin BP 75 mg.

Other ingredients: Flavours, lactose, maize starch, sodium saccharin.

Uses As a platelet antiaggregatory agent for the prevention of secondary myocardial infarction and in patients suffering from unstable angina.

Dosage and administration
Adults: Following myocardial infarction; two tablets to be taken once daily. Treatment should commence as soon as possible. Patients suffering from unstable angina; four tablets once daily.

Elderly patients: The risk/benefit ratios in the elderly have not been fully established.

Children: WARNING: Not recommended for children under 12 years old.

Contra-indications, warnings, etc
Contra-indications: Active peptic ulceration, haemophilia and other bleeding disorders, hypersensitivity to aspirin.

Use in pregnancy: There is clinical and epidemiological evidence of safety in human pregnancy.

Aspirin may prolong labour and contribute to maternal and neonatal bleeding, and should be avoided at term.

Precautions: Aspirin may enhance the effects of anticoagulants and may inhibit the action of uricosurics. Aspirins may precipitate bronchospasm and may induce attacks of asthma in susceptible subjects.

Warnings and adverse effects: Aspirin may induce gastro-intestinal haemorrhage, occasionally major. Patients with hypertension should be carefully monitored.

Overdose: Overdosage is unlikely due to the low level of aspirin in Angettes. If necessary gastric lavage, forced alkaline diuresis and supportive therapy may be employed. Restoration of acid/base balance may be required.

Pharmaceutical precautions Store at room temperature.

Legal category P.

Package quantities Original packs of 56 tablets.

Further information Nil.

Product licence number 0125/5020R.

BAXAN*

Presentation *Baxan Capsules:* white capsules containing cefadroxil monohydrate equivalent to 500 mg cefadroxil activity.

Other ingredients: Colloidal silicon dioxide, lactose, magnesium stearate; gelatin capsules contain titanium dioxide.

Baxan Suspension: supplied as a bottle containing powder for reconstitution to provide 125 mg, 250 mg or 500 mg per 5 ml.

Other ingredients: Flavours, polysorbate 40, sodium benzoate, sucrose, titanium dioxide, xanthan gum.

Uses Baxan is bactericidal in vitro against a wide range of Gram-positive and Gram-negative micro-organisms. Sensitive Gram-positive organisms include: penicillinase and non-penicillinase-producing staphylococci, β-haemolytic streptococci, *Streptococcus pneumoniae* and *Streptococcus pyogenes*. Sensitive Gram-negative organisms include *Escherichia coli, Klebsiella pneumoniae*, and some strains of *Proteus mirabilis, Haemophilus influenzae*, Salmonella spp. and Shigella spp.

Baxan is indicated in the treatment of the following infections when due to susceptible micro-organisms.

Respiratory tract infections: Tonsillitis, pharyngitis, lobar and bronchopneumonia, acute and chronic bronchitis, pulmonary abscess, empyema, pleurisy, sinusitis, laryngitis, otitis media.

Skin and soft-tissue infections: Lymphadenitis, abscesses, cellulitis, decubitus ulcers, mastitis, furunculosis, erysipelas.

Genitourinary tract infections: Pyelonephritis, cystitis, urethritis, gynaecological infections, including puerperal sepsis.

Other infections: Osteomyelitis, septic arthritis, septicaemia, peritonitis, typhoid.

Dosage and administration
Adults and children weighing more than 40 kg (88 lbs): 500 mg to 1 g twice a day, depending upon the severity of infection.

Alternatively, in skin and soft tissue and uncomplicated urinary tract infections, 1 g once a day.

Children weighing less than 40 kg (88 lbs):
Under 1 year: 25 mg/kg daily in divided doses, e.g. 2.5 ml of the 125 mg per 5 ml suspension twice a day for a 6 month old infant weighing 5 kg, or 5 ml of the 125 mg per 5 ml suspension twice a day for a 1 year old infant weighing 10 kg.
1–6 years: 250 mg twice a day
Over 6 years: 500 mg twice a day.

Elderly: Cefadroxil is excreted by the renal route, renal function should be assessed whenever possible and dosage adjusted as described under impaired renal function.

The bioavailability and consequent chemotherapeutic effects of cefadroxil are unaffected by food. It may, therefore, be taken with meals or on an empty stomach.

Note: In patients with renal impairment, the dosage should be adjusted according to creatinine clearance rates to prevent drug accumulation and serum levels should be monitored. A modified dosage schedule is unnecessary in patients with creatinine rates of greater than 50 ml/min. In those patients with creatinine clearance rates of 50 ml/min or less, the following reduced dosage schedule is recommended as a guideline, based upon the creatinine clearance rate (ml/min/1.73m^2).

Patients with renal insufficiency may be treated with an initial dose of 1000 mg of Baxan. Subsequent doses may be administered according to the following table:

Creatinine clearance	*Dose*	*Dose Interval*
0–10 ml/min/1.73m^2	1000 mg	36 hrs
11–25 ml/min/1.73m^2	1000 mg	24 hrs
26–50 ml/min/1.73m^2	1000 mg	12 hrs

Contra-indications, warnings, etc Baxan is contra-indicated in patients with a history of hypersensitivity to cephalosporins.

In patients with a history of penicillin allergy, Baxan should be used with caution. There is evidence of partial cross-allergenicity between the penicillins and the cephalosporins. Should an allergic reaction to Baxan occur, the drug should be discontinued and the patient treated with the usual agents (pressor amines, corticosteroids and/or antihistamines), depending on the severity of the reaction.

Use in pregnancy and lactation: Although animal studies and clinical experience have not shown any evidence of teratogenicity the safe use of Baxan during pregnancy has not been established. Baxan should be used with caution in lactating mothers.

Precautions: As experience in premature infants and neonates is limited, the use of Baxan in these patients should only be undertaken with caution.

There are not sufficient data available to indicate whether the concurrent use of Baxan and potential nephrotoxic agents such as aminoglycosides causes any alteration in their nephrotoxic effects.

A false-positive Coombs' reaction may occur in some patients receiving Baxan.

Urine from patients treated with Baxan may give a false-positive glycosuria reaction when tested with Benedict's or Fehling's solutions. This does not occur with enzyme based tests.

Adverse reactions: Rash, pruritus, urticaria and angioneurotic oedema may be observed infrequently. Side effects, including nausea, vomiting, diarrhoea, dyspepsia, abdominal discomfort, dizziness, headache, and monilial vaginitis may also occur. Reversible neutropenia may occur rarely, as may leucopenia, and minor elevations in serum transaminase.

Colitis, including rare instances of pseudo-membraneous colitis, has been reported.

Pharmaceutical precautions Store in a cool dry place.

Legal category POM.

Package quantities Capsules – Containers of 100. Suspension – Bottles containing 60 ml

Further information Nil.

Product licence numbers

Baxan 500 mg capsules	0125/0107
Baxan 125 mg/5 ml suspension	0125/0110
Baxan 250 mg/5 ml suspension	0125/0111
Baxan 500 mg/5 ml suspension	0125/0112

BiCNU*

Presentation *BiCNU Injection:* each package contains a 30 ml vial containing 100 mg carmustine and a 5 ml vial containing 3 ml sterile ethanol diluent.

Uses BiCNU is indicated as palliative therapy as a single agent or in established combination therapy with other approved chemotherapeutic agents in the following:

1. Brain tumours – Glioblastoma, brainstem glioma, medulloblastoma, astrocytoma, ependymoma, and metastatic brain tumours.
2. Multiple myeloma – In combination with prednisone.
3. Hodgkin's Disease – As secondary therapy in combination with other approved drugs in patients who relapse while being treated with primary therapy, or who fail to respond to primary therapy.
4. Non-Hodgkin's lymphomas – As secondary therapy in combination with other approved drugs in patients who relapse while being treated with primary therapy, or who fail to respond to primary therapy.

Dosage and administration

Intravenous administration: The recommended dose of BiCNU as single agent in previously untreated patients is 200 mg/m^2 intravenously every six weeks. This may be given as a single dose or divided into daily injections such as 100 mg/m^2 on two successive days.

When BiCNU is used in combination with other myelosuppressive drugs or in patients in whom bone marrow reserve is depleted the doses should be adjusted accordingly.

A repeat course of BiCNU should not be given until circulating blood elements have returned to acceptable levels (platelets above 100,000/mm^3; leucocytes above 4,000/mm^3) and this is usually in six weeks. Blood counts should be monitored frequently and repeat courses should not be given before six weeks because of delayed toxicity.

Doses subsequent to the initial dose should be adjusted according to the haematological response of the patient to the preceding dose. The following schedule is suggested as a guide to dosage adjustment.

Nadir after Prior Dose		*Percentage of prior dose to be given*
Leucocytes (/mm^3)	*Platelets (/mm^3)*	
>4000	>100,000	100
3000–3999	75,000–99,999	100
2000–2999	25,000–74,999	70
<2000	<25,000	50

Elderly: No dosage adjustment is required on the grounds of age.

Contra-indications, warnings, etc BiCNU should not be given to individuals who have demonstrated a previous hypersensitivity to it.

BiCNU should not be given to individuals with decreased circulating platelets, leucocytes, or erythrocytes either from previous chemotherapy or other causes.

Pregnancy and lactation: BiCNU should not normally be administered to patients who are pregnant or mothers who are breast-feeding. Male patients should be advised to use adequate contraceptive measures.

Safe use in pregnancy has not been established and therefore the benefit to risk of toxicity must be carefully weighed. BiCNU is embryotoxic and teratogenic in rats and embryotoxic in rabbits at dose levels equivalent to the human dose. BiCNU also affects fertility in male rats at doses somewhat higher than the human dose.

BiCNU is carcinogenic in rats and mice, producing a marked increase in tumour incidence in doses approximating those employed clinically.

BiCNU should be administered by individuals experienced in antineoplastic therapy. Since delayed bone marrow toxicity is the major toxicity, complete blood counts should be monitored frequently for at least six weeks after a dose. Repeat doses of BiCNU should not be given more frequently than every six weeks. The bone marrow toxicity of BiCNU is cumulative and therefore dosage adjustment must be considered on the basis of nadir blood counts from prior dose (see Dosage Adjustment Table under Dosage).

It is recommended that liver function tests also be monitored.

Adverse reactions: Haematological: The most frequent and most serious toxicity of BiCNU is delayed myelosuppression. It usually occurs four to six weeks after drug administration and is dose-related. Platelet nadirs occur at four to five weeks; leucocyte nadirs occur at five to six weeks post therapy. Thrombocytopenia is generally more severe than leucopenia. However both may be dose limiting toxicities. Anaemia also occurs, but is generally less severe. The occurrence of acute leukemia and bone marrow dysplasias have been reported in patients following long term nitrosourea therapy.

Gastro-intestinal: Nausea and vomiting after i.v. administration of BiCNU are noted frequently. This reaction appears within two hours of dosing, usually lasting four to six hours and is dose-related. Prior administration of anti-emetics is effective in diminishing and sometimes preventing this side-effect.

Hepatic: When high doses of BiCNU have been employed, a reversible type of hepatic toxicity, manifested by increased transaminase, alkaline phosphatase and bilirubin levels, has been reported in a small percentage of patients.

Pulmonary: Acute pulmonary toxicity characterised by pulmonary infiltrate and/or fibrosis has been reported in some patients receiving prolonged therapy with BiCNU. This may occur during treatment or within one or two years of therapy.

Very delayed onset pulmonary toxicity occurring up to 15 years after treatment has recently been reported in children following therapy with BiCNU at doses of 800 mg/sq meter or above.

The condition has been observed in children that were aged between 2 and 16 years when treated with BiCNU. Chest X-rays have demonstrated pulmonary hypoplasia with upper zone contraction, but gallium scans have been normal in all cases. Thoracic CT scans are often abnormal and have demonstrated an unusual pattern of upper zone fibrosis. There appears to be some late reduction of pulmonary function in a substantial percentage of these patients. This form of lung fibrosis may be slowly progressive, and has resulted in death in some cases.

Renal: Renal abnormalities consisting of decrease in kidney size, progressive azotaemia and renal failure have been reported in patients who receive large cumulative doses after prolonged therapy with BiCNU and related nitrosoureas. Kidney damage has also been reported in patients receiving lower total doses.

Local: Burning at the site of injection is common but true thrombosis is rare.

Other: Rapid i.v. infusion of BiCNU may produce intense flushing of the skin and suffusion of the conjunctiva within two hours, lasting about four hours.

Pharmaceutical precautions *Preparation of intravenous solution:* Dissolve BiCNU with 3 ml of the supplied sterile diluent (absolute ethanol) and then aseptically add 27 ml of sterile water for injection to the alcohol solution. Each ml of the resulting solution will contain 3.3 mg of BiCNU in 10% ethanol and has a pH of 5.6 to 6.0.

Reconstitution as recommended results in a clear colourless solution which may be further diluted with sodium chloride for injection, or 5% glucose for injection.

The reconstituted solution must be given intravenously and should be administered by i.v. drip over a one- to two-hour period. Injection of BiCNU over shorter periods of time may produce intense pain and burning at the site of injection.

Important note: The lyophilised dosage formulation contains no preservatives and is not intended as a multiple dose vial.

Stability: Unopened vials of the dry powder must be stored in a refrigerator (2°C–8°C).

After reconstitution as recommended, decomposition of BiCNU at room temperature is linear with time. After three hours, approximately 6% of the solution has decomposed and after six hours, approximately 8%. Refrigeration (4°C) of the reconstituted BiCNU significantly increases the stability of the solution. After 24 hours, when protected from light, there is only 4% decomposition. Further dilution of the reconstituted solution with 500 ml of sodium chloride for injection or 5% glucose for injection, results in a solution which is stable for 48 hours when protected from light and refrigerated.

Important note: BiCNU has a low melting point (approximately 30·5–32·0°C or 86·9–89·6°F). Exposure of the drug to this temperature or above will cause the drug to liquefy and appear as an oil film in the bottom of the vials. This is a sign of decomposition and vials should be discarded.

Guidelines for the safe handling of antineoplastic agents:

1. Trained personnel should reconstitute the drug.
2. This should be performed in a designated area.
3. Adequate protective gloves should be worn.
4. Precautions should be taken to avoid the drug accidentally coming into contact with the eyes. In the event of contact with the eyes, flush with copious amounts of water and/or saline.
5. The cytotoxic preparation should not be handled by pregnant staff.
6. Adequate care and precaution should be taken in the disposal of items (syringes, needles etc) used to reconstitute cytotoxic drugs. Excess material and body waste may be disposed of by placing in double sealed polythene bags and incinerating at a temperature of 1,000°C. Liquid waste may be flushed with copious amounts of water.
7. The work surface should be covered with disposable plastic-backed absorbent paper.
8. Use Luer-Lock fittings on all syringes and sets. Large bore needles are recommended to minimise pressure and the possible formation of aerosols. The latter may also be reduced by the use of a venting needle.

Legal category POM.

Package quantities BiCNU Injection packed in cartons of 10 units, each unit consisting of one vial of carmustine 100 mg and one vial of sterile absolute alcohol 3 ml.

Further information BiCNU alkylates DNA and RNA and has also been shown to inhibit several enzymes by carbamoylation of amino acids in proteins.

Intravenously administered BiCNU is rapidly degraded, with no intact drug detectable after 15 minutes. However, in studies with C^{14} labelled drug, prolonged levels of the isotope were observed in the plasma and tissue, probably representing radioactive fragments of the parent compound.

It is thought that the antineoplastic and toxic activities of BiCNU may be due to metabolites. Approximately 60 to 70% of a total dose is excreted in the urine in 96 hours and about 10% as respiratory CO_2. The fate of the remainder is undetermined.

Because of the high lipid solubility and the relative lack of ionisation at a physiological pH, BiCNU crosses the blood brain barrier.

Levels of radioactivity in the CSF are at least 50% higher than those measured concurrently in plasma.

Product licence number 0125/0108.

BUSPAR*

Presentation Buspar 5 mg tablets: white, pillow-shaped biconvex tablet engraved '5' on one face. Each tablet contains buspirone hydrochloride 5 mg.

Buspar 10 mg tablets; white, pillow-shaped biconvex tablet, engraved '10' and a scoreline on one face. Each tablet contains buspirone hydrochloride 10 mg.

Other ingredients: Colloidal silicon dioxide, lactose anhydrous, magnesium stearate, microcrystalline cellulose, sodium starch glycollate.

Uses Buspar is indicated for the short-term management of anxiety disorders and the relief of symptoms of anxiety with or without accompanying depression.

Dosage and administration Dosage should be adjusted according to response for maximum effect. The recommended initial dose is 5 mg two to three times daily and this may be increased every two to three days. The usual therapeutic dose is 15 to 30 mg daily in divided doses with a maximum recommended dose of 45 mg daily in divided doses.

Elderly: Although there is no evidence from kinetic and clinical studies that buspirone would behave differently in the elderly, there are limited data beyond 4 weeks and at doses above 30 mg/day in this age group. Therefore it is recommended that Buspar be used for short term treatment (up to 4 weeks) in the elderly patient, at a maximum dose normally not exceeding 30 mg daily.

Children: Use in children has not been established.

Contra-indications, warnings, etc
Contra-indications: Buspar should not be used in patients hypersensitive to buspirone hydrochloride. Buspar should not be used in patients with epilepsy. In patients with a history of renal or hepatic impairment buspirone should be used with caution. Buspar should not be used in patients with severe renal impairment, defined as a creatinine clearance of 20 ml/minute or below, or a plasma creatinine above 200 micromoles/litre. Buspar should not be used in patients with severe hepatic disease.

Use in pregnancy and lactation: In some studies, administration of high doses of buspirone to pregnant animals produced effects on survival, birth and weanling weights, although there was no effect on foetal development. Since the relevance of this finding in humans has not been established, Buspar is contra-indicated in pregnancy and in lactation.

Precautions: In controlled studies in healthy volunteers Buspar in single doses up to 20 mg caused no significant impairment of cognitive or psychomotor functions, unlike the benzodiazepines, diazepam or lorazepam. In studies in healthy volunteers, Buspar did not potentiate the psychomotor impairment produced by alcohol, in contrast to a comparative benzodiazepine. However no data is available on concomitant use of alcohol and Buspar at single doses greater than 20 mg. It is prudent therefore to avoid alcohol while taking Buspar.

As Buspar does not exhibit cross-tolerance with benzodiazepines and other common sedative/hypnotic agents, it will not block the withdrawal syndrome often seen with cessation of therapy with these compounds. Before starting therapy with Buspar, it is advisable to withdraw patients gradually from prior chronic treatment with these agents.

Drug interactions: The occurrence of elevated blood pressure in patients receiving both buspirone and monoamine oxidase inhibitors (phenelzine and tranylcypromine) has been reported. It is therefore recommended that Buspar should not be used concomitantly with a monoamine oxidase inhibitor.

In vitro studies have shown that buspirone does not displace warfarin, digoxin, phenytoin or propranolol from plasma proteins.

In a study in normal volunteers, no interaction with amitriptyline was seen. A similar study with diazepam showed a slight increase in metabolite (nordiazepam) levels.

Side-effects: Buspar is generally well tolerated. If side-effects occur they are normally observed at the beginning of treatment and usually subside with continued use and/or decreased dosage.

In controlled trials, the only side-effects that occurred with significantly greater frequency with buspirone treatment than with placebo were dizziness, headache, nervousness, light-headedness, excitement and nausea. Tachycardia, palpitations, chest pain, drowsiness, confusion, dry mouth, fatigue and sweating/clamminess have also been reported rarely.

Overdose: There is no specific antidote to Buspar. Buspar is not removed by haemodialysis. The stomach should be emptied as quickly as possible. Treatment should be symptomatic and supportive. The ingestion of multiple agents should be suspected.

Death by deliberate or accidental overdose has not been observed. A dose of 375 mg per day in healthy volunteers produced no significant adverse effects. As maximum dose levels are reached symptoms most commonly observed are: nausea, vomiting, dizziness, drowsiness and miosis.

Pharmaceutical precautions Buspirone tablets should be stored at room temperature.

Legal category POM.

Package quantities 5 mg: 100 tablet bottle; 6 × 21 tablet calendar pack. 10 mg: 100 tablet bottle.

Further information Buspar is an azaspirodecanedione. The exact mechanism of Buspar anxioselective action is not fully known. It does not act on benzodiazepine receptor sites and lacks sedative, anticonvulsant and muscle relaxant properties. From animal studies it is known to interact with serotonin, noradrenaline, acetylcholine and dopamine systems of the brain. Buspar enhances the activity of specific noradrenergic and dopaminergic pathways, whereas the activity of serotonin and acetylcholine are reduced.

Buspar is rapidly absorbed when given orally. It is then subject to considerable first-pass metabolism. Peak plasma levels occur 60–90 minutes after dosing. Plasma concentration is linearly related to dose. Following multiple dosing steady state plasma concentrations are achieved within 2 days. Buspar is 95% protein bound. Buspar is eliminated primarily by liver metabolism. In pharmacokinetic studies mean plasma half-lives have varied from 2 to 11 hours.

Product licence numbers

5 mg tablets	0125/0162.
10 mg tablets	0125/0163

ENKAID* ▼

Presentation White capsule containing encainide hydrochloride 25 mg.

Capsule with white body and yellow cap containing encainide hydrochloride 50 mg.

Other ingredients: lactose, magnesium stearate, sodium starch glycolate; gelatin capsules containing iron oxide (50 mg only) sulphurous anhydride, titanium dioxide.

Uses The product is indicated for the treatment of life-threatening ventricular arrhythmias, such as symptomatic sustained ventricular tachycardia, in patients who are intolerant of or unresponsive to other antiarrhythmic agents. Enkaid should not be used in patients with less severe ventricular arrhythmias, even if they are symptomatic.

Dosage and administration
Adults: It is recommended that treatment with Enkaid should be initiated in hospital following a full assessment of cardiac function.

The recommended initial dosing schedule for adults is 25 mg, 3 times daily, at 8 hourly intervals.

If necessary, after a period of 3 to 5 days, the dosage may be increased to 100 mg per day, then after a further period of 3 to 5 days, to 150 mg per day. Doses of more than 200 mg per day or a too rapid dose escalation should be avoided. Each single dose should not exceed 75 mg. Hospitalization is recommended if the dose is increased above 200 mg per day.

Dosage should be adjusted for each patient on the basis of therapeutic response and tolerance. ECG parameters and 24 hour Holter monitoring are a useful measure of treatment response and should be measured at intervals and when adjusting dosage.

Once therapeutic response is achieved patients may be maintained at a lower dosage than the maximum during titration.

Use of higher doses and rapid dosage adjustment have resulted in an increased incidence of proarrhythmic events particularly during the first days of dosing. With Enkaid, the concept of 'loading dose' must not be used.

As a general principle, when other antiarrhythmic therapy has been previously prescribed, it is recommended to wait for 2 to 4 plasma half lives before initiating Enkaid treatment.

If Enkaid is to be given to a patient taking cimetidine, dosing should be commenced at 25 mg twice daily.

Determination of plasma levels of Enkaid and its metabolites to guide the care of patients is not useful.

Children: Use in children has not been established.

Elderly: The dose is the same as for other adults.

Renal impairment: In patients with severe renal impairment (creatinine clearance between 10 and 30 ml/min), the elimination of Enkaid and its metabolites is reduced.

It is therefore recommended to:

(1) Start treatment with a daily dose of 25 mg for at least 7 days, to achieve steady-state.

(2) After 7 days, the daily dose of Enkaid may be increased by 25 mg increments every 7 days until adequate response is obtained. A dose of 25 mg three times daily should only be exceeded with extreme caution.

In cases of major renal insufficiency, (creatinine clearance below 10 ml/min) use of Enkaid is not recommended.

Hepatic impairment: Enkaid should be used cautiously in patients with elevated liver enzymes (greater than four times normal) with or without jaundice. Such patients treated with Enkaid should have frequent measurement of the enzyme levels.

Contra-indications, warnings, etc
Contra-indications: Enkaid is contra-indicated:

(i) in patients with a history of myocardial infarction who have either asymptomatic ventricular ectopics or asymptomatic non-sustained ventricular tachycardia.
(ii) in patients with known hypersensitivity to encainide hydrochloride.
(iii) in right bundle-branch block, complete left bundle-branch block, bifascicular block, and second or third degree atrioventricular block. These contra-indications do not apply if a pacemaker is present.
(iv) in cases of cardiogenic shock.

Precautions: Enkaid was included in the National Heart Lung and Blood Institute's Cardiac Arrhythmia Suppression Trial (CAST), a long-term, multi-centre, randomized, double-blind study in patients with asymptomatic non-life-threatening arrhythmias who had a myocardial infarction more than six days, but less than two years previously. An excessive mortality or non-fatal cardiac arrest rate was seen in patients treated with Enkaid compared with that seen in a carefully matched placebo-treated group. This rate was 2.7 times higher in the Enkaid group than in the placebo group. The average duration of treatment with Enkaid in this study was 10 months.

The applicability of the CAST results to other populations (e.g. those without myocardial infarction) is uncertain, but at present it is prudent to consider the risks of Enkaid therapy unacceptable in patients without life-threatening arrhythmias, even if the patients are experiencing unpleasant symptoms. In addition, although mortality has not been adequately studied outside of the CAST patient population, it may be assumed that any patient with a history of myocardial infarction, regardless of arrhythmia type, may be at significantly increased risk from Enkaid.

Enkaid, like other antiarrhythmics, can cause new or worsened arrhythmias in all patient populations, including those with life threatening arrhythmias. These precautions apply to all patients, including the latter group.

The risk of proarrhythmias is most frequent in patients with a history of ventricular fibrillation, sustained ventricular tachycardia, cardiomyopathy, congestive heart failure or previous history of myocardial infarction. Proarrhythmias cannot be predicted by age, sex or the ECG prior to or during treatment. These events occur most often at the beginning of treatment and are most common when doses exceed 200 mg per day. Therefore in subjects at risk treatment should be started with low doses and care should be taken to adjust dosage progressively.

Prior to commencing Enkaid therapy, a full assessment of cardiac function should be carried out.

Enkaid must be administered with caution in patients with sinus disease, SA block, first degree AV block, intra cardiac conduction disturbance (QRS >0.12 sec) or in life threatening arrhythmias, a left ventricular ejection fraction less than 40%.

In all of these cases dose increments should be made only after adequate patient evaluation including ECG and measurement of cardiac output as appropriate.

As with all drugs of this class, hypokalaemia or hyperkalaemia can alter the effects of antiarrhythmics. A metabolic disorder of this type must be corrected before administration of Enkaid.

The effects of Enkaid in patients with unstable angina have not been adequately studied. In patients with life-threatening arrhythmias, the effects of Enkaid on those with recent myocardial infarction (within six weeks) have not been adequately studied.

Since Enkaid has a limited potential for increasing pacemaker thresholds, it is advisable to establish the threshold before administration and at regular intervals during therapy.

Pregnancy and lactation: Although experimental studies in animals have not revealed any evidence of harm to the foetus, in the absence of human clinical data it is advised not to prescribe Enkaid during pregnancy. Fertility was reduced when both male and female rats received oral doses of 28 mg/kg/day (approximately 13 times the average human dose) prior to mating. This was not seen at lower doses or when each sex was treated separately at the same dose.

Enkaid is partially excreted in breast milk. A decision to continue treatment with Enkaid during lactation must take account of the risk/benefit ratio.

Effects on ability to drive vehicles or operate machines: The effect of Enkaid on ability to drive vehicles has not been evaluated.

Drug interactions: Enkaid should be used with caution with other antiarrhythmic agents or any agent that affects cardiac conduction because of the possibility of additive pharmacological effects. Treatment is compatible with digoxin, beta-blockers, calcium antagonists, diuretics and anticoagulants. Cimetidine at a dose of 300 mg four times daily increases plasma concentrations of Enkaid and its active metabolites so that if Enkaid is to be given to a patient taking cimetidine, dosing should be commenced at 25 mg twice daily. The dosage of Enkaid should also be reduced if cimetidine is to be given to a patient taking Enkaid.

Side-effects: In the CAST (see precautions), the incidence of total mortality and non-fatal cardiac arrest was 9.6% in the Enkaid group compared with 3.6% in the placebo group.

In pre-marketing clinical studies the following adverse events occurred more frequently in patients receiving Enkaid than in those receiving placebo and at a frequency of 1% or greater: abdominal pain, chest pains, death, pain in limbs, peripheral oedema, proarrhythmia, constipation, dyspepsia, nausea, vomiting, dizziness, insomnia, nervousness, rash, abnormal/blurred vision, anorexia, asthenia, dyspnoea, headache, palpitations, QRS prolongation, syncope.

Less common reactions include: paresthesia, congestive heart failure, diarrhoea, tremor, increased cough, taste perversion, increased or decreased blood pressure, confusion, ataxia, abnormal gait, dream disturbances, diplopia, photophobia, periorbital oedema.

There have also beeen rare reports of elevated blood glucose levels or increased insulin requirements in diabetic patients and of elevated serum liver enzymes and jaundice.

Overdosage
Symptoms: QRS widening, QT prolongation and atrio-ventricular dissociation. Ventricular tachycardia, ventricular flutter or fibrillation may develop. Also, hypotension, bradycardia, asystole and other conduction disturbances may occur. Overdosage has resulted in death.

Treatment: The patient should be hospitalized, managed in a coronary care unit and continuously monitored. An intravenous line should be established. Any arrhythmia which is life-threatening or produces haemodynamic instability should be treated in accordance with normal practice. The insertion of a pacemaker may be necessary for severe bradycardia or other significant conduction disturbances.

Acute overdosage should be managed by gastric lavage followed by activated charcoal. Treatment should be supportive.

No specific antidote has been identified although one report has suggested that hypertonic sodium bicarbonate may be useful for the management of cardiac toxicity. In this report, a solution containing 8.4% sodium bicarbonate was administered intravenously using the following regime: 100 ml given immediately, 50 ml 15 minutes later and 100 ml given over two minutes 2 hours after admission.

Pharmaceutical precautions Enkaid capsules should be stored at room temperature.

Legal category POM.

Package quantities Bottles of 100 capsules.

Further information Nil.

Product licence numbers
25 mg 0125/0202
50 mg 0125/0203

KERI* THERAPEUTIC LOTION

Presentation Keri Therapeutic Lotion is a white lotion containing mineral oil, 16%.

Other ingredients: Carbomer 934, glyceryl monostearate, lanolin oil, laureth 4, methyl hydroxybenzoate, perfume, polyethylene glycol, polyethylene glycol 40 stearate, propyl hydroxybenzoate, propylene glycol, quaternium 15, sodium doctyl sulphosuccinate, triethanolamine, water.

Uses Keri Therapeutic Lotion has emollient properties. It is indicated for the symptomatic treatment of dermatitis, eczema, ichthyosis, ammoniacal dermatitis (nappy rash), protection of raw and abraded skin areas, pruritus and related conditions where dry scaly skin is a problem. It is also indicated as an emollient before bathing for dry/ eczematous skin, to alleviate drying effects.

Dosage and administration Keri Therapeutic Lotion should be gently massaged into the skin three times daily or as often as required.

Elderly: No dosage adjustment is necessary.

Contra-indications, warnings, etc Keri Therapeutic Lotion contains lanolin oil and is therefore contra-indicated in those patients allergic to this ingredient.

Pharmaceutical precautions Store at room temperature.

Legal category P.

Package quantities Bottles containing 190 ml & 380 ml (original pack).

Further information Nil.

Product licence number 0125/0152

MEGACE*

Presentation Megace 40 mg tablets: White, circular, scored tablets, engraved '40' on one face, each tablet containing Megestrol Acetate BP 40 mg.

Other ingredients: Acacia, calcium hydrogen phosphate, lactose, magnesium stearate, maize starch, silicon dioxide.

Megace 160 mg tablets – off-white, oval scored tablets, engraved '160' on one face, each tablet containing Megestrol Acetate BP 160 mg.

Other ingredients: Colloidal silicon dioxide, lactose monohydrate, magnesium stearate, microcrystalline cellulose, povidone, sodium starch glycollate.

Uses Megace is a progestational agent, indicated for the treatment of certain hormone-dependent neoplasms, such as endometrial or breast cancer.

Dosage and administration Oral.

Breast cancer: 160 mg/day (40 mg qid or 160 mg taken once daily).

Endometrial cancer: 40–320 mg/day in divided doses (40–80 mg one to four times daily or one to two 160 mg tablets daily).

At least two months of continuous treatment is considered an adequate period for determining the efficacy of Megace.

Elderly: No dosage adjustment is necessary.

Contra-indications, warnings, etc Megace is contra-indicated in patients who have demonstrated hypersensitivity to the drug.

Precautions: Megace should be used with caution in patients with a history of thrombophlebitis.

Adverse reactions: The major side-effect experienced by patients while taking megestrol acetate, particularly at high doses, is weight gain, which is usually not associated with water retention, but which is secondary to an increased appetite and food intake. A rarely encountered side-effect of prolonged administration of megestrol acetate is urticaria, presumably an idiosyncratic reaction to the drug. An occasionally noted, usually transient, side-effect is nausea. Reports have been received of patients developing carpal tunnel syndrome, deep vein thrombophlebitis and alopecia while taking megestrol acetate. The drug is devoid of the myelosuppressive activity characteristic of many cytotoxic drugs and it causes no significant changes in haematology, blood chemistry or urinalysis.

Overdosage: No serious side effects have resulted from studies involving Megace (megestrol acetate) administered in dosages as high as 800 mg/day.

Pharmaceutical precautions Megace tablets should be stored at room temperature.

Legal category POM.

Package quantities 40 mg tablet – units of 100.
160 mg tablet – units of 30 tablets.

Further information Nil.

Product licence numbers
40 mg tablet 0125/0144
160 mg tablet 0125/0173

PARAPLATIN*

Presentation Vials containing 50 mg, 150 mg and 450 mg carboplatin [cis-diammine (1,1-cyclobutanedicarboxylato) platinum].

Other ingredients: Water for injection.

Uses Paraplatin is indicated for the treatment of:

1. advanced ovarian carcinoma of epithelial origin in:
   (a) first line therapy
   (b) second line therapy, after other treatments have failed.
2. small cell carcinoma of the lung.

Dosage and administration Paraplatin should be used by the intravenous route only. The recommended dosage of Paraplatin in previously untreated adult patients with normal kidney function is 400 mg/m^2 as a single i.v. dose administered by a short term (15 to 60 minutes) infusion. Therapy should not be repeated until four weeks after the previous Paraplatin course.

Reduction of the initial dosage by 20–25% is recommended for those patients who present with risk factors such as prior myelosuppressive treatment and low performance status (ECOG-Zubrod 2–4 or Karnofsky below 80).

Determination of the haematological nadir by weekly blood counts during the initial courses of treatment with Paraplatin is recommended for future dosage adjustment.

Impaired renal function: The optimal use of Paraplatin in patients presenting with impaired renal function requires adequate dosage adjustments and frequent monitoring of both haematological nadirs and renal function.

Combination therapy: The optimal use of Paraplatin in combination with other myelosuppressive agents requires dosage adjustments according to the regimen and schedule to be adopted.

Paediatrics: Sufficient usage of Paraplatin in paediatrics has not occurred to allow specific dosage recommendations to be made.

Elderly: Dosage adjustment, initially or subsequently, may be necessary dependent on the physical condition of the patient.

Dilution: The product may be diluted with 5% Glucose for Injection BP or 0.9% Sodium Chloride for Injection BP to concentrations as low as 0.5 mg/ml (500 micrograms/ml).

Contra-indications, warnings, etc

Contra-indications: Paraplatin should not be used in patients with severe pre-existing renal impairment (creatinine clearance at or below 20 ml/minute).

Paraplatin should not be employed in severely myelosuppressed patients. Paraplatin is also contra-indicated in patients with a history of severe allergic reactions to Paraplatin, other platinum containing compounds.

Warnings: Paraplatin should be administered by individuals experienced in the use of anti-neoplastic therapy.

Paraplatin myelosuppression is closely related to its renal clearance: patients with abnormal kidney function or receiving concomitant therapy with other drugs with nephrotoxic potential are likely to experience more severe and prolonged myelotoxicity. Renal function parameters should, therefore, be carefully assessed before and during therapy. Paraplatin courses should not be repeated more frequently than monthly under normal circumstances. Thrombocytopenia, leukopenia and anaemia occur after administration of Paraplatin. Frequent monitoring of peripheral blood counts is recommended throughout and following therapy with Paraplatin. Paraplatin combination therapy with other myelosuppressive compounds must be planned very carefully with respect to dosages and timing in order to minimise additive effects. Supportive transfusional therapy may be required in patients who suffer severe myelosuppression.

Paraplatin can cause nausea and vomiting. Premedication with anti-emetics has been reported to be useful in reducing the incidence and intensity of these effects.

Renal function impairment may be encountered with Paraplatin. Although no clinical evidence on compounding nephrotoxicity has been accumulated, it is recommended not to combine Paraplatin with aminoglycosides or other nephrotoxic compounds.

As for other platinum co-ordination compounds, allergic reactions to Paraplatin have been reported. These may occur within minutes of administration and should be managed with appropriate supportive therapy. Anaphylactic-like reactions may also occur as with other platinum co-ordination compounds.

Use in pregnancy: The safe use of Paraplatin during pregnancy has not been established; Paraplatin has been shown to be an embryotoxin and mutagen in several experimental systems.

Its carcinogenic potential has not been studied but compounds with similar mechanisms of action and mutagenicity have been reported to be carcinogenic.

Precautions: Peripheral blood counts and renal function tests should be monitored closely. Blood counts at the beginning of the therapy and weekly to assess haematological nadir for subsequent dose adjustment are recommended. Neurological evaluations should also be performed on a regular basis.

Adverse reactions: Incidences of adverse reactions reported hereunder are based on cumulative data obtained in a large group of patients with various pretreatment prognostic features.

Haematological toxicity: Myelosuppression is the dose-limiting toxicity of Paraplatin. At maximum tolerated dosages of Paraplatin administered as a single agent, thrombocytopenia, with nadir platelet counts of less than 50×10^9/L, occurs in about a third of the patients. The nadir usually occurs between days 14 and 21, with recovery within 35 days from the start of therapy. Leukopenia has also occurred in approximately 20% of patients but its recovery from the day of nadir (day 14–28) may be slower and usually occurs within 42 days from the start of therapy. A haemoglobin decrease may be observed in some patients.

Myelosuppression may be more severe and prolonged in patients with impaired renal function, extensive prior treatment, poor performance status and age above 65. Myelosuppression is also worsened by therapy combining Paraplatin with other compounds that are myelosuppressive.

Myelosuppression is usually reversible and not cumulative when Paraplatin is used as a single agent and at the recommended dosages and frequencies of administration.

Infectious complications have occasionally been reported. Haemorrhagic complications, usually minor, have also been reported.

Nephrotoxicity: Renal toxicity is usually not dose-limiting in patients receiving Paraplatin, nor does it require preventive measures such as high volume fluid hydration or forced diuresis. Nevertheless, increasing blood urea or serum creatinine levels can occur. Renal function impairment, as defined by a decrease in the creatinine clearance below 60 ml/min, may also be observed. The incidence and severity of nephrotoxicity may increase in patients who have impaired kidney function before Paraplatin treatment. It is not clear whether an appropriate hydration programme might overcome such an effect, but dosage reduction or discontinuation of therapy is required in the presence of severe alteration of renal function tests.

Decreases in serum electrolytes (magnesium, potassium and, rarely, calcium) have been reported after treatment with Paraplatin but have not been reported to be severe enough to cause the appearance of clinical signs or symptoms.

Gastrointestinal toxicity: Nausea without vomiting occurs in about a quarter of the patients receiving Paraplatin; vomiting has been reported in half of the patients and one-third of these suffer severe emesis. Nausea and vomiting usually disappear within 24 hours after treatment and are usually responsive to (and may be prevented by) anti-emetic medication. A quarter of patients experience no nausea or vomiting.

Allergic reactions: Infrequent allergic reactions to Paraplatin have been reported. These reactions are similar to those observed after administration of other platinum-containing compounds, i.e. erythematous rash, fever with no other apparent cause and pruritus.

Ototoxity: Subclinical decrease in hearing acuity, consisting of high-frequency (4000–8000 Hz) hearing loss determined by audiogram, has been reported in 15% of the patients treated with Paraplatin. However, only 1% of patients present with clinical symptoms, manifested in the majority of cases by tinnitus. In patients who have been previously treated with cisplatin and have developed hearing loss related to such treatment, the hearing impairment may persist, or worsen.

Neurotoxicity: The incidence of peripheral neuropathies after treatment with Paraplatin is 6%. In the majority of the patients neurotoxicity is limited to paraesthesia and decreased deep tendon reflexes. The frequency and intensity of this side effect increases in patients previously treated with cisplatin.

Paraesthesia present before commencing Paraplatin therapy, particularly if related to prior cisplatin treatment, may persist or worsen during treatment with Paraplatin.

Other: Abnormalities of liver function tests (usually mild to moderate) have been reported with Paraplatin in about one-third of the patients with normal baseline values. The alkaline phosphatase level is increased more frequently than SGOT, SGPT or total bilirubin. The majority of these abnormalities regress spontaneously during the course of treatment.

Rare events consisting of taste alteration, alopecia, fever and chills without evidence of infection or allergic reaction have occurred in less than 2% of the patients receiving Paraplatin.

Pharmaceutical precautions Paraplatin Solution should be stored at room temperature (15–20°C), protected from light.

Dilution: The product may be diluted with 5% Glucose for Injection BP, or 0.9% Sodium Chloride for Injection BP, to concentrations as low as 0.5 mg/ml (500 microgram/ml).

When diluted as directed, Paraplatin solutions are stable for eight hours stored at room temperature or 24 hours stored under refrigeration. Since no antibacterial preservatives are contained in the formulation, it is recommended that any Paraplatin solution be discarded after eight hours from dilution if stored at room temperature or after 24 hours if stored under refrigeration.

Guidelines for the safe handling of antineoplastic agents:

1. Trained personnel should reconstitute the drug.
2. This should be performed in a designated area.

3. Adequate protective gloves should be worn.

4. Precautions should be taken to avoid the drug accidentally coming into contact with the eyes. In the event of contact with the eyes, wash with water and/or saline.

5. The cytotoxic preparation should not be handled by pregnant staff.

6. Adequate care and precautions should be taken in the disposal of items (syringes, needles etc) used to reconstitute cytotoxic drugs. Excess material and body waste may be disposed of by placing in double sealed polythene bags and incinerating at a temperature of 1,000°C. Liquid waste may be flushed with copious amounts of water.

Dilution:

7. The work surface should be covered with disposable plastic-backed absorbent paper.

8. Use Luer-Lock fittings on all syringes and sets. Large bore needles are recommended to minimise pressure and the possible formation of aerosols. The latter may also be reduced by the use of a venting needle.

Legal category POM.

It is proposed to make Paraplatin available only on prescription and supplied to centres with experience in the chemotherapy of malignant diseases.

Package quantities Vials containing 50 mg, 150 mg 450 mg carboplatin as a 10 mg/ml solution.

Further information Paraplatin has biochemical properties similar to that of cisplatin, thus producing predominantly interstrand and intrastrand DNA crosslinks. Following administration of Paraplatin in man, linear relationships exist between dose and plasma concentrations of total and free ultrafilterable platinum. The area under the plasma concentration versus time curve for total platinum also shows a linear relationship with the dose.

Repeated dosing during four consecutive days did not produce an accumulation of platinum in plasma. Following the administration of Paraplatin reported values for the terminal elimination half-lives of free ultrafilterable platinum and Paraplatin in man are approximately 6 hours and 1.5 hours respectively. During the initial phase, most of the free ultrafilterable platinum is present as Paraplatin. The terminal half-life for total plasma platinum is 24 hours. Approximately 87% of plasma platinum is protein bound within 24 hours following administration. Paraplatin is excreted primarily in the urine, with recovery of approximately 70% of the administered platinum within 24 hours. Most of the drug is excreted in the first 6 hours. Total body and renal clearances of free ultrafilterable platinum correlate with the rate of glomerular filtration but not tubular secretion.

Product licence numbers

50 mg	0125/0179
150 mg	0125/0180
450 mg	0125/0181

QUESTRAN*
QUESTRAN A*

Presentation Questran sachets containing 9 g of orange-flavoured powder which produces a pale orange-coloured suspension when reconstituted with water. Each sachet supplies 4 g of anhydrous cholestyramine (a basic anion-exchange resin).

Other ingredients: Acacia, citric acid anhydrous, colloidal silicon dioxide, flavours, polysorbate 80, propylene glycol alginate, sucrose, sunset yellow.

Questran A sachets containing 5 g of orange-flavoured powder which produces a pale orange-coloured suspension when reconstituted with water. Each sachet supplies 4 g of anhydrous cholestyramine. The main sweetening agent in Questran A is aspartame rather than sucrose (as in Questran).

Other ingredients: Aspartame, citric acid anhydrous, colloidal silicon dioxide, flavours, propylene glycol alginate, quinoline yellow, sucrose, xanthan gum.

Uses Questran is used for:

1. Primary prevention of coronary heart disease in men between 35 and 59 years of age and with primary hypercholesterolaemia who have not responded to diet and other appropriate measures.

2. Reduction of plasma cholesterol in hypercholesterolaemia, particularly in those patients who have been diagnosed as Fredrickson's Type II (high plasma cholesterol with normal or slightly elevated triglycerides).

3. Relief of pruritus associated with partial biliary obstruction and primary biliary cirrhosis.

4. Relief of diarrhoea associated with ileal resection, Crohn's disease, vagotomy and diabetic vagal neuropathy.

5. Management of radiation-induced diarrhoea.

Dosage and administration *Adults:* As a precautionary measure, where concurrent drug therapy exists then such drugs should be administered at least one hour before or 4–6 hours after Questran.

1. For primary prevention of coronary heart disease and to reduce cholesterol: After initial introduction over a three to four week period, 3 to 6 Questran sachets per day, administered either as a single daily dose or in divided doses up to four times daily according to dosage requirements and patient acceptability. Dosage may be modified according to response and can be increased to 9 sachets per day if necessary.

Occasional slight gastro-intestinal upsets e.g. constipation, may occur when starting Questran. These usually pass with continued usage of Questran and are minimised by starting therapy gradually.

Final dose required	*Sachets per day*			
	Week 1	*Week 2*	*Week 3*	*Week 4*
3	1	2	3	3
4	1	2	3	4
6	1	2	3	6

2. To relieve pruritus: One or two sachets daily are usually sufficient.

3. To relieve diarrhoea: As for reduction of cholesterol but it may be possible to reduce this dosage.

Questran should not be taken in its dry form and should be administered mixed with water.

Children 6–12 years: The initial dose is determined by the following formula:

$$\frac{\text{child's weight in kg} \times \text{adult dose}}{70}$$

Subsequent dosage adjustment may be necessary where clinically indicated.

The dose has not been established in infants and children under 6 years.

Elderly: No dosage adjustment is necessary.

Contra-indications, warnings, etc

Contra-indications: Questran is likely to be ineffective in patients with complete biliary obstruction, since Questran cannot be effective where bile is not secreted into the intestine.

Side-effects: Since Questran may interfere with the absorption of fat soluble vitamins the diet may require supplementation with vitamins A, D and K during prolonged high dose administration.

Chronic use of Questran may be associated with increased bleeding tendency due to hypoprothrombinemia associated with Vitamin K deficiency. This will usually respond promptly to parenteral Vitamin K administration. Recurrences can be prevented by oral administration of Vitamin K.

Gastro-intestinal side effects are those most frequently reported. The principal complaint is constipation which may be controlled with the usual remedies, and frequently disappears on continued usage of Questran. Large doses of Questran can cause diarrhoea.

Use in pregnancy and lactation: As with other drugs,

Questran should not be given in pregnancy or lactation unless considered essential.

Interactions: Questran may delay or reduce the absorption of certain drugs (such as digitalis and its alkaloids, tetracycline, chlorothiazide, warfarin and thyroxine). The response to concomitant medication should be closely monitored and appropriate adjustments made if necessary.

Patients should take other drugs at least one hour before or 4–6 hours after Questran to minimise possible interference with their absorption.

Overdose: Overdosage with Questran has not been reported. The potential problem in overdosage would be obstruction of the gastro-intestinal tract.

Pharmaceutical precautions Questran should not be taken in its dry form. The powder should be prepared immediately prior to administration. Store in a dry place.

Legal category POM.

Package quantities Questran and Questran A are available in original packs containing 168 sachets.

Further information The correlation between high blood cholesterol levels and ischaemic heart conditions has prompted the dietary control of patients who have shown signs or symptoms of coronary artery disease. With Questran it is possible to reduce cholesterol levels without recourse to excessively stringent dietary measures or systemically absorbed drugs.

Questran (cholestyramine) is a basic anion exchange resin. It is not absorbed in the gut and its affinity for bile acids in the intestinal tract prevents their reabsorption. To compensate for the faecal loss of bile acids, their major precursor, cholesterol, is oxidised at an increased rate in the liver and plasma cholesterol levels are thus lowered.

Product licence numbers

Questran	0125/5009R.
Questran A	0125/0192.

SOTACOR*

Presentation *Sotacor tablets:* Sotacor 80 mg tablets – pink, circular, tablets, engraved 'SOTACOR 80' on one face, each tablet containing 80 mg sotalol hydrochloride.

Other ingredients: lactose, magnesium stearate, maize starch, Ponceau 40, talc.

Sotacor 160 mg tablets – blue, circular, tablets, engraved 'SOTACOR 160' on one face, each containing 160 mg sotalol hydrochloride.

Other ingredients: Indigo carmine, magnesium stearate, maize starch, microcrystalline cellulose, pregelatinised starch.

Sotacor injection: Ampoules containing sotalol hydrochloride 40 mg in each 4 ml of solution.

Other ingredients: Glacial acetic acid, sodium chloride, sodium hydroxide, water.

Uses Sotacor, the hydrochloride of 4-(2-isopropylamino-1-hydroxyethyl)-methanesulphonanilide, is a synthetic beta-adrenergic receptor blocking agent. Sotacor possesses Class III antiarrhythmic activity. It lengthens repolarisation and the effective refractory period in all cardiac tissues independently of its antiadrenergic activity. Sotacor exerts a significant antihypertensive effect and additionally protects the heart from undesirable sympathetic drive. It is devoid of intrinsic sympathomimetic and local anaesthetic activity.

1. *Hypertension:* Sotacor produces smooth and gradual reduction of blood pressure on a long-term basis.
2. *Angina pectoris:* Sotacor reduces the frequency and severity of anginal attacks and increases exercise tolerance.
3. *Thyrotoxicosis:* Sotacor relieves the effect of adrenergic over-activity.
4. *Cardiac arrhythmias:* Sotacor tablets may be used prophylactically and as maintenance therapy in the management of cardiac arrhythmias. Sotacor Injection is used in the management of acute cardiac arrhythmias, especially following myocardial infarction, to restore normal rate and rhythm.
5. *Myocardial Infarction:* Sotacor tablets may be used prophylactically to reduce the incidence of infarction following an acute myocardial infarct.

Dosage and administration When administering beta-blocking drugs to previously untreated patients it is desirable to start with a low dose and gradually increase the dose until optimum response has occurred. It is usually undesirable to reduce the heart rate below 55 beats per minute.

Sotacor Tablets: Sotacor may be administered daily in either single or divided doses.

Children: Sotacor is not intended for administration to children.

Adults: 1. *Hypertension:* Initial daily dose should be one 160 mg tablet. The majority of mild to moderate hypertensives will respond to one tablet daily and be adequately controlled at this level.

2. *Angina pectoris:* Initial daily dose should be one 160 mg tablet. The majority of anginal patients will be controlled at this dosage level.

N.B. A gradual transfer of therapy over a two-week period is recommended in patients receiving other anti-anginal therapy.

3. *Thyrotoxicosis:* Initial daily dose should be one 160 mg tablet.

4. *Arrhythmia:* In the management of cardiac arrhythmias, as prophylaxis or maintenance therapy, Sotacor dosage will normally be between 160 mg and 240 mg daily.

N.B. In all these indications dosage may be increased by increments of up to 160 mg per day – the rapidity with which this dosage increase takes place depends upon the patient's tolerance, particularly as measured by the degree of induced bradycardia and the clinical response.

Sotacor Injection should be administered slowly in doses of 20–60 mg intravenously over two to three minutes. Larger doses, up to 100 mg should be injected over three minutes or longer. Continuous ECG monitoring is recommended. Should repeated administrations be necessary, a 10-minute interval between injections is advised, remembering that additive effect and prolongation of effect may ensue.

5. *Myocardial Infarction:* As prophylaxis following an acute myocardial infarction, Sotacor dosage will normally be 320 mg once daily commenced 5–14 days after infarction.

Elderly: As sotalol is renally excreted dosage will need to be adjusted in patients with poor renal function and should be used with caution in patients with poor cardiac reserve.

Contra-indications, warnings, etc Sotacor should not be used where there is evidence of heart block; metabolic acidosis; history of bronchospasm; diabetic ketoacidosis. Beta-blockade may precipitate heart failure in subjects with poor cardiac reserve or may aggravate existing heart failure. Patients whose heart failure is well controlled with digitalis and diuretics may be given Sotacor.

Treated diabetes: Sotacor, like other beta-blocking drugs, may reduce or mask pre-hypoglycaemic warning signs.

Anaesthesia: It is not necessary to discontinue Sotacor prior to most forms of elective surgery, although there is some doubt as to whether beta-receptor blockers should be continued up to the time of surgery involving cardiopulmonary bypass. However, as with other beta-blockers, sudden withdrawal of Sotacor Tablets or Injection might expose the patient to severe angina, arrhythmias, and even myocardial infarction.

If the drug is to be discontinued prior to surgery, especially in patients with ischaemic heart disease, then the drug should be withdrawn over a period of one week. It is usual to discontinue Sotacor Injection 24 to 48 hours prior to elective surgery.

In the presence of Sotacor, anaesthesia may proceed

provided that vagal dominance is counteracted by an intravenous injection of atropine sulphate (0.5–2 mg) immediately prior to induction of anaesthesia. Some anaesthetic agents such as ether, cyclopropane, trichloroethylene, methoxyflurane and enflurane appear to cause impairment of myocardial contractility in the presence of beta-receptor blockade. Caution is advised in the use of these agents in patients receiving Sotacor. No evidence of serious interaction has been found between nitrous oxide, halothane or isoflurane and beta-receptor blockers. Raised pCO_2 levels should be avoided in patients receiving Sotacor.

Cases of torsade de pointes (atypical ventricular tachycardia) have been reported infrequently during treatment with Sotacor. Experience indicates that this can occur in hypokalaemic patients and in patients concomitantly treated with drugs which may cause torsade such as antidepressants and Class I antiarrhythmics. Thus, the patient's electrolyte balance, especially potassium levels, should always be checked and any abnormality corrected prior to initiation of Sotacor therapy. It is also important to monitor the electrolyte balance frequently during Sotacor treatment. Patients should be instructed to stop Sotacor therapy during episodes of diarrhoea or when encountering conditions that may result in hypokalaemia. Institution of concurrent therapy with drugs known to prolong the QT interval and/or to be associated with atypical ventricular tachycardia especially quinidine, disopyramide and tricyclic antidepressants should be done under close medical supervision.

Pregnancy: Notice should be taken of current views on the undesirability of administering drugs during pregnancy. Animal studies with sotalol hydrochloride have shown no evidence of teratogenicity or other harmful effects on the foetus.

Side-effects: There have been reports of skin rashes and/or dry eyes associated with the use of beta-adrenergic blocking drugs. The reported incidence is small and in most cases the symptoms have cleared when the treatment was withdrawn. Discontinuance of the drug should be considered if any such reaction is not otherwise explicable. Cessation of therapy with a beta-adrenergic blocker should be gradual.

Sotacor tablets: At the recommended dosage side effects are uncommon. However, minor side effects such as bradycardia, nausea, insomnia, lassitude and diarrhoea have been reported. These are usually transient and can be avoided by gradual introduction of treatment and usually remit on reduction of dosage.

Sotacor Injection is usually well tolerated. Side effects due to beta-blockade, manifested as bradycardia and hypotension, should be treated, if necessary, as for overdosage.

Overdosage: In the rare event of profound cardiovascular effects such as excessive bradycardia or hypotension, atropine sulphate, 0.5–2 mg intravenously, should be administered. It may also be necessary to administer isoprenaline 5 microgram per minute, up to 25 microgram, by slow intravenous injection in order to reverse beta-receptor blockade.

Pharmaceutical precautions Sotacor Tablets should be protected from light. Store in a cool dry place.

Legal category POM.

Package quantities Sotacor 80 mg and 160 mg tablets: Original packs of 28 – blister strips of 14 tablets with 2 strips to a carton.

Sotacor Injection is supplied as 40 mg sotalol hydrochloride in 4 ml ampoules, with 5 ampoules per box.

Further information The maximum dose of Sotacor is usually 320 mg daily. Where improved control of hypertension is required the addition of a diuretic will often give a more satisfactory response.

Product licence numbers

Sotacor 80 mg tablets	0125/0076
Sotacor 160 mg tablets	0125/0093
Sotacor Injection 40 mg/4 ml	0125/0123

SOTAZIDE*

Presentation *Sotazide tablets:* Pale blue, capsule-shaped, concave tablets containing 160 mg sotalol hydrochloride and 25 mg hydrochlorothiazide.

Other ingredients: Aluminium magnesium silicate, indigo carmine, lactose, magnesium stearate, microcrystalline cellulose, pregelatinised maize starch.

Uses In the management of mild or moderate hypertension. The combination product may be suitable for use when satisfactory control of arterial blood pressure cannot be obtained with either a diuretic or a beta-adrenoreceptor blocking drug used alone.

Dosage and administration *Initial dose:* One Sotazide tablet daily increasing to two if necessary.

The individual optimal dosage and the rapidity with which dosage increase occurs should be determined from blood pressure and pulse rate readings and by the degree of induced bradycardia.

Following a reduction in blood pressure the dosage should not be increased until the new blood pressure is stable.

A slight reduction in dosage will alleviate symptoms of weakness and dizziness if blood pressure continues to fall after a month or two on the maintenance dose.

Elderly: As sotalol is renally excreted dosage will need to be adjusted in patients with poor renal function and should be used with caution in patients with poor cardiac reserve.

Contra-indications, warnings, etc
Contra-indications: Sotazide should not be used where there is evidence of heart block; history of bronchospasm; diabetic keto-acidosis; impending or uncontrolled cardiac failure; anaesthesia that produces myocardial depression; hypersensitivity to sotalol, hydrochlorothiazide or sulphonamide derivatives.

Since thiazides appear in breast milk, patients should stop nursing if the use of Sotazide is essential.

Warnings: Pregnancy: In animal studies Sotazide has been shown to have no adverse teratogenic effects in doses up to 25 times the recommended human dose. However, its safe use in human pregnancy has not been fully established.

Treated diabetes: Hypoglycaemic therapy may have to be altered in diabetics; Sotazide may potentiate the insulin hypoglycaemic effects and mask the symptoms of hypoglycaemia.

Hepatic/renal disease: Sotazide should be used with caution in patients with impaired hepatic function, liver disease or severe renal disease, since they are particularly sensitive to alterations of fluid and electrolyte balance. Thiazides may precipitate azotaemia. Cumulative effects of the hydrochlorothiazide may develop in patients with impaired renal function.

Cases of torsade de pointes (atypical ventricular tachycardia) have been reported infrequently during treatment with Sotazide. Experience to date indicates that this can occur in hypokalaemic patients and in patients concomitantly treated with drugs which may cause torsade such as antidepressants and Class I antiarrhythmics. Thus, the patient's electrolyte balance, especially potassium levels, should always be checked and any abnormality corrected prior to initiation of Sotazide therapy. It is also important to monitor the electrolyte balance frequently during Sotazide treatment. Patients should be instructed to stop Sotazide therapy during episodes of diarrhoea or when encountering conditions that may result in hypokalaemia. Institution of concurrent therapy with drugs known to prolong the QT interval and/or to be associated with atypical ventricular tachycardia especially quinidine, disopyramide and tricyclic antidepressants should be done under close medical supervision.

Anaesthesia: It is not necessary to discontinue Sotazide prior to most forms of elective surgery, although there is some doubt as to whether beta-receptor blockers should be continued up to the time of surgery involving cardiopulmonary bypass. However, sudden withdrawal of Sotazide might expose the patient to severe angina, arrhythmias, and even myocardial infarction.

If the drug is to be discontinued prior to surgery, especially in patients with ischaemic heart disease, then the drug should be withdrawn over a period of one week.

In the presence of Sotazide, anaesthesia may proceed provided that vagal dominance is counteracted by an intravenous injection of atropine sulphate (0.5–2 mg) immediately prior to induction of anaesthesia. Some anaesthetic agents such as ether, cyclopropane, trichloroethylene, methoxyflurane and enflurane appear to cause impairment of myocardial contractility in the presence of beta-receptor blockade. Caution is advised in the use of these agents in patients receiving Sotazide. No evidence of serious interaction has been found between nitrous oxide, halothane, or isoflurane and beta-receptor blockers. Raised pCO_2 levels should be avoided in patients receiving Sotazide.

Precautions: In view of the minimal myocardial depressant effect of sotalol and the lack of myocardial effect of hydrochlorothiazide, Sotazide has only a remote potential for precipitation or exacerbation of cardiac failure. Nevertheless, Sotazide should not be given to patients with cardiac decompensation unless incipient or established heart failure is controlled. At the first sign of impending cardiac failure or the progression of failure, Sotazide dosage should be reduced or discontinued.

The dosage of Sotazide should be decreased or therapy discontinued if the pulse rate falls below 50 beats/minute. Following a reduction in blood pressure, the dosage of Sotazide should not be increased before a stable level of blood pressure is attained.

Institution of concurrent therapy with drugs known to prolong the QT interval and/or to be associated with atypical ventricular tachycardia (AVT, torsade de pointes), especially quinidine, disopyramide, tricyclic antidepressants should be under close medical supervision.

Sudden withdrawal of treatment with beta-blockers in hypertensive patients with angina pectoris has induced severe and continuous angina in some cases. Although this effect has not been observed with Sotazide, should such a reaction occur, Sotazide treatment should be reinstituted and then withdrawn gradually by reducing the dosage over a period of weeks.

All patients receiving hydrochlorothiazide (as in Sotazide) therapy should be checked periodically for clinical signs of fluid or electrolyte imbalance: hyponatraemia, hypochloraemic alkalosis and hypokalaemia. Hypokalaemia can sensitise or exaggerate the response of the heart to the toxic effects of cardiac glycosides. With the lower dose of hydrochlorothiazide present in Sotazide, the possibility of any imbalance becomes less likely.

With the use of hydrochlorothiazide (as in Sotazide), serum protein-bound iodine may decrease without producing symptoms of thyroid disturbance.

Side-effects: The overall incidence of side-effects with Sotazide is low. The few reported adverse reactions were largely the pharmacological effects seen with the use of beta-blocking agents and diuretics. These reactions are mild, or moderate in intensity, most often transitory, and usually do not require interruption or withdrawal of therapy.

Sotalol, when used alone, is generally well tolerated. Dyspnoea, tiredness, dizziness, light-headedness, headache, fever and excessive bradycardia have been reported. Most of these side-effects are transient or disappear when the dosage is reduced.

There have been reports of skin rashes and/or dry eyes associated with the use of beta-adrenergic blocking drugs. The reported incidence is small and in most cases the symptoms have cleared when the treatment was withdrawn. Discontinuance of the drug should be considered if any such reaction is not otherwise explicable. Cessation of therapy with a beta-adrenergic blocker should be gradual.

Hyperuricaemia has been observed with thiazides but clinical gout is rare. Other side-effects for thiazides are documented but uncommon. Photosensitivity, anaphylactic reactions and depression of the formed elements of the blood have been reported.

The relevance of these observations to Sotazide therapy has not yet been determined.

Overdosage: If excessive bradycardia (and/or hypotension) occurs, atropine 0.5–2.0 mg should be given intravenously, immediately followed, if necessary, by a beta-receptor stimulating agent, such as isoprenaline, intravenously, 5 microgram/minute up to 25 microgram total dose.

Pharmaceutical precautions Store in a cool dry place. Protect tablets from light.

Legal category POM.

Package quantities Original packs of 28 – blister strips of 14 tablets with 2 strips per carton.

Further information Sotazide is an effective anti-hypertensive which combines sotalol hydrochloride, a beta-adrenergic blocking agent, and hydrochlorothiazide, a diuretic/antihypertensive. The concomitant use of these agents frequently produces a more pronounced anti-hypertensive effect than if either is used alone. By using lower doses than would be required if each agent were used alone, side-effects, especially the hypokalaemia associated with diuretics, are minimised. In hypertensive patients, where sodium and water retention is frequently a problem, the diuretic component will help control fluid imbalance.

Product licence number 0125/0113.

TOLERZIDE*

Presentation Tolerzide: circular, lilac, tablets containing 80 mg sotalol hydrochloride and 12.5 mg hydrochlorothiazide.

Other ingredients: Aluminium magnesium silicate, amaranth, lactose, magnesium stearate, microcrystalline cellulose, pregelatinised maize starch.

Uses In the management of mild or moderate hypertension particularly where a gradual fall in blood pressure is indicated such as in the elderly.

Dosage and administration Dose: one Tolerzide tablet daily.

Elderly: As sotalol is renally excreted dosage will need to be adjusted in patients with poor renal function and should be used with caution in patients with poor cardiac reserve.

Contra-indications, warnings, etc Tolerzide should not be used where there is evidence of heart block; history of bronchospasm; diabetic keto-acidosis; impending or uncontrolled cardiac failure; anaesthesia that produces myocardial depression; hypersensitivity to sotalol, hydrochlorothiazide or sulphonamide derivatives.

Since thiazides appear in breast milk, patients should stop nursing if the use of Tolerzide is essential.

Warnings:

Pregnancy: In animal studies Tolerzide has been shown to have no adverse teratogenic effects in doses up to 50 times the recommended human dose. However its safe use in human pregnancy has not been fully established.

Treated diabetes: Hypoglycaemic therapy may have to be altered in diabetics; Tolerzide may potentiate insulin hypoglycaemic effects and mask the symptoms of hypoglycaemia.

Hepatic/renal disease: Tolerzide should be used with caution in patients with impaired hepatic function or severe renal disease; such patients are particularly sensitive to alterations in fluid and electrolyte balance.

Thiazides may precipitate azotaemia. Cumulative effects of hydrochlorothiazide may develop in patients with impaired renal function.

Anaesthesia: It is not necessary to discontinue Tolerzide prior to most forms of elective surgery, although there is some doubt as to whether beta-receptor blockers should be continued up to the time of surgery involving cardiopulmonary bypass. However, sudden withdrawal of Tolerzide might expose the patient to severe angina, arrhythmias, and even myocardial infarction.

If the drug is to be discontinued prior to surgery, especially in patients with ischaemic heart disease, then the drug should be withdrawn over a period of one week.

In the presence of Tolerzide, anaesthesia may proceed provided that vagal dominance is counteracted by an intravenous injection of atropine sulphate (0.5-2 mg) immediately prior to induction of anaesthesia. Some anaesthetic agents such as ether, cyclopropane, trichloroethylene, methoxyflurane and enflurane appear to cause impairment of myocardial contractility in the presence of beta-receptor blockade. Caution is advised in the use of these agents in patients receiving Tolerzide. No evidence of serious interaction has been found between nitrous oxide, halothane, or isoflurane and beta-receptor blockers. Raised pCO_2 levels should be avoided in patients receiving Tolerzide.

Precautions: In view of the minimal myocardial depressant effect of sotalol and the lack of myocardial effect of hydrochlorothiazide, Tolerzide has only a remote potential for precipitation or exacerbation of cardiac failure. Nevertheless, Tolerzide should not be given to patients with cardiac decompensation unless incipient or established heart failure is controlled. At the first sign of impending cardiac failure or the progression of failure, Tolerzide dosage should be reduced or discontinued.

The dosage of Tolerzide should be decreased or therapy discontinued if the pulse rate falls below 50 beats/minute.

Sudden withdrawal of treatment with beta-blockers in hypertensive patients with angina pectoris has induced severe and continuous angina in some cases. Although this effect has not been observed with Tolerzide, should such a reaction occur, Tolerzide treatment should be re-instituted and then withdrawn gradually by reducing the dosage over a period of weeks.

All patients receiving hydrochlorothiazide (as in Tolerzide) therapy should be checked periodically for clinical signs of fluid or electrolyte imbalance: hyponatraemia, hypochloraemic alkalosis and hypokalaemia. Hypokalaemia can sensitise or exaggerate the response of the heart to the toxic effects of cardiac glycosides. With the lower dose of hydrochlorothiazide present in Tolerzide, the possibility of any imbalance becomes less likely.

With the use of hydrochlorothiazide (as in Tolerzide), serum protein bound iodine may decrease without producing symptoms of thyroid disturbance.

Side effects: The overall incidence of side effects with Tolerzide is low. The few reported adverse reactions are largely the pharmacological effects seen with the use of beta-blocking agents and diuretics. These reactions are mild or moderate in intensity, most often transitory, and usually do not require interruption or withdrawal of therapy.

Sotalol, when used alone, is generally well tolerated. Dyspnoea, tiredness, dizziness, light-headedness, headache, fever and excessive bradycardia have been reported. Most of these side effects are transient or disappear when the dosage is reduced, eg with the use of Tolerzide.

There have been reports of skin rashes and/or dry eyes associated with the use of beta-adrenergic blocking drugs. The reported incidence is small and in most cases the symptoms have cleared when the treatment was withdrawn. Discontinuance of the drug should be considered if any such reaction is not otherwise explicable. Cessation of therapy with a beta-adrenergic blocker should be gradual.

Hyperuricaemia has been observed with thiazides but clinical gout is rare. Other side effects for thiazides are documented but uncommon. Photosensitivity, anaphylactic reactions and depression of the formed elements of the blood have been reported.

The relevance of these observations to Tolerzide therapy has not yet been determined.

Overdosage: If excessive bradycardia (and/or hypotension) occurs atropine 0.5 to 2.0 mg should be given intravenously, immediately followed, if necessary, by a beta-receptor stimulating agent such as isoprenaline, intravenously, 5 microgram/minute up to 25 microgram total dose. Patients experiencing this effect on initial administration of Tolerzide should be removed temporarily from therapy. Tolerzide could be reintroduced at a lower dosage and then gradually increased.

Pharmaceutical precautions Store at room temperature.

Legal category POM.

Package quantities Tolerzide tablets: Original packs of 28 – blister strips of 14 tablets with 2 strips per carton.

Further information Tolerzide is an effective anti-hypertensive which combines sotalol hydrochloride, a beta-adrenergic blocking agent, and hydrochlorothiazide, a diuretic/anti-hypertensive. The concomitant use of these agents frequently produces a more pronounced antihypertensive effect than if either is used alone. By using lower doses than would be required if each agent were used alone, side effects, especially the hypokalaemia associated with diuretics, are minimised. In hypertensive patients where sodium and water retention is frequently a problem, the diuretic component will help control fluid imbalance.

Product licence number
Tolerzide tablets: 0125/0133

VEPESID* CAPSULES
VEPESID* INJECTION

Presentation Vepesid Injection-vials containing 100 mg etoposide in 5 ml.

Other ingredients: Benzyl alcohol, citric acid anhydrous, dehydrated ethanol, polyethylene glycol, polysorbate 80.

Vepesid Capsules-soft gelatin, pale pink capsules containing 50 mg and 100 mg etoposide.

Other ingredients: citric acid, glycerol, polyethylene glycol 400, water; gelatin capsules containing glycerol, iron oxide, sodium hydroxybenzoic acid, ethyl ester, sodium propyl hydroxybenzoate, titanium dioxide, water.

Uses Vepesid is an anti-neoplastic drug for intravenous or oral use, which can be used alone or in combination with other oncolytic drugs.

Present data indicate that Vepesid is applicable in the therapy of: small cell lung cancer, resistant non-seminomatous testicular carcinoma.

Dosage and administration The recommended course of Vepesid Injection is 60–120 mg/m², i.v., daily for five consecutive days. As Vepesid produces myelosuppression, courses may not be repeated more frequently than at 21 day intervals. In any case, repeat courses of Vepesid should not be given until the blood picture has been checked for evidence of myelosuppression and found to be satisfactory

Immediately before administration, the required dose of Vepesid Injection must be diluted with 0.9% saline solution for injection to give a solution concentration of not more than 0.25 mg/ml of etoposide; it should then be given by intravenous infusion over a period of not less than 30 minutes.

Care should be taken to avoid extravasation.

If oral dosing is preferred, twice the relevant i.v. dose should be given daily, for five consecutive days. As Vepesid produces myelosuppression, courses may not be repeated more frequently than at 21 day intervals. In any case, repeat courses of Vepesid should not be given until the blood picture has been checked for evidence of myelosuppression and found to be satisfactory.

Elderly: No dosage adjustment is necessary.

Paediatric use: Safety and effectiveness in children have not been established.

Contra-indications, warnings, etc Vepesid is contra-indicated in patients with severe hepatic dysfunction or in those patients who have demonstrated hypersensitivity to the drug.

Vepesid must not be given by intra-cavity injection.

Warnings

Use in pregnancy: Vepesid should not normally be administered to patients who are pregnant or to mothers who are breast feeding. Safe use in pregnancy has not been established.

Vepesid is teratogenic in rats at dose levels equivalent to those employed clinically.

The influence of Vepesid on human reproduction has not been determined.

In-vitro tests indicate that Vepesid is mutagenic.

Precautions: Vepesid should be administered by individuals experienced in the use of antineoplastic therapy.

When Vepesid is administered intravenously care should be taken to avoid extravasation.

If radiotherapy and/or chemotherapy has been given prior to starting Vepesid treatment, an adequate interval should be allowed to enable the bone marrow to recover. If the leucocyte count falls below 2,000/mm^3, treatment should be suspended until the circulating blood elements have returned to acceptable levels (platelets above 100,000 mm^3, leucocytes above 4,000/mm^3), this is usually within 10 days.

Peripheral blood counts and liver function should be monitored. (See Adverse Reactions.)

Bacterial infections should be brought under control before treatment with Vepesid commences.

Adverse reactions: Haematological: The dose limiting toxicity of Vepesid is myelosuppression, predominantly leucopenia and thrombocytopenia. Anaemia occurs infrequently.

The leucocyte count nadir occurs approximately 21 days after treatment.

Alopecia: Alopecia occurs in approximately 66% of patients and is reversible on cessation of therapy.

Gastrointestinal: Nausea and vomiting are the major gastrointestinal toxicities and occur in approximately 30–40% of patients. Anti-emetics are useful in controlling these side effects. Abdominal pain, diarrhoea and anorexia occur infrequently.

Other Toxicities: Hypotension may occur following an excessively rapid infusion and may be reversed by slowing the infusion rate.

Anaphylactic-like reactions have been reported rarely following administration of Vepesid. Reactions respond to cessation of therapy and administration of an anti-histamine.

Vepesid has been shown to reach high concentrations in the liver and kidney, thus presenting a potential for accumulation in cases of functional impairment. Fever, pigmentation, pruritus, dysphagia and transient cortical blindness have also been reported following the administration of Vepesid.

Pharmaceutical precautions Vepesid injection should be stored at room temperature. The injection should be protected from light. Vepesid capsules should be stored between 10°–25°C. Do not open any blister in which there is evidence of capsule leakage.

Preparation of intravenous solution: Immediately before administration the required dose of Vepesid Injection must be diluted with 0.9% saline solution for injection to give a solution concentration of not more than 0.25 mg/ml of etoposide; it should then be given by intravenous infusion over a period of not less than 30 minutes. The infusion solution should be kept at room temperature and should be used within six hours of preparation. Solutions of concentration greater than 0.25 mg/ml may show signs of precipitation, and are therefore not recommended. Any solutions showing signs of precipitation should be discarded.

The intravenous solution is suitable for infusion in glass or PVC containers.

Vepesid should not be physically mixed with any other drug.

Guidelines for the safe handling of antineoplastic agents:

1. Trained personnel should reconstitute the drug.
2. This should be performed in a designated area.
3. Adequate protective gloves should be worn.
4. Precautions should be taken to avoid the drug accidentally coming into contact with the eyes. In the event of contact with the eyes, irrigate with large amounts of water and/or saline.
5. The cytotoxic preparation should not be handled by pregnant staff.
6. Adequate care and precautions should be taken in the disposal of items (syringes, needles etc) used to reconstitute cytotoxic drugs. Excess material and body waste may be disposed of by placing in double sealed polythene bags and incinerating at a temperature of 1,000°C. Liquid waste may be flushed with copious amounts of water.
7. The work surface should be covered with disposable plastic-backed absorbent paper.
8. Use Luer-Lock fittings on all syringes and sets. Large bore needles are recommended to minimise pressure and the possible formation of aerosols. The latter may also be reduced by the use of a venting needle.

Legal category POM.

Package quantities Vepesid injection is packed in cartons of 10 vials, each vial containing 100 mg etoposide in 5 ml of solution.

Vepesid 100 mg capsules are packed in blister packs of 10 capsules, each capsule containing 100 mg etoposide.

Vepesid 50 mg capsules are packed in blister packs of 20 capsules, each capsule containing 50 mg etoposide.

Further information Etoposide is a semisynthetic derivative of podophyllotoxin.

Experimental data indicate that etoposide arrests the cell cycle in the G_2 phase. Etoposide differs from the vinca alkaloids in that it does not cause an accumulation of cells in metaphase, but prevents cells from entering mitosis or destroys cells in the G_2 phase. The incorporation of thymidine into DNA is inhibited in-vitro by etoposide. Etoposide does not interfere with microtubule assembly. Etoposide is approximately 94% protein-bound in human serum. Plasma decay kinetics follow a bi-exponential curve and correspond to a two compartmental model. The mean volume of distribution is approximately 32% of body weight. Etoposide demonstrates relatively poor penetration into the cerebrospinal fluid. Urinary excretion is approximately 45% of an administered dose, 29% being excreted unchanged in 72 hours.

An information sheet on the storage, preparation and handling of the product is available

Product licence numbers

Vepesid 50 mg Capsules	0125/0153
Vepesid 100 mg Capsules	0125/0124
Vepesid Injection	0125/0121

**Trade Mark*

Britannia Pharmaceuticals Limited

Forum House
41–51 Brighton Road
Redhill
Surrey RH1 6YS

ELDEPRYL*

Presentation White, scored, uncoated tablets 6 mm diameter containing 5 mg selegiline hydrochloride.

Uses
Properties: Eldepryl is a selective MAO-B inhibitor which prevents dopamine breakdown in the brain. It also inhibits the re-uptake of dopamine at the pre-synaptic dopamine receptor. These effects potentiate dopaminergic function in the brain and help to even out and prolong the effect of exogenous or endogenous dopamine.

Recent studies have demonstrated that use of selegiline in previously untreated patients can delay the development of disability and prolong the time before levodopa therapy is required. Eldepryl potentiates and prolongs the effect of levodopa in the treatment of parkinsonism. The addition of Eldepryl to levodopa (with or without decarboxylase inhibitor) therapy helps to alleviate dose related fluctuations and end-of-dose deterioration. At a later stage in the disease it can also smooth the symptoms of the on/off effect.

Unlike conventional MAO inhibitors, which inhibit both the MAO-A and MAO-B enzyme, Eldepryl is a specific MAO-B inhibitor and can be given safely with levodopa. There are no dietary restrictions associated with Eldepryl treatment, i.e. it does not cause the so called 'cheese effect'.

Indications: Eldepryl is indicated for the treatment of Parkinson's disease, or symptomatic parkinsonism. Eldepryl may be used alone in early Parkinson's disease to delay the need for levodopa (with or without decarboxylase inhibitor). Eldepryl may also be used as an adjunct to levodopa (with or without decarboxylase inhibitor).

Dosage and administration Eldepryl 10 mg (2 tablets) daily either alone or as an adjunct to levodopa or levodopa/peripheral decarboxylase inhibitor.

Eldepryl may be administered either as a single dose in the morning or in two divided doses of 5 mg taken at breakfast and lunch.

When Eldepryl is added to a levodopa regimen it is possible to reduce the levodopa dosage by an average of 30 per cent.

Contra-indications, warnings, etc
Contra-indications: None.

Interactions: Selegiline should not be given in conjunction with non-specific monoamine oxidase inhibitors.

Use in pregnancy: Eldepryl is indicated for parkinsonism. This tends to be a disease of the elderly past child-bearing age. No work has been done to assess the effects of selegiline on pregnancy and lactation, thus it should not be used in such cases.

Precautions: Because Eldepryl potentiates the effects of levodopa the side effects of levodopa might be emphasised, particularly when the patient is on a very high dosage of levodopa. The addition of Eldepryl to maximal doses of levodopa may cause involuntary movement and/or agitation. Such side effects disappear when the levodopa dosage is decreased. Levodopa treatment can be reduced by an average of 30 per cent when Eldepryl is added to the treatment. When an optimal levodopa dose has been established, the side effects of the combination have been found to be fewer than for levodopa alone.

Side effects: Hypotension and nausea have been reported as isolated symptoms associated with Eldepryl treatment. Confusion or psychosis have also been reported.

Treatment of overdosage: Eldepryl has such a low toxicity that no overdosage problems have been encountered. Selegiline hydrochloride is rapidly metabolised and the metabolites rapidly excreted. In cases of suspected overdosage the patient should be kept under observation for 24–48 hours.

Pharmaceutical precautions Protect from heat, moisture and light.

Legal category POM.

Package quantities 100 tablets.

Further information Nil.

Product licence number 4483/0024.

RIMSO-50*

Presentation Sterile aqueous solution containing dimethyl sulphoxide 50% w/w in water.

Uses Indicated only for the symptomatic relief of patients with interstitial cystitis (Hunner's Ulcer).
For bladder instillation only.
Not for IM or IV injection.

Dosage and administration Instillation of 50 ml of Rimso-50 (dimethyl sulphoxide) directly into the bladder may be accomplished by catheter or bladder syringe and allowed to remain for 15 minutes. Application of an analgesic lubricant gel such as lignocaine jelly to the urethra is suggested prior to the insertion of the catheter to avoid spasm. The medication is expelled by spontaneous voiding. It is recommended that treatment be repeated every two weeks until maximum symptomatic relief is obtained. Thereafter, time intervals between therapy may be increased appropriately. In selected cases where symptomatic relief is not complete, the bladder may be gently distended by gravity instillation with up to 500 ml of a solution prepared immediately prior to instillation in a glass bottle, with one part Rimso-50 and one part sterile water prior to the instillation of the standard dose of 50 ml of Rimso-50. After retention of Rimso-50 for 15 minutes the medication is again expelled by spontaneous voiding. Administration of oral analgesic medication prior to instillation of Rimso-50 can reduce bladder spasm in particularly sensitive patients.

In patients with very sensitive bladders, the treatment should be done under anaesthesia (preferably saddle block type).

Rimso-50 is recommended for bladder instillation only.

Contra-indications, warnings, etc
Contra-indications: None.

Precautions: Changes in the refractive index and lens opacities have been seen in monkeys, dogs and rats given dimethyl sulphoxide chronically. No ophthalmic changes attributable to intravesical instillation of dimethyl sulphoxide have been reported in patients carefully followed for up to 17 months; nevertheless, full eye evaluations, including slit lamp examinations, are recommended prior to and at six months intervals during treatment.

Along with the ophthalmological examinations, patients should be investigated with respect to biochemical parameters, particularly renal and hepatic function, at six month intervals.

Intravesical instillation of Rimso-50 may be harmful to patients with urinary tract malignancy because of dimethyl sulphoxide-induced vasodilation.

Warnings: Dimethyl sulphoxide can initiate the liberation of histamine and there has been an occasional hypersensitivity reaction with topical administration of dimethyl sulphoxide. This hypersensitivity has not occurred in patients receiving intravesical Rimso-50; however, the physician should be cognizant of this possibility in prescribing Rimso-50. If anaphylactoid symptoms develop, appropriate therapy should be instituted. Some data indicates that dimethyl sulphoxide potentiates other concomitantly administered medications.

Use in pregnancy: The safety of dimethyl sulphoxide for the human foetus has not been established, hence it should be given to pregnant women only when the potential benefits to the mother have been weighed against possible hazards to the child.

Pharmaceutical precautions Store in a cool place protected from light.

Legal category POM.

Package quantities Bottles of 50 ml.

Further information Nil.

Product licence number 4047/0001.

VIRAZID*

Presentation Virazid is a sterile lyophilised powder of ribavirin to be reconstituted for aerosol administration. Each 100 ml glass vial contains 6 g of ribavirin and, when reconstituted to the correct volume of 300 ml with Water for Injections BP, the solution will contain 20 mg/ml ribavirin at a pH of approximately 5.5.

Uses Virazid is indicated in the treatment of infants and children with severe respiratory syncytial virus (RSV) bronchiolitis.

Dosage and administration Aerosol administration or nebulisation should be carried out in a small particle aerosol generator (SPAG). Before use read the SPAG Operator's Manual for instructions.

Dosage: Ribavirin aerosol is only recommended for use in infants and children.

Treatment is carried out for 12–18 hours per day for at least 3 and no more than 7 days and is part of a total treatment programme.

The concentration of ribavirin in the reservoir is 20 mg/ml in the SPAG unit and the average concentration for a 7 hour period is 190 micrograms/l of air.

Administration: By aseptic technique dissolve the powder in Water for Injections BP in the 100 ml vial. The solution should be adequately mixed to ensure complete dissolution. It is not recommended that this solution is heated during dissolution. Transfer to the clean sterilised 500 ml flask and dilute to a final volume of 300 ml with Water for Injections BP. The final concentration should be 20 mg/ml.

The aerosol is delivered to an infant oxygen hood from the SPAG aerosol generator. Administration by face mask or oxygen tent may be necessary if a hood cannot be employed (See SPAG Operator's Manual).

However, the volume of distribution and condensation area are larger in a tent and the efficacy of this method of administration has been evaluated only in a small number of patients.

Important: Ribavirin aerosol is more effective when instituted within the first 3 days of the treatment of bronchiolitis. Treatment early in the course of the disease may be necessary to achieve efficacy.

Treatment with Virazid must be accompanied by, and does not replace, standard supportive respiratory and fluid management for infants and children with severe respiratory tract infection.

Nebulised bronchodilators, when clinically indicated, should be administered with the SPAG generator turned off.

The Water for Injections BP used to make up the Virazid solution should not have any antimicrobial agent or any other substance added and all solutions should be inspected for particulate matter and discolouration prior to administration.

Contra-indications, warnings, etc *Contra-indications:* Ribavirin is contra-indicated in females who are or may become pregnant and it should be noted that ribavirin can be detected in human blood even four weeks after oral administration has ceased.

Warnings: Precipitation of the drug in respiratory equipment and consequent accumulation of fluid in the tubing has caused difficulties for patients requiring assisted ventilation.

In infants requiring assisted ventilation Virazid should only be used when there is constant monitoring of both patients and equipment.

Directions for use during assisted ventilation are given in the SPAG manual which should be read carefully before such administration.

Side-effects: Several serious adverse events occurred in severely ill infants with life-threatening underlying disease many of whom required assisted ventilation. These events included worsening of respiratory status, bacterial pneumonia and pneumothorax. The role of ribavirin aerosol in these events has not been determined.

Anaemia has been reported with oral and intravenous administration but no such incidents have been reported with aerosol administration. Reticulocytosis has been reported with aerosol use.

Overdoses: No overdoses have been reported.

Pharmaceutical precautions Vials containing the lyophilised powder should be stored in a cool dry place at room temperature (15–25°C). Newly reconstituted solutions should be used within 24 hours. After administration during any 24 hour period any remaining solution must be discarded.

Legal category POM.

Package quantities Virazid is supplied as a tri-pack containing three 6 g vials of ribavirin lyophilised powder.

Further information Virazid is intended for use as an aerosol only.

Nebulised Virazid may potentially escape into the hospital environment during therapy. However ribavirin was not detected in the erythrocytes, plasma or urine of subjects exposed for a mean of 25 hours during 5 consecutive days.

Although there are no pertinent human data, oral ribavirin has been found to be teratogenic in tested rodent species. Pregnant baboons given up to 120 mg/kg/day orally over a four day period and within twenty days of gestation failed to exhibit any teratogenic effects.

Ribavirin is active *in vitro* against a wide spectrum of viruses, including influenzae and herpes viruses.

In inhibitory activity of ribavirin on RSV in cell cultures is selective. The mechanism of action is unknown but there is evidence that ribavirin interferes with protein translation by mRNA, possibly the result of interference with formation of the 5′ cap structure of mRNA.

Product licence number 4657/0004.

**Trade Mark*

Brocades (Great Britain) Limited
Brocades House
Pyrford Road
West Byfleet, Surrey

AMFIPEN* CAPSULES
AMFIPEN* SYRUP
AMFIPEN* SYRUP FORTE

Presentation Amfipen Capsules (Ampicillin Capsules BP) are presented as grey and red capsules each containing 250 mg or 500 mg Ampicillin BP, imprinted 'Amfipen 250' or 'Amfipen 500'. The inactive ingredients of Amfipen Capsules include lactose.

Amfipen Syrup (Ampicillin Mixture BPC) and Amfipen Syrup Forte (Strong Ampicillin Mixture BPC) are presented as bottles containing dry powder for the preparation of 100 ml of an orange-pink or pink-coloured suspension. On reconstitution with 50 ml or 48 ml purified water respectively each 5 ml dose contains 125 mg or 250 mg Ampicillin BP respectively. The inactive ingredients of Amfipen Syrup include sodium benzoate, propyl and methyl paraben, amaranth, sunset yellow, and sucrose; those of Amfipen Syrup Forte include, in addition, amaranth.

Uses Amfipen is a broad-spectrum penicillin for the treatment of a wide range of infections caused by ampicillin-sensitive organisms.

Dosage and administration
Usual oral dosage for adults:

Ear, nose and throat infections: 250 mg four times a day.

Bronchitis in infections exacerbations of chronic obstructive airways disease: usually 250 mg four times a day in routine therapy; 1 g four times a day in high-dosage regimes.

Pneumonia: 500 mg four times a day.

Gastro-intestinal infection: 500–750 mg three or four times daily.

Urinary tract infections: 500 mg four times daily.

Enteric fevers: in acute cases 1–2 g four times a day for 14 days; carriers should be treated with this dosage for 4–12 weeks.

In the treatment of gonorrhoea 2 g should be given with 1 g probenecid as a single dose. In the treatment of females repeated doses are recommended.

Usual oral dosage for the elderly: As for adults; reduced doses may be required in those with impaired renal function.

Usual children's oral dosage: Half of the adult dosage.

The above oral dosages are recommended dosages only, as a guide. In severe infections the dosages may be increased. Amfipen should be given orally a half to one hour before meals.

Administration: Amfipen may be administered orally as capsules or syrup or syrup forte.

Contra-indications, warnings, etc
Contra-indications: Contra-indicated in patients with penicillin/cephalosporin hypersensitivity and glandular fever.

Interactions: As with all ampicillins, Amfipen may reduce the efficacy of oral contraceptives and patients should be warned accordingly.

Allopurinol increases ampicillin induced skin reactions. Tetracyclines, erythromycin and chloramphenicol antagonise the action of ampicillin.

Side-effects: Pseudomembranous colitis may rarely occur. Skin reactions may occur rarely, and be due to either penicillin hypersensitivity (urticarial rash) or specific ampicillin sensitivity (erythematous rash); treatment should be discontinued if a rash occurs. Occasionally, diarrhoea may occur. Superinfection by resistant organisms may occur following prolonged use.

Use in pregnancy and lactation: Ampicillin crosses the placenta. Cord blood levels may equal those in the maternal circulation and ampicillin is detectable in the amniotic fluid for 24–36 hours after injection of the mother. Complete safety in all stages of pregnancy has not been established.

Concentrations in breast milk in the region of 70 mcg/ml follow a 500 mg dose. The amount likely to be taken by a feeding infant would be well below the paediatric dose.

Overdosage: Although ampicillin is usually safe, some toxic effects associated with the central nervous system occasionally occur. Apart from allergic reactions (skin rashes, eosinophilia, fever etc.) diarrhoea, vomiting and abdominal pains may occur.

From a theoretical consideration, oral overdose would perhaps best be treated by gastric lavage. Renal dialysis has been found effective in lowering ampicillin blood levels and would therefore be indicated in cases of both oral and parenteral overdosage.

Pharmaceutical precautions Amfipen preparations should be stored in a cool dry place. On reconstitution with 50 ml or 48 ml respectively of purified water, Amfipen Syrup and Amfipen Syrup Forte should be used within seven days if stored in a cool place.

In order to obtain a homogeneous suspension it is recommended that the bottle be well shaken before reconstitution of the syrup.

Legal category POM.

Package quantities *Amfipen Capsules 250 mg:* Bottles of 250.

Amfipen capsules 500 mg: Bottles of 250.

Amfipen Syrup and Syrup Forte: Bottles for the preparation of 100 ml (OP).

Further information Each 5 ml of the syrup presentation contains ca 4.1 g sucrose.

Product licence numbers

Amfipen Capsules 250 mg	0166/0065
Amfipen Capsules 500 mg	0166/0066
Amfipen Syrup	0166/0067
Amfipen Syrup Forte	0166/0068
Amfipen Injection 250 mg	0166/0069
Amfipen Injection 500 mg	0166/0070

BICILLIN* INJECTION

Presentation Bicillin Injection is presented as vials of dry powder for the preparation of Fortified Procaine Penicillin Injection BP. Each vial contains 1.8 mega units (1.8 g) procaine penicillin EP and 0.6 mega unit (0.36 g) benzylpenicillin sodium EP. The inactive ingredients of Bicillin are polyoxyethylene, sorbitan mono-oleate, sodium citrate, and citric acid.

Uses Antibiotic for the treatment of infections due to penicillin-sensitive organisms, where prolonged release is desired.

Dosage and administration For intramuscular injection only.

Adults and the elderly: 400,000 units (300 mg procaine penicillin and 60 mg benzylpenicillin sodium) 24-hourly or 12-hourly, or as directed by the physician.

Children: Over 25 kg as for adults; under 25 kg proportionally to body weight, or as directed by the physician.

In acute uncomplicated gonorrhoea: Up to 12 ml, as a single dose, or as directed by the physician.

In early syphilis: 3 ml (4 ml in heavier patients), or as directed by the physician.

Contra-indications, warnings, etc
Contra-indications: Hypersensitivity to penicillin or procaine.

Interactions: Probenecid delays the excretion of penicillin.

Side-effects: Skin reactions may occur but usually resolve on cessation of therapy. Generalised, systemic reactions are rare and usually associated with a history of allergy or penicillin intolerance.

Use in pregnancy and lactation: The safety of Bicillin Injection in these circumstances has not been established.

Overdosage: General supportive measures may be indicated.

Pharmaceutical precautions Store in a cool place. Upon constitution the preparation is for single-dose use only. It may be kept at 2°C–8°C for up to 24 hours after constitution, but must be discarded after the first usage or at the end of that period of 24 hours.

Legal category POM.

Package quantities Boxes of 10 vials each containing 2.4 mega units (1.8 g procaine penicilllin and 0.36 g benzylpenicillin sodium) per vial.

Further information Reconstitution with 4.6 ml Water for Injections BP produces 6 ml; each ml of suspension contains 300,000 units (300 mg) procaine penicillin and 100,000 units (60 mg) benzylpenicillin sodium.

Product licence number 0166/0147.

BROCADOPA* CAPSULES

Presentation Brocadopa is presented as clear colourless hard gelatine capsules each containing 125 mg, 250 mg or 500 mg Levodopa BP, imprinted 'Brocadopa 125', '250' or '500'. Brocadopa Capsules comply with the monograph for Levodopa Capsules BP. Brocadopa Capsules contain no inactive ingredients which require disclosure.

Uses Dopaminergic, for the treatment of all forms of Parkinsonism, except drug-induced (neuroleptic syndrome).

Dosage and administration By oral administration.
Adults: Initially 250 mg daily in divided doses, increasing by 250 mg every three to four days until optimal response is obtained. This may occur at any level between 1 g and 8 g daily in divided doses after a period of four to six weeks.

Elderly: Generally as for adults; levodopa tolerance is less in the elderly, and more severe hypotensive side-effects are produced, especially in those with a history of myocardial infarction.

Children: No recommendation made.

Contra-indications, warnings, etc
Contra-indications: Narrow-angle glaucoma, presence of severe psychoses or neuroses, or malignant melanoma, administration with, or within 2 weeks of, monoamineoxidase inhibitors, or with anti-psychotic drugs.

Interactions: Pyridoxine blocks the action of levodopa. Concurrent administration of hypotensive agents (e.g. resperine and methyldopa), phenothiazines, butyrophenones, thioxanthines, amphetamines, and tricyclic anti-depressants, is to be avoided or approached with caution.

Side-effects: Gastro-intestinal disturbances, such as nausea, vomiting and anorexia, are the commonest side-effects and occur early. They may be diminished by administration after food and by finer fractionation of the daily dose. A non-phenothiazine anti-emetic drug may be given half an hour before each dose.

Hypotension, generally postural in type, may occur, usually unaccompanied by symptoms or change in pulse rate. Smaller dosage increments will reduce the incidence.

Involuntary movements usually occur at higher dosage level, and may be alleviated by a small reduction in dosage of 0.5–1 g daily or by fractionation of dosage.

Psychic manifestations such as restlessness and nervousness may occur with some disturbance of sleep. More rarely, agitation or mania with hallucinations have been reported. Psychiatric side-effects are more likely to occur in patients with a pre-existing psychosis but may be diminished or abolished by reduction or cessation of dosage.

Cardiac disturbances, e.g. paroxysmal tachycardia and arrhythmias, have been reported. It may be advisable to stop dosage and recommence at a lower level.

Rarely, headache and peripheral neuropathy have been reported.

Use in pregnancy: Levodopa is not recommended in pregnancy. There is no evidence of harmful effect in pregnancy in animals but inadequate evidence of the safety of the drug in human pregnancy. It has been in wide use for many years without apparent ill consequence, but should not be used unless absolutely indicated.

Other warnings and precautions: Administer with caution in patients with endocrine, renal, hepatic, pulmonary or cardiac disease, or peptic ulcer. Periodic evaluation of hepatic, haemopoietic, renal and cardiac functions are advisory.

Overdosage: Overdosage would be associated with symptomatology of side-effects; gastric lavage, airway maintenance and surveillance for arrhythmias by ECG may be needed. IV fluids may be required and if necessary anti-arrythmic therapy.

Pharmaceutical precautions Normal pharmaceutical storage and handling are indicated.

Legal category POM.

Package quantities *Capsules:* 250 × 125 mg, 250 × 250 mg, and 250 × 500 mg.

Further information Nil.

Product licence numbers

Brocadopa Capsules 125 mg	0166/5013
Brocadopa Capsules 250 mg	0166/5014
Brocadopa Capsules 500 mg	0166/5015

CONDYLINE*

Presentation Condyline is presented as a clear colourless alcoholic solution containing 0.5% podophyllotoxin in vials of 3.5 ml, with a suitable quantity of special applicators.

Uses For the topical treatment of condylomata acuminata affecting the penis or the female external genitalia.

Dosage and administration By topical administration.

Adults and the elderly: Apply twice daily for three days directly to the warts. Allow to dry after treatment.

Use the applicator provided, applying not more than 50 applicators-full for each application.

This three-day treatment may be repeated, if necessary, at weekly intervals, for a total of five weeks of treatment.

Lesions in the female, and lesions greater than 4 cm^2 in the male, should be treated under direct medical supervision.

Children: Not recommended.

Contra-indications, warnings, etc
Contra-indications: Hypersensitivity to podophyllotoxin.

Special precautions: Avoid contact with healthy skin; lesions in the female, and lesions greater than 4 cm^2 in the male, should be treated under direct medical supervision. Do not use on open wounds following surgical procedures.

Side-effects: Local irritation, usually mild, may occur.

Overdosage: In topical overdosage, wash well with soap and water; if the eyes are involved bathe thoroughly with water. If accidentally ingested give stomach washout and monitor electrolyte balance, blood gases, liver function and blood picture.

Pharmaceutical precautions Normal pharmaceutical storage and handling are indicated.

Legal category POM.

Package quantities 3.5 ml, in an amber glass vial, fitted with a child-proof cap, together with a suitable quantity of special applicators (OP).

Further information The product should be discarded six weeks after first opening the vial. Keep away from naked flames.

Product licence number 0166/0142.

CYCLOSPASMOL* SUSPENSION

Presentation Cyclospasmol Suspension is presented as a dry powder, ready for reconstitution at the time of dispensing by the addition of 375 ml distilled water. The resulting suspension provides 90 doses each of 5 ml, each 5 ml dose containing 400 mg cyclandelate. The inactive ingredients in Cyclospasmol Suspension include methyl paraben, sodium paracombin, and sucrose.

Uses For the treatment of organic vasospastic peripheral and cerebrovascular diseases associated with impaired circulation, especially in the long-term management of chronic insufficiency and in the sequelae of strokes, and in the improvement of mental function, dementia, confusion etc., and in intermittent claudication, Raynaud's phenomenon, chilblains, night cramps, acrocyanosis, cold hands and feet, etc.

Dosage and administration By oral administration.

Adults and the elderly: 1,600 mg (20 ml) daily in 2 or 4 divided doses.

Children: A dosage for children has not been established.

Contra-indications, warnings, etc Contra-indicated in the acute phase of a cerebrovascular accident.

Special precautions: None.

Side-effects: At very high dosage, nausea, gastro-intestinal distress or flushing may occur.

Overdosage: Gross overdosages have not been reported; theoretically circulatory collapse could occur and treatment would be gastric lavage and, if necessary, vasopressors.

Pharmaceutical precautions Normal pharmaceutical storage and handling are indicated. Upon reconstitution, Cyclospasmol suspension carries an expiry date of 3 months from the date of reconstitution.

Legal category P.

Package quantities Each bottle, after reconstitution, provides 90 doses each of 400 mg cyclandelate in 5 ml, as an original pack (OP).

Further information Each 5 ml dose contains approximately 500 mg sucrose. For maximum therapeutic effect it is recommended that the daily dose of 1,600 mg be given; maximal therapeutic response may not be seen within the first one or two months of treatment.

Product licence number 0166/0062.

CYCLOSPASMOL* TABLETS
CYCLOSPASMOL* CAPSULES

Presentation Cyclospasmol is presented as pink sugar-coated tablets each containing 400 mg cyclandelate, imprinted 'Cyclospasmol'; and as pink/grey hard gelatine capsules each containing 400 mg cyclandelate, imprinted 'Cyclospasmol'. The inactive ingredients in Cyclospasmol tablets include sucrose; those in Cyclospasmol capsules do not require disclosure.

Uses For the treatment of organic vasospastic peripheral and cerebrovascular diseases associated with impaired circulation, especially in the long-term management of chronic insufficiency and in the sequelae of strokes, and in the improvement of mental function, dementia, confusion, etc., and in intermittent claudication, Raynaud's phenomenon, chilblains, night cramps, acrocyanosis, cold hands and feet, etc.

Dosage and administration By oral administration.

Adults and the elderly: 1,600 mg daily in 2 or 4 divided doses.

Children: A dosage for children has not been established.

Contra-indications, warnings, etc
Contra-indicated in the acute phase of a cerebrovascular accident.

Special precautions: None.

Side-effects: At very high dosages, nausea, gastro-intestinal distress or flushing may occur.

Overdosage: Gross overdosages have not been reported; theoretically circulatory collapse could occur and treatment would be gastric lavage and, if necessary, vasopressors.

Pharmaceutical precautions Normal pharmaceutical storage and handling are indicated.

Legal category P.

Package quantities
Cyclospasmol Tablets: Treatment pack of 112 tablets as an original pack (OP).
Cyclospasmol Capsules: Treatment pack of 112 capsules as an original pack (OP).

Further information For maximum therapeutic effect, it is recommended that the daily dosage of 1,600 mg be given; maximal therapeutic response may not be seen within the first one or two months of treatment. Cyclospasmol tablets contain ca 170 mg sucrose per tablet.

Product licence numbers

Cyclospasmol Capsules	0166/0021
Cyclospasmol Tablets	0166/0052

DE-NOL*

Presentation De-Nol is presented as a clear red liquid containing 120 mg tri-potassium di-citrato bismuthate (calculated as Bi_2O_3) in each 5 ml. The inactive ingredients in De-Nol include ethanol and sucrose.

Uses Ulcer healing agent. For the treatment of gastric and duodenal ulcers.

Dosage and administration By oral administration. Each dose is to be diluted with 15 ml of water.

Adults and the elderly: Two 5 ml spoonsful twice daily (half an hour before breakfast and half an hour before the evening meal). Alternatively, one 5 ml spoonful four times a day (half an hour before each of the three main meals of the day and two hours after the evening meal). The treatment course should be taken for the full 28-day period and it is important that a dose is not missed. If necessary, one further course of therapy may be given. Maintenance therapy with De-Nol is not indicated, but treatment may be repeated after an interval of one month.

Children: Not recommended.

Milk should not be drunk by itself during the course of treatment as this can prevent the medicine from working properly. Small quantities of milk on breakfast cereal or in tea or coffee taken with meals are permissible. Antacids should not be taken for half an hour before or half an hour after taking a dose of De-Nol as these can interfere with the action of the drug.

Contra-indications, warnings, etc
Contra-indications: De-Nol should not be administered to patients with renal disorders, and on theoretical grounds is contra-indicated in pregnancy.

Interactions: De-Nol may inhibit the efficacy of orally administered tetracyclines.

Side effects: Blackening of the stool usually occurs; darkening of the tongue, nausea and vomiting have been reported.

Overdosage: Extremely few cases of overdosage have occurred; contact the company for further information.

Pharmaceutical precautions Normal pharmaceutical storage and handling are indicated.

Legal category P.

Package quantities Treatment pack of 560 ml as an original pack (OP).

Further information Some patients with an associated gastritis may experience an initial discomfort whilst taking De-Nol. Each 5 ml dose contains ca 100 mg ethanol and 500 mg sucrose.

Product licence number 0166/5024.

DE-NOLTAB*

Presentation De-Noltab is presented as a round white film-coated tablet, marked gbr 152, each tablet containing 120 mg tri-potassium di-citrato bismuthate (calculated as Bi_2O_3). De-Noltab contains no inactive ingredients which require disclosure.

Uses Ulcer healing agent. For the treatment of gastric and duodenal ulcers.

Dosage and administration By oral administration. Each dose is to be swallowed with half a tumblerful of water.

Adults: Two tablets twice daily (half an hour before breakfast and half an hour before the evening meal). Alternatively, one tablet four times a day (half an hour before each of the three main meals of the day and two hours after the evening meal). The treatment course should be taken for the full 28-day period and it is important that a dose is not missed. If necessary, one further course of therapy may be given. Maintenance therapy with De-Noltab is not indicated, but treatment may be repeated after an interval of one month.

Children: Not recommended.

Milk should not be drunk by itself during the course of treatment as this can prevent the medicine from working properly. Small quantities of milk on breakfast cereal or in tea or coffee taken with meals are permissible. Antacids should not be taken for half an hour before or half an hour after taking a dose of De-Noltab as these can interfere with the action of the drug.

Contra-indications, warnings, etc
Contra-indications: De-Noltab should not be administered to patients with renal disorders, and on theoretical grounds is contra-indicated in pregnancy.

Interactions: De-Noltab may inhibit the efficacy of orally administered tetracyclines.

Side effects: Blackening of the stool usually occurs; nausea and vomiting have been reported.

Overdosage: Extremely few cases of overdosage have occurred; contact the company for further information.

Pharmaceutical precautions Normal pharmaceutical storage and handling are indicated.

Legal category P.

Package quantities Treatment pack of 112 tablets, in foil strips of eight, as an original pack (OP).

Further information Nil.

Product licence number 0166/0124.

DISIPAL* TABLETS

Presentation Disipal Tablets are presented as yellow sugar-coated tablets each containing 50 mg Orphenadrine Hydrochloride BP, imprinted 'Disipal'. Disipal Tablets comply with the monograph for Orphenadrine Hydrochloride Tablets BP. The inactive ingredients in Disipal Tablets include lactose, sucrose, amaranth, tartrazine and sunset yellow.

Uses Anticholinergic, for the treatment of all forms of Parkinsonism, including drug-induced (neuroleptic syndrome).

Dosage and administration *By oral administration: Adults and the elderly:* Initially 150 mg daily in divided doses, increasing by 50 mg every two or three days until maximum benefit is obtained. Optimal dosage is usually 250–300 mg daily in divided doses in idiopathic and post-encephalitic Parkinsonism, 100–150 mg daily in divided doses in arteriosclerotic Parkinsonism, and 150–300 mg daily in divided doses in the neuroleptic syndrome. Maximal dosage, 400 mg daily in divided doses. The elderly may be more susceptible to side-effects at doses which are clinically optimal.

Children: A dosage for children has not been established.

Contra-indications, warnings, etc
Contra-indications: Contra-indicated in patients with tardive dyskinesia, glaucoma or prostatic hypertrophy.

Special precautions: Use with caution in patients with micturition difficulties or in pregnancy, and in the presence of cardiovascular disease and hepatic or renal impairment. Avoid abrupt discontinuation of treatment. For some patients orphenadrine may be a drug of abuse.

Side-effects: Occasionally dry mouth, disturbances of visual accommodation, gastro-intestinal disturbances, dizziness and micturition difficulties may occur; these usually disappear spontaneously or may be controlled by a slight reduction in dosage. Less commonly, tachycardia, hypersensitivity, nervousness, euphoria and insomnia may be seen.

Overdosage: Toxic effects are anticholinergic in nature and the treatment is gastric lavage, cholinergics such as carbachol, anticholinesterases such as physostigmine and general non-specific treatment.

Pharmaceutical precautions Normal pharmaceutical storage and handling are indicated.

Legal category POM.

Package quantities 100 × 50 mg, 250 × 50 mg, 1,000 × 50 mg, 10,000 × 50 mg.

Further information Although very rarely reported, there may be provocation of dextropropoxyphene side-effects when that drug is administered concurrently with orphenadrine. Patients on Disipal may show spuriously elevated values for the T_3 test using a Sephadex method, but these are not indicative of hyperthyroidism. Each tablet contains ca 60 mg sucrose.

Product licence number 0166/5001

LIPOBASE*

Presentation Lipobase is the bland cream base as used in Locoid Lipocream. The inactive constituents in Lipobase are cetostearyl alcohol, cetomacrogol, liquid paraffin, white soft paraffin, methyl paraben, sodium citrate, citric acid, and purified water.

Uses For topical use where it is desired by the physician to reduce gradually the topical dosage of Locoid Lipocream. It may also be used where a continuously alternating application of the active product and the base is required e.g. in prophylactic therapy. Application of Lipobase is also recommended where it is felt by the physician that the use of a bland emollient base is preferable to the cessation of therapy with the active product. Lipobase may also be used as diluent for the active product in those cases where dilution is regarded as necessary by the prescriber.

Lipobase may also be used, other than in conjunction with a topical corticosteroid, for its emollient action, and for the treatment of mild skin lesions such as pruritus or dry, scaly skin, where topical corticosteroid therapy is not warranted.

Dosage and administration
Adults, children and the elderly: Lipobase may be used either by replacing an application of the active product or alternating the application of the active product and the base, gradually diminishing the application of active product until therapy ceases.

When used for its emollient activity or for the treatment of mild skin lesions such as pruritus or dry, scaly skin, the product should be applied three or four times a day or as directed by the physician.

Contra-indications, warnings, etc None.

Pharmaceutical precautions Store at room temperature (15–25°C).

Legal category P.

Package quantities Tubes of 50 g as an original pack (OP).

Further information Lipobase is a high fat content oil in water emulsion, the oily phase constituting 70% by weight of the finished product.

Product licence number 0166/0125.

LOCOID* CREAM
LOCOID* OINTMENT

Presentation Locoid Cream, containing 0.1% hydrocortisone 17-butyrate in a cream base. The inactive constituents in Locoid Cream are cetostearyl alcohol, cetomacrogol, liquid paraffin, white soft paraffin, methyl paraben, citric acid, sodium citrate, and purified water.

Locoid Ointment, containing 0.1% hydrocortisone 17-butyrate in an ointment base. The inactive constituents in Locoid Ointment are liquid paraffin and polyethylene.

Uses Eczema and dermatitis of all types including atopic eczema, photodermatitis, primary irritant and allergic dermatitis, lichen planus, lichen simplex, prurigo nodularis, discoid lupus erythematosus, necrobiosis lipoidica, pretibial myxoedema and erythematosus psoriasis of the scalp, chronic plaque psoriasis of the palms and soles, and other forms of psoriasis (excluding widespread plaque psoriasis).

Dosage and administration Apply a small quantity to the affected part two or three times daily. Application may be made under occlusion in the more resistant lesions such as thickened psoriatic plaques on elbows and knees.

Contra-indications, warnings, etc
Contra-indications: Facial rosacea, acne vulgaris, perioral dermatitis, perianal and genital pruritus, napkin eruptions, bacterial (e.g. impetigo), viral (e.g. herpes simplex) and fungal (e.g. candida or dermatophyte) infections.

Side-effects: Local and systemic toxicity is common especially following long continued use on large areas of damaged skin, in flexures and with polythene occlusion. If used in childhood, or on the face, courses should be limited to 5 days and occlusion should not be used. Local irritation may occur in those with a hypersensitivity to parabens.

Use in pregnancy and lactation: There is inadequate evidence of safety in human pregnancy. Topical administration of corticosteroids to pregnant animals can cause abnormalities of fetal development including cleft plate and intra-uterine growth retardation. There may therefore be a very small risk of such effects in the human fetus.

Other warnings and precautions: Long term continuous therapy should be avoided in all patients irrespective of age. Application under occlusion should be restricted to dermatoses involving limited areas.

Topical corticosteroids may be hazardous in psoriasis for a number of reasons including rebound relapses following development of tolerance, risk of generalised pustular psoriasis and local and systemic toxicity due to impaired barrier function of the skin. Steroids may have a place in psoriasis of the scalp and chronic plaque psoriasis of the hands and feet. Careful patient supervision is important.

Overdosage: Overdosage would result in the topical and systemic signs and symptoms associated with high corticosteroid dosage. If overdosage should occur, treatment should not stop immediately but be gradually withdrawn. Adrenal insufficiency may need therapy with intravenous hydrocortisone. It should be noted that overdosage of this topical corticosteroid product would be unlikely to occur other than as a result of severe and prolonged abuse of product.

Pharmaceutical precautions Store at room temperature (15–25°C).

Legal category POM.

Package quantities *Locoid Cream:* Tubes of 30 g and 100 g as original packs (OP).

Locoid Ointment: Tubes of 30 g and 100 g as original packs (OP).

Further information Locoid is a non-fluorinated topical steroid. Whilst clinical trials have shown it to be as effective as the potent fluorinated steroids, in clinical practice there is a low incidence of reported clinical side-effects.

Product licence numbers
Locoid Cream 0166/0058
Locoid Ointment 0166/0059

LOCOID LIPOCREAM*

Presentation Locoid Lipocream, containing 0.1% hydrocortisone 17-butyrate in a high fat content cream base. The inactive constituents in Locoid Lipocream are cetostearyl alcohol, cetomacrogol, liquid paraffin, white soft paraffin, methyl paraben, sodium citrate, citric acid, and purified water.

Uses The product is recommended for clinical use in the treatment of conditions responsive to topical corticosteroids, e.g. eczema, dermatitis and psoriasis. The product is intended for topical application.

Dosage and administration
Adults, children and the elderly: A small quantity to be applied two or three times a day, only sufficient to cover the affected area. The formulation of the product makes it suitable for use in both for scaly lesions and for moist, weeping lesions.

Contra-indications, warnings, etc
Contra-indications: Contra-indicated in the presence of bacterial (e.g. impetigo), viral (e.g. herpes simplex), or fungal (e.g. candida or dermatophyte), infections.

Side-effects: Locoid Lipocream is usually well tolerated; if signs of hypersensitivity do occur, treatment should be ceased.

In naturally occluded or moist areas of the skin, especially in small children, where absorption may be favoured, unduly prolonged therapy may give rise to systemic side-effects.

Use in pregnancy and lactation: There is inadequate evidence of safety in human pregnancy. Topical administration of corticosteroids to pregnant animals can cause abnormalities of fetal development including cleft palate and intra-uterine growth retardation. There may therefore be a very small risk of such effects in the human fetus. The use of topical corticosteroids during lactation is unlikely to present a hazard to infants being breast-fed.

Other warnings and precautions: Although generally regarded as safe, even for long-term administration in adults, there is a potential for overdosage in infancy. Extreme caution is required in dermatoses of infancy including napkin eruption. In such patients, courses of treatment should not normally exceed 7 days.

Overdosage: Overdosage would result in the topical and systemic signs and symptoms associated with high corticosteroid dosage. If overdosage should occur, treatment should not stop immediately but be gradually withdrawn. Adrenal insufficiency may need therapy with intravenous hydrocortisone. It should be noted that overdosage of this topical corticosteroid product would be unlikely to occur other than as a result of severe and prolonged abuse of the product.

Pharmaceutical precautions Store at room temperature (15–25°C).

Legal category POM.

Package quantities Tubes of 30 g and 100 g as original packs (OP).

Further information Locoid, a non-fluorinated topical steroid has been shown to be as effective as the potent fluorinated steroids, yet in clinical practice there is a low incidence of reported side-effects. The oily phase constitutes 70% by weight of the product.

Product licence number 0166/0112.

LOCOID* C CREAM LOCOID* C OINTMENT

Presentation Locoid C cream, containing 0.1% hydrocortisone 17-butyrate and 3% chlorquinaldol, in a cream base. The inactive constituents in Locoid C Cream are cetostearyl alcohol, cetomacrogol, liquid paraffin, white soft paraffin, sodium citrate, citric acid, and purified water.

Locoid C ointment, containing 0.1% hydrocortisone 17-butyrate and 3% chlorquinaldol, in an ointment base. The inactive constituents in Locoid C Ointment are liquid paraffin and polyethylene.

Uses The products are recommended for clinical use in the treatment of conditions responsive to topical corticosteroids, e.g. eczema, dermatitis and psoriasis, where secondary bacterial or fungal infection by a microorganism susceptible to chlorquinadol is present or is to be prevented.

The products are intended for topical application.

Dosage and administration
Adults, children and the elderly: To be applied to the affected part two to four times a day, or as directed by the physician.

Contra-indications, warnings, etc Topical corticosteroids are contra-indicated in the presence of viral, tubercular or syphilitic lesions and in bacterial or fungal infections other than those at the site of inunction responsive to topical chlorquinaldol. Contact with the eye should be avoided.

In pregnant animals, administration of corticosteroids can cause abnormalities of foetal development. The relevance of this finding to human beings has not been established. However, topical steroids should not be used extensively in pregnancy, i.e. in large amounts or for long periods.

In infants, long-term continuous topical therapy shold be avoided. Adrenal suppression can occur, even without occlusion.

Occlusive dressings are not recommended in the presence of infections.

Pharmaceutical precautions Store at room temperature (15–25°C).

Legal category POM.

Package quantities *Locoid C Cream:* Tubes of 30 g as an original pack (OP).

Locoid C Ointment: Tubes of 30 g as an original pack (OP).

Further information Locoid is a non-fluorinated topical steroid. Whilst clinical trials have shown it to be as effective as the potent fluorinated steroids, in clinical practice there is a low incidence of reported side-effects.

Chlorquinaldol is an effective topical antibacterial and antimycotic.

Product licence numbers
Locoid C Cream 0166/0056
Locoid C Ointment 0166/0057

LOCOID* SCALP LOTION

Presentation Locoid Scalp Lotion contains 0.1% hydrocortisone 17-butyrate in an alcohol/water base, specially formulated for the treatment of skin disorders of the scalp. The inactive constituents of Locoid Scalp Lotion are glycerin, povidone, citric acid, sodium citrate, iso-propyl alcohol, and purified water.

Uses In the treatment of steroid-responsive dermatoses of the scalp, including seborrhoea capitis with or without an associated severe dandruff; psoriasis of the scalp (excluding widespread plaque psoriasis).

Dosage and administration
Adults, children and the elderly: Apply a small quantity 2 to 3 times daily to the affected area of the scalp, or as directed.

Contra-indications, warnings, etc *Contra-indications:* Facial rosacea, acne vulgaris, perioral dermatitis, perianal and genital pruritus, napkin eruptions, bacterial (e.g. impetigo), viral (e.g. herpes simplex) and fungal (e.g. candida or dermatophyte) infections, known hypersensitivity to the product.

Side-effects: Local and systemic toxicity is common especially following long continued use on large areas. Local irritation may occur.

Use in pregnancy and lactation: There is inadequate evidence of safety in human pregnancy. Topical administration of corticosteroids to pregnant animals can cause abnormalities of fetal development including cleft palate and intra-uterine growth retardation. There may therefore be a very small risk of such effects in the human fetus.

Other warnings and precautions: Long term continuous therapy should be avoided in all patients irrespective of age. Application under occlusion should be restricted to dermatoses involving limited areas.

Topical corticosteroids may be hazardous in psoriasis for a number of reasons including rebound relapses following development of tolerance, risk of generalised pustular psoriasis and local and systemic toxicity due to impaired barrier function of the skin. Steroids may have a place in psoriasis of the scalp and chronic plaque psoriasis of the hands and feet. Careful patient supervision is important.

Overdosage: Overdosage would result in the topical and systemic signs and symptoms associated with high corticosteroid dosage. If overdosage should occur, treatment should not stop immediately but be gradually withdrawn. Adrenal insufficiency may need therapy with intravenous hydrocortisone. It should be noted that overdosage of this topical corticosteroid product would be unlikely to occur other than as a result of severe and prolonged abuse of product.

Pharmaceutical precautions Store at room temperature (15–25°C).

Legal category POM.

Package quantities Plastic squeeze bottles of 30 ml and 100 ml as original packs (OP).

Further information Locoid lotion should be kept

away from the eyes, and not used near a fire or naked flame.

Product licence number 0166/0060.

MILDISON* LIPOCREAM

Presentation Mildison Lipocream is presented as an oil-in-water high-lipid content emollient base containing Hydrocortisone BP 1% w/w. The inactive ingredients of Mildison Lipocream are cetostearyl alcohol, cetomacrogol, liquid paraffin, white soft paraffin, methyl paraben, citric acid, sodium citrate, and purified water.

Uses By topical administration in the treatment of eczema and dermatitis of all types, including atopic eczema, photodermatitis, otitis externa, primary irritant and allergic dermatitis, intertrigo, prurigo nodularis, seborrhoeic dermatitis, and insect bite reactions.

Dosage and administration
For adults, children and the elderly: Apply a small quantity only sufficient to cover the affected area two or three times a day. The formulation of the product makes it suitable for use both for dry scaly lesions, and for moist or weeping lesions.

Contra-indications, warnings, etc
Contra-indications: Contra-indicated in the presence of bacterial (e.g. impetigo), viral (e.g. herpes simplex), or fungal (e.g. candida or dermatophyte), infections.

Side-effects: Mildison 1% is usually well tolerated. If signs of hypersensitivity do occur, treatment should cease.

In naturally occluded or moist areas of the skin, especially in small children, where absorption may be favoured, unduly prolonged therapy may give rise to systemic side-effects.

Use in pregnancy and lactation: There is inadequate evidence of safety in human pregnancy. Topical administration of corticosteroids to pregnant animals can cause abnormalities of fetal development including cleft palate and intra-uterine growth retardation. There may therefore be a very small risk of such effects in the human fetus. The use of topical corticosteroids during lactation is unlikely to present a hazard to infants being breast-fed.

Other warnings and precautions: Although generally regarded as safe, even for long-term administration in adults, there is a potential for overdosage in infancy. Extreme caution is required in dermatoses of infancy including napkin eruption. In such patients, courses of treatment should not normally exceed 7 days.

Overdosage: Overdosage would result in the topical and systemic signs and symptoms associated with high corticosteroid dosage. If overdosage should occur, treatment should not stop immediately but be gradually withdrawn. Adrenal insufficiency may need therapy with intravenous hydrocortisone. It should be noted that overdosage of this topical corticosteroid product would be unlikely to occur other than as a result of severe and prolonged abuse of the product.

Pharmaceutical precautions Store at room temperature (15–25°C).

Legal category POM.

Package quantities Tubes of 30 g as an original pack (OP).

Further information Hydrocortisone is a topical steroid well known for its efficacy and safety. The Lipocream base promotes both hydration of the stratum corneum and suppleness of dry, scaly, excoriated skin, with greater patient acceptability than an ordinary ointment. The product is particularly suited for use on dry, subacute and chronic lesions and for those patients presenting with mixed lesions.

Product licence number 0166/0131.

PREFERID* CREAM
PREFERID OINTMENT

Presentation Preferid cream contains budesonide 0.025% w/w in a cream base of white soft paraffin, liquid paraffin, cetostearyl alcohol, cetomacrogol 1000, sorbic acid, citric acid, sodium citrate and purified water. Preferid ointment contains budesonide 0.025% in an ointment base of propylene glycol, white beeswax, liquid paraffin and white soft paraffin.

Uses By topical administration in the treatment of eczema and dermatitis of all types including atopic eczema, photodermatitis, primary irritant and allergic dermatitis, lichen planus, lichen simplex, prurigo nodularis, discoid lupus erythematosus, necrobiosis lipoidica, pretibial myxoedema and erythroderma; psoriasis of the scalp, chronic plaque psoriasis of the palms and soles, and other forms of psoriasis (excluding widespread plaque psoriasis).

Dosage and administration For adults, children and the elderly, apply a small quantity to the affected part two or three times daily. Application may be made under occlusion in the more resistant lesions such as thickened psoriatic plaques on elbows and knees.

Contra-indications, warnings, etc
Contra-indications: Contra-indicated in the presence of bacterial (e.g. impetigo), viral (e.g. herpes simplex) and fungal (e.g. candida or dermatophyte) infections. Also in facial rosacea, acne vulgaris, perioral dermatitis, perianal and genital pruritus and napkin eruptions.

Side-effects: Local and systemic toxicity with topical corticosteroids is common, especially following long continued use on large areas of damaged skin, in flexures and with polythene occlusion. If used in childhood, or on the face, courses should be limited to 5 days and occlusion should not be used.

Use in pregnancy and lactation: There is inadequate evidence of safety in human pregnancy. Topical administration of corticosteroids to pregnant animals can cause abnormalities of foetal development including cleft palate and intra-uterine growth retardation. There may therefore be a very small risk of such effects in the human foetus.

Other warnings and precautions: Long term continuous therapy should be avoided in all patients irrespective of age. Application under occlusion should be restricted to dermatoses involving limited areas.

Topical corticosteroids may be hazardous in psoriasis for a number of reasons including rebound relapses following development of tolerance, risk of generalised pustular psoriasis and local and systemic toxicity due to impaired barrier function of the skin. Steroids may have a place in psoriasis of the scalp and chronic plaque psoriasis of the hands and feet. Careful patient supervision is important.

Overdosage: Overdosage would result in the topical and systematic signs and symptoms associated with high corticosteroid dosage. If overdosage should occur, treatment should not stop immediately but be gradually withdrawn. Adrenal insufficiency may need therapy with intravenous hydrocortisone. It should be noted that overdosage of this topical corticosteroid product would be unlikely to occur other than as a result of severe and prolonged abuse of the product.

Legal category POM.

Package quantities Tubes of 30 and 100 grams (OP).

Further information Preferid is a non-fluorinated topical steroid.

Product licence numbers
Preferid Ointment 0166/0122.
Preferid Cream 0166/0123.

STAFOXIL* CAPSULES

Presentation Hard gelatin capsule with cream cap and light brown body, inscribed gbr 191 (250 mg capsule) or gbr 192 (500 mg capsule, containing 250 mg or 500 mg flucloxacillin as Flucoxacillin Sodium BP. Stafoxil Capsules contain no inactive ingredients which require disclosure.

Uses Stafoxil is indicated in the treatment of infections caused by flucloxacillin sensitive micro-organisms, in particular penicillinase-producing staphylococci, as in respiratory tract infections, infections of the skin and soft tissues and generalised infections.

Dosage and administration
Adults and the elderly: In mild to moderately severe infections, usually 250 mg four times daily, half to one hour before food.

Children: 2–12 years, usually half the daily adult dose or 50 mg/kg body weight per 24 hours divided into four doses, half to one hour before food.

In serious infections the dosages may be doubled.

In chronic relapsing and severe infections parenteral administration is to be preferred.

Contra-indications, warnings, etc Contra-indicated in penicillin hypersensitivity. There are no contra-indications for the use of Staxofil during pregnancy. Flucloxacillin is secreted in mothers milk and may occasionally cause a sensitisation of the infant. In patients with infectious mononucleosis and lymphatic leukaemia, exanthema is common. Cross-allergy and cross-resistance between the penicillins and cephalosporins may exist.

Probenecid slows down the excretion of flucloxacillin.

Gastrointestinal side effects have been reported such as nausea, vomiting and diarrhoea. Although transient and not severe, macular and maculopapular skin reactions may occur. Typical allergic reactions have been observed such as urticaria and purpora. Anaphylaxis has occasionally resulted from the oral use of penicillin or one of its derivatives. With high, chiefly parenteral, doses, neurotoxicity may develop.

Pharmaceutical precautions Store under normal pharmaceutical conditions.

Legal category POM.

Package quantities Both strengths of capsule are available in 28's and 100's. The 250 mg capsule is also available in 500's.

Further information Nil.

Product licence numbers
Stafoxil Capsules 250 mg 0166/0116
Stafoxil Capsules 500 mg 0166/0117

ZINERYT*

Presentation Zineryt is presented as a pack of two bottles, one containing a solution and the other a powder, together with a special applicator and protective cap. The contents of the two bottles are intended to be admixed by the pharmacist at the time of dispensing, and the applicator and cap fitted. When constituted, the 30 ml of topical application produced contains 40 mg/ml erythromycin and 12 mg/ml zinc acetate, as an erythromycin-zinc complex.

Uses By topical administration, for the treatment of acne vulgaris.

Dosage and administration
For adults, children, and the elderly: Apply twice daily over the whole of the affected areas for a period of 10 to 12 weeks.

Contra-indications, warnings, etc
Contra-indications: Contra-indicated in patients who are hypersensitive to erythromycin or other macrolide antibiotics, or to zinc, di-isopropyl sebacate or ethanol.

Side-effects: Occasionally a slight burning sensation or a slight redness of the skin may be observed; this is due to the alcohol base of Zineryt, and is transient and of minor clinical significance.

Use in pregnancy and lactation: There is no contra-indication to the use of Zineryt in pregnancy, or while breast-feeding.

Other warnings and precautions: Cross-resistance may occur with other antibiotics of the macrolide group, and with lincomycin or clindamycin. Contact with the eyes or the mucous membrane of the nose and mouth should be avoided.

Overdosage: It is not expected that overdosage would occur in normal use. Patients showing idiosyncratic hypersensitivity should wash the treated area with copious water and simple soap.

Legal category POM.

Package quantities Pack to make 30 ml on constitution.

Further information After constitution by the pharmacist, the application is stable for a period of 5 weeks at room temperature.

Product licence number 0166/0109

**Trade Mark*

Charwell Pharmaceuticals Ltd

Charwell House
Wilsom Road
Alton, Hampshire GU34 2TJ

CHARWELL PHARMACEUTICALS

MIGRALEVE*

Presentation *Pink Migraleve:* Blister-packed, pink, capsule-shaped, film-coated tablets, engraved 'MGE' on one face, each containing:

Buclizine hydrochloride	6.25 mg
Paracetamol PhEur	500 mg
Codeine Phosphate PhEur	8 mg

Yellow Migraleve: Blister-packed, yellow, capsule-shaped, film-coated tablets, engraved 'MGE' on one face, each containing:

Paracetamol PhEur	500 mg
Codeine Phosphate PhEur	8 mg

Uses For the treatment of migraine attacks which can include the symptoms of migraine headache, nausea and vomiting.

Dosage and administration *Adult: Treatment:* 2 Pink Migraleve immediately it is known that a migraine attack has started or is imminent. If symptoms persist, 2 Yellow Migraleve every four hours. Maximum 8 tablets (2 Pink and 6 Yellow) in 24 hours.

Children 10–14 years: One Pink Migraleve initially. If required, 1 Yellow Migraleve every four hours. Maximum 4 tablets (1 Pink and 3 Yellow) in 24 hours.

Elderly (over 65 years): As for adults. No clinical or pharmacokinetic data specific to this age group is available. However at normal dosages no problems have been reported.

Contra-indications, warnings, etc *Side-effects:* Drowsiness is an occasional feature of migraine attacks. It may, theoretically, also be caused by the small antihistamine content of Pink Migraleve, but this has never been apparent from clinical observations.

Use in pregnancy: Migraleve has been in wide use for many years without apparent ill consequence. Although experiments in some species gave rise to adverse effects following the administration of buclizine to pregnant animals e.g. foetal abnormalities and maternal deaths, these occurred at doses in excess of 120 times the human daily dose. Whilst there are no specific reasons for contra-indicating Migraleve during pregnancy, as with all drugs it is recommended that Migraleve be used in pregnancy only when the physician has considered the need in respect of the patients' welfare.

Insignificant levels of the active ingredients pass into breast milk; therefore Migraleve is not contra-indicated in breast-feeding mothers.

Precautions: Migrainous patients suffering from high blood pressure should first be treated for this condition independently. Because of the possibility of drowsiness, consideration should be given to patients involved in hazardous occupations.

Treatment of overdosage: In the event of overdosage the toxic effects of codeine may be reversed by injection of naloxone. Symptoms of paracetamol overdosage are often delayed for at least 24 hours but to prevent hepatic damage treatment should be given as soon as possible and within 10 hours of ingestion. Treatment is by the administration of oral methionine or i.v. acetylcysteine.

Pharmaceutical precautions Nil.

Legal category P.

Package quantities 48 (32 Pink and 16 Yellow) tablets. Also continuation packs of 48 Pink and 48 Yellow tablets.

Further information Nil.

Product licence number 0232/5008R.

PANCREOLAURYL* TEST

Presentation Two blue capsules each containing: 174.25 mg (=0.25 mmol) fluorescein dilaurate. One red capsule containing: 188.14 mg (=0.50 mmol) Fluorescein Sodium BP.

Uses For the assessment of exocrine pancreatic function. The Pancreolauryl Test is used to detect abnormally low pancreatic digestive function. Symptoms associated with disturbances of pancreatic digestive function include recurrrent diarrhoea, increased flatulence, fat intolerance and recurrent upper abdominal pain.

Principle: The test compound, fluorescein dilaurate, is administered orally in capsules. Pancreas-specific cholesterol ester hydrolase from pancreatic juice hydrolyses the fluorescein dilaurate into lauric acid and free, water-soluble fluorescein. The fluorescein can then be absorbed and excreted in the urine. The urine is collected and there is a simple procedure to measure quantitatively the fluorescein excreted. This is directly proportional to the action of esterases and therefore proportional to the digestive ability of the exocrine pancreas.

Fluorescein dilaurate has low water solubility and will pass through the gastrointestinal tract unchanged if not acted upon by pancreatic secretions. In order to assess pancreatic function, the secretion must be stimulated. This is achieved by means of a standard meal taken with 2 blue test capsules which will activate the endogenous secretin-pancreozymin mechanisms.

To assess the absorption and excretion characteristics for individual patients, a repeat test using the control capsule is carried out the next day. The control capsule is red and contains unesterified fluorescein (fluorescein sodium).

The quantity of fluorescein excreted from the test capsules is expressed as a percentage of the quantity of fluorescein excreted from the control capsule. This value is termed the T/K ratio, and is used as a parameter of exocrine pancreatic function.

The following is a schematic representation of the test principle:

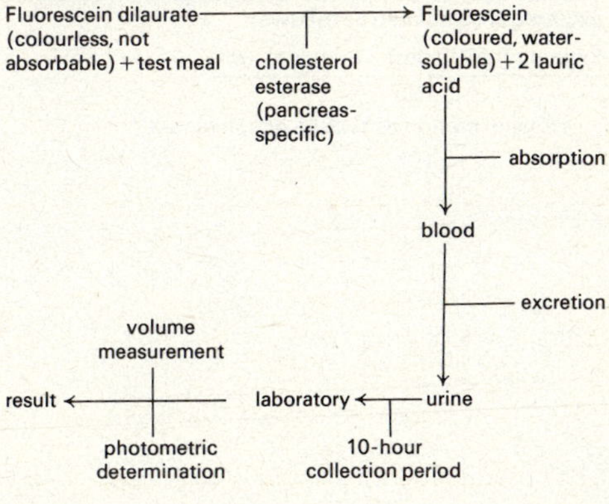

Dosage and administration *Adults:* The 2 blue capsules containing fluorescein dilaurate are taken on day 1 following an overnight fast. The capsules are swallowed with a simple roll and butter standard breakfast which is taken to stimulate exocrine pancreatic secretion. Urine is collected for 10 hours following the administration of the capsules. The patient must drink 500 ml of non-interfering liquid such as water, dilute orange or lemon squash (not fruit juice) or tea or coffee (without sugar or milk), half an hour before the start of the test, a further cup of liquid with the standard breakfast and one litre of liquid from three to five hours following administration of the capsules. Following this, patients can eat and drink as desired.

On the following day (day 2) this procedure is repeated using the red control capsule which contains fluorescein sodium.

Children: Although satisfactory results have been obtained in children, the test in its present form is not recommended for children.

The following sequence has proved suitable for carrying out the Pancreolauryl Test. The patient can eat and drink as usual on the evening prior to the test, but no medicines containing vitamins or digestive aids should be taken.

		***IMPORTANT** The *only* liquids allowed between 6.30 am and 12.00 mid-day are: water, dilute fruit squash (not fruit juice), weak tea or coffee (no milk or sugar).
	6.30 am	Pass urine and discard. Drink 500 ml (1 pint) liquid.*
collect urine (7.00 am to 5.00 pm)	7.00 am	Eat 50 g of bread spread with 20 g (¾ oz) of butter. The capsule(s) should be swallowed and not chewed during the middle of the test meal. Drink one cup of liquid.* Collect all urine from now onwards.
	10.00 am	Drink 1 litre (2 pints) of liquid* between 10 am and mid-day.
	12.00 mid-day	After mid-day, eat and drink as desired but vitamins and digestive aids are not to be taken. Continue to collect all urine.
	5.00 pm	The bladder should be emptied as completely as possible. (Note: If less than 600 ml of urine is collected, results become less reliable).

Laboratory measurement of fluorescein in urine: The urine collected during the 10 hour period is shaken well and the volume measured accurately using a graduated measuring cylinder (graduated collection bottles are not sufficiently accurate).

0.5 ml of urine is added to 4.5 ml of 0.1 N sodium hydroxide solution. To hydrolyse fluorescein glucuronides (colourless conjugation products formed in the liver), the sample is immersed in a water bath at 65°–70°C for 10 minutes, cooled and centrifuged. The supernatant liquid is compared photometrically at 492 nm against water. The percentage of fluorescein excreted is calculated as follows:

$$\frac{\text{Extinction (492 nm)} \times \text{urine vol. (ml)}}{35}$$

= Dye excretion as % dose administered

Evaluation: Individual T/K ratios are used for evaluation.

T = Excretion of dye from test capsule
K = Excretion of dye from control capsule

Calculate T and K from the above calculation and obtain the T/K ratio

$$\frac{(T \times 100)}{K}$$

The T/K ratio is a parameter of exocrine pancreatic function. T/K ratios of 30 and above are found in normal exocrine pancreatic function. With pancreatic insufficiency the ratio is below 20.

If a T/K ratio between 20 and 30 is found, the test should be repeated in order to exclude false results. If it is suspected that the patient suffers intermittent attacks of chronic pancreatitis, then a series of tests should be carried out to monitor the T/K ratio.

Contra-indications, warnings, etc Acute necrotizing pancreatitis. Although satisfactory results have been obtained in children, the test in its present form is not recommended for children. Use during pregnancy is contra-indicated.

Side-effects and interactions with other drugs: No side-effects have been reported and no reactions are known other than those which could interfere with the test results, i.e. concomitant use of digestive aids, or vitamins. False negative results may arise if patients take pancreatic enzyme preparations during the course of the test; any such treatment therefore should be stopped on the evening prior to the test.

Sulphasalazine which is used for ulcerative colitis and Crohn's disease can interfere with photometric measurements.

Pharmaceutical precautions Store in a cool, dry place.

Legal category POM.

Package quantities Each pack contains 2 blue test capsules and 1 red control capsule. These are required for a single test.

Further information *False results:* Currently available clinical data indicate a negative predictive value approaching 100%; this means that in patients with a normal result, it is usually unnecessary to carry out additional pancreatic function tests. Positive predictive values have varied with groups of patients used and a meaningful figure cannot be quoted; however 1 in 20 patients showing a possible false positive is typical. A positive result invariably merits further investigation. False results may be due to pathophysiological conditions in which asynchrony of the G.I. tract interferes with normal substrate and enzyme interaction or because of test error.

False positive results: May be due to insufficient diuresis, where total volume of urine collected is less than 600 ml. Other reasons could be incomplete collection of urine or failure to take the test meal and capsules simultaneously.

False negative results: May arise if pancreatic enzyme preparations are taken during the course of the test.

Product licence number 0232/0039.

**Trade Mark*

Ciba Consumer Pharmaceuticals
Horsham
West Sussex RH12 4AB

BRADOSOL* PLUS

Presentation Lozenges containing 0.5 mg Domiphen Bromide BP and 5.0 mg Lignocaine Hydrochloride BP. The lozenges are flat, round and pink with a diameter of approximately 16 mm and impressed 'CIBA' on one side and 'BRADOSOL PLUS' on the other. They contain sucrose.

Uses Symptomatic relief of sore throat. Bradosol Plus alleviates soreness of throat and associated difficulty in swallowing.

Mode of action: Domiphen bromide has an antimicrobial and fungicidal action on a wide range of pathogenic organisms including those most commonly associated with upper respiratory tract infection.

Lignocaine hydrochloride is a local anaesthetic, with a rapid onset of action that has been widely used to anaesthetise mucous membranes.

Pharmacokinetics: The limited data available suggests that systemic absorption of domiphen bromide occurs only on an insignificant scale.

Lignocaine hydrochloride is readily absorbed through the mucous membrane and is extensively metabolised. The products of metabolism are excreted in the urine.

Dosage and administration
Adults and elderly: One lozenge to be sucked every 2–3 hours and no more than eight lozenges per day. Duration of use 4–5 days.

Children: Not recommended for children under 12 years.

Contra-indications, warnings, etc
Use in pregnancy and lactation: Domiphen bromide: No animal data on teratogenic effects have been reported, nor has therapeutic experience extending over many years yielded evidence of any harmful influence on development of the embryo and/or foetus. Nevertheless, during the first three months of pregnancy, Bradosol Plus, like all medication should only be employed for compelling reasons. It is not necessary to contraindicate the use of Bradosol Plus in lactating mothers.

Contra-indications: Known hypersensitivity to domiphen bromide or lignocaine hydrochloride.

Precautions: In the unlikely event of a hypersensitivity reaction occurring with Bradosol Plus, the treatment should be discontinued.

Where Bradosol Plus is being taken as self-medication, the patient should consult a doctor if the symptoms are still present after about five days of treatment or are severe, or are accompanied by fever, headache, nausea or vomiting.

Patients should not eat or drink for one hour after sucking a lozenge.

Drug interactions: None clinically important.

Side-effects: Only in very rare cases have there been reports of local hypersensitivity reactions in the form of local reddening of the mucous membranes and swelling of the pharyngeal mucosa giving rise to difficulty in swallowing.

Overdosage: No cases of overdosage have been reported to date.

Pharmaceutical precautions Protect from heat and moisture.

Legal category P.

Package quantities Cartons of 24 lozenges consisting of blister pack modules each containing 12 lozenges.

Further information Nil.

Product licence number 0001/0123.

OTRIVINE* CHILDREN'S FORMULA NASAL DROPS

Presentation Clear, colourless odourless solution containing 0.05% w/v Xylometazoline Hydrochloride BP.

The nasal drops also contain sodium acid phosphate, sodium phosphate, sodium chloride, disodium edetate, domiphen bromide and thiomersal.

Uses
Indications: For the symptomatic relief of nasal congestion, perennial and allergic rhinitis (including hay fever), sinusitis.

Mode of action: A sympathomimetic agent with marked alpha-adrenergic activity. It is a vasoconstrictor with a rapid and prolonged action used for the relief of nasal congestion.

Pharmacokinetics: Systemic absorption may occur following nasal application of xylometazoline hydrochloride solutions. It is not used systemically.

Dosage and administration
Children under 12: 1 or 2 drops of the Otrivine Children's Formula Nasal Drops in each nostril once or twice daily. Not to be used in infants less than 3 months.

Contra-indications, warnings, etc
Contra-indications: Patients with trans-sphenoidal hypophysectomy or surgery exposing the dura mater.

Warnings: Each Otrivine pack should be used by one person only to prevent any cross-infection.

Precautions: Patients are advised not to take decongestants for more than seven consecutive days. Excessive use or abuse of Otrivine may cause rebound congestion or drug-induced rhinitis. Systemic cardiovascular effects have occurred, and this should be kept in mind when giving Otrivine® to patients with cardiovascular diseases.

Drug interactions: No drug interactions have been reported.

Side-effects: Side effects are infrequent with Otrivine and are generally mild, but some patients who have sensitive nasal passages may feel some local discomfort at the time of application, including stinging, sneezing, dryness of the nose and also headache. Occasionally small children may show restlessness or sleep disturbance when Otrivine is used. If this occurs Otrivine should be stopped.

Overdosage: Symptoms of overdose include elevated blood pressure, drowsiness and respiratory depression or irregularity. There is no specific treatment and appropriate supportive treatment should be initiated.

Pharmaceutical precautions Protect from heat. For reasons of hygiene do not use the bottle more than 28 days after first opening it.

Legal category GSL.

Package quantities Otrivine Children's Formula Nasal Drops 10 ml.

Further information Nil.

Product licence number 0008/5022

**Trade Mark*

CIBA Laboratories
Horsham
West Sussex RH12 4AB

CIBA

APRESOLINE*

Presentation Tablets containing 25 mg Hydralazine Hydrochloride BP, circular, polished, sugar-coated, pale yellow in colour marked CIBA on one side and the letters GF on the other.

Tablets containing 50 mg Hydralazine Hydrochloride BP, circular, polished, sugar-coated, violet-red in colour, marked CG on one side and the letters HG on the other.

Ampoules for intravenous use containing 20 mg hydralazine hydrochloride, as a white or yellowish lyophilised powder (requiring reconstitution before use – see 'Dosage' below).

The tablets also contain sucrose and gluten (wheat starch). The 50 mg tablets also contain erythrosine.

Uses
Indications: Hypertension – *Oral:* Moderate to severe hypertension usually as an adjunct to other anti-hypertensive agents. Use in combination with long acting nitrates in moderate to severe chronic congestive cardiac failure in patients in whom optimal doses of diuretics and cardiac glycosides have proved insufficient. *Intravenous:* Hypertensive emergencies, particularly those associated with pre-eclampsia and toxaemia of pregnancy and in hypertension with renal complications.

Mode of action: Hydralazine is a direct acting vasodilator which exerts its effects principally on the arterioles. Its precise mode of action is not known. Administration of hydralazine produces a fall in peripheral resistance and a decrease in arterial blood pressure, effects which induce reflex sympathetic cardiovascular responses. The concomitant use of a beta-blocker will reduce these reflex effects and enhance the anti-hypertensive effect. The use of hydralazine can result in sodium and fluid retention, producing oedema and reduced urinary volume. These effects can be prevented by concomitant administration of a diuretic.

Pharmacokinetics: Orally administered Apresoline is rapidly and completely absorbed but is subject to a dose-dependent first pass effect (systemic bioavailability: 26–55%) which is dependent upon the individuals acetylator status. Peak plasma concentrations are attained after 0.5 to 1.5 hours. Apresoline appears in the plasma chiefly in the form of a readily hydrolysable conjugate with pyruvic acid. Plasma half-life averages 2–3 hours but is prolonged up to 16 hours in severe renal failure (creatinine clearance less than 20 ml/min) and shortened to approximately 45 minutes in rapid acetylators. Apresoline is rapidly distributed in the body and displays a particular affinity for the blood-vessel walls. Plasma protein binding is of the order of 90%. Within 24 hours after an oral dose, the quantity recovered in the urine averages 80% of the dose. The bulk of the dose is excreted as acetylated and hydroxylated metabolites, some of which are conjugated with glucuronic acid.

Dosage and administration SEE 'PRECAUTIONS' BEFORE USE.

Adults
Hypertension: The dose should be adjusted to the individual requirements of the patient. Treatment should begin with low doses of Apresoline which, depending on the patients response should be increased stepwise to achieve optimal therapeutic effect whilst keeping unwanted effects to a minimum. Oral: Initially 25 mg twice daily. This can be increased gradually to a dose not exceeding 200 mg daily. The dose should not be increased beyond 100 mg daily without first checking the patients acetylator status (see 'Warnings'). Parenteral: Initially 5 to 10 mg by slow intravenous injection, to avoid precipitous decreases in arterial pressure with a critical reduction in cerebral or utero-placental perfusion. If necessary a repeat injection can be given after an interval of 20–30 minutes, throughout which blood pressure and heart rate should be monitored. A satisfactory response can be defined as a decrease in diastolic blood pressure to 90/100 mmHg. The contents of the vial should be reconstituted by dissolving in 1 ml of Water for Injection BP. This should then be further diluted with 10 ml of Sodium Chloride Injection BP 0.9% and be administered by slow intravenous injection. The injection must be given immediately and any remainder discarded. Apresoline may also be given by continuous intravenous infusion, beginning with a flow rate of 200–300 µg/min. Maintenance flow rates must be determined individually and are usually within the range 50–150 µg/min. The product reconstituted as for direct iv injection may be added via the infusion container to 500 ml of Sodium Chloride Injection BP 0.9% and given by continuous infusion. The addition should be made immediately before administration and the mixture should not be stored. Apresoline for infusion can also be used with 5% sorbitol solution or isotonic inorganic infusion solutions such as Ringer's solution.

Incompatibility: Dextrose infusion solutions are not compatible because contact between hydralazine and glucose causes hydralazine to be rapidly broken down.

Chronic congestive heart failure.

Treatment with Apresoline should always be initiated in hospital, where the patients' individual haemodynamic values can be reliably determined with the help of invasive monitoring. It should then be continued in hospital until the patient has become stabilised on the requisite maintenance dose. Doses vary greatly between individual patients and are generally higher than those used for treating hypertension. After progressive titration (initially 25 mg tid or qid increasing every second day) the maintenance dosage averages 50–75 mg qid.

Children: Not recommended.

Elderly: Clinical evidence would indicate that no special dosage regime is necessary. Advancing age does not affect either blood concentration or systemic clearance. Renal elimination may however be affected insofar as kidney function diminishes with age.

Use in pregnancy and lactation: Use of Apresoline in pregnancy, before the third trimester should be avoided but the drug may be employed in later pregnancy if there is no safer alternative or when the disease itself carries serious risks for the mother or child eg pre-eclampsia and/or eclampsia.

Hydralazine has been found to be teratogenic in mice producing a small incidence of cleft palate and certain other bony malformations, in oral doses ranging from 20–120 mg/kg ie 20–30 times the maximum human daily dose. It was not teratogenic in rats or rabbits.

No serious adverse effects in human pregnancy have been reported to date with Apresoline, although experience in the third trimester is extensive.

Hydralazine passes into breast milk but reports available so far have not shown adverse effects on the infant. Mothers in whom use of Apresoline proves unavoidable may breast feed their infant provided that the infant is observed for possible adverse effects.

Contra-indications, warnings, etc

Contra-indications: Known hypersensitivity to hydralazine or dihydralazine. Idiopathic systemic lupus erythematosus (SLE) and related diseases. Severe tachycardia and heart failure with a high cardiac output (eg in thyrotoxicosis).

Myocardial insufficiency due to mechanical obstruction (eg in the presence of aortic or mitral stenosis or constrictive pericarditis).

Isolated right ventricular failure due to pulmonary hypertension (cor pulmonale).

Dissecting aortic aneurysm.

Warnings: The overall "hyperdynamic" state of the circulation induced by hydralazine may accentuate certain clinical conditions. Myocardial stimulation may provoke or aggravate angina pectoris. Patients with suspected or confirmed coronary artery disease should therefore be given Apresoline only under cover of a beta-blocker or in combination with other suitable sympatholytic agents. It is important that the beta-blocker medication should be commenced a few days before the start of treatment with Apresoline.

Patients who have survived a myocardial infarction should not receive Apresoline until a post-infarction stabilisation phase has been achieved.

Prolonged treatment with hydralazine (ie usually for more than 6 months) may provoke a lupus erythematosus (LE) like syndrome, especially where doses exceed 100 mg daily. First symptoms are likely to be arthralgia, sometimes associated with fever and rash and are reversible after withdrawal of the drug. In its more severe form it resembles acute SLE, and in rare cases renal and ocular involvement have been reported. Long term treatment with corticosteroids may be required to reverse these changes. Since such reactions tend to occur more frequently the higher the dose and the longer its duration, and since they are also more common in slow acetylators, it is recommended that for maintenance therapy the lowest effective dose should be used. If 100 mg daily fails to elicit an adequate clinical effect, the patient's acetylator status should be evaluated. Slow acetylators and women run a greater risk of developing the LE-like syndrome and every effort should therefore be made to keep the dosage below 100 mg daily and a careful watch kept for signs and symptoms suggestive of this syndrome. If such symptoms do develop the drug should be gradually withdrawn. Rapid acetylators often respond inadequately even to doses of 100 mg daily and therefore the dose can be raised with only a slightly increased risk of an LE-like syndrome.

During long-term treatment with Apresoline it is advisable to determine the antinuclear factors and conduct urine analysis at intervals of approximately 6 months. Microhaematuria and/or proteinuria, in particular together with positive titres of ANF, may be initial signs of immune-complex glomerulonephritis associated with the SLE-like syndrome. If overt clinical signs or symptoms develop, the drug should be withdrawn immediately.

In high (cyto-) toxic concentrations, Hydralazine induces gene mutations in single cell organisms and in mammalian cells *in-vitro.* No unequivocally mutagenic effects have been detected *in-vivo* in a great number of test systems.

Hydralazine, in lifetime carcinogenicity studies, caused, towards the end of the experiments, small but statistically significant increases in lung tumours in mice and in hepatic and testicular tumours in rats. These tumours also occur spontaneously with fairly high frequency in aged rodents.

With due consideration of these animal and *in-vitro* toxicological findings, hydralazine in therapeutic doses does not appear to bear a risk that would necessitate a limitation of its administration. Many years of clinical experience have not suggested that human cancer is associated with hydralazine use.

Apresoline may impair the patient's reactions, especially at the start of treatment. The patient should be warned of the hazard when driving or operating machinery.

Precautions: In patients with renal impairment (creatinine clearance < 30 ml/min or serum creatinine concentrations > 2.5 mg/100 ml or 221 μmol/l) and in patients with hepatic dysfunction the dose or interval between doses should be adjusted according to clinical response, in order to avoid accumulation of the "apparent" active substance.

Apresoline should be used with caution in patients with coronary artery disease (since it may increase angina) or cerebrovascular disease.

When undergoing surgery, patients treated with Apresoline may show a fall in blood pressure, in which case one should not use adrenaline to correct the hypotension, since it enhances the cardiac-accelerating effects of hydralazine.

When initiating therapy in heart failure, particular caution should be exercised and the patient kept under surveillance and/or haemodynamic monitoring for early detection of postural hypotension or tachycardia. Where discontinuation of therapy in heart failure is indicated, Apresoline should be withdrawn gradually (except in serious situations, such as SLE-like syndrome or blood dyscrasias) in order to avoid precipitation and/or exacerbation of heart failure.

Drug interactions: Potentiation of effects: Concurrent therapy with other antihypertensives (vasodilators, calcium antagonists, ACE inhibitors, diuretics), anaesthetics, tricyclic antidepressants, major tranquillisers or drugs exerting central depressant actions (including alcohol). Administration of Apresoline shortly before or after diazoxide may give rise to marked hypotension.

MAO inhibitors should be used with caution in patients receiving Apresoline.

Concurrent administration of Apresoline with beta-blockers subject to a strong first-pass effect (eg propranolol) may increase their bioavailability. Downward adjustment of these drugs may be required when they are given concomitantly with Apresoline.

Side-effects: Some of the adverse effects listed below eg tachycardia, palpitation, anginal symptoms, flushing, headache, dizziness, nasal congestion and gastrointestinal disturbances are commonly seen at the start of treatment, especially if the dose is raised quickly. However such effects generally subside in the further course of treatment.

Cardiovascular system: Frequently: tachycardia, palpitation. Occasionally: flushing, hypotension, anginal symptoms. Rarely: oedema, heart failure. Isolated cases: paradoxical pressor responses.

Central and peripheral nervous system: Frequently: headache. Rarely: dizziness. Isolated cases: peripheral neuritis, polyneuritis, paraesthesiae (these unwanted effects may be reversed by administering pyridoxine).

Musculo-skeletal system: Occasionally: arthralgia, joint swelling, myalgia.

Skin and appendages: Rarely: rash.

Urogenital system: Rarely: proteinuria, increased plasma creatinine, haematuria sometimes in association with glomerulonephritis. Isolated cases: acute renal failure, urinary retention.

Gastro-intestinal tract: Occasionally: gastro-intestinal disturbances, diarrhoea, nausea, vomiting. Rarely: jaundice, liver enlargement, abnormal liver function sometimes in association with hepatitis. Isolated cases: paralytic ileus.

Blood: Rarely: anaemia, leucopenia, neutropenia, thrombocytopenia with or without purpura. Isolated cases: haemolytic anaemia, leucocytosis, lymphadenopathy, pancytopenia, splenomegaly, agranulocytosis.

Psyche: Rarely: agitation, anorexia, anxiety. Isolated cases: depression, hallucinations.

Sense organs: Rarely: increased lacrimation, conjunctivitis, nasal congestion.

Hypersensitivity reactions: Occasionally: SLE-like syndrome (see under "Warnings"). Rarely: hypersensitivity reactions such as pruritus, urticaria, vasculitis, eosinophilia, hepatitis.

Respiratory tract: Rarely: dyspnoea, pleural pain.

Miscellaneous: Rarely: fever, weight decrease, malaise. Isolated cases: exophthalmos.

Overdosage: Symptoms include hypotension, tachycardia, myocardial ischaemia, dysrrhythmias and coma.

Gastric lavage should be instituted as soon as possible. Supportive measures including intravenous fluids are also indicated. If hypotension is present, an attempt should be made to raise the blood pressure without increasing the tachycardia. Adrenaline should therefore be avoided.

Pharmaceutical precautions The tablets should be protected from heat and moisture. The ampoules should be protected from heat and light.

Legal category POM.

Package quantities Apresoline tablets: Securitainers of 100. Apresoline ampoules: Boxes of 5.

Further information Nil.

Product licence numbers
Apresoline tablets 25 mg: 0008/5002R
Apresoline tablets 50 mg: 0008/0029R
Apresoline ampoules 20 mg: 0008/5065R

AREDIA* ▼

Presentation Ampoules containing 15 mg pamidronate disodium (calculated as anhydrous form) dissolved in 5 ml Water for Injections PhEur. The aqueous concentrate is for intravenous infusion. The ampoules also contain mannitol and phosphoric acid.

Uses
Indication: For the treatment of tumour-induced hypercalcaemia.

Mode of action: Aredia (pamidronate disodium) is a bisphosphonate. It is known to be a potent inhibitor of bone resorption but the exact mechanism of action has not been fully elucidated. There is evidence that Aredia can inhibit osteoclastic activity, and the formation and dissolution of calcium apatite crystals *in vitro*. The physico-chemical interaction between the drug and the apatite crystals accounts for its avid binding to bone.

Pharmacokinetics: It has not yet been possible to define the detailed pharmacokinetics of Aredia in man, although it is clear that the drug displays a very strong affinity for bone.

Experimental work in rats using radiolabelled pamidronate disodium has shown that after intravenous administration, approximately 50% of the dose (10 mg/kg) is retained in bone. The apparent elimination half-life from bone is estimated to be about 300 days. Biliary excretion accounts for less than 0.1% of the administered dose. Pamidronate disodium is not metabolised in rats to a measurable degree.

Dosage and administration Aredia must never be given as a bolus injection (see 'Warnings'). Following appropriate parenteral/oral rehydration, Aredia should be diluted in a calcium-free infusion solution (e.g. 0.9% w/v Sodium Chloride Intravenous Infusion BP or 5% Glucose Intravenous Infusion BP) and infused *slowly*.

Use in adults and the elderly: It is recommended that the total dosage of Aredia used be determined by the patient's initial plasma calcium level.

The following guidelines are derived from clinical data on uncorrected calcium values. However, doses in the ranges given would also be applicable for calcium corrected for total protein or albumin:

Initial plasma calcium (mmol/l)	*(mg %)*	*Recommended total dose (mg)*
up to 3.0	up to 12.0	15–30
3.0–3.5	12.0–14.0	30–60
3.5–4.0	14.0–16.0	60–90
>4.0	>16.0	90

The total dosage of Aredia may be given as a single infusion or in divided doses as convenient. The maximum dose per treatment course of Aredia is 90 mg for both initial and repeat courses. Higher doses bring no increased clinical benefit.

Single intravenous infusions:
15 mg Aredia given in 125 ml infusion solution over 2 hours.
30 mg Aredia given in 250 ml infusion solution over 4 hours.
60 mg Aredia given in 500 ml infusion solution over 8 hours.

In severe cases, a dose of 90 mg may be necesary and until further experience is gained, this should be given in at least one litre of infusion solution over 24 hours.

Multiple intravenous infusions:
The total dosage may be given in divided doses over 2–4 consecutive days. The recommended dilution volumes and infusion times are as described above for single infusions.

A total dose of 30 mg: 15 mg Aredia given on 2 consecutive days
A total dose of 60 mg: 15 mg Aredia given on 4 consecutive days
or
30 mg Aredia given on 2 consecutive days.

Serum calcium levels start to decrease 24–48 hours after drug administration and maximum lowering can be expected after 4–5 days. If normocalcaemia is not achieved within this time period, a further dose may be given. The duration of the response varies considerably from patient to patient and treatment can be repeated whenever hypercalcaemia recurs. Clinical experience to date suggests that Aredia may be less effective as the number of treatments increases.

Transient asymptomatic hypocalcaemia is not uncommon, but symptomatic hypocalcaemia is rare.

Use in children: There is no clinical experience of Aredia in children.

Contra-indications, warnings, etc
Contra-indications: Known hypersensitivity to pamidronate disodium.

Warnings: Aredia must never be given as a bolus injection since severe local reactions and thrombophlebitis may occur. Aredia should always be diluted and given as a slow intravenous infusion over at least 2 hours (see 'Dosage and administration').

Aredia should not be co-administered with other bisphosphonates or plicamycin (mithramycin).

There is a possibility of precipitating convulsions in some patients due to the electrolyte changes associated with tumour-induced hypercalcaemia and its effective treatment.

Precautions: There is very little experience of the use of Aredia in patients with severe renal insufficiency. Therefore Aredia should be used with caution in such patients, i.e. it is recommended that the chosen dose be administered as multiple doses rather than as a single administration. Aredia has been used successfully in patients with moderate renal insufficiency (i.e. plasma creatinine levels of at least twice the normal value).

Oliguria has been seen with bisphosphonates in general, although to date there is little evidence of Aredia causing severe impairment of renal function.

Use in pregnancy: There is no clinical experience in pregnant women and therefore the drug should only be used if considered to be essential.

Drug interactions: No specific drug interactions have been reported to date although the additive effects of other hypocalcaemic therapies (e.g. calcitonin, steroids) should be recognised. (Also see 'Warnings'.)

Side-effects: The following effects have been observed frequently:

A mild, transient rise in body temperature of 1–2°C at the onset of treatment; this generally lasts for 1–2 days.

A transient reduction in lymphocyte count lasting for 1–7 days after the infusion.

These effects do not appear to be clinically relevant.

Overdosage: There is no experience on overdosage with Aredia.

Symptoms: Overdosage would be clinically manifested as the signs and symptoms of hypocalcaemia, i.e. paraesthesia and carpopedal spasm.

Treatment: In the event of clinically significant hypocalcaemia, reversal may be achieved with an infusion of calcium gluconate.

Pharmaceutical precautions
Storage: Store ampoules in a refrigerator at 2–8°C. Do not store the diluted infusion solution before use.

Incompatibilities: Aredia must not be admixed with calcium-containing infusion solutions, e.g. Ringer, Hartmann's solution.

Legal category POM.

Package quantities Aredia is available in packs of 4 ampoules. Ampoules contain 15 mg pamidronate disodium in 5 ml Water for Injection PhEur.

Further information Changes in biochemical parameters which reflect a decrease in bone resorption and improvements secondary to the normalisation of serum calcium include decreased urinary hydroxyproline, urinary calcium and urinary phosphate excretion.

Aredia has no direct effect on any renal component of hypercalcaemia. However, a consequence of its hypocalcaemic effect is an improvement in renal function and decreased serum creatinine levels in most patients.

Product licence number 0001/0138.

DESFERAL*

Presentation A sterile, lyophilised powder available in vials containing 500 mg of Desferrioxamine Mesylate BP.

Uses
Indications: Iron overload—Acute iron poisoning; primary and secondary haemochromatosis including thalassaemia and transfusional haemosiderosis; in patients in whom concomitant disorders (e.g. severe anaemia, hypoproteinaemia, renal failure) preclude phlebotomy; for the treatment of corneal rust stains and ocular siderosis; and for the diagnosis of iron storage disease and certain anaemias.

Aluminium overload—in patients on maintenance dialysis for end stage renal failure where preventative measures (eg reverse osmosis) have failed and with proven aluminium-related bone disease and/or anaemia, dialysis encephalopathy; and for diagnosis of aluminium overload.

Mode of action: Desferal is a chelating agent for trivalent iron and aluminium ions; the resulting chelates (ferrioxamine and aluminoxamine) are stable and non-toxic. Neither chelate undergoes intestinal absorption, and any formed systemically as a result of parenteral administration is rapidly excreted via the kidneys without deleterious effects. Desferal takes up iron either free or bound to ferritin and haemosiderin. Similarly it mobilises and chelates tissue bound aluminium. It does not remove iron from haemin containing substances including haemoglobin and transferrin. Since both ferrioxamine and aluminoxamine are completely excreted, Desferal promotes the excretion of iron and aluminium in urine and faeces thus reducing pathological iron or aluminium deposits in the organs and tissues.

Pharmacokinetics: Desferrioxamine mesylate is rapidly absorbed following intramuscular or subcutaneous administration. In healthy volunteers peak plasma concentrations of desferrioxamine (15.5 μmol/litre – 8.7 μg/ml) and ferrioxamine (3.7 μmol/litre – 2.3 μg/ml) were observed at 30 minutes and 1 hour respectively, following an injection (10 mg/kg) of desferrioxamine.

Serum protein binding of desferrioxamine is less than 10% *in vitro*.

In healthy subjects elimination is biphasic, first phase half-lives for desferrioxamine and ferrioxamine are 1 hour and 2.4 hours, respectively. In the second phase both compounds have a half-life of 6 hours. Of the injected dose 22% appears in the urine as desferrioxamine and 1% as ferrioxamine, after 6 hours.

In patients with haemochromatosis peak plasma levels of 7.0 μmol/litre (3.9 μg/ml) were measured for desferrioxamine, and 15.7 μmol/litre (9.6 μg/ml) for ferrioxamine, 1 hour after intramuscular injection of 10 mg/kg desferrioxamine. These patients eliminated desferrioxamine and ferrioxamine with half-lives of 5.6 and 4.6 hours, respectively. Six hours after the injection 17% of the dose was excreted in the urine as desferrioxamine and 12% as ferrioxamine.

In patients dialysed for renal failure who received 40 mg/kg desferrioxamine infused i.v. within 1 hour, the plasma concentration at the end of the infusion was 152 μmol/litre (85.2 μg/ml) when the infusion was given between dialysis sessions. Plasma concentrations of desferrioxamine were between 13% and 27% lower when the infusion was administered during dialysis. Concentrations of ferrioxamine were in all cases approx. 7.0 μmol/litre (4.3 μg/ml) with concomitant aluminoxamine levels of 2–3 μmol/litre (1.2–1.8 μg/ml). After the infusion was discontinued, the plasma concentration of desferrioxamine decreased rapidly with a half-life of 20 minutes. A smaller fraction of the dose was eliminated with a longer half-life of 14 hours. Plasma concentrations of aluminoxamine continued to increase for up to 48 hours post-infusion and reached values of approx. 7 μmol/litre (4 μg/ml). Following dialysis the plasma concentration of aluminoxamine fell to 2.2 μmol/litre (1.3 μg/ml), indicating that the aluminoxamine complex is dialysable.

During peritoneal dialysis desferrioxamine is absorbed if administered in the dialysis fluid.

Dosage and administration Desferal may be administered parenterally, orally (for acute iron poisoning only) or by ocular instillation (for treatment of corneal rust stains and ocular siderosis).

Preparation
For parenteral administration: The drug should be employed in the form of a 10% solution, e.g. by dissolving the contents of one vial (500 mg) in 5 ml of Water for Injection. The 10% Desferal solution can be diluted with routinely employed infusion solutions (saline, glucose, dextrose or dextrose-saline), although these should not be used as solvent for the dry substance. Dissolved Desferal can also be added to dialysis fluid and given intraperitoneally to patients on continuous ambulatory peritoneal dialysis (CAPD) or continuous cyclic peritoneal dialysis (CCPD).

Only clear Desferal solutions should be used. Heparin is pharmaceutically incompatible with Desferal solutions.

For oral administration: 5–10 g Desferal should be dissolved in 50–100 ml of water.

For ocular instillation: Method of preparation of eye drops.

1. Preparation of solvent: Formula:

Methyl cellulose 4,000 cps	25 mg	0.5%
Benzyl alcohol	50 mg	1.0%
Water for Injection q.s.	5.0 ml	100%

Method: The methyl cellulose is dispersed in Water for Injection at 90°C. This is cooled with continuous stirring. When the temperature reaches 35°C, benzyl alcohol is added and the solution diluted to volume with Water for Injection. The solution should be filtered through a No 1, then No 2 sintered glass filter. 5 ml of this solution are filled into brown/amber eye drop bottles, stoppered and autoclaved at 110°C for 20 minutes.

2. Preparation of drops: To be carried out under aseptic conditions.

(a) Remove foil disc from Desferal vial containing 500 mg Desferal.
(b) Unscrew eye drop bottle cap and take up 5 ml of solvent into a sterile syringe; replace cap.
(c) Inject solvent into vial and shake to dissolve the Desferal. Care should be taken to dissolve all the Desferal.
(d) Withdraw the solution into the sterile syringe;

remove cap from bottle; transfer solution to bottle and replace cap.

The drops are now ready for use.

Treatment

Acute iron poisoning: Desferal may be administered both orally and parentally. It is important to initiate treatment as soon as possible.

Gastric lavage should be carried out as quickly as possible using, if readily available, 1% sodium bicarbonate solution. This should be followed by oral administration of Desferal which will chelate any iron remaining in the stomach and prevent any further absorption. Further measures, e.g. sodium bicarbonate, sedatives, oxygen etc., may be given as necessary.

To eliminate the iron that has already been absorbed Desferal should be given either intramuscularly or – particularly if the patient is seriously ill and already in a state of shock or hypotensive – intravenously. The dosage and route of administration should be adapted to the severity of the poisoning, preferably by reference to the serum iron levels and total iron binding capacity, which should be regularly monitored.

Dosage: The normal dose is:

Adults: 2 g given as a single i.m. dose
Children: 1 g given as a single i.m. dose

If the patient is hypotensive, the i.v. route of administration is recommended. It is recommended that the maximum rate of i.v. administration 15 mg/kg/hr, should be reduced after 4–6 hours so that the total i.v. dose does not exceed 80 mg/kg/24 hours. However in the absence of adverse effects, much larger doses may be tolerated.

Therapy should be continued until serum iron levels are less than the total iron binding capacity.

The effectiveness of treatment is dependent on an adequate urine output in order that the iron complex (ferrioxamine) is excreted from the body. Therefore, if oliguria or anuria develop, peritoneal dialysis or haemodialysis may become necessary to remove ferrioxamine.

It should be noted that the serum iron level may rise sharply when the iron is released from the tissues.

Theoretically 100 mg Desferal can chelate 8.5 mg of ferric iron.

Primary and secondary haemochromatosis including thalassaemia, in patients in whom concomitant disorders (e.g. severe anaemia, hypoproteinaemia) preclude phlebotomy: Treatment of chronic iron overload with Desferal is designed to achieve: (i) an iron balance and prevent haemosiderosis in young patients, (ii) to produce a negative iron balance to slowly deplete iron stores and to prevent the toxic effects of iron in those with established disease.

Dosage:

Adults and children: The dosage schedules should be individually adapted according to the degree of iron overload.

To assess the chelation therapy, 24 hour urinary iron excretion should be monitored daily. Starting with a dose of 500 mg daily the dose should be raised until a plateau of iron excretion is reached. Once the appropriate dose has been established, urinary iron excretion can be determined at longer intervals, the maximum recommended interval is once every 2 weeks.

Chelation therapy is considered to be satisfactory when serum ferritin levels are close to normal (less than or equal to 300 μg/l).

Although the dosage and route of administration should be determined for each individual, in most patients daily doses of 20–40 mg/kg body weight are usually adequate. The lowest dose effective in producing a negative iron balance should be used. Higher doses should only be employed if the benefit for the patient outweighs the risk of unwanted effects.

Although Desferal can be given by intramuscular injection, in most cases it exerts a considerably greater effect when administered – preferably with the aid of a portable, light-weight, infusion pump – by continuous intravenous or subcutaneous infusions, which are particularly suitable for ambulant patients. The dose is delivered over a period of 8–12 hours. In some patients it is possible to achieve a further increase in iron excretion by infusing the same daily dose over a 24 hour period. Patients should be treated 3–7 times a week depending on the degree of iron overload.

For intramuscular treatment the average initial dose is 500 mg–1.0 g daily, given in 1–2 injections. The maintenance dose to be selected will depend on the patient's iron excretion rate.

Corneal rust stains and ocular siderosis: The eye drops should be administered 4–6 times daily.

Diagnosis of iron storage disease and certain anaemias: The Desferal test for iron overload is based on the principle that normal subjects do not excrete more than a fraction of a milligram of iron in their urine daily and a standard intramuscular injection of 500 mg of Desferal does not increase this above 1 mg. In iron storage diseases, however, the increase may be well over 1.5 mg. The test yields reliable results only when renal function is normal.

Procedure:

1. The haemoglobin, serum iron and total iron binding capacity are estimated.

2. 500 mg of Desferal are given intramuscularly and 400 ml of water are drunk.

3. All urine is collected over the next six hours.

4. The urinary iron is estimated in the six hour urine specimen.

An excretion of 1–1.5 mg (18–27 μmol) of iron during this 6-hour period is suggestive of an iron-storage disease; values of more than 1.5 mg (27 μmol) can be regarded as pathological.

Patients with terminal renal failure: In such patients receiving haemodialysis, serum iron should be determined before and after administration of Desferal (500 mg i.m.). A continuous increase in serum iron during the hours following is suggestive of iron overload.

Use in the elderly: No special dosage regime is necessary but concurrent renal insufficiency should be taken into account.

Use in children: The dosage recommendations are the same as for adults.

Treatment for aluminium overload in patients with terminal renal failure: The precise dosage should be individually determined and adapted during the course of treatment.

Theoretically 100 mg Desferal can bind 4.1 mg $A1^{+++}$.

Patients on maintenance haemodialysis or haemofiltration: In patients with moderate aluminium overload (without concomitant iron overload) 1 g given i.v. during the last hour of every third dialyses should produce a maximal increase in serum aluminium which will then be eliminated during subsequent dialyses as chelate. In cases of severe aluminium overload, plasma aluminium levels should be determined before and after administration of different doses so that the lowest effective dose level can be selected.

Patients on CAPD or CCPD: 1 g once or twice per week; Desferal is equally effective administered i.v. (by slow infusion), i.m., s.c. or intraperitoneally. The mode of administration should be individually determined and the dosage adapted during the course of therapy.

Diagnosis of aluminium overload: Serum aluminium values should be determined before and after Desferal administration (1 g i.v.). A continuous increase in serum aluminium during the 24 to 48 hour period following administration is suggestive of aluminium overload.

Use in children: Little clinical experience has been gained to date on the use of desferrioxamine in aluminium-overloaded children, the condition being rare in the very young. Until further data are available it is recommended that dosage be adapted at the discretion of the physician from the adult dose adjusted for bodyweight (ie 15 to 20 mg/kg).

Contra-indications, warnings, etc

Contra-indications: Hypersensitivity to desferrioxamine mesylate unless the patient can be desensitized.

Precautions: Desferal should be used with caution in

patients with renal dysfunction, since the metal complexes are excreted mainly via the kidneys. In these patients, dialysis will increase the elimination of chelated iron and aluminium.

Used alone Desferal may exacerbate neurological dysfunction in patients with aluminium-related encephalopathy. This deterioration (manifest as seizures) is probably related to an acute increase in brain aluminium secondary to elevated circulating levels. Pretreatment with clonazepam has been shown to afford protection against such dysfunction.

Treatment with Desferal by the intravenous route should only be administered in the form of *slow* infusions. If an intramuscular injection is accidentally given intravenously, this may lead to circulatory collapse.

Patients suffering from iron overload are particularly susceptible to infection. There have been reports of Desferal promoting some infections such as Yersinia enterocolitica and Y. pseudotuberculosis. If patients develop fever with pharyngitis, diffuse abdominal pain or enteritis/enterocolitis, Desferal therapy should be stopped, and appropriate treatment with antibiotics should be instituted. Desferal therapy may be resumed once the infection has cleared.

In patients undergoing haemodialysis while receiving Desferal, there have been rare reports of severe fungal infection (i.e. cases of mucormycosis). However no causal link with the use of the drug has been established.

Disturbances of vision and hearing have been reported during prolonged Desferal therapy. In particular this has occurred in patients on higher than recommended therapy or in patients with low serum ferritin levels. Therefore, ophthalmological and audiological tests should be carried out both prior to the institution of long-term therapy with Desferal and at 3-monthly intervals during treatment. A detailed ophthalmological assessment is recommended (visual field measurements, funduscopy, colour vision testing using pseudiosochromatic plates and the Farnsworth D-15 colour test, slit lamp investigation, visual evoked potential studies).

If disturbances of vision or hearing do occur, treatment with Desferal should be stopped. Such disturbances may be reversible. If Desferal therapy is re-instituted later at a lower dosage, close monitoring of ophthalmological/auditory function should be carried out with due regard to the risk-benefit ratio.

Use in pregnancy and lactation: Desferal has caused teratogenic effects in animals when given during pregnancy, particularly in the first trimester.

In rabbits, desferrioxamine caused skeletal malformations. However, these teratogenic effects in the foetuses were observed at doses which were toxic to the mother. In mice and rats desferrioxamine appears to be free of teratogenic activity.

It is not known whether Desferal is excreted into the breast milk.

Desferal should not be given to pregnant or lactating women unless in the judgement of the physician, the expected benefits to the mother outweigh the potential risk to the child.

Drug interactions: Oral administration of vitamin C in the standard dosage (150–250 mg daily, given in fractional doses) may serve to enhance excretion of the iron complex in response to Desferal; larger doses of vitamin C fail to produce an additional effect. Vitamin C should not be administered within 1–2 weeks of starting Desferal therapy. In patients with severe chronic iron-storage disease undergoing combined treatment with Desferal and high doses of vitamin C (more than 500 mg daily) impairment of cardiac function has been encountered; this proved reversible when the vitamin C was withdrawn. Monitoring of cardiac function is indicated during such combined therapy.

Desferal should not be used in combination with prochlorperazine (a phenothiazine derivative) since prolonged unconsciousness may result.

There is evidence that aluminium intoxication causes reduced erythropoiesis. In dialysed patients with aluminium and/or iron overload treated with desferrioxamine and erythropoietin some dosage adjustment of the latter may be necessary. Regular monitoring of iron stores should also be carried out.

Side-effects: There have been rare reports of allergic skin reactions, cardiovascular (e.g. hypotension, cardiac arrhythmias), neurological (e.g. dizziness, convulsions), and gastro-intestinal disturbances, impairment of hepatic and renal function, changes in the blood picture (e.g. thrombocytopenia), anaphylactoid reactions and leg cramps.

Disturbances of hearing and vision have been reported including opacities of the lens (see 'Precautions').

Retinal changes have been described in patients on higher than recommended, intensive Desferal therapy and also in predisposed patients (e.g. in patients with impaired glucose tolerance and those with increased vascular permeability) receiving the recommended therapeutic dose. Initial symptoms include night blindness, loss of colour vision, field defects and blurred vision. If eye symptoms in any way suggestive of a retinopathy occur, Desferal should be discontinued. In patients considered at risk, examination of the retina is essential prior to and during treatment.

Some of the side effects mentioned above must be considered as signs and symptoms of the underlying disease. Local pain may occur after intramuscular injection. Excretion of the iron complex during treatment with Desferal may cause reddish-brown discolouration of the urine.

Overdosage: Desferal is usually administered parenterally and acute poisoning is unlikely to occur, (daily doses of 16 g Desferal given by i.v. infusion have been well tolerated).

Signs and symptoms: Tachycardia, hypotension and gastrointestinal symptoms have occasionally occurred in patients who received an overdose of Desferal.

Treatment: There is no specific antidote to Desferal but signs and symptoms may be eliminated by reducing the dosage and Desferal is dialysable. Appropriate supportive therapy should be instituted.

Pharmaceutical precautions
Storage: Desferal should be stored in a cool place (8–15°C).

Dilution: The reconstituted solution should not be stored for longer than 24 hours at room temperature (23°C or below).

The eye drop solution should be discarded at the end of one week from the date of preparation.

Legal category POM.

Package quantities Packs of 10 vials containing 500 mg Desferal.

Further information Nil.

Product licence number 0008/5073R

ESIDREX*

Presentation Tablets containing 25 mg Hydrochlorothiazide BP, circular, flat, white, with bevelled edges, impressed with the monogram CIBA on one side and the letters CE and a break line on the other.

Tablets containing 50 mg of Hydrochlorothiazide BP, circular, flat, white, with bevelled edges impressed with the monogram CIBA on one side and the letters UT and a break line on the other.

The tablets also contain lactose and gluten (wheat starch).

Uses *Mode of action;* Esidrex is a thiazide diuretic which exerts its diuretic effect in inhibiting the re-absorption of sodium, chloride and water, probably at the proximal renal tubules.

Indications: It is indicated for the treatment of oedema associated with acute and chronic heart failure, various hepatic conditions, renal disorders; such as chronic glomerular nephritis and nephrotic syndrome, the pre-menstrual syndrome and fluid retention associated with obesity, diabetes insipidus or drug therapy (e.g. with corticosteroids.) It is also recommended for the treatment of hypertension, including hypertension occurring during pregnancy. It is also used to potentiate other antihypertensives such as guanethidine and reserpine.

Dosage and administration Esidrex is given orally. The dosage for adults is:

In acute and chronic heart failure – initially 50–100 mg daily, reducing to a maintenance dose of 25–50 mg three or four days weekly.

Chronic glomerular nephritis, nephrotic syndrome, ascites and hepatic cirrhosis, initially 50–75 mg daily. This may be reduced to a maintenance dose of 25–50 mg on alternate days.

Pre-menstrual oedema – 25 mg daily from the onset of symptoms until menstruation begins.

Drug-induced oedema, 25–50 mg on alternate days.

Hypertension – 25 mg increasing gradually to 75 mg daily according to the response.

Hypertension and oedema of pregnancy, mild symptoms, 25–50 mg daily, moderate hypertension – 50–100 mg daily initially and then reducing to a lower dose when control is achieved.

In all indications the total daily dose may be given as a single dose after breakfast. As Esidrex increases salt excretion it is usually possible to relax dietary salt restrictions.

Children: At the discretion of the physician.

Use in the elderly: No special dosage regime is necessary (also see 'Precautions').

Contra-indications, warnings, etc

Contra-indications: Esidrex, in common with other thiazides is contra-indicated in the presence of precoma associated with hepatic cirrhosis, or Addison's disease or advanced renal failure.

Precautions: In patients with some degree of renal impairment, a rise in blood urea can occur and in extreme cases result in an oliguric crisis. In such cases, either the dose should be reduced or the treatment interrupted temporarily.

Prolonged doses may bring about a decrease in glucose tolerance and precipitate a diabetic condition. In known diabetics the addition of Esidrex to the treatment regime will almost certainly alter the insulin requirement.

In common with other thiazide diuretics hyperuricaemia may be induced by Esidrex. Gout may be exacerbated in patients with a previous history or family history of this condition.

Patients who are being treated with this preparation may require regular monitoring of fluid and electrolyte balance particularly when diuresis is substantial or in patients suffering from renal impairment. Potassium supplements may be required. Particular caution is needed with this preparation in the elderly since electrolyte balance is more likely to be precarious due to bowel or renal dysfunction. Also urinary retention is more likely.

Esidrex should only be used during pregnancy if considered essential by the physician.

The concomitant administration of this preparation with cardiac glycosides or hypotensive agents may necessitate adjustment of the dosage of those drugs.

Drug interactions; The action of tricyclic antidepressants and MAO inhibitors may be potentiated by Esidrex.

Side-effects: Side-effects such as mild anorexia, nausea, constipation and diarrhoea, skin rashes and photosensitivity may occur. There have been reports of blood dyscrasias including thrombocytopenia, but these are rare.

Overdosage: Esidrex is self-limiting in its action and toxic effects have not been observed.

Pharmaceutical precautions Esidrex should be protected from moisture and should preferably be dispensed in a moisture-proof container.

Legal category POM.

Package quantities Esidrex 25 mg and 50 mg Tablets are available in Securitainers of 100.

Further information Esidrex has a powerful saluretic and diuretic action, is well tolerated and remains effective when administered for long periods.

Esidrex acts on the renal tubules, inhibiting the reabsorption of sodium and chloride. Low-salt diets may therefore be relaxed during Esidrex therapy.

Esidrex reduces high blood pressure and potentiates the action of other antihypertensives but has no effect on the blood pressure in normotensive individuals.

Product licence numbers

Esidrex Tablets 25 mg 0008/5045
Esidrex Tablets 50 mg 0008/5046

ESTRADERM* TTS

Presentation Estraderm TTS is a self-adhesive, transparent, transdermal therapeutic system, containing a drug reservoir of 17β-oestradiol. It is available in three sizes:

Estraderm TTS 25 with an absorption rate of approximately 25 micrograms of oestradiol in 24 hours (active surface area 5 cm^2, oestradiol content 2 mg).

Estraderm TTS 50 with an absorption rate of approximately 50 micrograms of oestradiol in 24 hours (active surface area 10 cm^2, oestradiol content 4 mg).

Estraderm TTS 100 with an absorption rate of approximately 100 micrograms of oestradiol in 24 hours (active surface area 20 cm^2 oestradiol content 8 mg).

The drug reservoir contains ethanol.

Uses

Indications: Oestrogen replacement therapy for patients with disorders due to natural or surgically induced menopause e.g. vasomotor symptoms (hot flushes and nocturnal sweating), urogenital conditions such as atrophic vaginitis/vulvitis, and/or atrophic urethritis and trigonitis.

Oestrogen therapy must not be used in patients with an intact uterus unless an appropriate dose of progestogen is administered for twelve days per month.

Mode of action: Oestrogen substitution effectively prevents the characteristic symptomatic, metabolic and trophic changes associated with loss of ovarian function due to natural or surgical menopause.

Estraderm TTS is a dosage form designed to achieve release of 17β-oestradiol, via intact skin to the systemic circulation for several days at a low rate.

Pharmacokinetics: Within four hours after application of the first system, plasma oestradiol levels reach the therapeutic range and these are maintained throughout the dose interval (for up to four days).

After removal of the last system plasma oestrogen levels return to baseline values in less than 24 hours and urinary oestrogen conjugates within 2–3 days.

Absorption rate may vary between individual patients. However, the plasma oestradiol levels achieved with different sized systems has been shown to be proportional to the drug-releasing area of the dosage form.

Dosage and administration

Adults and elderly: Therapy should be initiated with one Estraderm TTS 50 and the dose adjusted after the first treatment month depending on efficacy and signs of overdosage (e.g. breast tenderness). For maintenance therapy the lowest effective dose should be used; a maximum dose of 100 micrograms per day should not be exceeded. Unopposed oestrogen therapy should not be used unless the patient has had a hysterectomy. Where a progestogen is considered necessary, the appropriate dose should be administered for 12 days per month.

Estraderm TTS should be applied twice weekly on a continuous basis, each used system being removed after 3–4 days and a fresh system applied to a slightly different site. Recommended application sites are clean, dry and intact areas of skin on the trunk below the waistline. Estraderm TTS should *NOT* be applied on or near the breasts.

Children: Estraderm TTS is not indicated in children.

Use in pregnancy and lactation: Estraderm TTS is not indicated.

Contra-indications, warnings, etc
Contra-indications: Cancer of the breast, genital tract or other oestrogen-dependant neoplasia; severe hepatic, renal or cardiac disease; undiagnosed vaginal bleeding; history of thrombosis or thromboembolic disease; endometriosis.

Precautions and warnings: Before commencing any oestrogen replacement therapy it is recommended that the patient should have a thorough physical and gynaecological examination. This should be repeated at regular intervals.

Close monitoring of patients with the following conditions is recommended: Mastopathy, or strong family history of mammary cancer; hypertension – regular monitoring of blood pressure should be carried out; cholelithiasis.

Prior to surgery, discontinuation should be considered.

Side-effects: Although side-effects are rare, headaches, nausea and breast tenderness may occur. (If breast tenderness is continual a dosage reduction should be considered.)

Some patients experience mild and transient local erythema at the site of patch application, with or without itching. This usually disappears 3–4 days after patch removal and is similar to the effect sometimes observed after occlusion of the skin with household medical adhesive plasters. Very infrequently local swelling, papules/vesicles and scaling have been reported, which also resolved spontaneously and did not result in permanent skin damage.

If unacceptable topical side-effects do occur discontinuation of treatment with Estraderm TTS should be considered.

Overdosage: This is not likely due to the mode of administration, but can if necessary be rapidly reversed by removal of the patch(es).

Pharmaceutical precautions Store below 25°C.

Legal category POM.

Package quantities Cartons containing eight Estraderm TTS patches, each individually sealed in a protective pouch (sufficient for one month's treatment) (OP).

Further information Estraderm TTS represents an easy and efficient method of administering 17β-oestradiol in a manner which gives oestradiol blood levels similar to those in the early follicular phase. The transdermal route achieves similar oestradiol plasma levels to those obtained with oral therapy, but at much lower daily doses and with restoration of the natural physiological oestrone/oestradiol ratio. Unlike oral oestrogens, transdermal therapy results in a low total oestrogen load on the liver, and Estraderm TTS does not increase renin substrate levels. Dose adjustments can easily be made as accumulation of oestrogen metabolites does not occur.

Product licence numbers

Estraderm TTS 25	0001/0112
Estraderm TTS 50	0001/0113
Estraderm TTS 100	0001/0114

ESTRAPAK* 50

Presentation Estrapak 50 is a calendar pack comprising:

(i) 8 self-adhesive, transparent, transdermal therapeutic systems (patches), containing a drug reservoir of 17β-oestradiol with an absorption rate of approximately 50 micrograms of oestradiol per day (active surface area 10 cm^2, oestradiol content 4 mg). The drug reservoir also contains ethanol.

(ii) 12 red tablets containing 1 mg Norethisterone Acetate BP. The tablets are round, have slightly convex faces, slightly bevelled edges, approximately 6.2 mm diameter, imprinted CG on one side and LK on the other. The tablets also contain lactose and polyethoxylated castor oils.

Uses
Indications: Hormone replacement therapy for patients with disorders due to natural or surgically induced menopause, e.g. vasomotor symptoms (hot flushes and nocturnal sweating), urogenital conditions such as atrophic vaginitis/vulvitis, and/or atrophic urethritis and trigonitis.

Mode of action: Oestrogen substitution effectively prevents the characteristic symptomatic, metabolic and trophic changes associated with loss of ovarian function due to the menopause.

The transdermal oestrogen patch is a dosage form designed to achieve release of 17β-oestradiol, via intact skin to the systemic circulation for several days, at a low rate.

An oral progestogen is included for 12 days in each cycle in order to prevent endometrial hyperstimulation. A withdrawal bleed can be expected to start on day 24–26 of treatment.

Pharmacokinetics: Within four hours after application of the first transdermal oestrogen patch, plasma oestradiol levels reach the therapeutic range and these are maintained throughout the dose interval (for up to four days).

After removal of the last patch, plasma oestradiol levels return to baseline values in less than 24 hours and urinary oestrogen conjugates within 2–3 days.

Absorption rate may vary between individual patients.

Norethisterone acetate is rapidly absorbed from the gastrointestinal tract and converted to norethisterone, which has a half-life of 7.5–8 hours.

Dosage and administration
Adults and elderly: Transdermal oestrogen administration is continued without a break in therapy; oral progestogen is included in the dosage regime for 12 days out of each month of oestrogen replacement.

The transdermal oestrogen patch should be applied twice weekly on a continuous basis, each used patch being removed after 3–4 days and a fresh patch applied to a slightly different site. Recommended application sites are clean, dry and intact areas of skin on the trunk below the waistline. The oestrogen patches should *not* be applied on or near the breasts. One norethisterone acetate tablet should be taken by mouth daily for days 15–26 of each 28 days of oestrogen replacement therapy.

In women with an intact uterus for whom hormone replacement is required, Estrapak 50 should be administered in preference to unopposed oestrogen therapy. This may be particularly important in those who are obese or who have diabetes, low parity or a familial history of endometrial carcinoma.

Estrapak 50 contains oestrogen and a progestogen to induce withdrawal bleeding, thereby avoiding endometrial hyperstimulation. Most patients will bleed towards the end of progestogen therapy.

If patients have regular periods, treatment with Estrapak 50 should be started within 5 days of onset of menstruation. If patients have no periods, or irregular periods, treatment may be started at any time. Some breakthrough bleeding or spotting may be seen until therapy has become established.

Children: Estrapak 50 is not indicated in children.

Use in pregnancy and lactation: Estrapak 50 is not indicated.

Contra-indications, warnings, etc
Contra-indications: Cancer of the breast, genital tract or other oestrogen-dependent neoplasia; severe hepatic, renal or cardiac disease; undiagnosed vaginal bleeding; history of thrombosis or thromboembolic disease; endometriosis; otosclerosis.

Precautions and warnings: Before commencing any oestrogen replacement therapy it is recommended that the patient should have a thorough physical and gynaecological examination. This should be repeated at regular intervals. Breakthrough bleeding is an indication for endometrial assessment, which may include biopsy.

Close monitoring of patients with the following

conditions is recommended: benign breast disease, or strong family history of mammary cancer; hypertension – regular monitoring of blood pressure should be carried out; cholelithiasis.

Prior to surgery, discontinuation should be considered. Estrapak 50 is not an oral contraceptive.

Side-effects: Although side effects are rare, headaches, nausea and breast tenderness may occur.

Some patients experience mild and transient local erythema at the site of patch application, with or without itching. This usually disappears 3–4 days after patch removal and is similar to the effect sometimes observed after occlusion of the skin with household medical adhesive plasters. Very infrequently local swelling, papules/vesicles and scaling have been reported, which also resolved spontaneously and did not result in permanent skin damage.

If unacceptable side effects do occur, discontinuation of treatment with Estrapak 50 should be considered.

Overdosage: Oestrogen overdosage is not likely, due to the mode of administration, but can if necessary be rapidly reversed by the removal of the patch(es).

Progestogen overdosage may be manifested by nausea, vomiting, breast enlargement and vaginal bleeding. There is no specific antidote and treatment should be symptomatic. Gastric lavage may be employed if the overdosage is large and the patient is seen sufficiently early (within 4 hours).

Pharmaceutical precautions Store below 25°C.

Legal category POM.

Package quantities Calendar pack containing 8 transdermal oestrogen patches (each individually sealed in a protective pouch) and 12 norethisterone acetate tablets (in a blister pack) (OP).

Further information The transdermal oestrogen patches included in Estrapak 50 represent an easy and efficient method of administering 17β-oestradiol in a manner which gives oestradiol blood levels similar to those in the early follicular phase of the menstrual cycle. The transdermal route achieves similar oestradiol plasma levels to those obtained with oral therapy, but at much lower daily doses and with restoration of the natural physiological oestrone/oestradiol ratio. Unlike oral oestrogens, transdermal therapy results in a low total oestrogen load on the liver, and does not increase renin substrate levels.

Norethisterone acetate 1.0 mg daily is included for 12 days in each cycle to minimise the risk of endometrial hyperplasia and carcinoma which can occur with unopposed oestrogen therapy.

Product licence number 0001/0121.

ISMELIN* AMPOULES

Presentation Ismelin ampoules each containing 10 mg/ml, colourless solution of Guanethidine Monosulphate BP in a clear glass 1 ml ampoule for intramuscular administration. However if Ismelin is given by intravenous infusion, the contents of the ampoule should be added to saline or dextrose saline.

The ampoules also contain sodium chloride, sulphuric acid and water.

Uses

Indications: For control of hypertensive crises, and to obtain more rapid blood pressure control.

Mode of action: Ismelin is a peripheral sympathetic blocking drug which lowers blood pressure by depleting and inhibiting reformation of noradrenaline in postganglionic nerve endings. Ismelin active substance, guanethidine, being highly polar does not cross the blood-brain barrier and is unlikely therefore to exert any effect on the central nervous system. In addition, guanethidine has no effect on the parasympathetic nervous system.

Pharmacokinetics: Guanethidine may be excreted more slowly in those patients with moderate to severely compromised renal function. Therefore the potential for accumulation of the drug will be higher.

Dosage and administration

Adults: In the management of hypertensive crises including toxaemia of pregnancy, Ismelin should be given by intramuscular injection. One injection of 10–20 mg will generally cause a fall in blood pressure within 30 minutes which reaches a maximum in one to two hours and is maintained for four to six hours. If a further dose of 10–20 mg is deemed necessary, then three hours should be allowed to elapse between doses.

In hypertensive patients with moderate renal insufficiency, the intervals between dosing should be extended or the dosage reduced to avoid accumulation as the drug is renally excreted. (For patients with renal failure, see 'Contra-indications').

Use in children: Ismelin is not recommended for use in children.

Use in the elderly: Clinical evidence would indicate that no special dosage regime is necessary, but concurrent coronary or cerebral insufficiency should be taken into account.

Contra-indications, warnings, etc

Contra-indications: Ismelin is contra-indicated in cases of phaechromocytoma and in patients previously treated with monoamine oxidase inhibitors (see 'Drug Interactions'); in such cases, Ismelin may lead to the release of large quantities of catecholamines which may cause a hypertensive crisis.

Ismelin is also contra-indicated in patients with known hypersensitivity to guanethidine and related derivatives, in heart failure due to causes other than hypertension, and in those patients with renal failure (creatinine clearance 10–40 ml/min).

Warnings: Intravenous injections of Ismelin may provoke a hypertensive response, hence if the iv route is preferred it should be by slow iv infusion.

Heat and physical exertion may increase the antihypertensive effect of Ismelin.

Ismelin may cause drowsiness. If affected, the patient should not drive or operate machinery.

Precautions: Ismelin should be used with caution in patients with moderate renal insufficiency (creatinine clearance 41–65 ml/min), or with coronary and/or cerebral arteriosclerosis; abrupt lowering of blood pressure should be avoided. Caution should be exercised in asthmatic patients or in patients with a history of gastro-intestinal ulceration.

The concurrent administration of guanethidine and β-blockers may provoke severe bradycardia.

When patients have to undergo surgery, it is recommended that treatment with Ismelin be withdrawn a few days before the operation. To avoid excessive bradycardia during anaesthesia, it is advisable to premedicate with larger than usual doses of atropine.

After prolonged treatment with Ismelin, latent heart failure may develop. This is due to salt and water retention, and mild negative inotropic and chronotropic effects. Concomitant administration of diuretics can readily correct this condition.

If patients develop fever, the dose of Ismelin should be lowered.

Use in pregnancy and lactation: No foetal toxicity or fertility studies have been carried out in animals. Therefore the drug should only be used if there is no safer alternative. However, in particular, it should not be used during the first trimester of pregnancy nor within at least two weeks prior to the birth or during labour since it may induce paralytic ileus in the newborn infant.

In mothers receiving Ismelin in therapeutic doses, the active substance passes into the breast milk, but in quantities so small that no undesirable effects on the infant are to be expected.

Side-effects: Side-effects are often an indication of excessive dosage. The following effects may occur:

Central nervous system: Particularly at the start of treatment: dizziness, tiredness, lethargy, paraesthesia and headache. Occasionally: blurred vision and depression. Rarely: myalgia and muscular tremor.

Cardiovascular system: Postural hypotension (which may be associated with cerebral or myocardial ischaemia in severe cases) especially when getting up in the morning or after physical exertion, sick-sinus syndrome, oedema, exacerbation of intermittent claudication and bradycardia. Occasionally: heart failure. Rarely: angina pectoris.

Gastro-intestinal tract: Diarrhoea and gaseous distension. Occasionally: vomiting, nausea and dry mouth. Rarely: swelling of parotid glands.

Respiratory tract: Nasal congestion. Rarely: asthma.

Urogenital system: Raised BUN levels or uraemia in patients with latent or manifest renal failure, and ejaculation disturbances.

Skin and hair: Occasionally: dermatitis. Rarely: hair loss.

Blood: Isolated reports of anaemia, leucopenia, and/or thrombocytopenia.

Drug interactions: Monoamine oxidase inhibitors should be withdrawn at least fourteen days before starting treatment with Ismelin (see 'Contra-indications').

Concurrent administration of Ismelin with anti-arrhythmic agents and digitalis may lead to sinus bradycardia.

The anti-hypertensive action of Ismelin may be enhanced by other anti-hypertensive agents such as reserpine, methyldopa, vasodilators (especially minoxidil), calcium antagonists, β-blockers, ACE inhibitors and alcohol.

The anti-hypertensive action of Ismelin may be reduced by chlorpromazine, phenothiazine derivatives, tricyclic anti-depressants and related anti-psychotic drugs, and oral contraceptives. Consequently if larger doses of Ismelin are prescribed, care must be taken upon the withdrawal of any of the drugs listed as severe hypotension may ensue if the dose of Ismelin is not adjusted in advance.

After prolonged treatment with Ismelin, it may be necessary to adjust the dosage of insulin or oral anti-diabetic drugs.

Patients on Ismelin may become hypersensitive to adrenaline, amphetamines or other sympathomimetic agents. Therefore caution should be exercised when taking or using preparations containing these drugs.

Overdosage

Symptoms may include postural hypotension which may cause syncope, sinus bradycardia although tachycardia has been observed, tiredness, dizziness, blurring of vision, muscular weakness, nausea, vomiting, severe diarrhoea and oliguria.

Postural hypotension may be overcome by keeping the patient recumbent, or by instituting fluid and electrolyte replacement, and if necessary, by cautious administration of pressor agents (see Drug Interactions). Sinus bradycardia can be treated with atropine, and diarrhoea with an anti-cholinergic agent.

Pharmaceutical precautions Protect from light.

Legal category POM.

Package quantities Ampoules of 1 ml containing 10 mg: Boxes of 5.

Further information Nil.

Product licence number 0008/5077.

ISMELIN* TABLETS

Presentation Ismelin tablets each containing 10 mg Guanethidine Monosulphate BP. Circular, flat, white tablets with bevelled edges, impressed with the monogram CIBA on one side and Ismelin 10 on the other.

Ismelin Tablets each containing 25 mg Guanethidine Monosulphate BP. Circular, flat pale red tablets, with bevelled edges, impressed with the monogram CIBA on one side and Ismelin 25 on the other.

The tablets also contain lactose and gluten (wheat starch).

Uses

Indications: Recommended in cases of moderate to severe hypertension which have failed to respond adequately to other anti-hypertensive agents.

Mode of action: Ismelin is a peripheral sympathetic blocking drug which lowers blood pressure by depleting and inhibiting reformation of noradrenaline in postganglionic nerve endings. Ismelin active substance, guanethidine, being highly polar does not cross the blood-brain barrier and is unlikely therefore to exert any effect on the central nervous system. In addition, guanethidine has no effect on the parasympathetic nervous system.

The onset of action of guanethidine is slow; maximum hypotensive effects are usually seen after 2–3 days, and may persist for up to 10 days following drug withdrawal.

Pharmacokinetics: Following oral administration of guanethidine, between 35–50% of the dose is slowly absorbed from the gastro-intestinal tract. In hypertensive patients without renal disease, peak plasma concentrations are reached within 2–4 hours of a single oral dose. Following absorption, guanethidine is widely distributed in the tissues. No binding to serum proteins has been demonstrated. Within 3 days, 35% of a single oral dose is excreted in the urine, mostly as inactive metabolites (65%). Renal clearance amounts to 130–220 ml/min. Only traces of guanethidine are found in the bile. Drug levels plateau only after at least a week of repeated daily administration. Following discontinuation of the drug, the initial elimination half-life is 1.5 days and this rises to 4–8 days 72 hours after drug cessation.

Guanethidine may be excreted more slowly in those patients with moderate to severely compromised renal function. Therefore the potential for accumulation of the drug will be higher.

Dosage and administration Ismelin should be used in combination with other anti-hypertensive agents, i.e. diuretics or vasodilators.

Adults: The dosage of Ismelin should be individually titrated to give the lowest effective dose. Blood pressure should be measured both when the patient is standing, and after exercise.

Ismelin can be given as a single daily dose usually in the morning. The following recommendations are useful in practice: Initially dosage should be 10 mg daily. The dosage can be raised by 10 mg at weekly intervals until the desired reduction in blood pressure is attained. Usual daily dosages range from 25–50 mg.

In hypertensive patients with moderate renal insufficiency, the intervals between dosing should be extended or the dosage reduced to avoid accumulation as the drug is renally excreted. (For patients with renal failure, see 'Contra-indications').

Use in children: Ismelin is not recommended for use in children.

Use in the elderly: Clinical evidence would indicate that no special dosage regime is necessary, but concurrent coronary or cerebral insufficiency should be taken into account.

Contra-indications, warnings, etc

Contra-indications: Ismelin is contra-indicated in cases of phaechromocytoma and in patients previously treated with monoamine oxidase inhibitors (see 'Drug Interactions'); in such cases, Ismelin may lead to the release of large quantities of catecholamines which may cause a hypertensive crisis.

Ismelin is also contra-indicated in patients with known hypersensitivity to guanethidine and related derivatives, in heart failure due to causes other than hypertension, and in those patients with renal failure (creatinine clearance 10–40 ml/min).

Warnings: Heat and physical exertion may increase the anti-hypertensive effect of Ismelin.

Ismelin may cause drowsiness. If affected, the patient should not drive or operate machinery.

Precautions: Ismelin should be used with caution in patients with moderate renal insufficiency (creatinine clearance 41–65 ml/min), or with coronary and/or cerebral arteriosclerosis; abrupt lowering of blood pressure should be avoided. Caution should be exercised in asthmatic patients or in patients with a history of gastro-intestinal ulceration.

The concurrent administration of guanethidine and β-blockers may provoke severe bradycardia.

When patients have to undergo surgery, it is recommended that treatment with Ismelin be withdrawn a few days before the operation. To avoid excessive bradycardia during anaesthesia, it is advisable to premedicate with larger than usual doses of atropine.

After prolonged treatment with Ismelin, latent heart failure may develop. This is due to salt and water retention, and mild negative inotropic and chronotropic effects. Concomitant administration of diuretics can readily correct this condition.

If patients develop fever, the dose of Ismelin should be lowered.

Use in pregnancy and lactation: No foetal toxicity or fertility studies have been carried out in animals. Therefore the drug should only be used if there is no safer alternative. However, in particular, it should not be used during the first trimester of pregnancy nor within at least two weeks prior to the birth or during labour since it may induce paralytic ileus in the newborn infant.

In mothers receiving Ismelin in therapeutic doses, the active substance passes into the breast milk, but in quantities so small that no undesirable effects on the infant are to be expected.

Side-effects: Side-effects are often an indication of excessive dosage. The following effects may occur:

Central nervous system: Particularly at the start of treatment: dizziness, tiredness, lethargy, paraesthesia and headache. Occasionally: blurred vision and depression. Rarely: myalgia and muscular tremor.

Cardiovascular system: Postural hypotension (which may be associated with cerebral or myocardial ischaemia in severe cases) especially when getting up in the morning or after physical exertion, sick-sinus syndrome, oedema, exacerbation of intermittent claudication and bradycardia. Occasionally: heart failure. Rarely: angina pectoris.

Gastro-intestinal tract: Diarrhoea and gaseous distension. Occasionally: vomiting, nausea and dry mouth. Rarely: swelling of parotid glands.

Respiratory tract: Nasal congestion. Rarely: asthma.

Urogenital system: Raised BUN levels or uraemia in patients with latent or manifest renal failure, and ejaculation disturbances.

Skin and hair: Occasionally: dermatitis. Rarely: hair loss.

Blood: Isolated reports of anaemia, leucopenia, and/or thrombocytopenia.

Drug interactions: Monoamine oxidase inhibitors should be withdrawn at least fourteen days before starting treatment with Ismelin (see 'Contra-indications').

Concurrent administration of Ismelin with anti-arrhythmic agents and digitalis may lead to sinus bradycardia.

The anti-hypertensive action of Ismelin may be enhanced by other anti-hypertensive agents such as reserpine, methyldopa, vasodilators (especially minoxidil), calcium antagonists, β-blockers, ACE inhibitors and alcohol.

The anti-hypertensive action of Ismelin may be reduced by chlorpromazine, phenothiazine derivatives, tricyclic anti-depressants and related anti-psychotic drugs, and oral contraceptives. Consequently if larger doses of Ismelin are prescribed, care must be taken upon the withdrawal of any of the drugs listed as severe hypotension may ensue if the dose of Ismelin is not adjusted in advance.

After prolonged treatment with Ismelin, it may be necessary to adjust the dosage of insulin or oral anti-diabetic drugs.

Patients on Ismelin may become hypersensitive to adrenaline, amphetamines or other sympathomimetic agents. Therefore caution should be exercised when taking or using preparations containing these drugs.

Overdosage

Symptoms may include postural hypotension which may cause syncope, sinus bradycardia although tachycardia has been observed, tiredness, dizziness, blurring of vision, muscular weakness, nausea, vomiting, severe diarrhoea and oliguria.

Treatment: To reduce absorption, emesis, or gastric lavage and administration of activated charcoal should be instituted initially.

Postural hypotension may be overcome by keeping the patient recumbent, or by instituting fluid and electrolyte replacement, and if necessary, by cautious administration of pressor agents (see Drug Interactions). Sinus bradycardia can be treated with atropine, and diarrhoea with an anti-cholinergic agent.

Pharmaceutical precautions Protect from moisture.

Legal category POM.

Package quantities Tablets 10 mg and 25 mg: Blister packs of 100 (5 strips of 20 tablets).

Further information Nil.

Product licence numbers
Ismelin tablets 10 mg 0008/5006
Ismelin tablets 25 mg 0008/5007

LIORESAL*

Presentation Lioresal tablets each containing 10 mg baclofen; circular, flat, white to faintly yellowish tablets, uncoated, with bevelled edges, having the monogram CG on one side and the letters KJ and a break line on the other.

Lioresal liquid containing 5 mg/5 ml baclofen; clear, very slightly yellow solution with a raspberry flavour.

The tablets also contain gluten (wheat starch) and the liquid contains methyl hydroxybenzoate and propyl hydroxybenzoate.

Uses

Indications: Lioresal is indicated for the relief of spasticity of voluntary muscle resulting from such disorders as: multiple sclerosis, other spinal lesions e.g. tumours of the spinal cord, syringomyelia, motor neurone disease, transverse myelitis, traumatic partial section of the cord.

Lioresal is also indicated in adults and children for the relief of spasticity of voluntary muscle arising from e.g. cerebrovascular accidents, cerebral palsy, meningitis, traumatic head injury.

Patient selection is important when initiating Lioresal therapy; it is likely to be of most benefit in patients whose spasticity constitutes a handicap to activities and/or physiotherapy. Treatment should not be commenced until the spastic state has become stabilised.

Mode of action: Lioresal is an antispastic agent acting at the spinal level. A gamma-aminobutyric acid (GABA) derivative, Lioresal is chemically unrelated to other antispastic agents.

Lioresal depresses monosynaptic and polysynaptic reflex transmission, probably by stimulating the $GABA_B$-receptors, this stimulation in turn inhibiting the release of the excitatory amino acids glutamate and aspartate. Neuromuscular transmission is unaffected by Lioresal.

The major benefits of Lioresal stem from its ability to reduce painful flexor spasms and spontaneous clonus thereby facilitating the mobility of the patient, increasing his independence and helping rehabilitation.

Lioresal also exerts an antinociceptive effect. General well being is often improved and sedation is less often a problem than with centrally acting drugs.

Pharmacokinetics: Lioresal (baclofen) is rapidly and completely absorbed from the gastrointestinal tract. Following oral administration of single doses (10–30 mg) peak plasma concentrations are recorded after 0.5 to 1.5 hours and areas under the serum concentration curves are proportional to the dose.

In cerebrospinal fluid active substance concentrations are approximately 8.5 times lower than in the plasma.

The plasma elimination half-life of baclofen averages

3 to 4 hours. The serum protein binding rate is approximately 30%.

Baclofen is eliminated largely in unchanged form. Within 72 hours, about 75% of the dose is excreted via the kidneys with about 5% of this amount as metabolites.

Dosage and administration Lioresal is given orally in either tablet or liquid form. These two formulations are bioequivalent. The liquid may be particularly suitable for children or those adults who are unable to take tablets. Dosage titration can be more precisely managed with the liquid.

Before starting treatment with Lioresal it is prudent to realistically assess the overall extent of clinical improvement that the patient may be expected to achieve. Careful titration of dosage is essential (particularly in the elderly) until the patient is stabilised. If too high a dose is initiated or if dosage is increased too rapidly side effects may occur. This is particularly relevant if the patient is ambulant in order to minimise muscle weakness in the unaffected limbs or where spasticity is necessary for support.

Adults: The following gradually increasing dosage regime is suggested, but should be adjusted to suit individual patient requirements.

5 mg three times a day for three days
10 mg three times a day for three days
15 mg three times a day for three days
20 mg three times a day for three days

Satisfactory control of symptoms is usually obtained with doses up to 60 mg daily, but a careful adjustment is often necessary to meet the requirements of each individual patient. The dose may be increased slowly if required, but a maximum daily dose of more than 100 mg is not advised unless the patient is in hospital under careful medical supervision. Small frequent dosage may prove better in some cases than larger spaced doses. Also some patients benefit from the use of Lioresal only at night to counteract painful flexor spasm. Similarly a single dose given approximately 1 hour prior to the performance of specific tasks such as washing, dressing, shaving, physiotherapy, will often improve mobility.

Once the maximum recommended dose has been reached, if the therapeutic effect is not apparent within 6 weeks a decision whether to continue Lioresal should be taken.

Elderly: Elderly patients may be more susceptible to side-effects, particularly in the early stages of introducing Lioresal. Small doses should therefore be used at the start of treatment, the dose being titrated gradually against the response, under careful supervision. There is no evidence that the eventual average maximum dose differs from that in younger patients.

Children: A dosage range of 0.75–2 mg/kg body weight should be used. In children over 10 years of age, however a maximum daily dosage of 2.5 mg/kg body weight may be given. Treatment is usually started with 2.5 mg given 4 times daily. The dosage should be cautiously raised at about 3 day intervals, until it becomes sufficient for the child's individual requirements. The recommended daily dosages for maintenance therapy are as follows:

Children aged, 12 months–2 years: 10–20 mg;
2 years–6 years: 20–30 mg;
6 years–10 years: 30–60 mg

Patients with impaired renal function: In patients with impaired renal function or undergoing chronic haemodialysis, a particularly low dosage of Lioresal should be selected i.e. approx. 5 mg daily.

Patients with spastic states of cerebral origin: Unwanted effects are more likely to occur in these patients. It is therefore recommended that a very cautious dosage schedule be adopted and that patients be kept under appropriate surveillance.

Contra-indications, warnings and precautions
Contra-indications: Hypersensitivity to baclofen, peptic ulceration.

Precautions: Psychotic disorders, schizophrenia or confusional states may be exacerbated by treatment with Lioresal. Patients suffering from these conditions should therefore be treated cautiously and kept under close surveillance.

Lioresal may also exacerbate epileptic manifestations but can be employed provided appropriate supervision and adequate anticonvulsive therapy are maintained. Lioresal should be used with extreme care in patients already receiving antihypertensive therapy (see 'Interactions').

Lioresal should be used with caution in patients suffering from cerebrovascular accidents or from respiratory, hepatic or renal impairment.

Since under treatment with Lioresal neurogenic disturbances affecting emptying of the bladder may show an improvement, whereas in patients with pre-existing sphincter hypertonia acute retention of urine may occur, the drug should be used with caution in such patients.

Anxiety and confusional states, hallucinations, psychotic, manic or paranoid states, convulsions (status epilepticus), tachycardia and as rebound phenomenon temporary aggravation of spasticity have been reported with abrupt withdrawal of Lioresal, especially after long term medication. Treatment should, always (unless serious adverse effects occur) therefore, be gradually discontinued by successively reducing the dosage over a period of about 1–2 weeks.

The patient's reactions may be adversely affected by Lioresal-induced sedation or decreased alertness, patients should therefore exercise due caution. Operating equipment or machinery may be hazardous.

Since in rare instances elevated SGOT, alkaline phosphatase and glucose levels in serum have been recorded, appropriate laboratory tests should be performed in patients with liver diseases or diabetes mellitus in order to ensure that no drug induced changes in these underlying diseases have occurred.

Use in pregnancy and lactation: Baclofen increases the incidence of omphaloceles (ventral hernias) in the foetuses of rats at high doses. No teratogenic effects have been noted in mice or rabbits.

A dose related increase in the incidence of ovarian cysts, and a less marked increase in enlarged and/or haemorrhagic adrenals have been observed in female rats treated for 2 years. The clinical relevance of these findings is not known.

During pregnancy, especially in the first 3 months, Lioresal should only be employed if its use is of vital necessity. The benefits of the treatment for the mother must be carefully weighed against the possible risks for the child. Baclofen crosses the placental barrier.

In mothers taking Lioresal in therapeutic doses, the active substance passes into the breast milk, but in quantities so small that no undesirable effects on the infant are to be expected.

Interactions: Where Lioresal is taken concomitantly with other drugs acting on the CNS or with alcohol, increased sedation may occur.

Lioresal may produce severe aggravation of hyperkinetic symptoms in patients receiving lithium.

Pretreatment with Lioresal may prolong the duration of fentanyl induced analgesia.

During concurrent treatment with tricyclic antidepressants, the effect of Lioresal may be potentiated, resulting in pronounced muscular hypotonia.

Since concomitant treatment with Lioresal and antihypertensives is likely to increase the fall in blood pressure, the dosage of antihypertensive medication should be adjusted accordingly.

Drugs which may produce renal insufficiency e.g. ibuprofen may reduce baclofen excretion leading to toxic effects.

In patients with Parkinson's disease receiving treatment with Lioresal and levodopa plus carbidopa, there have been reports of mental confusion, hallucinations and agitation.

Side-effects: Unwanted effects occur mainly at the start of treatment, if the dosage is raised too rapidly, if large doses are employed, or in elderly patients. They are often transitory and can be attenuated or eliminated by reducing the dosage; they are seldom severe enough to necessitate withdrawal of the medication.

Central nervous system: Particularly at the start of treatment, unwanted effects such as daytime sedation, drowsiness, and nausea may frequently occur. Also occasionally encountered are dryness of the mouth, respiratory depression, light-headedness, lassitude, exhaustion, mental confusion, dizziness, retching, vomiting, headache, and insomnia.

Should nausea persist following a reduction in dosage, it is recommended that Lioresal be ingested with food or a milk beverage.

Neurological and/or psychiatric manifestations which have occasionally or rarely been reported include: euphoria, depressive states, paraesthesiae, myalgia, muscular weakness, ataxia, tremor, nystagmus, accommodation disorders, hallucinations, nightmares. It is often difficult to distinguish between these manifestations and those of the disease under treatment. Lowering of the convulsion threshold and attacks of convulsions may possibly occur, particularly in epileptic patients.

Gastro-intestinal tract: Occasionally, mild gastro-intestinal disturbances (constipation, diarrhoea).

Cardiovascular system: Occasionally, hypotension, respiratory or cardiovascular depression.

Urogenital system: Occasionally or rarely, dysuria, frequency of micturition, enuresis. It is often difficult to distinguish between these manifestations and those of the diseases under treatment.

Miscellaneous unwanted effects: In rare or isolated cases visual disturbances, alterations in the taste sensation, hyperhidrosis, skin rash, deterioration in liver function tests.

Certain patients have shown increased spasticity as a paradoxical reaction to the medication.

An undesirable degree of muscular hypotonia – making it more difficult for patients to walk or fend for themselves – may occur and can usually be relieved by re-adjusting the dosage (i.e. by reducing the doses given during the day and possibly increasing the evening dose).

Overdosage

Symptoms: Prominent features are signs of central nervous depression: drowsiness, impairment of consciousness, respiratory depression, coma. Also liable to occur are: confusion, hallucinations, agitation, accommodation disorders, absent pupillary reflex; generalised muscular hypotonia, myoclonia, hyporeflexia or areflexia; convulsions; peripheral vasodilatation, hypotension, bradycardia; hypothermia; nausea, vomiting, diarrhoea, hypersalivation; elevated LDH, SGOT and AP values.

A deterioration in the condition may occur if various substances or drugs acting on the central nervous system (e.g. alcohol, diazepam, tricyclic antidepressants) have been taken at the same time.

Treatment: No specific antidote is known.

Elimination of the drug from the gastro-intestinal tract (induction of vomiting, gastric lavage; comatose patients should be intubated prior to gastric lavage), administration of activated charcoal; if necessary, saline aperient; in respiratory depression, administration of artificial respiration, also measures in support of cardiovascular functions. Since the drug is excreted chiefly via the kidneys, generous quantities of fluid should be given, possibly together with a diuretic. In the event of convulsions diazepam should be administered cautiously i.v.

Pharmaceutical precautions Lioresal tablets should be protected from heat. Lioresal liquid should be protected from heat and light and should not be refrigerated.

Dilution: Lioresal liquid may be diluted with Purified Water BP and stored at room temperature for up to 14 days.

Legal category POM.

Package quantities
Tablets 10 mg: Blister packs of 100.
Tablets 10 mg: Securitainer of 200.
Liquid 5 mg/5 ml: Bottles of 300 ml with child proof closures.

Further information Lioresal liquid contains no sucrose and is therefore suitable for diabetics and children.

Product licence numbers

Tablets 10 mg	0008/0053
Liquid 5 mg/5 ml	0008/0195

LUDIOMIL*

Presentation Ludiomil tablets each containing 10 mg maprotiline hydrochloride, pale yellow, circular, film-coated tablets with CIBA on one side and the letters CO on the reverse.

Ludiomil tablets each containing 25 mg maprotiline hydrochloride, greyish-red, circular, film-coated tablets with CIBA on one side and the letters DP on the reverse.

Ludiomil tablets each containing 50 mg maprotiline hydrochloride; light orange, circular, film-coated tablets with CIBA on one side and the letters ER on the reverse.

Ludiomil tablets each containing 75 mg maprotiline hydrochloride; brownish-orange, circular, film-coated tablets with CIBA on one side and the letters FS and a break line on the reverse.

The tablets also contain lactose and gluten (wheat starch). The 10 mg tablets also contain an azo-dye.

Uses *Indications:* Symptoms of depressive illness, especially where sedation is required.

Mode of action: Maprotiline is a tetracyclic antidepressant with similar basic therapeutic properties to the tricyclic antidepressants. It has a potent and selective inhibitory effect on the re-uptake of noradrenaline. Maprotiline has a weak affinity for the central $alpha_1$-adrenoceptors but exerts little inhibitory effect on re-uptake of serotonin. It displays marked antihistaminic activity and a moderate anticholinergic effect.

Pharmacokinetics: Maprotiline is completely absorbed from Ludiomil film coated tablets, peak levels in the blood occurring within 8 hours. Maprotiline is eliminated from blood with a mean half-life of 43 hours (range 27–58 hrs).

Within 21 days 57% of a single dose is excreted in the urine and 30% in the faeces. Excretion is as unchanged drug and metabolite (mainly glucuronides). Only 2–4% of the dose is excreted unchanged in the urine.

Steady state concentrations in the blood are attained during the second week of treatment and are linearly proportional to dose but tend to be higher in elderly patients.

Impairment of renal function does not affect maprotiline elimination half life provided that hepatic function is normal.

In therapeutically relevant and higher plasma concentration, 88–89% of the drug is protein bound. The apparent volume of distribution is 23 litres/kg.

Dosage and administration The optimum dose depends on the severity of the depression and the individual patient response to treatment. The aim should be to slowly raise the dosage and achieve a therapeutic effect with the lowest possible dose. This is particularly important for elderly patients with an unstable autonomic nervous system as these patients show a more marked response to Ludiomil than younger patients. A daily dosage of 150 mg should not be exceeded.

Adults: The usual dose range is 25–75 mg daily which may be given either in one dose or in three divided doses.

For moderate or severe depression, treatment should start with 75 mg daily, increasing step-wise, if necessary, to a maximum of 150 mg daily. Initially the patient should be closely monitored and dosage adjusted after 1 to 2 weeks according to response. Treatment will need to be maintained until natural remission of the depression permits gradual weaning off Ludiomil or the use of a lower dose for maintenance.

Use in the elderly: It may be advisable in elderly patients, or those who may be sensitive to this type of drug, to start treatment with lower doses such as 30 mg once a day or 10 mg three times a day. This should then be adjusted in a stepwise fashion over one to two weeks up to 25 mg tid or 75 mg once a day, depending on the patient's response. In the majority of cases half the normal dose would be sufficient.

Use in children: Not recommended.

Contra-indications, warnings, etc

Contra-indications: Ludiomil is contraindicated in: patients who are known or suspected to be epileptic or have a lowered convulsion threshold, recent myocardial infarction, in the presence of defects in bundle-branch conduction, narrow angle glaucoma, retention of urine (eg prostatic disease), severe liver or renal disease, mania.

Known hypersensitivity to maprotiline.

Ludiomil should not be employed or should be withdrawn in cases of acute poisoning with alcohol, hypnotics, analgesics or psychotropic drugs.

Warnings: In some patients improvement may not occur for 2–3 weeks. The patients' reactions, eg as a road user, may be impaired to a varying degree depending on dosage and individual susceptibility. Patients should be warned of the possible hazard when driving or operating machinery.

Precautions: Caution should be exercised when drugs which lower the convulsion threshold, eg phenothiazine derivatives, are prescribed concomitantly. Convulsions have been reported in patients with and without a history of epilepsy (see drug interactions and side effects).

When benzodiazepines, prescribed concomitantly with Ludiomil are to be withdrawn this should also be done with special care.

Combined treatment with Ludiomil and a monoamine oxidase inhibitor should be avoided, see drug interactions.

In common with other substances in this therapeutic group, Ludiomil should be used with caution and under surveillance in patients with cardiovascular disease such as any degree of heart block or other cardiac arrhythmias, or a case history of myocardial infarction: monitoring of cardiac function and if necessary, ECG are indicated.

Caution is also called for in patients with hyperthyroidism, or when administering thyroid hormone preparations, in view of the possibility of an increase in unwanted cardiac effects.

The elderly are particularly liable to experience side effects especially agitation, confusion and postural hypotension. The initial dosage should, therefore be increased with caution and the patients kept under close supervision (see dosage).

When starting treatment with Ludiomil frequent monitoring of blood pressure is advisable particularly in elderly patients and other patients showing a tendency to postural hypotension.

Psychotic crises have occasionally become manifest in schizophrenic patients treated with tricyclic antidepressants and should be borne in mind when using Ludiomil.

Although reductions in the white blood cell count have been reported with Ludiomil only in isolated cases, it is known that antidepressants may lead to changes in the blood picture. An appropriate watch for symptoms suggestive of leucopenia (eg fever and sore throat, white cell count) should be kept on patients treated with Ludiomil, especially during the first few months of treatment.

Patients showing a high suicidal risk require close initial and continuing supervision.

Pregnancy and lactation: Use of Ludiomil during pregnancy should be avoided unless it is essential and there is no safer alternative.

As a general rule no drugs should be taken during the first 3 months of pregnancy, and the benefits and risks of taking drugs should be carefully considered throughout the whole of pregnancy.

Experience with Ludiomil in pregnancy is limited. Isolated cases suggesting a possible association between Ludiomil and adverse effects on the foetus have been reported. There is no evidence as to drug safety in human pregnancy; nor is there evidence that it is free from hazard.

Withdrawal symptoms in neonates whose mothers received tri/tetracyclic antidepressants during the third trimester have been reported.

Nursing mothers should be advised to cease breast feeding, although reports available so far have shown no adverse effects on the infant.

Maprotiline passes into breast milk. After repeated administration of 150 mg daily for 5 days, the concentration measured in the breast milk exceeds that in the blood by a factor of 1.3–1.5.

Drug interactions: Concomitant treatment with Ludiomil and major tranquillisers may give rise to elevated concentrations of maprotiline in the serum, to lowering of the convulsion threshold and to seizures.

The following drug interactions although not necessarily reported with Ludiomil, have been reported with tri/tetracyclic antidepressants.

Combined treatment with Ludiomil and monoamine oxidase inhibitor should be avoided. Where Ludiomil is to be employed following treatment with a monoamineoxidase inhibitor, this should be done only after an interval of at least 14 days. The same caution should be observed when administering an MAO inhibitor after previous treatment with Ludiomil. In both instances, Ludiomil or the MAO inhibitor should initially be given in small, gradually increasing doses and its effect monitored until onset of the therapeutic response.

It is advisable to review all antihypertensive therapy during treatment with tri/tetracyclic antidepressants. If required concomitant treatment for hypertension with vasodilators, diuretics or beta-blockers which do not undergo pronounced biotransformation is advised. Administration of Ludiomil with drugs which undergo pronounced biotransformation may result in increased plasma levels of maprotiline.

Neuroleptics and methylphenidate may also increase plasma levels of Ludiomil.

Ludiomil should be used with caution in patients receiving sympathomimetic agents.

Tri/tetracyclic antidepressants are known to potentiate the cardiovascular effects of sympathomimetic agents, eg noradrenaline, adrenaline, amphetamine, methylphenidate, ephedrine, isoprenaline, phenylephrine and phenylpropanolamine. Tri/tetracyclic antidepressants may also potentiate the effects of alcohol, CNS depressant drugs, anticholinergic agents, eg atropine, biperiden and levodopa.

Hepatic enzyme inducing drugs may accelerate maprotiline metabolism weakening the antidepressive effect of Ludiomil.

Coadministration of tri/tetracyclic antidepressants and phenytoin may lead to elevated plasma levels of phenytoin. Plasma levels should be monitored to prevent phenytoin produced side effects and on withdrawal of maprotiline a possible fall in phenytoin levels resulting in convulsions.

Combinations of Ludiomil with benzodiazepines may cause increased sedation.

It is known that administration of cimetidine together with tricyclic antidepressants may lead to a rise in the latters serum concentration and may cause unwanted effects (eg very severe dryness of the mouth, disturbances of vision).

Anaesthetics given during tri/tetracyclic antidepressant therapy may increase the risk of arrhythmias and hypotension. If surgery is necessary, the anaesthetist should be informed that a patient is being so treated.

Side-effects: Various unwanted effects of Ludiomil are of a mild and transient nature and usually disappear in the further course of treatment or following a decrease in the dosage. Convulsions have been reported as occurring in patients both with and without a history of epilepsy. The rare occurrence of convulsions may increase at higher doses. Skin rashes are not uncommon, an incidence of 3% has been reported.

Elderly patients are particularly sensitive to adverse

anticholinergic, neurological, psychiatric or cardiovascular reactions.

The following adverse effects, although not necessarily reported with Ludiomil, have occurred with tri/tetracyclic antidepressants.

Central nervous system: Neurological – occasional or frequent: lightheadedness, headache, dizziness; extrapyramidal disturbances (eg tremor, akathisia, myoclonus), ataxia; isolated or rare cases: dysarthria, weakness, paraesthesiae (numbness, tingling).

Psychiatric – occasional or frequent: transient tiredness, daytime sedation, drowsiness; rare: sleep disturbances, agitation, anxiety; isolated cases: nightmares, restlessness, confusional states, delirium, hallucinations, hypomania, mania.

Liver: Rare: increases in serum transaminases; isolated cases of hepatitis with or without jaundice.

Blood: Isolated cases: leucopenia, agranulocytosis, eosinophilia.

Sense organs: Isolated cases of tinnitus, taste disturbances.

Anticholinergic effects: Occasional or frequent: dryness of the mouth; rare: blurring of vision; rare or occasional: retention of urine; isolated cases of stomatitis.

An increased incidence of dental caries has been reported in patients under long term treatment with antidepressants; regular dental inspections are therefore advisable during long term therapy.

Skin: Occasional: skin reactions (rash, urticaria), sometimes with fever; isolated cases: cutaneous vasculitis, angio-oedema, itching, purpura, photosensitivity, oedema.

Gastrointestinal tract: Occasional: nausea, vomiting; rare or occasional: constipation.

Cardiovascular system: Rare or occasional: postural hypotension, tachycardia, cardiac arrhythmias; isolated cases: disturbances of cardiac conduction (eg A-V block), palpitation, hypertension, syncope.

Respiratory tract: Isolated cases: allergic alveolitis with or without eosinophilia.

Endocrine system: Isolated cases: breast enlargement, galactorrhoea.

Miscellaneous: Occasional or frequent: sweating; occasional: weight gain; rare: sexual disturbances; isolated cases: flushing, losing of hair or alopecia.

Withdrawal symptoms may occur on abrupt cessation of therapy and include insomnia, irritability and excessive perspiration.

Overdosage

Signs and symptoms: Poisoning may exert either a depressant or an excitant action on the central nervous system and give rise to severe anticholinergic and cardiotoxic effects. The following signs are characteristic of an acute overdosage.

Drowsiness, restlessness, ataxia, convulsions, stupor, hyperpyrexia, coma, tachycardia, cardiac arrhythmia, hypotension and respiratory depression.

Treatment: There is no specific antidote to Ludiomil. Gastric lavage and forced emesis should be employed immediately to reduce the absorption of the drug. Patients presenting with major symptoms of overdosage should be nursed in an intensive care unit where full support of vital functions is possible. Any serious overdose requires continuous cardiac monitoring for at least 48 hours and dysrhythmias treated on an individual basis. Respiratory insufficiency may necessitate intubation and ventilation. In the event of hypotension and circulatory collapse administer a plasma expander and if there is acidosis give sodium bicarbonate. In the presence of reduced myocardial function, treatment with dopamine or dobutamine by drip infusion should be considered. Correction of metabolic acidosis and low serum potassium concentrations by means of bicarbonate i.v. and potassium supplementation has proved effective treatment for arrhythmias. Temporary insertion of a cardiac pacemaker should be considered for bradyarrhythmia or A-V block. Convulsions may be controlled with intravenous diazepam. Physostigmine should not be used following an overdosage of Ludiomil. There have been reports that physostigmine increases the risk of seizures.

Pharmaceutical precautions Nil.

Legal category POM.

Package quantities Ludiomil tablets are available in four strengths, 10 mg, 25 mg, and 50 mg in containers of 100 tablets, 75 mg in containers of 28 tablets. All tablets are packed in PVC/foil bubble packs.

Further information Nil.

Product licence numbers
Ludiomil tablets 10 mg 0008/0117
Ludiomil tablets 25 mg 0008/0118
Ludiomil tablets 50 mg 0008/0119
Ludiomil tablets 75 mg 0008/0129

METOPIRONE*

Presentation Metopirone Capsules each containing 250 mg metyrapone in an opaque cylindrical soft gelatine capsule, coloured white.

The capsules also contain sodium salts of ethyl hydroxybenzoate and propyl hydroxybenzoate.

Uses *Mode of action:* Metopirone inhibits the enzyme responsible for the 11 β-hydroxylation stage in the biosynthesis of cortisol and to a lesser extent aldosterone.

The fall in plasma concentration of circulating glucocorticoids stimulates ACTH secretion, via the feedback mechanism which accelerates steroid biosynthesis. As a result, 11-deoxycortisol, the precursor of cortisol, is released into the circulation, metabolised by the liver and excreted in the urine. Unlike cortisol, 11-deoxycortisol does not suppress ACTH secretion and its urinary metabolites may be measured.

Indications: As a diagnostic aid in the differential diagnosis of ACTH-dependent Cushing's syndrome. For the management of patients with Cushing's syndrome.

In conjunction with glucocorticoids, in the treatment of resistant oedema due to increased aldosterone secretion in patients suffering from cirrhosis, nephrosis and congestive heart failure.

Pharmacokinetics: Metyrapone, the active substance of Metopirone, is rapidly absorbed and eliminated from the plasma. Peak plasma levels usually occur one hour after ingestion of Metopirone; after a dose of 750 mg Metopirone, plasma drug levels average 3.7 micrograms/ml. Plasma drug levels decrease to a mean value of 0.5 micrograms/ml 4 hours after dosing. The half-life of elimination of Metopirone from the plasma is 20–26 minutes.

Seventy-two hours after a first daily dose of 4.5 g Metopirone (750 mg every 4 hours), 5.3% of the total dose was excreted in the urine as metyrapone (9.2% in free form and 90.8% conjugated with glucuronic acid), and 38.5% in the form of metyrapol, the principal active metabolite (8.1% in free and 91.9% conjugated with glucuronic acid).

Dosage and administration The capsules should be taken with milk or after a meal to minimise nausea and vomiting which can lead to impaired absorption.

For use as a diagnostic aid: Urinary 17-oxygenic steroid excretion is measured over 24 hours on each of 4 consecutive days. The first 2 days serve as a control period. On the third day, 750 mg Metopirone (3 capsules) must be given at four-hourly intervals to give a total of 6 doses (i.e. 4.5 g). Maximum urine steroid excretion may occur on the fourth day. If urinary steroid excretion increases in response to Metopirone, this suggests the high levels of circulatory cortisol are due to adrenocortical hyperplasia following excessive ACTH production rather than a cortisol-producing adrenal tumour.

Use in children: Children should be given a smaller amount based upon 6 four-hourly doses of 15 mg per kg, with a minimum dose of 250 mg every four hours.

For therapeutic use: For the management of Cushing's

syndrome, the dosage must be adjusted to meet the patients requirements; a daily dose from 250 mg to 6 g may be required to restore normal cortisol levels.

For the treatment of resistant oedema, 2.5 g to 4.5 g (10–18 capsules) should be given daily in divided doses in conjunction with a glucocorticoid.

Use in the elderly: Clinical evidence would indicate that no special dosage regimen is necessary.

Contra-indications, warnings, etc
Contra-indications: Adrenocortical insufficiency. Hypersensitivity to Metopirone.

Pregnancy and lactation: Metopirone should not be administered during pregnancy since the drug can impair the biosynthesis of foetal-placental steroids. It is not known whether metyrapone passes into the breast milk, therefore nursing mothers should refrain from breastfeeding their infants during treatment with Metopirone.

Precautions
In relation to use as a diagnostic aid: Anticonvulsants (eg phenytoin, barbiturates), anti-depressants and neuroleptics (eg amitripyline, chlorpromazine), hormones that affect the hypothalamo-pituitary axis and antithyroid agents may influence the results of the Metopirone test. If these drugs cannot be withdrawn, the necessity of carrying out the Metopirone test should be reviewed.

Patients with liver cirrhosis often show a delayed response to Metopirone due to liver damage delaying the metabolism of cortisol.

In cases of thyroid hypofunction, urinary steroid levels may rise very slowly, or not at all, in response to Metopirone.

Side-effects: Nausea, vomiting, dizziness, headache, hypotension and allergic reactions have occasionally been reported.

Treatment of Overdosage: The clinical picture of acute Metopirone poisoning is characterised by gastro-intestinal symptoms and acute adreno-cortical insufficiency. Gastric lavage and forced emesis should be employed to reduce the absorption of the drug. A large dose of hydrocortisone should be administered, together with i.v. saline and glucose. This should be repeated as necessary in accordance with the patient's clinical condition.

Pharmaceutical precautions The capsules should be protected from heat and moisture.

Legal category POM.

Package quantities 250 mg capsules of Metopirone in Securitainers of 100.

Further information Nil.

Product licence number 0008/5078.

MONASPOR*

Presentation Vials containing cefsulodin sodium dry active substance corresponding to 0.5 g, 1 g cefsulodin free acid for intramuscular and intravenous use.

Uses *Mode of action:* Monaspor is a semi-synthetic bactericidal beta-lactam antibiotic for parenteral use which displays marked activity against Pseudomonas aeruginosa. The minimum inhibitory concentrations (MIC) are very low, lying within the range of 0.25–8 mcg/ml for 88% of the Pseudomonas strains investigated.

Monaspor is stable against the majority of relevant beta-lactamases and is also active against most strains of Pseudomonas aeruginosa resistant to carbenicillin and gentamicin.

Indications: Monaspor is indicated for the treatment of infections caused by sensitive strains of Pseudomonas aeruginosa. These include:

Chronic recurrent urinary tract infections e.g. pyelonephritis, infections accompanying obstructions of the urinary tract (e.g. in the presence of neoplasms; calculi of the urinary tract, or following surgery), prostatitis.

Respiratory tract infections e.g. pneumonia, chronic purulent bronchitis and infections associated with mucoviscidosis.

A number of cases of Pseudomonas infection of bone and soft tissue, such as osteomyelitis, and infected wounds and burns have been treated successfully with Monaspor.

Dosage and administration *Adults:* In adults with normal renal function the usual daily dose is 1–4 grams daily in 2–4 fractional doses.

In urinary tract infections, and chronic bronchitis, 1–3 grams daily in 2–4 fractional doses usually suffices.

In critical cases (e.g. severe pneumonia, osteomyelitis) daily doses of 6 grams or more may be necessary.

Elderly: No specific information on use in the elderly is available. Concurrent renal insufficiency should be taken into account.

Children: The recommended daily dose is 20–50 mg/kg bodyweight.

Administration: Intramuscular: The dry powder should be dissolved using 0.5% lignocaine solution before intramuscular administration.

Intravenous: The dry powder should be reconstituted with Water for Injection to a concentration of 1 g in 10 ml and slowly injected either directly into a vein or into the tube of an intravenous drip.

Infusion: Monaspor can be dissolved in the routinely employed solutions e.g. Sodium Chloride Intravenous Infusion BP, Ringer's Injection USP, Dextrose Intravenous Infusion BP, Dextran 40 Intravenous Infusion BP (10%). It must not be mixed with sodium bicarbonate.

When administering an infusion lasting more than 30–60 minutes and in order to obtain high initial blood levels, it is advisable to inject the first dose as a slow bolus injection.

If Monaspor is infused intermittently via a Y-attachment to another infusion, administration of the latter should be interrupted while the Monaspor infusion is in progress.

Monaspor can be administered in combination with other antibiotics such as gentamicin or carbenicillin. They can either be infused together or injected in the same syringe (diluted with Water for Injection to a total volume of 10 ml). Monaspor, however, should not be pre-mixed with tobramycin but they may be administered separately.

Aqueous solutions of the drug take on a yellow colouration. This has no effect on the drug's antibiotic activity.

Solutions displaying clouding or precipitation after admixing of the drug should not be used.

Only freshly prepared Monaspor solutions should be employed. Monaspor infusion solutions should not be used if they have been stored for longer than 24 hours in a refrigerator (5°C) or 12 hours at room temperature (23°C). Mixtures containing Monaspor and other drugs in the same syringe should not be stored for more than 4 hours at room temperature. The stability of Monaspor solutions is greatest between pH 4–7. Solutions with a pH of greater than 7 should be administered immediately after they have been prepared.

Contra-indications, warnings, etc *Contra-indications:* Hypersensitivity to cephalosporins.

Precautions: In chronic infections it is important that the treatment should be of sufficiently long duration to obtain a successful clinical result.

In cases where lengthy treatment with large doses of Monaspor is required, blood counts and tests of renal function should be performed.

As with any type of antibiotic therapy, it is advisable to determine the sensitivity of the causative micro-organisms before initiating treatment.

In patients known to be allergic to penicillin, caution should be exercised when employing Monaspor, since cross-sensitivity with cephalosporins may be encountered. If allergic reactions occur, Monaspor should be withdrawn and suitable countermeasures taken.

In patients with renal failure, the priming dose should be the same as in patients without renal disease. Repeat doses, however, must be reduced in size or the interval between them prolonged. The recommendations in the following table may be used as a guide. The elimination of the drug in dialysis fluid is about 45% of the dose and it is suggested that a normal dose be given at the beginning and end of the dialysis period.

Creatinine clearance	*Maintenance doses in % of normal doses at following intervals:*			
ml/min	*6 h*	*8 h*	*12 h*	*24 h*
50	90	90	95	—
30	75	80	90	—
20	65	70	80	—
10	55	60	70	—
5	45	55	65	—
2.5	40	45	60	—
0	—	—	—	75

In patients suffering from severe liver damage and in those allergic to local anaesthetics, Monaspor should be given intramuscularly with sterile Water for Injection or intravenously (i.e. without lignocaine).

When determining urinary sugar levels, enzymatic methods should be used because other techniques may yield false positive results.

Pregnancy: As with other drugs, the use of Monaspor during pregnancy is advised only if there are compelling reasons.

Side-effects: Monaspor is generally well tolerated. The following have been observed as rare side effects: nausea, dizziness, allergic skin reactions, and eosinophilia, as well as occasional increases in the values for transaminases, alkaline phosphatase, non-protein nitrogen, and serum creatinine. Intravenous injections of Monaspor are usually painless when administered slowly. Local pain occurring as a reaction to intramuscular injections can be prevented by using 0.5% lignocaine solution.

Pharmaceutical precautions The vials should be stored below 25°C and protected from light.

Legal category POM.

Package quantities Vials containing 0.5 g or 1 g of active substance.

Further information Nil.

Product licence numbers
500 mg vials 0008/0159
1 g vials 0008/0162

NAVIDREX*

Presentation Navidrex Tablets containing 0.5 mg of Cyclopenthiazide BP as white, flat, circular tablets with bevelled edges, bearing the monogram CIBA on one side, and the letters AO on each side of a breakline on the other.

The tablets also contain lactose and gluten (wheat starch).

Uses *Mode of action:* Navidrex is a thiazide diuretic which exerts its diuretic effect by inhibiting the reabsorption of sodium, chloride and water, probably at the distal renal tubules.

Indications: Navidrex is indicated for the treatment of mild to moderate hypertension, in more severe hypertension it may be used in conjunction with other antihypertensive agents. It is also indicated for the treatment of acute and chronic heart failure and oedema associated with renal disease, pre-menstrual tension and liver disease.

Dosage and administration The dosage should be individually adjusted according to the clinical picture and patient response. Navidrex may be given as a single daily dosage, preferably in the morning, or in divided doses. During long term therapy the lowest effective dosage should be employed, particularly in the elderly.

Adults: Hypertension 0.25 mg to 0.5 mg daily, increasing rarely to a maximum of 1.5 mg. For best results in hypertension doses should be given seven days a week, the entire dose being taken in the morning.

In acute and chronic heart failure, oedema associated with renal or liver disease, an initial dose of 0.5 mg to 1 mg until a satisfactory clinical response is attained. The maximum effective dose is 1.5 mg daily although this is rarely required. When a satisfactory clinical response is achieved a dose of 0.5 mg on alternate days is usually adequate.

Pre-menstrual tension 0.25 mg to 0.5 mg daily from the onset of symptoms until menstruation begins.

Since Navidrex increases salt excretion it is usually possible to relax dietary salt restriction.

Children: Extensive clinical experience in children is lacking.

Elderly: Particular caution should be exercised in the elderly since they are more susceptible to electrolyte imbalance (see *Precautions*).

Contra-indications, warnings, etc

Side-effects: Navidrex is generally well tolerated at the recommended dosage. However, the following side effects may occasionally be observed, particularly with higher doses:

Skin: Allergic urticaria (nettle rash) and other forms of skin rash, photosensitisation. In very rare cases: necrotising vasculitis.

Gastro-intestinal tract: Loss of appetite, mild nausea, vomiting, gastrospasm, diarrhoea or possibly constipation, pancreatitis.

Central nervous system: Headache, muzziness, dizziness. Occasionally: sleep disturbances, depression, paraesthesiae.

Blood: Thrombocytopenia. In isolated cases: leucopenia, agranulocytosis, anaemia, purpura, and very rarely bone marrow depression.

Electrolytes: Hypokalaemia, hyponatraemia, hypomagnesaemia. In isolated cases: hypochloraemic alkalosis and hypercalcaemia. If hypercalcaemia occurs, further diagnostic clarification is necessary (eg possibility of hyperparathyroidism).

Liver: In rare cases: intrahepatic cholestasis or jaundice.

Miscellaneous: Idiosyncracy (pulmonary oedema); occasionally impotence.

Metabolism: Hyperuricaemia, hyperglycaemia, glycosuria. Gout or diabetes may be precipitated or aggravated. Increased blood lipid levels in response to higher doses.

Cardiovascular system: Postural hypotension and cardiac arrhythmias; postural hypotension may be aggravated by alcohol, anaesthetics, or sedatives.

Contra-indications: Anuria, severe renal and hepatic failure, hypersensitivity to cyclopenthiazide or other sulphonamide derivatives, refractory hypokalaemia and hyponatraemia, hypercalcaemia, symptomatic hyperuricaemia, Addison's disease, concurrent lithium therapy.

Precautions: Renal function should be monitored in patients taking thiazide diuretics. In the presence of impaired renal function, accumulation of thiazides occurs and uraemia may become more marked. In extreme cases an oliguric crisis can occur, when the dose should either be reduced or treatment interrupted temporarily. Creatinine clearance, urea, and electrolytes should be monitored. At creatinine clearance levels of <30 ml/min (or at serum creatinine levels of >2.5 mg/100 ml $=$ >221 μmol/litre), thiazides no longer exert an adequate diuretic effect. In such cases, loop diuretics are indicated.

Thiazides may raise the serum uric acid level and provoke attacks of gout in predisposed patients. Glucose tolerance may be adversely affected, and diabetes mellitus can occasionally occur under treatment with thiazides. In patients with hyperlipidaemia, the serum lipids should be regularly monitored. In the event of a rise in the serum lipids, withdrawal of the thiazide medication should be considered.

Disturbances in the serum electrolyte balance, in particular hypokalaemia, may occur during treatment. Since the excretion of electrolytes is increased, an excessively strict low-salt diet should be avoided. Periodic serum electrolyte determinations should be carried out, especially in digitalised patients. If signs of potassium depletion appear (eg muscular weakness, cardiac arrhythmias, or corresponding ECG changes) or if additional loss of potassium occurs (due to vomiting, diarrhoea, malnutrition, nephrosis, liver cirrhosis, hyperaldosteronism, or to treatment with ACTH or corticosteroids), potassium medication will need to be given under surveillance. Alternatively, a potassium-sparing diuretic may be appropriate.

Patients receiving relatively high doses of thiazides may develop hypomagnesaemia accompanied by signs and symptoms such as nervousness, muscle spasms, and cardiac arrhythmias.

The elderly, especially those suffering from chronic disease, and patients with liver cirrhosis, are more susceptible to regulatory disorders affecting the electrolyte and fluid balance. During treatment with thiazides, hyponatraemia accompanied by neurological symptoms (nausea, debility, progressive disorientation, apathy) has been observed in isolated cases. In the elderly and patients with liver cirrhosis, the serum electrolytes should be monitored at more frequent intervals.

Lupus erythematosus may possibly become activated under treatment with thiazides.

Pregnancy: Diuretics are best avoided for the management of oedema or hypertension in pregnancy as their use may be associated with hypovolaemia, increased blood viscosity and reduced placental perfusion. There have been reports of foetal bone marrow depression, thrombocytopenia, and foetal and neonatal jaundice associated with the use of thiazide diuretics.

Lactation: Cyclopenthiazide passes into breast milk. Navidrex should therefore be avoided during breast feeding.

Interactions: Thiazides potentiate the action of curare derivatives and antihypertensive drugs (eg guanethidine, methyldopa, beta-blockers, vasodilators, calcium antagonists, ACE inhibitors).

The hypokalaemic effect of thiazides may be increased by corticosteroids, ACTH, amphotericin, and carbenoxolone.

It may prove necessary to adjust the dosage of insulin and of oral antidiabetic agents.

Hypokalaemia or hypomagnesaemia possibly occurring as unwanted effects favour the onset of digitalis-induced cardiac arrhythmias.

Concomitant administration of certain non-steroidal anti-inflammatory drugs (eg indomethacin) may weaken the diuretic and antihypertensive activity of thiazides, and there have been isolated reports of a deterioration in renal function in predisposed patients.

Overdosage

Signs and Symptoms: The following may occur: dizziness, nausea, somnolence, hypovolaemia, hypotension, and electrolyte disturbances associated with cardiac arrhythmias and muscle spasms.

Treatment: Induction of vomiting or gastric lavage and administration of activated charcoal. Blood pressure, and fluid and electrolyte balance should be monitored and appropriate corrective measures taken. Intravenous fluid and electrolyte replacement may be indicated.

Pharmaceutical precautions Protect from heat and moisture.

Legal category POM.

Package quantities Navidrex is available in Securitainers of 100.

Further information After a single oral dose diuresis starts within one or two hours reaching a maximum in four to eight hours, lasting up to 12 hours. If taken in the morning the clearly defined duration of action ensures that the patient can sleep undisturbed at night. It is important that the patient be encouraged to take a potassium rich diet during treatment with Navidrex.

Product licence number 0008/5047.

NAVISPARE*

Presentation Navispare tablets containing 0.25 mg Cyclopenthiazide BP and 2.5 mg Amiloride Hydrochloride BP, as orange-yellow, round film-coated tablets marked 'CIBA' on one face and 'RC' on the other. The tablets also contain gluten (wheat starch), lactose and polyethoxylated castor oils.

Uses Navispare contains a thiazide diuretic in combination with a potassium-sparing diuretic, and is indicated for the treatment of mild to moderate hypertension.

Mode of action: Cyclopenthiazide is a thiazide diuretic which exerts its diuretic effect by inhibiting the reabsorption of sodium, chloride and water, probably at the distal renal tubules.

Amiloride hydrochloride is a mild diuretic that acts mainly on the distal part of the renal tubule. It increases the excretion of sodium and chloride and reduces the excretion of potassium. The presence of amiloride hydrochloride in the combination minimises the likelihood of potassium loss.

Dosage and administration

Adults: Usually 1 or 2 Navispare tablets taken once a day in the morning.

Elderly: Although no special dosage regime is necessary in the elderly, particular caution should be exercised in the elderly, since they are more susceptible to electrolyte imbalances.

Children: Navispare is not suitable for use in children.

Contra-indications, warnings, etc

Contra-indications: Navispare is contra-indicated in patients hypersensitive to cyclopenthiazide or other sulphonamide derivatives; Addison's disease; hyperkalaemia; in the presence of other potassium-conserving agents or potassium supplements; anuria; severe renal and hepatic failure; diabetic nephropathy; concurrent lithium therapy; refractory hypokalaemia and hyponatraemia; hypercalcaemia; symptomatic hyperuricaemia.

Precautions

Diabetes mellitus: Hyperkalaemia has occurred in diabetic patients receiving amiloride hydrochloride, especially those with chronic renal disease or prerenal azotaemia. The status of renal function should therefore be determined before use in a known or suspected diabetic patient. Navispare should be discontinued for at least three days before a glucose tolerance test. Prolonged doses may bring about a decrease in glucose tolerance and precipitate a diabetic condition. In known diabetics the addition of a thiazide to the treatment regime may alter their antidiabetic requirement.

Metabolic or respiratory acidosis: Potassium-conserving therapy should be initiated with caution in patients in whom metabolic or respiratory acidosis may occur; eg in patients with cardiopulmonary disease or decompensated diabetes. Shifts in acid-base balance alter the balance of extracellular-intracellular potassium and the development of acidosis may be associated with rapid increases in plasma potassium.

Electrolyte considerations: In patients with renal impairment, a rise in blood urea can occur. In such cases, either the dose should be reduced or the treatment interrupted temporarily. Thiazides may precipitate an attack of gout in patients predisposed to this condition.

The elderly, especially those suffering from chronic disease, and patients with hepatic cirrhosis are more susceptible to a lack of electrolyte and fluid balance homeostasis. During treatment with thiazides hyponatraemia accompanied by neurological symptoms has been observed in isolated cases. In the elderly and patients with hepatic cirrhosis, the serum electrolytes should be monitored at more frequent intervals.

Patients receiving relatively high doses of thiazides may develop hypomagnesaemia accompanied by signs

and symptoms such as nervousness, muscle spasms and cardiac arrhythmias.
Miscellaneous: In patients with hyperlipidaemia, the serum lipids should be regularly monitored. In the event of a rise in the serum lipids, withdrawal of the thiazide medication should be considered.

Lupus erythematosus may possibly become activated under treatment with thiazides.

Use in pregnancy and lactation: Diuretics are best avoided for the management of hypertension in pregnancy, as their use may be associated with hypovolaemia, increased blood viscosity and reduced placental perfusion. There is inadequate evidence of safety in human pregnancy and there have been reports of foetal bone marrow depression, thrombocytopenia, and foetal and neonatal jaundice reported with the use of thiazide diuretics.

As cyclopenthiazide passes into breast milk, Navispare should be avoided in mothers who wish to breast-feed. It is not known whether amiloride hydrochloride passes into breast milk.

Drug interactions: The concomitant administration of thiazides with other antihypertensive agents (eg beta-blockers, vasodilators, calcium antagonists) may necessitate adjustment of the dosage of those drugs. The concomitant administration of potassium-sparing agents such as amiloride or ACE inhibitors may increase serum potassium levels and is not to be recommended. However, if the concomitant use of these agents is deemed appropriate, they should be used with caution and with frequent monitoring of plasma potassium.

NSAIDs may attenuate the antihypertensive effect of thiazide diuretics. Thiazide-containing drugs may increase the responsiveness to tubocurarine.

Orthostatic hypotension may occur, and may be potentiated by alcohol, barbiturates and narcotics.

Side-effects: Navispare is generally well tolerated. Reported side-effects of the combination include dizziness, headache, light-headedness, tiredness, nausea and vomiting, discomfort/pain in the chest. However, the following side-effects of cyclopenthiazide and amiloride as single agents have been reported:

Cyclopenthiazide
Skin: Allergic urticaria (nettle rash) and other forms of skin rash, photosensitisation. In very rare cases: necrotising vasculitis.
Gastro-intestinal tract: Loss of appetite, mild nausea, vomiting, gastrospasm, diarrhoea or possibly constipation, pancreatitis.
Central nervous system: Headache, muzziness, dizziness. Occasionally: sleep disturbances, depression, paraesthesiae.
Blood: Thrombocytopenia. In isolated cases: leucopenia, agranulocytosis, anaemia, purpura, and very rarely bone marrow depression.
Electrolytes: Hypokalaemia, hyponatraemia, hypomagnesaemia. In isolated cases: hypochloraemic alkalosis and hypercalcaemia. If hypercalcaemia occurs, further diagnostic clarification is necessary (eg possibility of hyperparathyroidism).
Liver: In rare cases: intrahepatic cholestasis or jaundice.
Miscellaneous: Occasionally impotence.
Metabolic: Hyperuricaemia, hyperglycaemia, glycosuria. Gout or diabetes may be precipitated or aggravated. Increased blood lipid levels in response to higher doses.
Cardiovascular system: Postural hypotension and cardiac arrhythmias; postural hypotension may be aggravated by alcohol, anaesthetics, or sedatives.

Amiloride
Gastro-intestinal tract: Anorexia, nausea, vomiting, diarrhoea, constipation, abdominal pain, GI bleeding, jaundice, thirst, dyspepsia, heartburn, flatulence.
Central nervous system: Dizziness, vertigo, paraesthesiae, tremors, encephalopathy, nervousness, mental confusion, insomnia, decreased libido, depression, somnolence.
Cardiovascular system: Angina pectoris, orthostatic hypotension, arrhythmias, palpitation.
Respiratory: Cough, dyspnoea.
Special senses: Nasal congestion, visual disturbances, increased intra-ocular pressure, tinnitis.
Urogenital: Impotence, polyuria, dysuria, frequency of micturition.
Musculoskeletal: Muscle cramps, joint pain.
Skin and appendages: Pruritus, rash, dryness of mouth, alopecia.

Overdosage: Signs: In cases of overdosage the following signs and symptoms may occur: dizziness, nausea, somnolence, hypovolaemia, hypotension and electrolyte disturbances associated with cardiac arrhythmias and muscle spasms.

Treatment: Emesis should be induced or gastric lavage performed. Intravenous fluid and electrolyte replacement may be indicated.

Pharmaceutical precautions Protect from heat and moisture.

Legal category POM.

Package quantities Blister packs of 28 tablets (OP).

Further information Nil.

Product licence number 0001/0135.

ORIMETEN*

Presentation Tablets containing 250 mg aminoglutethimide. White to yellowish white, round with slightly convex faces and slightly bevelled edges, printed 'CG' on one side and 'GG' with score on the other.

Uses *Mode of action:* Orimeten inhibits several cytochrome P450 mediated hydroxylation steps in the adrenal cortex, including the initial step of cholesterol side chain cleavage to $\Delta 5$ pregnenolone. It further inhibits the extra-adrenal aromatisation of androgens to oestrogens.

The mode of action of Orimeten in prostatic carcinoma is not fully understood, and the concurrent use of a corticosteroid is at present recommended.

Pharmacokinetics: Orimeten is well absorbed and peak plasma levels are attained within 1–2 hours. The drug is 21–25% bound to plasma proteins and during long term therapy plasma half-life averages 7 hours (during the first 7–14 days of therapy auto-induction occurs). Approximately 40% of the dose is excreted in the urine unchanged and up to 25% in the form of N-acetylaminoglutethimide.

Indications: Advanced carcinoma of the breast in postmenopausal or oophorectomised women (especially where the tumours are oestrogen-sensitive), including in particular patients who have previously responded to endocrine therapy or have painful bony metastases.

Advanced carcinoma of the prostate as palliative treatment. Subjective improvement and pain relief have been noted in up to 50% of patients.

Cushing's syndrome due to malignant disease, e.g. adrenocortical carcinoma or ectopic ACTH syndrome, in place of or in conjunction with surgery.

Dosage and administration Orimeten tablets should be administered orally.

Adults:
Advanced carcinoma of the breast and of the prostate: Starting at one tablet daily the dose should be increased each week by one tablet per day to the maximum tolerated dose, not exceeding 1000 mg daily e.g. Week 1 – 250 mg once daily, Week 2 – 250 mg twice daily, Week 3 – 250 mg three times daily, Week 4 – 250 mg four times daily.

In the majority of patients treated for carcinoma of the prostate the effective dose has not exceeded 750 mg daily.

Supplementary therapy: In order to provide physiological replacement, a glucocorticoid should be given in conjunction with Orimeten.

20 mg hydrocortisone twice daily is suitable at all Orimeten dose levels. Orimeten accelerates the metabolism of dexamethasone to a variable extent, therefore

individual titration to a relatively high dose (up to 3 mg daily) may be required if this glucocorticoid is used.

Cushings syndrome due to malignant disease: Initially 250 mg daily, increasing gradually according to response up to 1 g daily in divided doses. In some cases, especially ectopic ACTH syndrome, higher dosages (of up to 1.5–2 g daily) may occasionally prove necessary to achieve adequate suppression.

Supplementary therapy: During initial treatment no corticosteroids should be necessary. Plasma cortisol levels should be regularly monitored and dosage adapted accordingly. In some cases, an 'escape' phenomenon may occur, i.e. the plasma cortisol concentration may rise again after a certain time; in other cases – especially in patients with adrenocortical tumours, who possibly respond more sensitively to Orimeten – it may show excessive decrease. Should adrenocortical insufficiency occur supplementary glucocorticoids may be given.

Use in the elderly: There is no evidence to suggest that dosage should be different in the elderly.

Use in children: Dosage not established.

Contra-indications, warnings, etc
Precautions: In some patients the suppression of aldosterone synthesis may lead to hyponatraemia, hyperkalaemia, hypotension and dizziness, in which case a mineralocorticoid (e.g. fludrocortisone 0.1–0.15 mg daily or on alternate days) should be given.

The patients blood count and plasma electrolytes should be checked regularly particularly during the first 2–3 months when blood counts should be carried out every two to three weeks. If, during treatment with aminoglutethimide, signs of Cushing's Syndrome (due to concomitant glucocorticoid medication) appear, the dosage of the glucocorticoid should be reduced.

Treatment with Orimeten and steroids may impair the adrenal response to stress.

Drug interactions: Orimeten may increase the rate of metabolism and therefore necessitate dosage adjustment of some drugs e.g. coumarin anti-coagulants, oral anti-diabetic agents and synthetic glucocorticoids.

Contra-indications:
Use in pregnancy and lactation: Since foetal abnormalities have been observed in animals and there have been cases of pseudohermaphroditism in newborn infants of women treated with Orimeten, use during pregnancy and lactation is contra-indicated.

Side-effects: The tolerability of Orimeten varies greatly from patient to patient and after the first 6–8 weeks of treatment side-effects diminish or abate completely.

Central nervous side effects, such as dizziness, somnolence and lethargy are not uncommon, but unsteadiness occurs only in the higher dosage range. Gastrointestinal effects such as nausea, vomiting or diarrhoea, are less frequent. All these effects are dose dependent.

Drug rash – accompanied sometimes by fever – may develop after 7–14 days; it usually subsides within 7–10 days despite continued treatment, but if it fails to do so, the treatment must be reduced or temporarily withdrawn or the dosage of the concomitant glucocorticoid raised.

Isolated cases of allergic alveolitis (eosinophilic pulmonary infiltrates) have been reported. Where such alveolitis is suspected, Orimeten should be withdrawn immediately.

Blood dyscrasias such as leucopenia, agranulocytosis, pancytopenia and thrombocytopenia may be encountered.

Occasionally, Orimeten has been found to interfere with thyroid function by inhibiting thyroxine biosynthesis.

Overdosage: Clinical experience with Orimeten in overdose is limited. However, it may reduce the production of steroids from the adrenal cortex to a degree which is clinically relevant. Overdosage may lead to hypotension, central nervous system depression, impaired consciousness, electrolyte disturbances, respiratory depression and hypoventilation.

Removal of the tablets from the gastro-intestinal tract is recommended. Supportive treatment to maintain fluid and electrolyte balance and treatment with iv steroids may be needed. The chemical structure of Orimeten indicates that it may have a great affinity for fatty tissue and symptoms may therefore recur.

Pharmaceutical precautions Protect from heat, light and moisture.

Legal category POM.

Package quantities Securitainers of 100 tablets.

Further information In many cases of carcinoma of the breast, metastases or recurring tumours diminish in size or even disappear during treatment with Orimeten. Such remission may be maintained for several years. Bone metastases attributable to breast cancer respond particularly well, the patient often experiencing marked relief of pain.

In advanced carcinoma of the prostate, patients may also benefit from marked relief of bone pain. Objective tumour regression has been seen in some patients.

Product licence number 0008/0147.

PRESCAL* ▼

Presentation The active ingredient, isradipine, is presented as: 2.5 mg yellow, flat circular angled scored tablets (designed to be easily divided), 6 mm diameter, marked NM on one face and CIBA on the other.

The tablets also contain lactose.

Uses
Indication: Prescal is recommended for the treatment of essential hypertension.

Mode of action: Isradipine is a dihydropyridine calcium antagonist with a higher affinity for calcium channels in arterial smooth muscle than for those in the myocardium. Thus it produces vasodilation of peripheral, coronary, and cerebral arteries without notably depressing cardiac function. As a result of the vasodilation of peripheral arteries, the arterial blood pressure is lowered; the attendant afterload reduction improves myocardial contractility and increases cardiac output, while myocardial oxygen consumption decreases. In animal studies isradipine has been observed to exert a cardioprotective effect against ischaemic injury without cardiodepression.

Pharmacokinetics: Following oral administration of Prescal, isradipine is almost completely absorbed (90–95%) from the gastro-intestinal tract and undergoes extensive first pass metabolism, resulting in a bioavailability of about 15–24%. Single oral doses are detectable in the plasma within 20 minutes and peak plasma concentrations are reached approximately 2 hours after intake. Isradipine is approximately 95% bound to plasma proteins.

No clear correlation between renal function and pharmacokinetic parameters has been found; both an increase and decrease in bioavailability has been observed in patients with impaired renal function. The bioavailability of isradipine was increased in elderly patients with impaired liver function.

Dosage and administration Prescal can be administered with or without food.

The recommended dosage is 2.5 mg twice a day (morning and evening). Treatment for 3–4 weeks is required for the maximum effect to develop. If blood pressure is not adequately controlled after this period patients may require a dosage of 5 mg twice a day, or if more appropriate, the addition of a low dose of another antihypertensive agent, i.e. thiazide diuretic or beta-blocker. Exceptionally, some patients may require up to 10 mg twice a day. Prescal can also be added to an ongoing regimen of other antihypertensive agents.

Use in the elderly and patients with impaired hepatic or renal function: In elderly patients, or where hepatic or renal function is impaired, a more suitable starting dose is 1.25 mg twice a day for hypertension. However, the dosage may be increased according to the requirements of the individual patient. Once-daily maintenance treatment with 2.5 mg or 5 mg may be sufficient in some hypertensive patients.

Use in children: The efficacy and safety of Prescal have not been established in children, and it is therefore not recommended in these patients.

Contra-indications, warnings, etc
Precautions: If hypersensitivity occurs, Prescal should be discontinued. As for other calcium antagonists Prescal does not give protection against the danger of abrupt beta-blocker withdrawal in angina pectoris. Beta-blockers should therefore be withdrawn gradually, preferably over 8–10 days.

Extreme caution should be used in patients with tight aortic stenosis. Caution should be taken when treating patients with documented or strongly suspected sick sinus syndrome who are not fitted with a pacemaker.

Care is recommended when treating patients with a low systolic blood pressure.

There is no evidence that Prescal interferes with glucose metabolism; however, diabetic patients should be initially monitored in accord with good clinical practice.

Use in pregnancy and lactation: Although some dihydropyridine compounds have been found to be teratogenic in animals, animal data in the rat and rabbit on isradipine provide no evidence for a teratogenic or embryotoxic effect. There is no clinical experience with Prescal in pregnant women. Therefore unless the potential benefit to the mother is expected to outweigh any potential risk to the offspring, Prescal should not be administered during pregnancy. Pre-natal observations in animals suggest that high doses of isradipine may cause prolongation of labour.

Care should be taken in the treatment of nursing mothers with Prescal since animal data indicate that small quantities of isradipine may be excreted in the breast milk.

Drug interactions: The bioavailability of Prescal is not affected by co-administration of food. However, the lag time to absorption and time to peak plasma concentration may be delayed by about one hour.

The pharmacokinetics of isradipine are not modified by the concomitant administration of digoxin, propranolol, or hydrochlorothiazide. Nor are the kinetics of digoxin or hydrochlorothiazide altered by the concomitant administration of Prescal. However, Prescal increases the bioavailability of propranolol, but this does not appear to be of any clinical significance. Isradipine is non-specifically bound to proteins. Enzyme inducing anticonvulsants may be associated with reduced levels of isradipine.

Side-effects: Clinical studies indicate that Prescal is well tolerated, with an overall incidence of adverse effects similar to that of placebo when used in doses up to 2.5 mg twice a day. Generally, side-effects are mild, dose-dependent and tend to disappear or decrease in intensity as treatment is continued. Discontinuation of therapy is generally not required. Those side-effects mentioned most often are related to the vasodilating properties of Prescal: headache, flushing, dizziness, tachycardia and palpitations, and localised peripheral oedema of non-cardiac origin; hypotension is uncommon and there have been no reports of orthostatic hypotension.

Non-specific side-effects are rare and include: weight gain, fatigue, abdominal discomfort, and skin rash.

Elevations of serum transaminases have been observed on very rare occasions; these changes were reversible both spontaneously and following Prescal withdrawal.

Overdosage
Symptoms: Available data on calcium antagonists suggest that overdosage would result in marked and prolonged systemic hypotension requiring cardiovascular support, with monitoring of cardiac and respiratory functions and attention to possible cerebral ischaemia (elevation of the lower extremities) and to circulating blood volume (intravenous fluid or plasma volume expanders).

Management: In cases of severe hypotension, vasoconstrictors could be beneficial provided there is no contra-indication to their use. Intravenous calcium may help to reverse the effect of calcium entry blockade. Animal data suggest the risk for cardiodepression with Prescal should be minimal, but depression of the sinus node may occur, in which case temporary pacemaker treatment may be useful.

Since isradipine is bound to plasma proteins to a very large extent, dialysis cannot be expected to be of benefit.

Pharmaceutical precautions The tablets should be protected from light.

Legal category POM.

Package quantities Calendar packs of 56 tablets (OP).

Further information Prescal is effective in both Negroid and Caucasian hypertensive patients, requiring no alteration of dose. Additionally, no potential deleterious first dose effects have been observed.

In asthmatic patients a single dose of isradipine has been found to blunt the bronchospastic response to exercise.

In patients with congestive heart failure, single oral doses of Prescal improved cardiac performance in terms of increasing cardiac output and decreasing pulmonary capillary venous pressure.

Prescal has not been shown to be arrhythmogenic and does not depress the atrioventricular node.

Product licence number 0001/0132.

RIMACTANE*

Presentation Rimactane Capsules each containing 150 mg rifampicin. An opaque, two-piece, hard gelatine capsule size 2, reddish-brown in colour, marked with the monogram CG on each half and the code JZ 150. The capsule has a diameter of 6.3 mm approx. and is 17.5 mm approx. in length.

Rimactane Capsules each containing 300 mg rifampicin. An opaque, two-piece, hard gelatine capsule size 1, coloured reddish-brown and dark brown, marked with the monogram CG on each half and the code CS 300. The capsule is approx. 6.7 mm in diameter and 18.9 mm approx. in length.

Rimactane Syrup: An opaque, red-coloured suspension having the odour and taste of raspberry; each 5 ml contains 100 mg rifampicin.

The capsules also contain lactose. The syrup contains sucrose, potassium sorbate, methyl hydroxybenzoate and propylhydroxybenzoate.

Uses Rimactane is a major drug in the management of tuberculosis (all forms) and certain opportunistic mycobacterial infections. It is effective in cases resistant to other anti-tuberculous agents and shows no cross-resistance outside the rifamycin group of drugs. In the treatment of tuberculosis Rimactane must always be combined with at least one other anti tuberculous agent. It is effective in combination with isoniazid, streptomycin, pyrazinamide, ethambutol and the majority of second line drugs.

Rimactane is also indicated for the chemoprophylaxis of meningococcal meningitis.

Mode of action: Rimactane is a rifamycin antibiotic which exerts, both *in vitro* and *in vivo* bactericidal effects on Mycobacterium tuberculosis. It also exhibits variable activity against other atypical species of Mycobacterium.

In vivo it exerts its bactericidal effect not only on micro-organisms in the extracellular spaces but also on those located intracellularly.

Mechanism of action: Rifampicin inhibits the DNA-dependent RNA polymerase of sensitive bacterial strains, but without affecting the corresponding mammalian enzyme.

Pharmacokinetics: Rifampicin is rapidly and completely absorbed. Following a single dose taken on an empty stomach (600 mg) the peak serum concentrations (approx 10 μg/ml) are observed after about 2 hours. Ingestion with food may adversely affect the absorption of rifampicin.

The plasma protein-binding rate is approximately 80%.

The active substance quickly penetrates into the various body fluids and tissue, including the bones and central nervous system.

The plasma elimination half-life, which is dose-dependent, amounts to approx. 2.5 hours after a single dose of 300 mg, to approx. 3–4 hours after one of 600 mg, and to approx. 5 hours after one of 900 mg.

Repeated administration of rifampicin reduces its bioavailability, owing to enzyme induction in the liver eg its half-life falls to 1–2 hours following repeat doses of 600 mg. During oral administration, induction of extra-hepatic enzymes – very probably in the intestinal wall – also plays a role. Consequently, the plasma concentrations show a more marked decline after repeated oral than after repeated intravenous administration of the same doses.

The principal metabolite of rifampicin produced in the liver is 25-0-deacetylrifampicin, which is microbiologically active and, like unchanged rifampicin, subject to enterohepatic circulation.

The bulk of the drug is eliminated in the bile, in which approx. 80% of the quantity excreted is accounted for by the deacetylrifampicin metabolite.

Rifampicin also appears in the urine; 4–18% of a dose is excreted, depending on dose, in the urine in unchanged form (dosage range 150–900 mg).

In patients with severe hepatic dysfunction the dosage may have to be adjusted as plasma concentrations are raised and half-life prolonged.

Excretion in the urine is dose-dependent, approximately 8% of a 600 mg dose is excreted as unchanged rifampicin in the 36-hour urine.

In the presence of impaired renal function, the half-life becomes prolonged only at doses exceeding 600 mg. Provided that hepatic excretory function is normal, the dosage in patients with impaired renal function does not need to be reduced below 600 mg daily.

In elderly patients, renal clearance is reduced, but, owing to the large scale on which the drug is eliminated via the liver, the plasma concentrations are similar to those in young patients.

Dosage and administration Rimactane should be given as a single dose, preferably on an empty stomach, at least 30 minutes before breakfast to ensure a high peak serum concentration. Dosage should be adjusted according to patients body weight.

For the management of tuberculosis and certain opportunistic mycobacterial infections: Rimactane must always be given in association with at least one and preferably two other anti-tuberculosis drugs, to prevent emergence of resistant strains. Especially good results have been reported when Rimactane has been used in combination with isoniazid and ethambutol. Whilst it is not generally recommended that rifampicin is used in combination with para-aminosalicyclic acid (PAS), if for any reason this regimen is used, the drugs should be given not less than eight hours apart to ensure satisfactory blood levels.

Use in adults: 450–600 mg daily as a single dose (based on approximately 10 mg per kg body weight). (Those patients 50 kg (8 stone) and over should take 600 mg rifampicin daily, whilst patients under 50 kg should take 450 mg).

The following chemotherapeutic agents are employed today as combined therapy for tuberculosis: Rifampicin (Rimactane) (RMP), isoniazid (INH), pyrazinamide (PZA), ethambutol (EMB), streptomycin (STM).

The dosages recommended by the IUAT and WHO are as follows:

Preparation	*Daily*		*2 or 3 times a week*	
	mg/kg	*Max. mg*	*mg/kg*	*Max. mg*
RMP	10	600	10	600
INH	8	400	15	750
PZA	30	2,000	50	3,500
EMB	20	1,200	40	2,000
STM	15	1,000	15	1,000

For the treatment of sputum-positive pulmonary tuberculosis, preference is given to the following regimens:

Daily for a total of 9 months
For 2 months: RMP 450 or 600 mg+INH 300 mg+EMB 1,200 mg or STM 1 g
For 7 months: RMP 450 or 600 mg+INH 300 mg
Daily for a total of 6 months.
For 2 months: RMP 450 or 600 mg+INH 300 mg+PZA 1.5–2.5 g (depending on body weight)+EMB 1,200 mg or STM 1 g
For 4 months: RMP 450 or 600 mg+INH 300 mg.

Use in children: Up to 20 mg per kg body weight daily to a maximum of 600 mg as a single dose.

Use in premature and newborn infants: 10 mg/kg once daily. Premature and newborn infants should be treated only in cases of emergency and with extreme caution since their liver enzyme system may not be fully developed.

Use in elderly: No special dosage regime is necessary but concurrent hepatic insufficiency should be taken into account (see Pharmacokinetics).

For the chemoprophylaxis of meningococcal meningitis: Note: Rimactane should not be used to treat overt meningococcal meningitis.

Use in adults: 600 mg twice daily (12 hourly) for 2 days.

Use in children: (aged 1–12 years): 10 mg/kg twice daily (12 hourly) for 2 days. Children at the lower end of this age range may metabolise rifampicin more rapidly and produce significantly lower serum levels than newborns or adults. In such cases doses up to 15 mg/kg 12 hourly may be required.

Use in infants (up to 1 year): 5 mg/kg twice daily (12 hourly) for 2 days.

Use in the elderly: There is no evidence to suggest that dose adjustments are necessary.

This prophylactic administration should be started as soon as possible. It is recommended that Rimactane is only given for 2 days in this indication since resistance to this class of antibacterial agent may develop.

Contra-indications, warnings, etc

Contra-indications: Hypersensitivity to rifamycins; jaundice.

Warnings: Patients receiving Rimactane for the chemoprophylaxis of meningococcal meningitis should be kept under close surveillance. Special attention should be paid to signs of overt infection.

Rimactane should not be used to treat an overt meningococcal infection.

To prevent the emergence of resistant bacteria, Rimactane must always be combined with other antibiotics/chemotherapeutic agents when used to treat infections.

Precautions: When resuming treatment with Rimactane after a temporary or a prolonged interval, the drug should be given in small, gradually increasing doses and adequate surveillance should be maintained. In adults an initial dose of 75 mg daily should be administered, raised subsequently by 75 mg per day until the desired dosage level is attained. If, as may happen in exceptional cases, the patient develops renal failure, thrombocytopenia, purpura or haemolytic anaemia, treatment with Rimactane should be stopped at once and not reinstated at a later date.

As Rimactane is excreted principally by the biliary

tract, caution should be excercised in treating patients with hepatic disorders.

In patients with or likely to have liver function abnormalities including those with chronic liver disease, chronic alcoholism, the elderly and the undernourished, the benefit of combined treatment with rifampicin must be weighed against the possible risks. This applies particularly to combination of isoniazid and/or pyrazinamide with rifampicin. In the presence of severely impaired liver function the dosage may have to be reduced.

During prolonged treatment and in patients with hepatic disorders, blood counts and liver function tests should be performed periodically.

Owing to its enzyme-inducing effect, rifampicin must be employed with extreme caution in patients with porphyria, because activation of delta-aminolaevulinic acid synthetase may lead to an acute manifestation of porphyria.

To preclude all possibility of pregnancy during treatment with Rimactane, non-hormonal means of contraception must be employed (see Interactions).

Use in pregnancy and lactation: In female mice of a strain known to be susceptible to hepatomas, a significant increase in such tumours was observed after 1 year of treatment with rifampicin in quantities equivalent to 2–10 times the maximum clinical doses.

In mice of another strain treated for 1 year, and in rats treated for 2 years, no significant increase was noted in the incidence of any type of tumour. Studies with various mammalian models, as well as with bacteria, yielded no evidence that rifampicin has a mutagenic effect.

In daily doses of 150–250 mg/kg, rifampicin proved teratogenic in mice and rats, insofar as an increased occurrence of spina bifida and cleft palate was observed. In rabbits it had no teratogenic effect. In all three animal species, unspecific embryotoxic effects occurred after doses > 150 mg/kg.

In women of childbearing age, the possibility of pregnancy should be excluded prior to treatment with Rimactane, and pregnancy should be avoided during the treatment. During the first 3 months of pregnancy, Rimactane must only be employed in life-threatening conditions and where no suitable alternative drug is available. In the remaining 6 months, the possible risk for the foetus must be weighed against the benefits of the treatment for the mother.

Administration of Rimactane during the last few weeks of pregnancy can cause post-natal haemorrhage in the mother and newborn infant. This may necessitate treatment with vitamin K preparations.

Rifampicin passes into the breast milk but no adverse effects on breast fed infants have been observed. Therefore nursing mothers may continue to breast feed their infants.

Drug interactions: Antacids, opiates, and anticholinergic drugs reduce the bioavailability of rifampicin when given concomitantly by mouth. The same applies to PAS preparations containing bentonite. To avoid this interaction, rifampicin must be administered a few hours before these preparations.

Rifampicin is a potent inducer of liver enzymes which may increase the metabolism of concomitantly administered drugs such as those listed below. The activity of the following drugs may be impaired and their dosage must be reassessed during and after treatment with rifampicin.

Corticosteroids (Addison patients may develop a crisis; exacerbation of pemphigus may occur; treatment for corticosteroid dependent asthma may become more difficult or impossible); sex hormones (menstrual disorders may appear); oral contraceptives (their effect can no longer be relied upon); oral anticoagulants; oral antidiabetic agents; dapsone; phenytoin; digitalis preparations; quinidine; mexiletine; methadone (withdrawal symptoms may appear), theophylline; chloramphenicol, ketoconozole; cyclosporin A; azathioprine (transplants may be rejected); beta blockers, verapamil; cimetidine.

Rifampicin can delay the biliary excretion of contrast media employed to X-ray the gall bladder.

Microbiological techniques for assaying folic acid and vitamin B_{12} in the serum are unsuitable for use during treatment with Rimactane.

Side-effects:

Dermatological: Occasionally flushing, itching with or without skin rash, and reddening of the eyes. Severe signs and symptoms, such as exudative conjunctivitis or generalised hypersensitivity reactions involving the skin, occur only in isolated instances.

Gastrointestinal tract: Occasionally anorexia, nausea, abdominal pains, gaseous distension; rarely vomiting or diarrhoea; isolated occurrences of pseudomembranous colitis.

Hepatic: Frequently an asymptomatic increase in liver enzymes; rarely hepatitis or jaundice; here account should also be taken of the liver toxicity of chemotherapeutic agents, eg isoniazid or pyrazinamide, employed in combination with rifampicin. Induction of porphyria in isolated cases.

Central and peripheral nervous system: Occasionally tiredness, drowsiness, headache, light-headedness, dizziness; rarely ataxia, mental confusion; muscular weakness (myopathy) in isolated cases.

Haematological: Isolated occurrences of transient leucopenia; eosinophilia; thrombocytopenia and thrombocytopenic purpura.

Endocrine: In rare instances disturbances in the menstrual cycle (in extreme cases amenorrhoea); induction of a crisis in Addison patients (see Interactions).

Effects following intermittent or interrupted therapy: Side-effects to rifampicin, probably of immunological/allergic origin have been reported, particularly in connection with intermittent, interrupted or repeated treatment eg influenza-like symptoms and rarely skin rashes, fever, dyspnoea have occurred. If serious complications arise such as thrombocytopenia, purpura, acute renal failure, haemolytic anaemia, shock, or asthma attacks, rifampicin should be stopped at once and never restarted.

Overdosage:

Signs and symptoms: Nausea, vomiting, abdominal pains; enlargement of the liver, jaundice, elevated liver enzyme levels, possibly acute pulmonary oedema, lethargy, clouding of consciousness, convulsions.

Treatment: Gastric lavage together with instillation of an activated charcoal suspension; general supportive measures to maintain vital functions; forced diuresis; haemodialysis; in the presence of severe liver damage, cholecystotomy if necessary. Bear in mind that other drugs used in combination with Rimactane may also have been taken in an overdosage and necessitate additional specific measures.

Pharmaceutical precautions This product should be protected from heat and moisture.

The syrup should be stored below 25°C.

Legal category POM.

Package quantities Capsules of 150 mg Rimactane and 300 mg in securitainers of 100.

Syrup containing 100 mg in 5 ml; in bottles of 100 ml.

Further information Rimactane is orally active, very well tolerated and its activity is comparable with that of isoniazid. In combination, these two agents are commonly used as first-line treatment of tuberculosis and offer the greatest chance of rapid eradication of the infection. It is usual, however, to employ a third drug during the first two months of treatment, or at least until the results of sensitivity tests are known. The orange-red colour imparted to the urine, sputum and tears by rifampicin is a valuable guide to adherence to the drug regime. Rifampicin may also permanently discolour soft contact lenses.

Product licence numbers

Rimactane Capsules 150 mg 0008/5080

Rimactane Capsules 300 mg 0008/5081

Rimactane Syrup 0008/0106

RIMACTANE* INFUSION

Presentation 10 ml vial containing 300 mg rifampicin BP (red lyophilised powder) with an accompanying 5 ml ampoule of Water for Injections BP.

The vials also contain sodium formaldehyde sulphoxylate (pyrogen free).

Uses

Indications: Rimactane is a major drug in the management of tuberculosis (all forms) and certain opportunistic mycobacterial infections. It is effective in cases resistant to other anti-tuberculous agents and shows no cross-resistance outside the rifamycin group of drugs. In the treatment of tuberculosis Rimactane must always be combined with at least one other anti-tuberculous agent. It is effective in combination with isoniazid, streptomycin, pyrazinamide, ethambutol and the majority of second line drugs.

Rimactane infusion is indicated in patients with all forms of tuberculosis who are unable to tolerate oral therapy, eg post-operative or comatose patients or patients in whom gastrointestinal absorption is impaired.

Mode of action: Rimactane is a rifamycin antibiotic which exerts, both *in vitro* and *in vivo* bactericidal effects on Mycobacterium tuberculosis. It also exhibits variable activity against other atypical species of Mycobacterium.

In vivo it exerts its bactericidal effect not only on micro-organisms in the extracellular spaces but also on those located intracellularly.

Mechanism of action: Rifampicin inhibits the DNA-dependent RNA polymerase of sensitive bacterial strains, but without affecting the corresponding mammalian enzyme.

Pharmacokinetics: An intravenous drip infusion of rifampicin (600 mg) lasting 3 hours produces peak plasma concentrations of approx. 10 μg/ml. The plasma profiles are similar to those obtained following the administration of the same dose in capsules.

The plasma protein-binding rate is approximately 80%.

The active substance quickly penetrates into the various body fluids and tissues, including the bones and central nervous system.

The plasma elimination half-life, which is dose-dependent, amounts to approx. 2.5 hours after a single dose of 300 mg, to approx. 3–4 hours after one of 600 mg, and to approx. 5 hours after one of 900 mg.

Repeated administration of rifampicin reduces its bioavailability, owing to enzyme induction in the liver eg its half-life falls to 1–2 hours following repeated doses of 600 mg. During oral administration, induction of extrahepatic enzymes – very probably in the intestinal wall – also plays a role. Consequently, the plasma concentrations show a more marked decline after repeated oral than after repeated intravenous administration of the same doses.

The principal metabolite of rifampicin produced in the liver is 25-0-deacetylrifampicin, which is microbiologically active and, like unchanged rifampicin, subject to enterohepatic circulation.

The bulk of the drug is eliminated in the bile, in which approx. 80% of the quantity excreted is accounted for by the deacetylrifampicin metabolite.

In patients with severe hepatic dysfunction the dosage may have to be adjusted as plasma concentrations are raised and half-life prolonged.

Excretion in the urine is dose-dependent, approximately 8% of a 600 mg dose is excreted as unchanged rifampicin in the 36-hour urine.

In the presence of impaired renal function, the half-life becomes prolonged only at doses exceeding 600 mg. Provided that hepatic excretory function is normal, the dosage in patients with impaired renal function does not need to be reduced below 600 mg daily.

In elderly patients, renal clearance is reduced, but, owing to the large scale on which the drug is eliminated via the liver, the plasma concentrations are similar to those in young patients.

Dosage and administration

For the management of tuberculosis and certain opportunistic mycobacterial infections.

Use in adults: 450–600 mg daily as a single dose (based on approximately 10 mg per kg body weight). A daily dose of 600 mg given in an intravenous infusion over two to three hours has been found to be effective and well tolerated for the majority of adult patients. Serum levels following this regimen are similar to those obtained following oral administration. Lower doses are recommended for small or frail patients. Patients 50 kg (8 stone) and over should receive 600 mg rifampicin daily, patients under 50 kg should receive 450 mg.

The following chemotherapeutic agents are employed as combined therapy for tuberculosis:

Rifampicin (Rimactane) (RMP), isoniazid (INH), pyrazinamide (PZA), ethambutol (EMB), streptomycin (STM).

The dosages recommended by the IUAT and WHO are as follows:

Preparation	*Daily*		*2 or 3 times a week*	
	mg/kg	*Max. mg*	*mg/kg*	*Max. mg*
RMP	10	600	10	600
INH	8	400	15	750
PZA	30	2,000	50	3,500
EMB	20	1,200	40	2,000
STM	15	1,000	15	1,000

For the treatment of sputum-positive pulmonary tuberculosis, preference is given to the following regimens:

Daily for a total of 9 months
For 2 months: RMP 450 or 600 mg+INH 300 mg+EMB 1,200 mg or STM 1 g
For 7 months: RMP 450 or 600 mg+INH 300 mg
Daily for a total of 6 months.
For 2 months: RMP 450 or 600 mg+INH 300 mg+PZA 1.5–2.5 g (depending on body weight)+EMB 1,200 mg or STM 1 g
For 4 months: RMP 450 or 600 mg+INH 300 mg.

Use in children: Paediatric usage has not yet been established. However, the following regimen is suggested. In tuberculosis, a single daily dose of up to 20 mg/kg body weight is recommended, although total daily dose should not usually exceed 600 mg.

Use in premature and newborn infants: 10 mg/kg once daily. Premature and newborn infants should be treated only in cases of emergency and with extreme caution since their liver enzyme system may not be fully developed.

Use in elderly: No special dosage regimen is necessary but concurrent hepatic insufficiency should be taken into account (see Pharmacokinetics).

Transfer to oral therapy: When patients are able to accept oral medication, they should be transferred to Rimactane capsules or syrup. Oral dosage would be expected to be the same as that used with the infusion (see oral Rimactane data sheet).

Preparation of infusion: (see 'Warnings'). Rimactane infusion is prepared for use by aseptically adding the solvent to the vial of dry rifampicin powder and shaking vigorously and continuously for 30–60 seconds.

When the powder is completely dissolved, the solution should be immediately diluted in 250 ml of 5% glucose solution or other suitable infusion fluid (see Pharmaceutical Precautions). Freshly prepared solutions must be used within 6 hours. It is recommended that the infusion be administered over a period of 2–3 hours.

Contra-indications, warnings, etc

Contra-indications: Hypersensitivity to rifamycins; jaundice.

Warnings: To prevent the emergence of resistant bacteria, Rimactane must always be combined with other antibiotics/chemotherapeutic agents when used to treat infections.

Staff preparing and setting up infusions may develop

hypersensitivity reactions affecting the hands and face. It is recommended that the procedure be carried out in a vertical lamina flow cabinet and gloves should be worn.

Rifampicin may colour the urine, sputum and tears orange-red. Rifampicin may also permanently discolour soft contact lenses.

Precautions: When resuming treatment with Rimactane after a temporary or a prolonged interval, the drug should be given in small, gradually increasing doses and adequate surveillance should be maintained. In adults an initial dose of 75 mg daily should be administered, raised subsequently by 75 mg per day until the desired dosage level is attained. If, as may happen in exceptional cases, the patient develops renal failure, thrombocytopenia, purpura or haemolytic anaemia, treatment with Rimactane should be stopped at once and not reinstated at a later date.

As Rimactane is excreted principally by the biliary tract, caution should be exercised in treating patients with hepatic disorders.

In patients with or likely to have liver function abnormalities including those with chronic liver disease, chronic alcoholism, the elderly and the undernourished, the benefit of combined treatment with rifampicin must be weighed against the possible risks. This applies particularly to combination of isoniazid and/or pyrazinamide with rifampicin. In the presence of severely impaired liver function the dosage may have to be reduced.

During prolonged treatment and in patients with hepatic disorders, blood counts and liver function tests should be performed periodically.

Owing to its enzyme-inducing effect, rifampicin must be employed with extreme caution in patients with porphyria, because activation of delta-aminolaevulinic acid synthetase may lead to an acute manifestation of the porphyria.

To preclude all possibility of pregnancy during treatment with Rimactane, non-hormonal means of contraception must be employed (see Interactions).

Use in pregnancy and lactation: In female mice of a strain known to be susceptible to hepatomas, a significant increase in such tumours was observed after 1 year of treatment with rifampicin in quantities equivalent to 2–10 times the maximum clinical doses.

In mice of another strain treated for 1 year, and in rats treated for 2 years, no significant increase was noted in the incidence of any type of tumour. Studies with various mammalian models, as well as with bacteria, yielded no evidence that rifampicin has a mutagenic effect.

In daily doses of 150–250 mg/kg, rifampicin proved teratogenic in mice and rats, insofar as an increased occurrence of spina bifida and cleft palate was observed. In rabbits it has no teratogenic effect. In all three animal species, unspecific embryotoxic effects occurred after doses > 150 mg/kg.

In women of childbearing age, the possibility of pregnancy should be excluded prior to treatment with Rimactane, and pregnancy should be avoided during the treatment. During the first 3 months of pregnancy, Rimactane must only be employed in life-threatening conditions and where no suitable alternative drug is available. In the remaining 6 months, the possible risk for the foetus must be weighed against the benefits of the treatment for the mother.

Administration of Rimactane during the last few weeks of pregnancy can cause post-natal haemorrhage in the mother and newborn infant, which may necessitate treatment with vitamin K preparations.

Rifampicin passes into the breast milk but no adverse effects on breast fed infants have been observed. Therefore nursing mothers may continue to breast feed their infants.

Drug interactions: Rifampicin is a potent inducer of liver enzymes which may increase the metabolism of concomitantly administered drugs such as those listed below. The activity of the following drugs may be impaired and their dosage must be reassessed during and after treatment with Rifampicin.

Coticosteroids (Addison patients may develop a crisis; exacerbation of pemphigus may occur; treatment for corticosteroid dependent asthma may become more difficult or impossible); sex hormones (menstrual disorders may appear); oral contraceptives (their effect can no longer be relied upon); oral anticoagulants; oral antidiabetic agents; dapsone; phenytoin; digitalis preparations; quinidine; mexiletine; methadone (withdrawal symptoms may appear), theophylline; chloramphenicol, ketoconozole; cyclosporin A; azathioprine (transplants may be rejected); beta blockers, verapamil; cimetidine.

Rifampicin can delay the biliary excretion of contrast media employed to X-ray the gall bladder.

Microbiological techniques for assaying folic acid and vitamin B_{12} in the serum are unsuitable for use during treatment with Rimactane.

Side-effects

Effects relating to intravenous administration: During prolonged (more than 30 days) administration i.v., local thrombophlebitis occasionally occurs.

Dermatological: Occasionally flushing, itching with or without skin rash, and reddening of the eyes. Severe signs and symptoms, such as exudative conjunctivitis or generalised hypersensitivity reactions involving the skin, occur only in isolated instances.

Gastrointestinal tract: Occasionally anorexia, nausea, abdominal pains, gaseous distension; rarely vomiting or diarrhoea; isolated occurrences of pseudomembranous colitis.

Hepatic: Frequently an asymptomatic increase in liver enzymes; rarely hepatitis or jaundice; here account should also be taken of the liver toxicity of chemotherapeutic agents, eg isoniazid or pyrazinamide, employed in combination with rifampicin. Induction of porphyria in isolated cases.

Central and peripheral nervous system: Occasionally tiredness, drowsiness, headache, light-headedness, dizziness; rarely ataxia, mental confusion; muscular weakness (myopathy) in isolated cases.

Haematological: Isolated occurrences of transient leucopenia; eosinophilia; thrombocytopenia and thrombocytopenic purpura.

Endocrine: In rare instances disturbances in the menstrual cycle (in extreme cases amenorrhoea); induction of a crisis in Addison patients (see 'Interactions').

Effects following intermittent or interrupted therapy: Side-effects to rifampicin, probably of immunological/allergic origin have been reported, particularly in connection with intermittent, interrupted or repeated treatment eg influenza-like symptoms and rarely skin rashes, fever, dyspnoea have occurred. If serious complications arise such as thrombocytopenia, purpura, acute renal failure, haemolytic anaemia, shock, or asthma attacks, rifampicin should be stopped at once and never restarted.

Overdosage:

Signs and symptoms: Nausea, vomiting, abdominal pains; enlargement of the liver, jaundice, elevated liver enzyme levels, possibly acute pulmonary oedema, lethargy, clouding of consciousness, convulsions.

Treatment: General supportive measures to maintain vital functions; forced diuresis; haemodialysis; in the presence of severe liver damage, cholecystotomy if necessary. Bear in mind that other drugs used in combination with Rimactane may also have been taken in an overdosage and necessitate additional specific measures.

Pharmaceutical precautions Rimactane Infusion should be freshly prepared. The vials should be protected from heat and light.

Compatibility: Rimactane infusion is compatible with the following infusion solutions: NaCl 0.9%, Ringer's solution (lactate or acetate), dextrose 5% or 10%, mannitol 10% or 20%, sodium bicarbonate 1.4%, Macrodex with saline solution, Macrodex with glucose solution, Rheomacrodex and Fructose 5% and 10%.

Incompatibility: Rimactane infusion is incompatible with the following infusion solutions: sodium bicarbonate 5%, Ringer's solution (acetate) plus glucose, Perfudex and sodium lactate 0.167M.

Rimactane infusion diluted in glucose or saline is not

compatible with: cephamandole, tetracycline, rolitetracycline, doxycycline.

Rimactane infusion should not be mixed with other drugs if there is a possibility that precipitation may occur; concurrent intravenous therapy should be administered via a different site of injection.

Legal category POM.

Package quantities Combined pack of 1 vial + 1 × 5 ml solvent ampoule.

Product licence number 0008/0151.

RIMACTAZID* COMBINED TABLETS

Presentation Rimactazid 150 Tablets each containing 150 mg Rifampicin BP (Rimactane*) and 100 mg Isoniazid BP, pink, round, bi-convex, sugar-coated tablets, marked with the monogram CG on one side and the letters EI on the other.

Rimactazid 300 Tablets each containing 300 mg Rifampicin BP (Rimactane*) and 150 mg Isoniazid BP; brownish orange, capsule-shaped, bi-convex, sugar-coated tablets marked with the monogram CG on one side and the letters DH on the other.

Uses *Indications:* Rimactane and isoniazid are both major drugs in the management of tuberculosis and in certain opportunist mycobacterial infections. Rifampicin is effective in cases resistant to other anti-tuberculous agents and shows no cross-resistance outside the rifamycin group of drugs. Extensive UK experience has led to the routine use of Rimactane and isoniazid as basic therapy supported in the first six to eight weeks, or until cultures are negative, by a third drug, eg streptomycin, pyrazinamide, ethambutol and the majority of second-line drugs.

Mode of action: Rifampicin: Rifampicin is a rifamycin antibiotic which exerts, both *in vitro* and *in vivo* bactericidal effects on Mycobacterium tuberculosis. It also exhibits variable activity against other atypical species of Mycobacterium.

In vivo it exerts its bactericidal effect not only on micro-organisms in the extracellular spaces but also on those located intracellularly.

Mechanism of action: Rifampicin inhibits the DNA-dependent RNA polymerase of sensitive bacterial strains, but without affecting the corresponding mammalian enzyme.

Isoniazid: Isoniazid is a specific antituberculous agent exerting a strong bactericidal effect mainly on rapidly growing populations of *Mycobacterium tuberculosis*. Its mechanism of action is probably based chiefly on inhibition of mycolic acid synthesis, mycolic acid being an important constituent of the mycobacterial cell wall.

Pharmacokinetics: Rifampicin and isoniazid penetrate rapidly into the various body fluids and tissues, including the central nervous system.

Absorption/serum concentration:

Rifampicin single dose (600 mg) maximum concentration 9.4 μg/ml at 2–3 hours.

Isoniazid single dose (300 mg) maximum concentration 6.1 μg/ml at 0.5–2 hours.

Distribution/elimination half-life ($t_{\frac{1}{2}}$) from plasma:

$t_{\frac{1}{2}}$ rifampicin – dependent upon dose, approximately 2.5–5 hours after 300–900 mg

— Repeated administration of rifampicin reduces its bioavailability, owing to enzyme induction in the liver, eg its half life falls to 2–3 hours after repeated doses of 900 mg.

$t_{\frac{1}{2}}$ isoniazid – 0.6–1.8 hours (rapid acetylators)
1.8–6.7 hours (slow acetylators).

Protein binding: Rifampicin 89%, isoniazid 0%.

Metabolism: Rifampicin: rifampicin is metabolised in the liver, its principal metabolite being 25-0-deacetylrifampicin which is microbiologically active. Rifampicin induces its own metabolism.

Isoniazid: isoniazid is acetylated and hydrolysed in the liver. Acetylation is the most important metabolic step, the rate being dependent on whether or not the patient is a rapid or slow acetylator, see above. The metabolites are microbiologically inactive.

Excretion: Rifampicin: though eliminated mainly in the bile rifampicin also appears in the urine; 4–18% of a dose is excreted, depending on dose, in the urine in unchanged form (dosage range 150–900 mg).

Isoniazid: N-acetylisoniazid is eliminated in the urine together with other metabolites. Within 24 hours 75%–95% of the dose is excreted, mainly as metabolites, in the urine. The amount of unchanged isoniazid appearing in the urine amounts to 12% of dose in rapid acetylators and 27% of the dose in slow acetylators.

In the presence of impaired renal function the half-life of elimination of rifampicin becomes prolonged only at doses exceeding 600 mg. Provided that hepatic excretory function is normal, the dosage in patients with impaired renal function does not need to be reduced below 600 mg daily.

In slow acetylators with severely impaired renal function, some accumulation of isoniazid may occur. In such cases serum concentrations of isoniazid should be monitored and if necessary the dosage reduced.

In the presence of impaired liver function the half-lives of rifampicin and isoniazid may be prolonged and to avoid unwanted effects it may be necessary to adapt the dosage accordingly.

In elderly patients renal clearance of rifampicin is reduced but owing to the large scale on which the drug is eliminated by the liver, the plasma concentrations are similar to those in young patients. The rate of elimination of isoniazid in elderly patients is not significantly different from that in other patients.

Dosage and administration Rimactazid should be given as a single dose, preferably on an empty stomach, at least 30 minutes before breakfast to ensure a high peak serum concentration. Dosage should be adjusted according to patient body weight. Whilst it is not generally recommended that rifampicin be used in combination with PAS, if for any reason this regimen is used, the drugs should be given not less than eight hours apart to ensure satisfactory blood levels.

Adults: The combined tablets of Rimactazid provide Rimactane and isoniazid in the accepted ratios to provide the currently recommended adult dose of these two drugs. Thus, 2 tablets of Rimactazid 300 once daily are recommended for patients of 50 kg (8 stone) or over and 3 tablets of Rimactazid 150 for patients under 50 kg, (ie the usual daily dosage of 600 mg or 450 mg Rimactane, each with 300 mg isoniazid).

Duration of treatment and combined medication
Total duration 9 months
For 2 months: Rimactazid 300, 2 tablets daily or
Rimactazid 150, 3 tablets daily plus
ethambutol 1.2 g or streptomycin 1 g daily
For 7 months: Rimactazid 300, 2 tablets daily or
Rimactazid 150, 3 tablets daily
Total duration 6 months
For 2 months: Rimactazid 300, 2 tablets daily or
Rimactazid 150, 3 tablets daily plus
pyrazinamide 1.5–2.5 g daily plus
ethambutol 1.2 g or streptomycin 1 g daily
For 4 months: Rimactazid 300, 2 tablets daily or
Rimactazid 150, 3 tablets daily

Children: The ratios of Rimactane and isoniazid present in Rimactazid 150 and 300 make it difficult for both components to be administered in a dosage suitable for children. Rimactazid tablets are therefore not recommended for paediatric use.

Elderly: No special dosage regime is necessary but concurrent hepatic insufficiency should be taken into account (see pharmacokinetics).

Contra-indications, warnings, etc

Contra-indications: Known hypersensitivity to rifampicin and/or to isoniazid, a history of drug induced hepatitis, acute liver disease regardless of their origin, peripheral neuritis.

Precautions: When resuming treatment with rifampicin after a temporary interruption or a prolonged interval, the drug should be given in small gradually increasing doses and adequate surveillance should be maintained. For this purpose, rifampicin and isoniazid should temporarily be administered in free combination. In adults an initial dose of rifampicin 75 mg daily should be administered, raised subsequently by 75 mg per day until the desired dosage level is attained. During this period, renal function should be closely monitored. If, as may happen in exceptional cases, the patient develops renal failure, thrombocytopenia, purpura, dyspnoea, shock or haemolytic anaemia, treatment with rifampicin should be stopped at once and not re-instituted at a later date. Normal dosage of isoniazid should be continued over this period.

If other signs of hypersensitivity appear, such as fever or skin reactions, Rimactazid should be withdrawn. For safety reasons, treatment should not be continued with rifampicin. Where isoniazid is considered essential, treatment should be resumed in low doses and under strict surveillance.

As rifampicin and isoniazid are metabolised in the liver, patients with impaired liver function should be treated with caution. Patients with hepatic disorders or undergoing prolonged treatment should have blood counts and liver function tests performed periodically. Any deterioration in liver function in these patients is an indication for stopping treatment.

The occurrence of liver function abnormalities is more common when rifampicin and isoniazid are used in combination and special care is therefore required in patients with pre-existing liver impairment or malnourished patients.

In patients with chronic liver disease, as well as in chronic alcoholics and undernourished patients, the therapeutic benefits of treatment with Rimactazid must be weighed against the possible risks. If the treatment is considered necessary, the dosage of both components must be correspondingly reduced. In such cases it is only possible to adapt the dosage by administering rifampicin and isoniazid separately.

Owing to its enzyme-inducing effect, rifampicin must be employed with extreme caution in patients with porphyria, because activation of delta-aminolaevulinic acid synthetase may lead to an acute manifestation of porphyria.

To preclude the possibility of pregnancy during treatment with rifampicin, additional non-hormonal means of contraception must be employed (see interactions).

Owing to the neurotoxic action of isoniazid, patients suffering from convulsive disorders must be kept under special observation during treatment with Rimactazid.

Pyridoxine may be useful in preventing the occurrence of peripheral neuritis and should be given in a dose of 10 mg daily from the start of treatment with Rimactazid.

Doses of 10 mg/kg or greater, of isoniazid may produce adverse reactions of the nervous system, eg peripheral neuropathy and thus impair the patients ability to drive or operate machinery.

Patients should abstain from alcohol while under treatment with Rimactazid.

Use in pregnancy and lactation:

Rifampicin: In female mice of a strain known to be susceptible to hepatomas, a significant increase in such tumours was observed after 1 year of treatment with rifampicin in quantities equivalent to 2–10 times the maximum clinical doses.

In mice of another strain treated for 1 year, and in rats treated for 2 years, no significant increase was noted in the incidence of any type of tumour. Studies with various mammalian models, as well as with bacteria, yielded no evidence that rifampicin has a mutagenic effect.

Daily doses of 150–250 mg/kg rifampicin increased the occurrence of spina bifida and cleft palate in mice and rats. No teratogenic effect was seen in rabbits. In all three species embryotoxic effects were observed at doses of greater than 150 mg/kg.

Isoniazid – No teratogenic effects due to isoniazid have been observed in mice, rats or rabbits.

Since Rimactazid contains rifampicin, in women of child bearing age the possibility of pregnancy should be excluded prior to treatment with it, and pregnancy should be avoided during treatment. During the first 3 months of pregnancy rifampicin must only be employed in life threatening conditions and where no suitable alternative drug is available. In the remaining 6 months, the possible risk to the foetus must be weighed against the benefits of the treatment for the mother.

Isoniazid has been found to entail relatively little risk during pregnancy but since it is theoretically possible for the drug to produce neurotoxic effects in the child, it is recommended that the mother should take pyridoxine during her pregnancy.

Administration of rifampicin during the last few weeks of pregnancy can cause post natal haemorrhage in the mother and newborn infant, which may necessitate treatment with vitamin K preparations.

Although rifampicin and isoniazid pass into the breast milk, no adverse effects on breast fed infants have been observed. It is not, therefore, absolutely necessary to wean the infant but in view of the theoretical possibility of neurotoxic effects due to isoniazid, breast fed infants should be kept under careful surveillance. Prophylactic administration of pyridoxine to the mother and child is recommended.

Drug interactions

Rifampicin: Antacids, opiates, and anticholinergic drugs reduce the bioavailability of rifampicin when it is given concomitantly by mouth. The same applies to PAS preparations containing bentonite. To avoid this interaction, rifampicin must be administered a few hours before these preparations.

Rifampicin is a potent inducer of liver enzymes which may increase the metabolism of concomitantly administered drugs such as those listed below. The activity of the following drugs may be impaired and their dosage must be reassessed during and after treatment with rifampicin.

Corticosteroids (patients with Addison's disease may develop a crisis; exacerbation of pemphigus may occur; treatment for corticosteroid dependent asthma may become more difficult or impossible); sex hormones (menstrual disorders may appear); oral contraceptives (their effect can no longer be relied upon); oral anticoagulants; oral antidiabetic agents; dapsone; p-henytoin (see also isoniazid); digitalis preparations; quinidine; mexiletine; methadone (withdrawal symptoms may appear), theophylline; chloramphenicol, ketoconozole; cyclosporin A; azathioprine (transplants may be rejected); beta blockers, verapamil; cimetidine.

Rifampicin can delay the biliary excretion of contrast media employed to X-ray the gall bladder.

Microbiological techniques for assaying folic acid and vitamin B_{12} in the serum are unsuitable for use during treatment with Rimactane.

Isoniazid: Isoniazid retards the metabolism of various concomitantly administered drugs, including phenytoin, carbamazepine, primidone and valproic acid. The dosages of these drugs may have to be reduced. It is not advisable to administer disulphiram concomitantly with isoniazid as this may lead to mental disturbances, the mechanism of this interaction is not known.

Side-effects: associated with rifampicin:

Dermatological: Occasionally: flushing, itching with or without skin rash, and reddening of the eyes. Isolated cases: severe signs and symptoms such as, exudative conjunctivitis or generalised hypersensitivity reactions involving the skin.

Gastrointestinal: Occasionally: anorexia, nausea, abdominal pain, gaseous distension. Rarely: vomiting or diarrhoea. Isolated cases: pseudomembranous colitis.

Hepatic: Frequently: asymptomatic increase in liver enzymes. Rarely: hepatitis or jaundice. Isolated cases: porphyria.

Central and peripheral nervous system: Occasionally: tiredness, drowsiness, headache, light-headedness, dizziness. Rarely: ataxia, mental confusion. Isolated cases: muscular weakness (myopathy).

Blood: Isolated cases: transient leucopenia, eosinophilia, thrombocytopenia and thrombocytopenic purpura.
Endocrine: Rarely: disturbances to the menstrual cycle, induction of a crisis in Addison's Disease (see drug "interactions").
Immunopathological: In patients taking rifampicin other than daily or in those resuming treatment with the drug after temporary interruption, an influenza like syndrome may set in, which is probably of immunopathological origin. It is characterised by fever, shivering and headache, dizziness, and pain in the limbs. In rare cases the 'flu syndrome' may be folllowed by thrombocytopenia, purpura, dyspnoea, asthma-like attacks, haemolytic anaemia, shock and acute renal failure. These symptoms may also occur without the preceding 'flu syndrome', again chiefly following when treatment is resumed after an interruption.

Associated with isoniazid
Central nervous system: Frequently: peripheral neuropathy (dose dependent and more common in undernourished patients, alcoholics and diabetics).

Rarely: Damage to the optic nerve, convulsions, psychoses, dizziness, light-headedness, headache. High doses may increase seizure frequency in epileptics.
Gastrointestinal: Occasionally: nausea, vomiting, epigastric distress.
Hepatic: Frequently: disturbances of liver function (usually transient). Rarely: hepatitis. Isolated cases: severe hepatitis. The incidence of hepatitis increases with the patient's age.
Blood: Isolated cases: agranulocytosis, eosinophilia, thrombocytopenia, anaemia (haemolytic, hypoplastic).
Allergic and miscellaneous reactions: Occasional: drug rash, fever. Rarely: dryness of the mouth, heartburn, disorders of micturition, rheumatic syndrome, lupus erythematosis-like signs and symptoms, pellagra.

Overdosage
Signs and symptoms: (Rifampicin) Nausea, vomiting, abdominal pain, enlargement of the liver, jaundice, elevated liver enzymes, possible acute pulmonary oedema, lethargy, clouding of consciousness, convulsions. (Isoniazid) In mild poisoning – ataxia, symptoms of polyneuritis, disturbed articulation, vertigo. In severe poisoning – hallucinations, epileptiform tonic-clonic attacks, respiratory depression, coma, severe metabolic acidosis, hyperglycaemia, acetonuria.
Treatment: General supportive measures to maintain vital functions; intravenous administration of anti-convulsants and pyridoxine in large doses; control of metabolic acidosis, gastric lavage together with instillation of an activated charcoal suspension; forced diuresis; haemodialysis, in the presence of severe liver damage, cholecystotomy if necessary.

Pharmaceutical precautions Protect from heat and moisture.

Legal category POM.

Package quantities Rimactazid 150 tablets and Rimactazid 300 tablets in securitainers of 100. Rimactazid 150 tablets blister packs of 84. Rimactazid 300 tablets blister packs of 56.

Further information Rimactane is orally active, very well tolerated and its activity is comparable with that of isoniazid. In combination, these two agents are commonly used as first-line therapy and offer the greatest chance of rapid eradication of the infection. It is usual, however, to employ a third drug during the first two months of treatment or at least until the results of sensitivity tests are known. Continuation therapy with rifampicin and isoniazid has been shown to eradicate the infection in almost all patients faster and with a lower relapse rate than any alternative regime. The combined tablets of Rimactazid thus make the most effective combination simpler to take. The orange-red colour imparted to the urine, sputum and tears by rifampicin is a valuable guide to drug adherence; rifampicin may also permanently discolour soft contact lenses.

Product licence numbers
Rimactazid 150 mg 0008/0121
Rimactazid 300 mg 0008/0120

ROGITINE*

Presentation Clear glass ampoules each containing 10 mg phentolamine mesylate presented as a colourless to pale yellow solution in 1 ml Water for Injection. The ampoules also contain water, sodium metabisulphite and glucose for injection.

Uses
Mode of Action: Acute, severe cardiac insufficiency is often characterised by a high degree of sympathico-adrenergic stimulation which leads to a pronounced increase in the myocardial oxygen requirement. Marked peripheral vasoconstriction and a rise in left-ventricular filling pressure, accompanied by pulmonary congestion or pulmonary oedema, are usually also present.

Rogitine acts directly on vascular smooth muscle, by blocking the alpha-receptors, and by indirectly stimulating the beta-receptors. Rogitine exerts a rapid and potent vasodilator effect which also extends to the venous system. Systemic and pulmonary vascular resistance, as well as left, ventricular filling pressure, are reduced thus reducing the workload of the heart. In addition stroke volume and cardiac output are increased, limiting the fall in blood pressure.

Rogitine has a positive inotropic action but does not unduly increase the heart rate. In addition to the direct haemodynamic effect, Rogitine also stimulates secretion of insulin, which is reduced in the presence of severe cardiac insufficiency; this stimulant action tends to have a favourable influence on myocardial metabolism.

Indications: Acute left ventricular failure (cardiogenic shock) particularly following myocardial infarction.

Paroxysmal hypertension associated with phaeochromocytoma or interaction of foodstuffs with MAOI's; and as prophylactic treatment (in combination with a beta-blocker) before and during surgical removal of phaeochromocytoma.

As a diagnostic agent in cases of suspected phaeochromocytoma.

Pharmacokinetics: Rogitine has a half-life in the blood of 19 minutes following intravenous administration. Approximately 13% of a single intravenous dose appears in the urine as unchanged drug.

Dosage and administration *Adults.*
Cardiogenic Shock: The dosage should be individually adapted to the patient's requirements and will depend on the severity of the cardiac insufficiency and on the blood pressure.

Rogitine should be administered in the form of an intravenous infusion in 5% sterile glucose, saline or dextrose saline solution. A dose of 5–60 mg Rogitine should be given over a period of 10–30 minutes at an infusion rate of 0.2–2 mg per minute. If necessary, especially in cases where the systemic arterial blood pressure is elevated, the infusion rate during the first minute can be raised up to 5 mg per minute.

Systolic blood pressure should be carefully monitored during the infusion and a fall below 100 mm Hg is an indication for reducing the infusion rate (see Precautions).

Depending on the patient's response, the treatment can either be continued for several hours or repeated at intervals.

Paroxysmal hypertension: 5–10 mg intramuscularly or intravenously to be repeated if necessary. When used prior to surgical removal of phaeochromocytoma, administer the injection 2 hours before surgery and repeat if necessary during the operation.
As a diagnostic test for phaeochromocytoma: This test is based upon the fact that Rogitine produces a fall in blood pressure when it is caused by excess circulating adrenaline and/or noradrenaline, so it is of value only in the hypertensive phase.

The initial step in the test is to determine the basal blood pressure of the patient – this is essential for the correct interpretation of the test. An intravenous injection of 5 mg of Rogitine is then administered. As the insertion of the needle may involve a pressor response the blood pressure should be allowed to drop back to within 3 to 4 mm Hg of the basal level before injecting Rogitine.

An immediate marked drop in both systolic and diastolic blood pressure is the typical positive response in patients having a phaeochromocytoma which is discharging adrenaline or noradrenaline at the time of the test. The maximum depressor effect usually occurs within two minutes and usually involves a marked fall in systolic pressure and the fall in diastolic pressure usually exceeds 25 mm Hg. The blood pressure remains low for only a relatively short time and may return to pre-injection levels within 10–15 minutes. Positive results should be confirmed by either estimation of catecholamines in the urine or by another diagnostic procedure. Blood pressure measurements should be made at 30 second intervals for 3 minutes and then at one minute intervals until the baseline reading is reached.

False positive results may be seen in patients with uraemia and those having taken sedatives or narcotics during the 24 hours prior to the test and also false negative results may be seen:

(a) if at the time of injection the tumour is not discharging sufficient adrenaline or noradrenaline to elevate the blood pressure significantly;
(b) when a phaeochromocytoma is present in a patient also having essential hypertension, the test may not cause such a marked fall in blood pressure.

Addditional clinical findings and investigations would usually assist in the interpretation of such results.

The intravenous administration of Rogitine may cause tachycardia in rare instances, weakness, dizziness or flushing.

Children: During surgery for the removal of phaeochromocytoma, the dosage is 1 mg to 5 mg given intravenously according to age.

When performing the diagnostic test for phaeochromocytoma an intravenous injection of 1 mg Rogitine is administered.

Elderly: In elderly patients the possibility of concurrent coronary insufficiency should be considered. In such patients it is advisable to use a low dose or a slow infusion rate, under careful supervision.

Contra-indications, warnings, etc
Contra-indication: Hypotension.

Precautions: Monitoring of the patient's blood pressure, heart rate and clinical condition is necessary not only to ensure correct selection of cases suitable for treatment with Rogitine but also to decide upon the appropriate dosage and duration of parenteral therapy. As a general rule, a systolic blood pressure of 80 mmHg should be regarded as the lowest limit for using the drug.

Use in pregnancy and lactation: There is inadequate evidence of safety to assess the use of Rogitine in human pregnancy. Rogitine should be used during pregnancy only if there are compelling reasons and no safer alternative exists. The potential benefit to the mother must justify the potential risk to the foetus.

It is not known whether Rogitine is excreted in breast milk. Therefore nursing mothers should be advised to discontinue the drug, or cease breast feeding.

Side-effects: When administered in the recommended dosages, Rogitine is generally well tolerated but the following effects may occur.

Central nervous system: Dizziness.

Cardiovascular system: Hypotension (flushing, sweating, feelings of apprehension), tachycardia.

Gastro-intestinal tract: Nausea and diarrhoea have been reported in response to fairly high doses, but they usually subside again following discontinuation of the infusion.

Respiratory tract: Nasal congestion has been reported in response to moderate and high doses but should subside again following discontinuation of the infusion.

Treatment of overdosage

Symptoms: Overdosage with Rogitine is characterised chiefly by cardiovascular disturbances, such as arrhythmias, tachycardia and hypotension. The following effects may also occur: hyperexcitation, headache, sweating, pupillary constriction, visual disturbances, nausea, vomiting, diarrhoea and hypoglycaemia.

Treatment: There is no specific antidote for Rogitine. In the event of overdosage it is normally sufficient to discontinue the infusion. Signs and symptoms usually abate rapidly as Rogitine has a short duration of action. If necessary the effect of Rogitine can be attenuated by giving noradrenaline, and appropriate supportive therapy should be instituted.

Pharmaceutical precautions Protect from heat and light.

Legal category POM.

Package quantities Ampoules each containing 10 mg Rogitine in 1 ml Water for Injection. Boxes of 5.

Further information Nil.

Product licence number 0008/5070.

SCOPODERM TTS*

Presentation Scopoderm TTS is a transdermal drug delivery system consisting of a self-adhesive, pink-coloured system containing a drug reservoir of hyoscine. The average amount of hyoscine absorbed from each system in 72 hours is 500 micrograms. Each system has a contact surface area measuring 2.5 cm^2 and hyoscine content of 1.5 mg.

Uses
Indications: For the prevention of symptoms of motion sickness such as nausea, vomiting and vertigo.

Mode of action: The transdermal therapeutic system (TTS) is a novel form of drug delivery designed to achieve a continuous release of hyoscine through the intact skin to the systemic circulation for up to 72 hours.

Hyoscine has anticholinergic properties. It acts as a competitive antagonist to acetylcholine and other parasympathomimetic agents. Its mechanism of action in the central nervous system in preventing motion sickness has yet to be elucidated. Hyoscine produces classical symptoms of parasympathetic blockade.

Pharmacokinetics: Following Scopoderm TTS administration, measurement of the urinary excretion has shown the equilibrium between absorption and elimination to be reached within about 6 hours. Steady plasma concentrations or hyoscine in the range of 0.17–0.33 nmol/litre are produced. Provided the system is not removed, this equilibrium is maintained and plasma hyoscine levels are within the therapeutic range for up to 72 hours.

After removal of Scopoderm TTS, the plasma concentration diminishes slowly to approximately one third over the following 24 hours because hyoscine in the skin continues to enter the blood stream.

Dosage and administration
Adults: To achieve the optimum protective effect, one system should be applied about 5–6 hours before embarking on a journey (or on the evening before). The system should be placed onto a clean, dry, hairless area of skin behind the ear, taking care to avoid any cuts or irritation. One system can provide protection for up to 72 hours. Should protection be required for longer periods of time, a fresh system should be placed behind the other ear after 72 hours (no more than one system should be used at a time). Conversely, if protection is only required for shorter periods of time, the system should be removed at the end of the journey.

Patients should wash their hands thoroughly after handling the system. In addition, after removal of the system, the site of application should also be washed. These precautions are necessary to minimise any chance of hyoscine accidentally being transferred to the eyes (see 'Side-effects').

Limited contact with water (i.e. during bathing or

swimming) should not affect the system, although it should be kept as dry as possible.

If the Scopoderm TTS becomes accidentally detached, it should be replaced by a fresh system.

Use in elderly: Scopoderm TTS may be used in the elderly (see dosage recommendations for adults) although the elderly may be more prone to suffer from the side-effects of hyoscine (see 'Precautions').

Use in children: Scopoderm TTS can be used in children aged 10 years or over (see dosage recommendations for adults). Insufficient data are available to recommend the use of Scopoderm TTS for younger children.

Contra-indications, warnings, etc

Contra-indications: Scopoderm TTS is contra-indicated in patients with glaucoma or with a history of the condition, and in patients with known hypersensitivity to hyoscine.

Warnings: Scopoderm TTS may cause drowsiness, dizziness, confusion or visual disturbance in certain individuals. Patients using the system must not drive, operate machinery, pilot an aircraft, dive or engage in any other activities in which such symptoms could be dangerous (see 'Side-effects').

Care should be taken after removal of the system, as side-effects may persist for up to 24 hours or longer.

Patients should not consume alcohol whilst using Scopoderm TTS.

Precautions: Scopoderm TTS should be used with caution in patients with pyloric stenosis, those who have bladder outflow obstruction, or in patients with intestinal obstruction.

Scopoderm TTS should also be used with caution in elderly patients, and in patients with impaired hepatic or renal function.

In rare cases, confusional states and visual hallucinations may occur. In such cases, Scopoderm TTS should be removed immediately. If severe symptoms persist, appropriate therapeutic measures should be taken (see 'Overdosage' section).

Idiosyncratic reactions may occur with ordinary therapeutic doses of hyoscine.

In isolated cases an increase in seizure frequency in epileptic patients has been reported.

Use in pregnancy and lactation: Teratogenic studies have been performed in pregnant rats and rabbits with hyoscine administered by daily intravenous injection. No adverse effects were noted in rats. In rabbits, the drug had a marginal embryotoxic effect at a high dose (at drug plasma levels approximately 100 times those observed in humans using Scopoderm TTS).

Scopoderm TTS should only be used during pregnancy if the expected benefits to the mother outweigh the potential risks to the foetus.

It is not known if hyoscine passes into the breast milk. Therefore nursing mothers should refrain from breast-feeding their infants whilst using Scopoderm TTS.

Drug interactions: Scopoderm TTS should be used with caution in patients being treated with drugs that act on the central nervous system (including alcohol) or drugs with anticholinergic properties.

Side-effects: The following side-effects may occur:

Eyes: In isolated cases pupillary dilatation may precipitate acute glaucoma, particularly narrow angle glaucoma (see 'Contra-indications').

Occasional: irritation of the eyelids. If traces of hyoscine on the hands enter the eyes, transient cycloplegia and pupillary dilatation (occasionally unilateral) frequently occur.

Mouth: Frequent: transient dryness of the mouth.

Central nervous system: Occasional: drowsiness.

Rare: impairment of memory and concentration, restlessness, dizziness, disorientation, confusion and visual hallucination (see 'Precautions').

Skin: Occasional: local irritation.

In isolated cases: a generalised skin rash.

Urogenital system: Rare: disturbances of micturition (i.e. urine retention).

Side-effects after removal of Scopoderm TTS: Rare: unwanted effects, including headache and disturbance of balance occurring after removal of the system. In such cases, patients shoud not drive or engage in other activities requiring concentration (see 'Warnings').

Overdosage

Symptoms: Initially, restlessness, excitation and confusion may be observed. Higher doses may provoke delirium, hallucinations and convulsions. At very high doses, coma and respiratory paralysis may occur.

Treatment: If symptoms of overdosage occur, the system(s) should be removed immediately. Physostigmine is the most effective antidote. Depending on the severity of poisoning, physostigmine should be given by slow intravenous injection in doses of 1–4 mg (0.5 mg in children). Repeated injections may be necessary since physostigmine is rapidly metabolised. Diazepam may be used to counter excitation and convulsions, although at higher doses it may cause respiratory depression. In severe cases, artificial respiration may be necessary.

If hyperthermia occurs, immediate action should be taken to dissipate heat.

Pharmaceutical precautions Store below 25°C. Do not freeze.

Legal category POM.

Package quantities Cartons containing 2 Scopoderm TTS systems, each individually sealed in a protective pouch (OP).

Further information Scopoderm TTS contains hyoscine, which is a potent anticholinergic agent.

Instructions for use: Tear open the pouch and remove the system. Peel off the transparent hexagonal protective foil, taking care not to touch the silver adhesive side. Press the system (silver adhesive side downwards) firmly onto a clean, dry area of skin behind the ear. Undue pressure should not be applied to the system. Once the system has been fixed in place, it should not be touched again until it is necessary to remove it. Wash hands after applying or removing the system. The system should be disposed of carefully and out of the reach of children.

Product licence number 0001/0099.

SLOW-FE*

Presentation A circular, biconvex, yellowish-white tablet, impressed with the letters CG 503 on one side and plain on the other side. The tablets have a thin, transparent film coat and contain 160 mg of dried ferrous sulphate in a special slow-release wax core (equivalent to 50 mg elemental iron).

The tablets also contain lactose.

Uses As a haematinic for the treatment of, or prophylaxis of iron deficiency anaemia, including that associated with post-gastrectomy and other malabsorption syndromes.

Dosage and administration The preparation is intended for oral administration.

Adults: For prophylaxis, one tablet daily. For the treatment of iron deficiency anaemia, two tablets only.

Children: For treatment, one tablet daily for children over the age of six years.

The tablets should be swallowed whole with fluid and may be taken at any time of the day.

Contra-indications, warnings, etc

Contra-indications: Known hypersensitivity to ferrous sulphate. Iron therapy is contra-indicated in the presence of haemochromatosis, haemosiderosis and haemolytic anaemia.

Precautions: As with all iron preparations, Slow-Fe should be used with care in patients with known or suspected gastro-intestinal strictures or diverticulae.

Use in pregnancy and lactation: Slow Fe can be used in the iron deficiency anaemia of pregnancy, with or without additional folic acid as appropriate.

Interactions: Concurrent administration of antacids may

reduce absorption of iron preparations. Iron chelates with tetracyclines and absorption of both agents may be impaired. Iron may reduce the absorption of penicillamine and zinc salts.

Side-effects: As with all iron containing preparations gastro-intestinal side effects such as abdominal discomfort, nausea, vomiting, constipation, diarrhoea and dark stools may occur.

Overdosage

Symptoms: Abdominal pain, nausea and vomiting, diarrhoea and haematemesis.

Treatment: Gastric lavage or emesis should be carried out immediately. To chelate excess free iron in the gastro-intestinal tract, 5 g desferrioxamine dissolved in 50 ml water should be introduced into the stomach. To chelate excess free iron in the blood, desferrioxamine may be given parenterally; depending on the patients condition, 1 g desferrioxamine given every three hours intramuscularly may be appropriate.

Pharmaceutical precautions Tablets should be protected from heat and moisture.

Legal category P.

Package quantities Blister packs of 150 tablets.

Further information The precision release principle of Slow-Fe ensures that the iron is released evenly over a period of 1 to 2 hours. Complete release therefore occurs before the tablet has left the duodenum or upper jejunum, and maximum iron absorption can take place.

The incidence of side effects would appear to be lower than with plain ferrous sulphate.

Product licence number 0008/5040R.

SLOW-FE FOLIC*

Presentation A circular biconvex yellowish-white tablet impressed with the monogram CIBA on one side and the letters TP on the other. The tablets have a thin transparent film-coat and contain dried ferrous sulphate 160 mg (equivalent to 50 mg elemental iron) in a special slow-release core and folic acid 0.4 mg.

These tablets also contain lactose.

Uses Slow-Fe Folic is indicated during the second and third trimesters of pregnancy for prophylaxis of iron and folic acid deficiency. Slow-Fe folic is designed to minimise the problems of gastro-intestinal disturbances associated with most oral iron preparations, and contains 0.4 mg of folic acid, a daily supplement which prevents the occurrence of megaloblastic anaemia due to folate deficiency.

Dosage and administration The product is intended for oral administration, one tablet to be taken daily throughout pregnancy. In the case of a multiple pregnancy, the dosage should be increased to two tablets daily. The tablets should be swallowed whole and for preference taken after food.

Contra-indications, warnings, etc

Contra-indications: Iron therapy is contra-indicated in the presence of haemochromatosis, haemosiderosis and haemolytic anaemia.

Side-effects: Slow-Fe Folic is particularly well tolerated although gastro-intestinal side effects such as nausea, vomiting, constipation or diarrhoea may occur infrequently. On very rare occasions, skin rashes have been reported.

Precautions: Concurrent administration of antacids may reduce absorption of iron preparations. Iron chelates with tetracyclines and absorption of both agents may be impaired.

Iron may reduce the absorption of penicillamine and zinc salts. In epileptic patients who have become folate deficient (for instance during phenytoin treatment) folic acid supplementation can result in decreased anticonvulant serum concentrations, which (unless the anticonvulsant dosage is adjusted), can lead to loss of seizure control.

Overdosage

Symptoms: Symptoms include abdominal pain, nausea and vomiting, diarrhoea and haematemesis.

Treatment: Gastric lavage or emesis should be carried out immediately. To chelate excess free iron in the gastro-intestinal tract, 5 g desferrioxamine dissolved in 50 ml water should be introduced into the stomach. To chelate excess free iron in the blood desferrioxamine may be given parenterally; depending on the patients condition, 1 g desferrioxamine given every 3 hours intramuscularly may be appropriate.

Pharmaceutical precautions Tablets should be protected from heat and moisture.

Legal category POM.

Package quantities Slow-Fe folic tablets are available form-packed in quantities of 150.

Further information The precision-release principle of Slow-Fe folic ensures that the iron is released evenly over a period of 1½ to 2 hours. Complete release therefore occurs before the tablet has left the duodenum or upper jejunum, and maximum iron absorption can take place. This avoids wastage, and associated side effects, whilst producing an effective haematinic response from a relatively low dose of iron.

The incidence of side effects is comparable with placebo levels and considerably lower than with plain ferrous sulphate.

Product licence number 0008/5041

SLOW-K*

Presentation Pale orange, polished, sugar-coated tablets about 12 mm in diameter, printed with the name Slow-K, containing 600 mg (8.06 mmol) of Potassium Chloride BP.

The tablets also contain sucrose.

Uses

Mode of action: The potassium chloride in Slow-K is finely distributed in a neutral wax base, from which it is gradually released over a period of 3–6 hours during its passage through the digestive tract. This special form of potassium substitution therapy is designed to avoid high localised concentrations of potassium chloride which might irritate or damage the mucosa. The potassium chloride present in Slow-K is completely absorbed in the intestinal tract.

Indications: Slow-K is indicated for the correction and/or prevention of hypokalaemia in those patients who cannot tolerate and/or refuse to take liquid or effervescent potassium chloride, or when there is a problem of compliance with these preparations.

Dosage and administration It is important that the tablets should be swallowed whole, with fluid during meals, whilst the patient is sitting upright.

Adults: The dosage of Slow-K should be adapted to the cause, degree and duration of potassium depletion. 2–6 tablets are usually an adequate supplement. In states of severe potassium deficiency, a higher dose of 9–12 tablets daily may be needed. If the dosage exceeds 16 mmol K^+ (2 tablets) it should be taken in divided doses. Where intermittent diuretic therapy is being used, it is advisable to give Slow-K on intervening days between administration of the diuretic. The response to treatment should preferably be monitored by repeat determination of plasma potassium and Slow-K continued until the hypokalaemia has been corrected.

Children: Not recommended.

Use in the elderly: No special dosage adjustment is usually necessary, but concurrent renal insufficiency should be taken into account (also see 'Precautions').

Contra-indications, warnings, etc

Side-effects: Side-effects are rare with Slow-K, as any excess potassium is rapidly excreted in the urine.

Gastro-intestinal tract: In rare cases, oral potassium preparations may provoke gastro-intestinal disturbances (nausea, vomiting, abdominal pains, diarrhoea) necessitating either a reduction in dosage or withdrawal of medication (see Precautions).

In isolated cases; obstruction, bleeding and ulceration, with or without perforation of the upper or lower GIT, have been reported, usually associated with other factors known to predispose a patient to these effects (eg delayed GIT transit time, obstruction of GIT).

Skin: Rare: Pruritis and/or skin rash, urticaria.

Electrolytes: Hyperkalaemia may develop in patients having difficulty with either renal potassium excretion or potassium metabolism.

Contra-indications: Hypersensitivity to potassium administration eg hyperkalaemic periodic paralysis, congenital paramyotonia. Marked renal failure (even when not yet associated with manifest hyperkalaemia), untreated Addison's disease, hyporeninaemic hypoaldosteronism, acute dehydration, hyperkalaemia and conditions involving extensive cell destruction (eg severe burns).

All solid forms of potassium medication are contraindicated in the presence of obstructions in the digestive tract (e.g. resulting from compression of the oesophagus due to dilation of the left atrium or from stenosis of the gut).

In cases of metabolic acidosis, the hypokalaemia should be treated not with potassium chloride but with an alkaline potassium salt (e.g. potassium bicarbonate). Concomitant treatment with potassium sparing diuretics (eg spironolactone, triamterene, amiloride).

Precautions: If a patient under treatment with Slow-K develops severe vomiting, severe abdominal pains or flatulence, or gastro-intestinal haemorrhage, the preparation should be withdrawn at once, because in the presence of an obstruction it could conceivably give rise to ulceration or perforation.

Oral potassium preparations should be prescribed with particular caution in patients with a history of peptic ulcer.

Caution should be exercised when prescribing solid oral potassium preparations, particularly in high dosage, in patients concurrently receiving anticholinergics because of their potential to slow gastro-intestinal motility.

Patients with ostomies may have altered intestinal transit times and are better treated with other forms of potassium salts.

In patients suffering from impaired renal function, special care should be exercised when prescribing potassium salts owing to the risk of their producing hyperkalaemia. Monitoring of the serum electrolytes is particularly necessary in patients with diseases of the heart or kidneys.

In some patients diuretic induced magnesium deficiency will prevent restoration of intracellular deficits of potassium so that hypomagnesaemia should be corrected at the same time as hypokalaemia.

Drug interactions: Combined treatment with the following increase the risk of hyperkalaemia: Angiotensin-converting enzyme inhibitors, cyclosporin, NSAIDs, beta blockers, heparin, digoxin, potassium sparing diuretics (see 'Contra-indications').

Use in pregnancy: As a general rule, no drugs should be taken during the first three months of pregnancy and the risks and benefits of taking drugs should be carefully considered throughout pregnancy.

Because of gastrointestinal hypomotility associated with pregnancy, solid forms of oral potassium preparations should be given to pregnant women only if clearly needed.

The normal K^+ content of human milk is about 13 mmol/litre. Since oral potassium becomes part of the body's potassium pool, provided this is not excessive, Slow K can be expected to have little or no effect on the potassium level in human milk.

Overdosage

Signs and symptoms: Mainly cardiovascular (hypotension, shock, ventricular arrhythmias, bundle-branch block, ventricular fibrillation leading possibly to cardiac arrest) and neuromuscular (paraesthesiae, convulsions, areflexia, flaccid paralysis of striated muscle leading possibly to respiratory paralysis). Beside elevation of serum potassium concentration, typical ECG changes are also encountered (increasing amplitude and peaking of T waves, disappearance of P wave, widening of QRS complex and S-T depression).

Treatment: Gastric lavage, administration of cation-exchange agents, infusion of glucose and insulin, forced diuresis and possibly peritoneal dialysis or haemodialysis.

Pharmaceutical precautions Slow-K tablets should be protected from heat and moisture. The tablets should be dispensed in moisture-proof containers.

Legal category P.

Package quantities Slow-K Tablets (600 mg Potassium Chloride BP in a special slow-release core, equivalent to 8.06 mmol K^+) Securitainers of 500, and containers of 5000.

Further information Slow-K has been successfully used in those patients who cannot tolerate liquid potassium chloride preparations or who find their taste unacceptable.

Product licence number 0008/5039.

SLOW SODIUM*

Presentation White, biconvex, polished, coated tablets about 11.4 mm in diameter, printed "CIBA" on one side, containing 600 mg (10 mmol) of Sodium Chloride BP.

Uses *Mode of action:* Slow Sodium tablets release sodium chloride gradually from a special sustained release formulation, maximum plasma concentrations occurring 4–6 hours after administration. This method of delivery is designed to avoid high localised concentrations of sodium chloride which might irritate or damage the gut mucosa. The sodium chloride present in Slow Sodium is completely absorbed in the G.I. tract.

Indications: For the treatment and prophylaxis of sodium chloride deficiency.

Dosage and administration It is important that the tablets should be swallowed whole with water (approx. 70 ml per tablet where kidney function is normal to avoid hypernatraemia), and not chewed.

Adults: For prophylaxis 4–8 tablets per day. For treatment dosage to be adjusted to individual needs up to a maximum of 20 tablets per day in cases of severe salt depletion.

For control of muscle cramps during routine maintenance haemodialysis usually 10–16 tablets per dialysis. In cases of chronic renal salt-wasting up to 20 tablets per day may be required with appropriate fluid intake.

Children: Dosage should be adjusted to individual needs.

Use in the elderly: No special dosage adjustment.

Contra-indications, warnings, etc

Contra-indications: Slow Sodium is contra-indicated in any situation where salt retention is undesirable, such as oedema, heart disease, cardiac decompensation and primary or secondary aldosteronism; or where therapy is being given to produce salt and water loss.

Side-effects: No side-effects have been reported with Slow Sodium at the recommended dosage.

Precautions: Use of Slow Sodium without adequate water supplementation can produce hypernatraemia. The matrix (ghost) is often eliminated intact and owing to the risk of obstruction Slow Sodium should not be given to patients suffering from Crohn's disease or any other intestinal condition where strictures or diverticula may form.

Interactions: In hypertensive patients with chronic renal failure Slow Sodium may tend to impair the efficacy of antihypertensive drugs.

Use in pregnancy: No additional precautions required.

Overdosage: Excessive intake of sodium chloride can result in hypernatraemia. Symptoms of hypernatraemia include restlessness, weakness, thirst, reduced salivation and lacrymation, swollen tongue, flushing of the skin, pyrexia, dizziness, headache, oliguria, hypertension, tachycardia, delerium, hyperpnoea and respiratory arrest.

Treatment requires the use of sodium-free liquids and the cessation of excessive sodium intake. In the event of a significant overdose serum sodium levels should be evaluated as soon as possible and appropriate steps taken to correct any abnormalities. The use of a loop diuretic eg frusemide (with potassium supplementation as required) may be appropriate in severe cases of hypernatraemia. Levels should be monitored until they return to normal.

Pharmaceutical precautions Protect from heat and moisture. The tablets should be dispensed in moisture proof containers.

Legal category GSL.

Package quantities The tablets are available as a pack size of 500, consisting of five Securitainers of 100 tablets.

Further information Slow Sodium has been successfully used by those patients unable to tolerate sodium chloride in capsules, compressed salt tablets or saline solution.

Product licence number 0008/0101R.

SLOW-TRASICOR*

Presentation Slow-Trasicor tablets each containing 160 mg Oxprenolol Hydrochloride BP in a special sustained-release formulation. Circular, slightly bi-convex, white film-coated tablets, having the monogram CIBA impressed on one side and Slow-Trasicor on the other.

The tablets also contain lactose.

Uses *Mode of action:* Slow-Trasicor tablets release oxprenolol hydrochloride (a non-selective beta-adrenergic receptor blocking drug with intrinsic sympathomimetic activity) gradually from a special sustained release formulation, thus prolonging the pharmacological action.

Indications: Hypertension: All grades of hypertension in once-daily dosage. The concomitant use of a thiazide diuretic will enhance the antihypertensive effect of Slow-Trasicor, resulting in better control from reduced dosage.

Angina pectoris: For continuous prophylaxis in once-daily dosage to improve exercise tolerance and reduce the frequency and severity of anginal attacks.

Dosage and administration Slow-Trasicor tablets release oxprenolol gradually from a special sustained-release formulation. This provides a considerably longer pharmacological action from a given dose, thus allowing once-daily dosage.

Adults: Hypertension: Initially one tablet daily, given in the morning. If necessary, this dose can be raised to two or more tablets, usually given once daily until satisfactory blood pressure control is achieved. However, when used as monotherapy, dosage should not exceed 3 tablets daily, i.e. 480 mg Slow-Trasicor, since experience has shown that hardly any increase in the response can be achieved by this means. Usually, patients respond to a dose of one or two tablets of Slow-Trasicor in combination with a diuretic and most of the antihypertensive effect is achieved within 2–3 days.

Angina pectoris: Initially one tablet daily, given in the morning. This can be increased to two or three tablets, usually given once daily depending on patient response. An evening dose may be beneficial in nocturnal angina. Increased dosage is related to increased exercise tolerance, but doses higher than three tablets should not normally be required.

Use in the elderly: No special dosage regime is necessary but concurrent hepatic insufficiency should be taken into account.

Children: The administration of Slow-Trasicor to children is not recommended.

Contra-indications, warnings, etc

Side-effects: Slow-Trasicor is well tolerated. However, dizziness, drowsiness, headache, insomnia, excitement, dry mouth, disturbances of vision, keratoconjunctivitis, loss of libido and gastro-intestinal disturbance may occur particularly at the start of treatment. Isolated cases of excessive bradycardia hypotension, A-V conduction disorders and thrombocytopenia, have been reported. As with other beta-blockers, bronchospasm and heart failure may occasionally be precipitated in susceptible patients (see Precautions) and exertional tiredness and feelings of coldness in the extremities have been reported on rare occasions. However, the incidence of these side-effects is low.

Slow-Trasicor possess antihypertensive effects but these are unlikely to be noted in normotensive subjects.

There have been reports of skin rashes and/or dry eyes associated with the use of beta-adrenergic blocking drugs. The reported incidence is small, and in most cases the symptoms have cleared when the treatment was withdrawn. Discontinuance of the drug should be considered if any such reaction is not otherwise explicable. Cessation of therapy with a beta-adrenergic blocker should be gradual.

Contra-indications: Slow-Trasicor is contra-indicated in patients with second or third degree atrio-ventricular block, marked bradycardia, uncontrolled heart failure, cardiogenic shock, hypersensitivity to oxprenolol and related derivatives, sick-sinus syndrome, bronchial asthma and anaesthesia with chloroform or ether.

Precautions: As with other beta-blockers, when discontinuing treatment with oxprenolol the drug should be withdrawn gradually, because abrupt interruption of the medication, particularly in cases of ischaemic heart disease, may lead to an acute deterioration in the patients condition.

If there is evidence of cardiac failure, this must be controlled by digitalis and/or diuretics before and during Slow Trasicor therapy.

Should the pulse rate fall before 50 per minute, then treatment should be withdrawn and restarted at a lower dose.

Caution should be observed when treating patients with chronic bronchitis, emphysema as well as in those with a case history of asthmatic disorders. Additional treatment with a beta-2-stimulant may be necessary; alternatively the dosage of bronchodilator medication may need to be readjusted when starting treatment with Trasicor.

In rare cases, a pre-existing A-V conduction disorder of moderate degree may become aggravated (possibly leading to A-V block). As a rule, no worsening of peripheral conduction disorders (left and/or right bundle branch block) occurs.

Treatment with a beta-blocker is liable to mask the symptoms of hypoglycaemia and also to affect carbohydrate metabolism. In patients with labile or insulin-dependent diabetes in particular, it may therefore be necessary to readjust the dosage of anti-diabetic medication. In patients who have been fasting for any length of time, hypoglycaemia may be increased or its symptoms masked.

Beta-blockers may mask the signs and symptoms of a thyrotoxic crisis.

Beta-blockers may aggravate the signs and symptoms of peripheral vascular disorders (Raynaud's disease).

In patients with phaeochromocytoma a beta-blocker should only be given together with an alpha-blocker.

Beta-blockers may diminish liver function and thus effect the metabolism of other drugs. In the presence of liver cirrhosis, the bioavailability of oxprenolol may be increased. No major alteration in its bioavailability is likely to occur in patients with compensated renal failure.

Depending on the individual concerned, beta-blockers may adversely affect the patients reactions as a road user or as an operator of machinery, particularly if he also consumes alcohol.

Pregnancy and Lactation: Beta-blockers may cause bradycardia in the foetus which can also persist after birth. During pregnancy, in the course of labour and during lactation beta-blockers should only be employed after the needs of the mother have been weighed against the possible risks to the foetus or infant.

Treatment of overdosage: Overdosage with Slow-Trasicor may lead to excessive bradycardia, hypotension, heart failure, cardiogenic shock or even cardiac arrest. In addition dyspnoea, bronchospasm, vomiting, impairment of consciousness and also generalised convulsions may occur. It should also be noted that severe toxicity may develop rapidly and that there may be severe hypotension and bradycardia despite a normal ECG. For sinus bradycardia and hypotension 0.5–2.0 mg of atropine should be slowly administered by intravenous infusion. If this does not raise the heart rate sufficiently isoprenaline hydrochloride may be necessary. The dose of isoprenaline needs to be sufficient to reverse the blockade and should be assessed by the clinical response. A reasonable starting dose would be 25 mcg of isoprenaline hydrochloride.

In severe cardiogenic shock the treatment of choice appears to be glucagon. The initial dose should be 5–10 mg intravenously, further boluses or an infusion can be used according to the patient's condition. Transvenous pacing has been used, sometimes with success. If bronchospasm develops bronchodilators should be used. Patients should be monitored for several days as the beta-blocking effects of Slow-Trasicor exceed its plasma half-life.

Pharmaceutical precautions The tablets have no special storage requirements.

Legal category POM.

Package quantities Cartons of 28 Slow-Trasicor Tablets consisting of two reminder calendar foils of 14. (Each carton of 28 represents 2–4 weeks' treatment, depending on whether dosage is one or two tablets daily) (OP).

Further information Slow-Trasicor is a sustained release preparation specifically designed to release oxprenolol over an extended period, resulting in a prolonged pharmacological action, and the elimination of high peak plasma concentrations.

Product licence number 0008/0130.

SYNACTHEN*

Presentation Tetracosactrin Acetate β^{1-24} corticotrophin (Tetracosactide INN) BP as a clear, colourless, sterile solution containing the equivalent of 250 micrograms of tetracosactrin per ml. This preparation is available in 1 ml ampoules.

The ampoules contain acetic acid, sodium acetate, sodium chloride and water.

Uses
Mode of action: Tetracosactrin, the active substance of Synacthen consists of the first 24 amino acids occurring in the natural corticotrophic hormone (ACTH) sequence and displays the same physiological properties as ACTH. In the adrenal cortex, it stimulates the biosynthesis of glucocorticoids, mineralocorticoids and, to a lesser extent, androgens.

Indications: As a diagnostic test for the investigation of adrenocortical insufficiency.

Pharmacokinetics: Tetracosactrin has an apparent volume of distribution of approximately 0.4 litres/kg.

Following an intravenous injection, elimination of the compound from the plasma consists of 3 phases. The half-lives of these phases are approximately 7 minutes (0–1 hour), 37 minutes (1–2 hours) and 3 hours thereafter. In the serum, tetracosactrin is broken down by serum endopeptidases into inactive oligopeptides and then by aminopeptidases into free amino acids. The rapid elimination from plasma is probably not attributable to this relatively slow cleavage process, but rather to the rapid concentration of the active substance in the adrenal glands and kidneys. Following an intravenous dose of ^{131}I-labelled tetracosactrin, 95–100% of the radioactivity is excreted in the urine within 24 hours.

Dosage and administration This preparation of Synacthen is intended for administration for diagnostic purposes only as a single intramuscular or intravenous dose; it is not to be used for repeated therapeutic administration.

The 30-minute Synacthen diagnostic test: This test is based on measurement of the plasma cortisol concentration immediately before and exactly 30 minutes after an intramuscular or intravenous injection of 250 micrograms (1 ml) Synacthen. Adrenocortical function can be regarded as normal if the post-injection rise in plasma cortisol concentration amounts to at least 200 nmol/litre (70 micrograms/litre).

Where the 30-minute test has yielded inconclusive results, or where it is desired to determine the functional reserve of the adrenal cortex, a 5-hour test can be performed with Synacthen Depot (see separate data sheet). Furthermore, a three-day test with Synacthen Depot may be used to differentiate between primary and secondary adrenocortical insufficiency.

Use in the elderly: There is no evidence to suggest that dosage should be different in the elderly.

Use in children: An intravenous dose of 250 micrograms/1.73 m^2 body surface area has been suggested. Thus for children aged 5–7 years, approximately half the adult dose will be adequate. For more accurate dosing of other ages, standard body surface area tables should be consulted.

Use in pregnancy: The Synacthen test should not be utilised during pregnancy unless there are compelling reasons for doing so.

Contra-indications, warnings, etc
Contra-indications: History of hypersensitivity to ACTH, Synacthen or Synacthen Depot. Synacthen is contra-indicated in patients with allergic disorders (e.g. asthma).

Precautions: Before using Synacthen, the doctor should make every effort to find out whether the patient is suffering from, or has a history of allergic disorders (see 'Contra-indications'). In particular, he should enquire whether the patient has previously experienced adverse reactions to ACTH, Synacthen or other drugs.

Synacthen should only be administered under the supervision of appropriate senior hospital medical staff (e.g. consultants).

If local or systemic hypersensitivity reactions occur after the injection (for example, marked redness and pain at the injection site, urticaria, pruritis, flushing, faintness or dyspnoea), Synacthen or other ACTH preparations should be avoided in the future. Hypersensitivity reactions tend to occur within 30 minutes of an injection. The patient should therefore be kept under observation during this time.

Preparation should be made in advance to combat any anaphylactic reaction that may occur after an injection of Synacthen. In the event of a serious anaphylactic reaction occurring, despite these precautions, the following measures must be taken immediately: administer adrenaline (0.4–1 ml of a 0.1% solution intramuscularly or 0.1–0.2 ml of a 0.1% solution in 10 ml physiological saline *slowly* intravenously) as well as a large intravenous dose of a corticosteroid (for example 1–2 g prednisolone as prednisolone Sodium Phosphate BP) repeating the dose if necessary.

Side-effects: Synacthen may provoke hypersensitivity reactions, which in patients suffering from, or susceptible to, allergic disorders (especially asthma) may take the form of anaphylactic shock (see 'Contra-indications').

Treatment of overdosage: Overdosage is unlikely to be a problem.

Pharmaceutical precautions Synacthen should be protected from light and stored in a refrigerator (2–8°C).

Legal category POM.

Package quantities Synacthen ampoules 250 micrograms per ml in boxes of 5.

Further information Nil.

Product licence number 0008/0034.

SYNACTHEN* DEPOT

Presentation Tetracosactrin Acetate (β^{1-24} corticotrophin) BP is absorbed on to zinc phosphate. A sterile, white suspension, which settles on standing, containing 1 mg of tetracosactrin acetate per ml and 10 mg benzyl alcohol per ml. This preparation is available in 1 ml ampoules and 2 ml multi-dose vials.

The ampoules contain zinc, sodium phosphate, benzyl alcohol, sodium chloride, sodium hydroxide and water.

Uses

Mode of action: Tetracosactrin, the active substance of Synacthen consists of the first 24 amino acids occurring in the natural corticotrophic hormone (ACTH) sequence and displays the same physiological properties as ACTH. In the adrenal cortex, it stimulates the biosynthesis of glucocorticoids, mineralocorticoids and, to a lesser extent, androgens.

Indications: Therapeutic use: Synacthen Depot should normally only be used for short-term therapy in conditions for which glucocorticoids are indicated in principal, for example, in ulcerative colitis and Crohn's disease, juvenile rheumatoid arthritis, or as adjunct therapy in patients with rheumatoid arthritis and osteoarthrosis. Synacthen Depot may be particularly useful in patients unable to tolerate oral glucocorticoid therapy or in patients where normal therapeutic doses of glucocorticoids have been ineffective.

Diagnostic use: As a diagnostic aid for the investigation of adrenocortical insufficiency.

Pharmacokinetics: Tetracosactrin is absorbed on to a zinc phosphate complex which ensures the sustained release of the active substance from the intramuscular injection site. After an intramuscular injection of 1 mg Synacthen Depot, plasma cortisol levels remain elevated for 24–32 hours. After 12 hours, plasma levels of tetracosactrin are between 200–300 pg/ml.

Tetracosactrin has an apparent volume of distribution of approximately 0.4 litres/kg.

In the serum, tetracosactrin is broken down by serum endopeptidases into inactive oligopeptides and then by aminopeptidases into free amino acids.

Following an intravenous dose of ^{131}I-labelled tetracosactrin, 95–100% of the radioactivity is excreted in the urine within 24 hours.

Dosage and administration Synacthen Depot is intended for intramuscular injection. The ampoule should be shaken before use.

Therapeutic use: Initially, daily doses of Synacthen Depot should be given but after approximately 3 days, intermittent doses may be given.

Adults: Initially 1 mg intramuscularly daily or 1 mg every 12 hours in acute cases. After the acute symptoms of the disease have disappeared, treatment may be continued at a dose of 1 mg every 2–3 days; in patients who respond well, the dosage may be reduced to 0.5 mg every 2–3 days or 1 mg per week.

Infants aged 1 month–2 years: Initially 0.25 mg intramuscularly daily; the maintenance dose is 0.25 mg every 2–8 days.

Children aged 2–5 years: Initially 0.25–0.5 mg intramuscularly daily; the maintenance dose is 0.25–0.5 mg every 2–8 days.

Children aged 5–12 years: Initially 0.25–1 mg intramuscularly daily; the maintenance dose is 0.25–1 mg every 2–8 days.

Elderly: There is no evidence to suggest that dosage should be different in the elderly.

Diagnostic use: In cases of suspected adrenocortical insufficiency, where the 30 minute diagnostic test with Synacthen ampoules (see Synacthen data sheet) has yielded inconclusive results or where it is desired to determine the functional reserve of the adrenal cortex, a 5-hour test with Synacthen Depot may be performed.

Adults: This test is based on measurement of the plasma cortisol concentration before and exactly 30 minutes, 1, 2, 3, 4 and 5 hours after an intramuscular injection of 1 mg Synacthen Depot. Adrenocortical function can be regarded as normal if the post-injection rise in plasma cortisol concentration increases 2-fold in the first hour, and continues to rise steadily. The values expected would be 600–1,250 nmol/l in the first hour increasing slowly up to 1,000–1,800 nmol/l by the fifth hour. Lower concentrations of plasma cortisol may be attributable to Addison's disease, secondary adrenocortical insufficiency due to a disorder of hypothalamo-pituitary function or overdosage of corticosteroids.

A 3-day test with Synacthen Depot may be used to differentiate between primary and secondary adrenocortical insufficiency.

Children: No paediatric dosage has been established.

Elderly: There is no evidence to suggest that dosage should be different in the elderly.

Use in pregnancy: Synacthen Depot is contra-indicated during pregnancy and should not be used unless there are compelling reasons for doing so.

Contra-indications, warnings, etc

Contra-indications: History of hypersensitivity to ACTH, Synacthen or Synacthen Depot. Synacthen Depot therapy is also contra-indicated in acute psychoses, in infectious diseases, in Cushing's syndrome, in patients with peptic ulcer, refractory heart failure, adrenogenital syndrome and for therapeutic use in adrenocortical insufficiency.

In view of the increased risk of anaphylactic reactions, Synacthen Depot should not be used for the treatment of asthma or other allergic disorders.

Synacthen Depot is contra-indicated for use in neonates (especially premature infants) since it contains benzyl alcohol which can cause severe poisoning.

Synacthen Depot must not be administered intravenously.

Warnings: Synacthen Depot should only be used in patients who, in addition to the disease being treated, are suffering from, or have a history of allergic disorders (especially asthma) if other therapeutic treatment has failed and if the severity of the condition warrants such treatment.

Precautions: Before using Synacthen Depot, the doctor should make every effort to find out whether the patient is suffering from, or has a history of allergic disorders. In particular, he should enquire whether the patient has previously experienced adverse reactions to ACTH, Synacthen Depot or other drugs.

Synacthen Depot should only be administered under medical supervision.

If local or systemic hypersensitivity reactions occur during or after an injection (for example, marked redness and pain at the injection site, urticaria, pruritus, flushing, faintness or dyspnoea), Synacthen Depot or other ACTH preparations should be avoided in the future. Hypersensitivity reactions tend to occur within 30 minutes of the injection. The patient should therefore be kept under observation during this time.

In the event of a serious anaphylactic reaction occurring, despite these precautions, the following measures must be taken immediately: administer adrenaline (0.4–1 ml of a 0.1% solution intramuscularly or 0.1–0.2 ml of a 0.1% solution in 10 ml physiological saline *slowly* intravenously) as well as a large intravenous dose of a corticosteroid (for example 1–2 g prednisolone as Prednisolone Sodium Phosphate BP) repeating the dose if necessary.

Salt and water retention caused by Synacthen Depot can often be avoided or eliminated by prescribing a low-salt diet. Potassium supplements may be required if prolonged treatment is necessary.

Patients receiving concomitant medication for diabetes mellitus or moderate to severe hypertension are likely to need their dosage regimen adjusted when treatment with Synacthen Depot is instituted.

Provided the dose is chosen to meet the individual's needs, Synacthen Depot is unlikely to inhibit growth in children. Nevertheless, growth should be monitored in children undergoing long-term treatment. In infants and children aged up to 5 years, reversible myocardial hypertrophy may occur in rare cases following long-term treatment with high doses. Therefore echocardiographic recordings should be made regularly.

Side-effects: Synacthen Depot may provoke hypersensitivity reactions, which in patients suffering from, or susceptible to allergic disorders (especially asthma) may take the form of anaphylactic shock.

In rare cases, the benzyl alcohol in Synacthen Depot may provoke hypersensitivity reactions.

Since Synacthen Depot stimulates the adrenal cortex to increase the output of glucocorticoids and mineralocorticoids, side-effects associated with excessive adrenocorticotrophic activity may be encountered.

Treatment of overdose: Relating to therapeutic usage of Synacthen Depot: Overdosage may lead to fluid retention and signs of excessive adrenocorticotrophic activity (Cushing's Syndrome). In such cases, Synacthen Depot should either be withdrawn temporarily, given in lower doses or the interval between injections should be prolonged (e.g. 5–7 days).

Pharmaceutical precautions Synacthen Depot should be protected from light and stored in a refrigerator (2–8°C).

Legal category POM.

Package quantities Ampoules of 1 mg in 1 ml packed in boxes of 10.

Multi-dose vials of 2 mg in 2 ml packed singly.

Further information Nil.

Product licence number

Ampoules 1 mg	0008/5071
Vials 2 mg	0008/5072

TRANSIDERM*-NITRO 5 and 10

Presentation Transiderm-Nitro is a transdermal drug delivery system, comprising a self-adhesive, pink coloured patch, containing a drug reservoir of glyceryl trinitrate.

For each Transiderm-Nitro 5, the average amount of glyceryl trinitrate absorbed per patch in 24 hours is 5 mg. Each patch has a contact surface measuring 10 cm^2, and a glyceryl trinitrate content of 25 mg.

For Transiderm-Nitro 10, the average amount of glyceryl trinitrate absorbed per patch in 24 hours is 10 mg. Each patch has a contact surface measuring 20 cm^2, and a glyceryl trinitrate content of 50 mg.

The drug reservoir contains lactose.

Uses

Indications: Prophylactic treatment of attacks of angina pectoris, as monotherapy or in combination with other anti-anginal agents. Transiderm-Nitro 5 only: Prophylactic treatment of phlebitis and extravasation secondary to venous cannulation for intravenous fluid and drug administration when the duration of treatment is expected to last for 2 days or longer.

Mode of action: Transiderm-Nitro is a novel drug delivery system designed to achieve a prolonged and constant release of glyceryl trinitrate.

Glyceryl trinitrate acts by venous and arterial vasodilatation and redistribution of myocardial blood flow.

Following the application of Transiderm-Nitro the plasma level of glyceryl trinitrate reaches a constant plateau within two hours, which is maintained throughout the day until patch removal. During the first hour after removal of the patch the plasma level falls rapidly.

Dosage and administration

Adults: Angina: Treatment should be initiated with one Transiderm-Nitro 5 patch daily. If a higher dosage is required a Transiderm-Nitro 10 patch may be substituted. The dosage may be increased to a maximum of two Transiderm-Nitro 10 patches daily in resistant cases. Transiderm-Nitro may be given either continuously, or intermittently with a patch-off period of 8–12 hours, usually at night, during each 24 hour period. Development of tolerance or attenuation of therapeutic effect commonly occurs with prolonged or frequent administration of all long-acting nitrates. Recent evidence suggests that intermittent therapy with Transiderm-Nitro may reduce the incidence of tolerance.

Prior to the use of intermittent therapy, the clinical benefits to the patient should be weighed against the risks of angina in the patch-free interval. In patients considered to be at risk, concomitant anti-anginal therapy should be implemented (see 'Precautions').

It is recommended that the patch is applied to the lateral chest wall. The replacement patch should be applied to a new area of skin. Allow several days to elapse before applying a fresh patch to the same area of skin. If acute attacks of angina pectoris occur, rapidly acting nitrates may be required.

Phlebitis and extravasation: One Transiderm-Nitro 5 patch is to be applied distal to the site of intravenous cannulation at the time of venepuncture. The patch should be removed after 3–4 days and a new replacement patch applied to a different area of skin. Treatment with Transiderm-Nitro should be discontinued once intravenous therapy has stopped.

Use in the elderly: No specific information on use in the elderly is available, however, no evidence exists to suggest that an alteration in dosage is required.

Use in children: There is insufficient knowledge of the effects of Transiderm-Nitro in children and therefore recommendations for its use cannot be made.

Contra-indications, warnings, etc

Contra-indications: Transiderm-Nitro should not be prescribed to patients hypersensitive to nitrates. Severe hypotension. Increased intracranial pressure. Myocardial insufficiency due to obstruction (eg in the presence of aortic or mitral stenosis or of constrictive pericarditis).

Precautions: In recent myocardial infarction or acute heart failure, Transiderm-Nitro should be employed only under careful surveillance.

As with all anti-anginal nitrate preparations, withdrawal of long-term treatment should be gradual, by replacement with decreasing doses of long-acting oral nitrates.

The system should be removed before cardioversion or DC defibrillation is attempted. This is to avoid the possibility of arcing between the patch and the electrodes. Also the system should be removed before diathermy treatment.

Caution should be exercised in patients with arterial hypoxaemia due to severe anaemia because, in such patients the biotransformation of nitroglycerin is reduced. Similarly, caution is called for in patients with hypoxaemia and a ventilation/perfusion imbalance due to lung disease or ischaemic heart failure.

Postural hypotension has been reported rarely following initiation of treatment with Transiderm-Nitro and care is advised when driving or operating machinery.

Nitrate therapy may aggravate the angina caused by hypertrophic cardiomyopathy.

The possibility of increased frequency of angina during patch-off periods should be considered. In such cases, the use of concomitant anti-anginal therapy is desirable.

If tolerance to nitroglycerin patches develops, the effect of sublingual nitroglycerin on exercise tolerance may be partially diminished.

Pregnancy and lactation: As with all drugs, Transiderm-Nitro should not be prescribed during pregnancy, particularly during the first trimester, unless there are compelling reasons for doing so.

It is not known whether the active substance passes into the breast milk. The benefits for the mother must be weighed against the risks for the child.

Drug interactions: Concomitant treatment with other vasodilators, calcium antagonists, ACE inhibitors, beta-blockers, diuretics, antihypertensives, tricyclic antidepressants and major tranquillisers, as well as the consumption of alcohol, may potentiate the blood pressure lowering effects of Transiderm-Nitro.

Concurrent administration of Transiderm-Nitro with dihydroergotamine may increase the bioavailability of dihydroergotamine and lead to coronary vasoconstriction.

The possibility that the ingestion of acetylsalicylic acid and non-steroidal anti-inflammatory drugs might diminish the therapeutic response to Transiderm-Nitro cannot be excluded.

Side-effects

Central nervous system: Like other preparations, Transiderm-Nitro may give rise to headache, which is due to cerebral vasodilation and is dose-dependent. Such headaches, however, may regress after a few days despite continuation of the therapy. If they do not disappear, they should be treated with mild analgesics. In cases where headaches are unresponsive to treatment, the dosage of nitroglycerin should be reduced or use of the product discontinued.

Skin: Reddening of the skin, with or without local itching or burning sensation, as well as allergic contact dermatitis may occasionally occur. Upon removal of the patch, any slight reddening of the skin will usually disappear within a few hours. The application site should be changed on patch replacement to prevent local irritation.

Cardiovascular: Facial flushing, faintness, dizziness or lightheadedness, and postural hypotension, which may be associated with reflex-induced tachycardia, have been reported rarely. Reflex tachycardia can be controlled by concomitant treatment with a beta-blocker.

Gastro-intestinal: Rarely nausea, vomiting.

Treatment of overdosage

Signs: High dose of glyceryl trinitrate are known to cause pronounced systemic side effects, eg a marked fall in blood pressure and reflex tachycardia resulting in collapse and syncope. Methaemoglobinaemia has also been reported following accidental overdosage of nitroglycerin. However, with Transiderm-Nitro, the release membrane will reduce the likelihood of overdosage occurring.

Management: In contrast to long acting oral nitrate preparations, the effect of Transiderm-Nitro can be rapidly terminated simply by removing the system. Any fall in blood pressure or signs of collapse that may occur, may be managed by general resuscitative measures.

Pharmaceutical precautions Store below 25°C.

Legal category P.

Package quantities Boxes of 30 patches (OP).

Further information Transiderm-Nitro gives a controlled release of glyceryl trinitrate over at least 24 hours, and thereby avoids high peaks of blood levels, minimising the incidence of side-effects.

Although glyceryl trinitrate is volatile, resulting, in the case of most products, in a loss of the drug after relatively short storage, the design of the Transiderm-Nitro patch ensures that the dosage to the patient is maintained even after 2 years storage.

Product licence numbers
Transiderm-Nitro 5 0001/0094
Transiderm-Nitro 10 0001/0095.

TRASICOR*

Presentation Trasicor tablets each containing 20 mg Oxprenolol Hydrochloride BP. Circular, flat, white, film-coated tablets with bevelled edges, having the monogram CIBA impressed on one side and Trasicor 20 on the other.

Trasicor tablets each containing 40 mg Oxprenolol Hydrochloride BP. Circular, flat, white, film-coated tablets with bevelled edges, having the monogram CIBA impressed on one side and Trasicor 40 on the other.

Trasicor tablets each containing 80 mg Oxprenolol Hydrochloride BP. Circular, pale yellow, slightly bi-convex, film-coated tablets having the monogram CIBA impressed on one side and Trasicor 80 on the other.

Trasicor tablets each containing 160 mg Oxprenolol Hydrochloride BP. Circular, pale orange, slightly bi-convex, film-coated tablets, having the monogram CIBA impressed on one side and Trasicor 160 on the other.

The 20 mg and 40 mg tablets also contain sucrose and gluten (wheat starch).

Uses *Mode of action:* Trasicor is a beta-adrenergic receptor blocking drug with intrinsic sympathomimetic activity.

Indications: For the treatment of angina pectoris, all grades of hypertension and sympathetically induced cardiac arrhythmias.

Short-term relief of sympathomimetic symptoms of anxiety.

Subsidiary indications include functional heart disorders, hypertrophic obstructive cardiomyopathy and dysrhythmias associated with anaesthesia.

Dosage and administration *Adults: Angina pectoris:* Most patients respond to 40–160 mg three times daily. Individual patients may require more, but only rarely are doses above 480 mg daily required.

Hypertension: Initially 80 mg twice daily. If necessary, this daily dose can be increased at convenient intervals (e.g. weekly or fortnightly) until satisfactory blood-pressure control is achieved. When used as monotherapy, doses of 480 mg/day should not be exceeded, since experience has shown that hardly any increase in the response can be achieved by this means. Usually, patients respond to 80–320 mg Trasicor in combination with a diuretic and most of the antihypertensive effect is achieved within 2–3 days.

Cardiac arrhythmias: Initial dose 20–40 mg three times daily. This may be increased if necessary to achieve the desired effect.

Anxiety states: The sympathomimetic syptoms of anxiety are alleviated by Trasicor. An initial dose of 40 mg twice daily is suggested, increasing to a total daily dose of 160 mg, if necessary. Although no evidence of habituation or tolerance has been observed with Trasicor, its effectiveness in the long term treatment of anxiety has not been established. Symptoms of anxiety occurring in transient situations may be alleviated by a single dose of 40–80 mg Trasicor.

Elderly: No special dosage regime is necessary but concurrent hepatic insufficiency should be taken into account.

Children: The administration of Trasicor to children is not recommended. However, occasionally Trasicor has been given to children and infants to control arrhythmias. No dosage scheme has been worked out but oral Trasicor has been given empirically on a body-weight basis of approximately 1 mg/kg.

Use in pregnancy and lactation: Beta-blockers may cause bradycardia in the foetus which can also persist after birth. During pregnancy, in the course of labour and during lactation, beta-blockers should only be employed if the benefits to the mother outweigh the possible risks to the foetus or infant.

Contra-indications, warnings, etc

Side-effects: Trasicor is well tolerated. However dizziness, drowsiness, headache, insomnia, excitement, dry mouth, disturbances of vision, keratoconjunctivitis, loss of libido and gastro-intestinal disturbances may occur, particularly at the start of treatment. Isolated cases of excessive bradycardia, hypotension, A-V conduction disorders and thrombocytopenia have been reported.

As with other beta-blockers, bronchospasm, dyspnoea and heart failure may occasionally be precipitated in susceptible patients (see 'Precautions') and exertional tiredness and feelings of coldness in the extremities have been reported on rare occasions. However, the incidence of these side-effects is low.

Trasicor possesses antihypertensive effects, but these are unlikely to be noted in normotensive subjects.

There have been reports of skin rashes and/or dry eyes associated with the use of beta-adrenergic blocking drugs. The reported incidence is small, and in most cases the symptoms have cleared when the treatment was withdrawn. Discontinuance of the drug should be considered if any such reaction is not otherwise explicable. Cessation of therapy with a beta-adrenergic blocker should be gradual.

Contra-indications: Trasicor is contra-indicated in patients with second or third degree atrioventricular block, marked bradycardia, uncontrolled heart failure, cardiogenic shock, hypersensitivity to oxprenolol and related derivatives, sick-sinus syndrome, bronchial asthma and anaesthesia with chloroform or ether.

Precautions: As with other beta-blockers, when discontinuing treatment with oxprenolol the drug should be withdrawn gradually, because abrupt interruption of the medication, particularly in cases of ischaemic heart disease, may lead to an acute deterioration in the patients condition.

If there is evidence of cardiac failure, this must be controlled by digitalis and/or diuretics before and during Trasicor therapy.

Should the pulse rate fall below 50 per minute, then treatment should be withdrawn and started at a lower dose.

Caution should be observed when treating patients with chronic bronchitis, emphysema as well as in those with a case history of asthmatic disorders. Additional treatment with a beta-2-stimulant may be necessary; alternatively the dosage of bronchodilator medication may need to be readjusted when starting treatment with Trasicor.

In rare cases, a pre-existing A-V conduction disorder of moderate degree may become aggravated (possibly leading to A-V block). As a rule, no worsening of peripheral conduction disorders (left and/or right bundle-branch block) occurs.

Treatment with a beta-blocker is liable to mask symptoms of hypoglycaemia and also to affect carbohydrate metabolism. In patients with labile or insulin dependent diabetes in particular, it may therefore be necessary to readjust the dosage of antidiabetic medication. In patients who have been fasting for any length of time, hypoglycaemia may be increased or its symptoms masked.

Beta-blockers may mask the signs and symptoms of a thyrotoxic crisis.

Beta-blockers may aggravate the signs and symptoms of peripheral vascular disorders (Raynaud's disease).

In patients with phaeochromocytoma a beta-blocker should only be given together with an alpha-blocker.

Beta-blockers may diminish liver function and thus affect the metabolism of other drugs. In the presence of liver cirrhosis the bioavailability of oxprenolol may be increased. No major alteration in its bioavailability is likely to occur in patients with compensated renal failure.

Depending on the individual concerned, beta-blockers may adversely affect the patients reactions as a road user or as a operator of machinery, particularly if he also consumes alcohol.

Drug interactions: The antihypertensive effect of oxprenolol is enhanced by concomitant treatment with other antihypertensives.

The central depressant effect of alcohol, analgesics, antihistamines and tricyclic antidepressants is potentiated.

A watch should be kept for possible additive effects if oxprenolol is given together with calcium antagonists and/or anti-arrhythmic agents; particularly after intravenous administration of verapamil, the possibility of hypotension and cardiac arrhythmia or arrest cannot be excluded.

Beta-blockers may potentiate the negative inotropic and dromotropic effect of anti-arrhythmic agents of the quinidine type and amiodarone.

Adrenaline or other substances with sympathomimetic activity may lead to hypertensive reactions in patients under treatment with oxprenolol and other non-cardioselective beta-blockers.

If combined treatment with clonidine has to be interrupted, the beta-blocker medication should be withdrawn several days before clonidine.

The hypoglycaemic effects of insulin or oral antidiabetic agents may be potentiated.

During concurrent treatment with indomethacin, a decrease in the antihypertensive effects of oxprenolol has been observed.

Cimetidine increases the bioavailability of beta-blockers which are mainly metabolised by the liver; the effect of oxprenolol may therefore be potentiated by concomitant treatment with cimetidine.

Patients under treatment with preparations which deplete the catecholamine depots (e.g. reserpine, guanethidine) or with MAO inhibitors should be kept under careful surveillance during concurrent beta-blocker medication.

A deterioration in peripheral blood flow has been reported in predisposed patients receiving concomitant treatment with ergot alkaloids and beta-blockers.

Attention should be paid to the cardiodepressant effect of inhalation anaesthetics in patients receiving beta-blocker therapy. In a patient under beta-blockade, the anaesthetic selected should be one exhibiting as little negative inotropic activity as possible eg halothane/nitrous oxide. If on the other hand, inhibition of sympathetic tone during the operation is regarded as undesirable, the beta-blocker can be withdrawn gradually prior to surgery.

Treatment of overdosage: Overdosage with Trasicor may lead to excessive bradycardia, hypotension, heart failure, cardiogenic shock or even cardiac arrest. In addition dyspnoea, bronchospasm, vomiting, impairment of consciousness and also generalised convulsions may occur. It should also be noted that severe toxicity may develop rapidly and that there may be severe bradycardia despite a normal ECG.

For sinus bradycardia and hypotension 0.5–2.0 mg of atropine should be administered slowly by intravenous infusion. If this does not control the heart rate sufficiently isoprenaline hydrochloride may be necessary. The dose of isoprenaline needs to be sufficient to reverse the blockade and should be assessed by the clinical response. A reasonable starting dose would be 25 micrograms of isoprenaline hydrochloride.

In severe cardiogenic shock the treatment of choice appears to be glucagon. The initial dose should be 5–10 mg intravenously, further boluses or an infusion can be used according to the patient's condition. Transvenous pacing has been used, sometimes with success. If bronchospasm develops bronchodilators should be used. Patients should be monitored for several days as the beta-blocking effects of Trasicor exceed its plasma half-life.

Pharmaceutical precautions The tablets should be protected from moisture.

Legal category POM.

Package quantities Tablets: All strengths in blister packs of 100.

Further information Nil.

Product licence numbers

Trasicor Tablets 20 mg	0008/0124
Trasicor Tablets 40 mg	0008/0125
Trasicor Tablets 80 mg	0008/0122
Trasicor Tablets 160 mg	0008/0123

TRASIDREX

Presentation Trasidrex tablets each contain 160 mg Oxprenolol Hydrochloride BP in a sustained release core and 0.25 mg Cyclopenthiazide BP in the coat. The tablets are circular, with a red sugar coat, and printed CIBA on one side and TRASIDREX on the other, both words in black.

Trasidrex tablets also contain sucrose and an azo-dye.

Uses *Mode of action:* Trasicor* (oxprenolol) is a non-selective beta-adrenergic receptor blocking drug with antihypertensive properties. It exerts a competitive and reversible blockade of the beta-adrenergic receptors, thereby protecting the cardiovascular system against excessive adrenergic stimuli, such as those produced by emotional stress and environmental factors. Oxprenolol also has partial agonist activity (PAA) also known as intrinsic sympathomimetic activity (ISA). This property means that some degree of stimulation of the beta receptors is maintained. Under conditions of rest this tends to counter-balance the negative chronotropic and negative inotropic effects of beta-blockade.

The gradual release of oxprenolol from a special sustained release core in Trasidrex prolongs its pharmacological action to 24 hours.

Navidrex* (cyclopenthiazide) is a thiazide diuretic with sustained antihypertensive activity.

The combination of cyclopenthiazide and a slow-release formulation of oxprenolol in a single tablet has a number of advantages:

1. Since oxprenolol and cyclopenthiazide have different modes of antihypertensive activity their therapeutic actions are complementary.
2. Once daily dosage with the combination improves patient compliance.
3. Trasicor inhibits the rise in renin caused by diuretics alone. Conversely Navidrex may be expected to improve the response in low renin hypertensives.
4. The addition of Navidrex to Trasicor further reduces the minimal risk of cardiac failure.

Indications: In the treatment of mild and moderate hypertension.

Dosage and administration *Adults:* Initially 1 tablet daily, usually given in the morning. Most of the antihypertensive effect of the combination is achieved within two to three days. If necessary, the dose can be increased to 2 or more tablets given once daily, until satisfactory blood pressure control is achieved. Most patients should respond to 1 or 2 tablets.

Trasidrex can be successfully combined with other single antihypertensive drugs having a different pharmacological effect. In particular, a free combination with a vasodilator will often be beneficial.

Use in the elderly: No special dosage regime is necessary but concurrent hepatic insufficiency should be taken into account (also see 'Precautions').

Contra-indications, warnings, etc *Side-effects:* Trasidrex is well tolerated. However dizziness, drowsiness, headache, insomnia, excitement and gastrointestinal disturbances may occur, particularly at the start of treatment. Like other beta-blockers, there have been isolated reports of bradycardia and thrombocytopenia.

As with other beta-blockers, bronchospasm, and heart failure may occasionally be precipitated in susceptible patients (see precautions) and exertional tiredness and feelings of coldness in the extremities have been reported on rare occasions. However, the incidence of these side-effects is low, possibly due to the partial protection afforded by the sympathomimetic effect of Trasicor.

There have been reports of skin rashes and/or dry eyes associated with the use of beta-adrenergic blocking drugs. The reported incidence is small, and in most cases the symptoms have cleared when the treatment was withdrawn. Discontinuance of the drug should be considered if any such reaction is not otherwise explicable. Cessation of therapy with a beta-adrenergic blocker should be gradual.

Like other diuretics with a similar mode of action, cyclopenthiazide may cause latent gout or latent diabetes mellitus to become manifest. In a few cases, allergic skin reactions, mild anorexia, nausea, constipation and diarrhoea have been reported. In common with other thiazides, there have been isolated reports of thrombocytopenia.

Contra-indications: Trasidrex is contra-indicated in patients with atrio-ventricular block, marked bradycardia, uncontrolled heart failure and cardiogenic shock. Because of the cyclopenthiazide content, it is contra-indicated in patients with marked renal insufficiency.

An antidiuretic effect has been reported following concomitant treatment with thiazide diuretics and lithium. As with all products which contain thiazide diuretics Trasidrex is contra-indicated during lithium treatment.

Pregnancy: Beta-blockers may cause bradycardia in the foetus, which can also persist after birth. During pregnancy, in the course of labour and during lactation beta-blockers should only be employed after the needs of the mother have been weighed against the possible risks to the foetus.

Precautions: If there is evidence of cardiac failure, this must be controlled by digitalis before and during Trasidrex therapy. Should the pulse rate fall below 50 per minute, treatment should be re-started at a lower dose, if feasible. Particular caution should be observed when treating asthmatics, chronic bronchitics or other individuals where bronchospasm may be provoked.

Trasidrex should be given cautiously to patients with metabolic acidosis or anaesthesia with ether or chloroform. For anaesthesia the agent selected should be one exhibiting as little negative inotropic activity as possible e.g. halothane, nitrous oxide.

Treatment with a beta-blocker is liable to mask the symptoms of hypoglycaemia and also to affect carbohydrate metabolism. In patients with labile or insulin-dependent diabetes in particular, it may therefore be necessary to readjust the dosage of anti-diabetic medication. Navidrex, a thiazide diuretic, may also decrease glucose tolerance.

Like other beta-blockers, Trasidrex should not be given in combination with calcium-antagonists of the verapamil type, because their concomitant use may result in bradycardia, hypotension or even cardiac arrest.

As with other beta-blocking drugs, sudden withdrawal of treatment with Trasidrex may induce severe and continuous angina. Patients should, therefore, be advised to avoid interruption of established therapy and if withdrawal becomes necessary it should be done gradually.

Because of its Navidrex content, Trasidrex should be used with care in patients with some degree of renal impairment, as a rise in blood urea can occur and in extreme cases result in an oliguric crisis.

During long-term treatment with Trasidrex, salt restriction is unnecessary.

The potassium sparing action of Trasicor may obviate the necessity of giving potassium supplements to counter the effects of the thiazide.

Treatment of overdosage: Overdosage with Trasidrex may lead to excessive bradycardia, hypotension, coma and convulsions. It should also be noted that severe toxicity may develop rapidly and that there may be severe hypotension and bradycardia despite a normal ECG. For sinus bradycardia and hypotension 0.5–2.0 mg of atropine should be administered slowly by intravenous infusion. If this does not raise the heart rate sufficiently isoprenaline may be necessary. The dose of isoprenaline needs to be sufficient to reverse the blockade and should be assessed by the clinical response. A reasonable starting dose would be 25 mcg of isoprenaline hydrochloride.

In severe cardiogenic shock the treatment of choice appears to be glucagon. The initial dose should be 5–10 mg intravenously, further boluses or an infusion can be used according to the patient's condition. Transvenous pacing has been used, sometimes with success. If bronchospasm develops bronchodilators should be used. Patients should be monitored for several days as the beta-blocking effects of Trasidrex exceed its plasma half-life. Because Trasidrex is a slow-release formulation, it is likely that the effects of overdosage will be more persistent than following conventional oxprenolol. Further information may be obtained from CIBA Laboratories, Horsham.

Pharmaceutical precautions The tablets should be protected from heat, light and moisture.

Legal category POM.

Package quantities Cartons of 28 tablets consisting of two reminder calendar foils of 14 tablets (each carton of 28 represents two to four weeks' treatment depending on whether dosage is 1 or 2 tablets daily) (OP).

Further information By combining a beta-blocker (Trasicor*) and a thiazide diuretic (Navidrex*) in a single tablet in a calendar pack, the management of hypertension can be greatly simplified for the majority of patients. Compliance will be improved and many of the pharmacological actions of the two components produce beneficial complementary effects.

Product licence number 0008/0138.

**Trade Mark*

Cilag Limited
PO Box 79, Saunderton
High Wycombe
Buckinghamshire HP14 4HJ.

ACI-JEL* THERAPEUTIC VAGINAL JELLY

Presentation Acetic Acid BP 0.92% w/w in a buffered (pH 4) gel base.

Uses In any case where the restoration and maintenance of vaginal acidity is desirable, as in the treatment of non-specific vaginal infection and in the milder forms of simple cervicitis. Aci-Jel Therapeutic Vaginal Jelly is also useful as an adjunct to systemic therapy in trichomoniasis, and prophylactically after courses of other, more specific therapy.

Dosage and administration One applicatorful intravaginally in the morning and upon retiring. The frequency of the application and duration of treatment depend upon the type of case and the degree of progress.

Contra-indications, warnings, etc
Contra-indications: None known.

Warnings: Rarely, local irritation and inflamation have been reported.

Precautions: Use during pregnancy: In view of the nature of the active ingredients Aci-Jel can be used with caution during pregnancy.

Overdosage: Aci-Jel Therapeutic Vaginal Jelly is intended for intravaginal use. If accidental ingestion of large quantities of the product occurs, an appropriate method of gastric emptying may be used if considered desirable.

Pharmaceutical precautions Store at room temperature.

Legal category GSL.

Package quantities Tube containing 85 g. with the ORTHO* Plastic Vaginal Applicator.

Further information Nil.

Product licence number 0076/5015.

ALIMIX* ▼

Presentation White, biconvex, scored tablets, engraved J/Y on one side and C on the reverse. Each tablet contains cisapride monohydrate equivalent to 10 mg of cisapride. The tablets contain lactose.

Uses
Properties: Alimix is a gastrointestinal prokinetic agent which stimulates lower oesophageal, gastric, small intestinal and colonic motility.

Alimix probably acts by enhancing the release of acetylcholine at the level of the myenteric plexus in the gut wall, and therefore its effects on motility can largely be abolished by atropine. The mechanism by which acetylcholine release is enhanced is unclear. Alimix is devoid of antidopaminergic and direct cholinergic effects, and has no effect on prolactin release or gastric secretion.

In patients with gastro-oesophageal reflux, Alimix increases the resting tone of the lower oesophageal sphincter, and increases the amplitude of lower oesophageal contractions. Alimix has also been shown, by pH monitoring, to reduce the duration of reflux episodes.

Alimix accelerates gastric emptying of liquid and solid meals, and shortens mouth to caecum transit time. It also stimulates colonic propulsive peristalsis and accelerates colonic transit.

Indications: Treatment of symptoms (e.g. heartburn, regurgitation) and mucosal lesions associated with gastro-oesophageal reflux.

Relief of symptoms (e.g. nausea, early sateity, anorexia, bloating, epigastric pain) of impaired gastric motility secondary to disturbed and delayed emptying associated with diabetes, systemic sclerosis and autonomic neuropathy.

The management of symptoms of dyspepsia e.g. epigastric pain or burning, early satiety or bloating, where peptic ulcer or other lesions have been excluded from the diagnosis.

Dosage and administration Alimix should preferably be taken 15–30 minutes before a meal in order to ensure maximum plasma levels immediately after food intake. When an additional dose is required to control night time symptoms, the tablet should be taken at bedtime.

Adults and children aged 12 years and over. Gastro-oesophageal reflux: 10 mg Alimix three or four times daily, depending upon the symptoms being treated and the clinical response. Healing of oesophageal lesions has been reported following treatment with 10 mg q.d.s. for 12 weeks.

A 12 week course of treatment is recommended to obtain maximum benefit.

Impaired gastric motility: 10 mg Alimix three or four times daily. An initial course of six weeks is recommended, but longer periods of treatment may be required.

Dyspepsia: 10 mg Alimix three times daily. The usual course of treatment is four weeks.

Use in children: Clinical experience with Alimix in children younger than 12 years is limited. Hence the drug can only be recommended for use in children aged 12 years and older.

Use in elderly: Repeated dosing in elderly patients with Alimix produced steady state plasma levels, which were generally higher than those reported in younger patients, due to a moderate prolongation of the elimination half life. Therapeutic doses, however, are similar to those used in younger patients. Therefore it is recommended that when Alimix is used in elderly patients, a starting dose similar to that used in other adults is prescribed initially. This can then be adapted depending on the therapeutic effects or possible side-effects of the treatment.

Abnormal renal or liver function: Because of the importance of the hepatic metabolism and renal excretion of Alimix, the dosage should initially be halved in patients with hepatic or renal insufficiency. Subsequently the dose can be adapted depending on individual clinical response.

Contra-indications, warnings, etc
Contra-indications: Alimix is contra-indicated in pregnancy (see 'Use in pregnancy' section) and in patients in whom gastro-intestinal stimulation might be dangerous, e.g. gastrointestinal haemorrhage, mechanical obstruction or perforation.

Warnings: Abnormal renal or liver function (see Dosage Section)

Drug interactions: Since Alimix accelerates gastric emptying, the absorption from the stomach of concomitantly administered drugs may be diminished, whereas absorption of drugs from the small intestine may be accelerated. For drugs that require careful individual titration, such as anticonvulsants, it may be useful to measure their plasma concentration.

Alimix does not affect psychomotor performance nor does it induce sedation or drowsiness. However, the sedative effects of benzodiazepines and alcohol may be accelerated when administered concomitantly with Alimix.

The beneficial effects of Alimix on gastrointestinal motility are largely antagonised by anticholinergic drugs.

Concomitant treatment with H_2 antagonists increases the bioavailability of Alimix, and decreases that of the H_2 antagonist. The difference is unlikely to be clinically significant.

In patients receiving anticoagulants, the prothrombin time may be increased. It is advisable to check the prothrombin time one week after initiation or discontinuation of Alimix treatment, and to adapt the dose of anticoagulant if necessary.

The drug exhibits extensive binding to plasma proteins, mainly to albumin.

Use in pregnancy: In animals Alimix has shown no teratogenic or primary foetotoxic effects. Nevertheless, the safety of Alimix in human pregnancy has not been established and therefore, as with other new drugs, it is contra-indicated in pregnancy.

Use in lactation: Although the excretion of Alimix in human breast milk is minimal (milk to serum ratio of 0.045), it is not advisable to breastfeed while taking Alimix.

Side-effects: The most frequent side-effects reported with Alimix are gastrointestinal: abdominal cramps, borborygmi and diarrhoea. They are mainly transient and rarely require discontinuation of treatment.

Infrequent side-effects include headaches and light-headedness. Reports of convulsions and extrapyramidal effects have been received.

Overdosage: There has been one reported overdosage with cisapride. An adult took 540 mg and for 2 hours experienced retching, borborygmi, flatus, stool frequency and urinary frequency. There were no neurological, cardiovascular (including ECG), respiratory, biochemical or haematological effects.

Treatment should include gastric lavage, close observation and general supportive measures.

Pharmaceutical precautions Store at room temperature and protect from light.

Legal category POM.

Package quantities 10 mg tablets: pack of 120 tablets.

Further information Alimix is rapidly absorbed, with peak plasma levels 1 to 2 hours after dosing, and an elimination half-life of approximately 10 hours.

It undergoes extensive first-pass metabolism in the liver and gut wall, with the main metabolic pathways being oxidative N-dealkylation and aromatic hydroxylation. Excretion is mainly as metabolites (90%) with approximately equal amounts in both urine and faeces.

Product licence number 0076/0144.

DERMONISTAT* CREAM

Presentation A smooth, white non-staining cream containing Miconazole Nitrate PhEur 2% w/w.

Uses A potent antimycotic cream for the treatment of fungal infections of the skin, hair and nails.

Dosage and administration May be applied topically to both adults and children.

Fungal infections of the skin: The cream should be applied to the lesions twice daily and continued for 10 days after the lesions have disappeared.

Fungal infections of the nail: The cream should be applied thinly to the infected nail once daily and the nail covered with a non-perforated plastic bandage. Nails should be clipped short at regular intervals and treatment continued until the growth of the new nail is established and a definite cure can be observed.

Contra-indications, warnings, etc Hypersensitivity to the product.

Side-effects: Isolated cases of sensitisation and irritation have been reported. If this occurs administration of the product should be discontinued.

Precautions: Dermonistat Cream is only absorbed in small amounts following application to the skin. Hence no special precautions are necessary in elderly patients. In view of the low level of absorption and the lack of teratogenic effects in animals, Dermonistat can be used with caution during pregnancy.

Overdosage: Dermonistat Cream is intended for topical use. If accidental ingestion of large quantities of the product occurs, an appropriate method of gastric emptying may be used if considered desirable.

Pharmaceutical precautions None known.

Legal category P.

Package quantities 30 g tubes. A patient-instruction leaflet is enclosed in each package.

Further information Nil.

Product licence number 0076/0041.

FORMULIX*

Presentation Formulix is an amber coloured, cherry flavoured elixir containing 120 mg paracetamol and 12 mg codeine phosphate in each 5 ml.

Uses Formulix is indicated for the relief of mild to moderate pain.

Dosage and administration Formulix is given orally. The usual doses in children are:

3–6 years: 1 teaspoonful (5 ml) 3 or 4 times daily.
7–12 years: 2 teaspoonsful (10 ml) 3 or 4 times daily.

Contra-indications, warnings, etc

Precautions: Patients receiving other central nervous system depressants (including other opioid analgesics, tranquillisers, sedative hypnotics and alcohol) concomitantly with this drug may exhibit an additive depressant effect. When such therapy is contemplated, the dose of one or both agents should be reduced.

Formulix is not recommended during pregnancy or lactation since safety in pregnant women or nursing mothers has not been established.

Because safety and effectiveness in the administration of Formulix in infants under 3 years of age have not been established, such use is not recommended.

Warnings: Codeine can produce drug dependence of the morphine type and therefore has the potential for being abused.

Side-effects: The most frequently observed adverse reactions include lightheadedness, dizziness, sedation, nausea and vomiting. These effects seem to be more prominent in ambulatory than in non-ambulatory patients and some of these adverse reactions may be alleviated if the patient lies down.

Overdosage: In serious overdosage of codeine, respiratory depression, bradycardia and hypotension may occur. Primary attention should be given to maintain vital functions. Opioid antagonists may be employed. Patients receiving a severe overdosage of Formulix may also be susceptible to the hepatic toxicity of paracetamol overdosage and appropriate measures such as gastric lavage and antidotal therapy should be taken.

Pharmaceutical precautions Protect from light.

Legal category POM.

Package quantities Bottle containing 500 ml.

Further information Nil.

Product licence number 0076/0106.

GYNO-PEVARYL* CREAM

Presentation A white non-perfumed cream containing 1% w/w econazole nitrate.

Uses For the treatment of vulvitis associated with candidal vaginitis. Balanitis.

Dosage and administration The cream should be applied to the vulva and perianal region and/or to the sexual partner's penis, including under the foreskin for 14 days.

Contra-indications, warnings, etc
Contra-indications: None known.

Side-effects: Rarely, transient local mild irritation may occur immediately after application.

Precautions: Hypersensitivity has rarely been recorded, if it should occur, administration should be discontinued. Gyno-Pevaryl Cream is only absorbed in small amounts following topical application. Hence, no special precautions are necessary in elderly patients.

In animals, econazole nitrate has shown no teratogenic effects, but is foetotoxic at high doses. The significance of this to man is unknown as there is no evidence of increased risk when taken in human pregnancy. However, as with other imidazoles, econazole should only be used in pregnancy if the practitioner considers it to be necessary.

Overdosage: Gyno-Pevaryl Cream is intended for intravaginal use. If accidental ingestion of large quantities of the product occurs, an appropriate method of gastric emptying may be used if considered desirable.

Pharmaceutical precautions Store in a cool place.

Legal category POM.

Package quantities Tubes of 15 g and 30 g.

Further information Anogenital hygiene is important to help prevent reinfection.

Product licence number 0076/0060.

GYNO-PEVARYL* 1 VAGINAL PESSARY
GYNO-PEVARYL* 1 VAGINAL PESSARY AND CREAM C.P. PACK

Presentation
Pessary: White egg-shaped pessary containing 150 mg econazole nitrate in a polysaccharide containing base and melting at 37°C.

C.P. Pack: A combination pack comprising a Gyno-Pevaryl 1 Vaginal Pessary (containing 150 mg econazole nitrate in a polysaccharide containing base) plus a 15 g tube of Gyno-Pevaryl Cream (containing 1% econazole nitrate).

Uses
Pessary: Vaginitis due to *Candida albicans* and other yeasts.

C.P. Pack: Pessary for vaginitis; cream for associated vulvitis and to treat sexual partner to help prevent re-infection.

Dosage and administration
Pessary: The pessary should be inserted as high as possible into the vagina in the evening prior to retiring.

C.P. Pack: Pessary as above. The cream should be applied to the vulva and perianal region and/or to the sexual partner's penis, including under the foreskin.

Contra-indications, warnings, etc
Contra-indications: None known.

Side-effects: Rarely, transient local mild irritation may occur immediately after application.

Precautions: Hypersensitivity has rarely been recorded, if it should occur, administration of the product should be discontinued.

In animals econazole nitrate has shown no teratogenic effects, but is foetotoxic at high doses. The significance of this in man is unknown as there is no evidence of an increased risk when taken in human pregnancy. However, as with other imidazoles, econazole should be used in pregnancy only if the practitioner considers it to be necessary.

Overdosage: Gyno-Pevaryl 1 Vaginal Pessary and Cream are intended for intravaginal use. If accidental ingestion of large quantities of the product occurs, an appropriate method of gastric emptying may be used if considered desirable.

Pharmaceutical precautions Store in a cool place.

Legal category POM.

Package quantities *Pessaries:* Each pack contains one pessary with a plastic vaginal applicator and a patient instruction leaflet. The pessary is individually sealed in a white plastic strip marked Gyno-Pevaryl 1.

C.P. Pack: Each pack contains one pessary, a 15 g tube of cream and a patient instruction leaflet.

Further information Anogenital hygiene is important to help prevent re-infection.

Due to the differing nature of the pessary base of Gyno-Pevaryl 1, substitution of a single Gyno-Pevaryl 150 pessary from the three pessary treatment must not be made.

Product licence numbers

Pessaries	0076/0097
C.P. Pack	0076/0097 and 0076/0060

GYNO-PEVARYL*150 VAGINAL PESSARIES
GYNO-PEVARYL*150 VAGINAL PESSARIES AND CREAM COMBIPACK

Presentation *Pessaries:* White egg-shaped pessaries each containing 150 mg econazole nitrate and melting at 37°C.

Combipack: A combination pack comprising 3 Gyno-Pevaryl vaginal pessaries (each containing 150 mg econazole nitrate) plus a 15 g tube of Gyno-Pevaryl cream (containing 1% econazole nitrate).

Uses *Pessaries:* Vaginitis due to *Candida albicans* and other yeasts.

Combipack: Pessaries for vaginitis; cream for associated vulvitis and to treat the sexual partner to help prevent re-infection.

Dosage and administration *Pessaries:* One pessary should be inserted high into the vagina each evening for three consecutive days.

Combipack: Pessaries as above. The cream should be applied to the vulva and perianal region and/or to the sexual partner's penis, including under the foreskin.

Contra-indications, warnings, etc
Contra-indications: None known.

Side-effects: Rarely, transient local mild irritation may occur immediately after application.

Precautions: Hypersensitivity has rarely been recorded, if it should occur, administration should be discontinued. Gyno-Pevaryl Pessaries and Cream are only absorbed in small amounts following topical application. Hence no special precautions are necessary in elderly patients.

In animals econazole nitrate has shown no teratogenic effects, but is foetotoxic at high doses. The significance of this in man is unknown as there is no evidence of an increased risk when taken in human pregnancy. However, as with other imidazoles, econazole should be used in pregnancy only if the practitioner considers it to be necessary.

Overdosage: Gyno-Pevaryl Vaginal Pessaries and Cream are intended for intravaginal use. If accidental ingestion of large quantities of the product occurs, an appropriate method of gastric emptying may be used if considered desirable.

Pharmaceutical precautions Store in a cool place.

Legal category POM.

Package quantities *Pessaries:* Each pack contains 3 pessaries and a patient instruction leaflet. The pessaries are individually sealed in a white plastic strip marked Gyno-Pevaryl 150 at regular intervals.

Combipack: Each pack contains 3 pessaries, a 15 g tube of cream and a patient instruction leaflet.

Further information Anogenital hygiene is important to help prevent re-infection.

Product licence numbers
Pessaries 0076/0058
Combipack 0076/0058 and 0076/0060

MASSE* BREAST CREAM

Presentation A white oil in water cream containing glycerin, lanolin, arachis oil, sorbitan monostearate, glyceryl monostearate, cetyl alcohol, stearic acid, polysorbate 60, propyl p-hydroxybenzoate, methyl-p-hydroxybenzoate, sodium benzoate, purified water.

Uses For pre-natal and post-natal nipple care. Use prenatally for preparing the nipples for breast feeding including the massage of flat and inverted nipples. Use post-natally for routine application to the nipples of lactating women.

Dosage and administration *Pre-natal nipple care:* Masse Breast Cream is applied once or twice daily during the last two or three months of pregnancy. A 1″ ribbon of cream is massaged gently into the nipples and the surrounding pigmented area with the fingertips until the cream is absorbed. The massage should be with gentle outward motion from the areola to the apex of the nipple.

Post-natal nipple care: Masse Breast Cream is massaged gently around the nipple and areola after the breast has been cleansed after each nursing.

Contra-indications, warnings, etc Acute mastitis or breast abscess. Lanolin sensitivity.

Hypersensitivity to the product: In cases of excess soreness or irritation consult your physician.

Local irritation has been reported in rare cases.

Overdosage: Masse Breast Cream is intended for topical use. If accidental ingestion of large quantities of the product occurs, an appropriate method of gastric emptying may be used if considered desirable.

Pharmaceutical precautions None known.

Legal category GSL.

Package 28 g tubes.

Further information Nil.

Product licence number 0076/5009.

MONISTAT* CREAM
MONISTAT* PESSARIES

Presentation *Cream:* A white, water-miscible cream containing Miconazole Nitrate PhEur 2% w/w.

Pessaries: White egg-shaped pessaries each containing 100 mg Miconazole Nitrate PhEur and melting at 37°C.

Uses A potent antimycotic agent for the local treatment and rapid symptomatic relief of vulvovaginal moniliasis and balanitis.

Dosage and administration *Cream:* One applicatorful (approx. 5 g) intravaginally, with additional cream smeared onto other affected areas, once daily, preferably at night, for 14 days.

Pessaries: One pessary should be inserted high into the vagina at night for the same period.

Patients should be instructed not to discontinue treatment upon relief of symptoms, but to complete the prescribed course. The simultaneous treatment of the partner with Monistat Cream is advisable.

Contra-indications, warnings, etc Hypersensitivity to the product.

Side-effects: Isolated cases of vulvo-vaginal burning, itching and irritation have been reported after using the product. If this occurs, administration of the product should be discontinued.

Precautions: Monistat Cream and Pessaries are only absorbed in small amounts following topical application. Hence no special precautions are necessary in elderly patients.

In animals, miconazole nitrate has shown no teratogenic effects, but is foetotoxic at high doses. The significance of this to man is unknown as there is no evidence of an increased risk when taken in human pregnancy. However, as with other imidazoles, miconazole should be used in pregnancy only if the practitioner considers it to be necessary.

The base containing the pessary formulation may interact with certain latex products, such as that in vaginal contraceptive diaphragms. Concurrent use is not recommended.

Overdosage: Monistat Cream and Pessaries are intended for intravaginal use. If accidental ingestion of large quantities of the product occurs, an appropriate method of gastric emptying may be used if considered desirable.

Pharmaceutical precautions Cream – none known. Pessaries – store in a cool place.

Legal category POM.

Package quantities *Cream:* 78 g tube with Ortho* Plastic Vaginal applicator.

Pessaries: Each pessary is completely sealed in PVC strips with seven pessaries to a strip. Each carton contains two strips of seven pessaries.

Both packs contain full patient instructions.

Further information Monistat Cream or Pessaries are particularly useful in the treatment of those patients with predisposing conditions for monilial vulvovaginitis, diabetes and those taking oral contraceptives or broad-spectrum antibiotics.

Product licence numbers
Cream 0076/0040
Pessaries 0076/0048

PANCREASE* CAPSULES

Presentation Hard, white, gelatin capsules printed 0095 on the body, containing enteric coated microspheres of porcine Pancrelipase USP. Each capsule has a protease activity of not less than 330 BP Units, an amylase activity of not less than 2,900 BP Units and lipase activity of not less than 5,000 BP Units.

Uses Exocrine pancreatic enzyme deficiency as in cystic fibrosis, chronic pancreatitis, post-pancreatectomy, post-gastrointestinal bypass surgery (e.g. Billroth II gastroenterostomy), ductal obstruction from neoplasm (e.g. of the pancreas or common bile duct).

The enzymes catalyse the hydrolysis of fats into glycerol and fatty acids, protein into proteoses and derived substances and starch into dextrins and sugars.

Dosage and administration For adults and children 1 or 2 capsules during each meal and one capsule with snacks. Occasionally a third capsule with meals may be required depending upon individual requirements. Where swallowing of capsules is difficult, they may be opened and the microspheres taken with liquids or soft foods which do not require chewing. To protect the enteric coating the microspheres should not be crushed or chewed.

Contra-indications, warnings, etc Hypersensitivity to pork protein. The safety of Pancrease during pregnancy has not yet been established. Such use is not recommended.

The most frequently reported adverse reactions to Pancrease Capsules are gastrointestinal in nature. Less frequently allergic-type reactions have also been observed.

Extremely high doses of exogenous pancreatic enzymes have been associated with hyperuricosuria and hyperuricaemia.

Contact of the microspheres with food having a pH higher than 5.5 can dissolve the protective enteric shell.

Pharmaceutical precautions Keep bottle tightly closed. Store at room temperature in a dry place. Do not refrigerate.

Legal category P.

Package quantities Containers of 100 capsules.

Further information The enteric coated Pancrease microspheres resist gastric inactivation and deliver predictable, high levels of biologically active enzymes into the duodenum.

Product licence number 0076/0129.

PEVARYL* CREAM
PEVARYL* LOTION
PEVARYL* SPRAY POWDER

Presentation *Cream:* A white cream containing 1% econazole nitrate.

Lotion: A white water-miscible lotion containing 1% econazole nitrate.

Spray Powder: A white powder containing 1% econazole nitrate, emitted as a spray by means of an aerosol container.

Uses Econazole nitrate is a broad-spectrum antifungal agent.

Cream: All fungal skin infections due to dermatophytes (e.g., Trichophyton species), yeasts (e.g., Candida species), moulds and other fungi. These include ringworm (tinea) infections, athlete's foot, paronychia, pityriasis versicolor, erythrasma and vulvitis, balanitis and napkin rash due to Candida.

Lotion: As Pevaryl Cream, but particularly suitable for hairy and moist areas and for fungal otitis externa.

Spray Powder: As Pevaryl Cream, but particularly suitable in intertriginous areas.

Dosage and administration *Cream:* Apply to the affected area 2-3 times daily and rub in gently.

In nail infections, apply once daily and cover with an occlusive dressing.

Lotion: As for Pevaryl* Cream.

Spray Powder: Apply to the affected area twice daily until the lesions have healed.

In order to prevent relapse, treatment should be continued for 2 weeks after clinical cure.

Contra-indications, warnings, etc *Contra-indications:* None known.

Side effects: Rarely, transient local mild irritation may occur immediately after application.

Precautions: Cream and Lotion: Hypersensitivity has rarely been recorded, if it should occur, administration of the product should be discontinued.

Spray Powder: As for Pevaryl Cream and Pevaryl Lotion. The spray should be kept away from the eyes and mucous membranes. Care should be taken in the presence of eczematous dermatitis.

Pevaryl Cream, Lotion and Spray Powder are only absorbed in small amounts following application to the skin. Hence no special precautions are necessary in elderly patients. In view of the low level of absorption and the lack of teratogenic effects in animals, the products can be used with caution during pregnancy.

Overdosage: Pevaryl Cream, Lotion and Spray Powder are intended for topical use. If accidental ingestion of large quantities of the product occurs, an appropriate method of gastric emptying may be used if considered desirable.

Pharmaceutical precautions
Cream and Lotion: None.

Spray Powder: Shake well before use. Contents are under pressure. Store in a cool place away from heat and sunlight; do not burn or puncture, even when empty.

Legal category
Cream: P.
Lotion: P.
Spray Powder: P.

Package quantities *Cream:* Each tube contains 30 g.

Lotion: Each bottle contains 30 ml.

Spray Powder: 200 g aerosol can contains 20 g econazole nitrate powder 1%.

Further information The infected area should be kept clean and dry during treatment.

Pevaryl Spray Powder is suitable for use in conjunction with Pevaryl Cream or Pevaryl Lotion. It is also useful for the treatment of clothing such as shoes and socks in cases of tinea pedis.

Product licence numbers

Cream:	0076/0059
Lotion:	0076/0066
Spray powder	0076/0063

PEVARYL* TC CREAM

Presentation Pevaryl TC cream is a white cream containing 1% w/w Econazole Nitrate BP and 0.1% w/w Triamcinolone Acetonide BP.

Uses For the topical treatment of inflammatory dermatomycoses and inflammatory skin conditions complicated by or threatened by bacterial or fungal skin infection.

Econazole nitrate is a broad spectrum antifungal agent with activity against many gram positive bacteria.

Triamcinolone acetonide is a potent corticosteroid with anti-inflammatory, antipruritic and antiallergic activity.

Dosage and administration The cream should be applied by gently rubbing it into the affected area twice daily for 14 days. Following disappearance of the inflammation, consideration should be given to continuing treatment with antifungal therapy alone until two weeks after clinical cure has been achieved.

Contra-indications, warnings, etc Like all preparations containing corticosteroids, Pevaryl TC cream should not be used on tubercular or luetic skin infections or in viral diseases (e.g. herpes, vaccinia, varicella). Pevaryl TC cream should not be administered to patients who have previously exhibited hypersensitivity to imidazoles or corticosteroids.

Long-term continuous steroid therapy should be avoided since adrenal suppression can occur, particularly when infants or children are treated or when occlusive dressings are applied. In addition, long term therapy with corticosteroids can cause skin lesions such as atrophy, telangiectasia and striae.

Topical administration of corticosteroids to pregnant animals can cause foetal abnormalities. The relevance of this finding to human beings has not been established. Nevertheless, the product should not be administered during pregnancy unless the possible risks involved have been carefully considered.

Introduction of the product into the eye should be avoided. If accidental instillation occurs, the eye and conjunctival sac should immediately be thoroughly rinsed under a thin jet of running water with the eye wide open. Subsequent referral to a specialist is indicated.

No specific precautions are necessary in the elderly.

Side-effects: Transient local mild irritation at the application site has been reported. Hypersensitivity has rarely been reported. Discontinuation of therapy usually results in cessation of the symptoms.

Overdosage: If accidental ingestion of large quantities of the product occurs, an appropriate method of gastric emptying may be used if considered desirable, followed by symptomatic therapy. Topical application of large quantities of corticosteroids, especially under occlusion, may result in sufficient absorption to produce systemic effects.

Pharmaceutical precautions Protect from light.

Legal category POM.

Package quantities 15 g tube.

Further information Nil.

Product licence number 0076/0062.

RETIN-A* LOTION, GEL, CREAM

Presentation Retin-A is available as either a clear yellow solution of 0.025% w/w Tretinoin BP supplied in amber bottles or in tubes of Tretinoin BP gel 0.01% w/w or Tretinoin BP cream 0.025% w/w.

Retin-A Forte is available in tubes of Tretinoin BP gel 0.025% w/w and cream 0.05% w/w.

Uses For topical application in the treatment of acne vulgaris in which comedones, papules and pustules predominate.

Retin-A Lotion is best suited for large areas such as the back.

Retin-A Gel is best suited for severe acne, for initial therapy and for oily and dark skin.

Retin-A Cream is best suited for use on dry and fair skin.

Dosage and administration Retin-A should be applied once or twice daily to the area of skin where acne lesions occur. Only apply sufficient to cover the affected area lightly, using a gauze swab, cotton wool or the tips of clean fingers. Avoid over-saturation to the extent that excess medication could run into the eyes, angles of the nose or other areas where treatment is not intended.

Initial application may cause transitory stinging and a feeling of warmth. The correct frequency of administration should produce a slight erythema similar to that of mild sunburn. In patients with sensitive skin, application once daily may be sufficient. In patients with normal skin, increasing the frequency of application to twice daily is usually necessary.

It is also possible to apply Retin-A and benzoyl peroxide alternately. The suggested regimens are either benzoyl peroxide in the morning and Retin-A in the evening or the preparations could be used on alternate days.

If Retin-A is applied excessively, no more rapid or better results will be obtained and marked redness, peeling or discomfort may occur. Should this occur accidentally or through over enthusiastic use, application should be discontinued for a few days.

Patience is needed in this treatment, since therapeutic effects will not usually be observed until after 6-8 weeks of treatment. During the early weeks of treatment, an apparent exacerbation of inflammatory lesions may occur. This is due to the action of the medication on deep, previously unseen comedones and papules. Once the acne lesions have responded satisfactorily, it should be possible to maintain the improvement with less frequent applications.

Cosmetics may be used, but the areas to be treated should be thoroughly washed beforehand. Astringent toiletries should be avoided.

Contra-indications, warnings, etc Use of the product should be discontinued if hypersensitivity to any of the ingredients should occur. Retin-A should be kept away from the eye and eyelids, the mouth and other mucous membranes. Care should also be taken not to let the medication accumulate in folds of the skin and the angles of the nose. Retin-A should not be applied to eczematous skin, nor to cuts and abrasions.

Retin-A should not be applied at the same time as other skin medications, particularly those containing peeling agents such as sulphur, resorcinol, benzoyl peroxide or salicyclic acid.

Following prolonged use of a peeling agent it is advisable to 'rest' a patients' skin until the effects of the peeling agent subside before the use of Retin-A is begun. When Retin-A and peeling agent therapy are alternated, contact dermatitis may result and the frequency of application may have to be reduced.

Recent studies in mice treated with the active ingredient (tretinoin) of Retin-A and exposed to artificial sunlight suggest that tretinoin may speed up the appearance of sunlight induced skin tumours. Laboratory mice treated with tretinoin but not exposed to sunlight did not develop skin tumours. The significance of these studies as related to human beings is unknown. However it is important to avoid or minimise exposure of Retin-A treated areas to sunlight or sunlamps during the course of treatment. Patients with sunburn should be advised not to use the product until fully recovered because of heightened susceptibility to sunlight as a result of the use of tretinoin. Weather extremes such as wind or cold, also may be irritating to patients under treatment with tretinoin.

Retin-A should not be used in patients with a personal or family history of cutaneous epithelioma.

High oral doses of tretinoin (retinoic acid), like Vitamin A, are teratogenic in animals. However, reproduction studies performed in rats and rabbits at dermal doses up to 50 times the human dose (assuming the human dose to be 500 mg of gel per day) have revealed no evidence of impaired fertility or harm to the foetus due to tretinoin (retinoic acid). There was, however, a slightly higher incidence of irregularly contoured or partially ossified skull bones in some rat and rabbit foetuses. The use of Retin-A should be avoided in pregnancy.

Side effects: The application of excessive amounts of Retin-A to the skin may cause severe erythema, irritation and discomfort. Should this occur, the frequency of application should be reduced or the use of Retin-A discontinued temporarily. Temporary hypo or hyperpigmentation has been reported in a few individuals treated with Retin-A. All side effects so far reported have been reversible upon discontinuation of Retin-A therapy.

Overdosage: Retin-A is intended for topical use only. Excessive use is dealt with under side-effects. Taken orally by mischance Retin-A is liable to taste unpleasant. Unless the amount is small an appropriate method of gastric emptying should be used as soon as possible.

Pharmaceutical precautions Store in a cool place. The 100 ml bottle of lotion should be protected from light and any remaining medicine discarded on completion of treatment.

Legal category POM.

Package quantities *Lotion:* Amber glass bottle containing 100 ml.

Gel and Cream: Tubes containing 60 g.

Further information Nil.

Product licence numbers

Lotion	0076/0037
Gel	0076/0051
Cream	0076/0057
Gel Forte	0076/0050
Cream Forte	0076/0056

SULTRIN* TRIPLE SULFA CREAM

Presentation A white, non-staining cream containing Sulphathiazole BP 3.42% w/w, Sulphacetamide 2.86% w/w and Sulphabenzamide 3.70% w/w.

Uses For the treatment of infections caused by *Haemophilus Vaginalis* and non-specific bacterial vaginitis and cervicitis. It may also be used in the prevention of bacterial complications following cervical and vaginal surgery and vulvectomy and as an anti-infective in the post-partum state.

Dosage and administration One applicatorful intravaginally twice daily for 10 days. The dosage may then be reduced to once a day if necessary.

Contra-indications, warnings, etc Sulphonamide sensitivity and renal disease.

There is no evidence as to the safety of Sultrin in human pregnancy nor is there evidence from animal work that sulphonamides administered vaginally are free from hazard. Therefore, although no reports of adverse effects of Sultrin in pregnancy have been documented, as with any drug in this category, use in pregnancy should be avoided.

The safety and effectiveness for use in children have not been established.

The most frequent adverse reaction to Sultrin is localised irritation and/or allergy.

Precautions: Since the primary route of excretion of sulphonamides is renal, caution should be used in prescribing the product to elderly patients who potentially may have impaired renal function.

Overdosage: Sultrin Triple Sulfa Cream is intended for intravaginal use. If accidental ingestion of large quantities of the product occurs, an appropriate method of gastric emptying may be used if considered desirable. Elimination of sulphonamides in the urine may be assisted by giving alkalis such as sodium bicarbonate and increasing fluid intake.

Pharmaceutical precautions Store at room temperature, avoid excessive heat.

Legal category POM.

Package quantities Tube containing 78 g with the ORTHO* Plastic Vaginal Applicator.

Further information The three sulphonamides exert optimal bacteriostatic action at different specific pH levels. The point of optimal activity for each drug is:

Sulphathiazole	pH 7.0
Sulphacetamide	pH 5.2
Sulphabenzamide	pH 4.6

Product licence number 0076/5012R.

SULTRIN* VAGINAL TABLETS

Presentation Sultrin Vaginal Tablets are white, non-staining, water-dispersible, lozenge-shaped tablets engraved on one side with the Ortho shield design and on the reverse with C. Each tablet contains:

Sulphathiazole BP	172.5 mg
Sulphacetamide	143.75 mg
Sulphabenzamide	184.0 mg

in a rapidly disintegrating base.

Uses For the treatment of infections caused by *Haemophilus Vaginalis* and non-specific bacterial vaginitis and cervicitis. It may also be used in the prevention of bacterial complications following cervical and vaginal surgery and vulvectomy and as an anti-infective in the post-partum state.

Dosage and administration One tablet placed high in the vagina twice daily for 10 days. Repeat if necessary.

Contra-indications, warnings, etc Sulphonamide sensitivity; renal disease.

There is no evidence as to the safety of Sultrin in human pregnancy nor is there evidence from animal work that sulphonamides administered vaginally are free from hazard. Therefore, although no reports of adverse reactions of Sultrin in pregnancy have been documented, as with any drug in this category, use in pregnancy should be avoided.

The safety and effectiveness for use in children have not been established.

The most frequent adverse reaction to Sultrin is localised irritation and/or allergy.

Precaution: Since the primary route of excretion of sulphonamides is renal, caution should be used in prescribing the product to elderly patients who potentially may have impaired renal function.

Overdosage: Sultrin Vaginal Tablets are intended for intravaginal use. If accidental ingestion of large quantities of the product occurs, an appropriate method of gastric emptying may be used if considered desirable. Elimination of sulphonamides in the urine may be assisted by giving alkalis such as sodium bicarbonate and increasing fluid intake.

Pharmaceutical precautions None known.

Legal category POM.

Package quantities Packages of 20 foil-wrapped tablets with vaginal applicator.

Further information The three sulphonamides exert optimal bacteriostatic action at different specific pH levels. The point of optimal activity for each drug is:

Sulphathiazole	pH 7.0
Sulphacetamide	pH 5.2
Sulphabenzamide	pH 4.6

Product licence number 0076/5013R.

TOLECTIN* 200 mg CAPSULES

Presentation A size '1' hard gelatin capsule with an ivory opaque body and an orange opaque cap printed 'T-200', containing a yellow powder. For oral administration.

Tolectin (tolmetin sodium) 200 mg capsules each containing 246 mg of tolmetin sodium dihydrate, which is equivalent to 200 mg of tolmetin. Each capsule contains 18 mg (0.784 mEq) of sodium.

Uses Tolectin is a non-steroidal anti-inflammatory agent with analgesic and antipyretic properties. It is indicated for: Rheumatoid arthritis; osteoarthritis; ankylosing spondylitis; peri-articular disorders such as fibrositis and bursitis.

Dosage and administration The usual dosage is 600–1800 mg daily in 2, 3 or 4 divided doses depending on patient response and the severity of the disease. In juvenile rheumatoid arthritis the dosage is 20–25 mg/kg/day in 3–4 divided doses. The maximum dose is 30 mg/kg/day or 1800 mg/day whatever the body weight.

Contra-indications, warnings, etc
Contra-indications: Active peptic ulcer; previous sensitivity to Tolectin, aspirin, or other non-steroidal anti-inflammatory agents which have induced symptoms of asthma, rhinitis or urticaria.

As with other non-steroidal anti-inflammatory drugs, allergic reactions, including anaphylactoid reactions, have been reported with Tolectin. Patients who have anaphylactoid reactions on Tolectin should be treated with conventional therapy, such as adrenaline, antihistamines and/or steroids. A patient who exhibits sensitivity to Tolectin should be withdrawn from therapy.

Warnings: Tolectin should be used with caution in patients with a history of upper gastro-intestinal tract disease. Tolectin prolongs bleeding time and patients who may be adversely affected should be carefully monitored during Tolectin therapy.

No teratogenic effects have been found in animals, but, as in the case of all drugs, caution should be exercised in the prescribing of Tolectin to pregnant women. Safety for use during pregnancy or lactation has not been established.

Renal papillary necrosis has occurred in animals after long term administration although there has been no evidence of renal toxicity in clinical trials. However, since Tolectin is eliminated primarily by the kidneys, caution should be observed and patients with impaired renal function, such as the elderly, should be closely monitored and may require lower doses.

In patients with rheumatoid arthritis who have received certain anti-rheumatic drugs, eye changes have been observed. During clinical studies of up to 2 years with Tolectin, no such changes have occurred.

Side-effects: Epigastric discomfort, headache (rare), water and sodium retention, skin rash. Gastro-intestinal disturbance may occur but blood loss due to Tolectin is rare.

Small and transient decreases in haemoglobin and haematocrit not associated with gastro-intestinal bleeding have occurred. A few cases of granulocytopenia have been observed.

Management of overdosage: In the event of overdosage, the stomach should be emptied by inducing vomiting or by gastric lavage followed by the administration of activated charcoal. Studies in rats indicate that the urinary excretion of the drug is enhanced when the urine is made alkaline with sodium bicarbonate.

Pharmaceutical precautions Extremes of temperature and humidity should be avoided.

Legal category POM.

Package quantities Container of 90 capsules.

Further information In clinical trials Tolectin has shown no interaction with concomitantly administered drugs, such as gold, corticosteroids and paracetamol.

Preliminary studies indicate that Tolectin does not interact with anticoagulant drugs.

In adult diabetic patients under treatment with either sulphonylureas or insulin no changes have been observed in the clinical effects of either Tolectin or the hypoglycaemic agents.

The metabolites of tolmetin in urine have been found to give positive tests for proteinuria using tests which rely on acid precipitation as their endpoint. No interference is seen in the tests for proteinuria using dye-impregnated commercially available reagent strips.

Product licence number 0076/0084.

TOLECTIN* 400 mg CAPSULES

Presentation A size 'O' hard gelatin capsule with an orange opaque body and an orange opaque cap printed T-400 containing a yellow powder. For oral administration.

Tolectin (tolmetin sodium) 400 mg capsules each contain 490 mg of tolmetin sodium dihydrate, which is equivalent to 400 mg of tolmetin. Each capsule contains 36 mg (1.568 m Eq) of sodium.

Uses Tolectin is a non-steroidal anti-inflammatory agent with analgesic and antipyretic properties. It is indicated for: Rheumatoid arthritis; osteoarthritis; ankylosing spondylitis; peri-articular disorders such as fibrositis and bursitis.

Dosage and administration The initial adult dosage is 400 mg three times daily. This may be adjusted within the range 800–1600 mg daily in 2, 3 or 4 divided doses depending on patient response and the severity of the disease. Doses of larger than 2000 mg/day have not been studied and are not recommended.

Tolectin is rapidly and completely absorbed with peak plasma levels being reached within 30–60 minutes after an oral therapeutic dose.

Contra-indications, warnings, etc *Contra-indications:* active peptic ulcer; previous sensitivity to Tolectin, aspirin, or other non-steroidal anti-inflammatory agents, which have induced symptoms of asthma, rhinitis or urticaria. As with other non-steroidal anti-inflammatory drugs, allergic reactions, including anaphylactoid reactions, have been reported with Tolectin. Patients who have anaphylactoid reactions on Tolectin should be treated with conventional therapy, such as adrenaline, antihistamines and/or steroids. A patient who exhibits sensitivity to Tolectin should be withdrawn from therapy.

Warnings: Tolectin should be used with caution in patients with a history of upper gastrointestinal tract disease. Peptic ulceration and gastrointestinal bleeding have been reported in patients receiving Tolectin therapy. Tolectin, like salicylates, inhibits platelet function and prolongs bleeding time. In clinical studies an effect on prothrombin time in subjects stabilised on warfarin was not detected: however, in clinical use, cases of increased prothrombin time have been reported. Therefore, patients with coagulation disorders and those stabilised on warfarin should be closely monitored when Tolectin is administered.

No teratogenic effects have been found in animals, but, as in the case of all new drugs, caution should be exercised in the prescribing of Tolectin to pregnant women. Safety for use during pregnancy or lactation has not been established.

Renal papillary necrosis has occurred in animals after long term administration although there has been no evidence of renal toxicity in clinical trials. However, since Tolectin is eliminated primarily by the kidneys, caution should be observed and patients with impaired renal function, such as the elderly, should be closely monitored and may require lower doses.

In patients with rheumatoid arthritis who have received certain anti-rheumatic drugs, eye changes have been observed. During clinical studies of up to 2 years with Tolectin no such changes have occurred. Because the safety and effectiveness have not been established in infants under two years of age, use of Tolectin in infants is not recommended.

Side effects: Adverse reactions observed in clinical trials were usually mild. The most frequently observed reactions occurring with Tolectin administration are nausea, gastrointestinal distress, dizziness, diarrhoea, elevated blood pressure, oedema and allergic reactions.

Small and transient decreases in haemoglobin and haematocrit not associated with gastrointestinal bleeding have occurred. A few cases of granulocytopenia have been observed.

Overdosage: In the event of overdosage, the stomach should be emptied by inducing vomiting or by gastric lavage followed by the administration of activated charcoal.

Pharmaceutical precautions Extremes of temperature and humidity should be avoided.

Legal category POM.

Package quantities Containers of 90 capsules.

Further information Clinical studies have shown that when added to a regimen of gold salts or corticosteroids Tolectin has produced added benefit.

In adult diabetic patients under treatment with either sulphonylureas or insulin no changes have been observed in the clinical effects of either Tolectin or the hypoglycaemic agents.

The metabolites of tolmetin in urine have been found to give positive tests for proteinuria using tests which rely on acid precipitation as their endpoint. No interference is seen in the tests for proteinuria using dye-impregnated commercially available reagent strips.

Product licence number 0076/0075.

TYLEX* CAPSULES

Presentation Tylex Capsules are size 0 hard gelatin capsules imprinted C30 with a white body and red cap. Each capsule contains 500 mg of Paracetamol PhEur and 30 mg Codeine Phosphate PhEur.

Uses For the relief of severe pain.

Dosage and administration Tylex Capsules are given orally. The usual adult dose is one or two capsules every four hours as required. The total daily dose should not exceed 240 mg codeine phosphate.

Dosage should be adjusted according to the severity of the pain and the response of the patient. However, it should be kept in mind that tolerance to codeine can develop with continued use and that the incidence of untoward effects is dose related. Doses of codeine higher than 60 mg fail to give commensurate relief of pain but merely prolong analgesia and are associated with an appreciably increased incidence of undesirable side effects.

Contra-indications, warnings, etc Tylex Capsules should not be administered to patients who have previously exhibited hypersensitivity to either paracetamol or codeine.

Tylex Capsules are not recommended during pregnancy or lactation since safety in pregnant women or nursing mothers has not been established.

Not recommended for children under 12 years.

Precautions: The capsules contain sodium metabisulphite, a sulphite that may cause allergic-type reactions including anaphylactic symptoms and life threatening or less severe asthmatic episodes in certain susceptible people. The overall prevalence of sulphite sensitivity in the general population is unknown and probably low. Sulphite sensitivity is seen more frequently in asthmatic than non-asthmatic people.

Tylex should be used with caution in patients with head injuries, increased intracranial pressure, acute abdominal conditions, the elderly and debilitated, and those with severe impairment of hepatic or renal function, hypothyroidism, Addison's disease, and prostatic hypertrophy or urethral stricture.

At high doses codeine has most of the disadvantages of morphine, including respiratory depression. Patients receiving other central nervous system depressants, including other narcotic analgesics, antipsychotics, antianxiety agents and alcohol, concomitantly with Tylex may exhibit an additive depressant effect. When such therapy is contemplated, the dose of one or both agents should be reduced. Concurrent use of MAO inhibitors or tricyclic antidepressants with codeine may increase the effect of either the antidepressant or codeine. Concurrent use of anticholinergics and codeine may produce paralytic ileus.

Codeine can produce drug dependence of the morphine type, and therefore has the potential for being abused. Codeine may impair the mental and/or physical abilities required for the performance of potentially hazardous tasks.

Side-effects: The most frequently observed reactions include light headedness, dizziness, sedation, shortness of breath, nausea and vomiting. These effects seem more prominent in ambulatory than non-ambulatory patients and some of these adverse reactions may be alleviated if the patient lies down. Other adverse reactions include allergic reactions, euphoria, dysphoria, constipation, abdominal pain and pruritus.

Overdose: Early symptoms following a potential hepatotoxic overdose with paracetamol may include nausea, vomiting, diaphoresis and general malaise. Clinical laboratory evidence of hepatic toxicity may not be apparent until 48 to 72 hours post-ingestion. If paracetamol overdose is suspected, antidotal therapy with N-acetylcysteine should be administered as early as possible.

Serious overdose with codeine is characterised by respiratory depression, extreme somnolence progressing to stupor or coma, skeletal muscle flaccidity, cold and clammy skin and sometimes bradycardia and hypotension. In severe overdose with codeine, apnoea, circulatory collapse, cardiac arrest and death may occur. Primary attention should be given to the re-establishment of adequate respiratory exchange through the provision of a patent airway and the institution of assisted or controlled ventilation. Oxygen, intravenous fluids, vasopressors and other supportive measures should be employed as indicated. Opioid antagonists may be employed.

Gastric lavage should be considered.

Pharmaceutical precautions Protect from light.

Legal category CD (Sch 5), POM.

Package quantities Containers of 100 capsules.

Further information Nil.

Product licence number 0076/0109.

**Trade Mark*

Cilag Biotech
A division of Cilag Limited
PO Box 79, Saunderton
High Wycombe
Buckinghamshire HP14 4HJ

EPREX* ▼

Presentation Eprex is a sterile, clear, colourless aqueous solution for intravenous or subcutaneous injection, containing 2,000, or 4,000 U/ml epoetin alfa (a recombinant human erythropoietin) and 2.5 mg/ml human serum albumin in 1 ml vials.

Uses Eprex is indicated for the treatment of anaemia associated with chronic renal failure in patients on dialysis.

Eprex is also indicated for the treatment of severe anaemia of renal origin accompanied by clinical symptoms in patients with renal insufficiency not yet undergoing dialysis.

Dosage and administration
Dialysis patients: The recommended starting dose is 50 U/kg body weight, three times per week (total 150 U/kg per week) administered as an intravenous injection over one to two minutes. Further dose increments will depend upon the initial response. Dose adjustments in steps of 25 U/kg in intervals of four weeks are recommended. If the rate of haemoglobin rise exceeds 2 g/dl per month at 50 U/kg three times per week, downward dosage adjustments should be made by omitting one of the weekly doses. The maximum dose should generally not exceed 200 U/kg three times per week (total 600 U/kg per week). When an Hb level of 10–12 g/dl (HCT 30–35%) has been achieved, the total maintenance dose (average 100–300 U/kg) should be divided into two or three injections. The optimal level of Hb should be judged by the doctor. Available data indicate that patients starting treatment at very low levels (<6 g/dl) may require higher maintenance doses than those starting therapy with an Hb of 8 g/dl or above.

Pre-dialysis patients: The recommended starting dose is 50 U/kg, three times per week (total 150 U/kg per week). The subcutaneous route of administration should be preferred over the intravenous route of administration. For the subcutaneous route, a maximum volume of 1 ml at one injection site should generally not be exceeded. In the case of larger volumes, more than one site should be chosen for the injection. Dosage may be increased in 25 U/kg increments (3 times weekly) until the desired response, 10–12 g/dl (HCT 30–35%) is achieved. A maintenance dose of btween 50 and 100 U/kg per week divided into three injections may be administered to maintain haemoglobin values at the desired level. The maximum dosage should not exceed 200 U/kg body weight three times a week.

Parenteral drug products should be visually inspected for particulate matter and discolouration prior to administration.

Prepare Eprex for injection by drawing solution into a syringe from a single use vial. Attach needle for injection.

For dialysis patients, administration is by i.v. injection over one to two minutes. In patients on dialysis the injection should follow the dialysis procedure. Slow injection over five minutes may be beneficial to those who experience flu-like symptoms.

For pre-dialysis patients the subcutaneous route of administration should be preferred over the intravenous route of administration.

Do not administer by intravenous infusion or in conjunction with other drug solutions.

Paediatric use: Safety and efficacy in children have not been established.

Contra-indications, warnings, etc
Contra-indications: Eprex is contra-indicated in uncontrolled hypertension.

Warnings and precautions: Iron status should be evaluated for all patients prior to and during treatment and iron supplementation administered if necessary. In most cases, serum ferritin values fall simultaneously with the rise in packed cell volume. Therefore, oral iron substitution of 200–300 mg/day is recommended for all patients whose serum ferritin levels are below 100 mg/ml.

In addition, hyperkalaemia has been observed in isolated cases.

Other causes of anaemia, such as vitamin B_{12} or folate deficiency should be excluded before instituting therapy with Eprex.

Eprex should be used with caution in the presence of untreated, inadequately treated or poorly controllable hypertension (close monitoring is required to detect any changes in blood pressure and serum electrolytes). It may be necessary to add or increase anti-hypertensive treatment. If blood pressure cannot be controlled, Eprex treatment should be discontinued.

Eprex should also be used with caution in those patients with ischaemic vascular disease, or history of seizures, and in the presence of malignant tumours, epilepsy, thrombocytosis, chronic liver failure, and known hypersensitivity to the medication.

A gradual increase in Hb of less than 2 g/dl per month is recommended. All patients receiving Eprex should have the level of their haemoglobin measured frequently (weekly) until it is stable at 10–12 g/dl. Thereafter the level should be measured periodically. When Eprex is discontinued, the haemoglobin concentration decreases by approximately 0.5 g/dl weekly.

Non-response to Eprex therapy should prompt a search for causative factors which include: iron, folate, or Vitamin B12 deficiency; aluminium intoxication; intercurrent infections, inflammatory or traumatic episodes; occult blood loss; haemolysis; bone marrow fibrosis.

Increase in pre-dialysis urea and creatinine may occur in individual patients as a result of increased protein intake, in which case dialysis regimen modification may be necessary.

Based on information available to date, correction of anaemia with Eprex in pre-dialysis patients does not accelerate the rate of progression of renal insufficiency.

Pregnancy and lactation: Eprex has been shown to decrease foetal body weight, delay ossification and increase mortality in animals when given in weekly doses of approximately 20 times the recommended human weekly dose. These changes are believed to be secondary to decreased maternal body weight gain.

There are no adequate and well controlled studies in pregnant women, Eprex should be used in pregnancy and lactation only if the potential benefit justifies the potential risk to the foetus.

The following adverse events have been reported:
- 'Flu-like' symptoms such as headaches, joint pains, feelings of weakness, dizziness, tiredness and chills may occur, especially at the start of treatment.
- The most frequent adverse reaction during treatment

is a dose dependent increase in blood pressure or aggravation of existing hypertension. These increases in blood pressure can be treated with drugs. Moreover, monitoring of blood pressure is recommended, particularly at the start of therapy.

- The following reactions may also occur in isolated patients with normal or low blood pressure: hypertensive crisis with encephalopathy-like symptoms (e.g. headaches, confused state) and generalised tonoclonal seizures, requiring the immediate attention of a physician and intensive medical care. Particular attention should be paid to sudden stabbing migraine-like headaches as a possible warning signal.
- Serum potassium levels should be regularly monitored during Eprex therapy. Potassium elevation has been exhibited in a few predialysis patients receiving Eprex though causality has not been established. If an elevated (or rising) serum potassium level is observed then consideration should be given to ceasing Eprex administration until hyperkalaemia has been corrected.
- There may be a moderate dose-dependent rise in the platelet count within the normal range during treatment with Eprex. This regresses during the course of continued therapy. Development of thrombocytosis is very rare. It is recommended that the platelet count is regularly monitored during the first eight weeks of therapy.
- Shunt thromboses may occur, particularly in patients with a tendency to hypotension or whose arteriovenous fistulae exhibit complications (e.g. stenoses, aneurysms, etc). Early shunt revision and thrombosis prophylaxis by administration of acetylsalicylic acid for example is recommended in these patients.
- An increase in heparin dose during dialysis is frequently required during the course of therapy with Eprex as a result of the increased packed cell volume. Occlusion of the dialysis system is possible if heparinisation is not optimum.
- The following adverse effects have also been occasionally observed; – seizures, skin reactions, palpebral oedema, possibly allergic in nature.

Interactions: Eprex should not be administered by intravenous infusion or in conjunction with other drug solutions.

No evidence exists indicating that treatment with Eprex alters the metabolism of other drugs. However, since cyclosporine is bound by red blood cells there is potential for drug interaction. If Eprex is given concomitantly with cyclosporin, blood levels of cyclosporin should be monitored, and the dose of cyclosporin adjusted as the haematocrit rises.

The efficacy of Eprex would be potentiated by the simultaneous administration of a haematinic agent where a deficiency state existed.

Overdosage: The therapeutic margin of Eprex is very wide. Even at very high serum levels, no symptoms of poisoning have been observed.

Incompatibilities: Do not administer by intravenous infusion or in conjunction with other drug solutions. See 'Injections' above.

Further information: Erythropoietin is an endogenous glycoprotein hormone that regulates red blood cell production. Its production primarily occurs in, and is regulated by, the kidney in response to changes in tissue oxygenation.

Measurement of epoetin alfa following multiple dose intravenous administration revealed a half life of approximately four hours in normal patients and five hours in renal failure patients.

Following subcutaneous injection, serum levels are much lower than those achieved by intravenous injection. The levels increase slowly, reaching a peak between twelve and eighteen hours post dosing. The peak is always well below the peak achieved using the i.v. route. There is no accumulation, levels remaining the same whether determined twenty four hours after the first or last injection.

The half life is difficult to evaluate for the subcutaneous route and is estimated at about twenty four hours. The bioavailability of subcutaneously injected erythropoeitin is approximately 20% that of the drug when administered intravenously.

Pharmaceutical precautions Store at 2° to 8°C. Do not freeze or shake. Protect from light. Eprex is a sterile but unpreserved product. Under no circumstances should more than one dose be administered per vial.

Legal category POM.

Package quantities Packages of 6 vials each containing 2,000 or 4,000 U/ml of epoetin alfa.

Product licence numbers

Eprex 2,000 U/ml	0076/0150
Eprex 4,000 U/ml	0076/0151

**Trade Mark*

Consolidated Chemicals Limited

Abbey Road
The Industrial Estate
Wrexham
Clwyd LL13 9PW

APP* STOMACH POWDER

Presentation A white powder.

Powder: Contains in 100 g:

Calcium Carbonate BP	37.9%
Magnesium Carbonate BP	37.0%
Magnesium Trisilicate BP	20%
Bismuth Carbonate BP	2.0%
Aluminium Hydroxide Gel USP	3.0%
Homatropine Methyl Bromide USP	0.1%

Uses The symptomatic relief of dyspepsia, excess acidity, gastric and intestinal spasms, symptomatic treatment of gastric and duodenal ulcer.

Dosage and administration
Adults including the elderly and children 12 years and above: 1 × 5 ml (teaspoonful) in water or milk, 3–4 times daily after meals.

Children: Not recommended for children under 12 years old.

Contra-indications, warnings, etc APP Stomach Powder is contra-indicated in glaucoma and myasthenia gravis because of the anticholinergic effects of homatropine.

Side-effects: Diarrhoea, constipation and flatulence may occur.

Use in pregnancy and lactation: There are no animal data on the effects of APP Stomach powder in pregnancy or lactation and there are no specific human data, therefore APP Stomach Powder should only be used if there is no safer alternative.

Drug interactions: The calcium carbonate content may enhance the action of digitalis glycosides and calcium carbonate may reduce the absorption of tetracycline. The preparation is incompatible with alkalis and halide compounds.

Overdosage: Symptoms would reflect the toxic effects of anticholinergic agents. These include flushing and dry skin, tachycardia, rapid respiration, hyperpyrexia, restlessness, confusion and excitement. In severe intoxication, depression of the CNS may occur with hypertension or circulatory failure and respiratory depression.

Treatment: Empty the stomach by aspiration and lavage. Administer charcoal to prevent absorption of homatropine. Physostigmine can be administered parenterally to counteract the central and peripheral effects. Excitement may be controlled by diazepam.

Pharmaceutical precautions Store in air-tight container in a dry place.

Legal category P.

Package quantities Containers of 100 g.

Further information Postprandial administration ensures the preparation resides for a longer period of time in the stomach enabling its neutralising potential to be achieved. Absorption of active ingredients into the bloodstream will occur, but side effects which result from high oral doses of a simple antacid are unlikely in this formulation.

Product licence number 0183/5033R.

APP* STOMACH TABLETS

Presentation A plain flat white tablet.

Tablets: Each tablet contains:

Calcium Carbonate BP	183.0 mg
Magnesium Carbonate BP	180.0 mg
Magnesium Trisilicate BP	108.0 mg
Bismuth Carbonate BP	12.5 mg
Aluminium Hydroxide Gel BP	15.0 mg
Homatropine Methyl Bromide USP	1.5 mg

Uses The symptomatic relief of dyspepsia, excess acidity, gastric and intestinal spasm, symptomatic treatment of gastric and duodenal ulcer.

Dosage and administration
Adults including the elderly and children 12 years and above: One tablet to be chewed three or four times daily after meals.

Children: Not recommended for children under 12 years.

Contra-indications, warnings, etc APP Stomach Tablets are contra-indicated in glaucoma and myasthenia gravis because of the anticholinergic effects of homatropine.

Side-effects: Diarrhoea, constipation and flatulence may occur.

Use in pregnancy and lactation: There are no animal data on the effects of APP Stomach powder in pregnancy or lactation and there are no specific human data, therefore APP Stomach Tablets should only be used if there is no safer alternative.

Drug interactions: The calcium carbonate content may enhance the action of digitalis glycosides and calcium carbonate may reduce the absorption of tetracycline. The preparation is incompatible with alkalis and halide compounds.

Overdosage: Symptoms would reflect the toxic effects of anticholinergic agents. These include flushing and dry skin, tachycardia, rapid respiration, hyperpyrexia, restlessness, confusion and excitement. In severe intoxication, depression of the CNS may occur with hypertension or circulatory failure and respiratory depression.

Treatment – empty the stomach by aspiration and lavage. Administer charcoal to prevent absorption of homatropine. Physostigmine can be administered parenterally to counteract the central and peripheral effects. Excitement may be controlled by diazepam.

Pharmaceutical precautions Store in air-tight container in a dry place.

Legal category P.

Package quantities Containers of 50 and 250.

Further information The tablets contain lactose. Chewing or sucking of the tablet increases the surface area of antacid available to the gastric acid, thereby increasing its neutralising activity. Postprandial administration ensures the preparation resides for a longer period of time in the stomach enabling its neutralising potential to be achieved. Absorption of active ingredients into the bloodstream will occur, but side effects which result from high oral doses of a single antacid are unlikely in this formulation.

Product licence number 0183/5013R.

CARDIACAP* CAPSULES

Presentation Sustained release capsules. Each capsule contains pentaerythritol tetranitrate (PETN) 30 mg. Blue/yellow capsule size 2 containing white and cream granules.

Uses Sustained symptomatic relief of angina pectoris.

Dosage and administration
Adults including the elderly: One capsule to be taken every 12 hours.

Children: There is no data specific to children to recommend a dose.

Contra-indications, warnings, etc Contra-indicated in patients who are sensitive to nitrates, or in patients with cerebral haemorrhage or acute myocardial infarction. It should be used with caution in glaucoma.

Use in pregnancy: due to the nature of the indication, experience in pregnancy is limited. There is no evidence of the safety of PETN in human pregnancy nor is there any relevant animal work. Use in pregnancy should be avoided unless there is no safer alternative.

Side-effects: nitrate headaches, transient dizziness and weakness may occur. These may affect the ability to drive and operate machines. Skin rashes are occasionally reported.

Overdosage: symptoms include dizziness, flushing, hypotension and methaemoglobinaemia. Treatment: gastric lavage may be used to remove any capsules remaining in the stomach. Bed rest with head lowered. Give oxygen and maintain respiration. methylene blue 1 or 2 mg/kg body weight may be given iv for methaemoglobinaemia.

Drug interactions: pentaerythritol tetranitrate can antagonise adrenaline, noradrenaline, acetylcholine and histamine. Alcohol can accentuate cerebral ischaemia associated with postural hypotension.

Pharmaceutical precautions Store in a cool place, protected from light in a sealed container.

Legal category P.

Package quantities 30 capsules.

Further information Cardiacap capsules release their active principle by diffusion. This process ensures a constant release of PETN over approximately 12 hours. The process is independent of pH, enzymatic activity and gastric motility. No excessively high peak blood levels are attained, therefore the product tends to be devoid of associated side effects.

Product licence number 0183/5018R.

FERROCAP* CAPSULES

Presentation Slow release capsules. Each capsule contains:

Ferrous fumarate 330 mg
(equivalent to 110 mg elemental iron)

Green/orange capsule, size 0, containing brown and white granules.

Uses Ferrocap Capsules are recommended for treatment of anaemia from iron deficiency or chronic blood loss, and in all cases where dietary iron supplementation is desired.

Dosage and administration
Adults including the elderly: One capsule daily.

Children: Not recommended.

Contra-indications, warnings, etc
Contra-indications and precautions: None known.

Use in pregnancy: Iron preparations are frequently used in pregnancy and there is no evidence to suggest a hazard to the foetus.

Side-effects: Nausea and other gastrointestinal side effects are associated with oral iron therapy. However, these are less likely to occur with Ferrocap because of the special release mechanism.

Overdosage: Symptoms of overdosage with iron salts include epigastric pain, nausea and vomiting, haematemesis and circulatory collapse. In severe cases, encephalopathy, acute hepatic necrosis and acute renal failure may develop after a latent period. Treatment: induce vomiting. Administer 2 g desferrioxamine mesylate parenterally then carry out gastric lavage. A solution of 5 g desferrioxamine in 100 ml fluid may be left in the stomach.

Drug interactions: iron preparations interact with tetracyclines reducing the absorption of both. Oral iron may also reduce the absorption of penicillamine. Magnesium trisilicate and zinc salts may reduce the absorption of iron salts.

Pharmaceutical precautions None.

Legal category P.

Package quantities 30 and 200 capsules.

Further information Ferrocap releases its active principle by diffusion. This process ensures gradual release over four hours which is independent of pH, gastric enzymatic activity or agitation. This avoids the risk of high initial concentrations in the blood stream.

Product licence number 0183/5014R.

FERROCAP*-F 350 CAPSULES

Presentation Slow release capsules. Each capsule contains:

Ferrous fumarate 330 mg
(equivalent to 110 mg elemental iron)
Folic acid 350 micrograms

Standard pink capsule, size 0, containing brown, white and yellow granules.

Uses Ferrocap-F 350 Capsules are recommended in the management of anaemia in pregnancy, for folate deficiency and where iron intolerance is a factor.

Dosage and administration
Adults including the elderly: One capsule daily.

Children: Not recommended.

Contra-indications, warnings, etc None known.

Use in pregnancy: Iron preparations are frequently used in pregnancy and there is no evidence to suggest a hazard to the foetus.

Side-effects: nausea and other gastrointestinal side effects are associated with oral iron therapy.

Overdosage: Symptoms of overdosage with iron salts include epigastric pain, nausea and vomiting, haematemesis and circulatory collapse. In severe cases, encephalopathy, acute hepatic necrosis and acute renal failure may develop after a latent period. Treatment: induce vomiting. Administer 2 g desferrioxamine mesylate parenterally then carry out gastric lavage. A solution of 5 g desferrioxamine in 100 ml fluid may be left in the stomach.

Drug interactions: iron preparations interact with tetracyclines reducing the absorption of both. Oral iron may also reduce the absorption of penicillamine. Magnesium trisilicate and zinc salts may reduce the absorption of iron salts.

Pharmaceutical precautions None.

Legal category P.

Package quantities 30 and 200 capsules.

Further information Ferrocap-F 350 releases its active principle by diffusion rather than disintegration. This process ensures gradual release over four hours which is independent of pH, gastric enzymatic activity or agitation. This avoids the risk of high initial concentrations in the blood stream.

Product licence number 0183/5017R.

NU-K*

Presentation Pale blue opaque hard gelatin slow release capsule size 0 containing 600 mg Potassium Chloride BP equivalent to approx. 8 mEq of K^+.

Uses Treatment or prevention of potassium depletion or hypokalaemia from any cause eg. prolonged treatment with diuretics (especially thiazides or frusemide) or corticosteroids, cirrhosis, malabsorption, conditions associated with chronic diarrhoea.

Dosage and administration
Adults: Dosage depends on the degree of potassium depletion. In most adult patients one to six capsules per day (8–48 mEqK^+), preferably one at a time after food. It should be remembered that the degree of depletion of tissue potassium is not accurately reflected by the serum potassium level.

Where oesophageal transit may be delayed, the outer hard gelatin capsule should be opened and the enclosed micro-encapsulated granules swallowed with a draught of fluid.

The same procedure can be applied whenever a patient experiences difficulty in swallowing the capsules. The Nu-K capsule should be opened and the contents can then be taken on a spoonful of honey or jam, or taken with a draught of fluid.

Elderly: It is not usually necessary to adjust the dosage but concurrent renal insufficiency should be taken into account.

Children: Not recommended.

Contra-indications, warnings, etc Obstruction of the alimentary tract, advanced renal failure and conditions associated with hyperkalaemia, such as untreated Addison's disease. In the presence of impaired renal function, the serum potassium level should be monitored to adjust dosage.

Side-effects: The risk of gastro-intestinal irritation or ulceration inherent in oral administration of potassium preparations is minimised by the mode of action of the time release granules. If symptoms of obstruction or ulceration occur, oral potassium preparations should be withdrawn.

Use in pregnancy and lactation: Solid forms of oral potassium preparations should not be given to pregnant women because of reduced gastro-intestinal motility associated with pregnancy.

Interactions: Caution should be exercised when used with potassium sparing diuretics such as aldosterone antagonists or triamerene.

Overdosage: Hypotension, cardiac arrhythmias, mental confusion, aesthenia and paraesthesia may occur with characteristic EGG changes (widening of the QRS complex and peaked T waves). Treatment should be directed to the removal of ingested material by induced emesis or gastric lavage as appropriate. Fluid intake and output should be monitored and measures directed to the restoration of fluid and electrolyte balance. Measures to combat hypotension should be taken if required.

Pharmaceutical precautions Store in a cool dry place.

Legal category P.

Package quantities 100 capsules and 500 capsules.

Further information Nil.

Product licence number 0183/0018.

**Trade Mark*

Cox Pharmaceuticals
A. H. Cox & Co. Limited
Whiddon Valley
Barnstaple
North Devon EX32 8NS

COBADEX*

Presentation Cobadex Cream is a white cream available in two strengths containing Hydrocortisone BP 0.5% w/w or Hydrocortisone BP 1.0% w/w; and Dimethicone 350 BPC 20% w/w.

Uses Cobadex Cream is formulated to include volatile and skin-penetrating solvents. This enables the hydrocortisone to be carried into the skin by the organic solvent vehicle, and at the same time evaporation of water will take place from the external surface of the cream, leaving a water-repellent silicone film in contact with the air. Cobadex is indicated, therefore, in all steroid responsive dermatoses wherever water, soap, chemicals, etc. cause irritation, e.g. contact dermatitis (especially of hands and body).

Dosage and administration A thin layer of cream should be applied to the affected area two or three times daily.

Contra-indications, warnings, etc
Contra-indications: Bacterial (impetigo), viral (herpes simplex) or fungal (candida or dermatophyte) infections. The cream should not be used on raw, weeping surfaces because it tends to hold back any exudate. The area of skin around the eye should be avoided.

Use in pregnancy and lactation: There is inadequate evidence of safety in human pregnancy. Topical administration of corticosteroids to pregnant animals can cause abnormalities of foetal development including cleft palate and intra-uterine growth retardation. There may therefore be a very small risk of such effects in the human foetus.

Other undesirable effects: Discontinue treatment should sensitisation occur.

Other special warnings and precautions: Steroid therapy in infants should not exceed seven days, since adrenal suppression may occur, even without occlusion.

Pharmaceutical precautions Cobadex should be stored in a cool place; avoid freezing.

Legal category POM.

Package quantities Both strengths of Cobadex are available in 20 g tubes.

Further information Cobadex Cream also contains propylene glycol, cetostearyl alcohol, paraffin, isopropyl myristate, cetomacrogol, polysorbate, methyl and propyl hydroxy benzoates, isobornyl acetate and disodium edetate.

Product licence numbers

0.5% cream	0142/0200
1% cream	0142/0201

COSALGESIC* (CO-PROXAMOL)

Presentation White, film-coated oval tablets impressed with the word "COX" on one face and the letters "CC" on the reverse; each containing Dextropropoxyphene Hydrochloride BP 32.5 mg (equivalent to approximately 30 mg dextropropoxyphene base) and Paracetamol BP 325 mg.

Uses Analgesic. For the relief of mild to moderate pain.

Dosage and administration *Adults:* Two tablets, three or four times daily.

Dosage in the elderly: Initial dosage of one tablet, two or three times daily.

Children: Not recommended for children.

Contra-indications, warnings, etc
Contra-indications: Hypersensitivity to dextropropoxyphene or paracetamol.

Interactions: Isolated reports suggest that dextropropoxyphene may inhibit the metabolism of some concurrently administered drugs. Patients receiving anticonvulsants, antidepressants or warfarin-like drugs should be monitored during therapy.

Cosalgesic is an analgesic with CNS depressing properties. It should be used with great caution in patients taking other CNS depressants, including alcohol.

Other undesirable effects: Dizziness, drowsiness, headache, nausea and vomiting are all possible side-effects and appear to be more likely to occur in ambulatory than in non-ambulatory patients, therefore alleviation of these side-effects can sometimes be produced by lying down after taking the tablets.

Other reported side-effects are constipation, abdominal pain, skin rashes, euphoria, lightheadedness and minor visual disturbances.

Use in pregnancy and lactation: The safety of dextropropoxyphene has not been established in pregnancy.

Other special warnings and precautions: Cosalgesic should be administered with caution to patients with severe renal or hepatic impairment as delayed elimination or elevated serum levels may result.

The patient should be advised that alcohol should be avoided when taking Cosalgesic.

Care should be exercised in prescribing Cosalgesic for patients with a psychological or personality disorder.

An overdosage of paracetamol can cause hepatic necrosis.

Dextropropoxyphene may impair the mental and/or the physical abilities required for the performance of potentially hazardous tasks such as driving a car or operating machinery.

Tolerance: Psychological and physical dependence may occur rarely.

Overdosage: An overdose of paracetamol can cause hepatic necrosis. A chronic ingestion of dextropropoxyphene in doses exceeding 720 mg as base (equivalent to 780 mg as hydrochloride) per day has caused toxic psychoses and convulsions.

The symptoms of acute toxicity may be rapid in onset with the danger of respiratory arrest. Symptoms exhibited are similar to those experienced with morphine and other narcotics. These are respiratory depression (a decrease in respiratory rate and/or tidal volume), Cheyne-Stokes respiration, cyanosis, extreme somnolence (progressing to stupor or coma), constriction of the pupil, circulatory collapse and other characteristic symptoms of narcotic poisoning. Cardiac arrhythmias and pulmonary oedema have been reported.

Fatalities due to apnoea and cardiac arrest have occurred on rare occasions.

Treatment of overdosage: Firstly, adequate respiratory

exchange should be re-established by provision of an adequate airway and assisted or controlled ventilation.

The narcotic antagonist naloxone is a specific antidote against the respiratory depression produced by dextropropoxyphene. An initial dose of 0.4–2 mg should be administered intravenously with simultaneous efforts at respiratory resuscitation. If the desired degree of improvement is not obtained, the dose should be repeated at two to three minute intervals. Subsequent doses of naloxone may be necessary for up to 24 hours due to the slow elimination of dextropropoxyphene. Naloxone may also be administered by infusion.

In addition to the use of a narcotic antagonist, the patient may require careful titration with an anticonvulsant to control seizures. Analeptic drugs (e.g. caffeine or amphetamines) should not be used because of their tendency to precipitate convulsions.

Early assessment of the severity of paracetamol poisoning by measurement of plasma paracetamol levels is essential if treatment, which should be instituted within ten hours of ingestion, is to be effective. Present evidence suggests that cysteamine, methionine or N-acetylcysteine given within this period are effective in greatly reducing the toxic effects of paracetamol. Oxygen, intravenous fluids, vasopressors and other supportive measures should be employed as indicated.

Gastric lavage may be helpful. Activated charcoal can adsorb a significant amount of ingested dextropropoxyphene.

Pharmaceutical precautions Store in a cool, dry place.

Legal category CD (Sch 5), POM.

Package quantities Cartons of 100 tablets containing 10 blisters of 10 tablets.

Further information Cosalgesic also contains maize starch, stearic acid, colloidal silica, magnesium stearate, cellulose, polysorbate and titanium dioxide (E171).

Product licence number 0142/0187.

KLOREF*

Presentation White, effervescent, lemon and lime flavoured tablets impressed 'Kloref' on one face; each tablet contains Potassium Bicarbonate BPC, Potassium Chloride BP, potassium benzoate and Betaine Hydrochloride BPC 1949, which provides 6.7 mmol potassium (K^+) and 6.7 mmol chloride (Cl^-) (equivalent to 500 mg potassium chloride) when dissolved in water.

Uses Kloref is indicated in all cases of potassium depletion resulting from prolonged or intensive diuretic therapy, an inadequate dietary potassium intake, and those receiving digitalis – here the elderly population are a special risk. A lack of cellular potassium in the latter can increase the toxic effect of digitalis.

Other indications are corticosteroid therapy, use of carbenoxolone sodium, advanced hepatic cirrhosis, chronic renal disease, Cushing's syndrome, diabetic ketosis, patients on a low-salt diet and in conditions requiring potassium supplementation due to prolonged or chronic diarrhoea or vomiting.

Dosage and administration Each tablet should be fully dissolved in at least 100 ml of cold or refrigerated water before drinking. The tablets themselves should not be swallowed.

Adults: In most cases 1–2 tablets three times daily (20–40 mmol K^+ and Cl^-). A few patients may need considerably bigger doses.

Children and pregnant women: Treatment should only be initiated under close medical supervision in hospital, with frequent monitoring of serum electrolytes.

Elderly: The elderly also require monitoring of serum electrolytes.

Contra-indications, warnings, etc
Contra-indications: Hyperchloraemia; renal tubular or metabolic acidosis.

Use in pregnancy and lactation: Potassium may be indicated as replacement therapy for pregnant women with low potassium levels such as those receiving diuretics. Serum levels should be closely monitored.

Administration of potassium during lactation is considered to be safe providing that maternal serum levels are maintained in the physiological range.

Other special warnings and precautions: Cautious administration is required in cases of chronic renal disease.

Overdosage: Hyperkalaemia. Poisoning is usually minimal below 6.5 mmol/l, moderate between 6.5 and 8 mmol/l and severe above that level. The absolute toxicity is governed by both pH and associated sodium levels.

Hyperkalaemic symptoms and particularly the ECG effects, may be transiently controlled by calcium gluconate, administration of glucose or glucose and insulin, sodium bicarbonate or hypertonic sodium infusions, cation exchange resins or by haemodialysis and peritoneal dialysis. Caution should be exercised in patients who are digitalised and who may experience acute digitalis intoxication in the course of potassium removal.

Pharmaceutical precautions Kloref Tablets should be stored in a tightly closed container in a cool dry place. Avoid storing at temperatures in excess of 25°C.

Legal category P.

Package quantities Kloref is available in packs of 50 tablets.

Further information The addition of each tablet to water brings about a reaction between the betaine hydrochloride and potassium bicarbonate; effervescence results from the liberation of carbon dioxide.

Betaine is a naturally occurring substance found in beet, and is metabolised by the body.

Kloref also contains citric acid, povidone, macrogol, saccharin calcium and dioctyl sodium sulphosuccinate.

Product licence number 0142/0275.

KLOREF-S*

Presentation Lemon and lime flavoured effervescent granules in individual sachets; each sachet contains Potassium Bicarbonate BPC, Potassium Chloride BP and Betaine Hydrochloride BPC 1949, which provide 20 mmol potassium (K^+) and 20 mmol chloride (Cl^-) (equivalent to 1.5 g potassium chloride) when dissolved in water.

Uses Kloref-S is indicated in all cases of potassium depletion resulting from intensive or prolonged diuretic therapy, an inadequate potassium dietary intake, and those receiving digitalis – here the elderly population are a special risk. A lack of cellular potassium in the latter can increase the toxic effect of digitalis.

Other indications are corticosteroid therapy, use of carbenoxolone sodium, advanced hepatic cirrhosis, chronic renal disease, Cushing's syndrome, diabetic ketosis, patients on a low-salt diet and in conditions requiring potassium supplementation due to prolonged or chronic diarrhoea or vomiting.

Dosage and administration *Adults:* In most cases 1 or 2 sachets daily (20–40 mmol K^+ and Cl^-) preferably after meals. A few patients may need considerably bigger doses. Each sachet should be dissolved in at least 200 ml of cold water.

Children and pregnant women: Treatment should only be initiated under close medical observation in hospital, with frequent monitoring of serum electrolytes.

Elderly: The elderly also require monitoring of serum electrolytes.

Contra-indications, warnings, etc
Contra-indications: Contra-indicated in hyperchloraemia, renal tubular or metabolic acidosis.

Use in pregnancy and lactation: Potassium may be indicated as replacement therapy for pregnant women with low potassium levels such as those receiving diuretics. Serum levels should be closely monitored.

Administration of potassium during lactation is considered to be safe providing that maternal serum levels are maintained in the physiological range.

Other special warnings and precautions: Cautious administration is required in cases of chronic renal disease.

Overdosage: Hyperkalaemia. Poisoning is usually minimal below 6.5 mmol/l, moderate between 6.5 and 8 mmol/l and severe above that level. The absolute toxicity is governed by both pH and associated sodium levels.

Hyperkalaemic symptoms and particularly the ECG effects, may be transiently controlled by calcium gluconate, administration of glucose or glucose and insulin, sodium bicarbonate or hypertonic sodium infusions, cation exchange resins or by haemodialysis and peritoneal dialysis. Caution should be exercised in patients who are digitalised and who may experience acute digitalis intoxication in the course of potassium removal.

Pharmaceutical precautions Kloref-S should be stored in a cool dry place. Avoid storing at temperatures in excess of 25°C.

Legal category P.

Package quantities Kloref-S is available in boxes of 30 sachets.

Further information The addition of each sachet to water brings about a reaction between the betaine hydrochloride and potassium bicarbonate; effervescence results from the liberation of carbon dioxide.

Betaine is a naturally occurring substance found in beet, and is metabolised by the body.

Kloref-S also contains citric acid and saccharin calcium.

Product licence number 1866/0001.

**Trade Mark*

CP Pharmaceuticals Limited
Incorporating Weddel Pharmaceuticals
Ash Road North
Wrexham
Clwyd LL13 9UF

ANTABUSE 200*

Presentation White scored tablet marked $\frac{\text{ANT}}{200}$ on one side and CP on reverse. Each tablet contains 200 mg Disulfiram BP. Antabuse tablets contain lactose.

Uses Alcoholic deterrant compound. Antabuse 200 is indicated as an adjuvant in the treatment of carefully selected and co-operative patients with drinking problems. Its use should be supported by appropriate supportive treatment.

Dosage and administration
Adults and the elderly: It is recommended that treatment with Antabuse 200 should be initiated only in a hospital or specialised clinic and by physicians experienced in its use. The patient should have adequate social and family support to avoid ingestion of alcohol. Suitable patients should not have ingested alcohol for at least 24 hours and must be warned that an Antabuse-alcohol reaction is potentially dangerous.

On the first day of treatment, the patient should be given no more than 4 tablets of Antabuse 200 in one dose (800 mg). The next day the patient should take 3 tablets followed on the third day by 2 tablets and on the fourth and fifth days by 1 tablet. Subsequently, daily dosing should continue at 1 or half a tablet daily for as long as advised by the physician but no longer than six months without review.

In the routine management of the alcoholic it is not recommended to carry out an alcohol challenge test. If the clinician feels an alcohol challenge test is essential for the success of the therapy, full information on the procedure and risks of this test can be obtained from the company. As severe reactions can occur any alcohol challenge should be carried out in specialized units by physicians acquainted with the procedure. Full resuscitation facilities must be immediately available.

Children: Not applicable.

Contra-indications, warnings, etc
Contra-indications: Antabuse 200 is contra-indicated in the presence of cardiac failure, coronary artery disease, previous history of CVA, hypertension, severe personality disorder, suicidal risk or psychosis.

Precautions/Warnings: Caution should be exercised in the presence of renal failure, hepatic or respiratory disease, diabetes mellitus and epilepsy.

Before initiating treatment it is advised that appropriate examinations should be carried out to establish the suitability of the patient for treatment. Patients must not ingest alcohol during or for 1 week after ceasing Antabuse therapy. Patients must be warned of the unpredictable and potentially severe nature of an Antabuse-alcohol reaction as, in rare cases deaths have been reported following the drinking of alcohol by patients receiving Antabuse 200.

Many liquid medicines, remedies, tonics and foods contain sufficient alcohol to elicit an Antabuse-alcohol reaction and patients should be made aware of this. All personnel involved in the administration of Antabuse to the patient must know that disulfiram should not be given during a drinking episode.

Use in pregnancy and lactation: The use of disulfiram in the first trimester of pregnancy is not advised. The risk/benefit ratio in assessing adverse effects of alcoholism in pregnancy should be taken into account when considering the use of disulfiram in pregnant patients.

There have been rare reports of congenital abnormalities in infants whose mothers have received disulfiram in conjunction with other medicines.

No information is available on whether disulfiram is excreted in breastmilk. Its use during breast feeding is not advised especially where there is a possibility of inter-action with medicines that the baby may be taking.

Drug interactions: Antabuse 200 may potentiate the toxic effects of warfarin, antipyrine, phenytoin, chlordiazepoxide and diazepam by inhibiting their metabolism. Animal studies have indicated similar inhibition of metabolism of pethidine, morphine and amphetamines. A few case reports of increase in confusion and changes in affect behaviour have been noted with the concurrent administration of metronidazole, isoniazid or paraldehyde. Potentation of organic brain syndrome with amitriptyline and choreoathetosis following pimozide have occurred very rarely. The intensity of the Antabuse-alcohol reaction may be increased by chlorpromazine and amitriptyline and decreased by diazepam and certain components decreased by chlorpromazine. Disulfiram inhibits the oxidation and renal excretion of rifampicin.

Side-effects: During initial treatment, drowsiness and fatigue may occur. Nausea, vomiting, halitosis and reduction in libido have been reported. If side-effects are marked the dosage may be reduced.

Psychotic reactions, including depression, paranoia, schizophrenia and mania occur rarely in patients receiving Antabuse 200. There are occasional reports of allergic dermatitis, peripheral neuritis and hepatic cell damage.

Treatment of Antabuse-alcohol reaction: Antabuse 200 blocks the metabolism of alcohol and leads to an accumulation of acetaldehyde in the blood stream. The Antabuse-alcohol reaction can occur within 10 minutes of ingestion of alcohol and may last several hours. It is characterised by violent flushing, dyspnoea, headache, palpitations, tachycardia, nausea and vomiting.

Intensive supportive therapy should be available in the event of severe reaction to alcohol. Oxygen should be available and supportive measures may be necessary to counteract hypotension. Severe vomiting may occur and may require administration of intravenous fluids.

Overdosage and treatment of overdose: Antabuse alone has low toxicity. Reports of the ingestion of quantities of up to 25 g refer to central and peripheral neurological symptoms which have resolved without sequelae. Treatment should be symptomatic; gastric lavage and observation are recommended.

Pharmaceutical precautions Keep tightly closed, protect from light.

Legal category POM.

Package quantities Pack of 50 Tablets.

Further information Antabuse 200 is rapidly absorbed from the gastro-intestinal tract but is very slowly eliminated and may be detected in body fluids up to seven days after cessation of administration.

Patient information booklets and patient warning cards are available from CP Pharmaceuticals on request.

Product licence number 0495/5900.

ARTHROXEN*

Presentation Arthroxen Tablets contain Naproxen BP 250 mg or 500 mg. Arthroxen Tablets 250 mg are white circular, flat faced tablets with bevelled edges with CP on one face and NXN with a break-line on the other. Arthroxen Tablets 500 mg are white, elongated tablets with CP on one face and NXN 500 with a break-line on the other. Arthroxen tablets also contain Lactose BP, Maize Starch BP, Povidone BPC, Pre-Gelatinised Maize Starch USNF XV and Magnesium Stearate BP.

Uses Arthroxen Tablets are indicated for the treatment of rheumatoid arthritis, juvenile rheumatoid arthritis, osteoarthritis, ankylosing spondylitis, acute gout, and acute musculoskeletal disorders.

Dosage and administration
Adults: In rheumatoid arthritis, osteoarthritis and ankylosing spondylitis: 500 mg to 1 g daily in two doses at 12 hourly intervals.

For acute gout: 750 mg at once then 250 mg every eight hours until the attack has passed. In the treatment of acute musculoskeletal disorders: 500 mg initially followed by 250 mg at 6 to 8 hour intervals with a maximum daily dose after the first day of 1250 mg.

Use in the elderly: As with other drugs used in the elderly, it is prudent to use the lowest effective dose.

Children over 5 years: For the treatment of juvenile rheumatoid arthritis the usual dosage is 10 mg/kg/day taken in two doses at 12 hour intervals.

Contra-indications, warnings, etc
Contra-indications: Naproxen is contra-indicated in active peptic ulceration or hypersensitivity to naproxen. Since there is a potential for cross-sensitivity reactions it is important that naproxen should not be given to patients in whom aspirin or other NSAIDs induce asthma, rhinitis or urticaria.

Precautions and warnings: Patients with a history of gastro-intestinal disease should be closely supervised during naproxen therapy because of the potential for gastro-intestinal bleeding. Arthroxen should be used with care in asthmatics or patients with allergic disease as bronchospasm may be precipitated.

Assessment of renal function before and during naproxen therapy is advised for those patients in whom renal blood flow may be compromised. As naproxen is eliminated mainly by urinary excretion via glomerular filtration it should be used with great caution in patients with impaired renal function. Monitoring of serum creatinine and/or creatinine clearance is advised in these patients. Naproxen should not be used in patients having a baseline creatinine clearance less than 20 ml/minute.

Chronic liver disease reduces the total plasma concentration of naproxen while increasing the concentration of unbound drug. It is therefore prudent to use the lowest effective dose in patients with impaired hepatic function.

As naproxen is strongly bound to plasma proteins, patients receiving concurrent treatment with hydantoins, anti-coagulants or highly protein-bound sulphonamides should be observed for overdosage of these drugs. Naproxen decreases platelet count and a prolongation of bleeding time may be observed. Naproxen and other NSAIDs can reduce the antihypertensive effect of propranolol and other beta-blockers. The natriuretic effect of frusemide has been reported to be inhibited by some drugs of this class. Renal lithium clearance may be inhibited leading to increased plasma lithium concentrations. Naproxen plasma levels are increased and its plasma half life extended by the concurrent administration of probenecid. Naproxen delays the excretion of methotrexate thereby enhancing the toxicity of the latter.

Side-effects: Nausea, vomiting, abdominal discomfort and epigastric distress may be encountered. More serious reactions that may occur occasionally are gastro-intestinal bleeding and peptic ulceration, sometimes with haemorrhage and perforation. Skin rashes, urticaria and angio-oedema have been reported. More serious dermatological and hypersensitivity reactions may occur rarely. These include anaphylactic reactions, eosinophilic pneumonia, alopecia, erythema multiforme, Stevens-Johnson syndrome, epidermal necrolysis, and photosensitive dermatitis. Headache, insomnia, inability to concentrate and cognitive disfunction have been reported.

Thrombocytopenia, granulocytopenia, aplastic anaemia and haemolytic anaemia may occur rarely. Other rarely encountered side-effects that have been reported include tinnitus, hearing impairment, vertigo, mild peripheral oedema, jaundice, fatal hepatitis, nephropathy, haematuria, visual disturbances, vasculitis and ulcerative stomatitis.

Pregnancy and lactation: There is inadequate evidence of safety of the drug in human pregnancy. As with other drugs of this type naproxen delays parturition in animals but the relevance of this finding to human patients is not known. It also affects the human foetal cardiovascular system by causing closure of the ductus arteriosus. It should be used in pregnancy only when no safer alternative is available. Particular caution should be exercised in the first and third trimesters. Naproxen should be avoided in patients who are breast feeding.

Overdosage: Overdosing with naproxen may lead to drowsiness, heartburn, indigestion, nausea or vomiting. It is not exceptionally toxic and up to 25 g have been ingested as a single dose, resulting in transient gastro-intestinal distress. In the event of a large overdose it is suggested that the stomach be emptied and supportive measures employed.

Pharmaceutical precautions Arthroxen Tablets should be stored in a cool dry place protected from light.

Legal category POM.

Package quantities Arthroxen Tablets are available in blister packs containing 60 tablets (OP).

Further information Nil.

Product licence numbers
Arthroxen Tablets 250 mg 4543/0260
Arthroxen tablets 500 mg 4543/0261

CARDINOL*

Presentation Cardinol Tablets are available in four strengths containing Propranolol Hydrochloride BP 10 mg, 40 mg, 80 mg and 160 mg. The tablets are pink film-coated and biconvex having on one face 'CP' and on the other a break-line with PRP10, PRP40, PRP80 or PRP160 according to strength. Cardinol Tablets also contain Lactose BP, Maize Starch BP, Povidone BPC, Formocasein, Magnesium Stearate BP and Hydroxypropyl Methyl Cellulose (E120).

Uses Cardinol Tablets are indicated in:

(a) the control of essential and renal hypertension.
(b) the management of angina pectoris.
(c) the long-term prophylaxis after recovery from acute myocardial infarction.
(d) the control of most forms of cardiac dysrhythmias.
(e) the prophylaxis of migraine.
(f) the management of essential tremor.
(g) the control of anxiety and anxiety tachycardia.
(h) the adjunctive management of thyrotoxicosis.
(i) the management of phaeochromocytoma (with an alpha blocker).

Dosage and administration
Adults
Hypertension: 80 mg twice a day increased at weekly intervals according to patient response. The usual dose range is 160–320 mg per day. A further reduction of blood pressure may be obtained with the addition of diuretic or other antihypertensive agents.

Angina, anxiety, migraine and essential tremor: Initially 40 mg two or three times daily increased at weekly intervals according to patient response. The effective dose is usually seen in the range 80–160 mg/day and in angina in the range 120–240 mg/day.

Dysrhythmias, anxiety tachycardia and thyrotoxicosis: The required response is usually achieved by a dosage in the range 10–40 mg three or four times a day.

Post myocardial infarction: Treatment should start between days 5 and 21 after myocardial infarction, with an initial dose of 40 mg four times a day for 2 or 3 days. In order to improve compliance the total daily dosage may thereafter be given as 80 mg twice a day.

Phaeochromocytoma: (Used only in conjunction with an alpha-receptor blocking drug.) Pre-operative: 60 mg daily for three days is recommended. Non-operable malignant cases: 30 mg daily.

Children
Dysrhythmias, phaeochromocytoma, thyrotoxicosis: As a guide 0.25–0.5 mg/kg three or four times daily as required. The dose of Cardinol should be determined according to the cardiac status of the patient and the circumstances necessitating treatment. These doses are only a guide. Alternative therapy should be used whenever possible and treatment with Cardinol should be with the lowest clinically effective dose.

Migraine: Under the age of 12: 20 mg two or three times daily. Over the age of 12: the adult dose.

Elderly: Evidence concerning the relationship between blood level and age is conflicting. In elderly patients, the optimum dose should be individually determined according to clinical response. Impaired renal and/or hepatic function may necessitate dosage reduction.

Contra-indications, warnings, etc
Contra-indications: Cardinol Tablets are contra-indicated:

(1) In the presence of second or third degree heart block.
(2) If there is a history of bronchospasm or poor respiratory function.
(3) After prolonged fasting.
(4) In metabolic acidosis (and therefore in some diabetics).
(5) Severe bradycardia.
(6) Heart failure.
(7) Hypotension.
(8) Intermittent claudication.

Interactions: Propranolol absorption is adversely affected by aluminium hydroxide and alcohol; it is displaced from plasma binding sites by heparin. Propranolol is eliminated at an increased rate by concurrent administration of phenytoin, phenobarbitone and rifampicin.

Its elimination is reduced by chlorpromazine, cimetidine and hydralazine. Currently evidence concerning the effects of frusemide and alcohol on elimination rate is equivocal. Propranolol may adversely affect the metabolism of co-administered drugs including antipyrine, chlorpromazine, theophylline, thyroxine and lignocaine. In general, beta-adrenoceptor blocking agents should not be given concomitantly with adrenaline, amphetamines, sympathomimetic amines, local anaesthetic-type antiarrhythmic agents, clonidine and calcium channel blocking agents, such as nifedipine and verapamil. Excessive hypotension may occur if certain inhalation anaesthetics are administered to patients taking propranolol.

Precautions and warnings: Special care should be taken with patients whose cardiac reserve is poor. Heart failure following myocardial infarction must have been controlled before treatment with propranolol is started. The dose of propranolol should be reduced in hepatic and renal failure. It should be used with caution in diabetic patients in whom the response to insulin or hypoglycaemic agents may be altered. The symptoms of hypoglycaemia and thyrotoxicosis may be masked by propranolol. Therapy should not be discontinued abruptly, particularly in patients with evidence of coronary ischaemia and should be tailed off over 4–7 days.

Pregnancy: The safety of propranolol in pregnancy has not been established and its use should be avoided. Propranolol is not significantly excreted into breast milk, and its use is not therefore absolutely contra-indicated in breast feeding women.

Side-effects: These include gastrointestinal disturbances, fatigue, depression, dizziness, confusion, sleep disturbances, hallucinations, flushing, skin rashes, dry mouth, fluid retention, pulmonary oedema, weight gain and muscle cramps.

In addition congestive heart failure, bradycardia, heartblock, hypotension, bronchospasm, dyspnoea, cold extremities and paraesthesia have been reported. These effects are probably related to the β-blocking action of propranolol. Blood disorders and constipation have also been reported. Cessation of therapy with a beta-adrenergic blocker should be gradual. In the rare event of intolerance, manifested as bradycardia and hypotension, the drug should be withdrawn and, if necessary, treatment for overdosage instituted.

Current evidence on the effects of propranolol on the ability to drive and to use machines is conflicting, but patients should be advised not to drive or operate machinery if affected.

Overdosage: Excessive bradycardia may be countered with atropine 1–2 mg intravenously, followed, if necessary, by a beta-adrenoceptor stimulant such as isoprenaline 25 micrograms initially or orciprenaline 0.5 mg given by slow intravenous injection. Glucagon has also been reported to be useful as a cardiac stimulant in a dose of 10 mg intravenously.

Pharmaceutical precautions Store in a cool dry place protected from light and moisture.

Legal category POM.

Package quantities Each strength of Cardinol tablets is available in blister packs containing:

Strength	*Number of tablets per pack*
10 mg	100 (OP)
40 mg	100 (OP)
80 mg	60 (OP)
160 mg	60 (OP)

Further information Nil.

Product licence numbers

Cardinol Tablets	10 mg	4543/0266
Cardinol Tablets	40 mg	4543/0267
Cardinol Tablets	80 mg	4543/0268
Cardinol Tablets	160 mg	4543/0269

CHENDOL-250*
CHENDOL-125*

Presentation *Tablets:* Round orange-coloured, film-coated tablets embossed on one surface with 'CHENDOL' and on the reverse with '250'. The reverse side is scored. Each tablet contains 250 mg chenodeoxycholic acid.

The filmcoat is coloured with sunset yellow (E110).

Capsules: Each orange and pearl capsule marked 'CHENDOL' contains 125 mg of chenodeoxycholic acid. Chendol capsules contain lactose. Colours in the capsule shell include Erythrosine (E127) and Quinoline Yellow (E104).

Uses *Indications:* For dissolution of radiolucent cholesterol-rich gallstones in functioning gallbladders. Cholesterol stones coated with calcium, or stones composed of bile pigments are not dissolved by chenodeoxycholic acid. It has a particular place in the treatment of patients in whom surgery is contra-indicated or who are anxious to avoid surgery.

Pharmacology: Chenodeoxycholic acid is a normal constituent of human bile. It is known as a primary bile acid since it is one of the main acids synthesised by the liver. Its possible main mechanism of action is that it reduces the output of cholesterol secreted into the bile by inhibiting the enzyme HMG CoA reductase. A secondary mechanism of action is the expansion in the bile acid pool which accompanies taking exogenous chenodeoxycholic acid.

Dosage and administration The present clinical evidence suggests that optimum results will be obtained on a dose level of 10–15 mg per kg body weight daily, either as a single night-time dose or in divided doses.

Duration of treatment appears to be correlated with size of stone. Generally speaking the smaller the stones, the shorter the treatment – dissolution may occur after only three months. On the other hand, larger stones may require up to two years treatment. It is recommended that treatment continues for three months after dissolution.

Contra-indications, warnings, etc Chendol should not be administered to patients with radio-opaque calcified gallstones nor to patients with non-functioning gallbladders.

Chendol should not be administered to women who may become pregnant, nor to patients with chronic liver disease, nor with inflammatory diseases of the small intestine and colon.

Chendol is generally well tolerated; the only side-effects reported to date are diarrhoea and pruritus. It has been found that after a slight reduction in dose for a few days, diarrhoea ceases and the dose can then gradually be increased to the former level.

The clinician's discretion should be applied to the necessity, in individual cases, for laboratory monitoring.

Chenodeoxycholic acid given in long-term studies at doses of 600 mg/kg/day to rats and 1000 mg/kg/day to mice, induced malignant liver cell tumours in female rats and benign liver cell tumours in female rats and male mice. The clinical significance of these findings is not known.

Children: Not recommended.

Elderly: No current evidence for alteration of recommended dose.

Pharmaceutical precautions Store in a well closed container.

Legal category POM.

Package quantities 112 tablets (OP). 224 capsules (OP).

Further information Nil.

Product licence numbers

Tablets 4543/0215.
Capsules 4543/0229.

DEXTRAVEN* 110 IN SALINE

Presentation Dextraven 110 in Saline: a clear, almost colourless slightly viscous liquid. Dextran 110 Injection BP in 0.9% sodium chloride. A sterile solution containing 6% w/v dextrans of weight average molecular weight 110,000 in Sodium Chloride Injection BP.

Uses For the restoration and maintenance of blood volume where this has been reduced as a result of haemorrhage, extravasation of blood or plasma, accidental or surgical wounds, and in burns. Prophylactically, in major surgery to maintain blood volume and pressure during prolonged operations.

Dosage and administration

Haemorrhage: In moderate blood loss 500 ml are infused rapidly, taking 15 minutes. A further 500 ml are given more slowly, taking 30–45 minutes. In severe haemorrhage, 1000 ml are infused as rapidly as possible. A further 500 ml may be given more slowly, depending on the clinical condition of the patient and the availability of cross-matched blood.

Crush injuries: The loss of plasma proteins into injured tissues and the consequent attraction of water out of the circulation may be combated by the infusion of 500–1,500 ml of Dextraven 110. The rate of infusion is dictated by the degree of shock. Where this is severe, rapid infusion is necessary.

Burns: As a guiding principle up to 3,000 ml of Dextraven 110 may be given in the first 36–48 hours. Electrolytes, dextrose and possibly blood will also be required according to the clinical situation.

Prophylaxis: Prior to major surgery a Dextraven 110 drip at the rate of 10–20 drops a minute is set up as soon as the patient is anaesthetised. The drip rate may be adjusted to maintain the blood pressure during the operation. It is seldom necessary to continue the infusion after the operation is complete.

Elderly patients: No current evidence for alteration of the recommended dose schedules.

Contra-indications, warnings, etc Anaphylactoid reactions occur rarely. They are more common and may be more severe in patients with a history of asthma.

The most frequently observed signs of such reactions are hypotension and bronchospasm, progressing on very rare occasions to cardiac arrest. In addition, skin manifestations such as erythema and urticaria may be seen.

In view of the above it is essential to observe patients closely throughout the infusion, particularly during the first few minutes. If there is any suspicion of an anaphylactoid reaction, treatment with Dextraven should be discontinued *immediately* and appropriate resuscitative measures instituted.

In continuing haemorrhage, whole blood or packed cells may be indicated after 1,000–1,500 ml of Dextraven 110 have been infused. This prevents over-dilution of clotting factors and maintains oxygen-carrying capacity. Where clotting factors are already reduced (e.g. in hypofibrinogenaemia or thrombocytopenia) correction of this condition must be undertaken prior to or concomitantly with the Dextraven infusion.

Pharmaceutical precautions Do not store in excess of 25°C or expose to undue fluctuations in temperature. Do not use if cloudy or if a deposit is present. Discard any unused solution.

Legal category POM.

Package quantity 500 ml.

Further information If blood samples are required for grouping and cross-matching, they should be taken when possible before infusion.

Product licence number 0113/5059.
Product Licence held by Fisons plc, Loughborough.

DIAZEPAM INJECTION B.P.

Presentation Amber ampoules each containing 10 mg in 2 ml of a clear, colourless to yellow solution of diazepam 5 mg/ml. The formulation includes benzoic acid, benzyl alcohol, ethanol, propylene glycol and sodium benzoate.

Uses Diazepam has anticonvulsant, sedative and muscle relaxant properties. It is used in the treatment of severe anxiety and tension states, as a sedative and premedicant, in the control of muscle spasm and in the management of alcohol withdrawal symptoms.

Dosage and administration In severe anxiety or acute muscle spasm, diazepam 10 mg may be given intravenously or intramuscularly and repeated after 4 hours. Patients with tetanus may be given 100 to 300 micrograms per kg body-weight intravenously and repeated every 1 to 4 hours: alternatively, a continuous infusion of 3 to 10 mg per kg every 24 hours may be used or similar doses may be given by nasoduodenal tube. In status epilepticus 150 to 250 micrograms per kg is given by intramuscular or intravenous injection and repeated if required after 30 to 60 minutes. Once the patient is controlled, recurrence of seizures may be prevented by a slow infusion providing 3 mg per kg over 24 hours. The usual dose in minor surgical procedures and dentistry is 200 micrograms per kg by injection adjusted to the patient's requirements.

Children: A suggested initial dose is 100 to 200 micrograms per kg body weight daily by mouth, but up to 800 micrograms per kg daily has been given. If either intramuscular or intravenous injection is required Diazepam Injection up to 200 micrograms per kg may be given.

Diazepam Injection is not recommended for premature infants.

Elderly patients: Doses should not exceed half those normally recommended.

In order to reduce the likelihood of untoward effects during intravenous sedation the injection should be given slowly (1.0 ml solution per minute).

Intravenous injections should be given into a large vein of the antecubital fossa. It is advisable to keep the patient supine for at least an hour after administration.

Where continuous intravenous infusion is necessary it is suggested that 2 ml Diazepam Injection is mixed with at least 200 ml of infusion fluid such as Sodium Chloride Injection or Dextrose Injection and that such solutions should be used immediately. There is evidence that diazepam is absorbed onto plastic infusion bags and giving sets. It is therefore recommended that glass bottles should be used for the administration of diazepam by intravenous infusion.

Contra-indications, warnings, etc *Contra-indications:* Known sensitivity to diazepam. Acute pulmonary insufficiency; respiratory depression.

Use in pregnancy: There is no evidence as to drug safety in human pregnancy, nor is there evidence from animal work that it is free from hazard. Do not use during pregnancy, especially during the first and last trimesters unless there are compelling reasons.

Warnings: Diazepam Injection should not be used in phobic or obsessional states as there is insufficient evidence of efficacy and safety in this situation, nor should it be used alone in the treatment of depression or anxiety associated with depression due to the risk of suicide being precipitated in this patient group. Diazepam Injection should not be used in the treatment of chronic psychosis. In common with other benzodiazepines the use of diazepam may be associated with amnesia and Diazepam Injection should not be used in cases of loss or bereavement as psychological adjustment may be inhibited.

As with other benzodiazepines extreme caution should be used if prescribing Diazepam Injection for patients with personality disorders. The disinhibiting effects of benzodiazepines may be manifested as the precipitation of suicide in patients who are depressed and aggressive behaviour towards self and others.

Withdrawal symptoms occur with benzodiazepines following normal therapeutic doses given for short periods of time and may be associated with physiological and psychological sequelae including depression.

Precautions: Diazepam Injection should be used with caution in patients with renal or hepatic dysfunction, chronic pulmonary insufficiency, closed-angle glaucoma or organic brain changes, particularly arteriosclerosis.

Elderly or debilitated patients are particularly susceptible to side-effects and may require lower doses.

Alertness and performance at skilled tasks may be impaired. Patients should be warned not to drive or operate machinery. Alcohol may potentiate these effects.

Alcohol may alter the response to diazepam.

In labour, high single doses or repeated low doses have been reported to produce hypotonia, poor suckling and hypothermia in the neonate and irregularities in the foetal heart.

Diazepam is excreted in breast milk and therefore its use during lactation should be avoided.

Drug interactions: If diazepam is combined with centrally-acting drugs such as neuroleptics, antidepressants, hypnotics, analgesics and anaesthetics the sedative effect may be intensified.

Furthermore, if such centrally-acting depressant drugs are given parenterally in conjunction with intravenous diazepam, severe respiratory and cardiovascular depression may occur.

When intravenous diazepam is to be administered concurrently with a narcotic analgesic agent, e.g. in dentistry, it is recommended that diazepam be given after the analgesic and that the dose be carefully titrated to meet the patient's needs.

Diazepam may potentiate the effect of phenytoin when taken concurrently. Valproate displaces protein bound diazepam and inhibits its metabolism. Occasionally diazepam has been reported to antagonise the effect of levodopa. Cimetidine may potentiate the effect of diazepam because of decreased hepatic metabolism.

Adverse effects: Intravenous injection may be associated with local reactions and thrombophlebitis and venous thrombosis may occur.

The most common side-effects are drowsiness, lightheadedness, unsteadiness and ataxia.

Elderly patients are particularly susceptible to these effects.

Other rare side-effects include hypotension, apnoea, gastrointestinal and visual disturbances, skin rashes, urinary retention, headaches, confusion, vertigo, changes in libido, blood dyscrasias and jaundice.

Paradoxical reactions to benzodiazepines have been reported, provoking excitement instead of sedation.

Pharmaceutical precautions The recommended maximum storage temperature is 30°. Protect from light. Diazepam Injection should not be mixed with other drugs in the same infusion solution or in the same syringe.

Legal category CD (Sch 4), POM.

Package quantities Boxes of ten 2 ml ampoules.

Further information As with a number of other medicaments, intramuscular injection of diazepam (but not intravenous administration) can lead to a rise in serum creatine phosphokinase activity, with a maximum between 12 and 24 hours after the injection. This fact should be taken into account in the differential diagnosis of myocardial infarction.

Diazepam is a long-acting benzodiazepine, it is one of the main metabolites of medazepam and is itself metabolised to active metabolites n-desmethyl-diazepam and oxazepam. Repeated doses will lead to cumulation of the whole drug and its metabolites. It may take 2 weeks for N-desmethyldiazepam to reach steady state and the concentration after chronic administration may exceed that of diazepam.

Product licence number 4543/0179.

DIAZEPAM RECTAL TUBES (STESOLID*)

Presentation White, polyethylene rectal tubes containing a clear, colourless to slightly yellowish solution of 2 mg/ml or 4 mg/ml diazepam. The formulation includes benzoic acid, benzyl alcohol, ethanol, propylene glycol and sodium benzoate. Approximately 2.5 ml can be squeezed from each tube, giving an individual dose of 5 mg or 10 mg diazepam.

Uses Diazepam has anticonvulsant, sedative and muscle relaxant properties. It is used in the treatment of severe anxiety and tension states, as a sedative and premedicant, in the control of muscle spasm and in the management of alcohol withdrawal symptoms.

Diazepam Rectal Tubes (Stesolid) may be used in acute severe anxiety and agitation, epileptic and febrile convulsions, tetanus, as a sedative in minor surgical and dental procedures or other circumstances in which a rapid effect is required but where intravenous injection is impracticable or undesirable.

Diazepam Rectal Tubes (Stesolid) may be of particular value for the immediate treatment of convulsions in infants and children.

Dosage and administration Sensitivity to diazepam varies with age.

Children: 1 to 3 years of age – one 5 mg tube. Over 3 years of age – one 10 mg tube.

Adults: One 10 mg tube.

Elderly patients: One 5 mg tube.

If no effect is seen after five minutes, one further tube (5 mg or 10 mg diazepam respectively) can be administered. Further doses of Diazepam Rectal Tubes (Stesolid) should be administered only after consultation with a physician.

If convulsions are still not controlled, then other anticonvulsive measures should be instituted.

Diazepam Rectal Tubes (Stesolid) should be used, as required, only as an acute treatment.

Contra-indications, warnings, etc Known sensitivity to diazepam. Acute pulmonary insufficiency; respiratory depression.

Warnings: Diazepam Rectal Tubes (Stesolid) should not be used in phobic or obsessional states as there is insufficient evidence of efficacy and safety in this situation, nor should they be used alone in the treatment of depression or anxiety associated with depression due to the risk of suicide being precipitated in this patient group. Diazepam Rectal Tubes (Stesolid) should not be used in the treatment of chronic psychosis. In common with other benzodiazepines the use of diazepam may be associated with amnesia and Diazepam Rectal Tubes (Stesolid) should not be used in cases of loss or bereavement as psychological adjustment may be inhibited.

As with other benzodiazepines extreme caution should be used if prescribing Diazepam Rectal Tubes (Stesolid) for patients with personality disorders. The disinhibiting effects of benzodiazepines may be manifested as the precipitation of suicide in patients who are depressed and aggressive behaviour towards self and others.

Withdrawal symptoms occur with benzodiazepines following normal therapeutic doses given for short periods of time and may be associated with physiological and psychological sequelae including depression.

Precautions: Diazepam Rectal Tubes (Stesolid) should be used with caution in patients with renal or hepatic dysfunction, chronic pulmonary insufficiency or closed-angle glaucoma.

Elderly or debilitated patients are particularly susceptible to side-effects and may require lower doses.

Alertness and performance at skilled tasks may be impaired. Patients should be warned not to drive or operate machinery. Alcohol may potentiate these effects.

Diazepam may enhance the effects of other CNS depressants. Their concurrent use should be avoided.

Alcohol may alter the response to diazepam.

There is no evidence as to the safety of diazepam in human pregnancy. It should not be used, especially during the first and last trimesters, unless the benefit is considered to outweight the potential risk.

In labour, high single doses or repeated low doses have been reported to produce hypotonia, poor sucking and hypothermia in the neonate and irregularities in the foetal heart.

Diazepam is excreted in breast milk and therefore its use during lactation should be avoided.

Side-effects: The side-effects of diazepam are usually mild and infrequent.

The most common side-effects are drowsiness, lightheadedness, unsteadiness and ataxia.

Elderly patients are particularly susceptible to these effects.

Other rare side-effects include hypotension, apnoea, gastro-intestinal and visual disturbances, skin rashes, urinary retention, headache, confusion, vertigo, changes in libido, blood dyscrasias and jaundice.

Paradoxical reactions to benzodiazepines have been reported, provoking excitement instead of sedation.

Pharmaceutical precautions Diazepam Rectal Tubes (Stesolid) should be stored in a cool place, preferably under refrigeration.

Legal category CD (Sch 4), POM.

Package quantities Packs of 5 tubes.

Further information Nil.

Product licence numbers

5 mg rectal tube	4543/0180
10 mg rectal tube	4543/0181

HEPARIN INJECTION B.P. (MONOPARIN*, MONOPARIN*-Ca, MULTIPARIN*, UNIPARIN*, UNIPARIN*-Ca and UNIPARIN* FORTE)

Presentation A sterile, pyrogen-free, clear colourless or slightly straw coloured solution of the sodium or calcium salt of porcine mucosal Heparin BP in Water for Injections BP adjusted to a pH of 5 to 8. Multiparin preparations include 0.15% chlorocresol as preservative.

Uses Heparin is an anticoagulant and acts by inhibiting thrombin and by potentiating the naturally occurring inhibitors of activated factor X (Xa).

Monoparin and Multiparin are used in the treatment of arterial and venous thrombosis. They may also be used in the prophylaxis against post-operative venous thrombosis; in extra-corporeal circulation (heart-lung and dialysis machines); in blood transfusions; and in coronary thrombosis as a cover for the first 36–48 hours of oral anticoagulant therapy.

Monoparin 5,000 international units in 0.2 ml, Monoparin-Ca, Uniparin and Uniparin-Ca: Low blood levels of heparin produced by subcutaneous injections (5,000 international units every twelve hours) exert an antithrombotic effect by inactivating factor Xa.

Monoparin 5,000 international units in 0.2 ml, Monaparin-Ca, Uniparin and Uniparin-Ca are used in prophylaxis of venous thrombosis and thrombo-embolism in surgical patients. Their use may also be considered in prophylaxis of thrombo-embolism in other medical or obstetrical situations in which there is considered to be increased risk of thrombo-embolism.

Uniparin Forte is for use in the prophylaxis of venous thrombosis and pulmonary embolism in those patients who require an increased dose of heparin, e.g. in pregnancy, where it has been shown that the anticoagulant response is diminished.

Dosage and administration

Treatment: Monoparin, Multiparin: Adults: An initial intravenous injection of 12,500 units may be given, followed by maintenance doses of about 6,000 to 12,000 units every 4 hours. The dose should, however, be adjusted to individual response, monitored by anticoagulation tests. For continuous infusion, 10,000 to 20,000 units are given in Dextrose Injection or Sodium Chloride Injection over 12 hours. In an emergency, heparin may be given subcutaneously in doses of 10,000 to 12,500 units at 6 to 12 hour intervals. The intramuscular route of administration is not recommended. The intravenous injection volume of Multiparin should not exceed 15 ml.

Prophylaxis: Monoparin 5,000 iu in 0.2 ml, Monoparin-Ca, Uniparin and Uniparin-Ca: Prophylactic administration consists of the subcutaneous injection of 5,000 iu every 12 hours. In the case of prophylactic administration to surgical patients, the first dose should be given 2 hours before operation and continued for at least 10 days post-operatively.

In other conditions where anticoagulation is required doses of 5,000 to 40,000 iu/24 hours may be used. Patients show individual responses to heparin, therefore consideration should be given to monitoring individual clotting times especially where higher doses are used.

Uniparin Forte: Prophylactic administration of Uniparin Forte consists of the subcutaneous injection of 10,000 iu every 12 hours.

Monoparin 5,000 iu in 0.2 ml, Monoparin-Ca, Uniparin, Uniparin-Ca and Uniparin Forte should be injected into the subcutaneous tissue of the lateral abdominal wall, inserting the needle vertically into a pinched-up fold of skin.

Children: The initial dose is 50 units per kg bodyweight by intravenous infusion, increased to about 100 units per kg every 4 hours. Clotting times should be monitored.

Elderly: There is some evidence to suggest that elderly patients, especially women, have an increased tendency to bleed when given heparin. This has usually been associated with treatment doses of heparin. Consideration should be given to reducing dosage and monitoring coagulation times during treatment or prophylaxis with heparin preparations in these patients.

Contra-indications, warnings, etc
Contra-indications: Heparin is contra-indicated in surgery of the brain, spinal cord and eye, because of the special hazard of post-operative haemorrhage in these patients which could cause significant disability. The relative risks and benefits of heparin should be carefully assessed in patients with a bleeding tendency or those patients with an actual or potential bleeding site, e.g. hiatus hernia, peptic ulcer, neoplasm, bacterial endocarditis, retinopathy, bleeding haemorrhoids, suspected intra-cranial haemorrhage, cerebral thrombosis or threatened abortion. Neither menstruation nor pregnancy is a contra-indication. Heparin does not cross the placenta or appear in breast milk.

Warnings: In patients with advanced renal or hepatic disease, a reduction in dosage may be necessary. Although heparin hypersensitivity is rare, it is advisable to give a trial dose of 1,000 units in patients with a history of allergy.

In most patients the recommended low-dose regimen produces no alteration in clotting time. However, patients show an individual response to heparin, and it is therefore essential that the effect of therapy on coagulation time should be monitored in patients undergoing major surgery. Drugs that interfere with platelet aggregation, e.g. aspirin, dextran solutions, should be used with care.

Thrombocytopenia has been observed occasionally. There is some evidence that prolonged dosing with heparin (i.e. over many months) may cause alopecia and osteoporosis. Hypersensitivity reactions occur but are extremely rare.

Overdose information: The chief danger of heparin therapy is haemorrhage, but this is usually due to overdosage and the risk is minimised by strict laboratory control. In addition, the Uniparin, Uniparin-Ca and Uniparin Forte syringes are designed to minimise the risk of overdose. Slight haemorrhage can usually be treated by withdrawing the drug. If bleeding is more severe, clotting time and platelet count should be determined. Prolonged clotting time will indicate the presence of an overtly anticoagulant effect requiring neutralisation by intravenous protamine sulphate, at a dosage of 1 mg for every 100 units of heparin to be neutralised. The bolus dose of protamine sulphate should be given slowly over about 10 minutes and not exceed 50 mg.

Pharmaceutical precautions Monoparin, Multiparin and Uniparin preparations should be stored at a temperature not exceeding 25°C when they can be expected to maintain potency for at least 3 years from the date of manufacture.

Monoparin, Multiparin and Uniparin preparations should not be frozen. Heparin should be stored protected from light.

Other preparations should not be mixed with Uniparin, Uniparin-Ca or Uniparin Forte in the disposable syringe.

Heparin is incompatible with many injectable preparations. Further information is available from CP Pharmaceuticals.

Legal category POM.

Package quantities Multiparin Vials—Packs of ten. Monoparin Ampoules—Packs of ten. Uniparin and Uniparin Forte—Packs of fifty prefilled disposable syringes. Uniparin-Ca packs of ten and packs of fifty prefilled syringes.

Further information Nil.

Product licence numbers

Without preservative	
Monoparin 1,000 iu/ml (1 ml, 5 ml, 10 ml)	0495/5015
Monoparin 5,000 iu/ml (1 ml, 5 ml)	0495/0028
Monoparin 25,000 iu/ml (0.2 ml, 1 ml)	0495/0009
Monoparin-Ca 25,000 iu/ml (0.2 ml)	0495/0032
With preservative	
Multiparin 1,000 iu/ml (5 ml)	0495/5001
Multiparin 5,000 iu/ml (5 ml)	0495/5002
Multiparin 25,000 iu/ml (5 ml)	0495/5003
Pre-filled syringe without preservative	
Uniparin 25,000 iu/ml (0.2 ml)	0495/0009
Uniparin-Ca 25,000 iu/ml (0.2 ml, 0.5 ml)	0495/0032
Uniparin-Forte 25,000 iu/ml (0.4 ml)	4543/0230

HEPSAL*

Presentation A sterile, pyrogen-free, clear, colourless solution, of Heparin Sodium (Mucous) BP in Sodium Chloride Injection BP adjusted to pH 5 to 8. The solution is preservative free. Each 5 ml ampoule contains 50 units Heparin Sodium (10 units per ml).

Uses Heparin is an anticoagulant. It is believed to act by enhancing the effects of antithrombin III, thereby inactivating several activated clotting factors, including activated Factor X (Xa).

Hepsal is indicated in any clinical circumstances in which it is desired to maintain the patency of indwelling, intravascular catheters/cannulae, attendant lines or heparin locks.

Hepsal is not recommended for systemic use.

Dosage and administration Flush with 5 mls (50 units) every 4 hours or as required.

Children/elderly: No current evidence for alteration of the recommended adult dose.

Contra-indications, warnings, etc The very rare occurrence of established hypersensitivity to heparin is the only contra-indication to Hepsal.

Used as directed, it is extremely unlikely that the low levels of heparin reaching the blood will have any systemic effect.

Rigorous aseptic technique should be observed at all times in its use.

Use in pregnancy: There is no documented evidence for the safety of Hepsal in pregnancy but the dose of heparin involved would not be expected to constitute a hazard.

Pharmaceutical precautions Heparin may be incompatible with solutions of certain other drugs. Hepsal should be stored at a temperature not exceeding 25°C when it can be expected to retain its potency for at least three years after the date of manufacture.

Legal category POM.

Package quantities Packs of 10 × 5 ml Ampoules.

Further information Nil.

Product licence number 0495/0014.

HYALASE*

Presentation A white, fluffy, odourless powder. Each ampoule contains 1,500 international units of Hyaluronidase BP (Ovine).

Uses Hyaluronidase has a temporary and reversible depolymerising action on the polysaccharide hyaluronic acid which is present in the intra-cellular matrix of connective tissue. This action allows the rapid dispersal and absorption of substances given by subcutaneous or intra-muscular injection. Hyaluronidase also facilitates the dispersal of extravasated fluid and haematomatous swellings.

Dosage and administration *Adults:* In hypodermoclysis – a two-way subcutaneous infusion set is required with the fluid container supported about one metre above the patient. Suitable hypodermic needles are attached to the connecting tubes after any contained air has been expelled. The needles are then inserted into the subcutaneous tissues at selected sites and the fluid allowed to run in by gravity. The contents of one ampoule of Hyalase (1,500 international units), dissolved in one ml of water for injections, are injected through the rubber tubing about 2 cm from each needle, at the beginning of the infusion.

When this method is employed, approximately 200 ml of fluid can be administered in 20 minutes.

Repeated infusions may be given as required, but it is advisable to change the site of injection.

Injection may alternatively be given from a syringe directly into a site into which one ml water for injections containing 1,500 international units of Hyalase has previously been injected. The needle should be maintained in the site adopted throughout the procedure which, in this case, should not be unduly prolonged.

It is not advisable to raise the temperature of the fluid prior to infusion since this has been observed to reduce the rate of absorption.

Site of injection: The possible sites of administration are numerous, irrespective of the position of the patient. Choice may be made, for example, from the axillae pectoral regions, subscapular and trunk areas, thighs and calves.

In general 1,500 international units of Hyalase are sufficient for the administration of 500–1,000 ml of most fluids. In the case of whole blood, however, 3,000 units may be required.

Obstetric anaesthesia: The anaesthetic mixture is prepared as follows:
Hyalase 1,500 international units.
Adrenaline hydrochloride 0.5 ml of 1:1,000 dilution.
Procaine hydrochloride 30 ml of 1% solution.

Heins' method is as follows: 'The needle is passed horizontally to the ischial spine, and 5 ml of the solution is deposited here to anaesthetise the pudendal nerve as it enters Alcock's canal. Next, 5 ml of the mixture is infiltrated in the superior portion of the labia minora to anaesthetise the perineal branches of the ilioinguinal nerve. The same procedure is carried out on both sides of the perineum.'

Prevention of post partum haemorrhage: 1,500 international units of Hyalase are dissolved in one ml of a solution containing 0.5 mg ergometrine for intramuscular injection. The injection is given in the thigh at the moment of crowning or delivery of the foetal head. When ergometrine is given with Hyalase in this way, the oxytocic effect is apparent 3–4 minutes earlier than when ergometrine is given alone and the effect is approximately that of intravenous ergometrine.

As an aid to local anaesthesia in ophthalmology: The solution employed consists of a 2% solution of procaine hydrochloride and 0.4% potassium sulphate. One drop of adrenaline hydrochloride (1:1,000) and approximately 150 international units of Hyalase are added to each 5 ml of the solution.

Two further drops of adrenaline are added for cone injections if this is not contra-indicated.

As an aid to local anaesthesia in fracture reduction
For Colles fracture: 20 ml of 1% procaine are mixed with 1,500 international units of Hyalase. Two injections are made: the bulk of the solution is put directly into the fracture haematoma from the extensor aspect of the forearm, and 2–3 ml are infiltrated around the ulnar styloid process. The anaesthetic solution diffuses rapidly all around the injured area and the fracture can be manipulated as soon as the needle is withdrawn.

For Potts fracture: 40 ml of 1% procaine are mixed with 1,500 international units of Hyalase.

Radiography: The contents of one ampoule of Hyalase are dissolved in one ml water for injections (a fresh solution must be prepared on each occasion).

Half a millilitre of Hyalase solution is then added to 5.0 ml of 35 per cent diodone solution and made up to 15.0 ml with water for injections.

Fifteen millilitres of the mixture are injected subcutaneously in the scapular region and are followed immediately by a further 15.0 ml at another site, e.g. the contralateral scapular region.

The area of injection is massaged vigorously to aid dispersion. Normally renal secretion commences five minutes after injection; adequate concentration is obtained in 24–25 minutes and is equal to that obtained by the intravenous method.

Note – The volumes stated are also applicable to children aged from a few weeks to five years and to elderly patients provided that renal function is not grossly impaired.

Contra-indications, warnings, etc
Contra-indications: Not to be used to reduce the swelling of bites or stings, or at sites where infection or malignancy is present. Not to be used for intravenous injections.

Pharmaceutical precautions Store in a cool, dry place. Solutions of Hyalase rapidly lose activity and should be used within 12–24 hours of preparation.

Legal category POM.

Package quantities Boxes of 10 ampoules.

Further information Nil.

Product licence number 0113/5021.
Product Licence held by Fisons plc, Loughborough.

HYPURIN NEUTRAL*
HYPURIN ISOPHANE*
HYPURIN LENTE*
HYPURIN PROTAMINE ZINC*

Presentation *Hypurin Neutral:* Complies with the requirements of the British Pharmacopoeia for Neutral Insulin Injection. It is a clear, neutral solution of highly purified bovine insulin adjusted to a pH of 7.4 to 7.6. The solution includes m-cresol and Phenol BP as preservatives and a phosphate buffer.

Hypurin Isophane: Complies with the requirements of the British Pharmacopoeia for Isophane Insulin Injection. It is a white, neutral suspension of highly purified bovine insulin complexed with protamine adjusted to a pH of 6.9 to 7.3. The aqueous vehicle includes m-cresol and Phenol BP as preservatives, Glycerol BP and a phosphate buffer.

Hypurin Lente: Complies with the requirements of the British Pharmacopoeia for Insulin Zinc Suspension (Mixed). It is a white, neutral suspension of highly purified bovine insulin with zinc chloride; consisting of 30% insulin zinc suspension (amorphous) and 70% insulin zinc suspension (crystalline) adjusted to a pH of 6.9 to 7.5. The aqueous vehicle includes methylparahydroxybenzoate as a preservative and an acetate buffer.

Hypurin Protamine Zinc: Complies with the requirements of the British Pharmacopoeia for Protamine Zinc Insulin Injection. It is a white, neutral suspension of highly purified bovine insulin complexed with an excess of protamine adjusted to a pH of 6.9 to 7.3. The aqueous vehicle includes Phenol BP as a preservative, Glycerol BP and a phosphate buffer.

Uses The treatment of insulin dependent diabetes mellitus.

Hypurin Neutral: May be used for diabetics who require an insulin of prompt onset and short duration. It is a suitable preparation for admixture with longer acting insulins. It is particularly useful where intermittent, short term or emergency therapy is required, during initial stabilisation and in the treatment of labile diabetes.

Hypurin Isophane: May be used for diabetics requiring a depot insulin of medium duration. Where a more rapid, intense onset is desirable it may be mixed with Hypurin Neutral.

Hypurin Lente: May be used for diabetics requiring a depot insulin of medium to extended duration. Where a more rapid, intense onset is desirable it may be mixed with Hypurin Neutral.

Hypurin Protamine Zinc: May be used for diabetics requiring a depot insulin of extended duration. It is characteristically slow in onset and is commonly used in conjunction with Hypurin Neutral.

Dosage and administration The dosage is determined by the physician according to the needs of the patient.

Hypurin Neutral: Is usually administered subcutaneously but, where necessary it may be given intramuscularly or for very rapid effect intravenously. Onset of action occurs within 30–60 minutes after subcutaneous injection with an overall duration of 6–8 hours. Maximum effect is exerted over the mid range.

Hypurin Isophane: It is usually administered subcutaneously but where necessary it may be given intramuscularly in which case onset is more rapid and overall duration shorter. It should not be given intravenously. Onset of action occurs within 2 hours after subcutaneous injection with an overall duration of 18–24 hours. Maximum effect is exerted between the sixth and twelfth hours.

Hypurin Lente: Is usually administered subcutaneously but where necessary it may be given intramuscularly in which case onset is more rapid and overall duration shorter. It should not be given intravenously. Onset of action occurs approximately 2 hours after subcutaneous injection with an overall duration extending towards 30 hours. Maximum effect is exerted between the eighth and twelfth hours.

Hypurin Protamine Zinc: Is administered subcutaneously, it is not recommended for intramuscular use and should not be given intravenously. Onset of action occurs after 4–6 hours with an overall duration of 24–36 hours. Maximum effect is exerted between the tenth and twentieth hours.

Contra-indications, warnings, etc
Contra-indications: Insulin is contra-indicated in hypoglycaemia.

Precautions: Insulin requirements may increase during illness, puberty, pregnancy, emotional upsets or if drugs with hyperglycaemic activity are being taken. Insulin requirements may decrease during periods of increased activity, in liver or kidney diseases or when drugs with hypoglycaemic activity are being taken.

Patients transferred to Hypurin insulins from other commercially available preparations may require dosage adjustment. Patients whose blood glucose control is greatly improved e.g. by intensified insulin therapy, may lose some or all of the warning symptoms of hypoglycaemia and should be advised accordingly.

Overdosage: An overdosage of insulin causes hypoglycaemia. The patient should take sugar and rest. If the patient is comatose Strong Dextrose Injection BPC should be given intravenously.

Pharmaceutical precautions Hypurin Isophane, Hypurin Lente and Hypurin Protamine Zinc should be shaken gently before the dose is withdrawn. In no circumstances should they be given intravenously. Hypurin Isophane or Hypurin Lente may be mixed with Hypurin Neutral in the syringe, in which case Hypurin Neutral should be the first dose to be withdrawn. The mixing of Hypurin Protamine Zinc and Hypurin Neutral in the syringe is inadvisable. Injections should be made immediately.

Hypurins should be stored between 2°C and 8°C. They should not be frozen.

Legal category P.

Package quantities 10 × 10 ml vials each containing 100 i.u./ml.

Further information Nil.

Product licence numbers

Hypurin Neutral	4543/0203
Hypurin Isophane	4543/0196
Hypurin Lente	4543/0214
Hypurin Protamine Zinc	4543/0199

LITAREX*

Presentation Oval, white, biconvex, controlled-release tablets of diameter 16 mm and 8 mm. Each tablet contains lithium citrate 564 mg equivalent to 6 mmol lithium.

Uses Litarex is a source of lithium ions in a controlled-release dosage form. Lithium may act by competing with sodium ions at various sites in the body. It changes the electrolyte composition of body fluids and increases the intracellular and total body water volume. The mechanism of action in affective disorders is not known. It is used for the treatment of acute mania and for the prophylaxis of recurrent affective disorders.

Dosage and administration
Adults: Prophylactic long term treatment with Litarex should be started with a low dosage and then increased step-wise over a period of several weeks. Treatment is managed by measuring serum lithium concentration and monitoring clinical symptoms.

The initial dose is one tablet (6 mmol Li^+) each morning and evening. Estimation of plasma-lithium concentration should be carried out after 48 hours and then at weekly intervals, and the dosage adjusted to produce a concentration of about 0.80 mmol/litre. In some patients effective serum lithium levels may lie within the wider range 0.4 to 1.0 mmol/litre. Toxic symptoms are usually associated with serum lithium exceeding 1.2 mmol/litre. When the dosage is stabilised plasma lithium estimations should be carried out weekly for one month and thereafter at monthly intervals.

Blood samples for estimation of lithium should be taken exactly 12 hours after the evening dose.

There is considerable biological variation in renal lithium clearance and thus the number of Litarex tablets required by individual patients to reach their particular effective plasma concentration is variable. Tablets should be taken in two or three divided doses. Treatment of acute mania should be initiated in hospital. The required initial dose may be high, for example 48 mmol lithium daily in four divided doses and access to immediate examination of plasma lithium level is necessary. Lithium concentrations should not exceed 1.2 mmol/litre.

Use in elderly: Elderly patients may require smaller doses. Toxic symptoms are likely with serum concentrations above 1.0 mmol/litre.

Use in children: Not recommended.

Contra-indications, warnings, etc *Contra-indications:* Lithium is contra-indicated in patients with renal disease, cardiovascular disease or Addison's disease, and in women who are breast feeding.

Precautions: Lithium therapy should not be initiated unless adequate facilities for monitoring serum concentrations are available.

The use of lithium for long-term prophylactic treatment requires careful supervision. Serum lithium concentration should be monitored regularly and determined from a blood sample drawn 12 hours after the last dose. Frequent monitoring is advisable after a change in dose; during an intercurrent illness provoking fluid loss; after starting a slimming diet; in the treatment of elderly patients; if signs of lithium toxicity or of mania or depressive relapse occur.

As bioavailability varies from product to product, a change of product should be regarded as initiation of new treatment. Blood levels should therefore be monitored weekly until restabilisation is achieved.

ECG, renal function and thyroid function should be determined prior to treatment. Patients should be euthyroid before starting treatment.

Use in pregnancy: The lithium ion crosses the placenta. It is, therefore, advisable that a pregnancy test should be carried out prior to treatment; and that women treated with lithium should adopt adequate contraceptive methods; and that treatment should be withdrawn for the first trimester of pregnancy. Treatment with lithium throughout pregnancy is associated with an incidence of congenital abnormality greater than that for the general population. Lithium dosage requirements may vary during pregnancy and after delivery; serum lithium concentrations should be monitored closely.

Lithium is excreted in breast milk, and therefore lithium treated patients should not breast feed.

Drug interactions: Lithium should be given with great care to patients taking diuretics as lithium clearance is reduced. A low sodium intake facilitates lithium reabsorption in the renal tubules and may lead to lithium accumulation.

Raised plasma levels of ADH may occur during treatment.

Symptoms of nephrogenic diabetes are particularly prevalent in patients receiving concurrent treatment with tri/tetracyclic antidepressants.

Serum lithium concentrations may increase during concomitant therapy with indomethacin or tetracycline.

Long-term treatment with lithium may result in permanent changes in the kidney and impairment of renal function. High serum concentrations of lithium, including episodes of acute lithium toxicity may enhance these changes. The minimum clinically effective dose of lithium should always be used. Patients should be maintained on lithium after 3–5 years only if, on assessment, benefit persists.

Renal function should be routinely monitored in patients with polyuria and polydypsia. Clear instructions regarding the symptoms of impending toxicity should be given by the doctor to all patients receiving long-term lithium therapy. Patients should also be warned to report if polyuria or polydypsia develop. Episodes of nausea and vomiting or other conditions leading to salt/water depletion should also be reported. Patients should be advised to maintain their usual salt and fluid intake.

Overdosage: Symptoms of severe lithium poisoning include hyper-reflexia, attacks of hyper-extension of the limbs, epileptic seizures, toxic psychosis, syncope, oliguria, circulatory failure and coma. Deaths have been reported. Gross overdosage with serum concentration of 3 mmol per litre is managed by haemodialysis or peritoneal dialysis.

Side-effects: Thirst and polyuria, fine tremor of the hands, muscular weakness, nausea and loose stools are the commonest side-effects during the first days or weeks of treatment. These often subside as treatment progresses.

During maintenance therapy fine hand tremor, weight gain, oedema, polyuria, hypothyroidism and goitre may occur.

More serious side-effects which may signal imminent lithium toxicity include loss of appetite, slurred speech, drowsiness, coarse hand tremor, vomiting, diarrhoea, fasiculation, vertigo and confusion.

Mild cognitive impairment may occur during long-term use.

Hypercalcaemia, hypermagnesaemia, hyperparathyroidism and an increase in antinuclear antibodies have also been reported.

Exacerbation of psoriasis may occur.

Pharmaceutical precautions: Tablets should be swallowed whole.

Legal category POM.

Package quantities Containers of 100.

Further information The lithium citrate in Litarex tablets is distributed in a plastic/lipid matrix from which the lithium salt is released over a period of four to five hours during passage through the gastro-intestinal tract. The tablets are formulated in such a way as to give absorption which is slow and even, so that rapid increases and high peak levels in serum lithium concentrations are avoided.

Product licence number 4543/0249.

LOMODEX* 40 IN DEXTROSE
LOMODEX* 40 IN SALINE

Presentation *Lomodex 40 in Dextrose:* a clear, almost colourless, slightly viscous liquid. Dextran 40 Injection BP in 5% dextrose. A sterile solution containing 10% w/v dextrans of weight average molecular weight 40,000 in 5% w/v Dextrose Injection BP.

Lomodex 40 in Saline: a clear, almost colourless, slightly viscous liquid. Dextran 40 Injection BP in 0.9% sodium chloride. A sterile solution containing 10% w/v dextrans of weight average molecular weight 40,000 in Sodium Chloride Injection BP.

Uses Lomodex 40 solutions are given by intravenous infusion for the prevention and treatment of intravascular 'sludging'.

1. In the management of the crush syndrome, fat embolism, severe burns and mesenteric infarction.
2. In vascular surgery.
3. In extra-corporeal circulation procedures.
4. Before angiography.
5. In plastic surgery e.g. skin grafts.
6. Vascular insufficiency.
7. Peripheral vascular disorders.
8. Short-term plasma expander in shock.

Dosage and administration *Crush syndrome, fat embolism, severe burns and mesenteric infarction:* 1st day: 500–1,000 ml Lomodex 40 should be given by IV infusion, followed by a further 1,000–2,000 ml given slowly over the next 24 hours. 2nd day: 1,000–2,000 ml by slow infusion. 3rd day: 500–1,000 ml by slow infusion (N.B. larger doses may be required in burns).

Vascular surgery: Before surgery: 500 ml by continuous infusion. During surgery: a further 500 ml. After surgery: 500 ml daily for at least three days.

Extra-corporeal circulation procedures: Lomodex 40 is added to the perfusion fluid (not more than 20 ml Lomodex 40/kg body weight).

Before angiography: e.g. aortography: 10–15 ml Lomodex 40/kg body weight is administered by intravenous infusion over 30 minutes.

Plastic surgery and vascular insufficiency: The rate of infusion and dosage will depend on clinical circumstances, bearing in mind the precautions indicated below.

Peripheral vascular disorders: 500 ml are given every 12 hours until 2,000 ml have been infused. Repeat infusions are required two to four times a year.

Shock: A rapid infusion of 500 ml followed by a further 500–1,000 ml over the next three to five hours, depending on the degree of shock.

Elderly patients: No current evidence for alteration of the recommended adult dose.

Contra-indications, warnings, etc Anaphylactoid reactions occur rarely. They are more common and may be more severe in patients with a history of asthma.

The most frequently observed signs of such reactions are hypotension and bronchospasm, progressing on very rare occasions to cardiac arrest. In addition, skin manifestations such as erythema and urticaria may be seen.

In view of the above, it is essential to observe patients closely throughout the infusion, particularly during the first few minutes. If there is any suspicion of an anaphylactoid reaction, treatment with Lomodex should be discontinued *immediately* and appropriate resuscitative measures instituted.

Lomodex 40 should not be used in patients with renal failure, with blood urea levels above 10 mmol/litre (60 mg/100 ml) or whose urine output cannot be maintained above 1,500 ml/day.

Renal function should be monitored, especially when treatment is prolonged for more than two to three days consecutively. Lomodex 40 should be withdrawn if the specific gravity of the urine rises above 1.045 or if there is a reduced output of urine. If oliguria occurs, urine output should be stimulated with diuretics and intravenous fluids as appropriate.

Dehydration should preferably be corrected prior to, or at least concomitantly with, the infusion, of Lomodex 40. Until dehydration is corrected, the infusion rate should not exceed 500 ml/hour.

In surgery, dosage for any one infusion should not exceed 20 ml Lomodex 40/kg body weight because of the risk of capillary oozing. When clotting factors are already reduced (e.g. in hypofibrinogenaemia or thrombocytopenia) correction of the condition must be undertaken prior to, or concomitantly with, infusion of Lomodex 40.

With Lomodex 40 there is no necessity to take blood for cross-matching prior to infusion as there is no interference if a sample is subsequently required.

Pharmaceutical precautions Do not store in excess of 25°C or expose to undue fluctuations in temperature. Do not use if cloudy or if a deposit is present. Discard any unused solution.

Legal category POM.

Package quantity Bags of 500 ml.

Further information Nil.

Product licence numbers
Lomodex 40 in Dextrose 0113/5062
Lomodex 40 in Saline 0113/5063
Product licences held by Fisons plc.

LOMODEX* 70 IN DEXTROSE
LOMODEX* 70 IN SALINE

Presentation *Lomodex 70 in Dextrose:* a clear, almost colourless, slightly viscous liquid. Dextran 70 Injection BP in 5% Dextrose. A sterile solution containing 6% w/v dextrans of weight average molecular weight, 70,000 in 5% w/v Dextrose Injection BP.

Lomodex 70 in Saline: a clear, almost colourless, slightly viscous liquid. Dextran 70 Injection BP in 0.9% sodium chloride. A sterile solution containing 6% w/v dextrans of weight average molecular weight 70,000 in Sodium Chloride Injection BP.

Uses 1. Prevention of post-operative deep vein thrombosis.
2. Short-term blood volume expansion.

Dosage and administration
Prevention of post-operative deep vein thrombosis: Continuous infusion before, during and after surgery. A total infusion of 1,000 ml over a period of six hours.

Short-term blood volume expansion: Haemorrhage: In moderate blood loss 500 ml are infused rapidly, taking 15 minutes. A further 500 ml are given more slowly taking 30–45 minutes. In severe haemorrhage 1,000 ml are infused as rapidly as possible. A further 500 ml may be given more slowly, depending on the clinical condition of the patient and the availability of cross-matched blood.

Crush injuries: The loss of plasma proteins into injured tissues and the consequent attraction of water out of the circulation may be combated by the infusion of 500–1,500 ml of Lomodex 70. The rate of infusion is dictated by the degree of shock. Where this is severe, rapid infusion is necessary.

Burns: As a guiding principle, up to 3,000 ml of Lomodex 70 may be given in the first 36–48 hours. Electrolytes, dextrose and possibly blood will also be required according to the clinical situation.

Elderly patients: No current evidence for alteration of the recommended adult dose.

Contra-indications, warnings, etc Anaphylactoid reactions occur rarely. They are more common and may be more severe in patients with a history of asthma. The most frequently observed signs of such reactions are hypotension and bronchospasm, progressing on very rare occasions to cardiac arrest. In addition, skin manifestations such as erythrema and urticaria may be seen.

In view of the above, it is essential to observe the patients closely throughout the infusion, particularly during the first few minutes. If there is any suspicion of an anaphylactoid reaction, treatment with Lomodex should be discontinued *immediately* and appropriate resuscitative measures instituted.

In continuing haemorrhage, whole blood or packed cells may be indicated after 1,000–1,500 ml of Lomodex 70 have been infused. This prevents over-dilution of clotting factors and maintains oxygen-carrying capacity. Where clotting factors are already reduced (e.g. in hypofibrinogenaemia or thrombocytopenia) correction of this condition must be undertaken prior to or concomitantly with the infusion.

Pharmaceutical precautions Do not store in excess of 25°C or expose to undue fluctuations in temperature. Do not use if cloudy or if a deposit is present. Discard any unused solution.

Legal category POM.

Package quantity Bags of 500 ml.

Further information Nil.

Product licence numbers
Lomodex 70 in Dextrose 0013/5060
Lomodex 70 in Saline 0113/5061
Product licence held by Fisons plc, Loughborough.

PROSULF*
Protamine Sulphate Injection BP

Presentation A sterile, pyrogen-free, clear, colourless 1% solution of Protamine Sulphate (Salmine) in Sodium Chloride Intravenous Infusion BP (0.9% w/v) adjusted to a pH of 2.5 to 3.5 and supplied in 5 ml glass ampoules.

Uses Protamine is a basic protein which combines with heparin to form a stable, inactive complex. It is used to counteract the anticoagulant effect of heparin; before surgery; after renal dialysis; after open-heart surgery; if excessive bleeding occurs and when an overdose has inadvertently been given.

Dosage and administration *Adults:* Prosulf Injection should be administered by slow intravenous injection over a period of about 10 minutes. The dose is dependent on the amount of heparin to be neutralised. 1 mg of protamine will usually neutralise at least 100 international units of mucous heparin or 80 units of lung heparin. Since heparin is being continuously excreted the dose of Prosulf should be reduced if more than 15 minutes have elapsed since the heparin injection. Ideally, the dose required to neutralise the action of heparin should be calculated from the results of determinations of the amount required to produce an acceptable blood clotting time in the patient. In gross excess, protamine itself acts as an anticoagulant.

Children/elderly: No current evidence for alteration of the recommended adult dosage.

Contra-indications, warnings, etc Not more than 50 mg Protamine (5 ml) should be given at any one time. Protamine is not suitable for reversing the effect of oral anticoagulants.

A sudden fall in blood pressure, bradycardia, dyspnoea,

transitory flushing and a feeling of warmth have been observed following injection of protamine.

Caution should be observed when administering Prosulf to patients who may be at increased risk of allergic reaction to protamine. These patients include those who have previously undergone procedures, such as coronary angioplasty or cardio-pulmonary bypass, which may include use of protamine, diabetics who have been treated with protamine-insulin, patients allergic to fish and men who have had a vasectomy.

Pregnancy and lactation: Prosulf should be avoided in pregnant or breast feeding women unless, in the opinion of the physician, any risk to the foetus/infant is outweighed by the benefit to the mother.

Pharmaceutical precautions Store between 15°C and 25°C.

Legal category POM.

Package quantities 5 ml × 10 ampoules.
10 ml × 10 ampoules.

Further information Nil.

Product licence number 0495/5000.

PUR-IN*

Presentation
Pur-in Neutral is a clear colourless solution containing 100 iu/ml of highly purified human insulin (emp), glycerol, sodium dihydrogenphosphate, and m-cresol as preservative.

Pur-in Isophane is a neutral suspension containing 100 iu/ml of highly purified isophane human insulin (emp), protamine sulphate, zinc chloride, glycerol, sodium dihydrogenphosphate, and phenol and m-cresol as preservatives.

Pur-in Mix 15/85 is a neutral suspension containing 100 iu/ml of highly purified human insulin (emp) comprising 15% Neutral Insulin Injection and 85% Isophane Insulin Injection.

Pur-in Mix 25/75 is a neutral suspension containing 100 iu/ml of highly purified human insulin (emp) comprising 25% Neutral Insulin Injection and 75% Isophane Insulin Injection.

Pur-in Mix 50/50 is a neutral suspension containing 100 iu/ml of highly purified human insulin (emp) comprising 50% Neutral Insulin Injection and 50% Isophane Insulin Injection.

The insulin is available in 10 ml vials and 3 ml cartridges. The latter are for use in the Pur-in Pen* dosage system.

Uses The treatment of insulin dependent diabetes mellitus.

Pur-in Neutral: May be used in patients with diabetes who require an insulin of prompt onset and short duration of action. It may be mixed with Pur-in Isophane.

Pur-in Neutral is particularly suitable in the treatment of diabetic coma, during initial patient stabilisation and in the treatment of brittle (labile) diabetes.

Pur-in Isophane: May be used in patients with diabetes who require a depot injection of insulin of medium duration of action. It may be mixed with Pur-in Neutral when a more rapid onset of action is required.

Pur-in Mix 15/85, Pur-in Mix 25/75, Pur-in Mix 50/50: May be used in patients with diabetes, once or twice daily as required. They are particularly suited to those patients who find difficulty mixing insulins and for whom the clinician considers one of these mixtures to be the appropriate ratio of neutral and isophane insulin.

Dosage and administration
Adults and children: The dosage of insulin depends upon the severity of the diabetes and will vary from patient to patient. The amount required may range from less than 10 to more than 100 units per day but the minimum necessary to maintain the patient normoglycaemic on a diet of adequate energy value must be determined for each patient individually. Larger doses may be necessary during illness and infection, in accidental or surgical trauma, in emotional stress and in pregnancy.

All Pur-in insulins can be given by subcutaneous or intramuscular injection. Recommended injection sites include the upper arms, thighs, buttocks and lower abdominal wall. A different site should be used each time and having chosen a general area, the point of entry should also be varied. After injection the site should not be massaged. When the intramuscular route is used, onset of action is more rapid and the overall duration of effect will be shorter. Only Pur-in Neutral may be administered intravenously.

Time action profiles for the Pur-in range are given in the table below.

Time action profiles for Pur-in insulins

Presentation	*Onset of action (hours after s/c admin)*	*Duration of action (hours after s/c admin)*	*Peak activity (hours after s/c admin)*
Pur-in Neutral	½	5–8	1–2
Pur-in Isophane	1½	11–24	4–6
Pur-in Mix 15/85	½ to ¾	11–20	3–5
Pur-in Mix 25/75	½	12–18	1½–2
Pur-in Mix 50/50	½	10–16	1–2

Prior to use Pur-in Isophane and the Pur-in mixes should be shaken gently or rolled slowly between the fingers to mix the contents adequately.

Elderly: Due to the potential in the elderly for poor renal function, their dosage should be reviewed regularly since there may be a prolongation of the effect of the insulin.

Use in pregnancy: Insulin requirements are likely to vary during pregnancy. Insulin requirements usually fall during the first trimester and rise in the second and third trimesters. Regular review of dosage requirements is essential.

Contra-indications, warnings, etc
Contra-indications: The Pur-in Pen system, Pur-in Isophane, and the mixtures 15/85, 25/75, 50/50 should not be used for intravenous administration.

Pur-in insulins are contra-indicated in hypoglycaemia.

Precautions: Patients whose blood glucose control is greatly improved e.g. by intensified insulin therapy may lose some or all of the warning symptoms of hypoglycaemia and should be advised accordingly.

Insulin requirements may be increased during illness or emotional disturbances, or by concurrent administration of drugs with hyperglycaemic activity e.g. oral contraceptives, corticosteroids or thyroid replacement therapy.

Insulin requirements may be reduced by the concurrent administration of drugs with hypoglycaemic activity e.g. MAOIs and beta-adrenergic blockers, or in the presence of renal or hepatic impairment. A change in diet or increased physical activity may also necessitate an adjustment in insulin dosage.

Allergic reactions to human insulin are very rare and usually take the form of erythema. Very occasionally severe erythema, wheals and itching may occur. Intolerability reactions to be phenol and m-cresol contained as preservatives may occur; in such cases the preparation may need to be changed.

Patients should be adequately stabilised on their insulin therapy in order to drive or operate machines with safety.

Transferring from other insulins: A small number of patients transferring from insulins of animal origin may require a reduced dosage and/or change in the ratio of soluble to intermediate preparations, especially if they are tightly controlled and bordering on hypoglycaemia. The dosage reduction may occur immediately after transfer or be a gradual process over several weeks. The risk can be considered minimal if the daily dosage is less than 40 units. Insulin resistant patients receiving more than 100 units daily should be referred to hospital for transfer. A few patients who became hypoglycaemic after transfer to human insulin have reported that their early warning symptoms were less pronounced or different from those experienced with their previous insulin.

Side-effects: Lipodystrophy (atrophy or hypertrophy of the fat issue), or oedema at the injection site, and insulin hypersensitivity can occur with animal insulins. There is minimal evidence that such side-effects occur with Pur-in and due to the highly purified form of the human insulin it is likely that such effects will be seen only rarely.

Drug interactions: The hypoglycaemic effects of insulin may be potentiated by such drugs as: alpha-adrenergic receptor blockers, amphetamine, anabolic steroids, Beta-adrenergic receptor blockers, clofibrate, cyclophsophamide, ifosfamide, fenfluramine, MAO inhibitors, methyldopa, tetracyclines, clonidine or sulphonamides.

The effects of insulin may be reduced by such drugs as: chlorprothixene, oral contraceptives, corticosteroids, diazoxide, isoniazid, lithium salts, nicotinic acid, phenothiazine derivatives, phenytoin, diuretics, sympathomimetics, thyroid hormones, and tricyclic antidepressants. Alcohol tolerance may be reduced.

Treatment with reserpine and salicylates may cause an imbalance of the insulin therapy.

Overdosage: Overdosage with Pur-in will cause hypoglycaemia. Typical symptoms may include listlessness, confusion, headache, palpitations, sweating and vomiting. Mild episodes will respond to oral glucose or sugar and rest followed by oral carbohydrate. Moderately severe hypoglycaemia can be corrected by the intramuscular or subcutaneous administration of glucagon. If the patient fails to respond to glucagon injection or is comatose, they may require s.c., i.m. or possibly i.v. Dextrose Injection.

Pharmaceutical precautions Pur-in should not be exposed to extremes of either heat or cold. When stored between 2 and 8°C, shelf life is 2 years. When stored at ambient temperature, shelf life is 3 weeks. Do not allow to freeze. Human Insulin that has been frozen should not be used.

Mixing of Pur-in insulins: When mixing Pur-in insulins, Pur-in Neutral should be drawn into the syringe first so as to avoid contamination of the vial contents by the longer acting preparation. When mixed, Pur-in insulins should be injected immediately.

Legal category P.

Package quantities 10 ml glass vials. 3 ml cartridges for use in Pur-in Pen devices.

Further information Nil.

Product licence numbers

	Vials	*Cartridges*
Pur-in Neutral	4543/0275	4543/0294
Pur-in Isophane	4543/0274	4543/0298
Pur-in Mix 15/85	4543/0276	4543/0295
Pur-in Mix 25/75	4543/0277	4543/0296
Pur-in Mix 50/50	4543/0278	4543/0297

RUSYDE*

Presentation Rusyde Tablets are available in two strengths containing Frusemide BP 20 mg and 40 mg. The tablets are white and circular with a bevelled edge, marked 'CP' on one face and F20 or F40 with a break-line on the other. Rusyde tablets also contain Lactose BP, Maize Starch BP and Magnesium Stearate BP.

Uses Rusyde tablets are indicated in all conditions requiring prompt diuresis, including cardiac, pulmonary, hepatic, renal and peripheral oedema.

Dosage and administration
Adults: The usual initial daily dose is 40 mg orally. This may be increased or decreased until the effective dose is achieved.

Children: Dosage ranges from 1 to 3 mg/kg body weight daily.

Elderly: Frusemide is generally eliminated more slowly in the elderly. The dose should be titrated until the required response is achieved.

Contra-indications, warnings, etc
Contra-indications: Frusemide is contra-indicated in pre-comatose states associated with liver cirrhosis, in electrolyte deficiency and in patients with hypersensitivity to sulphonamides.

Precautions and warnings: Cephaloridine nephrotoxity may be increased by concomitant administration of potent diuretics. Serum lithium levels may rise when frusemide is given with lithium. Salicylates and certain other non-steroidal anti-inflammatory agents may antagonise the action of diuretics. The effects of curariform muscle relaxants may be increased by frusemide. The dosage of concurrently administered cardiac glycosides or antihypertensive agents may require adjustment.

Mental alertness may be reduced and ability to drive or operate dangerous machinery may be affected.

Patients with prostatic hypertrophy or impairment of micturation have an increased risk of developing acute retention. Caution is required in patients liable to electrolyte deficiency.

Use in pregnancy and lactation: Frusemide should not be used in pregnancy unless strictly necessary. Frusemide may inhibit lactation and is therefore not recommended in nursing mothers.

Side-effects: Side-effects are generally minor and include nausea, malaise or gastric upset. Calcium depletion may occur. Incidence of allergic reactions, e.g. skin rash, is low. Hyperuricaemia may occur. Bone marrow depression occurs rarely.

Overdosage: Treatment of overdose consists of fluid replacement and correction of the electrolyte imbalance.

Pharmaceutical precautions Store in a cool dry place protected from light.

Legal category POM.

Package quantities Rusyde Tablets are available in blister packs containing 28 tablets (OP).

Further information Nil.

Product licence numbers

Rusyde Tablets 20 mg	4543/0073
Rusyde Tablets 40 mg	4543/0074

TOTAMOL* TABLETS

Presentation Totamol Tablets are orange film coated biconvex tablets containing either 50 mg or 100 mg Atenolol BP. The tablets are coded ATL 50 or ATL 100 and 'CP' on the reverse. Totamol tablets also contain Maize Starch BP, Heavy Magnesium Carbonate BP, Povidone BP, Sodium Starch Glycollate BP, Magnesium Stearate BP, Hydroxypropylmethyl Cellulose BP, Polyethylene Glycol 400 and the colouring agents E171, E110 and E104.

Uses Totamol tablets are indicated for the management of hypertension, angina pectoris, and cardiac dysrhythmias. They are also indicated for early intervention in the acute phase of myocardial infarction.

Mode of action: Atenolol is a cardioselective beta-adrenoceptor blocking drug having no sympathomimetic or membrane stabilising properties. It crosses the blood brain barrier only to a negligible degree.

The efficacy of Atenolol in the treatment of angina is probably due to its ability to reduce cardiac rate and contractility. Its mode of action in the treatment of hypertension has not been fully elucidated.

Dosage and administration
Adults:
Hypertension: Usually 100 mg daily as a single dose. Some patients may respond to 50 mg daily. Full therapeutic effect is established during the first 2 weeks.

Further reduction of blood pressure may be achieved by combining Totamol with other anti-hypertensive agents.

Angina: The usual dose is 100 mg once daily or 50 mg twice daily.

Dysrhythmias: Following control of the dysrhythmias with intravenous atenolol, a single daily oral maintenance dose of 50 or 100 mg may be given.

Myocardial infarction: For patients suitable for treatment with intravenous beta-blockade and presenting within 12 hours of the onset of the chest pain. Atenolol 5–10 mg should be given by slow intravenous injection (1 mg/minute) followed by Totamol 50 mg orally about 15 minutes later provided no untoward effects occur from the intravenous dose. This should be followed by a further 50 mg orally 12 hours after the intravenous dose and then 12 hours later by 100 mg orally to be given once daily. If bradycardia and/or hypotension requiring treatment, or any other untoward effects occur, Totamol should be discontinued.

Elderly patients: Dosage requirements may be reduced, especially in patients with impaired renal function.

Children: Totamol is not recommended for use in children under 12 years of age.

Contra-indications, warnings, etc
Contra-indications: Totamol is contra-indicated in patients with severe bradycardia, second degree or third degree heart block, heart failure and in intermittent claudication.

Although cardioselective beta-blockers may have less effect on lung function than non-selective beta-blockers, as with all beta-blockers these should be avoided in patients with reversible obstructive airways disease unless there are compelling clinical reasons for their use.

Precautions: Care should be taken when using beta-blockers in patients with poor cardiac reserve. Totamol should be avoided in overt heart failure but may be used in patients whose signs of failure have been adequately controlled.

Totamol reduces heart rate. In instances when symptoms may be attributable to the slow heart rate, the dose may be reduced.

Totamol modifies the tachycardia of hypoglycaemia. If the use of Totamol in patients with asthma or a history of obstructive airways disease is unavoidable the risk of inducing bronchospasm should be appreciated and appropriate precautions taken. If bronchospasm occurs this may usually be reversed by dosage of commonly used bronchodilators such as salbutamol or isoprenaline.

In patients suffering from ischaemic heart disease, treatment should not be discontinued abruptly.

In patients with renal impairment Totamol should be used with caution and reduction of dosage should be considered. The dose should be reduced if GFR is less than 20 ml/min.

In general, beta-adrenoceptor blocking agents should not be given concomitantly with adrenaline, amphetamines, sympathomimetic amines, ergotamine indomethacin, local anaesthetic-type anti-arrhythmic agents, clonidine and calcium channel blocking agents such as nifedipine and verapamil. Reduced absorption may occur if calcium or aluminium hydroxide is administered concurrently.

Pregnancy: The safety of Totamol if given in early pregnancy has not been established and its use should therefore be avoided. Atenolol has however been used effectively under close supervision for the treatment of hypertension associated with pregnancy. The use of Atenolol in late pregnancy may lead to signs of beta blockade in the new born. There is an accumulation of Atenolol in breast milk. However, detrimental effects in the baby during breast feeding have not been reported.

Side-effects: Side-effects reported include coldness of the extremities, isolated cases of bradycardia, and muscular fatigue. Sleep disturbances of the type noted with other beta-blockers have rarely been reported.

There have been reports of skin rashes and/or dry eyes associated with the use of beta-adrenergic blocking agents. Withdrawal of the drug should be considered if any such reaction is not otherwise explicable. Discontinuation of therapy with a beta-blocker should be gradual.

Overdosage: Treatment should be symptomatic. It is suggested that excessive bradycardia may be countered by atropine, 1–2 mg intravenously, and if necessary, this may be followed by a beta-stimulant, such as isoprenaline 25 micrograms initially, or orciprenaline 0.5 mg given by slow intravenous injection. Care must be taken to ensure that the blood pressure does not fall too low if the dose of the beta-receptor agonist has to be increased.

Glucagon has also been reported to be useful as a cardiac stimulant in a single dose of 10 mg intravenously.

Pharmaceutical precautions Totamol Tablets should be stored in a cool dry place protected from light.

Legal category POM.

Package quantities Totamol Tablets 50 mg and 100 mg are available in calendar blister packs of 28 tablets (OP).

Further information Nil.

Product licence numbers
50 mg 4543/0264
100 mg 4543/0265

**Trade Mark*

Cutter Biological
Bayer House
Strawberry Hill
Newbury
Berkshire RG13 1JA

Cutter

GAMIMUNE* N

Presentation Gamimune N is a sterile, 5% intravenous solution (pH 4.25) of unmodified human immunoglobulin stabilised with 10% maltose.

Uses
Mode of action: Gamimune N is a stable preparation of unmodified normal immunoglobulin. It retains the functional activities of the IgG molecule and has a very low level of spontaneous anticomplementary activity.

The precise mode of action in idiopathic thrombocytopenic purpura has yet to be elucidated.

Indications: Replacement therapy for congenital agammaglobulinaemia and hypogammaglobulinaemia.

Treatment of idiopathic thrombocytopenic purpura.

Dosage and administration
Dosage:
Replacement therapy for congenital agammaglobulinaemia and hypogammaglobulinaemia: The usual dose of Gamimune N for prophylaxis in immunodeficiency syndromes is 100 mg to 200 mg/kg (2–4 ml/kg) bodyweight, administered once a month by intravenous infusion. The dose may be given more frequently or increased to 400 mg/kg (8 ml/kg) bodyweight if the clinical response is inadequate or the level of IgG achieved in the circulation is felt to be insufficient.

Idiopathic thrombocytopenic purpura: The treatment dose is 400 mg/kg bodyweight daily by intravenous infusion for five successive days. A maintenance dose of 400 mg/kg bodyweight may be administered as a single dose every few weeks as required to maintain the platelet count.

Administration: Gamimune N should be infused intravenously at an initial rate of 0.01 to 0.02 ml/kg bodyweight per minute for 30 minutes. If well tolerated, the rate may be gradually increased to a maximum of 0.08 ml/kg bodyweight per minute for the remainder of the infusion. If side-effects occur, the rate should be reduced or the infusion interrupted until symptoms subside. The infusion may then be resumed at the rate which is comfortable for the patient.

Contra-indications, warnings, etc
Contra-indications: Gamimune N is contra-indicated in individuals who are known to have had an anaphylactic or severe systemic response to Immune Serum Globulin (Human).

Individuals with IgA deficiencies should not receive Gamimune N or any immunoglobulin preparation.

Warnings: Gamimune N should be administered only intravenously.

On rare occasions, Gamimune N may cause a precipitous fall in blood pressure and the clinical picture of anaphylaxis, even when the patient has shown no sensitivity to previous administration of immunoglobulin preparations. These reactions appear to be related to the rate of infusion. Accordingly, the infusion rate given under 'Dosage and administration' should be closely followed, at least until the physician has had sufficient experience with a given patient. Patients should be monitored closely and careful observation made for any symptoms throughout the infusion period. Adrenaline should be readily available for treatment of any acute anaphylactoid reaction.

Gamimune N should be administered during pregnancy only if clearly needed. Animal reproduction studies have not been conducted.

The risk of transmission of infection, in particular Non-A, Non-B hepatitis, by intravenous immunoglobulin preparations cannot be entirely excluded.

Precautions: Although Gamimune N may be diluted with 5% dextrose no other drug interactions or compatibilities have been evaluated.

Gamimune N should be infused via a separate line and not mixed with other intravenous fluids or medications.

Gamimune N should be used promptly after entering vial.

Side-effects: Reported side-effects include chills, headache, nausea, and mild back or hip pain during infusion.

Overdosage: Overdosage with Gamimune N has not been reported but any adverse effects would be expected to be similar to those which may occur on rare occasions with normal doses.

Pharmaceutical precautions Store at 2°C to 8°C. Do not freeze. Partially used vials must be discarded.

Legal category POM.

Package quantities Gamimune N is supplied in 0.5 g: 10 ml, 2.5 g: 50 ml or 5.0 g: 100 ml single dose vials.

Further information Gamimune N is prepared by cold alcohol fractionation of large pools of human venous plasma. Each individual unit of plasma has been tested and found non-reactive for hepatitis B surface antigen and antibody to human immunodeficiency virus 1 (HIV-1) by approved FDA tests. Each unit used in the manufacture of this product has been found to have an ALT level less than twice the upper limit of normal for the test. The immunoglobulin has not been chemically modified.

Not less than 90% of the gammaglobulin is monomer. The rest is dimer and not more than 5% fragments and 5% aggregates. Also present are traces of IgA and IgM. The distribution of subclasses is similar to that found in normal serum.

Gamimune N has a buffer capacity of 16.5 mEq/l (approximately 0.3 mEq/g of protein). A dose of 150–400 mg/kg (3–8 ml/kg) therefore represents an acid load of 0.0495–0.1320 mEq/kg.

Product licence number 0055/0109.

**Trade Mark*

Davis + Geck
(A Division of Cyanamid of Great Britain Limited)
Fareham Road
Gosport, Hampshire PO13 0AS

DAVIS + GECK

DEXON* 'S'
DEXON* PLUS

Presentation Dexon 'S' and Dexon Plus sutures are Synthetic Absorbable Sutures made of polyglycolic acid. Dexon Plus sutures are coated with Poloxamer 188, an absorbable surfactant which is inert, non-collagenous, non-antigenic and non-pyrogenic. Dexon 'S' and Dexon Plus are available undyed, with a natural beige colour, or coloured green to enhance visibility in tissues.

Uses Dexon 'S' or Dexon Plus may be used for suturing surgical and traumatic wounds and for ligating blood vessels.

Polyglycolic acid is a synthetic absorbable material which provokes minimal tissue reaction and may therefore be used where an absorbable suture is indicated.

Absorption characteristics: Absorption studies of Dexon 'S' and Dexon Plus in rabbits revealed minimal absorption at 7 to 15 days, significant absorption at 30 days and essentially complete absorption in 60–90 days. There have been occasional reports of its persistence within tissues for a longer period.

Dosage and administration As indicated in the surgical procedure.

Contra-indications, warnings, etc
Contra-indications: Dexon 'S' and Dexon Plus are contra-indicated where a non-absorbable suture is needed to provide prolonged wound support. The safe use of Dexon 'S' and Dexon Plus in neural tissue and in cardiovascular surgery has not been established.

Precautions: When tying Dexon 'S' special care is needed in placing the first knot.

Dexon Plus sutures are coated to enhance surface smoothness and may therefore require additional knot throws if indicated by surgical circumstances and the experience of the surgeon.

Adverse reactions: Although there have been a few reports of foreign body giant cell reactions, these are not considered to be specific to Dexon 'S' or Dexon Plus. As with all suture materials, inflammation at the site of absorption can occur although its incidence is less than with catgut. Wound dehiscence and bleeding have occasionally occurred.

Pharmaceutical precautions Discard opened, unused sutures. Do not re-sterilise.

Legal category P.

Package quantities Sealed envelopes containing sterile sutures in size 9.0 USP (0.3 metric) to 2 USP (5 metric), either as non-needled pre-cut lengths or attached to needles of varying types and sizes. These envelopes are sealed within a clear peel-apart secondary envelope, with the interspace being sterile. The sales unit is boxes of 1 dozen or 3 dozen envelopes.

Further information Radioisotope studies show that less than 3% of the coating of Dexon Plus sutures remains on the suture or within 1 gram of the surrounding tissue at 7 hours after implantation. Absorption studies in rabbits have shown that 80% to 97% of the coating was excreted in the urine during the first three days following implantation, with the remainder being excreted within 40 days.

Product licence numbers

Dexon 'S' (undyed beige)	0095/5092
Dexon 'S' (dyed green)	0095/0023
Dexon Plus (undyed beige)	0095/0082
Dexon Plus (dyed green)	0095/0083

HISTOACRYL*

Presentation The tissue adhesive Histoacryl (Enbucrilate) blue is an n-butyl 2-cyanoacrylate monomer, which is supplied as a sterile liquid in sealed plastic vials. Histoacryl (Enbucrilate) contains a blue dye to indicate clearly the thickness of the adhesive film applied. The plastic vials are packed in cylindrical plastic tubes with plastic overseals to demonstrate product integrity.

Uses Histoacryl (Enbucrilate) blue is a tissue adhesive especially suitable for the closure of minor skin wounds without suturing, and sealing sutured skin wounds.

Dosage and administration Histoacryl (Enbucrilate) blue tissue adhesive is supplied in plastic vials as a monomeric substance. It polymerises very rapidly into a firm adhesive bond in the presence of anions especially hydroxyl ions, as is the case when contact is made with water or tissue moisture.

Clean and dry the tissue area and approximate the tissue surfaces accurately. The Histoacryl (Enbucrilate) blue should be applied in spots or evenly in a thin layer along the length of the wound. The edges of the wound should be pressed together for one minute, caution must be taken to approximate the wound edges exactly, as polymerisation time is only 20 seconds and mistakes cannot be corrected later. Wounds which are subject to tension should be secured by tension sutures. Skin wounds more than 3 cm long may also be secured by additional sutures.

Contra-indications, warnings, etc
Contra-indications: Histoacryl (Enbucrilate) blue should not be used for gluing wounds of inner organs. In use, this product results in an exothermic reaction. Histoacryl (Enbucrilate) blue must not be applied to the surface of the brain and parts of the central and peripheral nervous system as tissue damage and scar formation may occur with resulting functional disturbances.

The application of Histoacryl (Enbucrilate) blue on blood vessels should be avoided because a thrombosis can originate from the exothermic polymerisation. Care must always be taken when using Histoacryl (Enbucrilate) blue to ensure that it does not come into contact with the cornea or conjunctiva as conglutination will occur.

Warnings: As a basic rule, Histoacryl (Enbucrilate) blue tissue adhesive should be applied sparingly as a very thin film. Heavy application may cause thermal damage to the surrounding tissue disturbing healing.

Instruments, clothes, swabs or gloves that come into contact with Histoacryl (Enbucrilate) blue tissue adhesive will adhere to it.

It is extremely important that such objects do not come into contact with the adhesive during the polymerisation period. Instruments which have been contaminated with the adhesive can be cleaned with dimethyl formamide or acetone.

Pharmaceutical precautions Histoacryl (Enbucrilate) blue tissue adhesive must be stored in the refrigerator or freezer, and must be protected from light if removed from the packaging for long periods. A shelf-life of 2 years is given under the recommended conditions of storage.

Histoacryl (Enbucrilate) blue tissue adhesive is a single use product only and once vials are opened must be discarded.

Histoacryl (Enbucrilate) blue tissue adhesive must not be resterilised.

Legal category P.

Package quantities 1 Box of Histoacryl contains 5 vials. Each vial contains 0.5 g of monomer.

Further information Nil.

Product licence number 3551/0001.

KIEL BONE GRAFT

Presentation Kiel Bone Graft, prepared by the method of Maatz and Bauermeister, is a mineral and collagenous matrix specially processed from calf bone, purified and gamma-ray-sterilised. According to the nature of the materials selected, Kiel Bone Graft consists of spongy or cortical tissue or a combination of both in various proportions. The grafts are packed in sterile double plastic bags in an outer box.

Uses The usual indications for Kiel Bone Graft are replacement of bone cysts, intervertebral locking, reparation of bone surface defects and the use as osteotomy wedges.

Dosage and administration As indicated in the surgical procedure.

Contra-indications, warnings, etc Kiel Bone Graft should not be implanted into a potentially infected host site. If the nature of the implant bed precludes the resorption process and the ingrowth of new bone, Kiel Bone Graft should not be used.

Pharmaceutical precautions Store in a dry place at room temperature. Opened and unused packages should be discarded and Kiel Bone Graft should not be resterilised.

Kiel Bone Graft cannot be resterilised. Autoclaving will soften the bone and resterilising with ethylene oxide may raise the ethylene glycol residue beyond admissible levels.

Legal category P.

Package quantities Kiel Bone Graft is available in various sizes and types. Boxes contain 1 to 33 packages.

Further information Nil.

Product licence number 3551/5900.

LYODURA*

Presentation Lyodura is a sterile transplant material consisting of a mesh-like texture of collagenous fibres, which is developed from homologous human dura mater cerebri by special processing, lyophilised and gamma-ray sterilised.

Uses Lyodura is a patch material which is substituted after implantation by connective tissue. Lyodura is used in the repair of defects, lesions and as a reinforcement of body tissues, e.g. for covering and sealing defects and for sheathing and securing sutures, in neuro-thoracic and general surgery.

Restrictions for use: Procedures in which the use of human dura is essential, consideration having been given to autologous tissue or synthetic materials.

Dosage and administration As indicated in the surgical procedure.

Prior to use of Lyodura, physicians must become familiar with the surgical technique(s) and specific applications and characteristics of Lyodura use in vivo. Physicians are therefore strongly advised to carefully read and review all medical literature associated with the use of lyophilised dura mater allografts, prior to use. This literature is available on request.

The use of absorbable sutures to affix Lyodura material to connective tissue is not advised. The absorption time of an absorbable suture may be shorter than the absorption time of the Lyodura material.

Tri- or bi-cutting edge suture needles are not advised for suturing Lyodura material. Atraumatic round-bodied suture needles or trocar-point needles enable less damage to the allograft material.

The Lyodura may be rehydrated prior to implantation (before or after trimming) by soaking the allograft material in a sterile physiological aqueous solution until the graft is supple and fully compliant.

The Lyodura is then sutured in place by the appropriate suture technique with suitable atraumatic suture material.

Contra-indications, warnings, etc Lyodura is contra-indicated:

As a transplant graft in the presence of infection.
As a vascular graft material.
As a heart wall graft material.
As a replacement of tendons and ligaments.

Adjacent tissue adhesions in situ to the allograft transplant can occur postoperatively.

A single case record indicated a delayed immune response in conjunction with 'freeze-dried cadaveric dural graft' transplant material.

Calcification of Lyodura when used as an allograft, can occur.

In a single isolate reported case, a patient who had received a Lyodura allograft transplant developed Creutzfeldt-Jakob Disease (CJD). The report suggested that the disease may possibly have been related to the implantation of Lyodura.

During the manufacturing of Lyodura, the Dura Mater Cerebri is treated for one hour with 1 N sodium hydroxide (NaOH). This treatment according to most recent reports in the literature is effective in inactivation of slow viruses. (These being responsible for a Jakob-Creutzfeldt infection).

In spite of a strictly controlled modern manufacturing process an absolute guarantee of Lyodura free of Jakob-Creutzfeldt virus cannot be given.

There have been no reported incidence of hepatitis A, hepatitis B or AIDS (HIV/LAV/HTLV) associated with the transplantation of lyophilised dura mater. In accordance with our manufacturing process, which includes a treatment with hydrogen peroxide (H_2O_2) and sodium hydroxide solution (NaOH) as well as gamma-sterilisation with 25 kGy (2.5 Mrad) from a cobalt 60 source. AIDS viruses are inactivated.

Pharmaceutical precautions Lyodura packaging must be visually inspected prior to use. If the package(s) appears to have been damaged, opened or tampered, do not use the allograft contained therein.

Opened or unused Lyodura material cannot be resterilised and must be discarded.The reason for this is that a resterilisation can result in a change of structure of the material and the biological behaviour with negative influence of Lyodura.

Lyodura material should be stored at room temperature up to 80°F (up to 27°C).

Lyodura from unopened and undamaged original packaging must be used only.

Lyodura must not be used after the expiry date which is mentioned on the outer packaging.

Legal category P.

Package quantities Lyodura is available in the following dimensions:

(1) 6 × 14 cm package containing 1 piece
(2) 4 × 10 cm package containing 1 piece
(3) 2 × 10 cm package containing 2 pieces
(4) 4 × 5 cm package containing 2 pieces
(5) 1.5 × 3 cm package containing 5 pieces
(6) 1.5 × 3 cm package containing 5 pieces perforated

(7) Patches 9 and 14 mm packages with 3 pieces each.

Further information Nil.

Product licence number 3551/0004.

LYOSTYPT* COLLAGEN HAEMOSTATIC FELT

Presentation Lyostypt is a gamma-ray sterilised, absorbable, fluid-stabilised haemostatic agent of natural collagen fibres.

Lyostypt is supplied in sterile peel pouches in several sizes.

Uses The application of sterile Lyostypt is indicated in the control capillary bleeding, parenchymatous haemorrhages, oozing wound haemorrhage and as an ancillary aid to other haemostatic techniques.

Dosage and administration As indicated in the surgical procedure, Lyostypt is usually used in dry state.

Contra-indications, warnings, etc Lyostypt must not be used in infected areas since it may intensify the infection. Abscess formation in the abdominal or thoracic cavities may result.

Lyostypt should not be used for arresting haemorrhages from bone wounds if a prosthesis is to be fixed with methylmethycrylate adhesive as its bonding strength is considerably reduced by collagen.

In spite of the excellent haemostatic properties of Lyostypt, this material is not intended to replace conventional haemostatic procedures such as ligation or direct compression.

Pharmaceutical precautions Store in dry place at room temperature. Opened and unused packages should be discarded and material must not be resterilised.

Legal category P.

Package quantities Lyostypt is available in the following dimensions:

	Dimension	*Cat. No.*
1 Box of 6 pieces	3×5 cm	106910/1
1 Box of 6 pieces	5×8 cm	106915/2
1 Box of 4 pieces	10×12 cm	106920/9
1 Box of 2 pieces	20×30 cm	106925/0
1 Box of 4 pieces	5×30 cm	106930/6

Further information Nil.

Product licence number 3551/0009.

MAXON* ▼

Presentation Maxon (polyglyconate) monofilament synthetic absorbable suture is prepared from a copolymer of glycolic acid and trimethylene carbonate. The empirical formula of the copolymer is $(C_4H_4O_4)_m\ (C_4H_6O_3)_n$. The sutures are available undyed or coloured green with D & C Green No 6 to enhance visibility during surgery.

Action: Three important characteristics describe the *in vivo* performance of absorbable sutures: tensile strength retention, absorption and tissue reaction.

Implantation studies in rats revealed that approximately 70% of the original suture strength remains 2 weeks after implantation and approximately 55% of original suture strength remains 3 weeks after implantation. Animal data also indicate that suture absorption for Maxon (loss of suture bulk) is minimal until about the 60th day post implantation. Absorption is essentially complete six months after implantation.

Maxon sutures are sterile, non-collagenous, non-antigenic, and non-pyrogenic. They elicit only a mild tissue reaction during absorption.

Uses Maxon (polyglyconate) sutures are intended for use where an absorbable suture or ligature is indicated.

Dosage and administration As indicated in the surgical procedure.

Contra-indications, warnings, etc
Contra-indications: The use of Maxon sutures is contra-indicated in neural, cardiovascular and ocular tissues.

Maxon sutures, being absorbable, should not be used where extended tissue approximation is required.

Precautions, Warnings: Care should be exercised when selecting absorbable sutures for tissue approximation in particular where wound healing may be abnormally extended or unduly compromised. As with all monofilament suture materials, handling with surgical instruments may cause reduction in the strength of the strand. Do not grip the strand with surgical instruments, such as needle holders or forceps, except when grasping the free end of the suture during an instrument tie. Use is not recommended in procedures in which instrumental gripping of the suture along its length is anticipated. Particular care is necessary in continuous mass or layered closure of the abdomen and any situation where tissues are approximated under tension.

Non-slip lock knots should be used at both ends of a continuous closure. Likewise following continuous closure with a looped suture a non-slip locking knot should be employed for maximum security.

As with other absorbable sutures, vaginal mucosal sutures and skin sutures remaining in place for extended periods may be associated with localized irritation and should be removed as indicated.

Maxon did not enhance infection in animal and in-vitro studies; however, since any foreign material in the presence of bacterial contamination may increase the incidence of infectivity, standard drainage and closure procedures should be followed with infected wounds.

Pharmaceutical precautions Discard opened, unused sutures. Do not re-sterilise.

Legal category P.

Package quantities Sealed envelopes containing dyed or undyed monofilament sutures in size 7–0 USP (0.5 metric) to size 02 USP (5 metric) with a variety of needles attached. The envelopes are sealed within a clear peel-apart secondary envelope, with the interspace being sterile.

Further information Nil.

Product licence numbers
Clear 0095/0100
Green 0095/0101.

SOFTGUT*

Presentation Uniform, firmly twisted strands of collagen prepared from healthy mammals, purified, softened, dry packed and sterilised. Available as both plain and chromic sutures.

Uses Softgut is sterile catgut used for suturing surgical and traumatic wounds and for ligating blood vessels. It may be used in practically all tissues. Softgut Plain is relatively rapidly absorbed and should therefore be used only where short term wound support is required. It is generally considered advisable to use Softgut Chromic where somewhat more prolonged wound support is desired.

Dosage and administration As indicated in the surgical procedure.

Contra-indications, warnings, etc Softgut is contra-indicated in situations where a non-absorbable suture is needed.

Adverse reactions may include tissue reaction or inflammation.

Wound dehiscence and bleeding may occasionally occur.

Pharmaceutical precautions Discard opened unused sutures. Do not re-sterilise. Store at room temperature.

Legal category P.

Package quantities Sutures are available in varying

sizes, in non-needled pre-cut lengths or swaged to needles of varying types and sizes in packages of one dozen and/or two dozen and/or three dozen sutures.

Further information Nil.

Product licence numbers

Softgut Plain	0095/0096
Softgut Chromic	0095/0097

STERILISED SURGICAL CATGUT

Presentation Uniform, firmly twisted strands of collagen prepared from healthy mammals, purified, wet packed and sterilised. Available as both plain and chromic sutures. Sterilised surgical catgut is wet packed in a solution of isopropanol, water and triethanolamine.

Uses Sterilised Surgical Catgut may be used for suturing surgical and traumatic wounds and for ligating blood vessels. It may be used in practically all tissues. Catgut is relatively rapidly absorbed and should therefore be used only where short-term wound support is required. It is generally considered advisable to use Chromic Catgut where somewhat more prolonged wound support is desired.

Dosage and administration As indicated in the surgical procedure.

Contra-indications, warnings, etc Sterilised Surgical Catgut is contra-indicated where a non-absorbable suture is needed to provide prolonged wound support.

Opened and unused sutures should be discarded and material must not be re-sterilised. Adverse reactions may include tissue reaction or inflammation. Wound dehiscence and bleeding may occasionally occur.

Pharmaceutical precautions Store in a cool dry place. Discard opened unused sutures.

Legal category P.

Package quantities Sutures are available in varying sizes (Plain 6/0 to 3; Mild Chromic 7/0 to 4/0; and Chromic 5/0 to 3) in non-needled pre-cut lengths or swaged to Atraumatic* carbon steel needles of varying types and sizes in three dozen packages (N.B. certain ophthalmic sutures are available in one dozen packages).

Further information Nil.

Product licence numbers

Sterilised Surgical Catgut (Plain)	0095/5090
Sterilised Surgical Catgut (Mild Chromic)	0095/5091
Sterilised Surgical Catgut (Chromic)	0095/5091

**Trade Mark*

Degussa Pharmaceuticals Limited

Asta House
Cowley Road
Cambridge CB4 4DL

BRONCHODIL* AEROSOL BRONCHODIL* TABLETS

Presentation Aerosol dispenser with metered-dose unit, containing 20 ml suspension. Each metered dose provides 0.5 mg reproterol hydrochloride.

White, half-scored, oval, film-coated tablets, each containing 20 mg reproterol hydrochloride.

Uses Bronchodil, a selective β_2-adrenergic stimulant with very little action on cardiac receptors, is indicated for the treatment of conditions involving reversible airways obstruction, such as bronchial asthma, including that of an allergic origin, acute and chronic bronchitis and emphysema.

It is effective in the prophylaxis of acute attacks of bronchospasm.

Because of its selective action on the bronchi, Bronchodil may be used in the treatment of bronchospasm in patients with co-existing heart disease or hypertension.

Dosage and administration
Inhalation – Aerosol
Adults: For acute attacks of bronchospasm, the usual dose is 1 or 2 inhalations, repeated every 3–6 hours as required.

For chronic reversible obstruction of the airways, and the prophylaxis of recurrent attacks of acute bronchospasm, the usual dose is 2 inhalations three times a day.

Children: 6–12 years: No more than 1 inhalation every 3–6 hours for acute attacks, or three times a day for prophylaxis.

Oral – Tablets
Adults: The usual adult dose is one tablet three times daily. If side-effects occur, the dosage should be reduced to half a tablet three times daily.

Children: 6–12 years: Usually half a tablet three times daily. *Over 12 years:* usually half to one tablet 3 times daily, according to bodyweight.

Contra-indications, warnings, etc
Contra-indications: There are no known contra-indications.

Interactions: Potentially serious hypokalaemia may result from $beta_2$ agonist therapy. Particular caution is advised in severe asthma as this effect may be potentiated by concomitant treatment with xanthine derivatives, steroids, diuretics and by hypoxia. It is recommended that serum potassium levels are monitored in such situations.

Side-effects: Bronchodil is generally well tolerated but, as with other β-adrenergic stimulants, digital tremor, palpitations, slight tachycardia and restlessness may occur. Potentially serious hypokalaemia may result from $beta_2$ agonist therapy.

Precautions: Care should be taken with patients suffering from myocardial infarction, thyrotoxicosis or phaeochromocytoma. Bronchodil should be used with caution in patients already receiving sympathomimetic agents. Bronchodil should not be prescribed with β-blocking drugs. Although no teratogenic effects have been observed in animal experiments, caution is recommended during the first trimester of pregnancy.

Exceeding the stated dose does not produce an enhanced therapeutic effect, and should be avoided.

Overdosage: Reversal of the therapeutic action on the bronchi is never required, since excessive bronchodilatation cannot result from overdosage. General blockade of the β-adrenergic stimulus is therefore never appropriate, and if a β-blocker is used, it should be of the cardioselective type. Such a drug is the recommended antidote. However, β-blockade is not mandatory unless there is severe tachycardia or cardiac arrhythmia threatens, and β-blockers should be used with caution in patients with existing or potential cardiac failure, which may be precipitated by the negative inotropic effect of β-blockade on the myocardium. Muscle tremor and restlessness can be treated with benzodiazepines, which are particularly useful in children.

Pharmaceutical precautions Store in a cool, dry place.

Shelf-lives: tablets 5 years, aerosol 3 years.

The aerosol canister should be kept away from heat, and must not be punctured or incinerated, even when empty.

Legal category POM.

Package quantities Each aerosol canister provides 400 metered doses.

The tablets are supplied as blister packs of 100.

Further information Nil.

Product licence numbers

Aerosol	8336/0026
Tablets	8336/0025

DIUMIDE*-K CONTINUS* TABLETS

Presentation White and orange film-coated bi-layered tablets, bi-convex in shape embossed DK on one side and with the logo DPL on the other. Each tablet contains Frusemide BP 40 mg and Potassium Chloride BP 600 mg (8m Eq), the latter incorporated within a patented controlled release system.

Uses Diumide-K Continus tablets are indicated in patients requiring diuresis and concomitant potassium supplementation.

Indications include cardiac oedema, pulmonary oedema, hepatic oedema, renal oedema and peripheral oedema of various aetiologies.

Dosage and administration The usual adult dose is one tablet daily, normally in the morning. This may be adjusted depending on the condition.

N.B. The tablets should be swallowed whole with water preferably prior to or during a meal. The tablets should not be chewed so as not to destroy the controlled release system constituting the potassium chloride layer.

Children: Diumide-K Continus Tablets are not suitable for paediatric use.

Elderly: Normal adult dose.

Contra-indications, warnings, etc
Contra-indications: Diumide-K Continus tablets are contra-indicated in porphyria, hyperkalaemia, precomatose states associated with liver cirrhosis, Addison's disease and concomitant administration of potassium sparing diuretics. Although the controlled release system minimises the likelihood of oesophageal ulceration, all solid forms of potassium medication are contra-indicated in the presence of obstructions in the digestive tract (e.g. resulting from compression of the oesophagus due to dilation of the left atrium or from stenosis of the gut).

Warnings: Patients with prostatic hypertrophy or impairment of micturition have an increased risk of developing acute urinary retention.

Latent diabetes may become manifest or the insulin requirements of diabetic patients may increase.

Precautions: Care should be taken in patients being concurrently administered cardiac glycosides, hypotensive agents and cephaloridine. Care should also be exercised in patients with renal insufficiency where there is a risk of hyperkalaemia. Non steroidal anti-inflammatory drugs antagonise the diuretic effect. As with all medicines, keep out of the reach of children.

Use in pregnancy: Specific experience is unavailable with Diumide-K Continus Tablets. Rat studies have shown that the administration of frusemide (37.5–300 mg/kg twice daily) on days 6–17 of gestation produced dose related increases in wavy ribs. When providing potassium chloride during the dosing period, the incidence of wavy ribs reduced by 90% indicating that the teratogenicity was probably related to hypokalaemia.

In humans, frusemide crosses the placenta. Oral doses of 25 to 40 mg have produced peak cord serum concentrations after approximately 9 hours. Maternal and cord levels were equal at approximately 8 hours. Increased foetal urine production after maternal frusemide therapy has been observed in newborns exposed to frusemide shortly before birth. Urinary sodium and potassium in treated neonates have been found to be significantly greater than in non exposed controls. Neonatal electrolyte disturbances may occur.

Whilst potassium chloride is a natural constituent of tissues and fluids, high or low levels can be detrimental to maternal and foetal cardiac function and serum levels should therefore be monitored closely. Frusemide has been used in pregnancy, in labour and in the puerperium in cases of excessive weight gain, oedema, hypertension and toxaemia of pregnancy with satisfactory results and with no embryofoetotoxic or teratogenic effects.

Diumide-K Continus Tablets should not be administered during the first trimester. Diuretics may reduce placental perfusion. After the first trimester, Diumide-K Continus Tablets should not be administered if the adequacy of placental perfusion is suspect.

Nursing mothers: Lactation may be inhibited due to maternal fluid depletion. Frusemide is excreted into breast milk, therefore Diumide-K Continus Tablets should be used with caution.

Side-effects: Frusemide is generally well tolerated and the patented controlled release tablet ensures virtual absence of gastro-intestinal side-effects often associated with potassium administration.

In rare instance of allergic reaction treatment should be discontinued. Hyperuricaemia may occur with frusemide therapy. Bone marrow depression has also been reported as a rare complication and therapy should be withdrawn.

Overdosage: Overdosage is characterised by excessive diuresis. Treatment of overdosage should be aimed at fluid replacement and correction of the resulting electrolyte imbalance.

Pharmaceutical precautions Diumide-K Continus tablets should be stored in a cool, dry place protected from light.

Legal category POM.

Package quantities Blister packs of 30 (OP) and containers of 250 tablets or 1000 tablets.

Further information Frusemide produces a rapid and sustained diuresis which lasts for approximately four hours following administration. The potassium chloride content is released from the patented controlled release tablet over a prolonged period ensuring maximum absorption, the avoidance of 'flushing out' of the potassium by the action of the diuretic, and virtual freedom from side-effects.

Product licence number 8336/0001.

DIUREXAN* TABLETS

Presentation Tablets each containing 20 mg Xipamide. The tablets are white, round, with bisecting score on one side and debossed A on the other, and have a diameter of 6 mm.

Uses Diurexan is a diuretic and antihypertensive agent having a gentle onset of action and gradual, prolonged effect. Whereas the main diuretic activity lasts for up to 12 hours, the antihypertensive effect is evident for 24 hours or more.

Hypertension: All grades of hypertension respond to treatment with Diurexan. It is an effective treatment on its own in mild to moderate hypertension, and may be used alone or combined with other antihypertensive agents in severe hypertension.

Oedema: Diurexan is indicated whenever diuretic therapy is required including congestive cardiac failure, hepatic oedema, renal oedema, peripheral oedema due to venous insufficiency and oedema of pregnancy in the second and third trimesters.

Dosage and administration For oral administration.

Hypertension: Adults: The usual dose is 1 tablet (20 mg) daily, as a single early morning dose. In more severe grades of hypertension, 2 tablets daily, as a single early morning dose, may be required. When using Diurexan in combination with other antihypertensive therapy, the initial dose should not exceed 1 tablet daily.

Elderly: See 'Precautions'.

Children: No dose recommended.

Oedema: Adults: In the initial phase of treatment the usual dose is 2 tablets (40 mg) daily in a single early morning dose. Depending on the patient's response, the dose may be lowered to 1 tablet daily when sufficient control of oedema has been achieved. Higher doses, up to 4 tablets daily (80 mg), may be employed in resistant cases.

Elderly: See 'Precautions'.

Children: No dose recommended.

Contra-indications, warnings, etc

Contra-indications: Diurexan is contra-indicated in severe electrolyte deficiency, precomatose states associated with liver cirrhosis and severe renal insufficiency.

Side-effects: Diurexan is generally well tolerated. Slight gastro-intestinal disturbances have been reported in a few cases as have episodes of mild dizziness.

Precautions: Like other diuretics, Diurexan may induce hypokalaemia in long-term therapy. Potassium supplements may be necessary particularly in the elderly where dietary potassium intake may be inadequate.

Animal experiments have indicated that Diurexan is devoid of teratogenic properties or effects on fertility and reproduction. Nevertheless, discretion is required before permitting therapy in pregnant patients. As with all drugs, treatment should be avoided in the first trimester of pregnancy.

Warnings: The dosage of other hypotensive drugs and cardiac glycosides may require adjustment when used in conjunction with Diurexan. In common with other diuretics, Diurexan may induce hyperuricaemia or changed glucose metabolism in patients predisposed to these conditions. Diabetic patients will probably require an adjustment of insulin dosage, or other hypoglycaemic agent therapy.

An increased risk of developing acute urinary retention may arise in patients with prostatic hypertrophy.

Treatment of overdosage: General measures should be aimed at the maintenance of blood pressure, restoration of blood volume and correction of electrolyte imbalance.

Pharmaceutical precautions Store in a cool dry place.

Legal category POM.

Package quantities Cartons of 140 tablets in blister packs of 14 tablets.

Further information Nil.

Product licence number 8336/0008.

ENDOXANA* INJECTION ENDOXANA* TABLETS

Presentation

Tablets: White, sugar-coated tablets containing Cyclophosphamide BP 50 mg.

Injection: White powder for injection in vials containing Cyclophosphamide BP 107 mg, 214 mg, 535 mg or 1,069 mg (equivalent to 100 mg, 200 mg, 500 mg or 1,000 mg anhydrous cyclophosphamide respectively) and sodium chloride sufficient to render isotonic when diluted with Water for Injections using the volume recommended for each strength.

Uses

Action: Cyclophosphamide is inert until activated by microsomal enzymes. This occurs mainly in the liver, producing potent alkylating cytotoxic metabolites.

Indications: Endoxana is a cytotoxic drug for the treatment of malignant disease. As a single agent it has successfully produced an objective remission in a wide range of malignant conditions. Endoxana is also frequently used in combination with other cytotoxic drugs.

Dosage and administration Endoxana should only be used by clinicians experienced in the use of cancer chemotherapy.

Dosage: The dose, route of administration and frequency of administration should be determined by the tumour type, tumour stage, the general condition of the patient and whether other chemotherapy or radiotherapy is to be administered concurrently.

A guide to the dosage regimens used for most indications is given below:

Conventional dose: 100–300 mg daily as a single i.v. or oral dose, or 500 mg–1 g as a single i.v. dose weekly.

High dose: 20–40 mg/kg as a single i.v. dose or short infusion, given at 10–20 day intervals.

Administration: Endoxana is inert until activated by enzymes in the liver. However, as with all cytotoxics, it is suggested that reconstitution should be performed by trained personnel, in a designated area. Those handling the preparation should wear protective gloves. Care should be taken to avoid splashing material into the eyes. The material should not be handled by women who are pregnant. Adequate care and precautions should be taken in the disposal of items (syringes, needles etc.) used to reconstitute cytotoxic drugs. The dry contents of a vial should be dissolved in sterile water (5 ml per 100 mg Endoxana) and used within eight hours. The pH of an aqueous solution is between 4.0 and 6.0.

Endoxana is usually given directly into the vein over one or two minutes or directly into the tubing of a fast running i.v. infusion with the patient supine. Care should be taken that extravasation does not take place, however, should it occur, no specific measures need be taken. Endoxana injection may also be given intraperitoneally or intrapleurally but these routes offer no therapeutic advantages over the i.v. route. For further information contact Degussa Pharmaceuticals Limited. Endoxana has been given intra-arterially and by local perfusion. These routes should be used by clinicians experienced in these procedures.

A minimum urine output of 100 ml/hr should be maintained during therapy with conventional doses. If the larger doses are used an output of at least this level should be maintained for 24 hours following administration, if necessary by a forced diuresis. Alkalinisation of the urine is not recommended. Endoxana should be given early in the day and the bladder voided frequently. The patient should be well hydrated and maintained in fluid balance. Mesna (Uromitexan*) can be used concurrently to reduce urotoxic effects (see Uromitexan data sheet). Anti-emetics given before and during therapy may reduce nausea and vomiting.

If the leucocyte count is below 4,000/mm^3 or the platelet count is below 100,000/mm^3, treatment with Endoxana should be temporarily withheld until the blood count returns to normal levels.

An elixir may be prepared by dissolving the contents of the dry powder vials in Aromatic Elixir USP shortly before oral administration. No specific information on the use of this product in the elderly is available. Clinical trials have included patients over 65 years and no adverse reactions specific to this age group have been reported.

Contra-indications, warnings, etc

Contra-indications: Endoxana should only be administered where there are facilities for regular monitoring of clinical, biochemical and haematological parameters before during and after administration and under the direction of a specialist oncology service.

Endoxana is contra-indicated in patients with known hypersensitivity, with acute infections, with bone marrow aplasia, with acute urinary tract infection or with acute urothelial toxicity from cytotoxic chemotherapy or radiation therapy.

Endoxana should not be used in the management of non-malignant disease, except for immuno-suppression in life-threatening situations. Contraception in both sexes is advised during Endoxana therapy. Patients should receive counselling with respect to subsequent pregnancies. Endoxana should not be used in pregnancy, especially the first trimester, unless the expected benefit is thought to outweigh the substantial risk to the foetus. Mothers should not breast-feed while being treated with Endoxana.

Precautions: Care should be exercised in patients who are elderly, debilitated, have diabetes mellitus or evidence of myelosuppression or who have recently received or are receiving concurrent treatment with radiotherapy or cytotoxic agents.

Cardiotoxicity may be induced in patients who have had or are receiving mediastinal irradiation or doxorubicin.

Endoxana is not recommended in patients with plasma creatinine greater than 120 μmol/l (1.5 mg/100 ml), bilirubin greater than 17 μmol/l (1 mg/100 ml), or with transaminases or alkaline phosphatase more than 2–3 times the normal value.

Increased myelosuppression may be seen following concurrent administration of other marrow depressant drugs.

Endoxana potentiates the hypoglycaemic effects of the sulphonylurea compounds. An alteration in carbohydrate metabolism may be seen in patients on Endoxana; hyperglycaemia has been reported.

Side-effects: Nausea and vomiting. This may be reduced by the prior administration of an anti-emetic agent.

Alopecia occurs to some degree in about 20% of patients receiving over 100 mg daily and is inevitable following high doses. Epilation commences usually after the first three weeks of treatment but regrowth is evident after three months in most patients even though they remain on treatment.

The reticulo-endothelial system is depressed, granulopoiesis and lymphopoiesis being more affected than thrombopoiesis and erythropoiesis but this depression is reversible. When a single dose is given, the fall in the peripheral white cell count reaches its nadir within 5 to 10 days. Recovery is seen at 10–14 days following administration, with full recovery in most cases by 21–28 days. The fall in the peripheral count and the time taken to recover may increase with increasing doses of Endoxana. If the peripheral white cell count is very low, an increased risk of infection should be considered but since recovery is usually spontaneous, steroids are not recommended. Haematuria may occur during or after therapy with Endoxana. An adequate output of urine (2–3 L/day) should be maintained. Adequate hydration with frequent emptying of the bladder is recommended. The administration of a diuretic may sometimes be necessary to achieve this, particularly when higher doses of Endoxana are used. Mesna (Uromitexan) may be considered to reduce the urotoxicity and if used, frequent emptying of the bladder should be avoided. Endoxana should be withheld from patients with cystitis from whatever cause, until it has been treated.

Amenorrhoea and azoospermia often occur but can be reversible. Endoxana may have an effect on pre-pubertal gonads and appropriate counselling should be given.

Cardiotoxicity has been observed with high doses of Endoxana. Endoxana should be discontinued and appropriate treatment given. Other side-effects such as pigmentation, macrocytosis, water retention, and induction of hyperglycaemia or hypoglycaemia have been reported. Following large doses ECG changes and elevation of LDH, SGOT and CPK have been reported in some patients. Pneumonitis and pulmonary fibrosis have also occasionally been associated with Endoxana therapy. Side-effects have occasionally occurred after cessation of treatment.

Endoxana has been shown to be mutagenic, teratogenic and carcinogenic in certain laboratory tests, and, as with other cytotoxic agents, there have been reports of possible drug-induced neoplasia.

Overdosage: The most serious consequences of overdosage are myelosuppression and haemorrhagic cystitis. The former usually recovers spontaneously, but until it does, administration of a broad spectrum antibiotic may be advisable. Transfusion of whole-blood, platelets or white cells are rarely necessary.

If the overdose is recognised within the first 24 hours and possibly up to 48 hours, i.v. mesna may be beneficial in ameliorating damage to the urinary system. Normal supportive measures such as analgesics and maintenance of fluid balance should be instituted. If despite these measures the cystitis does not resolve, more intensive treatment may be necessary and a urological opinion should be sought. No further courses should be given until the patient has fully recovered.

Pharmaceutical precautions Store below 25°C; protect from light. The solution for parenteral use should be used within eight hours of preparation.

Legal category POM.

Package quantities Cartons containing 10 blister packs, each of 10 × 50 mg tablets.
100 mg dry vials, in packs of 10.
200 mg dry vials, in packs of 10.
500 mg dry vials, singles.
1,000 mg dry vials, singles.

Further information The dosage regimen for Uromitexan varies according to the dose of Endoxana administered. In general, Uromitexan is given as 60% w/w of the dose of i.v. Endoxana in three equal doses of 20% at 0, 4 and 8 hours. With the higher doses of Endoxana, the dose and frequency of administration may need to be increased. Full prescribing information is available on the Uromitexan data sheet.

Product licence numbers

Tablets of 50 mg	8336/0016
Vials of 100 mg	8336/0011
Vials of 200 mg	8336/0012
Vials of 500 mg	8336/0013
Vials of 1,000 mg	8336/0014

FERROCONTIN* CONTINUS* TABLETS

Presentation Red, film-coated, bi-convex tablets. Each tablet contains the equivalent of 100 mg ferrous iron in the form of ferrous glycine sulphate within a patented controlled release system.

Uses Ferrocontin Continus Tablets are indicated for the treatment and prophylaxis of iron deficiency anaemia.

Dosage and administration One tablet to be taken daily, or as directed by the physician. Ferrocontin Continus tablets should be swallowed whole and not chewed.

Children: Not suitable for children under 10 years.

Elderly: Normal adult dose.

Contra-indications, warnings, etc Tetracyclines will chelate with iron, impairing the absorption of both agents. Concurrent administration reduces the absorption of penicillamine and zinc. As with all medicines keep out of the reach of children.

Use in pregnancy: When administering ferrous sulphate to pregnant mice and rats in dosages of up to 100 times (1200 mg/kg/day) the human adult dose, no influence on survival of dams, survival, development and abnormality, appearance of foetuses and offspring was observed. Experimental studies have not been described on the use of glycine in pregnancy in laboratory animals.

There are conflicting reports on the tendency of ferrous sulphate to induce congenital malformations in the foetuses of women receiving iron containing preparations during the first trimester. Harmful effects on the foetus, the mother or the pregnancy have not been reported for the ingestion of glycine.

Ferrocontin Continus Tablets should be used with caution during the first trimester of pregnancy.

Nursing mothers: Iron salts are excreted into breast milk which may be of benefit when there is iron deficiency in the neonate.

Treatment of overdosage: Symptoms of overdosage may include gastro-intestinal irritation, haematemesis and diarrhoea. Empty the stomach immediately, preferably by vomiting. Inject Desferrioxamine 2 g intramuscularly. Lavage stomach with 1% sodium bicarbonate. Administer 5 g Desferrioxamine per os. Maintain fluid and electrolyte balance. The physician should be aware that tablets in the intestine will continue to release ferrous glycine sulphate for a period of hours.

Pharmaceutical precautions Store in a cool dry place protected from light.

Legal category P.

Package quantities Containers of 30 (OP, child resistant) and 250 tablets.

Further information The amino acid-iron chelate ferrous glycine sulphate prevents oxidation to the ferric form in the gastro-intestinal tract, thus enhancing absorption. The use of a patented controlled release system optimises the bioavailability of ferrous iron and minimises the likelihood of side-effects. The symptoms of nausea and gastrointestinal irritation often associated with iron therapy are unlikely to occur with Ferrocontin Continus Tablets.

Product licence number 8336/0004.

FERROCONTIN* FOLIC CONTINUS* TABLETS

Presentation Pale orange, film-coated bi-convex tablets. Each tablet contains the equivalent of 100 mg ferrous iron in the form of ferrous glycine sulphate within a patented controlled release system and 0.5 mg Folic Acid BP.

Uses Ferrocontin Folic Continus Tablets are indicated for the prophylaxis of iron and folic acid deficiencies during pregnancy.

Dosage and administration One tablet to be taken daily, or as directed by the physician. Ferrocontin Folic Continus tablets should be swallowed whole and not chewed. Not appropriate for children and the elderly.

Contra-indications, warnings, etc The tablets should not be given to patients with B_{12} deficiency without concomitant B_{12} supplementation.

Tetracyclines will chelate with iron impairing the absorption of both agents. Concurrent administration reduces the absorption of penicillamine and zinc. Folate administration may reduce serum anticonvulsant levels.

As with all medicines keep out of the reach of children.

Use in pregnancy: When administering ferrous sulphate to pregnant mice and rats in dosages of up to 100 times

(1200 mg/kg/day) the human adult dose, no influence on survival of dams, survival, development and abnormality, appearance of foetuses and offspring was observed. Experimental studies have not been described on the use of glycine in pregnancy in laboratory animals.

Studies in pregnant rats have confirmed that the administration of folic acid antagonists results in embryo destruction and foetal abnormalities. Co-administration of folic acid has been shown to safeguard against these effects. Very high doses of folic acid have been shown to cause foetal abnormalities in rats.

There are conflicting reports on the tendency of ferrous sulphate to induce congenital malformations in the foetuses of women receiving iron containing preparations during the first trimester. Harmful effects on the foetus, the mother or the pregnancy have not been reported for the ingestion of glycine.

Folic acid deficiency during pregnancy and especially multiple pregnancy may lead to the appearance of foetal malformations. Imbalance in folate requiring trophoblast cells may also lead to detachment of the placenta.

Harmful effects on the foetus, the mother or the pregnancy have not been reported for the ingestion of folic acid.

Ferrocontin Folic Continus Tablets should be used with caution during the first trimester of pregnancy.

Nursing mothers: Iron salts and folic acid are excreted into breast milk which may be of benefit when there is iron or folic acid deficiency in the neonate.

Treatment of overdosage: Symptoms of severe overdosage may include gastrointestinal irritation, haematemesis, and diarrhoea. Empty the stomach immediately, preferably by vomiting. Inject Desferrioxamine 2 g intramuscularly. Lavage stomach with 1% sodium bicarbonate. Administer 5 g Desferrioxamine per os. Maintain fluid and electrolyte balance. The physician should be aware that tablets in the intestine will continue to release ferrous glycine sulphate for a period of hours.

Pharmaceutical precautions Store in a cool dry place protected from light.

Legal category P.

Package quantities Containers of 30 (OP, child resistant) and 250 tablets.

Further information The amino acid-iron chelate ferrous glycine sulphate prevents oxidation to the ferric form in the gastrointestinal tract, thus enhancing absorption. The use of a patented controlled release system optimises the bioavailability of ferrous iron and minimises the likelihood of side-effects. The folic acid content of 1 tablet is unlikely to mask the presence of pernicious anaemia. The symptoms of nausea and gastrointestinal irritation often associated with iron therapy are unlikely to occur with Ferrocontin Folic Continus Tablets.

Product licence number 8336/0005.

MITOXANA*

Presentation White powder for injection in vials containing ifosfamide 500 mg, 1 g or 2 g for dissolving in Water for Injections using the volume recommended for each strength.

Uses

Action: Mitoxana is an alkylating agent which is inert until activated by microsomal enzymes. This occurs mainly in the liver, producing antitumour metabolites.

Indications: Clinical experience so far has shown Mitoxana to be effective in tumors of lung, ovary, cervix, breast and testis and in soft tissue sarcoma. Responses have also been reported in osteosarcoma, malignant lymphomas, carcinoma of the pancreas, and in head and neck tumours.

Mitoxana has been used as a single agent and in combination with radiotherapy, surgery and other cytotoxic agents.

Dosage and administration Mitoxana should only be used by clinicians experienced in the use of cytotoxic drugs. Mitoxana is inert until activated by enzymes in the liver. However, as with all cytotoxics, it is suggested that reconstitution should be performed by trained personnel, in a designated area. Those handling the preparation should wear protective gloves. Care should be taken to avoid splashing material into the eyes. The material should not be handled by women who are pregnant. Adequate care and precautions should be taken in the disposal of items (syringes, needles, etc.) used to reconstitute cytotoxic drugs.

Dosage: Mitoxana should not be used without the concurrent administration of mesna (Uromitexan). The dosage of mesna is discussed under Further information.

The dose of Mitoxana varies considerably depending on the clinical indication and the regimen employed. The usual total dose for each course is either 8-10 g/m^2, which is equally fractionated as single daily doses over five days, or 5-6 g/m^2 (maximum 10 g) given as a twenty-four hour infusion. Courses are normally repeated at intervals of 2-4 weeks for intermittent therapy or 3-4 weeks for 24-hour infusions depending on the haematological and biochemical status of the patient. The white cell count should not be less than 4000/mm^3 or the platelet count less than 100,000/mm^3 before the start of each course. There should be no signs or symptoms of urothelial toxicity or renal or hepatic impairment.

The usual number of courses given is four but up to seven (six by 24-hour infusion) courses have been given. Re-treatment has been given following relapse.

Experience in children is limited and involves the five day regimen only.

Administration: The dry contents of a vial should be dissolved in Water for Injections as follows:

500 mg vial:	add 6.5 ml of Water for Injections.
1 g vial:	add 12.5 ml of Water for Injections.
2 g vial:	add 25 ml of Water for Injections.

The resultant solution of 8% ifosfamide should not be injected directly into the vein. The solution may be:

1. diluted to less than a 4% solution and injected directly into the vein, with the patient supine, or
2. infused in 5% dextrose-saline or normal saline over 30-120 mins or
3. injected directly into a fast-running infusion or
4. made up in 3 litres of dextrose-saline or normal saline and infused over 24 hours. Each litre should be given over eight hours, and should be freshly made up immediately before infusion.

Should the drug accidently be given extravenously, local tissue damage is unlikely and no specific measures need be to be taken.

Repeated intravenous injections of large doses of Mitoxana have resulted in local irritation.

Mesna (Uromitexan) should be used to prevent urothelial toxicity.

Where Mitoxana is used as an i.v. bolus, increased dosages of mesna are recommended in children, patients whose urothelium may be damaged from previous therapies and those who are not adequately protected by the standard dose of mesna.

Patients should be maintained in fluid balance, replacement fluids being given as necessary to achieve this. The fluid intake of patients on the intermittent regimen should not be less than 2L in 24 hours. As Mitoxana may exert an antidiuretic effect, a diuretic may be necessary to ensure an adequate urinary output.

Urine should be sent for laboratory analysis before, and at the end of, each course of treatment, and the patient should be monitored for output and evidence of proteinuria and haematuria at regular intervals (4-hourly if possible) throughout the treatment period. The patient should be instructed to report any signs or symptoms of cystitis. Antiemetics administered before and during treatment may reduce nausea and vomiting. Oral hygiene is important.

No specific information on the use of this product in the elderly is available. Clinical trials have included patients over 65 years and no adverse reactions specific to this age group have been reported.

Contra-indications, warnings, etc

Contra-indications: Mitoxana is contra-indicated in patients with known hypersensitivity, bone marrow aplasia, myelosuppression, infections including urinary tract infections or acute urothelial toxicity, renal impairment (serum creatinine above 120 μmol/l i.e. 1.5 mg/100 ml), or hepatic impairment (bilirubin above 17 μmol/l i.e. 1 mg/100 ml, with alkaline phosphatase or transaminases more than 2-3 times normal).

Contraception in both sexes is advised during Mitoxana therapy. Patients should receive counselling with respect to subsequent pregnancies. Mitoxana should not be given in pregnancy, especially the first trimester, unless the expected benefit is thought to outweigh the substantial risk to the foetus. Mothers should not breastfeed whilst being treated with Mitoxana.

Precautions: Mitoxana has been shown to be mutagenic, teratogenic and carcinogenic in laboratory tests and there is a risk of drug-induced neoplasia following long-term treatment. Amenorrhoea and azoospermia can occur. Patients should be warned of a potential risk to future progeny.

Mitoxana is a potent immunosuppressive drug and the increased risk to a patient should be borne in mind.

The concomitant use of Mitoxana with anticoagulants, especially Warfarin, may result in disturbance of anticoagulant control and an increased risk of bleeding.

Care should be exercised in patients who are elderly, debilitated, have diabetes mellitus or evidence of myelosuppression or who have recently received radiotherapy or cytotoxic drugs. Caution is necessary in patients who have previously received platinum compounds or undergone a nephrectomy. In children, high cumulative doses of ifosfamide and continued treatment in the presence of renal tubular dysfunction may be associated with increased frequency or severity of renal damage.

Side-effects: Urothelial toxicity is the usual dose-limiting factor. This can be largely prevented by the concurrent administration of mesna. Urotoxicity can affect the efferent urinary tract as well as the bladder. The usual symptoms are frequency, dysuria, or haematuria.

Nephrotoxicity may occur with oliguria, raised uric acid, increased blood urea and serum creatinine and decreased creatinine clearance. Glycosuria, proteinuria, aminoaciduria and renal rickets have been reported with changes in serum proteins and electrolytes. Nephrotoxicity is usually reversible, especially in the early stages but severe cases are recorded, including Fanconi's syndrome and diabetes insipidus.

Nausea and vomiting. Anti-emetic administration before and during treatment may reduce this.

Large doses of Mitoxana give rise to a predictable marrow toxicity. The white cell count reaches its nadir 5-10 days after commencing treatment, recovery commencing after 10-14 days and usually returning to normal within 2-3 weeks. About 30% of patients would be expected to have a fall in haemoglobin of greater than 2 g/100 ml and a white cell count less than 2000/mm^3 but only 5% would be expected to have a platelet count less than 100,000/mm^3. There have been only occasional reports of coagulation disorders.

Central nervous system side effects may occur. Confusion and lethargy have been most commonly reported but tonic-clonic spasms, motor unrest, emotional lability and disorientation have been noted. These resolve spontaneously 1-2 days after cessation of the therapy.

A much rarer event involving EEG changes, fever, tachycardia, confusion, echolalia, disorientation, some aggression and depression of consciousness has been reported. Occasionally this has been fatal. If such effects occur, the drug should be stopped and supportive therapy given.

Alopecia occurs frequently but is usually reversible.

Hepatic as well as cardiac dysfunction has been observed in rare cases and jaundice has occurred in one patient.

Other side-effects reported are stomatitis, diarrhoea, pulmonary fibrosis, allergy, dermatitis, and venous irritation.

Overdosage: The most serious consequences of overdosage are haemorrhagic cystitis and myelosuppression. The latter usually recovers spontaneously but until it does, administration of a broad spectrum antibiotic may be advisable. Transfusions of whole blood should be given as necessary.

If the overdose is recognised within the first 24 hours and possibly up to 48 hours, i.v. mesna may be beneficial in ameliorating damage to the urinary system.

Normal supportive measures such as analgesics and maintenance of fluid balance should be instituted. If despite these measures the cystitis does not resolve, more intensive treatment may be necessary and a urological opinion should be sought. No further courses should be given until the patient has fully recovered.

Pharmaceutical precautions Store below 25°C; protect from light.

Legal category POM.

Package quantities 500 mg, 1 g and 2 g dry vials, singles.

Further information Mitoxana is not recommended for use in non-malignant conditions. The dosage of mesna (Uromitexan) varies according to its route of administration and the dose and route of administration of Mitoxana. The Uromitexan data sheet should be consulted for full prescribing information before commencing treatment. Further information is available from Degussa Pharmaceuticals Ltd.

Product licence numbers

Vials of 500 mg	8336/0030
Vials of 1 g	8336/0031
Vials of 2 g	8336/0032

NITROCONTIN* CONTINUS* TABLETS

Presentation Nitrocontin Continus Tablets 2.6 mg are flat, bevelled, pink, controlled release tablets containing Glyceryl Trinitrate BP 2.6 mg and embossed NC on one side and with the logo DPL on the other.

Nitrocontin Continus Tablets 6.4 mg are flat, bevelled, pink, controlled release tablets containing Glyceryl Trinitrate BP 6.4 mg and embossed $\frac{NC}{64}$ on one side and with the logo DPL on the other.

Uses For the prophylaxis and continued treatment of angina pectoris, whether or not associated with previous history of myocardial infarction. Nitrocontin Continus Tablets are indicated in all cases in which sublingual nitroglycerin has provided temporary relief, whether these be cases of classical angina pectoris or the anginal pain subsequent to myocardial infarction.

Dosage and administration *Adults including elderly:* The tablets must be swallowed whole and not chewed. Dosage should always be adjusted according to the response obtained by the individual patient and the severity of the angina pain. Initially, the recommended dosage is one 2.6 mg tablet morning and evening.

If symptoms have not been adequately controlled after a week on this regimen, the dosage should be increased to one 6.4 mg tablet morning and evening.

An increase in dosage to 6.4 mg three times daily may be found necessary in severe cases of angina pectoris which have not fully responded to the lesser recommended dosage.

Children: No recommended dose.

Contra-indications, warnings, etc

Contra-indications: As with all nitrates, cerebral haemorrhage and brain trauma, incipient glaucoma, pronounced anaemia.

Interactions: Nitrocontin Continus Tablets may be co-prescribed with beta-blocking agents for enhanced prophylaxis from Angina. Co-prescribing nitrates with antihypertensive drugs and vasodilators carries the risk of inducing hypotension.

Other undesirable effects: Facial flushing, tachycardia and postural hypotension.

An infrequent side-effect of a transient nature which occurs with all nitrate administration is 'nitrate headache'. This disappears with continued treatment since patients develop tolerance to this symptom. However, such side-effects are virtually absent or substantially diminished with Nitrocontin Continus Tablet therapy due to the patented controlled release system.

Side-effects affecting the ability to drive include severe headache and dizziness: patients so affected should not drive if symptoms are severe.

Use in pregnancy and lactation: Nitrocontin Continus Tablets are not contra-indicated in pregnancy, however, experience in pregnant women is limited as angina pectoris rarely occurs in young women. There have been no reports of harmful effects on the human foetus, mother or pregnancy. The muscle relaxant effects of glyceryl trinitrate affect uterine muscle. Glyceryl trinitrate may reduce systemic blood pressure and therefore blood flow to the placenta could be reduced. These actions represent potential hazard to the foetus.

For these reasons it is recommended that Nitrocontin Continus Tablets should be avoided in pregnancy, particularly in the first trimester unless the potential benefits outweigh the risks in a particular patient. Safety in lactation has not been established.

Special warnings and precautions: Although tolerance has not been demonstrated to occur in clinical trials with Nitrocontin Continus Tablets, the possibility of tolerance to the drug should be considered if symptoms of angina recur on high or more frequent dosing schedules.

Overdosage: Symptoms of overdosage include vomiting, hypotension, restlessness, syncope, cyanosis and methaemoglobinaemia. Treatment should include gastric lavage and attention to circulatory symptoms and signs. In severe cases, oxygen and other symptomatic and supportive respiratory and cardiovascular measures should be provided.

Methaemoglobinaemia may be treated with intravenous methylene blue in the dose of 1-4 mg/kg body weight. The Physician should be aware that tablets in the intestine will release glyceryl trinitrate for a period of hours.

Pharmaceutical precautions Store in a cool dry place protected from light.

Legal category P.

Package quantities
Tablets 2.6 mg: 100 tablets
Tablets 6.4 mg: 100 tablets

Further information Glyceryl trinitrate has a twofold action in relieving angina pectoris. It reduces cardiac work and dilates the coronary arteries. Thus, not only is the arterial oxygen requirement of the myocardium lessened, but the amount of oxygenated blood reaching the ischaemic heart is increased.

Nitrocontin Continus Tablets provide adequate and continuous activity throughout the day and night on a simple b.d. dosage. The need for sublingual glyceryl trinitrate is substantially reduced as the frequency and severity of anginal attacks are decreased.

Nitrocontin Continus Tablets actively prevent anginal episodes and reduce heavy dependance on multiple doses of sublingual glyceryl trinitrate administration.

Product licence numbers
Tablets 2.6 mg 8336/0002
Tablets 6.4 mg 8336/0003

PENDRAMINE*

Presentation Tablets each containing 125 mg or 250 mg D-penicillamine base. The 125 mg tablets are white, elongated, film coated with bisecting score on one side, and have a length of 11 mm and a width of 5.5 mm. The 250 mg tablets are white, elongated, film coated with bisecting score on one side, debossed HB on the same side, and have a length of 16 mm and a width of 7 mm.

Uses Pendramine is indicated for the treatment of severe active rheumatoid arthritis, Wilson's disease, cystinuria, heavy metal poisoning and active chronic hepatitis.

Dosage and administration *For oral administration.*
1. Severe active rheumatoid arthritis

Adults: A dose of 125–250 mg daily for the initial 4 week period, then increasing at intervals of not less than four weeks by similar amounts. The ultimate maintenance dose will depend on the response obtained in individual patients. The usual maintenance dose is 500–750 mg in divided dosages. Improvement may not occur for some months.

A few patients may require up to 2000 mg daily to obtain benefit.

The minimum maintenance dose to achieve suppression of symptoms should be used. Treatment should be discontinued if no benefit is obtained within 12 months.

When clinical assessment shows that suppression of disease activity has been achieved, the dose should be kept at this maintenance level for six months, thereafter reducing the daily dosage by 250 mg at intervals of two or three months. Relapse may occur following withdrawal or when an inadequate dose level is reached, usually within three months, but most patients respond to further courses of Pendramine.

The Elderly: Increased toxicity unrelated to renal function occurs in the elderly. A maximum initial dose of 50–125 mg daily for 4–8 weeks should be used, increased at intervals of not less than 4 weeks by similar amounts. The maximum recommended dose is 1000 mg daily.

Children: 15–20 mg/kg/day is considered appropriate in the majority of cases. It is suggested that the initial dose is lower and increased at four-weekly intervals over a period of three to six months.

2. Wilson's disease: D-penicillamine is a copper-chelating agent, and is most effectively used in conjunction with a low-copper diet (below 1 mg of copper per day).

Adults: 1500 to 2000 mg daily in divided doses, to be taken 30 minutes before food. The dose may be reduced to 750–1000 mg daily when disease control is achieved as evidenced by urinary copper excretion. (Twenty-four hour urine samples should be examined at 3-monthly intervals). A dose of 2000 mg daily should not be continued for more than one year.

The Elderly: Up to 20 mg per kg body weight daily in divided doses before food. The dosage should be adjusted to achieve disease control.

Children: Up to 20 mg per kg body weight daily in divided doses before food. Maximum dose 500 mg/day.

3. Cystinuria: Prevention and treatment of cystine stones.

Treatment of stones:

Adults: For the treatment of cystine stones, 750 mg daily in divided doses and especially at bedtime, increasing to 1500–2000 mg daily. The dose is adjusted to maintain urinary excretion of cystine below 100 mg per day. Maintain adequate fluid intake of 3 litres/day to provide a urine flow of 2 ml/min.

The Elderly: The minimum dose which maintains urinary excretion of cystine below 100 mg per day.

Children: Up to 30 mg per kg body weight daily in divided doses and especially at bedtime. The dose should be adjusted to maintain urine cystine levels below 100 mg/day.

Prophylaxis:

Adults: (No history of stone formation but a cystine output in excess of 300 mg per day) 250–750 mg at night before retiring. The dose is adjusted to maintain overnight urine cystine excretion below 100 mg/day.

Fluid intake should not be less than 3 litres/day.

Safety in pregnancy is not established but if treatment is unavoidable should not exceed a dose of 1000 mg/24 hours.

The Elderly: The minimum dose required to maintain

urinary excretion of cystine below 100 mg per day should be used.

Children: Paediatric dosage not yet established.

4. Heavy metal poisoning (lead)

Adults: Daily oral dose of 1500–2000 mg in divided doses until urinary lead is stabilised at 0.5 mg/day.

The Elderly: 20 mg per kg body weight until urinary lead is stabilised at 0.5 mg/day.

Children: 20–25 mg per kg body weight daily in divided doses before food.

5. Active chronic hepatitis

Adults: Pendramine is intended for the maintenance treatment of active chronic hepatitis. The diagnosis should be based on a history of at least three months duration with features of chronic aggressive hepatitis, with or without cirrhosis. Treatment with Pendramine should not be commenced until the disease process has been brought under control, initially by treatment with corticosteroids (e.g. 30 mg prednisone daily, sometimes with 75 mg azathioprine daily added to the regime). Disease control should be evidenced by biochemical analysis of liver function to include evaluation of serum bilirubin and transaminase activity.

Pendramine therapy should be commenced with 500 mg daily, in divided doses, increasing gradually over three months to the maintenance dose of 1250 mg daily. Concurrently, the dosage of corticosteroids should be reduced and phased out over a three-month period. Throughout therapy, liver function tests should be carried out at suitable intervals for assessment of disease status.

The Elderly: Not recommended.

Children: Not recommended.

Contra-indications, warnings, etc Renal insufficiency; lupus erythematosus; hypersensitivity to D-penicillamine particularly if nephrotic syndrome or bone marrow depression has previously occurred.

Interactions with other medicaments and other forms of interaction: Concomitant oral iron therapy should not be given within 2 hours of taking penicillamine.

Effects on ability to drive and to use machinery: Not known.

Other undesirable effects: Both the frequency and severity of many side-effects and adverse reactions to D-penicillamine are found to be dose-related, hence the importance of initiating therapy at low doses and gradually increasing the quantity of drug given to optimum level.

Nausea and vomiting may occur.

D-penicillamine may cause allergic reactions such as urticaria and erythema accompanied by hyperpyrexia. Transient rashes and fever may occur early in therapy; if persistent, temporary withdrawal of treatment with or without a short course of steroids may be necessary. Penicillamine may be re-introduced at a lower dosage. If steroids are given, penicillamine should be reintroduced before steroid withdrawal.

A late rash, described as "Epidermolysis Bullosa" and "Penicillamine Dermopathy" may occur, after several months or years of therapy and may necessitate discontinuation of treatment.

Goodpastures syndrome, haemolytic anaemia and anorexia have been reported.

Other disorders of later onset and attributed to D-penicillamine are rheumatoid-like reactions, stomatitis and taste impairment. Reversible loss of taste occurs frequently. Reactions involving the appearance of thrombocytopenia, neutropenia or proteinuria may occur, particularly with higher dose levels. Less common are nephrotic syndrome and haematuria, purpura and increased skin friability due to increased collagen. Haematuria is rare, but if it occurs, treatment should be stopped immediately.

Serious complications include myasthenia gravis, pemphigus, nephrotic syndrome, Stevens–Johnson-like syndrome and lupus erythematosus. Deaths from agranulocytosis and aplastic anaemia have been recorded.

Pendramine should not be given concurrently with iron or other heavy metals with which it may form complexes.

Use in pregnancy and lactation – warning: The safety of penicillamine in pregnancy and lactation has not been established. It has been shown to be teratogenic in rats when given in doses several times higher than those administered to humans.

Other special warnings and precautions: Known sensitivity to penicillamine. Throughout pregnancy.

Penicillamine should not be used in patients who are receiving concurrent gold therapy, antimalarial or cytotoxic drugs, oxyphenbutazone or phenylbutazone since these drugs have a propensity to cause similar serious haematologic and/or renal adverse reactions.

Establish the lowest effective dose of D-penicillamine by quantitative amino acid chromatography on urine. Urine protein estimations should be carried out initially weekly for the first three months of therapy and thereafter monthly. Renal function should be assessed monthly for 6 months and 3 monthly thereafter.

The observation of proteinuria necessitates repeated quantitative estimations. Heavy or steadily increasing proteinuria or significant haematuria necessitates withdrawal of Pendramine.

With the exception of Wilson's disease patients (see later) platelet and white cell counts must be normal before commencing treatment. Because of the risk of blood dyscrasias and renal disturbances, full blood counts and urine examinations are essential during treatment. Weekly tests are recommended after each increase in dose as well as during the first eight weeks of therapy to monitor thrombocytopenia and neutropenia then monthly when dosage regimes have been stabilised.

Platelet counts below 120,000 mm^{-3} or leucocyte counts below 2,500 mm^{-3} necessitate withdrawal of D-penicillamine with resumption at a reduced dosage when counts return to normal. Recurrence of thrombocytopenia or leucopenia are indications for cessation of treatment.

A low platelet or white cell count is not a contra-indication to commence treatment of Wilson's disease. Treatment should be discontinued however, if a low initial count falls further and/or excessive bruising or petechial haemorrhages occur.

Iron deficiency may occur in menstruating women.

Allergic phenomena occurring early, unless severe, respond to cyproheptadine and temporary reductions of dose of D-penicillamine. Copper supplements may be necessary for alleviating taste impairment when treating conditions other than Wilson's disease.

In the treatment of rheumatoid arthritis, response to Pendramine is often slow and the use of existing analgesics, anti-inflammatories or steroids should be continued and later gradually withdrawn, subject to patient improvement.

Overdosage: Treatment of overdosage is symptomatic and withdrawal of the drug is necessary if serious side effects as mentioned above occur.

Incompatibilities: Not known.

Pharmaceutical precautions Store in a dry place below 25°C. Keep containers tightly closed.

Legal category POM.

Package quantities *Tablets:* 125 mg, plastic bottles of 100

Tablets: 250 mg, plastic bottles of 100

Further information Pendramine may be considered as an alternative to prednisone in the treatment of active chronic hepatitis when the latter drug causes complications such as diabetes, osteoporosis, etc. Occasionally, patients with rheumatoid arthritis who have responded to a particular dose begin to relapse. Most of these will respond to a dose increase which should be gradual.

Product licence numbers
Pendramine 125 mg 0493/0080
Pendramine 250 mg 0493/0081

Product licence holder: E. Merck Limited, Four Marks, Alton, Hampshire.

UROMITEXAN*

Presentation Clear, glass ampoules containing a clear, colourless, aqueous solution of mesna (sodium 2-mercapto-ethanesulphonate) 400 mg in 4 ml and 1000 mg in 10 ml.

Uses

Action: Mesna is a sulphydryl-containing compound which is excreted in the urine. Co-administration with oxazaphosphorine alkylating agents such as ifosfamide (Mitoxana)and cyclophosphamide (Endoxana) significantly reduces the troublesome urotoxic effects of these by reacting with the causal metabolites, including acrolein, in the urinary system. No reduction in the antitumour activity of these oxazaphosphorine compounds has been detected.

Indications: For the prophylaxis of urothelial toxicity in patients treated with ifosfamide and cyclophosphamide.

Dosage and administration Sufficient mesna must be given to protect the patient adequately from the urotoxic effects of the oxazaphosphorine. When calculating the dose of mesna the quantity should be rounded up to the nearest whole ampoule. Urinary output should be maintained and the urine monitored for haematuria and proteinuria throughout the treatment period.

Where ifosfamide or cyclophosphamide is used as an i.v. bolus: Mesna is given by intravenous injection over 15-30 minutes as 20% of the simultaneously administered oxazaphosphorine on a weight for weight basis (w/w). The same dose of mesna is repeated after 4 and 8 hours. The total dose of mesna is 60% (w/w) of the oxazaphosphorine dose. This is repeated on each occasion that the cytotoxic agents are used.

If necessary the dose of mesna can be increased to 40% of the oxazaphosphorine dose given four times at three hourly intervals (0, 3, 6 and 9 hours). (Total dose = 160% (w/w) of the oxazaphosphorine dose). This larger dose is recommended in children, in patients whose urothelium may be damaged from previous treatment with oxazaphosphorine or pelvic irradiation, or in patients who are not adequately protected by the standard dose of mesna.

Where ifosfamide is used as a 24-hour infusion: Mesna can be used as a concurrent infusion. An initial 20% (w/w) of the total ifosfamide dose is given as an i.v. bolus, then an infusion of 100% (w/w) of the ifosfamide over 24 hours, followed by a further 12-hour infusion of 60% (w/w) of the ifosfamide dose. (Total mesna dose = 180% of the ifosfamide dose).

The final 12-hour infusion of mesna may be replaced by boluses at 28, 32 and 36 hours, each of 20% (w/w) of the ifosfamide dose, or by oral mesna (see below). Mesna can be mixed in the same infusion bag as the ifosfamide.

Oral use of mesna: Mesna has been shown to be effective when taken orally with intermittent oxazaphosphorine therapy or following the 24-hour infusion of ifosfamide and mesna. The first dose of 40% (w/w) of the oxazaphosphorine is given with the oxazaphosphorine or as the infusion is stopped, and repeated after 4 and 8 hours. Mesna should be taken immediately the ampoule is opened, in a soft drink (e.g. orange juice).

No specific information on the use of this product in the elderly is available. Clinical trials have included patients over 65 years and no adverse reactions specific to this age group have been reported.

Contra-indications, warnings, etc

Contra-indications: There are no absolute contra-indications to the use of mesna.

Precautions: As mesna counteracts only the urotoxic side-effects of cyclophosphamide and ifosfamide, other side-effects of cytotoxic therapy e.g. myelosuppression, nausea, vomiting, alopecia, may still be expected. No other interaction between mesna and these alkylating agents has been demonstrated.

Side-effects: Because patients receive potent cytotoxic agents concurrently, the side-effect profile of mesna is difficult to define. However, in healthy volunteers the following side-effects occurred at single doses of 60-70 mg/kg per day, nausea, vomiting, colic diarrhoea, fatigue, headache, limb pains, depression, irritability, lack of energy and rash.

Overdose: There is no clinical experience of overdosage. Standard supportive measures should be adopted.

Pharmaceutical precautions Protect from light, store below 30°C. Mesna is stable for up to 24-hours in a solution of sodium chloride 0.9% and of ifosfamide in sodium chloride 0.9%.

Legal category POM.

Package quantities 4 ml ampoules in boxes of 15. 10 ml ampoules in boxes of 15.

Further information There is evidence that the long term urothelial toxicity of the oxazaphosphorines can be almost totally prevented by the concurrent administration of mesna in the appropriate dosage.

A false positive test for urinary ketones (e.g. Rothera's test, N-Multistix reagent strip) may arise in patients treated with mesna. The colour is red-violet rather than violet and it will fade immediately on the addition of glacial acetic acid.

Product licence numbers

Ampoules of 4 ml	8336/0033
Ampoules of 10 ml	8336/0033

**Trade Mark*

Delandale Laboratories Limited
Delandale House
37 Old Dover Road
Canterbury, Kent, CT1 3JF

BIOPHYLLINE* SYRUP

Presentation A clear yellow coloured, cherry menthol flavoured, sugar-free syrup containing 250 mg theophylline sodium glycinate, equivalent to 125 mg Theophylline Hydrate BP per 5 ml.

Uses Biophylline Syrup is indicated for the prophylaxis and relief of bronchospasm in the treatment of asthma and bronchitis.

Dosage and administration The following recommended dosage should be taken orally, preferably after food.

Adults: 5–10 ml (equivalent to 125–250 mg Theophylline Hydrate BP) every six to eight hours.

Children: 7–12 years: 2.5 ml–5 ml (equivalent to 62.5 – 125 mg Theophylline Hydrate BP) every six to eight hours.

2–6 years: 2.5 ml (equivalent to 62.5 mg Theophylline Hydrate BP) every six to eight hours.

Under 2 years: Not recommended.

It is suggested that treatment is commenced at the lower end of the recommended range and dosage increased gradually until steady-state blood levels in the range 10–20 micrograms/ml theophylline are achieved. Elderly patients may require lower, less frequent doses due to reduced theophylline clearance.

Contra-indications, warnings, etc
Contra-indications: None known.

Precautions: Theophylline should be administered with caution to the elderly or patients with cardiac or liver disease and those with a history of peptic ulceration. Theophylline clearance may be significantly reduced during intercurrent illness. Smokers tend to have increased theophylline clearance and may require higher doses. Patients with renal failure may be given usual doses; serum concentrations are reduced by dialysis. Rifampicin may impair theophylline absorption. Theophylline blood levels may be increased with concurrent administration of erythromycin, triacetyloleandomycin, propranolol, cimetidine and corticosteroids.

Barbiturates may increase theophylline clearance. Sympathomimetic agents and other xanthines may cause enhanced bronchodilation and increased toxic effects when given with theophylline. Xanthines can potentiate hypokalaemia resulting from beta agonist therapy, steroids, diuretics and hypoxia. Particular caution is advised in severe asthma. It is recommended that serum potassium levels are monitored in such situations. Theophylline crosses the placenta, apparently without teratogenic effects in humans but medication is best avoided during the first trimester of pregnancy. Excretion occurs into breast milk and may cause irritability in the infant.

Side-effects: Biophylline treatment may be associated with the usual side-effects of theophylline, namely gastrointestinal irritation and central nervous system stimulation.

Overdosage: Serum concentrations of theophylline above 20 micrograms/ml are likely to give rise to toxic effects. Overdosage is characterised by vomiting, impaired consciousness, hyperreflexia, hyperventilation, hypokalaemia, tachycardia, arrhythmias, hypotension and convulsions. Treatment of overdosage is by gastric lavage followed by symptomatic measures. Fluid and electrolyte balance should be maintained and oxygen given if required. Convulsions may be controlled with intravenous diazepam or thiopentone sodium. Dialysis or haemoperfusion may be used.

Pharmaceutical precautions Store in a cool place. Protect from direct sunlight. Dilution of Biophylline Syrup is not recommended.

Legal category P

Package quantities Biophylline Syrup is available in bottles of 250 ml.

Further information Nil.

Product licence number 0357/0027.

BIOPHYLLINE* TABLETS

Presentation Biophylline tablets 500 mg: Each white capsule-shaped tablet, embossed BIO 500 one side with a breakmark on the other, contains 500 mg Theophylline PhEur in a controlled release formulation.

Biophylline tablets 350 mg: Each white capsule-shaped tablet, embossed BIO 350 one side with a breakmark on the other, contains 350 mg Theophylline PhEur in a controlled release formulation.

Uses Biophylline tablets are indicated for the treatment of reversible obstructive airways disease.

Dosage and administration The following recommended dosage should be taken orally. Tablets should not be crushed or chewed.

As response to theophylline may vary between patients, dosage should be individually titrated in order to achieve an optimum clinical response. Once stabilised on Biophylline Tablets, patients should not be changed to another preparation without careful restabilisation.

Adults and children over 12 years:

Over 70 kg:	The usual maintenance dose is one 500 mg tablet taken every 12 hours
Under70 kg:	The usual maintenance dose is one 350 mg tablet taken every 12 hours
Children under 12 years:	Not recommended
Elderly patients:	Elderly patients may require lower, less frequent doses due to reduced theophylline clearance

Smokers tend to have increased theophylline clearance and may require higher doses.

It is suggested that treatment is commenced with one tablet once daily and dosage increased gradually until steady-state blood levels in the range 10–20 micrograms/ml theophylline are achieved. Biophylline tablets are scored, therefore they can be divided to provide dosage increments of 175 mg or 250 mg.

Contra-indications, warnings, etc
Contra-indications: None known.

Precautions: Theophylline should be administered with caution to the elderly or patients with cardiac or liver disease and those with a history of peptic ulceration. Theophylline clearance may be significantly reduced during intercurrent illness. Patients with renal failure may be given ususal doses; serum concentrations are reduced by dialysis. Rifampicin may impair theophylline absorption. Theophylline blood levels may be increased with concurrent administration of erythromycin, triacetyloleandomycin, propranolol, cimetidine and corticosteroids. Barbiturates may increase theophylline clearance. Sympathomimetic agents and other xanthines may cause enhanced bronchodilation and increased toxic effects when given with theophylline. Xanthines can potentiate hypokalaemia resulting from beta agonist therapy, steroids, diuretics and hypoxia. Particular caution is advised in severe asthma. It is recommended that serum potassium levels are monitored in such situations. Theophylline crosses the placenta, apparently without teratogenic effects in humans but medication is best avoided during the first trimester of pregnancy. Excretion occurs into breast milk and may cause irritability in the infant.

Side-effects: Biophylline treatment may be associated with the usual side-effects of theophylline, namely gastrointestinal irritation and central nervous system stimulation.

Overdosage: Serum concentrations of theophylline above 20 micrograms/ml are likely to give rise to toxic effects. Overdosage is characterised by vomiting, impaired consciousness, hyperreflexia, hyperventilation, hypokalaemia, tachycardia, arrthythmias, hypotension and convulsions. Treatment of overdosage is by gastric lavage followed by symptomatic measures. Fluid and electrolyte balance should be maintained and oxygen given if required. Convulsions may be controlled with intravenous diazepam or thiopentone sodium. Dialysis or haemoperfusion may be used.

Pharmaceutical precautions Store in a cool, dry place.

Legal category P.

Package quantities Biophylline tablets are blister packed into cartons of 56 tablets.

Further information nil.

Product licence numbers
Biophylline Tablets 350 mg 0357/0030
Biophylline Tablets 500 mg 0357/0031

DICYNENE* 500 TABLETS

Presentation Dicynene 500 Tablets. Each white, scored, capsule-shaped tablet contains 500 mg ethamsylate and is engraved 'D500' one side, with a breakmark on the other.

Mode of action: Dicynene is a non-hormonal agent which reduces capillary exudation and blood loss. Dicynene does not affect the normal coagulation mechanism since administration is without effect on prothrombin time, fibrinolysis, platelet count or function.

Dicynene is thought to act by increasing capillary vascular wall resistance and platelet adhesiveness in the presence of a vascular lesion, by inhibiting the biosynthesis and actions of those prostaglandins which cause platelet disaggregation, vasodilation and increased capillary permeability and does not have a vasoconstricting action.

Uses Dicynene is used clinically for the short term treatment of blood loss in primary and IUCD-induced menorrhagia.

Dosage and administration The normal dosage is 500 mg four times daily from the start of bleeding until menstruation ceases.

Contra-indications, warnings, etc Treatment should only be undertaken following exclusion of other pelvic pathology, in particular the presence of fibroids.

Precautions: In patients receiving Dicynene for menorrhagia the use of the product before onset of bleeding is not recommended.

Use in pregnancy and lactation: Studies in animals have revealed no teratogenic effect of Dicynene, but since there is inadequate evidence of safety in human pregnancy, clinical use in pregnancy is not recommended.

Dicynene is secreted in breast milk and administration to nursing mothers is not recommended.

Side-effects: Occasional headaches or skin rashes may occur which usually disappear on reduced dosage. A few patients may experience nausea, however this may be overcome by administering the dose after food.

Pharmaceutical precautions Dicynene tablets should be stored in a cool, dry place. Dispense in airtight containers offering adequate protection from light and moisture.

Legal category POM.

Package quantities Securitainers of 100 tablets.

Further information Dicynene is fully absorbed when given orally and is excreted unchanged, largely by the urinary route.

Product licence number 0357/5003R.

DICYNENE* INJECTION

Presentation Each clear glass 2 ml ampoule, printed DICYNENE, contains 250 mg ethamsylate.

Mode of action: Dicynene is a non-hormonal agent which reduces capillary exudation and blood loss. Dicynene does not affect the normal coagulation mechanism since administration is without effect on prothrombin time, fibrinolysis, platelet count or function.

Dicynene is thought to act by increasing capillary vascular wall resistance and platelet adhesiveness in the presence of a vascular lesion, by inhibiting the biosynthesis and actions of those prostaglandins which cause platelet disaggregation, vasodilation and increased capillary permeability and does not have a vasoconstricting action.

Uses Dicynene injection is used for the prophylaxis and treatment of periventricular haemorrhage in low birth weight infants.

Dosage and administration The normal dosage is 12.5 mg/kg given by intravenous or intramuscular route every six hours.

Contra-indications, warnings, etc

Precautions: Dicynene Injection is intended for neonatal use only.

Side-effects: Dicynene is well tolerated. However, occasional headaches, nausea or skin rashes may occur which usually disappear on reduced dosage.

Pharmaceutical precautions Dicynene Injection should be stored in a cool place, protected from light. If the contents of the ampoules become coloured they should not be administered.

Dicynene Injection is incompatible with solutions of sodium bicarbonate and compound sodium lactate. When Dicynene Injection is mixed with saline it should be used immediately.

Legal category POM.

Package quantities Boxes containing 10 × 2 ml ampoules.

Further information Following intravenous administration maximum blood levels of ethamsylate are achieved in 2–3 minutes, while after intramuscular injection, maximum blood levels of ethamsylate are achieved after about one hour. Ethamsylate is excreted unchanged, largely by the urinary route.

Product licence number 0357/5001R.

KIDITARD*

Presentation Hard gelatin capsules, size 0, with clear light blue and clear dark blue shell. Each capsule contains 250 mg quinidine bisulphate (equivalent to 200 mg quinidine sulphate) in the form of sustained release micro-pellets.

Uses Sustained release quinidine therapy. The active ingredient is absorbed from the gastro-intestinal tract over a 12 hour period. An even pattern of release of the drug is established which prevents excessively high initial blood levels and therefore limits undesirable side effects. The capsules permit a twice daily dosage regime and prevent wide fluctuation in plasma quinidine levels.

Kiditard capsules are used clinically for: extra-systoles; paroxysmal atrial tachycardia; nodal tachycardia; atrial fibrillation; atrial flutter; paroxysmal ventricular tachycardia; maintenance of sinus rhythm following restoration by electro-conversion.

Dosage and administration Kiditard dosage should be individually adapted to each patient. As a rule, treatment should commence with two capsules every 10–12 hours, after a test dose of 1 capsule to test for patient sensitivity.

Kiditard capsules are not recommended for use in children.

Contra-indications, warnings, etc Acute infections, atrio-ventricular block and idiosyncrasy to quinidine form absolute contra-indications to Kiditard therapy. Special care must be taken with heavily digitalised patients and in patients with congestive heart failure, hypotension or ventricular tachycardia due to possible overdosage with quinidine. Special care is also needed in patients on prolonged anti-coagulant treatment since cases of quinidine-induced hypoprothrombinaemic haemorrhage have been recorded. Patients should be carefully observed for their reactions to the first dose of the drug since idiosyncrasy is a possible response to quinidine. The following allergic reactions to quinidine have been reported: urticaria, purpura, asthma, thrombocytopaenia. Gastro-intestinal upset, commonly associated with quinidine therapy, is largely avoided through the use of Kiditard. There are reports of hepatitis due to quinidine; none has been fatal and signs and symptoms disappear on withdrawal. Cardiotoxic side-effects (ventricular extra systole, A-V block, increased QRS complex above 50%, ventricular tachycardia) may occur; repeated high doses may lead to cinchonism.

If overdosage occurs treatment should be as for quinidine. Gastric lavage and a saline purgative should be employed. Promote excretion by acidifying urine with ammonium chloride. Maintain fluid balance and blood pressure. Assist respiration and monitor cardiac rhythm.

Pharmaceutical precautions Protect from light and moisture.

Legal category POM.

Package quantities Containers of 100 capsules.

Further information Nil.

Product licence number 0357/0012.

PRIADEL*

Presentation Controlled release lithium carbonate tablets.

Priadel: White, circular, bi-convex tablets engraved PRIADEL one side, scored on the other side. Each containing 400 mg Lithium Carbonate PhEur in a controlled release formulation.

Priadel 200: White, scored, capsule-shaped tablets engraved P200 on one side. Each containing 200 mg Lithium Carbonate PhEur in a controlled release formulation.

Uses 1. Treatment of mania and hypomania.

2. Lithium may also be tried in the treatment of some patients with recurrent bipolar depression, where treatment with other antidepressants has been unsuccessful.

3. Prophylactic treatment of recurrent affective disorders.

4. Control of aggressive or self-mutilating behaviour.

Dosage and administration A simple treatment schedule has been evolved which except for some minor variations should be followed whether using Priadel therapeutically or prophylactically. The minor variations to this schedule depend on the elements of the illness being treated and these are described later.

1. In patients of average weight (70 kg) an initial dose of 400–1,200 mg may be given as a single daily dose in the morning or on retiring. Alternatively, the dose may be divided and given morning and evening. The tablets should not be crushed or chewed. When changing from other lithium preparations serum lithium levels should first be checked, then Priadel therapy commenced at a daily dose as close as possible to the dose of the other form of lithium. As bioavailability varies from product to product (particularly with regard to retard or slow release preparations) a change of product should be regarded as initiation of new treatment.

2. Four to five days after starting treatment (and never longer than one week) a blood sample should be taken for the estimation of serum lithium level.

3. The objective is to adjust the Priadel dose so as to maintain the serum lithium level permanently within the diurnal range of 0.5–1.5 mmol/l. In practice, the blood sample should be taken between 12 and 24 hours after the previous dose of Priadel. 'Target' serum lithium concentrations at 12 and 24 hours are shown in the table below.

	'Target' serum lithium concentration (mmol/l)	
	At 12 hours	*At 24 hours*
Once daily dosage	0.7–1.0	0.5–0.8
Twice daily dosage	0.5–0.8	

Both strengths of tablet are scored, therefore they can be divided accurately to provide dosage adjustments as small as 100 mg. Serum lithium levels should be monitored weekly until stabilisation is achieved.

4. Lithium therapy should not be initiated unless adequate facilities for routine monitoring of serum concentrations are available. Following stabilisation of serum lithium levels, the period between subsequent estimations can be increased gradually but should not normally exceed three months. Additional measurements should be made following alteration of dosage, on development of intercurrent disease, signs of manic or depressive relapse, following significant change in sodium or fluid intake, or if signs of lithium toxicity occur.

5. Whilst a high proportion of acutely ill patients may respond within three to seven days of the commencement of Priadel therapy, Priadel should be continued through any recurrence of the affective disturbance. This is important as the full prophylactic effect may not occur for 6 to 12 months after the initiation of therapy.

6. In patients who show a positive response to Priadel therapy, treatment is likely to be long term. Careful clinical appraisal of the patient should be exercised throughout medication (see Precautions).

Prophylactic treatment of recurrent affective disorders and control of aggressive or self-mutilating behaviour: It is recommended that the described treatment schedule is followed.

Treatment of acute mania, hypomania and recurrent bipolar depression: It is likely that a higher than normal Priadel intake may be necessary during an acute phase and divided doses would be required here. Therefore as soon as control of mania or depression is achieved, the serum lithium level should be determined and it may be necessary, dependent on the results, to lower the dose of Priadel and re-stabilise serum lithium levels. In all other details the described treatment schedule is recommended.

Use in elderly: In elderly patients or those below 50 kg in weight, it is recommended that the starting dose be 400 mg. Elderly patients may be more sensitive to undesirable effects of lithium and also may require lower doses in order to maintain normal serum lithium levels. It follows therefore that long term patients often require a reduction in dosage over a period of years.

Use in children and adolescents: Not recommended.

Contra-indications, warnings, etc
Contra-indications. Renal insufficiency, cardiovascular insufficiency, Addison's disease and untreated hypothyroidism are all contra-indications to lithium therapy.

Use in pregnancy: There is epidemiological evidence that lithium may be harmful to the foetus in human pregnancy.

Total no. 'lithium babies' reported	*Total malformed infants*	*Ebstein's anomaly and other major cardiovascular malformations*
225	25 (11%)	18 (8%)

It is strongly recommended that lithium be discontinued before a planned pregnancy. If it is considered essential to maintain Priadel treatment during pregnancy, serum lithium levels should be monitored closely since renal function changes gradually during pregnancy and suddenly at parturition, requiring dosage adjustments. It is recommended that lithium be discontinued shortly before delivery and recommenced a few days postpartum.

Babies may show signs of lithium toxicity necessitating fluid therapy in the neonatal period. Babies born with low serum lithium concentrations may have a flaccid appearance which returns to normal without any treatment. Lithium is secreted in breast milk, therefore bottle feeding is recommended.

Precautions: When considering Priadel therapy, it is necessary to ascertain whether patients are receiving lithium in any other form. If so, check serum levels before proceeding. It is important to ensure that renal function is normal – if necessary a creatinine clearance test or other renal function test should be performed. Cardiac and thyroid function should be assessed before commencing lithium treatment. Patients should be euthyroid before the initiation of lithium therapy. Renal function, cardiac function and thyroid function should be reassessed periodically.

Clear instructions regarding the symptoms of impending toxicity should be given by the doctor to all patients receiving long term lithium therapy (see Toxic effects). Patients should also be warned to report if polyuria or polydipsia develop. Episodes of nausea and vomiting or other conditions leading to salt/water depletion (including severe dieting) should also be reported. Elderly patients are particularly liable to lithium toxicity.

Caution should be exercised to ensure that diet and fluid intake are normal thus maintaining a stable electrolyte balance. This may be of special importance in very hot weather or work environment. Infectious diseases including colds, influenza, gastro-enteritis and urinary infections may alter fluid balance and thus affect serum lithium levels. Treatment should be discontinued during any intercurrent infection and should only be reinstituted after the patient's physical health has returned to normal.

Drug interactions: Concurrent use of lithium and diuretics may cause reduced lithium clearance, leading to intoxication. If a diuretic has to be prescribed for a lithium patient, the lithium dosage should first be lowered and the patient re-stabilised with frequent monitoring. Similar precautions should be exercised on diuretic withdrawal. Other drugs affecting electrolyte balance e.g. steroids, may alter lithium excretion and should be avoided in patients on lithium. If other psychotropic drugs are used they should be initiated at a lower dosage than usual, as their side effects may be potentiated by the use of lithium. This has been shown to be of particular importance for the concurrent use of lithium and haloperidol or flupenthixol.

There have been isolated reports of possible interactions between lithium and diazepam (resulting in hypothermia), methyldopa, tetracyclines, phenytoin, carbamazepine, indomethacin and other prostaglandin-synthetase inhibitors.

Warnings and adverse effects: Side effects are usually related to serum lithium concentrations and are infrequent at levels below 1.0 mmol/l.

Mild gastrointestinal effects, nausea, vertigo, muscle weakness and a dazed feeling may occur initially, but frequently disappear after stabilisation. Fine hand tremors, polyuria and mild thirst may persist. Weight gain or oedema may present in some patients but should not be treated with diuretics.

Hypercalcaemia, hypermagnesaemia and hyperparathyroidism have been reported. Skin conditions including acne, psoriasis, generalised pustular psoriasis, rashes and leg ulcers have occasionally been reported as being aggravated by lithium treatment.

Long term treatment with lithium may be associated with disturbances of thyroid function, including goitre, hypothyroidism and thyrotoxicosis. Lithium-induced hypothyroidism may be managed successfully with concurrent thyroxine.

Memory impairment may occur during long term use.

Nephrotoxicity: Up to one third of patients on lithium may develop polyuria with a urinary output of up to three litres per day. This is usually due to lithium blocking the effect of ADH and is reversible on lithium withdrawal. However, long term treatment with lithium may also result in permanent changes in kidney histology and impairment of renal function. High serum concentrations of lithium including episodes of acute lithium toxicity may aggravate these changes. The minimum clinically effective dose of lithium should always be used. In patients who develop polyuria or polydipsia, renal function should be monitored, e.g. with measurement of blood urea, serum creatinine and urinary protein levels in addition to the routine serum lithium estimations.

After a period lasting 3–5 years, patients should be carefully assessed to ensure that benefit persists.

Toxic effects: Such effects are indicative of impending lithium intoxication and fall into two groups:

1. Gastro-intestinal: increasing anorexia, diarrhoea and vomiting.
2. Central nervous system: muscle weakness, lack of co-ordination, drowsiness or lethargy progressing to giddiness with ataxia, tinnitus, blurred vision, dysarthria, coarse tremor and muscle twitching.

At blood levels above 2–3 mmol/l there may be a large output of dilute urine, with increasing disorientation, seizures, coma and death.

Patients should be instructed to stop taking their tablets if toxic symptoms appear and to report immediately for a serum lithium estimation.

Lithium intoxication: There is no specific antidote to lithium poisoning. In the event of accumulation, lithium should be stopped and serum estimations should be carried out every six hours.

Under no circumstances should a diuretic be used. Osmotic diuresis (mannitol or urea infusion) or alkalinisation of the urine (sodium lactate or sodium bicarbonate infusion) should be initiated.

If the serum lithium level is over 4.0 mmol/l, if there is a deterioration in the patient's condition, or if the serum lithium concentration is not falling at a rate corresponding to a half-life of under 30 hours, peritoneal or haemodialysis should be instituted promptly. This should be continued until there is no lithium in the serum or dialysis fluid. Serum lithium levels should be monitored for at least a further week to take account of any possible rebound in serum lithium levels as a result of delayed diffusion from body tissues.

Pharmaceutical precautions Store in a cool, dry place. Dispense in airtight containers.

Legal category POM.

Package quantities Priadel (400 mg): Securitainers of 100 and 1,000 tablets and Hospital Packs of 50 and 100 tablets.
Priadel 200: Securitainers of 100 and 500 tablets.

Further information Nil.

Product licence numbers
Priadel (400 mg) 0357/5000R
Priadel 200 0357/0028

PRIADEL* LIQUID

Presentation A clear, yellow coloured, pineapple flavoured sugar free syrup containing 520 mg lithium citrate (equivalent to 200 mg lithium carbonate) per 5 ml.

Uses
1. Treatment of mania and hypomania.
2. Lithium may also be tried in the treatment of some patients with recurrent bipolar depression, where treatment with other antidepressants has been unsuccessful.
3. Prophylactic treatment of recurrent affective disorders.
4. Control of aggressive or self-mutilating behaviour.

Dosage and administration A simple treatment schedule has been evolved which except for some minor variations should be followed whether using Priadel Liquid therapeutically or prophylactically. The minor variations to this schedule depend on the elements of the illness being treated and these are described later.

1. In patients of average weight (70 kg) an initial total daily dose of 10–30 ml of Priadel Liquid (equivalent to 400–1200 mg lithium carbonate) should be given in divided doses, ideally twice a day.

When changing between lithium preparations serum lithium levels should first be checked, then Priadel Liquid therapy commenced at a daily dose as close as possible to that of the other form of lithium. As bioavailability varies from product to product (particularly with regard to slow release preparations) a change of product should be regarded as initiation of new treatment.

2. Four to five days after starting treatment (and never longer than one week) a blood sample should be taken for the estimation of serum lithium level.

3. The objective is to adjust the Priadel Liquid dose so as to maintain the serum lithium level permanently within the diurnal range of 0.5–1.5 mmol/l. In practice, the blood sample should be taken 12 hours after the previous dose of Priadel Liquid. 'Target' serum lithium concentration at 12 hours should be 0.5–0.8 mmol/l.

Priadel Liquid is supplied with a 2.5/5 ml double ended spoon to provide dosage adjustments equivalent to 100 mg and 200 mg lithium carbonate respectively. Serum lithium levels should be monitored weekly until stabilisation is achieved.

4. Lithium therapy should not be initiated unless adequate facilities for routine monitoring of serum concentrations are available. Following stabilisation of serum lithium levels, the period between subsequent estimations can be increased gradually but should not normally exceed three months. Additional measurements should be made following alteration of dosage, on development of intercurrent disease, signs of manic or depressive relapse, following significant change in sodium or fluid intake, or if signs of lithium toxicity occur.

5. Whilst a high proportion of acutely ill patients may respond within three to seven days of the commencement of therapy with Priadel Liquid, it should be continued through any recurrence of the affective disturbance. This is important as the full prophylactic effect may not occur for 6 to 12 months after the initiation of therapy.

6. In patients who show a positive response to therapy with Priadel Liquid, treatment is likely to be long term. Careful clinical appraisal of the patient should be exercised throughout medication (see Precautions).

Prophylactic treatment of recurrent affective disorders: It is recommended that the described treatment schedule is followed.

Treatment of acute mania, hypomania and recurrent bipolar depression: It is likely that a higher than normal intake of Priadel Liquid may be necessary during an acute phase. As soon as control of mania or depression is achieved, the serum lithium level should be determined and it may be necessary, dependent on the results, to lower the dose of Priadel Liquid and to re-stabilise serum lithium levels.

Use in elderly: In elderly patients or those below 50 kg in weight, it is recommended that a starting dose of 5 ml (equivalent to 200 mg lithium carbonate) taken twice daily. Elderly patients may be more sensitive to undesirable effects of lithium and also may require lower doses in order to maintain normal serum lithium levels. It follows therefore that long term patients often require a reduction in dosage over a period of years.

Use in children and adolescents: Not recommended.

Contra-indications, warnings, etc
Contra-indications. Renal insufficiency, cardiovascular insufficiency, Addison's disease and untreated hypothyroidism are all contra-indications to lithium therapy.

Use in pregnancy: There is epidemiological evidence that lithium may be harmful to the foetus in human pregnancy.

Total no. 'lithium babies' reported	*Malformed infants*	*Ebstein's anomaly and other major cardiovascular malformations*
225	25 (11%)	18 (8%)

It is strongly recommended that lithium be discontinued before a planned pregnancy. If it is considered essential to maintain treatment with Priadel Liquid during pregnancy, serum lithium levels should be monitored closely since renal function changes gradually during pregnancy and suddenly at parturition, requiring dosage adjustments. It is recommended that administration of Priadel Liquid be discontinued shortly before delivery and recommenced a few days post-partum.

Babies may show signs of lithium toxicity necessitating fluid therapy in the neonatal period. Babies born with low serum lithium concentrations may have a flaccid appearance which returns to normal without any treatment. Lithium is secreted in breast milk, therefore bottle feeding is recommended.

Precautions: When considering therapy with Priadel Liquid, it is necessary to ascertain whether patients are receiving lithium in any other form. If so, check serum levels before proceeding. It is important to ensure that renal function is normal – if necessary a creatinine clearance test or other renal function test should be performed. Cardiac and thyroid function should be assessed before commencing lithium treatment. Patients should be euthyroid before the initiation of lithium therapy. Renal function, cardiac function and thyroid function should be re-assessed periodically.

Clear instructions regarding the symptoms of impending toxicity should be given by the doctor to all patients receiving long term lithium therapy (see Toxic effects). Patients should also be warned to report if polyuria or polydipsia develop. Episodes of nausea and vomiting or other conditions leading to salt/water depletion (including severe dieting) should also be reported. Elderly patients are particularly liable to lithium toxicity.

Caution should be exercised to ensure that diet and fluid intake are normal thus maintaining a stable electrolyte balance. This may be of special importance in very hot weather or work environment. Infectious diseases including colds, influenza, gastro-enteritis and urinary infections may alter fluid balance and thus affect serum lithium levels. Treatment should be discontinued during any intercurrent infection and should only be reinstituted after the patient's physical health has returned to normal.

Drug interactions: Concurrent use of lithium and diuretics may result in reduced lithium clearance, leading to intoxication. If a diuretic has to be prescribed for a lithium patient, the lithium dosage should first be lowered and the patient re-stabilised with frequent monitoring. Similar precautions should be exercised on diuretic withdrawal. Other drugs affecting electrolyte balance e.g. steroids, may alter lithium excretion and should be avoided in patients on lithium. If other psychotropic drugs are used they should be initiated at a lower dosage than usual, as their side effects may be potentiated by the use of lithium. This has been shown to be of particular importance for the concurrent use of lithium and haloperidol or flupenthixol.

There have been isolated reports of possible interactions between lithium and diazepam (resulting in hypothermia), methyldopa, tetracyclines, phenytoin, carbamazepine, indomethacin and other prostaglandin-synthetase inhibitors.

Warnings and adverse effects
Side effects: Side effects are usually related to serum lithium concentrations and are infrequent at levels below 1.0 mmol/l.

Mild gastrointestinal effects, nausea, vertigo, muscle weakness and a dazed feeling may occur initially, but frequently disappear after stabilisation. Fine hand tremors, polyuria and mild thirst may persist. Weight gain or oedema may present in some patients but should not be treated with diuretics.

Hypercalcaemia, hypermagnesaemia and hyperparathyroidism have been reported. Skin conditions including acne, psoriasis, generalised pustular psoriasis, rashes and leg ulcers have occasionally been reported as being aggravated by lithium treatment.

Long term treatment with lithium may be associated with disturbances of thyroid function, including goitre, hypothyroidism and thyrotoxicosis. Lithium-induced hypothyroidism may be managed successfully with concurrent thyroxine.

Memory impairment may occur during long term use.

Nephrotoxicity: Up to one third of patients on lithium may develop polyuria with a urinary output of up to three litres per day. This is usually due to lithium blocking the effect of ADH and is reversible on lithium withdrawal. However, long term treatment with lithium may also result in permanent changes in kidney histology and impairment of renal function. High serum concentrations of lithium including episodes of acute lithium toxicity may aggravate these changes. The minimum clinically effective dose of lithium should always be used. In patients who develop polyuria or polydipsia, renal function should be monitored, e.g. with measurement of blood urea, serum creatinine and urinary protein levels in addition to the routine serum lithium estimations.

After a period lasting 3–5 years, patients should be carefully assessed to ensure that benefit persists.

Toxic effects: Such effects are indicative of impending lithium intoxication and fall into two groups:

(a) Gastro-intestinal: increasing anorexia, diarrhoea and vomiting.

(b) Central nervous system: muscle weakness, lack of co-ordination, drowsiness or lethargy progressing to giddiness with ataxia, tinnitus, blurred vision, dysarthria, coarse tremor and muscle twitching.

At blood levels above 2–3 mmol/l there may be a large output of dilute urine, with increasing disorientation, seizures, coma and death.

Patients should be instructed to stop taking their Priadel Liquid if toxic symptoms appear and to report immediately for a serum lithium estimation.

Lithium intoxication: There is no specific antidote to lithium poisoning. In the event of accumulation, lithium should be stopped and serum estimations should be carried out every six hours.

Under no circumstances should a diuretic be used. Osmotic diuresis (mannitol or urea infusion) or alkalinisation of the urine (sodium lactate or sodium bicarbonate infusion) should be initiated.

If the serum lithium level is over 4.0 mmol/l, if there is a deterioration in the patient's condition, or if the serum lithium concentration is not falling at a rate corresponding to a half-life of under 30 hours, peritoneal or haemodialysis should be instituted promptly. This should be continued until there is no lithium in the serum or dialysis fluid. Serum lithium levels should be monitored for at least a further week to take account of any possible rebound in serum lithium levels as a result of delayed diffusion from body tissues.

Pharmaceutical precautions Store in a cool place. Protect from direct sunlight. Dilution of Priadel Liquid is not recommended.

Legal category POM.

Package quantities Priadel Liquid is available in bottles of 150 ml.

Further information Nil.

Product licence number 0357/0032.

**Trade Mark*

Dermal Laboratories Limited
Tatmore Place
Gosmore, Hitchin
Herts, SG4 7QR

ANHYDROL FORTE*

Presentation Colourless evaporative solution containing 20% w/v Aluminium Chloride Hexahydrate.

Ingredients: Aluminium Chloride Hexahydrate; Industrial Methylated Spirit BP.

Uses For the topical treatment of hyperhidrosis specifically involving axillae, hands or feet.

Dosage and administration Apply to the affected sites at night, as required, and allow to dry. Wash off in the morning.

Contra-indications, warnings, etc Care should be taken to restrict the application to the affected sites only. Do not bathe immediately before use and, if the axillae are treated, do not shave or use depilatories on this area within 12 hours before or after use.

Keep away from the eyes and mucous membranes.

Care should be taken to avoid Anhydrol Forte coming into direct contact with clothing, polished surfaces, jewellery or metal.

Do not use if sensitive to any of the ingredients.

Pharmaceutical precautions Highly flammable, store upright in a cool place away from flames. Replace cap tightly after use.

Legal category POM.

Package quantity Anhydrol Forte is supplied in a glass roll-on bottle containing 10 ml. This is supplied as an original pack (OP).

Further information The formulation of Anhydrol Forte has been tested in widespread clinical practice, and has been shown to be effective when used in accordance with the recommended instructions. Should irritation occur, reduce the frequency of application and if necessary apply mild hydrocortisone cream.

Product licence number 0173/0030.

CALLUSOLVE*

Presentation Clear orange/brown coloured paint containing 25% w/v Benzalkonium Chloride Bromine.

Ingredients: Benzalkonium Chloride Bromine; Liquid Paraffin BP; Chloroform.

Uses For topical use in the treatment of warts, especially multiple or mosaic warts.

Dosage and administration Gently rub the surface of the wart with a piece of pumice stone or manicure emery board, or pare down any hard skin. Using the applicator provided, carefully apply a few drops of the paint to the wart, taking care to localise the application to the affected area. Allow each drop to dry before the next is applied. Cover with an adhesive plaster and leave for 24 hours. On subsequent days, remove the plaster and repeat the above instructions.

Contra-indications, warnings, etc Keep away from the eyes and mucous membranes. Not to be used on the face, anal or perineal region. Not to be used by diabetics or individuals with impaired peripheral blood circulation. Not to be used on moles or on any other skin lesion for which it is not indicated. Avoid inhaling vapour. Avoid spreading onto surrounding uninvolved skin. If the treated area becomes inflamed or painful, treatment should be suspended until the inflammation resolves.

Do not use if sensitive to any of the ingredients.

Accidental oral ingestion should be treated immediately by gastric lavage with 2 to 5% aqueous sodium bicarbonate solution. Fluid and electrolyte balance should be monitored and appropriate supportive measures should be provided. Symptoms include headache, nausea, vomiting, diarrhoea and respiratory depression.

Pharmaceutical precautions Store upright in a cool place. Replace cap tightly after use. Avoid spillage.

Legal category P.

Package quantity Callusolve is supplied in an amber glass bottle containing 10 ml, incorporating a spatula for ease of application. This is supplied as an original pack (OP).

Further information Benzalkonium chloride bromine is an adduct of benzalkonium chloride with bromine, which is dissolved in a non-aqueous volatile solvent. When applied to the wart, a slow release of bromine attacks the immature keratin, fragmenting the lesion and killing the virus.

Product licence number 0173/5005R.

CAPASAL* THERAPEUTIC SHAMPOO

Presentation Brown coloured foaming shampoo containing 0.5% w/w Salicylic Acid BP, 1.0% w/w Coconut Oil BP and 1.0% w/w Distilled Coal Tar.

Ingredients: Salicylic Acid BP; Coconut Oil BP; Distilled Coal Tar; Lauric Acid Diethanolamide; Coco Amido Propyl Dimethyl Betaine; Triethanolamine Lauryl Sulphate; Phenoxyethanol BP; Water.

Uses For use as a shampoo in the treatment of dry, scaly scalp conditions such as seborrhoeic eczema, seborrhoeic dermatitis, pityriasis capitis, psoriasis, and cradle cap in children. It may also be used to remove any previous scalp applications.

Dosage and administration Use as a shampoo, daily if necessary. Wet hair thoroughly. Massage a small amount of the shampoo into the scalp, ideally leaving on for a few minutes before washing out. Repeat, producing a rich lather. Rinse hair well and dry.

Contra-indications, warnings, etc Keep undiluted shampoo away from the eyes. Keep out of the reach of children. In case of irritation, discontinue treatment.

Do not use if sensitive to any ingredient.

Use in pregnancy: No known side-effects.

Use in children: No known side-effects.

Pharmaceutical precautions Store in a cool dark place. Avoid spillage.

Legal category P.

Package quantity Capasal Therapeutic Shampoo is supplied in a polythene bottle containing 250 ml. This is supplied as an original pack (OP).

Further information The effectiveness of salicylic acid, coconut oil and coal tar in the topical treatment of scaly scalp conditions has been confirmed in widespread clinical practice, for example in Coconut Oil Compound Ointment (Ung.Cocois Co). Capasal Therapeutic Shampoo contains these three active ingredients in an advanced formulation specifically developed for better patient compliance.

Product licence number 0173/0048.

CAPITOL*

Presentation Clear aqueous gel containing 0.5% w/w Benzalkonium Chloride BP.

Ingredients: Benzalkonium Chloride BP; Sodium Lauryl Ether Sulphate; Coconut Diethanolamide; Phenoxyethanol BP; Dilute Hydrochloric Acid BP; Sodium Chloride BP; Purified Water BP.

Uses For the topical treatment of pityriasis capitis and other seborrhoeic scalp conditions, where there is scaling and dandruff.

Dosage and administration Wet the hair. Apply a liberal quantity of the shampoo to the scalp and, with the tips of the fingers, rub in thoroughly. Rinse. Repeat application and massage to produce a rich lather. Remove as much lather as possible with the hands, before rinsing thoroughly under running water.

Contra-indications, warnings, etc Keep away from the eyes.

Do not use if sensitive to any of the ingredients.

Pharmaceutical precautions Store in a cool place. Replace cap after use.

Legal category P.

Package quantity Capitol is supplied in a glass jar containing 120 g. This is supplied as an original pack (OP).

Further information Capitol contains both a cationic quaternary germicide to lift scales from the scalp and an anionic foaming agent to remove them from the hair.

Product licence number 0173/5008R.

DIODERM*

Presentation White aqueous cream containing 0.1% w/w Hydrocortisone BP.

Ingredients: Hydrocortisone BP; Citric Acid BP; Emulsifying Ointment BP; Propylene Glycol BP; Purified Water BP.

Uses Topical treatment of eczema and dermatitis.

Dosage and administration Apply to the affected areas twice daily.

Contra-indications, warnings, etc As with all topical steroids, Dioderm is contra-indicated where there is a bacterial, viral or fungal infection. It should not be applied to open wounds, ulcers or broken skin. It may also be hazardous in psoriasis for a number of reasons including rebound relapses following development of tolerance, risk of generalised pustular psoriasis and local and systemic toxicity due to impaired barrier function of the skin. In such patients, careful patient supervision is important. Dioderm should not normally be used under occlusion.

Use in pregnancy: There is inadequate evidence of safety in human pregnancy. Topical administration of corticosteroids to pregnant animals can cause abnormalities of fetal development including cleft palate and intra-uterine growth retardation. There may therefore be a very small risk of such effects in the human fetus.

Use in infants: Although generally regarded as safe, even for long-term administration in adults, there is a potential for overdosage in infancy. Extreme caution is required in dermatoses of infancy including napkin eruption. In such patients, courses of treatment should not normally exceed 7 days.

Keep away from the eyes.

Do not use if sensitive to any of the ingredients.

Pharmaceutical precautions Store in a cool place. Replace cap tightly after use.

Legal category POM.

Package quantity Dioderm is supplied in a collapsible tube containing 30 g. This is supplied as an original pack (OP).

Further information Although Dioderm contains the relatively low concentration of 0.1% hydrocortisone, the formulation is designed to provide clinical activity at least equivalent to the usual strength of 1.0% Hydrocortisone Cream BP.

Product licence number 0173/0047.

DITHROCREAM*

Presentation Dithrocream is presented as a pale yellow aqueous cream containing 0.1%, 0.25%, 0.5% (Forte), 1.0% (HP) or 2.0% w/w Dithranol BP, supplied in a collapsible tube containing 50 g.

Ingredients: Dithranol BP; White Soft Paraffin BP; Salicylic Acid BP; Cetostearyl Alcohol BP; Chlorocresol BP; Ascorbic Acid BP; Sodium Lauryl Sulphate BP; Purified Water BP.

Dithrocream 2.0% also contains Liquid Paraffin BP.

The packs are colour coded as follows:

0.1%	pale blue
0.25%	red
0.5%	purple
1.0%	brown
2.0%	yellow

Uses Dithrocream is recommended for the topical treatment of sub-acute and chronic psoriasis, including psoriasis of the scalp. Dithrocream 0.5% (Forte), Dithrocream 1.0% (HP) and Dithrocream 2.0% should only be used for those patients who have failed to respond to lower strengths of dithranol. Dithrocream 1.0% and 2.0% should normally only be applied for 'short contact' periods.

Dosage and administration Where the response to Dithrocream has not previously been established, always commence treatment with Dithrocream 0.1%, continuing for at least one week and then, if necessary, increase to the 0.25% followed by the 0.5% (Forte), the 1.0% (HP), and finally the 2.0% strength. Dithrocream 0.5%, Dithrocream 1.0% and Dithrocream 2.0% should always be used under medical supervision.

Dithrocream should be applied once every 24 hours, at any convenient time of the day or evening, and then removed by washing off, usually no more than one hour after application. Alternatively, it may be applied at night before retiring and washed off in the morning.

Dithrocream should be applied sparingly, only to the affected areas. Rub the cream gently and carefully into the skin until completely absorbed. It is most important to avoid applying an excessive amount of the cream, which may cause unnecessary soiling and staining of clothing and/or bed linen. After each period of treatment, a bath/shower should be taken to remove any residual cream. To prevent the possibility of discolouration, particularly where Dithrocream 1.0% or 2.0% has been used, always rinse the bath/shower with hot water immediately after washing/showering and then use a suitable cleanser to remove any deposit on the surface of the bath or shower.

For use on the scalp, first comb the hair to remove scalar debris and, after suitably parting, rub the cream well into the affected areas.

Treatment should be continued until the skin is entirely clear, i.e. when there is nothing to feel with the fingers and the texture is normal.

By gradually increasing the strength of cream applied it should be possible to clear psoriasis patches within 4 to 6 weeks.

Contra-indications, warnings, etc Not to be used for acute or pustular psoriasis.

If the initial treatment produces excessive soreness, or if the lesions spread, reduce frequency of application, and, in extreme cases, stop treatment. Exercise care when using Dithrocream on the face and intertriginous areas, and do not use high strengths on these sites. Keep away from the eyes and mucous membranes. Always wash the hands after use.

As long term use of topical corticosteroids is known to destabilise psoriasis, and withdrawal may give rise to a rebound phenomenon, an interval of at least one week should be allowed between the discontinuance of such steroids and the commencement of Dithrocream therapy. A suitably bland emollient may usefully be applied in the intervening period.

Contact with fabrics, plastics and other materials may cause permanent staining and should be avoided.

Dithrocream may cause temporary staining of the skin and/or hair.

Use in pregnancy: Although there is no experimental evidence to support the safety of the drug in pregnancy, no adverse effects have been reported.

Use in children: No evidence of any adverse effects. However, use cautiously with regular supervision.

Accidental ingestion: Dithranol is a cathartic (laxative) and if accidentally swallowed should be removed by gastric lavage.

Do not use if sensitive to any of the ingredients.

Pharmaceutical precautions Store in a cool place. Replace cap tightly after use.

Legal category P except for Dithrocream 2.0% (POM).

Package quantities All strengths of Dithrocream are supplied in collapsible tubes containing 50 g. These are supplied as original packs (OP).

Further information Dithrocream has been developed as a cream formulation of dithranol for particular convenience for home treatment, and is especially suitable for the exposed surfaces and hairy regions of the body, including psoriasis of the scalp.

Product licence numbers

Dithrocream 0.1%	0173/0029
Dithrocream 0.25%	0173/0028
Dithrocream 0.5% (Forte)	0173/0027
Dithrocream 1.0% (HP)	0173/0039
Dithrocream 2.0%	0173/0045

DITHROLAN*

Presentation Stiff yellow ointment containing 0.5% w/w Dithranol BP, 0.5% w/w Salicylic Acid BP, in equal quantities of hard and soft paraffin.

Ingredients: Dithranol BP; Salicylic Acid BP; Hard Paraffin BP; White Soft Paraffin BP.

Uses For the topical treatment of quiescent psoriasis.

Dosage and administration Apply accurately to the psoriatic lesions, commencing treatment on a few of the thicker lesions. Aim for a localised feeling of warmth; a sensation of burning can be controlled by varying the quantity and frequency of application.

At first, the ointment should only be left in contact with the skin for a few hours, e.g. during the evening whilst watching television, before removal by bathing. The duration of contact can later be extended to intensify the response. As resting aids the response to treatment, the ointment may conveniently be applied before retiring to bed and removed by bathing the next morning.

Bathing is necessary to remove residual ointment, and to control the reaction to treatment by preventing a build-up of dithranol in the skin.

The lesions will reduce in thickness as a red-brown stain develops. This is indicative of an effective response. No attempt should be made to remove the stain, which will disappear completely following cessation of treatment. In view of the staining of clothing and bed linen which can occur as part of dithranol therapy, it is advisable to utilise old pyjamas, under garments, bed linen and towels.

In the treatment of thinner lesions and flexures, a smaller amount of ointment should be applied accurately once or twice weekly.

Treatment should be continued until the skin is entirely clear, i.e. when there is nothing to feel with the fingers and the texture is normal. When in doubt, continue treatment for a further week, leaving the ointment on the skin for shorter periods.

During treatment, the ointment may be stored in a warm place to reduce stiffness and assist ease of application.

Contra-indications, warnings, etc Not to be used for acute or pustular psoriasis.

In view of the rebound effect which may be experienced, after the use of potent topical steroids, it is recommended that patients be treated with a bland emollient preparation for approximately two weeks after cessation of steroid treatment. Treatment may then be commenced, using Dithrolan diluted with four parts of yellow soft paraffin, reducing the dilution as tolerance develops.

If the initial treatment produces soreness, or if the lesions spread (particularly when potent topical steroids have recently been used), reduce frequency of application and, in extreme cases, stop treatment. Cautiously resume treatment, commencing with a few of the thicker lesions, alternating application of the ointment with yellow soft paraffin. Do not use Dithrolan on the face and intertriginous areas.

Keep away from the eyes and mucous membranes. Always wash the hands after use.

Contact with fabrics, plastics and other materials may cause permanent staining and should be avoided.

Dithrolan may cause temporary staining of the skin and/or hair.

Use in pregnancy: Although there is no experimental evidence to support the safety of the drug in pregnancy, no adverse effects have been reported.

Use in children: No evidence of any adverse effects. However, use cautiously with regular supervision.

Accidental ingestion: Dithranol is a cathartic (laxative) and if accidentally swallowed should be removed by gastric lavage.

Do not use if sensitive to any of the ingredients.

Pharmaceutical precautions Store in a dark place. Do not expose to direct heat. Replace cap after use.

Legal category P.

Package quantity Dithrolan is supplied in an amber glass jar containing 90 g. This is supplied as an original pack (OP).

Further information Dithrolan provides the clinical efficacy of the dithranol paste which has been established as part of the Ingram regime. It is, however, easier to apply and remove, whilst retaining adequate stiffness.

Product licence number 0173/0024.

EMULSIDERM*

Presentation Pale blue/green liquid emulsion containing 0.5% w/w Benzalkonium Chloride BP, 25% w/w Liquid Paraffin BP, 25% w/w Isopropyl Myristate BP.

Ingredients: Benzalkonium Chloride BP; Liquid Paraffin BP; Isopropyl Myristate BP; Sorbitan Monostearate BP; Polysorbate 60 BP; Methylene Blue; Industrial Methylated Spirit BP; Water.

Uses An aid in the treatment of dry skin conditions, especially those associated with eczema, ichthyosis or xeroderma. It permits re-hydration of the keratin by replacing lost lipids, and its antiseptic properties assist in overcoming secondary infection.

Dosage and administration Shake bottle before use.

For use in the bath: Add 30 ml to a 6–8 inch bath of warm water. For infant bathing use 15 ml. Soak for 5–10 minutes. Pat dry.

For application to the skin: Rub a small amount of undiluted emollient into the dry areas of skin until absorbed.

Contra-indications, warnings, etc Keep away from the eyes. Take care to avoid slipping in the bath.

Do not use if sensitive to any of the ingredients.

Pharmaceutical precautions Store in a cool place. Replace cap after use.

Legal category P.

Package quantities Emulsiderm is supplied in polythene bottles; a 250 ml with a measuring cap, and a 1 litre with a measuring cup. These are supplied as original packs (OP).

Further information Emulsiderm contains the antiseptic benzalkonium chloride in an emulsion system which permits rapid dispersion of its oil content in the bathwater.

Product licence number 0173/0036.

EXOLAN* CREAM

Presentation Pale yellow aqueous cream containing 1% w/w 1, 8, 9-Triacetoxyanthracene (Dithranol Triacetate).

Ingredients: 1,8,9-Triacetoxyanthracene (Dithranol Triacetate); Emulsifying Wax BP; White Soft Paraffin BP; Liquid Paraffin BP; Chlorocresol BP; Purified Water BP.

Uses For the topical treatment of sub-acute and chronic psoriasis, including psoriasis of the scalp.

Dosage and administration Gently rub the cream into the lesions until completely absorbed, taking care to localise the application to the affected areas. The following morning, a bath should be taken to remove any residue of the cream.

For use on the scalp, shampoo to remove scalar debris and any previous application. Dry the hair and, after suitably parting, rub the cream well into the lesions.

Contra-indications, warnings, etc Not to be used for acute or pustular psoriasis. If the initial treatment produces excessive soreness, or if the lesions spread, reduce the frequency of application and, in extreme cases, stop treatment. Exercise care when using Exolan Cream on the face and intertriginous areas. Keep away from the eyes and mucous membranes. Always wash the hands after use. Contact with fabrics, plastics and other materials may cause permanent staining and should be avoided.

Exolan Cream may cause temporary staining of the skin and/or hair.

Use in pregnancy: Although there is no experimental evidence to support the safety of the drug in pregnancy, no adverse effects have been reported.

Use in children: No evidence of any adverse effects. However use cautiously with regular supervision.

Accidental ingestion: Triacetoxyanthracene is a cathartic (laxative) and if accidentally swallowed should be removed by gastric lavage.

Do not use if sensitive to any of the ingredients.

Pharmaceutical precautions Store in a cool place. Replace cap tightly after use.

Legal category P.

Package quantity Exolan Cream is supplied in a collapsible tube containing 50 g. This is supplied as an original pack (OP).

Further information Triacetoxyanthracene has a similar mode of action to dithranol whilst minimising the problems of irritation and staining.

Product licence number 0173/5004R.

EXTEROL*

Presentation Viscous solution containing 5% w/w Urea Hydrogen Peroxide.

Ingredients: Urea Hydrogen Peroxide; 8-Hydroxyquinoline; Glycerol BP.

Uses An aid in the removal of hardened ear wax.

Dosage and administration Remove the protective cap, invert the pipette above the opening of the affected ear and, with the head tilted sideways, gently squeeze 5–10 drops into the ear. Retain drops in ear for several minutes by keeping head tilted and then wipe away any surplus.

Repeat once or twice daily for at least 3–4 days, or as required.

Contra-indications, warnings, etc Keep away from the eyes. Do not use if eardrum is known or suspected to be perforated. Stop usage if irritation or pain occurs.

Do not use if sensitive to any of the ingredients.

Pharmaceutical precautions Store in a cool place, but do not refrigerate. Replace cap after use, and return bottle to carton.

Legal category P.

Package quantity Exterol is supplied in an amber glass bottle containing 12 ml, incorporating a specially designed pipette enclosed in a protective cap. This is supplied as an original pack (OP).

Further information After insertion of the drops into the ear, the urea hydrogen peroxide liberates oxygen which acts to break up the hardened wax. Subsequently, the glycerol and urea assist in the softening of the wax in order that it may more easily be removed from the ear, either with or without syringing. Due to the release of oxygen, patients may experience a mild, temporary effervescence in the ear.

Product licence number 0173/0037.

GLUTAROL*

Presentation Colourless evaporative solution containing 10% w/v Glutaraldehyde.

Ingredients: Glutaraldehyde; Bitrex; Industrial Methylated Spirit BP; Purified Water BP.

Uses For the topical treatment of warts, especially plantar warts.

Dosage and administration Gently rub the surface of the wart with a piece of pumice stone or manicure emery board, or pare down any hard skin. Using the applicator provided, carefully apply a few drops of the solution to the wart, taking care to localise the application to the affected area. Allow each drop to dry before the next is applied. Repeat twice daily. On subsequent days, repeat the above instructions. It is not necessary to cover the treated wart(s) with an adhesive plaster.

Contra-indications, warnings, etc Keep away from the eyes and mucous membranes. Not to be used on the face, anal or perineal region. Not to be used on moles or on any other skin lesion for which it is not indicated. Avoid inhaling vapour. Avoid spreading onto surrounding uninvolved skin.

Do not use if sensitive to any of the ingredients.

Accidental oral ingestion should be treated immediately by gastric lavage with 2 to 5% aqueous sodium bicarbonate solution. Fluid and electrolyte balance should be monitored and appropriate supportive measures should be provided. Symptoms include headache, nausea, vomiting, diarrhoea, and respiratory depression.

Pharmaceutical precautions Flammable, store upright in a cool place away from flames. Replace cap tightly after use. Avoid spillage.

Legal category P.

Package quantity Glutarol is supplied in an amber

glass bottle containing 10 ml, incorporating a specially designed spatula, for ease of application. This is supplied as an original pack (OP).

Further information Glutaraldehyde is virucidal and thus inactivates the wart virus. On the skin, it also acts as an anhidrotic, drying the warts and surrounding skin, thus reducing the spread of lesions and simplifying the removal of persistent warts by curettage.

As glutaraldehyde stains the outer layers of the skin brown, treatment can be seen to be carried out. This stain soon disappears after cessation of treatment.

Product licence number 0173/0022.

PSORIDERM* BATH EMULSION

Presentation Buff coloured liquid emulsion containing 40% w/v Distilled Coal Tar.

Ingredients: Distilled Coal Tar; Polysorbate 20 BP; Triethanolamine BP; Phenoxyethanol BP; Water.

Uses An aid in the treatment of sub-acute and chronic psoriasis.

Dosage and administration Add 30 ml of the emulsion to a standard bath of warm water. Soak for 5 minutes, pat dry.

Contra-indications, warnings, etc Keep away from the eyes.

Do not use if sensitive to any of the ingredients.

Pharmaceutical precautions Store in a cool, dark place. Replace cap after use. Avoid spillage.

Legal category P.

Package quantity Psoriderm Bath Emulsion is supplied in an amber glass bottle containing 200 ml. This is supplied as an original pack (OP).

Further information The use of coal tar has long been advocated as a therapeutic agent in the management of psoriasis. Psoriderm Bath Emulsion conveniently provides a coal tar bath which may be used alone, or as part of a more extensive treatment regime.

Product licence number 0173/5003R.

PSORIDERM* CREAM

Presentation Buff coloured aqueous cream containing 6% w/w Distilled Coal Tar, 0.4% w/w Lecithin.

Ingredients: Distilled Coal Tar; Lecithin; Stearic Acid BPC; Isopropyl Palmitate; Phenoxyethanol BP; Propylene Glycol BP; Triethanolamine BP; Purified Water BP.

Uses For the topical treatment of sub-acute and chronic psoriasis, including psoriasis of the scalp and flexures.

Dosage and administration Apply to the affected areas twice daily, or as required.

Contra-indications, warnings, etc Not to be used for acute psoriasis. Keep away from the eyes and mucous membranes. Wash the hands after use.

Do not use if sensitive to any of the ingredients.

It has been reported that in rare instances coal tar may cause irritation, acne-like eruptions and/or photosensitisation of the skin.

Pharmaceutical precautions Store in a cool, dark place. Replace cap after use. Avoid spillage.

Legal category P.

Package quantity Psoriderm Cream is supplied in an amber glass jar containing 225 ml. This is supplied as an original pack (OP).

Further information The use of coal tar has long been advocated as a therapeutic agent in the management of psoriasis. Psoriderm Cream may be used alone, or as part of a more extensive treatment regime, and is particularly suitable for treating the hair bearing areas of the body and the flexures.

Product licence number 0173/5000R.

PSORIDERM* SCALP LOTION

Presentation Golden brown coloured foaming shampoo containing 2.5% w/v Distilled Coal Tar, 0.3% w/v Lecithin.

Ingredients: Distilled Coal Tar; Lecithin; Triethanolamine Lauryl Sulphate; Lauric Acid Diethanolamide; Disodium Edetate BP; Sodium Chloride BP; Phenoxyethanol BP; Water.

Uses For the topical treatment of psoriasis of the scalp.

Dosage and administration Wet the hair thoroughly. Apply a small amount of the shampoo to the scalp, and massage gently until a rich lather has been generated. Retain on the scalp for a few minutes. Remove excess lather with the hands, before rinsing with warm water. Repeat the above procedure.

Contra-indications, warnings, etc Not to be used for acute psoriasis. Keep away from the eyes and mucous membranes.

Do not use if sensitive to any of the ingredients.

Pharmaceutical precautions Store in a cool, dark place. Replace cap after use. Avoid spillage.

Legal category P.

Package quantities Psoriderm Scalp Lotion is supplied in a polythene bottle containing 250 ml. This is supplied as an original pack (OP).

Further information The use of coal tar has long been advocated as a therapeutic agent in the management of psoriasis. Psoriderm Scalp Lotion may be used alone as a coal tar shampoo, or as part of a more extensive treatment regime.

Product licence number 0173/5001R.

SALACTOL*

Presentation Colourless or pale yellow/brown evaporative paint containing 16.7% w/w Salicylic Acid BP, 16.7% w/w Lactic Acid BP, 66.6% w/w Flexible Collodion.

Ingredients: Salicylic Acid BP; Lactic Acid BP; Flexible Collodion.

Uses For the topical treatment of warts, verrucae, corns and calluses.

Dosage and administration Soak the affected site in warm water and pat dry. Gently rub the surface with a pumice stone or manicure emery board to remove any hard skin. Using the applicator provided, carefully apply a few drops of the paint to the lesion, taking care to localise the application to the affected area. Cover with an adhesive plaster, if a plantar wart. Leave for 24 hours. Repeat this procedure daily, removing old Collodion on each occasion.

Contra-indications, warnings, etc Keep away from the eyes and mucous membranes. Not to be used on the face, anal or perineal region. Not to be used by diabetics or individuals with impaired peripheral blood circulation. Not to be used on moles or on any other skin lesion for which it is not indicated. Avoid inhaling vapour. Avoid spreading onto surrounding uninvolved skin.

If the treated area becomes inflamed or painful, treatment should be suspended until the inflammation resolves.

Do not use if sensitive to any of the ingredients.

Accidental oral ingestion: should be treated immediately by gastric lavage with a 2 to 5% aqueous sodium bicarbonate solution. Fluid and electrolyte balance should be monitored and appropriate supportive measures should be provided. Symptoms include headache, nausea, vomiting, diarrhoea and respiratory depression.

Pharmaceutical precautions Extremely flammable, store upright in a cool place, away from flames. Replace cap tightly after use. Avoid spillage.

Legal category P.

Package quantity Salactol is supplied in an amber glass bottle containing 10 ml, incorporating a specially designed spatula for ease of application. This is supplied as an original pack (OP).

Further information The effectiveness of Salactol has been confirmed in a clinical study on 76 patients with plantar warts. 84% of warts resolved at 12 weeks, without any reported side-effects.

Product licence number 0173/5006R.

SALATAC* GEL

Presentation Clear, viscous gel containing 12% w/w Salicylic Acid BP, 4% w/w Lactic Acid BP.

Ingredients: Salicylic Acid BP; Lactic Acid BP; Camphor BP; Pyroxylin BP; Ethanol (96%) BP; Ethyl Acetate.

Uses For the topical treatment of warts, verrucae, corns and calluses.

Dosage and administration Once daily application.

1. Every night, soak the affected site in warm water for 2–3 minutes.
2. Dry thoroughly with the patient's own towel.
3. Apply one or two drops of the gel carefully to the lesion and allow to dry over its surface. Take care to avoid spreading onto surrounding normal skin. No adhesive plaster is necessary.
4. The following evening, carefully remove and discard the elastic film formed from the previous application, and re-apply the gel.
5. Once a week, gently rub away the treated surface using an emery board, as provided, or pumice stone, before re-applying the gel.
6. The wart, corn or callus may take up to twelve weeks to disappear, and it is necessary to persevere with the treatment. Some mild transient irritation may be expected, but treatment should be discontinued in cases of more severe irritation.

Contra-indications, warnings, etc Keep away from the eyes and mucous membranes.

Not to be used on the face or anogenital regions, or by diabetics or individuals with impaired peripheral blood circulation.

Not to be used on moles or on any other skin lesions for which the gel is not indicated.

Avoid spreading onto surrounding uninvolved skin.

If the treated area becomes inflamed or painful, treatment should be suspended until the inflammation resolves.

Do not use if sensitive to any of the ingredients.

Avoid inhaling vapour, and keep applicator cap firmly closed when not in use.

Contact with clothing, fabrics, plastics and other materials may cause damage, and should be avoided.

Pharmaceutical precautions The gel is highly flammable. Store in a cool place, away from flames.

Legal category P.

Package quantity Salatac Gel is supplied in a collapsible tube containing 8 g, complete with special applicator, emery board and instructions. This is supplied as an original pack (OP).

Further information Salatac Gel has been specially formulated to provide the optimum effectiveness of salicylic acid and lactic acid in a convenient film-forming gel which is ideally suited for patient compliance.

Product licence number 0173/0046.

VARICLENE*

Presentation Green aqueous gel containing 0.5% w/w Brilliant Green, 0.5% w/w Lactic Acid BP.

Ingredients: Lactic Acid BP; Brilliant Green; Methyl Cellulose 10,000; Industrial Methylated Spirit BP; Purified Water BP.

Uses An aid in the topical treatment of venous and other types of skin ulcers.

Dosage and administration Ensure that the area of skin to be treated is as clean and dry as possible. Using a disposable applicator (e.g. cotton wool bud, wooden spatula or gauze pad), gently apply and smooth the Variclene gel over the affected area, until the ulcer site is completely covered. For extensive ulceration, the gel may be spread initially over a sterile dressing, which is then applied to the affected area. Minimise spreading onto surrounding skin and avoid direct contact between the nozzle of the tube and the ulcer.

The treated area should then be dressed using an impregnated paste bandage such as Viscopaste* PB7 or Quinaband*, followed by stockinette or, in the case of a venous ulcer, pressure bandaging. This allows a clean granulating bed to develop.

If the dressings become soaked in exudate, a layer of cotton wool, or lint or gamgee may be 'sandwiched' between the paste and stockinette/pressure bandaging to absorb exudate.

The dressing should be changed at regular intervals (usually 48 to 72 hours) and not left longer than 7 days.

Contra-indications, warnings, etc Avoid contact with clothing and linen. Some patients may experience transient stinging on application. In cases of arterial or extensive, painful venous ulceration, this may be prolonged, when treatment should be discontinued until greater tolerance has been achieved.

Keep away from the eyes.

Do not use if sensitive to any of the ingredients.

Pharmaceutical precautions Store in a cool place. Always replace cap after use. Avoid spillage.

Legal category P.

Package quantity Variclene is supplied in a collapsible tube containing 50 g. This is supplied as an original pack (OP).

Further information As with all open wounds, care should be taken to keep the affected area clean and, as far as possible, free from contamination.

Where appropriate, Variclene should be used in conjunction with a treatment regime involving the use of pressure bandaging.

Product licence number 0173/0015.

**Trade Mark*

Dispersa
10 West Street
Alderley Edge
Cheshire SK9 7XP

DISPERSA

TEOPTIC* EYE-DROPS

Presentation A clear colourless odourless sterile solution containing carteolol hydrochloride 1% or 2% w/v with benzalkonium chloride as a preservative.

Also contains: sodium chloride, dibasic sodium phosphate, monobasic sodium phosphate and water.

Uses Teoptic is a beta-adrenergic-receptor-blocking agent possessing intrinsic sympathomimetic activity. Teoptic Eye-Drops are a topical treatment for the reduction of intra-ocular pressure, e.g. in ocular hypertension, chronic open angle glaucoma, some secondary glaucomas.

Dosage and administration Teoptic Eye-Drops are for local administration to the eye. Initially, the recommended adult dose is one drop of Teoptic 1% Eye-Drops instilled twice daily in each affected eye. If the clinical response is not adequate, the dosage may be altered to one drop of Teoptic 2% Eye-Drops instilled twice daily in each affected eye.

Teoptic Eye-Drops may, if necessary, be used in association with pilocarpine, adrenaline, carbachol and carbonic anhydrase inhibitors.

Children: Teoptic Eye-Drops have not been studied in children. Their use in these patients is therefore not recommended.

Use in the elderly: In clinical trials, the efficacy and tolerability profiles of Teoptic Eye-Drops were similar in elderly patients and in the general adult patient population. The usual recommended adult dose may therefore be considered suitable for elderly patients.

Contra-indications, warnings, etc
Contra-indications: Unsatisfactorily controlled cardiac insufficiency; bronchospasm, including bronchial asthma or chronic obstructive pulmonary disease; pregnancy; hypersensitivity to any of the components of the formulation.

Precautions: Teoptic has not been detected in plasma following ocular instillation of the eye-drops. However, as with other topically applied ophthalmic preparations, Teoptic may be absorbed systemically. Teoptic Eye-Drops should therefore be used with caution in patients receiving systemic beta-adrenergic-receptor-blocking therapy and in patients with known contra-indications to systemic beta-blockers, e.g. sinus bradycardia, second and third degree atrioventricular block, cardiogenic shock, right ventricular insufficiency due to pulmonary hypertension and congestive heart failure, unsatisfactorily controlled diabetes mellitus.

As with all ophthalmic preparations containing benzalkonium chloride, soft contact lenses (hydrophilic lenses) and gas-permeable contact lenses should not be worn during treatment with Teoptic Eye-Drops.

Side-effects: Local ocular reactions such as irritation, burning, itching and pain, blurred vision, photophobia, xerosis, conjunctival hyperaemia, conjunctival discharge and corneal disorders such as diffuse superficial keratitis may occasionally develop. As with all beta-blocking agents, bradycardia, dyspnoea, headache, lassitude and vertigo have occasionally been reported.

Use in pregnancy and lactation: Teoptic Eye-Drops have not been studied in human pregnancy and lactation. Use during pregnancy is therefore contra-indicated. In animal studies, orally administered carteolol has been shown to penetrate the breast milk and the use of Teoptic Eye-Drops in lactating mothers should therefore only be used at the discretion of the physician.

Overdosage: There is no experience of overdosage with Teoptic Eye-Drops. However, potential symptoms (typical of β-blocking agents) which may occur after accidental oral ingestion include bradycardia, severe hypotension, acute cardiac failure, bronchospasm, hypoglycaemia, delirium and unconsciousness. Initially, treatment should be by removal of any unabsorbed drug (e.g. gastric lavage) and general supportive measures, i.e. marked bradycardia should be treated in the first instance by intravenous atropine sulphate at a dose of 500 micrograms–2.0 mg depending on severity; intravenous glucagon and cardiac pacemakers may be required in more severe cases; bronchospasm should be treated with appropriate bronchodilators, including β_2-agonists and aminophylline where necessary. Patients should be monitored for several days as the beta-blocking effects of Teoptic may exceed its plasma half-life.

Pharmaceutical precautions Protect from heat. Teoptic Eye-Drops are sterile until the seal is broken. The container should not be accepted for initial use if the seal is damaged. The drops should not be used later than one month after first breaking the seal.

Legal category POM.

Package quantities 1% Eye-Drops: 5 ml dropper-bottle (OP). 2% Eye-Drops: 5 ml dropper-bottle (OP).

Further information Unlike miotics, Teoptic Eye-Drops reduce intra-ocular pressure without altering accommodation or pupil diameter. A slight increase in pupil diameter may be noted, however, if patients are transferred from miotic therapy to Teoptic Eye-Drops.

Product licence numbers
1% Eye-Drops: 0030/0040.
2% Eye-Drops: 0030/0041.

*Trade Mark

Dista Products Limited

Kingsclere Road,
Basingstoke,
Hants. RG21 2XA

DISTA

ALLEGRON*

Presentation Tablets each containing Nortriptyline Hydrochloride BP equivalent to 25 mg nortriptyline. The tablets are orange, scored and have a diameter of 8 mm. They are marked 'DISTA'.

Tablets each containing Nortriptyline Hydrochloride BP equivalent to 10 mg nortriptyline. The tablets are white, unscored and have a diameter of 5.5 mm. They are marked 'DISTA'.

Uses Allegron is indicated for the relief of symptoms of depression. It may also be used for the treatment of some cases of nocturnal enuresis.

Dosage and administration For oral administration.

Adults: The usual adult dose is 25 mg three or four times daily. Dosage should begin at a low level and be increased as required. Alternatively, the total daily dose may be given once a day. When doses above 100 mg daily are administered, plasma levels of nortriptyline should be monitored and maintained in the optimum range of 50 to 150 ng/ml. Doses above 150 mg per day are not recommended.

Lower than usual dosages are recommended for elderly patients and adolescents. Lower dosages are also recommended for outpatients than for hospitalised patients who will be under close supervision. The physician should initiate dosage at a low level and increase it gradually, noting carefully the clinical response and any evidence of intolerance. Following remission, maintenance medication may be required for a longer period of time at the lowest dose that will maintain remission.

If a patient develops minor side-effects, the dosage should be reduced. The drug should be discontinued promptly if adverse effects of a serious nature or allergic manifestations occur.

The elderly: 30 to 50 mg/day in divided doses.

Adolescent patients: 30 to 50 mg/day in divided doses.

Plasma levels: Optimal responses to nortriptyline have been associated with plasma concentrations of 50 to 150 ng/ml. Higher concentrations may be associated with more adverse experiences. Plasma concentrations are difficult to measure, and physicians should consult the laboratory professional staff.

Older patients have been reported to have larger plasma concentrations of the active nortriptyline metabolite 10-hydroxynortriptyline. In one case, this was associated with apparent cardiotoxicity despite nortriptyline concentrations within the 'therapeutic range'. Clinical findings should predominate over plasma concentrations as primary determinants of dosage changes.

Children: (for nocturnal enuresis only).

Age (years)	*Weight*		*Dose (mg)*
	kg	*lbs*	
6–7	20–25	44–55	10
8–11	25–35	55–77	10–20
>11	35–54	77–119	25–35

The dose should be administered thirty minutes before bedtime.

The maximum period of treatment should not exceed three months. A further course of treatment should not be started until a full physical examination, including an ECG, has been made.

Contra-indications, warnings, etc

Contra-indications: Hypersensitivity to nortriptyline.

Recent myocardial infarction, any degree of heart block or other cardiac arrhythmias.

Severe liver disease. Mania.

Nortriptyline is contra-indicated for the nursing mother and for children under the age of six years.

Please also refer to 'Drug interactions' section.

Warnings: As improvement may not occur during the initial weeks of therapy, patients, especially those posing a high suicidal risk, should be closely monitored during this period.

Withdrawal symptoms, including insomnia, irritability and excessive perspiration, may occur on abrupt cessation of therapy.

The use of nortriptyline in schizophrenic patients may result in an exacerbation of the psychosis or may activate latent schizophrenic symptoms. If administered to overactive or agitated patients, increased anxiety and agitation may occur. In manic-depressive patients, nortriptyline may cause symptoms of the manic phase to emerge.

Cross sensitivity between nortriptyline and other tricyclic antidepressants is a possibility.

Patients with cardiovascular disease should be given nortriptyline only under close supervision because of the tendency of the drug to produce sinus tachycardia and to prolong the conduction time. Myocardial infarction, arrhythmia and strokes have occurred. Great care is necessary if nortriptyline is administered to hyperthyroid patients or to those receiving thyroid medication, since cardiac arrhythmias may develop.

The use of nortriptyline should be avoided, if possible, in patients with a history of epilepsy. If it is used, however, the patients should be observed carefully at the beginning of treatment, for nortriptyline is known to lower the convulsive threshold.

Nortriptyline may impair the mental and/or physical abilities required for the performance of hazardous tasks, such as operating machinery or driving a car; therefore the patient should be warned accordingly.

Drug interactions: Under no circumstances should nortriptyline be given concurrently with, or within two weeks of cessation of, therapy with monoamine oxidase inhibitors. Hyperpyretic crises, severe convulsions and fatalities have occurred when similar tricyclic antidepressants were used in such combinations.

Nortriptyline should not be given with sympathomimetic agents such as adrenaline, ephedrine, isoprenaline, noradrenaline, phenylephrine and phenylpropanolamine.

Nortriptyline may decrease the antihypertensive effect of guanethidine, debrisoquine, bethanidine and possibly clonidine. Concurrent administration of reserpine has been shown to produce a 'stimulating' effect in some depressed patients. It would be advisable to review all antihypertensive therapy during treatment with tricyclic antidepressants.

Barbiturates may increase the rate of metabolism of nortriptyline.

Anaesthetics given during tricyclic antidepressant therapy may increase the risk of arrhythmias and hypotension. If surgery is necessary, the drug should be discontinued, if possible, for several days prior to the procedure, or the anaesthetist should be informed if the patient is still receiving therapy.

Tricyclic antidepressants may potentiate the CNS depressant effect of alcohol.

The potentiating effect of excessive consumption of alcohol may lead to increased suicidal attempts or overdosage, especially in patients with histories of emotional disturbances or suicidal ideation.

Steady-state serum concentrations of the tricyclic antidepressants are reported to fluctuate significantly as cimetidine is either added to or deleted from the drug regimen. Higher than expected steady-state serum concentrations of the tricyclic antidepressant have been observed when therapy is initiated in patients already taking cimetidine. A decrease may occur when cimetidine therapy is discontinued.

Greater than two-fold increases in previously stable plasma levels of nortriptyline have occurred when fluoxetine was administered concomitantly. Fluoxetine and its active metabolite, norfluoxetine, have long half-lives (7–9 days for norfluoxetine).

Supervision and adjustment of dosage may be required when nortriptyline is used with other anticholinergic drugs.

Usage in pregnancy: The safety of nortriptyline for use during pregnancy has not been established, nor is there evidence from animal studies that it is free from hazard; therefore the drug should not be administered to pregnant patients or women of childbearing age unless the potential benefits clearly outweigh any potential risk.

Usage in nursing mothers: See 'Contra-indications'.

Precautions: The elderly are particularly liable to experience adverse reactions, especially agitation, confusion and postural hypotension.

Troublesome hostility in a patient may be aroused by the use of nortriptyline.

Behavioural changes may occur in children receiving therapy for nocturnal enuresis.

If possible, the use of nortriptyline should be avoided in patients with narrow angle glaucoma or symptoms suggestive of prostatic hypertrophy.

The possibility of a suicide attempt by a depressed patient remains after the initiation of treatment. This possibility should be considered in relation to the quantity of drug dispensed at any one time.

When it is essential, nortriptyline may be administered with electroconvulsive therapy, although the hazards may be increased.

Both elevation and lowering of blood sugar levels have been reported. Significant hypoglycaemia was reported in a Type II diabetic patient maintained on chlorpropamide (250 mg/day), after the addition of nortriptyline (125 mg/day).

Side-effects: Included in the following list are a few adverse reactions that have not been reported with this specific drug. However, the pharmacological similarities among the tricyclic antidepressant drugs require that each of the reactions be considered when nortriptyline is administered.

Cardiovascular: Hypotension, hypertension, tachycardia, palpitation, myocardial infarction, arrhythmias, heart block, stroke.

Psychiatric: Confusional states (especially in the elderly) with hallucinations, disorientation, delusions; anxiety, restlessness, agitation; insomnia, panic, nightmares; hypomania; exacerbation of psychosis.

Neurological: Numbness, tingling, paraesthesia of extremities; inco-ordination, ataxia, tremors; peripheral neuropathy; extrapyramidal symptoms; seizures, alteration of EEG patterns; tinnitus.

Anticholinergic: Dry mouth and, rarely, associated sublingual adenitis or gingivitis; blurred vision, disturbance of accommodation, mydriasis; constipation, paralytic ileus; urinary retention, delayed micturition, dilation of the urinary tract.

Allergic: Rash, petechiae, urticaria, itching, photosensitisation (avoid excessive exposure to sunlight); oedema (general or of face and tongue), drug fever, cross-sensitivity with other tricyclic drugs.

Haematological: Bone-marrow depression, including agranulocytosis; aplastic anaemia; eosinophilia; purpura; thrombocytopenia.

Gastro-intestinal: Nausea and vomiting, anorexia, epigastric distress, diarrhoea; peculiar taste, stomatitis, abdominal cramps, black tongue, constipation, paralytic ileus.

Endocrine: Gynaecomastia in the male; breast enlargement and galactorrhoea in the female; increased or decreased libido, impotence; testicular swelling; elevation or depression of blood sugar levels; syndrome of inappropriate secretion of antidiuretic hormone.

Other: Jaundice (simulating obstructive); altered liver function, hepatitis and liver necrosis; weight gain or loss; sweating; flushing; urinary frequency, nocturia; drowsiness, dizziness, weakness, fatigue; headache; parotid swelling; alopecia.

Withdrawal symptoms: Though these are not indicative of addiction, abrupt cessation of treatment after prolonged therapy may produce nausea, headache and malaise.

Overdose

Signs and symptoms: 50 mg of a tricyclic antidepressant can be an overdose in a child. Of patients who are alive at presentation, mortality of 0–15% has been reported. Symptoms may begin within several hours and may include blurred vision, confusion, restlessness, dizziness, hypothermia, hyperthermia, agitation, vomiting, hyperactive reflexes, dilated pupils, fever, rapid heart rate, decreased bowel sounds, dry mouth, inability to void, myoclonic jerks, seizures, respiratory depression, myoglobinuric renal failure, nystagmus, ataxia, dysarthria, choreoathetosis, coma, hypotension and cardiac arrhythmias. Cardiac conduction may be slowed, with prolongation of QRS complex and QT intervals, right bundle branch and AV block, ventricular tachyarrhythmias (including Torsade de pointes and fibrillation) and death. Prolongation of QRS duration to more than 100 msec is predictive of more severe toxicity. The absence of sinus tachycardia does not ensure a benign course. Hypotension may be caused by vasodilatation, central and peripheral alpha-adrenergic blockade and cardiac depression. In a healthy young person, prolonged resuscitation may be effective; one patient survived 5 hours of cardiac massage.

Treatment: Symptomatic and supportive therapy is recommended. Activated charcoal may be more effective than emesis or lavage to reduce absorption.

Ventricular arrhythmias, especially when accompanied by lengthened QRS intervals, may respond to alkalinisation by hyperventilation or administration of sodium bicarbonate. Serum electrolytes should be monitored and managed. Refractory arrhythmias may respond to propranolol, bretylium or lignocaine. Quinidine and procainamide usually should not be used because they may exacerbate arrhythmias and conduction already slowed by the overdose.

Seizures may respond to diazepam. Phenytoin may treat seizures and cardiac rhythm disturbances. Physostigmine may antagonise atrial tachycardia, gut immotility, myoclonic jerks and somnolence. The effects of physostigmine may be short-lived.

Diuresis and dialysis have little effect. Haemoperfusion is unproven. Monitoring should continue, at least until the QRS duration is normal.

Pharmaceutical precautions Store below 25°C.

Legal category POM.

Package quantities
Tablets 25 mg: Bottles of 100.
Tablets 10 mg: Bottles of 100.

Further information Nil.

Product licence numbers
Tablets 25 mg 0006/5003
Tablets 10 mg 0006/5002

CAPASTAT*

Presentation Capreomycin sulphate as sterile white powder for intramuscular injection only, in sealed vials each containing 1,000,000 units (approximately equivalent to 1 g capreomycin base).

Uses

Actions: Capreomycin is active against human strains of *Mycobacterium tuberculosis.*

Frequent cross-resistance occurs between capreomycin and viomycin. Varying degrees of cross-resistance between capreomycin and kanamycin and neomycin have been reported. No cross-resistance has been observed between capreomycin and isoniazid, aminosalicylic acid, cycloserine, streptomycin, ethionamide or ethambutol.

Indications: Capastat should be used concomitantly with other appropriate antituberculous agents for the treatment of pulmonary infections caused by capreomycin-susceptible strains of *Mycobacterium tuberculosis* when the primary agents (isoniazid, rifampicin, streptomycin and ethambutol) have been ineffective or cannot be used because of toxicity or the presence of resistant tubercle bacilli.

Dosage and administration The usual dose is 1 g daily (but 20 mg/kg/day should not be exceeded) given by deep intramuscular injection only for 60 to 120 days, followed by 1 g intramuscularly two or three times a week. Capastat is always administered in combination with at least one other antituberculous agent to which the patient's strain of tubercle bacillus is susceptible.

Capastat should be dissolved in 2 ml of 0.9% Sodium Chloride Intravenous Infusion BP or Water for Injections PhEur. Two to three minutes should be allowed for complete solution.

For administration of a 1 g dose, the entire contents of the vial should be given. For dosages of less than 1 g the following dilution table may be used:

Diluent to be added (ml)	*Approximate volume of Capastat solution (ml)*	*Approximate average concentration (mg/ml) in terms of mg of capreomycin activity*
2.15	2.85	350
2.63	3.33	300
3.3	4.0	250
4.3	5.0	200

The elderly: As for adults. Reduce dosage if renal function is impaired.

Patients with reduced renal function: A reduced dosage should be given based on creatinine clearance using the guidance given in the following table. These dosages are designed to achieve a mean steady-state capreomycin level of 10 micrograms/ml, at various levels of renal function:

Creatinine clearance (ml/min)	*Capreomycin clearance (l/kg/h × 10⁻²)*	*Half life (hours)*	*Dose for these dosing intervals (mg/kg)*		
			24 h	*48 h*	*72 h*
0	0.54	55.5	1.29	2.58	3.87
10	1.01	29.4	2.43	4.87	7.30
20	1.49	20.0	3.58	7.16	10.70
30	1.97	15.1	4.72	9.45	14.20
40	2.45	12.2	5.87	11.70	
50	2.92	10.2	7.01	14.00	
60	3.40	8.8	8.16		
80	4.35	6.8	10.40		
100	5.31	5.6	12.70		
110	5.78	5.2	13.90		

Infants and children: Not for paediatric use since the safety of capreomycin for use in infants and children has not been established.

Contra-indications, warnings, etc

Contra-indication: Hypersensitivity to capreomycin.

Warnings: The use of capreomycin in patients with renal insufficiency or pre-existing auditory impairment must be undertaken with great caution, and the risk of additional eighth cranial nerve impairment or renal injury should be weighed against the benefits to be derived from treatment.

Simultaneous administration of other antituberculous drugs which also have ototoxic and nephrotoxic potential (e.g. streptomycin, viomycin) is not recommended. Also, use with other drugs that are not given for the treatment of tuberculosis but have ototoxic or nephrotoxic potential (e.g. polymyxin, colistin sulphate, amikacin, gentamicin, tobramycin, vancomycin, kanamycin and neomycin) should also be undertaken only with great caution.

Pregnancy: The safety of capreomycin for use during pregnancy has not been established. Capreomycin has been shown to be teratogenic in rats when given at 3.5 times the human dose. There are no adequate and well controlled studies in pregnant women. Capastat should be used during pregnancy only if the potential benefit justifies the potential risk to the fetus.

Studies have not been performed to determine potential for carcinogenicity, mutagenicity, or impairment of fertility.

Nursing mothers: It is not known whether capreomycin is excreted in human milk. Caution should be exercised when administering to a nursing woman.

Precautions: As capreomycin is potentially ototoxic, audiometry and assessment of vestibular function should be performed before starting treatment and at regular intervals during treatment.

Regular tests of renal function should be made throughout the period of treatment, and reduced dosage should be used in patients with known, or suspected, renal impairment (see 'Dosage and administration').

Since hypokalaemia may occur during capreomycin therapy, serum potassium levels should be determined frequently.

A partial neuromuscular block can occur after large doses of capreomycin.

Capreomycin should be administered cautiously to patients with a history of allergy, particularly to drugs.

Side-effects

Renal: Elevation of serum creatinine or blood urea and abnormal urine sediment have been observed. Toxic nephritis was reported in one patient with tuberculosis and portal cirrhosis who was treated with capreomycin (1 g) and aminosalicylic acid daily for one month. This patient developed renal insufficiency and oliguria and died. The post-mortem showed subsiding acute tubular necrosis.

Electrolyte disturbances resembling Bartter's syndrome have been reported in one patient.

Hepatic: A decrease in bromsulphthalein excretion without change in serum enzymes has been noted in the presence of pre-existing liver disease. Abnormal results in liver function tests have occurred in many patients receiving capreomycin in combination with other antituberculous agents which are also known to cause changes in hepatic function. Periodic determinations of liver function are recommended.

Haematological: Leucocytosis and leucopenia have been observed. Rare cases of thrombocytopenia have been reported. Most patients receiving daily capreomycin have had eosinophilia exceeding 5%, but this has subsided with the reduction of capreomycin dosage to two or three times weekly.

Hypersensitivity: Urticaria and maculopapular rashes associated in some cases with febrile reactions have been reported when capreomycin and other antituberculous drugs were given concomitantly.

Otic: Clinical and subclinical auditory loss has been noted. Some audiometric changes have proved reversible and others, with permanent loss have not been progressive following withdrawal of capreomycin. Tinnitus and vertigo have occurred.

Injection site reactions: Pain and induration at injection sites have been observed. Excessive bleeding and sterile abscesses have also been reported at these sites.

Overdosage
Signs and symptoms: Hypokalaemia, hypocalcaemia, hypomagnesaemia and an electrolyte disturbance resembling Bartter's syndrome have been reported to occur in patients with capreomycin toxicity. Nephrotoxicity, including acute tubular necrosis; and ototoxicity, including dizziness, tinnitus, vertigo and loss of high-tone acuity (see 'Warnings' and 'Precautions'). Neuromuscular blockage or respiratory paralysis may occur following rapid intravenous administration.

If capreomycin is ingested, toxicity is unlikely because less than 1% is absorbed from an intact gastro-intestinal system.

Treatment: Symptomatic and supportive therapy is recommended. Activated charcoal may be more effective than emesis or lavage in reducing absorption.

Patients who have received an overdose of capreomycin and have normal renal function should be hydrated to maintain a urine output of 3–5 ml/kg/hr. Fluid balance electrolytes and creatinine clearance should be monitored.

Haemodialysis is effective in patients with significant renal disease.

Pharmaceutical precautions
Dry powder: Store in a cool, dry place.

After reconstitution: The solution may acquire a pale straw colour and darken with time, but this is not associated with loss of potency or the development of toxicity. Solutions of Capastat may be stored for 48 hours at room temperature (15°–25°C) and up to 14 days under refrigeration (2°–8°C).

Legal category POM.

Package quantities Vials of 1,000,000 units (1 g base approximately): Pack of 5 vials.

Further information Capastat must be used only in conjunction with adequate doses of other antituberculous drugs. The use of Capastat alone allows the rapid development of strains resistant to it.

Product licence number 0006/5005.

DISTALGESIC*

Approved name: Co-proxamol

Presentation Tablets each containing 32.5 mg Dextropropoxyphene Hydrochloride BP (equivalent to approximately 30 mg dextropropoxyphene base) with 325 mg Paracetamol PhEur. The tablets are white, pillow-shaped, film coated, 14 mm in length and marked 'DG'.

Uses *Actions:* Dextropropoxyphene is a mild narcotic analgesic structurally related to methadone.

Indication: For the management of mild to moderate pain.

Dosage and administration For oral administration to adults only. The usual dose is 2 tablets three or four times daily and should not normally be exceeded.

Consideration should be given to a reduced total daily dosage in patients with hepatic or renal impairment.

The elderly: There is evidence of prolonged half-life in the elderly, so reduction in dosage should be considered.

Children: Distalgesic is not recommended for use in children.

Contra-indications, warnings, etc
Contra-indications: Hypersensitivity to dextropropoxyphene or paracetamol. Use in patients who are suicidal or addiction-prone.

Warnings:
PATIENTS SHOULD BE ADVISED NOT TO EXCEED THE RECOMMENDED DOSE AND TO AVOID ALCOHOL.

Dextropropoxyphene products in excessive doses, either alone or in combination with other CNS depressants, including alcohol, are a major cause of drug-related deaths. Fatalities within the first hour of overdosage are not uncommon and can occur within 15 minutes. Some deaths have occurred as a consequence of the accidental ingestion of excessive quantities of Distalgesic alone, or in combination with other drugs.

Overdosage may damage the liver, due predominantly to the accumulation of intermediate metabolites of paracetamol which cause hepatic necrosis.

Distalgesic should be prescribed with caution for those patients whose medical condition requires the concomitant administration of sedatives, tranquillisers, muscle relaxants, antidepressants or other CNS-depressant drugs; patients should be advised of the additive depressant effects of these combinations. Distalgesic should also be prescribed with caution in patients who use alcohol in excess.

Drug dependence: Dextropropoxyphene, when taken in higher than recommended doses over long periods of time, can produce drug dependence.

Ambulatory patients: Dextropropoxyphene may impair abilities required for tasks such as driving a car or operating machinery. The patient should be cautioned accordingly.

Pregnancy: Safety in pregnancy has not been established relative to possible adverse effects on fetal development. Withdrawal symptoms in neonates have been reported following use during pregnancy. Therefore, Distalgesic should not be used in pregnant women unless, in the judgement of the physician, the potential benefits outweigh the possible hazards.

Nursing mothers: Low levels of dextropropoxyphene have been detected in human milk. In postpartum studies involving nursing mothers who were given dextropropoxyphene, no adverse effects were noted in the infants.

Precautions: Distalgesic should be administered with caution to patients with hepatic or renal impairment since higher serum concentrations or delayed elimination may occur.

Drug interactions: The CNS-depressant effect of dextropropoxyphene is additive with that of other CNS depressants, including alcohol.

Dextropropoxyphene may interfere with the metabolism of antidepressants, anticonvulsants and warfarin-like drugs. Severe neurological signs, including coma, have occurred with concomitant use of carbamazepine.

Side-effects: The most frequently reported have been dizziness, sedation, nausea and vomiting. Some of these side-effects may be alleviated if the patient lies down.

Other side-effects include constipation, abdominal pain, rashes, light-headedness, headache, weakness, euphoria, dysphoria, hallucinations and minor visual disturbances.

Dextropropoxyphene therapy has been associated with abnormal liver function tests and, more rarely, with instances of reversible jaundice.

Hepatic necrosis may result from acute overdose of paracetamol. In chronic alcohol abusers, this has been reported rarely with short-term use of paracetamol dosages of 2.5 to 10 g/day. Fatalities have occurred. Renal papillary necrosis may result from chronic paracetamol use, particularly when the dosage is greater than recommended and when combined with aspirin.

Subacute painful myopathy has occurred following chronic dextropropoxyphene overdosage.

Chronic ingestion of dextropropoxyphene in doses exceeding 720 mg per day has caused toxic psychoses and convulsions.

Overdosage: Initial consideration should be given to the management of the CNS effects of dextropropoxyphene overdosage. Resuscitative measures should be initiated promptly.

Dextropropoxyphene: In the acute phase dextropropoxyphene produces symptoms typical of narcosis, with somnolence or coma and respiratory depression, sometimes with convulsions. Blood pressure falls and cardiac performance deteriorates. Cardiac arrhythmias and conduction delay may be present. A combined respiratory-metabolic acidosis occurs, which may be severe if large amounts of salicylates have also been ingested. Death may occur.

Naloxone will reduce the respiratory depression and

0.4–2 mg iv should be administered promptly. (This may be repeated at 2–3 minute intervals, but if there is no response after 10 mg of naloxone the diagnosis should be questioned.) The duration of antagonism may be brief and need repeating for up to 24 hours. Mechanical ventilation, with oxygen may be required, and PEEP ventilation is desirable if pulmonary oedema is present.

Blood gases, pH and electrolytes should be monitored and electrocardiographic monitoring is essential. Ventricular fibrillation or cardiac arrest may occur. Respiratory acidosis rapidly subsides as ventilation is restored and hypercapnoea eliminated, but lactic acidosis may require iv bicarbonate for prompt correction. In addition to the use of a narcotic antagonist, the patient may require titration with an anticonvulsant to control convulsions. Gastric lavage may be useful and activated charcoal can absorb a significant amount of ingested dextropropoxyphene.

Treatment of dextropropoxyphene overdose in children: See general comments above. Naloxone at 0.01 mg/kg body weight iv should be administered promptly. If there is no response a dose of 0.1 mg/kg iv may be used.

Paracetamol: Overdose symptoms may not become apparent until later but early measurement of paracetamol levels is essential. N-acetylcysteine given as early as possible is effective in reducing the toxic effects of paracetamol. Treatment should be instituted within 16 hours of ingestion. Initial symptoms may be anorexia, nausea, vomiting, profuse sweating, malaise and abdominal pain, but the patient may have no symptoms. Subsequent evidence of liver dysfunction may be apparent up to 72 hours after ingestion, and if severe lead to irreversible hepatic necrosis and death within 3–7 days.

In adults, hepatic toxicity has rarely been reported with acute overdoses of less than 10 g and fatalities with less than 15 g.

Acute renal failure may accompany the hepatic dysfunction and can occur without signs of fulminant hepatic failure. Typically renal impairment is more apparent 6–9 days after overdose.

Pharmaceutical precautions Nil.

Legal category CD (Sch 5), POM.

Package quantities Blister packs of 100 (10 strips of 10 tablets).

Further information Nil.

Product licence number 0006/5000.

DISTAMINE*

Presentation Tablets each containing 50 mg, 125 mg or 250 mg D-penicillamine base. The 50 mg tablets are white, coated, scored and have a diameter of 5.5 mm. The 125 mg tablets are white, coated and have a diameter of 8 mm. They are marked 'DS' on one face and '125' on the other. The 250 mg tablets are white, coated and have a diameter of 10 mm. They are marked 'DM' on one face and '250' on the other.

Uses
(a) Severe active rheumatoid arthritis, including juvenile forms.
(b) Wilson's disease (hepatolenticular degeneration).
(c) Cystinuria – Dissolution and prevention of cystine stones.
(d) Lead poisoning.
(e) Chronic active hepatitis.

Dosage and administration For oral administration.

(a) Rheumatoid arthritis: Adults: 125–250 mg daily for the first month. Increase by the same amount every 4 to 12 weeks until remission occurs. The minimum maintenance dose to achieve suppression of symptoms should be used and treatment should be discontinued if no benefit is obtained within twelve months. Improvement may not occur for some months.

The usual maintenance dose is 500–750 mg daily. Up to 1.5 g daily may be required. If possible, penicillamine should be taken at least half an hour before meals, or on retiring.

If remission is established and has been sustained for six months, gradual reduction by 125–250 mg amounts every 12 weeks may be attempted.

The elderly: Increased toxicity has been observed in this patient population regardless of renal function. Initial dose should not exceed 50–125 mg daily for the first month, increasing by similar increments every 4 to 12 weeks until the minimum maintenance dose to suppress symptoms is reached. Daily dosage should not exceed 1 g.

Children: 15–20 mg/kg/day as a maintenance dose, starting with 50 mg daily for one month and increasing at four-weekly intervals.

(b) Wilson's disease: Adults: 1.5–2 g daily in divided doses 30 minutes before food. Dose may be reduced to 750 mg–1 g daily when control of the disease is achieved. Patients must be maintained in negative copper balance and the minimum dosage of penicillamine required to achieve this should be given.

It is advisable that a dose of 2 g/day should not be continued for more than a year.

The elderly: 20 mg/kg/day in divided doses. Adjust dosage to control disease and maintain negative copper balance.

Children: Up to 20 mg/kg/day in divided doses before food. Minimum dose 500 mg/day.

(c) Cystinuria: Ideally, establish the lowest effective dose by quantitative amino acid chromatography of urine.

(i) *Dissolution of cystine stones: Adults:* 1–3 g daily in divided doses 30 minutes before food, where possible.

Urine cystine levels of not more than 200 mg/l should be maintained.

(ii) *Prevention of cystine stones: Adults:* 500 mg–1 g on retiring. Fluid intake should be not less than 3 litres/day.

Urine cystine levels of not more than 300 mg/l should be maintained.

The elderly: Use the minimum dose to maintain urinary cystine levels below 200 mg/l.

Children: No dose range established, but urinary cystine levels must be kept below 200 mg/l. The minimum dose of penicillamine required to achieve this should be given.

(d) Lead poisoning: Adults: 1–1.5 g daily in divided doses before food until urinary lead is stabilised at less than 0.5 mg/day.

The elderly: 20 mg/kg/day in divided doses until urinary lead is stabilised at less than 0.5 mg/day.

Children: 20 mg/kg/day.

(e) Chronic active hepatitis: Adults: For maintenance treatment after the disease process has been brought under control with corticosteroids. The initial dosage of 500 mg daily, in divided doses, should be increased gradually over three months to a maintenance dose of 1.25 g daily. During this period, the dosage of corticosteroids should be phased out. Throughout therapy, liver function tests should be carried out periodically to assess the disease status.

The elderly: Not recommended.

(f) Desensitisation: No fixed dose regimen. An initial dose of 25 mg daily is suggested, this to be gradually increased in accordance with the response of the patient. Higher initial doses have been employed in cystinuric patients.

Contra-indications, warnings, etc

Contra-indications: Hypersensitivity to penicillamine, except in a life-threatening situation, when desensitisation should be attempted (see 'Dosage and Administration'). Agranulocytosis or severe thrombocytopenia due to penicillamine. Lupus erythematosus.

Warnings

Usage in pregnancy: The safety of penicillamine for use during pregnancy has not been established. It has been shown to be teratogenic in rats when given in doses several times higher than those recommended for human use.

Wilson's disease: There has been one case reported of reversible cutis laxa in an infant born to a mother taking 1.5 g penicillamine daily throughout pregnancy. Although there have been no controlled studies on the use of penicillamine during pregnancy, two retrospective studies have reported the successful delivery of 43 normal infants to 28 women receiving between 0.5 g and 2 g of penicillamine daily.

Cystinuria: There have been reports of patients delivered of normal infants, and one report of a severe connective tissue abnormality in the infant of a mother who received 2 g penicillamine daily throughout pregnancy. Whenever possible, penicillamine should be withheld during pregnancy, but if stones continue to form, the benefit of resuming treatment must be weighed against the possible risk to the fetus.

Rheumatoid arthritis or chronic active hepatitis: Penicillamine should not be administered to patients who are pregnant, and therapy should be stopped when pregnancy is diagnosed or suspected, unless considered to be absolutely essential by the physician.

Side-effects: NB: The incidence and severity of some of the adverse reactions, noted below, varies according to the dosage and nature of the disease under treatment.

Nausea, anorexia, fever and rash may occur early in therapy, especially when full doses are given from the start. Antihistamines, steroid cover, or temporary reduction of dose will control urticarial reactions.

Reversible loss of taste may occur. Mineral supplements to overcome this are not recommended.

Thrombocytopenia occurs commonly and neutropenia less often. These reactions may occur at any time during treatment and are usually reversible. Deaths from agranulocytosis and aplastic anaemia have occurred. Full blood counts should be carried out weekly or fortnightly during the first eight weeks of therapy, in the week after any increase in dose, and otherwise monthly thereafter. In cystinuria or Wilson's disease, longer intervals may be adequate.

Withdrawal of treatment should be considered if platelets fall below 120,000 or white blood cells below 2,500/mm^3, or if three successive falls are noted within the normal range. Treatment may be restarted at a reduced dosage when counts return to normal, but should be permanently withdrawn on recurrence of neutropenia or thrombocytopenia.

Proteinuria occurs in up to 30 per cent of patients and is partially dose-related. Urine should be tested weekly at first and after each increase in dose, then monthly, though again longer intervals may be adequate with cystinuria and Wilson's disease. Increasing proteinuria may necessitate withdrawal of treatment.

Haematuria is rare, but if it occurs in the absence of renal stones or other known cause, treatment should be stopped immediately.

Other complications have included haemolytic anaemia, nephrotic syndrome, drug induced lupus erythematosus, and conditions closely resembling myasthenia gravis, pemphigus, Goodpasture's syndrome, Stevens-Johnson syndrome and rheumatoid arthritis.

A late rash, described as acquired epidermolysis bullosa and penicillamine dermopathy, may occur after several months or years of therapy. This may necessitate a reduction in dosage.

Precautions: Full blood and platelet counts should be performed and renal function should be assessed prior to treatment with penicillamine. Monitoring of blood and platelet counts should be carried out at appropriate intervals, together with urinalysis for detection of haematuria and proteinuria.

If concomitant oral iron therapy is indicated, this should not be given within two hours of taking penicillamine.

Caution should be observed when anti-inflammatory or other drugs with known propensity for causing marrow injury are taken concurrently with penicillamine.

Care should be exercised in patients with renal insufficiency; modification of dosage may be necessary.

Treatment of overdosage: No instances of adverse reactions to an overdose of penicillamine have been recorded and no specific measures are indicated.

Further information Nil.

Pharmaceutical precautions Store in a dry place below 25°C. Keep containers tightly closed.

Legal category POM.

Package quantities Tablets 50 mg: Bottles of 100
Tablets 125 mg: Bottles of 100
Tablets 250 mg: Bottles of 100

Product licence numbers

Tablets	50 mg	0006/0105
Tablets	125 mg	0006/0090
Tablets	250 mg	0006/5008

DISTAQUAINE* V-K

Presentation *Phenoxymethylpenicillin Potassium Tablets BP:* Containing the equivalent of 250 mg phenoxymethylpenicillin (400,000 units). The tablets are white, scored, 10.5 mm in diameter and marked 'DD KF'.

Syrup: Granules for the preparation of Phenoxymethylpenicillin Elixir BP, 125 mg/5 ml (200,000 units). The granules are pale pink, converting to orange liquid on reconstitution.

The potassium content is 14.03 mg (0.36 mEq) in 125 mg, and 28.06 mg (0.72 mEq) in 250 mg.

Uses Penicillin exerts high activity *in vitro* against staphylococci (except penicillinase-producing strains), streptococci (groups A, C, G, H, L, and M), pneumococci, *Corynebacterium diphtheriae, Bacillus anthracis, Actinomyces bovis, Streptobacillus moniliformis, Listeria monocytogenes, Neisseria gonorrhoeae, Treponema pallidum, Clostridium* species and Leptospira.

Phenoxymethylpenicillin and potassium phenoxymethylpenicillin are indicated in the treatment of mild to moderately severe infections associated with microorganisms whose susceptibility to penicillin is within the range of serum levels attained with these dosage forms.

The following infections will usually respond to adequate doses:

Streptococcal infections (without bacteraemia): Mild to moderate infections of the upper respiratory tract, scarlet fever and mild erysipelas.

Pneumococcal infections: Mild to moderately severe infections of the respiratory tract.

Staphylococcal infections sensitive to penicillin: Mild infections of the skin and soft tissues.

Fusospirochaetosis (Vincent's gingivitis and pharyngitis): Mild to moderately severe infections of the oropharynx usually respond to therapy with oral penicillin.

Note: Severe empyema, bacteraemia, pericarditis, meningitis and arthritis should not be treated with penicillin V during the acute phase.

Prophylactic use: Prophylaxis with oral penicillin has proved effective in preventing recurrence of rheumatic fever and chorea.

Patients with a past history of rheumatic fever receiving continuous prophylaxis may harbour penicillin-resistant organisms. In these patients, the use of another prophylactic agent should be considered.

Note: Oral penicillin should not be used as adjunctive prophylaxis for genito-urinary instrumentation or surgery, lower intestinal tract surgery, sigmoidoscopy and childbirth.

Dosage and administration For oral administration.

Adults: 125 mg or 250 mg every four to six hours, depending on the severity of the condition.

The elderly: As for adults. Reduce dosage if renal function is markedly impaired.

Children over 5 years: The adult dose.

Children 5 years or less: 125 mg every six hours.

Infants (up to 1 year): 62.5 mg every six hours.

In all but the most serious cases, the last dose of the day may be doubled to avoid disturbing sleep. Ideally, each dose should be given half an hour before (or at least three hours after) a meal.

Prophylactic use: 125 mg twice daily is recommended for long term prophylaxis of rheumatic fever.

Contra-indications, warnings, etc
Contra-indication: A previous hypersensitivity reaction to any penicillin.

Warnings: All degrees of hypersensitivity, including fatal anaphylaxis, have been observed with oral penicillin. These reactions are more likely to occur in individuals with a history of sensitivity to penicillins, cephalosporins and other allergens. Enquiry should be made for such a history before therapy with a penicillin is begun. If an allergic reaction occurs, the drug should be discontinued and the patient treated with the usual agents (e.g. adrenaline and other pressor amines, antihistamines and corticosteroids).

Usage in pregnancy: Although laboratory and clinical studies have shown no evidence of teratogenicity, caution should be exercised when prescribing for the pregnant patient.

Precautions: Penicillin should be used with caution in individuals with histories of significant allergies and/or asthma.

Oral therapy should not be relied upon in patients with severe illness, or with nausea, vomiting, gastric dilatation, cardiospasm or intestinal hypermotility.

Occasionally patients do not absorb therapeutic amounts of orally administered penicillin.

Administer with caution in the presence of markedly impaired renal function, as safe dosage may be lower than that usually recommended.

Streptococcal infections should be treated for a minimum of 10 days, and post-therapy cultures should be performed to confirm the eradication of the organisms.

Prolonged use of antibiotics may promote the overgrowth of non-susceptible organisms, including fungi. If superinfection occurs, appropriate measures should be taken.

Side-effects: Although reactions have been reported much less frequently after oral than after parenteral therapy, it should be remembered that all degrees of hypersensitivity, including fatal anaphylaxis, have been observed with oral penicillin.

The most common reactions to oral penicillin are nausea, vomiting, epigastric distress, diarrhoea and black, hairy tongue. The hypersensitivity reactions noted are skin eruptions (ranging from maculopapular to exfoliative dermatitis); urticaria; reactions resembling serum sickness, including chills, fever, oedema, arthralgia and prostration; laryngeal oedema; and anaphylaxis. Fever and eosinophilia may frequently be the only reactions observed. Haemolytic anaemia, leucopenia, thrombocytopenia, neuropathy and nephropathy are infrequent reactions and are usually associated with high doses of parenteral penicillin.

Overdosage
Signs and symptoms: A large oral overdose of penicillin may cause nausea, vomiting, stomach pain, diarrhoea and, rarely, major motor seizures. If other symptoms are present consider the possibility of an allergic reaction.

Hyperkalaemia may result from overdosage, particularly in patients with renal insufficiency.

Treatment: No specific antidote is known. Symptomatic and supportive therapy is recommended. Activated charcoal with a cathartic, such as sorbitol, may hasten drug elimination. Penicillin may be removed by haemodialysis.

Pharmaceutical precautions *Tablets:* Protect from moisture.

Syrup: Protect from moisture. Reconstituted preparations may be stored for seven days at room temperature (15°–25°C) or 14 days in a refrigerator (2°–8°C).

Legal category POM.

Package quantities
Tablets 250 mg: Bottles of 100 and 500.
Syrup Granules 125 mg/5 ml: Bottles of 100 ml.

Further information Nil.

Product licence numbers

Tablets 250 mg	0006/5032
Syrup 125 mg/5 ml	0006/5121

FENOPRON 300*
FENOPRON 600*

Presentation Fenoprofen Calcium Tablets BP, each containing fenoprofen calcium equivalent to 300 mg or 600 mg fenoprofen.

Fenopron 300 tablets are orange, elliptical, 14 mm long and marked DISTA 4019.

Fenopron 600 tablets are orange, para-capsule, 20 mm long and marked DISTA 4021.

Uses For the treatment of osteoarthritis, rheumatoid arthritis and ankylosing spondylitis.

For the relief of mild/moderate pain.

Dosage and administration For oral administration to adults only, and not recommended for administration to children.

Dosage: 300–600 mg three or four times per day.

Fenopron 300: Recommended initial dosage is 2 tablets three times per day, then adjusted to the needs of the patient.

Fenopron 600: Recommended initial dosage is 1 tablet three times per day, plus one at night if necessitated by a more severe condition. The dosage may then be adjusted to the needs of the patient.

The maximum daily dose should not exceed 3 g.

If fenoprofen is administered with meals the total amount absorbed is not affected, although peak blood levels are delayed and diminished.

The elderly: There is no difference in the metabolism or pharmacokinetics of fenoprofen in the elderly. However, it may be advisable to start therapy with a low dose, as side-effects of non-steroidal anti-inflammatory drugs are more pronounced in this patient population.

Contra-indications, warnings, etc
Contra-indications: Hypersensitivity to the drug. Active, or a history of, peptic or intestinal ulceration.

Fenoprofen should not be given to patients in whom aspirin and other non-steroidal anti-inflammatory drugs induce the symptoms of asthma, rhinitis, or urticaria, because cross-sensitivity to these drugs occurs in a high proportion of patients.

Patients with a history of significantly impaired renal function.

Warnings
Gastro-intestinal: Serious toxicity, such as bleeding, ulceration and perforation, can occur at any time, without warning symptoms, in patients treated chronically. Elderly or debilitated patients tolerate ulceration or bleeding less well than other individuals and most spontaneous reports of fatal gastro-intestinal events are in this population. Minor upper gastro-intestinal problems, such as dyspepsia, are common, usually developing early in therapy.

Fenoprofen should only be given under close supervision to patients with a history of upper gastro-intestinal disease or peptic ulcer risk factors.

Genito-urinary: The most frequently reported problems have been episodes of dysuria, cystitis, haematuria, interstitial nephritis and nephrotic syndrome. This syndrome may be preceded by the appearance of fever, rash, arthralgia, oliguria and uraemia, and may progress to anuria. Early recognition of the syndrome and withdrawal of the drug have been followed by rapid recovery. Patients who have had similar reactions with other non-steroidal anti-inflammatory drugs should not be given fenoprofen. Patients likely to have compromised renal function should be monitored periodically.

Bronchospasm may be precipitated in patients suffering from, or with a previous history of, bronchial asthma or allergic disease.

Usage in pregnancy: The safety of fenoprofen for use during pregnancy has not been established; therefore it should not be used during pregnancy unless considered essential by the physician. Animal studies showed prolongation of parturition, but no evidence of teratogenicity.

Usage in nursing mothers: Safety has not been established, therefore administration to nursing mothers is not recommended.

Precautions: In patients with conditions leading to reduction in renal blood flow or blood volume, administration of non-steroidal anti-inflammatory drugs may precipitate overt renal decompensation. Patients at greatest risk of this reaction are those with impaired renal function, heart failure, liver dysfunction, those taking diuretics, and the elderly. Discontinuation of therapy is typically followed by recovery to the pre-treatment state.

Since fenoprofen is eliminated primarily by the kidneys, patients with possibly compromised renal function (such as the elderly) should be closely monitored; a lower daily dosage should be anticipated to avoid excessive drug accumulation.

Some patients have developed elevation of serum transaminase, LDH and alkaline phosphatase and it is recommended that fenoprofen be discontinued if any significant liver abnormalities occur. Borderline elevations of one or more liver function tests may occur in up to 15% of patients. Severe hepatic reactions, including jaundice and cases of fatal hepatitis, have been reported.

Patients with initial low haemoglobin values who are receiving long-term therapy with fenoprofen should have a haemoglobin determination at reasonable intervals.

Peripheral oedema has been observed in some patients taking fenoprofen, therefore it should be used with caution in patients with compromised cardiac function or hypertension. The possibility of renal involvement should be considered.

Studies to date have not shown changes in the eyes attributable to the administration of fenoprofen. However, adverse ocular effects have been observed with other anti-inflammatory drugs, so eye examinations should be performed if visual disturbances occur in patients taking fenoprofen.

Caution should be exercised by patients whose activities require alertness if they experience central nervous system side-effects.

Since the safety of fenoprofen has not been established in patients with impaired hearing, these patients should have periodic tests of auditory function during chronic therapy.

Fenoprofen decreases platelet aggregation and may prolong bleeding time.

Laboratory test interactions: Values of total and free triiodothyronine in patients receiving fenoprofen have been reported as falsely elevated. Thyroid stimulating hormones, total thyroxine and thyrotropin releasing hormone response are not affected.

Drug interactions: The concurrent use of fenoprofen and salicylates is not recommended.

Chronic administration of phenobarbitone may be associated with a decrease in the plasma half-life of fenoprofen. Dosage adjustment of fenoprofen may be required.

Patients treated with fenoprofen may be resistant to the effects of loop diuretics.

In vitro studies have shown that fenoprofen may displace other drugs, for example hydantoins, sulphonamides, or sulphonylureas, from their binding sites and this may lead to drug interaction. Theoretically, fenoprofen could likewise be displaced. In patients receiving coumarin-type anticoagulants, the addition of fenoprofen could prolong the prothrombin time.

Side-effects:

Gastro-intestinal: These are the most commonly observed side-effects and include dyspepsia, constipation, diarrhoea, nausea, vomiting, anorexia, ulceration of the buccal mucosa, abdominal pain, flatulence, dry mouth, gastritis, metallic taste, pancreatitis and occult blood in the stool. Cases of peptic ulceration, including some complicated by bleeding or perforation have occurred.

Renal: Cases of acute renal insufficiency, in association with interstitial nephritis, nephrotic syndrome or papillary necrosis, have been reported. Episodes of dysuria, cystitis and haematuria, oliguria, azotaemia and anuria have occurred.

Hepatic: Severe hepatic reactions, including jaundice and fatal hepatitis, have been reported rarely. Increases in alkaline phosphatase, LDH and AST have been observed.

Haematological: Various syndromes involving the bone marrow have been reported rarely; thrombocytopenia, pancytopenia and aplastic anaemia have occurred. Purpura, bruising, haemorrhage, haemolytic anaemia and agranulocytosis have also been reported.

Allergic/skin: Pruritus, rash, urticaria, anaphylaxis, Stevens-Johnson syndrome, angioneurotic oedema, increased sweating, exfoliative dermatitis, toxic epidermal necrolysis and alopecia have been reported.

Neurological: Reactions reported include headache, somnolence, dizziness, tremor, confusion and insomnia, depression, disorientation, seizures and trigeminal neuralgia.

Cardiovascular: Palpitations, tachycardia, atrial fibrillation, pulmonary oedema, ECG changes and supraventricular tachycardia have been reported.

Miscellaneous: Tinnitus, hearing decrease, amblyopia, blurred vision, diplopia, optic neuritis, nervousness, peripheral oedema, asthenia, dyspnoea, fatigue, malaise, burning tongue, personality change, lymphadenopathy, mastodynia, fever, upper respiratory infection and nasopharyngitis have been reported.

Overdosage: Symptoms of overdose appear within several hours and generally involve the gastro-intestinal and central nervous systems. They include dyspepsia, nausea, vomiting, abdominal pain, dizziness, headache, ataxia, tinnitus, tremor, drowsiness and confusion. Hyperpyrexia, tachycardia, hypotension and acute renal failure may occur rarely following overdose. Respiratory depression and metabolic acidosis have also been reported following overdose with certain non-steroidal anti-inflammatory drugs.

Treatment: Standard therapy to evacuate gastric contents and to support vital functions should be employed. Alkalinisation of the urine, forced diuresis, peritoneal dialysis, haemodialysis and charcoal haemoperfusion do not enhance systemic drug elimination.

Pharmaceutical precautions Nil.

Legal category POM.

Package quantities
Fenopron 300: Bottles of 100 tablets
Fenopron 600: Bottles of 100 tablets

Further information Nil.

Product licence numbers
Fenopron 300 0006/0101
Fenopron 600 0006/0104

HAELAN*
HAELAN-X*

Presentation *Haelan:* Collapsible tubes containing 0.0125% flurandrenolone in cream or ointment base. The cream is white in colour and the ointment is translucent.

Haelan-X: Collapsible tubes containing 0.05% flurandrenolone in cream or ointment base. The cream is white in colour and the ointment is translucent.

Uses *Adults and children:* Eczema and dermatitis of all types including childhood and adult atopic eczema, photodermatitis, primary irritant and allergic dermatitis, lichen planus, lichen simplex, prurigo nodularis, discoid lupus erythematosus, necrobiosis lipoidica, pretibial myxoedema and erythroderma.

Dosage and administration For topical administration.

Cream: For moist weeping lesions, the cream should be applied gently to the affected area two or three times daily.

Ointment: For dry, scaly lesions, the ointment should be applied as a thin film to the affected area two or three times daily.

The elderly: As the skin is likely to be thin, apply sparingly to avoid development of atrophy.

Dilution is not recommended, but if considered necessary Aqueous Cream BP may be used for the creams and White Soft Paraffin BP for the ointments.

Contra-indications, warnings, etc

Contra-indications: Tuberculosis of the skin. Facial rosacea. Acne vulgaris. Perioral dermatitis. Perianal and genital pruritus. Dermatoses in infancy including eczema, dermatitic napkin eruption, bacterial (impetigo), viral (herpes simplex) and fungal (candida or dermatophyte) infections. Use in patients with a history of hypersensitivity to any of the components in the preparation.

Warnings and precautions: Preparations of Haelan are not intended for ophthalmic use.

Local and systemic toxicity is common especially following long-term continuous use, continued use on large areas of damaged skin, flexures and with polythene occlusion.

Systemic absorption of topical corticosteroids has produced reversible hypothalamic-pituitary-adrenal (HPA) axis suppression (see 'Side-effects'). Therefore, patients receiving a large dose of a potent topical steroid applied to a large surface area or under an occlusive dressing should be evaluated periodically for evidence of HPA axis suppression by using urinary-free cortisol and ACTH stimulation tests. If HPA axis suppression is noted, an attempt should be made to withdraw the drug, to reduce the frequency of application or to substitute a less potent steroid. Recovery of HPA axis function is generally prompt and complete on discontinuation of the drug. Infrequently, signs and symptoms of steroid withdrawal may occur, so that supplemental systemic corticosteroids are required.

Long-term continuous therapy should be avoided in all patients irrespective of age.

Application under occlusion should be restricted to dermatoses in very limited areas.

If used on the face, courses should be limited to five days and occlusion should not be used.

In the presence of skin infections, the use of an appropriate antifungal or antibacterial agent should be instituted. If a favourable response does not occur promptly, flurandrenolone should be discontinued until the infection has been adequately controlled.

Usage in children: If used in childhood, courses should be limited to five days and occlusion should not be used.

Children may absorb proportionally larger amounts of topical corticosteroids and thus may be more susceptible to systemic toxicity. Children may also demonstrate greater susceptibility to topical corticosteroid induced HPA axis suppression and Cushing's syndrome than do mature patients because of a larger skin surface to body weight ratio. Administration of topical corticosteroids to children should be limited to the least amount compatible with an effective therapeutic regimen. Chronic corticosteroid therapy may interfere with the growth and development of children.

Usage in pregnancy: There is inadequate evidence of safety in human pregnancy. There may be a very small risk of cleft palate and intra-uterine growth retardation as well as suppression of the neonatal HPA axis. There is evidence of harmful effects in animals.

Use in pregnancy only when there is no safer alternative and when the disease itself carries risks for mother and child.

Usage in nursing mothers: It is not known whether topical administration of corticosteroids could result in sufficient systemic absorption to produce detectable quantities in the breast milk of nursing mothers. Systemically administered corticosteroids are secreted into breast milk in quantities not likely to have a deleterious effect on the infant. Nevertheless, caution should be exercised when topical corticosteroids are administered to nursing mothers.

Side-effects: The following local adverse reactions are reported infrequently with topical corticosteroids but may occur more frequently with the use of occlusive dressings. These reactions are listed in an approximate decreasing order of occurrence: burning, itching, irritation, dryness, folliculitis, hypertrichosis, acneform eruptions, hypopigmentation, perioral dermatitis, allergic contact dermatitis, maceration of the skin, secondary infection, skin atrophy, miliaria, striae and thinning and dilatations of superficial blood vessels producing telangiectasia.

Prolonged use of large doses to extensive areas can result in sufficient systemic absorption to produce generalised manifestations of steroid toxicity and may result in depression of HPA function on discontinuing treatment.

Manifestations of Cushing's syndrome, hyperglycaemia and glycosuria have occurred in some patients.

Manifestations of adrenal suppression in children include linear growth retardation, delayed weight gain, low plasma cortisol levels and absence of response to ACTH stimulation. Intracranial hypertension including bulging fontanelles, headaches and bilateral papilloedema have also been reported in children receiving topical corticosteroids.

Infected skin lesions, viral, bacterial or fungal may be substantially exacerbated by topical steroid therapy. Wound healing is significantly retarded.

Hypersensitivity reactions may occur.

Overdosage: Topically applied corticosteroids can be absorbed in sufficient amounts to produce systemic effects (see 'Warnings and precautions').

Pharmaceutical precautions Ointments: Do not store above 25°C.

Creams: No special pharmaceutical precautions.

See 'Administration' for diluents.

Legal category POM.

Package quantities

Haelan Cream: (0.0125% flurandrenolone) Tubes of 60 g.

Haelan Ointment: (0.0125% flurandrenolone) Tubes of 60 g.

Haelan-X Cream: (0.05% flurandrenolone) Tubes of 15 g.

Haelan-X Ointment: (0.05% flurandrenolone) Tubes of 15 g.

Further information As with all topical steroids, the activity can be enhanced by the use of occlusive dressings. Preparations of Haelan are recommended only as a supplement to, and not as a substitute for, preparations (lotions, wet dressings, etc.) used in the conventional management of skin lesions.

Haelan and Haelan-X preparations do not contain parahydroxybenzoates or lanolin.

Product licence numbers

Haelan Cream	0006/5012
Haelan Ointment	0006/5011
Haelan-X Cream	0006/5020
Haelan-X Ointment	0006/5039

HAELAN-C*

Presentation Collapsible tubes containing 0.0125% flurandrenolone with the addition of 3% Clioquinol BP in cream or ointment base. The cream is white in colour and the ointment is translucent.

Uses *Adults and children:* Topical steroid with antibacterial added, for use in exudative and secondarily infected eczema and dermatitis, including atopic eczema, primary irritant dermatitis, allergic and seborrheic dermatitis, infected insect bite reactions and genital or perianal intertrigo.

If there is little evidence of improvement after about seven days' use, cultural isolation of the offending organism(s) should be followed by appropriate local or systemic antibiotic therapy.

Dosage and administration For topical administration.

Cream: For moist weeping lesions, the cream should be applied gently to the affected area two or three times daily.

Ointment: For dry, scaly lesions, the ointment should be applied as a thin film to the affected area two or three times daily.

The elderly: As the skin is likely to be thin, apply sparingly to avoid development of atrophy.

Dilution is not recommended, but if considered necessary Aqueous Cream BP may be used for the creams and White Soft Paraffin BP for the ointments.

Contra-indications, warnings, etc

Contra-indications: Tuberculosis of the skin. Facial rosacea. Acne vulgaris. Perioral dermatitis. Perianal and genital pruritus. Dermatoses in infancy including eczema, dermatitic napkin eruption, bacterial (impetigo), viral (herpes simplex) and fungal (candida or dermatophyte) infections.

Hypersensitivity to iodine. Primary skin infections (impetigo, furunculosis, pyoderma, cutaneous candidiasis). Secondary infection due to yeasts.

Warnings and precautions: Preparations of Haelan-C are not intended for ophthalmic use.

Local and systemic toxicity is common especially following long-term continuous use, continued use on large areas of damaged skin, flexures and with polythene occlusion.

Systemic absorption of topical corticosteroids has produced reversible hypothalamic-pituitary-adrenal (HPA) axis suppression (see 'Side-effects'). Therefore, patients receiving a large dose of a potent topical steroid applied to a large surface area or under an occlusive dressing should be evaluated periodically for evidence of HPA axis suppression by using urinary-free cortisol and ACTH stimulation tests. If HPA axis suppression is noted, an attempt should be made to withdraw the drug, to reduce the frequency of application or to substitute a less potent steroid. Recovery of HPA axis function is generally prompt and complete on discontinuation of the drug. Infrequently signs and symptoms of steroid withdrawal may occur, so that supplemental systemic corticosteroids are required.

Long-term continuous therapy should be avoided in all patients irrespective of age.

Application under occlusion should be restricted to dermatoses in very limited areas.

If used on the face, courses should be limited to five days and occlusion should not be used.

Haelan-C may cause staining of the hair, clothing and many fabrics.

Usage in children: If used in childhood, courses should be limited to five days and occlusion should not be used.

Children may absorb proportionally larger amounts of topical corticosteroids and thus may be more susceptible to systemic toxicity. Children may also demonstrate greater susceptibility to topical corticosteroid induced HPA axis suppression and Cushing's syndrome than do mature patients because of a larger skin surface to body weight ratio. Administration of topical corticosteroids to children should be limited to the least amount compatible with an effective therapeutic regimen. Chronic corticosteroid therapy may interfere with the growth and development of children.

Usage in pregnancy: There is inadequate evidence of safety in human pregnancy. There may be a very small risk of cleft palate and intra-uterine growth retardation as well as suppression of the neonatal HPA axis. There is evidence of harmful effects in animals.

Use in pregnancy only when there is no safer alternative and when the disease itself carries risks for mother and child.

Usage in nursing mothers: It is not known whether topical administration of corticosteroids could result in sufficient systemic absorption to produce detectable quantities in the breast milk of nursing mothers. Systemically administered corticosteroids are secreted into breast milk in quantities not likely to have a deleterious effect on the infant. Nevertheless, caution should be exercised when topical corticosteroids are administered to nursing mothers.

Side-effects: The following local adverse reactions are reported infrequently with topical corticosteroids but may occur more frequently with the use of occlusive dressings. These reactions are listed in an approximate decreasing order of occurrence: burning, itching, irritation, dryness, folliculitis, hypertrichosis, acneform eruptions, hypopigmentation, perioral dermatitis, allergic contact dermatitis, maceration of the skin, secondary infections, skin atrophy, miliaria, striae and thinning and dilatations of superficial blood vessels producing telangiectasia.

Prolonged use of large doses to extensive areas can result in sufficient systemic absorption to produce generalised manifestations of steroid toxicity and may result in depression of HPA function on discontinuing treatment.

Manifestations of Cushing's syndrome, hyperglycaemia and glycosuria have occurred in some patients.

Manifestations of adrenal suppression in children include linear growth retardation, delayed weight gain, low plasma cortisol levels and absence of response to ACTH stimulation. Intracranial hypertension including bulging fontanelles, headaches and bilateral papilloedema have also been reported in children receiving topical corticosteroids.

Infected skin lesions, viral, bacterial or fungal may be substantially exacerbated by topical steroid therapy. Wound healing is significantly retarded.

Hypersensitivity reactions may occur.

Overdosage: Topically applied corticosteroids can be absorbed in sufficient amounts to produce systemic effects (see 'Warnings and precautions').

Pharmaceutical precautions Ointments: Do not store above 25°C.

Creams: No special pharmaceutical precautions.

See 'Administration' for diluents.

Legal category POM.

Package quantities

Haelan-C Cream: (0.0125% flurandrenolone with 3% Clioquinol BP) Tubes of 30 g.

Haelan-C Ointment: (0.0125% flurandrenolone with 3% Clioquinol BP) Tubes of 30 g.

Further information When secondary bacterial and fungal infection of the skin is present or suspected in an otherwise steroid responsive skin condition, Haelan-C should be used and treatment resumed with Haelan after the infection has been controlled. Such patients must be under constant medical observation.

Product licence numbers

Haelan-C Cream 0006/5018

Haelan-C Ointment 0006/5021

HAELAN* Tape

Presentation A translucent, polythene adhesive film impregnated with 4 micrograms flurandrenolone per square centimetre and protected by a removable paper liner.

Uses Occlusive topical steroid. Adjunctive therapy for chronic, localised, recalcitrant dermatoses that may respond to topical corticosteroids, and particularly dry, scaling lesions.

Dosage and administration For application to the skin, which should be clean, dry and shorn of hair. In most instances the tape need only remain in place for 12 out of 24 hours.

Cosmetics may be applied over the tape.

Application: The tape is cut so as to cover the lesion and a quarter inch margin of normal skin. Corners should be rounded off. After removing the lining paper, the tape is applied to the centre of the lesion with gentle pressure and worked to the edges, avoiding excessive tension of the skin. If longer strips of tape are to be applied, the lining paper should be removed progressively.

If irritation or infection develops, remove tape and consult a physician.

Contra-indications, warnings, etc

Contra-indications: Chicken pox. Vaccinia. Tuberculosis of the skin. Hypersensitivity to any of the components. Facial rosacea. Acne vulgaris. Perioral dermatitis. Perianal and genital pruritus. Dermatoses in infancy including eczema, dermatitic napkin eruption, bacterial (impetigo), viral (herpes simplex) and fungal (candida or dermatophyte) infections.

Warnings and precautions: Not advocated for acute and weeping dermatoses.

Local and systemic toxicity of medium and high potency topical corticosteroids is common, especially following long-term continuous use, continued use on large areas of damaged skin, flexures and with polythene occlusion.

Systemic absorption of topical corticosteroids has produced reversible hypothalamic-pituitary-adrenal (HPA) axis suppression (see 'Side-effects'). Therefore, patients receiving a large dose of a potent topical steroid applied to a large surface area or under an occlusive dressing should be evaluated periodically for evidence of HPA axis suppression by using urinary-free cortisol and ACTH stimulation tests. If HPA axis suppression is noted, an attempt should be made to withdraw the drug, to reduce the frequency of application or to substitute a less potent steroid. Recovery of HPA axis function is generally prompt and complete on discontinuation of the drug. Infrequently, signs and symptoms of steroid withdrawal may occur, so that supplemental systemic corticosteroids are required.

Long-term continuous therapy should be avoided in all patients irrespective of age.

Application under occlusion should be restricted to dermatoses in very limited areas.

If used on the face, courses should be limited to five days and occlusion should not be used.

In the presence of skin infections, the use of an appropriate antifungal or antibacterial agent should be instituted. If a favourable response does not occur promptly, flurandrenolone should be discontinued until the infection has been adequately controlled.

Usage in children: If used in childhood, courses should be limited to five days and occlusion should not be used.

Children may absorb proportionally larger amounts of topical corticosteroids and thus may be more susceptible to systemic toxicity. Children may also demonstrate greater susceptibility to topical corticosteroid induced HPA axis suppression and Cushing's syndrome than do mature patients because of a larger skin surface to body weight ratio. Administration of topical corticosteroids to children should be limited to the least amount compatible with an effective therapeutic regimen. Chronic corticosteroid therapy may interfere with the growth and development of children.

Usage in pregnancy: There is inadequate evidence of safety in human pregnancy. There may be a very small risk of cleft palate and intra-uterine growth retardation as well as suppression of the neonatal HPA axis. There is evidence of harmful effects in animals.

Use in pregnancy only when there is no safer alternative and when the disease itself carries risks for mother and child.

Usage in nursing mothers: It is not known whether topical administration of corticosteroids could result in sufficient systemic absorption to produce detectable quantities in the breast milk of nursing mothers. Systemically administered corticosteroids are secreted into breast milk in quantities not likely to have a deleterious effect on the infant. Nevertheless, caution should be exercised when topical corticosteroids are administered to nursing mothers.

Side-effects: The following local adverse reactions are reported infrequently with topical corticosteroids but may occur more frequently with the use of occlusive dressings. These reactions are listed in an approximate decreasing order of occurrence: burning, itching, irritation, dryness, folliculitis, hypertrichosis, acneform eruptions, hypopigmentation, perioral dermatitis, allergic contact dermatitis, maceration of the skin, secondary infection, skin atrophy, miliaria, striae and thinning and dilatations of superficial blood vessels producing telangiectasia.

Prolonged use of large doses to extensive areas can result in sufficient systemic absorption to produce generalised manifestations of steroid toxicity and may result in depression of HPA function on discontinuing treatment.

Manifestations of Cushing's syndrome, hyperglycaemia and glycosuria have occurred in some patients.

Manifestations of adrenal suppression in children include linear growth retardation, delayed weight gain, low plasma cortisol levels and absence of response to ACTH stimulation. Intracranial hypertension including bulging fontanelles, headaches and bilateral papilloedema have also been reported in children receiving topical corticosteroids.

Infected skin lesions, viral, bacterial or fungal, may be substantially exacerbated by topical steroid therapy. Wound healing is significantly retarded.

Hypersensitivity reactions may occur.

Overdosage: Topically applied corticosteroids can be absorbed in sufficient amounts to produce systemic effects (see 'Warnings and precautions').

Pharmaceutical precautions Store in a dry place, below 25°C.

Legal category POM.

Package quantities
Single rolls of tape, 7.5 cm wide, 50 cm long.
Single rolls of tape, 7.5 cm wide, 200 cm long.

Further information Nil.

Product licence number 0006/5158.

ILOSONE*

Presentation Capsules each containing the equivalent of 250 mg erythromycin base as Erythromycin Estolate BP. The capsules are ivory/red, marked 'DISTA' and are 2.1 cm long.

Tablets each containing the equivalent of 500 mg erythromycin base as Erythromycin Estolate BP. The tablets are pink, para-capsule shaped, 1.9 cm long and coded DISTA DI.

Ready-mixed suspension, each 5 ml containing the equivalent of 125 mg erythromycin base as Erythromycin Estolate BP. The suspension is orange coloured.

Ready-mixed suspension forte, each 5 ml containing the equivalent of 250 mg erythromycin base as Erythromycin Estolate BP. The suspension is orange coloured.

Uses Antibiotic. Erythromycin is indicated in the treatment of the following infections when due to susceptible organisms:

Upper and lower respiratory tract infections
Otitis media
Skin and soft-tissue infections, including erythrasma and acne
Dental infections
Genito-urinary infections, including gonorrhoea, syphilis and chlamydial infections
Intestinal amoebiasis (extra-enteric amoebiasis requires treatment with other agents)

Erythromycin is also indicated for the following:

Endocarditis: Continuous or short-term prophylaxis against bacterial endocarditis, especially prior to dental or other operative procedures, in patients with a history of rheumatic fever or congenital heart disease and who are hypersensitive to penicillin. Erythromycin is not suitable for prophylaxis prior to genito-urinary or gastro-intestinal tract surgery.

Diphtheria: As an adjunct to antitoxin, to prevent establishment of carriers, and to eradicate the organism in carriers.

Whooping cough: When given early after exposure, erythromycin may reduce the risk of development of classical symptoms.

Legionnaires' disease: Limited clinical experience would suggest that erythromycin may be effective in treating Legionnaires' disease.

Erythromycin is active against the following organisms *in-vitro*: *Streptococcus pyogenes*; *Str. pneumoniae*; Alpha-haemolytic streptococci (viridans group); *Staphylococcus aureus*; *Haemophilus influenzae*; *Mycoplasma pneumoniae*; Corynebacterium spp.; *Listeria monocytogenes*; *Bordetella pertussis*; *Legionella pneumophila*; Campylobacter spp.; *Neisseria gonorrhoeae*; *Treponema pallidum*; *Chlamydia trachomatis*; anaerobic bacteria including *Bacteroides* spp., *Clostridium* spp. and *Propionibacterium acnes*; *Entamoeba histolytica*.

Dosage and administration For oral administration.

Adults: The usual dose is 250 mg every six hours. This may be increased up to 4 g per day according to the severity of the infection. Dosage should be limited to a maximum of 1.5 g daily in patients with severe renal impairment.

The elderly: As for adults.

Children: Age, weight, and severity of the infection are important factors in determining the correct dosage. The usual range is 20–50 mg/kg/day in divided doses.

For mild to moderate infections:

Body weight	*Total daily dose*
10 kg or less	250 mg
10–18 kg	375 mg
18–25 kg	500 mg
25–36 kg	750 mg
More than 36 kg	1000 mg (adult dose)

For more severe infections these dosages may be doubled.

If administration on a twice daily schedule is desirable, one-half of the total daily dose may be given every 12 hours. Twice daily dosing is not recommended when doses larger than 1 g daily are administered.

Streptococcal infections: For streptococcal pharyngitis and tonsillitis, the usual dosage range is 20–50 mg/kg/day in divided doses. In the treatment of group A beta-haemolytic streptococcal infections, a therapeutic dosage of erythromycin should be administered for at least 10 days. In continuous prophylaxis of streptococcal infections in persons with a history of rheumatic heart disease, the dosage is 250 mg twice daily.

When Ilosone is used prior to surgery to prevent endocarditis caused by alpha-haemolytic streptococci (viridans group) a recommended schedule for adults is 1 g pre-operatively (20 mg/kg for children) and 500 mg (10 mg/kg for children) 6 hours later.

Pertussis: Doses of erythromycin estolate utilised in reported clinical studies were 40–50 mg/kg/day, given in divided doses for 5 to 14 days.

Gonorrhoea: For disseminated infection, 500 mg four times daily for 7 days.

Syphilis: A regimen of 20 g of erythromycin estolate in divided doses over a period of 10 days has been shown to be effective.

Amoebic dysentery: Dosage for adults is 250 mg four times daily for 10 to 14 days: for children, 30–50 mg/kg/day in divided doses for 10 to 14 days.

Legionnaires' disease: Although optimum regimens have not been established, 1–4 g daily in divided doses has been utilised in reported clinical studies.

Conjunctivitis of the newborn caused by C. trachomatis: 50 mg/kg/day, in four divided doses, for at least two weeks.

Pneumonia of infancy caused by C. trachomatis: 50 mg/kg/day, in four divided doses, for at least three weeks.

Urogenital infections during pregnancy due to C. trachomatis: 500 mg four times a day for at least seven days. For women who cannot tolerate this regimen, a decreased dose of 250 mg four times a day should be used for at least fourteen days.

For adults with uncomplicated urethral, endocervical, or rectal infections caused by *C. trachomatis* in whom tetracyclines are contra-indicated or not tolerated: 500 mg four times a day for at least seven days.

Contra-indications, warnings, etc

Contra-indications: Hypersensitivity to erythromycin.

Patients who have previously developed jaundice or who have pre-existing liver disease or dysfunction.

Warnings: The administration of erythromycin estolate has been associated with the infrequent occurrence of reversible cholestatic hepatitis. Hepatic dysfunction with or without jaundice has occurred, chiefly in adults. It may be accompanied by malaise, nausea, vomiting, abdominal colic and fever. In some instances severe abdominal pain may simulate the pain of biliary colic, pancreatitis, perforated ulcer, or an acute abdominal surgical problem. In other instances, clinical symptoms and results of liver function tests have resembled findings in extrahepatic obstructive jaundice. Laboratory findings have been characterised by abnormal hepatic function test values, peripheral eosinophilia and leucocytosis. If the above findings occur, discontinue Ilosone promptly.

Initial symptoms have developed in some cases after a few days of treatment, but generally have followed one or two weeks of continuous therapy. Symptoms reappear promptly, usually within 48 hours, after the drug is re-administered to sensitive patients. The syndrome seems to result from a form of sensitisation, occurs chiefly in adults, and has been reversible when medication is discontinued.

The diagnosis of pseudomembranous colitis should be considered should diarrhoea develop. Mild cases usually respond to drug discontinuation alone. Additional measures will be required in more severe cases, which may be life-threatening.

Usage in pregnancy: Reproduction studies in rats, mice and rabbits, with doses several times the usual human dose, have revealed no evidence of impaired fertility or fetal harm related to erythromycin. There are no adequate studies in pregnant women. Because animal reproductive studies are not always predictive of human response, this drug should be used during pregnancy only if clearly needed.

Usage in nursing mothers: Erythromycin is excreted in breast milk. Caution should be exercised when it is administered to a nursing woman.

Precautions: The antibacterial activity of erythromycin is markedly greater in alkaline than in neutral or acid media. Urinary alkalinisation shold be considered when treating urinary infections.

Laboratory tests: Erythromycin interferes with some clinical laboratory tests, for example, high SGOT values may be artifacts and may not necessarily reflect changes in liver function.

Drug interactions: Since probenecid inhibits tubular reabsorption of erythromycin in animals, it prolongs maintenance of plasma levels.

Erythromycin and lincomycin or clindamycin may, under some conditions, be antagonistic. Lincomycin or clindamycin therapy should be avoided in treatment of infections due to erythromycin-resistant organisms.

The use of erythromycin in patients who are receiving concomitant high doses of theophylline may be associated with an increase in serum theophylline levels and potential theophylline toxicity. If symptoms of toxicity or elevated serum theophylline levels develop, the dose of theophylline should be reduced.

Concomitant administration of erythromycin and digoxin has been reported to result in elevated digoxin serum levels.

There have been reports of increased anticoagulant effects when erythromycin and oral anticoagulants were used concomitantly. Increased anticoagulation effects due to this drug interaction may be more pronounced in the elderly.

Concurrent use of erythromycin and ergotamine or dihydroergotamine has been associated in some patients with acute ergot toxicity characterised by severe peripheral vasospasm and dysaesthesia.

Erythromycin has been reported to decrease the clearance of triazolam and thus may increase the pharmacological effect of triazolam.

The use of erythromycin in patients concurrently taking drugs metabolised by the cytochrome P450 system may be associated with elevation in serum levels of these other drugs.

Elevated serum concentrations of the following drugs have been reported when administered concurrently with erythromycin: carbamazepine, cyclosporin, hexobarbitone, phenytoin, alfentanil, disopyramide, lovastatin and bromocriptine. Serum concentrations of such drugs should be monitored closely in patients concurrently receiving erythromycin.

During prolonged or repeated therapy, there is a possibility of overgrowth of non-susceptible bacteria or fungi. If such infections arise, the drug should be discontinued and appropriate therapy instituted.

Side-effects: The most frequent side-effects of erythromycin preparations are gastro-intestinal (e.g. abdominal cramping and discomfort) and are dose-related. Nausea, vomiting and diarrhoea occur infrequently with usual oral doses.

Mild allergic reactions, such as urticaria and other skin rashes, have occurred. Serious allergic reactions, including anaphylaxis, have been reported.

There have been isolated reports of hearing loss and/or tinnitus occurring chiefly in patients with renal or hepatic insufficiency and in patients receiving high doses of erythromycin. Ototoxic effects are usually reversible upon discontinuation, but in rare instances, involving intravenous administration, the ototoxic effect has been irreversible.

Rarely, erythromycin has been associated with ventricular arrhythmias, including ventricular tachycardia and torsade des pointes, in individuals with prolonged QT intervals.

Overdosage:

Symptoms: nausea, vomiting and dose-related epigastric distress and diarrhoea. Reversible mild acute pancreatitis has been reported. Hearing loss, with or without tinnitus and vertigo, may occur (see 'Side-effects').

Treatment: Unless 5 times the normal single dose has been ingested gastro-intestinal decontamination should not be necessary. Consider activated charcoal instead of, or in addition to, gastric emptying.

Forced diuresis, peritoneal dialysis, haemodialysis, or charcoal haemoperfusion have not been established as beneficial.

Pharmaceutical precautions
Capsules and tablets: Keep container tightly closed.
Suspensions: Keep container tightly closed and protect from light. Shake well before use. For dilution, use Syrup BP and when diluted use within 14 days.

Legal category POM.

Package quantities
Capsules 250 mg: Bottles of 100
Tablets 500 mg: Bottles of 12
Ready-mixed Suspension 125 mg/5 ml: Bottles of 100 ml
Ready-mixed Suspension 250 mg/5 ml: Bottles of 100 ml

Strengths expressed are base equivalent as Erythromycin Estolate BP.

Further information Nil.

Product licence numbers

Capsules 250 mg	0006/5022
Tablets 500 mg	0006/5015
Suspension 125 mg/5 ml	0006/5023
Suspension 250 mg/5 ml	0006/5024

KEFADOL*

Presentation 10 ml vials containing cefamandole nafate for injection equivalent to 500 mg or 1 g cefamandole.

100 ml vials containing cefamandole nafate for injection equivalent to 2 g cefamandole.

The vials also contain 63 mg Sodium Carbonate USP per gram of cefamandole. The total sodium content is approximately 77 mg per gram of cefamandole activity.

Uses Cefamandole is indicated in the treatment of infections of the lower respiratory tract, genito-urinary tract, bones and joints, bloodstream (septicaemia), skin and soft tissue, gall bladder and peritoneum, and pelvic inflammatory disease in women, when due to susceptible micro-organisms.

Prophylactic use: Perioperative administration of cefamandole may reduce the incidence of postoperative infections in patients undergoing contaminated or potentially contaminated surgical procedures associated with a high risk of infection, or where the occurrence of a postoperative infection could be especially serious.

Cefamandole is usually active against the following organisms *in vitro* and in clinical infections:

Gram-positive
Staphylococci, including coagulase-positive, coagulase-negative (e.g. *Staphylococcus epidermidis*) and penicillinase-producing strains

Beta-haemolytic and other streptococci (most strains of enterococci, e.g. *Enterococcus faecalis*, are resistant)

Streptococcus pneumoniae

Gram-negative
Escherichia coli
Klebsiella spp.
Enterobacter spp. (initially susceptible organisms occasionally may become resistant during therapy)
Haemophilus influenzae
Proteus mirabilis
Providencia rettgeri
Morganella morganii
Proteus vulgaris (some strains of *P. vulgaris* have been shown by *in vitro* tests to be resistant to cefamandole and certain other cephalosporins)

Anaerobic organisms
Gram-positive and gram-negative cocci (including *Peptococcus* and *Peptostreptococcus* spp.)

Gram-positive bacilli (including *Clostridium* spp.)

Gram-negative bacilli (including *Bacteroides*)
Most strains of *Bacteroides fragilis* are resistant

Pseudomonas, Acinetobacter calcoaceticus and most *Serratia* strains are resistant to cefamandole and certain other cephalosporins. Cefamandole is resistant to degradation by β-lactamases from certain members of the *Enterobacteriaceae*.

Dosage and administration Cefamandole nafate may be given intravenously or by deep intramuscular injection into a large muscle mass to minimise pain.

Adults and the elderly: The dosage range for cefamandole is 500 mg to 2 g every four to eight hours, depending on the severity and site of infection.

Impaired renal function: When renal function is impaired, a reduced dosage must be employed and serum concentrations should be monitored when feasible. After an initial dose of 1 to 2 g (depending on the severity of infection), a maintenance dosage schedule should be followed (see table). Continued dosage should be determined by degree of renal impairment, severity of infection and susceptibility of the causative organism.

Maintenance dosage of cefamandole in patients with impaired renal function

Creatinine clearance ml/min/1.73 m^2	Life-threatening infections	Severe infections	Less severe infections
80–50	2 g q 6 h	1.5 g q 6 h	0.75 g q 6 h
50–25	2 g q 8 h	1.5 g q 8 h	0.75 g q 8 h
25–10	1.25 g q 8 h	1.0 g q 8 h	0.5 g q 8 h
10–2	1 g q 12 h	0.75 g q 12 h	0.5 g q 12 h
<2	0.75 g q 12 h	0.5 g q 12 h	0.25 g q 12 h

Intramuscular administration: Each gram of cefamandole should be reconstituted with 3 ml of Water for Injections PhEur or Sodium Chloride Intravenous Infusion BP. However, the 500 mg vial should be reconstituted in 2 ml of diluent. Shake well until dissolved.

Intravenous administration: Intravenous route may be preferable for bacterial septicaemia, localised parenchymal abscesses, peritonitis, or other severe or life-threatening infections.

1. *For direct intermittent intravenous administration,* each gram of cefamandole should be reconstituted with 10 ml of Water for Injections PhEur, 5% Dextrose Intravenous Infusion BP, or Sodium Chloride Intravenous Infusion BP. Slowly inject directly into the vein over a period of three to five minutes or give through the tubing of an administration set while the patient is also receiving one of the following intravenous fluids:

   Sodium Chloride Intravenous Infusion BP
   5% Dextrose Intravenous Infusion BP
   10% Dextrose Intravenous Infusion BP
   5% Dextrose and 0.9% Sodium Chloride Intravenous Infusion BP
   5% Dextrose and 0.45% Sodium Chloride Intravenous Infusion BP
   Sodium Lactate Intravenous Infusion BP

2. *Intermittent intravenous infusion with a Y-type administration set or volume control set* can also be accomplished while any of the above mentioned intravenous fluids are being infused. However, during infusion of the solution containing cefamandole, it is desirable to discontinue the other solution. When this technique is employed, careful attention should be paid to the volume of the solution containing cefamandole so that the calculated dose will be infused. When a Y-tube connection is used, 100 ml of an appropriate diluent should be added to the 2 g (100 ml) vial. If Water for Injections PhEur is used as the diluent, reconstitute with approximately 20 ml per g to avoid a hypotonic solution.

3. *For continuous intravenous infusion,* each gram of cefamandole should be diluted with 10 ml of Water for Injections PhEur. An appropriate quantity of the resulting solution may be added to an i.v. bottle containing one of the previously mentioned intravenous fluids.

If combination therapy with cefamandole and an aminoglycoside is indicated, each of these should be administered at separate sites.

Infants and children: Administration of 50 to 100 mg/kg/day in equally divided doses every four to eight hours has been effective for most infections susceptible to cefamandole. This may be increased to a total daily dose of 150 mg/kg (not to exceed the maximum adult dose) for serious infections.

Infants: Cefamandole has been effectively used in this age group, but all laboratory parameters have not been extensively studied in infants between 1 and 6 months of age. Safety of this product has not been established in prematures and infants under 1 month of age; therefore, if cefamandole is to be administered to infants, the physician should determine whether the potential benefits outweigh the possible risks involved. Accumulation of cephalosporins (with resulting prolongation of drug half-life) has been reported in neonates.

Prophylactic use:
The following schedules are recommended for peri-operative use:

Adults and the elderly: 1 or 2 g intravenously or intramuscularly one-half to one hour prior to surgical incision, followed by 1 or 2 g every six hours for 24 to 48 hours.

For patients undergoing procedures involving implantation of prosthetic devices, administration for up to 72 hours is recommended.

Children (more than three months of age): 50–100 mg/kg/day in equally divided doses by the same routes and schedule designated for adults.

If signs of infection occur, cultures should be obtained and appropriate therapy instituted.

Kefadol should be continued for a minimum of 48 to 72 hours after the patient becomes asymptomatic or bacterial eradication has occurred. A minimum of 10 days treatment is recommended in infections caused by group A beta-haemolytic streptococci. In chronic urinary tract infection, frequent bacteriological and clinical appraisal is necessary during therapy and possibly for several months after completion. Persistent infections may require treatment for several weeks.

Contra-indications, warnings, etc

Contra-indication: Cefamandole is contra-indicated in patients with known allergy to the cephalosporin group of antibiotics.

Warnings: Before cefamandole therapy is instituted, careful enquiry should be made concerning previous hypersensitivity reactions to cephalosporins, penicillins or other drugs. Kefadol should be given cautiously to penicillin-sensitive patients.

There is some clinical and laboratory evidence of partial cross-allergenicity of the penicillins and the cephalosporins. Patients have been reported to have had severe reactions (including anaphylaxis) to both drugs.

Antibiotics should be administered with caution to any patient who has demonstrated some form of allergy, particularly to drugs.

Pseudomembranous colitis has been reported with most broad-spectrum antibiotics. Its diagnosis should be considered in patients who develop diarrhoea with antibiotics. Such colitis may range from mild to life-threatening.

Usage in pregnancy: Reproduction studies in rats given doses of 500 or 1000 mg/kg/day (approximately 5 times the maximum clinical dose) revealed no evidence of impaired fertility or harm to the fetus due to cefamandole nafate. There are, however, no adequate and well-controlled studies in pregnant women. Because animal studies are not always predictive of human response, this drug should be used during pregnancy only if clearly needed.

Nursing mothers: Caution should be exercised.

Precautions: Although cefamandole rarely produces alteration in kidney function, evaluation of renal status is recommended, especially in seriously ill patients receiving maximum doses. Patients with impaired renal function should be placed on the dosage schedule recommended under 'Dosage and administration'. Usual doses in such individuals may result in excessive serum concentrations.

Nephrotoxicity has been reported following concomitant administration of aminoglycoside antibiotics and cephalosporins.

The results of experimental studies in animals suggest that the concurrent use of potent diuretics such as frusemide or ethacrynic acid may also increase the risk of renal toxicity with cephalosporin antibiotics.

As with other broad-spectrum antibiotics, hypoprothrombinaemia with or without bleeding has been reported rarely, but it has been promptly reversed by administration of vitamin K. Such episodes have usually occurred in elderly, debilitated or otherwise compromised patients with deficient stores of vitamin K. Prophylactic administration of vitamin K may be indicated in such patients, especially when intestinal sterilisation and surgical procedures are performed.

In a few patients receiving cefamandole, nausea, vomiting and vasomotor instability with hypotension and peripheral vasodilatation, has occurred following the ingestion of alcohol. Cefamandole inhibits the enzyme acetaldehyde dehydrogenase in laboratory animals. This causes accumulation of acetaldehyde when ethanol is administered concurrently.

Broad-spectrum antibiotics should be prescribed with caution in individuals with a history of gastro-intestinal disease, particularly colitis.

Prolonged use of cefamandole may result in the overgrowth of non-susceptible organisms. Careful observation of the patient is essential. If superinfection occurs during therapy, appropriate measures should be taken.

A false positive reaction for glucose in the urine may occur with Benedict's or Fehling's solutions or with Clinitest tablets. A false positive test for proteinuria may occur with acid and denaturisation precipitation tests.

Impairment of fertility: Very high doses of cefamandole (equivalent to approximately 5 times the maximum clinical dose) have been found to delay maturation of the testicular germinal epithelium in rats. This effect was seen only when cefamandole was given to neonatal rats during initial spermatogenic development. The clinical significance of this finding is unknown due to differences in the time of initiation of spermatogenesis, rate of spermatogenic development and duration of puberty.

Side-effects: Hypersensitivity: Anaphylaxis, maculopapular rash, urticaria, eosinophilia and drug fever have been reported. These reactions are more likely to occur in patients with a history of allergy, particularly to penicillin.

Haematological: Thrombocytopenia has been reported rarely. Neutropenia has been reported, especially in long courses of treatment. Some individuals have developed positive direct Coombs' tests during treatment with the cephalosporin antibiotics.

Gastro-intestinal: Nausea and vomiting occur rarely. Colitis, including rare instances of pseudomembranous colitis, has been reported.

Liver: Transient rise in AST, ALT and ALP levels have been noted. Transient hepatitis and cholestatic jaundice have been reported rarely.

Kidney: Decreased creatinine clearance has been reported in patients with prior renal impairment. As with some other cephalosporins, transitory elevations of blood urea have occasionally been observed; their frequency increases in patients over 50 years of age. In some of these cases, there was also a mild increase in serum creatinine.

Local reactions: Pain on intramuscular injection is infrequent. Thrombophlebitis occurs rarely.

Overdosage: The administration of inappropriately large doses of parenteral cephalosporins may cause seizures, particularly in patients with renal impairment. Dosage reduction is necessary when renal function is impaired (see 'Dosage and Administration'). If seizures occur, the drug should be promptly discontinued; anticonvulsant therapy may be administered if clinically indicated.

In the event of serious overdosage, general supportive care is recommended, with monitoring of haematological, renal and hepatic functions, and coagulation status, until the patient is stable. Haemodialysis may be considered in cases of overwhelming overdosage.

Pharmaceutical precautions *Unreconstituted vials:* Store below 25°C. Protect from light.

It is good practice to reconstitute immediately before use. If this is not feasible, reconstituted solutions may be stored in a refrigerator (2°–8°C) and used within 96 hours. If kept below 25°C, use within 24 hours. During storage at room temperature, carbon dioxide develops inside the vial after reconstitution. This pressure may be dissipated prior to withdrawal of the vial contents, or it may be used to aid withdrawal if the vial is inverted over the syringe needle and the contents are allowed to flow into the syringe.

The pH of freshly reconstituted solutions usually ranges from 6.0 to 8.5.

Do not mix an aminoglycoside with cefamandole in the same intravenous fluid container.

Legal category POM.

Package quantities

Vials 500 mg:	Individual vials in packs of 10.
Vials 1 g:	Individual vials in packs of 10.
Vials 2 g:	Individual vials.

Further information Solutions of cefamandole range from light yellow to amber, depending upon a variety of factors, including concentration and the diluent used.

Product licence number 0006/0111.

PROZAC* ▼

Presentation Capsules (green and off-white, coded 3105) each containing 20 mg fluoxetine hydrochloride.

Uses
Depression: Prozac is indicated for the treatment of the symptoms of depressive illness, especially where sedation is not required.

Bulimia nervosa: Prozac is indicated for the reduction of binge-eating and purging activity.

Dosage and administration For oral administration to adults only.

Depression—adults and the elderly: A dose of 20 mg/day is recommended.

Bulimia nervosa—adults and the elderly: A dose of 60 mg/day is recommended.

Fluoxetine has a half-life of 2 to 3 days, and its major active metabolite has a half life of 7 to 9 days. Steady state plasma concentrations are only achieved after continuous dosing for weeks. When dosing is stopped, active drug substance will persist in the body for weeks. This should be borne in mind when starting or stopping treatment.

Children: The use of Prozac in children is not recommended, as safety and efficacy have not been established.

Patients with renal and/or hepatic dysfunction: See 'Contra-indications' and 'Precautions' sections.

Contra-indications, warnings, etc
Contra-indications: Hypersensitivity to fluoxetine.

Fluoxetine should not be administered to patients with severe renal failure (GFR <10 ml/min) because accumulation may occur in these patients during chronic treatment.

Usage in nursing mothers: Prozac should not be prescribed to nursing mothers. In one breast milk sample the concentration of fluoxetine, plus norfluoxetine, was 70.4 ng/ml, compared to 295.0 ng/ml in the mother's plasma. No adverse effects on the infant were noted.

Monoamine oxidase inhibitors: At least 14 days should elapse between discontinuation of an MAOI and initiation of treatment with Prozac. At least five weeks should elapse between discontinuation of Prozac and initiation of therapy with an MAOI.

Serious, sometimes fatal, reactions (including hyperthermia, rigidity, myoclonus, autonomic instability with possible rapid fluctuations of vital signs, and mental status changes that include extreme agitation progressing to delirium and coma) have been reported with concomitant use or when fluoxetine had been recently discontinued and an MAOI started. Cyproheptadine or dantrolene may benefit patients experiencing such reactions.

Warnings
Rash and allergic reactions: Upon the appearance of rash or of other allergic phenomena for which an alternative aetiology cannot be identified, Prozac should be discontinued.

Pregnancy: The safety of fluoxetine in human pregnancy has not been established; accordingly, the drug should be avoided in pregnancy unless there is no safer alternative. There was no evidence of teratogenicity from animal studies but full testing was limited by maternal toxicity.

Lactation: See 'Contra-indications'.

Precautions: Prozac should be discontinued in any patient who develops seizures. Prozac should be avoided in patients with unstable epilepsy; patients with controlled epilepsy should be carefully monitored. There have been rare reports of prolonged seizures in patients on fluoxetine receiving ECT treatment.

Fluoxetine is extensively metabolised by the liver and excreted by the kidneys. A lower dose, e.g. alternate day dosing, is recommended in patients with significant hepatic dysfunction or mild to moderate renal failure (GFR 10–50 ml/min).

Clinical experience in acute cardiac disease is limited, therefore caution is advisable. However, the ECG of 312 patients who received fluoxetine in double-blind trials were retrospectively evaluated; no conduction abnormalities that resulted in heart block were observed.

Prozac may cause weight loss which may be undesirable in underweight depressed patients. Only rarely have depressed or bulimic patients been discontinued for weight loss when treated with fluoxetine.

In patients with diabetes, fluoxetine may alter glycaemic control. Hypoglycaemia has occurred during therapy with fluoxetine and hyperglycaemia has developed following discontinuation. Insulin and/or oral hypoglycaemic dosage may need to be adjusted.

There have been reports of abnormal bleeding in several patients, but causal relationship to fluoxetine and clinical importance are unclear.

Although fluoxetine has been shown not to affect psychomotor performance in healthy volunteers, any psychoactive drug may impair judgement or skills. Therefore patients should be cautioned that their ability to perform potentially hazardous tasks (e.g. driving, operating machinery) may be impaired.

As improvement may not occur during the first two or more weeks of treatment, patients should be closely monitored during this period. The possibility of a suicide attempt is inherent in depression and may persist until significant remission occurs.

Drug interactions: Monoamine oxidase inhibitors (see 'Contra-indications').

Caution is advised if the concomitant administration of Prozac and CNS active drugs, including lithium, is required.

There have been reports of both increased and decreased lithium levels when used concomitantly with fluoxetine. Cases of lithium toxicity have been reported. Lithium levels should be monitored.

Greater than two-fold increases of previously stable plasma levels of cyclic antidepressants have been observed when Prozac has been administered in combination.

Agitation, restlessness and gastro-intestinal symptoms have been reported in a small number of patients receiving fluoxetine in combination with tryptophan.

The long elimination half-lives should be borne in mind (see 'Dosage and Administration') when considering pharmacodynamic or pharmacokinetic drug interactions.

In formal testing, no drug interaction of clinical significance has been observed between fluoxetine and chlorothiazide, ethanol, secobarbital, tolbutamide and warfarin.

Fluoxetine is bound to plasma protein and concurrent administration may alter plasma concentrations of other plasma protein bound drugs, or conversely fluoxetine.

Fluoxetine does not appear to potentiate the effects of alcohol.

Adverse effects:

Body as a whole: asthenia, fever

Digestive system: nausea, diarrhoea, dry mouth, appetite loss, dyspepsia, vomiting.

Nervous system: headache, nervousness, insomnia, drowsiness, anxiety, tremor, dizziness, fatigue, decreased libido, seizures (see 'Precautions'). Hypomania or mania occurred in approximately one per cent of fluoxetine treated trial patients.

Respiratory system: pharyngitis, dyspnoea. Pulmonary events (including inflammatory processes of varying histopathology and/or fibrosis) have been reported rarely. Dyspnoea may be the only preceding symptom.

Skin and appendages: a small percentage of patients developed rash and/or urticaria (see 'Warnings'). Serious systemic reactions, possibly related to vasculitis, have developed in patients with rash, and rarely death has been reported. Excessive sweating, serum sickness and anaphylactoid reactions have also been reported.

Urinogenital system: sexual dysfunction (delayed or inhibited orgasm).

Hyponatraemia (including serum sodium below 110 mmol/l) has been rarely reported and appeared to be reversible when Prozac was discontinued. Some cases were possibly due to the syndrome of inappropriate antidiuretic hormone secretion. The majority of reports were associated with older patients, and patients taking diuretics or otherwise volume depleted.

The following have been reported in association with fluoxetine but no causal relationship has been established: cerebral vascular accident, confusion, dyskinesia, ecchymoses, gastro-intestinal haemorrhage, hyperprolactinaemia, pancreatitis, suicidal ideation, thrombocytopenia, thrombocytopenic purpura, vaginal bleeding after drug withdrawal and violent behaviour.

Overdose: On the evidence available, fluoxetine has a wide margin of safety in overdose. Since introduction, a single death, attributed to a large overdose of fluoxetine alone, has been reported.

One patient who reportedly took 3000 mg of fluoxetine experienced 2 grand mal seizures that remitted spontaneously. Nausea and vomiting were prominent in overdoses involving higher fluoxetine doses. Agitation, restlessness, hypomania and other signs of CNS excitation were also observed.

Management: No specific antidote is known.

An airway should be established. Cardiac and vital signs monitoring is recommended, along with general symptomatic and supportive measures.

Based on experience with animals, fluoxetine-induced seizures which fail to remit spontaneously may respond to diazepam. Due to the large volume of distribution of fluoxetine, forced diuresis, dialysis, haemoperfusion and exchange transfusion are unlikely to be of benefit. Activated charcoal, which may be used with sorbitol, may be as or more effective than emesis or lavage.

Pharmaceutical precautions Store at room temperature (15°–25°C).

Legal category POM.

Package quantities Calendar packs of 28 capsules: 2 strips of 14 capsules.

Further information Fluoxetine is chemically unrelated to tricyclic and tetracyclic antidepressant agents. It is a specific serotonin (5-hydroxytryptamine, 5-HT) reuptake inhibitor, whose specificity is unaltered by its major metabolite.

Product licence number 0006/0195.

**Trade Mark*

Dumex Limited
Longwick Road
Princes Risborough
Aylesbury
Bucks HP17 9UZ

DUMEX

DIAZEMULS*

Presentation Ampoules of a white, opaque emulsion containing Diazepam BP 10 mg in 2 ml.

Uses *Action:* Diazepam is a potent anxiolytic, anticonvulsant and central muscle relaxant mediating its effects mainly via the limbic system as well as the polysynaptic spinal reflexes. The formulation of diazepam in an oil-in-water emulsion similar to Intralipid reduces the incidence of local pain and thrombophlebitis after injection.

Indications:

1. Sedation prior to procedures such as endoscopy, dentistry, cardiac catheterisation and cardioversion.
2. Premedication prior to anaesthesia.
3. Control of acute muscle spasm due to tetanus or poisoning.
4. Control of convulsions; status epilepticus.
5. Management of severe acute anxiety or agitation including delirium tremens.

Dosage and administration Diazemuls may be administered by slow intravenous injection (1 ml per min), or by continuous infusion. Diazemuls should be drawn up into the syringe immediately prior to administration.

1. *Sedation:* 0.1–0.2 mg diazepam/kg body weight by iv injection. The normal adult dose is 10–20 mg, but dosage should be titrated to the patient's response.
2. *Premedication:* 0.1–0.2 mg diazepam/kg body weight by iv injection. Dosage should be titrated to the patient's response. In this indication, prior treatment with diazepam leads to a reduction in fasciculations and postoperative myalgia associated with the use of suxamethonium.
3. *Tetanus:* 0.1–0.3 mg diazepam/kg body weight by iv injection repeated every 1–4 hours as required. Alternatively, a continuous infusion (see below) of 3–10 mg/kg body weight every 24 hours may be used.
4. *Status epilepticus:* An initial dose of 0.15–0.25 mg/kg body weight by iv injection repeated in 30 to 60 minutes if required, and followed if necessary by infusion (see below) of up to 3 mg/kg body weight over 24 hr.
5. *Anxiety and tension, acute muscle spasm, acute states of excitation, delirium tremens:* The usual dose is 10 mg repeated at intervals of 4 hours, or as required.

Elderly or debilitated patients: Elderly or debilitated patients are particularly sensitive to benzodiazepines. Dosage should initially be reduced to one half of the normal recommendations.

If a continuous infusion is required Diazemuls may be added to dextrose solution 5% or 10% to achieve a final diazepam concentration within the range 0.1–0.4 mg/ml (i.e. 2–8 ml Diazemuls per 100 ml dextrose solution). A dextrose solution containing added Diazemuls should be used within 6 hours of the admixture. Diazemuls can be mixed in all proportions with Intralipid 10% or 20% but not with saline solutions. It can be injected into the infusion tube during an ongoing infusion of isotonic saline or dextrose solution 5% or 10%. As with other diazepam injections, adsorption may occur to plastic infusion equipment. This adsorption occurs to a lesser degree with Diazemuls than with aqueous diazepam injection preparations when mixed with dextrose solutions.

Contra-indications, warnings, etc As with other benzodiazepine preparations:

1. Should not be used in phobic or obsessional states since there is inadequate evidence of efficacy and safety.
2. Should not be used in the treatment of chronic psychosis.

Warnings and precautions:

1. Treatment with diazepam may cause drowsiness and increase the patient's reaction time. This should be considered in situations where alertness is required, e.g. driving a car.
2. Use with caution in patients with impairment of renal or hepatic function and in patients with pulmonary insufficiency or myasthenia gravis.
3. Should not be used alone to treat depression or anxiety associated with depression.
4. Amnesia may occur. In cases of loss or bereavement psychological adjustment may be inhibited by benzodiazepines.
5. Disinhibiting effects may be manifested in various ways. Suicide may be precipitated in patients who are depressed and aggressive behaviour toward self and others may be precipitated. Extreme caution should therefore be used in prescribing benzodiazepines in patients with personality disorders.
6. Physiological and psychological symptoms of withdrawal including depression may be associated with discontinuation of benzodiazepines even after normal therapeutic doses for short periods of time.

Interactions with other medicaments: Concomitant use of central nervous system depressants, e.g. alcohol, general anaesthetics, narcotic analgesics, or antidepressants, including MAOI's will result in accentuation of their sedative effects. When Diazemuls is combined with centrally depressant drugs administered parenterally, severe respiratory and cardiovascular depression may occur. It is recommended that Diazemuls is administered following the analgesic, and that the dose should be carefully titrated to the patient's response. Diazepam clearance is increased by concomitant administration of phenobarbitone, and is decreased by administration of cimetidine.

Pregnancy: Diazepam crosses the placenta and should not be used during pregnancy. Maternal doses administered during delivery may produce clinical effects in the newborn, for example hypotonia and hypothermia.

Lactation: Diazepam can be transmitted in breast milk and clinical effects may occur in the breast-fed infant. Diazemuls should be administered during lactation only if considered essential.

Side-effects: This formulation may rarely cause local pain or thrombophlebitis in the vein used for administration.

Rare instances have been reported of a local painless erythematous rash around the site of injection, which has resolved in 1–2 days. Urticaria and, rarely, anaphylaxis have been reported following the injection of Diazemuls.

Overdosage: CNS depression and coma. Treatment symptomatic.

Pharmaceutical precautions For full information on admixture see dosage and administration. Diazemuls should only be mixed in the same container or syringe with dextrose solution 5% or 10% or Intralipid 10% or 20%. The contents of the ampoule should not be mixed with any drugs other than the infusion solutions mentioned above. Store at room temperature. Do not freeze.

Legal category CD (Sch 4), POM.

Package quantities Boxes of 10 × 2 ml ampoules.

Further information During prolonged administration, for example in the treatment of tetanus, the plasma concentration of desmethyldiazepam, the main (and similarly potent) active metabolite of diazepam, may exceed that of the parent compound. Accordingly, there is a risk of accumulation and prolonged CNS depression if the dosage is not reduced following continuous administration for 5–7 days.

The clinician should be aware that intravenous sedation is associated with a significant incidence of anterograde and retrograde amnesia.

Product licence number 10183/0001.

**Trade Mark*

Duncan, Flockhart Division
A Division of Glaxo Laboratories Limited
Stockley Park West
Uxbridge, Middlesex UB11 1BT

BETA-CARDONE*

Presentation *Beta-Cardone Tablets 200 mg:* White, circular, scored tablets engraved DF/BC20, each containing sotalol hydrochloride 200 mg.

Beta-Cardone Tablets 80 mg: Pink, circular, scored tablets engraved DF/BC8, each containing sotalol hydrochloride 80 mg.

Beta-Cardone Tablets 40 mg: Green, circular, scored tablets engraved DF/BC4, each containing sotalol hydrochloride 40 mg.

Uses Beta-Cardone is a β-adrenoceptor blocking agent which is devoid of intrinsic sympathomimetic and local anaesthetic activity. Its major therapeutic effect is to protect the heart from undesirable sympathetic activity. Beta-Cardone reduces the rate and force of contraction of the heart; cardiac work and oxygen consumption are diminished.

In angina pectoris: Beta-Cardone reduces the frequency and severity of anginal attacks and increases exercise tolerance.

In hypertension: Beta-Cardone reduces blood pressure without the side-effects usually associated with peripherally acting hypotensive drugs.

In cardiac arrhythmias: Beta-Cardone is used to restore normal rate and rhythm or to reduce the rate of ventricular contraction, particularly in arrhythmias of supraventricular origin.

In thyrotoxicosis: Beta-Cardone is recommended for short-term symptomatic relief of sympathetic overactivity as an adjunct to specific anti-thyroid therapy.

Dosage and administration *Oral administration in adults:*

General instructions: When administering Beta-Cardone to a patient for the first time, it is desirable to start with a low dose and gradually increase the dose until the desired response is obtained; as a general rule the heart rate should not be reduced to less than 55 beats per minute.

No special precautions, other than the observance of the contra-indications listed below, are required when transferring patients to Beta-Cardone from other β-blockers. Beta-Cardone can be administered in conjunction with diuretic agents (see *'Warnings'*), digitalis, lignocaine and specific anti-thyroid drugs such as carbimazole. The following are guidelines for oral administration.

The Elderly: Since elderly patients may have renal insufficiency, a low initial dose and cautious titration of the effects of incremental doses are recommended.

Dosage in angina pectoris: The optimum dosage is usually found to be between 200 mg and 600 mg per day in a single or divided dose.

Treatment should be initiated with 80 mg twice daily for the first 7 to 10 days. The patient may then be given 200 mg once daily, preferably on rising in the morning. Further increments of 200 mg may thereafter be given, if necessary, at intervals of two or more weeks but, in angina pectoris, it is rarely found necessary to administer more than 400 mg per day.

Dosage in hypertension: The optimum dosage is usually found to be between 200 mg and 600 mg per day in a single or divided dose.

Again treatment should be initiated with 80 mg twice daily for the first 7 to 10 days. The patient may then be given 200 mg once daily, preferably on rising in the morning. Further increments of 200 mg may thereafter be given, if necessary, at intervals of two or more weeks and, in hypertension, there have been occasional reports of up to 4,000 mg being administered daily in divided doses.

Dosage in cardiac arrhythmia: The optimum dosage is usually found to be between 120 mg and 240 mg per day in a single or divided dose.

Dosage in Thyrotoxicosis: In most cases it has been found that a dosage of between 120 mg and 240 mg per day, in a single or divided dose, will reduce sympathetic overactivity.

In cardiac arrhythmia and thyrotoxicosis, treatment should be commenced with a dose of 40 mg, three times daily for the first 7 to 10 days. Once the maintenance phase is reached a single dose of 200 mg daily, preferably on rising in the morning, may be adequate.

Contra-indications, warnings, etc
Heart block and bronchospasm: Beta-Cardone should not be given to patients suffering from heart block or who have a history of bronchospasm.

In patients with poor cardiac reserve β-blockade can precipitate heart failure; in such cases, Beta-Cardone therapy should not be commenced until the patient has been controlled by cardiac glycosides and, if necessary, diuretic therapy.

Warning: There have been reports of skin rashes and/or dry eyes associated with the use of β-adrenoceptor-blocking drugs. The reported incidence is small and in most cases the symptoms have cleared when the treatment was withdrawn. Discontinuance of the drug should be considered if any such reaction is not otherwise explicable. Cessation of therapy with a β-blocker should be gradual.

Diabetic keto-acidosis and metabolic acidosis: Beta-Cardone should not be given to patients suffering from diabetic keto-acidosis or metabolic acidosis; therapy with Beta-Cardone can be commenced or resumed when the metabolic condition has been corrected.

Treated diabetes: Beta-Cardone, like other β-blocking agents, may reduce or mask the usual pre-hypoglycaemic warning signs. It may be necessary to adjust the dose of antidiabetic therapy.

General anaesthesia: If desired, Beta-Cardone may be stopped four days prior to surgery. However, where sudden withdrawal might expose the patient to severe angina or arrhythmias, anaesthesia can proceed provided that the following precautions are taken.

1. Vagal dominance is counteracted by premedication with atropine sulphate (0.25 to 2.0 mg) administered intravenously.
2. Ether, chloroform, cyclopropane and trichlorethylene are not used.

Pregnancy: Animal studies with sotalol hydrochloride have shown no evidence of teratogenicity or other harmful effects to the fetus, nevertheless its use throughout pregnancy should be avoided unless it is absolutely necessary. It crosses the placenta and may cause fetal bradycardia.

Breast milk: Infants should not be fed with breast milk from mothers being treated with Beta-Cardone.

Alcoholism: β-adrenoceptor blocking drugs may precipitate cardiac failure in alcoholic patients.

Renal insufficiency: Since Beta-Cardone is mainly excreted unchanged in the urine, accumulation may be avoided by reduction in dosage.

Serum sotalol levels increase in renal insufficiency and correlate with prolongation of the Q-Tc interval (see *Overdosage* below).

Upper respiratory infections: In these conditions patients without a history of airways obstruction may suffer bronchospasm from β-blockade.

Hypokalaemia/hypomagnesaemia: Ventricular tachycardia, including torsade de pointes, has been reported infrequently in patients treated with sotalol who were hypokalaemic secondary to the use of potassium-losing diuretics or who were also on drugs that prolong the QT interval e.g. disopyramide, Class I antiarrhythmics or tricyclic antidepressants (see *Drug Interactions*).

Patients' plasma electrolyte concentrations should be measured prior to initiating therapy with Beta-Cardone and monitored frequently during the course of treatment. Patients should be advised to stop Beta-Cardone therapy if severe or persistent diarrhoea should occur or if other potential for hypokalaemia/hypomagnesaemia exists.

Side-effects: Beta-Cardone is usually well tolerated. Beta-blockers, even those with apparent cardioselectivity should not be used in patients with asthma or a history of obstructive airways disease unless no alternative treatment is available. In such cases, the risk of inducing bronchospasm should be appreciated and appropriate precautions taken. If bronchospasm should occur after the use of Beta-Cardone it can be treated with a $beta_2$-agonist by inhalation e.g. salbutamol (the dose of which may need to be greater than the usual dose in asthma) and, if necessary, intravenous atropine 1 mg.

Interactions: In combined therapy, clonidine should not be discontinued until several days after withdrawal of Beta-Cardone. Use with great caution with drugs that also prolong the QT interval, e.g. disopyramide, amiodarone, Class I anti-arrhythmic agents, calcium antagonists of the verapamil type or tricyclic antidepressants.

Overdosage: Overdosage causes excessive bradycardia and hypotension; to counteract this atropine sulphate (0.25 to 2.0 mg) should be administered intravenously and, if need be, isoprenaline (about 5 micrograms per minute) by slow intravenous injection.

In severe overdose, intravenous glucagon may be preferred: an initial bolus dose of 5 to 10 mg in dextrose or saline should be followed by an intravenous infusion of 4 mg/hour or as sufficient to maintain cardiac output.

Prolongation of the Q-Tc interval has been reported. Transvenous pacing may be required.

Pharmaceutical precautions Beta-Cardone Tablets should be protected from light.

Legal category POM.

Package quantities *Beta-Cardone Tablets 200 mg* are available in containers of 30 tablets (OP).

Beta-Cardone Tablets 80 mg are available in containers of 100 tablets (OP).

Beta-Cardone Tablets 40 mg are available in containers of 100 tablets (OP).

Further information Beta-Cardone is not metabolised and, in the main, is excreted in the urine. After oral administration the plasma half life has been shown to be 17 hours; the lipid solubility is very low.

Product licence numbers

Beta-Cardone Tablets 200 mg	0021/0056
Beta-Cardone Tablets 80 mg	0021/0055
Beta-Cardone Tablets 40 mg	0021/0054

CYTACON* LIQUID AND TABLETS

Presentation Cytacon Tablets are white, film-coated and engraved 'Cytacon' on one side. Each contains 50 micrograms Cyanocobalamin BP.

Cytacon Liquid is red coloured and contains 35 micrograms Cyanocobalamin BP in each 5 ml.

Uses *Post-gastrectomy deficiency:* As many as 50% of patients who have had a partial gastrectomy are likely to develop abnormally low serum vitamin B_{12} levels within five years of the operation unless supplementary vitamin B_{12} is given. Megaloblastic anaemia is not uncommon and subacute degeneration of the cord has been reported. After total gastrectomy, it is better to administer vitamin B_{12} by injection (e.g. Hydroxocobalamin Injection BP) rather than orally. Diseases of the alimentary tract, such as 'blind-loop' syndrome and small bowel diverticula, may also be associated with vitamin B_{12} deficiency.

Nutritional deficiency: Low serum vitamin B_{12} levels may occur in strict vegetarians and in old people subsisting on limited diets. The diagnosis of pernicious anaemia should be excluded before administering oral vitamin B_{12}.

Tropical sprue: Both folic acid and vitamin B_{12} may be needed: in some cases oral vitamin B_{12} may be sufficiently well absorbed to avoid the need for injections.

Pernicious anaemia: If injections of vitamin B_{12} cannot be used, large daily oral doses may be substituted (see Dosage below) but the blood must be examined at least every three months for 18 months until stabilised and then annually.

Dosage and administration *Adults:* 1 to 3 tablets or more daily at the discretion of the physician. Alternatively, one or two 5 ml spoonfuls Cytacon Liquid 2 or 3 times daily or at the discretion of the physician. In pernicious anaemia, intramuscular therapy is preferable for initial correction of vitamin B_{12} deficiency. However, if necessary, the oral route may be used to follow this, in which case at least 300 micrograms should be given daily.

Children: One 5 ml spoonful Cytacon Liquid 2 to 3 times daily or one Cytacon Tablet twice daily or at the discretion of the physician.

Where possible, doses should be taken between meals.

Contra-indications, warnings, etc
Contra-indications: Hypersensitivity to the product.

Precautions: In pernicious anaemia, an adequate dose must be used and the blood picture must be examined regularly at least every three months for 18 months until stabilised and then annually.

Indiscriminate administration may mask precise diagnosis.

Long-term treatment with Cytacon Liquid may increase the risk of dental caries. It is important that adequate dental hygiene is maintained.

Medicines containing sugar should be administered with care to patients with diabetes mellitus.

Pregnancy: Cytacon should not be used for the treatment of megaloblastic anaemia of pregnancy since this is always due to folate deficiency.

Side-effects: Sensitisation to cyanocobalamin is rare but it may present as an itching exanthema, and exceptionally as anaphylactic shock. Acneiform and bullous eruptions have been reported rarely.

Persons who have become sensitised to cyanocobalamin by injection are often able to take it by the oral route without trouble.

Interactions: Absorption of Cytacon may be reduced by para-aminosalicylic acid, colchicine, biguanides, neomycin, cholestyramine, potassium chloride, methyldopa and cimetidine. Chloramphenicol treated patients may respond poorly to Cytacon. Serum concentrations of cyanocobalamin may be lowered by oral contraceptives. These interactions are unlikely to have clinical significance.

Antimetabolites and most antibiotics invalidate vitamin B_{12} assays by microbiological techniques.

Overdosage: Treatment is unlikely to be needed in cases of overdosage.

Pharmaceutical precautions Protect from light. Store in well closed containers.

Legal category P.

Package quantities *Tablets:* packs of 50.
Liquid: bottles of 200 ml and 2 litres.

Further information Nil.

Product licence numbers
Cytacon Tablets 0021/5909R
Cytacon Liquid 0021/5908R

CYTAMEN* (Cyanocobalamin Injection BP)

Presentation Cytamen '1000' is a clear, red solution containing 1,000 micrograms cyanocobalamin per millilitre.

Cytamen complies with the specification for Cyanocobalamin Injection BP.

Uses Addisonian pernicious anaemia. Prophylaxis and treatment of other macrocytic anaemias associated with vitamin B_{12} deficiency. Schilling test.

Dosage and administration The following dosage schemes are suitable for adults and children.

Addisonian pernicious anaemia and other macrocytic anaemias without neurological involvement: Initially: 250 to 1,000 micrograms intramuscularly on alternate days for one to two weeks, then 250 micrograms weekly until the blood count is normal.

Maintenance: 1,000 micrograms monthly.

Addisonian pernicious anaemia and other macrocytic anaemias, anaemias with neurological complications: Initially: 1,000 micrograms intramuscularly on alternate days as long as improvement is occurring.

Maintenance: 1,000 micrograms monthly.

Prophylaxis of macrocytic anaemia associated with vitamin B_{12} deficiency resulting from gastrectomy, some malabsorption syndromes and strict vegetarianism: 250 to 1,000 micrograms monthly.

Schilling test: An intramuscular injection of 1,000 micrograms cyanocobalamin is an essential part of this test.

Contra-indications, warnings, etc
Contra-indications: Hypersensitivity to cyanocobalamin.

Not indicated for treatment of toxic amblyopias – use Neo-Cytamen.

Precautions: The dosage schemes given above are usually satisfactory, but regular examination of the blood is advisable. If megaloblastic anaemia fails to respond to Cytamen, folate metabolism should be investigated.

Doses in excess of 10 micrograms daily may produce a haematological response in patients with folate deficiency. Indiscriminate administration may mask the true diagnosis. Cardiac arrhythmias secondary to hypokalaemia during initial therapy have been reported. Plasma potassium should therefore be monitored during this period.

Pregnancy: Cytamen should not be used for the treatment of megaloblastic anaemia of pregnancy.

Side-effects: Sensitisation to cyanocobalamin is rare but it may present as an itching exanthema, chills, fever, hot flushes, nausea and dizziness, and exceptionally as anaphylactic shock. Acneiform and bullous eruptions have been reported rarely.

Interactions: Chloramphenicol-treated patients may respond poorly to Cytamen. Serum concentrations of cyanocobalamin may be lowered by oral contraceptives.

These interactions are unlikely to have clinical significance.

Antimetabolites and most antibiotics invalidate vitamin B_{12} assays by microbiological techniques.

Overdosage: Treatment is unlikely to be needed in cases of overdosage.

Pharmaceutical precautions Protect from light.

Legal category POM.

Package quantities Ampoules of 1 ml in boxes of 5.

Further information Nil.

Product licence numbers
Cytamen '1000' 0021/0118

DINDEVAN* TABLETS

Presentation *Dindevan Tablets 10 mg:* White tablets engraved DF/D10, each tablet containing Phenindione BP 10 mg.

Dindevan Tablets 25 mg: Green tablets engraved DF/D25, each tablet containing Phenindione BP 25 mg.

Dindevan Tablets 50 mg: White tablets engraved DF/D50, each tablet containing Phenindione BP 50 mg.

Uses Dindevan (Phenindione BP) is a synthetic anticoagulant which acts by interfering with the formation of clotting factors II, VII, IX and X. It produces its effect in 36 to 48 hours after the initial dose: the effect wanes over a period of 48 to 72 hours after Dindevan is stopped.

Anticoagulant therapy can be initiated with heparin and Dindevan together.

Indications: Prophylaxis of systemic embolisation in patients with rheumatic heart disease and atrial fibrillation.

Prophylaxis after insertion of prosthetic heart valves. Prophylaxis and treatment of venous thrombosis and pulmonary embolism.

Dosage and administration *Initial loading dose:* Usually 200 mg, followed on the second day with a dose of 100 mg.

Maintenance therapy: Dosage must be adjusted, from the third day, in accordance with the results of appropriate coagulation tests. Concomitant heparin therapy affects the results of control tests and should be discontinued at least six hours before the first test is carried out.

Control tests must be made at regular intervals and the dosage further adjusted according to the results obtained. As a general guide, a maintenance dosage of between 50 to 150 mg per day will prove satisfactory in most cases. Occasionally, a resistant patient may need 200 mg or more per day; on the other hand a sensitive patient may need less than 50 mg per day.

Contra-indications, warnings, etc
Contra-indications: Pregnancy. Infants should not be fed with breast milk from mothers being treated with Dindevan. Known hypersensitivity to phenindione. Dindevan should not be given in the presence of severe hepatic or renal disease, bacterial endocarditis, actual or potential haemorrhagic conditions, or to patients with uncontrolled hypertension. Its use within 24 hours following surgery or labour should be undertaken with caution, if at all.

Precautions: (See *Drug interactions*) The following factors may exaggerate the effects of Dindevan and necessitate a reduction in dosage: loss of weight; elderly subject; acute illness, impaired renal function; decreased dietary intake of vitamin K and administration of certain drugs (see 'Drug interactions').

Factors which may call for an increase in maintenance dosage include weight gain, diarrhoea and vomiting, increased intake of vitamin K, fats and oils and administration of certain drugs (see 'Drug interactions').

Administration of vitamin K can lead to resistance to the action of Dindevan for some days. For this reason, fresh-frozen plasma should be administered to patients with prosthetic heart valves where haemorrhage has occurred.

Pregnancy: Oral anticoagulants should not be used in pregnancy particularly because of possible teratogenicity and the risk of fetal haemorrhage near term. It is therefore suggested that heparin (which does not cross the placenta) be used during the first trimester and after 37 weeks' gestation. However, the use of heparin in pregnancy is not absolutely safe and specialist guidance is advisable for those who are pregnant and who need anti-coagulant therapy. Women of child-bearing age who are receiving treatment with Dindevan should be cautioned about the possible complications of pregnancy.

Side-effects: The following effects have been reported: hypersensitivity including skin rashes, alopecia, enanthema, skin necrosis, exfoliative dermatitis, fever, leucopenia and agranulocytosis, diarrhoea, vomiting, hepatitis and renal damage with tubular necrosis. Micro-adenopathy, jaundice, albuminuria, eosinophilia, a leukaemoid blood picture or cytopenia or haemothorax may also be observed. If any of these are observed administration of Dindevan should stop immediately and full investigations of blood and of liver and kidney function should be carried out. Possible sensitivity to other drugs should be considered. Other anticoagulants, such as warfarin, are usually tolerated by patients sensitive to Dindevan. If therapy is controlled as recommended then bleeding due to overdosage of anticoagulant is rare. An episode of bleeding occurring during anticoagulant therapy must therefore be investigated fully and not regarded automatically as a manifestation of overdosage.

N.B. The metabolites of Dindevan often colour the urine pink or orange. This may be distinguished from discoloration caused by haemoglobin by the addition of a few drops of dilute acetic acid to the urine. If the colour is due to Dindevan it will disappear immediately.

Drug interactions: Care is required in the concomitant use of all drugs in patients receiving oral anticoagulant therapy. The following may exaggerate the effects of Dindevan: ACTH, allopurinol, amiodarone, amitriptyline/nortriptyline, anabolic steroids, azapropazone, broad spectrum antibiotics, cimetidine, clofibrate, corticosteroids, co-trimoxazole, dextropropoxyphene, diflunisal, dipyridamole, disulfiram, feprazone, flurbiprofen, glucagon, hepato-toxic drugs, indomethacin, metronidazole, oxyphenbutazone, phenformin, phenylbutazone, quinidine, salicylates, sulindac, sulphinpyrazone, thyroid compounds, tolbutamide. Monitoring and reduction of the dose of Dindevan may be necessary.

The following may reduce the effects of Dindevan: alcohol in large amounts, carbamazepine, cholestyramine, dichloralphenazone, glutethimide, griseofulvin, phenobarbitone, phenytoin, rifampicin. Monitoring and increase of the dose of Dindevan may be necessary.

Overdosage: If haemorrhage occurs or a potential bleeding state arises, excessive depression of the coagulation activity can be corrected by temporary withdrawal of Dindevan accompanied, if necessary, by infusion of fresh-frozen plasma or whole blood. Vitamin K_1, 5 to 10 mg intravenously, may be required to supplement specific treatment with factor concentrates.

Pharmaceutical precautions No special requirements or precautions.

Legal category POM.

Package quantities Dindevan Tablets 10 mg, 25 mg and 50 mg are each available in containers of 100 tablets (OP).

Further information Nil.

Product licence numbers

Dindevan Tablets 10 mg	0021/5064R
Dindevan Tablets 25 mg	0021/5065R
Dindevan Tablets 50 mg	0021/5066R

FERSADAY* TABLETS

Presentation Fersaday Tablets are ochre, film-coated tablets engraved 'Fersaday' on one side. Each tablet contains Ferrous Fumarate BP equivalent to 100 mg ferrous iron.

These tablets comply with the specification for Ferrous Fumarate Tablets BP.

Uses Prophylaxis and treatment of iron deficiency states.

Dosage and administration The usual adult dose is one tablet daily. (The foil enclosing the tablets is printed with the days of the week in sequence.) In severe or refractory iron deficiency one Fersaday Tablet may be given twice daily.

This presentation of ferrous fumarate is not intended for the treatment of children.

Contra-indications, warnings, etc

Contra-indications: Known hypersensitivity to the product. Paroxysmal nocturnal haemoglobinuria, haemosiderosis, haemochromatosis, active peptic ulcer, repeated blood transfusions, regional enteritis and ulcerative colitis.

Fersaday must not be used in anaemias other than those due to iron deficiency.

Precautions: Some post-gastrectomy patients show poor absorption of iron. Care is needed when treating iron deficiency anaemia in patients with treated or controlled peptic ulceration.

Duration of treatment of uncomplicated iron deficiency anaemia should not usually exceed 6 months (or 3 months after reversal of the anaemia has been achieved).

Since anaemia due to combined iron and vitamin B_{12} or folate deficiencies may be microcytic in type, patients with microcytic anaemia resistant to therapy with iron alone should be screened for vitamin B_{12} or folate deficiency.

Fersaday Tablets should be kept out of the reach of children.

Pregnancy: Administration of Fersaday during the first trimester of pregnancy may be undesirable.

Side-effects: Gastro-intestinal disorders have been reported including gastro-intestinal discomfort, anorexia, nausea, vomiting, constipation, diarrhoea. Darkening of the stools may occur.

Interactions: Iron reduces the absorption of penicillamine. Absorption of both iron and antibiotic may be reduced if Fersaday is given with a tetracycline.

Concurrent administration of antacids may reduce absorption of iron.

Chloramphenicol delays plasma iron clearance, incorporation of iron into red blood cells and interferes with erythropoiesis. Some inhibition of iron absorption may occur if it is taken with cholestyramine, tea, eggs, or milk.

Overdosage: Acute overdosage of oral iron requires emergency treatment as described below. In young children, 200 to 250 mg/kg ferrous fumarate is considered to be extremely dangerous.

Symptoms and signs of abdominal pain, vomiting and diarrhoea appear within 60 minutes. Cardiovascular collapse with coma may follow. Some improvement may occur after this phase which in some patients, is followed by recovery. In others, after about 16 hours, deterioration may occur involving diffuse vascular congestion, pulmonary oedema, convulsions, anuria, hypothermia, severe shock, metabolic acidosis, coagulation abnormalities or hypoglycaemia.

Vomiting should be induced immediately, followed as soon as possible by parenteral injection of desferrioxamine mesylate and then gastric lavage. In the meantime it is helpful to give milk and/or 5% sodium bicarbonate solution by mouth.

Dissolve 2 grams desferrioxamine mesylate in 2 or 3 ml of Water for Injections and give intramuscularly. A solution of 5 grams desferrioxamine in 50 to 100 ml of fluid may be left in the stomach. If desferrioxamine is not available, leave 300 ml of 1% to 5% sodium bicarbonate solution in the stomach. Fluid replacement is essential.

Recovery may be complicated by long-term sequelae such as hepatic necrosis, pyloric stenosis or acute toxic encephalitis which may lead to CNS damage.

Pharmaceutical precautions Protect from light.

Legal category P.

Package quantities Cartons of two calendar blister packs of 14 tablets (OP).

Further information Nil.

Product licence number 0021/5912R.

FERSAMAL* TABLETS AND SYRUP

Presentation Fersamal Tablets are small, light brown tablets engraved 'Fersamal' on one side. Each tablet contains Ferrous Fumarate BP equivalent to 65 mg ferrous iron. These tablets comply with the specification for Ferrous Fumarate Tablets BP.

Fersamal Syrup is a brown, aqueous suspension containing Ferrous Fumarate BP equivalent to 45 mg ferrous iron per 5 ml.

Uses Prophylaxis and treatment of iron-deficiency states.

For prophylaxis during pregnancy, a combination of iron and folic acid is usually recommended, e.g. Pregaday* Tablets.

Dosage and administration *Adults and the elderly:* 1 tablet three times a day or two 5 ml spoonfuls of syrup twice a day. The dose may be doubled if required. The tablets are easily swallowed but may also be crushed or chewed being almost tasteless.

Full term infants and young children: Half to one 5 ml spoonful of syrup twice a day.

Premature infants: The usual dosage is 0.6 ml/kg/day but some may require 2.4 ml/kg/day.

Contra-indications, warnings, etc
Contra-indications: Known hypersensitivity to the product. Paroxysmal nocturnal haemoglobinuria, haemosiderosis, haemochromatosis, active peptic ulcer, repeated blood transfusions, regional enteritis, and ulcerative colitis. Fersamal must not be used in anaemias other than those due to iron deficiency.

Precautions: Some post-gastrectomy patients show poor absorption of iron. Care is needed when treating iron deficiency anaemia in patients with treated or controlled peptic ulceration.

Duration of treatment of uncomplicated iron deficiency anaemia should not usually exceed 6 months (or 3 months after reversal of the anaemia has been achieved).

Since anaemia due to combined iron and vitamin B_{12} or folate deficiency may be microcytic in type, patients with microcytic anaemia resistant to therapy with iron alone should be screened for vitamin B_{12} or folate deficiency.

Long-term treatment with Fersamal Syrup may increase the risk of dental caries. It is important that adequate dental hygiene is maintained.

Medicines containing sugar should be administered with care to patients with diabetes mellitus.

Fersamal should be kept out of the reach of children.

Pregnancy: Administration of Fersamal during the first trimester of pregnancy may be undesirable.

Side-effects: Gastro-intestinal disorders have been reported including gastro-intestinal discomfort, anorexia, nausea, vomiting, constipation, diarrhoea. Darkening of the stools may occur.

Rarely, allergic reactions may occur to metabisulphite in the vehicle of the syrup e.g. urticaria and breathing difficulties.

Interactions: Iron reduces the absorption of penicillamine.

Absorption of both iron and antibiotic may be reduced if Fersamal is given with a tetracycline.

Concurrent administration of antacids may reduce absorption of iron.

Chloramphenicol delays plasma iron clearance, incorporation of iron into red blood cells and interferes with erythropoiesis.

Some inhibition of iron absorption may occur if it is taken with cholestyramine, tea, eggs or milk.

Overdosage: Acute overdose of oral iron requires emergency treatment as described below. In young children, 200 to 250 mg/kg ferrous fumarate is considered to be extremely dangerous.

Symptoms and signs of abdominal pain, vomiting and diarrhoea appear within 60 minutes. Cardiovascular collapse with coma may follow. Some improvement may occur after this phase which in some patients, is followed by recovery. In others, after about 16 hours, deterioration may occur involving diffuse vascular congestion, pulmonary oedema, convulsions, anuria, hypothermia, severe shock, metabolic acidosis, coagulation abnormalities or hypoglycaemia.

Vomiting should be induced immediately, followed as soon as possible by parenteral injection of desferrioxamine mesylate, and then gastric lavage. In the meantime, it is helpful to give milk and/or 5% sodium bicarbonate solution by mouth.

Dissolve 2 grams desferrioxamine mesylate in 2 to 3 ml of Water for Injections and give intramuscularly. A solution of 5 grams desferrioxamine in 50 to 100 ml of fluid may be left in the stomach. If desferrioxamine is not available, leave 300 ml of 1% to 5% sodium bicarbonate solution in the stomach. Fluid replacement is essential.

Recovery may be complicated by long-term sequelae such as hepatic necrosis, pyloric stenosis or acute toxic encephalitis which may lead to CNS damage.

Pharmaceutical precautions Protect from light.

Legal category P.

Package quantities Tablets: packs of 100 (OP) and 1,000.
Syrup: bottles of 150 ml (OP).

Further information Fersamal Syrup may be diluted with Syrup BP at the time of dispensing if required.

Product licence numbers

Fersamal Tablets:	0021/5910R
Fersamal Syrup:	0021/5911R

ILUBE* EYE DROPS

Presentation Ilube Eye Drops: a clear, colourless, sterile solution containing Acetylcysteine BP 5% w/v and Hypromellose 0.35% w/v, preserved with benzalkonium chloride 0.01% w/v. It is presented in a 15 ml glass bottle with a separate polycarbonate dropper.

Uses Ilube Eye Drops are artificial tears with mucolytic and lubricant properties, suitable for the relief of dry eye syndromes associated with deficient tear secretion, impaired or abnormal mucous production.

Acetylcysteine has marked mucolytic properties which reduce the viscosity and tenacity of mucus in the eyes. This, combined with the emollient properties of hypromellose, ensures lubrication and soothing relief for dry eye syndromes.

Dosage and administration The usual dosage is one or two drops instilled into the affected eye three or four times daily.

Contra-indications, warnings, etc
Contra-indications: Known hypersensitivity to any component is a contra-indication to the use of Ilube Eye Drops.

Precautions: Ilube Eye Drops contain benzalkonium chloride as preservative and therefore should not be used to treat patients who wear soft contact lenses.

Discontinue use if discomfort, increased reddening or irritation occurs and persists.

Pharmaceutical precautions Store below 25°C. Protect from light. Avoid touching tip of dropper to prevent contamination. The contents should be discarded 4 weeks after first opening the bottle.

Legal category POM.

Package quantities Amber glass bottle containing 15 ml with separate polycarbonate dropper.

Further information Nil.

Product licence number 0021/0116.

JEXIN*

Presentation Jexin is Tubocurarine Injection BP and is a clear colourless, or faintly coloured sterile solution containing Tubocurarine Chloride BP 10 mg per ml.

Uses Jexin produces paralysis of voluntary muscle by interfering with transmission across the neuromuscular junction. It acts by competitive blockade of motor end-plates. Paralysis appears in the muscles of the face and neck, of the limbs and of the abdomen, in that order, the intercostal muscles and diaphragm being affected last. The paralysis reaches its maximum two to five minutes after intravenous injection and lasts for about 30 minutes. There is, however, a residual action lasting for as long as 24 hours, and during this time smaller doses are required to reproduce the effect of the initial dose.

Jexin is mainly indicated as an adjunct to anaesthesia to secure muscular relaxation in surgery and obstetrics. It can also be used in tetanus.

Dosage and administration *Adults:* The dose-response varies in individual patients but an initial dose of 15 to 30 mg intravenously is commonly used for profound muscular relaxation accompanied by apnoea, which may be maintained by supplementary doses of 5 to 10 mg. Smaller initial doses, e.g. 10 to 15 mg, may be used, according to the depth of muscular relaxation needed. The action can be reversed by injection of neostigmine preceded by atropine. Recovery may be monitored by the use of a nerve stimulator.

Children: An average initial dose for infants and children above 1 year of age is 300 to 500 micrograms/kg; for premature infants and neonates it is 200 to 250 micrograms/kg.

Elderly: The requirements for initial doses are unchanged but maintenance doses should be reduced and the intervals between them increased.

Contra-indications, warnings, etc

Contra-indications: Jexin is contra-indicated in patients with respiratory insufficiency or in the presence of renal or hepatic impairment, in patients with hypersensitivity to curare-like drugs and in patients in whom histamine release is a definite hazard e.g. those with asthma.

Precautions: Jexin should be used only when there are facilities for endotracheal intubation and administration of oxygen by intermittent positive pressure ventilation.

In patients with myasthenia gravis or myasthenic syndrome, Jexin should be administered in very small doses and with extreme caution; a reduction in dosage is also advisable in cases of gross obesity, myopathy and after poliomyelitis.

Care is also necessary in patients with endocrine dysfunction. If labour occurs during Jexin administration to the mother, curare-like effects may occur in the newborn infant. Neonates may be particularly sensitive to Jexin.

Tubocurarine has been reported to be a possible cause of malignant hyperpyrexia. In the majority of patients with an inherited predisposition, there is an elevated serum creatine phosphokinase (CPK) concentration. Particular care is needed in patients with a family history of hyperpyrexia.

Care is necessary if Jexin has to be given to a patient on two occasions within 24 hours.

Rarely, anaphylactoid reactions may occur following the use of tubocurarine. Particular caution should be exercised in administering Jexin to patients with a history of atopy or of previous drug reactions.

Hypokalaemia may enhance the effects of Jexin. Plasma potassium concentration should be measured prior to its administration.

Pregnancy: Safety for use during pregnancy has not been established. Use during early pregnancy only when clearly needed and when potential benefits outweigh the unknown potential hazards to the fetus. Large and repeated doses of tubocurarine might cause fetal bone deformities if given during early pregnancy, or diminished skeletal muscle activity of the newborn if given near delivery.

Lactation: It is not known whether the drug is excreted in human milk. Exercise caution when administering to a nursing mother.

Side-effects: The dosage recommended produces few side-effects; a transient fall in blood pressure may occur.

Jexin may cause erythema of the chest and neck or at the injection site. Some patients may be pharmacologically hypersensitive to Jexin and may suffer from the following side-effects: profound muscle relaxation with prolonged apnoea, circulatory depression, ganglionic block, histamine release.

Drug interactions: The effects of Jexin are enhanced by ether, halothane methoxyflurane, enflurane and isoflurane. Jexin increases the hypotension produced by halothane which itself increases the effects of Jexin. A reduced dose of Jexin should be used.

Jexin may be potentiated by diazepam and by clindamycin, colistin, kanamycin, neomycin, polymyxins, streptomycin, tobramycin, framycetin amikacin, gentamicin and other amino-glycoside antibiotics, by quinidine, tetracyclines, magnesium salts (including parenteral magnesium sulphate), trimetaphan, potassium-depleting diuretics and by amphotericin. Many drugs may modify plasma concentrations of calcium and, under these circumstances, altered reactions to muscle relaxants have been reported, including prolonged curarisation in hypocalcaemia.

Anticholinesterases, such as neostigmine, antagonise the action of Jexin. Atropine should be administered before neostigmine to counter bradycardia that would otherwise occur. Atropine has been given together with tubocurarine prior to induction of shock in electroconvulsive therapy. Apnoea may occur if aprotinin is administered concomitantly with or during recovery from Jexin. Pre-treatment with azathioprine/mercaptopurine or lymphocytic antiglobulin can reduce the effect of Jexin. Narcotics augment the depression of respiratory function.

Synergistic or antagonistic effects may result when a depolarising and a non-depolarising muscle relaxant are given simultaneously or immediately in sequence and the resulting neuromuscular block may be irreversible by neostigmine. When used following succinylcholine for intubation, the administration of Jexin should be delayed until the effects of succinylcholine begin to diminish.

Overdosage: Following overdosage, apnoea, cardiovascular collapse and histamine release may occur. The treatment is positive pressure artificial respiration with oxygen. Recovery of normal respiration can be hastened by intravenous neostigmine preceded by atropine to counter bradycardia. Neostigmine may aggravate the hypotension. Monitor cardiovascular, respiratory and electrolyte status. Apply other supportive and symptomatic treatment as indicated.

Pharmaceutical precautions No special requirements or precautions.

Legal category POM.

Package quantities Jexin is supplied in 1.5 ml ampoules in boxes of 5.

Further information Although Jexin should not normally be mixed with thiopentone, this can be done if prepared immediately prior to injection and used only if the solution remains perfectly clear.

Product licence number 0021/5025R.

MAREVAN* TABLETS

Presentation Marevan Tablets are Warfarin Tablets BP.

Marevan Tablets 1 mg: Brown tablets engraved DF/M1, each tablet containing Warfarin Sodium BP 1 mg.

Marevan Tablets 3 mg: Blue tablets engraved DF/M3, each tablet containing Warfarin Sodium BP 3 mg.

Marevan Tablets 5 mg: Pink tablets engraved DF/M5, each tablet containing Warfarin Sodium BP 5 mg.

Uses Marevan is a synthetic anti-coagulant of the coumarin series and acts by inhibiting the formation of active clotting factors II, VII, IX and X. An effect on prothrombin time is produced in 24 to 36 hours after the initial dose. This reaches a maximum in 36 to 48 hours and is maintained for 48 hours or more after administration is stopped.

Indications: Prophylaxis of systemic embolisation in patients with rheumatic heart disease and atrial fibrillation.

Prophylaxis after insertion of prosthetic heart valves. Prophylaxis and treatment of venous thrombosis and pulmonary embolism.

Transient cerebral ischaemic attacks.

Dosage and administration 10 to 15 mg daily, according to age and body weight, and adjusted with relation to the results of daily control tests until the desired level of anticoagulant activity is achieved – usually three to six days after the initiation of treatment.

In emergencies, anticoagulant therapy should be initiated with heparin and Marevan together. Where there is less urgency, as in patients disposed to or at special risk of thromboembolism, anticoagulant therapy may be initiated with Marevan alone.

Concomitant heparin therapy affects the results of control tests and should be discontinued at least six hours before the first test is carried out.

Control tests should be made at regular intervals and Marevan maintenance dosage further adjusted according to the results obtained.

Contra-indications, warnings, etc
Contra-indications: Pregnancy (*see below*). Known hypersensitivity to warfarin. Marevan should not be given in the presence of severe hepatic or renal disease, bacterial endocarditis, actual or potential haemorrhagic conditions, e.g. peptic ulcer, or to patients with uncontrolled hypertension. Its use within 24 hours following surgery or labour should be undertaken with caution, if at all.

Precautions: The following factors may exaggerate the effects of Marevan and necessitate a reduction in dosage; loss of weight, elderly subject, acute illness, deficient renal function, decreased dietary intake of vitamin K, administration of certain drugs (see 'Drug interactions').

Factors which may call for an increase in maintenance dosage include weight gain, diarrhoea and vomiting, increased intake of vitamin K, fats and oils, and the administration of certain drugs (see 'Drug interactions').

Careful additional laboratory control is necessary if the patient is to be changed from one formulation to another.

Reversal of warfarin anticoagulation by vitamin K takes several days. In emergency situations fresh-frozen plasma should be given.

Pregnancy: Oral anticoagulants should not be used in pregnancy particularly because of possible teratogenicity and the risk of fetal haemorrhage near term. It is therefore suggested that heparin (which does not cross the placenta) be used during the first trimester and after 37 weeks' gestation. However, the use of heparin in pregnancy is not absolutely safe and specialist guidance is advisable for those who are pregnant and who need anticoagulant therapy. Women of child bearing age who are receiving treatment with Marevan should be cautioned about the possible complications of pregnancy.

Side-effects: The following effects have been reported: hypersensitivity, skin rashes, alopecia, diarrhoea, an unexplained drop in haematocrit, and a 'purple toes' syndrome.

Skin necrosis within a few days of starting treatment has been infrequently reported. Most subjects are obese, elderly women. The first sign is an erythematous swollen patch. Administration of vitamin K_1 at this stage may prevent the development of ecchymosis and infarction.

Purpura, fever, nausea and vomiting, pancreatitis, haemothorax and epistaxis may also be observed. If any of these are observed administration of Marevan should stop immediately. Possible sensitivity to other drugs should be considered. Other anticoagulants are often tolerated by patients sensitive to Marevan. If therapy is controlled as recommended then bleeding due to overdosage of anticoagulant is rare. An episode of bleeding occurring during anticoagulant therapy must therefore be investigated fully and not regarded automatically as a manifestation of overdosage.

Drug interactions: Care is required in the concomitant use of all drugs in patients receiving oral anticoagulant therapy.

The activity of warfarin may be potentiated by anabolic steroids (e.g. ethylestranol, methandrostenolone, norethandrolone), amiodarone, amitriptyline/nortriptyline, azapropazone, bezafibrate, cephamandole, chloral hydrate, chloramphenicol, cimetidine, clofibrate, co-trimoxazole, danazol, dextropropoxyphene, dextrothyroxine, erythromycin, feprazone, glucagon, latamoxef, metronidazole, miconazole, neomycin, oxyphenbutazone, phenformin, phenylbutazone, phenyramidol, quinidine, salicylates, tolbutamide, sulphonamides (e.g. sulphaphenazole, sulphinpyrazone), dipyramidole, tamoxifen and triclofos.

Potentiation may also occur with the following drugs, diflunisal, flurbiprofen, indomethacin, mefenamic acid, piroxicam, sulindac and possibly other anti-inflammatory analgesics, ketoconazole, nalidixic acid, norfloxacin, tetracyclines and other broad spectrum antibiotics.

Anticoagulant activity may be possibly increased by allopurinol, disulfiram, methylphenidate, paracetamol, thyroid drugs, and any potentially hepatoxic drug.

Both potentiation and inhibition of anticoagulant effect have been reported with phenytoin, ACTH & corticosteroids.

Anticoagulant activity may also be increased with large amounts or chronic ingestion of alcohol, particularly in patients with impaired liver function.

Warfarin absorption is impaired and activity decreased by cholestyramine and sucralfate. Cholestyramine, however, may also decrease absorption of vitamin K and thus increase coumarin anticoagulant activity. Anticoagulant effect may be decreased by administration of vitamin K (e.g. as a constituent of some enteral feeds).

The anticoagulant activity of warfarin may be inhibited by drugs which induce liver enzymes such as aminoglutethimide barbiturates, carbamazepine, ethchlorvynol, glutethimide, primidone, griseofulvin, dichloralphenazone, rifampicin and oral contraceptives.

Overdosage: If haemorrhage occurs or a potential bleeding state arises, excessive depression of the coagulation activity can be corrected by temporary withdrawal of Marevan accompanied, if necessary, by infusion of fresh-frozen plasma or whole blood. Vitamin K_1, 5 to 10 mg orally or intravenously, may be required to supplement specific treatment with factor concentrates.

Pharmaceutical precautions Replace cap securely and protect from light.

Legal category POM.

Package quantities Marevan Tablets 1 mg are available in containers of 100 (OP) and 500.
Marevan Tablets 3 mg are available in containers of 100 (OP) and 500.
Marevan Tablets 5 mg are available in containers of 100 (OP) and 500.

Further information Nil.

Product licence numbers

Marevan Tablets 1 mg	0021/5071R
Marevan Tablets 3 mg	0021/5072R
Marevan Tablets 5 mg	0021/5073R

MAXEPA* CAPSULES AND LIQUID

Presentation Maxepa Capsules are clear, self-coloured gelatin capsules containing 1 g (approx. 1.1 ml) of oil comprising, as a percentage of total fatty acid composition, 18% w/w eicosapentaenoic acid and 12% w/w docosahexaenoic acid.

Maxepa Liquid is a clear, golden-coloured oil containing, as a percentage of total fatty acid composition, 18% w/w eicosapentaenoic acid and 12% w/w docosahexaenoic acid.

Maxepa Capsules and Liquid contain Vitamin A (less than 100 I.U./g) and Vitamin D (less than 10 I.U./g). A sufficient amount, 0.74 mg (1 I.U./g) of d-alpha tocopheryl acetate is added as a natural anti-oxidant.

Uses Maxepa Capsules or Liquid are indicated for the reduction of plasma triglycerides in patients with severe hypertriglyceridaemia who are judged to be at special risk of ischaemic heart disease and/or pancreatitis.

Maxepa Liquid or Capsules should be used in conjunction with appropriate dietary measures and after diet alone has failed to produce an adequate response. Other risk factors such as hypertension and smoking should be dealt with.

Dosage and administration
Adults: Maxepa Capsules: Five capsules to be taken orally twice daily, with food.

Liquid: One 5 ml spoonful to be taken orally twice daily, with food.

Children: The use of Maxepa Capsules or Liquid has not been established in children.

Elderly: The normal adult dosage is appropriate for elderly patients.

Contra-indications, warnings, etc
Contra-indications: There are no absolute contra-indications to the use of Maxepa Capsules or Liquid.

Precautions: On theoretical grounds it is advisable to monitor patients with bleeding disorders such as haemophilia, and also those receiving anticoagulant therapy or other drugs affecting coagulation.

Pregnancy: There has been no reported experience of the use of Maxepa in pregnancy or breast feeding.

Side-effects: No major side-effects have been reported although, in some patients, occasional nausea and eructation have been reported.

Overdosage: Maxepa is composed entirely of constituents which are found as a normal part of the diet and, as such, may be regarded as harmless at the proposed dosage levels. Deleterious effects due to overdosage have been shown to be unlikely and studies in rats have shown no upper toxic levels of administration.

Pharmaceutical precautions Store in unopened containers until required. Protect from heat, light and moisture. Maxepa Liquid should be dispensed in the original pack and once opened should be used within one month.

Legal category P.

Package quantities Maxepa Capsules – Containers of 200 capsules (OP).

Maxepa Liquid – Bottles of 150 ml (OP).

Further information Epidemiological studies have shown that populations consuming a diet, rich in marine oil lipids have a lower incidence of cardiovascular disease, compared to populations consuming diets high in saturated fats or those with a high intake of monoenoic acids. A regular intake of concentrated oils such as Maxepa has been shown to lead to a sustained reduction in plasma triglycerides and a relative increase in high density lipoprotein levels.

Studies in patients with Type IIB and Type V hyperlipidaemias have shown that diets supplemented with Maxepa led to decreases in triglycerides, plasma cholesterol and very low density lipoproteins.

Product licence numbers
Maxepa Capsules 1932/0002
Maxepa Liquid 1932/0003

Product licence holder: Marfleet Refining Company Limited, Marfleet, Kingston-upon-Hull HU9 5NJ.

Distributor: Duncan, Flockhart & Co. Limited.

NEO-CYTAMEN* (Hydroxocobalamin Injection BP)

Presentation Ampoules containing a clear, red solution which provides 1,000 micrograms (Neo-Cytamen '1000') of hydroxocobalamin per millilitre. Neo-Cytamen Injection complies with the specification for Hydroxocobalamin Injection BP.

Uses Addisonian pernicious anaemia. Prophylaxis and treatment of other macrocytic anaemias associated with vitamin B_{12} deficiency. Tobacco amblyopia and Leber's optic atrophy.

Dosage and administration The following dosage schemes are suitable for adults and children.

Addisonian pernicious anaemia and other macrocytic anaemias without neurological involvement: Initially: 250 to 1,000 micrograms intramuscularly on alternate days for one to two weeks, then 250 micrograms weekly until the blood count is normal.

Maintenance: 1,000 micrograms every two or three months.

Addisonian pernicious anaemia and other macrocytic anaemias with neurological involvement: Initially: 1,000 micrograms on alternate days as long as improvement is occurring.

Maintenance: 1,000 micrograms every two months.

Prophylaxis of macrocytic anaemia associated with vitamin B_{12} deficiency resulting from gastrectomy, some malabsorption syndromes and strict vegetarianism: 1,000 micrograms every two or three months.

Tobacco amblyopia and Leber's optic atrophy: Initially: 1,000 micrograms or more daily by intramuscular injection for two weeks then twice weekly as long as improvement is occurring.

Maintenance: 1,000 micrograms monthly.

Contra-indications, warnings, etc
Contra-indications: Hypersensitivity to any ingredient in the preparation.

Precautions: The dosage schemes given above are usually satisfactory, but regular examination of the blood is advisable. If megaloblastic anaemia fails to respond to Neo-Cytamen, folate metabolism should be investigated. Doses in excess of 10 micrograms daily may produce a haematological response in patients with folate deficiency. Indiscriminate administration may mask the true diagnosis.

Cardiac arrhythmias secondary to hypokalaemia during initial therapy have been reported. Plasma potassium should therefore be monitored during this period.

Pregnancy: Neo-Cytamen should not be used for the treatment of megaloblastic anaemia of pregnancy.

Side-effects: Sensitisation to hydroxocobalamin is rare but may manifest itself as itching exanthema, chills, fever, hot flushes, nausea and dizziness and exceptionally, anaphylaxis. Acneiform and bullous eruptions have been reported rarely.

Interactions: Chloramphenicol-treated patients may respond poorly to Neo-Cytamen. Serum concentrations of hydroxocobalamin may be lowered by oral contraceptives.

These interactions are unlikely to have clinical significance.

Antimetabolites and most antibiotics invalidate vitamin B_{12} assays by microbiological techniques.

Overdosage: Treatment is unlikely to be needed in cases of overdosage.

Pharmaceutical precautions Protect from light.

Legal category POM.

Package quantities Ampoules of 1 ml in boxes of 5.

Further information An intramuscular injection of hydroxocobalamin produces higher serum levels than the same dose of cyanocobalamin, and these levels are well maintained.

Product licence number
Neo-Cytamen '1000' 0021/0121

NEO-NACLEX*

Presentation Small white tablets engraved 'Neo-NaClex' on one side and scored on the reverse. Each tablet contains 5 mg bendrofluazide and complies with the specification for Bendrofluazide Tablets BP.

Uses *Essential hypertension:* The mechanism whereby the thiazides exert their antihypertensive effect has not been clearly established. In non-oedematous patients there may be little noticeable diuretic effect. Neo-NaClex may be used as the sole antihypertensive agent, or as an adjunct to other drugs whose action it may enhance.

Oedema: Neo-NaClex inhibits the renal tubular absorption of salt and water by its action at the beginning of the distal convoluted tubule. Sodium and chloride ions are excreted in equivalent proportions. Because potassium excretion is promoted, metabolic alkalosis may occur secondary to hypokalaemia. There is no important effect upon carbonic anhydrase. Neo-NaClex causes a steady diuresis lasting for about 12 hours. It is indicated in the treatment of oedema associated with conditions such as congestive heart failure, nephrotic syndrome, and cirrhosis of the liver.

Dosage and administration
Adults: When Neo-NaClex is added to other antihypertensive drugs, the dosage of the latter can usually be reduced gradually as Neo-NaClex takes effect.

Essential hypertension: 2.5 to 10 mg once daily, alone or in conjunction with other antihypertensive agents.

Oedema: 5 mg given orally once daily in the morning usually produces the desired effect without diuresis interfering with sleep but this dose can be increased to 10 mg if required. During the first few days of treatment there is usually a large increase in urinary volume which diminishes as treatment continues.

Maintenance: Many patients will respond adequately to a daily dose of 2.5 mg or 5 mg on only two or three days in the week.

Children: For children up to 12 years of age, 50 to 100 micrograms/kg bodyweight daily.

Elderly: (See 'Precautions').

Contra-indications, warnings, etc
Contra-indications: Severe renal or hepatic failure, hypersensitivity to the product or other sulphonamide-like drugs, Addison's disease, diabetic keto-acidosis and hypercalcaemia. Neo-NaClex should not be administered concurrently with lithium carbonate.

Precautions: When treatment with the Neo-NaClex is intensive or continuous, periodic estimations of serum electrolyte should be done. Some loss of potassium may occur and, in these circumstances, potassium chloride supplements are recommended. If the patient is vomiting, has diarrhoea or is suffering from an acute febrile or chronic illness (especially cirrhosis of the liver or heart failure) supplementary potassium may be particularly important. Supplementary potassium to prevent hypokalaemia and the danger of arrhythmias and other ECG changes is strongly recommended if patients receiving digitalis require prolonged diuretic treatment. In concurrent therapy with carbenoxolone or corticosteroids, potassium supplements are recommended. Patients at risk of myocardial infarction and patients admitted for cardiac surgery also need potassium supplements.

Potassium depletion may cause polyuria, malaise, muscle weakness or cramp, decreased tendon reflexes, anorexia, dizziness, nausea or vomiting. Also, sensitivity to digitalis may increase and signs of overdosage appear. Prolonged potassium deficiency may induce chronic pyelonephritis. Renal function should be monitored. Potassium supplements must not be given in renal insufficiency complicated by hyperkalaemia.

In addition, in prolonged therapy it is necessary to test for glycosuria and investigate polyuria. In renal insufficiency, renal function should be monitored. The possibility of magnesium depletion should also be considered.

In cirrhosis of the liver, thiazides may precipitate hepatic encephalopathy.

Thiazides may aggravate existing diabetes mellitus and cause symptoms in patients with latent disease. Neo-NaClex may impair control of diabetes in patients receiving sulphonylureas. Thiazides should be used with caution in systemic lupus erythematosus.

Serum uric acid levels may be raised, with or without gout, in some patients. Thiazides may cause or aggravate hyperlipidaemia; pancreatitis may occur.

The elderly: The elderly are sensitive to the effects of thiazides on blood pressure and electrolyte. Administration of supplementary potassium is particularly important in the elderly. Patients with prostatic hypertrophy may develop acute urinary retention.

Pregnancy: Diuretics are best avoided in the management of oedema of pregnancy or hypertension in pregnancy as their use may be associated with hypovolaemia, increased blood viscosity and reduced placental perfusion. There is inadequate evidence of safety in human pregnancy. There are reports of fetal and neonatal bone marrow depression, thrombocytopenia, electrolyte imbalance, hypoglycaemia and jaundice. Expectant mothers who receive thiazide diuretics may be at increased risk from acute haemorrhagic pancreatitis. In parturition, thiazides may cause uterine inertia and delay the onset of labour. Thiazides are only indicated in pregnancy if oedema complicates a pathological lesion and, even then, after assessing risk versus benefit including the undesirability of administering drugs in the first trimester. As thiazide diuretics are secreted in mothers' milk, breast feeding should be avoided.

Side-effects: The following have been reported: disturbances of electrolyte, acid-base balance, lipids, glucose and uric acid levels; thirst, polyuria, weakness, dizziness, muscle cramps and reversible impotence; nausea, vomiting, mild anorexia, gastric irritation, diarrhoea or constipation; rashes, skin reactions, purpura and blood dyscrasias including thrombocytopenia; hypocalciuria, precipitation of gout, pancreatitis, hepatic encephalopathy and postural hypotension.

Interactions:
Diabetes mellitus: Thiazides may impair control in diabetics receiving sulphonylureas.

Lithium toxicity: The renal clearance of lithium carbonate is reduced; concomitant use is contra-indicated.

Anaesthesia: Halothane's hypotensive effect is increased by thiazides.

Sensitivity to tubocurarine is increased in hypokalaemia. Plasma potassium should be monitored prior to its use in thiazide-treated patients.

Antagonism and hypokalaemia: Carbenoxolone, indomethacin, phenylbutazone, and corticosteroids may both antagonise thiazides' hypotensive effect and increase potassium loss. Monitoring and potassium supplements are recommended.

Hypotension: Enhanced hypotensive effects may follow the concomitant use of thiazides and barbiturates, alcohol, other antihypertensives (e.g. beta-blocking agents, ACE inhibitors, calcium antagonists), MAOIs or narcotics.

Hypersensitivity: Use of allopurinol and a thiazide in patients with renal dysfunction should be avoided: severe hypersensitivity vasculitis has been reported.

Hypokalaemic effects: Hypokalaemia secondary to the use of thiazides may increase the toxicity of cardiac glycosides and antagonise the effect of anti-arrhythmics.

Potassium imbalance: Caution is required in the use of thiazides with any drug/disease state which has a potential for producing potassium imbalance.

Overdosage: CNS depression (e.g. drowsiness, lethargy and coma) may occur without cardiovascular or respiratory depression. Hypovolaemia, hypokalaemia and mild hypoglycaemia are likely to be present. In the case of recent ingestion, gastric lavage should be carried out; activated charcoal may help reduce absorption. Treatment should be symptomatic and directed at fluid and electrolyte replacement which should be monitored together with the blood pressure and renal function. Hyponatraemia should be treated with water deprivation rather than by the administration of NaCl. Cathartics should be avoided.

Pharmaceutical precautions Protect from light.

Legal category POM.

Package quantities Containers of 100 and 500 tablets.

Further information Nil.

Product licence number 0021/5906R.

NEO-NACLEX*-K

Presentation Neo-NaClex-K is a film-coated, two-layered tablet containing bendrofluazide in the white layer and potassium chloride in the pink layer. The white side is engraved 'Neo-NaClex-K'. The potassium chloride is in a special matrix which provides gradual release of the electrolyte, so minimising gastro-intestinal irritation. Each tablet contains 2.5 mg Bendrofluazide BP and 630 mg Potassium Chloride BP, providing 330 mg elemental potassium (8.4 mEq). Neo-NaClex-K is not directly interchangeable with Neo-NaClex because of the difference in bendrofluazide content.

Uses The potassium chloride contained in Neo-NaClex-K provides a useful supplement to help offset the potassium-losing effect of bendrofluazide.

Essential hypertension: The mechanism whereby the thiazides exert their antihypertensive effect has not been clearly established. In non-oedematous patients there may be little noticeable diuretic effect. Neo-NaClex-K may be used as the sole antihypertensive agent, or as an adjunct to other drugs whose action it may enhance.

Oedema: Neo-NaClex-K inhibits the renal tubular absorption of salt and water by its action at the beginning of the distal convoluted tubule. Sodium and chloride ions are excreted in equivalent proportions. Because potassium excretion is promoted, metabolic alkalosis may occur secondary to hypokalaemia. There is no important effect upon carbonic anhydrase. Neo-NaClex-K causes a steady diuresis lasting for about 12 hours. It is indicated in the treatment of oedema associated with conditions such as congestive heart failure, nephrotic syndrome, and cirrhosis of the liver.

Dosage and administration *Adults:* Neo-NaClex-K tablets should be swallowed whole with water.

When Neo-NaClex-K is added to other antihypertensive drugs, the dosage of the latter can usually be reduced gradually as the Neo-NaClex-K takes effect.

Essential hypertension: One to 4 tablets once daily, alone or in conjunction with other antihypertensive agents.

Oedema: Two tablets given orally once daily in the morning usually produce the desired effect without diuresis interfering with sleep, but this dose can be increased to 4 tablets if required. During the first few days of treatment there is usually a large increase in urinary volume, which diminishes as treatment continues.

Maintenance: Many patients will respond adequately to a daily dose of 1 or 2 tablets on only two or three days in the week.

Children: Neo-NaClex-K is not recommended for children.

Elderly: (See 'Precautions').

Contra-indications, warnings, etc
Contra-indications: Severe renal or hepatic failure, hypersensitivity to the product or other sulphonamide-like drugs, Addison's disease, diabetic keto-acidosis, hyperkalaemia and hypercalcaemia. Neo-NaClex-K is a solid potassium-containing preparation and is therefore contra-indicated in conditions of the gastro-intestinal tract where strictures may form. Neo-NaClex-K should not be administered concurrently with lithium carbonate.

Precautions: When treatment is prolonged and intensive, potassium depletion can develop insidiously. Periodic estimations of serum electrolyte should be done. Neo-NaClex-K Tablets usually provide sufficient potassium to maintain the serum concentration in hypertension, but it is sometimes advisable to give potassium chloride in addition to that contained in Neo-NaClex-K. If the patient is vomiting, has diarrhoea or is suffering from an acute febrile or chronic illness (especially cirrhosis of the liver or heart failure) supplementary potassium may be particularly important. Additional potassium chloride to prevent hypokalaemia and the danger of arrhythmias and other ECG changes is strongly recommended if patients receiving digitalis require prolonged treatment. In concurrent therapy with carbenoxolone or corticosteroids, additional potassium supplements are recommended. Patients at risk of myocardial infarction and patients admitted for cardiac surgery also need potassium supplements.

Potassium depletion may cause polyuria, malaise, muscle weakness or cramp, decreased tendon reflexes, anorexia, dizziness, nausea or vomiting. Also sensitivity to digitalis may increase and signs of overdosage appear. Prolonged potassium deficiency may induce chronic pyelonephritis. Renal function should be monitored. Neo-NaClex-K and additional potassium supplements must not be given in renal insufficiency complicated by hyperkalaemia.

In addition, in prolonged therapy, it is necessary to test for glycosuria and investigate polyuria. In renal insufficiency, renal function should be monitored. The possibility of magnesium depletion should also be considered.

In cirrhosis of the liver, thiazides may precipitate hepatic encephalopathy.

Thiazides may aggravate existing diabetes mellitus and cause symptoms in patients with latent disease. Neo-NaClex-K may impair control of diabetes in patients receiving sulphonylureas. Thiazides should be used with caution in systemic lupus erythematosus.

Serum uric acid levels may be raised, with or without gout, in some patients. Thiazides may cause or aggravate hyperlipidaemia; pancreatitis may occur.

The elderly: The elderly are sensitive to the effects of thiazides on blood pressure and electrolyte. Administration of supplementary potassium is particularly important in the elderly. Patients with prostatic hypertrophy may develop acute urinary retention.

Pregnancy: Diuretics are best avoided in the management of oedema of pregnancy or hypertension in pregnancy as their use may be associated with hypovolaemia, increased blood viscosity and reduced placental perfusion. There is inadequate evidence of safety in human pregnancy. There are reports of fetal and neonatal bone marrow depression, thrombocytopenia, electrolyte imbalance, hypoglycaemia and jaundice. Expectant mothers who receive thiazide diuretics may be at increased risk from acute haemorrhagic pancreatitis. In parturition, thiazides may cause uterine inertia and delay the onset of labour. Thiazides are only indicated in pregnancy if oedema complicates a pathological lesion and, even then, after assessing risk versus benefit including the undesirability of administering drugs in the first trimester. As thiazide diuretics are secreted in mothers' milk, breast feeding should be avoided.

Side-effects: If abdominal pain, distension, nausea, vomiting or gastro-intestinal bleeding occur during the administration of tablets containing potassium salts, they should be discontinued immediately. Small bowel lesions are usually associated with enteric-coated tablets and are less likely to occur with Neo-NaClex-K.

The following have been reported: disturbances of electrolyte, acid-base balance, lipids, glucose and uric acid levels; thirst, polyuria, weakness, dizziness, muscle cramps and reversible impotence; nausea, vomiting, mild anorexia, gastric irritation, diarrhoea or constipation; rashes, skin reactions, purpura and blood dyscrasias including thrombocytopenia; hypocalciuria, precipitation of gout, pancreatitis, hepatic encephalopathy and postural hypotension.

Interactions:

Diabetes mellitus: Thiazides may impair control in diabetics receiving sulphonylureas.

Lithium toxicity: The renal clearance of lithium carbonate is reduced; concomitant use is contra-indicated.

Anaesthesia: Halothane's hypotensive effect is increased by thiazides.

Sensitivity to tubocurarine is increased in hypokalaemia. Plasma potassium should be monitored prior to its use in thiazide-treated patients.

Antagonism and hypokalaemia: Carbenoxolone, indomethacin, phenylbutazone, and corticosteroids may both antagonise thiazides' hypotensive effect and increase potassium loss. Monitoring and potassium supplements are recommended.

Hypotension: Enhanced hypotensive effects may follow the concomitant use of thiazides and barbiturates, alcohol, other antihypertensives (e.g. beta-blocking agents, ACE inhibitors, calcium antagonists), MAOIs or narcotics.

Hypersensitivity: Use of allopurinol and a thiazide in patients with renal dysfunction should be avoided: severe hypersensitivity vasculitis has been reported.

Hypokalaemic effects: Hypokalaemia secondary to the use of thiazides may increase the toxicity of cardiac glycosides and antagonise the effect of anti-arrhythmics.

Potassium imbalance: Caution is required in the use of Neo-NaClex-K with any drug/disease state which has a potential for producing potassium imbalance.

Vitamin B_{12}: Potassium chloride, as in Neo-NaClex-K, may reduce absorption of oral vitamin B_{12}.

Overdosage: CNS depression (e.g. drowsiness, lethargy and coma) may occur without cardiovascular or respiratory depression. Hypovolaemia, hyperkalaemia and mild hypoglycaemia are likely to be present. In the case of recent ingestion, gastric lavage should be carried out; activated charcoal may help reduce absorption. Treatment should be symptomatic and directed at fluid replacement and correction of imbalance of electrolyte which should be monitored together with the blood pressure and renal function.

Severe hyperkalaemia following overdose with potassium-containing thiazide combinations is rare. Lethargy, confusion, muscle weakness, paralysis, arrhythmia or cardiac arrest may occur. Measurement of plasma potassium, ECG monitoring and correction of any abnormalities is required. Other treatment depends on the plasma potassium concentration.

When this is less than 6.5 mEq/L, fluid replacement with oral calcium polystyrene sulphonate is recommended. For levels of 6.5 mEq/L or greater urgent treatment is required with intravenous insulin, glucose, sodium bicarbonate and/or calcium gluconate, oral calcium polystyrene sulphonate and possibly haemodialysis.

Hyponatraemia should be treated with water deprivation rather than by the administration of NaCl. Cathartics should be avoided.

Pharmaceutical precautions Protect from light and moisture.

Legal category POM.

Package quantities Containers of 100 and 500 tablets.

Further information Nil.

Product licence number 0021/5907R.

PARVOLEX*

Presentation Parvolex is a clear, colourless, sterile, pyrogen-free, aqueous solution of 20% w/v Acetylcysteine BP (N-acetyl-3-mercapto-alanine) adjusted to pH 7.0 with sodium hydroxide. Parvolex contains 200 mg acetylcysteine in each ml i.e., each 10 ml ampoule contains 2 g.

Uses Acetylcysteine is a derivative of the naturally-occurring amino acid L-cysteine.

In paracetamol overdosage the observed hepatotoxicity is due to the formation of a toxic metabolite which is thought to cause liver cell damage and necrosis. Hepatic-reduced glutathione inactivates the toxic metabolite by conjugation but glutathione stores are rapidly depleted with hepatotoxic doses of paracetamol. Acetylcysteine, being a sulphydryl (SH) group donor, protects the liver possibly by restoring depleted hepatic-reduced glutathione or by acting as an alternative substrate for the toxic paracetamol metabolite.

Indications: Paracetamol overdosage.

Dosage and administration An initial dose of 150 mg/kg body weight of acetylcysteine is infused in 200 ml of 5% dextrose intravenously over 15 minutes, followed by an intravenous infusion of 50 mg/kg body weight in 500 ml of 5% dextrose over the next four hours, and 100 mg/kg body weight in 1 litre of 5% dextrose over the next 16 hours. (This gives a total dose of 300 mg/kg body weight of acetylcysteine in 20 hours.)

NOTE: Parvolex contains 200 mg acetylcysteine per ml; i.e., each 10 ml ampoule contains 2 g.

Children: The quantity of intravenous fluid used in children should be modified to take into account age and weight.

Critical times: Parvolex is very effective when administered up to eight hours after paracetamol overdosage. The protective effect falls off slowly between eight and ten hours, more rapidly after ten hours and increasingly between twelve and fifteen hours. Parvolex is ineffective after fifteen hours and its use after this time may be associated with harmful effects.

Contra-indications, warnings, etc Hypersensitivity to any ingredient in the preparation.

Precautions: Administer with caution in asthma or a history of bronchospasm. Acetylcysteine is not compatible with rubber and metals, particularly, iron, copper and nickel. Silicone rubber and plastic are satisfactory for use with Parvolex.

Pregnancy: The safety of Parvolex in pregnancy has not been established.

Side-effects: Rash and anaphylaxis have been reported. These have occurred between fifteen minutes and one hour after the start of the infusion.

Hypokalaemia and ECG changes have been noted in patients with paracetamol poisoning irrespective of the treatment given. Monitoring of plasma potassium concentration is therefore recommended.

Overdosage: There is a theoretical risk of hepatic encephalopathy. There is no specific treatment and general supportive measures should be carried out.

Pharmaceutical precautions Store below 25°C.

Legal category POM.

Package quantities Parvolex is supplied in ampoules of 10 ml. 10 × 10 ml ampoules are packed in printed cartons.

Further information Nil.

Product licence number 0021/0086.

PREGADAY* TABLETS

Presentation Pregaday Tablets are reddish brown, film-coated tablets engraved 'Pregaday' on one face. Each tablet contains Ferrous Fumarate BP equivalent to 100 mg ferrous iron and 350 micrograms (0.35 mg) anhydrous folic acid.

Uses There is evidence that a daily intake of 100 mg of elemental iron in the ferrous form is adequate to prevent development of iron deficiency in expectant mothers. If a mild iron deficiency is present when Pregaday administration is started, this will be corrected by increased absorption of iron. The daily folate requirement rises steeply during the final trimester of pregnancy, and evidence of maternal depletion may be found. To ensure normal tissue folate levels in the mother after delivery, a daily supplement of about 300 micrograms is required during the second and third trimester of pregnancy. This dose does not obscure the blood picture of Addisonian pernicious anaemia. Pregaday is indicated during the second and third trimester of pregnancy for prophylaxis against iron deficiency and megaloblastic anaemia of pregnancy. Pregaday is not intended as a treatment for established megaloblastic anaemia of pregnancy.

Dosage and administration It is usual to begin therapy with Pregaday about the thirteenth week of pregnancy (see Precautions) either as routine prophylaxis or selectively if the haemoglobin concentration is less than 11 grams/100 ml (less than 75% of normal).

One tablet daily by mouth (the foil enclosing the tablets is printed with the days of the week in sequence).

Contra-indications, warnings, etc
Contra-indications: Vitamin B_{12} deficiency.

Known hypersensitivity to the product. Paroxysmal nocturnal haemoglobinuria, haemosiderosis, haemochromatosis, active peptic ulcer, repeated blood transfusion, regional enteritis and ulcerative colitis.

Pregaday must not be used in the treatment of anaemias other than those due to iron deficiency.

Precautions:
Pregnancy: Administration of Pregaday during the first trimester of pregnancy may be undesirable.

A minority of pregnant women are not protected by physiological doses of folic acid. The development of anaemia despite prophylaxis with Pregaday calls for investigation.

Some post-gastrectomy patients show poor absorption of iron. Care is needed when treating iron deficiency anaemia in patients with treated or controlled peptic ulceration.

Caution should be exercised when administering folic acid to patients who may have folate dependent tumours.

Since anaemia due to combined iron and Vitamin B_{12} or folate deficiencies may be microcytic in type, patients with microcytic anaemia resistant to therapy with iron alone should be screened for Vitamin B_{12} or folate deficiency.

Pregaday Tablets should be kept out of the reach of children.

Side-effects: Gastro-intestinal disorders have been reported including gastro-intestinal discomfort, anorexia, nausea, vomiting, constipation, diarrhoea. Darkening of the stools may occur.

Rarely, allergic reactions may occur.

Interactions: Iron reduces the absorption of penicillamine. Absorption of both iron and antibiotic may be reduced if Pregaday is given with a tetracycline.

Concurrent administration of antacids may reduce absorption of iron.

Co-trimoxazole, chloramphenicol or sulphasalazine may interfere with folate metabolism. Serum levels of anticonvulsant drugs may be reduced by administration of folate. Oral chloramphenicol delays plasma iron clearance, incorporation of iron into red blood cells and interferes with erythropoiesis.

Some inhibition of iron absorption may occur if it is taken with cholestyramine, tea, eggs or milk.

Overdosage: Acute overdosage of oral iron requires emergency treatment. In young children, 200 to 250 mg/kg ferrous fumarate is considered to be extremely dangerous.

Symptoms and signs of abdominal pain, vomiting and diarrhoea appear within 60 minutes. Cardiovascular collapse with coma may follow. Some improvement may occur after this phase which in some patients, is followed by recovery. In others, after about sixteen hours, deterioration may occur involving diffuse vascular congestion, pulmonary oedema, convulsions, anuria, hypothermia, severe shock, metabolic acidosis, coagulation abnormalities or hypoglycaemia.

Vomiting should be induced immediately, followed as soon as possible by parenteral injection of desferrioxamine mesylate, and then gastric lavage. In the meantime, it is helpful to give milk and/or 5% sodium bicarbonate solution by mouth.

Dissolve 2 grams desferrioxamine mesylate in 2 to 3 ml of Water for Injections and give intramuscularly. A solution of 5 grams desferrioxamine in 50 to 100 ml of fluid may be left in the stomach. If desferrioxamine is not available, leave 300 ml of 1% to 5% sodium bicarbonate solution in the stomach. Fluid replacement is essential.

Recovery may be complicated by long-term sequelae such as hepatic necrosis, pyloric stenosis or acute toxic encephalitis which may lead to CNS damage.

Pharmaceutical precautions Protect from light.

Legal category P.

Package quantities Cartons of two calendar blister packs of 14 tablets (OP).

Further information Nil.

Product licence number 0021/0119.

SCOLINE*

Presentation A clear, colourless, sterile solution containing Suxamethonium Chloride (succinylcholine chloride) BP 50 mg per ml. This is equivalent to 36.5 mg of active cation.

Uses Scoline is a depolarising, short-acting neuromuscular blocking agent for intravenous administration. It is suitable for brief procedures in which profound muscular relaxation is required such as tracheal intubation, short operations, orthopaedic manipulations, electroconvulsive therapy and closure of the peritoneum. Prolonged muscular relaxation in surgery can be attained by means of repeated injections of the drug or by continuous intravenous drip.

Dosage and administration Scoline must not be administered to the conscious patient. It is given intravenously after anaesthesia has been induced (e.g. after thiopentone and from a different syringe) and should be accompanied by assisted respiration. The dosage for children and adults depends on body weight and is 0.6 mg/kg (range 0.3 to 1.1 mg/kg depending on the degree of relaxation required) i.v. over 10 to 30 seconds. The maximum total dose is 100 mg. It ranges from 20 mg (0.4 ml) to 100 mg (2 ml) according to the body weight of the patient and the degree of muscular relaxation required. In adults the dosage for intubation is from 50mg (1 ml) to 80 mg (1.6 ml), for electroconvulsive therapy 40 mg (0.8 ml) to 75 mg (1.5 ml) and for manipulation 80 mg (1.6 ml). For administration by continuous intravenous drip, a 0.1% solution may be prepared by mixing 10 ml injection of Scoline with 500 ml of 5% glucose or isotonic sodium chloride. The adult dose ranges from 2 to 5 mg per minute.

Contra-indications, warnings, etc
Contra-indications: Scoline should not be used in patients known to have atypical serum pseudocholinesterase or low serum levels of pseudocholinesterase. Deficiency of this serum enzyme may occur as a very rare inherited characteristic or result from liver disease, severe anaemia, malnutrition or poisoning with an organo-phosphorus insecticide.

Patients with myasthenia gravis are resistant to Scoline and a state of dual block may develop rapidly.

Patients with the myasthenic (Eaton-Lambert) syndrome are relatively sensitive to Scoline and the dose should be reduced.

If eye drops containing long-acting cholinesterase inhibitor drugs, such as ecothiopate iodide (Phospholine iodide* Ayerst Laboratories Ltd) or demecarium bromide (Tosmilen* Sinclair), are used within a period of one month prior to an operation, then decreased plasma cholinesterase levels may preclude the use of Scoline.

Scoline should not be used in ophthalmic cases including those with penetrating wounds of the eye or when the anterior chamber of the eye is open. Nor must it be used in cases of hyperkalaemia, severe burns, massive trauma, tetanus, myotonia or muscular rigidity, muscular disease or neurological disorders.

Precautions: Neostigmine and other anticholinesterase drugs are not antidotes to Scoline but would normally have the effect of intensifying the depolarisation effect. However, in some cases of prolonged apnoea following Scoline, a state of 'dual block' may be responsible. In dual block the muscle relaxation is due to non-depolarising blockade and is reversible with neostigmine. To investigate this possibility the short-acting anticholinesterase drug, edrophonium, should be given and a transitory return of muscle power confirms the presence of dual block, which can then be reversed with neostigmine. In seriously burnt children Scoline can precipitate gross cardiac arrhythmias and cardiac arrest. This can be prevented by the administration of tubocurarine 6 mg five minutes before giving Scoline. Sinus tachycardia and rise in blood pressure has occurred after the continuous infusion of suxamethonium chloride. Care should be taken with patients currently receiving systemic antibiotics such as streptomycin, neomycin, kanamycin, tobramycin, framycetin, amikacin, gentamicin, colistin and the polymyxins, as they can potentiate the action of Scoline. Renal failure, trauma and mild burns may increase the risk of hyperkalaemia with Scoline.

Since the initial contractions caused by Scoline are painful, Scoline should not be administered until the anaesthetic has taken full effect. Suxamethonium chloride is fairly quickly hydrolysed by thiopentone therefore, when this anaesthetic is used, Scoline should be injected after thiopentone using a different syringe.

The Elderly: Caution is required because of the possible cardiovascular effects of depolarising agents.

Pregnancy: The drug should not be administered to pregnant women unless the potential benefit outweighs the possible hazard.

When given in high doses Scoline may pass the placental barrier.

Since neonates have low pseudocholinesterase activity, caution is required if Scoline is used during Caesarean Section.

It should also be noted that during pregnancy and for some days post-partum, maternal pseudocholinesterase activity is also low.

Side-effects: Muscle pain (particularly in the muscles of the chest, abdomen and shoulder girdle) can occur following the use of Scoline. It occurs most frequently in patients who are ambulant in the early post-operative period and can be avoided by the prior administration of any of the non-depolarising muscle relaxants. Bradyarrhythmias are common when Scoline is used with halothane or cyclopropane anaesthesia. Thiopentone may protect against the effects. Its use is inadvisable in patients with phaeochromocytoma.

Malignant hyperpyrexia is a rare, possibly fatal, complication in patients anaesthetised with general anaesthetic agents and has been increasingly associated with concomitant administration of suxamethonium chloride. It occurs in apparently healthy individuals genetically predisposed to this syndrome.

Myoglobinuria has been reported, either alone or associated with malignant hyperpyrexia.

Other side-effects which have been reported include hypertension, fever, hypersensitivity reactions and bronchospasm.

Suxamethonium chloride causes a transient rise in intra-ocular pressure and salivary gland enlargement. There may be some increase in bowel movements and in gastric and salivary secretions due to the muscarinic action of suxamethonium chloride.

Interactions: The effect of Scoline may be reduced by: diazepam and propranolol and enhanced by: oxytocin (prolonged, but less intense); procainamide; procaine; lignocaine; the phenothiazines, promazine, propanidid; phenelzine; cytotoxic alkylating agents; whole body irradiation; lithium carbonate, quinidine; meturedepa; amphotericin; aminoglycoside antibiotics, e.g. streptomycin, neomycin, kanamycin, tobramycin, framycetin, amikacin, and gentamicin; other antibiotics, e.g. colistin, polymyxins, rolitetracycline and oxytetracycline.

The time to 25% twitch-height recovery is not changed in women taking oral contraceptives.

Hexafluorenium bromide has been used to prolong the relaxant effects of Scoline.

Overdosage: Because Scoline is usually administered by an anaesthetist, overdosage is unlikely. However, the unsuspected presence of low pseudocholinesterase levels in the serum, or this being replaced by the atypical enzyme, or the occurrence of dual block, can lead to a similar situation: prolonged apnoea. Management first consists of maintaining light anaesthesia and continued mechanical respiration to ensure an adequate supply of oxygen whilst the cause is determined. Dual block can be recognised by the response to edrophonium, and treatment then consists of reversal with neostigmine. Subsequently, the patient should remain under observation as the dual block may outlast the duration of action of neostigmine (at least 20 minutes) and if apnoea recurs a further dose of neostigmine is indicated. Apnoea due to atypical or low serum cholinesterase levels can be corrected by intravenous administration of a highly concentrated preparation of pseudocholinesterase or transfusion of plasma or whole blood.

Pharmaceutical precautions Scoline should be stored at as low a temperature as possible above its freezing point and not exceeding 4°C; under these conditions it may be expected to retain its potency for at least two years from the date of preparation.

Scoline Injection should not be re-sterilised.

Legal category POM.

Package quantities Scoline is available in boxes of five 2 ml ampoules.

Further information Nil.

Product licence number 0021/5024R.

TRANDATE* INJECTION

Presentation Trandate Injection: 20 ml ampoules each containing 100 mg (5 mg/ml) labetalol hydrochloride in an aqueous colourless solution.

Labetalol hydrochloride is 2-hydroxy-5-[1-hydroxy-2-(1-methyl-3-phenyl-propylamino) ethyl] benzamide hydrochloride.

Uses *Indications:* Trandate Injection is indicated when rapid control of blood pressure is essential in severely hypertensive patients including severe hypertension of pregnancy and for use in anaesthesia where a hypotensive technique is indicated.

It is also indicated in hypertensive episodes following acute myocardial infarction.

Mode of action: Trandate lowers the blood pressure primarily by blocking alpha-adrenoceptors in peripheral arterioles and thereby reducing the peripheral resistance. Concurrent beta-blockade protects the heart from reflex sympathetic drive normally induced by peripheral vasodilatation. Cardiac output is not significantly reduced at rest or after moderate exercise. Increases in systolic pressure during exercise are, however, reduced after Trandate; corresponding changes in diastolic pressure are essentially normal. All these effects would be expected to benefit hypertensive patients.

Dosage and administration

Adults: Trandate Injection is intended for intravenous use in hospitalised patients. The plasma concentrations achieved after intravenous doses of Trandate in severe hypertension are substantially greater than those following oral administration of the drug and provide the greater degree of blockade of alpha-adrenoceptors necessary to control the more severe disease. Patients should, therefore, always receive the drug whilst in the supine or left lateral position. Raising the patient into the upright position, within three hours of intravenous Trandate administration, should be avoided since excessive postural hypotension may occur.

Bolus injection: If it is essential to reduce the blood

pressure quickly, as, for example, in hypertensive encephalopathy, a dose of 50 mg of Trandate should be given by intravenous injection over a period of at least one minute. If necessary, doses of 50 mg may be repeated at five minute intervals until a satisfactory response occurs. The total dose should not exceed 200 mg. After bolus injection, the maximum effect usually occurs within five minutes and the effective duration of action is usually about six hours but may be as long as eighteen hours.

Intravenous infusion: An alternative method for administering Trandate is intravenous infusion of a solution made by diluting the contents of two ampoules (200 mg) to 200 ml with Sodium Chloride and Dextrose Injection BP or 5% Dextrose Intravenous Infusion BP. The resultant infusion solution contains 1 mg/ml of Trandate. It should be administered using a paediatric giving set fitted with a 50 ml graduated burette to facilitate dosage.

In the hypertensions of pregnancy, the infusion can be started at the rate of 20 mg per hour and this dose may be doubled every thirty minutes until a satisfactory reduction in blood pressure has been obtained or a dosage of 160 mg per hour is reached. Occasionally, higher doses may be necessary.

In hypertensive episodes following acute myocardial infarction, infusion should be commenced at 15 mg per hour and gradually increased to a maximum of 120 mg per hour, depending on the control of blood pressure.

In hypertension due to other causes the rate of infusion of Trandate should be about 2 mg (2 ml of infusion solution) per minute, until a satisfactory response is obtained; the infusion should then be stopped. The effective dose is usually in the range of 50 to 200 mg, depending on the severity of the hypertension. For most patients it is unnecessary to administer more than 200 mg but larger doses may be required especially in patients with phaeochromocytoma. The rate of infusion may be adjusted according to the response, at the discretion of the physician. The blood pressure and pulse rate should be monitored throughout the infusion.

It is desirable to monitor the heart rate after injection and during infusion. In most patients, there is a small decrease in the heart rate; severe bradycardia is unusual but may be controlled by injecting atropine 1 to 2 mg intravenously. Respiratory function should be observed particularly in patients with any known impairment.

Once the blood pressure has been adequately reduced, maintenance therapy with Trandate Tablets should be instituted with a starting dose of one 100 mg tablet twice daily. (See Trandate Tablets Data Sheet for further details.) Trandate Injection has been administered to patients with uncontrolled hypertension already receiving other hypotensive agents, including beta-blocking drugs, without adverse effects.

In hypotensive anaesthesia induction should be with standard agents (e.g. sodium thiopentone) and anaesthesia maintained with nitrous oxide and oxygen with or without halothane. The recommended starting dose of Trandate Injection is 10 to 20 mg intravenously depending on the age and condition of the patient. Patients for whom halothane is contra-indicated usually require a higher initial dose of Trandate (25 to 30 mg). If satisfactory hypotension is not achieved after five minutes, increments of 5 to 10 mg should be given until the desired level of blood pressure is attained.

Halothane and Trandate act synergistically therefore the halothane concentration should not exceed 1 to 1.5% as profound falls in blood pressure may be precipitated. Following Trandate Injection the blood pressure can be quickly and easily adjusted by altering the halothane concentration and/or adjusting table tilt. The mean duration of hypotension following 20 to 25 mg of Trandate is fifty minutes.

Hypotension induced by Trandate Injection is readily reversed by atropine 0.6 mg and discontinuation of halothane.

Tubocurarine and pancuronium may be used when assisted or controlled ventilation is required. IPPV may further increase the hypotension resulting from Trandate Injection and/or halothane.

Children: Safety and efficacy have not been established.

Contra-indications, warnings, etc *Contra-indications:* Hypersensitivity to labetalol, second or third degree heart block, cardiogenic shock and other conditions associated with severe and prolonged hypotension or severe bradycardia.

Where peripheral vasoconstriction suggests low cardiac output, the use of Trandate Injection to control hypertensive episodes following acute myocardial infarction is contra-indicated.

Precautions: There have been rare reports of severe hepatocellular injury with labetalol therapy. The hepatic injury is usually reversible and has occurred after both short-term and long-term treatment. Appropriate laboratory testing should be done at the first sign or symptom of liver dysfunction. If there is laboratory evidence of liver injury or the patient is jaundiced, labetalol should be stopped and not re-started.

Where cardiac reserve is poor, control with a cardiac glycoside and a diuretic should be obtained prior to cautious use of Trandate Injection.

Beta-blockers, even those with apparent cardioselectivity, should not be used in patients with asthma or a history of obstructive airways disease unless no alternative treatment is available. In such cases, the risk of inducing bronchospasm should be appreciated and appropriate precautions taken. If bronchospasm should occur after the use of Trandate, it can be treated with a beta$_2$-agonist by inhalation e.g. salbutamol (the dose of which may need to be greater than the usual dose in asthma) and if necessary intravenous atropine 1 mg.

It is not necessary to discontinue Trandate therapy in patients requiring anaesthesia but they should be given intravenous atropine prior to induction; the effect of halothane on blood pressure may be enhanced by Trandate. During anaesthesia Trandate may mask the compensatory physiological responses to sudden haemorrhage (tachycardia and vasoconstriction). Close attention must therefore be paid to blood loss and the blood volume maintained.

Care should be taken in the concomitant use of labetalol and either Class I antiarrhythmic agents or calcium antagonists of the verapamil type.

Risk of anaphylactic reaction: While taking beta-blockers, patients with a history of severe anaphylactic reaction to a variety of allergens may be more reactive to repeated challenge, either accidental, diagnostic or therapeutic. Such patients may be unresponsive to the usual doses of adrenaline used to treat allergic reaction.

Pregnancy: Although no teratogenic effects have been demonstrated in animals, Trandate should only be used during the first trimester of pregnancy if the potential benefit outweighs the potential risk. Trandate crosses the placental barrier and the possibility of the consequences of alpha- and beta-adrenoceptor blockade in the fetus and neonate should be borne in mind.

Perinatal and neonatal distress (bradycardia, hypotension, respiratory depression, hypoglycaemia, hypothermia) has been rarely reported. Sometimes these symptoms developed a day or two after birth. Response to supportive measures (e.g. intravenous fluids and glucose) is usually prompt but with severe pre-eclampsia, particularly after prolonged intravenous labetalol, recovery may be slower. This may be related to diminished liver metabolism in premature babies. Intra-uterine and neonatal deaths have been reported but other drugs (e.g. vasodilators, respiratory depressants) and the effects of pre-eclampsia, intra-uterine growth retardation and prematurity were implicated.

Such clinical experience warns against unduly prolonging high dose labetalol and delaying delivery and against co-administration of hydralazine.

Trandate is excreted in breast milk. No adverse effects in breast feeding infants have been reported.

Side-effects: Trandate Injection is usually well tolerated. Excessive postural hypotension may occur if patients are allowed to assume the upright position within three hours of receiving Trandate Injection.

There have been a few reports of nasal congestion and

rare reports of hypersensitivity: rash, pruritus, angio-edema and dyspnoea.

There are rare reports of raised liver function tests, jaundice (both hepatocellular and cholestatic), hepatitis and hepatic necrosis. The signs and symptoms are usually reversible on withdrawal of the drug.

There are rare reports of bradycardia and heart block.

Overdosage: Profound cardiovascular effects are to be expected, e.g. excessive, posture-sensitive hypotension and sometimes bradycardia. Patients should be laid supine with the legs raised. Use a cardiac glycoside and a diuretic in cardiac failure; for bronchospasm, administer a beta$_2$-agonist per aerosol. Intravenous atropine 0.25 to 3 mg should be given to relieve bradycardia. Intravenous noradrenaline 5 to 10 micrograms initially, repeated according to response, may be preferable to isoprenaline to improve the circulation. Alternatively, noradrenaline may be infused at a rate of 5 micrograms per minute until the response is satisfactory.

In severe overdose, intravenous glucagon may be preferred: an initial bolus dose of 5 to 10 mg in dextrose or saline should be followed by an intravenous infusion of 5 mg/hour or as sufficient to maintain cardiac output. Transvenous pacing may be required.

Oliguric renal failure has been reported after massive overdose of labetalol orally. In one case, the use of dopamine to increase the blood pressure may have aggravated the renal failure.

Haemodialysis removes less than 1% labetalol HCl from the circulation.

Pharmaceutical precautions Protect from light.

Trandate Injection is incompatible with Sodium Bicarbonate Injection BP 4.2% w/v.

Legal category POM.

Package quantities *Trandate Injection 20 ml ampoules:* Boxes of 5.

Further information Trandate does not adversely affect renal function and is a particularly suitable drug for use in hypertensive patients with renal disease. The metabolites of Trandate are excreted in the faeces as well as in the urine and so the drug is unlikely to accumulate in the body even in renal failure.

The plasma half-life of Trandate is about four hours. Only about 50% of Trandate in the blood is protein bound.

Trandate fluoresces in alkaline solution at an excitation wavelength of 334 nm and a fluorescence wavelength of 412 nm and may therefore interfere with the assays of certain fluorescent substances.

The presence of labetalol metabolites in the urine may result in falsely elevated levels of urinary catecholamines, metanephrine, normetanephrine, and vanillylmandelic acid (VMA) when measured by fluorimetric or photometric methods. In screening patients suspected of having a phaeochromocytoma and being treated with Trandate a specific method, such as a high performance liquid chromatographic assay with solid phase extraction (e.g. J. Chromatogr. 385, 241, 1987) should be employed in determining levels of catecholamines.

Product licence number 0021/0130.

TRANDATE* TABLETS

Presentation

Trandate Tablets: Circular, orange-coloured, film-coated, biconvex tablets marked TRANDATE and the strength in milligrams on one face.

Trandate Tablets 50 mg: each containing labetalol hydrochloride 50 mg

Trandate Tablets 100 mg: each containing labetalol hydrochloride 100 mg

Trandate Tablets 200 mg: each containing labetalol hydrochloride 200 mg

Trandate Tablets 400 mg: each containing labetalol hydrochloride 400 mg

Labetalol hydrochloride is 2-hydroxy-5-[1-hydroxy-2 (1-methyl-3-phenyl-propylamino) ethyl] benzamide hydrochloride.

Uses

Indications: Trandate Tablets are indicated in mild, moderate and severe hypertension including the hypertensions of pregnancy, when oral therapy is desirable.

Trandate Tablets are also indicated in angina pectoris with existing hypertension.

Actions: Trandate lowers blood pressure by blocking peripheral arteriolar alpha-adrenoceptors, thus reducing peripheral resistance, and by concurrent beta-blockade, protects the heart from reflex sympathetic drive that would otherwise occur. Cardiac output is not significantly reduced at rest or after moderate exercise. Increases in systolic blood pressure during exercise are reduced but corresponding changes in diastolic pressure are essentially normal.

In patients with angina pectoris co-existing with hypertension, the reduced peripheral resistance decreases myocardial after-load and oxygen demand. All these effects would be expected to benefit hypertensive patients and those with co-existing angina.

Dosage and administration Trandate Tablets should be taken with food.

Adults

Hypertension: Treatment should start with 100 mg twice daily. In patients already being treated with antihypertensives and in those of low body weight this may be sufficient to control blood pressure. In others, increases in dosage of 100 mg twice daily should be made at fortnightly intervals. Many patients' blood pressure is controlled by 200 mg twice daily and up to 800 mg daily may be given as a twice daily regimen. In severe, refractory hypertension, daily doses up to 2,400 mg have been given. Such doses should be divided into a three or four times a day regimen.

Elderly: In elderly patients, an initial dose of 50 mg twice daily is recommended. This has provided satisfactory control in some cases.

In hypertensions of pregnancy: The initial dosage of 100 mg twice daily may be increased, if necessary, at weekly intervals by 100 mg twice daily. During the second and third trimesters, the severity of the hypertension may require further dose titration to a three times daily regimen, ranging from 100 mg t.d.s. to 400 mg t.d.s. A total daily dose of 2,400 mg should not be exceeded.

Hospital in-patients with severe hypertension, particularly of pregnancy, may have daily increases in dosage.

General: If rapid reduction of blood pressure is necessary, see the data sheet for Trandate Injection. If long-term control of hypertension following the use of Trandate Injection is required, oral therapy with Trandate Tablets should start with 100 mg twice daily.

Additive hypotensive effects may be expected if Trandate Tablets are administered together with other antihypertensives, e.g. diuretics, methyldopa etc. When transferring patients from such agents, Trandate Tablets should be introduced with a dosage of 100 mg twice daily and the previous therapy gradually decreased. Abrupt withdrawal of clonidine or beta-blocking agents is undesirable.

Angina co-existing with hypertension: In patients with angina pectoris co-existing with hypertension, the dose of Trandate will be that required to control the hypertension.

Children: Safety and efficacy in children have not been established.

Contra-indications, warnings, etc

Contra-indications: Trandate Tablets are contra-indicated in second or third degree heart block, cardiogenic shock and other conditions associated with severe and prolonged hypotension or severe bradycardia.

Labetalol is contra-indicated for patients known to have a hypersensitivity to the drug.

Warnings: There have been reports of skin rashes and/or dry eyes associated with the use of beta-adrenoceptor blocking drugs. The reported incidence is small and in most cases the symptoms have cleared when the treatment was withdrawn. Gradual discontinuance of the drug should be considered if any such reaction is not otherwise explicable.

There have been rare reports of severe hepatocellular injury with labetalol therapy. The hepatic injury is usually reversible and has occurred after both short-term and long-term treatment. Appropriate laboratory testing should be done at the first sign or symptom of liver dysfunction. If there is laboratory evidence of liver injury or the patient is jaundiced, labetalol should be stopped and not re-started.

Precautions: Special care should be taken with patients whose cardiac reserve is poor and heart failure should be controlled with a cardiac glycoside and diuretic before starting Trandate therapy.

Beta-blockers, even those with apparent cardioselectivity, should not be used in patients with asthma or a history of obstructive airways disease unless no alternative treatment is available. In such cases, the risk of inducing bronchospasm should be appreciated and appropriate precautions taken. If bronchospasm should occur after the use of Trandate, it can be treated with a beta$_2$-agonist by inhalation e.g. salbutamol (the dose of which may need to be greater than the usual dose in asthma) and, if necessary, intravenous atropine 1 mg.

Trandate Tablets need not be discontinued prior to anaesthesia but patients should receive intravenous atropine prior to induction. Trandate may enhance the hypotensive effect of halothane. Care should be taken if labetalol is used concomitantly with Class I anti-arrhythmic agents or calcium antagonists of the verapamil type.

Patients, particularly those with ischaemic heart disease, should not interrupt/discontinue abruptly Trandate therapy.

Risk of anaphylactic reaction: While taking betablockers, patients with a history of severe anaphylactic reaction to a variety of allergens may be more reactive to repeated challenge, either accidental, diagnostic or therapeutic. Such patients may be unresponsive to the usual doses of adrenaline used to treat allergic reaction.

Pregnancy: Although no teratogenic effects have been demonstrated in animals, Trandate should only be used during the first trimester of pregnancy if the potential benefit outweighs the potential risk. Trandate crosses the placental barrier and the possibility of the consequences of alpha- and beta-adrenoceptor blockade in the fetus and neonate should be borne in mind.

Perinatal and neonatal distress (bradycardia, hypotension, respiratory depression, hypoglycaemia, hypothermia) has been rarely reported. Sometimes these symptoms developed a day or two after birth. Response to supportive measures (e.g. intravenous fluids and glucose) is usually prompt but with severe pre-eclampsia, particularly after prolonged intravenous labetalol, recovery may be slower. This may be related to diminished liver metabolism in premature babies. Intra-uterine and neonatal deaths have been reported but other drugs (e.g. vasodilators, respiratory depressants) and the effects of pre-eclampsia, intra-uterine growth retardation and prematurity were implicated. Such clinical experience warns against unduly prolonging high dose labetalol and delaying delivery and against co-administration of hydralazine.

Trandate is excreted in breast milk. No adverse effects in breast feeding infants have been reported.

Side-effects: Most side-effects are transient and occur during the first few weeks of treatment. They include headache, tiredness, dizziness, depressed mood, lethargy, nasal congestion, sweating and, rarely, ankle oedema. Postural hypotension is uncommon except at very high doses or if the initial dose is too high or doses are increased too rapidly. A tingling sensation in the scalp, usually transient, also may occur in a few patients early in treatment. Tremor has been reported in the treatment of hypertensions of pregnancy. Acute retention of urine, difficulty in micturition, ejaculatory failure, epigastric pain, nausea and vomiting have been reported. There have been rare reports of positive anti-nuclear antibodies unassociated with disease as well as rare cases of systemic lupus erythematosus and very rarely drug fever. There have been very rare reports of toxic myopathy. Rare reports of hypersensitivity: rash, pruritus, angioedema and dyspnoea. A reversible lichenoid rash has occurred rarely. Blurred vision, eye irritation and cramps have been reported but were not necessarily related to Trandate.

There are rare reports of raised liver function tests, jaundice (both hepatocellular and cholestatic), hepatitis and hepatic necrosis. The signs and symptoms are usually reversible on withdrawal of the drug.

There are rare reports of bradycardia and heart block.

Drug interactions: Concomitant use of tricyclic anti-depressants may increase the incidence of tremor. Cimetidine may increase the bio-availability of labetalol and care is required in the oral dosing of the latter.

Overdosage: Profound cardiovascular effects are to be expected, e.g. excessive, posture-sensitive hypotension and sometimes bradycardia. Patients should be laid supine with the legs raised. Gastric lavage or induced emesis is warranted for a few hours after ingestion; use a cardiac glycoside and a diuretic in cardiac failure; for bronchospasm, administer a beta$_2$-agonist per aerosol. Intravenous atropine 0.25 to 3 mg should be given to relieve bradycardia. Intravenous noradrenaline 5 to 10 micrograms initially, repeated according to response, may be preferable to isoprenaline to improve the circulation. Alternatively, noradrenaline may be infused at a rate of 5 micrograms per minute until the response is satisfactory.

In severe overdose, intravenous glucagon may be preferred: an initial bolus dose of 5 to 10 mg in dextrose or saline should be followed by an intravenous infusion of 5 mg/hour or as sufficient to maintain cardiac output. Transvenous pacing may be required.

Oliguric renal failure has been reported after massive overdose of labetalol orally. In one case, the use of dopamine to increase the blood pressure may have aggravated the renal failure.

Haemodialysis removes less than 1% labetalol HCl from the circulation.

Pharmaceutical precautions No special storage precautions are required.

Legal category POM.

Package quantities
Trandate Tablets 100 mg and 200 mg are available in containers of 250;
Trandate Tablets 400 mg in containers of 50 (OP) and 250;
Trandate Tablets 50 mg, 100 mg and 200 mg are also available in calendar blister packs of 56 tablets (OP).

Further information Trandate does not adversely affect renal function and is particularly suitable for use in hypertensive patients with renal disease. Its metabolites are excreted in faeces as well as urine and the drug is unlikely to accumulate in the body even in renal failure.

The plasma half-life of Trandate is about 4 hours. Only about 50% of labetalol in the blood is protein bound. It fluoresces in alkaline solution at an excitation wavelength of 334 nm and a fluorescence wavelength of 412 nm and may therefore interfere with the assays of certain fluorescent substances including catecholamines.

The presence of labetalol metabolites in the urine may result in falsely elevated levels of urinary catecholamines, metanephrine, normetanephrine, and vanillylmandelic acid (VMA) when measured by fluorimetric or photometric methods. In screening patients suspected of having a phaeochromocytoma and being treated with Trandate a specific method, such as a high performance liquid chromatographic assay with solid phase extraction (e.g. J. Chromatogr. 385, 241, 1987) should be employed in determining levels of catecholamines.

Product licence numbers
Trandate Tablets 50 mg 0021/0131
Trandate Tablets 100 mg 0021/0132

Trandate Tablets 200 mg 0021/0133
Trandate Tablets 400 mg 0021/0134

VOLMAX* TABLETS

Presentation Volmax Tablets 8 mg: White hexagonal controlled release tablets each containing 8 mg salbutamol as Salbutamol Sulphate BP. Printed 8 on one side.

Volmax Tablets 4 mg: White hexagonal controlled release tablets each containing 4 mg salbutamol as Salbutamol Sulphate BP. Printed 4 on one side.

The tablet consists of an outer semi-permeable membrane and an inner core containing salbutamol sulphate. There is a hole in the outer coat which allows osmotically controlled release of the drug.

Uses Salbutamol is a beta-adrenergic stimulant which has a highly selective action on the β_2-receptors in bronchial smooth muscle and, in therapeutic dosage, little or no action on the cardiac β_1-receptors. Volmax Tablets are indicated for the treatment of reversible airways obstruction of all types including bronchial asthma, chronic bronchitis and emphysema.

Dosage and administration Volmax Tablets must be swallowed whole with a glass of water and not chewed or crushed.

Adults: The recommended dose is one 8 mg tablet twice daily.

Elderly: There is no need to adjust the dose in the elderly.

Children: In children aged 3 to 12 years, the recommended dose is one 4 mg tablet twice daily.

Contra-indications, warnings, etc
Contra-indications: Although intravenous salbutamol and occasionally salbutamol tablets are used in the management of premature labour uncomplicated by conditions such as placenta praevia or ante-partum haemorrhage, or toxaemia of pregnancy. Presentations containing salbutamol should not be used for threatened abortion during the first or second trimesters of pregnancy.

Volmax Tablets are contra-indicated in patients with a history of hypersensitivity to any of their components.

Precautions: Volmax Tablets should be administered cautiously to patients suffering from thyrotoxicosis.

Salbutamol and non-selective beta-blocking drugs, such as propranolol, should not usually be prescribed together.

Potentially serious hypokalaemia may result from beta$_2$-agonist therapy. Particular caution is advised in acute severe asthma as this effect may be potentiated by concomitant treatment with xanthine derivatives, steroids, diuretics and hypoxia. It is recommended that serum potassium levels are monitored in such situations.

Pregnancy: Administration of drugs during pregnancy should only be considered if the expected benefit to the mother is greater than any possible risk to the fetus.

Salbutamol has been in widespread use for many years in human beings without apparent ill consequence; this includes its well established use in management of premature labour. However, as with the majority of drugs there is little published evidence of its safety in the early stages of human pregnancy. In animal studies there was evidence of some harmful effects on the fetus at very high dose levels.

Lactation: As salbutamol is probably secreted in breast milk its use in nursing mothers is not recommended unless the expected benefits outweigh any potential risk. It is not known whether salbutamol has a harmful effect on the neonate.

Side-effects: Volmax Tablets may cause a fine tremor of skeletal muscle in some patients; usually the hands are most obviously affected. This effect is common to all beta-adrenergic stimulants. The incidence of tremor with this preparation is similar to that seen with standard salbutamol tablets. A few patients experience feelings of tension; this is also due to the effects on skeletal muscle and not to direct CNS stimulation. In patients who are unusually sensitive to beta-adrenergic stimulants, peripheral vasodilatation and a compensatory small increase in heart rate may occur. Occasionally headaches have been reported.

There have been very rare reports of transient muscle cramps. Hypersensitivity reactions including angioedema, urticaria, bronchospasm, hypotension and collapse have been reported very rarely.

Potentially serious hypokalaemia may result from beta$_2$-agonist therapy.

Overdosage: The preferred antidote for overdosage with Volmax Tablets is a cardio-selective beta-blocking agent, but beta-blocking drugs should be used with caution in patients with a history of bronchospasm.

Pharmaceutical precautions *Storage:* Volmax Tablets should be stored at a temperature not exceeding 30°C.

Volmax Tablets should not be removed from their foil pack until required for administration.

Legal category POM.

Package quantities Volmax Tablets, 8 mg and 4 mg, are supplied in double foil blisters of 14 in cartons of 56 (OP).

Further information Volmax does not cause difficulty in micturition because, unlike sympathomimetic drugs such as ephedrine, it does not stimulate alpha-adrenoceptors.

Volmax is not contra-indicated in patients under treatment with monoamine oxidase inhibitors (MAOIs).

Product licence numbers
Volmax Tablets 8 mg 0021/0129
Volmax Tablets 4 mg 0021/0128

**Trade Mark*

Duphar Laboratories Limited
Gaters Hill
West End
Southampton SO3 3JD

ALGESAL*

Presentation Off white, lavender-scented cream containing diethylamine salicylate 10% w/w. Excipients include stearates, triethanolamine, liquid and white soft paraffins, microcrystalline wax and lavender oil.

Uses An analgesic cream for the symptomatic relief of rheumatic and minor musculo-skeletal conditions including lumbago, fibrositis, sciatica, bruises and sprains.

Dosage and administration
Adults (including the elderly) and children over 6 years: Apply three times daily to the affected area, massaging until cream is fully absorbed.

Children under 6 years: Not recommended.

Contra-indications, warnings, etc Algesal should not be used if the surface of the skin is broken. This product contains a salicylate which is related to aspirin.

Use in pregnancy: There is inadequate evidence of safety in human pregnancy, but it has been in wide use for many years without apparent ill consequence. However, it should only be used in pregnancy where there is no safer alternative.

Treatment of overdosage: Adverse systemic effects are unlikely even after accidental oral ingestion. No special measures are necessary.

Pharmaceutical precautions Store at room temperature.

Legal category P.

Package quantities Tube containing 50 g.

Further information Nil.

Product licence number 0512/0066.

COLOFAC*

Presentation
Tablets: White, round, sugar-coated tablets with no superficial markings each containing 135 mg mebeverine hydrochloride. Excipients include lactose and sucrose.

Liquid: Yellow, banana-flavoured, sugar-free suspension containing mebeverine pamoate equivalent to 50 mg mebeverine hydrochloride per 5 ml. Excipients include sodium benzoate.

Uses Mebeverine is a musculotropic antispasmodic with a direct action on the smooth muscle of the gastrointestinal tract, relieving spasm without affecting normal gut motility. Since this action is not mediated by the autonomic nervous system, anticholinergic side-effects are absent. Mebeverine is suitable for patients with prostatic hypertrophy and glaucoma.

Indications:

1. For the symptomatic treatment of irritable bowel syndrome and other conditions usually included in this grouping such as: chronic irritable colon, spastic constipation, mucous colitis, spastic colitis. Colofac is effectively used to treat the symptoms of these conditions, such as: colicky abdominal pain and cramps, persistent non-specific diarrhoea (with or without alternating constipation) and flatulence.
2. For the symptomatic treatment of gastro-intestinal spasm secondary to organic diseases.

Dosage and administration
Adults (including the elderly) and children 10 years and over: Tablets: One tablet three times a day, preferably 20 minutes before meals.

Suspension: 15 ml (150 mg) three times a day, preferably 20 minutes before meals.

After a period of several weeks when the desired effect has been obtained, the dosage may be gradually reduced.

Children under 10 years: Not applicable.

Contra-indications, warnings, etc
Contra-indications: None known.

Warnings: Animal experiments have failed to show any teratogenic effects. However, the usual precautions concerning the administration of any drug during pregnancy should be observed.

Treatment of overdosage: On theoretical grounds it may be predicted that CNS excitability will occur in cases of overdosage. No specific antidote is known; gastric lavage and symptomatic treatment is recommended.

Pharmaceutical precautions Tablets: Store in a dry place, at room temperature, protected from light.

Suspension: Store at room temperature. Shake well before use. Dilution and subsequent storage not recommended.

Legal category POM.

Package quantities Tablets: Available in packs of 100 (5 strips of 20 blister-packed tablets).

Suspension: Available in bottles of 300 ml.

Further information Mebeverine does not produce false positive reactions in standard diagnostic urine tests.

Product licence numbers

Tablets	0512/0044
Suspension	0512/0061

CREON*

Presentation Brown/yellow hard gelatin capsules containing buff coloured enteric coated granules of pancreatin, equivalent to:

8,000 BP units of lipase
9,000 BP units of amylase
210 BP units of protease

Uses Replacement therapy in pancreatic enzyme deficiency states.

Indications: Pancreatic exocrine insufficiency.

Dosage and administration *Adults (including the elderly) and children:* Initially one to two capsules with meals, then adjust according to response. Clinical experience indicates that the effective dose may lie between 5–15 capsules daily.

The capsules can be swallowed whole, or for ease of administration they may be opened and the granules taken with fluid or soft food, but without chewing. If the granules are mixed with food it is important that they are taken immediately, otherwise dissolution of the enteric coating may result.

Contra-indications, warnings, etc
Contra-indications: Substitution with pancreatic enzymes is contra-indicated in the early stages of acute pancreatitis.

Use in pregnancy: There is inadequate evidence of safety in use during pregnancy.

Warnings:

The product is of porcine origin.

Rarely cases of hyper-uricosuria and hyper-uricaemia have been reported with very high doses of pancreatin.

Overdosage could precipitate meconium ileus equivalent.

Perianal irritation could occur, and rarely, inflammation when large doses are used.

Pharmaceutical precautions Store at room temperature.

Legal category P.

Package quantities Available in packs of 100 capsules.

Further information Nil.

Product licence number 5727/0001.

Product licence holder: Kali Chemie Pharma GmbH, Postfach 220, D-3000, Hannover 1, West Germany.

DUPHASTON*

Presentation White, flat, round tablet scored on one side with the imprint '155' on each half of the tablet and imprinted 'DUPHAR' on the reverse, each containing 10 mg Dydrogesterone BP. Excipients include lactose.

Uses Dydrogesterone is an orally active progestogen which produces a complete secretory endometrium in an oestrogen-primed uterus. It is indicated in all cases of endogenous progesterone deficiency.

Indications: To counteract the effects of unopposed oestrogen in Hormone Replacement Therapy, premenstrual syndrome, endometriosis, dysmenorrhoea, infertility, irregular cycles, functional bleeding (with added oestrogen), secondary amenorrhoea (with added oestrogen), threatened and habitual abortion (associated with proven progesterone deficiency).

Dosage and administration *Adults*

Hormone replacement therapy: When continuous oestrogen is given, 10 mg dydrogesterone twice daily for the first 12–14 days of each calendar month.

Premenstrual syndrome: 10 mg twice daily from day 12 to 26 of the cycle. The dosage may be increased if necessary.

Endometriosis: 10 mg two to three times daily from day 5 to 25 of the cycle, or continuously.

Dysmenorrhoea: 10 mg twice daily from day 5 to 25 of the cycle.

Infertility or irregular cycles: 10 mg twice daily from day 11 to day 25 of the cycle. Treatment should be maintained for at least six consecutive cycles. If the patient conceives, it is advisable to continue treatment for the first few months of pregnancy as described under 'habitual abortion'.

Functional bleeding – to arrest bleeding: 10 mg twice daily together with an oestrogen once daily for five to seven days.

Functional bleeding – to prevent bleeding: 10 mg twice daily together with an oestrogen once daily from day 11 to 25 of the cycle.

Amenorrhoea: An oestrogen once daily from day 1 to 25 of the cycle, together with 10 mg dydrogesterone twice daily from day 11 to 25 of the cycle.

Threatened abortion: 40 mg at once then 10 mg every eight hours until symptoms remit. If symptoms persist or return during treatment the dose can be increased by one tablet every eight hours. The effective dose must be maintained for a week after symptoms have ceased and can then be gradually decreased unless symptoms return.

Habitual abortion: Treatment should be started as early as possible, preferably before conception. 10 mg should be given twice daily from day 11 to day 25 of the cycle until conception and then continuously (10 mg twice daily) until the twentieth week of pregnancy, then dosage may be gradually reduced.

Elderly: Hormone replacement therapy: Standard adult dosage is recommended.

Children: Primary dysmenorrhoea: 10 mg twice daily at the discretion of the physician.

Contra-indications, warnings, etc

Contra-indications: None known.

Warning: Breakthrough bleeding may occur in a few patients. It can, however, be prevented by increasing the dosage.

Treatment of overdosage: No reports of ill effects from overdosage have been recorded and remedial action is generally unnecessary. If a large overdosage is discovered within 2–3 hours and treatment seems desirable, gastric lavage is recommended. There are no special antidotes and treatment should be symptomatic.

Pharmaceutical precautions Store in a dry place, at room temperature, protected from light.

Legal category POM.

Package quantities Available in packs of 60 (4 strips of 15 blister-packed tablets).

Further information Duphaston is non-androgenic, non-oestrogenic, non-thermogenic, non-corticoid, non-anabolic and is not excreted as pregnanediol.

Dydrogesterone does not produce false positive reactions in standard diagnostic urine tests.

Product licence number 0512/5004R.

FAVERIN*

Presentation Round, yellow, enteric-coated tablets each containing 50 mg fluvoxamine maleate, imprinted with 'Duphar 291'.

Oval, yellow, enteric-coated tablets each containing 100 mg fluvoxamine maleate, imprinted with 'Duphar 313'.

Uses The treatment of symptoms of depressive illness.

Dosage and administration The tablets should be swallowed without chewing and with water.

Adults (including the elderly): The effective daily dose usually varies between 100 mg and 200 mg and should be adjusted to the individual response of the patient up to a maximum of 300 mg. The minimum recommended starting dose is 100 mg given in the evening. A total daily dosage in excess of 100 mg should be given in divided doses.

Children: There are insufficient data to recommend the use of Faverin in children.

Contra-indications, warnings, etc Although studies in animals have not shown any direct teratogenic effect, the safety of Faverin in human pregnancy has not been established. On basic principles its use during pregnancy and in nursing mothers should be avoided, unless there are compelling reasons.

Faverin should not be given together with or within two weeks of terminating treatment with monoamine-oxidase inhibitors.

Faverin has been used in combination with lithium in the treatment of patients with severe drug-resistant depression. However, lithium (and possibly tryptophan) enhances the serotonergic effects of Faverin and the combination should therefore be used with caution.

Patients with hepatic or renal insufficiency should begin treatment with a low dose and be carefully monitored. Rarely treatment with Faverin has been associated with an increase in hepatic enzymes, usually accompanied by symptoms. The drug should be withdrawn in such subjects.

The effects of alcohol may be potentiated by Faverin.

As improvement may sometimes be delayed for two or more weeks, patients should be closely monitored during this initial treatment period.

Interactions with other drugs: Faverin can prolong the elimination of drugs metabolised by oxidation in the liver. A clinically significant interaction is possible with drugs with a narrow therapeutic index (e.g. warfarin, phenytoin and theophylline).

Actually, in interaction studies increased plasma levels of propranolol and warfarin were seen during concurrent administration of Faverin. It may therefore be advisable to lower the dose of these drugs when prescribing Faverin. Although not recommended, Faverin has been used together with other antidepressants. It has been reported that in combination Faverin can increase previously stable plasma levels of tricyclic antidepressants. No interactions were seen with digoxin or with atenolol.

Side-effects: The commonest side-effects associated with the administration of Faverin are gastrointestinal; nausea, vomiting and diarrhoea being the most frequently reported. In some patients who report nausea, vomiting may occur. Caution should therefore be exercised when administering Faverin to patients with a medical condition likely to be exacerbated by vomiting. Other adverse effects reported include dizziness, somnolence, agitation, headache and tremor. Anxiety has been reported less often.

Convulsions have been reported and Faverin should be avoided in patients with a history of epilepsy. If convulsions occur Faverin therapy should be discontinued.

Other reported effects are often associated with the illness and their incidence in controlled trials is comparable to that experienced with placebo.

Faverin may cause a decrease in heart rate. During treatment, limited changes in repolarisation were observed in the ECG, but no causal relationship could be demonstrated. Hypotension has been rarely reported.

Treatment of overdosage: No specific antidote is known. The stomach should be emptied as soon as possible after tablet ingestion and symptomatic treatment should be given. The use of medicinal charcoal is also recommended. Seventy-seven percent of fluvoxamine maleate is bound to plasma proteins.

Pharmaceutical precautions Store at room temperature.

Legal category POM.

Package quantities 50 mg tablets: available in packs of 60 (3 strips of 20 blister-packed tablets).

100 mg tablets: available in packs of 30 (3 strips of 10 blister-packed tablets).

Further information The mechanism of action of Faverin is thought to be related to its selective serotonin re-uptake inhibition in brain neurones, whilst there is minimum interference with noradrenergic processes. Faverin is chemically unrelated to other currently available antidepressants.

If required, benzodiazepines may be prescribed with Faverin.

Faverin is indicated for short term and maintenance treatment.

Faverin is rapidly and completely absorbed after oral administration. The plasma half-life is approximately 15 hours. It is transformed in the liver into pharmacologically inactive metabolites which are excreted by the kidney. Steady-state levels are attained within two weeks of treatment with a constant dose.

The pharmacokinetic profile in the elderly is similar to that in the general population.

Product licence number

50 mg:	0512/0070
100 mg:	0512/0072

INFLUVAC* SUB-UNIT

Presentation Single-dose disposable syringes of a colourless opalescent suspension of Influenza Vaccine (Surface Antigen) BP containing the purified haemagglutinin and neuraminidase antigens prepared from influenza virus. The product contains appropriate quantities of the A and B strains currently recommended by the WHO. The aqueous buffered medium contains traces of sucrose.

Uses Prophylaxis of influenza. Particularly recommended in:

- Chronic pulmonary disease, e.g. chronic bronchitis and emphysema, asthma, bronchiectasis, pulmonary tuberculosis and fibrosis.
- Chronic heart disease, e.g. valvular and hypertensive heart disease.
- Chronic renal disease, e.g. chronic nephritis, including patients with renal disease on immunosuppressive drugs.
- Diabetes and possibly other less common endocrine disorders.
- Elderly people.
- Key personnel.
- Chronic furunculosis or other chronic staphylococcal infections.
- Persons living in residential establishments in which rapid spread is likely following the introduction of infection.

Dosage and administration

Adults (including the elderly) and children (over 13 years): 0.5 ml.

Children (4–13 years): 0.5 ml, followed by a second injection of 0.5 ml after an interval of 4–6 weeks, unless previously primed with H_1N_1 antigen, in which case one dose of 0.5 ml is sufficient.

To be given by intramuscular or deep subcutaneous injection after allowing the vaccine to reach room temperature.

Contra-indications, warnings, etc

Contra-indications: Persons with hypersensitivity to eggs, chicken proteins or feathers and influenza viral proteins should not be vaccinated.

Immunisation should be postponed in patients with febrile illness.

Use in pregnancy: Although there is no evidence that influenza vaccine has any harmful effect during pregnancy, careful consideration should be given to the use of the vaccine.

Other undesirable effects (frequency and seriousness): Systemic effects, such as pyrexia, fatigue and headache may be experienced. Local effects, such as transient erythema and swelling at the site of injection may also occur, but reactions of both types are usually less frequent than those associated with the administration of whole virus vaccine.

Neurological disorders such as encephalomyelitis and neuritis after influenza vaccination have been rarely reported. An association has not been established except in the case of Guillain Barré Syndrome (U.S.A. Mass-vaccination programme 1976).

The vaccine contains a maximum per dose of 0.00625 IU polymyxin and 0.00625 micrograms neomycin. Use with caution in patients hypersensitive to these antibiotics.

Other special warnings and precautions: The unit cartons contain the following statements:

'This vaccine has been prepared in eggs'.

'Allow the vaccine to reach room temperature before injection'.

The package insert contains the following statement: In the rare event of an unexpected, severe immediate hypersensitivity reaction, Adrenaline Injection BP should be ready for use.

Overdose (symptoms, emergency procedures, antidotes): In view of the nature of the product, overdose is unlikely to have any untoward effect. Accidental administration of ten times the normal dose has occurred without adverse effect.

Incompatibilities (major): None.

Pharmaceutical precautions Store between +2 and +8°C, protected from light. Do not freeze.

Legal category POM.

Package quantities Single-dose (0.5 ml) disposable syringes.

Further information Non-essential viral components have been removed thus decreasing the reactogenicity. Studies have shown that the purified haemagglutinin and neuraminidase antigens contained in Influvac Sub-Unit produce a protective antibody level in a high percentage of patients.

Product licence number 0512/0093.

LACTULOSE SOLUTION BP

Presentation A colourless to brownish yellow, clear or not more than slightly opalescent solution containing lactulose 3.35 g/5 ml. Also contains lactose 0.3 g/5 ml, galactose 0.55 g/5 ml. The product complies with the specification for Lactulose Solution BP.

Uses The action of lactulose in treating constipation depends on the inability of the enzymes in the small intestine to hydrolyse this synthetic disaccharide into its component molecules of fructose and galactose. Therefore, as lactulose is virtually unabsorbed, it passes into the large bowel chemically unchanged and forms a substrate for commensal saccharolytic bacteria.

The resulting breakdown products, simple organic compounds like lactic and acetic acid, give rise to increased intra-colonic osmotic pressure, with consequent increased faecal bulk, and stimulate peristalsis. The growth of saccharolytic bacteria is favoured and the normal colonic flora restored.

A soft stool is formed, and normal bowel action encouraged without irritation or direct interference with the gut mucosa.

In patients with hepatic encephalopathy larger doses of lactulose are used; a significant reduction in the pH of the colonic contents results, which reduces markedly the formation and absorption of ammonium ions and other nitrogenous toxins into the portal circulation. Rapid decrements in blood ammonia concentration have been reported following lactulose treatment.

Indications: 1. Constipation.

2. Hepatic encephalopathy (Portal systemic encephalopathy): hepatic coma.

Dosage and administration *Constipation:* Initially lactulose may be given twice daily. In due course the dose should be adjusted to the needs of the individual, but the following serves as a guide.

Starting dose

Adults (including the elderly)	15 ml twice daily
Children 5 to 10 years	10 ml twice daily
Children under 5 years	5 ml twice daily
Babies under 1 year	2.5 ml twice daily

Each dose of lactulose may, if necessary, be taken with water or fruit juices, etc.

Hepatic encephalopathy

Adults (including the elderly): Initially 30–50 ml. (6–10 × 5 ml spoonfuls) three times a day. Subsequently adjust the dose to produce two or three soft stools each day.

Children: No dosage recommendations for this indication.

Contra-indications, warnings, etc

Contra-indications: Galactosaemia. In common with other preparations used for the treatment of constipation, lactulose should not be used when there is evidence of gastro-intestinal obstruction.

Precaution: Lactose intolerance.

Use in pregnancy: Wide clinical experience, together with data from animal reproduction studies has not revealed any increase in embryotoxic hazard to the fetus, if used in the recommended dosage during pregnancy. If drug therapy is needed in pregnancy the use of this drug is acceptable.

Side-effects: During the first few days of treatment meteorism and increased flatulance may occur. These symptoms usually disappear under continued therapy. Diarrhoea may occur especially when using higher dosages, e.g. during treatment of PSE. Dosage should then be adjusted to obtain two or three formed stools per day.

Treatment of overdosage: No specific antidote. Symptomatic treatment should be given.

Pharmaceutical precautions Store below 20°C. Do not freeze. Dilution and subsequent storage not recommended.

Legal category P.

Package quantities Available in bottles of 300 ml, 500 ml, 1 litre and plastic containers of 5 litres.

Further information Because of lactulose's physiological mode of action it may take up to 48 hours before effects are obtained. However, clinical experience has shown that this medicament does exhibit a 'carry-over' effect which may enable the patient to reduce the effective dose gradually over a period of time.

A maintenance dose of 15 ml per day provides only 58 kJ (14 kcals), and is therefore, unlikely to adversely affect diabetics.

Product licence number 0512/5001R.

MONOTRIM*

Presentation *Tablets:* White, flat, round, with bevelled edges, imprinted with the manufacturer's symbol on one face, with a single break bar and coded on the reverse.

Each tablet contains either 100 mg or 200 mg Trimethoprim BP. Excipients include lactose.

100 mg tablets coded $\frac{\text{AE}}{2}$.

200 mg tablets coded $\frac{\text{DE}}{5}$.

Suspension: White, sugar free, aniseed flavoured suspension containing 50 mg trimethoprim per 5 ml. The formulation includes methyl parahydroxy benzoate.

Uses Trimethoprim is active *in-vitro* against most Gram-positive and Gram-negative aerobic organisms. The antimicrobial activity is due to selective inhibition of bacterial dihydrofolate reductase.

Indications: Treatment of susceptible infections caused by trimethoprim-sensitive organisms including urinary and respiratory tract infections and for the prophylaxis of recurrent urinary tract infections.

Dosage and administration

Acute infections:

Tablets:

Adults and children over 12 years: 200 mg twice daily
Children 6 years to 12 years: 100 mg twice daily
Children 6 months to 5 years: 50 mg twice daily

Suspension:

Adults and children over 12 years: 200 mg (20 ml) twice daily
Children 6 years to 12 years: 100 mg (10 ml) twice daily
Children 6 months to 5 years: 50 mg (5 ml) twice daily
Children 6 weeks to 5 months: 25 mg (2.5 ml) twice daily
Elderly: Depending on kidney function, see special dosage schedule.

Treatment should continue for at least one week but not last longer than two weeks. The first dose can be doubled. The approximate dosage in children is 8 mg trimethoprim per kg body weight per day.

Long-term treatment and prophylactic therapy:

Tablets:

Adults and children over 12 years: 100 mg at night
Children 6 years to 12 years: 50 mg at night

Suspension:
Adults and children over 12 years: 100 mg (10 ml) at night
Children 6 years to 12 years: 50 mg (5 ml) at night
Children 6 months to 5 years: 25 mg (2.5 ml) at night

The approximate dosage in children is 2 mg trimethoprim per kg body weight per day.
Elderly: Depending on kidney function, see special dosage schedule.

Dosage advised where there is reduced kidney function:

Creatinine clearance (ml/sec)	*Plasma creatinine (micromol/l)*		*Dosage advised*
Over 0.45	men women	<250 <175	normal
0.25–0.45	men women	250–600 175–400	normal for 3 days then half dose
Under 0.25	men women	>600 >400	half the normal dose

Contra-indications, warnings, etc
Contra-indications: Pregnancy, trimethoprim hypersensitivity, blood dyscrasias, severe renal insufficiency where blood levels cannot be monitored.

Interactions: Bone marrow depressants – Trimethoprim may increase the potential for bone marrow aplasia. Rifampicin may increase the elimination and shorten the elimination half-life of trimethoprim. Phenytoin and digoxin: The patients should be carefully controlled as trimethoprim may increase the elimination half-life of phenytoin and digoxin.

Use in pregnancy and lactation: Pregnancy is a contraindication. Although trimethoprim is excreted in breast milk, it is not a contraindication for short-term therapy in lactating mothers.

Precautions: Caution should be exercised in the administration of trimethoprim to patients with actual or potential folate deficiency (e.g. elderly) and administration of folate supplement should be considered. Although an effect on folic acid metabolism is possible, interference with haematopoiesis rarely occurs at the recommended dose. If any such change is seen, folinic acid should reverse the effect. Elderly people may be more susceptible and a lower dose may be advisable. In neonates, trimethoprim should be used under careful medical supervision.

In patients with impairment of renal function, care should be taken to avoid accumulation.

Side-effects: Skin rashes, nausea and vomiting have been reported in rare instances.

Treatment of overdosage: Symptomatic treatment, gastric lavage and forced diuresis can be used. Depression of haematopoiesis by trimethoprim can be counteracted by intramuscular administration of calcium folinate.

Pharmaceutical precautions Monotrim suspension should be stored below 25°C. It may be diluted with water or sorbitol solution BP. The diluted suspension is stable for 14 days.

Legal category POM.

Package quantities
Tablets: 200 mg containers of 100 and 500 tablets
100 mg containers of 100 and 500 tablets
Suspension: Bottle of 100 ml.

Further information Trimethoprim is effective *in-vitro* against most Gram-positive and Gram-negative aerobic organisms, including enterobacteria – *E. coli, Proteus, Klebsiella pneumoniae; Streptococcus faecalis; Streptococcus pneumoniae; Haemophilus influenzae;* and *Staphylococcus aureus.*

It is not active against *Mycobacterium tuberculosis, Neisseria gonorrhoeae, Pseudomonas aeruginosa, Treponema pallidum,* or anaerobic bacteria.

Product licence numbers
Tablets: 200 mg 4012/0003
Tablets: 100 mg 4012/0001
Suspension: 100 ml 4012/0002

Product licence holder: GEA Limited, DK-2000, Copenhagen F, Denmark.

MONOTRIM* INJECTION

Presentation Ampoules containing a sterile, clear, colourless, aqueous solution (pH=4.0), containing trimethoprim lactate equivalent to 20 mg trimethoprim base per ml. Each ampoule contains 5 ml corresponding to 100 mg of trimethoprim base.

Uses Trimethoprim is active *in-vitro* against most Gram-positive and Gram-negative aerobic organisms. The antimicrobial activity is due to selective inhibition of bacterial dihydrofolate reductase.

Indications: Treatment of susceptible infections caused by trimethoprim-sensitive organisms, particularly Gram-negative infections.

Dosage and administration
Dosage: Adults (including the elderly) and children over 12 years: 200 mg every 12 hours.

Children under 12 years: The approximate dosage in children is 8 mg trimethoprim per kg body weight per day, divided into two or three equal doses.

In severely ill patients, the initial doses may be higher or given more frequently.

Dosage advised where there is reduced kidney function:

Creatinine clearance (ml/sec)	*Plasma creatinine (micromol/l)*		*Dosage advised*
Over 0.45	men women	<250 <175	normal
0.25–0.45	men women	250–600 175–400	normal for 3 days then half dose
Under 0.25	men women	>600 >400	half the normal dose

Administration: Monotrim Injection may be administered:

1. By direct intravenous injection, or
2. Via the tubing of an established intravenous infusion.

It is compatible with the following commonly used infusion fluids:
Dextran 40 Injection BP 10% w/v in normal saline
Dextran 70 Injection BP 6% w/v in normal saline
Dextrose Injection BP 5% w/v
Laevulose Injection BP 5% w/v
Ringer's Injection USP
Sodium Chloride Injection BP 0.9% w/v
Sodium Chloride 0.45% w/v and Dextrose 2.5% w/v Injection BP
Sodium Lactate Injection BP
Compound Sodium Lactate Injection BP

Contra-indications, warnings, etc
Contra-indications: Pregnancy, known hypersensitivity to trimethoprim, blood dyscrasias, severe renal insufficiency where blood levels cannot be monitored.

Interactions: Bone marrow depressants: Trimethoprim may increase the potential for bone marrow aplasia. Rifampicin may increase the elimination and shorten the elimination half-life of trimethoprim. Phenytoin and digoxin: The patients should be carefully controlled as trimethoprim may increase the elimination half-life of phenytoin and digoxin.

Use in pregnancy and lactation: Pregnancy is a contraindication. Although trimethoprim is excreted in breast milk, it is not a contraindication for short-term therapy in lactating mothers.

Precautions: Caution should be exercised in the administration of trimethoprim to patients with actual or potential folate deficiency (e.g. elderly) and administration of folate supplement should be considered. Although an effect on folic acid metabolism is possible, interference with haematopoiesis rarely occurs at the recommended dose. If any such change is seen, folinic acid should reverse the effect. Elderly people may be more susceptible and a lower dose may be advisable. In neonates, trimethoprim should be used under careful medical supervision.

In patients with impairment of renal function, care should be taken to avoid accumulation.

Side effects: Skin rashes, nausea and vomiting have been reported in rare instances.

Treatment of overdosage: Symptomatic treatment and forced diuresis can be used. Depression of haematopoiesis by trimethoprim can be counteracted by intramuscular administration of calcium folinate.

Pharmaceutical precautions Store below 25°C, protected from light.

Monotrim Injection is incompatible with solutions of sulphonamides and should not be mixed with such preparations.

Legal category POM.

Package quantities Boxes of 5 × 5 ml ampoules.

Further information Trimethoprim is effective *in-vitro* against most Gram-positive and Gram-negative aerobic organisms, including enterobacteria – *E. coli, Proteus, Klebsiella pneumoniae; Streptococcus faecalis; Streptococcus pneumoniae; Haemophilus influenzae;* and *Staphylococcus aureus.*

It is not active against *Mycobacterium tuberculosis, Neisseria gonorrhoeae, Pseudomonas aeruginosa, Treponema pallidum,* or anaerobic bacteria.

Monotrim Injection may be given in conjunction with, but separately from, other parenterally administered antibacterials, for example, aminoglycosides, metronidazole or sulphonamides whenever such a combination seems suitable.

Product licence number 4012/0008.

Product licence holder: GEA Limited, DK-2000, Copenhagen F, Denmark.

SERC*
SERC* – 16

Presentation A white, flat, round tablet, imprinted '256' on one side and 'DUPHAR' on the reverse, each tablet containing 8 mg betahistine dihydrochloride.

A white, flat, round tablet imprinted '267' on one face, 'DUPHAR' on the reverse, each tablet containing 16 mg betahistine dihydrochloride.

Uses Betahistine is an orally effective treatment for Ménière's syndrome, which appears to exert its effect by reducing endolymphatic pressure. It is a histamine analogue which was developed following the successful parenteral use of histamine in patients with Ménière's syndrome. Animal studies have confirmed its specific effect. Clinical experience has demonstrated the efficacy of betahistine on all the principal symptoms of Ménière's syndrome, not only reducing vertiginous episodes and tinnitus but also arresting hearing loss.

Indications: Vertigo, tinnitus and hearing loss associated with Ménière's syndrome.

Dosage and administration *Adults (including the elderly):* Initially 16 mg three times daily, taken preferably with meals. Maintenance doses are generally in the range 24–48 mg daily.

Children: No dosage recommendations are made for children.

Contra-indications, warnings, etc
Contra-indication: Phaeochromocytoma.

Precautions: Clinical intolerance to Serc in bronchial asthma patients has not been shown, but caution should be exercised when administering this histamine analogue to bronchial asthma patients.

Though an antagonism between Serc and antihistamines could be expected on a theoretical basis, no such interactions have been reported.

Use in pregnancy: High dosage animal tests have shown no teratogenic properties, but the usual precautions should be observed when administering Serc to patients during pregnancy.

Side-effects: There have been a small number of reports of gastric upset.

Treatment of overdosage: No specific antidote. Gastric lavage and symptomatic treatment is recommended.

Pharmaceutical precautions Store at room temperature.

Legal category POM.

Package quantities 8 mg: Available in packs of 120 tablets (8 strips of 15 blister packed tablets).

16 mg: Available in calendar packs of 84 tablets (4 strips of 21 blister packed tablets).

Further information Betahistine does not produce false positive reactions in standard diagnostic urine tests.

Product licence numbers

8 mg:	0512/0076
16 mg:	0512/0088

YUTOPAR*

Presentation *Tablets* – Round, flat, yellow with bevelled edges, inscribed 'YUTOPAR' on one face and a breakline on the reverse. Each tablet contains 10 mg ritodrine hydrochloride. Excipients include lactose.

Injection – Clear, aqueous solution containing 10 mg/ml of ritodrine hydrochloride. Aqueous buffered vehicle contains sodium chloride and sodium metabisulphite.

Uses Yutopar is a betamimetic drug developed for obstetric use. It mainly stimulates the beta$_2$-receptors, thereby decreasing uterine contractility. However, some chronotropic cardiac effect and peripheral vasodilation are also seen at therapeutic doses. Yutopar is active after oral, intramuscular and intravenous administration, and inhibits frequency and intensity of uterine contractions.

Indications:
The management of:
Uncomplicated pre-term labour.
Fetal Asphyxia in labour where it is desired to obtain uterine relaxation.

Dosage and administration *Adults. Pre-term labour: I/V:* To be administered as early as possible at the onset of pre-term labour. Initial dose 50 micrograms per minute to be gradually increased according to the response by 50 micrograms/minute every 10 minutes until the desired result is obtained, or the maternal heart rate reaches 140 beats per minute. The effective dosage usually lies between 150 micrograms and 350 micrograms/minute. The infusion should be continued for 12 to 48 hours after the uterine contractions have ceased.

The recommended infusion fluid is dextrose.

I/M: If intravenous administration is considered to be inappropriate, intramuscular administration may be substituted, giving 10 mg intramuscularly every three to eight hours. The intramuscular regime should be continued for 12–48 hours following arrest of labour.

Oral: One tablet (10 mg) may be given approximately 30 minutes before the termination of intravenous therapy. The usual dosage schedule for the first 24 hours of oral maintenance is one tablet (10 mg) every two hours. Thereafter, the usual dose is one or two tablets (10–20 mg) every four to six hours depending on uterine activity and unwanted effects.

The total daily dose of oral ritodrine should not exceed 120 mg. The treatment may be continued as long as the physician considers it desirable to prolong pregnancy.

Fetal asphyxia: I/V: This treatment scheme is only

recommended as a means of improving the condition of the fetus, so that intervention may be carried out under better conditions for the baby.

The recommended starting dose is 50 micrograms per minute by intravenous infusion rapidly increasing the infusion rate until the uterine activity is suppressed, or the maternal heart rate reaches 140 beats per minute. The required dose is unlikely to exceed 350 micrograms per minute. Whilst the infusion is given preparations should be made for the assisted delivery of the baby. Fifteen to 20 minutes after starting the infusion a fetal scalp blood sample should be taken. If the fetal scalp pH has not improved during the 15–20 minutes of infusion then the planned assisted delivery should be carried out. If the pH has significantly risen, the obstetrician may decide to continue the infusion for a further 15–30 minutes, with continued careful observation before proceeding with the delivery.

Elderly: Not applicable.
Children: Not applicable.

Contra-indications, warnings, etc
Contra-indications:

1. Antepartum haemorrhage which demands immediate delivery.
2. Eclampsia and severe pre-eclampsia.
3. Intra-uterine fetal death.
4. Chorioamnionitis.
5. Maternal cardiac disease.
6. Cord compression.

Precautions: Maternal pulmonary oedema has been reported in patients treated concomitantly with betamimetics and corticosteroids. Therefore, close monitoring of the patients state of hydration is advised and if pulmonary oedema develops during administration treatment should be discontinued.

Careful monitoring is required in patients with suspected heart disease, or those receiving other drugs, in particular those which could interact with ritodrine such as monoamine oxidase inhibitors, tricyclic antidepressants, corticosteroids, sympathomimetic amines, beta-adrenergic blocking drugs, anaesthetics used in surgery and potassium-depleting diuretics, as intravenous administration of Yutopar has been shown to decrease plasma potassium levels.

Experiments in animals have shown that even in high dosage Yutopar has no teratogenic properties. Nevertheless, in view of the limited available information from human studies, the administration of Yutopar is not recommended during the first 16 weeks of pregnancy.

In diabetic patients, glucose levels should be closely monitored and insulin requirements adjusted accordingly during intravenous treatment. On oral treatment no alterations have been reported. It is also advisable to screen patients with potential cardiac risk before deciding on ritodrine treatment.

The drug should not be administered to patients with mild to moderate pre-eclampsia, hypertension or hyperthyroidism unless the attending physician considers that the benefits clearly outweigh the risks.

Side-effects: In appropriate dosage Yutopar is well tolerated. In particular no hypotension occurs if the recommended administration schedule is followed and the patient is maintained in the left lateral position. It is only rarely that side-effects call for discontinuation of the treatment. The maternal pulse rate may progressively increase, usually to a moderate degree. This may lead to palpitations.

Any pronounced tachycardia that may arise during an intravenous infusion of Yutopar disappears shortly after decreasing the dosage or after the infusion is stopped. Whether the maternal tachycardia is considered acceptable must be determined from case to case, but it is recommended that, in healthy patients, a heart rate of more than 140/min should be avoided.

Flushing, sweating, tremor, nausea and vomiting have been reported in a few cases.

Treatment of overdosage: In cases of overdosage of Yutopar, a non-selective beta-sympatholytic agent may be given as an antidote.

Pharmaceutical precautions *Tablets:* Store in a cool dry place, protected from light.

Injection: Store in a cool place, protected from light. Do not use if solution is discoloured or contains a precipitate.

Legal category POM.

Package quantities *Tablets* – Packs of 90 (6 strips of 15 blister packed tablets) each containing 10 mg ritodrine hydrochloride.
Injection – Boxes of 10 × 5 ml ampoules containing ritodrine hydrochloride 10 mg/ml.

Further information Less effect can be expected if the membranes are ruptured or the dilation of the cervix exceeds 4 cm.

Ritodrine does not produce false positive reactions in standard diagnostic urine tests.

Product licence numbers

Tablets	0512/0018R
Injection	0512/0020R

**Trade Mark*

Du Pont Pharmaceuticals Limited
Wedgwood Way
Stevenage
Herts SG1 4QN

BREVIBLOC* ▼

Presentation 10 ml ampoules containing 2.5 g esmolol hydrochloride (250 mg/ml) in a sterile aqueous solution to be diluted before intravenous administration.

Uses Brevibloc is indicated for the short-term treatment of:

(a) Supraventricular tachyarrhythmias, including atrial fibrillation, artrial flutter and sinus tachycardia.

(b) Tachycardia and hypertension occurring in the perioperative period.

Mode of action: Brevibloc is a beta$_1$-selective (cardioselective) adrenergic receptor blocking agent with rapid onset, a very short duration of action and no significant intrinsic sympathomimetic or membrane stabilising activity at therapeutic doses. Its elimination half-life after intravenous infusion is approximately 9 minutes. Brevibloc is metabolised by esterases in the red blood cells.

Dosage and administration Brevibloc is not compatible with sodium bicarbonate.

Brevibloc must be diluted before infusion. Dilute the contents of two ampoules to 500 ml with an appropriate intravenous fluid to give a final concentration of 10 mg/ml. See 'Pharmaceutical precautions' for appropriate diluents. For administration by continuous infusion at the required rate, use a suitable constant infusion control device.

Supraventricular tachycardia: The effective dose of Brevibloc for treatment of supraventricular tachycardia is 50 to 200 mcg/kg/min, although doses as high as 300 mcg/kg/min have been used. In a few patients a dosage of 25 mcg/kg/min has been adequate. Brevibloc dosage in supraventricular tachycardia must be individualised by titration in which each step consists of a loading dosage followed by a maintenance dose.

Flow chart for initiation and maintenance of treatment

Loading dosage infusion of 500 micrograms/kg/min for 1 minute

THEN maintenance infusion of 50 micrograms/kg/min for 4 minutes*

Response
Maintain infusion at 50 micrograms/kg/min

Inadequate response within 5 minutes
Repeat 500 micrograms/kg/min for 1 minute
Increase maintenance infusion to 100 micrograms/kg/min for 4 minutes

Response
Maintain infusion at 100 micrograms/kg/min

Inadequate response within 5 minutes
Repeat 500 micrograms/kg/min for 1 minute
Increase maintenance infusion to 150 micrograms/kg/min for 4 minutes

Response
Maintain infusion at 150 micrograms/kg/min

Inadequate response
Repeat 500 micrograms/kg/min for 1 minute
Increase maintenance infusion to 200 micrograms/kg/min and maintain

* As the desired heart rate safety end-point (e.g. lowered blood pressure) is approached, *OMIT* the loading infusion and *reduce* the *incremental* dose in the maintenance infusion from 50 micrograms/kg/min to 25 micrograms/kg/min or lower. If necessary, the interval between titration steps may be increased from 5 to 10 minutes.

NB. Maintenance doses above 200 micrograms/kg/min have not been shown to have significantly increased benefits, and the safety of doses above 300 micrograms/kg/min has not been studied.

In the event of an adverse reaction, the dosage of Brevibloc may be reduced or discontinued. Pharmacological adverse reactions should resolve within 30 minutes. If a local infusion site reaction develops, an alternative infusion site should be used and caution should be taken to prevent extravasation.

Abrupt discontinuation of Brevibloc in patients has not been reported to produce the withdrawal effects which may occur with abrupt withdrawal of beta-blockers following chronic use in coronary artery disease (CAD) patients. However, caution should still be used in discontinuing Brevibloc infusions abruptly in CAD patients.

After achieving an adequate control of the heart rate and a stable clinical status in patients with supraventricular tachycardia, transition to alternative antiarrhythmic agents such as verapamil, propranolol or metoprolol, digoxin or quinidine may be accomplished. A recommended guideline for such a transition is given below but the physician should carefully consider the labelling instructions for the alternative agent selected:

Alternative agent	*Dosage*
Propranolol hydrochloride	10–20 mg 4–6 hourly p.o.
Digoxin	0.125–0.5 mg 6 hourly (p.o. or i.v.)
Verapamil	80 mg 6 hourly p.o.
Quinidine	200 mg 2 hourly p.o.

The dosage of Brevibloc should be reduced as follows:

(1) Within the first hour after the first dose of the alternative agent, reduce the Brevibloc infusion rate by one-half (50%).

(2) Following the second dose of the alternative agent, monitor the patient's response and if satisfactory control is maintained for the first hour, discontinue the Brevibloc infusion.

The use of Brevibloc infusions for longer than 24 hours has not been thoroughly evaluated. Infusion durations greater than 24 hours should only be used with caution.

Perioperative tachycardia and hypertension: When treating tachycardia and/or hypertension in the perioperative setting, the following dose regimens may be used:

(a) For intraoperative treatment – during anaesthesia when immediate control is required, give an 80 mg loading bolus over 15–30 seconds followed by a 150 mcg/kg/min infusion. Titrate the infusion rate as required up to 300 mcg/kg/min.

(b) Upon awakening from anaesthesia, administer an infusion of 500 mcg/kg/min for four minutes followed by a 300 mcg/kg/min infusion.

(c) For postoperative situations when time for titration is available give the 500 mcg/kg/min loading dose over one minute before each titration step to produce a rapid onset of action. Use titration steps of 50, 100, 150, 200, 250 and 300 mcg/kg/min given over four minutes, stopping at the desired therapeutic effect.

Additional dosing information: as the desired therapeutic effect or a safety endpoint (e.g. lowered blood pressure) is approached, omit the loading dose and reduce the incremental infusion to 12.5 to 25 mcg/kg/min. Also, if desired, increase the interval between titration steps from five to ten minutes. Brevibloc should be discontinued when heart rate or blood pressure rapidly approach or exceed a safety limit, and then restarted without a loading infusion at a lower dose after the heart rate or blood pressure has returned to an acceptable level.

Contra-indications, warnings, etc
Contra-indications: Brevibloc is contra-indicated in patients with sinus bradycardia, heart block greater than first degree, cardiogenic shock and overt heart failure.

Use in pregnancy: There is no experience with Brevibloc in pregnancy and, although animal tests have shown no teratogenic effect, the use of Brevibloc in women where pregnancy is suspected or confirmed should be avoided.

It is not known whether Brevibloc is excreted in human milk; however, administration of Brevibloc in nursing mothers should be avoided.

Warnings: Patients with bronchospastic disease should, in general, not receive beta blockers. Because of its relative beta$_1$ selectivity and titratability, Brevibloc should be used with caution in patients with bronchospastic diseases. However, since beta$_1$ selectivity is not absolute, Brevibloc should be carefully titrated to obtain the lowest possible effective dose. In the event of bronchospasm, the infusion should be terminated immediately and a beta$_2$ agonist should be administered if necessary.

There exist no data on the interactions of esmolol with calcium channel blockers; however, in common with other beta-adrenoceptor antagonists it is recommended that esmolol be used with caution in combination with verapamil in patients with impaired ventricular function. The combination should not be given to patients with conduction abnormalities and esmolol should not be administered within 48 hours of discontinuing verapamil.

Continued depression of the myocardium with beta-blocking agents over a period of time can, in some cases, lead to cardiac failure. At the first sign or symptom of impending cardiac failure, the dosage should be reduced or Brevibloc should be withdrawn and specific treatment should also be considered.

In clinical trials the most frequently observed side effect was hypotension which was rapidly reversible with dosage reduction or discontinuation. Thus, it is recommended that all patients receiving esmolol should have blood pressure frequently monitored; in the event of a hypotensive episode the infusion rate should be lowered or if necessary the infusion stopped.

Brevibloc should be administered with caution to patients with impaired renal function because the acid metabolite of Brevibloc is primarily excreted unchanged by the kidney.

The use of Brevibloc infusions for longer than 24 hours has not been thoroughly evaluated. Infusion durations greater than 24 hours should only be used with caution.

Use in children: The safety and effectiveness of Brevibloc in children have not been established.

Use in the elderly: Special studies in the elderly have not been conducted. However, analysis of data from 252 patients over 65 years of age indicated that no variations in pharmacodynamic effects occurred as compared with data from patients under 65.

Precautions: Infusion concentrations of 20 mg/ml have been associated with significant venous irritation and thrombophlebitis in animals and man. Extravasation of 20 mg/ml may lead to a serious local reaction and possible skin necrosis. Concentrations greater than 10 mg/ml or infusion into small veins or through a butterfly catheter should be avoided.

Brevibloc should be used with caution in diabetic patients.

Patients with low pre-treatment systolic pressures should be carefully observed during titration and maintenance infusion with Brevibloc.

Drug interactions: Catecholamine-depleting drugs, e.g. reserpine, may have an additive effect when given with beta-blocking agents. Patients treated concurrently with Brevibloc and a catecholamine depletor should therefore be closely observed for evidence of hypotension or marked bradycardia, which may result in vertigo, syncope, or postural hypotension.

Data from an interaction study between Brevibloc and warfarin showed that concomitant administration of Brevibloc and warfarin does not alter warfarin plasma levels. Brevibloc concentrations, however, were equivocally higher when given with warfarin.

When digoxin and Brevibloc were concomitantly administered intravenously to normal volunteers, there was a 10–20% increase in digoxin blood levels at some time points. Digoxin did not affect Brevibloc pharmacokinetics.

When intravenous morphine and Brevibloc interaction was studied in normal subjects, no effect on morphine blood levels was seen. The Brevibloc steady-state blood levels were increased by 46% in the presence of morphine, but no other pharmacokinetic parameters were changed.

The effect of Brevibloc on the duration of succinylcholine-induced neuromuscular blockade has been studied in patients undergoing surgery. The onset of neuromuscular blockade by succinylcholine was unaffected by Brevibloc, but the duration of neuromuscular blockade was prolonged from 5 minutes to 8 minutes.

Although the interactions observed in these studies are not of major clinical importance, Brevibloc should be titrated with caution in patients being treated concurrently with digoxin, morphine, succinylcholine or warfarin.

The hypotensive effects of inhalation anaesthetic agents may be increased in the presence of Brevibloc. The dosage of either agent may be modified as needed to maintain the desired haemodynamics.

Adverse effects: In the event of an adverse reaction, the dosage of Brevibloc may be reduced or discontinued.

Pharmacological adverse reactions should resolve within thirty minutes of discontinuing the infusion.

The most frequently observed side effect has been hypotension.

Less frequently observed were sweating, nausea, peripheral ischaemia, confusion, somnolence, dizziness, fatigue, agitation, headache, vomiting, inflammation, induration or infiltration at the infusion site, skin discoloration, burning at the infusion site, thrombophlebitis and local skin necrosis from extravasation.

Rarely seen are oedema, wheezing, dyspnoea, anxiety, anorexia, constipation, urinary retention, speech disorder, abnormal vision, rigor and fever.

In the perioperative situation, bradycardia and bronchospasm have also been observed.

Overdose: Because of its approximately 9-minute elimination half-life, the first step in the event of toxicity should be to discontinue Brevibloc administration. Then general supportive measures should be instituted as appropriate.

Pharmaceutical precautions Brevibloc is not compatible with sodium bicarbonate.

Brevibloc has been shown to be compatible with the following commonly used intravenous fluids, in both glass and PVC containers, at a final concentration of 10 mg esmolol hydrochloride per ml:

Dextrose 5% Injection
Dextrose 5% in Ringer's Injection
Dextrose 5% and Sodium Chloride 0.45% Injection
Dextrose 5% and Sodium Chloride 0.9% Injection
Dextrose 5% in Lactated Ringer's Injection
Lactated Ringer's Injection

Sodium Chloride (0.45%) Injection
Sodium Chloride (0.9%) Injection
Potassium Chloride (40 mEq/l) in Dextrose Injection

Diluted Brevibloc injection is compatible with commonly used PVC giving sets.

There is no information on compatibility of other drugs mixed with Brevibloc infusion.

Store at room temperature (15°–30°C).

Exposure to elevated temperatures should be avoided.

After dilution Brevibloc is stable for 24 hours when stored at 2° to 8°C.

Legal category POM.

Package quantities Brevibloc 250 mg/ml, 10 ml ampoule, is supplied individually packed.

Further information Nil.

Product licence number 4524/0025.

Product licence holder: Du Pont (U.K.) Limited, Wedgwood Way, Stevenage, Hertfordshire SG1 4QN.

HESPAN*

Presentation Hespan is a 6% colloidal solution for plasma volume expansion.

Composition:

Each 100 ml contains:

Hetastarch	6.0 g
Sodium Chloride BP	0.9 g
Water for Injections BP	qs

pH adjusted with Sodium Hydroxide. Concentration of Electrolytes (mEq/litre): Sodium 154, Chloride 154. pH: Approx. 5.5.

Calculated Osmolarity: Approx. 310 mOsm/litre

Weight average molecular weight	450,000
Number average molecular weight	70,000
Degree of substitution	0.7

Description: Hetastarch is an artificial colloid derived from a waxy starch composed almost entirely of amylopectin. Hydroxyethyl ether groups are introduced into the glucose units of the starch and the resultant material is hydrolyzed to yield a product with a molecular weight suitable for use as a plasma expander. Clinical Hetastarch is characterized by its molecular weight and its degree of substitution. The weight average molecular weight is approximately 450,000 with 90% of the polymer units falling within the range of 10,000 to 1,000,000. The degree of substitution is 0.7 which means Hetastarch has 7 hydroxyethyl groups for every 10 glucose units. The polymerized glucose units in Hetastarch are joined primarily by 1–4 linkages with hydroxyethyl groups being attached primarily at the No. 2 position. The polymer closely resembles glycogen.

The Hetastarch dosage form is a clear, pale yellow to amber solution. Exposure to prolonged adverse storage conditions (temperatures above 25°C or below freezing) may result in a change to turbid deep brown or the formation of a crystalline precipitate. Do not use the solution if these conditions are evident.

Uses *Actions:* The colloidal properties of 6% Hetastarch approximate those of human albumin. Intravenous infusion of Hetastarch results in expansion of plasma volume slightly in excess of the volume infused, which decreases from this maximum over the succeeding 24 to 36 hours. This expansion of plasma volume may improve the haemodynamic status for 24 hours and longer.

Hetastarch molecules below 50,000 molecular weight are rapidly eliminated by renal excretion with approximately 40% of a given total dose appearing in the urine in 24 hours. This is a variable process but generally results in an intravascular Hetastarch concentration of less than 1% of the total dose injected by two weeks. The hydroxyethyl group is not cleaved by the body, but remains intact and attached to glucose units when excreted.

The addition of Hetastarch to whole blood increases the erythrocyte sedimentation rate. Therefore, Hetastarch is used to improve the efficiency of granulocyte collection by centrifugal means.

Indications:

(1) As a plasma volume expander in cases of hypovolaemia due to:
- (a) Haemorrhage
- (b) Acute trauma
- (c) Burns
- (d) Sepsis
- (e) Water and electrolyte loss in acute gastrointestinal disturbances
- (f) Surgery

(2) Leucapheresis
(3) Extracorporeal circulation

Contra-indications, warnings, etc There are no absolute contraindications to the use of Hespan but Hespan should be used with caution in patients with established renal failure since Hespan is excreted primarily in the urine. In common with all plasma volume expanders, Hespan can produce dilutional effects on fibrinogen and prothrombin activity. In large volumes Hespan may alter the coagulation mechanism and produce a transient prolongation of the clotting time. Hespan should be used with caution in patients with severe bleeding disorders.

Hespan should be used with caution in patients vulnerable to vascular overloading (congestive cardiac failure, renal disease, etc.). Caution should be observed before administering Hespan to patients with a history of liver disease in view of slightly raised indirect bilirubin levels observed on very rare occasions in volunteers.

Hespan is non-antigenic, nor is its administration associated with raised plasma histamine levels. Mild allergic or sensitivity reactions have been occasionally reported consisting of peri-orbital oedema, urticaria or wheezing. If such reactions occur, they are readily controlled by discontinuation of the drug and, if necessary, administration of an antihistaminic agent.

Use in pregnancy: Reproduction studies have been done in mice with no evidence of fetal damage. Relevance to humans is not known since Hetastarch has not been given to pregnant women. Therefore, it should not be used in pregnant women, particularly during early pregnancy, unless in the judgement of the physician the potential benefits outweigh the potential hazards.

Use in Children: No data available pertaining to use in children.

Dosage and administration

Plasma volume expansion: Hespan should be administered by intravenous infusion only, in an initial volume approximately equal to half the estimated blood loss.

In adults the amount usually administered is 500 ml to 1,000 ml. Total dosage does not usually exceed 1,500 ml per day or 20 ml per kg of bodyweight for a typical 70 kg patient, but in common with other colloids, the limiting dose will depend on circulating volume and haematocrit.

In acute haemorrhagic shock, an initial administration rate approximately 20 ml/kg/hr may be recommended; in burns or septic shock, it is usually administered at slower rates. However, both the rate of infusion and the total dosage will be dependent upon the condition of the patient.

Leucapheresis: In leucapheresis procedures 250–700 ml Hespan is typically added to the Y junction just above the bleed out in the ratio of 1 part citrated Hespan to at least 8 parts whole blood; ratios of 1:20 have been used. On rare occasions, 500 ml Hespan has been infused into the donors 15–30 minutes before collection.

Multiple leucapheresis procedures using Hespan of up to 2 per week or a total of 7–10 have been reported to be safe and effective. The safety of more frequent or a greater number of procedures has not yet been established.

Pharmaceutical precautions The safety and compatability of additives have not been established.

Handling and Storage: Follow instructions for use of Steriflex bags: (instruction leaflet enclosed with package insert/data sheet).

Do not freeze. Store between 2 and 25°C.

Legal category POM.

Package quantities Hespan is supplied in 500 ml Steriflex bags, in boxes of 10.

Further information Intravenous infusion of Hydroxethyl starch results in expansion of plasma volume slightly in excess of the volume infused which decreases from this maximum over the succeeding 24–36 hours.

Isovolaemic substitution with Hespan up to 20% does not interfere with cross-matching determinations. Higher dilutions may lead to rouleaux formation which can easily be distinguished from agglutination by the addition of isotonic saline solution.

Product licence number 4524/0022.

Product licence holder: Du Pont (UK) Limited, Wedgwood Way, Stevenage, Herts SG1 4QN.

INTROPIN*

Presentation Ampoules containing a clear and practically colourless sterile solution of 200 mg dopamine hydrochloride and 50 mg sodium metabisulphite in 5 ml.

Uses *Actions:* Intropin exerts its beneficial haemodynamic effects by its action on different receptors. In relatively low doses Intropin dilates the renal and mesenteric vascular beds by its unique action on 'dopaminergic' receptors, causing increases in glomerular filtration rate, renal blood flow, sodium excretion, and urine output.

As the dosage is increased Intropin exerts a direct inotropic effect on the myocardium causing dose related increases in cardiac output with minimal effect on heart rate. Blood pressure usually rises and further increases in the urine output are seen.

With larger doses there are further increases in cardiac output and Intropin raises blood pressure by its alpha adrenergic action on peripheral blood vessels; however, even at these doses renal blood flow is higher than prior to therapy.

Preparation: Transfer 800 mg Intropin by aseptic technique to 500 ml of one of the following sterile intravenous solutions:

1. Sodium Chloride Injection
2. 5% Dextrose Injection
3. 5% Dextrose and 0.9% Sodium Chloride Injection
4. 5% Dextrose in 0.45% Sodium Chloride Solution
5. 5% Dextrose in Lactated Ringer Solution
6. Sodium Lactate (1/6 Molar) Injection
7. Lactated Ringer's Injection.

This gives a concentration of 1,600 micrograms/ml of Intropin.

Intropin is stable for 24 hours after dilution in the above solutions, however dilution should be made just before administration.

Do NOT add Intropin to 5% sodium bicarbonate or other alkaline solution since the drug is inactivated.

Administration: Intropin, after dilution, is administered intravenously through an intravenous catheter or needle in as large a vein as possible. An I.V. drip chamber or infusion pump is essential for controlling the infusion rate in drops/minute. The infusion rate should be titrated to the optimum patient response and constantly evaluated in terms of patient's changing condition.

Indications: Intropin is indicated for the correction of poor perfusion, low cardiac output, impending renal failure and shock associated with: Myocardial infarction, trauma, endotoxic septicaemia, open heart surgery, heart failure.

Dosage and administration *Warning:* This is a potent drug. It must be diluted before administration.

Dosage: Where appropriate, restoration of blood volume with a suitable plasma expander should be started or completed before Intropin therapy.

Begin infusion of Intropin therapy at 2 mcg/kg/min in patients who are likely to respond to modest increments in heart force and renal perfusion. In more seriously ill patients begin infusion of Intropin at 5 mcg/kg/min and in both cases the infusion rate should be titrated upwards in 5–10 mcg/kg/min increments up to 20–50 mcg/kg/min if needed. The majority of patients can be satisfactorily maintained on doses of dopamine less than 20 micrograms/kg/minute.

Contra-indications, warnings, etc

Contra-indications: Intropin should not be used in patients with phaeochromocytoma. Hypovolaemia should be corrected where necessary prior to Intropin infusion.

Intropin should not be used in the presence of uncorrected tachyarrhythmias or ventricular fibrillation.

Hyperthyroidism.

Precautions and warnings: Intropin contains sodium metabisulphite, a sulphite that may cause allergic-type reactions including anaphylactic symptoms and life-threatening or less severe asthmatic episodes in certain susceptible people. The overall prevalence of sulphite sensitivity in the general population is unknown, and probably low. Sulphite sensitivity is seen more frequently in asthmatic than in non-asthmatic people.

The degree of response to dopamine is reduced the longer the interval between onset of haemodynamic deterioration and treatment.

Dopamine should only be used under the direct supervision of physicians to whom facilities for regular, intensive monitoring of cardiovascular and renal parameters, in particular blood volume, myocardial contractility, cardiac output, electrocardiography, urine flow rate, blood and pulse pressure are available.

Extravasation of Intropin at the infusion site can cause local vasoconstriction, hence the desirability of infusion into a large vein. The resulting ischaemia can be reversed by infiltration of the affected area with 10–15 ml of saline containing 5–10 mg phentolamine mesylate. A syringe with a fine hypodermic needle should be used to liberally infiltrate the ischaemic area as soon as extravasation is noted.

Vasoconstriction can occur due to the alpha adrenergic actions of Intropin, especially in patients with a history of occlusive vascular disease. If desired, this condition can be rapidly reversed by dose reduction or discontinuing the infusion, since Intropin has a half-life of less than 2 minutes in the body.

Since the effect of dopamine on impaired renal and hepatic function is not known, close monitoring is advisable.

The appearance of unwarranted increase in blood pressure or decrease in urine output requires a reduction in quantity of drug infused.

Interactions: Use of dopamine in patients who are receiving, or have received within two weeks, monoamine oxidase inhibitors will require reduction of dosage to avoid potentiation. The starting dose should be one tenth (1/10) of the usual dose.

The cardiac effects of dopamine are antagonised by beta-adrenergic blocking agents such as propranolol and metoprolol.

Dopamine should only be used with extreme caution in patients receiving cyclopropane or halogenated hydrocarbon anaesthetics because of potential for arrhythmias.

Use in children: The safety and efficacy of Intropin use in children have not been established.

Use in pregnancy: Animal studies have shown no evidence of teratogenic effects with Intropin. The drug should only be used in pregnant women when the expected benefits outweigh the potential risk to the foetus.

Adverse reactions: The most frequently reported reactions to Intropin have been ectopic beats, tachycardia, anginal pain, palpitations, dyspnoea, nausea, vomiting, hypotension and vasoconstriction. Very rarely reported reactions include aberrant conduction, bradycardia, piloerection, widened QRS complex, azotaemia and hypertension. Vomiting is rare with Intropin, but should it occur, electrolytic replacement should be given.

Overdosage: Accidental overdosage as evidenced by excessive blood pressure elevation can be controlled by dose reduction or discontinuing the Intropin infusion for a short period, since the duration of action of Intropin is short.

Should these measures fail, an infusion of phentolamine mesylate should be considered.

Pharmaceutical precautions Do not add Intropin to 5% sodium bicarbonate or other alkaline solution since the drug is inactivated. Protect from light, do not use if discoloured. Avoid contact with solutions of alkalis.

Legal category POM.

Package quantities Ampoules containing 200 mg dopamine hydrochloride, 20 ampoules per outer carton.

Further information Nil.

Product licence number
Intropin 200 mg Ampoule 4524/0033

Product licence holder: Du Pont (UK) Limited, Wedgwood Way, Stevenage, Herts SG1 4QN.

MODURET 25*

Presentation Moduret 25 is available as off-white, diamond-shaped tablets, marked 'MSD 923', containing Amiloride Hydrochloride BP equivalent to 2.5 mg anhydrous amiloride hydrochloride and 25 mg Hydrochlorothiazide BP.

Uses Potassium-conserving diuretic and antihypertensive.

Moduret 25 is indicated alone or as an adjunct to other antihypertensive agents in: hypertension, congestive heart failure, hepatic cirrhosis with ascites and oedema.

Moduret 25 is intended for the treatment of patients in whom potassium depletion might be suspected or anticipated. The presence of amiloride hydrochloride minimises the likelihood of potassium loss during vigorous diuresis for long term maintenance therapy. The combination is thus indicated especially in conditions where potassium balance is particularly important.

Dosage and administration
Hypertension: Usually two or four Moduret 25 tablets given once a day or in divided doses. Some patients may require only one Moduret 25 Tablet a day. The dosage may be increased if necessary, but must not exceed eight Moduret 25 tablets a day.

Congestive heart failure: Initially two or four tablets of Moduret 25 a day, subsequently adjusted if required, but not exceeding eight Moduret 25 tablets a day. Optimal dosage is determined by the diuretic response and the plasma potassium level. Once an initial diuresis has been achieved, reduction in dosage may be attempted for maintenance therapy. Maintenance therapy may be on an intermittent basis.

Hepatic cirrhosis with ascites: Initiate therapy with a low dose. A single daily dose of two Moduret 25 tablets may be increased gradually until there is an effective diuresis. Dosage should not exceed eight Moduret 25 tablets a day. Maintenance dosages may be lower than those required to initiate diuresis; dosage reduction should therefore be attempted when the patient's weight is stabilised. A gradual weight reduction is especially desirable in cirrhotic patients to reduce the likelihood of untoward reactions associated with diuretic therapy.

Paediatric use: Moduret 25 is not recommended for children (see 'Contra-indications').

Use in the elderly: Particular caution is needed in the elderly because of their susceptibility to electrolyte imbalance; the dosage should be carefully adjusted to renal function and clinical response.

Contra-indications, warnings, etc
Contra-indications: Hyperkalaemia (plasma potassium over 5.5 mmol/l); other potassium-conserving diuretics. Potassium supplements or potassium-rich food (except in severe and/or refractory cases of hypokalaemia under careful monitoring); concomitant use with spironolactone or triamterene; anuria; acute renal failure, severe progressive renal disease, severe hepatic failure, precoma associated with hepatic cirrhosis, Addison's disease, hypercalcaemia, concurrent lithium therapy, diabetic nephropathy; patients with blood urea over 10 mmol/l, patients with diabetes mellitus, or those with serum creatinine over 130 umol/l in whom serum electrolyte and blood urea levels cannot be monitored carefully and frequently. Prior hypersensitivity to amiloride hydrochloride, hydrochlorothiazide or other sulphonamide derived drugs. Because the safety of amiloride hydrochloride for use in children has not been established, Moduret 25 is not recommended for children. For 'Use in pregnancy' and 'Use in breast-feeding mothers', see 'Precautions'.

Precautions: Hyperkalaemia has been observed in patients receiving amiloride hydrochloride, either alone or with other diuretics, particularly in the aged or in hospital patients with hepatic cirrhosis or congestive heart failure with renal involvement, who were seriously ill, or were undergoing vigorous diuretic therapy. Such patients should be carefully observed for clinical, laboratory, and ECG evidence of hyperkalaemia (not always associated with an abnormal ECG).

Neither potassium supplements nor a potassium-rich diet should be used with Moduret 25 except under careful monitoring in severe and/or refractory cases of hypokalaemia.

Some deaths have been reported in this group of patients.

Treatment of hyperkalaemia: Should hyperkalaemia develop, discontinue treatment immediately and, if necessary, take active measures to reduce the plasma potassium to normal.

Impaired renal function: Renal function should be monitored because the use of Moduret 25 in impaired renal function may result in the rapid development of hyperkalaemia. Thiazide diuretics become ineffective when creatinine levels fall below 30 ml/min.

Electrolyte imbalance: Although the likelihood of electrolyte imbalance is reduced by Moduret 25, careful check should be kept for such signs of fluid and electrolyte imbalance as hyponatraemia, hypochloraemic alkalosis, hypokalaemia and hypomagnesaemia. It is particularly important to make serum and urine electrolyte determinations when the patient is vomiting excessively or receiving parenteral fluids. Warning signs or symptoms of fluid or electrolyte imbalance include: dryness of the mouth, weakness, lethargy, drowsiness, restlessness, seizures, muscle pains or cramps, muscular fatigue, hypotension, oliguria, tachycardia, and gastro-intestinal disturbances such as nausea and vomiting.

Hypokalaemia may develop, especially as a result of brisk diuresis, after prolonged therapy or when severe cirrhosis is present. Hypokalaemia can sensitise or exaggerate the response of the heart to the toxic effects of digitalis (e.g. increased ventricular irritability).

Diuretic-induced hyponatraemia is usually mild and asymptomatic. It may become severe and symptomatic in a few patients who will then require immediate attention and appropriate treatment.

Thiazides may decrease urinary calcium excretion. Thiazides may cause intermittent and slight elevation of serum calcium in the absence of known disorders of calcium metabolism. Therapy should be discontinued before carrying out tests for parathyroid function.

Azotaemia may be precipitated or increased by hydrochlorothiazide. Cumulative effects of the drug may develop in patients with impaired renal function. If increasing azotaemia and oliguria develop during treatment of renal disease, Moduret 25 should be discontinued.

Hepatic disease: Thiazides should be used with caution in patients with impaired hepatic function or progressive liver disease (see 'Contra-indications'), since minor alterations of fluid and electrolyte balance may precipitate hepatic coma.

Metabolic: Hyperuricaemia may occur, or gout may be precipitated or aggravated, in certain patients receiving thiazides. Thiazides may impair glucose tolerance. Diabetes mellitus may be precipitated or aggravated by therapy with Moduret 25 (see 'Contra-indications'). Dosage adjustment of antidiabetic agents, including insulin, may be required.

Increases in cholesterol and triglyceride levels may be associated with thiazide diuretic therapy.

To minimise the risk of hyperkalaemia in diabetic or suspected diabetic patients, the status of renal function should be determined before initiating therapy with Moduret 25. Therapy should be discontinued at least three days before giving a glucose tolerance test. Potassium-conserving therapy should be initiated only with caution in severely ill patients in whom metabolic or respiratory acidosis may occur, e.g. patients with cardiopulmonary disease or patients with inadequately controlled diabetes.

Shifts in acid-base balance alter the balance of extracellular/intracellular potassium, and the development of acidosis may be associated with rapid increases in plasma potassium.

Sensitivity reactions: The possibility that thiazides may activate or exacerbate systemic lupus erythematosus has been reported.

Use in pregnancy: The routine use of diuretics in otherwise healthy pregnant women with or without mild oedema is not indicated, because they may be associated with hypovolaemia, increased blood viscosity, and decreased placental perfusion. Diuretics do not prevent the development of toxaemia of pregnancy and there is no satisfactory evidence that they are useful for its treatment.

Since thiazides cross the placental barrier and appear in cord blood, use where pregnancy is present or suspected requires that the benefits of the drug be weighed against possible hazards to the fetus. These hazards include fetal or neonatal jaundice, thrombocytopenia, bone marrow depression and possibly other side effects that have occurred in the adult.

Use in breast-feeding mothers: Although it is not known whether amiloride hydrochloride thiazides do appear in breast milk. If use of the drug combination is deemed essential, the patient should stop breast-feeding.

Drug interactions: When amiloride hydrochloride is administered concomitantly with an ACE inhibitor, the risk of hyperkalaemia may be increased. Therefore, if concomitant use of these agents is indicated because of demonstrated hypokalaemia, they should be used with caution and with frequent monitoring of serum potassium.

When given concurrently, the following drugs may interact with thiazide diuretics:

Alcohol, barbiturates or narcotics: Co-administration may potentiate orthostatic hypotension. Oral and parenteral antidiabetic drugs may require adjustment of dosage with concurrent use. Other antihypertensive drugs may have an additive effect. Therefore the dosage of these agents, especially adrenergic-blockers, may need to be reduced when Moduret 25 is added to the regimen. Diuretic therapy should be discontinued for 2–3 days prior to initiation of therapy with an ACE inhibitor to reduce the likelihood of first dose hypotension. Corticosteroids or ACTH may intensify any thiazide-induced electrolyte depletion, particularly hypokalaemia. Pressor amines such as adrenaline may show decresed arterial responsiveness when used with Moduret 25 but this reaction is not enough to preclude their therapeutic usefulness. Non-depolarising muscle relaxants such as tubocurarine may possibly interact with Moduret 25 to increase muscle relaxation. Lithium may accumulate as a result of reduced renal clearance. Non-steroidal anti-inflammatory drugs may attenuate the diuretic, natriuretic and antihypertensive effects of diuretics. Chlorpropamide: Moduret 25 can act synergistically with chlorpropamide to increase the risk of hyponatraemia. Drug/laboratory tests: Because thiazides may affect calcium metabolism, Moduret 25 may interfere with tests for parathyroid function.

Side-effects: Although minor side effects are relatively common, significant side effects are infrequent.

Reported side effects are generally associated with diuresis, thiazide therapy, or with the underlying disease.

No increase in the risk of adverse reactions has been seen over those of the individual components.

The reported adverse reactions of the combination:

Body as a whole: headache, weakness, fatigue, malaise, chest pain, back pain, syncope.

Cardiovascular: arrhythmias, tachycardia, digitalis toxicity, orthostatic hypotension, angina pectoris.

Digestive: anorexia, nausea, vomiting, diarrhoea, constipation, abdominal pain, GI bleeding, appetite changes, abdominal fullness, flatulence, thirst, hiccups.

Metabolic: elevated plasma potassium levels (above 5.5 mmol/l), electrolyte imbalance, hyponatraemia, gout, dehydration, symptomatic hyponatraemia.

Integumentary: rash, pruritis, flushing, diaphoresis.

Musculoskeletal: leg ache, muscle cramps, joint pain.

Nervous: dizziness, vertigo, paraesthesiae, stupor.

Psychiatric: insomnia, nervousness, mental confusion, depression, sleepiness.

Respiratory: dyspnoea.

Special senses: bad taste, visual disturbance, nasal congestion.

Urogenital: impotence, dysuria, nocturia, incontinence, renal dysfunction including renal failure.

The reported adverse reactions of amiloride:

Body as a whole: neck/shoulder ache, a pain in extremities.

Digestive: abnormal liver function, activation of probable pre-existing peptic ulcer, dyspepsia, jaundice.

Integumentary: dry mouth, alopecia, diaphoresis.

Nervous: tremors, encephalopathy.

Haematological: aplastic anaemia, neutropenia.

Cardiovascular: one patient with partial heart block developed complete heart block, palpitation.

Psychiatric: decreased libido, somnolence.

Respiratory: cough.

Special senses: tinnitus, increased intra-ocular pressure.

Urogenital: polyuria, urinary frequency, bladder spasm.

The reported adverse reactions of hydrochlorothiazide:

Body as a whole: anaphylactic reaction, fever.

Cardiovascular: necrotising angiitis (vasculitis, cutaneous vasculitis).

Digestive: jaundice (intrahepatic cholestatic jaundice), pancreatitis, cramping, gastric irritation.

Endocrine/Metabolic: glycosuria, hyperglycaemia, hyperuricaemia.

Integumentary: photosensitivity, sialadenitis, urticaria.

Haematological: agranulocytosis, aplastic anaemia, haemolytic anaemia, leucopenia, purpura, thrombocytopenia.

Psychiatric: restlessness.

Renal: interstitial nephritis.

Respiratory: respiratory distress, including pneumonitis, pulmonary oedema.

Special senses: transient blurred vision, xanthopsia.

Overdosage: No specific data are available on overdosage with Moduret 25. No specific antidote is available, and it is not known whether the drug is dialysable.

Treatment should be symptomatic and supportive. Therapy should be discontinued and the patient watched closely. Emesis should be induced and/or gastric lavage performed. The most common signs and symptoms of overdosage with amiloride hydrochloride are dehydration and electrolyte imbalance. Blood pressure should be monitored and corrected where necessary. If hyperkalaemia occurs, active measures should be taken to reduce the plasma potassium levels.

Electrolyte depletion (hypokalaemia, hypochloraemia, hyponatraemia) and dehydration are the most common signs and symptoms of hydrochlorothiazide overdosage. If digitalis has been administered, hypokalaemia may accentuate cardiac arrhythmias.

The plasma half-life of hydrochlorothiazide is 5.6 hours with a subsequent longer terminal half-life: the plasma half-life of amiloride is about six hours.

Pharmaceutical precautions Store in a dry place below 25°C, protected from light.

Legal category POM.

Package quantities Cartons of four calendar packs, each pack holding 7 tablets.

Further information The combination of amiloride with hydrochlorothiazide has been shown to cause less magnesium excretion than either the thiazides or the loop diuretics when used alone.

Onset of diuretic action begins within two hours after administration, and reaches a peak at about the fourth hour; there is detectable activity for about 24 hours.

Product licence number 0025/0178.

Product licence holder: Merck Sharp & Dohme Limited, Hertford Road, Hoddesdon, Hertfordshire, EN11 9BU.

MODURETIC*

Presentation Moduretic is available as peach-coloured, half-scored, diamond shaped tablets, marked 'MSD 917', containing amiloride hydrochloride BP, equivalent to 5 mg anhydrous amiloride hydrochloride and 50 mg hydrochlorothiazide BP.

Moduretic is also available as aniseed/peppermint-flavoured solution containing amiloride hydrochloride BP, equivalent to 5 mg anhydrous amiloride hydrochloride, and 50 mg hydrochlorothiazide BP in each 5 ml.

Uses Potassium-conserving diuretic and antihypertensive.

Moduretic is indicated in patients with: hypertension, congestive heart failure, hepatic cirrhosis with ascites and oedema. In hypertension, Moduretic may be used alone or in conjunction with other antihypertensive agents.

Moduretic is intended for the treatment of patients in whom potassium depletion might be suspected or anticipated. The presence of amiloride hydrochloride minimises the likelihood of potassium loss during vigorous diuresis for long term maintenance therapy. The combination is thus indicated especially in conditions where potassium balance is particularly important.

Dosage and administration

Hypertension: Usually one or two Moduretic tablets given once a day or in divided doses. Some patients may require only half a Moduretic tablet a day. The dosage may be increased if necessary, but must not exceed four Moduretic tablets (or equivalent) a day.

Congestive heart failure: Initially one or two tablets of Moduretic a day, subsequently adjusted if required, but not exceeding four Moduretic tablets (or equivalent) a day. Optimal dosage is determined by the diuretic response and the plasma potassium level. Once an initial diuresis has been achieved, reduction in dosage may be attempted for maintenance therapy. Maintenance therapy may be on an intermittent basis.

Hepatic cirrhosis with ascites: Initiate therapy with a low dose. A single daily dose of one Moduretic tablet or equivalent may be increased gradually until there is an effective diuresis. Dosage should not exceed four Moduretic tablets (or equivalent) a day. Maintenance dosages may be lower than those required to initiate diuresis; dosage reduction should therefore be attempted when the patient's weight is stabilised. A gradual weight reduction is especially desirable in cirrhotic patients to reduce the likelihood of untoward reactions associated with diuretic therapy.

Paediatric use: Moduretic is not recommended for children (see 'Contra-indications').

Use in the elderly: Particular caution is needed in the elderly because of their susceptibility to electrolyte imbalance; the dosage should be carefully adjusted to renal function and clinical response.

Contra-indications, warnings, etc

Contra-indications: Hyperkalaemia (plasma potassium over 5.5 mmol/l); other potassium-conserving diuretics. Potassium supplements or potassium-rich food (except in severe and/or refractory cases of hypokalaemia under careful monitoring); concomitant use with spironolactone or triamterene; anuria; acute renal failure, severe progressive renal disease, severe hepatic failure, precoma associated with hepatic cirrhosis, Addison's disease, hypercalcaemia, concurrent lithium therapy, diabetic nephropathy; patients with blood urea over 10 mmol/l, patients with diabetes mellitus, or those with serum creatinine over 130 umol/l in whom serum electrolyte and blood urea levels cannot be monitored carefully and frequently. Prior hypersensitivity to amiloride hydrochloride, hydrochlorothiazide or other sulphonamide derived drugs. Because the safety of amiloride hydrochloride for use in children has not been established, Moduretic is not recommended for children. For 'Use in pregnancy' and 'Use in breast-feeding mothers', see 'Precautions'.

Precautions: Hyperkalaemia has been observed in patients receiving amiloride hydrochloride, either alone or with other diuretics, particularly in the aged or in hospital patients with hepatic cirrhosis or congestive heart failure with renal involvement, who were seriously ill, or were undergoing vigorous diuretic therapy. Such patients should be carefully observed for clinical, laboratory, and ECG evidence of hyperkalaemia (not always associated with an abnormal ECG).

Neither potassium supplements nor a potassium-rich diet should be used with Moduretic except under careful monitoring in severe and/or refractory cases of hypokalaemia.

Some deaths have been reported in this group of patients.

Treatment of hyperkalaemia: Should hyperkalaemia develop, discontinue treatment immediately and, if necessary, take active measures to reduce the plasma potassium to normal.

Impaired renal function: Renal function should be monitored because the use of Moduretic in impaired renal function may result in the rapid development of hyperkalaemia. Thiazide diuretics become ineffective when creatinine levels fall below 30 ml/min.

Electrolyte imbalance: Although the likelihood of electrolyte imbalance is reduced by Moduretic, careful check should be kept for such signs of fluid and electrolyte imbalance as hyponatraemia, hypochloraemic alkalosis, hypokalaemia and hypomagnesaemia. It is particularly important to make serum and urine electrolyte determinations when the patient is vomiting excessively or receiving parenteral fluids. Warning signs or symptoms of fluid or electrolyte imbalance include: dryness of mouth, weakness, lethargy, drowsiness, restlessness, seizures, muscle pains or cramps, muscular fatigue, hypotension, oliguria, tachycardia, and gastro-intestinal disturbances such as nausea and vomiting.

Hypokalaemia may develop, especially as a result of brisk diuresis, after prolonged therapy or when severe cirrhosis is present. Hypokalaemia can sensitise or exaggerate the response of the heart to the toxic effects of digitalis (e.g. increased ventricular irritability).

Diuretic-induced hyponatraemia is usually mild and asymptomatic. It may become severe and symptomatic in a few patients who will then require immediate attention and appropriate treatment.

Thiazides may decrease urinary calcium excretion. Thiazides may cause intermittent and slight elevation of serum calcium in the absence of known disorders of calcium metabolism. Therapy should be discontinued before carrying out tests for parathyroid function.

Azotaemia may be precipitated or increased by hydrochlorothiazide. Cumulative effects of the drug may develop in patients with impaired renal function. If increasing azotaemia and oliguria develop during treatment of renal disease, Moduretic should be discontinued.

Hepatic disease: Thiazides should be used with caution in patients with impaired hepatic function or progressive liver disease (see 'Contra-indications'), since minor alterations of fluid and electrolyte balance may precipitate hepatic coma.

Metabolic: Hyperuricaemia may occur, or gout may be precipitated or aggravated, in certain patients receiving thiazides. Thiazides may impair glucose tolerance. Diabetes mellitus may be precipitated or aggravated by therapy with Moduretic (see 'Contra-indications'). Dosage adjustment of antidiabetic agents, including insulin, may be required.

Increases in cholesterol and triglyceride levels may be associated with thiazide diuretic therapy.

To minimise the risk of hyperkalaemia in diabetic or suspected diabetic patients, the status of renal function should be determined before initiating therapy with Moduretic. Therapy should be discontinued at least three days before giving a glucose tolerance test. Potassium-conserving therapy should be initiated only with caution in severely ill patients in whom metabolic or respiratory acidosis may occur, e.g. patients with cardiopulmonary disease or patients with inadequately controlled diabetes.

Shifts in acid-base balance alter the balance of extracellular/intracellular potassium, and the development of acidosis may be associated with rapid increases in plasma potassium.

Sensitivity reactions: The possibility that thiazides may activate or exacerbate systemic lupus erythematosus has been reported.

Use in pregnancy: The routine use of diuretics in otherwise healthy pregnant women with or without mild oedema is not indicated, because they may be associated with hypovolaemia, increased blood viscosity, and decreased placental perfusion. Diuretics do not prevent the development of toxaemia of pregnancy and there is no satisfactory evidence that they are useful for its treatment.

Since thiazides cross the placental barrier and appear in cord blood, use where pregnancy is present or suspected requires that the benefits of the drug be weighed against possible hazards to the foetus. These hazards include foetal or neonatal jaundice, thrombocytopenia, bone marrow depression and possibly other side effects that have occurred in the adult.

Use in breast-feeding mothers: Although it is not known whether amiloride hydrochloride is excreted in human milk, it is known that thiazides do appear in breast milk. If use of the drug combination is deemed essential, the patient should stop breast-feeding.

Drug interactions: When amiloride hydrochloride is administered concomitantly with an ACE inhibitor, the risk of hyperkalaemia may be increased. Therefore, if concomitant use of these agents is indicated because of demonstrated hypokalaemia, they should be used with caution and with frequent monitoring of serum potassium.

When given concurrently, the following drugs may interact with thiazide diuretics:

Alcohol, barbiturates or narcotics: Co-administration may potentiate orthostatic hypotension. Oral and parenteral antidiabetic drugs may require adjustment of dosage with concurrent use. Other antihypertensive drugs may have an additive effect. Therefore the dosage of these agents, especially adrenergic-blockers, may need to be reduced when Moduretic is added to the regimen. Diuretic therapy should be discontinued for 2–3 days prior to initiation of therapy with an ACE inhibitor to reduce the likelihood of first dose hypotension. Corticosteroids or ACTH may intensify any thiazide-induced electrolyte depletion, particularly hypokalaemia. Pressor amines such as adrenaline may show decresed arterial responsiveness when used with Moduretic but this reaction is not enough to preclude their therapeutic usefulness. Non-depolarising muscle relaxants such as tubocurarine may possibly interact with Moduretic to increase muscle relaxation. Lithium may accumulate as a result of reduced renal clearance. Non-steroidal anti-inflammatory drugs may attenuate the diuretic, natriuretic and antihypertensive effects of diuretics. Chlorpropamide: Moduretic can act synergistically with chlorpropramide to increase the risk of hyponatraemia. Drug/laboratory tests: Because thiazides may affect calcium metabolism, Moduretic may interfere with tests for parathyroid function.

Side-effects: Although minor side effects are relatively common, significant side effects are infrequent.

Reported side effects are generally associated with diuresis, thiazide therapy, or with the underlying disease.

No increase in the risk of adverse reactions has been seen over those of the individual components.

The reported adverse reactions of the combination:

Body as a whole: headache, weakness, fatigue, malaise, chest pain, back pain, syncope.

Cardiovascular: arrhythmias, tachycardia, digitalis toxicity, orthostatic hypotension, angina pectoris.

Digestive: anorexia, nausea, vomiting, diarrhoea, constipation, abdominal pain, GI bleeding, appetite changes, abdominal fullness, flatulence, thirst, hiccups.

Metabolic: elevated plasma potassium levels (above 5.5 mmol/l), electrolyte imbalance, hyponatraemia, gout, dehydration, symptomatic hyponatraemia.

Integumentary: rash, pruritis, flushing, diaphoresis.

Musculoskeletal: leg ache, muscle cramps, joint pain.

Nervous: dizziness, vertigo, paraesthesiae, stupor.

Psychiatric: insomnia, nervousness, mental confusion, depression, sleepiness.

Respiratory: dyspnoea.

Special senses: bad taste, visual disturbance, nasal congestion.

Urogenital: impotoence, dysuria, nocturia, incontinence, renal dysfunction including renal failure.

The reported adverse reactions of amiloride:

Body as a whole: neck/shoulder ache, a pain in extremities.

Digestive: abnormal liver function, activation of probable pre-existing peptic ulcer, dyspepsia, jaundice.

Integumentary: dry mouth, alopecia, diaphoresis.

Nervous: tremors, encephalopathy.

Haematological: aplastic anaemia, neutropenia.

Cardiovascular: one patient with partial heart block developed complete heart block, palpitation.

Psychiatric: decreased libido, somnolence.

Respiratory: cough.

Special senses: tinnitus, increased intra-ocular pressure.

Urogenital: polyuria, urinary frequency, bladder spasm.

The reported adverse reactions of hydrochlorothiazide:

Body as a whole: anaphylactic reaction, fever.

Cardiovascular: necrotising angiitis (vasculitis, cutaneous vasculitis).

Digestive: jaundice (intrahepatic cholestatic jaundice), pancreatitis, cramping, gastric irritation.

Endocrine/Metabolic: glycosuria, hyperglycaemia, hyperuricaemia.

Integumentary: photosensitivity, sialadenitis, urticaria.

Haematological: agranulocytosis, aplastic anaemia, haemolytic anaemia, leucopenia, purpura, thrombocytopenia.

Psychiatric: restlessness.

Renal: interstitial nephritis.

Respiratory: respiratory distress, including pneumonitis, pulmonary oedema.

Special senses: transient blurred vision, xanthopsia.

Overdosage: No specific data are available on overdosage with Moduretic. No specific antidote is available, and it is not known whether the drug is dialysable.

Treatment should be symptomatic and supportive. Therapy should be discontinued and the patient watched closely. Emesis should be induced and/or gastric lavage performed. The most common signs and symptoms of overdosage with amiloride hydrochloride are dehydration and electrolyte imbalance. Blood pressure should be monitored and corrected where necessary. If hyperkalaemia occurs, active measures should be taken to reduce the plasma potassium levels.

Electrolyte depletion (hypokalaemia, hypochloraemia, hyponatraemia) and dehydration are the most common signs and symptoms of hydrochlorothiazide overdosage. If digitalis has been administered, hypokalaemia may accentuate cardiac arrhythmias.

The plasma half-life of hydrochlorothiazide is 5.6 hours with a subsequent longer terminal half-life: the plasma half-life of amiloride is about six hours.

Pharmaceutical precautions Store in a dry place

below 25°C, protected from light. Moduretic Solution should not be diluted.

Legal category POM.

Package quantities
Moduretic Tablets: Bottles of 100 and 500 tablets.
Moduretic Solution: Bottles of 200 ml solution.

Further information The combination of amiloride with hydrochlorothiazide has been shown to cause less magnesium excretion than either the thiazides or the loop diuretics when used alone.

Onset of diuretic action begins within two hours after administration, and reaches a peak at about the fourth hour; there is detectable activity for about 24 hours.

Product licence numbers

Moduretic Tablets	0025/5016.
Moduretic Solution	0025/0165.

Product licence holder: Merck Sharp & Dohme Limited, Hertford Road, Hoddesdon, Hertfordshire, EN11 9BU.

NALOREX*

Presentation Pale orange mottled tablets, round, flat faced, bevelled edge, scored on one side, containing 50 mg naltrexone hydrochloride.

Uses Nalorex is indicated as an adjunctive therapy in the maintenance of detoxified, formerly opioid-dependent patients.

Dosage and administration Nalorex treatment should be initiated in a drug addiction centre and supervised by suitably qualified physicians.

The initial dose of Nalorex should be 25 mg (half a tablet) followed by 50 mg (one tablet) daily.

A three-times a week dosing schedule may be considered if it is likely to result in better compliance, e.g. 100 mg on Monday, 100 mg on Wednesday and 150 mg on Friday.

Treatment with Nalorex should be considered only in patients who have remained opioid-free for a minimum of 7–10 days.

Narcan* (Naloxone hydrochloride) challenge is recommended to minimise the chance of a prolonged withdrawal syndrome precipitated by Nalorex (see also 'Warnings').

As Nalorex is a prophylactic agent and full recovery from opioid dependence is variable, no standard duration of therapy can be recommended; an initial period of three months should be considered. However, prolonged administration may be necessary.

Contra-indications, warnings, etc
Contra-indications: Nalorex should not be given to patients currently dependent on opioids since an acute withdrawal syndrome may ensue.

Nalorex should not be given to patients who are hypersensitive to it.

Nalorex should not be given to patients with acute hepatitis or liver failure.

Warnings: It is not uncommon for opioid abusing individuals to have impaired liver functions. Liver function test abnormalities have been reported in obese and elderly patients taking naltrexone who have no history of drug abuse. Liver function tests should be carried out both before and during treatment.

A withdrawal syndrome may be precipitated by Nalorex* in opioid dependent patients; signs and symptoms may develop within 5 minutes and last up to 48 hours.

Treatment should be symptomatic and may include opioid administration.

Narcan (Naloxone hydrochloride) challenge is recommended to screen for presence of opioid use; a withdrawal syndrome precipitated by Narcan* will be of shorter duration than one precipitated by Nalorex*.

The recommended procedure is as follows:

- i.v. injection of 0.2 mg Narcan
- if after 30 seconds no adverse reactions occur, a further i.v. injection of 0.6 mg Narcan may be administered.
- continue to observe the patient for withdrawal effects for a further 30 minutes.

If doubt exists that the patient is opioid-free, the challenge may be repeated with a Narcan dose of 1.6 mg.

If there is no evidence of a reaction, Nalorex administration may be initiated with 25 mg by mouth (half a tablet).

Concomitant administration of Nalorex with an opioid containing medication should be avoided. Patients should be warned that attempts to overcome the blockade may result in acute opioid intoxication which may be life threatening. In an emergency requiring opioid analgesia an increased dose of opioid may be required to control pain. The patient should be closely monitored for evidence of respiratory depression or other adverse symptoms and signs.

Use in pregnancy: As with all new drugs, Nalorex should not be used during the first three months of pregnancy.

Because of absence of documented clinical experience Nalorex should only be given to pregnant or breast-feeding women when, in the judgement of the attending physician, the potential benefits outweigh the possible risks.

Use in children: Safe use in children has not been established.

Precautions: Since Nalorex* is extensively metabolised by the liver and excreted predominantly in the urine, caution should be observed in administering the drug to patients with impaired hepatic or renal function.

Adverse effects: The following adverse reactions have been reported before and during naltrexone medication: an incidence of more than 10% in detoxified opioid abusers; difficulty in sleeping, anxiety, nervousness, abdominal pain/cramps, nausea and/or vomiting, low energy, joint and muscle pain, and headache: an incidence of less than 10%; loss of appetite, diarrhoea, constipation, increased thirst, increased energy, feeling down, irritability, dizziness, skin rash, delayed ejaculation, decreased potency, chills, chest pain, increased sweating, and increased lacrimation. Occasional liver function abnormalities have also been reported. One case of reversible idiopathic thrombocytopenic purpura has occurred in a patient taking Nalorex*.

Overdose: There is no clinical experience with Nalorex* overdose in patients. There was no evidence of toxicity in volunteers receiving 800 mg/day for seven days, however, in case of overdose, patients should be monitored and treated symptomatically in a closely supervised environment.

Pharmaceutical precautions Store at room temperature. Protect from light.

Legal category POM.

Package quantities Amber glass bottles, 50 tablets.

Further information The development of tolerance and dependence have not been observed with Nalorex.

Product licence number 4524/0006.

Product licence holder: Du Pont (UK) Limited, Wedgwood Way, Stevenage, Herts SG1 4QN.

NARCAN*
NARCAN* NEONATAL

Presentation A sterile, clear, colourless solution of naloxone hydrochloride in clear, colourless ampoules.

Narcan (1 ml ampoules): each 1 ml of solution contains 400 micrograms naloxone hydrochloride.

Narcan (1 ml pre-filled syringes): each 1 ml of solution contains 400 micrograms naloxone hydrochloride.

Narcan (2 ml ampoules): each 1 ml of solution contains 1 milligram naloxone hydrochloride.

Narcan Neonatal (2 ml ampoules): each 1 ml of solution contains 20 micrograms naloxone hydrochloride.

Uses Narcan may be used for the complete or partial reversal of opioid depression, including mild to severe respiratory depression induced by natural and synthetic opioids, the agonist/antagonists nalbuphine and pentazocine, or dextropropoxyphene. It may also be used for the diagnosis of suspected acute opioid overdosage. Narcan Neonatal may be used to counteract respiratory and other CNS depression in the new-born resulting from the administration of analgesics to the mother during childbirth.

Dosage and administration Narcan is for intravenous, intramuscular or subcutaneous injection or intravenous infusion.

Intravenous infusion: Narcan may be diluted for intravenous infusion in normal saline (0.9%) or 5% dextrose in water or saline: the addition of 2 mg of Narcan in 500 ml of either solution provides a concentration of 4 micrograms/ml. Mixtures should be used within 24 hours. After 24 hours, the remaining unused solution must be discarded. The rate of administration should be titrated in accordance with the patient's response to both the Narcan infusion and to any previous bolus doses administered.

Parenteral drug products should be inspected visually for particulate matter and discoloration prior to administration whenever solution and container permit. Narcan should not be mixed with preparations containing bisulphite, metabisulphite, long-chain or high molecular weight anions or any solution having an alkaline pH. No drug or chemical agent should be added to Narcan unless its effect on the chemical and physical stability of the solution has first been established.

Adults:

Opioid overdosage (known or suspected): An initial dose of 400 to 2000 micrograms of Narcan may be administered intravenously. If the desired degree of counteraction and improvement in respiratory function is not obtained it may be repeated at 2 to 3 minute intervals. If no response is observed after 10 mg of Narcan have been administered the diagnosis of opioid-induced or partial opioid-induced toxicity should be questioned. Intramuscular or subcutaneous administration may be necessary if dosing by the intravenous route is not feasible.

N.B. The duration of action of certain opioids can outlast that of an IV bolus of Narcan, e.g. dextropropoxyphene (present in commonly prescribed analgesics which in over-dosage have been associated with suicide), dihydrocodeine and methadone. In situations where one of these opioids is known or suspected it is recommended that an infusion of Narcan (see above) be used to produce sustained antagonism to the opioid without repeated injection.

Post-operative use: When Narcan is used post-operatively, the dose should be titrated for each patient in order to obtain optimum respiratory response while maintaining adequate analgesia. Intravenous doses of 100–200 micrograms (1.5–3 micrograms/kg body weight) are usually sufficient, but a full two minutes should be allowed between each 100 micrograms increment of Narcan administered. Further intramuscular doses may be needed within one to two hours, depending on the interval since the last opioid administration and the amount and type (i.e. long or short-acting) of drug used. Alternatively Narcan may be administered as an intravenous infusion (see above).

Children: The usual initial dose in children is 10 micrograms per kg body weight given IV. If this dose does not result in the desired degree of clinical improvement, a subsequent dose of 100 micrograms per kg of body weight may be administered. Narcan may be required by infusion as described above. If an IV route of administration is not feasible, Narcan may be administered IM or SC in divided doses.

Neonatal use: An adequate airway should be established in the apnoeic infant before Narcan is administered. The usual dose for opioid-induced depression is 10 micrograms/kg body weight administered IV, IM or SC. If the desired degree of counteraction and improvement in respiratory function is not obtained it may be repeated at 2 to 3 minute intervals. Alternatively, a single dose of 200 micrograms (approximately 60 micrograms/kg body weight) may be given intramuscularly at birth. It should, however, be noted that onset of action is slower following IM injection.

Contra-indications, warnings, etc Narcan should not be given to patients who are known to be hypersensitive to it. It should be administered cautiously to patients who have received large doses of opioids or to those physically dependent on opioids since too rapid reversal of opioid effects by Narcan may precipitate an acute withdrawal syndrome in such patients. The same caution is needed when giving Narcan to neonates delivered of such patients.

Although animal reproduction studies have not demonstrated any teratogenic or embryotoxic effects, Narcan should, like all drugs, be used with caution during pregnancy. However, Narcan may be administered to the mother during the second stage of labour to correct respiratory depression in the new-born caused by opioids used to provide obstetrical analgesia.

Patients who have responded satisfactorily to Narcan should be kept under observation. Repeated doses of Narcan may be necessary since the duration of action of some opioids may exceed that of Narcan.

Narcan is not effective against respiratory depression caused by non-opioid drugs.

Two patients with ventricular irritability have developed tachycardia or fibrillation following the administration of naloxone. Although a direct relationship has not been established, it is suggested that Narcan be used with caution in patients with cardiac irritability.

Adverse effects: Occasionally, nausea and vomiting have been reported in post-operative patients who have received Narcan in doses higher than those recommended; however, a cause and effect relationship has not been established.

Overdosage: There have been no reports of acute overdosage with Narcan. Single doses of 10 mg intravenously and subcutaneous doses of 15 mg every four hours for two weeks have been administered without producing either respiratory depression or psychotomimetic effects.

Pharmaceutical precautions Protect from light.

Legal category POM.

Package quantities Narcan ampoules each containing 400 micrograms in 1 ml are supplied in boxes of 3 or 10 ampoules.

Narcan ampoules each containing 2 milligrams in 2 ml are supplied in boxes of 3 ampoules.

Narcan single dose pre-filled syringes each containing 400 micrograms in 1 ml are supplied in boxes of one syringe.

Narcan Neonatal ampoules each containing 40 micrograms in 2 ml are supplied in boxes of 10 ampoules.

Further information Nil.

Product Licence Numbers

Narcan (400 micrograms/ml)	
1 ml Ampoule	4524/0014
1 ml Syringe	4524/0027
Narcan (1 milligram/ml)	
2 ml Ampoule	4524/0021
Narcan Neonatal (20 micrograms/ml)	
2 ml Ampoule	4524/0002

Product licence holder: Du Pont (UK) Limited, Wedgwood Way, Stevenage, Herts SG1 4QN.

NUBAIN*

Presentation Ampoules containing a clear colourless sterile aqueous solution of 20 mg nalbuphine hydrochloride in 2 ml or 10 mg nalbuphine hydrochloride in 1 ml.

Uses Nubain injection is indicated for the relief of moderate to severe pain. It can also be used as a premedication, for pre- and post-operative analgesia, and as a component of balanced anaesthesia. It can also be used in the management of pain due to suspected myocardial infarction.

Dosage and administration Nubain injection may be administered subcutaneously, intramuscularly or intravenously. It may also be administered by patient-controlled on demand intravenous infusion, using a delivery system which is appropriately calibrated and does not interact with the drug.

The usual recommended dosage is 10 mg–20 mg for a 70 kg individual. The dosage should be adjusted according to the severity of pain, physical status of the patient and other medications the patient may be receiving.

Balanced anaesthesia

Induction: 0.3 mg/kg to 1 mg/kg I.V. over a 10–15 minute period.

Maintenance: 0.25–0.5 mg/kg at 30 minute intervals.

Premedication: 0.1–0.2 mg/kg.

Suspected myocardial infarction: Usual dose 20 mg by slow intravenous injection. Some patients may be successfully managed on 10 mg while others may need to have the dose increased to 30 mg. In the absence of pain relief a repeat dose of 20 mg may be given within 30 minutes.

Children: An initial dose of up to 0.3 mg/kg IV, IM or SC which may be repeated once or twice as necessary.

Contra-indications, warnings, etc

Contra-indications: Nubain should not be administered to patients who are hypersensitive to it.

Warnings: Drug dependence: Nubain has low abuse potential. However, caution should be observed in prescribing it for emotionally unstable patients or for patients with a history of opioid abuse.

When Nubain is selected for the control of chronic pain, its suggested prolonged activity may delay the need for larger or more frequent doses.

Abrupt discontinuation of Nubain following prolonged use has been followed by symptoms of opioid withdrawal.

Use in ambulatory patients: Nubain may impair the mental or physical abilities required by the performance of potentially dangerous tasks such as driving a car or operating machinery. Therefore, Nubain should be administered with caution to ambulatory patients who should be warned to avoid such hazards.

Use in pregnancy: Safe use of Nubain in pregnancy (including labour) has not been established.

Although animal studies have not revealed teratogenic or embryotoxic effects, nalbuphine should only be administered to pregnant women when, in the judgement of the physician, the potential benefits outweigh the possible hazards.

Nubain should be used to provide analgesia in patients with head injury and increased intracranial pressure only when essential, and then should be administered with extreme caution.

Patients receiving an opioid analgesic, general anaesthetic, phenothiazine or other tranquillizer, sedative, hypnotic or other CNS depressant (including alcohol) concomitantly with Nubain may exhibit an additive effect. When such combined therapy is contemplated, the dose of one or both agents should be reduced.

Precautions: Nubain used as a premedication causes some respiratory depression. Caution should be observed in administering the drug to patients with impaired respiration, or with other medications which produce respiratory depression.

During evaluation of Nubain in anaesthesia, a higher incidence of bradycardia has been reported in patients not administered pre-operative atropine.

In the presence of bronchial asthma, uraemia, severe infection, cyanosis or respiratory obstruction, Nubain should be administered with caution and in reduced doses.

Nubain should be used with caution and administered in reduced amounts in patients with impaired renal or hepatic function.

Adverse effects: The most frequently seen reaction to Nubain is sedation. Less frequent are sweating, nausea, vomiting, dizziness, dry mouth, vertigo and headache. Rarely seen are CNS effects such as nervousness, depression, confusion and dysphoria. Also reported have been hyper- and hypotension, bradycardia, tachycardia, urticaria, speech difficulty, blurred vision and flushing.

Management of overdosage: The immediate intravenous administration of Narcan* (naloxone hydrochloride) is a specific antidote. Oxygen, intravenous fluids, vasopressors and other supportive measures should be used as indicated.

Pharmaceutical precautions Protect from light. Store at room temperature (15–30°C).

Legal category POM.

Package quantities

Nubain 2 ml ampoules are supplied in boxes of 10.
Nubain 1 ml ampoules are supplied in boxes of 10.

Further information Nubain is compatible with 0.9% sodium chloride, 5% dextrose, 4.3% dextrose/0.18% saline and Hartmann's solution used in glass, PVC and polyethylene infusion containers.

Product licence number 4524/0003.

Product licence holder: Du Pont (UK) Limited, Wedgwood Way, Stevenage, Herts SG1 4QN.

PENTASPAN* ▼

Presentation Pentaspan is a 10% sterile, non-pyrogenic, colloidal solution for plasma volume expansion and leucapheresis.

Composition: Each 100 ml contains:

Pentastarch	10.0 g
Sodium Chloride PhEur	0.9 g
Water for Injection PhEur	qs
pH adjusted with Sodium Hydroxide	qs
Concentration of Electrolytes (mEq/litre)	Sodium 154, Chloride 154
Calculated osmolarity	Approx 320 mOsm/litre
pH	Approx 5.0
Weight average molecular weight	250,000
Degree of substitution	0.45

Description: Pentastarch is a colloid derived from waxy starch composed almost entirely of amylopectin. Hydroxyethyl ether groups are introduced into the glucose units of the starch and the resultant material is hydrolysed to yield a product with a molecular weight suitable for use as a plasma volume expander or as an erythrocyte sedimenting agent. Pentastarch is characterised by its molar substitution, and also by its molecular weight. The molar substitution is 0.45 which means pentastarch has 45 hydroxyethyl groups for every 100 glucose units. The weight average molecular weight of the pentastarch polydispersion is approximately 250,000 with a range of 150,000 to 300,000 with 80% of the polymers falling between 15,000 and 1,500,000. Hydroxyethyl groups are attached by an ether linkage primarily at C-2 of the glucose unit and to a lesser extent at C-3 and C-6. The polysaccharide resembles glycogen.

Pentaspan is a clear, pale yellow to amber solution. Exposure to prolonged adverse storage conditions (temperatures above 40°C or below freezing) may result in a change to a turbid deep brown or the formation of a crystalline precipitate. Do not use the solution if these conditions are evident.

Uses

Actions: The colloidal properties of Pentaspan (10% pentastarch in 0.9% sodium chloride) are moderately greater than the related product Hespan (6% hetastarch in 0.9% sodium chloride) and those of 5% human albumin. Pentaspan administrations resulted in 1.5 times greater volume expansion when compared to equal volumes of Hespan. The plasma volume expansion resulting from intravenous infusion of Pentaspan persists for approximately 18 to 24 hours. This expansion of plasma volume may improve the haemodynamic status for 12–18 hours.

Pentastarch molecules below 50,000 molecular weight are rapidly eliminated by renal excretion. A single dose of approximately 500 ml of Pentaspan (approximately 50 g) results in elimination in the urine of approximately 70% of a given dose within 24 hours and approximately 80% of the dose within one week. 14–15% (approximately 6–8 g) of an administered dose is quantitatively eliminated at a slower rate.

This elimination process generally results in an intravascular pentastarch concentration below the level of detection by one week. The hydroxyethyl group remains attached to glucose units when excreted.

In leucapheresis 5–6% of the pentastarch dose is recovered in the collection bags.

The addition of Pentaspan to whole blood increases the erythrocyte sedimentation rate. Therefore, Pentaspan is used to improve the efficiency of leucocyte collection by centrifugal means.

Volume expansion may be expected to occur following use of Pentaspan in leucapheresis procedures.

Indications: Plasma volume expansion in cases of hypovolaemia due to haemorrhage, surgery, sepsis, burns or other trauma. Leucapheresis.

Dosage and administration

Plasma volume expansion: Pentaspan is administered by intravenous infusion only. Total dosage and rate of infusion depend upon the amount of blood or plasma lost. In adults the amount usually administered is 500–2000 ml. Total daily dosage does not usually exceed 2000 ml for a typical 70 kg patient or 28 ml per kg of body weight. In acute haemorrhagic shock an administration rate approaching 20 ml/kg/hr may be used. Use beyond 72 hours has not been studied.

Leucapheresis: 250 to 700 ml Pentaspan injection to which citrate anticoagulant has been added is typically administered by the aseptic addition to the input line of the centrifugation apparatus at a ratio of 1:8 to 1:134 to venous whole blood. The bottle containing Pentaspan and citrate should be thoroughly mixed to assure effective anticoagulation of blood as it flows through the leucapheresis machine.

The safety and compatibility of other additives have not been established.

Contra-indications, warnings, etc

Contra-indications: In patients with known hypersensitivity to hydroxyethyl starch.

In patients with severe bleeding disorders or in patients with severe congestive heart failure where volume overload is a potential problem.

In patients with renal failure with oliguria or anuria not related to hypovolaemia.

In patients with acute cerebral infarction where cerebral oedema is a potential problem.

Warnings

Usage in plasma volume expansion: Haematocrit and haemoglobin may be decreased and plasma proteins diluted excessively by administration of large volumes of Pentaspan.

Like most plasma volume expanders, large volumes of Pentaspan may slightly alter the coagulation mechanism, i.e., there may be transient prolongation of prothrombin time and partial thromboplastin clotting time, therefore the physician should be alert to the possibility of transient prolongation of bleeding time.

Isovolaemic substitution with Pentaspan up to 20% does not interfere with cross-matching determinations. Higher dilutions may lead to rouleaux formation (this is not agglutination as the addition of a drop of saline will disperse the rouleaux formation).

Usage in leucapheresis: Platelet counts and haemoglobin levels have been observed to decrease slightly in donors undergoing repeated leucapheresis procedures using Pentaspan due to the dilutional effect of plasma volume expansion and the collection of platelets and erythrocytes. Haemoglobin levels usually return to normal within 24 hours. Haemodilution by Pentaspan and saline may also result in a slight decrease of total protein, albumin, calcium and fibrinogen values. None of these effects pose clinically significant risks to healthy donors.

Precautions: Pentaspan should be given with caution to patients at risk from vascular overloading, e.g. congestive cardiac failure and renal disease, etc.

Care should be exercised in patients with primary renal impairment as Pentaspan is excreted primarily in the urine.

Pentaspan should be used with caution in patients with a history of liver disease in view of slightly raised indirect bilirubin levels observed on very rare occasions in volunteers.

There is no evidence from clinical trials that Pentaspan is antigenic. Pentaspan has been reported to produce sensitivity reactions such as wheezing and urticaria. If such reactions occur, they are readily controlled by discontinuation of Pentaspan and, if necessary, administration of an antihistaminic agent.

Elevated serum amylase levels may be observed temporarily following administration of Pentaspan although no association with pancreatitis has been demonstrated.

Regular and frequent clinical evaluation including complete blood counts (CBC) are necessary for monitoring during leucapheresis using Pentaspan. If leucapheresis is frequent, the following additional tests may be helpful: platelet count, prothrombin time (PT) and partial thromboplastin time (PTT).

Pentaspan is not suitable as a replacement for the fresh components of plasma or the cellular components of blood.

Use in pregnancy: High doses (40 ml/kg/day) of Pentaspan increased the number of resorptions and minor visceral abnormalities in rabbits and reduced nidation in mice.

Pentaspan has not been given to pregnant women: therefore it should not be used, particularly during early pregnancy, unless in the judgement of the physician the potential benefits outweigh the potential hazards.

It is not known whether Pentaspan is excreted in human milk therefore caution should be exercised in administering it to nursing mothers.

Use in children: The safety and efficacy of Pentaspan in children have not been established.

Use in the elderly: No specific dosage recommendations.

Adverse reactions: The following have been reported in association with use of Pentaspan. Plasma volume replacement or expansion: coagulation disorders or haemorrhage. Leucapheresis: headache, diarrhoea, nausea, weakness, temporary weight gain, insomnia, fatigue, fever, oedema, paraesthesia, acne, malaise, shakiness, dizziness, chest pain, chills, nasal congestion, anxiety and increased heart rate. For either indication it is uncertain whether any of these adverse experiences are attributable to the drug, the leucapheresis or surgical procedures, concurrent adjunctive medication, or a combination of these factors.

Pharmaceutical precautions Store at 2–25°C. Do not freeze. The safety and compatibility of additives, other than citrate anticoagulant, have not been established.

Parenteral drug products should be inspected for particulate matter and turbid brown discoloration prior to administration whenever solution and container permit.

Legal category POM.

Package quantities Pentaspan is supplied in 250 and 500 ml PVC Intraflex bags, in boxes of 10.

Product licence number 4524/0038.

Product licence holder: Du Pont (UK) Limited, Wedgwood Way, Stevenage, Hertfordshire SG1 4QN

SINEMET*

Presentation

Sinemet-LS is available as yellow, half-scored, oval tablets, marked 'SINEMET LS', containing 12.5 mg carbidopa (as carbidopa monohydrate) and 50 mg levodopa.
Sinemet-110 is available as dapple-blue, half-scored, oval tablets, marked 'MSD 647' containing 10 mg carbidopa (as carbidopa monohydrate) and 100 mg levodopa.
Sinemet-Plus is available as yellow, half-scored, oval tablets, marked 'SINEMET PLUS', containing 25 mg carbidopa (as carbidopa monohydrate) and 100 mg levodopa.
Sinemet-275 is available as dapple-blue, half-scored, oval tablets, marked 'MSD 654', containing 25 mg carbidopa (as carbidopa monohydrate) and 250 mg levodopa.

Uses Antiparkinsonian agent.

For treatment of Parkinson's disease and syndrome. Sinemet is useful in relieving many of the symptoms of parkinsonism, particularly rigidity and bradykinesia. It is frequently helpful in the management of tremor, dysphagia, sialorrhoea, and postural instability associated with Parkinson's disease and syndrome.

When response to levodopa alone is irregular, and signs and symptoms of Parkinson's disease are not controlled evenly throughout the day, substitution of Sinemet usually reduces fluctuations in response. By reducing some of the adverse reactions produced by levodopa alone, Sinemet permits more patients to obtain adequate relief of the symptoms of Parkinson's disease.

Sinemet may be given to patients with Parkinson's disease and syndrome who are taking vitamin preparations that contain pyridoxine hydrochloride (Vitamin B6).

Dosage and administration The optimum daily dosage of Sinemet must be determined by careful titration for each patient.

Sinemet Tablets are available in a ratio of 1:4 or 1:10 of carbidopa to levodopa to provide facility for fine dosage titration for each patient.

General considerations: Studies show that the peripheral enzyme dopa-decarboxylase is fully inhibited (saturated) by carbidopa at doses between 70 and 100 mg a day. Patients receiving less than this amount of carbidopa are more likely to experience nausea and vomiting.

Because both therapeutic and adverse effects are seen more rapidly with Sinemet than with levodopa, patients should be carefully monitored during the dosage adjustment period. Involuntary movements, particularly blepharospasm, is a useful early sign of excess dosage in some patients.

If general anaesthesia is required, therapy with Sinemet may be continued for as long as the patient is permitted to take fluids and medicines by mouth. If therapy has to be stopped temporarily, Sinemet may be restarted as soon as oral medication can be taken at the same daily dosage as before.

Patients not receiving levodopa: Dosage may be best initiated with one tablet of Sinemet-Plus three times a day. This dosage schedule provides 75 mg of carbidopa per day. Dosage may be increased by one tablet of Sinemet-LS or Sinemet-Plus every day or every other day, as necessary, until a dosage equivalent of eight tablets of Sinemet-Plus a day is reached.

If Sinemet-110 or Sinemet-LS is used, dosage may be initiated with one tablet three or four times a day. Titration upward may be required in some patients to achieve optimum dosage of carbidopa. The dosage may be increased by one tablet every day or every other day until a total of eight tablets (two tablets q.d.s.) is reached. For patients starting with Sinemet-275, the initial dose is one-half tablet taken once or twice daily. However, this may not provide the optimal amount of carbidopa needed by many patients. If necessary, add one-half tablet every day or every other day until optimal response is reached.

Response has been observed in one day, and sometimes after one dose. Fully effective doses usually are reached within seven days as compared to weeks or months with levodopa alone.

Sinemet-LS or Sinemet-110 may be used to facilitate dosage titration according to the needs of the individual patient.

Patients receiving levodopa: Discontinue levodopa at least 12 hours (24 hours for slow-release preparations) before starting therapy with Sinemet. The easiest way to do this is to give Sinemet as the first morning dose after a night without any levodopa. The dose of Sinemet should be approximately 20% of the previous daily dosage of levodopa.

Patients taking less than 1,500 mg levodopa a day should be started on one tablet of Sinemet-Plus three or four times a day dependent on patient need. The suggested starting dose for most patients taking more than 1,500 mg levodopa a day is one tablet of Sinemet-275 three or four times a day.

Maintenance: Therapy with Sinemet should be individualised and adjusted gradually according to response. When a greater proportion of carbidopa is required, each tablet of Sinemet-110 may be replaced with a tablet of Sinemet-Plus or Sinemet-LS.

When more levodopa is required, Sinemet-275 should be substituted at a dosage of one tablet three or four times a day. If necessary, the dosage of Sinemet-275 may be increased by half to one tablet every other day to a maximum of eight tablets a day. Experience with a total daily dosage greater than 200 mg carbidopa is limited.

Patients receiving other antiparkinsonian agents: The combination of Sinemet with MAO-B-inhibitors (e.g. selegiline) has been reported to improve the efficacy of Sinemet in controlling episodes of akinesia and/or dyskinesia.

Use in children: The safety of Sinemet in patients under 18 years of age has not been established.

Use in the elderly: There is wide experience in the use of this product in elderly patients. The recommendations set out above reflect the clinical data derived from this experience.

Contra-indications, warnings, etc
Contra-indications: MAO-inhibitors (except low doses of selective MAO-B-inhibitors) and Sinemet should not be given concomitantly (these must be discontinued at least two weeks before starting Sinemet); narrow-angle glaucoma; known hypersensitivity to this medication. Because levodopa may activate a malignant melanoma, it should not be used in patients with suspicious undiagnosed skin lesions or a history of melanoma. See also 'Pregnancy and lactation', under 'Precautions'.

Precautions: Sinemet is not recommended for the treatment of drug-induced extrapyramidal reactions.

Sinemet should be administered cautiously to patients with severe cardiovascular or pulmonary disease, bronchial asthma, renal, hepatic or endocrine disease.

Care should be exercised when Sinemet is administered to patients with a history of myocardial infarction who have atrial, nodal, or ventricular arrhythmias. Cardiac function should be monitored with particular care in such patients during the period of initial dosage adjustment.

All patients should be monitored carefully for the development of mental changes, depression with suicidal tendencies, and other serious antisocial behaviour. Patients with current psychoses should be treated with caution.

As with levodopa, Sinemet may cause involuntary movements and mental disturbances. Patients with a history of severe involuntary movements or psychotic episodes when treated with levodopa alone should be observed carefully when Sinemet is substituted. These reactions are thought to be due to increased brain dopamine following administration of levodopa, and use of Sinemet may cause a recurrence. A syndrome resembling the neuroleptic malignant syndrome including muscular rigidity, elevated body temperature, mental changes and increased serum creatine phosphokinase has been reported with the abrupt withdrawal of antiparkinsonian agents. Therefore, any abrupt dosage reduction or withdrawal of Sinemet should be carefully observed, particularly in patients who are also receiving neuroleptics.

Concomitant administration of psycho-active drugs such as phenothiazines or butyrophenones should be carried out with caution, and the patients carefully observed for loss of antiparkinsonian effect. Patients with a history of convulsions should be treated with caution.

Patients with chronic wide-angle glaucoma may be treated cautiously with Sinemet, provided the intra-ocular pressure is well controlled and the patient monitored carefully for changes in intra-ocular pressure during therapy.

As with levodopa, there is a possibility of upper gastro-intestinal haemorrhage in patients with a history of peptic ulcer.

Laboratory tests: Commonly, levels of blood urea, creatinine and uric acid are lower during administration of Sinemet than with levodopa. Transient abnormalities include elevated levels of blood urea, AST (SGOT), ALT (SGPT), LDH, bilirubin, alkaline phosphatase, and protein-bound iodine.

Positive Coombs tests have been reported, both with Sinemet and levodopa alone, but haemolytic anaemia is extremely rare.

Sinemet may cause a false positive result when a dipstick is used to test for urinary ketone; and this reaction is not altered by boiling the urine. The use of glucose oxidase methods may give false negative results for glycosuria.

Drug interactions: Postural hypotension can occur when Sinemet is added to the treatment of patients already receiving antihypertensive drugs. Dosage adjustments of the antihypertensive agent may be required. Rarely, reactions including hypertension and dyskinesia have been reported with the concomitant use of tricyclic antidepressants. (See the Contra-indications for patients receiving MAOIs.)

Phenothiazines, butyrophenones, phenytoin and papaverine may reduce the therapeutic effect of levodopa. Patients taking these drugs with Sinemet should be carefully observed for loss of therapeutic response.

Since levodopa competes with certain amino acids, the absorption of Sinemet may be impaired in some patients on a high protein diet.

Pregnancy and lactation: Although the effects of Sinemet on human pregnancy and lactation are unknown, both levodopa and combinations of carbidopa and levodopa have caused visceral and skeletal malformations in rabbits. Therefore, use of Sinemet in women of child-bearing potential requires that the anticipated benefits of the drug be weighed against possible hazards should pregnancy occur. Sinemet should not be given to brest-feeding mothers.

Side-effects: Side-effects that occur frequently with Sinemet are those due to the central neuropharmacological activity of dopamine. These reactions can usually be diminished by dosage reduction. The most common are dyskinesias including choreiform, dystonic, and other involuntary movements. Muscle twitching and blepharospasm may be taken as early signs to consider dosage reduction.

Other serious side-effects are mental changes, including paranoid ideation and psychotic episodes; depression, with or without development of suicidal tendencies; and dementia. A common but less serious side effect is nausea.

Less frequent side-effects are cardiac irregularities and/or palpitations, orthostatic hypotensive episodes, bradykinetic episodes (the 'on-off' phenomenon), anorexia, vomiting, dizziness, and somnolence.

Gastro-intestinal bleeding, development of duodenal ulcer, hypertension, phlebitis, leucopenia, haemolytic and non-haemolytic anaemia, thrombocytopenia, agranulocytosis, chest pain, dyspnoea and paraesthesia have occurred rarely.

Other side-effects that have been reported with levodopa include:

Neurological: ataxia, numbness, increased hand tremor, muscle twitching, blepharospasm, muscle cramp, trismus, activation of latent Horner's syndrome.

Psychiatric: confusion, sleepiness, insomnia, nightmares, hallucinations, delusions, agitation, anxiety, euphoria.

Gastro-intestinal: dry mouth, bitter taste, sialorrhoea, dysphagia, bruxism, hiccups, abdominal pain and distress, constipation, diarrhoea, flatulence, burning sensation of the tongue.

Metabolic: weight gain or loss, oedema.

Integumentary: flushing, incresed sweating, dark sweat, rash, hair loss.

Genito-urinary: urinary retention, urinary incontinence, dark urine, priapism.

Special senses: diplopia, blurred vision, dilated pupils, oculogyric crises.

Miscellaneous: weakness, faintness, fatigue, headache, hoarseness, malaise, hot flushes, sense of stimulation, bizarre breathing patterns, neuroleptic malignant syndrome, malignant melanoma (see 'contra-indications').

Overdosage: Management of acute overdosage with Sinemet is basically the same as management of acute overdosage with levodopa; however, pyridoxine is not effective in reversing the actions of Sinemet. General supportive measures should be employed, along with immediate gastric lavage. Intravenous fluids should be administered judiciously, and an adequate airway maintained. ECG monitoring should be instituted, and the patient carefully observed for the possible development of arrhythmias; if required, appropriate anti-arrhythmic therapy should be given.

The possibility that the patient may have taken other drugs as well as Sinemet should be taken into consideration. To date, no experience has been reported with dialysis, and hence its value in the treatment of overdosage is not known. Pyridoxine has no effect in reversing the effects of Sinemet.

The terminal half-life of levodopa is about two hours in the presence of carbidopa.

Pharmaceutical precautions Keep container tightly closed; store in a cool place, protected from light.

Legal category POM.

Package quantities
Sinemet-LS in bottles of 84.
Sinemet-110 in bottles of 100.
Sinemet-Plus in bottles of 100.
Sinemet-275 in bottles of 100.

Further information Levodopa relieves the symptoms of Parkinson's disease presumably by being decarboxylated to dopamine in the brain. Carbidopa, which does not cross the blood-brain barrier, inhibits only the extra-cerebral decarboxylation of levodopa, making more levodopa available for transport to the brain and subsequent conversion to dopamine. This obviates the need for large doses of levodopa at frequent intervals. The lower dosage reduces or eliminates many adverse reactions, some of which are attributed to dopamine being formed in extra-cerebral tissues.

Product licence numbers

Sinemet-LS	0025/0226
Sinemet-110	0025/0084
Sinemet-Plus	0025/0150
Sinemet-275	0025/0085

Product licence holder: Merck, Sharp and Dohme Limited, Hertford Road, Hoddesdon, Hertfordshire EN11 9BU

TRIDIL*

Presentation Tridil 50 mg is supplied as a sterile, non-pyrogenic, practically colourless solution containing 5 mg/ml glyceryl trinitrate in 30% v/v Alcohol BP and 30% v/v propylene glycol and Water for Injections PhEur. Each 10 ml ampoule contains 50 mg glyceryl trinitrate for intravenous infusion.

Tridil 5 mg is supplied as a sterile, non-pyrogenic solution containing 0.5 mg/ml glyceryl trinitrate stabilized by alcohol BP 10% v/v, lactose and monobasic sodium phosphate. Each 10 ml glass ampoule contains 5 mg glyceryl trinitrate for intravenous use.

Actions: Glyceryl trinitrate causes relaxation of vascular smooth muscle. In a dose related manner glyceryl trinitrate produces dilatation of both the arterial and venous vascular beds, however, the venous effects predominate. Dilatation of the post capillary vessels including large veins results in peripheral pooling and a reduction in venous return. Therapeutic doses of Tridil given intravenously produce a reduction in left ventricular end diastolic volume, left ventricular end diastolic pressure and myocardial wall tension. Myocardial oxygen consumption, as measured by the rate pressure product and tension time index is decreased.

Pulmonary vascular resistance, systemic vascular resistance and arterial pressure are all reduced by Tridil administration. Although the predominant clinical benefits result from the peripheral venodilating effects and the resultant reduction in myocardial oxygen demand, some effect on oxygen supply may occur by direct coronary vasodilatation. A re-distribution of blood from normal to ischaemic areas of the myocardium has been demonstrated.

Uses *Surgery:* Tridil may be used for the prompt control of hypertension encountered during cardiac surgery.

Tridil may be used to reduce blood pressure and maintain controlled hypotension during surgical procedures.

Tridil may be used to control myocardial ischaemia during and after cardiovascular surgery.

Unresponsive Congestive Cardiac Failure Secondary to Acute Myocardial Infarction: Tridil may be used to reduce elevated left ventricular filling pressure in patients with unresponsive congestive cardiac failure secondary to acute myocardial infarction.

Unstable Angina: Tridil infusion can reduce myocardial oxygen demand in proportion to the reduction in preload and after-load. Tridil may be indicated for the control of anginal episodes in patients with unstable angina who are refractory to treatment with standard therapy.

Patients with recurrent myocardial ischaemia not responsive to beta-blockers or sublingual nitrates may benefit from the intravenous Tridil infusion prior to surgery or angiography.

Frequent monitoring of blood pressure and pulse rate are recommended during the infusion.

Dosage and administration Tridil is a concentrated pharmacological drug which should be diluted in 5% Dextrose in Water or 0.9% Sodium Chloride prior to its infusion.

It is recommended that the drug is diluted to give a final concentration of 400 micrograms/ml or less according to the dosage requirements of the patient. Most patients respond to doses between 10–200 micrograms/min, although doses up to 400 micrograms/min may be required during some surgical procedures.

Dosage: The recommended dosage range is 10–200 micrograms/min. Doses in excess of these have been used and up to 400 micrograms/min may be required during some surgical procedures.

Clinical assessment and frequent monitoring of blood pressure are essential to maintain the appropriate infusion rate. Where available, measurement of pulmonary capillary wedge pressure and cardiac output can be used to titrate dosage to response.

Surgery: For the control of hypertensive episodes the recommended starting dose is 25 micrograms/min increasing in steps of 25 micrograms/min at 5 minute intervals until the desired drop in B.P. is achieved. Although most patients respond to doses between 10–200 micrograms/min, doses up to 400 micrograms/min have been required during some surgical procedures. In the treatment of perioperative myocardial ischaemia, the recommended starting dose is 15–20 micrograms/min increasing in steps of 10–15 micrograms/min until the desired effect is achieved.

Unresponsive Congestive Cardiac Failure Secondary to Acute Myocardial Infarction: The recommended starting dose is 20–25 micrograms/min which can be decreased to 10 micrograms/min or increased in steps of 20–25 micrograms/min at 15–30 minute intervals until the desired effect is achieved.

Unstable angina: The recommended starting dose is 10 micrograms/min increasing in steps of 5–10 micrograms/min at approximately 30 minute intervals.

Children: The safety and efficacy of Tridil have not been established in children.

Contra-indications, warnings, etc
Contra-indications: Tridil should not be given to patients with known hypersensitivity to nitrates.

Tridil should not be used in patients with marked anaemia, head trauma, cerebral haemorrhage, severe hypotension or hypovolaemia.

Precautions and warnings: Tridil should be used with caution in patients suffering from hypothyroidism, malnutrition, severe liver or renal disease or hypothermia.

Safety for intracoronary injection has not been shown.

As with all vasodilators, Tridil should be used with caution in patients predisposed to closed angle glaucoma.

Clinical assessment and frequent monitoring of blood pressure is essential and measurements of pulmonary artery wedge pressure or cardiac output where available are desirable to maintain the appropriate infusion rate adjusted to the patients response.

Tridil should be administered by means of a micro-drip set infusion pump or similar device which permits maintenance of a constant infusion rate. The giving set should be composed of glass or rigid polyethylene. Infusion systems composed of PVC may absorb up to 50% of the glyceryl trinitrate from solution, thus reducing the potency of the infusion. (See 'Pharmaceutical precautions'.)

Use in children: The safety and efficacy of Tridil have not been established in children.

Use in pregnancy: As the safety of Tridil during pregnancy, and lactation, has not been established, it should not be used unless considered essential by the physician.

Adverse reactions: Adverse reactions to nitrates may include hypotension, tachycardia, nausea, retching, diaphoresis, apprehension, headache, restlessness, muscle twitching, retrosternal discomfort, palpitations, dizziness, and abdominal pain. Paradoxical bradycardia has occasionally been observed.

Overdosage: Mild overdosage usually resulting in hypotension and tachycardia can be reversed by elevating the legs or decreasing or terminating the infusion. If severe, intravenous administration of methoxamine or phenylephrine is recommended.

Pharmaceutical precautions Opened ampoules should be used immediately and any unused diluted drug should be discarded.

Tridil solution is stable for at least 24 hours at room temperature in glass or recommended plastic containers (see compatibility). Considerable losses of glyceryl trinitrate will occur if Tridil is in contact with polyvinylchloride (PVC) plastic infusion bags and therefore contact with PVC should be avoided. Tridil should therefore be administered in the recommended infusion bottles/packs or via a syringe pump.

Protect from strong light. Do not use if discoloured.

Compatibility: Tridil is compatible with glass infusion bottles. Tridil has also been shown to be compatible with certain rigid infusion packs made of polyethylene; these include the polyfusor from Kendall or bottlepak and flatpak from Braun, Dublin. Tridil can be administered as an infusion using one of these recommended infusion bottles/packs.

Tridil is not compatible with infusion bags made from PVC and loss of activity in excess of 40% may occur if contact between glyceryl trinitrate and polyvinylchloride is prolonged. It is therefore recommended that contact with PVC bags is avoided. Some loss of activity can also occur through the infusion sets but the clinical response should be used to determine the rate of infusion and thus the dosage of the drug required by the patient.

An alternative method of administration is via syringe pump. Tridil can be infused slowly via a syringe pump using a glass syringe or rigid plastic syringe (Gillette Sabre syringe, Brunswick Disposable, BD Plastipak syringes). A high pressure polyethylene tubing known to be compatible with glyceryl trinitrate is the Lectrocath tubing, Vygon Gloucester.

The chosen method of administration should ensure that the drug is given at the constant infusion rate.

Legal category POM.

Package quantities Tridil 50 mg is available in a box containing four 10 ml ampoules.

Tridil 5 mg is available in a box containing twenty 10 ml ampoules.

Further information Experience so far has shown that when given by slow infusion, the onset of action occurs within approximately 3–5 minutes.

Glyceryl trinitrate is also known as nitroglycerin, trinitroglycerin and trinitrin.

Product licence numbers

Tridil 5 mg 4524/0035
Tridil 50 mg 4524/0036

Product licence holder: Du Pont (UK) Limited, Wedgwood Way, Stevenage, Herts SG1 4QN.

**Trade Mark*

Ethicon Limited
PO Box 408
Bankhead Avenue
Edinburgh EH11 4HE

ABSELE* STERILE ABSORBABLE BONE SEALANT

Presentation A paste of putty-like consistency composed of:

Stabilised bovine fibrin	17.5% w/w
Solubilised bovine collagen	17.5% w/w
Dextran 70	8.0% w/w
Glycerol	30.0% w/w
Water	to100

Physically it is a yellowish brown to brown, slightly sticky paste having a distinctive odour. It is malleable and adheres to wet cut bone surfaces. Complete absorption of the paste has been shown experimentally in rats in 14 to 21 days. The general mechanism by which *in vivo* degradation occurs is proteolytic enzymatic action. Absele Bone Sealant provokes initially a mild inflammatory reaction which quickly subsides. The bone sealant is sterilised by gamma irradiation.

Uses To control bleeding from the divided, drilled or chipped edges of bone by physically plugging the osseous canals which contain the bleeding capillaries.

Dosage and administration By implantation and application to bone as required to control haemorrhage.

Contra-indications, warnings, etc To date there have been no contra-indications to the use of this product.

Use only as much bone sealant as is necessary for haemostasis. It should be applied with the fingers or with a suitable spatulated instrument until bleeding stops. Remove any excess bone sealant before surgical closure.

Pharmaceutical precautions The product remains in optimum condition when stored at low temperatures. The shelf-life is two years when stored at 15°C; the expiry date is shown on each pack. Storage under refrigeration will extend the expected shelf-life. Exposure to temperatures in excess of 30°C may cause irreversible adverse changes to the product. Do not re-sterilise the contents of the pack. Unused product from opened packs should be discarded.

Legal category P.

Package quantities Flat discs of approximately 2 grams in weight are packaged in a sealed aluminium foil pack and peel-apart overwrap pouch. The sales unit is a film-wrapped box containing 12 packs.

Further information Absorbable bone sealant will harden if left exposed to the atmosphere for long periods, particularly under the heat of operating lights. The package should, therefore, only be opened immediately before use.

Product licence number 0508/0006.

ABSOLOK* EXTRA
Sterile Polydioxanone Absorbable Ligating Clips

Presentation Absolok Extra Ligating Clips are absorbable, 'V' shaped ligating clips available in four sizes, prepared from the polyester p-dioxanone. The empirical molecular formula of the polymer is $(C_4H_6O_3)_n$. Absolok Extra (polydioxanone) clips are dyed with D & C Violet No 2 during polymerisation. Sterilisation is by ethylene oxide gas.

Absolok Extra clips are relatively inert, non-antigenic, non-pyrogenic and elicit only a mild tissue reaction during absorption.

Action: The absorption characteristics of polydioxanone have been extensively studied. The general mechanism by which *in vivo* degradation of polydioxanone occurs is hydrolysis. The *in vivo* hydrolysis of polydioxanone cleaves the ester linkages and initially results in the loss of strength. Ultimately, the hydrolysed polymer is eliminated from the body, primarily in urine.

The results of implantation studies of polydioxanone clips in animals indicate that the clips retained their strength longer than necessary for a thrombus or clot to occur in a vessel.

Data obtained from implantation studies in rats indicate that the absorption of these clips is minimal until about the 90th post-implantation day. Absorption is essentially complete within 210 days.

Uses Absolok Extra clips are intended for use as absorbable ligatures. These clips are designed to offer a rapid, efficient means of ligation. Unlike cautery, the vessel and/or tissue is occluded with no thermal destruction. Unlike conventional metallic haemostatic clips, the absorbable clips are radiotransparent. Therefore, they will not interfere with interpretations of postoperative X-ray, CT or NMR scans.

The Absolok Extra clip applier, designed for use specifically with Absolok Extra clips optimises visibility of the clip at the ligation site and facilitates access to virtually all vessels and/or tissues.

Dosage and administration By implantation.

Contra-indications, warnings, etc Absolok Extra clips should not be used where prolonged or permanent ligation of tissues or vessels is required.

The use of the Absolok Extra Clip in vasectomy procedures and tubal ligation procedures is contra-indicated. The safety and effectiveness of the Absolok Extra Clip in contact with neural tissues have not been established.

Use only with an Absolok Extra clip applier of the appropriate size. Identification for each size is facilitated by the matching colour on the clip cartridge and the handle of the applier.

The clip must be latched to ensure proper ligation of the vessel or tissue.

Tissue must be compliant enough to allow latch to engage securely. Depending on the toughness of the surrounding tissue, the latch may not displace the tissue enough to latch. Some dissection of tissue from vessel surface may then be necessary.

As with any ligating device, the surgeon should inspect the ligation site following placement of the clip to ensure proper haemostasis and ligation has been achieved.

Do not re-sterilise the clips or clip cartridge.

Pharmaceutical precautions The recommended storage conditions are below 25°C, away from moisture and direct heat. Shelf life is 5 years; the expiry date is shown on each pack.

Legal category Not applicable.

Package quantities Clips are available in four sizes as follows:

Product code	*Colour coding*	*Approximate vessel sizes*
AP100	Blue	0.5–2.0 mm
AP200	White (silver handle on applier)	1.5–3.0 mm
AP300	Green	2.5–4.0 mm
AP400	Yellow	3.5–5.5 mm

Each colour coded cartridge contains ten clips. Each cartridge is sealed in an aluminium foil pack and peel apart overwrap pouch. The sales unit is a filmwrapped box containing 6 packs.

Further information No clip-related adverse reactions were reported during clinical trials.

Based upon the experience of the surgeon, Absolok Extra ligating clips sizes and corresponding applier selection should be consistent with the vessel being ligated.

Closed clips have minimal gap ensuring even the smallest vessels in the appropriate size range will be properly latched.

The latch of Absolok Extra clips is designed to allow direct application to vessels with little or no tissue dissection.

Product licence number 0508/0015.

BIETHIUM* STERILE ABSORBABLE OX FIBRIN PROSTHESIS

Presentation Moulded pliable implants in various shapes and sizes, sterilised by gamma irradiation and contained in a sealed foil sachet, which is in turn contained in a sterilised overwrap. The implant is composed of 65% heat treated bovine fibrin and 35% glycerol. Physically, it is a yellowish brown translucent product with a distinctive honey-like odour. It is pliable and resilient and has a specific gravity of 1.2. Absorption of the implant as observed experimentally in rats is approximately six weeks. However, if the implant is treated with a buffered formaldehyde solution prior to gamma irradiation, the absorption period can be extended for up to five months.

Uses

1. A bean-shaped prosthesis is used for the surgical correction of female stress incontinence. The bean is placed surgically at the urethro-vesical junction to reconstruct the normal angle of exit of the urethra from the bladder.

2. The buffer is rectangular and, used in pairs, effectively compresses the liver substance, following biopsy or liver resection, again by broadening the surface area of pressure of the ligating suture.

3. The rod shaped prosthesis provides support for exteriorising the loop of large bowel during a defunctioning colostomy.

Dosage and administration One bean only is required in stress incontinence, one rod for a defunctioning colostomy, while the liver buffers are used in pairs. Administration is by implant at a surgical procedure.

Contra-indications, warnings, etc Biethium Ox Fibrin Prosthesis are supplied sterile and should not be resterilised.

Pharmaceutical precautions Store under normal shelf conditions. Observe expiry date.

Legal category Not applicable.

Package quantities One bean per foil pack, with five foil packs per box. Two buffers per foil pack, with five foil packs per box. One rod per foil pack with five foil packs per box. Each foil pack is overwrapped in a peel-open container. The boxes containing the foil packs are film overwrapped.

Further information *Storage:* Two years' shelf life. Avoid storing beside caustics, chlorides and mercurials which could damage the aluminium foil pack.

Product licence number 0508/0003R.

COATED VICRYL* (Polyglactin 910) Sterile Braided Synthetic Absorbable Suture

Presentation Vicryl (Polyglactin 910) Suture is prepared from a copolymer of glycolide and lactide in the ratio 90/10. The substances are derived respectively from glycolic and lactic acids. The empirical formula of the copolymer is $(C_2H_2O_2)m(C_3H_4O_2)n$.

Coated Vicryl (Polyglactin 910) Sutures are obtained by coating the braided Vicryl (Polyglactin 910) suture material with a mixture composed of a copolymer of lactide and glycolide in the ratio of 65/35 and an equal amount of calcium stearate. This coating does not affect the biological properties of the suture.

Vicryl (Polyglactin 910) Sutures are coloured by adding D & C Violet No 2 during polymerisation of the lactide and glycolide. Sutures may also be manufactured in the undyed form.

Coated Vicryl (Polyglactin 910) is available in non-needled lengths or attached to stainless steel needles of varying types and sizes, and is sterilised by ethylene oxide gas.

These sutures are relatively inert, nonantigenic, non-pyrogenic and elicit only a mild tissue reaction during absorption.

Action: Two important characteristics describe the *in vivo* behaviour of absorbable sutures. The first of these is tensile strength retention and the second absorption rate or loss of mass.

The general mechanism by which *in vivo* degradation of Vicryl (Polyglactin 910) occurs is hydrolysis.

Subcutaneous tissue implantation studies of Coated Vicryl (Polyglactin 910) Suture in rats show at 14 days post-implantation approximately 65% of the original tensile strength remains. At 21 days approximately 40% of the original strength is retained for gauge sizes Metric 0.7 (6/0) and larger, and approximately 30% of the original strength is retained for gauge sizes Metric 0.5 (7/0) and smaller. All of the original tensile strength is lost between 28 and 35 days post implantation.

Intramuscular implantation studies in rats show that the absorption of these sutures occurs thereafter and is complete between the 56th and 70th day.

Uses Coated Vicryl (Polyglactin 910) synthetic absorbable Sutures are intended for use where an absorbable suture or ligature is indicated.

Dosage and administration By implantation.

Contra-indications, warnings, etc These sutures, being absorbable, should not be used where extended approximation of tissues under stress is required.

Sutures placed in skin and conjunctiva may cause localised irritation if left in place for longer than 7 days.

The safety and effectiveness of Coated Vicryl (Polyglactin 910) in neural tissue and in cardiovascular tissue have not been established.

At the discretion of the surgeon, appropriate non-absorbable sutures may be used to provide additional wound support when Coated Vicryl (Polyglactin 910) Sutures are used in ophthalmic procedures.

Under certain circumstances, notably orthopaedic procedures, immobilisation by external support may be employed at the discretion of the surgeon.

Coated Vicryl (Polyglactin 910) sutures, which are treated to enhance handling characteristics, require the standard surgical technique of flat and square ties with additional throws if indicated by surgical circumstances and the experience of the operator.

Acceptable surgical practice must be followed with respect to drainage and closure of infected wounds.

Pharmaceutical precautions Recommended storage conditions: Below 25 deg C, away from moisture and direct heat. Shelf life is 5 years, the expiry date is shown on each pack. Do not re-sterilise the pack contents. Unused product from opened packs should be discarded.

As with all sutures care should be taken to avoid damage when handling. Avoid the crushing or crimping application of surgical instruments, such as needle holders and forceps to the strand, except when grasping the free end of the suture during an instrument tie.

Legal category Not applicable.

Package quantities Coated Vicryl (Polyglactin 910) is available in various lengths in gauge sizes 0.4 to 5.0 Metric (8/0 to 2) and 3 metre lengths on Ligapak* reels 2.0 to 4.0 Metric (3/0 to 1). All products are sealed in aluminium foil packs and peel-apart overwrap pouches. The sales unit is a film wrapped box containing 10, 12 or 24 packs.

Further information No suture related adverse reactions were reported during clinical trials, although a number of minor reactions were classified as being of unknown cause.

Product licence number 0508/0009.

PDS* and PDS II (Polydioxanone) Sterile Synthetic Absorbable Suture

Presentation PDS and PDS II (Polydioxanone) Monofilament Synthetic Absorbable Sutures are prepared from the polyester poly (p-dioxanone). The empirical molecular formula of the polymer is $(C_4H_6O_3)n$. PDS (Polydioxanone) sutures are coloured by adding D & C Blue No 6 during polymerisation. PDS II sutures are coloured by adding D & C Violet No 2. PDS II sutures may also be manufactured undyed (clear). PDS and PDS II (Polydioxanone) are available attached to stainless steel needles of various types and sizes and are sterilised by ethylene oxide gas.

PDS and PDS II (Polydioxanone) sutures are relatively inert, non-antigenic, non-pyrogenic and elicit only a mild tissue reaction during absorption.

Action: Two important characteristics describe the *in vivo* behaviour of absorbable sutures. The first of these is tensile strength retention and the second absorption rate or loss of mass. The general mechanism by which *in vivo* degradation of polydioxanone occurs is hydrolysis.

Data obtained from implantation studies in rats show the following absorption profile:
14 days post implantation – 70% strength remaining
28 days post implantation – 50% strength remaining
56 days post implantation – 14% strength remaining

This indicates a significantly longer period of wound support than previously available with an absorbable suture.

The absorption or loss of mass is minimal until about the 90th post implantation day and is essentially complete within 180 days.

Uses PDS and PDS II (Polydioxanone) monofilament sutures are intended for use where an absorbable suture or ligature is indicated. They may have particular application where longer wound support is required. See strength retention data above.

Dosage and administration By implantation.

Contra-indications, warnings, etc These sutures, being absorbable, should not be used where extended approximation of tissues under stress is required or in conjunction with prosthetic devices eg heart valves or synthetic grafts.

As with all monofilament synthetic sutures, care should be taken to ensure proper knot security.

Conjunctival, cuticular and vaginal epithelium sutures could cause localised irritation if left in place for longer than 10 days. Superficial placement of subcuticular sutures may also be associated with erythema and reaction during the course of absorption.

The safety and effectiveness of PDS and PDS II (Polydioxanone) sutures in neural and cardiac tissue have not been established.

Pharmaceutical precautions Recommended storage conditions are below 25 deg C away from moisture and direct heat. Shelf life is 5 years, the expiry date is shown on each pack. Do not re-sterilise the pack contents. Unused product from opened packs should be discarded.

As with all sutures care should be taken to avoid damage when handling. Avoid the crushing or crimping application of surgical instruments, such as needle holders and forceps to the strand, except when grasping the free end of the suture during an instrument tie.

Legal category Not applicable.

Package quantities PDS is available in various lengths in gauge sizes 0.2 to 0.4 Metric (10/0 to 8.0). PDS II is available in various lengths in gauge sizes 0.5 to 5.0 Metric (7/0 to 2). The sutures are packaged in sealed aluminium foil packs and peel apart overwrap pouches. The sales unit is a film wrapped box containing 12 or 24 packs.

Further information No suture related adverse reactions were reported during clinical trials, although a number of minor reactions were classified as being of unknown cause.

Product licence numbers
0508/0020 PDS II – Undyed.
0508/0021 PDS II – Violet Dyed.
0508/0022 PDS – Blue Dyed.

STERILE POLYTEF PASTE FOR INJECTION

Presentation A sterile, white, injectable paste in tin tubes within a see-through, peel-apart overwrap. Polytef Paste contains 50% of polytetrafluoroethylene powder (which has been pyrolised to purify it) in Glycerin USP containing polyoxyethylene sorbitan monolaurate (Tween 20).

Uses Polytef Paste for Injection is used for intravocal cord injection of the paralysed vocal cord. It is administered by injection directly into the cord.

Dosage and administration By injection. Dose varies according to size of cord, but should not exceed 0.6 cc per site of injection.

Contra-indications, warnings, etc Contra-indicated until at least six months have elapsed following the onset of paralysis, and/or until an intensive trial of rehabilitation by voice therapy has been given since many patients are capable of overcoming their vocal disability.

In bilateral laryngeal paralysis. In vocal disorders of psychogenic origin. In the presence of foreign bodies in the larynx (e.g. fragments of shells or bullets).

In the presence of an acute inflammation, infection or inadequately controlled malignancy, or a rapidly advancing disease, especially when these are in the laryngeal or upper respiratory tract area.

Warnings: Intra-cordal injection is a delicate procedure and should be conducted with precision and great caution. This product should be used only by trained ENT surgeons.

General anaesthesia is not advisable. Over-sedation may lead to an unco-operative patient and difficult airway problems. Intravascular injections must be avoided. Likewise, over-injection should be avoided.

It is safer to under-inject the involved cord than to over-inject because treatment may be repeated at a later time. If the procedure is followed by upper respiratory tract inflammatory changes in excess of the reaction expected at the site of injection, diagnostic and therapeutic procedures should be implemented. In acute fulminating reactions, steroid and antibiotic therapy may be indicated. This therapy should be at the discretion of the surgeon.

Pharmaceutical precautions Recommended storage conditions are below 25°C away from moisture and direct heat. Discard unused paste. Do not re-sterilise.

Legal category POM.

Package quantities Polytef Paste for Injection is packaged in tin tubes containing 7 ml and contained in a peel-apart overwrap, 1 per sales unit box.

Further information Nil.

Product licence number 0508/0002.

STERILE SURGICAL BONE WAX

Presentation A white solid wax in slab form comprising: White Beeswax BP 75% w/w; Paraffin Wax BP 15% w/w; isopropyl palmitate 10% w/w.

Bone wax is sterilised by gamma irradiation. This material is non-absorbable. Mild inflammatory reactions have been reported in tissue immediately adjacent to the site of implantation.

Uses The wax is used to control bleeding from the divided, drilled or chipped edges of bone by physically plugging the osseous canals which contain the bleeding capillaries.

Dosage and administration By implantation and application to bone as required to control haemorrhage.

Contra-indications, warnings, etc Bone wax should not be used where rapid osseous regeneration and fusion are desired.

Bone wax should be used sparingly and any excess removed from the operative site.

Bone wax may inhibit osteogenesis and may act as a physical barrier to the reparative process.

Pharmaceutical precautions Recommended storage conditions are below 25°C, away from moisture and direct heat. Shelf-life is 5 years, the expiry date is shown on each pack. Do not resterilise. Unused bone wax from opened packs should be discarded.

The package containing bone wax should be opened just prior to use to minimise the possibility of contamination and excessive drying.

Bone wax should be used immediately after removal from the package and, using an aseptic technique, warmed to the desired consistency by manipulation with the fingers.

Legal category P.

Package quantities Slabs (5 × 2 × 0.3 cm) of approximately 2.5 g in weight packed in an envelope and a peel apart overwrap pouch. The sales unit is a film-wrapped box containing 12 packs.

Further information Nil.

Product licence number 0508/5001R.

STERILE SURGICAL CATGUT BP

Presentation An absorbable strand consisting of collagen derived from gut of healthy mammals uniformly twisted to produce virtually a monofilament strand which conforms to the requirements set out in the European Pharmacopoeia and British Pharmacopoeia.

Plain catgut is Sterilised Surgical Catgut which has not been treated to prolong its resistance to digestion. It is straw coloured.

Chromic catgut is material which has been tanned by treatment with chromium salts in trivalent form and with oxidised pyrogallol (oxidised pyrogallic acid) to prolong its resistance to absorption. It is brown coloured.

Surgical Catgut is packed in conditioning fluid containing various proportions of Sodium Benzoate, 2-Diethylaminoethanol, Isopropanol and Water. It is available in non-needled lengths or attached to Stainless Steel Needles of varying types and sizes. It is sterilised by gamma irradiation.

Uses Surgical Catgut is intended for use where an absorbable suture or ligature is indicated.

Dosage and administration By implantation.

Contra-indications, warnings, etc These sutures, being absorbable, should not be used where extended approximation of tissues under stress is required.

Pharmaceutical precautions It is recommended that rinsing or soaking in fluids other than the conditioning fluid is not carried out. Recommended storage conditions are below 25 deg C away from moisture and direct heat. Shelf life 5 years, an expiry date is shown on each pack. Do not re-sterilise the contents of the pack. Unused product from opened packs should be discarded.

As with all sutures, care should be taken to avoid damage when handling. Avoid the crushing or crimping application of surgical instruments such as needle holders and forceps to the strand, except when grasping the free end of the suture during an instrument tie.

Legal category Not applicable.

Package quantities Various lengths, in gauge sizes Metric 1.0 to 7.0 (6/0 to 3) in aluminium foil packs and peel-apart overwrap pouches. The sales unit is a film-wrapped box containing 12 packs.

Further information None.

Product licence numbers
Chromic 0508/0017
Plain 0508/0018

VICRYL* MESH (Polyglactin 910) Sterile Absorbable Mesh

Presentation Vicryl (Polyglactin 910) Mesh is prepared from a copolymer of glycolide and lactide. These substances are derived respectively from glycolic and lactic acids. The mesh is composed of undyed fibre identical in composition to that used in Vicryl (Polyglactin 910) Synthetic Absorbable Suture and is sterilised by ethylene oxide gas. This material, when used as a suture has been found to be relatively inert, non-antigenic, non-pyrogenic and to elicit only a mild tissue reaction during absorption. Vicryl (Polyglactin 910) mesh is intended for use as a buttress to provide temporary support during the healing process.

Actions: Two important characteristics describe the *in vivo* function and behaviour of Vicryl (Polyglactin 910) Absorbable Mesh; first, reinforced wound strength and second, the rate of absorption (loss of mass).

The dehiscence force values of healing abdominal wounds in rats closed with size 1.5 metric (4/0) absorbable sutures were compared with the healing abdominal wounds closed with size 1.5 metric (4/0) absorbable sutures and reinforced with Vicryl (Polyglactin 910) Mesh. In this animal model the strength of the incision, when supported by the mesh, was significantly stronger than unsupported incisional wound. Explanted Vicryl (Polyglactin 910) Mesh, which before implantation had an initial average burst strength of 63 lb, was found to have 80% of its original burst strength remaining after 14 days *in vivo*.

Subcutaneous implantation studies in rats indicate that the absorption of Vicryl (Polyglactin 910) Mesh is minimal until about the forty-second post implantation day. Absorption is essentially complete between 60 and 90 days. The general mechanism by which *in vivo* degradation of Vicryl (Polyglactin 910) occurs is hydrolysis.

Uses
1. Prevention of post-operative eventration in the absence of infection.
2. Salvage of injured solid tissue organs in the absence of infection.

Dosage and administration By implantation.

Contra-indications, warnings, etc Vicryl (Polyglactin 910) Mesh should not be used where extended reinforcement or support of tissue is required.

Apart from the areas of prevention and treatment listed under 'Uses' no other areas of use have been satisfactorily investigated. The use of Vicryl (Polyglactin 910) mesh in situations other than the approved areas is contra-indicated.

Do not re-sterilise the mesh.

Pharmaceutical precautions Recommended storage conditions are below 25°C away from moisture and direct heat. Shelf life is 5 years; the expiry date is shown on each pack.

Legal category Not applicable.

Package quantities Undyed mesh in sheet sizes of approximately 30 × 30 cm and 15 × 15 cm, inside sealed aluminium foil packs and peel-apart overwrap pouches. The sales unit is a box containing 1 pack.

Further information It is recommended that absorbable or nonabsorbable sutures be placed 6 mm to 12 mm apart at a distance approximately 6 mm from the edge of the mesh. Some surgeons prefer to suture mesh larger than the defect into position over the defect, starting on one side of the mesh. The opposite sides are then sutured to assure proper closure under correct tension. When the margin sutures have all been placed, the extra mesh is trimmed away, leaving approximately 6 mm of mesh extending beyond the suture line.

Product licence number 0508/0016.

ZENODERM* STERILE CORIUM IMPLANT

Presentation A white biscuit-like matrix of enzyme treated, glutaraldehyde tanned, lyophilised or air dried dermal collagen. All non-collagenous elements are removed by immersion in a proteolytic enzyme whilst glutaraldehyde treatment tans the collagen. Individual sheets are cut to various sizes and thicknesses depending upon their ultimate clinical application. The material is sterilised by gamma irradiation.

Studies have shown that after implantation into rats Zenoderm Corium Implant is gradually replaced by host tissue. The absorption time varies from 6 to 12 months depending on size, tissue and site. The general mechanism by which *in vivo* degradation occurs is proteolytic enzymatic action.

Uses As a biological implant for tissue replacement in areas where tissue is weak, deficient or absent, e.g. in: Dural Replacement, Fascia Lata Substitute, Bladder Sling, Oro Antral Fistulae, Repair of Herniae, Perforations of the Tympanic Membrane.

Dosage and administration By implantation.

Contra-indications, warnings, etc No situation has presented, to date, in the areas listed above, where the use of the material is contra-indicated.

Pharmaceutical precautions Recommended storage conditions are below 25°C, away from moisture and direct heat. Shelf life is 5 years. An expiry date is shown on each pack. Do not re-sterilise. Unused product from opened packs should be discarded.

Legal category Not applicable.

Package quantities Supplied sterile in double peel apart overwrap pouches. Zenoderm Corium Implant is available in the following sizes. The sales unit is a film-wrapped box containing 5 packs.

25 cm × 12 cm × 0.6 mm	(ZD 6251)
10 cm × 10 cm × 0.3 mm	(ZD 3101)
30 cm × 2 cm × 0.6 mm	(ZD 6301)
20 cm × 1.5 cm × 0.6 mm	(ZD 6201)
10 cm × 5 cm × 0.6 mm	(ZD 6101)
3 cm × 3 cm × 0.3 mm	(ZD 3033)
2 cm × 2 cm × 0.1 mm	(ZD 1021)

Further information Nil.

Product licence number 0508/0007.

**Trade Mark*

Evans Medical Limited
Langhurst
Horsham
West Sussex RH12 4QD

EVANS

ADSORBED DIPHTHERIA AND TETANUS VACCINE BP (DT/Vac/Ads)

Presentation Adsorbed Diphtheria and Tetanus Vaccine is a mixture of diphtheria formol toxoid and tetanus formol toxoid adsorbed on aluminium hydroxide. Each 0.5 ml dose has an immunising potency of not less than 30 units of diphtheria toxoid, and not less than 40 units of tetanus toxoid.

Uses Active immunisation against diphtheria and tetanus in infants and children. Reinforcement of immunity to diphtheria and tetanus in children under the age of 10 years.

Dosage and administration *Children under 10 years:* The vaccine is administered by deep subcutaneous or intramuscular injection. The container should be shaken before withdrawing the prescribed dose.

Primary immunisation: A course consists of three doses each of 0.5 ml, and in line with the current DoH recommendation, the course is started at two months with an interval of one month between each dose. This will increase the degree of patient compliance compared to the previous regime. If the course is interrupted it should be resumed where it left off, without starting at the beginning again.

Reinforcing doses: Children under the age of 10 years immunised in infancy with adsorbed diphtheria and tetanus vaccine or diphtheria, tetanus and pertussis vaccine should receive a reinforcing dose of diphtheria and tetanus vaccine immediately prior to school entry.

Contra-indications, warnings, etc
Contra-indications: Presence of acute infectious disease.

Warnings: A sterile syringe and adrenaline injection should be ready for use in case the need arises for emergency treatment of an allergic reaction.

Side-effects: Local reactions including pain, redness and swelling may occur at the injection site and last for several days. Systemic reactions may include headache, malaise, lethargy, myalgia and pyrexia. A small painless nodule may form at the injection site. Severe anaphylactoid reactions are rare. Neurological symptoms have been reported occasionally.

Pharmaceutical precautions Protect from light. Store in a refrigerator between 2 and 8°C (36 and 46°F). Do not freeze.

Partly used multidose containers should be discarded within 4 hours of withdrawal of the first dose.

Legal category POM.

Package quantities Carton of 10 × 0.5 ml ampoules and carton of 1 × 5 ml vial.

Further information Nil.

Product licence number 0039/0114.

CLoSTET* (Adsorbed Tetanus Vaccine BP)

Presentation Adsorbed Tetanus Vaccine is a suspension of purified formol toxoid, prepared by formalin detoxification of *Clostridium tetani* exotoxin, adsorbed on aluminium hydroxide. Each 0.5 ml dose has an immunising potency of not less than 40 units.

Uses Active immunisation against tetanus. Reinforcement of immunity to tetanus.

Dosage and administration The vaccine is administered by deep subcutaneous or intramuscular injection. The container should be shaken before withdrawing the prescribed dose.

Primary immunisation: A course consists of three doses each of 0.5 ml and in line with the current DoH recommendation the interval between each dose is one month. This will increase the degree of patient compliance compared to the previous regime. If the course is interrupted it should be resumed where it left off, without starting at the beginning again.

Reinforcing doses: A reinforcing dose of 0.5 ml should be given 10 years after the basic course, and another around 10 years later provides a satisfactory degree of protection.

After a basic course has been given, a single reinforcing dose will provide protection in the event of an injury which is considered might give rise to tetanus. Reinforcing doses should not be given at too frequent intervals as they may provoke hypersensitivity reactions.

Tetanus vaccine should not routinely be given to any patient who has received a reinforcing dose in the preceding 5 years, unless the wound is regarded as carrying an unusually high risk of tetanus, and even then vaccine is not necessary if a reinforcing dose has been given during the preceding year.

Patients presenting with a tetanus prone wound who have not received a primary course, or whose immunisation status is not known, should receive one injection of antitetanus immunoglobulin at one site, and the first dose of a primary course of adsorbed tetanus vaccine at another site.

Patients who have completed a primary course or received a reinforcing dose more than 10 years previously should receive one injection each of antitetanus immunoglobulin and adsorbed tetanus vaccine.

Contra-indications, warnings, etc
Contra-indications: Acute infection is a contra-indication to routine tetanus immunisation, except in the presence of a tetanus-prone wound.

Warnings: A sterile syringe and adrenaline injection should be ready for use, in case the need arises for emergency treatment of an allergic reaction.

Side-effects: Local reactions including pain, redness and swelling may occur at the injection site and last for several days. Systemic reactions may include headache, malaise, lethargy, myalgia and pyrexia. A small painless nodule may form at the injection site. Severe anaphylactoid reactions are rare. Neurological symptoms have been reported occasionally.

Pharmaceutical precautions Protect from light. Store in a refrigerator between 2 and 8°C (36 and 46°F). Do not freeze.

Legal category POM.

Package quantities Carton of one 0.5 ml pre-filled syringe and of 10 × 0.5 ml prefilled syringes.

Further information Nil.

Product licence number 0039/0115.

INTRADERMAL BCG VACCINE BP

Presentation Intradermal BCG Vaccine contains a live attenuated strain derived from *Mycobacterium bovis*, and known to protect man against tuberculosis. It is presented as a multidose vial containing a white freeze-dried plug which easily disperses to form an opalescent liquid on reconstitution.

The potency of this vaccine is of the order of one tenth that of Percutaneous BCG Vaccine, and contains between 8 and 26 million colony forming units per 10 dose vial, and between 40 and 130 million colony forming units per 50 dose vial.

Development of special culture conditions has resulted in a vaccine which, in the dry state, resists the effects of heat. No batch of vaccine is released until it has been shown to resist a temperature of 37°C for 28 days.

This vaccine complies with the specifications for Bacillus Calmette-Guérin Vaccine BP, and Vaccinum Tuberculosis (BCG) Cryodesiccatum (Ph Eur), and is of standardised potency.

It also complies with WHO Requirements for Dried BCG Vaccine – Revised 1985.

Uses Intradermal BCG Vaccine induces active immunity to tuberculosis. Vaccinated persons normally become Mantoux-positive after eight weeks, but sometimes up to 14 weeks are needed.

Dosage and administration *Adults and children over 3 months of age:* 0.1 ml *strictly by* ***intradermal*** *injection* (subcutaneous injection must be avoided).

Infants under 3 months of age: 0.05 ml *strictly by* ***intradermal*** *injection.*

The inoculation should be given in the arm, over the insertion of the deltoid muscle. Administration in the leg has been associated with more severe reactions in neonates and should be avoided.

The vaccine must not be contaminated with any antiseptic or detergent. If alcohol is used to swab the skin, it must be allowed to evaporate before the vaccine is injected. Similarly if alcohol is used to swab the rubber bung of the vial, it must be allowed to evaporate before the bung is penetrated with the syringe needle.

The vaccine suspension is prepared by adding 1 ml of Water for Injections BP or Sodium Chloride Injection BP to the 10 dose vial. When using the 50 dose vial, 5 ml of Sodium Chloride Injection BP (not Water for Injections BP) should be added. Do NOT shake as this causes frothing. Allow to stand for one minute, then draw into the syringe twice to ensure homogeneity. Once the liquid vaccine has been prepared, it should be protected from light and used in the same session, i.e. within 4 hours.

The injection site is best left uncovered to facilitate healing.

Contra-indications, warnings, etc
Contra-indications: BCG Vaccine should NOT be given to persons receiving systemic corticosteroids or immunosuppressive treatment, those suffering from malignant conditions (e.g. lymphoma, leukaemia, Hodgkins Disease), those in whom normal immunological mechanism is impaired (e.g. hypogammaglobulinaemia), those known to be HIV positive, and persons with pyrexia or generalised infected dermatoses. The effect of Intradermal BCG Vaccine may be exaggerated in these patients, and a more generalised infection is possible. Eczema is not a contra-indication, but the vaccine site must be lesion free.

Intradermal BCG Vaccine should not be given to patients who are receiving prophylactic doses of anti-tuberculous drugs.

Tuberculin-positive persons, i.e. those with induration of 6 mm or greater in diameter in the Mantoux test, or those in Heaf grades 2 to 4, do not require the vaccine. Its administration to these persons may result in an accelerated local reaction of larger size than normal.

Pregnancy: Vaccination should be avoided in early pregnancy, and if possible delayed until after delivery.

Warnings: Intradermal BCG Vaccine may be given at the same time as oral poliomyelitis vaccine. An interval of three weeks should be allowed between administration of BCG and any other live vaccine, but the interval can be reduced to 10 days if a longer period is not available.

No further vaccination should be given for at least three months in the arm used for BCG vaccination, because of the risk of regional lymphadenitis.

Any prepared vaccine remaining at the end of the session (maximum 4 hours) should be discarded, and preferably incinerated or treated with a disinfectant such as strong hypochlorite solution.

Side-effects: Rash, fever, local induration, pain and lymphadenopathy may occur.

Occasionally an excessive response to Intradermal BCG Vaccine results in a discharging ulcer. This may be attributable to inadvertent subcutaneous injection, or to excessive dosage. The ulcer should be encouraged to dry and abrasion avoided, e.g. by tight clothes. Waterproof dressings should not be used. If the ulcer persists, it can be treated by application of a mild corticosteroid cream with or without a topical antibiotic, or with the latter alone. Isoniazid powder has also been used topically.

In the rare cases of severe local reaction with abscess formation, aspiration should be carried out, perhaps with streptomycin replacement. Enlargement of axillary lymph glands is unlikely, except occasionally in young infants.

Overdosage: If gross overdosage occurs, and there is reason to suspect the development of a more generalised infection with BCG, systemic treatment with isoniazid or any other suitable anti-tuberculous drug should be given.

Pharmaceutical precautions Protect from light and store in a refrigerator between 2 and 8°C (36 and 46°F) but avoid freezing ampoules of diluent.

Legal category POM.

Package quantities Carton of 10 × 10 dose vials.

Composite pack of 5 × 10 dose vials with 5 × 1 ml ampoules of Water for Injections BP.

Composite pack of 5 × 50 dose vials with 5 × 5 ml ampoules of Sodium Chloride Injection BP.

All packs are available to United Kingdom Health Authorities and hospitals through Department of Health contract.

Further information Measles or rubella infection can cause tuberculin positive patients to revert temporarily and become tuberculin negative.

The administration of Intradermal BCG Vaccine should preferably be carried out with a syringe fitted with a short bevel gauge 25 needle.

The use of jet injectors to administer the vaccine is not recommended.

Isoniazid Resistant Intradermal BCG Vaccine is available on request direct from Evans Medical (Customer Services, Dunstable. Tel. 0582 608308).

Product licence number 0039/0110.

PERCUTANEOUS BCG VACCINE BP

Presentation Percutaneous BCG Vaccine contains a live attenuated strain derived from *Mycobacterium bovis*, and known to protect man against tuberculosis. It is presented as a multidose vial containing a white freeze-dried plug which easily disperses to form an opalescent suspension on reconstitution.

The potency of this vaccine is of the order of ten times that of Intradermal BCG Vaccine, each vial containing between 50 and 250 million colony forming units.

This vaccine complies with the specification for Percutaneous BCG Vaccine BP, and is of standardised potency.

Uses Percutaneous BCG Vaccine induces active immunity to tuberculosis. Vaccinated persons normally become Mantoux-positive after eight weeks, but sometimes up to 14 weeks are needed.

Dosage and administration Percutaneous BCG Vaccine is used with a multiple puncture apparatus equipped with not less than 20 needles giving reliable penetration of the skin to a depth of 2 mm. Alcohol may be used to prepare the skin, which must be dry before the vaccine is used. If alcohol is used to swab the rubber bung of the vial, it must be allowed to evaporate before the bung is penetrated with the syringe needle.

With a dry syringe add 0.3 ml of water for injections or sodium chloride injection to the multidose vial and allow to stand for about one minute to allow a suspension to form. Do NOT shake, as this causes frothing. A small amount (about 0.03 ml) is transferred onto the skin by means of a glass rod, platinum loop or spatula. The treated area of skin is then immediately punctured with the multiple puncture apparatus.

Once the liquid vaccine has been prepared, it should be protected from light and used in the same session i.e. within 4 hours.

The injection site is best left uncovered to facilitate healing. The multiple puncture apparatus must be properly sterilised each time after use, according to the maker's instructions. Alternatively a disposable head may be used each time. Any alcohol used should be burnt off before the apparatus is used, which must be allowed to cool before use. Detergents or antiseptics should not be used.

Contra-indications, warnings, etc
Contra-indications: BCG vaccine should NOT be given to persons receiving systemic corticosteroids or immunosuppressive treatment, those suffering from malignant conditions (e.g. lymphoma, leukaemia, Hodgkins Disease), those in whom normal immunological mechanism is impaired (e.g. hypogammaglobulinaemia), those known to be HIV positive, and persons with pyrexia or generalised infected dermatoses. The effect of Percutaneous BCG Vaccine may be more exaggerated in these patients, and a more generalised infection is possible. Eczema is not a contra-indication, but the vaccination site must be lesion free.

Percutaneous BCG Vaccine should not be given to patients who are receiving prophylactic doses of anti-tuberculous drugs.

Tuberculin positive persons, i.e., those with induration of 6 mm or greater in diameter with the Mantoux test, or those in Heaf grades 2 to 4, do not require the vaccine. Its administration to these persons may result in an accelerated local reaction of larger size than normal.

Pregnancy: Vaccination should be avoided in early pregnancy, and if possible delayed until after delivery.

Warnings: Percutaneous BCG Vaccine must NOT be given by intradermal injection.

Percutaneous BCG Vaccine may be given at the same time as oral poliomyelitis vaccine. An interval of three weeks should be allowed between administration of BCG and any other live vaccine, but the interval can be reduced to 10 days if a longer period is not available.

No further vaccination should be given for at least three months in the arm used for BCG vaccination, because of the risk of regional lymphadenitis.

Any prepared vaccine remaining at the end of the session (maximum 4 hours) should be discarded, and preferably incinerated or treated with a disinfectant such as stong hypochlorite solution.

Side-effects: Rash, fever, local induration, pain and lymphadenopathy may occur.

Occasionally an excessive response to Percutaneous BCG Vaccine results in a discharging ulcer. This should be encouraged to dry and abrasion avoided, e.g. by tight clothes. Waterproof dressings should not be used. If the ulcer persists, it can be treated by application of a mild corticosteroid cream with or without a topical anti biotic, or with the latter alone. Isoniazid powder has also been used topically.

In the rare cases of severe local reaction with abscess formation, aspiration should be carried out, perhaps with streptomycin replacement. Enlargement of axillary lymph glands is unlikely, except occasionally in young infants.

Overdosage: If gross overdosage occurs, and there is reason to suspect the development of a generalised infection with BCG, systemic treatment with isoniazid or any other suitable anti-tuberculous drug should be given.

Pharmaceutical precautions Protect from light and store in a refrigerator between 2 and 8°C (36 and 46°F).

Legal category POM.

Package quantities Carton of 10 multidose vials.

Further information Measles or rubella infection can cause tuberculin positive patients to revert temporarily and become tuberculin negative.

Product licence number 0039/0112.

CORACTEN* CAPSULES

Presentation Opaque, brownish-pink capsules, opaque reddish-brown capped, marked with a white heart-shaped monogram on both cap and body, and filled with yellow pellets. Each capsule contains 20 mg nifedipine in sustained-release form designed to prolong therapeutic blood concentrations.

Uses Nifedipine is a potent calcium-channel blocker which, by dilating peripheral arterial smooth muscle, decreases cardiac work and myocardial oxygen requirement. It also dilates coronary arteries, thereby improving myocardial perfusion and reducing coronary artery spasm. In hypertension, it reduces blood pressure but has little or no effect in normotensive subjects. It has no therapeutic antiarrhythmic effect.

Coracten capsules are indicated in the prophylactic treatment of angina pectoris such as exercise-induced angina, angina at rest including Prinzmetal angina, unstable angina, and angina following myocardial infarction, and in the treatment of hypertension.

Dosage and administration
Adults only: In angina pectoris and hypertension: Normally one Coracten capsule every 12 hours. If necessary, the dosage may be increased to up to 2 capsules every 12 hours.

Elderly: Nifedipine is generally well tolerated in the elderly, but as with other agents caution should be exercised when treating older patients.

Caution should be exercised in treating patients with hepatic impairment. In these patients a reduced dose of sustained-release nifedipine should be used, together with careful monitoring.

Dosage adjustments are not usually required in patients with renal impairment.

The capsules should be swallowed whole with a little fluid.

Contra-indications, warnings, etc
Contra-indications: Known hypersensitivity to nifedipine. Cardiogenic shock. Women who are or who may become pregnant (see 'Use in pregnancy and lactation').

Precautions: Use with caution in patients who are hypotensive; in patients with poor cardiac reserve; in diabetic patients as they may require adjustment of their diabetic therapy; and in dialysis patients with malignant hypertension and irreversible renal failure with hypovolaemia, since a significant drop in blood pressure may occur due to the vasodilator effects of nifedipine.

Since nifedipine has no beta-blocking activity, it gives no protection against the dangers of abrupt withdrawal of beta-blocking drugs. Withdrawal of any previously prescribed beta-blockers should be gradual, preferably over 8 to 10 days.

Nifedipine may be used in combination with beta-blockers and other antihypertensive agents, but the possibility of an additive effect resulting in postural hypotension and/or cardiac failure must be borne in mind.

Cardiac ischaemic pain has been reported in a minority of patients within 30 minutes of giving nifedipine; such patients should stop treatment.

Increased plasma levels of nifedipine have been reported during concominent use of H_2-receptor antagonists, but no clinically significant effects have been reported. Whilst most studies have shown no clinically significant effect on plasma digoxin concentration, the possibility of an interaction must be borne in mind. When used in combination with nifedipine, serum quinidine levels have been shown to be suppressed regardless of dosage of quinidine.

Use in pregnancy and lactation: Because animal studies show embryotoxicity and teratogenicity, Coracten is contra-indicated during pregnancy (see also Contra-indications). Embryotoxicity was noted at 6 to 20 times the maximum recommended dose for Coracten given to rats, mice and rabbits, and teratogenicity was noted in rabbits given 20 times the maximum recommended dose for Coracten. Coracten is not recommended during lactation.

Adverse reactions: Side-effects are generally transient and mild, and usually occur at the start of treatment only. They include headache, flushing and, usually at higher dosages, nausea, dyspepsia, heartburn, dizziness, lethargy, skin reactions, paraesthesia, hypotension, palpitation, tachycardia and dependent oedema. There have been very rare reports of allergic hepatitis and of reversible gingival hyperplasia.

Overdosage: Hypotension is likely to predominate and tachycardia or bradycardia may also occur. Treatment consists of gastric lavage followed by oral activated charcoal together with supportive and symptomatic measures, principally intravenous fluids to maintain circulating blood volume. If the latter is not sufficient, dopamine or dobutamine may be given. Intravenous calcium gluconate may be considered as an antidote.

Pharmaceutical precautions Store in original pack at a temperature not exceeding 30°C and protect from light.

Legal category POM.

Package quantities Coracten capsules are available in blister packs of 100.

Further information Inactive ingredients include lactose.

Product licence number 0002/0159.

DIAMORPHINE HYDROCHLORIDE BP FOR INJECTION

Presentation Ampoules containing 5, 10, 30, 100 and 500 mg of pure diamorphine hydrochloride as a white freeze-dried plug. The colour of the plugs in the larger strength ampoules is off-white, and occasionally the integral plug may break up to produce a crystalline powder.

Uses Diamorphine is a powerful narcotic analgesic which is more potent than morphine and more likely to produce euphoria and addiction, but relatively less nausea, constipation and hypotension.

It is readily absorbed after injection and rapidly hydrolysed to 6-monoacetylmorphine in the blood, and then more slowly metabolised to morphine the major active metabolite. Up to 80% of a dose is excreted in the urine in 24 hours, mainly as morphine-3-glucuronide together with about 5 to 7% of the dose as free morphine.

Diamorphine is used to control severe pain, such as that associated with cancer, acute myocardial infarction and acute pulmonary oedema.

Dosage and administration
Administration: The drug may be given by the intramuscular, subcutaneous or intravenous routes, the latter two routes using either bolus injection or infusion.

Its solubility in water is 1 in 1.6, and the small volume of diluent required is of obvious benefit in treating an emaciated patient. Presentations up to 100 mg will readily dissolve in 1 ml of diluent. Because of the bulk of material in the 500 mg ampoule, 2 ml of diluent is required to effect solution and it is recommended that the plug be tapped down, thoroughly wetted and the ampoule gently shaken until the plug dissolves. It is compatible with glucose and sodium chloride intravenous infusions, and an aqueous solution has maximum stability of several days at pH 3.8 to 4.4, the stability reducing as the pH rises. For this reason glucose intravenous infusion is the preferred diluent, particularly when the drug is administered by a continuous infusion pump over 24 to 48 hours. The occurrence of nausea and vomiting may require the concurrent administration of an anti-emetic. If given together with diamorphine as a bolus injection, IV infusion or in a continuous infusion pump, hyoscine hydrobromide, metoclopramide and methotrimeprazine are stable and compatible with Diamorphine. Chlorpromazine and prochlorperazine are compatible with diamorphine but should not be given by the SC route. Cyclizine and haloperidol have also been used. (Allwood M C, B J Pharm Practice Mar 1984, 88–90; Regnard C et al B J Pharm Practice Aug 1986, 218–220).

Dosage: It is important that the dosage be suited to the individual patient, taking into account the properties of the drug, the nature of the pain, the total condition of the patient and previous or concurrent medication.

Cancer: Use of Diamorphine or other narcotic analgesics although very important, should be only one part of the comprehensive approach to total pain control, which ideally should include non-drug measures and psychosocial support. Diamorphine may be used parenterally when oral administration of narcotic analgesics is no longer possible because of the dosage required, impaired absorption, intestinal disorders, nausea and vomiting or difficulty in swallowing. An initial dosage of 5 to 10 mg every 4 hours may be suitable, but higher doses are reported in the literature (Dover SB, BMJ 1987, 294, 553–555). The dosage will usually depend on the dose and drug given previously to the patient orally. The persistent pain is controlled by titrating the dose against the degree of pain, until the smallest dose required to remove the pain is reached. This dose is maintained and the patient's condition continually re-assessed, the dose being increased or decreased as necessary. The therapeutic objective must be to control the pain by regular administration of the correct dose when this is determined, and continuous infusion may be preferred to intermittent therapy.

Acute myocardial infarction: A dose of 5 mg may be given by slow intravenous injection (1 mg per minute), followed by 2.5 to 5 mg if necessary.

Acute pulmonary oedema: A dose of 2.5 to 5 mg may be given by slow intravenous injection.

Use in children and the elderly: Mainly because of its respiratory depressant effect, caution should be exercised when giving the drug to the very young and the elderly, and a lower starting dose than normal should be used.

Contra-indications, warnings, etc
Contra-indications: Acute respiratory depression, obstructive airways disease and concurrent administration of monoamine oxidase inhibitors or within two weeks of their discontinuation.

Warnings: Administration to patients with head injuries or raised intracranial pressure increases the risk of respiratory depression and further elevation of CSF pressure. The sedation and pupillary changes produced may interfere with accurate monitoring of the patient.

The drug can cause hypotension in patients who already have conditions or drug therapy that interfere with the ability to maintain normal blood pressure.

Concurrent administration of other CNS sedative/hypnotic drugs may have an additive effect necessitating their dosage reduction. Administration of drugs having anti-muscarinic activity (atropine and synthetic anticholinergics) may increase the risk of severe constipation and/or urinary retention.

Precautions: Tolerance and physical dependence on the drug is likely to develop in most patients after a few weeks of treatment, but this does not prevent reduction of dosage or discontinuation when considered necessary, and drug abuse is not normally a problem in patients with severe pain. Great caution should be exercised however, in using the drug in patients with a known tendency to, or history of, drug abuse.

Care should be exercised in treating the elderly, debilitated patients, and those with hepatic or renal impairment. It is recommended that a lower than normal initial dose is given to these patients.

Careful consideration should be given before treating patients with myxoedema or hypothyroidism, adrenocortical insufficiency, toxic psychoses, CNS depression, prostatic hypertrophy or urethral stricture, kyphoscoliosis, acute alcoholism and delirium tremens, severe inflammatory bowel disease and severe diarrhoea.

Use in pregnancy: There is no, or inadequate, evidence of safety in human pregnancy but the drug has been widely used for many years without apparent ill consequences.

Side-effects: The most serious hazards of therapy are respiratory depression and arrest, although circulatory depression, shock and cardiac arrest can occur.

The most common side effects are sedation, nausea and vomiting, constipation and sweating.

Other side effects include tachycardia, postural hypotension, palpitations, faintness and syncope; euphoria, dysphoria, weakness, insomnia, dizziness, confusional symptoms and occasionally hallucinations; dry mouth, anorexia, cramps, taste alterations; urinary retention, reduced libido or potency; pruritus, urticaria and other skin rashes.

Overdosage: The symptoms of serious overdosage are respiratory depression, stupor or coma, muscle flaccidity, cold clammy skin, constricted pupils and occasionally bradycardia and hypotension.

The specific antidote naloxone is indicated if coma or bradypnoea are present. A dose of 0.4 to 2 mg may be given by SC, IM or IV injection repeated at intervals of 2–3 minutes up to a maximum of 10 mg if respiratory function does not improve. The dosage for children is 10 micrograms per kilogram body weight. Alternatively naloxone may be given by continuous IV infusion, 2 mg diluted in 500 ml intravenous solution, at a rate adjusted to the patient's response.

Pharmaceutical precautions Diamorphine is incompatible with mineral acids and alkalis. Store below 25°C.

Legal category CD (Sch 2), POM.

Package quantities Ampoules of 5, 10, 30 mg in cartons of 5 and boxes of 100. Ampoules of 100 mg and 500 mg in cartons of 5.

Further information Nil.

Product licence numbers

5 mg	0039/5662
10 mg	0039/5663
30 mg	0039/5665
100 mg	0039/0154
500 mg	0039/0163

MEVILIN*-L
Measles Vaccine, Live BP (Schwarz strain) Meas/Vac (Live)

Presentation Mevilin-L is a freeze-dried preparation of living attenuated virus of the Schwarz strain. It must be reconstituted with Water for Injections immediately prior to injection. The reconstituted vaccine may vary in colour from pale straw to pink, but this variation is not indicative of deterioration.

Uses Prophylaxis against measles and, given within 72 hours of contact, to prevent development of infection.

Dosage and administration One 0.5 ml dose by deep subcutaneous or intramuscular injection (contains not less than 1,000 plaque forming units of measles virus). Mevilin-L should be administered to infants at between 12 and 15 months of age. There is no upper age limit for measles vaccination.

To reconstitute Mevilin-L inject 0.5 ml Water for Injections BP from the ampoule provided into the vial containing the freeze-dried vaccine, allow to stand for about a minute then mix the suspension by withdrawing into the syringe and expelling back into the vial. The use of a 2 ml disposable syringe is recommended.

Contra-indications, warnings, etc

Contra-indications: Mevilin-L should not be given to children below the age of one year unless at special risk of contracting measles. If this is the case, a second dose should be given at a later date as interference from maternally derived antibodies may cause a failure to respond.

Vaccination should be delayed in children suffering from a febrile illness.

Mevilin-L should NOT be given to children receiving systemic corticosteroids or immunosuppressive treatment, those suffering from malignant conditions (.e.g. lymphoma, leukaemia, Hodgkin's Disease), or those in whom normal immunological mechanism is impaired (e.g. hypogammaglobulinaemia). These children should be given an injection of immunoglobulin as soon as possible after exposure to measles. Siblings and close contacts of such children must be immunised against measles.

The vaccine should not be given within 3 months of receiving immunoglobulin, in pregnancy, or to persons who are hypersensitive to neomycin or polymyxin.

Allergy to hens' eggs is no longer considered to be a contra-indication to the vaccine except in children with a history of anaphylactoid reaction to egg ingestion. Children who have allergies to egg that are not of an anaphylactoid nature and those with allergies to chicken feathers may be vaccinated in the usual manner.

Human Normal Immunoglobulin with a specific content of measles antibody is available for those children in whom Mevilin-L is contra-indicated. This is available in 1.7 ml ampoules containing 250 mg and 5 ml ampoules containing 750 mg, and is given by intramuscular injection. Dosage is as follows:

	Age	*Dose*
To prevent an attack	Under 1 year	250 mg
	1–2 years	500 mg
	3 years and over	750 mg
To allow an attenuated attack	Under 1 year	100 mg
	1 year and over	250 mg

This immunoglobulin must NOT be given with Mevilin-L.

Children with a personal history of convulsions, or whose parents or siblings have a history of idiopathic epilepsy, SHOULD receive the vaccine, and simultaneous injection of specially diluted immunoglobulin is NO LONGER considered necessary. The parents of such children should be given advice on prophylaxis of febrile convulsions.

Precautions: Live measles vaccine is quickly killed by alcohol and detergents, and these agents should not be used for sterilising syringes prior to immunisation. Alcohol used to clean the skin prior to injection should be allowed to dry before the vaccine is given.

Warnings: A sterile syringe and adrenaline injection should be ready for use, in case the need arises for emergency treatment of an allergic reaction.

Mevilin-L must not be given intravenously and should not normally be given within 3 months of a transfusion of blood or plasma. If these have been used near to the time of vaccination, a test for the presence of measles antibody should be made at a later date.

The vaccine should not normally be given less than 3 weeks before or after immunisation with other live virus vaccines.

Measles vaccine may depress tuberculin skin sensitivity for 4 weeks or longer.

The attenuated vaccine virus is not excreted after vaccination and thus there is no risk of infection from vaccine recipients.

Management of measles outbreaks: The spread of measles infection can be contained by giving the vaccine within 3 days to susceptible children who have been in contact with an infected child. If the child's measles immunity is in doubt, the vaccine should be given since there is no greater risk than that associated with giving the vaccine for the first time.

Side-effects: The most common reactions occurring in 10–15% of children are malaise and fever, with or without rash, occurring some 5–10 days after vaccination and usually resolve within 48 hours. Convulsions may accompany the fever.

Severe reactions are uncommon and encephalitis has been reported on rare occasions.

Pharmaceutical precautions Mevilin-L should be protected from light and stored in a refrigerator between 2 and 8°C (36 and 46°F). Do not freeze.

The reconstituted vaccine should be used as soon as possible and certainly within one hour.

Legal category POM.

Package quantities Single dose vial with 0.5 ml ampoule of Water for Injections BP, in packs of 1, 10 and 50.

Further information It is important to recognise that children with chronic conditions affecting physical development (e.g. cystic fibrosis, congenital heart disease), and those in residential or day care over the age of one year are at special risk of contracting measles.

Human Normal Immunoglobulin with a specific content of measles antibody is available from: Central Public Health Laboratory (Tel: 081-200-6868); Blood Products Laboratory, Elstree (Tel: 081-953-6191).

Product licence number 0039/0144.

MICRALAX* MICRO-ENEMA

Presentation A disposable plastic tube with a 2-inch pliable plastic nozzle, which contains 5 ml of a colourless viscous liquid incorporating 450 mg sodium citrate, 45 mg sodium alkylsulphoacetate and 5 mg sorbic acid, together with glycerin, sorbitol and purified water.

Uses Micralax combines the action of sodium citrate, a peptizing agent which can displace bound water present in the faeces; sorbitol, which enhances this action; and sodium alkylsulphoacetate, a wetting agent.

Micralax is indicated whenever an enema is necessary to relieve constipation: in dyschezia, especially in bedridden patients; in geriatrics, paediatrics and obstetrics; and in preparation for X-ray examination, proctoscopy and sigmoidoscopy.

Dosage and administration
Adults and children aged 3 years and over: Administer the contents of one micro-enema rectally, inserting the full length of the nozzle. No lubricant is needed as a drop of the mixture is sufficient.

Contra-indications, warnings, etc
Contra-indication: Do not use in patients with inflammatory bowel disease.

Adverse reactions: Excessive use may cause diarrhoea and fluid loss, which should be treated symptomatically.

Pharmaceutical precautions Store below 25°C.

Legal category P.

Package quantities Packs of 12 and 100.

Further information Inactive ingredients include sorbic acid.

Product licence number 0002/5037R.

STREPTOMYCIN SULPHATE BP

Presentation Streptomycin sulphate is presented as a white sterile powder for preparation of Streptomycin Sulphate Injection BP.

Uses Streptomycin has antibacterial activity particularly against *Mycobacterium tuberculosis, Klebsiella pneumoniae* and *Escherichia coli*.

Streptomycin may be used in the treatment of: tuberculosis; non-tuberculous infections, including chronic respiratory infections, septicaemia and bacterial endocarditis (usually in conjunction with penicillin); pneumonia due to *Klebsiella pneumoniae*; infections with *Escherichia coli*, particularly of the urinary tract; tularaemia and plague; brucellosis (normally in conjunction with a tetracycline).

Dosage and administration *Tuberculosis: Adults:* Usually 1 g daily, but in patients over 40 years of age, 0.75 g daily by intramuscular injection may be appropriate. Streptomycin is always given together with other antituberculosis drugs. The injection should be given deeply into muscle, and the site changed for each injection. A 1 g dose is usually dissolved in 2 or 3 ml of water for injections. The displacement volume of 1 gram is approximately 0.75 ml.

Children: Usually 30 mg/kg (13.6 mg/lb) body weight daily up to 1 g a day by intramuscular injection.

Tuberculous meningitis: Intramuscular dosage 30–40 mg/kg (13.6–18 mg/lb) body weight up to 1 g a day. In addition to this streptomycin may be given intrathecally: adults, 50 mg a day; infants and children, 1 mg per kilogram body weight daily. The antibiotic is dissolved in sodium chloride injection, using 5 ml for infants and 10 ml or more for children and adults. The concentration of streptomycin in the injection must not exceed 5 mg per ml. After withdrawal of an equal volume of cerebrospinal fluid, the solution is injected slowly, taking at least 10 minutes. An injection may be given once a day for 10 days, perhaps followed by a dose on three alternate days.

Use of a sterile disposable membrane filter of 0.45 micron pore size is convenient to ensure clarity of the solution.

Non-tuberculous infections. Adults: Usually 1 g a day by intramuscular injection for three to seven days.

Children: 22–40 mg/kg (10–18 mg/lb) body weight daily. Divided doses are often used.

N.B. In urinary-tract infections the urine should be kept alkaline.

Contra-indications, warnings, etc
Contra-indications: Allergy to streptomycin, diseases of the ear, particularly suppurative otitis media and labyrinthine disturbances, pregnancy and myasthenia gravis.

Precautions: In the presence of actual or suspected renal insufficiency, treatment may start with a dose of 250–500 mg streptomycin. No further dose should be given until the blood level has fallen to 20 mcg/ml or less (*Brit. Med. J.* 1963, **1**, 1393). If the 24 hour serum level exceeds 3 micrograms per ml, the dosage should be reduced.

In tuberculous patients over 60 years of age, the serum level of streptomycin 24 hours after injection should not exceed 1 microgram per ml. It is important to repeat this estimation several times in the early weeks of treatment (*Brit. Med. J.* 1963, **1**, 1527).

To avoid increases in plasma levels, care should be taken with diuretics.

Skin sensitisation may occur in persons handling the antibiotic and care should be taken to avoid contact with the substance. Use of rubber gloves is recommended.

Side-effects: Ototoxicity: Some impairment of vestibular function (less often of auditory function) can occur, particularly with prolonged or intensive therapy, in the presence of renal dysfunction, and in the elderly patient.

Nephrotoxicity.

Sensitivity: Occasional allergic-type reaction, rarely severe, often responding to antihistamine treatment. Anaphylactic reaction is rarely reported.

Overdosage: Streptomycin can be removed from the body by haemodialysis.

Pharmaceutical precautions Sterile solutions of streptomycin should be used as soon as possible after reconstitution. Although presented as a single dose vial, where less than a 1 gram dose is required, the solution may be kept below 4°C in a refrigerator for a few days.

Although solutions may discolour slightly on keeping, their potency is not decreased.

Legal category POM.

Package quantities Carton of 10 vials each containing 1 g Streptomycin base as sulphate.

Further information Nil.

Product licence number 0039/6002.

TUBERCULIN PURIFIED PROTEIN DERIVATIVE (PPD) BP

Presentation Sterile aqueous solutions for intradermal injection containing Tuberculin PPD BP prepared from human strains of *Mycobacterium tuberculosis*.

Use As a diagnostic test for hypersensitivity to tubercle bacilli.

Dosage and administration

1. *Mantoux Test:* The Mantoux test enables an estimate to be obtained of the degree of hypersensitivity of a particular person. It consists of injecting intradermally ready diluted Tuberculin PPD.

Clean the skin of the volar surface of the left forearm with alcohol. Then using a disposable syringe inject 0.1 ml intradermally so that a weal 7 mm in diameter is raised.

It is normal to give one dose of 0.1 ml of 100 units per ml Tuberculin dilution (10 units). If there is any doubt about interpretation of the zone size produced, a second dose of 0.1 ml of 1000 units per ml Tuberculin dilution (100 units) may be given 2 days later. If that reading is negative, the patient is normally assessed as tuberculin negative.

Young children under 5 years of age are usually given half of the above doses.

If there is concern about a person being hypersensitive to tuberculin, or his or her tuberculous status is in doubt, a dose of 0.1 ml of 10 units per ml Tuberculin dilution (1 unit) or even less should be given.

A positive reaction is characterised by an area of 6 mm or greater of palpable induration, which may sometimes be surrounded by erythema. The results should be read after 72 hours, but usually a valid reading can be obtained up to 96 hours.

Control solution may be used at the same time but at a different site, to assess an individual patient's response to the vehicle used.

2. *Heaf test:* This test is performed using undiluted Tuberculin PPD 100,000 units per ml.

Clean the skin as for the Mantoux test and allow to dry, then transfer undiluted tuberculin using a syringe needle or loop and smooth over a circular area of about 1 cm in diameter. Using the Heaf multiple puncture apparatus set the apparatus to give a puncture of 1 mm for children under the age of two years or 2 mm for older children and adults. Holding the apparatus at right angles to the skin, place the end plate firmly and evenly in the centre of the film of tuberculin and press the handle to release the needles. No dressing need be applied. It is very important that the gun is properly sterilised after each application, or a disposable end plate used.

The test should be read at 3 to 10 days. A positive result should be recorded only when there is palpable induration around at least four puncture points. The induration is best felt by passing the finger lightly over the punctures, and if no resistance is felt, a negative result should be recorded.

Four grades of positive response are recognised.

Grade 1 – at least 4 small indurated papules.

Grade 2 – an indurated ring formed by confluent papules.

Grade 3 – a solid induration 5 to 10 mm wide.

Grade 4 – induration over 10 mm wide.

Contra-indications, warnings, etc Caution should be exercised in giving tuberculin to persons who have, or are suspected of having, active tuberculosis.

Temporary diminution of skin sensitivity to tuberculin may occur after ultra-violet light treatment, during treatment with corticosteroids or immunosuppressive agents, and for 4 weeks or longer following measles or measles vaccination.

Tuberculin can cause a severe acute local reaction in some individuals if the solution is allowed to come into contact with open cuts, the eyes and the mouth. The affected area should be washed with copious quantities of water followed, if necessary, by a topical corticosteroid.

The potency of tuberculins may be affected if they are diluted with diluents which differ in composition from the vehicle used in their preparation.

Where it is necessary to dilute one of the tuberculin presentations, Control Solution for Mantoux Test should be used.

The Heaf multiple puncture apparatus should be checked at regular intervals to ensure the points are sufficiently sharp to penetrate the skin.

Pharmaceutical precautions The British Pharmacopoeia directs that Tuberculin presentations should be stored in a refrigerator between 2 and 8°C. Data is available however which shows that the potency remains unaffected even after storage at temperatures up to 37°C for one month.

Protect from light and do not allow to freeze.

Use contents of ampoule as soon as possible and certainly within 4 hours of opening, provided adequate aseptic precautions are taken. Care should be taken to avoid contamination of the ampoule contents. Any unused solution at the end of the session (maximum 4 hours) should be disposed of by flushing away to waste with copious water.

Legal category POM.

Package quantities *Undiluted, Dilutions* and *Control Solution:* All in carton of 5 × 1 ml ampoules.

Tuberculin undiluted and Tuberculin 100 units per ml are available to United Kingdom Health Authorities and hospitals through Department of Health contract.

Further information 1 ml of each dilution is normally sufficient for 5 or 6 Mantoux tests, and 1 ml of undiluted Tuberculin is normally sufficient for up to 50 Heaf tests.

Product licence numbers

Tuberculin PPD BP undiluted 100,000 units per ml for Heaf Multiple Puncture Test	0039/5975
Tuberculin PPD BP dilutions for Mantoux Test	
10 units per ml	0039/5976
100 units per ml	0039/5977
1,000 units per ml	0039/5978
Control Solution for Mantoux Test	0039/5984

**Trade Mark*

Farmitalia Carlo Erba Limited
Italia House
23 Grosvenor Road,
St Albans,
Hertfordshire AL1 3AW

AMINOGLUTETHIMIDE

Presentation Practically white, round, scored tablets, containing 250 mg aminoglutethimide.

Uses Aminoglutethimide is indicated for treatment of metastatic carcinoma of the breast in post-menopausal or oophorectomised women.

Aminoglutethimide is also indicated in Cushing's syndrome due to malignant disease, where surgical treatment is inappropriate or as an adjunct to surgery, either pre-operatively in the management of metabolic disturbances or post-operatively for the treatment of relapse.

Dosage and administration
Adults: Metastatic carcinoma of the breast: administration should start at 250 mg twice daily for two weeks. In the absence of severe side-effects the dose may be increased to 250 mg four times daily.

Cushing's syndrome due to malignant disease: treatment should be started at 250 mg daily, increasing gradually up to 1 g daily. In some cases, especially ectopic ACTH syndrome, higher doses may be necessary to achieve adequate suppression.

Elderly: The adult dosage schedules may be given without modification.

Children: Not recommended.

Contra-indications, warnings, etc
Contra-indications: Use during pregnancy and lactation is contra-indicated as foetal abnormalities have been seen in animal studies and cases of pseudohermaphroditism have been reported in neonates of women treated with aminoglutethimide.

Warnings: Aminoglutethimide suppresses production of glucocorticoids and in patients with breast carcinoma supplementary glucocorticoids will be needed.

During initial treatment of Cushing's syndrome due to malignant disease, no corticosteroids should be necessary. Plasma cortisol levels should be monitored regularly and if adrenocortical insufficiency occurs supplementary glucocorticoids may be given.

The suppression of aldosterone synthesis may lead to hyponatraemia, hyperkalaemia, hypotension and dizziness, in which case a mineralocorticoid should be given.

Blood count and plasma electrolytes should be checked regularly. Aminoglutethimide has been found occasionally to diminish thyroid function. If, during treatment of breast carcinoma signs of Cushing's syndrome appear which are due to concomitant glucocorticoid medication, the dosage of the glucocorticoid should be reduced.

Aminoglutethimide may increase the rate of metabolism of some drugs such as coumarin anticoagulants, oral hypoglycaemic agents and dexamethasone and dosage of these may need adjustment.

Side-effects: Aminoglutethimide tolerability varies greatly and CNS side-effects such as dizziness, somnolence and lethargy are relatively common and dose dependent; unsteadiness occurs only in the highest dosage range. Gastrointestinal effects are less frequent but usually dose-dependent. A drug rash, sometimes accompanied by fever, may develop after 7–14 days. This usually subsides within 7–10 days even though treatment is continued: if it should not subside, treatment should be stopped temporarily. Alternatively the dose of concomitant glucocorticoid may be increased. Rarely pancytopenia, leucopenia and agranulocytosis have been reported.

Overdosage: Following overdosage of aminoglutethimide, no serious outcome has been reported. However, gastric lavage should be performed as soon as possible and full supportive measures should be employed. In severe cases, haemodialysis or charcoal haemoperfusion may be useful. Steroid replacement should be maintained or initiated, as necessary.

Pharmaceutical precautions Protect from heat, light and moisture.

Legal category POM.

Package quantities Cartons of 100 tablets.

Further information Aminoglutethimide inhibits steroid biosynthesis in the adrenal cortex causing a chemical adrenalectomy. This inhibition occurs at an early stage in the biosynthesis. Suppression of oestrogen production in peripheral tissue may also occur.

Product licence number 3433/0104.

CISPLATIN

Presentation Cisplatin powder for injection: Yellowish-white freeze-dried cake in vials containing 10 mg and 50 mg cisplatin (cis-diamminedichloroplatinum). The formulation also contains sodium chloride and mannitol.

Uses Cisplatin has antitumour activity either as a single agent or in combination chemotherapy particularly in the treatment of testicular and metastatic ovarian tumours, also cervical tumours, lung carcinoma and bladder cancer.

Dosage and administration Cisplatin powder should be dissolved in Water for Injections such that the reconstituted solution contains 1 mg/ml of cisplatin. Cisplatin reconstituted powder should be diluted in 2 litres of 0.9% saline or a dextrose/saline solution (to which 37.5 g of mannitol may be added) and administration should be over a 6–8 hour period.

Single agent therapy
Adults and children: The usual dose regimen given as a single agent is 50–120 mg/m^2 by infusion once every 3 to 4 weeks or 15–20 mg/m^2 by infusion daily for five consecutive days, every 3 to 4 weeks.

Combination chemotherapy
Dosage may be adjusted if the drug is used in combination with other anti-tumour chemotherapy.

With multiple drug treatment schedules cisplatin is usually given in doses from 20 mg/m^2 upward every 3 to 4 weeks.

Dosage should be reduced for patients with renal impairment or depressed bone marrow function (see Contra-indications, Warnings etc).

Pre-treatment hydration with 1 to 2 litres of fluid infused for 8 to 12 hours prior to the cisplatin will initiate diuresis. Adequate subsequent hydration should maintain diuresis during the 24 hours following administration.

Contra-indications, warnings, etc
Contra-indications: Cisplatin is contra-indicated in patients who have had previous allergic reactions to cisplatin or other platinum compounds as anaphylactic-like reactions have been reported. Relative contra-indications are pre-existing renal impairment, hearing disorders and depressed bone marrow function which may increase toxicity (see Warnings).

Warnings: This agent should only be administered under the direction of physicians experienced in cancer chemotherapy.

Nephrotoxicity of cisplatin is cumulative and serum creatinine, BUN and creatinine clearance should be measured before starting each course of therapy. Repeat courses of cisplatin should not be given unless levels of serum creatinine are below 1.5 mg/100 ml (100 mcmol/l) or blood urea below 55 mg/100 ml (9 mmol/l) and circulating blood elements are at an acceptable level.

Diuresis should be controlled and serum electrolyte levels monitored regularly. Adequate pre-treatment and 'during treatment' hydration should be ensured and such agents as mannitol given to minimise hazards of renal toxicity. In addition, adequate post-treatment hydration and urinary output should be monitored. Concomitant use of nephrotoxic drugs may seriously impair kidney function.

Ototoxicity is cumulative and occurs with high dose regimens. Hearing function should be evaluated before, and regularly during, therapy (see Adverse Reactions).

Haematologic toxicity is dose-related and may be cumulative; RBC, WBC and platelet counts should be monitored.

The nephrotoxicity, ototoxicity and myelosuppression induced by cisplatin will be additive to existing impairment or to the similar toxicity of agents such as cephaloridine, frusemide, aminoglycosides, etc. administered concurrently.

Anaphylactic-like reactions to cisplatin have been observed. These reactions can be controlled by administration of antihistamines, adrenaline and/or glucocorticoids.

Neurotoxicity secondary to cisplatin administration has been reported and therefore neurological examinations are recommended (see Adverse Reactions). Cisplatin has been shown to be mutagenic. It may also have an anti-fertility effect. Other antineoplastic substances have been shown to be carcinogenic and this possibility should be borne in mind in long term use of cisplatin.

Cisplatin has been shown to be teratogenic and embryotoxic in animals. The use of the drug should be avoided in pregnant or nursing women if possible.

Adverse reactions:
Nephrotoxicity: Immediate renal toxicity is greatly reduced when extensive saline hydration is used but cumulative toxicity may remain a problem and requires careful monitoring when repeat courses of cisplatin are administered.

Renal function impairment is evidenced by an increase in blood urea nitrogen, creatinine and serum uric acid levels and by a decreased creatinine clearance.

Cisplatin induces pathological lesions in the distal renal tubules and the collecting ducts.

Gastrointestinal toxicity: Nausea and vomiting occur in the majority of patients, usually starting within 1 hour of treatment and lasting up to 24 hours. Anorexia, nausea and occasional vomiting may persist for up to a week.

Myelosuppression: Cisplatin can cause suppression of all three blood elements.

Leucopenia is dose-related, possibly cumulative, usually reversible. The onset of leucopenia occurs usually between days 6 and 26 and the time of recovery ranges from 21 to 45 days. Thrombocytopenia is also a dose-limiting effect of cisplatin but is usually reversible. The onset of thrombocytopenia is usually from days 10 to 26 and the time of recovery ranges from about 28 to 45 days.

The incidence of cisplatin-induced anaemia (haemoglobin drop of 2 g/100 ml) ranges from 9% to 40%, although this is a difficult toxic effect to assess because it may have a complex aetiology in cancer patients.

Ototoxicity: Unilateral or bilateral tinnitus, which is usually reversible, and/or hearing loss in the high frequency range may occur.

The overall incidence of audiogram abnormalities is 24%, but large variations exist. These abnormalities usually appear within 4 days after drug administration and consist of at least a 15 decibel loss in pure tone threshold. The damage seems to be cumulative and is not reversible. The audiogram abnormalities are most common in the 4000–8000 Hz frequencies.

Neurotoxicity: Peripheral neuropathies with paraesthesia in both upper and lower extremities, tremor and loss of taste have been observed in some patients, generally those treated with repeated courses.

Anaphylactic-like reactions: Anaphylactic-like reactions such as flushing, facial oedema, wheezing, tachycardia and hypotension may occur within a few minutes after intravenous administration. Antihistamines, adrenaline and/or glucocorticoids control all these reactions.

Hyperuricaemia: Hyperuricaemia occurring with cisplatin is more pronounced with doses greater than 50 mg/m^2. Allopurinol effectively reduces uric acid levels.

Hypomagnesaemia: Asymptomatic hypomagnesaemia has been documented in a certain number of patients treated with cisplatin, symptomatic hypomagnesaemia has been observed in a limited number of cases.

Pharmaceutical precautions The unopened vials of the freeze-dried powder should be stored at room temperature protected from light. Solutions of cisplatin must not be cooled or refrigerated as cooling may result in precipitation; they should be stored at room temperature protected from light and used within 20 hours. It is recommended that diluted infusion solutions of cisplatin be protected from light during administration.

Any unused solution should be discarded.

Cisplatin is degraded on contact with aluminium. Aluminium containing equipment should not be used for administration of cisplatin.

It is recommended that personnel handling cisplatin wear protective gloves. Spillage or leakage should be mopped up wearing protective gloves and all cleaning materials should be placed in high-risk, waste-disposal bags and then incinerated. Contaminated surfaces should be washed with copious amounts of water.

Legal category POM.

Package quantities Cisplatin Powder 10 and 50 – Individual vials.

Further information Nil.

Product licence numbers

Cisplatin 10	3433/0061
Cisplatin 50	3433/0063

CYCLOPHOSPHAMIDE

Presentation Pink, biconvex, sugar-coated tablets containing 53.5 mg Cyclophosphamide BP (equivalent to 50 mg anhydrous cyclophosphamide).

Cyclophosphamide for injection is a sterile white powder in clear glass vials, with rubber caps and aluminium seals, containing 107 mg, 214 mg, 535 mg or 1070 mg Cyclophosphamide BP (equivalent to 100 mg, 200 mg, 500 mg or 1000 mg anhydrous cyclophosphamide) with sodium chloride.

Uses Alkylating, antineoplastic agent. Cyclophosphamide has been used successfully to induce and maintain regressions in a wide range of neoplastic conditions, including leukaemias, lymphomas, soft tissue and osteogenic sarcomas, paediatric malignancies and adult solid tumours; in particular, breast and lung carcinomas.

Cyclophosphamide is frequently used in combination chemotherapy regimens involving other cytotoxic drugs.

Dosage and administration The dosage regimen should be tailored to the individual requirements of the patient, depending on his general condition, concurrent therapy, the type and state of tumour, and the patient's response. Three sample regimens may serve as guides:

Low dose	80 to 240 mg/m^2 (2 to 6 mg/kg) as a single dose weekly i.v., or in divided doses orally.
Medium dose	400 to 600 mg/m^2 (10 to 15 mg/kg) as a single dose weekly i.v.
High dose	800 to 1,600 mg/m^2 (20 to 40 mg/kg) as a single dose i.v. at 10–20 day intervals.

Higher doses should be used only at the discretion of a physician experienced in cytotoxic chemotherapy.

It is recommended that the calculated dose of cyclophosphamide be reduced when it is given in combination with other anti-neoplastic agents or radiotherapy, and in patients with bone marrow depression.

Cyclophosphamide tablets should be swallowed whole, preferably on an empty stomach, but if gastric irritation is severe, they may be taken with meals.

Cyclophosphamide injection should be reconstituted with Water for Injections, 5 ml for each 100 mg of anhydrous cyclophosphamide. After reconstitution the solution will remain stable at room temperature for 2–3 hours. It should be given by slow intravenous injection over a period of 2–3 minutes or into the tubing of a freely running intravenous infusion over a period of 2–3 minutes.

Contra-indications, warnings, etc Cyclophosphamide should be used only under the direction of physicians experienced in cytotoxic or immunosuppressant therapy.

Contra-indications: Hypersensitivity and haemorrhagic cystitis.

Warnings: Cyclophosphamide should be withheld in the presence of severe bone marrow depression and reduced doses should be used in the presence of lesser degrees of bone marrow depression. Single doses will produce a leucopenia which may be severe but usually returns to normal within 21 days. Regular blood counts should be performed in patients receiving cyclophosphamide. This product should not normally be administered to patients who are pregnant or to mothers who are breast-feeding. It should not normally be given to patients with severe infections and should be withdrawn if such infections become life-threatening.

Cyclophosphamide should be used with caution in debilitated patients and those with renal and/or hepatic failure. In all such cases, dosage should be reduced. Oral hypoglycaemic agents may be potentiated by cyclophosphamide.

Amenorrhoea and azoospermia often occur during treatment with cyclophosphamide but in most cases are reversible. Alkylating agents, including cyclophosphamide, have been shown to possess mutagenic, teratogenic and carcinogenic potential. Pregnancy should therefore be avoided during cyclophosphamide therapy and for three months thereafter.

Cyclophosphamide is excreted mainly in the urine, largely in the form of active metabolites. These may give rise to a chemical cystitis which may be haemorrhagic. Because of this, a high fluid intake should be maintained with frequent emptying of the bladder. However, cyclophosphamide may give rise to fluid retention with subsequent water intoxication. Should this arise, a diuretic may be given. Cyclophosphamide may cause myocardial toxicity, especially at high dosage.

Cyclophosphamide may induce permanent sterility in children.

Adverse reactions: In addition to those noted above, the following may accompany cyclophosphamide therapy: hair loss, which may be total, although generally reversible; mucosal ulceration, anorexia, nausea and vomiting, pigmentation typically affecting the palms and nails of the hands and the soles of the feet, and interstitial pulmonary fibrosis.

Overdosage: Myelosuppression (particularly granulocytopenia) and haemorrhagic cystitis are the most serious consequences of overdosage. Recovery from myelosuppression will occur by the 21st day after the overdose in the great majority of patients (at doses up to 200 mg/kg iv) while granulocytopenia is usually seen by day 6 and lasts for a mean period of 12 days (up to 18 days). A broad spectrum antibiotic may be administered until recovery occurs. Transfusion of whole-blood, platelets or white cells and reverse barrier nursing may be necessary.

If the drug has been taken in the form of tablets, early gastric lavage may reduce the amount of drug absorbed. During the first 24 hours and possibly up to 48 hours after overdosage, i.v. mesna may be beneficial in ameliorating damage to the urinary system. Normal supportive measures such as analgesics and maintenance of fluid balance should be instituted. If the cystitis does not resolve, more intensive treatment may be necessary. No further courses should be given until the patient has fully recovered.

Pharmaceutical precautions *Tablets:* Store in a cool dry place and protect from light.

Injection: Store in a cool place and protect from light.

If heated above 32°C, cyclophosphamide may decompose to a damp-looking gel. It is, therefore, recommended that this product is never stored where heat build-up may occur such as near radiators, etc.

Legal category POM.

Package quantities

Tablets: Containers of 100 and 250 tablets of 50 mg.

Injection:
Vials of 100 mg in packs of 6.
Vials of 200 mg in packs of 6.
Vials of 500 mg in packs of 6.
Vials of 1,000 mg in packs of 6.
Each vial contains dry powder for reconstitution.

Further information Nil.

Product licence numbers

Cyclophosphamide Tablets 50 mg	3433/0036
Cyclophosphamide Injection 100 mg	3433/0037
Cyclophosphamide Injection 200 mg	3433/0038
Cyclophosphamide Injection 500 mg	3433/0039
Cyclophosphamide Injection 1,000 mg	3433/0040

DOXORUBICIN RAPID DISSOLUTION

Presentation Sterile, pyrogen-free, orange-red, freeze-dried powder in vials containing 10 and 50 mg of doxorubicin hydrochloride with lactose and hydroxybenzoate.

Uses Antimitotic and cytotoxic. Doxorubicin has been used successfully to produce regression in a wide range of neoplastic conditions including acute leukaemia, lymphomas, soft-tissue and osteogenic sarcomas, paediatric malignancies and adult solid tumours, in particular breast and lung carcinomas.

Doxorubicin is frequently used in combination chemotherapy regimens involving other cytotoxic drugs. Doxorubicin cannot be used as an antibacterial agent.

Dosage and administration For reconstitution the contents of the 10 mg vial may be dissolved in 5 ml Water for Injections or Sodium Chloride Injection and those of the 50 mg vial in 25 ml of the same solvents.

After adding the diluent, the vial contents will dissolve with gentle shaking, without inversion, within 30 seconds. The approximate displacement value of the contents of a 50 mg vial, after 25 ml of solvent have been added, is 0.15 ml.

Adults and children:

Intravenous administration: This is the most frequently used route of administration. The reconstituted solution is given via the tubing of a freely-running intravenous infusion, taking 2–3 minutes over the injection. This technique minimises the risk of thrombosis or perivenous extravasation which can lead to severe cellulitis and vesication. Commonly used acceptable solutions are

Sodium Chloride Injection, Dextrose Injection 5% or Sodium Chloride and Dextrose Injection.

Dosage is usually calculated on the basis of body surface area. On this basis, 60–75 mg/m^2 may be given every three weeks when doxorubicin is used alone. If it is used in combination with other antitumour agents having overlapping toxicity, the dosage of doxorubicin may need to be reduced to 30–40 mg/m^2 every three weeks. If dosage is to be calculated on the basis of body weight, 1.2–2.4 mg/kg should be given as a single dose every three weeks.

It has been shown that giving doxorubicin as a single dose every three weeks greatly reduces the distressing toxic effect, mucositis; however, there are still some who believe that dividing the dose over three successive days (0.4–0.8 mg/kg or 20–25 mg/m^2 on each day) gives greater effectiveness even though at the cost of higher toxicity.

Administration of doxorubicin in a weekly regimen has been shown to be as effective as the 3-weekly regimen. The recommended dosage is 20 mg/m^2 weekly although objective responses have been seen at 6–12 mg/m^2. Weekly administration leads to a reduction in cardiotoxicity.

Dosage may need to be reduced for patients who have had prior treatment with other cytotoxic agents.

Dosage may also need to be reduced in children and the elderly.

If hepatic function is impaired, doxorubicin dosage should be reduced according to the following table:

Serum bilirubin levels	*BSP retention*	*Recommended dose*
1.2–3.0 mg/100 ml	9–15%	50% normal dose
>3.0 mg/100 ml	>15%	25% normal dose

Intra-arterial administration: Intra-arterial injection has been used in attempts to produce intense local activity while keeping the total dose low and therefore reducing general toxicity. It should be emphasised that this technique is potentially extremely hazardous and can lead to widespread necrosis of the perfused tissue unless due precautions are taken.

Intra-arterial injection should only be attempted by those fully conversant with this technique.

Intravesical administration: Doxorubicin is being increasingly used by intravesical administration for the treatment of transitional cell carcinoma, papillary bladder tumours and carcinoma-in-situ. It should not be employed in this way for the treatment of invasive tumours which have penetrated the bladder wall. It has also been found useful to instil doxorubicin into the bladder at intervals after transurethral resection of a tumour in order to reduce the probability of recurrence. While at present many regimens are in use, making interpretation difficult, the following may be helpful guides: The concentration of doxorubicin in the bladder should be 50 mg per 50 ml. To avoid undue dilution with urine, the patient should be instructed not to drink any fluid in the 12 hours prior to instillation. This should limit urine production to approximately 50 ml per hour. The patient should be rotated a quarter turn every 15 minutes while the drug is in situ. Exposure to the drug solution for one hour is generally adequate and the patient should be instructed to void at the end of this time.

Contra-indications, warnings, etc Doxorubicin Rapid Dissolution is intended for use under the direction of those experienced in cytotoxic therapy.

Hypersensitivity to hydroxybenzoates is a contra-indication.

Dosage should not be repeated in the presence of bone-marrow depression or buccal ulcerations. The latter may be preceded by premonitory buccal burning sensations and repetition in the presence of this symptom is not advised.

Haematological monitoring should be undertaken regularly in both haematological and non-haematological conditions, because of the possibility of bone-marrow depression which may become evident around ten days from the time of administration.

Cardiotoxicity may be manifested in tachycardia, including supra-ventricular tachycardia and ECG changes. Routine ECG monitoring is recommended and caution should be exercised in patients with impaired cardiac function.

A cumulative dose of 450–550 mg/m^2 should only be exceeded with extreme caution. Above this level, the risk of irreversible congestive cardiac failure increases greatly. The total dose of doxorubicin administered to the individual patient should also take account of any previous or concomitant therapy with other potentially cardiotoxic agents such as high-dose i.v. cyclophosphamide, mediastinal irradiation or related anthracycline compounds such as daunorubicin. Administration of doxorubicin weekly has been shown to be associated with reduced cardiotoxicity compared with a 3-weekly schedule allowing patients to be treated to a higher cumulative dose. It should be noted that cardiac failure may also occur several weeks after administration and may not respond to treatment.

Baseline and follow-up ECGs during and immediately after drug administration are advisable. Transient ECG changes, such as T-wave flattening, S-T segment depression and arrhythmias, are not considered indications for the suspension of doxorubicin therapy. A reduction of the QRS wave is considered more indicative of cardiac toxicity. If this change occurs, the benefit of continued therapy must be carefully evaluated against the risk of producing irreversible cardiac damage.

Severe cardiac failure may occur suddenly, without premonitory ECG changes.

Doxorubicin Rapid Dissolution may impart a red colour to the urine, particularly to the first specimen passed after the injection, and patients should be advised that this is no cause for alarm.

Alopecia occurs frequently, including the interruption of beard-growth, but all hair growth normally resumes after treatment is stopped.

Nausea, vomiting and diarrhoea may also occur.

The risk of thrombophlebitis at the injection site may be minimised by following the procedure for administration recommended above. A stinging or burning sensation at the site of administration signifies a small degree of extravasation and the infusion should be stopped and re-started in another vein.

Pregnancy and lactation: There is no conclusive information as to whether doxorubicin may adversely affect human fertility or cause teratogenesis. Experimental data, however, suggest that doxorubicin may harm the foetus and should, therefore, not be administered to pregnant women or to mothers who are breast-feeding.

Overdosage: Single doses of 250 mg and 500 mg of doxorubicin have proved fatal. Such doses may cause acute myocardial degeneration within 24 hours and severe myelosuppression, the effects of which are greatest between 10 and 15 days after administration. Treatment should aim to support the patient during this period and should utilise such measures as blood transfusions and reverse barrier nursing. Delayed cardiac failure may occur up to six months after the overdose. Patients should be observed carefully and should signs of cardiac failure arise, be treated along conventional lines.

Pharmaceutical precautions The vial contents are under a negative pressure to minimise aerosol formation during reconstitution; particular care should be taken when the needle is inserted. Inhalation of any aerosol produced during reconstitution must be avoided.

The following protective recommendations are given due to the toxic nature of this substance:

— Personnel should be trained in good technique for reconstitution and handling.

— Pregnant staff should be excluded from working with this drug.

— Personnel handling Doxorubicin Rapid Dissolution should wear protective clothing: goggles, gowns and disposable gloves and masks.

— A designated area should be defined for reconstitution (preferably under a laminar flow system). The work

surface should be protected by disposable, plastic-backed, absorbent paper.
— All items used for reconstitution, administration or cleaning, including gloves, should be placed in high-risk, waste-disposal bags for high-temperature incineration.

The reconstituted solution is stable when stored for up to 48 hours at room temperature in normal artificial light, however, in line with good pharmaceutical practice it is recommended that it should normally be stored at 2°–8°C, protected from light and used within 24 hours. The reconstituted solution is chemically stable for at least 24 hours at room temperature in strong sunlight.

The reconstituted solution contains 0.02% hydroxybenzoate. This is not a preservative solution. Discard any unused solution.

Prolonged contact with any solution of an alkaline pH should be avoided as it will result in hydrolysis of the drug. Doxorubicin Rapid Dissolution should not be mixed with heparin as a precipitate may form and it is not recommended that Doxorubicin Rapid Dissolution be mixed with other drugs.

Accidental contact with the skin or eyes should be treated immediately by copious lavage with water, or soap and water, or sodium bicarbonate solution: medical attention should be sought.

Spillage or leakage should be treated with dilute sodium hypochlorite (1% available chlorine) solution, preferably by soaking, and then water. All cleaning materials should be disposed of as indicated previously.

Legal category POM.

Package quantities 10 mg and 50 mg vials for injection.

Further information Nil.

Product licence numbers
10 mg 3433/0110
50 mg 3433/0112

DOXORUBICIN SOLUTION FOR INJECTION

Presentation Sterile, red, mobile solution in vials containing 10 mg and 50 mg of doxorubicin hydrochloride as a 2 mg/ml solution in 0.9% Sodium Chloride Injection.

Uses Antimitotic and cytotoxic. Doxorubicin has been used successfully to produce regression in a wide range of neoplastic conditions, including acute leukaemia, lymphomas, soft-tissue and osteogenic sarcomas, paediatric malignancies and adult solid tumours; in particular, breast and lung carcinomas.

Doxorubicin is frequently used in combination chemotherapy regimens with other cytotoxic drugs. Doxorubicin cannot be used as an antibacterial agent.

Dosage and administration Adults and children.
Intravenous administration: The solution is given via the tubing of a freely-running intravenous infusion, taking 2–3 minutes over the injection. This technique minimises the risk of thrombosis or perivenous extravasation which can lead to severe cellulitis and vesication.

Dosage is usually calculated on the basis of body surface area. On this basis, 60–75 mg/m^2 may be given every three weeks when doxorubicin is used alone. If it is used in combination with other antitumour agents having overlapping toxicity, the dosage of doxorubicin may need to be reduced to 30–40 mg/m^2 every three weeks. If dosage is calculated on the basis of body weight, 1.2–2.4 mg/kg should be given as a single dose every three weeks.

It has been shown that giving doxorubicin as a single dose every three weeks greatly reduces the distressing toxic effect, mucositis; however there are still some who believe that dividing the dose over three successive days (0.4–0.8 mg/kg or 20–25 mg/m^2 on each day) gives greater effectiveness though at the cost of higher toxicity.

Administration of doxorubicin in a weekly regimen has been shown to be as effective as the 3-weekly regimen. The recommended dosage is 20 mg/m^2 weekly although objective responses have been seen at 6–12 mg/m^2. Weekly administration leads to a reduction in cardiotoxicity.

Dosage may need to be reduced for patients who have had prior treatment with other cytotoxic agents.

Dosage may also need to be reduced in children and the elderly.

If hepatic function is impaired, doxorubicin dosage should be reduced according to the following table:

Serum bilirubin levels	*BSP retention*	*Recommended dose*
1.2–3.0 mg/100 ml	9–15%	50% normal dose
>3.0 mg/100 ml	>15%	25% normal dose

Contra-indications, warnings, etc Doxorubicin Solution for Injection is intended for use under the direction of those experienced in cytotoxic therapy.

Dosage should not be repeated in the presence of bone-marrow depression or buccal ulcerations. The latter may be preceded by premonitory buccal burning sensations and repetition in the presence of this symptom is not advised.

Haematological monitoring should be undertaken regularly in both haematological and non-haematological conditions, because of the possibility of bone-marrow depression which may become evident around ten days from the time of administration.

Cardiotoxicity may be manifested in tachycardia, including supraventricular tachycardia, and ECG changes. Routine ECG monitoring is recommended and caution should be exercised in patients with impaired cardiac function.

A cumulative dose of 450–550 mg/m^2 should only be exceeded with extreme caution. Above this level, the risk of irreversible congestive cardiac failure increases greatly. The total dose of doxorubicin administered to the individual patient should also take account of any previous or concomitant therapy with other potentially cardiotoxic agents such as high-dose i.v. cyclophosphamide, mediastinal irradiation or related anthracycline compounds such as daunorubicin.

Administration of doxorubicin weekly has been shown to be associated with reduced cardiotoxicity compared with a 3-weekly schedule allowing patients to be treated to a higher cumulative dose.

It should be noted that cardiac failure may also occur several weeks after administration and may not respond to treatment.

Baseline and follow-up ECGs during and immediately after drug administration are advisable. Transient ECG changes, such as T-wave flattening, S-T segment depression and arrhythmias, are not considered indications for the suspension of doxorubicin therapy. A reduction of the QRS wave is considered more indicative of cardiac toxicity. If this change occurs, the benefit of continued therapy must be carefully evaluated against the risk of producing irreversible cardiac damage.

Severe cardiac failure may occur suddenly, without premonitory ECG changes.

Doxorubicin Solution for Injection may impart a red colour to the urine, particularly to the first specimen passed after the injection and patients should be advised that this is no cause for alarm.

Alopecia occurs frequently, including the interruption of beard growth, but all hair growth normally resumes after treatment is stopped.

Nausea, vomiting and diarrhoea may also occur.

The risk of thrombophlebitis at the injection site may be minimised by following the procedure for administration recommended above. A stinging or burning sensation at the site of administration signifies a small degree of extravasation and the infusion should be stopped and re-started in another vein.

Pregnancy and lactation: There is no conclusive information as to whether doxorubicin may adversely affect human fertility, or cause teratogenesis. Experimental data, however, suggest that doxorubicin may harm the foetus and should, therefore, not be administered to pregnant women or to mothers who are breast-feeding.

Overdosage: Single doses of 250 mg and 500 mg of doxorubicin have proved fatal. Such doses may cause acute myocardial degeneration within 24 hours and severe myelosuppression, the effects of which are greatest between 10 and 15 days after administration. Treatment should aim to support the patient during this period and should utilise such measures as blood transfusions and reverse barrier nursing. Delayed cardiac failure may occur up to six months after the overdose. Patients should be carefully observed and should signs of cardiac failure arise, be treated along conventional lines.

Pharmaceutical precautions The following protective recommendations are given due to the toxic nature of this substance:

—Personnel should be trained in good technique for handling.

—Pregnant staff should be excluded from working with this drug.

—Personnel handling Doxorubicin Solution for Injection should wear protective clothing: goggles, gowns and disposable gloves and masks.

—All items used for administration or cleaning, including gloves, should be placed in high-risk, waste-disposal bags for high-temperature incineration.

Discard any unused solution.

Prolonged contact with any solution of an alkaline pH should be avoided as it will result in hydrolysis of the drug. Doxorubicin Solution for Injection should not be mixed with heparin as a precipitate may form and it is not recommended that Doxorubicin Solution for Injection be mixed with other drugs.

Accidental contact with the skin or eyes should be treated immediately by copious lavage with water, or soap and water, or sodium bicarbonate solution: medical attention should be sought.

Spillage or leakage should be treated with dilute sodium hypochlorite (1% available chlorine) solution, preferably by soaking, and then water. All cleaning materials should be disposed of as indicated previously.

Legal category POM.

Package quantities 10 mg and 50 mg vials for injection.

Further information Doxorubicin Solution for Injection is adjusted to pH 3 with 0.5 N hydrochloric acid.

Product licence number 3433/0127.

FARLUTAL*

Presentation *Injection:* White, sterile suspension for i.m. injection, which settles on standing and readily disperses on shaking, containing 500 mg of medroxyprogesterone acetate in 2.5 ml, or 1000 mg in 5.0 ml.

Tablets: White, uncoated, round, biconvex, scored tablets, diameter 9 mm (100 mg) or 11 mm (250 mg), stamped '100' or '250' diametrically and containing 100 mg or 250 mg of medroxyprogesterone acetate, respectively.

White, uncoated, capsule-shaped tablets, measuring about 22 mm × 7 mm, scored on both faces and stamped 'FCE' and '500' on one face, containing 500 mg of medroxyprogesterone acetate.

Uses Palliative treatment of hormone-sensitive malignancies. Farlutal has been successfully used to produce regressions in breast, endometrial, prostatic and renal cell carcinoma. High dose Farlutal therapy has proved especially useful in breast carcinoma and in achieving subjective improvements in terminally ill patients, notably pain relief and improved performance status.

Dosage and administration Suggested dosage schemes are as follows:

Breast carcinoma

Initial dose	500–1000 mg/day i.m. for 4 weeks.
Maintenance	500 mg i.m. twice a week.

Alternatively, 1000–1500 mg daily, orally, is recommended, although doses of up to 2000 mg daily have been used. Daily oral administration, to be effective, must be at least 2–3 times the recommended i.m. dosage.

Endometrial carcinoma

Initial dose	500 mg i.m. twice weekly for 3 months.
Maintenance	500 mg i.m. weekly.
Alternatively	100–500 mg/day orally.

Renal adenocarcinoma

Initial dose	500 mg i.m. on alternate days for 30 days.
Maintenance	500 mg i.m. twice weekly until 60th day, then 250 mg i.m. weekly.
Alternatively	100–500 mg/day orally.

Prostatic adenocarcinoma

Initial dose	500 mg i.m. twice weekly.
Maintenance	500 mg i.m. weekly.
Alternatively	100–500 mg/day orally.

Intramuscular administration should be by deep injection into alternate gluteal muscles using a long wide-bore needle such as 21 G × $1\frac{1}{2}$" (8/10 40 mm). Narrow-bore or short needles must not be used.

Large tablets, and in this case particularly Farlutal 500, should be taken while sitting or standing and with copious amounts of liquid. The tablets may be broken in half before administration, if necessary.

Contra-indications, warnings, etc

Contra-indications: Thrombophlebitis, thrombo-embolic disorders, severe hepatic insufficiency and hypercalcaemia as may occur in patients with osseous metastases; also, suspected or early breast carcinoma, missed abortion, metrorrhagia, pregnancy and known hypersensitivity to medroxyprogesterone acetate or, for the injectable formulation, hydroxybenzoates (excipients).

Warnings: Farlutal should be used under the direction of those experienced in cancer chemotherapy.

Since medroxyprogesterone acetate appears to enhance blood clotting potential, treatment should be discontinued upon the appearance of thrombo-embolic episodes, migraine or associated ocular problems such as sudden partial or total loss of vision, diplopia or vascular lesions of the retina.

In the event of vaginal bleeding occurring, an accurate diagnosis should be made. If a histological examination is indicated, the laboratory should be informed that the patient has been receiving a progestogen.

Precautions: Animal studies have shown that medroxyprogesterone acetate possesses adrenocorticoid activity and this effect has also been observed in humans. Patients treated with high doses continuously over long periods should be carefully observed for signs normally associated with adrenocorticoid therapy, such as hypertension, sodium retention, oedema, etc, and care is needed in treating patients with diabetes and/or arterial hypertension.

Farlutal may raise plasma calcium levels; some cases of hypercalcaemia have been reported in the treatment of breast carcinoma.

Administration of progesterone during the first months of pregnancy may possibly be associated with the occurrence of congenital cardiac malformations in the neonate. In addition, instances of masculinisation of female foetuses have been reported following high dose therapy during pregnancy. For these reasons, Farlutal is contra-indicated during pregnancy.

It should be noted that long term administration of medroxyprogesterone acetate to beagle dogs has resulted in the development of mammary nodules which were occasionally found to be malignant. The relevance of these findings to humans has, however, not been established.

Adverse reactions: As is generally found after intramuscular administration of large volumes of suspension, the i.m. preparation may cause local lesions at the injection site, such as sterile abscesses or inflammatory infiltrates. The suspension should, therefore, be well shaken before use and injected deeply into healthy gluteal muscle.

In common with other progestogens, Farlutal may cause mastodynia, galactorrhoea, vaginal bleeding, changes in menstrual flow, amenorrhoea, cervical erosions and modifications of cervical secretions. Farlutal also exerts a corticoid-like effect which may lead to facies lunaris, Cushingoid syndrome and weight changes; and an adrenergic-like action which may result in fine hand tremors, sweating and cramps in the calves at night. Cholestatic jaundice has occasionally been reported.

Pharmaceutical precautions The vials for injection should be well shaken before use and the contents should not be mixed with other agents. The vials are for single dose administration only, should be stored between 15°–30°C and should not be frozen.

The tablets should be stored in a dry place.

Package quantities

Farlutal 100	Cartons containing blister packs of 100 tablets
Farlutal 250	Cartons containing blister packs of 50 tablets
Farlutal 500	Cartons containing calendar blister packs of 56 tablets
Farlutal 500 for Injection	Vials in individual cartons
Farlutal 1000 for Injection	Vials in individual cartons

Legal category POM.

Further information Analysis of the various i.m. dosage schedules so far employed indicates that higher response rates may be obtained by attainment and maintenance of high plasma levels. The intramuscular injection of Farlutal as a 20% suspension of medroxyprogesterone acetate, enables these levels to be achieved while minimising the local side effects associated with high dose therapy using formulations of lower concentrations.

After oral administration of medoxyprogesterone acetate, absorption is rapid. The plasma half life is of the order of 2 days and with repeated dosing once daily a steady state concentration is reached in about 10 days. Plasma concentrations are usually proportional to the administered dose, but considerable individual variation occurs. In general, to obtain concentrations comparable to those achieved after 4 weeks i.m. administration, at least twice the daily i.m. dose should be given.

Product licence numbers

Farlutal 100	3433/0056
Farlutal 250	3433/0058
Farlutal 500	3433/0080
Farlutal 500 for Injection and Farlutal 1000 for Injection	3433/0045

GASTROMAX*

Presentation Opaque orange/yellow capsules containing white to light beige pellets. Each capsule contains 30 mg Metoclopramide Hydrochloride BP in a pH sensitive controlled release delivery system.

Uses For the relief of upper gastro-intestinal symptoms in patients aged over 20 years including heartburn, dyspepsia and flatulence associated with such conditions as peptic ulcer, reflux oesophagitis, gastric reflux, gastritis, duodenitis and hiatus hernia.

For the relief of nausea and vomiting due to gastrointestinal disorders. Also for use as an anti-emetic for nausea and vomiting associated with cytotoxic drugs.

Dosage and administration
Adults over 20 years of age: Gastromax should be taken without chewing, with liquid, preferably before a meal. Dosage is one capsule, once daily either morning or evening dependent upon the timing of symptoms.

For example, in cases of nocturnal reflux and heartburn, the capsule should be taken in the evening. If symptoms are mainly associated with daytime activity e.g. after meals, bending, stooping etc., the capsule should be taken in the morning.

Under 20 years of age: Not recommended.

Elderly: As for adults. The dose should be strictly adhered to and if long-term, treatment should be regularly reviewed.

Contra-indications, warnings, etc Gastromax should not be administered to patients under 20 years of age. Contra-indicated in patients with phaeochromocytoma.

Use in pregnancy: Gastromax should only be used where there are compelling reasons and not during the 1st trimester. Not recommended during lactation.

Precautions: Patients with renal insufficiency should be observed carefully; treatment should be discontinued immediately if side-effects occur.

Warnings and adverse effects: Various extrapyramidal reactions usually of the dystonic type have been reported. Symptoms which can occur include spasm of facial, extra-ocular or cervical muscles which may be constant or rhythmic. There may also be a generalised increase in muscle tone. Anti-Parkinsonian drugs of the anticholinergic type may be used to counteract these reactions.

Rarely fatigue, dizziness and restlessness have been reported. Reaction times may be affected; in such cases the control of vehicles and machinery may be impaired. Mammary engorgement and galactorrhoea may occur after long-term administration. These symptoms disappear on discontinuation of therapy.

Tardive dyskinesia may occur, principally in the elderly, after prolonged treatment. The dose in the elderly should be strictly adhered to and treatment should be regularly reviewed.

Interactions with other drugs: Anticholinergic drugs can reduce the effects of Gastromax. Concomitant administration of Gastromax with phenothiazines should be avoided. The effects of tricyclic antidepressants, MAOIs and sympathomimetic drugs can be affected. The absorption of digoxin may be reduced and that of paracetamol, various antibiotics and alcohol accelerated.

Overdosage: Gastric lavage and intensive supportive therapy should be initiated. Dystonic symptoms should be treated with atropine, benztropine or other anticholinergic agents.

Pharmaceutical precautions Nil.

Legal category POM.

Package quantities Blister packs of 28 capsules.

Further information Nil.

Product licence number 0232/0060.

KELFIZINE W*

Presentation White, uncoated tablets each containing sulfametopyrazine 2 g stamped 'Kelfizine W' obverse, and 'Weekly Dose' reverse.

Uses The treatment of infections due to sulphonamide-sensitive organisms. Kelfizine W is recommended in the management of chronic bronchitis (including prophylaxis), it is also indicated for use in urinary tract infections.

Dosage and administration
Adults: 2 g once weekly by mouth.

Children: Not recommended.

Elderly: As hepatic conjugation and renal clearance occur at a reduced rate in the elderly, caution is advised when prescribing the drug for long periods of time, to avoid accumulation.

The tablet should be stirred into half a tumblerful of water or orange squash.

Contra-indications, warnings, etc
Contra-indications: Not to be taken by persons sensitive to sulphonamides.

Warnings: Occasionally severe reactions such as erythema multiforme and the Stevens–Johnson syndrome, epidermal necrolysis, eosinophilia, agranulocytosis, granulocytopenia, purpura and leucopenia have been reported in patients treated with sulphonamides.

Sulphonamides, and thus sulfametopyrazine, may potentiate the effects of coumarin derivatives, some oral antidiabetic agents (sulphonylureas) and some diaminopyrimidine derivatives (trimethoprim, pyrimethamine). Paraminobenzoic acid can antagonize the antibacterial activity of sulfametopyrazine.

Adverse reactions: Other side-effects reported with the use of sulphonamides include nausea, vomiting and rashes: these are usually mild and transient with Kelfizine W.

Precautions: Sulfametopyrazine should be used with caution in patients with renal or hepatic dysfunction, dehydration, or blood dyscrasias.

Use in pregnancy and lactation: There is no evidence of the drug's safety in human pregnancy nor is there evidence from animal work that it is free from hazard. Kelfizine W is contra-indicated during the third trimester of pregnancy and during breast-feeding.

Overdosage: Doses up to 8 g have been taken over 36 hours without evidence of ill effects. To increase excretion a high fluid intake should be maintained for seven days and the urine rendered alkaline with Potassium Citrate mixture BP or sodium bicarbonate. The sulphonamide will then be retained in the urine in higher concentrations in the form of the alkali metal salt.

Legal category POM.

Package quantities Pack of 5 tablets individually foil wrapped.

Further information Sulfametopyrazine has a long half-life. This is due not to a high degree of serum protein binding (which is only 60%) but to a high degree of renal tubular re-absorption coupled with a low rate of hepatic metabolism of the drug.

Product licence number 3433/5916R.

KEMICETINE* SUCCINATE

Presentation Individual glass vials of chloramphenicol sodium succinate for injection containing the equivalent of 1 g of chloramphenicol.

Uses Kemicetine (chloramphenicol) is a broad-spectrum antibiotic and is active against many gram-positive and gram-negative organisms, spirillae and rickettsia. Kemicetine should not be used for trivial infections due to the possibility of severe blood dyscrasias, which may prove fatal.

Kemicetine succinate is indicated for typhoid, meningitis caused by *H. influenzae* infections and other serious infections. It is also indicated wherever chloramphenicol is deemed the antibiotic of choice and oral administration is not possible, or higher than usual blood concentrations are required.

Dosage and administration
In order to ensure rapid attainment of high blood levels, Kemicetine succinate is best administered by i.v. injection. Where this is not possible, however, intramuscular administration may be used, although it should be borne in mind that absorption may be slow and unpredictable.

The injection should be reconstituted with Water for Injections, Sodium Chloride Injection, or Dextrose Injection 5%. The following dilution table may be useful for the administration of a proportion of the contents of a vial:

Concentration	*Solution strength*	*Volume of diluent to be added*	*Total volume after dilution*
40%	400 mg/ml	1.7 ml	2.5 ml
25%	250 mg/ml	3.2 ml	4.0 ml
20%	200 mg/ml	4.2 ml	5.0 ml
10%	100 mg/ml	9.2 ml	10.0 ml

The dose administered and the concentration used is dependent on the severity of the infection. The recommended standard dosage is as follows:

Adults: The equivalent of 1 g chloramphenicol every 6–8 hours.

Children: The equivalent of 50 mg/kg chloramphenicol, according to body weight, daily in divided doses every 6 hours (this dose should not be exceeded). The patient should be carefully observed for signs of toxicity.

Elderly: The usual adult dosage should be given subject to normal hepatic and renal function.

Neonates and premature infants: 25 mg/kg in divided doses.

Certain infections, such as meningitis or septicaemia, may require substantially higher doses.

The 10% solution should be given by intravenous injection over a period of about a minute, or in a larger volume of fluid, by slow intravenous infusion.

The concurrent administration of i.v. Kemicetine succinate with topical treatment has been found to be very effective in the treatment of osteomyelitic foci, abscesses, empyema and skin and urinary infections.

Contra-indications, warnings, etc Kemicetine succinate is contra-indicated in patients with a previous history of sensitivity and/or toxic reaction to chloramphenicol. It is also contra-indicated in pregnancy and whilst breast feeding. Kemicetine is to be administered only under the direction of a medical practitioner. Chloramphenicol may cause severe bone marrow depression which may lead to agranulocytosis, thrombocytopenic purpura or aplastic anaemia. These effects on the haemopoietic system are usually associated with a high dose, prolonged administration, or repeated courses, but they may occur at relatively low doses. Chloramphenicol should not be used in the treatment of any infection for which a less toxic antibiotic is available. It is also advisable to perform blood tests in the case of prolonged or repeated administration. Evidence of any detrimental effect on blood elements is an indication to discontinue therapy immediately.

Other adverse reactions which may become apparent after chloramphenicol treatment are: dryness of the mouth, nausea and vomiting, diarrhoea, urticaria, optic neuritis with blurring, or temporary loss of vision, peripheral neuritis, headache and depression. Superinfection by fungi, e.g. *C. albicans* in the gastro-intestinal tract, or vagina, may also occur due to the disturbance of normal bacterial flora.

Chloramphenicol has been shown to interact with, and enhance the effects of: coumarin anticoagulants, some hypoglycaemic agents (e.g. tolbutamide) and phenytoin. When given concurrently, a dose reduction of these agents may, therefore, be necessary. Plasma concentrations of chloramphenicol may be reduced with concomitant usage of phenobarbitone and rifampicin. Chloramphenicol may also impede the development of immunity and should therefore not be given during active immunisation.

The drug should be used with great caution in patients with impairment of hepatic or renal function. The dosage should be reduced in these patients. 'The Grey Syndrome' may occur after administration, in patients with immature hepatic metabolic capacity, i.e. infants and neonates, usually in those treated with doses substantially in excess of those recommended.

Because of its toxic nature, it is important to monitor serum levels of this antibiotic particularly in newborn and premature infants, in the elderly, in patients with renal or hepatic disease and in those receiving other drugs with which chloramphenicol may interact.

Overdosage: General supportive therapy should be given.

Pharmaceutical precautions Any Kemicetine succinate solution remaining in the vial after use should be discarded, as chloramphenicol sodium succinate is not bactericidal or bacteriostatic.

Legal category POM.

Package quantities Cartons containing 25 individual vials.

Further information Nil.

Product licence number 3433/5903R.

MAXTREX*

Presentation *Maxtrex tablets:* Round, uncoated, convex tablets diameter 6 mm, containing 2.5 mg (pale yellow tablets marked 'M2.5' on one side and 'F' on the other) and 10 mg (deep yellow tablets marked 'M10' on one side and scored on the other) methotrexate.

Uses Methotrexate is a folic acid antagonist and is classified as an antimetabolite cytotoxic agent.

Methotrexate has been used to produce regression in a wide range of neoplastic conditions including acute leukaemias, non-Hodgkin's lymphoma, soft-tissue and osteogenic sarcomas, and solid tumours particularly breast, lung, head and neck, bladder, cervical, ovarian, and testicular carcinoma.

Methotrexate has also been used in the treatment of severe, uncontrolled psoriasis which is not responsive to other therapy.

Dosage and administration Single doses, not exceeding 30 mg/m^2, on not more than 5 successive days. A rest period of at least two weeks is recommended between treatments, in order to allow the bone marrow to return to normal.

Methotrexate has been used both alone and in combination chemotherapy with radiotherapy and surgery. Dosage regimens may therefore vary considerably. Leucovorin rescue regimens are discussed briefly under 'Further information'.

If methotrexate is administered in combination chemotherapy regimens, the dosage should be reduced, taking into consideration any overlapping toxicity of the other drug components.

Dosage for psoriasis: For the treatment of severe psoriasis 10–25 mg orally, once weekly, is recommended. Dosage should be adjusted according to the patient's response and the haematological toxicity.

Contra-indications, warnings, etc Maxtrex is usually intended for use under the direction of those experienced in cytotoxic therapy.

Contra-indications: Methotrexate is contra-indicated in the presence of severe renal or hepatic impairment and serious anaemia, leucopenia or thrombocytopenia.

Warnings: Methotrexate should be used with extreme caution in patients with haematological depression, renal impairment, diarrhoea, ulcerative disorders of the G.I. tract and psychiatric disorders and in the elderly and very young. Hepatic toxicity has been observed. Renal lesions may develop if the urinary flow is impeded and urinary pH is low, especially if large doses have been administered.

The administration of low doses of methotrexate for prolonged periods may give rise, in particular, to hepatic toxicity. Liver function tests should be periodically carried out and abnormalities are an indication for discontinuing treatment for at least a period of 2 weeks.

Particular care and possible cessation of treatment are indicated if stomatitis or G.I. toxicity occurs as haemorrhagic enteritis and intestinal perforation may result.

After intrathecal administration, leucoencephalopathies have been observed, especially with concomitant cerebral radiotherapy.

Reversible eosinophilic pulmonary reactions and treatment-resistant, interstitial fibrosis may occur, particularly after long-term treatment.

Methotrexate is teratogenic and should not ordinarily be administered to patients who are pregnant or to mothers who are breast-feeding. The drug affects spermatogenesis and oogenesis and may therefore decrease fertility. The effect appears to be reversible after discontinuation of therapy. Conception should be prevented for at least 6 months after administration has ceased.

There are isolated reports in the literature of tumours occurring in patients following treatment with methotrexate, and in some studies in animals. However controlled animal studies and human epidemiological surveys have not demonstrated carcinogenicity. Nevertheless, the possibility of such an effect should be borne in mind when designing long-term management.

Methotrexate is immunosuppressive and may therefore reduce immunological response to concurrent vaccination. Severe antigenic reactions may occur if a live vaccine is given concurrently.

Precautions: Before, during and after treatment with methotrexate a complete haematological analysis should be performed, together with renal and hepatic function tests. Haemopoietic depression may occur suddenly even with low doses. A severe reduction of any blood element requires immediate cessation of treatment and suitable supportive measures such as blood transfusion and reverse barrier nursing. During therapy urine should be kept alkaline, if necessary, by giving oral or i.v. sodium bicarbonate, to prevent crystal deposition.

The disappearance of methotrexate from plasma should be monitored, if possible. This is recommended in particular when high, or very high doses are administered, in order to permit calculation of an adequate dose of leucovorin rescue. (See under 'Further information'.)

Radiotherapy to the CNS should not be given concomitantly with intrathecally administered methotrexate.

After intrathecal administration the drug is transported into the general circulation and may therefore still give rise to systemic toxicity, particularly myelosuppression.

Drug interactions: Methotrexate is extensively protein bound and may displace, or be displaced by, other acidic drugs. The concurrent administration of agents such as aminobenzoic acid, chloramphenicol, phenytoin, propionic acid anti-inflammatory agents, salicylates, sulphonamides, tetracyclines, thiazide diuretics, probenecid or sulphinpyrazone will decrease the methotrexate transport function of renal tubules, thereby reducing excretion and almost certainly increasing methotrexate toxicity.

Side-effects: Common side-effects are leucopenia and thrombocytopenia (which are usually reversible), nausea and vomiting, diarrhoea and stomatitis. Other side-effects include G.I. ulceration, alopecia, erythematous skin reactions and suppression of ovarian and testicular function.

Megaloblastic anaemia has been reported. Renal and hepatic damage may occur, particularly after high doses or prolonged administration, respectively. Reversible, eosinophilic pulmonary reactions and treatment-resistant interstitial fibrosis have been recorded.

CNS side-effects that may follow intrathecal or intraventricular use are headache, drowsiness, blurred vision, ataxia and, rarely, dementia and convulsions.

Overdosage: Leucovorin is a specific antidote for methotrexate and, following accidental overdosage, should be administered within one hour at a dosage equal to, or greater than, the methotrexate dose. It may be administered by i.v. bolus or infusion. Further doses may be required. The patient should be observed carefully and blood transfusions, renal dialysis and reverse barrier nursing may be necessary.

Pharmaceutical precautions Maxtrex should be stored at room temperature protected from light.

Legal category POM.

Package quantities
Maxtrex 2.5 tablets: Bottles of 100.
Maxtrex 10 tablets: Bottles of 100.

Further information Methotrexate is a folic acid antagonist and its major site of action is the enzyme dihydrofolate reductase. Its main effect is inhibition of DNA synthesis, but it also acts directly both on RNA and protein synthesis. Methotrexate is a phase specific substance, the main effect being directed during the S-phase of cell division.

The inhibition of dihydrofolate reductase can be circumvented by the use of leucovorin (folinic acid; citrovorum factor) and protection of normal tissues can be carried out by properly timed administration of leucovorin calcium. Dosage regimens for leucovorin rescue vary, depending on the dose of methotrexate administered. Up to 120 mg are generally given (as the calcium salt), usually in divided doses over 12–24 hours, by i.m., or i.v. bolus, or intravenous infusion in normal saline. This is followed by 12–15 mg i.m. or 15 mg orally every 6 hours for 48 hours.

Product licence numbers

Maxtrex 2.5	3433/0071
Maxtrex 10	3433/0072

MINODIAB*

Presentation Minodiab is available as white, biconvex, 8 mm tablets containing 2.5 or 5 mg of glipizide. The 5 mg tablets are scored.

Uses Minodiab is an orally active hypoglycaemic sulphonylurea and has been shown to be effective in the treatment of diabetes mellitus Type II. In certain patients receiving insulin, the concurrent use of Minodiab allows a reduction in the daily dose of insulin.

Dosage and administration The usual dose range of Minodiab is 2.5–30 mg daily but if control is not achieved within this range then it may be increased to a total daily dose of 40 mg, although the additional proportion of patients responding to this higher dosage may not be large.

Patients previously untreated: The initial dose is 2.5–5 mg daily. Doses of 2.5 mg daily should be taken as a single dose before breakfast. Doses of 5 mg daily may be taken as a single dose before breakfast or as two doses; one in the morning and one in the evening before meals.

Patients changing from other oral antidiabetics: The recommended starting dose is 5 mg daily taken as a single dose or in two divided doses.

Dosage adjustments in all patients, either upwards or downwards, should be in 2.5–5 mg steps at weekly intervals until good control is achieved. The maximum recommended single dose is 15 mg. Doses above 15 mg should ordinarily be taken in 2 divided doses before meals. Multiple divided doses (2 or 3 daily) are recommended for patients who experience particularly high post-prandial blood glucose peaks.

Concomitant food intake may delay absorption and administration should therefore be 15–20 minutes before a main meal: therapeutic effects are usually seen within 30 minutes and peak at about 60 minutes. Glipizide is rapidly metabolised and excreted mainly in the urine and therefore it is unlikely that delayed hypoglycaemic episodes will occur.

When administered in divided daily doses glipizide can be considered as having a physiological action as its peak effect coincides with post-prandial peak blood-sugar levels.

A biguanide may be added to the treatment if control is not achieved with Minodiab.

Contra-indications, warnings, etc

Contra-indications: Minodiab is contra-indicated in pregnancy, juvenile diabetes, diabetic ketoacidosis, diabetic coma, severe renal or hepatic insufficiency, infections and febrile conditions, gangrene and in severe trauma and major surgical procedures.

Warnings: Concurrent use of MAOIs, phenylbutazone, β-blockers, sulphonamides, coumarin derivatives or salicylates may enhance the hypoglycaemic effect. Conversely the effect may be diminished in the presence of adrenaline, corticosteroids, oral contraceptives and thiazide diuretics.

Patients should be instructed to take their meals regularly and not to exercise excessively without additional calorie intake. Failure to do so may result in a hypoglycaemic episode. The hypoglycaemia is controlled by giving carbohydrates.

Adverse reactions: Side-effects are not common with Minodiab. Those that do occur are associated with the gastro-intestinal tract, and include nausea, vomiting, anorexia, gastric pain, etc. Skin reactions have been reported, e.g. rash, urticaria, pruritus, etc. Other reactions include headache, dizziness and vertigo.

Overdosage: Gastric lavage should be performed as soon as possible. Hypoglycaemia should be treated as it occurs with appropriate measures including oral or i.v. glucose.

Pharmaceutical precautions None.

Legal category POM.

Package quantities Cartons containing 60 tablets.

Further information Glipizide is almost completely absorbed from the GI tract and appears to act by stimulating insulin secretion from pancreatic β cells, but may also act by potentiating peripheral insulin action. Peak concentrations in blood are achieved within 60 minutes and the half-life is approximately 3½ hours.

Product licence numbers

Minodiab 2.5	3433/0022.
Minodiab 5	3433/0023.

NAXOGIN* 500

Presentation Naxogin 500 is available as white or slightly yellow bi-convex tablets scored on one side and plain on the other. Each tablet contains 500 mg nimorazole.

Uses Naxogin is a trichomonacidal agent. It is indicated for the systemic treatment of trichomonal vaginitis. Sexual partners should also be treated even if they are free of symptoms.

Naxogin is also effective against other protozoa and may be used for the treatment of giardiasis, amoebiasis and acute ulcerative gingivitis.

Dosage and administration *For the treatment of trichomoniasis:* 2 g (4 tablets) to be taken together as a single dose with a main meal. This may be repeated if there is no clinical improvement.

For acute ulcerative gingivitis: 500 mg twice daily for two days.

For giardiasis or amoebiasis: Adults: 500 mg twice daily for five days.

Children (over 10 kg body weight): 500 mg daily for five days.

Children (under 10 kg body weight): 250 mg daily for five days.

Contra-indications, warnings, etc Like all nitroimidazoles, Naxogin 500 is contra-indicated for nursing mothers as it is excreted in breast milk and the effect on the neonate is unknown. Also this group of drugs should not be given in the presence of active CNS disease. Treatment should be discontinued if ataxia or other CNS symptoms appear.

Naxogin 500 should be given with caution during pregnancy although there is no known teratogenicity. Naxogin should only be given during pregnancy if no other suitable drug is available.

As Naxogin 500 is excreted principally via the kidneys, overt renal insufficiency is also a contra-indication.

Unwanted effects are rare and may comprise transient gastro-intestinal effects such as nausea and vomiting. No blood dyscrasias have been reported. Intolerance to alcohol, similar to that induced by disulfiram, has been observed with the nitroimidazoles.

Overdosage: There is no specific treatment but gastric lavage should be performed as soon as possible. Supportive measures should be instituted as required and a high fluid intake maintained.

Pharmaceutical precautions None.

Legal category P.

Package quantities Bottles of 8 and 100 tablets.

Further information Naxogin 500 is well absorbed after oral administration, achieving blood levels of 32 mcg/ml within two hours and 1.9 mcg/ml at 24 hours. The metabolites of the drug are trichomonacidal and are excreted mainly by the kidney so that there are high urinary concentrations. Concentrations are high in vaginal and salivary secretions.

Naxogin 500 is also recommended for the treatment of acute ulcerative gingivitis in patients hypersensitive to penicillin.

Product licence number 3433/5914R.

OLBETAM*

Presentation Red-brown/dark-pink, hard gelatin capsules stamped 'Farmitalia Carlo Erba' containing acipimox 250 mg (capsule size No. 1) as a white to cream powder.

Uses Olbetam is indicated for the treatment of lipid disorders characterised, according to Fredrickson, by elevated plasma levels of triglycerides (Type IV hyperlipoproteinaemia), or cholesterol (Type IIa hyperlipoproteinaemia), and of both triglycerides and cholesterol (Type IIb hyperlipoproteinaemia).

Olbetam inhibits the release of fatty acids from adipose tissue and reduces the blood concentration of very low density lipoproteins (VLDL or pre-beta) and low density lipoproteins (LDL or beta) with a subsequent overall reduction in triglyceride and cholesterol levels.

The drug also has a favourable effect on high density lipoproteins (HDL or alpha) which increase during treatment.

Dosage and administration The daily dosage should be adjusted individually depending on plasma triglyceride and cholesterol levels.

The dosage most frequently used is between 500 and 750 mg/day; in particular, the lower dose is advised in Type IV and the higher dose in Types IIa and IIb hyperlipoproteinaemias. The daily dose should be divided and taken with main meals.

Daily dosages of up to 1200 mg have been safely administered for long periods. Improvement in the plasma lipids' picture is usually seen within the first month of therapy.

In patients with renal impairment it is advisable to reduce the dosage on the basis of creatinine clearance values. For guidance the following is suggested:

Clearance between 60 and 30 ml/min – 150 mg twice daily.

Clearance between 30 and 10 ml/min – 150 mg once daily.

Clearance below 10 ml/min – 150 mg every other day.

(Capsules containing 150 mg are available on request.)

Contra-indications, warnings, etc

Contra-indications: Olbetam is contra-indicated in patients who are hypersensitive to the drug and those with peptic ulceration.

Warnings and precautions: Modification of hyperlipidaemia is recommended only for patients with hyperlipidaemia of a degree and type considered appropriate for treatment. Low-cholesterol and low-fat diets, together with cessation of alcohol consumption, are preferable therapeutic approaches to be tried before starting treatment with Olbetam.

The absorption of Olbetam is not affected by the concomitant administration of cholestyramine.

Evidence of clinical efficacy in the prevention of heart disease has not been established.

The possible beneficial, and adverse, long-term consequences of some drugs used in the hyperlipidaemias are still the subject of scientific discussion.

Pregnancy and lactation: There is no evidence from the animal studies that acipimox is teratogenic. However, a higher incidence of immature and underweight foetuses was seen in pregnant animals given high doses of acipimox. This effect may be due to maternal toxicity.

There is only limited experience to date of administration of acipimox to humans therefore epidemiological data are not available.

Taking into account the present experience of administration to humans of acipimox and that the safety of acipimox in human pregnancy has not yet been ascertained it is recommended, therefore, that acipimox not be administered to women who are, or may be, pregnant.

In the absence of animal data on the levels of acipimox excreted in milk, Olbetam should not be administered to women who are breast-feeding.

Adverse reactions: The drug may induce skin vasodilation giving rise to a sensation of heat, flushing or itching, especially at the beginning of therapy and also rash and erythema. These reactions usually disappear rapidly during the first days of treatment. Moderate gastric disturbances (heartburn, epigastric pain, nausea and diarrhoea) have been reported occasionally, as well as headache and malaise. On rare occasions patients have developed urticaria, angioedema and bronchospasm; anaphylactoid reactions have also been reported.

Overdosage: If toxic effects are observed, supportive care and symptomatic treatment should be administered.

Pharmaceutical precautions Store below 30°C in a dry place.

Legal category POM.

Package quantities Blister packs of 100 capsules.

Further information Acipimox is rapidly and completely absorbed orally, reaching peak plasma levels within two hours. The half-life is about two hours. It does not bind to plasma proteins, it is not significantly metabolised and is eliminated almost completely intact by the urinary route.

Product licence number 3433/0097

PHARMORUBICIN* RAPID DISSOLUTION

Presentation Sterile, pyrogen-free, red, freeze-dried powder in vials containing 10 mg, 20 mg and 50 mg of epirubicin hydrochloride with lactose and hydroxybenzoate.

Uses Antimitotic and cytotoxic.

Epirubicin as a single agent has produced regression in a wide range of neoplastic conditions, including breast, ovarian, gastric and colorectal carcinomas, lymphomas, leukaemias and multiple myeloma. Intravesical administration of epirubicin has been found to be beneficial in the treatment of superficial bladder carcinoma. Pharmorubicin Rapid Dissolution may be used in combination chemotherapy regimens involving other cytotoxic drugs. Comparative studies on the effects of epirubicin with doxorubicin in inducing remission and estimating cardiotoxicity have only been performed in breast cancer.

Dosage and administration For reconstitution the contents of the 10 mg vial should be dissolved in 5 ml of Water for Injections or Sodium Chloride Injection, the 20 mg vial in 10 ml of Water for Injections or Sodium Chloride Injection and the 50 mg vial in 25 ml of Water for Injections or Sodium Chloride Injection.

After adding the diluent the vial contents will dissolve with gentle shaking, without inversion, within 30 seconds. The approximate displacement value of the contents of a 50 mg vial after 25 ml of solvent have been added is 0.15 ml.

Intravenous administration: The reconstituted solution should be given via the tubing of a freely running intravenous infusion of Sodium Chloride Injection taking 3–5 minutes over the injection. This technique minimises the risk of thrombosis or perivenous extravasation which can lead to severe cellulitis and necrosis. Venous sclerosis may result from injection into small veins or repeated injections into the same vein.

Dosage is usually calculated on the basis of body surface area.

Single agent: The dose range most commonly used in clinical trials has been 75–90 mg/m^2. The dose should be repeated at 21-day intervals; the total dose for the cycle may be divided over two successive days. The dosage schedule should however, take into account the haematological status of the patient. In particular, a lower dose is recommended for patients whose bone marrow function has been impaired by previous chemotherapy or radiotherapy and in the elderly.

Combination chemotherapy: When Pharmorubicin Rapid Dissolution is used in combination with other antitumour agents the dosage should be reduced. A comparative combination study in advanced breast carcinoma has shown that the combination FEC (5-FU, epirubicin, cyclophosphamide) is as efficacious as FAC (5-FU, Adriamycin, cyclophosphamide) when the Pharmorubicin (epirubicin) and Adriamycin components are both given at 50 mg/m^2.

Since the major excretory route is the hepatobiliary system the dosage should also be reduced in patients with impaired liver function to avoid an increase of overall toxicity. Moderate liver impairment (bilirubin 1.2–3 mg/100 ml or BSP retention 9–15%), requires a dose reduction of the order of 50%, while severe impairment (bilirubin >3 mg/100 ml or BSP retention >15%) necessitates a dose reduction of the order of 75%.

Pharmorubicin Rapid Dissolution can be administered on a weekly regimen, particularly for the palliative treatment of poor risk patients for whom the toxicity of a conventional three-weekly treatment regimen would be unacceptable. For these patients the dosage most commonly used is 20 mg per week.

Intravesical administration: Pharmorubicin Rapid Dissolution can be given by intravesical administration for the treatment of papillary transitional cell carcinoma of the bladder and carcinoma-in-situ. It should not be used in this way for the treatment of invasive tumours which have penetrated the bladder wall where systemic therapy or surgery is more appropriate. Epirubicin has also been successfully used intravesically as a prophylactic agent after transurethral resection of superficial tumours in order to prevent recurrences.

While many regimens have been used, the following may be helpful as a guide: for therapy, 8 × weekly instillations of 50 mg per 50 ml of saline or distilled sterile water. In the case of local toxicity (chemical cystitis), a dose reduction to 30 mg per 50 ml is advised. For carcinoma-in-situ, depending on the individual tolerability of the patient, the dose may be increased up to 80 mg per 50 ml. For prophylaxis, 4 × weekly administrations of 50 mg per 50 ml followed by 11 × monthly instillations at the same dosage, is the schedule most commonly used.

The solution should be retained intravesically for 1 hour. To avoid undue dilution with urine, the patient should be instructed not to drink any fluid in the 12 hours prior to instillation. During the instillation, the patient should be rotated occasionally and should be instructed to void at the end of the instillation time.

Contra-indications, warnings, etc Pharmorubicin is intended for use under the direction of those experienced in cytotoxic therapy.

The drug should not be given to patients with marked myelosuppression induced by previous drug therapy or radiotherapy. Administration is normally contra-indicated in patients with a current or previous history of cardiac impairment and in patients already treated with maximum cumulative doses of other anthracyclines such as doxorubicin or daunorubicin.

During the first cycles of treatment with Pharmorubicin Rapid Dissolution patients must be carefully and frequently monitored.

Haematological monitoring should be undertaken regularly in both haematological and non-haematological conditions in view of the possibility of bone-marrow depression. Leucopenia is usually transient with the recommended dosage schedules, reaching a nadir between 10 and 14 days after administration. A return to normal blood values usually occurs within 21 days from administration.

Before starting treatment, and if possible during therapy, liver function should be evaluated [SGOT (AST), SGPT (ALT), alkaline phosphatase, bilirubin, BSP].

The data obtained in different animal species and the results of clinical trials have consistently indicated that epirubicin is less cardiotoxic than doxorubicin. A cumulative dose of 900–1000 mg/m^2 should only be exceeded with extreme caution. Above this level the risk of irreversible congestive cardiac failure increases greatly. However, there is objective evidence that cardiac toxicity may occur rarely below this range.

A lower cumulative dose of Pharmorubicin Rapid Dissolution is recommended in patients with prior or concomitant mediastinal radiation or therapy with related anthracycline compounds such as doxorubicin or daunorubicin or anthracene derivatives. In particular, patients who have received prior cumulative doses of more than 450 mg/m^2 of doxorubicin or daunorubicin are at a high risk of developing congestive heart failure (CHF). CHF and/or cardiomyopathy may occur several weeks after discontinuation of epirubicin therapy.

Cardiac function should be carefully monitored during treatment in order to minimise the risk of cardiac failure of the type described for other anthracycline compounds. It is recommended that an ECG be taken before and after each treatment cycle. Alterations of the ECG, such as flattening or inversion of the T wave, depression of the S-T segment, or the onset of arrhythmias, are generally transient and reversible and need not necessarily indicate that treatment should be stopped. Cardiomyopathy induced by anthracyclines, and by doxorubicin in particular, is associated with persistent QRS voltage reduction, prolongation beyond normal limits of the systolic interval (PEP/LVET) and a reduction of the ejection fraction. It is also advisable to assess cardiac function by non-invasive techniques such as ECG, echocardiography and, if necessary, measurement of the ejection fraction by radionuclide angiography.

Early clinical diagnosis of drug induced heart failure appears to be essential for successful treatment with digitalis, diuretics, peripheral vasodilators, a low salt diet and bed rest.

Alopecia is common and nausea, vomiting and diarrhoea may occur. Alopecia and lack of beard growth in males are usually reversible. Mucositis may appear 5–10 days after starting treatment and usually involves stomatitis with painful erosions, often along the sides of the tongue and on the sublingual mucosa. The frequency and severity of these side-effects is, however, lower than that described with other anthracycline compounds, such as doxorubicin.

The risk of thrombophlebitis at the injection site may be minimised by following the recommended procedure for administration.

Pharmorubicin Rapid Dissolution may impart a red colour to the urine and patients should be advised that this is no cause for alarm.

There is no conclusive information as to whether epirubicin may adversely affect human fertility, or cause teratogenesis. Experimental data, however, suggest that epirubicin may harm the foetus. This product should not normally be administered to patients who are pregnant or to mothers who are breast-feeding. Like most other anticancer agents, epirubicin has shown mutagenic and carcinogenic properties in animals.

Overdosage: Very high single doses of epirubicin may be expected to cause acute myocardial degeneration within 24 hours and severe myelosuppression within 10–14 days. Treatment should aim to support the patient during this period and should utilise such measures as blood transfusions and reverse barrier nursing. Delayed cardiac failure has been seen with the anthracyclines up to 6 months after the overdose. Patients should be observed carefully and should, if signs of cardiac failure arise, be treated along conventional lines.

Pharmaceutical precautions The vial contents are

under a negative pressure to minimise aerosol formation during reconstitution; particular care should be taken when the needle is inserted. Inhalation of any aerosol produced during reconstitution must be avoided.

The following protective recommendations are given due to the toxic nature of this substance:

— Personnel should be trained in good technique for reconstitution and handling.
— Pregnant staff should be excluded from working with this drug.
— Personnel handling Pharmorubicin Rapid Dissolution should wear protective clothing: goggles, gowns and disposable gloves and masks.
— A designated area should be defined for reconstitution (preferably under a laminar flow system). The work surface should be protected by disposable, plastic-backed, absorbent paper.
— All items used for reconstitution, administration or cleaning, including gloves, should be placed in high-risk, waste-disposal bags for high temperature incineration.

The reconstituted solution is chemically stable when stored for up to 48 hours at 2° to 8°C or 24 hours at room temperature; however, it is recommended that, in line with good pharmaceutical practice, the solution should not normally be stored for longer than 24 hours at 2° to 8°C. Avoid exposure of the product to sunlight or direct light.

The reconstituted solution contains 0.04% hydroxybenzoate. This is not a preservative solution.

Discard any unused solution.

Prolonged contact with any solution of an alkaline pH should be avoided as it will result in hydrolysis of the drug. Pharmorubicin Rapid Dissolution should not be mixed with heparin as a precipitate may form and it is not recommended that Pharmorubicin Rapid Dissolution be mixed with other drugs.

Accidental contact with the skin or eyes should be treated immediately by copious lavage with water, or soap and water, or sodium bicarbonate solution; medical attention should be sought.

Spillage or leakage should be treated with dilute sodium hypochlorite (1% available chlorine) solution, preferably by soaking, and then water.

All cleaning materials should be disposed of as indicated previously.

Legal category POM.

Package quantities 10 mg, 20 mg and 50 mg vials for injection.

Further information In patients with normal hepatic and renal function, plasma levels, after i.v. injection of 75–90 mg/m^2 of the drug, follow a tri-exponential decrease with a very fast first phase and a slow terminal phase corresponding to a half-life of about 40 hours. Plasma levels of the main metabolite, the 13-OH derivative, are constantly lower and virtually parallel those of the unchanged drug. Epirubicin is mainly eliminated via the hepatobiliary system; high plasma clearance values (0.9 l/min) indicate that the slow elimination is due to extensive tissue distribution. Epirubicin does not cross the blood–brain barrier.

After intravesical administration of 30–50 mg/ml of epirubicin, absorption through the basement membrane of the transitional cell epithelium into the capillary plexus of the bladder is minimal, rarely leading to Cmax > 10 ng/ml.

Product licence number 3433/0082

PHARMORUBICIN* SOLUTION FOR INJECTION

Presentation Sterile, red, mobile solution in vials containing 10 mg, 20 mg and 50 mg of epirubicin hydrochloride as a 2 mg/ml solution in 0.9% Sodium Chloride Injection.

Uses Antimitotic and cytotoxic. Pharmorubicin as a single agent has produced regression in a wide range of neoplastic conditions, including breast, ovarian, gastric and colorectal carcinomas, lymphomas, leukaemias and multiple myeloma. Pharmorubicin may be used in combination chemotherapy regimens involving other cytotoxic drugs. Comparative studies on the effects of Pharmorubicin compared with doxorubicin in inducing remission and estimating cardiotoxicity have only been performed in breast cancer.

Dosage and administration Pharmorubicin should be administered only by the intravenous route and the solution should be given via the tubing of a freely running intravenous infusion of Sodium Chloride Injection taking 3–5 minutes over the injection. This technique minimises the risk of thrombosis or perivenous extravasation which can lead to severe cellulitis and necrosis. Venous sclerosis may result from injection into small veins or repeated injections into the same vein.

Dosage is usually calculated on the basis of body surface area.

Single agent: The dose range most commonly used in clinical trials has been 75–90 mg/m^2. The dose should be repeated at 21 day intervals; the total dose for the cycle may be divided over two successive days. The dosage schedule should however, take into account the haematological status of the patient. In particular, a lower dose is recommended for patients whose bone marrow function has been impaired by previous chemotherapy or radiotherapy and in the elderly.

Combination chemotherapy: When Pharmorubicin is used in combination with other antitumour agents the dosage should be reduced.

Since the major excretory route is the hepatobiliary system the dosage should also be reduced in patients with impaired liver function to avoid an increase of overall toxicity. Moderate liver impairment (bilirubin 1.2–3 mg/100 ml or BSP retention 9–15%), requires a dose reduction of the order of 50%, while severe impairment (bilirubin > 3 mg/100 ml or BSP retention > 15%) necessitates a dose reduction of the order of 75%.

Pharmorubicin can be administered on a weekly regimen, particularly for the palliative treatment of poor risk patients for whom the toxicity of a conventional three-weekly treatment regimen would be unacceptable. For these patients the dosage most commonly used is 20 mg per week.

Contra-indications, warnings, etc Pharmorubicin Solution for Injection is intended for use under the direction of those experienced in cytotoxic therapy.

The drug should not be given to patients with marked myelosuppression induced by previous drug therapy or radiotherapy. Administration is normally contra-indicated in patients with a current or previous history of cardiac impairment and in patients already treated with maximum cumulative doses of other anthracyclines such as doxorubicin or daunorubicin.

During the first cycles of treatment with Pharmorubicin, patients must be carefully and frequently monitored. Haematological monitoring should be undertaken regularly in both haematological and non-haematological conditions in view of the possibility of bone-marrow depression. Leucopenia is usually transient with the recommended dosage schedules, reaching a nadir between 10 and 14 days after administration. A return to normal blood values usually occurs within 21 days from administration. Before starting treatment, and if possible during therapy, liver function should be evaluated [SGOT (AST), SGPT (ALT), alkaline phosphatase, bilirubin, BSP].

The data obtained in different animal species and the results of clinical trials have consistently indicated that Pharmorubicin is less cardiotoxic than doxorubicin.

A cumulative dose of 900–1000 mg/m^2 by the intravenous route should only be exceeded with extreme caution. Above this level the risk of irreversible congestive cardiac failure increases greatly. However, there is objective evidence that cardiac toxicity may occur rarely below this range.

A lower cumulative dose of Pharmorubicin is recommended in patients with prior or concomitant mediastinal radiation or therapy with related anthracycline compounds such as doxorubicin or daunorubicin or anthracene derivatives. In particular, patients who have received prior cumulative doses of more than 450 mg/m^2 of doxorubicin or daunorubicin are at a high risk of developing congestive heart failure (CHF). CHF and/or cardiomyopathy may occur several weeks after discontinuation of Pharmorubicin therapy.

Cardiac function should be carefully monitored during treatment in order to minimise the risk of cardiac failure of the type described for other anthracycline compounds. It is recommended that an ECG be taken before and after each treatment cycle. Alterations of the ECG, such as flattening or inversion of the T wave, depression of the S-T segment, or the onset of arrhythmias, are generally transient and reversible and need not necessarily indicate that treatment should be stopped. Cardiomyopathy induced by anthracyclines, and by doxorubicin in particular, is associated with persistent QRS voltage reduction, prolongation beyond normal limits of the systolic interval (PEP/LVET) and a reduction of the ejection fraction. It is also advisable to assess cardiac function by non-invasive techniques such as ECG, echocardiography and, if necessary, measurement of the ejection fraction by radionuclide angiography.

Early clinical diagnosis of drug induced heart failure appears to be essential for successful treatment with digitalis, diuretics, peripheral vasodilators, a low salt diet and bed rest.

Alopecia is common and nausea, vomiting and diarrhoea may occur. Alopecia and lack of beard growth in males are usually reversible. Mucositis may appear 5–10 days after starting treatment and usually involves stomatitis with painful erosions, often along the sides of the tongue and on the sublingual mucosa. The frequency and severity of these side-effects is, however, lower than that described with other anthracycline compounds, such as doxorubicin.

The risk of thrombophlebitis at the injection site may be minimised by following the recommended procedure for administration. Pharmorubicin Solution for Injection may impart a red colour to the urine and patients should be advised that this is no cause for alarm.

There is no conclusive information as to whether Pharmorubicin may adversely affect human fertility, or cause teratogenesis. Experimental data, however, suggest that Pharmorubicin may harm the foetus. This product should not normally be administered to patients who are pregnant or to mothers who are breast-feeding. Like most other anticancer agents, epirubicin has shown mutagenic and carcinogenic properties in animals.

Overdosage: Very high single doses of Pharmorubicin may be expected to cause acute myocardial degeneration within 24 hours and severe myelosuppression within 10–14 days. Treatment should aim to support the patient during this period and should utilise such measures as blood transfusions and reverse barrier nursing. Delayed cardiac failure has been seen with the anthracyclines up to 6 months after the overdose. Patients should be observed carefully and should, if signs of cardiac failure arise, be treated along conventional lines.

Pharmaceutical precautions The following protective recommendations are given due to the toxic nature of this substance:

— Personnel should be trained in good technique for handling.
— Pregnant staff should be excluded from working with this drug.
— Personnel handling Pharmorubicin should wear protective clothing: goggles, gowns and disposable gloves and masks.
— All items used for administration or cleaning, including gloves, should be placed in high-risk, waste-disposal bags for high temperature incineration.

Pharmorubicin Solution for Injection should be stored at 2°C–8°C.

Discard any unused solution.

Use within 24 hours of first penetration of the rubber stopper.

Prolonged contact with any solution of an alkaline pH should be avoided as it will result in hydrolysis of the drug. Pharmorubicin should not be mixed with heparin as a precipitate may form and it is not recommended that Pharmorubicin be mixed with other drugs.

Accidental contact with the skin or eyes should be treated immediately by copious lavage with water, or soap and water, or sodium bicarbonate solution: medical attention should be sought.

Spillage or leakage should be treated with dilute sodium hypochlorite (1% available chlorine) solution, preferably by soaking, and then water. All cleaning materials should be disposed of as indicated previously.

Legal category POM.

Package quantities 10 mg, 20 mg and 50 mg vials for injection.

Further information In patients with normal hepatic and renal function, plasma levels, after iv injection of 75–90 mg/m^2 of the drug, follow a tri-exponential decrease with a very fast first phase and a slow terminal phase corresponding to a half-life of about 40 hours. Plasma levels of the main metabolite, the 13-OH derivative, are constantly lower and virtually parallel to those of the unchanged drug. Pharmorubicin is mainly eliminated via the hepatobiliary system; high plasma clearance values (0.9 l/min) indicate that the slow elimination is due to extensive tissue distribution. Epirubicin does not cross the blood–brain barrier.

Product licence number 3433/0135.

REFOLINON*

Presentation Clear, pale yellow liquid for injection containing leucovorin 3 mg/ml (as the calcium salt) in ampoules of 2 ml and 10 ml.

Pale yellow, round, convex, scored, uncoated tablet marked with an 'F' on one side and 'CF' on the other; diameter 9 mm containing 15 mg leucovorin (as the calcium salt).

Uses Leucovorin (folinic acid) is the formyl derivative of tetrahydrofolic acid and is an intermediate product of the metabolism of folic acid. Leucovorin is used in cytotoxic therapy as an antidote to folic acid antagonists such as methotrexate. Leucovorin is effective in the treatment of megaloblastic anaemia due to folate deficiency.

Dosage and administration (Adults and children)

Leucovorin rescue: Depending upon the dose of methotrexate administered, dosage regimens of leucovorin calcium vary. Up to 120 mg leucovorin calcium are generally given, usually in divided doses over 12–24 hours by intramuscular injection, bolus intravenous injection or intravenous infusion in normal saline. This is followed by 12–15 mg intramuscularly or 15 mg orally every 6 hours for 48 hours. Rescue therapy is usually started 24 hours after the commencement of methotrexate administration.

If overdosage of methotrexate is suspected, the dose of leucovorin calcium should be equal to or greater than the dose of methotrexate and should be administered within one hour of the methotrexate administration.

Megaloblastic anaemia (folate deficiency): 15 mg (one tablet) leucovorin per day.

Contra-indications, warnings, etc Calcium folinate should not be used for the treatment of pernicious anaemia or other megaloblastic anaemia where vitamin B12 is deficient.

Leucovorin should not be given simultaneously with a folic acid antagonist, for the purpose of reducing or preventing clinical toxicity, as the therapeutic effect of the antagonist may be nullified.

High-dose methotrexate therapy together with leucovorin rescue should only be carried out under the direction of physicians experienced in antitumour chemotherapy.

Adverse reactions to leucovorin calcium are rare, but

following parenteral administration occasional pyrexial reactions have been reported.

Pharmaceutical precautions Protect from light.

Refolinon for injection has been shown to be compatible with 0.9% sodium chloride solution. Under normal light conditions and at room temperature solutions of calcium folinate in 0.9% sodium chloride have been shown to be stable for 24 hours.

Legal category POM.

Package quantities

Refolinon for Injection	10 × 2 ml ampoules
	10 × 10 ml ampoules
Refolinon Tablets	Containers of 30 tablets

Further information Nil.

Product licence numbers

Refolinon for Injection	3433/0079
Refolinon Tablets	3433/0078

SINTISONE*

Presentation White, scored tablets each containing 6.65 mg of prednisolone steaglate, therapeutically equivalent to prednisolone 5 mg.

Uses Sintisone is a synthetic glucocorticoid and is indicated in all conditions that respond to corticosteroid treatment, such as: allergy and anaphylaxis including bronchial asthma and angioneurotic oedema; blood disorders in particular leukaemia and malignant lymphoma; endocrine disorders including primary and secondary adrenal insufficiency; gastro-intestinal disorders including Crohn's disease and ulcerative colitis; ocular disorders including scleritis, posterior uveitis and giant cell arteritis; rheumatic disorders including rheumatoid arthritis, systemic lupus erythematosus and rheumatic fever with severe carditis and skin disorders including pemphigus vulgaris and bullous pemphigoid.

Dosage and administration *Adults:* The average initial dose for adults is 2–4 tablets, orally, twice daily, gradually reducing this to a maintenance dose of 1–3 tablets daily.

Elderly: Whilst no special dosage is required for the elderly it should be borne in mind that, where long term therapy is planned, they are more susceptible to the common side-effects of corticosteroid therapy and to those diseases for which corticosteroid therapy is contra-indicated.

Children: Initial dose: 0.6–2 mg/kg body weight, orally in divided doses. Maintenance dose: 1 mg/kg body weight, orally in divided doses (see 'Warnings').

Treatment may be given in short (6–10 day) courses for the alleviation of the symptoms of acute inflammatory episodes.

Alternate-day corticosteroid therapy is known to reduce the incidence of unwanted effects. Sintisone may be used with advantage in this manner by giving twice the normal daily dose every other day.

Treatment with corticosteroids should not terminate abruptly but should be withdrawn gradually.

Contra-indications, warnings, etc

Contra-indications: The contra-indications are those common to other corticosteroids. Corticosteroids are usually also contra-indicated in the presence of acute bacterial or viral infections.

Warnings: Conditions where caution is necessary include active or previous history of tuberculosis, peptic ulceration, steroid psychosis; Cushing's disease, osteoporosis particularly in post-menopausal females, hypertension, diabetes mellitus (or a family history of diabetes), glaucoma (or a family history of glaucoma), previous steroid myopathy, epilepsy or a tendency to thromboembolic episodes.

Patients receiving corticosteroids or who have been prescribed them during the preceding two years should be given supplementary corticosteroids for one to two days before surgery and continued until stress has ceased before tapering off the dose.

Use in pregnancy: There is inadequate evidence of safety in human pregnancy and there may be a very small risk of cleft palate and intra-uterine growth retardation in the foetus: there is evidence of harmful effects on pregnancy in animals. Sintisone should therefore, be used with caution in pregnancy, especially during the first trimester.

Use in children: Corticosteroids cause growth retardation in infancy, childhood and adolescence. Treatment should be limited to the minimum dosage for the shortest possible time. In order to minimise suppression of the hypothalamo-pituitary adrenal axis and growth retardation, treatment should be administered where possible as a single dose on alternate days.

Use in the elderly: Treatment of elderly patients, particularly if long term, should be planned bearing in mind the more serious consequences of the common side effects of corticosteroids in old age, especially osteoporosis, diabetes, hypertension, susceptibility to infection and thinning of the skin.

Side-effects: Adverse effects in systemic use and important sequalae to treatment are as follows:

Gastro-intestinal: Dyspepsia, peptic ulceration with perforation and haemorrhage, abdominal distension, oesophageal ulceration, oesophageal candidiasis, acute pancreatitis.

Musculo-skeletal: Proximal myopathy, osteoporosis, vertebral and long bone fractures, avascular osteonecrosis, tendon rupture.

Fluid and electrolyte disturbance: Sodium and water retention, hypertension, hypokalemic alkalosis.

Dermatological: Impaired healing, skin atrophy, bruising, striae, telangiectasis, acne.

Endocrine/metabolic: Suppression of the hypothalamo-pituitary adrenal axis, growth suppression in childhood and adolescence, menstrual irregularity and amenorrhoea. Cushingoid facies, hirsutism, weight gain, impaired carbohydrate tolerance with increased requirement for antidiabetic therapy, negative nitrogen balance.

Neuropsychiatric: Euphoria, psychological dependence, depression, insomnia. Intracranial hypertension in children. Aggravation of schizophrenia.

Ophthalmic: Increased intra-ocular pressure, glaucoma, papilloedema, cataracts, corneal or scleral thinning, exacerbation of ophthalmic viral disease.

General: Opportunistic infection, recurrence of dormant tuberculosis, leucocytosis, hypersensitivity, thromboembolism, increased appetite, nausea, malaise.

Withdrawal symptoms: Fever, myalgia, arthralgia, adrenal insufficiency.

Teratogenicity: See 'Use in pregnancy'.

Sintisone, however, circulates in the blood as prednisolone steaglate which is slowly metabolised to prednisolone, therefore there is a reduced tendency to the side-effects associated with corticosteroid therapy.

Overdosage: There is no specific treatment but gastric lavage should be performed as soon as possible. Supportive measures should be instituted as required.

Pharmaceutical precautions Store protected from light.

Legal category POM.

Package quantities Bottles of 100 tablets.

Further information Sintisone is a lipid soluble ester of prednisolone which is absorbed intact from the gut more completely than prednisolone.

Product licence number 3433/5906R.

TEMAZEPAM GELTHIX* CAPSULES

Presentation

Temazepam Gelthix Capsules 10 mg: Green, gel-filled, soft gelatin capsules marked '10' in white on one side and 'Gelthix' on the other, containing temazepam 10 mg.

Temazepam Gelthix Capsules 15 mg: Green, gel-filled,

soft gelatin capsules marked '15' in white on one side and 'Gelthix' on the other, containing temazepam 15 mg.

Temazepam Gelthix Capsules 20 mg: Green, gel-filled, soft gelatin capsules marked '20' in white on one side and 'Gelthix' on the other, containing temazepam 20 mg.

Temazepam Gelthix Capsules 30 mg: Green, gel-filled, soft gelatin capsules marked '30' in white on one side and 'Gelthix' on the other, containing temazepam 30 mg.

Uses Temazepam Gelthix Capsules 10, 15, 20 and 30 mg are indicated for the short-term treatment of sleep disturbances considered severe or disabling or where insomnia is subjecting the individual to extreme distress. These products are especially useful in those patients for whom the persistance of hypnotic effect after rising would be undesirable.

Products in the temazepam range are particularly suitable for patients with transient sleep disorders in whom the re-establishment of normal sleep patterns is expected following the resolution of precipitating factors.

They are also indicated for pre-medication for minor surgical and investigative procedures, especially in the case of out-patients.

Dosage and administration
Adults: Temazepam Gelthix Capsules 10 mg – *Insomnia:* One to three capsules on retiring. A dose of two capsules will be found satisfactory for most patients. This may be increased to four or six capsules in patients who do not respond to the lower dose. *Premedication:* 2 to 4 capsules from half an hour to one hour prior to surgery or investigative procedures.

Temazepam Gelthix Capsules 15 mg – *Insomnia:* One to two capsules on retiring. *Premedication:* 1 to 2 capsules from half an hour to one hour prior to surgery or investigative procedures.

Temazepam Gelthix Capsules 20 mg – *Insomnia:* For those patients resistant to low hypnotic dosage, two or three capsules before retiring. *Premedication:* 1 to 2 capsules from half an hour to one hour prior to surgery or investigative procedures.

Temazepam Gelthix Capsules 30 mg – *Insomnia:* For those patients resistant to low hypnotic dosage 1 or 2 capsules before retiring. *Premedication:* 1 capsule from half an hour to one hour prior to surgery or investigative procedures.

Elderly: Elderly patients or those suffering from cerebral vascular changes such as arteriosclerosis are likely to respond to smaller doses. Half the normal dose may be sufficient for a therapeutic response.

Children: Not recommended.

Treatment should if possible be intermittent.

The lowest dose which can control symptoms should be used. It should not be continued beyond 4 weeks.

Long-term chronic use is not recommended.

Treatment should always be tapered off gradually. Patients who have taken benzodiazepines for a long time may require a longer period during which doses are reduced.

Contra-indications, warnings, etc
Contra-indications: Known sensitivity to benzodiazepines. Acute pulmonary insufficiency.

Warnings: Although hangover effect is uncommon, patients should be warned against driving or operating dangerous machinery if so affected. Doses of 30 mg and above of temazepam are more likely to cause hangover effects to persist into the following day than lower doses, particularly in patients unused to hypnotics and in the elderly. As with all compounds which have an effect on the CNS, patients should be advised not to consume alcohol whilst taking temazepam.

Use in pregnancy: There is no evidence as to drug safety in human pregnancy, nor is there evidence from animal work that the drug is free from hazard. Do not use during pregnancy, especially during the first and last trimesters unless there are compelling reasons.

Adverse effects: Amnesia may occur. In cases of loss or bereavement psychological adjustment may be inhibited by benzodiazepines.

Common adverse effects of benzodiazepines include drowsiness, sedation, blurring of vision and unsteadiness and ataxia. These symptoms are liable to be potentiated by alcohol. The elderly are more liable to experience such effects. (See also under Dependence potential and withdrawal symptoms.) Abnormal psychological reactions to benzodiazepines have been reported. Rare behavioural adverse effects include paradoxical aggressive outbursts, excitement, confusion and the uncovering of depression with suicidal tendencies. Extreme caution should therefore be used in prescribing benzodiazepines in patients with personality disorders.

Other rare adverse effects, including hypotension, gastro-intestinal and visual disturbances, skin rashes, urinary retention, headache, vertigo, changes in libido, blood dyscrasias and jaundice have been reported.

Precautions: An underlying cause for insomnia should be sought before deciding upon the use of benzodiazepines for symptomatic relief.

Give with caution to patients with chronic pulmonary insufficiency, or renal or hepatic dysfunction. Avoid benzodiazepines if possible during lactation.

The concurrent use of other CNS depressants such as alcohol, general anaesthetics, narcotic analgesics, monoamine oxidase inhibitors and antidepressants should be avoided as it will result in an accentuation of their effects.

Where temazepam is used as medication before surgical or investigative procedures, patients should be accompanied home.

Dependence potential and withdrawal symptoms: In general, the dependence potential of benzodiazepines is low, but this increases when high dosage is used, especially when given over long periods. This is particularly so in patients with a history of alcoholism, drug abuse or in patients with marked personality disorders. Regular monitoring of treatment in such patients is essential, and routine repeat prescriptions should be avoided.

Treatment in all patients should be withdrawn gradually as symptoms such as depression, nervousness, rebound insomnia, irritability, sweating and diarrhoea have been reported following abrupt cessation of treatment with benzodiazepines in patients receiving even normal therapeutic doses for short periods of time.

Abrupt withdrawal following excessive dosage may produce confusion, toxic psychosis, convulsions or a condition resembling delirium tremens.

Overdosage: Doses substantially in excess of those recommended have been taken without ill effect. As with other benzodiazepines, treatment of overdosage should be symptomatic with general supportive measures as required. Although temazepam in this formulation is rapidly absorbed, gastric lavage may be useful if performed shortly after ingestion.

Pharmaceutical precautions
Dispense in glass or plastic containers.

Legal category CD (Sch 4), POM.

Package quantities
Temazepam Gelthix Capsules 10 mg: Containers of 500 and 1000 capsules.

Temazepam Gelthix Capsules 15 mg: Containers of 60 capsules.

Temazepam Gelthix Capsules 20 mg: Containers of 250 and 500 capsules.

Temazepam Gelthix Capsules 30 mg: Containers of 60 capsules.

Further information The formulation of temazepam as a gel in soft gelatin capsules ensures rapid and complete absorption which, with its short half life and lack of active metabolites, results in prompt induction of sleep and a low incidence of hangover effects.

Temazepam is a short-acting benzodiazepine. As accumulation tends not to occur, patients are less likely to experience excessive drowsiness or impairment in the performance of skilled tasks. The short half-life of this drug may offer advantages in the treatment of the elderly, in patients with impaired renal or liver function, and in situations where day-time alertness is desirable.

Product licence numbers

Temazepam Gelthix Capsules 10 mg	3433/0094
Temazepam Gelthix Capsules 15 mg	3433/0105
Temazepam Gelthix Capsules 20 mg	3433/0095
Temazepam Gelthix Capsules 30 mg	3433/0106

TEMAZEPAM ELIXIR

Presentation A clear, green, lemon-mint flavoured elixir containing 10 mg temazepam per 5 ml in a sugar-free base.

Uses Temazepam elixir is indicated for the short-term treatment of sleep disturbances considered severe or disabling or where insomnia is subjecting the individual to extreme distress. This product is especially useful in those patients for whom particularly rapid onset of hypnotic action is required and for whom the persistence of hypnotic effect after rising would be undesirable.

Temazepam elixir is indicated particularly where a liquid formulation is preferable.

Temazepam is particularly suitable for patients with transient sleep disorders in whom the re-establishment of normal sleep patterns is expected following the resolution of precipitating factors. It is also indicated for pre-medication for minor surgical and investigative procedures, especially in the case of out-patients.

Dosage and administration
Adults:

Insomnia: Each 5 ml dose of temazepam elixir is equivalent to 10 mg temazepam. The usual dose is 5–15 ml orally on retiring; a dose of 10 ml will be found to be satisfactory for most patients and is equivalent to 20 mg temazepam in capsule form. This may be increased to 20 or 30 ml (40–60 mg temazepam) in patients who do not respond to the lower dose. Lower doses may be adequate for some patients, as for the elderly.

Premedication: 10 to 20ml from half an hour to one hour prior to surgery or investigative procedures.

Elderly: Elderly patients or those suffering from cerebral vascular changes such as arteriosclerosis are likely to respond to smaller doses. Half the normal dose, 2.5 to 7.5 ml (5 to 15 mg), may be sufficient for a therapeutic response.

Children:
Insomnia: Not recommended.

Premedication: 1 mg (0.5 ml)/kg one hour prior to surgery or investigative procedures.

Treatment should if possible be intermittent.

The lowest dose which can control symptoms should be used. It should not be continued beyond 4 weeks.

Long-term chronic use is not recommended.

Treatment should always be tapered off gradually. Patients who have taken benzodiazepines for a long time may require a longer period during which doses are reduced.

Contra-indications, warnings, etc
Contra-indications: Known sensitivity to benzodiazepines. Acute pulmonary insufficiency.

Warnings: Although hangover effect is uncommon, patients should be warned against driving or operating dangerous machinery if so affected. Doses of 30 mg and above of temazepam are more likely to cause hangover effects to persist into the following day than lower doses, particularly in patients unused to hypnotics and in the elderly. As with all compounds which have an effect on the CNS, patients should be advised not to consume alcohol whilst taking temazepam.

Use in pregnancy: There is no evidence as to drug safety in human pregnancy, nor is there evidence from animal work that the drug is free from hazard. Do not use during pregnancy, especially during the first and last trimesters unless there are compelling reasons.

Adverse effects: Amnesia may occur. In cases of loss or bereavement psychological adjustment may be inhibited by benzodiazepines.

Common adverse effects of benzodiazepines include drowsiness, sedation, blurring of vision and unsteadiness and ataxia. These symptoms are liable to be potentiated by alcohol. The elderly are more liable to experience such effects. (See also under: Dependence potential and withdrawal symptoms). Abnormal psychological reactions to benzodiazepines have been reported. Rare behavioural adverse effects include paradoxical aggressive outbursts, excitement, confusion and the uncovering of depression with suicidal tendencies. Extreme caution should therefore be used in prescribing benzodiazepines in patients with personality disorders.

Other rare adverse effects, including hypotension, gastro-intestinal and visual disturbances, skin rashes, urinary retention, headache, vertigo, changes in libido, blood dyscrasias and jaundice have been reported.

Precautions: An underlying cause for insomnia should be sought before deciding upon the use of benzodiazepines for symptomatic relief.

Give with caution to patients with chronic pulmonary insufficiency, or those with renal or hepatic dysfunction. Avoid benzodiazepines if possible during lactation.

The concurrent use of other CNS depressants such as alcohol, general anaesthetics, narcotic analgesics, monoamine oxidase inhibitors and antidepressants should be avoided as it will result in an accentuation of their effects.

Where temazepam is used as medication before surgical or investigative procedures, the patients should be accompanied home.

Dependence potential and withdrawal symptoms: In general, the dependence potential of benzodiazepines is low, but this increases when high dosage is used, especially when given over long periods. This is particularly so in patients with a history of alcoholism, drug abuse or in patients with marked personality disorders. Regular monitoring of treatment in such patients is essential and routine repeat prescriptions should be avoided.

Treatment in all patients should be withdrawn gradually as symptoms such as depression, nervousness, rebound insomnia, irritability, sweating and diarrhoea have been reported following abrupt cessation of treatment with benzodiazepines in patients receiving even normal therapeutic doses for short periods of time. Abrupt withdrawal following excessive dosage may produce confusion, toxic psychosis, convulsions or a condition resembling delirium tremens.

Overdosage: Doses substantially in excess of those recommended, have been taken without ill effect. As with other benzodiazepines, treatment of overdosage should be symptomatic with general supportive measures as required. Although temazepam in this formulation is rapidly absorbed, gastric lavage may be useful if performed shortly after ingestion.

Pharmaceutical precautions Store below 25°C and protect from direct light. Temazepam elixir is sugar-free being based on a glycerol vehicle. If dilution of the elixir is required, Glycerol BP is a suitable diluent.

Legal category CD (Sch 4), POM.

Package quantities
Single dose containers of 5 ml (10 mg) and 10 ml (20 mg) in packs of 15.
Bottles of 300 ml.

Further information The formulation of temazepam as an elixir ensures rapid and complete absorption which, with its short half life and lack of active metabolites, results in prompt induction of sleep and a low incidence of hangover effects.

Temazepam is a short-acting benzodiazepine. As accumulation tends not to occur, patients are less likely to experience excessive drowsiness or impairment in the performance of skilled tasks. The short half-life of this drug may offer advantages in the treatment of the elderly, in patients with impaired renal or liver function, and in situations where day-time alertness is desirable.

Product licence number 3433/0054.

TETRALYSAL* 300

Presentation Tetralysal 300 is available as white, hard gelatin capsules marked Farmitalia Carlo Erba containing 408 mg of Lymecycline BP, equivalent to 300 mg tetracycline base.

Uses Tetralysal 300 is a broad spectrum antibiotic and is recommended for the treatment of all infections caused by tetracycline-sensitive organisms and may be utilised in all conditions where tetracycline therapy is indicated. In common with other tetracyclines, it is indicated in penicillin-sensitive patients for the treatment of staphylococcal infections.

Typical indications include: Ear, nose and throat infections; acute and chronic bronchitis (including prophylaxis); infections of the gastro-intestinal and urinary tracts; non-gonoccocal urethritis of chlamydial origin and other chlamydial infections such as trachoma; acne; rickettsial fevers; soft tissue infections.

Dosage and administration The usual recommended dose is 1 capsule b.d. If higher doses are required, 3–4 capsules may be given over 24 hours. Lower doses may be given for prophylaxis and for the chronic treatment of acne: in such cases treatment should be continued for at least 8 weeks. In the management of sexually transmitted disease both partners should be treated.

Contra-indications, warnings, etc Tetracyclines are selectively absorbed by developing bones and teeth and may cause dental staining and enamel hypoplasia. In addition, these compounds readily cross the placental barrier and therefore Tetralysal 300 should not be administered to pregnant women or to children below the age of 8 years.

As Tetralysal 300 is mainly excreted by the kidneys, it should not be administered to patients with overt renal insufficiency.

Its use is also contra-indicated in patients hypersensitive to tetracyclines.

The absorption of tetracyclines may be affected by the simultaneous administration of antacids and iron preparations.

It should also be borne in mind that the prolonged use of broad spectrum antibiotics may result in the appearance of resistant organisms and superinfection.

Bulging fontanelles in infants and benign intracranial hypertension in adults has been reported during treatment with tetracyclines. Therefore treatment should cease if evidence of raised intracranial pressure develops during treatment with Tetralysal.

Overdosage: There is no specific treatment, but gastric lavage should be performed as soon as possible. Supportive measures should be instituted as required and a high fluid intake maintained.

Pharmaceutical precautions The capsules should be stored in air-tight containers in a cool place protected from light.

Legal category POM.

Package quantities Containers of 20 and 100 capsules.

Further information Tetralysal 300 (lymecycline) is tetracycline chemically bonded to the amino-acid L-lysine. It has been estimated that 408 mg of lymecycline (containing the equivalent of 300 mg of tetracycline base) is equivalent in its action to 500 mg of tetracycline hydrochloride. Lymecycline is approximately 5000 times more soluble than tetracycline base and unlike tetracycline hydrochloride it is soluble at all physiological pH values (a 5% aqueous solution does not precipitate in the presence of serum).

Product licence number 3433/0044

ZAVEDOS* ▼

Presentation Sterile, pyrogen-free, orange-red, freeze-dried powder in vials containing 5 and 10 mg of idarubicin hydrochloride with 50 mg and 100 mg of lactose, respectively.

Uses Antimitotic and cytotoxic agent. Acute non-lymphocytic leukemia (ANLL) in adults for remission induction in untreated patients or for remission induction in relapsed or refractory patients.

Acute lymphocytic leukemia (ALL) as second line treatment in adults and children.

Zavedos may be used in combination chemotherapy regimens involving other cytotoxic agents.

Dosage and administration For reconstitution, the contents of the 5 mg vial should be dissolved in 5 ml of Water for Injections (PhEur) and the 10 mg vial in 10 ml of Water for Injections. Zavedos must be administered only by the intravenous route and the reconstituted solution should be given via the tubing of a freely running intravenous infusion of 0.9% Sodium Chloride Injection taking 5 to 10 minutes over the injection. This technique minimises the risk of thrombosis or perivenous extravasation which can lead to severe cellulitis and necrosis. Venous sclerosis may result from injection into small veins or repeated injections into the same vein.

Dosage is usually calculated on the basis of body surface area.

Acute non-lymphocytic leukemia (ANLL): In adult ANLL the dose schedule suggested is 12 mg/m^2 i.v. daily for 3 days in combination with cytarabine.

Another dose-schedule which has been used in ANLL as a single agent and in combination is 8 mg/m^2 i.v. daily for 5 days.

Acute lymphocytic leukemia (ALL): As single agent in ALL the suggested dose in adults is 12 mg/m^2 i.v. daily for 3 days and in children is 10 mg/m^2 i.v. daily for 3 days.

All of these dosage schedules should, however, take into account the haematological status of the patient and the dosages of other cytotoxic drugs when used in combination.

Contra-indications, warnings, etc
Contra-indications: Zavedos therapy should not be started in patients with severe renal and liver impairment or patients with uncontrolled infections. See also 'Use during pregnancy and lactation'.

Warnings: Zavedos is intended for use under the direction of those experienced in leukemia chemotherapy. The drug should not be given to patients with pre-existing bone marrow suppression induced by previous drug therapy or radiotherapy unless the benefit warrants the risk. Pre-existing heart disease and previous therapy with anthracyclines at high cumulative doses or other potentially cardiotoxic agents are co-factors for increased risk of idarubicin-induced cardiac toxicity and the benefit to risk ratio of Zavedos therapy in such patients should be weighed before starting treatment with Zavedos.

Like most other cytotoxic agents, idarubicin has mutagenic properties and it is carcinogenic in rats.

Bone marrow: Zavedos is a potent bone marrow suppressant. Myelosuppression, primarily of leukocytes, will therefore occur in all patients given a therapeutic dose of this agent and careful haematologic monitoring including granulocytes, red cells and platelets is required. Facilities with laboratory and supportive resources adequate to monitor drug tolerability and protect and maintain a patient compromised by drug toxicity should be available. It must be possible to treat rapidly and effectively a severe haemorrhagic condition and/or a severe infection.

Cardiac effects: Myocardial toxicity as manifested by potentially fatal congestive heart failure, acute life-threatening arrhythmias or other cardiomyopathies may occur during therapy or several weeks after termination of therapy. Treatment with digitalis, diuretics, sodium restriction and bed-rest is indicated.

Cardiac function should be carefully monitored during

treatment in order to minimise the risk of cardiac toxicity of the type described for other anthracycline compounds. The risk of such myocardial toxicity may be higher following concomitant or previous radiation to the mediastinal-pericardial area or treatment with other potentially cardiotoxic agents or in patients with a particular clinical situation due to their disease (anaemia, bone marrow depression, infections, leukemic pericarditis and/or myocarditis).

On the basis of the recommended dosage schedules the total cumulative dose administered over two courses can be expected to reach 60–80 mg/m². Although a cumulative dose limit cannot yet be defined, a specific cardiological evaluation in cancer patients showed no significant modifications of cardiac function in patients treated with Zavedos at a mean cumulative dose of 93 mg/m².

While there is no reliable method for predicting acute congestive heart failure, cardiomyopathy induced by anthracyclines is usually associated with persistent QRS voltage reduction, increase beyond normal limits of the systolic time interval (PEP/LVET) and decrease of the left ventricular ejection fraction (LVET) from pretreatment baseline values. An electrocardiogram or echocardiogram and a determination of left ventricular ejection fraction should be performed prior to starting therapy and during treatment with Zavedos. Early clinical diagnosis of drug-induced myocardial damage appears to be important for pharmacological treatment to be useful.

Evaluation of hepatic and renal function: Since hepatic and/or renal function impairment can affect the disposition of idarubicin, liver and kidney function should be evaluated with conventional clinical laboratory tests (using serum bilirubin and serum creatinine as indicators) prior to, and during, treatment. In a number of Phase III clinical trials, treatment was not given if bilirubin and/or creatinine serum levels exceeded 2 mg%. With other anthracyclines, a 50% dose reduction is generally employed if bilirubin and creatinine levels are in the range 1.2–2.0 mg%.

Precautions: Therapy with Zavedos requires close observation of the patient and laboratory monitoring. Patients aged over 55 years should be given vigorous supportive treatment during the aplastic period.

Hyperuricemia secondary to rapid lysis of leukemic cells may be induced: blood uric acid levels should be monitored and appropriate therapy initiated if hyperuricemia develops. Appropriate measures must be taken to control any systemic infection before beginning therapy.

Extravasation of Zavedos at the site of i.v. injection can cause severe local tissue necrosis. The risk of thrombophlebitis at the injection site may be minimised by following the recommended procedure for administration. A stinging or burning sensation at the site of administration signifies a small degree of extravasation and the infusion should be stopped and re-started in another vein.

Adverse reactions: Severe myelosuppression and cardiac toxicity are the two major adverse effects. Other adverse reactions include: reversible alopecia in most patients; acute nausea and vomiting; mucositis, usually involving the oral mucosa and appearing 3–10 days after starting treatment; oesophagitis and diarrhoea; fever, chills, skin rash; elevation of liver enzymes and bilirubin in about 20–30% of cases. Severe and sometimes fatal infections have been associated with Zavedos alone or in combination with cytarabine.

Zavedos may impart a red colour to the urine for 1–2 days after administration and patients should be advised that this is no cause for alarm.

Use in pregnancy and lactation: There is no information as to whether idarubicin may adversely affect human fertility, or cause teratogenesis. However, in rats (but not rabbits) it is teratogenic and embryotoxic. Women of child bearing potential should be advised to avoid pregnancy.

If Zavedos is to be used during pregnancy, or if the patient becomes pregnant during therapy, the patient should be informed of the potential hazard to the foetus. Mothers should be advised not to breast-feed while undergoing chemotherapy with this drug.

Interactions: Zavedos is a potent myelosuppressant and combination chemotherapy regimens which contain other agents having a similar action may be expected to lead to additive myelosuppressive effects.

Overdose: Very high doses of Zavedos may be expected to cause acute myocardial toxicity within 24 hours and severe myelosuppression within one or two weeks. Treatment should aim to support the patient during this period and should utilise such measures as blood transfusions and reverse-barrier nursing. Delayed cardiac failure has been seen with the anthracyclines up to several months after the overdose. Patients should be observed carefully and if signs of cardiac failure arise, should be treated along conventional lines.

Pharmaceutical precautions The vial contents are under a negative pressure to minimise aerosol formation during reconstitution: particular care should be taken when the needle is inserted. Inhalation of any aerosol produced during reconstitution must be avoided.

The following protective recommendations which are valid for all cytotoxic agents are given:

—Personnel should be trained in good technique for reconstitution and handling.
—Pregnant staff should be excluded from working with this drug.
—Personnel handling the drug should wear protective clothing: goggles, gowns and disposable gloves and masks.
—A designated area should be defined for reconstitution (preferably under a vertical laminar flow system). The work surface should be protected by disposable, plastic-backed, absorbent paper.
—All items used for reconstitution, administration or cleaning, including gloves, should be placed in high-risk, waste disposal bags for high temperature incineration.

Accidental contact with the skin or eyes should be treated immediately by copious lavage with water: medical attention should be sought.

Spillage or leakage should be treated with dilute sodium hypochlorite (1% available chlorine) solution, preferably by soaking, and then water. All cleaning materials should subsequently be disposed of as indicated previously.

The reconstituted solution is chemically stable when stored for at least 48 hours at 2°–8°C and 24 hours at room temperature; however, it is recommended that, in line with good pharmaceutical practice, the solution should not normally be stored for longer than 24 hours at 2°–8°C.

Discard any unused solution.

Prolonged contact with any solution of an alkaline pH should be avoided as it will result in degradation of the drug. Zavedos should not be mixed with heparin as a precipitate may form and it is not recommended that it be mixed with other drugs.

Legal category POM.

Package quantities 5 mg and 10 mg vials for injection.

Further information Nil.

Product licence numbers
Zavedos 5 mg 3433/0133
Zavedos 10 mg 3433/0134

**Trade Mark*

Ferring Pharmaceuticals Ltd
11 Mount Road
Feltham
Middlesex TW13 6AR

FERRING
PHARMACEUTICALS

DESMOSPRAY*

Presentation Metered-dose, pre-compression atomiser delivering 50 doses of 10 micrograms desmopressin per spray.

Uses Desmopressin is a structural analogue of the natural antidiuretic hormone vasopressin, with two chemical changes, namely desamination of the N-terminal and replacement of 8-L-arginine by 8-D-arginine. These changes have increased the antidiuretic activity and prolonged the duration of action. The pressor activity is reduced to 0.01% of the natural peptide as a result of which side-effects are rarely seen.

Desmospray is indicated in the treatment of primary nocturnal enuresis.

Desmospray is also indicated for the diagnosis and treatment of vasopressin-sensitive cranial diabetes insipidus.

Desmospray may also be used to establish the renal concentration capacity.

Dosage and administration
Primary nocturnal enuresis: Adults and children (from 5 years of age) with normal urine concentrating ability who have primary nocturnal enuresis should take one spray in each nostril (20 micrograms) before retiring. The dose may be increased up to two sprays in each nostril (40 micrograms) if the lower dose is not sufficiently effective. The need for continued treatment should be reassessed after 3 months by means of a period of at least 1 week without Desmospray.

Treatment of diabetes insipidus: Dosage is individual but clinical experience has shown that the average maintenance dose in adults and children is one or two sprays (10 to 20 micrograms) once or twice daily. If a dose of two sprays is required, this should be taken as one spray in each nostril.

Diagnosis of diabetes insipidus: The diagnostic dose in adults and children is two sprays (20 micrograms).

Failure to elaborate a concentrated urine after water deprivation, followed by the ability to do so after the administration of Desmospray confirms a diagnosis of cranial diabetes insipidus. Failure to concentrate after the administration suggests nephrogenic diabetes insipidus.

Renal function testing: Recommended doses for the renal concentration test:
Adults: Two sprays in each nostril (40 micrograms).
Children (1–15 years): One spray in each nostril (20 micrograms).
Infants (to 1 year): One spray (10 micrograms).

Adults and children with normal renal function can be expected to achieve concentrations above 700 mOsm/kg in the period of 5 to 9 hours following administration of Desmospray. It is recommended that the bladder should be emptied at the time of administration.

In normal infants a urine concentration of 600 mOsm/kg should be achieved in the 5 hour period after administration of Desmospray. The fluid intake at the two meals following the administration should be restricted to 50 per cent of the ordinary intake in order to avoid water overload.

Contra-indications, warnings, etc
Contra-indications: When used to control primary nocturnal enuresis Desmospray should only be used in patients with normal blood pressure.

Precautions: Desmospray should be given with caution to pregnant patients, although the oxytocic effect of desmopressin is very low.

Care should be taken with patients who have reduced renal function and/or cardiovascular disease or cystic fibrosis.

Following diagnostic testing for diabetes insipidus or renal concentration, care should be taken to prevent fluid overload. Fluid should not be forced, orally or parenterally, and patients should only take as much fluid as they require to satisfy thirst.

Pharmaceutical precautions Desmospray should be stored in the refrigerator at 4 to 8°C and must be protected from light.

Legal category POM.

Package quantities 5 ml bottle (50 doses of 10 micrograms desmopressin per spray).

Further information Children requiring doses of less than 10 micrograms should use DDAVP desmopressin intranasal solution which employs a small plastic calibrated catheter to administer doses of 5 to 20 micrograms.

Product licence number 3194/0024.

PENTASA* MESALAZINE ENEMA▼

Presentation Individually foil-wrapped unit dose plastic enema bottles with protective sleeve. Each bottle contains 100 ml suspension containing 1 g mesalazine.

Uses Treatment of ulcerative colitis affecting the distal colon and rectum.

Dosage and administration *Adults:* The recommended dosage is one enema at bedtime.
Children: Not recommended.

Contra-indications, warnings, etc *Contra indications:* Known sensitivity to salicylates.

Precautions and warnings: Although no renal toxicity has been reported in patients taking Mesalazine, large doses given intravenously to rats have resulted in tubular and glomerular toxicity. Therefore, Pentasa is not recommended in patients with renal impairment. Patients with raised blood urea or proteinuria should be treated with caution.

Use during pregnancy: Pentasa should be used with caution during pregnancy and lactation and only if the potential benefit outweighs the possible hazards in the opinion of the physician. No data are available on teratogenicity but negligible quantities of Mesalazine cross the placenta and none can be detected in breast milk during sulphasalazine therapy.

Use in the Elderly: Pentasa should be used with caution in the elderly and should only be used in those patients with normal renal function.

Adverse reactions: Adverse reactions including nausea, headache and abdominal pain may occur in a small proportion of patients.

Pentasa may be associated with the exacerbation of the symptoms of colitis in patients who have previously had this problem with sulphasalazine.

Treatment of overdosage: There is no specific antidote;

intravenous infusion of electrolytes may be used to promote diuresis.

Pharmaceutical precautions Store at room temperature. Protect from light. Use immediately after opening the individual foil pack.

Legal category POM.

Package quantities Cartons containing seven individually foil-wrapped 100 ml enemas.

Further information A plastic sleeve bearing administration instructions is provided for each enema bottle. The sleeve also facilitates hygienic application of the enema and disposal after use.

Product licence number 3194/0027.

PENTASA* SLOW RELEASE TABLETS

Presentation Round, white to light grey mottled tablets with a break line on one side. Each tablet contains 250 mg mesalazine in a slow release presentation.

Uses For the maintenance of remission in mild to moderate ulcerative colitis.

Dosage and administration *Adults:* the usual dose is two tablets, three times daily.
Children: Not recommended.
Elderly patients: Pentasa is not recommended in patients with renal impairment. Otherwise, the usual adult dose applies.

Contra-indications, warnings, etc *Contra indications:* Children under the age of 15 years. Known sensitivity to salicylates.

Precautions, warnings etc: Although no renal toxicity has been reported in patients taking Pentasa, large doses of mesalazine given intravenously to rats have resulted in tubular and glomerular toxicity. Therefore, Pentasa is not recommended in patients with renal impairment. Patients with raised blood urea or proteinuria should be treated with caution.

Use during pregnancy and lactation: Pentasa should be used with caution during pregnancy and lactation and only if the potential benefit outweighs the possible hazards in the opinion of the physician. No data are available on teratogenicity but negligible quantities of mesalazine cross the placenta and none can be detected in breast milk.

Adverse reactions: Headache, diarrhoea and dyspepsia may occur in a small proportion of patients. Exacerbation of the symptoms of colitis may arise in patients who have previously had this problem with sulphasalazine.

Treatment of overdose: There is no specific antidote; intravenous infusion of electrolytes may be used to promote diuresis.

Pharmaceutical precautions Store at room temperature. Protect from sunlight.

Legal category POM.

Package quantities Amber glass screw top bottles each containing 200 tablets

Further information Pentasa Slow Release Tablets disintegrate in the stomach to yield coated slow release granules which are conveyed into the intestinal tract. The release of mesalazine from the granulation takes place at all physiological pH values but is slower in the acidic conditions found in the upper gastrointestinal tract. This approach ensures that mesalazine is available in the lumen of the intestine for topical activity in ulcerative colitis. Plasma levels of mesalazine and its metabolites are similar to those observed during therapy with sulphasalazine.

Product licence number 3194/0043.

**Trade Mark*

Fisons plc
Pharmaceutical Division
12 Derby Road
Loughborough, Leics LE11 0BB

FISONS Pharmaceuticals

ASPELLIN*

Presentation A clear, almost colourless liquid with slight yellow tinge and characteristic odour.

Active ingredients:
Aspellin is manufactured using:

Menthol BP	1.4% w/v
Aspirin BP	1.2% w/v
Camphor BP	0.6% w/v
Methyl Salicylate BP	0.6% w/v

and the finished product contains:

Menthol	1.4% w/v
Camphor	0.6% w/v
Ammonium salicylate	1.0% w/v
Salicylic acid (as methyl and ethyl esters)	0.54% w/v

Inactive ingredients: Citronella Oil BPC, Glycerol BP, industrial methylated spirit, ammonia, and water.

Uses For the symptomatic relief of muscular and rheumatic pain, sciatica, lumbago, fibrositis, sprains and strains of ligaments and tendons, bruises, muscle stiffness.

Dosage and administration For external use only.

Sprinkle Aspellin on the affected part and use gentle massage until the pain is relieved. If necessary repeat once more after 10–15 minutes. Thereafter apply three times daily. When convenient use after a warm bath. When acute symptoms have subsided apply Aspellin morning and evening.

Contra-indications, warnings, etc Not to be used on children under six years of age.

Do not apply to skin abrasions, and if used on tender skin do not cover immediately after application. Do not apply to irritated skin and if an adverse reaction occurs discontinue use immediately. If symptoms persist consult your doctor.

Keep away from eyes and other sensitive areas.

Keep out of reach of children.

Use in pregnancy and lactation: There is no or inadequate evidence of safety in human pregnancy. Use in pregnancy only when there is no safer alternative. Use in lactation is acceptable.

Pharmaceutical precautions Flammable. Do not use near naked flame or hot surface.

Should not be placed on or used near polished or painted surfaces.

Aspellin spray: Do not expose to sun or excessive heat. Contents under pressure. Do not puncture or burn even when empty. Do not force open or use in confined spaces, and avoid inhaling the spray.

Keep in a tightly closed container and store in a cool place.

Legal category GSL.

Package quantities Bottles of 100 ml, 500 ml and 2 litres. Spray can of 150 ml.

Further information Nil.

Product licence numbers Liniment 0339/5000R
Spray 0339/0008R

BARQUINOL* HC

Presentation Smooth, buff cream containing:

Active ingredients:

Hydrocortisone Acetate BP	0.5% w/w
Clioquinol BP	3.0% w/w

Inactive ingredients: Glyceryl monostearate, Collone Wax SE, Wool Fat BP, Liquid Paraffin BP, Glycerol BP, Methylhydroxybenzoate BP, Purified Water BP.

Uses Exudative or secondarily infected eczema (including infantile, nummular, allergic or stasis type), dermatitis (seborrhoeic, atopic or contact), anogenital intertrigo and secondarily infected insect bite reactions.

Dosage and administration Apply directly to the affected area as a smear or spread on a dressing.

Adults and children: Apply two or three times daily for up to 7 days.

Not more than 25 g to be used daily.

Infants: Apply sparingly for short courses up to 7 days. Occlusion should not be used.

Elderly: No current evidence for alteration of the dose.

Contra-indications, warnings, etc
Contra-indications: Acne rosacea, primary skin infections (e.g. Herpes simplex and impetigo) and secondary infections which are infected with yeasts.

Precautions:

If no improvement is noted after 7 days of the normal recommended dose, then cultural investigation of the causative organisms should be undertaken to identify the specific infective agent.

Use in pregnancy: There is inadequate evidence of safety in human pregnancy. Topical administration of corticosteroids to pregnant animals can cause abnormalities of foetal development including cleft palate and intrauterine growth retardation. There may therefore be a very small risk of such effects in the human foetus and so topical corticosteroids should not be used extensively during pregnancy.

Use in lactating women: Steroids are known to be excreted in milk and therefore mothers using large doses of topical steroids should be advised not to breast-feed their infants.

Use in infants: Long-term continuous topical therapy should be avoided. Adrenal suppression can occur even without occlusion.

Side-effects: Clioquinol may occasionally cause severe irritation. Long-term use of topical corticosteroids may cause changes in the skin, particularly on the face, including striae, thinning and telangiectasia, particularly when occlusive dressings are used.

Warnings: Topical clioquinol should not be used by patients with liver disease, thyroid dysfunction or iodine sensitivity. It is best avoided by patients with neurological disorders. Clioquinol stains clothing and linen yellow and may discolour skin or fair hair.

Pharmaceutical precautions Nil.

Legal category POM.

Package quantities Tube of 15 g.

Further information Topical clioquinol treatment may interfere with tests for thyroid function. This effect may persist for several weeks after the end of treatment.

Product licence number 0113/5004R

DIMYRIL* LINCTUS
Approved name: Isoaminile cough linctus

Presentation Faintly opalescent, red liquid, each 5 ml of which contains 40 mg isoaminile citrate.

Amaranth, benzoic acid, dextrose and sucrose are included in the formulation.

Uses Cough suppressant for the treatment of cough associated with acute and chronic bronchitis, influenza, common cold, laryngitis and measles.

Dosage and administration *Oral: Adults:* 5 ml three to five times per day.

Children 6–12 years: 2.5–5 ml three to five times per day.

Children 3–6 years: 2.5 ml three to five times per day.

Children below 3 years: As recommended by the physician.

Elderly: No current evidence for alteration of the adult dose.

Contra-indications, warnings, etc *Side-effects:* Dizziness, nausea and constipation occur rarely.

Precautions: Use in pregnancy: while isoaminile citrate does not appear to be teratogenic in animals, there is inadequate evidence of the safety of Dimyril in human pregnancy and its use is not recommended.

Overdosage: Symptoms: Hallucinations and mania. Treatment: Withdrawal of drug; induction of vomiting/gastric lavage if large quantities have been taken; medical observation and supportive measures as necessary.

Warning: Do not exceed the stated dose.

Pharmaceutical precautions Nil.

Legal category POM.

Package quantities Bottle of 150 ml.

Further information Dimyril contains a single active ingredient and hence is reimbursible under the NHS if prescribed generically as Isoaminile Cough Linctus.

Product licence number 0113/5012R.

DOPACARD* ▼

Presentation A clear glass ampoule containing 5 ml of a 1% aqueous colourless solution of dopexamine hydrochloride (50 mg). The solution is adjusted to pH 2.5 and contains 0.01% Disodium Edetate BP as stabiliser.

Uses *Pharmacological action:* The primary actions of Dopacard (dopexamine hydrochoride) are the stimulation of adrenergic β_2-receptors and peripheral dopamine receptors of DA_1 and DA_2 subtypes. In addition, Dopacard is an inhibitor of neuronal re-uptake of noradrenaline (Uptake 1). These pharmacological actions result in an increase in cardiac output mediated by afterload reduction (β_2, DA_1) and positive inotropism (β_2, Uptake 1 inhibition) together with an increase in blood flow to vascular beds (DA_1) such as the renal and mesenteric beds. Dopacard is not an α-adrenergic agonist and does not cause vasoconstriction.

Indications: Dopacard is indicated for short term intravenous administration to patients who require peripheral vasodilator (afterload reduction), renal vasodilator and mild positive inotropic therapy in the treatment of heart failure associated with cardiac surgery.

Dosage and administration Dopacard must be diluted before use.

Preparation: The contents of four ampoules should be injected aseptically into one of the following

0.9% Sodium Chloride Injection	500 or 250 ml
5% Dextrose Injection	500 or 250 ml

These dilutions given a concentration for administration as follows:

4 ampoules of Dopacard in 500 ml = 400 micrograms (µg)/ml

4 ampoules of Dopacard in 250 ml = 800 micrograms (µg)/ml

Administration: Dopacard should only be administered intravenously by infusion through a cannula or catheter in a central or large peripheral vein. Contact with metal parts in infusion apparatus should be minimised. A device which provides accurate control of the rate of flow is essential.

Recommended dosage for adults including the elderly: Infusion should begin at a dose of 0.5 micrograms/kg/min and may be increased to 1 microgram/kg/min and then in increments (1 microgram/kg/min) up to 6 micrograms/kg/min at 10–15 minute intervals.

The rate of administration and duration of therapy should be adjusted according to the patient's response as determined by heart rate, blood pressure, urine output and, if possible, measurement of cardiac output.

Where invasive haemodynamic monitoring is available, titration of dose and the selection of an optimal dose of Dopacard is readily determined. When however, cardiac output measurements are not available, it is recommended that a starting dose of 0.5 microgram/kg/min is administered. This may be increased, if necessary, within the limits of the dosage recommendation and acceptable effects on heart rate. The benefit of the infusion to the patient should be assessed by reference to urine flow and clinical evaluation of peripheral perfusion. Although Dopacard is not a vasoconstrictor agent, small increases in blood pressure may occur in hypotensive patients due to an increase in cardiac output. The absence of an effect on blood pressure does not exclude a marked improvement in cardiac output and peripheral perfusion.

It is recommended that the infusion of Dopacard is reduced gradually rather than withdrawn abruptly.

Contra-indications, warnings, etc

Contra-indications: Patients who are receiving monoamine oxidase inhibitors (MAOI's).

Patients with left ventricular outlet obstruction such as hypertrophic obstructive cardiomyopathy or aortic stenosis.

Phaeochromocytoma

Thrombocytopenia

Precautions: If any correction of hypovolaemia is required, this should be achieved before the administration of Dopacard.

Warnings: Dopacard should be administered with caution to patients with acute myocardial infarction or recent episodes of angina pectoris since any significant increases in heart rate may increase myocardial oxygen demand and may intensify ischaemia.

As has been observed with some other β-adrenergic agonists, a fall in circulation platelet numbers has been observed in some patients. No adverse experiences attributable to alterations in platelets in platelet count have been seen in clinical studies.

Care should be used when administering Dopacard in the presence of hypokalaemia or hyperglycaemia. In common with other β_2-agonists, Dopacard depresses plasma potassium and raises blood glucose. These effects are mild and reversible. The monitoring of potassium and glucose is advisable in patients likely to be at risk from such changes e.g. diabetics, patients with myocardial infarction or patients being treated with diuretics or cardiac glycosides.

There is no evidence to suggest that Dopacard has significant arrhythmogenic potential. However, if a cardiac arrhythmia occurs during administration, a reduction or temporary discontinuation of the infusion should be considered.

In patients with a marked reduction in systemic vascular resistance, Dopacard should not be used as a direct substitute for pressor agents or other inotropes.

The safety and efficacy of Dopacard for use in children has not been established.

Use in pregnant and lactating women: There is no experience of the use of Dopacard in pregnant or lactating women and therefore its safety in these situations has not been established. There is insufficient evidence from animal studies to indicate it is free from hazard. Therefore Dopacard is not currently recommended for use in pregnant and lactating women.

Side-effects: Increases in heart rate may occur during infusion of Dopacard; in most cases these are not clinically significant. Occasionally excessive tachycardia or ventricular ectopic beats have been noted during the infusion. Tachycardia may be more pronounced in patients with pre-existing atrial fibrillation. In these situations, the infusion should be reduced or temporarily discontinued.

The following side-effects have been reported infrequently, in most cases at high dosage, nausea, vomiting, anginal pain, and tremor.

Interactions: As Dopacard inhibits Uptake 1, it may potentiate the effects of exogenous noradrenaline or dopamine. Caution is recommended when these agents are administered concomitantly with Dopacard or soon after discontinuation of its use.

Concomitant use with β_2-adrenergic and dopamine receptor antagonists requires caution since attenuation of the pharmacological effects of Dopacard may occur.

Overdosage: The half-life of Dopacard in blood is short (approximately 6–7 mins). Consequently, the effects of overdosage are likely to be short-lived provided that administration is discontinued.

Effects of overdosage are likely to be related to the pharmacological actions and include tachycardia, tremulousness and tremor, nausea and vomiting, and anginal pain. Treatment should be supportive and directed to these symptoms.

Pharmaceutical precautions Store below 25°C, protect from light.

Dopacard, in common with other catecholamines, may turn slightly pink in prepared solutions during the recommended storage period (up to 24 hours at room temperature). There is no significant loss of potency associated with this change.

Ampoules should be discarded if contents are discoloured.

Dopacard should only be diluted with 0.9% Sodium Chloride Injection or 5% Dextrose Injection and should not be added to 5% Sodium Bicarbonate or any other strongly alkaline solutions as inactivation will occur.

Prepared intravenous solutions in 0.9% Sodium Chloride Injection or 5% Dextrose Solution are stable for 24 hours at room temperature.

Dopacard should not be mixed with any other active agents before administration.

Contact with metal parts, in infusion apparatus for example, should be minimised.

Legal category POM.

Package quantities Box of 10 clear glass ampoules each containing 5 ml of 1% solution of dopexamine hydrochloride (50 mg per ampoule).

Further information The main haemodynamic effects of Dopacard consist of an increase in cardiac output associated with a large reduction in systemic vascular resistance and a smaller decrease of left ventricular filling pressure. Heart rate effects are variable but there is a general tendency for a small increase particularly at high doses. There is little effect on arterial blood pressure.

Dopacard is rapidly eliminated from blood with a half-life of approximately 6–7 minutes. Subsequent elimination of the metabolites is by urinary and biliary excretion. The response to Dopacard is rapid in onset and effects subside rapidly on discontinuation of the infusion. Increases in dose may be made at intervals of not less than 10–15 minutes.

Experience in clinical trials has shown that Dopacard can increase cardiac output by over 100% within the recommended dose range and increases of the order of 50% are frequently achieved at doses of 1–2 micrograms/kg/min without a clinically significant effect on heart rate.

Product licence number 0113/0126.

FRUSENE*

Presentation Pale yellowish, scored tablets 9 mm diameter. Each tablet containing 40 mg frusemide and 50 mg triamterene.

Lactose is included in the formulation.

Uses
Indications: Cardiac or hepatic oedema.

Properties: Frusene contains frusemide and triamterene, thus minimising the possible hypokalaemia produced by frusemide and the hyperkalaemia produced by triamterene. It has been demonstrated that when Frusene is used no decrease in serum potassium level is observed whilst the diuretic response is similar to an equivalent dose of frusemide.

Frusene does not raise the creatinine level in patients with normal renal function. If the patient has an elevated creatinine level at initiation of therapy the use of Frusene may further raise it.

The fact that Frusene prevents hypokalaemia is of importance when treating out-patients with severe cardiac insufficiency or other patients needing potent diuretic therapy. In geriatric patients who are especially sensitive to the development of hypokalaemia the use of Frusene should be considered even when diuretics are only needed every other day. In hypertensive patients the use of Frusene may be more advisable than frusemide alone.

Potassium replacement during Frusene treatment should only be considered in special cases and is not normally required.

Dosage and administration The dosage will depend on individual requirements.

The usual adult dose is ½–2 tablets daily, taken in the morning. Maximum daily dosage: 6 tablets.

Contra-indications, warnings, etc
Contra-indications: Frusene is contra-indicated in severe renal or hepatic failure or if the serum potassium level is elevated.

Precautions: Frusene should be used with caution during the first trimester of pregnancy.

In patients with mild renal failure serum creatinine and electrolytes should be monitored regularly.

Side effects: Frusene is a combination of frusemide and triamterene and side effects due to either component are possible. Reported side effects are as follows:

Triamterene: nausea, diarrhoea, fatigue, headache, dry mouth or rash have been reported. If renal function is impaired triamterene has been reported to cause elevation of BUN and the uric acid level. Some leukopaenia cases have been reported due to triamterene.

Frusemide: Frusemide is generally well tolerated. Side effects of a minor nature such as nausea, malaise or gastric upset may occur but are not usually severe enough to cause withdrawal of treatment. The incidence of allergic reactions such as skin rashes is very low but when these occur treatment should be withdrawn. In common with other sulphonamide-based diuretics hyperuricaemia may occur and in rare cases, clinical gout may be precipitated. Bone marrow depression has been reported as a rare complication and necessitates withdrawal of treatment.

Drug interactions: Hyperkalaemia may occur if Frusene is used in combination with other drugs which raise serum potassium levels, including ACE-inhibitors, potassium sparing diuretics or potassium supplements.

Pharmaceutical precautions Frusene should be stored in a dry place protected from light.

Legal category POM.

Package quantities Frusene is available in calendar packs, each containing 56 tablets. Packs of 100 tablets and hospital packs of 1,000 tablets are also available.

Further information Nil.

Product licence number 0339/0018.

GENISOL*

Presentation A clear, golden-yellow liquid containing sodium sulphosuccinated undecylenic monoalkylolamide 1% w/v, purified coar-tar fractions 0.25% w/v designed to be therapeutically equivalent to 2% Prepared Coal Tar BP and comprising:

Phenol	8% w/w	o-Cresol	8% w/w
Quinoline	4% w/w	Pyridine	2% w/w
α-Picoline	2% w/w	Toluene	16% w/w
Xylene	8% w/w	Phenanthrene	32% w/w
Carbazole	20% w/w		

Inactive ingredients: Isopropyl alcohol, detergent, Anhydrous Citric Acid BP, Sunset Yellow FCF, perfume.

Uses Seborrhoeic dermatitis of the scalp (dandruff) and psoriasis of the scalp.

Dosage and administration *Adults and children:* To be used once per week or more frequently if required, in the manner of a shampoo. Stir about 10 ml of Genisol into half a tumblerful of warm water. Wet the hair thoroughly, apply half the solution and work into the scalp with the fingers. Rinse and repeat the application. Finally, rinse the hair thoroughly in clean water.

Elderly: No current evidence for alteration of the dose.

Contra-indications, warnings, etc When washing the hair, care should be taken to keep the solution away from the eyes.

Use during pregnancy or lactation: There is inadequate evidence of safety in pregnant or lactating women but Genisol has been in use for many years without apparent ill-consequence.

Overdosage: There is no evidence that overuse of topical Genisol would be harmful other than possibly inducing a hypersensitivity to coal tar. Ingestion of Genisol may require gastric lavage depending on the quantity taken and should be treated symptomatically.

Pharmaceutical precautions Nil.

Legal category P.

Package quantities Bottles of 58 ml, 250 ml and 600 ml.

Further information Nil.

Product licence number 0113/5020R.

IMFERON*

Presentation Imferon is dark brown, slightly viscous, sterile liquid complex of ferric hydroxide and low molecular weight dextran in a 0.9% sodium chloride solution for injection. It contains the equivalent of 50 mg elemental iron (as iron dextran) per ml.

Uses Imferon is indicated for the parenteral treatment of proven severe iron deficiency anaemia. Imferon is administered by intramuscular injection for patients who cannot tolerate, do not respond to oral iron, or cannot be relied upon to take oral iron, e.g. because of gastro-intestinal intolerance or resistant malabsorption conditions. It may also be given by intravenous injection or total dose infusion: such use must be confined to the hospital treatment of patients for whom the intramuscular route or other forms of therapy such as blood transfusion are inappropriate or are not available.

Dosage and administration *Dosage: Adults:* The dose of Imferon is determined by the haemoglobin level, bodyweight and sex of the patient. The following table provides a convenient means of determining the dose. This dose is intended to provide sufficient iron to restore haemoglobin levels to a normal level (14.8 g/dl) and to replenish depleted iron stores. The table takes account of the higher iron stores in men. In pregnancy, a further 10 ml should be added to the dose.

Alternatively the total dose required may be calculated. If the patient's bodyweight in kilograms is W and the haemoglobin level is H g/dl.

Dose of Imferon in ml required for women = $[0.0476 \times W \times (14.8 - H)] + 6$

Dose of Imferon in ml required for men = $[0.0476 \times W \times (14.8 - H)] + 14.0$

The dose may also be calculated if the bodyweight in kilograms (W) and the percentage haemoglobin deficit (D) are known.

Dose of Imferon in ml required for women = $0.00705 \times W \times D + 6$

Dose of Imferon in ml required for men = $0.00705 \times W \times D + 14$.

Children up to 15 years: A separate entry is provided in the dosage table for children up to 15 years of age which takes account of lower iron stores. Imferon should not normally be given in the first four months of life. Alternatively the total dose may be calculated. If the child's bodyweight in kilograms is W and the haemoglobin level is H g/dl:

Dose of Imferon required in ml = $0.0476 \times W \times (14.8 - H)$.

The dose may also be calculated if the bodyweight in kilograms (W) and the percentage haemoglobin deficit (D) are known.

Dose of Imferon in ml required = $0.00705 \times W \times D$.

Administration: Imferon may be given intramuscularly or intravenously. The intramuscular route is to be used unless there are valid reasons for intravenous administration. The intravenous administration of Imferon by the Total Dose Infusion method should be restricted to hospital usage only.

Intramuscular administration: The total amount of Imferon required is determined either from the dosage table or by calculation. It is administered as a series of injections: the volume of each is ordinarily determined by the patient's bodyweight. Infants below 10 lb (5 kg) should receive 0.5 ml; children below 20 lb (9 kg) 1.0 ml; adults normally 2.0 ml up to a maximum of 5.0 ml. If the patient is moderately active, injections may be given daily into alternate buttocks. In inactive or bed-ridden patients, the frequency of injections should be reduced to once or twice weekly.

Imferon must be given by deep intramuscular injection to minimise the risk of subcutaneous staining. It should be injected only into the muscle mass of the upper outer quadrant of the buttock – never into the arm or other exposed areas. A 20–21 gauge needle at least 50 mm long should be used for normal adults. For obese patients the length should be 80–100 mm, while for children and small adults a shorter and smaller needle (23 gauge × 32 mm) is used. The patient should be lying in the lateral position with the injection site uppermost, or standing bearing their weight on the leg opposite the injection site. To avoid injection or leakage into the subcutaneous tissue, a Z-track technique (displacement of the skin laterally prior to injection) is recommended. Imferon is injected slowly and smoothly. It is important to wait for a few seconds before withdrawing the needle to allow the muscle mass to accommodate the injection volume. To minimise leakage up the injection track the patient shoud be encouraged not to rub the injection site.

Intravenous administration: Imferon may be administered in large volumes intravenously, either diluted as in the Total Dose Infusion technique or undiluted, for the hospital treatment of patients for whom the intramuscular route or other forms of therapy are inappropriate or are not available.

Whenever Imferon is given intravenously, it is *essential* that one of the test-dose procedures described below is followed in full. Anaphylactoid reactions to Imferon are usually evident within a few minutes, and close observation is necessary to ensure early recognition. *If at any time during the intravenous administration of Imferon, any signs of a hypersensitivity reaction or intolerance are detected, administration must be stopped immediately.* Resuscitative equipment should be available, and anaphylactoid reactions should be treated with 0.5 ml of aqueous adrenaline 1:1000 given subcutaneously with general supportive measures. This should be followed by

Total dose of Imferon in millilitres

Bodyweight		*Observed haemoglobin levels*								
kg	*lb*	*3.0 g/dl 20%*			*4.4 g/dl 30%*			*5.9 g/dl 40%*		
		Man	*Woman*	*Child*	*Man*	*Woman*	*Child*	*Man*	*Woman*	*Child*
5	11	—	—	3	—	—	2	—	—	2
10	22	—	—	6	—	—	5	—	—	4
15	33	—	—	8	—	—	7	—	—	6
20	44	—	—	11	—	—	10	—	—	8
25	55	—	—	14	—	—	12	—	—	11
30	66	31	23	17	29	21	15	27	19	13
35	77	34	26	20	31	23	17	29	21	15
40	88	37	29	23	34	26	20	31	23	17
45	99	39	31	25	36	28	22	33	25	19
50	110	42	34	28	39	31	25	35	27	21
55	121	45	37	31	41	33	27	37	29	23
60	132	48	40	34	44	36	30	39	31	25
65	143	51	43	—	46	38	—	41	33	—
70	154	53	45	—	49	41	—	44	36	—
75	165	56	48	—	51	43	—	46	38	—
80	176	59	51	—	53	45	—	48	40	—
85	187	62	54	—	56	48	—	50	42	—
90	198	65	57	—	58	50	—	52	44	—
95	209	68	60	—	61	53	—	54	46	—
100	220	70	62	—	63	55	—	56	48	—
105	231	73	65	—	66	58	—	58	50	—
110	242	76	68	—	68	60	—	61	53	—
115	253	79	71	—	71	63	—	63	55	—
120	264	82	74	—	73	65	—	65	57	—
		7.4 g/dl 50%			*8.9 g/dl 60%*			*10.4 g/dl 70%*		
		Man	*Woman*	*Child*	*Man*	*Woman*	*Child*	*Man*	*Woman*	*Child*
5	11	—	—	2	—	—	1	—	—	1
10	22	—	—	4	—	—	3	—	—	2
15	33	—	—	5	—	—	4	—	—	3
20	44	—	—	7	—	—	6	—	—	4
25	55	—	—	9	—	—	7	—	—	5
30	66	25	17	11	22	14	8	20	12	6
35	77	26	18	12	24	16	10	21	13	7
40	88	28	20	14	25	17	11	22	14	8
45	99	30	22	16	27	19	13	24	16	10
50	110	31	23	17	28	20	14	25	17	11
55	121	33	25	19	30	22	16	26	18	12
60	132	35	27	21	31	23	17	27	19	13
65	143	37	29	—	32	24	—	28	20	—
70	154	39	31	—	34	26	—	29	21	—
75	165	40	32	—	35	27	—	30	22	—
80	176	42	34	—	37	29	—	31	23	—
85	187	44	36	—	38	30	—	32	24	—
90	198	46	38	—	39	31	—	33	25	—
95	209	47	39	—	41	33	—	34	26	—
100	220	49	41	—	42	34	—	35	27	—
105	231	51	43	—	44	36	—	36	28	—
110	242	53	45	—	45	37	—	37	29	—
115	253	55	47	—	46	38	—	38	30	—
120	264	56	48	—	47	39	—	39	31	—

either oral or parenteral antihistamines and/or corticosteroids.

The intravenous route should not be used for patients with a history of asthma. If it is judged necessary to use the intravenous route for patients with a history of allergy, effective antihistamine cover should be given before administration of Imferon.

1. *Total Dose Infusion (TDI) Technique:* The total amount of Imferon required, determined from the dosage table or by calculation, is added aseptically immediately before administration to the required volume, usually 500 ml, of sterile normal saline or 5% dextrose solution. *The initial rate of infusion must not exceed 5 drops per minute for 10 minutes* and the patient must be kept under close medical supervision during this period. If the test dose is well tolerated, the rate of infusion may be increased *progressively* to 45–60 drops per minute. Patients should be observed carefully during the infusion and for at least one hour after it is completed.

2. *Undiluted Imferon Administration:* The total amount of Imferon is determined from the dosage table or by calculation: it may be given as a single dose or divided and given as a series of two or more intravenous injections. Before receiving the therapeutic dose of Imferon, *all patients must be given a slowly-administered test dose of 0.5 ml Imferon* diluted with 4–5 ml or more of the patient's own blood. The patient should then be observed carefully for at least 30 minutes and the therapeutic dose given only if the test dose is well tolerated. The therapeutic dose should be given as a

slow intravenous injection: *the rate must not exceed 1 ml per minute* and the patient must be under strict medical supervision throughout the injection. Careful observation should continue for at least one hour thereafter.

Contra-indications, warnings, etc
Contra-indications: Imferon is contra-indicated in patients who have shown hypersensitivity to iron dextran. It should not be used during the acute phase of infectious kidney disease. It should not be given intravenously to patients with a history of asthma.

It should not be used during the first trimester of pregnancy.

Warnings: The use of Imferon, as with the parenteral use of other iron-carbohydrate complexes, carries a risk of immediate and potentially severe anaphylactoid reactions. Patients should be closely observed during and immediately after administration. Resuscitative equipment, adrenaline, antihistamines and corticosteroids should be available for immediate treatment of reactions.

Imferon should be used with extreme care in patients with serious impairment of liver function. Caution should be used when Imferon is given to patients suffering from an acute infection, or with a history of allergy or chronic infection. The intramuscular route should be used, and a graded series of injections is strongly recommended, starting with 0.5 ml, 1.0 ml, then 2.0 ml. Should it be judged necessary to use the intravenous route for patients with a history of allergy, effective antihistamine cover should be given before administration of Imferon.

An increased incidence of sepsis, primarily due to *E.coli,* has been reported when Imferon is given to neonates in Polynesian populations. The association with Imferon remains unclear. Iron supplementation is rarely necessary in the first four months of life and Imferon should not normally be given during this period.

A high incidence of post-infusion arthralgia has been reported in patients with rheumatoid arthritis treated by the intravenous route. This route should be used *only* when all other methods of treatment have been shown to be unsuccessful in these patients.

The intramuscular and subcutaneous injection of iron-carbohydrate complexes in very large doses under experimental conditions in animals produced sarcoma in rats, mice, rabbits, possibly hamsters but not in guinea-pigs. Cumulative information and independent assessment indicate that the risk of sarcoma formation in man is minimal.

Overdosage: Overdosage with Imferon is unlikely and is not known to be associated with any acute manifestations. Excessive doses beyond the requirements for haemoglobin restoration and replenishment of iron stores may lead to haemosiderosis. Such iron overload is more likely to occur in patients with haemoglobinopathies and other refractory anaemias which might erroneously be diagnosed as iron deficiency anaemia. Periodic monitoring of serum ferritin levels should be helpful in recognising a deleterious progressive accumulation of iron.

Adverse effects: Anaphylactoid reactions occur rarely with both intravenous and intramuscular administration. They may be severe, and fatalities have been reported. They occur usually within the first few minutes of administration, and are generally characterised by the sudden onset of respiratory difficulty and/or cardiovascular collapse. Other manifestations of immediate hypersensitivity include urticaria, rashes, itching, nausea and shivering. Administration must be stopped *immediately* when signs of an anaphylactoid reaction are seen.

Delayed reactions are well described and may be severe. These reactions, of unknown aetiology, are seen more frequently when large doses are given intravenously. They are characterised by arthralgia, myalgia and sometimes fever. The onset varies from several hours up to four days after administration. Symptoms usually last two to four days and settle spontaneously or following the use of simple analgesics.

Other reactions reported include: soreness and inflammation at or near injection site, sterile abscess (IM); brown skin discoloration (IM); local phlebitic reaction (IV); peripheral vascular flushing and hypotension (IV); lymphadenopathy; exacerbation of joint pain in rheumatoid arthritis.

Use in pregnancy: Imferon has been shown to be teratogenic and embryocidal in non-anaemic pregnant animals at high single doses above 2.5 ml/kg. The highest dose in clinical use is approximately 1 ml/kg. Iron deficiency anaemia occurring in the first trimester of pregnancy can normally be adequately treated with oral iron. If the benefit of Imferon treatment is judged to outweigh the potential risk to the foetus, it is recommended that treatment should be confined to the second and third trimester.

There is no information available on the excretion of iron dextran in human breast milk.

Pharmaceutical precautions Protect from heat: do not freeze. Intravenous infusions containing Imferon should be prepared immediately before use. Solutions of Imferon in 5% dextrose must not be autoclaved, because precipitation may occur. Other agents should not be added to Imferon infusions, nor is it recommended that Imferon is added to blood for transfusion.

Imferon has a particle size of 2–3 nm and will pass through the usual particulate filters. It does not cross the membranes commonly used in haemodialysis.

Legal category POM.

Package quantities
Ampoules of 2 ml (100 mg Fe) in boxes of 10 and 100.

Ampoules of 5 ml (250 mg Fe) in boxes of 5 and 50.

Ampoules of 20 ml for Total Dose Infusion (hospital use only) in boxes of 5.

Further information After intramuscular injection, iron dextran is taken up into the capillaries and the lymphatic system. Circulating iron dextran is gradually removed from the plasma by the reticuloendothelial cells, primarily of the liver and spleen. The complex is split into its components of iron and dextran, and the iron is immediately bound to the available protein moieties to form haemosiderin or ferritin and to a lesser extent transferrin. This iron, which is subject to physiological control, replenishes haemoglobin and depleted iron stores.

Laboratory Investigations: Evidence of a therapeutic response can be seen within a few days of administration of Imferon as an increase in the reticulocyte count. Serum ferritin levels usually provide a good guide to the replenishment of iron stores. In renal dialysis patients receiving Imferon, this correlation may not be valid.

Caution should be used in interpreting the results of serum iron determinations for up to 3 weeks after the administration of large doses of Imferon intravenously. Brown discoloration of serum has been reported after intravenous doses of 5 ml or more. Bone scans with radiolabelled technetium diphosphonate (^{99M}Tc) have been reported to show a dense crescentic area of activity in the buttocks visualised 1–6 days after intramuscular injection of Imferon.

Product licence number 0113/5073.

INTAL*

Presentation Intal is a presentation for inhalation of Sodium Cromoglycate BP 20 mg in micronised powder form. It is presented in a yellow/colourless, transparent, hard gelatin cartridge, bearing the overprint 'FISONS INTAL P'.

Uses Intal is indicated for the preventive treatment of bronchial asthma which may be due to allergy, exercise, cold air or chemical and occupational irritants. Sodium cromoglycate inhibits the release from sensitised mast cells of mediators of the allergic reaction. In the lung this inhibition of mediator release prevents both the immediate and late asthmatic response to immunological stimuli. Sodium cromoglycate also prevents the bronchoconstriction caused by exercise, cold air and chemical irritants.

Dosage and administration Intal is presented in a single dose cartridge, the 'Spincap', for use in the 'Spinhaler'. Inhalation of the drug is controlled by the patient's inspiratory effort. Intal is not effective if the 'Spincap' is swallowed because the prevention of the asthmatic attack depends upon local application to the lung.

Dosage: Since Intal therapy is essentially preventive, it is important that the patient is instructed to maintain regular dosage, as distinct from inhaling the drug intermittently to relieve symptoms.

Adults and children: The normal dose is one 'Spincap' four times daily, i.e. one night and morning and at intervals of 3–6 hours in between. It may be necessary to increase this to 6–8 times daily in more severe cases or during periods of severe antigen challenge. Additional doses may be taken before exertion to prevent exercise induced asthma or before exposure to other trigger factors.

When the asthmatic condition is stabilised, it may be possible to reduce the dosage provided that adequate control of the asthma is maintained.

Elderly: No current evidence for alteration of the adult dose.

Concomitant steroid therapy: In patients currently treated with steroids, the addition of Intal to the regime may make it possible to reduce the maintenance dose or to discontinue steroids completely. The patient must be carefully supervised while steroid dose is reduced; a rate of reduction of 10% weekly is suggested. An increase in steroid dosage may be necessary if symptoms increase and at times of infection, severe antigen challenge or stress. If reduction in steroid dosage has been possible Intal should not be withdrawn until steroid cover has been re-instituted.

Concomitant bronchodilator therapy: If bronchodilators are used concomitantly patients may find that the frequency of bronchodilator usage can be reduced as their asthma is stabilised with Intal.

Contra-indications, warnings, etc
Contra-indications: There are no specific contra-indications.

Side-effects: Mild throat irritation, coughing and transient bronchospasm may occur. This may be overcome by changing to Intal Compound. Very rarely severe bronchospasm associated with a marked fall in pulmonary function has been reported. In such cases treatment should be stopped and should not be reintroduced.

Overdosage: No action other than medical observation should be necessary.

Withdrawal of Intal therapy: Since Intal acts prophylactically, it is important to continue treatment in those patients who benefit. If it is necessary to withdraw Intal, this should be done progressively over a period of one week. Symptoms of asthma may recur.

Use in pregnancy: As with all medications, particular caution must be exercised during the first trimester of pregnancy.

Pharmaceutical precautions Store in a cool, dry place protected from light.

Intal Spincaps can be adversely affected by moisture ingress. To prevent possible deterioration of the product, it is essential that the Spincaps are always kept in their original container.

It is acceptable for upto four of the Spincaps to be stored in the Spinhaler Carrying Case for upto 24 hours.

Legal category POM.

Package quantities Original packs containing 112 Spincaps. 'Spinhaler' Insufflators are supplied in individual containers. Instructions for use are supplied with each pack.

Further information Nil.

Product licence number 0113/5022R.

INTAL* AUTOHALER

Presentation A breath-actuated pressurised aerosol delivering 112 inhalations each containing a total of 5 mg Sodium Cromoglycate BP.

Inactive ingredients: Dichlorotetrafluoroethane BP, Dichlorodifluoromethane BP, sorbitan trioleate.

Uses Intal Autohaler is indicated for the treatment of bronchial asthma, including the prevention of exercise-induced asthma.

Dosage and administration Since Intal Autohaler therapy is essentially preventative it is important that the patient is instructed to maintain regular dosage, as distinct from inhaling the drug intermittently to relieve symptoms.

Adults and children: Initial dose is two inhalations of the aerosol four times daily. Once adequate control of symptoms has been achieved it may be possible to reduce to a maintenance dose of one inhalation four times daily. However, the dose may be increased to two inhalations six or eight times daily in more severe cases or during periods of severe antigen challenge. Additional doses before exercise may also be taken.

Elderly patients: No current evidence for alteration of the recommended adult dosage.

Concomitant bronchodilator therapy: Where a concomitant aerosol bronchodilator is prescribed, it is recommended that this be administered prior to the Intal Autohaler.

Concomitant steroid therapy: In patients currently treated with steroids the addition of Intal Autohaler to the regimen may make it possible to reduce the maintenance dose or to discontinue steroids completely. The patient must be carefully supervised while the steroid dose is reduced; a rate of reduction of 10% weekly is suggested. If reduction of a steroid dosage has been possible Intal Autohaler should not be withdrawn until steroid cover has been re-instituted.

Contra-indications, warnings, etc
Contra-indications: There are no specific contra-indications.

Side-effects: Mild throat irritation, coughing and transient bronchospasm may occur. Very rarely severe bronchospasm associated with a marked fall in pulmonary function has been reported. In such cases treatment should be stopped and should not be reintroduced.

Overdosage: No action other than medical observation should be necessary.

Withdrawal of Intal Autohaler therapy: Since the therapy is essentially prophylactic it is important to continue therapy in those patients who benefit. If it is necesary to withdraw this treatment it should be done progressively over a period of one week. Symptoms of asthma may recur.

Use in pregnancy: As with all medication particular caution must be exercised during the first trimester of pregnancy.

Pharmaceutical precautions Store the inhaler in a cool place. The aerosol inhaler canister is pressurised. The canister should be protected from direct sunlight and must not be punctured or burnt, even when empty.

Legal category POM.

Package quantities Each pack contains a canister delivering 112 metered inhalations of sodium cromoglycate in an Autohaler device. Instructions for use are supplied with each pack.

Further information Nil.

Product licence number 0113/0138.

INTAL* COMPOUND

Presentation Intal Compound is a presentation for inhalation of Sodium Cromoglycate BP 20 mg (micronised) and Isoprenaline Sulphate BP 100 micrograms in powder form. It is presented in an orange/colourless, transparent, hard gelatin cartridge bearing the overprint 'FISONS INTAL PC'.

Uses Intal Compound is indicated for the preventive treatment of bronchial asthma which may be due to allergy, exercise, cold air or chemical and occupational irritants. Sodium cromoglycate inhibits the release from sensitised mast cells of mediators of the allergic reaction. In the lung this inhibition of mediator release prevents both the immediate and late asthmatic response to immunological stimuli. Sodium cromoglycate also prevents the bronchoconstriction caused by exercise, cold air and chemical irritants. Isoprenaline sulphate is included to offset the transient bronchospasm which occurs in some patients on inhalation of a fine dry powder.

Dosage and administration Intal Compound is presented in a single dose cartridge, the 'Spincap', for use in the 'Spinhaler'. Inhalation of the drug is controlled by the patient's inspiratory effort. Intal Compound is not effective if the 'Spincap' is swallowed because prevention of the asthmatic attack depends upon local application to the lung.

Dosage: Since Intal Compound therapy is essentially preventive, it is important that the patient is instructed to maintain regular dosage, as distinct from inhaling the drug intermittently to relieve symptoms.

Adults and children: The normal dose is one 'Spincap' four times daily, i.e. one night and morning and at intervals of 3–6 hours in between. It may be necessary to increase this to 6–8 times daily in more severe cases or during periods of severe antigen challenge. Additional doses may be taken before exertion to prevent exercise induced asthma or before exposure to other trigger factors.

When the asthmatic condition is stabilised, it may be possible to reduce the dosage provided that adequate control of the asthma is maintained.

Elderly: No current evidence for alteration of the adult dose.

Concomitant steroid therapy: In patients currently treated with steroids, the addition of Intal Compound to the regime may make it possible to reduce the maintenance dose or discontinue steroids completely. The patient must be carefully supervised while the steroid dose is reduced: a rate of reduction of 10% weekly is suggested. An increase in steroid dosage may be necessary if symptoms increase and at times of infection, severe antigen challenge or stress.

If reduction of steroid dosage has been possible Intal Compound should not be withdrawn until steroid cover has been re-instituted.

Concomitant bronchodilator therapy: If additional bronchodilators are used concomitantly, patients may find that the frequency of bronchodilator usage can be reduced as their asthma is stabilised with Intal Compound.

Contra-indications, warnings, etc
Contra-indications: There are no specific contra-indications.

Side-effects: Mild throat irritation, coughing and transient bronchospasm may occur. Very rarely severe bronchospasm associated with a marked fall in pulmonary function has been reported. In such cases treatment should be stopped and should not be reintroduced.

Precautions: The precautions normally applying to isoprenaline should be observed. Where concomitant bronchodilator therapy is prescribed, the possibility of isoprenaline overdosage should be remembered.

Overdosage: No action other than medical observation should be necessary.

Withdrawal of Intal Compound therapy: Since Intal Compound acts prophylactically, it is important to continue treatment in those patients who benefit. If it is necessary to withdraw Intal Compound, this should be done progressively over a period of one week. Symptoms of asthma may recur.

Use in pregnancy: As with all medications, particular caution must be exercised during the first trimester of pregnancy.

Pharmaceutical precautions Store in a cool, dry place protected from light.

Intal Compound Spincaps can be adversely affected by moisture ingress. To prevent possible deterioration of the product it is essential that the Spincaps are always kept in their original container.

It is acceptable for upto four of the Spincaps to be stored in the Spinhaler Carrying Case for upto 24 hours.

Legal category POM.

Package quantities Original packs containing 112 Spincaps. 'Spinhaler' Insufflators are supplied in individual containers. Instructions for use are supplied with each pack.

Further information Nil.

Product licence number 0113/5023R.

INTAL* INHALER

Presentation Metered dose pressurised aerosol delivering 112 inhalations each containing a total of 5.0 mg Sodium Cromoglycate BP.

Inactive ingredients: Dichlorotetrafluoroethane BPC, Dichlorodifluoromethane BPC, sorbitan trioleate.

Uses Intal Inhaler is indicated for the treatment of bronchial asthma, including the prevention of exercise-induced asthma.

Dosage and administration Since Intal Inhaler therapy is essentially preventative it is important that the patient is instructed to maintain regular dosage, as distinct from inhaling the drug intermittently to relieve symptoms.

Adults and children: Initial dose is two inhalations of the aerosol four times daily. Once adequate control of symptoms has been achieved it may be possible to reduce to a maintenance dose of one inhalation four times daily. However, the dose may be increased to two inhalations six or eight times daily in more severe cases or during periods of severe antigen challenge. Additional doses before exercise may also be taken.

Elderly patients: No current evidence for alteration of the recommended adult dosage.

Concomitant bronchodilator therapy: Where a concomitant aerosol bronchodilator is prescribed, it is recommended that this be administered prior to the Intal Inhaler.

Concomitant steroid therapy: In patients currently treated with steroids the addition of Intal Inhaler to the regimen may make it possible to reduce the maintenance dose or to discontinue steroids completely. The patient must be carefully supervised while the steroid dose is reduced; a rate of reduction of 10% weekly is suggested.

If reduction of a steroid dosage has been possible Intal Inhaler should not be withdrawn until steroid cover has been re-instituted.

Contra-indications, warnings, etc
Contra-indications: There are no specific contra-indications.

Side-effects: Mild throat irritation, coughing and transient bronchospasm may occur. Very rarely severe bronchospasm associated with a marked fall in pulmonary function has been reported. In such cases treatment should be stopped and should not be reintroduced.

Overdosage: No action other than medical observation should be necessary.

Withdrawal of Intal Inhaler therapy: Since the therapy is

essentially prophylactic it is important to continue therapy in those patients who benefit. If it is necessary to withdraw this treatment, it should be done progressively over a period of one week. Symptoms of asthma may recur.

Use in pregnancy: As with all medication particular caution must be exercised during the first trimester of pregnancy.

Pharmaceutical precautions Store the inhaler in a cool place. The aerosol inhaler canister is pressurised. The canister should be protected from direct sunlight and must not be punctured or burnt, even when empty.

Legal category POM.

Package quantities Each pack contains a canister delivering 112 metered inhalations of sodium cromoglycate and a plastic mouthpiece. Instructions for use are supplied with each pack.

Further information Nil.

Product licence number 0113/0109.

INTAL* NEBULISER SOLUTION

Presentation Intal Nebuliser Solution is presented in plastic ampoules containing Sodium Cromoglycate BP 20 mg in 2 ml of a clear colourless sterile aqueous solution.

Uses Intal Nebuliser Solution is indicated for the preventive treatment of bronchial asthma which may be due to allergy, exercise, cold air or chemical and occupational irritants. Sodium cromoglycate inhibits the release from sensitised mast cells of mediators of the allergic reaction. In the lung this inhibition of mediator release prevents both the immediate and late asthmatic response to immunological stimuli. Sodium cromoglycate also prevents the bronchoconstriction caused by exercise, cold air and chemical irritants.

Dosage and administration Intal Nebuliser Solution should be administered from a power-operated nebuliser at an adequate flow rate, *via* a face mask or mouthpiece. Information on suitable power operated nebulisers is available on request. Hand operated nebulisers are not suitable for the administration of Intal Nebuliser Solution.

Dosage: Since Intal Nebuliser Solution therapy is essentially preventive, it is important that regular dosage is maintained, as distinct from intermittent use to relieve symptoms.

Adults and children: The contents of one ampoule are administered by nebulisation four times a day, i.e. night and morning and at intervals of 3–6 hours. In severe cases frequency of administration may be increased to 5 or 6 times daily.

Elderly: No current evidence for alteration of the adult dose.

Concomitant steroid therapy: In patients currently treated with steroids the addition of Intal Nebuliser solution to the regime may make it possible to reduce the maintenance dose or discontinue steroids completely. The patient must be carefully supervised while the steroid dose is reduced; a rate of reduction of 10% weekly is suggested. An increase in steroid dosage may be necessary if symptoms increase and at times of infection, severe antigen challenge or stress.

If reduction of steroid dosage has been possible, Intal Nebuliser Solution should not be withdrawn until steroid cover has been re-instituted.

Concomitant bronchodilator therapy: If bronchodilators are used concomitantly, patients may find that the frequency of bronchodilator usage can be reduced as their asthma is stabilised with Intal Nebuliser Solution.

Contra-indications, warnings, etc
Contra-indications: There are no specific contra-indications. Intal Nebuliser Solution must not be given by injection.

Side-effects: Mild throat irritation, coughing and transient bronchospasm may occur. Very rarely severe bronchospasm associated with a marked fall in pulmonary function has been reported. In such cases treatment should be stopped and should not be reintroduced.

Overdosage: No action other than medical observation should be necessary.

Withdrawal of Intal Nebuliser Solution therapy: Since sodium cromoglycate acts prophylactically, it is important to continue treatment in those patients who benefit. If it is necessary to withdraw Intal Nebuliser Solution this should be done progressively over a period of one week. Symptoms of asthma may recur.

Use in pregnancy: As with all medication, particular caution must be exercised during the first trimester of pregnancy.

Pharmaceutical precautions Store in a cool place protected from sunlight. Should the physician decide to mix Intal Nebuliser Solution with other agents, the mixture should be prepared just prior to use and discarded if any turbidity develops. Any unused solution should be discarded immediately and the chamber of the nebuliser thoroughly cleaned.

Legal category POM.

Package quantities Box containing 60 × 2 ml ampoules.

Further information Nil.

Product licence number 0113/0068R.

MIRAXID* TABLETS
MIRAXID* 450 TABLETS
MIRAXID* PAEDIATRIC SUSPENSION

Presentation *Miraxid Tablets:* White, film-coated tablets each containing: Pivampicillin 125 mg and Pivmecillinam hydrochloride 100 mg.

Miraxid 450 Tablets: White, film-coated tablets each containing: Pivampicillin 250 mg and Pivmecillinam hydrochloride 200 mg.

Miraxid Paediatric Suspension: Unit dose foil sachets, each containing Pivampicillin 62.5 mg and pivmecillinam 46.2 mg.

The suspension contains sucrose.

Uses Miraxid contains the orally active derivatives of ampicillin and mecillinam – pivampicillin and pivmecillinam respectively. Following oral administration, Miraxid is absorbed rapidly. Pivampicillin and pivmecillinam are hydrolysed in the body by non-specific enzymes present in blood and other tissues, liberating ampicillin and mecillinam. Both drugs produce maximum plasma levels at 15 mins to 1 hour after administration. Ampicillin and mecillinam are both mainly excreted unchanged in the urine within the first 8 hours after administration. Smaller amounts of both drugs are excreted in bile.

Miraxid shows high anti-bacterial activity against most commonly occurring Gram-positive and Gram-negative pathogens. Sensitive organisms include: Gram-positive: penicillin-sensitive *Staph. aureus, Strep. pyogenes, Strep. faecalis, Strep. viridans, Strep. pneumoniae* and Clostridia species.

Gram-negative: *Neisseria meningitidis, Neisseria gonorrhoeae, Haemophilus influenzae, Escherichia coli, Proteus mirabilis, Proteus vulgaris, Klebsiella pneumoniae,* Enterobacter and Citrobacter species, *Salmonella typhi, Salmonella paratyphi,* other Salmonella species and species of Serratia, Shigella and Yersinia.

The anti-bacterial effect of Miraxid is further enhanced by the synergistic action of ampicillin and mecillinam, which has been demonstrated with many of the Gram-negative organisms.

Penicillinase-producing staphylococci and *Pseudomonas aeruginosa* are resistant to Miraxid.

Indications: Miraxid is indicated for the treatment of acute bronchitis, pneumonia, acute exacerbations of chronic bronchitis, otitis media, sinusitis, tonsillitis, tracheitis, laryngitis, pharyngitis and urinary tract infections due to organisms sensitive to the combination.

Dosage and administration Both the tablets and the suspension should be taken preferably with or immediately after a meal or with bland fluids such as water or milk. The tablets must be taken with at least half a glass of water.

Suspension: Mix the contents of the sachet in a little water (5–10 mls) and stir well before drinking. The suspension should be taken immediately.

For acute uncomplicated infections
Adults and children over 10 years: Two Miraxid tablets or one Miraxid 450 tablet twice daily.

Children aged 6–10 years: One Miraxid tablet or 2 sachets of Miraxid Paediatric Suspension twice daily.

Children under 6 years: One sachet of Miraxid Paediatric Suspension twice daily.

For severe infections
Adults and children over 10 years: Three Miraxid tablets twice daily. Dosages of up to 4 Miraxid tablets (equivalent to 2 Miraxid 450 tablets), twice daily, have been given to adults.

Children aged 6–10 years: Three sachets of Miraxid Paediatric Suspension twice daily.

Children under 6 years: Two sachets of Miraxid Paediatric Suspension twice daily.

Dosage in the elderly: Renal excretion of mecillinam and ampicillin is delayed in the elderly but significant accumulation of the drug is not likely at the recommended adult dosage.

Contra-indications, warnings, etc
Contra-indications: Penicillin and cephalosporin hypersensitivity. Because of the frequency of exanthemata associated with ampicillin therapy in infectious mononucleosis, treatment with Miraxid is contra-indicated in this disease.

Precautions: During long-term usage, it is advisable to carry out routine liver and kidney function tests. As with other antibiotics which are excreted mainly by the kidneys, raised blood levels of ampicillin and mecillinam may occur if repeated doses are given to patients with impaired renal function.

Caution is urged if patients with lymphatic leukaemia are treated with Miraxid, because of the frequency of exanthemata associated with ampicillin therapy.

Pregnancy: Although tests in two animal species have shown no teratogenic effect, in keeping with current practice, use during the first trimester of pregnancy should be avoided. The drug, as ampicillin and mecillinam, crosses the placenta. Ampicillin has been detected in breast milk.

Adverse reactions: Side-effects are rare and usually of a mild and transitory nature. Urticaria, erythematous rash and pruritus may occur. Upper gastro-intestinal disturbances in the form of dyspepsia, nausea and vomiting have been observed but can generally be avoided by administration with meals. Diarrhoea has been reported infrequently. Anaphylactic reactions, though not yet reported, may occur.

Overdosage: There has been no experience with Miraxid. However, excessive dosage is likely to induce nausea, vomiting and gastritis. Treatment should be restricted to symptomatic and supportive measures.

Pharmaceutical precautions Miraxid Tablets and Miraxid 450 Tablets – nil.

Miraxid Paediatric Suspension: store below 15°C. Once reconstituted, use the suspension immediately.

Legal category POM.

Package quantities Miraxid and Miraxid 450 tablets: Bottles of 100 tablets.

Miraxid Paediatric Suspension: Boxes of 10 sachets.

Further information Nil.

Product licence numbers
Miraxid Tablets 0043/0069
Miraxid 450 Tablets 0043/0070
Miraxid Paediatric Suspension 0043/0098.

Product licence holder:
Leo Laboratories Limited, Longwick Road, Princes Risborough, Aylesbury, Bucks, HP17 9RR.

NALCROM*

Presentation Nalcrom is a presentation of sodium cromoglycate for oral use. It is presented in clear/clear hard gelatin capsules printed Fisons 101 in black. Each capsule contains 100 mg sodium cromoglycate as a white powder.

Uses Food allergy (where adequate investigations have been performed to determine sensitivity to one or more ingested allergens) in conjunction with restriction of main causative allergens.

Sodium cromoglycate inhibits the release from mast cells of mediators of the allergic reaction. In gastro-intestinal disease the release of mediators causes a local inflammation which can either result in gastrointestinal symptoms or may allow absorption of antigenic material leading to systemic allergic reactions.

Dosage and administration
Initial dose: Adults: 2 capsules four times daily before meals.

Children: From 2–14 years: 1 capsule four times daily before meals.

For adults and children if satisfactory control is not achieved within two to three weeks the dosage may be doubled but should not exceed 40 mg/kg/day.

Maintenance dose: Once a therapeutic response has been achieved the dose may be reduced to the minimum required to maintain the patient free of symptoms.

Patients who are unable to avoid allergenic foods under certain circumstances (e.g. school meals, restaurants) may be able to protect themselves against the effect of these foods by taking a single dose of Nalcrom 15 minutes before the meal. The optimum dosage will need to be determined for each patient and a suitable starting dose would be 200 mg in adults and 100 mg in children.

Elderly: No current evidence for alteration of the adult dose.

Administration: The capsules may be swallowed whole or the powder contents may be dissolved in a small quantity of very hot water and diluted with cold water to drink. Administration as a solution in water is probably the method of choice.

Contra-indications, warnings, etc
Contra-indications: There are no specific contra-indications.

Warnings: The safety of Nalcrom in pregnancy and for the treatment of children under two years has not yet been established.

Side-effects: Nausea, skin rashes and joint pains have been reported in a few cases.

Overdosage: As Nalcrom is absorbed only to a very limited extent, no action other than medical observation should be necessary.

Pharmaceutical precautions Store in a dry place. Reclose the container tightly after use.

Legal category POM.

Package quantities Containers of 100 capsules.

Further information If oral steroid therapy is to be reduced or withdrawn this should be done cautiously and not more rapidly than 10% per week.

Product licence number 0113/0073.

OPTICROM* AQUEOUS EYE DROPS

Presentation A clear colourless aqueous solution of Sodium Cromoglycate BP 2% w/v, with benzalkonium chloride 0.01% w/v.

Inactive ingredients: Benzalkonium chloride, Disodium Edetate BP.

Uses For the relief and treatment of acute allergic conjunctivitis such as hay fever, chronic allergic conjunctivitis and vernal kerato conjunctivitis. Sodium cromoglycate inhibits the release from sensitised mast cells of mediators of the allergic reaction.

Dosage and administration One or two drops into each eye four times daily.

Elderly: No current evidence for alteration of the dose.

Contra-indications, warnings, etc Known hypersensitivity to benzalkonium chloride.

Pharmaceutical precautions Store below 30°C. Protect from direct sunlight.

Legal category POM.

Package quantities 13.5 ml.

Further information Discard any remaining contents four weeks after opening the bottle. As with other ophthalmic solutions containing benzalkonium chloride, soft contact lenses should not be worn during the treatment period.

Product licence number 0113/0039R.

OPTICROM* EYE OINTMENT

Presentation Opticrom Eye Ointment is a cream coloured opaque sterile ointment containing 4% w/w Sodium Cromoglycate BP.

Inactive ingredients: Liquid Paraffin BP, Yellow Soft Paraffin BP, Modulan.

Uses For the relief and treatment of allergic conjunctivitis such as hay fever, chronic allergic conjunctivitis and vernal kerato conjunctivitis. Sodium cromoglycate inhibits the release from sensitised mast cells of mediators of the allergic reaction.

Dosage and administration *Adults and children:* To be applied to the eye two to three times daily.

Elderly patients: no current evidence for alteration of the dose.

Care should be taken to avoid direct contact between the eye and the tube nozzle.

Contra-indications, warnings, etc
Contra-indications: nil.

Warnings: As with other ophthalmic ointments, transient blurring of vision may occur. The ointment should not be used if contact lenses are being worn.

Pharmaceutical precautions Store below 25°C. Protect from direct sunlight. It is desirable that the contents should be discarded four weeks after opening.

Legal category POM.

Package quantities 5 g.

Further information Patients may prefer to use Opticrom Aqueous Eye Drops during the day and Opticrom Eye Ointment at night.

Product licence number 0113/0103.

PARACODOL*
Approved name: Co-codamol Eff, Co-codamol Disp

Presentation Large, white, soluble, effervescent tablets each containing:

Paracetamol BP	500 mg
Codeine Phosphate BP	8 mg

Formulation includes Sodium Benzoate BP.

Uses For the treatment of pain, including muscular and rheumatic pains, headache, migraine, neuralgia, toothache, sore throat, period pains, aches and pains. Discomfort associated with influenza, feverishness and feverish colds.

Dosage and administration The tablets are to be dissolved in water before oral administration.

Adults: 1–2 tablets, which may be repeated every four to six hours with a maximum of 8 in 24 hrs.

Children: Aged 6–12 years: ½–1 tablet. Not more than 4 doses to be taken in 24 hours. The tablets are not scored and care should be taken to halve them accurately. Discard the unused half of the tablet.

Under 6 years: Not recommended.

Elderly: No current evidence for alteration of the adult dose except where there is impaired hepatic function when dosage reduction may be necessary.

Contra-indications, warnings, etc *Precautions:* The tablet base is designed to be equivalent to 1.5 g Sodium Citrate BP equivalent to 352 mg or 15.3 millimole Na^+. It should therefore be prescribed with caution in long term treatment of patients in whom a restricted salt intake is indicated.

Preparations containing paracetamol should be given with care to patients with impaired liver function.

Use in pregnancy and lactation: There is inadequate evidence of safety of the drug in human pregnancy, but it has been in wide use for many years without apparent ill consequence, although there is evidence that exposure to codeine during pregnancy may have a higher incidence of respiratory malformations. If drug therapy is needed in pregnancy, this drug can be used if there is no safer alternative. At normal doses, low levels of paracetamol and codeine are present in breast milk. Use of this product during lactation is acceptable.

Overdosage: It is unlikely that a toxic dose of large, effervescent tablets would be ingested. In the event of an overdose, the toxic effects of codeine may be reversed by the administration of naloxone injection. Symptoms of paracetamol overdose are often delayed for at least 24 hours but to prevent hepatic damage, treatment should be given as soon as possible and within 10 hours of ingestion. Treatment is by the administration of oral methionine, oral or intravenous acetylcysteine.

Pharmaceutical precautions Store in a cool dry place.

Legal category CD (Sch 5), P.

Package quantities Boxes of 100 tablets.

Further information Under the limited list regulations, NHS prescriptions for Paracodol will not be reimbursed. However, Paracodol complies with the specification for Co-codamol dispersible or effervescent tablets and if supplied against generic prescriptions is eligible for reimbursement under the NHS.

Product licence number 0113/5076R.

RYNACROM*

Presentation *Nasal Spray:* A metered dose presentation of a clear aqueous solution of sodium cromoglycate 2% w/v. The pack contains a bottle of solution and pump, ready assembled.

Inactive ingredients: Benzalkonium chloride, Disodium Edetate BP.

Nasal Drops: a plastic dropper bottle containing a clear, aqueous solution of Sodium Cromoglycate BP, 2.0% w/v.

Inactive ingredients: Benzalkonium chloride, Disodium Edetate BP.

Cartridges: pink, transparent hard gelatin cartridges, each bearing the overprint 'RYNACROM'. Each cartridge contains 10 mg Sodium Cromoglycate BP in powder form for nasal insufflation.

Inactive ingredients: Lactose BP.

Uses Rynacrom is indicated for the preventive treatment of allergic rhinitis (seasonal and perennial). Sodium cromoglycate inhibits the release from sensitised mast cells of mediators of the allergic reaction. In the nose this inhibition of mediator release prevents the symptoms of rhinitis.

Dosage and administration Since therapy with Rynacrom is essentially preventive, it is important that the patient is instructed to maintain regular dosage, as distinct from using the drug intermittently to relieve symptoms.

Adults and children: Rynacrom Nasal Spray – 1 spray to each nostril four or six times daily.

One spray delivers approximately 2.6 mg of sodium cromoglycate from the metered dose device.

Rynacrom Nasal Drops: Instil 2 drops into each nostril six times daily.

Rynacrom Cartridges: The contents of one cartridge are insufflated into each nostril up to four times daily. The first dose should be insufflated on rising and the last one immediately before retiring.

Elderly: No current evidence for alteration of the adult dose.

Contra-indications, warnings, etc There are no specific contra-indications.

Side-effects: Occasional irritation of the nasal mucosa may occur during the first days of use. In rare cases wheezing or tightness of the chest have been reported by patients.

Use in pregnancy and lactation: Cumulative experience from the widespread use of sodium cromoglycate in the recommended dose has revealed no adverse effects on mother or child. If drug therapy is needed in pregnancy, the use of the drug is acceptable.

Sodium cromoglycate is excreted in the breast milk in trace amounts only. No evidence exists to suggest any adverse consequences on its use to the infant.

Overdosage: No action other than medical supervision should be necessary.

Pharmaceutical precautions Store below 30°C. Rynacrom Nasal Spray and Nasal Drops should be protected from direct sunlight. Rynacrom Cartridges should be protected from light and kept dry.

Legal category P.

Package quantities Rynacrom Nasal Spray: 26 ml bottle with pump.

Rynacrom Nasal Drops: bottle of 15 ml.

Rynacrom Cartridges: containers of 100 cartridges.

Rynacrom Insufflators are supplied in separate containers. Instructions for use are supplied with each pack.

Further information A reduction in concomitant antihistamine therapy will often be possible.

Product licence numbers

Rynacrom Nasal Spray:	0113/0066R
Rynacrom Nasal Drops:	0113/0040R
Rynacrom Cartridges:	0113/5032R

RYNACROM* COMPOUND

Presentation A metered-dose presentation of a clear aqueous solution of Sodium Cromoglycate BP 2% w/v and Xylometazoline Hydrochloride BP 0.025% w/v. The pack contains a bottle of solution and a pump unit ready assembled.

Inactive ingredients: Benzalkonium chloride, Disodium Edetate BP.

Uses Rynacrom Compound is indicated for the prophylaxis, relief and treatment of allergic rhinitis (such as hayfever and perennial rhinitis) where this is accompanied by nasal congestion.

Sodium cromoglycate inhibits the release of mediators of the allergic reaction from sensitised mast cells. In the nose, this inhibition of mediator release prevents the symptoms of rhinitis.

Xylometazoline hydrochloride is a sympathomimetic agent with alpha-adrenergic activity. It produces vasoconstriction thus reducing nasal congestion.

Dosage and administration *Adults and children:* One spray to each nostril four times daily.

One spray delivers approximately 2.6 mg of sodium cromoglycate and 0.0325 mg of xylometazoline hydrochloride from the metered-dose device.

Elderly: No current evidence for alteration of the adult dose.

Contra-indications, warnings, etc

Contra-indications: There are no specific contra-indications.

Side-effects: No serious side effects have been reported. Occasional irritation of the nasal mucosa may occur during the first days of use. In rare cases with sodium cromoglycate solutions alone wheezing and tightness of the chest have been reported. Because a lower dose of xylometazoline is employed in this presentation than in other formulations, the side-effects usually attributed to this drug are expected to be minimal or absent.

Exposure to higher doses of xylometazoline than are likely with the correct use of Rynacrom Compound are reported to cause mild side-effects such as nasal irritation, dryness of the nose, sneezing, headache, insomnia, drowsiness and palpitations.

Precautions: The prolonged use or abuse of decongestants in general may lead to rebound congestion or drug induced rhinitis. This is reported to be less likely with xylometazoline.

Use in pregnancy: As with all medicines, caution should be exercised during pregnancy, especially in the first trimester.

Overdosage: Adults: Generally no action other than medical supervision should be necessary.

Infants and children: Overdosage of decongestants may cause sedation; uneventful recovery is usual, although medical supervision is recommended. Should accidental overdosage lead to convulsions or respiratory depression, gastric lavage and symptomatic therapy should be instituted.

Pharmaceutical precautions Store below 30°C. Protect from direct sunlight.

Legal category P.

Package quantities Bottle of 26 ml and pump unit.

Further information Nil.

Product licence number 0113/0097.

TILADE*

Presentation Metered dose pressurised aerosol delivering 112 actuations, each containing 2 mg of nedocromil sodium.

Inactive ingredients: Dichlorotetrafluoroethane BPC, Dichlorodifluoromethane BPC, sorbitan trioleate.

Uses

Indications: Tilade is indicated in the management of Reversible Obstructive Airways Disease (ROAD) in patients of a wide age range. Tilade is intended for regular prophylactic treatment and not for symptomatic relief. ROAD includes bronchial asthma, whether extrinsic or intrinsic in nature; asthmatic bronchitis; late onset asthma; exercise induced asthma; and bronchospasm provoked by a variety of stimuli such as cold air, inhaled allergens, atmospheric pollutants and other irritants.

In the management of ROAD Tilade improves pulmonary function, reduces the frequency and severity of attacks and reduces bronchospasm, cough and bronchial hyper-reactivity.

In patients already receiving treatment for their ROAD,

Tilade can be given in addition to all existing therapies and will in many cases provide added therapeutic benefit. Having established this benefit of Tilade, it may be possible to eliminate or reduce concomitant therapy.

Pharmacology: Nedocromil sodium markedly inhibits the release of inflammatory mediators from a variety of cell types which occur in the lumen and in the mucosa of the bronchial tree. When it is administered topically to the bronchi it displays specific anti-inflammatory properties. Laboratory experiments have shown that Tilade prevents the release of inflammatory, chemotactic and smooth muscle contracting mediators which are preformed or derived from arachidonic acid metabolism by both the lipoxygenase and cyclo-oxygenase pathways in a range of human and animal leucocytes.

Dosage and administration
Adults (including the elderly) and children over 12 years of age: In initial and maintenance therapy two actuations (4 mg of nedocromil sodium) twice daily. Where necessary this may be increased to two actuations four times daily.
Children below 12 years: It is recommended that Tilade should not be used since the profile of Tilade is still under investigation.

Tilade is intended for regular daily usage and should not be used for the relief of symptoms in an acute attack.

After inhalation Tilade is deposited in the lungs, absorbed and excreted unchanged in the bile and urine. Any of the drug which is deposited in the orophyarynx is swallowed and excreted via the alimentary tract. Tilade is poorly absorbed from the gastro-intestinal tract, and it is not metabolised. The drug does not accumulate on long-term dosing nor is it retained in any tissues.

Contra-indications, warnings, etc
Contra-indications: There are no specific contra-indications.

Side-effects: Few side-effects have been reported, principally headache and nausea, which have been mild and transient, insufficient to cause withdrawal from a trial in nearly all cases. Some patients have reported a bitter taste.

Uses in pregnancy and lactating women: Studies in pregnant and lactating animals have failed to reveal a hazard. However, as with all new medicines caution should be exercised, especially during the first trimester of pregnancy.

Overdosage: Animal studies have not shown evidence of toxic effects of Tilade even at high dosage, nor have extended human studies revealed any safety hazard with the drug. Overdosage is unlikely, therefore, to cause problems. However, if overdosage is suspected, treatment should be supportive and directed to the control of the relevant symptoms.

Pharmaceutical precautions Store below 30°C away from direct sunlight. The canister is pressurised and must not be punctured or burnt even when empty.

Legal category POM.

Package quantities Each pack contains a canister delivering 112 actuations, in an adaptor mouthpiece. Instructions for use are included in each pack.

Further information Tilade offers an effective treatment in a wide range of patients suffering from ROAD where inflammation of allergic or non-allergic origin and bronchial hyper-reactivity are significant factors.

A single dose of Tilade confers protection against the immediate effects of specific and non-specific stimuli. The therapeutic benefits of repeated doses of Tilade will be apparent in most patients within one week of starting treatment. Continuous administration of Tilade reduces the bronchial hyper-reactivity characteristic of ROAD.

Product licence number 0113/0117.

**Trade Mark*

Fournier Pharmaceuticals Limited
116–120 London Road
Oxford OX3 9AT

FOURNIER PHARMACEUTICALS

LIPANTIL* ▼

Presentation White, hard gelatin capsules each containing 100 mg fenofibrate.

Uses Lipantil reduces elevated serum cholesterol and triglycerides and is of benefit in the treatment of severe hyperlipidaemias found in some patients, in whom dietary measures alone have failed to produce an adequate response. Lipantil is therefore indicated in appropriate cases of type IIa, IIb, III, IV and V hyperlipidaemia (Fredrickson classification).

Type	*Major lipid elevated*	*Lipoproteins elevated*
IIa	Cholesterol	LDL
IIb	Cholesterol, triglycerides	LDL, VLDL
III	Cholesterol, triglycerides	LDL, Chylomicrons
IV	Triglycerides	VLDL
V	Triglycerides	Chylomicrons, VLDL

Lipantil should only be used in patients in whom a full investigation has been performed to define their abnormality, in whom the long-term risks associated with their condition warrant treatment, and whose disease is unresponsive to dietary control. Other risk factors, such as hypertension and smoking may also require management.

Epidemiological studies have demonstrated a positive correlation between abnormally increased serum lipid levels and an increased risk of coronary heart disease. The control of such dyslipidaemias forms the rationale for treatment with Lipantil. However, the possible beneficial and adverse long-term consequences of drugs used in the hyperlipidaemias are still the subject of scientific discussion. Therefore the presumptive beneficial effect of Lipantil on cardiovascular morbidity and mortality is as yet unproven.

Studies with Lipantil on lipoprotein fractions show decreases in levels of LDL- and VLDL-cholesterol. HDL-cholesterol levels are frequently increased. LDL- and VLDL-triglycerides are reduced. The overall effect is a decrease in the ratio of low and very low density lipoproteins to high density lipoprotein, which epidemiological studies have correlated with a decrease in atherogenic risk. Apolipoprotein-A and apolipoprotein-B levels are altered in parallel with HDL, and LDL and VLDL levels respectively.

Regression of xanthomata has been observed during Lipantil therapy.

Plasma uric acid levels are increased in approximately 20% of hyperlipidaemic patients, particularly in those with type IV disease. Lipantil has a uricosuric effect and is therefore of additional benefit in such patients.

Dosage and administration The recommended initial dose of Lipantil is 300 mg daily, taken in divided doses. The normal adult dose is recommended in the elderly. In children the dose level is 5 mg/kg/day. Since it is less well absorbed from an empty stomach, Lipantil should always be taken with food. Dietary restrictions instituted before therapy should be continued.

Response to therapy should be monitored by determination of serum lipid values, and dosage altered within the range 200–400 mg daily as necessary. Rapid reduction of serum lipid levels usually follows Lipantil treatment, but treatment should be discontinued if an adequate response has not been achieved within three months.

Contra-indications, warnings, etc Lipantil is contra-indicated in patients with severe liver dysfunction, existing gallbladder disease, severe renal disorders and in patients hypersensitive to Lipantil. Lipantil has not been shown to be teratogenic in animals. However, signs of embryotoxicity have been seen in rats and it is therefore recommended that Lipantil should not be administered to women who are pregnant or are breast-feeding.

In renal dysfunction the dose of Lipantil may need to be reduced, depending on the rate of creatinine clearance (for example to 200 mg daily for a creatinine clearance of 60 ml/minute, and to 100 mg daily for a creatinine clearance of 20 ml/minute).

Dose reduction should be considered in elderly patients with impaired renal function.

In common with other hypolipidaemic drugs, chronic administration of Lipantil to rodents has been associated with hepatic tumour formation. However, liver studies in Lipantil-treatment patients show no evidence of related effects.

In patients receiving anti-coagulant therapy the dose of anti-coagulant should be reduced by about one-third at the commencement of treatment and then gradually adjusted if necessary. No proven clinical interactions of Lipantil with other drugs have been reported, although in vitro interaction studies suggest displacement of phenylbutazone from plasma protein binding sites. In common with other fibrates, Lipantil induces microsomal mixed-function oxidases involved in fatty acid metabolism in rodents and may interact with drugs metabolised by these enzymes. Possible interactions with oral hypoglycaemic agents should also be considered.

Adverse reactions observed during Lipantil treatment are infrequent; they are generally minor, transient and do not interfere with treatment. Most commonly reported are mild gastro-intestinal disturbances, skin reactions, headache, fatigue and vertigo. Sexual asthenia and muscle cramps are less frequently reported. There is no evidence of an increased incidence of gallstones. Moderately elevated levels of serum transaminases may be found in some patients but rarely interfere with treatment.

No reports of ill effects from overdosage have been reported. There are no specific antidotes and treatment of acute overdosage should be symptomatic. Gastric lavage and appropriate supportive care may be instituted if necessary.

Pharmaceutical precautions Lipantil capsules should be stored at room temperature protected from light.

Legal category POM.

Package quantities Lipantil is available in blister packs of 21 capsules (hospital pack) and 84 capsules.

Further information Nil.

Product licence number 5159/0001.

Product licence holder: Laboratoires Fournier, France.

Trade Mark

Galderma (U.K.) Ltd
Imperial Way
Watford
Hertfordshire, WD2 4YR

UNITED KINGDOM GALDERMA

ALCODERM* CREAM/LOTION

Presentation *Cream:* A white, thick smooth cream.

Lotion: A creamy white, smooth, viscous lotion.

Alcoderm contains liquid paraffin, purified water, cetylalcohol, stearyl alcohol, sodium lauryl sulphate, carbomer, triethanolamine, methylparaben, propylparaben, sorbitan monostearate, isopropyl palmitate, Sorbitol USP, spermaceti, silicone fluid.

Uses Dry, chafed or irritated skin – Alcoderm is indicated in any condition where the moisture content of the horny layer has decreased below the normal level and the skin is no longer soft and pliable.

Also recommended:
(a) in acute inflammatory conditions where the skin is intact, such as sunburn and windburn.
(b) as a smoothing, hydrating agent in certain inflammatory skin conditions where there is dryness and scaling, such as ichthyosis, atopic eczema, winter itch etc.
(c) as a vehicle for other active constituents.

Additional information: Alcoderm is a specially formulated emulsion with a double acting moisturising effect. The lotion is suitable for large areas of skin, the cream for smaller drier areas. Alcoderm has a double moisturising action which can be provided only by oil-in-water emulsions. It hydrates rapidly the surface layers of the skin, and at the same time the oil droplets form a thin, protective layer on the skin. This film gives Alcoderm its special characteristics; it is highly hydrostatic and protects the skin against excessive evaporation of the water. Only 0.6% of the film-forming surface active agents in Alcoderm are water-soluble. No other oil-in-water emulsion contains such a small quantity of water soluble ingredients.

Administration Apply topically to the skin as required.

Contra-indications, warnings, etc Avoid contact with the eyes.

Legal category P.

Package quantities
Cream: 60 g
Lotion: 120 ml

Further information Nil.

Product licence numbers
0649/0004 Cream
0649/0005 Lotion

IONAX* SCRUB

Presentation A pale yellow semi-translucent abradant gel with a fresh odour of lemon. The active ingredients are polyethylene granules, benzalkonium chloride, macrogol (4) lauryl ether, macrogol (23) lauryl ether and alcohol in a foaming, aqueous gel base containing propylene glycol, potassium sorbate, silica, lauramine oxide.

Uses An abradant cleanser for the control and hygiene of acne. Use Ionax Scrub to cleanse skin prior to acne or oily skin treatment.

Administration Apply to wet face. Massage on the skin for one or two minutes, then rinse thoroughly.

Use once or twice daily.

Contra-indications, warnings, etc *Caution:* Avoid contact with the eyes.

Upon accidental contact, flush with water and avoid rubbing.

If the skin gets too dry or too reddened discontinue use temporarily.

Pharmaceutical precautions There are no special pharmaceutical precautions.

Legal category P.

Package quantities 60 g packs in plastic collapsible tubes with plastic screw caps.

Further information Nil.

Product licence number 0649/0006.

IONIL T* SHAMPOO

Presentation A clear brown liquid shampoo with a slight odour of coal tar. It contains salicylic acid, benzalkonium chloride, coal tar solution 4.25% with polyoxyethylene ethers in an hydro-alcoholic shampoo base containing disodium edetate.

Uses For seborrhoeic dermatitis of the scalp.

Administration Massage Ionil T Shampoo into wet hair.

Do not expect much initial lather as the shampoo is formulated for low foaming.

Rinse, and then apply Ionil T shampoo again and massage into a lather. Allow to remain in the hair for about five minutes before rinsing.

Repeat treatment once or twice weekly.

For best results do not use soap, detergent or other shampoo on the hair immediately before or after using Ionil T.

Contra-indications, warnings, etc *Caution:* Avoid contact with the eyes.

Upon accidental contact, flush with clear water.

Pharmaceutical precautions Store away from internal preparations and foods.

Legal category P.

Package quantities 200 ml in cylindrical plastic containers with plastic screw caps.

Further information Nil.

Product licence number 10590/0003.

NUTRAPLUS* Cream

Presentation A smooth white, unperfumed cream. It contains 10% urea, purified water, blend of light mineral oil, glyceryl monostearate, propylene glycol, methylparaben, propylparaben ethylhexyl palmitate, promulgin D.

Uses An emollient, moisturising and protective cream for the treatment of dry or damaged skin. The presence of 10% urea in the product assists in providing a 'moisturising' effect lasting 5-6 hours, as shown by experiments measuring 'trans-epidermal water loss', in addition to providing the recognised actions of urea for dermatological purposes.

Dosage and administration Apply evenly to dry skin areas 2 to 3 times daily, or as necessary.

Contra-indications, warnings, etc If irritation occurs to any ingredient, discontinue use temporarily. Avoid contact with eyes.

Pharmaceutical precautions Store in a cool place. Replace cap after use.

Legal category P.

Package quantities 60 g.

Further information Nil.

Product licence number 10590/0002.

PSORIGEL*

Presentation A clear thin brown gel with a slight characteristic odour of tar. It contains solution of coal tar 7.5%, 33% alcohol, carbomer 940, propylene glycol, denatured alcohol, laureth 4, diisopropanolamine, and purified water. The hydroalcoholic gel base which is emollient, provides a moist film with the minimum of tar odour and staining potential.

Uses For use on the skin and the scalp. For the relief and treatment of inflammatory manifestations of tar responsive dermatoses. Among these are eczema, psoriasis, inflammation, erythema, scaling, pruritus and induration that accompanies various forms of dermatitis.

It also helps to relieve the itching that accompanies psoriasis, and eczema, and helps control flaking and scaling.

Dosage and administration Rub into the affected areas once or twice daily. The gel may be applied more frequently if necessary.

Rub in well, allow to dry and remove any excess by patting with a paper tissue.

Contra-indications, warnings, etc *Caution:* Avoid contact with eyes. Upon accidental contact, flush with water.

After using, avoid exposure to direct sunlight, unless its action is specifically required.

Do not use on highly inflamed or broken skin.

The product contains alcohol.

If undue irritation develops, reduce the frequency of use, or suspend use until irritation subsides.

The staining potential of the product is minimal, but if it does occur, standard laundry procedure will remove most stains.

Pharmaceutical precautions There are no special pharmaceutical precautions.

Legal category GSL.

Package quantities 90 g in plastic collapsible tubes.

Further information Nil.

Product licence number 10590/0001.

**Trade Mark*

Geigy Pharmaceuticals
Horsham
West Sussex
RH12 4AB

ANAFRANIL*
ANAFRANIL SR*

Presentation The active ingredient, clomipramine hydrochloride, is presented as:

Pink, film coated tablets, round, slightly biconvex with slightly bevelled edges, imprinted 'GEIGY' on one face and GD on the other, diameter approximately 8 mm, thickness approximately 4.3 mm, each containing 75 mg in a sustained release formulation.

Two-tone blue/caramel-coloured capsules, hard gelatin size No. 4, imprinted GEIGY, each containing 50 mg.

Two-tone orange/caramel-coloured capsules, hard gelatin size No. 4, imprinted GEIGY, each containing 25 mg.

Two-tone yellow/caramel-coloured capsules, hard gelatin size No. 4, imprinted GEIGY, each containing 10 mg.

Orange flavoured and coloured syrup containing the equivalent of 25 mg clomipramine hydrochloride in 5 ml.

Ampoules of clear glass containing 25 mg clomipramine hydrochloride in 2 ml.

SR tablets contain polyethoxylated castor oils. The 10 mg, 25 mg and 50 mg capsules also contain lactose. The syrup also contains sucrose, azo-dyes, methyl hydroxybenzoate and propyl hydroxybenzoate. Ampoules also contain glycerol and water.

Uses Antidepressant: Symptoms of depressive illness especially where sedation is required. Obsessive and phobic states. Cataplexy associated with narcolepsy.

Dosage and administration
Dosage: Adults: Oral – 10 mg/day initially, increasing gradually to 30–150 mg/day, if required, in divided doses throughout the day or as a single dose at bedtime. Many patients will be adequately maintained on 30–50 mg/day. Higher doses may be needed in some patients, particularly those suffering from obsessional or phobic disorders. Where a higher dosage is required, the 75 mg S.R. formulation may be preferable.

Elderly: 10 mg/day initially. The initial dose should be increased with caution under close supervision to 30–75 mg daily. Half the normal maintenance dose may be sufficient to produce a satisfactory clinical response.

Children: not recommended.

Intramuscular administration: Treatment may be commenced with intramuscular injections of up to 6 × 25 mg ampoules daily. Once therapy has started to be effective, a change to oral dosing should be made as soon as possible.

Dosage: Intravenous infusion: Any standard giving set may be used but a cannula or fine needle with a flange which can be strapped in position should be chosen. Anafranil ampoules may be diluted with either physiological saline or 5% Dextrose BP. The required dose of Anafranil should be introduced into the infusion fluid with a sterile syringe and the contents should be agitated to ensure even distribution of the drug before infusion is commenced, into a forearm vein.

In the first instance a small dose of Anafranil (25 mg or 50 mg) should be diluted in 200–500 ml of infusion fluid and infused over a period of two hours to assess tolerance. If satisfactory, the dose may be increased by 25 mg daily until an optimum therapeutic dose has been achieved. At the same time the bulk of fluid may be reduced (to a minimum of 125 ml) and the duration of infusion decreased (to a minimum of 45 minutes).

On average the optimum therapeutic dose will be in the region of 100 mg but higher doses may be required in more severe depressions or in obsessional and phobic states.

Length of treatment: Infusions should be given only to patients who are unable to take the drug orally. Oral therapy should be substituted once therapy has started to be effective, usually after 7–10 days.

Changeover to oral therapy: Following a satisfactory response to infusion, the quantity of intravenous Anafranil should be gradually reduced and oral therapy substituted. It is advisable to give double the maximum intravenous dosage orally until the patient's response is assured. Thereafter, a suitable maintenance dose, if considered necessary, can be selected.

Monitoring during treatment: During the course of infusion, patients should be carefully monitored for adverse effects. Particular attention should be paid to blood pressure recording, especially if there are any changes of position after conclusion of the infusion, as hypotension may occur. Patients often feel pleasantly drowsy during treatment and not infrequently fall asleep.

Contra-indications, warnings, etc
Contra-indications: Recent myocardial infarction, cardiac failure, any degree of heart block or other cardiac arrhythmias. Severe liver disease. Concurrent administration with monoamine oxidase inhibitors. Narrow angle glaucoma. Retention of urine. Mania.

Precautions: The elderly are particularly liable to experience adverse effects, especially agitation, confusion and postural hypotension. (See dosage).

Avoid if possible in patients with a history of epilepsy or with symptoms of bladder neck obstruction, e.g. prostatic hypertrophy.

Patients posing a high suicide risk require close initial supervision.

Tricyclic antidepressants potentiate the central nervous depressant action of alcohol.

Anaesthetics given during tri/tetracyclic antidepressant therapy may increase the risk of arrhythmias and hypotension. If surgery is necessary, the anaesthetist should be informed that a patient is being so treated.

As improvement may not occur during the first 2–4 weeks of treatment, patients should be closely monitored during this period.

Clomipramine may initially impair alertness. Patients should be warned of the possible hazard when driving or operating machinery.

Use in pregnancy and lactation: Do not use during pregnancy, especially during the first and last trimesters, unless there are compelling reasons. There is no evidence as to drug safety in human pregnancy; animal work has not shown clomipramine to be free from hazard.

Anafranil is excreted in breast milk. Do not use during lactation unless considered essential; in this case nursing mothers should be advised to cease breast feeding.

Withdrawal symptoms in neonates whose mothers receive tri/tetracyclic antidepressants during the third trimester have also been reported and include respiratory depression, convulsions and jitteriness.

Drug interactions: Clomipramine should not be given concurrently, or within 3 weeks of cessation of therapy, with monoamine oxidase inhibitors.

Clomipramine may decrease the antihypertensive effect of guanethidine, debrisoquine, bethanidine and possibly clonidine and methyldopa. It would be advisable to review all antihypertensive therapy during treatment with tricyclic antidepressants.

Clomipramine should not be given with sympathomimetic agents such as adrenaline, ephedrine, isoprenaline, noradrenaline, phenylephrine and phenylpropanolamine.

Barbiturates may decrease and methylphenidate and neuroleptics may increase the plasma level of clomipramine.

Side-effects: The following adverse effects, although not necessarily all reported with Anafranil have occurred with other tri/tetracyclic antidepressants:

Atropine-like side effects including dry mouth, disturbances of accommodation, tachycardia, constipation and hesitancy of micturition may occur early in treatment, but usually lessen.

Other possible adverse effects include nausea, drowsiness, sweating, postural hypotension, hypomania, tremor, paraesthesia, ataxia and, rarely, skin rashes.

Male patients may occasionally experience ejaculation disorders and, more rarely, impotence. Women occasionally experience orgasmic impotence.

Epileptiform convulsions have been experienced in a small number of patients.

Serious adverse effects are rare; these include impaired liver function and jaundice, bone marrow depression, including leucopenia, eosinophilia and thrombocytopenia. Agranulocytosis has occasionally occurred in patients receiving tricyclic antidepressants. It is advisable to perform blood counts during treatment with Anafranil especially if the patient develops fever, sore throat or other signs of infection. Cardiac arrhythmias and severe hypotension are likely to occur with high dosage or in deliberate overdosage. They may also occur in patients with pre-existing heart disease taking normal dosage.

Although not indicative of addiction, withdrawal symptoms may occur on abrupt cessation of therapy and include insomnia, irritability and excessive perspiration.

Psychotic manifestations, including mania and paranoid delusions, may be exacerbated during treatment with tricyclic antidepressants.

Overdosage:
Signs and Symptoms: Major symptoms of overdosage include coma, convulsions, respiratory depression and disturbances in cardiac rate and rhythm.

Treatment: There is no specific antidote to Anafranil. Gastric lavage and forced emesis should be employed immediately to reduce absorption of the drug. Patients presenting with major symptoms of overdosage should be nursed in an intensive care unit where full support of vital functions is possible. Any serious overdosage requires continuous cardiac monitoring for at least 48 hours and dysrhythmias treated on an individual basis. Respiratory insufficiency may necessitate intubation and ventilation, and convulsions may be controlled with intravenous diazepam. Physostigmine should not be used following an overdosage of Anafranil. There have been reports that physostigmine increases the risk of seizures.

Pharmaceutical precautions *Storage: Tablets* – protect from moisture. *Capsules* – protect from heat and moisture. *Syrup* – protect from heat. Keep containers tightly closed. *Ampoules* – protect from heat and light.

Dilutions: Syrup – dilutions down to 15 mg/5 ml can be prepared with boiled, distilled or de-ionised water. For dilutions below 15 mg/5 ml the recommended diluent is equal parts simple Syrup BP and freshly prepared Tragacanth Mucilage BPC 1973. After dilution the solution should be used within a few days.

Legal category POM.

Package quantities
Tablets 75 mg SR.: Blister packs of 100.
Capsules 50 mg: Blister packs of 100.
Capsules 25 mg: Blister packs of 100.
Capsules 10 mg: Blister packs of 100.
Syrup 25 mg/5 ml: Bottles of 150 ml.
Ampoules 25 mg/2 ml: Boxes of 10.

Further information Nil.

Product licence numbers

Tablets 75 mg S.R.	0001/0087
Capsules 50 mg	0001/0068
Capsules 25 mg	0001/5000
Capsules 10 mg	0001/0037
Syrup 25 mg/5 ml	0001/5001
Ampoules 25 mg/2 ml	0001/5036

ANTURAN*

Presentation Tablets containing 200 mg Sulphinpyrazone BP, light yellow, sugar coated, round, biconvex, approximately 10.6 mm diameter printed GEIGY on one side. Tablets containing 100 mg Sulphinpyrazone BP, pale yellow, sugar coated, round, biconvex, approximately 8.5 mm diameter printed GEIGY on one side.

The tablets also contain lactose and sucrose.

Uses *Mode of action:* Anturan lowers serum urate levels by blocking tubular reabsorption, thereby increasing renal excretion of uric acid. As a result of increased excretion, serum urate deposits are mobilised and tophi are no longer formed.

Indication: Chronic, including tophaceous gout; recurrent gouty arthritis; hyperuricaemia.

Dosage and administration Anturan is administered orally in tablet form with meals or milk.

Dosage: Adults: 100–200 mg daily increasing gradually (over the first two or three weeks) to 600 mg daily, and maintained until the serum urate level has fallen within the normal range. Subsequent dosage should be reduced, to the lowest level which maintains serum urate within the normal range. Maintenance dose may be as low as 200 mg daily. Reduced dose required in renal impairment. Not to be used in severe renal impairment.

Children: Paediatric usage not established.

Contra-indications, warnings, etc
Contra-indications: Active peptic ulcer. Sensitivity to phenylbutazone or other pyrazole derivatives. Severe hepatic disease.

In the treatment of chronic gout salicylates antagonise the action of Anturan and should not be given concurrently.

Precautions: Use with caution in patients with impaired renal function, and with healed peptic ulcer as well as in those in whom attacks of asthma have been precipitated by acetylsalicylic acid or by other drugs with prostaglandin synthesis inhibiting activity.

In patients with an elevated plasma uric acid level and/or with a history of nephrolithiasis or renal colic, and also when resuming treatment after interruption of the medication, a cautious incremental dosage schedule should be adopted. As with any form of long-term uricosuric medication, renal function tests should be performed regularly, particularly in cases where there is pre-existing evidence of renal failure.

Since Anturan may lead to sodium and water retention caution is indicated in patients with latent heart failure.

Since Anturan may potentiate the action of coumarin-type anticoagulants, frequent estimation of prothrombin time should be undertaken when these drugs are given concurrently, and the dosage of anticoagulant adjusted accordingly.

Anturan may also potentiate the action of other plasma protein binding drugs such as hypoglycaemic agents and sulphonamides, which may necessitate a modification in dosage.

Anturan should be used with caution in pregnant women, weighing the potential risk against the possible benefits.

Warnings and side-effects: During the early stages of treatment in patients with hyperuricaemia or gout, acute attacks of gout may be precipitated. To help prevent episodes of urolithiasis or renal colic, ensure adequate fluid intake and alkalinisation of the urine during initial stages of therapy.

Gastro-intestinal bleeding has been reported; transient gastro-intestinal side-effects may occur and are usually of a mild nature.

Impairment of renal function may occur, with changes in the electrolyte balance; as a rule the respective values revert to normal after the drug has been withdrawn; occasional cases of renal failure have also been reported, although no clear-cut causal relationship has been established. Rash or blood dyscrasias may occur, and are contra-indications to further treatment; onset may be sudden or gradual, and occur after small doses or after long periods of treatment.

For the early detection of a haematological abnormality, careful clinical supervision and full blood count should be done before and at regular intervals during treatment.

Accidental overdosage: There is no antidote to Anturan, and treatment is symptomatic. Immediate treatment consists of forced emesis to recover undigested tablets. This is followed by gastric lavage preferably with mild alkaline solution such as sodium bicarbonate solution and supportive therapy as indicated.

Pharmaceutical precautions *Storage:* Protect from heat and moisture.

Legal category POM.

Package quantities Tablets 100 mg: Containers of 100. Tablets 200 mg: Cartons of 112 consisting of 4 calendar reminder foils of 28 (OP).

Product licence numbers
Tablets 100 mg 0001/5002
Tablets 200 mg 0001/0080

BUTACOTE*

Presentation The active ingredient, Phenylbutazone BP is presented as sugar-coated, enteric tablets, biconvex, approximately 7.8 mm in diameter, pale violet coloured and imprinted GEIGY on one side and DM on the other, each tablet containing 100 mg.

The tablets also contain sucrose and an azo-dye.

Uses Ankylosing spondylitis. Butacote should only be used where other therapies have been found unsuitable.

Dosage and administration The dosage selected should be as low as possible, and duration of treatment should be as short as possible; when long term treatment is unavoidable, special precautions should be taken (see Precautions), and the dosage should be adjusted to the needs of each patient taking account of the patient's age and general condition.

Butacote tablets should be swallowed whole with a meal together with liquid.

Adults: For the initial 48 hr 400–600 mg daily in divided doses. Thereafter, reduce to the minimum amount necessary, usually 200–300 mg daily in divided doses.

Elderly: In the elderly, always use the minimum effective dose (see Precautions).

Children: Not recommended for children under 14 years.

Contra-indications, warnings, etc
Contra-indications: History, however remote, of peptic ulcer, gastrointestinal haemorrhage, or blood dyscrasia. Haemorrhagic diathesis (thrombocytopenia, disorders of blood coagulation), severe cardiac, hepatic or renal insufficiency, oedema or hypertension, where there is danger of cardiac decompensation, thyroid disease, Sjogren's syndrome and previous adverse reactions to pyrazoles.

Like other non-steroidal anti-inflammatory agents, Butacote is also contra-indicated in asthmatic patients in whom attacks of asthma, urticaria or acute rhinitis are precipitated by acetylsalicylic acid or other drugs with prostaglandin synthetase inhibiting activity.

Last trimester of pregnancy.

Precautions and warnings: Like all potent drugs, Butacote should be used only under close medical supervision.

In elderly patients who are generally more prone to side-effects, particular caution should be exercised.

History of dyspepsia.

As blood dyscrasias may occur suddenly after a small dose, or insidiously after prolonged therapy, particularly in the elderly, blood counts should be monitored before and regularly during therapy, if it is anticipated that treatment may continue for more than one week. If significant changes occur e.g. decrease in leucocyte and/or platelet count or in the haematocrit, the drug should be withdrawn. Therapy should also be stopped if symptoms suggestive of these complications arise (e.g. bruising, fever, sore throat, rash, mouth ulceration) and patients should be advised accordingly.

Sodium retention and oedema may occur, and this should be considered in patients with cardiovascular disease.

Butacote may aggravate or acutely exacerbate systemic lupus erythematosus. If allergic reactions, fever, sore throat, salivary gland swelling or jaundice occur, or if blood appears in the stools, the medication should be discontinued at once.

Butacote should not be administered during the last 3 months of pregnancy, as it may lead to premature closure of the ductus arteriosus in the foetus. During the first six months of pregnancy, Butacote should be used with caution, especially in the first trimester, weighing the potential risks against the possible benefits. Since phenylbutazone passes into breast milk, albeit in small quantities, nursing mothers taking Butacote should not breast feed their infants.

Side-effects: Allergic reactions, rash and gastro-intestinal disorders (dyspepsia, epigastric pain, bleeding, recurrence of peptic ulcer) may occur. There have also been very occasional reports of headache, muzziness, nausea, vomiting, oedema due to sodium retention, stomatitis, salivary gland swelling, disturbances of vision, goitre, hepatitis, pancreatitis, and nephritis, and as rare complications, Stevens-Johnson syndrome, Lyells syndrome, leucopenia, thrombocytopenia, agranulocytosis and aplastic anaemia.

Isolated occurrences of an 'acute pulmonary syndrome' – marked by dyspnoea, fever, shadows in radiographs of the lungs and sometimes also by eosinophilia – have been reported. Although a causal relationship has not been proven, the drug should be withdrawn at first signs of this potentially serious syndrome, for the treatment of which corticosteroids and supportive cardiotherapy may be necessary.

Drug interactions: By competitively displacing them from their serum-protein binding sites, phenylbutazone may increase the activity and duration of effects of other drugs, e.g. other anti-inflammatory agents, oral anticoagulants, oral antidiabetic drugs, phenytoin and sulphonamides. Phenylbutazone may also accelerate the metabolism of dicoumarol, digitoxin and cortisone by inducing hepatic microsomal enzymes. Conversely it may inhibit the metabolic degradation of phenytoin and potentiate the effect of insulin. In patients previously treated with drugs which activate the hepatic microsomal enzyme system, e.g. barbiturates, chlorpheniramine, rifampicin, promethazine and corticosteroids (e.g. prednisone) the elimination half life of phenylbutazone is shortened. When phenylbutazone is given together with methylphenidate the serum concentration of metabolite oxyphenbutazone rises and the elimination half life of phenylbutazone is prolonged.

During concomitant administration of anabolic steroids and phenylbutazone, the serum concentration of metabolite oxyphenbutazone rises.

Since phenylbutazone may potentiate the effect of methotrexate, caution is indicated in cases where the two drugs are given concomitantly. Concomitant administration of cholestyramine reduces the enteral absorption of phenylbutazone. Phenylbutazone displaces thyroid hormone from its serum protein-binding sites and may thus make it more difficult to interpret tests of thyroid function.

When given together with lithium preparations, phenylbutazone causes increased tubular reabsorption of lithium, thereby raising the latter's serum concentration.

Overdosage: Where the recommended dosage has been appreciably exceeded, the following are the chief complications liable to be encountered: nausea, retching, gastro-intestinal pains or ulceration, respiratory depression, hypotension, coma, convulsions, hepatic and renal failure, thrombocytopenia, leucopenia and elevated transaminase values.

Treatment: Evacuation of the stomach (induction of vomiting, gastric lavage), and activated charcoal. If necessary, saline purgatives, artificial respiration, measures to support the circulation, anticonvulsants (e.g. diazepam iv) and haemodialysis. Haemoperfusion may be useful.

Pharmaceutical precautions Protect from heat and moisture.

Legal category POM.

Package quantities Containers of 100 and 500

Further information Butacote tablets are available through hospitals only.

Product licence number 0001/0024.

HYGROTON*

Presentation Pale yellow compressed tablets, containing 50 mg Chlorthalidone BP, approximately 7 mm diameter, flat with bevelled edges and impressed GEIGY on one side, breakline and ZA on the other.

Uses *Indications:* Hygroton is indicated for the treatment of mild to moderate hypertension. Hygroton is also indicated for the treatment of diabetes insipidus and oedema associated with cardiac failure, renal or hepatic disease.

Mode of action: Hygroton is a sulphonamide derivative. It exerts diuretic and antihypertensive effects by inhibiting the reabsorption of sodium, chloride and water, probably at the distal renal tubules. In renal diabetes insipidus, Hygroton paradoxically reduces polyuria.

Pharmacokinetics: Chlorthalidone is absorbed slowly with peak drug concentrations attained approximately 12 hours after ingestion. Chlorthalidone is extensively bound to carbonic anhydrase of erythrocytes, and the plasma and blood elimination half-life is approximately 50 hours. In response to repeated daily doses steady-state blood concentrations are achieved after 1–2 weeks. Chlorthalidone is excreted mainly in the urine in unchanged form.

After a single oral dose a marked salt and water diuresis is evident within 2 hours and a maximum effect reached within 12 hours. This natriuretic activity of Hygroton persists for 48–72 hours.

Dosage and administration The dosage of Hygroton should be individually titrated to give the lowest effective dose; this is particularly important in the elderly. Hygroton should be taken orally preferably as a single daily dose at breakfast time.

Adults: Hypertension: In mild to moderate hypertension, 25 mg daily increasing to 50 mg if necessary. If a further reduction in blood pressure is required, other antihypertensive therapy may be added to the dosage regime.

Oedema: Initially 100–200 mg on alternate days or if preferred, 50 mg daily; in severe cases, 100–200 mg daily may be given. A maintenance dose should be the minimum effective dose which may be as low as 50–100 mg three times a week.

Diabetes insipidus: Initially 100 mg twice daily but reducing where possible to a daily maintenance dose of 50 mg.

Use in children: A dosage of up to 2 mg/kg daily may be appropriate but is dependent on the diagnosis.

Use in the elderly: Chlorthalidone may be excreted more slowly in the elderly and therefore a reduction in the recommended adult dosage may be necessary. Particular caution should be exercised since the elderly are more susceptible to electrolyte imbalances (see 'Precautions').

Contra-indications, warnings, etc *Contra-indications:* Anuria, severe renal or hepatic insufficiency, hypersensitivity to chlorthalidone and other sulphonamide derivatives, refractory hypokalaemia and hyponatraemia, hypercalcaemia, symptomatic hyperuricaemia, untreated Addison's disease and concomitant lithium therapy.

Precautions: As with the use of other thiazide diuretics, glucose intolerance may occur; this is manifest as hyperglycaemia and glycosuria. Hygroton may very seldom aggravate or precipitate diabetes mellitus; this is usually reversible on stopping therapy.

Chlorthalidone can cause hyperuricaemia and thus provoke attacks of gout in predisposed patients. In cases where prolonged elevation of serum uric acid occurs, the concurrent use of a uricosuric agent will reverse the hyperuricaemia without loss of therapeutic effect.

As with other thiazide diuretics, Hygroton may cause disturbances in the serum electrolyte balance during prolonged treatment. Since the excretion of electrolytes is increased, a very strict low-salt diet should be avoided.

Periodic serum electrolyte determinations should be carried out, particularly in digitalised patients. If signs of potassium depletion occur, such as muscular weakness or cardiac arrhythmias, oral potassium supplements (16–40 mEq/day) should be used. Supplementary potassium medication is also indicated in cases where additional potassium loss occurs, such as vomiting, diarrhoea, malnutrition, nephrosis, hepatic cirrhosis, hyperaldosteronism or in patients receiving concomitant treatment with digitalis, glucorticoids or ACTH. Alternatively a potassium-sparing diuretic may be appropriate.

As with all antihypertensive agents, a cautious dosage schedule is indicated in patients with severe coronary or cerebral arteriosclerosis.

Since chlorthalidone is excreted largely unchanged in the urine, the drug may accumulate in patients with impaired renal function. At creatinine clearance levels of less than 30 ml/min (or at serum creatinine levels of greater than 2.5 mg/100 ml which is greater than or equal to 220 μmol/litre) chlorthalidone will not exert an adequate diuretic effect. In such cases, loop diuretics are indicated.

The elderly, in particularly those suffering from chronic disease and patients with hepatic cirrhosis, are very susceptible to electrolyte and fluid imbalance. There have been isolated reports of hyponatraemia with neurological symptoms (eg nausea, debility, progressive disorientation and apathy) following thiazide treatment. Serum electrolyte levels should be monitored particularly in the elderly and those with hepatic cirrhosis.

In patients with hyperlipidaemia, serum lipids should be monitored regularly. Withdrawal of Hygroton should be considered if serum lipids rise further.

Pregnancy and lactation: Diuretics are best avoided for the management of oedema or hypertension in pregnancy as their use may be associated with hypovolaemia, increased blood viscosity and reduced placental perfusion. There have been reports of foetal bone marrow depression, thrombocytopenia, and foetal and neonatal jaundice associated with the use of thiazide diuretics.

Chlorthalidone passes into the breast milk and thus mothers taking Hygroton should refrain from breast-feeding their infants.

Side-effects: Hygroton is generally well tolerated in the recommended dosage. The following unwanted effects may occur with higher dosages:

Electrolytes: Hypokalaemia, hyponatraemia, hypomagnesaemia. In isolated cases, hypochloraemic alkalosis and hypercalcaemia.

Skin: Allergic urticaria and other forms of skin rash, photosensitisation.

Liver: Rarely intrahepatic cholestasis or jaundice.

Cardiovascular system: Postural hypotension and cardiac arrhythmias.

Central nervous system: Dizziness and rarely, paraesthesia.

Gastrointestinal tract: Loss of appetite, mild nausea, vomiting, gastrospasm, diarrhoea or constipation, pancreatitis.

Metabolism: Hyperuricaemia, hyperglycaemia, glycosuria, worsening of glucose intolerance (see Precautions), elevated blood lipids.

Blood: Thrombocytopenia and rarely leucopenia, agranulocytosis and eosinophilia.

Other effects: Idiosyncratic effects (eg pulmonary oedema), and occasionally impotence and disturbances of vision.

Interactions: Diuretics potentiate the action of curare derivatives and antihypertensive drugs (eg guanethidine, methyldopa, beta-blockers, vasodilators, calcium antagonists and ACE inhibitors).

The hypokalaemic effect of diuretics may be potentiated by corticosteroids, ACTH, amphotericin and carbenoxolone.

It may prove necessary to adjust the dosage of insulin and oral anti-diabetic agents.

Hypokalaemia or hypomagnesaemia possibly occurring as unwanted effects may cause onset of digitalis-induced cardiac arrhythmias.

Concomitant administration of certain non-steroidal anti-inflammatory drugs (eg indomethacin) may reduce the diuretic and antihypertensive activity of Hygroton; there have been isolated reports of a deterioration in renal function in predisposed patients.

Overdosage: Symptoms: Dizziness, nausea, somnolence, hypovolaemia, hypotension and electrolyte disturbances associated with cardiac arrhythmias and muscle spasms.

Treatment: There is no specific antidote to Hygroton. Gastric lavage, emesis or activated charcoal should be employed to reduce absorption. Blood pressure and fluid and electrolyte balance should be monitored and appropriate corrective measures taken. Intravenous fluid and electrolyte replacement may be indicated.

Pharmaceutical precautions None.

Legal category POM.

Package quantities Tablets 50 mg: Containers of 100 and 500.

Further information Nil.

Product licence number 0001/5011

HYGROTON K*

Presentation Round, red, sugar coated tablets of approximately 11.3 mm diameter and imprinted GEIGY on one side, containing 25 mg Chlorthalidone BP and 500 mg Potassium Chloride BP–6.7 mEq K (controlled release).

Hygroton-K also contains lactose, gluten (wheat starch), sucrose and azo-dyes.

Uses *Mode of action:* Hygroton K contains a diuretic (chlorthalidone) in combination with a potassium chloride core. Chlorthalidone is a sulphonamide derivative. It exerts a diuretic effect by inhibiting the reabsorption of sodium, chloride and water, probably at the distal renal tubules.

Indications: Hygroton K is for use only when diuretic therapy in combination with potassium supplementation is indicated.

Hygroton K may be used in the treatment of:

- Mild to moderate hypertension.
- Oedema associated with cardiac failure, renal or hepatic disease.

Pharmacokinetics: Chlorthalidone is absorbed relatively slowly with peak drug concentrations attained approximately 12 hours after ingestion. Chlorthalidone is extensively bound to carbonic anhydrase of erythrocytes, and the plasma and blood elimination half-life is approximately 50 hours. In response to repeated daily doses steady-state blood concentrations are achieved after 1–2 weeks. Chlorthalidone is excreted mainly in the urine in unchanged form.

After a single oral dose a marked salt and water diuresis is evident within 2 hours and a maximum effect reached within 12 hours. This natriuretic activity of Hygroton K persists for 48–72 hours.

Potassium chloride is contained in a specially formulated matrix and its release is largely independent of local pH within the gastrointestinal tract. During its passage through the gastro-intestinal tract, the potassium chloride is slowly and steadily released and completely absorbed. In subjects with a normal potassium balance, approximately 90% of the potassium thus administered is excreted in the urine.

Dosage and administration The dosage should be individually adjusted according to the clinical picture and patient response. Hygroton K may be given as a single daily dose, preferably in the morning, or in divided doses. During long-term therapy the lowest effective dosage should be employed, particularly in the elderly. Hygroton K tablets should be swallowed whole with a glass of water and not chewed.

Adults

Hypertension: In mild to moderate hypertension, 1 tablet daily. If necessary 1 tablet may be given twice daily. If a further reduction in blood pressure is required, other antihypertensive therapy may be added to the dosage regimen.

Oedema: Initially, conventional chlorthalidone in doses of 100–200 mg on alternate days or if preferred, 50 mg daily (see separate data sheet). The patient should then be transferred to a maintenance dose of Hygroton K, usually 2 to 4 tablets, three times a week or 1 to 2 tablets daily.

Use in children: Hygroton K is contra-indicated for use in children.

Use in the elderly: Chlorthalidone may be excreted more slowly in the elderly and therefore a reduction in the recommended adult dosage may be necessary. Particular caution should be exercised since the elderly are more susceptible to electrolyte imbalances (see 'Precautions').

Contra-indications, warnings, etc *Contra-indications:* Anuria, severe renal or hepatic failure, hypersensitivity to chlorthalidone or other sulphonamide derivatives, refractory hypokalaemia and hyponatraemia, hypercalcaemia, symptomatic hyperuricaemia, untreated Addison's disease and concomitant lithium therapy.

Solid dosage forms of potassium salts are contra-indicated in patients suffering from inflammation or obstruction of the oesophagus or gastro-intestinal tract and in cases of hyperkalaemia.

Pregnancy and lactation: Hygroton K is contra-indicated in pregnant or nursing mothers.

Warnings: If severe nausea, vomiting, persistent abdominal pain, flatulence or diarrhoea occur or if gastro-intestinal ulceration or haemorrhage is suspected, Hygroton K should be withdrawn at once until a definitive diagnosis has been made.

Hygroton K alone is not considered to be effective therapy for hypokalaemia from any cause.

Hygroton K should not be given concomitantly with either potassium-sparing diuretics or ACE inhibitors due to the possibility of provoking hyperkalaemia.

Precautions: As with thiazide diuretics, disturbances in the serum electrolyte balance may occur during treatment, especially in patients with liver cirrhosis, digitalised patients and the elderly. Periodic serum electrolyte determinations should be carried out. If there is evidence of clinically significant hypokalaemia, if signs of potassium depletion occur, or if additional potassium loss occurs, (due to vomiting, diarrhoea, malnutrition, nephrosis, liver cirrhosis, hyperaldosteronism or due to treatment with ACTH, or glucocorticoids), additional potassium supplementation will need to be given under surveillance.

Chlorthalidone can cause hyperuricaemia and thus provoke attacks of gout in predisposed patients. In cases where prolonged elevation of serum uric acid occurs, the concurrent use of a uricosuric agent will reverse the hyperuricaemia without loss of therapeutic effect. As with the use of thiazide diuretics, glucose intolerance may occur; this is manifest as hyperglycaemia and glycosuria. Hygroton K may very seldom aggravate or precipitate diabetes mellitus; this is usually reversible on stopping therapy. In patients with hyperlipidaemia, serum lipids should be monitored regularly. In the event of a further rise in serum lipids, withdrawal of Hygroton K should be considered.

As with all antihypertensive agents a cautious dosage schedule is indicated in patients with severe coronary or cerebral arteriosclerosis.

Since chlorthalidone is excreted largely unchanged in the urine, the drug may accumulate in patients with impaired renal function. At creatinine clearance levels of < 30 ml/min (or at serum creatinine levels of > 2.5 mg/100 ml = > 221 μmol/litre) chlorthalidone will not exert an adequate diuretic effect. In extreme cases, an oliguric crisis can occur, when the drug should be stopped; in such cases, loop diuretics may be indicated.

Drug interactions: Diuretics potentiate the action of curare derivatives and antihypertensive drugs (eg guanethidine, methyldopa, beta-blockers, vasodilators, calcium antagonists). Combined treatment with potassium-containing diuretics or ACE inhibitors may lead to potassium retention.

The hypokalaemic effect of diuretics may be potentiated by corticosteroids, ACTH, amphotericin and carbenoxolone.

It may prove necessary to adjust the dosage of insulin and oral antidiabetic agents.

Hypokalaemia or hypomagnesaemia possibly occurring as unwanted effects may favour the onset of digitalis-induced cardiac arrhythmias.

Concomitant administration of certain non-steroidal anti-inflammatory drugs (eg indomethacin) may reduce the diuretic and antihypertensive activity of diuretics; there have been isolated reports of a deterioration in renal function in predisposed patients.

Side-effects: Hygroton K is generally well tolerated at the recommended dosage. However, the following side effects may occasionally be observed, particularly with higher doses:

Electrolytes: Hypokalaemia (e.g. muscular weakness, cardiac arrhythmias or corresponding ECG changes), hyponatraemia (usually accompanied by neurological symptoms e.g. nausea, debility, progressive disorientation, apathy), hypomagnesaemia (e.g. nervousness, muscle spasms and cardiac arrhythmias). In isolated cases, hypochloraemic alkalosis and hypercalcaemia. If hypercalcaemia occurs, further diagnostic clarification is necessary (e.g. possibility of hyperparathyroidism).

Skin: Allergic urticaria (nettle rash) and other forms of skin rash, photosensitisation.

Liver: In rare cases intrahepatic cholestasis or jaundice.

Cardiovascular system: Postural hypotension and cardiac arrhythmias; postural hypotension may be aggravated by alcohol, anaesthetics or sedatives.

Central nervous system: Dizziness and rarely, paraesthesia.

Gastro-intestinal tract: Loss of appetite, mild nausea, vomiting, gastrospasm, diarrhoea or possibly constipation, pancreatitis. Rarely, solid dosage forms of potassium salts may lead to haemorrhage, ulceration and cicatricial stenosis in the gastro-intestinal tract (see Warnings).

Metabolism: Hyperuricaemia, hyperglycaemia, glycosuria, gout or diabetes may be precipitated or aggravated (see Precautions). Increased blood lipids in response to higher doses.

Blood: Thrombocytopenia. In isolated cases: leucopenia, agranulocytosis and eosinophilia.

Other effects: Idiosyncratic effects (eg pulmonary oedema), and occasionally impotence and disturbances of vision.

Overdosage

Signs and symptoms: The following may occur: anorexia, nausea, vomiting, diarrhoea, profound diuresis, dehydration, dizziness and hypotension.

Treatment: Treatment should be symptomatic and directed at correction of fluid loss and electrolyte balance. In acute overdosage, gastric lavage should be performed and ECG and electrolyte monitoring instituted. The potassium content may cause hyperkalaemia with associated cardiac arrhythmias and muscular hypotonia and management should be dictated by serial potassium levels. If this is less than 6.5 mEq/l then fluid replacement with intravenous glucose/saline is usually sufficient. For levels above 6.5 mEq/l, ECG changes occurring in order of severity include: – tenting of T waves, diminution of P waves, widening of the QRS complex and slurring of the ST segment. Active measures to lower potassium levels including administration of intravenous glucose/insulin and oral ion exchange resins should be instituted. If the level is greater than 8 mEq/l an intravenous injection of 10–30 mls of 10% calcium gluconate should be given in addition to the previous measures and dialysis considered.

Chronic administration may cause significant electrolyte disturbance. Hypokalaemia may occur if diuresis is significant with associated cardiac arrhythmias and impaired urinary concentrating ability due to hypokalaemic nephropathy. Potassium levels should be monitored and if below 3.5 mEq/l, consideration given to potassium supplements or cessation of therapy.

Pharmaceutical precautions Protect from heat and moisture.

Legal category POM.

Package quantities Containers of 100 and 250 tablets.

Further information The potassium chloride in Hygroton K is dispersed in a matrix. After the potassium chloride is completely absorbed, the undissolved matrix may be excreted in a softened form in the faeces.

Product licence number 0001/0059R.

LAMPRENE*

Presentation Red-brown, soft gelatin capsules each containing 100 mg of the active substance, clofazimine. Lamprene is presented as a microcrystalline suspension in an oil-wax base.

The capsules also contain the sodium salts of ethyl hydroxybenzoate and propyl hydroxybenzoate.

Uses

Mode of action: Lamprene exerts a bacteriostatic and mild bactericidal effect on *Mycobacterium leprae* (Hansen's bacillus). Lamprene also possesses anti-inflammatory properties. No cross-resistance occurs between Lamprene and either dapsone or rifampicin.

Indications: Lamprene, given in combination with dapsone and rifampicin, can be used to treat the multibacillary forms of leprosy. These include lepromatous, borderline lepromatous and mid-borderline leprosy. In addition, this combination of drugs may be used to treat the lepra reaction, erythema nodosum leprosum. Combined chemotherapy should be employed to prevent the emergence of resistant strains of *M. leprae*.

Pharmacokinetics: Lamprene is absorbed rather slowly, with peak plasma concentrations of unchanged active substance reached 8–12 hours after a single oral dose. The bioavailability of the drug increases if given with food.

In patients with leprosy, minimal plasma concentrations of Lamprene were 910 pmol/g, 42 days after daily treatment with 100 mg; steady state conditions were not reached at this time. The calculated elimination half-life is 15–20 days.

Lamprene is strongly lipophilic and accumulates primarily in fatty tissue and in macrophages of the reticulo-endothelial system. Lamprene has not been found in the brain, even after prolonged treatment.

Lamprene is excreted mainly in the faeces. An average of 35% (range of 9–74%) of the administered dose was recovered within 3 days, some of which may be attributable to biliary excretion of the drug.

Dosage and administration Lamprene should be taken at meal-times or together with milk.

Lamprene should be used in combination with rifampicin and dapsone. The following dosage regimen is recommended by the World Health Organisation:

Adults: The dosage of Lamprene should be adjusted according to body weight, but for adults weighing approximately 60 kg, the following doses are recommended:

For the treatment of multibacillary forms of leprosy:
Lamprene: 300 mg once a month under surveillance and 100 mg once every 2 days.
Rifampicin: 600 mg once a month under surveillance.
Dapsone: 100 mg once a day.

This combined therapy should be given for at least 2 years, and whenever possible, until such time the skin smears become negative.

For the treatment of erythema nodosum leprosum:
Lamprene: a maximum of 300 mg once a day for not longer than 3 months.
Rifampicin: 600 mg once a month under surveillance.
Dapsone: 100 mg once a day.

Elderly: Clinical evidence would indicate that no special dosage regime is necessary but concurrent renal or hepatic insufficiency should be taken into account.

Children: Children should receive lower doses according to their body weight.

Contra-indications, warnings, etc
Use in pregnancy and lactation: Unless the use of the drug is thought essential, Lamprene should not be administered during pregnancy and lactation. Embryotoxicity has been shown at high doses in animals. Lamprene crosses the placental barrier, and is also excreted in breast milk; new-born infants of women under treatment may therefore show relatively pronounced discolouration due to the drug.

Contra-indications: Hypersensitivity to clofazimine.

Precautions: Lamprene should not be used to treat leprosy patients suffering from repeated attacks of abdominal pain and diarrhoea, or in patients with renal or hepatic damage, unless absolutely necessary.

Patients should be kept under medical supervision when treated with daily doses of Lamprene exceeding 100 mg; this dosage should not be continued for longer than 3 months.

If gastro-intestinal symptoms develop during treatment, the dosage should be reduced or the interval between doses, prolonged. Patients suffering from persistent diarrhoea or vomiting should be confined to hospital.

Side-effects: The following side-effects have been observed:

Dryness of the skin, ichthyosis, pruritus, photosensitivity, acneform eruptions and non-specific skin rashes. Nausea, vomiting, abdominal pains, diarrhoea, anorexia, loss of weight and eosinophilic enteropathy.

Reddish to dark-brown discolouration of the skin and of leprous lesions, particularly in lighter-skinned patients at sites exposed to light; discolouration of the hair, the conjunctiva and cornea, lacrimal fluid, sweat, sputum, urine and faeces. This discolouration is reversible, although skin discolouration may only disappear some months after stopping treatment.

Overdosage: There is no specific antidote to Lamprene overdose and treatment is symptomatic.

Pharmaceutical precautions Protect from heat and moisture.

Legal category POM.

Package quantities Capsules: Containers of 100.

Further information Nil.

Product licence number 0001/5041.

LOPRESOR*

Presentation The active ingredient metoprolol tartrate is presented as: pale red, round, slightly biconvex, film-coated tablets with slightly bevelled edges: approximately 9 mm diameter, engraved GEIGY on one side and scored on the other side. Each tablet contains 50 mg.

Lopresor is also available as: light blue, round, slightly biconvex, film-coated tablets with slightly bevelled edges: approximately 10 mm diameter, engraved GEIGY on one side and scored on the other. Each tablet contains 100 mg. The 100 mg tablets also contain indigocarmine.

Uses Beta-adrenergic receptor blocking agent.

Indications: Hypertension and angina pectoris, cardiac arrhythmias, especially supraventricular tachyarrhythmias.

Adjunct to treatment of thyrotoxicosis.

Early intervention with Lopresor in acute myocardial infarction reduces infarct size and the incidence of ventricular fibrillation. Pain relief may also decrease the need for opiate analgesics.

Lopresor has been shown to reduce mortality when administered to patients with acute myocardial infarction.

Prophylaxis of migraine.

Dosage and administration *Administration:* Lopresor tablets should be administered orally and swallowed unchewed.

Dosage: The dose must always be adjusted to the individual requirements of the patient. The following are guidelines.

Adults: Hypertension: Initially a dose of 100 mg per day should be prescribed either as single or divided doses.

Depending upon the response the dosage may be increased by 100 mg per day at weekly intervals to 400 mg daily given in single or divided doses. Over the dosage range most patients may be expected to respond rapidly and satisfactorily. A further reduction in blood pressure may be achieved if Lopresor is used in conjunction with an antihypertensive diuretic or other hypotensive agent.

Lopresor may be administered with benefit both to previously untreated patients with hypertension and to those in whom the response to previous therapy is inadequate. In the latter type of patient the previous therapy may be continued and Lopresor added in to the regime with adjustment of the previous therapy if necessary.

Angina pectoris: 50–100 mg, twice or three times daily.

In general a significant improvement in exercise tolerance and reduction of anginal attacks may be expected with a dose of 50–100 mg twice daily.

Cardiac arrhythmias: A dosage of 50 mg two or three times daily is usually sufficient. If necessary the dose can be increased up to 300 mg per day administered in divided doses.

If the treatment has been initiated with metoprolol injection continuation therapy with Lopresor tablets should be initiated 4–6 hours later. In such cases, the initial oral dose should not exceed 50 mg three times daily.

Hyperthyroidism: 50 mg four times daily. The dosage should be progressively reduced as euthyroid state is slowly achieved.

Myocardial infarction: Early intervention.

Oral therapy should commence 15 minutes after administration of metoprolol injection, at a dose of 50 mg every 6 hours for 48 hours. Patients who fail to tolerate intravenous therapy should be given half the suggested oral dose.

Maintenance: The usual maintenance dose is 200 mg daily.

Prophylaxis of migraine: 100–200 mg daily, given in divided doses (morning and evening).

Elderly: There is no evidence to suggest that dosage requirements are different in otherwise healthy elderly patients. However, caution is indicated in elderly patients as an excessively pronounced decrease in blood pressure or pulse rate may cause the blood supply to vital organs to fall to inadequate levels.

In patients with significant hepatic dysfunction the lower dosage recommendations will be more appropriate.

Children: Not recommended.

Contra-indications, warnings, etc

Contra-indications: Known hypersensitivity to metoprolol and related derivatives, severe asthma, atrioventricular block of second or third degree, uncontrolled heart failure, clinically relevant sinus bradycardia, sick-sinus syndrome, severe peripheral arterial disease, cardiogenic shock. Metoprolol is also contra-indicated when myocardial infarction is complicated by significant bradycardia, first degree heart block, systolic hypotension (less than 100 mmHg) and/or severe heart failure.

Precautions: Metoprolol may aggravate bradycardia, symptoms of peripheral arterial circulatory disorders and anaphylactic shock.

Abrupt cessation of therapy with a beta-blocker should be avoided. When possible, Lopresor should be withdrawn gradually over a period of 10 days, the doses diminishing to 25 mg for the last 6 days. During its withdrawal the patient should be kept under close surveillance.

Lopresor may be administered when heart failure has been controlled. Digitalisation and/or diuretic therapy should also be considered for patients with a history of heart failure or patients known to have a poor cardiac reserve.

Although cardioselective beta-blockers may have less effect on lung function than non selective beta-blockers these should be avoided in patients with reversible obstructive airways disease unless there are compelling clinical reasons for their use. Therapy with a beta$_2$-stimulant may become necessary or current therapy require adjustment.

In labile and insulin-dependent diabetes it may be necessary to adjust the hypoglycaemic therapy.

In patients with a phaeochromocytoma, an alpha-blocker should be given concomitantly.

In patients with significant hepatic dysfunction it may be necessary to adjust the dosage because metoprolol undergoes biotransformation in the liver.

The addition of adrenaline to patients undergoing beta-blockade can result in an increase in blood pressure and bradycardia although this is less likely to occur with beta$_1$-selective drugs.

Lopresor should be given cautiously to patients with metabolic acidosis.

Lopresor therapy should be brought to the attention of the anaesthetist prior to general anaesthesia. In a patient under beta-blockade, the anaesthetic selected should be one exhibiting as little negative inotropic activity as possible (halothane/nitrous oxide).

Use during pregnancy and lactation: Lopresor should not be used in pregnancy or lactation unless it is considered that the benefit outweighs the possible risk to the foetus/infant. Metoprolol has, however, been used in pregnancy associated hypertension under close supervision after 20 weeks gestation. Although the drug crosses the placental barrier and is present in cord blood no evidence of foetal abnormalities have been reported. Animal experiments have shown neither teratogenic potential nor other adverse events on the embryo and/or foetus relevant to the safety assessment of the product.

The amount of metoprolol ingested via breast milk seems to be negligible with regard to its beta-blocking effects if the mother is treated in doses within the therapeutic range.

If Lopresor is used during pregnancy and lactation special attention should be paid to the foetus, neonate and breast fed infant for undesirable effects of the drug's beta-blocking action (e.g. bradycardia, hypoglycaemia).

Drug interactions: The effects of metoprolol and other antihypertensive drugs on blood pressure are usually additive, and care should be taken to avoid hypotension. As with all beta-blockers particular caution is called for when metoprolol is administered together with prazosin for the first time. However, combinations of antihypertensive drugs may often be used with benefit to improve control of hypertension.

Metoprolol can reduce myocardial contractility and impair intracardiac conduction. Care should be exercised when drugs with similar activity e.g. antiarrhythmic agents, general anaesthetics, are given concurrently. Like all other beta-blockers, metoprolol should not be given in combination with verapamil since this may cause bradycardia, hypotension and asystole.

Care should also be exercised when beta-blockers are given in combination with sympathetic ganglion blocking agents, other beta-blockers (also in the form of eye drops) or MAO inhibitors.

If combination treatment with clonidine is to be discontinued metoprolol should be withdrawn several days before clonidine.

As beta-blockers may affect the peripheral circulation, care should be exercised when drugs with similar activity e.g. ergotamine are given concurrently.

Metoprolol will antagonise the beta$_1$ effects of sympathomimetic agents but should have little influence on the bronchodilator effects of beta$_2$-agonists at normal therapeutic doses.

Enzyme inducing agents (e.g. rifampicin) may reduce plasma concentrations of metoprolol, whereas enzyme inhibitors (e.g. cimetidine) may increase plasma concentrations.

During concomitant ingestion of alcohol and metoprolol the concentration of blood alcohol may reach higher levels and may decrease more slowly.

Metoprolol may impair the elimination of lignocaine.

Indomethacin may reduce the antihypertensive effect of beta-blockers.

Side-effects:

Central and peripheral nervous system: Occasionally fatigue, dizziness, headache. Rarely paraesthesiae, muscle cramps, depression, decreased mental alertness, somnolence or insomnia, nightmares. In isolated cases personality disorder.

Cardiovascular system: Occasionally bradycardia, postural disorders (occasionally with syncope). Rarely heart failure, cardiac arrhythmias, oedema, palpitation, Raynaud's phenomenon. In isolated cases disturbances of cardiac conduction, precordial pain, gangrene in patients with pre-existing severe peripheral circulatory disorders.

Gastro-intestinal tract: Occasionally nausea and vomiting, abdominal pain. Rarely diarrhoea or constipation. In isolated cases dryness of the mouth, liver function test abnormalities.

Skin and appendages: Rarely skin rash (in the form of urticaria, psoriasiform and dystrophic skin lesions), occurrence of antinuclear antibodies (not associated with SLE). In isolated cases photosensitivity, increased sweating, loss of hair.

Respiratory tract: Occasionally exertional dyspnoea. Rarely bronchospasm, also in patients without a history of obstructive lung disease. In isolated cases rhinitis.

Endocrine system and metabolism: In isolated cases weight gain.

Urogenital system: There are isolated reports on disturbances of libido and potency.

Sense organs: In isolated cases disturbances of vision, dry and/or irritated eyes, tinnitus.

Blood: In isolated cases thrombocytopenia.

The reported incidence of skin rashes and/or dry eyes associated with the use of beta-blockers is small and in most cases the symptoms have cleared when treatment was withdrawn. Discontinuation of the drug should be considered if any such reaction is not otherwise explicable.

Overdosage:

Signs: In more severe cases an overdosage of metoprolol may lead to severe hypotension, sinus bradycardia, atrioventricular block, heart failure, cardiogenic shock, cardiac arrest, bronchospasm, impairment of consciousness, coma, nausea, vomiting, cyanosis, hypoglycaemia and occasionally hyperkalaemia. The first manifestations usually appear 20 minutes to 2 hours after drug ingestion.

Treatment: Treatment should include close monitoring of cardiovascular, respiratory and renal functions, and blood glucose and electrolytes. Further absorption may be prevented by induction of vomiting, gastric lavage or administration of activated charcoal if ingestion is recent. Cardiovascular complications should be treated symptomatically which may require the use of sympathomimetic agents (e.g. noradrenaline, metaraminol), atropine or inotropic agents (e.g. dopamine, dobutamine). Temporary pacing may be required for AV block. Glucagon can reverse the effects of excessive beta-blockade given in a dose of 1–10 mg intravenously. Intravenous $beta_2$-stimulants may be required to relieve bronchospasm. Metoprolol cannot be effectively removed by haemodialysis.

Pharmaceutical precautions *Storage:* Protect from moisture.

Legal category POM.

Package quantities *Lopresor 50 mg:* Securitainers of 100 tablets.
Lopresor 100 mg: Securitainers of 100 tablets. Calendar packs of 56 tablets.

Further information Metoprolol is well absorbed after oral administration, peak plasma concentrations occurring 1.5–2 hours after dosing. The bioavailability of a single dose is approximately 50%, increasing to approximately 70% during repeated administration. The bioavailability also increases if metoprolol is given with food.

Elimination is mainly by hepatic metabolism and the average elimination half-life is 3.5 hours (range 1 to 9 hours). Rates of metabolism vary between individuals, with poor metabolisers (approximately 10%) showing higher plasma concentrations and slower elimination than extensive metabolisers. Within individuals, however, plasma concentrations are stable and reproducible.

Because of variation in rates of metabolism, the dose of metoprolol should always be adjusted to the individual requirements of the patient. As the therapeutic response, adverse effects and relative cardioselectivity are related to plasma concentration, poor metabolisers may require lower than normal doses. Dosage adjustment is not routinely required in the elderly or in patients with renal failure, but dosage may need to be reduced in patients with significant hepatic dysfunction when metoprolol elimination may be impaired.

Product licence numbers

Tablets 50 mg	0001/0065
Tablets 100 mg	0001/0066

LOPRESOR* SR

Presentation The active ingredient metoprolol tartrate is presented as pale yellow, round, film-coated tablets with slightly convex faces; approximately 10.1 mm diameter, imprinted GEIGY on one side and CDC on the other. Each tablet contains 200 mg metoprolol tartrate in a sustained release formulation.

Uses Selective beta-adrenergic receptor blocking agent.

Indications: Hypertension and angina pectoris. Prophylaxis of migraine.

Dosage and administration *Administration:* Lopresor SR tablets should be administered orally.

Dosage: Hypertension: Initially one Lopresor SR tablet should be given in the morning. Most patients may be expected to respond satisfactorily within 14 days to one or two tablets once daily. Further antihypertensive effect may be achieved by the addition of a diuretic such as chlorthalidone or a vasodilator such as hydralazine.

Lopresor SR may be administered with benefit to both previously untreated patients with hypertension and to those in whom the response to previous therapy is inadequate. In the latter type of patient therapy may be continued and Lopresor SR added to the regime with adjustment of previous therapy if necessary.

Angina pectoris: Initially, one Lopresor SR tablet daily. The dose may be increased to two tablets once daily if required. In general a significant improvement in exercise tolerance and a reduction of anginal attacks may be expected with a dose of one Lopresor SR tablet daily.

Prophylaxis of migraine: One tablet daily given in the morning.

Use in the elderly: There is no evidence to suggest that dosage requirements are different in the elderly.

Contra-indications, warnings, etc
Contra-indications: Atrioventricular block of second or third degree, uncontrolled heart failure, severe bradycardia, cardiogenic shock, severe asthma.

Precautions: Although cardioselective beta-blockers may have less effect on lung function than non selective beta-blockers, as with all beta-blockers these should be avoided in patients with reversible obstructive airways disease unless there are compelling clinical reasons for their use. Therapy with a beta-2-stimulant may become necessary or current therapy require adjustment.

Lopresor SR must not be used in patients with untreated heart failure, but may be administered when the failure has been brought under control. Where heart failure appears during treatment with Lopresor SR the drug may be temporarily withdrawn until the failure has been controlled.

Lopresor SR may mask some of the symptoms of hypoglycaemia. Since treatment with a beta-blocker may affect carbohydrate metabolism, it may be necessary to adjust the dose of the hypoglycaemic agent in labile and insulin dependent diabetics.

Lopresor SR should be given cautiously to patients with metabolic acidosis.

Lopresor SR therapy should be brought to the attention of the anaesthetist prior to general anaesthesia. In a patient under beta-blockade, the anaesthetic selected should be one exhibiting as little negative inotropic activity as possible, (e.g. halothane/nitrous oxide).

There have been reports of skin rash and/or dry eyes associated with the use of beta-adrenergic blocking drugs. The reported incidence is small and in most cases the symptoms have cleared when treatment was withdrawn. Discontinuance of the beta-adrenoceptor blocking drug should be considered if any such reaction is not otherwise explicable. Cessation of therapy with a beta-blocker should be gradual.

Like other beta-blockers, Lopresor SR should not be given in combination with antiarrhythmic agents of the verapamil type because their concomitant use may result in bradycardia, hypotension or even cardiac arrest.

If it becomes necessary to discontinue treatment with a beta-blocker, one should withdraw the drug gradually i.e. over a period of 8–10 days, because abrupt interruption of the medication – particularly in cases of ischaemic heart disease – may be followed by an acute deterioration in the patient's condition.

Pregnancy: The administration of Lopresor SR during pregnancy as with other drugs is advised only if there are compelling reasons. If Lopresor SR is used during pregnancy and lactation special attention should be paid to the foetus, neonate and breast fed infant for undesirable effects of the drug's beta-blocking action (e.g. slowing of heart rate).

Side-effects: Gastro-intestinal upsets, sleep disturbances and exertional tiredness may occasionally occur. In most cases these effects have been transient or have disappeared after a reduction in dosage. In rare cases, feelings of coldness in the extremities may occur.

As with other beta-blockers excessive bradycardia may occasionally occur, bronchospasm and heart failure may occasionally be precipitated in susceptible patients.

Overdosage: The symptoms of overdosage will be marked bradycardia and possible hypotension.

Bradycardia may be overcome by the administration of intravenous atropine sulphate (0.25–2.0 mg) which will decrease vagal tone. If bradycardia persists, sympathomimetic drugs such as metaraminol or noradrenaline should be employed. These drugs have a pressor effect which may also help to overcome hypotension. The positive inotropic and chronotropic properties of glucagon may be useful when it is given in doses of 1–5 mg (maximum 10 mg).

Pharmaceutical precautions No special precautions.

Legal category POM.

Package quantities Lopresor SR packs of 28 tablets (2 × 14 calendar pack foils) (OP).

Further information Lopresor SR is a sustained release preparation of Lopresor (metoprolol tartrate) designed to release this selective beta-adrenergic receptor blocking drug so that maximal response is obtained within 4–6 hours while the pharmacological action is sustained for 24 hours. This formulation reduces peak serum concentration which, in turn, minimises unwanted side-effects of beta-blockade.

Lopresor SR is a cardioselective beta-adrenergic blocking agent. It has relatively greater blocking effects on β_1 receptors (i.e. those mediating adrenergic stimulation of heart rate and contractility and release of free fatty acids from fat stores) than on β_2 receptors which are chiefly involved in broncho- and vasodilation.

Lopresor SR therefore possesses the therapeutically desirable effect of shielding the heart and blood vessels from the harmful effects of extensive adrenergic challenge during stress or exercise with minimal interference with respiratory function or vascular tone.

In hypertension, Lopresor SR is effective during the first few days of treatment and reaches its full effect in fourteen days. No orthostatic hypotension or tendency has been observed even with fairly high doses.

Because of its cardioselectivity, Lopresor SR may be administered even to patients with obstructive respiratory disorders, provided that adequate precautions are taken.

Product licence number 0001/0081.

LOPRESORETIC*

Presentation Off-white, round, bi-convex film-coated tablets with slightly bevelled edges, approximately 10 mm diameter, with a breakline on one face and GEIGY impressed on the other. Each tablet contains metoprolol tartrate (active ingredient of Lopresor*) 100 mg and Chlorthalidone BP (active ingredient of Hygroton*) 12.5 mg.

Uses Antihypertensive agent.

Principal therapeutic actions: Lopresor (metoprolol tartrate) is a beta-adrenergic receptor blocking agent which is relatively more selective for beta-1-receptors which mediate heart rate and force of contraction, free fatty acid release and renin production, than for beta-2-receptors which mediate bronchodilation and peripheral vascular dilation. Consequently Lopresor protects the heart and cardiovascular system from excessive sympathetic stimulation caused by either physical or emotional activity while having relatively little effect on the airways or on peripheral vascular responses. The attenuation of the effects of excessive sympathetic drive on the heart result in a fall in myocardial work and oxygen consumption. Systolic pressure is reduced and this is most noticeable in hypertensive subjects, in whom the diastolic pressure is also reduced significantly.

Hygroton (chlorthalidone BP) is a long acting diuretic which lowers both systolic and diastolic pressures in hypertensive patients. In general the higher the initial blood pressure, the greater the fall brought about by Hygroton. The addition of Hygroton enhances the antihypertensive effect of the selective beta-blocker thus resulting in a better control in a higher proportion of patients. This is probably the result of the two active ingredients having different sites of action, Lopresor acting on the heart and possibly also centrally while Hygroton reduces peripheral resistance.

Indications: In the treatment of mild and moderate hypertension.

Dosage and administration *Dosage:* Lopresoretic tablets should be administered orally. Initial starting dose, one tablet in the morning. However, in patients who have not been successfully controlled by a diuretic or beta-blocking drug used alone, a dose of two tablets in the morning would be appropriate. Most patients may be expected to respond within 14 days.

Occasionally the response may be unsatisfactory in which case it may be found beneficial to raise the dosage to 3–4 tablets given in single or divided doses and/or to add a vasodilator such as hydralazine at an initial dose of 25 mg twice daily, increasing as necessary.

Use in the elderly: No specific information available.

Contra-indications, warnings, etc
Contra-indications: Atrioventricular block of second or third degree, uncontrolled heart failure, severe bradycardia, cardiogenic shock and marked renal insufficiency. Severe asthma. Anti-diuretic effect has been reported following concomitant treatment with diuretics and lithium. As with all products which contain diuretics, Lopresoretic tablets are contra-indicated during lithium therapy.

Precautions: Although cardioselective beta-blockers may have less effect on lung function than non-selective beta-blockers, as with all beta-blockers these should be avoided in patients with reversible obstructive airways disease unless there are compelling clinical reasons for their use. Therapy with a beta-2-stimulant may become necessary or current therapy require adjustment.

As with other preparations containing beta-blockers, Lopresoretic tablets must not be used in patients with untreated heart failure, but may be administered when the failure has been brought under control. Where heart failure appears during treatment with Lopresoretic the drug may be temporarily withdrawn until the failure has been controlled.

Lopresoretic may mask some of the symptoms of hypoglycaemia. Since treatment with a beta-blocker may affect carbohydrate metabolism, it may be necessary to adjust the dose of the hypoglycaemic agent in labile and insulin dependent diabetics. Chlorthalidone may also decrease glucose tolerance.

Hyperuricaemia may occasionally occur and acute attacks of gout may be precipitated. Where prolonged elevation of serum uric acid occurs the concurrent use of a uricosuric agent will reverse the hyperuricaemia without loss of therapeutic effect.

Lopresoretic tablets should be given cautiously to patients with metabolic acidosis.

Lopresoretic therapy should be brought to the attention of the anaesthetist prior to general anaesthesia. In a patient under beta-blockade, the anaesthetic selected should be one exhibiting as little negative inotropic activity as possible, (e.g. halothane/nitrous oxide).

If it becomes necessary to discontinue treatment with a beta-blocker one should withdraw the drug gradually i.e. over a period of 8–10 days, because abrupt interruption of the medication – particularly in cases of ischaemic heart disease – may be followed by an acute deterioration in the patient's condition.

Like other beta-blockers, Lopresoretic should not be given in combination with antiarrhythmic agents of the verapamil type because their concomitant use may result in bradycardia, hypotension or even cardiac arrest.

There have been reports of skin rashes and/or dry eyes associated with the use of beta-adrenoceptor blocking drugs. The reported incidence is small and in most cases the symptoms have cleared when treatment was withdrawn. Discontinuance of the beta-adrenoceptor blocking drug should be considered if any such reaction is not otherwise explicable. Cessation of therapy with a beta-blocker should be gradual.

Because of their chlorthalidone content, Lopresoretic tablets should be used with care in patients with some degree of renal impairment.

Pregnancy: The administration of Lopresoretic during pregnancy as with other drugs is advised only if there are compelling reasons. If Lopresoretic is used during pregnancy and lactation special attention should be paid to the foetus, neonate and breast fed infant for undesirable effects of the drug's beta-blocking action (e.g. slowing of the heart).

Side-effects: Gastro-intestinal upsets; sleep disturbances and exertional tiredness may occasionally occur.

In most cases these effects have been transient or have disappeared after a reduction in dosage. In rare cases, feelings of coldness in the extremities may occur.

As with other beta-blockers excessive bradycardia may occasionally occur; bronchospasm and heart failure may occasionally be precipitated in susceptible patients.

Like other diuretics with a similar mode of action, chlorthalidone may cause latent gout or latent diabetes mellitus to become manifest. In a few cases, allergic skin reactions, mild anorexia, nausea, constipation and diarrhoea have been reported. There have been isolated reports of leucopenia, but these are rare.

Overdosage: The symptoms of overdosage will be marked bradycardia and possible hypotension. Bradycardia may be overcome by the administration of intravenous atropine sulphate (0.25–2.0 mg) which will decrease vagal tone. If bradycardia persists – sympathomimetic drugs such as metaraminol or noradrenaline should be employed. These drugs have a pressor effect which may also help to overcome hypotension. The positive inotropic and chronotropic properties of glucagon may be useful when it is given in doses of 1–5 mg (max. 10 mg). Supportive treatment aimed at maintaining normal fluid and electrolyte balance is essential.

Pharmaceutical precautions Protect from moisture.

Legal category POM.

Package quantities Cartons of 56 tablets consisting of blister pack modules each containing 14 tablets (each carton represents 2–8 weeks treatment depending on the dose) (OP).

Further information Lopresoretic tablets simplify the management of hypertension since they combine two effective antihypertensive agents which act together in a complementary manner. In addition to the two modes of action already described, the Lopresor component prevents the increase in plasma renin which occurs as a result of diuretic therapy.

Lopresoretic tablets contain a selective beta-blocker and thus can be administered to patients with obstructive respiratory disease provided they have access to a beta-2-stimulant bronchodilator; being a selective agent, Lopresoretic is less likely to interfere with the action of beta-2-stimulants.

Product licence number 0001/0085.

PERTOFRAN*

Presentation The active ingredient, Desipramine Hydrochloride BP, is presented as: pale apricot-pink, sugar-coated tablets, bi-convex, 5.6 mm diameter and imprinted CG on one side and EW on the other. Containing 25 mg Desipramine Hydrochloride BP in each tablet.

The tablets also contain lactose and sucrose.

Uses *Antidepressant:* Symptoms of depressive illness.

Dosage and administration Pertofran is given orally in tablet form.

Adult dosage: 1 × 25 mg tablet three times a day for the first three days, increasing to 2 tablets three or four times daily. It will often be possible for the daily dose to be given as a single dose at night.

Elderly: Patients over 60 years of age may respond to lower doses of Pertofran than those recommended, usually 25 mg daily initially. The initial dose should be increased with caution under close supervision.

Children: Not recommended.

Contra-indications, warnings, etc

Contra-indications: Recent myocardial infarction. Any degree of heart block or other cardiac arrhythmias. Mania. Severe liver disease. Narrow angle glaucoma. Retention of urine.

Precautions: The elderly are particularly liable to experience adverse reactions, especially agitation, confusion and postural hypotension. Avoid if possible in patients with a history of epilepsy or with symptoms of bladder neck obstruction e.g. prostatic hypertrophy. Patients posing a high suicide risk require close initial supervision. Tricyclic anti-depressants potentiate the central nervous depressant action of alcohol.

Anaesthetics given during tri/tetracyclic antidepressant therapy may increase the risk of arrhythmias and hypotension. If surgery is necessary, the anaesthetist should be informed that a patient is being so treated.

As improvement in depression may not occur during the first four weeks of treatment, patients should be closely monitored during this period.

Pertofran may cause drowsiness. Patients should be warned of the possible hazard when driving or operating machinery.

Cardiac arrhythmias and severe hypotension are likely to occur with high dosage or in deliberate overdosage. They may also occur in patients with pre-existing heart disease taking normal dosage.

Do not use during pregnancy, especially during the first and last trimesters, unless there are compelling reasons. There is no evidence as to drug safety in humans; evidence from animal work has shown that desipramine is not totally free from hazard.

Pertofran is excreted in breast milk. Do not use during lactation unless essential; nursing mothers should be advised to cease breast feeding.

Drug interactions: Pertofran should not be given concurrently with, or within 2 weeks of cessation of therapy with monoamine oxidase inhibitors.

Pertofran may decrease the antihypertensive effect of guanethidine, debrisoquine, bethanidine and possibly clonidine. It would be advisable to review all antihypertensive therapy during treatment with tricyclic antidepressants.

Pertofran should not be given with sympathomimetic agents such as adrenaline, ephedrine, isoprenaline, noradrenaline, phenylephrine and phenylpropanolamine.

Barbiturates may decrease and neuroleptics and methylphenidate may increase respectively the plasma level of tricyclic antidepressants. Such changes may alter the clinical response to tricyclic antidepressants but clinical data on this is inconclusive.

Side-effects: The following adverse effects, although not necessarily all reported with Pertofran, have occurred with other tricyclic antidepressants:

Atropine-like side effects including dry mouth, disturbances of accommodation, tachycardia, constipation and hesitancy of micturition are common early in treatment, but usually lessen.

Serious adverse effects are rare; the following have been reported: Impaired liver function and jaundice, hypomania, epileptiform convulsions. Bone marrow depression, including leucopenia, eosinophilia and thrombocytopenia. Agranulocytosis has occasionally occurred in patients receiving tricyclic antidepressants. It is advisable to perform blood counts during treatment with tri/tetracyclic antidepressants, especially if the patient develops fever, sore throat or other signs of infection.

Other possible adverse effects include sweating, postural hypotension, tremor and skin rashes. Interference with sexual function may occur.

Psychotic manifestations, including mania and paranoid delusion, may be exacerbated during treatment with tricyclic antidepressants.

Although not indicative of addiction, withdrawal symptoms may occur on abrupt cessation of therapy and include insomnia, irritability and excessive perspiration.

Adverse effects such as withdrawal symptoms, respiratory depression and agitation have been reported in neonates whose mothers had taken Pertofran during the last trimester of pregnancy.

Overdosage:

Signs and symptoms: Major symptoms of overdosage include coma, convulsions, respiratory depression and disturbances in cardiac rate and rhythm.

Treatment: There is no specific antidote to Pertofran. Gastric lavage and forced emesis should be employed immediately to reduce absorption of the drug. Patients presenting with major symptoms of overdosage should be nursed in an intensive care unit where full support of vital functions is possible. Any serious overdosage requires continuous cardiac monitoring for at least 48 hours and any dysrhythmias treated on an individual basis. Respiratory insufficiency may necessitate intubation and ventilation and convulsions may be controlled with intravenous diazepam. Physostigmine should not be used following an overdosage of Pertofran. There have been reports that physostigmine increases the risk of seizures.

Pharmaceutical precautions *Storage:* Protect from moisture.

Legal category POM.

Package quantities Blister packs of 100 tablets.

Further information Nil.

Product licence number 0001/5019.

SINTHROME*

Presentation The active ingredient, Nicoumalone BP, is presented as:

White, compressed, scored tablets, approximately 7 mm diameter, impressed GEIGY on one side containing 4 mg in each tablet.

Pink, compressed tablets, approximately 5 mm diameter, containing 1 mg in each tablet.

The tablets also contain lactose. The 1 mg tablets also contain an azo-dye.

Uses Sinthrome is an oral anticoagulant for the treatment and prevention of thromboembolic diseases.

Mode of action: To initiate blood clotting, vitamin K causes γ-carboxylation of certain glutamic acid molecules on the coagulation factors II, VII, IX and X. Coumarin derivatives such as Sinthrome prevent γ-carboxylation of these proteins by vitamin K although the precise nature of this antagonism has yet to be established.

Depending on the initial dosage, Sinthrome prolongs the thromboplastin time within approximately 36–72 hours. Following withdrawal of Sinthrome, the thromboplastin time usually reverts to normal after a few days.

Pharmacokinetics: Following oral administration, Sinthrome is rapidly absorbed; at least 60% of the administered dose is systemically available. Peak plasma concentrations are achieved within 1–3 hours after a single dose of 10 mg and AUC values are proportional to the size of the dose over a dosage range of 8–16 mg.

No correlation between plasma concentrations of Sinthrome active substance (nicoumalone) and the apparent prothrombin levels can be established due to the variation of plasma drug concentrations between patients.

Plasma drug concentrations are generally higher in patients of 70 years or over when compared with younger patients, after the same dose.

Over 98% of nicoumalone is protein-bound, mainly to albumin. The calculated apparent volume of distribution is 0.16–0.18 l/kg for the R(+) enantiomer and 0.22–0.34 l/kg for the S(−) enantiomer.

Nicoumalone is extensively metabolised although the metabolites appear to be pharmacologically inactive in man.

The elimination half-life of nicoumalone from the plasma is 8–11 hours. Less than 0.2% of the dose is renally excreted unchanged with 60% being excreted in the urine and 29% in the faeces.

Dosage and administration Sensitivity to anticoagulants varies from patient to patient and may also fluctuate during the course of treatment. Therefore it is essential to perform regular coagulation tests and to adjust the patients dosage accordingly. If this is not possible, Sinthrome should not be used.

Sinthrome should be given in a single dose at the same time every day.

Initial dosage: If the thromboplastin time before starting treatment is within the normal range, the following dosage schedule is recommended:

First day	8–12 mg
Second day	4–8 mg

If the initial thromboplastin time is abnormal, treatment should be instituted with caution.

Maintenance therapy: The maintenance dose of Sinthrome varies from patient to patient and must be determined on the basis of regular laboratory estimations of the patient's blood coagulation time.

Adjustment of the maintenance dose can only be made by monitoring the Quick value or International Normalised Ratio (INR) at regular intervals so that dosage remains within the therapeutic range. Depending on the individual, the maintenance dose generally lies between 1–8 mg daily.

Before the start of treatment, up to the time when the coagulation valency is stabilised within the optimum range, routine measurement of the thromboplastin time should be carried out daily in hospital. Blood samples for laboratory tests should always be taken at the same time of day.

The INR is the ratio of the patient's plasma thromboplastin time and the normal thromboplastin time raised to a power determined for a reference thromboplastin. As the Quick value decreases, the patient's thromboplastin time increases and the INR is greater. The therapeutic range generally lies between INR values of 2–4.5.

Generally after withdrawal of Sinthrome, there is usually no danger of reactive hypercoagulability and therefore it is not necessary to give gradually diminishing doses. However, in extremely rare cases in some high risk patients (e.g. after myocardial infarction) withdrawal should be gradual.

Use in the elderly: A dose lower than the recommended adult dose may be sufficient in elderly patients (see 'Precautions').

Contra-indications, warnings, etc

Use in pregnancy and lactation: Sinthrome, like other coumarin derivatives may be associated with congenital malformations of the embryo. Therefore Sinthrome is contra-indicated for use in pregnancy. Women of child-bearing potential should take contraceptive measures during treatment with Sinthrome.

Sinthrome active substance passes into the breast milk of lactating mothers, but in quantities so small that no undesirable effects on the infant are to be expected. However, as a precaution, the infant should be given 1 mg vitamin K_1 per week as a prophylactic measure.

Contra-indications: Sinthrome is contra-indicated in patients with a known hypersensitivity to nicoumalone and related coumarin derivatives, and in patients unable to co-operate (e.g. unsupervised and senile patients, alcoholics and patients with psychiatric disorders).

Sinthrome is also contra-indicated in all conditions where the risk of haemorrhage exceeds possible clinical benefit, e.g. haemorrhagic diathesis and/or blood dyscrasia, immediately prior to, or after surgery on the central nervous system or eyes and traumatising surgery involving extensive exposure of the tissues, peptic ulceration or haemorrhage in the gastro-intestinal tract, urogenital tract or respiratory system, cerebrovascular haemorrhages, pericarditis, pericardial effusion, subacute bacterial endocarditis, severe hypertension (due to occult risks), severe hepatic or renal disease, and in cases of increased fibrinolytic activity following operations on the lung, prostate and uterus.

Precautions: Strict medical supervision should be given in cases where the disease or condition may reduce the protein binding of Sinthrome (e.g. thyrotoxicosis, tumours, renal diseases, infections and inflammation).

Particular care should be taken in patients with hepatic dysfunction since the synthesis of blood coagulation factors may be impaired. Disorders affecting gastro-intestinal absorption may alter the anticoagulant activity of Sinthrome. In severe heart failure, a very cautious dosage schedule must be adopted, since hepatic congestion may reduce the activation or γ-carboxylation of coagulation factors. However with reversal of the hepatic congestion, it may be necessary to raise the dosage.

In elderly patients, anticoagulation medication should be monitored with special care (see 'Pharmacokinetics' and 'Dosage' recommendations).

Since nicoumalone is extensively metabolised by the liver, impaired renal function will not greatly affect the elimination of the drug although care should be taken due to the possibility of underlying platelet dysfunction.

During treatment with anticoagulants, intramuscular injections may cause haematomas and should be avoided. Subcutaneous and intravenous injections may be given without such complications.

Meticulous care should be taken where it is necessary to shorten the thromboplastin time for diagnostic or therapeutic procedures (e.g. angiography, lumbar puncture, minor surgery, tooth extractions, etc.).

Drug interactions: There are many possible interactions between coumarins and other drugs; the interactions of clinical relevance are given below. The mechanisms of these interactions include disturbances of absorption, inhibition or induction of liver microsomal enzyme systems and reduced availability of vitamin K necessary for γ-carboxylation of coagulation factors. Every form of therapy may involve the risk of an interaction although not all will be significant. Thus careful surveillance is important and frequent coagulation tests (e.g. twice weekly) should be carried out when initially prescribing any drug in combination with Sinthrome or withdrawing a concomitantly administered drug.

The anticoagulation effect may be potentiated by concomitant administration of the following drugs: Allopurinol, anabolic steroids, androgens, anti-arrhythmic agents (e.g. amiodarone, quinidine), antibiotics (e.g. erythromycin, tetracyclines, neomycin, chloramphenicol), clofibric acid, its derivatives and structural analogues, disulfiram, ethacrynic acid, glucagon, histamine H_2-receptor antagonists, imidazole derivatives (e.g. metronidazole and, even when administered locally, miconazol), long-acting sulphonamides (including co-trimoxazoles), oral antidiabetics, thyroid hormones (incl. dextrothyroxine), sulphinpyrazone.

Drugs altering haemostasis may potentiate the anticoagulant activity of Sinthrome, and thereby increase the risk of gastro-intestinal haemorrhage. Consequently, Sinthrome should not be prescribed with such drugs, which include heparin, salicylic acid and its derivatives.

When Sinthrome is prescribed in combination with NSAIDs, coagulation tests should be performed more frequently.

The anticoagulant effect may be diminished by concomitant administration of the following drugs: Aminoglutethimide, barbiturates, carbamazepine, cholestyramine (see below), griseofulvin, oral contraceptives, rifampicin, and thiazide diuretics.

During concomitant treatment with hydantoin derivatives, the serum hydantoin concentration may rise.

Sinthrome may potentiate the hypoglycaemic effect of sulphonylurea derivatives.

Patients being treated with Sinthrome (especially those suffering from hepatic dysfunction), should limit their alcohol intake since it is not possible to predict the severity of any drug interactions nor identify any early signs of such interactions.

Side-effects: Haemorrhage, in various organs, is the most common side-effect associated with Sinthrome; its occurrence is related to the dosage of the drug, the patient's age and the nature of the underlying disease (but not the duration of treatment).

Possible sites of haemorrhage include the gastro-intestinal tract, brain, urogenital tract, uterus, liver, gall bladder and the eye.

If haemorrhage occurs in a patient with a thromboplastin time within the therapeutic range, diagnosis of their condition must be clarified.

Rare effects noted with similar coumarin derivatives include gastro-intestinal disorders (loss of appetite, nausea, vomiting), allergic reactions (urticaria, dermatitis and fever) and reversible alopecia.

Isolated cases of haemorrhagic skin necrosis (usually associated with congenital protein C deficiency) and liver damage have also been reported.

Overdosage: Clinical manifestations of overdosage are unlikely with large single doses but more likely following prolonged use of daily doses exceeding those required therapeutically.

Symptoms: The onset and severity of the symptoms are dependent on the individual's sensitivity to oral anticoagulants, the size of the overdose and the duration of treatment.

Haemorrhage is the prominent feature of an overdose and may occur within 1–5 days after ingestion. Nosebleeds, haematemesis, haemoptysis, gastro-intestinal haemorrhage, vaginal bleeding, haematuria (with renal colic), cutaneous haemorrhages, bleeding into the joints or menorrhagia may be experienced.

Further symptoms include tachycardia, hypotension, peripheral circulatory disorders due to loss of blood, nausea, vomiting, diarrhoea, and abdominal pains.

Laboratory tests will show an extremely low Quick value (or high INR value) pronounced prolongation of the recalcification time or thromboplastin time and disturbed γ-carboxylation of factors II, VII, IX and X.

Treatment: If, at the time of overdosage, the patient's thromboplastin time was normal, drug absorption may be reduced by emesis or gastric lavage in combination with giving activated charcoal or a fast-acting laxative. Cholestyramine may markedly enhance the drug's elimination by inhibiting the enterohepatic circulation.

A temporary reduction of the dose of Sinthrome is often sufficient to control slight bleeding.

Vitamin K_1 may antagonise the effect of Sinthrome within 3–5 hours. In cases of moderate haemorrhage, 2–5 mg vitamin K_1 should be given orally; in severe haemorrhage, 1–10 mg vitamin K_1 should be injected *very slowly* (at a rate less than 1 mg/min) intravenously. Additional doses (up to a maximum dose of 40 mg daily) should be given at 4-hour intervals. Vitamin K_1 should not be given by intramuscular injection.

Doses of vitamin K_1 in excess of 5 mg can cause resistance to further anticoagulant therapy for several days. If an anticoagulant is required, heparin may be used temporarily, although oral anticoagulant therapy should be resumed at the same time and heparin withdrawn once the therapeutic range has been reached.

In the case of life-threatening haemorrhage, intravenous transfusions of fresh frozen plasma or whole blood can abolish the effects of Sinthrome.

Pharmaceutical precautions Sinthrome is light-sensitive. Store and dispense in the original or a dark container.

Legal category POM.

Package quantities
Tablets 1 mg: Containers of 200.
Tablets 4 mg: Containers of 100.

Further information Nil.

Product licence number
Tablets 1 mg 0001/5021
Tablets 4 mg 0001/5022.

SYMMETREL* CAPSULES

Presentation The active ingredient, amantadine hydrochloride, is presented as: brownish-red hard gelatin capsules, imprinted GEIGY in white on both cap and body, each containing 100 mg amantadine hydrochloride.

The capsules also contain lactose and an azo-dye.

Uses Parkinson's disease. Herpes zoster. Prophylaxis and treatment of A_2, A/NJ/1/76, A/Moscow/77, A/Hong Kong/77, A/Brazil/11/78 and A/Alaska/78 influenza.

Note: Herpes zoster: It is recommended that the drug be given to elderly or debilitated patients in whom the physician suspects that a severe and painful rash could occur.

A_2 Influenza: It is suggested that Symmetrel be given to patients suffering from clinical influenza in whom complications might be expected to occur. In addition, Symmetrel is recommended prophylactically in cases particularly at risk, for example those with chronic respiratory disease or debilitating conditions, the elderly, those living in crowded conditions and for individuals in families where influenza has already been diagnosed, or those in essential services who are unvaccinated.

Dosage and administration *Parkinson's disease:* Initially one capsule daily for the first week, increasing to one capsule twice daily. In combination therapy, Symmetrel may be administered at these same doses. In many cases it will be possible after a few days to reduce the dosage of the other anti-Parkinson drug without loss of benefit.

Herpes zoster: Treatment should be started as soon as possible after the diagnosis has been made. The dosage is 1 capsule twice daily for 14 days. If post-herpetic pain persists after this period it is recommended that treatment be continued for a further 14 days.

Treatment of A_2 influenza: Adults: 1 capsule to be taken twice daily for five to seven days or at the discretion of the physician.

Prophylaxis of A_2 influenza: Adults: 1 capsule twice daily for as long as protection from influenza infection is required. In most instances this is expected to be for 7–10 days.

Treatment and prophylaxis in children: 10–15 years: 1 capsule every morning for the recommended period or at the discretion of the physician.

Below 10 years: As a reduced dosage is unavailable, it is not recommended that the drug be prescribed for this age group.

It is not recommended that the dosage be increased above that stated.

It may be found convenient to administer the drug at about 8 a.m. and 4 p.m.

Use in the elderly: No special dose regime is necessary but concurrent cardiovascular, renal or hepatic insufficiency should be taken into account.

Contra-indications, warnings, etc

Contra-indications: It is not recommended that Symmetrel be used to treat individuals who are subject to convulsions, or who have a history of gastric ulceration.

Symmetrel should not be used in patients with severe renal disease.

Although there are no specific contra-indications to the drug being administered to a person who has received a recent dose of influenza vaccine, such administration would be considered unnecessary.

Precautions: Symmetrel should be used with caution in patients with confusional or hallucinatory states.

As Symmetrel is excreted by the kidneys a cautious dosage scheme is recommended in the presence of impaired renal function. Care should be exercised when administering Symmetrel to patients with liver disease.

Patients who note central nervous system effects or blurring of vision should be advised to avoid situations where alertness is essential.

When employing Symmetrel in combination with other anti-Parkinson drugs, a watch should be kept for the latter's side-effects. Symmetrel may aggravate central nervous, gastro-intestinal or other side-effects provoked by anticholinergic drugs or L-dopa.

Although no incompatibilities with other drugs have become known, caution should be exercised if dextroamphetamine or other central nervous stimulants are used during Symmetrel therapy.

Peripheral oedema thought to be due to an alteration in the responsiveness of peripheral vessels may occur in some patients during treatment with Symmetrel. This should be considered when the drug is prescribed for those with congestive heart failure.

Use in pregnancy: Symmetrel has not been studied in pregnant women. The use of this drug in women of child-bearing age should be undertaken only after weighing the possible risks to the foetus against benefit to the patient. Symmetrel has been reported to be embryotoxic and teratogenic in rats at 50 mg/kg/day, about 12 times the recommended human dose, but not at 37 mg/kg/day. Embryotoxic and teratogenic effects were not seen in rabbits which received up to 25 times the usual recommended adult human dose.

Side-effects: Symmetrel is well tolerated. Nevertheless, side-effects may occur in some patients. Livedo reticularis and peripheral oedema have been noted. In addition central nervous system effects such as nervousness, insomnia, dizziness and convulsions or psychic reactions such as hallucinations, or feeling of detachment have occurred. Skin rash has occurred rarely in patients sensitive to the drug.

Accidental overdosage: There is no specific antidote to Symmetrel. Supportive therapeutic measures aimed at those symptoms arising from excessive central stimulation should be instituted.

Pharmaceutical precautions *Storage:* Protect from heat and moisture.

Legal category POM.

Package quantities *Capsules 100 mg:* Containers of 100.

Further information Symmetrel warrants serious consideration in the management of herpes zoster. This has been confirmed by a large double-blind study involving 100 patients which showed that Symmetrel can significantly reduce the proportion of patients experiencing pain of long duration.

Symmetrel has been shown to have an antiviral activity predominantly against A_2 influenza. When administered as a treatment to patients with clinical influenza, it results in a reduction of the duration of fever and symptoms of the infection. Used prophylactically, Symmetrel will provide rapid cover against influenza infection which will last for as long as therapy is continued.

The majority of studies have shown that Symmetrel does not interfere with normal antibody production.

Product licence number 0001/0006.

SYMMETREL* SYRUP

Presentation A clear, citrus flavoured syrup containing 50 mg/5 ml of the active ingredient amantadine hydrochloride.

The syrup also contains methyl hydroxybenzoate and propyl hydroxybenzoate.

Uses Parkinson's disease. Herpes zoster.

Note: Herpes zoster: It is recommended that the drug be given to elderly or debilitated patients in whom the physician suspects that a severe and painful rash could occur.

Dosage and administration *Parkinson's disease:* Initially 100 mg daily for the first week, increasing to 100 mg twice daily. In combination therapy, Symmetrel may be administered at these same doses. In many cases it will be possible after a few days to reduce the dosage of the other anti-Parkinson drug without loss of benefit.

Herpes zoster: The treatment should be started as soon as possible after the diagnosis has been made. The dosage is 100 mg Symmetrel twice daily for 14 days. If post-herpetic pain persists after this period it is recommended that treatment be continued for a further 14 days.

It is not recommended that the dosage be increased above that stated.

It may be found convenient to administer the drug at about 8 a.m. and 4 p.m.

Use in the elderly: No special dose regime is necessary but concurrent cardiovascular, renal or hepatic insufficiency should be taken into account.

Contra-indications, warnings, etc
Contra-indications: It is not recommended that Symmetrel be used to treat individuals who are subject to convulsions, or who have a history of gastric ulceration.

Symmetrel should not be used in patients with severe renal disease.

Precautions: Symmetrel should be used with caution in patients with confusional or hallucinatory states.

As Symmetrel is excreted by the kidneys a cautious dosage scheme is recommended in the presence of impaired renal function. Care should be exercised when administering Symmetrel to patients with liver disease.

Patients who note central nervous system effects or blurring of vision should be advised to avoid situations where alertness is essential.

When employing Symmetrel in combination with other anti-Parkinson drugs, a watch should be kept for the latter's side-effects. Symmetrel may aggravate central nervous, gastro-intestinal or other side-effects provoked by anticholinergic drugs or L-dopa.

Although no incompatibilities with other drugs have become known, caution should be exercised if dextroamphetamine or other central nervous stimulants are used during Symmetrel therapy.

Peripheral oedema thought to be due to an alteration in the responsiveness of peripheral vessels may occur in some patients during treatment with Symmetrel. This should be considered when the drug is prescribed for those with congestive heart failure.

Use in pregnancy: Symmetrel has not been studied in pregnant women. The use of this drug in women of child-bearing age should be undertaken only after weighing the possible risks to the foetus against benefit to the patient. Symmetrel has been reported to be embryotoxic and teratogenic in rats at 50 mg/kg/day, about 12 times the recommended human dose, but not at 37 mg/kg/day. Embryotoxic and teratogenic effects were not seen in rabbits which received up to 25 times the usual recommended adult human dose.

Side-effects: Symmetrel is well tolerated. Nevertheless, side-effects may occur in some patients. Livedo reticularis and peripheral oedema have been noted. In addition central nervous system effects such as nervousness, insomnia, dizziness and convulsions or psychic reactions such as hallucinations, or feeling of detachment have occurred. Skin rash has occurred rarely in patients sensitive to the drug.

Accidental overdosage: There is no specific antidote to Symmetrel. Supportive therapeutic measures aimed at those symptoms arising from excessive central stimulation should be instituted.

Pharmaceutical precautions *Storage:* Protect from heat and light.

Legal category POM.

Package quantities 150 ml bottles.

Further information Symmetrel warrants serious consideration in the management of herpes zoster. This has been confirmed by a large double-blind study involving 100 patients which showed that Symmetrel can significantly reduce the proportion of patients experiencing pain of long duration.

Product licence number 0001/0067.

TEGRETOL*
TEGRETOL CHEWTABS*

Presentation The active ingredient, Carbamazepine BP, is presented as: 100 mg white, compressed tablets, 9 mm diameter, impressed TEGRETOL 100 on one side, breakline on the other.

200 mg white, scored, compressed tablets, 9 mm diameter, impressed TEGRETOL 200 on one side, breakline on the other.

400 mg white, rod shaped, flat faced tablets with bevelled edges, 17 mm long, 5.5 mm wide and 5.5 mm thick, impressed GEIGY/GEIGY on one face with breakline. Other face impressed TEGRETOL with breakline.

Chewtabs containing 100 mg Carbamazepine BP in a chewable formulation, pale orange, square tablets, width 10.0 mm, height 4.2 mm, first side embossed with 'T', second side impressed TEGRETOL 100.

Chewtabs containing 200 mg Carbamazepine BP in a chewable formulation, pale orange, square tablets, width 12.5 mm, height 5.4 mm, first side embossed with 'T', second side impressed with TEGRETOL 200.

White liquid with a flavour of caramel, containing 100 mg/5ml Carbamazepine BP.

Tegretol liquid also contains polyethoxylated castor oils, methyl hydroxybenzoate and propyl hydroxybenzoate. Tegretol Chewtabs also contain sorbitol.

Uses
Indications: Epilepsy – generalised tonic – clonic and partial seizures.

NOTE: Tegretol is not usually effective in absences (petit mal). Moreover, anecdotal evidence suggests that seizure exacerbation may occur in patients with atypical absences.

The paroxysmal pain of trigeminal neuralgia.

Conventional tablets and liquid only: For the prophylaxis of manic-depressive psychosis in patients unresponsive to lithium therapy.

Dosage and administration Tegretol is given orally in either tablet or liquid form.

Chewtabs should be chewed before swallowing and taken after a meal.

The chewtabs and liquid are particularly suitable for children and adults who have difficulty in swallowing tablets.

Epilepsy:
Adults: Use a gradually increasing dosage scheme and adjust to suit the needs of the patient. It may be helpful to monitor the plasma concentration of carbamazepine to ensure adequate therapeutic levels; in most cases the optimum therapeutic plasma level ranges from 3–10 microgram/ml (13–42 micromoles/L).

Tegretol should be taken in a number of divided doses although initially 100–200 mg once or twice daily is recommended. This may be followed by a slow increase until the best response is obtained, often 800–1200 mg daily. In some instances, 1,600 mg daily may be necessary.

Elderly: There is no evidence to suggest that dosage requirements are different in the elderly but it is recommended that the initial dose be small and the increments titrated against the patients clinical condition.

Children: Use a gradually increasing dosage scheme and adjust to suit the needs of the patient. It may be helpful to monitor the plasma concentration of carbamazepine to ensure adequate therapeutic levels; in most cases the optimum therapeutic plasma level ranges from 3–10 micrograms/ml (13–42 micromoles/L).

Usual dosage 10–20 mg/kg bodyweight daily to be taken in several divided doses.

Tegretol tablets are not recommended for very young children.

Age up to 1 year: for flexibility of dosage use Tegretol liquid: 5–10 ml per day,

1–5 years:	10–20 ml liquid per day, or 2–4 × 100 mg chewtabs per day where appropriate.
5–10 years:	2–3 × 200 mg tablets or 20–30 ml liquid per day.
10–15 years:	3–5 × 200 mg tablets or 30–50 ml liquid per day,

to be taken in several divided doses.

Whenever possible antiepileptic agents should be prescribed as the sole drug therapy (monotherapy) but in patients already receiving other antiepileptic agents the same incremental dosage pattern for Tegretol should be followed, as above.

Trigeminal neuralgia: The individual dosage requirements of Tegretol vary considerably, depending on the age and weight of the patient. It is recommended that the initial dose be small, particularly in the frail and elderly, and that 100 mg tablets or liquid are used in the first instance.

The dose may be increased gradually until a satisfactory clinical response is obtained, which in some instances necessitates 1,600 mg Tegretol daily. It has been found that in the majority of patients a dosage of 200 mg three or four times a day is sufficient to maintain a pain-free state. It is suggested that Tegretol is taken only during acute stage of the condition and not as a prophylactic measure.

For the prophylaxis of manic-depressive psychosis in patients unresponsive to lithium therapy: Initial starting dose of 400 mg daily in divided doses, increasing gradually until symptoms are controlled or a total daily dose of 1,600 mg, given in divided doses is reached. The usual dosage range is 400–600 mg, in divided doses.

Contra-indications, warnings, etc

Contra-indications: Previous drug sensitivity to Tegretol.

Because Tegretol depresses AV-conduction, it is inadvisable to administer this drug to patients with atrioventricular conduction abnormalities unless paced.

Precautions: In patients with severe cardiovascular diseases, or with hepatic or renal disorders and in elderly patients the initial dosage should be small and the increments titrated against the patients condition. Blood counts and liver function tests should be performed before commencing treatment. Blood counts should then be repeated at weekly intervals during the first month of treatment and subsequently at monthly intervals; liver function tests should also be undertaken periodically. If allergic skin reactions occur, or if tests reveal a deterioration in liver function, Tegretol should be withdrawn.

Non-progressive or fluctuating asymptomatic leucopenia, which is quite often encountered, does not generally call for withdrawal of Tegretol. However treatment with Tegretol should be discontinued if the patient develops leucopenia which is severe, progressive or accompanied by clinical manifestations, e.g. fever or sore throat.

If treatment with Tegretol has to be withdrawn abruptly, the changeover to another anti-epileptic drug should if necessary be effected under the cover of benzodiazepines.

The patients' reactions, e.g. as a road user, may be impaired by Tegretol, especially in the early stages of treatment. Patients should be warned of the possible hazards when driving or operating machinery.

In rats treated with carbamazepine for two years, the incidence of tumours of the liver was found to be increased. There is, however, no evidence to indicate that this observation has any significant bearing on the therapeutic use of the drug.

NOTE: In keeping with current opinion it is suggested that the level of serum folic acid is observed during anticonvulsant therapy.

Use in pregnancy and lactation: In animal reproduction studies, very high doses of carbamazepine (above 200 mg/kg body weight) caused maternal toxicity in rodents, with an increase in embryolethality. Growth retardation in the rat foetus was observed at a maternal toxic dose (above 200 mg/kg body weight) and in mice this led to an increased rate of absorption. In a single study using mice, carbamazepine (40–240 mg/kg body weight) caused defects in 4.7% of foetuses compared with 1.3% in controls. However, overall there is no strong evidence of a teratogenic potential and clinical experience indicates that the risk of teratogenesis with Tegretol therapy is low. In women of child-bearing potential, the need to control seizures in the mother should be carefully weighed against possible risks to the foetus. This is particularly important during the first three months of pregnancy.

The incidence of congenital abnormalities in the offspring of women being treated with a combination of anti-convulsants is greater than in those mothers receiving monotherapy. Therefore, in women of child-bearing potential, Tegretol should be prescribed as monotherapy wherever possible.

Carbamazepine passes into breast milk in concentrations of about 25–60% of the plasma level. This is not believed to present a significant hazard to the infant, which is likely to receive at most 10% of an appropriate therapeutic dose of carbamazepine for an infant with epilepsy. However, as with all drugs, the benefits of breast feeding should be weighed against the remote possibility of an adverse effect occurring in the infant. Mothers taking Tegretol may nurse their infant provided the infant is observed for possible adverse reactions. There is one report of a severe skin (hypersensitivity) reaction in a breast fed baby.

Drug interactions: Induction of hepatic enzymes in response to Tegretol may have the effect of diminishing the activity of certain drugs that are metabolised in the liver, this should be borne in mind particularly when prescribing other drugs concomitantly, e.g. anti-epileptic agents.

In patients receiving oral anticoagulant medication, it may be necessary to adjust the dosage when Tegretol is prescribed.

Tegretol may also reduce the activity of those hormones contained in the combined oral contraceptive pill. This may present clinically as breakthrough bleeding or spotting. Patients taking Tegretol and requiring oral contraception should receive a preparation containing not less than 50 mcg of oestrogen or use some alternative non-hormonal method of contraception.

Tegretol should not be administered with, or within two weeks of cessation of MAOI therapy.

Certain drugs have been shown to elevate carbamazepine levels: macrolide antibiotics (e.g. erythromycin), isoniazid, some calcium antagonists (i.e. verapamil, diltiazem), dextropropoxyphene, viloxazine and possibly cimetidine.

The combination of lithium and carbamazepine may cause enhanced toxicity in spite of lithium plasma concentrations being within the therapeutic range.

Alcohol may exacerbate the CNS side-effects of psychoactive drugs including Tegretol; it is therefore advisable that the patient abstain from alcohol during treatment.

Side-effects: Provided a gradually increasing dosage scheme is followed, Tegretol is generally well tolerated but side-effects may occur particularly at the start of treatment. These effects usually disappear spontaneously after 7–14 days or following a temporary reduction in dosage.

Central nervous system: Occasionally dizziness, diplopia (usually dose dependent), headache, somnolence, ataxia, disorders of visual accommodation, states of confusion and agitation (in elderly patients).

Gastro-intestinal tract: Occasionally dry mouth, nausea, diarrhoea or constipation, loss of appetite.

Metabolism: In rare cases hyponatraemia due to the anti-diuretic effect of Tegretol, (possibly accompanied by vomiting, headache and mental confusion), has been reported in patients on higher doses of Tegretol. The effect is reversible upon reduction in dosage.

Skin: Generalised erythematous rash, in some cases severe, has been reported in about 3% of cases. This has been found to disappear leaving no sequelae on stopping therapy.

Isolated occurrences of exfoliative dermatitis, Stevens-Johnson syndrome, toxic epidermal necrolysis and hair loss have been reported.

Blood: Occasionally: Leucopenia, thrombocytopenia, isolated cases of agranulocytosis, aplastic anaemia and thrombo-embolism have been reported.

It is suggested that the blood count is checked at regular intervals particularly during the early stages of treatment.

Miscellaneous: Oedema has occasionally been noted but it is reversible upon reduction of dosage. Fever has also occasionally been reported. Isolated cases of proteinuria, lymph-node enlargement and acute renal failure have been reported. Rare cases of disturbance to cardiac impulse conduction, hepatitis also have been reported.

Overdosage
Signs and symptoms: Overdosage may give rise to the following, tremor, excitation, convulsions, changes in blood pressure (hypotension, or at times hypertension), impairment of consciousness and coma. EEG and ECG changes including for example cardiac arrhythmias may also occur.

Treatment: There is no specific antidote to Tegretol. Measures to monitor and safeguard vital functions should be undertaken and appropriate supportive therapy should be instituted e.g. measures to limit drug absorption (aspiration of gastric contents, activated charcoal may be left in the stomach to further reduce absorptions) and where necessary administration of benzodiazepines.

Pharmaceutical precautions
Storage: Liquid – Protect from heat, keep container tightly closed. Chewtabs – Protect from heat and moisture.

Dilutions: Tragacanth Mucilage BPC 1973 is suitable when used in a 1:1 ratio with Tegretol Liquid. After dilution the liquid should be used within 14 days.

Legal category POM.

Package quantities
Tablets 100 mg: Blister packs of 100 and containers of 500.
Tablets 200 mg: Blister packs of 100 and containers of 500.
Tablets 400 mg: Blister packs of 100.
Chewtabs 100 mg: Blister packs of 100.
Chewtabs 200 mg: Blister packs of 100.
Liquid 100 mg/5 ml: Bottles of 300 ml.

Further information Tegretol Chewtabs and liquid contain no sucrose and are therefore suitable for diabetics and children.

No problems would be expected if Chewtabs were allowed to disintegrate in the mouth i.e. sucked.

Pharmacokinetic studies have shown that Chewtabs also perform well if inadvertently swallowed whole.

Product licence numbers

Tablets 100 mg	0001/5027
Tablets 200 mg	0001/5028
Tablets 400 mg	0001/0088
Chewtabs 100 mg	0001/0125
Chewtabs 200 mg	0001/0126
Liquid 100 mg/5 ml	0001/0050

TEGRETOL RETARD*

Presentation Retard Divitabs containing 200 mg Carbamazepine BP, in a formulation to reduce peak plasma levels, beige-orange, capsule shaped, convex faces, with deep break-score on both sides, 13.2 mm long, 5.2 mm wide, 5.0 mm thick, impressed CG/CG on one side and HC/HC on the other side.

Retard Divitabs containing 400 mg Carbamazepine BP, in a formulation to reduce peak plasma levels, brown-orange, capsule shaped, convex faces, with deep break-score on both sides, 17.2 mm long, 6.6 mm wide, 6.0 mm thick, impressed CG/CG score on one side and ENE/ENE on the other side.

The tablets also contain polyethoxylated castor oils.

Uses
Indications: Epilepsy – generalised tonic-clonic and partial seizures. Tegretol Retard is indicated in newly diagnosed patients with epilepsy and in those patients who are uncontrolled or unable to tolerate their current anti-convulsant therapy.

NOTE: Carbamazepine is not usually effective in absences (petit mal). Moreover, anecdotal evidence suggests that seizure exacerbation may occur in patients with atypical absences.

The paroxysmal pain of trigeminal neuralgia.

Dosage and administration Tegretol Retard is given orally in tablet form. Tegretol Retard is a formulation which reduces the peak concentration of active substances in the plasma thus allowing a greater unit dose to be administered. Fluctuations in plasma concentration are also reduced throughout the day. These properties make it possible as a rule to administer Tegretol Retard twice daily.

The Divitab presentation enables flexibility of dosing to be achieved. Tegretol Retard (either the whole or half Divitab as prescribed) should *not* be chewed but should be swallowed with a little liquid during or after a meal.

Epilepsy
Adults: Use a gradually increasing dosage scheme and adjust to suit the needs of the patient. It may be helpful to monitor the plasma concentration of carbamazepine to ensure adequate therapeutic levels; in most cases the optimum therapeutic plasma level ranges from 3–10 micrograms/ml (13–42 micromoles/L).

Initially: 100–200 mg once or twice a day, followed by a slow increase until the best response is obtained, often 800–1200 mg daily. In some instances, 1600 mg daily may be necessary.

Elderly: There is no evidence to suggest that dosage requirements are different in the elderly but it is recommended that the initial dose be small and the increments titrated against the patient's clinical response.

Children: Use a gradually increasing dosage scheme and adjust to suit the needs of the patient. It may be helpful to monitor the plasma concentration of carbamazepine to ensure adequate therapeutic levels; in most cases the optimum therapeutic plasma level ranges from 3–10 micrograms/ml (13–42 micromoles/L).

Usual dosage 10–20 mg/kg bodyweight daily in two divided doses.
Age up to 5 years: Tegretol Retard tablets are not recommended. For flexibility of dosage use Tegretol Liquid – see separate data sheet.
5–10 years: 400–600 mg daily.
10–15 years: 600–1000 mg daily.

Wherever possible antiepileptic agents should be prescribed as the sole drug therapy (monotherapy) but in patients already receiving other antiepileptic agents the same incremental dosage pattern for Tegretol Retard should be followed as above.

Trigeminal neuralgia: The individual dosage requirements of Tegretol Retard vary considerably, depending on the age and weight of the patient. It is recommended that the initial dose be small, particularly in the frail and elderly.

The dose may be increased gradually until a satisfactory clinical response is obtained, which in some instances necessitates 1600 mg Tegretol Retard daily. It has been found that in the majority of patients doses of 600–800 mg daily are sufficient to maintain a pain-free state. It is suggested that Tegretol Retard is taken only during the acute stage of the condition and not as a prophylactic measure.

Contra-indications, warnings, etc
Contra-indications: Previous drug sensitivity to carbamazepine.

Because carbamazepine depresses AV-conduction, it is inadvisable to administer Tegretol Retard to patients with atrioventricular conduction abnormalities unless paced.

Precautions: In patients with severe cardiovascular diseases, or with hepatic or renal disorders and in elderly patients the initial dose should be small and the increments titrated against the patients condition.

Blood counts and liver function tests should be performed before commencing treatment. Blood counts should then be repeated at weekly intervals during the first month of treatment and subsequently at monthly intervals; liver function tests should also be undertaken periodically. If allergic skin reactions occur, or if tests reveal a deterioration in liver function, Tegretol Retard should be withdrawn.

Non-progressive or fluctuating asymptomatic leucopenia, which is quite often encountered, does not generally call for withdrawal of Tegretol Retard. However treatment with Tegretol Retard should be discontinued if the patient develops leucopenia which is *severe*, progressive or accompanied by clinical manifestations, e.g. fever or sore throat.

If treatment with Tegretol Retard has to be withdrawn abruptly, the changeover to another antiepileptic drug should if necessary be effected under the cover of benzodiazepines.

The patients' reactions, e.g. as a road user, may be impaired by Tegretol Retard, especially in the early stages of treatment. Patients should be warned of the possible hazard when driving or operating machinery.

In rats treated with carbamazepine for two years, the incidence of tumours of the liver was found to be increased. There is, however, no evidence to indicate that this observation has any significant bearing on the therapeutic use of the drug.

NOTE: In keeping with current opinion it is suggested that the level of serum folic acid is observed during anticonvulsant therapy.

Use in pregnancy and lactation: In animal reproduction studies, very high doses of carbamazepine (above 200 mg/kg body weight) caused maternal toxicity in rodents, with an increase in embryolethality. Growth retardation in the rat foetus was observed at a maternal toxic dose (above 200 mg/kg body weight) and in mice this led to an increased rate of abortion. In a single study using mice, carbamazepine (40–240 mg/kg body weight) caused defects in 4.7% of foetuses compared with 1.3% in controls. However, overall there is no strong evidence of a teratogenic potential and clinical experience indicates that the risk of teratogenesis with Tegretol Retard therapy is low. In women of child-bearing potential, the need to control seizures in the mother should be carefully weighed against possible risks to the foetus. This is particularly important during the first three months of pregnancy.

The incidence of congenital abnormalities in the offspring of women being treated with a combination of anti-convulsants is greater than in those mothers receiving monotherapy. Therefore, in women of child-bearing potential, Tegretol Retard should be prescribed as monotherapy wherever possible.

Carbamazepine passes into breast milk in concentrations of about 25–60% of the plasma level. This is not believed to present a significant hazard to the infant, which is likely to receive at most 10% of an appropriate therapeutic dose of carbamazepine for an infant with epilepsy. However, as with all drugs, the benefits of breast feeding should be weighed against the remote possibility of an adverse effect occurring in the infant. Mothers taking Tegretol may nurse their infant provided the infant is observed for possible adverse reactions. There is one report of a severe skin (hypersensitivity) reaction in a breast fed baby.

Drug interactions: Induction of hepatic enzymes in response to Tegretol Retard may have the effect of diminishing the activity of certain drugs that are metabolised in the liver, this should be borne in mind particularly when prescribing other drugs concomitantly, e.g. anti-epileptic agents.

In patients receiving oral anticoagulant medication, it may be necessary to adjust the dosage when Tegretol Retard is prescribed.

Tegretol Retard may also reduce the activity of those hormones contained in the combined oral contraceptive pill. This may present clinically as breakthrough bleeding or spotting. Patients taking Tegretol Retard and requiring oral contraception should receive a preparation containing not less than 50 mcg of oestrogen or use some alternative non-hormonal method of contraception.

Tegretol Retard should not be administered with, or within two weeks of cessation of MAOI therapy.

Certain drugs have been shown to elevate carbamazepine levels: macrolide antibiotics (e.g. erythromycin), isoniazid, some calcium antagonists (i.e. verapamil, diltiazem), dextropopoxyphene, viloxazine and possibly cimetidine.

The combination of lithium and carbamazepine may cause enhanced toxicity in spite of lithium plasma concentrations being within the therapeutic range.

Alcohol may exacerbate the CNS side effects of psychoactive drugs including carbamazepine; it is therefore advisable that the patient abstain from alcohol during treatment.

Side-effects: Provided a gradually increasing dosage scheme is followed, Tegretol Retard is generally well tolerated but side effects may occur particularly at the start of treatment. These effects usually disappear spontaneously after 7–14 days or following a temporary reduction in dosage.

Central nervous system: Occasionally dizziness, diplopia (usually dose dependent), headache, somnolence, ataxia, disorders of visual accommodation, states of confusion and agitation (in elderly patients).

Gastro-intestinal tract: Occasionally dry mouth, nausea, diarrhoea or constipation, loss of appetite.

Metabolism: In rare cases hyponatraemia due to the anti-diuretic effect of Tegretol Retard, (possibly accompanied by vomiting, headache and mental confusion), has been reported in patients on higher doses of Tegretol Retard. The effect is reversible upon reduction in dosage.

Skin: Generalised erythematous rash, in some cases severe, has been reported in about 3% of cases. This has been found to disappear leaving no sequelae on stopping therapy.

Isolated occurrences of exfoliative dermatitis, Stevens-Johnson syndrome, toxic epidermal necrolysis and hair loss have been reported.

Blood: Occasionally: leucopenia, thrombocytopenia. Isolated cases of agranulocytosis, aplastic anaemia and thromboembolism have been reported.

It is suggested that the blood count is checked at regular intervals particularly during the early stages of treatment.

Miscellaneous: Oedema has occasionally been noted but it is reversible upon reduction of dosage. Fever has also occasionally been reported.

Isolated cases of proteinuria, lymph node enlargement and acute renal failure have been reported. Rare cases of disturbance to cardiac impulse conduction and hepatitis also have been reported.

Overdosage

Signs and symptoms: Overdosage may give rise to tremor, excitation, convulsions, changes in blood pressure, (hypotension, or at times hypertension), impairment of consciousness and coma. EEG and ECG changes including for example cardiac arrhythmias may also occur.

Treatment: There is no specific antidote to Tegretol Retard. Measures to monitor and safeguard vital functions should be undertaken and appropriate supportive therapy should be instituted e.g. measures to limit drug absorption (aspiration of gastric contents, activated charcoal may be left in the stomach to further reduce absorption) and where necessary administration of benzodiazepines.

Pharmaceutical precautions Store below 25°C and protect from moisture.

Legal category POM.

Package quantities
Retard Divitabs 200 mg: Blister packs of 100.
Retard Divitabs 400 mg: Blister packs of 100.

Further information Nil.

Product licence numbers
Retard Divitabs 200 mg 0001/0118
Retard Divitabs 400 mg 0001/0119

TOFRANIL*

Presentation The active ingredient, Imipramine Hydrochloride BP, is presented as: red-brown, sugar-coated tablets, round bi-convex, 5.6 mm diameter, imprinted GEIGY on one side, each containing 25 mg.

Red-brown, sugar-coated, triangular-shaped tablets, 5.8 mm diameter, imprinted GEIGY on one side, each containing 10 mg.

White, viscous syrup with a vanilla flavour containing

the equivalent of 25 mg/5 ml Imipramine Hydrochloride BP.

The tablets also contain lactose and sucrose. The syrup also contains sucrose, methyl hydroxybenzoate and propyl hydroxybenzoate.

Uses Symptoms of depressive illness. Relief of nocturnal enuresis in children.

Mode of action: Imipramine is a tricyclic antidepressant and its pharmacological action includes alpha-adrenolytic, anti-histaminic, anticholinergic and 5HT-receptor blocking properties. However the therapeutic activity of imipramine is believed to be based mainly on its ability to inhibit the neuronal re-uptake of noradrenaline and 5HT. It inhibits their re-uptake to approximately the same extent.

Pharmacokinetics: Imipramine is absorbed quickly and completely following oral administration. The intake of food has no effect on its absorption and bioavailability. During its first passage through the liver, orally administered imipramine becomes partly converted to desmethylimipramine, a metabolite which likewise exhibits antidepressant activity.

During oral administration of 50 mg 3 times daily for 10 days, the mean steady-state plasma concentrations of imipramine and desmethylimipramine were 33–85 ng/ml and 43–109 ng/ml respectively. Owing to lower clearance in the plasma, resulting in increased systemic availability, elderly patients require lower doses of imipramine than patients in intermediate age groups. Renal impairment is not expected to have any influence on the kinetics of unchanged imipramine and its desmethyl metabolite since both are excreted only in small amounts by the kidneys.

The mean plasma half-life of imipramine is approximately 20 hours, mean plasma protein binding 86% and mean distribution volume 21 L/kg. The quantity of unchanged imipramine and active metabolite desmethylimipramine excreted is low, most excretion being as inactive metabolites in urine (approximately 80%) and faeces (approximately 20%).

Dosage and administration

Depression

Adults: 1 × 25 mg up to three times daily, increasing stepwise to 150–200 mg. This should be reached by the end of the first week and maintained until definite improvement has occurred. The subsequent maintenance dose should be individually determined by gradually reducing the dosage, usually to about 50–100 mg daily.

In hospitalised patients i.e. severe cases the dose may be increased to 100 mg three times daily until a distinct improvement has been achieved. Again the subsequent maintenance dose should be determined individually by reducing the dosage, usually to about 100 mg daily.

Elderly: Patients over 60 years of age may respond to lower doses of Tofranil than those recommended above. Treatment should be initiated with 10 mg daily, gradually increasing to 30–50 mg daily. The optimum dose should be reached after about 10 days and then continued until the end of treatment.

Children (for nocturnal enuresis only).

Not for use in children under 6 years.

6–7 years (weight 20–25 kg or 44–55 lbs) 25 mg

8–11 years (weight 25–35 kg or 55–77 lbs) 25–50 mg

Over 11 years (weight 35–54 kg or 77–119 lbs) 50–75 mg

A daily dosage of 2.5 mg/kg should not be exceeded in children. The dose should be taken just before bedtime. The maximum period of treatment should not exceed three months and withdrawal should be gradual. Should a relapse occur, a further course of treatment should not be started until a full physical examination has been made.

Contra-indications, warnings, etc

Contra-indications: Known hypersensitivity to tricyclic antidepressants of the dibenzazepine group. Recent myocardial infarction. Any degree of heart block or other cardiac arrhythmias, mania, severe liver disease, narrow angle glaucoma. Infants and children under 6 years old. Retention of urine. Concurrent use in patients receiving, or within 3 weeks of cessation of therapy with, monoamine oxidase inhibitors.

Warnings: As improvement in depression may not occur for the first two to four weeks treatment, patients should be closely monitored during this period. Tofranil may initially impair alertness. Patients should be warned against engaging in activities, such as driving motor vehicles and operating machinery, which require quick reactions.

Precautions: Caution is called for when employing Tofranil in:

- Patients with a low convulsion threshold
- Patients with severe hepatic or renal disease
- Patients receiving steroid hormones
- Patients with tumours of the adrenal medulla (eg phaeochromocytoma, neuroblastoma), in whom the drug may provoke hypertensive crises.

Concomitant treatment of Tofranil and electroconvulsive therapy should only be resorted to under careful supervision.

Many patients with panic disorders experience intensified anxiety symptoms at the start of the treatment with antidepressants. This paradoxical initial increase in anxiety is most pronounced during the first few days of treatment and generally subsides within two weeks.

Caution is indicated in patients with hyperthyroidism or during concomitant treatment with thyroid preparations, since aggravation of unwanted cardiac effects may occur.

Before initiating treatment it is advisable to check the patient's blood pressure, because individuals with hypotension or a labile circulation may react to the drug with a fall in blood pressure.

The blood count should also be monitored during treatment with Tofranil (especially if the patient develops fever, sore throat, or other symptoms such as are associated with influenzal infections), since isolated cases of agranulocytosis have been associated with the use of tricyclic antidepressants.

It is advisable to monitor cardiac and hepatic function during long-term therapy with Tofranil.

Avoid if possible in patients with symptoms of bladder neck obstruction eg prostatic hypertrophy.

Patients posing a high suicide risk require close initial supervision.

Tricyclic antidepressants potentiate the central nervous depressant action of alcohol.

Anaesthetics given during tri/tetracyclic antidepressant therapy may increase the risk of arrhythmias and hypotension. If surgery is necessary, the anaesthetist should be informed that a patient is being so treated.

Lengthy treatment with tricyclic antidepressants can lead to an increased incidence of dental caries.

Tofranil may cause anxiety, feelings of unrest, and hyperexcitation in agitated patients and patients with accompanying schizophrenic symptoms.

In predisposed and elderly patients, Tofranil may, particularly at night, provoke pharmacogenic (delirious) psychoses, which disappear without treatment within a few days of withdrawing the drug. Agitation, confusion and postural hypotension may occur.

A swing from depression to hypomania or mania is possible in patients with bipolar affective disorders. In such cases it may be necessary to withdraw Tofranil and administer drugs to control the mania. After such episodes have subsided, low-dose therapy with Tofranil may be resumed if required.

Behavioural changes may occur in children receiving Tofranil for treatment of nocturnal enuresis.

Use during pregnancy and lactation: Treatment with Tofranil should be avoided during pregnancy, unless there are compelling reasons. There is no, or inadequate, evidence of safety of the drug in human pregnancy.

Neonates whose mothers had taken Tofranil up till delivery have developed dyspnoea, lethargy, colic, irritability, hypotension or hypertension, tremor or spasms, during the first few hours or days. Tofranil should

– if this is at all justifiable – be withdrawn at least 7 weeks before the calculated date of confinement.

The active substance of Tofranil and its metabolite desmethylimipramine pass into the breast milk in small quantities. Since nothing is known about the clinical relevance of this, it may be advisable to withdraw the medication or use a breast milk substitute.

Drug interactions: Tofranil should not be given concurrently with, or within 3 weeks of cessation of therapy with monoamine oxidase inhibitors. The same precaution should be taken when administering an MAO inhibitor after previous treatment with Tofranil. In either instance, medication should be initiated cautiously and the dosage slowly raised stepwise until the patient is optimally stabilised.

Antihypertensive therapy should be reviewed and if possible avoided when using Tofranil due to possible interactions.

Tofranil should not be given with sympathomimetic agents such as adrenaline, ephedrine, isoprenaline, noradrenaline, phenylephrine, and phenylpropanolamine (including nasal drops and local anaesthetic containing sympathomimetics) as the cardiovascular effects may be potentiated.

Tricyclic antidepressants may also increase the effect of alcohol and central depressant drugs (eg barbiturates, benzodiazepines or general anaesthetics) as well as that of anticholinergic agents (eg atropine, biperiden, levodopa).

When tricyclic antidepressants are given in combination with anticholinergics or antipsychotics with an anticholinergic action, hyperexcitation states or delirium may occur, as well as attacks of glaucoma.

Tricyclic antidepressants should not be employed in combination with anti-arrhythmic agents of the quinidine type.

Substances which activate the hepatic mono-oxygenase enzyme system (eg carbamazepine, barbiturates, phenytoin, nicotine) may lower the plasma concentration of tricyclic antidepressants and so reduce their antidepressive effect.

In addition, concomitant administration of imipramine and phenytoin may lead to elevated serum phenytoin concentrations.

Many antipsychotic agents may increase the plasma concentration of imipramine. No such effects are known to occur in combination with diazepam, but it might be necessary to reduce the dosage of imipramine if administered concomitantly with alprazolam or disulfiram.

Since cimetidine raises the plasma concentration of imipramine, the dosage of imipramine should be reduced if the two drugs are administered concurrently; by contrast, ranitidine does not alter the kinetics of imipramine.

If administered concomitantly with oestrogens, the dose of imipramine should be reduced, since steroid hormones inhibit the metabolism of imipramine.

Side-effects:
Anticholinergic effects: Frequently dryness of the mouth, constipation, sweating, hot flushes, disorders of visual accommodation and blurred vision. Occasionally disturbances of micturition. Isolated cases of mydriasis, glaucoma and paralytic ileus.
Central nervous system:
Psychic effects: Occasionally fatigue, drowsiness, sleep disturbances, increased anxiety, feelings of unrest and agitation, swings from depression to hypomania or mania, delirium, confusion, disorientation and hallucinations (particularly in geriatric patients and those suffering from Parkinson's disease), activation of psychotic symptoms. In isolated cases, aggressiveness.
Neurological effects: Frequently fine tremor. Occasionally paraesthesiae symptoms suggestive of peripheral neuropathy, headache, dizziness. Rarely, epileptic seizures. Isolated cases of EEG changes, myoclonus, weakness, extrapyramidal symptoms, ataxia, speech disorders.
Cardiovascular system: Frequently sinus tachycardia and clinically irrelevant ECG changes (T and ST changes) in patients of normal cardiac status, postural hypotension. Occasionally arrhythmias, conduction disorders (widening of QRS complex and PR interval, bundle-branch block), palpitations. Isolated cases of increased blood pressure, cardiac decompensation, peripheral vasospastic reactions.
Respiratory tract: Isolated cases of allergic alveolitis with or without eosinophilia.
Gastro-intestinal tract: Occasionally nausea, vomiting, anorexia. Isolated cases of stomatitis, tongue lesions, abdominal disorders.
Hepatic effects: Impaired liver function, rarely: elevated transaminases, isolated cases of hepatitis with or without jaundice.
Skin: Occasionally allergic skin reactions. Isolated cases of pruritus, petechiae, photosensitivity, oedema (local or generalised) loss of hair.
Endocrine system and metabolism: Frequently weight gain. Occasionally disturbances of libido and potency. Isolated cases of enlarged mammary glands, galactorrhoea, SSIADH (syndrome of inappropriate antidiuretic hormone secretion), increase or decrease in blood sugar, weight loss.
Blood: Isolated cases of eosinophilia, leucopenia, agranulocytosis and thrombocytopenia.
Miscellaneous: Occasional withdrawal symptoms following abrupt discontinuation of treatment: nausea, vomiting, abdominal pain, diarrhoea, insomnia, headache, nervousness and anxiety.

Isolated cases of tinnitus, drug fever.

Overdosage: Children react more sensitively than adults to acute overdosages of tricyclics, and some fatalities have been reported.

Signs and Symptoms: The first signs and symptoms of poisoning with tricyclic antidepressants generally take the form of severe anticholinergic reactions, which set in about 1/2–2 hours after the drug has been taken. The following may be encountered: Central nervous system: drowsiness, stupor, coma, ataxia, restlessness, agitation, enhanced reflexes, muscular rigidity, athetoid and choreiform movements, convulsions.

Cardiovascular System: Hypotension, tachycardia, arrhythmia, conduction disorders, heart failure; in very rare cases, cardiac arrest.

In addition, respiratory depression, cyanosis, shock, vomiting, fever, hydriasis, sweating and oliguria or anuria may occur.

Treatment: There is no specific antidote. Physostigmine should not be used since it may increase the risk of epileptic seizures.

Where the drug has been taken by mouth, try to induce vomiting; otherwise the stomach must be irrigated. Activated charcoal should be administered.

Severe poisoning with tricyclic drugs requires immediate hospitalisation and continuous cardiovascular monitoring for at least 48 hours.

In all patients with ECG abnormalities, cardiac function should – even after the ECG tracings have reverted to normal – be kept under close observation for at least another 72 hours, because relapses may occur.

The following measures should be taken in cases of overdosages:
– In respiratory failure: intubation and artificial respiration.
– In severe hypotension: the patient should be placed in an appropriate position and be given a plasma expander, dopamine, or dobutamine by intravenous drip.
– Cardiac arrhythmias must be treated according to the requirements of the case.
– Implantation of a cardiac pacemaker should be considered.
– Low potassium values and acidosis should be corrected.
– In convulsions: diazepam should be given i.v., or another anticonvulsant such as phenobarbitone or paraldehyde (these substances may exacerbate existing respiratory failure, hypotension, or coma).
– Dialysis and haemodialysis are of no use.

Pharmaceutical precautions *Storage:* Syrup – protect from heat; keep containers tightly closed. Tablets: protect from moisture.

Dilutions: Syrup – for dilutions down to 15 mg/5 ml, boiled, distilled or de-ionised water can be used. For dilutions below 15 mg/5 ml, the recommended diluent is equal parts simple Syrup BPC and freshly prepared Tragacanth Mucilage BPC 1973. After dilution the solution should be used within a few days.

Legal category POM.

Package quantities Tablets 25 mg: Blister packs of 100.
Tablets 10 mg: Blister packs of 100.
Syrup 25 mg/ml: Bottles of 150 ml.

Further information Nil.

Product licence numbers

Tablets 25 mg	0001/5029
Tablets 10 mg	0001/5030
Syrup 25 mg/5 ml	0001/5032

VOLTAROL*
VOLTAROL RETARD*
VOLTAROL DISPERSIBLE*

Presentation Tablets containing 25 mg diclofenac sodium, circular, slightly biconvex with bevelled edges, yellow enteric coated, approximately 7 mm diameter, imprinted 'GEIGY' on one side and 'VOLTAROL 25' on the other.

Tablets containing 50 mg diclofenac sodium, circular, slightly biconvex with bevelled edges, light brown enteric coated, approximately 8 mm diameter, imprinted 'GEIGY' on one side and 'VOLTAROL 50' on the other.

Dispersible tablets containing 46.5 mg diclofenac (equivalent to 50 mg diclofenac sodium) triangular, pink, imprinted GEIGY on one side, and with a raised 'V' on the other.

Retard tablets containing 100 mg diclofenac sodium in a sustained release formulation, circular, slightly biconvex, pale red, approximately 9 mm diameter, imprinted 'VOLTAROL R' on one side, 'GEIGY' on the other.

Suppositories, containing 100 mg diclofenac sodium in a yellowish-white, torpedo shaped, waxy base, weighing approximately 2.00 g.

Suppositories containing 12.5 mg diclofenac sodium in an off-white, torpedo shaped, waxy base, weighing approximately 900 mg.

Ampoules for intramuscular injection containing 75 mg/3 ml diclofenac sodium.

The 25 mg and 50 mg tablets contain lactose, and polyethoxylated castor oils. The Dispersible tablets contain erythrosine. Retard tablets contain sucrose. Ampoules contain mannitol, sodium metabisulphite, benzyl alcohol, propylene glycol, sodium hydroxide and water.

Uses
Tablets and suppositories.

Adults: Rheumatoid arthritis; osteoarthrosis; low back pain; acute musculo-skeletal disorders and trauma such as periarthritis (especially frozen shoulder), tendinitis, tenosynovitis, bursitis, sprains, strains and dislocations; relief of pain in fractures; ankylosing spondylitis; acute gout; control of pain and inflammation in orthopaedic, dental and other minor surgery.

Children: Juvenile chronic arthritis.

Ampoules for injection: Acute exacerbations of rheumatoid arthritis and osteoarthrosis; acute back pain; acute gout; post-operative pain; relief of pain in acute trauma and fractures; and renal colic.

Mode of action: Voltarol is a non-steroidal agent with marked analgesic/anti-inflammatory properties. It is an inhibitor of prostaglandin synthetase (cyclo-oxygenase).

Diclofenac sodium *in vitro* does not suppress proteoglycan biosynthesis in cartilage at concentrations equivalent to the concentrations reached in humans.

Pharmacokinetics: Diclofenac sodium is rapidly absorbed from the gut and is subject to first-pass metabolism. Tablets give peak plasma concentrations after 1–4 hours, suppositories within 1 hour and ampoules within half an hour. Voltarol Dispersible tablets give peak plasma concentrations after approximately 1–2 hours. The active substance is 99.7% protein bound and plasma half-life for the terminal elimination phase is 1–2 hours. Approximately 60% of the administered dose is excreted via the kidneys in the form of metabolites and less than 1% in unchanged form. The remainder of the dose is excreted via the bile in metabolised form. In patients with impaired renal function, no accumulation of Voltarol has been reported.

Dosage and administration
Adults: Tablets 25 and 50 mg: 75–150 mg daily in two or three divided doses. The Voltarol Dispersible tablet should be dropped into a glass of water, and the liquid stirred to aid dispersion, before swallowing.

Voltarol Retard: One tablet daily, taken whole with liquid, preferably at meal times. If necessary, the daily dosage can be increased to 150 mg by supplementation with conventional Voltarol tablets. For milder cases, where a lower dosage is sufficient, other dosage forms of Voltarol may be used.

Suppositories: One 100 mg suppository daily, usually administered at night. In more severe cases, combined therapy with 25 or 50 mg tablets is recommended. The total daily dose should not exceed 150 mg.

Injection: One ampoule once (or in severe cases twice) daily intramuscularly by deep intragluteal injection into the upper outer quadrant. If two injections daily are required it is advised that the alternate buttock be used for the second injection. Voltarol ampoules should not be given for more than 2 days; if necessary, treatment can be continued with tablets or suppositories. Voltarol should not be administered by intravenous injection. Renal colic: 1 × 75 mg ampoules intramuscularly. A further ampoule may be administered after 30 minutes if necessary. As with oral Voltarol the total daily dose should not exceed 150 mg.

Children (1 year or over): 1–3 mg/kg per day in divided doses. The following dosage forms are not suitable for children: tablets 50 mg, suppositories 100 mg, ampoules 75 mg, Voltarol Retard and Voltarol Dispersible.

Elderly: Although the pharmacokinetics of Voltarol are not impaired to any clinically relevant extent in elderly patients non-steroidal anti-inflammatory drugs should be used with particular caution in such patients who are generally more prone to adverse reactions. In particular it is recommended that the lowest effective dosage be used in frail elderly patients or those with a low body weight (see also precautions).

Contra-indications, warnings, etc
Use in pregnancy and lactation: Although animal studies have not demonstrated teratogenic effects, Voltarol should not be prescribed during pregnancy, unless there are compelling reasons for doing so. If employed, the lowest effective dosage should be used.

Use of prostaglandin synthetase inhibitors may result in premature closure of the ductus arteriosus or uterine inertia; such drugs are therefore not recommended during the last trimester of pregnancy.

Following oral doses of 50 mg every 8 hours, traces of active substance have been detected in breast milk, but in quantities so small that no undesirable effects on the infant are to be expected.

Ampoules: due to insufficient data these cannot be recommended during pregnancy or lactation.

Contra-indications: Active or suspected peptic ulcer or gastro-intestinal bleeding. Previous sensitivity to Voltarol. Patients in whom attacks of asthma, urticaria or acute rhinitis are precipitated by aspirin or other non-steroidal anti-inflammatory agents. Use of Voltarol suppositories in ulcerative or acute inflammatory conditions of the anus, rectum and sigmoid colon (e.g. proctitis).

Ampoules: hypersensitivity to the excipients sodium metabisulphite, benzyl alcohol, propylene glycol, mannitol.

Precautions: Gastro-intestinal ulceration, haematemesis or melaena (which may occur with or without warning symptoms or a previous history) and are generally more serious in the elderly, ulcerative colitis, Crohn's disease, bleeding diathesis or haematological abnormalities.

Patients with severe hepatic, cardiac or renal insufficiency or the elderly should be kept under close surveillance.

All patients who are receiving long-term treatment with non-steroidal anti-inflammatory agents should be monitored as a precautionary measure e.g. renal, hepatic function (elevation of liver enzymes may occur) and blood counts.

If abnormal liver function tests persist or worsen, clinical signs or symptoms consistent with liver disease develop or if other manifestations occur (eosinophilia, rash), Voltarol should be discontinued.

Use of Voltarol in patients with hepatic porphyria may trigger an attack.

The importance of prostaglandins in maintaining renal blood flow should be taken into account in patients with impaired cardiac or renal function, those being treated with diuretics or recovering from major surgery. Effects on renal function are usually reversible on withdrawal of Voltarol.

Voltarol, in common with other NSAIDs, can reversibly inhibit platelet aggregation.

Drug interactions: Voltarol may increase plasma concentrations of lithium and digoxin.

Clinical investigations do not appear to indicate that Voltarol affects the activity of anticoagulants but there have been isolated reports of an increased risk of haemorrhage with the combined use of these agents. Close monitoring is therefore recommended. Clinical studies have shown that Voltarol can be given together with oral antidiabetic agents without influencing their clinical effect. However there have been isolated reports of hypoglycaemic and hyperglycaemic effects which have required adjustments to the dosage of hypoglycaemic agents.

Cyclosporin nephrotoxicity may be increased by the effect of non-steroidal anti-inflammatory drugs on renal prostaglandins.

Caution should be exercised if NSAIDs and methotrexate are administered within 24 hours of each other, since NSAIDs may increase methotrexate plasma levels, resulting in increased toxicity.

Concomitant therapy with other systemic NSAIDs may increase the frequency of side-effects.

Various NSAIDs are liable to inhibit the activity of diuretics. Concomitant treatment with potassium-sparing diuretics may be associated with increased serum potassium levels, hence serum potassium should be monitored.

Side-effects: If serious side-effects occur, Voltarol should be withdrawn.

Gastro-intestinal tract: Occasional: epigastric pain, other gastro-intestinal disorders (e.g. nausea, vomiting, diarrhoea, abdominal cramps, dyspepsia, flatulence, anorexia).

Rare: gastro-intestinal bleeding, peptic ulcer (with or without bleeding or perforation), bloody diarrhoea.

In isolated cases: lower gut disorders (e.g. non-specific haemorrhagic colitis and exacerbations of ulcerative colitis or Crohn's proctocolitis), pancreatitis, aphthous stomatitis, glossitis, oesophageal lesions, constipation.

Suppositories only: Occasional: local reactions (e.g. itching, burning and increased bowel movement); in isolated cases: exacerbation of haemorrhoids.

Central nervous system: Occasional: headache, dizziness, or vertigo. Rare: drowsiness, tiredness. In isolated cases: disturbances of sensation (paraesthesia, memory disturbance, disorentation, disturbance of vision (blurred vision, diplopia), impaired hearing, tinnitus, insomnia, irritability, convulsions, depression, anxiety, nightmares, tremor, psychotic reactions. Taste alteration disorders.

Skin: Occasional: rashes or skin eruptions. Rare: urticaria. In isolated cases: bullous eruptions, eczema, erythema multiforme, Stevens-Johnson syndrome, Lyell's syndrome, (acute toxic epidermolysis), erythrodema (exfoliative dermatitis), loss of hair, photosensitivity reactions, purpura including allergic purpura.

Kidney: In isolated cases: acute renal insufficiency, urinary abnormalities (e.g. haematuria, proteinuria), interstitial nephritis, nephrotic syndrome, papillary necrosis.

Liver: Occasional: elevation of serum aminotransferase enzymes (SGOT, SGPT). Rare: liver function disorders including hepatitis (in isolated cases fulminant) with or without jaundice.

Blood: In isolated cases: thrombocytopenia, leucopenia, agranulocytosis, haemolytic anaemia, aplastic anaemia.

Other organ systems: Rare: oedema, hypersensitivity reactions (e.g. bronchospasm, anaphylactic/anaphylactoid systemic reactions including hypotension). Isolated cases: impotence (association with Voltarol intake is doubtful), palpitation, chest pain, hypertension.

Ampoules only: Rare: injection site disorders e.g. local pain and induration; in isolated cases: abscesses and local necrosis.

Overdosage: Management of acute poisoning with NSAIDs essentially consists of supportive and symptomatic measures. There is no typical clinical picture resulting from Voltarol overdosage. The therapeutic measures to be taken are: absorption should be prevented as soon as possible after overdosage by means of gastric lavage and treatment with activated charcoal; supportive and symptomatic treatment should be given for complications such as hypotension, renal failure, convulsions, gastro-intestinal irritation, and respiratory depression; specific therapies such as forced diuresis, dialysis or haemoperfusion are probably of no help in eliminating NSAIDs due to their high rate of protein binding and extensive metabolism.

Pharmaceutical precautions The ampoules should not be mixed with other injection solutions.

Storage precautions: Tablets 25 and 50 mg – protect from heat and moisture.

Voltarol Dispersible 46.5 mg – protect from heat and moisture.

Voltarol Retard tablets 100 mg – protect from moisture.

Suppositories 12.5 mg and 100 mg – protect from heat.

Ampoules for injection – protect from heat and light.

Legal category POM.

Package quantities
Tablets: Blister packs of 100.
Voltarol Dispersible tablets: aluminium blister packs of 21 (OP).
Voltarol Retard tablets: Blister packs of 28 (OP).
Suppositories 12.5 mg and 100 mg: packs of 10.
Injection: packs of 10 ampoules.

Further information Nil.

Product licence numbers

Tablets 25 mg	0001/0036
Tablets 50 mg	0001/0082
Voltarol Dispersible (equivalent to 50 mg diclofenac sodium).	0001/0134
Suppositories 100 mg	0001/0083
Suppositories 12.5 mg	0001/0102
Ampoules for injection 75 mg/3 ml	0001/0091
Voltarol Retard 100 mg	0001/0101

VOLTAROL EMULGEL*

Presentation Voltarol Emulgel is a white, pleasantly perfumed, non-greasy emulsion in an aqueous gel. Each 100 g contains 1.16 g diclofenac diethylammonium salt (which corresponds to 1 g diclofenac sodium). The gel also contains diethylamine, carbopol, cetomacrogol, a caprylic/capric acid fatty alcohol ester, isopropanol, liquid paraffin, perfume, propylene glycol and water.

Uses *Mode of action:* Voltarol Emulgel is an anti-inflammatory and analgesic preparation designed for external application. Due to an aqueous-alcoholic base it exerts a soothing and cooling effect.

When Voltarol Emulgel is applied locally, the active substance is absorbed through the skin. In healthy volunteers approximately 6% of the dose applied is absorbed when determined by urinary excretion of diclofenac and its hydroxylated metabolites. Findings in patients confirm that diclofenac penetrates inflamed areas following local application of Voltarol Emulgel.

Indications: For the local symptomatic relief of pain and inflammation in:
- trauma of the tendons, ligaments, muscles and joints, e.g. due to sprains, strains and bruises.
- localised forms of soft tissue rheumatism.

It is recommended that treatment be reviewed after 14 days.

Dosage and administration *Adults:* Voltarol Emulgel should be rubbed gently into the skin. Depending on the size of the affected site to be treated 2–4 g (a circular shaped mass approximately 2.0–2.5 cm in diameter) should be applied 3–4 times daily. After application, the hands should be washed unless they are the site being treated.

Use in the elderly: The usual adult dosage may be used.

Children: not recommended.

Contra-indications, warnings, etc
Contra-indications: Hypersensitivity to diclofenac, acetylsalicylic acid or other non-steroidal anti-inflammatory drugs. Hypersensitivity to propylene glycol or isopropanol.

Precautions: Voltarol Emulgel should be applied only to intact, non-diseased skin and not to skin wounds or open injuries. It should not be used with occlusion. It should not be allowed to come into contact with the eyes or mucous membranes, and should never be taken by mouth.

Interactions: No drug interactions during treatment with Voltarol Emulgel have been reported.

Pregnancy and lactation: Since no experience has been acquired with Voltarol Emulgel in pregnancy or lactation, it is not recommended for use in these circumstances.

During the last trimester of pregnancy the use of prostaglandin synthetase inhibitors may result in premature closure of the ductus arteriosus, or in uterine inertia.

Side-effects:

Local: Voltarol Emulgel is usually well tolerated. Local irritation, erythema, pruritus or dermatitis may occasionally occur. Skin photosensitivity, desquamation, atrophy, discoloration and bullous or vesicular eruptions have been reported in isolated cases.

General: Systemic absorption of Voltarol Emulgel is low compared with plasma levels obtained following oral forms of Voltarol. However, where Voltarol Emulgel is applied to a relatively large area of skin and over a prolonged period, the possibility of systemic side-effects cannot be completely excluded.

The following additional side-effects have been observed with *oral* forms of Voltarol:

Gastro-intestinal tract: Occasional: epigastric pain, other gastro-intestinal disorders (e.g. nausea, vomiting, diarrhoea). Rare: gastro-intestinal bleeding, peptic ulcer. In isolated cases: peptic ulcer with perforation, lower gut disorders (e.g. non-specific haemorrhagic colitis and exacerbations of ulcerative colitis).

Central nervous system: Occasional: headache, dizziness or vertigo. Rare: drowsiness, tiredness. In isolated cases: disturbances of sensation or vision (blurred vision, diplopia), tinnitus, insomnia, irritability, convulsions.

Skin: Rare: urticaria. In isolated cases: bullous eruptions, eczema, erythema multiforme, Stevens-Johnson syndrome, Lyell's syndrome, loss of hair.

Kidney: In isolated cases: acute renal insufficiency, urinary abnormalities (e.g. haematuria), interstitial nephritis, nephrotic syndrome.

Liver: Rare: liver function disorders including hepatitis (in isolated cases fulminant) with or without jaundice.

Blood: In isolated cases: thrombocytopenia, leucopenia, agranulocytosis, haemolytic anaemia, aplastic anaemia.

Other organ systems: Rare: oedema, hypersensitivity reactions (e.g. bronchospasm, anaphylactic/anaphylactoid systemic reactions including hypotension).

Overdosage: The low systemic absorption of topical diclofenac renders overdosage extremely unlikely. In the event of accidental ingestion, resulting in significant systemic side-effects, general therapeutic measures normally adopted to treat poisoning with non-steroidal anti-inflammatory drugs should be used.

Management of overdosage with NSAIDs essentially consists of supportive and symptomatic measures. There is no typical clinical picture resulting from Voltarol overdosage. Supportive and symptomatic treatment should be given for complications such as hypotension, renal failure, convulsions, gastro-intestinal irritation, and respiratory depression; specific therapies such as forced diuresis, dialysis or haemoperfusion are probably of no help in eliminating NSAIDs due to their high rate of protein binding and extensive metabolism.

Pharmaceutical precautions Protect from heat.

Legal category POM.

Package quantities Tubes containing 100 g

Further information Nil.

Product licence number 0001/0131.

**Trade Mark*

Geistlich Sons Limited
Newton Bank
Long Lane
Chester CH2 3QZ

AMINOPLEX* 5

Presentation A clear, colourless to yellowish coloured, sterile, pyrogen-free solution for central intravenous infusion, containing synthetic L-form amino acids in combination with calorie supplement. The solution is contained in 1000 ml glass infusion bottles.

Active ingredients per litre: Synthetic-L-form amino acids:

L-Isoleucine	1.53 g
L-Leucine	2.33 g
L-Lysine HCl	2.74 g*
L-Methionine	1.93 g
L-Phenylalanine	2.77 g
L-Threonine	1.29 g
L-Tryptophan	0.56 g
L-Valine	1.80 g
L-Arginine	3.70 g
L-Histidine	0.89 g
L-Alanine	4.03 g
L-Glutamic acid	0.80 g
Glycine	1.77 g
L-Proline	4.83 g
L-Ornithine-L-Aspartate	0.80 g
L-Serine	0.97 g

(*2.19 g as free base)

Calorie source:

Sorbitol	125 g
Ethanol	50 g

Electrolytes:

Sodium	35 mmol
Potassium	28 mmol
Magnesium	4 mmol
Chloride	43 mmol
Acetate	28 mmol

Additional nutrient:

L-Malic acid	1.85 g

Providing: 5 g/litre of utilisable nitrogen. Total energy content 4.2 MJ (1000 kcal). Non-nitrogen energy content: 3.5 MJ (845 kcal). Hypertonic solution: Osmolality approximately 2415 mosmol/kg. pH 7.4 ± 0.2.

Uses For intravenous feeding, providing in a utilisable form, basic body requirements for amino acids, calories and certain electrolytes in one solution. This provides a simple regime for short-term total intravenous feeding, or alternatively a basis for more complex nutritional programmes tailored to specific clinical requirements.

Aminoplex 5 can be used in the correction of protein depletion and the maintenance of adequate nitrogen and electrolyte balance in clinical situations where oral feeding is impossible or contra-indicated, including pre- and post-operative feeding and gastro-intestinal disturbances, such as malaborptive states.

Dosage and administration The quantity and rate of administration is dependent on the age, weight, clinical state and degree of deficiency of the patient and must be determined on an individual basis.

General recommendations

Adults (70 kg bodyweight): 1000–3000 mL in 24 hours by central intravenous infusion. Infusion rate should be commenced slowly at 20 mL/kg/day on the first day. For the second day and thereafter, the infusion rate may be increased to a maximum of 40 mL/kg/day; a constant infusion rate over the full 24 hours of each day should be maintained. Infusion rate: maximum 40–50 drops per minute corresponding to an infusion time of 8 hours per litre.

Elderly: As adult dose.

Children: Up to 1 year: not recommended for neonates (first month) or preterm or ill infants due to the relatively high phenylalanine content. Dosage of all other infants at the clinician's discretion, but phenylalanine levels should be monitored.

Over 1 year: At clinician's discretion.

Utilisable nitrogen is provided as synthetic L-form amino acids, 1 g nitrogen being administered with each 175 non-nitrogen kcal. In cases with greatly increased requirements, e.g. sepsis or complications of surgery, where glucose may be a more appropriate energy source, patients may benefit from an alternative intravenous regimen involving glucose (with or without insulin) and a more concentrated source of L-amino acids.

Contra-indications, warnings, etc

Contra-indications

1. Advanced or irreversible hepatocellular disease and advanced liver disease or advanced renal disease when dialysis facilities are not available.
2. Severe renal insufficiency and use in hyperkalaemia such as is associated with adrenal insufficiency or severe renal insufficiency.
3. Disturbed protein metabolism and inherited disorders of amino acid metabolism.
4. Manifest cardiac insufficiency.
5. Hyperhydration.
6. Acidosis.

Precautions and warnings

1. Before commencing infusion with Aminoplex 5, it is important to exclude conditions which may promote the risk of acidosis. For this reason certain patient selection criteria should be applied. These are:

a. adequate circulating volume
b. adequate liver function
c. adequate renal function
d. absence of acidosis or hypoxaemia.

Aminoplex 5 should not be given to patients not conforming to these criteria, who may have elevated lactate levels, or where the requirements for nitrogen and calories cannot be met within the maximum recommended infusion rate of 40 mL/kg/day.

2. Where shock, metabolic acidosis or severe dehydration is present, the condition should be corrected before the commencement of intravenous feeding.
3. Administration should be carried out only under specialist surveillance. Plasma electrolyte levels should be monitored during use, especially in patients with pre-existing imbalances, in renal failure or hepatic disease.
4. Potassium replacement therapy is critical and must be guided by electrocardiography. Plasma levels may not be directly related to tissue levels. Potassium replacement should be used with extreme caution in patients with cardiac disease, renal dysfunction, digitalisation or hepatic insufficiency. Administration of potassium chloride in glucose solutions will yield lower levels of serum potassium than if given without glucose.
5. Great care should be exercised in renal insufficiency and blood urea nitrogen levels monitored. Routine monitoring of serum electrolytes, water and acid-base should be conducted in these patients.

6. Aminoplex 5 should be administered with great care to patients with diabetes mellitus, liver disease or myocardial insufficiency. Volume overload leading to cardiac failure must be avoided.

7. Caution should be exercised when administering Aminoplex 5 to patients with irreversible liver damage or cardiac failure.

8. Depending on the patient's clinical state and electrolyte balance, there may be a need for supplementary electrolyte replacement based on biochemical montoring. Routine supplementation with vitamins and trace elements should also be undertaken when necessary. Amino acid mixtures may precipitate acute folate deficiency, and folic acid should be given daily. Vitamin B_{12} status should be checked and prophylaxis given if necessary.

9. Abnormalities of liver function tests, cholestasis and portal tract fibrosis have been observed in patients, including infants, receiving total parenteral nutrition.

10. Hypercalciuria and osteomalacia have been reported during total intravenous feeding.

11. Potentially toxic hyperphenylalaninaemia (plasma levels greater than 600 µmol/L) has been reported in association with use of some amino acid solutions. When this solution is used in infants, plasma phenylalanine levels should be monitored and kept within the range 200–500 µmol/L.

12. Patients receiving central amino acid/hypertonic glucose solutions may develop hyperglycaemia. Pancreatitis, liver disease and sepsis may predispose to its development. Hypoglycaemia may also occur rarely.

13. Central venous feeding catheters should be placed using strict aseptic technique with proper fixation and dressing and X-ray confirmation where possible. Asepsis should be maintained during changes of tubing and dressing and use of the catheter should be confined to intravenous feeding alone.

14. Patients receiving these infusions may suffer from air embolism, pneumothorax, central venous thrombosis, brachial plexus or thoracic duct injury, catheter-linked sepsis, subdural haematomata (due to anti-coagulants) or infusion thrombophlebitis. Care should be taken to avoid these complications. Immunosuppressed patients are particularly prone to infection.

15. As Aminoplex 5 contains ethanol and sorbitol, care should be taken when considering the administration of drugs which interfere with their pathways of metabolism.

16. The addition of other medicaments or substances to amino acid solutions should be avoided unless compatibility is known.

Use in pregnancy and lactation: Amino acids, sorbitol and electrolyte administration are not precluded in pregnancy and lactation, but the effect of ethanol on intrauterine growth and other potential deleterious effects has not been determined and therefore the use of the solution is not recommended.

Side-effects: Side-effects are notably absent at the recommended infusion rates and provided the contra-indications are observed.

Overdosage: Nausea, vomiting, flushing, sweating or tachycardia may occur if the recommended infusion rate is exceeded. These symptoms will rapidly resolve on immediate reduction or cessation of infusion with uneventful outcome.

Within the recommended infusion rates and patient selection criteria, lactic acidosis is a rare complication of treatment with Aminoplex 5. If an acidosis does occur, it has been shown that immediate cessation of infusion followed by continued glucose/insulin treatment together with 4.2% sodium bicarbonate (125 mmol in total) will result in lactate concentration and lactate; pyruvate ratio rapidly falling to normal with a rapid rise in arterial pH and standard bicarbonate despite the relatively small dose of sodium bicarbonate.

Pharmaceutical precautions Check that the solution is clear, and the container undamaged. Discard if not fully used at one injection. Store below 25°C. Keep away from light.

There are no major incompatibilities, but the admixture of antibiotics to amino acid solutions can result in a significant decrease of antimicrobial activity of most of the major classes of antibiotics. Data on compatibility and levels of permissible additions of vitamins and trace elements are available from the manufacturer.

Legal category POM.

Package quantities Glass bottles of 1000 ml.

Further information Owing to optical sensitivity of the ingredients, some colour variation of the solution may be anticipated.

Product licence number 0184/0036.

AMINOPLEX* 12

Presentation A clear, colourless to yellowish coloured, sterile, pyrogen-free solution of synthetic L-form amino acids and electrolytes. The solution is contained in 250 ml, 500 ml or 1000 ml glass infusion bottles.

Active ingredients per litre: Synthetic L-form amino acids:

L-Isoleucine	3.80 g
L-Leucine	5.80 g
L-Lysine HCl*	6.80 g*
L-Methionine	4.80 g
L-Phenylalanine	6.88 g
L-Threonine	3.20 g
L-Tryptophan	1.40 g
L-Valine	4.48 g
L-Arginine	9.20 g
L-Histidine	2.20 g
L-Alanine	10.00 g
L-Glutamic acid	2.00 g
Glycine	4.40 g
L-Proline	12.00 g
L-Ornithine-L-Aspartate	2.00 g
L-Serine	2.40 g

(*5.44 g as base)

Electrolytes:

Sodium	35 mmol
Potassium	30 mmol
Magnesium	2.5 mmol
Chloride	67 mmol
Acetate	5 mmol

Additional nutrient:

L-Malic acid	4.60 g

Providing: 12.44 g/l of utilisable nitrogen. Total energy content 1.3 MJ (315 kcal).

Hypertonic solution. Osmolality approximately 830 mosmol/kg. pH 7.4 ± 0.2.

Uses A synthetic L-form amino acid and electrolyte mixture for intravenous feeding when a high intake of protein amino acids is required in a low fluid volume and also in situations where flexibility of choice of calorific substrate is preferred. Administration of Aminoplex 12 should always be accompanied by concurrent administration of a suitable energy source.

Aminoplex 12 can be used in the correction of protein depletion and the maintenance of adequate nitrogen and electrolyte balance in clinical situations where oral feeding is impossible or contra-indicated.

In cases with greatly increased requirements, e.g. sepsis or complications of surgery and trauma, glucose is considered the appropriate energy source and patients may benefit from Aminoplex 12 plus glucose (with or without insulin).

Dosage and administration In order to obtain an optimal metabolic effect and promote positive nitrogen balance, additional calories such as glucose with or without insulin and/or lipid emulsion should be administered concurrently. Approximately 75–250 calories/g nitrogen are required depending on the clinical state. The usual nitrogen load for patients requiring simple protein replacement is 0.15 g nitrogen/kg/day. In catabolic post-operative and post-trauma patients approximately 0.25 g nitrogen/kg/day are needed. In severely catabolic and glucose intolerant patients, especially in the early stages of recovery, 0.35 g nitrogen/kg/day may be needed. Nitrogen requirements should be determined on an individual basis by clinical assessment and biochemical monitoring.

The quantity and rate of administration is dependent on the age, weight, clinical state and degree of deficiency of the patient and must be determined on an individual basis.

General recommendations

Adults (70 kg bodyweight): 500–2000 mL in 24 hours by central intravenous infusion. Infusion rate: maximum 40–50 drops per minute corresponding to an infusion time of 8 hours per litre.

Elderly: As adult dose.

Children: Up to 1 year: not recommended for infants due to the relatively high phenylalanine content.

Over 1 year: At clinician's discretion.

Contra-indications, warnings, etc

Contra-indications

1. Advanced or irreversible hepatocellular disease and advanced liver disease or advanced renal disease when dialysis facilities are not available.
2. Severe renal insufficiency and use in hyperkalaemia such as is associated with adrenal insufficiency or severe renal insufficiency.
3. Disturbed protein metabolism and inherited disorders of amino acid metabolism.
4. Manifest cardiac insufficiency.
5. Hyperhydration.

Precautions and warnings

1. Where shock, metabolic acidosis or severe dehydration is present, the condition should be corrected before the commencement of intravenous feeding.
2. Administration should be carried out only under specialist surveillance. Plasma electrolyte levels should be monitored during use, especially in patients with pre-existing imbalances, in renal failure or hepatic disease.
3. Potassium replacement therapy is critical and must be guided by electrocardiography. Plasma levels may not be directly related to tissue levels. Potassium replacement should be used with extreme caution in patients with cardiac disease, renal dysfunction, digitalisation or hepatic insufficiency. Administration of potassium chloride in glucose solutions will yield lower levels of serum potassium than if given without glucose.
4. Great care should be exercised in renal insufficiency and blood urea nitrogen levels monitored. Routine monitoring of serum electrolytes, water and acid-base should be conducted in these patients.
5. Aminoplex 12 should be administered with great care to patients with diabetes mellitus, liver disease or myocardial insufficiency. Volume overload leading to cardiac failure must be avoided.
6. Caution should be exercised when administering Aminoplex 12 to patients with irreversible liver damage or cardiac faiure.
7. Depending on the patient's clinical state and electrolyte balance, there may be a need for supplementary electrolyte replacement based on biochemical monitoring. Routine supplementation with vitamins and trace elements should also be undertaken when necessary. Amino acid mixtures may precipitate acute folate deficiency, and folic acid should be given daily. Vitamin B_{12} status should be checked and prophylaxis given if necessary.
8. Abnormalities of liver function tests, cholestasis and portal tract fibrosis have been observed in patients, including infants, receiving total parenteral nutrition.
9. Hypercalciuria and osteomalacia have been reported during total intravenous feeding.
10. Potentially toxic hyperphenylalaninaemia (plasma levels greater than 600 μmol/L) has been reported in association with use of some amino acid solutions.
11. Patients receiving central amino acid/hypertonic glucose solutions may develop hyperglycaemia. Pancreatisis, liver disease and sepsis may predispose to its development. Hypoglycaemia may also occur rarely.
12. Central venous feeding catheters should be placed using strict aseptic technique with proper fixation and dressing and X-ray confirmation where possible. Asepsis should be maintained during changes of tubing and dressing and use of the catheter should be confined to intravenous feeding alone.
13. Patients receiving these infusions may suffer from air embolism, pneumothorax, central venous thrombosis, brachial plexus or thoracic duct injury, catheter-linked sepsis, subdural haematoma (due to anti-coagulants) or infusion thrombophlebitis. Care should be taken to avoid these complications. Immunosuppressed patients are particularly prone to infection.
14. The addition of other medicaments or substances to amino acid solutions should be avoided unless compatibility is known.

Use in pregnancy and lactation: The administration of amino acids and electrolytes is neither deleterious nor precluded in pregnancy and lactation, but dosage and administration should be at the discretion of the physician.

Side-effects: Side-effects are notably absent at the recommended infusion rates and provided the contra-indications are observed.

Overdosage: Nausea, vomiting, flushing, sweating or tachycardia may occur if the recommended infusion rate is exceeded. These symptoms will rapidly resolve on immediate reduction or cessation of infusion with uneventful outcome.

Pharmaceutical precautions Check that the solution is clear and the container undamaged. Discard if not fully used at one injection. Store between 15 and 25°C. Keep away from light.

There are no major incompatibilities, but the admixture of antibiotics to amino acid solutions can result in a significant decrease of antimicrobial activity of most of the major classes of antibiotics. Data on compatibiity and levels of permissible additions of lipid emulsions, vitamins and trace elements are available from the manufacturer.

Legal category POM.

Package quantities Glass bottles of 250 ml, 500 ml and 1000 ml.

Further information Owing to optical sensitivity of the ingredients, some colour variation of the solution may be anticipated. Slight deposition of amino acids may occur if inadvertently stored at below 15°C which will dissolve on shaking the container.

Product licence number 0184/0030.

AMINOPLEX* 24

Presentation A clear, colourless to slightly yellow coloured, sterile, pyrogen-free solution of concentrated synthetic L-form amino acids. The solution is contained in 250 ml or 500 ml glass infusion bottles.

Active ingredients per litre: Synthetic L-form amino acids:

L-Isoleucine	7.60 g	
L-Leucine	11.60 g	
L-Lysine HCl	6.80 g	} *
L-Lysine-L-Malate	10.44 g	
L-Methionine	9.60 g	
L-Phenylalanine	13.76 g	
L-Threonine	6.40 g	
L-Tryptophan	2.80 g	
L-Valine	8.96 g	
L-Arginine	18.40 g	
L-Histidine	4.40 g	
L-Alanine	20.00 g	
L-Glutamic Acid	4.00 g	
Glycine	8.80 g	
L-Proline	24.00 g	
L-Ornithine-L-Aspartate	4.00 g	

L-Serine	4.80 g
(*10.88 g as base)	
Electrolytes:	
Sodium	35 mmol
Potassium	30 mmol
Magnesium	2.5 mmol
Chloride	67 mmol
Acetate	5 mmol
Additional nutrient:	
L-Malic acid	4.50 g

Providing: 24.9 g/l of utilisable nitrogen. Total energy content 2.6 MJ (630 kcal).

Hypertonic solution. Osmolality approximately 1570 mosmol/kg. pH 7.4 ± 0.2.

Uses A synthetic L-form amino acid and electrolyte mixture for intravenous feeding, for the correction of protein depletion and the maintenance of adequate nitrogen and electrolyte balance when sufficient oral feeding is not possible in patients with conditions leading to protein breakdown requiring a high nitrogen load and/or a low infusion volume. In cases of renal and liver failure where amino acid therapy is indicated the low fluid volume of Aminoplex 24 may be advantageous, but caution (see contra-indications, warnings and precautions) should be exercised.

In cases of greatly increased requirements, e.g. sepsis or complications of surgery and trauma, glucose is considered the appropriate energy source and patients may benefit from a regimen of Aminoplex 24 plus glucose (with or without insulin).

Dosage and administration In order to obtain an optimal metabolic effect and promote positive nitrogen balance, additional calories such as glucose with or without insulin and/or lipid emulsion should be administered concurrently. Approximately 75–250 calories/g nitrogen are required depending on the clinical state. The usual nitrogen load for patients requiring simple protein replacement is 0.15 g nitrogen/kg/day. In catabolic post-operative and post-trauma patients approximately 0.25 g nitrogen/kg/day are needed. In severely catabolic and glucose intolerant patients, especially in the early stages of recovery, 0.35 g nitrogen/kg/day may be needed. Nitrogen requirements should be determined on an individual basis by clinical assessment and biochemical monitoring.

The quantity and rate of administration is dependent on the age, weight, clinical state and degree of deficiency of the patient and must be determined on an individual basis.

General recommendations

Adults (70 kg bodyweight): 250–1000 mL in 24 hours by slow central intravenous infusion over the full 24 hour period. Infusion rate: maximum 20–25 drops per minute.

Elderly: As adult dose.

Children: Up to 5 years: not recommended for infants due to the relatively high phenylalanine content.

Over 5 years: At clinician's discretion.

Contra-indications, warnings, etc

Contra-indications

1. Advanced or irreversible hepatocellular disease and advanced liver disease or advanced renal disease when dialysis facilities are not available.
2. Severe renal insufficiency and use in hyperkalaemia such as is associated with adrenal insufficiency or severe renal insufficiency.
3. Disturbed protein metabolism and inherited disorders of amino acid metabolism.
4. Manifest cardiac insufficiency.
5. Hyperhydration.

Precautions and warnings

1. Where shock, metabolic acidosis or severe dehydration is present, the condition should be corrected before the commencement of intravenous feeding.
2. Administration should be carried out only under specialist surveillance. Plasma electrolyte levels should be monitored during use, especially in patients with pre-existing imbalances, in renal failure or hepatic disease.
3. Potassium replacement therapy is critical and must be guided by electrocardiography. Plasma levels may not be directly related to tissue levels. Potassium replacement should be used with extreme caution in patients with cardiac disease, renal dysfunction, digitalisation or hepatic insufficiency. Administration of potassium chloride in glucose solutions will yield lower levels of serum potassium than if given without glucose.
4. Great care should be exercised in renal insufficiency and blood urea nitrogen levels monitored. Routine monitoring of serum electrolytes, water and acid-base should be conducted in these patients.
5. Aminoplex 24 should be administered with great care to patients with diabetes mellitus, liver disease or myocardial insufficiency. Volume overload leading to cardiac failure must be avoided.
6. Caution should be exercised when administering Aminoplex 24 to patients with irreversible liver damage hypoxaemia or cardiac faiure.
7. Depending on the patient's clinical state and electrolyte balance, there may be a need for supplementary electrolyte replacement based on biochemical monitoring. Routine supplementation with vitamins and trace elements should also be undertaken when necessary. Amino acid mixtures may precipitate acute folate deficiency, and folic acid should be given daily. Vitamin B_{12} status should be checked and prophylaxis given if necessary.
8. Abnormalities of liver function tests, cholestasis and portal tract fibrosis have been observed in patients receiving total parenteral nutrition.
9. Hypercalciuria and osteomalacia have been reported during total intravenous feeding.
10. Potentially toxic hyperphenylalaninaemia (plasma levels greater than 600 μmol/L) has been reported in association with use of some amino acid solutions.
11. Patients receiving central amino acid/hypertonic glucose solutions may develop hyperglycaemia. Pancreatitis, liver disease and sepsis may predispose to its development. Hypoglycaemia may also occur rarely.
12. Central venous feeding catheters should be placed using strict aseptic technique with proper fixation and dressing and X-ray confirmation where possible. Asepsis should be maintained during changes of tubing and dressing and use of the catheter should be confined to intravenous feeding alone.
13. Patients receiving these infusions may suffer from air embolism, pneumothorax, central venous thrombosis, brachial plexus or thoracic duct injury, catheter-linked sepsis, subdural haematomata (due to anti-coagulants) or infusion thrombophlebitis. Care should be taken to avoid these complications. Immunosuppressed patients are particularly prone to infection.
14. The addition of other medicaments or substances to amino acid solutions should be avoided unless compatibility is known.

Use in pregnancy and lactation: The administration of amino acids and electrolytes is neither deleterious nor precluded in pregnancy and lactation, but dosage and administration should be at the discretion of the physician.

Side-effects: Side-effects are notably absent at the recommended infusion rates and provided the contra-indications are observed.

Overdosage: Nausea, vomiting, flushing, sweating or tachycardia may occur if the recommended infusion rate is exceeded. These symptoms will rapidly resolve on immediate reduction or cessation of infusion with uneventful outcome.

Pharmaceutical precautions Check that the solution is clear and the container undamaged. Discard if not fully used at one injection. Store between 15 and 25°C. Keep away from light.

There are no major incompatibilities, but the admixture of antibiotics to amino acid solutions can result in a significant decrease of antimicrobial activity of most of the major classes of antibiotics. Data on compatibiity and levels of permissible additions of lipid emulsions, vitamins and trace elements are available from the manufacturer.

Legal category POM.

Package quantities Glass bottles of 250 ml and 500 ml.

Further information Owing to optical sensitivity of the ingredients, some colour variation of the solution may be anticipated. Slight deposition of amino acids may occur if inadvertently stored below 15°C, and will dissolve on shaking the container.

Product licence number 0184/0042.

ANAFLEX* CREAM

Presentation A smooth white water-miscible cream with a pleasant odour containing 10% Polynoxylin.

Uses An antibacterial and antifungal preparation for use in a wide variety of dermatological conditions including athlete's foot, nappy rash, pressure sores, boils, stasis ulcers, pruritus ani, pruritus vulvae.

The product has proved of value in promoting wound healing and for the control of tissue reaction following radiotherapy.

Anaflex Cream is indicated also for the treatment of a wide range of aural and nasal infections including otitis externa.

Dosage and administration By application to the affected site once or twice daily.

For the treatment of infected ears the cream should be applied daily by means of a ½-inch ribbon gauze wick.

Contra-indications, warnings, etc Nil.

Pharmaceutical precautions Store below 25°C.

Legal category P.

Package quantities Tubes of 50 g.

Further information Nil.

Product licence number 0184/5006.

GLUCOPLEX* 1000

Presentation A clear, colourless to yellow, sterile, pyrogen-free solution of 24% glucose pre-mixed with electrolytes and trace elements. The solution is contained in 500 mL or 1000 mL glass infusion bottles.

Active ingredients per litre:

Sodium	50.0 mmol
Potassium	30.0 mmol
Magnesium	2.5 mmol
Zinc	45.6 μmol
Dihydrogen phosphate	18.0 mmol
Chloride	67.0 mmol
Anhydrous glucose	240.0 g

Providing: 4.2 MJ (1000 kcal) per litre.
Hypertonic solution
Osmolality approximately 1750 mosmol/kg.

Uses Prophylactic and replacement therapy requiring a solution providing calories from glucose, with electrolytes and trace elements in clinical situations where oral feeding is impossible or contra-indicated. Glucoplex 1000 may be administered concurrently with amino acid solutions.

Dosage and administration When Glucoplex 1000 is administered with an amino acid solution, approximately 75–250 kcal/g nitrogen are required to obtain an optimal metabolic effect and promote positive nitrogen balance. The quantity and rate of administration is dependent on the age, weight, clinical state and degree of deficiency of the patient and must be determined on an individual basis. General recommendations are:

Adult Dose (70 kg bodyweight): 1000–3000 ml in 24 hours by central intravenous infusion.

Infusion Rate: Maximum infusion 50 drops per minute.

Children's Dose: At physicians' discretion.

Elderly: As adult dose.

Contra-indications, warnings, etc
Contra-indications:

1. Administration in congestive heart failure, or in conditions of severe impairment of renal function.
2. Use in hyperkalaemia such as is associated with adrenal insufficiency or severe renal insufficiency.
3. Administration to patients with glucose/galactose malabsorption syndrome.
4. Use of a solution which is cloudy, contains sediment or is in any way unusual.

Precautions and warnings:

1. Where shock, metabolic acidosis or severe dehydration is present, the condition should be stabilised before the commencement of intravenous feeding.
2. Administration of intravenous feeding regimens should be carried out only under specialist surveillance with comprehensive biochemical monitoring e.g. fluid balance and plasma electrolyte levels – particularly in patients with pre-existing imbalances, renal failure or hepatic disease.
3. Glucoplex 1000 should only be administered with great care to patients with diabetes mellitus, diabetes insipidus, hyperosmotic coma, renal insufficiency, water intoxication, liver disease and myocardial insufficiency.
4. Administration must be continuous to avoid osmotic and hence volume overload leading to cardiac failure. Rapid infusion may invoke hyperglycaemia, hyperosmolar states, osmotic diuresis and resultant dehydration if used in inappropriately high doses or in patients with impaired glucose metabolism.
5. Because GluCoplex 1000 contains potassium, hyperkalaemia may be induced on rapid infusion. Potassium replacement therapy is critical and must be guided by electrocardiography. Plasma levels may not be directly related to tissue levels and potassium replacement should be used with extreme caution in patients with cardiac disease, renal dysfunction, digitalisation or hepatic insufficiency. Administration of potassium chloride in glucose solutions will yield lower levels of serum potassium than if given without glucose.
6. Due to the likely occurrence of thrombophlebitis induced by hypertonic glucose, administration should be through a silicone rubber venous catheter, preferably directly into the left subclavian vein and placed by an experienced operator. Central venous feeding catheters should be placed using strict aseptic technique with proper fixation and dressings and X-ray confirmation where possible. Asepsis should be maintained during changes of tubing and dressing and use of the catheter should be confined to intravenous feeding alone.
7. The addition of other medicaments or substances should be avoided unless compatibility is known.

Use in pregnancy and lactation: Administration of glucose and electrolytes/trace elements is neither deleterious or precluded in pregnancy and lactation. However, as the foetus utilises only glucose and since the renal threshold for glucose is lowered in pregnancy and infused glucose is lost via the kidneys, dosage and administration should be at the discretion of the clinician.

Side-effects: Side-effects are notably absent at recommended infusion rates and provided the contra-indications and precautions/warnings are observed.

Overdosage: If glucose solutions are given at a rate which exceeds their metabolism, a hyperosmolar condition with a rising serum sodium may occur. In such cases there may be hypernatraemia and a rise in the MCV which must be differentiated from iatrogenic sodium overload. Alternatively the respiratory quotient (RQ) may rise above one, giving a high CO_2 production. These complications are more common in severely ill patients. The appropriate glucose load for the patient may be judged from the patient's clinical state, biochemical response to glucose or by assessment of resting metabolic expenditure.

The glucose infusion should be slowly reduced and 0.5% saline alternated with 0.9% saline commenced. Insulin is required at the rate of 1 unit per hour and should be doubled every hour until the blood glucose is controlled between 6–10 mmol/L. As the glucose is taken up into the cell accompanied by water, intracellular volume will increase at the expense of ECF. As the patient improves following rehydration, insulin requirements will fall and usually within 2–3 days, endogenous insulin production will be adequate. Re-institution of glucose administration should then be commenced with careful monitoring of blood glucose and recommencement of insulin if necessary to contain the blood glucose below 10 mmol/L.

Pharmaceutical precautions Check that the solution is clear and the container undamaged. Discard if not fully used at one injection. Store between 15 and 25°C. Keep away from light.

Data on compatibility and levels of permissible additions of lipid emulsions, vitamins and trace elements are available from the manufacturers.

Legal category POM.

Package quantities Clear glass bottles of 500 ml and 1000 ml.

Further information Nil.

Product licence number 0184/0032.

GLUCOPLEX* 1600

Presentation A clear, colourless to yellow coloured, sterile, pyrogen-free solution of 40% glucose pre-mixed with electrolytes and trace elements. The solution is contained in 500 mL or 1000 mL glass infusion bottles.

Active ingredients per litre:

Sodium	50.0 mmol
Potassium	30.0 mmol
Magnesium	2.5 mmol
Zinc	45.6 µmol
Dihydrogen phosphate	18.0 mmol
Chloride	67.0 mmol
Anhydrous glucose	400.0 g

Providing: 6.72 MJ (1600 kcal) per litre.
Hypertonic solution
Osmolality approximately 2900 mosmol/kg.

Uses Prophylactic and replacement therapy requiring a solution providing calories from glucose, with electrolytes and trace elements in clinical situations where oral feeding is impossible or contra-indicated. Glucoplex 1600 may be administered concurrently with amino acid solutions.

Dosage and administration When Glucoplex 1600 is administered with an amino acid solution, approximately 75–250 kcal/g nitrogen are required to obtain an optimal metabolic effect and promote positive nitrogen balance.

The quantity and rate of administration is dependent on the age, weight, clinical state and degree of deficiency of the patient and must be determined on an individual basis. General recommendations are:

Adult Dose (70 kg bodyweight): 1000–3000 ml in 24 hours by central intravenous infusion.

Infusion Rate: Maximum infusion 50 drops per minute.

Children's Dose: At physicians' discretion.

Elderly: As adult dose.

Contra-indications, warnings, etc
Contra-indications

1. Administration in congestive heart failure, or in conditions of severe impairment of renal function.
2. Use in hyperkalaemia such as is associated with adrenal insufficiency or severe renal insufficiency.
3. Administration to patients with glucose/galactose malabsorption syndrome.
4. Use of a solution which is cloudy, contains sediment or is in any way unusual.

Precautions and warnings:

1. Where shock, metabolic acidosis or severe dehydration is present, the condition should be stabilised before the commencement of intravenous feeding.
2. Administration of intravenous feeding regimens should be carried out only under specialist surveillance with comprehensive biochemical monitoring e.g. fluid balance and plasma electrolyte levels, particularly in patients with pre-existing imbalances, renal failure or hepatic disease.
3. Glucoplex 1600 should only be administered with great care to patients with diabetes mellitus, diabetes insipidus, hyperosmotic coma, renal insufficiency, water intoxication, liver disease and myocardial insufficiency.
4. Administration must be continuous to avoid osmotic and hence volume overload leading to cardiac failure. Rapid infusion may invoke hyperglycaemia, hyperosmolar states, osmotic diuresis and resultant dehydration if used in inappropriately high doses or in patients with impaired glucose metabolism.
5. Because GluCoplex 1600 contains potassium, hyperkalaemia may be induced on rapid infusion. Potassium replacement therapy is critical and must be guided by electrocardiography. Plasma levels may not be directly related to tissue levels and potassium replacement should be used with extreme caution in patients with cardiac disease, renal dysfunction, digitalisation or hepatic insufficiency. Administration of potassium chloride in glucose solutions will yield lower levels of serum potassium than if given without glucose.
6. Due to the likely occurrence of thrombophlebitis induced by hypertonic glucose administration should be through a silicone rubber venous catheter, preferably directly into the left subclavian vein and placed by an experienced operator. Central venous feeding catheters should be placed using strict aseptic technique with proper fixation and dressings and X-ray confirmation where possible. Asepsis should be maintained during changes of tubing and dressing and use of the catheter should be confined to intravenous feeding alone.
7. The addition of other medicaments or substances should be avoided unless compatibility is known.

Use in pregnancy and lactation: Administration of glucose and electrolytes/trace elements is neither deleterious nor precluded in pregnancy and lactation. However, as the foetus utilizes only glucose and since the renal threshold for glucose is lowered in pregnancy and infused glucose is lost via the kidneys, dosage and administration should be at the discretion of the clinician.

Side-effects: Side-effects are notably absent at recommended infusion rates and provided the contra-indications and precautions/warnings are observed.

Overdosage: If glucose solutions are given at a rate which exceeds their metabolism, a hyperosmolar condition with a rising serum sodium may occur. In such cases there may be hypernatraemia and a rise in the MCV which must be differentiated from iatrogenic sodium overload. Alternatively the respiratory quotient (RQ) may rise above one, giving a high CO_2 production. These complications are more common in severely ill patients. The appropriate glucose load for the patient may be judged from the patient's clinical state, biochemical response to glucose or by assessment of resting metabolic expenditure.

The glucose infusion should be slowly reduced and 0.5% saline alternated with 0.9% saline commenced. Insulin is required at the rate of 1 unit per hour and should be doubled every hour until the blood glucose is controlled between 6–10 mmol/L. As the glucose is taken up into the cell accompanied by water, intracellular volume will increase at the erxpense of ECF. As the patient improves following rehydration, insulin requirements will fall and usually within 2–3 days, endogenous insulin production will be adequate. Re-institution of glucose administration should then be commenced with careful monitoring of blood glucose and recommencement of insulin if necessary to contain the blood glucose below 10 mmol/L.

Pharmaceutical precautions Check that the solution is clear and the container undamaged. Discard if not fully used at one injection. Store between 15 and 25°C. Keep away from light.

Data on compatibility and levels of permissible additions of lipid emulsions, vitamins and trace elements are available from the manufacturers.

Legal category POM.

Package quantities Clear glass bottles of 500 ml and 1000 ml.

Further information Nil.

Product licence number 0184/0033.

HEPANUTRIN*

Presentation A concentrated solution of synthetic L-form amino acids containing a high percentage of branched-chain amino acids and a low percentage of aromatic amino acids and methionine. Sterile and pyrogen free.

Active ingredients per litre: Synthetic L-form amino acids:

L-Isoleucine	11.1 g
L-Leucine	13.5 g
L-Lysine	7.5 g
L-Methionine	1.2 g
L-Phenylalanine	1.2 g
L-Threonine	5.6 g
L-Tryptophan	0.8 g
L-Valine	10.4 g
L-Arginine	9.6 g
L-Histidine	3.0 g
L-Alanine	9.2 g
L-Proline	9.8 g
L-Serine	6.1 g
Glycine	11.0 g
Additional nutrient:	
D, L-Malic acid	7.8 g

Providing 15.6 g/l of utilisable nitrogen. Hypertonic solution pH 6.4–6.9
Osmolarity approximately 933 mosmol/kg.

Uses Hepanutrin provides nutritional support for patients with diseases of the liver (pre-coma and hepatic coma, pre and postoperative) who require intravenous feeding and are intolerant of general purpose amino acid formulations.

Dosage and administration
Adult dose: 500–1500 ml in 24 hours by continuous central intravenous infusion.

Infusion rate: 1.0 ml per kg body weight per hour, corresponding to 20 drops per minute.

Children's dose at clinician's discretion.

Contra-indications, warnings, etc Hepanutrin is not recommended in patients with inborn errors of amino acid metabolism – especially those involving branched chain amino acid metabolism (e.g. maple syrup urine disease). Care should be exercised in renal insufficiency (particularly in the elderly) with careful monitoring of blood urea nitrogen levels.

Routine monitoring of serum electrolytes, water and acid-base levels is essential.

Simultaneous administration of an appropriate energy source is required, together with electrolyte supplementation where necessary. Amino acid mixtures may precipitate acute folate deficiency, and folic acid should be given daily. Vitamin B_{12} status should be checked and prophylaxis given if necessary.

Specific reproduction studies in animals have not been undertaken with Hepanutrin but amino acid solutions have been safely used during pregnancy in the human. If clinically indicated, dosage and administration should be at the discretion of the clinician.

Side-effects: Hepanutrin is well-tolerated. As with all amino acid solutions, nausea may occasionally occur in a sensitive patient. If the recommended rate of infusion is exceeded, nausea, vomiting, flushing and sweating may occur.

Pharmaceutical precautions Check that the solution is clear, and the container undamaged.

Discard if not fully used at one injection.

The addition of other medications or substances to this solution should be avoided unless compatibility is known.

Store below 25°C. Keep away from light.

Legal category POM.

Package quantities Glass bottles of 500 ml.

Further information Due to optical sensitivity of the ingredients, some colour variation of the solution may be anticipated. Sodium metabisulphite is added as a stabiliser (approx. 30 mg/L).

Product licence number 0184/0040.

KAY-CEE-L* SYRUP

Presentation A clear red cherry flavoured sugar-free syrup containing Potassium Chloride BP 7.50% w/v providing Potassium – 1 mmol per ml (39 mg per ml).

Uses Indicated in all situations where oral potassium supplementation is required. Typical examples—diuretic therapy, Cushing's syndrome, megaloblastic anaemia, diabetic ketosis; during intensive steroid, corticotrophin and carbenoxolone therapy. Primary aldosteronism, metabolic alkalosis.

Dosage and administration *Adults:* 10–50 ml per day at clinician's discretion.

Children: At clinician's discretion.

Doses should be given in divided amounts, after food.

Contra-indications, warnings, etc Impaired renal function, dehydration, and hyperkalaemia.

High doses taken inadvertently will act as an emetic.

Pharmaceutical precautions Store below 25°C.

Legal category P.

Package quantities Bottles of 500 ml.

Further information Potassium chloride in an oral syrup form has recently been cited as potentially more effective than tablets because of its rapid absorption from the stomach. The syrup is also without risk of causing small bowel haemorrhage, ulceration, and stricture formation. It is also important to recognise the use of the chloride salt of potassium, due to the effect of the chloride moiety in controlling metabolic alkalosis. Contains Sorbitol.

Product licence number 0184/0031.

NOXYFLEX* 'S'

Presentation A white crystalline powder containing 2.5 g Noxythiolin.

Uses Noxythiolin has a wide spectrum of antifungal and antibacterial activity for the prevention and eradication of infection from the body surface and specified accessible cavities. Intraperitoneally, it is an effective anti-endotoxin and anti-adhesion agent.

Dosage and administration Noxyflex 'S' Solution is most commonly used at concentrations of 1% and 2.5% as specified below.

When possible pre-warm the Solution to 37°C prior to instillation/irrigation and ensure contact of the Solution on the body surface or in specified body cavities for at least 30 minutes.

Duration of treatment will vary according to the clinical/bacteriological situation, but will normally be 3 to 7 days. Thereafter clinical/bacteriological assessments should be undertaken and the prescribed treatment regimen either repeated or modified accordingly.

Intermittent catheterisation: 100 ml of a 2.5% Solution is pre-warmed to 37°C and slowly instilled into the bladder. The catheter is clamped and the Solution allowed to remain in situ for 30–60 minutes before draining. The procedure is repeated at each catheterisation.

Indwelling catheterisation:

Prophylaxis: 100 ml of a 2.5% Solution is pre-warmed to 37°C and slowly instilled into the bladder. The catheter is clamped and the Solution allowed to remain in situ for 30–60 minutes before draining. The procedure should be carried out 2–3 times per week, although for patients with a past history of recurrent infection daily instillations are preferable.

Treatment of existing infection: 100 ml of a 2.5% Solution is pre-warmed to 37°C and slowly instilled into the bladder. The catheter is clamped and the Solution allowed to remain in situ for 30–60 minutes before draining. This procedure should be carried out twice daily.

In cases of particularly heavy infections, perhaps with associated catheter obstruction, the two instillations should be consecutive. Here, the first instillation is allowed to remain in situ for a minimum of 40 minutes; drainage is immediately followed by the second instillation which is retained for a further 40 minutes.

Whichever treatment regimen is chosen, the duration of therapy should be 5–7 days, following which routine clinical/microbiological assessments should be carried out and the prescribed regimen either repeated or modified accordingly.

If infection is slow to clear:

Check concentration of Noxyflex 'S' Solution used is correct.

Check that Noxyflex 'S' Solution is allowed to remain in the bladder for the correct length of time.

Check for systemic involvement; if present, supplement Noxyflex 'S' instillations with an appropriate course of systemic therapy.

Peritonitis

Noxyflex 'S' is used locally in the peritoneal cavity as an adjunct to the routine treatment of peritonitis and its accompanying shock.

Treatment is based on the following five principles:

- Removal of the cause of peritoneal soiling by surgical exploration.
- Mechanical cleansing of the peritoneal cavity by irrigation with saline.
- Treatment of systemic infection by appropriate antibiotics, such as an aminoglycoside or third generation cephalosporin plus metronidazole.
- Supportive therapy with blood transfusion, intravenous electrolyte solutions and steroids if required to combat shock.
- Intraperitoneal instillation of Noxyflex 'S':

As a single instillation at the time of laparotomy in straightforward bacterial infection. As a repeated instillation or by per- and postoperative irrigation in severe peritonitis, *or* where it is anticipated there may be an accumulation of toxic products such as blood or pus, *or* continuing soiling of the peritoneum.

Technique of single instillation: Following laparotomy and toilet of the peritoneum, the wound is closed after instillation of 5.0 g of Noxyflex 'S' in 200 ml of Water for Injections BP or saline, at the site of maximum contamination. If a drain is left in situ it should be clamped for two hours to prevent drainage of the Noxyflex 'S' Solution.

Technique of repeated instillation: At laparotomy a fine No 9 umbilical catheter is inserted through a stab wound in the upper abdomen to lie in relation to the right lobe of the liver. A tube drain down to the site of maximum contamination is brought out through a stab wound in the lower abdomen. 5.0 g of Noxyflex 'S' in 200 ml of Water for Injections BP or saline is instilled into the abdomen before closing the wound. Thereafter, 2.5 g Noxyflex 'S' in 100 ml of Water for Injections BP or saline is injected twice daily through the umbilical catheter for five days postoperatively. The lower drain should be clamped for two hours after each instillation.

Technique of per- and postoperative irrigation: At laparotomy the peritoneal cavity is lavaged with 5.0 g of Noxyflex 'S' in 500 ml of Water for Injections BP or saline until the returning fluid is clear. In severe contamination a second 500 ml aliquot is used. Following conclusion of the operative procedure, a Ryles tube is inserted via a stab wound into the peritoneal cavity to lie in relation to the site of maximum contamination. Two corrugated drains are introduced by separate stab incisions to permit free egress of the drainage fluid. The Ryles tube is connected to a conventional drip arrangement, and 5.0 g of Noxyflex 'S' in 500 ml of Water for Injections BP or saline is dripped in continuously every 12 hours for one to three days depending on the estimated degree of contamination.

Empyema

Acute: 100 ml of a 1% or 2.5% Solution instilled daily for a minimum of five days leaving the intercostal drain clamped for a minimum period of 30 minutes.

Chronic: Begin with four-hourly irrigations of 100 ml of 1% Solution and after 12–24 hours alternate these with one or more four-hourly cycles of normal saline.

Infected wounds and fistulae: Irrigate with a 1%–2.5% Solution twice daily for five days.

Infected burns: 1%–2.5% Solution as a wet dressing twice daily.

Abscess cavities: Irrigate with a 2.5% Solution via polythene tube, twice daily.

Radiotherapy (*Ca Bladder*): 50 ml of 2.5% Solution instilled via catheter during planning.

Contra-indications, warnings, etc The use of Noxyflex 'S' in conjunction with other pharmaceutical agents for combined irrigation/instillation therapy is not recommended and Solution preparation should be carried out as stated under 'Pharmaceutical preparation'. The normal daily usage of Noxyflex 'S' in adults should not exceed 10 g for either accumulative (ie. repeated) instillation regimens or continuous irrigation regimens. Solutions are not intended for intravenous use.

Pharmaceutical precautions *Storage of powder:* The powder vials should be stored below 25°C.

Storage of Solution: Solution should be kept at 2–10°C and used within 7 days. Containers of prepared Solution are intended for single use only.

Solution Preparation (20 ml vial): The powder should be dissolved completely in a sufficient quantity of Water for Injections BP or Sodium Chloride Intravenous Infusion BP (0.9 per cent w/v) by an aseptic technique. Slight difficulty may be experienced in preparing Solutions.

To make a 2.5% Solution: Add contents of one vial (2.5 g) to 100 ml of Water for Injections BP or Sodium Chloride Intravenous Infusion BP (0.9 per cent w/v) and shake for a half to two minutes.

To make a 1% Solution: Add contents of one vial (2.5 g) to 250 ml of Water for Injections BP or Sodium Chloride Intravenous Infusion BP (0.9 per cent w/v) and shake for a half to two minutes.

Solution preparation (100 ml vial): Reconstitution procedure to produce 100 ml Noxyflex 'S' Solution (e.g. 2.5%):

Materials: Transfer needle; 100 ml of Water for Injections BP or Sodium Chloride Intravenous Infusion BP (0.9% w/v); Alcohol Swabs; IVA additive seal.

Procedure:

1. Using aseptic technique, expose rubber stoppers of Noxyflex 'S' 100 ml vial and diluent vial. Swab exposed surfaces.
2. Remove transfer needle set from wrapping.
3. Remove protective sheath from one end of transfer set and insert spike *fully* into stopper of Noxyflex 'S' vial.
4. Remove protective sheath from other end of transfer set and insert spike *fully* into stopper of diluent vial.
5. Invert assembly so that the vial of diluent is uppermost and allow fluid to drain into Noxyflex 'S' vial. (Briefly shake assembly if flow is reluctant to start.)
6. Withdraw transfer spike from Noxyflex 'S' vial.

7. Swab stopper of Noxyflex 'S' vial.
8. Remove protective backing from IVA seal and apply IVA seal to stopper of Noxyflex 'S' vial.
9. Ensure Noxyflex 'S' has completely dissolved; if necessary, shake vial until solution is clear.

Legal category POM.

Package quantities
20 ml vials containing 2.5 g:
Boxes of 10 vials
Individually-cartoned vials

100 ml vials containing 2.5 g:
Boxes of 8 vials with transfer-needle sets and additive seals.
Individually cartoned vials with transfer-needle set and additive seal.

Further information Where desirable, the discretionary use of a suitable local anaesthetic may be used.

Product licence number 0184/5012

**Trade Mark*

Glaxo Laboratories Limited
Stockley Park West
Uxbridge, Middlesex UB11 1BT

Glaxo

BETNELAN* TABLETS

Presentation Small white tablets engraved 'Betnelan Glaxo' on one side and scored on the reverse. Each tablet contains 500 micrograms (0.5 mg) betamethasone.

The product complies with the specification for Betamethasone Tablets BP.

Uses Betamethasone is a glucocorticosteroid which is about eight to ten times as active as prednisolone on a weight-for-weight basis.

A wide variety of diseases may sometimes require corticosteroid therapy. Some of the principal indications are: Bronchial asthma, severe hypersensitivity reactions, anaphylaxis; rheumatoid arthritis, systemic lupus erythematosus, dermatomyositis, mixed connective tissue disease (excluding systemic sclerosis), polyarteritis nodosa;

Inflammatory skin disorders, including pemphigus vulgaris, bullous pemphigoid and pyoderma gangrenosum;

Minimal change nephrotic syndrome, acute interstitial nephritis; ulcerative colitis, Crohn's disease;

Sarcoidosis;

Rheumatic carditis;

Haemolytic anaemia (auto-immune), acute and lymphatic leukaemia, malignant lymphoma, multiple myeloma, idiopathic thrombocytopenic purpura;

Immuno-suppression in transplantation.

Dosage and administration The lowest dosage that will produce an acceptable result should be used; when it is possible to reduce the dosage, this must be accomplished by stages. During prolonged therapy, dosage may need to be increased temporarily during periods of stress or in exacerbations of illness.

Adults: The dose used will depend upon the disease, its severity, and the clinical response obtained. The following regimens are for guidance only. Divided dosage is usually employed.

Short-term treatment: 2 to 3 mg daily for the first few days, subsequently reducing the daily dosage by 250 or 500 micrograms (0.25 or 0.5 mg) every two to five days, depending upon the response.

Rheumatoid arthritis: 500 micrograms (0.5 mg) to 2 mg daily. For maintenance therapy the lowest effective dosage is used.

Most other conditions: 1.5 to 5 mg daily for one to three weeks, then reducing to the minimum effective dosage.

Larger doses may be needed for mixed connective tissue diseases and ulcerative colitis.

Children: Fractions of the adult dosage may be used (e.g. 75% at twelve years, 50% at seven years and 25% at one year) but clinical factors must be given due weight.

Contra-indications, warnings, etc

Contra-indications: Systemic infections, unless specific anti-infective therapy is employed.

Live virus immunisation. Hypersensitivity to any component of the tablets.

Precautions: Administration of corticosteroids may impair the ability to resist and counteract infection e.g. where there is a previous history of tuberculosis; in addition, clinical signs and symptoms of infection are suppressed.

Corticosteroid treatment is likely to reduce the response of the pituitary-adrenal axis to stress, and relative insufficiency may persist for up to a year after withdrawal of prolonged therapy.

Because of the possibility of fluid retention, care must be taken when corticosteroids are administered to patients with congestive heart failure.

Corticosteroids may worsen diabetes mellitus, osteoporosis, hypertension, glaucoma and epilepsy.

Care should be taken when there is a history of severe affective disorders (especially a previous history of steroid psychosis), previous steroid myopathy or peptic ulceration.

Since corticosteroids are secreted in breast milk, the advisability of breast feeding should be considered in women on high dosage.

Steroids may reduce the effects of anticholinesterases in myasthenia gravis, cholecystographic X-ray media and salicylates.

The effect of steroids may be reduced by phenytoin, phenobarbitone, ephedrine and rifampicin.

The dosage of concomitantly administered anticoagulants may have to be altered (usually decreased).

In patients with liver failure, blood levels of corticosteroids may be increased, as with other drugs which are metabolised in the liver.

Systemic corticosteroids may cause growth retardation in infancy, childhood and adolescence. Treatment should be limited to the minimum dosage for the shortest possible time. In order to minimise suppression of the HPA axis and growth retardation, consideration should be given to administration of a single dose on alternate days.

Treatment of elderly patients, particularly if long-term, should be planned bearing in mind the more serious consequences of the common side-effects of corticosteroids in old age, especially osteoporosis, diabetes, hypertension, susceptibility to infection and thinning of the skin.

When treatment is to be discontinued, the dose should be reduced gradually over a period of several weeks or months depending on the dosage and duration of the therapy.

Pregnancy: There is inadequate evidence of safety in human pregnancy. Administration of corticosteroids to pregnant animals can cause abnormalities of fetal development including cleft palate and intra-uterine growth retardation. There may therefore be a very small risk of such effects in the human fetus.

Depression of hormone levels has been described in pregnancy but the significance of this finding is not clear.

Side-effects: Prolonged treatment with corticosteroids in high dosage is occasionally associated with subcapsular cataract, skin thinning and glaucoma. In addition, any of the features of hypercorticism, such as suppression of the HPA axis, may occur. Aseptic osteonecrosis, particularly of the femoral head, may occur after prolonged corticosteroid therapy or after repeated short courses involving high dosage. Peptic ulceration may develop, or be aggravated.

In children, prolonged therapy may retard growth.

In patients on long-term therapy, fluid and electrolyte balance may be altered. Other rare side-effects which have been reported include benign intracranial hypertension and psychic instability.

Drug interactions: Steroids may reduce the effects of anticholinesterases in myasthenia gravis, cholecystographic X-ray media and non-steroidal anti-inflammatory agents. It should also be remembered that the effects of steroids may be reduced by phenytoin, phenobarbitone, ephedrine and rifampicin.

Overdosage: Treatment is unlikely to be needed in cases of acute overdosage.

Pharmaceutical precautions Protect from light.

Legal category POM.

Package quantities Bottles of 100 (OP) or 500 tablets.

Further information Betnelan does not normally cause retention of salt and water, and the risk of inducing oedema and hypertension is almost negligible.

Product licence number 0004/5134R.

Product licence holder: Glaxo Operations UK Limited, Greenford, Middlesex UB6 0HE.

BETNESOL* EYE, EAR AND NOSE PREPARATIONS

Presentation Betnesol Drops contain betamethasone sodium phosphate 0.1% w/v, and benzalkonium chloride 0.02% w/v in a clear, colourless to pale yellow aqueous solution that is sterile until the bottle is opened. This product complies with the BPC specification for Betamethasone Eye Drops.

Betnesol Eye Ointment contains betamethasone sodium phosphate 0.1% w/w in a bland, soft paraffin base of white, translucent appearance. Sterile until opened.

Uses Short-term treatment of steroid responsive inflammatory conditions of the eye after clinical exclusion of bacterial, viral and fungal infections.

Non-infected inflammatory conditions of the ear or nose.

Dosage and administration *Adults (and the Elderly) and Children: Eyes:* 1 or 2 drops instilled into the eye every one or two hours until control is achieved, when the frequency may be reduced. An extrusion of the ointment about ¼ inch long may be introduced beneath the lower lid two or three times daily and/or at night.

Ears: 2 or 3 drops instilled into the ear every two or three hours until control is achieved, when the frequency can be reduced.

Nose: 2 or 3 drops instilled into each nostril two or three times daily.

Contra-indications, warnings, etc

Contra-indications: Bacterial, viral, fungal, tuberculous or purulent conditions of the eye. Use is contra-indicated if glaucoma is present, or herpetic keratitis (e.g. dendritic ulcer) is considered a possibility.

Use of topical steroids in the latter condition can lead to the extension of the ulcer and marked visual deterioration.

Hypersensitivity to the preparation.

Betnesol Drops contain benzalkonium chloride as a preservative and therefore should not be used as eye drops to treat patients who wear soft contact lenses.

Precautions: Topical corticosteroids should never be given for an undiagnosed "red eye" as inappropriate use is potentially blinding.

Ophthalmological treatment with corticosteroid preparations should not be repeated or prolonged without regular review to exclude raised intra-ocular pressure, cataract formation, or unsuspected infections.

Prolonged use may lead to the risk of adrenal suppression in infants.

Pregnancy and Lactation: Safety for use in pregnancy and lactation has not been established. There is inadequate evidence of safety in human pregnancy. Topical administration of corticosteroids to pregnant animals can cause abnormalities of fetal development including cleft palate and intra-uterine growth retardation. There may, therefore, be a very small risk of such effects in the human fetus.

Side-effects: Hypersensitivity reactions, usually of the delayed type, may occur leading to irritation, burning, stinging, itching and dermatitis.

Topical steroid use may increase intra-ocular pressure leading to optic nerve damage, reduced visual acuity and visual field defects.

Intensive or prolonged use of topical corticosteroids may lead to formation of posterior subcapsular cataracts.

In those diseases causing thinning of the cornea or sclera, corticosteroid therapy may result in thinning of the globe leading to perforation.

Excessive and prolonged intranasal usage above the recommended dose may induce systemic side effects.

Overdosage: Oral ingestion of the contents of one bottle (up to 10 ml) of drops, or one tube (3 g) of ointment is unlikely to lead to any serious adverse effects.

Pharmaceutical precautions It is desirable that the contents should not be used more than four weeks after first opening the bottle or tube.

Legal category POM.

Package quantities *Betnesol Drops:* Plastic dropper bottles containing 10 ml.

Betnesol Eye Ointment: Narrow-nozzle tubes containing 3 g.

Further information Nil.

Product licence numbers

Betnesol Drops 0004/5135R
Betnesol Eye Ointment 0004/5137R

Product licence holder: Glaxo Operations UK Limited, Greenford, Middlesex UB6 0HE.

BETNESOL*-N EYE, EAR AND NOSE PREPARATIONS

Presentation Betnesol-N Drops contain betamethasone sodium phosphate 0.1% w/v, neomycin sulphate 0.5% w/v and thiomersal 0.005% w/v in a clear, colourless to pale yellow aqueous solution. Sterile until opened.

Betnesol-N Eye Ointment contains betamethasone sodium phosphate 0.1% w/w and neomycin sulphate 0.5% w/w in a bland, soft paraffin base of white translucent appearance. Sterile until opened.

Uses Betamethasone has topical corticosteroid activity. The presence of neomycin should prevent the development of bacterial infection.

Eye: For the short-term treatment of steroid responsive conditions of the eye when prophylactic antibiotic treatment is also required, after excluding the presence of fungal and viral disease.

Ear: Otitis externa or other steroid responsive conditions where prophylactic antibiotic treatment is also required.

Nose: Steroid responsive inflammatory conditions where prophylactic antibiotic treatment is also required.

Dosage and administration *Adults (and the Elderly) and Children:*

Eyes: 1 or 2 drops applied to each affected eye up to six times daily or more frequently if required. An extrusion of the ointment about ¼ inch long may be introduced beneath the lower lid two or three times daily and/or at night.

Ear: 2 or 3 drops instilled into the ear three to four times daily.

Nose: 2 or 3 drops instilled into each nostril two or three times daily.

Contra-indications, warnings, etc

Contra-indications: Viral, fungal, tuberculous or purulent conditions of the eye. Use is contra-indicated if glaucoma is present or herpetic keratitis (e.g., dendritic ulcer) is considered a possibility. Use of topical steroids in the latter condition can lead to extension of the ulcer and marked visual deterioration.

Otitis externa should not be treated when the eardrum is perforated because of the risk of ototoxicity.

Hypersensitivity to the preparation.

Betnesol-N Drops contain benzalkonium chloride as a preservative and should not be used as eye drops to treat patients who wear soft contact lenses.

Precautions: Topical corticosteroids should never be given for an undiagnosed "red eye" as inappropriate use is potentially blinding.

Treatment with corticosteroid/antibiotic combinations should not be continued for more than 7 days in the absence of any clinical improvement, since prolonged use may lead to occult extension of infection due to the masking effect of the steroid. Prolonged use may also lead to skin sensitisation and the emergence of resistant organisms.

Prolonged use may lead to the risk of adrenal suppression in infants.

Treatment with corticosteroid preparations should not be repeated or prolonged without regular review to exclude raised intra-ocular pressure, cataract formation or unsuspected infections.

Aminoglycoside antibiotics may cause irreversible, partial or total deafness when given systemically or when applied topically to open wounds or damaged skin. This effect is dose related and is enhanced by renal or hepatic impairment. Although this effect has not been reported following topical ocular use, the possibility should be considered when high dose topical treatment is given to small children or infants.

Pregnancy and lactation: Safety for use in pregnancy and lactation has not been established. There is inadequate evidence of safety in human pregnancy. Topical administration of corticosteroids to pregnant animals can cause abnormalities of fetal development including cleft palate and intra-uterine growth retardation. There may therefore be a very small risk of such effects in the human fetus. There is a risk of fetal ototoxicity if aminoglycoside antibiotic preparations are administered during pregnancy.

Side-effects: Hypersensitivity reactions, usually of the delayed type, may occur leading to irritation, burning, stinging, itching and dermatitis.

Topical steroid use may result in increased intra-ocular pressure leading to optic nerve damage, reduced visual acuity and visual field defects.

Intensive or prolonged use of topical corticosteroids may lead to formation of posterior subcapsular cataracts.

In those diseases causing thinning of the cornea or sclera, corticosteroid therapy may result in thinning of the globe leading to perforation.

Overdosage: Long-term intensive topical use may lead to systemic effects.

Oral ingestion of the contents of one bottle (up to 10 ml) of drops, or one tube (3 g) of ointment is unlikely to lead to any serious adverse effects.

Pharmaceutical precautions It is desirable that the contents should not be used more than four weeks after first opening the bottle or tube.

Legal category POM.

Package quantities *Betnesol-N Drops:* Plastic dropper bottles containing 10 ml.

Betnesol-N Eye Ointment: Tubes containing 3 g.

Further information Nil.

Product licence numbers

Betnesol-N Drops	0004/5136R
Betnesol-N Eye Ointment	0004/5138R

Product licence holder: Glaxo Operations UK Limited, Greenford, Middlesex UB6 OHE.

BETNESOL* INJECTION

Presentation Each ampoule of ready-prepared Betnesol Injection contains 4 mg betamethasone as the sodium phosphate ester in 1 ml of sterile aqueous solution. The injection is clear and colourless or pale yellow, and complies with the specification for Betamethasone Sodium Phosphate Injection BP.

Uses Betamethasone is a glucocorticosteroid which is about eight to ten times as active as prednisolone on a weight-for-weight basis. It may be indicated in the following conditions:

Status asthmaticus and acute allergic reactions, including anaphylactic reaction to drugs. Betnesol Injection supplements the action of adrenaline.

Severe shock arising from surgical or accidental trauma or overwhelming infection.

Acute adrenal crisis caused by abnormal stress in Addison's disease, Simmonds' disease, hypopituitarism following adrenalectomy, and when adrenocortical function has been suppressed by prolonged corticosteroid therapy.

Soft tissue lesions such as tennis elbow, tenosynovitis and bursitis.

N.B. Betnesol Injection does not replace other forms of therapy for the treatment of shock and status asthmaticus.

Dosage and administration *Systemic therapy in adults:* 4 to 20 mg betamethasone (1 to 5 ml) administered by intravenous injection over half to one minute. This dose can be repeated three or four times in 24 hours, or as required, depending upon the condition being treated and the patient's response. Alternatively, Betnesol Injection may be given in an intravenous infusion. The same dose can be given by intramuscular injection, but the response is likely to be less rapid, especially in shock.

This dose can be repeated three or four times in 24 hours, depending upon the condition being treated and the patient's response.

Systemic therapy in children: Infants up to 1 year may be given 1 mg betamethasone intravenously; children aged 1 to 5 years, 2 mg; 6 to 12 years, 4 mg (1 ml).

This dose can be repeated three or four times in 24 hours, depending upon the condition being treated and the patient's response.

Other routes: Local injections of 4 to 8 mg Betnesol may be used when treating soft tissue lesions in adults; children may require smaller doses. This dose can be repeated on two or three occasions depending on the patient's response.

Betnesol Injection has also been administered subconjunctivally as a single injection of 0.5 to 1 ml.

Intrathecal use is not recommended.

Contra-indications, warnings, etc

Contra-indications: Systemic infections, unless specific anti-infective therapy is employed. Live virus immunisation.

Betnesol Injection contains sodium metabisulphite (0.1% w/v) as a preservative and therefore should not be used to treat patients with known hypersensitivity to bisulphite, metabisulphite or any other component of the injection.

Betnesol Injection should not be injected directly into tendons.

Precautions: Administration of corticosteroids may impair the ability to resist and counteract infection e.g., where there is a previous history of tuberculosis; in addition, clinical signs and symptoms of infection are suppressed.

Corticosteroid treatment is likely to reduce the response of the pituitary adrenal axis to stress, and relative insufficiency may persist for up to a year after withdrawal of prolonged therapy.

Because of the possibility of fluid retention, care must be taken when corticosteroids are administered to patients with congestive heart failure.

Corticosteroids may worsen diabetes mellitus, osteoporosis, hypertension, glaucoma and epilepsy.

Care should be taken where there is a history of severe affective disorders (especially a previous history of steroid psychosis), previous steroid myopathy or peptic ulceration.

Since corticosteroids are secreted in breast milk, the advisability of breast feeding should be considered in women on high dosage.

Steroids may reduce the effects of anticholinesterases in myasthenia gravis, cholecystographic X-ray media and salicylates.

The effect of steroids may be reduced by phenytoin, phenobarbitone, ephedrine and rifampicin.

The dosage of concomitantly administered anti-coagulants may have to be altered (usually decreased).

In patients with liver failure, blood levels of corticosteroid may be increased, as with other drugs which are metabolised in the liver.

Systemic corticosteroids may cause growth retardation in infancy, childhood and adolescence. Treatment should be limited to the minimum dosage for the shortest possible time. In order to minimise suppression of the HPA axis and growth retardation consideration should be given to administration of a single dose on alternate days.

Treatment of elderly patients, particularly if long-term, should be planned bearing in mind the more serious consequences of the common side effects of corticosteroids in old age, especially osteoporosis, diabetes, hypertension, susceptibility to infection and thinning of the skin.

When treatment is to be discontinued, the dose should be reduced gradually over a period of several weeks or months depending on the dosage and duration of the therapy.

Pregnancy: There is inadequate evidence of safety in human pregnancy. Administration of corticosteroids to pregnant animals can cause abnormalities of fetal development including cleft palate and intra-uterine growth retardation. There may therefore be a very small risk of such effects in the human fetus.

Depression of hormone levels has been described in pregnancy but the significance of this finding is not clear.

Side-effects: Prolonged treatment with corticosteroids in high dosage is occasionally associated with subcapsular cataract, skin thinning, osteoporosis and glaucoma. In addition, any of the features of hypercorticism, such as suppression of the HPA axis may occur. Aseptic osteonecrosis, particularly of the femoral head, may occur after prolonged corticosteroid therapy, or after repeated short courses involving high dosage. Peptic ulceration may develop, or be aggravated.

In children, prolonged therapy may retard growth.

In patients on long-term therapy, fluid and electrolyte balance may be altered. Other rare side effects which have been reported include benign intracranial hypertension and psychic instability.

Drug interactions: Steroids may reduce the effects of anticholinesterases in myasthenia gravis, cholecystographic X-ray media and non-steroidal anti-inflammatory agents. It should also be remembered that the effects of steroids may be reduced by phenytoin, phenobarbitone, ephedrine and rifampicin.

Overdosage: Treatment is unlikely to be needed in cases of acute overdosage.

Pharmaceutical precautions Protect from light.

Legal category POM.

Package quantities 1 ml ampoules in box of 5.

Further information There is a lack of evidence that use of corticosteroids in septic shock affects mortality in the long term.

Product licence number 0004/5139R.

Product licence holder: Glaxo Operations UK Limited, Greenford, Middlesex UB6 0HE.

BETNESOL* TABLETS

Presentation Small, soluble pink tablets engraved 'Betnesol Glaxo' on one side and scored on the reverse. Each tablet contains 500 micrograms (0.5 mg) betamethasone as the sodium phosphate ester.

The tablets comply with the specification for Betamethasone Sodium Phosphate Tablets BP.

Uses Betamethasone is a glucocorticosteroid which is about eight to ten times as active as prednisolone on a weight-for-weight basis.

Betamethasone sodium phosphate is very soluble in water, and is therefore less likely to cause local gastric irritation than corticosteroids which are only slightly soluble. This is important when high dosages are required, as in immuno-suppressive therapy.

Betnesol does not normally cause retention of salt and water and the risk of inducing oedema and hypertension is almost negligible.

A wide variety of diseases may sometimes require corticosteroid therapy. Some of the principal indications are:

Bronchial asthma, severe hypersensitivity reactions, anaphylaxis, rheumatoid arthritis, systemic lupus erythematosus, dermatomyositis, mixed connective tissue disease (excluding systemic sclerosis), polyarteritis nodosa;

Inflammatory skin disorders, including pemphigus vulgaris, bullous pemphigoid and pyoderma gangrenosum; minimal change nephrotic syndrome, acute interstitial nephritis; ulcerative colitis, Crohn's disease; sarcoidosis;

Rheumatic carditis;

Haemolytic anaemia (auto-immune), acute and lymphatic leukaemia, malignant lymphoma, multiple myeloma, idiopathic thrombocytopenic purpura;

Immuno-suppression in transplantation.

Dosage and administration Betnesol Tablets are best taken dissolved in water, but they can be swallowed whole without difficulty. The lowest dosage that will produce an acceptable result should be used; when it is possible to reduce the dosage, this must be accomplished by stages. During prolonged therapy, dosage may need to be increased temporarily during periods of stress or in exacerbations of illness.

Adults: The dose used will depend upon the disease, its severity and the clinical response obtained. The following regimens are for guidance only. Divided dosage is usually employed.

Short-term treatment: 2 to 3 mg daily for the first few days, subsequently reducing the daily dosage by 250 or 500 micrograms (0.25 mg or 0.5 mg) every two to five days, depending upon the response.

Rheumatoid arthritis: 500 micrograms (0.5 mg) to 2 mg daily. For maintenance therapy the lowest effective dosage is used.

Most other conditions: 1.5 to 5 mg daily for one to three weeks, then reducing to the minimum effective dosage.

Larger doses may be needed for mixed connective tissue diseases and ulcerative colitis.

Children: Fractions of the adult dosage may be used (e.g. 75% at twelve years, 50% at seven years and 25% at one year) but clinical factors must be given due weight.

Contra-indications, warnings, etc

Contra-indications: Systemic infections, unless specific, anti-infective therapy is employed. Live virus immunisation. Hypersensitivity to any component of the tablets.

Precautions: Administration of corticosteroids may impair the ability to resist and counteract infection e.g. where there is a previous history of tuberculosis; in addition, clinical signs and symptoms of infection are suppressed.

Corticosteroid treatment is likely to reduce the response of the pituitary-adrenal axis to stress, and relative insufficiency may persist for up to a year after withdrawal of prolonged therapy.

Because of the possibility of fluid retention, care must be taken when corticosteroids are administered to patients with congestive heart failure.

Corticosteroids may worsen diabetes mellitus, osteoporosis, hypertension, glaucoma and epilepsy.

Care should be taken when there is a history of severe affective disorders (especially a previous history of steroid psychosis), previous steroid myopathy or peptic ulceration.

Since corticosteroids are secreted in breast milk, the

advisability of breast feeding should be considered in women on high dosage.

Steroids may reduce the effects of anticholinesterases in myasthenia gravis, cholecystographic X-ray media and salicylates.

The effect of steroids may be reduced by phenytoin, phenobarbitone, ephedrine and rifampicin.

The dosage of concomitantly administered anti-coagulants may have to be altered (usually decreased).

In patients with liver failure, blood levels of corticosteroid may be increased, as with other drugs which are metabolised in the liver.

Systemic corticosteroids may cause growth retardation in infancy, childhood and adolescence. Treatment should be limited to the minimum dosage for the shortest possible time. In order to minimise suppression of the HPA axis and growth retardation, consideration should be given to administration of a single dose on alternate days.

Treatment of elderly patients, particularly if long-term, should be planned bearing in mind the more serious consequences of the common side-effects of corticosteroids in old age, especially osteoporosis, diabetes, hypertension, susceptibility to infection and thinning of the skin.

When treatment is to be discontinued, the dose should be reduced gradually over a period of several weeks or months depending on the dosage and duration of the therapy.

Pregnancy: There is inadequate evidence of safety in human pregnancy. Administration of corticosteroids to pregnant animals can cause abnormalities of fetal development including cleft palate and intra-uterine growth retardation. There may therefore be a very small risk of such effects in the human fetus.

Depression of hormone levels has been described in pregnancy but the significance of this finding is not clear.

Side-effects: Prolonged treatment with corticosteroids in high dosage is occasionally associated with subcapsular cataract, skin thinning, osteoporosis and glaucoma. In addition, any of the features of hypercorticism, such as suppression of the HPA axis may occur. Aseptic osteonecrosis, particularly of the femoral head, may occur after prolonged corticosteroid therapy, or after repeated short courses involving high dosage. Peptic ulceration may develop, or be aggravated.

In children, prolonged therapy may retard growth.

In patients on long-term therapy, fluid and electrolyte balance may be altered. Other rare side-effects which have been reported include benign intracranial hypertension and psychic instability.

Drug interactions: Steroids may reduce the effects of anticholinesterases in myasthenia gravis, cholecystographic X-ray media and non-steroidal anti-inflammatory agents. It should also be remembered that the effects of steroids may be reduced by phenytoin, phenobarbitone, ephedrine and rifampicin.

Overdosage: Treatment is unlikely to be needed in cases of acute overdosage.

Pharmaceutical precautions Nil.

Legal category POM.

Package quantities The tablets are strip-packed in cartons of 100 (OP).

Further information Betnesol Tablets do not contain carbohydrates.

Product licence number 0004/5140R.

Product licence holder: Glaxo Operations UK Limited, Greenford, Middlesex UB6 0HE.

BETNOVATE* RECTAL OINTMENT

Presentation Betnovate Rectal Ointment is a white, translucent preparation containing 0.05% w/w betamethasone valerate, 0.1% w/w phenylephrine hydrochloride, and 2.5% w/w lignocaine hydrochloride.

Uses The clinical effectiveness of Betnovate Rectal Ointment is attributable to the marked local anti-inflammatory property of the corticosteroid betamethasone valerate, the analgesic effect of lignocaine, and the vasoconstrictor effect of phenylephrine.

Betnovate Rectal Ointment is indicated for: relief of the symptoms of itching, irritation, discomfort or pain associated with local non-infective anal or peri-anal conditions such as external haemorrhoids.

Dosage and administration A course of treatment should be limited to seven days.

Apply a small amount of ointment two or three times a day initially, using the applicator if internal administration is required. When inflammation is subsiding, once-daily application is sufficient in most cases.

Contra-indications, warnings, etc

Contra-indications: Primary cutaneous viral infections (e.g. herpes simplex, chickenpox). Hypersensitivity to any component of the preparation.

The use of Betnovate Rectal Ointment is not indicated in the treatment of primarily infected skin lesions caused by infection with fungi (e.g. candidiasis, tinea); or bacteria (e.g. impetigo); dermatoses in children under 1 year of age, including dermatitis and napkin eruptions.

Pregnancy: There is inadequate evidence of safety in human pregnancy. Topical administration of corticosteroids to pregnant animals can cause abnormalities of fetal development including cleft palate and intra-uterine growth retardation. There may therefore be a very small risk of such effects in the human fetus.

Side-effects: As with all topical corticosteroids, if the Betnovate preparations are used for prolonged periods, the consequences of systemic absorption, e.g. suppression of the HPA axis, should be considered, especially in children.

Prolonged and intensive treatment with active corticosteroid preparations may cause local atrophic changes in the skin.

Pharmaceutical precautions Nil.

Legal category POM.

Package quantities Tube of 30 g with applicator nozzle.

Further information Nil.

Product licence number
Betnovate Rectal Ointment 0004/5128R

Product licence holder: Glaxo Operations UK Limited, Greenford, Middlesex UB6 0HE.

BETNOVATE* SCALP APPLICATION

Presentation Betnovate Scalp Application is a transparent, slightly gelled solution containing 0.1% w/w betamethasone as valerate. The vehicle contains 50% of isopropyl alcohol, which has antibacterial activity. This preparation complies with the specification for Betamethasone Valerate Scalp Application, BP.

Uses Steroid-responsive dermatoses of the scalp, such as psoriasis and seborrhoeic dermatitis.

Dosage and administration A small quantity of Betnovate Scalp Application should be applied to the scalp night and morning until improvement is noticeable. It may then be possible to sustain improvement by applying once a day, or less frequently.

Contra-indications, warnings, etc

Contra-indications: Infections of the scalp. Hypersensitivity to the preparation.

Dermatoses in children under one year of age, including dermatitis.

Precautions: Care must be taken to keep the preparation away from the eyes. Do not use near a naked flame.

Long-term continuous topical therapy should be avoided where possible, particularly in infants and children, as adrenal suppression can occur even without occlusion.

Topical corticosteroids may be hazardous in psoriasis for a number of reasons including rebound relapses, development of tolerance, risk of generalised pustular psoriasis and development of local or systemic toxicity due to impaired barrier function of the skin. If used in psoriasis careful patient supervision is important.

Development of secondary infection requires withdrawal of topical corticosteroid therapy and commencement of appropriate systemic antimicrobial therapy.

Pregnancy: There is inadequate evidence of safety in human pregnancy. Topical administration of corticosteroids to pregnant animals can cause abnormalities of fetal development including cleft palate and intra-uterine growth retardation. There may therefore be a very small risk of such effects in the human fetus.

Side-effects: Betnovate preparations are usually well tolerated, but if signs of hypersensitivity appear, application should be stopped immediately.

As with other topical corticosteroids, prolonged use of large amounts or treatment of extensive areas can result in sufficient systemic absorption to produce the features of hypercorticism and suppression of the HPA axis. These effects are more likely to occur in infants and children, and if occlusive dressings are used. Local atrophy may occur after prolonged treatment, under occlusion.

In rare instances, treatment of psoriasis with corticosteroids (or its withdrawal) is thought to have provoked the pustular form of the disease (see 'Precautions').

Overdosage: Acute overdosage is very unlikely to occur, however, in the case of chronic overdosage or misuse the features of hypercorticism may appear and in this situation topical steroids should be discontinued.

Pharmaceutical precautions Nil.

Legal category POM.

Package quantities Plastic squeeze bottles of 30 and 100 ml.

Further information The least potent corticosteroid which will control the disease should be selected. The viscosity of the scalp application has been adjusted so that the preparation spreads easily without being too fluid. The specially-designed bottle and nozzle allow easy application direct to the scalp through the hair.

Product licence number 0004/5133R.

Product licence holder: Glaxo Operations UK Limited, Greenford, Middlesex UB6 0HE.

BETNOVATE* SKIN PREPARATIONS

Presentation The Betnovate skin preparations contain 0.1% betamethasone as the valerate ester. The Betnovate R.D. (Ready Diluted) skin preparations contain 0.025% betamethasone as the valerate ester.

Betnovate Cream is a smooth, white, water-miscible preparation. It complies with the specification for Betamethasone Valerate Cream BP.

Betnovate Ointment is a white preparation based on soft paraffin. It complies with the specification for Betamethasone Valerate Ointment BP.

Betnovate Lotion is a white, translucent, aqueous fluid. It complies with the specification for Betamethasone Valerate Lotion BP.

Betnovate R.D. Cream and Ointment are ready-diluted 1 in 4 preparations.

Uses Betamethasone valerate is an active topical corticosteroid which produces a rapid response in those inflammatory dermatoses that are normally responsive to topical corticosteroid therapy, and is often effective in the less responsive conditions such as psoriasis.

Betnovate preparations are indicated for the treatment of: eczema in children and adults, including atopic and discoid eczemas; prurigo nodularis; psoriasis (excluding widespread plaque psoriasis); neurodermatoses, including lichen simplex, lichen planus; seborrhoeic dermatitis; contact sensitivity reactions; discoid lupus erythematosus and they may be used as an adjunct to systemic steroid therapy in generalised erythroderma.

Betnovate R.D. preparations are indicated for maintenance treatment when control has been achieved with Betnovate.

Dosage and administration A small quantity of Betnovate should be applied to the affected area two or three times daily until improvement occurs. It may then be possible to maintain improvement by applying once a day, or even less often, or by using the appropriate ready-diluted (1 in 4) preparation Betnovate R.D. If no improvement is seen within two or four weeks, reassessment of the diagnosis, or referral, may be necessary.

Betnovate and Betnovate R.D. Creams are especially appropriate for moist or weeping surfaces and Betnovate and Betnovate R.D. Ointments for dry, lichenified or scaly lesions, but this is not invariably so. Betnovate Lotion is particularly suitable when a minimal application to a large area is required.

In the more resistant lesions, such as the thickened plaques of psoriasis on elbows and knees, the effect of Betnovate can be enhanced, if necessary, by occluding the treatment area with polythene film. Overnight occlusion only is usually adequate to bring about a satisfactory response in such lesions; thereafter, improvement can usually be maintained by regular application without occlusion.

Contra-indications, warnings, etc

Contra-indications: Rosacea, acne vulgaris and peri-oral dermatitis. Primary cutaneous viral infections (e.g. herpes simplex, chickenpox). Hypersensitivity to the preparation.

The use of Betnovate skin preparations is not indicated in the treatment of primarily infected skin lesions caused by infection with fungi (e.g. candidiasis, tinea), or bacteria (e.g. impetigo); primary or secondary infections due to yeast; peri-anal and genital pruritus; dermatoses in children under 1 year of age, including dermatitis and napkin eruptions.

Precautions: Long-term continuous topical therapy should be avoided where possible, particularly in infants and children, as adrenal suppression can occur even without occlusion.

The face, more than other areas of the body, may exhibit atrophic changes after prolonged treatment with potent topical corticosteroids. This must be borne in mind when treating such conditions as psoriasis, discoid lupus erythematosus and severe eczema. If applied to the eyelids, care is needed to ensure that the preparation does not enter the eye, as glaucoma might result.

If used in childhood or on the face, courses should be limited if possible to five days and occlusion should not be used.

Topical corticosteroids may be hazardous in psoriasis for a number of reasons including rebound relapses, development of tolerance, risk of generalised pustular psoriasis and development of local or systemic toxicity due to impaired barrier function of the skin. If used in psoriasis careful patient supervision is important.

Appropriate antimicrobial therapy should be used whenever treating inflammatory lesions which have become infected. Any spread of infection requires withdrawal of topical corticosteroid therapy and systemic administration of antimicrobial agents. Bacterial infection is encouraged by the warm, moist conditions induced by occlusive dressings, and so the skin should be cleansed before a fresh dressing is applied.

Pregnancy: There is inadequate evidence of safety in human pregnancy. Topical administration of corticosteroids to pregnant animals can cause abnormalities of fetal development including cleft palate and intra-uterine growth retardation. There may therefore be a very small risk of such effects in the human fetus.

Side-effects: Prolonged and intensive treatment with highly active corticosteroid preparations may cause local atrophic changes in the skin such as striae, thinning, and dilatation of the superficial blood vessels, particularly when occlusive dressings are used or when skin folds are involved.

As with other topical corticosteroids, prolonged use of large amounts or treatment of extensive areas can result in sufficient systemic absorption to produce the features of hypercorticism and suppression of the HPA axis. These effects are likely to occur in infants and children, and if occlusive dressings are used. In infants the napkin may act as an occlusive dressing.

In rare instances, treatment of psoriasis with corticosteroids (or its withdrawal) is thought to have provoked the pustular form of the disease (see Precautions).

The Betnovate and Betnovate R.D. preparations are usually well tolerated but, if signs of hypersensitivity appear, application should stop immediately.

Pharmaceutical precautions Nil.

Legal category POM.

Package quantities Betnovate Cream and Ointment are supplied in 30 and 100 g tubes.

Betnovate R.D. Cream and Ointment are supplied in 100 g tubes.

Betnovate Lotion is supplied in 100 ml bottles.

Further information The least potent corticosteroid which will control the disease should be selected. None of these preparations contain lanolin. Betnovate Cream and Ointment and the corresponding R.D. preparations, do not contain parabens. Betnovate Lotion contains parabens.

Product licence numbers

Betnovate Cream	0004/5121R
Betnovate Ointment	0004/5124R
Betnovate R.D. Cream	0004/0277
Betnovate R.D. Ointment	0004/0278
Betnovate Lotion	0004/5130R

Product licence holder: Glaxo Operations UK Limited, Greenford, Middlesex UB6 0HE.

BETNOVATE*-C SKIN PREPARATIONS

Presentation The Betnovate-C skin preparations contain 0.1% betamethasone as the valerate ester and 3% clioquinol.

Betnovate-C Cream is a smooth, straw-coloured water-miscible cream.

Betnovate-C Ointment is a pale, straw-coloured to yellow paraffin-based ointment.

Uses Betamethasone valerate is an active topical corticosteroid which produces a rapid response in those inflammatory dermatoses that are normally responsive to topical corticosteroid therapy, and is often effective in the less responsive conditions such as psoriasis.

Clioquinol is an anti-infective agent which has both antibacterial and anticandidal activity.

Betnovate-C preparations are indicated for the treatment of the following conditions where secondary bacterial and/or fungal infection is present, suspected or likely to occur: eczema in children and adults, including atopic and discoid eczemas; prurigo nodularis; psoriasis (excluding widespread plaque psoriasis); neurodermatoses; seborrhoeic dermatitis; contact sensitivity reactions, and discoid lupus erythematosus.

Betnovate-C can also be used in the management of secondarily infected insect bites and anal and genital intertrigo.

Dosage and administration A small quantity should be applied gently to the affected area two or three times daily until improvement occurs. It may then be possible to maintain improvement by applying once a day, or even less often.

Betnovate-C Cream is often appropriate for moist or weeping surfaces and Betnovate-C Ointment for dry, lichenified or scaly lesions, but this is not invariably so.

Contra-indications, warnings, etc

Contra-indications: Rosacea, acne and peri-oral dermatitis. Primary cutaneous viral infections (e.g. herpes simplex, chickenpox). Hypersensitivity to the preparation or to iodine.

Use of Betnovate-C skin preparations is not indicated in the treatment of primarily infected skin lesions caused by infection with fungi (e.g. candidiasis, tinea); or bacteria (e.g. impetigo); primary or secondary infections due to yeast; dermatoses in children under 1 year of age, including dermatitis and napkin eruptions.

Precautions: Long-term continuous topical therapy should be avoided where possible, particularly in infants and children, as adrenal suppression can occur even without occlusion.

The face, more than other areas of the body, may exhibit atrophic changes after prolonged treatment with potent topical corticosteroids. This must be borne in mind when treating such conditions as psoriasis, discoid lupus erythematosus and severe eczema with Betnovate. If applied to the eyelids, care is needed to ensure that the preparation does not enter the eye, as glaucoma might result.

If used in childhood, or on the face, courses should be limited to five days and occlusion should not be used.

Topical corticosteroids may be hazardous in psoriasis for a number of reasons including rebound relapses, development of tolerance, risk of generalised pustular psoriasis and development of local or systemic toxicity due to impaired barrier function of the skin. If used in psoriasis careful patient supervision is important.

If infection persists, systemic chemotherapy is required. Any spread of infection requires withdrawal of topical corticosteroid therapy. Bacterial infection is encouraged by the warm, moist conditions induced by occlusive dressings, and the skin should be cleansed before a fresh dressing is applied.

Do not continue for more than seven days in the absence of clinical improvement, since occult extension of infection may occur due to the masking effect of the steroid.

Betnovate-C may stain hair, skin or fabric, and the application should be covered with a dressing to protect clothing.

Products which contain antimicrobial agents should not be diluted.

Pregnancy: There is inadequate evidence of safety in human pregnancy. Topical administration of corticosteroids to pregnant animals can cause abnormalities of fetal development including cleft palate and intra-uterine growth retardation. There may therefore be a very small risk of such effects in the human fetus.

Side-effects: Prolonged and intensive treatment with highly active corticosteroid preparations may cause local atrophic changes in the skin such as thinning, striae, and dilatation of the superficial blood vessels, particularly when occlusive dressings are used or when skin folds are involved.

As with other topical corticosteroids, prolonged use of large amounts or treatment of extensive areas can result in sufficient systemic absorption to produce the features of hypercorticism and suppression of the HPA axis. These effects are likely to occur in infants and children, and if occlusive dressings are used. In infants the napkin may act as an occlusive dressing.

In rare instances, treatment of psoriasis with corticosteroids (or its withdrawal) is thought to have provoked the pustular form of the disease (see Precautions).

The Betnovate preparations are usually well tolerated, but if signs of hypersensitivity appear, application should be stopped immediately.

Pharmaceutical precautions Nil.

Legal category POM.

Package quantities Betnovate-C Cream and Ointment are supplied in 30 g tubes.

Further information The least potent corticosteroid which will control the disease should be selected. These preparations do not contain lanolin or parabens.

Product licence numbers
Betnovate-C Cream 0004/5122R
Betnovate-C Ointment 0004/5126R

Product licence holder: Glaxo Operations UK Limited, Greenford, Middlesex UB6 0HE.

BETNOVATE*-N SKIN PREPARATIONS

Presentation The Betnovate-N skin preparations contain 0.1% betamethasone as the valerate ester and 0.5% neomycin sulphate (3,500 units per gram or per millilitre).

Betnovate-N Cream is a smooth, white, water-miscible cream.

Betnovate-N Ointment is a white, paraffin-based ointment.

Uses Betamethasone valerate is an active topical corticosteroid which produces a rapid response in those inflammatory dermatoses that are normally responsive to topical corticosteroid therapy, and is often effective in the less responsive conditions such as psoriasis.

Neomycin sulphate is a broad-spectrum, bactericidal antibiotic effective against the majority of bacteria commonly associated with skin infections.

Betnovate-N preparations are indicated for the treatment of the following conditions where secondary bacterial infection is present, suspected, or likely to occur: eczema in children and adults, including atopic and discoid eczema; prurigo nodularis; psoriasis (excluding widespread plaque psoriasis), neurodermatoses, seborrhoeic dermatitis; contact sensitivity reactions and they may be used as an adjunct to systemic steroid therapy in generalised erythroderma.

Betnovate-N preparations can also be used in the management of secondarily infected insect bites and anal and genital intertrigo.

Dosage and administration A small quantity should be applied gently to the affected area two or three times daily until improvement occurs. It may then be possible to maintain improvement by applying once a day, or even less often.

Betnovate-N Cream is especially appropriate for moist or weeping surfaces, and Betnovate-N Ointment for dry, lichenified or scaly lesions, but this is not invariably so.

Contra-indications, warnings, etc
Contra-indications: Rosacea, acne vulgaris and peri-oral dermatitis. Primary cutaneous viral infections (e.g. herpes simplex, chickenpox). Hypersensitivity to the preparation.

Application to large areas especially during pregnancy, in the elderly and in patients with impaired renal function due to a risk of ototoxicity.

Use of Betnovate-N skin preparations is not indicated in the treatment of primarily infected skin lesions caused by infection with fungi (e.g. candidiasis, tinea), or bacteria (e.g. impetigo); primary or secondary infections due to yeast.

Dermatoses in children under 1 year of age, including dermatitis and napkin eruptions.

Preparations containing neomycin should not be used for the treatment of otitis externa when the ear drum is perforated, because of the risk of ototoxicity.

Precautions: Long-term continuous topical therapy should be avoided where possible, particularly in infants and children, as adrenal suppression can occur even without occlusion.

The face, more than other areas of the body, may exhibit atrophic changes after prolonged treatment with potent topical corticosteroids. This must be borne in mind when treating such conditions as psoriasis, discoid lupus erythematosus and severe eczema with Betnovate. If applied to the eyelids, care is needed to ensure that the preparation does not enter the eye, as glaucoma might result.

If used in childhood, or on the face, courses should be limited to five days and occlusion should not be used.

Topical corticosteroids may be hazardous in psoriasis for a number of reasons including rebound relapses, development of tolerance, risk of generalised pustular psoriasis and development of local or systemic toxicity due to impaired barrier function of the skin. If used in psoriasis careful patient supervision is important.

Do not continue for more than seven days in the absence of clinical improvement, since occult extension of infection may occur due to the masking effect of the steroid.

If bacterial infection persists, systemic chemotherapy is required. Any spread of infection requires withdrawal of topical corticosteroid therapy. Bacterial infection is encouraged by the warm, moist conditions induced by occlusive dressings, and the skin should be cleansed before a fresh dressing is applied.

Extended or recurrent application may increase the risk of contact sensitisation.

Products which contain antimicrobial agents should not be diluted.

Pregnancy: There is inadequate evidence of safety in human pregnancy. Topical administration of corticosteroids to pregnant animals can cause abnormalities of fetal development including cleft palate and intra-uterine growth retardation. There may therefore be a very small risk of such effects in the human fetus.

The use of neomycin may be associated with a theoretical risk of fetal ototoxicity (see Contra-indications).

Side-effects: Prolonged and intensive treatment with highly active corticosteroid preparations may cause local atrophic changes in the skin such as thinning, striae, and dilatation of the superficial blood vessels, particularly when occlusive dressings are used or when skin folds are involved.

As with other topical corticosteroids, prolonged use of large amounts or treatment of extensive areas can result in sufficient systemic absorption to produce the features of hypercorticism and suppression of the HPA axis. These effects are likely to occur in infants and children, and if occlusive dressings are used. In infants the napkin may act as an occlusive dressing.

In rare instances, treatment of psoriasis with corticosteroids (or its withdrawal) is thought to have provoked the pustular form of the disease (see Precautions).

The Betnovate preparations are usually well tolerated, but if signs of hypersensitivity appear, application should stop immediately.

Overdosage: Acute overdosage is very unlikely to occur. However, in the case of chronic overdosage or misuse the features of hypercorticism may appear and in this situation topical steroids should be discontinued.

Pharmaceutical precautions Nil.

Legal category POM.

Package quantities Betnovate-N Cream and Ointment are supplied in 30 and 100 g tubes.

Further information The least potent corticosteroid which will control the disease should be selected. These preparations do not contain lanolin or parabens.

Product licence numbers
Betnovate-N Cream 0004/5123R
Betnovate-N Ointment 0004/5127R

Product licence holder: Glaxo Operations UK Limited, Greenford, Middlesex UB6 0HE.

CEPOREX*

Presentation Ceporex Tablets are pink, film-coated tablets, each containing 250 mg, 500 mg or 1 g cephalexin. They are engraved 'Ceporex 250' or 'Ceporex 500' respectively on one side and 'Glaxo' on the reverse. Ceporex Tablets 1 g are engraved with a breakline on one side and 'Glaxo' on the reverse. They comply with the BP specification for Cephalexin Tablets.

Ceporex Capsules are caramel and grey, hard gelatin capsules, each containing 250 mg or 500 mg cephalexin. They are marked 'Ceporex 250' or 'Ceporex 500' respectively, and 'Glaxo'. They comply with the BP specification for Cephalexin Capsules.

Ceporex Syrups are prepared by adding water to the granules to give orange-flavoured and coloured suspensions containing 125 mg, 250 mg or 500 mg cephalexin in each 5 ml. All strengths comply with the BP specification for Cephalexin Mixture.

Ceporex Paediatric Drops are prepared by adding water to give 10 ml of orange-flavoured and coloured suspension containing 125 mg cephalexin in each 1.25 ml. The dropper is calibrated at 125 mg and 62.5 mg.

Ceporex Suspension is a ready-prepared, yellow, banana-flavoured suspension of cephalexin in vegetable oil. Each 5 ml contains 125 mg or 250 mg cephalexin.

Uses

Indications: Ceporex is a bactericidal antibiotic of the cephalosporin group which is active against a wide range of Gram-positive and Gram-negative organisms. It is indicated for treatment of the following conditions, when caused by susceptible bacteria.

Respiratory tract infections: acute and chronic bronchitis and infected bronchiectasis.

Ear, nose and throat infections: otitis media; mastoiditis; sinusitis; follicular tonsillitis and pharyngitis.

Urinary tract infections: acute and chronic pyelonephritis, cystitis and prostatitis. Prophylaxis of recurrent urinary tract infection.

Gynaecological and obstetric infections.

Skin, soft-tissue and bone infections.

Gonorrhoea (when Penicillin is unsuitable).

Dental procedures: treatment of dental infections. As prophylaxis treatment for patients with heart disease undergoing dental treatment as an alternative to penicillin.

Dosage and administration Many infections in adults will respond to oral dosage of 1 gram to 2 grams per day in divided doses; however, for most infections, the following simple dosage scheme will be found satisfactory:

Adults and children over 12 years 1 g b.d.

The following additional information should also be considered:

Adults: For severe or deep-seated infections, especially when less sensitive organisms are involved, the dosage should be increased to 1 g t.d.s. or 3 g b.d.

For prophylaxis of recurrent urinary tract infections in adults, a dose of 125 mg each night is recommended and may be continued for several months. (The 125 mg/5 ml Suspension is suitable for this purpose.)

Children: Ideally, dosage should be calculated on a body-weight basis, particularly in infants. The following dosage recommendations for children are derived from a normal dosage of 25 to 60 mg/kg/day. For chronic, severe or deep-seated infections, this should be increased to 100 mg/kg/day (maximum 4 g/day).

Children under 1 year	(25 to 60 mg/kg/day) 62.5 to 125 mg b.d.
Children 1 to 6 years	250 mg to 500 mg b.d.
Children 7 to 12 years	500 mg to 1 g b.d.

Notes: For most acute infections, treatment should continue for at least two days after signs have returned to normal and symptoms have subsided, but in chronic, recurrent or complicated urinary tract infections treatment for two weeks (giving 1 g b.d.) is recommended. For gonorrhoea, a single dose of 3 g with 1 g probenecid for males or 2 g with 0.5 g probenecid for females is usually effective. Concurrent administration of probenecid delays excretion of cephalexin and raises the serum levels by 50 to 100%.

Ceporex has not been shown to have a toxic effect on the kidney, but as with other antibiotics which are excreted mainly by the kidneys, unnecessary accumulation may occur in the body when renal function is below about half of normal. Therefore, the maximum recommended dosages (i.e., adults 6 g/day, children 4 g/day) should be reduced proportionately in these patients.

In elderly patients the possibility of renal impairment should be considered.

Adult patients receiving intermittent dialysis should be given an additional 500 mg Ceporex after each dialysis, i.e., a total dosage of up to 1 g on that day. Children should receive an additional 8 mg per kg.

Contra-indications, warnings, etc *Contra-indications:* Hypersensitivity to any ingredient of the preparation.

Precautions: Ceporex is usually well tolerated by patients allergic to penicillin, but cross-reaction has been encountered rarely.

As with other broad-spectrum antibiotics, prolonged use may result in the overgrowth of non-susceptible organisms (e.g. Candida, Enterococci, *Clostridium difficile*), which may require interruption of treatment. Pseudomembranous colitis has been reported with the use of broad-spectrum antibiotics, therefore, it is important to consider its diagnosis in patients who develop severe diarrhoea during or after antibiotic use.

As with other antibiotics that are excreted mainly by the kidneys, when renal function is poor, dosage of Ceporex should be suitably reduced (see 'Dosage and administration'). Laboratory experiments and clinical experience show no evidence of teratogenicity, but it would be wise to proceed with caution during the early months of pregnancy, as with all drugs.

In patients receiving Ceporex, a false-positive reaction for glucose in the urine may be given, with Benedict's or Fehling's solution, or with 'Clinitest' tablets, but not with enzyme-based tests.

There are reports of positive Coomb's test.

Ceporex can interfere with the alkaline picrate assay for creatinine, giving a falsely high reading, but the degree of elevation is unlikely to be of clinical importance.

Side-effects: A small proportion of patients receiving Ceporex experience gastro-intestinal disturbances such as nausea, vomiting and diarrhoea.

As with other broad-spectrum antibiotics, there have been rare reports of pseudomembranous colitis.

As with other antibiotics, prolonged use may result in the overgrowth of non-susceptible organisms e.g. Candida. This may present as vulvo-vaginitis.

Reversible neutropenia has occurred in a few patients, but is very rare. Drug rashes, both urticarial and maculopapular, are uncommon.

Interactions: Concurrent treatment with high doses of cephalosporins and nephrotoxic drugs such as aminoglycosides or potent diuretics (e.g. Frusemide, ethacrynic acid and piretamide) may adversely effect renal function. Clinical experience has shown that it is not likely to be a problem with Ceporex at the recommended dosage levels.

Overdosage: Serum levels of cephalexin can be reduced greatly by peritoneal dialysis or haemodialysis.

Pharmaceutical precautions Ceporex Tablets and Capsules should be protected from light. Ceporex Suspension should not be refrigerated.

The reconstituted syrups retain their potency for 10 days when kept in a cool place, preferably a refrigerator. The reconstituted syrups may be diluted with water (not Syrup BP), after which they should be used within seven days. Ceporex Suspension must not be diluted with water or syrup.

Legal category POM.

Package quantities *Tablets 250 mg and 500 mg:* Bottles of 28 (OP), 100 and 500.

Tablets 1 g: Containers of 14 (OP).

Capsules 250 mg and 500 mg: Bottles of 28 (OP), 100 and 500.

Syrup 125 mg/5 ml, 250 mg/5 ml and 500 mg/5 ml: Bottles of 100 ml (OP).

Paediatric Drops 125 mg/1.25 ml: Bottles of 10 ml (OP).

Suspension 125 mg/5 ml and 250 mg/5 ml: Bottles of 100 ml (OP).

Further information Ceporex is resistant to the action of staphylococcal penicillinase, and is therefore active against strains of *Staph. aureus* that are insensitive to penicillin (or ampicillin) through production of that enzyme. Ceporex is also active against the majority of ampicillin-resistant *E. coli*.

Absorption of Ceporex is almost complete, even in the presence of food, and is not adversely affected by coeliac disease, partial gastrectomy, achlorhydria, jaundice or diverticulosis (duodenal or jejunal). Ceporex is excreted in the urine in high concentration.

The serum half-life is normally about one hour, but is longer in the newborn (see 'Dosage and administration'). Ceporex has a wide margin of safety.

Product licence numbers

Ceporex Tablets 250 mg	0004/5046R
Ceporex Tablets 500 mg	0004/5047R
Ceporex Tablets 1 g	0004/0337
Ceporex Capsules 250 mg	0004/5041R
Ceporex Capsules 500 mg	0004/5042R
Ceporex Syrup 125 mg	0004/5043R
Ceporex Syrup 250 mg	0004/5044R
Ceporex Syrup 500 mg Ceporex Paediatric Drops	0004/5045R
Ceporex Suspension 125 mg	0004/0268
Ceporex Suspension 250 mg	0004/0269

Product licence holder: Glaxo Operations UK Limited, Greenford, Middlesex UB6 0HE.

CORLAN* PELLETS

Presentation Small white pellets engraved 'Corlan Glaxo' on one side. Each pellet contains 2.5 mg hydrocortisone in the form of the water-soluble ester hydrocortisone sodium succinate. The pellets comply with the specification for Hydrocortisone Lozenges BPC.

Uses Local use in aphthous ulceration of the mouth, whether simple or occurring as a complication in diseases such as sprue, idiopathic steatorrhoea and ulcerative colitis.

Dosage and administration *Adults and children:* Corlan Pellets should not be sucked, but kept in the mouth and allowed to dissolve slowly in close proximity to the ulcers. One pellet should be used in this way four times a day. When ulcers recur quickly after withdrawal of treatment, maintenance therapy with reduced dosage is desirable for a period.

Contra-indications, warnings, etc
Contra-indications: Corlan Pellets should not be used in the presence of oral infection unless effective chemotherapy is also employed. Hypersensitivity to any component of the product.

Precautions: If aphthous ulceration is severe or recurring, serious underlying disease should be excluded.

There is inadequate evidence of safety in human pregnancy. Topical administration of corticosteroids to pregnant animals can cause abnormalities of fetal development including cleft palate and intra-uterine growth retardation. There may, therefore, be a very small risk of such effects in the human fetus.

Side-effects: Corticosteroids may worsen diabetes.

Occasionally, topical steroid therapy may result in an exacerbation of local infection.

Overdosage: Treatment is unlikely to be needed in cases of acute overdosage.

Pharmaceutical precautions Replace cap firmly after use.

Legal category POM.

Package quantities Container of 20 pellets (OP).

Further information Nil.

Product licence number 0004/5077R.

Product licence holder: Glaxo Operations UK Limited, Greenford, Middlesex UB6 0HE.

CRYSTAPEN* INJECTION

Presentation Vials containing 600 mg (1 mega unit) sodium benzylpenicillin (penicillin G) as a white, crystalline water-soluble powder for the preparation of Benzylpenicillin Injection BP.

Uses Crystapen has bactericidal activity in infections due to penicillin-sensitive organisms, particularly streptococci, pneumococci *(Streptococcus pneumoniae)*, meningococci, gonococci and staphylococci (excluding penicillinase-producing strains). Crystapen is indicated for most wound infections, pyogenic infections of the skin, soft tissue infections and infections of the nose, throat, nasal sinuses, respiratory tract and middle ear, etc.

Generalised infections, septicaemia and pyaemia from susceptible bacteria. Acute and chronic osteomyelitis, subacute bacterial endocarditis, and meningitis caused by susceptible organisms. Gonorrhoea.

Dosage and administration The following dosages apply to both intramuscular and intravenous injection.

Adults: Usually 600 to 1,200 mg (1 to 2 mega units) daily, divided into 2 to 4 doses. In bacterial endocarditis, 8 mega units or more may be given daily in divided doses by the intravenous route, often by infusion. Intravenous doses in excess of 1.2 g (2 mega units) should be given slowly, taking at least one minute for each 300 mg (0.5 mega unit) to avoid high levels causing irritation of the central nervous system. High dosage of sodium benzylpenicillin may result in hypernatraemia and hypokalaemia unless the sodium content is taken into account.

Children aged 1 month to 12 years: 10 to 20 mg (17,000 to 34,000 units) per kilogram body weight in 24 hours, usually divided into 4 doses. In meningitis the dosage may be doubled.

Newborn infants: 30 mg/kg/day (50,000 units) in divided doses, usually twice daily in the first few days of life, then three or four times a day. In meningitis the systemic dosage may be increased to 60 to 90 mg/kg/day (100,000 to 150,000 units) divided into 3 or 4 doses.

PREPARATION OF SOLUTIONS
Intramuscular injection: A 600 mg (1 mega unit) dose is usually dissolved in 1.6 to 2.0 ml of Water for Injections BP.

Intravenous injection: A suitable concentration is 600 mg (1 mega unit) dissolved in 4 to 10 ml of Water for Injections BP.

Intravenous infusion: It is recommended that 600 mg (1 mega unit) should be dissolved in at least 10 ml of Sodium Chloride Injection BP or other transfusion solution.

OTHER ROUTES OF ADMINISTRATION

These usually supplement systemic dosage.

Subconjunctival injection: 300 or 600 mg dissolved in 0.5 to 1 ml of Water for Injections BP.

Intrathecal injection: Must be diluted by hospital pharmacy. Only freshly prepared solutions should be used. For adults, 6 mg (10,000 units) dissolved in 10 ml of Sodium Chloride Injection BP. Maximum dose, 12 mg (20,000 units). For infants and children, 0.1 mg/kg (170 units/kg) is suitable. The concentration of penicillin in the injection should not exceed 0.6 mg/ml (1,000 units/ml).

Overdosage can cause convulsions, paralysis and may be fatal.

Use of a disposable membrane filter of 0.45 micron pore size is convenient for ensuring clarity of the solution.

Contra-indications, warnings, etc
Contra-indications: Allergy to penicillins. Hypersensitivity to any ingredient of the preparation.

Precautions: Massive doses of sodium penicillin can cause hypokalaemia and sometimes hypernatraemia. Use of a potassium-sparing diuretic may be helpful.

If renal function is very poor, large doses of penicillin (e.g. 12 mega units or more) can cause cerebral irritation and fits.

Overdosage by the intrathecal route can cause convulsions, paralysis and may be fatal (see Preparation of Solutions).

Skin sensitisation may occur in persons handling the antibiotic, and care should be taken to avoid contact with the substance.

It should be recognised that any patient with a history of allergy, especially to drugs, is more likely to develop a hypersensitivity reaction to penicillin.

Pregnancy: Crystapen has been taken by a large number of pregnant women and women of child-bearing age without an increase in malformations or other direct or indirect harmful effects on the fetus having been observed.

Side-effects: Occasionally hypersensitivity to penicillin, in the form of urticarial rash, may occur; it may be treated with antihistamine drugs. More rarely, anaphylactic reactions have been reported.

Haemolytic anaemia and granulocytopenia have been reported in patients receiving prolonged high dosage of benzylpenicillin sodium (e.g. in subacute bacterial endocarditis).

Overdosage: Excessive blood levels of penicillin G can be corrected by haemodialysis.

In the event of overdosage by the intrathecal route, CSF lavage to reduce the toxic concentration of Penicillin G may be considered.

Pharmaceutical precautions Store below 25°C.

Reconstituted solutions of penicillin are intended for immediate administration but may be stored for up to 24 hours at 2 to 8°C if necessary. For intrathecal injection *only freshly prepared* solutions should be used.

Legal category POM.

Package quantities *Vials:* 600 mg (1,000,000 units) unbuffered, box of 100.

Further information 600 mg Crystapen in solution displaces 0.4 ml. Each mega unit of unbuffered Crystapen represents 1.68 mmol of sodium.

Product licence number
Crystapen 600 mg 0004/5070.

Product licence holder: Glaxo Operations UK Limited, Greenford, Middlesex UB6 0HE.

DERMOVATE* CREAM AND OINTMENT

Presentation Dermovate Cream and Ointment each contain 0.05% w/w clobetasol propionate. The water-miscible cream and the paraffin-based ointment are both white in appearance.

Uses Clobetasol propionate is a very active topical corticosteroid which is of particular value when used in short courses for the treatment of more resistant dermatoses such as psoriasis (excluding widespread plaque psoriasis), recalcitrant eczemas, lichen planus, discoid lupus erythematosus, and other conditions which do not respond satisfactorily to less active steroids.

Dosage and administration Apply sparingly to the affected area once or twice daily until improvement occurs. As with other highly-active topical steroid preparations, therapy should be discontinued when control is achieved. In the more responsive conditions this may be within a few days. If no improvement is seen within two to four weeks, reassessment of the diagnosis, or referral, may be necessary.

Repeated short courses of Dermovate may be used to control exacerbations. If continuous steroid treatment is necessary, a less potent preparation should be used.

In very resistant lesions, especially where there is hyperkeratosis, the anti-inflammatory effect of Dermovate can be enhanced, if necessary, by occluding the treatment area with polythene film. Overnight occlusion only is usually adequate to bring about a satisfactory response. Thereafter, improvement can usually be maintained by application without occlusion.

Contra-indications, warnings, etc
Contra-indications: Rosacea, acne vulgaris and peri-oral dermatitis.

Primary cutaneous viral infections (e.g. herpes simplex, chickenpox).

Hypersensitivity to the preparation.

The use of Dermovate skin preparations is not indicated in the treatment of primarily infected skin lesions caused by infection with fungi (e.g. candidiasis, tinea), or bacteria (e.g. impetigo); peri-anal and genital pruritus. Dermatoses in children under one year of age, including dermatitis and napkin eruptions.

Precautions: Long-term continuous topical therapy should be avoided where possible, particularly in infants and children, as adrenal suppression can occur readily even without occlusion.

If used in childhood or on the face, courses should be limited if possible to five days and occlusion should not be used.

The face, more than other areas of the body, may exhibit atrophic changes after prolonged treatment with potent topical corticosteroids. This must be borne in mind when treating such conditions as psoriasis, discoid lupus erythematosus and severe eczema.

If applied to the eyelids, care is needed to ensure that the preparation does not enter the eye, as glaucoma might result.

Topical corticosteroids may be hazardous in psoriasis for a number of reasons including rebound relapses, development of tolerance, risk of generalised pustular psoriasis and development of local or systemic toxicity due to impaired barrier function of the skin. If used in psoriasis careful patient supervision is important.

Appropriate antimicrobial therapy should be used whenever treating inflammatory lesions which have become infected. Any spread of infection requires withdrawal of topical corticosteroid therapy and systemic administration of antimicrobial agents.

Bacterial infection is encouraged by the warm, moist conditions induced by occlusive dressings, and so the skin should be cleansed before a fresh dressing is applied.

Pregnancy: There is inadequate evidence of safety in human pregnancy. Topical administration of corticosteroids to pregnant animals can cause abnormalities of fetal development including cleft palate and intra-uterine growth retardation. There may therefore be a very small risk of such effects in the human fetus.

Side-effects: As with other topical corticosteroids, prolonged use of large amounts, or treatment of extensive areas can result in sufficient systemic absorption to produce the features of hypercorticism. Provided the weekly dosage is less than 50 grams in adults, any suppression of the HPA axis is likely to be transient with a rapid return to normal values once the short course of steroid therapy has ceased. The same applies to children given proportionate dosage. Use of occlusive dressing increases the absorption of topical corticosteroids. In infants, the napkin may act as an occlusive dressing.

Prolonged and intensive treatment with a highly active corticosteroid preparation may cause local atrophic changes in the skin such as thinning, striae, and dilatation of the superficial blood vessels, particularly when occlusive dressings are used or when skin folds are involved.

In rare instances, treatment of psoriasis with corticosteroids (or its withdrawal) is thought to have provoked the pustular form of the disease (see 'Precautions').

Dermovate is usually well tolerated, but if signs of hypersensitivity appear, application should be stopped immediately.

Overdosage: Acute overdosage is very unlikely to occur. However, in the case of chronic overdosage or misuse the features of hypercorticism may appear and in this situation topical steroids should be discontinued.

Pharmaceutical precautions None.

Legal category POM.

Package quantities Tubes of 30 and 100 grams.

Further information The least potent corticosteroid which will control the disease should be selected. Dermovate preparations do not contain lanolin or parabens.

Product licence numbers
Dermovate Cream 0004/0219
Dermovate Ointment 0004/0220

Product licence holder: Glaxo Operations UK Limited, Greenford, Middlesex UB6 0HE.

DERMOVATE* SCALP APPLICATION

Presentation Dermovate Scalp Application is a transparent, slightly gelled solution containing 0.05% w/w clobetasol propionate. The vehicle contains 50% isopropyl alcohol, which has antibacterial activity.

Uses Psoriasis and recalcitrant eczemas of the scalp. Clobetasol propionate is a highly-active topical corticosteroid which is indicated for use in short courses for conditions which do not respond satisfactorily to less active steroids.

Dosage and administration Apply sparingly to the scalp night and morning until improvement occurs. As with other highly-active topical steroid preparations, therapy should be discontinued when control is achieved. Repeated short courses of Dermovate Scalp Application may be used to control exacerbations. If continuous steroid treatment is necessary, a less potent preparation should be used.

Contra-indications, warnings, etc
Contra-indications: Infections of the scalp.
Hypersensitivity to the preparation.
Dermatoses in children under one year of age, including dermatitis.

Precautions: Care must be taken to keep the preparation away from the eyes. Do not use near a naked flame.
Long-term continuous topical therapy should be avoided, particularly in infants and children, as adrenal suppression can occur readily even without occlusion.
Development of secondary infection requires withdrawal of topical corticosteroid therapy and commencement of appropriate systemic antimicrobial therapy.
Topical corticosteroids may be hazardous in psoriasis for a number of reasons including rebound relapses, development of tolerance, risk of generalised pustular psoriasis and development of local or systemic toxicity due to impaired barrier function of the skin. If used in psoriasis careful patient supervision is important.

Pregnancy: There is inadequate evidence of safety in human pregnancy. Topical administration of corticosteroids to pregnant animals can cause abnormalities of fetal development including cleft palate and intra-uterine growth retardation. There may therefore be a very small risk of such effects in the human fetus.

Side-effects: Dermovate preparations are usually well tolerated, but if signs of hypersensitivity appear, application should be stopped immediately.
As with other topical corticosteroids, prolonged use of large amounts or treatment of extensive areas can result in sufficient systemic absorption to produce the features of hypercorticism and suppression of the HPA axis. These effects are more likely to occur in infants and children, and if occlusive dressings are used. Local atrophy may occur after prolonged treatment particularly if occlusive dressings are used.
In rare instances, treatment of psoriasis with corticosteroids (or its withdrawal) is thought to have provoked the pustular form of the disease (see 'Precautions').

Overdosage: Acute overdosage is very unlikely to occur, however, in the case of chronic overdosage or misuse the features of hypercorticism may appear and in this situation topical steroids should be discontinued.

Pharmaceutical precautions None.

Legal category POM.

Package quantities Plastic squeeze bottle with elongated nozzle containing 30 or 100 ml.

Further information The least potent corticosteroid which will control the disease should be selected. The viscosity of the scalp application has been adjusted so that the preparation spreads easily without being too fluid. The specially-designed bottle and nozzle allow easy application direct to the scalp through the hair.

Product licence number 0004/0242.

Product licence holder: Glaxo Operations UK Limited, Greenford, Middlesex UB6 0HE.

DERMOVATE*-NN SKIN PREPARATIONS

Presentation Dermovate-NN skin preparations contain clobetasol propionate 0.05% w/w, neomycin sulphate 0.5% and nystatin 100,000 units per gram.
Dermovate-NN Ointment is a buff, paraffin-based ointment.
Dermovate-NN Cream is buff in colour.

Uses Clobetasol propionate is a highly active topical corticosteroid which is of particular value when used in short courses for the treatment of recalcitrant eczemas, neurodermatoses, and other conditions which do not respond satisfactorily to less active steroids.
Dermovate-NN is indicated in more resistant dermatoses such as recalcitrant eczemas and psoriasis (excluding widespread plaque psoriasis) where secondary bacterial or candidal infection is present, suspected or likely to occur, as when using occlusive dressings.

Dosage and administration Apply sparingly to the affected area once or twice daily until improvement occurs. As with other highly-active topical steroid preparations therapy should be discontinued when control is achieved. In the more responsive conditions this may be within a few days.
If a longer course is necessary, it is recommended that treatment should not be continued for more than four weeks without the patient's condition being reviewed.
Repeated short courses of Dermovate-NN may be used to control exacerbations. If continuous steroid treatment is necessary, a less potent preparation should be used.
In very resistant lesions, especially where there is hyperkeratosis, the anti-inflammatory effect of Dermovate-NN can be enhanced, if necessary, by occluding the treatment area with polythene. Overnight occlusion only is usually adequate to bring about a satisfactory response, thereafter improvement can usually be maintained by application without occlusion.

Contra-indications, warnings, etc
Contra-indications: Rosacea, acne vulgaris and peri-oral dermatitis.
Primary cutaneous viral infections (e.g. herpes simplex, chickenpox).
Hypersensitivity to the preparations.
Use of Dermovate-NN skin preparations is not indicated in the treatment of primarily infected skin lesions caused by infection with fungi (e.g. candidiasis, tinea), bacteria (e.g. impetigo), or yeast.
Dermatoses in children under one year of age, including dermatitis and napkin eruptions.
Preparations containing neomycin should not be used for the treatment of otitis externa when the ear drum is perforated, because of the risk of ototoxicity.
Application to large areas especially during pregnancy, in the elderly and in patients with impaired renal function due to a risk of ototoxicity.

Precautions: Long-term continuous topical therapy should be avoided where possible, particularly in infants and children, as adrenal suppression can occur readily even without occlusion.
If used in childhood, or on the face, courses should be limited to five days and occlusion should not be used.

The face, more than other areas of the body, may exhibit atrophic changes after prolonged treatment with potent topical corticosteroids. This must be borne in mind when treating such conditions as psoriasis and severe eczema with Dermovate-NN. If applied to the eyelids, care is needed to ensure that the preparation does not enter the eye, as glaucoma might result.

Topical corticosteroids may be hazardous in psoriasis for a number of reasons, including rebound relapses, development of tolerance, risk of generalised pustular psoriasis and development of local or systemic toxicity due to impaired barrier function of the skin. If used in psoriasis, careful patient supervision is important.

Do not continue for more than seven days in the absence of clinical improvement, since occult extension of infection may occur due to the masking effect of the steroid.

If infection persists, systemic chemotherapy is required. Any spread of infection requires withdrawal of topical corticosteroid therapy. Bacterial infection is encouraged by the warm, moist conditions induced by occlusive dressings, and the skin should be cleansed before a fresh dressing is applied.

Extended or recurrent application may increase the risk of contact sensitisation.

Products which contain antimicrobial agents should not be diluted.

Pregnancy: There is inadequate evidence of safety in human pregnancy. Topical administration of corticosteroids to pregnant animals can cause abnormalities of fetal development including cleft palate and intra-uterine growth retardation. There may therefore be a very small risk of such effects in the human fetus.

The use of neomycin may be associated with a theoretical risk of fetal ototoxicity. (See 'Contra-indications'.)

Side-effects: As with other topical corticosteroids prolonged use of large amounts or treatment of extensive areas can result in sufficient systemic absorption to produce the features of hypercorticism.

Provided the weekly dosage is less than 50 g in adults, any suppression of the HPA axis is likely to be transient with a rapid return to normal values once the short course of steroid therapy has ceased. The same applies to children given proportionate dosage. Use of occlusive dressings increases the absorption of topical corticosteroids. In infants the napkin may act as an occlusive dressing.

Prolonged and intensive treatment with highly active corticosteroid preparations may cause local atrophic changes in the skin such as thinning, striae, and dilatation of the superficial blood vessels, particularly when occlusive dressings are used, or when skin folds are involved.

In rare instances, treatment of psoriasis with corticosteroids (or its withdrawal) is thought to have provoked the pustular form of the disease (see 'Precautions').

Dermovate-NN is usually well tolerated, but if signs of hypersensitivity appear, application should be stopped immediately.

Overdosage: Acute overdosage is very unlikely to occur. However, in the case of chronic overdosage or misuse the features of hypercorticism may appear and in this situation topical steroids should be discontinued.

Pharmaceutical precautions None.

Legal category POM.

Package quantities Tubes of 30 grams.

Further information The least potent corticosteroid which will control the disease should be selected. Dermovate-NN preparations contain neither lanolin nor parabens.

Product licence numbers

Dermovate-NN Ointment	0004/0237
Dermovate-NN Cream	0004/0255

Product licence holder: Glaxo Operations UK Limited, Greenford, Middlesex UB6 0HE.

EFCORTELAN* SKIN PREPARATIONS

Presentation Efcortelan Cream contains 0.5%, 1% or 2.5% hydrocortisone in a smooth, white, water-miscible cream base.

Efcortelan Ointment contains 0.5%, 1% or 2.5% hydrocortisone in an off-white paraffin-based ointment.

Efcortelan Cream 1% complies with the specification for Hydrocortisone Cream BP.

Efcortelan Ointments comply with the specification for Hydrocortisone Ointment BP.

Uses Hydrocortisone has topical anti-inflammatory activity of value in the treatment of a wide variety of dermatological conditions, including the following: eczema, including atopic, infantile, discoid and stasis eczemas; prurigo nodularis, neurodermatoses, seborrhoeic dermatitis, intertrigo, contact sensitivity reactions.

Efcortelan preparations can also be used in the management of insect bites and otitis externa.

Efcortelan 0.5% preparations can be used as continuation therapy in mild cases of seborrhoeic or atopic eczema once the acute inflammatory phase has passed.

Dosage and administration A small quantity should be applied to the affected area two or three times daily.

Efcortelan Cream is often appropriate for moist or weeping surfaces, and Efcortelan Ointment for dry, lichenified or scaly lesions, but this is not invariably so.

Contra-indications, warnings, etc

Contra-indications: Skin lesions caused by infection with viruses (e.g., herpes simplex, chickenpox), fungi (e.g., candidiasis, tinea) or bacteria (e.g., impetigo).

Hypersensitivity to the preparations.

Precautions: In infants and children, long-term continuous topical therapy should be avoided where possible, as adrenal suppression can occur even without occlusion. In infants, the napkin may act as an occlusive dressing, and increase absorption. Treatment should therefore be limited if possible, to a maximum of seven days.

Appropriate antimicrobial therapy should be used whenever treating inflammatory lesions which have become infected. Any spread of infection requires withdrawal of topical corticosteroid therapy, and systemic administration of antimicrobial agents.

As with all corticosteroids, prolonged application to the face is undesirable.

Pregnancy: There is inadequate evidence of safety in human pregnancy. Topical application of corticosteroids to pregnant animals can cause abnormalities of fetal development including cleft palate and intra-uterine growth retardation. There may, therefore, be a very small risk of such effects in the human fetus.

Side-effects: Efcortelan preparations are usually well tolerated, but if signs of hypersensitivity appear, application should stop immediately.

Local atrophic changes may occur where skin folds are involved, or in areas such as the nappy area in small children, where constant moist conditions favour the absorption of hydrocortisone. Sufficient systemic absorption may also occur in such sites to produce the features of hypercorticism and suppression of the HPA axis after prolonged treatment. This effect is more likely to occur in infants and children, and if occlusive dressings are used.

Pharmaceutical precautions None.

Legal category POM.

Package quantities Efcortelan Cream and Ointment are supplied in 30 gram tubes.

Further information The least potent corticosteroid which will control the disease should be selected. None of these preparations contain lanolin or parabens.

Product licence numbers

Efcortelan Cream 0.5%	0004/5080R
Efcortelan Cream 1%	0004/5081R
Efcortelan Cream 2.5%	0004/5082R

Efcortelan Ointment 0.5%	0004/5085R
Efcortelan Ointment 1%	0004/5086R
Efcortelan Ointment 2.5%	0004/5087R

Product licence holder: Glaxo Operations UK Limited, Greenford, Middlesex UB6 0HE.

EFCORTELAN* SOLUBLE

Presentation Vials of Efcortelan Soluble contain freeze-dried hydrocortisone sodium succinate as a white plug. Each vial contains 100 mg hydrocortisone as the sodium succinate ester; this readily dissolves in the 2 ml ampoule of Water for Injections supplied with the vial. When prepared as directed, this preparation complies with the specification for Hydrocortisone Sodium Succinate Injection BP.

Uses Status asthmaticus and acute allergic reactions, including anaphylactic reaction to drugs. Efcortelan Soluble supplements the action of adrenaline.

Severe shock arising from surgical or accidental trauma or overwhelming infection.

Acute adrenal insufficiency caused by abnormal stress in Addison's disease, hypopituitarism, following adrenalectomy, and when adrenocortical function has been suppressed by prolonged corticosteroid therapy.

Soft-tissue conditions such as tennis elbow, tenosynovitis and bursitis.

Note: Efcortelan Soluble does not replace other forms of therapy for the treatment of shock and status asthmaticus.

Dosage and administration For intravenous injection, 100 mg Efcortelan Soluble may be dissolved in 2 ml Water for Injections immediately before administration. Efcortelan Soluble may also be given as an intravenous infusion.

A clinical effect is seen in two to four hours, and it persists for up to eight hours after intravenous injection.

Efcortelan Soluble can be given by intramuscular injection, but the response is likely to be less rapid, especially in shock.

Systemic therapy in adults: 100 to 500 mg administered by slow intravenous injection taking half to one minute. This dose can be repeated three or four times in 24 hours, depending upon the condition being treated and the patient's response.

Systemic therapy in children: Infants up to 1 year may be given 25 mg hydrocortisone intravenously; children 1 to 5 years, 50 mg; 6 to 12 years, 100 mg.

This dose can be repeated three or four times in 24 hours depending upon the condition being treated and the patient's response.

Other uses: Local treatment of soft-tissue lesions – 100 to 200 mg. This daily dose can be repeated on two or three occasions depending on the patient's response.

Contra-indications, warnings, etc
Contra-indications: Systemic infections, unless specific anti-infective therapy is employed. Live virus immunisation. Hypersensitivity to any component of the injection.

Efcortelan Soluble should not be injected directly into tendons.

Precautions: Administration of corticosteroids may impair the ability to resist and counteract infection; in addition, clinical signs and symptoms of infection are suppressed.

Steroids may reduce the effects of anticholinesterases in myasthenia gravis, cholecystographic X-ray media and salicylates.

The effect of steroids may be reduced by phenytoin, phenobarbitone, ephedrine and rifampicin.

Pregnancy: There is inadequate evidence of safety in human pregnancy. Administration of corticosteroids to pregnant animals can cause abnormalities of fetal development including cleft palate and intra-uterine growth retardation. There may therefore be a very small risk of such effects in the human fetus.

Side-effects: In the short-term, high levels of hydrocortisone involve little risk of adverse reactions, except that peptic ulceration may occur, or be aggravated and there may be a small but significant increase in the risk of infection. With continued use, signs of hypercorticism may become apparent.

Pharmaceutical precautions Protect from light.

Legal category POM.

Package quantities Vials of 100 mg hydrocortisone with a 2 ml ampoule of Water for Injections.

Further information Each vial provides 8.5 mg (0.37 mmol) of sodium and 0.45 mmol of phosphate (PO_4).

There is a lack of evidence that use of corticosteroids in septic shock affects mortality in the long term.

Product licence number 0004/5088R.

Product licence holder: Glaxo Operations UK Limited, Greenford, Middlesex UB6 0HE.

EFCORTESOL* INJECTION

Presentation Ampoules of Efcortesol Injection contain an aqueous, ready-prepared buffered solution of hydrocortisone sodium phosphate. Each millilitre contains 100 mg hydrocortisone as the sodium phosphate ester. The solution is clear and colourless or pale yellow. Efcortesol Injection complies with the specification for Hydrocortisone Sodium Phosphate Injection BP.

Uses This presentation permits rapid use in emergency situations involving the following conditions:

Status asthmaticus and acute allergic reactions, including anaphylactic reaction to drugs. Efcortesol supplements the action of adrenaline.

Severe shock arising from surgical or accidental trauma or overwhelming infection.

Acute adrenal insufficiency caused by abnormal stress in Addison's disease, hypopituitarism, following adrenalectomy, and when adrenocortical function has been suppressed by prolonged corticosteroid therapy.

Soft-tissue lesions such as tennis elbow, tenosynovitis and bursitis.

Note: Efcortesol does not replace other forms of therapy for the treatment of shock and status asthmaticus.

Dosage and administration *Systemic therapy in adults:* 100 to 500 mg hydrocortisone (1 to 5 ml) administered by slow intravenous injection, taking at least half to one minute. This dose can be repeated three or four times in 24 hours, depending upon the condition being treated and the patient's response. Alternatively, Efcortesol Injection may be given as an intravenous infusion. A clinical effect is seen in two to four hours, and it persists for up to eight hours after intravenous injection. The same dose can be given by intramuscular injection, but the response is likely to be less rapid, especially in shock.

Systemic therapy in children: As a guide, infants up to 1 year may be given 25 mg hydrocortisone intravenously; children 1 to 5 years, 50 mg; 6 to 12 years, 100 mg (1 ml). This dose can be repeated three or four times in 24 hours depending upon the condition being treated and the patient's response.

Other uses: Local treatment of soft-tissue lesions – 100 to 200 mg. This daily dose may be repeated on two or three occasions depending upon the patient's response.

Efcortesol Injection is not recommended for intrathecal use.

Contra-indications, warnings, etc
Contra-indications: Systemic infections, unless specific anti-infective therapy is employed. Live virus immunisation. Hypersensitivity to any component.

Efcortesol Injection should not be injected directly into tendons.

Precautions: Administration of corticosteroids may impair the ability to resist and counteract infection; in addition, clinical signs and symptoms of infection are suppressed.

Steroids may reduce the effects of anticholinesterases in myasthenia gravis, cholecystographic X-ray media and salicylates.

The effect of steroids may be reduced by phenytoin, phenobarbitone, ephedrine and rifampicin.

Pregnancy: There is inadequate evidence of safety in human pregnancy. Administration of corticosteroids to pregnant animals can cause abnormalities of fetal development including cleft palate and intra-uterine growth retardation. There may therefore be a very small risk of such effects in the human fetus.

Side-effects: Paraesthesia may occur following intravenous administration and is probably related to the rate of injection. It is often localised to the genital area but in some cases may radiate over the entire body. The unpleasant and sometimes painful sensation usually passes off within a few minutes and no sequelae have been reported. The effect seems to be related to the sodium phosphate salt of hydrocortisone and is unlikely to occur with Efcortelan Soluble Injection (hydrocortisone sodium succinate).

In the short-term, high dosage of hydrocortisone involves little risk of adverse reactions, except that peptic ulceration may occur, or be aggravated and there may be a small but significant increase in the risk of infection. With continued use, signs of hypercorticism, may become apparent.

Pharmaceutical precautions Protect from light.

Legal category POM.

Package quantities Ampoules 1 ml (100 mg) in box of 5.

Ampoules 5 ml (500 mg) in box of 10.

Further information It should be noted that 10 ml Efcortesol Injection contains 152 mg (6.6 mmol) sodium and 298 mg (28.2 mmol) phosphate (PO_4). There is a lack of evidence that use of corticosteroids in septic shock affects mortality in the long term.

Product licence number 0004/5089R.

Product licence holder: Glaxo Operations UK Limited, Greenford, Middlesex UB6 0HE.

ELTROXIN* TABLETS

Presentation Small white tablets engraved 'Eltroxin 50 Glaxo' or 'Eltroxin 100 Glaxo' containing 50 micrograms (0.05 mg) or 100 micrograms (0.1 mg) anhydrous thyroxine sodium respectively. The lower-strength tablets are scored. Eltroxin Tablets comply with the specification for Thyroxine Tablets BP.

Uses Hypothyroidism.

Dosage and administration *Adults:* Initially 50 to 100 micrograms daily, preferably taken before breakfast, and adjusted at three to four week intervals by 50 micrograms until normal metabolism is steadily maintained; this may require doses of 100 to 200 micrograms daily. With patients aged over 50 years, it is not advisable to exceed 50 micrograms a day initially, and where there is cardiac disease, 25 micrograms daily, or 50 micrograms on alternate days, is more suitable. In this condition the daily dosage may be increased by 25 micrograms at intervals of perhaps four weeks.

In younger patients, and in the absence of heart disease, a serum thyroxine (T4) level of about 70 to 160 nanomols per litre, or a serum thyrotrophin level of less than 5 milli-units per litre, should be aimed at. In those aged over 50, and/or in the presence of heart disease, clinical response is probably a more acceptable criterion of dosage than serum levels.

A pre-therapy ECG is valuable, as changes induced by hypothyroidism may be confused with ECG evidence of ischaemia. If too rapid an increase of metabolism is produced (causing diarrhoea, nervousness, rapid pulse, insomnia, tremors and sometimes anginal pain where there is latent myocardial ischaemia), dosage must be reduced or withheld for a day or two, then begun again at a lower level.

Congenital hypothyroidism and juvenile myxoedema: The largest dose consistent with freedom from toxic effects should be given. The dosage is guided by clinical response, growth assessment and appropriate thyroid function tests – clinically, normal pulse rate and absence of diarrhoea or constipation are the most useful indicators.

Thyrotrophin levels may remain elevated during the first year of life in children with neonatal hypothyroidism due to re-setting of the hypothalamic-pituitary axis. For infants with congenital hypothyroidism, a suitable starting dose is 25 micrograms Eltroxin daily, with increments of 25 micrograms every two to four weeks until mild toxic symptoms appear. Dosage is then slightly reduced. The same applies to juvenile myxoedema, except that the starting dose for children older than one year may be 2.5 to 5 micrograms/kg/day.

Contra-indications, warnings, etc
Contra-indications: Thyrotoxicosis. Hypersensitivity to any component.

Precautions: Patients with panhypopituitarism or other causes predisposing to adrenal insufficiency may react unfavourably to thyroxine treatment, and it is advisable to initiate corticosteroid therapy before giving thyroxine in these cases.

Especial care is needed in the elderly and in patients with symptoms of myocardial insufficiency or ECG evidence of myocardial infarction and also those with diabetes mellitus or insipidus.

Use in pregnancy and lactation: The safety of Eltroxin during pregnancy has not been established but the risk of congenital abnormalities should be weighed up against the risk to the fetus of untreated hypothyroidism.

Thyroxine is excreted into breast milk in low concentrations and this may be sufficient to interfere with neonatal screening for hypothyroidism.

Side-effects: The following effects are indicative of excessive dosage, and usually disappear on reduction of dosage or withdrawal of treatment for a few days. Anginal pain, cardiac arrhythmias, palpitation, and cramps in skeletal muscle; also tachycardia, diarrhoea, vomiting, tremors, restlessness, excitability, insomnia, headache, flushing, sweating, excessive loss of weight and muscular weakness.

Drug interactions: Thyroxine increases the effect of anticoagulants and it may be necessary to reduce the dose of anticoagulant if excessive hypoprothrombinaemia and bleeding are to be avoided. Cholestyramine given concurrently reduces the gastrointestinal absorption of thyroxine. Phenytoin levels may be increased by thyroxine. Thyroxine enhances the toxicity of digitalis and therefore if thyroxine therapy is initiated in digitalised patients the dose of digitalis may require adjustment. Thyroxine raises blood sugar levels and this may upset the stability of patients receiving anti-diabetic agents. Thyroxine increases receptor sensitivity to catecholamines thus accelerating the response to tricyclic antidepressants. The effects of sympathomimetic agents are also enhanced.

A number of drugs may affect thyroid function tests and this should be borne in mind when monitoring a patient on thyroxine therapy.

Overdosage: Gastric lavage or emesis is required if the patient is seen within several hours of taking the dose. In addition to exaggeration of side effects the following symptoms may be seen: agitation, confusion, irritability, hyperactivity, sweating, mydriasis, tachycardia, arrhythmias, tachypnoea, pyrexia and convulsions. The appearance of clinical hyperthyroidism may be delayed for up to five days.

Treatment is symptomatic, and tachycardia has been controlled in an adult by 40 mg doses of propranolol given every six hours and other symptoms by diazepam and/or chlorpromazine as appropriate.

Pharmaceutical precautions Protect from light.

Legal category POM.

Package quantities Bottles of 100 and 1,000 tablets.

Further information 100 micrograms thyroxine is equivalent in activity to 20 to 30 micrograms liothyronine or 60 mg Thyroid BP.

Product licence numbers

Tablets 50 micrograms	0004/5018R
Tablets 100 micrograms	0004/5019R

Product licence holder: Glaxo Operations UK Limited, Greenford, Middlesex UB6 0HE.

EUMOVATE* CREAM AND OINTMENT

Presentation Eumovate Cream and Ointment contain 0.05% clobetasone butyrate, and are white in appearance. The emollient cream is water-miscible, whilst the ointment has a paraffin base.

Uses Clobetasone butyrate is a topically active corticosteroid which provides an exceptional combination of activity and safety. When formulated as Eumovate, it is more effective in the treatment of eczemas than 1% hydrocortisone, or the less-active synthetic steroid preparations that are in common use, yet has little effect on hypothalamic-pituitary-adrenal function. This has been so even when Eumovate was applied to adults in large amounts under whole-body occlusion. All topical corticosteroids can cause cutaneous atrophy if grossly misused. However, studies in animal and human models indicate that Eumovate and hydrocortisone cause less thinning of the epidermis than the other topical steroids tested.

Eumovate is suitable for the treatment of eczema and dermatitis of all types including atopic eczema, photodermatitis, otitis externa, primary irritant and allergic dermatitis (including napkin rash), intertrigo, prurigo nodularis, seborrhoeic dermatitis and insect bite reactions.

Eumovate may be used as maintenance therapy between courses of one of the more active topical steroids.

Dosage and administration Eumovate should be applied to the affected area up to four times a day until improvement occurs, when the frequency of application may be reduced.

Contra-indications, warnings, etc

Contra-indications: Skin lesions caused by infection with viruses (e.g., herpes simplex, chickenpox), fungi (e.g., candidiasis, tinea) or bacteria (e.g., impetigo).

Hypersensitivity to the preparations.

Precautions: Although generally regarded as safe, even for long-term administration in adults, there is a potential for overdosage, and in infants and children this may result in adrenal suppression. Extreme caution is required in dermatoses in such patients including napkin eruption (as the napkin may act as an occlusive dressing and increase absorption) and treatment should not normally exceed seven days.

Appropriate antimicrobial therapy should be used whenever treating inflammatory lesions which have become infected. Any spread of infection requires withdrawal of topical corticosteroid therapy, and systemic administration of antimicrobial agents.

As with all corticosteroids, prolonged application to the face is undesirable.

Topical corticosteroids may be hazardous in psoriasis for a number of reasons including rebound relapses, development of tolerance, risk of generalised pustular psoriasis and development of local or systemic toxicity due to impaired barrier function of the skin. If used in psoriasis, careful patient supervision is important.

Pregnancy: There is inadequate evidence of safety in human pregnancy. Topical administration of corticosteroids to pregnant animals can cause abnormalities of fetal development including cleft palate and intra-uterine growth retardation. There may therefore be a very small risk of such effects in the human fetus.

Side-effects: In the unlikely event of signs of hypersensitivity appearing, application should stop immediately. When large areas of the body are being treated with Eumovate, it is possible that some patients will absorb sufficient steroid to cause transient adrenal suppression despite the low degree of systemic activity associated with clobetasone butyrate.

Local atrophic changes could possibly occur in situations where moisture increases absorption of clobetasone butyrate, but only after prolonged use.

Pharmaceutical precautions Nil.

Legal category POM.

Package quantities Tubes of 30 and 100 grams.

Further information The least potent corticosteroid which will control the disease should be selected. Neither of these preparations contain lanolin or parabens.

Product licence numbers

Eumovate Cream	0004/0233
Eumovate Ointment	0004/0254

Product licence holder: Glaxo Operations UK Limited, Greenford, Middlesex UB6 0HE.

EUMOVATE* EYE DROPS

Presentation Eumovate Eye Drops contain clobetasone 17-butyrate 0.1% w/v, with benzalkonium chloride 0.01% w/v as a preservative, as an off-white suspension that is sterile until the bottle is opened.

Uses For short-term treatment of steroid responsive inflammatory conditions of the eye after clinical exclusion of bacterial, viral and fungal infections. In these conditions it has been shown to have comparable anti-inflammatory activity to Betamethasone Sodium Phosphate Eye Drops.

Eumovate Eye Drops have less adverse effect on intra-ocular pressure than hydrocortisone (1%), betamethasone sodium phosphate (0.1%), prednisolone sodium phosphate (0.5%), or dexamethasone (0.1%) eye drops.

Dosage and administration The usual dosage is one or two drops four times a day; for severe inflammatory conditions one or two drops should be instilled into the eye every one or two hours until signs of improvement are apparent, when the frequency may be reduced.

Contra-indications, warnings, etc

Contra-indications: Bacterial, viral, fungal, tuberculous or purulent conditions of the eye.

Use is contra-indicated if glaucoma is present, or where herpetic keratitis (e.g. dendritic ulcer) is considered a possibility. Inadvertent use of topical steroids in the latter condition can lead to extension of the ulcer and marked visual deterioration.

Hypersensitivity to the preparation.

Eumovate Eye Drops contain benzalkonium chloride as a preservative and therefore should not be used to treat patients who wear soft contact lenses.

Precautions: Steroids should not be administered to 'red eyes' until a definitive diagnosis has been made.

Although Eumovate Eye Drops have been shown to have little effect on intra-ocular pressure in most patients, ophthalmological treatment with steroid preparations should not be repeated or prolonged without regular review to exclude raised intra-ocular pressure or unsuspected infections.

Cataract is reported to have occurred after unduly prolonged treatment with some topical corticosteroids and in those diseases which cause thinning of the cornea, perforation has been known to occur.

Pregnancy: There is inadequate evidence of safety in human pregnancy. Administration of corticosteroids to pregnant animals can cause abnormalities of fetal development including cleft palate and intra-uterine growth retardation. There may therefore be a very small risk of such effects in the human fetus.

Side-effects: Rises in intra-ocular pressure have been reported in susceptible patients but these are generally much less than with other corticosteroid eye preparations, including hydrocortisone.

Pharmaceutical precautions The contents should not be used more than four weeks after first opening the bottle.

Legal category POM.

Package quantities Plastic dropper bottles containing 10 ml.

Further information Nil.

Product licence number 0004/0260.

Product licence holder: Glaxo Operations UK Limited, Greenford, Middlesex UB6 0HE.

EUMOVATE*-N EYE DROPS

Presentation Eumovate-N Eye Drops contain clobetasone 17-butyrate 0.1%, and neomycin sulphate 0.5% w/v, with benzalkonium chloride 0.01% w/v as a preservative, as an off-white suspension that is sterile until the bottle is opened.

Uses For the short-term treatment of steroid responsive conditions of the eye when prophylactic antibiotic treatment is also required, after excluding the presence of fungal and viral disease. In these conditions it has been shown to have comparable anti-inflammatory activity to Betamethasone Sodium Phosphate with Neomycin Eye Drops.

Dosage and administration
Adults (and the Elderly) and Children: The usual dosage is one or two drops four times a day; for severe inflammatory conditions one or two drops should be applied to each affected eye up to six times daily or more frequently if required.

Contra-indications, warnings, etc
Contra-indications: Viral, fungal, tuberculous or purulent conditions of the eye. Use is contra-indicated if glaucoma is present or herpetic keratitis (e.g. dendritic ulcer) is considered a possibility. Use of topical steroids in the latter condition can lead to extension of the ulcer and marked visual deterioration.

Hypersensitivity to the preparation.

Eumovate-N Drops contain benzalkonium chloride as a preservative and therefore should not be used to treat patients who wear soft contact lenses.

Precautions: Topical corticosteroids should never be given for an undiagnosed "red eye" as inappropriate use is potentially blinding.

Treatment with corticosteroid/antibiotic combinations should not be continued for more than 7 days in the absence of any clinical improvement, since prolonged use may lead to occult extension of infection due to the masking effect of the steroid. Prolonged use may also lead to skin sensitisation and the emergence of resistant organisms.

Prolonged use may lead to the risk of adrenal suppression in infants.

Treatment with corticosteroid preparations should not be repeated or prolonged without regular review to exclude raised intra-ocular pressure, cataract formation or unsuspected infections.

Aminoglycoside antibiotics may cause irreversible, partial or total deafness when given systemically or when applied topically to open wounds or damaged skin. This effect is dose related and is enhanced by renal or hepatic impairment. Although this effect has not been reported following topical ocular use, the possibility should be considered when high dose topical treatment is given to small children or infants.

May cause transient blurring of vision on instillation. Warn patients not to drive or operate hazardous machinery unless vision is clear.

Pregnancy and lactation: Safety for use in pregnancy and lactation has not been established. There is inadequate evidence of safety in human pregnancy. Topical administration of corticosteroids to pregnant animals can cause abnormalities of fetal development including cleft palate and intra-uterine growth retardation. There may, therefore, be a very small risk of such effects in the human fetus. There is a risk of fetal ototoxicity if aminoglycoside antibiotic preparations are administered during pregnancy.

Side-effects: Hypersensitivity reactions, usually of the delayed type, may occur leading to irritation, burning, stinging, itching and dermatitis.

Topical steroid use may result in increased intra-ocular pressure leading to optic nerve damage, reduced visual acuity and visual field defects.

Intensive or prolonged use of topical corticosteroids may lead to formation of posterior subcapsular cataracts.

In those diseases causing thinning of the cornea or sclera, corticosteroid therapy may result in thinning of the globe leading to perforation.

Overdosage: Long-term intensive topical use may lead to systemic effects.

Oral ingestion of the contents of one bottle (up to 10 ml) is unlikely to lead to any serious adverse effects).

Pharmaceutical precautions The contents should not be used more than four weeks after first opening the bottle.

Legal category POM.

Package quantities Plastic dropper bottles containing 10 ml.

Further information Nil.

Product licence number 0004/0276.

Product licence holder: Glaxo Operations UK Limited, Greenford, Middlesex UB6 0HE.

FORTUM FOR INJECTION

Presentation Fortum for Injection is supplied as a white to faintly yellow powder in vials containing 250 mg, 500 mg, 1 g and 2 g ceftazidime (as pentahydrate) with sodium carbonate (118 mg per gram of ceftazidime). On the addition of Water for Injections, Fortum for Injection dissolves with effervescence to produce a solution for injection.

Fortum for Injection contains approximately 52 mg (2.3 mEq) of sodium per gram of ceftazidime. 116 mg ceftazidime pentahydrate is equivalent to 100 mg ceftazidime free acid. For laboratory tests associated with ceftazidime administration, use ceftazidime pentahydrate obtainable on request from Glaxo.

Uses Ceftazidime is a bactericidal cephalosporin antibiotic which is resistant to most beta-lactamases and is active against a wide range of Gram-positive and Gram-negative bacteria.

It is indicated for the treatment of single infections and for mixed infections caused by two or more susceptible organisms.

Ceftazidime, because of its broad antibacterial spectrum, may be used alone as first choice drug, pending sensitivity test results.

In meningitis it is recommended that the results of a sensitivity test are known before treatment with ceftazidime as a single agent. It may be used for infections caused by organisms resistant to other antibiotics including aminoglycosides and many cephalosporins. When appropriate, however, it may be used safely in combination with an aminoglycoside or other beta-lactam antibiotic, for example in the presence of severe neutropenia, or with an antibiotic active against anaerobes when the presence of *Bacteroides fragilis* is suspected (see Pharmaceutical precautions).

Indications include:

Severe infections in general: for example, septicaemia, bacteraemia, peritonitis, meningitis, infections in immunosuppressed patients with haematological or solid

malignancies, and in patients in intensive care units with specific problems, e.g., infected burns.
Respiratory tract infections: for example, pneumonia, bronchopneumonia, infected pleurisy, empyema, lung abscess, infected bronchiectasis and bronchitis and in lung infections in patients with cystic fibrosis.
Ear, nose and throat infections: for example, otitis media, malignant otitis externa, mastoiditis, sinusitis and other severe ear and throat infections.
Urinary tract infections: for example, acute and chronic pyelonephritis, pyelitis, prostatitis, cystitis, urethritis (bacterial only), renal abscess, and infections associated with bladder and renal stones.
Skin and soft tissue infections: for example, erysipelas, abscesses, cellulitis, infected burns and wounds, mastitis, skin ulcers.
Gastrointestinal, biliary and abdominal infections: for example, cholangitis, cholecystitis, empyema of gall bladder, intra-abdominal abscesses, peritonitis, diverticulitis, enterocolitis, post-partum and pelvic inflammatory conditions.
Bone and joint infections: for example, osteitis, osteomyelitis, septic arthritis, infected bursitis.
Dialysis: infections associated with haemo- and peritoneal dialysis and with continuous ambulatory peritoneal dialysis (CAPD).

Bacteriology:
Ceftazidime is bactericidal in action, exerting its effect on target cell wall proteins and causing inhibition of cell wall synthesis. A wide range of pathogenic strains and isolates associated with hospital-acquired infections are susceptible to ceftazidime *in vitro*, including strains resistant to gentamicin and other aminoglycosides. It is highly stable to most clinically important beta-lactamases produced by both Gram-positive and Gram-negative organisms and consequently is active against many ampicillin- and cephalothin-resistant strains. Ceftazidime has high intrinsic activity *in vitro* and acts within a narrow MIC range for most genera with minimal changes in MIC at varied inoculum levels. Ceftazidime has been shown to have *in vitro* activity against the following organisms:
Gram-negative:
Pseudomonas aeruginosa, Pseudomonas spp. (other), *Klebsiella pneumoniae*, Klebsiella spp. (other), *Proteus mirabilis, Proteus vulgaris, Morganella morganii* (formerly *Proteus morganii*), *Proteus rettgeri*, Providencia spp., *Escherichia coli*, Enterobacter spp., Citrobacter spp., Serratia spp., Salmonella spp., Shigella spp., *Yersinia enterocolitica, Pasteurella multocida*, Acinetobacter spp., *Neisseria gonorrhoeae, Neisseria meningitidis, Haemophilus influenzae* (including ampicillin-resistant strains), *Haemophilus parainfluenzae* (including ampicillin-resistant strains).
Gram-positive:
Staphylococcus aureus (methicillin-sensitive strains), *Staphylococcus epidermidis* (methicillin-sensitive strains), Micrococcus spp., *Streptococcus pyogenes*, Streptococcus Group B, *Streptococcus pneumoniae, Streptococcus mitis*, Streptococcus spp. (excluding *Streptococcus faecalis*).
Anaerobic strains:
Peptococcus spp., Peptostreptococcus spp., Streptococcus spp., Propionibacterium spp., *Clostridium perfringens*, Fusobacterium spp., Bacteroides spp. (many strains of *Bact. fragilis* are resistant).

Ceftazidime is not active *in vitro* against methicillin-resistant staphylococci, *Streptococcus faecalis* and many other Enterococci, *Listeria monocytogenes*, Campylobacter spp. or *Clostridium difficile*.

In vitro the activities of ceftazidime and aminoglycoside antibiotics in combination have been shown to be at least additive; there is evidence of synergy in some strains tested. This property may be important in the treatment of febrile neutropenic patients.

Dosage and administration *General dosage recommendations:* Ceftazidime is to be used by the parenteral route, the dosage depending upon the severity, sensitivity and type of infection and the age, weight and renal function of the patient.

Recommended maintenance doses of ceftazidime in renal insufficiency

Creatinine clearance ml/min	*Approx. Serum creatinine* µmol/l (mg/dl)*	*Recommended Unit dose of ceftazidime g*	*Frequency of dosing hourly*
50–31	150–200 (1.7–2.3)	1.0	12
30–16	200–350 (2.3–4.0)	1.0	24
15–6	350–500 (4.0–5.6)	0.5	24
<5	>500 (>5.6)	0.5	48

*These values are guide-lines and may not accurately predict renal function in all patients especially in the elderly in whom the serum creatinine concentration may overestimate renal function.

Adults: The adult dosage range for ceftazidime is 1 to 6 g per day: for instance, 500 mg, 1 g or 2 g given 12 or 8-hourly by i.v. or i.m. injection. In urinary tract infections and in many less serious infections, 500 mg or 1 g 12-hourly is usually adequate. In the majority of infections, 1 g 8-hourly or 2 g 12-hourly should be given. In very severe infections, especially in immunocompromised patients, including those with neutropenia, 2 g 8 or 12-hourly should be administered.

Elderly: In view of the reduced clearance of ceftazidime in acutely ill elderly patients, the daily dosage should not normally exceed 3 g, especially in those over 80 years of age.

Cystic fibrosis: In fibrocystic adults with normal renal function who have pseudomonal lung infections, high doses of 100 to 150 mg/kg/day as three divided doses should be used. In adults with normal renal function 9 g/day has been used safely.

Infants and children: The usual dosage range for children aged over two months is 30 to 100 mg/kg/day, given as two or three divided doses.

Doses up to 150 mg/kg/day (maximum 6 g daily) in three divided doses may be given to infected immunocompromised or fibrocystic children or children with meningitis.

Neonates and children up to 2 months of age: Whilst clinical experience is limited, a dose of 25 to 60 mg/kg/day given as two divided doses has proved to be effective. In the neonate the serum half-life of ceftazidime can be three to four times that in adults.

Dosage in impaired renal function: Ceftazidime is excreted by the kidneys almost exclusively by glomerular filtration. Therefore, in patients with impaired renal function it is recommended that the dosage of ceftazidime should be reduced to compensate for its slower excretion, except in mild impairment, i.e., glomerular filtration rate (GFR) greater than 50 ml/min. In patients with suspected renal insufficiency, an initial loading dose of 1 g of ceftazidime may be given. An estimate of GFR should be made to determine the appropriate maintenance dose.

Recommended maintenance doses are shown above.

In patients with severe infections, especially in neutropenics, who would normally receive 6 g of ceftazidime daily were it not for renal insufficiency, the unit dose given in the table above may be increased by 50% or the dosing frequency increased appropriately. In such patients it is recommended that ceftazidime serum levels should be monitored and trough levels should not exceed 40 mg/litre.

When only serum creatinine is available, the following formula (Cockcroft's equation) may be used to estimate creatinine clearance. The serum creatinine should represent a steady state of renal function:

Preparation of Solution

Vial Size		*Amount of Diluent to be added (ml)*	*Approximate Concentration (mg/ml)*
250 mg	intramuscular	1.0 ml	210
250 mg	intravenous	2.5 ml	90
500 mg	intramuscular	1.5 ml	260
500 mg	intravenous	5 ml	90
1 g	intramuscular	3 ml	260
1 g	intravenous	10 ml	90
2 g	intravenous bolus	10 ml	170
2 g	intravenous infusion	50 ml*	40

*NOTE: Addition should be in two stages (see text).

Males:
Creatinine clearance (ml/min) =

$$\frac{\text{Weight (kg)} \times (140 - \text{age in years})}{72 \times \text{serum creatinine (mg/dl)}}$$

Females:
0.85 × above value.
To convert serum creatinine in μmol/litre into mg/dl divide by 88.4.

In children the creatinine clearance should be adjusted for body surface area or lean body mass and the dosing frequency reduced in cases of renal insufficiency as for adults.

The serum half-life of ceftazidime during haemodialysis ranges from 3 to 5 hours. The appropriate maintenance dose of ceftazidime should be repeated following each haemodialysis period.

Dosage in peritoneal dialysis: Ceftazidime may also be used in peritoneal dialysis and continuous ambulatory peritoneal dialysis (CAPD). As well as using ceftazidime intravenously, it can be incorporated into the dialysis fluid (usually 125 to 250 mg for 2 L of dialysis fluid).

Administration: Ceftazidime may be given intravenously or by deep intramuscular injection into a large muscle mass such as the upper outer quadrant of the gluteus maximus or lateral part of the thigh.

Instructions for reconstitution: See table above for addition volumes and solution concentrations, which may be useful when fractional doses are required.

All sizes of vials as supplied are under reduced pressure. As the product dissolves, carbon dioxide is released and a positive pressure develops. For ease of use, it is recommended that the following techniques of reconstitution are adopted.

250 mg i.m./i.v., 500 mg i.m./i.v., 1 g i.m./i.v. and 2 g i.v. bolus vials:

1. Insert the syringe needle through the vial closure and inject the recommended volume of diluent. The vacuum may assist entry of the diluent. Remove the syringe needle.
2. Shake to dissolve: carbon dioxide is released and a clear solution obtained in about 1 to 2 minutes.
3. Invert the vial. With the syringe plunger fully depressed, insert the needle through the vial closure and withdraw the total volume of solution into the syringe (the pressure in the vial may aid withdrawal). Ensure that the needle remains within the solution and does not enter the headspace. The withdrawn solution may contain small bubbles of carbon dioxide; they may be disregarded.

2 g i.v. infusion vial:
This vial may be reconstituted for short intravenous infusion (e.g., up to 30 minutes) as follows:

1. Insert the syringe needle through the vial closure and inject 10 ml of diluent. The vacuum may assist entry of the diluent. Remove the syringe needle.
2. Shake to dissolve; carbon dioxide is released and a clear solution obtained in about 1 to 2 minutes.
3. Insert a gas relief needle through the vial closure to relieve the internal pressure and, with the gas relief in position, add a further 40 ml of diluent. Remove the gas relief needle and syringe needle; shake the vial and set up for infusion use in the normal way.

NOTE: To preserve product sterility, it is important that a gas relief needle is *not* inserted through the vial closure before the product has dissolved.

These solutions may be given directly into the vein or introduced into the tubing of a giving set if the patient is receiving parenteral fluids. Ceftazidime is compatible with the most commonly used intravenous fluids (see Pharmaceutical precautions).

Contra-indications, warnings, etc

Contra-indications: Ceftazidime is contra-indicated in patients with known hypersensitivity to cephalosporin antibiotics.

Warnings: As with other beta-lactam antibiotics, before therapy with ceftazidime is instituted, careful inquiry should be made for a history of hypersensitivity reactions to ceftazidime, cephalosporins, penicillins, or other drugs. Ceftazidime should be given only with special caution to patients with type I or immediate hypersensitivity reactions to penicillin. If an allergic reaction to ceftazidime occurs, discontinue the drug. Serious hypersensitivity reactions may require epinephrine (adrenaline), hydrocortisone, antihistamine or other emergency measures.

Precautions: Cephalosporin antibiotics at high dosage should be given with caution to patients receiving concurrent treatment with nephrotoxic drugs, e.g., aminoglycoside antibiotics, or potent diuretics such as frusemide, as these combinations are suspected of affecting renal function adversely. Clinical experience with ceftazidime has shown that this is not likely to be a problem at the recommended dose levels. There is no evidence that ceftazidime adversely affects renal function at normal therapeutic doses: however, as for all antibiotics eliminated via the kidneys, it is necessary to reduce the dosage according to the degree of reduction in renal function to avoid the clinical consequences of elevated antibiotic levels, e.g., neurological sequelae, which have occasionally been reported when the dose has not been reduced appropriately (see Dosage in Impaired Renal Function).

There is no experimental evidence of embryopathic or teratogenic effects attributable to ceftazidime but, as with all drugs, it should be administered with caution during the early months of pregnancy and in early infancy. Use in pregnancy requires that the anticipated benefit be weighed against the possible risks. Ceftazidime is excreted in human milk in low concentrations and consequently caution should be exercised when ceftazidime is administered to a nursing mother.

Ceftazidime does not interfere with enzyme-based tests for glycosuria. Slight interference with copper reduction methods (Benedict's, Fehling's, Clinitest) may be observed. Ceftazidime does not interfere in the alkaline picrate assay for creatinine.

The development of a positive Coombs' test associated with the use of ceftazidime in about 5% of patients may interfere with the cross-matching of blood.

As with other broad spectrum antibiotics, prolonged use of ceftazidime may result in the overgrowth of non-susceptible organisms (e.g., Candida, Enterococci) which may require interruption of treatment or adoption of appropriate measures. Repeated evaluation of the patient's condition is essential.

Chloramphenicol is antagonistic *in vitro* with ceftazidime and other cephalosporins. The clinical relevance of this finding is unknown, but if concurrent administration of ceftazidime with chloramphenicol is proposed, the possibility of antagonism should be considered.

Side-effects: Clinical trial experience has shown that ceftazidime is generally well tolerated.

Adverse reactions are infrequent and include:
Local: phlebitis or thrombophlebitis with i.v. administration; pain and/or inflammation after i.m. injection.
Hypersensitivity: maculopapular or urticarial rash, fever, pruritus, and very rarely angioedema and anaphylaxis (bronchospasm and/or hypotension).

Gastrointestinal: diarrhoea, nausea, vomiting, abdominal pain, and very rarely oral thrush or colitis. As with other cephalosporins, colitis may be associated with *Clostridium difficile* and may present as pseudomembranous colitis.

Other adverse events which may be related to ceftazidime therapy or of uncertain aetiology include:
Genito-urinary: Candidiasis, vaginitis.
Central Nervous System: headache, dizziness, paraesthesiae and bad taste. There have been reports of neurological sequelae including tremor, myoclonica, convulsions and encephalopathy in patients with renal impairment in whom the dose of ceftazidime has not been appropriately reduced.

Laboratory test changes noted transiently during ceftazidime therapy include: eosinophilia, positive Coombs' test without haemolysis, thrombocytosis and slight elevations in one or more of the hepatic enzymes, ALT (SGPT), AST (SGOT), LDH, GGT and alkaline phosphatase.

As with some other cephalosporins, transient elevation of blood urea, blood urea nitrogen and/or serum creatinine have been observed occasionally. Very rarely, transient leucopenia, neutropenia, agranulocytosis, thrombocytopenia and lymphocytosis have been seen.

Overdosage: Overdosage can lead to neurological sequelae including encephalopathy, convulsions and coma.

Serum levels of ceftazidime are reduced by dialysis.

Pharmaceutical precautions Vials of Fortum for Injection as supplied are under reduced pressure; a positive pressure is produced on reconstitution due to the release of carbon dioxide. See Administration section above for recommended techniques of reconstitution.

Vials of Fortum for Injection should be stored at a temperature below 25°C. Occasional storage at temperatures not higher than 30°C for up to 2 months is not detrimental to the product.

Vials of Fortum for Injection do not contain any preservatives and should be used as single-dose preparations.

In keeping with good pharmaceutical practice it is preferable to use freshly constituted solutions of Fortum for Injection. If this is not practicable, satisfactory potency is retained for 24 hours in the refrigerator (2–8°C) when prepared in Water for Injection BP or any of the injections listed below.

At ceftazidime concentrations between 1 mg/ml and 40 mg/ml in:

0.9% Sodium Chloride Injection BP
M/6 Sodium Lactate Injection BP
Compound Sodium Lactate Injection BP (Hartmann's Solution)
5% Dextrose Injection BP
0.225% Sodium Chloride and 5% Dextrose Injection BP
0.45% Sodium Chloride and 5% Dextrose Injection BP
0.9% Sodium Chloride and 5% Dextrose Injection BP
0.18% Sodium Chloride and 4% Dextrose Injection BP
10% Dextrose Injection BP
Dextran 40 Injection BP 10% in 0.9% Sodium Chloride Injection BP
Dextran 40 Injection BP 10% in 5% Dextrose Injection BP
Dextran 70 Injection BP 6% in 0.9% Sodium Chloride Injection BP
Dextran 70 Injection BP 6% in 5% Dextrose Injection BP

(Ceftazidime is less stable in Sodium Bicarbonate Injection than in other intravenous fluids. It is not recommended as a diluent.)

At concentrations of between 0.05 mg/ml and 0.25 mg/ml in Intraperitoneal Dialysis Fluid (Lactate) BPC 1973.

When reconstituted for intramuscular use with:
0.5% or 1% Lignocaine Hydrochloride Injection BP

When admixed at 4 mg/ml with (both components retain satisfactory potency):

Hydrocortisone (hydrocortisone sodium phosphate) 1 mg/ml in 0.9% Sodium Chloride Injection BP or 5% Dextrose Injection BP
Cefuroxime (cefuroxime sodium) 3 mg/ml in 0.9% Sodium Chloride Injection BP
Cloxacillin (cloxacillin sodium) 4 mg/ml in 0.9% Sodium Chloride Injection BP
Heparin 10 u/ml or 50 u/ml in 0.9% Sodium Chloride Injection BP
Potassium Chloride 10 mEq/l or 40 mEq/l in 0.9% Sodium Chloride Injection BP

The contents of a 500 mg vial of Fortum for Injection, reconstituted with 1.5 ml Water for Injections, may be added to metronidazole injection (500 mg in 100 ml) and both retain their activity. Ceftazidime and aminoglycosides should not be mixed in the same giving set or syringe.

Precipitation has been reported when vancomycin has been added to ceftazidime in solution. Therefore, it would be prudent to flush giving sets and intravenous lines between administration of these two agents.

Solutions range from light yellow to amber depending on concentration, diluent and storage conditions used. Within the stated recommendations, product potency is not adversely affected by such colour variations.

Protect from light.

Legal category POM.

Package quantities Individually cartoned vials containing 250 mg, 500 mg or 1 g ceftazidime (as pentahydrate) for intramuscular or intravenous use in packs of 5.

Individually cartoned vials containing 2 g ceftazidime (as pentahydrate) for intravenous injection in packs of 5.

Individually cartoned vials containing 2 g ceftazidime (as pentahydrate) for intravenous infusion in packs of 5.

Further information Ceftazidime administered by the parenteral route reaches high and prolonged serum levels. In man after intramuscular administration of 500 mg and 1 g, serum mean peak levels of 18 and 37 mg/litre respectively are rapidly achieved. Five minutes after an intravenous bolus injection of 500 mg, 1 g and 2 g, serum mean levels are respectively 46, 87 and 170 mg/litre.

Therapeutically effective concentrations are still found in the serum 8 to 12 hours after both intravenous and intramuscular administration. The serum half-life is about 1.8 hours in normal volunteers and about 2.2 hours in patients with apparently normal renal function. The serum protein binding of ceftazidime is low at about 10%.

Ceftazidime is not metabolised in the body and is excreted unchanged in the active form into the urine by glomerular filtration. Approximately 80 to 90% of the dose is recovered in the urine within 24 hours. Less than 1% is excreted via the bile, significantly limiting the amount entering the bowel.

Concentrations of ceftazidime in excess of the minimum inhibitory levels for common pathogens can be achieved in tissues such as bone, heart, bile, sputum, aqueous humour, synovial and pleural and peritoneal fluids. Transplacental transfer of the antibiotic readily occurs. Ceftazidime penetrates the intact blood brain barrier poorly and low levels are achieved in the CSF in the absence of inflammation. Therapeutic levels of 4 to 20 mg/litre or more are achieved in the CSF when the meninges are inflamed.

Product licence numbers

250 mg vials	0004/0304
500 mg vials	0004/0292
1 gram vials	0004/0293
2 gram vials	0004/0294

Product licence holder: Glaxo Operations UK Limited, Greenford, Middlesex UB6 0HE.

GRISOVIN* TABLETS

Presentation Grisovin Tablets contain 125 mg or 500 mg of the antibiotic griseofulvin in fine particle form.

Both are white, film-coated, bi-convex tablets engraved 'Grisovin 125' or 'Grisovin 500' on one side as appropriate and 'Glaxo' on the other. They comply with the specification for Griseofulvin Tablets BP, BNF.

Uses The treatment of fungal infections of the skin, scalp, hair or nails where topical therapy is considered inappropriate or has failed. When griseofulvin is given orally for systemic treatment of ringworm infections, it enables newly formed keratin of the skin, hair and nails to resist attack by the fungi. As the new keratin extends, the old infected keratin is shed.

Grisovin is effective against the dermatophytes causing ringworm (tinea), including: *Microsporum canis*, and *T. verrucosum*.

Grisovin is not effective in infections caused by *Candida albicans* (monilia), Aspergilli, *Malassezia furfur (Pityriasis versicolor)* and Nocardia species.

Dosage and administration Doses should be taken after meals, otherwise absorption is likely to be inadequate.

Adults: Normally 500 to 1,000 mg daily, but not less than 10 mg/kg body weight daily. A single dose daily is often satisfactory, but divided doses may be more effective in patients who respond poorly.

Children: Usually 10 mg per kg (5 mg/lb) body weight daily in divided doses.

Duration of treatment: This depends upon the thickness of keratin at the site of infection. For hair or skin at least four weeks' treatment is required, whereas toe or finger nails may need six to twelve months' treatment. Therapy should be continued for at least two weeks after all signs of infection have disappeared.

Contra-indications, warnings, etc
Contra-indications: Porphyria or severe liver disease. Griseofulvin may cause liver disease to deteriorate, and liver function should be monitored in such conditions.

Systemic lupus erythematosus: Griseofulvin has been reported to exacerbate the condition.

Hypersensitivity to any ingredient of the preparation.

Contraception/pregnancy: Concurrent treatment with griseofulvin may reduce the effectiveness of oral contraceptives, so additional contraceptive precautions should be taken during griseofulvin treatment and for a month after stopping griseofulvin.

There is no evidence of its safety in human pregnancy. Griseofulvin is teratogenic in animals and some case-reports suggest that it produces human fetal abnormalities. Griseofulvin should not be used in pregnancy.

Precautions: Griseofulvin may decrease the effect of the coumarin anticoagulants.

Absorption of griseofulvin is inhibited when phenobarbitone is taken concurrently. The blood level, and hence efficacy, of griseofulvin may also be impaired as the result of concurrent administration of substances such as phenylbutazone and sedative and hypnotic drugs which induce metabolising enzymes.

Photosensitivity reactions can occur on exposure to intense natural or artificial sunlight.

In those rare cases where individuals are affected by drowsiness while taking griseofulvin, they should not drive vehicles or operate machinery. Patients should be warned that an enhancement of the effects of alcohol by griseofulvin has been reported.

Long-term administration of high doses of griseofulvin with food has been reported to induce hepatomas in mice and thyroid tumours in rats but not hamsters. The clinical significance of these findings is not known. In view of these data, griseofulvin tablets should not be used prophylactically.

Side-effects: Headache and gastric discomfort sometimes occur, but usually disappear as treatment continues. On rare occasions urticarial reactions, erythematous rashes and precipitation of systemic lupus erythematosus have been reported.

Toxic epidermal necrolysis and erythema multiforme have been reported.

There have been reports of central nervous system effects e.g. confusion, dizziness, impaired co-ordination and peripheral neuropathy.

Overdosage: Treatment is unlikely to be required in cases of acute overdosage.

Pharmaceutical precautions None.

Pharmacokinetics: The absorption of griseofulvin from the gastrointestinal tract is variable and incomplete. On average, less than 50% of the oral dose is absorbed, but fatty foods and a reduction in particle size will increase the rate and extent of the absorption.

After oral dosing there is a phase of rapid absorption followed by slower prolonged absorption. Peak plasma levels (0.5–1.5 micrograms after a 500 mg oral dose) are achieved by 4 hours and are maintained for 10–20 hours. The terminal plasma half-life ranges from 9.5–21 hours, there being considerable intersubject variability. In plasma, griseofulvin is approximately 84% bound to plasma proteins, predominantly albumin.

The absorbed griseofulvin is excreted in the urine mainly as 6-desmethylgriseofulvin or its glucuronide conjugate.

There is selective deposition of griseofulvin in newly-formed keratin of hair, nails and skin, which gradually moves to the surface of these appendages.

Legal category POM.

Package quantities *125 mg tablets:* Bottles of 100 tablets (OP).

500 mg tablets: Bottles of 100 tablets (OP).

Further information Customary hygienic measures should be adopted to minimise the risk of re-infection, and concurrent use of a topical fungicide may be helpful to minimise any spread of infective material.

Product licence numbers
Grisovin Tablets 125 mg 0004/5060R
Grisovin Tablets 500 mg 0004/5061R

Product licence holder: Glaxo Operations UK Limited, Greenford, Middlesex UB6 0HE.

PREDNESOL* TABLETS

Presentation Small, pink, soluble tablets engraved 'Prednesol Glaxo' on one side and scored on the reverse. Each tablet contains 5 mg prednisolone as the sodium phosphate ester.

Uses Prednisolone is a glucocorticosteroid which is about four times as active as hydrocortisone on a weight-for-weight basis.

Prednisolone sodium phosphate is very soluble in water, and is therefore less likely to cause local gastric irritation than prednisolone alcohol, which is only slightly soluble. This is important when high dosages are required, as in immuno-suppressive therapy.

A wide variety of diseases may sometimes require corticosteroid therapy. Some of the principal indications are: bronchial asthma, severe hypersensitivity reactions, anaphylaxis; rheumatoid arthritis, systemic lupus erythematosus, dermatomyositis, mixed connective tissue disease (excluding systemic sclerosis), polyarteritis nodosa; inflammatory skin disorders, including pemphigus vulgaris, bullous pemphigoid and pyoderma gangrenosum; minimal change nephrotic syndrome, acute interstitial nephritis; ulcerative colitis, Crohn's disease; sarcoidosis; rheumatic carditis; haemolytic anaemia (auto-immune), acute and lymphatic leukaemia, malignant lymphoma, multiple myeloma, idiopathic thrombocytopenic purpura; immuno-suppression in transplantation.

Dosage and administration Prednesol Tablets are best taken dissolved in water, but they can be swallowed whole without difficulty.

The lowest dosage that will produce an acceptable result should be used; when it is possible to reduce the dosage, this must be accomplished by stages. During prolonged therapy, dosage may need to be increased temporarily during periods of stress or in exacerbations of illness.

Adults: The dose used will depend upon the disease, its severity and the clinical response obtained. The following regimens are for guidance only. Divided dosage is usually employed.

Short-term treatment: 20 to 30 mg daily for the first few days, subsequently reducing the daily dosage by 2.5 or 5 mg every two to five days, depending upon the response.

Rheumatoid arthritis: 7.5 to 10 mg daily. For maintenance therapy the lowest effective dosage is used.

Most other conditions: 10 to 100 mg daily for one to three weeks, then reducing to the minimum effective dosage.

Children: Fractions of the adult dosage may be used (e.g. 75% at 12 years, 50% at 7 years and 25% at one year), but clinical factors must be given due weight.

Contra-indications, warnings, etc
Contra-indications: Systemic infections, unless specific anti-infective therapy is employed. Live virus immunisation. Hypersensitivity to any component of the tablet.

Precautions: Administration of corticosteroids may impair the ability to resist and counteract infection e.g. where there is a previous history of tuberculosis; in addition, clinical signs and symptoms of infection are suppressed.

Corticosteroid treatment is likely to reduce the response of the pituitary-adrenal axis to stress, and relative insufficiency may persist for up to a year after withdrawal of prolonged therapy.

Because of the possibility of fluid retention, care must be taken when corticosteroids are administered to patients with congestive heart failure.

Corticosteroids may worsen diabetes mellitus, osteoporosis, hypertension, glaucoma and epilepsy.

Care should be taken when there is a history of severe affective disorders (especially a previous history of steroid psychosis), previous steroid myopathy or peptic ulceration.

Since corticosteroids are secreted in breast milk, the advisability of breast feeding should be considered in women on high dosage.

Steroids may reduce the effects of anticholinesterases in myasthenia gravis, cholecystographic X-ray media and salicylates.

The effect of steroids may be reduced by phenytoin, phenobarbitone, ephedrine and rifampicin.

The dosage of concomitantly administered anti-coagulants may have to be altered (usually decreased).

In patients with liver failure, blood levels of corticosteroid may be increased, as with other drugs which are metabolised in the liver.

Systemic corticosteroids may cause growth retardation in infancy, childhood and adolescence. Treatment should be limited to the minimum dosage for the shortest possible time. In order to minimise suppression of the HPA axis and growth retardation, consideration should be given to administration of a single dose on alternate days.

Treatment of elderly patients, particularly if long-term, should be planned bearing in mind the more serious consequences of the common side-effects of corticosteroids in old age, especially osteoporosis, diabetes, hypertension, susceptibility to infection and thinning of the skin.

When treatment is to be discontinued, the dose should be reduced gradually over a period of several weeks or months depending on the dosage and duration of the therapy.

Pregnancy: There is inadequate evidence of safety in human pregnancy. Administration of corticosteroids to pregnant animals can cause abnormalities of fetal development including cleft palate and intra-uterine growth retardation. There may therefore be a very small risk of such effects in the human fetus.

Depression of hormone levels has been described in pregnancy but the significance of this finding is not clear.

Side-effects: Prolonged treatment with corticosteroids in high dosage is occasionally associated with subcapsular cataract, skin thinning, osteoporosis and glaucoma. In addition, any of the features of hypercorticism, such as suppression of the HPA axis, may occur. Aseptic osteonecrosis, particularly of the femoral head, may occur after prolonged corticosteroid therapy, or after repeated short courses involving high dosage. Peptic ulceration may develop, or be aggravated.

In children, prolonged therapy may retard growth.

In patients on long-term therapy, fluid and electrolyte balance may be altered. Other rare side-effects which have been reported include benign intracranial hypertension and psychic instability.

Drug interactions: Steroids may reduce the effects of anticholinesterases in myasthenia gravis, cholecystographic X-ray media and non-steroidal anti-inflammatory agents. It should also be remembered that the effects of steroids may be reduced by phenytoin, phenobarbitone, ephedrine and rifampicin.

Overdosage: Treatment is unlikely to be needed in cases of acute overdosage.

Pharmaceutical precautions Protect from light.

Legal category POM.

Package quantities The tablets are strip-packed in cartons of 100 (OP).

Further information Prednesol Tablets do not contain carbohydrates.

Product licence number 0004/5091R.

Product licence holder: Glaxo Operations UK Limited, Greenford, Middlesex UB6 0HE.

PREDSOL* DROPS FOR EYE AND EAR

Presentation Predsol Drops contain prednisolone sodium phosphate 0.5% w/v and benzalkonium chloride 0.02% w/v in a sterilised clear and colourless aqueous solution. The product complies with the specification for Prednisolone Sodium Phosphate Eye Drops BPC.

Uses Short-term treatment of steroid responsive inflammatory conditions of the eye after clinical exclusion of bacterial, viral and fungal infections.

Non-infected inflammatory conditions of the ear.

Dosage and administration *Eyes:* 1 or 2 drops instilled into the eye every one or two hours until control is achieved, when the frequency may be reduced.

Ears: 2 or 3 drops instilled into the ear every two or three hours until control is achieved, when the frequency can be reduced.

Contra-indications, warnings, etc
Contra-indications: Bacterial, viral, fungal, tuberculous or purulent conditions of the eye. Use in the eye is contra-indicated if glaucoma is present or where herpetic keratitis (e.g. dendritic ulcer) is considered a possibility. Inadvertent use of topical steroids in the latter condition can lead to the extension of the ulcer and marked visual deterioration.

Hypersensitivity to any component of the preparation.

Predsol Eye Drops contain benzalkonium chloride as a preservative and therefore should not be used to treat patients who wear soft contact lenses.

Precautions: Steroids should not be administered to 'red eyes' until a definitive diagnosis has been made. Ophthalmological treatment with steroid preparations should not be repeated or prolonged without regular review to exclude raised intra-ocular pressure or unsuspected infections.

Pregnancy: There is inadequate evidence of safety in human pregnancy. Administration of corticosteroids to pregnant animals can cause abnormalities of fetal development including cleft palate and intra-uterine growth retardation. There may, therefore, be a very small risk of such effects in the human fetus.

Side-effects: Eye Drops containing corticosteroids cause a serious rise in intra-ocular pressure in a small percentage of the population, which includes most of those with a family history of glaucoma. A milder rise may be experienced by a larger proportion of subjects if treatment is continued for longer than a few weeks. Thinning of the cornea leading to perforation has occurred with the use of topical corticosteroids. Cataract is reported to have occurred after unduly prolonged treatment of eye conditions with topical corticosteroids.

Pharmaceutical precautions It is desirable that the contents should not be used more than four weeks after first opening the bottle.

Legal category POM.

Package quantities Plastic dropper bottles containing 10 ml.

Further information Nil.

Product licence number 0004/5092R.

Product licence holder: Glaxo Operations UK Limited, Greenford, Middlesex UB6 0HE.

PREDSOL*-N DROPS FOR EYE OR EAR

Presentation Predsol-N Drops contain prednisolone sodium phosphate 0.5% w/v, neomycin sulphate 0.5% w/v and benzalkonium chloride 0.01% w/v in a clear, colourless, aqueous solution. Sterile until opened.

Uses *Eye:* For the short-term treatment of steroid responsive conditions of the eye when prophylactic antibiotic treatment is also required, after excluding the presence of fungal and viral disease.

Ear: Otitis externa or other steroid responsive conditions where prophylactic antibiotic treatment is also required.

Dosage and administration
Adults (and the Elderly) and Children:
Eyes: 1 or 2 drops applied to each affected eye up to six times daily or more frequently if required.

Ears: 2 or 3 drops instilled into the ear three to four times daily.

Contra-indications, warnings, etc
Contra-indications: Viral, fungal, tuberculous or purulent conditions of the eye. Use is contra-indicated if glaucoma is present, or herpetic keratitis (e.g. dendritic ulcer) is considered a possibility. Use of topical steroids in the latter condition can lead to extension of the ulcer and marked visual deterioration.

Otitis externa should not be treated when the eardrum is perforated because of the risk of ototoxicity.

Hypersensitivity to the preparation.

Predsol-N Eye Drops contain benzalkonium chloride as a preservative and, therefore, should not be used to treat patients who wear soft contact lenses.

Precautions: Topical corticosteroids should never be given for an undiagnosed 'red eye' as inappropriate use is potentially blinding.

Treatment with corticosteroid/antibiotic combinations should not be continued for more than 7 days in the absence of any clinical improvement, since prolonged use may lead to occult extension of infection due to the masking effect of the steroid. Prolonged use may also lead to skin sensitisation and the emergence of resistant organisms.

Prolonged use may lead to the risk of adrenal suppression in infants.

Treatment with corticosteroid preparations should not be repeated or prolonged without regular review to exclude raised intra-ocular pressure, cataract formation or unsuspected infections.

Aminoglycoside antibiotics may cause irreversible, partial or total deafness when given systemically or when applied topically to open wounds or damaged skin. This effect is dose related and is enhanced by renal or hepatic impairment. Although this effect has not been reported following topical ocular use, the possibility should be considered when high dose topical treatment is given to small children or infants.

Pregnancy and lactation: Safety for use in pregnancy and lactation has not been established. There is inadequate evidence of safety in human pregnancy. Topical administration of corticosteroids to pregnant animals can cause abnormalities of fetal development including cleft palate and intra-uterine growth retardation. There may therefore be a very small risk of such effects in the human fetus. There is a risk of fetal ototoxicity if aminoglycoside antibiotic preparations are administered during pregnancy.

Side-effects: Hypersensitivity reactions, usually of the delayed type, may occur leading to irritation, burning, stinging, itching and dermatitis.

Topical steroid use may result in increased intra-ocular pressure leading to optic nerve damage, reduced visual acuity and visual field defects.

Intensive or prolonged use of topical corticosteroids may lead to formation of posterior subcapsular cataracts.

In those diseases causing thinning of the cornea or sclera, corticosteroid therapy may result in thinning of the globe leading to perforation.

Overdosage: Long-term intensive topical use may lead to systemic effects.

Oral ingestion of the contents of one bottle (up to 10 ml) is unlikely to lead to any serious adverse effects.

Pharmaceutical precautions It is desirable that the contents should not be used more than four weeks after first opening the bottle.

Legal category POM.

Package quantities Plastic dropper bottles containing 10 ml.

Further information Nil.

Product licence number 0004/5093.

Product licence holder: Glaxo Operations UK Limited, Greenford, Middlesex UB6 0HE.

PREDSOL* RETENTION ENEMA

Presentation 100 ml disposable plastic bags, each containing 20 mg prednisolone as the sodium phosphate ester in a buffered solution. The product complies with the specification for Prednisolone Sodium Phosphate Enema BPC.

Uses Predsol Retention Enema provides local corticosteroid treatment for rectal and recto-sigmoidal disease in ulcerative colitis and Crohn's disease.

Dosage and administration *Adults:* 1 enema used nightly, for two to four weeks. Treatment may be continued in patients showing progressive improvement, but it should not be persisted with if the response has been inadequate. Some patients may relapse after an interval but are likely to respond equally well to a repeated course of treatment.

Predsol Retention Enema as packed is not suitable for use in children.

The enema is used each night on retiring. It may be warmed before administration by placing the bag in a vessel of hot water for a few minutes. When in bed and lying on the left side with knees drawn up, the patient should remove the stopper from the bag, lubricate the nozzle with petroleum jelly and gently insert about half the length of the nozzle into the rectum. The bag should then be slowly rolled up like a tube of toothpaste until it is emptied, taking a minute or two to do so. The nozzle should then be removed, with the bag still rolled up, and the whole unit discarded. The patient should then roll over to lie face down for three to five minutes but may sleep in any comfortable position.

Contra-indications, warnings, etc
Contra-indications: Hypersensitivity to the preparation. The use of Predsol Retention Enema is not indicated in primary infection by viruses or other micro-organisms.

Pregnancy: There is inadequate evidence of safety in human pregnancy. Topical administration of corticosteroids to pregnant animals can cause abnormalities of fetal development including cleft palate and intra-uterine growth retardation. There may therefore be a very small risk of such effects in the human fetus.

Side-effects: The consequences of systemic absorption e.g. suppression of the HPA axis, should be considered if Predsol Retention Enema is used over long periods or in high dosage.

Pharmaceutical precautions Protect from light.

Legal category POM.

Package quantities Boxes of seven 100 ml disposable bags (instructions to patients enclosed).

Further information The volume of the enema is considered to be the optimum to ensure maximum coverage of the affected area.

Product licence number 0004/5094R.

Product licence holder: Glaxo Operations UK Limited, Greenford, Middlesex UB6 0HE.

PREDSOL* SUPPOSITORIES

Presentation Predsol Suppositories are white and opaque. Each suppository contains 5 mg prednisolone as the sodium phosphate ester.

Uses Prednisolone is a glucocorticosteroid which is about four times as potent as hydrocortisone on a weight-for-weight basis.

Predsol Suppositories are indicated for the treatment of haemorrhagic and granular proctitis and the rectal complications of Crohn's disease.

Dosage and administration One suppository inserted at night and one in the morning after defaecation for adults or children. When the response is good, treatment is usually continued for some months. If symptoms recur later, treatment should be resumed.

Contra-indications, warnings, etc
Contra-indications: Hypersensitivity to the preparation. The use of Predsol Suppositories is not indicated in primary infection by viruses or other micro-organisms.

Pregnancy: There is inadequate evidence of safety in human pregnancy. Topical administration of corticosteroids to pregnant animals can cause abnormalities of fetal development including cleft palate and intra-uterine growth retardation. There may therefore be a very small risk of such effects in the human fetus.

Side-effects: As with all topical corticosteroids, if Predsol Suppositories are used for prolonged periods the consequences of systemic absorption, e.g. suppression of the HPA axis, should be considered, especially in children.

Pharmaceutical precautions Nil.

Legal category POM.

Package quantities Cartoned plastic moulds each containing 10 suppositories.

Further information Nil.

Product licence number 0004/5095R.

Product licence holder: Glaxo Operations UK Limited, Greenford, Middlesex UB6 0HE.

PROPADERM* CREAM AND OINTMENT

Presentation Propaderm Cream and Ointment are topical preparations of Beclomethasone Dipropionate BP. Beclomethasone Dipropionate BP is a potent anti-inflammatory steroid when applied topically to the skin.

Propaderm Cream: Beclomethasone Dipropionate BP 0.025% in a cream base.

Propaderm Ointment: Beclomethasone Dipropionate BP 0.025% in an ointment base.

Propaderm Cream is white in colour; Propaderm Ointment is yellowish.

Uses Propaderm Cream and Ointment are indicated for the treatment of the various forms of eczema in children and adults including atopic and discoid eczemas; primary irritant and allergic dermatitis; psoriasis (excluding widespread plaque psoriasis); neurodermatoses including lichen simplex; intertrigo; discoid lupus erythematosus.

Propaderm Cream is often appropriate for moist or weeping surfaces and Propaderm Ointment for dry, lichenified or scaly lesions but this is not invariably so.

Dosage and administration Propaderm preparations should be applied thinly over the whole of the affected area and gently rubbed in. Initially, application should be made twice daily, but when improvement is seen, the intervals between applications may be extended and treatment eventually stopped. If no improvement is seen within two to four weeks, reassessment of the diagnosis, or referral may be necessary. After cessation of treatment, should the condition recur, twice daily treatment should be re-instituted. However, when improvement is seen again, the intervals between application may be gradually extended until maintenance dosing of application every third or fourth day is achieved. This is likely to avoid subsequent reappearance of the condition. The beneficial effects may be enhanced by preliminary use of hot soaks, or by intermittent applications of occlusive dressings.

Contra-indications, warnings, etc
Contra-indications: Propaderm should not be applied to the eyes. Rosacea, acne vulgaris; peri-oral dermatitis. Primary cutaneous viral infections (e.g. herpes simplex, chickenpox). Hypersensitivity to the preparation. Varicose ulcers or any other stasis ulcers.

Use of Propaderm preparations is not indicated in the treatment of primarily infected skin lesions caused by infection with fungi (e.g. candidiasis, tinea) or bacteria (e.g. impetigo); primary or secondary infections due to yeasts; peri-anal and genital pruritus; dermatoses in children under 1 year of age, including dermatitis and napkin eruptions.

Precautions: Long-term continuous therapy should be avoided where possible, particularly in infants and children, as adrenal suppression can occur even without occlusion.

The face, more than the other areas of the body, may exhibit atrophic changes after prolonged treatment with potent topical corticosteroids. This must be borne in mind when treating such conditions as psoriasis, discoid lupus erythematosus and severe eczema. If applied to the eyelids, care is needed to ensure that the preparation does not enter the eye, as glaucoma might result.

If used in childhood, or on the face, courses should be limited if possible to five days and occlusion should not be used.

Topical corticosteroids may be hazardous in psoriasis for a number of reasons including rebound relapses, development of tolerance, risk of generalised pustular psoriasis and development of local or systemic toxicity due to impaired barrier function of the skin. If used in psoriasis careful patient supervision is important.

Appropriate antimicrobial therapy should be used whenever treating inflammatory lesions which have become infected. Any spread of infection requires withdrawal of topical corticosteroid therapy and systemic administration of antimicrobial agents.

Bacterial infection is encouraged by the warm, moist conditions induced by occlusive dressings, and so the skin should be cleansed before a fresh dressing is applied.

Pregnancy: There is inadequate evidence of safety in human pregnancy. Topical administration of corticosteroids to pregnant animals can cause abnormalities of fetal development including cleft palate and intra-uterine growth retardation. There may therefore be a very small risk of such effects in the human fetus.

Side-effects: Prolonged and intensive treatment with

highly active corticosteroid preparations may cause local atrophic changes in the skin such as thinning, striae, and dilatation of the superficial blood vessels, particularly when occlusive dressings are used or when skin folds are involved.

As with other topical corticosteroids, prolonged use of large amounts, or treatment of extensive areas, can result in sufficient systemic absorption to produce the features of hypercorticism. The effect is more likely to occur in infants and children, and if occlusive dressings are used. In infants, the napkin may act as an occlusive dressing.

Should systemic corticosteroid effects arise from application of Propaderm preparations topical treatment should be discontinued. If adrenal function is impaired the patient will need to be protected from any harmful effects of stress with oral corticosteroid preparations until normal adrenal function is established.

In rare instances, treatment of psoriasis with corticosteroids (or its withdrawal) is thought to have provoked the pustular form of the disease (see 'Precautions').

Propaderm Cream and Ointment are usually well tolerated, but if signs of hypersensitivity appear, application should stop immediately.

Overdosage: Acute overdosage is very unlikely to occur. However, in the case of chronic overdosage or misuse the features of hypercorticism may appear and in this situation topical steroids should be discontinued.

Pharmaceutical precautions
Storage: All Propaderm preparations should be stored at a temperature below 25°C and protected from light.

Dilution: Propaderm Cream may be diluted, if necessary, with Cetomacrogol Cream Formula A BPC. For Propaderm Ointment, dilution can be effected with White Soft Paraffin BP.

Legal category POM.

Package quantities Propaderm Cream is available in tubes of 30 g; Propaderm Ointment in tubes of 30 g.

Further information No Propaderm preparation contains lanolin or parabens.

Product licence numbers

Propaderm Cream	0045/5000R
Propaderm Ointment	0045/5005R

Product licence holder: Allen & Hanburys Limited, Greenford, Middlesex UB6 0HE.

PROPADERM*-A OINTMENT

Presentation Propaderm-A Ointment contains Beclomethasone Dipropionate BP 0.025% and Chlortetracycline Hydrochloride BP 3.0%. It is pale yellow in colour.

Beclomethasone Dipropionate BP is a potent anti-inflammatory steroid when applied topically to the skin. Chlortetracycline Hydrochloride BP is a broad-spectrum antibiotic unlikely to cause skin sensitisation reactions.

Uses Propaderm-A Ointment is indicated for the treatment of the following conditions where secondary bacterial infection is present, suspected, or likely to occur; eczema in children and adults, including atopic and discoid eczema, prurigo nodularis; psoriasis (excluding widespread plaque psoriasis), neurodermatoses, seborrhoeic dermatitis; contact sensitivity reactions and it may be used as an adjunct to systemic steroid therapy in generalised erythroderma.

Propaderm-A Ointment can also be used in the management of secondary infected insect bites and anal and genital intertrigo.

Dosage and administration Propaderm-A Ointment should be applied thinly over the whole of the affected area and gently rubbed in. Initially, application should be twice daily, but when improvement is seen the intervals between applications may be extended and treatment eventually stopped. After cessation of treatment, should the condition recur, twice daily treatment should be reinstituted. However, when improvement is seen again, the intervals between applications may be gradually extended until maintenance dosing of application every third or fourth day is achieved. This is likely to avoid subsequent reappearance of the condition.

Contra-indications, warnings, etc
Contra-indications: Propaderm-A Ointment should not be applied to the eyes. Rosacea, acne vulgaris and perioral dermatitis. Primary cutaneous viral infections (e.g. herpes simplex, chickenpox). Hypersensitivity to the preparation. Varicose ulcers or any other stasis ulcer. Use of Propaderm-A Ointment is not indicated in the treatment of primarily infected skin lesions caused by infection with fungi (e.g. candidiasis, tinea) or bacteria (e.g. impetigo); primary or secondary infections due to yeasts or Pseudomonas or Proteus species; dermatoses in children under 1 year of age, including dermatitis and napkin eruptions.

Precautions: Long-term continuous topical therapy should be avoided where possible, particularly in infants and children, as adrenal suppression can occur even without occlusion.

The face, more than other areas of the body, may exhibit atrophic changes after prolonged treatment with potent topical corticosteroids. This must be borne in mind when treating such conditions as psoriasis, discoid lupus erythematosus and severe eczema. If applied to the eyelids, care is needed to ensure that the preparation does not enter the eye, as glaucoma might result. If used in childhood, or on the face, courses should be limited to five days and occlusion should not be used.

Topical corticosteroids may be hazardous in psoriasis for a number of reasons including rebound relapses, development of tolerance, risk of generalised pustular psoriasis, and development of local or systemic toxicity due to impaired barrier function of the skin. If used in psoriasis careful patient supervision is important.

If bacterial infection persists, systemic chemotherapy is required. Any spread of infection requires withdrawal of topical corticosteroid therapy.

Bacterial infection is encouraged by the warm, moist conditions induced by occlusive dressings, and the skin should be cleansed before a fresh dressing is applied.

Do not continue for more than seven days in the absence of clinical improvement, since occult extension of infection may occur due to the masking effect of the steroid.

Extended or recurrent application may increase the risk of contact sensitisation.

Chlortetracycline is ineffective against Pseudomonas and Proteus species which are recognised secondary infecting organisms in exudative dermatoses, and therefore preliminary identification of organisms and determination of antibiotic sensitivity is important. Propaderm-A Ointment may stain hair, skin or fabric, and the application should be covered with a non-occlusive dressing to protect clothing.

Products which contain antimicrobial agents should not be diluted.

Pregnancy: There is inadequate evidence of safety in human pregnancy. Topical administration of corticosteroids to pregnant animals can cause abnormalities of fetal development, including cleft palate and intra-uterine growth retardation. There may therefore be a very small risk of such effects in the human fetus.

Side-effects: Prolonged and intensive treatment with highly active corticosteroid preparations may cause local atrophic changes in the skin, such as thinning, striae and dilatation of the superficial blood vessels, particularly when occlusive dressings are used or when skin folds are involved.

As with other topical corticosteroids, prolonged use of large amounts, or treatment of extensive areas, can result in sufficient systemic absorption to produce the features of hypercorticism. The effect is more likely to occur in infants and children, and if occlusive dressings are used. In infants, the napkin may act as an occlusive dressing.

Should systemic corticosteroid effects arise from application of Propaderm preparations, topical treatment should be discontinued. If adrenal function is impaired the patient will need to be protected from any harmful effects of stress with oral corticosteroid preparations until normal adrenal function is established.

In rare instances, treatment of psoriasis with corticosteroids (or its withdrawal) is thought to have provoked the pustular form of the disease (see Precautions).

The Propaderm-A Ointment is usually well tolerated, but if signs of hypersensitivity appear application should be stopped immediately.

Overdosage: Acute overdosage is very unlikely to occur. However, in the case of chronic overdosage or misuse the features of hypercorticism may appear and in this situation topical steroids should be discontinued.

Pharmaceutical precautions Store at a temperature not exceeding 25°C and protect from light.

Legal category POM.

Package quantities Propaderm-A Ointment is available in tubes of 30 g.

Further information No lanolin or parabens included in the formula of Propaderm-A Ointment.

Product licence number 0045/5006.

Product licence holder: Allen & Hanburys Limited, Greenford, Middlesex UB6 0HE.

TERTROXIN* TABLETS

Presentation Small, white, uncoated tablets engraved 'Tertroxin Glaxo' on one side and scored on the other. Each tablet contains 20 micrograms (0.02 mg) liothyronine sodium and complies with the specification for Liothyronine Tablets BP.

Uses Liothyronine (L-triiodothyronine) sodium is a naturally occurring thyroid hormone. Its biological action is qualitatively similar to that of thyroxine, but the effect develops in a few hours and disappears within 24 to 48 hours of stopping treatment.

Tertroxin may be preferred for treating severe and acute hypothyroid states because of its rapid and more potent effect, but thyroxine sodium is normally the drug of choice for routine replacement therapy.

It is indicated in the treatment of: coma due to myxoedema; management of severe chronic thyroid deficiency; hypothyroid states arising in treatment of thyrotoxicosis.

Tertroxin can also be used therapeutically in the treatment of thyrotoxicosis as an adjunct to carbimazole in order to prevent subclinical hypothyroidism developing during treatment.

Dosage and administration *Thyroid deficiency:* Treatment of adults may be begun with 10 or 20 micrograms every eight hours increasing, if necessary, after one week to the usual recommended dosage of 60 micrograms daily in divided doses.

For children and elderly patients it is suggested that the initial dosage should be 5 micrograms daily. (To obtain small doses, tablets may be crushed and triturated with lactose for administration as a powder.)

Tertroxin should be given in divided doses two or three times daily.

Myxoedema coma: 60 micrograms may be given by stomach tube, then 20 micrograms every eight hours, although it is more usual to start treatment with intravenous liothyronine.

As therapy for thyrotoxicosis with carbimazole: In adults, 20 micrograms of liothyronine every eight hours.

Contra-indications, warnings, etc
Contra-indications: Tertroxin is contra-indicated in patients with angina of effort or cardiovascular disorders.

Precautions: In myxoedema, care must be taken to avoid imposing excessive burden on cardiac muscle affected by prolonged severe thyroid depletion.

Pregnancy: Use in pregnancy has not been documented. There is, however, very limited placental transfer of thyroid hormones.

Side-effects: The following effects are indicative of excessive dosage, and usually disappear on reduction of dosage or withdrawal of treatment for a day or two. Anginal pain, cardiac arrhythmias, palpitation, and cramps in skeletal muscle; also tachycardia, diarrhoea, restlessness, excitability, headache, flushing, sweating, excessive loss of weight and muscular weakness.

Overdosage: Gastric lavage or emesis is required if the patient is seen within several hours of taking the dose. Treatment is symptomatic; tachycardia has been controlled in an adult by 40 mg doses of propranolol given every six hours.

Pharmaceutical precautions Protect from light.

Legal category POM.

Package quantities Bottles of 100 tablets (OP).

Further information 20 micrograms liothyronine is equivalent in activity to 60 to 100 micrograms thyroxine or to 60 mg Thyroid BP.

Product licence number 0004/5032R.

Product licence holder: Glaxo Operations UK Limited, Greenford, Middlesex UB6 0HE.

TRIIODOTHYRONINE INJECTION

Presentation A freeze-dried sterile white plug containing 20 micrograms sodium triiodothyronine (Liothyronine Sodium, BP) with dextran. The plug is dissolved in Water for Injections for preparation of an intravenous injection.

Uses Treatment of myxoedema coma, usually in conjunction with other measures, including intravenous injection of a corticosteroid. For lesser degrees of myxoedema and for maintenance therapy, orally administered thyroxine should be used.

Dosage and administration Triiodothyronine injection is usually given by the intravenous route, as the alkalinity of the solution might cause irritation of the tissues if given by deep intramuscular injection. The solution is prepared by adding 1 ml or 2 ml of Water for Injections and shaking the ampoule gently until the substance has dissolved.

The dosage may be 5 to 20 micrograms given by slow intravenous injection and repeated at intervals of 12 hours, or sometimes more frequently. The minimum interval between doses is four hours. Some authorities have advocated an initial dose of 50 micrograms intravenously, followed by further intravenous injections of 25 micrograms every eight hours until improvement occurs. The dosage may then be reduced to 25 micrograms intravenously twice daily.

Contra-indications, warnings, etc
Contra-indications: No absolute contra-indication is known.

Precautions: Triiodothyronine must be given with extreme caution in myxoedema coma, as too large a dose can precipitate heart failure, especially in elderly patients and in those with ischaemic heart disease. Electrocardiographic monitoring can give a useful indication of impending ischaemia, but the ST changes of hypothyroidism may be confused with ECG evidence of ischaemia.

Use of sedatives may cause respiratory depression.

Side-effects: The following effects are indicative of excessive dosage, and usually disappear on reduction of dosage or withdrawal of treatment for a day or two. Anginal pain, cardiac arrhythmias, palpitation, and/or cramps in skeletal muscle. Also tachycardia, diarrhoea, restlessness, excitability, headache, flushing, sweating and muscular weakness.

Overdosage: Treatment of overdosage is symptomatic; tachycardia has been controlled in an adult by 40 mg doses of propranolol given every six hours.

Pharmaceutical precautions Protect from light.

Legal category POM.

Package quantities Ampoules containing 20 micrograms sterile Liothyronine Sodium BP. Boxes of 3 ampoules.

Further information 20 micrograms liothyronine are equivalent in activity to 60 to 100 micrograms thyroxine.

Product licence number 0004/5033R.

Product licence holder: Glaxo Operations UK Limited, Greenford, Middlesex UB6 0HE.

TRIMOVATE* CREAM AND OINTMENT

Presentation Trimovate Cream is a yellow water-miscible cream, containing clobetasone butyrate 0.05% w/w, oxytetracycline 3.0% w/w as calcium oxytetracycline and nystatin 100,000 units per gram.

Trimovate Ointment is a yellow ointment containing clobetasone butyrate 0.05% w/w, chlortetracycline hydrochloride 3.0% w/w and nystatin 100,000 units per gram in soft paraffin base.

Uses Clobetasone butyrate is a topically active corticosteroid which provides an exceptional combination of activity and safety. Topical formulations have been shown to be more effective in the treatment of eczemas than 1% hydrocortisone, yet to have little effect on hypothalamic-pituitary-adrenal function.

The combination of the topically active antibiotics, nystatin and a tetracycline, provides a broad spectrum of antibacterial and anticandidal activity against many of the organisms associated with infected dermatoses.

Trimovate is indicated for the treatment and management of steroid-responsive dermatoses where candidal or bacterial infection is present, suspected, or likely to occur, and the use of a more potent topical corticosteroid is not required. These include infected eczemas, intertrigo, napkin rash, anogenital pruritus and seborrhoeic dermatitis.

Dosage and administration Apply to the affected area up to four times a day.

Suitable for treating infants, children and adults.

Contra-indications, warnings, etc

Contra-indications: Primary cutaneous infections caused by viruses, fungi and bacteria. Secondary infections due to dermatophytes, Pseudomonas or Proteus species.

Hypersensitivity to the preparation.

Precautions: Although generally regarded as safe, even for long-term administration in adults, there is a potential for overdosage, and in children this may result in adrenal suppression. Extreme caution is required in dermatoses in such patients and treatment should not normally exceed seven days. In infants, the napkin may act as an occlusive dressing, and increase absorption.

If infection persists, systemic chemotherapy is likely to be required. Any spread of infection requires withdrawal of topical corticosteroid therapy. Bacterial infection is encouraged by the warm, moist conditions induced by occlusive dressings, and the skin should be cleansed before a fresh dressing is applied.

Do not continue for more than seven days in the absence of clinical improvement, since occult extension of infection may occur due to the masking effect of the steroid.

With all corticosteroids, prolonged application to the face is undesirable.

Trimovate may cause slight staining of hair, skin or fabric, but this can be removed by washing. The application may be covered with a non-occlusive dressing to protect clothing.

Extended or recurrent application may increase the risk of contact sensitisation.

Products which contain antimicrobial agents should not be diluted.

Pregnancy: There is inadequate evidence of safety in human pregnancy. Topical administration of corticosteroids to pregnant animals can cause abnormalities of fetal development including cleft palate and intra-uterine growth retardation. There may, therefore, be a very small risk of such effects in the human fetus.

Side-effects: In the unlikely event of signs of hypersensitivity appearing, application should be stopped immediately.

If large areas of the body were to be treated with Trimovate, it is possible that some patients would absorb sufficient steroid to cause transient adrenal depression despite the low degree of systemic activity associated with clobetasone butyrate.

Local atrophic changes could possibly occur in situations where moisture increases absorption of clobetasone butyrate, but only after prolonged use.

Overdosage: Acute overdosage is very unlikely to occur, however, in the case of chronic overdosage or misuse the features of hypercorticism may appear and in this situation topical steroids should be discontinued.

Pharmaceutical precautions Nil.

Legal category POM.

Package quantities Tubes of 30 grams.

Further information The least potent corticosteroid which will control the disease should be selected. Trimovate Cream and Ointment do not contain lanolin or parabens.

The low systemic activity of clobetasone butyrate has been demonstrated in adults under conditions of whole body occlusion. In animal and human models, preparations of clobetasone butyrate and of hydrocortisone caused less thinning of the epidermis than the other topical corticosteroids tested.

Product licence numbers

Trimovate Cream	0004/0266
Trimovate Ointment	0004/0265

Product licence holder: Glaxo Operations UK Limited, Greenford, Middlesex UB6 0HE.

TRIPLOPEN*

Presentation Each single-dose vial contains a white, sterile powder consisting of:

Benethamine penicillin	475 mg (500,000 units)
Procaine penicillin	250 mg (250,000 units)
Sodium benzyl penicillin	300 mg (500,000 units)

A suspension for intramuscular injection (Benethamine Penicillin Injection Fortified, BPC; Triple Penicillin Injection BNF) is formed on addition of Water for Injections.

Uses The dose of sodium benzyl penicillin gives a prompt, high blood level which supplements the lower but more prolonged level of the procaine penicillin. The therapeutic level is further maintained by the benethamine penicillin. Altogether, the effect lasts for two or three days.

Triplopen is of value in the following infections: acute localised infections such as boils, carbuncles and cellulitis; many infections caused by the more sensitive bacteria, e.g., haemolytic streptococci and pneumococci; prophylaxis against infections after accident or surgery; treatment of gonorrhoea and syphilis.

Dosage and administration To prepare the suspension for intramuscular administration, inject 1.3 ml Water for Injections into the inverted vial. On shaking, a very fluid suspension is formed which may be injected with a 23 SWG needle.

General infections in adults: Effective treatment can be carried out conveniently by a single injection of Triplopen, which can be repeated every two or three days. Triplopen is given only by deep intramuscular injection, preferably into the thigh or buttocks.

Gonorrhoea:

Four vials as a single dose given once (divided between two sites), together with 1 g of oral Probenecid.

Syphilis:
Early, i.e., less than one year duration (primary, secondary or latent): two vials given once.

Late, i.e., more than one year duration or cardiovascular syphilis: two vials given weekly for three weeks.

Neurosyphilis: Two vials given daily plus oral Probenecid 500 mg four times daily for ten days.

Congenital syphilis: 50,000 units Penicillin/kg given daily for at least ten days.

Because of the frequency of the Jarisch-Herxheimer reaction following treatment, patients should be reassured that this is an expected, benign, self-limiting reaction.

General infections in infants and children:
Age 0 to 6 years: A quarter vial
Age 7 to 12 years: A half vial
13 years and over: One vial.

Any suspension remaining after giving a fractional dose should be discarded unless it can be used promptly.

Contra-indications, warnings, etc
Contra-indications: Hypersensitivity to penicillins.

Precautions: Inadvertent intravascular administration or injection of penicillin in preparations adjacent to an artery has resulted in severe neurovascular damage including transverse myelitis, gangrene requiring amputation and necrosis and sloughing at and around the injection site. These events have most often been reported in infants and small children. Prompt consultation with an appropriate specialist is indicated if any evidence of impairment of blood supply occurs near or distal to the site of injection. The risk can usually be avoided by attempting to aspirate blood before injecting the antibiotics.

It should be recognised that a patient with a history of allergy, especially to drugs, is more likely to develop a hypersensitivity reaction.

Pregnancy: Triplopen has been taken by a large number of pregnant women and women of childbearing age without an increase in malformations or other direct or indirect harmful effects on the fetus having been observed.

Side-effects: Penicillin hypersensitivity usually takes the form of an urticarial rash which can be treated with systemic antihistamine drugs. Occasionally anaphylactic reactions to penicillin occur, and resuscitative measures, including subcutaneous injection of adrenaline and use of an intravenous corticosteroid should be employed.

Skin sensitisation may occur in persons handling penicillin, and appropriate protective measures should be taken to avoid contact with the substance.

Transient bizarre behavioural and neurological reactions (e.g. confusion or convulsions) may rarely occur within a few minutes of the intramuscular injection of high doses of procaine penicillin. These are probably attributable to the procaine component.

Granulocytopenia has been reported in patients receiving prolonged high dosage of benzylpenicillin sodium (e.g. in subacute bacterial endocarditis).

Overdosage: Excessive blood levels of penicillin G can be corrected by haemodialysis.

Pharmaceutical precautions As this product does not contain a bacteriostat, it should be used without undue delay after reconstitution.

Legal category POM.

Package quantities Single-dose vial in box of 10.

Further information If 1.3 ml of water are used to suspend Triplopen, the total volume will be 2.27 ml, but the full amounts of antibiotics are contained in 2 ml of suspension. Each vial contains 27 mg sodium (1.2 mEq).

Product licence number 0004/5076.

Product licence holder: Glaxo Operations UK Limited, Greenford, Middlesex UB6 0HE.

ZANTAC* INJECTION

Presentation Zantac Injection: 2 ml ampoules each containing 50 mg ranitidine (as hydrochloride) in 2 ml aqueous solution for intravenous or intramuscular administration.

2 ml Zantac Injection contains 2.82 mg (0.122 mmol) sodium.

Uses *Indications:* Zantac Injection is indicated for the treatment of duodenal ulcer, benign gastric ulcer, post-operative ulcer, reflux oesophagitis, Zollinger-Ellison syndrome, and the following conditions where reduction of gastric secretion and acid output is desirable: the prophylaxis of gastrointestinal haemorrhage from stress ulceration in seriously ill patients, the prophylaxis of recurrent haemorrhage in patients with bleeding peptic ulcers and before general anaesthesia in patients considered to be at risk of acid aspiration (Mendelson's Syndrome), particularly obstetric patients during labour.

For appropriate cases, Zantac Tablets are also available (see separate Data Sheet).

Mode of action: Zantac is a specific, rapidly acting histamine H_2-antagonist. It inhibits basal and stimulated secretion of gastric acid, reducing both the volume and the acid and pepsin content of the secretion.

Dosage and administration *Adults:* Zantac Injection may be given either as a slow (over a period of at least two minutes) intravenous injection of 50 mg, after dilution to a volume of 20 ml per 50 mg dose, which may be repeated every six to eight hours; or as an intermittent intravenous infusion at a rate of 25 mg per hour for two hours; the infusion may be repeated at six to eight hour intervals; or as an intramuscular injection of 50 mg (2 ml) every six to eight hours.

In the prophylaxis of haemorrhage from stress ulceration in seriously ill patients or the prophylaxis of recurrent haemorrhage in patients bleeding from peptic ulceration, parenteral administration may be continued until oral feeding commences. Patients considered to be still at risk may then be treated with Zantac Tablets 150 mg twice daily (see separate Data Sheet).

In the prophylaxis of upper gastro-intestinal haemorrhage from stress ulceration in seriously ill patients a priming dose of 50 mg as a slow intravenous injection followed by a continuous intravenous infusion of 0.125 to 0.250 mg/kg/hour may be preferred.

In patients considered to be at risk of developing acid aspiration syndrome Zantac Injection 50 mg may be given intramuscularly or by slow intravenous injection 45 to 60 minutes before induction of general anaesthesia.

Children: The use of Zantac Injection in children has not been evaluated.

Contra-indications, warnings, etc
Contra-indications: Ranitidine is contra-indicated for patients known to have hypersensitivity to the drug.

Precautions: Treatment with a histamine H_2-antagonist may mask the symptoms associated with carcinoma of the stomach and therefore may delay diagnosis of the condition. Accordingly, where gastric ulcer is suspected the possibility of malignancy should be excluded before therapy with Zantac is instituted.

Ranitidine is excreted via the kidney and so plasma levels of the drug are increased in patients with severe renal impairment. Accordingly, it is recommended in such patients that Zantac be administered in doses of 25 mg.

Bradycardia in association with rapid administration of Zantac Injection has been reported rarely, usually in patients with factors predisposing to cardiac rhythm disturbances. Recommended rates of administration should not be exceeded.

It has been reported that use of higher than recommended doses of intravenous H_2-antagonists has been associated with rises in liver enzymes when treatment has been extended beyond five days.

Zantac crosses the placenta but therapeutic doses administered to obstetric patients in labour or undergoing caesarean section have been without any adverse effect on labour, delivery or subsequent neonatal progress.

Zantac is also excreted in human breast milk. Like other drugs, Zantac should only be used during pregnancy and nursing if considered essential.

Side-effects: The following have been reported as events in clinical trials or in the routine management of patients treated with ranitidine. The relationship to ranitidine therapy has not been established in many cases.

Transient and reversible changes in liver function tests can occur. There have been occasional reports of hepatitis (hepatocellular, hepatocanalicular or mixed) with or without jaundice. These were usually reversible.

Leucopenia and thrombocytopenia have occurred rarely in patients. These are usually reversible. Rare cases of agranulocytosis or of pancytopenia, sometimes with marrow hypoplasia, or aplasia have been reported.

Hypersensitivity reactions (urticaria, angioneurotic oedema, fever, bronchospasm, hypotension, anaphylactic shock) have been seen rarely following the parenteral and oral administration of ranitidine. These reactions have occasionally occurred after a single dose.

As with other H_2-receptor antagonists there have been rare reports of bradycardia, A-V Block and asystole.

Headache, sometimes severe, and dizziness have been reported in a very small proportion of patients. Rare cases of reversible mental confusion and hallucinations have been reported, predominantly in severely ill and elderly patients.

Skin rash has been rarely reported.

No clinically significant interference with endocrine or gonadal function has been reported. There have been a few reports of breast symptoms (swelling and/or discomfort) in men taking ranitidine; some cases have resolved on continued ranitidine treatment. Discontinuation of therapy may be necessary in order to establish the underlying cause.

Overdosage: Zantac is very specific in its action and accordingly no particular problems are expected following overdosage with the drug. Symptomatic and supportive therapy should be given as appropriate. If need be, the drug may be removed from the plasma by haemodialysis.

Pharmaceutical precautions Zantac Injection has been shown to be compatible with the following intravenous infusion fluids: 0.9% Sodium Chloride BP, 5% Dextrose BP, 0.18% Sodium Chloride BP and 4% Dextrose BP, 4.2% Sodium Bicarbonate BP and Hartmann's Solution. Although compatibility studies have only been undertaken in polyvinyl chloride infusion bags (in glass for Sodium Bicarbonate BP) and a polyvinyl chloride administration set it is considered that adequate stability would be conferred by the use of a polyethylene infusion bag. All unused admixtures of Zantac Injection with infusion fluids should be discarded 24 hours after preparation.

Store below 25°C. Protect from light. Zantac Injection should not be autoclaved.

Legal category POM.

Package quantities Zantac Injection: 2 ml ampoules, boxes of five.

Further information *Drug interactions:* Ranitidine does not inhibit the hepatic cytochrome P450-linked mixed function oxygenase enzyme system. Accordingly, ranitidine does not potentiate the actions of drugs which are inactivated by this enzyme; these include diazepam, lignocaine, phenytoin, propranolol, theophylline and warfarin.

Pharmacokinetics: Absorption of ranitidine after intramuscular injection is rapid and peak plasma concentrations are usually achieved within 15 minutes of administration. The elimination half-life of ranitidine is approximately two hours. Ranitidine is excreted via the kidneys mainly as the free drug and in minor amounts as metabolites. Its major metabolite is an N-oxide and there are smaller quantities of S-oxide and desmethyl ranitidine. The 24-hour urinary recovery of free ranitidine and its metabolites is about 75% after intravenous administration.

Use in renal transplants: Zantac has been used in patients with renal transplants.

Product licence number 0004/0289.

Product licence holder: Glaxo Operations UK Limited, Greenford, Middlesex UB6 OHE.

ZANTAC* TABLETS AND SYRUP

Presentation Zantac Tablets 150 mg: White, round, film-coated tablet, engraved ZANTAC 150 on one face and GLAXO on the other. Each tablet contains ranitidine 150 mg (as hydrochloride).

Zantac Tablets 300 mg: White, capsule-shaped, film-coated tablet, engraved ZANTAC 300 on one face and GLAXO on the other. Each tablet contains ranitidine 300 mg (as hydrochloride).

Zantac Dispersible Tablets: White, capsule-shaped, film-coated tablet with a breakline on one face. Each tablet contains ranitidine 150 mg (as hydrochloride).

Zantac Syrup: A peppermint-flavoured, sugar-free syrup, free from artificial colouring. Each 10 ml contains ranitidine 150 mg (as hydrochloride).

Uses
Indications: Zantac Tablets and Syrup are indicated for the treatment of duodenal ulcer and benign gastric ulcer, including that associated with non-steroidal anti-inflammatory agents.

Zantac Tablets and Syrup are also indicated for the treatment of post-operative ulcer, oesophageal reflux disease and Zollinger-Ellison Syndrome. Other patients with chronic episodic dyspepsia, characterised by pain (epigastric or retrosternal) which is related to meals or disturbs sleep but is not associated with the preceding conditions may benefit from ranitidine treatment. Zantac Tablets and Syrup are indicated for the following conditions where reduction of gastric secretion and acid output is desirable: the prophylaxis of gastrointestinal haemorrhage from stress ulceration in seriously ill patients, the prophylaxis of recurrent haemorrhage in patients with bleeding peptic ulcers and before general anaesthesia in patients considered to be at risk of acid aspiration (Mendelson's Syndrome), particularly obstetric patients during labour. For appropriate cases, Zantac Injection is also available (see separate Data Sheet).

Mode of action: Zantac is a specific, rapidly acting histamine H_2-antagonist. It inhibits basal and stimulated secretion of gastric acid, reducing both the volume and the acid and pepsin content of the secretion. Zantac has a relatively long duration of action and so a single 150 mg dose effectively suppresses gastric acid secretion for twelve hours.

Dosage and administration Zantac Dispersible Tablets should be placed in half a glass of water (minimum 75 ml) and stirred until dispersed before swallowing.

Adults: The usual dosage is 150 mg twice daily, taken in the morning and evening. Alternatively, patients with duodenal ulceration, gastric ulceration or oesophageal reflux disease may be treated with a single bedtime dose of 300 mg. It is not necessary to time the dose in relation to meals. In most cases of duodenal ulcer, benign gastric ulcer and post-operative ulcer, healing occurs in four weeks. Healing usually occurs after a further four weeks of treatment in those patients whose ulcers have not fully healed after the initial course of therapy.

In ulcers following non-steroidal anti-inflammatory drug therapy or associated with continued non-steroidal anti-inflammatory drugs, eight weeks treatment may be necessary.

In duodenal ulcer 300 mg twice daily for 4 weeks results in healing rates which are higher than those at 4 weeks with ranitidine 150 mg twice daily or 300 mg nocte. The increased dose has not been associated with an increased incidence of unwanted effects.

Maintenance treatment at a reduced dosage of 150 mg at bedtime is recommended for patients who have responded to short-term therapy, particularly those with a history of recurrent ulcer. In the management of oesophageal reflux disease, the recommended course of treatment is either 150 mg twice daily or 300 mg at bedtime for up to eight weeks.

In patients with severe oesophagitis, and those who fail to respond to standard doses of ranitidine, the dosage of ranitidine may be increased to 300 mg four times daily for up to eight weeks. The increased dose has not been associated with an increased incidence of unwanted effects.

In patients with Zollinger-Ellison syndrome, the starting dose is 150 mg three times daily and this may be increased as necessary. Patients with this syndrome have been given increasing doses up to 6 grams per day and these doses have been well tolerated.

For patients with chronic episodic dyspepsia the recommended course of treatment is 150 mg twice daily for up to six weeks. Anyone not responding or relapsing shortly afterwards should be investigated.

In the prophylaxis of haemorrhage from stress ulceration in seriously ill patients or the prophylaxis of recurrent haemorrhage in patients bleeding from peptic ulceration, treatment with Zantac Tablets or Syrup 150 mg twice daily may be substituted for Zantac Injection (see separate Data Sheet) once oral feeding commences in patients considered to be still at risk from these conditions.

In patients thought to be at risk of acid aspiration syndrome an oral dose of 150 mg can be given 2 hours before induction of general anaesthesia, and preferably also 150 mg the previous evening. Alternatively, Zantac Injection for intravenous and intramuscular use is also available (see separate Data Sheet).

In obstetric patients at commencement of labour, an oral dose of 150 mg may be given followed by 150 mg at six hourly intervals. It is recommended that since gastric emptying and drug absorption are delayed during labour, any patient requiring emergency general anaesthesia should be given, in addition, a non-particulate antacid (e.g. sodium citrate) prior to induction of anaesthesia. The usual precautions to avoid acid aspiration should also be taken.

Children: Experience with Zantac in children is limited and such use has not been fully evaluated in clinical studies. It has however been used successfully in children aged 8 to 18 years in doses up to 150 mg (2 mg/kg) twice daily.

Contra-indications, warnings, etc
Contra-indications: Ranitidine is contra-indicated for patients known to have hypersensitivity to the drug.

Precautions: Treatment with a histamine H_2-antagonist may mask symptoms associated with carcinoma of the stomach and may therefore delay diagnosis of the condition. Accordingly, where gastric ulcer has been diagnosed or in patients of middle age and over with new or recently changed dyspeptic symptoms the possibility of malignancy should be excluded before therapy with Zantac Tablets or Syrup is instituted.

Ranitidine is excreted via the kidney and so plasma levels of the drug are increased in patients with severe renal impairment. Accordingly, it is recommended that the therapeutic regimen for Zantac in such patients be 150 mg at night for four to eight weeks. The same dose should be used for maintenance treatment should this be deemed necessary. If an ulcer has not healed after treatment the standard dosage regimen of 150 mg twice daily should be instituted, followed, if need be, by maintenance treatment at 150 mg at night.

Regular supervision of patients with peptic ulcer and on non-steroidal anti-inflammatory drugs is recommended, especially if elderly.

Zantac crosses the placenta but therapeutic doses administered to obstetric patients in labour or undergoing caesarean section have been without any adverse effect on labour, delivery or subsequent neonatal progress. Zantac is also excreted in human breast milk.

Like other drugs, Zantac should only be used during pregnancy and nursing if considered essential.

Side-effects: The following have been reported as events in clinical trials or in the routine management of patients treated with ranitidine. The relationship to ranitidine therapy has not been established in many cases.

Transient and reversible changes in liver function tests can occur. There have been occasional reports of hepatitis (hepatocellular, hepatocanalicular or mixed) with or without jaundice. These were usually reversible.

Leucopenia and thrombocytopenia have occurred rarely in patients. These are usually reversible. Rare cases of agranulocytosis or of pancytopenia, sometimes with marrow hypoplasia, or aplasia have been reported.

Hypersensitivity reactions (urticaria, angioneurotic oedema, fever, bronchospasm, hypotension, anaphylactic shock) have been seen rarely following the parenteral and oral administration of ranitidine. These reactions have occasionally occurred after a single dose.

As with other H_2-receptor antagonists, there have been rare reports of bradycardia and A-V block.

Headache, sometimes severe, and dizziness have been reported in a very small proportion of patients. Rare cases of reversible mental confusion and hallucinations have been reported, predominantly in severely ill and elderly patients.

Skin rash has been rarely reported.

No clinically significant interference with endocrine or gonadal function has been reported. There have been a few reports of breast symptoms (swelling and/or discomfort) in men taking ranitidine; some cases have resolved on continued ranitidine treatment. Discontinuation of therapy may be necessary in order to establish the underlying cause.

Use in elderly patients: Rates of healing of ulcers in clinical trial patients aged 65 and over have not been found to differ from those in younger patients. Additionally, there was no difference in the incidence of adverse effects.

Overdosage: Zantac is very specific in action and accordingly no particular problems are expected following overdosage with the drug. Symptomatic and supportive therapy should be given as appropriate. If need be, the drug may be removed from the plasma by haemodialysis.

Pharmaceutical precautions Zantac Syrup should be stored at a temperature not exceeding 25°C. Zantac Syrup should not be diluted or admixed with other liquid preparations.

Legal category POM.

Package quantities Zantac Tablets (150 mg): Carton of 60 tablets, foil-wrapped (OP).

Zantac Tablets (300 mg): Carton of 30 tablets, foil-wrapped (OP).

Zantac Dispersible Tablets (150 mg): Carton of 60 tablets, foil-wrapped (OP).

Zantac Syrup: Bottles of 300 ml (OP).

Further information *Drug interactions:* Ranitidine does not inhibit the hepatic cytochrome P450-linked mixed function oxygenase system. Accordingly, ranitidine does not potentiate the actions of drugs which are inactivated by this enzyme; these include diazepam, lignocaine, phenytoin, propranolol, theophylline and warfarin.

Pharmacokinetics: Absorption of ranitidine after oral administration is rapid and peak plasma concentrations are usually achieved within two hours of administration. Absorption is not significantly impaired by food or antacids. The elimination half-life of ranitidine is approximately two hours. Ranitidine is excreted via the kidneys mainly as the free drug and in minor amounts as metabolites. Its major metabolite is an N-oxide and there are smaller quantities of S-oxide and desmethyl ranitidine. The 24-hour urinary recovery of free ranitidine and its metabolites is about 40% with orally administered drug.

Use in renal transplants: Zantac has been used in patients with renal transplants.

Zantac Syrup contains 7.5% w/v ethanol.

Product licence numbers
Zantac Tablets (150 mg): 0004/0279
Zantac Tablets (300 mg): 0004/0302
Zantac Dispersible Tablets (150 mg): 0004/0298
Zantac Syrup: 0004/0310

Product licence holder: Glaxo Operations UK Limited, Greenford, Middlesex UB6 0HE.

ZINACEF*

Presentation Vials containing 250 mg, 750 mg or 1.5 g cefuroxime as cefuroxime sodium.

Cefuroxime is a white to faintly yellow powder to which appropriate amounts of water are added to prepare an off-white suspension for intramuscular use or a yellowish solution for intravenous administration. Variations in the intensity of this colour do not indicate any change in either the efficacy or safety of the product.

Uses Zinacef is a bactericidal cephalosporin antibiotic which is resistant to most β-lactamases and is active against a wide range of Gram-positive and Gram-negative organisms. It is indicated for the treatment of infections before the infecting organism has been identified or when caused by sensitive bacteria. In addition, it is an effective prophylactic against post-operative infection in a variety of operations. Usually Zinacef will be effective alone, but when appropriate it may be used in combination with an aminoglycoside antibiotic, or in conjunction with metronidazole, orally or by suppository or injection (see Pharmaceutical precautions). In situations where mixed aerobic and anaerobic infections are encountered or suspected (e.g. peritonitis, aspiration pneumonia, abscesses in the lung, pelvis and brain), or are likely to occur (e.g. in association with colorectal or gynaecological surgery) it is appropriate to administer Zinacef in combination with metronidazole. Most of these infections will respond to an i.v. regimen of Zinacef (750 mg) plus metronidazole injection (500 mg/100 ml) administered eight-hourly. In more severe or well established mixed infections, an i.v. regimen of Zinacef (1.5 g) plus metronidazole injection (500 mg/100 ml) eight-hourly may be indicated. For the prophylaxis of infection in surgery (e.g. colorectal and gynaecological) a single dose of 1.5 g Zinacef plus metronidazole injection (500 mg/100 ml) is appropriate. Alternatively, this may be followed by two 750 mg doses of Zinacef plus metronidazole.

Indications include:

Respiratory tract infections for example, acute and chronic bronchitis, infected bronchiectasis, bacterial pneumonia, lung abscess and post-operative chest infections.

Ear, nose and throat infections for example, sinusitis, tonsillitis and pharyngitis.

Urinary tract infections for example, acute and chronic pyelonephritis, cystitis and asymptomatic bacteriuria.

Soft-tissue infections for example, cellulitis, erysipelas, peritonitis and wound infections.

Bone and joint infections for example, osteomyelitis and septic arthritis.

Obstetric and gynaecological infections pelvic inflammatory diseases.

Gonorrhoea particularly when penicillin is unsuitable.

Other infections including septicaemia and meningitis.

Prophylaxis against infection in abdominal, pelvic, orthopaedic, cardiac, pulmonary, oesophageal and vascular surgery where there is increased risk from infection.

Bacteriology: Zinacef is highly active against *Staphylococcus aureus,* including strains which are resistant to penicillin (but not the rare methicillin resistant strains), *Staph. epidermidis, Haemophilus influenzae,* Klebsiella spp., Enterobacter spp., *Streptococcus pyogenes, Escherichia coli, Str. mitis* (viridans group), Clostridium spp., *Proteus mirabilis, Pr. rettgeri, Salmonella typhi, S. typhimurium* and other Salmonella spp. Shigella spp., Neisseria spp. (including β-lactamase producing strains of *N. gonorrhoeae)* and *Bordetella pertussis.* It is also moderately active against strains of *Pr. vulgaris, Pr. morganii* and *Bacteroides fragilis.*

The following organisms are not susceptible to cefuroxime: *Clostridium difficile,* Pseudomonas spp., Campylobacter spp., *Acinetobacter calcoaceticus,* Legionella spp., and Methicillin-resistant strains of *Staph. aureus* and *Staph. epidermidis.*

Some strains of the following genera have also been found not to be susceptible to Zinacef: *Strep. faecalis, Morganella morganii, Proteus vulgaris,* Enterobacter spp., Citrobacter spp., Serratia spp., and *Bacteroides fragilis. In vitro* the activities of Zinacef and aminoglycoside antibiotics in combination have been shown to be at least additive with occasional evidence of synergy.

Dosage and administration *General dosage recommendations: Adults:* Many infections will respond to 750 mg t.i.d. by i.m. or i.v. injection. For more severe infections, this dose should be increased to 1.5 g t.i.d. i.v. The frequency of i.m. or i.v. injections can be increased to six-hourly if necessary, giving total doses of 3 g to 6 g daily.

Infants and children: Doses of 30 to 100 mg/kg/day, given as three or four divided doses. A dose of 60 mg/kg/day will be appropriate for most infections.

Neonates: Doses of 30 to 100 mg/kg/day, given as two or three divided doses. In the first weeks of life the serum half-life of cefuroxime can be three to five times that in adults.

Other recommendations: Gonorrhoea: 1.5 g should be given as a single dose. This may be given as 2 × 750 mg injections into different sites, e.g., each buttock.

Meningitis: Zinacef is suitable for sole therapy of bacterial meningitis due to sensitive strains. The following dosages are recommended.

Infants and children: 200 to 240 mg/kg/day i.v. in three or four divided doses. This dosage may be reduced to 100 mg/kg/day i.v. after three days or when clinical improvement occurs.

Neonates: The initial dosage should be 100 mg/kg/day i.v. A reduction to 50 mg/kg/day i.v. may be made when clinically indicated.

Adults: 3 g i.v. every eight hours. Data are not yet sufficient to recommend a dose for intrathecal administration.

Prophylaxis: The usual dose is 1.5 g i.v. with induction of anaesthesia for abdominal, pelvic and orthopaedic operations, but may be supplemented with two 750 mg i.m. doses eight and sixteen hours later. In cardiac, pulmonary, oesophageal and vascular operations, the usual dose is 1.5 g i.v. with induction of anaesthesia continuing with 750 mg i.m. t.i.d. for a further 24 to 48 hours.

In total joint replacement, 1.5 g cefuroxime powder may be mixed dry with each pack of methyl methacrylate cement polymer before adding the liquid monomer.

Dosage in impaired renal function: Cefuroxime is excreted by the kidneys. Therefore, as with all such antibiotics, in patients with markedly impaired renal function it is recommended that the dosage of Zinacef should be reduced to compensate for its slower excretion. However, it is not necessary to reduce the dose until the creatinine clearance falls below 20 ml/min. In adults with marked impairment (creatinine clearance 10 to 20 ml/min) 750 mg b.d. is recommended and with severe impairment (creatinine clearance < 10 ml/min) 750 mg once daily is adequate. For patients on haemodialysis a further 750 mg dose should be given at the end of each dialysis. When continuous peritoneal dialysis is being used, a suitable dosage is usually 750 mg twice daily.

Administration: Intramuscular: Add 1 ml Water for Injections to 250 mg Zinacef or 3 ml Water for Injections to 750 mg Zinacef. Shake gently to produce an opaque suspension.

Intravenous: Dissolve Zinacef in Water for Injections using at least 2 ml for 250 mg, at least 6 ml for 750 mg, or 15 ml for 1.5 g. For short intravenous infusion (e.g., up to 30 minutes), 1.5 g may be dissolved in 50 ml Water for Injections. These solutions may be given directly into the vein or introduced into the tubing of the giving set if the patient is receiving parenteral fluids.

Zinacef is compatible with the more commonly used intravenous fluids (see Pharmaceutical precautions.)

Contra-indications, warnings, etc
Contra-indications: Hypersensitivity to cephalosporin antibiotics.

Precautions: Cephalosporin antibiotics may in general be given safely to patients who are hypersensitive to penicillins, although cross-reactions have been reported. Especial care is indicated in patients who have experienced an anaphylactic reaction to penicillin.

Cephalosporin antibiotics at high dosage should be given with caution to patients receiving concurrent treatment with potent diuretics such as frusemide and aminoglycosides, as these combinations are suspected of adversely affecting renal function. Clinical experience with Zinacef has shown that this is not likely to be a problem at the recommended dose levels.

There is no experimental evidence of embryopathic or teratogenic effects attributable to Zinacef but, as with all drugs, it should be administered with caution during the early months of pregnancy.

Cefuroxime is excreted in human milk, and consequently caution should be exercised when Zinacef is administered to a nursing mother.

Zinacef does not interfere in enzyme-based tests for glycosuria. Slight interference with copper reduction methods (Benedict's, Fehling's, Clinitest) may be observed. However, this should not lead to false-positive results, as may be experienced with some other cephalosporins.

It is recommended that either the glucose oxidase or hexokinase methods are used to determine blood/plasma glucose levels in patients receiving Zinacef. This antibiotic does not interfere in the alkaline picrate assay for creatinine.

Side-effects: Adverse reactions to Zinacef have occurred relatively infrequently and have been generally mild and transient in nature.

Hypersensitivity reactions have been reported: these include skin rashes (maculopapular and urticarial); drug fever and very rarely anaphylaxis. As with other antibiotics, prolonged use may result in the overgrowth of non-susceptible organisms, e.g. Candida.

Gastro-intestinal disturbance, including, very rarely, symptoms of pseudomembranous colitis may occur during or after treatment.

The principal changes in haematological parameters seen in some patients have been decreased haemoglobin concentration and of eosinophilia, leukopenia and neutropenia. A positive Coombs' test has been found in some patients treated with cefuroxime – this phenomenon can interfere with the cross-matching of blood. Although there are sometimes transient rises in serum liver enzymes or serum bilirubin, particularly in patients with pre-existing liver disease there is no evidence of hepatic involvement.

There may be some variation in the results of biochemical tests of renal function, but these do not appear to be of clinical importance. As a precaution, renal function should be monitored if this is already impaired.

Transient pain may be experienced at the site of intramuscular injection. This is more likely to occur with higher doses. However, it is unlikely to be a cause of discontinuation of treatment.

Occasionally, thrombophlebitis may follow intravenous injection.

Overdosage: Overdosage of cephalosporins can cause cerebral irritation leading to convulsions. Serum levels of cefuroxime can be reduced by haemodialysis or peritoneal dialysis.

Pharmaceutical precautions Protect from light.

Zinacef should not be mixed in the syringe with aminoglycoside antibiotics.

In keeping with good pharmaceutical practice, it is preferable to use freshly constituted suspensions or solutions of Zinacef for Injection. If this is not practicable, suspensions or solutions may be stored for up to 24 hours in the refrigerator (2 to 8°C) when prepared in Water for Injection BP. Solutions may also be stored for up to 24 hours in the refrigerator (2 to 8°C) when prepared in any of the injections listed below:

0.9% w/v Sodium Chloride Injection BP.

5% Dextrose Injection BP.

0.18% w/v Sodium Chloride plus 4% Dextrose Injection BP.

Sodium Lactate Injection BP (Hartmann's solutions).

Zinacef (5 mg/ml) may be constituted in 5% xylitol injection.

1.5 g Zinacef constituted with 15 ml Water for Injection BP may be added to metronidazole injection (500 mg/100 ml), or azlocillin (1 g/15 ml) or (5 g/50 ml).

The pH of 2.74% w/v Sodium Bicarbonate Injection BP considerably affects the colour of solutions and therefore this solution is not recommended for the dilution of Zinacef. However, if required, for patients receiving Sodium Bicarbonate Injection by infusion the Zinacef may be introduced into the tube of the giving set.

Legal category POM.

Package quantities Vials containing 250 mg or 750 mg cefuroxime as the sodium salt (for use by intramuscular or intravenous injection) in packs of 5.

Vials containing 1.5 g cefuroxime as the sodium salt (for use by intravenous injection), packed singly.

Vials containing 1.5 g cefuroxime as the sodium salt (for use by intravenous infusion), packed singly.

Further information Peak levels of cefuroxime are achieved within 30 to 45 minutes after intramuscular administration. The serum half-life after either intramuscular or intravenous injection is approximately 70 minutes. Concurrent administration of probenecid prolongs the excretion of the antibiotic and produces an elevated peak serum level. There is almost complete recovery of unchanged cefuroxime in the urine within 24 hours of administration, the major part being eliminated in the first six hours. Approximately 50% is excreted through the renal tubules and approximately 50% by glomerular filtration. Concentrations of cefuroxime in excess of the minimum inhibitory levels for common pathogens can be achieved in bone, synovial fluid and aqueous humour. Cefuroxime passes the blood-brain barrier when the meninges are inflamed.

Each 750 mg vial contains 42 mg sodium (1.8 mEq). When dissolved, the contents of a 750 mg vial displace 0.53 ml on average.

Cefuroxime is also available as the axetil ester (Zinnat*) for oral administration. This permits parenteral therapy with cefuroxime to be followed by oral therapy in situations where a change from parenteral to oral is clinically indicated.

Product licence number 0004/0263.

Product licence holder: Glaxo Operations UK Limited, Greenford, Middlesex UB6 0HE.

ZINNAT* TABLETS

Presentation Zinnat Tablets 125 mg: white, film-coated, capsule-shaped tablets engraved with 'Glaxo' on one side and '125' on the other. Each tablet contains cefuroxime 125 mg (as cefuroxime axetil).

Zinnat Tablets 250 mg: white, film-coated, capsule-shaped tablets engraved with 'Glaxo' on one side and '250' on the other. Each tablet contains cefuroxime 250 mg (as cefuroxime axetil).

Uses Cefuroxime axetil is an oral prodrug of the bactericidal cephalosporin antibiotic cefuroxime, which is resistant to most beta-lactamases and is active against a wide range of Gram-positive and Gram-negative organisms. It is indicated for the treatment of infections caused by sensitive bacteria.

Indications include:

Lower respiratory tract infections for example, acute and chronic bronchitis, and pneumonia.

Upper respiratory tract infections for example, ear,

nose and throat infections, such as otitis media, sinusitis, tonsillitis and pharyngitis.

Genito-urinary tract infections for example, pyelonephritis, cystitis and urethritis.

Skin and soft-tissue infections for example, furunculosis, pyoderma and impetigo.

Gonorrhoea acute, uncomplicated gonococcal urethritis, and cervicitis.

Microbiology: Cefuroxime axetil owes its *in vivo* bactericidal activity to the parent compound, cefuroxime. Cefuroxime is a well-characterised and effective antibacterial agent which has broad-spectrum bactericidal activity against a wide range of common pathogens, including beta-lactamase-producing strains. Cefuroxime has good stability to bacterial beta-lactamase and, consequently, is active against many ampicillin-resistant or amoxycillin-resistant strains. The bactericidal action of cefuroxime results from inhibition of cell-wall synthesis by binding to essential target proteins.

Cefuroxime is usually active against the following organisms *in vitro:*

Aerobes, Gram-negative: *Haemophilus influenzae* (including ampicillin-resistant strains); *Haemophilus parainfluenzae; Branhamella catarrhalis; Escherichia coli;* Klebsiella species; *Proteus mirabilis; Proteus inconstans;* Providencia species; *Proteus rettgeri* and *Neisseria gonorrhoeae* (including penicillinase- and non-penicillinase-producing strains).

Some strains of *Morganella morganii*, Enterobacter species and Citrobacter species have been shown by *in vitro* tests to be resistant to cefuroxime and other beta-lactam antibiotics.

Aerobes, Gram-positive: *Staphylococcus aureus* (including penicillinase-producing strains but excluding methicillin-resistant strains); *Staphylococcus epidermidis, Streptococcus pneumoniae* (and other beta-haemolytic streptococci); Streptococcus Group B (*Streptococcus agalactiae*) and Propionibacterium species. Certain strains of enterococci, e.g. *Streptococcus faecalis*, are resistant.

Anaerobes, Gram-positive and Gram-negative cocci (including Peptococcus and Peptostreptococcus species); Gram-positive bacilli (including Clostridium species) and Gram-negative bacilli (including Bacteroides and Fusobacterium species). Most strains of *Bacteroides fragilis* are resistant.

Pseudomonas species, Campylobacter species, *Acinetobacter calcoaceticus* and most strains of Serratia and *Proteus vulgaris* and *Clostridium difficile* are resistant to many cephalosporins including cefuroxime.

Dosage and administration

Adults: Most infections will respond to 250 mg b.d. In mild to moderate lower respiratory tract infections e.g., bronchitis 250 mg b.d. should be given. For more severe lower respiratory tract infections, or if pneumonia is suspected then 500 mg b.d. should be given. For urinary tract infections a dose of 125 mg b.d. is usually adequate; in pyelonephritis the recommended dose is 250 mg b.d. A single dose of 1 g is recommended for the treatment of uncomplicated gonorrhoea.

Children: The usual dose is 125 mg b.d. In children with otitis media, 250 mg b.d. may be used. Cefuroxime axetil Tablets should not be crushed and are therefore unsuitable for children under five years of age.

No special precautions are necessary in patients with renal impairment or on renal dialysis or in the elderly at dosages up to the normal maximum of 1 g per day.

The usual course of therapy is seven days. Cefuroxime axetil should be taken after food for optimum absorption.

Contra-indications, warnings, etc

Contra-indications: Hypersensitivity to cephalosporin antibiotics.

Precautions: Cephalosporin antibiotics may in general be given safely to patients who are hypersensitive to penicillins, although cross-reactions have been reported.

Special care is indicated in patients who have experienced an anaphylactic reaction to penicillins.

As with other antibiotics, prolonged use of cefuroxime axetil may result in the overgrowth of non-susceptible organisms (e.g. Candida, Enterococci, *Clostridium difficile*), which may require interruption of treatment. Pseudomembranous colitis has been reported with the use of broad-spectrum antibiotics, therefore, it is important to consider its diagnosis in patients who develop serious diarrhoea during or after antibiotic use. There is no experimental evidence of embryopathic or teratogenic effects attributable to cefuroxime axetil but, as with all drugs, it should be administered with caution during the early months of pregnancy. Cefuroxime is excreted in human milk and, consequently, caution should be exercised when cefuroxime axetil is administered to a nursing mother.

Cefuroxime axetil tablets should not be crushed and are, therefore, unsuitable for children under the age of five years.

It is recommended that either the glucose oxidase or hexokinase methods are used to determine blood/plasma glucose levels in patients receiving cefuroxime axetil. This antibiotic does not interfere in the alkaline picrate assay for creatinine.

Side-effects: Adverse reactions to cefuroxime axetil have been generally mild and transient in nature.

A small proportion of patients receiving cefuroxime axetil have experienced gastrointestinal disturbances, including diarrhoea, nausea and vomiting.

As with other broad-spectrum antibiotics, there have been rare reports of pseudomembranous colitis.

Headache has also been reported.

There have been rare reports of hypersensitivity reactions including skin rashes.

Eosinophilia and transient increases of hepatic enzyme levels [ALT (SGPT) and AST (SGOT)] have been noted during Zinnat therapy. A positive Coombs' test has been reported during treatment with cephalosporins – this phenomenon can interfere with cross-matching of blood.

Overdosage: Overdosage of cephalosporins can cause cerebral irritancy leading to convulsions.

Serum levels of cefuroxime can be reduced by haemodialysis or peritoneal dialysis.

Pharmaceutical precautions Zinnat Tablets should be stored below 25°C. Occasional storage at temperatures not higher than 30°C for up to two months is not detrimental to the product.

Legal category POM.

Package quantities All strengths of tablets are supplied in foil strips of 14 (OP) and 50.

Further information After oral administration, cefuroxime axetil is absorbed from the gastrointestinal tract and rapidly hydrolysed in the intestinal mucosa and blood to release cefuroxime into the circulation. Optimum absorption occurs when it is administered after a meal. Peak serum cefuroxime levels occur approximately two to three hours after oral dosing. The serum half-life is about 1.2 hours. Approximately 50% of serum cefuroxime is protein bound. Cefuroxime is not metabolised and is excreted by glomerular filtration and tubular secretion. Concurrent administration of probenecid increases the area under the mean serum concentration time curve by 50%. Serum levels of cefuroxime are reduced by dialysis.

Cefuroxime is also available as the sodium salt (Zinacef) for parenteral administration. This permits parenteral therapy with cefuroxime to be followed by oral therapy in situations where a change from parenteral to oral treatment is clinically indicated.

Product licence numbers
Zinnat Tablets (125 mg): 0004/0317
Zinnat Tablets (250 mg): 0004/0318

Product licence holder: Glaxo Operations UK Limited, Greenford, Middlesex UB6 0HE.

ZOFRAN* INJECTION AND TABLETS ▼

Presentation *Zofran Injection 2 mg/ml:* Ampoules each containing 4 mg ondansetron (as hydrochloride dihydrate) in 2 ml aqueous solution for intravenous administration. Ampoules each containing 8 mg ondansetron (as hydrochloride dihydrate) in 4 ml aqueous solution for intravenous administration.

Zofran Tablets 4 mg: Yellow, oval, film-coated tablet engraved "GLAXO" on one face and "4" on the other. Each tablet contains ondansetron 4 mg (as hydrochloride dihydrate).

Zofran Tablets 8 mg: Yellow, oval, film-coated tablet engraved "GLAXO" on one face and "8" on the other. Each tablet contains ondansetron 8 mg (as hydrochloride dihydrate).

Uses Zofran is indicated for the management of nausea and vomiting induced by cytotoxic chemotherapy and radiotherapy.

Mode of action: Ondansetron is a potent, highly selective $5HT_3$ receptor-antagonist. Its precise mode of action in the control of nausea and vomiting is not known. Chemotherapeutic agents and radiotherapy may cause release of 5HT in the small intestine initiating a vomiting reflex by activating vagal afferents via $5HT_3$ receptors. Ondansetron blocks the initiation of this reflex. Activation of vagal afferents may also cause a release of 5HT in the area postrema, located on the floor of the fourth ventricle, and this may also promote emesis through a central mechanism. Thus, the effect of ondansetron in the management of the nausea and vomiting induced by cytotoxic chemotherapy and radiotherapy is due to antagonism of $5HT_3$ receptors on neurons located both in the peripheral and central nervous system.

In psychomotor testing ondansetron does not impair performance nor cause sedation.

Ondansetron does not alter plasma prolactin concentrations.

Dosage and administration

Adults: Highly emetogenic chemotherapy e.g. regimens containing cisplatin: initially Zofran may be given as a slow intravenous injection or 15 minute infusion of 8 mg immediately before chemotherapy, followed by a continuous intravenous infusion of 1 mg/hour for up to 24 hours or by a further two doses of 8 mg, given by slow intravenous injection or 15 minute infusion four hours apart. Either regimen is then followed by 8 mg orally every eight hours for up to 5 days.

Less emetogenic chemotherapy e.g. regimens containing cyclophosphamide, doxorubicin, carboplatin: Zofran may be given as a slow intravenous injection or 15 minute infusion of 8 mg, immediately before chemotherapy, or 8 mg orally one to two hours before chemotherapy, followed by 8 mg orally every eight hours for up to 5 days.

Radiotherapy induced nausea and vomiting: Zofran may be given orally, 8 mg every eight hours. The first dose should be taken one to two hours before radiotherapy. The duration of treatment will depend upon the length of the course of radiotherapy.

Children: Experience is currently limited but ondansetron was effective and well tolerated in children over the age of four years, when given intravenously at a dose of 5 mg/m^2 over 15 minutes, immediately before chemotherapy, followed by oral therapy at doses of 4 mg every eight hours for up to 5 days.

Elderly patients: Efficacy and tolerance in patients aged over 65 years was similar to that seen in younger adults, indicating no need to alter dosage or route of administration in the elderly.

Contra-indications, warnings, etc

Contra-indications: Hypersensitivity to any component of the preparation.

Precautions

Pregnancy: Zofran is not teratogenic in animals. There is no experience in humans. As with other medications, Zofran should not be used during pregnancy, especially during the first trimester, unless the expected benefit to the patient is thought to outweigh any possible risk to the fetus.

Lactation: Tests have shown that ondansetron is excreted in the breast milk of rats. It is therefore recommended that mothers receiving Zofran should not breast-feed their babies.

Side-effects: Ondansetron is known to increase large bowel transit time and may cause constipation in some patients. The following side effects can occur: headache, a sensation of flushing or warmth in the head and epigastrium, and occasional transient, asymptomatic increases in aminotransferases. There have been rare reports of immediate hypersensitivity reactions.

Overdosage: Little is at present known about overdosage with ondansetron. However two patients who received doses of 84 mg and 145 mg intravenously reported only mild side effects and required no active therapy. In cases of suspected overdose, symptomatic and supportive therapy should be given as appropriate.

Pharmaceutical precautions Zofran Injection should be protected from light. No other special storage conditions are necessary.

Dilutions of Zofran Injection in compatible intravenous infusion fluids are stable under normal room lighting conditions or daylight for at least 24 hours, thus no protection from light is necessary while infusion takes place.

Zofran Injection should not be administered in the same syringe or infusion as any other medication.

Zofran Injection ampoules should not be autoclaved.

Compatibility with intravenous fluids: Zofran Injection should only be admixed with those infusion solutions which are recommended:

Sodium Chloride Intravenous Infusion BP 0.9% w/v.

Glucose Intravenous Infusion BP 5% w/v.

Mannitol Intravenous Infusion BP 10% w/v.

Ringer's Intravenous Infusion.

Potassium Chloride 0.3% w/v and Sodium Chloride 0.9% w/v Intravenous Infusion BP.

Potassium Chloride 0.3% w/v and Glucose 5% w/v Intravenous Infusion BP.

In keeping with good pharmaceutical practice, dilutions of Zofran Injection in intravenous fluids should be prepared at the time of infusion or stored at 2 to 8°C for no more than 24 hours before the start of administration.

Compatibility studies have been undertaken in polyvinyl chloride infusion bags and polyvinyl chloride administration sets. It is considered that adequate stability would also be conferred by the use of polyethylene infusion bags or type 1 glass bottles. Dilutions of Zofran in sodium chloride 0.9% w/v or in glucose 5% w/v have been demonstrated to be stable in polypropylene syringes. It is considered that Zofran Injection diluted with other compatible infusion fluids would be stable in polypropylene syringes.

Compatibility with other drugs: Zofran may be administered by intravenous infusion at 1 mg/hour, e.g. from an infusion bag or syringe pump. The following drugs may be administered via the Y-site of the Zofran giving set for ondansetron concentrations of 16 to 160 micrograms/ml (e.g. 8 mg/500 ml and 8 mg/50 ml respectively):

Cisplatin: Concentrations up to 0.48 mg/ml (e.g. 240 mg in 500 ml) administered over one to eight hours.

5-fluorouracil: Concentrations up to 0.8 mg/ml (e.g. 2.4 g in 3 litres or 400 mg in 500 ml) administered at a rate of at least 20 ml per hour (500 ml per 24 hours). Higher concentrations of 5-fluorouracil may cause precipitation of ondansetron. The 5-fluorouracil infusion may contain up to 0.045% w/v magnesium chloride in addition to other excipients shown to be compatible.

Carboplatin: Concentrations in the range 0.18 mg/ml to 9.9 mg/ml (e.g. 90 mg in 500 ml to 990 mg in 100 ml), administered over ten minutes to one hour.

Etoposide: Concentrations in the range 0.14 mg/ml to 0.25 mg/ml (e.g. 72 mg in 500 ml to 250 mg in 1 litre), administered over thirty minutes to one hour.

Ceftazidime: Doses in the range 250 mg to 2,000 mg reconstituted with Water for Injections BP as recommended by the manufacturer (e.g. 2.5 ml for 250 mg and 10 ml for 2 g ceftazidime) and given as an intravenous bolus injection over approximately five minutes.

Cyclophosphamide: Doses in the range 100 mg to 1 g, reconstituted with Water for Injections BP, 5 ml per 100 mg cyclophosphamide, as recommended by the manufacturer and given as an intravenous bolus injection over approximately five minutes.

Doxorubicin: Doses in the range 10 mg to 100 mg reconstituted with Water for Injections BP, 5 ml per 10 mg doxorubicin, as recommended by the manufacturer and given as an intravenous bolus injection over approximately five minutes.

Legal category POM.

Package quantities Zofran Injection: 2 ml and 4 ml ampoules in boxes of five.
Zofran Tablets (4 mg): Containers of 30 tablets.
Zofran Tablets (8 mg): Containers of 30 tablets.

Further information *Pharmacokinetics and metabolism:* The bioavailability of oral ondansetron is approximately 60%. The drug is extensively metabolised and metabolites are excreted in faeces and urine. Following oral administration the time to peak concentration is approximately 1.6 hours. The elimination half-life is approximately 3 hours, though this may be prolonged to approximately 5 hours in the elderly. Plasma protein binding is 70 to 76%.

Product licence numbers
Zofran Injection (2 mg/ml): 0004/0375
Zofran Tablets (4 mg): 0004/0376
Zofran Tablets (8 mg): 0004/0377

Product licence holder: Glaxo Operations UK Limited, Greenford, Middlesex UB6 0HE.

**Trade Mark*

Glenwood Laboratories Ltd

Jenkins Dale
Chatham
Kent ME4 5RD

MYOTONINE*

Presentation Bethanechol chloride tablets: 10 mg – pale blue, scored; 25 mg – pale blue, cross scored.

Uses
Mode of Action: Myotonine is a choline ester which produces the effects of stimulation of the parasympathetic nervous system. Myotonine is not hydrolysed by cholinesterase. The muscarinic effects are exerted mainly on the urinary bladder, the gastro-intestinal tract and the eye. The pharmacological effect is usually apparent within 30 to 90 minutes of administration and lasts about an hour.

Indications: Reflux oesophagitis. Urinary retention (post operative, postpartum and neurogenic). Adynamic ileus. Gastric atony and retention. Megacolon.

Dosage and administration
Adults: The therapeutic dose of Myotonine should be individualised by titrating the dose to the response of the patient. In many cases a satisfactory response can be obtained with 10 mg to 25 mg Myotonine, three or four times a day. Occasionally it may be felt necessary to initiate therapy with a 50 mg dose. Myotonine tablets should be administered when the stomach is empty as nausea and vomiting may occur when they are taken soon after eating.

Children: Experience with Myotonine tablets in children is limited. The dose of Myotonine should be adjusted on a weight basis.

Contra-indications, warnings, etc Parasympathomimetic or cholinergic drugs are contraindicated in patients with asthma or susceptibility to asthmatic attacks, hyperthyroid states, marked vagotonia, pronounced vasomotor instability, severe bradycardia and hypotension, recent myocardial infarction, epilepsy, parkinsonism or during pregnancy. Parasympathomimetic or cholinergic drugs should not be used in patients with urinary or gastro-intestinal obstruction or where increased muscular activity of the urinary bladder or gastro-intestinal tract may prove harmful.

Side effects: Untoward reactions are rare following oral administration of therapeutic doses of bethanechol chloride. Nausea and vomiting may occur if the drug is taken immediately after the ingestion of food. Reported side effects include frequency of micturition, lower abdominal cramps, blurred vision.

Antidote: The pharmacological effects of bethanechol chloride can be promptly abolished by the administration of atropine sulphate.

Pharmaceutical precautions No special storage conditions are necessary. For oral use only.

Legal category POM.

Package quantities Myotonine tablets 10 mg 100 tablets. Myotonine tablets 25 mg 100 tablets.

Further information Nil.

Product licence numbers
10 mg 0245/5009
25 mg 0245/5010

POTABA*

Presentation Potaba is pure potassium para-aminobenzoate. It is available in the following presentations:
Potaba envules. Single dose sachets, each containing 3 g Potaba.
Potaba tablets – White concave tablets each containing 500 mg Potaba.
Potaba capsules – Red/white capsules each containing 500 mg Potaba.

Uses
Mode of Action: Potaba is an antifibrosis agent. It has been suggested that the antifibrosis activity of Potaba is brought about by the drug increasing oxygen uptake at the tissue level. Fibrosis is believed to occur from either too much serotonin or too little monoamine oxidase activity over a period of time. The activity of monoamine oxidase is dependent upon an adequate oxygen supply. By increasing oxygen supply at the tissue level Potaba enhances monoamine oxidase activity thereby preventing or bringing about regression of fibrosis.

Indications: Scleroderma. Peyronie's disease (Induratio penis plastica).

Dosage and administration The usual dose of Potaba is 3 g, four times a day. This dosage is best achieved by the administration of one Potaba Envule four times a day taken with food. The contents of the envule is dissolved in any desired drink. Citrus juices are excellent vehicles. Alternatively, six Potaba tablets or capsules may be taken four times a day with food.

Contra-indications, warnings, etc Potaba should not be administered to patients taking sulphonamides, as it will inactivate this medication.

Precautions: Treatment with Potaba should be interrupted during periods of low food intake (eg, during fasting, anorexia, nausea). This is to avoid the possible development of hypoglycaemia.

Potaba should be given cautiously to patients with renal impairment.

Potaba treatment should be discontinued if a hypersensitivity reaction occurs.

Side effects: No serious adverse effects have been reported in patients treated with Potaba. Anorexia, nausea, fever and rash occur infrequently and subside with omission of the drug. Desensitisation can often be accomplished and treatment with Potaba resumed.

Overdose: No particular problems are expected following overdosage with Potaba. Symptomatic and supportive therapy should be given as appropriate.

Pharmaceutical precautions Potaba preparations should be stored in a cool place.

Legal category P.

Package quantities Potaba Envules – Box of 40 envules. Potaba tablets – Containers of 120 and 1000 tablets. Potaba capsules – Containers of 240 and 1000 capsules.

Further information It is necessary to continue treatment with Potaba at the full recommended dose (12 g daily) for up to twelve months or longer to effect regression of the fibrous plaque in the penis. Patients should be instructed not to interrupt treatment, except during periods of low food intake (see precautions above).

p–Aminobenzoate is considered to be a member of the vitamin B complex. Small amounts are found in yeast, cereal, eggs, milk and meats. Detectable amounts are normally present in human blood and other biological fluids.

Product licence numbers

Envules	0245/5000
Capsules	0245/5001
Tablets	0245/5002

**Trade Mark*

Gold Cross Pharmaceuticals
Division of G. D. Searle & Company Limited
PO Box 53
Lane End Road
High Wycombe
Bucks HP12 4HL

ALDACTIDE* 50
ALDACTIDE* 25

Presentation
Aldactide 50: Buff, film-coated tablets engraved 'SEARLE 180' on one side containing Spironolactone B.P. 50 mg and Hydroflumethiazide B.P. 50 mg.

Aldactide 25: Buff, film-coated tablets engraved 'SEARLE 101' on one side containing Spironolactone B.P. 25 mg and Hydroflumethiazide B.P. 25 mg.

Uses Congestive cardiac failure.

Dosage and administration Administration of Aldactide once daily with a meal is recommended.

Adults: Most patients will require an initial dosage of four tablets Aldactide 25 or two tablets Aldactide 50 daily. The dosage should be adjusted as necessary and may range from one tablet Aldactide 25 to eight tablets Aldactide 25 or four tablets Aldactide 50 daily.

Elderly: It is recommended that treatment is started with the lowest dose and titrated upwards as required to achieve maximum benefit. Care should be taken in severe hepatic and renal impairment which may alter drug metabolism and excretion.

Children: Although clinical trials using Aldactide have not been carried out in children, as a guide, a daily dosage providing 1.5 to 3 mg of spironolactone per kilogram body weight, given in divided doses, may be employed.

Contra-indications, warnings, etc
Contra-indications: Aldactide is contra-indicated in patients with anuria, acute renal insufficiency, rapidly deteriorating or severe impairment of renal function, hyperkalaemia, significant hypercalcaemia, Addison's disease and in patients who are hypersensitive to spironolactone, thiazide diuretics or to other sulphonamide derived drugs.

Aldactide should not be administered concurrently with other potassium-conserving diuretics and potassium supplements should not be given routinely with Aldactide as hyperkalaemia may be induced.

Warnings: Carcinogenicity: Spironolactone has been shown to produce tumours in rats when administered at high doses over a long period of time. The significance of these findings with respect to clinical use is not certain. However, the long term use of spironolactone in young patients requires careful consideration of the benefits and the potential hazard involved.

Sulphonamide derivatives, including thiazides, have been reported to exacerbate or activate systemic lupus erythematosus.

Precautions: Fluid and electrolyte balance: Fluid and electrolyte status should be regularly monitored, particularly in the elderly, in those with significant renal and hepatic impairment and in patients receiving digoxin and drugs with pro-arrhythmic effects.

Hyperkalaemia may occur in patients with impaired renal function or excessive potassium intake and can cause cardiac irregularities which may be fatal. Should hyperkalaemia develop Aldactide should be discontinued, and if necessary, active measures taken to reduce the serum potassium to normal.

Hypokalaemia may develop as a result of profound diuresis, particularly when Aldactide is used concomitantly with loop diuretics, glucocorticoids or ACTH.

Hyponatraemia may be induced, especially when Aldactide is administered in combination with other diuretics.

Hepatic impairment: Caution should be observed in patients with acute or severe liver impairment as vigorous diuretic therapy may precipitate encephalopathy in susceptible patients. Regular estimation of serum electrolytes is essential in such patients.

Reversible hyperchloraemic metabolic acidosis usually in association with hyperkalaemia has been reported to occur in some patients with decompensated hepatic cirrhosis, even in the presence of normal renal function.

Urea and uric acid: Reversible increases in blood urea have been reported, particularly accompanying vigorous diuresis or in the presence of impaired renal function.

Thiazides may cause hyperuricaemia and precipitate attacks of gout in some patients.

Diabetes mellitus: Thiazides may aggravate existing diabetes and the insulin requirements may alter. Diabetes mellitus which has been latent may become manifest during thiazide administration.

Hyperlipidaemia: Caution should be observed as thiazides may raise serum lipids.

Drug interactions: Spironolactone has been reported to increase serum digoxin concentration and to interfere with certain serum digoxin assays. In patients receiving digoxin and spironolactone the digoxin response should be monitored by means other than serum digoxin concentrations, unless the digoxin assay used has been proven not to be affected by spironolactone therapy. If it proves necessary to adjust the dose of digoxin patients should be carefully monitored for evidence of enhanced or reduced digoxin effect.

Potentiation of the effect of antihypertensive drugs occurs and their dosage may need to be reduced when Aldactide is added to the treatment regime, and then adjusted as necessary.

Since ACE inhibitors decrease aldosterone production they should not routinely be used with Aldactide, particularly in patients with marked renal impairment.

As carbenoxolone may cause sodium retention and thus decrease the effectiveness of Aldactide, concurrent use should be avoided.

Nonsteroidal anti-inflammatory drugs may attenuate the natriuretic efficacy of diuretics due to inhibition of intrarenal synthesis of prostaglandins.

Concurrent use of lithium and thiazides may reduce lithium clearance leading to intoxication.

Spironolactone and thiazides may reduce vascular responsiveness to noradrenaline. Caution should be exercised in the management of patients subjected to regional or general anaesthesia while they are being treated with Aldactide.

In fluorimetric assays spironolactone may interfere with the estimation of compounds with similar fluorescence characteristics.

The absorption of a number of drugs including thiazides

is decreased when co-administered with cholestyramine and colestipol.

Thiazides co-administered with calcium and/or vitamin D may increase the risk of hypercalcaemia.

Thiazides may delay the elimination of quinidine.

Pregnancy: Spironolactone or its metabolites may, and hydroflumethiazide does, cross the placental barrier. With spironolactone feminisation has been observed in male rat foetuses. Thiazides may decrease placental perfusion, increase uterine inertia and inhibit labour. In the foetus or neonate thiazides may cause jaundice, thrombocytopenia, hypoglycaemia, electrolyte imbalance and death from maternal complications. The use of Aldactide in pregnant women requires that the anticipated benefit be weighed against the possible hazards to the mother and foetus.

Nursing mothers: Metabolites of spironolactone, and hydroflumethiazide, have been detected in breast milk. If use of Aldactide is considered essential, an alternative method of infant feeding should be instituted.

Adverse effects: Gynaecomastia may develop in association with the use of spironolactone. Development appears to be related to both dosage level and duration of therapy and is normally reversible when the drug is discontinued. In rare instances some breast enlargement may persist. Other adverse reactions reported in association with spironolactone include: gastrointestinal intolerance, drowsiness, lethargy, headache, mental confusion, ataxia, drug fever, skin rashes, menstrual irregularities, breast soreness, impotence and mild androgenic effects.

Adverse reactions reported in association with thiazides include: gastrointestinal upset, skin rashes, photosensitivity, blood dyscrasias, raised serum lipids, aplastic anaemia, purpura, muscle cramps, weakness, restlessness, headache, dizziness, vertigo, jaundice, orthostatic hypotension, impotence, paraesthesia, and rarely pancreatitis, necrotising vasculitis and xanthopsia. Rarely hypercalcaemia has been reported in association with thiazides, usually in patients with pre-existing metabolic bone disease or parathyroid dysfunction.

Overdosage: Acute overdosage may be manifested by drowsiness, mental confusion, nausea, vomiting, dizziness or diarrhoea. Hyponatraemia, hypokalaemia or hyperkalaemia may be induced, or hepatic coma may be precipitated in patients with severe liver disease, but these effects are unlikely to be associated with acute overdosage. Symptoms of hyperkalaemia may manifest as paraesthesia, weakness, flaccid paralysis or muscle spasm and may be difficult to distinguish clinically from hypokalaemia. Electrocardiographic changes are the earliest specific signs of potassium disturbances. No specific antidote has been identified. Improvement may be expected after withdrawal of the drug. General supportive measures including replacement of fluids and electrolytes may be indicated.

Pharmaceutical precautions Store in a dry place below 30°C (86°F).

Legal category POM.

Package quantities *Aldactide 50*: Calendar blister pack of 28 tablets (OP); blister pack of 100 tablets; plastic bottle of 500 tablets. *Aldactide 25*: Blister pack of 100 tablets; plastic bottle of 500 tablets.

Further information Hydroflumethiazide induces diuresis usually within two hours, which lasts for 12–18 hours.

Spironolactone, as a competitive aldosterone antagonist, increases sodium excretion whilst reducing potassium loss at the distal renal tubule. It has a gradual and prolonged action. The renal action of single doses of spironolactone reaches its peak after 7 hours, and activity persists for at least 24 hours.

Product licence numbers
Aldactide 50 0020/0082
Aldactide 25 0020/5001

CONOVA* 30

Presentation White, film-coated tablets engraved 'SEARLE 930' on one side containing Ethynodiol Diacetate BP 2 mg and Ethinyloestradiol PhEur 30 micrograms.

Uses Oral contraception.

Dosage and administration One tablet daily for 21 days, starting on Day 5 of the menstrual cycle (where Day 1 is the first day of bleeding). The next course of tablets should be started after seven tablet free days. This 'three weeks on, one week off' regimen is continued for as long as contraception is required. Women should be advised to use an additional form of contraception (a sheath or a cap plus spermicide) for the first 14 days of the first pack.

Women switching from another combined oral contraceptive should start Conova 30 seven days after finishing their current pack.

After pregnancy oral contraception is usually started as soon as spontaneous menstruation has been resumed. However, if thought appropriate, oral contraception can be started within 7–12 days of vaginal delivery provided the woman is ambulant and there are no puerperal complications. An additional form of contraception (a sheath or a cap plus spermicide) should be used for the first 14 days of the first pack.

Missed tablets: Women who miss a single tablet should be instructed to take the missed tablet as soon as they remember, even though this may mean taking two tablets on one single day. The regular tablet for that day should be taken at the usual time. An additional method of contraception (a sheath or a cap plus spermicide) should be used for the remainder of the cycle. If two consecutive tablets are missed, women should be instructed to take two tablets each day for the next two days and use an additional method of contraception for the rest of the cycle. Those who miss more than two tablets should resume as soon as they remember, ignoring those tablets they have missed, and should use additional contraceptive precautions for the rest of the cycle.

Vomiting or diarrhoea: Vomiting or diarrhoea may reduce the effectiveness of the tablets, particularly if this should occur at or around the time of ovulation. The woman should be advised to use an additional form of contraception for the rest of the cycle when an episode of vomiting and/or diarrhoea occurs.

Contra-indications, warnings, etc
Contra-indications: The contra-indications for combined oral contraceptives are: thrombophlebitis, thromboembolic disorders, cerebral vascular disease, myocardial infarction, coronary artery disease, or a past history of these conditions; known, suspected or a past history of breast, genital or hormone dependent cancer; past or present, benign or malignant liver tumours; impaired liver function; active liver disease; history during pregnancy of idiopathic jaundice or severe pruritus; disorders of lipid metabolism; haemoglobinopathies; undiagnosed abnormal vaginal bleeding or amenorrhoea; known or suspected pregnancy.

Warnings: Combined oral contraceptives have been associated with an increase in the risk of thromboembolic and thrombotic disease including cerebral and myocardial infarction, subarachnoid haemorrhage, pulmonary embolism, deep vein thrombosis and transient ischaemic attacks. Risk has been reported to be related to both oestrogenic and progestogenic activity. The risk of arterial thrombosis associated with combined oral contraceptives increases with age, and this risk is aggravated by cigarette smoking. The use of combined oral contraceptives by women in the older age group, especially those who are cigarette smokers, should therefore be discouraged, and alternative methods advised.

Certain factors may predispose to the development of coronary artery disease, e.g. smoking, obesity, diabetes, hypertension, hypercholesterolaemia, history of pre-eclamptic toxaemia, regardless of whether or not oral contraceptives are used. The suitability of a combined oral contraceptive should be judged according to the severity of such conditions in the individual case and should be discussed with the woman before she decides to take it.

An increase in blood pressure has been reported in women receiving oral contraceptives. The amount of increase may correlate directly with increasing progestogenic activity.

Persistence of risk after discontinuation of oral contraceptives has been reported for circulatory disease including non-rheumatic heart disease and cerebrovascular disease such as subarachnoid haemorrhage, cerebral thrombosis and transient ischaemic attacks.

Conova 30 should be discontinued at least six weeks before elective surgery or during periods of prolonged immobilisation. It would be reasonable to resume oral contraceptives two or three weeks after surgery provided the woman is ambulant. Every woman however, should be considered individually with regard to the nature of the operation, the extent of immobilisation, the presence of additional risk factors and the chance of unwanted conception.

Conova 30 should be discontinued if there is a gradual or sudden, partial or complete loss of vision or any evidence of ocular changes, onset or aggravation of migraine or development of headache of a new kind which is recurrent, persistent or severe, suspicion of thrombosis or infarction, significant rise in blood pressure or if jaundice occurs.

Malignant hepatic tumours have been reported on rare occasions in long term users of oral contraceptives. Benign hepatic tumours have also been associated with oral contraceptive usage. A hepatic tumour should be considered in the differential diagnosis when upper abdominal pain, enlarged liver or signs of intra-abdominal haemorrhage occur.

Numerous epidemiological studies have been reported on the risks of ovarian, endometrial, cervical and breast cancer in women using combined oral contraceptives. The evidence is clear that combined oral contraceptives offer substantial protection against both ovarian and endometrial cancer.

An increased risk of cervical cancer in long term users of combined oral contraceptives has been reported in some studies, but there continues to be controversy about the extent to which this is attributable to the confounding effects of sexual behaviour and other factors.

The evidence linking combined oral contraceptive use and breast cancer remains inconclusive. The results of some studies suggest an increased risk of breast cancer presenting below the age of about 35, the risk rising with duration of use. Any possible increased risk of breast cancer with combined oral contraceptives is however likely to be small, and may be expected to be less with low dosage pills. This possible risk should be weighed against the many benefits of combined oral contraceptives, including their protective effects against ovarian and endometrial cancers.

Precautions: Women receiving treatment with oestrogen or progestogen or both, should be kept under regular surveillance.

Caution should be exercised where there is the possibility of an interaction between a pre-existing disorder and a known or suspected side-effect. The use of Conova 30 in women suffering from epilepsy, or with a history of migraine, or cardiac or renal dysfunction may result in exacerbation of these disorders, because of fluid retention. Caution should also be observed in women who wear contact lenses, women with impaired carbohydrate tolerance, hypertension, asthma, depression, gallstones, chloasma, varicose veins, or any disease that is prone to worsen during pregnancy, and in young women in whom the growth period has not yet ended.

Drug interactions: Conova 30 may be rendered less effective and increased incidence of breakthrough bleeding may occur by virtue of drug interactions. At present, drugs suspected to interact in this way include rifampicin, barbiturates, anticonvulsants and antibiotics. Ascorbic acid (Vitamin C) has been reported to increase the bioavailability of ethinyloestradiol resulting in increased plasma concentrations.

Pregnancy: Several reports suggest an association between foetal exposure to female sex hormones, including oral contraceptives, and congenital anomalies. Pregnancy should be excluded before continuing treatment in women who have missed two consecutive periods.

Nursing mothers; Active ingredients of oral contraceptives have been detected in the milk of mothers taking such drugs. The effect of Conova 30 on breast-fed infants has not been determined. Oral contraceptives may diminish lactation when given immediately postpartum.

Adverse effects: In addition to those mentioned under Warnings and Precautions other known or suspected side effects of oral contraceptives include nausea, vomiting, other gastro-intestinal symptoms (e.g., abdominal cramps and bloating), irregular vaginal bleeding, amenorrhoea, dysmenorrhoea, increase in size of uterine myofibromata, change in cervical erosion and secretion, endocervical hyperplasia, vaginal candidiasis, skin disorders including chloasma, breast and weight changes, ocular changes, headache, hypertension, Raynaud's disease, migraine, depression, change in libido and appetite, fluid retention, infertility after discontinuation, and changes in carbohydrate, lipid and vitamin metabolism.

The use of oral contraceptives has also been associated with a possible increased incidence of gallbladder disease.

Tests of endocrine, hepatic and thyroid function, as well as coagulation tests, may be affected by this preparation.

There is evidence of an association between the use of oral contraceptives and mesenteric thrombosis, Budd-Chiari syndrome, neuro-ocular lesions (e.g., retinal thrombosis and optic neuritis), although confirmatory studies have not been done.

Haemolytic uraemic syndrome, premenstrual-like syndrome, cystitis-like syndrome, dizziness, allergic rhinitis, hirsutism, erythema, malignant hypertension, pulmonary hypertension, arthritis and related disorders such as systemic lupus erythematosus, pituitary tumour, malignant melanoma and rarely chorea, haemorrhagic eruption, purpura, pancreatitis, colitis, gingivitis and dry socket have been reported in users of combined oral contraceptives.

Overdosage: Serious ill-effects have not been reported following acute ingestion of large doses of oral contraceptives by young children. Nausea and vomiting may occur and vaginal withdrawal bleeding may present in pre-pubertal girls. In general, treatment of overdosage is not necessary. However if thought appropriate, as there is no specific antidote, treatment should be symptomatic.

Pharmaceutical precautions Store in a dry place below 30°C (86°F).

Legal category POM.

Package quantities Carton containing one strip of 21 tablets, with instructions. (OP)

Further information Nil.

Product licence number 0020/0066.

FEMULEN*

Presentation White tablets engraved 'SEARLE' on both sides, containing Ethynodiol Diacetate BP 500 micrograms.

Uses Oral contraception.

Dosage and administration Starting on the first day of menstruation, one tablet every day without a break in medication for as long as contraception is required. Additional contraceptive precautions (a sheath or a cap plus spermicide) should be taken for the first 14 days of the first pack. Tablets should be taken at the same time each day.

Missed tablets: If the woman misses one tablet or takes it later than the usual time, contraceptive efficacy may be reduced and additional contraceptive precautions (a sheath or a cap plus spermicide) should be used until the next period occurs. Women who miss a single tablet should be instructed to take the missed tablet as soon as they remember, even though this may mean taking two tablets on one single day. The regular tablet for that day should be taken at the usual time. If two or more consecutive tablets are missed Femulen should be discontinued and alternative contraceptive measures should be taken until menstruation occurs and the possibility of pregnancy is excluded.

Vomiting or diarrhoea: Vomiting or diarrhoea may reduce the effectiveness of Femulen, particularly if this should occur at or around the time of ovulation. If an episode of vomiting and/or diarrhoea occurs the woman should be advised to use an additional form of contraception (a sheath or a cap plus spermicide) until the next menstrual period occurs.

Contra-indications, warnings, etc

Contra-indications: The contra-indications for progestogen-only oral contraceptives are: known, suspected, or a past history of breast, genital or hormone dependent cancer; past or present, benign or malignant liver tumours; impaired liver function; active liver disease; history during pregnancy of idiopathic jaundice or severe pruritus; disorders of lipid metabolism; undiagnosed abnormal vaginal bleeding or amenorrhoea; known or suspected pregnancy.

Combined oestrogen/progestogen preparations have been associated with an increase in the risk of thromboembolic and thrombotic disease. Risk has been reported to be related to both oestrogenic and progestogenic activity. In the absence of long term epidemiological studies with progestogen-only oral contraceptives, it is required that the existence or history of thrombophlebitis, thromboembolic disorders, cerebral vascular disease, myocardial infarction, coronary artery disease, or a haemoglobinopathy be described as a contra-indication to Femulen as it is to oestrogen containing oral contraceptives.

Warnings: Femulen should be discontinued if there is a gradual or sudden, partial or complete loss of vision or any evidence of ocular changes, onset or aggravation of migraine or development of headache of a new kind which is recurrent, persistent or severe, suspicion of thrombosis or infarction, significant rise in blood pressure or if jaundice occurs.

Malignant hepatic tumours have been reported on rare occasions in long term users of oral contraceptives. Benign hepatic tumours have also been associated with oral contraceptive usage. A hepatic tumour should be considered in the differential diagnosis when upper abdominal pain, enlarged liver or signs of intra-abdominal haemorrhage occur.

Progestogen-only oral contraceptives may offer less protection against ectopic pregnancy, than against intrauterine pregnancy.

Precautions: Women receiving treatment with Femulen should be kept under regular medical surveillance.

Femulen should be discontinued at least 6 weeks before elective surgery or during periods of prolonged immobilisation. It would be reasonable to resume Femulen two or three weeks after surgery provided the woman is ambulant. Every woman, however, should be considered individually with regard to the nature of the operation, the extent of immobilisation, the presence of additional risk factors and the chance of unwanted conception.

Caution should be exercised where there is the possibility of an interaction between a pre-existing disorder and a known or suspected side-effect. The use of Femulen in women suffering from epilepsy, or with a history of migraine or cardiac or renal dysfunction may result in exacerbation of these disorders because of fluid retention. Caution should also be observed in women who wear contact lenses, women with impaired carbohydrate tolerance, depression, gallstones, varicose veins, hypertension, asthma or any disease that is prone to worsen during pregnancy.

Pregnancy: Several reports suggest an association between foetal exposure to female sex hormones, including oral contraceptives, and congenital anomalies.

If a woman does not have a menstrual period within 45 days of her last menstrual period, the possibility of pregnancy should be excluded.

Drug interactions: Femulen may be rendered less effective and increased incidence of breakthrough bleeding may occur by virtue of drug interaction. At present, drugs suspected to interact in this way include rifampicin, barbiturates, anticonvulsants, and antibiotics.

Nursing mothers: There is no evidence that progestogen-only oral contraceptives diminish the yield of breast milk. In a study of nursing mothers taking Femulen, the median percentage of norethisterone, the principal metabolite of ethynodiol diacetate given to the mother which was ingested by the infant was 0.02%. No adverse effect of the drug on the infants was noted.

Adverse effects: Women taking progestogen-only oral contraceptives for the first time may initially experience menstrual irregularity. This may include amenorrhoea, prolonged bleeding and/or spotting and should decrease with time. Clinical investigations with Femulen indicate that side-effects are infrequent and tend to decrease as treatment continues. Known or suspected side-effects of progestogen-only oral contraceptives include nausea, vomiting, other gastrointestinal symptoms, skin disorders including chloasma, breast and weight changes, ocular changes, headache, migraine, depression, change in libido and appetite, increase in size of uterine myofibromata, and changes in carbohydrate, lipid or vitamin metabolism. Rarely dizziness, hirsutism, haemorrhagic eruption and colitis have been reported in users of progestogen-only oral contraceptives.

The use of oral contraceptives has also been associated with a possible increased incidence of gallbladder disease.

Tests of endocrine, hepatic and thyroid function, as well as coagulation tests may be affected by this preparation.

Overdosage: Serious ill-effects have not been reported following acute ingestion of large doses of oral contraceptives by young children. Nausea and vomiting may occur and vaginal withdrawal bleeding may present in pre-pubertal girls. In general, treatment of overdosage is not necessary. However, if thought appropriate, as there is no specific antidote, treatment should be symptomatic.

Pharmaceutical precautions Store in a dry place below 30°C (86°F).

Legal category POM.

Package quantities Carton of 28 tablets with instructions (OP).

Further information Femulen does not necessarily inhibit ovulation but it is believed to discourage implantation of the fertilised ovum by altering the endometrium. Cervical mucus viscosity is also changed which may render the passage of sperm less likely.

Product licence number 0020/0054.

GRAVIGARD*
MINI-GRAVIGARD*

Gravigard and Mini-Gravigard were discontinued in 1990 and the following prescribing information was current on December 31 1990. It is included for the continued management of women using these intrauterine devices.

Presentation Gravigard – transverse arm 26 mm; vertical arm 36 mm.
Mini-Gravigard – transverse arm 22 mm; vertical arm 28 mm.

Each device consists of pure electrolytic copper wire, surface area approximately 200 mm^2, wound onto the vertical arm of a plastic carrier which approximates the shape of the number 7. The plastic carrier is composed of polypropylene homopolymer impregnated with barium sulphate to render it radio-opaque, with a monofilament thread attached to the base of the vertical arm. Each device is presented partially loaded in its inserter tube and instructions for use are included with each sterile pack.

Uses Intrauterine contraception

Dosage and administration Gravigard is recommended for women with a uterine size measurement from external os to fundus greater than 6.5 cm. Mini-Gravigard is recommended for women with a uterine size measurement from external os to fundus of 5.5 to 6.5 cm. Gravigard and Mini-Gravigard should be replaced every three years. The procedure for insertion is fully detailed in the instructions for use leaflet included with each sterile pack. Insertion is not recommended if uterine size from external os to fundus measures less than 5.5 cm.

Although IUCDs may be inserted at any time during the menstrual cycle, insertion during or shortly after the menstrual period reduces the possibility of an existing undiagnosed pregnancy. Postpartum insertion is usually delayed until involution of the uterus is complete. The benefits of immediate post abortion insertion should be weighed against the risks due to the relatively soft structure of the uterus.

Contra-indications, warnings, etc
Contra-indications: Contra-indications are pregnancy; history of ectopic pregnancy; postpartum endometritis or septic abortion within the past three months; abnormalities of the uterine cavity including developmental abnormalities; large or multiple fibroids; acute pelvic inflammatory disease; a history of repeated, recent or severe pelvic inflammatory disease; acute cervicitis; cervical dysplasia; endometrial disease such as hyperplasia or uterine polyps; suspected or proven malignancy of the genital organs, including unresolved abnormal Papanicolaou smear; severe dysmenorrhoea; menorrhagia and/or intermenstrual bleeding; significant anaemia; heart disease; leukaemia; use of chronic corticosteroid therapy because of the increased susceptibility to infection with certain microorganisms which may possibly be introduced at the time of an IUCD insertion; Wilson's disease or a hypersensitivity to copper.

Medical diathermy to the abdominal and sacral regions is contraindicated in Gravigard or Mini-Gravigard users because of the possibility of heat injury to the surrounding tissue.

Warnings: An increased incidence of pelvic inflammatory disease and menorrhagia associated with the use of IUCDs has been reported. Pelvic infection may result in future infertility. Women with certain known or suspected heart diseases are more susceptible to development of subacute bacterial endocarditis. Use of an IUCD in these women may represent a potential source of septic emboli. Appropriate precautions including administration of antibiotics should be observed when inserting an IUCD in such cases.

Syncope or bradycardia may occur in some women during insertion or removal of an IUCD. In the event of early signs of vasovagal attack, insertion may need to be abandoned or the device removed. The woman should be kept supine, the head lowered and the legs elevated to the vertical position if necessary in order to restore cerebral blood flow. A clear airway must be maintained; an airway should always be at hand. Persistent bradycardia may be controlled with intravenous atropine in a dose of 600 micrograms. If oxygen is available it may be administered by using an Ambu bag. In the very rare emergency situation where the woman fails to regain consciousness she should be transferred to hospital intensive care.

Post-insertion cramps are usually of only a few minutes duration, but some women may experience cramps for several hours or days. Spotting, intermenstrual bleeding or increased menstrual flow may occur. If heavy or persistent bleeding or persistent abdominal cramps occur, removal of the device may be indicated.

Gravigard or Mini-Gravigard should be removed in the event of partial expulsion and a new device inserted. If perforation of the uterus or cervix is suspected, the device should be removed as soon as medically feasible. Adhesions, foreign body reactions and intestinal obstruction may result if an IUCD is left within the peritoneal cavity. Removal is also indicated in cases of pelvic infection resistant to treatment, menorrhagia producing significant anaemia, or intractable pain.

Precautions: A complete gynaecological examination, including measurement of the uterus, should precede insertion of the device. Ideally the woman should be re-examined within the first three months after insertion and annually thereafter. After insertion the woman should be taught to examine herself to ascertain the continued presence of the retrieval thread. Advise her to consult her doctor if pregnancy is suspected.

Intrauterine devices should be used with caution in women with anaemia, menorrhagia, hypermenorrhoea, a history of a previous uterine incision or perforation of the uterus and those receiving anticoagulants, steroid therapy or having a coagulopathy.

The possibility of seizure being precipitated in an epileptic at or shortly after the insertion of an IUCD should also be borne in mind.

It has been reported that IUCDs may be less effective in insulin-dependent diabetics.

Lost threads: If the retrieval thread is not visible at the cervix on follow-up examination, it may have been drawn up into the uterus or cervical canal and may reappear during the next menstrual period. The thread may usually be located by gently probing with a suitable instrument. If it cannot be found, it may have broken off, or the device may be expelled. Ultrasound or X-ray may be used to locate the device.

Pregnancy: The risk of ectopic pregnancy is reported to be greater in women who conceive with an IUCD in situ than in those without an IUCD. Therefore, if a woman becomes pregnant with an IUCD in situ, she should be carefully evaluated for possible ectopic pregnancy.

There have been reports of an increased incidence of septic abortion, associated in some instances with septicaemia, septic shock and death, in women who become pregnant with an IUCD in situ. Women who are pregnant with an IUCD in situ should be closely observed and told to report immediately all abnormal symptoms such as 'flu-like symptoms, fever, cramp-like pain, bleeding or excessive discharge, as the onset of septicaemia associated with septic abortion may be insidious with general symptoms rather than initial signs of spontaneous abortion. Also, the incidence of spontaneous abortion appears to be increased over that in unprotected women when conception occurs with an IUCD in situ. If pregnancy occurs with an IUCD in situ and the thread is visible then the device should be removed. If the thread is not visible or device removal would be difficult, the IUCD may be left in situ until the pregnancy goes to term or until a decision is made to terminate the pregnancy. If the woman elects to continue the pregnancy, careful observation is required. The long term effects of intrauterine copper on the foetus are unknown.

Adverse effects: Uterine or cervical perforation, vaginal discharge, embedment and allergic reactions have been reported.

Pharmaceutical precautions Gravigard and Mini-Gravigard are supplied in sterile packs which should not be opened until required for insertion. Each device should be handled with aseptic precautions and should not be left folded in its inserter tube for more than two minutes, as this may prevent the transverse arm from reassuming its correct position.

Care should be taken not to damage the sterile package which should be stored in a cool dry place.

Legal category POM.

Package quantities Gravigard: Pack containing one sterile device. Outer containing five packs. Pack containing ten sterile devices.

Mini-Gravigard: Pack containing one sterile device. Outer containing five packs. Pack containing ten sterile devices.

Further information The average amount of copper eluted from copper IUCDs is well below the daily dietary intake of copper. Small increases of endometrial copper levels have been noted in the presence of copper IUCDs, but these are not cumulative. No changes in blood levels of copper have been detected.

LOMOTIL* TABLETS
LOMOTIL* LIQUID

Presentation *Lomotil Tablets:* White tablets engraved SEARLE on one side. Each tablet contains Diphenoxylate Hydrochloride BP 2.5 mg with Atropine Sulphate PhEur 25 micrograms.

Lomotil Liquid: Red, cherry flavoured liquid. Each 5 ml measure contains Diphenoxylate Hydrochloride BP 2.5 mg with Atropine Sulphate PhEur 25 micrograms.

Uses Adjunctive therapy to appropriate rehydration in diarrhoea.

Control of stool formation after colostomy or ileostomy.

Relief of symptoms in chronic mild ulcerative colitis (see Warnings)

Dosage and administration *Caution:* The recommended dosage should not be exceeded. Once satisfactory control is achieved, dosage should be reduced to suit the requirements of the individual patient.

Adults: The recommended starting dose is four tablets, or four 5 ml measures, followed by two tablets or two 5 ml measures every six hours.

Elderly: Consideration should be given to the presence of other disease and concomitant drug therapy (see *Precautions*).

Children: Recommended dosage guide:
Under 4 years: Not recommended.
4-8 years: 1 tablet or one 5 ml measure three times daily.
9-12 years: 1 tablet or one 5 ml measure four times daily.
13-16 years: 2 tablets or two 5 ml measures three times daily.

Contra-indications, warnings, etc Lomotil is contra-indicated in patients with a known hypersensitivity to diphenoxylate hydrochloride or atropine, in patients with jaundice or intestinal obstruction, acute ulcerative colitis, and in the treatment of diarrhoea associated with pseudomembranous enterocolitis.

Appropriate fluid and electrolyte therapy should be given to protect against dehydration. If severe dehydration or electrolyte imbalance is present, Lomotil should be withheld until appropriate corrective therapy has been initiated.

In some patients with ulcerative colitis, agents which inhibit intestinal motility or delay intestinal transit time have been reported to induce toxic megacolon. Patients with ulcerative colitis should be observed carefully and Lomotil therapy should be discontinued promptly if abdominal distension or other untoward symptoms develop.

Lomotil should be used with extreme caution in patients with advanced hepatorenal disease and in all patients with abnormal liver function since hepatic coma may be precipitated.

Precautions: Because a subtherapeutic dose of atropine is added to Lomotil, atropinic effects may occur in susceptible individuals or in overdosage. Individuals with Down's syndrome appear to have an increased susceptibility to the actions of atropine.

Drug interactions: Since the chemical structure of diphenoxylate hydrochloride resembles that of meperidine hydrochloride, concurrent use with MAO inhibitors could precipitate hypertensive crisis. Close observation is required when these medications are given concomitantly with diphenoxylate hydrochloride.

Diphenoxylate hydrochloride may potentiate the action of central nervous system depressants such as barbiturates, tranquillisers and alcohol.

Pregnancy: Animal teratology and reproduction studies have demonstrated no adverse effects. The safety of Lomotil in pregnancy has not been established. However, as with all drugs, caution is recommended when used in early pregnancy.

Nursing mothers: Diphenoxylate hydrochloride and atropine sulphate may be excreted in human milk. If a nursing mother is taking Lomotil, the infant may exhibit some effects of the drug.

Adverse effects:
Adverse reactions reported include: *Central nervous system:* malaise/lethargy/sedation/somnolence, confusion, dizziness, restlessness, depression, euphoria, hallucinations, headache.

Allergic: anaphylaxis, angioedema, urticaria, pruritus.

Gastrointestinal system: paralytic ileus, toxic megacolon, gastrointestinal intolerance such as nausea and vomiting, anorexia, abdominal discomfort.

Atropine effects, such as flushing, dryness of skin and mucous membranes, tachycardia, hyperthermia and urinary retention may occur, especially in children.

Overdosage: Accidental overdosage may produce narcosis with respiratory depression or atropine poisoning or both, particularly in children. Symptoms of overdosage include dryness of the skin and mucous membranes, flushing, hyperthermia and tachycardia, nystagmus, pinpoint pupils, hypotonic reflexes, lethargy, coma and severe respiratory depression. The onset of symptoms of overdosage may be considerably delayed and respiratory depression may not become evident until as late as 12 to 30 hours after ingestion, and may recur in spite of an initial response to narcotic antagonists. Continuous observation should be maintained for at least 48 hours.

If respiratory depression develops, naloxone, a specific antidote, should be administered. The duration of action of naloxone hydrochloride is considerably shorter than that of diphenoxylate hydrochloride and repeated injections of the antidote may be required. Establishment of a patent airway and artificial ventilation may be needed. If the patient is not comatose gastric lavage and administration of a slurry of activated charcoal may be indicated.

Pharmaceutical precautions Store in a dry place below 30°C (86°F).

Legal category POM.

Package quantities

Lomotil Tablets:	Carton containing blister strips of 100, 500 and 1,000 tablets.
Lomotil Liquid:	Bottles containing 100 ml (with 5 ml measure) (OP).

Further information Nil.

Product licence numbers

Lomotil Tablets:	0020/5014
Lomotil Liquid:	0020/5015

PRO-BANTHINE*

Presentation Pink, sugar coated, biconvex tablets, printed "SEARLE" on one side. Each tablet contains Propantheline Bromide BP 15 mg.

Actions: Pro-Banthine is an anticholinergic.

Uses Symptomatic treatment of irritable bowel syndrome. Adjunctive therapy for peptic ulcer together with antacids. Hyperhidrosis. Enuresis.

Dosage and administration *Caution:* Food has been reported to reduce the bioavailability of Pro-Banthine. Tablets should be taken at least one hour before meals.

Adults: A dosage up to eight tablets daily in divided doses may be required. In peptic ulcer the recommended initial starting dose is one tablet before each meal, and two tablets at bedtime. Subsequently, dosage should be adjusted according to the patient's individual response and tolerance.

Elderly: Elderly patients may be more susceptible to anticholinergic side-effects; glaucoma and urinary retention may occur. Consideration should be given to the presence of other disease and concomitant drug therapy (see "Contra-indications, warnings, etc").

Children: Safety and efficacy in children have not been established.

Contra-indications, warnings, etc
Contra-indications: Pro-Banthine is contra-indicated in patients with obstructive diseases of the gastrointestinal or urinary tract, pyloric stenosis, intestinal atony, severe ulcerative colitis or toxic megacolon, hiatus hernia associated with reflux oesophagitis, unstable cardiovascular adjustment in acute haemorrhage, myasthenia gravis, glaucoma and in patients who are hypersensitive to propantheline bromide.

Warnings: In some patients, especially those with ileostomy or colostomy, diarrhoea may be a symptom of incomplete intestinal obstruction. Pro-Banthine therapy should be avoided in such patients.

Patients with severe heart disease in whom an increase in heart rate is undesirable should be observed closely if Pro-Banthine is administered.

Pro-Banthine may produce drowsiness or blurred vision. Patients should not drive or operate machinery if affected in this way.

Precautions: Patients with prostatic hypertrophy may experience some urinary hesitancy. This may be minimised if such patients are advised to micturate at the time the medication is taken.

Patients with ulcerative colitis should be treated with caution, since Pro-Banthine may suppress intestinal motility to the point of producing paralytic ileus, thus precipitating or aggravating toxic megacolon.

Pro-Banthine should be used with caution in the elderly and in all patients with autonomic neuropathy, hepatic or renal disease, hyperthyroidism, coronary heart disease, congestive heart failure, cardiac arrhythmias or hypertension.

Drug interactions: Concurrent use of Pro-Banthine with slow-dissolving tablets of digoxin may cause increased serum digoxin levels.

Since anticholinergics tend to delay gastric emptying they may alter the absorption of other medication given concomitantly.

Excessive cholinergic blockade may occur if Pro-Banthine is given concomitantly with belladonna alkaloids, synthetic and semisynthetic anticholinergic agents or other drugs with anticholinergic activity.

Pregnancy: Animal reproduction and teratology studies have not been performed. Cohort data on parasympatholytics indicate a possible association with minor malformations. In view of this Pro-Banthine should not be administered in pregnancy unless considered essential.

Nursing mothers: It is unknown whether propantheline bromide is excreted in human breast milk. No animal studies have been conducted. In view of this Pro-Banthine should not be administered during breast feeding unless considered essential. Suppression of lactation may occur with parasympatholytics.

Adverse effects: Side-effects of anticholinergics include dryness of the mouth with difficulty in swallowing and thirst, dilatation of the pupils with loss of accommodation and sensitivity to light, increased intra-ocular pressure, flushing, dryness of the skin, decreased sweating, heat stroke, bradycardia followed by tachycardia, palpitations and arrhythmias, urinary hesitancy and retention and constipation.

Overdosage: Intensification of the usual side-effects may occur. In severe intoxication disturbances of the central nervous system may occur resulting in convulsion, coma, circulatory failure, respiratory depression, delirium, hallucinations and restlessness.

In the event of overdosage, empty the stomach and give activated charcoal. Excitement may be controlled by diazepam. Supportive treatment may require oxygen, assisted ventilation and the administration of fluids. In severe cases (convulsions, hyperpyrexia, respiratory depression) the use of intravenous physostigmine (500 micrograms to 2 mg) should be considered. Since it has a brief duration of action of about 1 to 2 hours, it may be necessary to repeat injections up to a total dose of 5 mg.

Pharmaceutical precautions Store in a dry place below 30°C (86°F).

Legal category POM.

Package quantities Carton of 100 tablets containing 10 × 10 blister strips. Bottles containing 1,000 tablets.

Further information Propantheline bromide is extensively metabolised in man. Some enzymic hydrolysis of the drug may occur in the gastrointestinal tract prior to its absorption.

Studies in healthy men demonstrated that peak plasma levels of unchanged drug were reached within 2 hours of a single, oral dose of propantheline bromide. Following single oral dosing the plasma elimination half-life was about 2–3 hours and some 1–10% of propantheline bromide was excreted in urine as unchanged drug.

In healthy men studies have shown onset of anticholinergic effects within 1 hour of oral administration. Effects persisted for up to 6 hours after oral dosing.

Product licence number 0020/5026.

**Trade Mark*

Hoechst UK Limited
Pharmaceutical Division
Hoechst House, Salisbury Road
Hounslow, Middlesex TW4 6JH

ARELIX* CAPSULES

Presentation Arelix Capsules each contain 6 mg piretanide in a sustained release formulation. The capsules have a light green body and an orange cap.

Excipients include sucrose and liquid glucose.

Uses Arelix is a diuretic for the treatment of mild to moderate hypertension.

Dosage and administration One or two capsules daily. The capsules should be taken with food as a single dose in the morning.

Children: There is at present insufficient experience of the use of this product in children to enable dosage recommendations to be made.

Elderly: Piretanide may be excreted more slowly in the elderly.

Contra-indications, warnings, etc

Contra-indications: Arelix is contra-indicated in patients with severe electrolyte imbalance, hypovolaemia or hypotension. It should not be used in patients who are hypersensitive to piretanide or sulphonamides.

Warnings: Patients with impaired micturition or prostatic hypertrophy may develop retention of urine after Arelix administration.

Cephalosporin nephrotoxicity and aminoglycoside ototoxicity have been reported to be increased by the concomitant administration of intravenous or large oral doses of diuretics.

In common with all thiazide and loop diuretics, Arelix can cause hypokalaemia. Corticosteroids and laxatives may exacerbate potassium loss. In patients with severe liver disease, Arelix may precipitate hepatic coma; the use of potassium-sparing diuretics may be preferable in the first instance in these patients.

There have been reports that diuretics may cause latent diabetes to become manifest or may necessitate adjustment of the dosage of concurrently administered hypoglycaemic agents.

The dosage of concurrently administered anti-hypertensive agents, cardiac glycosides and agents used in the treatment of gout may require adjustment. Combination therapy with ACE inhibitors should be monitored carefully at the start of treatment.

The action of salicylates and muscle relaxants may be increased, while the action of pressor amines may be decreased.

In common with other diuretics, serum lithium levels may be increased when lithium is given concomitantly with Arelix, necessitating adjustment of the lithium dosage.

Certain non-steroidal anti-inflammatory agents have been shown to antagonise the action of diuretics such as Arelix.

Precautions: Arelix should not be used during the first trimester of pregnancy. Sufficient experience is not yet available to assess the safety of its use during the later stages of pregnancy; however, there is no evidence of an adverse effect from animal studies.

Serum electrolytes should be regularly monitored in patients with severely impaired renal function or pre-comatose states associated with liver cirrhosis.

Caution should be observed in patients liable to electrolyte imbalance; the levels of serum potassium should be monitored where cardiac glycosides or corticosteroids are to be administered and in patients with liver disease.

Nursing mothers: Arelix may inhibit lactation in nursing mothers; piretanide and its metabolites appear in the breast milk of animals. It should not be used during lactation.

Overdosage: In cases of overdose there is a danger of dehydration and electrolyte depletion due to excessive diuresis. Treatment should therefore be aimed at fluid replacement and correction of the electrolyte imbalance.

Side-effects: Arelix is generally well tolerated. Reactions such as gastro-intestinal upset (nausea, vomiting or diarrhoea) or allergic reactions such as skin rashes are very rare.

Side-effects associated with increased excretion of water and electrolytes may occur, particularly following prolonged treatment with high doses; circulatory disturbance due to fluid loss may occur, especially in the elderly.

There may be an aggravation of pre-existing metabolic alkalosis.

In isolated instances, serum creatinine, urea and uric acid concentrations may rise during Arelix treatment.

Thrombocytopenia has been observed in isolated instances.

Muscle cramps have been reported following the administration of high doses of Arelix but not when used within the dose range recommended for the treatment of hypertension.

Pharmaceutical precautions Arelix should be stored in a cool dry place, protected from light, in containers similar to those of the manufacturer.

Legal category POM.

Package quantities Arelix capsules are supplied in original calendar packs containing 28 capsules.

Further information The diuretic effect of Arelix capsules begins about two hours after administration and lasts for about eight hours. The diuretic effect is gradual and exhibits no marked peak effect.

Product licence number 0086/0092.

CYCLOGEST*

Presentation White pessaries, suitable for vaginal or rectal insertion. Each 1.85 g pessary contains either 200 mg or 400 mg Progesterone BP.

Uses Treatment of the symptoms of premenstrual syndrome, including premenstrual tension and depression, treatment of puerperal depression.

Dosage and administration 200 mg daily to 400 mg twice a day, by vaginal or rectal insertion. For premenstrual syndrome commence treatment on day 14 of menstrual cycle and continue treatment until onset of menstruation. If symptoms are present at ovulation commence treatment on day 12.

Children: Not applicable.

Elderly: Not applicable.

Contra-indications, warnings, etc Cyclogest contains the hormone progesterone which is present in significant concentrations in women during the second half of the menstrual cycle and during pregnancy. This should be borne in mind when treating patients with conditions that may be hormone-sensitive.

Contra-indications: Undiagnosed vaginal bleeding.

Warnings: Use rectally if barrier methods of contraception are used.

Precautions: Use vaginally if patients suffer from colitis or faecal incontinence. Use rectally if patients suffer from vaginal infection (especially moniliasis) or recurrent cystitis. Use rectally in patients who have recently given birth.

Progesterone is metabolised in the liver and should be used with caution in patients with hepatic dysfunction.

Use in pregnancy and lactation: Due to indications of the product it is anticipated that it will not be administered to pregnant women. As progesterone is a natural hormone, it is not expected to have adverse effects; however, no evidence is available to this effect.

Side-effects: Menstruation may occur earlier than expected, or, more rarely, may be delayed. Soreness, diarrhoea and flatulence may occur with rectal administration.

As with other vaginal or rectal preparations, some leakage of the pessary base may occur.

Overdosage: There is a wide margin of safety with Cyclogest pessaries, but overdosage may produce euphoria or dysmenorrhoea.

Pharmaceutical precautions Store in a cool, dry place.

Legal category POM.

Package quantities
Packs of 15 pessaries 200 mg (OP)
Packs of 15 pessaries 400 mg (OP)

Further information It is recommended that the diagnosis and evaluation of the treatment of premenstrual syndrome be monitored using premenstrual charts.

Product licence numbers
Cyclogest Pessaries 200 mg 2343/0001
Cyclogest Pessaries 400 mg 2343/0002

Product Licence Holder: L. D. Collins & Co Ltd. Sunray House, 9 Plantagenet Road, New Barnet, Herts. EN5 5JG.

DANERAL* SA TABLETS

Presentation Daneral SA Tablets each contain 75 mg Pheniramine Maleate BP in a sustained release formulation. Daneral SA is presented as unmarked pink, sugar-coated tablets 10.3 mm in diameter. Excipients include lactose and sucrose (as part of the sugar coating).

Uses Allergic conditions such as hay fever, vasomotor rhinitis, acute rhinitis, urticaria, allergic dermatoses, pruritus.

Dosage and administration One tablet at bedtime will be sufficient for most patients. In more severe cases two tablets may be taken one at night and one in the morning (or both at night). The tablet should be swallowed whole and not sucked or chewed.

Children: This formulation is not suitable for children.

Elderly: As pheniramine is excreted by the kidney a reduced dose (or dose frequency) may be necessary in the elderly.

Contra-indications, warnings, etc
Contra-indications: Daneral SA must not be used in patients hypersensitive to pheniramine. Daneral SA should not be taken by patients with prostatic hypertrophy and urinary frequency suggesting a large residual volume.

Warnings: Daneral SA Tablets may cause drowsiness. Those affected should not drive or operate machinery.

In common with all antihistamines, the sedative effect of other central nervous system depressant agents, e.g. alcohol, tranquillisers, sedatives, neuroleptic agents and MAO inhibitors, may be potentiated.

In infants and children antihistamines may act as central stimulants.

Precautions: Use in pregnancy. There is little evidence of the safety of Daneral SA in human or animal pregnancy, although the drug has been in wide, general use for many years without apparent ill consequence. However, as a precaution, it should not be taken during pregnancy or lactation.

Overdosage: The primary symptom is sedation. Following doses of 300–1,800 mg cerebral stimulation, convulsions and hyperpyrexia may occur. If an overdose has been taken recently by mouth the stomach should be emptied by aspiration and lavage. Peritoneal dialysis is not effective. The patient should be kept quiet, diazepam i.v. may be given to prevent paroxysms and excessive hyperkinesia.

Side-effects: The following symptoms have occasionally been experienced: dryness of the mouth, urine retention, increase in intraocular pressure, gastro-intestinal upset, palpitations and after high dose, hallucinations, agitation and disorientation.

Pharmaceutical precautions Daneral SA Tablets should be stored in a dry place, at ambient temperature, protected from light, in containers similar to those of the manufacturer.

Legal category P.

Package quantities Daneral SA Tablets are available in original packs of 30.

Further information In patients with narrow angle glaucoma, treatment with Daneral SA must be carried out under ophthalmological supervision. Blood dyscrasias that very occasionally occur with antihistamines have so far not been observed with pheniramine.

Product licence number 0086/5001.

DAONIL* TABLETS SEMI-DAONIL* TABLETS

Presentation Daonil Tablets each contain 5 mg Glibenclamide BP. Daonil is presented as white oblong tablets, scored in the middle, one half bearing the Hoechst insignia, the other bearing the letters LDI. The tablet is 10 mm in length and 5 mm wide.

Semi-Daonil Tablets each contain 2.5 mg Glibenclamide BP. Semi-Daonil is presented as white circular biplanar tablets, 6 mm in diameter, one side bearing the Hoechst insignia, the other scored and bearing the letters LBG on either side of the score mark.

Excipients include lactose.

Uses Daonil is a hypoglycaemic agent, indicated for the oral treatment of patients with non-insulin dependent diabetes who respond inadequately to dietary measures alone.

Dosage and administration
1. *Treatment of previously untreated diabetics:* Stabilisation can be started with one 5 mg tablet of Daonil daily. The dose should be taken by mouth, with or immediately after breakfast or the first main meal. Where control is satisfactory, 1 tablet is continued as the maintenance dose. If control is unsatisfactory, the dose can be adjusted by increments of 2.5 or 5 mg at weekly intervals. The total daily dosage rarely exceeds 15 mg and increasing the daily dosage above this does not generally produce any additional effect. The total daily requirement should normally be administered as a single dose at breakfast, or with the first main meal; due consideration should be given to the patient's dietary habits and daily activity in apportioning the dosage.

Elderly: In debilitated or aged patients, who may be more liable to hypoglycaemia, treatment should be initiated with one Semi-Daonil tablet daily.

2. *Change-over from other oral anti-diabetics:* The change over to Daonil from other drugs with a similar mode of action can be carried out without any break in therapy.

Daonil treatment should be started with one 5 mg tablet daily and adjusted by increments of 2.5–5 mg to achieve control. For patients not adequately controlled on other oral agents, treatment is commenced with the equivalent dose of Daonil, without exceeding an initial dose of 10 mg. If response is inadequate, the dose can be raised in a stepwise fashion to 15 mg daily. One 5 mg tablet of Daonil is approximately equivalent to 1 g tolbutamide or glymidine, 250 mg chlorpropamide or tolazamide, 500 mg acetohexamide, 25 mg glibornuride or 5 mg glipizide.

3. *Change-over from biguanides:* Daonil treatment should be started with 1 tablet of Semi-Daonil (2.5 mg) and the biguanide withdrawn. The dosage should then be adjusted by increments of 2.5 mg to achieve control.

Combination with biguanides: If adequate control is not possible with diet and 15 mg of Daonil, control can often be re-established by combined administration of Daonil and a biguanide derivative.

4. *Change-over from insulin:* While it is appreciated that most patients who are on insulin therapy will continue to need it, there may be a few patients, particularly those on low daily doses, who will remain stablilised if transferred from insulin to Daonil.

The tablets should always be taken with, or immediately after, the first main meal.

Children: As non-insulin dependent diabetes is not usually a disease of childhood, Daonil is not recommended for use in children.

Contra-indications, warnings, etc
Contra-indications: Daonil should not be used in patients who have or have ever had diabetic ketoacidosis or those who have insulin-dependent diabetes mellitus, serious impairment of renal, hepatic or adrenocortical function, in patients who are hypersensitive to glibenclamide, or in circumstances of unusual stress, e.g. surgical operations or during pregnancy, when dietary treatment and insulin are essential.

Warnings: The hypoglycaemic effect of glibenclamide may be enhanced by dicoumarol, monoamine oxidase inhibitors, beta-adrenergic blocking agents, sulphonamides, phenylbutazone, chloramphenicol, cyclophosphamide, benzafibrate, clofibrate, fenfluramine, sulphinpyrazone, tetracycline compounds and salicylates or diminished by adrenaline, corticosteroids, oral contraceptives, phenothiazine derivatives, thyroid hormones, nicotinic acid (high dose), diuretics and abuse of laxatives.

There is no information on the use of Daonil in human pregnancy but it has been in wide, general use for many years without apparent ill consequence. Animal studies have shown no hazard.

Nursing mothers: It has not yet been established whether glibenclamide is transferred to human milk. However, other sulphonylureas have been found in milk and there is no evidence to suggest that glibenclamide differs from the group in this respect.

Overdosage: Hypoglycaemia may be treated in the conscious patient by the administration of glucose, or three to four lumps of table sugar with water. This may be repeated as necessary.

If the patient is comatose, glucose should be administered as an intravenous infusion and the patient monitored. Bolus glucose injections are not recommended because of the possibility of rebound hypoglycaemia which may be delayed. Alternatively, glucagon may be administered in a dose of 1 mg subcutaneously or intramuscularly to restore consciousness.

Side-effects: Adverse reactions serious enough to warrant discontinuation of treatment are uncommon, but mild gastro-intestinal or allergic skin reactions have occurred. Reversible leucopenia and thrombocytopenia have been reported but are rare. Treatment with sulphonylureas has been associated with occasional disturbances of liver function and cholestatic jaundice. If hepatitis or cholestatic jaundice occurs, glibenclamide should be discontinued. Hypoglycaemic symptoms have occasionally been reported when the dose has been administered without due regard to the patients' dietary habits.

Pharmaceutical precautions Daonil Tablets should be stored in a cool, dry place protected from light and in containers similar to those of the manufacturer.

Legal category POM.

Package quantities Daonil and Semi-Daonil Tablets are available in blister packs of 28 (OP).

Further information Orally administered Daonil is rapidly absorbed. It is substantially metabolised prior to its excretion in urine and bile. Some of the metabolites have hypoglycaemic activity, markedly reduced in comparison with the parent compound and usually without clinical significance.

Product licence numbers

Daonil Tablets 5 mg	0086/5002.
Semi-Daonil Tablets 2.5 mg	0086/0068.

FERTIRAL*

Presentation Fertiral contains Gonadorelin BP (luteinising hormone releasing hormone) 500 micrograms in 1 ml aqueous solution presented as a 2 ml ampoule containing 1000 micrograms. The solution also contains sodium chloride, sodium dihydrogen phosphate and benzyl alcohol as excipients.

Uses Amenorrhoea and infertility associated with:
1. Hypogonadotrophic hypogonadism.
2. Multifollicular ovaries: where this finding implies that pulse frequency and amplitude of endogenous LHRH are abnormal, e.g. in patients in whom weight related amenorrhoea has been corrected.

Dosage and administration Gonadorelin is given by means of an intermittent pulsatile pump, a pulse being delivered every 90 minutes over the entire 24 hour period. Treatment should be initiated by subcutaneous infusion but in some patients intravenous therapy may be required. Dosage should be determined individually but a starting dose of 10–20 micrograms given over 1 minute every 90 minutes is recommended. Treatment should be continued until conception occurs, or for a maximum of 6 months. Ultrasound of ovary or oestradiol or urinary oestrogen levels or basal body temperature measurements may be used to monitor treatment. (*See also Pharmaceutical Precautions*).

Contra-indications, warnings, etc Gonadorelin should not be used in patients with endometriotic cysts or polycystic disease of the ovaries. Treatment with gonadorelin should not be started in women with weight related amenorrhoea until the weight has been corrected and the ponderal index is above 19.5. Gonadorelin may be discontinued once evidence of conception has been obtained. Pituitary adenoma is a relative contra-indication.

Side-effects: Side-effects are very rare. A skin rash has been reported at the infusion site. The following reactions have been reported after treatment with the high dose diagnostic preparation of gonadorelin: Abdominal pain, nausea, headache and increased menstrual bleeding.

Overdosage: Treatment of overdose should be symptomatic.

Pharmaceutical precautions Gonadorelin should be infused using a pulsatile pump e.g. Graseby MS 27 with an infusion set of minimum volume e.g. Butterfly 25 or Butterfly 19 cannulae (Abbott). For intravenous administration heparin is added to the gonadorelin solution at a concentration of 150 IU/ml.

Store in a cool dark place. Use normal saline to dilute if necessary; use immediately after dilution. The solution is stable in the pump, at about body temperature, for 4 days.

Fertiral contains benzyl alcohol 1% as a preservative.

Legal category POM.

Package quantities Fertiral is available in packs of 5 × 2 ml ampoules.

Further information Results from clinical studies show a rate of multiple pregnancy very similar to that of the normal population.

Product licence number 0086/0093.

FIBROGAMMIN P*

Presentation Fibrogammin P, heat treated Factor XIII Concentrate, is presented in clear glass vials, each containing approximately 85 mg lyophilised concentrate, having Factor XIII activity equivalent to at least 250 ml fresh pooled citrated plasma. Each vial is provided with an ampoule containing 4 ml Water for Injections for reconstitution of the lyophilisate. The concentrate also contains albumin, glucose and sodium chloride as excipients.

Uses Factor XIII Concentrate is indicated for replacement therapy in congenital Factor XIII deficiency.

Dosage and administration The contents of one vial should be dissolved in 4 ml of Water for Injections and the solution should be administered by slow intravenous injection.

When reconstituted, the dosage for congenital Factor XIII deficiency is as follows:

1. *Prophylaxis of haemorrhages:* 8–12 ml at intervals of 4 weeks. The interval is to be shortened if spontaneous haemorrhages develop.
2. *Before surgical operations:* In the case of adults 40 ml immediately before the operation, and 8–12 ml on each of the following 5 days. Children receive a correspondingly lower dose.
3. *Therapy:* In the case of severe haemorrhages and extensive haematomas, 8–20 ml daily until the bleeding has stopped.

In the case of larger operations and severe haemorrhages the aim is to maintain normal values. It is advisable to monitor the substitution therapy with a Factor XIII determination.

Children: In children under the age of 14 years, the dose is normally half the adult dose.

Contra-indications, warnings, etc Factor XIII Concentrate is contra-indicated for patients with fresh thrombosis because of its fibrin-stabilising effect.

In rare cases allergic reactions and a rise in temperature may be observed. In very rare cases the development of Factor XIII inhibitors may occur.

Pharmaceutical precautions Factor XIII Concentrate should be stored at 4°C. Prepared solutions of Factor XIII Concentrate should be used immediately and any remainder discarded. No additives or diluents should be used other than pyrogen-free Water for Injections.

Legal category POM.

Package quantities The product is supplied as single vials each with an ampoule containing Water for Injections.

Further information Fibrogammin P, Factor XIII Concentrate, is a purified standardised and concentrated preparation of human coagulation factor XIII, fibrin-stabilising factor. The method of production of Factor XIII Concentrate has been shown to inactivate experimental artificial contamination with DNA viruses (EBV, CMV, HSV) and RNA viruses (HIV−1, Rous sarcoma-, measles-, mumps-, rubella- and polio-virus). In addition, every batch is routinely tested for freedom from HB_sAg. However, no procedure has been shown to be totally effective in removing hepatitis infectivity.

Fibrogammin P prepared from starting material experimentally infected with hepatitis B virus was given to chimpanzees, and an inactivation rate of $10^{4.5}$ was demonstrated.

Product licence number 0086/0047.

FRISIUM*

Presentation Frisium capsules each contain 10 mg clobazam. Frisium is presented as hard gelatin capsules coloured powder blue opaque with 'Frisium' printed on both cap and body. Excipients include lactose.

Uses Frisium is a 1,5-benzodiazepine indicated for the short-term relief (2–4 weeks) only of anxiety that is severe, disabling or subjecting the individual to unacceptable distress, occurring alone or in association with insomnia or short-term psychosomatic, organic or psychotic illness. The use of Frisium to treat short-term 'mild' anxiety is inappropriate and unsuitable. Frisium may be used as adjunctive therapy in epilepsy.

Dosage and administration The usual anxiolytic dose for adults is 20–30 mg daily in divided doses or as a single dose given at night. Doses of up to 60 mg daily have been used in the treatment of adult in-patients with severe anxiety.

The lowest dose that can control symptoms should be used. It should not be used for longer than 4 weeks. Long term chronic use as an anxiolytic is not recommended. Treatment should always be withdrawn gradually. Patients who have taken Frisium for a long time may require a longer period during which doses are reduced.

Epilepsy: In epilepsy a starting dose of 20–30 mg/day is recommended, increasing as necessary up to a maximum of 60 mg daily. A break in therapy may be beneficial if drug exhaustion develops, recommencing therapy at a low dose.

Elderly: Doses of 10–20 mg daily in anxiety may be used in the elderly, who are more sensitive to the effects of psychoactive agents.

Children: When prescribed for children over three years of age, dosage should not exceed half the recommended adult dose. There is insufficient experience of the use of Frisium in children under three years of age to enable any dosage recommendation to be made.

Contra-indications, warnings, etc
Contra-indications: Frisium should not be used in patients known to be hypersensitive to benzodiazepines.

Frisium should not be used in phobic and obsessional states or for the treatment of chronic psychosis. It should not be used alone to treat depression or anxiety associated with depression as suicide may be precipitated in such patients.

Precautions, warnings: Frisium is a benzodiazepine derivative and, in common with other members of this group, may potentiate the effects of central nervous system depressant drugs, such as alcohol, analgesics, hypnotics and neuroleptics.

Addition of Frisium to established anticonvulsant medication may cause a change in plasma levels of these drugs. If used as an adjuvant in epilepsy the dosage of Frisium should be determined by monitoring the EEG and the plasma levels of the drugs checked.

The ability to drive or operate machinery may be impaired in individuals who are particularly sensitive to the effects of Frisium or in patients taking high doses.

Amnesia may occur with benzodiazepines. In cases of loss or bereavement psychological adjustment may be inhibited by benzodiazepines.

Disinhibiting effects may be manifested in various ways. Suicide may be precipitated in patients who are depressed and aggressive behaviour towards self and others may be precipitated. Extreme caution should therefore be used in prescribing benzodiazepines in patients with personality disorders.

Benzodiazepines should be used in reduced doses in patients with impaired renal or hepatic function.

Withdrawal from benzodiazepines may be associated with physiological and psychological symptoms. Withdrawal symptoms occur with benzodiazepines following normal therapeutic doses given for short periods of time.

Respiratory function should be monitored in patients with acute severe respiratory insufficiency.

Pregnancy: There is little information on the use of Frisium in early pregnancy but no untoward effects have been found in animal studies. However, there are reports of a possible association between malformations in infants and the administration of other benzodiazepines in early pregnancy. Frisium should not be used in the first trimester of pregnancy and in the later stages only if there are strong indications for its use.

Nursing mothers: Clobazam has been detected in the breast milk of nursing mothers, but the effect on the neonate is not known. However, breast feeding should be stopped during clobazam treatment.

Overdosage: Muscle weakness, ataxia, drowsiness and sedation may occur and, after very high doses, the patient may lose consciousness. The treatment of overdosage is symptomatic. The stomach should be emptied as soon as possible by gastric lavage and general supportive measures should be undertaken as necessary.

Side-effects: Side-effects such as drowsiness, dizziness or dryness of the mouth, constipation, loss of appetite, nausea, or a fine tremor of the fingers have been reported. These are more likely to occur at the beginning of treatment and often disappear with continued treatment or a reduction in dose. Paradoxical reactions, such as restlessness or irritability, may occur. Isolated cases of skin reactions, such as rashes or urticaria, have been observed.

After prolonged use of benzodiazepines, impairment of consciousness, sometimes combined with respiratory disorders, has been reported in very rare cases, particularly in elderly patients: it sometimes persists for some length of time. These disorders have not been seen so far under clobazam treatment.

When used as an adjuvant in the treatment of epilepsy, this preparation may in rare cases cause restlessness and muscle weakness.

As with other benzodiazepines, the therapeutic benefit must be balanced against the risk of habituation and dependence during prolonged use.

Pharmaceutical precautions Frisium capsules should be stored in a cool, dry place in the original container or in containers similar to those of the manufacturer.

Legal category CD (Sch 4), POM.

Package quantities Frisium is available as 10 mg capsules packed in blister packs of 30 capsules (original packs).

Further information Experimental evidence shows that, in general, when given as a single dose of up to 20 mg or in divided doses of up to 30 mg Frisium does not affect psychomotor function, skilled performance, memory or higher mental function. However, individuals who are sensitive to the effects of Frisium may be adversely affected, particularly at the beginning of treatment.

Clobazam may be supplied at NHS expense if prescribed for epilepsy and prescription is endorsed 'S3B' (or 'S2B' in Scotland).

Product licence number 0086/0065.

HAEMACCEL* INFUSION SOLUTION

Presentation 3.5% colloidal infusion solution for plasma substitution.

Composition:

Haemaccel contains	*Per 500 ml bottle*	*Per 1,000 ml*
Polygeline (degraded and modified gelatin of average molecular weight 35,000)	17.50 g	35.00 g
Cations		
Na^+	72.50 mmol	145.00 mmol
K^+	2.55 mmol	5.10 mmol
Ca^{++}	3.13 mmol	6.25 mmol
Anions		
Cl^-	72.50 mmol	145.00 mmol
PO_4^{---} and SO_4^{--}	traces	traces

Isoionic equilibrium is made up by the polypeptides. There are no preservatives.

Physico-Chemical Properties:

Viscosity ratio	1.7–1.8
Dynamic viscosity (at 37°C)	1.15–1.20 kPa.s (cP)
The iso-electric point is at	pH 4.7 ± 0.3
pH of the infusion solution	7.3 ± 0.3
Colloid osmotic pressure (at 37°C)	3.432–3.824 kPa (350–390 mmH_2O)
Gel point	below +3°C
Appearance	straw-coloured
Nitrogen equivalent of polygeline	3.15 g in 500 ml

Uses

1. As a plasma volume substitute in the initial treatment of hypovolaemic shock due to:
   (a) Haemorrhage (visible or concealed)
   (b) Burns, peritonitis, pancreatitis, crush injuries
2. Fluid replacement in plasma exchange.
3. Extra-corporeal circulation.
4. Isolated organ perfusion.
5. As a carrier solution for insulin.

Dosage and administration Haemaccel should be administered intravenously in a volume approximately equal to the estimated blood loss.

In common with all intravenous infusion solutions, Haemaccel should, if possible, be warmed to body temperature before use. However, in emergencies, it may be infused at ambient temperatures.

Infusion rate: The rate of infusion is determined by the condition of the patient. Normally 500 ml will be infused in not less than 60 minutes, but in emergencies Haemaccel can be rapidly infused. Losses of up to 25% of the blood volume can be replaced by Haemaccel alone.

Plastic infusion bottle: It is advisable to disinfect the bottle top then pull out the plastic ring. A hole will be exposed through which the piercing needle of an infusion set can be pushed. There is no need to disinfect the cap further.

Hypovolaemic shock: 500–1,000 ml Haemaccel should be infused intravenously initially. Up to 1,500 ml blood loss can be replaced entirely by Haemaccel. For between 1,500 ml and 4,000 ml blood loss, fluid replacement should be with equal volumes of Haemaccel and blood, given separately (see Pharmaceutical precautions). For losses over 4,000 ml the separate infusions should be in the ratio of two parts blood to one part Haemaccel. The haematocrit should not be allowed to fall below 25%.

Burns: It is suggested that at least 1 ml Haemaccel be infused per kg body weight, multiplied by the % of body surface burned for each 24 hours for two days, e.g. if a 70 kg person has burns covering 10% of body surface, then the dosage of Haemaccel should be at least 1 (ml) × 70 (kg) × 10(%) = 700 ml/24 hours. Additional crystalloid solutions should be given to cover the normal fluid loss, i.e. about 2,000 ml per 24 hours. In severe burns, additional protein and vitamin therapy may be required. The volume of colloid and crystalloid given should be varied according to the clinical response of the patient, the urine volume, its specific gravity and osmolality, etc.

Plasma exchange: Haemaccel should be given either alone or in combination with other replacement fluids in a volume adequate to replace the plasma removed. Up to 2 litres have been given as sole replacement fluid.

Contra-indications, warnings, etc There are no absolute contra-indications to the use of Haemaccel. However, caution should be used in infusing Haemaccel in any patient likely to develop circulatory overloading (e.g. severe congestive cardiac failure). Inappropriately rapid administration of Haemaccel, especially to normovolaemic patients, may cause the release of vasoactive substances. The exact mechanism of such histamine release has not been clearly defined. Histamine release may be especially hazardous in patients with known allergic conditions such as asthma. In these cases prophylaxis with H_1 or H_2 receptor antagonists is advisable. In the event of histamine release, the infusion should be discontinued and appropriate action taken with antihistamines, etc.

In the event of anaphylactic shock, the infusion should be discontinued and adrenalin (5–10 ml of 1:10,000 by slow intravenous injection or 0.5–1.0 ml of 1:1,000 by i.m./s.c. injection) should immediately be given. Administration of adrenalin should be repeated every 15 minutes until improvement occurs. Circulatory collapse requires volume replacement, preferably monitored by a central venous pressure line. Large volumes of electrolyte solution may be necessary, because in severe anaphylactic shock, plasma loss may constitute up to 40% of the plasma volume. A slow intravenous injection of an H_1 antagonist such as 10–20 mg chlorpheniramine may be given.

Haemaccel contains calcium ions and caution should be observed in patients being treated with cardiac glycosides.

Pregnancy: Haemorrhage around the time of childbirth or blood loss during other obstetric or gynaecological procedures may necessitate plasma volume replacement. Haemaccel has been used for many years for the initial treatment in such cases without apparent ill consequence. If plasma volume replacement is needed during pregnancy, Haemaccel may be used if blood is not available.

Pharmaceutical precautions There are no special storage requirements. Haemaccel will gel below 3°C; however, warming will reverse this. Freezing does not alter its physico-chemical characteristics in any way. Haemaccel contains no preservatives; any unused fluid should be discarded once a bottle has been opened.

Haemaccel may be mixed with other infusion solutions (e.g. saline, dextrose, Ringer's solution, etc.) or with heparinised blood. Sterility must be maintained. Compatible water-soluble drugs may be infused in Haemaccel, e.g. insulin, streptokinase, etc. Any additive should be injected into the bottle through the small hole located next to the pull-ring.

Citrated blood should *not* be mixed with Haemaccel since clotting of the blood may occur due to the presence of calcium ions in Haemaccel. However, citrated blood may be infused before or after Haemaccel provided that there is adequate flushing of the infusion set.

Do not use Haemaccel if the seal has been broken or if the contents are cloudy.

Haemaccel has a shelf life of five years at storage temperatures of up to 25°C.

Legal category POM.

Package quantities Available in 500 ml plastic bottles.

Further information Haemaccel is of particular value as a volume replacement as it promotes a demonstrable osmotic diuresis, thereby protecting the kidneys. Provided that the recipient's red cells are suspended in saline rather than serum it does not interfere with subsequent blood grouping and cross matching, nor does it interfere with the coagulation system. It is non-immunogenic and does not induce antibody formation.

Product licence number 0086/0040.

HAEMATE P* ▼

Presentation Haemate P (Factor VIII HS, heat treated) is presented in clear glass vials containing 250 or 500 units of Factor VIII as a lyophilised concentrate. When reconstituted with the vial of solvent provided, the solution will contain 25 IU Factor VIII per ml.

Uses Prophylaxis and therapy of haemorrhages in Hemophilia A and other diseases with Factor VIII deficiency.

Dosage and administration Unless prescribed otherwise the dosage should depend on the degree of Factor VIII deficiency and the extent and location of the bleeding. The amount of Factor VIII required can be estimated as follows: On administration of 1 IU/kg bodyweight a rise in Factor VIII activity by about 1% of the normal is to be expected.

In the case of the following haemorrhagic events, the Factor VIII activity should not fall below the given level (in per cent of normal) in the corresponding period:

Hemorrhagic event	*Therapeutically necessary blood level of Factor VIII*	*Period during which it is necessary to maintain the therapeutic blood level*
1. Hemorrhages into joints; Gastro-intestinal hemorrhages; Bite injuries in the oral cavity; Slighter injuries (where local therapy is unsuccessful)	10–20%	2–3 days
2. Hemorrhages into muscles; Larger injuries; Minor operations; (Teeth extractions)	20–30%	3–4 days
3. Intracranial, intra-abdominal or intrathoracic hemorrhages; Medium operations; Fractures	30–50%	4–14 days or until wound completely healed
4. Major operations	over 50%	14–21 days or until wound completely healed

The amount to be administered should always be oriented to the clinical effectiveness in the individual case. Under certain circumstances larger amounts than those calculated can be required, especially in the case of the initial dose.

In the case of major surgical interventions in particular, a precise monitoring of the substitution therapy by means of coagulation analyses is indispensable.

Administration: The contents of one vial should be dissolved, by slow swirling of the vial, in the appropriate amount of water for injection previously brought to 20°–37°C. The material will dissolve in less than 10 minutes to give a clear to slightly opalescent solution.

Injection: Using a filter needle, withdraw solution from the vial into a syringe. Inject the solution slowly (maximum 4 ml per minute) intravenously. Administration may be effected with the infusion set or with a suitable injection needle. Do not use the filter needle for injection.

Infusion: Dissolve the preparation as described and infuse slowly by means of a disposable transfusion set (with filter inset).

Contra-indications, warnings, etc
Contra-indications: None known.

Warnings: In the case of patients with known allergic diathesis, antihistamines and corticosteroids should be administered as prophylaxis. Caution should be observed in cases of impaired liver or kidney function.

In the case of massive therapy, symptoms of hypervolaemia and – in rare cases – haemolytic reactions through blood-group isoagglutinins should be watched for.

The therapeutic effect may not be achieved if the blood of the patient contains a high level of inhibitors for Factor VIII ('inhibitor hemophilia'). In such cases an attempt must be made to override the inhibitors by administration of large amounts of Factor VIII.

This concentrate has been prepared from large pools of human plasma non-reactive for hepatitis B surface antigen (HbsAg). However, such plasma may contain one or more causative agents of viral hepatitis. Haemate -P is heated to 60°C for 10 hours in solution form.

However, no procedure has been shown to be totally effective in removing hepatitis infectivity from Antihemophilic Factor (Human).

Side-effects: Haemate P is usually tolerated without reaction. Rare cases of allergic reactions and rise in temperature have been observed. Therapeutic countermeasures depend on nature and severity of the side-effect. In the case of slight reactions, corticosteroids and antihistamines may be used.

In the case of severe reactions (anaphylactic shock), immediate discontinuation of the preparation and injection of adrenalin slowly iv supplemented by high doses of corticosteroids slowly iv.

Pharmaceutical precautions Haemate P should be stored in a refrigerator at +2°C to +8°C and used on or before the expiry date given on the pack. The dissolved preparation should be used within 3 hours of reconstitution.

Legal category POM.

Package quantities The product is supplied as a single vial with an ampoule containing Water for Injections.

Further information Haemate P is a specific hemostatic agent for intravenous application in hemophilia A. The lyophilised preparation is sterile and pyrogen-free and does not contain any preservative. No fibrinogen can be detected by the Clauss method.

Haemate P is obtained from HB_sAg-negative and anti HIV-negative plasma of healthy donors. In addition the ALT in the plasma is determined and donations with pathological values are rejected. The pasteurisation process, heating to 60°C for 10 hours in solution form, has been shown to inactivate several DNA viruses (Epstein Barr, cytomegalovirus, herpes simplex and hepatitis B) and RNA viruses (rubella, mumps, measles, poliomyelitis and HIV), and the pathogens of hepatitis non-A/non-B (Hutchison Pool).

Haemate P prepared from cryoprecipitate experimentally infected with Hepatitis B virus was given to chimpanzees. After 6 and 9 months follow-up the test animals remained serologically negative.

Product licence number 0086/0100.

LASIKAL* TABLETS

Presentation Lasikal Tablets each contain 20 mg Frusemide BP and 750 mg (10 mmol K^+) slow-release potassium chloride. They are presented as film-coated, biconvex, twin-layered tablets, 12.5 mm in diameter, marked 'LK' on one side. The frusemide layer is white and the slow-release potassium chloride layer is yellow.

Excipients include lactose and Sunset Yellow.

Uses Lasikal contains a short-acting diuretic and a slow-release potassium supplement. It is intended for the treatment of oedema in patients who require potassium supplementation.

Dosage and administration The recommended initial adult dose is 2 tablets (40 mg frusemide and 20 mmol K^+) to be taken each morning. This may be increased to four tablets daily, to be taken as 2 tablets each morning and evening, or may be decreased to 1 tablet each morning, according to clinical response.

Lasikal tablets must be swallowed whole.

Children: Lasikal tablets cannot be sub-divided and are unsuitable for paediatric use.

Elderly: Frusemide and potassium may both be excreted more slowly in the elderly.

Contra-indications, warnings, etc

Contra-indications: Lasikal is contra-indicated in anuria, hyperkalaemia, precomatose states associated with liver cirrhosis, Addison's disease and in patients taking potassium-sparing diuretics. Hypersensitivity to frusemide or sulphonamides is also a contra-indication.

Warnings: Patients with prostatic hypertrophy or impairment of micturition have an increased risk of developing acute retention.

Where indicated, steps should be taken to correct hypotension or hypovolaemia before commencing therapy.

The dosage of concurrently administered cardiac glycosides or antihypertensive agents may require adjustment.

ACE inhibitors should not be used in combination with Lasikal as serum potassium levels may be increased.

The toxic effects of nephrotoxic antibiotics may be increased by concomitant administration of potent diuretics such as frusemide.

Latent diabetes may become manifest or the insulin requirements of diabetic patients may increase.

Care should be exercised when treating patients with renal insufficiency because of the risk of hyperkalaemia.

In common with other diuretics, serum lithium levels may be increased when lithium is given concomitantly with frusemide, necessitating adjustment of the lithium dosage.

Certain non-steroidal anti-inflammatory agents (e.g. indomethacin, acetyl salicyclic acid) may attenuate the action of frusemide and may cause renal failure in cases of pre-existing hypovolaemia.

Frusemide may sometimes attenuate the effects of other drugs (e.g. the effects of antidiabetics and of pressor amines) and sometimes potentiate them (e.g. the effects of salicylates, theophylline, lithium and curare-type muscle relaxants).

Interactions have also been reported with ototoxic antibiotics. In caes of concomitant glucocorticoid therapy or abuse of laxitives, the risk of an increased potassium loss should be borne in mind.

Precautions: Results of animal work, in general, show no hazardous effect of frusemide in pregnancy. There is clinical evidence of safety of the drug in the third trimester of human pregnancy; however, frusemide should be used in pregnancy only if strictly indicated and for short term treatment.

Nursing mothers: As frusemide may inhibit lactation or pass into breast milk, it should be used with caution in nursing mothers.

Overdosage: In cases of overdose there is a danger of dehydration and electrolyte depletion due to excessive diuresis. Treatment should therefore be aimed at fluid replacement and correction of the electrolyte imbalance.

Side-effects: Lasikal is generally well tolerated. Side-effects of a minor nature such as nausea, malaise or gastric upset may occur but are not usually severe enough to necessitate withdrawal of treatment.

As with other diuretics, electrolytes and water balance may be disturbed as a result of diuresis after prolonged therapy. This may cause symptoms such as headache, hypotension or muscle cramps.

Serum calcium levels may be reduced; in very rare cases tetany has been observed. Nephrocalcinosis has been reported in premature infants.

Isolated cases of acute pancreatitis have been reported after long-term diuretic (including frusemide) treatment. Disorders of hearing after frusemide are rare and, in most cases reversible. They may occur if frusemide is injected too rapidly, particularly in patients with renal insufficiency.

As with other diuretics a transient rise in creatinine and urea levels has also been reported with frusemide.

The incidence of allergic reactions, such as skin rash, photosensitivity, vasculitis, fever or interstitial nephritis, is very low, but when these occur treatment should be withdrawn.

In common with other sulphonamide-based diuretics, hyperuricaemia may occur and, in rare cases, clinical gout may be precipitated.

Serum cholesterol and triglyceride levels may rise during frusemide treatment but will usually return to normal within 6 months.

Bone marrow depression has been reported as a rare complication and necessitates withdrawal of treatment.

Pre-existing metabolic alkalosis (e.g. in decompensated cirrhosis of the liver) may be aggravated by frusemide treatment.

Reduced mental alertness may impair ability to drive or operate dangerous machinery.

Pharmaceutical precautions Lasikal should be stored in a cool dry place, protected from light, in the original container or in containers similar to those of the manufacturer. Lasikal tablets should be dispensed in moisture-tight containers which offer protection from light.

Legal category POM.

Package quantities Lasikal is available in containers of 100 tablets.

Further information Frusemide produces a prompt and effective diuresis which lasts for approximately four hours following oral administration. The potassium chloride in Lasikal tablets is contained in an inert matrix which allows slow release of potassium ions, thereby helping to avoid high local K^+ ion concentrations in the intestine.

Ghost tablets may appear in the patient's faeces.

Product licence number 0086/0060.

LASILACTONE* CAPSULES

Presentation Lasilactone Capsules each contain 20 mg of Frusemide BP and 50 mg Spironolactone BP. They are presented as hard gelatin capsules with a light blue opaque cap and white opaque body. Excipients include lactose.

Uses Lasilactone contains a short-acting diuretic and a long-acting aldosterone antagonist. It is indicated in the treatment of resistant oedema where this is associated with secondary hyperaldosteronism; conditions include chronic congestive cardiac failure and hepatic cirrhosis.

Treatment with Lasilactone should be reserved for cases refractory to a diuretic alone at conventional dosage.

This fixed ratio combination should only be used if titration with the component drugs separately indicates that this product is appropriate.

The use of Lasilactone in the management of essential hypertension should be restricted to patients with demonstrated hyperaldosteronism. It is recommended that in these patients also, this combination should only be used if titration with the component drugs separately indicates that this product is appropriate.

Dosage and administration In accordance with the recommendations on usage given above the dosage of Lasilactone will normally be in the range of 1 to 4 capsules daily (20–80 mg Lasix and 50–200 mg spironolactone).

Children: The product is not suitable for use in children.

Elderly: Frusemide and spironolactone may both be excreted more slowly in the elderly.

Contra-indications, warnings, etc

Contra-indications: Lasilactone should not be given in renal insufficiency (creatinine clearance <30 ml/minute $\equiv$ serum creatinine of about 1.8–2.0 mg/100 ml), anuric states, hyperkalaemia or Addison's disease. Hypersensitivity to frusemide, spironolactone or sulphonamides.

Warnings: Patients with prostatic hypertrophy or impairment of micturition have an increased risk of developing acute retention. Caution should also be exercised in the presence of liver disease as hepatic coma may be precipitated in susceptible cases. Administration of Lasilactone should be avoided in the presence of hyperkalaemia and hyponatraemia. Concomitant administration of triamterene, amiloride or potassium supplements is not recommended as hyperkalaemia may result. Where indicated, steps shoud be taken to correct hypotension, hypovolaemia and severe hypokalaemia before starting therapy.

The dosage of concurrently administered cardiac glycosides or hypotensive agents may require adjustment.

ACE inhibitors should not be used in combination with Lasilactone as serum potassium levels may be increased.

The toxic effects of nephrotoxic antibiotics may be potentiated by concurrent administration of potent diuretics such as frusemide.

Latent diabetes may become manifest; the insulin requirements of diabetic patients may increase.

In common with other diuretics, serum lithium levels may be increased when lithium is given concomitantly with frusemide, necessitating adjustment of the lithium dosage.

Certain non-steroidal anti-inflammatory agents have been shown to antagonise the action of diuretics such as frusemide and may cause renal failure in cases of pre-existing hypovolaemia. Frusemide may sometimes attenuate the effects of other drugs (e.g. the effects of antidiabetics and of pressor amines) and sometimes potentiate them (e.g. the effects of salicylates, theophylline, lithium and curare-type muscle relaxants). Salicylates may attenuate the effect of spironolactone.

Concomitant glucocorticoid medication or abuse of laxatives may lead to potassium deficiency. In the presence of potassium deficiency the effect of cardiac glycosides may be enhanced.

Interactions have also been reported with carbenoxolone and with ototoxic antibiotics.

Carcinogenicity: Spironolactone has been shown to produce tumours in rats when administered at high doses over a long period of time. The significance of these findings with respect to clinical use is not certain. However, the long-term use of spironolactone in young patients requires careful consideration of the benefits and the potential hazard involved.

Precautions: Caution should be observed in patients liable to electrolyte deficiency.

Results of animal work, in general, show no hazardous effect of frusemide in pregnancy. There is clinical evidence of the safety of the drug in the third trimester of human pregnancy; however, frusemide should be used in pregnancy only if strictly indicated and for short term treatment.

Spironolactone or its metabolites may cross the placental barrier.

Nursing mothers: Lasilactone is contra-indicated in nursing mothers because canrenone, a metabolite of the spironolactone component of this preparation, appears in breast milk. (Frusemide may inhibit lactation or pass into breast milk).

Overdosage: In cases of overdosage with Lasilactone there is a danger of severe electrolyte disturbance and dehydration due to excessive diuresis. Signs of overdosage may include drowsiness, mental confusion, nausea, vomiting, dizziness or diarrhoea. Electrolyte disturbances such as hyperkalaemia and hyponatraemia may be induced. Hyperkalaemia may be manifested clinically by paraesthesia, weakness, flaccid paralysis or muscle spasm and may be difficult to distinguish from hypokalaemia. Electrocardiographic changes may be the earliest signs of potassium disturbances.

Treatment should be aimed at the replacement of fluid and the correction of any electrolyte imbalance.

Side-effects: Frusemide is generally well tolerated. Side-effects of a minor nature such as nausea, malaise or gastric upset may occur but are not usually severe enough to necessitate withdrawal of treatment.

As with other diuretics, electrolytes and water balance may be disturbed as a result of diuresis after prolonged therapy. This may cause symptoms such as headache, hypotension or muscle cramps.

Calcium depletion may occur. Nephrocalcinosis has been reported in premature infants treated with frusemide.

The incidence of allergic reactions, such as skin rashes (including photosensitivity reactions), vasculitis, fever or interstitial nephritis, is very low, but when these occur treatment should be withdrawn.

Auditory disorders and acute pancreatitis have been reported with high dose parenteral frusemide.

A transient rise in creatinine and urea levels has also been reported.

In common with other sulphonamide-based diuretics, the administration of frusemide may induce a rise in serum uric acid; in rare cases, clinical gout may be precipitated.

Serum cholesterol and triglyceride levels may rise during frusemide treatment but will usually return to normal within six months.

Bone marrow depression has been reported as a rare complication of Lasix therapy and necessitates withdrawal of treatment.

Spironolactone has been reported to induce gastrointestinal intolerance and also drowsiness, headache, ataxia, lethargy and mental confusion. Mastodynia and reversible gynaecomastia may occur. Maculopapular or erythematous cutaneous eruptions have been reported rarely. In women, menstrual irregularities and hirsuitism may be seen and in men impairment of potency. Spironolactone may cause vocal changes in the form of hoarseness and deepening of the voice in women and increase in pitch in men. These vocal changes in both sexes may be irreversible. Therefore the risk should be carefully considered for patients whose voice is of professional importance e.g. singers, teachers, actors.

Reduced mental alertness may impair the ability to drive or operate dangerous machinery.

Pharmaceutical precautions Lasilactone should be stored at ambient temperature, protected from light, in the original container or in containers similar to those of the manufacturer.

Legal category POM.

Package quantities Lasilactone is available in blister strips packed in cartons of 28 capsules (original packs).

Further information Lasix is an effective short-acting diuretic; diuresis usually commences within one hour and lasts for four to six hours.

Spironolactone is a competitive inhibitor of aldosterone and thus increases sodium excretion whilst reducing potassium loss at the distal renal tubule. It has a slow and prolonged action, maximum response being usually attained after 2-3 days' treatment.

Product licence number 0086/0039.

LASIPRESSIN*

Presentation Lasipressin Tablets each contain 20 mg Frusemide BP and 40 mg penbutolol sulphate. They are presented as yellowish-white, oblong, film-coated tablets, with a score mark on both sides. Excipients include lactose.

Uses In the management of mild or moderate hypertension.

Dosage and administration The normal dose is one tablet each morning. This can be increased, if necessary, to one tablet twice daily.

Children: Lasipressin is not suitable for use in children.

Elderly: Frusemide may be excreted more slowly in the elderly. Penbutolol undergoes metabolism in the liver and is predominantly excreted by the kidney.

Contra-indications, warnings, etc
Contra-indications: Severe bradycardia (pulse rates below 50/minute), conduction defects (2nd and 3rd degree AV block, sinoatrial block, sick-sinus syndrome), digitalis refractory heart failure, cardiogenic shock, metabolic acidosis, bronchial asthma, chronic obstructive airways disease, allergic rhinitis, peripheral circulatory disorders, concurrent administration of general anaesthetics with myocardial depressant activity, anuria, hepatic coma, uncompensated hypokalaemia, hyponatraemia and hypovolaemia with or without hypotension, the terminal stages of renal failure, phaeochromocytoma not treated with alpha-adrenergic receptor blockers, hypersensitivity to frusemide or sulphonamides.

Warnings: Cessation of therapy with all beta-blockers should be gradual. Close observation is recommended when Lasipressin is administered to patients receiving catecholamine-depleting drugs such as reserpine and guanethidine or other negatively inotropic drugs. The dosage of concurrently administered cardiac glycosides or antihypertensive agents or drugs causing bradycardia may require adjustment. Simultaneous administration of anti-arrhythmic agents and calcium antagonists of the verapamil type increases the risk of conduction disorders of the heart or bradycardia. If nifedipine is administered concomitantly with Lasipressin there may be a marked fall in blood pressure.

A marked fall in blood pressure may be seen when ACE inhibitors are added to frusemide therapy. The dose of frusemide should be reduced, or the drug stopped, before initiating the ACE inhibitor.

The toxic effects of nephrotoxic antibiotics may be increased.

Patients with diabetes or a predisposition to diabetes should be carefully monitored. Frusemide may cause latent diabetes to become manifest or the insulin requirements of diabetics to increase. Penbutolol may mask the symptoms of hypoglycaemia.

Patients with prostatic hypertrophy or impairment of micturition have an increased risk of developing acute retention when taking frusemide.

Serum lithium levels may be increased when lithium is given concomitantly with frusemide, necessitating adjustment of the lithium dosage.

Certain non-steroidal anti-inflammatory agents (e.g. indomethacin, acetyl salicylic acid) may attenuate the action of frusemide and may cause renal failure in pre-existing hypovolaemia.

Frusemide may sometimes attenuate the effects of other drugs (e.g. the effects of antidiabetics and of pressor amines) and sometimes potentiate them (e.g. the effects of salicylates, theophylline, lithium and curare-type muscle relaxants). Interactions have also been reported with ototoxic antibiotics. Corticosteroids may cause sodium retention and exacerbate potassium loss. If during combined treatment with clonidine, medication has to be discontinued, the Lasipressin should be withdrawn first to prevent an excessive rise in blood pressure after withdrawal of the clonidine.

Precautions: Caution should be observed in patients liable to or sensitive to electrolyte deficiency.

Pregnancy: Studies in animals with the component drugs have not shown any evidence of teratogenicity. However, it is recommended that Lasipressin should not be given in pregnancy.

Nursing mothers: As frusemide may inhibit lactation or may pass into the breast milk, Lasipressin should be used with caution in nursing mothers.

Overdosage: Excessive bradycardia or hypotension may be counteracted with 1–2 mg atropine intravenously followed, if necessary, by a beta-receptor stimulant such as isoprenaline 25 micrograms intravenously. Excessive diuresis may cause dehydration and electrolyte (sodium, potassium and calcium) depletion, treatment should be aimed at fluid replacement and the correction of electrolyte imbalance.

Side-effects: Penbutolol: There have been occasional reports of dizziness, drowsiness, headache, sweating, cold extremities, insomnia, mental disorders (e.g. depressive moods, anxiety, hallucinations) and gastro-intestinal disturbance. Rare isolated cases of bradycardia, which could lead to atrioventricular conduction disorders and myocardial insufficiency, have been observed.

As with other beta-blocking agents, penbutolol may precipitate bronchospasm and heart failure in susceptible patients. However, the incidence of these side-effects is low, possibly due to the partial protection afforded by the intrinsic sympathomimetic effect of penbutolol. Anginal attacks may be aggravated and triggered in Prinzmetal angina. The incidence of skin rash and/or dry eyes associated with the use of beta-blockers is small, and, in most cases, symptoms have cleared when treatment was withdrawn. Discontinuation of the drug should be considered if there is no adequate explanation for such a reaction.

Impairment of male potency may occur.

An increase in blood lipids (triglycerides) is possible.

Frusemide: Generally well tolerated. Side-effects of a minor nature such as nausea, malaise or gastric upset may occur but are not usually severe enough to necessitate withdrawal of treatment.

Side-effects related to electrolyte and water excretion may be encountered. Potassium, calcium or sodium depletion may occur. Headaches or hypotension may occur.

If salt intake is too severely restricted sodium deficiency may result in an acute fall in blood pressure, calf cramps, loss of appetite, a feeling of weakness, dizziness, drowsiness, vomiting or confusion.

Auditory disorders and acute pancreatitis have been reported with high dose parenteral frusemide. As with other diuretics a transient rise in creatinine and urea levels has also been reported with frusemide.

The incidence of allergic reactions, such as skin rashes, photosensitivity, vasculitis, fever or intestitial nephritis, is very low, but when these occur treatment should be withdrawn. Hyperuricaemia may occur and, in rare cases, clinical gout may be precipitated.

Serum cholesterol and triglyceride levels may rise during frusemide treatment but will usually return to normal within six months.

Bone marrow depression has been reported as a rare complication with Lasix and necessitates withdrawal of treatment.

Reduced mental alertness may impair ability to drive or operate dangerous machinery.

Pharmaceutical precautions Lasipressin tablets should be stored in a cool, dry place in containers similar to those of the manufacturer.

Legal category POM.

Package quantities Lasipressin tablets are available in blister packs of 30 (original packs).

Further information Nil.

Product licence number 0086/0087.

LASIX* TABLETS 20 mg
LASIX* TABLETS 40 mg

Presentation Lasix Tablets 20 mg each contain 20 mg Frusemide BP. They are presented as white, circular, biplanar tablets, 6 mm in diameter, one side bearing the Hoechst insignia, the other scored and bearing the letters DLF on either side of the score mark.

Lasix Tablets 40 mg each contain 40 mg Frusemide BP. They are presented as white, circular, biplanar tablets, 8 mm in diameter, one side bearing the Hoechst insignia, the other scored and bearing the letters DLI on one side of the score mark and '40' on the other.

Excipients include lactose.

Uses Lasix is a diuretic recommended for use in all indications when a prompt and effective diuresis is required. Indications for Lasix Tablets 40 mg include cardiac, pulmonary, hepatic and renal oedema, peripheral oedema due to mechanical obstruction or venous insufficiency and hypertension.

Lasix Tablets 20 mg are indicated for the maintenance therapy of mild oedema of any origin.

Dosage and administration Lasix has an exceptionally wide therapeutic range, the effect being proportional to the dosage. Lasix is best given as a single dose either daily or on alternate days.

The usual initial daily dose is 40 mg. This may require adjustment until the effective dose is achieved. In mild cases, 20 mg daily or 40 mg on alternate days may be sufficient, whereas in cases of resistant oedema, daily doses of 80 mg and above may be used.

Children: Oral doses for children range from 1 to 3 mg/kg body weight daily up to a maximum total dose of 40 mg/day.

Elderly: In the elderly, frusemide is generally eliminated more slowly. Dosage should be titrated until the required response is achieved.

Contra-indications, warnings, etc

Contra-indications: Lasix is contra-indicated in anuria, electrolyte deficiency and pre-comatose states associated with liver cirrhosis. Hypersensitivity to frusemide or sulphonamides.

Warnings: Patients with prostatic hypertrophy or impairment of micturition have an increased risk of developing acute retention.

Where indicated, steps should be taken to correct hypotension or hypovolaemia before commencing therapy.

The dosage of concurrently administered cardiac glycosides or anti-hypertensive agents may require adjustment. A marked fall in blood pressure may be seen when ACE inhibitors are added to frusemide therapy. The dose of frusemide should be reduced, or the drug stopped, before initiating the ACE inhibitor.

The toxic effects of nephrotoxic antibiotics may be increased by concomitant administration of potent diuretics such as frusemide.

Latent diabetes may become manifest or the insulin requirements of diabetic patients may increase.

In common with other diuretics, serum lithium levels may be increased when lithium is given concomitantly with frusemide, necessitating adjustment of the lithium dosage.

Certain non-steroidal anti-inflammatory agents (e.g. indomethacin, acetyl salicylic acid) may attenuate the action of frusemide and may cause renal failure in cases of pre-existing hypovolaemia. Frusemide may sometimes attenuate the effects of other drugs (e.g. the effects of antidiabetics and of pressor amines) and sometimes potentiate them (e.g. the effects of salicylates, theophylline, lithium and curare-type muscle relaxants).

Interactions have also been reported with ototoxic antibiotics. In cases of concomitant glucocorticoid therapy or abuse of laxatives, the risk of an increased potassium loss should be borne in mind.

Precautions: Caution should be observed in patients liable to electrolyte deficiency.

Results of animal work, in general, show no hazardous effect of Lasix in pregnancy. There is clinical evidence of safety of the drug in the third trimester of human pregnancy; however, Lasix should be used in pregnancy only if strictly indicated and for short term treatment.

Nursing mothers: As Lasix may inhibit lactation or may pass into the breast milk it should be used with caution in nursing mothers.

Overdosage: In cases of overdose there is a danger of dehydration and electrolyte depletion due to excessive diuresis. Treatment should therefore be aimed at fluid replacement and correction of the electrolyte imbalance.

Side-effects: Lasix is generally well tolerated. Side-effects of a minor nature such as nausea, malaise or gastric upset may occur but are not usually severe enough to necessitate withdrawal of treatment.

As with other diuretics, electrolytes and water balance may be disturbed as a result of diuresis after prolonged therapy. This may cause symptoms such as headache, hypotension or muscle cramps.

Serum calcium levels may be reduced; in very rare cases tetany has been observed. Nephrocalcinosis has been reported in premature infants.

Isolated cases of acute pancreatitis have been reported after long-term diuretic (including frusemide) treatment. Disorders of hearing after frusemide are rare and, in most cases reversible. They may occur if frusemide is injected too rapidly, particularly in patients with renal insufficiency.

As with other diuretics a transient rise in creatinine and urea levels has also been reported with frusemide.

The incidence of allergic reactions, such as skin rashes, photosensitivity, vasculitis, fever or interstitial nephritis, is very low, but when these occur treatment should be withdrawn.

In common with other sulphonamide-based diuretics,

hyperuricaemia may occur and, in rare cases, clinical gout may be precipitated.

Serum cholesterol and triglyceride levels may rise during frusemide treatment but will usually return to normal within six months.

Bone marrow depression has been reported as a rare complication and necessitates withdrawal of treatment.

Pre-existing metabolic alkalosis (e.g. in decompensated cirrhosis of the liver) may be aggravated by frusemide treatment.

Reduced mental alertness may impair ability to drive or operate dangerous machinery.

Pharmaceutical precautions Lasix tablets should be stored in a cool dry place, protected from light, in containers similar to those of the manufacturer.

Legal category POM.

Package quantities Lasix Tablets 20 mg are available in packs of 28. Lasix Tablets 40 mg are available in packs of 28 and 250 (The pack size of 28 is an original pack).

Further information Lasix produces a prompt and effective diuresis which lasts for approximately four hours following oral administration. Therefore the time of administration can be adjusted to suit the patient's requirements.

Product licence numbers
Lasix Tablets 20 mg 0086/0017.
Lasix Tablets 40 mg 0086/5011.

LASIX* INJECTION 20 mg/2 ml
LASIX* INJECTION 50 mg/5 ml

Presentation Lasix Injection 20 mg contains 20 mg Frusemide BP in 2 ml aqueous solution. Lasix Injection 50 mg contains 50 mg Frusemide BP in 5 ml aqueous solution. The solutions also contain sodium chloride and sodium hydroxide as excipients.

Uses Lasix is a diuretic recommended for use when a prompt and effective diuresis is required. The intravenous formulation is appropriate for use in emergencies or when oral therapy is precluded. Indications include cardiac, pulmonary, hepatic and renal oedema.

Dosage and administration Lasix injection *must* always be given slowly. The diuretic effect of Lasix is proportional to the dosage. Doses of 20–50 mg intramuscularly or intravenously may be given initially. If larger doses are required, they should be given by slow infusion and titrated according to the response. In such cases the use of Lasix 250 mg ampoules should be considered.

Children: Parenteral doses for children range from 0.5–1.5 mg/kg body weight daily up to a maximum total daily dose of 20 mg.

Elderly: In the elderly, frusemide is generally eliminated more slowly. Dosage should be titrated until the required response is achieved.

Contra-indications, warnings, etc Intravenous injections of Lasix *must* always be given slowly, i.e. at a rate not exceeding 4 mg/minute.

Contra-indications: Lasix is contra-indicated in anuria, electrolyte deficiency and pre-comatose states associated with liver cirrhosis. Hypersensitivity to frusemide or sulphonamides.

Warnings: Patients with prostatic hypertrophy or impairment of micturition have an increased risk of developing acute retention.

Where indicated, steps should be taken to correct hypotension or hypovolaemia before commencing therapy.

The dosage of concurrently administered cardiac glycosides or antihypertensive agents may require adjustment. A marked fall in blood pressure may be seen when ACE inhibitors are added to frusemide therapy. The dose of frusemide should be reduced, or the drug stopped, before initiating the ACE inhibitor.

The toxic effects of nephrotoxic antibiotics may be increased by concomitant administration of potent diuretics such as frusemide.

Latent diabetes may become manifest or the insulin requirements of diabetic patients may increase.

In common with other diuretics, serum lithium levels may be increased when lithium is given concomitantly with frusemide, necessitating adjustment of the lithium dosage.

Certain non-steroidal anti-inflammatory agents (e.g. indomethacin, acetyl salicylic acid) may attenuate the action of frusemide and may cause renal failure in cases of pre-existing hypovolaemia. Frusemide may sometimes attenuate the effects of other drugs (e.g. the effects of antidiabetics and of pressor amines) and sometimes potentiate them (e.g. the effects of salicylates, theophylline, lithium and curare-type muscle relaxants).

Interactions have also been reported with ototoxic antibiotics. In cases of concomitant glucocorticoid therapy or abuse of laxatives, the risk of an increased potassium loss should be borne in mind.

Precautions: Caution should be observed in patients liable to electrolyte deficiency.

Results of animal work, in general, show no hazardous effect of Lasix in pregnancy. There is clinical evidence of safety of the drug in the third trimester of human pregnancy; however, Lasix should be used in pregnancy only if strictly indicated and for short term treatment.

Nursing mothers: As Lasix may inhibit lactation or may pass into breast milk, it should be used with caution in nursing mothers.

Overdosage: In cases of overdose there is a danger of dehydration and electrolyte depletion due to excessive diuresis. Treatment should therefore be aimed at fluid replacement and correction of the electrolyte imbalance.

Side-effects: Lasix is generally well tolerated. Side-effects of a minor nature such as nausea, malaise or gastric upset may occur but are not usually severe enough to necessitate withdrawal of treatment. Serum calcium levels may be reduced; in very rare cases tetany has been observed. Nephrocalcinosis has been reported in premature infants.

The incidence of allergic reactions, such as skin rashes, photosensitivity, vasculitis, fever, interstitial nephritis or shock, is very low but when these occur, treatment should be withdrawn. Standard measures for the treatment of shock should be taken if necessary.

Isolated cases of acute pancreatitis have been reported after long-term diuretic (including frusemide) treatment. Disorders of hearing after frusemide are rare and, in most cases reversible. They may occur if frusemide is injected too rapidly, particularly in patients with renal insufficiency.

As with other diuretics a transient rise in creatinine and urea levels has been reported with frusemide.

In common with other sulphonamide-based diuretics hyperuricaemia may occur and, in rare cases, clinical gout may be precipitated.

Bone marrow depression has been reported as a rare complication and necessitates withdrawal of treatment.

Pre-existing metabolic alkalosis (e.g. in decompensated cirrhosis of the liver) may be aggravated by frusemide treatment.

Reduced mental alertness may impair ability to drive or operate dangerous machinery.

Pharmaceutical precautions Lasix injections should be stored in a cool dry place, protected from light. Injections of Lasix should not be mixed with any other preparations. Opened ampoules should be used immediately and any remainder discarded.

Legal category POM.

Package quantities Lasix ampoules 20 mg are available in packs of 5 × 2 ml. Lasix ampoules 50 mg are available in packs of 5 × 5 ml.

Further information Lasix 20 mg and 50 mg injections contain approximately 0.14 mmol Na^+/ml.

Product licence numbers
Lasix injection 20 mg 0086/5012.
Lasix injection 50 mg 0086/0054.

LASIX* TABLETS 500 mg

Presentation Lasix Tablets 500 mg each contain 500 mg of Frusemide BP. They are presented as yellow, circular, biplanar, uncoated tablets, 13 mm in diameter, one side bearing the Hoechst insignia; the other is quarter-scored bearing the letters DLX, one in each of three of the four quarters.

Excipients include lactose and ultra-amylopectin.

Uses Lasix 500 mg is a diuretic for the management of oliguria due to acute or chronic renal insufficiency with a GFR below 20 ml/minute.

Dosage and administration In patients with chronic renal insufficiency, an initial daily dose of 250 mg (½ tablet) is employed. If a satisfactory diuresis is not produced then the dose may be increased in steps of 250 mg at four to six hourly intervals up to a maximum daily dose of 1,500 mg (3 tablets) in 24 hours. In exceptional cases up to 2,000 mg (4 tablets) in 24 hours may be given.

In cases of acute renal failure which have been initially controlled using Lasix Injection 250 mg, oral therapy may be substituted for parenteral therapy, regarding one 500 mg tablet as approximately equal to one 250 mg ampoule. Appropriate dosage adjustments may then be made according to the observed clinical response.

Children: Lasix Tablets 500 mg are unlikely to be suitable for use in children.

Elderly: In the elderly, frusemide is generally eliminated more slowly. Dosage should be titrated until the required response is achieved.

Contra-indications, warnings, etc During treatment with high-dosage forms of Lasix, fluid balance should be carefully controlled. In the particular case of patients with shock, steps should be taken to correct the blood pressure and circulating blood volume before commencing therapy. Regular checks of plasma electrolytes, particularly sodium, potassium, chloride and bicarbonate, should be carried out and electrolyte replacement therapy instituted accordingly.

Contra-indications: Lasix Tablets 500 mg are contra-indicated in renal failure with anuria or renal failure as a result of poisoning by nephrotoxic or hepatotoxic agents and in renal failure associated with hepatic coma.

Hypersensitivity to frusemide or sulphonamides is also a contra-indication.

Lasix tablets 500 mg should not be given to patients with normal renal function.

Warnings: Patients with prostatic hypertrophy or impairment of micturition have an increased risk of developing acute retention.

The dosage of concurrently administered cardiac glycosides or antihypertensive agents may require adjustment.

A marked fall in blood pressure may be seen when ACE inhibitors are added to frusemide therapy. The dose of frusemide should be reduced, or the drug stopped, before initiating the ACE inhibitor.

The toxic effects of nephrotoxic antibiotics may be increased by concomitant administration of potent diuretics such as frusemide.

Latent diabetes may become manifest or the insulin requirements of diabetic patients may increase.

In common with other diuretics, serum lithium levels may be increased when lithium is given concomitantly with frusemide, necessitating adjustment of the lithium dosage.

Certain non-steroidal anti-inflammatory agents (e.g. indomethacin, acetyl salicylic acid) may attenuate the action of frusemide and may cause renal failure in cases of pre-existing hypovolaemia. Frusemide may sometimes attenuate the effects of other drugs (e.g. the effects of antidiabetics and of pressor amines) and sometimes potentiate them (e.g. the effects of salicylates, theophylline, lithium and curare-type muscle relaxants).

Interactions have also been reported with ototoxic antibiotics and parenteral cisplatin. In cases of concomitant glucocorticoid therapy or abuse of laxatives, the risk of an increased potassium loss should be borne in mind.

Precautions: There is little evidence of safety of high-dose Lasix in human pregnancy, although the results of animal work, in general, show no hazardous effects. However, Lasix should be used in pregnancy only if strictly indicated and for short term treatment.

Nursing mothers: As Lasix may inhibit lactation or may pass into breast milk, it should be used with caution in nursing mothers.

Overdosage: In cases of overdosage there is a danger of dehydration and electrolyte depletion due to excessive diuresis. Treatment should therefore be aimed at fluid replacement and correction of the electrolyte imbalance.

Side-effects: Lasix Tablets 500 mg are generally well tolerated. Side-effects of a minor nature such as nausea, malaise or gastric upset may occur but are not usually severe enough to necessitate withdrawal of treatment.

The incidence of allergic reactions, such as skin rashes, photosensitivity, vasculitis, fever, interstitial nephritis or shock, is very low but, when these occur, treatment should be withdrawn. Standard measures for the treatment of shock should be taken if necessary.

As with other diuretics, electrolytes and water balance may be disturbed as a result of diuresis after prolonged therapy. This may cause symptoms such as headache, hypotension or muscle cramps.

Serum calcium levels may be reduced; in very rare cases tetany has been observed. Nephrocalcinosis has been reported in premature infants.

As with other diuretics a transient rise in creatinine and urea levels has also been reported with frusemide.

Isolated cases of acute pancreatitis have been reported after long-term diuretic (including frusemide) treatment. Disorders of hearing after frusemide are rare and, in most cases reversible. They may occur if frusemide is injected too rapidly, particularly in patients with renal insufficiency.

In common with other sulphonamide-based diuretics, hyperuricaemia may occur and, in rare cases, clinical gout may be precipitated.

Serum cholesterol and triglyceride levels may rise during frusemide treatment but will usually return to normal within six months.

Bone marrow depression has been reported as a rare complication and necessitates withdrawal of treatment.

Pre-existing metabolic alkalosis (e.g. in decompensated cirrhosis of the liver) may be aggravated by frusemide treatment.

Reduced mental alertness may impair ability to drive or operate dangerous machinery.

Pharmaceutical precautions Lasix tablets should be stored in a cool dry place, protected from light, in the original container or in containers similar to those of the manufacturer.

Legal category POM.

Package quantities Lasix Tablets 500 mg are available in packs of 100.

Further information Diuresis commences within one hour of taking the tablets and the effect lasts for approximately four hours.

Product licence number 0086/5013.

LASIX* INJECTION 250 mg/25 ml

Presentation Lasix 250 mg ampoules contain 250 mg Frusemide BP in 25 ml aqueous solution, The solution also contains mannitol and sodium hydroxide as excipients.

Uses Lasix Injection 250 mg is a diuretic for the management of oliguria due to acute or chronic renal insufficiency with a GFR below 20 ml/minute.

Dosage and administration Lasix 250 mg should be

administered by intravenous injection at a rate not exceeding 4 mg/minute.

The recommended initial dose is one 25 ml ampoule (250 mg) diluted in approximately 225 ml Sodium Chloride Injection BP or Ringer's Solution for Injection administered over one hour. This gives an approximate drip rate of 80 drops/minute, ensuring that the infusion is at the level of 4 mg/minute.

If a satisfactory increase in urine output, such as 40–50 ml/hour, is not attained within the next hour, a second infusion of two 25 ml ampoules (500 mg) in an appropriate infusion fluid should be given, the total volume of the infusion being governed by the patient's state of hydration. If a satisfactory output is still not achieved within one hour of the end of the second infusion, a third infusion consisting of four 25 ml ampoules (1,000 mg) can be given. The rate of infusion should not exceed 4 mg/minute.

If the third infusion using the maximum intravenous dose of 1,000 mg over four hours is not effective, then dialysis will probably be required.

In oliguric or anuric patients with significant fluid overload, it may not be practicable to administer high-dose Lasix injection by the method suggested above. Under these circumstances, the use of a constant-rate infusion pump (e.g. Sage pump) with micrometer screw-gauge adjustment may be considered for direct administration of the injection into the vein. The rate of administration should not exceed 4 mg/minute.

If the Lasix infusion produces a satisfactory response of 40–50 ml/hour, then the effective dose (up to 1,000 mg) can be repeated every 24 hours. Alternatively, maintenance therapy can be continued with oral Lasix 500 mg Tablets when one 500 mg tablet may be regarded as being approximately equal to one 250 mg ampoule. Appropriate dosage adjustments may then be made according to the observed clinical response.

Children: Doses for children can only be determined on the basis of the severity of the renal insufficiency and clinical response to initial doses.

Elderly: In the elderly, frusemide is generally eliminated more slowly. Dosage should be titrated until the required response is achieved.

Contra-indications, warnings, etc During treatment with high-dosage forms of Lasix, fluid balance should be carefully controlled. In the particular case of patients with shock, steps should be taken to correct the blood pressure and circulating blood volume before commencing therapy. Regular checks of plasma electrolytes, particularly sodium, potassium, chloride and bicarbonate, should be carried out, and electrolyte replacement therapy instituted accordingly.

Intravenous injections of Lasix *must* be given slowly.

If the recommended infusion rate of 4 mg/minute is exceeded, transient deafness may occur.

Contra-indications: Lasix Injection 250 mg is contra-indicated in renal failure with anuria or in renal failure as a result of poisoning by nephrotoxic or hepatotoxic agents and in renal failure associated with hepatic coma.

Hypersensitivity to frusemide or sulphonamides is also a contra-indication.

Lasix Injection 250 mg should not be given to patients with normal renal function.

Warnings: Patients with prostatic hypertrophy or impairment of micturition have an increased risk of developing acute retention.

The dosage of concurrently administered cardiac glycosides or antihypertensive agents may require adjustment.

A marked fall in blood pressure may be seen when ACE inhibitors are added to frusemide therapy. The dose of frusemide should be reduced, or the drug stopped, before initiating the ACE inhibitor.

The toxic effects of nephrotoxic antibiotics may be increased by concomitant administration of potent diuretics such as frusemide.

Latent diabetes may become manifest or the insulin requirements of diabetic patients may increase.

In common with other diuretics, serum lithium levels may be increased when lithium is given concomitantly with frusemide, necessitating adjustment of the lithium dosage.

Certain non-steroidal anti-inflammatory agents (e.g. indomethacin, acetyl salicylic acid) may attenuate the action of frusemide and may cause renal failure in cases of pre-existing hypovolaemia. Frusemide may sometimes attenuate the effects of other drugs (e.g. the effects of antidiabetics and of pressor amines) and sometimes potentiate them (e.g. the effects of salicylates, theophylline, lithium and curare-type muscle relaxants).

Interactions have also been reported with ototoxic antibiotics and parenteral cisplatin. In cases of concomitant glucocorticoid therapy or abuse of laxatives, the risk of an increased potassium loss should be borne in mind.

Precautions: There is little evidence of safety of high-dose Lasix in human pregnancy although the results of animal work, in general, show no hazardous effects. However, Lasix should be used in pregnancy only if strictly indicated and for short term treatment.

Nursing mothers: As Lasix may inhibit lactation or may pass into breast milk, it should be used with caution in nursing mothers.

Overdosage: In cases of overdose there is a danger of dehydration and electrolyte depletion due to excessive diuresis. Treatment should therefore be aimed at fluid replacement and correction of the electrolyte imbalance.

Side-effects: Lasix injection 250 mg is generally well tolerated. Side-effects of a minor nature such as nausea, malaise or gastric upset may occur but are not usually severe enough to necessitate withdrawal of treatment.

As with other diuretics, electrolytes and water balance may be disturbed as a result of diuresis after prolonged therapy. This may cause symptoms such as headache, hypotension or muscle cramps.

Serum calcium levels may be reduced; in very rare cases tetany has been observed. Nephrocalcinosis has been reported in premature infants.

The incidence of allergic reactions, such as skin rashes, photosensitivity, vasculitis, fever, interstitial nephritis or shock is very low but, when these occur, treatment should be withdrawn. Standard measures for the treatment of shock should be taken if necessary.

Isolated cases of acute pancreatitis have been reported after long-term diuretic (including frusemide) treatment. Disorders of hearing after frusemide are rare and, in most cases reversible. They may occur if frusemide is injected too rapidly, particularly in patients with renal insufficiency.

In common with other sulphonamide-based diuretics, hyperuricaemia may occur and, in rare cases, clinical gout may be precipitated.

As with other diuretics a transient rise in creatinine and urea levels has also been reported with frusemide.

Serum cholesterol and triglyceride levels may rise during frusemide treatment but will usually return to normal within six months.

Bone marrow depression has been reported as a rare complication and necessitates withdrawal of treatment.

Pre-existing metabolic alkalosis (e.g. in decompensated cirrhosis of the liver) may be aggravated by frusemide treatment.

Reduced mental alertness may impair ability to drive or operate dangerous machinery.

Pharmaceutical precautions Lasix Injection 250 mg should be stored in a cool place protected from light. Frusemide may precipitate in solutions of low pH and therefore dextrose solutions are not suitable infusion fluids for Lasix injections. The injection solution should not be mixed with other drugs in the infusion bottle.

Opened ampoules should be used immediately and any remainder of either the ampoule content or the prepared infusion solution should be discarded.

Legal category POM.

Package quantities Lasix Injections 250 mg are available in packs of 5 × 25 ml.

Further information Diuresis should commence within a few minutes and last for approximately two hours. A diuretic effect is seen during the infusion and its duration is related to the infusion time.

Lasix Injection 250 mg contains approximately 0.04 mmol Na^+/ml.

Product licence number 0086/5014.

LASIX* + K COMBINATION PACK

Presentation Lasix Tablets 40 mg each contain 40 mg of Frusemide BP. They are presented as white, circular, biplanar tablets measuring 8 mm in diameter. On one side they bear the Hoechst insignia. The other side is scored and bears the letters DLI on one side of the score mark and '40' on the other. Excipients include lactose.

The potassium chloride slow-release tablets each contain 750 mg (10 mmol) of potassium chloride. They are presented as yellow, circular, biconvex tablets, 12 mm in diameter, and have no superficial markings. Excipients include Sunset Yellow.

These tablets are presented together in a calendar pack as Lasix + K.

Uses Lasix + K contains a short-acting diuretic and a slow-release potassium supplement. The calendar pack is designed for patients who require a fixed dose comprising 40 mg of Lasix (1 tablet) and 20 mmol of potassium (2 tablets) each day. It is not intended for patients who require individual titration of dosage.

Dosage and administration Lasix + K is supplied in calendar packs bearing directions for use. The instructions state that the Lasix 40 mg tablet is taken in the morning, that one potassium chloride tablet is taken at noon, and one in the evening. This ensures that the release of the latter occurs outside the diuretic phase, at a time when conditions are optimal for absorption and retention.

Children: Lasix + K is not suitable for paediatric use.

Elderly: Frusemide and potassium may both be excreted more slowly in the elderly.

Contra-indications, warnings, etc
Contra-indications: Lasix + K is contra-indicated in anuria, hyperkalaemia, precomatose states associated with liver cirrhosis and Addison's disease, and in patients taking potassium-sparing diuretics. Hypersensitivity to frusemide or sulphonamides.

Warnings: Patients with prostatic hypertrophy or impairment of micturition have an increased risk of developing acute retention.

Where indicated, steps should be taken to correct hypotension or hypovolaemia before commencing therapy.

The dosage of concurrently administered cardiac glycosides or antihypertensive agents may require adjustment.

ACE inhibitors should not be used in combination with Lasix + K as serum potassium levels may be increased.

The toxic effects of nephrotoxic antibiotics may be increased by concomitant administration of potent diuretics such as frusemide.

Latent diabetes may become manifest or the insulin requirements of diabetic patients may increase.

Care should be exercised when treating patients with renal insufficiency because of the risk of hyperkalaemia.

In common with other diuretics, serum lithium levels may be increased when lithium is given concomitantly with frusemide, necessitating adjustment of the lithium dosage.

Certain non-steroidal anti-inflammatory agents (e.g. indomethacin, acetyl salicylic acid) may attenuate the action of frusemide and may cause renal failure in cases of pre-existing hypovolaemia. Frusemide may sometimes attenuate the effects of other drugs (e.g. the effects of antidiabetics and of pressor amines) and sometimes potentiate them (e.g. the effects of salicylates, theophylline, lithium and curare-type muscle relaxants).

Interactions have also been reported with ototoxic antibiotics. In cases of concomitant glucocorticoid therapy or abuse of laxatives, the risk of an increased potassium loss should be borne in mind.

Precautions: Results of animal work, in general, show no hazardous effect of Lasix in pregnancy. There is clinical evidence of safety of the drug in the third trimester of human pregnancy; however, Lasix should be used in pregnancy only if strictly indicated and for short-term treatment.

Nursing mothers: As Lasix may inhibit lactation or pass into breast milk it should be used with caution in nursing mothers.

Overdosage: In cases of overdose there is a danger of dehydration and electrolyte depletion due to excessive diuresis. Treatment should therefore be aimed at fluid replacement and correction of the electrolyte imbalance.

Side-effects: Lasix + K is generally well tolerated. Side-effects of a minor nature such as nausea, malaise or gastric upset may occur but are not usually severe enough to necessitate withdrawal of treatment.

As with other diuretics, electrolytes and water balance may be disturbed as a result of diuresis after prolonged therapy. This may cause symptoms such as headache, hypotension or muscle cramps.

Serum calcium levels may be reduced; in very rare cases tetany has been observed. Nephrocalcinosis has been reported in premature infants.

Isolated cases of acute pancreatitis have been reported after long-term diuretic (including frusemide) treatment. Disorders of hearing after frusemide are rare and, in most cases reversible. They may occur if frusemide is injected too rapidly, particularly in patients with renal insufficiency.

As with other diuretics a transient rise in creatinine and urea levels has been reported with frusemide.

The incidence of allergic reactions, such as skin rashes, photosensitivity, vasculitis, fever or interstitial nephritis, is very low, but when these occur treatment should be withdrawn.

In common with other sulphonamide-based diuretics, hyperuricaemia may occur and, in rare cases, clinical gout may be precipitated.

Serum cholesterol and triglyceride levels may rise during frusemide treatment but will usually return to normal within 6 months.

Bone marrow depression has been reported as a rare complication and necessitates withdrawal of treatment.

Pre-existing metabolic alkalosis (e.g. in decompensated cirrhosis of the liver) may be aggravated by frusemide treatment.

Reduced mental alertness may impair ability to drive or operate dangerous machinery.

Pharmaceutical precautions Lasix + K should be stored in a cool dry place, protected from light, in the original container or in containers similar to those of the manufacturer.

Legal category POM.

Package quantities Lasix + K is packed in blister strips, each containing 10 Lasix tablets and 20 potassium chloride tablets. It is supplied in boxes of three blister strips (original packs).

Further information Lasix produces a prompt and effective diuresis which lasts for approximately four hours following oral administration. The potassium chloride is contained in an inert matrix allowing sustained release over a period of six to eight hours.

If the prescribing instructions are followed, this ensures potassium release outside the diuretic phase at a time when conditions are optimal for absorption and retention.

Ghost tablets may appear in the patient's faeces.

Product licence number 0086/0037.

LASIX* PAEDIATRIC LIQUID

Presentation Lasix Paediatric Liquid is presented as a granulate for reconstitution. The granulate is reconstituted with distilled water to produce a solution containing 1 mg/ml Frusemide BP in a volume of 150 ml. Excipients include disodium edetate, Nipasept sodium and sodium sulphite.

Uses Lasix Paediatric Liquid is a diuretic which is indicated for the treatment of oedema in children. It may also be used in elderly patients or other patients unable to take solid oral dose forms of Lasix.

Dosage and administration The recommended daily dose of Lasix Paediatric Liquid for children is 1–3 mg/kg body weight (1–3 ml/kg as the reconstituted liquid).

When Lasix Paediatric Liquid is used as a substitute for tablet therapy in adults, the normal dose range is 20–80 mg (20–80 ml) daily (see 'Side-effects' section).

Elderly: In the elderly, frusemide is generally eliminated more slowly. Dosage should be titrated until the required response is achieved.

Reconstitution: Lasix Paediatric Liquid is supplied in a 150 ml bottle containing granules for reconstitution. The granules are reconstituted by the addition of 142 ml distilled water to the bottle which is then shaken vigorously to dissolve the granulate before oral administration. Tap water should not be used.

Contra-indications, warnings, etc

Contra-indications: Lasix Paediatric Liquid is contra-indicated in anuria, electrolyte deficiency and pre-comatose states associated with liver cirrhosis. Hypersensitivity to frusemide or sulphonamides.

Warnings: Lasix Paediatric Liquid contains sorbitol and may cause flatulence, abdominal distension or diarrhoea if given in large quantities to adults who are unable to take solid oral dose forms of Lasix.

Patients with prostatic hypertrophy or impairment of micturition have an increased risk of developing acute retention.

Where indicated, steps should be taken to correct hypotension or hypovolaemia before commencing therapy.

The dosage of concurrently administered cardiac glycosides or hypotensive agents may require adjustment.

A marked fall in blood pressure may be seen when ACE inhibitors are added to frusemide therapy. The dose of frusemide should be reduced, or the drug stopped, before initiating the ACE inhibitor.

The toxic effects of nephrotoxic antibiotics may be increased by concomitant administration of potent diuretics such as frusemide.

Latent diabetes may become manifest or the insulin requirements of diabetic patients may increase.

In common with other diuretics, serum lithium levels may be increased when lithium is given concomitantly with frusemide, necessitating adjustment of the lithium dosage.

Certain non-steroidal anti-inflammatory agents (e.g. indomethacin, acetyl salicylic acid) may attenuate the action of frusemide and may cause renal failure in cases of pre-existing hypovolaemia. Frusemide may sometimes attenuate the effects of other drugs (e.g. the effects of antidiabetics and of pressor amines) and sometimes potentiate them (e.g. the effects of salicylates, theophylline, lithium and curare-type muscle relaxants).

Interactions have also been reported with ototoxic antibiotics. In cases of concomitant glucocorticoid therapy or abuse of laxatives, the risk of an increased potassium loss should be borne in mind.

Precautions: Caution should be exercised in patients liable to electrolyte deficiency.

Results of animal work, in general, show no hazardous effect of Lasix in pregnancy. There is clinical evidence of safety of the drug in the third trimester of human pregnancy; however, Lasix should be used in pregnancy only if strictly indicated and for short term treatment.

Nursing mothers: As Lasix may inhibit lactation or may pass into breast milk it should be used with caution in nursing mothers.

Overdosage: In cases of overdose there is a danger of dehydration and electrolyte depletion due to excessive diuresis. Treatment should therefore be aimed at fluid replacement and correction of the electrolyte imbalance.

Side-effects: Lasix is generally well tolerated. Side-effects of a minor nature such as nausea, malaise or gastric upset may occur but are not usually severe enough to necessitate withdrawal of treatment.

As with other diuretics, electrolytes and water balance may be disturbed as a result of diuresis after prolonged therapy. This may cause symptoms such as headache, hypotension or muscle cramps.

Flatulence, abdominal distension or diarrhoea may occur following the ingestion of large quantities of Lasix Paediatric Liquid, due to its sorbitol content.

Serum calcium levels may be reduced; in very rare cases tetany has been observed. Nephrocalcinosis has been reported in premature infants.

Isolated cases of acute pancreatitis have been reported after long-term diuretic (including frusemide) treatment. Disorders of hearing after frusemide are rare and, in most cases reversible. They may occur if frusemide is injected too rapidly, particularly in patients with renal insufficiency.

As with other diuretics a transient rise in creatinine and urea levels has been reported with frusemide.

The incidence of allergic reactions, such as skin rashes, photosensitivity, vasculitis, fever or interstitial nephritis is very low but, when these occur, treatment should be withdrawn.

In common with other sulphonamide-based diuretics, hyperuricaemia may occur and, in rare cases, clinical gout may be precipitated.

Serum cholesterol and triglyceride levels may rise during frusemide treatment but will usually return to normal within 6 months.

Bone marrow depression has been reported as a rare complication and necessitates withdrawal of treatment.

Pre-existing metabolic alkalosis (e.g. in decompensated cirrhosis of the liver) may be aggravated by frusemide treatment.

Reduced mental alertness may impair ability to drive or operate dangerous machinery.

Pharmaceutical precautions Lasix Paediatric Liquid granulate should be stored in a cool dry place, protected from light, in the original container.

The granulate should be reconstituted only with 142 ml of distilled water. When reconstituted the liquid should be stored in a cool place, preferably in a refrigerator at 5°C, protected from light.

Under these conditions, reconstituted Lasix Paediatric Liquid may be used for up to 30 days, after which any remaining solution must be discarded.

The shelf-life of the granulate prior to reconstitution is three years. The use of sterile distilled water is recommended when the product is intended for administration to neonates.

Legal category POM.

Package quantities Lasix Paediatric Liquid is available in 150 ml bottles.

Further information Lasix produces a prompt and effective diuresis which lasts for approximately four hours following oral administration. Therefore, the time of administration can be adjusted to suit the patient's requirements. Lasix Paediatric Liquid does not contain sucrose.

Product licence number 0086/0063.

LASORIDE* (co-amilofruse)

Presentation Yellow tablets 8 mm in diameter, with Hoechst name and logo on one side, containing 40 mg Frusemide BP and 5 mg Amiloride Hydrochloride BP. Excipients include lactose.

Uses Lasoride is indicated where a prompt diuresis is required and where potassium conservation is important.

Dosage and administration The adult dose is one to two tablets, to be taken in the morning.

Elderly: The elderly are more likely to experience hyperkalaemia since renal reserve may be reduced. The dosage should be adjusted according to renal function, blood electrolytes and diuretic response.

Children: Not recommended for use in children.

Contra-indications, warnings, etc

Contra-indications: Hyperkalaemia (serum potassium >5.3 mmol/litre), Addison's disease, acute renal failure, anuria, severe progressive renal disease, electrolyte imbalance, precomatose states associated with cirrhosis, concomitant potassium supplements, known sensitivity to frusemide or amiloride.

Lasoride is contra-indicated in children as safety in this age group has not been established.

Warnings: Hyperkalaemia has been observed in patients receiving amiloride hydrochloride.

Frusemide may cause latent diabetes to become manifest. It may be necessary to increase the dose of hypoglycaemic agents in diabetic patients.

Lasoride should be discontinued before a glucose tolerance test.

Patients with prostatic hypertrophy or impairment of micturition have an increased risk of developing acute urinary retention during diuretic therapy.

Serum uric acid levels may rise during treatment with Lasoride and acute attacks of gout may be precipitated.

The dosage of concurrently administered cardiac glycosides or antihypertensive agents may require adjustment.

The toxic effects of nephrotoxic antibiotics may be increased by concomitant administration of potent diuretics such as Lasoride.

In common with other diuretics, serum lithium levels may be increased when lithium is given concomitantly with frusemide, necessitating adjustment of the lithium dosage.

ACE inhibitors should not be used in combination with Lasoride as serum potassium levels may be increased.

Certain non-steroidal anti-inflammatory agents (e.g. indomethacin, acetyl salicylic acid) may attenuate the action of frusemide and may cause renal failure in cases of pre-existing hypovolaemia. Frusemide may sometimes attenuate the effects of other drugs (e.g. the effect of antidiabetics and of pressor amines) and sometimes potentiate them (e.g. the effects of salicylates, theophylline, lithium and curare-type muscle relaxants).

Interactions have also been reported with ototoxic antibiotics. In cases of concomitant glucocorticoid therapy or abuse of laxatives, the risk of an increased potassium loss should be borne in mind.

Precautions: Patients who are being treated with the preparation require regular supervision, with monitoring of fluid and electrolyte states to avoid excessive loss of fluid.

Lasoride should be used with particular caution in elderly patients or those with potential obstruction in the urinary tract or disorders rendering electrolyte balance precarious.

Hyponatraemia, hypochloraemia and raised blood urea nitrogen may occur during vigorous diuresis, especially in seriously ill patients or the elderly. Careful monitoring of serum electrolytes and urea should therefore be undertaken in these patients.

Pregnancy and lactation: The safety of Lasoride use during pregnancy and lactation has not been established.

Overdosage: Treatment of overdosage should be aimed at reversing dehydration and correcting electrolyte imbalance, particularly hyperkalaemia. Emesis should be induced or gastric lavage performed. Treatment is symptomatic and supportive. If hyperkalaemia is seen, appropriate measures to reduce serum potassium must be instituted.

Side-effects: Malaise, gastric upset, nausea, vomiting, diarrhoea, and constipation may occur.

If skin rashes or pruritus occur, treatment should be withdrawn.

Serum calcium levels may be reduced; in very rare cases tetany has been observed.

Serum cholesterol and triglyceride levels may arise during frusemide treatment but will usually return to normal within six months.

Rare complications may include minor psychiatric disturbances and disturbances in liver function tests. Isolated cases of acute pancreatitis have been reported after long-term diuretic (including frusemide) treatment. Disorders of hearing after frusemide are rare and, in most cases reversible. They may occur if frusemide is injected too rapidly, particularly in patients with renal insufficiency.

Bone marrow depression occasionally complicates treatment, necessitating withdrawal of the product. The haematopoietic state should be regularly monitored during treatment.

Reduced mental alertness may impair ability to drive or operate dangerous machinery.

Pharmaceutical precautions Store at ambient temperature. Protect from light.

Legal category POM.

Package quantities Cartons of 28 tablets consisting of 2 calendar foils of 14 tablets (original packs) and a hospital ward bottle of 100 tablets.

Further information Lasoride is particularly suitable for patients at risk from hypokalaemia and causes significantly less potassium excretion than frusemide during the 12 hours after administration. The daily loss of potassium with Lasoride is equivalent to normal potassium excretion.

Product licence number 0086/0120.

METENIX* 5 TABLETS

Presentation Metenix 5 Tablets each contain 5 mg metolazone. They are presented as blue flat uncoated round tablets, 7 mm in diameter, marked with a figure '5' on one side and the Hoechst insignia on the other side.

Uses Metenix 5 is a diuretic for use in the treatment of mild and moderate hypertension. Metenix 5 may be used in conjunction with non-diuretic antihypertensive agents and, in these circumstances, it is usually possible to achieve satisfactory control of blood pressure with a reduced dose of the non-diuretic agent. Patients who have become resistant to therapy with these agents may respond to the addition of Metenix 5 to their antihypertensive regimen.

Metenix 5 may also be used for the treatment of cardiac, renal and hepatic oedema, ascites or toxaemia of pregnancy.

Dosage and administration

Hypertension: The recommended initial dose in mild and moderate hypertension is 5 mg daily. After three to four weeks, the dose may be reduced if necessary to 5 mg on alternate days as maintenance therapy.

Oedema: In oedematous conditions, the normal recommended dose is 5–10 mg daily, given as a single dose. In resistant conditions, this may be increased to 20 mg daily or above. However, no more than 80 mg should be given in any 24-hour period.

Children: There is insufficient knowledge of the effects of Metenix 5 in children for any dosage recommendations to be made.

Elderly: Metolazone may be excreted more slowly in the elderly.

Contra-indications, warnings, etc

Contra-indications: Metenix 5 is contra-indicated in electrolyte deficiency states, anuria, coma or precomatose states associated with liver cirrhosis; also in patients with known allergy or hypersensitivity to metolazone.

Warnings: The dosage of concurrently administered cardiac glycosides may require adjustment. Metenix 5 may aggravate the increased potassium excretion associated with steroid therapy or diseases such as cirrhosis or severe ischaemic heart disease.

Latent diabetes may become manifest or the insulin requirements of diabetic patients may increase.

Precautions: Because of the antihypertensive effects of metolazone the dosage of concurrently administered non-diuretic antihypertensive agents may need to be reduced.

Caution should be exercised during Metenix 5 therapy in patients liable to electrolyte deficiency.

Fluid and electrolyte balance should be carefully monitored during therapy especially if Metenix 5 is used concurrently with other diuretics. In particular, Metenix 5 may potentiate the diuresis produced by frusemide and, if the two agents are used concurrently, patients should be carefully monitored. This combination of drugs has been used in the treatment of resistant oedema.

Prolonged therapy with Metenix 5 may result in hypokalaemia. Serum potassium levels should be determined at regular intervals and, if necessary, potassium supplementation should be instituted.

Chloride deficit, hyponatraemia and a low salt syndrome may also occur, particularly when the patient is also on a diet with restricted salt intake. Hypomagnesaemia has been reported as a consequence of prolonged diuretic therapy.

There is little evidence of safety of the drug in human pregnancy, but it has been in wide, general use for many years without apparent ill consequence, animal studies having shown no hazard.

Nursing mothers: If Metenix 5 is given to nursing mothers, metolazone may be present in the breast milk.

Overdosage: In cases of overdose there is a danger of dehydration and electrolyte depletion. Treatment should therefore be aimed at fluid replacement and correction of the electrolyte imbalance.

Side-effects: Metenix 5 is generally well tolerated. There have been occasional reports of headache, anorexia, vomiting, abdominal discomfort, muscle cramps and dizziness. There have been isolated reports of urticaria, leucopenia, tachycardia, chills and chest pain.

Hyperuricaemia or azotaemia may occur during treatment with Metenix 5, particularly in patients with impaired renal function. On rare occasions, clinical gout has been reported.

Pharmaceutical precautions Metenix 5 Tablets should be stored in a cool dry place, protected from light, in the original container or in containers similar to those of the manufacturer.

Legal category POM.

Package quantities Metenix 5 Tablets are available in blister strips packed in cartons of 100 tablets.

Further information Metolazone is a substituted quinazolinone diuretic.

Diuresis and saluresis begin within one hour of administration of Metenix 5 Tablets, reaching a maximum in two hours and continuing for 12–24 hours according to dosage.

Product licence number 0086/0056.

RASTINON* TABLETS 500 mg

Presentation Rastinon Tablets each contain 500 mg Tolbutamide BP. They are presented as uncoated white, circular, scored tablets, 13 mm in diameter, one side bearing the Hoechst insignia, the other bearing the marks 'Rastinon' above and '0.5' below the score mark.

Uses Rastinon is a hypoglycaemic agent, indicated for the oral treatment of patients with non-insulin dependent diabetes who respond inadequately to dietary treatment alone. Rastinon is particularly suitable for elderly patients.

Dosage and administration

1. *Treatment of previously untreated diabetics:* Stabilisation can be achieved by commencing with 2 tablets daily. The subsequent dosage must depend on the patient's individual response. The average daily dose is 1–3 tablets which can be taken as a single or divided dose as required. Generally, patients who do not respond to 4 tablets (2 g) daily will not respond to higher doses.

2. *Change-over from other oral antidiabetics:* The change-over to Rastinon, from other drugs with a similar mode of action, can be carried out without any break in therapy, even with chlorpropamide despite the long persistence of this agent in the body.

Stabilisation can be achieved by commencing with 2 tablets daily, subsequent dosage depending on the patient's individual response.

3. *Combination with biguanides:* If adequate control is not possible with diet and 4 tablets of Rastinon daily, control can often be re-established by combined administration of Rastinon and a biguanide derivative.

4. *Change-over from insulin:* Some cases of non-insulin dependent diabetes, previously treated with insulin, can be changed to Rastinon. Low insulin doses (less than 20 units) can be replaced immediately. With higher doses a gradual change is advisable by giving insulin and Rastinon concurrently and reducing the dose of insulin.

The tablets may be taken by mouth as a single dose with or immediately after the first main meal of the day, or as a divided dose.

Children: As non-insulin dependent diabetes is not usually a disease of childhood, Rastinon is not recommended for use in children.

Elderly: Rastinon is particularly suitable for elderly patients. However, since this patient group may be more liable to sulphonylurea-induced hypoglycaemia, treatment should be initiated at lower dosage.

Contra-indications, warnings, etc

Contra-indications: Rastinon should not be used in patients who have or have ever had diabetic ketoacidosis, who have insulin-dependent diabetes mellitus, serious impairment of renal, hepatic, adrenocortical or thyroid function or in circumstances of unusual stress, e.g. surgical operations or during pregnancy, when dietary treatment and insulin are essential.

Rastinon should not be used during the first trimester of pregnancy. There is some evidence of harmful effects in pregnancy in animals and isolated reports which suggest a hazard in human pregnancy.

Nursing mothers: Tolbutamide has been detected in breast milk in small quantities; the effect of this low dose on the neonate is unknown.

Warnings: Debilitated or aged patients may be more liable to hypoglycaemia. Rastinon may be used in mild to moderate renal impairment at a reduced dose. The hypoglycaemic effect of tolbutamide may be enhanced by dicoumarol, monoamine oxidase inhibitors, beta-adrenergic blocking agents, sulphonamides, phenylbutazone, chloramphenicol, cyclophosphamide and salicylates, or diminished by adrenaline, lithium, rifampicin, corticosteroids, oral contraceptives or thiazide diuretics.

Overdosage: Hypoglycaemia may be treated in the conscious patient by the administration of glucose or 3–4 lumps of table sugar with water. This may be repeated as necessary.

If the patient is comatose, up to 50 ml of a 50% glucose solution should be given as a rapid intravenous injection. This may be followed by a continuous infusion of a more dilute (10%) glucose solution at a rate that will maintain the blood glucose at a level about 5.6 mmol/l (100 mg/dl). The patient should be monitored closely for 24–48 hours for any recurrence of hypoglycaemia. Alternatively, glucagon may be administered in a dose of 1 mg subcutaneously or intramuscularly to restore consciousness.

Side-effects: Adverse reactions serious enough to warrant discontinuation of treatment are uncommon but mild gastro-intestinal and allergic skin reactions have occurred. There have been reports of anaemia, pancytopenia and transient changes in liver enzyme concentrations and liver function tests during treatment with tolbutamide, but these effects are not known to be directly attributable to the drug. Haemolytic anaemia and cholestatic jaundice, though not common, have been reported. Hypoglycaemic symptoms have occasionally been reported when the dose has been administered without due regard to the patient's dietary habits.

Pharmaceutical precautions Rastinon tablets should be stored at ambient temperature in a dry place, protected from light, in the original container or in containers similar to those of the manufacturer.

Legal category POM.

Package quantities Rastinon is available in packs of 100 tablets.

Further information Orally administered Rastinon is rapidly absorbed. It is extensively metabolised in the liver prior to excretion in the urine. Both of its metabolites possess some hypoglycaemic activity; this, however, is less pronounced than that of the parent compound.

Product licence number 0086/5016.

RELEFACT* LH-RH INJECTION

Presentation Each ampoule contains 100 microgram Gonadorelin BP (luteinizing hormone releasing hormone) in 1 ml aqueous solution. The solution also contains mannitol, sodium dihydrogen phosphate and sodium chloride as excipients.

Uses Intravenous injection of Relefact LH-RH causes release of LH (luteinizing hormone) and FSH (follicle-stimulating hormone) from the pituitary gland. It provides a means of assessing the reserve of LH and FSH in the pituitary glands of patients with suspected pituitary impairment. In addition, Relefact LH-RH may be of value in the differential diagnosis of delayed puberty and hypogonadism.

Dosage and administration Relefact LH-RH should be administered intravenously to adults or children as a single dose of 100 microgram. The test is based upon the pituitary response to this dose measured as serum LH and FSH levels. Qualitative data may be obtained from a single test but each laboratory must establish its own normal range for values of serum LH and FSH to obtain quantitative assessment of pituitary reserve.

Test procedure:

1. Obtain venous blood sample for control value of LH and, if facilities are available for its measurement, FSH.
2. Rapid intravenous injection of 100 microgram Relefact LH-RH.
3. Obtain venous blood sample 20 minutes after injection for measurement of LH/FSH response.

Interpretation of results:

1. *Normal response:* Following the administration of Relefact LH-RH there is a rise in serum LH within two minutes of injection; the response is dose-dependent. Peak levels are achieved 20–30 minutes after injection and baseline levels are approached six hours after a dose of 100 microgram. The FSH response is similar but of lesser magnitude (except (a) prior to puberty when, in both sexes, the FSH response is higher than the LH response and (b) in some patients with hypothalamic-pituitary dysfunction, e.g. anorexia nervosa). The normal female response to Relefact LH-RH shows cyclical variation, the response in the luteal phase being about twice that seen in the early follicular phase.

It is important for each laboratory to establish its own normal ranges of LH and FSH according to the time of the menstrual cycle before attempting to obtain quantitative results.

2. *Assessment of pituitary function:* Relefact LH-RH is a very sensitive index of pituitary function. Consequently, many patients with pituitary tumours, who do not respond to other dynamic tests of pituitary function (such as the growth hormone response to hypoglycaemia), will show a normal response to Relefact LH-RH; others will show an impaired or absent response. A normal response to the Relefact LH-RH test in clinically hypogonadal patients with pituitary abnormalities indicates that their pituitary glands are capable of producing LH and FSH in response to therapy. Similar responses may be seen in patients with hypothalamic tumours such as craniopharyngiomas.

3. *Assessment of primary and secondary hypogonadism:* Patients with primary hypogonadism resulting from gonadal failure or gonadal dysgenesis will have an exaggerated response to Relefact LH-RH. The majority of these patients will also have elevated basal values. The test is of particular value in those cases where basal levels are normal.

The majority of patients with congenital hypogonadotrophic hypogonadism with or without hyposmia (Kallman's syndrome) show a normal or impaired response to single doses of Relefact LH-RH.

These results indicate that, in most cases of isolated pituitary gonadotrophin deficiency, there is a reduced output of hypothalamic hormone releasing factor. An absent response to a single injection, however, is not necessarily indicative of pituitary failure, as more than one injection may be required in order to produce a response.

4. *Assessment of delayed puberty:* In simple delayed puberty the LH and FSH responses are within the normal range, whereas patients with hypogonadotrophic hypogonadism or hypopituitarism have an absent or impaired response. Patients with primary gonadal failure will have an exaggerated response.

Contra-indications, warnings, etc Relefact LH-RH should not be administered in pregnancy. There is a theoretical possibility of induction of ovulation following the administration of LH-RH. Pituitary adenoma is a relative contra-indication.

Side-effects: Side-effects of any description are rare, but the following reactions have been reported in isolated cases in healthy women: abdominal pain, nausea, headache and increased menstrual bleeding.

Overdosage: Overdosage with Relefact LH-RH has never been reported and is unlikely to be a problem.

Pharmaceutical precautions Store in a cool dark place. Do not dilute or administer with any additive.

Legal category POM.

Package quantities Relefact LH-RH is available in packs of 10 ampoules.

Further information Relefact LH-RH (luteinizing hormone-releasing hormone) is a synthetic decapeptide. It has also been referred to in the literature as LRF (luteinizing hormone/releasing factor), as LH/FSH-RH (luteinizing hormone/follicle stimulating hormone-releasing hormone) and as luliberin.

Product licence number 0086/0019.

RELEFACT* LH-RH/TRH INJECTION

Presentation Each ampoule contains 100 microgram Gonadorelin BP (luteinizing hormone-releasing hormone) and 200 microgram protirelin (thyrotrophin-releasing hormone) in 1 ml aqueous solution. The solution also contains sodium chloride, sodium biphosphate and mannitol as excipients.

Uses Intravenous injection of Relefact LH-RH/TRH causes the release of LH (luteinizing hormone), FSH (follicle-stimulating hormone) and TSH (thyroid-stimulating hormone) from the pituitary gland. In addition, TRH is also known to cause the release of prolactin.

The use of a combined releasing hormone preparation provides a means of simultaneous assessment of anterior pituitary reserve of these hormones in patients with suspected pituitary impairment.

Dosage and administration The contents of 1 ampoule of LH-RH/TRH should be administered intravenously to adults and children as a single dose (100 microgram LH-RH and 200 microgram TRH). The test is based upon the pituitary response to this dose measured as serum TSH, LH and FSH levels. Qualitative data may be obtained from a single combined test but each laboratory must establish its own normal range for the serum level of these hormones to obtain a quantitative assessment of pituitary function.

Test procedure:

1. Obtain venous blood sample for control measurements of TSH, LH and, if required, FSH.
2. Rapid intravenous injection of one ampoule LH-RH/TRH.
3. Obtain venous blood sample 20 minutes after injection to give peak LH, FSH and TSH values.
4. A further venous blood sample may be taken at 60 or 90 minutes to detect a delayed or prolonged response.

Interpretation of results:

LH-RH

1. *Normal response:* Following the administration of LH-RH there is a rise of serum LH within two minutes of injection; the response is dose-dependent. Peak levels are achieved 20–30 minutes after injection and baseline levels are approached six hours after a dose of 100 mcg. The FSH response is similar but of lesser magnitude (except (a) prior to puberty when, in both sexes, the FSH response is higher than the LH response and (b) in some patients with hypothalamic-pituitary dysfunction, e.g. anorexia nervosa). The normal female response to LH-RH shows cyclical variation, the response in the luteal phase being about twice that seen in the early follicular phase.

It is important for each laboratory to establish its own normal ranges of LH and FSH according to the time of the menstrual cycle before attempting to obtain quantitative results.

2. *Assessment of pituitary function:* LH-RH response is a very sensitive index of pituitary function. Consequently, many patients with pituitary tumours who do not respond to other dynamic tests of pituitary function (such as the growth hormone response to hypoglycaemia) will show a normal response to LH-RH; others will show an impaired or absent response. A normal response to the LH-RH test in clinically hypogonadal patients with pituitary abnormalities indicates that their pituitary glands are capable of producing LH and FSH in response to therapy. Similar response may be seen in patients with hypothalamic tumours such as craniopharyngiomas.

3. *Assessment of primary and secondary hypogonadism:* Patients with primary hypogonadism resulting from gonadal failure or gonadal dysgenesis will have an exaggerated response to LH-RH. Most of these patients will also have elevated basal values. The test is of particular value in those cases where basal levels are normal.

The majority of patients with congenital hypogonadotrophic hypogonadism with or without hyposmia (Kallman's syndrome) show a normal or impaired response to single doses of LH-RH.

These results indicate that, in most cases of isolated pituitary gonadotrophin deficiency, there is a reduced output of hypothalamic hormone-releasing factor. An absent response to a single injection, however, is not necessarily indicative of pituitary failure, as more than one injection may be required in order to produce a response.

4. *Assessment of delayed puberty:* In simple delayed puberty the LH and FSH responses are within the normal range, whereas patients with hypogonadotrophic hypogonadism or hypopituitarism have an absent or impaired response. Patients with primary gonadal failure will have an exaggerated response.

TRH

1. *Normal response:* In normal subjects, intravenous injection of TRH causes a prompt rise (within five minutes) in serum TSH. This increases to a maximum at about 20 minutes and is declining at 60 minutes. Basal levels are reached about four hours after TRH administration.

2. *Thyroid disease:* **Hyperthyroidism.** Diagnosis is based upon the measurement of two parameters.

(a) the increase in TSH values from basal levels, 20 minutes after TRH administration ($\triangle$TSH).
(b) the ratio of 20 minute TSH value to its basal value (TSH_{20}/TSH_0).

The usual hyperthyroid response is as follows:

(a) increase in TSH 20 minutes after injection will be less than 2 mcU/ml ($\triangle TSH < 2$).
(b) the ratio of 20 minute TSH to its basal value will be equal to or less than 1.5 ($TSH_{20}/TSH_0 \leqslant 1.5$).

Primary hypothyroidism. Primary hypothyroidism is characterised by a high basal TSH level and an exaggerated and prolonged rise in serum TSH following the administration of TRH.

3. *Hypothalamic or pituitary disease:* **Pituitary disease.** An absent or impaired TSH response indicates a reduction in pituitary reserve (although failure to respond to TRH is also found in patients with hyperthyroidism, this will not usually cause diagnostic difficulty).

Hypothalamic disease. Patients with hypothyroidism caused by hypothalamic disease may have a normal TSH response to TRH. However, more usually, a delayed response is found.

Note: The administration of TRH together with LH-RH may cause slightly greater FSH release in males than that caused by LH-RH alone.

Contra-indications, warnings, etc Relefact LH-RH/TRH should not be used in patients with bronchial asthma or obstructive airways disease. Care should be exercised in patients with myocardial ischaemia. Pituitary adenoma is a relative contra-indication.

LH-RH/TRH should not be administered in pregnancy; there is a theoretical possibility of induction of ovulation following the administration of LH-RH/TRH.

Side-effects: The following minor transient side-effects have been reported in patients given TRH: desire to micturate, sensation of heat, slight dizziness and a peculiar taste. There have been isolated reports of transient amaurosis, severe headache, unconsciousness, convulsions and hypotension.

LH-RH administration has been associated with the following reactions in isolated cases in healthy women: abdominal pain, nausea, headache and increased menstrual bleeding.

Overdosage: Overdosage with LH-RH/TRH should be treated symptomatically.

Pharmaceutical precautions Store in a cool dark place; do not dilute or administer with any additive.

Legal category POM.

Package quantities Relefact LH-RH/TRH is available in packs of 10 ampoules.

Further information LH-RH, TRH and insulin have been administered at the same time for a full and rapid assessment of anterior pituitary function. Such combined administration does not appreciably affect the various hormone responses (LH, FSH, TSH, growth hormone, ACTH, corticosteroids and prolactin).

Note: The mixing of insulin and LH-RH/TRH in the same syringe is not recommended.

Product licence number 0086/0059.

STREPTASE* INJECTION

Presentation Streptase (Streptokinase Injection BP) is presented as a freeze-dried powder in vials containing 250,000 Units, 750,000 Units and 1,500,000 Units of purified streptokinase. Excipients include albumin, polysolin and sodium glutamate.

Uses Streptase is a fibrinolytic agent which may be used for:

(a) The treatment of acute myocardial infarction.

(b) Intravascular dissolution of thrombi and emboli in: extensive deep venous thrombosis; pulmonary embolism; acute or sub-acute occlusion of peripheral arteries; central retinal venous or arterial thrombosis.

Dosage and administration Streptase should be given by intravenous infusion in 50–200 ml physiological saline, 5% glucose or Haemaccel.

(a) Acute myocardial infarction: A single dose of 1.5 million IU streptokinase may be infused intravenously over one hour for the treatment of acute myocardial infarction.

Control of therapy: No laboratory controls are necessary for the one hour intravenous lysis in myocardial infarction.

Adjuvant treatment: Treatment with aspirin (150 mg daily), for at least 4 weeks is recommended for prophylaxis after streptokinase therapy for acute myocardial infarction.

Children: There are no recommendations for the use of Streptase in acute myocardial infarction in children.

(b) Intravascular dissolution of thrombi and emboli: The initial dosage is given by infusion. Maintenance dosage is given thereafter by slow infusion.

Loading dose: Since human exposure to streptococci is common, antibodies to streptokinase (streptokinase resistance) are found normally. Thus, a loading dose of Streptase sufficient to neutralize the resistance is required when relatively small doses are used. A dose of 250,000 Units of Streptase infused into a peripheral vein over 30 minutes has been found appropriate in over 90% of patients.

Maintenance dose: A maintenance dose infusion of 100,000 Units/hour is given following the loading dose. Administer the maintenance dose of 100,000 Units per hour for 72 hours for the treatment of deep vein thrombosis, for 24 hours for the treatment of pulmonary embolism (up to 72 hours if concurrent deep vein thrombosis is suspected) and for 24–72 hours for the treatment of arterial thrombosis.

Control of therapy: If the thrombin time or any other parameter of lysis after 4 hours of therapy is less than approximately 1.5 times the normal control value, discontinue Streptase as excessive resistance to streptokinase is present.

Children: In children, in whom it is always advisable to estimate the initial dose by means of the streptokinase resistance test, the recommended maintenance dose per hour is 20 Units/ml blood volume.

Patient monitoring: Before commencing thrombolytic therapy, it is desirable to obtain a thrombin time (TT), pro-thrombin time (PT), haematocrit and platelet count to obtain the haemostatic status of the patient. If heparin has been given it should be discontinued, and the TT should be less than twice the normal control value before thrombolytic therapy is started.

During the infusion, decreases in the plasminogen and fibrinogen levels and an increase in the level of fibrin degradation products (FDP) (the latter two serving to prolong the clotting times of coagulation tests) will generally confirm the existence of a lytic state. Therefore, therapy can be monitored by performing the TT or PT approximately 4 hours after initiation of therapy.

Following the infusion, before instituting heparin, the TT should be less than twice the normal control value.

Anticoagulation after terminating intravenous streptokinase treatment: At the end of Streptase therapy, treatment with heparin by continuous intravenous infusion is recommended to prevent recurrent thrombosis. Heparin treatment (without a loading dose) should not begin until the thrombin time has decreased to less than twice the normal control value (approximately 3 to 4 hours). (See manufacturer's prescribing information for proper use of heparin.) This should be followed by oral anticoagulation in the conventional manner.

Contra-indications, warnings, etc

Contra-indications: Existing or very recent haemorrhage:

- all forms of reduced blood coagulability, in particular spontaneous fibrinolysis and uncontrollable clotting disorders (with the exception of consumption coagulopathy)
- local lesions with risk of bleeding (e.g. gastrointestinal conditions with existing haemorrhage, previous translumbar aortography, puncture of large arteries, intramuscular injections, indwelling catheters or endotracheal tubes)
- recent operations (up to the 6th post-operative day, depending on the extent of the procedure) and recent severe trauma
- recent abortion or delivery
- diseases of the urogenital tract with existing or potential sources of bleeding.

Recent streptococcal infections which have produced high anti-streptokinase titres (e.g. acute rheumatic fever, acute glomerulonephritis), or recent streptokinase therapy more than 5 days and less than 12 months previously.

Previous allergic reactions, including vasculitic purpura, to streptokinase or streptokinase-containing products.

Subacute bacterial endocarditis.

Severe hypertension with systolic values over 200 mm Hg or diastolic values over 100 mm Hg or hypertensive retinal changes Grades III/IV.

Severe liver or kidney damage.

Disorders of cerebral blood flow or recent cerebral haemorrhage.

Pulmonary disease with cavitation (e.g. open tuberculosis) or severe bronchitis.

Acute pancreatitis or severe diabetes mellitus.

Advanced age with suspicion of arteriosclerotic degeneration.

Pregnancy (see 'Precautions').

Warnings: There is an increased risk of haemorrhage in patients who are receiving or who have recently been treated with anticoagulants or any drugs which affect platelet formation or function (e.g. acetylsalicyclic acid, allopurinol, anabolic steroids, androgens, dipyridamole, thyroid hormones, volatile oils, quinidine, clofibric acid derivatives, phenylbutazone, indomethacin, aryl acetic acid and aryl propionic acid derivatives, tetracyclines, valproic acid, thiouracils and sulphonamides). Simultaneous treatment with dextrans also increases the danger of haemorrhage. The effects of drugs which act upon platelet formation or function should be allowed to subside before starting long-term systemic lysis with Streptase.

If the patient has previously been receiving heparin, its effects can be neutralized by giving protamine sulphate.

In patients previously treated with coumarin derivatives, the pro-thrombin index must not be less than 50% and should have a rising trend before starting streptokinase infusion.

Precautions: Streptase is contra-indicated in pregnancy.

There is no evidence of the drug's safety in pregnancy nor is there evidence from animal work that it is free from hazard. Bleeding and anaphylactic reactions might cause abortion and fetal death, especially when Streptase is given within the first 18 weeks of pregnancy. Use only when there is no safer alternative and when the disease (as, for example, in individual cases of massive pulmonary embolism) carries a high degree of risk for the mother.

Caution is necessary in patients with mitral valve defects or atrial fibrillation, because of the danger of cerebral embolization from the left side of the heart.

The risks of therapy must be weighed against the dangers of the disease.

In the following conditions streptokinase is unlikely to be effective:

- Deep vein thrombosis more than 14 days old
- Central retinal vessels: occlusion of central retinal arteries more than 6–8 hours old, and thrombosis of central retinal vein more than 10 days old.

Side-effects:

Early reactions: Headaches, pain in the back and allergic-anaphylactic reactions with flushing and dyspnoea may occur. Allergic reactions can be largely avoided by giving the initial intravenous dose slowly. Corticosteroids can also be given prophylactically (e.g. 100–250 mg methylprednisolone 10 minutes before starting streptokinase treatment). If an allergic reaction occurs the infusion should be discontinued and the patient should be given corticosteroids intravenously, together with adrenaline and an antihistamine. Once the symptoms have subsided, treatment can be continued with Streptase or urokinase.

Treatment of anaphylactic shock: Discontinue Streptase immediately. Adrenaline should be given immediately by slow intravenous injection. In addition, high doses of corticosteroids by slow intravenous injection may be given.

Pyrexia, chills and rashes: Chills with or without pyrexia may occur during treatment. In most cases fever responds promptly and lastingly to antipyretics. Generalized rashes can be treated by giving methylprednisolone i.v.

Haemorrhages: If haemorrhages occur they are usually confined to puncture sites. In such a case discontinuation of treatment is not necessary.

In serious haemorrhagic complications, streptokinase therapy should be discontinued and a proteinase inhibitor, e.g. aprotinin should be given in the following dosages:

Initially 500,000 KIU to one million KIU by slow intravenous injection or infusion (maximum rate 5 ml/min). If necessary this should be followed by 200,000 KIU four-hourly until the bleeding stops. In addition, combination with synthetic antifibrinolytics is recommended. If necessary, clotting factors can be substituted.

Other reactions: In a few sporadic cases, neuroallergic symptoms (polyneuropathy) have been reported in temporal coincidence with Streptase administration.

Serum sickness has been reported but is rare.

Arrhythmias and transient hypotension have been noted, particularly after high-dose, short-term therapy.

The risk of pulmonary embolism in patients with deep vein thrombosis is not greater during treatment with streptokinase than during treatment with heparin alone. If acute or recurrent pulmonary embolism occurs during treatment, the course of streptokinase therapy should be continued as originally planned, so as to lyse the emboli.

A transient increase in serum enzymes has been reported following Streptase therapy.

Overdosage:
Long-term overdosage of streptokinase may induce the risk of rethrombosis by prolonged decrease of plasminogen. See also 'Side-effects (haemorrhages)'.

Pharmaceutical precautions Streptase is stable for at least 3 years when stored at +2 to +25°C.

After being dissolved in 5 ml of sterile physiological saline, Streptase can be stored in a refrigerator at +2 to +8°C for 24 hours without loss of activity.

To ensure that the contents of the vial are rapidly and completely dissolved, 5 ml of physiological saline should be injected into the vial, and the residual vacuum abolished by briefly loosening the needle from the syringe.

For administration with an infusion pump, physiological saline, Ringer-lactate solution, 5% glucose or fructose solution can be used as diluent. For higher dilutions, Haemaccel* may be used as diluent.

Legal category POM.

Package quantities Available in vials in the following packs:
1 × 250,000 IU.
1 × 750,000 IU.
1 × 1,500,000 IU.

Further information Streptase activates the intrinsic fibrinolytic system by the formation of a linkage compound between streptokinase and the proactivator plasminogen molecule. This complex possesses activator properties and brings about the conversion of plasminogen into the fibrinolytic enzyme plasmin. Plasminogen absorbed on to the fibrin clot is also activated, therefore lysis can take place internally as well as externally.

When thrombolytic therapy is necessary and a high antibody concentration against streptokinase is present, or when recent streptokinase therapy has been given (more than 5 days and less than 12 months previously), urokinase can be used.

Product licence numbers

Streptase 250,000 Units	0086/5020
Streptase 750,000 Units	0086/5021
Streptase 1,500,000 Units	0086/0127

SUPREFACT* INJECTION
SUPREFACT* NASAL SPRAY

Presentation Suprefact injection contains 1.00 mg buserelin as buserelin acetate in 1 ml aqueous solution contining benzyl alcohol as preservative. The solution also contains sodium chloride, sodium dihydrogen phosphate and sodium hydroxide as excipients.

Suprefact nasal spray contains 100 micrograms buserelin as buserelin acetate in one spray dose (100 mg) of aqueous solution containing benzylkonium chloride as preservative. The solution also contains citric acid, sodium chloride and sodium citrate.

1.00 mg buserelin is equivalent to 1.05 mg buserelin acetate.

Uses For the treatment of advanced prostatic carcinoma (stage C or stage D according to the classification of Murphy et al. in Cancer, 45, p 1889–95, 1980) in which suppression of testosterone is indicated. Buserelin acts by blockade and subsequent down-regulation of pituitary LHRH receptor synthesis. Gonadotrophin release is consequently inhibited. As a result of this inhibition there is reduced stimulation of testosterone secretion and serum testosterone levels fall to the castration range. Before inhibition occurs there is a brief stimulatory phase during which testosterone levels may rise.

Dosage and administration

1. Initiation of therapy: is most conveniently carried out in hospital; 0.5 ml Suprefact injection should be injected subcutaneously at 8 hourly intervals for 7 days.
2. Maintenance therapy: on the 8th day of treatment the patient is changed to intranasal administration of Suprefact. One spray dose is introduced into each nostril 6 times a day according to the following schedule:

1st dose before breakfast
2nd dose after breakfast
3rd and 4th doses before and after midday meal
5th and 6th doses before and after evening meal.

This dosage regimen is to ensure adequate absorption of the material and to distribute the dose throughout the day.

Contra-indications, warnings, etc
Contra-indications: Suprefact should not be used if the tumour is found to be insensitive to hormone manipulation or after surgical removal of the testes. It is contraindicated in cases of known hypersensitivity to benzalkonium chloride (nasal spray) or benzyl alcohol (injection) or buserelin.

Precautions and warnings: Monitoring of the clinical effect of Suprefact is carried out by the methods generally used in prostatic carcinoma. Initially serum testosterone levels rise and a clinical effect will not be seen until levels start to fall into the therapeutic (castration) range. Disease flare (temporary deterioration of patient's condition) has been reported at the beginning of treatment. The incidence is variable, but of the order of 10%. Symptoms are usually confined to transient increase in pain, but the exact nature depends on the site of the lesions. Neurological sequelae have been reported where secondary deposits impinge upon the spinal cord or CNS. Disease flare is prevented by the prophylactic use of an anti-androgen, e.g. cyproterone acetate, 300 mg daily. It is recommended that treatment should be started at least 3 days before the first dose of Suprefact and continued for at least 3 weeks after commencement of Suprefact therapy.

Once testosterone levels have started to fall below their baseline concentration clinical improvement should start to become apparent. If testosterone levels do not reach the therapeutic range within 4 weeks (6 weeks at the latest) the dose schedule should be checked to be sure that it is being followed exactly. It is unlikely that a patient who is taking the full dose will not show a suppression of testosterone to the therapeutic range. If this is the case, alternative therapy should be considered.

After the initial determination, testosterone levels should be monitored at 3-monthly intervals. A proportion of patients will have tumours that are not sensitive to hormone manipulation. Absence of clinical improvement in the face of adequate testosterone suppression is diagnostic of this condition, which will not benefit from further therapy with buserelin.

Patients not known to suffer from depression should be carefully monitored during treatment with Suprefact.

Side-effects: Suprefact is generally well tolerated. Side-effects consequent upon the suppression of testosterone secretion are hot flushes and loss of potency and libido. These occur in most patients.

Gynaecomastia may occur rarely, but is usually not painful. Depressive moods have been noted in rare cases.

Headaches have been reported to occur in up to 10% of patients receiving buserelin. These tend to occur at the start of treatment and are seldom severe enough to necessitate the discontinuation of buserelin therapy.

Transient nasal irritation and nosebleeds have been reported after nasal application but are rare.

Hypersensitivity reactions, including reddening of the skin, urticaria and difficulty in breathing, have been reported on rare occasions. Anaphylactic reactions are very rare.

Isolated cases of thrombosis with pulmonary embolism have been reported. The causality of these events is uncertain.

Gastro-intestinal disorders (eg nausea, vomiting and diarrhoea) have been observed. Dizziness may occur.

Overdosage: No adverse effects due to overdosage have been reported. Animal studies have not revealed any hazard. Treatment should be symptomatic.

Pharmaceutical precautions Store at room temperature. The spray solution should last for 1 week of treatment. Any residual material after this time should be discarded.

Legal category POM.

Package quantities
Suprefact for Injection: Box of 2 × 5.5 ml multidose vials each containing 1.05 mg buserelin acetate per 1 ml, corresponding to 1.00 mg buserelin per 1 ml.

Suprefact Nasal Spray: Outer of 4 bottles each containing 10 g solution, and 4 spray pumps.

Further information The therapeutic effect of Suprefact can only be achieved if the dosage is conscientiously adhered to. It is, therefore, advisable to administer Suprefact nasal spray before and after meals. It can also be used at other times provided uniform intervals are maintained between doses.

If used correctly, reliable absorption of the active substance takes place via the nasal mucous membrane. Suprefact nasal spray is absorbed even if the patient has a cold.

Product licence numbers

Suprefact Nasal Spray	0086/0101.
Suprefact Injection	0086/0102.

TARIVID* ▼

Presentation Tarivid tablets each contain 200 mg ofloxacin. They are yellowish-white oblong tablets, 14 × 7 mm, biconvex with a score mark on one side. Excipients include lactose.

Uses Ofloxacin is a synthetic 4-fluoroquinolone antibacterial agent with bactericidal activity against a wide range of Gram-negative and Gram-positive organisms. It is indicated for the treatment of the following infections when caused by sensitive organisms: Upper and lower urinary tract infections; lower respiratory tract infections; uncomplicated urethral and cervical gonorrhoea; non-gonococcal urethritis and cervicitis.

Microbiological results indicate that the following pathogens may be regarded as sensitive: *Staphylococcus aureus* (including methicillin resistant staph.), *Staphylococcus epidermidis*, Neisseria species, *Escherichia coli*, Citrobacter, Klebsiella, Enterobacter, Hafnia, Proteus (indole-negative and indole-positive strains), *Pseudomonas aeruginosa*, *Haemophilus influenzae*, Chlamydiae, Mycoplasmas, Legionella, Gardnerella.

Variable sensitivity is shown by Streptococci, *Serratia marcescens*, Bacteroides species.

Anaerobic bacteria (e.g. Fusobacterium species, Eubacterium species, Peptococci, Peptostreptococci), *Treponema pallidum*, are normally resistant.

Dosage and administration General dosage recommendations: The dose of ofloxacin is determined by the type and severity of the infection. The dosage range for adults is 200 mg to 800 mg daily. Up to 400 mg may be given as a single dose, preferably in the morning, larger doses should be given as two divided doses. Tarivid tablets should be swallowed with liquid; they should not be taken within two hours of magnesium/aluminium containing antacids or iron preparations since reduction of absorption of ofloxacin can occur.

Lower urinary tract infection: 200 –400 mg daily.

Upper urinary tract infection: 200–400 mg daily increasing, if necessary, to 400 mg twice a day.

Lower respiratory tract infection: 400 mg daily increasing, if necessary, to 400 mg twice daily.

Uncomplicated urethral and cervical gonorrhoea: A single dose of 400 mg.

Non-gonococcal urethritis and cervicitis: 400 mg daily in single or divided doses.

Impaired renal function: Following a normal initial dose, dosage should be reduced in patients with impairment of renal function. When creatinine clearance is 20–50 ml/minute (serum creatinine 1.5–5.0 mg/dl) the dosage should be reduced by half (100–200 mg daily). If creatinine clearance is less than 20 ml/minute (serum creatinine greater than 5 mg/dl) 100 mg should be given every 48 hours.

In patients undergoing haemodialysis or peritoneal dialysis, 100 mg should be given every 48 hours.

Elderly: No adjustment of dosage is required in the elderly, other than that imposed by consideration of renal function.

Children: Ofloxacin is not indicated for use in children or growing adolescents.

Duration of treatment: Duration of treatment is dependent on the severity of the infection and the response to treatment. The usual treatment period is 5–10 days except in uncomplicated gonorrhoea, where a single dose is recommended.

Treatment should not exceed 2 months duration.

Contra-indications, warnings, etc
Contra-indications: Ofloxacin should not be used in patients with known hypersensitivity to 4-quinolone antibacterials.

Ofloxacin, like other 4-quinolones, is contra-indicated in patients with a history of epilepsy or with a lowered seizure threshold.

Ofloxacin is contra-indicated in children or growing adolescents, and in pregnant or breast-feeding women, since animal experiments do not entirely exclude the risk of damage to the cartilage of joints in the growing subject.

Warnings and precautions: Patients being treated with ofloxacin should not expose themselves unnecessarily to strong sunlight and should avoid UV rays (sunlamps, solarium). Caution is recommended if the drug is to be used in psychotic patients or in patients with a history of psychiatric disease.

Use in pregnancy and lactation: Reproduction studies performed in rats and rabbits did not reveal any evidence of teratogenicity, impairment of fertility or impairment of peri-/post-natal development. However, as with other quinolones, ofloxacin has been shown to cause arthropathy in immature animals and therefore its use during pregnancy is not recommended. Studies in rats have indicated that ofloxacin is secreted in milk. It should therefore not be used during lactation.

Interactions: Co-administered magnesium/aluminium antacids or iron preparations can reduce absorption.

Side-effects: Hypersensitivity reactions, immediate or delayed, usually involving the skin but occasionally with other signs of anaphylaxis, shock, dyspnoea, vasculitic reactions, oedema of the glottis, face or tongue, tachycardia, may occur. Treatment should be stopped immediately, and supportive treatment given. There have been a few cases of skin reactions on exposure to strong sunlight and occasionally other severe skin reactions have occurred.

There have been occasional disturbances of the central nervous system, e.g. sleep disorders, headaches, dizziness, nightmares, unsteady gait and tremor, neuropathy, numbness and paraesthesia, visual disturbances, disturbances of taste and smell. Restlessness, agitation, anxiety and confusion have been reported, as have hallucinations and psychotic reactions. These reactions have occurred in some patients after the first dose of ofloxacin. In such cases, discontinue treatment immediately.

There have been rare reports of pain in joints and muscles.

There have been rare reports of bone marrow depression (leukopenia, agranulocytosis, thrombocytopenia and anaemia). Transient increases in liver enzymes and/or bilirubin have been reported, as have disturbances of kidney function including increases in serum creatinine.

As with other antimicrobials, gastrointestinal symptoms may occur (gastric symptoms, abdominal pain, loss of appetite, nausea, vomiting, diarrhoea). Pseudomembranous colitis has also been reported.

Ability to drive: Since there have been occasional reports of dizziness and visual disturbances, patients should know how they react to Tarivid before they drive or operate machinery.

Overdosage: Information on overdosage is not available. Routine measures such as gastric lavage should be carried out as soon as possible.

Pharmaceutical precautions Keep medicines out of the reach of children. Store in a dry place.

Legal category POM.

Package quantities Blister packs of 10, 20 and 100 tablets.

Further information Crystalluria has not been reported with ofloxacin. Interactions with theophylline metabolism and caffeine are unlikely because of the lack of metabolism of ofloxacin.

Product licence number 0086/0139.

TRENTAL* 400

Presentation Trental 400 tablets each contain 400 mg oxpentifylline in a slow-release formulation. They are presented as oblong, pink, sugar-coated tablets, 17.5 mm long, 8.75 mm wide and 6 mm thick. Excipients include sucrose (as part of the sugar coating).

Uses Trental is indicated in the treatment of peripheral vascular disease, including intermittent claudication and rest pain.

Dosage and administration The recommended initial dose is 1 tablet (400 mg) three times daily; two tablets daily may prove sufficient in some patients, particularly for maintenance therapy. Tablets should be taken with or immediately after meals, and swallowed whole with plenty of water.

Elderly: No special dosage requirements.

Children: Trental 400 is not suitable for use in children.

Contra-indications, warnings, etc

Contra-indications: Trental 400 is contra-indicated in cases where there is known hypersensitivity to the active constituent, oxpentifylline.

Warnings: High doses of Trental injection have been shown, in rare cases, to intensify the hypoglycaemic action of insulin and oral hypoglycaemic agents. However, no effect on insulin release has been observed with Trental following oral administration.

Trental 400 may potentiate the effect of anti-hypertensive agents and the dosage of the latter may need to be reduced.

In patients with hypotension or severe coronary artery disease, Trental 400 should be used with caution, as a transient hypotensive effect is possible and, in isolated cases, might result in a reduction in coronary artery perfusion.

In patients with a creatinine clearance of less than 10 ml/min it may be necessary to adjust the daily dose of oxpentifylline to avoid accumulation.

Precautions: There is no information on the use of Trental in pregnancy but no untoward effects have been found in animal studies. Trental 400 should not be administered during pregnancy.

Nursing mothers: There is no information on the use of Trental 400 in nursing mothers.

Overdosage: The treatment of overdosage should be symptomatic with particular attention to supporting the cardiovascular system.

Side-effects: Gastrointestinal side-effects (e.g. nausea, vomiting, diarrhoea), headache or dizziness may occur which, in individual cases, could necessitate discontinuation of treatment.

There have been very rare reports of flushing, tachycardia, angina pectoris and hypotension, particularly if using high doses of oxpentifylline. In such cases a discontinuation of the medication or a reduction of the daily dosage is required.

Hypersensitivity reactions such as pruritus, rash, urticaria or angioneurotic edema are extremely rare and usually disappear rapidly after discontinuation of the drug treatment.

A few very rare events of bleeding (e.g. skin, mucosa) have been reported in patients treated with Trental with and without anticoagulants or platelet aggregation inhibitors. The serious cases are predominantly concentrated in the gastrointestinal, genitourinary, multiple site and surgical wound areas and are associated with bleeding risk factors. A causal relationship between Trental therapy and bleeding has not been established. Thrombocytopenia occurred in a few cases.

Pharmaceutical precautions Trental 400 should be stored at ambient temperature in a dry place in the original container or in containers similar to those of the manufacturer.

Legal category POM.

Package quantities Trental 400 tablets are available in packs of 90 (original pack) and 250 (hospital pack).

Further information Nil.

Product licence number 0086/0058.

TRITACE* ▼

Presentation Yellow opaque/white opaque hard gelatin capsules each containing 1.25 mg ramipril.

Orange opaque/white opaque hard gelatin capsules each containing 2.5 mg ramipril.

Crimson opaque/white opaque hard gelatin capsules each containing 5.0 mg ramipril.

Uses

Indications: Mild to moderate hypertension where standard therapy is ineffective or inappropriate because of adverse reactions.

Mechanism of action: Ramipril is a prodrug which, after absorption from the gastrointestinal tract, is hydrolysed in the liver to form the active angiotensin converting enzyme (ACE) inhibitor, ramiprilat which is a potent and long acting ACE inhibitor. Administration of ramipril causes an increase in plasma renin activity and a decrease in plasma concentrations of angiotensin II and aldosterone. The beneficial haemodynamic effects resulting from ACE inhibition are a consequence of the reduction in angiotensin II causing dilatation of peripheral vessels and reduction in vascular resistance. There is evidence suggesting that tissue ACE particularly in the vasculature, rather than circulating ACE, is the primary factor determining the haemodynamic effects.

Angiotensin converting enzyme is identical with kininase II, one of the enzymes responsible for the degradation of bradykinin. There is evidence that ACE inhibition by ramiprilat appears to have some effects on the kallikrein-kinin-prostaglandin systems. It is assumed that effects on these systems contribute to the hypotensive and metabolic activity of ramipril.

Administration of Tritace to hypertensive patients results in reduction of both supine and erect blood pressure. The antihypertensive effect is evident within one to two hours after the drug intake; peak effect occurs 3–6 hours after drug intake and has been shown to be maintained for at least 24 hours after usual therapeutic doses.

Dosage and administration The recommended initial dosage in patients not on diuretics and without congestive heart failure is 1.25 mg Tritace once a day. Dosage should be increased incrementally at intervals of 1–2 weeks, based on patient response, up to a maximum of 10 mg once a day.

A 1.25 mg dose will only achieve a therapeutic response in a minority of patients. The usual effective dose range is 2.5–5 mg as a single daily dose. If the patient response is still unsatisfactory at a dose of 10 mg Tritace, combination treatment is recommended.

Diuretic-treated patients: The diuretic should be discontinued 2–3 days before beginning therapy with Tritace to reduce the likelihood of symptomatic hypotension. It may be resumed later if required.

Cardiac failure: In hypertensive patients who also have congestive heart failure, with or without associated renal insufficiency, symptomatic hypotension has been observed after treatment with ACE inhibitors. In these patients therapy should be started at a dose of 1.25 mg under close medical supervision in hospital.

Dosage adjustment in renal impairment: The usual dose of Tritace is recommended for patients with a creatinine clearance >30 ml/min (serum creatinine <165 umol/l). For patients with a creatinine clearance <30 ml/min (serum creatinine >165 umol/l) the initial dose is 1.25 mg Tritace once daily and the maximum dose 5 mg Tritace once daily.

In patients with severe renal impairment (creatinine clearance <10 ml/min and serum creatinine of 400–650 umol/l), the recommended initial dose is also 1.25 mg Tritace once a day, but the maintenance dose should not exceed 2.5 mg Tritace once a day.

Dosage in hepatic impairment: In patients with impaired liver function the metabolism of the parent compound ramipril, and therefore the formation of the bioactive metabolite ramiprilat, is delayed due to diminished activity of esterases in the liver, resulting in elevated plasma ramipril levels. Treatment with Tritace should therefore be initiated at a dose of 1.25 mg under close medical supervision in patients with impaired liver function.

Elderly: Caution in elderly patients with concomitant use of diuretics, congestive heart failure or renal or hepatic insufficiency. The dose should be titrated according to need for the control of blood pressure.

Children: Tritace has not been studied in children, and therefore use in this age group is not recommended.

Tritace should be taken with plenty of liquid with or after food. Food intake has no marked effect on the extent of absorption.

Contra-indications, warnings, etc

Contra-indications: Hypersensitivity to ramipril. History of angioneurotic oedema. Pregnancy. Lactation.

Warnings: Tritace should not be used in patients with aortic stenosis or outflow obstruction.

Precautions: Assessment of renal function: Evaluation of the patient should include assessment of renal function prior to initiation of therapy and during treatment.

Impaired renal function: Patients with renal insufficiency may require reduced or less frequent doses of Tritace; their renal function should be closely monitored. In the majority, renal function will not alter. There is a risk of impairment of renal function, particularly in patients with renal insufficiency, congestive heart failure, bilateral renal artery stenosis and unilateral renal artery stenosis in the single kidney as well as after renal transplantation. If recognised early, such impairment of renal function is reversible upon discontinuation of therapy.

Some hypertensive patients with no apparent pre-existing renal disease, may develop minor and usually transient increases in blood urea nitrogen and serum creatinine when Tritace is given, in particular concomitantly with a diuretic. Dosage reduction of Tritace and/or discontinuation of the diuretic may be required. Additionally, in patients with renal insufficiency, there is a risk of hyperkalaemia.

Impaired liver function: As ramipril is a prodrug metabolised to its active moiety in the liver, particular caution and close monitoring should be applied to patients with impaired liver function. The metabolism of the parent compound, and therefore the formation of the bioactive metabolite ramiprilat, may be diminished resulting in markedly elevated plasma levels of the parent compound (due to the reduced activity of esterases in the liver).

Symptomatic hypotension: In patients with uncomplicated hypertension, symptomatic hypotension has been observed rarely after the initial dose of Tritace as well as after increasing the dose of Tritace. It is more likely to occur in patients who have been volume-and salt-depleted by prolonged diuretic therapy, dietary salt restriction, dialysis, diarrhoea or vomiting. Therefore, in these patients, diuretic therapy should be discontinued and volume and/or salt depletion should be corrected before initiating therapy with Tritace.

If symptomatic hypotension occurs, the patient should be placed in a supine position and, if necessary, receive an intravenous infusion of physiological saline. Intravenous atropine may be necessary if there is associated bradycardia. Treatment with Tritace may usually be continued following restoration of effective blood volume and blood pressure.

Surgery/anaesthesia: In patients undergoing surgery or during anaesthesia with agents producing hypotension, Tritace may block angiotensin II formation secondary to compensatory renin release. If hypotension occurs and is considered to be due to this mechanism, it can be corrected by appropriate treatment.

Agranulocytosis and bone marrow depression: In patients on angiotensin converting enzyme inhibitors agranulocytosis and bone marrow depression have been seen rarely. They are more frequent in patients with renal impairment, especially if they have a collagen vascular disease. However, regular monitoring of white blood cell counts and protein levels in urine should be considered in patients with collagen vascular disease (e.g. lupus erythematosus and scleroderma), especially associated with impaired renal function and concomitant therapy particularly with corticosteroids and antimetabolites.

Hyperkalaemia: Elevated serum potassium has been observed very rarely in hypertensive patients. Risk factors for the development of hyperkalaemia include renal insufficiency, potassium sparing diuretics and the concomitant use of agents to treat hypokalaemia.

Use during pregnancy and lactation: Pregnancy should be excluded before start of treatment with Tritace and avoided during treatment; exposure of the mother to ACE inhibitors in mid or late pregnancy has been associated with oligohydramnios and neonatal hypotension with anuria or renal failure.

From animal experiments it is known that use of ramipril may cause a decreased utero-placental perfusion. There is also a potential risk of fetal or post-natal effect as ACE inhibitors also influence the local renin-angiotensin system. In peri-post natal studies increased renal pelvic dilatation was observed in the first generation offspring. However, ramipril was not fetotoxic in our studies although ACE inhibitors have shown fetotoxicity in some species.

Tritace should not be used during lactation.

Influence on driving ability and handling machinery: In individual cases, treatment with Tritace may affect the ability to drive and operate machinery. This occurs especially at the start of treatment, when changing over from other preparations and during concomitant use of alcohol. After the first dose or subsequent increases in dose it is not advisable to drive or operate machinery for several hours.

Drug interactions: Combination with diuretics or other antihypertensive agents may potentiate the antihypertensive response to Tritace. Adrenergic-blocking drugs should only be combined with ramipril under careful supervision.

Potassium sparing diuretics (spironolactone, amiloride, triamterene) or potassium supplements may increase the risk of hyperkalaemia. Tritace may attenuate the potassium loss caused by thiazide-type diuretics. If concomitant use of these agents is indicated, they should be given with caution and serum potassium should be monitored regularly.

If Tritace is given with lithium, an increase in serum lithium concentration may occur.

The protein binding of ramipril is about 73% and of ramiprilat about 56%.

Side-effects: In clinical trials the frequency of Tritace-related adverse reactions was low. Generally, adverse reactions have been mild and transient, and have not required discontinuation of therapy. The most frequently reported adverse reactions are nausea, dizziness and headache.

Cardiovascular: Symptomatic hypotension accompanied by dizziness, weakness and nausea may occur after the initial dose of Tritace and after an increase in the dose of Tritace. It has been rarely observed, but may occur in severely salt/volume-depleted patients such as those treated with diuretics, patients on dialysis and in patients with severe congestive heart failure. Syncope has also been observed rarely.

Renal: Treatment with Tritace may impair renal function.

Gastrointestinal: Nausea, vomiting, abdominal pain and diarrhoea may occur, but these reactions are often transient. In very rare cases, taste disturbances may occur.

Allergic: Hypersensitivity reactions accompanied by pruritus, rash, shortness of breath and sometimes fever may occur, but usually resolve spontaneously after withdrawal of Tritace.

Angioneurotic oedema: In very rare cases angioneurotic oedema has occurred during therapy with ACE inhibitors including Tritace. If laryngeal stridor or angioedema of the face, tongue or glottis occurs, treatment with Tritace must be discontinued and appropriate therapy instituted immediately.

Other: Headache, fatigue and aesthenia, dizziness and dry cough may occur.

Laboratory test findings: Increases in blood urea nitrogen and serum creatinine may occur, in particular with renal insufficiency or in patients pretreated with a diuretic.

Serum sodium levels may decrease. Elevation of serum potassium may occur, since Tritace leads to a decrease in aldosterone secretion; potassium-sparing diuretics (spironolactone, amiloride, triamterene) or potassium supplements should therefore be avoided.

Overdosage: In case of overdosage prolonged hypotension is to be expected. Treatment with an intravenous infusion of physiological saline and/or angiotensin II may be required.

Pharmaceutical precautions
Stability: The expiry date is indicated on the package.

Storage: Tritace capsules should be stored below 25°C. They should be kept away from children.

Legal category POM.

Package quantities Tritace is available in blister packs of 28 capsules.

Further information
Pharmacokinetics and metabolism: Following oral administration ramipril is rapidly absorbed from the gastrointestinal tract, peak plasma concentrations of ramipril are reached within one hour. Peak plasma concentrations of the active metabolite, ramiprilat, are reached within 2–4 hours.

Plasma concentrations of ramiprilat decline in a polyphasic manner. The effective half-life of ramiprilat after multiple once daily administration of ramipril is 13–17 hours for 5–10 mg ramipril and markedly longer for lower doses, 1.25–2.5 mg ramipril. This difference is related to the long terminal phase of the ramiprilat concentration time curve observed at very low plasma concentrations. This terminal phase is independent of the dose, indicating a saturable capacity of the enzyme to bind ramiprilat. Steady-state plasma concentrations of ramiprilat after once daily dosing with the usual doses of ramipril are reached by about the fourth day of treatment.

Ramipril is almost completely metabolised and the metabolites are excreted mainly via the kidneys. In addition to the bioactive metabolite, ramiprilat, other, inactive, metabolites have been identified, including diketopiperazine ester, diketopiperazine acid and conjugates.

Product licence numbers

1.25 mg	capsule	0086/0130.
2.50 mg	capsule	0086/0131.
5 mg	capsule	0086/0132.

**Trade Mark*

Hough, Hoseason & Company Limited
Chapel Street
Levenshulme
Manchester M19 3PT

AQUASEPT* SKIN CLEANSER

Presentation An antiseptic skin cleanser containing 2% w/v triclosan in a blue, perfumed tenside solution.

Uses Pre-operative surgical hand disinfection.
As an antiseptic skin cleanser (for ward hand disinfection).
To help to eliminate pathogens by whole body bathing.
For the prevention of cross infection.

Dosage and administration
Pre-operative hand disinfection: Wet hands and forearms with water. Apply about 5 ml Aquasept and wash for one minute. Clean finger nails. Rinse. Repeat the wash for two minutes. Rinse thoroughly. Dry on a sterile towel.

As an antiseptic skin cleanser: Wet the hands and wrists. Apply about 5 ml Aquasept and wash for one minute. Dry on a disposable towel.

Pre-operative skin care prior to surgery: By whole body bathing in bath or shower on three occasions prior including once on the day of the operation. 28.5 ml Aquasept should be used as a liquid soap, applying it to the wet skin and paying particular attention to the flexures, perineum, groin and hair. Bedridden patients may be washed with Aquasept using the normal bed washing protocol.

Contra-indications, warnings, etc For external use only. Avoid contact with eyes. If swallowed, gastric lavage and symptomatic treatment.

Legal category GSL.

Package quantities 28.5 ml, 100 ml, 250 ml, 500 ml and 5 l.

Further information Aquasept is resistant to contamination in use.

Product licence number 0423/0009.

MANUSEPT*

Presentation A clear, blue coloured solution containing 70% v/v Isopropyl Alcohol BP, 0.5% w/v Triclosan.

Uses For the disinfection of intact skin.
For preoperative disinfection of physically clean hands.
For skin disinfection prior to surgery, injection or venepuncture.

Dosage and administration
For the disinfection of physically clean hands: Dispense approximately 3 ml of Manusept into the palm of one hand. Rub both hands, wrists and forearms together vigorously, paying particular attention to the area around the fingernails. Continue rubbing until dry. Repeat this procedure once more for the preoperative disinfection.

For the disinfection of intact skin before surgery, injection or venepuncture: Apply a quantity of Manusept with a sterile swab. Rub vigorously until dry. Repeat this procedure once more.

Contra-indications, warnings, etc *Treatment of overdosage:* If swallowed, gastric aspiration and lavage avoiding pulmonary aspiration. Apomorphine should not be used.
Avoid contact with eyes. For external use only.

Pharmaceutical precautions Store at or below normal ambient temperatures. Do not use in the vicinity of naked flames.

Legal category GSL.

Package quantities 500 ml, 250 ml and 5 Litre.

Further information Triclosan is compatible with soap, which can be used to obtain physically clean hands.

Product licence number 0423/0008.

STER-ZAC* BATH CONCENTRATE

Presentation A clear solution containing 2% Triclosan.

Uses Ster-Zac Bath Concentrate has an antibacterial effect in bath water.
For the prevention of cross-infection and secondary infection.

Dosage and administration *Baths:* Add 28.5 ml of Ster-Zac Bath Concentrate to a bathful of water (approx. 140 litres) immediately prior to the patient entering the water.

For washing: Add 1 ml of Ster-Zac Bath Concentrate to 5 litres of water prior to use.

Contra-indications, warnings, etc Avoid contact with the eyes. For external use only.

Pharmaceutical precautions For external use only. Store in a cool dry place.

Legal category P.

Package quantities 28.5 ml, 500 ml and 2 litres.

Further information Nil.

Product licence number 0423/5001.

STER-ZAC* DC SKIN CLEANSER

Presentation A white cream. Contains 3% Hexachlorophane BP.

Uses Ster-Zac DC has an antibacterial effect and is used for the pre-operative preparation of the hands.

Indications For the pre-operative disinfection of the hands of surgical personnel.

Dosage and administration For external use only. Apply 3 ml to 5 ml to pre-moistened hands and wash for up to three minutes. Rinse and repeat.

Contra-indications To be administered to children under two years of age on medical advice only. Do not use for whole body bathing. Do not apply to burns or badly damaged skin. For external use only.

Pharmaceutical precautions No special requirements.

Legal category POM.

Package quantities 150 ml 4.5 litres.

Further information Ster-Zac DC skin cleanser is resistant to contamination in use.

Product licence number 0423/0007.

STER-ZAC* POWDER

Presentation A white dusting powder containing 0.33% Hexachlorophane BP.

Uses For the prevention of neo-natal staphylococcal cross infection.

As an adjunct for the treatment of recurrent furunculosis.

For routine whole trunk application for ward use in maternity hospitals and in domiciliary midwifery.

Dosage and administration
For the prevention of neonatal staphylococcal cross infection: Immediately after ligature, dust the cord and surrounding area and apply the powder to the perineum, buttocks, flexures and axillae. Repeat at each napkin change until the cord stump has dropped away and the wound has healed.

For the treatment of furunculosis: Dust the affected area and surrounds regularly.

Contra-indications, warnings, etc The product should be administered to children under two years of age on medical advice only. Because of the absence of evidence to the contrary the product should not be administered during pregnancy. For external use only. Do not use on badly excoriated skin.

Pharmaceutical precautions No special requirements.

Legal category P.

Package quantities Sprinkler tins of 30 g.

Further information May be used on full term and premature infants and low birth weight infants provided that the skin is undamaged.

Product licence number 0423/5000.

TERPOIN* ANTITUSSIVE

Presentation A yellow clear syrupy solution with a predominant menthol odour and taste. Each 5 ml contains: Codeine Phosphate BP 15.0 mg.

Uses For the treatment of cough.
Indications: Terpoin is indicated in the treatment of persistent cough.

Dosage and administration *Adults:* 5 ml in a little water (if necessary) every three hours.

Children: Not recommended for children under 16 years of age.

Contra-indications, warnings, etc Severe respiratory depression. Not recommended for children under 16 years of age. Should not be used during pregnancy unless the physician considers it necessary.

Treatment for overdosage: Gastric lavage and aspiration with supporting therapy.

Pharmaceutical precautions No special requirements.

Legal category CD (Sch. 5), P.

Package quantities 100 ml, 225 ml, 2.25 l.

Further information Also contains Menthol BP and Eucalyptol BPC Terpoin may not be prescribed under the NHS.

Product licence number 0423/5005.

TRICLOSEPT* ANTIBACTERIAL CREAM

Presentation A white cream containing 1% w/w triclosan.

Uses To help prevent infection. For rapid disinfection of the skin.

Dosage and administration
For hand disinfection: apply approximately 1 g Triclosept to dry the palm of one hand. Rub the hands together vigorously making sure that the areas around the fingernails and between the fingers are treated. Rub until the cream has been absorbed into the skin.

Other skin areas: Apply about 1 g Triclosept per 100 square inches of skin. Rub vigorously until the cream has been absorbed.

Contra-indications, warnings, etc For external use only. Avoid contact with eyes.

Pharmaceutical precautions Do not freeze.

Legal category GSL.

Package quantities 100 ml.

Further information Triclosept contains stearic acid monoethanolamide to enhance cosmetic acceptability.

Product licence number 0423/0010.

**Trade Mark*

ICI Pharmaceuticals
King's Court
Water Lane
Wilmslow, Cheshire SK9 5AZ

ATROMID*-S

Presentation Atromid-S is presented as red, soft gelatin capsules, each containing 500 mg Clofibrate BP. Inactive ingredients are gelatin, glycerol, ink, Ponceau 4R, sodium ethyl hydroxybenzoate and sodium propyl hydroxybenzoate.

Uses

Atromid-S is indicated in the treatment of severe hyperlipoproteinaemia where full investigation has been performed to define the abnormality. It should be used in conjunction with appropriate dietary measures and after diet alone has failed to produce an adequate response. Other risk factors such as hypertension and smoking should be dealt with. Examples of abnormal lipid patterns are:

Frederickson type	*Lipoprotein elevated*	*Major lipid elevations*
I (very rare)	Chylomicrons	Triglycerides
IIa	β(LDL)	Cholesterol
IIb	pre-β+β (LDL+VLDL)	Cholesterol+ Triglycerides
III (rare)	abnormal β(LDL)	Chol.+TG
IV	pre-β(VLDL)	Triglycerides
V (rare)	Chylomicrons +pre-β(VLDL)	Triglycerides+ Cholesterol

Atromid-S is effective in patients with Type III hyperlipidaemia and in patients with severe hypertriglyceridaemia found in some patients in Types IIb, IV and V.

Mode of action: Atromid-S is a lipid-lowering drug, being a member of the fibric acid class of hypolipidaemic agents. It lowers serum cholesterol and triglyceride levels by reducing very low density lipoprotein (VLDL) and low-density lipoprotein (LDL).

Atromid-S is readily absorbed following oral dosage and is hydrolysed to the active acid. The plasma half-life is typically 18–22 hours and the drug is excreted via the kidneys. Some 91–97% is bound to serum albumin with a volume of distribution of 5–9 litres; none enters the cerebrospinal fluid. Concomitant administration of cholestyramine does not impair absorption of Atromid-S.

Dosage and administration A dose of 20–30 mg/kg body weight is given daily. This should be divided into 2 or 3 doses after meals. The effective dose level must be maintained. Examples of dosage:

Patients over 65 kg: 2 g daily (4 × 500 mg capsules).

Patients 50–65 kg: 1.5 g daily (3 × 500 mg capsules).

The biochemical response to clofibrate is variable, and it is not always possible to predict from the lipoprotein type or other factors which patients will obtain favourable results. It is essential that lipid levels be measured and that the drug be discontinued in any patient in whom lipids do not show significant improvement within three months of initiating therapy.

Elderly patients: There are no special dosage recommendations for the elderly, but it may be advisable to monitor elderly patients so that optimum dosage can be individually determined.

Contra-indications, warnings, etc Because of its effect on cholesterol metabolism, Atromid-S may enhance the lithogenicity of bile and increase the frequency of gallstone formation. Accordingly, clofibrate should not be used in patients with a history of, or existent gallbladder disease, or stones.

Also, it is contra-indicated in patients with impairment of renal or hepatic function (e.g. biliary cirrhosis).

In patients with low serum albumin levels, for example those with nephrotic syndrome, high levels of unbound Atromid-S may give rise to myalgia with raised serum creatinine kinase levels. Caution is advised in treating such patients.

Patients taking anticoagulants and Atromid-S together should have their dose of anticoagulant halved and adjusted later as necessary.

Atromid-S may also displace other acidic drugs, such as phenytoin or tolbutamide, from protein binding sites and thereby potentiate the effect of such drugs.

Clofibrate has been shown to produce liver tumours in rats and mice. The liver changes found in rodents have not been seen in other species, including sub-human primates and man. The relevance of this finding to man has not been established.

Pregnancy: The significance of the rise in maternal cholesterol levels during late pregnancy is unclear. Also, the effect of Atromid-S, which is secreted in breast milk, on the infant has not been studied. Therefore, Atromid-S should not be given during pregnancy or lactation.

Side-effects: Atromid-S has been in clinical use since 1963 and has been subjected to many long-term studies. Side-effects are seldom seen but include transient slight upper abdominal discomfort, nausea and looseness of the bowels and impotence. It is usually unnecessary to discontinue treatment. Very occasionally myalgia and alopecia have been reported. Due to its action on bile there is an increased incidence of gallstones (see 'Contra-indications and warnings' above).

At therapeutic doses Atromid-S does not enter the liver cell. In some cases slight and usually transient increases in serum transaminase levels have been observed. It is considered that these reflect adaptive responses of the liver. In large, long-term studies, even transient increases in transaminase levels have seldom been reported. Atromid-S has not been shown to affect serum bilirubin or bromosulphthalein tests. Serial liver biopsy studies in patients undergoing long-term treatment have confirmed the absence of hepatotoxicity in man.

There has been a published report of ventricular arrhythmia associated with Atromid-S treatment. However, the patient had an unstable rhythm prior to treatment.

Atromid-S normally has no effect on the blood picture. Isolated cases of adverse effects include slight fluctuation in haemoglobin values and occasional reduction in white cell counts. There is no evidence of marrow toxicity, but one case of agranulocytosis has been reported in a patient undergoing multiple drug therapy which included Atromid-S.

Overdosage: No adverse biochemical or clinical effects have been observed upon overdosage with Atromid-S, but should these occur, symptomatic treatment should be administered.

One case of a 15-year-old boy has been recorded who took 12.25 g of Atromid-S with no resulting adverse effects.

Pharmaceutical precautions Store at room temperature, protected from light and moisture.

Legal category POM.

Package quantities Containers of 100 capsules (OP).

Further information
Effect on ability to drive or operate machinery: Clofibrate does not enter the CNS and therefore Atromid-S is unlikely to have any effect on the ability to drive or operate machinery.

Product licence number 0029/5022.

AVLOCLOR* TABLETS

Presentation Avloclor Tablets are presented as white, bi-convex tablets, each with a bisecting line and bearing the ICI roundel. The tablets each contain 250 mg Chloroquine Phosphate BP which is equivalent to 155 mg chloroquine base. Inactive ingredients are magnesium stearate and maize starch.

Uses Avloclor is an antimalarial drug of the 4-aminoquinoline group. It is indicated for the following:

(a) Treatment of malaria;
(b) Prophylaxis and suppression of malaria;
(c) Treatment of amoebic hepatitis and abscess;
(d) Treatment of discoid and systemic lupus erythematosus;
(e) Treatment of rheumatoid arthritis.

Dosage and administration
(a) Treatment of malaria

P. falciparum infection

Partially immune subjects

Adults: A single dose of four tablets. In severe attacks, continue with two tablets six hours later and then two tablets a day for two days.

Children: A single dose of 10 mg/kg bodyweight. In severe attacks, continue with 5 mg base/kg six hours later and then 5 mg base/kg a day for two days.

Non-immune subjects
Adults: The initial dose is four tablets which is followed by two tablets six hours later and then two tablets a day for two days.

Children: A single dose of 10 mg base/kg, followed six hours later by 5 mg base/kg and 5 mg base/kg a day for two days.

Age (years)	*Initial dose*	*Second dose 6 hrs after first*	*Dose on each of the two subsequent days*
1–4	1 tablet	½ tablet	½ tablet
5–8	2 tablets	1 tablet	1 tablet
9–14	3 tablets	1½ tablets	1½ tablets

P. vivax, P. ovale and P. malariae infections

Adults: A single dose of four tablets followed by a course of treatment with primaquine phosphate (15 mg base daily for fourteen days).

Children: A single dose of 10 mg base/kg followed by a course of primaquine phosphate (0.2–0.3 mg base/kg daily for fourteen days).

(b) Prophylaxis and suppression of malaria

Adults: Two tablets taken once a week, on the same day each week, during exposure to risk and continued for four weeks after leaving the malarious area.

Children: A single dose of 5 mg chloroquine base/kg per week, on the same day each week during exposure to risk and continued for four weeks after leaving the malarious area.

For practical purposes, children aged over 14 years may be treated as adults. The dose given to infants and children should be calculated on their body weight and must not exceed the adult dose regardless of weight.

1–4 years:	½ tablet
5–8 years:	1 tablet
9–14 years:	1½ tablets

(c) Amoebic hepatitis

Adults: Four tablets daily for two days followed by one tablet twice daily for two or three weeks.

(d) Lupus erythematosus

Adults: One tablet twice daily for one to two weeks followed by a maintenance dosage of one tablet daily.

(e) Rheumatoid arthritis

Adults: The usual dosage is one tablet daily, at bedtime.

Elderly patients: There are no special dosage recommendations for the elderly, but it may be advisable to monitor elderly patients so that optimum dosage can be individually determined.

Contra-indications, warnings, etc
Contra-indications: There are no absolute contra-indications to the use of Avloclor.

Precautions: Caution is necessary when giving Avloclor to patients with porphyria who also have hepatic dysfunction or cirrhosis as the drug may precipitate severe constitutional symptoms and an increase in the amount of porphyrins excreted in the urine. This reaction is especially apparent in alcoholics.

Caution is necessary when giving Avloclor to patients with renal disease.

The most serious toxic hazard of prolonged therapy with high doses is the occasional development of irreversible retinal damage.

Considerable caution is needed in the use of Avloclor for long-term high dosage therapy and such use should only be considered when no other drug is available.

Patients receiving Avloclor continuously at higher dose levels for periods longer than 12 months should undergo ophthalmic examination at three monthly intervals. This also applies to patients receiving Avloclor at weekly intervals for a period of more than 3 years as a prophylactic against malarial attacks or if the total consumption exceeds 1.6 g/kg.

Defects in visual accommodation may occur on first taking Avloclor and patients should be warned regarding driving or operating machinery.

The use of chloroquine in patients with psoriasis may precipitate a severe attack of psoriasis.

Pregnancy: As with all drugs, the use of Avloclor during pregnancy should be avoided if possible unless, in the case of life threatening infections, in the judgement of the physician, potential benefit outweighs the risk. There is evidence to suggest that Avloclor given to women in high doses throughout pregnancy can give rise to foetal cochlear damage.

Lactation: Although Avloclor is excreted in breast milk, the amount is insufficient to confer any benefit on the infant. Separate chemoprophylaxis for the infant is required.

In any locality where drug resistant malaria is known or suspected, it is essential to take local medical advice on what prophylactic regimen is appropriate.

Side-effects: When used at the standard dosage regimens recommended for the control of malaria, Avloclor is well tolerated and side effects such as headache and gastro-intestinal disturbances which may occur are not of a serious nature. Where prolonged high dosage is required, side effects can be of greater severity and patients may develop skin eruptions, pruritus, occasional depigmentation or loss of hair, neurological and electrocardiographic changes, difficulty in accommodation, blurring of vision, corneal opacities and, less often, retinal degeneration. Corneal opacities disappear completely when the drug is stopped. Rarely, thrombocytopenia, agranulocytosis and aplastic anaemia have been reported.

Overdosage: In the event of gross overdosage with Avloclor prompt measures will be required to counteract the depressant effect of the drug on the cardiovascular and respiratory systems. Vomiting should be induced or gastric lavage carried out as soon as possible, followed by appropriate resuscitative measures, such as tracheal intubation with artificial respiration and the administration of vasopressor agents or intravenous fluids. Intravenous molar sodium lactate solution 30–50 ml has been used to counteract the quinidine-like action of chloroquine on the myocardium.

Early intraveneous diazepam therapy has been shown to be of value in the management of severe chloroquine overdosage.

Pharmaceutical precautions Store at room temperature. When in plastic containers, protect from light and moisture.

Legal category POM.
P. for prevention of malaria.

Package quantities Containers of 20 and 100 (OP) tablets.

Further information Nil.

Product licence number 0029/5053.

CETAVLEX* CREAM

Presentation A white water-miscible cream containing 0.5% w/w cetrimide (incorporated as Strong Cetrimide Solution BP). Inactive ingredients are cetostearyl alcohol, liquid paraffin, methyl parahydroxybenzoate, propyl parahydroxybenzoate and water.

Uses Cetavlex is an antiseptic cream for skin disorders such as minor wounds, burns, abrasions and napkin rash.

Dosage and administration Apply liberally to the affected area. In some cases it may be necessary to cover the wound or burn with a clean dressing.

Contra-indications, warnings, etc Cetavlex is contra-indicated for patients who have previously shown a hypersensitivity reaction to cetrimide preparations.

For topical application only. Keep out of the eyes and avoid contact with the brain, meninges or middle ear. Do not use in body cavities or as an enema.

Side-effects: Irritative skin reactions can occasionally occur. Hypersensitivity to cetrimide preparations has been reported, usually developing after repeated application, but is rare. Should such a reaction occur stop application of the product.

Accidental ingestion: The toxicity of Cetavlex arises from the content of cetrimide. It seems unlikely that systemic toxicity will occur from accidental ingestion of the cream. However, in the event of large quantities being swallowed carry out gastric lavage with milk, gelatin or mild soap. Do not induce vomiting. Do not give alcohol in any form. Employ supportive measures as appropriate.

Pharmaceutical precautions Store at room temperature and use undiluted. Cetrimide is incompatible with anionic agents.

Legal category GSL.

Package quantities Tubes of 50 g (OP).

Further information Nil.

Product licence number 0029/5015.

CORSODYL* DENTAL GEL

Presentation Corsodyl Dental Gel is presented as a clear colourless gel containing 1% w/w chlorhexidine gluconate (equivalent to 5% v/w Chlorhexidine Gluconate Solution BP). Inactive ingredients are hydroxypropylcellulose, isopropyl alcohol, menthol, peppermint oil, polyoxyethylene hydrogenated castor oil, sodium acetate and water.

Uses Corsodyl Dental Gel inhibits the formation of dental plaque. It is indicated as an aid in the treatment and prevention of gingivitis and in the maintenance of oral hygiene.

Dosage and administration Brush the teeth thoroughly with 1 inch of gel on a moistened toothbrush, once or twice daily for about one minute. For the treatment of gingivitis, a course of treatment of about one month is advisable.

Corsodyl is incompatible with anionic agents which are usually present in conventional dentifrices. These should therefore be used before Corsodyl (rinsing the mouth *and* toothbrush between applications) or at a different time of day.

Contra-indications, warnings, etc Corsodyl is contra-indicated for patients who have previously shown a hypersensitivity reaction to chlorhexidine. However, such reactions are extremely rare.

For oral use only, keep out of the eyes and avoid contact with the brain, meninges and middle ear.

Side-effects: Irritative skin reactions to chlorhexidine preparations can occasionally occur. Generalised allergic reactions to chlorhexidine have also been reported but are extremely rare.

A superficial discolouration of the tongue may occur, this disappears after treatment is discontinued. Discolouration of the teeth and silicate or composite restorations may also occur. This stain is not permanent and can largely be prevented by brushing with a conventional toothpaste daily before using the gel. However, in certain cases, scaling and polishing may be necessary to remove this stain completely.

Transient disturbances of taste sensation and a burning sensation of the tongue may occur on initial use. These usually diminish with continued use.

Overdosage: This has not been reported.

Chlorhexidine taken orally is poorly absorbed. Systemic effects are unlikely even if large amounts are ingested. However, gastric lavage may be advisable using milk, gelatin or mild soap. Employ supportive measures as appropriate.

Pharmaceutical precautions Hypochlorite bleaches may cause brown stains to develop in fabrics which have previously been in contact with chlorhexidine preparations.

Store at room temperature.

Legal category P.

Package quantities Tubes of 50 g (OP).

Further information Corsodyl Dental Gel has an antiplaque action. The effect on gingivitis is maximal after removal of subgingival deposits by scaling.

Product licence number 0029/0080.

CORSODYL* MOUTHWASH
CORSODYL* MINT MOUTHWASH

Presentation A clear aniseed-flavoured pink solution and a clear colourless mint-flavoured solution containing 0.2% w/v chlorhexidine gluconate (equivalent to 1% v/v Chlorhexidine Gluconate Solution BP). The inactive ingredients of 'Corsodyl' Mouthwash are anise oil, ethanol, peppermint oil, polyoxyethylene hydrogenated castor oil, Ponceau 4R and water. The inactive ingredients of 'Corsodyl' Mint Mouthwash are ethanol, peppermint oil, polyoxyethylene hydrogenated castor oil, sorbitol and water.

Uses Corsodyl Mouthwash is an antibacterial solution which inhibits the formation of dental plaque. It is indicated as an aid in the treatment and prevention of gingivitis, and in the maintenance of oral hygiene, particularly in situations where toothbrushing cannot be adequately employed (e.g. following oral surgery or in mentally or physically-handicapped patients). It may also be used in a post-periodontal surgery regimen to promote gingival healing. It is useful in the management of aphthous ulceration and oral candidal infections, (e.g. denture stomatitis and oral thrush).

Dosage and administration Thoroughly rinse the mouth for about one minute with 10 ml twice daily. In the dental surgery the patient should be instructed to rinse the mouth with 10 ml for one minute prior to surgery.

Corsodyl is incompatible with anionic agents which are usually present in conventional dentifrices. These should therefore be used before Corsodyl (rinsing the mouth between applications) or at a different time of day.

For the treatment of gingivitis, a course of about a month is advisable although some variation in response is to be expected. In the case of aphthous ulceration and oral candidal infections, treatment should be continued for 48 hours after clinical resolution. For the treatment of denture stomatitis the dentures should be cleansed and soaked in Corsodyl Mouthwash for 15 minutes twice daily.

Contra-indications, warnings, etc Corsodyl is contra-indicated for patients who have previously shown a hypersensitivity reaction to chlorhexidine. However, such reactions are extremely rare.

For oral use only, keep out of the eyes and avoid contact with the brain, meninges and middle ear.

Side-effects: Irritative skin reactions to chlorhexidine preparations can occasionally occur. Generalised allergic reactions to chlorhexidine have also been reported but are extremely rare.

A superficial discolouration of the dorsum of the tongue may occur, this disappears after treatment is discontinued. Discolouration of the teeth and silicate or composite restorations may also occur. This stain is not permanent and can largely be prevented by brushing with a conventional toothpaste daily before using the mouthwash, or in the case of dentures, cleaning with a conventional denture cleanser. However, in certain cases, scaling and polishing may be required to remove this stain completely. Similarly where normal toothbrushing is not possible, as for example with intermaxillary fixation, or with extensive orthodontic appliances, scaling and polishing may be required once the underlying condition has resolved.

Transient disturbances of taste sensation and a burning sensation of the tongue may occur on initial use of the mouthwash. These effects usually diminish with continued use.

In cases where oral desquamation occurs, dilution of the mouthwash (5 ml mouthwash with 5 ml tap water freshly mixed) and instructions to rinse less vigorously will often allow continued use of the mouthwash.

Very occasionally, swelling of the parotid glands during use of chlorhexidine mouthwash has been reported. In all cases spontaneous resolution has occurred on discontinuing treatment.

Overdosage: This has not been reported.

Chlorhexidine taken orally is poorly absorbed. Systemic effects are unlikely even if large volumes are ingested. However, gastric lavage may be advisable using milk, gelatin or mild soap. Employ supportive measures as appropriate.

Pharmaceutical precautions Hypochlorite bleaches may cause brown stains to develop in fabrics which have previously been in contact with chlorhexidine solutions.

Store at room temperature.

Legal category P.

Package quantities 300 ml bottle (OP).

Further information Nil.

Product licence number

Corsodyl Mouthwash	0029/0124
Corsodyl Mint Mouthwash	0029/0201.

DIPRIVAN* ▼

Presentation White, aqueous and isotonic emulsion for intravenous injection containing 10 mg propofol per 1 ml. The vehicle contains glycerol, purified egg phosphatide, sodium hydroxide, soybean oil and water.

Uses Diprivan is a short-acting intravenous anaesthetic agent suitable for induction and maintenance of general anaesthesia for surgical procedures which generally do not exceed one hour in duration.

Dosage and administration

Adults:

Induction: In unpremedicated and in premedicated patients, it is recommended that Diprivan should be titrated (approximately 4 ml [40 mg] every 10 seconds in an average healthy adult) against the response of the patient until the clinical signs show the onset of anaesthesia. Most adult patients aged less than 55 years are likely to require 2.0 to 2.5 mg/kg of Diprivan. Over this age, the requirement will generally be less. In patients of ASA Grades 3 and 4, lower rates of administration should be used (approximately 2 ml [20 mg] every 10 seconds).

Maintenance: Anaesthesia can be maintained by administering Diprivan either by continuous infusion or by repeat bolus injections to prevent the clinical signs of light anaesthesia. Experience in procedures lasting more than one hour is limited.

Infusion

The average rate of administration varies considerably between patients but rates in the region of 0.1 to 0.2 mg/kg/min (6 to 12 mg/kg/hr) usually maintain satisfactory anaesthesia. Slightly higher rates of administration may be required for 10 to 20 minutes after induction of anaesthesia. Diprivan can be used for infusion undiluted or diluted with 5% Dextrose (Intravenous Infusion BP) only, in PVC infusion bags or glass infusion bottles. Dilutions, which must not exceed 1 in 5 (2 mg propofol per ml) should be prepared immediately before administration and must be used within 6 hours of preparation. It is recommended that when using diluted Diprivan the volume of 5% Dextrose removed from the infusion bag during the dilution process is totally replaced in volume by Diprivan emulsion.

The dilution may be used with a variety of infusion control techniques but a giving set used alone will not avoid the risk of accidental, uncontrolled infusion of large volumes of diluted Diprivan. A burette, drop counter or volumetric pump must be included in the infusion line. The risk of uncontrolled infusion must be taken into account when deciding the maximum amount of Diprivan in the burette.

When Diprivan is used undiluted to maintain anaesthesia, it is recommended that drop counters, syringe pumps or volumetric infusion pumps should always be used to control infusion rates.

Repeat Bolus Injections

If a technique involving repeat bolus injections is used, increments of 25 mg (2.5 ml) to 50 mg (5.0 ml) may be given according to clinical need.

General

Diprivan may be administered via a Y-piece close to the injection site, into infusions of Dextrose 5% (Intravenous Infusion BP), Sodium Chloride 0.9% (Intravenous Infusion BP), or Dextrose 4% with Sodium Chloride 0.18% (Intravenous Infusion BP).

Supplementary analgesic agents are generally required in addition to Diprivan. Diprivan has been used in association with spinal and epidural anaesthesia and with commonly used premedicants, neuromuscular blocking drugs, inhalational agents and analgesic agents; no pharmacological incompatibility has been encountered.

Diprivan should not be mixed prior to administration with injections or infusion fluids other than 5% Dextrose (Intravenous Infusion BP).

Elderly patients: Diprivan should be titrated against the response of the patient. Patients over the age of about 55 years may require lower doses of Diprivan for induction of anaesthesia (approximately 20% less).

Paediatric usage: At this stage, there is no experience of Diprivan in children or in mothers who are breast feeding.

Contra-indications, warnings, etc

Contra-indications: Known allergy to Diprivan.

Precautions: Diprivan should be given by those trained in anaesthesia and facilities for maintenance of a patent airway, artificial ventilation, and oxygen enrichment should be available. During induction of anaesthesia, hypotension and transient apnoea may occur depending on the dose and use of premedicants and other agents. Occasionally, hypotension may require use of intravenous fluids and reduction of the rate of administration of Diprivan during the period of anaesthetic maintenance.

An adequate period is needed prior to discharge of the patient to ensure full recovery after general anaesthesia.

As .vith other anaesthetic agents, when Diprivan is administered to an epileptic patient, there may be an increased risk of convulsion.

As with other intravenous anaesthetic agents, caution should be applied in patients with cardiac, respiratory, renal or hepatic impairment or in hypovolaemic or debilitated patients. Diprivan lacks vagolytic activity and has been associated with reports of bradycardia, occasionally profound. The intravenous administration of an anticholinergic agent before induction, or during maintenance of anaesthesia should be considered, especially in situations where vagal tone is likely to predominate or when Diprivan is used in conjunction with other agents likely to cause a bradycardia. Appropriate care should be applied in patients with disorders of fat metabolism and in other conditions where lipid emulsions must be used cautiously.

Pregnancy: On general principles, Diprivan should not be used in pregnancy. Diprivan has been used, however, during termination of pregnancy.

Additional precautions: Diprivan should be inspected for particulate matter and discolouration before administration.

Aseptic techniques must be applied to handling of the drug. Diprivan contains no antimicrobial preservatives and the vehicle supports growth of microorganisms.

Diprivan is for use in a single patient only. When Diprivan is to be aspirated, it should be drawn into a sterile syringe or giving set immediately after opening the ampoule or breaking the vial seal. Administration should commence without delay. The syringe or giving set and any unused portion of Diprivan or solution containing Diprivan must be discarded at the end of the surgical procedure.

Side effects: General. Induction of anaesthesia is generally smooth with minimal evidence of excitation. Other side-effects during induction, maintenance and recovery occur uncommonly. Epileptiform movements, including convulsions, and opisthotonus have occurred rarely in a temporal relationship to Diprivan. During the recovery phase nausea, vomiting and headache occur in only a small proportion of patients. Rarely, discolouration of urine has been reported following prolonged administration of Diprivan. Very rarely, clinical features of anaphylaxis, which may include bronchospasm, erythema and hypotension, occur following Diprivan administration. There have been reports of fever occurring.

Local. The local pain which may occur during intravenous injection of Diprivan can be minimised when the larger veins of the forearm and antecubital fossa are used. Thrombosis and phlebitis are rare. Accidental clinical extravasation and animal studies showed minimal tissue reaction. Intra-arterial injection in animals did not induce local tissue effects.

Overdosage: Accidental overdosage is likely to cause cardiorespiratory depression. Respiratory depression should be treated by artificial ventilation with oxygen. Cardiovascular depression would require lowering of the patient's head and, if severe, use of plasma expanders and pressor agents.

Pharmaceutical precautions
Storage precautions: Diprivan should be stored between 2°C and 25°C; it must not be frozen.

In-use precautions: Containers should be shaken before use.

Any portion of the contents remaining after use should be discarded.

Diprivan should not be mixed prior to administration with injections or infusion fluids other than 5% Dextrose (see 'Dosage and administration').

Legal category POM.

Package quantities Ampoules of 20 ml in boxes of 5. Vials of 50 ml.

Further information Diprivan is distributed rapidly with a half-life between 1.8 and 8.3 minutes. Diprivan is metabolised by conjugation probably in the liver (half-life between 34 and 64 minutes) and this facilitates control of anaesthetic depth during maintenance as well as promoting rapid, clear-headed recovery. Inactive metabolites are excreted by the kidney. Under the usual maintenance regimens, significant accumulation of propofol does not occur.

In vitro studies have shown that Diprivan, at the concentrations likely to occur clinically, does not inhibit the synthesis of adrenocortical hormones.

Product licence number 0029/0190.

EXELDERM* CREAM

Presentation Exelderm is a white to off-white cream containing 1% w/w sulconazole nitrate. The inactive ingredients are ascorbyl palmitate, cetyl alcohol, glycerol stearate, PEG 100 stearate, isopropyl myristate, polysorbate 60, propylene glycol, sodium hydroxide, sorbitan monostearate, stearyl alcohol and water.

Uses Exelderm Cream is designed for topical application and contains an imidazole antimycotic with a broad spectrum of activity against the causative organisms of tinea pedis, tinea corporis and tinea cruris, pityriasis versicolor and candidiasis.

Dosage and administration Exelderm Cream should be gently massaged into the affected and surrounding skin areas twice daily (morning and evening). For less severe cases once daily administration may be sufficient.

Often clinical improvement with relief of symptoms occurs within one week. However, treatment should be continued for 2 to 3 weeks after clinical cure to prevent relapse.

Contra-indications, warnings, etc Exelderm is contra-indicated in patients with hypersensitivity to the formulated product or imidazoles.

Precautions: The treatment should be discontinued if a reaction suggesting sensitivity or irritation occurs. If the patient shows no clinical improvement after 4 weeks of treatment the diagnosis should be reviewed. Avoid the introduction of Exelderm into the eyes. Lens changes were seen in one animal species following very high repeated oral doses.

Pregnancy: Reproductive toxicology studies produced no evidence of teratogenicity in laboratory animals, although some more general toxicological effects were seen in the dams and foetuses in these studies. Therefore this product should not be used in pregnancy unless considered essential to the welfare of the patient.

Side-effects: Occasional itching, burning, erythema, stinging and blistering have been reported.

Accidental ingestion: The 30 g tube of Exelderm contains 300 mg of sulconazole nitrate. Toxic effects are very unlikely even if the full contents are ingested but if they occur symptomatic treatment should be given.

Pharmaceutical precautions Store at room temperature.

Legal category POM.

Package quantities Exelderm Cream is supplied in 30 g tubes (OP).

Further information Nil.

Product licence number 0029/0185.

FLUOTHANE*

Presentation Fluothane is a colourless, volatile liquid, non-explosive and non-flammable in the concentrations usually used. Chemically it is 2-bromo-2-chloro-1,1,1-

trifluoroethane stabilised with thymol 0.01% w/w (Halothane PhEur).

Uses Fluothane is a volatile anaesthetic which is suitable for the induction and maintenance of anaesthesia for all types of surgery and in patients of all ages.

Mode of action: When inhaled, Fluothane is absorbed through the alveoli into the bloodstream. In the bloodstream Fluothane circulates through the body to the principal site of action, the brain. Here Fluothane causes a progressive depression of the central nervous system, beginning with the higher centres (cerebral cortex) and spreading to the vital centres in the medulla. This depression is reversible. However, its mode of action, like all anaesthetic agents, is unknown.

Fluothane has a relatively low solubility in blood and therefore alveoli/blood concentrations equilibrate rapidly. The triexponential decline in Fluothane blood concentrations following the end of administration is thought to represent distribution into three compartments; the vessel rich group (brain/heart/liver), the musculature and adipose tissue. Approximately 80% of the inhaled Fluothane is eliminated unchanged by the lungs. The remaining 20% is metabolised in the liver by oxidative and, under hypoxic conditions, reductive pathways. The main metabolites are trifluoroacetic acid, bromide and chloride salts (via the oxidative pathway) and fluoride salts (via the reductive pathway). The concentrations of metabolites peak 24 hours post-operatively and are eliminated by renal excretion during the following week.

Dosage and administration A number of anaesthetic vaporisers specially designed for use with Fluothane are available. Open, semi-open, semi-closed and closed circuit systems have all been used with good results.

For induction of anaesthesia in the adult patient a concentration of 2–4% Fluothane in oxygen or oxygen/nitrous oxide may be used. In children a concentration of 1.5–2% Fluothane in oxygen or oxygen/nitrous oxide is used. A concentration of 0.5–2% is usually adequate for maintenance of anaesthesia in both adults and children. The lower concentration is usually most suitable for elderly patients.

Contra-indications, warnings, etc Fluothane can induce liver damage; however, the incidence of severe liver damage (jaundice, which may lead to hepatic failure as a consequence of massive hepatic cell necrosis) is unknown. The risk of developing hepatic failure appears to be increased by repeated exposure. Although short intervals of time between exposures are likely to increase the risk of hepatotoxicity, even long intervals between exposure may not eliminate the risks, since some patients have developed severe reactions following Fluothane given many years after the previous exposure. On the information which is available at the present time, it is advised that the following precautions be taken:

(i) A careful anaesthetic history should be taken prior to use, to determine previous exposure and previous reactions following Fluothane anaesthesia.

(ii) Repeated exposure to Fluothane within a period of at least 3 months should be avoided unless there are overriding clinical circumstances.

(iii) History of unexplained jaundice and pyrexia in a patient following exposure to Fluothane is a contraindication to its future use in that patient unless absolutely essential.

(iv) Patients should be informed if they have developed a reaction possibly related to Fluothane anaesthesia; such patients should be provided with a medical alert card stating the problem.

As Fluothane causes relaxation of the uterine muscle it is advisable that anaesthesia should be maintained in the lightest plane possible during obstetric operations.

The use of moderate hyperventilation during neurosurgery is recommended to counteract the rise in cerebrospinal fluid pressure which may occur with Fluothane.

Malignant hyperpyrexia has been reported in some patients receiving Fluothane. This syndrome occurs with other anaesthetic agents, and may respond to intravenous dantrolene sodium.

During the induction of Fluothane anaesthesia a moderate fall in blood pressure commonly occurs. The pressure tends to rise when the vapour concentration is reduced to maintenance levels, but it usually remains steady below the pre-operative level. This hypotensive effect is useful in providing a clear operating field and a reduction in haemorrhage. However, if necessary, intravenous doses of methoxamine (5 mg are usually adequate) can be given to counteract the fall in blood pressure.

Cardiac arrhythmias have been reported during anaesthesia.

Fluothane augments the action of non-depolarising muscle relaxants.

Caution should be exercised during the administration of adrenaline to patients anaesthetised with Fluothane as dysrhythmias may be precipitated. For this reason the dose of adrenaline should be restricted and beta-receptor antagonists administered if necessary.

Ensure adequate room ventilation when Fluothane is being used. Keep the concentration of Fluothane in air as low as possible.

Pregnancy: Although the data from experimental investigations in animals cannot be directly related to man, it would be prudent to avoid general anaesthesia with inhalation agents during early pregnancy, except where such use is essential.

Lactation: There are no well controlled studies with Fluothane in lactating women. Fluothane has been detected in breast milk of lactating women, but the effects of Fluothane on breast fed neonates has not been established. However, Fluothane has been in wide use for over 30 years without apparent ill consequence.

Effect on ability to drive or operate machinery: Patients should be advised that performance at skilled tasks, such as driving and operating machinery, may be impaired for some time after general anaesthesia.

Accidental ingestion: Cases of ingestion must be treated symptomatically.

Pharmaceutical precautions Bottles of Fluothane must be securely closed and stored at room temperature, protected from light. Fluothane must be kept in the original container until immediately prior to its use.

Whilst in the liquid phase, Fluothane must not be diluted or contaminated; however, in the vapour phase it may be administered together with oxygen or a mixture of nitrous oxide and oxygen.

Legal category P.

Package quantities Fluothane is supplied in bottles of 250 ml.

Further information *Spillage:* Absorb spillage using a suitable absorbent material and transfer to a closed container for disposal. In case of insufficient ventilation wear suitable respiratory equipment.

Disposal: Disposal is normally carried out by incineration under carefully controlled conditions.

Product licence number 0029/5058.

FULCIN* 500 TABLETS
FULCIN* 125 TABLETS
FULCIN* ORAL SUSPENSION

Presentation Fulcin is griseofulvin in a fine-particle form designed to give optimal absorption when taken orally.

Fulcin 500 is presented as white, film-coated, bi-convex tablets, one side plain, the obverse marked with the ICI roundel. Each contains 500 mg Griseofulvin Ph. Eur. Inactive ingredients are calcium carboxymethylcellulose, ethylcellulose, glycerol, magnesium stearate, methylhydroxypropyl cellulose, maize starch, povidone, stearic acid and titanium dioxide. Fulcin 125 Tablets are white, bi-convex, one side bisected, the obverse marked with the ICI roundel. Each contains 125 mg Griseofulvin PhEur. Inactive ingredients are calcium carboxymethylcellulose, magnesium stearate, maize starch and povidone.

Fulcin Oral Suspension is a brown aqueous suspension which contains 2.5% w/v Griseofulvin PhEur. Inactive ingredients are calcium chloride, chocolate flavour, cocoa powder, methyl hydroxybenzoate, peppermint oil, propyl hydroxybenzoate, sodium alginate, sodium carboxymethylcellulose, sodium citrate, sucrose, vanillin and water.

Uses Fulcin is effective against the dermatophytes causing ringworm (tinea), including *Microsporum canis, Trichophyton rubrum* and *Trichophyton verrucosum*.

Fulcin is indicated for the treatment of fungal infections of the skin, hair and nails when topical therapy has failed or is considered inappropriate.

Mode of action: Griseofulvin inhibits fungal cell mitosis by causing disruption of the mitotic spindle structure, thereby arresting the metaphase of cell division. It is deposited in varying degrees in the keratin precursor cells of skin, hair and nails, rendering the keratin resistant to fungal invasion. As the infected keratin is shed, it is replaced with healthy tissue.

Following oral administration, griseofulvin is absorbed principally from the duodenum. Peak plasma concentrations of the drug (approx 1–2 micrograms/ml) occur about 4 hours after dosing. Concentrations of approximately 12–25 micrograms/g are maintained in skin during long term administration, whilst concurrent serum levels remain at 1–2 micrograms/ml. When the drug is discontinued, the drug is not detectable after 2 days in the skin and after 4 days in the plasma. The drug has an elimination half-life of 9–24 hours and it is metabolised in the liver, the major metabolite being 6-demethylgriseofulvin which is microbiologically inactive. The metabolites are excreted mainly in the urine whilst unchanged griseofulvin is excreted mainly in the faeces. Griseofulvin is also excreted in perspiration.

Dosage and administration The adult dosage is normally 500 mg daily, but in severe conditions up to twice this amount may be given, reducing to the lower level when a clinical response has occurred. The normal dosage may be given as one 125 mg tablet or 5 ml of suspension four times a day, or as one 500 mg tablet once daily after food.

For children the most suitable form is the pleasantly flavoured Fulcin Oral Suspension. The daily dosage is 10 mg griseofulvin per kg body weight daily, i.e. 5 ml of suspension for every 12.5 kg in single or divided doses after food.

Elderly patients: There are no special dosage recommendations for the elderly, but it may be advisable to monitor elderly patients so that optimum dosage can be individually determined.

The duration of treatment depends on the type of infection and the time required for normal replacement of infected tissues.

For complete eradication of the infection, Fulcin treatment should be combined with general measures of care and hygiene. Reservoirs of infection may include clothing, footwear and bedding as well as the patient's hair.

Contra-indications, warnings, etc
Fulcin should not be used for prophylaxis.

Fulcin should not be administered to patients who have established porphyria or hepatocellular failure or to patients with systemic lupus erythematosus.

Fulcin is contra-indicated in pregnancy. Griseofulvin administered to rats during pregnancy has been associated with foetotoxicity and tail deformities at high dosages.

Fulcin may decrease the response to coumarin anticoagulants administered concomitantly.

Liver enzyme inducing drugs, such as barbiturates, may reduce the effectiveness of Fulcin therapy.

Barbiturates can reduce the effectiveness of Fulcin therapy by interfering with gastrointestinal absorption of the drug.

Breakthrough bleeding, amenorrhoea and failure of contraceptive therapy have been reported in patients taking griseofulvin and oral contraceptive steroids. It may be advisable to consider additional contraceptive precautions during Fulcin therapy and for up to one month afterwards.

Patients should be warned that an enhancement of the effects of alcohol by griseofulvin has been reported.

Long-term administration of high doses of griseofulvin with food has been reported to induce hepatomas in mice and thyroid tumours in rats but not in hamsters. The clinical significance of this finding for man is not known.

Lactation: it is not known if griseofulvin is excreted in breast milk. Safety in children of nursing mothers has not been established.

Effect on ability to drive or operate machinery: Fulcin may impair the ability of some individuals to drive and operate machinery. There have been occasional reports of dizziness and confusion with impaired coordination and griseofulvin has been reported to enhance the effects of alcohol.

Side-effects: Fulcin is generally well tolerated. Urticarial reactions and erythematous rashes have been noted in a few cases. There have been occasional complaints of headache and gastric discomfort which, in most cases, have regressed during treatment. Dizziness, fatigue, granulocytopenia and leucopenia have also been reported. Photosensitivity associated with griseofulvin therapy has been recorded and there have been rare reports of precipitation of systemic lupus erythematosus, confusion with impaired co-ordination and of oral candidiasis.

Overdosage: Treatment of overdosage should be symptomatic.

Pharmaceutical precautions *Fulcin tablets:* Store at room temperature, protected from moisture.

Fulcin Oral Suspension: Store at room temperature.

Legal category POM.

Package quantities *Fulcin 500 tablets:* Containers of 100 tablets (OP).
Fulcin 125 Tablets: Containers of 100 tablets (OP).
Fulcin Oral Suspension: Bottles of 100 ml (OP).

Further information A suitable diluent for Fulcin Oral Suspension is Syrup BP which has been preserved with methylhydroxybenzoate. The dilution should be used within 14 days of preparation.

Product licence numbers

Fulcin 500 Tablets	0029/5061
Fulcin 125 Tablets	0029/5060
Fulcin Oral Suspension	0029/5059

HIBIDIL*

Presentation Hibidil is presented as a pink aqueous solution containing 0.05% w/v chlorhexidine gluconate (equivalent to 0.25% v/v Chlorhexidine Gluconate Solution BP). Inactive ingredients are carmoisine, ethanol, nonyl phenol/ethylene oxide condensate and water.

Uses Hibidil is an antimicrobial agent active against a wide range of organisms. It is recommended for swabbing wounds and burns and in obstetrics.

Dosage and administration Apply undiluted.

Contra-indications, warnings, etc Hibidil is contra-indicated for patients who have previously shown a hypersensitivity reaction to chlorhexidine.

For external use only. Keep out of the eyes and avoid contact with brain, meninges or middle ear. Not for injection. Do not use in body cavities.

If chlorhexidine solutions come into contact with eyes, wash out promptly and thoroughly with water.

Discard any surplus solution immediately after use.

Side-effects: Irritative skin reactions can occasionally

occur. Generalised allergic reactions to chlorhexidine have also been reported but are extremely rare.

Accidental ingestion: Chlorhexidine taken orally is poorly absorbed. Treat with a gastric lavage using milk, gelatin or mild soap. Employ supportive measures as appropriate.

Accidental intravenous transfusion: Blood transfusion may be necessary to counteract haemolysis.

Pharmaceutical precautions Hypochlorite bleaches may cause brown stains to develop in fabrics which have previously been in contact with preparations containing chlorhexidine.

Chlorhexidine is incompatible with anionic agents.

Store at room temperature.

Legal category P.

Package quantities Packs of 250 × 25 ml and 60 × 100 ml individual sachets.

Further information The British Pharmaceutical Codex (1973) recommends that antiseptics applied to broken skin should be sterile. The use of Hibidil complies with this recommendation.

Product licence number 0029/0143.

HIBISCRUB*

Presentation Hibiscrub is presented as a red detergent solution containing 4% w/v chlorhexidine gluconate (equivalent to 20% v/v Chlorhexidine Gluconate Solution BP). Inactive ingredients are d-glucono lactone, isopropyl alcohol, lauryl dimethyl amine oxide, perfume, polyoxyethylene-polyoxypropylene block copolymer, Ponceau 4R and water.

Uses Hibiscrub is an antimicrobial preparation for pre-operative surgical hand disinfection, antiseptic hand-washing on the ward and pre-operative and post-operative skin antisepsis for patients undergoing elective surgery.

Dosage and administration *Pre-operative surgical hand preparation:* Wet the hands and forearms, apply 5 ml of Hibiscrub and wash for one minute cleaning the fingernails with a brush or scraper. Rinse, apply a further 5 ml of Hibiscrub and continue washing for a further two minutes. Rinse thoroughly and dry.

Antiseptic handwash on the ward: Wet the hands and forearms, apply 5 ml of Hibiscrub and wash for one minute. Rinse thoroughly and dry.

Pre-operative skin preparation for the patient: The patient washes his whole body in the bath or shower on at least two occasions, usually the day before and the day of operation as follows:

The day before the operation, the patient washes with 25 ml of Hibiscrub beginning with the face and working downwards paying particular attention to areas around the nose, axillae, umbilicus, groin and perineum. The body is then rinsed and the wash repeated with a further 25 ml, this time including the hair. Finally the patient rinses his entire body thoroughly and dries on a clean towel. This procedure should be repeated the following day. Patients confined to bed can be washed with Hibiscrub using a standard bed-bath technique.

Conventional disinfection of the operation site will then be performed when the patient is in theatre.

Post-operative skin antisepsis for the patient: The patient washes his whole body, excluding the operation wound in the bath or shower usually on the third day after the operation using the procedure described above.

Contra-indications, warnings, etc Hibiscrub is contra-indicated for persons who have previously shown a hypersensitivity reaction to chlorhexidine. However, such reactions are extremely rare.

For external use only. Keep out of the eyes and avoid contact with brain, meninges and middle ear. In patients with head or spinal injuries or perforated ear drum, the benefit of use in pre-operative preparation should be evaluated against the risk of contact.

If chlorhexidine solutions come into contact with eyes, wash out promptly and thoroughly with water.

Side-effects: Irritative skin reactions can occasionally occur. Generalised allergic reactions to chlorhexidine have also been reported but are extremely rare.

Accidental ingestion: Chlorhexidine taken orally is poorly absorbed. Treat with gastric lavage using milk, gelatin or mild soap. Employ supportive measures as appropriate.

Pharmaceutical precautions Hypochlorite bleaches may cause brown stains to develop in fabrics which have previously been in contact with preparations containing chlorhexidine.

Chlorhexidine is incompatible with anionic agents.

Store at room temperature protected from light.

Legal category GSL.

Package quantities Containers of 100 ml, 250 ml (OP), 500 ml, 5 litres. Dispensing brackets and pumps are available.

Further information Nil.

Product licence number 0029/0127.

HIBISOL*

Presentation Hibisol is presented as an alcoholic solution containing 0.5% w/v chlorhexidine gluconate (equivalent to 2.5% v/v Chlorhexidine Gluconate Solution BP) in 70% w/w Isopropyl Alcohol BP with emollients. Inactive ingredients are castor oil, glycerol, isopropyl alcohol and water.

Uses Hibisol is a rapid-acting antimicrobial preparation for the disinfection of clean intact skin. It is used for pre-operative surgical hand disinfection, hand disinfection on the ward prior to aseptic procedures or after handling contaminated material, and for disinfection of patients' skin prior to surgery or other invasive procedures.

Dosage and administration
Pre-operative surgical hand disinfection: Dispense 5 ml of Hibisol and spread thoroughly over both hands and forearms, rubbing vigorously. When dry apply a further 5 ml and repeat the procedure.

NB. Before the first operation on a list or subsequently when hands are soiled the hands should be cleansed and disinfected with an effective antiseptic/detergent handwash.

Antiseptic hand disinfection on the ward: Dispense 3 ml of Hibisol and spread thoroughly over the hands and wrists rubbing vigorously until dry.

NB. If the hands are soiled, cleanse and *dry* before using Hibisol or alternatively use an effective antiseptic/detergent handwash.

Disinfection of patients skin: Prior to surgery, apply Hibisol to a sterile swab and rub vigorously over the operation site for a minimum of two minutes. Hibisol is also used for preparation of the skin prior to invasive procedures such as venepuncture.

Contra-indications, warnings, etc Hibisol is contra-indicated for persons who have previously shown a hypersensitivity reaction to chlorhexidine. However, such reactions are extremely rare.

For external use only. Keep out of the eyes and avoid contact with brain, meninges or middle ear. Not for injection. Do not use in body cavities.

If chlorhexidine solutions come into contact with the eyes, wash out promptly and thoroughly with water.

Flammable. This preparation contains alcohol. When use is to be followed by diathermy do not allow pooling of the fluid to occur, and ensure that the skin and surrounding drapes are dry.

Side-effects: Irritative skin reactions can occasionally occur. Generalised allergic reactions to chlorhexidine have also been reported but are extremely rare.

Accidental ingestion: Chlorhexidine taken orally is poorly absorbed. Treat with gastric lavage using milk, gelatin or mild soap avoiding pulmonary aspiration. Do not use apomorphine. Assist respiration if necessary and keep patient warm. Intravenous laevulose can accelerate alcohol metabolism. In severe cases, haemodialysis or peritoneal dialysis may be necessary.

Pharmaceutical precautions Flammable.
Hypochlorite bleaches may cause brown stains to develop in fabrics which have previously been in contact with preparations containing chlorhexidine.
Chlorhexidine is incompatible with anionic agents.
Store at room temperature.

Legal category GSL.

Package quantities Containers of 250 ml (OP) and 500 ml.

Further information A suitable antiseptic-detergent preparation which is compatible with Hibisol is Hibiscrub.

Product licence number 0029/0134.

HIBITANE* OBSTETRIC CREAM

Presentation Hibitane Obstetric Cream is presented as a water-miscible cream containing 1% w/w chlorhexidine gluconate (equivalent to 5% v/w Chlorhexidine Gluconate Solution BP). Inactive ingredients are cetostearyl alcohol, cetostearyl alcohol/ethylene oxide condensate, isopropyl alcohol, linalyl acetate, liquid paraffin, water and white soft paraffin.

Uses Hibitane Obstetric Cream is an antimicrobial preparation for use as an antiseptic and lubricant in obstetric and gynaecological practice.

Dosage and administration Apply liberally to the skin around the vulva and perineum of the patient, and to the hands of the midwife or doctor.

Contra-indications, warnings, etc Hibitane preparations are contra-indicated for patients who have previously shown a hypersensitivity reaction to chlorhexidine. However, such reactions are extremely rare.
For topical application only. Keep out of the eyes and avoid contact with the brain, meninges and middle ear.

Side-effects: Irritative skin reactions can occasionally occur. Generalised allergic reactions to chlorhexidine have also been reported but are extremely rare.

Accidental ingestion: Chlorhexidine taken orally is poorly absorbed. Treat with gastric lavage using milk, gelatin or mild soap. Employ supportive measures as appropriate.

Pharmaceutical precautions Hypochlorite bleaches may cause brown stains to develop in fabrics which have previously been in contact with preparations containing chlorhexidine.
Chlorhexidine is incompatible with anionic agents.
Store at room temperature.

Legal category GSL.

Package quantities Polythene dispenser pack 250 ml (OP).

Further information Nil.

Product licence number 0029/5019.

HIBITANE* 5% CONCENTRATE

Presentation Hibitane 5% Concentrate is presented as a red aqueous solution containing 5% w/v chlorhexidine gluconate (equivalent to 25% v/v Chlorhexidine Gluconate Solution BP). Inactive ingredients are carmoisine, d-gluconolactone, isopropyl alcohol, linalyl acetate, nonyl phenol/ethylene oxide condensate and water.

Uses Hibitane 5% Concentrate is an antimicrobial agent for general antiseptic purposes. A surface active agent is present to inhibit precipitation when dilutions are made with hard water.

Dosage and administration

Method of preparation	*Concentration of active ingredient required (chlorhexidine gluconate)*	*Use*
10 ml made up to 1 litre with water (1 in 100)	1 in 2,000 (0.05%) Aqueous	Swabbing in obstetrics, wounds and burns† Storage of sterile instruments
10 ml with 15 ml water made up to 100 ml with 95% alcohol (1 in 10)	1 in 200 (0.5%) in 70% Alcohol	Pre-operative skin disinfection. Emergency instrument disinfection (2 minutes' immersion). (Excluding endoscopes containing cemented glass components)

† Sterilise the dilution by autoclaving at 115–116°C for 30 minutes or 121–123°C for 15 minutes.

Contra-indications, warnings, etc Hibitane preparations are contra-indicated for patients who have previously shown a hypersensitivity reaction to chlorhexidine. However, such reactions are extremely rare.
For external use only.
Dilute before use.
Keep out of the eyes and avoid contact with brain, meninges and middle ear. Not for injection. Do not use in body cavities.
If chlorhexidine solutions come into contact with eyes, wash out promptly and thoroughly with water.
Solutions applied to wounds, burns or broken skin should be sterile.
Syringes, needles and instruments which have been immersed in Hibitane solutions should be thoroughly rinsed in sterile water or saline before use.
Hibitane 5% Concentrate contains a surfactant and therefore instruments containing cemented glass components should not be disinfected with solutions prepared from Hibitane 5% Concentrate.

Side-effects: Irritative skin reactions can occasionally occur. Generalised allergic reactions to chlorhexidine have also been reported but are extremely rare.

Accidental ingestion: Chlorhexidine taken orally is poorly absorbed. Treat with gastric lavage using milk, gelatin or mild soap. Employ supportive measures as appropriate.

Accidental intravenous transfusion: Blood transfusion may be necessary to counteract haemolysis.

Pharmaceutical precautions Dilute with freshly distilled water, tap water of an acceptable bacteriological standard or alcohol (ethanol, Industrial Methylated Spirit or isopropranol).
As a precaution against bacterial contamination, stock aqueous solutions should contain at least 4% v/v of isopropranol or 7% v/v of ethanol, which may be denatured (for example, Industrial Methylated Spirit).
Aqueous dilutions of Hibitane used for instrument storage should contain 0.1% sodium nitrite to inhibit metal corrosion. Such solutions must be changed every 7 days.
As cork may protect certain Gram-negative organisms from the action of antiseptics, Hibitane solutions must be stored in bottles with glass, plastic or rubber closures.
Store at room temperature.
Hypochlorite bleaches may cause brown stains to develop in fabrics which have previously been in contact with Hibitane solutions.
Chlorhexidine is incompatible with anionic agents.

Legal category GSL.

Package quantities Containers of 5 litres and dispensers are available.

Further information Nil.

Product licence number 0029/5032.

HIBITANE* GLUCONATE 20% SOLUTION
(Chlorhexidine Gluconate Solution BP)

Presentation Hibitane Gluconate 20% Solution is presented as an aqueous solution containing 20% w/v chlorhexidine gluconate.

Uses Hibitane Gluconate is an antimicrobial agent for general antiseptic purposes. This presentation is an aqueous solution without additives which, when diluted allows use on body tissues where other antiseptics may prove too irritant. It may also be used for the chemical disinfection of delicate instruments such as cystoscopes.

Dosage and administration

Method of preparation	*Concentration of active ingredient required (chlorhexidine gluconate)*	*Use*
1.0 ml made up to 1 litre with water (1 in 1,000)	1 in 5,000 (0.02%) Aqueous	Bladder irrigation† Pleural or peritoneal irrigation† Cystoscopy medium†
2.5 ml made up to 1 litre with water (1 in 400)	1 in 2000 (0.05%) Aqueous	Eye irrigation† Dip bowls† Clean instrument disinfection including endoscopes (30 minutes' immersion)
2.5 ml of sterile solution made up to 1 litre with sterile glycerin and mixed aseptically (1 in 400)	1 in 2,000 (0.05%) in glycerin	Urethral disinfection and catheter lubrication
25 ml with 225 ml water made up to 1 litre with 95% alcohol (1 in 40)	1 in 200 (0.5%) in 70% alcohol	Emergency disinfection of clean instruments (2 minutes' immersion)

† Sterilise the dilution by autoclaving at 115°–116°C for 30 minutes or 121°–123°C for 15 minutes.

Contra-indications, warnings, etc Hibitane preparations are contra-indicated for patients who have previously shown a hypersensitivity reaction to chlorhexidine. However, such reactions are extremely rare.

Dilute before use.

Keep concentrated solutions out of the eyes. Avoid contact with the brain, meninges and middle ear. Not for injection.

If concentrated chlorhexidine solutions come into contact with the eyes, wash out promptly and thoroughly with water.

Solutions introduced into body cavities, eyes, or on to broken skin should be sterile.

Syringes, needles and instruments which have been immersed in Hibitane solutions should be thoroughly rinsed in sterile water or saline before use.

The low solubility of inorganic salts of chlorhexidine may cause precipitation and consequent loss of activity if Hibitane Gluconate 20% Solution is diluted with a solution containing inorganic anions, for example, saline or peritoneal dialysis fluid. This precipitation may occur when Hibitane Gluconate 20% Solution is used to disinfect catheters intended for use in peritoneal dialysis. Inadvertent repeated exposure of peritoneal membranes to precipitated material has been claimed as a possible predisposing factor for peritoneal fibrosis.

Side-effects: Irritative skin reactions can occasionally occur. Generalised allergic reactions to chlorhexidine have also been reported but are extremely rare.

Accidental ingestion: Chlorhexidine taken orally is poorly absorbed. Treat with gastric lavage using milk, gelatin or mild soap. Employ supportive measures as appropriate.

Accidental intravenous transfusion: Blood transfusion may be necessary to counteract haemolysis.

Pharmaceutical precautions Dilute with freshly distilled water, alcohol (ethanol, Industrial Methylated Spirit, or isopropanol) or glycerin. Mix well before use.

As a precaution against bacterial contamination, aqueous stock solution should contain at least 4% v/v of isopropanol or 7% v/v of ethanol which may be denatured, for example, Industrial Methylated Spirit.

Aqueous dilutions of Hibitane used for instrument storage should contain 0.1% sodium nitrite to inhibit metal corrosion. Such solutions must be changed every 7 days.

As cork may protect certain Gram-negative organisms from the action of antiseptics, Hibitane solutions must be stored in bottles with glass, plastic or rubber closures.

Store at room temperature.

Hypochlorite bleaches may cause brown stains to develop in fabrics which have previously been in contact with Hibitane solutions.

Chlorhexidine is incompatible with anionic agents.

Legal category GSL.

Package quantities Containers of 500 ml (OP) and 5 litres are available. Dispensers to fit 5L are available.

Further information Nil.

Product licence number 0029/5031.

IMPERACIN* TABLETS

Presentation Yellow, biconvex, film-coated tablets marked with IMPERACIN on one side. Each tablet contains 250 mg of Oxytetracycline Dihydrate PhEur. Inactive ingredients are alginic acid, calcium carboxymethylcellulose, gelatin, glycerol, magnesium stearate, methylhydroxypropyl cellulose, microcrystalline cellulose, tartrazine and titanium dioxide.

Uses Imperacin is a bacteriostatic broad-spectrum antibiotic well absorbed after oral administration. It is active against a variety of Gram-positive and Gram-negative bacteria, spirochaetes, certain mycoplasma species, rickettsiae, protozoa and the psittacosislymphogranuloma-venereum-trachoma group (Chlamydia). It is indicated in the treatment of the following conditions when they are caused by susceptible organisms.

The acute infective exacerbations of chronic bronchitis.

Venereal diseases, including penicillin-resistant gonorrhoea, non-gonococcal urethritis and lymphogranuloma venereum.

Brucellosis, typhus, amoebic dysentery and psittacosis.

Tetracyclines are of value in the treatment of staphylococcal and streptococcal infections in penicillin-sensitive patients where tetracycline resistance is not a problem.

Mode of action: Imperacin is a member of the tetracycline group of antibiotics with a wide range of activity against Gram-negative and Gram-positive organisms. Imperacin inhibits bacterial protein synthesis and thus checks their further multiplication.

Tetracyclines are incompletely and irregularly absorbed from the gastrointestinal tract. Absorption is reduced by calcium, aluminium, magnesium, iron, milk and food.

Oxytetracycline is 20–35% protein-bound and has a half-life of approximately 10 hours. Seventy per cent of the absorbed dose is excreted unchanged in the urine. High levels are achieved in the bile and the drug undergoes enterohepatic recirculation. Oxytetracycline is widely distributed in body tissues and fluids. It crosses the placenta and is present in significant concentrations in breast milk.

Dosage and administration
Adults: 250 to 500 mg four times daily.

Children: 25 to 50 mg/kg bodyweight daily, divided into four equal doses.

Elderly patients: There are no special dosage recommendations for the elderly, but it may be advisable to monitor elderly patients so that optimum dosage can be individually determined.

Doses are best given either 1 hour before or 2 hours after food.

Therapy should be continued for at least 24 to 48 hours after symptoms and fever have subsided.

In the treatment of streptococcal infections, a therapeutic dose should be administered for at least 10 days.

Contra-indications, warnings, etc Imperacin is contra-indicated in persons who have previously shown hypersensitivity to any of the tetracyclines.

Imperacin is contraindicated in chronic renal failure.

In the presence of renal impairment, normal doses may lead to excessive systemic accumulation of the drug and possible liver toxicity. Under such circumstances, lower than usual total doses are indicated and, if therapy is prolonged, serum level determinations of the drug may be advisable.

The combination of tetracyclines with diuretics may be detrimental to renal function.

The antianabolic action of the tetracyclines may cause an increase in BUN. While this is not a problem in those with normal renal function, in patients with significantly impaired renal function, higher serum levels of tetracycline may lead to azotaemia, hyperphosphataemia and acidosis.

Imperacin should be used with caution in the presence of hepatic dysfunction.

High doses of tetracyclines have been associated with a syndrome involving fatty liver degeneration and pancreatitis.

The use of tetracyclines during tooth development (last half of pregnancy, infancy and childhood to the age of eight years) may cause permanent discolouration of the teeth. This adverse reaction is more common during long term use but has been observed following repeated short term courses. Enamel hypoplasia has also been reported. Tetracycline drugs, therefore, should not be used in this age group unless other drugs are not likely to be effective or are contra-indicated.

As with other antibiotic preparations, Imperacin may result in overgrowth of non-susceptible organisms. If superinfection occurs, appropriate measures should be taken.

Antacids containing aluminium, calcium or magnesium impair absorption and should not be given to patients taking Imperacin.

Antidiarrhoeal preparations such as kaolin-pectin and bismuth subsalicylate hinder the absorption of tetracyclines.

Simultaneous oral administration of tetracycline preparations with iron leads to poor absorption of both substances.

Food and some dairy products also interfere with absorption.

Tetracyclines have been shown occasionally to depress plasma prothombin activity and patients who are on anticoagulant therapy may require an adjustment of their anticoagulant dosage.

Since bacteriostatic drugs may interfere with the bactericidal action of penicillin, it is advisable to avoid giving Imperacin in conjunction with penicillin.

Photosensitivity, manifested by an exaggerated sunburn reaction has been observed in some patients taking tetracyclines.

Hypersensitivity reactions and anaphylaxis are rarely seen during treatment with Imperacin. Treatment of anaphylaxis includes the immediate administration of adrenaline (0.5 ml Adrenaline Injection BP subcutaneously), oxygen and artificial respiration.

Treatment of severe bronchospasm includes administration of aminophylline, or salbutamol and antihistamines. General measures include administration of plasma, blood, vasopressor drugs (noradrenaline) and hydrocortisone (100 mg i.v.).

Pregnancy: It is known that tetracyclines cross the placental barrier and may have a toxic effect on the foetus. Special care should be exercised if administered during pregnancy.

Lactation: Levels of up to 60% of those found in maternal blood have been measured in breast milk. The use of tetracyclines in lactating women should be avoided, if possible.

Tetracyclines form a stable calcium complex in any bone forming tissue. A decrease in the fibula growth rate has been observed in prematures given oral tetracycline in doses of 25 mg/kg evey six hours. This reaction was shown to be reversible when the drug was discontinued.

Bulging fontanelles in infants and benign intracranial hypertension in adults has been reported. Treatment should cease if evidence of raised intracranial pressure develops.

Side-effects: These are uncommon in the recommended dosage. However, nausea, dysphagia, diarrhoea, maculopapular and erythematous rashes, morbilliform skin reactions and exfoliative dermatitis have been reported. Haemolytic anaemia, thrombocytopenia, neutropenia, eosinophilia, pericarditis and exacerbation of systemic lupus erythematosus have also been reported. Overgrowth of resistant organisms e.g. Candida, may occur and cause glossitis and rectal and vaginal irritation. Similarly, resistant staphylococci may cause enterocolitis. Pseudomembranous colitis has been associated with the use of tetracyclines.

Overdosage: Serious symptoms are unlikely. Gastric lavage might be beneficial in the first hours after ingestion followed by conservative management. Milk will reduce absorption.

Pharmaceutical precautions Store at room temperature, protected from light and moisture.

Legal category POM.

Package quantities *Tablets:* Containers of 100 (OP).

Further information
Effect on ability to drive or operate machinery: No special precautions are required.

Product licence number
Imperacin Tablets 0029/5087.

INDERAL* TABLETS AND INJECTION

Presentation

1. Tablets each containing 10 mg Propranolol Hydrochloride PhEur. Pink, round, bi-convex, film coated tablets, impressed with the legend 'INDERAL' 10 on one face and ICI on the other. The impressions are highlighted in white.
2. Tablets each containing 40 mg Propranolol Hydrochloride PhEur. Pink, round, bi-convex, film coated tablets, impressed with the legend 'INDERAL' 40 on one face and ICI on the other. The impressions are highlighted in white.
3. Tablets each containing 80 mg Propranolol Hydrochloride PhEur. Pink, round, bi-convex, film coated tablets, impressed with the legend 'INDERAL' 80 on one face and ICI on the other. The impressions are highlighted in white.

Inactive ingredients of Inderal Tablets are calcium carboxymethylcellulose, carmine, gelatin, glycerol, lactose, magnesium carbonate, magnesium stearate, methylhydroxypropyl cellulose and titanium dioxide.

4. Injection – a solution containing Propranolol Hydrochloride PhEur. 1 mg per 1 ml in glass ampoules of 1 ml. Inactive ingredients are citric acid and water.

Uses Inderal, a beta-adrenoceptor blocking drug, is indicated in:

(a) the control of hypertension
(b) the management of angina pectoris
(c) the long term prophylaxis against reinfarction after recovery from acute myocardial infarction
(d) the control of most forms of cardiac dysrhythmia

(e) the prophylaxis of migraine
(f) the management of essential tremor
(g) relief of situational anxiety and generalised anxiety symptoms, particularly those of somatic type.
(h) prophylaxis of upper gastro-intestinal bleeding in patients with portal hypertension and oesophageal varices
(i) the adjunctive management of thyrotoxicosis and thyrotoxic crisis
(j) management of hypertrophic obstructive cardiomyopathy
(k) management of phaeochromocytoma perioperatively (with an alpha blocker)

Dosage and administration *Adults: Oral: Hypertension:* A starting dose of 80 mg twice a day may be increased at weekly intervals according to response. The usual dose range is 160–320 mg per day. With concurrent diuretic or other antihypertensive drugs a further reduction of blood pressure is obtained.

Angina, migraine and essential tremor: A starting dose of 40 mg two or three times daily may be increased by the same amount at weekly intervals according to patient response. An adequate response in migraine and essential tremor is usually seen in the range 80–160 mg/day and in angina in the range 120–240 mg/day.

Situational and generalised anxiety: A dose of 40 mg daily may provide short term relief of acute situational anxiety. Generalised anxiety, requiring longer term therapy, usually responds adequately to 40 mg twice daily which, in individual cases, may be increased to 40 mg three times daily. Treatment should be continued according to response. Patients should be reviewed after six to twelve months' treatment.

Dysrhythmias, anxiety tachycardia, hypertrophic obstructive cardiomyopathy and thyrotoxicosis: A dosage range of 10–40 mg three or four times a day usually achieves the required response.

Post myocardial infarction: Treatment should start between days 5 and 21 after myocardial infarction, with an initial dose of 40 mg four times a day for 2 or 3 days. In order to improve compliance the total daily dosage may thereafter be given as 80 mg twice daily.

Portal hypertension: Dosage should be titrated to achieve approximately 25% reduction in resting heart rate. Dosing should begin with 40 mg twice daily, increasing to 80 mg twice daily depending on heart rate response. If necessary, the dose may be increased incrementally to a maximum of 160 mg twice daily.

Phaeochromocytoma: (Used only with an alpha-receptor blocking drug). Pre-operative: 60 mg daily for three days is recommended. Non-operable malignant cases: 30 mg daily.

Intravenous; The intravenous injection is intended for the emergency treatment of cardiac dysrhythmias and thyrotoxic crisis only. The initial dose of Inderal is 1 mg (1 ml) injected over one minute. This may be repeated at two-minute intervals until a response is observed or to a maximum dose of 10 mg in conscious patients or 5 mg in patients under anaesthesia.

Children: Dysrhythmias, phaeochromocytoma, thyrotoxicosis; Dosage should be individually determined and the following is only a guide: *Oral:* 250–500 micrograms/kg three or four times daily as required. *Intravenous:* 25–50 micrograms/kg injected slowly under ECG control and repeated three or four times daily as required.

Migraine: Oral: Under the age of 12: 20 mg two or three times daily.

Over the age of 12: the adult dose.

Fallot's Tetralogy: The value of Inderal in this condition is confined mainly to the relief of right-ventricular outflow tract shut-down. It is also useful for treatment of associated dysrhythmias and angina. Dosage should be individually determined and the following is only a guide: *Oral:* Up to 1mg/kg repeated three or four times daily as required. *Intravenous:* Up to 100 micrograms/kg injected slowly under ECG control, repeated three or four times daily as required.

Elderly patients: Evidence concerning the relation between blood level and age is conflicting. With regard to the elderly, the optimum dose should be individually determined according to clinical response.

Contra-indications, warnings, etc
Contra-indications: Inderal should not be used:

1. In the presence of second or third degree heart block.
2. In patients with cardiogenic shock.
3. If there is a history of bronchospasm.
4. After prolonged fasting.
5. In metabolic acidosis (e.g. in some diabetics).

Precautions: The intravenous injection is intended for the emergency treatment of cardiac dysrhythmias and thyrotoxic crisis only.

Special care should be taken with patients whose cardiac reserve is poor. Beta-adrenoceptor blocking drugs should be avoided in overt heart failure. However, they may be used in patients whose signs of failure have been controlled.

Heart failure due to thyrotoxicosis often responds to Inderal alone, but if other adverse factors co-exist myocardial contractility must be maintained and signs of failure controlled with digitalis and diuretics.

One of the pharmacological actions of Inderal is to reduce heart rate. In the rare instance when symptoms may be attributable to the slow heart rate, the dose may be reduced.

Inderal modifies the tachycardia of hypoglycaemia. Caution should be exercised in the concurrent use of Inderal and hypoglycaemic therapy in diabetic patients. Propranolol may prolong the hypoglycaemic response to insulin.

Liver function will deteriorate in patients with portal hypertension and hepatic encephalopathy may develop. There have been some reports suggesting that treatment with propranolol may increase the risk of developing hepatic encephalopathy.

In patients suffering from ischaemic heart disease, as with other beta-adrenoceptor blocking agents, treatment should not be discontinued abruptly. Either the equivalent dosage of another beta-adrenoceptor blocker may be substituted or the withdrawal of Inderal should be gradual.

Care should be taken in the parenteral administration of preparations containing adrenaline to patients taking beta-adrenoceptor blocking drugs as, in rare cases, vasoconstriction, hypertension and bradycardia may result.

Caution should be exercised when transferring patients from clonidine to beta-adrenoceptor blocking drugs. If beta-adrenoceptor blocking drugs and clonidine are given concurrently, clonidine should not be discontinued until several days after withdrawal of the beta-adrenoceptor blocking drug (see also prescribing information on clonidine).

Care should be taken in prescribing a beta-adrenoceptor blocking drug with Class 1 antidysrhythmic agents such as disopyramide.

Beta-adrenoceptor blocking drugs should be used with caution in combination with verapamil in patients with impaired ventricular function. The combination should not be given to patients with conduction abnormalities. Neither drug should be administered intravenously within 48 hours of discontinuing the other.

Anaesthesia: Care should be taken when using anaesthetic agents with Inderal. The anaesthetist should be informed and the choice of anaesthetic should be the agent with as little negative inotropic activity as possible.

Interference with laboratory tests: Inderal has been reported to interfere with the estimation of serum bilirubin by the diazo method and with the determination of catecholamines by methods using fluorescence.

Pregnancy: As with all other drugs, Inderal should not be given in pregnancy unless its use is essential. There is no evidence of teratogenicity with Inderal.

Lactation: There is some accumulation of propranolol in breast milk. However, a breast feeding child receives only small amounts of drug so that adverse effects are unlikely.

Side-effects: Inderal is usually well tolerated. Minor side-effects such as cold extremities, nausea, diarrhoea, sleep disturbances, lassitude and muscle fatigue are often transient. Isolated cases of paraesthesia of the hands have been reported. Rare cases of bradycardia, thrombocytopenia and purpura have been recorded. A low incidence of CNS symptoms including hallucinations have been reported.

There have been reports of skin rashes and/or dry eyes associated with the use of beta-adrenergic blocking drugs. The reported incidence is small and in most cases the symptoms have cleared when treatment was withdrawn. Discontinuance of the drug should be considered if any such reaction is not otherwise explicable. Cessation of therapy with a beta-adrenergic blocker should be gradual. In the rare event of intolerance, manifested as bradycardia and hypotension, the drug should be withdrawn and, if necessary, treatment for overdosage instituted.

Overdosage: Excessive bradycardia can be countered with atropine 1–2 mg intravenously. If necessary this may be followed by a bolus dose of glucagon 10 mg intravenously. If required this may be repeated or followed by an intravenous infusion of glucagon 1–10 mg/hr i.v. depending on response. If no response to glucagon occurs, or if glucagon is unavailable, a beta-adrenoceptor stimulant such as isoprenaline 25 micrograms initially or orciprenaline 500 micrograms may be given by slow intravenous injection.

Pharmaceutical precautions Inderal tablets should be stored at room temperature, protected from light and moisture. Inderal injection should be stored at room temperature, protected from light.

Legal category POM.

Package quantities *Tablets 10 mg:* Containers of 100 (OP).
Tablets 40 mg: Containers of 100 (OP).
Tablets 80 mg: Containers of 60 (OP).
Injection: 1 ml ampoules in boxes of 10.

Further information *Compatibility with intravenous infusion fluids:* Inderal Injection is compatible with 0.9% w/v sodium chloride and 5% w/v dextrose.

Details of a suitable formula for the extemporaneous preparation of a paediatric oral suspension of Inderal are available on request to the manufacturer.

Effect on ability to drive or operate machinery: Propranolol has no overall effect on car driving and machinery operation.

Product licence numbers

Inderal Tablets	10 mg	0029/5063
Inderal Tablets	40 mg	0029/5064
Inderal Tablets	80 mg	0029/5065
Inderal Injection		0029/5062

INDERAL* LA HALF-INDERAL* LA

Presentation Inderal LA and Half-Inderal LA capsules contain spheroids of the beta-adrenoceptor blocking drug propranolol hydrochloride which have a sustained release coating to provide long action.

Inderal LA capsules each contain 160 mg Propranolol Hydrochloride PhEur. Inderal LA is presented as size 1 gelatin capsules with a clear pink body and opaque, lavender cap bearing the ICI Roundel and marked Inderal LA in white.

Half-Inderal LA capsules each contain 80 mg Propranolol Hydrochloride PhEur. Half-Inderal LA is presented as size 3 gelatin capsules with a clear pink body and opaque, pale lavender cap bearing the ICI Roundel and marked Half-Inderal LA in black.

Inactive ingredients are erythrosine, ethylcellulose, gelatin, glycerol, iron oxide, methylhydroxypropylcellulose, microcrystalline cellulose, and titanium dioxide.

Uses Inderal LA and Half-Inderal LA are indicated in the management of angina, essential tremor, relief of situational anxiety and generalised anxiety symptoms, particularly those of somatic type, prophylaxis of upper gastro-intestinal bleeding in patients with portal hypertension and oesophageal varices, the adjunctive management of thyrotoxicosis, and the prophylaxis of migraine.

Inderal LA is indicated in the control of hypertension.

One Half-Inderal LA capsule daily is unlikely on its own to be sufficient to treat hypertension, but it may be used as a starting dose in appropriate patients (e.g. the elderly) or to provide a convenient method of gradual dosage alteration.

Dosage and administration *Adults: Hypertension:* The usual starting dose is one 160 mg Inderal LA capsule daily, taken either morning or evening. An adequate response is seen in most patients at this dosage. If necessary, it can be increased in 80 mg Half-Inderal LA increments until an adequate response is achieved. A further reduction in BP can be attained if a diuretic or other antihypertensive agent is given in addition to Inderal LA and Half-Inderal LA.

Angina, essential tremor, thyrotoxicosis and the prophylaxis of migraine: One Half-Inderal LA capsule daily taken either morning or evening may be sufficient to provide adequate control in many patients. If necessary the dose may be increased to one Inderal LA capsule per day and an additional Half-Inderal LA increment may be given.

Situational and generalised anxiety: One Half-Inderal LA capsule taken daily should be sufficient to provide short term relief of acute situational anxiety. Generalised anxiety, requiring longer term therapy, usually responds adequately at the same dosage. In individual cases, the dosage may be increased to one Inderal LA capsule per day. Treatment should be continued according to response. Patients should be reviewed after six to twelve months' treatment.

Portal hypertension: Dosage should be titrated to achieve approximately 25% reduction in resting heart rate. Dosing should begin with one 80 mg Half-Inderal LA capsule daily, increasing to one 160 mg Inderal LA capsule daily depending on heart rate response. Further 80 mg Half-Inderal LA increments may be added up to a maximum dose of 320 mg once daily.

Patients who are already established on equivalent daily doses of Inderal tablets should be transferred to the equivalent doses of Half-Inderal LA or Inderal LA daily taken either morning or evening.

Children: Inderal LA and Half-Inderal LA are not intended for use in children.

Elderly patients: Evidence concerning the relation between blood level and age is conflicting. It is suggested that treatment should start with one Half-Inderal LA capsule once daily. The dose may be increased to one Inderal LA daily or higher as appropriate.

Contra-indications, warnings, etc
Contra-indications: Inderal LA and Half-Inderal LA should not be used:

1. In the presence of second or third degree heart block.
2. In patients with cardiogenic shock.
3. If there is a history of bronchospasm.
4. After prolonged fasting.
5. In metabolic acidosis (e.g. in some diabetics).

Precautions: Special care should be taken with patients whose cardiac reserve is poor. Beta-adrenoceptor blocking drugs should be avoided in overt heart failure. However, they may be used in patients whose signs of failure have been controlled.

Heart failure due to thyrotoxicosis often responds to Inderal LA alone, but if other adverse factors co-exist myocardial contractility must be maintained and signs of failure controlled with digitalis and diuretics.

One of the pharmacological actions of Inderal LA or Half-Inderal LA is to reduce the heart rate. In the rare instance when symptoms may be attributable to the slow heart rate the dose may be reduced.

Inderal LA and Half-Inderal LA modify the tachycardia of hypoglycaemia. Caution should be exercised in the concurrent use of Inderal LA or Half-Inderal LA and hypoglycaemic therapy in diabetic patients. Propranolol may prolong the hypoglycaemic response to insulin.

Liver function will deteriorate in patients with portal hypertension and hepatic encephalopathy may develop. There have been some reports suggesting that treatment with propranolol may increase the risk of developing hepatic encephalopathy.

In patients suffering from ischaemic heart disease, as with other beta-adrenoceptor blocking agents, treatment should not be discontinued abruptly. Either the equivalent dosage of another beta-adrenoceptor blocker may be substituted or the withdrawal should be gradual. This can be achieved by first substituting the daily Inderal LA dose by the equivalent in Half-Inderal LA capsules and then gradually reducing the number of capsules.

Care should be taken in the parenteral administration of preparations containing adrenaline to patients taking beta-adrenoceptor blocking drugs as, in rare cases, vasoconstriction, hypertension and bradycardia may result.

Caution should be exercised when transferring patients from clonidine to beta-adrenoceptor blocking drugs. If beta-adrenoceptor blocking drugs and clonidine are given concurrently, clonidine should not be discontinued until several days after withdrawal of the beta-adrenoceptor blocking drug (see also prescribing information on clonidine).

Care should be taken in prescribing a beta-adrenoceptor blocking drug with Class 1 antidysrhythmic agents such as disopyramide.

Beta-adrenoceptor blocking drugs should be used with caution in combination with verapamil in patients with impaired ventricular function. The combination should not be given to patients with conduction abnormalities. Neither drug should be administered intravenously within 48 hours of discontinuing the other.

Anaesthesia: Care should be taken when using anaesthetic agents with Inderal LA. The anaesthetist should be informed and the choice of anaesthetic should be the agent with as little negative inotropic activity as possible.

Interference with laboratory tests: Inderal LA has been reported to interfere with the estimation of serum bilirubin by the diazo method and with the determination of catecholamines by methods using fluorescence.

Pregnancy: As with all other drugs, neither Inderal LA nor Half-Inderal LA should be given in pregnancy unless their use is essential. There is no evidence of teratogenicity with Inderal.

Lactation: There is some accumulation of propranolol in breast milk. However, a breast feeding child receives only small amounts of drug so that adverse effects are unlikely.

Side-effects: Inderal LA and Half-Inderal LA are usually well tolerated. Minor side effects, such as cold extremities, nausea, diarrhoea, sleep disturbances, lassitude and muscle fatigue are often transient. Isolated cases of paraesthesia of the hands have been reported. Rare cases of bradycardia, thrombocytopenia and purpura have been recorded. A low incidence of CNS symptoms including hallucinations have been reported.

There have been reports of skin rashes and/or dry eyes associated with the use of beta-adrenergic blocking drugs. The reported incidence is small and in most cases the symptoms have cleared when treatment was withdrawn. Discontinuance of the drug should be considered if any such reaction is not otherwise explicable. Cessation of therapy with a beta-adrenergic blocker should be gradual. In the rare event of intolerance, manifested as bradycardia and hypotension, the drug should be withdrawn and, if necessary, treatment for overdosage instituted.

Overdosage: Excessive bradycardia can be countered with atropine 1–2 mg intravenously. If necessary this may be followed by a bolus dose of glucagon 10 mg intravenously. If required this may be repeated or followed by an intravenous infusion of glucagon 1–10 mg/hr i.v. depending on response. If no response to glucagon occurs, or if glucagon is unavailable, a beta-adrenoceptor stimulant such as isoprenaline 25 micrograms initially or orciprenaline 500 micrograms may be given by slow intravenous injection.

Pharmaceutical precautions Store at room temperature, protected from light and moisture.

Legal category POM.

Package quantities Patient Calendar Pack of 28 capsules (OP).

Further information Inderal LA and Half-Inderal LA capsules provide controlled release of propranolol hydrochloride such that blood levels are maintained for over 24 hours following a single oral dose and, unlike therapy with conventional tablets, irregular peaks and troughs of blood level are avoided.

Effect on ability to drive or operate machinery: Propranolol has no overall effect on car driving and machinery operation.

Product licence numbers

Inderal LA	0029/0128.
Half-Inderal LA	0029/0173

INDERETIC*

Presentation White, opaque capsules, printed with Inderetic and the ICI Roundel. Each capsule contains 80 mg Propranolol Hydrochloride PhEur and 2.5 mg Bendrofluazide PhEur. Inactive ingredients are gelatin, iron oxide, lactose, magnesium stearate, shellac and titanium dioxide.

Uses The management of hypertension.

Dosage and administration *Adults:* One capsule twice daily should prove effective in most cases.

For new patients a maximum response is achieved usually within two weeks. If a greater antihypertensive effect is desired, Inderetic is compatible with most other antihypertensives which may be added (see *Warnings* below).

Children: There is no paediatric experience with Inderetic and for this reason it is not recommended for children.

Elderly patients: Evidence concerning the relation between blood level and age is conflicting. The optimum dose should be individually determined.

Contra-indications, warnings, etc

Contra-indications: Inderetic should not be used:

1. In the presence of second or third degree heart block.
2. In patients with cardiogenic shock.
3. If there is a history of bronchospasm.
4. In patients with anuria, renal failure, or with a history of sensitivity to thiazides.
5. After prolonged fasting.
6. In patients with metabolic acidosis (e.g. in some diabetics).

Precautions: Special care should be taken with patients whose cardiac reserve is poor. Beta-adrenoceptor blocking drugs should be avoided in overt heart failure. However, they may be used in patients whose signs of failure have been controlled.

One of the pharmacological actions of beta-adrenoceptor blocking drugs is to reduce heart rate. In the rare instance when symptoms may be attributable to the slow heart rate, the dose may be reduced.

In patients suffering from ischaemic heart disease, as with other beta-adrenoceptor blocking agents, treatment should not be discontinued abruptly.

Care should be taken in the parenteral administration of preparations containing adrenaline to patients taking beta-adrenoceptor blocking drugs, as, in rare cases, vasoconstriction, hypertension and bradycardia may result.

Caution should be exercised when transferring patients from clonidine to beta-adrenoceptor blocking drugs. If beta-adrenoceptor blocking drugs and clonidine are given concurrently, clonidine should not be discontinued until several days after withdrawal of the beta-adrenoceptor blocking drug (see also prescribing information on Clonidine).

Care should be taken in prescribing a beta-adrenoceptor blocking drug with Class 1 antidysrhythmic agents such as disopyramide.

Beta-adrenoceptor blocking drugs should be used with caution in combination with verapamil in patients with impaired ventricular function. The combination should not be given to patients with conduction abnormalities. Neither drug should be administered intravenously within 48 hours of discontinuing the other.

Inderetic contains a thiazide diuretic which may decrease glucose tolerance. Care is necessary when Inderetic is administered to patients with a known predisposition to diabetes.

Inderetic modifies the tachycardia of hypoglycaemia. Caution should be exercised in the concurrent use of Inderetic and hypoglycaemic therapy in diabetic patients. Propranolol may prolong the hypoglycaemic response to insulin.

As with other combinations of beta-adrenoceptor blocking drugs and diuretics, Inderetic may be associated with minor changes in potassium status. Potassium depletion may be dangerous in patients receiving digitalis or those with hepatic cirrhosis with ascites.

Preparations containing lithium generally should not be given with diuretics because they may reduce its renal clearance.

Anaesthesia: Care should be taken when using anaesthetic agents with Inderetic. The anaesthetist should be informed and the choice of anaesthetic should be the agent with as little negative inotropic activity as possible.

Interference with laboratory tests: Inderetic has been reported to interfere with the estimation of serum bilirubin by the diazo method and with the determination of catecholamines by methods using fluorescence.

Pregnancy: Although there is no evidence of teratogenicity, both constituents cross the placental barrier and Inderetic is, therefore, considered to be unsuitable for pregnant patients.

Lactation: As diuretics pass into breast milk, they should be avoided in mothers who wish to breast feed.

Side-effects: Propranolol hydrochloride is usually well tolerated. Minor side-effects, such as cold extremities, nausea, diarrhoea, sleep disturbances, lassitude and muscle fatigue are often transient. Isolated cases of paraesthesia of the hands have been reported. Rare cases of bradycardia, thrombocytopenia and purpura have been recorded. A low incidence of CNS symptoms, including hallucinations have been reported.

There have been reports of skin rashes and/or dry eyes associated with the use of beta-adrenergic blocking drugs. The reported incidence is small and in most cases the symptoms have cleared when treatment was withdrawn. Discontinuance of the drug should be considered if any such reaction is not otherwise explicable. Cessation of therapy with a beta-adrenergic blocker should be gradual. In the rare event of intolerance to the propranolol hydrochloride in Inderetic, manifested as bradycardia and hypotension, the drug should be withdrawn and, if necessary, treatment for overdosage instituted.

Adverse effects of bendrofluazide are uncommon in the small dose contained in Inderetic. Hypokalaemia may occur and may be dangerous in patients receiving digitalis or in those with hepatic cirrhosis when coma may be precipitated. Hyperuricaemia sometimes occurs, but an attack of gout is rare. The thiazide diuretics increase blood urea and they should be used with care in patients with renal failure. Reports of other adverse reactions to thiazides are rare. They include skin rashes with associated photosensitivity, necrotising vasculitis, acute pancreatitis, blood dyscrasias and aggravation of pre-existing myopia.

Overdosage: Excessive bradycardia can be countered with atropine 1–2 mg intravenously. If necessary this may be followed by a bolus dose of glucagon 10 mg intravenously. If required this may be repeated or followed by an intravenous infusion of glucagon 1–10 mg/hr i.v. depending on response. If no response to glucagon occurs, or if glucagon is unavailable, a beta-adrenoceptor stimulant such as isoprenaline 25 micrograms initially or orciprenaline 500 micrograms may be given by slow intravenous injection. Excessive diuresis should be countered by maintaining normal fluid and electrolyte balance.

Pharmaceutical precautions Store at room temperature, protected from light and moisture.

Legal category POM.

Package quantities Containers of 100 capsules (OP).

Further information Inderetic is designed to aid drug compliance by providing a convenient presentation of the standard beta-adrenoceptor blocking drug Inderal, propranolol hydrochloride, with the diuretic bendrofluazide for the treatment of hypertension. Concurrent use of propranolol and bendrofluazide produces a more pronounced and consistent antihypertensive response than when either component is used alone.

Effect on ability to drive or operate machinery: Propranolol has no overall effect on car driving and machinery operation. Studies to investigate the effects of bendrofluazide have not been carried out. There have been no published reports of impaired performance of such tasks.

Product licence number 0029/0138.

INDEREX*

Presentation Capsules, having opaque pink caps and opaque grey bodies printed with the name Inderex and the ICI Roundel. Each capsule contains 160 mg Propranolol Hydrochloride PhEur in the form of spheroids having a sustained release coating to provide long action, and 5 mg Bendrofluazide PhEur. Inactive ingredients are erythrosine, ethyl cellulose, gelatin, iron oxide, lactose, maize starch, methylhydroxypropyl cellulose, microcrystalline cellulose, Patent Blue V, stearic acid, talc and titanium dioxide.

Uses The management of hypertension.

Dosage and administration *Adults:* One capsule daily should prove effective in most cases.

For new patients a maximum response is achieved usually within two weeks. If a greater antihypertensive effect is desired, Inderex is compatible with most other antihypertensives which may be added (see Warnings below).

Children: There is no paediatric experience with Inderex and for this reason it is not recommended for children.

Elderly patients: Evidence concerning the relation between blood level and age is conflicting. The optimum dose should be individually determined.

Contra-indications, warnings, etc

Contra-indications: Inderex should not be used:

1. In the presence of second or third degree heart block.
2. In patients with cardiogenic shock.
3. If there is a history of bronchospasm.
4. In patients with anuria, renal failure, or with a history of sensitivity to thiazides.
5. After prolonged fasting.
6. In patients with metabolic acidosis (e.g. in some diabetics).

Precautions: Special care should be taken with patients whose cardiac reserve is poor. Beta-adrenoceptor blocking drugs should be avoided in overt heart failure. However, they may be used in patients whose signs of failure have been controlled.

One of the pharmacological effects of beta-adrenoceptor blockade is a reduction in heart rate. If this falls much below 50–55 beats/minute, the dose should not be increased further.

In patients suffering from ischaemic heart disease, it is important that treatment with a beta-adrenoceptor blocking agent is not discontinued abruptly.

Care should be taken in the parenteral administration of preparations containing adrenaline to patients taking beta-adrenoceptor blocking drugs as, in rare cases, vasoconstriction, hypertension and bradycardia may result.

Caution should be exercised when transferring patients from clonidine to beta-adrenoceptor blocking drugs. If beta-adrenoceptor blocking drugs and clonidine are given concurrently, clonidine should not be discontinued until several days after withdrawal of the beta-adrenoceptor blocking drug (see also prescribing information on clonidine).

Care should be taken in prescribing a beta-adrenoceptor blocking drug with Class 1 antidysrhythmic agents such as disopyramide.

Beta-adrenoceptor blocking drugs should be used with caution in combination with verapamil in patients with impaired ventricular function. The combination should not be given to patients with conduction abnormalities. Neither drug should be administered intravenously within 48 hours of discontinuing the other.

Inderex contains a thiazide diuretic which may decrease glucose tolerance. Care is necessary when Inderex is administered to patients with a known predisposition to diabetes.

Inderex modifies the tachycardia of hypoglycaemia. Caution should be exercised in the concurrent use of Inderex and hypoglycaemic therapy in diabetic patients. Propranolol may prolong the hypoglycaemic response to insulin.

As with other combinations of beta-adrenoceptor blocking drugs and diuretics, Inderex may be associated with minor changes in potassium status. Potassium depletion may be dangerous in patients receiving digitalis or those with hepatic cirrhosis with ascites.

Preparations containing lithium generally should not be given with diuretics because they may reduce its renal clearance.

Anaesthesia: Care should be taken when using anaesthetic agents with Inderex. The anaesthetist should be informed and the choice of anaesthetic should be the agent with as little negative inotropic activity as possible.

Intereference with laboratory tests: Inderex has been reported to interfere with the estimation of serum bilirubin by the diazo method and with the determination of catecholamines by methods using fluorescence.

Pregnancy: Although there is no evidence of teratogenicity, both constituents cross the placental barrier and Inderex is, therefore, considered to be unsuitable for pregnant patients.

Lactation: As diuretics pass into breast milk, they should be avoided in mothers who wish to breast feed.

Side-effects: Propranolol hydrochloride is usually well tolerated. Minor side effects, such as cold extremities, nausea, diarrhoea, sleep disturbances, lassitude and muscle fatigue are often transient. Isolated cases of paraesthesia of the hands have been reported. Rare cases of bradycardia, thrombocytopenia and purpura have been recorded. A low incidence of CNS symptoms, including hallucinations have been reported.

There have been reports of skin rashes and/or dry eyes associated with the use of beta-adrenergic blocking drugs. The reported incidence is small and in most cases the symptoms have cleared when treatment was withdrawn. Discontinuance of the drug should be considered if any such reaction is not otherwise explicable. Cessation of therapy with a beta-adrenergic blocker should be gradual. In the rare event of intolerance to the propranolol hydrochloride in Inderex, manifested as bradycardia and hypotension, the drug should be withdrawn and, if necessary, treatment for overdosage instituted.

Adverse effects of bendrofluazide are uncommon in the small dose contained in Inderex. Hypokalaemia may occur and may be dangerous in patients receiving digitalis or in those with hepatic cirrhosis when coma may be precipitated. Hyperuricaemia sometimes occurs, but an attack of gout is rare. The thiazide diuretics increase blood urea and they should be used with care in patients with renal failure. Reports of other adverse reactions to thiazides are rare. They include skin rashes with associated photosensitivity, necrotising vasculitis, acute pancreatitis, blood dyscrasias and aggravation of pre-existing myopia.

Overdosage: Excessive bradycardia can be countered with atropine 1–2 mg intravenously. If necessary this may be followed by a bolus dose of glucagon 10 mg intravenously. If required this may be repeated or followed by an intravenous infusion of glucagon 1–10 mg/hr i.v. depending on response. If no response to glucagon occurs, or if glucagon is unavailable, a beta-adrenoceptor stimulant such as isoprenaline 25 micrograms initially or orciprenaline 500 micrograms may be given by slow intravenous injection. Excessive diuresis should be countered by maintaining normal fluid and electrolyte balance.

Pharmaceutical precautions Store at room temperature, protected from light and moisture.

Legal category POM.

Package quantities Patient calendar pack of 28 capsules (OP).

Further information Inderex is designed to aid drug compliance by providing a convenient presentation of a sustained release formulation of propranolol hydrochloride with the diuretic bendrofluazide for the treatment of hypertension. Concurrent use of propranolol and bendrofluazide produces a more pronounced and consistent antihypertensive response than when either component is used alone.

Effect on ability to drive or operate machinery: Propranolol has no overall effect on car driving and machinery operation. Studies to investigate the effects of bendrofluazide have not been carried out. There have been no published reports of impaired performance of such tasks.

Product licence number 0029/0157.

MYSOLINE* TABLETS
MYSOLINE* ORAL SUSPENSION

Presentation Mysoline tablets are round, white, biconvex, marked with a parallel line on each side of the bisecting line on one face and the ICI roundel on the obverse, and contain 250 mg Primidone Ph Eur. Inactive ingredients are calcium carboxymethylcellulose, gelatin, magnesium stearate, povidone and stearic acid.

Mysoline Oral Suspension is a white, pleasantly flavoured aqueous suspension which contains 250 mg Primidone Ph Eur per 5 ml. Inactive ingredients are aluminium magnesium silicate, cetostearyl alcohol/ethylene oxide condensate, methyl hydroxybenzoate, propyl hydroxybenzoate, sodium carboxymethylcellulose, sucrose, vanilla flavouring and water.

Uses Mysoline is indicated in the management of grand mal and psychomotor (temporal lobe) epilepsy. It is also of value in the management of focal or Jacksonian seizures, petit mal, myoclonic jerks and akinetic attacks.

Mysoline is also indicated in the management of essential tremor.

Dosage and administration *Epilepsy:* Treatment must always be planned on an individual basis. In many patients it will be possible to use Mysoline alone, but in some, Mysoline will need to be combined with other anticonvulsants or with supporting therapy.

Mysoline is usually given twice daily. Begin with 125 mg once daily late in the evening. Every three days increase the daily dosage by 125 mg until the patient is receiving 500 mg daily. Thereafter, every three days increase the daily dosage by 250 mg in adults or 125 mg in children under 9 years – until control is obtained or the maximum tolerated dosage is being given. This may be as much as 1.5 g a day in adults; 1 g a day in children.

Average daily maintenance doses:

	Tablets (250 mg) or 5 ml measures of suspension (250 mg/5 ml)	*Milligrams*
Adults and children over 9 years	3–6	750–1,500
Children 6–9 years	3–4	750–1,000
Children 2–5 years	2–3	500–750
Children up to 2 years	1–2	250–500

The total daily dose is usually best divided and given in two equal amounts, one in the morning and the other in the evening. In certain patients, it may be considered advisable to give a larger dose when the seizures are more frequent. For instance: 1) if the attacks are nocturnal then all or most of the day's dose may be given in the evening; 2) if the attacks are associated with some particular event such as menstruation, a slight increase in the appropriate dose is often beneficial.

When it is necessary to give 125 mg of Mysoline Suspension to a small child, it is advisable to dilute the suspension and administer a 5 ml dose.

A suitable diluent is:

Sodium carboxymethyl cellulose (50 cp)	1% w/v
Sucrose	20%
Methylhydroxybenzoate	0.15%
Propylhydroxybenzoate	0.015%
Water	to 100%

Elderly patients: It is advisable to monitor elderly patients with reduced renal function who are receiving primidone.

Patients on other Anticonvulsants: Where a patient's attacks are not sufficiently well controlled with other anticonvulsants, or disturbing side effects have arisen, 'Mysoline' may be used to augment or replace existing treatment. First add 'Mysoline' to the current anticonvulsant treatment by the method of gradual introduction described previously. When a worthwhile effect has been achieved and the amount of 'Mysoline' being given has been built up to at least half the estimated requirement, withdrawal of the previous treatment can then be attempted. This should be done gradually over a period of two weeks, during which time it may be necessary to increase the 'Mysoline' dosage to maintain control. Withdrawal of previous treatment should not be too rapid or status epilepticus may occur. Where phenobarbitone formed the major part of the previous treatment, however, both its withdrawal and 'Mysoline' substitution should be made earlier, so as to prevent excessive drowsiness from interfering with accurate assessment of the optimum dosage of 'Mysoline'.

Essential tremor: Initially a dose of 50 mg daily should be introduced using Mysoline Suspension. The daily dose should be increased gradually over a 2–3 week period until remission of symptoms or the highest dose tolerated up to a maximum of 750 mg daily.

Patients with essential tremor who have not previously been exposed to anticonvulsants, or other drugs known to induce increased hepatic enzyme activity, may experience acute symptoms of intolerance to Mysoline, frequently characterised by vertigo, unsteadiness and nausea. It is, therefore, essential to start such patients at a low dosage (initially 50 mg daily) increasing very slowly up to the maximum tolerated dose or that which produces remission of tremor (up to 750 mg daily).

Contra-indications, warnings, etc Patients who exhibit hypersensitivity or an allergic reaction to primidone should not receive the drug. Primidone should not be administered to patients with acute intermittent porphyria.

Mysoline should be given with caution, and may be required in reduced dosage, in children, the elderly, debilitated patients or those with impaired renal, hepatic or respiratory function.

Primidone is a potent CNS depressant and is partially metabolised to phenobarbitone. After prolonged administration there is a potential for tolerance, dependence and a withdrawal reaction on abrupt cessation of treatment.

Both primidone and its major metabolite phenobarbitone induce liver enzyme activity. This may lead to altered pharmacokinetics in concomitantly administered drugs including other anticonvulsants such as phenytoin and coumarin anticoagulants. Blood levels of both Mysoline and any additional anticonvulsant agent may be altered by concomitant administration. Breakthrough bleeding and failure of contraceptive therapy have been noted in patients taking anticonvulsant drugs and oral contraceptive steroids. This is usually assumed to be due to induction of liver enzymes by the anticonvulsant with accelerated breakdown of the hormones.

As with most other anticonvulsants, patients who drive vehicles or operate machinery should be aware of the possibility of impaired reaction time.

Pregnancy: There is some evidence of a higher than average incidence of congenital abnormalities in infants born of epileptic mothers. The factors influencing this are unknown, but the possibility that anticonvulsant therapy may be involved and the very slight risk of an abnormal foetus must be weighed against the risks of withholding treatment during pregnancy.

Long-term anticonvulsant therapy can be associated with decreased serum folate levels. As folic acid requirements are also increased during pregnancy, regular screening of patients at risk is advised, and treatment with folic acid and vitamin B_{12}, although controversial, should be considered.

Anticonvulsant therapy in pregnancy has occasionally been associated with coagulation disorders in the neonates. For this reason pregnant patients should be given Vitamin K_1 through the last month of pregnancy up to the time of delivery. In the absence of such pretreatment then 10 mg Vitamin K_1 may be given to the mother at the time of delivery, and 1 mg should be given immediately to the neonate at risk.

During breast feeding the baby should be monitored for sedation.

Side-effects: If side-effects do appear they are generally confined to the early stages of treatment when patients frequently feel drowsy and listless.

Symptoms of neurotoxicity such as visual disturbances, nausea, headache, vomiting, nystagmus and ataxia have been reported but are usually transient even when pronounced. On occasions an idiosyncratic reaction may occur which involves these symptoms in an acute and severe form necessitating withdrawal of treatment. Dermatological reactions are infrequent and usually occur at the onset of therapy. Rarely personality changes, which may include psychotic reactions have been reported.

Exceptionally, as with phenytoin and phenobarbitone, megaloblastic anaemia may develop requiring discontinuation of primidone. This condition may respond to treatment with folic acid and/or Vitamin B_{12}. There have been isolated reports of other blood dyscrasias.

Overdosage: Primidone is metabolised extensively to phenobarbitone and overdosage leads to varying degrees of CNS depression which, depending on the dose ingested, may include ataxia, loss of consciousness, respiratory depression and coma. Treatment should include aspiration of stomach contents and general supportive measures. There is no specific antidote.

Pharmaceutical precautions Store at room temperature.

Legal category POM.

Package quantities *Tablets 250 mg:* Containers of 100 (OP).
Suspension (250 mg/5 ml): Bottles of 250 ml (OP).

Further information Nil.

Product licence numbers
Mysoline Tablets 0029/5074
Mysoline Oral Suspension 0029/5072

NASEPTIN*

Presentation Naseptin is presented as a non-greasy, white, water-miscible cream containing 0.1% w/w Chlorhexidine Hydrochloride BP and 0.5% w/w Neomycin Sulphate PhEur. Inactive ingredients are arachis oil, cetostearyl alcohol, cetostearyl alcohol/ethylene oxide condensate, liquid paraffin and water.

Uses Naseptin is an antimicrobial cream, intended for application to the nares. It is used for eradicating nasal carriage of staphylococci.

Dosage and administration
Adults (including the elderly) and children: A small amount of Naseptin is placed on the little finger and applied to the inside of each nostril.

For prophylaxis: Naseptin is applied as above, twice daily, to prevent patients from becoming carriers and to inhibit the dispersion of staphylococci.

For eradication of infection: Naseptin is applied four times daily for 10 days to eliminate organisms from the nares.

Contra-indications, warnings, etc Naseptin is contra-indicated for patients who have previously shown an hypersensitivity reaction to neomycin.

Naseptin is contra-indicated for patients who have previously shown a hypersensitivity reaction to chlorhexidine. However, such reactions are extremely rare.

For nasal application only. Keep out of the eyes and ears.

Prolonged use of neomycin preparations can lead to skin sensitisation, ototoxicity and nephrotoxicity.

Side-effects: Irritative skin reactions and hypersensitivity can occasionally occur. Generalised allergic reactions to chlorhexidine have also been reported but are extremely rare. In such cases the use of Naseptin must be discontinued and if necessary symptomatic treatment given.

Accidental ingestion: Accidental ingestion of the contents of a Naseptin tube is not likely to have any adverse effect on the patient.

Pharmaceutical precautions
Hypochlorite bleaches may cause brown stains to develop in fabrics which have previously been in contact with preparations containing chlorhexidine.
Chlorhexidine is incompatible with anionic agents.
Store at room temperature.

Legal category POM.

Package quantities Tubes of 15 g (OP).

Further information Nil.

Product licence number 0029/5009.

NOLVADEX*
NOLVADEX-D TABLETS
NOLVADEX-FORTE TABLETS

Presentation *Nolvadex:* White, round, bi-convex tablets, each tablet containing Tamoxifen Citrate BP equivalent to 10 mg of tamoxifen, marked with Nolvadex 10 on one face and ICI on the other.

Nolvadex-D: White, octagonal, biconvex tablets, each containing Tamoxifen Citrate BP equivalent to 20 mg of tamoxifen, marked with Nolvadex-D on one face and ICI on the other.

Nolvadex-Forte: White, elongated octagonal tablets, each containing Tamoxifen Citrate BP equivalent to 40 mg of tamoxifen, marked with Nolvadex-Forte on one face and bisected on the other side with the letters ICI in each segment.

Inactive ingredients are croscarmellose sodium, gelatin, lactose, macrogol, magnesium stearate, maize starch, methylhydroxypropylcellulose, and titanium dioxide.

Uses At the recommended dosage Nolvadex has anti-oestrogenic properties and competes with oestrogen for binding sites in target organs. It does not have androgenic properties.

Nolvadex is indicated for:

1. The treatment of breast cancer. The proportion of patients with breast cancer who respond to Nolvadex is similar to that seen with oestrogens or androgens. However, because Nolvadex produces fewer serious side-effects it is more acceptable to the patient.
2. The treatment of anovulatory infertility.

Mode of action: Nolvadex (tamoxifen) is a non-steroidal antioestrogen. In man Nolvadex acts primarily as an antioestrogen, inhibiting the effects of endogenous oestrogen, probably by binding with cytoplasmic oestrogen receptors. However, clinical results have shown some benefit in oestrogen receptor negative tumours which may indicate other mechanisms of action.

After oral administration, tamoxifen is absorbed rapidly with maximum serum concentrations attained within 4–7 hours. Steady state concentrations (about 300 ng/ml) are achieved after four weeks treatment. The drug is highly protein bound to serum albumin (>99%). Metabolism is by hydroxylation, demethylation and conjugation, giving rise to several major metabolites which have a similar pharmacological profile to the parent compound and thus contribute to the therapeutic effect. Excretion occurs primarily via the faeces and an elimination half-life of approximately seven days has been calculated for the drug itself, whereas that for N-desmethyltamoxifen, the principal metabolite, is 14 days.

Dosage and administration
1. *Breast cancer:* The dose range is 20 to 40 mg daily given either in divided doses twice daily or as a single dose once daily.

Elderly patients: Similar dosage regimens of Nolvadex have been used in elderly patients with breast cancer and in some of these patients it has been used as sole therapy.

2. *Infertility:* Before commencing any course of treatment, whether initial or subsequent, the possibility of pregnancy must be excluded. In women who are menstruating regularly, but with anovular cycles, the initial course of treatment consists of 20 mg of Nolvadex daily on the second, third, fourth and fifth days of the menstrual cycle. If unsatisfactory basal temperature records or poor pre-ovulatory cervical mucus indicate that this initial course of treatment has been unsuccessful, further courses may be given during subsequent menstrual periods, increasing the dosage to 40 mg and then to 80 mg daily.

In women who are not menstruating regularly the initial course may begin on any day. If no signs of ovulation are demonstrable then a subsequent course of treatment may start 45 days later, with dosage increased as above. If a patient responds with menstruation, then the next course of treatment is commenced on the second day of the cycle.

Contra-indications, warnings, etc *Pregnancy:* Nolvadex must not be given during pregnancy. Premenopausal patients must be carefully examined before treatment for breast cancer or infertility to exclude the possibility of pregnancy.

Menstruation is suppressed in a proportion of premenopausal women receiving Nolvadex for the treatment of breast cancer. Cystic ovarian swellings have occasionally been observed in premenopausal women receiving Nolvadex.

A small number of patients with bony metastases have developed hypercalcaemia on initiation of therapy.

When Nolvadex is used in combination with coumarin-type anticoagulants, a significant increase in anticoagulant effect may occur. Where such co-administration is initiated, careful monitoring of the patient is recommended.

A small number of cases of endometrial hyperplasia,

endometrial polyps and endometrial carcinoma have been reported in association with Nolvadex treatment. A definitive relationship to Nolvadex therapy has not been established.

Tamoxifen was not mutagenic in a range of in vitro and in vivo mutagenicity tests. Gonadal tumours in mice and liver tumours in rats receiving tamoxifen have been reported in long-term studies. The clinical relevance of these findings has not been established.

Lactation: It is not known if Nolvadex is excreted in human milk and therefore the drug is not recommended during lactation. The decision either to discontinue nursing or discontinue Nolvadex should take into account the importance of the drug to the mother.

Side-effects: During long-term treatment side-effects are not as numerous or as serious with Nolvadex as with the androgens and oestrogens which are also used to treat breast cancer. Those that have been reported can be classified as either due to the anti-oestrogenic action of the drug, e.g. hot flushes, vaginal bleeding, and pruritus vulvae, or as more general effects, e.g. gastro-intestinal intolerance, tumour flare, light-headedness and, occasionally, fluid retention.

When side-effects are severe it is sometimes possible to control them by a simple reduction of dosage without loss of control of the disease. If side-effects do not respond to this measure, it may be necessary to stop the treatment.

Transient falls in platelet count, usually only to 80 000–90 000 per cu mm but occasionally lower, have been reported in patients taking tamoxifen for breast cancer. No haemorrhagic tendency has been reported and the platelet counts have recovered even though treatment with the drug has continued.

A number of cases of visual disturbance including corneal changes, cataracts and retinopathy, have been described in patients receiving Nolvadex therapy.

There have been infrequent reports of thromboembolic events occurring during Nolvadex therapy. As an increased incidence of these events is known to occur in patients with malignant disease, a causal relationship with Nolvadex has not been established.

Overdosage: On theoretical grounds overdosage would be expected to cause enhancement of the anti-oestrogenic side-effects mentioned above. Observations in animals show that extreme overdosage (100–200 times recommended daily dose) may produce oestrogenic effects.

There is no specific antidote to overdosage, and treatment must be symptomatic.

Pharmaceutical precautions Store at room temperature protected from light.

Legal category POM.

Package quantities Nolvadex tablets are blister packed in containers of 30 tablets (OP).

Nolvadex-D tablets are blister packed in containers of 30 tablets (OP).

Nolvadex-Forte tablets are blister packed in containers of 30 tablets (OP).

Further information *Effect on ability to drive or operate machinery:* There is no evidence that Nolvadex results in impairment of these activities.

Product licence numbers

Nolvadex	0029/0064
Nolvadex-D	0029/0155
Nolvadex-Forte	0029/0176

PALUDRINE* TABLETS

Presentation White, bi-convex tablets marked with the ICI roundel on one side and bisected on the other side with a letter P in each segment. Each tablet contains 100 mg of Proguanil Hydrochloride BP. Inactive ingredients are calcium carbonate, gelatin, magnesium stearate and maize starch.

Uses Paludrine is an effective antimalarial agent. It is recommended for the prevention and suppression of malaria.

Paludrine is effective against the tissue forms of some strains of *P. falciparum* and acts through an active metabolite cycloguanil. The mechanism of action is probably due to inhibition of dihydrofolate reductase. The effect of this action is to prevent schizogony and its main effect is against the developing primary tissue schizonts.

Proguanil is well absorbed in man with peak plasma concentrations of approximately 140 ng/ml occurring around four hours after an oral dose of 200 mg to an adult. The active triazine metabolite cycloguanil peaks at approximately 75 ng/ml one hour later. The elimination half-lives for proguanil and cycloguanil are reported to be of the order of 20 hours.

There is a low degree of drug accumulation after repeat doses, leading to steady state conditions after approximately three days. When daily doses are not taken, blood levels fall sharply but do not disappear completely until at least two or three doses are missed.

Dosage and administration Non-immune subjects entering a malarious region are advised to begin treatment with Paludrine at least 24 hours before arrival. The daily dose of Paludrine should be continued throughout exposure to risk and for four weeks after leaving the area.

Adults: 2 tablets (200 mg) daily.

Children: Under 1 year: $\frac{1}{4}$ tablet (25 mg) daily.

1–4 years: $\frac{1}{2}$ tablet (50 mg) daily.

5–8 years: 1 tablet (100 mg) daily.

9–14 years: $1\frac{1}{2}$ tablets (150 mg) daily.

Over 14 years: Adult dose daily.

The daily dose is best taken with water, after food, at the same time each day.

Provided the tablet fragment gives the minimum amount specified, precise accuracy in children's dosage is not essential since the drug possesses a wide safety margin. For a young child, the dose may be administered crushed and mixed with milk, honey or jam.

Elderly patients: There are no special dosage recommendations for the elderly, but it may be advisable to monitor elderly patients so that optimum dosage can be individually determined.

Contra-indications, warnings, etc Paludrine should be used with caution in patients with severe renal failure.

Pregnancy: Pregnancy increases the risks from malaria. It is generally accepted that all drug treatment should be avoided if possible during the first trimester of pregnancy. Paludrine has been widely used for over 40 years and a causal connection between its use and any adverse effect on mother or foetus has not been established.

Lactation: Although Paludrine is excreted in breast milk, the amount is insufficient to confer any benefit on the infant. Separate chemoprophylaxis for the infant is required.

Effect on ability to drive or operate machinery: There is no evidence to suggest that Paludrine causes sedation or is likely to affect concentration.

Side-effects: At normal dosage levels the side-effect most commonly encountered is mild gastric intolerance. This usually subsides as treatment is continued. Mouth ulceration and stomatitis have on occasion been reported. Isolated cases of skin reaction and reversible hair loss have been reported in association with the use of proguanil.

Overdosage: The following effects have been reported in cases of overdosage: haematuria, renal irritation, epigastric discomfort and vomiting.

There is no specific antidote, and symptoms should be treated as they arise.

Pharmaceutical precautions Store at room temperature.

Legal category P.

Package quantities Containers of 100 (OP).

Further information In any locality where drug-resistant malaria is known or suspected, it is essential to take local medical advice on what prophylactic regimen is appropriate.

Product licence number 0029/5079.

PEPTAVLON*

Presentation Peptavlon (Pentagastrin Injection BP) is a clear, colourless, sterile, isotonic solution containing 250 micrograms/ml of Pentagastrin BP. It is packed in neutral, clear glass ampoules which each contain 500 micrograms of Pentagastrin BP in 2 ml of solution. Inactive ingredients are sodium chloride, ammonium chloride and water.

Uses Peptavlon is used for the diagnostic testing of gastric secretion.

Mode of action: Pentagastrin is a synthetic pentapeptide containing the carboxyl terminal tetrapeptide responsible for the actions of natural gastrins. The most prominent action of pentagastrin is to stimulate the secretion of gastric acid, pepsin and intrinsic factor. Additionally, it stimulates pancreatic secretion, inhibits absorption of water and electrolytes from the ileum, contracts the smooth muscle of the lower oesophageal sphincter and stomach (but delays gastric emptying time), relaxes the sphincter of Oddi and increases blood flow in the gastric mucosa.

Pentagastrin stimulates gastric acid secretion approximately ten minutes after subcutaneous injection, with peak response occurring in most cases twenty to thirty minutes after administration. Duration of activity is usually between sixty and eighty minutes.

Pentagastrin is rapidly absorbed after administration. Pentagastrin has a short half life (10 minutes or less) in the circulation. It is metabolised primarily in the liver and excretion is mainly by the kidneys.

Dosage and administration The following procedure is adopted for testing gastric secretion with Peptavlon.

The patient receives no medication (e.g. antacids, etc.) that might affect the results of the tests for 24 hours and no food for 12 hours before the test. On the morning of the test a radio-opaque tube (Leven No. 7 or Ryle's 12-16Fr) is passed into the patient's stomach by way of the nose. Radiological observation is used to ensure that the tube is correctly positioned in the lower part of the body of the stomach.

The tube is securely fastened to the patient's nose and forehead with adhesive tape to ensure that it is not displaced. The patient lies on his left side.

The gastric juices are then collected by applying continuous suction (at 30–50 mm Hg below atmospheric pressure) to this tube, supplemented by manual suction. The patient takes occasional deep breaths to improve collection. The basal secretion is obtained by collecting samples at 15 minute intervals over an hour.

Peptavlon is then given, either at a dose of (a) 6 micrograms/kg body weight subcutaneously, or (b) 0.6 micrograms/kg/hour as a continuous intravenous infusion. A Tuberculin syringe is used to give a dose correct to 0.01 ml.

Specimens of the gastric juice are again collected, over periods of 10 or 15 minutes. The volume of the sample is measured and it is immediately filtered through gauze into a bottle. The acidity of each sample is determined by titration. The same doses and method may be used in both adults, including the elderly, and children. If dilution is required normal saline may be used.

Contra-indications, warnings, etc When the patient has previously shown a severe idiosyncratic response to the drug, Peptavlon should not be administered.

Pregnancy: Peptavlon should not be administered during pregnancy.

As pentagastrin stimulates gastric acid secretion it should be used with caution in patients with acute or bleeding peptic ulcer disease, though there is no clinical evidence to contra-indicate use.

Side-effects: At the recommended dosage the incidence of side-effects is extremely small, although very occasionally an individual may respond with hypotension and associated faintness. Other unwanted effects reported are mild abdominal discomfort, abdominal cramps, nausea, vomiting, sweating, headaches, drowsiness or exhaustion, heaviness or weakness of the legs, allergic reactions, bradycardia, tachycardia. These effects disappear once administration of Peptavlon has ceased.

Overdosage; The form of presentation makes it unlikely that overdosage will occur, and no such occurrence has been reported. As maximal secretory response is produced by the normal dosage, increased dosage would be expected to have no sequel other than an accentuation of the known side-effects.

Pharmaceutical precautions Peptavlon ampoules must be kept at or below 4°C but above freezing point and protected from light. If dilution is required Sodium Chloride Injection BP may be used. This solution should be prepared immediately before it is required for use.

Legal category POM.

Package quantities Ampoules containing 2 ml Peptavlon, supplied in boxes of 5.

Further information *Lactation:* No special precautions are required.

Effect on ability to drive or operate machinery: No precautions are required.

Product licence number 0029/5013.

PRIMAQUINE PHOSPHATE TABLETS

Presentation Primaquine phosphate is presented as brown, bi-convex, sugar-coated tablets, which each contain 13.2 mg of Primaquine Phosphate BP (equivalent to 7.5 mg of base). Inactive ingredients are acacia, gelatin, iron oxide, lactose, magnesium stearate, maize starch, shellac, sucrose, talc, tartaric acid and titanium dioxide.

Uses Primaquine phosphate is indicated for the radical cure of *Plasmodium vivax* or *Plasmodium ovale* malaria.

Mode of action: Primaquine is highly effective against the exoerythrocytic (liver) stages of *P. vivax* and *P. ovale* and is used to prevent relapse. The exact mechanism of antimalarial activity of primaquine has not been determined, but the drug appears to interfere with the function of plasmodial DNA and also inhibits mitochondrial respiration.

Primaquine is well absorbed from the gastro-intestinal tract. Following oral administration, peak plasma concentrations of the drug are generally attained within 6 hours; plasma concentrations are generally negligible after 24 hours. Primaquine is widely distributed in the body following oral administration. Primaquine is a low clearance compound (systemic clearance is approximately 24 litres per hour) and it has an apparent volume of distribution of about 150–250 litres in healthy adults.

Primaquine has a plasma half-life of 3.7–9.6 hours in healthy adults. Primaquine is rapidly metabolised in the liver and only a small amount (less than 5%) of the drug is excreted unchanged in urine. The principal metabolite is carboxyprimaquine and plasma concentrations of the metabolite greatly exceed those of unchanged primaquine. Carboxyprimaquine persists at elevated levels in the plasma and it is subjected to further bio-transformation prior to excretion.

Dosage and administration Primaquine should be given after a short intensive course with a blood schizonticidal agent such as chloroquine, to achieve a radical cure. Where possible, the glucose-6-phosphate dehydrogenase status of the patient should be determined before starting primaquine treatment.

Adults: A daily dose of 2 tablets is given for 10–14 days

(equivalent to 15 mg of primaquine base per day). Curative dosages of primaquine may vary from 10 to 30 mg administered daily for 10–14 days.

Children: A daily dose of 0.2–0.3 mg primaquine base per kg bodyweight is given for 10–14 days.

Elderly patients: There are no special dosage recommendations for the elderly.

Patients with known or suspected glucose-6-phosphate dehydrogenase deficiency: A regimen of weekly dosage may be considered. Adults may receive 30–45 mg primaquine base (4–6 tablets) and children 0.5–0.75 mg per kg bodyweight primaquine base, once weekly for eight weeks.

Alternatively, low doses should be given initially and further increments made to reach the therapeutic dose. During this period frequent blood examinations should be made to detect the possible occurrence of haemolytic anaemia or methaemoglobinaemia.

Contra-indications, warnings, etc Primaquine should be administered with caution to patients with any serious systemic disease characterised by a tendency to granulocytopenia (e.g. rheumatoid arthritis, lupus erythematosus) and is contra-indicated in such patients when they are acutely ill.

Primaquine should be given with caution to people with known or suspected glucose-6-phosphate dehydrogenase deficiency as the drug may cause haemolysis in patients who are deficient in the enzyme.

If methaemoglobinaemia or haemolysis occurs, primaquine treatment should be stopped.

Primaquine should not be administered with other drugs liable to induce haemolysis or bone marrow depression.

Pregnancy and lactation: If vivax malaria occurs during pregnancy a curative course of chloroquine should be given and radical cure with primaquine delayed until after delivery and until breast feeding has been completed.

Side-effects: Abdominal pain, nausea, vomiting, methaemoglobinaemia and haemolysis have been reported at the recommended dosage.

Overdosage; The symptoms of overdosage include anorexia, nausea, epigastric pain, abdominal cramps, occasional vomiting, weakness, cyanosis, haemolytic anaemia and jaundice, bone marrow depression and methaemoglobinaemia.

There is no specific antidote and treatment must therefore be symptomatic.

Pharmaceutical precautions Store at room temperature, protected from light and moisture.

Legal category P.

Package quantities Containers of 1,000 tablets.

Further information *Effect on ability to drive or operate machinery:* There is no evidence to suggest that primaquine will produce sedation. Therefore no precautions are suggested concerning the ability of the patient to drive and operate machinery.

Product licence number 0029/5081.

RAZOXIN*

Presentation Razoxin Tablets, each containing 125 mg razoxane, are white to pale cream, and marked on one side with the ICI roundel and a bisection line on the other. Inactive ingredients are alginic acid, magnesium stearate, microcrystalline cellulose and povidone.

Uses In contrast to most anti-cancer agents Razoxin interferes with cell division at the G_2M phase of the cycle.

Razoxin in combination with radiotherapy may be used for all forms of soft-tissue, chondro- and osteosarcomas. In comparison with radiotherapy alone, this combination may increase the response rate and reduce recurrence. Razoxin can produce remissions in previous radio-resistant lesions.

Razoxin may be useful alone or in combination with other antimitotic agents in the treatment of malignant lymphomas, including mycosis fungoides, acute leukaemias, especially the acute blast cell-crisis of chronic myeloid leukaemia, and Kaposi's sarcoma. Experience to date has been in open studies which indicated that the product is of value in patients in whom previous therapies have been unsuccessful.

Dosage and administration *Note:* Because of an association between administration of Razoxin and the development of acute myeloid leukaemia or skin epitheliomata, the drug should only be used in the above malignant conditions and then when its administration is essential such as when other treatments have failed.

Adults and children: Razoxin is administered orally. The following guidelines are based on the regimens with which responses have been obtained. In all regimens, if unacceptable degrees of leucopenia, thrombocytopenia or gastrointestinal disturbance occur, the dosage of Razoxin should be reduced or temporarily withdrawn to allow recovery.

Soft-tissue, Osteo- and Chondro-sarcomata: 125 mg (1 tablet) twice daily 3 days before the start of radiotherapy, continued throughout that therapy. On days when radiation is given, 1 tablet of Razoxin should be taken 1–4 hours before radiotherapy; the other tablet in the evening. The dosage of radiation should be selected and administered using normal criteria.

Malignant lymphomas (including mycosis fungoides): 0.5 to 1.5g/m²/week should be administered orally as long as a remission is maintained. For example the dosage can be given as:

(a) 125 mg (1 tablet) twice daily on 3–5 days/week
or
(b) three doses of 375 mg (3 tablets) given eight hours apart and repeated weekly

If an inadequate response is obtained the dosage may be increased, provided that the white cell count permits.

Acute leukaemias (including blast cell crisis of chronic myeloid leukaemia): 150–500 mg/m²/day for 3–5 days. Treatment should be repeated at 14–28 day intervals, depending on the peripheral blood count. Allopurinol may also be given to prevent uric acid deposition.

Kaposi's sarcoma: 333 mg/m² three times daily for 3 days every 3 weeks, and adjusted as necessary according to peripheral blood count.

Elderly patients: There are no special dosage recommendations for the elderly, but it may be advisable to monitor elderly patients so that optimum dosage can be individually determined.

Contra-indications, warnings, etc Razoxin is contra-indicated in the treatment of non-malignant conditions such as psoriasis.

Mice and rats developed tumours following long term intraperitoneal administration of Razoxin. There is an association between the development of acute myeloid leukaemia or skin epitheliomata and the administration of Razoxin in man.

Razoxin is contra-indicated in pregnancy because of its action on cell division. Animal studies have revealed abnormalities of foetal development. It should not normally be administered to mothers who are breast feeding.

The peripheral blood count should be monitored throughout Razoxin therapy. Unacceptable degrees of leucopenia or thrombocytopenia are quickly reversed on cessation of treatment. Unacceptable degrees of myelosuppression are more likely to occur in patients who have received extensive chemotherapy previously.

Side-effects: The principal reported side-effects include leucopenia, thrombocytopenia, nausea, vomiting, diarrhoea, skin reactions and alopecia. Early skin reactions in patients receiving Razoxin plus radiotherapy may be more marked than those expected from radiotherapy alone. Severe late subcutaneous fibrosis has been reported in some patients receiving the combined therapy. There appears to be an increased likelihood of oesophagitis and pneumonitis in patients who require radiotherapy for thoracic lesions.

Overdosage: In cases of overdosage, signs and symptoms are likely to be qualitatively similar to side-effects; there is no specific antidote and treatment must be symptomatic.

Pharmaceutical precautions Store at room temperature, protected from light and moisture.

It is recommended that adequate protective gloves be worn when handling Razoxin Tablets and that Razoxin tablets should not be handled by pregnant staff.

Legal category POM.

Package quantities Containers of 30 tablets (OP).

Further information In contrast to most anti-cancer agents, Razoxin interferes with cell division at the G_2M phase of the cell cycle and in multiple-drug chemotherapy regimens, it is logical to combine razoxane with agents acting at the other phases in the cell cycle.

Product licence number 0029/0065.

SAVLOCLENS*

Presentation Savloclens is presented as an amber yellow aqueous solution containing 0.05% w/v chlorhexidine gluconate (equivalent to 0.25% v/v Chlorhexidine Gluconate Solution BP) and 0.5% w/v cetrimide (incorporated as Strong Cetrimide Solution BP). Inactive ingredients are ethanol, industrial methylated spirits, Sunset Yellow FCF and water.

Uses Savloclens is an antimicrobial preparation with cleansing properties for cleansing and disinfecting contaminated wounds and burns.

Dosage and administration Apply undiluted.

Contra-indications, warnings, etc Savloclens is contra-indicated for patients who have previously shown a hypersensitivity reaction to either chlorhexidine or cetrimide. However, such reactions are extremely rare.

For external use only. Keep out of the eyes and avoid contact with the brain, meninges and middle ear. Not for injection. Do not use in body cavities or as an enema.

If cetrimide/chlorhexidine solutions come into contact with the eyes, wash out promptly and thoroughly with water.

Discard any surplus solution immediately after use.

Side-effects: Irritative skin reactions can occasionally occur and rare hypersensitivity to cetrimide preparations, usually developing after repeated application, has been reported. Generalised allergic reactions to chlorhexidine have also been reported but are extremely rare.

Accidental ingestion: Do not give alcohol in any form. Carry out a gastric lavage with milk, gelatin or mild soap. Do not induce vomiting. Employ supportive measures as appropriate.

Accidental intravenous transfusion: Blood transfusion may be necessary to counteract haemolysis.

Pharmaceutical precautions Use contents immediately after opening.

Discard any surplus solution.

Hypochlorite bleaches may cause brown stains to develop in fabrics which have previously been in contact with chlorhexidine solutions.

Chlorhexidine and cetrimide are incompatible with anionic agents.

Store at room temperature.

Legal category P.

Package quantities Packs of 60 × 100 ml individual sachets.

Further information The British Pharmaceutical Codex (1973) recommends that antiseptics applied to broken skin should be sterile. The use of Savloclens complies with this recommendation.

Product licence number 0029/0142.

SAVLODIL*

Presentation Savlodil is presented as a clear yellow aqueous solution containing 0.015% w/v chlorhexidine gluconate (equivalent to 0.075% v/v Chlorhexidine Gluconate Solution BP) and 0.15% w/v cetrimide (incorporated as Strong Cetrimide Solution BP). Inactive ingredients are ethanol, quinoline yellow and water.

Uses Savlodil is an antimicrobial agent with cleansing properties for the antiseptic treatment of wounds and burns and swabbing in obstetrics.

Dosage and administration Apply undiluted.

Contra-indications, warnings, etc Savlodil is contra-indicated for patients who have previously shown a hypersensitivity reaction to either chlorhexidine or cetrimide. However, such reactions are extremely rare.

For external use only. Keep out of the eyes and avoid contact with the brain, meninges and middle ear. Not for injection. Do not use in body cavities or as an enema.

If cetrimide/chlorhexidine solutions come into contact with the eyes, wash out promptly and thoroughly with water.

Discard any surplus solution immediately after use.

Side-effects: Irritative skin reactions can occasionally occur and rare hypersensitivity to cetrimide preparations, usually developing after repeated application, has been reported. Generalised allergic reactions to chlorhexidine have also been reported but are extremely rare.

Accidental ingestion: Do not give alcohol in any form. Carry out gastric lavage with milk, gelatin or mild soap. Do not induce vomiting. Employ supportive measures as appropriate.

Accidental intravenous transfusion: Blood transfusion may be necessary to counteract haemolysis.

Pharmaceutical precautions Use contents immediately after opening.

Discard any surplus solution.

Hypochlorite bleaches may cause brown stains to develop in fabrics which have previously been in contact with chlorhexidine solutions.

Chlorhexidine and cetrimide are incompatible with anionic agents.

Store at room temperature.

Legal category P.

Package quantities Packs of 250 × 25 ml and 60 × 100 ml individual sachets.

Further information The British Pharmaceutical Codex (1973) recommends that antiseptics applied to broken skin should be sterile. The use of Savlodil complies with this recommendation.

Product licence number 0029/0114.

SAVLON* HOSPITAL CONCENTRATE

Presentation Savlon Hospital Concentrate is presented as a deep orange aqueous solution containing 1.5% w/v chlorhexidine gluconate (equivalent to 7.5% v/v Chlorhexidine Gluconate Solution BP) and 15% w/v cetrimide (incorporated as Strong Cetrimide Solution BP). Inactive ingredients are benzyl benzoate, isopropyl alcohol, liquid deodoriser, Sunset Yellow FCF, terpineol and water.

Uses Savlon Hospital Concentrate is an antimicrobial preparation with cleansing properties for general antiseptic purposes.

Dosage and administration

Method of preparation	*Dilution rate*	*Use*
10 ml made up to 1 litre with water	1 in 100 (1%) Aqueous	Cleansing/antiseptic treatment of wounds and burns.† Swabbing in obstetrics, gynaecology and urology. Cleansing/disinfectant soak for used metal instruments. Clean instrument disinfection where no means of sterilisation is available (30 minutes' immersion).‡ Cleansing/disinfection of equipment, furniture and fittings in the vicinity of the patient. Storage of clinical thermometers and sterile instruments.
35 ml made up to 1 litre with water	1 in 30 (approx) Aqueous	Cleansing/antiseptic treatment of wounds and burns where greater cleansing/antisepsis is required.† Cleansing/disinfectant soak for soiled instruments.
35 ml with 200 ml water made up to 1 litre with 95% alcohol	1 in 30 (approx) in 70% Alcohol	Rapid skin antisepsis before operation and other invasive procedures. Disinfection of clean instruments and equipment (two minutes immersion).† Disinfection of clinical thermometers.

† Sterilise the dilution by autoclaving at 115–116°C for 30 minutes or 121–123°C for 15 minutes.
‡ Endoscopes should not be placed in solutions of Savlon.

Contra-indications, warnings, etc Savlon preparations are contra-indicated for patients who have previously shown a hypersensitivity reaction to chlorhexidine or cetrimide. However, such reactions are extremely rare.

For external use. Dilute before use. Keep out of the eyes and avoid contact with brain, meninges and middle ear. Not for injection. Do not use in body cavities or as an enema.

If cetrimide/chlorhexidine solutions come into contact with the eyes, wash out promptly and thoroughly with water.

If concentrated cetrimide solutions come into contact with the skin, rinse promptly and thoroughly with water.

Solutions applied to wounds, burns or broken skin should be sterile.

Syringes, needles and instruments which have been immersed in Savlon solutions should be thoroughly rinsed in sterile water or saline before use.

Savlon solutions may affect glass cement and therefore are not suitable for the disinfection of endoscopes.

Side-effects: Irritative skin reactions can occasionally occur and rare hypersensitivity to cetrimide preparations, usually developing after repeated application, has been reported. There have been rare reports of severe burn-like reactions to concentrated cetrimide solutions. Should such a reaction occur treat as a chemical burn. Generalised allergic reactions to chlorhexidine have also been reported but are extremely rare.

Accidental oral or rectal administration: Fatal poisoning may arise due to the presence of cetrimide when the only pathological signs are visceral congestion, cloudy swelling, mild pulmonary oedema or varying degrees of gastro-intestinal irritation. Severe CNS depression, sometimes preceded by excitement and convulsions can cause death from respiratory paralysis.

Specific antidotes: Soap, anionic surfactants.

General measures: Do not give alcohol in any form. If the product is swallowed give large quantities of milk, gelatin or mild soap. Avoid vomiting or lavage if it is believed that a concentrated solution has been ingested.

Central paralysis cannot be countered by curare antagonists or CNS stimulants but sympathomimetic drugs have been given.

Mechanically assisted ventilation with oxygen may be necessary. Persistent convulsions may be controlled with cautious doses of a short-acting barbiturate.

Accidental intravenous infusion: Massive haemolysis can occur which will require blood transfusion.

Accidental intra-uterine administration: Introduction into the uterus can lead to haemolysis and pulmonary embolism.

Pharmaceutical precautions Dilute with tap water of an acceptable bacteriological standard or alcohol (ethanol, Industrial Methylated Spirit or isopropanol). Add diluent slowly to prevent excessive foaming.

As a precaution against bacterial contamination, aqueous stock solutions should contain at least 4% v/v of isopropanol or 7% v/v of ethanol which may be denatured (i.e. Industrial Methylated Spirit).

Savlon solutions used for instrument storage should contain 0.4% sodium nitrite to inhibit metal corrosion. Such solutions must be changed every 7 days. Prolonged immersion of rubber appliances in Savlon solutions is undesirable.

As cork may protect certain Gram-negative organisms from the action of antiseptics, Savlon solutions must be stored in bottles with glass, plastic or rubber closures.

Hypochlorite bleaches may cause brown stains to develop in fabrics which have previously been in contact with chlorhexidine.

Chlorhexidine and cetrimide are incompatible with anionic agents.

Store at room temperature.

Legal category GSL.

Package quantities Containers of 1 litre and 5 litres. Dispensers to fit 5L packs are also available.

Further information Nil.

Product licence number 0029/5012.

SIOPEL* CREAM

Presentation A white water-repellant barrier cream which contains 0.3% w/w cetrimide (incorporated as Strong Cetrimide Solution BP) and 10% w/w Dimethicone 1,000 PhEur. Inactive ingredients are Arachis oil, butylated hydroxytoluene, cetostearyl alcohol, citric acid, methyl hydroxybenzoate and water.

Uses Siopel Cream combines the antiseptic properties of cetrimide with the water-repellant properties of the silicone dimethicone. It is useful whenever the skin needs to be protected from water-soluble irritants.

Dosage and administration Wash and dry the skin. Apply Siopel sparingly and massage well into the skin. Apply three to five times daily for three to four days then once or twice daily.

Contra-indications, warnings, etc Siopel is contra-indicated for patients who have previously shown a hypersensitivity reaction to cetrimide preparations.

For topical application only. Keep out of the eyes and avoid contact with the brain, meninges and middle ear. Do not use in body cavities or as an enema. Do not use on skin that is acutely inflamed or weeping, or before the skin has been cleansed of contaminating irritants.

Side-effects: Irritative skin reactions can occasionally occur and hypersensitivity to cetrimide preparations has been reported, usually developing after repeated application, but is rare. Should such a reaction occur stop application of the product.

Accidental ingestion: It seems unlikely that systemic toxicity will occur from accidental ingestion of the cream. However, in the event of large quantities being swallowed, carry out gastric lavage with milk, gelatin or mild soap and apply supportive measures as appropriate. Do not induce vomiting. Do not give alcohol in any form.

Pharmaceutical precautions Store at room temperature and use undiluted. Cetrimide is incompatible with anionic agents.

Legal category GSL.

Package quantities Containers of 50 g.

Further information Nil.

Product licence number 0029/5014.

SYNALAR* CREAM
SYNALAR* OINTMENT

Presentation Synalar is presented as a white, water-miscible cream and a greasy ointment. Both preparations contain 0.025% w/w Fluocinolone Acetonide BP. The inactive ingredients in Synalar Cream are benzyl alcohol, cetostearyl alcohol, citric acid, liquid paraffin, polysorbate, propylene glycol, sorbitan monostearate and water. The inactive ingredients in Synalar Ointment are citric acid, lanolin, propylene glycol and white soft paraffin.

Uses Synalar Cream and Ointment contain an effective topical corticosteroid, and are suitable for treating a wide variety of local inflammatory, pruritic and allergic disorders of the skin. Synalar is particularly suitable for topical application in:

Eczema and dermatitis; atopic eczema, seborrhoeic eczema, discoid eczema, otitis externa, contact dermatitis, neurodermatitis.

Prurigo.

Psoriasis (excluding widespread plaque psoriasis). Lichen planus. Discoid lupus erythematosus.

Mode of action: Fluocinolone acetonide is a synthetic anti-inflammatory corticosteroid. Its mechanisms of action are related to vasoconstriction and suppression of membrane permeability, mitotic activity, the immune response and release of inflammatory mediators.

The extent of percutaneous absorption of fluocinolone acetonide is determined by many factors including the vehicle, the integrity of the epidermal barrier and the use of occlusive dressings. Following absorption, fluocinolone acetonide is metabolised primarily in the liver and excreted by the kidneys.

Dosage and administration A small quantity of Synalar is applied lightly to the affected area two or three times a day, and massaged gently and thoroughly into the skin. These recommendations apply to both children and adults, including the elderly.

When an occlusive dressing is required, the affected area should first be thoroughly cleansed. Synalar is then applied and covered with a suitable plastic dressing. Occlusion should not be used for children or for the face.

In some cases the application of hot, moist compresses may be an advantage. The creams are particularly suitable for moist or weeping surfaces and for flexures of the body. The ointments are suitable for dry, scaly lesions.

Contra-indications, warnings, etc Synalar is contra-indicated in primary infections of the skin caused by bacteria, fungi or viruses and in rosacea, acne, perioral dermatitis, anogenital pruritus and napkin eruption.

Long-term continuous topical steroid therapy can produce local atrophic skin changes. Prolonged use of topical steroids or treatment of extensive areas, even without occlusion, can result in sufficient absorption of the steroid to produce the features of adrenal suppression, especially in infants and children.

It is recommended that treatment on the face and for children should not normally be extended beyond five days, and occlusion in such cases should not be used.

When there is an infection associated with an inflammatory skin condition, Synalar should only be administered if adequate anti-infective cover is given.

When using topical corticosteroids to treat psoriasis there are risks both of rebound relapse following the development of tolerance, and of generalised pustular psoriasis. Impairment of the barrier function of the skin may lead to local and systemic toxicity. Careful patient supervision is important.

Treatment should be discontinued if unfavourable reactions are seen.

Pregnancy: There is inadequate evidence of safety in human pregnancy. Topical administration of corticosteroids to pregnant animals can cause abnormalities of foetal development, including cleft palate and intrauterine growth retardation. There may therefore be a very small risk of such effects on the human foetus.

Lactation: When topical steroid treatment is considered necessary during breast feeding, both the amount applied and the length of treatment should be minimised.

Side-effects: With Synalar, side-effects are extremely rare, but, as with all topical corticosteroids, the occasional patient may show an adverse reaction such as hypersensitivity. Irritation at the site of application may occur infrequently. Extensive treatment can result in both local atrophic changes, such as striae, skin thinning and telangiectasia and systemic effects such as adrenal suppression.

The use of topical steroids on infected lesions, without the addition of appropriate anti-infective therapy, can result in the spread of opportunist infections.

Accidental ingestion: The 50 g tube of Synalar contains 12.5 mg of the steroid, other tubes containing proportionately less. No toxic effects are likely to occur even if the full contents of a 50 g tube are ingested. Similarly the ingredients of the base are unlikely to have any toxic effect in the quantities in which they occur. Therefore no remedial action is required in the event of accidental ingestion.

Pharmaceutical precautions Store at room temperature and use undiluted.

Legal category POM.

Package quantities Synalar Cream and Ointment are supplied in tubes of 15 g, 30 g (OP) and 50 g.

Further information *Effect on ability to drive or operate machinery:* No precautions are necessary.

Product licence numbers

Synalar Cream	0029/5037
Synalar Ointment	0029/5041

SYNALAR* CREAM 1 IN 4 DILUTION
SYNALAR* OINTMENT 1 IN 4 DILUTION

Presentation Synalar Cream 1 in 4 dilution is presented as a white, water-miscible cream. Synalar Ointment 1 in 4 dilution is a greasy ointment. Both contain 0.00625% w/w Fluocinolone Acetonide BP. The inactive ingredients of Synalar Ointment 1 in 4 dilution are citric acid, lanolin, propylene glycol and white soft paraffin. The inactive ingredients of Synalar Cream 1 in 4 dilution are benzyl alcohol, cetostearyl alcohol, citric acid, liquid paraffin, polysorbate, propylene glycol, sorbitan monostearate and water.

Uses Synalar Cream and Ointment dilutions contain an effective topical corticosteroid and are suitable for treating the milder forms of a wide variety of local inflammatory, pruritic and allergic disorders of the skin. Synalar Cream and Ointment dilutions are particularly suitable for topical application in:

Eczema and dermatitis: atopic eczema, seborrhoeic eczema, discoid eczema, otitis externa, contact dermatitis, neurodermatitis.

Prurigo.

Psoriasis (excluding widespread plaque psoriasis). Lichen planus. Discoid lupus erythematosus.

Synalar Cream and Ointment dilutions are indicated for milder forms of these conditions; for maintenance therapy when control has been achieved with Synalar; for use under occlusive dressings; and for paediatric dermatology, e.g.: infantile eczema.

Mode of action: Fluocinolone acetonide is a synthetic anti-inflammatory corticosteroid. Its mechanisms of action are related to vasoconstriction and suppression of membrane permeability, mitotic activity, the immune response and release of inflammatory mediators.

The extent of percutaneous absorption of fluocinolone acetonide is determined by many factors including the vehicle, the integrity of the epidermal barrier and the use of occlusive dressings. Following absorption, fluocinolone acetonide is metabolised primarily in the liver and excreted by the kidneys.

Dosage and administration A small quantity of the Synalar Cream or Ointment dilution is applied lightly to the affected area two or three times a day, and massaged gently and thoroughly into the skin. These recommendations apply to both children and adults, including the elderly.

When an occlusive dressing is required, the affected area should first be thoroughly cleansed; the Synalar Cream or Ointment dilution is then applied and covered with a suitable plastic dressing. Occlusion should not be used for children or for the face.

The Cream dilution is particularly suitable for moist or weeping surfaces and for flexures of the body. The Ointment dilution is suitable for dry, scaly lesions.

Contra-indications, warnings, etc Synalar Cream and Ointment dilutions are contra-indicated in primary infections of the skin caused by bacteria, fungi or viruses and in rosacea, acne, peri-oral dermatitis, anogenital pruritus and napkin eruption.

Long-term continuous topical steroid therapy can produce local atrophic skin changes. Prolonged use of topical steroids or treatment of extensive areas, even without occlusion, can result in sufficient absorption of the steroid to produce the features of adrenal suppression, especially in infants and children. It is recommended that treatment on the face and for children should not normally be extended beyond five days, and occlusion in such cases should not be used. When there is an infection associated with an inflammatory skin condition, Synalar preparations should only be administered if adequate anti-infective cover is given.

When using topical corticosteroids to treat psoriasis there are risks both of rebound relapse following the development of tolerance, and of generalised pustular psoriasis. Impairment of the barrier function of the skin may lead to local and systemic toxicity. Careful patient supervision is important.

Treatment should be discontinued if unfavourable reactions are seen.

Pregnancy: There is inadequate evidence of safety in human pregnancy. Topical administration of corticosteroids to pregnant animals can cause abnormalities of foetal development, including cleft palate and intrauterine growth retardation. There may therefore be a very small risk of such effects on the human foetus.

Lactation: When topical steroid treatment is considered necessary during breast feeding, both the amount applied and the length of treatment should be minimised.

Side-effects: With Synalar preparations, side-effects are extremely rare, but, as with all topical corticosteroids, the occasional patient may show an adverse reaction such as hypersensitivity. Irritation at the site of application may occur infrequently. Extensive treatment can result in both local atrophic changes, such as striae, skin thinning and telangiectasia and systemic effects such as adrenal suppression.

The use of topical steroids on infected lesions, without the addition of appropriate anti-infective therapy, can result in the spread of opportunist infections.

Accidental ingestion: Toxic effects are not likely jto occur following accidental ingestion of the contents of a 50 g tube. If greater quantities are ingested and toxicity develops, symptomatic treatment should be given.

Pharmaceutical precautions Store at room temperature and use undiluted.

Legal category POM.

Package quantities Synalar Cream and Ointment dilutions 1 in 4 are supplied in 50 g tubes (OP).

Further information *Effect on ability to drive or operate machinery:* No precautions are necessary.

Product licence numbers

Synalar Cream 1 in 4 dilution	0029/0151
Synalar Ointment 1 in 4 dilution	0029/0196

SYNALAR* CREAM 1 IN 10 DILUTION

Presentation Synalar Cream 1 in 10 dilution is presented as a white, water-miscible cream which contains 0.0025% w/w Fluocinolone Acetonide BP. The inactive ingredients of Synalar Cream 1 in 10 dilution are benzyl alcohol, cetostearyl alcohol, citric acid, liquid paraffin, polysorbate, propylene glycol, sorbitan monostearate and water.

Uses Synalar Cream 1 in 10 dilution contains an effective topical corticosteroid and is suitable for treating the milder forms of a wide variety of local inflammatory, pruritic and allergic disorders of the skin. Synalar Cream 1 in 10 Dilution is particularly suitable for topical application in:

Eczema and dermatitis: atopic eczema, seborrhoeic eczema, discoid eczema, otitis externa, contact dermatitis, neurodermatitis.

Prurigo, Psoriasis (excluding widespread plaque psoriasis). Lichen planus. Discoid lupus erythematosus.

Synalar Cream 1 in 10 dilution is indicated for milder forms of these conditions; for maintenance therapy when control has been achieved with Synalar; for use under occlusive dressings; and for paediatric dermatology, e.g. infantile eczema.

Mode of action: Fluocinolone acetonide is a synthetic anti-inflammatory corticosteroid. Its mechanisms of action are related to vasoconstriction and suppression of membrane permeability, mitotic activity, the immune response and release of inflammatory mediators.

The extent of percutaneous absorption of fluocinolone acetonide is determined by many factors including the vehicle, the integrity of the epidermal barrier and the use of occlusive dressings. Following absorption, fluocinolone acetonide is metabolised primarily in the liver and excreted by the kidneys.

Dosage and administration A small quantity of Synalar Cream 1 in 10 dilution is applied lightly to the affected area two or three times a day, and massaged gently and thoroughly into the skin. These recommendations apply to both children and adults including the elderly.

When an occlusive dressing is required, the affected area should first be thoroughly cleansed; Synalar Cream 1 in 10 dilution is then applied and covered with a suitable plastic dressing. Synalar Cream 1 in 10 dilution is particularly suitable for moist or weeping surfaces and for flexures of the body.

Contra-indications, warnings, etc Synalar Cream 1 in 10 dilution is contra-indicated in primary infections of the skin caused by bacteria, fungi or viruses and in rosacea, acne, peri-oral dermatitis, anogenital pruritus and napkin eruptions.

Long-term continuous topical steroid therapy can produce local atrophic skin changes. Prolonged use of topical steroids or treatment of extensive areas, even without occlusion, can result in sufficient absorption of the steroid to produce the features of adrenal suppression, especially in infants and children. It is recommended that treatment on the face and for children should not normally be extended beyond five days and occlusion in such cases should not be used.

When there is an infection associated with an inflammatory skin condition, Synalar preparations should only be administered if adequate anti-infective cover is given.

When using topical corticosteroids to treat psoriasis there are risks both of rebound relapse following the development of tolerance, and of generalised pustular psoriasis. Impairment of the barrier function of the skin may lead to local and systemic toxicity. Careful patient supervision is important.

Treatment should be discontinued if unfavourable reactions are seen.

Pregnancy: There is inadequate evidence of safety in human pregnancy. Topical administration of corticosteroids to pregnant animals can cause abnormalities of foetal development, including cleft palate and intrauterine growth retardation. There may therefore be a very small risk of such effects on the human foetus.

Lactation: When topical steroid treatment is considered necessary during breast feeding, both the amount applied and the length of treatment should be minimised.

Side-effects: With Synalar preparations, side-effects are extremely rare, but, as with all topical corticosteroids, the occasional patient may show an adverse reaction such as hypersensitivity. Irritation at the site of application may occur infrequently. Extensive treatment can result in both local atrophic changes, such as striae, skin thinning and telangiectasia and systemic effects such as adrenal suppression.

The use of topical steroids on infected lesions, without the addition of appropriate anti-infective therapy, can result in the spread of opportunist infections.

Accidental ingestion: Toxic effects are not likely to occur following accidental ingestion of the contents of a 50 g tube. If greater quantities are ingested and toxicity develops, symptomatic treatment should be given.

Pharmaceutical precautions Store at room temperature and use undiluted.

Legal category POM.

Package quantities Synalar Cream dilution 1 in 10 is supplied in 50 g tubes (OP).

Further information *Effect on ability to drive or operate machinery:* No precautions are necessary.

Product licence number 0029/0152.

SYNALAR* GEL

Presentation Synalar Gel consists of Fluocinolone Acetonide BP 0.025% w/w, presented as a clear, water-miscible gel. The inactive ingredients are carboxy polymethylene, citric acid, disodium edetate, industrial methylated spirits, methyl parahydroxybenzoate, propyl parahydroxybenzoate, propylene glycol, triethanolamine and water.

Uses Synalar Gel is an effective topical corticosteroid formulated as a clear, non-greasy gel. It is designed for application to the scalp and other hairy regions, but can equally well be applied elsewhere on the body. Specific indications for Synalar Gel are seborrhoea, seborrhoeic dermatitis and psoriasis of the scalp, but it may be applied satisfactorily to inflammatory dermatoses on other parts of the body.

Mode of action: Fluocinolone acetonide is a synthetic anti-inflammatory corticosteroid. Its mechanisms of action are related to vasoconstriction and suppression of membrane permeability, mitotic activity, the immune response and release of inflammatory mediators.

The extent of percutaneous absorption of fluocinolone acetonide is determined by many factors including the vehicle, the integrity of the epidermal barrier and the use of occlusive dressings. Following absorption, fluocinolone acetonide is metabolised primarily in the liver and excreted by the kidneys.

Dosage and administration A small quantity of Synalar Gel is massaged into the scalp night and morning using the finger tips. For maintenance therapy, treatment should be repeated once or twice weekly.

These recommendations apply to both children and adults, including the elderly.

Contra-indications, warnings, etc Synalar Gel is contra-indicated in primary infections of the skin caused by bacteria, fungi or viruses and in rosacea, acne, perioral dermatitis and napkin eruptions.

Long-term continuous topical steroid therapy can produce local atrophic skin changes. Prolonged use of topical steroids or treatment of extensive areas, even without occlusion, can result in sufficient absorption of the steroid to produce the features of adrenal suppression, especially in infants and children. It is recommended that treatment on the face and for children should not normally be extended beyond five days, and occlusion in such cases should not be used.

Where there is an infection associated with an inflammatory skin condition, Synalar preparations should only be administered if adequate anti-infective cover is given.

When using topical corticosteroids to treat psoriasis there are risks both of rebound relapse following the development of tolerance, and of generalised pustular psoriasis. Impairment of the barrier function of the skin may lead to local and systemic toxicity. Careful patient supervision is important.

Treatment should be discontinued if unfavourable reactions are seen.

Pregnancy: There is inadequate evidence of safety in human pregnancy. Topical administration of corticosteroids to pregnant animals can cause abnormalities of foetal development, including cleft palate and intrauterine growth retardation. There may therefore be a very small risk of such effects on the human foetus.

Lactation: When topical steroid treatment is considered necessary during breast feeding, both the amount applied and the length of treatment should be minimised.

Side-effects: With Synalar preparations, side-effects are extremely rare, but, as with all topical corticosteroids, the occasional patient may show an adverse reaction such as hypersensitivity. Irritation at the site of application may occur infrequently. Extensive treatment can result in both local atrophic changes, such as striae, skin thinning and telangiectasia and systemic effects such as adrenal suppression.

The use of topical steroids on infected lesions, without the addition of appropriate anti-infective therapy, can result in the spread of opportunist infections.

Accidental ingestion: The 30 g tube of Synalar Gel contains 7.5 mg of the steroid. No toxic effects are likely to occur, even if the full contents of a 30 g tube are ingested. Similarly the ingredients of the base are unlikely to have any toxic effects in the quantities in which they occur. Therefore no remedial action is required in the event of ingestion.

Pharmaceutical precautions Store at room temperature and use undiluted.

Legal category POM.

Package quantities Synalar Gel is supplied in 30 g tubes (OP).

Further information *Effect on ability to drive or operate machinery:* No precautions are necessary.

Product licence number 0029/5039.

SYNALAR* C CREAM AND OINTMENT

Presentation These products contain 0.025% w/w of the steroid Fluocinolone Acetonide BP and 3% w/w of Clioquinol BP (chinoform, iodochlorhydroxyquinoline). Synalar C is presented as an off-white, water-miscible cream and as a greasy ointment. The inactive ingredients of Synalar C cream are cetostearyl alcohol, citric acid, disodium edetate, liquid paraffin, methyl parahydroxybenzoate, polysorbate, propyl parahydroxybenzoate, propylene glycol, sorbitan monostearate and water. The inactive ingredients of Synalar C Ointment are citric acid, lanolin, liquid paraffin, propylene glycol and white soft paraffin.

Uses Synalar C combines the effective topical corticosteroid Synalar with the effective antibacterial and antifungal agent Clioquinol BP.

It is indicated for inflammatory dermatoses – including eczema, dermatitis, seborrhoea and intertrigo – where secondary bacterial and/or fungal infection is present or is likely to occur.

Mode of action: Fluocinolone acetonide is a synthetic anti-inflammatory corticosteroid. Its mechanisms of action are related to vasoconstriction and suppression of membrane permeability, mitotic activity, the immune response and release of inflammatory mediators.

Clioquinol is a broad-spectrum antibacterial and antifungal agent. Its precise mechanism of action is unknown.

The extent of percutaneous absorption of fluocinolone acetonide is determined by many factors including the vehicle, the integrity of the epidermal barrier and the use of occlusive dressings. Following absorption, fluocinolone acetonide is metabolised primarily in the liver and excreted by the kidneys.

Dosage and administration A small quantity of the Synalar C preparation is applied lightly to the affected area two or three times a day, and massaged gently and thoroughly into the skin. These recommendations apply to both children and adults, including the elderly.

Treatment should not normally be for longer than seven days and it is preferable to identify the causative organism.

If used in childhood or on the face, courses should be limited to five days, and occlusion should not be used.

If an occlusive dressing is indicated, the affected area is first thoroughly cleansed, the Synalar C preparation is then applied and covered with a suitable plastic dressing. Synalar C Cream is particularly suitable for very inflamed or weeping surfaces and for flexures of the body, whilst Synalar C Ointment is more suitable for dry scaly lesions.

Contra-indications, warnings, etc Synalar C preparations are contra-indicated in primary infections of the skin caused by bacteria, fungi or viruses and in rosacea, acne, peri-oral dermatitis and napkin eruptions.

Long-term continuous topical steroid therapy can produce local atrophic skin changes. Prolonged use of topical steroids or treatment of extensive areas, even without occlusion, can result in sufficient absorption of the steroid to produce the features of adrenal suppression, especially in infants and children.

In the presence of a viral infection, the use of an appropriate agent should be instituted. If a favourable response does not occur promptly Synalar C should be discontinued until the infection has been adequately controlled.

Treatment should be discontinued if unfavourable reactions are seen. This product should not be used by patients with known iodine-sensitivity.

Pregnancy: There is inadequate evidence of safety in human pregnancy. Topical administration of corticosteroids to pregnant animals can cause abnormalities of foetal development, including cleft palate and intra-uterine growth retardation. There may therefore be a very small risk of such effects on the human foetus.

Lactation: When topical steroid treatment is considered necessary during breast feeding, both the amount applied and the length of treatment should be minimised.

Side-effects: With Synalar preparations, side-effects are extremely rare, but, as with all topical corticosteroids, the occasional patient may show an adverse reaction such as hypersensitivity. Irritation at the site of application may occur infrequently. Extensive treatment can result in both local atrophic changes, such as striae, skin thinning and telangiectasia and systemic effects such as adrenal suppression.

Local application of clioquinol in creams or ointments may occasionally cause severe irritation, which may be less marked because of the fluocinolone acetonide.

Staining may occur due to breakdown of the clioquinol. A protective covering may be placed over the application to prevent staining of clothing or linen.

Accidental ingestion: The 15 g tube of Synalar C contains 3.75 mg of steroid and 0.45 g of Clioquinol BP. No toxic effects are likely to occur, even if the full contents of a tube are ingested. Similarly the ingredients of the base are unlikely to have any toxic effects in the quantities in which they occur. Therefore no remedial action is required in the event of ingestion.

Pharmaceutical precautions Store at room temperature and use undiluted.

Legal category POM.

Package quantities Synalar C Cream and Ointment are available in tubes of 15 g (OP).

Further information *Effect on ability to drive or operate machinery:* No precautions are necessary.

Product licence numbers

Synalar C Ointment	0029/5043
Synalar C Cream	0029/5042

SYNALAR* N CREAM AND OINTMENT

Presentation These products contain 0.025% w/w of the steroid Fluocinolone Acetonide BP and 0.5% w/w of Neomycin Sulphate PhEur. Synalar N is presented as a white, water-miscible cream and as a greasy ointment. The inactive ingredients of Synalar N Cream are cetostearyl alcohol, liquid paraffin, methyl parahydroxybenzoate, polysorbate, propylene glycol, propyl parahydroxybenzoate, sorbitan monostearate and water. The inactive ingredients of Synalar N Ointment are lanolin, liquid paraffin, propylene glycol and white soft paraffin.

Uses Synalar N combines the effective topical corticosteroid Synalar with an effective antibacterial agent, Neomycin Sulphate PhEur.

It is indicated for inflammatory dermatoses – including eczema, dermatitis, seborrhoea and intertrigo – where secondary bacterial infection is present or is likely to occur.

Mode of action: Fluocinolone acetonide is a synthetic anti-inflammatory corticosteroid. Its mechanisms of action are related to vasoconstriction and suppression of membrane permeability, mitotic activity, the immune response and release of inflammatory mediators.

Neomycin sulphate is an aminoglycoside antibacterial agent which inhibits bacterial protein synthesis.

The extent of percutaneous absorption of fluocinolone acetonide is determined by many factors including the vehicle, the integrity of the epidermal barrier and the use of occlusive dressings. Following absorption, fluocinolone acetonide is metabolised primarily in the liver and excreted by the kidneys.

Neomycin is not absorbed through intact skin. It is readily absorbed from large denuded, burned, or granulating areas. Excretion is then as unchanged drug.

Dosage and administration A small quantity of the Synalar N preparation is applied lightly to the affected area two or three times a day, and massaged gently and thoroughly into the skin. These recommendations apply to both children and adults, including the elderly.

Treatment should not normally be for longer than seven days and it is preferable to identify the causative organism.

If used in childhood or on the face, courses should be limited to five days, and occlusion shold not be used.

If an occlusive dressing is indicated, the affected area is first thoroughly cleansed, the Synalar N preparation is then applied and covered with a suitable plastic dressing. Synalar N Cream is particularly suitable for very inflamed or weeping surfaces and for flexures of the body, whilst Synalar N Ointment is more suitable for dry, scaly lesions.

Contra-indications, warnings, etc Synalar N preparations are contra-indicated in primary infections of the skin caused by bacteria, fungi or viruses and in rosacea, acne, peri-oral dermatitis and napkin eruptions. Synalar N is contra-indicated in those patients with a history of hypersensitivity to neomycin. Topical neomycin preparations should not be applied to the external auditory canal of patients with perforated eardrums.

Long-term continuous topical steroid therapy can produce local atrophic skin changes. Prolonged use of topical steroids or treatment of extensive areas, even without occlusion, can result in sufficient absorption of the steroid to produce the features of adrenal suppression, especially in infants and children.

In the presence of a viral or fungal infection, the use of an appropriate agent should be instituted. If a favourable response does not occur promptly, Synalar N should be discontinued until the infection has been adequately controlled.

Because of the potential hazard of nephrotoxicity and ototoxicity associated with neomycin, prolonged use or use of large amounts of the product should be avoided in conditions where absorption of neomycin is possible. Care is particularly needed in elderly or renally-impaired patients.

These preparations are not for ophthalmic use.

Treatment should be discontinued if unfavourable reactions are seen.

Pregnancy: There is inadequate evidence of safety in human pregnancy. Topical administration of corticosteroids to pregnant animals can cause abnormalities of foetal development, including cleft palate and intrauterine growth retardation. There may therefore be a very small risk of such effects on the human foetus.

Lactation: When topical steroid treatment is considered necessary during breast feeding, both the amount applied and the length of treatment should be minimised.

Side-effects: With Synalar preparations, side-effects are extremely rare, but, as with all topical corticosteroids, the occasional patient may show an adverse reaction such as hypersensitivity. Irritation at the site of application may occur infrequently. Extensive treatment can result in both local atrophic changes, such as striae, skin thinning and telangiectasia and systemic effects such as adrenal suppression.

Accidental ingestion: The 30 g tube of Synalar N contains 7.5 mg of steroid and 150 mg of neomycin. No toxic effects are likely to occur, even if the full contents of a 30 g tube are ingested. Similarly the ingredients of the base are not likely to have any toxic effects in the quantities in which they occur. Therefore no remedial action is required in the event of ingestion.

Pharmaceutical precautions Store at room temperature and use undiluted.

Legal category POM.

Package quantities Synalar N Cream and Ointment are available in tubes of 15 g and 30 g (OP).

Further information *Effect on ability to drive or operate machinery:* No precautions are necessary.

Product licence numbers

Synalar N Cream	0029/5044
Synalar N Ointment	0029/5046

TETMOSOL* SOAP

Presentation Tetmosol Soap is a yellow perfumed soap tablet containing 5% w/w Monosulfiram BP (Sulfiram INN).

Uses Tetmosol is a parasiticide, active against the burrowing mite *Sarcoptes scabiei*. It is indicated for the treatment and prophylaxis of scabies. The soap is especially useful for prophylaxis in hospitals and schools, etc.

Dosage and administration *Application:* Tetmosol Soap is used in place of ordinary toilet soap for the prophylaxis of scabies. Ideally, the person should bathe in hot water and soap themselves liberally with Tetmosol Soap paying particular attention to the folded areas of the skin. After bathing, the body should be allowed to dry naturally or dried with a towel using a 'blotting' action. Tetmosol Soap should be used daily for as long as the danger of infection remains.

Contra-indications, warnings, etc Tetmosol is contra-indicated when the patient has previously shown an idiosyncratic response to its application.

Side-effects: Very few side-effects occur with Tetmosol. A few cases of erythematous rash have been reported, but these are rare enough to be considered as idiosyncratic responses of the patients concerned.

Overdosage: Over application is unlikely to have any adverse effect. In the event of the soap being ingested, symptomatic treatment should be given.

Legal category P.

Pharmaceutical precautions Tetmosol Soap must be stored in the manufacturer's original wrapper, at room temperature.

Package quantities 75 g (2.6 oz) (OP).

Further information Nil.

Product licence number 0029/5006.

TETMOSOL* SOLUTION

Presentation Tetmosol Solution is a clear, brown liquid, forming a fine suspension when diluted with water. It contains Monosulfiram BP (Sulfiram INN) as a 25% w/w solution in industrial methylated spirit. The inactive ingredients are acetone, industrial methylated spirits, polyglyceryl ricinoleate.

Uses Tetmosol Solution is a parasiticide active against the burrowing mite *Sarcoptes scabiei*. It is indicated for the treatment and prophylaxis of scabies.

Dosage and administration Before application Tetmosol Solution should be diluted with two to three parts of water. The patient's body should be liberally washed with soap and water and thoroughly dried. Apart from the face and scalp, the entire body should be painted with the dilute solution, which is rubbed well in and left to dry. About ten minutes is allowed for the skin to dry naturally and the patient then dresses. Application is suitable for use in clinics dealing with children. In difficult cases this routine may be repeated successively for two or three days. These instructions are applicable to adults and children.

Contra-indications, warnings, etc Tetmosol Solution is contra-indicated when the patient has previously shown an idiosyncratic response to its application. The solution is flammable and should not be applied near a naked flame. Because of the close chemical relationship between monosulfiram and disulfiram, it is considered advisable to abstain from alcohol before and for at least 48 hours after the application of Tetmosol.

Side-effects; Very few side-effects occur with Tetmosol Solution, even in cases of undiluted application. A few cases of erythematous rash have been reported, but these are rare enough to be considered as idiosyncratic responses of the patients concerned.

Overdosage: The solution contains alcohol and monosulfiram, and if ingested this combination will produce a severe reaction, with flushing, dyspnoea, headache, dizziness, nausea, vomiting, drowsiness or sleep. Tachycardia and hypotension may also occur and the resultant myocardial ischaemia may be fatal.

Symptomatic measures are required – oxygen, if dyspnoea is excessive, and control of the blood pressure. Other treatment which has been found useful includes cardiac stimulants, intravenous iron, ascorbic acid and nicotinamide, adenine and intravenous sodium thiosulphate.

Pharmaceutical precautions Tetmosol Solution should not be stored in a cold place as this causes deposition of crystals. These can be redissolved by immersing the bottle in warm water. The solution is flammable and should not be kept near a naked flame. Water is a suitable diluent for Tetmosol.

Legal category P.

Package quantities Bottles of 100 ml (OP).

Further information Nil.

Product licence number 0029/5011.

VIVALAN*

Presentation Tablets each containing viloxazine hydrochloride equivalent to 50 mg viloxazine. Round, biconvex, white, film-coated tablets marked V on one face and the ICI roundel on the other. The inactive ingredients are calcium phosphate, glycerol, magnesium stearate, maize starch, methylhydroxypropyl cellulose, microcrystalline cellulose, sodium starch glycollate and titanium dioxide.

Uses Symptoms of depressive illness, especially where sedation is not required.

Dosage and administration *Adults:* Most patients respond to 300 mg/day preferably taken as 200 mg in the morning and 100 mg at lunchtime. Total daily dose should not exceed 400 mg and the last dose of the day should not be taken later than 6.00 pm.

Elderly: 100mg/day initially. The initial dose should be increased with caution under close supervision. Half the normal maintenance dose may be sufficient to produce a satisfactory clinical response.

Children: Vivalan is not recommended in children under 14 years of age.

Contra-indications, warnings, etc
Contra-indications: Mania, severe liver disease, history of peptic ulcer, recent myocardial infarction, during breast feeding.

Pregnancy: There is no evidence as to the drug's safety in human pregnancy; do not use during pregnancy, especially during the first and third trimesters, unless there are compelling reasons.

Precautions: Vivalan should be used with caution in patients with ischaemic heart disease and congestive cardiac failure, or any degree of heart block.

Caution is advised when administering Vivalan to patients with epilepsy, especially those receiving phenytoin (see below).

Patients posing a high suicidal risk require close initial supervision.

If surgery is necessary during therapy, the anaesthetist should be informed that the patient has received Vivalan.

Drug interactions: Vivalan should not be given concurrently with, or within two weeks of cessation of therapy with monoamine oxidase inhibitors.

Vivalan may decrease the antihypertensive effect of guanethidine, debrisoquine, bethanidine, and possibly clonidine.

When Vivalan is coadministered with drugs which undergo hepatic metabolism via oxidative pathways, there is a possibility of an interaction. It may be necessary therefore to adjust the dose of such coadministered drugs which have narrow therapeutic margins, for example the dosage of phenytoin, carbamazepine and theophylline may need to be reduced.

On theoretical grounds, caution is advised when patients receiving L-DOPA are treated with Vivalan.

Most antidepressants have been shown to potentiate the central nervous depressant action of alcohol, and, therefore, patients should be advised of the risks involved in drinking alcohol whilst on antidepressant medication.

Warnings and adverse effects: Nausea is frequently observed, but may be transient. Headache and vomiting may also occur.

As improvement may not occur during the first two weeks of treatment, patients should be closely monitored during this period.

Vivalan initially may impair alertness, and patients should be advised of the possible hazard when driving or operating machinery.

Anticholinergic side-effects, such as dry mouth, disturbance of accommodation, tachycardia, constipation and hesitancy of micturition have been reported less frequently with viloxazine than with tricyclic antidepressants.

Cardiac arrhythmias and severe hypotension are less likely to occur with viloxazine than with tricyclic antidepressants in high dosage or in deliberate overdosage.

Adverse effects which have been reported rarely with viloxazine include exacerbation of anxiety and agitation, drowsiness, confusion, ataxia, dizziness, insomnia, tremor, paraesthesia, sweating, musculo-skeletal pain, mild hypertension and skin rashes.

Psychotic manifestations, including hypomania and aggressive behaviour may be exacerbated.

Two serious adverse effects possibly associated with Vivalan have been reported:

(a) jaundice with elevated transaminases
(b) convulsions

Withdrawal symptoms are rare, but may include malaise, headache and vomiting.

Overdosage: Vivalan is rapidly absorbed and gastric lavage should be carried out with minimum delay. Overdosage should be treated on general principles with careful monitoring of vital functions, together with intensive supportive therapy where necessary. As the drug is almost exclusively excreted in urine, forced diuresis may be performed to reduce blood levels. There is no specific antidote.

Pharmaceutical precautions Store at room temperature.

Package quantities Tablets 50 mg: Containers of 100.

Further information Vivalan is an oxazine and is chemically distinct from the tri- and tetracyclic antidepressants, while retaining the biogenic amine reuptake inhibitory properties in the central nervous system. Pharmacologically, it differs from these drugs in its decreased sedative and anticholinergic properties, and its lesser effect on the cardiovascular system.

Legal category POM.

Product licence number
Vivalan Tablets 50 mg 0029/0074

ZESTRIL*

Presentation White, round, biconvex uncoated tablets, impressed with a heart shape plus a number denoting tablet strength on one side and a company logo on the other side, containing 2.5 mg lisinopril as the dihydrate. The inactive ingredients are calcium hydrogen phosphate, magnesium stearate, maize starch and mannitol.

Pink, round, biconvex uncoated tablets, impressed with a heart shape plus a number denoting the tablet strength on one side and a bisecting line impressed on the other, containing 5 mg lisinopril as the dihydrate. The inactive ingredients are calcium hydrogen phosphate, iron oxide, magnesium stearate, maize starch and mannitol.

Pink, round, biconvex uncoated tablets, impressed with a heart shape plus a number denoting the tablet strength and the trademark on one side and a company logo on the other side, containing 10 mg lisinopril as the dihydrate. The inactive ingredients are calcium hydrogen phosphate, iron oxide, magnesium stearate, maize starch and mannitol.

Red, round, biconvex uncoated tablets, impressed with a heart shape plus a number denoting the tablet strength and the trademark on one side and a company logo on the other side, containing 20 mg lisinopril as the dihydrate. The inactive ingredients are calcium hydrogen phosphate, iron oxide, magnesium stearate, maize starch and mannitol.

Uses *Indications:*
Hypertension: All grades of essential hypertension and

renovascular hypertension. Zestril may be used alone or with other anti-hypertensive agents.

Congestive heart failure: In the treatment of congestive heart failure as adjunctive therapy with non-potassium sparing diuretics and, where appropriate, digitalis. Treatment with Zestril should always be initiated in hospital under close medical supervision.

Mode of action: Zestril is an orally active specific inhibitor of angiotensin I converting enzyme, a membrane-bound enzyme which catalyses the conversion of the inactive decapeptide angiotensin I to the active octapeptide angiotensin II. Zestril thus reduces levels of angiotensin II, a very powerful vasoconstrictor substance. As a consequence, blood pressure may be reduced in hypertensive patients and cardiac workload may be reduced in patients with congestive heart failure. The onset of action begins gradually, with the maximum effect usually occurring four to six hours after the first dose, with effects persisting for 24 hours after a single daily dose.

Dosage and administration The absorption of Zestril is not affected by food.

Hypertension: The need for dosage titration should be determined by measurement of the blood pressure just before the next dose.

Essential and Renovascular Hypertension: Treatment should be started with 2.5 mg once daily and titrated upwards to achieve optimal blood pressure control. A 2.5 mg dose seldom achieves a therapeutic response. The usual effective dose range is 10–20 mg once daily. The maximum recommended dose is 40 mg once daily.

Diuretic treated patients: If possible, the diuretic should be discontinued, or the dose reduced, 2 to 3 days before beginning therapy with Zestril (see 'Precautions') and may be resumed later if required.

Use in the elderly: Age alone does not appear to affect the efficacy or safety profile of Zestril. Thus, elderly patients should start treatment with Zestril as directed above.

Congestive heart failure: Zestril may be used as adjunctive therapy with non-potassium sparing diuretics with or without digitalis.

Initial dosage: Treatment should be initiated in hospital, under close medical supervision, with a recommended starting dose of 2.5 mg with subsequent dose titration. If possible, the dose of diuretic should be reduced before beginning treatment.

Blood pressure and renal function should be monitored closely both before and during treatment because severe hypotension and, more rarely, consequent renal failure have been reported with angiotensin-converting enzyme (ACE) inhibitors. The appearance of hypotension after the initial dose of Zestril does not preclude subsequent careful dose adjustment with the drug, following effective treatment of the hypotension.

Maintenance dosage: The dose should be gradually increased, depending on the patient's response, to the usual maintenance dose (5–20 mg). This dose adjustment may be performed over a two to four week period, or more rapidly if clinically indicated.

Impaired renal function: Zestril is excreted by the kidney and should be used with caution in patients with renal insufficiency.

Zestril is dialysable. Dialysis patients may be given the usual dose of Zestril on dialysis days. On the days when patients are not on dialysis the dosage should be tailored to the blood pressure response.

Paediatric use: Zestril has not been studied for use in children.

Contra-indications, warnings, etc

Contra-indications: Zestril has been shown to be fetotoxic in rabbits during middle and late pregnancy.

Effects of exposure of the fetus to ACE inhibitors during the first trimester of human pregnancy are unknown. Fetal exposure during the second and third trimesters of pregnancy has been associated with fetal and neonatal morbidity and mortality.

ACE inhibitors in human pregnancy have been associated with oligohydramnios. Hypotension and renal failure have occurred in the newborn. Because of these findings Zestril is contra-indicated in pregnancy.

Hypersensitivity to Zestril and in patients with a history of angioneurotic oedema relating to previous ACE-inhibitor therapy.

Precautions:

Assessment of renal function: Evaluation of the patient should include assessment of renal function prior to initiation of therapy and during treatment.

Impaired renal function: Zestril should be used with caution in patients with renal insufficiency, as they may require reduced or less frequent doses (see 'Dosage and administration'). Close monitoring of renal function during therapy should be performed as deemed appropriate in those with renal insufficiency. In the majority, renal function will not alter, or may improve.

Renal failure has been reported in association with ACE inhibitors and has been mainly in patients with severe congestive heart failure or underlying renal disease, including renal artery stenosis. If recognised promptly and treated appropriately, renal failure is usually reversible.

Some hypertensive patients, with no apparent preexisting renal disease, have developed increases in blood urea and creatinine when Zestril has been given concurrently with a diuretic. Dosage reduction of Zestril and/or discontinuation of the diuretic may be required. This situation should raise the possibility of underlying renal artery stenosis (see 'Renovascular hypertension').

Symptomatic hypotension: symptomatic hypotension was seen rarely in uncomplicated hypertensive patients. It is more likely to occur in patients who have been volume-depleted by diuretic therapy, dietary salt restriction, dialysis, diarrhoea, or vomiting. In these patients, by discontinuing diuretic therapy or significantly reducing the diuretic dose 2 to 3 days prior to initiating Zestril, the possibility of this occurrence is reduced.

Similar caution and close supervision may apply also to patients with ischaemic heart or cerebrovascular disease in whom severe hypotension could result in a myocardial infarct or cerebrovascular accident.

Severe hypotension has been reported with ACE inhibitors mainly in patients with severe heart failure. Many of these patients were on high doses of loop diuretics, and some had hyponatraemia or functional renal impairment. If hypotension develops, the patient should be placed in a supine position. Volume repletion with oral fluids or intravenous normal saline may be required. Intravenous atropine may be necessary if there is associated bradycardia. Treatment with Zestril may be restarted with careful dose titration following restoration of effective blood volume and pressure.

In some patients with congestive heart failure who have normal or low blood pressure, additional lowering of systemic blood pressure may occur with Zestril. If such hypotension becomes symptomatic, a reduction of dose or discontinuation of Zestril may become necessary.

The appearance of hypotension after the initial dose of Zestril does not preclude subsequent careful dose adjustment with the drug after effective management of hypotension.

Renovascular hypertension: Zestril can be used when surgery is not indicated, or prior to surgery. In some patients with bilateral renal artery stenosis or stenosis of the artery to a solitary kidney, increases of blood urea and creatinine, reversible upon discontinuation of therapy, have been seen. This is especially likely in patients treated with diuretics and/or those with renal insufficiency.

Surgery/anaesthesia: In patients undergoing major surgery or during anaesthesia with agents that produce hypotension, Zestril blocks angiotensin II formation secondary to compensatory renin release. This may lead to hypotension which can be corrected by volume expansion.

General: Zestril should not be used in patients with aortic stenosis, cor pulmonale or outflow tract obstruction.

Where Zestril is used as a single agent in hypertension,

Afro-Caribbean patients may show a reduced therapeutic response.

Drug interactions: Combination with other antihypertensive agents such as beta-blockers and diuretics may increase the antihypertensive efficacy. Zestril minimises the development of thiazide-induced hypokalaemia and hyperuricaemia. Indomethacin may reduce the antihypertensive efficacy of Zestril.

Zestril has been used with nitrates without significant clinical interaction.

As Zestril may reduce the elimination of lithium, serum levels of lithium should be monitored if lithium salts are administered.

Plasma potassium: Usually remains within normal limits. If Zestril is given with a diuretic, the likelihood of diuretic-induced hypokalaemia may be lessened. Zestril may elevate plasma potassium levels in patients with renal failure. Potassium supplements, potassium-sparing diuretics and potassium containing salt substitutes are not recommended.

Breast-feeding mothers: Because it is not known whether Zestril is excreted in human milk, caution should be exercised if Zestril is given to nursing mothers.

Side-effects: Hypotension has occurred in association with therapy with Zestril. This appears to occur in certain specific sub-groups (see 'Precautions').

Angioneurotic oedema: It has been reported with ACE inhibitors, including Zestril. In such cases, Zestril should be discontinued immediately and the patient observed. Where swelling is confined to the face, lips and mouth, the condition will usually resolve without further treatment, although antihistamines may be useful in relieving symptoms. These patients should be followed carefully until the swelling has resolved. However, where there is involvement of the tongue, glottis or larynx, likely to cause airways obstruction, subcutaneous adrenaline (0.5 ml 1:1000) should be administered promptly when indicated.

Other hypersensitivity reactions have been reported.

Other adverse reactions: Dizziness, headache, diarrhoea, cough, nausea and fatigue are the most frequent. Other less frequent side effects include rash and asthenia. Palpitation and impotence have been observed rarely.

Laboratory test findings: Increases in blood urea and creatinine, reversible on discontinuation of Zestril, are most likely in the presence of bilateral renal artery stenosis, especially in patients with renal insufficiency. Increases in blood urea and creatinine may occur without evidence of pre-existing renal impairment, especially in patients taking diuretics. In this event, undiagnosed renal artery stenosis should be suspected. Dosage reduction of Zestril and/or discontinuation of the diuretic should be considered.

Decreases in haemoglobin and haematocrit have been reported in a few patients, but a causal relationship to Zestril has not been established.

Increases in liver enzymes and serum bilirubin have occurred which are usually reversible on discontinuation of Zestril. Hyperkalaemia has occurred in a few cases.

Overdosage: Available data are limited. The most likely manifestation of overdosage would be hypotension, which can be treated, if necessary, by intravenous infusion of normal saline solution. Zestril can be removed by haemodialysis.

Pharmaceutical precautions Store at room temperature.

Legal category POM.

Package quantities
Tablets 20 mg: Calendar packs of 28 tablets (OP), bottles of 60 tablets.
Tablets 10 mg: Calendar packs of 28 tablets (OP), bottles of 60 tablets.
Tablets 5 mg: Calendar packs of 28 tablets (OP), bottles of 60 tablets.
Tablets 2.5 mg: Calendar packs of 28 tablets (OP), bottles of 60 tablets.

Further information Nil.

Product licence numbers

Zestril Tablets 2.5 mg	0029/0208
Zestril Tablets 5 mg	0029/0204
Zestril Tablets 10 mg	0029/0205
Zestril Tablets 20 mg	0029/0206

ZOLADEX*

Presentation A sterile, white to cream coloured cylindrical depot in which goserelin acetate (equivalent to 3.6 mg of goserelin) is dispersed in a biodegradable matrix of lactide-glycolide co-polymer. It is supplied in a single dose syringe applicator.

Uses Zoladex, an LHRH analogue is indicated in prostate cancer suitable for hormonal manipulation.

Dosage and administration *Adults: Male:* One 3.6 mg depot of Zoladex injected subcutaneously into the anterior abdominal wall, every 28 days. Local anaesthetic may be used if desired. No dosage adjustment is necessary for patients with renal failure or in the elderly.

Contra-indications, warnings, etc
Initially, Zoladex, like other LHRH agonists, transiently increases serum testosterone. Some patients may experience a temporary increase in bone pain, which can be managed symptomatically. The use of Zoladex in patients at particular risk of developing ureteric obstruction or spinal cord compression should be considered carefully and the patients monitored closely during the first month of therapy. Consideration should be given to the initial use of an anti-androgen (e.g. cyproterone acetate 300 mg daily for 3 days before and 3 weeks after commencement of Zoladex) at the start of LHRH analogue therapy, since this has been reported to prevent the possible sequelae of the initial rise in serum testosterone. If spinal cord compression or renal impairment due to ureteric obstruction are present or develop, specific standard treatment of these complications should be instituted.

Following long-term repeated dosing with Zoladex, an increased incidence of benign pituitary tumours has been observed in male rats. Whilst this finding is similar to that previously noted in this species following surgical castration, any relevance to man has not been established.

Side-effects
Pharmacological effects include hot flushes and a decrease in libido, seldom requiring withdrawal of therapy. Breast swelling and tenderness are noted infrequently.

Skin rashes are generally mild, often regressing without discontinuation of therapy.

Occasional local reactions include mild bruising at the subcutaneous injection site.

Overdosage: There is no human experience of overdosage. Animal tests suggest that no effect other than the intended therapeutic effects on sex hormone concentrations and on the reproductive tract will be evident with higher doses of Zoladex. If overdosage occurs, this should be managed symptomatically.

Pharmaceutical precautions Store below 25°C.

Legal category POM.

Package quantities Boxes of 1.

Further information Nil.

Product licence number 0029/0198.

**Trade Mark*

IMMUNO Ltd
Arctic House, Rye Lane
Dunton Green, Nr. Sevenoaks,
Kent, TN14 5HB

ENDOBULIN*
Immune Globulin (Human) Intravenous

Presentation Endobulin is a freeze-dried concentrate of functionally intact, aggregate free immunoglobulin G. It is produced from pooled human venous plasma. Only plasma units which are non reactive in tests for HBsAg and antibody to HIV are used in the manufacture of Endobulin. All plasma units are further tested for ALT.

Following reconstitution with Water for Injections it has the following composition:

Functionally intact IgG	50 mg/ml
Total protein	55 mg/ml
Sodium Chloride	3 mg/ml
Glucose	50 mg/ml

Only traces of IgA and IgM are present. The preparation does not contain any preservative.

Uses Endobulin is recommended for replacement therapy in primary antibody deficiency syndrome, for the treatment of idiopathic thrombocytopenic purpura and Kawasaki syndrome.

Dosage and administration Endobulin must be administered intravenously immediately after reconstitution. Reconstituted vials should be inspected visually for particulate matter and discolouration prior to administration. Any vials found to contain either particles or discolouration should not be used. Partially used bottles should be discarded.

The usual rate of administration of Endobulin is 1 ml per minute up to a maximum of 2 ml per minute for the 5% strength.

The following is also appropriate for children and the elderly.

Replacement therapy in primary immunodeficiency: Initially 600–1,000 mg (12–20 ml) per kg bodyweight in up to five individual doses within the first two weeks of treatment until the IgG level 1–4 days after the last application has risen to at least 800 mg/100 ml.

Subsequently 100–600 mg (2–12 ml) per kg bodyweight per month in one or more doses.

If a higher dose than that given above is required the dose may be increased to 1,000 mg/kg.

It is advisable to use doses and treatment intervals which ensure that a preinfusion level of at least 400 mg/100 ml is reached and maintained.

Idiopathic thrombocytopenic purpura: 400 mg (8 ml) per kg bodyweight on each of five consecutive days. If the platelet count rises to 100,000/mm^3 and then drops a renewed increase may be attempted by repeating the dose on one or more occasions.

Kawasaki Syndrome: 400 mg (8 ml) per kg bodyweight daily on 4 consecutive days as soon as possible after onset of the disease.

Use in the elderly: No specific precautions need to be observed during the use of Endobulin in the elderly.

Use in pregnancy: See interactions with live vaccines (e.g. rubella).

Animal reproduction studies have not been carried out with this product. Also it is not known whether Endobulin can cause fetal harm when administered to a pregnant woman or whether it can affect the reproduction capacity. The product should only be given to a pregnant woman if absolutely essential. According to present knowledge, no influence on the administration of Anti D (Rh_o) immunoglobulin can be proved. It may be assumed that intravenously administered immunoglobulin G will cross the placenta.

Contra-indications, warnings, etc No contra-indications are known.

Endobulin should only be administered intravenously.

Endobulin should be administered with caution to patients who have a history of adverse reactions to immunoglobulin preparations.

Although moderate and severe anaphylactoid reactions have not been observed in any of the clinical studies with Endobulin their occurrence cannot be ruled out. As these reactions are sometimes related to the rate of infusion, the recommended infusion rate should be closely followed.

If reactions occur (flushing of the face oppression, hypotension, etc) immediately discontinue. Intravenous antihistamines, steroids and/or sympathomimetics are effective treatments and should always be available.

Severe incompatibility reactions should be treated according to the guidelines of modern shock therapy.

After slight incompatibility reactions have subsided treatment may be started again using diluted solutions.

To prevent adverse reactions in patients with hypersensitivity to human immunoglobulins, patients with agammaglobulinaemia or selective IgA deficiency, it is advisable to start treatment using low doses, diluted solutions, low infusion rates or infusions given at shorter intervals (e.g. apply the lower dose in two infusions a day).

The administration of high doses of Endobulin may cause a temporary increase in serum glucose in diabetics.

The risk of transmission of virus infection in particular Non A Non B hepatitis by intravenous immunoglobulin preparations cannot be entirely excluded.

Treatment of overdosage: Overdosage need not be expected to lead to more frequent or more severe adverse reactions than the recommended dose.

Pharmaceutical precautions Endobulin should be stored at +2 to +8°C protected from light. The shelf life is three years.

Legal category POM.

Package quantities Endobulin is available in packs of 500 mg, 1,000 mg, 2,500 mg, 5,000 mg, 7,500 mg and 10,000 mg complete with Water for Injections and necessary needles for reconstitution. The 2,500 mg, 5,000 mg, 7,500 mg and 10,000 mg sizes also contain equipment for infusion.

Further information

Interactions: Endobulin may be given in conjunction with electrolyte solutions. In all other cases Endobulin is administered as a separate injection or infusion.

Active immunisation with live vaccines should be postponed until six months after the last administration of Endobulin as the efficacy of the live virus vaccine may be impaired.

If possible an interval of two weeks should be observed after administration of live virus vaccines prior to Endobulin administration.

Effect on laboratory tests: Antibody determination may be influenced by Endobulin administration in that an increased level or new appearance of various types of antibodies (e.g. antibacterial, antiviral or antitoxic) may occur.

With very high doses serum complement determination may give reduced values due to complement consumption. Phagocytosis (Phagocytosis index) may be increased. Endobulin does not have any influence on the immunoregulatory T cells. High doses may cause a temporary rise in serum glucose in diabetics.

Product licence number 0215/0023.

GAMMABULIN*
Normal Immunoglobulin Injection BP.

Presentation Gammabulin is a concentrate of antibodies present in the IgG fraction of human plasma and is available in liquid or lyophilised forms. It is produced from pooled human plasma of venous origin. Only plasma units which are non reactive in tests for HBsAg and antibody to HIV are used in the manufacture of Gammabulin.

Gammabulin liquid is a clear pale yellow to light brown solution. Gammabulin lyophilised is a white to slightly yellowish powder or friable mass completely soluble in Water for Injections BP.

Gammabulin has a protein content of 16% of which 90% is gamma globulin. Glycine is added as a stabiliser at a concentration of 2.25% for the liquid and 6% for the lyophilised forms.

There is no preservative added to the product.

Uses Gammabulin is used in the treatment of:

Antibody deficiency syndrome and recurring bacterial infections in dys-, hypo- and agammaglobulinaemia.

Hepatitis A prophylaxis.

Prevention or modification of measles infection.

Treatment of susceptible pregnant women exposed to Rubella infection in whom continuing pregnancy places the fetus at risk.

Dosage and administration Gammabulin must be administered by the intramuscular route.

All recommendations and doses given below refer to the 16% solution and are expressed in ml.

Antibody deficiency syndrome in dys-, hypo- and agammaglobulinaemia: By intramuscular administration of Gammabulin antibody concentrate the frequency and severity of recurring bacterial infections can be reduced. For treatment of immunoglobulin deficiency, it is necessary to achieve and maintain an immunoglobulin level of approximately 200 mg per 100 ml serum.

Initial dosage: 1.8 ml per kg bodyweight e.g. in three single administrations of 0.6 ml/kg bodyweight each at intervals of 24 hours.

Maintenance dose: 0.6 ml per kg bodyweight, monthly.

Hepatitis A: Gammabulin is an efficient agent for the prevention or modification of hepatitis A. It must be pointed out that after immunoglobulin administration an anicteric course of hepatitis has been observed. Because of this, regular monitoring of transaminase levels may be warranted.

Dosage for children: 0.02–0.04 ml per kg bodyweight. If exposure continues, repeat the dose after 4–6 months.

Dosage for adults:

(a) for a short period of exposure of less than 2 months: 0.02 to 0.04 ml per kg bodyweight.
(b) for longer periods of exposure 0.08 to 0.12 ml per kg bodyweight. If exposure continues, repeat the dose after 4 to 6 months

Note: No benefit may be expected if administered after the onset of clinical symptoms.

Measles: Gammabulin should be given as soon as possible at a dose of 0.25 ml/kg to prevent or modify measles in a susceptible person exposed less than six days previously. Gammabulin may be especially indicated for susceptible household contacts of measles patients, particularly with children under one year of age or children who are immunosuppressed or have an immune deficiency disease and should not receive measles vaccine or any other live viral vaccine.

Prophylaxis: 0.2 ml per kg bodyweight with continued or repeated exposure repeat after 3 weeks.

Mitigation without influence on the immunising effect: 0.04 ml per kg bodyweight.

Rubella: (German Measles) The routine use of Gammabulin prophylaxis of Rubella in early pregnancy is of dubious value and cannot be justified. Some studies suggest that the use of Gammabulin in exposed, susceptible women can lessen the likelihood of infection and fetal damage, therefore, 20 ml of Gammabulin may benefit those women in whom continuing pregnancy places the fetus at risk.

Use in the elderly: No special precautions need to be observed in the elderly.

Use in pregnancy: See interactions with live vaccines e.g. Rubella. According to present knowledge, no influence of immunoglobulin administrations in temporal connection with Rh_0-prophylaxis with anti-D immunoglobulin can be proved. The diaplacental passage of administered immunoglobulin G into the fetus may be assumed.

Contra-indications, warnings, etc Gammabulin is generally well tolerated without reactions. On very rare occasions (e.g. in special forms of a- or hypogammaglobulinaemia) anaphylactoid reactions may occur in patients who have antibodies against immunoglobulin A (IgA) or who have shown atypical reaction after blood transfusion or following administration of blood derivatives.

Gammabulin must not be administered intravenously.

Treatment of overdosage: Gammabulin is a homologous protein the antibody spectrum and protein structure of which corresponds qualitatively to that of an average donor population. Overdosage need not be expected to lead to more frequent or more severe adverse reactions than the recommended dose.

Pharmaceutical precautions Gammabulin liquid should be stored between +2° and +8°C when it will have a shelf life of 3 years.

Gammabulin lyophilised should be stored at room temperature (+2° to +25°C) when it will have a shelf life of 5 years.

Both preparations should be protected from the light.

Legal category POM.

Package quantities *Gammabulin liquid:* Rubber capped vials containing 2 ml, 5 ml or 10 ml.

Gammabulin lyophilised: Rubber capped vial containing 320 mg lyophilised powder. A 2 ml ampoule of Water for Injections BP is also enclosed.

Further information Gammabulin Lyophilised should be used immediately after reconstitution and Gammabulin Liquid immediately after drawing up the vial contents. Gammabulin vials are intended for single dose use only.

Effect on laboratory tests: Laboratory tests as far as antibody determinations are concerned are influenced inasmuch as the application of Gammabulin may lead to an increased or new appearance of types of antibodies (e.g. antibacterial, antiviral or antitoxic antibodies). In case of very high doses, determinations of serum complement may give reduced values (consumption). Phagocytosis (phagocytosis index) may be increased.

Interactions: Active immunization with live virus vaccines (e.g. measles, mumps or rubella) should be postponed until 3 months after the last administration of Gammabulin, as the efficacy of the live virus vaccines may be impaired.

Administration of Gammabulin should be postponed until 2–4 weeks after the first complete cycle of immunization with live virus vaccines and 2 weeks after booster injection.

Product licence numbers
Liquid 0215/0018
Lyophilised 0215/0019

HEPARIN – INJECT 5,000 IMMUNO

Presentation A sterile pyrogen-free, clear, colourless or slightly straw coloured solution of Heparin Sodium BP (mucous) in Water for Injections BP. It is available in pre-filled sterile unit-dose syringes containing 5,000 I.U. in 0.3 ml. Each pre-loaded syringe contains 2.7 mg of Sodium Chloride in 0.3 ml of injection.

Uses Prevention of thrombosis following surgery and for prophylactic treatment of other patients at risk from thromboembolic events.

Dosage and administration Heparin – Inject 5,000 must be administered by the subcutaneous route preferably through the adipose tissue of the abdominal wall. The following dosage is recommended:

Heparin-Inject 5000 is not normally intended for use in children and juveniles.

Pre-operative administration: 1 pre-loaded syringe containing Heparin – Inject 5,000 to be given two hours before surgery.

Post-operative administration: 1 pre-loaded syringe containing Heparin – Inject 5,000 to be given at intervals of 8–12 hours up to the 7th–12th day.

Other patients: 1 pre-loaded syringe containing Heparin – Inject 5,000 to be given at intervals of 8–12 hours.

Use in the elderly: Generally, the above dosage schedules apply also to elderly patients. Special care should be taken however in the elderly (patients over sixty) who are generally more sensitive to the anticoagulant effect of Heparin.

Use in pregnancy: Heparin crosses membranes poorly because of its polarity and large molecular size. It is thus not absorbed from gastrointestinal and sublingual sites. Its passage both across the placenta and into maternal milk is also hindered. Nevertheless pregnant women and nursing mothers should be carefully monitored under Heparin therapy.

Contra-indications, warnings, etc Heparin should not be used in patients with the following conditions:

1. Heparin allergy.
2. Surgery carried out on the central nervous system and the eye.
3. Haemorrhagic diatheses including haemophilia, thrombocytopenia and when linked with endocarditis.
4. Advanced stages of kidney, liver or pancreatic disease.
5. Post-operative seeping haemorrhage.

Precautions are necessary in patients with potential bleeding sites such as peptic ulcer and ulcerative colitis. Also in pregnancy and in patients with persistent hypertension or cerebral thrombosis; and during simultaneous administration of Warfarin, Aspirin, other salicylates or other medicaments having an impact on blood coagulation. Experience indicates that Heparin can be used with very little risk in the prophylaxis of thrombosis. If, however, bleeding complications occur during or after an operation, the patient's thrombin time or partial thromboplastin time should be determined. If the results of these tests are within the normal range it is unlikely that heparinisation is the cause.

It must, however, be borne in mind that on very rare occasions Heparin can cause thrombocytopenia and could therefore be the cause of the haemorrhage.

Treatment of overdosage: Slight haemorrhage caused by overdosage can usually be controlled by withdrawing the drug. In case of severe bleeding neutralisation of heparin by administration of protamine sulphate is recommended. Protamine Sulphate Injection BP (10 mg in 1 ml) must be given by slow (10 min) intravenous injection. Ideally, the dose required should be accurately determined by titration. If there is insufficient time to titrate the dose, the following dosage scale is recommended:

Time interval following dose of 5,000 i.u. Heparin	*Dose of Protamine Sulphate injection 10 mg in 1 ml*
Immediately after	5.0 ml
Half an hour after	2.5 ml
One hour after	1.25 ml

Pharmaceutical precautions It should be stored at a temperature not exceeding 25°C when it will have a shelf life of three years.

Legal category POM.

Package quantities Pre-loaded syringes containing 0.3 ml solution of 5,000 i.u. Heparin Sodium supplied in packs of 10.

Further information An increased tendency towards haemorrhage must be carefully avoided during the operation period and any error of dosage excluded.

Heparin – Inject 5,000 is packed in a pre-loaded syringe which enables an accurate dose to be administered. The hazard of overdosage can therefore be avoided.

Effect on laboratory tests: Heparin causes a dose-dependent prolongation of the following clotting times: thrombin time; activated PTT (partial thromboplastin time); to some extent also the prothrombin time; whole blood clotting time. High dose heparin treatment may result in decreased AT III values.

Product licence number 0215/0017.

HUMAN ALBUMIN SOLUTION 4.5% BP IMMUNO

Presentation Human Albumin Solution 4.5% BP Immuno is a sterile solution of protein for intravenous administration prepared from human plasma of venous origin. Only plasma units which are non reactive in tests for HBsAg and antibody to HIV are used in the manufacture of Human Albumin Solution 4.5% BP Immuno. It is heat treated for 10 hours at 60°C in the final container in accordance with international guidelines. The product contains a minimum of 96% albumin and is stabilised with 3.6 mmol/l sodium caprylate and sodium acetyltryptophanate.

Uses Human Albumin Solution 4.5% BP Immuno is indicated for volume replacement in hypovolaemic shock, as a replacement fluid during therapeutic plasmapheresis and in hypoalbuminaemia associated with an oncotic deficit.

Dosage and administration
Hypovolaemic shock: The dosage is largely determined by the duration and severity of hypovolaemia.

Adults: 500 ml/hour (125 drops/min) in severe shock up to 1000 ml/hour (rapid infusion).

Children: For shock due to hypovolaemia and/or dehydration 20–30 ml/kg bodyweight infused at a rate of 5–10 ml/min.

If the haematocrit drops below 25% packed red cells or whole blood should be given in conjunction with Human Albumin Solution 4.5% BP Immuno to maintain the oxygen transport capacity of the blood.

Hypoalbuminaemia with oncotic deficit
Adults: 3.5–7.0 ml/kg bodyweight daily infused at a rate of 250–500 ml/hr.

Children: 5–10 ml/kg bodyweight per day given slowly.

Use in the elderly: In elderly patients careful haemodynamic and respiratory monitoring is essential throughout the administration of Human Albumin Solution 4.5% BP Immuno as a circulatory overload may lead to decompensation of the haemodynamic system.

In dehydrated patients only low concentrated protein

solutions (up to 5% protein content) should be administered.

Use in pregnancy: As some patients show renal insufficiency during pregnancy concentrated human albumin should be administered only when absolutely indicated and with utmost caution. Based on a persisting hypertension careful haemodynamic monitoring is essential to avoid an overloading syndrome which may lead to cardiac decompensation.

Contra-indications, warnings, etc Do not use if the solution is cloudy or contains a deposit.

Once the container has been penetrated the contents should be used within three hours and any unused preparation discarded.

Adequate precautions should be taken against circulatory overload. If symptoms of hypervolaemia develop the rate of infusion should be slowed or even halted.

Though side effects are extremely rare, such reactions as flushing, chills, fever, tachycardia, hypotension, urticarial skin rash and nausea may occur.

In these cases, the infusion of Human Albumin Solution 4.5% BP Immuno should be interrupted (or replaced by Ringer's solution) and antihistamines and/or corticosteroids should be administered intravenously (e.g. 50–200 mg prednisolone).

Treatment of overdosage: Interrupt infusion immediately and carefully watch the patient's haemodynamic parameters.

The half life of human albumin in the tissue is approximately 16–18 days. The disappearance rate of intravascular albumin depends on the permeability of the vascular system and on the catabolic rate.

Pharmaceutical precautions Human Albumin Solution 4.5% BP Immuno should be stored between +2° and +25°C. It must be protected from light. The shelf life is 5 years.

Legal category POM.

Package quantities Human Albumin Solution 4.5% BP Immuno is supplied in 50 ml, 100 ml, 250 ml, and 400 ml infusion bottles.

Further information Human Albumin Solution 4.5% BP Immuno is compatible with whole blood or packed red cells as well as the usual electrolyte and carbohydrate solutions intended for intravenous use. However, it should not be mixed with protein hydrolysates, amino acid mixtures or solution containing alcohol. Human Albumin Solution 4.5% BP Immuno must not be given through infusion sets which have been used, or are intended, for simultaneous infusion of protein hydrolysates, amino acid mixtures, or solutions containing alcohol. Only clear solutions of slightly yellowish colour should be administered.

Effects on laboratory tests: As a consequence of haemodilution patients' blood samples taken during or shortly after infusion show lower laboratory test results (e.g. haematocrit) corresponding to the amount of Human Albumin Solution 4.5% BP Immuno administered to the patient (calculation based on isotonic solutions). Human Albumin Solution 4.5% BP Immuno does not interfere with the determination of patients' Rh-factors nor is there any adverse effect on thrombocyte function or blood coagulation.

Product licence number 0215/0002.

HUMAN ALBUMIN SOLUTION 20% BP IMMUNO

Presentation Human Albumin Solution 20% BP Immuno is a solution in water of human albumin containing a low proportion of salt and is described as Salt Poor Albumin. It is a clear liquid varying in colour from amber to orange-brown and is presented as a solution for intravenous injection or infusion. It is prepared from pooled plasma of venous origin. Only plasma units which are non reactive in tests for HBsAg and antibody to HIV are used in the manufacture of Human Albumin Solution 20% BP Immuno. The product contains 20% protein of which at least 96% is albumin, the rest being thermostable alpha and beta globulins.

It is stabilised with 16 mmol/L sodium caprylate and 16 mmol/L sodium acetyltryptophanate and heat treated for 10 hours at 60°C in the final container in accordance with international guidelines. There is no preservative added to the solution.

Uses Human Albumin Solution 20% BP Immuno is administered as an injection or an infusion in the treatment of acute oedema; hypoalbuminaemia. For the treatment of the acute phase of burns or haemorrhagic shock, Human Albumin Solution 20% BP Immuno is diluted 1:4 with dextrose 5%, or isotonic electrolyte solutions and the resulting 5% solution administered by infusion.

Dosage and administration

Acute oedema

There is an increased tendency for oedema to occur in patients with hypoalbuminaemia. Attempts should be made to bring about diuresis using the appropriate dose of Human Albumin Solution 20% BP Immuno. A reduction in oedema may then result.

Recommended dosage – Adults: 100 ml Human Albumin Solution 20% BP Immuno (20 g).

Children: 2 ml Human Albumin Solution 20% BP Immuno (0.4 g) per kg bodyweight.

Pre- and post-operative hypoproteinaemia

In debilitated patients stabilisation of the protein balance with Human Albumin Solution 20% BP Immuno may considerably improve the pre-operative condition of the patient. The catabolism of albumin can be severely disturbed after operations on the gastro-intestinal tract and hypoproteinaemia may result. The normal average albumin breakdown of 70 g per week may be enhanced under pathological conditions. Additional loss of protein and diminished albumin synthesis might lead to severe albumin deficiency.

Repeated post-operative infusions of Human Albumin Solution 20% BP Immuno can be most valuable in such cases.

Recommended dosage for pre- and post-operative hypoproteinaemia: Adults: 100–200 ml Human Albumin Solution 20% BP Immuno (20 to 40 g) daily in concentrated or diluted form depending on the plasma volume and serum albumin level of the patient. The dosage and duration of this substitution therapy depends on the amount of protein lost and should be continued until the serum concentration returns to normal.

Children: 1.5 to 3 ml Human Albumin Solution 20% BP Immuno (0.3 to 0.6 g) per kg bodyweight daily in concentrated form or diluted to a 5% solution. In hypoproteinaemia multiple administration of albumin might be necessary until the plasma protein level has returned to normal.

Attention must be paid to the oncotic activity of albumin which may lead to an increased blood volume.

See 'Precautions'.

Other hypoalbuminaemia

(a) Hepatic cirrhosis with diffuse loss of parenchyma leads to diminished production of albumin and a resulting hypoalbuminaemia which, as a consequence, enhances the formation of ascites and oedema. Treatment with albumin results in the disappearance of oedema and a reduction of ascites.

Recommended dosage: Adults: 100 to 200 ml Human Albumin Solution 20% BP Immuno (20 to 40 g) daily.

Children and infants: 1.5 to 3 ml Human Albumin Solution 20% BP Immuno (0.3 to 0.6 g) per kg bodyweight.

(b) Nephrotic syndrome – In cases of nephrotic syndrome particularly with patients who do not respond at all, or only slightly, to diuretics, the administration of Human Albumin Solution 20% BP Immuno will induce diuresis and, therefore, bring about a reduction of the oedema.

Recommended dosage: Adults: 200 to 400 ml Human Albumin Solution 20% BP Immuno (40 to 80 g) daily.

Children and infants: 3 to 6 ml Human Albumin Solution 20% BP Immuno (0.6 to 1.2 g) per kg bodyweight in concentrated form.

The dose should be infused over a period of 60 to 90 minutes.

Shock

Shock due to blood loss should be treated with whole blood, red cell concentrates, fresh frozen plasma or with albumin diluted with isotonic electrolyte and/or dextrose solution 5%.

Adults: 50 to 200 ml Human Albumin Solution 20% BP Immuno (10 to 40 g) diluted 1:4 with isotonic electrolyte and/or dextrose solution 5%.

Children: 1 to 2 ml Human Albumin Solution 20% BP Immuno (0.2 g to 0.4 g) per kg bodyweight diluted 1:4 with isotonic electrolyte and/or dextrose solution 5%.

Burns

Return of fluid from the extravascular compartment to the circulation must be ensured in cases of burns with associated hypoalbuminaemia.

In these cases hyperoncotic Human Albumin Solution 20% BP Immuno can be used with careful control of the oncotic pressure and the haemodynamic parameters.

Recommended dosage: Adults: 50 to 200 ml Human Albumin Solution 20% BP Immuno (10 to 40 g).

Children: 1 to 2 ml Human Albumin Solution 20% BP Immuno (0.2 to 0.4 g) per kg bodyweight.

The initial dose should be infused over a period of 5 to 15 minutes.

In cases of extensive and severe burns with an increased haematocrit value, normalisation of the circulatory conditions can be achieved very effectively with Human Albumin Solution 20% BP Immuno diluted with 5% dextrose or isotonic electrolyte solutions.

Recommended initial dosage: Adults: 200 to 400 ml Human Albumin Solution 20% BP Immuno (40 to 80 g) diluted 1:4 corresponding to 800 to 1600 ml of a 5% albumin solution.

Children: 4 ml Human Albumin Solution 20% BP Immuno per kg bodyweight diluted 1:4 corresponding to 16 ml of a 5% albumin solution.

The total dosage over the first 24 hours can be determined in accordance with the formula:

2 ml × bodyweight (kg) × % of surface burned + 1500 ml

After the acute stage has been brought under control, considerable protein deficiency, largely of albumin, may occur. This hypoalbuminaemia can be corrected by administration of the following doses:

Adults: 50 ml Human Albumin Solution 20% BP Immuno (10 g) twice a day.

Children: 1 ml Human Albumin Solution 20% BP Immuno (0.2 g) per kg bodyweight twice a day.

Use in the elderly: In elderly patients careful haemodynamic and respiratory monitoring is essential throughout the administration of Human Albumin Solution 20% BP Immuno as a circulatory overload may lead to decompensation of the haemodynamic system.

In dehydrated patients only low concentrated protein solutions (up to 5% protein content) should be administered.

Use in pregnancy: As some patients show renal insufficiency during pregnancy concentrated human albumin should be administered only when absolutely indicated and with utmost caution. Based on a persisting hypertension monitoring is essential to avoid an overloading syndrome which may lead to cardiac decompensation.

Contra-indications, warnings, etc

1. Human Albumin Solution 20% BP Immuno must not be used if the solution is cloudy or contains a deposit.

Once the container has been penetrated, the contents must be used within 3 hours and any unused preparation discarded.

2. With patients suffering from hypertension or in cases of latent or manifest cardiac insufficiency, caution is indicated in the administration of Human Albumin Solution 20% BP Immuno. The single doses should be reduced to relatively small amounts and the infusion given slowly. A careful watch must be kept for the possible development of pulmonary oedema. If pulmonary oedema occurs, the infusion must be stopped immediately.

3. In all cases of considerable blood loss, whole blood or packed red cells must be given in addition to Human Albumin Solution 20% BP Immuno.

4. Intolerance reactions are extremely rare with Human Albumin Solution 20% BP Immuno.

Treatment of overdosage: Interrupt infusion immediately and carefully watch the patient's haemodynamic parameters.

The half life of human albumin in the tissue is approximately 16–18 days. The disappearance rate of intravascular albumin depends on the permeability of the vascular system and on the catabolic rate.

Pharmaceutical precautions Human Albumin Solution 20% BP Immuno should be stored between +2°C and +25°C. It must be protected from light. The shelf life is 3 years.

Legal category POM.

Package quantities Human Albumin Solution 20% BP Immuno is supplied in rubber capped vials of 10 ml, 50 ml and 100 ml.

Further information Human Albumin Solution 20% BP Immuno is compatible with whole blood or packed red cells as well as the usual electrolyte and carbohydrate solutions intended for intravenous use. However, it should not be mixed with protein hydrolysates, amino acid mixtures or solutions containing alcohol. Human Albumin Solution 20% BP. Immuno must not be given through infusion sets which have been used, or are intended, for simultaneous infusion of protein hydrolysates, amino acid mixtures, or solutions containing alcohol. Only clear solutions of slightly yellowish colour should be administered.

Effect on laboratory tests: As a consequence of haemodilution patients' blood samples taken during or shortly after infusion show lower laboratory test results (e.g. haematocrit) corresponding to the amount of Human Albumin Solution 20% BP Immuno administered to the patient (calculation based on isotonic solutions). Human Albumin Solution 20% BP Immuno does not interfere with the determination of patients' Rh-factors nor is there any adverse effect on thrombocyte function or blood coagulation.

Product licence number 0215/0009.

PARTOBULIN*
Anti-D (Rh_o) Immunoglobulin Injection B.P.

Presentation Partobulin is a clear liquid varying in colour from pale yellow to light brown. Each vial or preloaded syringe contains 1,250 iu (250 micrograms) Anti-D in 1 ml of solution. It is prepared from pooled human venous plasma with a high content of Anti-D antibodies. Only plasma units which are non reactive in tests for HBsAg and antibody to HIV are used in the manufacture of Partobulin.

Glycine and sodium chloride are added as stabilisers. There is no preservative added to the product.

Uses Partobulin is used for the prevention of Rh_o(D) sensitisation in susceptible individuals following abortion or miscarriage, parturition or an Rh_o(D) incompatible blood transfusion.

Dosage and administration Partobulin must be administered by the intramuscular route.

(a) Abortion and miscarriage: Following every abortion or miscarriage where Rh_o(D) sensitisation may be expected, i.e.

(1) When the mother is Rh_o(D) negative, and

(2) When the fetus is Rh_o(D) positive (or D^u positive) or the rhesus factor cannot be determined or is unknown.

1,250 iu should be administered immediately or at the latest within seventy two hours.

(b) Parturition: Following all deliveries where $Rh_o(D)$ sensitisation may be expected, i.e.

(1) When the mother is $Rh_o(D)$ negative, and

(2) When the child is $Rh_o(D)$ positive (or D^u positive) or the rhesus factor cannot be determined or is unknown.

1,250 iu should be administered immediately, or at the latest within seventy two hours.

(c) Macrotransfusion: In all deliveries or miscarriages with a transplacental haemorrhage of more than 25 ml fetal blood (1% of fetal erythrocytes according to Kleihauer and Betke elution method) into the maternal circulation and a rhesus incompatibility exists, i.e.

(1) When the mother is $Rh_o(D)$ negative, and

(2) When the child is $Rh_o(D)$ positive (or D^u positive) or when the rhesus factor cannot be determined or is unknown.

A dose of 5,000 iu (i.e. 4 vials or syringes of Partobulin) or 50 iu per ml of fetal blood is recommended.

Macroinfiltration occurs in less than 1% of cases.

(d) $Rh_o(D)$ incompatible blood transfusion: Following transfusion of incompatible blood:

(1) When the recipient is $Rh_o(D)$ negative, and

(2) When the transfused blood is $Rh_o(D)$ positive (or D^u positive).

A dose of 50 to 100 iu per ml transfused blood is recommended.

Use in the elderly: Use in the elderly is normally limited to the prevention of sensitisation following incompatible transfusion. Under these circumstances no special precautions or dosage amendments need to be observed in the elderly.

Use in pregnancy: Partobulin is not licensed for use in pregnancy. However, the administration of anti-D immunoglobulin during pregnancy has been described for prevention of antenatal sensitisation. This does not usually produce antibody titres in the maternal circulation that might threaten the fetus. Exceptions are possible, for example, if anti-D immunoglobulin is given repeatedly at short intervals. In general, the antibody titre in the maternal blood should not exceed 1:2 (Coombs Test).

Contra-indications, warnings, etc Partobulin must not be administered intravenously.

Partobulin must not be administered to $Rh_o(D)$ positive individuals or neonates.

Partobulin is generally well tolerated without reactions. On very rare occasions (e.g. in special forms of a- or Hypo-gammaglobulinaemia), anaphylactoid reactions may occur in people who have antibodies against immune globulin A (IgA) or have shown atypical reaction after blood transfusion or following administration of blood derivatives.

Active Immunisation with live virus vaccines (e.g. measles, mumps or rubella) should be postponed until 3 months after the last administration of Partobulin, as the efficacy of the live virus vaccine may be impaired.

If Partobulin needs to be administered within 2–4 weeks of a live virus vaccination, then the efficacy of such a vaccination may be impaired.

Treatment of overdosage: In rhesus negative individuals overdosage need not be expected to lead to more frequent or more severe adverse reactions than the normal dose. It has been observed that even an accidental injection of the preparation into the newborn does not necessarily lead to adverse reaction.

Pharmaceutical precautions Partobulin should be stored between +2 and +8 degrees Centigrade when it will have a shelf life of three years.

Legal category POM.

Package quantities Rubber capped vials or preloaded syringes containing 1,250 iu (250 micrograms) in 1 ml.

Further information
Partobulin should be administered immediately following removal of the protective needle cover (preloaded syringe) or after drawing up the vial contents. Partobulin syringes and vials are intended for single dose use only.

Effect on laboratory tests: Passively introduced $Rh_o(D)$ antibodies may be detected in the blood of the mother several weeks and even months after an injection of Partobulin. Therefore, any previous administration of Partobulin must be taken into account when examining maternal blood for its content of $Rh_o(D)$ antibody and when evaluating these tests.

The presence of additional antibodies (e.g. Rubella) in Partobulin may lead to false positive reactions in tests for such antibodies.

Product licence numbers 0215/0024, 0215/0026.

**Trade Mark*

Innovex Medical
A division of Innovex Medical Products Ltd
Innovex House
Reading Road
Henley-on-Thames
Oxfordshire, RG9 1EL

INNOVEX MEDICAL

NORMAX*

Presentation Normax Capsules (Co-danthrusate Capsules), containing 50 mg danthron and 60 mg docusate sodium. Dark brown capsules, overprinted with the product name 'Normax'.

Uses
Principal action: Danthron is a mild peristaltic stimulant acting on the lower bowel to encourage normal bowel movement without causing irritation. Docusate sodium is a softening agent which prevents excessive colonic dehydration and hardening of stools.

Indications: Constipation in geriatric practice.

Analgesic induced constipation in terminally ill patients of all ages.

Constipation in cardiac failure and coronary thrombosis (conditions in which defecation must be free of strain).

Dosage and administration For oral administration only.

Adults (including elderly patients): 1–3 capsules taken at bedtime. Children (6–12 years): 1 capsule at bedtime.

Prolonged use is not recommended.

Contra-indications, warnings, etc
Contra-indications: In common with all laxatives, Normax is contra-indicated in cases of non-specific abdominal pain and when intestinal obstruction is suspected.

Use in pregnancy and lactation: Normax should not be used during pregnancy or lactation.

Precautions: In experimental animals, danthron has been associated with adenocarcinomas in the bowel and tumours in the liver.

Side-effect: The griping often found with other types of laxative is not an appreciable problem with Normax. Occasionally, an orange tint in the urine may be observed due to the danthron component.

Overdosage: The patient should be encouraged to drink fluids. An anticholinergic preparation may be used to ease excessive intestinal motility if necessary.

Pharmaceutical precautions Store in a dry place.

Legal category POM.

Package quantities Normax is available in blister packs of 63 capsules.

Further information Nil.

Product licence number 0038/0092.

Product licence holder: Beecham Group plc, Great West Road, Brentford, Middlesex TW8 9BD.

TOPAL*

Presentation Round, pale cream tablets with a fragrant odour and sweet, slightly gelatinous taste containing dried aluminium hydroxide gel 30 mg, light magnesium carbonate 40 mg, alginic acid 200 mg, plus excipients to 1.65 g. The inactive ingredients are citric acid, flavour, lactose, magnesium stearate, polyvinylpyrrolidone, silica, sodium bicarbonate, sugar, vanillin and water.

Uses Relief of discomfort and heartburn due to reflux oesophagitis, hiatus hernia, gastritis and hyperacidity.

Dosage and administration
Adults including the elderly: One to three tablets chewed four times a day after meals and at bedtime.

Children: Half the adult dose.

Contra-indications, warnings, etc No specific contra-indications, but care should be observed if used by diabetics because of the sugar content (see 'Further information').

Topal is not recommended in patients who are severely debilitated or on low phosphorus diets and in patients with severe renal insufficiency, alkalosis or hypermagnesaemia.

Antacids, may interfere with the absorption of some drugs, especially tetracyclines.

Pregnancy: It is probably wise to avoid any drug during first trimester of pregnancy unless there are compelling reasons for its use.

Side-effects: Topal is well tolerated and any side effects which occur are likely to be mild and transient.

Overdosage: Treatment should be symptomatic.

Pharmaceutical precautions Store in room temperature protected from moisture.

Legal category GSL.

Package quantities Blister packs of 42 tablets (OP).

Further information Each tablet also contains 40 mg sodium bicarbonate, 880 mg of sucrose and 220 mg lactose, but no added colouring.

Product licence number 0029/0197

Product licence holder: ICI Pharmaceuticals, South Bank, Alderley Park, Macclesfield, Cheshire SK10 4TF.

**Trade Mark*

International Laboratories Limited
Floats Road
Wythenshawe
Manchester M23 9NF

DERBAC*-M LIQUID

Presentation A white, creamy, aqueous liquid containing malathion 0.5% w/w. Inactive ingredients include preservative—parabens.

Uses Eradication of head lice, crab lice and their eggs. Treatment of scabies.

Dosage and administration
Adults, children six months of age and above, elderly:

1. *Treatment of head lice:* Rub the liquid gently into the scalp until all hair and scalp is thoroughly moistened.

Leave the hair to dry naturally in a warm but well ventilated room. After 12 hours, or the next day if preferred, shampoo the hair in the normal way.

Rinse the hair and comb whilst wet to remove dead lice and eggs (nits) using the Derbac Nit comb.

2. *Treatment of crab lice:* Apply Derbac-M Liquid to the entire skin surface. Pay particular attention to all hairy areas including beards and moustaches. Avoid any other areas above the neck.

Leave on for at least one hour before washing but preferably Derbac-M Liquid should be left on overnight.

Wash off or bathe in the usual manner.

3. *Treatment of scabies:* Apply Derbac-M Liquid to the entire skin surface. In adults it may not be necessary to apply above the neck but children under the age of two years should have a thin film of Derbac-M liquid applied to the scalp, face and ears avoiding the eyes and mouth. Do not wash or bathe for 24 hours. If hands or any other parts must be washed during this period, the treatment must be re-applied to those areas immediately.

The infection is cleared by the treatment. However the itching and rash may persist for up to seven days. An anti-irritant cream can be applied if necessary.

Clothing and bedding may be washed or dry cleaned in the normal way.

Contra-indications, warnings, etc
Contra-indications: Known sensitivity to malathion. Not to be used on infants less than six months old except on medical advice.

Warnings and precautions: Avoid contact with the eyes. It is advisable that nursing staff in regular contact with the product should wear rubber gloves when carrying out treatment.

Derbac-M Liquid is for external use only and should be kept out of the reach of children.

Continued prolonged treatment with Derbac-M Liquid should be avoided. It should not be used more than once a week for three weeks at a time.

Side-effects: Very rarely, skin irritation has been reported.

Pregnancy and lactation: No known effects. However, as with all medicines, Derbac-M Liquid should be used with caution.

Accidental ingestion: It is most unlikely that a toxic dose of malathion will be ingested. Treatment consists of gastric lavage, assisted respiration and, if necessary in the event of massive ingestion, administration of atropine.

Pharmaceutical precautions Store below 25°C, away from direct sunlight.

Legal category P.

Package quantities Bottles of 50 ml and 200 ml.

Further information Family members and close contacts should be treated simultaneously. For areas where official policy is to alternate between malathion and carbaryl, in the treatment of head lice, Derbac-C with carbaryl is available.

Product licence number 8452/0006.

DERBAC*-C SHAMPOO

Presentation A yellow opalescent, aqueous liquid containing carbaryl 0.5% w/w (Carbaril INN) in a shampoo base. Inactive ingredients include colouring—E104 and preservative—parabens.

Uses Treatment of head lice.

Dosage and administration
Adults, children six months of age and above, elderly: Wet hair thoroughly with tepid (not hot) water and massage Derbac-C shampoo into the scalp. Rinse with clean water, apply a further quantity of shampoo and work into a rich lather ensuring that areas around the ears and the back of the neck are thoroughly treated. Allow to remain on the head for at least five minutes. Rinse with clean water and remove dead lice with the Derbac Nit comb. The treatment should be repeated twice more at three day intervals (giving a total of three treatments over a period of one week).

Contra-indications, warnings, etc
Contra-indications: Known sensitivity to carbaryl. Not to be used on infants under six months old except on medical advice.

Warnings and precautions: As with all medicated shampoo products, keep out of the eyes, as some irritation may occur.

It is advisable that nursing staff in regular contact with this product should wear rubber gloves when carrying out treatment.

Derbac-C Shampoo is for external use only and should be kept out of the reach of children.

Continued prolonged treatment with Derbac-C Shampoo should be avoided.

Side-effects: Very rarely, skin irritation has been reported.

Pregnancy and lactation: No known effects. However, as with all medicines, Derbac-C Shampoo should be used with caution.

Accidental ingestion: It is most unlikely that a toxic dose of carbaryl will be ingested. Treatment consists of gastric lavage, assisted respiration and, if necessary in the event of massive ingestion, administration of atropine.

Pharmaceutical precautions Store below 25°C, away from direct sunlight.

Legal category P.

Package quantities Bottles of 75 ml.

Further information For areas where official policy is to alternate between carbaryl and malathion, Derbac-M Liquid with Malathion is available. Family members and close contacts should be treated simultaneously.

Product licence number 8452/0008.

SULEO*-C LOTION

Presentation A clear blue alcohol-based lotion containing carbaryl 0.5% w/v (Carbaril INN). Inactive ingredients include colouring—E131.

Uses Eradicates head lice infection.

Dosage and administration
Adults, children six months of age and above, elderly: Rub the lotion gently into the scalp until all hair and scalp is thoroughly moistened. Allow to dry naturally in a well ventilated room. Do not use a hair dryer or other artificial heat. Live lice will be eradicated after a minimum treatment period of two hours. However the lotion should be left on the head for a further period of eight to ten hours to ensure that all lice eggs are totally eradicated.

Shampoo in normal manner. Rinse and comb the hair while wet to remove the dead lice.

In the event of early re-infection, Suleo-C lotion may be applied again provided seven days have elapsed since the first application.

Residual protective effect is variable and of short duration and should not be relied upon.

Contra-indications, warnings, etc
Contra-indications: Known sensitivity to carbaryl. Not to be used on infants under six months of age except on medical advice.

Warnings and precautions: Avoid contact with the eyes. Do not cover the head until the hair has dried completely. It is advisable that nursing staff involved in repeated applications should wear gloves when carrying out treatment.

Suleo-C lotion is for external use only and should be kept out of reach of children.

Keep away from exposed flame or lighted objects (eg cigarettes, gas and electric fires) during application and while hair is wet.

Continued prolonged treatment with Suleo-C lotion should be avoided. It should not be used more than once a week for three weeks at a time.

Alcohol-based products may cause a stinging sensation on patients with sensitive skin.

Side-effects: Very rarely, skin irritation has been reported with carbaryl products.

Pregnancy and lactation: No known effects. However, as with all medicines, Suleo-C lotion should be used with caution.

Accidental ingestion: Gastric lavage, assisted respiration and, if necessary, administration of atropine.

Pharmaceutical precautions Store below 25°C, away from direct sunlight.

Legal category P.

Package quantities Bottles of 50 ml and 200 ml (family pack).

Further information For areas where official policy is to alternate between malathion and carbaryl, Suleo-M lotion with malathion is available. Family members and close contacts should be treated simultaneously.

Product licence number 8452/0004.

SULEO*-C SHAMPOO

Presentation A clear green shampoo containing carbaryl 0.5% w/w (Carbaril INN). Inactive ingredients include colouring—E131, E102 and preservative—formaldehyde.

Uses Eradicates head lice infection.

Dosage and administration
Adults, children six months of age and above, elderly: Wet hair thoroughly with tepid (not hot) water and massage Suleo-C shampoo into the scalp (the same quantity as used for ordinary shampoo). Rinse out thoroughly. Apply a second measure of Suleo-C shampoo and work into a rich lather ensuring that areas around the ears and at the back of the neck are thoroughly treated.

Allow to remain on the head for at least five minutes and then rinse off with clean water. Comb out hair with a fine-toothed comb. Apply as directed at three day intervals for a total of three applications.

Contra-indications, warnings, etc
Contra-indications: Known sensitivity to carbaryl. Not to be used on infants less than six months old except on medical advice.

Warnings and precautions: As with all shampoos, avoid contact with the eyes as some irritation may occur.

It is advisable that nursing staff involved in repeated applications should wear gloves when carrying out treatment.

Suleo-C Shampoo is for external use only and should be kept out of the reach of children.

Continued prolonged treatment with Suleo-C shampoo should be avoided.

Side-effects: Very rarely, skin irritation has been reported with carbaryl products.

Pregnancy and lactation: No known effects. However, as with all medicines, Suleo-C shampoo should be used with caution.

Accidental ingestion: Gastric lavage, assisted respiration and, if necessary, administration of atropine.

Pharmaceutical precautions Store below 25°C, away from direct sunlight.

Legal category P.

Package quantities Bottles of 75 ml.

Further information For areas where official policy is to alternate between carbaryl and malathion, Suleo-M lotion with malathion is available. Family members and close contacts should be treated simultaneously.

Product licence number 8452/0005.

SULEO*-M LOTION

Presentation A clear colourless alcohol-based lotion containing malathion 0.5% w/v.

Uses Eradicates head lice infection.

Dosage and administration
Adults, children six months of age and above, elderly: Rub the lotion gently into the scalp until all hair and scalp is thoroughly moistened. Allow to dry naturally in a well ventilated room. Do not use hair dryer or other artificial heat. Live lice will be eradicated after a minimum treatment period of two hours. However the lotion should be left on the head for a further period of eight to ten hours to ensure that all lice eggs are totally eradicated.

Shampoo in normal manner. Rinse and comb the hair while wet to remove the dead lice.

In the event of early re-infection, Suleo-M Lotion may be applied again provided seven days have elapsed since the first application.

Residual protective effect is variable and of short duration and should not be relied upon.

Contra-indications, warnings, etc
Contra-indications: Known sensitivity to malathion. Not to be used on infants under six months of age except on medical advice.

Warnings and precautions: Avoid contact with the eyes. Do not cover the head until the hair has dried completely. It is advisable that nursing staff involved in repeated applications should wear gloves when carrying out treatment.

Suleo-M lotion is for external use only and should be kept out of reach of children.

Keep away from exposed flame or lighted objects (eg cigarettes, gas and electric fires) during application and while hair is wet.

Continued prolonged treatment with Suleo-M lotion should be avoided. It should not be used more than once a week for three weeks at a time.

Alcohol-based products may cause a stinging sensation on patients with sensitive skin.

Side-effects: Very rarely, skin irritation has been reported with malathion products.

Pregnancy and lactation: No known effects. However, as with all medicines, Suleo-M lotion should be used with caution.

Accidental ingestion: Gastric lavage, assisted respiration and, if necessary, administration of atropine.

Pharmaceutical precautions Store below 25°C, away from direct sunlight.

Legal category P.

Package quantities Bottles of 50 ml and 200 ml (family pack).

Further information For areas where official policy is to alternate between malathion and carbaryl, Suleo-C lotion with carbaryl is available.

Family members and close contacts should be treated simultaneously.

Product licence number 8452/0003.

**Trade Mark*

Invicta Pharmaceuticals
A division of Pfizer Limited
Sandwich
Kent CT13 9NJ

CARDURA*

Presentation Cardura is available as white tablets containing doxazosin mesylate to the equivalent of 1, 2, and 4 mg of the active constituent doxazosin as below:

1 mg pentagonal tablets: marked DXP1 on one side and 'PFIZER' on the other
2 mg ovoid tablets: marked DXP2 on one side and 'PFIZER' on the other
4 mg square tablets: marked DXP4 on one side and 'PFIZER' on the other

Inactive excipients: These include lactose. All strengths of the tablets are gluten free.

Uses
Actions: Doxazosin exerts its vasodilator effect via selective and competitive blockade of post-junctional alpha$_1$-adrenoceptors.

Following oral administration, doxazosin is well absorbed with peak blood levels occurring 2 hours post-dose. Plasma elimination is biphasic with a mean terminal half-life of 22 hours providing the basis for once daily dosing. Doxazosin is extensively metabolised in the liver and excreted mainly via the intestinal tract with $<5\%$ excreted as the unchanged drug.

Studies in the elderly have shown no major pharmacokinetic differences.

Administration of Cardura reduces blood pressure due to a decrease in systemic vascular resistance. With once daily dosing, clinically significant reductions in blood pressure are maintained throughout the day and at 24 hours post-dose. During the onset of therapy, a gradual reduction in blood pressure occurs, and orthostatic effects are comparable with those of other antihypertensives. Maximum reduction in blood pressure normally occurs two to six hours after dosing, and is similar in both supine and standing positions. Unlike non-selective alpha-adrenoceptor blocking agents, tolerance has not been observed in long-term Cardura therapy. Tachycardia is seen infrequently in sustained therapy.

Cardura has been shown to be free of adverse metabolic effects and is suitable for use in patients with asthma, gout and in elderly patients.

Indications: Cardura is indicated for the first-line treatment of hypertension and may be used as the sole agent to control blood pressure in the majority of patients. In patients inadequately controlled on single antihypertensive therapy, Cardura may be used in combination with a thiazide diuretic or a beta-blocking drug.

Dosage and administration
Adults: Cardura is used in a once daily regimen. The initial dose is 1 mg. Dosage may then be increased after 1 or 2 weeks of therapy to 2 mg and thereafter, if necessary, to 4 mg. The majority of patients who respond to Cardura will do so at a dose of 4 mg or less. Dosage can be further increased, if necessary, to 8 mg or the maximum recommended dose of 16 mg.

Use in children: There is insufficient experience to recommend the use of Cardura in children.

Use in the elderly: Normal adult dosage is recommended.

Use in renal insufficiency: Since there is no change in pharmacokinetics in patients with impaired renal function, the usual dosage is recommended. Doxazosin is not dialysable.

Contra-indications, warnings, etc
Contra-indications: Cardura is contra-indicated in patients with a known hypersensitivity to quinazolines.

Use during lactation: Animal studies have shown that doxazosin accumulates in breast milk. The clinical safety of Cardura during lactation has not been established, consequently Cardura is contra-indicated in nursing mothers.

Warnings:
Use during pregnancy: Although animal tests have shown no evidence of teratogenic effects, the clinical safety of Cardura during pregnancy has not yet been established. Accordingly, Cardura should be used only when, in the opinion of the physician, potential benefit outweighs potential risk.

Drug interactions: Doxazosin is highly bound to plasma proteins (98%). *In vitro* data in human plasma indicates that doxazosin has no effect on protein binding of the drugs tested (digoxin, phenytoin, warfarin or indomethacin).

No adverse drug interactions have been observed with thiazide diuretics, frusemide, beta-blocking agents, non-steroidal anti-inflammatory drugs, antibiotics, oral hypoglycaemic drugs, uricosuric agents, or anticoagulants.

Side-effects: In patients with hypertension, the most common reaction associated with Cardura therapy is postural hypotension, rarely associated with fainting. Other reactions include: dizziness, vertigo, headache, fatigue, asthenia and oedema.

Rat studies at high doses have shown a reversible effect (reduction in ejaculation rate) on male fertility. The significance of this to man is currently unknown but is considered unlikely.

Overdosage: Should overdosage lead to hypotention, the patient should be immediately placed in a supine, head down position. Other supportive measures may be appropriate in individual cases. Since doxazosin is highly protein bound, dialysis is not indicated.

Pharmaceutical precautions Store below 30°C.

Legal category POM.

Package quantities
1 mg: Calendar packs of 28 tablets (Original pack).
2 mg: Calendar packs of 28 tablets (Original pack).
4 mg: Calendar packs of 28 tablets (Original pack).

Further information Cardura, in addition to its antihypertensive effect has in short term studies produced a modest reduction in plasma total cholesterol and LDL cholesterol concentrations.

Product licence numbers
Cardura tablets 1 mg 0057/0276
Cardura tablets 2 mg 0057/0277
Cardura tablets 4 mg 0057/0278

HYPOVASE*

Presentation Hypovase is available in tablets containing Prazosin Hydrochloride BP equivalent to the following quantities of prazosin:

500 microgram white tablets, unscored: marked 'Pfizer' on one side.
1 mg scored orange tablets: marked HYP/1 on one side.

2 mg scored white tablets: marked HYP/2 on one side and 'Pfizer' on the other.
5 mg scored white tablets: marked HYP/5 on one side and 'Pfizer' on the other.

Inactive excipients: The 1 mg tablet contains the azo dye sunset yellow.

All strengths of the tablets are free of gluten, lactose and other sugars.

Uses

Actions: Hypovase causes a decrease in total peripheral vascular resistance thought to be mediated by selective inhibition of post-synaptic alpha-1-adrenoceptors in vascular smooth muscle. The results of forearm plethysmographic studies in humans demonstrate that the resultant peripheral vasodilatation is a balanced effect on both resistance vessels (arterioles) and capacitance vessels (veins).

In hypertensive patients, blood pressure is lowered in both the supine and standing positions; this effect is more pronounced on the diastolic blood pressure. Tolerance to the antihypertensive effect has not been observed in long-term clinical use; relatively little tachycardia or change in renin levels has been noted. Rebound elevation of blood pressure does not occur following abrupt cessation of Hypovase therapy.

The therapeutic efficacy of Hypovase in patients with congestive heart failure is ascribed to a reduction in left ventricular filling pressure, reduction in cardiac impedance and an augmentation of cardiac output. The use of Hypovase in congestive heart failure does not provoke a reflex tachycardia and blood pressure reduction is minimal in normotensive patients.

Hypovase has been found to successfully reduce the severity of the signs, symptoms, frequency and duration of attacks, in patients with Raynaud's disease.

Clinical studies have shown that Hypovase therapy is not associated with adverse changes in the serum lipid profile.

Following oral administration in normal volunteers and hypertensive patients, plasma concentrations reach a peak in one to two hours, with a plasma half-life of two to three hours. Pharmacokinetic data in a limited number of patients with congestive heart failure, most of whom showed evidence of hepatic congestion, indicates that peak plasma concentrations are reached in 2.5 hours and plasma half-life is approximately 7 hours. Hypovase is highly bound to plasma protein. Studies indicate that Hypovase is extensively metabolised, primarily by demethylation and conjugation, and excreted mainly via bile and faeces.

Renal blood flow and glomerular filtration rate are not impaired by long term oral administration and thus Hypovase can be used with safety in hypertensive patients with impaired renal function.

Indications:
Hypertension: Hypovase is indicated in the treatment of all grades of essential (primary) hypertension and of all grades of secondary hypertension of varied aetiology. It can be used as the initial and sole agent or it may be employed in a treatment regimen in conjunction with a diuretic and/or other antihypertensive drug as needed for proper patient response.

Congestive heart failure: Hypovase may be used alone or added to the therapeutic regimen in those patients with congestive heart failure who are resistant or refractory to conventional therapy with diuretics, and/or cardiac glycosides.

Raynaud's phenomenon and Raynaud's disease: Hypovase is indicated for the symptomatic treatment of patients with Raynaud's Phenomenon and Raynaud's Disease.

Benign prostatic hyperplasia: See additional data sheet.

Dosage and administration

Hypertension: The dosage range is from 500 micrograms–20 mg daily. It is recommended that therapy be initiated at the lowest dose, 500 micrograms, twice or three times daily for three to seven days, with the starting dose administered in the evening. This dose should be increased to 1 mg twice or three times daily for a further three to seven days. Thereafter, the daily dose should be increased gradually as determined by the patients response to the blood pressure lowering effect. Most patients are likely to be maintained on a dosage regimen of Hypovase alone of up to 15 mg daily in divided doses. Maximum recommended daily dosage: 20 mg in divided doses.

The b.d. starter pack is available for the convenience of prescribers to initiate treatment up to 2 mg twice daily.

Patients receiving other antihypertensive therapy but with inadequate control: The dosage of the other drug should be reduced to a maintenance level and Hypovase initiated at 500 micrograms in the evening, then continuing with 500 micrograms twice or three times daily. Subsequent dosage increase, should be made gradually depending upon the patient's response.

There is evidence that adding Hypovase to angiotensin converting enzyme inhibitor, beta-adrenergic antagonist or calcium antagonist therapy may bring about a substantial reduction in blood pressure. Therefore, the low initial dosage regimen is recommended.

Congestive cardiac failure: The recommended starting dose is 500 micrograms two, three or four times daily, increasing to 4 mg in divided doses. Dosage should be adjusted according to the patient's clinical response, based on careful monitoring of cardiopulmonary signs and symptoms, and when indicated, haemodynamic studies. Dosage may be adjusted as often as every two to three days in patients under close medical supervision. In severely ill, decompensated patients, rapid dosage adjustment over one to two days may be indicated and is best done when haemodynamic monitoring is available. In clinical studies, the therapeutic dosages ranged from 4 mg to 20 mg daily in divided doses. Adjustment of dosage may be required in the course of Hypovase therapy in some patients to maintain optimal clinical improvement.

Usual daily maintenance dosage: 4 mg to 20 mg in divided doses.

Raynaud's phenomenon and Raynaud's disease: The recommended starting dosage is 500 micrograms twice daily given for a period of three to seven days and should be adjusted according to the patient's clinical response. Usual maintenance dosage 1 mg or 2 mg twice daily.

Patients with moderate to severe grades of renal impairment: Evidence to date shows that Hypovase does not further compromise renal function when used in patients with renal impairment. As some patients in this category have responded to small doses of Hypovase, it is recommended that therapy be initiated at 500 micrograms daily and that dosage increases be instituted cautiously.

Patients with hepatic dysfunction: No information is available on the use of Hypovase in this patient group. However, since Hypovase normally undergoes substantial first pass metabolism and subsequent metabolism and excretion by the liver, it is recommended that therapy be initiated at 500 micrograms daily and that dosage increases be instituted cautiously.

Use in the elderly: Since the elderly may be more susceptible to hypotension, therapy should be initiated with the lowest possible dose.

Use in children: Hypovase is not recommended for the treatment of children under the age of 12 years since safe conditions for its use have not been established.

Contra-indications, warnings, etc

Contra-indications: Sensitivity to Hypovase or related quinazolines.

Warnings:
Use in pregnancy or lactation: Although no teratogenic effects were seen in animal testing, the safety of Hypovase during pregnancy has not yet been established. The use of prazosin and a beta-blocker for the control of severe hypertension in 44 pregnant women revealed no drug-related foetal abnormalities or adverse effects. Therapy with prazosin was continued for as long as 14 weeks.

Prazosin has also been used alone or in combination with other hypotensive agents in severe hypertension of pregnancy. No foetal or neonatal abnormalities have been reported with the use of prazosin.

Studies to date are inadequate to establish the safety of Hypovase in pregnancy, accordingly, it should be used only when, in the opinion of the physician, potential benefit outweighs potential risk. Hypovase has been shown to be excreted in small amounts in human milk. Caution should be exercised when Hypovase is administered to nursing mothers.

In patients with congestive cardiac failure: Hypovase is not recommended in the treatment of congestive cardiac failure due to mechanical obstruction such as aortic valve stenosis, mitral valve stenosis, pulmonary embolism and restrictive pericardial disease. Adequate data are not yet available to establish efficacy in patients with heart failure due to recent myocardial infarction.

Precautions:

In patients with hypertension: A very small percentage of patients may respond in an abrupt and exaggerated manner to the initial dose of Hypovase. Postural hypotension evidenced by dizziness and weakness, or rarely loss of consciousness, has been reported, particularly with the commencement of therapy, but this effect is readily avoided by initiating treatment with a low dose of Hypovase and with small increases in dosage during the first one to two weeks of therapy. The effect when observed, is not related to the severity of hypertension, is self-limiting and in most patients does not recur after the initial period of therapy or during subsequent dosage increments.

When instituting therapy with any effective antihypertensive agent, the patient should be advised how to avoid symptoms resulting from postural hypotension and what measures to take should they develop. The patient should be cautioned to avoid situations where injury could result should dizziness or weakness occur during the initiation of Hypovase therapy (e.g. driving or operating machinery).

In patients with congestive cardiac failure: When Hypovase is initially administered to patients with congestive cardiac failure who have undergone vigorous diuretic or other vasodilator treatment, particularly in higher than the recommended starting dose, the resultant decrease in left ventricular filling pressure may be associated with a significant fall in cardiac output and systemic blood pressure. In such patients, observance of the recommended starting dose of Hypovase followed by gradual dosage increase is particularly important (see 'Dosage and administration').

The clinical efficacy of Hypovase in congestive cardiac failure has been reported to diminish after several months of treatment, in a proportion of patients. In these patients there is usually evidence of weight gain or peripheral oedema indicating fluid retention. Since spontaneous deterioration may occur in such severely ill patients a causal relationship to prazosin therapy has not been established. Thus, as with all patients with congestive cardiac failure, careful adjustment of diuretic dosage according to the patient's clinical condition is required to prevent excessive fluid retention and consequent relief of symptoms.

In those patients without evidence of fluid retention, when clinical improvement has diminished, an increase in the dosage of Hypovase will usually restore clinical efficacy.

Raynaud's phenomenon and Raynaud's disease: Because Hypovase decreases peripheral vascular resistance, careful monitoring of blood pressure during initial administration and during subsequent dosage increments of Hypovase is suggested. Close observation is especially recommended for patients already taking medications that are known to lower blood pressure.

Drug interactions: Hypovase has been administered without any adverse drug interaction in clinical experience to date with the following:

(1) cardiac glycosides – digitalis and digoxin;
(2) hypoglycaemic agents – insulin, chlorpropamide, phenformin, tolazamide and tolbutamide;
(3) tranquilizers and sedatives – chlordiazepoxide, diazepam and phenobarbitone;
(4) agents for treatment of gout – allopurinol, colchicine and probenecid;
(5) anti-arrhythmic agents – procainamide and quinidine;
(6) analgesic, antipyretic, and anti-inflammatory agents – dextropropoxyphene, aspirin, indomethacin and phenylbutazone;

There is evidence that adding Hypovase to beta-adrenergic antagonist or calcium antagonist therapy may produce a substantial reduction in blood pressure. Therefore, the low initial dosage regimen is recommended.

Drug/laboratory test interactions: False positive results may occur in screening tests for phaeochromocytoma (urinary vanillylmandelic acid (VMA) and methoxyhydroxyphenyl glycol (MHPG) metabolites of noradrenaline) in patients who are being treated with Hypovase.

Side-effects: In patients with hypertension: The most common side-effects associated with Hypovase therapy are: dizziness, headache, drowsiness, lack of energy, weakness, nausea, and palpitations. In most instances side-effects will disappear with continued therapy or may be tolerated with no decrease in dosage of the drug.

In addition, the following reactions have been associated with Hypovase therapy: vomiting, diarrhoea, constipation, abdominal discomfort and/or pain, liver function abnormalities, pancreatitis, oedema, dyspnoea, faintness, transient temporary loss of consciousness, tachycardia, nervousness, vertigo, hallucinations, depression, paraesthesia, rash, pruritus, alopecia, lichen planus, urinary frequency, impotence, incontinence, priapism, blurred vision, reddended sclera, epistaxis, tinnitus, dry mouth, nasal congestion, diaphoresis, fever, positive ANA titre and arthralgia.

Some of these reactions have occurred rarely, and in many instances the exact causal relationships have not been established.

Literature reports exist associating Hypovase therapy with a worsening of pre-existing narcolepsy. A causal relationship is uncertain in these cases.

In patients with congestive cardiac failure: The following side-effects have been observed when Hypovase is used in conjunction with cardiac glycosides and diuretics: drowsiness, dizziness, postural hypotension, blurred vision, oedema, dry mouth, palpitations, nausea, diarrhoea, impotence, headache, and nasal congestion. In most instances these occurrences have been mild to moderate in severity and have resolved with continued therapy or have been tolerated with no decrease in drug dosage.

Raynaud's phenomenon and Raynaud's disease: The most common, although infrequently reported side-effect, is mild dizziness.

Overdosage: Should overdosage lead to hypotension, support of the cardiovascular system is of first importance. Restoration of blood pressure and normalisation of heart rate may be accomplished by keeping the patient in the supine position. If this measure is inadequate, shock should first be treated with volume expanders. If necessary, vasopressors including angiotensin should then be used. Renal function should be monitored and supported as needed. Laboratory data indicate Hypovase is not dialysable because it is protein bound.

Pharmaceutical precautions Store below 30°C.

Legal category POM.

Package quantities b.d. starter pack, for the convenience of patients initiating Hypovase therapy, containing 8 × 500 micrograms Hypovase tablets and 32 × 1 mg Hypovase tablets (see 'Further information').

Hypovase 500 microgram: Original packs of 56 tablets (in blister strips of 4 × 14 tablets).
Hypovase 1 mg: Original packs of 56 tablets (in blister strips of 4 × 14 tablets).
Hypovase 2 mg: Original packs of 56 tablets (in blister strips of 4 × 14 tablets).

Hypovase 5 mg: Original packs of 56 tablets (in blister strips of 4 × 14 tablets).

Further information The two week b.d. starter pack has the following instructions to the patient:

"Step 1 (500 micrograms tablets) – evening day 1 to morning day 5
Step 2 (1 mg tablets) – evening day 5 to morning day 9
Step 3 (2 × 1 mg tablets) – evening day 9 to morning day 15"
Your doctor will wish you to follow further dosage instructions beyond Step 3 and you should follow those instructions or see your doctor before the end of Step 3.

The tablets (500 micrograms and 1 mg) are carefully packed in sequence, in blister strips to ensure correct usage.

Product licence numbers

500 microgram tablet	0057/0149R
1 mg tablet	0057/0106R
2 mg tablet	0057/0107R
5 mg tablet	0057/0108R

HYPOVASE* (BENIGN PROSTATIC HYPERTROPHY)

Presentation Hypovase is available in tablets containing Prazosin Hydrochloride BP equivalent to the following quantities of prazosin:
500 microgram white tablets, unscored: marked 'Pfizer' on one side.
1 mg scored orange tablets: marked HYP/1 on one side.
2 mg scored white tablets: marked HYP/2 on one side and 'Pfizer' on the other.

Inactive excipients: The 1 mg tablet contains the azo dye sunset yellow.

All strengths of the tablets are free of gluten, lactose and other sugars.

Uses Hypovase is a selective postsynaptic alpha-1-adrenoceptor antagonist and a recognised treatment for all grades of hypertension of varied aetiology. In low dosage, antagonism of alpha-1-receptors on prostatic and urethral smooth muscle has been shown to improve the urinary pressure profile in men and to improve symptoms of benign prostatic hypertrophy.

Hypovase is indicated as an adjunct in the symptomatic treatment of urinary obstruction caused by benign prostatic hyperplasia, and may therefore be of value in patients awaiting prostatic surgery.

Dosage and administration Benign prostatic hyperplasia: The recommended dosage is 500 micrograms twice daily for a period of 3 to 7 days, with the initial dose administered in the evening. The dosage should then be adjusted according to clinical response. The usual maintenance dosage is 2 mg twice daily. This dose should not be exceeded, unless the patient requires Hypovase as antihypertensive therapy.

Use in the elderly: Since the elderly may be more susceptible to hypotension, therapy should be initiated with the lowest possible dose.

Patients with moderate to severe grades of renal impairment: Evidence to date shows that Hypovase does not further compromise renal function when used in patients with renal impairment. As some hypertensive patients with renal impairment have responded to small doses of Hypovase, it is recommended that therapy be initiated at 500 micrograms daily and that dosage be increased cautiously.

Patients receiving antihypertensive therapy: It is recommended that patients receiving antihypertensive therapy are administered Hypovase only under supervision of the practitioner responsible for treating the patient's hypertension.

Contra-indications, warnings, etc
Contra-indications: Sensitivity to Hypovase or related quinazolines.

Warnings: Hypovase is not recommended for patients with a history of micturition syncope.

Precautions: Hypovase decreases peripheral vascular resistance and since many patients with this disorder are elderly, careful monitoring of blood pressure during initial administration and during adjustment of dosage is recommended. The possibility of postural hypotension, or rarely, loss of consciousness, as reported in other patient groups should be borne in mind. Hypovase may augment the efficacy of antihypertensive therapy, consequently, close observation is especially recommended for patients taking medications that are known to lower blood pressure. Hypovase should not normally be administered to patients already receiving another alpha-1-antagonist.

In patients with hypertension or congestive heart failure, it is recommended that the full Hypovase data sheet is referred to.

The patient should be cautioned to avoid situations where injury could result should dizziness or weakness occur during the initiation of Hypovase therapy (e.g. driving or operating machinery).

Drug interactions: Hypovase has been administered without any adverse drug interaction in clinical experience to date with the following:
(1) cardiac glycosides – digitalis and digoxin;
(2) hypoglycaemic agents – insulin, chlorpropamide, phenformin, tolazamide and tolbutamide;
(3) tranquillizers and sedatives – chlordiazepoxide, diazepam and phenobarbitone;
(4) agents for treatment of gout – allopurinol, colchicine and probenecid;
(5) anti-arrhythmic agents – procainamide and quinidine;
(6) analgesic, antipyretic, and anti-inflammatory agents – dextropropoxyphene, aspirin, indomethacin and phenylbutazone;

Drug/laboratory test interactions: False positive results may occur in screening tests for phaeochromocytoma (urinary vanillylmandelic acid (VMA) and methoxyhydroxyphenyl glycol (MHPG) metabolites of noradrenaline) in patients who are being treated with Hypovase.

Side-effects: The most common, although infrequently reported side-effect in patients with benign prostatic hypertrophy is dizziness.

The most common side-effects observed in patients with hypertension are dizziness, headache, drowsiness, lack of energy, weakness, nausea, and palpitations. In most instances side-effects will disappear with continued therapy or may be tolerated with no decrease in dosage of the drug.

In addition, the following reactions have rarely been associated with Hypovase therapy and in many instances the exact causal relationships have not been established: vomiting, diarrhoea, constipation, abdominal discomfort and/or pain, liver function abnormalities, pancreatitis, oedema, dyspnoea, faintness, transient temporary loss of consciousness, tachycardia, nervousness, vertigo, hallucinations, depression, paraesthesia, rash, pruritus, alopecia, urinary frequency, impotence, incontinence, priapism, blurred vision, reddened sclera, lichen planus, epistaxis, tinnitus, dry mouth, nasal congestion, diaphoresis, fever, positive ANA titre and arthralgia.

Overdosage: Should overdosage lead to hypotension, support of the cardiovascular system is of first importance. Restoration of blood pressure and normalisation of heart rate may be accomplished by keeping the patient in the supine position. If this measure is inadequate, shock should first be treated with volume expanders. If necessary vasopressors including angiotensin should then be used. Renal function should be monitored and supported as needed. Laboratory data indicate Hypovase is not dialysable because it is protein bound.

Pharmaceutical precautions Store below 30°C.

Legal Category: POM.

Package quantities Hypovase b.d. starter pack, for the convenience of patients initiating Hypovase therapy, containing 8 × 500 microgram Hypovase tablets and 32 × 1 mg Hypovase tablets (see 'Further information').

Hypovase 500 microgram, 1 mg and 2 mg: Original packs of 56 tablets, (in blister strips of 4 × 14 tablets).

Further information The two week b.d. starter pack has the following instructions to the patient:

"Step 1 (500 microgram tablets) – evening day 1 to morning day 5
Step 2 (1 mg tablets) – evening day 5 to morning day 9
Step 3 (2 × 1 mg tablets) – evening day 9 to morning day 15"
Your doctor will wish you to follow further dosage instructions beyond Step 3 and you should follow those instructions or see your doctor before the end of Step 3.

The tablets (500 microgram and 1 mg) are carefully packed in sequence, in blister strips to ensure correct usage.

Product licence numbers

500 microgram tablet	0057/0270
1 mg tablet	0057/0271
2 mg tablet	0057/0272

LUSTRAL* ▼

Presentation Lustral is available as tablets containing sertraline hydrochloride equivalent to 50 mg or 100 mg sertraline.

50 mg white capsular shaped tablets coded 'LTL-50' on one side and marked 'PFIZER' on the other.

100 mg white capsular shaped tablets coded 'LTL-100' on one side and marked 'PFIZER' on the other.

The tablets are free of gluten, lactose and other sugars.

Uses

Actions: Sertraline is a potent and specific inhibitor of neuronal 5-HT uptake *in vitro* and *in vivo*, but is without affinity for muscarinic, serotonergic, adrenergic or GABA receptors.

After oral administration of sertraline in man, peak blood levels occur at about 6–8 hours. Sertraline has a plasma half-life of approximately 26 hours and is approximately 98% bound to plasma proteins. The principal metabolite, desmethylsertraline is inactive in *in vivo* tests and has a half-life of approximately 62–109 hours. Sertraline and desmethylsertraline are both extensively metabolised in man and the resultant metabolites excreted in faeces and urine in equal amounts. Only a small amount of unchanged sertraline is excreted in the urine.

Since bioavailability is increased in the presence of food it is recommended that Lustral be administered with a meal.

Indications: Lustral is indicated for the treatment of symptoms of depressive illness. Following satisfactory response, continuation with Lustral therapy is effective in preventing relapse of the initial episode of depression or recurrence of further depressive episodes.

Dosage and administration

Adults: Lustral tablets should be given as a single daily dose with food. The starting dose is 50 mg daily and the usual therapeutic dose is 50 or 100 mg daily.

Dosage adjustments, in 50 mg increments over a period of weeks, from 100 mg to a maximum of 200 mg, may be considered in patients with incomplete response but good toleration at lower doses. Once optimal therapeutic response is achieved the dose should be reduced to the lowest effective level. Doses of 150 mg or more should not be used for periods exceeding 8 weeks. The onset of therapeutic effect may be seen within 7 days, although 2–4 weeks are usually necessary for full antidepressant activity. Dosage during prolonged maintenance therapy should be kept at the lowest effective level, with subsequent adjustments depending on therapeutic response.

Use in children: The use of Lustral in children is not recommended, as safety and efficacy have not been established.

Use in the elderly: No special precautions are required. The usual adult dosage is recommended.

Contra-indications, warnings, etc

Contra-indications: Lustral is contra-indicated in patients with a known hypersensitivity to sertraline.

Use in hepatic insufficiency: Sertraline is extensively metabolised by the liver. The pharmacokinetics of sertraline have not been studied in patients with significant hepatic dysfunction nor have patients with significant hepatic dysfunction been evaluated during treatment with sertraline. Accordingly, Lustral should not be administered to such patients.

Use in renal insufficiency: Until the pharmacokinetics of sertraline have been studied in patients with renal impairment, Lustral should not be administered to such patients.

Warnings: Monoamine oxidase inhibitors: Because no clinical data are available on the effects of the combined use of Lustral and monoamine oxidase inhibitors (MAOI), their combined use should be avoided. Based on experience with combined administration of MAOI and tricyclic antidepressants, at least 14 days should elapse between discontinuation of an MAOI and initiation of treatment with Lustral. At least 7 days should elapse before starting any MAOI following discontinuation of Lustral.

Use in pregnancy: Fertility studies conducted in rats at doses approximately 20 times the maximum human dose, indicated that sertraline had no adverse effects on fertility. There was, however, decreased neonatal survival following maternal administration of sertraline at doses approximately 5–6 times the maximum human dose. Similar effects on neonatal survival have been described for other antidepressant drugs.

Reproduction studies have been performed in rats and rabbits at doses up to 20 times the maximum daily human dose. There was no evidence of teratogenicity or embryotoxicity at any dose level. At the dose level corresponding to 5–6 times the maximum daily human dose, however, sertraline caused maternal toxicity which in turn delayed ossification processes in foetuses.

There are no adequate and well-controlled studies in pregnant women. Since animal reproduction studies are not always predictive of human response, Lustral should be used during pregnancy only if clearly needed. Women of childbearing potential should employ an adequate method of contraception if taking Lustral.

Use during lactation: No data containing sertraline levels in breast milk are available, hence use in nursing mothers is not recommended.

Precautions: Electroconvulsive therapy (ECT): In patients receiving ECT, concomitant administration of Lustral should be avoided due to the lack of experience in this situation.

Driving/use of machinery: Since antidepressants may impair ability to perform potentially hazardous tasks, such as driving a car or operating machinery, the patient should be cautioned accordingly. Lustral should not be administered with benzodiazepines or other tranquillisers in patients who drive or operate machinery.

Seizures: Seizures are a potential risk with antidepressant drugs. Lustral should be avoided in patients with unstable epilepsy; patients with controlled epilepsy should be carefully monitored. The drug should be discontinued in any patient who develops seizures.

Drug interactions:

Alcohol: In 11 healthy subjects administered sertraline (200 mg daily) for 9 days, there was no adverse effect on cognitive or psychomotor performance relative to placebo following a single dose of 500 mg/kg alcohol. However, the concomitant use of Lustral and alcohol in depressed patients is not recommended.

Centrally active medication: Caution is advised if Lustral is administered with other centrally active medication. Co-administration with lithium or tryptophan may lead to a higher incidence of 5-HT associated side-effects. There is no experience of concomitant use of Lustral with lithium or tryptophan in depressed patients.

Other drug interactions: Since sertraline is bound to plasma proteins, the potential of Lustral to interact with other plasma protein bound drugs should be borne in mind. The potential of Lustral to interact with e.g. digoxin, warfarin, propranolol and phenytoin, has not been fully assessed.

Side-effects: In multiple dose studies involving dose escalation based on the patient's response, side-effects which occurred significantly more frequently with Lustral than placebo were: dry mouth, nausea, diarrhoea/loose stools, ejaculatory delay, tremor, increased sweating and dyspepsia.

Asymptomatic elevations of serum transaminases resulting in discontinuation of therapy have occurred infrequently in clinical trials. These occurred predominantly at doses greater than 100 mg (approximately 1.3 per cent of patients). These have resolved on cessation of therapy.

Overdosage: In three patients who took overdoses of up to 2 g of sertraline, there were no reported changes in vital signs, cardiovascular toxicity, level of consciousness nor unwanted symptomatology; each patient recovered without sequelae.

No specific therapy is recommended and there are no specific antidotes to sertraline. Gastric lavage should be considered if large amounts of sertraline are known or suspected to have been swallowed within the preceding twelve hours. Forced diuresis and haemodialysis are not recommended due to the high degree of protein binding.

Pharmaceutical precautions Lustral tablets should be stored below 30°C.

Legal category POM.

Package quantities
50 mg: Calendar pack of 28 tablets
100 mg: Calendar pack of 28 tablets.

Further information Nil.

Product licence numbers
Lustral Tablets 50 mg 0057/0308
Lustral Tablets 100 mg 0057/0309

VIBRAMYCIN* CAPSULES VIBRAMYCIN* 50 CAPSULES VIBRAMYCIN*-D DISPERSIBLE TABLETS

Presentation

Vibramycin Capsules are green capsules containing 100 mg doxycycline as the hydrochloride, coded 'Pfizer' and 'VBM 100'. Inactive excipients: These include lactose and the dyes quinoline yellow, patent blue V and titanium dioxide.

Vibramycin 50 Capsules are green and ivory capsules containing 50 mg doxycycline as the hydrochloride, coded 'Pfizer' and 'VBM 50'. Inactive excipients: These include lactose and the dyes quinoline yellow, patent blue V, indigotine, titanium dioxide and yellow iron oxide.

Vibramycin-D Dispersible Tablets are off white-buff tablets coded D 9 on one side and 'Pfizer' on the other, each containing 100 mg doxycycline as the monohydrate.

The Vibramycin range is free of gluten and azo dyes.

Vibramycin is a broad-spectrum antibiotic synthetically derived from oxytetracycline.

Vibramycin has a high degree of lipid solubility and a low affinity for calcium. It is highly stable in normal human serum. Vibramycin will not degrade into an epianhydro form.

Uses

Actions: Vibramycin is primarily bacteriostatic and is believed to exert its antimicrobial effect by the inhibition of protein synthesis. Vibramycin is active against a wide range of Gram-positive and Gram-negative bacteria and certain other micro-organisms.

Tetracyclines are readily absorbed and are bound to plasma proteins in varying degrees. They are concentrated by the liver in the bile and excreted in the urine and faeces at high concentrations and in a biologically active form. Vibramycin is virtually completely absorbed after oral administration. Studies reported to date indicate that the absorption of Vibramycin, unlike certain other tetracyclines, is not notably influenced by the ingestion of food or milk.

Following a 200 mg dose, normal adult volunteers averaged peak serum levels of 2.6 micrograms/ml of doxycycline at 2 hours decreasing to 1.45 micrograms/ml at 24 hours. Studies have shown no significant difference in serum half-life of Vibramycin (range 18 to 22 hours) in individuals with normal or severely impaired renal function.

Indications: Vibramycin has been found clinically effective in the treatment of a variety of infections caused by susceptible strains of Gram-positive and Gram-negative bacteria and certain other micro-organisms.

Respiratory tract infections: Pneumonia and other lower respiratory tract infections due to susceptible strains of *Streptococcus pneumoniae, Haemophilus influenzae, Klebsiella pneumoniae* and other organisms. *Mycoplasma pneumoniae* pneumonia. Treatment of chronic bronchitis. Sinusitis.

Urinary tract infections: Infections caused by susceptible strains of the *Klebsiella* species, *Enterobacter* species, *Escherichia coli, Streptococcus faecalis* and other organisms.

Sexually Transmitted Diseases: Infections due to *Chlamydia trachomatis* including uncomplicated urethral, endocervical or rectal infections. Non-gonococcal urethritis caused by *Ureaplasma urealyticum* (T-mycoplasma).

Vibramycin is also indicted in chancroid and infections due to *Calymmatobacterium granulomatis.*

Vibramycin is an alternative drug in the treatment of gonorrhoea and syphilis.

Dermatological infections: Acne vulgaris when antibiotic therapy is considered necessary.

Since Vibramycin is a member of the tetracycline series of antibiotics, it may be expected to be useful in the treatment of infections which respond to other tetracyclines, such as:

Ophthalmic infections: Due to susceptible strains of gonococci, staphylococci, and *Haemophilus influenzae*. Vibramycin is indicated in the treatment of trachoma, although the infectious agent is not always eliminated, as judged by immunofluorescence. Inclusion conjunctivitis may be treated with oral Vibramycin alone or in combination with topical agents.

Rickettsial infections: Rocky Mountain spotted fever, typhus group, Q fever and Coxiella endocarditis and tick fevers.

Miscellaneous: Psittacosis, cholera, meliodosis, leptospirosis, other infections due to susceptible strains of *Yersinia* species, *Brucella* species (in combination with Streptomycin), *Clostridium* species, *Francisella tularensis* and chloroquine-resistant falciparum malaria.

Vibramycin is indicated for prophylaxis in the following conditions: Scrub typhus, travellers' diarrhoea (enterotoxigenic *Escherichia coli*), leptospirosis.

Dosage and administration

Adults: The usual dose of Vibramycin for the treatment of acute infections in adults is 200 mg on the first day (administered as a single dose or divided into two equal doses with a 12 hour interval), followed by a maintenance dose of 100 mg/day. In the management of more severe infections (particularly chronic infections of the urinary tract), 200 mg daily should be given throughout the treatment period.

Vibramycin capsules should be administered with adequate amounts of fluid. This should be done in the sitting or standing position and well before retiring for the night.

Vibramycin-D tablets are administered by drinking a suspension of the tablet in a small amount of water.

If gastric irritation occurs, it is recommended that Vibramycin be given with food or milk. Studies indicate that the absorption of Vibramycin is not notably influenced by simultaneous ingestion of food or milk.

Exceeding the recommended dosage may result in an increased incidence of side effects. Therapy should be continued at least 24 to 48 hours after symptoms and fever have subsided. When used in streptococcal infections, therapy should be continued for 10 days to prevent the development of rheumatic fever or glomerulonephritis.

Specific infections

Acne vulgaris: 50 mg daily with food or fluid for 6 to 12 weeks.

Sexually transmitted diseases: 100 mg twice daily for 7 days is recommended in the following infections: uncomplicated gonococcal infections (except anorectal infections in men); uncomplicated urethral, endocervical or rectal infection caused by *Chlamydia trachomatis*; non-gonococcal urethritis caused by *Ureaplasma urealyticum*.

Acute epididymo-orchitis caused by *Chlamydia trachomatis* or *Neisseria gonorrhoeae* 100 mg twice daily for 10 days.

Primary and secondary syphilis: 300 mg a day in divided doses for at least 10 days.

Louse- and tick-borne relapsing fevers: A single dose of 100 or 200 mg according to severity.

Chloroquine-resistant falciparum malaria: 200 mg daily for at least 7 days. Due to the potential severity of the infection, a rapid-acting schizonticide such as quinine should always be given in conjunction with Vibramycin; quinine dosage recommendations vary in different areas.

For the prevention of scrub typhus: 200 mg as a single dose.

For the prevention of travellers' diarrhoea in adults: 200 mg on the first day of travel (administered as a single dose or as 100 mg every 12 hours) followed by 100 mg daily throughout the stay in the area. Data on the use of the drug prophylactically are not available beyond 21 days.

For the prevention of leptospirosis: 200 mg once each week throughout the stay in the area and 200 mg at the completion of the trip. Data on the use of the drug prophylactically are not available beyond 21 days.

Use in children: See "Contra-indications".

Use in the elderly: Vibramycin may be prescribed in the usual dose with no special precautions. No dosage adjustment is necessary in the presence of renal impairment. The Vibramycin-D dispersible tablet may be preferred for the elderly since it is less likely to be associated with oesophageal irritation and ulceration.

Use in renal impairment: Studies to date have indicated that administration of Vibramycin at the usual recommended doses does not lead to excessive accumulation of the antibiotic in patients with renal impairment.

The anti-anabolic action of the tetracyclines may cause an increase in blood urea. Studies to date indicate that this does not occur with the use of Vibramycin in patients with impaired renal function.

Haemodialysis does not alter the serum half-life of Vibramycin.

Contra-indications, warnings, etc

Contra-indications: Vibramycin is contra-indicated in persons who have shown hypersensitivity to any of the tetracyclines.

The use of drugs of the tetracycline class during tooth development (pregnancy, infancy and childhood to the age of 12 years) may cause permanent discolouration of the teeth (yellow-grey-brown). This adverse reaction is more common during long term use of the drugs but has been observed following repeated short term courses. Enamel hypoplasia has also been reported. Vibramycin is, therefore, contra-indicated in these groups of patients.

Pregnancy: Vibramycin is contra-indicated in pregnancy.

Results of animal studies indicate that tetracyclines cross the placenta, are found in foetal tissues and can have toxic effects on the developing foetus (often related to retardation of skeletal development). Evidence of embryotoxicity has also been noted in animals treated early in pregnancy. (See above about use during tooth development.)

Nursing mothers: Tetracyclines are present in the milk of lactating women who are taking a drug of this kind and should therefore not be used in nursing mothers. (See above about use during tooth development.)

Children: Vibramycin is contra-indicated in children under the age of 12 years. As with other tetracyclines, Vibramycin forms a stable calcium complex in any bone-forming tissue. A decrease in the fibula growth rate has been observed in premature infants given oral tetracycline in doses of 25 mg/kg every 6 hours. This reaction was shown to be reversible when the drug was discontinued. (See above about use during tooth development.)

Warnings: Photosensitivity manifested by an exaggerated sunburn reaction has been observed in some individuals taking tetracyclines. Patients likely to be exposed to direct sunlight or ultraviolet light should be advised that this reaction can occur with tetracycline drugs and treatment should be discontinued at the first evidence of skin erythema.

Vibramycin should be administered with caution to patients with hepatic impairment or those receiving potentially hepatotoxic drugs.

Precautions: The use of antibiotics may occasionally result in over-growth of non-susceptible organisms. Constant observation of the patient is essential. If a resistant organism appears, the antibiotic should be discontinued and appropriate therapy instituted.

When treating venereal disease, where co-existent syphilis is suspected, proper diagnostic procedures, including dark-field examinations, should be utilised. In all such cases monthly serological tests should be made for at least four months.

Infections due to group A beta-haemolytic streptococci should be treated for at least 10 days.

Drug interactions: Because the tetracyclines have been shown to depress plasma prothrombin activity, patients who are on anticoagulant therapy may require downward adjustment of their anticoagulant dosage.

Since bacteriostatic drugs may interfere with the bactericidal action of penicillin, it is advisable to avoid giving Vibramycin in conjunction with penicillin.

Absorption of tetracyclines is impaired by antacids containing aluminium, calcium, magnesium or zinc, and iron-containing preparations.

Barbiturates, carbamazepine, and phenytoin decrease the half-life of doxycycline.

The concurrent use of tetracyclines and methoxyflurane has been reported to result in fatal renal toxicity.

Although not reported for Vibramycin, a few cases of pregnancy or breakthrough bleeding have been attributed to the concurrent use of tetracycline or oxytetracycline with oral contraceptives.

Side-effects: Due to virtually complete absorption of Vibramycin gastro-intestinal side-effects are infrequent. The following adverse reactions have been observed in patients receiving tetracyclines.

Gastro-intestinal: Anorexia, nausea, vomiting, diarrhoea, glossitis, dysphagia, enterocolitis, and inflammatory lesions (with monilial overgrowth) in the anogenital region. Oesophagitis and oesophageal ulceration have been reported in patients receiving Vibramycin. A significant proportion of these cases has occurred with the hydrochloride salt in the capsule form. Most of these patients took medication immediately before going to bed.

Skin: Maculopapular and erythematous rashes. Exfoliative dermatitis has been reported but is uncommon. Photosensitivity is discussed in the 'Warnings' section.

Renal toxicity: Rise in blood urea has been reported with tetracyclines and is apparently dose related.

Hypersensitivity reactions: Urticaria, angioneurotic oedema, anaphylaxis, anaphylactoid purpura, pericarditis, and exacerbation of systemic lupus erythematosus.

Bulging fontanelles in infants and benign intracranial hypertension in adults have been reported in some individuals receiving full therapeutic dosages. These conditions disappeared rapidly when the drug was discontinued.

Blood: Haemolytic anaemia, thrombocytopenia, neutropenia and eosinophilia have been reported with tetracyclines.

When given over prolonged periods, tetracyclines have been reported to produce brown-black microscopic discolouration of thyroid tissue. No abnormalities of thyroid function are known to occur.

Overdosage: Acute overdosage with antibiotics is rare. In the event of overdosage, gastric lavage plus appropriate supportive treatment is indicated.

Pharmaceutical precautions Storage: Store below 25°C.

Legal category POM.

Package quantities Vibramycin 100 mg capsules in blister strip of 8 capsules (original pack).

Vibramycin 50: 50 mg capsules in calendar packs of 28 (original pack).

Vibramycin D: 100 mg Dispersible tablets in blister strip of 8 (original pack).

Further information Nil.

Product licence numbers

Capsules 100 mg	0057/5059R
Capsules 50 mg	0057/0238
Dispersible tablets 100 mg	0057/0188

**Trade Mark*

Janssen Pharmaceutical Limited
Grove
Wantage
Oxfordshire OX12 0DQ

ANQUIL*

Presentation White, uncoated tablets marked 'JANSSEN' on one side and 'A' above '0.25' on the reverse. Each tablet contains 0.25 mg benperidol. The tablets also contain lactose.

Uses Anquil is a neuroleptic of the butyrophenone series for the control of deviant anti-social sexual behaviour.

Dosage and administration Anquil is intended for oral administration to adults only. The recommended daily dose is 0.25–1.5 mg in divided doses. Dosage is best initiated and adjusted under close clinical supervision, as individual response to neuroleptic drugs is variable.

In determining dosage, consideration should be given to the patient's age, severity of symptoms and previous response to other neuroleptic drugs.

In adolescents a lower dose may be advisable.

Use in elderly: Patients who are elderly or debilitated, or those with previously reported adverse reactions to neuroleptic drugs, may require less Anquil, and half the normal starting dose may be sufficient for therapeutic response.

Contra-indications, warnings, etc
Contra-indications: Comatose state, patients with extrapyramidal symptoms.

Use in pregnancy: The safety of Anquil in pregnancy has not been established, although studies in animals have not demonstrated teratogenic effects. As with other drugs, it is not advisable to administer Anquil in pregnancy.

Warnings: In common with all neuroleptics, Anquil can increase the central nervous system depression produced by other CNS-depressant drugs, including alcohol, hypnotics, sedatives, or strong analgesics, and may antagonise the action of adrenaline and other sympathomimetic agents.

Anquil may impair the anti-Parkinson effects of levodopa. The dosage of anti-convulsants may need to be increased to take account of the lowered seizure threshold.

Enhanced CNS effect, when combined with methyldopa, has been reported for some butyrophenones.

Acute withdrawal symptoms, including nausea, vomiting and insomnia, have very rarely been described after abrupt cessation of high doses of anti-psychotic drugs. Relapse may also occur and gradual withdrawal is advisable.

Precautions: Butyrophenones are excreted in breast milk and are not recommended during lactation. If the use of Anquil is considered essential, breast feeding should be discontinued.

Where prolonged treatment with Anquil is envisaged, it would be a reasonable precaution to carry out regular blood counts and tests of liver function.

Caution is advised in patients with liver disease, renal failure, Parkinson's disease, epilepsy, and conditions predisposing to epilepsy or convulsions.

Adverse effects: Some degree of sedation or impairment of alertness may occur, particularly with higher doses, and at the start of treatment, and may be potentiated by alcohol. Patients should be advised not to drive or operate machinery during treatment, until their susceptibility is known.

In common with all neuroleptics, extrapyramidal symptoms may occur. Acute dystonias may occur early in treatment. Parkinsonian rigidity, tremor and akathisia tend to appear less rapidly. Oculogyric crises and laryngeal dystonias have been reported.

Anti-Parkinson agents should only be given as required; they should not be prescribed routinely because of the possible risk of impairing Anquil's therapeutic efficacy.

Tardive dyskinesia may occur during administration or after withdrawal of neuroleptic drugs, including Anquil. The syndrome is common among patients treated with moderate to high doses of anti-psychotic drugs for prolonged periods of time and may prove irreversible, particularly in patients over the age of 50.

It is unlikely to occur in the short-term when low or moderate doses of Anquil are used as recommended, but since its occurrence may be related to duration of treatment as well as daily dose, Anquil should be given in the minimal effective dose for the minimum possible time.

The potential seriousness and unpredictability of tardive dyskinesia and the fact that it has occasionally been reported to occur when neuroleptic anti-psychotic drugs have been prescribed for relatively short periods in low dosage, means that the prescribing of such agents requires especially careful assessments of risks versus benefit. Tardive dyskinesia can be precipitated or aggravated by anti-Parkinson drugs. Tardive dyskinesias may occur after abrupt drug withdrawal.

Gastrointestinal symptoms, nausea, loss of appetite and dyspepsia have been reported.

Hormonal effects of anti-psychotic neuroleptic drugs include hyper-prolactinaemia, which may cause galactorrhoea, gynaecomastia and oligo- or amenorrhoea.

Weight changes may occur.

Dose-related hypotension is uncommon, but can occur, particularly in the elderly, who are more susceptible to the sedative and hypotensive effects.

Anquil, even in low dosage in susceptible (especially non-psychotic) individuals, may cause unpleasant subjective feelings of being mentally dulled or slowed down, dizziness, headache, or paradoxical effects of excitement, agitation or insomnia.

Jaundice, or transient abnormalities of liver function in the absence of jaundice, have been reported.

The following effects have been reported rarely: oedema, skin rashes or reactions, confusional or agitated states, epileptic fits.

Blood dyscrasias, including granulocytopenia, have been reported very rarely.

Overdosage: There have been no serious toxic effects attributed to Anquil and fatal overdosage has not been reported. Treatment of overdosage consists of supportive measures combined with sedative or anti-Parkinsonian drugs, as required.

Pharmaceutical precautions Protect from light.

Legal category POM.

Package quantities Anquil tablets, each containing 0.25 mg benperidol, are supplied in packs of 100.

Further information Nil.

Product licence number 0242/0014R.

DAKTACORT*

Presentation *Cream:* White, non-staining, water-miscible cream containing Miconazole Nitrate BP 2% w/w and Hydrocortisone PhEur 1% w/w. The cream also contains pegoxol stearate, polyoxyethylene glycol glycerides, mineral oil, benzoic acid, disodium edetate, butylated hydroxyanisole, purified water.

Ointment: White, odourless, fatty ointment containing Miconazole Nitrate BP 2.0% w/w and Hydrocortisone PhEur 1.0% w/w. The ointment also contains plastibase.

Uses For the topical treatment of inflamed dermatoses where infection by susceptible organisms and inflammation coexist e.g. intertrigo and infected eczema. For moist or dry eczema or dermatitis including atopic eczema, primary irritant or contact allergic eczema or seborrhoeic eczema including that associated with acne. Also for intertriginous eczema including inframammary intertrigo, perianal and genital dermatitis.

Organisms which are susceptible to miconazole are dermatophytes and pathogenic yeasts (e.g. Candida spp). Also many Gram-positive bacteria including many strains of Streptococcus and Staphylococcus.

Daktacort's properties indicate it particularly for the initial stages of treatment. Once the inflammatory symptoms have disappeared (after about 7 days), treatment can be continued where necessary with Daktarin* cream or powder.

Dosage and administration Daktacort cream and ointment should be applied topically to the affected area two or three times daily. The same dosage applies to both adults and children. In infants, long term continuous topical corticosteroid therapy should be avoided.

Occlusive dressing is usually only necessary in the case of nail lesions.

If after about 7 days of treatment no improvement has occurred, cultural isolation of the infecting organism should be followed by appropriate local or systemic antimicrobial therapy.

Use in the elderly: Natural thinning of the skin occurs in the elderly; hence corticosteroids should be used sparingly and for short periods of time.

Contra-indications, warnings, etc
Contra-indications; True hypersensitivity to any of the ingredients. Tubercular or viral infections of the skin or those caused by Gram-negative bacteria.

Precautions: As with any topical corticosteroid, care is advised with infants and children when Daktacort is to be applied to extensive surface areas or under occlusive dressings including baby napkins. Application to the face should be avoided.

Warning: In infants, long term continuous topical corticosteroid therapy should be avoided. Adrenal suppression can occur even without occlusion.

Use in pregnancy: In animals, miconazole nitrate has shown no teratogenic effects but is foetotoxic at high oral doses. Administration of corticosteroids to pregnant animals can cause abnormalities of foetal development. The relevance of these findings to humans has not been established. However, combinations of topical steroids with imidazoles should be used in pregnant women only if the practitioner considers them to be necessary.

Side-effects: Rarely, local sensitivity may occur requiring discontinuation of treatment.

Overdosage: Topically applied corticosteroids can be absorbed in sufficient amounts to produce systemic effects. If accidental ingestion of large quantities of the product occurs, an appropriate method of gastric emptying may be used if considered to be necessary.

Pharmaceutical precautions Store at room temperature.

Legal category POM.

Package quantities Daktacort ointment is supplied in 30 g tubes. Daktacort cream is supplied in 30 g tubes.

Further information Nil.

Product licence numbers

Daktacort Cream	0242/0042
Daktacort Ointment	0242/0130

DAKTARIN* CREAM, POWDER AND TWIN PACK

Presentation
Cream: White, non-staining, water miscible cream containing Miconazole Nitrate BP 2% w/w. The cream also contains pegoxol stearate, polyoxyethylene glycol glycerides, mineral oil, benzoic acid, butylated hydroxyanisole and purified water.

Powder: White, non-staining powder containing Miconazole Nitrate BP 2% w/w. The powder also contains talc, zinc oxide and colloidal silicon dioxide.

Twin pack: White, non-staining, water miscible cream containing Miconazole Nitrate BP 2% w/w plus white, non-staining powder containing Miconazole Nitrate BP 2% w/w.

Uses Miconazole nitrate is a synthetic imidazole antifungal agent with a broad spectrum of activity against pathogenic fungi (including yeasts and dermatophytes) and Gram-positive bacteria (Staphylococcus and Streptococcus spp.). Daktarin cream and powder are used for the topical treatment of fungal infections of the skin and secondary infections due to Gram-positive bacteria.

These include athlete's foot, ringworm (tinea infections), intertrigo, candida nappy rash, paronychia, erythrasma, fungal infection of the outer ear and pityriasis versicolor. Daktarin cream may also be used for nail infections.

Dosage and administration The dosage is the same for all ages.

Cream: Apply to the affected area twice daily. In nail infections, apply to the infected nail(s) once daily.

Powder: Apply twice daily to skin lesions, separately or with the cream. Daktarin powder may also be dusted inside articles of clothing in contact with the affected areas.

To prevent relapse, treatment should be continued for ten days after all the lesions have disappeared.

Use in elderly: As above.

Contra-indications, warnings, etc
Contra-indications: Daktarin powder is not recommended for nail and hair infections.

Use in pregnancy: In animals, miconazole nitrate has shown no teratogenic effects but is foetotoxic at high oral doses. Only small amounts of miconazole nitrate are absorbed following topical administration. However, as with other imidazoles, miconazole nitrate should be used with caution during pregnancy.

Side-effects: Occasionally irritation has been reported. Rarely local sensitisation or hypersensitivity may occur in which case administration of the product should be discontinued.

Overdosage: Daktarin cream and powder are intended for topical use. If accidental ingestion of large quantities of the product occurs, an appropriate method of gastric emptying may be used if considered desirable.

Pharmaceutical precautions
Cream: Store away from direct heat.

Powder: Store at room temperature.

Legal category P.

Package quantities
Cream: 30 g tube.
Powder: 20 g 'puffer' pack.
Twin Pack: Daktarin cream 30 g tube plus Daktarin powder 30 g 'puffer' pack.

Further information Daktarin twin pack and powder are particularly indicated for those infections involving moist areas of the body, especially athlete's foot.

A leaflet outlining to the patient the hygiene routines to be observed and the correct method of application of

Daktarin is included in each pack of cream, powder and in the twin pack.

Product licence numbers

Daktarin cream	0242/0016
Daktarin powder	0242/0017

DAKTARIN* ORAL GEL

Presentation Sugar-free, orange-flavoured oral gel containing Miconazole base USP 2% w/w.

Uses Miconazole is a synthetic imidazole antifungal agent with a broad spectrum of activity against pathogenic fungi (including yeasts and dermatophytes) and Gram-positive bacteria (Staphylococcus and Streptococcus spp.).

Miconazole is incompletely absorbed from the gastrointestinal tract.

Daktarin oral gel is indicated for the treatment and prevention of fungal infections of the oropharynx and gastrointestinal tract and of superinfections due to Gram-positive bacteria. This includes oral candidosis and denture stomatitis. Daktarin oral gel may be used prophylactically in the management of patients at high risk from opportunistic fungal infection. Patients likely to benefit from this treatment include those who are immunosuppressed such as transplant patients, cancer patients (particularly those undergoing cytotoxic therapy) and patients suffering from congenital immunological abnormalities.

Daktarin oral gel may also be used for the eradication of fungi from gut reservoirs when necessary (such as prior to relevant surgery or as an adjunct to local treatment of vulvo-vaginitis).

Dosage and administration Daktarin oral gel should be taken after meals. Dosage is based on 15 mg/kg/day (one 5 ml spoonful contains 125 mg miconazole).

Adults: One to two spoonfuls (5–10 ml) of gel four times daily.

Children aged 6 years and over: One spoonful (5 ml) of gel four times daily.

Children aged 2–6 years: One spoonful of gel (5 ml) twice daily.

Infants under 2 years: Half spoonful (2.5 ml) of gel twice daily.

Alternatively, for localised lesions of the mouth, a small amount of gel may be applied directly to the affected area with a clean finger, two to four times a day.

For best results in the treatment of oral lesions, miconazole should be kept in contact with the affected area for as long as possible. This can be achieved by retaining the gel in the mouth for the maximum time possible.

Treatment should be continued for up to two days after symptoms have cleared.

Use in elderly: As for adults.

Contra-indications, warnings, etc

Contra-indications: There are no known contra-indications to the use of miconazole oral gel.

Warnings: Systemic miconazole may potentiate the activity of anticoagulants, anti-epileptics, or hypoglycaemic drugs, the dosage of which may require adjustment.

Use in pregnancy: In animals, miconazole has shown no teratogenic effects but is foetotoxic at high oral doses. The significance of this to man is unknown. However, as with other imidazoles, Daktarin oral gel should be avoided in pregnant women if possible.

Side-effects: No major side-effects have been recorded from the use of Daktarin oral gel. Mild gastrointestinal disturbances have occasionally been reported.

Overdosage: In the event of overdosage, diarrhoea, convulsions and possibly cardiac rhythm disorders may occur. Gastric lavage should be applied followed by a purgative and supportive treatment as appropriate.

Pharmaceutical precautions Nil.

Legal category POM.

Package quantities Daktarin oral gel is supplied in 80 g tubes with a 5 ml plastic spoon, marked with a 2.5 ml graduation.

Further information Oral miconazole is also available as Daktarin oral tablets, supplied in blister packs of 20 tablets each containing miconazole base 250 mg. For details of dosage and administration refer to separate data sheet. Daktarin oral gel contains alcohol and glycerine.

Product licence number 0242/0048.

DAKTARIN* ORAL TABLETS

Presentation White, cross-scored tablets marked with 'Janssen' and M250 containing Miconazole base USP 250 mg. The tablets also contain lactose and sucrose.

Uses Miconazole is a synthetic imidazole anti-fungal agent with a broad spectrum of activity against pathogenic fungi (including yeasts and dermatophytes) and Gram-positive bacteria (staphylococcus and streptococcus spp.).

Miconazole is incompletely absorbed from the gastrointestinal tract.

Daktarin oral tablets are for the treatment (including prophylaxis) of fungal infections of the oropharynx and gastrointestinal tract and of superinfections due to Gram-positive bacteria.

Daktarin oral tablets may be used prophylactically in the management of patients at high risk from opportunistic fungal infection. Patients likely to benefit from this treatment include those who are immunosuppressed such as transplant patients, cancer patients (particularly those undergoing cytotoxic therapy) and patients suffering from congenital immunological abnormalities. Daktarin oral tablets may also be used for the eradication of fungi from gut reservoirs when necessary (such as prior to relevant surgery).

Dosage and administration Daktarin oral tablets should be taken after meals.

Dosage is based on 15 mg/kg/day.

Adults: One 250 mg tablet four times/day for 10 days or for up to 2 days after the symptoms have cleared.

Children: Use Daktarin oral gel.

Use in elderly: As for adults.

Topical treatment of the oropharynx may be achieved by sucking the tablet, allowing it to dissolve slowly in the mouth.

Contra-indications, warnings, etc

Contra-indications: There are no known contra-indications to the use of miconazole.

Warnings: Systemic miconazole may potentiate the activity of anticoagulants, anti-epileptics or hypoglycaemic drugs, the dosage of which may require adjustment.

Use in pregnancy: In animals, miconazole has shown no teratogenic effects but is foetotoxic at high oral doses. The significance of this to man is unknown. However as with other imidazoles, Daktarin oral tablets should be avoided in pregnant women if possible.

Side effects: No major side effects have been recorded from the use of Daktarin oral tablets. Mild gastrointestinal disturbances have occasionally been reported.

Overdosage: In the event of overdosage vomiting, diarrhoea, convulsions and possibly cardiac rhythm disorders may occur. Gastric lavage should be applied followed by a purgative and supportive treatment as appropriate.

Pharmaceutical precautions Nil.

Legal category POM.

Package quantities Daktarin oral tablets are supplied in blister packs of 20.

Further information Oral miconazole is also available

as a sugar-free orange flavoured gel containing miconazole base 2% w/w (25 mg/ml). Daktarin Oral Gel is supplied in a 80 g tube. For details of dosage and administration refer to separate data sheet.

Product licence number
Daktarin Oral Tablets 0242/0047

DAKTARIN* INTRAVENOUS SOLUTION

Presentation Clear glass ampoules (20 ml), each containing a sterile solution of Miconazole (base) USP 200 mg. 10% of polyethyoxylated castor oil is included as solvent. Injection also contains lactic acid, methyl and propyl parabens and water for injection.

Uses *Indications:* Daktarin intravenous solution is indicated for the treatment of systemic mycoses, such as systemic candidosis, aspergillosis, coccidioidomycosis, cryptococcosis, blastomycosis.

Actions: Miconazole, a synthetic imidazole compound, has a broad spectrum of *in vitro* activity against fungi, yeasts and Gram-positive bacteria, including *Candida albicans, Candida tropicalis, Candida parapsilosis, Aspergillus fumigatus, Aspergillus niger, Cryptococcus neoformans, Coccidioides immitis, Paracoccidioides brasiliensis*, and a range of other less commonly occurring pathogens.

Intravenous infusion of doses above 9 mg/kg produces effective peak blood levels in excess of 1 microgram/ml. The drug is rapidly metabolised. The pharmacokinetics are unaffected in patients with renal insufficiency, including those on haemodialysis. Plasma levels, however, may be somewhat elevated. Clinical use has revealed no evidence of serious renal or hepatic toxicity associated with intravenous miconazole.

Dosage and administration Daktarin intravenous solution must be diluted with either physiological saline (Sodium Chloride Injection BP) or 5% Dextrose Injection BP and administered slowly *by intravenous infusion* over a period of at least 30 minutes. The usual adult dose is 600 mg (3 ampoules) three times daily; as an infusion of 200–500 ml infusion fluid. The incidence of side effects or the sensitivity of the fungal strain involved may require individual adjustment of this dose.

As a guide, clinically effective daily doses have ranged from as low as 600 mg/day, in a few patients, to as high as 3,600 mg/day.

In children a daily dose of about 40 mg/kg is recommended. A dose of 15 mg/kg per infusion should not be exceeded.

Duration of treatment is dictated by the rate of response of the infection to miconazole. Treatment should be continued until mycological evidence of remission or cure is obtained. Daktarin intravenous solution has been used without major side-effects or toxicity for periods of over 20 weeks.

Use in elderly: As for adults – the incidence of side effects may require individual adjustment of the dose.

Contra-indications, warnings, etc
Contra-indications: Patients who are hypersensitive to Daktarin intravenous solution, since in animal studies polyethoxylated castor oil has been shown to produce adverse effects associated with histamine release, and similar anaphylactoid reactions have been observed in rare cases following Daktarin i.v.

Warnings: Rapid injection of a bolus of undiluted drug can produce transient tachycardia and cardiac arrhythmias. These, if not spontaneously reversible, usually respond promptly to lignocaine. Daktarin intravenous solution is well tolerated (including by patients with pre-existing cardiovascular disorders) if given by intravenous infusion.

Systemic miconazole may potentiate the activity of anti-coagulant, anti-epileptic or hypoglycaemic drugs, the dosage of which may require adjustment. Antagonism of the *in vitro* activity of miconazole by amphotericin B has been reported.

Use in pregnancy: In animals, miconazole has shown no teratogenic effects but is foetotoxic at high oral doses. The safety of Daktarin intravenous solution in human pregnancy has not been established and its use in pregnant women should be avoided if possible.

Side-effects: Haematological and biochemical controls are recommended since the infusion of Daktarin intravenous solution in large volumes of fluid may produce a decrease in haemoglobin, haematocrit and serum sodium. When polyethoxylated castor oil is given to patients over a period of several days, it may cause hyperlipidemia and an abnormal plasma lipoprotein electrophoretic pattern, aggregation of erythrocytes or rouleaux formation on blood smears. These effects are reversible on discontinuation of treatment and are not usually sufficiently severe to warrant discontinuation of intravenous miconazole.

The adverse reactions reported during clinical investigations of Daktarin intravenous solution are phlebitis, pruritus, nausea and vomiting, febrile reactions, rash, drowsiness, diarrhoea, anorexia and flushes. Using a subclavian catheter or changing the sites of infusion every 48–72 hours reduces the incidence and severity of phlebitis. Nausea and vomiting can be prevented by giving an antiemetic drug before infusion, by reducing the dose, by slowing the rate of infusion or by avoiding mealtime administration.

Overdosage: Symptoms of accidental overdosage are likely to be vomiting, diarrhoea, convulsions and possibly cardiac rhythm disorders. There is no specific antidote. Treat effects symptomatically and monitor for 24 hours.

Pharmaceutical precautions Storage should be at room temperature. Shelf life is five years. Daktarin intravenous solution should be mixed only with the recommended diluents, Sodium Chloride Injection BP or 5% Dextrose Injection BP.

Legal category POM.

Package quantities Daktarin intravenous solution is supplied in 20 ml glass ampoules, packed in boxes of ten. Each ampoule contains Miconazole (base) USP 200 mg.

Further information Miconazole's broad spectrum of antifungal activity and its lack of serious toxicity suggest that Daktarin intravenous solution may be considered for treatment in cases of life-threatening systemic fungal infection.

Product licence number 0242/0052.

DROLEPTAN*

Presentation *Injection:* Clear, colourless, aqueous injection in 2 ml ampoules. Each millilitre contains 5 mg droperidol. Injection also contains lactic acid and water for injection.

Tablets: Yellow uncoated, scored tablets marked 'JANSSEN' on one side and D above 10 on the reverse. Each tablet contains 10 mg droperidol. Tablets also contain lactose and E104.

Liquid: Clear, colourless, odourless liquid containing 1 mg droperidol/ml for oral administration. Liquid also contains methyl and propyl parabens.

Uses Droleptan is a major tranquilliser of the butyrophenone series with the following indications:

1. In anaesthesia:
   (a) in conjunction with a narcotic analgesic in the technique of neuroleptanalgesia;
   (b) either alone or in combination with a narcotic analgesic for premedication;
   (c) for post-operative nausea and vomiting.
2. For treatment of chemotherapy-induced nausea and vomiting.
3. In psychiatry for rapidly calming the manic, agitated patient.

Dosage and administration

Neuroleptanalgesia

Adults: 5–15 mg iv at induction of anaesthesia with a narcotic analgesic.
Children: 0.2–0.3 mg/kg iv.

Premedication in anaesthesia

Adults: Up to 10 mg im or oral.
Children: 0.2–0.5 mg/kg im or 0.3–0.6 mg/kg oral.

Anti-emetic

Post-operative
Adults: 5 mg iv or im;
Children: Doses used have ranged between 0.02–0.075 mg/kg im or iv dependent on emetic stimulus.

In cancer chemotherapy

Adults: Out-patients or those on mildly emetic therapy should receive the lowest recommended dose. Patients on more aggressive chemotherapy may require doses in the upper range of those recommended. Dosage must always be determined individually.

A loading dose of 1–10 mg i.m. or i.v. should be given 30 minutes before commencement of therapy, followed either by a continuous infusion of 1–3 mg/hr or 1–5 mg im or iv every 1–6 hours as required.
Children: Doses used have ranged between 0.02–0.075 mg/kg im or iv depending on emetic stimulus. Dosage must be determined individually using minimum effective dose.

In psychiatry

Adults: 5–15 mg iv; up to 10 mg im; 5–20 mg oral. The dosage may be repeated at intervals of 4–6 hours (im or iv) or 4–8 hours (oral).
Children: 0.5–1 mg/day im or oral adjusted according to response.

In pyschiatry, dosage should be individually determined and is best initiated and titrated under close clinical supervision. To determine the initial dose, consideration should be given to the patient's age, severity of symptoms, and previous response to other neuroleptic drugs.

Patients who are elderly or debilitated or those with previously reported adverse reactions to neuroleptic drugs, may require less Droleptan and half the normal starting dose in psychiatry may be sufficient for therapeutic response. The optimal response in such patients is usually obtained with more gradual titration and at lower dose levels. In adolescents a lower starting dose may be advisable.

Contra-indications, warnings, etc

Contra-indications: Comatose states, severe depression.

Use in pregnancy: The safety of Droleptan in pregnancy has not been established, although studies in animals have not demonstrated teratogenic effects. As with other drugs, it is not advisable to administer Droleptan in pregnancy.

Precautions: Butyrophenones are excreted in breast milk and are not recommended during lactation. If the use of Droleptan is essential, breast feeding should be discontinued.

Caution is advised in patients with liver disease, renal failure, Parkinson's disease, epilepsy, and conditions predisposing to epilepsy or convulsions.

In anaesthesia, intravenous induction agents will generally be required in lower dosage where Droleptan is used as part of the anaesthetic technique, and the effects of heavy sedative premedication may be potentiated. When using Droleptan at induction of anaesthesia, provision should be made for rapid infusion of intravenous fluid to correct any large fall in blood pressure, which, if it occurs, is due to relative hypovolaemia and is more common in the elderly or untreated hypertensives.

Warnings: In common with all neuroleptics, Droleptan can increase the central nervous system depression produced by other CNS-depressant drugs, including alcohol, hypnotics, sedatives or strong analgesics; and may antagonise the action of adrenaline and other sympathomimetic agents.

Droleptan may impair the anti-Parkinson effects of levodopa. The dosage of anti-convulsants may need to be increased to take account of the lowered seizure threshold.

Enhanced CNS effects, when combined with methyldopa, have been reported for some butyrophenones.

Acute withdrawal symptoms, including nausea, vomiting and insomnia, have very rarely been described after abrupt cessation of high doses of anti-psychotic drugs. Relapse may also occur and gradual withdrawal is advisable.

Adverse effects: Some degree of sedation or impairment of alertness may occur, particularly with higher doses and at the start of treatment and may be potentiated by alcohol. Patients should be advised not to drive or operate machinery during treatment until their susceptibility is known, or on the day following administration if early discharge is envisaged.

In common with all neuroleptics, extrapyramidal symptoms may occur. Acute dystonias may occur early in treatment. Parkinsonian rigidity, tremor and akathisia tend to appear less rapidly. Oculogyric crises and laryngeal dystonias have been reported. Extrapyramidal symptoms are less common at the low single doses used in anaesthesia or as an anti-emetic.

Anti-Parkinson agents should only be given as required; they should not be prescribed routinely because of the possible risk of impairing the therapeutic efficacy of Droleptan.

Tardive dyskinesia may occur during administration or after withdrawal of neuroleptic drugs, including Droleptan, and can be precipitated or aggravated by anti-Parkinson drugs. Tardive dyskinesia has not been reported following anti-emetic or anaesthetic uses of Droleptan.

The syndrome is unlikely to occur in the short-term when low or moderate doses of Droleptan are used as recommended, but since its occurrence may be related to duration of treatment, as well as daily dose, Droleptan should be given in the minimum effective dose for the minimum possible time.

The potential seriousness and unpredictability of tardive dyskinesia, and the fact that it has occasionally been reported to occur when neuroleptic anti-psychotic drugs have been prescribed for relatively short periods in low doses, means that the prescribing of such agents requires especially careful assessment of risks versus benefits.

Gastrointestinal symptoms, nausea, loss of appetite and dyspepsia, have been reported.

Hormonal effects of anti-psychotic neuroleptic drugs include hyper-prolactinaemia, which may cause galactorrhoea, gynaecomastia and oligo- or amenorrhoea.

Dose-related hypotension is uncommon, but can occur, particularly in the elderly, who are more susceptible to the sedative and hypotensive effects.

Droleptan, even in low dosage in susceptible (especially non-psychotic) individuals, may cause unpleasant subjective feelings of being mentally dulled or slowed down, dizziness, headache, or paradoxical effects of excitement, agitation or insomnia.

In common with other antipsychotics, droperidol may be associated with rare cases of neuroleptic malignant syndrome, an idiosyncratic response characterised by hyperthermia, muscle rigidity, autonomic instability, altered consciousness and coma. Signs of autonomic dysfunction such as tachycardia, labile arterial pressure and sweating may precede the onset of hyperthermia, acting as early warning signs. Recovery usually occurs within five to seven days of antipsychotic withdrawal. Affected patients should be carefully monitored. Dantrolene sodium, bromocriptine mesylate and ECT have all been reported as offering benefit in some patients with neuroleptic malignant syndrome.

The following effects have been reported rarely: oedema, various skin rashes and reactions, hypersensitivity, jaundice or transient abnormalities of liver function in the absence of jaundice; anxiety or confusional states or epileptic fits, vision disturbances, sweating.

Blood dyscrasias have been reported very rarely.

Overdosage: There have been no serious toxic effects attributed to Droleptan and fatal over-dosage has not been reported. Treatment of overdosage consists of supportive measures combined with sedative or anti-Parkinsonian drugs, as required.

Pharmaceutical precautions Droleptan preparations should be protected from light.

If desired, Droleptan injection can be mixed with intravenous infusion solutions and with most agents commonly used in anaesthesia, but it is chemically incompatible with the induction agents thiopentone and methohexitone, because of the wide difference in pH.

Legal category POM.

Package quantities Droleptan injection is supplied in 2 ml ampoules (5 mg/ml) in packs of 10.

Droleptan tablets each containing 10 mg droperidol are supplied in packs of 50.

Droleptan liquid is supplied in amber glass bottles of 100 ml and 500 ml (1 mg/ml).

Further information Nil.

Product licence numbers

Droleptan injection	0242/5003R
Droleptan tablets	0242/5004R
Droleptan liquid	0242/0080

GYNO-DAKTARIN*

Presentation *Cream:* White, non-staining, water miscible cream containing Miconazole Nitrate BP 2% w/w. Cream also contains benzoic acid, butylated hydroxyanisole, mineral oil, pegoxol 7 stearate, polyoxyethylene glycol glycerides, and purified water.

Pessary: White, non-staining pessaries each containing 100 mg Miconazole Nitrate BP.

Combi-pack: White, non-staining pessaries each containing 100 mg Miconazole Nitrate BP plus white, non-staining, water miscible cream containing Miconazole Nitrate BP 2% w/w.

Tampons: Tampons, each coated with 100 mg Miconazole Nitrate BP.

Ovule: Soft white Scherer capsule containing white fatty mass. Each capsule contains 1200 mg Miconazole Nitrate BP.

Uses Miconazole is a synthetic imidazole antifungal agent with a broad spectrum of activity against pathogenic fungi (including yeasts and dermatophytes) and Gram-positive bacteria (Staphylococcus and Streptococcus spp).

Gyno-Daktarin is for the local treatment of vulvovaginal candidosis and superinfection due to susceptible Gram-positive bacteria.

Gyno-Daktarin cream may also be used for treatment of mycotic balanitis.

Dosage and administration Gyno-Daktarin cream may be used in both adults and children. Gyno-Daktarin pessaries, tampons and ovules are for use in adults only.

Vaginitis: 5 g of the cream, or one pessary should be inserted twice daily high into the vagina. Disposable applicators are provided for insertion of the cream. This procedure should be repeated for 7 days, even though symptomatic cure of the pruritus and leukorrhoea will have been noted within a few days of commencing therapy.

Gyno-Daktarin Tampons: One tampon should be inserted high into the vagina twice daily (morning and evening) for 5 days.

Gyno-Daktarin 1: A single 1200 mg ovule should be inserted high into the vagina as a single dose at night.

Vulvitis or balanitis: The cream should be applied topically twice daily.

Use in elderly: As above.

Contra-indications, warnings, etc
Contra-indications: None known.

Use in pregnancy: In animals miconazole nitrate has shown no teratogenic effects but is foetotoxic at high oral doses. The significance of this to man is unknown as there is no evidence of an increased risk when taken in human pregnancy. However as with other imidazoles, Gyno-Daktarin should be used in pregnant women only if the practitioner considers it to be necessary.

Side-effects: Occasionally, irritation has been reported. Rarely, local sensitisation may occur requiring discontinuation of treatment.

Precautions: Contact should be avoided between contraceptive diaphragms or sheaths and Gyno-Daktarin pessaries or Gyno-Daktarin ovules since the rubber may be damaged by the emollient base.

Overdosage: Gyno-Daktarin preparations are for intravaginal or topical use only. If accidental ingestion of large quantities occurs, an appropriate method of gastric emptying may be used if considered desirable.

Pharmaceutical precautions Store in a cool place.

Legal category POM.

Package quantities *Cream:* Gyno-Daktarin cream is supplied in 78 g tubes with disposable applicators – seven days' treatment.

Pessary: Gyno-Daktarin pessaries are supplied in packs each containing 14 pessaries – seven days' treatment.

Combi-pack: Gyno-Daktarin combi-pack consists of 14 pessaries plus 15 g topical cream.

Tampons: Gyno-Daktarin tampons are supplied in packs each containing 10 tampons.

Ovule: Gyno-Daktarin 1 is supplied in packs containing 1 ovule, with finger stall.

Further information Gyno-Daktarin may be used in 'problem vaginitis' as seen in diabetic patients and in women using oral contraceptives.

A leaflet instructing the patient on the correct use is included in each package of Gyno-Daktarin.

Product licence numbers

Gyno-Daktarin Cream	0242/0015
Gyno-Daktarin Pessaries	0242/0037
Gyno-Daktarin Combi-Pack	0242/0015 0242/0037
Gyno-Daktarin Tampons	0242/0056
Gyno-Daktarin 1	0242/0121

HALDOL*

Presentation Pale blue, scored, uncoated tablets, marked Janssen on one side and H/5 on the reverse, containing 5 mg Haloperidol BP. The tablets also contain lactose and E132 as inactive ingredients.

Yellow, scored, uncoated tablets, marked Janssen on one side and H/10 on the reverse, containing 10 mg Haloperidol BP. The tablets also contain E104 as an inactive ingredient.

Clear, colourless, odourless liquid containing 2 mg Haloperidol BP per ml for oral administration. The liquid also contains methyl paraben as an inactive ingredient.

Clear, colourless, odourless liquid containing 10 mg Haloperidol BP per ml for oral administration following dilution (see pack insert). The liquid also contains methyl and propyl parabens as inactive ingredients.

Amber glass ampoules containing 5 mg Haloperidol BP in 1 ml aqueous solution for injection also containing lactic acid and water for injections as inactive ingredients.

Amber glass ampoules containing 10 mg Haloperidol BP in 2 ml aqueous solution for injection also containing lactic acid and water for injections as inactive ingredients.

Uses Haldol is a neuroleptic butyrophenone drug with a wide range of actions indicated in the following conditions:

Adults:

- Schizophrenia: treatment of symptoms and prevention of relapse.
- Other psychoses, especially paranoid.
- Mania and hypomania.
- Mental or behavioural problems such as aggression,

hyperactivity and self-mutilation in the mentally retarded and in patients with organic brain damage.
- As an adjunct to short-term management of moderate to severe psychomotor agitation, excitement, violent or dangerously impulsive behaviour.
- Intractable hiccup.
- Restlessness and agitation in the elderly.
- Gilles de la Tourette syndrome and severe tics.
- Nausea and vomiting.

Children (oral administration only):
- Childhood behavioural disorders especially when associated with hyperactivity and aggression.
- Gilles de la Tourette syndrome.
- Childhood schizophrenia.

Dosage and administration Dosage for all indications should be individually determined and is best initiated and titrated under close clinical supervision. To determine the initial dose, consideration should be given to the patient's age, severity of symptoms and previous response to other neuroleptics.

Patients who are elderly or debilitated or those with previously reported adverse reactions to neuroleptic drugs may require less Haldol. The normal starting dose should be halved, followed by a gradual titration to achieve optimal response.

Oral administration

Adults

Schizophrenia, psychoses, mania and hypomania, mental or behavioural problems, psychomotor agitation, excitement, violent or dangerously impulsive behaviour, organic brain damage.

Initial dosage:

Moderate symptomatology 1.5–3.0 mg b.d. or t.d.s.

Severe symptomatology/resistant patients 3.0–5.0 mg b.d. or t.d.s.

In resistant schizophrenics, daily dosages up to 100 mg (or rarely 200 mg) may be necessary to achieve an optimal response.

The same starting doses may be employed in adolescents, who, in certain cases, may require up to 30 mg or, exceptionally, up to 60 mg/day.

Maintenance dosage: Once satisfactory control of symptoms has been achieved dosage should be gradually reduced to the lowest effective maintenance dose, often as low as 5 or 10 mg/day. Too rapid a dosage reduction should be avoided.

Restlessness or agitation in the elderly: Initial dose 1.5–3.0 mg b.d. or t.d.s. titrated as required, to attain an effective maintenance dose (1.5–50 mg daily).

Gilles de la Tourette syndrome, severe tics, intractable hiccup: Starting dose 1.5 mg t.d.s. adjusted according to response. A daily maintenance dose of 10 mg may be required in Gilles de la Tourette syndrome.

Children

Childhood behavioural disorders/schizophrenia: Total daily maintenance dose of 0.025–0.05 mg/kg/day. Half the total dose should be given in the morning and the other half in the evening, up to a maximum of 10 mg daily.

Gilles de la Tourette syndrome: Oral maintenance doses of up to 10 mg/day in most patients.

Parenteral administration

Adults

Schizophrenia, psychoses, mania and hypomania, mental or behavioural problems, psychomotor agitation, excitement, violent or dangerously impulsive behaviour, organic brain damage: For control of acutely agitated patients with moderate symptoms: 2–10 mg im.

Severely disturbed patients may require an initial dose of up to 30 mg.

Depending on the response of the patient, subsequent doses may be given every 4–8 hours, although it may be given every hour, if necessary.

Oral treatment should succeed intramuscular administration as soon as practicable. Bioavailability from the oral route is about 40% of that from the im route, and readjustment of dose may be required.

Haldol can also be administered by the iv route.

Nausea and vomiting: 1–2 mg im.

Children: Not recommended for parenteral use in children.

Contra-indications, warnings, etc

Contra-indications: Comatose states, patients with Parkinson's disease or a sensitivity to haloperidol.

Use in pregnancy and lactation: The safety of haloperidol in pregnancy has not been established. There is some evidence of harmful effects in some but not all animal studies. Human experience suggests there may be teratogenic effects, although a causal relationship has not been established.

Haloperidol is excreted in breast milk. If the use of haloperidol is considered essential, breast feeding should be discontinued.

Precautions and warnings: Please also refer to 'Drug interactions' section.

Caution is advised in patients with liver disease, renal failure, phaeochromocytoma, thyrotoxicosis, epilepsy, and conditions predisposing to epilepsy (eg alcohol withdrawal and brain damage) or convulsions.

Rare cases of sudden and unexplained death have been reported in psychiatric patients receiving antipsychotic drugs, including haloperidol. The nature of the evidence makes it impossible to determine the contributory role, if any, of the drug.

Acute withdrawal symptoms including nausea, vomiting and insomnia have very rarely been described after abrupt cessation of high doses of antipsychotic drugs. Relapse may also occur and gradual withdrawal is advisable.

In schizophrenia, the response to antipsychotic drug treatment may be delayed. If drugs are withdrawn, recurrence of symptoms may not become apparent for several weeks or months.

Some degree of sedation or impairment of alertness may occur, particularly with higher doses and at the start of treatment and may be potentiated by alcohol. Patients should be advised not to drive or operate machinery during treatment, until their susceptibility is known.

Drug interactions: In common with all neuroleptics, haloperidol can increase the central nervous system depression produced by other CNS-depressant drugs, including alcohol, hypnotics, sedatives or strong analgesics. An enhanced CNS effect, when combined with methyldopa, has been reported.

Haloperidol may antagonise the action of adrenaline and other sympathomimetic agents and reverses the blood pressure lowering effects of adrenergic-blocking agents such as guanethidine.

Haloperidol may impair the metabolism of tricyclic antidepressants (clinical significance unknown) and the antiparkinson effects of levodopa. The dosage of anticonvulsants may need to be increased to take account of the lowered seizure threshold.

Antagonism of the effect of phenindione has been reported.

Neurotoxic reactions during combined treatment with lithium and haloperidol have been reported, although there is no known mechanism for this effect. One report showing symptomless EEG abnormalities on the combination has suggested that EEG monitoring might be advisable. It is recommended that lithium levels should always be maintained below 1 mmol/l when combined with haloperidol. If unexplained pyrexia occurs in the presence of extrapyramidal side effects both lithium and haloperidol should be stopped immediately.

Adverse effects: In common with all neuroleptics, extrapyramidal symptoms may occur. Acute dystonias may occur early in treatment. Parkinsonian rigidity, tremor and akathisia tend to appear less rapidly. Oculogyric crises and laryngeal dystonias have been reported. Antiparkinson agents should not be prescribed routinely, but only be given as required, because of the possible risk of impairing the efficacy of Haldol.

Tardive dyskinesia may occur during administration or after withdrawal of neuroleptic drugs, including Haldol, and can be precipitated or aggravated by antiparkinson drugs. The syndrome is unlikely to occur in the short term when low or moderate doses of Haldol are used as recommended. However since its occurrence may be related to duration of treatment, as well as daily dose, Haldol should be given in the minimum effective dose for the minimum possible time, unless it is established that long term administration for the treatment of schizophrenia is required.

The potential seriousness and unpredictability of tardive dyskinesia, and the fact that it has occasionally been reported to occur when neuroleptic antipsychotic drugs have been prescribed for relatively short periods in low doses, means that the prescribing of such agents requires especially careful assessment of risks versus benefit.

In common with other antipsychotic drugs, haloperidol has been associated with rare cases of neuroleptic malignant syndrome (NMS), an idiosyncratic response characterised by hyperthermia, muscle rigidity, autonomic instability, altered consciousness, coma and elevated CPK. Signs of autonomic dysfunction such as tachycardia, labile arterial pressure and sweating may precede the onset of hyperthermia, acting as early warning signs. Antipsychotic treatment should be withdrawn immediately and appropriate supportive therapy and careful monitoring instituted. Dantrolene, bromocriptine, anticholinergics, amantadine or ECT have been used in the active treatment of NMS.

Gastrointestinal symptoms, nausea, loss of appetite and dyspepsia have been reported.

Hormonal effects of antipsychotic neuroleptic drugs include hyperprolactinaemia, which may cause galactorrhoea, gynaecomastia and oligo- or amenorrhoea.

Weight changes may occur.

Dose related hypotension is uncommon, but can occur, particularly in the elderly, who are more susceptible to the sedative and hypotensive effects. Cardiac effects such as ventricular arrhythmias have been reported very rarely.

Haloperidol, even in low dosage in susceptible (especially non-psychotic) individuals, may cause unpleasant subjective feelings of being mentally dulled or slowed down, dizziness, headache or paradoxical effects of excitement, agitation or insomnia.

The following effects have been reported rarely: oedema, various skin rashes and reactions, including exfoliative dermatitis and erythema multiforme; jaundice or transient abnormalities of liver function in the absence of jaundice; confusional states or epileptic fits; impairment of sexual function, including erection and ejaculation.

The following have been reported very rarely: blood dyscrasias, including agranulocytosis and transient leucopenia, and photosensitive skin reactions.

Autonomic effects such as blurring of vision are uncommon.

Overdose: In general, the signs and symptoms of overdosage would be an exaggeration of known pharmacological effects, the most prominent of which would be severe extrapyramidal symptoms, hypotension or sedation. The patient may appear comatose with respiratory depression and hypotension which could be severe enough to produce a shock-like state.

There is no specific antidote to haloperidol. Gastric lavage, establishment of a patent airway and, if necessary, mechanically assisted respiration are advised. Electrocardiographic monitoring should commence immediately and continue for as long as clinically indicated. Hypotension and circulatory collapse may be counteracted by the use of intravenous fluids and vasopressor agents such as noradrenaline. Adrenaline should NOT be used (see interactions).

Pharmaceutical precautions Store tablets in a cool dry place. Haldol liquid concentrate and oral solution should be stored at room temperature.

Dilution instructions for oral concentrate: Haldol oral liquid concentrate 10 mg/ml should be diluted before use. The recommended diluent is an aqueous solution of methyl paraben (0.5 mg/ml) and propyl paraben (0.05 mg/ml), which maintains the original concentrations of preservatives. Water should not be used to dilute the product. The diluted liquid should be stored in amber glass screw-cap bottles. When following these recommendations the diluted liquid may be stored for up to two months.

Legal catelgory POM.

Further information Nil.

Package quantities

5.0 mg tablet	: 100 in canisters
10.0 mg tablet	: 100 in canisters
5 mg/ml injectable solution	: 5 × 1 ml ampoules
10 mg/2 ml injectable solution	: 5 × 2 ml ampoules
2 mg/ml oral solution	: 100 ml amber glass bottles with calibrated pipette
10 mg/ml oral liquid	: 100 ml amber glass bottles with insert leaflet

Product licence numbers

5.0 mg tablet	0242/0031R
10.0 mg tablet	0242/0039R
5 mg/ml injectable solution	0242/0036R
10 mg/2 ml injectable solution	0242/0036R
2 mg/ml oral liquid	0242/0035R
10 mg/ml oral liquid	0242/0049

HALDOL* DECANOATE

Presentation Straw coloured, viscous solution presented in 1 ml brown glass ampoules equivalent to 100 mg/ml haloperidol (as decanoate ester) and in 1 ml brown glass ampoules containing haloperidol 50 mg/ml (as decanoate ester). Both solutions also contain benzyl alcohol and sesame oil as inactive ingredients.

Uses Haldol Decanoate is an ester of the potent butyrophenone neuroleptic, haloperidol. The active agent is slowly released from an intramuscular depot injection of Haldol Decanoate. Haldol Decanoate is indicated where long term maintenance treatment with a neuroleptic is required; for example in schizophrenia, other psychoses (especially paranoid), and other mental or behavioural problems where maintenance treatment is clearly indicated.

Dosage and administration Haldol Decanoate is for use in adults only and has been formulated to provide one month's therapy for most patients following a single deep intramuscular injection in the gluteal region.

Since individual response to neuroleptic drugs is variable, dosage should be individually determined and is best initiated and titrated under close clinical supervision.

The size of the initial dose will depend on both the severity of the symptomatology and the amount of oral medication required to maintain the patient before starting depot treatment.

An initial dose of 50 mg every four weeks is recommended, increasing if necessary by 50 mg increments to 300 mg every four weeks. If, for clinical reasons, two-weekly administration is preferred these doses should be halved.

In patients with severe symptomatology, or in those who required large oral doses as maintenance therapy, higher doses of Haldol decanoate will be required. However, clinical experience with Haldol decanoate at doses greater than 300 mg per month is limited.

Routine administration of volumes greater than 3 mls at any one injection site is not recommended as larger volumes of injection are uncomfortable for the patient.

Haldol decanoate should be administered deep intramuscularly with a 2–2.5 inch long needle of at least 21 gauge.

For patients previously maintained on oral neroleptics, an approximate guide to the starting dose of Haldol decanoate is as follows: 500 mg of chlorpromazine a day is equivalent to 100 mg of Haldol decanoate monthly.

The approximate equivalence for transferring patients previously maintained on fluphenazine decanoate or flupenthixol decanoate is as follows: 25 mg of fluphenazine decanoate 2-weekly or 40 mg of flupenthixol decanoate 2-weekly is equivalent to 100 mg of Haldol decanoate monthly. This dose should be adjusted to suit the individual patient's response.

Use in elderly: It is recommended to start with low doses, for example 12.5 mg–25 mg every four weeks, only increasing the dose according to the individual patient's response.

Contra-indications, warnings, etc
Contra-indications: Comatose states, patients with Parkinson's disease or a sensitivity to haloperidol.

Haloperidol is excreted in breast milk. If the use of haloperidol decanoate is considered essential, breast feeding should be discontinued.

Use in pregnancy and lactation: See 'Contra-indications'.

The safety of haloperidol in pregnancy has not been established. There is some evidence of harmful effects in some but not all animal studies. Human experience suggests there may be teratogenic effects, although a causal relationship has not been established.

Precautions and warnings: Please also refer to 'Drug interactions' section.

Caution is advised in patients with liver disease, renal failure, phaeochromocytoma, thyrotoxicosis, epilepsy and conditions predisposing to epilepsy (e.g. alcohol withdrawal and brain damage) or convulsions.

In schizophrenia, the response to antipsychotic drug treatment may be delayed. If drugs are withdrawn, recurrence of symptoms may not become apparent for several weeks or months.

Some degree of sedation or impairment of alertness may occur, particularly with higher doses and at the start of treatment. Patients should be advised not to drive or operate machinery during treatment, until their susceptibility is known.

Drug interactions: In common with all neuroleptics, haloperidol can increase the central nervous system depression produced by other CNS-depressant drugs, including alcohol, hypnotics, sedatives or strong analgesics. An enhanced CNS effect, when combined with methyldopa has been reported.

Haloperidol may antagonise the action of adrenaline and other sympathomimetic agents and reverses the blood pressure lowering effects of adrenergic-blocking agents such as guanethedine.

Haloperidol may impair the metabolism of tricyclic anti-depressants (clinical significance unknown) and the antiparkinson effects of levodopa. The dosage of anticonvulsants may need to be increased to take account of the lowered seizure threshold.

Antagonism of the effect of phenindione has been reported.

Whilst neurotoxic reactions to combined treatment with lithium and haloperidol have been reported, there have been no such reports relating to combined haloperidol decanoate and lithium. There is no known mechanism for this suggested neurotoxicity, however, one report showing EEG abnormalities alone on the combination has suggested that EEG monitoring might be advisable. In any case it is recommended that lithium levels should always be maintained below 1 mmol/L when combined with haloperidol. If unexplained pyrexia occurs in the presence of extrapyramidal side-effects, both lithium and haloperidol should be stopped immediately.

Adverse effects: In common with all neuroleptics, extrapyramidal symptoms may occur. Acute dystonias may occur early in treatment. Parkinsonian rigidity, tremor and akathisia tend to appear less rapidly. Oculogyric crises and laryngeal dystonias have been reported.

Antiparkinson agents should not be prescribed routinely, but only be given as required, because of the possible risk of impairing the efficacy of haloperidol. Preliminary results suggest that withdrawal of antiparkinson medication may be attempted following transfer from oral medication to monthly depot injections of Haldol Decanoate.

Tardive dyskinesia is common among patients treated with moderate to high doses of antipsychotic drugs for prolonged periods of time and may prove irreversible, particularly in patients over 50 years.

The potential seriousness and unpredictability of tardive dyskinesia and the fact that it has occasionally been reported to occur when neuroleptic antipsychotic drugs have been prescribed for relatively short periods in low doses means that the prescribing of such agents requires especially careful assessment of risk versus benefit. Tardive dyskinesia can be precipitated or aggravated by antiparkinson drugs.

In common with other antipsychotic drugs, haloperidol has been associated with rare cases of neuroleptic malignant syndrome (NMS), an idiosyncratic response characterised by hyperthermia, muscle rigidity, autonomic instability, altered consciousness, coma and elevated CPK. Signs of autonomic dysfunction such as tachycardia, labile arterial pressure and sweating may precede the onset of hyperthermia, acting as early warning signs. Antipsychotic treatment should be withdrawn immediately and appropriate supportive therapy and careful monitoring instituted. Dantrolene, bromocriptine, anticholinergics, amantadine or ECT have been used in the active treatment of NMS.

Gastrointestinal symptoms, nausea, loss of appetite and dyspepsia have been reported.

Hormonal effects of antipsychotic neuroleptic drugs include hyperprolactinaemia, which may cause galactorrhoea, gynaecomastia and oligo- or amenorrhoea.

Weight changes may occur.

Dose-related hypotension is uncommon, but can occur, particularly in the elderly, who are more susceptible to the sedative and hypotensive effects. Cardiac effects such as ventricular, arrhythmias have been reported very rarely.

Haloperidol, even in low dosage in susceptible (especially non-psychotic) individuals, may cause unpleasant subjective feelings of being mentally dulled or slowed down, dizziness, headache or paradoxical effects of excitement, agitation or insomnia.

The following effects have been reported rarely: oedema; various skin rashes and reactions, including exfoliative dermatitis and erythema multiforme; jaundice or transient abnormalities of liver function in the absence of jaundice; confusional states or epileptic fits; impairment of sexual function, including erection and ejaculation.

The following effects have been reported very rarely; blood dyscrasias, including agranulocytosis and transient leucopenia, and photosensitive skin reactions.

Autonomic effects such as blurring of vision are uncommon.

Occasional local reactions such as erythema, swelling or tender lumps have been reported.

Overdose: In general, the signs and symptoms of overdosage would be an exaggeration of known pharmacological effects, the most prominent of which would be severe extrapyramidal symptoms, hypotension or sedation. The patient may appear comatose with respiratory depression and hypotension which could be severe enough to produce a shock-like state.

There is no specific antidote to haloperidol. Establishment of a patent airway and, if necessary, mechanically assisted respiration are advised. Electrocardiographic monitoring should commence immediately and continue for as long as clinically indicated. Hypotension and circulatory collapse may be counteracted by the use of intravenous fluids, plasma or concentrated albumin and vasopressor agents such as noradrenaline. Adrenaline should not be used. (See 'Drug interactions' section).

In cases of severe extrapyramidal symptoms, antiparkinson medication should be administered.

Pharmaceutical precautions Haldol Decanoate should be protected from light and stored at room temperature. In common with other depot neuroleptics, if stored for long periods in the cold, precipitation may occur which may clear on storage at room temperature. If precipitate does not clear, the contents of the ampoule should be discarded. Do not store below room temperature.

Further information Nil.

Legal category POM.

Package quantities 100 mg/ml ampoules: 1 ml ampoules in packs of 5. 50 mg/ml ampoules: 1 ml ampoules in packs of 5.

Product licence numbers

50 mg/ml	0242/0094
100 mg/ml	0242/0095

HISMANAL*

Presentation White, biconvex, half-scored, uncoated tablets. Each tablet is marked 'Janssen' on one side and 'Ast/10' on the reverse, and contains astemizole 10 mg. Hismanal tablets also contain lactose. White suspension with a fruity flavour containing astemizole 1 mg/ml in 200 ml amber glass bottles. Hismanal suspension also contains sorbitol and alcohol.

Uses Hismanal is a long acting antihistamine (H_1-antagonist) characterised by a lack of sedative potential.

Hismanal is indicated for allergic rhinitis and conjunctivitis and other conditions normally responsive to antihistamines, including allergic skin reactions (urticaria).

Dosage and administration
Adults and children over 12 years: The daily dose is 10 mg as a single intake, which should not be exceeded.

Children 6–12 years: The daily dose is 5 mg (½ a tablet or 5 ml), which should not be exceeded.

Children under 6 years: There have been no specific studies in children under 6 years therefore the drug is not indicated in this age group.

Use in elderly: There have been no specific studies in the elderly.

Contra-indications, warnings, etc
Contra-indications: Hismanal is contra-indicated in women who are pregnant.

Precautions: Because of the risk of developing serious ventricular arrhythmias at very high doses, the recommended dose of Hismanal should not be exceeded.

Adequate contraceptive precautions should be taken by women of childbearing potential during therapy, and, in view of the prolonged half-life, for several weeks after stopping.

Specific studies of possible human liver enzyme induction have been carried out with negative results. There is, therefore, no reason to suggest any modification of oral contraceptive dosage in users of Hismanal.

Use in pregnancy: Like many other antihistamines, Hismanal has been associated with adverse effects on the maintenance of pregnancy in rats. No teratogenic effects were observed in animal studies with Hismanal.

The safety of Hismanal in human pregnancy has not been established. Therefore it is contra-indicated during pregnancy.

Since astemizole is excreted in breast milk, it should not be used by nursing mothers.

Adverse reactions: Ventricular arrhythmias have occurred at very high doses – see 'Overdose' section. As might be expected with Hismanal's lack of sedative potential, sedation has been reported extremely rarely. It should be recognised that, in controlled clinical trials, the incidence of sedation with Hismanal has been no greater than that with placebo. Weight gain has occasionally been reported.

Overdosage: In cases of overdosage, emesis and gastric lavage should be followed by close observation. In particular, ECG monitoring should be instituted as serious ventricular arrhythmias have occurred infrequently. Studies in patients with renal insufficiency suggest that haemodialysis does not increase clearance of the drug.

Pharmaceutical precautions Nil.

Legal category POM.

Package quantities Supplied in packs of 30 tablets. Amber glass bottles containing 200 ml suspension (1 mg/ml).

Further information Although clinical trials have shown no interaction between Hismanal and diazepam or alcohol, care should be taken to caution the patient against excessive alcohol intake while on medication. Controlled clinical trials with placebo and reference antihistamines have demonstrated that Hismanal is non-sedative, and should not therefore interfere with activities requiring mental alertness, for example, driving or operating machinery.

Nevertheless as with other medications, patients should exert caution when undertaking such activities following the first dose of Hismanal.

Product licence numbers

Hismanal tablets	0242/0086
Hismanal suspension	0242/0111

HYPNOMIDATE*

Presentation Clear, colourless solution containing 2 mg/ml etomidate. The aqueous vehicle contains 35% propylene glycol and water for injection.

Uses Hypnomidate is an intravenous induction agent.

Dosage and administration In adults and children a dose of 0.3 mg/kg given intravenously at induction of anaesthesia gives sleep lasting from 6 to 10 minutes.

Since Hypnomidate has no analgesic action, appropriate analgesics should be used in procedures involving painful stimuli. Hypnomidate is pharmacologically compatible with the muscle relaxants, premedicant drugs and inhalation anaesthetics in current clinical use.

Use in elderly: As for adults.

Contra-indications, warnings, etc
Contra-indications: There are no absolute contra-indications to the use of Hypnomidate.

Warnings: Reduced serum cortisol levels unresponsive to ACTH injections have been reported in some patients during maintenance of anaesthesia with etomidate; for this reason etomidate should not be used for maintenance. However, when etomidate is used for induction, the post-operative rise in serum cortisol which has been observed after thiopentone induction is delayed for approximately 3–6 hours.

Hypnomidate should not be administered to patients with evidence, or suggestion of, reduced adrenal cortical function. Convulsions may occur in unpremedicated patients.

Side-effects: The use of narcotic analgesics as premedication and during surgery will reduce the uncontrolled spontaneous muscle movements shown by some patients after Hypnomidate administration.

Pain can occur after injection into the small veins of the dorsum of the hand. Use of larger veins reduces pain on injection.

Other side-effects are rare.

Precautions: Hypnomidate by injection should be given slowly.

Use in pregnancy: Although animal studies have produced no evidence of any embryotoxic or teratogenic effects, safety in human pregnancy has not been established. As with other drugs, the possible risks should be weighed against the potential benefits before the drug is administered during pregnancy.

Overdosage: Overdosing is likely to result in prolonged anaesthesia. General supportive measures and close observation are recommended.

Pharmaceutical precautions Store at room temperature. Hypnomidate may be diluted with Sodium Chloride

Infusion BP or Dextrose Infusion BP but it is not compatible with compound Sodium Lactate Infusion BP (Hartmann's solution). Combinations with pancuronium bromide may show a very slight opalescence; for this reason the two should not be mixed together.

Legal category POM.

Package quantities Hypnomidate is supplied as 10 ml ampoules in packs of 10.

Further information Hypnomidate is rapidly metabolised and eliminated and recovery of consciousness from a single dose is rapid and complete.

Product licence number 0242/0019.

HYPNOMIDATE* CONCENTRATE

Presentation Concentrate for dilution: Clear, colourless liquid presented in 1 ml ampoules. Each millilitre contains etomidate hydrochloride equivalent to 125 mg etomidate base in dehydrated alcohol. One ampoule should be sufficient for 4–5 inductions.

Uses Hypnomidate is a short-acting intravenous hypnotic drug which may be used for induction of anaesthesia.

Dosage and administration
In adults (including the elderly): The contents of the ampoule should be withdrawn into a glass syringe and immediately added to a 50 ml glass bottle, containing Sodium Chloride or Dextrose Intravenous Infusion BP, and the contents thoroughly mixed. 8–10 ml of the solution should then be withdrawn for use as a bolus injection (approx dose 0.3 mg/kg).

Following withdrawal of the concentrate from the ampoule, the entire contents should be added to the diluent immediately. The diluted solution should be used within 12 hours.

In high risk patients, slow induction may be desirable, in which case, anaesthesia may be induced by up to 0.1 mg/kg/minute until anaesthesia is obtained. The patient should fall asleep after about 3 minutes. Some loss of activity can occur through infusion sets but the clinical response should be used to determine the rate of infusion and thus the dose of the drug required by the individual patient.

Since Hypnomidate has no analgesic action, appropriate analgesics should be used in procedures involving painful stimuli. Hypnomidate is pharmacologically compatible with the muscle relaxants, premedicant drugs and inhalation anaesthetics in current clinical use.

Use in children: Not recommended.

Contra-indications, warnings, etc
Contra-indications: There are no absolute contra-indications to the use of Hypnomidate.

Use in pregnancy: Safety in human pregnancy has not been established although studies in animals have not demonstrated teratogenic effects. As with other drugs, the risk should be weighed against potential benefit to the patient.

Warnings: The concentrate must be diluted before use. Hypnomidate should be given slowly.

Reduced serum cortisol levels, unresponsive to ACTH injections, have been reported in some patients during maintenance of anaesthesia with etomidate; for this reason etomidate should not be used for maintenance. However, when etomidate is used for induction, the post-operative rise in serum cortisol which has been observed after thiopentone induction is delayed for approximately 3–6 hours.

Hypnomidate should not be administered to patients with evidence, or suggestion, of reduced adrenal cortical function. Convulsions may occur in the unpremedicated patient.

Side-effects: The use of narcotic analgesics as premedication and during surgery will reduce the uncontrolled spontaneous muscle movement shown by some patients after Hypnomidate administration.

Pain can occur after administration into the small veins of the dorsum of the hand. Use of larger veins reduces pain on injection; venous irritation has also been occasionally reported following Hypnomidate infusions. Other side effects are rare.

Pharmaceutical precautions Store at room temperature. Hartmann's Solution is not recommended for use with Hypnomidate. Combinations with pancuronium bromide may show a very slight opalescence; for this reason the combination is not to be recommended. A pharmaceutical overfill of 0.1 ml is included in each 1 ml ampoule of the concentrate.

Since an interaction between Hypnomidate concentrate and syringes containing styrene/acrylonitrile copolymer has been reported, plastic syringes should not be used for withdrawal of the contents of the ampoule.

Only glass syringes should be used.

Once opened, the entire contents of the ampoule should be diluted immediately and once diluted, the solution should be used within 12 hours.

Legal category POM.

Package quantities Pack of 10 ampoules.

Further information Nil.

Product licence number 0242/0123.

IMODIUM*

Presentation *Capsules:* Hard gelatin capsules with a dark green, opaque cap and a standard grey opaque body. Each capsule contains loperamide hydrochloride 2 mg. Each capsule also contains lactose E132, E172, E171, E127.

Syrup: Red, fruity flavoured syrup containing loperamide hydrochloride 1 mg in 5 ml. The syrup also contains methyl and propyl parabens, alcohol and E120.

Uses
Mode of action: Imodium binds to the opiate receptor in the gut wall, reducing propulsive peristalsis, increasing intestinal transit time and enhancing resorption of water and electrolytes. Imodium does not change the physiological flora. Imodium increases the tone of the anal sphincter. Imodium does not act centrally because, due to its high affinity for the gut wall and its high first pass metabolism, very little reaches the systemic circulation.

Indications: Imodium is indicated for the symptomatic treatment of acute diarrhoea of any aetiology including acute exacerbations of chronic diarrhoea for periods of up to 5 days, in adults and children over 4 years, and chronic diarrhoea in adults. Since persistent diarrhoea can be an indicator of potentially more serious conditions, Imodium should not be used for prolonged periods until the underlying cause of the diarrhoea has been investigated.

Dosage and administration Imodium capsules and Imodium syrup are for oral administration.

Acute diarrhoea: Adults: Two capsules initially, followed by 1 capsule after every loose stool, for up to five days.

The usual dosage is 3 to 4 capsules a day; the maximum daily dose should not exceed 8 capsules.

Children: 9–12 years: Syrup 10 ml (or 1 capsule) four times daily until diarrhoea is controlled, for up to five days. *4–8 years:* Syrup 5 ml four times daily until diarrhoea is controlled, for up to three days. In children under 8 years, further investigation may be necessary if diarrhoea has not responded to three days' treatment. Not recommended for use in children under 4 years of age.

Chronic diarrhoea: Adults: Studies have shown that patients may need widely differing amounts of Imodium. The starting dosage should be between 2 and 4 capsules per day in divided doses, depending on severity. If required, this dose can be adjusted according to response.

Having established the patient's daily maintenance dose, the capsules may be administered on a twice daily regimen. Tolerance has not been observed and therefore subsequent dosage adjustment should be unnecessary.

Use of Imodium syrup: 10 ml is equivalent to 1 capsule.

Oral rehydration: In patients with diarrhoea, especially young children, fluid and electrolyte depletion may occur. Use of Imodium does not preclude the administration of appropriate fluid and electrolyte replacement therapy.

Use in elderly: As for adults.

Contra-indications, warnings, etc
Contra-indications: Imodium must not be used when inhibition of peristalsis is to be avoided, in particular when ileus or constipation are present or when abdominal distension develops particularly in severely dehydrated children or in patients with acute ulcerative colitis or pseudomembranous colitis associated with broad spectrum antibiotics.

Precautions: Imodium should not be used alone in acute dysentery, which is characterised by blood in stools and elevated body temperatures. Imodium must be used with caution when the hepatic function, necessary for the drug's metabolism, is defective (e.g. in cases of severe hepatic disturbance), as this might result in a relative overdose.

Use in pregnancy: Safety in human pregnancy has not been established, although studies in animals have not demonstrated any teratogenic effects. As with other drugs, it is not advisable to administer Imodium in pregnancy.

Use during lactation: Although the fraction of Imodium secreted in the human milk is extremely low, caution is advised if Imodium is to be administered to a nursing mother.

Side-effects: Abdominal cramps and skin reactions, including urticaria, have been reported.

On occasions paralytic ileus and abdominal bloating have been reported.

Overdosage: In case of overdosage the following effects may be observed; constipation, ileus and neurological symptoms (miosis, muscular hypertonia, somnolence and bradypnoea). If intoxication is suspected, naloxone may be given as an antidote. Since the duration of action of Imodium is longer than that of naloxone, the patient should be kept under constant observation for at least 48 hours in order to detect any possible depression of the central nervous system.

Pharmaceutical precautions No special storage requirements.

Legal category POM.

Package quantities Imodium is supplied in packs of 30 and 250. Imodium syrup is supplied in bottles of 100 ml.

Further information Water is a satisfactory diluent for Imodium syrup; dilutions are stable for at least two weeks at 20°C.

Imodium syrup is sugar-free

No drugs are known to be incompatible with Imodium.

The half-life of Imodium in man is 10.8 hours with a range of 9–14 hours. Studies on distribution in rats show high affinity for the gut wall with preference for binding to the receptors in the longitudinal muscle layer. Imodium is well absorbed from the gut, but is almost completely extracted and metabolised by the liver where it is conjugated and excreted via the bile. Due to this very high first pass effect, plasma concentrations of unchanged drug remain extremely low.

Excretion occurs mainly through the faeces.

Product licence numbers

Capsules	0242/0028
Syrup	0242/0040

NIZORAL*

Presentation White, flat, half-scored uncoated tablets. Each tablet is marked 'Janssen' on one side and K/200 on the reverse. Each tablet contains Ketoconazole USP 200 mg. Each tablet also contains lactose. Pink, cherry flavoured suspension in 100 ml amber glass bottles containing 20 mg Ketoconazole USP per ml. The suspension contains sucrose, sodium benzoate, saccharin and E127.

Uses Nizoral is an imidazole-dioxolane antimycotic which is effective after oral administration and has a broad spectrum of activity against dermatophytes, yeasts and other pathogenic fungi.

The indications for Nizoral are:

In adults and children

1. Systemic mycoses, e.g. systemic candidosis, paracoccidioidomycosis, coccidioidomycosis, histoplasmosis.
2. Serious chronic mucocutaneous candidosis (including exceptionally disabling paronychia) not responsive to other therapy or when the organism is resistant to other therapy.
3. Serious mycoses of the gastrointestinal tract not responsive to other therapy or when organisms are resistant to other therapy.
4. Chronic vaginal candidosis not responsive to other therapy.
5. Prophylactic treatment to prevent mycotic infection in patients with reduced immune responses, e.g. in cancer, during treatment with immunosuppressive medication, or with burns.
6. Culturally determined dermatophyte infections of skin or finger nails which have failed to respond to adequate dose regimes of conventional anti-dermatophyte agents (excluding fungus infection of toe nails).

Nizoral is not indicated for pityriasis versicolor, usually an asymptomatic skin rash.

Dosage and administration Nizoral is for oral administration and should always be taken with meals.

As the risk of hepatitis (see 'Warnings') may increase in relation to the duration of treatment, if therapy is continued for more than 14 days the benefits must be weighed against the possible risks.

In adults
Mycoses and dermatophyte infections (except vaginal candidosis):

1. One tablet or two teaspoonsful of suspension (200 mg) once daily usually for 14 days.
2. If an adequate response has not been achieved after 14 days, treatment can be continued until at least one week after symptoms have cleared and cultures have become negative. The dose may also be increased to 400 mg once daily.

As nail infections always require long term therapy they should only be treated when a clinical rather than a purely cosmetic problem exists and only after alternative treatment has failed.

Prophylaxis and maintenance treatment: One tablet or 2 teaspoonsful of suspension (200 mg) once daily.

Chronic vaginal candidosis: Two tablets or 4 teaspoonsful of suspension (400 mg) once daily for 5 days.

In Children: Dosage should be reduced to 50 or 100 mg depending on bodyweight (i.e. approximately 3 mg/kg), for example:

Age 1– 4 years— 50 mg
Age 5–12 years—100 mg

Use in elderly:
In the absence of specific data, chronic vaginal candidosis – as for adults; all other indications – 200 mg daily.

Contra-indications, warnings, etc
Contra-indications: Nizoral should not be used in patients with a known hypersensitivity to ketoconazole or to any other imidazole antifungal.

Since it cannot be excluded that patients with pre-existing liver disease may be at greater risk of developing hepatic damage, ketoconazole treatment is contraindicated in these patients.

In patients suspected of having pre-existing liver disease, liver function tests should be performed prior to treatment and ketoconazole should not be used if significant abnormalities are observed.

Nizoral is contra-indicated in pregnancy (see 'Use in pregnancy' section).

Warnings: Hepatitis has been reported. The risk of developing hepatitis is greater in patients on long term treatment (>14 days). In patients receiving long term treatment, the benefits must be weighed against possible risks.

In patients in whom long term treatment (i.e. >14 days) with ketoconazole is indicated, LFT's should be performed prior to starting treatment.

Asymptomatic elevations in serum transaminase can occur early during treatment with ketoconazole. These may either be insignificant and transient, or can represent early evidence of hepatotoxicity. Patients should therefore be monitored clinically and biochemically with serum transaminase determinations after the first 2 weeks of treatment, at 4 weeks and at monthly intervals thereafter. If significantly elevated levels are observed, liver function tests (LFT's) should be performed at weekly intervals until transaminase levels return to normal. If significant progressive elevation occurs or the patient develops symptoms of hepatitis (malaise, dark urine, pale stools or jaundice), treatment with ketoconazole should be stopped immediately. The patient should then be monitored both clinically and biochemically for at least 2 months or until enzyme levels return to normal. Patients should also be told to consult their doctor if any of the above symptoms develop.

Hepatic damage has usually been reversible on discontinuation of treatment. Rarely, however, fatalities have been reported following ketoconazole treatment, usually where therapy has been continued despite development of symptoms of hepatitis.

Precautions: Absorption of Nizoral is maximal when taken during a meal, as it depends on stomach acidity. Concomitant treatment with agents that reduce gastric secretion (anti-cholinergic drugs, antacids, H_2 blockers) should be avoided and, if indicated, such drugs should be taken not less than two hours after Nizoral.

Ketoconazole is extensively bound to plasma proteins.

Imidazole compounds like ketoconazole, may enhance the anticoagulant effect of coumarin-like drugs, thus if concomitant use is envisaged, the anti-coagulant effect should be carefully monitored and titrated.

Concomitant use of rifampicin with ketoconazole may reduce the blood levels of both drugs so if this combination is to be used, plasma levels should be carefully monitored.

Concomitant use of ketoconazole and phenytoin may alter the metabolism of one or both drugs.

Ketoconazole, when given together with cyclosporin A can result in increased blood levels of cyclosporin A. It is therefore important that blood levels of cyclosporin A are carefully monitored if the two drugs are to be given concomitantly.

Use in pregnancy: When administered in high doses (>80 mg/kg) to pregnant rats, Nizoral has been shown to cause abnormalities of foetal development. The relevance of this finding to humans has not been established and consequently Nizoral is contra-indicated in pregnancy.

Side-effects: Alterations in liver function tests have occurred in patients on ketoconazole; these changes may be transient. Cases of hepatitis have been reported (see 'Warnings' section).

In rare cases, anaphylactoid reactions have been reported after the first dose. Hypersensitivity reactions including urticaria and angio-oedema have also been reported. The most commonly observed side-effects are gastric upsets (nausea, vomiting, abdominal pain), rash, urticaria, pruritus and headache. Thrombocytopenia has been reported rarely.

Ketoconazole, 200 mg once daily, produces a transient decrease in plasma levels of testosterone during the first 4–6 hours after intake of the drug. During long term therapy at this dose, testosterone levels are usually not significantly different from controls. In rare instances, gynaecomastia has been reported. A few cases of menstrual irregularities associated with the oral contraceptive pill have been reported. Although impaired response of plasma cortisol to ACTH has been described, it is unlikely to occur at the recommended dosage. No symptoms of adrenal insufficiency have been reported.

Overdosage: In the event of overdosage, cases should be treated symptomatically with supportive measures or gastric lavage as necessary.

Pharmaceutical precautions Nil.

Legal category POM.

Package quantities Nizoral is supplied in packs of 30 tablets, and in 100 ml bottles of suspension.

Further information Nil.

Product licence numbers

Nizoral tablets	0242/0083
Nizoral suspension	0242/0101

NIZORAL* CREAM

Presentation White, non-staining, water miscible cream containing Ketoconazole USP 2% w/w.

Uses Nizoral has a potent antimycotic activity against dermatophytes and yeasts. Nizoral cream acts rapidly on pruritus which is commonly seen in dermatophyte and yeast infections. This symptomatic improvement often occurs before the first signs of healing are observed.

After topical application, Nizoral is not systemically absorbed and does not produce detectable plasma concentrations.

Nizoral cream is indicated for topical application in the treatment of dermatophyte infections of the skin such as tinea corporis, tinea cruris, tinea manus and tinea pedis infections due to Trichophyton spp., Microsporum spp. and Epidermophyton spp.

Nizoral cream is also indicated for the treatment of cutaneous candidosis (including external application in vulvitis), pityriasis versicolor, and seborrhoeic dermatitis caused by Pityrosporum spp.

Dosage and administration Nizoral cream should be applied to the affected areas once or twice daily, depending on the severity of the infection.

The treatment should be continued until a few days after the disappearance of all signs and symptoms. The usual duration of treatment is: pityriasis versicolor 2–3 weeks, tinea corporis 3–4 weeks, tinea pedis 4–6 weeks.

The diagnosis should be reconsidered if no clinical improvement is noted after 4 weeks. General measures in regard to hygiene should be observed to control sources of infection or reinfection.

Seborrhoeic dermatitis is a chronic condition and relapse is highly likely. If a potent topical corticosteroid has been used previously in the treatment of seborrhoeic dermatitis, a recovery period of 2 weeks should be allowed before using Nizoral cream, as an increased incidence of steroid induced skin sensitisation has been reported when no recovery period is allowed.

Contra-indications, warnings, etc

Contra-indications: Nizoral cream is contra-indicated in patients who have shown hypersensitivity to any of the ingredients (propylene glycol, cetyl alcohol, stearyl alcohol, sorbitan monostearate, polysorbates 60 and 80, sodium sulphite, isopropyl myristate) or to ketoconazole itself.

Warnings: Not for ophthalmic use.

Side-effects: A few instances of irritation, dermatitis, and burning sensation have been observed during treatment with Nizoral cream.

Use in pregnancy: After topical application, Nizoral cream is not systemically absorbed and does not produce detectable plasma concentrations. However as with any medication, Nizoral cream should only be used in pregnant women if its use is considered essential.

Overdosage: If accidental ingestion of Nizoral cream

occurs, an appropriate method of gastric emptying may be used if considered appropriate.

Pharmaceutical precautions Store away from direct heat.

Legal category POM.

Package quantities 30 g tubes.

Further information Nil.

Product licence number 0242/0107

NIZORAL* SHAMPOO

Presentation 100 ml viscous pink liquid in plastic bottles containing Ketoconazole USP 20 mg/ml. Nizoral shampoo also contains sodium laureth sulphate, disodium monolaureth sulphosuccinate, coconut fatty acid diethanolamide, laurdimonium hydrolysed animal collagen, macrogel 120 methyl glucose dioleate, perfume bouquet, imidurea, hydrochloric acid, E127 and purified water.

Uses Nizoral has a potent antimycotic activity against pathogenic dermatophytes and yeasts including Pityrosporum spp. Nizoral shampoo rapidly relieves the scaling and pruritus usually associated with seborrhoeic dermatitis, pityriasis capitis (dandruff) and pityriasis versicolor.

Nizoral shampoo is not systemically absorbed after topical administration. As blood levels are not detectable after chronic use, Nizoral shampoo is indicated for the prevention and treatment of seborrhoeic dermatitis of the scalp and hairline, dandruff and pityriasis versicolor in which the yeast Pityrosporum is involved.

Dosage and administration
Adults and children: Shake the bottle well. Wash the hair or affected areas of the skin with Nizoral shampoo. Leave in contact for 3–5 minutes before rinsing thoroughly.

Treatment: Seborrhoeic dermatitis and dandruff: Use Nizoral shampoo twice weekly for 2–4 weeks.

Pityriasis versicolor: Once daily for a maximum of 5 days.

Prophylaxis: Seborrhoeic dermatitis and dandruff: Use Nizoral shampoo once every 1–2 weeks.

Pityriasis versicolor: As patches of pityriasis versicolor become more apparent on tanning, Nizoral shampoo may be used once daily for a maximum of 3 days in a single treatment course before exposure to sunshine.

Contra-indications, warnings, etc
Contra-indications: Hypersensitivity to any of the ingredients.

Precautions: Irritation may occur when Nizoral shampoo is used immediately after prolonged treatment with topical corticosteroids on the same area. Therefore, it is recommended to wait about 2 weeks after stopping treatment with topical corticosteroids before using Nizoral shampoo.

Keep out of the eyes. If the shampoo should get into the eyes they should be bathed with cold water.

Use in pregnancy: Since no ketoconazole is detected in plasma following topical administration, pregnancy and lactation are not a contra-indication for the use of ketoconazole shampoo.

Side-effects: Irritation has been reported extremely rarely.

Accidental ingestion: In the event of accidental ingestion cases should be treated symptomatically with supportive measures or gastric lavage as necessary.

Pharmaceutical precautions Store between 15 and 30°C and protect from light.

Legal category POM.

Package quantities 100 ml bottles.

Further information Nil.

Product licence number 0242/0139.

OPERIDINE*

Presentation Clear colourless aqueous injection presented in 2 ml and 10 ml ampoules. Each millilitre contains 1 mg phenoperidine hydrochloride. Operidine also contains water for injection.

Uses Operidine is a narcotic analgesic. It is used:
(a) as an analgesic.
(b) in conjunction with a neuroleptic in neuroleptanalgesia.
(c) as a respiratory depressant/analgesic in patients requiring prolonged assisted ventilation in intensive care.

Dosage and administration Operidine, by the intravenous route, can be administered to both adults and children according to the following dosage regimen:

	Adults		
	initial	*supplemental*	*Children*
Spontaneous respiration	Up to 1 mg	0.5 mg	0.03–0.05 mg/kg
Assisted ventilation	2–5 mg	1.0 mg	0.1–0.15 mg/kg

Depending on the degree of pain stimulus and/or the depth of respiratory depression required, supplemental doses may be administered at intervals of 40–60 minutes.

In intensive care, Operidine may be administered by the intramuscular route at the above dosages.

Use in elderly: It is wise to reduce the dosage in the elderly.

Contra-indications, warnings, etc
Contra-indications: Obstructive airways disease; respiratory depression if not electively ventilating.

Concomitant administration with monoamine oxidase inhibitors or within 2 weeks of their discontinuation.

Warnings: Significant respiratory depression will occur following administration of phenoperidine in doses in excess of 1 mg. This and the other pharmacological effects of Operidine can be reversed with naloxone 0.1–0.2 mg i.m. or i.v. (to be repeated as required).

Bradycardia may occur and this may be antagonised with atropine. Muscular rigidity (morphine-like effect) may occur, in which case muscle relaxants have been found helpful.

If other narcotic or CNS depressant drugs are used concomitantly with Operidine, the effects of the drugs can be expected to be additive.

Precautions: It is wise to reduce the dosage in the elderly, in hypothyroidism and chronic liver disease.

As with other narcotic analgesics, administration in labour may cause respiratory depression in the newborn infant.

As with all potent opioids, profound analgesia is accompanied by marked respiratory depression, which may persist into or recur in the early post-operative period. Care should be taken after infusions or large doses of phenoperidine to ensure that adequate spontaneous breathing has been established and maintained before discharging the patient from the recovery area. Hyperventilation during anaesthesia may alter the patient's response to CO_2, thus affecting respiration postoperatively. Use of opioid premedication may enhance or prolong the respiratory depressant effects of phenoperidine. Where early discharge is envisaged patients should be advised not to drive or operate machinery.

Side-effects: Tolerance and dependence may occur. Nausea and vomiting may be troublesome. A few cases of jaundice have been reported.

Use in Pregnancy: Little human usage but no evidence of adverse effect in animals.

Overdosage: Overdosage should be treated with the antidotes mentioned above.

Pharmaceutical precautions If desired Operidine

can be mixed with 5% Dextrose Injection BP or 0.9% Sodium Chloride Injection BP and with most agents commonly used in anaesthesia, but the product is chemically incompatible with the induction agents thiopentone and methohexitone because of the wide difference in pH.

Legal category CD (Sch 2), POM.

Package quantities Operidine is supplied in 2 ml ampoules (1 mg/ml) in packs of 10 and in 10 ml ampoules (1 mg/ml) in packs of 5.

Further information Operidine does not contain preservatives.

Product licence number 0242/5000R.

ORAP*

Presentation White, scored, uncoated tablets marked 'JANSSEN' on one side and 0/2 on the other, each contains 2 mg pimozide. The tablets also contain lactose and sucrose as inactive ingredients.

Pale green, scored, uncoated tablets marked 'JANSSEN' on one side and 0/4 on the other, each contains 4 mg pimozide. The tablets also contain E132, E172 as inactive ingredients.

White, scored, uncoated tablets marked 'JANSSEN' on one side and 0/10 on the other, each contains 10 mg pimozide. The tablets also contain lactose, as an inactive ingredient.

Uses Orap is an anti-psychotic of the diphenylbutylpiperidine series and is indicated in:

Acute and chronic schizophrenia, for the treatment of symptoms and prevention of relapse.

Other psychoses, especially paranoid and monosymptomatic hypochondriacal psychoses (eg delusional parasitosis).

Mania and hypomania.

As an adjunct to the short-term management of moderate to severe psychomotor agitation and excitement.

Dosage and administration Orap is intended for once daily oral administration in adult and children over 12 years of age.

Since individual response to anti-psychotic drugs is variable, dosage should be individually determined and is best initiated and titrated under close clinical supervision. In determining the initial dose, consideration should be given to the patient's age, severity of symptoms and previous response to other neuroleptic drugs. Dose increases should be made at weekly intervals or longer, and by increments of 2–4 mg in the daily dose.

The patients should be reviewed regularly to ensure the minimum effective dose is being used.

Schizophrenia: Initial dose: In the acute episode, the starting dose is 10 mg. This may be gradually increased, if necessary, to a maximum of 20 mg daily.

Prevention of relapse: The dose ranges between 2 and 20 mg daily, with 2 mg as a starting dose. This may be increased according to response and tolerance to achieve an optimum dose.

Paranoid states and monosymptomatic hypochondriacal psychosis (MHP): An initial dose of 4 mg daily which may then be gradually increased, if necessary, according to response to a maximum of 16 mg daily.

Mania, hypomania, psychomotor agitation and excitement: An initial dose of 10 mg daily may be given. This may then be gradually increased, if necessary, to a maximum of 20 mg daily.

Use in elderly: Elderly patients require half the normal starting dose of pimozide.

Contra-indications, warnings, etc

Contra-indications: In common with several other neuroleptics, pimozide has been reported to prolong the QT interval. It is, therefore, contra-indicated in patients with a pre-existing congenital prolongation of QT and in patients with a history of cardiac arrhythmias.

Orap is also contra-indicated in patients with severe central nervous system depression and in patients with a known hypersensitivity to pimozide or other diphenylbutyl-piperidine derivatives.

Use in pregnancy and lactation: The safety of Orap in human pregnancy has not been established. Studies in animals have not demonstrated teratogenic effects. As with other drugs, it is not advisable to administer Orap in pregnancy.

Orap may be excreted in breast milk. If the use of Orap is considered essential, breast feeding should be discontinued.

Precautions and warnings: Please also refer to 'Drug interactions' section.

Caution is advised in patients with hepatic or renal dysfunction, Parkinson's disease, phaeochromocytoma, thyrotoxicosis, epilepsy and conditions predisposing to epilepsy (e.g. alcohol withdrawal and brain damage).

It is recommended that a baseline ECG is undertaken in all patients prior to commencing treatment with pimozide in view of the cardiac contraindications and in order to identify possible subsequent electrocardiographic changes.

Periodic assessment of cardiac function should be undertaken in those patients receiving pimozide in excess of 16 mg daily. If repolarisation changes (prolongation of QT interval, T-wave or U-wave changes) appear or arrhythmias develop, the need for treatment with pimozide in these patients should be reviewed. They should be closely monitored and their dose of pimozide should preferably be reduced.

Electrolyte disturbances, notably hypokalaemia, should also be considered a risk factor.

As with other neuroleptics, cases of sudden unexpected death have been rarely reported with pimozide (generally in doses in excess of the current recommended maximum of 20 mg per day). Whilst the cause of death in these cases is not known with certainty, it is postulated that the QT prolongation seen with pimozide in some patients may have made the patients susceptible to some form of fatal arrhythmia (e.g. Torsades de Pointes). Whilst some of these patients were taking pimozide as a sole therapy, the remainder were also taking other drugs, including neuroleptics, implicated in the aetiology of arrhythmias.

In schizophrenia, the response to antipsychotic drug treatment may be delayed. If drugs are withdrawn, recurrence of symptoms may not become apparent for several weeks or months.

Acute withdrawal symptoms, including nausea, vomiting and insomnia, have very rarely been described after abrupt cessation of high doses of antipsychotic drugs. Gradual withdrawal is advisable.

Orap may impair alertness, especially at the start of treatment. These effects may be potentiated by alcohol. Patients should be warned of the risks of sedation and advised not to drive or operate machinery during treatment until their susceptibility is known.

Drug interactions: As with all neuroleptics, Orap may increase the central nervous system depression produced by other CNS depressant drugs, including alcohol, hypnotics, sedatives or strong analgesics.

Orap may impair the antiparkinson effect of levodopa. The dosage of anticonvulsants may need to be increased to take account of the lowered seizure threshold.

The possible additive effects of concomitant use of other drugs known to prolong the QT interval (e.g. other antipsychotic drugs, cardioactive drugs) should be considered in patients receiving long-term pimozide treatment.

Side-effects: In common with all neuroleptics, extrapyramidal symptoms may occur. Antiparkinson agents should not be prescribed routinely because of the possible risk of impairing the efficacy of Orap. They should only be given as required.

Tardive dyskinesia is common among patients treated with moderate to high doses of antipsychotic drugs for prolonged periods of time and may prove irreversible, particularly in patients over 50 years of age.

The potential seriousness and unpredictability of tardive dyskinesia and the fact that it has occasionally been reported to occur when neuroleptic antipsychotic drugs have been prescribed for a relatively short period in low dosage means that the prescribing of such agents requires especially careful assessment of risk versus benefit. Tardive dyskinesia can be precipitated or aggravated by antiparkinson drugs. Short-term dyskinesias may occur after abrupt drug withdrawal.

Epileptic fits have been reported even in low dosage. The elderly may be more liable to experience adverse effects.

Dose-related side effects, including drowsiness, insomnia, anxiety, and gastrointestinal symptoms, such as nausea, constipation or dyspepsia may occur. Dry mouth, loss of libido, impotence and hypotension have been reported, but autonomic symptoms are infrequent. Skin rashes have rarely been reported.

Hormonal effects of antipsychotic neuroleptic drugs include hyperprolactinaemia, which may cause galactorrhoea, gynaecomastia and oligo- or amenorrhoea.

Glycosuria has been reported.

In common with other antipsychotics, pimozide has been associated with rare cases of neuroleptic malignant syndrome, an idiosyncratic response characterised by hyperthermia, muscle rigidity, autonomic instability, altered consciousness and coma. Signs of autonomic dysfunction such as tachycardia, labile arterial pressure and sweating may precede the onset of hyperthermia, acting as early warning signs. Recovery usually occurs within five to seven days of antipsychotic withdrawal. Affected patients should be carefully monitored. Dantrolene sodium, bromocriptine mesylate and ECT have all been reported as offering benefit in some patients with neuroleptic malignant syndrome.

Overdosage: In general, the signs and symptoms of overdosage with Orap would be an exaggeration of known pharmacological effects, the most prominent of which would be severe extrapyramidal symptoms, hypotension or sedation. The risk of cardiac arrhythmias should be considered. The patient may appear comatose with respiratory depression and hypotension which could be severe enough to produce a shock-like state.

Treatment: There is no specific antidote to pimozide. Gastric lavage, establishment of a patent airway and, if necessary, mechanically assisted respiration are advised. Electrocardiographic monitoring should commence immediately and continue until the ECG returns to normal. Hypotension and circulatory collapse may be counteracted by the use of intravenous fluids, plasma or concentrated albumin, and vasopressor agents such as noradrenaline. Adrenaline should not be used.

In cases of severe extrapyramidal symptoms, antiparkinson medication should be administered.

Because of the long half life of pimozide, patients who have taken an overdose should be observed for at least 4 days.

Pharmaceutical precautions Nil.

Legal category POM.

Package quantities Orap tablets each containing 2 mg pimozide are supplied in packs of 100.

Orap tablets each containing 4 mg pimozide are supplied in packs of 100.

Orap tablets each containing 10 mg pimozide are supplied in packs of 100.

Further information The mean serum elimination half-life of pimozide in schizophrenic patients is approximately 55 hours. This is highly variable and may be as long as 150 hours in some individuals. There is a 13-fold interindividual difference in the area under the serum pimozide concentration-time curve and an equivalent degree of variation in peak serum levels among patients studied. The significance of this is unclear since there are few correlations between plasma levels and clinical findings.

Product licence numbers

Orap 2 mg	0242/5010R
Orap 4 mg	0242/0038R
Orap 10 mg	0242/0069R

PREPULSID* ▼

Presentation White, biconvex, scored tablets, engraved CIS/10 on one side and JANSSEN on the reverse. Each tablet contains cisapride monohydrate equivalent to 10 mg of cisapride. The tablets contain lactose.

Uses

Properties: Prepulsid is a gastro intestinal prokinetic agent which stimulates lower oesophageal, gastric, small intestinal and colonic motility.

Prepulsid probably acts by enhancing the release of acetylcholine at the level of the myenteric plexus in the gut wall, and therefore its effects on motility can largely be abolished by atropine. The mechanism by which acetylcholine release is enhanced is unclear. There is no direct evidence of antidopaminergic or direct cholinergic effects. Prepulsid has no effect on prolactin release or gastric secretion.

In patients with gastro-oesophageal reflux, Prepulsid increases the resting tone of the lower oesophageal sphincter, and increases the amplitude of lower oesophageal contractions. Prepulsid has also been shown, by pH monitoring, to reduce the duration of reflux episodes.

In patients with dyspepsia, impaired gastric emptying and gastro-oesophagael reflux disease (GORD) Prepulsid improves gastric emptying of liquid and solid meals, and shortens mouth to caecum transit time.

Prepulsid also stimulates colonic propulsive peristalsis and accelerates colonic transit.

Indications: The management of symptoms of dyspepsia e.g. epigastric pain or burning, early satiety, bloating, where peptic ulcer or other lesions have been excluded from the diagnosis. Treatment of symptoms (e.g. heartburn, regurgitation) and mucosal lesions associated with gastro-oesophageal reflux.

Relief of symptoms (e.g. nausea, early satiety, anorexia, bloating, epigastric pain) of impaired gastric motility secondary to disturbed and delayed gastric emptying associated with diabetes, systemic sclerosis and autonomic neuropathy.

Dosage and administration Prepulsid should preferably be taken 15–30 minutes before a meal in order to ensure maximum plasma levels immediately after food intake.

Adults and children aged 12 years and over

Dyspepsia
10 mg Prepulsid three times daily. The usual course of treatment is 4 weeks.

Gastro-oesophageal reflux: 10 mg Prepulsid three times daily. Night time symptoms can be treated with an extra 10 mg dose at bedtime. Healing of oesophageal lesions has been reported following treatment with 10 mg q.d.s. A 12 week course of treatment is recommended to obtain maximum benefit.

Impaired gastric motility: 10 mg Prepulsid three or four times daily. An initial course of 6 weeks is recommended, but longer periods of treatment may be required.

Use in children: Clinical experience with Prepulsid in children younger than 12 years is limited. Hence the drug can only be recommended for use in children aged 12 years and older.

Use in elderly: Repeated dosing in elderly patients with Prepulsid produced steady state plasma levels, which were generally higher than those reported in younger patients, due to a moderate prolongation of the elimination half life. Therapeutic doses, however, are similar to those used in younger patients. Therefore it is recommended that when Prepulsid is used in elderly patients, a starting dose similar to that used in other adults is prescribed initially. This can then be adapted depending on the therapeutic effects or possible side effects of the treatment.

Abnormal renal or liver function: Because of the importance of the hepatic metabolism and renal excretion of Prepulsid, the dosage should initially be halved in patients with hepatic or renal insufficiency. Subsequently the dose can be adapted depending on individual clinical response.

Contra-indications, warnings, etc

Contra-indications: Prepulsid is contra-indicated in pregnancy (see 'Use in pregnancy' section) and in patients in whom gastrointestinal stimulation might be dangerous e.g. gastrointestinal haemorrhage, mechanical obstruction or perforation.

Warnings:

Abnormal renal or liver function: (see 'Dosage' section).

Drug interactions: Since Prepulsid accelerates gastric emptying, the absorption from the stomach of concomitantly administered drugs may be diminished, whereas absorption of drugs from the small intestine may be accelerated. For drugs that require careful individual titration, such as anticonvulsants, it may be useful to measure their plasma concentration.

Prepulsid does not affect psychomotor performance nor does it induce sedation or drowsiness. However, the sedative effects of benzodiazepines and alcohol may be accelerated when administered concomitantly with Prepulsid.

The beneficial effects of Prepulsid on gastrointestinal motility are largely antagonised by anticholinergic drugs.

Concomitant treatment with H_2 antagonists increases the bioavailability of Prepulsid, and decreases that of the H_2 antagonist. The level of change is unlikely to be clinically significant.

In patients receiving anticoagulants, the prothrombin time may be increased. It is advisable to check the prothrombin time one week after the initiation or discontinuation of Prepulsid treatment, and to adapt the dose of anticoagulant if necessary.

The drug exhibits extensive binding to plasma proteins, mainly to albumin.

Use in pregnancy: In animals Prepulsid has shown no teratogenic or primary foetotoxic effects. Nevertheless, the safety of Prepulsid in human pregnancy has not been established and therefore, as with other new drugs, it is contra-indicated in pregnancy.

Use in lactation: Although the excretion of Prepulsid in human breast milk is minimal (milk to serum ratio of 0.045), it is not advisable to breastfeed while taking Prepulsid.

Side-effects: The most frequent side-effects reported with Prepulsid are gastrointestinal: abdominal cramps, borborygmi and diarrhoea. They are mainly transient and rarely require discontinuation of treatment.

Infrequent side-effects include headaches and light-headedness. Reports of convulsions and extrapyramidal effects have been received.

Overdosage: There are few data available on overdosage of Prepulsid. In one case, an adult took 540 mg. No serious sequelae resulted; the patient experienced retching, borborygmi, flatus, stool frequency and urinary frequency for 2 hours. There were no neurological, cardiovascular (including ECG), respiratory, biochemical or haematological effects. Treatment should include gastric lavage, close observation and general supportive measures.

Pharmaceutical precautions Store at room temperature and protect from light.

Legal category POM.

Package quantities 10 mg tablets: packs of 112 tablets.

Further information Prepulsid is rapidly absorbed, with peak plasma levels 1 to 2 hours after dosing, and an elimination half-life of approximately 10 hours. It undergoes extensive first-pass metabolism in the liver and gut wall, with the main metabolic pathways being oxidative *N*-dealkylation and aromatic hydroxylation. Excretion is mainly as metabolites (90%) with approximately equal amounts in both urine and faeces.

Product licence number 0242/0136.

RAPIFEN*

Presentation Clear, colourless, aqueous injection presented in 2 ml and 10 ml ampoules. Each millilitre contains 500 microgram of alfentanil as the hydrochloride. Rapifen also contains sodium chloride and water for injection.

Uses Rapifen is a potent, narcotic analgesic with a very rapid and short-lived action. This makes it especially suitable for use as an adjunct to anaesthesia in short operative procedures and out-patient surgery, requiring spontaneous respiration.

Rapifen may also be administered to ventilated patients undergoing longer operative procedures, either as a bolus followed by i.v. increments or infusion, or as an i.v. infusion throughout.

Dosage: Rapifen by the intravenous route can be administered to both adults and children according to the following dosage regimen:

	Initial	*Supplemental*
Adults		
Spontaneous respiration	up to 500 micrograms (1 ml)	250 micrograms (0.5 ml)
Assisted ventilation	30–50 micrograms/kg	15 micrograms/kg
Children		
Assisted ventilation	30–50 micrograms/kg	15 micrograms/kg

Children may require higher or more frequent dosing owing to a shorter half life of Rapifen in this age group.

Use in elderly: The elderly may require lower or less frequent dosing owing to a longer half life.

In spontaneously breathing patients, the initial bolus dose should be given slowly over about 30 seconds (dilution may be helpful).

After intravenous administration in unpremedicated adult patients, 1 ml Rapifen may be expected to have a peak effect in 90 seconds and to provide analgesia for 5–10 minutes. Periods of more painful stimuli may be overcome by the use of small increments of Rapifen. For procedures of longer duration additional increments will be required.

In ventilated patients, the last dose of alfentanil should not be given later than about 10 minutes before the end of surgery to avoid the continuation of respiratory depression after surgery is complete.

In ventilated patients undergoing longer procedures, Rapifen may be infused at a rate of 0.5–1 microgram/kg/minute. Adequate plasma concentrations of alfentanil will only be achieved rapidly if this infusion is preceded by a loading dose of 50–100 microgram/kg given as a bolus or fast infusion over 10 minutes. Even lower doses may be adequate, for example, in geriatric patients or where anaesthesia is being supplemented by other agents. The infusion should be discontinued up to 30 minutes before the anticipated end of surgery. Increasing the infusion rate may prolong recovery. Supplementation of the anaesthetic if required is best managed by extra bolus doses of Rapifen (1–2 ml) or low concentrations of a volatile agent for brief periods.

The exact dose always depends on the length and type of surgery and on the individual patient.

Contra-indications, warnings, etc

Contra-indications: Obstructive airways disease or respiratory depression if not ventilating.

Concurrent administration with monoamine oxidase inhibitors or within 2 weeks of their discontinuation.

Administration in labour or before clamping of the cord during Caesarean section due to the possibility of respiratory depression in the newborn infant.

Patients with a known intolerance to alfentanil.

Warnings: Following administration of Rapifen, a transient fall in blood pressure may occur. The magnitude of this effect may be exaggerated in the hypovolaemic patient or in the presence of concomitant sedative medication.

Significant respiratory depression will occur following administration of alfentanil in doses in excess of 1000 microgram (2 ml). This and the other pharmacological effects of Rapifen are usually of short duration and can be reversed with naloxone 0.1–0.2 mg i.v. or i.m.

Like other opioids, alfentanil may cause bradycardia, an effect that may be marked and rapid in onset but which can be antagonised by atropine. Bradycardia may be more pronounced when alfentanil is combined with other anaesthetic agents which depress the heart or increase vagal activity. Heart rate should therefore be monitored carefully. As asystole has been reported on very rare occasions in non-atropinised patients, it is advisable to be prepared to administer an anticholinergic drug if the heart rate is considered low.

If other narcotic or CNS depressant drugs are used concurrently with alfentanil, the effects of the drugs can be expected to be additive.

Precautions: It is wise to reduce the dosage in the elderly, in hypothyroidism and in chronic liver disease.

As with all potent opioids, profound analgesia is accompanied by marked respiratory depression, which may persist into or recur in the early postoperative period. Care should be taken after infusions or large doses of alfentanil to ensure that adequate spontaneous breathing has been established and maintained in the absence of stimulation before discharging the patient from the recovery area. Hyperventilation during anaesthesia may alter the patient's response to CO_2, thus affecting respiration postoperatively. Use of opioid premedication may enhance or prolong the respiratory depressant effects of alfentanil.

Rapifen may induce muscle rigidity during induction. Rigidity may be avoided by the following measures:

- slow i.v. injection;
- premedication with a benzodiazepine;
- administration of a muscle relaxant just prior to administration of Rapifen.

The concomitant use of erythromycin with Rapifen can significantly inhibit alfentanil clearance and may increase the risk of prolonged or delayed respiratory depression. Therefore smaller doses may be required and the duration of action may be extended. Theoretically similar considerations may apply to other enzyme inhibitors.

Where early discharge is envisaged patients should be advised not to drive or operate machinery.

Side-effects: Nausea and vomiting and dizziness have been reported.

Use in pregnancy: Safety in human pregnancy has not been established although studies in animals have not demonstrated teratogenic effects. As with other drugs, risk should be weighed against potential benefit to the patient.

Overdosage: Symptoms and treatment are as follows:
Bradycardia: Anticholinergics such as atropine or glycopyrrolate.
Hypoventilation or apnoea: O_2 administration, assisted or controlled respiration may be required.
Muscle rigidity: intravenous neuromuscular blocking agent may be given.

Body temperature and adequate fluid intake should be maintained and the patient observed for 24 hours.

A specific narcotic antagonist (e.g. naloxone) should be available to treat respiratory depression.

Pharmaceutical precautions If desired, Rapifen can be mixed with Sodium Chloride Injection BP, Dextrose Injection BP or Compound Sodium Lactate Injection BP (Hartmann's Solution). Such dilutions are compatible with plastic bags and giving sets.

Legal category CD (Sch 2), POM.

Package quantities Rapifen is supplied in 2 ml ampoules (0.5 mg/ml) in packs of 10 and in 10 ml ampoules (0.5 mg/ml) in packs of 10.

Further information The analgesic potency of Rapifen is one quarter that of fentanyl. The duration of action of Rapifen is one third that of an equianalgesic dose of fentanyl and is clearly dose-related. Its depressant effects on respiratory rate and alveolar ventilation are also of shorter duration than those of fentanyl.

The onset of action of Rapifen is 4 times more rapid than that of an equianalgesic dose of fentanyl. The peak analgesic and respiratory depressant effects occur within 90 seconds.

Product licence number 0242/0091.

RAPIFEN* CONCENTRATE

Presentation Clear, colourless aqueous injection presented in 1 ml ampoules. Each millilitre contains 5 mg of alfentanil as the hydrochloride. Rapifen concentrate also contains sodium chloride and water for injection.

Uses Rapifen concentrate is a potent narcotic analgesic for use as an analgesic supplement at induction of and during, anaesthesia.

Rapifen concentrate is indicated for operative procedures of medium and long duration when given as an i.v. bolus followed by supplemental doses or by continuous i.v. infusion.

Dosage and administration Rapifen concentrate can be administered by the intravenous route to both adults and children with assisted ventilation according to the following dosage guidelines. It is recommended that Rapifen concentrate is diluted before use with Sodium Chloride Injection BP, Dextrose Injection BP or Compound Sodium Lactate Solution BP.

Adults and children

Initial	*Supplemental*
30–50 micrograms/kg	15 micrograms/kg

Children may require more frequent dosing because of the shorter half life of alfentanil in this age group.

Use in elderly: The elderly may require lower or less frequent dosing owing to a longer half life of alfentanil, thus in these patients Rapifen* (alfentanil 0.5 mg/ml) is to be preferred.

In ventilated patients undergoing longer procedures, steady state concentrations of alfentanil may be rapidly obtained by a bolus loading dose of 50–100 microgram/kg or by infusion at 5–10 microgram/kg/min over 10 minutes. Some stimulating procedures such as cholecystectomy may require an infusion of 10 microgram/kg/minute for up to 30 minutes. A maintenance infusion of 0.5–1.0 microgram/kg/minute may then be given until 20 minutes before the end of surgery. Increasing the infusion rate may prolong recovery, so periods of painful stimuli are best managed by extra bolus doses of Rapifen 500 microgram per ml (1–2 ml) or low concentrations of a volatile agent for brief periods if preferred.

The exact dose always depends on the length and the type of surgery and on the individual patient.

Rapifen concentrate should not be used in spontaneously breathing children.

Contra-indications, warnings, etc

Contra-indications: Obstructive airways disease or respiratory depression if not ventilating.

Concurrent administration with monoamine oxidase inhibitors or within 2 weeks of their discontinuation.

Administration in labour or before clamping of the cord during Caesarean section due to the possibility of respiratory depression in the newborn infant.

Patients with a known intolerance to alfentanil.

Warnings: Following administration of alfentanil, a transient fall in blood pressure may occur. The magnitude of this effect may be exaggerated in the hypovolaemic patient or in the presence of concomitant sedative medication.

Significant respiratory depression will occur following administration of Rapifen concentrate in doses in excess of 1000 micrograms (0.2 ml). The duration of respiratory depression is dose-related but usually of short duration and this and the other pharmacological effects of Rapifen concentrate can be reversed with naloxone 0.1–0.2 mg i.v. or i.m.

Rapifen concentrate may induce muscle rigidity during induction. Rigidity may be avoided by the following measures:

- slow i.v. injection;
- premedication with a benzodiazepine;
- administration of a muscle relaxant just prior to administration of Rapifen concentrate.

Like other opioids, alfentanil may cause bradycardia, an effect that may be marked and rapid in onset, but which can be antagonised by atropine. Bradycardia may be more pronounced when alfentanil is combined with other anaesthetic agents which depress the heart or increase vagal activity. Heart rate should therefore be monitored carefully. As asystole has been reported on very rare occasions in non-atropinised patients, it is advisable to be prepared to administer an anticholinergic agent if the heart rate is considered low.

If other narcotics or CNS depressant drugs are used concurrently with alfentanil, the effects of the drugs can be expected to be additive.

Precautions: It is wise to reduce the dosage in the elderly, in hypothyroidism and in chronic liver disease.

As with other narcotic analgesics, patients who have received Rapifen concentrate should remain under appropriate surveillance. Resuscitation equipment and a narcotic antagonist should be readily available to control significant respiratory depression.

As with all potent opioids, profound analgesia is accompanied by marked respiratory depression, which may persist into or recur in the early post-operative period. Care should be taken after infusions or large doses of alfentanil to ensure that adequate spontaneous breathing has been established and maintained in the absence of stimulation before discharging the patient from the recovery area. Hyperventilation during anaesthesia may alter the patient's response to CO_2, thus affecting respiration postoperatively. Use of opioid premedication may enhance or prolong the respiratory depressant effects of alfentanil.

The concomitant use of erythromycin with Rapifen concentrate can significantly inhibit alfentanil clearance and may increase the risk of prolonged or delayed respiratory depression. Therefore smaller doses may be required and the duration of action may be extended. Theoretically similar considerations may apply to other enzyme inhibitors.

Where early discharge is envisaged, patients should be advised not to drive or operate machinery.

Side-effects: Nausea and vomiting and dizziness have been reported.

Use in pregnancy: Safety in human pregnancy has not been established although studies in animals have not demonstrated teratogenic effects. As with other drugs, risk should be weighed against potential benefit to the patient.

There is no information on passage of alfentanil into breast milk.

Overdosage: Symptoms and treatment are as follows:

Bradycardia: Anticholinergics such as atropine or glycopyrrolate.
Hypoventilation or apnoea: O_2 administration, assisted or controlled respiration may be required
Muscle rigidity: intravenous neuromuscular blocking agent may be given

Body temperature and adequate fluid intake should be maintained and the patient observed for 24 hours.

A specific narcotic antagonist (e.g. naloxone) should be available to treat respiratory depression.

Pharmaceutical precautions Rapifen concentrate can be mixed with Sodium Chloride Intravenous Infusion BP, Glucose Intravenous Infusion BP or Compound Sodium Lactate Intravenous Infusion BP (Hartmann's solution). Such dilutions are compatible with plastic bags and giving sets.

Legal category CD (Sch 2), POM.

Package quantities Rapifen concentrate is supplied in 1 ml ampoules (5 mg/ml) in packs of 10.

Further information The analgesic potency of alfentanil is one quarter that of fentanyl. The duration of action of alfentanil is one third that of an equianalgesic dose of fentanyl and is clearly dose-related. Its depressant effects on respiratory rate and alveolar ventilation are also of shorter duration than those of fentanyl.

The onset of action of alfentanil is 4 times more rapid than that of an equianalgesic dose of fentanyl. The peak analgesic and respiratory depressant effects occur within 90 seconds.

Product licence number 0242/0131.

RAPIFEN* INTENSIVE CARE

Presentation Clear, colourless, aqueous injection presented in 1 ml ampoules. Each millilitre contains 5 mg of alfentanil as the hydrochloride.

Uses Rapifen Intensive Care is a potent, opioid analgesic with a very rapid onset of action. It is indicated for analgesia and suppression of respiratory activity and to provide analgesic cover for painful manoeuvres in mechanically ventilated patients on intensive care. It will aid compliance with mechanical ventilation, and tolerance of the endotracheal tube. Intravenous bolus doses of Rapifen (0.5 mg/ml) may be used to provide additional pain relief during brief painful procedures in intensive care such as physiotherapy, endotracheal suction etc.

Patients may appear to be awake in the presence of adequate analgesia. At the proposed doses, Rapifen Intensive Care has no sedative activity. Therefore supplementation with an appropriate hypnotic or sedative agent is recommended. As alfentanil and the sedative drug need to be titrated separately admixture of the two drugs is not recommended.

Alfentanil given by infusion should only be used in areas where facilities are available to deal with respiratory depression and where continuous monitoring is performed. Alfentanil should only be prescribed by physicians familiar with the use of potent opioids when given by continuous iv infusion.

Dosage and administration Once the patient has been intubated, mechanical ventilation can be initiated using the following dosage regimes:

The recommended initial infusion rate for mechanically ventilated adult patients is 2 mg per hour (equivalent to 0.4 mls per hour of undiluted Rapifen* Intensive Care). The product should be diluted using the standard infusion solutions. For a 70 kg patient, this corresponds to approximately 30 microgram per kilogram per hour. More rapid control may initially be gained by using a loading dose. For example, a dose of 5 mg may be given in divided doses over a period of 10 minutes, during which time careful monitoring of blood pressure and heart rate should be performed. If hypotension or bradycardia occur, the rate of administration should be reduced accordingly and other appropriate measures instituted.

The dose to produce the desired effects should then be individually determined and reassessed regularly to ensure that the optimum dose is being used. In clinical trials, patient requirements have generally been met with doses of 0.5 to 10 mg alfentanil per hour.

Additional bolus doses of 0.5–1.0 mg alfentanil may be given to provide analgesia during short painful procedures.

The elderly and those patients with significant liver impairment will require lower doses. Obese patients may require a dose based on their lean body mass.

Adolescents and young adults will require higher than average doses. There is little experience of use of alfentanil to treat children in intensive care.

The maximum recommended duration of treatment with alfentanil infusions is 4 days.

Present data suggest that clearance of alfentanil is unaltered in renal failure. However there is an increased free fraction and hence dosage requirements may be less than in the patient with normal renal function.

Contra-indications, warnings, etc
Contra-indications: None.

Warnings: Following administration of Rapifen Intensive Care, a transient fall in blood pressure may occur. The magnitude of this effect may be exaggerated in the hypovolaemic patient or in the presence of concomitant sedative medication. Like other opioids, alfentanil may cause bradycardia, an effect which may be marked and rapid in onset but which can be antagonised by atropine. Particular care must be exerted following pretreatment with drugs such as anaesthetic agents or beta blockers which may predispose to bradycardia or hypotension. Heart rate should therefore be monitored carefully. Asystole has been reported on very rare occasions in non-atropinised patients undergoing surgery; therefore an anti-cholinergic drug should be available for administration if clinically indicated.

If other narcotic or CNS depressant drugs are used concurrently with alfentanil, the effects of the drugs can be expected to be additive. Care must be taken if the patient has received monoamine oxidase inhibitors within the previous 2 weeks.

Significant respiratory depression will occur following administration of alfentanil in doses in excess of 1 mg. If necessary for assessment purposes, naloxone may be administered to reverse the respiratory depression and other pharmacological effects of alfentanil. More than one dose of naloxone may be required in view of its short half life.

Muscle rigidity (morphine-like effect) may occur, in which case neuromuscular blocking drugs may be helpful.

Precautions: It is wise to reduce the dosage in hypothyroidism and in chronic liver disease since alfentanil is metabolised in the liver.

As with all potent opioids, profound analgesia is accompanied by marked respiratory depression, which may persist into or recur in the early post infusion period. Care should therefore be taken throughout the weaning period and adequate spontaneous respiration should be established and maintained in the absence of stimulation or ventilatory support. Following cessation of the infusion the patient should be closely observed for at least six hours.

The concomitant use of cimetidine or erythromycin with Rapifen Intensive Care can significantly inhibit alfentanil clearance and may increase the risk of prolonged or delayed respiratory depression. Therefore smaller doses may be required and the duration of action may be extended.

Theoretically similar considerations may apply to other enzyme inhibitors.

Side-effects: Nausea and vomiting and dizziness have been reported.

Use in pregnancy: Safety in human pregnancy has not been established although studies in animals have not demonstrated teratogenic effects. As with other drugs possible risk should be weighed against potential benefit to the patient.

Overdosage: Symptoms and treatment are as follows:

Bradycardia: Anticholinergics such as atropine or glycopyrrolate.

Hypoventilation or apnoea: Oxygen administration, assisted or controlled respiration may be required.

Muscle rigidity: intravenous neuromuscular blocking agent may be given. Body temperature and adequate fluid intake should be maintained and the patient observed for 24 hours. A specific narcotic antagonist (e.g. naloxone) should be available to treat respiratory depression.

All the effects of alfentanil may be antagonised if necessary by a specific narcotic antagonist such as naloxone.

Pharmaceutical precautions Rapifen Intensive Care should be diluted with Sodium Chloride Intravenous Infusion BP, Glucose Intravenous Infusion BP or Compound Sodium Lactate Intravenous Infusion BP (Hartmann's solution). Such dilutions are compatible with plastic bags and giving sets.

Legal category CD (Sch2), POM.

Package quantities Rapifen Intensive Care 5 mg/ml is supplied in 1 ml ampoules in packs of 10 ampoules.

Further information Nil.

Product licence number 0242/0137.

SPORANOX*

Presentation Hard gelatin capsules (size 0) with opaque blue cap and pink transparent body. Each capsule contains 100 mg itraconazole as coated beads.

Uses
Mode of action: Sporanox is a substituted triazole antimycotic with a broad spectrum of activity against Candida spp. and other yeasts, dermatophytes and other pathogenic fungi. It acts by impairing the synthesis of ergosterol in fungal cell membranes.

Indications: Sporanox is indicated for the treatment of the following mycoses: vulvovaginal candidosis; oropharyngeal candidosis; pityriasis versicolor; dermatophytoses caused by organisms susceptible to itraconazole (Trichophyton spp, Microsporum spp, *Epidermophyton floccosum*) e.g. tinea pedis, tinea cruris, tinea corporis, tinea manuum.

Dosage and administration Sporanox is for oral administration and must be taken immediately after a meal for maximal absorption.

Treatment schedules in adults for each indication are as follows:

Vulvovaginal candidosis: 2 capsules (200 mg) b.d. for 1 day.

Oropharyngeal candidosis: 1 capsule (100 mg) o.d. for 15 days, in AIDS and neutropenic patients 2 capsules (200 mg) o.d. for 15 days is recommended due to impaired absorption.

Pityriasis versicolor: 2 capsules (200 mg) o.d. for 7 days.

Tinea corporis, tinea cruris: 1 capsule (100 mg) o.d. for 15 days.

Tinea pedis, tinea manuum: 1 capsule (100 mg) o.d. for 30 days.

Optimal clinical and mycological effects are reached 1–4 weeks after cessation of treatment, as elimination of itraconazole from skin and mucous membranes is slower than from plasma.

Sporanox should not be used for treatment periods longer than 1 month as insufficient data are available on efficacy or safety.

In children (below 12 years): There are inadequate data on Sporanox in children for its use to be recommended, unless the potential benefits outweigh the risks.

In elderly: As for use in children.

Contra-indications, warnings, etc
Contra-indications: When administered at high doses to pregnant rats (40 mg/kg/day) and mice (80 mg/kg/day), Sporanox was shown to cause abnormalities of foetal development. No data are available in human pregnancy, and Sporanox is therefore contra-indicated in pregnancy. Adequate contraceptive precautions should be taken by women of childbearing potential during therapy and for one menstrual cycle after stopping therapy. Sporanox is also contra-indicated in patients who have shown hypersensitivity to itraconazole, other azole antifungal agents or any of the excipients.

Warnings: Sporanox is predominantly metabolised in the liver. Although clinically it has not been associated with hepatic dysfunction, it is advisable not to give Sporanox to patients with a known history of liver disease, or to patients who have experienced liver toxicity with other drugs.

Studies in patients with impaired renal function have indicated that no dose adjustment is required.

It is recommended that patients should not breast feed whilst taking Sporanox.

Precautions: Sporanox should not be given concomitantly with rifampicin or phenytoin, as the latter drugs reduce blood levels of Sporanox.

Despite the fact that Sporanox is 99.8% bound to plasma proteins, there are no in vitro interactions on the plasma protein binding between Sporanox and imipramine, propranolol, diazepam, cimetidine, indomethacin, tolbutamide, sulfamethazine or warfarin, but Sporanox may possibly interact with drugs metabolised by oxidation e.g. cyclosporin.

There is no experience of concomitant administration of itraconazole with H_2 antagonists or antacids, but as absorption depends on gastric acidity it is possible that their concomitant administration will result in reduced absorption of the antifungal.

Side-effects: During clinical trials, minor side effects have been reported occasionally. The most frequently reported side effects were nausea, abdominal pain, dyspepsia and headache.

Overdosage: In the event of overdosage, patients should be treated symptomatically with supportive measures and gastric lavage as necessary.

Pharmaceutical precautions Store at room temperature. Protect from light.

Legal category POM.

Package quantities 4 and 15 capsules.

Further information Peak concentrations of Sporanox in keratinous tissues, especially skin, are up to 5 times higher than in plasma. Therapeutic levels in the skin and mucous membranes persist for up to 1–4 weeks after stopping treatment as elimination is related to epidermal regeneration, rather than redistribution into the systemic circulation. Sporanox is extensively metabolised by the liver to a large number of metabolites, which constitute 40% of the excreted dose. Faecal excretion of parent drug varies from 3–18% of the dose, and urinary excretion of unchanged drug is less than 0.03%.

Product licence number 0242/0142.

STUGERON* FORTE 75 mg

Presentation Hard gelatin capsules (No. 4) with an orange cap and cream body; each capsule contains cinnarizine 75 mg. The capsules also contain lactose and E110.

Uses Stugeron Forte is indicated for the long term management of the symptoms of peripheral arterial disease, including intermittent claudication, rest pain, muscular cramps and vasospastic disorders, e.g. Raynaud's disease.

Actions: Cinnarizine's action in the treatment of peripheral vascular disease are due to its anti-vasoconstrictor properties, its action on blood hyperviscosity and its anti-ischaemic effect. Anti-vasoconstriction is thought to be through a calcium blocker mechanism and is evident selectively in vascular smooth muscle. Increased peripheral muscle blood flow may be mediated by prevention of calcium entry into ischaemic erythrocytes, thereby preserving flexibility.

Dosage and administration Stugeron Forte is for oral administration to adults.

The recommended starting dose is 1 capsule three times daily. Maintenance dose is 1 capsule, two or three times daily according to response.

Peripheral arterial disease is slow to improve with any form of drug treatment. Maximum benefit with Stugeron Forte will not be seen until after several weeks of continuous treatment although significant improvement in blood flow has frequently been demonstrated after one month.

Use in elderly: As above.

Contra-indications, warnings, etc

Contra-indications: There are no specific contra-indications. Stugeron Forte has not been found to decrease blood pressure significantly. However, the drug should be used with reasonable caution in hypotensive patients.

Use in pregnancy: The safety of Stugeron Forte in human pregnancy has not been established although studies in animals have not demonstrated teratogenic effects. As with other drugs, it is not advisable to administer Stugeron Forte in pregnancy.

Warnings: Stugeron Forte may cause drowsiness; patients affected in this way should not drive or operate machinery. Avoid alcoholic drink.

Side-effects: Allergic skin reactions and fatigue have been reported on rare occasions. An aggravation or appearance of extrapyramidal symptoms has been reported extremely rarely in elderly people during prolonged therapy. The treatment should be reduced or stopped in such cases.

Overdosage: There is no specific antidote to Stugeron Forte and, in the event of overdosage, gastric lavage is recommended.

Pharmaceutical precautions Nil.

Legal category P.

Package quantities Stugeron Forte is supplied in packs of 100 capsules.

Further information No drug interactions have been seen with Stugeron Forte when administered concomitantly with antihypertensives, diuretics, anticoagulants or hypoglycaemics.

Animal studies have shown that cinnarizine protects the arterial wall from arteriosclerotic degeneration due to hypertension.

Product licence number 0242/0008.

SUBLIMAZE*

Presentation Clear, colourless, aqueous injection presented in 2 ml and 10 ml ampoules. Each millilitre contains 50 microgram fentanyl (as the citrate) in water for injection.

Uses Sublimaze is a narcotic analgesic. It is used in low doses to provide analgesia during short surgical procedures. In larger doses it is used as an analgesic/respiratory depressant in patients requiring assisted ventilation. In combination with a neuroleptic, Sublimaze is used in the technique of neuroleptanalgesia.

Dosage and administration Sublimaze, by the intravenous route, can be administered to both adults and children according to the following dosage regimen.

	Adults		*Children*	
	Initial micrograms	*Supplemental* micrograms	*Initial* micrograms/kg	*Supplemental* micrograms/kg
Spontaneous respiration	50–200	50	3–5	1
Assisted ventilation	300–3500	100–200	15	1–3

Doses in excess of 200 microgram are for use in anaesthesia only. As a premedicant, 1–2 ml Sublimaze may be given intramuscularly 45 minutes before induction of anaesthesia.

After intravenous administration in unpremedicated adult patients 2 ml Sublimaze may be expected to provide sufficient analgesia for 10–20 minutes in surgical procedures involving low pain intensity. 10 ml Sublimaze injected as a bolus gives analgesia lasting about one hour. The analgesia produced is sufficient for surgery involving moderately painful procedures. Giving a dose of 50 microgram/kg Sublimaze will provide intense analgesia for some four to six hours, for intensely stimulating surgery. When judging the dose it is important to assess the likely degree of surgical stimulation, the effect of premedicant drugs, and the duration of the procedure.

Use in elderly: It is wise to reduce the dosage in the elderly.

Contra-indications, warnings, etc Respiratory depression: obstructive airways disease.

Concurrent administration with monoamine oxidase inhibitors, or within two weeks of their discontinuation.

Warnings: Following intravenous administration of fentanyl, a transient fall in blood pressure may occur.

Significant respiratory depression will occur following the administration of fentanyl in doses in excess of 200 microgram. This, and the other pharmacological effects of fentanyl, can be reversed with naloxone 0.1–0.2 mg.

Bradycardia may occur and this can be antagonised by atropine. Muscular rigidity (morphine-like effect) may occur, in which case muscle relaxants have been found helpful.

If other narcotics or CNS depressant drugs are used concomitantly with fentanyl, the effects of the drugs can be expected to be additive. Tolerance and dependence may occur. Nausea and vomiting may be troublesome.

Precautions: As with all narcotic analgesics, care should be observed when administering fentanyl to patients with myasthenia gravis.

It is wise to reduce dosage in the elderly, in hypothyroidism, and chronic hepatic disease.

Administration in labour may cause respiratory depression in the new born infant.

As with all potent opioids, profound analgesia is accompanied by marked respiratory depression, which may persist into or recur in the early post-operative period. Care should be taken after large doses or infusions of fentanyl to ensure that adequate spontaneous breathing has been established and maintained before discharging the patient from the recovery area. Hyperventilation during anaesthesia may alter the patient's response to CO_2, thus affecting respiration postoperatively. Use of opioid premedication may enhance or prolong the respiratory depressant effects of fentanyl.

Where early discharge is envisaged patients should be advised not to drive or operate machinery.

Use in pregnancy: Little human usage but no adverse animal evidence.

Overdosage: Overdosage should be treated with the antidotes mentioned above.

Pharmaceutical precautions If desired Sublimaze can be mixed with i.v. infusion solutions and with most agents commonly used in anaesthesia, but the product is chemically incompatible with the induction agents thiopentone and methohexitone because of the wide differences in pH.

Legal category CD (Sch 2), POM.

Package quantities Sublimaze is supplied in 2 ml ampoules (0.05 mg/ml) in packs of 10 and in 10 ml ampoules (0.05 mg/ml) in packs of 10.

Further information Nil.

Product licence number 0242/5001 R.

THALAMONAL*

Presentation Clear, colourless, aqueous injection presented in 2 ml ampoules. Each millilitre contains 50 microgram fentanyl and 2.5 mg droperidol. Thalamonal also contains tartaric acid and water for injection.

Uses Thalamonal is a combination of a major tranquilliser and narcotic analgesic. It is used in the technique of neuroleptanalgesia or as a premedication. It can be used as an adjunct to general and regional anaesthesia in major, minor and diagnostic surgical procedures. Thalamonal can also be used in intractable labyrinthine vertigo, e.g. Ménière's disease, where rapid relief of symptoms can be expected.

Dosage and administration Thalamonal can be administered intravenously to adults or intramuscularly to both adults and children. The following dosage regimen is recommended:

Neuroleptanalgesia/Premedication:
Route: Intramuscular.
Adults: 1–2 ml.
Children: 0.03–0.045 ml/kg (approx 0.4–1.5 ml).
5–15 minutes pre-operatively.

At induction of anaesthesia:
Route: Intravenous.
Adults: 6–8 ml.
Followed by assisted ventilation.

Maintenance of anaesthesia:
Route: Intravenous.
Adults: 1–2 ml.
When signs of lightening of anaesthesia are observed.

Intractable labyrinthine vertigo:
Route: Intravenous.
Adults: 1–2 ml.
By slow injection.

Use in elderly: It is wise to reduce the dosage in the elderly.

Contra-indications, warnings, etc
Contra-indications: Severe depression, obstructive airways disease; respiratory depression if not ventilating.

Concurrent administration with monoamine oxidase inhibitors or within two weeks of discontinuation of them.

Warnings: Significant respiratory depression will occur following the administration of Thalamonal in doses in excess of 4 ml (200 microgram fentanyl). This may be reversed with naloxone 0.1–0.2 mg i.v. or i.m.

Intravenous induction agents will generally be required in lower dosages where Thalamonal is used as part of the anaesthetic technique, and the effects of heavy sedative premedication may be potentiated. When using Thalamonal at induction of anaesthesia, provision should be made for rapid infusion of intravenous fluid to correct any large fall in blood pressure, which, if it occurs, is due to relative hypovolaemia and is more common in the elderly or untreated hypertensives.

Bradycardia may occur and this may be antagonised by atropine. Muscular rigidity (morphine-like effect) may occur in which case muscle relaxants have been found helpful.

Extra-pyramidal effects have been seen and may be reversed by anti-Parkinson drugs.

If other narcotic or CNS depressant drugs are used concomitantly with Thalamonal, the effects can be expected to be additive.

Precautions: It is wise to reduce the dosage in the elderly, who are more sensitive to the sedative and hypotensive effects, in hypothyroidism and severe hepatic disease. Administration in labour may cause respiratory depression in the newborn infant.

Caution is advised in patients with liver disease, renal failure, Parkinson's disease, epilepsy, and conditions predisposing to epilepsy or convulsions.

As with all potent opioids, profound analgesia is accompanied by marked respiratory depression, which may persist into or recur in the early postoperative period. Care should be taken after infusions or large doses of Thalamonal to ensure that adequate spontaneous breathing has been established and maintained without stimulation before discharging the patient from the recovery area. Hyperventilation during anaesthesia may alter the patient's response to CO_2, thus affecting respiration postoperatively. Use of opioid premedication may enhance or prolong the respiratory depressant effects of Thalamonal.

Minor central effects can, in some instances, persist for up to 48 hours after administration. Hence where early discharge is envisaged, patients should be advised not to drive or operate machinery on the day following administration.

Use in pregnancy: The safety of Thalamonal in pregnancy has not been established, although studies in animals have not demonstrated teratogenic effects.

Side-effects: Tolerance and dependence may occur.

Overdosage: Overdosage should be treated with the antidotes mentioned above.

Pharmaceutical precautions Thalamonal should be protected from light. Thalamonal can be mixed with intravenous infusion solutions (Sodium Chloride Intravenous Infusion BP, Glucose Intravenous Infusion BP, or Compound Sodium Lactate Intravenous Infusion BP (Hartmann's Solution)) where slow administration is desired.

This product is chemically incompatible with thiopentone and methohexitone because of the wide difference in pH.

Legal category CD (Sch 2), POM.

Package quantities Thalamonal is supplied in 2 ml ampoules in packs of 10.

Further information Nil.

Product licence number 0242/5002R.

TINSET*

Presentation White biconvex scored tablets marked 'JANSSEN' on one side and OX/30 on the reverse; containing oxatomide 30 mg. Tinset tablets also contain lactose.

Uses Oxatomide is indicated for the symptomatic control of allergic rhinitis, conjunctivitis and urticaria and other conditions responsive to drugs with anti-histaminic properties. Food allergy.

Dosage and administration Twice daily oral administration (morning and evening after meals):

Adults and children over 14: 30 mg b.d. which may be increased to 60 mg b.d. if required (i.e. 1–2 tablets, twice daily).

Children aged 5–14: 15–30 mg b.d. ($\frac{1}{2}$–1 tablet, twice daily).

Use in elderly: 30 mg b.d.

Contra-indications, warnings, etc There are no specific contra-indications to the use of oxatomide.

Use in pregnancy: Although no teratogenic effects have been observed in experimental animals, the safety of oxatomide in pregnancy has not yet been established.

Side-effects: Oxatomide may cause drowsiness in some patients, who, if affected, should not drive or operate machinery. Avoid alcoholic drink. Increased appetite leading to weight gain has been occasionally reported in patients at higher dosage levels (above 60 mg b.d.), but is rare at the recommended dosage. This effect is reversible on discontinuation of treatment.

Overdosage: In event of accidental overdosage supportive measures and/or gastric lavage are recommended.

In children, acute dyskinetic reactions have been reported and anticholinergic drugs may be useful in controlling these.

Pharmaceutical precautions Nil.

Legal category POM.

Package quantities Packs of 25 tablets.

Further information Nil.

Product licence number 0242/0064.

VERMOX*

Presentation *Vermox tablets:* Pale orange, flat, scored, chewable tablets, approximately 10 mm in diameter, marked 'JANSSEN' on one side and Me/100 on the reverse. Each tablet contains mebendazole 100 mg. Vermox tablets also contain E110.

Vermox suspension: White, banana flavoured suspension of mebendazole 2% w/v. Each 5 ml contains mebendazole 100 mg. Vermox suspension also contains sucrose and methyl and propyl parabens.

Uses Vermox is a broad spectrum anthelmintic indicated for the treatment of:

Enterobius vermicularis / *Oxyuris vermicularis*	(Threadworm/Pinworm)
Trichuris trichiura	(Whipworm)
Ascaris lumbricoides	(Large Roundworm)
Ancylostoma duodenale	(Common Hookworm)
Necator americanus	(American Hookworm)

in single or mixed infestations.

Dosage and administration Vermox tablets and suspension are for oral administration. The tablets are orange flavoured and may be chewed or swallowed whole. Vermox suspension provides an alternative liquid formulation.

The same dosage applies to adults and children aged two years and above. No special procedures such as purging, use of laxatives and/or dietary changes are required.

(a) Threadworm *(Enterobius vermicularis)*
A single dose of one tablet, or 5 ml suspension. Care should be taken to avoid reinfection and it is strongly recommended that all members of the family are treated simultaneously.

(b) Whipworm *(Trichuris trichiura)*
Large Roundworm *(Ascaris lumbricoides)*
Common Hookworm *(Ancylostoma duodenale)*
American Hookworm *(Necator americanus)*
One tablet or 5 ml suspension twice daily (morning and evening) for three consecutive days.

Use in elderly: As above.

Contra-indications, warnings, etc *Pregnancy:* Vermox has shown embryotoxic and teratogenic activity in rats at single oral doses. No such findings have been reported in the rabbit, dog, sheep, or horse. Since there is a risk that Vermox could produce foetal damage if administered during pregnancy, *it is contra-indicated in pregnant women.*

Use in infants: Vermox has not been studied extensively in children under two years of age – for this reason it is not currently recommended in the treatment of children under two years.

Side-effects: Side-effects reported for Vermox have been minor. Transient abdominal pain and diarrhoea have been reported, only rarely, in cases of massive infestation and expulsion of worms.

Overdosage: No case of overdose has so far been reported for Vermox. In the event of overdosage, gastric lavage is recommended.

Pharmaceutical precautions Vermox suspension should be shaken before use.

Legal category POM.

Package quantities
Tablets: Blister pack of 6 tablets.
Suspension: 30 ml bottle.

Further information The efficacy of Vermox in threadworm *(Enterobius vermicularis)* infestations is such that treatment failures will be rare. However, the possibility of re-infection means that some patients may require a second treatment after two weeks.

Product licence numbers
Tablets 0242/0011
Suspension 0242/0050

**Trade Mark*

Kabi Pharmacia Limited
Davy Avenue
Knowhill
Milton Keynes
Bucks MK5 8PH

Kabi Pharmacia

ADDAMEL*

Presentation A straw coloured solution containing electrolytes and trace elements for addition to the Vamin amino acid solutions in the intravenous nutrition of adults. Addamel corresponds to the following formula:

Calcium chloride $2H_2O$	73.5 mg
Magnesium chloride $6H_2O$	30.42 mg
Ferric chloride $6H_2O$	1.35 mg
Zinc chloride	0.27 mg
Manganese chloride $4H_2O$	0.79 mg
Copper chloride $2H_2O$	85 micrograms
Sodium fluoride	0.21 mg
Potassium iodide	17 micrograms
Sorbitol	0.3 g
Water for injections to 1 ml	
pH 2.5	

One ampoule (10 ml of Addamel) contains the following amounts of electrolytes and trace elements:

Ca^{2+}	5 mmol
Mg^{2+}	1.5 mmol
Fe^{3+}	50 micromol
Zn^{2+}	20 micromol
Mn^{2+}	40 micromol
Cu^{2+}	5 micromol
F^-	50 micromol
I^-	1 micromol
Cl^-	13.3 mmol

One ampoule of Addamel contains less than 1 mmol of both potassium and sodium.

Uses Addamel is an integral part of a complete intravenous nutrition regimen. It should be used in conjunction with a Vamin solution, Intralipid and a suitable phosphate preparation containing potassium. This will provide the patient's basal requirements for electrolytes and trace elements. As the requirements for electrolytes and trace elements may vary in different clinical conditions these substances may have to be added as appropriate in the individual patient.

Dosage and administration *Recommended dosage for adults:* 1 ampoule (10 ml) of Addamel is added to 500 ml or 1,000 ml of a solution listed in the table. In this way the normal daily requirements of Ca, Mg, Fe, Zn, Mn, Cu, F, I and Cl can be supplied. Where higher amounts of trace elements are considered necessary, 2 ampoules of Addamel may be added to 1,000 ml of solution.

Recommended dosage for infants: For infants the trace element/electrolyte solution Ped-el should be used.

The requirements of potassium and sodium vary with different patient conditions. Addamel is not intended to meet these requirements. Potassium and sodium salts should be added as appropriate to the requirements of the individual patient. (Vamin 9, Vamin 9 Glucose and Vamin 14 contain potassium and sodium. See appropriate data sheet.)

Contra-indications, warnings, etc Should not be given undiluted. Care should be taken in the administration of Addamel to patients with impaired biliary or renal function.

One ampoule of Addamel contains 3 g sorbitol which is metabolised to fructose, and should therefore be given with caution to patients with fructose intolerance.

Overdosage: Overdosage, which may occur if the solution is injected undiluted, may result in temporary hyper-calcaemia causing bradycardia. Spontaneous reversal of this situation is likely to occur without the need for a specific antidote. If not, standard measures for treating bradycardia can be instituted.

Pharmaceutical precautions Addition of other drugs to be avoided due to the risk of precipitation.

1. Store below 25°C protected from light.
2. A cloudy solution or one containing a precipitate must not be used.
3. The following mixtures containing Vamin should be infused at an appropriate rate for the amino acid solution.

Infusion solution	*Volume to which 10 ml Addamel may be added (ml)*	*Infusion of admixture must be completed within: (hours)*
Vamin 9	500	12
Vamin 9	1000	24
Vamin 9 Glucose	500	24
Vamin 9 Glucose	1000	48
Vamin 14	500–1000	48
Vamin 14 Electro-lyte-Free	500–1000	48
Glucose 5–60%	250–1000	48

If Addamel is added to a solution other than those listed above, then ensure that the resulting solution is administered over a period of not less than 2 hours, so as to minimise renal losses.

Addamel should only be added to solutions where compatibility is known.

4. The addition of Addamel should be performed aseptically immediately before the start of the infusion and the mixtures infused before the time shown in the table. See under 'Dosage and administration'.

Legal category POM.

Package quantities Boxes of 10 × 10 ml ampoules.

Further information The manufacturer can be consulted for full information on complete and balanced intravenous nutrition regimens.

Product licence number 0022/0034.

ADDIPHOS*

Presentation Sterile colourless solution containing phosphate, potassium and sodium for addition to infusion fluids. Addiphos corresponds to the following formula:

Monobasic potassium phosphate	170.1 mg
Sodium phosphate $2H_2O$	133.5 mg
Potassium hydroxide	14.0 mg
Sorbitol	1.0 mg
Water for injections to 1 ml	
pH: 6.3–6.4	

One vial (20 ml Addiphos) provides the following:

Phosphate	40 mmol
Potassium	30 mmol
Sodium	30 mmol

Uses Addiphos may be added to infusion solutions such as Vamin solutions and glucose solutions to provide phosphate during complete intravenous nutrition. This also provides potassium and sodium. For precise details on compatibility with individual infusion solutions see Pharmaceutical precautions section.

Dosage and administration *Recommended dosage for adults:* A daily requirement for phosphate during complete intravenous nutrition would normally be within the range 10–40 mmol. This can be met by using 5–20 ml of Addiphos. 5–20 ml Addiphos also provides 7.5–30 mmol each of potassium and sodium. The infusion should be given intravenously at a rate corresponding to not more than 10 mmol K^+ per hour so as to avoid hyperkalaemia and also within the maximum infusion rate for the Vamin.

Recommended dosage for infants: Dosage should be reduced appropriately according to age and weight.

Contra-indications, warnings, etc This preparation must not be administered undiluted. For information on rate of infusion see dosage recommendations above. Addiphos should not be used in patients with hyperkalaemia such as is associated with adrenal insufficiency or severe renal insufficiency, nor should it be given in the presence of dehydration without fluid replacement.

Precautions: Care should be exercised in patients with cardiac disease, diabetes mellitus, renal dysfunction or hepatic insufficiency. Infusion of potassium may depress cardiac function and counteract the effects of digitalis. Simultaneous infusion of potassium and glucose will lower the serum potassium levels otherwise attainable. Plasma levels and clinical signs suggesting hyperkalaemia require discontinuation of the infusion.

Pharmaceutical precautions

1. Store at 5° to 25°C.
2. The addition of Addiphos should be performed aseptically immediately before the start of the infusion and should be used within 24 hours unless the mixture is refrigerated when it may be used within 48 hours of preparation.

Compatibility has been demonstrated with the following solutions up to the maximum levels indicated:

Infusion solution (500 ml volume)	*Maximum volume of Addiphos which may be added to 500 ml of infusion solution*
Vamin 9	30 ml
Vamin 9 Glucose	30 ml
Vamin 14	20 ml
Vamin 14 Electrolyte-Free	30 ml
Vamin 18 Electrolyte-Free	30 ml
Glucose 5–60%	30 ml

Addiphos must not be added to the foregoing undiluted solutions in the presence of Addamel/Additrace.

3. Addiphos must only be added to solutions where compatibility is known.
4. Each vial is for single use only. It should be mixed well immediately after addition to the infusion solution.
5. A cloudy solution or one containing a precipitate must not be used.

Legal category POM.

Package quantities Boxes of 10 × 20 ml vials.

Further information In regimens including Intralipid, it should be noted that 500 ml Intralipid provides approximately 7.5 mmol organic phosphate. The manufacturer can be consulted for full information on complete and balanced intravenous nutrition regimens.

Product licence number 0022/0050.

ADDITRACE*

Presentation A clear, almost colourless solution containing trace elements for addition to Vamin amino acid solutions in the intravenous nutrition of adults. Additrace corresponds to the following formula:

Ferric chloride $6H_2O$	0.54 mg
Zinc chloride	1.36 mg
Manganese chloride $4H_2O$	99.0 micrograms
Copper chloride $2H_2O$	0.34 mg
Chromic Chloride	5.33 micrograms
Sodium selenite $5H_2O$	10.5 micrograms
Sodium molybdate $2H_2O$	4.85 micrograms
Sodium fluoride	0.21 mg
Potassium iodide	16.6 micrograms
Sorbitol	300 mg
Water for injections to 1 ml	
pH 2.2	

One ampoule (10 ml Additrace) contains the following amounts of trace elements;

Fe^{3+}	20 micromol
Zn^{2+}	100 micromol
Mn^{2+}	5 micromol
Cu^{2+}	20 micromol
Cr^{3+}	0.2 micromol
Se^{4+}	0.4 micromol
Mo^{6+}	0.2 micromol
F^-	50 micromol
I^-	1 micromol

One ampoule of Additrace contains less than 1 mmol of both potassium and sodium.

Uses Additrace is used as part of a complete intravenous nutrition regimen and provides a source of trace elements during nutritional support.

Dosage and administration

Recommended dosage for adults: 1 ampoule (10 ml) of Additrace is added to either 500 ml or 1000 ml of a solution listed in the table below. Where higher amounts of trace elements are considered necessary, 2 ampoules of Additrace may be added to 1000 ml solution. Additrace should not be added to Vamin 9 amino acid solution. Where a regimen includes Vamin 9, Additrace should be added to the glucose infusion.

Additrace does not contain calcium, magnesium or phosphate. These minerals should be added to the intravenous nutrition regimen if appropriate. (Vamin 9 Glucose and Vamin 14 contain calcium and magnesium. See appropriate data sheet). Similarly Additrace does not contain significant amounts of potassium or sodium (see 'Presentation' above) since the requirements for these electrolytes vary with different clinical conditions. Potassium and sodium salts should therefore be added as appropriate to the individual patient. (Vamin 9 Glucose and Vamin 14 contain potassium and sodium. See appropriate data sheet).

Infusion solution	*Volume to which 10 ml Additrace may be added (ml)*	
Vamin 9 Glucose	500–1000	Infusion should be completed within 24 hours of addition.
Vamin 14	500–1000	
Vamin 14 Electrolyte-Free	500–1000	
Vamin 18 Electrolyte-Free	500–1000	
Glucose 5–50%	500–1000	

Additrace must only be added to solutions where compatibility is known.

The above mixtures containing Vamin should be infused at an appropriate rate for the amino acid solution and the infusion completed not more than 24 hours after preparation. If Additrace is added to a solution other than those listed above, then ensure that the solution is administered over a period of not less than 2 hours, so as to minimise renal losses.

Recommended dosage for infants: For infants the electrolyte solution Ped-el should be used.

Contra-indications, warnings, etc Should not be given undiluted.

Care should be taken in the administration of Additrace to patients with impaired biliary or renal function.

One ampoule of Additrace contains 3 g sorbitol which is metabolised to fructose and should therefore be given with caution to patients with fructose intolerance.

Pharmaceutical precautions No other additions should be made to solutions containing Additrace unless compatibility is known.

1. Store at room temperature.
2. The addition of Additrace should be performed aseptically immediately before the start of the infusion and should be used within 24 hours.

Legal category POM.

Package quantities Boxes of 10 × 10 ml ampoules.

Further information The manufacturer can be consulted for full information on complete and balanced intravenous nutrition regimens.

Product licence number 0022/0064.

CALMURID*

Presentation A white shiny cream containing Carbamide (urea) BP 10% and lactic acid 5% in a stabilising emulsified base containing betaine, cetyl diethanolamine phosphate, cholesterol, sodium chloride, mono, di- and tri-glycerides of saturated fatty acids, purified water.

Uses For correction of hyperkeratosis and dryness in ichthyosis and allied conditions characterised by dry, rough, scaly skin.

Dosage and administration A thick layer of Calmurid is applied twice daily after washing the affected area. The cream is left on the skin for three to five minutes and then lightly rubbed in. Excess cream can be wiped off with a tissue. Frequency of application can be reduced as patient progresses. In hyperkeratosis of the feet apply Calmurid as above after soaking the feet in warm water for 15 minutes and drying with a rough towel.

Elderly: No special instructions.

Contra-indications, warnings, etc *Adverse effects:* Calmurid is acidic and can cause smarting when applied to raw areas, fissures or mucous membranes. Where this is a barrier to therapy, use of Calmurid diluted 50% with Aqueous Cream BP for one week should result in freedom from smarting on application of Calmurid.

Pharmaceutical precautions Store in a cool place but do not freeze. Do not put in alloy containers.

Legal category GSL.

Package quantities Tube of 100 g. Pump-pack of 400 g.

Further information Calmurid, besides being keratolytic, replaces the small water-binding molecules of which dry skin may be deficient. It does not contain lanolin, steroids or preservatives.

Product licence number 0009/5009.

Product licence holder: Pharmacia Biosystems Ltd, Davy Avenue, Knowlhill, Milton Keynes MK5 8PH.

CALMURID* HC

Presentation A white shiny cream containing:

Carbamide (urea) BP	10%
Hydrocortisone	1%
Lactic acid	5%

in a stabilising emulsified base containing betaine, cetyl diethanolamine phosphate, cholesterol, sodium chloride, mono, di- and tri-glycerides of saturated fatty acids, purified water.

Uses Atopic eczema; Besnier's prurigo; acute and chronic allergic eczema; neurodermatitis and other hyperkeratotic skin conditions with accompanying inflammation.

Dosage and administration Apply the cream twice daily after washing and drying the lesion.

Elderly: No special instructions.

Contra-indications, warnings, etc *Adverse effects:* Because Calmurid HC is acidic it may cause smarting if applied to raw or fissured areas. Moist lesions should be encouraged to dry before beginning therapy.

Where smarting is a barrier to therapy, use of a mixture of Calmurid HC with an equal amount of Aqueous Cream BP for a week should result in freedom from smarting when undiluted Calmurid HC is applied.

In pregnant animals, administration of corticosteroids can cause abnormalities of foetal development. The relevance of this finding to human beings has not been established. However, topical steroids should not be used extensively in pregnancy, i.e. in large amounts or for long periods.

In infants, long-term continuous topical therapy should be avoided. Adrenal suppression can occur even without occlusion.

Contra-indications: Do not use in tubercular, viral or syphilitic skin infections. Antimycotic treatment should complement Calmurid HC in dermal fungal infections.

Pharmaceutical precautions Keep in a cool place but do not freeze. Do not pack in alloy containers.

Legal category POM.

Package quantities Tubes of 30 g and 100 g.

Further information Calmurid HC has keratolytic, antipruritic, anti-inflammatory and re-hydrating effects on the skin. It does not contain lanolin or preservatives.

Product licence number 0009/5003.

Product licence holder: Pharmacia Biosystems Ltd, Davy Avenue, Knowlhill, Milton Keynes MK5 8PH.

CALMURID* SOLUTION

Presentation Solution containing 20% urea, 5% lactic acid in a stabilising aqueous vehicle containing betaine, sodium chloride, Tween 20 and water.

Uses For the treatment of dry scalp conditions – seborrhoea, seborrhoeic eczema, atopic eczema, ichthyosis. As part of the treatment of psoriasis of the scalp.

Dosage and administration Apply the solution to the scalp twice a day.

Wash the hair every other day with a mild shampoo during the course of treatment.

Elderly and children: No special instructions.

Contra-indications, warnings, etc Calmurid Solution can cause smarting temporarily when applied to raw or fissured areas.

Over-use may cause matting of the hair. The dried lotion will readily dissolve off the hair.

A feeling of scalp dryness has occasionally been noted early in treatment, but it generally soon passes off. A persistent feeling of scalp dryness may be due to too frequent use or the use of a harsh shampoo when the hair is washed.

Pharmaceutical precautions Store in a cool place but do not freeze.

Legal category P.

Package quantities Plastic bottle of 125 ml.

Further information Calmurid Solution does not contain lanolin, steroids or preservatives.

Product licence number 0009/0017.

Product licence holder: Pharmacia Biosystems Ltd, Davy Avenue, Knowlhill, Milton Keynes MK5 8PH.

CYKLOKAPRON* INJECTION

Presentation Ampoules of 5 ml of colourless solution containing Tranexamic Acid BP 500 mg in each 5 ml.

Uses
Action: Tranexamic acid is an antifibrinolytic agent which competitively inhibits the activation of plasminogen to plasmin.

Indications: Local fibrinolysis – For short term use in prophylaxis and treatment in patients at high risk of per- and post-operative haemorrhage following
(a) Prostatectomy.
(b) Conisation of the cervix.
(c) Surgical procedures and dental extractions in haemophiliacs.

General fibrinolysis
(a) Haemorrhagic complications in association with thrombolytic therapy.
(b) Haemorrhage associated with disseminated intravascular coagulation with predominant activation of the fibrinolytic system (see Warnings below).

Dosage and administration
Local fibrinolysis: The recommended standard dose is 5–10 ml (500–1000 mg) by slow intravenous injection (1 ml/min), three times daily. If treatment continues for more than three days, consideration should be given to the use of Cyklokapron tablets or syrup. Alternatively, following an initial intravenous injection, subsequent treatment may proceed by intravenous infusion. Following addition to a suitable diluent (see Pharmaceutical precautions), Cyklokapron may be administered at a rate of 25–50 mg/kg body wt/day.

Children's dosage: According to body weight (10 mg/kg body wt/2–3 times daily).

Elderly patients: No reduction in dosage is necessary unless there is evidence of renal failure (see guidelines below).

General fibrinolysis: In disseminated intravascular coagulation with predominant activation of the fibrinolytic system, usually a single dose of 10 ml (1 g) is sufficient to control bleeding.

Neutralisation of thrombolytic therapy; 10 mg/kg body wt by slow intravenous injection.

Contra-indications, warnings, etc Cyklokapron is contra-indicated in patients with a history of thromboembolic disease.

Precautions:

1. In patients with renal insufficiency, because of the risk of accumulation. The dose should be reduced according to the following table:

Serum creatinine	*Dose i.v.*	*Dose frequency*
120–250 micromol/l	10 mg/kg	twice daily
250–500 micromol/l	10 mg/kg	every 24th hour
>500 micromol/l	5 mg/kg	every 24th hour

2. In massive haematuria from the upper urinary tract (especially in haemophilia) since, in a few cases, ureteric obstruction has been reported.

3. In patients with disseminated intravascular coagulation (DIC) treatment must be restricted to those in whom there is predominant activation of the fibrinolytic system with acute severe bleeding. Characteristically, the haematological profile approximates to the following: reduced euglobulin clot lysis time; prolonged prothrombin time; reduced plasma levels of fibrinogen, Factors V and VIII, plasminogen and alpha-2 macroglobulin; normal plasma levels of P and P complex, ie factors II (prothrombin), VII and X; increased plasma levels of fibrinogen degradation products; a normal platelet count. The foregoing presumes that the underlying disease state does not of itself modify the various elements in this profile. In such acute cases a single dose of 1 g tranexamic acid is frequently sufficient to control bleeding. The fibrinolytic activity in the blood will be reduced for about 4 hours if renal function is normal. Anticoagulation with heparin should be instigated in order to prevent further fibrin deposition. Administration of Cyklokapron in DIC should be considered only when appropriate haematological laboratory facilities and expertise are available. Cyklokapron must not be administered in DIC with predominant activation of the coagulation system.

Pregnancy: Although there is no evidence from animal studies of a teratogenic effect, the usual caution with the use of drugs in pregnancy should be observed.

Lactation: Tranexamic acid passes into breast milk to a concentration of approximately one hundredth of the concentration in the maternal blood. An antifibrinolytic effect in the infant is unlikely.

Side-effects: Gastro-intestinal disorders (nausea, vomiting, diarrhoea) may occur but disappear when the dosage is reduced. Rapid intravenous injection may cause dizziness and/or hypotension.

Antidote: No cases of overdosage have been reported. Symptoms may be nausea, vomiting, orthostatic symptoms and/or hypotension. Maintain a high fluid intake to promote renal excretion.

Pharmaceutical precautions The solution for injection may be mixed with the following solutions: isotonic sodium chloride; isotonic glucose; 20% fructose; 10% invertose; Dextran 40; Dextran 70; Ringer's solution.

Cyklokapron solution for injection may be mixed with heparin.

Cyklokapron solution for injection should NOT be added to blood for transfusion, or to injections containing penicillin.

Legal category POM.

Package quantities Boxes of 10 × 5 ml ampoules.

Further information Approximately 90% of an intravenously administered tranexamic acid dose is excreted, largely unchanged, in the urine within 24 hours. The plasma half-life is approximately 2 hours.

Product licence number 0022/0004R.

CYKLOKAPRON* SYRUP

Presentation A colourless or slightly yellow syrup containing Tranexamic Acid BP 500 mg in each 5 ml.

Uses
Action: Tranexamic acid is an antifibrinolytic agent which competitively inhibits the activation of plasminogen to plasmin.

Indications: Short-term use for haemorrhage or risk of haemorrhage in increased fibrinolysis or fibrinogenolysis.

1. Local fibrinolysis as occurs in the following conditions:

(a) Prostatectomy
(b) Menorrhagia
(c) Epistaxis
(d) Conisation of the cervix
(e) Traumatic hyphaema

2. Management of dental extraction in haemophiliacs.
3. Hereditary angioneurotic oedema.

Dosage and administration
Local fibrinolysis: The recommended standard dose is 15–25 mg/kg body wt, i.e. 10–15 ml syrup, two to three times daily. For the indications listed below the following doses may be used:

1a. *Prostatectomy:* Prophylaxis and treatment of haemorrhage in high risk patients should commence per- or post-operatively with Cyklokapron Injection; thereafter 10 ml syrup, three to four times daily until macroscopic haematuria is no longer present.

1b. *Menorrhagia:* 10–15 ml syrup three to four times daily for three to four days. Cyklokapron therapy is initiated only after heavy bleeding has started and its use should be restricted to not more than three menstrual cycles.

1c. *Epistaxis:* Where recurrent bleeding is anticipated oral therapy (10 ml syrup three times daily) should be administered for seven days.

1d. *Conisation of the cervix:* 15 ml syrup three times daily.

1e. *Traumatic hyphaema:* 10–15 ml syrup three times daily. The dose is based on 25 mg/kg three times a day.

2. *Haemophilia:* In the management of dental extractions 10–15 ml syrup every eight hours. The dose is based on 25 mg/kg.

3. *Hereditary angioneurotic oedema:* Some patients are aware of the onset of the illness; suitable treatment for these patients is intermittently 10–15 ml syrup two to three times daily for some days. Other patients are treated continuously at this dosage.

Children's dosage: This should be calculated according to body weight, at 25 mg/kg/2–3 times daily.

Elderly patients: No reduction in dosage is necessary unless there is evidence of renal failure (see guidelines below).

Contra-indications, warnings, etc Cyklokapron is contra-indicated in patients with a history of thromboembolic disease.

Precautions:

1. In patients with renal insufficiency, because of the risk of accumulation. By extrapolation from clearance data relating to the intravenous dosage form, the following reduction in the oral dosage is recommended.

Serum creatinine	*Oral dose*	*Dose frequency*
120–250 micromol/l	25 mg/kg	twice daily
250–500 micromol/l	25 mg/kg	every 24th hour
>500 micromol/l	12.5 mg/kg	every 24th hour

2. In massive haematuria from the upper urinary tract (especially in haemophilia) since, in a few cases, ureteric obstruction has been reported.

3. In the long-term treatment of patients with hereditary angioneurotic oedema regular eye examination (e.g. visual acuity, slit lamp, intra-ocular pressure, visual fields) and liver function tests should be performed.

Pregnancy: Although there is no evidence from animal studies of a teratogenic effect, the usual caution with use of drugs in pregnancy should be observed.

Lactation: Tranexamic acid passes into breast milk to a concentration of approximately one hundredth of the concentration in the maternal blood. An antifibrinolytic effect in the infant is unlikely.

Side-effects: Gastro-intestinal disorders (nausea, vomiting, diarrhoea) may occur but disappear when the dosage is reduced. Rare instances of transient colour vision disturbance have been reported.

Antidote: No cases of overdosage have been reported. Symptoms may be nausea, vomiting, orthostatic symptoms and/or hypotension. Initiate vomiting, then stomach lavage and charcoal therapy. Maintain a high fluid intake to promote renal excretion.

Pharmaceutical precautions Cyklokapron Syrup may be diluted with Syrup BP, and the resulting mixture may be stored for up to 14 days.

Legal category POM.

Package quantities Bottle of 300 ml Syrup.

Further information Absorption of tranexamic acid from the gastrointestinal tract is 30–40%. The plasma half-life is approximately 2 hours.

Product licence number 0022/0044.

CYKLOKAPRON* TABLETS

Presentation White, film-coated oblong tablets, 8 × 18 mm, engraved CY with an arc above and below the lettering. Each tablet contains Tranexamic Acid BP 500 mg.

Uses

Action: Tranexamic acid is an antifibrinolytic agent which competitively inhibits the activation of plasminogen to plasmin.

Indications: Short-term use for haemorrhage or risk of haemorrhage in increased fibrinolysis or fibrinogenolysis.

1. Local fibrinolysis as occurs in the following conditions:

(a) Prostatectomy
(b) Menorrhagia
(c) Epistaxis
(d) Conisation of the cervix
(e) Traumatic hyphaema

2. Management of dental extraction in haemophiliacs.
3. Hereditary angioneurotic oedema.

Dosage and administration

Local fibrinolysis: The recommended standard dose is 15–25 mg/kg body wt, i.e. 2–3 tablets two to three times daily. For the indications listed below the following doses may be used:

1a. *Prostatectomy:* Prophylaxis and treatment of haemorrhage in high risk patients should commence per- or post-operatively with Cyklokapron Injection; thereafter 2 tablets, three to four times daily until macroscopic haematuria is no longer present.

1b. *Menorrhagia:* 2–3 tablets three to four times daily for three to four days. Cyklokapron therapy is initiated only after heavy bleeding has started and its use should be restricted to not more than three menstrual cycles.

1c. *Epistaxis:* Where recurrent bleeding is anticipated oral therapy (2 tablets three times daily) should be administered for seven days.

1d. *Conisation of the cervix:* 3 tablets three times daily.

1e. *Traumatic hyphaema:* 2–3 tablets three times daily. The dose is based on 25 mg/kg three times a day.

2. *Haemophilia:* In the management of dental extractions 2–3 tablets every eight hours. The dose is based on 25 mg/kg.

3. *Hereditary angioneurotic oedema:* Some patients are aware of the onset of the illness; suitable treatment for these patients is intermittently 2–3 tablets two to three times daily for some days. Other patients are treated continuously at this dosage.

Children's dosage: This should be calculated according to body weight, at 25 mg/kg/2–3 times daily.

Elderly patients: No reduction in dosage is necessary unless there is evidence of renal failure (see guidelines below).

Contra-indications, warnings, etc Cyklokapron is contra-indicated in patients with a history of thromboembolic disease.

Precautions:

1. In patients with renal insufficiency, because of the risk of accumulation. By extrapolation from clearance data relating to the intravenous dosage form, the following reduction in the oral dosage is recommended.

Serum creatinine	*Oral dose*	*Dose frequency*
120–250 micromol/l	25 mg/kg	twice daily
250–500 micromol/l	25 mg/kg	every 24th hour
>500 micromol/l	12.5 mg/kg	every 24th hour

2. In massive haematuria from the upper urinary tract (especially in haemophilia) since, in a few cases, ureteric obstruction has been reported.

3. When disseminated intravascular coagulation is in progress.

4. In the long-term treatment of patients with hereditary angioneurotic oedema regular eye examination (e.g. visual acuity, slit lamp, intra-ocular pressure, visual fields) and liver function tests should be performed.

Pregnancy: Although there is no evidence from animal studies of a teratogenic effect, the usual caution with use of drugs in pregnancy should be observed.

Lactation: Tranexamic acid passes into breast milk to a concentration of approximately one hundredth of the concentration in the maternal blood. An antifibrinolytic effect in the infant is unlikely.

Side-effects: Gastro-intestinal disorders (nausea, vomiting, diarrhoea) may occur but disappear when the dosage is reduced. Rare instances of transient colour vision disturbance have been reported.

Antidote: No cases of overdosage have been reported.

Symptoms may be nausea, vomiting, orthostatic symptoms and/or hypotension. Initiate vomiting, then stomach lavage and charcoal therapy. Maintain a high fluid intake to promote renal excretion.

Legal category POM.

Package quantities Carton containing 5 blister strips of 12 tablets each.

Further information Absorption of tranexamic acid from the gastro-intestinal tract is 30–40%. The plasma half-life is approximately 2 hours.

Product licence number 0022/0003R.

DEBRISAN*

Presentation Sterile, straw-coloured spherical beads of dextranomer of 0.1–0.3 mm diameter, packed in plastic castors or single-use sachets.

Uses A dressing for moist wounds and indolent ulcers, whether clean or infected and small area burns.

Dosage and administration A 3 mm layer of Debrisan should be sprinkled onto the wound and kept in place by a pad of lint or a perforated plastic sheet. Debrisan is hydrophilic and the tissue exudate is drawn up into the layer. The Debrisan should be renewed before saturation occurs. Depending on the rate of exudation this may be necessary from one to five times a day. Once or twice daily is usually adequate. When Debrisan is changed the old material is readily rinsed off with water or saline and new material may then be sprinkled onto the wound.

Shallow wounds, or those in awkward positions, may be dressed more easily by using Debrisan Paste, or by mixing four parts of Debrisan with one part of sterile glycerol to form a stiff paste. This should be spread into the wound with a spatula to a depth of 3 mm or more. Dressing continues as above. The paste should be prepared freshly at each application. Once the wound is clean and poorly secreting, change therapy to an antiseptic dressing, e.g. chlorhexidine tulle, or a sterile pad.

Full instructions for use are enclosed with each pack. Treated in this manner the wound will remain soft and pliable during healing.

Elderly: No special instructions.

Contra-indications, warnings, etc

1. Do not leave Debrisan for more than 24 hours on wounds with a very low exudation rate as it may dry and form a crust which may be difficult to wash off.
2. Occlusive dressings may lead to maceration of skin round the wound under treatment.
3. When deep infected wounds are treated, care must be taken to wash Debrisan from the depths of the wound.
4. No side-effects have been reported.

Warning: Debrisan spillage can render surfaces very slippery. Clear spillages promptly.

Precautions:

1. Not to be used on dry wounds.
2. When exudate has been markedly removed by Debrisan alternative treatment should be substituted.
3. In order to avoid cross-infection it is recommended that the contents of a castor be confined to the treatment of a single patient for one day.

Pharmaceutical precautions Keep in a dry place in well-closed containers.

Package quantities Castors of 60 g.
Sachets of 4 g in boxes of ten sachets.

Legal category P.

Further information Each gram of Debrisan absorbs 4 grams of exudate. Capillary action carries debris and bacteria away from the wound surface. Local oedema is reduced so that the wound may look larger initially. Debrisan is non sensitising and controls malodour.

Product licence number 0009/0021.

Product licence holder: Pharmacia Biosystems Ltd, Davy Avenue, Knowlhill, Milton Keynes MK5 8PH.

DEBRISAN* ABSORBENT PAD

Presentation Foil sachet containing sterile off-white paste in textile bag. Paste consists of Dextranomer 90%, polyethylene glycol and water 10%. Dimensions 6 × 4 cm.

Uses For topical application to exudating or infected wounds, such as surgical wounds, post traumatic wounds, pressure sores and leg ulcers.

Dosage and administration Frequency of change of the pad will be dictated by the rate of exudation of the wound. This may vary from twice daily to every two days. The textile has little tendency to adhere to the wound, but when it does sterile saline should readily loosen it. No special regimes of age groups.

Contra-indications, warnings, etc
Precautions: Use with caution near the eyes.

Warnings: Transient pain may occur in the wound area. This can often be avoided by wetting the wound before pad application.

Pharmaceutical precautions None.

Legal category P.

Package quantities Box containing 7 × 3 g pads.

Further information Nil.

Product licence number 0009/0048.

Product licence holder: Pharmacia Biosystems Ltd, Davy Avenue, Knowlhill, Milton Keynes MK5 8PH.

DEBRISAN* PASTE

Presentation Foil-plastic laminate pouches containing 10 g of a sterile soft, white, granular paste consisting of: Dextranomer 6.4 g, polyethylene glycol 600 and water to 10 g.

Uses Treatment of exudative and infected wounds such as surgical or post-traumatic wounds, decubital ulcers and leg ulcers. As the paste is adherent it may be preferred to Debrisan beads on shallow wounds, or those where retention of the beads is a problem.

Dosage and administration After cleaning the wound with sterile water or saline the Paste is applied firmly with a spatula to a depth of not less than 3 mm. The wound is covered and the Paste changed at intervals governed by the exudation rate of the wound, the Paste being renewed before it is entirely discoloured and saturated with secretion and debris. Debrisan Paste should be changed from twice daily to every two days according to the rate of exudation. Stop Debrisan Paste once the wound is granulating and free of exudate, changing to sterile or antiseptic dressings.

Elderly: No special instructions.

Contra-indications, warnings, etc Use with caution: When applied near the eyes; in deep fistulae etc. with a narrow opening where paste removal might be difficult.

Occasionally pain may be experienced in the wound after application. This can be avoided by wetting the wound before applying the Paste.

Pharmaceutical precautions Stored at room temperature the shelf life is 3 years.

Legal category P.

Package quantities 6 × 10 g; 4 × 10 g.

Further information Nil.

Product licence number 0009/0044.

Product licence holder: Pharmacia Biosystems Ltd, Davy Avenue, Knowlhill, Milton Keynes MK5 8PH.

DIPENTUM*

Presentation Caramel coloured capsules containing 250 mg olsalazine sodium.

Uses Oral treatment of acute mild ulcerative colitis and the maintenance of remission. Olsalazine consists of two molecules of 5-amino-salicylic acid (5-ASA) joined through an azo-bond. The systemic absorption of olsalazine is minimal. 99% of an oral dose will reach the colon. Olsalazine is activated in the colon where it is converted into 5-ASA. The release of 5-ASA is neither pH nor time dependent. 5-ASA acts topically on the colonic mucosa and local colonic concentrations of 5-ASA are more than 1000 times that found in the serum.

Dosage and administration
Acute mild disease

Adults including the elderly: Commence on 1 g daily in divided doses and, depending upon the patient response, titrate the dose upwards to a maximum of 3 g daily over 1 week.

A single dose should not exceed 1 g.

Olsalazine should be taken with food.

Remission

Adults including the elderly: 2 capsules (0.5 g) twice daily taken with food.

Contra-indications, warnings, etc

Contra-indications: Hypersensitivity to salicylates.

There is no experience of the use of olsalazine in patients with significant renal impairment. Olsalazine is contra-indicated in patients with significant renal impairment.

Pregnancy: Comprehensive animal reproductive toxicity studies have not been performed. There is no experience with olsalazine treatment during pregnancy. Olsalazine is contra-indicated in pregnancy.

Lactation: There are no data on the excretion of olsalazine in breast milk.

Adverse reactions: Watery diarrhoea has been recorded in 15% of patients treated. In half of these patients the diarrhoea was either transient or overcome by dose reduction. In patients who do not respond to dose reduction the drug should be stopped.

As with sulphasalazine and mesalazine gastrointestinal side-effects are the most common. The most frequently reported adverse reactions are diarrhoea, abdominal cramps, headache, nausea, dyspepsia, arthralgia and rash.

Treatment of overdosage: There is no specific antidote to olsalazine. Treatment should be supportive.

Pharmaceutical precautions Store at room temperature in a dry place.

Legal category POM.

Package quantities Containers of 100 capsules.

Further information Olsalazine has been used concomitantly with glucocorticosteroids.

Product licence number 0009/0069

Product licence holder: Pharmacia Biosystems Ltd, Davy Avenue, Knowlhill, Milton Keynes MK5 8PH.

ESTRACYT* CAPSULES

Presentation Off-white gelatin capsules each containing 140 mg estramustine phosphate as the disodium salt.

Active ingredient: 140 mg estramustine phosphate – oestra-1,3,5(10)-triene-3,17β-diol-3-bis-(2-chloroethyl) carbamate-17-disodium phosphate.

Uses *Pharmacology:* Estracyt is a chemical compound of oestradiol and normustine and has both oestrogenic and cytotoxic activity. Its oestrogenic effect is weaker than that of oestradiol and this is reflected by the lower incidence of gynaecomastia and other feminising side-effects in patients treated with Estracyt for prostatic carcinoma. Estracyt also has antioestrogenic activity in that it antagonises the uterotrophic effect of oestrone in juvenile mice, antigonadotrophic activity in that it causes atrophy of the testes and accessory sex organs in rats, and anti-androgenic activity in that it inhibits testosterone-induced growth of the ventral prostate of castrated animals.

Estracyt's cytotoxic activity is weaker than that of conventional alkylating agents. It is concentrated ten times more efficiently than oestradiol in prostatic tissue and has a greater affinity for prostatic than for other tissue. Though active against experimental animal tumours (rat DMBA-induced mammary tumour and hepatoma AH130), Estracyt has weak general cytostatic effects and causes little or no marrow depression at conventional therapeutic dosage. It has no immunosuppressant effect.

Estracyt appears to lose its phosphate moiety in the gut, liver and in phosphatase-rich human tissue, and following breakage of the carbamate linkage the steroid and alkylating moieties are excreted independently. Absorption of Estracyt from the gut is about 75% complete.

Indications Carcinoma of the prostate, especially in cases unresponsive to, or relapsing after, treatment by conventional oestrogens (stilboestrol, polyoestradiol phosphate (Estradurin), etc) or by orchidectomy. The response rate to Estracyt in such oestrogen-resistant cases is about 30% to 50%.

Dosage and administration *Adults:* Dosage range may be from 1 to 10 capsules a day by mouth with meals. The capsules should not be taken with milk or milk products. Standard starting dosage is 4–8 capsules a day in divided doses with later adjustment according to response and gastrointestinal tolerance.

Children: Adenocarcinoma of the prostate is almost unknown in young boys and no relevant clinical studies of Estracyt have been carried out. Estracyt should not be administered to children.

Contra-indications, warnings, etc Peptic ulceration, severe liver disease and severe cardiac disease.

Precautions: Caution should be exercised in administering Estracyt to patients with moderate to severe bone marrow depression.

Adverse reactions: Adverse effects which may be encountered in treatment are gastrointestinal upset (most commonly transient nausea, but occasionally vomiting, and rarely diarrhoea); disturbance of liver function has been reported; rarely thrombocytopenia below 100,000 mm^3; gynaecomastia (seen in less than 5% of patients); cardiovascular (with an incidence of angina no greater than that encountered in patients treated with conventional oestrogens, but including rare drug-related deaths from myocardial infarction); and allergy (manifest as a rash and/or fever).

Overdosage: There is no specific antidote. In the event of dangerously low levels of red cell, white cell or platelet counts; cross-matched whole blood should be given as necessary. It may also be advisable to monitor liver function.

Pharmaceutical precautions Store at room temperature. The preparation has a shelf life of three years from the date of manufacture.

Legal category POM.

For use in hospitals and hospital clinics, and supplied to retail pharmacies for dispensing prescriptions for patients whose treatment has been initiated in hospital practice. Estracyt capsules are available on prescription only.

Package quantities Bottles of 100 capsules each containing 140 mg estramustine phosphate as the disodium salt.

Further information Nil.

Product licence number 0458/0016.

Product licence holder: Lundbeck Ltd, Hastings Street, Luton, Beds LU1 5BE.

ESTRADURIN* INJECTION

Presentation Estradurin Injection contains 40 mg or 80 mg polyoestradiol phosphate per vial, for reconstitution with water for injection.

Estradurin 40 mg vial:

Polyoestradiol phosphate	40 mg
Mepivacaine	5 mg
Nicotinamide	25 mg

Estradurin 80 mg vial:

Polyoestradiol phosphate	80 mg
Mepivacaine	5 mg
Nicotinamide	40 mg

Uses *Pharmacology:* Estradurin is a water-soluble polymer in which molecules of oestradiol-17β alternate with phosphate groups. After intramuscular injection it acts primarily as a long-acting form of oestradiol, but it also has an inhibitory action on acid and alkaline phosphatases.

The prolonged action of Estradurin is attributed to the slow progressive breakdown of the polymer by phosphatases *in vivo.* Since Estradurin has an inhibiting effect on phosphatases this breakdown is very slow, providing sustained oestrogen activity for up to four weeks after a single injection.

Indications: The treatment of oestrogen-responsive carcinoma of the prostate, particularly in men suspected of unreliability in the taking of conventional oral oestrogen.

Dosage and administration *Adults:* The recommended starting dose is 80–160 mg every four weeks for two to three months. Thereafter the dose may be reduced, in accordance with the patient's clinical and biochemical progress, to 40–80 mg every four weeks.

NB. Estradurin must be administered by *deep* intramuscular injection.

Children: Estradurin should not be administered to children.

Contra-indications, warnings, etc There are no contra-indications for Estradurin, but it should be used with caution in patients with serious liver impairment or thromboembolic cardiovascular disease.

Adverse reactions: Certain characteristic oestrogenic side-effects occur (e.g. gynaecomastia, feminisation), but their incidence and severity are considerably less than those encountered in patients receiving conventional stilboestrol therapy. Gastrointestinal disturbances have not been reported during treatment with Estradurin.

Overdosage: There is no specific antidote. Treatment should be purely symptomatic.

Pharmaceutical precautions Store at room temperature.

The product has a shelf life of five years from the date of manufacture. Estradurin solution is prepared by adding 2 ml water for injection to the vial and shaking until solution is complete.

It is recommended that solutions of Estradurin be prepared immediately before use.

Legal category POM.

Package quantities
10 × 40 mg vials: (with 10 × 2 ml ampoules water for injection.
10 × 80 mg vials: (with 10 × 2 ml ampoules water for injection).

Further information Mepivacaine, a local anaesthetic, is included to minimise discomfort at the site of injection.

Nicotinamide is included to enhance solubility of the polymer.

Product licence numbers
Estradurin 40 mg 0458/5000
Estradurin 80 mg 0458/5001

Product licence holder: Lundbeck Ltd, Hastings Street, Luton, Beds LU1 5BE

FRAGMIN* AMPOULES ▼

Presentation
Fragmin 10,000 iu/4 ml: Ampoules containing dalteparin sodium corresponding to 2,500 IU (anti-Factor Xa)/ml as a sterile, clear, colourless to straw coloured isotonic solution, for intravenous injection or intravenous infusion.

Fragmin 10,000 iu/1 ml: Ampoules containing dalteparin sodium, 10,000 IU (anti-Factor Xa) in 1 ml as a sterile, clear, colourless to straw coloured isotonic solution, for intravenous injection or intravenous infusion.

Uses
Actions: Dalteparin sodium is a physiological antithrombotic agent which acts mainly through potentiation of the inhibition of activated coagulation factors by antithrombin.

Indications: Prevention of clotting in the extracorporeal circulation during haemodialysis or haemofiltration, in patients with chronic renal insufficiency or acute renal failure.

Dosage and administration
Haemodialysis and haemofiltration
Adults: In chronic renal insufficiency for patients with no known additional bleeding risk, the dosage is:

(a) *Long-term haemodialysis or haemofiltration* – duration of haemodialysis/haemofiltration more than 4 hours.

An iv bolus injection of Fragmin 35 IU (anti-Factor Xa)/kg b.w., followed by an infusion of 13 IU (anti-Factor Xa)/kg b.w./hour.

(b) *Short-term haemodialysis or haemofiltration* – duration of haemodialysis/haemofiltration less than 4 hours.

Either as above, or, a single i.v. bolus injection of Fragmin 5000 IU (anti-Factor Xa).

Both for long and short-term haemodialysis and haemofiltration, the plasma anti-Factor Xa levels should be within the range 0.5–1.0 IU (anti-Factor Xa)/ml.

(c) *In acute renal failure, or chronic renal failure in patients with a high risk of bleeding, the dosage is* an i.v. bolus injection of Fragmin 8 IU (anti-Factor Xa)/kg b.w., followed by an infusion of 5 IU (anti-Factor Xa)/kg b.w./ hour.

The plasma anti-Factor Xa levels should be within the range 0.2–0.4 IU (anti-Factor Xa)/ml.

When necessary it is recommended that the antithrombotic effect of Fragmin may be monitored by means of analysing anti-Factor Xa activity using a suitable chromogenic substrate assay (see Further Information section).

Children: Not recommended for children.

Elderly: Fragmin has been used safely in elderly patients without the need for dosage adjustment.

Contra-indications, warnings, etc
Contra-indications: There are no known absolute contra-indications to Fragmin. However, caution should be exercised in patients in whom there is an increased risk of bleeding complications, e.g. following surgery or trauma, known haemorrhagic diathesis, haemorrhagic stroke, severe liver failure, thrombocytopenia or defective platelet function, use of concomitant haemostatic drugs, subacute endocarditis, severe hypertension, diabetes mellitus with retinopathy, and in patients receiving concurrent anticoagulant/antiplatelet agents (see Interactions section) and also in patients with known heparin hypersensitivity.

Precautions and warnings: Fragmin induces only a moderate prolongation of the APTT and thrombin time; prolongation of the APTT may be used only as a test of overdosage. Accordingly, dosage increments based upon prolongation of the APTT may cause overdosage and bleeding.

Anti-Factor Xa levels should be regularly monitored in new patients on haemodialysis during the first weeks, later less frequent monitoring is generally required. Patients undergoing acute haemodialysis have a narrower therapeutic dose range and should be monitored frequently in accordance with the individual course of the disease.

Patients with severely disturbed hepatic function may need a reduction in dosage and should be monitored accordingly.

Use in pregnancy and lactation: There has been little usage during pregnancy in humans but there has been no adverse animal evidence. Avoid in pregnancy if a better known and safer alternative is available.

It is not known whether Fragmin passes the placenta or is excreted in breast milk.

Side-effects: Bleeding may be provoked, especially at high dosages corresponding with anti-Factor Xa levels greater than 1.5 IU/ml. Transient, slight to moderate, elevation of liver transaminases (ASAT, ALAT) has been observed, but no clinical significance has been demonstrated.

The following side-effects of heparin have not been observed with Fragmin, however, they cannot be excluded as Fragmin is derived from heparin: thrombocytopenia; allergic reactions (urticaria, anaphylaxis, pruritus, hair loss and skin necrosis).

Long-term treatment with heparin has been associated with a risk of osteoporosis. Though this condition has not been observed with Fragmin the risk of osteoporosis cannot be excluded.

Overdosage or special warnings: The anticoagulant effect induced by Fragmin is inhibited by protamine. Since protamine itself has an inhibiting effect on primary haemostasis it should be used only in an emergency. The prolongation of the APTT induced by Fragmin is fully neutralised by protamine, but only about 25–50 per cent of the anti-Factor Xa activity is affected. 1 mg of protamine inhibits the effect of 100 IU (anti-Factor Xa) of Fragmin.

Interactions: Concomitant medication with anticoagulant/antiplatelet agents may enhance the anticoagulant effect of Fragmin, e.g. aspirin, vitamin-K antagonists and dextran.

The possibility of the following interactions should also be considered.

i. An enhancement of the anticoagulant effect by dipyridamole, indomethacin, sulphinpyrazone, probenecid, ethacrynic acid i.v. and cytostatics.
ii. A reduction of the anticoagulant effect may occur with concomitant administration of antihistamines, cardiac glycosides, tetracycline and ascorbic acid.

Pharmaceutical precautions Fragmin solution for injection 10,000 IU/4 ml (2500 IU/ml) and 10,000 IU/1 ml (anti-Factor Xa) is compatible with isotonic sodium chloride (9 mg/ml) or isotonic glucose (50 mg/ml) infusion solution in glass bottles and plastic containers, for up to 24 hours.

Fragmin should be stored at room temperature.

Legal category POM.

Package quantities
Fragmin 10,000 IU (anti-Factor Xa)/4 ml, 10 × 4 ml ampoules
Fragmin 10,000 IU (anti-Factor Xa)/1 ml, 10 × 1 ml ampoules

Further information Fragmin does not contain preservatives.

One unit of dalteparin sodium corresponds to the activity of one IU of the first International Standard for LMW Heparin with respect to the inhibition of coagulation Factor Xa in plasma.

Dalteparin sodium is a low molecular weight heparin fraction (average molecular weight 4000–6000 Daltons) produced from porcine-derived sodium heparin. Dalteparin sodium specifically inhibits the coagulation Factor Xa. The antithrombotic effect of dalteparin sodium correlates closely with the inhibition of Factor Xa.

The half life following i.v. injection is 2 hours. The bioavailability after s.c. injection is approximately 87 per cent and the pharmacokinetics are not dose dependent.

Compared with heparin, dalteparin sodium has a reduced effect on platelet function and adhesiveness, and thus has only a small effect on primary haemostasis.

The antithrombotic effect of Fragmin may be monitored by analysing anti-Factor Xa activity using a suitable chromogenic substrate assay. For further information contact Kabi Diagnostica.

Product licence numbers
10,000 IU/4 ml 0022/0074
10,000 IU/1 ml 0022/0075

FRAGMIN* 2500 and 5000 IU Syringes ▼

Presentation *Fragmin 2500 IU:* Single dose syringe containing dalteparin sodium 2500 IU (anti-Factor Xa) in 0.2 ml solution.

Fragmin 5000 IU: Single dose syringe containing dalteparin sodium 5000 IU (anti-Factor Xa) in 0.2 ml solution.

Fragmin contains no preservative.

Uses Actions: Dalteparin sodium is a physiological antithrombotic agent, which acts mainly through potentiation of the inhibition of activated coagulation factors by antithrombin.

Indications: Peri- and post-operative surgical thromboprophylaxis.

Dosage and administration
Route of administration: By subcutaneous injection into the abdominal wall.

Patients should be supine and the total length of the needle should be introduced vertically into a skin fold, which should be held throughout the procedure.

Adults:
(a) Surgical thromboprophylaxis in patients at *moderate risk of thrombosis.*

Fragmin 2500 IU (anti-Factor Xa) is administered subcutaneously 1–2 hours prior to the surgical procedure, and thereafter 2500 IU (anti-Factor Xa) s.c. daily for 5 days or until the patient is fully ambulant.

(b) Surgical thromboprophylaxis in patients at *high risk of thrombosis* (e.g. elective total hip replacement, hip fracture, or other extensive operations. Patients with malignant disease, a previous history of DVT, expected long immobilisation, or extreme age).

Fragmin 2500 IU (anti-Factor Xa) is administered subcutaneously 1–2 hours prior to the surgical procedure, and the same dosage is administered 12 hours later. Thereafter Fragmin 5000 IU (anti-Factor Xa) s.c. is administered daily for 5 days or until the patient is fully ambulant.

Children: Not recommended for children.

Elderly: Fragmin has been used safely in elderly patients without the need for dosage adjustment.

Contra-indications, warnings, etc
Contra-indications: There are no known absolute contra-indications to Fragmin.

Precautions and warnings: Caution should be exercised in patients in whom there is an increased risk of bleeding complications, eg.. following trauma, known haemorrhagic diathesis, haemorrhagic stroke, severe liver or renal failure, thrombocytopenia, or defective platelet function, subacute endocarditis, uncontrolled hypertension, diabetes mellitus with retinopathy, and in patients receiving concurrent anticoagulant/antiplatelet agents (see interactions section), and also patients with known heparin hypersensitivity.

As individual low molecular weight heparins have differing characteristics, switching to an alternative low molecular weight heparin should be avoided.

Fragmin when administered in a dose of 2500–5000 IU (anti-Factor Xa)/day does not generally accumulate, and therefore monitoring of the effect is not usually required. However, chromogenic substrate assays can be used to measure anti-Factor Xa activity, if considered necessary.

Pregnancy and lactation: There has been limited human usage and there has been no adverse animal evidence.

Avoid in pregnancy if a better known and safer alternative is available.

It is not known whether Fragmin passes the placenta or is excreted in breast milk.

Side-effects: Bleeding may be provoked, especially at high dosages corresponding with anti-Factor Xa levels greater than 1.5 IU/ml.

Transient, slight to moderate, elevation of liver transaminases (ASAT, ALAT) have been observed, but no clinical significance has been demonstrated.

The following side-effects of heparin have not been observed with Fragmin, however they cannot be excluded since Fragmin is derived from heparin: thrombocytopenia; allergic reactions (urticaria, anaphylaxis, pruritus, hair loss and skin necrosis).

Osteoporosis has been associated with long-term heparin treatment. Although this condition has not been observed with Fragmin, the risk of osteoporosis cannot be excluded.

Overdosage: The anticoagulant, ie. prolongation of the APTT effect induced by Fragmin is inhibited by protamine. Since protamine itself has an inhibitory effect on primary haemostasis it should be used only in an emergency. The prolongation of the clotting time induced by Fragmin may be fully neutralised by protamine, but only about 25–50% of the anti-Factor Xa activity is affected. 1 mg of protamine inhibits the effect of 100 IU (anti-Factor Xa) of Fragmin.

Interactions: Concomitant medication with anticoagulant/antiplatelet agents may enhance the anticoagulant effect of Fragmin, eg. aspirin, vitamin-K antagonists and dextran.

The possibility of the following interactions should also be considered:

i. An enhancement of the anticoagulant effect by dipyridamole, indomethacin, sulphinpyrazone, probenecid, ethacrynic acid and cytostatics.

ii. A reduction of the anticoagulant effect may occur with concomitant administration of antihistamines, cardiac glycosides, tetracycline and ascorbic acid.

Pharmaceutical precautions Fragmin should be stored at room temperature.

Legal category POM.

Package quantities Fragmin 2500 IU (anti-Factor Xa)/0.2 ml 10 × 0.2 ml single dose syringes.

Fragmin 5000 IU (anti-Factor Xa)/0.2 ml 10 × 0.2 ml single dose syringes.

Further information One unit of dalteparin sodium corresponds to the activity of one IU of the 1st International Standard for Low Molecular Weight Heparin with respect to the inhibition of coagulation Factor Xa in plasma.

Dalteparin sodium is a low molecular weight heparin fraction (average molecular weight 4000–6000 Daltons) produced from porcine-derived sodium heparin, and specifically inhibits the coagulation Factor Xa.

Pharmacokinetics: The half life following i.v. and s.c. administration is 2 hours and 3½–4 hours respectively, twice that of unfractionated heparin. The bioavailability following s.c. injection is approximately 87 per cent and the pharmacokinetics are not dose dependent.

Compared with standard, unfractionated heparin, dalteparin sodium has a reduced adverse effect on platelet function and thus has only a minimal effect on primary haemostasis.

Product licence numbers
2500 IU/0.2 ml 0022/0076
5000 IU/0.2 ml 0022/0077

GENOTROPIN* 4 IU ▼
GENOTROPIN 12 IU MULTIDOSE ▼

Presentation A single dose vial of sterile lyophilised powder of 4 IU somatropin (rbe) also containing aminoacetic acid and sodium phosphate as stabilisers. A 1 ml ampoule of Water for Injections is supplied for reconstitution.

A multidose vial of sterile lyophilised powder containing 12 IU somatropin (rbe) also containing aminoacetic acid and sodium phosphate as stabilisers. A 3 ml ampoule of Water for Injections with 0.25% m-cresol is supplied for reconstitution.

Uses The treatment of short stature caused by decreased or absent secretion of pituitary growth hormone. The diagnosis should be verified by a specialist medical practitioner.

The treatment of short stature in gonadal dysgenesis (Turner Syndrome).

Dosage and administration
Route of administration: By subcutaneous injection.

Recommended dosage: The dosage is individual. Generally a dose of 0.5–0.7 IU/kg body weight per week, or 12 IU/m² per week is recommended. In Turner Syndrome a dose of 1.0 IU/kg body weight per week (24 IU/m² per week) is recommended. Preferably the weekly dose should be divided into 6 or 7 subcutaneous injections. The injection site should be rotated to prevent lipoatrophy.

Preparation of solution: The solution is prepared by adding 1 ml of Water for Injections to the 4 IU vial or 3 ml of Water for Injections with 0.25% m-cresol to the 12 IU vial. Gently dissolve the drug with a slow swirling motion. Do not shake vigorously as this may cause denaturation of the active ingredient.

Contra-indications, warnings, etc Only patients with unfused epiphyses should be treated.

Precautions: Patients with diabetes mellitus may require adjustment of their antidiabetic therapy. Patients treated with Genotropin should be regularly assessed by a specialist in child growth. This assessment should include accurate determination of growth response and endocrinological status, as relative deficiencies of other pituitary hormones may be exposed or exacerbated by an adequate growth response. Hypothyroidism in particular is a reported occurrence.

Pregnancy and lactation: In the event of a pregnancy occurring during therapy with Genotropin, treatment should be discontinued, as there is no evidence from either human or animal studies of the safety of growth hormone treatment during pregnancy.

No information is available as to whether peptide hormones pass into breast milk, but the quantities involved would not have any clinical effect on the infant.

Overdosage: Acute overdosage is unlikely and does not represent a hazard to the patient. The consequences of long term administration of doses above the therapeutic range are unknown.

Side-effects: Recipients may develop antibodies to growth hormone and *E. coli* protein. However, as with pituitary derived hormone, only in very rare instances has growth retardation occurred. Reactions at the site of injection have been reported, such as itching, lumps, redness and lipoatrophy. Lipoatrophy can be prevented or minimised by varying the injection site. In Turner Syndrome temporary exacerbation of lymphoedema has been reported.

Pharmaceutical precautions Store at 2–8°C. Protect from light. Reconstituted Genotropin 12 IU Multidose should be stored in the refrigerator and protected from light. Under these conditions the reconstituted solution is stable for up to 21 days in use. Genotropin 4 IU is for single dose use only. When reconstituted it should be stored in the refrigerator and used within 24 hours.

Legal category POM.

Package quantities
Genotropin 4 IU: Two pack sizes are available.

Combined pack containing one vial of somatropin (rbe) 4 IU and one ampoule of 1 ml Water for Injections.

Combined pack containing ten vials of somatropin (rbe) 4 IU and ten ampoules of 1 ml Water for Injections.

Genotropin 12 IU Multidose: Combined pack containing one vial of somatropin (rbe) 12 IU and one ampoule of 3 ml Water for Injections with 0.25% m-cresol.

Further information Genotropin contains somatropin (rbe), which is produced using recombinant DNA technology and is identical in structure to endogenous human growth hormone. Somatropin (rbe) is the British Approved Name for recombinant human somatotropin.

Some cases of acute leukaemia have been reported in growth hormone deficient children untreated as well as treated with growth hormone and might possibly represent a slightly increased incidence compared with non growth hormone deficient children. A causal relationship to growth hormone therapy has not been established.

Intermittent dosage with human growth hormone has been associated with the appearance of hypoglycaemia, which has not been reported with the use of uninterrupted, i.e. daily, administration.

Product licence numbers

Genotropin 4 IU	0022/0071
Water for Injections	0022/0082
Genotropin 12 IU Multidose	0022/0079
Water for Injections with 0.25% m-cresol	0022/0081

GENOTROPIN* 16 IU KABIPEN* ▼

Presentation A two-compartment cartridge for reconstitution and injection of somatropin (rbe) using the KabiPen device. One compartment contains sterile lyophilised powder of 16 IU somatropin (rbe) with sodium dihydrogen phosphate, disodium phosphate, glycine and mannitol as stabilisers; the other compartment contains 1 ml of Water for Injections with mannitol and m-cresol 0.3%.

Uses The treatment of short stature due to decreased or absent secretion of growth hormone. The treatment of short stature in gonadal dysgenesis (Turner Syndrome). The diagnosis should be verified by a specialist medical practitioner.

Dosage and administration
Route of administration: By subcutaneous injection.

Recommended dosage: The dosage is individual. Generally a dose of 0.5–0.7 IU/kg body weight per week or 12 IU/m^2 per week is recommended. In Turner Syndrome a dose of 1.0 IU/kg body weight per week or 24 IU/m^2 per week is recommended. Preferably the weekly dose should be divided into 6 or 7 daily subcutaneous injections. The injection site should be varied to prevent lipoatrophy.

Preparation of solution: Somatropin (rbe) is reconstituted using the KabiPen device. Instructions on how to effect reconstitution are included with the device.

Contra-indications, warnings, etc Only patients with unfused epiphyses should be treated.

Precautions: Patients with diabetes mellitus may require adjustment of their antidiabetic therapy. Patients treated with Genotropin should be regularly assessed by a specialist in child growth. This assessment should include accurate determination of the growth response and endocrinological status, as relative deficiencies of other pituitary hormones may be exposed or exacerbated by an adequate growth response. Hypothyroidism in particular is a reported occurrence.

Pregnancy and lactation: Treatment should be discontinued in the event of a pregnancy occurring during therapy with Genotropin as there is no evidence from either human or animal studies of the safety of growth hormone treatment during pregnancy.

No information is available as to whether peptide hormones pass into breast milk, but the quantities involved would not have any clinical effect on the infant.

Overdosage: Acute overdosage is unlikely and does not represent a hazard to the patient. The consequences of long-term administration of doses above the therapeutic range are unknown.

Side-effects: Recipients may develop antibodies to growth hormone and *E. coli* protein. However, as with pituitary-derived hormone, only in very rare instances has growth retardation occurred. Reactions at the site of injection have been reported, such as itching, lumps, redness and lipoatrophy. Lipoatrophy can be prevented or minimised by varying the injection site. In Turner Syndrome temporary exacerbation of lymphoedema has been reported.

Pharmaceutical precautions Store at 2–8°C and protect from light. Once reconstituted, the cartridge in the device, may be stored in the refrigerator and used over a period of up to 2 weeks.

Legal category POM.

Package quantities Pack containing one refill cartridge for Genotropin 16 IU KabiPen.

Further information Genotropin contains somatropin (rbe), which is produced using recombinant DNA technology and is identical in structure to endogenous human growth hormone. Somatropin (rbe) is the British Approved Name for recombinant human somatotropin.

Some cases of acute leukaemia have been reported in growth hormone deficient children untreated as well as treated with growth hormone and might possibly represent a slightly increased incidence compared with non growth hormone deficient children. A causal relationship to growth hormone therapy has not been established.

Intermittent dosage with human growth hormone has been associated with the appearance of hypoglycaemia, which has not been reported with the use of uninterrupted, i.e. daily, administration.

Product licence number 0022/0085.

HEALONID*

Presentation Disposable single-use syringes containing Healonid of the following composition per ml:

Sodium hyaluronate	10 mg
Sodium chloride	8.5 mg
Disodium hydrogen phosphate dihydrate	0.28 mg
Sodium dihydrogen phosphate hydrate	0.04 mg
Water for injections	to 1 ml

The syringe membrane must be perforated before use, (see directions for use).

Uses Sodium hyaluronate is a visco-elastic polymer normally found in the aqueous and vitreous humour. Healonid, which contains sodium hyaluronate is a highly viscous clear solution at rest, yet it will readily flow through a fine cannula or needle under pressure. Introduction of Healonid into the anterior or posterior chamber keeps tissues separated during the operative procedure and protects them from trauma from other tissues or instruments. The anterior chamber depth is maintained, vitreous bulge can be reduced, and the loss of irreplaceable endothelial cells which inevitably accompanies surgery can be greatly reduced.

Indications: Surgical procedures on the eye, including intraocular lens insertion, intra and extra capsular lens extraction, glaucoma surgery, corneal graft, surgery for accidental trauma, retinal detachment and vitreal replacement procedures.

Dosage and administration The syringe is assembled and made ready for use according to the instruction sheet with each syringe. The indication governs the quantity of Healonid used.

It is recommended that Healonid be removed from the refrigerator to attain room temperature 30–60 mins before use.

Cataract surgery: A sufficient volume of Healonid is gently introduced into the anterior chamber at an early stage in the operation prior to lens extraction to protect the tissues from trauma.

Intraocular lens insertion: Healonid is introduced into the anterior chamber before lens extraction and is also used to coat the lens and instruments prior to introduction into the eye. Further Healonid may be injected to replace losses.

Glaucoma filtration surgery: Prior to trabeculectomy Healonid is injected slowly through a corneal paracentesis to maintain the anterior chamber volume. Injection may be continued to allow Healonid to flow through the sutured outer scleral flap to the conjunctival filtration site.

Corneal transplant surgery: After removal of the corneal button the anterior chamber is filled with Healonid. The donor graft is then placed on the bed of Healonid and sutured into place. Healonid may be put into the anterior chamber of the donor eye to protect the corneal endothelium.

Trauma: In various kinds of perforating trauma Healonid can be instilled to refill the anterior chamber, prevent prolapse of the iris and formation of synechiae. Blood contaminated Healonid should be replaced with new Healonid before closure.

Precautions: The anterior chamber should not be overfilled with Healonid, except in glaucoma surgery. At close of surgery some of the Healonid should be removed by irrigation or aspiration. Intraocular pressure should be monitored during the post operative period and any excessive rises treated with appropriate therapy.

Elderly: No special instructions.

Contra-indications, warnings, etc There are no known contra-indications to Healonid. Because the drug is extracted from avian tissues, despite rigorous purification procedures minute amounts of protein are present, and thus the remote possibility of idiosyncratic reactions remains.

Adverse reactions: The drug is very well tolerated and the only untoward effect reported has been a transient rise in intraocular pressure in a few cases.

Pharmaceutical precautions Healonid has a shelf life of 3 years when stored at 2–8°C protected from light and freezing. These conditions should be adhered to routinely. However, Healonid may be stored at room temperature for up to 4 weeks by the user.

Legal category POM.

Package quantities Disposable syringes containing 0.5 ml and 0.75 ml. A sterile single-use 27 g Rycroft cannula is supplied.

Further information Healonid does not interfere with the healing process. Its use may reduce incidence of synechiae and adhesions. Evidence from animal experiments indicates that Healonid is no longer present in the anterior chamber six days after introduction.

Product licence number 0009/0045.

Product licence holder: Pharmacia Biosystems Ltd, Davy Avenue, Knowlhill, Milton Keynes MK5 8PH.

HYSKON*

Presentation A sterile viscous aqueous solution of dextran 70 (M_w 70,000) and dextrose.
100 ml solution contains:

Dextran 70 (M_w 70,000) Pharmacia	32 g
Dextrose	10 g
Water for injections	to 100 ml

Viscosity at 20°C 220 cSt (255 cP).

Uses Hyskon is indicated for use with the hysteroscope. It is used both as a rinsing fluid and for dilatation of the uterus.

Dosage and administration *Dosage:* 50–100 ml for one examination. The amount of Hyskon required per patient depends on a number of factors, such as the type and length of the diagnostic procedure, whether or not manipulation or surgery is performed. Most often, however, the amount of Hyskon instilled into the uterus will be between 50 and 100 millilitres.

Administration: Hyskon should be introduced into the uterine cavity through the cannula of a hysteroscope under low pressure (approximately 100 mmHg) until the uterus is sufficiently distended to permit adequate visualisation. During the hysteroscopic examination, Hyskon should be infused at a rate that keeps the cavity suitably distended. To avoid injection of the fluid into the tissues of the uterus and parametria and to avoid having unnecessary amounts of the fluid pass into peritoneal cavity, pressures greater than 150 mmHg should be used with great care. Small amounts of fluid may occasionally escape into the peritoneal cavity.

Elderly: No special instructions.

Contra-indications, warnings, etc (1) Hyskon should not be used in patients known to be hypersensitive to dextran. Other contra-indications are those relative to the hysteroscopic procedure itself, such as pregnancy and upper genital tract infection.

(2) No other local or systemic reactions have been reported.

Pharmaceutical precautions (1) Use only if solution is clear.

(2) Store at an even temperature, preferably not exceeding 30°C.

Legal category POM.

Package quantities Carton containing 6 × 100 ml bottles.

Further information Hyskon has excellent optical properties.

The viscosity of Hyskon is adjusted to achieve optimum dilatation without too rapid escape of solution from the uterus. Its viscosity also prevents admixture with mucus and blood which would otherwise reduce visibility.

Thoroughly rinse the hysteroscope after use since dried Hyskon can seize the taps.

Product licence number 0009/0018.

Product licence holder: Pharmacia Biosystems Ltd, Davy Avenue, Knowlhill, Milton Keynes MK5 8PH.

INDOMOD*

Presentation

Indomod 25 mg: Hard gelatin orange capsules with the imprint AB27 in light type, containing 25 mg indomethacin, in modified release form (Repro-Dose).

Indomod 75 mg: Hard gelatin brown capsules with imprint AB26 in light type, containing 75 mg indomethacin, in modified release form (Repro-Dose).

Uses Inflammatory rheumatic diseases such as rheumatoid arthritis, ankylosing spondylitis and gout. Inflammatory phases in osteoarthrosis. Inflammatory conditions such as bursitis, tendinitis, and tenosynovitis.

Dosage and administration

Dosage: Use as directed by physician. The dose should be adjusted individually. In chronic rheumatoid disease the initial daily dose is normally 50–75 mg, which is increased by 25 mg or 50 mg at weekly intervals until a satisfactory effect is achieved. The daily dose should never exceed 200 mg.

In acute conditions, e.g. gouty arthritis, a dose of 100 mg is given initially, followed by 75 mg b.i.d. for controlling the pain. Then the dose is rapidly reduced and medication is discontinued. (See 'Further information').

Paediatric usage not established.

Contra-indications, warnings, etc

Contra-indications: Active peptic ulcer or a history of recurrent gastrointestinal lesions; ulcerative colitis.

Haemophilia and other bleeding disorders. Allergy to non-steroidal anti-inflammatory drugs (salicylates, etc.).

Warnings and precautions: To be used with caution in patients with psychiatric disturbances, parkinsonism, or epilepsy. NSAIDs have been reported to cause nephrotoxicity in various forms and their use can lead to interstitial nephritis, nephrotic syndrome and renal failure.

The symptoms of infection may be masked by indomethacin. The use of indomethacin is not recommended during pregnancy or lactation. Serum levels of indomethacin are raised by the concurrent administration of probenicid. Indomethacin reduces the natriuretic effect of frusemide.

Side-effects: Headache, dizziness, light-headedness, confusion and other reactions from the central nervous system are correlated to plasma concentrations and less likely to occur when high peak levels are avoided, as in the case with Indomod. Dyspepsia is another frequent side-effect of indomethacin likely to be modified by Indomod, due to the bypass of the stomach. Gastrointestinal bleeding and ulceration, fluid retention, disturbed renal or hepatic function, fatigue, tinnitus, drowsiness or insomnia may occur.

In patients with renal, cardiac or hepatic impairment caution is required since the use of NSAIDs may result in deterioration of renal function. The dose should be kept as low as possible and renal function should be monitored.

Anaphylactic reactions in hypersensitive patients.

Pharmaceutical precautions No special requirements or precautions.

Legal category POM.

Package quantities
Indomod 25 mg: Blister packs of 120 modified release capsules.
Indomod 75 mg: Blister packs of 30 modified release capsules.

Further information Due to the special indomethacin plasma profile obtained with Indomod, doses may be taken at intervals of 8–12 hours, and a capsule of 75 mg taken at bedtime can be expected to relieve the next day's morning stiffness.

Product licence numbers
Indomod 25 mg 4338/0006
Indomod 75 mg 4338/0007

Product licence holder: Benzon Pharma A/S, 29 Halmtorvet, DK-1700 Copenhagen, Denmark.

INTRALIPID* 10%
INTRALIPID* 20%

Presentation A white, oil in water emulsion containing:

	Intralipid 10%	*Intralipid 20%*
Fractionated soybean oil	50 g	100 g
Fractionated egg phospholipids	6 g	6 g
Glycerol	11 g	11 g
Water for injections to 500 ml		
pH 7.		

The emulsion is sterile and pyrogen free.

Uses

1. Intralipid is a concentrated source of energy for complete intravenous nutrition. Provision of a sufficient amount of energy in the form of carbohydrate is often restricted by such considerations as hypertonicity, hypervolaemia, tendency to thrombophlebitis and the limit beyond which further carbohydrate cannot be utilised. By the use of Intralipid it is possible to provide a high energy intake in a relatively small volume. One litre of Intralipid 20% provides 2,000 kcal (8.4 MJ) and one litre of Intralipid 10% 1,100 kcal (4.6 MJ).

2. Intralipid is a rich source of the essential fatty acids; linoleic and linolenic acids.

3. Intralipid has a protein-sparing effect when given in conjunction with amino acid and carbohydrate solutions.

4. Intralipid 20% has an osmolality of ~350 mosmol per kg water.

Intralipid 10% has an osmolality of ~300 mosmol per kg water. (Plasma ~290).

Therefore both these preparations are suitable for infusion into peripheral veins.

Indications: Intralipid should be used as part of a balanced intravenous feeding regimen in patients who are unable to receive sufficient amounts of nutrients enterally. Intralipid is especially valuable in providing a high energy intake to compensate for increased energy expenditure following trauma, infections, severe burns, etc.

Dosage and administration The dosage administered should be within the ranges recommended below and should be governed by the patient's ability to utilise fat.

Electrolyte, fluid, acid-base imbalance and shock should be corrected prior to commencement of intravenous nutrition. In the metabolic and nutritional management of the seriously ill patient, specific preliminary investigations and continuous monitoring are essential, particularly of electrolyte levels. Monitoring of vitamin and trace element levels should be included, especially in patients receiving long-term intravenous nutrition.

To achieve optimal nutritional support Intralipid should be given with amino acids (Vamin) and glucose, together with electrolytes (Addiphos), trace elements (Addamel/Additrace or Ped-el) and vitamins (Solivito N and Vitlipid N).

As with all infusions, care should be taken to avoid complications of catheterisation including air embolism and central venous thrombosis. The risk of serious thoracic complications can be avoided by the use of a peripheral catheter. The provision of intravenous nutrition via a peripheral catheter is facilitated by the near isotonicity of Intralipid. Strict asepsis should be maintained especially in the immunosuppressed patient.

Recommended dosage for adults: Intralipid 20%: 500–1000 ml per 24 hrs in conjunction with intravenous administration of amino acid and carbohydrate solutions. For lesser energy requirements Intralipid 10% 500–1500 ml per 24 hrs in conjunction with amino acid and carbohydrate solutions.

Intralipid 10% and 20% are administered by slow intravenous infusion. During the first 10 minutes the drip should be adjusted to 20 drops per minute and then gradually increased to a final rate after half an hour of 25–40 drops per minute for Intralipid 20% and 40–60 drops per minute for Intralipid 10%. 500 ml of Intralipid 20% should be given over a period of not less than five hours. 500 ml of Intralipid 10% should be given over a period of not less than three hours. On the first day of infusion it is advisable to administer 5 ml Intralipid 20% per kg body weight or 10 ml Intralipid 10% per kg body weight. Subsequently the dose is usually doubled and when a larger intake is indicated the dosage may be increased to 3 g fat per kg body weight per 24 hrs.

Recommended dosage for infants: Dosage is governed by the maturity and birth-weight of the infant. In mature infants dosage scheme 1. should be used. In small for gestational age and low birth-weight infants where the ability to handle fat may be impaired, dosage scheme 2. should be utilised.

In all cases the infant's ability to eliminate infused fat from the circulation should be checked daily as described in the fat elimination test in the precautions section. If lipaemia is present re-testing should be carried out after an interval of four hours.

When administered to infants Intralipid should, if possible, be infused continuously over twenty-four hours and to maintain a constant rate of infusion it is essential that an appropriate pump is used.

1. *Infants:* 0.5–4 g fat per kg body weight in 24 hrs. In practice 0.02–0.17 g/kg body weight should be administered each hour. The equivalent volumes of Intralipid are 10% 0.21–1.70 ml/kg/hr; 20% 0.10–0.85 ml/kg/hr. The dosage should be gradually increased during the first week of administration.

2. In small for gestational age and low birth-weight infants with impaired capacity to handle fat, commencing dosage should be 0.5 g fat per kg body weight in 24 hrs. In the absence of measurement of serum triglycerides

the dosage should not exceed 2 g fat per kg body weight in 24 hrs.

The rates given are maximum rates and no attempt should be made to exceed these in order to compensate for missed doses.

Contra-indications, warnings, etc Intralipid may be contraindicated in severe disorders of fat metabolism such as in severe liver damage and acute shock.

Precautions: Fat metabolism may be disturbed in conditions such as renal insufficiency, uncompensated diabetes, certain forms of liver insufficiency, metabolic disorders and sepsis. If intravenous administration of fat is considered in patients with the above mentioned disorders, the elimination of fat should be checked daily. In newborns with neonatal hyperbilirubinaemia Intralipid should be used with caution, especially in low birth weight infants, because of the risk of free fatty acids displacing bilirubin from albumin. Intralipid should be administered with caution to infants with known or suspected pulmonary hypertension.

Animal reproduction studies have not been carried out with Intralipid. There are, however, published reports of its successful and safe administration during pregnancy in the human.

Caution: Interference with certain laboratory measurements may occur if blood samples are taken before fat has been adequately cleared from the bloodstream.

Fat elimination test: In order to prevent the development of cumulative lipaemia the patient's capacity of fat elimination can be tested in the following manner. In the morning following the first day's infusion, a citrated blood sample is drawn, preferably when the patient is still in a fasting state. The blood sample is centrifuged at 1,200–1,500 rpm. If the plasma is found to be opalescent or milky, further infusion should be postponed. This test should be repeated at weekly intervals in patients in stable metabolic conditions. In the majority of patients, the plasma is completely clear 12 hours after the conclusion of an infusion of 2 g fat per kg body weight (corresponding to 10 ml of Intralipid 20% or 20 ml of Intralipid 10% per kg body weight). In patients with diagnosed or suspected metabolic disturbances (see precautions) the fat elimination capacity should be checked daily.

Side effects: In rare instances, initial administration of Intralipid has produced a rise in temperature with shivering. Infusion of Intralipid should be discontinued in such cases. Increased levels of transaminases, alkaline phosphatases and bilirubin have been observed in patients receiving intravenous nutrition. If the dosage is reduced values usually return to normal. Cholestasis has also been reported.

The infusion of Intralipid has been associated with an altered lipoprotein profile. The significance of these changes is not known.

Pharmaceutical precautions

1. Store below 25°C. Do not freeze. After long periods of storage the bottle of Intralipid should be gently inverted two or three times before use.
2. Do not use if the bottle is leaking.
3. Discard any unused contents.
4. Additives may only be added to Intralipid where compatibility is known. The following additions can be recommended:
   - (i) Vitlipid N Adult or Vitlipid N Infant.
   - (ii) Solivito N (see Solivito N data sheet for details on reconstitution).
   - (iii) Diazemuls.
   - (iv) Heparin.

Legal category POM.

Package quantities Intralipid 10% and 20%: 100 or 500 ml.

Further information Intralipid and Vamin solutions can be infused simultaneously, centrally or peripherally when the mixture reaches the vein through the same cannula. Intralipid can be mixed with other solutions in a single container (e.g. 3-litre bag). Such mixing must follow defined formulae and mixing techniques, details of which are available on request. The manufacturer can be consulted for full information on complete and balanced intravenous nutrition regimens.

Product licence numbers
Intralipid 10% 0022/0027R
Intralipid 20% 0022/0028R

KABIGLOBULIN*

Presentation Ampoules containing Human Normal Immunoglobulin solution 16%, a clear pale straw colour. The active constituent is gamma globulin.

Uses *Main pharmacological action:* The immunoglobulins present in Kabiglobulin may be used prophylactically and therapeutically to provide passive immunity against infectious diseases.

Indications: Prophylaxis against infectious hepatitis (Hepatitis A). Prophylaxis against Rubella following exposure during pregnancy. Prevention, or modification of symptoms, following measles exposure in susceptible individuals. Antibody deficiency syndromes; to reduce the incidence and severity of infections in agammaglobulinaemia, hypogammaglobulinaemia and dysgammaglobulinaemia. Following burns injury.

Dosage and administration *Route of administration:* By intramuscular injection only.

Recommended dosage: Infectious hepatitis (Hepatitis A): for prophylaxis against infectious hepatitis for up to 3 months, in adults and children, 0.02–0.04 ml per kg body weight is recommended by WHO. In massive exposure, e.g. to people visiting highly endemic areas, 0.06–0.12 ml per kg body weight is recommended. The effect of the larger injection lasts for a period of at least four months.

Rubella in pregnancy: 20 ml is administered as soon as possible following exposure. The effect of an injection lasts about 3 weeks and therefore the dosage should be repeated after this time in the case of renewed exposure to the disease.

Measles prevention: 0.2 ml per kg body weight is injected within five days of exposure. The preventive effect of an injection normally lasts three weeks. The dosage should therefore be repeated after that period of time in the case of renewed exposure to the disease.

Measles modification: 0.04 ml per kg body weight is injected within five days of exposure.

Antibody deficiency syndromes: agammaglobulinaemia, hypogammaglobulinaemia, dysgammaglobulinaemia. As an initial dosage, 1.3 ml per kg body weight (maximum 60 ml) injected in divided doses over 48 hours. Half this dosage, 0.65 ml per kg (maximum 30 ml), is then given every three to four weeks.

Burns injury: during the first week following the trauma a total of about 50 g gamma globulin in the form of Kabiglobulin should be given in addition to plasma and blood. From the third up to the tenth day, 15–30 ml (2.5–5.0 g gamma globulin) per day is administered.

Contra-indications, warnings, etc Kabiglobulin should not be given at the same time as live vaccines, such as measles, mumps, rubella and oral polio vaccines (Sabin). If Kabiglobulin (2 ml) has been administered these vaccines should not be given for 3 months. This period should be increased to 4 months for the 5 ml injection. Following administration of live vaccines a period of 2–3 weeks should elapse before giving Kabiglobulin. Kabiglobulin may be given at the same time as tetanus, typhoid, diphtheria, cholera, polio [the inactivated form (Salk)] and yellow fever; although a live vaccine, Kabiglobulin donors are unlikely to possess the antibody to yellow fever.

Pregnancy and lactation: There is no evidence of safety nor of toxicity of Kabiglobulin in human pregnancy or lactation, but it has been commonly used for many years without apparent ill consequence. If such therapy is needed in pregnancy or lactation, Kabiglobulin can be used if there is no alternative course of action.

Side-effects: In exceptional cases, intramuscular injections of gamma globulin may give rise to adverse reactions of the following types:

Local reactions: at the site of injection such as erythema, swelling, tenderness and induration, which generally subside within a few days after the injection.

General reactions: such as fever (38–40°C), chills and general malaise. These symptoms have appeared 6–8 hours after the injection and have generally subsided by the following day.

Hypersensitivity reactions: such as exanthema and pruritus. Flush, tachycardia and shock are rare. The reactions are more frequent in patients with hypogammaglobulinaemia or dysgammaglobulinaemia and may be delayed for some hours following administration.

Overdosage: There have been no reports of overdosage with Kabiglobulin. There is no specific antidote and in the unlikely event of any reactions occurring following overdosage, they should be treated symptomatically.

Pharmaceutical precautions Store between 2°C and 8°C.

Legal category POM.

Package quantities Ampoules of 2.0 and 5.0 ml.

Further information The IgA content of Kabiglobulin does not exceed 0.01% of the total protein content. Kabiglobulin contains no preservative agents. Based on results from model experiments and from clinical follow-up, several organisations such as the Food and Drug Administration, Centers for Disease Control and World Health Organisation have drawn the conclusion that immunoglobulin preparations, manufactured according to standard methods are safe with respect to transmission of HIV infectivity.

Product licence number 0022/5009.

KABIKINASE*

Presentation Vials containing a straw coloured lyophilised powder. Three preparations are available, vials of 100,000 iu, 250,000 iu and 600,000 iu of streptokinase. Human albumin and buffering agents are present as stabilisers.

Uses *Action:* By activating the fibrinolytic system streptokinase induces dissolution of intravascular thrombi and emboli.

Indications: Thrombolytic therapy by intravenous Kabikinase infusion is indicated in the treatment of deep vein thrombosis, acute major pulmonary embolism, acute arterial thromboembolism.

Additionally, thrombolytic therapy by local streptokinase administration is indicated in the treatment of myocardial infarction (see b, below) and in the clearance of clotted haemodialysis shunts (see c, below).

Dosage and administration *Routes of administration:* By intravascular infusion; intracoronary infusion.

Recommended dosage for adults:

(a) Standard intravenous infusion regimen: The standard intravenous dosage scheme includes a loading dose sufficient to neutralise circulating streptococcal antibody, followed by a maintenance dose to maintain an appropriate degree of fibrinolysis.

Loading dose: Streptokinase 600,000 iu is infused via a peripheral vein over a period of 30–60 minutes.

Maintenance dose: Streptokinase 100,000 iu/hour is infused for 72 hr. If further treatment is considered necessary it should be continued for not more than a further 3 days.

(b) Intracoronary administration in myocardial infarction: Intracoronary thrombolysis is performed using standard techniques for selective coronary angiography by either the brachial or femoral approach. Early intervention is recommended, ideally within 6 hours following onset of chest pain.

Using a standard 7 or 8 French catheter, angiography is used to identify the presence and location of the thrombus. Nitroglycerin (100–400 micrograms) is administered into the involved vessel, to relieve coronary artery spasm. Initially a bolus dose of streptokinase 10,000–25,000 iu is administered followed by a continuous infusion of 4,000 iu/minute, which is continued until vessel patency is restored, or for 60–75 minutes (total dose 240,000–300,000 iu). If reperfusion is achieved prior to this time then the infusion rate may be reduced when patency is restored, and infusion should continue for an additional 30–60 minutes (80,000–100,000 iu streptokinase) in order to lyse any remaining residual thrombus.

Subsequent anticoagulant treatment with heparin is necessary in order to prevent rethrombosis in the infarct-related coronary artery. However, in the majority of patients intracoronary streptokinase administration produces significant fibrinogen (and plasminogen) depletion. Additionally, circulating fibrin/fibrinogen degradation products exert an anticoagulant effect. Accordingly heparin should be administered incrementally and judiciously during the first 24 hr following treatment. The partial thromboplastin time should be monitored at regular intervals, and the heparin dosage adjusted to maintain the former within the range 2–2.5 times normal.

(c) Local application in occluded haemodialysis shunts: Kabikinase 100,000 iu is dissolved in normal saline 100 ml. 10,000–25,000 iu (10–25 ml) is deposited in the clotted portion of the shunt, which is then sealed on the venous side with forceps. A sterile single-dose syringe is attached on the arterial side to form an air cushion against which the artery can pulsate. If required, the treatment may be repeated after 30–45 minutes.

Recommended dosage for infants: Although the standard dosage scheme may be reduced proportionally to circulating volume, it may be preferable to titrate the initial dose followed by a maintenance dose of 1300–1400 iu/kg body weight/hr for 3 days. Response normally occurs within this period but if further therapy is considered it should not be for more than an additional 3 days.

Preparation of solution: The contents of a vial of Kabikinase are dissolved at room temperature in 5 ml water for injections carefully avoiding the formation of a foam. The concentrated solution thus obtained is transferred aseptically into an infusion bottle of glucose or saline of suitable volume, according to the needs of the patient. The rate of infusion is then adjusted to give the required dosage rate.

Standard intravenous infusion regimen: For the loading dose; a vial of 600,000 iu Kabikinase is made up in 100 ml 5% glucose or physiological saline and is administered over 30 minutes.

For the maintenance dose; a vial of 600,000 iu is made up in 500 ml 5% glucose or physiological saline, and is administered at a rate of 80 ml per hr (100,000 iu hourly). If desired, smaller volumes can be employed, to enable the use of a syringe pump.

Intracoronary administration: The contents of a reconstituted vial are added to a volume of 5% glucose or physiological saline in order to achieve a final streptokinase concentration of not less than 1,000 iu/ml.

Control of therapy (standard intravenous infusion regimen): Therapy is controlled by the thrombin clotting time performed at intervals and should be within the limits of two to four times the normal value.

Contra-indications, warnings, etc

Contra-indications: Kabikinase should not be administered intramuscularly. Since thrombolytic therapy increases the risk of bleeding, Kabikinase is contra-indicated in the following:

1. Surgery within the last 10 days.
2. Invasive procedures during the last 10 days.
3. Gastrointestinal bleeding within the last six months.
4. Thrombocytopenia or other evidence of defective haemostasis.
5. Liver or kidney disease.
6. Cerebrovascular accident.
7. Severe hypertension treated and untreated.

8. Parturition (within the last 10 days).
9. Ulcerative colitis.
10. Visceral carcinoma.
11. Menstrual bleeding.
12. During the first 18 weeks of pregnancy (see note below).

Precautions and warnings: Following 7–10 days' treatment with streptokinase, the patient's anti-streptokinase antibody titre increases considerably, and returns to normal only after up to 6 months. Normally, a second treatment with streptokinase should not be considered within 6 months of the first. If a second treatment is considered necessary within 6 months then the initial loading dose should be individually determined. The titrated initial dose may be calculated following determination of the smallest quantity of Kabikinase required to lyse a clot, formed from 1.0 ml of the patient's blood within 10 minutes.

If heparin or oral anticoagulants have been given before commencing Kabikinase thrombolytic therapy, further administration should cease (it is not advisable to give Kabikinase and heparin simultaneously). The Kabikinase infusion can then be started after 4 hours. If immediate Kabikinase therapy is required the heparin in the blood should be neutralised with protamine sulphate.

On termination of Kabikinase treatment, the patient should be given anticoagulants in an attempt to prevent rethrombosis. Preferably heparin should be used, starting four hours after the end of thrombolysis, and then oral anticoagulants may be introduced in the usual manner. Drugs which affect blood platelet function, such as salicylic acid preparations, pyrazolone, or indole derivatives, should not be administered concurrently with Kabikinase since the risk of bleeding will be increased.

Pregnancy: Thrombolytic therapy with Kabikinase during the first 18 weeks of pregnancy should be avoided, since there may be a risk of placental separation.

Negligible amounts of streptokinase cross the placenta. The foetal blood concentration reaches about one thousandth of the maternal blood concentration. Fibrinolytic effects in the foetus are unlikely.

Elderly patients: The incidence of cerebral haemorrhage resulting from thrombolytic therapy is increased in elderly patients. Therapy should be restricted to those patients in whom the benefit of treatment outweighs this additional hazard.

Side-effects: Kabikinase therapy may be accompanied by a slight to moderate elevation in body temperature. Mild allergic reactions such as urticaria occur uncommonly. Anaphylaxis occurs extremely rarely. These reactions may be controlled by the prior administration of corticosteroids (25 mg prednisolone or a corresponding amount of another glucocorticoid). Minor oozing or bleeding occurring at injection sites may be controlled by applying local pressure.

Exceptionally there may be severe haemorrhage, in which case administration of Kabikinase must be discontinued. If necessary, the antifibrinolytic agent Cylokapron (tranexamic acid-10 mg/kg body weight) should be given immediately by slow intravenous injection. Cryoprecipitate may be used to correct haemostatic deficiency.

Antidote: Tranexamic acid 10 mg/kg body weight by slow intravenous injection.

Pharmaceutical precautions Vials of Kabikinase should be stored below 25°C before reconstitution. Reconstituted vials may be stored for up to 24 hr when kept in a refrigerator. Kabikinase solutions diluted for infusion should be used within 12 hours of preparation.

Legal category POM.

Package quantities Vials of: 100,000 iu; 250,000 iu; 600,000 iu.

Further information Kabikinase is a highly purified streptokinase preparation. It is prepared from beta-haemolytic streptococci culture filtrates. Subsequent purification ensures that Kabikinase is virtually free from streptodornase, streptolysin, hyaluronidase and other enzymes. Kabikinase is soluble in water, is non-toxic and is non-pyrogenic, but is weakly antigenic. Kabikinase is stabilised with sterile human albumin and this imparts a faint straw colour to the preparation.

Product licence numbers
100,000 iu 0022/5013R
250,000 iu 0022/5012R
600,000 iu 0022/5006R

KABIKINASE* 1.5 Million IU ▼

Presentation Vial of straw coloured lyophilised powder containing 1.5 million iu of streptokinase. Human albumin and buffering agents are present as stabilisers.

Uses
Action: By activating the fibrinolytic system, streptokinase induces dissolution of intravascular thrombi and emboli.

Indication: Acute myocardial infarction.

Dosage and administration
Recommended dosage for adults: Streptokinase 1.5 million iu in physiological saline or dextrose 5% is administered as an intravenous infusion, at a constant rate, over 60 minutes.

Preparation of solution: Dissolve the contents of the vial by adding 10 ml Water for Injections.

The solution should be prepared at room temperature. Care should be taken to avoid the formation of foam. The concentrated solution thus obtained is transferred aseptically into an infusion bottle or PVC bag, containing 100 ml of physiological saline, or dextrose 5%.

Contra-indications, warnings, etc
Contra-indications: Kabikinase should not be administered intramuscularly. Since thrombolytic therapy increases the risk of bleeding, Kabikinase is contra-indicated in the following:

Invasive or traumatic procedures within the previous 10 days including the following: Surgery; central venous cannulation, or puncture of a non-compressible vessel; external cardiac compression; endotracheal intubation biopsy.

Defective haemostasis including: Thrombocytopenia or any other platelet disorder; coagulation disorders (including those caused by hepatic or renal impairment); acute systemic infection, bacteraemia or septicaemia; oral or intravenous anticoagulant therapy (see under 'Precautions', paragraph 2).

Potential for gastro-intestinal haemorrhage including: Oesophageal varices; history of peptic ulceration; visceral carcinoma; ulcerative colitis; diverticulitis.

Increased risk of cerebral haemorrhage/infarction as evidenced by any of the following: Stroke; cerebral tumour; hypertension (treated or untreated); hypertensive or diabetic retinopathy; transient ischaemic attacks.

Obstetric or gynaecological conditions likely to predispose to haemorrhage, including: Menstruation; pregnancy – see also 'Pregnancy' section; parturition within the previous 18 weeks.

Potential for cardiac thromboemboli, including: Active or recent infective endocarditis; atrial valve disease with atrial fibrillation.

Increased risk of pulmonary haemorrhage, including: Active tuberculosis; pneumothorax.

Previous streptokinase therapy, more than 5 days and up to 6 months previously, or recent streptococcal infection, since an elevated titre of anti-streptokinase antibody may render the treatment ineffective.

Coma.

Precautions: Patients should not receive streptokinase unless they will be managed within a hospital setting, under expert medical supervision. It is recommended that patients should be treated in a coronary care (or intensive care) unit.

1. The *diagnosis* of acute myocardial infarction should initially be based upon both clinical signs and ECG evidence. Specific ECG changes diagnostic of recent myocardial infarction should be present. The following

diagnoses, which can be associated with ECG changes, and in which administration of thrombolytic therapy might result in life-threatening haemorrhage **MUST** be excluded.

aortic dissection; acute pericarditis; oesophageal rupture; acute abdominal emergencies, including pancreatitis and perforation of the duodenum; intracranial haemorrhage; (see also (2) below).

A chest X-ray should be performed in order to assist in eliminating ruptured oesophagus (pneumomediastinum) of duodenum (air under the diaphragm) and aortic dissection (wide mediastinum). Aortic dissection should be suspected particularly when pain radiates into the back, aortic regurgitation is evident on auscultation or there are absent pulses. Pericarditis should be suspected when ST-segment elevation occurs in all ECG leads. Raised blood amylase is an indication of pancreatitis.

2. Thrombolytic therapy should be considered only in the case of patients for whom a well documented *medical history* is available. It is essential that thrombolytic therapy is not instituted in patients with co-existing medical conditions likely to exacerbate the risk of haemorrhage (e.g. peptic ulceration, history of cerebrovascular accident, cerebral tumour, visceral carcinoma, see also 'Contra-indications'). Additionally, caution should be exercised in patients who are receiving other drug therapies which are likely to predispose to increased risk of haemorrhagic complications.

3. In most patients, infarction probably is complete within 4–6 hrs and, accordingly, only patients in whom therapy can be iniated within this time interval should be considered for treatment. (But see statement on Q waves below.) *Myocardial salvage* is possible only when recanalisation of the infarct-related artery is effected within a critical time interval following coronary occlusion. The rate of progression of myocardial necrosis is inversely related to the extent of residual perfusion of the ischaemic myocardium. When infarction is due to subtotal coronary occlusion (ca 10–25% of patients) and there is some residual antegrade perfusion, the rate of necrosis is less than when infarction results from complete coronary occlusion. Similarly, in some patients (ca 5–10%) a well developed collateral circulation may retard the progress and reduce the severity of ischaemia. The maximum time delay commensurate with myocardial salvage and reduction in mortality is not known. In patients treated within one hour following symptomatic onset, the risk of death is halved. Generally, the presence of marked pathological Q waves in the ECG should be considered as evidence that transmural infarction is complete and that appreciable myocardial salvage is not possible.

Conversely, benefit may be derived up to 18 hours following symptoms onset, in patients in whom pathological Q waves are absent, or symptoms are intermittent.

4. *Hypokalaemia* predisposes to ventricular arrhythmias and, if present should be corrected.

5. If *venous access* is considered necessary (e.g. for cardiac pacing) the risk of haemorrhage from central venous cannulation must be considered, and preference should be given to the antecubital route.

6. Thrombolytic therapy with Kabikinase induces a *systemic fibrinolytic state*. The presence of circulating free plasmin results in consumption of fibrinogen and of coagulation factors (predominantly Factors V, VIII and XII). Additionally, circulating degradation products of fibrinogen and fibrin exert an anticoagulant effect. Accordingly thrombolytic therapy increases the risk of haemorrhage both throughout the period of streptokinase infusion, and for approximately 12–24 hours thereafter, i.e. until the serum fibrinogen exceeds 100 mg%.

7. Care should be exercised when moving the patient to avoid trauma-induced haematomas. Unnecessary venipunctures should be avoided.

8. *Reperfusion* is usually accompanied by relief of chest pain. Occasionally, reperfusion is preceded by a period of fluctuation in the severity of chest pain. Reperfusion is followed by resolution of the ischaemic ST segment changes. An ECG lead with distinct ST segment elevation should be selected for continuous monitoring, and the initial positions of the ST segment and the peak of the T waves marked. The time of reperfusion may then be recorded. In patients who have sustained minimal necrosis there may be no development of Q waves. However, development of Q waves may not imply complete necrosis, since myocardium subjected to prolonged ischaemia ('stunned myocardium') may take several days to recover.

9. In some patients with inferior wall infarction reperfusion is associated with *vagal reactions*, of nausea, vomiting, sinus bradycardia and hypotension. It has been proposed that these result from the triggering of the Bezold-Jarisch reflex by the restoration of perfusion to the inferior and posterior wall of the left ventricle. These vagal reactions usually respond to intravenous atropine.

10. Accelerated idioventricular rhythm occurs at the time of reperfusion or shortly thereafter in approximately 50–60% of patients. Reperfusion is also associated with ventricular ectopic beats occurring late in diastole. These may be single or may give rise to ventricular bigeminy or trigeminy, or may form fusion beats. These ventricular arrhythmias (frequently referred to as '*reperfusion arrhythmias*') are probably related to increased automaticity. Sustained ventricular tachycardia and ventricular fibrillation are rare, occurring no more commonly than in patients receiving standard management, and should be managed in the normal way.

11. The titre of circulating antistreptokinase antibody rises abruptly at 5–7 days following Kabikinase administration, and may reach levels sufficient to neutralise subsequent Kabikinase dosages administered within the following 6 months.

Accordingly,

(a) Information relating to the administration of Kabikinase therapy should be recorded clearly in the patient's notes.

(b) Kabikinase therapy should not be repeated within the period of 5 days to 6 months following the initial treatment.

(c) Patients with on-going, or recent, streptococcal infections may be resistant to Kabikinase therapy.

12. Subsequent *anticoagulant treatment* with heparin is generally considered necessary in order to prevent rethrombosis in the infarct-related coronary artery, since following thrombolysis, the thrombogenic segment is again exposed to circulating blood, and may again induce thrombosis in the affected artery. Reocclusion occurs in approximately 10–20% of successfully reperfused patients. If anticoagulant treatment is considered appropriate, then heparin should be administered incrementally and judiciously during the first 24 hr following treatment. The partial thromboplastin time should be monitored at regular intervals, and the heparin dosage adjusted to maintain the former within the range 2–2.5 times normal. The optimal duration of anticoagulant therapy is not known. The use of thrombolytic therapy should not necessarily lead to any change in the normal patient management of acute myocardial infarction.

13. Successful thrombolytic therapy will not obviate the requirement for further expert cardiological assessment and patient management.

Side-effects: Kabikinase therapy may be accompanied by a slight to moderate pyrexia. Mild allergic reactions such as uticaria are uncommon, particularly when the total duration of infusion is less than 2 hours. Anaphylaxis occurs extremely rarely (ca 0.1%). These reactions may be controlled by the prior intravenous administration of corticosteroids (e.g. hydrocortisone 100 mg, or prednisolone 25 mg). If streptokinase infusion is to be administered for more than 2 hours, or is to be repeated within 6 months, the prior administration of intravenous corticosteroid and/or an antihistamine should be considered, in order to reduce the incidence of allergic reactions.

Haemorrhagic complications largely result from inappropriate anticoagulant therapy, rather than from fibrinolysis *per se*. Minor bleeding, predominantly at puncture sites, occurs with an incidence of approximately 3–4%. Major haemorrhagic episodes requiring transfusion of 2 or more units of blood (gastro-intestinal and retroperitoneal haemorrhage) occur with an incidence of approximately 0.3%. Cerebral haemorrhage and stroke occurs with a frequency of approximately 0.1%. Though there is a theoretical risk of haemorrhagic infarction and haemorrhage into the pericardium, these are extremely rarely encountered. In cases of severe haemorrhage administration of Kabikinase must be discontinued. If necessary, the antifibrinolytic agent Cyklokapron, (tranexamic acid – 10 mg/kg body weight) should be given immediately by slow intravenous injection. Fresh frozen plasma, or preferably cryoprecipitate, should be administered, to correct haemostatic deficiencies.

Antidote: Tranexamic acid 10 mg/kg body weight by slow intravenous injection.

Pregnancy: Thrombolytic therapy with Kabikinase is contra-indicated during pregnancy, since there may be an increased risk of placental separation.

Elderly patients: The incidence of cerebral haemorrhage may be increased in elderly compared with young patients.

Children: Not recommended.

Pharmaceutical precautions Vials of Kabikinase should be stored below 25°C before reconstitution. The overall reconstituted shelf life is 12 hours. The concentrate should be stored at 2–8°C. Diluted material should be used as soon as possible and not longer than 12 hours after initial reconstitution.

Legal category: POM.

Package quantities Vials containing 1.5 million iu streptokinase.

Further information Kabikinase is a highly purified streptokinase preparation. It is prepared from beta-haemolytic streptococci culture filtrates. Subsequent purification ensures that Kabikinase is virtually free from streptodornase, streptolysin, hyaluronidase and other enzymes. Kabikinase is soluble in water, is non-toxic and is non-pyrogenic, but is weakly antigenic.

Kabikinase is stabilised with sterile human albumin and this imparts a faint straw colour to the preparation.

Product licence number 0022/0070.

MACRODEX* IN DEXTROSE

Presentation

Dextran of weight average molecular weight of 70,000	30 g
Dextrose	25 g
Water for Injections to	500 ml

Colourless, clear, slightly viscous solution. Bottle has a yellow seal. Complies with Dextran 70 Injection BP monograph.

Uses

Action: Dextran 70 molecules have a mean size approximating to albumin. The injection is thought to enhance blood flow and inhibit thromboembolism by:

1. Increasing blood volume
2. Decreasing blood viscosity
3. Reducing erythrocyte aggregation and platelet and leucocyte adhesiveness
4. Increasing capillary perfusion by combination of foregoing actions.

Indications: Macrodex is used for early fluid replacement or plasma volume expansion in the adjunctive treatment of certain types of shock or in impending shock including those resulting from burns, surgery, haemorrhage or trauma in which circulatory volume deficit is present.

Macrodex is not a substitute for whole blood or blood products when these are clearly indicated.

Macrodex may be used for prophylaxis of venous thrombosis and pulmonary embolism in patients at moderate or high risk of thromboembolism.

Macrodex is for intravenous administration only.

Dosage and administration The clinical dosage is dependent upon age, weight and clinical condition of the patient.

Volume replacement: The usual adult dose is 500–1000 ml per day administered at the rate of 20–40 ml per minute; however, the total dosage and rate of infusion depends upon the magnitude of fluid loss and the degree of haemoconcentration. It is recommended that the total dosage does not exceed 20 ml per kilogram of body weight during the first 24 hours.

In haemorrhagic emergency doses of greater than 1500 ml should be accompanied by equal volumes of blood. 500 ml infused expands circulating volume by about 500 ml: by 3 hours this has fallen to 430 ml, 6 hours – 380 ml and 12 hours – 330 ml.

In children, the best guide is body weight or surface area; the total dosage should not exceed 20 ml per kilogram.

In the elderly take care not to overload.

If therapy is continued beyond 24 hours, dosage should not exceed 10 ml/kg.

Treatment should not continue beyond 3 days.

For the prophylaxis of thromboembolism: Infuse 500 ml over 4–6 hours during or at the end of the surgery followed by 500 ml over 4–6 hours the next day. In high-risk patients the treatment may be continued with 500 ml over 4–6 hours on alternate days for a maximum of 10 days.

Contra-indications, warnings, etc

Contra-indications: Macrodex is contra-indicated in the presence of thrombocytopenia, hypofibrinogenaemia, severe congestive heart failure, renal disease with severe oliguria or anuria and where there is known intolerance to dextran.

Macrodex in dextrose should not be administered to patients in whom dextrose restriction is indicated. Macrodex in 0.9% sodium chloride is available.

Interactions: As with all parenterals, compatibilities should be checked when additives are used.

Thorough and careful mixing of any additives is mandatory.

Avoid storage of solutions so prepared.

Effect on ability to drive and use machinery: Not applicable.

Other undesirable effects: Allergic reactions, including urticaria, nasal congestion, wheezing and hypotension, rarely severe and fatal anaphylactoid reactions. Transient acidosis due to perfusion improvements may be noted.

Occasionally nausea, vomiting, fever and arthralgia may occur. Vomiting and involuntary defaecation have occurred in anaesthetised patients.

Use in pregnancy and lactation: Although anaphylactic reactions to Macrodex are rare, the product should only be used during pregnancy when strictly indicated, since anaphylactic reactions in the mother have been reported to cause anoxic brain damage which has resulted in death of the foetus in a number of cases.

Warnings: Macrodex is a colloidal solution and holds about 20 ml of water per gram of dextran. Care should be exercised in poorly hydrated patients to rectify fluid deficits with parenteral electrolyte or dextrose solutions and the Macrodex infusion limited to 500 ml per hour. Keep urine flow above 250 ml/6 hours and the S.G. below 1.065.

Recommended dosage of Macrodex effects only minor and transient changes in the coagulation of the blood. Excessive dosage may induce a prolonged bleeding time. Therefore, the physician should be aware of the possibility of a slight increase in blood loss.

It is strongly recommended that central venous pressure is frequently monitored during the initial infusion of Macrodex which should be immediately discontinued if there is a steep rise in central venous pressure. Without monitoring, the intravenous infusion should be slower and the patient carefully observed for signs of circulatory overloading.

Following the administration of Macrodex, an increase in urinary output usually occurs in oliguric patients. If no increase is observed after the administration of 500 ml, the infusion should be discontinued until adequate diuresis develops spontaneously or can be provoked by other means.

Macrodex infusion may depress plasma protein and haemoglobin levels. The amount of Macrodex given should not cause a depression of the haemoglobin concentration below 9 G% for more than a short time. Care should be taken to prevent a depression of the haematocrit below 30% volume.

Macrodex should be infused with caution in patients with cardiac, hepatic or renal dysfunction.

Precautions: Macrodex should not interfere with standard saline blood typing and cross matching techniques; however, cells should be washed with saline first. Enzymatic methods based on papain may be affected by the presence of dextran.

Strong acids in laboratory tests may liberate dextrose from dextran, yielding falsely elevated glucose assay results, while alcohol by precipitating dextran may give false readings in bilirubin assays and Biuret protein assays. Blood for such laboratory tests should be taken before therapy.

Patients should be closely observed for signs of anaphylaxis during the first few minutes and resuscitative measures should be readily available. Large doses may result in pulmonary oedema.

In patients in whom restriction of sodium is indicated, Macrodex in glucose should be used, and conversely, in patients in whom dextrose restriction is indicated, Macrodex in saline should be used.

Overdose: In the event of an accidental over infusion, treatment should temporarily be either discontinued or rate of infusion decreased significantly, depending on extent of over infusion. The patients should be observed for symptoms and signs of cardiorespiratory decompensation and hepatic and renal functions, and fluid and electrolyte balance should be carefully monitored together with any evidence of bleeding diathesis; other symptomatic and supportive measures should be provided.

Incompatibilities: The slightly acid pH of Macrodex despite negligible buffering capacity (<2 mEq/L) may precipitate salts of weak acids such as the various penicillins, unless they are buffered. Aminocaproic acid, dihydrallazine mesylate, warfarin sodium (dextrose vehicle only), 95% ethanol, dexamethasone sodium phosphate, isoxaprin hydrochloride and propantheline bromide have been reported incompatible.

Macrodex in Dextrose and blood or plasma should not be administered through the same set without first flushing with saline to prevent blood protein precipitation by the electrolyte-free dextran solution.

Pharmaceutical precautions Macrodex crystallizes occasionally due to swings of temperature causing expansion changes of meniscus level. Seed crystals form on the meniscus line which may grow into full crystals.

Store at steady room temperature not exceeding 25°C.

Crystals may be re-dissolved by heating for a short time, not exceeding 100°C. The solution should be cooled to 37°C before use.

Legal category POM.

Package quantities Infusion bottles of 500 ml.

Further information Nil.

Product licence number 0009/5001R.

Product licence holder: Pharmacia Biosystems Ltd, Davy Avenue, Knowlhill, Milton Keynes MK5 8PH.

MACRODEX* IN NORMAL SALINE

Presentation

Dextran of weight average molecular weight of 70,000	30 g
Sodium chloride	4.5 g
Water for Injections to	500 ml

Colourless, clear, slightly viscous solution. Bottle has a green seal. Complies with Dextran 70 Injection BP monograph.

Uses

Action: Dextran 70 molecules have a mean size approximating to albumin. The injection is thought to enhance blood flow and inhibit thromboembolism by:

1. Increasing blood volume
2. decreasing blood viscosity
3. Reducing erythrocyte aggregation and platelet and leucocyte adhesiveness
4. Increasing capillary perfusion by combination of foregoing actions.

Indications: Macrodex is used for early fluid replacement or plasma volume expansion in the adjunctive treatment of certain types of shock or in impending shock including those resulting from burns, surgery, haemorrhage or trauma in which circulatory volume deficit is present.

Macrodex is not a substitute for whole blood or blood products when these are clearly indicated.

Macrodex may be used for prophylaxis of venous thrombosis and pulmonary embolism in patients at moderate or high risk of thromboembolism.

Macrodex is for intravenous administration only.

Dosage and administration The clinical dosage is dependent upon age, weight and clinical condition of the patient.

Volume replacement: The usual adult dose is 500–1000 ml per day administered at the rate of 20–40 ml per minute; however, the total dosage and rate of infusion depends upon the magnitude of fluid loss and the degree of haemoconcentration. It is recommended that the total dosage does not exceed 20 ml per kilogram of body weight during the first 24 hours.

In haemorrhagic emergency doses of greater than 1500 ml should be accompanied by equal volumes of blood. 500 ml infused expands circulating volume by about 500 ml: by 3 hours this has fallen to 430 ml, 6 hours –380 ml and 12 hours –330 ml.

In children, the best guide is body weight or surface area: the total dosage should not exceed 20 ml per kilogram.

In the elderly take care not to overload.

If therapy is continued beyond 24 hours, dosage should not exceed 10 ml/kg.

Treatment should not continue beyond 3 days.

For the prophylaxis of thromboembolism: Infuse 500 ml over 4–6 hours during or at the end of the surgery followed by 500 ml over 4–6 hours the next day. In high-risk patients the treatment may be continued with 500 ml over 4–6 hours on alternate days for a maximum of 10 days.

Contra-indications, warnings, etc

Contra-indications: Macrodex is contra-indicated in the presence of thrombocytopenia, hypofibrinogenaemia, severe congestive heart failure, renal disease with severe oliguria or anuria and where there is known intolerance to dextran.

Macrodex in normal saline should not be administered to patients in whom sodium chloride restriction is indicated. Macrodex in 0.5% Dextrose is available.

Interactions: As with all parenterals, compatibilities should be checked when additives are used.

Thorough and careful mixing of any additives is mandatory.

Avoid storage of solutions so prepared.

Effect on ability to drive and use machinery: Not applicable.

Other undesirable effects: Allergic reactions, including urticaria, nasal congestion, wheezing and hypotension, rarely severe and fatal anaphylactoid reactions. Transient acidosis due to perfusion improvements may be noted.

Occasionally nausea, vomiting, fever and arthralgia may occur. Vomiting and involuntary defaecation have occurred in anaesthetised patients.

Use in pregnancy and lactation: Although anaphylactic reactions to Macrodex are rare, the product should only be used during pregnancy when strictly indicated, since anaphylactic reactions in the mother have been reported to cause anoxic brain damage which has resulted in death of the foetus in a number of cases.

Warnings: Macrodex is a colloidal solution and holds about 20 ml of water per gram of dextran. Care should be exercised in poorly hydrated patients to rectify fluid deficits with parenteral electrolyte or dextrose solutions and the Macrodex infusion limited to 500 ml per hour. Keep urine flow above 250 ml/6 hours and the S.G. below 1.065.

Recommended dosage of Macrodex effects only minor and transient changes in the coagulation of the blood. Excessive dosage may induce a prolonged bleeding time. Therefore, the physician should be aware of the possibility of a slight increase in blood loss.

It is strongly recommended that central venous pressure is frequently monitored during the initial infusion of Macrodex which should be immediately discontinued if there is a steep rise in central venous pressure. Without monitoring, the intravenous infusion should be slower and the patient carefully observed for signs of circulatory overloading.

Following the administration of Macrodex, an increase in urinary output usually occurs in oliguric patients. If no increase is observed after the administration of 500 ml, the infusion should be discontinued until adequate diuresis develops spontaneously or can be provoked by other means.

Macrodex infusion may depress plasma protein and haemoglobin levels. The amount of Macrodex given should not cause a depression of the haemoglobin concentration below 9 G% for more than a short time. Care should be taken to prevent a depression of the haematocrit below 30% volume.

Macrodex should be infused with caution in patients with cardiac, hepatic or renal dysfunction.

Precautions: Macrodex should not interfere with standard saline blood typing and cross matching techniques; however, cells should be washed with saline first. Enzymatic methods based on papain may be affected by the presence of dextran.

Strong acids in laboratory tests may liberate dextrose from dextran, yielding falsely elevated glucose assay results, while alcohol by precipitating dextran may give false readings in bilirubin assays and Biuret protein assays. Blood for such laboratory tests should be taken before therapy.

Patients should be closely observed for signs of anaphylaxis during the first few minutes and resuscitative measures should be readily available. Large doses may result in pulmonary oedema.

In patients in whom restriction of sodium is indicated, Macrodex in glucose should be used, and conversely, in patients in whom dextrose restriction is indicated, Macrodex in saline should be used.

Overdose: In the event of an accidental over infusion, treatment should temporarily be either discontinued or rate of infusion decreased significantly, depending on extent of over infusion. The patients should be observed for symptoms and signs of cardiorespiratory decompensation and hepatic and renal functions, and fluid and electrolyte balance should be carefully monitored together with any evidence of bleeding diathesis; other symptomatic and supportive measures should be provided.

Incompatibilities: The slightly acid pH of Macrodex despite negligible buffering capacity (<2 mEq/L) may precipitate salts of weak acids such as the various penicillins, unless they are buffered. Aminocaproic acid, dihydrallazine mesylate, warfarin sodium (dextrose vehicle only), 95% ethanol, dexamethasone sodium phosphate, isoxaprin hydrochloride and propantheline bromide have been reported incompatible.

Macrodex in Dextrose and blood or plasma should not be administered through the same set without first flushing with saline to prevent blood protein precipitation by the electrolyte-free dextran solution.

Pharmaceutical precautions Macrodex crystallizes occasionally due to swings of temperature causing expansion changes of meniscus level. Seed crystals form on the meniscus line which may grow into full crystals.

Store at steady room temperature not exceeding 25°C.

Crystals may be re-dissolved by heating for a short time, not exceeding 100°C. The solution should be cooled to 37°C before use.

Legal category POM.

Package quantities Infusion bottles of 500 ml.

Further information Nil.

Product licence number 0009/5000R.

Product licence holder: Pharmacia Biosystems Ltd, Davy Avenue, Knowlhill, Milton Keynes MK5 8PH.

MICTURIN* 12.5 and MICTURIN 25

Presentation

Micturin 12.5: white film-coated tablets 6 mm in diameter marked MC in arcs on one side. Each tablet contains terodiline hydrochloride 12.5 mg.

Micturin 25: white film-coated tablets 8 mm in diameter marked MT in arcs on one side. Each tablet contains terodiline hydrochloride 25 mg.

Uses Main pharmacological action: terodiline is a secondary amine which possesses anticholinergic and calcium antagonist properties. These properties are additive in effecting relaxation of the detrusor muscle of the urinary bladder. In patients with unstable bladder, terodiline increases bladder capacity and reduces the frequency of micturition. In patients with motor urge incontinence terodiline reduces the incidence of incontinent episodes. Terodiline is well absorbed following oral administration, is metabolised in the liver, and is excreted in the urine.

Adults: Urinary frequency, urgency and incontinence in patients with detrusor instability (motor urge incontinence) and neurogenic bladder disorders, e.g. uninhibited bladder and reflex bladder disease.

Dosage and administration

Route of administration: By mouth.

Recommended dosage: Adults 12.5–25 mg twice daily. The final dose will depend upon response and/or tolerance to side-effects. It will not normally be necessary to exceed 12.5 mg twice daily in the frail, elderly patient.

Children: Not recommended.

Contra-indications, warnings, etc Micturin is contra-indicated in the following groups of patients: those with bladder outflow obstruction; flaccid bladder or high residual urine; obstructive lesions particularly of the upper gastrointestinal tract; severe hepatic dysfunction or biliary tract dysfunction; glaucoma.

Precautions: As with other drugs with anticholinergic effects, caution should be observed in patients with gastric retention, incipient obstruction of the gastrointestinal tract, fever, thyrotoxicosis, or those with heart disease where an increase in heart rate is undesirable. Caution should also be observed in patients with hepatic dysfunction and in the frail, elderly patient. Potentiation of clinical effects may be expected when Micturin is administered to patients who also are receiving other drugs with anticholinergic or calcium antagonist effects.

Pregnancy: Although no teratogenic effects have been observed, use in pregnancy should be avoided, especially during the first trimester, unless the potential benefits are considered to outweigh the possible hazards.

Lactation: Administration to breast feeding mothers should be avoided unless considered essential.

Side-effects: As with other drugs with anticholinergic activity, Micturin may cause dryness of the mouth, visual accommodation disturbances, reduced lacrimation, constipation, dizziness, tachycardia and retention of urine. Rare instances of nausea and tremor have been reported.

Overdosage: Gastric lavage, symptomatic treatment. If atropine-like central anticholinergic side-effects predominate give physostigmine 1.0–2.0 mg by slow intravenous injection (ca 2 mins); in children give 0.02–0.04 mg/kg. Titrate to an effective dosage, which may be repeated in 30–60 minutes.

In cases of pronounced excitation or convulsions diazepam 10 mg should be administered intravenously (children 0.1–0.2 mg/kg). In respiratory insufficiency give artificial respiration. Tachycardia should be treated by administration of propranolol 1–5 mg by slow intravenous injection. Urinary retention may be treated by catheterisation. The patient should be placed in a dark, quiet room. If mydriasis is troublesome treatment with pilocarpine eye drops should be considered.

If calcium antagonist effects predominate, bradycardia and hypotension should be treated by intravenous infusion of 10 ml calcium gluconate solution 10 per cent, repeated if necessary, until the circulation improves. Adequate intravenous fluid substitution should be instituted.

Pharmaceutical precautions Nil.

Legal category POM.

Package quantities Micturin 12.5 and Micturin 25 are available in packs of 56 tablets, arranged in blister strips of 14 tablets.

Further information Steady state levels of terodiline are reached in the plasma only after 10–14 days administration, treatment should therefore be continued for two to three weeks when the optimal response will be obtained.

Product licence numbers
Micturin 12.5 0022/0065
Micturin 25 0022/0059

NOVAGARD*

Presentation Novagard is an intrauterine device consisting of pure copper wire with a silver core, surface area approximately 200 mm², wound on to the vertical arm of a T-shaped plastic carrier. The plastic carrier is composed of polyethylene impregnated with barium sulphate to render it radio-opaque, with a polyethylene thread attached to the base of the vertical arm. The device is presented partially loaded in its inserter tube and instructions for use are included with each sterile pack.

Novagard dimensions – Transverse arms 32 mm, Vertical arm 32 mm.

Uses Intrauterine contraception.

Dosage and administration Novagard is recommended for women with a uterine size measurement from external os to fundus greater than 5.5 cm. Novagard should be replaced at least every five years. The procedure for insertion is fully detailed in the instructions for use leaflet included with each sterile pack.

Although IUCDs may be inserted at any time during the menstrual cycle, insertion during or shortly after the menstrual period reduces the possibility of an existing undiagnosed pregnancy. Postpartum insertion is usually delayed until involution of the uterus is complete. The benefits of immediate post abortion insertion should be weighed against the risks due to the relatively soft structure of the uterus.

Contra-indications, warnings, etc
Contra-indications: Contra-indications are pregnancy; history of ectopic pregnancy; postpartum endometritis or septic abortion within the past three months; abnormalities of the uterine cavity including developmental abnormalities; large or multiple fibroids; acute pelvic inflammatory disease; a history of repeated, recent or severe pelvic inflammatory disease; acute cervicitis; cervical dysplasia; endometrial disease such as hyperplasia or uterine polyps; suspected or proven malignancy of the genital organs, including unresolved abnormal Papanicolaou smear; severe dysmenorrhoea; menorrhagia and/or intermenstrual bleeding; significant anaemia; heart disease; leukaemia; use of chronic corticosteroid therapy because of the increased susceptibility to infection with certain micro-organisms which may possibly be introduced at the time of an IUCD insertion; Wilson's disease or a hypersensitivity to copper.

Medical diathermy to the abdominal and sacral regions is contra-indicated because of the possibility of heat injury to the surrounding tissues.

Warnings: An increased incidence of pelvic inflammatory disease and menorrhagia associated with the use of IUCDs has been reported. Pelvic infection may result in future infertility. Women with certain known or suspected heart disease are more susceptible to development of subacute bacterial endocarditis. Use of IUCD in these women may represent a potential source of septic emboli. Appropriate precautions including administration of antibiotics should be observed when inserting an IUCD in such cases.

Syncope or bradycardia may occur in some women during insertion or removal of an IUCD. In the event of early signs of a vasovagal attack, insertion may need to be abandoned or the device removed. The woman should be kept supine, the head lowered and the legs elevated to the vertical position if necessary in order to restore cerebral blood flow. A clear airway must be maintained; an airway should always be at hand. Persistent bradycardia may be controlled with intravenous atropine in a dose of 0.6 mg. If oxygen is available it may be administered by using an Ambu bag. In the very rare emergency situation where the woman fails to regain consciousness she should be transferred to hospital intensive care.

Post-insertion cramps are usually of only a few minutes duration, but some women may experience cramps for several hours or days. Spotting, intermenstrual bleeding or increased menstrual flow may occur. If heavy or persistent bleeding or persistent abdominal cramps occur, removal of the device may be indicated.

Novagard should be removed in the event of partial expulsion and a new device inserted. If perforation of the uterus or cervix is suspected, the device should be removed as soon as medically feasible. Adhesions, foreign body reactions and intestinal obstruction may result if an IUCD is left within the peritoneal cavity. Removal is also indicated in cases of pelvic infection resistant to treatment, menorrhagia producing significant anaemia, or intractable pain.

Precautions: A complete gynaecological examination, including measurement of the uterus, should precede insertion of the device. Ideally the woman should be re-examined within the first three months after insertion and annually thereafter. After insertion the woman should be taught to examine herself to ascertain the continued presence of the retrieval thread. Advise her to consult her doctor if pregnancy is suspected.

Intrauterine devices should be used with caution in women with anaemia, menorrhagia, hypermenorrhoea, a history of a previous uterine incision or perforation of the uterus and those receiving anticoagulants, steroid therapy or having a coagulopathy.

The possibility of a seizure being precipitated in an epileptic, at or shortly after the insertion of an IUCD should also be borne in mind.

It has been reported that IUCDs may be less effective in insulin-dependent diabetics.

Lost threads: If the retrieval thread is not visible at the cervix on follow-up examination, it may have been drawn up into the uterus or cervical canal and may reappear during the next menstrual period. The thread may usually be located by gently probing with a suitable instrument. If it cannot be found, it may have broken off, or the device may have been expelled. Ultrasound or X-ray may be used to locate the device.

Pregnancy: The risk of ectopic pregnancy is reported to be greater in women who conceive with an IUCD in situ than in those without an IUCD. Therefore, if a woman becomes pregnant with an IUCD in situ, she should be carefully evaluated for possible ectopic pregnancy. There have been reports of an increased incidence of septic abortion, associated in some instances with septicaemia, septic shock and death, in women who become pregnant with an IUCD in situ. Women who are pregnant with an IUCD in situ should be closely observed and told to report immediately all abnormal symptoms such as 'flu-like symptoms, fever, cramp-like pain, bleeding or excessive discharge, as the onset of septicaemia associated with septic abortion may be insidious with general symptoms rather than initial signs of spontaneous abortion. Also, the incidence of spontaneous abortion appears to be increased over that in unprotected women when conception occurs with an IUCD in situ. If pregnancy occurs with an IUCD in situ and the thread is visible then the device should be removed. If the thread is not visible or device removal would be difficult, the IUCD may be left in situ until the pregnancy goes to term or until a decision is made to terminate the pregnancy. If the woman elects to continue the pregnancy, careful observation is required. The long term effects of intra-uterine copper on the foetus are unknown.

Adverse effects: Uterine or cervical perforation, vaginal discharge, embedment and allergic reactions have been reported.

Pharmaceutical precautions Novagard is supplied in a sterile pack which should not be opened until required for insertion. Each device should be handled with aseptic precautions and it is advisable that the folded device in the inserter tube should not be left for more than two minutes, as this may prevent the transverse arms from reassuming the correct position.

Care should be taken not to damage the sterile package which should be stored below 30°C (86°F).

Legal category POM.

Package quantities
Pack containing one sterile device.
Pack containing ten sterile devices.

Further information The average amount of copper eluted from copper IUCDs is well below the daily dietary intake of copper. Small increases of endometrial copper levels have been noted in the presence of copper IUCDs, but these are not cumulative. No changes in blood levels of copper have been detected.

Product licence number 0022/0046.

PED-EL*

Presentation A straw-coloured solution containing electrolytes and trace elements for addition to the Vamin Infant or Vamin 9 Glucose solutions in the intravenous nutrition of neonates and infants. Ped-el corresponds to the following formula:

Calcium chloride $2H_2O$	22.06 mg
Magnesium chloride $6H_2O$	5.08 mg
Ferric chloride $6H_2O$	135 micrograms
Zinc chloride	20.4 micrograms
Manganese chloride $4H_2O$	49.5 micrograms
Copper chloride $2H_2O$	12.8 micrograms
Sodium fluoride	31.5 micrograms
Potassium iodide	1.7 micrograms
Phosphoric acid	8.65 mg
Sorbitol	0.3 g
Water for injections to 1 ml	
pH 2.0	

1 ml of Ped-el contains the following amounts of electrolytes and trace elements:

Ca^{2+}	0.15 mmol
Mg^{2+}	25 micromol
Fe^{3+}	0.5 micromol
Zn^{2+}	0.15 micromol
Mn^{2+}	0.25 micromol
Cu^{2+}	0.075 micromol
F^-	0.75 micromol
I^-	0.01 micromol
P	75 micromol
Cl^-	0.35 mmol

1 vial of Ped-el contains less than 1 micromol potassium and less than 1.5 mmol sodium.

Uses Ped-el is an integral part of the complete intravenous nutrition of neonates and infants. It should be used in conjunction with Vamin Infant, Vamin 9 Glucose, Intralipid and a suitable phosphate preparation containing potassium. This will provide the infant's basal requirement of electrolytes and trace elements. As the requirements of electrolytes and trace elements may vary in different clinical conditions, these substances may have to be added as appropriate in the individual patient. Ped-el administration should not be started until kidney function is established – usually during the second day of life.

Dosage and administration *Recommended dosage for neonates and infants:* As part of a complete intravenous nutrition regimen 4 ml of Ped-el per kg body weight per day will cover the basal requirements of neonates and infants for electrolytes and trace elements and should be added to Vamin Infant or Vamin 9 Glucose. This infusion should be given at a very slow rate and is best done with an appropriate infusion pump or an automatic drop rate counter. The requirements of potassium and sodium vary with different patient conditions. Ped-el is not intended to meet these requirements.

Contra-indications, warnings, etc Should not be given undiluted.

Administration should be carried out only under specialist surveillance, especially in patients with pre-existing imbalances, in renal failure or in hepatic disease. The effects of digitalis on the heart may be enhanced by this preparation and digitalis intoxication may be precipitated. Care should be taken in the administration of Ped-el to patients with impaired or immature biliary or renal function when the excretion of trace elements may be significantly decreased. When given to neonates, monitoring of serum aluminium is recommended. Blood calcium levels will not approach cardiotoxic levels when Ped-el is administered slowly by adherence to the recommended infusion rate of the chosen diluent.

Ped-el contains sorbitol which is metabolised to fructose and should therefore be given with caution to patients with fructose intolerance.

Overdosage: Overdosage, which may occur if the solution is injected undiluted, may result in temporary hypercalcaemia causing bradycardia. Spontaneous reversal of this situation is likely to occur without the need for a specific antidote. If not, standard measures for treating bradycardia can be instituted.

Pharmaceutical precautions

1. Addition of other drugs to be avoided due to the risk of precipitation.
2. Store at 8° to 15°C.
3. A cloudy solution or one containing a precipitate must not be used.
4. The addition of Ped-el should be performed aseptically immediately before the start of the infusion and should be used within 24 hours unless the mixture is refrigerated when it may be used within 48 hours of preparation.

Legal category POM.

Package quantities Boxes of 10 × 20 ml vials.

Further information The manufacturer can be consulted for full information on complete and balanced intravenous nutrition regimens.

Product licence number 0022/0037.

RELAXIT*

Presentation A sterile viscous solution contained in a 5 ml applicator pack.

Relaxit contains:

Sodium citrate (dihydrate)	450 mg
Sodium lauryl sulphate	75 mg
Sorbic acid	5 mg
Glycerol and Sorbitol Solution to	5 ml

Uses Relaxit is a micro-enema for the relief of constipation.

Dosage and administration *Adults and children over the age of three:* The nozzle of the micro-enema is inserted fully into the rectum and the contents squeezed out.

Children under the age of three: Insert only half the length of the nozzle then squeeze the contents out.

Elderly: As adults.

Contra-indications, warnings, etc None.

Pharmaceutical precautions Store in a cool place.

Legal category P.

Package quantities Boxes of 4, 12 or 100.

Further information Relaxit liberates bound water in the faecal mass, thus producing a soft motion which may be easily evacuated. Defaecation usually occurs within 15 minutes.

Product licence number 0009/0019.

Product licence holder: Pharmacia Biosystems Ltd, Davy Avenue, Knowlhill, Milton Keynes MK5 8PH.

RHEOMACRODEX* IN DEXTROSE

Presentation

Dextran of weight average molecular weight of 40,000	50 g
Dextrose	25 g
Water for injection	500 ml

A colourless, clear slightly viscous solution. Bottle has a red seal. Complies with Dextran 40 Injection BP monograph.

Uses

Action: Dextran 40 is a colloidal polymer of glucose which may enhance blood flow by the following mechanisms.

1. Increase of blood volume.
2. Decreasing the viscosity of the blood.
3. Reduction of the aggregation of the erythrocytes and platelets by coating them, and maintenance of their electro-negative charge.
4. As the preparation is hyper-oncotic, extravascular fluid is drawn into the circulation.
5. Capillary flow is increased through the foregoing effects.

Indications: Rheomacrodex is used for early fluid replacement or for plasma volume expansion in the adjunctive treatment of certain types of shock or in impending shock, including those resulting from burns, surgery, haemorrhage or trauma in which circulatory volume deficit is present.

Rheomacrodex is not a substitute for whole blood or blood products where these are clearly indicated.

Rheomacrodex may be used in embolic episodes and for prophylaxis of venous thrombosis and pulmonary embolism in patients at moderate or high risk of thromboembolism.

Rheomacrodex is also used as a priming fluid during extra-corporeal circulation.

Rheomacrodex is used in conditions where improvement of circulatory flow is required.

Rheomacrodex is for intravenous administration only.

Dosage and administration

Dosage schedule: The recommended dosage is dependent upon the age, weight and clinical condition of the patient.

Infants: Up to 5 ml/kg body weight.

Children: Up to 10 ml/kg body weight.

Elderly: As adults but take extra care regarding dehydration, overloading and renal function.

The solution is hyperoncotic and draws extravascular fluid into the vascular space such that 500 ml infused rapidly into a normal hydrated patient may produce an expansion of almost one litre. This expansion is short lived due to excretion of smaller molecules, and by 3 hours expansion will have declined to about 520 ml, by 6 hours 430 ml and 12 hours 360 ml. Such expansion rapidly fills circulatory deficit, reduces haematocrit and concentration of clotting factors and may produce oozing from recent surgical incisions due to increase in capillary flow.

Dehydration must be corrected before giving the drug.

In shock the suggested total adult dose for the first 24 hours should not exceed 20 ml per kg of body weight. The first 10 ml per kg may be infused as rapidly as necessary to effect improvement. Monitoring central venous pressure is strongly recommended as a guide to infusion. Daily doses after the first 24 hours should not exceed 10 ml per kg and therapy should not be continued beyond 5 days.

For the treatment of thromboembolism: Initially 500–1000 ml over 4–6 hours on the first day followed by 500 ml over 4–6 hours on the next day. Then, the treatment may be continued with 500 ml over 4–6 hours on alternative days for a maximum of 10 days.

For the prophylaxis of thromboembolism: Infuse 500 ml over 4–6 hours during or at the end of the surgery followed by 500 ml over 4–6 hours the next day. In high-risk patients, the treatment may be continued with 500 ml over 4–6 hours on alternate days for a maximum of 10 days.

In extracorporeal perfusion the dose of Rheomacrodex will depend upon the volume needed to prime the pump oxygenator. Usually, a total dose of 10–20 ml per kg of body weight is added to the perfusion circuit. The total dose should not exceed 2 g per kg of body weight and this can be limited and controlled by adding other priming fluids.

In improvement of microcirculatory flow: Infuse 500–1000 ml in the first 24 hours. 500 ml is given the next day and then alternate days to a maximum of two weeks.

Contra-indications, warnings, etc

Contra-indications: Rheomacrodex is contra-indicated in the presence of thrombocytopenia, hypofibrinogenaemia, severe congestive heart failure, renal disease with severe oliguria or anuria and where there is known intolerance to dextran.

Rheomacrodex in sodium chloride should not be administered to patients in whom sodium restriction is indicated. Rheomacrodex in 5% dextrose is available.

Interactions: As with all parenterals, compatibilities should be checked when additives are used.

Thorough and careful mixing of any additives is mandatory.

Avoid storage of solutions so prepared.

Effects on ability to drive and to use machinery: Not applicable.

Other undesirable effects: Mild urticarial reaction, rarely severe anaphylactoid reactions, increase in viscosity and specific gravity of urine, reversible tubular vacuolisation, and occasionally transient acidosis due to improved tissue perfusion. Rarely renal failure has been reported.

Use in pregnancy and lactation: Although anaphylactic reactions to Rheomacrodex are rare, the product should only be used during pregnancy when strictly indicated, since anaphylactic reactions in the mother have been reported to cause anoxic brain damage which has resulted in death of the foetus in a number of cases.

Other special warnings: Because Rheomacrodex is a colloidal solution it withdraws water from the extravascular space and the resultant fluid shifts may become critical in poorly hydrated patients. The renal excretion of dextran is associated with elevations of the specific gravity of the urine and these may become significant in patients with reduced renal function. It is therefore, essential that the patient's state of hydration is assessed before Rheomacrodex is administered. If signs of dehydration are present, appropriate parenteral fluids should be administered and the infusion of Rheomacrodex limited to 500 ml per hour. An osmotic diuretic like Mannitol may be used to maintain urine excretion following adequate hydration. Urine flow should be kept above 250 ml/6 hours and the S.G. below 1.065.

Recommended dosage of Rheomacrodex effects only minor and transient changes in the coagulation of the blood. Excessive dosage may induce a prolonged bleeding time. Therefore, the physician should be aware of the possibility of a slight increase in blood loss.

It is strongly recommended that central venous pressure is frequently monitored during the initial infusion of Rheomacrodex. With monitoring, the first 500 ml may be administered rapidly, but should be immediately discontinued if there is a steep rise in central venous pressure. Without monitoring, the intravenous infusion should be slower and the patient carefully observed for signs of circulatory overload.

Following the administration of Rheomacrodex, an increase in urinary output usually occurs in oliguric patients. If no increase is observed after the administration of 500 ml, the infusion should be discontinued until adequate diuresis develops spontaneously or can be provoked by other means.

The amount of Rheomacrodex given should not cause a depression of the haemoglobin concentration below 9G% for more than a short time. Care should be taken to prevent a depression of the haematocrit below 30% volume.

Precautions: Although dextrans of higher molecular weight produce erythrocyte aggregation which may interfere with blood-typing and cross-matching, no such interference occurs with Rheomacrodex. Blood sugar determinations that employ high concentrations of acid may result in hydrolysis of dextran, yielding falsely elevated glucose assay results. This has been observed both with sulphuric acid and with acetic acid. In other laboratory tests, the presence of dextran in the blood may result in the development of turbidity, which can interfere with the assay. This has been observed in bilirubin assays in which alcohol is employed and in total protein assays employing Biuret reagent. Thus consideration should be given to withdrawal of blood for chemical laboratory tests prior to initiation therapy.

Patients should be closely observed for signs of anaphylaxis during the first few minutes and resuscitative measures should be readily available. Large doses may result in pulmonary oedema. Caution is advised in patients with poor cardiac function.

In patients in whom restriction of sodium is indicated Rheomacrodex in glucose should be used, and conversely, in patients in whom dextrose restriction is indicated, Rheomacrodex in saline should be used.

Overdose: In the event of an accidental over infusion, treatment should temporarily, be either discontinued or rate of infusion decreased significantly, depending on extent of over infusion. The patient should be observed for symptoms and signs of cardiorespiratory decompensation and hepatic and renal functions, and fluid and electrolyte balance should be carefully monitored together with any evidence of bleeding diathesis, other symptomatic and supportive measures should be provided.

Incompatibilities: The slightly acid ph of Rheomacrodex despite negligible buffering capacity (2 mEq/L) may precipitate salts of weak acids such as the various penicillins, unless they are buffered. Aminocaproic acid, dihydrallazine mesylate, warfarin sodium (dextrose vehicle only), 95% ethanol, dexamethasone sodium phosphate, isoxaprin hydrochloride and propantheline bromide have been reported incompatible.

Pharmaceutical precautions Rheomacrodex crystallises occasionally due to swings of temperature causing expansion changes of meniscus level. Seed crystals form on the meniscus line which may grow into full crystals. Storage should therefore be at a constant temperature not exceeding 25°C. If flakes of dextran appear, these can be redissolved by heating for a short time at a low temperature not to exceed 100°C. The solution should then be cooled to 37°C before infusion.

Legal category POM.

Package quantities Infusion bottles of 500 ml.

Further information Nil

Product licence number 0009/5005R.

Product licence holder: Pharmacia Biosystems Ltd, Davy Avenue, Knowlhill, Milton Keynes MK5 8PH.

RHEOMACRODEX* IN NORMAL SALINE

Presentation

Dextran of weight average molecular weight of 40,000	50 g
Sodium chloride	4.5 g
Water for injection	500 ml

A colourless, clear slightly viscous solution. Bottle has a blue seal. Complies with Dextran 40 Injection BP monograph.

Uses

Action: Dextran 40 is a colloidal polymer of glucose which may enhance blood flow by the following mechanisms.

1. Increase of blood volume.
2. Decreasing the viscosity of the blood.
3. Reduction of the aggregation of the erythrocytes and platelets by coating them, and maintenance of their electro-negative charge.
4. As the preparation is hyper-oncotic, extravascular fluid is drawn into the circulation.
5. Capillary flow is increased through the foregoing effects.

Indications: Rheomacrodex is used for early fluid replacement or for plasma volume expansion in the adjunctive treatment of certain types of shock or in impending shock, including those resulting from burns, surgery, haemorrhage or trauma in which circulatory volume deficit is present.

Rheomacrodex is not a substitute for whole blood or blood products where these are clearly indicated.

Rheomacrodex may be used in embolic episodes and for prophylaxis of venous thrombosis and pulmonary embolism in patients at moderate or high risk of thromboembolism.

Rheomacrodex is also used as a priming fluid during extra-corporeal circulation.

Rheomacrodex is used in conditions where improvement of circulatory flow is required.

Rheomacrodex is for intravenous administration only.

Dosage and administration

Dosage schedule: The recommended dosage is dependent upon the age, weight and clinical condition of the patient.

Infants: Up to 5 ml/kg body weight.

Children: Up to 10 ml/kg body weight.

Elderly: As adults but take extra care regarding dehydration, overloading and renal function.

The solution is hyperoncotic and draws extravascular fluid into the vascular space such that 500 ml infused rapidly into a normal hydrated patient may produce an expansion of almost one litre. This expansion is short lived due to excretion of smaller molecules, and by 3 hours expansion will have declined to about 520 ml, by 6 hours 430 ml and 12 hours 360 ml. Such expansion rapidly fills circulatory deficit, reduces haematocrit and concentration of clotting factors and may produce oozing from recent surgical incisions due to increase in capillary flow.

Dehydration must be corrected before giving the drug.

In shock the suggested total adult dose for the first 24 hours should not exceed 20 ml per kg of body weight. The first 10 ml per kg may be infused as rapidly as necessary to effect improvement. Monitoring central venous pressure is strongly recommended as a guide to infusion. Daily doses after the first 24 hours should not exceed 10 ml per kg and therapy should not be continued beyond 5 days.

For the treatment of thromboembolism: Initially 500–

1000 ml over 4–6 hours on the first day followed by 500 ml over 4–6 hours on the next day. Then, the treatment may be continued with 500 ml over 4–6 hours on alternative days for a maximum of 10 days.

For the prophylaxis of thromboembolism: Infuse 500 ml over 4–6 hours during or at the end of the surgery followed by 500 ml over 4–6 hours the next day. In high-risk patients, the treatment may be continued with 500 ml over 4–6 hours on alternate days for a maximum of 10 days.

In extracorporeal perfusion the dose of Rheomacrodex will depend upon the volume needed to prime the pump oxygenator. Usually, a total dose of 10–20 ml per kg of body weight is added to the perfusion circuit. The total dose should not exceed 2 g per kg of body weight and this can be limited and controlled by adding other priming fluids.

In improvement of microcirculatory flow: Infuse 500–1000 ml in the first 24 hours. 500 ml is given the next day and then alternate days to a maximum of two weeks.

Contra-indications, warnings, etc

Contra-indications: Rheomacrodex is contra-indicated in the presence of thrombocytopenia, hypofibrinogenaemia, severe congestive heart failure, renal disease with severe oliguria or anuria and where there is known intolerance to dextran.

Rheomacrodex in sodium chloride should not be administered to patients in whom sodium restriction is indicated. Rheomacrodex in 5% dextrose is available.

Interactions: As with all parenterals, compatibilities should be checked when additives are used.

Thorough and careful mixing of any additives is mandatory.

Avoid storage of solutions so prepared.

Effects on ability to drive and to use machinery: Not applicable.

Other undesirable effects: Mild urticarial reaction, rarely severe anaphylactoid reactions, increase in viscosity and specific gravity of urine, reversible tubular vacuolisation, and occasionally transient acidosis due to improved tissue perfusion. Rarely renal failure has been reported.

Use in pregnancy and lactation: Although anaphylactic reactions to Rheomacrodex are rare, the product should only be used during pregnancy when strictly indicated, since anaphylactic reactions in the mother have been reported to cause anoxic brain damage which has resulted in death of the foetus in a number of cases.

Other special warnings: Because Rheomacrodex is a colloidal solution it withdraws water from the extravascular space and the resultant fluid shifts may become critical in poorly hydrated patients. The renal excretion of dextran is associated with elevations of the specific gravity of the urine and these may become significant in patients with reduced renal function. It is therefore, essential that the patient's state of hydration is assessed before Rheomacrodex is administered. If signs of dehydration are present, appropriate parenteral fluids should be administered and the infusion of Rheomacrodex limited to 500 ml per hour. An osmotic diuretic like Mannitol may be used to maintain urine excretion following adequate hydration. Urine flow should be kept above 250 ml/6 hours and the S.G. below 1.065.

Recommended dosage of Rheomacrodex effects only minor and transient changes in the coagulation of the blood. Excessive dosage may induce a prolonged bleeding time. Therefore, the physician should be aware of the possibility of a slight increase in blood loss.

It is strongly recommended that central venous pressure is frequently monitored during the initial infusion of Rheomacrodex. With monitoring, the first 500 ml may be administered rapidly, but should be immediately discontinued if there is a steep rise in central venous pressure. Without monitoring, the intravenous infusion should be slower and the patient carefully observed for signs of circulatory overload.

Following the administration of Rheomacrodex, an increase in urinary output usually occurs in oliguric patients. If no increase is observed after the administration of 500 ml, the infusion should be discontinued until adequate diuresis develops spontaneously or can be provoked by other means.

The amount of Rheomacrodex given should not cause a depression of the haemoglobin concentration below 9G% for more than a short time. Care should be taken to prevent a depression of the haematocrit below 30% volume.

Precautions: Although dextrans of higher molecular weight produce erythrocyte aggregation which may interfere with blood-typing and cross-matching, no such interference occurs with Rheomacrodex. Blood sugar determinations that employ high concentrations of acid may result in hydrolysis of dextran, yielding falsely elevated glucose assay results. This has been observed both with sulphuric acid and with acetic acid. In other laboratory tests, the presence of dextran in the blood may result in the development of turbidity, which can interfere with the assay. This has been observed in bilirubin assays in which alcohol is employed and in total protein assays employing Biuret reagent. Thus consideration should be given to withdrawal of blood for chemical laboratory tests prior to initiation therapy.

Patients should be closely observed for signs of anaphylaxis during the first few minutes and resuscitative measures should be readily available. Large doses may result in pulmonary oedema. Caution is advised in patients with poor cardiac function.

In patients in whom restriction of sodium is indicated Rheomacrodex in glucose should be used, and conversely, in patients in whom dextrose restriction is indicated, Rheomacrodex in saline should be used.

Overdose: In the event of an accidental over infusion, treatment should temporarily, be either discontinued or rate of infusion decreased significantly, depending on extent of over infusion. The patient should be observed for symptoms and signs of cardiorespiratory decompensation and hepatic and renal functions, and fluid and electrolyte balance should be carefully monitored together with any evidence of bleeding diathesis, other symptomatic and supportive measures should be provided.

Incompatibilities: The slightly acid ph of Rheomacrodex despite negligible buffering capacity (2 mEq/L) may precipitate salts of weak acids such as the various penicillins, unless they are buffered. Aminocaproic acid, dihydrallazine mesylate, warfarin sodium (dextrose vehicle only), 95% ethanol, dexamethasone sodium phosphate, isoxaprin hydrochloride and propantheline bromide have been reported incompatible.

Pharmaceutical precautions Rheomacrodex crystallises occasionally due to swings of temperature causing expansion changes of meniscus level. Seed crystals form on the meniscus line which may grow into full crystals. Storage should therefore be at a constant temperature not exceeding 25°C. If flakes of dextran appear, these can be redissolved by heating for a short time at a low temperature not to exceed 100°C. The solution should then be cooled to 37°C before infusion.

Legal category POM.

Package quantities Infusion bottles of 500 ml.

Further information Nil

Product licence number 0009/5004R.

Product licence holder: Pharmacia Biosystems Ltd, Davy Avenue, Knowlhill, Milton Keynes MK5 8PH.

SALAZOPYRIN* TABLETS, ENEMAS, SUPPOSITORIES AND SUSPENSION

Presentation

Tablets: Yellow, 13.5 mm diameter tablets, tasteless, scored deeply on one side, with a Pharmacia logo on the other side, containing sulphasalazine (USP) 0.5 g. Excipients: Maize starch, PVP, magnesium stearate, colloidal silicon dioxide.

Enema: Soft plastic disposable enema bottles containing sulphasalazine 3 g, vehicle to 100 mls. Excipients: Normal saline, methyl and propyl parabens.

Suppositories: Yellow, odourless, torpedo-shaped containing sulphasalazine 0.5 g. Excipients: PVP, hard fat.

Suspension: Yellow suspension, orange-lemon flavour 250 mg/5 ml in polythene bottle with clic-loc cap. Excipients: Xanthan gum, microcrystalline cellulose, sucrose, orange/lemon flavouring, polysorbate 80, sodium benzoate, water.

Uses Treatment of ulcerative colitis and Crohn's disease.

Dosage and administration
Adults and elderly: The dose is adjusted according to the severity of the disease and the patient's tolerance to the drug, as detailed below.

1. Tablets: Induction and maintenance of remission of ulcerative colitis; treatment of active Crohn's disease.

Severe attack: Salazopyrin 2–4 tablets four times a day may be given in conjunction with steroids as part of an intensive management regime. Rapid passage of the tablets may reduce effect of the drug. Night-time interval between doses should not exceed eight hours.

Mild-moderate attack: 2–4 tablets four times a day may be given in conjunction with steroids.

Maintenance therapy: With induction of remission reduce the dose gradually to 4 tablets per day. This dosage should be continued indefinitely, since discontinuance even several years after an acute attack is associated with a four fold increase in risk of relapse.

2. Enemas: Treatment of ulcerative colitis and Crohn's colitis.

One enema should be given daily, preferably at bedtime.

3. Suppositories: Treatment of ulcerative colitis and Crohn's colitis affecting the rectum.

Two suppositories to be inserted in the morning and two at bedtime after defaecation. After three weeks it may be possible to gradually reduce the dosage as the patient improves.

Adjunct to oral therapy: In severe generalised disease affecting the rectum or rectosigmoid, and in cases slow to respond to oral therapy, one or two suppositories may be given morning and evening in addition.

4. Suspension: Dosage as for tablets, 10 ml being taken instead of each 0.5 g tablet.

Children

1. Tablets: The dose is reduced in proportion to body weight.

Severe attack:	40–60 mg/kg per day
Mild–moderate attack:	40–60 mg/kg per day
Maintenance:	20–30 mg/kg per day

2. Enema: The enema presentation contains an adult dose and is not recommended for children.
3. Suppositories: Reduce the adult dosage on the basis of body weight.
4. Suspension: 5 ml contains 250 mg sulphasalazine. Reduce adult dosage on the basis of body weight.

Severe attack:	0.8–1.2 ml/kg per day
Mild–moderate attack:	0.8–1.2 ml/kg per day
Maintenance therapy:	0.4–0.6 ml/kg per day

Contra-indications, warnings, etc
Contra-indications:

(a) History of sensitivity to sulphonamides or salicylates.
(b) Infants under 2 years of age.
(c) In the case of the Enema, subjects sensitive to methyl or propyl parabens.
(d) In the case of Suspension, subjects sensitive to sodium benzoate.

Precautions: Haematological and hepatic side effects may occur. Differential white cell, red cell and platelet counts should be performed initially and at monthly intervals for the first three months of treatment. Liver function tests should be carried out at monthly intervals for the first three months of treatment.

Patients with allergy, or renal or hepatic disease should be treated with caution. Patients with glucose-6-phosphate dehydrogenase deficiency should be closely observed for signs of haemolytic anaemia (Heinz body anaemia).

The uptake of digoxin and folate may be reduced. An acute attack may be precipitated in patients with porphyria.

Adverse effects: Since sulphasalazine is metabolised to sulphapyridine and 5-amino salicylic acid, side-effects of sulphonamides or salicylates may occur. Patients with slow acetylator status are more likely to experience adverse effects due to sulphapyridine. The most commonly encountered reactions are nausea, headache, rash, loss of appetite and raised temperature.

The following adverse reactions have been reported:

Haematological: Heinz body anaemia, methaemoglobinaemia, hypoprothrombinaemia, haemolytic anaemia, megaloblastic anaemia, thrombocytopenia.

Hypersensitivity reactions: Generalised skin eruptions, Stevens–Johnson syndrome, exfoliative dermatitis, epidermal necrolysis, pruritus, urticaria, photosensitisation, anaphylaxis, serum sickness, drug fever, periorbital oedema, conjunctival and scleral injection, arthralgia, allergic myocarditis, polyarteritis nodosa, LE-phenomenon and lung complications with dyspnoea, fever, cough, eosinophilia, fibrosing alveolitis.

Gastro-intestinal reactions: Stomatitis, parotitis, pancreatitis, hepatitis.

CNS reactions: Vertigo, tinnitus, peripheral neuropathy, ataxia, convulsions, insomnia, mental depression and hallucinations.

Fertility: Oligospermia, reversible on discontinuance of drug.

Renal reactions: Crystalluria, haematuria, proteinuria and nephrotic syndrome.

Overdosage: There is no specific antidote to Salazopyrin.

Pregnancy and lactation: Long term clinical usage and experimental studies have failed to reveal any teratogenic or icteric hazards. The amounts of drug present in the milk should not present a risk to a healthy infant.

Pharmaceutical precautions Store suppositories in a cool place.

Legal category POM.

Package quantities

Tablets:	Bottles of 100 and 500.
Suppositories:	Boxes of 10 and 50.
Enemas:	Boxes of 7 × 100 mls.
Suspension:	Bottles of 473 ml.

Further information The drug may colour the urine orange-yellow.

Extended-wear soft contact lenses (Bausch and Lomb 70) have been reported as being permanently stained during sulphasalazine treatment. Daily-wear soft contact and gas-permeable types should respond to standard cleansing.

When gastro-intestinal intolerance to Salazopyrin tablets occurs, Salazopyrin EN-tabs may be used instead. These film-coated enteric tablets are subject to a separate Data Sheet.

The suspension contains 33 g/100 ml sucrose.

Product licence numbers

Tablets:	0009/5006R
Suppositories:	0009/5008R
Enemas:	0009/0023
Suspension:	0009/0062

Product licence holder: Pharmacia Biosystems Ltd, Davy Avenue, Knowlhill, Milton Keynes MK5 8PH.

SALAZOPYRIN* EN-TABS

Presentation Yellow elliptical convex film coated enteric tablets, containing 0.5 g of sulphasalazine. One side of the tablet has Pharmacia logo on it. Excipients: maize starch, P.V.P., magnesium stearate, enteric coating, colloidal silicon dioxide.

Uses

1. The treatment of Rheumatoid Arthritis which has failed to respond to non-steroidal anti-inflammatory drugs (NSAIDs).
2. Induction and maintenance of remission of Ulcerative Colitis.
3. The treatment of active Crohn's disease.

Dosage and administration

Rheumatoid arthritis

Adults including the elderly: Commence treatment with 0.5 g daily (one tablet) for one week, thereafter increasing the dose by one tablet each week, to a maximum of 3 g/day (six tablets) as in the following table.

	1st Week	*2nd Week*	*3rd Week*	*4th Week*
Morning	—	1 tablet	1 tablet	2 tablets
Evening	1 tablet	1 tablet	2 tablets	2 tablets†

† etc to 3 g/day maximum.

Should a patient experience nausea, the dose should be reduced to a previously tolerated dose for one week and then increased. EN-tabs should not be broken or crushed. Alternatively, the total daily dose may be divided and taken three times or four times daily.

In rheumatoid arthritis Salazopyrin EN-tabs have a 'disease-modifying' action: clinical and haematological response is often seen after one month but may be delayed for up to 12 weeks following the commencement of treatment.

Salazopyrin EN-tabs do not possess analgesic activity, therefore NSAIDs or analgesic treatment should not be reduced or stopped abruptly until clinical response has been achieved.

Patients have been maintained on Salazopyrin EN-tabs for several years.

No recommendations are made for the treatment of children with rheumatoid arthritis.

Ulcerative colitis

Adults:

Severe: 2–4 tablets four times a day given in conjunction with steroids as part of an intensive management regime. The night-time interval between doses should not exceed eight hours. In severe disease rapid passage of the tablets may reduce the effect of the drug.

Mild–moderate: 2–4 tablets four times a day given in conjunction with steroids.

Maintenance: With induction of remission reduce the dose gradually to four tablets per day in divided doses. This dosage should be continued indefinitely, since discontinuance even several years after an acute attack has been shown to be associated with a four fold increase in the risk of relapse.

Salazopyrin EN-tabs should not be broken or crushed.

Children: The dose is reduced in proportion to body weight.

Severe:	40–60 mg/kg per day
Mild–Moderate:	40–60 mg/kg per day
Maintenance:	20–30 mg/kg per day

Crohn's Disease

In active Crohn's disease, Salazopyrin EN-tabs should be administered as for severe ulcerative colitis.

Contra-indications, warnings, etc

Contra-indications:

(a) History of sensitivity to sulphonamides or salicylates.
(b) Infants under 2 years of age.

Precautions: Haematological and hepatic side effects may occur. Differential white cell, red cell and platelet counts should be performed initially and at monthly intervals for the first three months of treatment. Liver function tests should be carried out at monthly intervals for the first three months of treatment.

Patients with allergy, or renal or hepatic disease should be treated with caution. Patients with glucose-6-phosphate dehydrogenase deficiency should be closely observed for signs of haemolytic anaemia (Heinz body anaemia).

The uptake of digoxin and folate may be reduced. An acute attack may be precipitated in patients with porphyria.

Adverse effects: Since sulphasalazine is metabolised to sulphapyridine and 5-amino salicylic acid, effects of sulphonamides or salicylates may occur. Patients with slow acetylator status are more likely to experience adverse effects due to sulphapyridine. The most commonly encountered reactions are nausea, headache, rash, loss of appetite and raised temperature.

The following adverse reactions have been reported:

Haematological: Heinz body anaemia, methaemoglobinaemia, hypoprothrombinaemia, haemolytic anaemia, leucopenia, agranulocytosis, aplastic anaemia, megaloblastic anaemia, thrombocytopenia.

Hypersensitivity reactions: Generalised skin eruptions, Stevens–Johnson syndrome, exfoliative dermatitis, epidermal necrolysis, pruritis, urticaria, photosensitisation, anaphylaxis, serum sickness, drug fever, periorbital oedema, conjunctival and scleral injection, arthralgia, allergic myocarditis, polyarteritis nodosa, LE-phenomenon and lung complications with dyspnoea, fever, cough, eosinophilia, fibrosing alveolitis.

Gastro-intestinal reactions: Stomatitis, parotitis, pancreatitis, hepatitis.

CNS reactions: Vertigo, tinnitus, peripheral neuropathy, ataxia, convulsions, insomnia, mental depression and hallucinations.

Fertility: Oligospermia, reversible on discontinuance of drug.

Renal reactions: Crystalluria, haematuria, proteinuria and nephrotic syndrome.

Overdosage: There is no specific antidote to Salazopyrin EN-tabs.

Pregnancy and lactation: Long term clinical usage and experimental studies have failed to reveal any teratogenic or icteric hazards. The amounts of drug present in the milk should not present a risk to a healthy infant.

Legal category POM.

Package quantities EN-tabs: Containers of 125 (special easily-opened pack for the disabled).

Further information The drug may colour the urine orange-yellow.

Extended-wear soft contact lenses (Bausch and Lomb 70) have been reported as being permanently stained during sulphasalazine treatment. Daily-wear soft contact and gas-permeable types should respond to standard cleansing.

Product licence number 0009/5007R.

Product licence holder: Pharmacia Biosystems Ltd, Davy Avenue, Knowlhill, Milton Keynes MK5 8PH.

SENTIAL E*

Presentation A white emollient oil in water cream containing: Urea BP 4%, Sodium Chloride PhEur 4% in a stabilising base containing cetyl alcohol, macrogol stearate, glycerylmonostearate, TRIS, stearic acid, liquid paraffin, parabens, water.

Uses For the relief of dryness, scaling and itching of the skin associated with conditions such as dry atopic eczema, pruritus senilis and ichthyosis.

Dosage and administration To be applied topically twice daily after washing or bathing. No special recommendations for age groups.

Contra-indications, warnings, etc Raw or very sensitive surfaces may smart on application of the cream. Avoid contact with the eyes.

Pregnancy and lactation: There is no evidence to suggest that the product may not be used.

Pharmaceutical precautions Store at or below room temperature but do not freeze.

Legal category GSL.

Package quantities Plastic tubes of 100 g.

Further information The cream is formulated to increase the concentration of natural water-binding substances in the skin surface, thereby improving the flexibility and softness of the skin.

Product licence number 0009/0064

Product licence holder: Pharmacia Biosystems Ltd, Davy Avenue, Knowlhill, Milton Keynes MK5 8PH.

SENTIAL HC*

Presentation Cream containing 4% urea, 4% sodium chloride, 0.5% hydrocortisone in a stabilising emulsified base containing cetyl alcohol, macrogol stearate, glyceryl monostearate, TRIS, stearic acid, liquid paraffin, sorbic acid, water.

Uses Atopic eczema and other dry eczemas of various genesis.

Dosage and administration Apply a thin layer twice daily to the affected areas.

Elderly and children: No special instructions.

Contra-indications, warnings, etc
Adverse effects: Sential may cause a smarting sensation of short duration when applied to the skin.

Contra-indications: Not to be used in the presence of skin infections unless effective specific therapy for the infection is being given.

Not to be used as a wound treatment.

Avoid contact with the eyes.

Pharmaceutical precautions Store in a cool place but do not freeze.

Legal category POM.

Package quantities Tubes of 30 g.

Further information Formerly called Sential.

Product licence number 0009/0051.

Product licence holder: Pharmacia Biosystems Ltd, Davy Avenue, Knowlhill, Milton Keynes MK5 8PH.

SOLIVITO* N

Presentation A yellow lyophilised mixture of water-soluble vitamins to be added, after reconstitution, to glucose solution or Intralipid for intravenous infusion. One vial of Solivito N corresponds to the following formula:

Thiamine mononitrate (B_1)	3.1 mg
Sodium riboflavine phosphate (B_2)	4.9 mg
Nicotinamide	40 mg
Pyridoxine hydrochloride (B_6)	4.9 mg
Sodium pantothenate	16.5 mg
Biotin	60 micrograms
Folic acid	0.4 mg
Cyanocobalamin (B_{12})	5.0 micrograms
Sodium ascorbate	113 mg
Glycine	300 mg
Sodium edetate	0.5 mg
Methyl hydroxybenzoate	0.5 mg

One vial of Solivito N contains the following quantities of water-soluble vitamins:

Vitamin B_1	3.2 mg
Vitamin B_2	3.6 mg
Nicotinamide	40 mg
Vitamin B_6	4.0 mg
Pantothenic acid	15.0 mg
Biotin	60 micrograms
Folic acid	0.4 mg
Vitamin B_{12}	5.0 micrograms
Vitamin C	100 mg

Uses Solivito N is intended as a supplement in intravenous nutrition in order to cover the daily requirements of the water-soluble vitamins in both adults and infants.

Dosage and administration The daily requirements of the majority of adult patients and children weighing 10 kg or more are met by the contents of one vial.

Children weighing less than 10 kg should receive 1/10 of the contents of one vial per kg bodyweight.

Recommended dosage for adults and children weighing 10 kg or more: The contents of one vial of Solivito N are dissolved by the aseptic addition of 10 ml of one of the following:

(i) Vitlipid N Adult or, for children under 11 years of age, Vitlipid N Infant
(ii) Intralipid 10% or 20%
(iii) Glucose intravenous infusion (5–60%)
(iv) Water for injections

The reconstituted mixtures (i) or (ii) should be aseptically transferred to Intralipid 10% or 20% for infusion. The reconstituted mixtures (iii) and (iv) should be added to either glucose solution (5–60%) or Intralipid 10% or 20%. In this way the basal requirements of the water-soluble vitamins are provided.

Recommended dosage for infants and children weighing under 10 kg: The contents of one vial are dissolved by the aseptic addition of 10 ml of one of the following:

(i) Vitlipid N Infant
(ii) Intralipid 10% or 20%
(iii) Glucose intravenous infusion (5–60%)
(iv) Water for injections

The basal requirements for water-soluble vitamins in children are provided by 1.0 ml of this reconstituted mixture per kg bodyweight.

The reconstituted mixtures (i) and (ii) should be aseptically transferred to Intralipid 10% or 20% for infusion. The reconstituted mixtures (iii) and (iv) should be added to either glucose solution (5–60%) or to Intralipid 10% or 20%.

1 vial of Solivito N should be infused over a minimum period of 2–3 hours in patients with normal renal function so as to minimise renal losses.

Contra-indications, warnings, etc Known hypersensitivity to any of the components, e.g. thiamine (vitamin B_1) or methyl hydroxybenzoate.

Pyridoxine (vitamin B_6) can reduce the effect of levodopa. Some of the optic neuropathies appear to respond to massive doses of hydroxocobalamin and have been claimed to be adversely affected by administration of cyanocobalamin. Folic acid may lower the serum concentration of phenytoin and obscure pernicious anaemia.

Pharmaceutical precautions Store the lyophilised powder before reconstitution below 15°C, protected from light. The addition of Solivito N should be performed aseptically immediately before the start of the infusion and the solution should be used within 24 hours of preparation.

Legal category POM.

Package quantities Boxes of 10 vials.

Further information The manufacturer can be consulted for full information on complete and balanced intravenous nutrition regimens.

Product licence number 0022/0061.

SPRILON*

Presentation An aerosol containing zinc oxide EP 12.5% and dimethicone 350 EP 1.04%. Base to 60 g (wool fat, wool alcohols, ceto stearyl alcohol, dextran, liquid paraffin, white soft paraffin, purified water). Propellant: butane/propane mix 4518.

Uses For prophylaxis and treatment of pressure sores, skin maceration due to faeces or urine, or around fistulae and ileostomies. Protection and treatment of fissures, leg ulcers, moist eczemas. Protection of skin beneath plaster casts.

Dosage and administration Shake can well. Spray surface at right angles from distance of eight inches. Two to three seconds should be sufficient for an area the size of the buttocks.

Elderly: No special instructions.

Contra-indications, warnings, etc *Precautions:* Protect the eyes. Keep out of the reach of children. Do not use on cases allergic to wool fat.

Warning: Do not puncture, incinerate or heat can over 50°C even when empty. Highly flammable.

Pharmaceutical precautions Nil.

Legal category GSL.

Package quantities 115 g.

Further information The spray rapidly forms a white, durable, flexible film which while protecting the skin and assisting healing also allows normal transepidermal water loss.

Product licence number 0009/5002R.

Product licence holder: Pharmacia Biosystems Ltd, Davy Avenue, Knowlhill, Milton Keynes MK5 8PH.

VAMIN* 9

Presentation A clear, colourless to straw-coloured solution of amino acids in the physiological L-form together with electrolytes for intravenous nutrition:

L-Alanine	3.0 g	
L-Arginine	3.3 g	
L-Aspartic acid	4.1 g	
L-Cysteine/cystine	1.4 g	
L-Glutamic acid	9.0 g	
Glycine	2.1 g	
L-Histidine	2.4 g	
L-Isoleucine	3.9 g	
L-Leucine	5.3 g	
L-Lysine	3.9 g	70.2 g
L-Methionine	1.9 g	
L-Phenylalanine	5.5 g	
L-Proline	8.1 g	
L-Serine	7.5 g	
L-Threonine	3.0 g	
L-Tryptophan	1.0 g	
L-Tyrosine	0.5 g	
L-Valine	4.3 g	
Sodium	50 mmol	
Potassium	20 mmol	
Calcium	2.5 mmol	
Magnesium	1.5 mmol	
Chloride	50 mmol	

in each 1,000 ml. pH 5.2. Free from antioxidant additives.

Osmolality: 700 mosmol per kg water.

Nitrogen per litre: 9.4 g corresponding to about 60 g of first-class protein.

Energy content per litre: 250 kcal (1.0 MJ).

Uses Vamin 9 provides a balanced mixture of all essential and non-essential amino acids. Electrolytes are present, but may need supplementing according to patient needs. Vamin 9 is indicated in conditions of protein depletion where sufficient enteral nutrition is impossible or impracticable.

Dosage and administration Electrolyte, fluid, acid-base imbalance and shock should be corrected prior to commencement of intravenous nutrition. In the metabolic and nutritional management of the seriously ill patient, specific preliminary investigations and continuous monitoring are essential, particularly of electrolyte levels. Monitoring of vitamin and trace element levels should be included, especially in patients receiving long-term intravenous nutrition.

To achieve an optimal utilisation of administered amino acids, adequate energy sources, e.g. glucose solutions and fat emulsions (Intralipid) should be provided, together with electrolytes, trace elements (Addamel) and vitamins (Solivito N and Vitlipid N).

Hypertonic preparations such as amino acid solutions and concentrated glucose solutions are commonly infused into a central vein. As with all infusions, care should be taken to avoid complications of catheterisation including air embolism and central venous thrombosis. The risk of serious thoracic complications can be avoided by the use of a peripheral catheter if Vamin 9 is given simultaneously with Intralipid through the same cannula, since the reduced osmolality of the overall mixture may reduce the risk of thrombophlebitis.

Strict asepsis should be maintained especially in the immunosuppressed patient. For safe administration of intravenous fluids from non-collapsible containers, a giving set with an integral airway is recommended.

Recommended dosage for adults: Depending upon patient requirements 0.5–2.0 litres intravenously per 24 hours.

Vamin 9 is administered by slow intravenous infusion at approx. 40–55 drops per minute (2.1–2.8 ml/min) corresponding to an infusion time of six to eight hours per litre. For long-term feeding (i.e. a period of longer than one week) or in short-term feeding if a deficiency of trace elements exists, a trace element solution should be added. Addamel has been specifically designed for this purpose and is compatible with Vamin 9 when used in the recommended proportions.

Recommended dosage for infants: 30 ml per kg body weight in 24 hours to be achieved gradually during first week of administration. (If a supply of trace elements and electrolytes is required, the recommended regimen is Ped-el with Vamin Infant or Vamin 9 Glucose).

Contra-indications, warnings, etc Vamin 9 is contra-indicated in patients with irreversible liver damage and in severe uraemia when dialysis facilities are not available. It should not be given to patients with hyperkalaemia – Vamin 14 Electrolyte-Free and Vamin 18 Electrolyte-Free may be suitable alternatives.

Care must be exercised in the administration of large volume infusion fluids to patients with cardiac insufficiency. Amino acid infusions must also be administered with caution to patients with disturbances in protein metabolism.

Precautions: Hyperkalaemia, hypernatraemia, and acidosis should be corrected prior to commencement of intravenous nutrition. Serum electrolytes, blood glucose levels and acid-base balance should be regularly monitored. Fluid balance should also be monitored since hypertonic dehydration may occur. Amino acid solutions may precipitate acute folate deficiency and folic acid should be given daily.

Vamin 9 should be given with caution to patients with electrolyte retention e.g. impaired renal function and to those with cardiac disease requiring electrolyte restriction or drug therapy e.g. Digitalis. Vamin 14 Electrolyte-Free or Vamin 18 Electrolyte-Free may be suitable in such patients. In particular, potassium replacement therapy should be carefully controlled as plasma potassium levels may not be directly related to tissue levels.

Animal reproduction studies have not been carried out with Vamin 9. There are, however, published reports on the successful and safe infusion of amino acid solutions during pregnancy in the human.

Side-effects: Vamin 9 is well tolerated. In exceptional cases, nausea may occur. As with all hypertonic infusion solutions, thrombophlebitis may occur when peripheral veins are used. The incidence could be reduced by the simultaneous infusion of Intralipid as described above.

Vomiting, flushing and sweating may occur if the recommended rate of infusion is exceeded. Abnormal liver function tests have been observed during intravenous nutrition but all values return to normal on cessation of artificial feeding. Cholestasis has been reported in some patients receiving intravenous nutrition.

Pharmaceutical precautions

1. Store at 5° to 25°C.
2. Do not use if the bottle is leaking or if the solution is cloudy or contains a precipitate.
3. Discard any unused contents.
4. For long-term feeding (i.e. a period of longer than one week) or in short-term feeding if a deficiency of

trace elements exists, a trace element solution should be added. Addamel and Ped-el have been specifically designed for this purpose and are compatible with Vamin 9 when used in the recommended proportions.

Additives may only be added to Vamin 9 where compatibility is known.

Legal category POM.

Package quantities Bottles of 500 ml and 1000 ml.

Further information The manufacturer can be consulted for full information on complete and balanced intravenous nutrition regimens.

Product licence number 0022/0031.

VAMIN* 9 GLUCOSE

Presentation A clear, pale yellow to yellow solution of amino acids in the physiological L-form together with glucose and electrolytes for intravenous nutrition:

L-Alanine	3.0 g	70.2 g
L-Arginine	3.3 g	
L-Aspartic acid	4.1 g	
L-Cysteine/cystine	1.4 g	
L-Glutamic acid	9.0 g	
Glycine	2.1 g	
L-Histidine	2.4 g	
L-Isoleucine	3.9 g	
L-Leucine	5.3 g	
L-Lysine	3.9 g	
L-Methionine	1.9 g	
L-Phenylalanine	5.5 g	
L-Proline	8.1 g	
L-Serine	7.5 g	
L-Threonine	3.0 g	
L-Tryptophan	1.0 g	
L-Tyrosine	0.5 g	
L-Valine	4.3 g	
Glucose anhydrous	100 g	
Sodium	50 mmol	
Potassium	20 mmol	
Calcium	2.5 mmol	
Magnesium	1.5 mmol	
Chloride	50 mmol	

in each 1,000 ml. pH 5.2. Free from antioxidant additives.

Osmolality: 1350 mosmol per kg water.

Nitrogen per litre: 9.4 g corresponding to about 60 g of first-class protein.

Energy content per litre: 650 kcal (2.7 MJ), of which 400 kcal (1.7 MJ) are provided by the glucose.

Uses Vamin 9 Glucose provides a balanced mixture of all essential and non-essential amino acids. Glucose is included to meet part of the carbohydrate requirements. Electrolytes are present, but may need supplementing according to patient needs. Vamin 9 Glucose is indicated in conditions of protein depletion where sufficient enteral nutrition is impossible or impracticable.

Dosage and administration Electrolyte, fluid, acid-base imbalance and shock should be corrected prior to commencement of intravenous nutrition. In the metabolic and nutritional management of the seriously ill patient, specific preliminary investigations and continuous monitoring are essential, particularly of electrolyte levels. Monitoring of vitamin and trace element levels should be included, especially in patients receiving long-term intravenous nutrition.

To achieve an optimal utilisation of administered amino acids, adequate energy sources, e.g. glucose solutions and fat emulsions (Intralipid) should be provided, together with electrolytes, trace elements (Addamel/Additrace) and vitamins (Solivito N and Vitlipid N).

Hypertonic preparations such as amino acid solutions and concentrated glucose solutions are commonly infused into a central vein. As with all infusions, care should be taken to avoid complications of catheterisation including air embolism and central venous thrombosis. The risk of serious thoracic complications can be avoided by the use of a peripheral catheter if Vamin 9 Glucose is given simultaneously with Intralipid through the same cannula, since the reduced osmolality of the overall mixture may reduce the risk of thrombophlebitis.

Strict asepsis should be maintained especially in the immunosuppressed patient. For safe administration of intravenous fluids from non-collapsible containers, a giving set with an integral airway is recommended.

Recommended dosage for adults: Depending upon patient requirements 0.5–2.0 litres intravenously per 24 hours.

Vamin 9 Glucose is administered by slow intravenous infusion at approx. 40–55 drops per minute (2.1–2.8 ml/min) corresponding to an infusion time of six to eight hours per litre.

Recommended dosage for infants: 30 ml per kg body weight in 24 hours to be achieved gradually during first week of administration.

Contra-indications, warnings, etc Vamin 9 Glucose is contra-indicated in patients with irreversible liver damage and in severe uraemia when dialysis facilities are not available. It should not be given to patients with hyperkalaemia – Vamin 14 Electrolyte-Free and Vamin 18 Electrolyte-Free may be suitable alternatives.

Care must be exercised in the administration of large volume infusion fluids to patients with cardiac insufficiency. Amino acid infusions must also be administered with caution to patients with disturbances in protein metabolism.

Precautions: Hyperkalaemia, hypernatraemia, and acidosis should be corrected prior to commencement of intravenous nutrition. Serum electrolytes, blood glucose levels and acid-base balance should be regularly monitored. Fluid balance should also be monitored since hypertonic dehydration may occur. Amino acid solutions may precipitate acute folate deficiency and folic acid should be given daily.

Vamin 9 Glucose should be given with caution to patients with electrolyte retention e.g. impaired renal function and to those with cardiac disease requiring electrolyte restriction or drug therapy e.g. Digitalis. Vamin 14 Electrolyte-Free or Vamin 18 Electrolyte-Free may be suitable in such patients. In particular, potassium replacement therapy should be carefully controlled as plasma potassium levels may not be directly related to tissue levels.

Animal reproduction studies have not been carried out with Vamin 9 Glucose. There are, however, published reports on the successful and safe infusion of amino acid solutions during pregnancy in the human.

Side-effects: Vamin 9 Glucose is well tolerated. In exceptional cases, nausea may occur. As with all hypertonic infusion solutions, thrombophlebitis may occur when peripheral veins are used. The incidence could be reduced by the simultaneous infusion of Intralipid as described above.

Vomiting, flushing and sweating may occur if the recommended rate of infusion is exceeded. Abnormal liver function tests have been observed during intravenous nutrition but all values return to normal on cessation of artificial feeding. Cholestasis has been reported in some patients receiving intravenous nutrition.

Pharmaceutical precautions

1. Store at 5° to 25°C.
2. Do not use if the bottle is leaking or if the solution is cloudy or contains a precipitate.
3. Discard any unused contents.
4. Additives may only be added to Vamin 9 Glucose where compatibility is known.

Legal category POM.

Package quantities Bottles of 100 ml, 500 ml and 1,000 ml.

Further information The manufacturer can be consulted for full information on complete and balanced intravenous nutrition regimens.

Product licence number 0022/0030.

VAMIN* 14

Presentation A clear, colourless to slightly yellow solution of amino acids in the physiological L-form with electrolytes, for intravenous nutrition:

L-Alanine	12.0 g	
L-Arginine	8.4 g	
L-Aspartic acid	2.5 g	
L-Cysteine/cystine	420 mg	
L-Glutamic acid	4.2 g	
Glycine	5.9 g	
L-Histidine	5.1 g	
L-Isoleucine	4.2 g	
L-Leucine	5.9 g	85 g
L-Lysine	6.8 g	
L-Methionine	4.2 g	
L-Phenylalanine	5.9 g	
L-Proline	5.1 g	
L-Serine	3.4 g	
L-Threonine	4.2 g	
L-Tryptophan	1.4 g	
L-Tyrosine	170 mg	
L-Valine	5.5 g	
Sodium	100 mmol	
Potassium	50 mmol	
Calcium	5 mmol	
Magnesium	8 mmol	
Chloride	100 mmol	
Sulphate	8 mmol	
Acetate	135 mmol	

in each 1,000 ml. pH 5.6. Free from antioxidant additives.

Osmolality: 1145 mosmol per kg water.

Nitrogen per litre: 13.5 g corresponding to about 84 g of protein.

Energy content per litre: 350 kcal (1.4 MJ).

Uses Vamin 14 provides a concentrated and balanced mixture of all essential and non-essential amino acids. Electrolytes are present, but may need supplementing according to patient needs. See under Dosage and administration for information on compatibility. Vamin 14 is indicated for the prophylaxis or therapeutic treatment of protein depletion, where sufficient enteral nutrition is impossible or impracticable. It is particularly suited to meet moderately increased requirements for nitrogen in patients in whom fluid intake is a limiting factor.

Dosage and administration Electrolyte, fluid, acid-base imbalance and shock should be corrected prior to commencement of intravenous nutrition. In the metabolic and nutritional management of the seriously ill patient specific preliminary investigations and continuous monitoring are essential, particularly of electrolyte levels. Monitoring of vitamin and trace element levels should be included, especially in patients receiving long-term intravenous nutrition.

To achieve an optimal utilisation of administered amino acids, adequate energy sources, e.g. glucose solutions and fat emulsions (Intralipid) should be provided, together with electrolytes, trace elements (Addamel/Additrace) and vitamins (Solivito N and Vitlipid N Adult).

Hypertonic preparations such as amino acid solutions and concentrated glucose solutions are commonly infused into a central vein. As with all infusions, care should be taken to avoid complications of catheterisation including air embolism and central venous thrombosis. The risk of serious thoracic complications can be avoided by the use of a peripheral catheter if Vamin 14 is given simultaneously with Intralipid through the same cannula, since the reduced osmolality of the overall mixture may reduce the risk of thrombophlebitis.

Strict asepsis should be maintained especially in the immuno-suppressed patient. For safe administration of intravenous fluids from non-collapsible containers, a giving set with an integral airway is recommended.

Recommended dosage for adults: Depending upon patient requirements, up to 1 litre intravenously per 24 hours. In severe catabolism, Vamin 18 Electrolyte-Free may be used. Vamin 14 is administered by slow intravenous infusion at a rate not exceeding 2 ml per minute corresponding to approximately 40 drops per minute or to an infusion time of at least 8 hours per litre.

Infant dosage: Can be administered at the physician's discretion. An amino acid solution containing larger amounts of cysteine/cystine and tyrosine may be considered more appropriate in infants.

Contra-indications, warnings, etc Vamin 14 is contra-indicated in patients with irreversible liver damage and in severe uraemia when dialysis facilities are not available. It should not be given to patients with hyperkalaemia – Vamin 14 Electrolyte-Free is a suitable alternative.

Care must be exercised in the administration of large volume infusion fluids to patients with cardiac insufficiency. Amino acid infusions must also be administered with caution to patients with disturbances in protein metabolism.

Precautions: Hyperkalaemia, hypernatraemia, and acidosis should be corrected prior to commencement of intravenous nutrition. Serum electrolytes, blood glucose levels and acid-base balance should be regularly monitored. Fluid balance should also be monitored since hypertonic dehydration may occur. Amino acid solutions may precipitate acute folate deficiency and folic acid should be given daily.

Vamin 14 should be given with caution to patients with electrolyte retention, e.g. impaired renal function and to those with cardiac disease requiring electrolyte restriction or drug therapy, e.g. Digitalis. Vamin 14 Electrolyte-Free is recommended in such patients. In particular, potassium replacement therapy should be carefully controlled as plasma potassium levels may not be directly related to tissue levels.

Animal reproduction studies have not been carried out with Vamin 14. There are, however, published reports on the successful and safe infusion of amino acid solutions during pregnancy in the human.

Side-effects: Vamin 14 is well tolerated. Rarely, nausea may occur. As with all hypertonic infusion solutions, thrombophlebitis may occur when peripheral veins are used. The incidence could be reduced by the simultaneous infusion of Intralipid as described above. Vomiting, flushing and sweating may occur if the recommended rate of infusion is exceeded. Abnormal liver function tests have been observed during intravenous nutrition but all values return to normal on cessation of artificial feeding. Cholestasis has been reported in some patients receiving intravenous nutrition.

Pharmaceutical precautions

1. Store at 5–25°C.
2. Do not use if the bottle is leaking or if the solution is cloudy or contains a precipitate.
3. Discard any unused contents.
4. Vamin 14 contains electrolytes, but additional electrolytes and trace elements may be required according to patient needs. Up to 20 ml Addamel/Additrace can be added to one litre Vamin 14 without risk of precipitation. Phosphate may be added to one litre Vamin 14 as up to 40 ml Addiphos (containing 80 mmol phosphate, 60 mmol Na^+ and 60 mmol K^+) provided Addamel/Additrace is not present. All additions should be performed aseptically immediately before the start of the infusion and should be used within 24 hours unless the mixture is refrigerated when it may be used within 48 hours of preparation.

Additives may only be added to Vamin 14 where compatibility is known.

Legal category POM.

Package quantities Bottles of 500 ml and 1000 ml.

Further information The manufacturer can be consulted for full information on complete and balanced intravenous nutrition regimens.

Product licence number 0022/0053.

VAMIN* 14 ELECTROLYTE-FREE

Presentation A clear, colourless to slightly yellow solution of amino acids in the physiological L-form for intravenous nutrition:

L-Alanine	12.0 g	85 g
L-Arginine	8.4 g	
L-Aspartic acid	2.5 g	
L-Cysteine/cystine	420 mg	
L-Glutamic acid	4.2 g	
Glycine	5.9 g	
L-Histidine	5.1 g	
L-Isoleucine	4.2 g	
L-Leucine	5.9 g	
L-Lysine	6.8 g	
L-Methionine	4.2 g	
L-Phenylalanine	5.9 g	
L-Proline	5.1 g	
L-Serine	3.4 g	
L-Threonine	4.2 g	
L-Tryptophan	1.4 g	
L-Tyrosine	170 mg	
L-Valine	5.5 g	

in each 1,000 ml. pH 5.6. Free from antioxidant additives.

Osmolality: 810 mosmol per kg water.

Nitrogen per litre: 13.5 g corresponding to about 84 g of protein.

Energy content per litre: 350 kcal (1.4 MJ).

Uses Vamin 14 Electrolyte-Free provides a concentrated and balanced mixture of all essential and non-essential amino acids. It is free from chlorides and other inorganic electrolytes, and electrolyte requirements can therefore be met by the addition of individually adjusted doses. See under Dosage and administration for information on compatibility. Vamin 14 Electrolyte-Free is indicated for the prophylaxis or therapeutic treatment of protein depletion, where sufficient enteral nutrition is impossible or impracticable. It is particularly suited to meet moderately increased requirements for nitrogen in patients in whom fluid intake is a limiting factor.

Dosage and administration Electrolyte, fluid, acid-base imbalance and shock should be corrected prior to commencement of intravenous nutrition. In the metabolic and nutritional management of the seriously ill patient, specific preliminary investigations and continuous monitoring are essential, particularly of electrolyte levels. Monitoring of vitamin and trace element levels should be included, especially in patients receiving long-term intravenous nutrition.

To achieve an optimal utilisation of administered amino acids, adequate energy sources, e.g. glucose solutions and fat emulsions (Intralipid) should be provided, together with electrolytes, trace elements (Addamel/Additrace) and vitamins (Solivito N and Vitlipid N Adult).

Hypertonic preparations such as amino acid solutions and concentrated glucose solutions are commonly infused into a central vein. As with all infusions, care should be taken to avoid complications of catheterisation including air embolism and central venous thrombosis. The risk of serious thoracic complications can be avoided by the use of a peripheral catheter if Vamin 14 Electrolyte-Free is given simultaneously with Intralipid through the same cannula, since the reduced osmolality of the overall mixture may reduce the risk of thrombophlebitis.

Strict asepsis should be maintained especially in the immunosuppressed patient. For safe administration of intravenous fluids from non-collapsible containers, a giving set with an integral airway is recommended.

Recommended dosage for adults: Depending upon patient requirements, up to 1 litre intravenously per 24 hours. In severe catabolism, Vamin 18 Electrolyte-Free may be used. Vamin 14 Electrolyte-Free is administered by slow intravenous infusion at a rate not exceeding 2 ml per minute corresponding to approximately 40 drops per minute or an infusion time of at least 8 hours per litre.

Recommended dosage for infants: Can be administered at the physician's discretion. An amino acid solution containing larger amounts of cysteine/cystine and tyrosine may be considered more appropriate in infants.

Contra-indications, warnings, etc Vamin 14 Electrolyte-Free is contra-indicated in patients with irreversible liver damage and in severe uraemia when dialysis facilities are not available.

Care must be exercised in the administration of large volume infusion fluids to patients with cardiac insufficiency. Amino acid infusions must also be administered with caution to patients with disturbances in protein metabolism.

Precautions: Hyperkalaemia, hypernatraemia and acidosis should be corrected prior to commencement of intravenous nutrition. Serum electrolytes, blood glucose levels and acid-base balance should be regularly monitored. Fluid balance should also be monitored since hypertonic dehydration may occur. Amino acid solutions may precipitate acute folate deficiency and folic acid should be given daily.

Animal reproduction studies have not been carried out with Vamin 14 Electrolyte-Free. There are, however, published reports on the successful and safe infusion of amino acid solutions during pregnancy in the human.

Side-effects: Vamin 14 Electrolyte-Free is well tolerated. Rarely, nausea may occur. As with all hypertonic infusion solutions, thrombophlebitis may occur when peripheral veins are used. The incidence could be reduced by the simultaneous infusion of Intralipid as described above. Vomiting, flushing and sweating may occur if the recommended rate of infusion is exceeded. Abnormal liver function tests have been observed during intravenous nutrition but all values return to normal on cessation of artificial feeding. Cholestasis has been reported in some patients receiving intravenous nutrition.

Pharmaceutical precautions

1. Store at 5–25°C.
2. Do not use if the bottle is leaking or if the solution is cloudy or contains a precipitate.
3. Discard any unused contents.
4. Vamin 14 Electrolyte-Free contains no electrolytes. Electrolyte and trace element requirements can be met by the addition of individually adjusted doses. Laboratory studies have shown that the maximum levels of electrolytes which are compatible with 1 litre of Vamin 14 Electrolyte-Free are as follows: 20 ml Addamel/Additrace, 480 mmol Na^+(as NaCl), 480 mmol K^+ (as KCl), 24 mmol Ca^{2+}(as calcium glubionate) and 48 mmol Mg^{2+} (as $MgSO_4$) which can be added either singly or in any combination. Phosphate may be added to 1 litre Vamin 14 Electrolyte-Free as up to 60 ml Addiphos (containing 120 mmol phosphate, 90 mmol Na^+ and 90 mmol K^+) with or without addition of up to 480 mmol Na^+ and 480 mmol K^+ as chlorides and 48 mmol Mg^{2+} as sulphate, provided Addamel/Additrace is not present. All additions should be performed aseptically immediately before the start of the infusion and should be used within 24 hours unless the mixture is refrigerated when it may be used within 48 hours of preparation.

Additives may only be added to Vamin 14 Electrolyte-Free where compatibility is known.

Legal category POM.

Package quantities Bottles of 500 ml and 1000 ml.

Further information The manufacturer can be consulted for full information on complete and balanced intravenous nutrition regimens.

Product licence number 0022/0052.

VAMIN* 18 ELECTROLYTE-FREE

Presentation A clear, colourless to slightly yellow solution of amino acids in the physiological L-form for intravenous nutrition:

L-Alanine	16.0 g	
L-Arginine	11.3 g	
L-Aspartic acid	3.4 g	
L-Cysteine/cystine	560 mg	
L-Glutamic acid	5.6 g	
Glycine	7.9 g	
L-Histidine	6.8 g	
L-Isoleucine	5.6 g	
L-Leucine	7.9 g	
L-Lysine	9.0 g	114 g
L-Methionine	5.6 g	
L-Phenylalanine	7.9 g	
L-Proline	6.8 g	
L-Serine	4.5 g	
L-Threonine	5.6 g	
L-Tryptophan	1.9 g	
L-Tyrosine	230 mg	
L-Valine	7.3 g	

in each 1,000ml. pH 5.6. Free from antioxidant additives.

Osmolality: 1130 mosmol per kg water.

Nitrogen per litre: 18.0 g corresponding to 112 g of protein.

Energy content per litre: 460 kcal (1.9 MJ).

Uses Vamin 18 Electrolyte-Free provides a concentrated and balanced mixture of all essential and non-essential amino acids. It is free from chlorides and other inorganic electrolytes, and electrolyte requirements can therefore be met by the addition of individually adjusted doses. See under Dosage and administration for information on compatibility.

Vamin 18 Electrolyte-Free is indicated for the prophylaxis or therapeutic treatment of protein depletion, where sufficient enteral nutrition is impossible or impracticable. It is particularly suited to meet increased requirements for nitrogen in patients in whom fluid intake is a limiting factor.

Dosage and administration Electrolyte, fluid, acid-base imbalance and shock should be corrected prior to commencement of intravenous nutrition. In the metabolic and nutritional management of the seriously ill patient, specific preliminary investigations and continuous monitoring are essential, particularly of electrolyte levels. Monitoring of vitamin and trace element levels should be included, especially in patients receiving long-term intravenous nutrition.

To achieve an optimal utilisation of administered amino acids, adequate energy sources, e.g. glucose solutions and fat emulsions (Intralipid) should be provided, together with electrolytes, trace elements (Additrace) and vitamins (Solivito N and Vitlipid N Adult).

Hypertonic preparations such as amino acid solutions and concentrated glucose solutions are commonly infused into a central vein. As with all infusions, care should be taken to avoid complications of catheterisation including air embolism and central venous thrombosis. The risk of serious thoracic complications can be avoided by the use of a peripheral catheter if Vamin 18 Electrolyte-Free is given simultaneously with Intralipid through the same cannula, since the reduced osmolality of the overall mixture may reduce the risk of thrombophlebitis.

Strict asepsis should be maintained especially in the immunosuppressed patient. For safe administration of intravenous fluids from non-collapsible containers, a giving set with an integral airway is recommended.

Recommended dosage for adults: Depending upon patient requirements, up to 1 litre intravenously per 24 hours. Vamin 18 Electrolyte-Free is administered by slow intravenous infusion at a rate not exceeding 2 ml per minute corresponding to approximately 40 drops per minute or an infusion time of at least 8 hours per litre.

Recommended dosage for infants: Can be administered at the physician's discretion. An amino acid solution containing larger amounts of cysteine/cystine and tyrosine may be considered more appropriate in infants.

Contra-indications, warnings, etc Vamin 18 Electrolyte-Free is contra-indicated in patients with irreversible liver damage and in severe uraemia when dialysis facilities are not available.

Care must be exercised in the administration of large volume infusion fluids to patients with cardiac insufficiency. Amino acid infusions must also be administered with caution to patients with disturbances in protein metabolism.

Precautions: Hyperkalaemia, hypernatraemia and acidosis should be corrected prior to commencement of intravenous nutrition. Serum electrolytes, blood glucose levels and acid-base balance should be regularly monitored. Fluid balance should also be monitored since hypertonic dehydration may occur. Amino acid solutions may precipitate acute folate deficiency and folic acid should be given daily.

Animal reproduction studies have not been carried out with Vamin 18 Electrolyte-Free. There are, however, published reports on the successful and safe infusion of amino acid solutions during pregnancy in the human.

Side-effects: Vamin 18 Electrolyte-Free is well tolerated. Rarely, nausea may occur. As with all hypertonic infusion solutions, thrombophlebitis may occur when peripheral veins are used. The incidence could be reduced by the simultaneous infusion of Intralipid as described above. Vomiting, flushing and sweating may occur if the recommended rate of infusion is exceeded. Abnormal liver function tests have been observed during intravenous nutrition but all values return to normal on cessation of artificial feeding. Cholestasis has been reported in some patients receiving intravenous nutrition.

Pharmaceutical precautions

1. Store at 5–25°C.
2. Do not use if the bottle is leaking or if the solution is cloudy or contains a precipitate.
3. Discard any unused contents.
4. Vamin 18 Electrolyte-Free contains no electrolytes. Electrolyte requirements can be met by the addition of individually adjusted doses. Laboratory studies have shown that the maximum levels of electrolytes which are compatible with 1 litre of Vamin 18 Electrolyte-Free are as follows: 20 ml Additrace, 480 mmol Na^+ (as NaCl), 480 mmol K^+ (as KCl), 24 mmol Ca^{2+} (as calcium glubionate) and 48 mmol Mg^{2+} (as $MgSO_4$) which can be added either singly or in any combination. Phosphate may be added to 1 litre Vamin 18 Electrolyte-Free as up to 60 ml Addiphos (containing 120 mmol phosphate, 90 mmol Na^+ and 90 mmol K^+) with or without addition of up to 480 mmol Na^+, and 480 mmol K^+ as chlorides and 48 mmol Mg^{2+} as sulphate providing Additrace is not present. Addamel should not be added to Vamin 18 Electrolyte-Free. All additions should be performed aseptically immediately before the start of the infusion and should be used within 24 hours unless the mixture is refrigerated when it may be used within 48 hours of preparation.

Additives may only be added to Vamin 18 Electrolyte-Free where compatibility is known.

Legal category POM.

Package quantities Bottles of 500 ml and 1000 ml.

Further information The manufacturer can be consulted for full information on complete and balanced intravenous nutrition regimens.

Product licence number 0022/0054.

VAMIN* INFANT

Presentation A clear, colourless to slightly yellow solution of amino acids in the physiological L-form for intravenous nutrition, specifically formulated for paediatric use.

L-Alanine	6.3 g	
L-Arginine	4.1 g	
L-Aspartic acid	4.1 g	
L-Cysteine/cystine	1.0 g	
L-Glutamic acid	7.1 g	
Glycine	2.1 g	
L-Histidine	2.1 g	
L-Isoleucine	3.1 g	
L-Leucine	7.0 g	65 g
L-Lysine	5.6 g	
L-Methionine	1.3 g	
L-Phenylalanine	2.7 g	
L-Proline	5.6 g	
L-Serine	3.8 g	
L-Threonine	3.6 g	
L-Tryptophan	1.4 g	
L-Tyrosine	0.5 g	
L-Valine	3.6 g	

in each 1000 ml. pH 5.2. Free from antioxidant additives.

Osmolality: 535 mosmol per kg water.

Nitrogen per litre: 9.3 g corresponding to 58 g of protein.

Energy content per litre: 240 kcal (1.0 MJ).

Uses Vamin Infant provides a balanced mixture of all essential and non-essential amino acids, with a profile similar to that of breast milk protein. This profile includes cysteine and tyrosine which seem to be essential for premature neonates. (The synthesis of cysteine from methionine also seems to be limited in adults when amino acid solutions free of cysteine are infused). Vamin Infant is indicated for the prophylaxis and therapeutic treatment of protein depletion in neonates and infants, where sufficient enteral nutrition is impossible or impracticable. It is free from chlorides and other inorganic electrolytes so as to allow administration in a dosage adjusted to the individual needs of the patient. (See under 'Pharmaceutical Precautions' for information on compatibility.)

Dosage and administration Electrolyte, fluid, acid-base imbalance and shock should be corrected prior to commencement of intravenous nutrition. In the metabolic and nutritional management of the seriously ill patient specific preliminary investigations and continuous monitoring are essential, particularly of electrolyte levels. Monitoring of vitamin and trace element levels should be included, especially in patients receiving long-term intravenous nutrition.

To achieve an optimal utilisation of administered amino acids, adequate energy sources, e.g. glucose solutions and fat emulsions (Intralipid) should be provided, together with electrolytes, trace elements (Ped-el or Addamel) and vitamins (Solivito N and Vitlipid N Infant or Vitlipid N Adult).

Hypertonic preparations such as amino acid solutions and concentrated glucose solutions are commonly infused into a central vein. Vamin Infant may also be infused into a peripheral vein when given simultaneously with Intralipid through the same cannula, since the reduced osmolality of the overall mixture may reduce the risk of thrombophlebitis.

As with all infusions, care should be taken to avoid complications of catheterisation including air embolism and central venous thrombosis. Strict asepsis should be maintained especially in the immuno-suppressed patient. For safe administration of intravenous fluids from non-collapsible containers, a giving set with an integral airway is recommended.

Recommended dosage for infants: The full dosage should be increased gradually during the first week of administration to a final daily dose of 30–35 ml Vamin Infant per kg body weight given as a continuous infusion over 24 hours using a suitable pump.

Recommended dosage for children: The full dosage should be increased gradually during the first week of administration to the final dose ranges indicated below and should be infused over 24 hours:

Weight (kg)	*Dosage (ml per kg body weight per 24 hours)*
10–20	18.5–24.0
20–30	16.0–18.5
30–40	14.5–16.0
>40	See adults

Recommended dosage for adults: Depending upon patient requirements, 0.5–2.0 litres by slow intravenous infusion per 24 hours or 0.8–1.6 g amino acids per kg body weight per day. The infusion should be at a rate of 2.0–2.8 ml per minute or approximately 40–55 drops per minute. This corresponds to an infusion time of between six to eight hours per litre.

Caution: The recommended infusion rate should not be exceeded.

Contra-indications, warnings, etc Vamin Infant is contra-indicated in patients with irreversible liver damage and in severe uraemia when dialysis facilities are not available.

Care must be exercised in the administration of large volume infusion fluids to patients with cardiac insufficiency. Amino acid infusions must also be administered with caution to patients with disturbances in protein metabolism.

Precautions: Hyperkalaemia, hypernatraemia and acidosis should be corrected prior to commencement of intravenous nutrition. Serum electrolytes, blood glucose levels and acid-base balance should be regularly monitored. Fluid balance should also be monitored since hypertonic dehydration may occur. Amino acid solutions may precipitate acute folate deficiency and folic acid should be given daily.

Side-effects: Vamin Infant is well tolerated. Rarely, nausea may occur. As with all hypertonic solutions, thrombophlebitis may occur when peripheral veins are used. The incidence could be reduced by the simultaneous infusion of Intralipid as described above. Abnormal liver function tests have been observed during intravenous nutrition but all values return to normal on cessation of artificial feeding. Cholestasis has been reported in some patients receiving intravenous nutrition.

Pharmaceutical precautions

1. Store at 5 to 25°C.
2. Do not use if the bottle is leaking or if the solution is cloudy or contains a precipitate.
3. Discard any unused contents.
4. Vamin Infant contains no electrolytes.

Electrolyte requirements should be individually assessed. Laboratory studies have shown the following electrolytes may be mixed with 500 ml Vamin Infant either singly or in any combination: up to 200 mmol Na^+ (as NaCl) up to 160 mmol K^+ (as KCl), up to 20 mmol Ca^{2+} (as $CaCl_2$ or calcium glubionate) and up to 9 mmol Mg^{2+} (as $MgCl_2$ or $MgSO_4$) together with either 66.7 ml Ped-el for infants or 5 ml Addamel for adults.

All additions should be performed aseptically immediately prior to infusion, and should be used within 24 hours. Additives may only be added to Vamin Infant where compatibility is known.

Legal category POM.

Package quantities Bottles of 100 ml and 500 ml.

Further information The manufacturer can be consulted for full information on complete and balanced intravenous nutrition regimens.

Product licence number 0022/0055.

VITLIPID* N ADULT

Presentation A white, oil in water emulsion containing the fat soluble vitamins A, D_2, E and K_1, in the oil phase of the emulsion with a composition corresponding to that of Intralipid 10%. Vitlipid N Adult is intended for addition to Intralipid 10% or 20% and for use in adults and children over 11 years of age receiving intravenous nutrition. One ampoule of Vitlipid N Adult contains:

Retinol palmitate corresponding to retinol	990 micrograms (3,300 i.u.)
Ergocalciferol	5 micrograms (200 i.u.)
dl-alpha-tocopherol	9.1 mg (10 i.u.)
Phytomenadione	150 micrograms
Fractionated soybean oil	1 g
Fractionated egg phospholipids	120 mg
Glycerol	225 mg
Water for injections to 10 ml	

Uses Vitlipid N Adult is indicated as a supplement to Intralipid 10% or 20% in intravenous nutrition of adults and older children in order to cover the daily requirements of the fat soluble vitamins A, D_2, E and K_1.

Dosage and administration *Recommended dosage for adults and children over 11 years of age:* One ampoule (10 ml) of Vitlipid N Adult is added to 500 ml of Intralipid 10% or 20%. After gentle shaking, the emulsion is infused as described for Intralipid. The daily maintenance dosages of the vitamins A, D_2, E and K_1 are thereby supplied.

Recommended dosage for infants and younger children: For patients under 11 years of age the preparation Vitlipid N Infant should be used.

Contra-indications, warnings, etc Should not be given undiluted. Vitlipid N Adult contains vitamin K_1 which may interact with anticoagulants of the coumarin type.

Pharmaceutical precautions Store at 2 to 8°C protected from light. The addition of Vitlipid N Adult should be performed aseptically immediately before the start of infusion and should be used within 24 hours.

Legal category POM.

Package quantities Boxes of 10 × 10 ml ampoules.

Further information Vitlipid N Adult is specially formulated for addition to Intralipid 10% or 20%. It may be used for the reconstitution of Solivito N before addition to Intralipid (see Solivito N data sheet for details).

The manufacturer can be consulted for full information on complete and balanced intravenous nutrition regimens.

Product licence number 0022/0062.

VITLIPID* N INFANT

Presentation A white, oil in water emulsion containing the fat soluble vitamins A, D_2, E and K_1, in the oil phase of the emulsion with a composition corresponding to that of Intralipid 10%. Vitlipid N Infant is intended for addition to Intralipid 10% or 20% and for use in infants and children receiving intravenous nutrition. One ml contains:

Retinol palmitate corresponding to retinol	69 micrograms (230 i.u.)
Ergocalciferol	1.0 micrograms (40 i.u.)
dl-alpha-tocopherol	0.64 mg (0.7 i.u.)
Phytomenadione	20 micrograms
Fractionated soybean oil	100 mg
Fractionated egg phospholipids	12 mg
Glycerol	22.5 mg
Water for injections to 1 ml	

Uses Vitlipid N Infant is indicated as a supplement to Intralipid 10% or 20% in intravenous nutrition of infants and children under 11 years of age in order to cover the daily requirements of the fat soluble vitamins A, D_2, E and K_1.

Dosage and administration *Recommended dosage for infants and children under 11 years of age:* Vitlipid N Infant in a dosage of 1 ml per kg bodyweight per day is added to Intralipid 10% or 20%. The daily dosage must not exceed 10 ml. After gentle shaking the emulsion is infused as stated for Intralipid.

Recommended dosage for adults and older children: The preparation Vitlipid N Adult is recommended for use in patients 11 years of age and older.

Contra-indications, warnings, etc Should not be given undiluted. Vitlipid N Infant contains vitamin K_1 which may interact with anticoagulants of the coumarin type.

Pharmaceutical precautions Store at 2 to 8°C protected from light. The addition of Vitlipid N Infant should be performed aseptically immediately before the start of the infusion and should be used within 24 hours.

Legal category POM.

Package quantities Boxes of 10 × 10 ml ampoules.

Further information Vitlipid N Infant is specially formulated for addition to either Intralipid 10% or 20%. It may be used for the reconstitution of Solivito N before addition to Intralipid (see Solivito N data sheet for details).

The manufacturer can be consulted for full information on complete and balanced intravenous nutrition regimens.

Product licence number 0022/0063.

VITRIMIX KV*

Presentation A combination pack containing a 250 ml bottle of Intralipid® 20% and a 1000 ml bottle partially filled with 750 ml of Vamin 9 Glucose which, when aseptically mixed via the transfer set provided, produces an intravenous nutrition mixture suitable for infusion via a peripheral or central vein.

The mixture contains:

L-Alanine	2.2 g
L-Arginine	2.5 g
L-Aspartic acid	3.1 g
L. Cysteine/cystine	1.0 g
L-Glutamic acid	6.8 g
Glycine	1.6 g
L-Histidine	1.8 g
L-Isoleucine	2.9 g
L-Leucine	4.0 g
L-Lysine	2.9 g
L-Methionine	1.4 g
L-Phenylalanine	4.1 g
L-Proline	6.1 g
L-Serine	5.6 g
L-Threonine	2.2 g
L-Tryptophan	0.75 g
L-Tyrosine	0.38 g
L-Valine	3.2 g
Glucose anhydrous	75 g
Fractionated soybean oil	50 g
Fractionated egg phospholipids	3.0 g
Glycerol	5.6 g
Sodium	38 mmol
Potassium	15 mmol
Calcium	1.9 mmol
Magnesium	1.1 mmol
Chloride	38 mmol

in each 1000 ml. pH 5.2. Free from antioxidant additives.

Osmolality: 1130 mosmol per kg. water.

Nitrogen per litre: 7.0 g corresponding to about 45 g of protein.

Energy content per litre: approximately 1000 kcal (4.18 MJ) of which 800 kcal (3.34 MJ) is provided as non-protein energy. Glucose provides 300 kcal (1.25 MJ) and Intralipid provides 500 kcal (2.09 MJ).

Uses The use of Vitrimix KV is indicated in conditions where sufficient enteral nutrition is impossible or impracticable and is likely to remain so for a short period of time. Vitrimix KV provides a balanced mixture of essential and non-essential amino acids together with energy in the form of Intralipid (62% of non-protein energy) and glucose (38% of non-protein energy). Electrolytes are present but may need supplementing according to patient needs, as will fluid. Electrolytes should not be added directly to the Vitrimix KV bottle but may be added to any additional fluid that is given.

Note: For conditions requiring intravenous nutrition as the sole source of nutrition for a longer period, complete intravenous nutrition including trace elements and vitamins will be more appropriate.

Dosage and administration Electrolyte, fluid, acid-base imbalance and shock should be corrected prior to commencement of intravenous nutrition. Vitrimix KV can be infused via a peripheral vein with reduced risk of thrombophlebitis. As with all infusions, strict asepsis should be maintained and care should be taken to avoid complications of catheterisation including air embolism and central venous thrombosis. For safe administration of intravenous fluids from non-collapsible containers, use of a giving set with an integral airway is recommended.

Recommended dosage for adults: 1–2 litres Vitrimix KV per 24 hours administered by slow intravenous infusion via either a peripheral or central vein at a rate of approximately 60 drops per minute (2.8 ml/min), corresponding to an infusion time of at least six hours per litre. Fluid intake may be supplemented by separate infusions; additional electrolytes and intravenous drugs may be given in these solutions if required.

Recommended dosage for infants: Not recommended.

Contra-indications, warnings, etc Vitrimix KV is a mixture of Vamin 9 Glucose and Intralipid 20%. The precautions which should be observed in its use are therefore similar to those required when these two preparations are simultaneously infused from individual containers, with the exception of considerations relevant to long term total parenteral nutrition (such as folate deficiency) which are not likely to be complicating factors in the short term use of Vitrimix.

Contra-indications: Vitrimix KV is contra-indicated in patients with severe or irreversible liver damage, acute shock or other severe disorders of fat metabolism, or severe uraemia, when dialysis facilities are not available.

Precautions: Hyperkalaemia, hypernatraemia and acidosis should be corrected prior to commencement of intravenous nutrition. Serum electrolytes, blood glucose levels and acid-base balance should be regularly monitored, as should fluid balance. In patients with electrolyte retention, e.g. impaired renal function, and to those with cardiac disease requiring electrolyte restriction or drug therapy, e.g. digitalis, alternative regimens incorporating electrolyte-free amino acid solutions may be more suitable.

Fat metabolism may be disturbed in conditions such as renal insufficiency, uncompensated diabetes, certain forms of hepatic insufficiency, metabolic disorders and sepsis. If intravenous administration of fat is considered in patients with these disorders, the elimination of fat should be checked daily. Care must be exercised in the administration of large volume infusion fluids to patients with cardiac insufficiency. Amino acid-containing infusions must also be administered with caution to patients with disturbances in protein metabolism.

Animal reproduction studies have not been carried out with Vitrimix KV or its components. There are, however, published reports on the successful and safe infusion of amino acid solutions and fat emulsions during pregnancy in the human.

Caution: Interference with certain laboratory measurements may occur if blood samples are taken before fat has been adequately cleared from the bloodstream.

Side-effects: The components of Vitrimix KV are well tolerated. In exceptional cases nausea may occur due to the Vamin 9 Glucose component and, rarely, initial administration of Intralipid has produced a rise in temperature with shivering. Infusion of Vitrimix KV should be discontinued in such cases.

Vomiting, flushing and sweating may occur if the recommended rate of infusion is exceeded. Abnormal liver function tests have been observed during intravenous nutrition but all values return to normal on cessation of artificial feeding. Cholestasis has been reported in some patients receiving intravenous nutrition. The infusion of Intralipid has been associated with an altered lipoprotein profile. The significance of these changes is not known.

Pharmaceutical precautions Store kit at 5–25°C. Do not freeze.

Do not use if either bottle is leaking or if the Vamin 9 Glucose solution is cloudy or contains a precipitate.

After long periods of storage the bottle of Intralipid 20% should be gently inverted two or three times before use.

Vitrimix KV should be prepared immediately prior to use and infusion should be completed within 24 hours.

No additions should be made to the individual Vamin 9 Glucose and Intralipid 20% bottles prior to mixing, nor should any additions be made to the final mixture.

Discard any unused contents.

Legal category POM.

Package quantities Combined pack consisting of one 250 ml bottle of Intralipid 20% and one 1000 ml bottle containing 750 ml of Vamin 9 Glucose, together with a sterile transfer set and directions for use, and a self-adhesive label for application to the bottle containing the final mixture.

Further information Vitrimix KV is intended to provide nutritional support for a limited period of time, where sufficient enteral nutrition is impossible or impracticable. The manufacturer can be consulted for full information on complete intravenous nutrition regimens suitable for patients requiring longer term intravenous nutritional support.

Product licence number 0022/0067.

WARTICON*

Presentation An acidic ethanolic solution of 0.5% w/v podophyllotoxin.

Uses For the treatment of penile warts (condylomata acuminata), located in the preputial space.

Dosage and administration The affected area should be thoroughly washed with soap and water, and dried prior to application.

Using the applicator provided, the warts should be painted twice daily for 3 days. The treated area should be allowed to dry.

If residual warts persist, further treatment may be repeated after 7 days.

The majority of patients will not require in excess of 30 loops for each application, however a maximum of 50 loops per application (equivalent to 250 μl of Warticon Solution) may be applied. Where lesions are greater in area than 4 cm^2, it is recommended that treatment takes place under the direct supervision of medical staff.

Contra-indications, warnings, etc Open wounds following surgical procedures should not be treated with podophyllotoxin. Hypersensitivity to podophyllotoxin is a contra-indication.

In the event of the preparation entering the eye, the eye should be thoroughly bathed in water.

Side-effects: Local irritation may occur on the second or third day of application associated with the start of wart necrosis. In the majority of cases the reactions are mild.

Overdosage: There have been no reported overdosages with Warticon Solution. No specific antidote is known. Following accidental spillage, wash the skin well with soap and water. In the event of accidental ingestion give emetic or stomach washout. Treatment should be symptomatic and in severe oral overdose ensure the airway is clear and give fluids, check and correct electrolyte balance, monitor blood gases and liver function. Blood count should be monitored for at least five days.

Pharmaceutical precautions Product should be stored at room temperature.

Legal category POM.

Package quantities Each bottle contains 3 ml of Warticon Solution. Plastic applicators are also enclosed in each pack. Each loop will carry a volume approximately 5 µl Warticon Solution.

Further information Warticon Solution contains highly purified podophyllotoxin of known potency. Podophyllotoxin is a classic inhibitor of cell division in the metaphase. Its therapeutic action in genital warts is associated with necrosis of epidermal cells.

Product licence number 0022/0093.

**Trade Mark*

Knoll Limited
Fleming House
71 King Street
Maidenhead
Berkshire SL6 1DU

knoll

AKINETON*

Presentation White tablets each containing 2 mg biperiden hydrochloride, quartered by score lines on one side with the Knoll logo on the reverse side.

Akineton is also available in 1 ml ampoules containing 5 mg of Biperiden Lactate BP.

Uses Akineton is an anticholinergic drug used for the treatment of drug-induced extrapyramidal symptoms and all other types of parkinsonism.

Dosage and administration
Adults
1. Tablets: Initially half tablet (1 mg) twice daily then increasing gradually to 1 tablet three times daily. After maintenance at this level for a few days, increase the dose gradually until no further symptomatic improvement is obtained. Decrease cautiously to lowest dose which adequately controls symptoms. The optimum maintenance dose varies from 3–12 mg daily. If reduction in salivation occurs, the tablets are best taken after meals. Otherwise, tablets should be taken during meals.
2. Ampoules: 0.5–1 ampoule as a single dose to a maximum of 4 ampoules in one day, by intramuscular or slow intravenous injection.

Children: Not recommended.

Contra-indications, warnings, etc
Contra-indications: Sensitivity to Akineton (biperiden hydrochloride/lactate). Narrow angle glaucoma. Intestinal obstruction and megacolon. Tardive dyskinesias (except where these appear in association with the indications under "Uses". See precautions).

Interactions with other medicaments and other forms of interaction: As with other drugs acting on the central nervous system, the consumption of alcohol should be avoided during Akineton therapy.

Effects on ability to drive and to use machines: Occasionally drowsiness may occur. These effects may possibly be enhanced by the additional administration of other anti-parkinsonism drugs, antihistamines, tricyclic antidepressants, neuroleptics or quinidine. Patients who drive a car or operate potentially dangerous machinery which requires concentration should be warned that side-effects of this type are a possibility.

Other undesirable effects (frequency and seriousness): Akineton is well tolerated and side-effects are minimal even with prolonged use. Dryness of the mouth, disturbances of accommodation, fatigue and vertigo may occur. In general, these symptoms disappear in a few days without change in the dose; in a few cases it may be necessary to reduce the dose, although complete withdrawal of Akineton is seldom required. Gastrointestinal symptoms can be prevented in most cases by administering Akineton during or after a meal. After parenteral administration blood pressure may decrease. Restlessness, confusion and euphoria may occur, but the incidence is low.

Use in pregnancy and lactation: As there is limited data available on the effect of biperiden on the foetus or the newborn, both in animals and the human, Akineton should not be used in pregnancy or in lactating mothers.

Other special warnings and precautions: Following parenteral administration, blood pressure may be decreased. An increase in extrapyramidal symptoms during treatment is a preliminary sign of intoxication due to excessive dosage and should be treated by a reduction of the dose. Caution should be exercised in patients who show an increased tendency to convulsions. Care should be taken when administering Akineton to patients with cardiac arrhythmias. Patients with recent myocardial infarction should be given Akineton only if the heart rate is well controlled. Tardive dyskinesias can be aggravated by anticholinergics. Therefore, in patients having only tardive dyskinesia, anticholinergics are contra-indicated. Patients with tardive dyskinesias who require continuing treatment with neuroleptics may develop Parkinsonian symptoms. As these symptoms are often more distressing to the patient than the tardive dyskinesia, treatment with anticholinergics may be necessary when the neuroleptic therapy cannot be discontinued. Treatment with Akineton should not be discontinued abruptly. Transfer of patients to Akineton from other anti-parkinsonism agents should be more gradual, the original agent being reduced in dose as Akineton is substituted. On rare occasions, particularly in patients with hypertrophy of the prostate, disturbances of micturition may occur and, even more rarely, retention of urine. Reduction of the dose will usually restore the bladder function to normal. As with other long-term medication, regular haematology and biochemistry are recommended.

Combined treatment: In some cases the response of tremor to Akineton alone may be inadequate. In such cases combined therapy with an additional preparation effective against tremor should be considered.

Overdosage (symptoms, emergency procedures, antidotes): The symptoms of overdose are anticholinergic effects such as mydriasis, dryness of mucous membranes, flushing, rise in heart rate, reduction of bowel motility, reduction in ureter and bladder tone, increased temperature, excitation, confusion, clouding of consciousness and/or hallucinations. In severe overdose, cardiac and respiratory depression may occur.

Treatment: Gastric lavage or emesis should be considered. Vital signs should be closely monitored and appropriate supportive measures taken. Artificial ventilation may be necessary. In the event of cardiac depression, a cardiac stimulant drug such as dobutamine may be considered.

Incompatibilities: None stated.

Pharmaceutical precautions Protect from light. Shelf-life 5 years.

Legal category POM.

Package quantities Akineton 2 mg tablets in blister packs of 100 tablets. Akineton 5 mg/ml ampoules in boxes of 5 × 1 ml ampoules.

Further information Metabolizable carbohydrate content: Approx. 0.16 g per tablet. Sodium content: 0.13 mmol per ampoule (0.13 mmol per ml).

Product licence numbers

Tablets	0169/0009
Ampoules	0169/0010

ARYTHMOL* ▼

Presentation White, film-coated tablets of 150 mg propafenone hydrochloride. White, scored, film-coated tablets of 300 mg propafenone hydrochloride.

Uses Arythmol is a Class IC antiarrhythmic drug with basic local anaesthetic and membrane-stabilising effects. It decreases the depolarisation velocity and slows conduction in the atria, atrioventricular node and especially in the His-Purkinje system with resulting lengthening of the PR interval and QRS complex duration on the surface ECG. It prolongs the refractory period in the atria and the ventricle dose-dependently. Arythmol also prolongs refractory period and slows conduction in accessory pathways in both directions. Some beta-blocking activity has been reported.

Arythmol is indicated for the prophylaxis and treatment of ventricular arrhythmias.

Dosage and administration The individual maintenance dose should be determined under cardiological surveillance including ECG monitoring and blood pressure control. It is recommended that Arythmol therapy should be initiated under hospital conditions. If the QRS interval is prolonged by more than 20%, the dose should be reduced or discontinued until the ECG returns to normal limits.

Adults: Initially 150 mg three times daily increasing at a minimum of three day intervals to 300 mg twice daily and, if necessary, to a maximum of 300 mg three times daily.

The tablets should be swallowed whole and taken with a drink after food. A reduction in the total daily dose is recommended for patients below 70 kg body weight.

Elderly patients: Higher plasma concentrations of propafenone have been noted during treatment. Elderly patients may therefore respond to a lower dose.

Children: A suitable dosage form of Arythmol for children is not available.

Dosage in impaired liver function: Arythmol is extensively metabolised via a saturable hepatic oxidative pathway. In view of the increased bioavailability and elimination half-life of propafenone, a reduction in the recommended dose may be necessary.

Dosage in impaired renal function: Although the elimination of propafenone and its major metabolite is not affected by renal impairment, Arythmol should be administered cautiously.

Contra-indications, warnings, etc

Contra-indications: Uncontrolled congestive heart failure, cardiogenic shock (except arrhythmia-induced), severe bradycardia, uncontrolled electrolyte disturbances, severe obstructive pulmonary disease, marked hypotension. Unless patients are adequately paced (see 'Precautions'), Arythmol should not be used in the presence of sinus node dysfunction, atrial conduction defects, second degree or greater atrioventricular block, bundle branch block or distal block. Minor prolongation of PR interval and intraventricular conduction defects (QRS duration of less than 20%) are to be expected during treatment with Arythmol and do not warrant dose reduction or drug withdrawal. Myasthenia gravis (there have been a few reported cases).

Interactions with other medicaments and other forms of interaction: Effects of Arythmol may be potentiated if it is given in combination with other local anaesthetic type agents or agents which depress myocardial activity.

Arythmol has been shown to increase the plasma levels of digoxin and caution should be exercised with regard to digitalis toxicity.

Arythmol has been shown to increase the plasma levels of warfarin with an accompanying increase in prothrombin time, which may require reduction of the dose of warfarin.

Plasma levels of propafenone may be increased by concomitant administration of cimetidine.

Increased propranolol and metoprolol plasma levels have been observed when these beta-blockers were used concurrently with Arythmol. Thus, dose reduction of these beta-blockers may be required. Details of interaction with other beta-blockers are not known.

Concomitant administation of propafenone and quinidine may result in decreased oral clearance with an increase in steady state plasma concentration of propafenone. There has been a report of the lowering of propafenone levels by rifampicin, via the hepatic mixed oxidase system. This reduction may lead to breakthrough arrhythmias.

Effects on ability to drive and to use machines: None known.

Other undesirable effects (frequency and seriousness): Arythmol may produce minor nervous system and cardiovascular side-effects but is generally well tolerated. Occasionally, particularly with higher doses, dizziness, nausea and vomiting, fatigue, bitter taste, constipation, diarrhoea, headache, blurred vision and dry mouth have been reported. Allergic skin reactions such as reddening, pruritis, exanthema or urticaria may occur infrequently. Postural hypotension is occasionally seen, particularly in the elderly. These effects disappear after reduction of the dose or discontinuation of the drug. Bradycardia, sino-atrial, atrioventricular or intraventricular blocks may occur (see 'Overdosage'). In common with other antiarrhythmic drugs there is a small risk of proarrhythmic effects. Rare cases of individual hypersensitivity reactions (manifested by cholestasis, blood dyscrasias, lupus syndrome) and seizures have been reported. All were reversible on discontinuation of treatment.

Use in pregnancy and lactation: Animal studies have not shown any teratogenic effects but as there is no experience of the use of the drug in human pregnancy, Arythmol should not be used during pregnancy.

Other special warnings and precautions: The weak negative inotropic effect of Arythmol may assume importance in patients predisposed to cardiac failure. In common with other anti-arrhythmic drugs Arythmol has been shown to alter sensitivity and pacing threshold. In patients with pacemakers, appropriate adjustment may be required. Because of the Beta-Blocking effect, care should be exercised in the treatment of patients with obstructive airways disease.

Overdosage (symptoms, emergency procedures, antidotes): Experience with overdosage is limited. No specific antidote is known. Procedures to enhance drug elimination from the body by haemodialysis or haemoperfusion are unlikely to succeed because of the large volume of drug distribution. The usual emergency measures for acute cardiovascular collapse should be applied. In severe conduction disturbance associated with a compromised cardiac function, atropine, isoprenaline or pacemaker therapy may be required. If electrical stimulation is not possible, an attempt should be made to shorten the QRS duration and increase the heart rate with high doses of isoprenaline: bundle branch block by itself is not an indication for isoprenaline. Hypotension may require inotropic support. Convulsions should be treated with i.v. diazepam.

Incompatibilities (major): None known.

Pharmaceutical precautions Store in a dry place at room temperature.

Legal category POM.

Package quantities Blister packs containing (150 mg) 90 tablets, (300 mg) 60 tablets.

Further information Nil.

Product licence numbers
150 mg 0169/0015
300 mg 0169/0016

SECURON*

Presentation Securon tablets containing 40 mg Verapamil Hydrochloride BP are white, film-coated tablets impressed with 40 on one side and △ on the other.

Securon tablets containing 80 mg Verapamil Hydrochloride BP are white, film-coated tablets impressed with SECURON 80 on one side and KNOLL above the score-line on the other.

Securon tablets containing 120 mg Verapamil Hydrochloride BP are white, film-coated tablets impressed with SECURON 120 on one side and KNOLL above the score-line on the other.

Securon tablets containing 160 mg Verapamil Hydrochloride BP are white, film-coated tablets impressed with SECURON 160 on one side and KNOLL above the score-line on the other.

Securon tablets contain lactose.

Uses Securon is a calcium antagonist which blocks the inward movement of calcium in cardiac muscle cells, in smooth muscle cells of the coronary and systemic arteries and in the cells of the intracardiac conduction system. Securon lowers peripheral vascular resistance with no reflex tachycardia. Its efficacy in reducing both raised systolic and diastolic blood pressure is thought to be primarily due to this mode of action.

The decrease in systemic and coronary vascular resistance and the sparing effect on intracellular oxygen consumption appear to explain the anti-anginal properties of the drug.

Because of its effect on the movement of calcium in the intracardiac conduction system, Securon reduces automaticity, decreases conduction velocity and increases the refractory period.

Securon is indicated for:

(1) The treatment of mild to moderate hypertension;

(2) the treatment and prophylaxis of chronic stable angina, vasospastic angina and unstable angina;

(3) the treatment and prophylaxis of paroxysmal supraventricular tachycardia; reduction of ventricular rate in atrial flutter/fibrillation. (Verapamil should not be used when atrial flutter/fibrillation complicates Wolff-Parkinson-White syndrome, see Precautions.)

Dosage and administration

Adults: Hypertension: Initially 120 mg b.d. increasing to 160 mg b.d. where necessary. In some cases dosages of up to 480 mg daily, in divided doses, have been used. A further reduction in blood pressure may be obtained by combining Securon with other antihypertensive agents, in particular diuretics. For concomitant administration with beta-blockers see Precautions.

Angina: 120 mg t.d.s. is recommended. 80 mg t.d.s. can be completely satisfactory in some patients with angina of effort. Less than 120 mg t.d.s. is not likely to be effective in variant angina.

Supraventricular tachycardias: 40–120 mg t.d.s. according to the severity of the condition.

Children: Up to 2 years: 20 mg, 2–3 times a day. Two years and above: 40–120 mg, 2–3 times a day, according to age and effectiveness.

Elderly patients: The adult dose is recommended unless liver or renal function is impaired (see Precautions).

Contra-indications, warnings, etc

Contra-indications: Cardiogenic shock; acute myocardial infarction complicated by bradycardia, hypotension, left ventricular failure; second or third degree atrioventricular block; sino-atrial block; sick sinus syndrome; uncompensated heart failure; bradycardia of less than 50 beats/minute; hypotension of less than 90 mmHg systolic.

Interactions with other medicaments and other forms of interaction: Verapamil hydrochloride has been shown to increase the serum concentration of digoxin and caution should be exercised with regard to digitalis toxicity.

The combination of Securon and beta-blockers, anti-arrhythmic agents or inhaled anaesthetics may lead to additive cardiovascular effects (e.g. AV block, bradycardia, hypotension, heart failure). Intra-venous beta-blockers should not be given to patients under treatment with Securon. The effects of Securon may be additive to other hypotensive agents.

Interactions with verapamil have been reported for carbamazepine (potentiated by verapamil) and rifampicin (effects of verapamil attenuated), cyclosporin and theophylline (increase of plasma levels by verapamil). Neurotoxic interactions have been reported with lithium. The effects of muscle relaxants employed in anaesthesia may be potentiated.

Effects on ability to drive and use machines: None stated.

Other undesirable effects (frequency and seriousness): Securon is generally well tolerated. Side-effects are usually mild and transient and discontinuation of therapy is rarely necessary. Constipation may occur. Flushing is observed occasionally and headaches, nausea, vomiting, dizziness, fatigue and ankle oedema have been reported rarely. Allergic reactions (e.g. erythema, pruritus) are very rarely seen. A reversible impairment of liver function, characterised by an increase of transaminase and/or alkaline phosphatase may occur on very rare occasions during verapamil treatment and is most probably a hypersensitivity reaction.

On very rare occasions, gynaecomastia has been observed in elderly male patients under long term verapamil treatment, which was fully reversible in all cases when the drug was discontinued.

Gingival hyperplasia may very rarely occur when the drug is administered over prolonged periods, and is fully reversible when the drug is discontinued.

Use in pregnancy and lactation: Although animal studies have not shown any teratogenic effects, verapamil hydrochloride should not be given during the first trimester of pregnancy unless, in the clinician's judgement, it is essential for the welfare of the patient. Verapamil is excreted into the breast milk in small amounts and is unlikely to be harmful. However, rare hypersensitivity reactions have been reported with verapamil and, therefore, it should only be used during lactation if, in the clinician's judgement, it is essential for the welfare of the patient.

Other special warnings and precautions: Since verapamil is extensively metabolised in the liver, careful dose titration of verapamil is required in patients with liver disease. The disposition of verapamil in patients with renal impairment has not been fully established and therefore careful patient monitoring is recommended. Verapamil is not removed during dialysis.

Verapamil may affect impulse conduction and therefore Securon should be used with caution in patients with first degree atrioventricular block. Patients with atrial flutter/fibrillation in association with an accessory pathway (e.g. WPW-syndrome) may develop increased conduction across the anomalous pathway and ventricular tachycardia may be precipitated. Securon may affect left ventricular contractility; this effect is small and normally not important but cardiac failure may be precipitated or aggravated. In patients with incipient cardiac failure, therefore, Securon should only be given after cardiac failure has been controlled with appropriate therapy, e.g. digitalis.

Overdosage: The symptoms of overdosage include hypotension, shock, loss of consciousness, first and second degree atrioventricular (AV) block (frequently as Wenckebach's phenomenon with or without escape rhythms), total AV block with total AV dissociation, escape rhythm, asystole, sinus bradycardia, sinus arrest.

Treatment of overdose depends upon the type and severity of symptoms. The specific antidote is calcium, e.g. 10–20 ml of 10% calcium gluconate solution i.v. (2.25–4.5 mmol), if necessary by repeated injection or continuous infusion (e.g. 5 mmol/hr). Gastric lavage, taking the usual precautionary measures, may be appropriate. The usual emergency measures for acute cardiovascular collapse should be applied, and followed by intensive care.

Similarly, in the case of second and third degree AV block, atropine, isoprenaline and, if required, pace-maker therapy should be considered.

If there are signs of myocardial insufficiency, dopamine, dobutamine, cardiac glycosides or calcium gluconate (10–20 ml of a 10% solution) should be administered. In the case of hypotension, after appropriately positioning the patient, dopamine, dobutamine, noradrenaline may be given.

Incompatibilities (major): None stated.

Pharmaceutical precautions Store in a dry place at room temperature. Shelf life five years.

Legal category POM.

Package quantities Securon 160 mg, 120 mg tablets: 28 day calendar pack of 56 tablets.

Securon 160 mg, 120 mg, 80 mg, 40 mg tablets: 100 tablets in plastic containers.

Further information Nil.

Product licence numbers

Securon Tablets 40 mg	0169/0003
Securon Tablets 80 mg	0169/0004
Securon Tablets 120 mg	0169/0005
Securon Tablets 160 mg	0169/0014

SECURON IV*

Presentation Securon IV is an aqueous solution of Verapamil Hydrochloride BP in a concentration of 2.5 mg/ml. Each syringe contains 2 ml (5 mg) of Verapamil Hydrochloride BP for intravenous injection.

Uses Securon is a calcium antagonist which blocks the inward movement of calcium in the cells of the intracardiac conduction system, in cardiac muscle cells and in the smooth muscle cells of the cardiovascular system. Through its effects on the movement of calcium in the intracardiac conduction system, Securon reduces automaticity, decreases conduction velocity, and increases the refractory period.

Securon IV is indicated in the treatment of paroxysmal supraventricular tachycardia; reduction of ventricular rate in atrial flutter/fibrillation. (Verapamil should not be used when atrial flutter/fibrillation complicates Wolff-Parkinson-White syndrome, see 'Precautions'.)

Dosage and administration

Adults: 5–10 mg by slow intravenous injection over a period of 2 minutes. The patient should be observed continuously preferably under ECG and blood pressure control. If necessary, e.g., in paroxysmal tachycardia, a further 5 mg may be given after 5–10 minutes.

Children: Securon IV must always be administered under ECG monitoring in young patients.

0–1 year	0.1–0.2 mg/kg body weight (Usual single dose range 0.75–2 mg)
1–15 years	0.1–0.3 mg/kg body weight (Usual single dose range 2–5 mg).

The dose may be repeated after 30 minutes if necessary.

Many cases are controlled by doses at the lower end of the range. The injection should be stopped at the onset of the desired effect.

Elderly: The dosage should be administered over 3 minutes to minimise the risk of adverse effects.

Dosage in impaired liver and renal function: Significant hepatic and renal impairment should not increase the effects of a single intravenous dose but may prolong its duration of action.

For use with beta-blocker therapy see 'Contra-indications' and 'Precautions.'

Contra-indications, warnings, etc

Contra-indications: Cardiogenic shock; acute myocardial infarction complicated by bradycardia, marked hypotension, left ventricular failure; second or third degree atrioventricular block; sino-atrial block; sick sinus syndrome; uncompensated heart failure; marked bradycardia of less than 50 beats/minute; marked hypotension of less than 90 mmHg systolic; patients with atrial flutter/fibrillation in the presence of an accessory pathway (e.g. WPW syndrome) may develop increased conduction across the anomalous pathway and ventricular tachycardia may be precipitated; simultaneous administration of intravenous beta-blockers.

Interactions with other medicaments and other forms of interaction: The effects of Securon IV, beta-blockers and anti-arrhythmic agents may be additive both with respect to conduction and contraction: Securon IV should not be given in combination with intravenous beta-blocker therapy and care must be exercised if Securon IV is combined with oral beta-blocker therapy or anti-arrhythmic agents by any route. Securon IV and inhaled anaesthetics may have additive cardiovascular effects. Securon IV may reduce blood pressure and an additive effect with antihypertensive drugs may be seen.

Verapamil hydrochloride has been shown to increase the serum concentration of digoxin and caution should be exercised with regard to digitalis toxicity.

Interactions with verapamil have been reported for carbamazepine (potentiated by verapamil) and rifampicin (effects of verapamil attenuated), cyclosporin and theophylline (increase of plasma levels by verapamil). Neurotoxic interactions have been reported with lithium. The effect of muscle relaxants employed in anaesthesia may be potentiated.

Effects on the ability to drive and use machines: None stated.

Other undesirable effects (frequency and seriousness): Securon IV is generally well tolerated but due to the drug's mode of action, undesired cardiovascular effects may occur, particularly at high doses and in patients with AV block and/or impaired myocardial function. Decreased heart rate, hypotension and decreased myocardial contractility have been reported. On rare occasions, second or third degree AV block may occur and, in extreme cases, this may lead to asystole. The asystole is usually of short duration and cardiac action returns spontaneously after a few seconds, usually in the form of sinus rhythm. If necessary, the procedures for the treatment of overdosage should be followed as described below. A slight transient fall in blood pressure, due to a reduction in peripheral resistance may be seen. In rare cases this may lead to severe hypotension. On rare occasions dizziness, headache, nausea, vomiting, nervousness and flushing have been reported. Allergic reactions (erythema, pruritus, urticaria, bronchospasm) are extremely rare. A reversible impairment of liver function, characterised by an increase of transaminase and/or alkaline phosphatase may occur on very rare occasions during verapamil treatment and is most probably a hypersensitivity reaction.

On very rare occasions, gynaecomastia has been observed in elderly male patients under long term verapamil treatment, which was fully reversible in all cases when the drug was discontinued.

Gingival hyperplasia may very rarely occur when the drug is administered over prolonged periods, and is fully reversible when the drug is discontinued.

Use in pregnancy and lactation: Although animal studies have not shown any teratogenic effects, verapamil HCl should not be given during the first trimester of pregnancy unless, in the clinician's judgement, it is essential for the welfare of the patient.

Verapamil is excreted into the breast milk in small amounts and is unlikely to be harmful. However, rare hypersensitivity reactions have been reported with verapamil and, therefore, it should only be used during lactation if, in the clinician's judgement, it is essential for the welfare of the patient.

Other special warnings and precautions: Securon IV may affect impulse conduction and should be used with caution in patients with first degree atrioventricular block. Securon IV may affect left ventricular contractility; this effect is small and normally not important but cardiac failure may be precipitated or aggravated. In patients with poor ventricular function, therefore, Securon IV should only be given after cardiac failure has been controlled with appropriate therapy, e.g. digitalis and/or diuretics.

Overdosage: The symptoms of overdosage include hypotension, shock, loss of consciousness, first and second degree atrioventricular (AV) block (frequently as Wenckebach's phenomenon with or without escape rhythms), total AV block with total AV dissociation, escape rhythm, asystole, sinus bradycardia, sinus arrest.

Treatment of overdosage depends on the type and severity of symptoms. The specific antidote is calcium, e.g. 10–20 ml of 10% calcium gluconate solution i.v. (2.25–4.5 mmol) if necessary by repeated injection or continuous infusion (e.g. 5 mmol/hr). The usual emergency measures for acute cardiovascular collapse should be applied and followed by intensive care. Similarly in the case of second and third degree AV block, atropine, isoprenaline and, if required, pace-maker therapy should be considered. If there are signs of myocardial insuffiency, dopamine, dobutamine, cardiac glycosides, or calcium gluconate (10–20 ml of a 10% solution) should be administered.

In the case of hypotension, after appropriately positioning the patient, dopamine, dobutamine, noradrenaline may be given.

Incompatibilities (major): None stated.

Pharmaceutical precautions Store at room temperature. Protect from light.

Legal category POM.

Package quantities 5 × 2 ml syringe in individual blister packs with a separate needle in each blister.

Further information Securon IV is incompatible with alkaline solutions.

Each ampoule contains 17 mg sodium chloride (8.5 mg/ml).

The syringe is graded in divisions of 0.25 ml.

Following intravenous infusion in man, verapamil is eliminated bioexponentially with a rapid distribution phase (half-life about 4 mins) and a slower terminal elimination phase (half-life 2–5 hours).

Product licence number 0169/0017.

SECURON SR*

Presentation Each Securon SR tablet contains 240 mg Verapamil Hydrochloride BP in a sustained release formulation. The tablets are pale green, film-coated, oblong shaped and scored on both sides with △ on one side.

Uses Securon SR is indicated for the treatment of mild to moderate hypertension, and the treatment and prophylaxis of angina pectoris. Securon SR is a sustained release preparation of Securon designed to release verapamil hydrochloride gradually thus prolonging the pharmacological action. Securon SR lowers peripheral vascular resistance with no reflex tachycardia.

Verapamil hydrochloride is a calcium antagonist which blocks the inward movement of calcium in cardiac muscle cells, in smooth muscle cells of the coronary and systemic arteries and in the cells of the intracardiac conduction system. Also, it has been shown to have therapeutic efficacy in various supraventricular dysrhythmias.

Dosage and administration

Adults: Hypertension: One tablet of Securon SR daily. However, verapamil may normalise raised blood pressure after one dose. Therefore, for patients new to verapamil therapy the physician should consider halving the initial dose to 120 mg. Most patients respond to 240 mg daily (one tablet) given as a single dose. If control is not achieved after a period of at least one week the dosage may be increased to a maximum of two tablets daily (one in the morning and one in the evening at an interval of about twelve hours). A further reduction in blood pressure may be achieved by combining Securon SR with other antihypertensive agents, in particular diuretics.

Angina pectoris: 240 mg twice daily. A small number of patients respond to a lower dose and where indicated, adjustment down to 240 mg once daily could be made.

The tablets should not be chewed.

Children: Securon SR is not recommended for children.

Elderly patients: The adult dose is recommended unless liver or renal function is impaired (see Precautions).

Contra-indications, warnings, etc

Contra-indications: Cardiogenic shock; acute myocardial infarction complicated by bradycardia, hypotension, left ventricular failure; second or third degree atrioventricular block; sino-atrial block; sick sinus syndrome; uncompensated heart failure; bradycardia of less than 50 beats/minute; hypotension of less than 90 mmHg systolic.

Interactions with other medicaments and other forms of interaction: Verapamil hydrochloride has been shown to increase the serum concentration of digoxin and caution should be exercised with regard to digitalis toxicity.

The combination of Securon SR and beta-blockers, anti-arrhythmic agents or inhaled anaesthetics may lead to additive cardiovascular effects (e.g. AV block, bradycardia, hypotension, heart failure). Intra-venous beta-blockers should not be given to patients under treatment with Securon SR. The effects of Securon SR may be additive to other hypotensive agents.

Interactions with verapamil have been reported for carbamazepine (potentiated by verapamil) and rifampicin (effects of verapamil attenuated), cyclosporin and theophylline (increase of plasma levels by verapamil). Neurotoxic interactions have been reported with lithium. The effects of muscle relaxants employed in anaesthesia may be potentiated.

Effects on ability to drive and use machines: None stated.

Other undesirable effects (frequency and seriousness): Securon SR is generally well tolerated. Side-effects are usually mild and transient and discontinuation of therapy is rarely necessary. Constipation may occur, flushing is observed occasionally and headache, nausea, vomiting, dizziness, fatigue and ankle oedema have been reported rarely. Allergic reactions (e.g. erythema, pruritus) are very rarely seen. A reversible impairment of liver function, characterised by an increase of transaminase and/or alkaline phosphatase may occur on very rare occasions during verapamil treatment and is most probably a hypersensitivity reaction.

On very rare occasions, gynaecomastia has been observed in elderly male patients under long term verapamil treatment, which was fully reversible in all cases when the drug was discontinued.

Gingival hyperplasia may very rarely occur when the drug is administered over prolonged periods, and is fully reversible when the drug is discontinued.

Use in pregnancy and lactation: Although animal studies have not shown any teratogenic effects, verapamil hydrochloride should not be given during the first trimester of pregnancy unless, in the clinician's judgement, it is essential for the welfare of the patient. Verapamil is excreted into the breast milk in small amounts and is unlikely to be harmful. However, rare hypersensitivity reactions have been reported with verapamil and, therefore, it should only be used during lactation if, in the clinician's judgement, it is essential for the welfare of the patient.

Other special warnings and precautions: Since verapamil is extensively metabolised in the liver, careful dose titration of verapamil is required in patients with liver disease. The disposition of verapamil in patients with renal impairment has not been fully established and therefore careful patient monitoring is recommended. Verapamil is not removed during dialysis.

Verapamil may affect impulse conduction and therefore Securon SR should be used with caution in patients with first degree atrioventricular block. Patients with atrial flutter/fibrillation in association with an accessory pathway (e.g. WPW-syndrome) may develop increased conduction across the anomalous pathway and ventricular tachycardia may be precipitated. Securon SR may affect left ventricular contractility: this effect is small and normally not important but cardiac failure may be precipitated or aggravated. In patients with incipient cardiac failure, therefore, Securon SR should be given only after such cardiac failure has been controlled with appropriate therapy, e.g. digitalis.

Overdosage (symptoms, emergency procedures, antidotes): The symptoms of overdosage include hypotension, shock, loss of consciousness, first and second degree atrioventricular (AV) block (frequently as Wenckebach's phenomenon with or without escape rhythms), total AV block with total AV dissociation, escape rhythm, asystole, sinus bradycardia, sinus arrest.

Treatment of overdose depends upon the type and

severity of symptoms. It should be remembered that Securon SR is a sustained release preparation, and that a portion of a tablet anywhere in the intestinal tract can act as an active drug depot. Release of active drug and absorption may take more than 48 hours. The specific antidote is calcium, e.g. 10–20 ml of 10% calcium gluconate solution i.v. (2.25–4.5 mmol), if necessary by repeated injection or continuous infusion (e.g. 5 mmol/hr). Gastric lavage, taking the usual precautionary measures, may be appropriate. The usual emergency measures for acute cardiovascular collapse should be applied, and followed by intensive care.

Similarly, in the case of second and third degree AV block, atropine, isoprenaline and, if required, pace-maker therapy should be considered.

If there are signs of myocardial insufficiency, dopamine, dobutamine, cardiac glycosides or calcium gluconate (10–20 ml of a 10% solution) should be administered.

In the case of hypotension, after appropriately positioning the patient, dopamine, dobutamine, noradrenaline may be given.

Incompatibilities: None stated.

Pharmaceutical precautions Store in a dry place at room temperature. Shelf life 5 years.

Legal category POM.

Package quantities Calendar packs of 28 Securon SR film-coated tablets.

Security containers of 100 film-coated tablets.

Further information Nil.

Product licence number 0169/0007

**Trade Mark*

Laboratories for Applied Biology Limited
91 Amhurst Park
London N16 5DR

CERUMOL* EAR DROPS

Presentation A clear oily preparation containing:

Arachis oil BP	57.3% w/v
Chlorbutol BP	5.0% w/v
p-Dichlorobenzene	2.0% w/v

Uses Occlusion or partial occlusion of external auditory meatus by either a collection of soft wax or a harder wax plug.

Dosage and administration *At home:* With the head inclined, 5 drops are put into the ear. This may cause a harmless tingling sensation. A plug of cotton wool moistened with Cerumol should then be applied to retain the liquid. One hour later, or the next morning, the plug is removed. The procedure is repeated twice a day for three days; the loosened wax may then come out on its own making syringing unnecessary. If any wax remains the doctor should be consulted so that syringing of the softened residue may be carried out.

At the surgery: If there has been no prior treatment with Cerumol, 5 drops are instilled as described above and left for at least 20 minutes. Then syringing or a probe tipped with cotton wool may be employed.

Contra-indications, warnings, etc Otitis externa, seborrhoeic dermatitis, eczema affecting the external ear and perforated ear drum.

Use in pregnancy: No side-effects have been reported.

Other special warnings: Not to be taken internally. Do not use for more than three days. If the condition persists consult your doctor.

Overdosage: As the product is applied topically, overdosage as such is not possible. In the case of accidental ingestion, the amounts of the majority of ingredients in the 11 ml bottle are too small to give rise to toxic effects. The 550 mg of chlorbutol in the whole bottle might cause excessive sedation in a child.

Pharmaceutical precautions No special storage precautions.

Legal category P

Package quantities 11 ml vial with separate dropper.

Further information Nil.

Product licence number 0118/0013.

EMESIDE* CAPSULES AND SYRUP

Presentation Soft orange gelatin capsules each containing 250 mg of Ethosuximide BP.

Blackcurrant or orange-flavoured syrup containing 250 mg of Ethosuximide BP per 5 ml.

Uses Emeside gives selective control of absence seizures (petit-mal) even when complicated by grand-mal. It is also indicated for myoclonic seizures. The reduction of seizure frequency is thought to be achieved by depression of the motor cortex and elevation of the threshold to convulsive stimuli as seen by the suppression of the characteristic spike and wave EEG pattern. Emeside may be prescribed together with other anticonvulsants such as phenobarbitone, phenytoin, primidone or sodium valproate where grandmal or other forms of epilepsy may require additional treatment.

Dosage and administration *Adults and children over 6 years:* Start with a small dose – 500 mg daily with increments of 250 mg every five to seven days until control is achieved usually with 1,000–1,500 mg (4–6 capsules) daily. Occasionally 2,000 mg daily in divided dose may be necessary.

The half life of ethosuximide in the plasma is about 60 hours in adults but the daily dose if large is more comfortably divided between morning and evening.

If Emeside is being substituted for another anti-epileptic drug the latter must not be withdrawn abruptly but the replacement made gradually with overlap of the preparations otherwise petit mal may break through; the slow withdrawal applies to Emeside when another drug is to replace it.

Children and infants under six years: Begin with a daily dose of 250 mg (5 ml syrup) and increase the dose gradually by small increments every few days until control is achieved, the maximum dose should be 1,000 mg.

Peak concentrations occur in plasma 1–7 hours after ingestion and the plasma half life is about 30 hours in children and 60 hours in adults. Plasma levels of ethosuximide to be effective lie between 40 and 85 microgram per ml but the clinical response should be the criterion for regulation of dosage. Because young children metabolise ethosuximide more rapidly than adults higher and more frequent doses may be necessary.

Contra-indications, warnings, etc Plasma concentrations are not accurately predictable and since compliance is variable, monitoring of plasma concentrations can be of value in unresponsive cases. Known hypersensitivity to succinimides. Exercise caution with regular appropriate tests in patients with hepatic or renal disease and monitor drug plasma concentrations. Porphyrias. Ethosuximide may be excreted into breast milk. Mothers receiving the drug should not breastfeed. There is a recognised small increase in the incidence of congenital malformations in children born to mothers receiving anticonvulsants. For women planning pregnancy or who are already pregnant the risk should be weighed carefully against the benefit of treatment.

As with all syrups it is advisable to brush the teeth or rinse the mouth after taking Emeside syrup.

Side Effects: Nausea, vomiting, anorexia and epigastric pain are common at first and generally subside. High dosage may cause sedation or confusion. Unusual symptoms are headache, fatigue, drowsiness, dizziness, ataxia, dyskinesia, hiccough, photophobia, depression and skin rash. Isolated reports have been made of erythema nodosum, erythema multiforme, agranulocytosis, aplastic anaemia and systemic lupus. In some instances, patients who become leucopenic on other anticonvulsant therapy have been treated satisfactorily with ethosuximide.

Drug Interaction: The plasma concentrations of ethosuximide are reduced by carbamazepine and increased by isoniazid, phenytoin and sodium valproate.

Overdosage: Where more than 2 g has been thought to be ingested gastric lavage may be employed, if the time lapse is less than four hours.

Routine observation of respiration and circulation will indicate the need for supportive measures.

Pharmaceutical precautions Store in a cool dry

place. Recommended diluent – unpreserved Syrup BP; use within 14 days.

Legal category POM.

Package quantities *Capsules:* 112 and 500.
Syrup (blackcurrant or orange flavour): Bottles of 200 ml and 1,000 ml.

Further information As with all syrups it is advisable to brush the teeth or rinse the mouth after taking Emeside syrup.

Product licence numbers

Emeside Capsules	0118/5002
Emeside Syrup orange	0118/5003
Emeside Syrup blackcurrant	0118/5004.

HALYCITROL* VITAMIN EMULSION

Presentation Orange flavoured emulsion containing 27,600 microgram (92,000 iu)/100 ml Vitamin A and 190 microgram (7,600 iu) Vitamin D per 100 ml. This is equivalent to 1,380 microgram (4,600 iu) of Vitamin A and 9.5 microgram (380 iu) of Vitamin D in a 5 ml daily dose.

Uses For prevention of vitamin A and D deficiency.

Dosage and administration *Adults and children above 6 months:* 5 ml daily.

Infants up to six months: 2.5 ml daily.

Contra-indications, warnings, etc Prolonged excessive ingestion of vitamins A and D can lead to hypervitaminosis states.

Hypervitaminosis A: Symptoms include dry rough skin, painful joint swellings, anorexia and vomiting.

Hypervitaminosis D: Infants already receiving vitamin D from such sources as vitaminised margarine and cereals can develop infantile hypercalcaemia from excessive vitamin D intake.

In children and adults the symptoms of hypercalcaemia are weakness, anorexia, abdominal pain, constipation, thirst and polyuria with the development of nephrocalcinosis, renal stones and renal failure. Individuals with renal disease and Sarcoidosis are particularly susceptible.

Pharmaceutical precautions Store in a cool place.

Legal category GSL.

Package quantities Bottles of 114 ml.

Further information This is a preparation of fish oil devoid of any fish odour or taste.

Product licence number 0118/0015.

LABITON* TONIC

Presentation A brown liquid containing vitamin B_1 0.75 mg, dried extract of kola nuts 6.05 mg, alcohol 2.8 ml, caffeine (total) 7 mg per 10 ml.

Uses The kola nut contains complex catechine-caffeinates which give central stimulation, increase muscular performance and reduce fatiguability. Vitamin B_1 is included to make up deficiency resulting from recent illness or anorexia. Labiton is indicated for use as a tonic for fatigue, anorexia and debility in convalescence after infections such as influenza and after operations.

Dosage and administration 10–20 ml twice daily, before or after meals, with or without water.

Not intended for administration to children.

Contra-indications, warnings, etc Undesirable in cases of hepatitis and patients taking sedatives. Car drivers should be made aware of the presence of alcohol and should be advised not to exceed the recommended dosage, especially if taking tranquillisers or remedies for allergies that have sedative side effects.

Drug interactions: With correct dosage, the alcohol content should give no interaction. With excessive dosage there could be potentiation of CNS depressants and potentiation of the hypoglycaemic effect of insulin.

Overdosage: Treatment is that for alcohol with correction of dehydration, attendance to the airway and other supportive measures for coma.

Pharmaceutical precautions Store in a cool place. Use within nine months of opening.

Legal category GSL.

Package quantities Supplied in bottles of 200 ml and 1 litre.

Further information Nil.

Product licence number 0118/5005.

LABOPHYLLINE* INJECTION

Presentation Ampoules each containing 10 ml of an aqueous solution of lysine and theophylline providing 200 mg of theophylline anhydride (and 122 mg of L-lysine), equivalent to 253 mg of aminophylline.

Uses Bronchodilator in acute asthma avoiding possible allergic reactions to aminophylline.

Dosage and administration The table gives guidance to dosage.

Loading doses:

1. Where patients have not taken theophyllines or other xanthines within the previous 24 hours:
Adults: by slow *intravenous injection* 200 mg (equivalent to 253 mg aminophylline) given over a period of 15 minutes. By *intravenous infusion* 4 mg/kg (equivalent to 5 mg/kg aminophylline) diluted in 100 ml of 0.9% Sodium Chloride Infusion or 5% Glucose Infusion given over 20 to 30 minutes.
Children: by slow *intravenous injection* 4 mg/kg given over a period of 15 minutes. By *intravenous infusion* dosage rate and procedure is as for adults.

2. Where patients have taken theophyllines or other xanthines during the previous 24 hours the initial doses given above may be inadvisable. If there are no signs of xanthine toxicity (see Overdosage), half the above doses may be given if theophylline treatment is considered to be essential.

Maintenance: For adults and children see the Table. Note that the elderly require caution in view of decreased metabolism of xanthines. Labophylline should be diluted in 500 ml of infusion fluid to run for 8 hours. Suitable fluids are 0.9% sodium chloride or 5% glucose.

Contra-indications, warnings, etc
Contra-indications: Known hypersensitivity to xanthine preparations.

Precautions: Special care must be taken if the patient has been receiving oral theophylline, aminophylline or other xanthine preparations. Due consideration must be given to the type and timing of the last dose (see Dosage).

Intravenous injections must be given slowly over not

Guide to dosage of theophylline given intravenously

Patient	*Loading dose* mg/kg*	*First 12 hours mg/kg/hr*	*Beyond 12 hours mg/kg/hr*
Adults†	4	0.5	0.4
Elderly	4	0.33	0.25
With heart failure	4	0.25	0.1
Children, 6 years and above	4	0.75	0.5
Children, 6 months to 6 years	4	1–0.8	0.6

* Where xanthines have not been taken in previous 24 hours.
† Otherwise healthy and non smoking.
Note: 4 mg of theophylline is equivalent to 5 mg aminophylline. Some authorities would regard these doses as low.

less than 5 minutes, if CNS and cardiovascular side-effects are to be avoided. As with all xanthines, theophylline must be administered with caution to all patients with cardiac disease or hepatic disease. The margin between therapeutic and toxic plasma levels of theophylline is small so that overdosage, as shown by tachycardia and fall in blood pressure, is easily reached. Monitoring of serum levels is now advised to overcome individual pharmacokinetic variations. This is particularly recommended in children and the elderly, who are faster and slower metabolisers of theophylline respectively. The optimal serum theophylline level is probably about 10 microgram/ml.

In pregnancy, theophylline is transferred to the foetus. Theophylline is secreted into breast milk and high levels may arise following intravenous injections. Breast feeding should be avoided for 6 to 8 hours following intravenous administration of theophylline.

Side-effects: Nausea and vomiting occur rarely.

Overdosage: The toxic effects of excessive treatment concern the cardiovascular system (tachycardia, hypertension) and the CNS (anxiety, insomnia and agitation, fits). Treatment is symptomatic. Serum potassium should be estimated and hypokalaemia treated. Peritoneal dialysis, haemodialysis and charcoal haemoperfusion have been used to supplement drug elimination.

Drug interactions: The bronchodilator and toxic effects of theophylline may be enhanced by sympathomimetics, including beta-adrenoceptor stimulants, and by other xanthines.

Xanthines can potentiate hypokalaemia resulting from beta-2 agonist therapy, steroids, diuretics and hypoxia. Particular caution is advised in severe asthma. It is recommended that serum potassium levels are monitored in such situations.

Erythromycin, quinolones especially ciprofloxacin, frusemide, interferon, allopurinol, thiabendazole, oral contraceptives and particularly cimetidine raise serum theophylline levels. Three patients have been reported to have had a rapid elevation of theophylline concentrations when given intravenous hydrocortisone while already receiving an infusion of theophylline. Monitoring for signs of theophylline toxicity is therefore advisable in similar circumstances. Theophylline toxicity has been described in children having a febrile viral illness and in individuals immunised with influenza vaccine. Smoking reduces the half life of theophylline, as do carbamazepine, phenytoin, rifampicin and sulphinpyrazone. The effects of phenytoin and lithium salts are reduced by concomitant theophylline. A low dose may provide safe antagonism to diazepam sedation.

Incompatibilities: Are similar to those of aminophylline. Theophylline is incompatible in infusion fluids with fructose, insulin, cimetidine, hydralazine, isoprenaline, noradrenaline, phenytoin sodium, and vitamin B and C injection. Theophylline is also incompatible with many antibiotics including benzylpenicillin, cephalothin, clindamycin, gentamicin, methicillin, tetracycline and vancomycin.

Pharmaceutical precautions Store at below 25 degrees; do not freeze.

Legal category POM.

Package quantities 10.

Further information Nil.

Product licence number 0118/0020.

LABOPRIN*

Presentation A round, scored tablet, white with brown flecks, containing 300 mg aspirin and 245 mg lysine.

Uses For the relief of headache, musculo-skeletal pains, arthralgia, pain and inflammation due to rheumatoid and other forms of arthritis.

Dosage and administration *Adults:* 1–3 tablets every 4–6 hours as necessary; maximum 12 tablets daily.

Children: Due to the possible development of Reye's Syndrome, Laboprin is not recommended in children under 12 years old except under close supervision, for example Still's disease.

Contra-indications, warnings, etc Peptic ulcer, dyspepsia, allergy to aspirin such as asthma, haemophilia, concurrent anticoagulant therapy.

Precautions: Use with care in patients with chronic renal insufficiency or hepatic disorder and in pregnancy, particularly avoiding large doses in late pregnancy and in lactation. There is an added risk of erosive gastritis if taken with alcohol, corticosteroids and nonsteroidal anti-inflammatory drugs.

Drug interaction: The activity of coumarin anticoagulants, heparin and hypoglycaemic agents is increased. The effects of other drugs may be altered, particularly uricosuric agents, methotrexate, spironolactone and corticosteroids. There is potentiation by metoclopramide and phenytoin is potentiated by aspirin.

Overdosage: Treatment is that of salicylate poisoning; gastric aspiration and lavage (gastric lavage is worthwhile even if there is delay in treating aspirin self-poisoning), correction of dehydration and of hypokalaemia; cautious use of sodium bicarbonate for the acidosis; intravenous vitamin K. If salicylate level exceeds 500 mg/l administer forced alkaline diuresis but if greater than 900 mg/l consider haemoperfusion and haemodialysis. Self-poisoning has been successfully treated by resin or charcoal haemoperfusion.

The above notes apply to all forms of oral aspirin.

Pharmaceutical precautions Laboprin tablets are extremely hygroscopic. They should be kept in the manufacturer's original container. The inner seal and screw cap should be replaced immediately after use. If discoloration or swelling takes place, the tablets should not be used.

Legal category GSL.

Package quantities 20 tablets per bottle.

Further information Nil.

Product licence number 0118/5006.

LABOSEPT* PASTILLES

Presentation Hexagonal red pastilles each containing Dequalinium Chloride BP 0.25 mg in a slow dissolving gelatine base.

Uses For bacterial and fungal infections of the mouth and throat.

Dosage and administration *Adults and children:* To be sucked slowly every three or four hours. For maximum benefit pastilles should be lodged comfortably between gum and cheek rather than be chewed. The daily dose should not exceed eight pastilles.

Contra-indications, warnings, etc Side effects and ill-effects from overdosage have not been reported.

Pharmaceutical precautions No special precautions.

Legal category P.

Package quantities Carton containing 20 pastilles.

Further information Contains no sugar.

Product licence number 0118/0012.

MONPHYTOL*

Presentation A colourless, rapidly drying, non-greasy paint containing chlorbutol 3%, methyl undecylenate 5%, propyl undecylenate 0.7%, salicylic acid 3%, methyl salicylate 25%, and propyl salicylate 5%.

Uses Monphytol is indicated for tinea pedis, tinea unguium, tinea circinata, erosio interdigitalis, intertrigo.

Dosage and administration *Adults over 12:* Twice daily moisten brush with Monphytol and apply to the affected parts, reaching gently into the folds of the skin. Treatment should be repeated from time to time after the condition has subsided to prevent reinfection.

Children under 12, pregnant and lactating women: The safety of this product has not been demonstrated for these groups. Its use must be at the physician's discretion.

Contra-indications, warnings, etc Monphytol may sting sensitive weeping areas of acutely inflamed skin. Other treatment (to reduce inflammation and exudation) may first be necessary. Monphytol should not be used on bleeding areas.

Pharmaceutical precautions Store away from heat.

Legal category P.

Package quantities Bottles containing 18 ml.

Further information Nil.

Product licence number 0118/5010R.

VOLITAL*

Presentation Round white, bi-convex tablets scored and marked P9 and containing 20 mg pemoline.

Uses As part of the treatment of hyperkinetic syndrome in children. Before prescribing Volital a positive diagnosis must be made based on careful documentation of mental state, behaviour assessment, past development, neurological and psychological function and family relationship, with symptom rating both from parents and teachers. Psychosis and severe mental retardation must be excluded and the accepted symptoms of restlessness, impaired attention, and impulsivity, must be present. The short term benefit of pemoline has been established; its value for longer periods of one or more years with trials comparing it with placebo remains undecided. There is no certainty that the future status of the patient will have been improved by medication in childhood. Medication alone is not sufficient treatment but must be accompanied by consideration of remedial education, parental counselling, and family therapy. The opinion of a child psychiatrist or specialist paediatrician should be sought.

The treatment is not recommended for children under 6 years old.

Dosage and administration Initially one tablet (20 mg) each morning, increasing by weekly increments of one tablet (20 mg) to a level of 60 mg but still given once daily. If there is no improvement at 60 mg then the dosage may be gradually increased to a maximum of 120 mg. Signs of improvement should occur by about six weeks. Reduction in dosage according to the development of side-effects may be needed.

Optimum clinical benefit is achieved with a wide range of dosage and serum concentrations of large variation. Hence routine serum monitoring is not useful.

Contra-indications, warnings, etc Glaucoma, extrapyramidal disorders, hyperexcitable states (thyrotoxicosis). Nervousness and tachycardia may result from large doses.

Side-effects: Dryness of the mouth, stomach ache, sweating, palpitations, nausea, headache, irritability, excitability, night terrors have been reported. Most of these were transient or subsided with reduction of dosage. Cessation of treatment was rarely required.

More common are anorexia and insomnia (4% and 5% respectively in one trial) which respond also to adjustment of dosage. A hallucinatory paranoid state has been reported in one patient treated for narcolepsy.

Drug interactions: The possibility of interaction with monamine-oxidase inhibitors to produce hypertensive crises has been suggested, but there are no reports of this.

Pregnancy: The safe use of pemoline during pregnancy has not been established and therefore the physician must use his judgment in prescribing it.

Adverse effects: There can be temporary retardation in weight and stature during treatment, with, it has been suggested, an inverse relationship between drug dosage and growth velocity. (In one series, following cessation of one year of successful treatment, catch-up in growth occurred). If the problem appears it can usually be overcome by drug holidays during the period of the normal school vacations. Drug holidays can also be taken at the beginning of the school term to allow assessment by the teachers. One study has shown no change in growth hormone or somatostatin levels. A growth chart should be kept and entries made at three-monthly intervals, and also when the drug is withheld, recommenced and discontinued. Decision can then be made whether any growth retardation is sufficient to justify reduction in dosage.

Chorea has been reported in two cases; one related to overdosage and the other in a hyperactive epileptic boy after seven months of treatment, soon ceasing when treatment was stopped. Tics of face, head and shoulders are rare and occur about two months after beginning treatment and cease within two weeks of dose reduction. Gilles de la Tourette disorder is aggravated by pemoline. If the diagnosis was overlooked in a dyskinetic child, pemoline might be held to have produced the disorder. The possibility of this diagnosis should be considered in any patient manifesting or having a history of tic.

There are isolated reports of mania and depression.

Addiction and tolerance: Addiction has not been described in children treated for hyperkinesia, nor has tolerance developed requiring increased dosage with time. Minor addiction in adolescents or adults, though so far not reported, might occur and therefore pemoline should not be prescribed for fatigue.

Abuse: There is one report of abuse by a 38-year-old physician who had abused other drugs from the age of twenty. Worries have been aired that adult patients might abuse the drug or sell it on the open market, but such fears have so far not materialised.

Toxic effects: Reports of liver enzyme abnormalities are conflicting; none occurring in some long term series or the incidence was no greater than observed in patients receiving placebo and found to be transient or reversible with cessation of treatment. There are reports of morbidity due to drug related hepatic disorders. Monitoring of the liver enzyme levels is not essential but values could be taken as a precaution before starting treatment.

Neutropenia has been reported once with recovery in six months.

A high level of prostatic acid phosphatase was found in a 63-year old male which returned to normal when pemoline was discontinued and then remained normal. He was being treated successfully for daytime sleepiness and was considered to have benign prostatic hypertrophy.

Accidental poisoning: There are two reports, one of a girl aged 23 months who suffered hyperactivity, tachycardia, hypertension and an epileptic fit; the other was a boy aged 35 months who become hyperactive, vomited and showed sucking of the tongue and choreiform movements, but no change in heart rate or blood pressure, remained co-operative and recovered in 4 days.

Gastric lavage may be undertaken up to 4 hours after ingestion. Treatment with diazepam and intravenous fluids should be given.

Pharmaceutical precautions To be kept cool and dry.

Legal category POM.

Further information Nil.

Product licence number 0118/5012R.

**Trade Mark*

Lagap Pharmaceuticals Ltd
Woolmer Way
Bordon
Hants GU35 9QE

CARBO DOME* CREAM

Presentation
Active ingredients: Coal Tar Solution BP 10% w/w.

Inactive ingredients: Dehydag Wax; Beeswax; White Soft Paraffin; Light Liquid Paraffin; Glycerol; Sodium Lauryl Sulphate; Methyl p-hydroxy benzoate.

Form and appearance: Carbo Dome Cream is a buff-coloured cream containing the active ingredient in a water-miscible base which is adjusted to the pH range of normal skin.

Uses
Actions: The coal tar solution in Carbo Dome Cream has a keratoplastic and antipruritic effect in psoriasis.

Indications: Psoriasis.

Dosage and administration For topical application only. Apply to the affected areas two or three times daily. This dosage is recommended for both children and adults.

Contra-indications, warnings, etc
Contra-indications: Known sensitivity to any of the ingredients.

Precautions: For external use only. Keep away from eyes.

Overdosage: Not applicable.

Main side-effects/adverse reactions: None reported.

Pharmaceutical precautions *Storage:* Store in a cool place.

Legal category P.

Package quantities 30 g and 100 g tubes.

Further information If sensitivity occurs, or if infection appears, discontinue use and institute appropriate therapy.

Carbo Dome Cream is a non-staining preparation of coal tar.

Product licence number 4416/0106.

Carbo Dome is a trade mark of Miles Inc, USA.

INDOLAR* SR

Presentation Blue/colourless capsules containing white sustained release beads. Each capsule containing 75 mg Indomethacin BP.

Inactive ingredients: Sucrose; Lactose.

Uses Non-steroidal analgesic and anti-inflammatory agent indicated in active rheumatoid arthritis, osteoarthritis, ankylosing spondylitis. Also indicated in periarticular disorders such as bursitis, tendinitis, synovitis, tenosynovitis and capsulitis. Also indicated in inflammation, pain and oedema following orthopaedic procedures.

Dosage and administration Indolar SR Capsules should always be given with food or milk to reduce the chance of gastro-intestinal disturbance.

Adults: One capsule once or twice daily, depending on patient needs and response.

Safety in children has not been established.

Particular care should be taken with older patients who are more susceptible to side-effects from indomethacin.

To minimise the evolution of unwanted reactions it is helpful in chronic conditions to start the therapy with a low dosage, increasing as required.

Contra-indications, warnings, etc
Contra-indications: Patients with angioneurotic oedema or who have, with aspirin or other non-steroidal anti-inflammatory drugs experienced acute asthmatic attacks, urticaria or rhinitis.

Active peptic ulcer, a history of recurrent gastro-intestinal lesions, sensitivity to indomethacin or to aspirin.

Not to be used during pregnancy or during lactation as indomethacin is secreted in breast milk.

Safety in children has not been established.

The most common side-effects are headache, dizziness and dyspepsia; patients should be warned that they may experience dizziness and should therefore avoid driving or undertaking other activities which require full alertness. If headache persists even after dosage reduction indomethacin should be withdrawn.

Gastro-intestinal disorders which occur can be reduced by giving indomethacin with food, milk or antacids. Ulceration of the oesophagus, stomach or duodenum may also occur, accompanied by haemorrhage and perforation (a few fatalities have been reported).

Intestinal ulceration has rarely been associated with stenosis and obstruction. Also, bleeding without obvious ulceration and perforation of pre-existing sigmoid lesions (such as a diverticulum or carcinoma) have occurred; and increased abdominal pain in patients with ulcerative colitis (or the development of this condition) and regional ileitis have been rarely reported. If gastro-intestinal bleeding does occur treatment with indomethacin should be discontinued.

Blood dyscrasias, particularly thrombocytopenia have been reported.

Oedema and increased blood pressure also sometimes occur, as does haematuria.

Hypersensitivity reactions include pruritus, urticaria, angiitis, erythema nodosum. Skin rash and hair loss may also occur.

Acute respiratory distress, including sudden dyspnoea and asthma, have been reported on rare occasions. Bronchospasm may be precipitated in patients suffering from, or with a previous history of, bronchial asthma or allergic disease.

Indomethacin should be used with caution in patients with hepatic or renal dysfunction. Hepatitis and jaundice have been reported rarely.

Non-steroidal anti-inflammatory drugs may precipitate renal decompensation in those with renal or hepatic dysfunction, diabetes mellitus, advanced age, extracellular volume depletion, congestive cardiac failure, sepsis or concomitant use of other nephrotoxic drugs. Also, there have been reports of acute interstitial nephritis with haematuria, proteinuria and occasionally the nephrotic syndrome in long-term therapy with indomethacin.

In common with other anti-inflammatory analgesic antipyretic agents, indomethacin may mask the signs and symptoms of infectious disease and this should be borne in mind in order to avoid delay in starting treatment for infection.

Indomethacin should be used with caution in patients with an existing, albeit controlled infection.

Particular care should be taken with older patients who are more susceptible to side-effects from indomethacin.

Interactions with other medicaments and other forms of interaction: Co-administration of diflunisal with Indomethacin increases the plasma level of Indomethacin by about a third with a concomitant decrease in renal clearance. Fatal gastro-intestinal haemorrhage has occurred. The combination should not be used.

Use of indomethacin with aspirin or other salicylates is not recommended because there is no enhancement of therapeutic effect while the incidence of gastro-intestinal side-effects is increased. Moreover, co-administration of aspirin may decrease the blood concentration of indomethacin.

Indomethacin may decrease the tubular secretion of methotrexate thus potentiating toxicity; simultaneous use should be undertaken with caution.

Patients receiving anticoagulants should be observed carefully for alteration of prothrombin time even though clinical studies suggest no influence from indomethacin on hypoprothrombinaemia induced by anticoagulants.

Indomethacin can inhibit platelet aggregation – an effect which disappears within 24 hours of discontinuation; the bleeding time may be prolonged and this effect may be exaggerated in patients with an underlying haemostatic defect.

Indomethacin and triamterine should not be administered together since reversible renal failure may be induced.

Co-administration of probenecid may increase plasma levels of Indomethacin.

Because Indomethacin may reduce the antihypertensive effect of beta-blockers, patients receiving dual therapy should have the antihypertensive effect of their therapy reassessed.

If the patient is receiving corticosteroids concomitantly, a reduction in dosage of these may be possible, but should only be affected slowly under supervision.

Indomethacin is an inhibitor of prostaglandin synthesis and therefore the following drug interactions may occur; Indomethacin may raise plasma lithium levels and reduce renal lithium clearance in subjects with steady state plasma lithium concentrations. At the onset of such combined therapy, plasma lithium concentration should be monitored more frequently.

Indomethacin may reduce the diuretic and antihypertensive effect of thiazides and frusemide in some patients. Indomethacin may cause blocking of the frusemide-induced increase in plasma renin activity.

It is reported that a few patients receiving non-steroidal anti-inflammatory drugs manifest borderline elevations in liver function test results; if these persist or worsen or symptoms of liver disease, a rash or eosinophilia develop, treatment with indomethacin should be stopped. Periodic assessments to detect, at an early stage, unwanted effects on peripheral blood (anaemia) and liver function are advisable. The dexamethasone suppression test may give false negative results. An increase in plasma potassium concentration (including hyperkalaemia) has been reported even in the absence of renal impairment. Since indomethacin is eliminated primarily by the kidney, patients with impaired renal function should be monitored closely and a lower daily dosage may be needed to avoid accumulation.

Warnings and adverse reactions:

CNS: Headache, dizziness or lightheadedness, depression, vertigo and fatigue are not uncommon; infrequently there may be confusion, anxiety or other psychiatric disturbance, drowsiness, convulsions, neuropathy or paraesthesia, involuntary movements, insomnia, aggravation of epilepsy or Parkinsonism. All are often transient and likely to abate or disappear with reduced or ceased dosage.

Gastro-intestinal: Nausea, anorexia, vomiting, epigastric discomfort or abdominal pain, constipation or diarrhoea all have been reported; more rarely, stomatitis, flatulence, ulceration at any point in the gastro-intestinal tract (even with resultant stenosis and obstruction), bleeding (even without obvious ulceration or from a diverticulum) and perforation of pre-existing sigmoid lesions have all been reported.

Hepatic: Rarely hepatitis and jaundice (some fatalities have been reported).

Cardiovascular/renal: Oedema, increased blood pressure, hypotension, tachycardia, chest pain, arrhythmia, palpitations, congestive cardiac failure, elevation of blood urea and haematuria all have been reported infrequently.

In patients with renal, cardiac or hepatic impairment caution is required since the use of non-steroidal anti-inflammatory drugs may result in deterioration of renal function. The dose should be kept as low as possible and renal function should be monitored.

Non-steroidal anti-inflammatory drugs have been reported to cause nephrotoxicity in various forms and their use can lead to interstitial nephritis, nephrotic syndrome and renal failure.

Dermatological/hypersensitivity: Itching, urticaria, angioneurotic oedema, angiitis, erythema nodosum, rash and exfoliative dermatitis all have been reported infrequently – as have Stevens Johnson syndrome erythema multiforme, toxic epidermal necrolysis, hair loss, acute anaphylaxis (including acute loss of blood pressure) and acute respiratory distress (including sudden dyspnoea, asthma and pulmonary oedema). There may be bronchospasm in patients with a history of bronchial asthma or other allergic disease.

Haematological: Blood dyscrasias (thrombocytopenia, leucopenia, petechiae, ecchymosis, purpura, aplastic or haemolytic anaemia, agranulocytosis and bone marrow depression, disseminated intravascular coagulation) may occur infrequently.

Ocular: Blurred vision and orbital and peri-orbital pain are seen infrequently. Corneal deposits and retinal disturbances have been reported in some patients with rheumatoid arthritis on prolonged therapy with indomethacin, and ophthalmic examinations are desirable in patients given prolonged treatment.

Aural: Tinnitus, or hearing disturbance (rarely deafness) have been reported.

Genito-urinary: Proteinuria, nephrotic syndrome, interstitial nephritis, renal insufficiency or failure all have been reported.

Other: Hyperglycaemia, glycosuria, hyperkalaemia, vaginal bleeding, epistaxis, breast changes (enlargement, tenderness, gynaecomastia), flushing, sweating and ulcerative stomatitis all have been reported rarely.

Overdosage: Many of the unwanted symptoms associated with indomethacin therapy may be seen. Treatment is symptomatic and supportive – emptying the stomach by induction of vomiting and/or lavage and use of activated charcoal. Antacid therapy may be useful. Close monitoring thereafter is required because intestinal ulceration may develop. It can be noted that indomethacin has a biphasic plasma elimination with the terminal phase showing a half-life ranging between 2 and 12 hours.

Pharmaceutical precautions Store in a cool, dry place and protect from light.

Legal category POM.

Package quantities 100 capsules.

Further information Nil.

Product licence number 4416/0066.

METROLYL*

Presentation *Metrolyl Tablets* containing 200 mg and 400 mg Metronidazole BP. 200 mg – white, breakline on one side, LAGAP on reverse. 400 mg – white, marked II breakline 400 on one side, LAGAP on reverse.

Metrolyl Suppositories containing 500 mg Metronidazole BP and 1 g Metronidazole BP.

Metrolyl Injection (for intravenous infusion) 0.5 per cent w/v in 100 ml PVC minibags (500 mg metronidazole per 100 ml).

Inactive ingredients: Metrolyl Tablets – Lactose; Metrolyl Injection – Sodium Chloride; Metrolyl Suppositories – Witepsol.

Oral dosage regime for Metrolyl

	Adults/Children over 10yrs	*Children 7–10 yrs*	*Children 3–7 yrs*	*Children 1–3 yrs*
Urogenital trichomoniasis (treat sexual partners concurrently)	200 mg tds × 7 d or 800 mg morning + 1200 mg evening × 2 d or 2 g once	100 mg tds × 7 d	100 mg bd × 7 d	50 mg tds × 7 d
Amoebiasis: (a) invasive intestinal disease in susceptible subjects	800 mg tds × 5 d	400 mg tds × 5 d	200 mg qds × 5 d	200 mg tds × 5 d
(b) intestinal disease in less susceptible subjects and chronic amoebic hepatitis	400 mg tds × 5–10 d	200 mg tds × 5–10 d	100 mg qds × 5–10 d	100 mg tds × 5–10 d
(c) amoebic liver abscess + other forms of extra-intestinal amoebiasis	400 mg tds × 5 d	200 mg tds × 5 d	100 mg qds × 5 d	100 mg tds × 5 d
(d) symptomless cyst passers	400 mg–800 mg tds × 5–10 d	200 mg–400 mg tds × 5–10 d	100 mg–200 mg qds × 5–10 d	100 mg–200 mg tds × 5–10 d
Giardiasis:	2000 mg od × 3 d	1000 mg od × 3 d	600 mg–800 mg od × 3 d	500 mg od × 3 d
Acute ulcerative gingivitis:	200 mg tds × 3 d	100 mg tds × 3 d	100 mg bd × 3 d	50 mg tds × 3 d
Acute dental infections:	200 mg tds × 3–7 d			

Proportionately smaller dosages should be given to children and babies weighing less than 10 kg.

Uses 1. Treatment of infections in which anaerobic bacteria have been identified or are suspected as pathogens, particularly *Bacteroides fragilis* and other species of bacteroides and including other species for which metronidazole is bactericidal e.g. fusobacteria, eubacteria, clostridia and anaerobic cocci.

Metrolyl can be used in septicaemia, bacteraemia, brain abscess, necrotising pneumonia, osteomyelitis, puerperal sepsis, pelvic abscess, peritonitis and post operative wound infection from which one or more of these anaerobes have been isolated.

2. Prevention of post operative infections due to anaerobic bacteria.
3. Use in treatment of acute ulcerative gingivitis and acute dental, pericoronitis and apical infections.
4. Trichomonas infections.
5. Amoebiasis.
6. Giardiasis.

Dosage and administration Seven days treatment should be satisfactory for most patients. Prolonged treatment can be used if the physician considers it to be necessary.

Metrolyl tablets should be swallowed with water, during or after a meal.

1. Treatment of anaerobic infections

A. Oral medication: Metrolyl tablets may be given alone or in association with other appropriate bactericidal agents. Adults and children over 10 years: 400 mg three times daily. Children under 10 years: 7.5 mg per kg body weight three times daily.

B. Rectal medication: Rectal administration using Metrolyl Suppositories can be used in patients for whom oral medication is not possible or is contra-indicated. The suppositories may be administered alone or concurrently with other bacteriologically appropriate antibacterial agents.

Treatment of anaerobic infections: Adults and children over 10 years: 1 gram suppository inserted into the rectum eight-hourly for three days. If rectal medication must be continued for more than three days the suppositories should be inserted at 12-hourly intervals. Children (5 to 10 years): As for adults *but* with 500 mg suppositories three times daily. Infants and children under five years: As for children of 5 to 10 years *but* with appropriate reduction in dosage of suppositories (one-half of a 500 mg suppository for one to five years and one-quarter of a 500 mg suppository for under one year).

C. Intravenous medication: Intravenous medication can be used in patients with severe anaerobic infections for whom oral medication is not possible: it is particularly useful in emergencies and is indicated in patients needing surgery who:

Have anaerobic sepsis such as septicaemia, peritonitis, subphrenic or pelvic abscesses.

At operation shown signs of established or impending anaerobic sepsis.

Undergo operations in which contamination occurs with anaerobes from the gastro intestinal or female genital tract or the oropharynx.

In infants and other patients maintained on intravenous fluids, Metrolyl Injection may be diluted with appropriate volumes of normal saline, dextrose-saline, dextrose 5% w/v or potassium chloride injections (20 mmol and 40 mmol.)

Treatment: Adults and children over 10 years: 100 ml (500 mg metronidazole) by intravenous injection eight hourly. Injection should be infused intravenously at the rate of 5 ml per minute but may be administered alone or concurrently (but separately) with other appropriate antibacterial agents in parenteral dosage forms. Oral medication (400 mg 3 times daily) should be substituted as soon as possible.

Children under 10 years: As for adults *but* single dose is based on 1.5 ml (7.5 mg metronidazole) per kg body weight every eight hours and the oral dose at 7.5 mg/kg body weight.

2. Prevention of anaerobic infections

A. Oral medication:

(a) Gynaecological surgery: Adults: 1 gram orally as a single dose followed by 200 mg orally 3 times daily until pre-operative witholding of solids and liquids by mouth becomes necessary. Oral medication with 200 mg 3 times daily should be resumed after the operation and for up to 7 days.

(b) Pre-operative medication for elective colonic surgery: Adults: 200 mg orally six hourly co-administered with an aminoglycoside antibiotic for 3 days before surgery; or 400 mg orally 8 hourly with phthalylsulphathiazole (2.5 g six hourly) for 4 days before surgery.

B. Rectal medication: In appendicectomy: Adults and

children over 10 years: 1 gram suppository inserted into the rectum two hours before surgery and repeated at eight-hourly intervals. If rectal medication is necessary after the third post-operative day, the frequency of administration should be reduced to 12-hourly.

Children (5 to 10 years): 500 mg suppositories administered as for adults.

C. Intravenous medication: Adults and children over 10 years: 100 ml (500 mg) by intravenous infusion immediately before, during or after operation, followed by the same dose eight hourly until oral medication (200 to 400 mg 3 times daily) can be given to complete a seven day course.

Children under 10 years: As for adults *but* the single intravenous dose is based on 1.5 ml (7.5 mg metronidazole) per kg body weight and the oral dose on 3.7 to 7.5 mg per kg body weight.

Contra-indications, warnings, etc There are no known absolute contra-indications for the use of Metrolyl. However, known sensitivity to metronidazole is an absolute contra-indication.

Precautions: Recommended doses are given as a guideline based on experience. If therapy is to continue for longer than 10 days clinical and laboratory monitoring is advised.

Clinicians considering continuous therapy for relief of chronic conditions are advised to consider the therapeutic benefit against risk of peripheral neuropathy.

Underlying gonococcal infection may persist after elimination of Trichomonas vaginalis.

Pregnancy: The safety of use of metronidazole in pregnancy has not been established and its uses should be avoided; if essential, short high-dose regimes should *not* be used. Metronidazole is excreted in milk and no adverse effects in the newborn have been reported; the intake by the suckling infant of a mother receiving normal dosage is less than a therapeutic dose for the infants.

No dose modification is needed in renal failure since the elimination half-life of metronidazole is unchanged in this condition. The clinical significance of retained metabolites is not known; their efficient removal occurs during dialysis so that metronidazole should be re-administered after haemodialysis. No dosage adjustment is needed for patients undergoing intermittent or continuous ambulatory peritoneal dialysis.

Impairment of metronidazole clearance may occur in patients with advanced hepatic insufficiency since the drug is mainly metabolized by hepatic oxidation. High concentrations of metronidazole may contribute to the symptoms of hepatic encephalopathy – a condition in which significant cumulation may occur. Dose reduction to one-third once daily may be needed.

The consumption of alcohol during metronidazole therapy should be avoided since there could be a disulfiram-like reaction.

Potentiation of warfarin-type (but not heparin) anticoagulant therapy has been reported so that dose adjustment of the anticoagulant may be needed.

Lithium retention with evidence of possible renal damage has been reported where this compound and metronidazole have been used concurrently; preferably, apart from monitoring lithium, creatinine and electrolyte concentrations, lithium therapy should be tapered and/or withdrawn before use of metronidazole.

The half-life of metronidazole is reduced from 7–8 hours to about 3 hours in patients receiving phenobarbitone.

In patients taking metronidazole, the assay of aspartate amino transferase may give spuriously low values; this depends on the method used.

Metronidazole has no activity against aerobic or facultative anaerobic bacteria.

Adverse effects: Serious reactions are rare.

An unpleasant taste in the mouth, furred tongue, nausea, vomiting or other gastro-intestinal disturbance have been reported.

Urticaria, skin rash, pruritis, angioedema and rarely anaphylaxis have occurred.

Drowsiness, dizziness, headache, ataxia and darkening of the urine (due to metabolites) have been reported rarely.

Peripheral neuropathy and/or transient epileptiform seizures have occurred during prolonged or intensive treatment but in most cases neuropathy disappears on cessation of therapy.

A moderate, reversible leucopenia has been reported in some patients.

Overdosage: There is no specific treatment and uneventful recovery has followed ingestion of up to 12 g.

Pharmaceutical precautions Store in a cool dry place, protect from light. The injection is not intended for multi-dose use.

Legal category POM.

Package quantities 200 mg tablets – packs of 250. 400 mg tablets – packs of 100. 500 mg suppository – packs of 10. 1 g suppository – packs of 10. 100 ml PVC minibag containing 500 mg metronidazole BP – packs of 10.

Product licence numbers

Metrolyl 200 mg Tablets	4416/0060
Metrolyl 400 mg Tablets	4416/0061
Metrolyl 500 mg suppository	4416/0053
Metrolyl 1 g suppository	4416/0054
Metrolyl Injection 500 mg/100 ml	4416/0010

PHASAL*

Presentation White sustained-release tablets marked on one side with 'P' inside a hexagon. Each Phasal tablet contains 300 mg Lithium Carbonate BP.

Inactive ingredient: Parabens.

Uses Lithium is an antimanic agent, it can also exert a stabilising influence on recurrent affective disorders.

Recommended uses: 1. Treatment of acute manic or hypomanic episodes. 2. Prophylaxis in manic-depressive disorders, recurrent mania or recurrent depression.

Dosage and administration Dosage may be adjusted in the individual patient according to clinical condition and the results of regular blood lithium determinations.

1. Acute episode: Initially 2 tablets b.d. Increase by 1 or 2 tablets per day if no response. Maintain blood lithium levels in the range 0.5–1.5 mmol. Dosage should be reduced rapidly once the initial attack subsides.

2. Prophylaxis: Usually 600–1,200 mg/day given in divided doses. Clinical improvement is usually associated with serum concentrations of 0.5 mmol or above. Toxic symptoms are usually associated with concentrations exceeding 1.5 mmol.

When starting directly on prophylactic therapy administer 2 tablets daily initially, with subsequent increments of 1 tablet until therapeutic blood levels are achieved.

Use in elderly: 500–1,000 mg/day given in divided doses. Toxic symptoms are likely with serum concentrations above 1.0 mmol.

Use in children: The use of lithium in children is not recommended.

Measurement of serum lithium concentrations: Lithium therapy should not be initiated unless adequate facilities for routine monitoring of serum concentrations are available. On initiation of therapy, serum concentrations should be measured weekly until stabilisation is achieved, then weekly for one month and at monthly intervals thereafter. Additional measurements should be made if signs of lithium toxicity occur (see below), on dosage alteration, development of significant intercurrent disease, signs of manic or depressive relapse and if significant change in sodium or fluid intake occurs. More frequent monitoring is required if patients are receiving diuretics. With Phasal maximum blood levels normally occur within two to four hours of dosing.

As bioavailability varies from product to product (particularly with regard to substained-release preparations) a change of product should be regarded as initiation of new treatment. Blood levels should therefore be monitored weekly until re-estabilisation is achieved.

Tablets must be swallowed whole, not chewed.

Contra-indications, warnings, etc
Contra-indications: Renal or cardiovascular disease, Addison's disease, hypothyroidism, sodium depletion or conditions requiring low sodium intake. Lithium should not be given to mothers who are breast feeding a child.

Use in pregnancy and lactation: There is epidemiological evidence that the drug may be harmful in human pregnancy. Should the use of lithium be unavoidable, close monitoring of serum concentrations should be made throughout the pregnancy and during parturition. Lithium should not be given to mothers who are breast feeding a child.

Precautions: Pre-treatment and periodic routine clinical monitoring is essential. This should include assessment of renal function, urine analysis, assessment of thyroid function and cardiac function, especially in patients with cardiovascular disease. Patients should be euthyroid before the initiation of lithium therapy. Clear instructions regarding the symptoms of impending toxicity should be given by the doctor to all patients receiving long-term lithium therapy (see Warnings and Adverse Effects). Patients should also be warned to report if polyuria or polydypsia develop. Episodes of nausea and vomiting or other conditions leading to salt/water depletion (including severe dieting) should also be reported. Patients should be advised to maintain their usual salt and fluid intake. Elderly patients are particularly liable to lithium toxicity.

Drug interactions: Lithium should only be given with great care to patients taking diuretics. Lower doses of lithium may be needed during diuretic therapy as lithium clearance is reduced. In some cases, a paradoxical antidiuretic effect leading to water retention has been reported following the use of diuretics during treatment with lithium salts. There is a possibility of water intoxication and lithium intoxication where diuretics and lithium salts are co-prescribed.

Raised plasma levels of the ADH may occur during lithium therapy. Symptoms of nephrotoxic diabetes are particularly prevalent in patients receiving concurrent treatment with tri/tetracyclic antidepressants. Serum lithium concentrations may increase during concomitant therapy with indomethacin or tetracycline.

Warnings and adverse effects: Long-term treatment with lithium may result in permanent changes in the kidney and impairment of renal function. High serum concentrations of lithium, including episodes of acute lithium toxicity may enhance these changes. The minimum clinically effective dose of lithium should always be used. Patients should be maintained on lithium after 3–5 years only if, on assessment, benefit persists.

Renal function should be routinely monitored in patients with polyuria and polydypsia.

Side-effects are usually related to serum lithium concentrations and are infrequent at levels below 1.0 mmol.

Mild gastrointestinal effects, nausea, vertigo, muscle weakness and a dazed feeling may occur, but frequently disappear after stabilisation. Fine hand tremors, polyuria and mild thirst may persist.

Long term treatment with lithium is frequently associated with disturbances of thyroid function including goitre, hypothyroidism and thyrotoxicosis.

Mild cognitive impairment may occur during long term use.

Hypercalcaemia, hypermagnesaemia, hyperparathyroidism and an increase in antinuclear antibodies have also been reported.

Exacerbation of psoriasis may occur.

Signs of impending toxicity: Appearance or aggravation of gastrointestinal symptoms, muscle weakness, lack of co-ordination, drowsiness or lethargy may be early signs of intoxication. With increasing toxicity there is ataxia, giddiness, tinnitus, blurred vision, coarse tremor, muscle twitching and a large output of dilute urine. At blood levels above 2–3 mmol/l, there is increasing disorientation, seizures, coma and death.

Overdosage: Early signs of toxicity usually respond to reduction or cessation of dosage.

There is no specific antidote for lithium poisoning. Treatment comprises general supportive measures and maintenance of electrolyte balance. Elimination of lithium may be facilitated by infusion of sodium bicarbonate, acetazolamide, urea or mannitol.

Prolonged continuous peritoneal dialysis may be more effective than haemodialysis.

Pharmaceutical precautions Store in a cool dry place.

Legal category POM.

Package quantities Securitainers of 60 tablets.

Further information Phasal is a sustained release preparation designed to facilitate control of blood lithium levels within the optimum range. The smaller diurnal variation provided by the use of a sustained release tablet: (i) reduces the risk of rapid and excessive absorption of lithium and thereby improves safety; (ii) maintains the desired blood levels and so provides continuous protection against relapse; (iii) improves convenience of dosing for the patient.

Product licence number 4416/0076

TRIPERIDOL*

Presentation Tablets 500 micrograms: White uncoated circular tablets, half-scored, marked T above 0.5 on one side, Janssen on the other side. Each tablet contains trifluperidol hydrochloride equivalent to 500 micrograms trifluperidol.
Tablets 1 mg: White uncoated circular tablets, half-scored, marked T above 1 on one side and Janssen on the other side. Each tablet contains trifluperidol hydrochloride equivalent to 1 mg trifluperidol.

Inactive ingredients include: Lactose, corn starch and magnesium stearate.

Uses Triperidol is a neuroleptic of the butyrophenone series and is indicated for the treatment of symptoms of schizophrenia and prevention of relapse, other psychoses, especially paranoid, mania and hypomania.

Dosage and administration Triperidol tablets are for oral administration to both adults and children.

Dosage for all indications should be individually determined and is best initiated and titrated under close clinical supervision. To determine the initial dose, consideration should be given to the patient's age, severity of symptoms and previous response to other neuroleptics.

Patients who are elderly or debilitated or those with previously reported adverse reactions to neuroleptic drugs may require less Triperidol. The normal starting dose should be halved, followed by a gradual titration to achieve optimum response.

Adults: Initially 0.5 mg daily, increasing by 0.5 mg every 3–4 days to a maximum of 6–8 mg daily. A large dose, e.g. 3 mg can be administered initially and adjusted up or down according to the patients' response.

In adolescents a lower dose may be advisable.

Children 5–12 years: 0.25 mg per day, increasing as necessary to a maximum of 2 mg per day. In general, a maintenance dose of 1 mg per day will be required.

Contra-indications, warnings, etc
Contra-indications: Comatose states.

Use in pregnancy and lactation: The safety of Triperidol in pregnancy has not been established. There is evidence of harmful effects in some, but not all, animal studies. As with other drugs, it is not advisable to administer Triperidol in pregnancy.

Butyrophenones are excreted in breast milk. If the use of Triperidol is considered essential, breast feeding should be discontinued.

Precautions and warnings: Please also refer to 'Drug interactions' section.

Caution is advised in patients with liver disease, renal failure, Parkinson's disease, epilepsy and conditions predisposing to epilepsy or convulsions.

In schizophrenia, the response to antipsychotic drug treatment may not become apparent for several weeks or months.

Acute withdrawal symptoms including nausea, vomiting and insomnia, have very rarely been described after abrupt cessation of high doses of antipsychotic drugs. Relapse may also occur and gradual withdrawal is advisable.

Some degree of sedation or impairment of alertness may occur, particularly with higher doses and at the start of treatment and may be potentiated by alcohol. Patients should be advised not to drive or operate machinery during treatment until their susceptibility is known.

Drug interactions: In common with all neuroleptics, Triperidol can increase the central nervous system depression produced by other CNS-depressant drugs, including alcohol, hypnotics, sedatives or strong analgesics. An enhanced CNS effect has been reported when methyldopa has been given concomitantly with some butyrophenones.

Triperidol may antagonise the action of adrenaline and other sympathomimetic agents and may impair the antiparkinson effects of levodopa.

The dosage of anticonvulsants may need to be increased to take account of the lowered seizure threshold.

Adverse effects: In common with all neuroleptics, extrapyramidal symptoms may occur. Acute dystonias may occur early in treatment. Parkinsonian rigidity, tremor and akathisia tend to appear less rapidly. Oculogyric crises and laryngeal dystonias have been reported.

Tardive dyskinesia may occur during administration or after withdrawal of neuroleptic drugs, including Triperidol, and can be precipitated or aggravated by antiparkinson drugs.

The syndrome is unlikely to occur in the short-term when low or moderate doses of Triperidol are used as recommended, but since its occurrence may be related to duration of treatment, as well as daily dose, Triperidol should be given in the minimum effective dose for the minimum possible time unless it is established that long-term administration for the treatment of schizophrenia is required.

The potential seriousness and unpredictability of tardive dyskinesia, and the fact that it has occasionally been reported to occur when neuroleptic antipsychotic drugs have been prescribed for relatively short periods in low doses, means that the prescribing of such agents requires especially careful assessment of risks versus benefits.

Gastrointestinal symptoms, nausea, loss of appetite and dyspepsia have been reported.

Hormonal effects of antipsychotic neuroleptic drugs include hyperprolactinaemia, which may cause galactorrhoea, gynaecomastia and oligo- or amenorrhoea.

Weight changes may occur.

Dose-related hypotension is uncommon, but can occur, particularly in the elderly, who are more susceptible to the sedative and hypotensive effects.

Triperidol, even in low dosage in susceptible (especially non-psychotic) individuals, may cause unpleasant subjective feelings of being mentally dulled or slowed down, dizziness, headache or paradoxical effects of excitement, agitation or insomnia.

The following effects have been reported rarely: various skin rashes and reactions, jaundice or transient abnormalities of liver function in the absence of jaundice, confusional states or epileptic fits. Blood dyscrasias have been reported very rarely.

Overdose: There have been no serious toxic effects attributed to Triperidol and fatal overdosage has not been reported. Treatment of overdosage consists of supportive mesures combined with sedative or antiparkinsonian drugs as required.

Pharmaceutical precautions Triperidol tablets should be stored at room temperature.

Legal category POM.

Package quantities

500 microgram tablets:	100 in canisters
1 mg tablets:	100 in canisters.

Further information Nil.

Product licence numbers

Triperidol Tablets 500 micrograms	0242/5006R
Triperidol Tablets 1 mg	0242/5007R

**Trade Mark*

Lederle Laboratories

Cyanamid of Great Britain Limited
Fareham Road
Gosport, Hants PO13 0AS

ACHROMYCIN* (ORAL PREPARATIONS)

Presentation *Capsules 250 mg:* Each opaque, orange capsule printed 'Lederle 4874' contains 250 mg tetracycline hydrochloride.

Tablets 250 mg: Each orange tablet printed 'Lederle 4745' contains 250 mg tetracycline hydrochloride.

Powder 25 g: Each bottle contains 25 g tetracycline hydrochloride.

Uses Achromycin is a broad-spectrum antibiotic used for the treatment of infections caused by tetracycline-sensitive organisms. Typical indications include: Ear, nose and throat infections. Acute and chronic bronchitis. Pneumonia. Gastro-intestinal Infections. Urinary tract infections. Soft tissue infections. Acne. Typhus fever. Psittacosis. Other infections due to Achromycin-sensitive organisms. Achromycin is also indicated for prophylaxis before or after surgical and dental procedures.

Dosage and administration *Adults: (tablets, capsules):* 1 tablet or capsule four times a day. This may be increased to 6 or 8 tablets or capsules daily in severe infections.

Children: Not recommended for children under 8 years of age. Information on dosage is available on request where specifically indicated.

Elderly: Achromycin should be used with caution in the treatment of elderly patients where accumulation is a possibility.

Administration: Achromycin should be taken an hour before or two hours after meals and therapy should be continued for up to three days after characteristic symptoms of the infection have subsided.

Contra-indications, warnings, etc
Contra-indications: A history of hypersensitivity to tetracyclines. Overt renal insufficiency. Systemic lupus erythematosus.

Warnings: Tetracyclines may cause a yellow to brown discoloration of the teeth in the developing foetus or child and therefore Achromycin should only be administered if considered essential to pregnant women and young children under eight years of age. Achromycin should be used with caution in patients with renal or hepatic dysfunction, or in conjunction with other potentially hepatotoxic drugs. Cross-resistance between tetracyclines may develop in micro-organisms and cross-sensitisation in patients.

Precautions: Absorption of Achromycin is impaired by the concomitant administration of calcium, magnesium, iron and particularly aluminium salts commonly used as antacids. Tetracyclines depress plasma prothrombin activity therefore reduced dosages of concurrent anticoagulants may be required. Lower doses are indicated in cases of renal impairment to avoid excessive systemic accumulation, and if therapy is prolonged, serum level determinations are advisable.

The concomitant use of oral tetracyclines may reduce the efficacy of oral contraceptives; an increased incidence of breakthrough bleeding may also be experienced.

Side-effects: Gastro-intestinal disturbances may occur and as with all antibiotics overgrowth of resistant organisms may cause glossitis, stomatitis, vaginitis, or staphylococcal enterocolitis. Photosensitivity and dermatological reactions are rare. Occurrences of enamel hypoplasia have been reported. Bulging fontanelles in infants and benign intracranial hypertension in adults has been reported. Treatment should cease if evidence of raised intracranial pressure develops.

Overdosage: No specific antidote. Gastric lavage plus oral administration of milk or antacids.

Pharmaceutical precautions Achromycin Capsules and Tablets should be stored at controlled room temperature (15–30°C) in the original pack.

Achromycin Powder should be stored in a cool, dry place (8–15°C) in the original pack.

Legal category POM.

Package quantities *Capsules 250 mg:* Bottles of 100 and 1,000.

Tablets 250 mg: Bottles of 100 and 1,000.

Powder: Bottle of 25 g.

Further information Nil.

Product licence numbers

Capsules 250 mg	0095/0041
Tablets 250 mg	0095/5026
Powder	0095/5037

ACHROMYCIN* (TOPICAL PREPARATIONS)

Presentation *Achromycin Ointment 3%:* Each gram of yellow ointment contains tetracycline hydrochloride 30 mg, methylparaben 2.4%, propylparaben 0.6%, in a white soft paraffin and wool-fat base.

Achromycin Eye and Ear Ointment 1%: Each gram of yellow ointment contains 10 mg tetracycline hydrochloride in a white soft paraffin and wool-fat base.

Uses Achromycin is a broad-spectrum antibiotic.

Achromycin Ointment 3% is indicated for the treatment of superficial pyogenic infections of the skin and for the prevention of infection in wounds, abrasions and after surgery. It is indicated for local infections caused by both Gram-positive and Gram-negative organisms including Streptococci, Staphylococci and the Coli-aerogenes group.

Achromycin Eye and Ear Ointment and Achromycin is indicated for the treatment of susceptible ocular infections caused by Staphylococci, Pneumococci, H. influenzae, Diplococcus of Morax-Axenfeld *(H. lacunatus)*, Streptococci, *A. aerogenes, Proteus vulgaris, Proteus morganii, E. coli, Alcaligenes faecalis* and *Pseudomonas aeruginosa.*

Achromycin Eye and Ear Ointment is also indicated in the treatment of external otitis due to tetracycline-susceptible organisms.

Dosage and administration *Adults and children: Achromycin Ointment 3%:* Apply the ointment directly to the involved area, preferably on sterile gauze once or more daily as the condition indicates. In severe local infections, local treatment should be supplemented by oral therapy.

Achromycin Eye and Ear Ointment 1%: Apply directly to the affected area every two hours. Severe ocular infections may require treatment for many days, and may also require oral therapy.

Contra-indications, warnings, etc
Contra-indications: Achromycin Ointment, Achromycin Eye and Ear Ointment are contra-indicated in patients with a history of hypersensitivity to tetracycline hydrochloride or any other ingredient.

Precautions: The use of antibiotics may result in overgrowth of non-susceptible organisms. Constant observation of the patient is essential. If new infections appear during therapy, appropriate measures should be taken.

The concomitant use of oral tetracyclines may reduce the efficacy of oral contraceptives; an increased incidence of breakthrough bleeding may also be experienced.

Side-effects: Some patients may be allergic to any of the components.

If adverse reaction or idiosyncrasy occurs, discontinue medication.

Pharmaceutical precautions The products should be stored in a cool place (8–15°C) in the original pack. Dilution is not recommended.

Achromycin Ointment may cause a yellow staining of clothes. Following extended use a similar local staining of the skin may occur which disappears on cessation of treatment.

Legal category POM.

Package quantities *Achromycin Ointment 3%:* Tubes of 30 g.

Achromycin Eye and Ear Ointment 1%: Tubes of 3.5 g.

Further information Nil.

Product licence numbers

Achromycin Ointment 3%	0095/5031
Achromycin Eye and Ear Ointment	0095/5032

ACHROMYCIN* INTRAMUSCULAR

Presentation Achromycin Intramuscular 100 mg. Each vial contains:

Tetracycline hydrochloride	100 mg
Procaine hydrochloride	40 mg
Magnesium chloride	46.84 mg
Ascorbic acid	250 mg

Uses Achromycin is a broad spectrum antibiotic indicated alone or adjunctively in the treatment of infections caused by tetracycline-sensitive organisms, and for prophylaxis before or after dental and surgical procedures.

For example, Achromycin is highly effective in the treatment of infections caused by *Borrellia recurrentis* (relapsing fever), *Calymmatobacterium granulinatis* (granuloma inguinale), *Chlamydia* species (psittacosis, lymphogranuloma venereum, trachoma, inclusion conjunctivitis), *Francisella tularensis* (tularaemia), *Haemophilus ducreyi* (chancroid), *Leptospira* (meningitis, jaundice), *Mycoplasma pneumoniae* (non-gonococcal urethritis), *Pseudomonas mallei* and *pseudomallei* (glanders and melioidosis), *Rickettsiae* (typhus fever, Q fever, rocky mountain spotted fever), *Vibrio* species (cholera). It is also highly effective alone or in combination with streptomycin, in the treatment of infections due to *Brucella* species (brucellosis), and *Yersinia pestis* (bubonic plague).

Other sensitive organisms include: *Actinomyces israelii, Bacillus anthracis* (pneumonia), *Bordetella pertussis* (whooping cough), *Clostridium* species (gas gangrene, tetanus), *Entamoeba histolytica* (dysentery), *Haemophilus influenzae* (pharyngitis, otitis media), *Listeria monocytogenes* (bacteraemia), *Neisseria gonorrhoeae, Shigella* species (acute gastroenteritis), *Streptococcus pyogenes, pneumoniae* and anaerobic species, *Treponema pallidum* and *pertenue* (syphilis and yaws).

Dosage and administration *Adults:* By intramuscular injection only.

100 mg two or three times a day. In severe infections 100 mg every four to six hours.

Children: 10 mg per kg of body weight per day, in divided doses, by intramuscular injection.

Administration: Dissolve the contents of each vial, immediately before use, by the addition of 2 ml of Water for Injections. The appropriate dose of the resulting solution (see Further Information) should be injected deeply into the gluteal region.

Oral Achromycin medication should replace parenteral as soon as practical, and be continued for up to three days after characteristic symptoms of the infection have subsided. Streptococcal infections should be treated for 10 days to prevent the development of rheumatic fever or glomerulonephritis, and acute staphylococcal infections for 10–14 days.

Contra-indications, warnings, etc
Contra-indications: Known hypersensitivity to tetracyclines or procaine hydrochloride. Overt renal insufficiency. Systemic lupus erythematosus.

Precautions: Achromycin may cause a yellow to brown discoloration of the teeth in the developing foetus or child and therefore should only be administered if considered essential to pregnant women and young children under eight years of age. Achromycin should be used with caution in patients with renal or hepatic dysfunction or in conjunction with other potentially hepatotoxic drugs. Lower doses are indicated in cases of renal impairment to avoid excessive systemic accumulation, and, if therapy is prolonged, serum level determinations are advisable. Patients who are pregnant or who have known liver disease should not receive more than 1 g daily. Tetracyclines depress plasma prothrombin activity therefore reduced dosages of concurrent anticoagulants may be required. Concurrent use with the anaesthetic methoxyflurane increases the risk of kidney failure.

The concomitant use of oral tetracyclines may reduce the efficacy of oral contraceptives; an increased incidence of breakthrough bleeding may also be experienced.

Warnings and adverse effects: As with all antibiotics, overgrowth of resistant or non-susceptible organisms may occur. Excessive systemic accumulation, due to renal impairment or other reasons, will cause a rise in blood urea nitrogen leading to uraemia, hyperphosphataemia and acidosis. Bulging fontanelles in infants and benign intracranial hypertension in adults has been reported. Treatment should cease if evidence of raised intracranial pressure develops. Enamel hypoplasia has been reported.

Cross-resistance between tetracyclines may develop in micro-organisms, and cross-sensitisation in patients.

Overdosage: No specific antidote. Gastric lavage plus oral administration of milk or antacids.

Pharmaceutical precautions Store in the original pack at controlled room temperature (15–30°C) and protect from light. The brown appearance of the vial is produced when the injection is sterilised by irradiation and does not indicate any degradation.

Legal category POM.

Package quantities 6 × 100 mg vials.

Further information When Achromycin Intramuscular is dissolved in 2 ml of Water for Injections, the injection volume is increased by approximately 15% due to displacement (i.e. the final volume is around 2.3 ml). The concentration of the resultant solution is therefore approximately 43.5 mg/ml.

Product licence number 0095/5033.

ACHROMYCIN* INTRAVENOUS/ INTRAPLEURAL

Presentation Achromycin Intravenous 250 mg and 500 mg. Each vial contains tetracycline hydrochloride 250 mg or 500 mg buffered with 625 mg or 1,250 mg of ascorbic acid respectively.

Uses

1. Achromycin is a broad spectrum antibiotic indicated alone or adjunctively in the treatment of infections caused by tetracycline-sensitive organisms, and for prophylaxis before or after dental and surgical procedures.

For example, Achromycin is highly effective in the treatment of infections caused by *Borrellia recurrentis* (relapsing fever), *Calymmatobacterium granulinatis* (granuloma inguinale), *Chlamydia* species (psittacosis, lymphogranuloma venereum, trachoma, inclusion conjunctivitis), *Francisella tularensis* (tularaemia), *Haemophilus ducreyi* (chancroid), *Leptospira* (meningitis, jaundice), *Mycoplasma pneumoniae* (non-gonococcal urethritis), *Pseudomonas mallei* and *pseudomallei* (glanders and melioidosis), *Rickettsiae* (typhus fever, Q fever, rocky mountain spotted fever), *Vibrio* species (cholera). It is also highly effective, alone or in combination with streptomycin, in the treatment of infections due to *Brucella* species (brucellosis), and *Yersinia pestis* (bubonic plague).

Other sensitive organisms include: *Actinomyces israelii, Bacillus* anthracis (pneumonia), *Bordetella pertussis* (whooping cough), *Clostridium* species (gas gangrene, tetanus), *Entamoeba histolytica* (dysentery), *Haemophilus influenzae* (pharyngitis, otitis media), *Listeria monocytogenes* (bacteraemia), *Neisseria gonorrhoeae, Shigella* species (acute gastroenteritis), *Streptococcus pyogenes, pneumoniae,* and anaerobic species, *Treponema pallidum* and *pertenue* (syphilis and yaws).

2. The treatment of recurrent pleural effusions, secondary to neoplastic disease or end stage cirrhosis, by intrapleural administration.

Dosage and administration

1. *For Antibiotic use by Intravenous Infusion: Adults:* 500 mg every 12 hours by intravenous infusion. Maximum daily dosage should not exceed 2 g.

Children: Up to 10 mg/kg body weight per day in divided doses by intravenous infusion.

Elderly: Achromycin should be used with caution in the treatment of elderly patients where accumulation is a possibility.

Administration: Achromycin should be reconstituted and diluted immediately before administration by intravenous infusion. The use of a terminal filter (suitable pore size 0.22 micron) in-line with the IV Giving Set is recommended. Reconstitute the injection by adding 5 ml of Water for Injections to the 250 mg vial (or 10 ml of Water for Injections to the 500 mg vial) and then dilute the resulting solution (50 mg/ml) to at least 100 ml (up to 1,000 ml) with any of the following diluents immediately before administration by intravenous infusion at a rate not exceeding 100 ml in five minutes: Sodium Chloride Intravenous Infusion BP 0.9%, Glucose Intravenous Infusion BP, Sodium Chloride and Glucose Intravenous Infusion BP, Compound Sodium Lactate Intravenous Infusion BP.

Oral Achromycin medication should replace parenteral as soon as practical, and be continued for up to three days after characteristic symptoms of the infection have subsided. Streptococcal infections should be treated for 10 days, to prevent the development of rheumatic fever or glomerulonephritis, and acute staphylococcal infections for 10–14 days.

2. *For Pleural Effusions by Intrapleural Administration: Adults:* A single dose of 500 mg by intrapleural administration.

Administration: The pleural space should first be completely drained with a thoracostomy tube which should be positioned to give optimum drainage. 500 mg of Achromycin in 30–50 ml of sterile saline is then instilled through the tube into the pleural space followed by flushing of the thoracostomy tube with more saline. The patient's position must then be altered frequently to ensure contact of the Achromycin with both the visceral and parietal pleural surfaces. It is recommended that initially the patient should be rotated to the left and right lateral decubitus, prone and supine positions for intervals of 2–3 minutes and then left in each of these positions for 30 minutes with the tube clamped. The thoracostomy tube should then be reconnected to negative pressure and the tube removed when drainage is complete or minimal. This can take up to 48–72 hours.

This procedure has been reported to produce pleural symphysis in up to 90% of cases.

Contra-indications, warnings, etc

Contra-indications: Known hypersensitivity to tetracyclines. Overt renal insufficiency. Systemic lupus erythematosus.

Precautions: Achromycin may cause a yellow to brown discoloration of the teeth in the developing foetus or child and therefore should only be administered if considered essential to pregnant women, during breast feeding or young children under eight years of age. The treatment period should be as short as feasible and repeated courses should be avoided. Achromycin should be administered with great caution in patients with hepatic insufficiency or in conjunction with other potentially hepatotoxic drugs. Parenteral administration, particularly during pregnancy or in cases of renal dysfunction may lead to severe hepatic damage. Patients who are pregnant or who have known liver disease should not receive more than 1 g daily and careful monitoring of dosage by serum levels is necessary. Lower doses are indicated in cases of renal impairment to avoid excessive systemic accumulation, and, if therapy is prolonged, serum level determinations are advisable. Tetracyclines depress plasma prothrombin activity therefore reduced dosages of concurrent anticoagulants may be required. Concurrent use with the anaesthetic methoxyflurane increases the risk of kidney failure.

The concomitant use of oral tetracyclines may reduce the efficacy of oral contraceptives; an increased incidence of breakthrough bleeding may also be experienced.

Warnings and adverse effects: As with all antibiotics, overgrowth of resistant or non-susceptible organisms may occur. Excessive systemic accumulation, due to renal impairment or other reasons, will cause a rise in blood urea nitrogen leading to uraemia, hyperphosphataemia and acidosis. Bulging fontanelles in infants and benign intracranial hypertension in adults has been reported. Treatment should cease if evidence of raised intracranial pressure develops. Enamel hypoplasia has been reported. Cross-resistance between tetracyclines may develop in micro-organisms, and cross-sensitisation in patients. Thrombophlebitis may occur at sites of injection. Photosensitivity and dermatological reactions are rare.

Intrapleural administration may be associated with transient local pain (which can be controlled by analgesics) and/or pyrexia.

Overdosage: No specific antidote. Use appropriate supportive treatment.

Pharmaceutical precautions Store in the original pack at controlled room temperature (15–30°C) and protected from light. The increase in injection volume, caused by displacement, during dissolution of the powder with Water for Injections, is clinically insignificant when calculating dosage and volume to be injected. The brown appearance of the vial is produced when the injection is sterilised by irradiation and does not indicate any degradation.

The following substances are incompatible in solution with Achromycin Intravenous, and should not be administered in the same drip:

Aminophylline, amphotericin, barbiturates, cephalothin, chloramphenicol, chlorothiazide, chlorpromazine, cyanocobalamin, dimenhydrinate, erythromycin, heparin, hydrocortisone, methicillin, methohexitone, methyldopa, nitrofurantoin, novobiocin, penicillins, phenytoin, polymixin B, prochlorperazine, riboflavine, sodium bicarbonate, sulphadiazine, sulphafurazole, thiopentone sodium, vitamin B complex, warfarin, various inorganic ions (Ca, Mg, Al, Mn, Fe) and donor blood.

Note: The use of solutions containing calcium should be avoided as these tend to form precipitates (especially in neutral to alkaline solution) and therefore should not be used unless necessary. However, Compound Sodium Lactate Intravenous Infusion BP may be used with caution since the calcium ion content in this diluent does not normally precipitate tetracycline in an acid medium.

Legal category POM.

Package quantities *Achromycin Intravenous 250 mg:* 6 × 250 mg vials.

Achromycin Intravenous 500 mg: 6 × 500 mg vials.

Further information Nil.

Product licence numbers
Achromycin Intravenous 250 mg 0095/5034
Achromycin Intravenous 500 mg 0095/5035

ACHROMYCIN* V

Presentation *Capsules 250 mg:* Each pink capsule, printed 'Lederle 4885', contains tetracycline equivalent to 250 mg of tetracycline hydrochloride buffered with sodium metaphosphate.

Uses Achromycin V is a broad-spectrum antibiotic used for the treatment of infections caused by tetracycline-sensitive organisms. Typical indications include: Ear, nose and throat infections. Acute and chronic bronchitis. Pneumonia. Venereal Diseases. Non-Gonococcal Urethritis. Gastro-intestinal Infections. Urinary tract infections. Soft tissue infections. Acne. Typhus fever. Psittacosis. Other infections due to Tetracycline-sensitive organisms. Achromycin V is also indicated for prophylaxis before or after surgical and dental procedures.

Dosage and administration *Adults:* One capsule four times a day. This may be increased to 6 or 8 capsules daily in severe infections.

Children: Not recommended for children under 8 years of age. Information on dosage is available on request where specifically indicated.

Elderly: Achromycin V should be used with caution in the treatment of elderly patients where accumulation is a possibility.

Administration: Achromycin V should be taken an hour before or two hours after meals and therapy should be continued for up to three days after characteristic symptoms of the infection have subsided.

Contra-indications, warnings, etc
Contra-indications: A history of hypersensitivity to tetracyclines. Overt renal insufficiency. Systemic lupus erythematosus.

Warnings: Tetracyclines may cause a yellow to brown discoloration of the teeth in the developing foetus or child and therefore Achromycin V should only be administered if considered essential to pregnant women and young children under eight years of age. Achromycin V should be used with caution in patients with renal or hepatic dysfunction, or in conjunction with other potentially hepatotoxic drugs. Cross-resistance between tetracyclines may develop in micro-organisms and cross-sensitisation in patients.

Precautions: Absorption of Achromycin V is impaired by the concomitant administration of calcium, magnesium, iron and particularly aluminium salts commonly used as antacids. Tetracyclines depress plasma prothrombin activity therefore reduced dosages of concurrent anticoagulants may be required. Lower doses are indicated in cases of renal impairment to avoid excessive systemic accumulation, and if therapy is prolonged, serum level determinations are advisable.

The concomitant use of oral tetracyclines may reduce the efficacy of oral contraceptives; an increased incidence of breakthrough bleeding may also be experienced.

Side-effects: Gastro-intestinal disturbances may occur and as with all antibiotics overgrowth of resistant organisms may cause glossitis, stomatitis, vaginitis, or staphylococcal enterocolitis. Phototoxicity, photosensitivity and dermatological reactions are rare but may occur. Occurrences of enamel hypoplasia have been reported. Bulging fontanelles in infants and benign intracranial hypertension in adults has been reported. Treatment should cease if evidence of raised intracranial pressure develops.

Overdosage: No specific antidote. Gastric lavage plus oral administration of milk or antacids.

Pharmaceutical precautions Achromycin V capsules should be stored at room temperature (15–30°C) in the original pack or in containers which prevent access of light and moisture.

Legal category POM.

Package quantities Bottles of 100 and 500.

Further information Nil.

Product licence number
Capsules 250 mg 0095/0061

ARTANE* TABLETS

Presentation *Tablets 2 mg:* Each white scored tablet coded 'Lederle 4434' contains benzhexol hydrochloride 2 mg.

Tablets 5 mg: Each white scored tablet coded 'Lederle 4436' contains benzhexol hydrochloride 5 mg.

Uses Artane is an antispasmodic drug which exerts a direct inhibitory effect on the parasympathetic nervous system. It also has a relaxing effect on smooth muscle.

It is indicated in all forms of Parkinsonism – post-encephalitic, arteriosclerotic and idiopathic – as well as to prevent and control extrapyramidal disorders due to central nervous system drugs such as reserpine and the phenothiazines. These disorders include tremor, rigidity and increased salivation as commonly encountered in Parkinson's disease; akathisia manifested by extreme restlessness; and dyskinesia characterised by spastic contractions and involuntary movements.

Artane is especially effective in reducing the rigidity of muscle spasm and is useful in relieving the depression and mental inertia characteristic of this syndrome. It decreases sialorrhoea and is a particularly valuable adjunct in the treatment of arteriosclerotic Parkinsonism.

Dosage and administration *Adults only:* Optimal dosage should always be determined empirically, usually by initiating therapy at a relatively low level and by subsequent graduated increments.

Normal dosage for Parkinsonism is 6–10 mg per day, although some patients chiefly in the post-encephalitic group may require an average total dose of 12–15 mg daily. It should be given orally either three or four times a day at mealtimes.

Normal dosage for drug-induced Parkinsonism is usually between 5 mg and 15 mg per day, although some cases have been controlled by 1 mg daily.

In all cases, Artane dosage should be increased or decreased only by small increments over a period of several days. In initial therapy the dose should be 1 mg the first day, 2 mg the second day with further increases of 2 mg per day at three to five-day intervals until the optimum dose is reached.

If patients are already being treated with other parasympathetic inhibitors, Artane should be substituted as part of the therapy.

Artane may be taken before or after meals according to the way the patient reacts. If Artane tends to dry the mouth excessively, it may be better to take it before meals, unless it causes nausea. If taken after meals, induced thirst can be allayed by peppermint, chewing gum or water.

Elderly: Patients over 65 years of age tend to be relatively more sensitive and require smaller amounts of the drug.

Contra-indications, warnings, etc
Precautions: Since the use of Artane must, of necessity, continue indefinitely, the patient should be under careful observation over the long term. It should be administered with care to avoid allergic or other untoward reactions.

Incipient glaucoma may be precipitated by parasympatholytic drugs such as Artane.

Hypertension, cardiac, liver or kidney disorders are not contra-indications, but such patients should be followed closely.

Artane should be used with caution in patients with glaucoma, obstructive disease of the gastro-intestinal or genito-urinary tracts, and in elderly males with possible prostatic hypertrophy.

Side-effects: Minor side-effects such as dryness of mouth, blurring of vision, dizziness, mild nausea or nervousness will be experienced by 30–50% of all patients. These reactions tend to become less pronounced as treatment continues.

Patients with arteriosclerosis or with a history of other drug idiosyncrasies may exhibit reactions of mental confusion, agitation, or nausea and vomiting. Such patients should be allowed to develop a tolerance using the smaller initial dose, with gradual increases until the effective level is reached.

Overdosage: No specific antidote. Gastric lavage, emetic, high enema. Usual general treatment plus cold compresses and forcing of fluid are mandatory. Atropine antagonists may be useful.

Pharmaceutical precautions The products should be stored at controlled room temperature (15–30°C) in either the original pack or in containers which prevent the access of moisture.

Legal category POM.

Package quantities *Artane Tablets 2 mg:* Bottles of 100 and 1,000.

Artane Tablets 5 mg: Bottles of 100 and 1,000.

Further information Nil.

Product licence numbers
Artane Tablets 2 mg 0095/5041
Artane Tablets 5 mg 0095/5042

ASENDIS*

Presentation
25 mg Tablets: White, flat, heptagonal-shaped tablets, each containing 25 mg of amoxapine and engraved 'LL25'.
50 mg Tablets: Orange, flat, scored, heptagonal-shaped tablets, each containing 50 mg of amoxapine and engraved 'LL50'.
100 mg Tablets: Blue, flat, scored, heptagonal-shaped tablets, each containing 100 mg of amoxapine and engraved 'LL100'.
150 mg Tablets: White, flat, scored, heptagonal-shaped tablets, each containing 150 mg of amoxapine and engraved 'LL150'.

Uses Asendis is an anti-depressant indicated for the symptomatic treatment of depressive illness.

Dosage and administration
Adults: Initially 100–150 mg daily increasing as necessary, according to clinical response, to 300 mg daily, in divided doses, or one dose which may be given at night.

Usual Maintenance Dose: 150 mg–250 mg daily.

Studies have demonstrated that the initial clinical effect of Asendis can occur within four to seven days. Treatment should be maintained for a minimum period of one month, and current psychiatric practice suggests that several months treatment may be necessary after initial clinical improvement.

Elderly: An initial dose of 25 mg twice a day is recommended. If necessary, dosage may be increased under close supervision after five to seven days to a maximum of 50 mg three times daily. Less than the normal dose may be sufficient to produce a satisfactory clinical response.

Children: Not recommended for use in children.

Contra-indications, warnings, etc
Contra-indications: Recent myocardial infarction. Heart block or other cardiac arrhythmias. Mania. Severe liver disease.

Precautions: Patients posing a high suicidal risk require close initial supervision. Asendis should be used with caution in patients with narrow angle glaucoma, urinary retention or epilepsy. In common with other anti-depressants, the elderly are liable to experience adverse reactions, especially agitation and confusion. The 150 mg tablet is not suitable for initial treatment in the elderly (see 'Dosage').

A minority of patients may not improve during the first 2–4 weeks of treatment. Patients should be closely monitored during this period.

Rarely, tardive dyskinesia has been reported, but symptoms subsided completely when treatment was discontinued.

Warnings and adverse effects: Side effects most often reported are sedative and anti-cholinergic effects such as drowsiness, dry mouth, constipation and blurred vision. Less commonly, sweating, tremor, and skin rash have been reported.

Reactions reported infrequently with Asendis include nausea, vomiting, diarrhoea, delayed micturition, menstrual irregularity, impotence, breast enlargement and galactorrhoea in the female.

Convulsions have occurred rarely and only in doses outside the recommended therapeutic range.

The following adverse effects, although not reported with Asendis, have occurred with other anti-depressants: depression of the bone marrow including agranulocytosis, cholestatic jaundice, hypomania, peripheral neuropathy, cardiac arrythmias and severe hypotension (with high dosage or in deliberate overdosage), withdrawal symptoms on abrupt cessation of long-term therapy. Psychotic manifestations may be exacerbated during treatment with tri/tetracyclic anti-depressants.

Asendis may initially impair alertness. Patients should be warned of the possible hazard when driving or operating machinery.

Drug interactions: Asendis should not normally be given concurrently with or within 2 weeks, of discontinuing therapy with monoamine oxidase inhibitors.

Asendis may decrease the anti-hypertensive effect of guanethidine, debrisoquine, bethanidine and possibly clonidine. It would be advisable to review all anti-hypertensive therapy during treatment.

Asendis should not be given with sympathomimetic agents such as adrenaline, ephedrine, isoprenaline, noradrenaline, phenylephrine and phenylpropanolamine.

Anaesthetics given during tri/tetracyclic anti-depressant therapy may increase the risk of arrhythmias and hypotension. If surgery is necessary, the anaesthetist should be informed that a patient is being so treated.

Barbiturates may increase the metabolism of tri/tetracyclic anti-depressants.

Asendis may potentiate the central nervous depressant action of alcohol.

Use in pregnancy and lactation: There is no evidence as to the drug safety in human pregnancy nor is there evidence from animal work that it is free from hazard.

Overdosage: There is no specific antidote to Asendis.

In general, treatment of overdosage should be symptomatic and supportive. If the patient is conscious, induced emesis followed by gastric lavage should be accomplished as soon as possible. Unconscious patients may require full support of vital functions and cardiac monitoring. Should convulsions occur, drugs which are known to potentiate any respiratory depression should be avoided.

Pharmaceutical precautions Store at controlled room temperature (15–30°C).

Legal category POM.

Package quantities Bottles containing 100 tablets.

Product licence numbers

Asendis 25 mg Tablets	0095/0056
Asendis 50 mg Tablets	0095/0057
Asendis 100 mg Tablets	0095/0058
Asendis 150 mg Tablets	0095/0070

AUDICORT*

Presentation Ear drops. Each millilitre contains:
Triamcinolone acetonide 1.0 mg
Neomycin undecylenate equivalent to Neomycin base 3.5 mg (3,500 units).

Uses Audicort is anti-inflammatory and antibacterial.

The preparation is indicated in the treatment of acute and chronic otitis externa due to or complicated by bacterial infection.

Dosage and administration *Adults and the elderly:* After careful cleansing of the ear, Audicort is administered in doses of 2–5 drops, usually three or four times daily. If desired, the drops may be used to saturate a gauze or cotton wick placed in the ear. This wick should be kept saturated by instilling 2–5 drops, three to four times a day, and should be replaced every 24–48 hours. Treatment should be reviewed after seven days with continuation of therapy up to 14 days if resolution has not occurred.

Contra-indications, warnings, etc
Contra-indications: Audicort is contra-indicated in infants and children and in patients with perforated tympanic membrane. Hypersensitivity to triamcinolone acetonide, neomycin or propylene glycol.

The preparation should not be used in the eyes.

Warnings and precautions
Use in pregnancy and lactation: Topical administration of corticosteroids to pregnant animals can cause abnormalities of foetal development including cleft palate and intra-uterine growth retardation. There may therefore be a very small risk of such effects in the human foetus. Audicort should only be used in pregnancy when there is no safer alternative.

Although corticosteroids appear in breast milk, the absorption of triamcinolone acetonide from Audicort is expected to be minimal so the risk to the baby is considered to be small.

Precautions: The tympanic membrane should be checked for integrity before Audicort drops are prescribed.

Use of an antibiotic may occasionally result in an overgrowth of non-susceptible micro-organisms, while the presence of an anti-inflammatory steroid may encourage their spread. If superinfection does occur, the drug should be stopped and appropriate therapy instituted.

Unlikely to produce any serious toxic effects if ingested.

Side-effects: Side effects from triamcinolone and neomycin in otic drops are rare, but neomycin has occasionally been responsible for localised skin sensitisation. Discomfort (stinging) may be experienced by some patients on application of the drops. If local reactions such as irritation or erythema occur, discontinue medication.

If absorbed systemically, neomycin is known to be ototoxic. However, during the course of treatment with Audicort, the maximum total exposure to neomycin is 35 mg and this is not thought to pose a significant clinical risk.

Overdose: Overdose of triamcinolone acetonide and neomycin undecylenate otic drops has not been reported. Excess drops can be removed from the ear by gentle washing.

Pharmaceutical precautions Audicort should be stored at controlled room temperature (25°C) in the original container. Excessive heating of the solution should be avoided.

Audicort should not be diluted.

Legal category POM.

Package quantities 10 ml of sterile solution in plastic dropper bottle.

Further information Nil.

Product licence number 0095/5069.

AUREOCORT* CREAM
AUREOCORT* OINTMENT

Presentation *Ointment:* Each gram of yellow ointment contains:

Chlortetracycline hydrochloride	30 mg
Triamcinolone acetonide	1 mg

in a greasy base of anhydrous wool fat and white soft paraffin, with 0.16% methylparaben and 0.04% propylparaben as preservative.

Cream: Each gram of yellow cream contains:

Chlortetracycline equivalent to chlortetracyline hydrochloride	30 mg
Triamcinolone acetonide	1 mg

in a smooth yellow water-miscible cream, with 0.2% chlorocresol as preservative.

Uses Aureocort combines the anti-inflammatory action of triamcinolone acetonide with the anti-infective properties of chlortetracycline.

It is indicated in the treatment of atopic dermatitis, contact dermatitis, eczema, neurodermatitis, otitis externa, seborrhoeic dermatitis, varicose eczema, vesiculopustular dermatitis. It may also be used in the treatment of infected insect bites.

Dosage and administration
Adults and children: Aureocort Ointment should be applied sparingly to the affected area either directly or on sterile gauze two or three times daily.

In varicose ulcers the ointment should be applied to the ulcer on sterile gauze, and the surrounding skin edges smeared thinly prior to dressing and pressure bandaging.

Aureocort Cream should be applied sparingly to the affected areas two or three times daily.

Contra-indications, warnings, etc
Contra-indications: The use of Aureocort is contra-indicated in tuberculous, fungal or viral lesions of the skin (herpes simplex, vaccinia and varicella).

Precautions: The use of antibiotics topically may result in overgrowth of non-susceptible organisms; if new infections appear during therapy appropriate measures should be taken.

The use of corticosteroids on infected areas should be continuously and carefully observed, bearing in mind the potential spreading of infection by anti-inflammatory corticosteroids (caused by organisms not sensitive to chlortetracycline) and the possible advisability of discontinuing corticosteroid therapy and/or initiating alternative antibacterial measures. Generalised dermatological conditions may require systemic corticosteroid therapy.

Topical administration of corticosteroids to pregnant animals can cause abnormalities of foetal development. The relevance of this finding to human beings has not been established; however, topical steroids should not be used extensively in early pregnancy, i.e. in large amounts or for long periods.

In infants, long term continous topical steroid therapy should be avoided. Adrenal suppression can occur even without occlusion.

Side-effects: A few patients may be allergic to any of the components. If adverse reaction or idiosyncrasy occurs discontinue medication.

The use of corticosteroids over extensive body areas, with or without occlusive non-permeable dressings, may result in systemic absorption of the corticosteroid, and the physician should be aware of such possible absorption and take appropriate precautions. When occlusive non-permeable dressings are used, miliaria, folliculitis and pyoderma may sometimes develop beneath the occlusive material. Localised atrophy and striae have been reported with the use of corticosteroids by the occlusive technique.

Pharmaceutical precautions Aureocort Ointment should be stored at controlled room temperature (15–30°C) in the original pack. Aureocort Cream should be stored in a cool place (8–15°C) in the original pack. Dilution of Aureocort Ointment and Cream is not recommended as it will affect the stability of the product.

Aureocort Cream and Ointment may cause a yellow staining of clothes. Following extended use a similar local staining of the skin may occur which disappears on cessation of treatment.

Legal category POM.

Package quantities
Aureocort Ointment: Tubes of 15 g.
Aureocort Cream: Tubes of 15 g.

Further information Nil.

Product licence numbers

Aureocort Ointment	0095/5076
Aureocort Cream	0095/0019

AUREOMYCIN* CAPSULES
AUREOMYCIN* POWDER

Presentation *Capsules 250 mg:* Each yellow capsule, printed 'Lederle 4739' contains chlortetracycline hydrochloride 250 mg.

Powder 25 g: Each bottle contains 25 g of chlortetracycline hydrochloride as a micropulverised yellow powder.

Uses Aureomycin is a broad-spectrum antibiotic used for the treatment of infections caused by chlortetracycline-sensitive organisms. Typical indications include:

Ear, nose and throat infections. Acute and chronic bronchitis. Pneumonia. Gastro-intestinal infections. Amoebic Hepatitis. Urinary tract infections. Soft tissue infections. Venereal diseases. Acne. Typhus fever.

Other infections due to Aureomycin-sensitive organisms.

Aureomycin is also indicated for prophylaxis before or after surgical and dental procedures.

Dosage and administration *Dosage: Adults:* 1 capsule four times a day. This may be increased to 6 or 8 capsules daily in severe infections.

In the treatment of amoebiasis, at least 2 capsules four times daily for 10–14 days is recommended.

Elderly: Aureomycin should be used with caution in the treatment of elderly patients where accumulation is a possibility.

Administration: Aureomycin should be taken an hour before or two hours after meals and therapy should be continued for up to three days after characteristic symptoms of the infection have subsided.

Contra-indications, warnings, etc
Contra-indications: A history of hypersensitivity to tetracyclines. Systemic lupus erythematosus.

Warnings: Tetracyclines may cause a yellow to brown discoloration of the teeth in the developing foetus or child and therefore Aureomycin should only be administered if considered essential to pregnant or lactating women and young children under eight years of age. Aureomycin should be used with caution in patients with renal or hepatic dysfunction, or in conjunction with other potentially hepatotoxic drugs. Cross-resistance beween tetracyclines may develop in micro-organisms and cross-sensitisation in patients.

Precautions: Absorption of Aureomycin is impaired by the concomitant administration of calcium, magnesium, iron and particularly aluminium salts commonly used as antacids. Tetracyclines depress plasma prothrombin activity therefore reduced dosages of concurrent anti-coagulants may be required. Lower doses may be required in cases of renal impairment to avoid excessive systemic accumulation, although this is unlikely due to the high biliary excretion of Aureomycin. If therapy in such cases, is prolonged, serum level determinations are advisable.

The concomitant use of oral tetracyclines may reduce the efficacy of oral contraceptives; an increased incidence of breakthrough bleeding may also be experienced.

Side-effects: Gastro-intestinal disturbances may occur and as with all antibiotics overgrowth of resistant organisms may cause glossitis, stomatitis, vaginitis, or staphylococcal enterocolitis. Photosensitivity and dermatological reactions are rare. Occurrences of enamel hypoplasia have been reported. Bulging fontanelles in infants and benign intracranial hypertension in adults has been reported. Treatment should cease if evidence of raised intracranial pressure develops.

Overdosage: No specific antidote. Gastric lavage plus oral administration of milk or antacids.

Pharmaceutical precautions Store at controlled room temperature (15–30°C).

Legal category POM.

Package quantities *Capsules:* Bottles of 100.
Powder: Bottles containing 25 g.

Further information Nil.

Product licence numbers

Capsules 250 mg	0095/0051
Powder 25 g	0095/5022

AUREOMYCIN* OINTMENT
AUREOMYCIN* CREAM
AUREOMYCIN* OPHTHALMIC OINTMENT

Presentation *Aureomycin Ointment 3%:* Each gram of yellow ointment contains chlortetracycline hydrochloride 30 mg in a greasy base of anhydrous wool fat and white soft paraffin with 2.4% methylparaben and 0.6% propylparaben as preservatives.

Aureomycin Cream 3%: Each gram of yellow cream contains chlortetracycline equivalent to chlortetracycline hydrochloride 30 mg in a smooth yellow water-miscible cream, with 0.2% chlorocresol as preservative.

Aureomycin Ophthalmic Ointment 1%: Each gram of yellow ointment contains chlortetracycline hydrochloride 10 mg in a greasy base of anhydrous wool fat and white soft paraffin.

Uses Aureomycin is a broad-spectrum antibiotic.

Aureomycin Ointment 3% and Aureomycin Cream 3%: Aureomycin topical preparations are indicated for the treatment of superficial pyogenic infections of the skin. They are effective against Gram-positive cocci (Streptococci, Staphylococci and Pneumococci) and Gram-negative bacteria (Coli-aerogenes group).

Aureomycin Ophthalmic Ointment 1%: Aureomycin Ophthalmic Ointment 1% is indicated in the treatment of susceptible ocular infections caused by Staphylococci, Pneumococci, *Haemophilus influenzae,* Diplococcus of Morax-Axenfeld, the Friedlander bacillus, Streptococci, *Aerobacter aerogenes, Proteus vulgaris, Proteus morganii, Escherichia coli, Alcaligenes faecalis, Pseudomonas aeruginosa,* and in the treatment of trachoma (in conjunction with oral therapy).

Dosage and administration
Adults and children: Aureomycin Ointment 3% and Cream 3%: In the treatment of local skin infections, apply the preparation directly to the involved area, preferably on sterile gauze, one or more times daily as the condition warrants. In severe local infection, topical application should be supplemented by oral administration.

Aureomycin Ophthalmic Ointment 1%: Aureomycin Ophthalmic Ointment should be applied to the infected eye every two hours or more often as the condition warrants and response indicates. Severe or stubborn infections may require treatment for many days and may also require oral therapy in addition to local treatment. Mild infections may respond in as little as 48 hours.

Contra-indications, warnings, etc
Contra-indications: Aureomycin topical preparations are contra-indicated in patients with a history of hypersensitivity to chlortetracycline hydrochloride or any other ingredient.

Precautions: The use of antibiotics may result in the overgrowth of non-susceptible organisms. If new infections appear during therapy appropriate measures should be taken.

The concomitant use of oral tetracyclines may reduce the efficacy of oral contraceptives; an increased incidence of breakthrough bleeding may also be experienced.

Side-effects: Some patients may be allergic to any of the components. If adverse reaction or idiosyncrasy occurs, discontinue medication.

Pharmaceutical precautions *Aureomycin Ointment 3%:* The product should be stored in a cool place (8–15°C). The ointment may be diluted with a base of 10% wool-fat in white soft paraffin.

Aureomycin Cream 3%: The product should be stored in a cool place (8–15°C). Dilution is not recommended.

Aureomycin Ophthalmic Ointment: The product should be stored in a cool place (8–15°C). Dilution of Aureomycin Ophthalmic Ointment is not recommended.

Aureomycin Cream and Ointment may cause a yellow staining of clothes. Following extended use a similar local staining of the skin may occur which disappears on cessation of treatment.

Legal category POM.

Package quantities
Aureomycin Ointment 3%: Tubes of 30 g.

Aureomycin Ophthalmic Ointment 1%: Tubes of 3.5 g.

Aureomycin Cream 3%: Tubes of 30 g.

Further information Nil.

Product licence numbers

Aureomycin Ointment 3%	0095/5019
Aureomycin Ophthalmic Ointment 1%	0095/5020
Aureomycin Cream 3%	0095/0018

CALCIUM LEUCOVORIN

Presentation *Injection 3 mg in 1 ml:* Ampoules containing 3 mg/ml folinic acid as the calcium salt.

Powder for Injection 15 mg and 30 mg: Vials containing a lyophilised powder of 15 mg or 30 mg folinic acid as the calcium salt.

Tablets 15 mg: Each yellowish-white scored tablet contains 15 mg of folinic acid respectively as the calcium salt.

Uses Calcium Leucovorin is the calcium salt of a formyl derivative of tetrahydrofolic acid, the metabolite of folic acid, and an essential coenzyme for nucleic acid synthesis. Calcium Leucovorin is used therefore to diminish the toxicity and counteract the action of folic acid antagonists such as Methotrexate in cytotoxic therapy. This procedure is commonly known as Calcium Leucovorin Rescue.

Calcium Leucovorin has also been demonstrated to be effective in producing amelioration of the blood picture in a number of megaloblastic anaemias due to folate deficiency.

Dosage and administration *Calcium Leucovorin Rescue: Adults and children:* Dosage regimes vary, depending upon the dose of Methotrexate administered. In general, up to 150 mg are usually given in divided doses, over 12–24 hours, by intramuscular injection, bolus intravenous injection, intravenous infusion or orally, followed by 12–15 mg intramuscularly or 15 mg (1 tablet) orally, every 6 hours for the next 48 hours. Rescue therapy is usually started following a delay of up to 8–24 hours, after the beginning of the Methotrexate infusion. One tablet (15 mg) of oral Calcium Leucovorin every 6 hours for 48–72 hours may be sufficient when lower doses (less than 100 mg) of Methotrexate have been given. Where overdosage of Methotrexate is suspected, the dose of Calcium Leucovorin should be equal to or higher than the offending dose of Methotrexate, and should be administered within the first hour.

In addition to Calcium Leucovorin, measures to assure the prompt excretion of Methotrexate are important. These measures include:

a. Alkalinization of urine so that the urinary pH is greater than 7.0 before Methotrexate infusion (to increase solubility of Methotrexate and its metabolites).

b. Maintenance of urine output of 1800–2000 cc/m^2/24 hr by increased oral or intravenous fluids on days 2, 3 and 4 following Methotrexate therapy.

c. Plasma Methotrexate concentration, BUN, and creatinine should be measured on days 2, 3 and 4.

These measures must be continued until the plasma Methotrexate level is less than 10–7 molar.

Because of the calcium content of the leucovorin solutions, no more than 160 mg of leucovorin should be injected intravenously per minute.

Treatment of Folate Deficiency:

Children up to 12 years of age: 0.25 mg/kg/day.

Adults: 10–20 mg daily. Oral therapy with one tablet of Calcium Leucovorin daily is more usual.

Contra-indications, warnings, etc
Contra-indications: Calcium Leucovorin should not be used for the treatment of pernicous anaemia or other megaloblastic anaemias due to vitamin B_{12} deficiency.

Precautions: Calcium Leucovorin should not be given simultaneously with an anti-neoplastic folic acid antagonist, e.g. Methotrexate to modify or abort clinical toxicity, as the therapeutic effect of the antagonist may be nullified. Concomitant Calcium Leucovorin will not however inhibit the antibacterial activity of other folic acid antagonists such as trimethoprim and pyrimethamine.

Side-effects: Adverse reactions to Calcium Leucovorin are rare, but occasional pyrexial reactions have been reported following parenteral administration.

Overdosage: Does not apply.

Pharmaceutical precautions Store at controlled room temperature (15–30°C) in the original package.

Each vial of Powder for Injection 15 mg and 30 mg should be reconstituted with 3 ml of Water for Injection to produce a solution for intramuscular or intravenous injection. Calcium Leucovorin is stable for at least 24 hours at controlled room temperature (15–30°C) when diluted with the following intravenous infusion fluids: Sodium Chloride 0.9%; Glucose 5%; Glucose 10%; Sodium Chloride 0.9% and Glucose 10%; Compound Sodium Lactate.

The powder for injection and the injection solution do not contain an antimicrobial preservative. The reconstituted powder for injection and the injection solution should be used immediately after opening or within 24 hours if stored in a refrigerator (2–8°C).

Legal category POM.

Package quantities *Injection 3 mg in 1 ml:* 10 × 1 ml ampoules.

Powder for Injection 15 mg and 30 mg: Boxes of one vial.

Tablets 15 mg: Bottles of 10 tablets.

Further information Further information, particularly on high-dosage regimes in conjunction with methotrexate, is available on request.

Product licence numbers

Injection 3 mg in 1 ml	0095/5053
Powder for Injection 15 mg and 30 mg	0095/0087
Tablets 15 mg	0095/0033

CISPLATIN* INJECTION CISPLATIN* POWDER FOR INJECTION

Presentation *Cisplatin Injection 10 mg, 25 mg and 50 mg:* Each vial contains 10 mg, 25 mg or 50 mg of Cisplatin in solution at a concentration of 1 mg Cisplatin in 1 ml.

Cisplatin Powder for Injection 10 mg, 50 mg: Each vial of lyophilised powder contains 10 mg or 50 mg Cisplatin.

Uses Cisplatin is indicated for use alone, or in addition to other modalities, or in established combination therapy with other chemotherapeutic agents in the management of neoplastic disease, especially:

Metastatic testicular tumours – In patients who have already received appropriate surgical and/or radiotherapeutic procedures. The combination of Cisplatin, bleomycin and vinblastine has been reported to be highly effective.

Metastatic ovarian tumours – As secondary therapy in patients refractory to standard chemotherapy.

Dosage and administration
Adults and children:
Single agent therapy: 50–120 mg/m^2 as a single IV dose every three to four weeks, or 15–20 mg/m^2 IV daily for five days every three to four weeks.

Combination therapy: In general, current multiple drug treatment schedules including Cisplatin employ lower doses ranging from 20 mg/m^2 upwards, administered IV every three to four weeks.

Directions for use: Pre-treatment hydration with 1–2 litres of fluid infused for 8–12 hours prior to a Cisplatin dose is recommended in order to initiate diuresis.

Cisplatin should be added to 2 litres of an intravenous infusion fluid prior to administration; either 0.9% Sodium Chloride or Sodium Chloride 0.9% and Glucose 5% are suitable.

For Cisplatin Powder for Injection, reconstitute the 10 mg vial contents with 10 ml, and the 50 mg vial contents with 50 ml of Water for Injection, before adding to the infusion fluid.

Cisplatin Injection should be added directly into the infusion fluid.

It is recommended that administration should be over a 6–8 hour period. Diuresis may be aided by the addition to the infusion solution of 37.5 g mannitol.

Adequate hydration and urinary output must be maintained during the 24 hours following infusion.

A repeat course of Cisplatin should not be given until the serum creatinine is below 1.5 mg/100 ml (130 μmol/L) and/or the blood urea below 55 mg/100 ml (9 mmol/L). A repeat course should not be given until circulating blood elements are at an acceptable level.

Subsequent doses of Cisplatin should not be given until an audiometric analysis indicates that auditory acuity is within normal limits.

Contra-indications, warnings, etc
Contra-indications: Cisplatin induces nephrotoxicity, myelosuppression, neurotoxicity and ototoxicity which may be additive to pre-existing dysfunctions. Consequently, the use of Cisplatin in patients with hearing or renal impairment, or depressed bone marrow function, may be associated with increased toxicities. Such conditions represent relative contra-indications.

Cisplatin is contra-indicated in patients with dehydration.

Cisplatin is contra-indicated in patients with a history of hypersensitivity to Cisplatin or other platinum-containing compounds.

Warnings: Cisplatin produces cumulative nephrotoxicity. The serum creatinine, BUN or creatinine clearance should be measured prior to initiating therapy and prior to each subsequent course.

Anaphylactic-like reactions to Cisplatin have been reported. These reactions have occurred within minutes of administration to patients with prior exposure to Cisplatin and have been alleviated by administration of adrenaline, steroids and antihistamines.

Safe use in pregnancy has not been established. Cisplatin should not be administered to patients who are pregnant or to mothers who are breast-feeding. In mice, high doses and doses approaching the maximum therapeutic dose for Cisplatin when used alone have been reported to be embryotoxic. The data concerning its teratogenic potential are inconclusive.

The influence of Cisplatin on human reproduction has not been determined. Cisplatin therapy might have an anti-fertility effect.

The carcinogenic potential in humans is unknown. The possibility of a carcinogenic effect should be kept in mind when planning long term therapy. When evaluated at high doses in mice by repeated intraperitoneal administration, Cisplatin increased the incidence of lung tumours. Cisplatin has been reported to be mutagenic in bacteria and produces chromosomal damage in animal and human cells in tissue culture.

Cisplatin causes immunosuppression. Concomitant use of live vaccines may lead to a generalised systemic reaction.

Precautions: Cisplatin should be administered under the supervision of a physician experienced in the use of cancer chemotherapeutic agents with adequate facilities available for patient monitoring. Since anaphylactic reactions may occur, appropriate supportive equipment should be available to control such reactions.

Neurotoxicity appears to be cumulative. Prior to each course, the absence of symptoms of peripheral neuropathy should be established. (See Adverse Reactions).

Since renal toxicity is cumulative, measurements of BUN, serum creatinine or creatinine clearance, should be performed prior to initiating therapy and prior to each subsequent course. At the recommended dosage Cisplatin should not be given more frequently than once every three to four weeks (see Adverse Reactions).

Since ototoxicity of Cisplatin is cumulative, audiometric testing should be performed prior to initiating therapy and prior to each subsequent course of the drug (see Adverse Reactions).

Concomitant administration of aminoglycoside antibiotics, cephaloridine or frusemide may result in increased ototoxicity or nephrotoxicity.

Peripheral blood counts should be monitored weekly. Liver function should be monitored periodically. Neurological examinations should also be performed regularly (see Adverse Reactions).

Adverse reactions
Nephrotoxicity: Renal toxicity has been noted in about one third of patients given a single dose of Cisplatin *when prior hydration has not been employed.* It is first noted during the second week after a dose and is manifested by elevations in BUN and serum creatinine, serum uric acid and/or a decrease in creatinine clearance.

Renal toxicity becomes more prolonged and severe with repeated courses of the drug. Renal function must return to normal before another dose of Cisplatin can be given. Renal function impairment has been associated with renal tubular damage. The administration of Cisplatin using a six to eight hour infusion with intravenous hydration and mannitol have been used to reduce nephrotoxicity. However, renal toxicity can still occur after utilisation of these procedures.

Neurotoxicity: Neurotoxicity, usually characterised by peripheral neuropathies, has occurred in some patients. Loss of taste and seizures have also been reported. Neuropathies resulting from Cisplatin treatment may occur after prolonged therapy (four to seven months); however, neurological symptoms have been reported to occur after a single dose.

Cisplatin therapy should be discontinued when the symptoms are first observed. Preliminary evidence suggests peripheral neuropathy may be irreversible in some patients.

Ototoxicity: Ototoxicity has been observed in patients treated with a single dose of Cisplatin, 50 mg/m^2 and is manifested by tinnitus and/or hearing loss in the high frequency range (4000 to 8000 Hz).

Decreased ability to hear normal conversational tones may occur occasionally. Ototoxic effects may be more severe in children receiving Cisplatin. Hearing loss can be unilateral or bilateral and tends to become more frequent and severe with repeated doses. It is unclear whether Cisplatin induced ototoxicity is reversible. Careful monitoring by audiometry should be performed prior to initiation of therapy and prior to subsequent doses of Cisplatin.

Ocular toxicity: Various degrees of visual loss have been reported rarely in the course of combination therapy including Cisplatin as part of the combination. Visual function was regained in those cases in which Cisplatin was immediately discontinued.

Haematological: Myelosuppression may occur in patients treated with Cisplatin. The nadirs in circulating platelets and leucocytes occur between days 18–23 (range 7.5–45) with most patients recovering by day 39 (13–62). Leucopenia and thrombocytopenia are more pronounced at higher doses. Anaemia (decrease in haemoglobin level by 2g/100ml blood) occurs at approximately the same frequency and with the same timing as leucopenia and thrombocytopenia.

Gastro-intestinal: Marked nausea and vomiting occur in almost all patients treated with Cisplatin and are occasionally so severe that the drug must be discontinued. Nausea and vomiting usually begin within one to four hours after treatment and last up to 24 hours. Various degrees of nausea and anorexia may persist for up to one week after treatment.

Other toxicities

Hyperuricaemia: Hyperuricaemia has been reported to occur at approximately the same frequency as the increases in BUN and serum creatinine. It is more pronounced after doses greater than 50 mg/m^2, and peak levels of uric acid generally occur between three to five days after the dose. Allopurinol therapy for hyperuricaemia effectively reduces uric acid levels.

Hypomagnesaemia: Asymptomatic hypomagnesaemia has been reported in a certain number of patients treated with Cisplatin; symptomatic hypomagnesaemia has been observed in a limited number of patients.

Anaphylactic-like reactions: Anaphylactic-like reactions, possibly secondary to Cisplatin therapy, have been occasionally reported in patients previously exposed to Cisplatin. The reactions consist of facial oedema, wheezing, tachycardia and hypotension within a few minutes of drug administration. All reactions may be controlled by intravenous adrenaline, corticosteroids or antihistamines. Patients receiving Cisplatin should be observed carefully for possible anaphylactic-like reactions and supportive equipment and medication should be available to treat such a complication.

Other toxicities reported to occur infrequently are cardiac abnormalities (including conduction defects and congestive heart failure), anorexia and elevated SGOT.

Overdosage: Overdosage can be expected to cause the toxic effects described above, but to an exaggerated degree. Adequate hydration and osmotic diuresis may help reduce the toxicity of Cisplatin if administered promptly following overdosage.

Convulsions may be treated with appropriate anticonvulsants. Renal function, cardiovascular function and blood counts should be monitored daily in order to assess the potential toxicity to these systems. Serum magnesium and calcium levels should be carefully monitored as should symptoms and signs of voluntary muscle irritability. If symptomatic tetany develops, electrolyte supplements should be administered. Serum liver enzymes and uric acid should also be monitored daily after an acute overdose.

If fever develops during prolonged myelosuppression, appropriate presumptive antibiotic coverage should be instilled after cultures have been obtained.

Pharmaceutical precautions

Storage: Cisplatin Injection and Cisplatin Powder for Injection should be stored at controlled room temperature (15–30°C) and protected from light.

Do not refrigerate Cisplatin Injection, or the reconstituted solution from Cisplatin Powder for Injection, as refrigeration will result in precipitation.

Preparations of intravenous injection: Cisplatin should be added to 2 litres of an intravenous infusion fluid prior to administration; either 0.9% Sodium Chloride or Sodium Chloride 0.9% and Glucose 5% are suitable.

For Cisplatin Powder for Injection, reconstitute the 10 mg vial contents with 10 ml, and the 50 mg vial contents with 50 ml of Water for Injection, before adding to the infusion fluid. The reconstituted solution is stable for 24 hours at controlled room temperature (15–30°C).

Cisplatin Injection should be added directly into the infusion fluid.

It is recommended that administration should be over a six to eight hour period. Diuresis may be added by the addition to the infusion solution of 37.5 g mannitol.

Cisplatin interacts with aluminium. Administration sets, cannulae and syringes containing aluminium must not be used with the product.

Handling of cytotoxic drugs: Trained personnel should reconstitute Cisplatin powder for injection in a designated area. The work surface should be covered with disposable plastic-backed absorbent paper.

Protective gloves should be worn and care should be taken to avoid the drug accidentally coming into contact with the eyes. Any contamination of the skin or eyes should immediately be thoroughly washed with water.

The cytotoxic preparation should not be handled by pregnant staff.

Any spillage or waste material may be disposed of by incineration. We do not make any specific recommendations with regards to the temperature of the incinerator.

Legal category POM.

Package quantities *Cisplatin Injection:*
10 mg in 10 ml: single vials
25 mg in 25 ml: single vials
50 mg in 50 ml: single vials

Cisplatin Powder for Injection:
10 mg vial: single vials
50 mg vial: single vials

Further information Cisplatin has biochemical properties similar to that of bifunctional alkylating agents producing inter-strand and intra-strand crosslinks in DNA. It is apparently cell-cycle non-specific. Following a single IV dose, Cisplatin concentrates in liver, kidneys and large and small intestine in animals and humans. Cisplatin apparently has poor penetration into CNS.

Plasma levels of radioactivity decay in a biphasic manner after an IV bolus dose of radioactive Cisplatin to patients. The initial plasma half-life is 25–49 minutes, and the post-distribution plasma half-life is 58–73 hours. During the post-distribution phase, greater than 90% of the radioactivity in the blood is protein-bound. Cisplatin is excreted primarily in the urine. However, urinary excretion is incomplete with only 27–43% of the radioactivity being excreted within the first 5 days post-dose in human beings. There are insufficient data to determine whether biliary or intestinal excretion occurs.

Product licence numbers

Cisplatin Injection	0095/0098
Cisplatin Powder for Injection	0095/0090

DETECLO* TABLETS

Presentation *Tablets 300 mg:* Each blue, film-coated tablet, embossed 'LL' on one side and '5422' on the reverse side, contains:

Tetracycline hydrochloride	115.4 mg
Chlortetracycline hydrochloride	115.4 mg

Demeclocycline hydrochloride 69.2 mg

Uses For the treatment of infections caused by tetracycline-sensitive organisms. For example, Deteclo is highly effective in the treatment of infections caused by Borrellia recurrentis (relapsing fever), Calymmatobacterium granulinatis (granuloma inguinale), Chlamydia species (psittacosis, lymphogranuloma venereum, trachoma, inclusion conjunctivitis), Francisella tularensis (tularaemia), Haemophilus ducreyi (chancroid), Leptospira (meningitis, jaundice), Mycoplasma pneumoniae (non-gonococcal urethritis), Pseumomonas mallei and pseudomallei (glanders and melioidosis), Rickettsiae (typhus fever, Q fever, rocky mountain spotted fever), Vibrio species (cholera). It is also highly effective, alone or in combination with streptomycin, in the treatment of infections due to Brucella species (brucellosis), and Yersinia pestis (bubonic plague). Severe acne vulgaris.

Other sensitive organisms include: Actinomyces israelii, Bacillus anthracis (pneumonia), Clostridium species (gas gangrene, tetanus), Entamoeba histolytica (dysentery), Neisseria gonorrhoeae, and anaerobic species, Treponema pallidum and pertenue (syphilis and yaws).

Dosage and administration *Dosage: Adults:* One tablet every 12 hours.

This may be increased to 3 or 4 tablets daily for short periods in more severe infections.

Gonorrhoea: 1,200 mg (4 tablets) followed by a similar dose six hours later.

Non-gonococcal urethritis: One tablet twice daily for 10–21 days.

Children: Not recommended for children under 12 years of age. Information on dosage is available on request where specifically indicated.

Elderly: Deteclo should be used with caution in the treatment of elderly patients where accumulation is a possibility.

Administration: Deteclo should be taken an hour before or two hours after meals and therapy should be continued for up to three days after characteristic symptoms of the infection have subsided.

Contra-indications, warnings, etc
Contra-indications: A history of hypersensitivity to tetracyclines. Overt renal insufficiency. Children under twelve years of age.

Warnings and precautions: Deteclo should be used with caution in patients with renal or hepatic dysfunction or in conjunction with other potentially hepatotoxic drugs. The anti-anabolic action of the tetracyclines may cause an increase in BUN.

Lower doses are indicated in cases of renal impairment to avoid excessive systemic accumulation, and if therapy is prolonged, serum level determinations are advisable. Patients who have known liver disease should not receive more than 1 g daily. In long term therapy, periodic laboratory evaluation of organ systems, including haematopoeitic, renal and hepatic studies should be performed.

Photoallergic reactions may occur in hypersensitive persons and such patients should be warned to avoid direct exposure to natural or artificial sunlight and to discontinue treatment at the first sign of skin discomfort.

Cross-resistance between tetracyclines may develop in micro-organisms and cross-sensitisation in patients. Deteclo should be discontinued if there are signs/symptoms of overgrowth of resistance organisms including candida, enteritis, glossitis, stomatitis, vaginitis, pruritis ani or staphylococcal enterocolitis.

Interactions: Deteclo should not be used with penicillins. Tetracyclines depress plasma prothrombin activity and reduced doses of concomitant anticoagulants may be required.

Absorption of Deteclo is impaired by the concomitant administration of iron, calcium, zinc, magnesium and particularly aluminium salts commonly used as antacids.

The concomitant use of oral tetracyclines may reduce the efficacy of oral contraceptives; an increased incidence of breakthrough bleeding may also be experienced.

Use in pregnancy: Results of animal studies indicate that tetracyclines cross the placenta, are found in foetal tissues and can have toxic effects on the developing foetus (often related to retardation of skeletal development). Evidence of embryotoxicity has also been noted in animals treated early in pregnancy. Deteclo therefore, should not be used in pregnancy unless considered essential, in which case the maximum daily dose should be 1 g.

The use of drugs of the tetracycline class during tooth development (last half of pregnancy) may cause permanent discoloration of the teeth (yellow-grey-brown). This adverse reaction is more common during long term use of the drugs but has been observed following repeated short term courses. Enamel hypoplasia has also been reported.

Use in lactation: Tetracyclines have been found in the milk of lactating women who are taking a drug in this class. Permanent tooth discoloration may occur in the developing infant and enamel hypoplasia has been reported. Therefore, Deteclo should not be administered to lactating women.

Use in children: The use of tetracyclines during tooth development in children under the age of 12 years may cause permanent discoloration (see above). Enamel hypoplasia has also been reported.

Side-effects: Gastro-intestinal disturbances including nausea, vomiting and diarrhoea may occur and, as with all antibiotics, overgrowth of resistant organisms may cause glossitis, stomatitis, vaginitis, or staphylococcal enterocolitis. Dermatological reactions are rare. Bulging fontanelles in infants and benign intracranial hypertension in adults has been reported. Treatment should cease if evidence of raised intracranial pressure develops. Hypersensitivity reactions including: urticaria, angioneurotic oedema, anaphylaxis, anaphylactoid purpura, pericarditis and exacerbation of systemic lupus erythematosus may occur. Haemolytic anaemia, thrombocytopenia, neutropenia and eosinophilia have been reported. When given over prolonged periods tetracyclines have been reported to produce brown-black microscopic discoloration of thyroid glands. No abnormalities of thyroid function are known to occur.

Overdosage: No specific antidote. Gastric lavage plus oral administration of milk or antacids.

Pharmaceutical precautions Store at controlled room temperature (15 to 30°C) in the original pack or in containers which prevent access of light and moisture.

Legal category POM.

Package quantities Bottles of 100 and 500.

Further information Deteclo is a unique combination of three effective tetracycline broad-spectrum antibiotics. The ratio of the different tetracyclines has been carefully chosen to ensure that high therapeutic blood levels are rapidly realised and maintained with a reduced potential for side-effects, on a twice daily dosage regime, because of their different rates of absorption and excretion.

Product licence number 0095/5070.

DIAMOX*

Presentation *Tablets 250 mg:* Each white scored tablet coded 'Lederle 4395' contains acetazolamide 250 mg.

Sodium Parenteral 500 mg: Each vial contains 500 mg of acetazolamide as the sodium salt with sodium hydroxide to adjust the pH to approximately 9.2.

Uses Diamox is an enzyme inhibitor and acts specifically on carbonic anhydrase. It is indicated in the treatment of:

1. *Glaucoma:* It is felt that Diamox is useful in glaucoma, because it acts on inflow, decreasing the amount of aqueous secretion.

2. *Abnormal retention of fluid:* Diamox is a diuretic

whose action is due to the effect on the reversible hydration of carbon dioxide and dehydration of the carbonic acid reaction in the kidney. The result is renal loss of HCO_3-ion which carries out sodium, water and potassium.

Diamox is therefore indicated in the treatment of oedema associated with pre-menstrual tension, drug-induced oedema, obesity, and congestive heart failure in each case where fluid retention is a problem.

3. *Epilepsy:* Best results with Diamox have been seen in petit mal in children. Good results, however, have been seen in patients, both children and adults, with other types of seizures such as grand mal, mixed seizure patterns, myoclonic jerk patterns, etc.

4. *Other fields:* Certain patients with Menière's disease have shown a good response, but this is probably limited to those patients who have a component of oedema in the labyrinth mechanism of the inner ear.

Similarly, there have been varying reports on the use of Diamox in hydrocephalus in the infant.

Dosage and administration *Tablets:*

1. *Glaucoma (acute congestive and secondary): Adults:* 250–1,000 mg (1–4 tablets) per 24 hours, usually in divided doses for amounts over 250 mg daily.

Children: 125–750 mg (½–3 tablets) daily in divided doses.

Elderly: See Contra-indications and warnings.

2. *Abnormal retention of fluid:* Congestive heart failure, drug-induced oedema. (Adults only.)

For diuresis, the starting dose is usually 1–1½ tablets (250–375 mg) once daily in the morning. If, after an initial response, the patient fails to continue to lose oedema fluid, do not increase the dose but allow for kidney recovery by omitting a day. Best results are often obtained on a regime of 1–1½ tablets daily for two days, rest a day, and repeat, or merely giving the Diamox every other day. The use of Diamox does not eliminate the need for other therapy, e.g. digitalis, bed rest and salt restriction in congestive heart failure and proper supplementation with elements such as potassium in drug-induced oedema.

For cases of pre-menstrual tension where fluid retention is a problem a daily dose (single) of 125–375 mg is suggested beginning 5–10 days prior to onset of menstruation, or at onset of symptoms. Therapy may be alternated with days of rest.

For obesity the recommended dosage is 250–375 mg daily. For some patients therapy may be on an alternate week basis. Diamox is not intended for use in curbing appetite.

3. *Epilepsy: Adults:* 250–1,000 mg daily in divided doses.

Children: 125–750 mg daily in divided doses.

The change from other medication to Diamox should be gradual.

Sodium Parenteral: Intravenous or intramuscular administration may be employed in the same dosage as indicated for oral use. The direct intravenous route is preferred as the intramuscular use is limited by the alkaline pH of the solution.

Each vial should be reconstituted with at least 5 ml of Water for Injection prior to use.

Contra-indications, warnings, etc

Contra-indications: Since Diamox may induce a mild acidosis, its use is contra-indicated in idiopathic renal hyperchloraemic acidosis. Because of the nature of its action, Diamox may be contra-indicated in conditions in which there is a known depletion of sodium and potassium at least until after successful preliminary medication with sodium and potassium salts. It is also contra-indicated in Addison's disease or all types of adrenal gland failure, precoma associated with hepatic cirrhosis, and renal insufficiency.

Long-term administration is contra-indicated in patients with chronic congestive angle-closure glaucoma since it may permit organic closure of the angle to occur while the worsening glaucoma is masked by lowered intra-ocular pressure. Diamox should not be used in patients hypersensitive to sulphonamides.

Uses in pregnancy and lactation: Acetazolamide has been reported to be teratogenic and embryotoxic in rats, mice, hamsters and rabbits at oral or parenteral doses in excess of ten times those recommended in human beings. Although there is no evidence of these effects in human beings, there are no adequate and well-controlled studies in pregnant women. Therefore, Diamox acetazolamide should not be used in pregnancy, especially during the first trimester, unless the potential benefit justifies the potential risk to the fetus.

Precautions: Patients who are being treated with Diamox require regular supervision with monitoring of fluid and electrolyte state. Increasing the dose does not increase the diuresis but may increase the incidence of drowsiness and/or paraesthesia. Less commonly, fatigue, excitement, gastro-intestinal upsets and increased polyuria have been reported. Disorientation has been observed in a few patients with oedema due to hepatic cirrhosis. Such cases should be under close supervision.

When Diamox is prescribed for long-term therapy, special precautions are advisable. The patient should be cautioned to report any unusual skin rash. Periodic blood cell counts are recommended. A precipitous drop in formed blood cell elements or the appearance of toxic skin manifestations should call for diminution or cessation of Diamox therapy. The transitory loss of hearing calls for immediate cessation of medication. Diamox should only be used with particular caution in elderly patients or those with potential obstruction in the urinary tract, or with disorders rendering their electrolyte balance precarious or with liver dysfunction. The concomitant administration of this preparation with cardiac glycosides or hypotensive agents may necessitate adjustment of the dosage of these drugs.

Side-effects: Instances of flushing, thirst, headache, drowsiness, dizziness, fatigue, irritability, excitement, polydipsia and polyuria, paraesthesia of extremities and face, ataxia, hyperpnoea, and gastro-intestinal upsets such as anorexia and vomiting have been reported. These side-effects have normally disappeared during continued medication or upon diminution or cessation of Diamox therapy.

However, Diamox is a sulphonamide derivative and therefore some side-effects similar to those caused by sulphonamides have occasionally been reported. These include fever, agranulocytosis, thrombocytopenia, thrombocytic purpura, leukopenia, and aplastic anaemia, skin toxicity, crystalluria, calculus formation, renal and ureteral colic, and renal lesions.

Transient myopia has been reported. This condition invariably subsides upon diminution or cessation of the medication.

Drug interactions: Possible potentiation of the effects of folic acid antagonists, hypoglycaemics and oral anticoagulants.

Overdosage: No specific antidote. Supportive measures with correction of electrolyte and fluid balance. Force fluids.

Pharmaceutical precautions The products should be stored at controlled room temperature (15–25°C) in either the original pack or in containers which prevent access of moisture.

Reconstituted solutions of Diamox Sodium Parenteral contain no preservative and should be used or discarded within 24 hours.

Legal category POM.

Package quantities *Diamox Tablets 250 mg:* Bottles of 100 and 1,000.

Diamox Sodium Parenteral: Vials, 500 mg.

Further information Diamox Sodium Parenteral contains 2.36 millimoles of sodium per vial.

Product licence numbers

Diamox Tablets 250 mg	0095/5075
Diamox Sodium Parenteral	0095/5073

DIAMOX* SUSTETS*

Presentation Each orange transparent capsule contains acetazolamide 500 mg.

Uses Diamox is an enzyme inhibitor which acts specifically on carbonic anhydrase, the enzyme which catalyses a reversible reaction involving the hydration of carbon dioxide and the dehydration of carbonic acid. In the eye, this inhibitory action of acetazolamide decreases the secretion of aqueous humor and results in a drop of intraocular pressure.

Indication: Glaucoma: (chronic simple (open angle) glaucoma, secondary glaucoma, and perioperatively in acute angle closure glaucoma where delay of surgery is desired in order to lower intraocular pressure) because acetazolamide acts on inflow, decreasing the amount of aqueous secrection.

Dosage and administration *Adults:* 1 Capsule at night and in the morning. The product is not intended for administration to children.

Elderly: Diamox should only be used with particular caution in elderly patients or those with potential obstruction in the urinary tract or with disorders rendering their electrolyte balance precarious or with liver dysfunction.

Contra-indications, warnings, etc

Contra-indications: Acetazolamide therapy is contraindicated in situations in which sodium and/or potassium blood serum levels are depressed, in cases of marked kidney and liver disease or dysfunction, suprarenal gland failure, and hyper-chloremic acidosis.

Long-term administration of Diamox acetazolamide is contra-indicated in patients with chronic noncongestive angle-closure glaucoma since it may permit organic closure of the angle to occur while the worsening glaucoma is masked by lowered intraocular pressure.

Diamox should not be used in patients hypersensitive to sulphonamides.

Warnings

Use in pregnancy: Acetazolamide has been reported to be teratogenic and embryotoxic in rats, mice, hamsters and rabbits at oral or parenteral doses in excess of ten times those recommended in human beings. Although there is no evidence of these effects in human beings, there are no adequate and well-controlled studies in pregnant women. Therefore, Diamox acetazolamide should not be used in pregnancy, especially during the first trimester.

Use in lactation: Diamox has been detected in low levels in the milk of lactating women who have taken Diamox. Although it is unlikely that this will lead to any harmful effects in the infant, extreme caution should be exercised when Diamox is administered to lactating women.

Precautions: Increasing the dose does not increase the diuresis and may increase the incidence of drowsiness and/or paraesthesia.

Increasing the dose often results in a decrease in diuresis. Under certain circumstances, however, very large doses have been given in conjunction with other diuretics in order to secure diuresis in complete refractory failure.

When Diamox is prescribed for long-term therapy, special precautions are advisable. The patient should be cautioned to report any unusual skin rash. Periodic blood cell counts and electrolyte levels are recommended. A precipitous drop in formed blood cell elements or the appearance of toxic skin manifestations should call for diminution or cessation of Diamox therapy.

In patients with pulmonary obstruction or emphysema where alveolar ventilation may be impaired, Diamox acetazolamide which may aggravate acidosis, should be used with caution.

Side-effects: Adverse reactions during short-term therapy are minimal. Those effects which have been noted include: paraesthesias, particularly a 'tingling' feeling in the extremities; some loss of appetite; polyuria, flushing, thirst, headache, dizziness, fatigue, irritability and occasional instances of drowsiness and confusion. Rarely, photosensitivity has been reported.

During long-term therapy, an acidotic state may occasionally supervene. This can usually be corrected by the administration of bicarbonate.

Transient myopia has been reported. This condition invariably subsides upon diminution or discontinuance of the medication.

However, Diamox is a sulphonamide derivative and therefore some side-effects similar to those caused by sulphonamides have occasionally been reported. These include fever, agranulocytosis, thrombocytopenia, thrombocytic purpura, leukopenia, and aplastic anaemia, rash (including erythema multiforme, Stevens-Johnson Syndrome, toxic epidermal necrolysis), anaphylaxis, crystalluria, calculus formation, renal and ureteral colic, and renal lesions.

Other occasional adverse reactions include: urticaria, melaena, haematuria, glycosuria, hepatic insufficiency, flaccid paralysis, and convulsions.

Drug interactions: Possible potentiation of the effects of folic acid antagonists, hypoglycaemics and oral anticoagulants. Concomitant administration with high-dose aspirin may potentiate the adverse reactions of Diamox. Adjustment of dose may be required when Diamox is given with cardiac glycosides or hypertensive agents.

Overdosage: No specific antidote. Supportive measures with correction of electrolyte and fluid balance. Force fluids.

Pharmaceutical precautions Store at controlled room temperature (15–25°C) in the original pack or in containers which prevent access of light and moisture.

Legal category POM.

Package quantities Bottles of 30, 100 and 500.

Product licence number 0095/5074.

LEDERCORT* CREAM AND OINTMENT

Presentation *Ledercort Cream 0.1%:* Each gram of white cream contains triamcinolone acetonide 1.0 mg in a water-miscible base with Benzyl alcohol 2.0% as a preservative.

Ledercort Ointment 0.1%: Each gram of pale yellow ointment contains triamcinolone acetonide 1.0 mg in a greasy base with methylparaben 0.16% and propylparaben 0.04% as preservatives.

Uses Triamcinolone acetonide is a corticosteroid with anti-inflammatory, antipruritic and anti-allergic effects.

Ledercort Cream 0.1% and Ledercort Ointment 0.1% are indicated in the treatment of inflammatory skin conditions such as atopic dermatitis; contact dermatitis; eczematous dermatitis; generalised erythrodermia; neurodermatitis; nummular eczema; otitis externa and seborrhoeic dermatitis.

Dosage and administration

Adults, children and the elderly: Apply in small quantities to the affected areas three or four times daily: the cream or ointment may be rubbed in or applied as a thin film.

Contra-indications, warnings, etc

Contra-indications: The use of Ledercort Cream 0.1% and Ledercort Ointment 0.1% is contra-indicated in bacterial (e.g. impetigo, tuberculous), fungal (e.g. candida or dermatophyte) or viral (e.g. herpes simplex, vaccinia and varicella) lesions of the skin and in those patients with a history of hypersensitivity to corticosteroids or any of the components of the preparations. It is also contra-indicated in facial rosacea, acne vulgaris, perioral dermatitis, perianal and genital pruritus, napkin eruptions.

Warnings
Use in pregnancy and lactation: Topical administration of corticosteroids to pregnant animals can cause abnormalities of foetal development. The relevance of this finding to human beings has not been established; however, topical steroids should not be used extensively in early pregnancy, ie in large amounts or for prolonged periods.

Ledercort Cream 0.1% and Ledercort Ointment should be used during pregnancy only if the potential benefit justifies the potential risk to the foetus. Caution should be exercised when topical corticosteroids are administered to nursing women.

Precautions: Children may absorb proportionately larger amounts of topical corticosteroids and thus be more susceptible to systemic toxicity. In infants long term continuous topical steroid therapy should be avoided. If used in childhood, or on the face, courses should be limited to 5 days and occlusion should not be used. Adrenal suppression can occur even without occlusion.

Long term continuous therapy should be avoided in all patients, irrespective of age. Application under occlusion should be restricted to dermatoses involving limited areas.

Topical corticosteroids may be hazardous in psoriasis for a number of reasons, including rebound relapses following development of tolerance, risk of generalised pustular psoriasis and local and systemic toxicity due to impaired barrier function of the skin. Careful patient supervision is important.

The use of corticosteroids over extensive body areas, with or without occlusive non-permeable dressings, may result in systemic absorption of the corticosteroid being used, and the physician should be aware of such possible absorption and take appropriate precautions. When occlusive non-permeable dressings are used, miliaria, folliculitis and pyoderma may sometimes develop beneath the occlusive material. Localised atrophy and striae have been reported with the use of corticosteroids by the occlusive technique.

Side-effects: A few patients may be allergic to any of the components. If adverse reactions or idiosyncrasy occurs, discontinue medication. Side-effects are not ordinarily encountered with topical application of corticosteroids; but as with all drugs some patients react unfavourably under certain conditions.

Pharmaceutical precautions
Ledercort Cream 0.1%: Ledercort cream should be stored in a cool place (8–15°C), in either the original pack or in containers with complete closure. The cream may be diluted, taking hygienic precautions, with aqueous cream. The diluted cream must be freshly prepared and not used more than one month after issue.

Ledercort Ointment 0.1%: Ledercort Ointment should be stored in a cool place (8–15°C), in either the original pack or in containers which prevent access of moisture. The ointment may be diluted with a basis consisting of one part wool fat and nine parts white soft paraffin.

Legal category POM.

Package quantities

Ledercort Cream 0.1%:	15 g tube.
Ledercort Ointment 0.1%:	15 g tube.

Further information Nil.

Product licence number

Ledercort Cream 0.1%	0095/0032
Ledercort Ointment 0.1%	0095/5005

LEDERCORT* TABLETS

Presentation *Tablets 2 mg:* Each blue, oblong tablet coded 'LLII' contains triamcinolone 2 mg.

Tablets 4 mg: Each white, oblong tablet coded 'LL9352' contains triamcinolone 4 mg.

Uses Ledercort is a potent glucocorticoid indicated in the treatment of rheumatoid arthritis; juvenile chronic arthritis; rheumatic fever with severe carditis; systemic lupus erythematosus and other collagen diseases (giant cell arteritis/polymyalgia rheumatica, mixed connective tissue disease, polyarteritis nodosa, poly-myositis); minimal change nephrotic syndrome; bronchial asthma; occupational asthma, pulmonary sarcoid; drug induced lung disease; serum sickness; allergic and inflammatory dermatoses (allergic contact dermatitis, bullous pemphigoid, exfoliative dermatitis (erythroderma), pemphigus vulgaris; Stevens-Johnson Syndrome); autoimmune haemolytic anaemia; idiopathic thrombocytopenic purpura; Crohn's Disease; ulcerative colitis.

Dosage and administration
1. *General. Adults and children:* Ledercort is administered orally in a wide range of dosages. The doctor should 'titrate' the dosage according to the condition. In adults and children over 75 lb (34 kg) body weight, the usual initial dose ranges from 8 mg to 16 mg per day in single or divided doses. For children under 75 lb (34 kg) the range is from 4 to 12 mg.

When a satisfactory response is obtained the initial dosage should be reduced gradually by 2 mg every two to three days until the smallest dosage is achieved which will adequately maintain the patient.

Elderly: Steroids should be used with caution in elderly patients.

2. *Dosage in specific conditions:*

(a) *Rheumatoid arthritis:* The initial suppressive dose usually ranges from 8 to 16 mg per day, although an occasional patient may require larger doses to suppress the disease adequately. Once the acute manifestations of the disease have subsided (usually within two to seven days) the dosage should gradually be reduced until the smallest maintenance dose is achieved. The daily maintenance dose has ranged from 2 to 16 mg per day, although an occasional patient may require more.

(b) *Rheumatic fever with severe carditis:* The initial dose is 16–20 mg daily; maintenance dosage is 6–20 mg daily. Dosage varies considerably according to the severity of the carditis and its complications.

(c) *Systemic lupus erythematosus:* The initial suppressive dose in collagen diseases should be 20–30 mg daily, reducing gradually to maintenance levels when the desired response is noted. Maintenance dosage varies from 3 to 30 mg daily. In severely ill patients, larger doses may be necessary to control the disease.

(d) *Minimal change nephrotic syndrome:* 16–20 mg daily should be administered until diuresis occurs, usually by the fourteenth day. After diuresis begins it is advisable to continue treatment until maximum or complete chemical and clinical remission occurs; then dosage should be reduced gradually and finally discontinued.

(e) *Bronchial asthma and respiratory allergy:* In acute bronchial asthma, initial suppressive doses of 8–16 mg should be given to bring the disease under control within 24–48 hours. Rarely, more than 16 mg may be necessary.

(f) *Dermatoses:* The initial suppressive dosage should be 8–16 mg daily, or higher in the rare case. The maintenance dose can be as little as 1–2 mg daily.

(g) *Haemolytic diseases:* Where steroid therapy is indicated in haemolytic diseases, the average initial dose of Ledercort is 12–24 mg daily.

3. *Change in maintenance from other glucocorticoids:* Because the variation in response to each glucocorticoid varies considerably with each type of disease, the following schedule should be adjusted according to individual response – 4 mg Ledercort for each:

25 mg cortisone
20 mg hydrocortisone
5 mg prednisone or prednisolone
4 mg methylprednisolone
0.75 mg dexamethasone
0.60 mg betamethasone

4. *Short-term therapy in asthma:* Ledercort can control exacerbations of asthma via a short-term dosage regimen that reduces as it progresses.

Short-term courses of either ten or four days duration may be prescribed, in the following schedules (using the 4 mg tablet):

	Number of tablets Ten-day course	Four-day course
1st day	4	4
2nd day	4	3
3rd day	4	2
4th day	3	1
5th day	3	
6th day	3	
7th day	2	
8th day	2	
9th day	1	
10th day	1	

Contra-indications, warnings, etc

Contra-indications: Tuberculosis and herpes simplex are usually considered to be absolute contra-indications. Active peptic ulcer, acute glomerulonephritis, myasthenia gravis, osteoporosis, fresh intestinal anastomoses, diverticulitis, thrombophlebitis, psychic disturbances, pregnancy and local or systemic infections, including fungal and exanthematous diseases, are relative contra-indications.

Precautions: General precautions common to all corticosteroid therapy should be observed. Daily doses over 32 mg are seldom indicated. Patients should be kept under careful observation because a few may react with side-effects under certain conditions; in such an event, the drug should be discontinued.

Corticosteroids should be used with caution in patients with diabetes mellitus (or a family history of diabetes), osteoporosis, hypertension, a history of severe affective disorders (especially previous history of steroid psychosis), glaucoma, previous steroid myopathy, or epilepsy. Since adrenal cortical function may be suppressed by glucocorticoids, it is important that therapy be withdrawn gradually after long-term treatment. Adequate supporting measures, ACTH supplementation or increase in dosage, are indicated when undue stress such as anaesthesia or surgical procedure occurs during or after Ledercort therapy. Ledercort is not the treatment of choice in adrenocortical insufficiency.

The possibility of development of infectious disease during glucocorticoid therapy requires careful observation of the patient, because initial signs of the infection may be obscured. Appropriate antibiotic therapy should be instituted in such cases. Concurrent administration of barbiturates, phenytoin, phenylbutazone may increase corticosteroid levels, while if anticoagulants are given with corticosteroids, adjustment of dosage of the former is usually necessary. The use of corticosteroids in the presence of other disorders or drugs with specific actions (e.g., hypoglycaemics) impinging on the effects of corticosteroids will result in imbalance of control. Withdrawal may result in acute rebound exacerbation of disease, acute adrenocortical insufficiency, polyarteritis.

Side-effects: Ledercort may produce the side-effects common to all cortisone-like drugs: moon face, striae, acne, buffalo hump, osteoporosis, spontaneous fractures, avascular osteonecrosis, tendon rupture, amenorrhoea, menstrual irregularity, aggravation of infection, psychic disturbances, (euphoria, psychological dependence, depression, aggravation of schizophrenia), thromboembolism, peptic ulcer, hypersensitivity, leucocytosis, increased appetite, nausea, malaise, gastro-intestinal haemorrhage, hyperglycaemia, increased intracranial pressure, headache, insomnia, fatigue, purpura, hirsutism, vertigo and leucopenia. Diminished lymphoid tissue and immune response may also occur. Caution is recommended during prolonged use in children because of the possibility of growth suppression. Subcapsular cataracts, increased ocular pressure, glaucoma, papilloedema, corneal or scleral thinning and exacerbation of ophthalmic viral disease may occur in patients on high dosage for long periods. Flushing of the face may occur. Necrotising angiitis is a rare possibility. Ulcerative oesophagitis, oesophageal candidiasis, abdominal distension, dyspepsia and acute pancreatitis have occurred during corticosteroid therapy and may be related to its administration.

The long-term administration of all anti-inflammatory steroids results in definite catabolic effects, as indicated by negative protein and calcium balance. This catabolic effect, coupled with anorexia, may produce weight loss, which is undesirable in some patients. A steroid myopathy with advanced muscle weakness may involve muscles of the thighs, pelvis and low back.

The effect of Ledercort on fluid and electrolyte balance differs from older corticosteroids in that it promotes mild sodium excretion. Patients with sodium retention and oedema, from underlying disease or from previous therapy with other corticosteroids, will frequently lose weight and show increased urinary output associated with sodium diuresis during the first three to seven days of therapy. This effect will not be seen in patients with decreased glomerular filtration.

Potassium balance is not affected under ordinary dosage circumstances, and potassium supplementation is not ordinarily necessary unless prolonged and/or high dosage is prescribed. Since hypertension and oedema are not commonly observed with Ledercort they should not be used as indications of overdosage.

Withdrawal symptoms include fever, myalgia, arthralgia and adrenal insufficiency.

Use in pregnancy: The use of Ledercort is contra-indicated in pregnancy. There is inadequate evidence of safety in human pregnancy and there may be a very small risk of cleft palate and intra-uterine growth retardation in the foetus; there is evidence of harmful effects on pregnancy in animals. Corticosteroids have been reported to be teratogenic in mice, rats, and rabbits when administered systemically at relatively low dosage levels. In monkeys, however, such effects have only been reported for excessively high doses of parenterally administered corticosteroids which were also toxic to the mother.

Use in children: Corticosteroids cause growth retardation in infancy, childhood and adolescence. Treatment should be limited to the minimum dosage for the shortest possible time. In order to minimise suppression of the hypothalamo-pituitary adrenal axis and growth retardation, treatment should be administered where possible as a single dose on alternate days.

Use in the elderly: Treatment of elderly patients, particularly if long term, should be planned bearing in mind the more serious consequences of the common side effects of corticosteroids in old age, especially osteoporosis, diabetes, hypertension, susceptibility to infection and thinning of the skin.

Overdosage: No specific antidote. Symptomatic treatment with electrolyte supplements.

Pharmaceutical precautions The product should be stored at controlled room temperature (15–30°C) in either the original pack or in containers which prevent access of moisture.

Legal category POM.

Package quantities *Tablets 2 mg:* Bottles of 100. *Tablets 4 mg:* Bottles of 100 and 500.

Further information Nil.

Product licence numbers

Ledercort Tablets 2 mg 0095/5006R
Ledercort Tablets 4 mg 0095/5007

LEDERFEN*

Presentation

300 mg tablets: Light blue, film coated, capsule shaped tablets each containing 300 mg of fenbufen and engraved 'Lederfen'.

300 mg capsules: Dark blue capsules, each containing 300 mg of fenbufen and printed 'Lederfen' on both the cap and body.

450 mg tablets: Light blue, film coated, lozenge shaped

tablets each containing 450 mg of fenbufen and engraved 'Lederfen' on one face and '450' on the other.

Lederfen F (450 mg effervescent tablets): Flat, round, white effervescent tablets each containing 450 mg of fenbufen. The effervescent tablets must be dissolved in half a glass of water.

Uses For the symptomatic treatment of rheumatoid arthritis, osteoarthritis, ankylosing spondylitis and acute musculoskeletal disorders.

Dosage and administration *Adults: 300 mg Tablets or Capsules:* One in the morning and two at night. *450 mg Tablets:* One in the morning and one at night. It is unnecessary to modify the dosage of Lederfen in cases of mild to moderate renal impairment. Lederfen may therefore be used in elderly patients in whom renal impairment commonly occurs.

Children: Not recommended for administration to children under the age of 14.

Contra-indications, warnings, etc
Contra-indications: Hypersensitivity to propionic acid anti-inflammatory drugs, or aspirin. Since the potential exists for cross-sensitivity, Lederfen should not be used in patients in whom attacks of asthma, urticaria or acute rhinitis are precipitated by aspirin or other NSAIDs.

Precautions: As with other non-steroidal anti-inflammatory agents, Lederfen should be used with great caution in patients with a history or evidence of active peptic or intestinal ulceration, and only when considered essential in pregnant and nursing women.

In common with other non-steroidal anti-inflammatory agents, fenbufen when administered concurrently with quinolone antibiotics may cause an increased incidence of quinolone CNS side-effects such as convulsions. Quinolones should not be administered concurrently with fenbufen.

Warnings and adverse effects: Skin rashes with an incidence of approximately 6% are the most commonly encountered adverse reactions. Serious reactions such as erythema multiforme and Stevens–Johnson syndrome have been reported. Lederfen treatment should be discontinued immediately on appearance of a rash.

Anti-histamine therapy may help any pruritus associated with the rash. The rash is commoner in women and in patients with the rare diagnosis of sero-negative rheumatoid arthritis and psoriatic arthritis. If rash does occur, it will most commonly be seen within the second week of therapy and is very unlikely to develop after two weeks of therapy. The median duration of therapy before a rash occurs is ten days. 80% of eruptions will have resolved after one week of discontinuation of therapy and by two weeks nearly 100% of eruptions will have resolved.

In common with other NSAIDs, allergic interstitial lung disorders (allergic alveolitis, or pulomonary eosinophilia) have been reported rarely; these reactions have resolved within 4–6 weeks of discontinuing therapy.

Other side effects reported include symptoms of gastro-intestinal intolerance such as vomiting, dyspepsia and nausea; signs of gastro-intestinal haemorrhage have been reported occasionally. Minor reactions including headache, dizziness and fatigue have also been reported.

Slight decreases in blood leucocytes, haemoglobin and haematocrit as well as slight increases in prothrombin time and eosinophilis have occasionally been recorded. Haematological effects such as agranulocytosis, thrombocytopenia, granulocytopenia and haemolytic anaemia have been reported rarely. Transient elevations in values of liver function tests have occurred in some patients.

Drug interactions: When single doses of aspirin 900 mg and Lederfen 500 mg were administered together, serum concentrations of Lederfen and its metabolites were reduced by 10–20%. Concomitant use of aspirin may require adjustment of dosage of Lederfen.

For interactions with quinolone antibiotics, see 'Precautions' section. Fenbufen produces minor prolongations of prothrombin time in patients taking warfarin. These changes are unlikely to be clinically significant. Lederfen is strongly protein bound; although no clinically significant interactions associated with protein-binding have been noted as yet, practitioners should be alert to this possibility.

Overdosage: Experience of Lederfen overdosage is limited. There is no specific antidote. Gastric lavage should be performed if appropriate. Otherwise, management should be symptomatic and supportive.

Pharmaceutical precautions Sore in the original container at controlled room temperature (15–30°C).

Legal category POM.

Package quantities
300 mg tablets and capsules: Blister calendar packs of 84 designated Lederfen CP.

450 mg tablets: Bottles of 56 designated Lederfen 450. Original pack boxes of 56 tablets in blister strips designated Lederfen 450.

450 mg effervescent tablets: Boxes containing 4 tubes of 14 effervescent tablets designated Lederfen F.

Further information Fenbufen is a pro-drug. It is converted to active metabolites following absorption.

Product licence numbers

Lederfen 300 mg tablets	0095/0081
Lederfen 300 mg capsules	0095/0043
Lederfen 450 mg tablets	0095/0092
Lederfen F tablets	0095/0111

LEDERMIX*

Presentation Ledermix combination kit consists of a package containing 4 units.

1. *Ledermix paste.* Each gram contains: Demeclocycline Calcium equivalent to Demeclocycline hydrochloride 30 mg. Triamcinolone acetonide 10 mg.

2. *Ledermix cement.* Each gram contains: Demeclocycline hydrochloride 20 mg. Triamcinolone acetonide 6.7 mg in combination with zinc oxide and calcium hydroxide.

3. *Hardener 'F' (fast setting time).* 85% w/w Eugenol USP in rectified turpentine oil.

4. *Hardener 'S' (slow setting time).* 85% w/w Eugenol USP and 10% w/w polyethylene glycol 4000 USP in rectified turpentine oil.

Uses Ledermix is a dental treatment which combines the antibiotic action of demeclocycline with the anti-inflammatory action of triamcinolone acetonide.

Ledermix is indicated in pulpitis, periodontitis, and hypersensitive dentine.

Dosage and administration *Adults and Children: Pulpitis:* In all instances of exposed pulp and in acute pulpitis (except total purulent pulpitis) Ledermix Paste is applied with a small cotton pledget to the dentine adjacent to the pulp or to the exposed pulp. The cavity is then closed with a temporary filling such as zinc oxide-eugenol. Approximately 3 to 6 days later the vitality of the tooth is determined, the cavity is reopened, and the cotton pledget is removed. The dentine close to the pulp, or the wound in the pulp, is covered with Ledermix Cement prepared in the following manner: To one drop of the Hardener (no more) add sufficient Ledermix Cement powder to obtain an homogeneous mixture of cream-like consistency. This cement, which hardens rapidly, may be applied with an amalgam plugger or blunt probe.

In small cavities with small areas of pulp exposure, Ledermix Cement suffices as a base. In larger cavities or more extensive pulp exposure, it is advisable to use Ledermix Cement as a lining cement only and then to cover it with a layer of zinc oxyphosphate cement before inserting the permanent amalgam filling. In certain instances of hyperaemia and partial serous pulpitis with closed pulp cavity, the use of Ledermix Paste may be eliminated and Ledermix Cement (mixed with the Hardener) applied in the first treatment period. However, as a general rule, and particularly in acute pulpitis and in teeth where the pulp is exposed, the prepared Ledermix Cement should *NOT* be applied without previous treatment with Ledermix Paste.

Periodontitis: In primary acute periodontitis and acute exacerbations of chronic periodontitis, the canal may be prepared to the apex at the first sitting. After irrigation, the canal may be filled completely with Ledermix Paste and sealed. This treatment can be repeated if necessary on the follow-up visit about one week later, or the canal may be irrigated to remove the paste and further treatment carried out according to one of the generally accepted methods. If an alveolar abscess is present, drainage should be effected before beginning treatment with Ledermix.

Hypersensitive Dentine: In instances of hypersensitive dentine following cavity or crown preparations, Ledermix Cement plus Hardener may be used as a lining for deep cavities.

Preparation of the cement: Ledermix Cement belongs to the class of zinc oxide-eugenol dental cements. The setting time of all such cements is greatly affected by temperature and humidity conditions and by the technique of the individual operator. Vigorous and prolonged mixing, or spreading the mix thinly over the slab leads to accelerated setting whilst lowering the temperature of the mixing slab will prolong the setting time. Under any given set of conditions, however, the operator may obtain a faster or slower setting of the paste by using the appropriate hardener. In general it will be found that the time required for the mixture to set, obtained by the use of Hardener "S", will be approximately 3 to 4 times that obtained with Hardener "F".

Under conditions of high temperature and humidity, care should be taken to blend rapidly a small amount of Ledermix Cement powder (taking no more than 10 to 15 seconds) into 1 drop of Hardener with 2 or 3 strokes of the spatula. All of the resultant mix should then be taken up at once on the spatula blade.

Contra-indications, warnings, etc
Contra-indications: Ledermix is contra-indicated in instances of *total* purulent pulpitis or in patients hypersensitive to any of the active ingredients.

Precautions: The suppression of the inflammatory process by the use of a corticosteroid may result in a temporary reduction of the resistance of the pulp to infection and reduced healing capacity. Prolonged or repeated use of an anti-infective may result in superinfection or development of resistant micro-organisms. Therefore, Ledermix Paste should not be in contact with the exposed pulp for too long. If the application of this water-soluble preparation is uncontrolled, or if the temporary filling fits loosely, the danger exists that the pulp may not survive. The tip of the Ledermix Paste tube should always be kept clean and tightly closed after use.

The Ledermix Cement Vial must be kept tightly closed after use.

If severe reactions or idiosyncrasies are encountered the filling should be removed and appropriate measures instituted. Although limited there is a possibility of systemic absorption of the anti-infective and corticosteroid resulting in the side effects associated with each component.

Side-effects: Since Ledermix is only administered locally, and the various constituents are drained from the site in minute amounts over a long period of time, the possibility of systemic side-effects is remote. Local side reactions are limited to paradental effects.

Pharmaceutical precautions The product should be stored in a cool place (8–15°C) in the original pack. Each container must be kept tightly closed.

Legal category POM.

Package quantities *Ledermix Combination Kit:* 2 g bottle of cement powder.

5.0 ml bottle with separate dropper of Hardener 'F' (fast setting time).

5.0 ml bottle with separate dropper of Hardener 'S' (slow setting time).

3 g tube of Ledermix Paste.

Ledermix Refill Kit No. II:
5 g Ledermix Paste.

Ledermix Refill Kit No. III:
3 g Ledermix Powder.

Ledermix Refill Kit No. IV:
5 ml bottle with separate dropper of Hardener 'F'.

Ledermix Refill Kit No. V:
5 ml bottle with separate dropper of Hardener 'S'.

Further information Nil.

Product licence number 0095/5014R.

LEDERMYCIN*

Presentation *Capsules 150 mg:* Each two-piece dark red/pale red hard shell capsule printed Lederle 9123 contains 150 mg of demeclocycline hydrochloride.

Tablets 300 mg: Each red, film-coated tablet printed Lederle 9157 contains 300 mg of demeclocycline hydrochloride.

Uses
1. For the treatment of infections caused by tetracycline-sensitive organisms. For example, Ledermycin is highly effective in the treatment of infections caused by *Borrellia recurrentis* (relapsing fever), *Calymmatobacterium granulinatis* (granuloma inguinale), Chlamydia species (psittacosis, lymphogranuloma venereum, trachoma, inclusion conjunctivitis), *Francisella tularensis* (tularaemia), *Haemophilus ducreyi* (chancroid), Leptospira (meningitis, jaundice), *Mycoplasma pneumoniae* (non-gonococcal urethritis), *Pseumomonas mallei* and *pseudomallei* (glanders and melioidosis), Rickettsiae (typhus fever, Q fever, rocky mountain spotted fever), Vibrio species (cholera). It is also highly effective, alone or in combination with streptomycin, in the treatment of infections due to Brucella species (brucellosis), and *Yersinia pestis* (bubonic plague). Severe acne vulgaris.

Other sensitive organisms include: *Actinomyces israelii, Bacillus anthracis* (pneumonia), Clostridium species (gas gangrene, tetanus), *Entamoeba histolytica* (dysentery), *Neisseria gonorrhoeae*, and anaerobic species, *Treponema pallidum* and pertenue (syphilis and yaws).

2. For the treatment of chronic hyponatraemia associated with the syndrome of inappropriate secretion of antidiuretic hormone (SIADH) secondary to malignant disease, where water restriction is ineffective, and the patient does not have concomitant cirrhosis.

Dosage and administration
1. *For antibiotic use: Adults (Capsules, Tablets):* 600 mg daily in two or four divided doses. For primary atypical pneumonia the average daily dose is 900 mg in 3 divided doses for six days.

Elderly: Use with caution in elderly patients. See contra-indications and warnings.

Children: Not recommended for children under 12 years of age. Information on dosage is available on request where specifically indicated.

2. *For the treatment of chronic hyponatraemia due to SIADH. (Adults only):* Initially: 900–1,200 mg daily in divided doses. Maintenance dose: 600–900 mg daily in divided doses.

Ledermycin should be taken an hour before or two hours after meals and antibiotic therapy should be continued for one to three days after characteristic symptoms or fever have subsided. The incidence of rheumatic fever or glomerulonephritis following streptococcal infections suggests that therapy of a streptococcal infection should be continued for eight full days even though symptoms have subsided.

Ledermycin therapy in the treatment of chronic hyponatraemia due to SIADH should not be withdrawn without commencing other methods of control.

Contra-indications, warnings, etc

Contra-indications: A history of hypersensitivity to tetracyclines. Overt renal insufficiency. Children under twelve years of age.

Warnings and precautions: Ledermycin should be used with caution in patients with renal or hepatic dysfunction, or in conjunction with other potentially hepatotoxic drugs. The anti-anabolic action of the tetracyclines may cause an increase in BUN. The treatment of chronic hyponatraemia may necessitate the administration of high doses of Ledermycin for prolonged periods, so increasing the potential for nephrotoxicity (manifested by rises in plasma urea and creatinine) and photoallergic reactions. Cross-resistance between tetracyclines may develop in micro-organisms and cross sensitisation in patients.

Lower doses are indicated in cases of renal impairment to avoid excessive systemic accumulation, and if therapy is prolonged, serum level determinations are advisable. Patients who have known liver disease should not receive more than 1 g daily. In long term therapy, periodic laboratory evaluation of organ systems, including haematopoietic, renal and hepatic studies should be performed.

Ledermycin has the greatest potential of the tetracycline analogues for causing photo-allergic reactions in hypersensitive persons. Such patients should be warned to avoid direct exposure to natural or artificial sunlight and to discontinue therapy at the first sign of skin discomfort.

Cross-resistance between tetracyclines may develop in micro-organisms and cross-sensitisation in patients. Ledermycin should be discontinued if there are signs/symptoms of overgrowth of resistant organisms including candida, enteritis, glossitis, stomatitis, vaginitis, pruritus ani or staphylococcal enterocolitis.

Interactions: Ledermycin should not be used with penicillins. Tetracyclines depress plasma prothrombin activity and reduced doses of concomitant anticoagulants may be required.

Absorption of Ledermycin is impaired by the concomitant administration of iron, calcium, zinc, magnesium and particularly aluminium salts commonly used as antacids.

The concomitant use of oral tetracyclines may reduce the efficacy of oral contraceptives; an increased incidence of breakthrough bleeding may also be experienced.

Use in pregnancy: Results of animal studies indicate that tetracyclines cross the placenta, are found in foetal tissues and can have toxic effects on the developing foetus (often related to retardation of skeletal development). Evidence of embryotoxicity has also been noted in animals treated early in pregnancy. Ledermycin therefore, should not be used in pregnancy unless considered essential.

The use of drugs of the tetracycline class during tooth development (last half of pregnancy and children to the age of 12 years) may cause permanent discoloration of the teeth (yellow-grey-brown). This adverse reaction is more common during long term use of the drugs but has been observed following repeated short term courses. Enamel hypoplasia has also been reported.

Use in lactation: Tetracyclines have been found in the milk of lactating women who are taking a drug in this class. Permanent tooth discoloration may occur in the developing infant and enamel hypoplasia has been reported. Therefore, Ledermycin should not be administered to lactating women.

Use in children: The use of tetracyclines during tooth development in children under the age of 12 years may cause permanent discoloration (see above). Enamel hypoplasia has also been reported.

Side-effects: Gastro-intestinal disturbances including nausea, vomiting and diarrhoea may occur and, as with all antibiotics, overgrowth of resistant organisms may cause glossitis, stomatitis, vaginitis, or staphylococcal enterocolitis. Dermatological reactions are rare. Bulging fontanelles in infants and benign intracranial hypertension in adults has been reported. Treatment should cease if evidence of raised intracranial pressure develops. Hypersensitivity reactions including: urticaria, angioneurotic oedema, anaphylaxis, anaphylactoid purpura, pericarditis and exacerbation of systemic lupus erythymatosus may occur. Haemolytic anaemia, thrombocytopenia, neutropenia and eosinophilia have been reported. When given over prolonged periods tetracyclines have been reported to produce brown black microscopic discoloration of thyroid glands. No abnormalities of thyroid function are known to occur. Reversible nephrogenic diabetes insipidus can occur especially if treatment is prolonged and/or at high dosages.

Overdosage: No specific antidote. Gastric lavage plus oral administration of milk or antacids. Maintain fluid and electrolyte balance.

Pharmaceutical precautions Ledermycin Capsules and Tablets should be stored at controlled room temperature (15–30°C), in either the original pack or in containers which prevent access of light and moisture.

Legal category POM.

Package quantities *Capsules 150 mg:* Bottles of 20 and 100.

Tablets 300 mg: Bottles of 100.

Further information Nil.

Product licence numbers

Capsules 150 mg	0095/0052
Tablets 300 mg	0095/5044

LEDERSPAN* INJECTION 20 mg/ml
LEDERSPAN* INJECTION 5 mg/ml

Presentation *Suspension 20 mg/ml:* Vials containing a sterile suspension of 20 mg or 100 mg of micronised triamcinolone hexacetonide in 1 ml or 5 ml respectively of an aqueous vehicle with 0.9% benzyl alcohol as a preservative.

Suspension 5 mg/ml: Vials containing a sterile suspension of 25 mg of micronised triamcinolone hexacetonide in 5 ml of an aqueous vehicle with 0.9% benzyl alcohol as a preservative.

Uses Triamcinolone hexacetonide is a relatively insoluble corticosteroid (0.0003% at 25°C in water). It has a prolonged effect on tissue at the local injection site, the duration usually ranging from a few weeks to several months.

Lederspan 20 mg/ml (*for intra-articular and intrasynovial administration*) is indicated in the treatment of rheumatoid arthritis; osteoarthritis; traumatic arthritis; gouty arthritis; synovitis and bursitis; fibrositis, tendinitis, and epicondylitis; intermittent hydrarthrosis; and other subacute or chronic diseases where glucocorticoids can be expected to be useful.

Lederspan 5 mg/ml (*for intralesional and sublesional administration*) is indicated in the treatment of cystic acne; alopecia areata, nummular and dyshidrotic eczema; granuloma annulare; keloids; lichen planus; discoid lupus erythematosus; localised neurodermatitis; prurigo nodularis; and psoriasis of the nails.

Dosage and administration *Adults and children:* For intra-articular and intrasynovial use, 2–30 mg (0.1–1.5 ml), depending on the size of the joint (or synovial space) to be injected, the degree of inflammation and the amount of fluid present. In general, large joints (such as knee, hips, shoulder), require 10–30 mg whereas small joints (such as interphalangeal, metacarpophalangeal) require 2–6 mg. When much synovial fluid is present, aspiration may be performed before administering Lederspan. Subsequent dosage and frequency of injection can best be judged by clinical response. Since Lederspan provides prolonged activity, injections into a single joint or synovial space more frequently than every three to four weeks are not recommended. Repeated intra-articular injections should be as infrequent as possible, consistent with adequate patient care.

For intralesional and sublesional use, the dosage is 0.5 mg or less per square inch of affected skin.

Strict asepsis is mandatory during administration. Topical ethyl chloride spray may be used locally before injection. Since micronised triamcinolone hexacetonide has been designed for ease of administration, a small-bore needle (including 24 gauge needles) may be used. The vial should be gently agitated to achieve uniform suspension before each use.

The optimum dilution (see under 'Pharmaceutical precautions') should be determined according to the nature of the lesion, its size, the depth of the injection, the volume needed, and the location of the lesion. In general, more superficial injections should be accomplished with more dilution. Certain conditions, such as keloids, require a less dilute suspension. Subsequent dose, dilution and frequency of injection should be determined on the basis of the clinical response. With the 20 mg/ml suspension, concentrations stronger than 1:4 should not be used intralesionally, since local subcutaneous atrophy may result.

Lederspan may be administered by Dermojet and the Porton Injector.

Elderly: Steroids should be used with caution in elderly patients.

Contra-indications, warnings, etc

Contra-indications: Although active, latent or questionably healed tuberculosis, ocular herpes simplex and acute psychosis are generally considered to be absolute contra-indications to glucocorticoid therapy, the minimal systemic activity of triamcinolone hexacetonide after local injection might permit cautious use when indicated. The drug should not be used when there is history of hypersensitivity to any of the components of the formulation or when previous injections have produced local atrophy. Infected joints should not be injected with corticosteroids.

As with other glucocorticoid agents, relative contra-indications are active peptic ulcer, acute glomerulonephritis, myasthenia gravis, osteoporosis, fresh intestinal anastomoses, diverticulitis, thrombophlebitis, psychic disturbances, pregnancy, diabetes mellitus, hyperthyroidism, acute coronary artery disease, hypertension, limited cardiac reserve and local or systemic infections, including fungal and exanthematous diseases. The minimal systemic activity of this preparation, however, reduces the risks involved in its use in the presence of these conditions.

Precautions and side-effects: As with all glucocorticoids, an exacerbation of symptoms or 'flare-up' may occur following intra-articular or intrasynovial injections. Local atrophy, burning, flushing, pain and swelling may occur. In addition, prolonged and repeated use in weight-bearing joints may result in further joint degeneration. This is probably related to premature use of still-diseased joints following relief of pain and other symptoms. Not more than two or three large joints should be treated simultaneously in the same patient.

In treating conditions such as tendinitis or tenosynovitis care should be taken that Lederspan is injected into the space between tendon sheath and tendon and not into the tendon itself.

Overdosage or excessive frequency of intralesional injections into the same site may produce local subcutaneous atrophy. If this occurs, recovery may be delayed for several months because of the prolonged action of the drug. Other local effects include abscess, erythema, pain, swelling and necrosis at the injection site.

Systemic effects are rare with Lederspan due to its slow release from the injection site. In addition to those common to all glucocorticoids, some effects particularly associated with triamcinolone therapy are anorexia, myopathy and depression of mood.

If severe reactions occur or an acute infection develops during therapy, use of the drug should be discontinued and appropriate measures taken.

Pharmaceutical precautions Lederspan should be stored at room temperature. Do not freeze.

It may be diluted with Water for Injections BP, Sodium Chloride Intravenous Infusion BP, Sodium Chloride and Glucose Intravenous Infusion BP, Lignocaine Hydrochloride Injection BP, immediately prior to injection.

Fluids containing methyl or propyl hydroxybenzoates or phenol should be avoided since these tend to cause flocculation of the steroid.

Legal category POM.

Package quantities *20 mg/ml:* Single vials containing 20 mg in 1 ml or 100 mg in 5 ml.

5 mg/ml: Single vials containing 25 mg in 5 ml.

Further information Nil.

Product licence numbers

Lederspan 20 mg/ml 0095/0008
Lederspan 5 mg/ml 0095/0009

LEUCOVORIN – see Calcium Leucovorin.

LOXAPAC* ▼

Presentation

10 mg Capsules: Two piece, hard shell, opaque capsules with a yellow body and a green cap, printed with script 'Lederle' over 'L2' on one half and '10 mg' on the other in grey ink, containing 10 mg loxapine as loxapine succinate. The capsules have a locking feature.

25 mg Capsules: Two piece, hard shell, opaque capsules with light green body and a dark green cap, printed with script 'Lederle' over 'L3' on one half and '25 mg' on the other in grey ink, containing 25 mg loxapine as loxapine succinate. The capsules have a locking feature.

50 mg Capsules: Two piece, hard shell, opaque capsules with a blue body and a dark green cap, printed with script 'Lederle' over 'L4' on one half and '50 mg' on the other in white ink, containing 50 mg loxapine as loxapine succinate. The capsules have a locking feature.

Uses The treatment of acute and chronic psychotic states.

Dosage and administration

Adults: Initially 20–50 mg/day in two doses. Dosage is then increased over 7–10 days to the range 60–100 mg/day in 2–4 doses, until there is effective control of psychotic symptoms.

Maximum daily dose: 250 mg.

Maintenance doses should be adjusted to the needs of the patient, usually in the range of 20–100 mg/day in divided doses.

Children: Not recommended for use in children.

Contra-indications, warnings, etc

Contra-indications: Use in comatose or semi-comatose patients or in severe drug-induced depressed states (alcohol, barbiturates, narcotics).

In individuals with known hypersensitivity to the drug.

Precautions: Loxapac may impair mental and/or physical abilities, especially during the first few days of therapy. Therefore, ambulatory patients should be warned about activities requiring alertness (e.g. operating machinery or vehicles), and about concomitant use of alcohol and other CNS depressants.

Loxapac should be used with extreme caution in patients with a history of convulsive disorders, since it lowers the convulsive threshold. Seizures have been reported in epileptic patients receiving Loxapac at antipsychotic dose levels, and may occur even with maintenance of routine anticonvulsant drug therapy.

Loxapac has an antiemetic effect in animals. Since this effect may also occur in man, Loxapac may mask signs of overdosage of toxic drugs and may obscure conditions such as intestinal obstruction and brain tumour.

Loxapac should be used with caution in patients with cardiovascular disease. Increased pulse rates have been reported in the majority of patients receiving antipsychotic doses; transient hypotension has been reported. In the presence of severe hypotension requiring vasopressor therapy, the preferred drugs may be noradrenaline or angiotensin. Usual doses of adrenaline may be ineffective because of inhibition of its vasopressor effect by Loxapac.

The possibility of ocular toxicity from Loxapac cannot be excluded at this time. Therefore, careful observation should be made for pigmentary retinopathy and lenticular pigmentation, since these have been observed in some patients receiving certain other antipsychotic drugs for prolonged periods.

Because of possible anticholinergic action the drug should be used cautiously in patients with glaucoma or a tendency to urinary retention, particularly with concomitant administration of anticholinergic type antiparkinson medication.

Warnings and adverse effects

CNS effects: Manifestations of adverse effects on the central nervous system other than extrapyramidal effects, have been seen infrequently. Drowsiness, usually mild, may occur at the beginning of therapy or when dosage is increased and usually subsides with continued Loxapac therapy. Dizziness, faintness, staggering gait, muscle twitching, weakness, and confusional states have been reported.

Extrapyramidal (Neuromuscular) reactions during the administration of Loxapac have been reported frequently, often during the first few days of treatment. In most patients, these reactions involved Parkinson-like symptoms such as tremor, rigidity, excessive salivation, and masked facies. Also, akathisia (motor restlessness) has been reported relatively frequently. These symptoms are usually not severe and can be controlled by reduction of dosage or by administration of anti-parkinson drugs in usual dosage. Dystonias include spasms of muscles of the neck and face, tongue protrusion, and oculogyric choreo-athetoid movements. These reactions sometimes require reduction or temporary withdrawal of Loxapac dosage in addition to appropriate counteractive drugs.

As with all antipsychotic agents, persistent tardive dyskinesia may appear in some patients on long term therapy or may appear after drug therapy has been discontinued. The risk appears to be greater in elderly patients on high-dose therapy, especially females. The symptoms are persistent and in some patients appear to be irreversible. The syndrome is characterised by rhythmical involuntary movement of the tongue, face, mouth or jaw (e.g. protrusion of tongue, puffing of cheeks, puckering of mouth, chewing movements). Sometimes these may be accompanied by involuntary movements of extremities.

There is no known effective treatment for tardive dyskinesia; anti-Parkinson agents usually do not alleviate the symptoms of this syndrome. It is suggested that all antipsychotic agents be discontinued if these symptoms appear. Should it be necessry to reinstitute treatment, or increase the dose of the agent, or switch to a different antipsychotic agent, the syndrome may be masked. It has been suggested that fine vermicular movements of the tongue may be an early sign of the syndrome, and, if the medication is stopped at that time, the syndrome may not develop.

Cardiovascular effects: Tachycardia, hypotension, hypertension, light-headedness, and syncope have been reported. A few cases of ECG changes similar to those seen with phenothiazines have been reported. It is not known whether these were related to administration.

Skin: Dermatitis, oedema (puffiness of face), pruritis, and seborrhea have been reported with Loxapac. The possibility of photosensitivity and/or phototoxicity occurring has not been excluded; skin rashes of uncertain aetiology have been observed in a few patients during hot summer months.

Endocrine effects: No endocrine abnormalities have been reported.

Anticholinergic effects: Dry mouth, nasal congestion, constipation, and blurred vision have occcurred; these are more likely to occur with concomitant use of anti-Parkinson agents.

Other adverse reactions: Nausea, vomiting, weight gain, weight loss, dyspnoea, ptosis, hyperpyrexia, flushed facies, headache, parasthesia, and polydipsia have been reported in some patients.

A case of neuroleptic malignant syndrome has been reported following the use of Loxapac. This syndrome is potentially fatal and presents with symptoms of hyperpyrexia, muscle rigidity, altered mental status and evidence of autonomic instability. If a patient is diagnosed as suffering from neuroleptic malignant syndrome, the management should include: (1) immediate discontinuation of antipsychotic drugs and other drugs not essential to concurrent therapy, (2) symptomatic treatment and monitoring of vital signs, and (3) treatment of any concomitant serious medical problems.

Drug interactions: Interaction with other central nervous system depressant drugs, anti-Parkinson drugs and alcohol may occur.

Use in pregnancy and lactation: Safe use of Loxapac during pregnancy and lactation has not been established; therefore, its use in pregnancy, in nursing mothers, or in women of childbearing potential, requires that the benefits of treatment be weighed against the possible risks to mother and child.

Overdosage: Signs and symptoms of overdosage might be expected to include convulsive seizures and range from mild depression of the CNS and cardiovascular systems to profound hypotension, respiratory depression and unconsciousness. Renal failure has been reported following Loxapac administration. Severe extrapyramidal reactions should be treated with anticholinergic anti-Parkinson agents or diphenhydramine hydrochloride, and anticonvulsant therapy should be initiated as indicated.

The treatment of overdosage would be essentially symptomatic and supportive. Early gastric lavage and extended dialysis might be expected to be beneficial. Centrally acting emetics may have little effect because of the antiemetic action of loxapine. Avoid analeptics, such as picrotoxin and pentylenetetrazole (pentetrazol), which may cause convulsions. Severe hypotension might be expected to respond to the administration of levarterenol or phenylephrine. ADRENALINE SHOULD NOT BE USED SINCE ITS USE IN A PATIENT WITH PARTIAL ADRENERGIC BLOCKADE MAY FURTHER LOWER THE BLOOD PRESSURE. Additional measures include oxygen and intravenous fluids.

Pharmaceutical precautions Store at controlled room temperature (15–30°C).

Legal category POM.

Package quantities Bottles containing 100 capsules.

Product licence numbers

Loxapac 10 mg Capsules	0095/0036
Loxapac 25 mg Capsules	0095/0037
Loxapac 50 mg Capsules	0095/0038

METHOTREXATE TABLETS METHOTREXATE INJECTION METHOTREXATE POWDER FOR INJECTION

Presentation *Tablets 2.5 mg:* Round, convex, scored, uncoated, yellow tablets embossed 'LL' and 'M1' containing methotrexate sodium equivalent to 2.5 mg of methotrexate per tablet.

Injection: A clear, yellow, sterile, aqueous, isotonic solution containing methotrexate sodium equivalent to 2.5 mg (ampoule), 5 mg, 25 mg, 50 mg, 100 mg, 200 mg, 500 mg, 1 g, or 5 g of methotrexate per vial together with sodium chloride and sodium hydroxide or hydrochloric acid to adjust the pH to approximately 8.5. The Injection does not contain an antimicrobial preservative.

Powder for Injection 500 mg: Vials containing a yellow, lyophilised powder of methotrexate sodium equivalent to 500 mg of methotrexate, which is reconstituted before use with 10 ml Water for Injection. Sodium hydroxide and, if necessary, hydrochloric acid are used during the manufacturing process to adjust the pH to approximately 8.5. The Powder for Injection does not contain any antimicrobial preservative.

Uses *Properties:* Methotrexate, a derivative of folic acid, belongs to the class of cytotoxic agents known as antimetabolites. It acts principally during the 'S' phase of cell division, by the competitive inhibition of the enzyme dihydrofolate reductase, thus preventing the reduction of dihydrofolate to tetrahydrofolate, a necessary step in the process of DNA synthesis and cellular replication.

Indications: The treatment of neoplastic disease. The treatment of severe cases of uncontrolled psoriasis, unresponsive to conventional therapy.

Dosage and administration *Adults and children:* Methotrexate may be given by oral, intramuscular, intravenous (bolus injection or infusion) intrathecal, intra-arterial and intraventricular routes of administration. Dosages are based on the patient's body weight or surface area except in the case of intrathecal or intraventricular administration when a maximum dose of 15 mg is recommended. Doses should be reduced in cases of haematological deficiency and hepatic or renal impairment. Larger doses (greater than 100 mg) are usually given by intravenous infusion over periods not exceeding 24 hours. Part of the dose may be given in an initial rapid intravenous injection.

All parenteral Methotrexate preparations are stable for 24 hours when diluted with the following infusion fluids:—0.9% Sodium Chloride; Glucose; Sodium Chloride and Glucose; Compound Sodium Chloride (Ringers Injection); Compound Sodium Lactate (Lactated Ringers Injection).

Methotrexate has been used with beneficial effects in a wide variety of neoplastic diseases, alone and in combination with other cytotoxic agents, hormones, immunotherapy, radiotherapy or surgery. Dosage schedules therefore vary considerably, depending on the clinical use, particularly when intermittent high-dose regimes are followed by the administration of Calcium Leucovorin (calcium folinate) in order to rescue normal cells from toxic effects.

Dosage regimes for Calcium Leucovorin rescue are discussed under Further Information.

Examples of doses of Methotrexate that have been used for particular indications are given below.

Choriocarcinoma and other trophoblastic tumours: Non-metastatic gestational trophoblastic neoplasms have been treated successfully with 0.25–1 mg/kg up to a maximum of 60 mg intramuscularly every 48 hours for four doses, followed by Calcium Leucovorin rescue. This course of treatment is repeated at seven day intervals until levels of urinary chorionic gonadotrophin hormone return to normal. Not less than four courses of treatment are usually necessary. Patients with complications, such as extensive metastases, may be treated with Methotrexate in combination with other cytotoxic drugs.

Methotrexate has also been used in similar doses for the treatment of hydatidiform mole and chorio-adenoma destruens.

Leukaemia in children: Remissions in acute lymphocytic leukaemia are usually best induced with a combination of corticosteroids and other cytotoxic agents.

Methotrexate 15 mg/m^2, given parenterally or orally once weekly, in combination with other drugs appears to be the treatment of choice for the maintenance of drug-induced remissions.

Meningeal leukaemia in children: The cerebro-spinal fluid (CSF) should be examined in all leukaemic patients in order to diagnose leukaemic invasion of the central nervous system. Doses up to 15 mg, intrathecally, at weekly intervals, until the CSF appears normal (usually 2–3 weeks), have been found useful for the treatment of meningeal leukaemia. It is now common practice because of the frequency of meningeal leukaemia to administer Methotrexate intrathecally, in similar doses, as prophylaxis in all cases of lymphocytic leukaemia.

Although intravenous doses of the order of 50 mg of Methotrexate do not appreciably penetrate the CSF, larger doses of the order of 500 mg/m^2 do produce cytotoxic levels of Methotrexate in the CSF. This type of therapy has been used in short courses, followed by administration of Calcium Leucovorin, as initial maintenance therapy to prevent leukaemic invasion of the central nervous system in children with poor prognosis lymphocytic leukaemia.

Lymphoma: Non-Hodgkin's lymphoma, e.g. childhood lymphosarcoma has recently been treated with 3–30 mg/kg (approximately 90–900 mg/m^2) of Methotrexate given by intravenous injection and infusion followed by administration of Calcium Leucovorin with the higher doses. Some cases of Burkitt's lymphoma, when treated in the early stages with courses of 15 mg/m^2 daily for five days have shown prolonged remissions. Combination chemotherapy is also commonly used in all stages of the disease, and a course of 15 mg/day of Methotrexate intrathecally for four days has been found useful for controlling episodes of invasion of the central nervous system.

Breast cancer: Methotrexate, in intravenous doses of 10–60 mg/m^2, is commonly included in cyclical combination regimes with other cytotoxic drugs in the treatment of advanced breast cancer. Similar regimes have also been used as adjuvant therapy in early cases following mastectomy and/or radiotherapy.

Osteogenic sarcoma: The use of Methotrexate alone and in cyclical combination regimes has recently been introduced as an adjuvant therapy to the primary treatment of osteogenic sarcoma by amputation with or without prosthetic bone replacement. This has involved the use of intravenous infusions of 20–300 mg/kg (approximately 600–9,000 mg/m^2) of Methotrexate followed by Calcium Leucovorin rescue. Methotrexate has also been used as the sole treatment in metastatic cases of osteogenic sarcoma.

Bronchogenic carcinoma: Intravenous infusions of 20–100 mg/m^2 of Methotrexate have been included in cyclical combination regimes for the treatment of advanced tumours. High doses with Calcium Leucovorin rescue have also been employed as the sole treatment.

Head and neck cancer: Intravenous infusions of 240–1,080 mg/m^2 with Calcium Leucovorin rescue have been used recently with encouraging results, both as pre-operative adjuvant therapy and in the treatment of advanced tumours. Intra-arterial infusions of Methotrexate have been used in the treatment of head and neck cancers.

Bladder carcinoma: Intravenous injections or infusions of Methotrexate in doses up to 100 mg every one or two weeks have been used in the treatment of bladder carcinoma with promising results, varying from only symptomatic relief to complete though unsustained regressions. Diuretics and hydration are employed in an attempt to reduce the excessive drug toxicity that has occurred in cases of renal impairment. The use of high doses of Methotrexate with Calcium Leucovorin rescue is currently being evaluated.

Psoriasis: In cases of severe uncontrolled psoriasis, unresponsive to conventional therapy, 10–25 mg orally once a week and adjusted by the patient's response is recommended.

Particular attention should be given to the appearance of liver toxicity by carrying out liver function tests before starting Methotrexate treatment and repeating these at two to four month intervals during therapy. Treatment should not be instituted or should be discontinued if any abnormality of liver function tests, or liver biopsy, is present or develops during therapy.

Such abnormalities should return to normal within two weeks after which treatment may be recommenced at the discretion of the physician.

The use of Methotrexate may permit the return to conventional topical therapy which should be encouraged.

Contra-indications, warnings, etc
Contra-indications: Profound impairment of renal or hepatic function. Serious cases of anaemia, leucopenia, or thrombocytopenia. Pregnancy.

Warnings: Methotrexate should not normally be administered to patients who are pregnant or to mothers who are breast-feeding. Methotrexate has been shown to be teratogenic. Methotrexate should be used with extreme caution in patients with haematological depression, renal impairment, peptic ulcer, ulcerative colitis, ulcerative stomatitis, diarrhoea, debility and in extreme young or old age.

Deaths have been reported with the use of Methotrexate in the treatment of malignancy and psoriasis. Serious adverse reactions including deaths have been reported with concomitant administration of Methotrexate (usually in high doses) along with some non-steroidal anti-inflammatory drugs (NSAIDs).

Symptoms of gastro-intestinal toxicity, usually first manifested by stomatitis, indicates interruption of therapy otherwise haemorrhagic enteritis and death from intestinal perforation may occur.

Methotrexate affects spermatogenesis and oogenesis during the period of its administration which may result in decreased fertility. To date this effect appears to be reversible on discontinuing therapy. Conception should be avoided for at least six months after treatment with Methotrexate has ceased. Patients receiving Methotrexate and their partners should be advised appropriately.

Methotrexate has some immunosuppressive activity and therefore the immunological response to concurrent vaccination may be decreased. In addition, concomitant use of a live vaccine could cause a severe antigenic reaction.

Precautions: Methotrexate should only be used by clinicians who are familiar with the various characteristics of the drug and its established clinical usage. It is essential that the following laboratory tests are included as part of the clinical evaluation and monitoring of patients receiving Methotrexate: complete haematological analysis, urinalysis, renal function tests, liver function tests and, when high doses are administered, determination of plasma levels of Methotrexate. These tests should be performed prior to, during and after termination of each course of therapy.

Haemopoietic suppression caused by Methotrexate may occur abruptly and with apparently safe dosages. Any profound drop in white-cell or platelet counts indicates immediate withdrawal of the drug and appropriate supportive therapy.

It should be noted that intrathecal doses are transported into the cardiovascular system and may give rise to unexpected systemic toxicity, as can the use of Methotrexate in patients with renal dysfunction, ascites, or other effusions due to a longer serum half-life.

High doses may cause the precipitation of Methotrexate or its metabolites in the renal tubules. Alkalinisation of the urine to pH 6.5–7.0 by the oral or intravenous administration of sodium bicarbonate (5 × 625 mg tablets every three hours) or Diamox (500 mg orally four times a day) is recommended as a preventative measure.

Drug interactions: Methotrexate is extensively protein bound and may be displaced by certain drugs such as salicylates, sulphonamides, diuretics, hypoglycaemics, diphenylhydantoins, tetracyclines, chloramphenicol, p-aminobenzoic acid, and the acidic anti-inflammatory agents, so causing a potential for increased toxicity when used concurrently. Concomitant use of other drugs with nephrotoxic or hepatotoxic potential (including alcohol) should be avoided.

Caution should be used when NSAIDs and salicylates are administered concomitantly with Methotrexate. These drugs have been reported to reduce the tubular secretion of Methotrexate in an animal model and thereby may enhance its toxicity. Renal tubular transport is also diminished by probenicid; use of Methotrexate with this drug should be carefully monitored.

Patients using constant dosage regimens of NSAIDs have received concurrent doses of Methotrexate problems. Therefore, until more is known about the NSAIDs/Methotrexate interaction, it is recommended that Methotrexate dosage be carefully controlled during treatment with NSAIDs.

Side-effects: These occur as a result of cytotoxic activity on rapidly reproducing normal cells of the haemopoietic system, gastro-intestinal tract, and sometimes skin. Consequently common adverse reactions are bone-marrow depression, leucopenia, anaemia, thrombocytopenia, nausea, vomiting, diarrhoea and ulcerative stomatitis. Upon prolonged treatment erythematous rashes, hepatic cirrhosis, acute liver atrophy and genitourinary toxicity manifested by renal failure, severe nephropathy, defective oogenesis or spermatogenesis may occur.

Adverse effects upon the central nervous system that may occur following intrathecal or intraventricular administration are headache, drowsiness, blurred vision, transient paresis, ataxia, and rarely, dementia and major convulsions. Other reactions such as pneumonitis, osteoporotic effects and photosensitivity have been attributed to the use of Methotrexate.

Overdosage: Calcium Leucovorin is the antidote for neutralising the immediate toxic effects of Methotrexate on the haemopoietic system. It may be administered orally, intramuscularly, or by an intravenous bolus injection or infusion. In cases of accidental overdosage, a dose of Calcium Leucovorin equal to or higher than the offending dose of Methotrexate should be administered within one hour and further doses as required. Other supporting therapy such as a blood transfusion and renal dialysis may be required.

Pharmaceutical precautions Methotrexate Powder for Injection 500 mg should be reconstituted immediately before use with 10 ml Water for Injection. The appropriate dose of the resulting solution (50 mg/ml) is then diluted for administration by intravenous infusion over periods not exceeding 24 hours. Part of the dose may be given by an initial bolus intravenous injection.

Parenteral Methotrexate preparations do not contain an antimicrobial preservative. Any unused injection or reconstituted solution from Powder for Injection should be discarded.

Parenteral Methotrexate preparations are stable for 24 hours when diluted with the following intravenous infusion fluids:—0.9% Sodium Chloride; Glucose; Sodium Chloride and Glucose; Compound Sodium Chloride (Ringers Injection); Compound Sodium Lactate (Lactated Ringers Injection).

Methotrexate preparations should be stored at controlled room temperature (15–30°C) and protected from direct sunlight. Other drugs should not be mixed with Methotrexate in the same infusion container.

Handling of cytotoxic drugs: Trained personnel should reconstitute Methotrexate powder for injection in a designated area. The work surface should be covered with disposable plastic-backed absorbent paper.

Protective gloves and goggles should be worn to avoid the drug accidentally coming into contact with the skin or eyes.

Methotrexate is not vesicant and should not cause harm if it comes in contact with the skin. It should, of course, be washed off with water immediately. Any transient stinging may be treated with bland cream. If there is any danger of systemic absorption of significant quantities of Methotrexate, by any route, Leucovorin cover should be given.

The cytotoxic preparation should not be handled by pregnant staff.

Any spillage or waste material may be disposed of by incineration. We do not make any specific recommendations with regards to the temperature of the incinerator.

Legal category POM.

Package quantities

Tablets 2.5 mg: Bottles of 100.

Tablets 10 mg: Bottles of 50.

Injection 2.5 mg in 1 ml: Boxes of 10 ampoules.

Injection 5 mg in 2 ml: Boxes of 5 vials.

Injection 25 mg in 1 ml: Boxes of 1 vial.

Injection 50 mg in 2 ml: Boxes of 1 vial.

Injection 100 mg in 4 ml: Boxes of 1 vial.

Injection 200 mg in 8 ml: Boxes of 1 vial.

Injection 500 mg in 20 ml: Boxes of 1 vial.

Injection 1 g in 40 ml: Boxes of 1 vial.

Injection 5 g in 200 ml: Boxes of 1 vial.

Powder for Injection 500 mg: Boxes of 1 vial.

Further information Dosage regimes for Calcium Leucovorin rescue vary, depending upon the dose of Methotrexate administered. In general, up to 150 mg are usually given in divided doses, over 12–24 hours, by intramuscular injection, bolus intravenous injection or intravenous infusion or orally, followed by 12–15 mg intramuscularly, IV, or 15 mg (one tablet) orally, every six hours for the next 48 hours. Rescue therapy is usually started following a delay of 8 to 24 hours from the beginning of the Methotrexate infusion. One tablet (15 mg) of Calcium Leucovorin every six hours for 48–72 hours may be sufficient when lower doses (less than 100 mg) of Methotrexate have been given.

Calcium Leucovorin is available as an injection (3 mg/ml) in 1 ml ampoules, as a vial of powder for injection (15 mg and 30 mg) and as tablets (15 mg) in bottles of 10.

The clinical use of high doses of Methotrexate with Calcium Leucovorin rescue in the treatment of a wide variety of previously resistant tumours remains the subject of intense research.

Further information on other formulations of Methotrexate, on results with particular cyclical regimes of combinations of cytotoxic drugs and other aspects of cancer chemotherapy with Methotrexate is available on request.

Product licence numbers

Tablets 2.5 mg	0095/5079
Injection 2.5 mg/ml	0095/0015
Injection 25 mg/ml	0095/0016
Powder for Injection 500 mg	0095/0054

MINOCIN* 50 and 100

Presentation *Tablets 100 mg:* Each orange, film-coated tablet, embossed LL on one face and M/100 on the reverse face, contains minocycline hydrochloride equivalent to 100 mg minocycline base.

Tablets 50 mg: Each beige film-coated tablet, embossed LL on one face and M/50 on the reverse face, contains minocycline hydrochloride equivalent to 50 mg minocycline base.

Uses Minocycline is a broad spectrum antibiotic used for the treatment of infections caused by tetracycline-sensitive organisms. Some tetracycline-resistant strains of Staphylococci are also sensitive.

Typical indications include: Gonorrhoea. Non-gonococcal urethritis. Prostatitis. Acne. Acute and chronic bronchitis. Bronchiectasis. Lung abscess. Pneumonia. Ear nose and throat infections. Urinary tract infections. Pelvic inflammatory disease (e.g. salpingitis, oophoritis). Skin and soft tissue infections caused by minocycline sensitive organisms. Ophthalmological infections. Nocardiosis. Prophylactic treatment of asymptomatic meningococcal carriers. Pre- and post-operative prophylaxis of infection.

Dosage and administration *Adults:*

1. Routine antibiotic use: 200 mg daily in divided doses.
2. Acne: 50 mg twice daily.
3. Gonorrhoea: In adult males: 200 mg initially followed by 100 mg every 12 hours for a minimum of 4 days with post-therapy cultures within 2–3 days. Adult females may require more prolonged therapy.
4. Prophylaxis of asymptomatic meningococcal carriers: 100 mg b.i.d. for five days, usually followed by a course of rifampicin.

Children: For children above 12 years of age the recommended dosage for Minocin is one 50 mg tablet every 12 hours. Minocin is not recommended for children under 12 years old.

Elderly: Minocin may be used at the normal recommended dosage in elderly patients even with mild to moderate renal impairment, however caution is advised in patients with severe renal impairment.

Administration: Unlike earlier tetracyclines, absorption of Minocin is not significantly impaired by food or moderate amounts of milk. Treatment of acne should be continued for a minimum of six weeks.

Contra-indications, warnings, etc

Contra-indications: Known hypersensitivity to tetracyclines, pregnancy, lactation, children under the age of 12 years, complete renal failure.

Warnings and precautions: Minocin should be used with caution in patients with hepatic dysfunction and in conjunction with alcohol and other hepatotoxic drugs. Clinical studies have shown that there is no significant drug accumulation in patients with renal impairment when they are treated with Minocin in the recommended doses. In cases of severe renal insufficiency, reduction of dosage and monitoring of renal function may be required.

Cross-resistance between tetracyclines may develop in micro-organisms and cross-sensitisation in patients. Minocin should be discontinued if there are signs/symptoms of overgrowth of resistant organisms, enteritis eg glossitis, stomatitis, vaginitis, pruritis ani or staphylococcal enteritis.

Interactions: Minocin should not be used with penicillins. Tetracyclines depress plasma prothrombin activity and reduced doses of concomitant anticoagulants may be necessary.

Absorption of Minocin is impaired by the concomitant administration of antacids, iron, calcium, magnesium and zinc salts. Unlike earlier tetracyclines, absorption of Minocin is not significantly impaired by food or moderate amounts of milk.

Use in pregnancy: Results of animal studies indicate that tetracyclines cross the placenta and are found in foetal tissues and can have toxic effects on the developing foetus (often related to retardation of skeletal development). Evidence of embryotoxicity has also been noted in animals treated early in pregnancy. Minocin therefore, should not be used in pregnancy unless considered essential.

The use of drugs of the tetracycline class during tooth development (last half of pregnancy) may cause permanent discoloration of the teeth (yellow-grey brown). This adverse reaction is more common during long term use of the drugs but has been observed following repeated short term courses. Enamel hypoplasia has also been reported.

Use in lactation: Tetracyclines have been found in the milk of lactating women who are taking a drug in this class. Permanent tooth discoloration may occur in the developing infant and enamel hypoplasia has been reported.

Use in children: The use of tetracyclines during tooth development in children under the age of 12 years may cause permanent discoloration (see above). Enamel hypoplasia has also been reported.

Side-effects: Gastrointestinal disturbances including nausea, vomiting and diarrhoea may occur. Dermatological reactions are rare. However, erythema multiforme, Stevens–Johnson syndrome, exfoliative dermatitis and photosensitivity have been reported. Hypersensitivity reactions including urticaria, angioneurotic oedema, anaphylaxis, anaphylactoid purpura, pericarditis and exacerbation of systemic lupus erythematosus have been reported.

Lightheadedness, dizziness and vertigo have occurred with Minocin and patients should be warned about the possible hazards of driving or operating machinery during treatment.

Bulging fontanelles in infants and benign intracranial hypertension in adults has been reported. Treatment should cease if evidence of raised intracranial pressure develops.

Blood: haemolytic anaemia, thrombocytopenia, neutropenia and eosinophilia have been reported with tetracyclines.

When given over prolonged periods, tetracyclines have been reported to produce brown-black microscopic discoloration of thyroid tissue. No abnormalities of thyroid function are known to occur.

Overdosage: No specific antidote. Gastric lavage plus appropriate supportive treatment.

Pharmaceutical precautions The product should be stored under normal room temperature conditions (15–30°C) in the original pack or in containers which prevent access of moisture. Protect from light.

Legal category POM.

Package quantities *100 mg Tablets:* Bottles of 20 and 50.

50 mg Tablets: Blister packs of 84.

Further information Nil.

Product licence numbers
100 mg Tablets 0095/0006
50 mg Tablets 0095/0062

MONOCOR* TABLETS

Presentation
Tablets 5 mg: Pink, round, scored, biconvex film-coated tablets marked 'LL' on one side and '5' on reverse, each containing 5 mg bisoprolol fumarate (2:1).
Tablets 10 mg: White, round biconvex film-coated tablets marked 'LL' on one side and '10' on reverse, each containing 10 mg bisoprolol fumarate (2:1).

Uses
Indications: The management of hypertension. The management of angina pectoris.

Mode of action: Monocor is a potent, highly cardioselective B_1–adrenoceptor blocking agent devoid of intrinsic sympathomimetic activity and without relevant membrane stabilising activity.

As with other beta-blocking agents, the mode of action in hypertension is not clear but it is known that Monocor reduces the heart rate and depresses plasma renin activity.

In patients with angina, blocking of cardiac B_1-receptors causes diminished cardiac oxygen demand because of the resulting reduced heart action. This makes Monocor effective in eliminating or reducing the symptoms.

Dosage and administration
Adults: The usual adult dose is 10 mg once daily with a maximum recommended dose of 20 mg per day. In some patients, 5 mg per day may be adequate.

It is not necessary to alter the dose in patients with mild to moderate hepatic or renal dysfunction. In patients with severe renal failure (creatinine clearance less than 20 ml/min) or in patients with severe hepatic dysfunction, the dosage should not exceed 10 mg Monocor once daily.

Experience of use of Monocor in renal dialysis patients is limited, however, there is no evidence that the dosage regimen needs to be altered.

Elderly: No dosage adjustment is normally required but 5 mg per day may be adequate in some elderly patients; as for other adults, the dosage may have to be reduced in cases of severe renal or hepatic dysfunction.

Children: There is no paediatric experience with bisoprolol, therefore its use cannot be recommended for children.

Contra-indications, warnings, etc
Contra-indications: As with other beta-adrenoceptor antagonists, Monocor should not be used in cases of untreated cardiac failure, cardiogenic shock, sinoatrial block, second or third degree AV block, marked bradycardia (less than 50 beats per minute), extreme hypotension or severe asthma.

Precautions: Monocor should be used with care in patients with a prolonged PR conduction interval, poor cardiac reserve and peripheral circulatory disturbances, such as Raynaud's phenomena.

In patients suffering ischaemic heart disease treatment should not be discontinued abruptly.

Due to the low affinity of Monocor for B_2-receptors, the drug does not appear to have a hypoglycaemic effect. However, it should be used with caution in diabetic patients since the symptoms of hypoglycaemia (in particular tachycardia) may be masked.

Although bisoprolol is a highly selective B_1-adrenoceptor blocking agent, it should be used with caution in patients with chronic obstructive airways diseases or a family history of asthma. In some asthmatic patients some increase in airways resistance may occur and this may be regarded as a signal to discontinue therapy. Bronchospasm can usually be reversed by commonly used bronchodilators such as salbutamol.

Pregnancy and lactation: No teratogenic effects have been demonstrated in animal studies but the safety of Monocor during human pregnancy has not been established. Like other beta-blockers, the benefits of use during pregnancy should be weighed against the possible hazards to mother and foetus. Studies in animals suggest that no clinically relevant levels of Monocor reach the breast milk. However, as in pregnancy, caution should be exercised for use during lactation.

Side-effects: Monocor is well tolerated. The reported side effects are generally attributable to its pharmacological actions and include lassitude, dizziness, mild headache, perspiration, aggravation of intermittent claudication or Raynaud's disease and paraesthesia of the extremities. A marked decrease in blood pressure and pulse rate or a disturbance of AV conduction, may be observed occasionally. As with other beta-blockers skin rashes and dry eyes have been reported although the incidence is low. Discontinuation of the drug is recommended if any such reaction is not otherwise explicable. Sleep disturbances of a type noted with othe beta-blockers have rarely been reported.

Drug interactions: Monocor may potentiate the effect of other concurrently administered anti-hypertensive drugs. Concomitant treatment with reserpine, alpha-methyldopa and clonidine may cause an exaggerated decrease in heart rate. In particular, if clonidine is to be discontinued this should not be done until Monocor treatment has been discontinued for several days.

Monocor should also be used with care when myocardial depressants, inhibitors of AV conduction such as calcium antagonists of the verapamil and diltiazem type, of Class I antidysrhythmic agents such as disopyramide are used concurrently.

The intravenous administration of calcium antagonists and antiarrhythmic agents is not recommended during Monocor therapy.

The concurrent use of rifampicin can reduce the elimination half-life of Monocor, although an increase in dose is generally not necessary. The effects of insulin or oral hypoglycaemic agents may be potentiated when used concurrently with Monocor.

Anaesthesia: Prior to anaesthesia, the anaesthetist should be informed if the patient is taking Monocor. In cases of severe ischaemic heart disease the risk/benefit of continuing treatment should be evaluated. Care should be taken when using either cyclopropane or trichloroethylene.

Overdosage: In the case of overdosage or a precipitous drop in pulse rate and/or blood pressure, treatment with Monocor must be discontinued. Excessive bradycardia may be countered by atropine 0.5–2.0 mg intravenously. If necessary this may be followed by a beta stimulant such as orciprenaline by slow intravenous injection. Glucagon may also be useful as a cardiac stimulant in a dose of 1 to 5 mg intravenously.

Pharmaceutical precautions No special requirements.

Legal category POM.

Package quantities Calendarised blister packs of 28

tablets in strips of 14. White plastic bottles containing 100 tablets.

Further information Bisoprolol is absorbed almost completely from the gastrointestinal tract. Together with the very small first pass effect in the liver, this results in a high bioavailability of approximately 90%. The drug is cleared equally by the liver and kidneys. The high bioavailability and the dual pathway of clearance lead to predictable blood levels. The long plasma half-life (10–12 hours) provides 24 hour efficacy following a once daily dosage. About 95% of the drug substance is excreted through the kidneys, half of this as unchanged Bisoprolol. There are no active metabolites in man.

Product licence numbers
Tablets 5 mg 0095/0177.
Tablets 10 mg 0095/0178.

MYAMBUTOL*

Presentation *Tablets 100 mg:* Each yellow, coated tablet contains 100 mg ethambutol hydrochloride.

Tablets 400 mg: Each grey, coated tablet contains 400 mg ethambutol hydrochloride.

Powder: Each bottle contains 50 g ethambutol hydrochloride.

Uses The primary treatment and re-treatment of tuberculosis and for prophylaxis in cases of inactive tuberculosis or large tuberculin-positive reaction. Myambutol should only be used in conjunction with other antituberculous drugs to which the patient's organisms are susceptible.

Dosage and administration The dosage of Myambutol must be adjusted according to the body weight of the patient.

Adults: For primary treatment and prophylaxis: Myambutol should be administered in a single daily oral dose of 15 mg/kg, concomitant drugs being used at their recommended dosage levels.

For re-treatment: For the first 60 days of treatment, Myambutol should be administered in a single daily oral dose of 25 mg/kg. Thereafter the dosage should be reduced to 15 mg/kg, concomitant drugs being maintained at their recommended dosage levels.

Children: For primary treatment and re-treatment: For the first 60 days of treatment, a single daily oral dose of 25 mg/kg. Thereafter the dosage should be reduced to 15 mg/kg, concomitant drugs being maintained at their recommended dosage levels.

For prophylaxis: A single daily oral dose of 15 mg/kg, concomitant drugs being used at their recommended dosage levels.

Elderly: As for adults. However, patients with decreased renal function may need to have the dosage adjusted as determined by blood levels of Myambutol.

Administration: In order to obtain maximum effect due to high serum levels, drug administration should be once daily. Absorption of Myambutol is not significantly altered by administration with food.

Paediatric doses can be given using an extemporaneously prepared syrup (see Further Information).

A table of dosages is given on the following page.

Contra-indications, warnings, etc

Contra-indications: Myambutol is contra-indicated in patients who are known to be hypersensitive to the drug. It is also contra-indicated in patients with known optic neuritis unless clinical judgement determines that it may be used.

Precautions: Patients with decreased renal function may need to have the dosage adjusted as determined by blood levels of Myambutol. Animal studies with Myambutol have shown some teratogenic potential. There have been several reports of the drug having been administered during pregnancy without untoward effect. Nevertheless, it is recommended that the possibility of such effects should be kept in mind when treating women of child-bearing age.

Because this drug has a unique effect on the eye, it is recommended that patients undergo a full ophthalmic examination before starting treatment. This should include visual acuity, colour vision, perimetry and ophthalmoscopy. Many physicians consider that routine ophthalmological examination for adults is not thereafter necessary, but patients should be informed of the importance of reporting any change in vision. However, routine ophthalmological examinations may be considered desirable when treating young children.

Side-effects: Myambutol may produce a unique type of visual impairment which is generally reversible and which appears to be due to optic neuritis and to be related to dose and duration of treatment. Less than 1% of patients undergoing treatment with the higher dose regimen of 25 mg/kg/day for two months, and 15 mg/kg/day thereafter, have exhibited decrease in visual acuity. The change may be unilateral or bilateral and hence both eyes must be tested individually. The effects are generally reversible when administration of the drug is discontinued promptly. In rare cases recovery may be delayed for up to one year or more and the effect may possibly be irreversible in these cases.

Recovery of visual acuity has usually occurred over a period of weeks to months after the drug was discontinued, and patients have then received Myambutol at lower dosages without toxicity. Test patients receiving Myambutol as sole therapy did not have gastro-intestinal

Dosage of Myambutol

15 mg/kg (7 mg/lb) schedule:

Weight range	*kg*	*Total daily dose (mg)*	*100 mg*		*400 mg*
Children	8	120			
	17	255			
	25	375			
	33	495			
Adults *lb*	*kg*		*Number of tablets* 100 mg		400 mg
85–94.5	38–42.5	600	2	+	1
95–109.5	43–49.5	700	3	+	1
110–124.5	50–56.5	800			2
125–139.5	57–63.5	900	1	+	2
140–154.5	64–70.5	1,000	2	+	2
155–169.5	71–78.5	1,100	3	+	2
170–184.5	79–83.5	1,200			3
185–199.5	84–89.5	1,300	1	+	3
200–214.5	90–96.5	1,400	2	+	3
215 and over	97 and over	1,500	3	+	3

25 mg/kg (11 mg/lb) schedule:

Weight range	*kg*	*Total daily dose (mg)*	*100 mg*		*400 mg*
Children	5	125			
	10	250			
	15	375			
	20	500			
	25	625			
	30	750			
	35	875			
Adults *lb*	*kg*		*Number of tablets* 100 mg		400 mg
85–92.5	38–41.5	1,000	2	+	2
93–101.5	42–44.5	1,100	3	+	2
102–109.5	45–49.5	1,200			3
110–118.5	50–53.5	1,300	1	+	3
119–128.5	54–57.5	1,400	2	+	3
129–136.5	58–61.5	1,500	3	+	3
137–146.5	62–66.5	1,600			4
147–155.5	67–70.5	1,700	1	+	4
156–164.5	71–74.5	1,800	2	+	4
165–173.5	75–78.5	1,900	3	+	4
174–182.5	79–82.5	2,000			5
183–191.5	83–86.5	2,100	1	+	5
192–199.5	87–90.5	2,200	2	+	5
200–209.5	91–94.5	2,300	3	+	5
210–218.5	95–98.5	2,400			6
219 and over	99 and over	2,500	1	+	6

disturbances (e.g. anorexia, nausea, vomiting, diarrhoea), transient impairment of liver function or allergic reactions, although these have been noted during multiple-drug antituberculous therapy in which Myambutol was employed. Numbness and paraesthesia of the extremities have been reported.

Overdosage: No specific antidote, but gastric lavage should be employed if necessary.

Pharmaceutical precautions Myambutol should be stored at controlled room temperature (15–30°C) in either the original pack or in containers which prevent access of moisture.

Legal category POM.

Package quantities *Myambutol 100 mg:* Bottles of 100 and 500.

Myambutol 400 mg: Bottles of 100 and 500.

Powder: Bottles of 50 g.

Further information Details of a formulation for ethambutol syrup suitable for paediatric use are available on request from the Medical Information Department. A mixture of ethambutol syrup and isoniazid elixir BPC should not be prepared as isoniazid is unstable in the presence of sugars.

Product licence numbers
Myambutol 100 mg 0095/0002
Myambutol 400 mg 0095/0003
Myambutol Powder 50 g 0095/5083

MYNAH*

Presentation *Mynah 200:* Each white tablet coded 'Lederle 5033' contains 200 mg ethambutol hydrochloride plus 100 mg isoniazid.

Mynah 250: Each yellow tablet coded 'Lederle 5133' contains 250 mg ethambutol hydrochloride plus 100 mg isoniazid.

Mynah 300: Each orange tablet coded 'Lederle 5137' contains 300 mg ethambutol hydrochloride plus 100 mg isoniazid.

Mynah 365: Each pink tablet coded 'Lederle 5134' contains 365 mg ethambutol hydrochloride plus 100 mg isoniazid.

Uses The primary treatment and re-treatment of tuberculosis and for prophylaxis in cases of inactive tuberculosis or large tuberculin-positive reaction.

Dosage and administration *Adults:* Dosage of Mynah is gauged according to the patient's body weight, which governs the included amount of ethambutol; the dosage of isoniazid is standardised at 100 mg per tablet.

For primary treatment and prophylaxis: Mynah should be administered in a single daily oral dose such that the patient receives 15 mg/kg of ethambutol plus 300 mg isoniazid, concomitant drugs being used at their recommended dosage levels.

For re-treatment: For the first 60 days of treatment Mynah should be administered in a single daily oral dose such that the patient receives 25 mg/kg of ethambutol plus 300 mg of isoniazid, concomitant drugs being used at their recommended dosage levels. Thereafter proceed as in 'Primary treatment' above.

Children: The quantities and proportions of the component drugs make Mynah tablets unsuitable for most children. (See Further Information).

Elderly: Patients with decreased renal function may need to have the dosage adjusted as determined by blood levels of ethambutol.

Administration: In order to obtain maximum effect due to high serum levels, drug administration should be once daily. As absorption of isoniazid but not ethambutol is significantly reduced by administration with food, it is recommended that Mynah be taken on an empty stomach.

A table of dosages is given above.

Contra-indications, warnings, etc
Contra-indications: Mynah is contra-indicated in patients who are known to be hypersensitive to ethambutol or isoniazid. It is also contra-indicated in patients with known optic neuritis unless clinical judgement determines that it may be used. Although no absolute contra-indications to the administration of isoniazid have been reported, care should be exercised in the administration of Mynah to epileptic patients since it may induce convulsions, or in psychotic states characterised by mania and hypomania, or in the presence of impaired renal function.

Precautions: Patients with decreased renal function may need to have the dosage adjusted as determined by blood levels of ethambutol. Animal studies with ethambutol have not demonstrated any teratogenic potential and there have been several reports of isoniazid or ethambutol having been administered during pregnancy without untoward effect. Nevertheless, it is recommended that the possibility of such effects should be kept in mind when treating women of childbearing age.

Because ethambutol has a unique effect on the eye, it is recommended that patients undergo a full ophthalmic examination before starting treatment. This should include visual acuity, colour vision, perimetry and ophthalmoscopy. Many physicians consider that routine ophthalmological examination is not thereafter necessary, but patients should be informed of the importance of reporting any change in vision.

Side-effects: For ethambutol: Ethambutol may produce a unique type of visual impairment which is generally reversible and which appears to be due to optic neuritis and to be related to dose and duration of treatment. Less than 1% of patients undergoing treatment with the higher dose regimen of 25 mg/kg/day for two months and 15 mg/kg/day thereafter, have exhibited decrease in visual acuity. The change may be unilateral or bilateral and hence both eyes must be tested individually. The effects are generally reversible when administration of the drug is discontinued promptly. In rare cases recovery may be delayed for up to one year or more and the effect may possibly be irreversible in these cases.

Recovery of visual acuity has usually occurred over a period of weeks to months after the drug is discontinued, and patients have then received ethambutol at lower dosages without toxicity. Test patients receiving ethambutol as sole therapy did not have gastro-intestinal disturbances (e.g. anorexia, nausea, vomiting, diarrhoea), transient impairment of liver function or allergic reactions, although these have been noted during multiple-drug antituberculous therapy in which ethambutol was employed. Numbness and paraesthesia of the extremities has been reported.

For isoniazid: Side-effects are infrequently encountered and are rarely serious. Peripheral neuritis is most often observed, and correlation exists between the dosage level and this reaction. When the dosage is 3 mg/kg/day, the incidence is approximately 1%; at 10 mg/kg/day, it rises to 15% or higher. Pyridoxine (vitamin B_6) has been used successfully for prophylaxis and treatment of isoniazid-induced peripheral neuritis.

Severe and sometimes fatal hepatitis associated with isoniazid therapy may occur and may develop even after many months of treatment. The risk of developing hepatitis is age related and is increased with daily consumption of alcohol.

CNS effects (insomnia, headache, restlessness, mental confusion, toxic psychoses, increased reflexes, muscle twitching, paraesthesia) may be encountered. Optic neuritis and optic atrophy have been reported. Ophthalmological examinations should be carried out wherever visual complaints occur, since the optic lesions are likely to be reversible if isoniazid is discontinued promptly. Extremely high dosages have produced convulsions in apparently normal individuals.

Urinary disturbances in the male (prostatic obstruction syndrome), constipation and dryness of the mouth have been reported. Allergic reactions occur infrequently. Agranulocytosis and exfoliative dermatitis have occasionally been reported.

Dosage of Mynah:

Table 1 Mynah tablets weight/dose schedule 15 mg/kg (7 mg/lb)

Body weight		Ingredients		
lb	*kg*	*INH mg*	*Ethambutol mg*	*Daily dose*
77–98	35–44.5	300	600	3 tablets Mynah 200
99–120	45–54.5	300	750	3 tablets Mynah 250
121–142	55–64.5	300	900	3 tablets Mynah 300
143–175	65–79.5	300	1095	3 tablets Mynah 365

Table 2 Mynah tablets weight/dose schedule 25 mg/kg (11 mg/lb)

Body weight		Ingredients		Daily dose	
lb	*kg*	*INH mg*	*Ethambutol mg*	*Mynah*	*Myambutol*
Under 77	Under 35	300	750	3×250	
77–83	35–37.8	300	900	3×300	
83.5–107	37.9–47	300	1095	3×365	
108–125	48–55	300	1300	3×300	+ 1×400 mg
126–143	56–63	300	1495	3×365	+ 1×400 mg
144–161	64–71	300	1700	3×300	+ 2×400 mg
162–180	72–79	300	1895	3×365	+ 2×400 mg
181–198	80–87	300	2100	3×300	+ 3×400 mg
199–216	88–94	300	2295	3×365	+ 3×400 mg
217–234	95–103	300	2500	3×300	+ 4×400 mg

Overdosage: No specific antidote, but gastric lavage should be employed if necessary.

Pharmaceutical precautions Mynah Tablets should be stored at controlled room temperature (15–30°C), in either the original pack or in containers which prevent access of moisture.

Legal category POM.

Package quantities *Mynah 200:* Bottles of 84.
Mynah 250: Bottles of 84.
Mynah 300: Bottles of 84.
Mynah 365: Bottles of 84.

Further information The quantities and proportions of the component drugs make Mynah tablets unsuitable for most children. Details of a formulation of ethambutol syrup suitable for paediatric use are available on request from the Medical Information Department. A mixture of ethambutol syrup and isoniazid elixir BPC should not be prepared as isoniazid is unstable in the presence of sugars.

Product licence numbers
Mynah 200 0095/0044
Mynah 250 0095/0045
Mynah 300 0095/0046
Mynah 365 0095/0047

NOLTAM*

Presentation White, round, biconvex film-coated tablets, containing Tamoxifen Citrate BP equivalent to 10 mg and 20 mg of Tamoxifen. 10 mg tablets are marked 'LL' on one face and 'T4' on the reverse face. 20 mg tablets are marked 'LL' on one face and 'T5' either side of a score line of the reverse face.

Uses At the recommended dosage, Noltam has anti-oestrogenic properties, probably because it competes with oestrogen for binding sites in target organs. It does not have androgenic properties.

Noltam is indicated for:

1. The treatment of breast cancer. The proportion of patients with breast cancer who respond to Noltam is similar to that seen with oestrogens or androgens. However, because Noltam produces fewer serious side effects, it is more acceptable to the patient.

2. The treatment of anovulatory infertility.

Dosage and administration

1. *Breast cancer:* The recommended initial dose of Noltam is 20 mg daily in single or divided doses. If no response is seen within one month, dosage should be increased to 40 mg daily in single or divided doses.

2. *Infertility:* Before commencing any course of treatment, whether initial or subsequent, the possibility of pregnancy must be excluded. In women who are menstruating regularly, but with anovular cycles, the initial course of treatment consists of 20 mg daily in single or divided doses given on the second, third, fourth and fifth days of the menstrual cycle. If unsatisfactory basal temperature records or poor pre-ovulatory cervical mucus indicate that this initial course of treatment has been unsuccessful, further courses may be given during subsequent menstrual periods, increasing the dosage to 40 mg and then to 80 mg daily in single or divided doses.

In women who are not menstruating regularly, the initial course may begin on any day. If no signs of ovulation are demonstrable, then a subsequent course of treatment may start 45 days later with dosage increased as above. If a patient responds with menstruation, then the next course of treatment is commenced on the second day of the cycle.

Contra-indications, warnings, etc Noltam must not be given during pregnancy. Pre-menopausal patients must be carefully examined before treatment for breast cancer or infertility to exclude the possibility of pregnancy.

Menstruation is suppressed in a proportion of pre-menopausal women receiving Noltam for the treatment of breast cancer. Reversible cystic ovarian swelling has very occasionally been observed when such women have been treated with 40 mg Noltam twice daily for short periods.

A small number of patients with bony metastases have developed hypercalcaemia on initiation of therapy.

During long-term treatment, side effects are not as numerous or as serious with Noltam as with the androgens and oestrogens which are also used to treat breast cancer. Those that have been reported can be classified as either due to the anti-oestrogenic action of the drug, e.g. hot flushes, vaginal bleeding, and pruritis vulvae, or as more general effects, e.g. gastro-intestinal intolerance, tumour pain, light-headedness and, occasionally, fluid retention.

When side effects are severe, it is sometimes possible to control them by a simple reduction of dosage without loss of control of the disease. If side effects do not respond to this measure, it may be necessary to stop the treatment.

Transient falls in platelet count, usually only to 80,000–90,000 but occasionally lower, have been reported in patients taking Noltam for breast cancer. No haemorrhagic tendency has been reported and the platelet counts have recovered even though treatment with Noltam has continued.

There have been infrequent reports of thromboembolic events occurring during Noltam therapy. As an increased incidence of these events is known to occur in patients with malignant disease, a causal relationship with Noltam has not been established.

A small number of endometrial hyperplasia, endometrial polyps and endometrial carcinomas have been reported in association with Noltam treatment. A definitive relationship to Noltam therapy has not been established.

A number of cases of visual disturbance including corneal changes, cataracts, and retinopathy, have been described in patients receiving Noltam therapy.

Drug interaction: coumarin anticoagulants: Patients taking coumarin-type anticoagulants require close monitoring during the introduction or withdrawal of tamoxifen. Serious over-anticoagulation may occur when tamoxifen is used in combination with warfarin; considerable reductions in the daily dose of warfarin may be required to maintain safe anticoagulation. Cases of life theatening interactions have been reported.

Overdosage: On theoretical grounds an overdosage would be expected to cause enhancement of the anti-oestrogenic side effects mentioned above. Observations in animals show that extreme overdosage (100–200 × recommended daily dose) may produce oestrogenic effects.

Corneal and macular changes resulting in blurred vision have been described in a small number of cases treated continuously with 12–16 times the recommended starting dose for periods in excess of 17 months.

There is no specific antidote to overdosage, and treatment must be symptomatic.

Pharmaceutical precautions Protect from light and store at controlled room temperature (15–30°C).

Legal category POM.

Package quantities Noltam is packed in containers of 30 and 250 tablets.

Further information Nil.

Product licence numbers
10 mg tablets 0095/0094
20 mg tablets 0095/0095

NOVANTRONE* INJECTION

Presentation Novantrone injection (2 mg/ml): Glass vials containing a sterile, dark blue aqueous isotonic solution of mitozantrone hydrochloride equivalent to 20 mg, 25 mg and 30 mg mitozantrone, together with sodium chloride and a buffer of sodium acetate and acetic acid to approximately pH3.

Uses Novantrone is an antineoplastic agent. Novantrone is indicated for the treatment of advanced breast cancer, non-Hodgkin's lymphoma and adult acute non-lymphocytic leukaemia. Novantrone has also been used in the palliation of non-resectable primary hepatocellular carcinoma.

Dosage and administration

1. Advanced breast cancer, non-Hodgkin's lymphoma, hepatoma:

(a) Single agent dosage – The recommended initial dosage of Novantrone used as a single agent is 14 mg/m² of body surface area, given as a single intravenous dose which may be repeated at 21-day intervals. A lower initial dosage (12 mg/m² or less) is recommended in patients with inadequate bone marrow reserves, e.g. due to prior chemotherapy or poor general condition.

Dosage modification and the timing of subsequent dosing should be determined by clinical judgement depending on the degree and duration of myelosuppression. For subsequent courses the prior dose can usually be repeated if white blood cell and platelet counts have returned to normal levels after 21 days.

The following table is suggested as a guide to dosage adjustment, in the treatment of advanced breast cancer, non-Hodgkin's lymphoma and hepatoma according to haematological nadir, (which usually occurs about 10 days after dosing):

Nadir after prior Dose WBC (per mm³)		Platelets (per mm³)	Time to recovery	Subsequent dose after adequate haematological recovery
> 1,500	and	> 50,000	≤ 21 days	Repeat prior dose after recovery, or increase by 2 mg/m² if myelosuppression is not considered adequate.
> 1,500	and	> 50,000	> 21 days	Withhold until recovery then repeat prior dose
< 1,500	or	< 50,000	Any duration	Decrease by 2 mg/m² from prior dose after recovery.
< 1,000	or	< 25,000	Any duration	Decrease by 4 mg/m² from prior dose after recovery.

(b) Combination therapy – Novantrone has been given as part of combination therapy. In advanced breast cancer, combinations of Novantrone with other cytotoxic agents including cyclophosphamide and 5-fluorouracil or methotrexate and mitomycin C have been shown to be effective. Reference should be made to the published literature for information on dosage modifications and administration. Novantrone has also been used in various combinations for non-Hodgkins lymphoma, however data are presently limited and specific regimens cannot be recommended.

As a guide, when Novantrone is used in combination chemotherapy with another myelosuppressive agent, the initial dose of Novantrone should be reduced by 2–4 mg/m² below the doses recommended above for single agent usage; subsequent dosing, as outlined in the table above, depends on the degree and duration of myelosuppression.

2. Acute non-lymphocytic leukaemia

(a) Single agent dosage in relapse – The recommended dosage for remission induction is 12 mg/m² of body surface area, given as a single intravenous dose daily for five consecutive days (total of 60 mg/m²).

In clinical studies with a dosage of 12 mg/m² daily for 5 days, patients who achieved a complete remission did so as a result of the first induction course.

(b) Combination therapy – Novantrone is commonly used in combination regimens for the treatment of ANLL. Most clinical experience has been with Novantrone combined with cytosine arabinoside. This combination has been used successfully for primary treatment of ANLL as well as in relapse.

An effective regimen for induction in previously untreated patients has been 10–12 mg/m² iv Novantrone for 3 days combined with Cytosine arabinoside 100 mg/m² iv for 7 days (by continuous infusion). This is followed by second induction and consolidation courses as though appropriate by the treating clinician. In clinical studies, duration of therapy in induction and consolidation courses with Novantrone have been reduced to 2 days and that of cytosine arabinoside to 5 days. However, modification to the above regimen should be carried out by the treating clinician depending on individual patient factors.

Efficacy has also been demonstrated with Novantrone in combination with Etoposide in patients who had relapsed or who were refractory to primary conventional chemotherapy. The use of Novantrone in combination with Etoposide as with other cytotoxics may result in greater myelosuppression than with Novantrone alone.

Reference should be made to the published literature for information on specific dosage regimens. Novantrone should be used by clinicians experienced in the use of chemotherapy regimens. Dosage adjustments should be made by the treating clinician as appropriate, taking into account toxicity, response and individual patient characteristics. As with other cytotoxic drugs, Novantrone should be used with caution in combination therapy until wider experience is available.

(c) Paediatric leukaemia–As experience with Novantrone in paediatric leukaemia is limited, dosage recommendations in this patient population cannot at present be given.

Method of intravenous administration: Care should be taken to avoid contact of Novantrone with the skin, mucous membranes, or eyes; see *Pharmaceutical Precautions* for further directions on handling.

Dilute the required volume of Novantrone injection to at least 50 ml in either of the following intravenous infusions: Sodium Chloride 0.9%, Glucose 5%, or Sodium Chloride 0.18% and Glucose 4%. Use Leur-lock fittings on all syringes and sets. Large bore needles are recommended to minimise pressure and the possible formation of aerosols. The latter may also be reduced by the use of a venting needle. Administer the resulting solution over not less than 3 minutes via the tubing of freely running intravenous infusion of the above fluids. Novantrone should not be mixed with other drugs in the same infusion.

If extravasation occurs the administration should be stopped immediately and restarted in another vein. The nonvesicant properties of Novantrone minimize the possibility of severe local reaction following extravasation.

Contra-indications, warnings, etc

Contra-indications: Demonstrated hypersensitivity to the drug.

Warnings: Novantrone should be used with caution in patients with myelosuppression (*see Dosage Section*) or poor general condition.

Cases of functional cardiac changes, including congestive heart failure and decreases in left ventricular ejection fraction have been reported. The majority of these cardiac events have occurred in patients who have had prior treatment with anthracyclines, prior mediastinal/thoracic radiotherapy, or with pre-existing heart disease. It is recommended that patients in these categories are treated with Novantrone at full cytotoxic dosage and schedule. However, added caution is required in these patients and careful regular cardiac examinations are recommended from the initiation of treatment.

As experience of prolonged treatment with Novantrone is presently limited, it is suggested that cardiac examinations also be performed in patients without identifiable risk factors during therapy exceeding a cumulative dose of 160 mg/m^2.

Careful supervision is recommended when treating patients with severe hepatic insufficiency.

The effects of Novantrone on human fertility or pregnancy have not been established. As with other antineoplastic agents, patients and their partners should be advised to avoid conception for at least six months after cessation of therapy. Novantrone should not normally be administered to patients who are pregnant or to mothers who are breast feeding.

Novantrone is mutagenic in vitro and in vivo in the rat. In the same species there was a possible association between administration of the drug and development of malignant neoplasia. The carcinogenic potential in man is unknown.

There is no experience with the administration of Novantrone other than by the intravenous route. Safety for intrathecal use has not been established.

Precautions: Novantrone is an active cytotoxic drug which should be used by clinicians familiar with the use of antineoplastic agents, and having the facilities for regular monitoring of clinical, haematological and biochemical parameters during and after treatment. Full blood counts should be undertaken serially during a course of treatment. Dosage adjustments may be necessary based on these counts (*see Dosage Section*).

Side-effects: Novantrone is clinically well tolerated demonstrating a low overall incidence of adverse events particularly those of a severe, irreversible, or life-threatening nature. Some degree of leucopenia is to be expected following recommended doses of Novantrone. With the single dose every 21 days, suppression of WBC count below 1000/mm^3 is infrequent; leucopenia is usually transient, reaching its nadir at about 10 days after dosing with recovery usually occurring by the 21st day. Thrombocytopenia can occur and anaemia occurs less frequently. Myelosuppression may be more severe and prolonged in patients having had extensive prior chemotherapy or radiotherapy or in debilitated patients.

When Novantrone is used as a single injection given every 21 days in the treatment of advanced breast cancer and lymphomas, the most commonly encountered side-effects are nausea and vomiting, although in the majority of cases these are mild and transient. Alopecia may occur, but is most frequently of minimal severity and reversible on cessation of therapy.

Other side-effects which have occasionally been reported include amenorrhoea, anorexia, constipation, diarrhoea, dyspnoea, fatigue and weakness, fever, gastrointestinal bleeding, stomatitis/mucositis and non-specific neurological side-effects. Tissue necrosis following extravasation has been reported rarely. In patients with leukaemia, the pattern of side-effects is generally similar, although there is an increase in both frequency and severity, particularly of stomatitis and mucositis.

Changes in laboratory test values have been observed infrequently e.g. elevated serum creatinine and blood urea nitrogen levels, increased liver enzyme levels (with occasional reports of severe impairment of hepatic function in patients with leukaemia).

Cardiovascular effects, which have only occasionally been of clinical significance, include decreased left ventricular ejection fraction, ECG changes and acute arrhythmia. Congestive heart failure has been reported and has generally responded well to treatment with digitalis and/or diuretics. In patients with leukaemia an increase in the frequency of adverse cardiac events has been observed; the direct role of Novantrone in these cases is difficult to assess as most patients had received prior therapy with anthracyclines and since the clinical course in leukaemic patients is often complicated by anaemia, fever, sepsis and intravenous fluid therapy.

Novantrone may impart a blue-green coloration to the urine for 24 hours after administration and patients should be advised that this is to be expected. A reversible blue coloration of the sclerae may be seen very rarely.

Overdosage: There is no known specific antidote for Novantrone. Haemopoietic, gastrointestinal, hepatic or renal toxicity may be seen depending on dosage given and the physical condition of the patient. In cases of overdosage the patient should be monitored closely and management should be symptomatic and supportive.

Pharmaceutical precautions Store at controlled room temperature (15–25°C). Do not freeze.

Novantrone injection does not contain an antimicrobial preservative. Therefore, in accordance with normal practice, dilutions for infusion should be used or discarded within 24 hours. Novantrone dilutions will maintain potency for 24 hours at room temperature in PVC or glass containers.

Novantrone must not be mixed in the same infusion as heparin since a precipitate may form. Because specific compatibility data are not available it is recommended that Novantrone should not be mixed in the same infusion with other drugs.

Handling of cytotoxic drugs: Novantrone, in common with other potentially hazardous cytotoxic drugs, should only be handled by adequately trained personnel. Pregnant staff should not be involved in the reconstitution or administration of Novantrone.

Care should be taken to avoid contact of Novantrone with the skin, mucous membranes, or eyes. The use of goggles, gloves and protective gowns is recommended during preparation, administration and disposal and the work surface should be covered with disposable plastic-backed absorbent paper.

Aerosol generation should be minimised. Novantrone can cause staining. Skin accidentally exposed to Novantrone should be rinsed copiously with warm water and if the eyes are involved standard irrigation techniques should be used.

Spillage disposal: The following clean-up procedure is recommended if Novantrone is spilled on equipment or environmental surfaces. Prepare a 50% solution of fresh concentrated bleach (any recognised proprietary brand containing either sodium or calcium hypochlorite) in water. Wet absorbent tissues in the bleach solution and apply the wetted tissues to the spillage. The spillage is deactivated when the blue colour has been fully discharged. Collect up the tissues with dry tissues. Wash the area with water and soak up the water with dry tissues. Appropriate protective equipment should be worn during the clean-up procedure. All Novantrone contaminated items (e.g., syringes, needles, tissues, etc.) should be treated as toxic waste and disposed of accordingly. Incineration is recommended.

Legal category POM.

Package quantities Novantrone injection is a sterile aqueous solution of mitozantrone hydrochloride, equivalent to 2 mg/ml mitozantrone. It is available in the following vial sizes:
20 mg in 10 ml – packs of 1 vial
25 mg in 12.5 ml – packs of 1 vial
30 mg in 15 ml – packs of 1 vial

Further information Although its mechanism of action has not been determined, Novantrone is a DNA-reactive agent. It has a cytocidal effect on proliferating and non-proliferating cultured human cells, suggesting activity against rapidly proliferating and slow-growing neoplasms.

Animal pharmacokinetic studies in rats, dogs and monkeys given radiolabelled Novantrone indicate rapid, extensive dose proportional distribution into most tissues. Novantrone does not cross the blood-brain barrier to any appreciable extent. Distribution into testes is relatively low. In pregnant rats the placenta is an effective barrier. Plasma concentrations decrease rapidly during the first two hours and slowly thereafter. Animal data established biliary excretion as the major route of elimination. In rats, tissue elimination half-life of radioactivity ranged from 20 days to 25 days as compared with plasma half-life of 12 days. Novantrone is not absorbed significantly in animals following oral administration.

Pharmacokinetic studies in patients following intravenous administration of Novantrone demonstrated a triphasic plasma clearance. Distribution to tissues is rapid and extensive. Elimination of the drug is slow with a mean half-life of 12 days (range 5–18) and persistent tissue concentrations. Similar estimates of half-life were obtained from patients receiving a single dose of Novantrone every 21 days and patients dosed on 5 consecutive days every 21 days.

Novantrone is excreted via the renal and hepatobiliary systems. Only 20–32% of the administered dose was excreted within the first five days after dosing (urine 6–11%, faeces 13–25%). Of the material recovered in the urine 65% was unchanged mitozantrone and the remaining 35% is primarily comprised of two inactive metabolites and their glucuronide conjugates. Approximately two thirds of the excretion occurred during the first day.

Product licence number 0095/0088.

PARFENAC*

Presentation Smooth white cream containing Bufexamac 5% in an aqueous base consisting of cetyl alcohol, glycerin, sodium lauryl sulphate, methyl paraben as a preservative.

Uses Parfenac is a synthetic non-steroidal anti-inflammatory agent for topical application.

It is intended for external use only in the treatment of various mild dermatoses such as contact dermatitis, atopic dermatitis, radiodermatitis (caused by sunburn and radiotherapy) and eczema.

Dosage and administration
Adults and children: Parfenac cream should be applied in small quantities to the affected areas two or three times daily and rubbed in gently until it disappears.

The cream is water-based and stains on clothing may be easily washed off.

Contra-indications, warnings, etc Parfenac is contra-indicated in patients with a history of hypersensitivity to any of its components.

If an infection is present an appropriate anti-infective agent should be prescribed. Parfenac should not be applied to broken skin. It should not be used on infants.

Local intolerance to Parfenac cream is manifested by burning and irritation which is rare and is attributable to the components of the cream vehicle. Bufexamac itself has not been found to have a sensitivity potential. If such a reaction occurs, the use of Parfenac should be discontinued.

Pharmaceutical precautions The product should be stored in a dry, cool place (8–15°C). It is not recommended that the product be diluted as this may affect its stability.

Legal category POM.

Package quantities 15 g and 30 g.

Further information Nil.

Product licence number 0095/0010R.

PIPRIL* INJECTION

Presentation Vials containing 1 g or 2 g of piperacillin as piperacillin sodium.

Infusion bottles containing 4 g of piperacillin as piperacillin sodium.

Infusion pack containing a 4 g piperacillin infusion bottle, a bottle of Water for Injections BP 50 ml and a sterile pyrogen free transfer needle.

Each 1 g vial of Pipril contains 1.94 mEq (44.5 mg) of sodium.

Uses Pipril is a broad spectrum bactericidal penicillin antibiotic indicated for the treatment of infections caused by sensitive organisms, and for peri-operative prophylaxis for example in patients undergoing abdominal surgery, vaginal hysterectomy, caesarian section.

Pipril is highly active against the following clinically important bacteria:

Gram-Negative:

Acinetobacter species	*Neisseria gonorrhoeae*
Citrobacter species	*Neisseria meningitidis*
Enterobacter species	*Proteus* sp. (indole positive and negative)
Escherichia coli	*Providencia* species
Haemophilus influenzae	*Pseudomonas aeruginosa* and other species
Klebsiella pneumoniae and other species	*Serratia marcescens* and other species
	Shigella species

Anaerobes:

Bacteroides fragilis	*Fusobacterium* species
Bacteroides species	*Peptococcus* species
Clostridium species	*Veillonella* species

Gram-Positive:

Enterococci	*Streptococcus (Diplococcus) pneumoniae*
Staphylococcus species (non-β-lactamase-producing)	*Streptococcus* species
	Other *Streptococcus* species

Because of its broad spectrum of activity, Pipril is indicated for the treatment of the following systemic and/or local infections in which one or more susceptible organisms have been detected or are suspected.

Systemic infections including bacterial septicaemia and endocarditis.

Urogenital tract infections including gonorrhoea.

Respiratory tract infections.

Ear, nose and throat and oral cavity infections.

Intra-abdominal infections including those of the biliary tract.

Gynaecological and obstetric infections.

Skin and soft tissue infections including infected wounds and burns.

Bone and joint infections.

Proven or suspected infections in patients with impaired or suppressed immunological status.

Peri-operative prophylaxis.

Pipril acts synergistically with aminoglycosides. Concurrent therapy with both drugs given in full therapeutic doses may be used in the treatment of life-threatening infections or in patients with impaired immune status. Pipril and aminoglycosides should not, however, be mixed in the same solution but administered separately.

Pipril may be used in combination with β-lactamase resistant penicillins in proven or suspected mixed infections involving β-lactamase producing *Staphylococcus aureus.*

Pipril may be administered (separately) with metronidazole in the treatment of mixed aerobic/anaerobic infections.

Cefoxitin should not be given with Pipril when *Pseudomonas* infections are suspected or confirmed as *in vitro* data have shown possible antagonism. However, Pipril may be administered concomitantly with other β-lactam antibiotics provided that an additive or synergistic antibacterial action is first ascertained through *in vitro* tests where appropriate.

Dosage and administration Pipril may be given by slow intravenous injection, by intravenous infusion or by intramuscular injection.

Intravenous Injection: Each gram of Pipril should be reconstituted with at least 5 ml of Water for Injection and given by slow intravenous injection over three to five minutes.

Intravenous Infusion: Each gram of Pipril should be reconstituted with at least 5 ml Water for Injection. The total dose should then be further diluted to at least 50 ml before infusion over 20–40 minutes. Suitable diluents are listed under Pharmaceutical Precautions.

Intramuscular Injection: Each gram of Pipril should be reconstituted with at least 2 ml of Water for Injection or 0.5–1% lignocaine. Administration should be by deep intramuscular injection. A single dose in adults should not exceed 2 g. A single dose in children should not exceed 0.5 g.

Adult dosage: Patients with normal renal function: Serious and complicated infections: 200–300 mg/kg/day. The usual dose is therefore 4 g every six or eight hours by IV administration. In life-threatening infections, particularly those caused by Pseudomonas and Klebsiella species a dosage of not less than 16 g/day is recommended.

Mild and uncomplicated infections: 100–150 mg/kg/day. The usual dose is therefore 2 g IV every six or eight hours; 4 g IV every twelve hours or 2 g IM every eight or twelve hours.

For peri-operative prophylaxis: 2 g just prior to surgery (or in caesarian section when the umbilical cord is clamped) followed by at least two doses of 2 g at four or six hour intervals.

Acute gonorrhoea: a single dose of 2 g IM.

Patients with renal insufficiency: In adults with renal impairment, intravenous or intramuscular dosage should be adjusted. Given below are the recommended maximum daily dosages of Pipril according to the degree of renal impairment as assessed by the physician.

Duration of Therapy: Pipril treatment in acute infections should be continued for three to four days after the disappearance of clinical signs and symptoms of the disease. However, the duration of treatment should be determined by the physician on the basis of the clinical course of infection.

Elderly: Pipril may be used at the same dose levels as adults except in cases of renal impairment when the dosage should be reduced.

Renal function	*Creatinine clearance (ml/min)*	*Maximum daily dosage (in divided doses)*	*Dose schedule*
Mild Impairment	40–80	16 grams	4 g q 6h
Moderate Impairment	20–40	12 grams	4 g q 8h
Severe Impairment	<20	8 grams	4 g q 12h
Patients on Haemodialysis*		6 grams	2 g q 8 h

* Haemodialysis removes 30% to 50% of the drug in four hours; an additional dose of 1 g of Pipril should be administered following each dialysis period.

Paediatric dosage: Children: Two months to twelve years of age: 100–300 mg/kg daily in three or four divided doses.

Neonates and Infants: Under two months of age: 100–300 mg/kg daily in two equally divided doses.

Contra-indications, warnings, etc

Contra-indications: Penicillin hypersensitivity or severe cephalosporin hypersensitivity.

Precautions: Safety for use in pregnant or lactating women has not yet been established. Use with caution in patients with infectious mononucleosis.

Warnings and side-effects: In common with other penicillins anaphylactic reactions have occasionally been reported in patients receiving piperacillin.

Side effects are uncommon and typical of other injectable penicillins.

Gastro-intestinal disturbances have been reported and transient leucopenia, neutropenia and/or eosinophilia can occur.

Dermatological manifestations such as erythema multiforme and Stevens–Johnson syndrome have been reported on rare occasions.

Interstitial nephritis may occur rarely.

In vitro, Pipril can be inactivated by β-lactamases produced by some strains of gram-negative and gram-positive bacteria.

Pain after intramuscular injections (rarely accompanied by induration) has been observed infrequently. This can be minimised by reconstituting Pipril with 0.5–1.0% lignocaine.

Overdosage: Other than general supportive treatment, no specific antidote is known. Excessive serum levels of piperacillin may be reduced by dialysis. Neuromuscular excitability or convulsions have been known to occur following large intravenous doses of penicillins. General supportive measures, including administration of appropriate anticonvulsant drugs, such as diazepam or barbiturates, may be indicated. Daily doses of piperacillin of 24 grams and above have been administered in man without observation of adverse effects.

Pharmaceutical precautions Pipril should be stored in a dry place at room temperature. Pipril should be freshly prepared prior to administration, any unused solution being discarded.

However, Pipril solutions are chemically stable for at least 24 hours at room temperature or 48 hours at 4°C.

Pipril may be administered in all commonly used infusion fluids including:

Dextrose 5%; Sodium Chloride 0.9%; Sodium Chloride 0.9% and Dextrose 5%; Compound Sodium Lactate (Lactated Ringer's Injection). The above fluids admixed with 40 mEq Potassium Chloride and/or 30 mEq Sodium Bicarbonate. Dextran 6% in Sodium Chloride 0.9%, Dextrose 30%, Mannitol 20%.

Because of chemical instability, Pipril should not be diluted with solutions containing only sodium bicarbonate.

Pipril should not be added to blood products or protein hydrolysates.

Pipril has also been shown to be compatible over 24 hours at room temperature when mixed with cephazolin sodium, flucloxacillin sodium, cefamandole nafate, or cefoxitin sodium in either Dextrose 5% or Saline 0.9% or Lactated Ringer's Injections.

Pipril should not be mixed in the same solution with aminoglycosides and should be administered separately from any other drugs unless compatibility is proven.

Legal category POM.

Package quantities Vials containing 1 g or 2 g Pipril, boxed singly. Infusion bottles containing 4 g Pipril, boxed singly. Pipril 4 g Infusion Packs containing a 4 g infusion bottle, a 50 ml bottle of Water for Injections BP and transfer needle.

Further information Pipril shows a pronounced activity against many clinically significant organisms resistant to other penicillins (including the acylureido group), cephalosporins and aminoglycosides. Some ampicillin-resistant *Escherichia coli* and *Proteus* and carbenicillin-resistant *Citrobacter, Klebsiella, Pseudomonas, Proteus* and *Serratia* are sensitive to piperacillin. Many ticarcillin-resistant *Pseudomonas, Klebsiella* and *Serratia*; cephalothin-resistant *Enterobacteriaceae* and many strains of *Pseudomonas* resistant to amikacin, gentamicin or tobramycin are susceptible to Pipril.

Pipril is widely distributed following parenteral administration into human tissues and body fluids, particularly bile. Pipril penetrates into cerebrospinal fluid in the presence of meningitis. It is not absorbed when given orally. As with other penicillins, Pipril is rapidly excreted, unchanged, by glomerular filtration and tubular secretion achieving high urinary concentrations for up to 12 hours after dosing. The binding of piperacillin to human serum protein is low (16%).

Product licence number 0095/0073.

PROSTAP* SR ▼

Presentation

Prostap SR Powder: Vial containing 3.75 mg (equivalent to 3.75 mg of base) leuprorelin acetate in a sterile, lyophilised, white, odourless PLGA (Copoly [DL-lactic acid/glycolic acid] 75:25 mol%) microcapsule powder.

Sterile vehicle: Prefilled syringes containing 2 ml of clear, colourless, slightly viscous, sterile vehicle for reconstitution of the microcapsules. Each 2 ml contains sodium carboxymethyl cellulose 10 mg, mannitol 100 mg, polysorbate 80 2 mg in water for injection.

Uses Prostap is a synthetic nonapeptide analogue of naturally occurring gonadotrophin releasing hormone (GnRH) which possesses greater potency than the natural hormone. Prostap is a peptide and therefore unrelated to the steroids. Chronic administration results in an inhibition of gonadotrophin production and subsequent suppression of ovarian and testicular steroid secretion.

The depot formulation is designed to provide, in a single subcutaneous injection, 3.75 mg leuprorelin acetate which is released at a constant rate over a period of one month. The constant release of drug provides for testosterone suppression equivalent to the daily subcutaneous injection of 1 mg leuprorelin acetate.

Prostap is indicated in the treatment of advanced prostatic cancer.

Dosage and administration

Dosage

Adults: The recommended dose is 3.75 mg administered as a single subcutaneous injection every 4 weeks. The majority of patients will respond to a 3.75 mg dose. Prostap therapy should not be discontinued when remission or improvement occurs. As with other drugs administered chronically by subcutaneous injection, the injection site should be varied periodically.

Elderly: As for adults.

Children: Safety and efficacy in children have not been established.

Response to Prostap therapy may be monitored by clinical parameters and by measuring serum levels to testosterone and acid phosphatase. Clinical studies have shown that testosterone levels increased during the first 4 days of treatment in the majority of non-orchidectomised patients. They then decreased and reached castrate levels by 2–4 weeks. Once attained, castrate levels were maintained as long as drug therapy continued. Transient increases in acid phosphatase levels sometimes occur early in the treatment period, but usually return to normal or near normal values by the 4th week of treatment.

Administration: The vial of Prostap SR microcapsule powder should be reconstituted immediately prior to administration by subcutaneous injection. Remove flip-cap from vial of Prostap SR Powder and cap from prefilled syringe of Sterile Vehicle. Fix 23 gauge needle to syringe and inject whole contents of syringe (2 ml) into vial of Prostap SR Powder using an aseptic technique. Remove the syringe/needle and keep aseptic. Shake vial gently for 15–20 seconds to produce a uniform cloudy suspension of Prostap. Immediately draw up suspension into syringe taking care to exclude air bubbles. Change 23 gauge needle on syringe and having cleaned appropriate injection site (eg abdominal wall), administer the suspension by subcutaneous injection taking care not to enter a blood vessel. Apply sterile dressing to injection site if required.

The injection should be given as soon as possible after mixing. If any settling of suspension occurs in vial or syringe, re-suspend by gentle shaking and administer immediately.

No other fluid can be used for reconstitution of Prostap SR Powder.

Contra-indications, warnings, etc There are no known contra-indications to the use of Prostap.

Warnings: In the initial stages of therapy, a transient rise in levels of testosterone, dihydrotestosterone and acid phosphatase may occur. In some cases, this may be associated with a 'flare' or exacerbation of the tumour growth resulting in temporary deterioration of the patient's condition. These symptoms usually subside on continuation of therapy. 'Flare' may manifest itself as systemic or neurological symptoms in some cases.

In order to reduce the risk of flare, an anti-androgen may be administered beginning 3 days prior to leuprorelin therapy and continuing for the first two to three weeks of treatment. This has been reported to prevent the sequelae of an initial rise in serum testosterone.

Patients at risk of ureteric obstruction or spinal cord compression should be considered carefully and closely supervised in the first few weeks of treatment. These patients should be considered for prophylactic treatment with anti-androgens. Should urological/neurological complications occur, these should be treated by appropriate specific measures.

If an anti-androgen is used over a prolonged period, due attention should be paid to the contra-indications and precautions associated with its extended use.

Whilst the development of pituitary adenomas has been noted in chronic toxicity studies at high doses in some animal species, this has not been observed in long term clinical studies with Prostap.

Precautions: Patients with urinary obstruction and patients with metastatic vertebral lesions should begin Prostap therapy under close supervision for the first few weeks of treatment.

Pregnancy: Prostap is not indicated for use in females.

Side-effects: Side effects seen with Prostap are due mainly to the specific pharmacological action, namely increases and decreases in certain hormone levels. In cases where a 'tumour flare' occurs after Prostap therapy, an exacerbation may occur in any symptoms or signs due to disease, for example, bone pain, urinary obstruction etc. These symptoms subside on continuation of therapy.

Impotence and decreased libido will be expected with Prostap therapy.

The administration of Prostap is often associated with hot flushes and sometimes sweating.

Other adverse events which have infrequently been

reported include peripheral oedema, fatigue, nausea and irritation at the injection site.

Overdosage: There is no clinical experience with the effects of an acute overdose of Prostap. In animal studies, doses of up to 500 times the recommended dose resulted in dyspnoea, decreased activity and local irritation at the injection site. In cases of overdosage, the patients should be monitored closely and management should be symptomatic and supportive.

Pharmaceutical precautions Store at room temperature (15–25°C), in the original container. Protect from light.

Legal category POM.

Package quantities Vials containing 3.75 mg leuprorelin acetate as microcapsule powder. Prefilled syringes containing 2 ml vehicle.

Further information Prostap is inactive when given orally. As an alternative route to subcutaneous administration, Prostap SR can be given by intramuscular injection.

Product licence numbers

Prostap SR Powder 3.75 mg vials	0095/0218
Sterile Vehicle prefilled syringes	0095/0220

STAPHLIPEN*

Presentation
Staphlipen Capsules: (Flucloxacillin Capsules BP) Light brown and grey capsules overprinted 'LL250' and '3832' each containing 250 mg of flucloxacillin as Flucloxacillin Sodium BP. Light brown and grey capsules overprinted 'LL500' and '3833' each containing 500 mg of flucloxacillin as Flucloxacillin Sodium BP.

Staphlipen Vials for Injection: (Flucloxacillin Injection BP); each vial contains the equivalent of 250 mg, 500 mg or 1 g of flucloxacillin as Flucloxacillin Sodium BP.

Uses Staphlipen is indicated for the treatment of infections due to Gram-positive organisms, including infections caused by penicillin-resistant staphylococci.

Typical indications include: Skin and soft tissue infections such as boils, abscesses and carbuncles. Infected skin conditions e.g. ulcer, eczema and acne. Furunculosis, cellulitis, impetigo and infected wounds. Otitis media and externa. Infected burns and for the protection of skin grafts.

Respiratory tract infections such as pneumonia, lung abscess and empyema.

Sinusitis, pharyngitis, tonsillitis and quinsy.

Other infections caused by flucloxacillin sensitive organisms e.g. urinary tract infection, endocarditis, enteritis, meningitis, osteomyelitis and septicaemia.

Dosage and administration
Adults and children over 12 years:
Oral: 250 mg four times a day.
Intramuscular and intravenous: The usual total daily dose is 750 mg to 1500 mg in divided doses.

Intrapleural:	250 mg once a day
Intra-articular:	250–500 mg once a day.
By nebuliser:	125–250 mg three times a day.

Paediatric dosage
2–10 years – half the adult dose.
Under 2 years – one quarter the adult dose.

Elderly dosage: In common with other penicillins, Staphlipen usage in patients with renal impairment does not usually require dosage reduction. However, in patients with severe renal failure a reduction of dose should be considered.

Administration
Intramuscular Injection: Add 1.5 ml Water for Injections BP to 250 mg vial or 2 ml Water for Injections to 500 mg vial.

Intravenous Injection: Dissolve 250–500 mg in 5–10 ml Water for Injections BP or 1 g in 15–20 ml Water for Injections BP. Administer by slow intravenous injection over 3–4 minutes.

Intravenous Infusion: Staphlipen may be added to the infusion fluids or injected, suitably diluted, into the drip tube over a period of 3–4 minutes. Suitable diluents are listed under Pharmaceutical Precautions.

Staphlipen may also be administered by other routes in conjunction with systemic flucloxacillin as follows:

Intrapleural Injection: Dissolve 250 mg in 5–10 ml Water for Injections BP.

Intra-articular: Dissolve 250–500 mg in up to 5 ml Water for Injections BP or 0.5% lignocaine hydrochloride solution.

Nebuliser solution: Dissolve 125–250 mg of the vial contents in 3 ml sterile water.

Contra-indications, warnings, etc
Contra-indications: Penicillin hypersensitivity. Ocular administration. Addition to blood, plasma or protein hydrolysates.

Precautions and warnings: Prolonged use of an anti-infective agent may occasionally result in overgrowth of non-susceptible organisms.

Staphlipen is excreted in a manner similar to that of benzyl penicillin, i.e. by glomerular filtration and tubular excretion. This should be borne in mind when designing therapy.

Cross-resistance and cross-sensitisation may occasionally occur with penicillins or cephalosporins.

The product should not be used during pregnancy unless considered essential by the physician. Pencillins are excreted in breast milk, presenting the risk of candiasis and also of central nervous system toxicity due to prematurity of the blood brain barrier. There is a theoretical possibility of later sensitisation.

Side-effects: Typical of other penicillins.

Pharmaceutical precautions Staphlipen capsules should be stored in a cool, dry place. Staphlipen should be used within 30 minutes after reconstitution. In aqueous solution Flucloxacillin injection is stable for up to 24 hours at room temperature and for 72 hours in a refrigerator. Reconstitution of the injection should be carried out under appropriate aseptic conditions if these extended storage periods are required.

Flucloxacillin injection has been shown to be stable over 24 hours at room temperature when administered with the following intravenous infusion fluids; Water for Injections BP, Sodium Chloride Intravenous Infusion 0.9% w/v BP, Glucose Intravenous Infusion 5% w/v BP, Sodium Chloride 0.18% w/v and Glucose 4% w/v, Intravenous Infusion BP, Dextran 40 Intravenous Infusion 10% in Sodium Chloride Intravenous Infusion 0.9%, Dextran 40 Intravenous Infusion 10% in Glucose Intravenous Infusion 5%, Sodium Lactate Intravenous Infusion BP (one-sixth molar), Compound Sodium Lactate Intravenous Infusion BP (Lactated Ringers Injection).

Flucloxacillin injection should not be added to intravenous lipids, blood products or other proteinaceous fluids e.g. protein hydrolysates.

Legal category POM.

Package quantities
Capsules 250 mg: Containers of 100.
Capsules 500 mg: Containers of 100.
Vials 250 mg, 500 mg and 1 g: Boxes of 10.

Further information Staphlipen has the same spectrum of activity as the earlier antistaphylococcal penicillins, methicillin and cloxacillin against Gram-positive organisms including penicillinase – producing strains.

Product licence numbers

Staphlipen Capsules 250 mg	0095/0109
Staphlipen Capsules 500 mg	0095/0110
Staphlipen Vials for Injection 250 mg	0095/0105
Staphlipen Vials for Injection 500 mg	0095/0106
Staphilipen Vials for Injection 1 g	0095/0107

SUPRAX* ▼

Presentation
Tablets 200 mg: Rectangular, white film-coated tablets with a break-line on each side and engraved 'SUPRAX' on one side and 'LL 200' on the other side. Each tablet contains 200 mg of cefixime.

Powder for Paediatric Oral Suspension: Bottles of powder for the preparation of suspension. When reconstituted each 5 ml volume contains 100 mg of cefixime. The suspension contains 2.5 mg of sucrose in 5 ml.

Uses Suprax is an orally active cephalosporin antibiotic which has marked in-vitro bactericidal activity against a wide variety of Gram-positive and Gram-negative organisms.

It is indicated for the treatment of the following acute infections when caused by susceptible micro-organisms.

Upper respiratory tract infections (URTI): For the treatment of otitis media; other URTI where the causative organism is known or suspected to be resistant to other commonly used antibiotics, or where treatment failure may carry significant risk.

Lower respiratory tract infections: e.g. bronchitis.

Urinary tract infections: e.g. cystitis, cystourethritis, uncomplicated pyelonephritis.

Clinical efficacy has been demonstrated in infections caused by commonly occurring pathogens including *Streptococcus pneumoniae, Streptococcus pyogenes, Escherichia coli, Proteus mirabilis, Klebsiella species, Haemophilus influenzae* (beta-lactamase positive and negative), *Branhamella catarrhalis* (beta-lactamase positive and negative) and *Enterobacter species*. Suprax is highly stable in the presence of beta-lactamase enzymes.

Most strains of enterococci (*Streptococcus faecalis*, group D *Streptococci*) and *Staphylococci* (including coagulase positive and negative strains and methicillin-resistant strains) are resistant to Suprax. In addition, most strains of *Pseudomonas, Bacteroides fragilis, Listeria monocytogenes* and *Clostridia* are resistant to Suprax.

Dosage and administration Absorption of Suprax is not significantly modified by the presence of food. The usual course of treatment is 7–14 days.

Adults and children over 12 years: The recommended adult dosage is 200–400 mg daily according to severity of the infection, given either as a single dose or in two divided doses.

The Elderly: Elderly patients may be given the same dose as recommended for adults. Renal function should be assessed and dosage should be adjusted in severe renal impairment (see 'Dosage in renal impairment').

Children (Use Paediatric Oral Suspension): The recommended dosage for children is 8 mg/kg/day administered as a single dose or in two divided doses. As a general guide for prescribing in children the following daily doses in terms of volume of Paediatric Oral Suspension are suggested.

6 months up to 1 year	:	3.75 ml daily
Children 1–4 years	:	5 ml daily
Children 5–10 years	:	10 ml daily
Children 11–12 years	:	15 ml daily

(A spoon is provided with the 37.5 ml bottle to aid correct dosing – see Package Quantities).

Children weighing more than 50 kg or older than 12 years should be treated with the recommended adult dose (200–400 mg daily depending on the severity of infection). The safety and efficacy of cefixime has not been established in children aged less than 6 months.

Dosage in renal impairment: Suprax may be administered in the presence of impaired renal function. Normal dose and schedule may be given in patients with creatinine clearance of 20 ml/min or greater. In patients whose creatinine clearance is less than 20 ml/min, it is recommended that a dose of 200 mg once daily should not be exceeded. The dose and regimen for patients who are maintained on chronic ambulatory peritoneal dialysis or haemodialysis should follow the same recommendation as that for patients with creatinine clearances of less than 20 ml/min.

Contra-indications, warnings, etc
Contra-indications: Patients with known hypersensitivity to cephalosporin antibiotics.

Warnings and precautions: Suprax should be given with caution to patients who have shown hypersensitivity to other drugs. Cephalosporins should be given with caution to penicillin-sensitive patients, as there is some evidence of partial cross-allergenicity between the penicillins and the cepthalosporins. Patients have had severe reactions (including anaphylaxis) to both classes of drugs. If an allergic effect occurs with Suprax, the drug should be discontinued and the patient treated with appropriate agents if necessary.

Suprax cefixime should be administered with caution in patients with markedly impaired renal function (see Dosage in renal impairment).

Treatment with broad spectrum antibiotics alters the normal flora of the colon and may permit overgrowth of clostridia. Studies indicate that a toxin produced by *Clostridium difficile* is a primary cause of antibiotic-associated diarrhoea. Pseudomembranous colitis is associated with the use of broad-spectrum antibiotics (including macrolides, sermi-synthetic penicillins, lincosamides and cephalosporins); it is therefore important to consider its diagnosis on patients who develop diarrhoea in association with the use of antibiotics. Symptoms of pseudomembranous colitis may occur during or after antibiotic treatment. Management of pseudomembranous colitis should include sigmoidoscopy, appropriate bacteriologic studies, fluids, electrolytes and protein supplementation. If the colitis does not improve after the drug has been discontinued, or if the symptoms are severe, oral vancomycin is the drug of choice for antibiotic-associated pseudomembranous colitis produced by *C. difficile*. Other causes of colitis should be excluded.

Use in pregnancy and breast feeding: Reproduction studies have been performed in mice and rats at doses up to 400 times the human dose and have revealed no evidence of impairment fertility or harm to the foetus due to cefixime. In the rabbit, at doses up to 4 times the human dose, there was no evidence of a teratogenic effect; there was a high incidence of abortion and maternal death which is an expected consequence of the known sensitivity of rabbits to antibiotic-induced changes in the population of the microflora of the intestine. There are no adequate and well-controlled studies in pregnant women. Suprax should therefore not be used in pregnancy or in nursing mothers unless considered essential by the physician.

Interactions: No significant drug interactions have been reported to date. A false positive reaction for glucose in the urine may occur with Benedict's or Fehling's solutions or with copper sulphate test tablets, but not with tests based on enzymatic glucose oxidase reactions. A false positive direct Coombs test has been reported during treatment with cephalosporin antibiotics, therefore it should be recognised that a positive Coombs test may be due to the drug.

Overdose: There is no experience with overdoses of Suprax. Adverse reactions seen at dose levels up to 2 g Suprax in normal subjects did not differ from the profile seen in patients treated at the recommended doses. Gastric lavage may be initiated in overdosage. No specific antidote exists. Suprax is not removed from the circulation in significant quantities by dialysis.

Side effects: Suprax is generally well tolerated. The majority of adverse reactions observed in clinical trials were mild and self limiting in nature.

Gastrointestinal disturbances: The most frequent side effects seen with Suprax cefixime are diarrhoea and stool changes. Some cases of moderate to severe diarrhoea have been reported; this has occasionally warranted cessation of therapy. Suprax should be discontinued if marked diarrhoea occurs. Other gastrointestinal side effects seen less frequently are nausea, abdominal pain, dyspepsia, vomiting and flatulence. Pseudomembranous colitis has been reported (see above).

Central nervous system: Headache and dizziness.

Hypersensitivity reactions: Allergies in the form of rash, pruritis, urticaria, drug fever and arthralgia have been observed. These reactions usually subsided upon discontinuation of therapy.

Haematological and clinical chemistry: Thrombocytopenia, leukopenia and eosinophilia have been reported. These reactions were infrequent and reversible. Mild transient changes in liver and renal function tests have been observed.

Miscellaneous: Other possible reactions include genital pruritis and vaginitis.

Pharmaceutical precautions
Tablets: Store at controlled room temperature (15–25°C) in the original pack or in containers which prevent access of light and moisture.

Powder for Paediatric Oral Suspension: Store unreconstituted product at controlled room temperature (15–25°C). To reconstitute, add 4 ml of water (5 ml bottle), 25 ml of water (37.5 ml bottle), 50 ml of water (75 ml bottle) in two portions shaking after each addition. After reconstitution, the suspension may be stored at room temperature (below 25°C) for 14 days without significant loss of potency. Do not freeze. Keep bottles tightly closed and shake well before use. Discard any unused portion after 14 days. Dilution of the suspension is not recommended.

Legal category POM.

Package quantities
Tablets 200 mg: Bottles containing 50 tablets.

Powder for Paediatric Oral Suspension (100 mg/5 ml: Bottles containing powder for preparation of 5 ml, 37.5 ml, and 75 ml of suspension. A double ended spoon (3.75 ml/5 ml) is supplied with the 37.5 ml bottle to enable correct dosing of the younger child (see 'Dosage and Administration').

Further information Nil.

Product licence numbers

Powder for Paediatric Oral Suspension	0095/0211
Tablets 200 mg	0095/0212

THIOTEPA

Presentation Vials of dry, white, sterile powder, requiring refrigeration (2–8°C). Each vial contains:

Thiotepa	15 mg
Sodium chloride	80 mg
Sodium bicarbonate	50 mg

Uses Thiotepa (N,N',N" triethylenethiophosphoramide) is a polyfunctional alkylating agent used alone or in combination with other cytotoxic drugs, hormones, radiotherapy or surgery in the treatment of neoplastic diseases. It is believed to exert its cytotoxic effects by alkylation of DNA.

Dosage and administration Thiotepa (15 mg) should be reconstituted with 1.5 ml water for injection immediately prior to use. Reconstituted solutions should be clear to slightly opaque. Solutions that are grossly opaque or precipitated should be discarded.

Thiotepa may be given by intravenous, intramuscular and intrathecal routes of injection; it may be given directly into pleural, pericardial or peritoneal cavities and as a bladder instillation.

Use Luer-Lock fittings on all syringes and sets. Large bore needles are recommended to minimise pressure and possible formation of aerosols, the latter may also be reduced by the use of a venting needle.

Adults and the Elderly: For intramuscular injection, bladder and intracavitary instillations: Up to 60 mg in single or divided doses. Doses should be reduced in cases of leucopenia as indicated in Table 1. Single dose administration of 90 mg Thiotepa as a bladder instillation is described under 'Bladder Cancer'.

Table 1

WBC Count (cells/mm^3)	*Dose of Thiotepa Adults and Children over 12 years*
6000	60 mg
5000–6000	45 mg
4500–5000	30 mg
4000–4500	20 mg
3500–4000	10 mg
3000–3500	5 mg
below 3000	omit dose

Children: Use in children is not recommended.

Intrathecal injection: Up to a maximum of 10 mg.

It is essential that a complete blood count should be performed 12–24 hours before each dose of Thiotepa. Thrombocytopenia in the absence of leucopenia has been noted.

Dosage schedules of Thiotepa vary widely according to the route of administration and the indication.

Examples of dosage schedules used according to specific tumour types are given below:

Breast cancer: Patients with advanced breast cancer have been treated with Thiotepa, as part of a combination regime, given intramuscularly in divided doses of 15–30 mg three times weekly for two weeks; this representing one course of treatment. An interval of six to eight weeks is recommended between courses to allow bone marrow recovery.

An alternative schedule employs Thiotepa as part of a combination regime, given as an initial priming dose of 15 mg intramuscularly or intravenously each day for four days. This may be followed in three weeks by maintenance doses of 15 mg I.M. every 14–21 days.

Bladder cancer: Instillations of Thiotepa have been used to treat multiple superficial tumours of the bladder, resulting in a complete clinical response in about one third of patients. Patients are dehydrated for 8–12 hours prior to treatment. Up to 60 mg Thiotepa dissolved in 60 ml sterile water is instilled into the bladder by catheter once a week for four weeks. During removal of the catheter following instillation, Thiotepa injection is continued to ensure bathing of the prostatic and pendulous urethra. The solution should be retained for up to two hours and the patient should be frequently repositioned to ensure maximum contact with the urothelium.

Patients are generally cystoscoped two weeks after a course of four instillations. If a response is observed a second course of four Thiotepa instillations may be given, generally at reduced dosage, e.g. 15–60 mg, with intervals of one to two weeks between instillations.

Instillations of Thiotepa have been used prophylactically as an adjunct to surgical resection of superficial tumours of the bladder, resulting in a marked decrease in the recurrence rate. It is recommended that there should be a minimum interval of one week between tumour resection and the commencement of prophylactic instillations of Thiotepa. 30–60 mg Thiotepa dissolved in 60 ml sterile water is instilled into the bladder for two hours and repeated at intervals of one to two weeks for a total of 4–8 instillations. This initial course may be followed by instillations of Thiotepa, 30–60 mg every four to six weeks for one year or longer.

Single dose Thiotepa instillations have been used prophylactically as an adjunct to surgical resection in the treatment of superficial tumours of the bladder. 90 mg Thiotepa dissolved in 100 ml sterile water is instilled into the bladder with the patient in the left lateral position. After 15 minutes the patient is transferred to the right lateral position and after a further 15 minutes the bladder is emptied. It is felt that such single dose administration decreases the incidence of systemic toxicity by decreasing the extent of systemic absorption of the drug.

Note: Patients who have had previous radiotherapy to the bladder are at increased risk of drug toxicity.

Malignant meningeal disease: Intrathecal injections of Thiotepa have been found to be useful for the palliative treatment of cases of meningeal infiltration by leukaemia and lymphoma. Clinical experience has shown Thiotepa to be effective in carcinomatous involvement of the meninges, but published data is limited. Thiotepa, at a concentration of 1 mg/ml in sterile water, is administered by injection through a lumbar theca in doses of up to 10 mg on alternate days until there is clearance of malignant cells from the cerebrospinal fluid (CSF). It is recommended that if no improvement occurs in the CSF after three courses of treatment, that treatment should be changed. Not more than four injections should be given on alternate days. Routine blood counts should be performed prior to each dose of Thiotepa.

Ovarian cancer: Ovarian cancer has been treated with Thiotepa as a single agent or as part of a combination regime in a variety of schedules. For example, 15 mg Thiotepa IV or IM may be given daily for four days initially and then continued with single doses administered at weekly or two weekly intervals.

Intracavitary instillation of Thiotepa: Instillations of Thiotepa have been used to treat malignant pleural effusions and abdominal ascites. The procedure recommended is first to aspirate as much fluid as possible and then to instil the dose of Thiotepa, 10–65 mg in 20–60 ml sterile water. This may be repeated at weekly or two weekly intervals.

Prevention of recurrence of Pterygium: A 1:2,000 solution of Thiotepa in sterile Ringer's solution (i.e. 15 mg powder in 30 ml Ringer's) applied topically as eye drops at three hourly intervals daily for up to six weeks after surgical removal of the pterygium, is effective in reducing the recurrence rate following surgery.

Condyloma Acuminata: Thiotepa applied topically or instilled intraurethrally in a gel has been successfully used to eradicate condyloma acuminata. The drug may be administered by first reconstituting 60 mg Thiotepa with 5 ml sterile water. This is diluted to 15 ml using a sterile mixture of water and lubricating jelly made to a consistency viscous enough to remain in the urethra and fluid enough to allow easy injection. This therapy may be repeated at weekly intervals.

Contra-indications, warnings, etc Thiotepa administration is contra-indicated in patients with a WBC count below 3,000 and/or a platelet count below 100,000. Thiotepa has been reported to possess mutagenic activity on the basis of bacterial, plant and mammalian mutagenicity tests. It has also been reported to be carcinogenic in mice and rats. These effects are consistent with its activity as an alkylating agent. The carcinogenic potential in humans has not been clearly established.

Use in pregnancy and lactation: Thiotepa is teratogenic and embryotoxic in mice and rats following intraperitoneal administration. In addition, it has been reported to interfere with spermatogenesis and ovarian function in rodent species. The drug, therefore, should not normally be administered to patients who are pregnant or to mothers who are breast feeding unless the benefit outweighs the risk to foetus or child.

Precautions: Thiotepa should only be used by clinicians who are familiar with the various characteristics of cytotoxic drugs and their clinical toxicity. WBC and platelet counts are recommended 12–24 hours before each dose of Thiotepa regardless of route of administration, except when used topically as eye drops or in the treatment of condyloma acuminata. Dosage should be reduced as indicated above in the presence of a compromised bone marrow as manifested by a reduced WBC count. Safe use in children has not been established.

Side-effects: The most serious side-effect is upon the blood forming elements and is a direct consequence of the cytotoxic action of the drug. In addition, Thiotepa may occasionally cause vomiting, headache and anorexia. Alopecia has been reported as a rare complication of therapy with Thiotepa. Local irritation, comparable to a mild radiation cystitis, may follow bladder instillations of Thiotepa, while haemorrhagic cystitis is rare. Depigmentation of periorbital skin has been reported rarely following the use of Thiotepa eye drops.

Overdosage: There is no specific antidote. Gastric lavage, forced fluids and general supportive measures are recommended. Blood counts should be carried out to estimate damage to the haematopoietic system and blood transfusions should be given as required.

Pharmaceutical precautions Thiotepa must be stored in a refrigerator (2–8°C). The occurrence of a precipitate on reconstitution (with 1.5 ml of water for injection) indicates that polymerisation has occurred with the formation of less active constituents and the injection must be discarded.

Reconstituted solutions may be stored in a refrigerator (2–8°C) for 24 hours. However, if a precipitate forms, the solution must be discarded.

Thiotepa may be mixed in the same syringe with Procaine Hydrochloride 2% or with adrenaline 1 in 1,000 or with both.

Handling of cytotoxic drugs: Trained personnel should reconstitute Thiotepa in a designated area. Adequate protective gloves and goggles should be worn and the work surface should be covered with disposable plastic-backed absorbent paper. Thiotepa is not vesicant and should not cause harm if it comes in contact with the skin. It should, of course, be washed off with water immediately. Any transient stinging may be treated with a bland cream.

The cytotoxic preparation should not be handled by pregnant staff.

Any spillage or waste material may be disposed of by incineration. We do not make any specific recommendations with regards to the temperature of the incinerator.

Legal category POM.

Package quantities Boxes of one vial.

Further information Thiotepa contains 1.97 millimoles of sodium per vial.

Product licence number 0095/5060.

TRAXAM* GEL

Presentation Clear, non-gresy, non staining gel containing 30 mg felbinac in each gram.

Uses Traxam Gel is a topical anti-inflammatory and analgesic. It is indicated for the relief of symptoms associated with soft tissue injury such as sprains, strains and contusions.

Dosage and administration Traxam Gel should be rubbed lightly into the affected area 2 to 4 times a day. If symptoms do not resolve within 14 days, the patient should be reviewed.

The total dose should not exceed 25 g per day regardless of the number of affected areas.

Elderly: No special dosage recommendations are made for elderly patients.

Children: Safe use in early childhood has not been established.

Contra-indications, warnings, etc
Contra-indications: Hypersensitivity to the ingredients. Patients in whom attacks of asthma, urticaria or acute rhinitis are precipitated by aspirin or other non-steroidal anti-inflammatory agents.

Warnings: Use of gel should be limited to intact skin. Contact with mucous membranes and the eyes should be avoided. Traxam Gel should not be applied with occlusive dressings.

Pregnancy and lactation: There is no evidence as to the safety of felbinac in human pregnancy or lactation. Its use should be avoided since dystocia and delayed parturition were observed in animal studies.

Interactions: Felbinac is highly protein bound. However,

serum levels following topical application are extremely low therefore clinical drug interactions are unlikely.

Side-effects: Mild local erythema, dermatitis and pruritus have been reported in less than 2% of patients. Spontaneous recovery occurs on cessation of treatment.

Overdosage: It is unlikely that Traxam Gel would cause adverse systemic effects even if accidental ingestion should occur. Patients shold consult a doctor if ingestion is suspected.

Pharmaceutical precautions Replace the cap after use. Dilution is not recommended.

Legal category POM.

Package quantities Tubes containing 50 g.

Further information Nil.

Product licence number 0095/0119.

TUBERCULIN, OLD, TINE TEST* (ROSENTHAL)

Presentation Each Tuberculin Tine Test unit consists of a stainless steel disc with four tines or prongs attached to a plastic handle. The tines have been dipped in Old Tuberculin, stabilised and dried. The entire unit has been sterilised. The reactivity of the Tuberculin Tine Test is comparable to the intermediate strength Mantoux test (5 T.U. or 0.0001 mg PPD).

Uses Tuberculin Tine Test is an intradermal test for the detection of tuberculin sensitivity, and is used for screening for tuberculosis. Tuberculin testing may be done during the first year of life. Frequency of repeated tuberculin tests depends on risk of exposure of the child and on the prevalence of tuberculosis in the population group; tuberculin testing may be repeated at intervals of a year or less.

Dosage and administration *Adults and children: Site:* for accurate, standardised tuberculin testing, the volar surface of the mid-forearm is the preferred site. The skin must be clean and dry. It may be cleansed with alcohol, acetone, ether, or soap and water. On other skin areas reactions are less reliable, and quantitatively do not bear the same significance to the standardised test. Hairy areas and areas without adequate subcutaneous tissue, such as concavities over a tendon or bone, should be avoided.

Method of application: Remove the Tuberculin Tine Test unit by levering or snapping the handle from the base of the container. Grasp the patient's arm firmly with one hand, stretching the skin of the forearm tightly, and apply the disc with the other hand. Hold for one second and withdraw. Sufficient pressure should be exerted to produce four visible puncture sites and a circular depression of the skin from the plastic base. The Tine Test should *never* be re-used. Local care of the skin site is not necessary.

Reading the reaction: Tests should be read at 48–72 hours. Induration is the only criterion. It is important to measure it exactly, by examining under adequate light and by thoroughly palpating the area. Identification of the application site is usually easy because of the distinct four-point pattern. A reaction of 2 mm or more of palpable induration around one or more puncture sites is clinically comparable to a zone of induration of 5 mm or more by the intermediate strength PPD (0.0001 mg PPD) Mantoux test. Recently, the interpretation of tuberculin test reactions as recommended by the National Tuberculosis and Respiratory Disease Association has been revised. Their recommendations for interpretation of the tine test are as follows:

5 mm or more of induration Positive Reaction.

The significance of the test and the management of the individual is the same as that for one who reacts with 10 mm or more of induration to the standard Mantoux test.

2 mm through 4 mm of induration Doubtful Reaction.

Even though such reactions may be due to M. tuberculosis, a significant proportion of them may not be confirmed by a positive standard Mantoux test. Therefore, a Mantoux test should be done on all individuals in this group, and management should be based on Mantoux reactions.

Less than 2 mm of induration Negative Reaction.

There is no need for retesting unless the individual is a contact to a case of tuberculosis or there is suggestive clinical evidence of the disease.

Contra-indications, warnings, etc
Contra-indications: None.

Precautions: Tuberculin testing should be done with caution in persons with active tuberculosis. However, activation of quiescent lesions is rare.

Although clinical allergy to acacia is very rare, Tine Test contains some acacia as a stabiliser and should be used with caution in patients with known allergy to this component.

Reactivity to the test may be suppressed in patients who are receiving corticosteroids or immunosuppressive agents, or those who have recently been vaccinated with live virus vaccine such as measles.

With a *large* positive reaction to the Tine Test, further diagnostic procedures must be considered. These may include X-ray of the chest, microbiological examinations of sputa and other specimens and confirmation of the positive Tine Test using the Mantoux method. Antituberculous therapy should not be instituted solely on the basis of a single positive Tine Test.

Side-effects: Vesiculation, ulceration, or necrosis may occur at the test site in highly sensitive persons. Pain, pruritus and discomfort at the test site may be relieved by cold packs or by a topical glucocorticoid ointment or cream. Transient bleeding may be observed at a puncture site and is of no significance.

Overdosage: Does not apply.

Pharmaceutical precautions Tuberculin Tine Test should be stored at controlled room temperature (15–30°C) in the original pack. DO NOT REFRIGERATE.

Legal category POM.

Package quantities Container of 24 tests.

Further information Nil.

Product licence number 0095/5002.

VARIDASE* TOPICAL

Presentation Each vial of dry, sterile powder which requires storage under refrigeration (2–8°C) contains; Streptokinase 100,000 units and Streptodornase at least 25,000 units.

The combi-pack contains a vial of Varidase Topical, a 20 ml vial of sterile Sodium Chloride 0.9% Solution BP (physiological saline) and a sterile transfer needle.

Uses Streptokinase acts indirectly upon a substrate of fibrin or fibrinogen by activating a fibrinolytic enzyme in human serum. Upon application of streptokinase in situ, the activation of this fibrinolytic system brings about rapid dissolution of blood clots and the fibrinous portion of exudates. Streptodornase liquefies the viscous nucleoprotein of dead cells or pus. Thus the action of the enzymes results in the liquefaction of the two main viscous substances resulting from inflammatory or infectious processes thereby facilitating cleansing and desloughing of wounds.

Varidase Topical has no effect on collagen or healthy tissue.

Indications: Varidase Topical is indicated wherever clotted blood, fibrinous or purulent accumulations are undesirably present, following trauma or infectious processes which have led to ulceration or abscess formation.

It is indicated in the treatment of suppurative surface lesions such as ulcers, pressure sores, amputation sites, diabetic gangrene, radiation necrosis, infected wounds, and surgical incisions until the wound is thoroughly cleansed of clots, fibrinous exudates and pus. It is also indicated in the treatment of burns and may be used prior to skin grafting.

Varidase Topical can be used to dissolve clots in the bladder or in urinary catheters.

Dosage and administration
Adults and children: Directions for use in the cleansing of necrotic and infected wounds.

Reconstitution: The contents of each vial should be gently mixed with 20 ml of sterile physiological saline or, if unavailable, 20 ml Water for Injection. Care should be taken to control the rate of addition of saline to the vial to avoid frothing. The resulting clear solution can then be withdrawn into a syringe.

As Varidase does not contain a preservative, multi-dose use is not recommended.

Standard methods of application: Pre-soak gauze with Varidase Topical solution then apply to the wound.

Following application a semi-occlusive dressing is necessary to prevent drying-out of the wound, e.g. a polythene film taped on two sides.

Alternatively the wound may be packed with dry gauze which is then soaked with Varidase Topical solution and dressed with a semi-occlusive dressing.

Alternative method of application: Where wounds are covered by a thick dry slough or eschar it is usually necessary to cross hatch the slough into approximately 3–5 mm squares and to a sufficient depth to allow the access of the enzymes to the underlying fibrinous and purulent material. Alternatively, Varidase Topical may be injected under the eschar, taking care that the solution enters only the cavity beneath and that the volume is not sufficient to cause pain through increased pressure. Injection of Varidase Topical in this way often results in the eschar becoming partly detached thus facilitating its mechanical removal.

Special technique of application: Varidase Topical may be applied in jelly form. This can be prepared by dissolving the contents of one vial in 5 ml of sterile water and mixing the resulting solution thoroughly but gently, with 15 ml of inert jelly, such as K–Y* or carboxymethylcellulose (CMC) jelly. This method can be particularly useful in cases of burns where dressings are not employed.

Frequency of application: Varidase Topical treatment should be repeated once or twice a day. Care should be taken to irrigate the lesion thoroughly with physiological saline and remove loosened material prior to the next application.

Duration of treatment: Treatment should be continued until healthy granulations are present and re-epithelialisation has begun, usually within one to two weeks.

Contra-indications, warnings, etc
Contra-indications: Active haemorrhage. Known hypersensitivity to Streptokinase or Streptodornase.

Pregnancy and lactation: Safe use of Varidase Topical during pregnancy and lactation has not been established.

Precautions: Varidase Topical is intended for local use only. **It should not be used intramuscularly or intravenously.**

In order to avoid cross-infection the contents of one vial of Varidase Topical and a separate sterile syringe and needle should be used for each individual patient.

Varidase Topical has been shown to be a sensitiser when administered at relatively low intradermal doses to guinea pigs. The relevance of these findings to humans is considered important only where prolonged repetitive treatment is anticipated. Under such circumstances, the potential to induce allergic reactions may be minimised as described under 'Side-effects'.

Side-effects: Allergic reactions to the topical application of Varidase Topical are infrequent and may be minimised by careful and frequent removal of exudate followed by thorough irrigation using physiological saline prior to retreatment with Varidase Topical.

Slight buring pain has been reported rarely after the use of Varidase Topical.

Overdosage: There is no specific antidote. Removal of the preparation by careful washing or by irrigation/suction drainage is recommended.

Pharmaceutical precautions Varidase Topical must be stored in a refrigerator (2–8°C) and should be reconstituted in 20 ml of sterile physiological saline or if unavailable Water for Injection. After preparation, the resulting solution should be used immediately or may be stored for up to 24 hours in a refrigerator (2–8°C).

The preparation is buffered to physiological pH. The enzymes of Varidase Topical can be inactivated by the concomitant use of other preparations of an acidic or alkaline pH. If the reconstituting fluid has a high calcium content, the solution becomes opalescent, but this does not affect the potency of the product.

Legal category POM.

Package quantities Single vials or combi-pack.

Further information Information on the intracavitary use of Varidase Topical in the treatment of, for example, haemothorax or thoracic empyema is available on request to the Medical Information Department.

Product licence number 0095/5038.

VINBLASTINE INJECTION BP 10 mg

Presentation A combination package consisting of (i) one vial of lyophilised powder consisting of 10 mg of Vinblastine sulphate for reconstitution before use with (ii) one ampoule of Diluting Solution, i.e. 10 ml of sodium chloride 0.9% with 2% benzyl alcohol as an antimicrobial preservative.

Uses The treatment of neoplastic disease.

Dosage and administration
Adults and Children: The dosage of Vinblastine must always be adjusted individually because of individual variations in the degree of leucopenia. Vinblastine is administered intravenously at intervals no more frequently than once a week, and has been used alone and in combination or sequence with other cytotoxic agents, radiotherapy or surgery in a wide variety of neoplastic diseases e.g. lymphomas including Hodgkin's disease, breast cancer unresponsive to appropriate endocrine, surgical, and hormonal therapy, testicular cancer, Methotrexate-resistant choriocarcinoma, reticulum cell sarcoma, mycosis fungoides, neuroblastoma and histiocytosis X (Letterer-Siwe disease).

Initial dosage is calculated by body weight or body surface area and varies according to the disease. However, in general, 0.1–0.2 mg/kg is given. Rarely, up to 0.5 mg/kg may be necessary. It is important to monitor the patients white blood cell count before each dose and the dose can be increased by increments of 0.05 mg/kg each week until an objective response is obtained or a nadir in the white cell count of approximately 3,000 cells/mm^3 is observed. A dose one increment smaller than this can then be administered at weekly or longer intervals for maintenance. It should be emphasised that, even if seven days have elapsed, the next dose of Vinblastine should not be given until the white cell count has returned to at least 4,000 cells/mm^3.

Administration: Vinblastine is irritant, particularly to the eyes and skin and it is recommended that goggles and gloves are worn during reconstitution and administration of the product. Following reconstitution, the calculated dose of Vinblastine is withdrawn from the vial and should only be injected either directly into a vein or into the tubing of a fast running intravenous infusion of Sodium Chloride 0.9%.

When reconstituted with the Diluting Solution provided, Vinblastine Injection may be stored in a refrigerator for 30 days without significant loss of potency.

Severe local pain and tissue damage will occur if Vinblastine injection extravasates during intravenous administration. The injection should be discontinued immediately and any remaining portion of the dose should then be introduced into another vein. Local injection of hyaluronidase and the application of moderate heat to the area of leakage help to disperse the drug and are thought to minimise discomfort and the possibility of cellulitis.

Care must be taken to avoid contamination of the eye with concentrations of Vinblastine used clinically. If accidental contamination occurs, severe irritation (or if the drug was delivered under pressure, even corneal ulceration) may result. The eye should be washed with water thoroughly and immediately.

Contra-indications, warnings, etc
Contra-indications: Vinblastine should not normally be administered to patients who are pregnant or to mothers who are breast-feeding. Leucopenia. Concurrent untreated infection. Intrathecal administration. Use in elderly cachectic patients.

Precautions: Vinblastine should be administered under the direction of a specialist oncology service having the facilities for regular monitoring of clinical, biochemical and haematological effects during and after administration.

The use of small amounts of Vinblastine daily for long periods is not advised. Little or no added therapeutic benefit compared with intermittent dosing has been demonstrated and convulsions, severe and permanent central nervous system damage and even death have occurred. If leucopenia with less than 2,000 white blood cells/mm^3 occurs following a dose of Vinblastine, the patient should be watched carefully for evidence of infection until the white blood cell count has returned to a safe level.

When cachexia or ulcerated areas of the skin surface are present, there may be a more profound leucopenic response to the drug. Its use should be avoided in older persons suffering from either of these conditions. In patients with malignant-cell infiltration of the bone marrow, the leucocyte and platelet counts have sometimes fallen precipitously after moderate doses of Vinblastine. Further use of the drug in such patients is inadvisable.

Vinblastine has been shown to be teratogenic. However, only limited information is available concerning the effect of Vinblastine on spermatogenesis. Although no abnormalities of the human foetus have been reported thus far, animal studies with Vinblastine would suggest that teratogenic effects may occur. Patients receiving Vinblastine and their partners should be advised to avoid conception.

There is a possibility that Vinblastine may exert a carcinogenic effect with long-term therapy, although to date no positive evidence is available.

Side-effects: Clinically, leucopenia is an expected effect of Vinblastine and the level of the leucocyte count is an important guide of treatment. Following therapy with Vinblastine, the nadir in the white blood cell count may be expected to occur five to ten days after the last day of drug administration, with complete recovery within another seven to fourteen days.

The effect of Vinblastine upon the thrombocyte count and/or red blood cell count is usually insignificant when other treatment does not complicate the picture.

Nausea and vomiting are common but are usually readily controlled by anti-emetic agents.

Stomatitis, constipation, diarrhoea, ileus, anorexia, abdominal pain, rectal bleeding, pharyngitis, bleeding from an old peptic ulcer and, rarely, haemorrhagic enterocolitis have also been observed.

Alopecia is uncommon and is frequently not total. Regrowth may occur during maintenance treatment.

Neurological side effects such as numbness, paraesthesiae, peripheral neuritis, mental depression, loss of deep tendon reflexes, headache or convulsions can occur but are much less common than with Vincristine.

Other adverse reactions that have been reported are malaise, weakness, dizziness, pain in the tumour site and vesiculation of the skin.

Toxicity is increased in patients with obstructive jaundice.

Overdosage: Side-effects following the use of Vinblastine are dose related. Therefore, following administration of more than the recommended dose, patients can be expected to experience these effects in an exaggerated fashion.

In addition, neurotoxicity similar to that seen with vincristine sulphate may be observed.

Treatment: Supportive care should include: (1) prevention of the side effects that result from the syndrome of inappropriate secretion of antidiuretic hormone. This includes restriction of fluid intake and perhaps the use of a diuretic acting on the loop of Henle and distal tubule function; (2) administration of an anticonvulsant; (3) prevention and treatment of ileus; (4) monitoring the patient's cardiovascular system; and (5) daily blood counts for guidance in transfusion requirement.

The major effect of excessive doses of Vinblastine will be on granulocytopoeisis, and this may be life-threatening.

Pharmaceutical precautions Vinblastine should be stored in a refrigerator (2–8°C). Injections reconstituted with the Diluting Solution provided contain an antimicrobial preservative and may be kept in a refrigerator for 30 days without significant loss of potency.

Handling of cytotoxic preparations: Vinblastine is irritant particularly to the eyes and skin. It is therefore recommended that gloves and goggles should be worn by trained personnel during reconstitution and administration of this drug. Accidental contamination of the eye may result in corneal ulceration if the drug is delivered under pressure. Any contamination should immediately be thoroughly washed with water. Reconstitution should be performed in a designated area and the work surface should be covered with disposable plastic-backed absorbent paper.

The cytotoxic preparation should not be handled by pregnant staff.

Any spillage or waste materials may be disposed of by incineration. We do not make any recommendations with regards to the temperature of the incinerator.

Legal category POM.

Package quantities Combination package consisting of one vial of Vinblastine 10 mg and one ampoule of Diluting Solution.

Further information Nil.

Product licence number 0095/0067.

VINCRISTINE INJECTION BP, 1 mg, 2 mg, 5 mg

Presentation A combination package consisting of (i) one vial of lyophilised powder consisting of 1 mg, 2 mg or 5 mg of Vincristine sulphate with 10 mg, 20 mg or 50 mg of lactose respectively, for reconstitution before use with (ii) one ampoule of Diluting Solution, i.e. 10 ml of sodium chloride 0.9% with 2% benzyl alcohol as an antimicrobial preservative.

Uses The treatment of neoplastic disease.

Dosage and administration
Adults and Children: The dosage must always be adjusted individually because of the narrow range between therapeutic and toxic levels and individual variations in response. Extreme care must be used in calculating and administering doses of Vincristine since overdosage may have a very serious or fatal outcome.

Vincristine is administered intravenously, usually at weekly or longer intervals and has been used alone and in combination or sequence with other cytotoxic agents, radiotherapy and/or surgery in a wide variety of neoplastic diseases, e.g. acute leukaemias, malignant lymphomas including Hodgkin's disease, sarcomas, neuroblastoma, Wilms's tumour and rhabdomyosarcoma. Vincristine may also be considered in the treatment of breast cancer, bronchial carcinoma, and gastro-intestinal cancer. Initial dosage is calculated by body surface area or body weight and varies according to the disease. However, in general,

1.0–2.0 mg/m^2 is given with a normal maximum weekly adult dose of 2 mg.

In children, remissions from acute leukaemia have been induced with weekly doses of 0.05–0.15 mg/kg of body weight.

In acute leukaemia of children the following incremental approach to dosage may be employed:

First dose: 0.05 mg/kg
Second dose: 0.075 mg/kg
Third dose: 0.1 mg/kg
and Fourth dose: 0.125 mg/kg up to a maximum of 0.15 mg/kg.

There is no need to advance the dosage beyond that level which produces therapeutic benefit. After remission has been obtained, the dosage may be reduced in some cases to a maintenance level of 0.05 to 0.075 mg/kg/week.

In adult leukaemia the suggested dosage is 0.025–0.075 mg/kg of body weight per weekly dose.

For malignancies other than leukaemia, a suggested dosage for Vincristine is 0.025 mg/kg/week intravenously until some beneficial effect is seen. Thereafter much smaller weekly doses in the range of 0.005–0.01 mg/kg may be employed for maintenance therapy for so long as an anti-tumour effect can be maintained.

Administration: Vincristine is irritant, particularly to the eyes and skin, and it is recommended that goggles and gloves are worn during reconstitution and administration of the product. Luer lock fittings should be used on all syringes and sets. Large bore needles are recommended to minimise pressure and the possible formation of aerosols. The latter may also be reduced by use of a venting needle. Following reconstitution, the calculated dose of Vincristine is withdrawn from the vial and should only be injected either directly into a vein or into the tubing of a fast running intravenous infusion of Sodium Chloride 0.9%.

When reconstituted with the Diluting Solution provided, Vincristine Injection may be stored in a refrigerator for 14 days without significant loss of potency.

Severe local pain and tissue damage will occur if Vincristine injection extravasates during intravenous administration. The injection should be discontinued immediately and any remaining portion of the dose should then be introduced into another vein. Local injection of hyaluronidase and the application of moderate heat to the area of leakage help to disperse the drug and are thought to minimise discomfort and the possibility of cellulitis.

Care must be taken to avoid contamination of the eye with concentrations of Vincristine used clinically. If accidental contamination occurs, severe irritation (or if the drug was delivered under pressure, even corneal ulceration) may result. The eye should be washed with water thoroughly and immediately.

Contra-indications, warnings, etc

Contra-indications: Vincristine should not normally be administered to patients who are pregnant or to mothers who are breast-feeding.
Intrathecal administration.
Use in the presence of untreated infection.

Precautions: Vincristine should only be administered under the direction of a specialist oncology service having the facilities for regular monitoring of clinical, biochemical and haematological effects during and after administration.

Effective Vincristine therapy does not normally result in leucopenia. Neuromuscular rather than bone-marrow toxicity is usually the dose-limiting factor. However, because of the possibility of leucopenia both physician and patient should remain alert for signs of any complicating infection. Although pre-existing leucopenia does not necessarily contra-indicate the administration of Vincristine the appearance of leucopenia during treatment warrants careful consideration before giving the next dose. Similarly, Vincristine should only be used with caution in patients with malignant infiltration of bone marrow.

Acute uric acid nephropathy has occurred following Vincristine treatment.

Vincristine has been shown to be teratogenic. However, no data are available concerning the effect of Vincristine on spermatogenesis. Patients receiving Vincristine and their partners should be advised to avoid conception.

Routine use of laxatives and enemas is recommended to ensure regular bowel function.

As Vincristine is excreted principally by the liver, it may be necessary to reduce initial doses in the presence of significantly impaired hepatic or biliary function.

When chemotherapy is being given in conjunction with radiation therapy through portals which include the liver, the use of Vincristine should be delayed until radiation therapy has been completed.

If central nervous system leukaemia is diagnosed, additional therapy, such as intrathecal Methotrexate, may be required, since Vincristine does not appear to cross the blood-brain barrier in adequate amounts. There is a possibility that Vincristine may exert a carcinogenic effect with long-term therapy, although to date no positive evidence is available.

Side-effects: In general, adverse reactions are reversible and are related to dosage. The most common side-effect is some degree of alopecia.

The main toxicity of Vincristine is neuropathy which may take any form but usually presents as a sensory motor peripheral neuropathy with paraesthesia, loss of tendon reflexes, muscle wasting and muscular weakness.

Frequently, there appears to be a sequence in the development of neuromuscular side-effects, in that initially sensory impairment and paraesthesia develop followed later by neuritic pain and motor difficulties. With single weekly doses, neuritic pain and difficulty in walking are usually of short duration (i.e. less than seven days). Other side-effects, such as sensory loss, paraesthesia, slapping gait, loss of deep tendon reflexes, and muscle wasting do not reverse so rapidly but persist for at least as long as treatment is continued. In most instances, these side-effects have disappeared by about the sixth week after discontinuing treatment, but in some patients neuromuscular difficulties may persist for prolonged periods.

No reports have yet been made of any agent that can reverse the neuromuscular manifestations of Vincristine. Discontinuation of treatment should be considered if neuromuscular effects continue to be a problem.

Vincristine commonly causes constipation which usually responds well to measures such as enemas and laxatives. Constipation may take the form of upper colon impaction and the rectum may be found to be empty on physical examination. Colicky abdominal pain, coupled with an empty rectum, may mislead the physician. A flat film of the abdomen is useful in demonstrating this condition. A routine prophylactic regimen against constipation is recommended for all patients receiving Vincristine.

On rare occasions intestinal necrosis and/or perforation have been reported when Vincristine is used in combination with a steroid.

Convulsions, frequently with hypertension, have been reported in a few patients receiving Vincristine.

Rare occurrences of the syndrome of inappropriate secretion of antidiuretic hormone have also been observed. With fluid deprivation, improvement occurs in the hyponatraemia and in the renal loss of sodium.

Other reported adverse reactions include abdominal cramps, ataxia, foot drop, weight loss, fever, cranial nerve manifestations, paraesthesiae and numbness of the digits, polyuria, dysuria, oral ulceration, headache, vomiting and diarrhoea.

Vincristine does not appear to have any constant or significant effect upon the platelets or the red blood cells. If thrombocytopenia is present when treatment with Vincristine is begun, it may actually improve before the appearance of marrow remission.

Overdosage: Side-effects following the use of Vincristine are dose related. Therefore, following administration of more than the recommended dose, patients can be expected to experience these effects in an exaggerated fashion.

Treatment: Supportive care should include: (a) prevention of side-effects that result from the syndrome of inappropriate secretion of antidiuretic hormone. This includes restriction of fluid intake and perhaps the use of a diuretic acting on the loop of Henle and distal tubule function; (b) administration of an anticonvulsant; (c) use of cathartics to prevent ileus; (d) monitoring the patients' cardiovascular system; and (e) daily blood counts for guidance in transfusion requirement. Animal studies indicate that folinic acid is effective in the treatment of overdosage. A suggested schedule is to administer 15 mg of folinic acid intravenously every 3 hours for 24 hours and then every 6 hours for at least 48 hours.

Pharmaceutical precautions Vincristine should be stored in a refrigerator (2–8°C). Injections, reconstituted with the Diluting Solution provided, contain an antimicrobial preservative and may be kept in a refrigerator for 14 days without significant loss of potency. Goggles and gloves should be worn during reconstitution and administration of Vincristine.

Handling of cytotoxic preparations: Vincristine is irritant particularly to the eyes and skin. It is therefore recommended that gloves and goggles should be worn by trained personnel during reconstitution and administration of this drug. Accidental contamination of the eye may result in corneal ulceration if the drug is delivered under pressure. Any contamination should immediately be thoroughly washed with water.

Reconstitution should be performed in a designated area and the work surface should be covered with disposable plastic-backed absorbent paper.

The cytotoxic preparation should not be handled by pregnant staff. Any spillage or waste materials may be disposed of by incineration. We do not make any recommendations with regards to the temperature of the incinerator.

Legal category POM.

Package quantities Combination packages consisting of one vial of Vincristine 1 mg, 2 mg or 5 mg and one ampoule of Diluting Solution.

Further information Nil.

Product licence numbers

Vincristine Injection BP 1 mg and 2 mg	0095/0065
Vincristine Injection BP 5 mg	0095/0066

ZADSTAT*

Presentation *Tablets 200 mg:* Each white, flat-faced, scored, uncoated tablet, embossed 'M200' on one side and 'LL' on the other side, contains 200 mg of Metronidazole BP.

Suppositories 500 mg and 1 g: Each suppository, containing 500 mg or 1 g of Metronidazole BP, is sealed in individual plastic suppository moulds.

Injection 500 mg in 100 ml: Each injection (for intravenous infusion) contains 500 mg of Metronidazole BP in a 100 ml Steriflex Minipack* container.

Uses Zadstat metronidazole is indicated for:

1. The treatment of infections due to anaerobic bacteria.

2. The prevention of post-operative infections due to anaerobic bacteria.

3. Urogenital trichomoniasis in the female (trichomonal vaginitis) and in the male. Sexual partners should be treated concurrently.

4. All forms of amoebiasis such as acute amoebic dysentery and amoebic liver abscess, and to eradicate cysts from asymptomatic cyst passers.

5. Giardiasis.

6. Acute ulcerative gingivitis.

7. Acute dental infections (e.g. acute pericoronitis and acute apical infections).

8. The treatment of anaerobically-infected leg ulcers and pressure sores.

Dosage and administration Zadstat metronidazole tablets should be taken with or after meals. The recommended dosage regimes (oral, rectal, intravenous) for the treatment and prevention of anaerobic infections are listed below. Oral dosage regimes used for all other indications are given in the table on following page.

1. Treatment of anaerobic infections: Treatment for seven days should be satisfactory for most patients. However, the duration of treatment should be determined by the physician on the basis of the clinical course of infection.

Oral therapy may be substituted for rectal or intravenous medication as soon as this becomes feasible.

A. Oral medication: Adults and children over 10 years: Two tablets (400 mg) three times daily.

Children and infants: 7.5 mg/kg body weight three times daily.

B. Rectal medication: The following doses should be given rectally every eight hours for three days, then every 12 hours therafter.

Adults and children over 10 years: 1 g

Children 5–10 years: 500 mg

Children 1–5 years: 250 mg

Children under 1 year: 125 mg

250 mg and 125 mg suppositories can be prepared by melting 500 mg suppositories and pouring into 1 g or 500 mg suppository moulds respectively.

C. Intravenous medication: Adults and children over 10 years: 100 ml (500 mg metronidazole) by intravenous infusion every eight hours.

Children under 10 years: 1.5 ml (7.5 mg metronidazole) per kg bodyweight every eight hours.

Zadstat metronidazole injection should be infused intravenously at the rate of 5 ml per minute and may be administered alone or concurrently (but separately) with other appropriate parenteral anti-bacterial agents.

2. Prevention of anaerobic infections: Oral and rectal therapy with Zadstat metronidazole is indicated both pre- and post-operatively for the prevention of post-operative infections due to anaerobic bacteria, for example in patients undergoing gynaecological surgery, elective colonic surgery, appendicectomy.

Intravenous medication with Zadstat metronidazole can be used in patients for whom oral or rectal therapy is inappropriate and is particularly indicated in emergencies, for example, in patients needing surgery who:

- have or are believed to have anaerobic sepsis such as septicaemia, peritonitis, subphrenic or pelvic abscesses;
- at operation show signs of established or impending anaerobic sepsis;
- undergo operation in which contamination occurs with anaerobes from the gastro-intestinal or female genital tracts or the oropharynx.

Oral therapy may be substituted for rectal or intravenous medication post-operatively as soon as this becomes feasible to complete a seven-day course.

A. Oral and rectal medication:

(i) *In gynaecological surgery in adults,* a single oral dose of 1 g followed by one tablet (200 mg) eight-hourly both before preoperative starvation, if possible, and soon as possible postoperatively for up to seven days.

(ii) *In elective colonic surgery in adults,* three regimes have been used sucessfully, i.e.:

(*a*) One tablet (200 mg) six-hourly with kanamycin (1 g orally six-hourly) for three days before surgery (without further medication).

(*b*) Two tablets (400 mg) eight-hourly with phthalylsulphathiazole (2.5 g orally six-hourly) for four days before surgery (without further medication).

(*c*) A single dose of 1 g suppository rectally and one tablet (200 mg) eight-hourly during the 24-hours period before pre-operative starvation followed by a 1 g suppository rectally two hours before

Oral dosage regimes for Zadstat tablets 200 mg

Indication	*Adults and children over 10 years*	*7–10 years*	*Children 3–7 years*	*1–3 years*
Urogenital trichomoniasis				
Sexual partners should be treated concurrently	1 tablet three times daily for seven days *OR* 4 tablets in the morning and 6 at night for two days *OR* 10 tablets as a single dose	$\frac{1}{2}$ tablet three times daily for seven days	$\frac{1}{2}$ tablet twice daily for seven days	$\frac{1}{4}$ tablet three times daily for seven days
Amoebiasis				
(a) Invasive intestinal disease in susceptible subjects	4 tablets three times daily for five days	2 tablets three times daily for five days	1 tablet four times daily for five days	1 tablet three times daily for five days
(b) Intestinal disease in susceptible subjects and 'chronic' amoebic hepatitis	2 tablets three times daily for five to ten days	1 tablet three times daily for five to ten days	$\frac{1}{2}$ tablet four times daily for five to ten days	$\frac{1}{2}$ tablet three times daily for five to ten days.
(c) Amoebic liver abscess and other forms of extra-intestinal amoebiasis	2 tablets three times daily for five days	1 tablet three times daily for five days	$\frac{1}{2}$ tablet four times daily for five days	$\frac{1}{2}$ tablet three times daily for five days
(d) Eradication of cysts from asymptomatic cyst passers	2 to 4 tablets three times daily for five to ten days	1 to 2 tablets three times daily for five to ten days	$\frac{1}{2}$ to 1 tablet four times daily for five to ten days	$\frac{1}{2}$ to 1 tablet three times daily for five to ten days
Giardiasis	10 tablets once daily for three days	5 tablets once daily for three days	3 to 4 tablets once daily for three days	500 mg once daily for three days
Acute ulcerative gingivitis	1 tablet three times daily for three days	$\frac{1}{2}$ tablet three times daily for three days	$\frac{1}{2}$ tablet twice daily for three days	$\frac{1}{4}$ tablet three times daily for three days
Acute dental infections	1 tablet three times daily for three to seven days			
Leg ulcers and pressure sores	2 tablets three times daily for seven days			

Immature children and babies weighing less than 10 kg should receive proportionately smaller dosages.

surgery and post-operatively every eight hours for three days, and thereafter every twelve hours to complete a seven day course. Oral medication (200–400 mg three times daily) may be substituted as soon as feasible.

(iii) *In elective colonic surgery in children pre-operative medication:*

	Oral metronidazole (8-hourly for 48 hours)	*Oral neomycin (6-hourly for 3 days)*
5–10 years	100 mg	500 mg
1–5 years	5 mg/kg	250 mg
Under 1 year	5 mg/kg	125 mg

post-operative medication:

	Metronidazole per rectum or via colostomy (8-hourly for 48 hours)
5–10 years	500 mg
1–5 years	250 mg
Under 1 year	125 mg

250 mg and 125 mg suppositories may be prepared by melting the 500 mg suppositories and pouring in 1g or 500 mg suppository moulds, respectively.

(iv) *In appendicectomy:* Adults and children over 10 years: a 1 g suppository rectally two hours before surgery and post-operatively every eight hours for three days and thereafter every 12 hours to complete a seven-day course. Oral medication (200–400 mg three times daily) may be substituted as soon as feasible. Children (5 to 10 years): 500 mg suppositories administered as for adults. Oral medication (3.7–7.5 mg/kg body weight three times daily) may be susbstituted as soon as feasible.

B. *Intravenous medication: Adults and children over 10 years:* 100 ml (500 mg metronidazole) by intravenous infusion immediately before, during or after operation and repeated eight-hourly until oral medication (200–400 mg three times daily) can be given to complete a seven-day course.

Children under 10 years: 1.5 ml (7.5 mg metronidazole) per kg body weight administered as for adults until oral medication (3.7 to 7.5 mg/kg bodyweight three times daily) can be given to complete a seven-day course.

Zadstat injection should be infused intravenously at the rate of 5 ml per minute and may be administered alone or concurrently (but separately) with other appropriate parenteral anti-bacterial agents.

Elderly: Zadstat may be used at the normal recommended dosage in elderly patients even with mild to moderate renal impairment. Regular monitoring should occur during long term treatment.

Contra-indications, warnings, etc

Contra-indications: A history of known allergy to metronidazole. Use in patients with disease of the peripheral nervous system.

Precautions: The recommended dosages, frequencies of administration and duration of medication have been found effective and well tolerated in nearly all cases. However, regular clinical and biological surveillance are advised if administration of metronidazole for more than 10 days is considered to be necessary.

Clinicians who contemplate continuous therapy, for the relief of chronic conditions, for periods longer than those recommended are advised to consider the possible therapeutic benefit against the risks of peripheral neuropathy.

Patients should be advised to avoid alcohol during therapy. Metronidazole may potentiate the action of anticoagulants and their activity should be routinely monitored. Metronidazole passes rapidly into the foetal circulation and into breast milk although no adverse effects on the new-born have been reported. As with all medicines, metronidazole should be used during pregnancy or lactation only when considered essential. In these circumstances the short high dosage regimens are not recommended.

Patients with limited degrees of renal impairment need no alteration in recommended dosage. Patients on haemodialysis should be dosed immediately following this procedure.

Metronidazole and a metabolite have been shown to be mutagenic in some tests with non mammanian cells.

Side-effects; There have been occasional reports of an unpleasant taste, furred tongue, nausea, urticaria and angio-oedema, and very rarely vomiting, drowsiness, dizziness, headache, ataxia, skin rashes, pruritus, incoordination of movement and darkening of the urine (due to a metronidazole metabolite). Anaphylaxis may occur rarely.

A few instances of peripheral neuropathy during intensive and/or prolonged therapy have been reported which usually resolved on withdrawing therapy or reducing dosage. Moderate transient leucopenia has also been reported.

High dosage regimes have been associated with transient epileptiform seizures. Caution is required with brain abscess.

Overdosage: There is no specific treatment but early gastric lavage is recommended following overdosage by mouth. Uneventful recovery has followed attempts at suicide with oral doses up to 12 g. Metronidazole is readily removed from plasma by haemodialysis.

Pharmaceutical precautions Protect from light. Zadstat metronidazole injection does not contain a preservative and is therefore not intended for multi-dose use. Zadstat metronidazole injection, if necessary, may be added to Sodium Chloride Injection BP 0.9%; Sodium Chloride 0.18% and Glucose 4% Injection BP; Glucose Injection BP 5%; Potassium Chloride Injection BP (20 mmol or 40 mmol).

Metronidazole injection is incompatible with Dextrose Injection 10%, Hartmann's solution (compound sodium lactate injection); protein hydrolysates, amino acid infusion or alkaline solutions.

Legal category POM.

Package quantities *Tablets:* Bottles of 250.
Suppositories: Boxes of 10 × 500 mg and 10 × 1 g.
Injection: Boxes containing 2 × 100 ml Steriflex Minipacks in sales packs of 5 boxes.

Further information Nil.

Product licence numbers

Tablets 200 mg	0095/0048
Suppositories 500 mg	0095/0084
Suppositories 1 g	0095/0085
Injection 500 mg in 100 ml	0095/0086.

**Trade Mark*

Leo Laboratories Limited
Longwick Road
Princes Risborough
Aylesbury
Bucks. HP17 9RR

L E O

BETIM*

Presentation White, flat circular tablets engraved with '102' on the scored face and with an Assyrian lion on the reverse. Each tablet contains Timolol Maleate PhEur 10 mg.

Uses
Mode of action: Betim is a beta-adrenergic receptor blocking agent. The competitive antagonism of adrenergic transmitters at beta receptors blocks beta-sympathomimetic activity particularly in the heart, the bronchi and blood vessels.

Betim has been shown to be a highly specific beta-adrenergic blocking drug and it does not block the chronotropic or inotropic effects of calcium, glucagon, theophylline or digitalis. It does not have significant local anaesthetic or direct myocardial depressant activity nor any significant intrinsic beta-adrenergic stimulant effect.

Betim reduces heart rate and force of myocardial contraction and therefore myocardial oxygen consumption. Modification of the cardiovascular responses to stress or exercise is therapeutically useful in the treatment of angina pectoris.

The beta blocking action of Betim is also of therapeutic value in hypertension although the exact mechanism of action is unclear.

Timolol maleate is rapidly and nearly completely absorbed following oral administration. Beta blocking activity is apparent within 30 minutes of administration and the duration of action, though dependent on dose, has been shown to last for up to 24 hours. Dose proportionality has been established. Plasma half life is approximately 2.7–5.0 hours with a peak plasma concentration occurring approximately 2 hours post dose. Timolol undergoes significant hepatic metabolism, but 'first pass metabolism' is low.

5% of timolol is excreted unchanged by the kidneys.

These pharmacokinetic parameters are unchanged in hypertensive patients and following multiple dosages.

The rate of timolol metabolism varies between individuals; poor metabolisers (approximately 10%) show higher plasma levels and slower elimination of timolol than extensive metabolisers. Within individuals, however, plasma concentrations and half-life are reproducible. As the therapeutic response and some adverse effects are related to plasma concentrations of timolol, poor metabolisers may require lower than normal doses.

Indications: Betim is indicated in angina pectoris due to ischaemic heart disease, for the treatment of hypertension and to reduce mortality and reinfarction in patients surviving acute myocardial infarction. Betim is also indicated in the prophylactic treatment of migraine in order to reduce the number of attacks.

Dosage and administration
For angina: The recommended dose range is 5–30 mg twice daily. The initial dose should be 5 mg twice daily, increasing the daily dose by 10 mg every 3–4 days to achieve optimum results.

Hypertension: The recommended dose range is 10–60 mg daily.

Most hypertensive patients will be controlled by 10–30 mg timolol which can be administered once daily or in two divided doses if preferred. Doses in excess of 30 mg daily should be given in two equally divided doses. The dose of Betim may need adjustment when used in conjunction with other antihypertensive drugs.

After myocardial infarction: Start with 5 mg (½ tablet) twice daily for two days. If there are no adverse effects, increase dosage to 10 mg twice daily and maintain at this dose.

For the prophylactic treatment of migraine: 10 to 20 mg once daily or in two divided doses.

Dosage in the elderly: Initiate treatment with lowest adult dose and thereafter adjust according to response.

Children: Safety and efficacy in children has not been established.

Contra-indications, warnings, etc
Contra-indications: Heart failure, unless adequately controlled. Sinus bradycardia or heart block. Cardiogenic shock. Bronchial asthma, chronic obstructive pulmonary disease. Patients receiving monoamine oxidase inhibitors. Pregnancy. Sick sinus syndrome, severe peripheral vascular disease or Raynaud's disease, hypersensitivity to timolol or any other ingredients.

Precautions: Although Betim has no direct myocardial depressant activity, the continued depression of sympathetic drive through beta blockade may lead to cardiac failure. All patients should be observed for evidence of cardiac failure; if it occurs, then treatment with beta blockers should be gradually withdrawn. If it is not possible to withdraw beta blocker treatment, then digitalisation and diuretic therapy should be considered.

Betim may be used safely in diabetes. It may however interfere with the cardiovascular and possibly the metabolic responses to hypoglycaemia and therefore should be used with caution in diabetic patients treated with insulin or oral hypoglycaemic agents as well as in patients subject to spontaneous hypoglycaemia.

Betim should be administered with caution to patients with impaired renal function or impaired hepatic function.

Drug interactions: Caution is recommended when Betim is administered to patients on catecholamine depleting drugs such as reserpine or guanethidine.

The bioavailability of Betim will be increased by co-administration with cimetidine and reduced with rifampicin.

Some non-steroidal anti-inflammatory agents have been shown to impair the anti-hypertensive effect of beta blocking drugs.

Betim may be prescribed with vasodilators, but increased gastro-intestinal blood flow may affect absorption and metabolism of timolol.

Betim should be used with caution in patients already receiving other hypotensive drugs, including clonidine.

The effect of sympathomimetic agents, eg isoprenaline, salbutamol, will be reduced by concomitant use of beta blockers.

The depressant effect of beta blocking drugs on myocardial contractility and on intracardiac conduction may be increased by concomitant use with other drugs having similar effects. Serious effects have been reported with verapamil, disopyramide, lignocaine and tocainide and may be anticipated with any of the Class 1 antiarrhythmic agents. Special care is necessary when any of these agents are given intravenously in patients who are beta blocked.

The adverse vasoconstrictor effects of ergot preparations may be potentiated during the treatment of migraine with beta blocking drugs.

Anaesthesia: The withdrawal of beta blocking drugs prior to surgery is not necessary in the majority of patients. However, anaesthetic agents such as ether, cyclopropane and trichloroethylene should not be used whereas halothane, isoflurane, nitrous oxide, intravenous induction agents, muscle relaxants, narcotic analgesics and local anaesthetic agents are all compatible with beta adrenergic blockade. Local anaesthetics with added vasoconstrictors, eg adrenaline, should be avoided.

Use in pregnancy: Betim is contraindicated in pregnancy. Timolol maleate appears in breast milk (milk: plasma ratio 0.8) and its use by nursing mothers requires caution. The neonate should be observed for any side-effects.

Side-effects: Betim is usually well tolerated in normal use. General symptoms resulting from beta blockade include fatigue and weakness.

Cardiovascular: bradycardia, heart failure, coldness of the limb extremities, hypotension, heart block.

Digestive: epigastric distress, nausea and vomiting.

CNS: dizziness, disorientation, vertigo, paraesthesiae, headache, hallucinations, nightmares, insomnia, somnolence, depression.

Respiratory: Dyspnoea, broncho-spasm.

Retroperitoneal fibrosis, allergic skin reactions, including erythematous or psoriaform rashes and arthralgia, have been rarely reported.

Warning: There have been reports of skin rashes and/or dry eyes associated with the use of beta-adrenergic blocking drugs. The reported incidence is rare and in most cases the symptoms have cleared when treatment was withdrawn.

Discontinuance of the drug should be considered if any such reaction is not otherwise explicable. Cessation of therapy with the beta-blocker should be gradual although withdrawal symptoms with timolol are infrequent.

Overdosage: Poisoning due to an overdose of Betim may lead to severe hypotension, sinus bradycardia, atrioventricular block, heart failure, cardiogenic shock, cardiac arrest, bronchospasm, impairment of consciousness, coma, occasionally, hyperkalaemia. The first manifestations usually appear 20 minutes to 2 hours after drug ingestion.

Treatment should include close monitoring of cardiovascular, respiratory and renal function, and blood glucose and electrolytes. Further absorption may be prevented by induction of vomiting, gastric lavage or administration of activated-charcoal if ingestion is recent. Cardiovascular complications should be treated symptomatically, which may require the use of sympathomimetic agents (eg noradrenaline, metariminol), atropine or inotropic agents, (eg dopamine, dobatamine). Temporary pacing may be required for AV block. Glucagon can reverse the effects of excessive beta-blockage, given in a dose of 1–10 mg intravenously. Intravenous B_2-stimulants, eg terbutaline may be required to relieve bronchospasm.

Timolol cannot be effectively removed by haemodialysis.

Pharmaceutical precautions Nil.

Legal category POM.

Package quantities Packs of 100 tablets.

Further information Nil.

Product licence number 0043/0035R.

BURINEX* TABLETS

Presentation *Tablets 1 mg:* Each tablet contains 1 mg bumetanide – a white, flat, circular, uncoated tablet marked with a score line and '1 mg' on one face.

Tablets 5 mg: Each tablet contains 5 mg bumetanide – a white, flat, circular, uncoated, bevelled-edge tablet marked with a score line and '5 mg' on one face.

Uses
Mode of action: Burinex (bumetanide) is a potent, high ceiling loop diuretic with a rapid onset and a short duration of action. The primary site of action is the ascending limb of the Loop of Henlé where it exerts inhibiting effects on electrolyte reabsorption causing the diuretic and natriuretic action observed.

After oral administration of 1 mg Burinex, diuresis begins within 30 minutes with a peak effect between one and two hours. The diuretic effect is virtually complete in three hours after a 1 mg dose.

Pharmacokinetics: Burinex is well absorbed after oral administration with the bioavailability reaching between 80 and 95%. The elimination half life ranges from between 0.75 to 2.6 hours. No active metabolites are known. Renal excretion accounts for approximately half the clearance with hepatic excretion responsible for the other half. There is an increase in half-life and a reduced plasma clearance in the presence of renal or hepatic disease. In patients with chronic renal failure the liver takes more importance as an excretory pathway although the duration of action is not markedly prolonged.

Indications: Burinex is indicated whenever diuretic therapy is required in the treatment of oedema, e.g. that associated with congestive heart failure, cirrhosis of the liver and renal disease including the nephrotic syndrome.

In oedema of cardiac or renal origin where high doses of a potent short acting diuretic are required, Burinex 5 mg tablets may be used.

Dosage and administration
Burinex 1 mg tablets: Most patients require a daily dose of 1 mg which can be given as a single morning or early evening dose. Depending on the patient's response, a second dose can be given six to eight hours later. In refractory cases, the dose can be increased until a satisfactory diuretic response is obtained, or infusions of Burinex can be given.

Burinex 5 mg tablets: The dose should be carefully titrated in each patient according to the patient's response and the required therapeutic activity. As a general rule, in patients not controlled on lower doses, dosage should be started at 5 mg daily and then increased by 5 mg increments every 12–24 hours until the required response is obtained or side-effects appear.

Consideration should be given to a twice daily dosage rather than once daily. Direct substitution of Burinex for frusemide in a 1:40 ratio at high doses should be avoided. Treatment should be initiated at a lower equivalent dose and gradually increased in 5 mg increments.

Children: Not recommended for children under 12 years of age.

Dosage in the elderly: Adjust dosage according to response; a dose of 0.5 mg bumetanide per day may be sufficient in some elderly patients.

Contra-indications, warnings, etc
Contra-indications: Although Burinex can be used to induce diuresis in renal insufficiency, any marked increase in blood urea or the development of oliguria or anuria during treatment of severe progressing renal disease are indications for stopping treatment with Burinex.

Burinex is contra-indicated in hepatic coma and care should be taken in states of severe electrolyte depletion.

As with other diuretics, Burinex should not be administered concurrently with lithium salts. Diuretics can reduce lithium clearance resulting in high serum levels of lithium.

Precautions: Excessively rapid mobilisation of oedema particularly in elderly patients, may give rise to sudden changes in cardiovascular pressure-flow relationships with circulatory collapse. This should be borne in mind when Burinex is given in high doses intravenously or orally. Electrolyte disturbances may occur particularly in those patients taking a low-salt diet. Regular checks of serum electrolytes, in particular sodium, potassium, chloride and bicarbonate should be performed and replacement therapy instituted where indicated.

Like other diuretics, Burinex shows a tendency to

increase the excretion of potassium which can lead to an increase in the sensitivity of the myocardium to the toxic effects of digitalis. Thus the dose may need adjustment when given in conjunction with cardiac glycosides.

Burinex may potentiate the effects of antihypertensive drugs. Therefore, the dose of the latter may need adjustment when Burinex is used to treat oedema in hypertensive patients.

As with other diuretics, Burinex may cause an increase in blood uric acid. Periodic checks on urine and blood glucose should be made in diabetics and patients suspected of latent diabetes.

Patients with chronic renal failure on high doses of Burinex should remain under constant hospital supervision.

Certain non-steroidal anti-inflammatory drugs have been shown to antagonise the action of diuretics.

Warnings: Encephalopathy may be precipitated in patients with pre-existing hepatic impairment.

Burinex should be used with caution in patients already receiving nephrotoxic or ototoxic drugs.

Use in pregnancy and lactation: Although tests in four animal species have shown no teratogenic effects, the ordinary precaution of avoiding use of Burinex in the first trimester of pregnancy should at present be observed.

Since it is not known whether bumetanide is distributed into breast milk, a nursing mother should either stop breast feeding or observe the infant for any adverse effects if the drug is absolutely necessary for the mother.

Adverse effects: Reported reactions include abdominal pain, vomiting, dyspepsia, diarrhoea, stomach and muscle cramps, arthralgia, dizziness, fatigue, hypotension, headache, nausea, encephalopathy (in patients with pre-existing hepatic disease), fluid and electrolyte depletion, dehydration, hyperuricaemia, raised blood urea and serum creatinine, hyperglycaemia, abnormalities of serum levels of hepatic enzymes, skin rashes, pruritis, urticaria, thrombocytopenia, gynaecomastia and painful breasts.

High dose therapy: In patients with severe chronic renal failure given high doses of Burinex, there have been reports of severe, generalised, musculoskeletal pain sometimes associated with muscle spasm, occurring one to two hours after administration and lasting up to 12 hours. The lowest reported dose causing this type of adverse reaction was 5 mg by intravenous injection and the highest was 75 mg orally in a single dose. All patients recovered fully and there was no deterioration in their renal function. The cause of this pain is uncertain but it may be a result of varying electrolyte gradients at the cell membrane level.

Experience suggests that the incidence of such reactions is reduced by initiating treatment at 5–10 mg daily and titrating upwards using a twice daily dosage regimen at doses of 20 mg per day or more.

Overdosage: Symptoms would be those caused by excessive diuresis. Empty stomach by gastric lavage or emesis. General measures should be taken to restore blood volume, maintain blood pressure and correct electrolyte disturbance.

Pharmaceutical precautions Burinex is presented in amber glass containers to protect against deterioration due to exposure to light.

Legal category POM.

Package quantities
1 mg tablets – bottles of 100 and 1,000.
5 mg tablets – bottles of 100.

Further information Burinex is also available as Burinex K tablets, each containing 0.5 mg bumetanide and 573 mg potassium chloride in a slow release core.

Product licence numbers
Burinex 1 mg 0043/0021R
Burinex 5 mg 0043/0043R

BURINEX* INJECTION
BURINEX* LIQUID

Presentation *Liquid:* An opalescent, pale green, viscous, aqueous solution for oral administration containing 1 mg bumetanide in 5 ml (0.2 mg per ml).

Injection: A solution containing 0.5 mg bumetanide per ml in amber glass ampoules of 2 ml, 4 ml and 10 ml, each ampoule containing 1 mg, 2 mg and 5 mg bumetanide respectively.

Uses *Mode of action:* Burinex (bumetanide) is a potent high ceiling diuretic with a rapid onset and a short duration of action. After oral administration of 1 mg Burinex, diuresis begins within 30 minutes with a peak effect between one and two hours. The diuretic effect is virtually complete in three hours after a 1 mg dose.

After intravenous injection, diuresis usually starts within a few minutes and ceases in about two hours.

In most patients 1 mg of Burinex produces a similar diuretic effect to 40 mg of frusemide.

Burinex is well absorbed after oral administration. Burinex excretion in the urine shows a good correlation with the diuretic response. In patients with chronic renal failure, the liver takes more importance as an excretory pathway, although the duration of action in such patients is not markedly prolonged.

Indications: Burinex is indicated whenever diuretic therapy is required in the treatment of oedema, e.g. that associated with congestive heart failure, cirrhosis of the liver and renal disease including the nephrotic syndrome.

For those oedematous conditions where a prompt diuresis is required, Burinex Injection may be used, e.g. acute pulmonary oedema, acute and chronic renal failure, salicylate or barbiturate poisoning. Burinex Injection can be given intravenously or intramuscularly to those patients who are unable to take Burinex tablets or who fail to respond satisfactorily to oral therapy. Burinex liquid may be more appropriate in patients who have difficulty swallowing tablets.

Dosage and administration *Burinex liquid:* Usually 1 mg (5 ml) as a single oral dose given morning or early evening. The dosage should be adjusted according to the patient's response.

Parenteral dosage: Pulmonary oedema: Initially 1–2 mg by intravenous injection. This can be repeated, if necessary, 20 minutes later.

In those conditions in which an infusion is appropriate, 2–5 mg may be given in 500 ml infusion fluid over 30–60 minutes. (See pharmaceutical precautions.)

When intramuscular administration is considered appropriate, a dose of 1 mg should be given initially and the dose then adjusted according to diuretic response.

Children: Not recommended for children under 12 years of age.

Dosage in the elderly: Adjust dosage according to response; a dose of 0.5 mg bumetanide per day may be sufficient in some elderly patients.

Contra-indications, warnings, etc
Contra-indications: Although Burinex can be used to induce diuresis in renal insufficiency, any marked increase in blood urea or the development of oliguria or anuria during treatment of severe progressing renal disease are indications for stopping treatment with Burinex.

Burinex is contra-indicated in hepatic coma and care should be taken in states of severe electrolyte depletion.

As with other diuretics, Burinex should not be administered concurrently with lithium salts. Diuretics can reduce lithium clearance resulting in high serum levels of lithium.

Precautions: Excessively rapid mobilisation of oedema particularly in elderly patients, may give rise to sudden changes in cardiovascular pressure-flow relationships with circulatory collapse. This should be borne in mind when Burinex is given in high doses intravenously or orally. Electrolyte disturbances may occur, particularly in those patients taking a low-salt diet. Regular checks of serum electrolytes, in particular sodium, potassium, chloride and bicarbonate should be performed and replacement therapy instituted where indicated.

Like other diuretics, Burinex shows a tendency to increase the excretion of potassium which can lead to an increase in the sensitivity of the myocardium to the toxic effects of digitalis. Thus the dose may need adjustment when given in conjunction with cardiac glycosides.

Burinex may potentiate the effects of antihypertensive drugs. Therefore, the dose of the latter may need adjustment when Burinex is used to treat oedema in hypertensive patients.

As with other diuretics, Burinex may cause an increase in blood uric acid. Periodic checks on urine and blood glucose should be made in diabetics and patients suspected of latent diabetes.

Patients with chronic renal failure on high doses of Burinex should remain under constant hospital supervision.

Pregnancy: Although tests in four animal species have shown no teratogenic effects, the ordinary precaution of avoiding use of Burinex in the first trimester of pregnancy should at present be observed.

Adverse Reactions: Reported reactions include skin rashes and muscular cramps in the legs, abdominal discomfort, thrombocytopenia and gynaecomastia.

High Dose Therapy: In patients with severe chronic renal failure given high doses of Burinex, there have been reports of severe, generalised, musculoskeletal pain sometimes associated with muscle spasm, occurring one to two hours after administration and lasting up to 12 hours. The lowest reported dose causing this type of adverse reaction was 5 mg by intravenous injection and the highest was 75 mg orally in a single dose. All patients recovered fully and there was no deterioration in their renal function.

The cause of this pain is uncertain but it may be a result of varying electrolyte gradients at the cell membrane level.

Experience suggests that the incidence of such reactions is reduced by initiating treatment at 5–10 mg daily and titrating upwards using a twice daily dosage regimen at doses of 20 mg per day or more.

Overdosage: Symptoms would be those caused by excessive diuresis. Empty stomach by gastric lavage or emesis. General measures should be taken to restore blood volume, maintain blood pressure and correct electrolyte disturbance.

Pharmaceutical precautions Burinex is presented in amber glass containers to protect against deterioration due to exposure to light.

Burinex Injection: When an intravenous infusion is required, Burinex Injection may be added to Dextrose Injection BP, Sodium Chloride Injection BP or Sodium Chloride and Dextrose Injection BP.

When 25 mg bumetanide (as Burinex Injection) was added to 1 litre of these infusion fluids, no evidence of precipitation was observed over a period of 72 hours. Higher concentrations of Burinex in these infusion fluids may cause precipitation. It is good practice to inspect all infusion fluids containing Burinex from time to time. Should cloudiness appear, the infusion should be discarded.

Burinex Liquid: Do not refrigerate.

Legal category POM.

Package quantities *Liquid:* Bottles of 150 ml (OP). A measure-spoon graduated at 2.5 ml and 5 ml is supplied. *Injection:* Packs of 5 × 2 ml, 5 × 4 ml and 5 × 10 ml.

Further information Burinex is also available as Burinex K tablets, each containing 0.5 mg bumetanide and 573 mg potassium chloride in a slow release core. Burinex liquid is sugar-free.

Product licence numbers

Burinex Injection	0043/0060
Burinex Liquid	0043/0075

BURINEX* A TABLETS

Presentation Cream, oval tablets, flat with bevelled edge, engraved with a number (149) on the scored face and with an Assyrian lion on the reverse. Each tablet contains 1 mg bumetanide and 5 mg amiloride hydrochloride.

Uses

Mode of action: Burinex A combines the potent loop diuretic bumetanide with the mild potassium sparing diuretic amiloride.

The action of bumetanide starts within 30 minutes and is virtually complete within 3 hours. The addition of amiloride will reduce any tendency towards hypokalaemia and its mild natriuretic effect will be additive to that of bumetanide.

Indications: Burinex A is indicated where a prompt diuresis is required. It is particularly of value in conditions where potassium conservation is important.

Dosage and administration The normal adult dose is 1 to 2 tablets daily. The dose may be adjusted according to response.

The elderly: The dose should be adjusted according to needs and serum electrolytes and urea should be monitored carefully.

Children: Not recommended for use in children.

Contra-indications, warnings, etc

Contra-indications: Hyperkalaemia, (serum potassium >5.3 mmol/litre), severe electrolyte imbalance, acute renal insufficiency, severe progressive renal disease, anuria, severe liver disease, adrenocortical insufficiency (Addison's Disease), precomatose states associated with cirrhosis, known sensitivity to bumetanide or amiloride. Burinex A should not be given concurrently with potassium supplements or potassium-sparing agents. Burinex A is contraindicated in children as safety in this age group has not been established.

Warnings: Serum uric acid levels may be increased and acute attacks of gout may be precipitated. Patients with prostatic hypertrophy or impaired micturition may be at risk of developing acute retention. Burinex A should be discontinued before a glucose tolerance test. Burinex A may cause latent diabetes to become manifest. It may be necessary to increase the dose of hypoglycaemic agents in diabetic patients.

Precautions: Patients who are being treated with this preparation require regular supervision with monitoring of fluid and electrolyte status to avoid excessive fluid loss.

In common with other potent diuretics, Burinex A should be used with caution in elderly patients or those with disorders rendering electrolyte balance precarious. Hyponatraemia, hypochloraemia and raised blood urea may occur during vigorous diuresis especially in seriously ill patients. Careful monitoring of serum electrolytes and urea should be undertaken in these patients.

Side-effects: Bumetanide and amiloride are generally well tolerated. Side effects which may occur include: Abdominal pain, nausea and vomiting, dyspepsia, diarrhoea, stomach and muscle cramps, arthralgia, dizziness, fatigue, hypotension, headache, encephalopathy (in patients with pre-existing hepatic disease), fluid and electrolyte depletion, dehydration, hyperuricaemia, increased blood urea and serum creatinine, hyperglycaemia, abnormalities of serum levels of hepatic enzymes, skin rashes, pruritis, urticaria, thrombocytopenia, gynaecomastia and painful breasts.

Use during pregnancy and lactation: The safety of the use of Burinex A during pregnancy and lactation has not been established.

Drug interactions: Hyperkalaemia has been observed in patients receiving amiloride and therefore concurrent use of Burinex A with potassium conserving diuretics is not recommended.

In common with other diuretics serum lithium levels may be increased when lithium is given concurrently with Burinex A necessitating adjustment of the lithium dosage. As ACE inhibitors may elevate serum potassium levels, especially in the presence of renal impairment, combination with Burinex A is best avoided in elderly patients or in those in whom renal function may be compromised. If use of the combination is considered essential the clinical condition and serum electrolytes must be carefully and continuously monitored.

Burinex A may enhance the nephrotoxicity of cephalosporin and aminoglycoside antibiotics. The dose of cardiac glycosides or hypotensive agents may require adjustment.

Overdosage: Symptoms would be those caused by excessive diuresis such as dehydration, electrolyte imbalance, particularly hyperkalaemia, and hypotension and treatment should be aimed at reversing these. No specific antidote is available. Emesis should be induced or gastric lavage performed. Treatment is symptomatic and supportive. If hyperkalaemia is present appropriate measures must be instituted to reduce serum potassium.

Pharmaceutical precautions Nil.

Legal category POM.

Package quantities Calendar pack of 2 × 14 tablets. Glass bottles of 100 tablets.

Further information Nil.

Product licence number 0043/0161.

BURINEX* K

Presentation White, ovoid, unmarked tablets each containing 0.5 mg bumetanide (Burinex) and 573 mg Potassium Chloride BP (7.7 mmol potassium in a slow release wax core).

Uses *Mode of Action:* Burinex K combines the very potent high-ceiling diuretic bumetanide, with a slow-release potassium chloride supplement. Bumetanide has a rapid onset and a short duration of action. As with most diuretics, long-term therapy may be associated with potassium depletion.

The potassium supplement in Burinex K will help to maintain normal levels of potassium, especially in those patients whose dietary intake of potassium is inadequate.

The formulation of Burinex K presents the following advantages. The diuretic is coated around the tablet, from which it is rapidly released. The diuretic and saluretic effects begin within 30 minutes after oral administration, peak at one to two hours, and are largely complete within three hours. In contrast, the potassium chloride, which is included in an inert wax core, is released only slowly after oral ingestion. This slow-release minimises the risk of gastro-intestinal intolerance as well as that of ulceration and stenosis resulting from localised high concentrations of potassium salts in the small bowel.

Indications: For the treatment of oedema where potassium supplementation is necessary.

Dosage and administration
Adults: The recommended initial dose is 2 tablets to be taken once daily (morning or evening). This may be increased up to 4 tablets daily (given as a single dose or in divided doses if preferred), or reduced to 1 tablet daily according to clinical response. If more than 4 tablets are to be taken daily, it is preferred to administer the diuretic and potassium supplement as two separate preparations.

Children: Not recommended in children under 12 years.

Elderly: Adjust dosage according to response. A dose of 1 tablet per day may be sufficient in some elderly patients.

Burinex K tablets must be swallowed whole and never chewed. The tablets should be swallowed with at least 100 mls of water.

Contra-indications, warnings, etc

Contra-indications: Burinex K should not be used with potassium-sparing diuretics (e.g. spironolactone, triamterene or amiloride) or in patients with renal insufficiency.

As with other diuretics, Burinex K should not be administered concurrently with lithium salts. Diuretics can reduce lithium clearance resulting in high serum levels of lithium.

All solid forms of potassium medication are contra-indicated in the presence of obstruction in the digestive tract (e.g. resulting from compression of the oesophagus due to dilation of the left atrium or from stenosis of the gut).

Anuria, Crohns disease, hyperkalaemia, precomatose states associated with liver cirrhosis, Addisons disease, known hypersensitivity to bumetanide.

Precautions: The 15.4 mmol of potassium included in the usual dose of Burinex K (2 tablets daily) should help to prevent hypokalaemia in many patients. Certain patients, however – as, for example, those with hepatic ascites or those on a very low potassium diet – may require considerably more potassium than this. Periodic checks should therefore be made on the serum potassium level in patients on long-term therapy.

The diuretic in Burinex K may potentiate the effect of antihypertensive drugs, increase blood uric acid and (though rarely) affect carbohydrate metabolism.

Certain non-steroidal anti-inflammatory drugs have been shown to antagonise the action of diuretics.

Non-specific small bowel lesions characterised by stenosis and possibly accompanied by ulceration have been associated with the oral administration of tablets and capsules containing potassium salts. Symptoms and signs which indicate ulceration or obstruction of the small bowel in patients taking tablets or capsules containing potassium salts are indications for stopping treatment with such preparations immediately.

Patients with prostatic hypertrophy or impairment of micturition have an increased risk of developing acute retention. Where indicated, steps should be taken to correct hypotension or hyperkalaemia before commencing therapy.

ACE inhibitors should not be used with combination diuretic potassium products, such as Burinex K, as serum potassium levels may be increased.

The toxic effects of nephrotoxic antibiotics may be increased by concomitant administration of potent diuretics such as bumetanide.

Adverse reactions: Reported reactions include skin rashes and muscular cramps in the legs, abdominal discomfort, thrombocytopenia and gynaecomastia.

As with other diuretics, fluid and electrolyte balance may be disturbed as a result of diuresis after prolonged therapy. This may cause symptoms such as headache, hypotension and myalgia.

Pregnancy: Although tests in four animal species have shown no teratogenic effects, the ordinary precaution of avoiding use of Burinex in the first trimester of pregnancy should at present be observed.

Overdosage: General methods should be taken to restore blood volume and maintain blood pressure. Any electrolyte imbalance should be corrected.

Pharmaceutical precautions Nil.

Legal category POM.

Package quantities Packs of 100, 500 and 1,000 tablets.

Further information Nil.

Product licence number 0043/0027.

CENTYL* TABLETS

Presentation *Tablets 2.5 mg:* Each contains 2.5 mg Bendrofluazide BP, white uncoated tablets, no coding marks.

Tablets 5 mg: Each contains 5 mg Bendrofluazide BP, white uncoated tablets, circular groove embossed on one face and score line on other.

Uses *Mode of Action:* Centyl contains the diuretic bendrofluazide, which is as effective as chlorothiazide at 100th the dose and produces a more prolonged diuresis. The diuresis is usually complete in 12–18 hours. In common with other thiazides, it increases the renal excretion of sodium, chloride and to a lesser extent potassium ions, together with an accompanying volume of water.

Indications: Hypertension: Control of blood pressure in mild to moderate hypertension.

Oedema: Oedema of cardiac, hepatic or renal origin. Pre-menstrual oedema. Oedema induced by use of steroids.

Dosage and administration *Adults and the elderly:* Initially, 5–10 mg bendrofluazide once daily. Maintain with 2.5–10 mg daily. Centyl should be taken in the morning to avoid nocturia.

Children: Not recommended.

Contra-indications, warnings, etc
Contra-indications: In common with other thiazide diuretics Centyl should not be used in patients with anuria, severe renal or hepatic failure, a history of hypersensitivity to thiazides and hypercalcaemia.

As with other diuretics, Centyl should not be administered concurrently with lithium salts. Diuretics can reduce lithium clearance resulting in high serum levels of lithium.

Warnings: As with other thiazide diuretics bendrofluazide may precipitate or aggravate diabetes mellitus. Thiazides may also precipitate or aggravate attacks of gout. Particular attention is required in elderly patients due to their susceptibility to electrolyte imbalance. Acute pancreatitis and blood dyscrasias may occur rarely.

Precautions: Thiazide diuretics should be used with caution in patients with renal or hepatic dysfunction. Renal function should be monitored. Fluid and electrolyte levels should be measured in patients undergoing prolonged or intense diuresis as potassium depletion may occur and potassium supplements may be needed. Potassium depletion is a particular danger to digitalised patients or those with hepatic cirrhosis with ascites.

Use in pregnancy and lactation: Diuretics are best avoided for the management of oedema of pregnancy or hypertension in pregnancy as their use may be associated with hypovolaemia, increased blood viscosity and reduced placental perfusion.

There is inadequate evidence on the safety of thiazide diuretics in human pregnancy. Foetal bone marrow depression and thrombocytopenia has been described together with foetal and neonatal jaundice. As diuretics pass into breast milk they should be avoided in mothers who wish to breast feed.

Interactions: Periodic testing for urine glucose is advisable in patients with diabetes. The dose of hypoglycaemic agents in diabetic patients may require adjustment. Thiazide diuretics are used for the treatment of hypertension, therefore, it may be necessary to reduce the dose of other hypotensive agents, e.g. reserpine, hydralazine, beta-blocking agents and ganglion blocking agents when used with Centyl. Interactions with non-steroidal anti-inflammatory drugs may occur.

Adverse Reactions: In common with other thiazide diuretics, impotence may occur. Thiazide diuretics may cause depletion of fluid and electrolytes during prolonged or intense use. Symptoms are muscle pain or fatigue, thirst, gastro-intestinal upset and oliguria. Hypokalaemia is most severe in patients already depleted of potassium as in renal or hepatic insufficiency. Coma may be precipitated in hepatic cirrhosis. The thiazide diuretics may induce hyperglycaemia and glycosuria in diabetic and other susceptible patients. This is usually reversible if the treatment is stopped. Hyperuricaemia sometimes occurs but an attack of gout is rare. The thiazide diuretics increase blood urea which is most pronounced in patients with renal disease and pre-existing retention of nitrogen.

Reports of other adverse reactions include skin rashes with associated photosensitivity, necrotising vasculitis and aggravation of pre-existing myopia.

Overdosage: Symptoms would be those caused by excessive diuresis. Gastric lavage should be performed together with symptomatic and supportive measures.

Blood pressure, fluid and electrolyte imbalance should be monitored and corrected where necessary.

Pharmaceutical precautions Nil.

Legal category POM.

Package quantities Bottles of 100 tablets.

Further information Nil.

Product licence numbers

Tablets 2.5 mg	0748/5901R
Tablets 5 mg	0748/5902R

Product licences held by Edwin Burgess Limited

CENTYL* K

Presentation Each tablet contains Bendrofluazide BP (Centyl) 2.5 mg and Potassium Chloride BP 573 mg (7.7 mmol potassium in a slow-release wax core). Green ovoid tablets. No identification marks.

Uses *Mode of Action:* Centyl K is a combination of the diuretic bendrofluazide with a potassium supplement.

Bendrofluazide is as effective as chlorothiazide at 100th the dose and produces a more prolonged diuresis, which is usually complete in 12–18 hours. In common with other thiazides, it increases the renal excretion of sodium, chloride and, to a lesser extent, potassium ions together with an accompanying volume of water. Potassium depletion is frequently associated with prolonged diuretic therapy; a potassium supplement is therefore included in Centyl K. This should minimise potassium depletion.

Because of the risk of localised high concentrations of potassium salts in the small bowel, potassium is included in an inert wax core, from which it is released slowly over several hours. Bendrofluazide is contained in a shell which surrounds the central core.

Indications: Oedema: Oedema of cardiac, hepatic or renal origin.

Hypertension: Control of blood pressure in mild to moderate hypertension.

Renal calcium stones: Prophylaxis against recurrent renal calcium stones.

Dosage and administration *Adults and the elderly: Oedema and Hypertension:* Initially 2–4 tablets daily. Maintain with 1–4 tablets daily or on alternate days. Centyl K should be taken in the morning to avoid nocturia.

For renal calcium stones: 2–3 tablets daily.

Children: Not recommended.

The tablets should be swallowed whole with at least 100 mls water.

Contra-indications, warnings, etc
Contra-indications: In common with thiazide diuretics Centyl K should not be used in patients wih anuria, severe renal or hepatic failure, a history of hypersensitivity to thiazides and hypercalcaemia.

As with other diuretics, Centyl K should not be administered concurrently with lithium salts. Diuretics can reduce lithium clearance resulting in high serum levels of lithium.

All solid forms of potassium medication are contraindicated in the presence of obstructions in the digestive tract (e.g. resulting from compression of the oesophagus due to dilation of the left atrium or from stenosis of the gut).

Warnings: As with other thiazide diuretics bendrofluazide may precipitate or aggravate diabetes mellitus. Thiazides may also precipitate or aggravate attacks of gout. Particular attention is required in elderly patients due to their susceptibility to electrolyte imbalance. As with other thiazide diuretics acute pancreatitis and blood dyscrasias may occur rarely.

Precautions: Thiazide diuretics should be used with

caution in patients with renal or hepatic dysfunction. Fluid and electrolyte levels should be measured in patients undergoing prolonged or intense diuresis. Even though Centyl K contains a potassium supplement, depletion may occur, which is a particular danger to digitalised patients or those with hepatic cirrhosis with ascites.

Non-specific small bowel lesions characterised by stenosis and possibly accompanied by ulceration have been associated with the oral administration of tablets and capsules containing potassium salts. Symptoms and signs which might indicate ulceration or obstruction of the small bowel in patients taking tablets or capsules containing potassium salts are indications for stopping treatment with such a preparation immediately.

Use in pregnancy and lactation: Diuretics are best avoided for the management of oedema of pregnancy or hypertension in pregnancy as their use may be associated with hypovolaemia, increased blood viscosity and reduced placental perfusion.

There is inadequate evidence on the safety of thiazides in human pregnancy and foetal bone marrow depression and thrombocytopenia has been described together with foetal and neonatal jaundice. As diuretics pass into breast milk they should be avoided in mothers who wish to breast feed.

Interactions: Periodic testing for urine glucose is advisable in patients with diabetes. The dose of hypoglycaemic agents in diabetic patients may require adjustment. Thiazide diuretics are used to treat hypertension, therefore, it may be necessary to reduce the dose of other hypotensive agents, eg hydralazine, beta-blocking agents and ganglion blocking agents when used with Centyl K. Interactions with non-steroidal anti-inflammatory drugs may occur.

Adverse Reactions: In common with other thiazide diuretics impotence may occur. Thiazide diuretics may cause excessive depletion of fluid and electrolytes during prolonged or intense use. Symptoms are muscle pain or fatigue, thirst, gastro-intestinal upset and oliguria. Hypokalaemia is most severe in patients already depleted of potassium, as in renal or hepatic insufficiency. Coma may be precipitated in hepatic cirrhosis. The thiazide diuretics may induce hyperglycaemia and glycosuria in diabetic and other susceptible patients. This is usually reversible if the treatment is stopped.

Hyperuricaemia sometimes occurs, but an attack of gout is rare. The thiazide diuretics may increase blood urea, which is most pronounced in patients with renal disease and pre-existing retention of nitrogen.

Reports of other adverse reactions include skin rashes with associated photosensitivity, necrotising vasculitis, and aggravation of pre-existent myopia.

Overdosage: Symptoms would be those caused by excessive diuresis. Gastric lavage should be performed together with symptomatic and supportive measures. Blood pressure, fluid and electrolyte imbalance should be monitored and corrected where necessary.

Pharmaceutical precautions Nil.

Legal category POM.

Package quantities Packs of 100, 500 and 1,000 tablets.

Further information Nil.

Product licence number 0748/5903R.
Product licence held by Edwin Burgess Limited

DICAPEN* INJECTION ▼

Presentation A white to off-white powder available in vials containing the equivalent of 1000 mg+2000 mg, 500 mg+1000 mg and 250 mg+500 mg of sulbactam and ampicillin, respectively.

Uses
Mode of action: Sulbactam has been shown to be an irreversible inhibitor of several important beta-lactamases that occur in resistant organisms, although it does not possess any useful anti-bacterial activity itself, except against *Neisseriaciae.* When given in combination with ampicillin, sulbactam displays marked synergistic effects against resistant bacteria, but has little or no effect on the activity of ampicillin against susceptible organisms.

The bactericidal component of Dicapen Injection is ampicillin which acts against sensitive organisms during the stage of active multiplication by the inhibition of biosynthesis of cell wall mucopeptide.

Dicapen Injection is effective against a wide range of Gram-positive and Gram-negative bacteria including: *Staphylococcus aureus* and *epidermidis* (including penicillin resistant and some methicillin-resistant strains); *Streptococcus pneumoniae*, *Streptococcus faecalis* and other *Streptococcus spp.*; *Haemophilus influenzae* and *parainfluenzae* (both beta-lactamase positive and negative strains); *Branhamella catarrhalis*; anaerobes, including *Bacteroides fragilis* and related species; *Escherichia coli*, *Klebsiella spp.*, *Proteus spp.* (both indole-positive and indole-negative), *Enterobacter spp.* and *Neisseria gonorrhoeae*.

Pharmacokinetics: Sulbactam/ampicillin diffuses readily into most body tissues and fluids. Penetration into brain and spinal fluid is low except when the meninges are inflamed. High concentrations of sulbactam and ampicillin are achieved in the blood following intravenous or intramuscular administration and both have a half life of approximately one hour. Most of the sulbactam/ampicillin is excreted unchanged in the urine.

Indications: Dicapen Injection is indicated for the treatment of infections caused by susceptible organisms. Typical indications include:

1. Upper and lower respiratory tract infections including sinusitis, otitis media and epiglottitis.
2. Bacterial pneumonias.
3. Urinary tract infections and pyelonephritis.
4. Intra-abdominal infections including peritonitis, endometritis and pelvic cellulitis.
5. Bacterial septicaemia.
6. Meningitis.
7. Skin, soft tissue, bone and joint infections.
8. Gonococcal infections.

Dicapen Injection may also be used prophylactically:

1. In patients undergoing abdominal surgery to reduce the incidence of wound sepsis.
2. In termination of pregnancy or caesarian section to reduce post-operative sepsis.

Administration of Dicapen Injection is by intravenous bolus injection or infusion or by deep intramuscular injection.

Dosage and administration Dicapen Injection can be administered by either intravenous or intramuscular routes. The following dilutions may be used:

Dose (g)	*Diluent volume* (ml)
0.75	1.6
1.5	3.2
3.0	6.4

For intravenous administration Dicapen Injection should be reconstituted with sterile water for injection or any compatible solution and allowed to stand to allow any foaming to dissipate to permit visual inspection for complete dissolution. The dose can be given by bolus injection over 3 minutes or can be used in greater dilutions as an intravenous infusion over 15–30 minutes. Dicapen Injection may also be administered by deep intramuscular injection; if pain is experienced, 0.5% sterile solution for injection of lignocaine hydrochloride anhydrous may be used for reconstitution of the powder.

Therapeutic use
Adult patients (including elderly patients): The recommended adult dosage of Dicapen Injection is 1.5–3 g (corresponding to sulbactam 0.5–1.0 g and ampicillin 1–2 g) usually 6 or 8 hourly up to a maximum daily dosage of sulbactam of 4 g according to the following indications:

Severity of infection	*Daily dose of Dicapen Injection*
Mild to moderate	Up to 6 g (2 g+4 g)
Severe	Up to 12 g (4 g+8 g)

Children, infants and neonates: The dosage of Dicapen Injection for most infections in children, infants and neonates is 150 mg/kg/day (corresponding to sulbactam 50 mg/kg/day and ampicillin 100/mg/kg/day). In children and infants the dose should be given 6 or 8 hourly. In neonates, dosing should be 12 hourly in accordance with the usual practice for ampicillin. Treatment is normally given for 5–14 days but may be extended in severely ill cases.

Prophylaxis: For the prophylaxis of surgical infections, 1.5–3 g of Dicapen Injection should be given at induction of anaesthesia, which allows sufficient time to achieve effective serum and tissue concentrations during the procedure; the dose may be repeated 6–8 hourly; administration is usually stopped 24 hours after the majority of surgical procedures unless a therapeutic course of Dicapen Injection is indicated.

In patients with severely impaired renal function the dose should be reduced or administered less frequently in accordance with the usual practice for ampicillin.

Contra-indications, warnings, etc

Contra-indications: The use of Dicapen Injection is contraindicated in individuals with a history of an allergic reaction to any of the penicillins.

Precautions: As with any antibiotic preparation, constant observation for signs of overgrowth of non-susceptible organisms, including fungi, is essential. Should superinfection occur, treatment should be discontinued and/or appropriate therapy instituted. As with any potent agent, it is advisable to check periodically for organ dysfunction during extended therapy; this includes renal, hepatic and haematopoietic systems. This is particularly important in prematures, neonates and other infants.

Warnings: Serious and occasionally fatal hypersensitivity (anaphylactic) reactions have been reported in patients on penicillin therapy. These reactions are more apt to occur in individuals with a history of penicillin hypersensitivity and/or hypersensitivity reactions to multiple allergens. There have been reports of individuals with a history of penicillin hypersensitivity who have experienced severe reactions when treated with cephalosporins. Before therapy with a penicillin, careful inquiry should be made concerning previous hypersensitivity reactions to penicillins, cephalosporins and other allergens.

If an allergic reaction occurs the drug should be discontinued and the appropriate therapy instituted. Serious anaphylactic reactions require immediate emergency treatment with adrenaline. Oxygen, intravenous steroids and airway management (including intubation) should be used as indicated.

Use in pregnancy and lactation: Animal reproduction studies have revealed no evidence of impaired fertility or harm to the foetus due to sulbactam and ampicillin. However, safety for use in human pregnancy and lactation has not been established.

Adverse effects: As with other parenteral antibiotics, the principal side effect observed is pain at the site of injection, especially associated with the intramuscular route of administration. A small number of patients may develop phlebitis after intravenous administration.

Gastrointestinal – nausea, vomiting and diarrhoea have been the most common.

Skin/skin structure – rash, itching and other skin reactions have been the most common.

Haematopoietic and lymphatic systems – anaemia, thrombocytopenia, eosinophilia and leukopenia have been reported during therapy and are believed to be sensitivity reactions.

Hepatic – transient elevations of alanine and aspartic aminotransferases (ALT, AST) have been observed.

It is expected that the adverse reactions associated with the use of ampicillin will be occasionally observed.

Overdosage: Since Dicapen Injection is a penicillin-type drug, problems of overdosage are unlikely to occur.

Pharmaceutical precautions Store dry powder below 30°C.

Stability and compatibility: Sulbactam sodium is compatible with most intravenous solutions but ampicillin sodium and hence Dicapen Injection is less stable in solutions containing dextrose or other carbohydrates and should not be mixed with blood products or protein hydrolysates.

The concentrated solution for intramuscular administration should be used within 1 hour of reconstitution.

Diluted solutions of sulbactam sodium/ampicillin sodium should be administered within 8 hours if stored at room temperature and within 24 hours if stored under refrigeration.

Time periods for use in different diluents for intravenous infusion are given in the package insert.

Legal category POM.

Package quantities

3 g	(bolus)	1 × 25 ml glass vials
1.5 g	(bolus)	5 × 10 ml glass vials
750 mg	(bolus)	5 × 10 ml glass vials

Further information Nil.

Product licence numbers

3 g	(bolus)	0043/0143
1.5 g	(bolus)	0043/0142
750 mg	(bolus)	0043/0141

DOVONEX* OINTMENT ▼

Presentation Dovonex Ointment contains 50 micrograms calcipotriol per g in a smooth, white, preservative-free ointment base.

Other ingredients: disodium edetate, disodium phosphate dihydrate, DL-α-tocopherol, liquid paraffin, polyoxyethylene-2-stearylether, propylene glycol, purified water, white soft paraffin.

Uses

Mode of action: Calcipotriol is a vitamin D derivative. *In vitro* data suggest that calcipotriol induces differentiation and suppresses proliferation of keratinocytes. This is the proposed basis for its effect in psoriasis.

Indications: Dovonex Ointment is indicated for the topical treatment of mild to moderate plaque psoriasis (psoriasis vulgaris) affecting up to 40% of skin area.

Dosage and administration

Adults: Dovonex Ointment should be applied to the affected area twice daily. Maximum weekly dose should not exceed 100 g and a course of treatment should not last longer than 6 weeks.

Children: There is no experience of the use of Dovonex Ointment in children.

Contra-indications, warnings, etc

Contra-indications: Dovonex Ointment is contra-indicated in patients with known disorders of calcium metabolism. As with other topical preparations, Dovonex Ointment is contra-indicated in patients wih hypersensitivity to any of its constituents.

Precautions: Dovonex Ointment should not be used on the face. Patients should be advised to wash their hands after applying the ointment and to avoid inadvertent transfer to other body areas, especially the face.

Side-effects: Transient local irritation may occur after application. Facial or perioral dermatitis may occur rarely.

Use during pregnancy and lactation: Safety for use during human pregnancy has not yet been established, although studies in experimental animals have not shown teratogenic effects. Avoid use in pregnancy unless there is no safer alternative. It is not known whether calcipotriol is excreted in breast milk.

Drug interactions: There is no interaction between calcipotriol and sunlight or UV light. There is no experience of concomitant therapy with other antipsoriatic products applied to the same skin area.

Overdosage: Hypercalcaemia does not occur at the usual

dose of Dovonex Ointment (up to 100 g per week). Excessive use (50–100 g Dovonex Ointment daily) may cause elevated serum calcium which rapidly subsides when the treatment is discontinued.

Pharmaceutical precautions Store at room temperature.

Legal category POM.

Package quantities Tubes of 30 g (OP) and 100 g (OP).

Further information Nil.

Product licence number 0043/0177.

FUCIDIN* TABLETS
FUCIDIN* SUSPENSION
FUCIDIN* FOR INTRAVENOUS INFUSION

Presentation *Fucidin Tablets:* White, oval, film coated tablet with an Assyrian lion on one side and the number 121 on the other. Each tablet contains 250 mg Sodium Fusidate BP (equivalent to 240 mg fusidic acid). Sodium fusidate is the sodium salt of fusidic acid.
Fucidin Suspension: Each 5 ml of white to off-white banana-flavoured aqueous suspension contains 250 mg Fusidic Acid BP (therapeutically equivalent to 175 mg Sodium Fusidate BP).
Fucidin for Intravenous Infusion: A pack of 2 vials. One vial contains Diethanolamine Fusidate BPC 1968, 580 mg (equivalent to 482 mg fusidic acid) as a dry powder. The second vial contains 50 ml sterile phosphate-citrate buffer solution (pH 7.4–7.6).

Uses *Mode of Action:* Fusidic acid and its salts are potent antistaphylococcal agents with unusual ability to penetrate tissue. Bactericidal levels have been assayed in bone and necrotic tissue. Blood levels are cumulative, reaching concentrations of 50–100 micrograms/ml after oral administration of 1.5 g daily for three to four days. Concentrations of 0.03–0.12 micrograms/ml inhibit nearly all strains of *Staphylococcus aureus*. Fusidic acid is active against *Staphylococcus epidermidis* and methicillin-resistant staphylococci.

Fucidin is excreted mainly in the bile, little or none being excreted in the urine.

In severe or deep-seated infections and when prolonged therapy may be required, systemic Fucidin should generally be given concurrently with other anti-staphylococcal antibiotic therapy.

Indications: Fucidin is indicated in the treatment of all staphylococcal infections due to susceptible organisms, such as: osteomyelitis; pneumonia; septicaemia; wound infections; endocarditis; superinfected cystic fibrosis; cutaneous infections.

Fucidin should be administered intravenously whenever oral therapy is inappropriate which includes cases where absorption from the gastro-intestinal tract is unpredictable.

Dosage and administration
Fucidin tablets: Adult: standard dose: 500 mg sodium fusidate (equivalent to 480 mg fusidic acid) three times daily. In severe or fulminating infections, this dosage may be doubled or appropriate combined therapy may be used.

Fucidin Suspension: Adult dose: 15 ml (737 mg* fusidic acid) three times daily.

Children: 0–1 year: 1 ml (49 mg* fusidic acid)/kg bodyweight daily divided into 3 equal doses.
1–5 years: 5 ml (246 mg* fusidic acid) three times daily.
5–12 years: 10 ml (492 mg* fusidic acid) three times daily.
*Owing to incomplete absorption of fusidic acid (approximately 70% of that observed with sodium fusidate) the effective dose is only 70% of the stated figure, i.e. 500 mg for adults. To avoid underdosing, recommendations must be adhered to.
Intravenous therapy: Adults weighing more than 50 kg: 580 mg diethanolamine fusidate three times daily.
Children and adults weighing less than 50 kg: 6 to 7 mg diethanolamine fusidate per kg bodyweight, three times daily.
Recommended procedure: To reconstitute, dissolve the contents of one vial containing 580 mg diethanolamine fusidate powder, (equivalent to 482 mg fusidic acid) in the 50 ml buffer provided. The enclosed needle may be used for this purpose.

1. For adults weighing more than 50 kg: Add the fusidate/buffer solution to 500 ml of infusion fluid and infuse slowly over a period of not less than six hours.
2. For children and adults weighing less than 50 kg: Each dose corresponds to approximately 0.6 ml of the fusidate/buffer solution per kg bodyweight. This volume should be further diluted, at least tenfold, with the appropriate infusion fluid, and infused slowly over a period of not less than six hours.

Since Fucidin is excreted in the bile, no dosage modifications are needed in renal impairment.

The dosage in patients undergoing haemodialysis needs no adjustment as Fucidin is not significantly dialysed.

Dosage in the elderly: No dosage alterations are necessary in the elderly.

If additional anti-bacterial therapy is to be employed, it is recommended that for parenteral administration, separate infusion fluids be used.

Contra-indications, warnings, etc
Contra-indications: Contra-indicated in patients with known hypersensitivity to fusidic acid and its salts. Intravenous Fucidin should not be infused with amino-acid solutions or in whole blood. Due to local tissue injury, Fucidin should not be administered intramuscularly or subcutaneously.
Precautions: Caution should be exercised with other antibiotics which have similar biliary excretion pathways, e.g. lincomycin and rifampicin.

Periodic liver function tests should be carried out when high oral doses are used, when the drug is given for prolonged periods and in patients with liver dysfunction.

Fucidin displaces bilirubin from its albumin binding site *in vitro*. The clinical significance of this finding is uncertain and kernicterus has not been observed in neonates receiving Fucidin. However, this observation should be borne in mind when the drug is given to preterm, jaundiced, acidotic or seriously ill neonates.
Intravenous Fucidin: In most cases Sodium Chloride Injection is used as an infusion fluid for intravenous Fucidin. It has also been given in plasma and occasionally in 5% dextrose, 40% dextrose, 20% fructose, and in Sodium Chloride and Dextrose Injection. Opalescence may be encountered with more acidic samples of dextrose, when the solution should be discarded. Infusion should be made into a wide bore vein with a good blood flow.

Each 50 ml of phosphate/citrate buffer for intravenous infusion contains 980 mg disodium hydrogen phosphate (equivalent to 5.5 mmols phosphate). Doses of intravenous Fucidin in excess of the recommended dose may result in hypocalcaemia due to the large amount of phosphate/citrate buffer administered. If more than the recommended dose is given for prolonged periods, the serum calcium should be closely monitored. Any hypocalcaemia occurring may be reversed by reducing the dosage of intravenous Fucidin to recommended levels and administering intravenous calcium gluconate.
Pregnancy and lactation: There is inadequate evidence of safety in human pregnancy. Animal studies and many years of clinical experience suggest that fusidic acid is devoid of teratogenic effects. There is evidence to suggest that when given systemically fusidic acid can cross the placental barrier. If the administration of Fucidin to pregnant patients is considered essential, its use requires that the potential benefits be weighed against the possible hazards to the foetus.

Safety in nursing mothers has not been established.

When fusidic acid (as the sodium salt) has been given systemically, levels have been detected in the breast milk. Caution is therefore required when Fucidin is used in mothers who wish to breast feed.

Adverse reactions: In some patients, given Fucidin, particularly the young and elderly, a reversible jaundice has been reported. Jaundice has been seen most frequently in patients receiving intravenous Fucidin in high dosage, or where the drug has been infused too rapidly or at too high a concentration in the infusion fluid. In some instances instituting oral therapy may be beneficial. If the jaundice persists Fucidin should be withdrawn, following which the serum bilirubin will invariably return to normal.

Overdosage: There has been no experience of overdosage with Fucidin. Treatment should be restricted to symptomatic and supportive measures. Dialysis is of no benefit, since the drug is not significantly dialysed.

Pharmaceutical precautions *Fucidin tablets:* Nil.

Fucidin Suspension: Protect from direct sunlight and heat. The Suspension should be shaken before use and dilution is not recommended.

Fucidin for intravenous infusion: Fucidin dry powder is stable for 3 years when stored below 25°C. When the buffer solution is transferred to the powder vial, this vial should be regarded as a unit dose. Although the Fucidin/buffer solution can be kept up to 24 hours, the required amount of solution should be withdrawn from the vial once only and any unused portion discarded.

Legal category POM.

Package quantities *Tablets:* Bottles of 100.
Suspension: Bottles of 50 ml (OP).
Infusion: Pack containing a single pair of vials, with transfer needle.

Further information Fucidin for intravenous infusion should be administered intravenously into a wide bore vein with a good blood flow. Excessive doses may cause venospasm, thrombophlebitis and haemolysis of erythrocytes.

Both oral and intravenous Fucidin have been given concurrently with other antibiotics e.g. cloxacillin, flucloxacillin, ampicillin, methicillin and erythromycin.

Fusidic acid and its salts exhibit no cross hypersensitivity or cross resistance with other antibiotics in clinical use.

Despite many years of clinical use, resistance to fusidic acid amongst *Staphylococcus aureus* remains low.

Product licence numbers
Tablets: 0043/5000R
Suspension: 0043/5014R
Infusion: 0043/5003R

FUCIDIN* CAVIJECT

Presentation Fucidin Caviject is a sterile, single-dose preparation containing Fusidic Acid BP 2% in a water miscible base (Fucidin Gel) fitted with an elongated flexible nozzle.

Uses
Mode of action: Fusidic acid is a potent topical antibacterial agent. Fusidic acid and its salts show fat and water solubility and strong surface activity and exhibit unusual ability to penetrate intact skin. Concentrations of 0.03–0.12 microgram/ml inhibit nearly all strains of *Staphylococcus aureus*. Topical application of fusidic acid is also effective against *Streptococci, Corynebacteria, Neisseria* and certain *Clostridia*.

Indications: Fucidin Caviject is indicated, either alone or in combination with systemic therapy, in the treatment of the following primary skin infections caused by sensitive strains of *Staphylococcus aureus* and *Streptococcus* spp.: Abscesses, hidradenitis axillaris, and carbuncles.

Dosage and administration The abscess should be incised and carefully curetted. The cavity is filled by injecting Fucidin Caviject and a dressing applied. The Caviject container should be used once only and then discarded.

Contra-indications, warnings, etc
Contra-indications: Infection caused by non-susceptible organisms, in particular, *Pseudomonas aeruginosa*.

Fucidin Caviject is contra-indicated in patients with hypersensitivity to fusidic acid and its salts.

Precautions: Bacterial resistance has been reported to occur with the use of fusidic acid applied topically. As with all topical antibiotics, extended or recurrent application may increase the risk of contact sensitisation and the development of antibiotic resistance.
Fusidic acid does not appear to cause conjunctival irritation in experimental animals. Caution should, however, still be exercised when using Fucidin Caviject near the eye.

Pregnancy and lactation: There is inadequate evidence of safety in human pregnancy. Animal studies and many years of clinical experience have suggested that fusidic acid is devoid of teratogenic effects. Safety in nursing mothers has not been established. There is evidence to suggest that when given systemically fusidic acid can penetrate the placental barrier. The use of topical Fucidin in pregnancy requires that the potential benefits be weighed against the possible hazards to the foetus. When fusidic acid (as the sodium salt) has been given systemically, levels have been detected in breast milk but with topical use the possible amount of drug present is unlikely to affect the infant.

Adverse reactions: Hypersensitivity reactions to the active ingredient in the form of skin rashes, mild stinging and irritation on application have been reported rarely.

Overdosage: Not applicable.

Pharmaceutical precautions Store below 25°C but do not freeze.

Legal category POM.

Package quantities Tubes of 7 g (OP).

Further information Fusidic acid and its salts exhibit no cross hypersensitivity with other antibiotics in clinical use.

Despite many years of clinical use, resistance to fusidic acid amongst *Staphylococcus aureus*, remains low.

The gel base is non-staining and contains no lanolin or other fatty constituents.

Product licence number 0043/0155R.

FUCIDIN* OINTMENT
FUCIDIN* GEL
FUCIDIN* INTERTULLE
FUCIDIN* CREAM

Presentation *Fucidin Ointment* contains Fusidic Acid, as the sodium salt, BP 2% in an ointment base (no preservative).

Fucidin Gel contains Fusidic Acid BP 2% in a water-miscible base; methylparaben 0.27% and propylparaben 0.03% as preservative.

Fucidin Intertulle: Sterile gauze squares each impregnated with Fusidic Acid, as the sodium salt, BP 2% (Fucidin Ointment) in an ointment base and enclosed between two leaves of sterile parchment in a sealed foil pack.

Fucidin Cream contains Fusidic Acid BP 2% in a cream base; potassium sorbate 0.27% as preservative.

Uses *Mode of Action:* Fusidic acid is a potent topical antibacterial agent. Fusidic acid and its salts show fat and water solubility and strong surface activity and exhibit unusual ability to penetrate intact skin. Concentrations of 0.03–0.12 microgram/ml inhibit nearly all strains of *Staphylococcus aureus*. Topical application of fusidic acid is also effective against Streptococci, Corynebacteria, Neisseria and certain Clostridia.

Indications: Indicated either alone or in combination with systemic therapy, in the treatment of primary and secondary skin infections caused by sensitive strains of *Staphylococcus aureus*, *Streptococcus spp* and *Corynebacterium minutissimum*. Primary skin infections that may be expected to respond to treatment with fusidic acid applied topically include: impetigo contagiosa, superficial folliculitis, furunculosis, sycosis barbae, hidradenitis axillaris, abscesses, carbuncles, paronychia and erythrasma; also such secondary skin infections as infected eczematoid dermatitis, infected contact dematitis, infected wounds, infected burns, infected ulcers and other bacterial superinfections.

Dosage and administration *Fucidin Gel, Fucidin Ointment and Fucidin Cream: Adults and children:* Uncovered lesions – apply gently, three or four times daily. Covered lesions – less frequent applications may be adequate.

Fucidin Intertulle: Usually, once a day application but frequency of application will vary with clinical circumstances. The intertulle should be covered with a suitable dressing which should be renewed frequently.

Contra-indications, warnings, etc
Contra-indications: Infection caused by non-susceptible organisms, in particular, *Pseudomonas aeruginosa*.

Fucidin Ointment, Gel, Intertulle and Cream are contra-indicated in patients with hypersensitivity to fusidic acid and its salts.

Precautions: Bacterial resistance has been reported to occur with the use of fusidic acid applied topically. As with all topical antibiotics extended or recurrent application may increase the risk of contact sensitisation and the development of antibiotic resistance.

Fusidic acid does not appear to cause conjunctival irritation in experimental animals. Caution should, however, still be exercised when using Fucidin Gel, or Cream near the eye. The sodium salt of fusidic acid has been shown to cause conjunctival irritation. The Ointment and Intertulle should not be used in or near the eye.

Pregnancy and lactation: There is inadequate evidence of safety in human pregnancy. Animal studies and many years of clinical experience have suggested that fusidic acid is devoid of teratogenic effects. There is evidence to suggest that when given systemically, fusidic acid can penetrate the placental barrier. The use of topical Fucidin in pregnancy requires that the potential benefits be weighed against the possible hazards to the foetus.

Safety in nursing mothers has not been established. When fusidic acid (as the sodium salt) has been given systemically, levels have been detected in breast milk but with topical use the possible amount of drug present is unlikely to affect the infant.

Adverse reactions: Hypersensitivity reactions to the active ingredient in the form of skin rashes and mild stinging and irritation on application, have been reported rarely.

Overdosage: Not applicable.

Pharmaceutical precautions *Fucidin Ointment and Cream:* Nil.

Fucidin Gel: Store below 25°C but do not freeze.

Fucidin Intertulle: Store below 25°C.

Legal category POM.

Package quantities *Fucidin Ointment, Fucidin Gel and Fucidin Cream:* Tubes of 15 g (OP) and 30 g (OP). *Fucidin Intertulle:* Box of 10 foil packs, each containing one tulle piece (10 cm × 10 cm) (OP).

Further information Fusidic acid and its salts exhibit no cross hypersensitivity with other antibiotics in clinical use.

Despite many years of clinical use, resistance to fusidic acid amongst *Staphylococcus aureus*, remains low.

The ointment base contains lanolin.

The gel base is non-staining and contains no lanolin or other fatty constituents.

The cream base is a vanishing base and contains no lanolin.

Product licence numbers

Fucidin Ointment	0043/5005R
Fucidin Gel	0043/5018R
Fucidin Intertulle	0043/5007R
Fucidin Cream	0043/0065

FUCIDIN* H OINTMENT
FUCIDIN* H GEL
FUCIDIN* H CREAM

Presentation Fucidin H Ointment contains Fusidic Acid, as the sodium salt, BP 2% and Hydrocortisone Acetate BP 1% in an ointment base.

Fucidin H Gel contains Fusidic Acid BP 2% and Hydrocortisone Acetate BP 1% in a water-miscible gel base; methylparaben 0.27% and propylparaben 0.03% as preservative.

Fucidin H cream contains Fusidic Acid BP 2% and Hydrocortisone Acetate BP 1% in a cream base; potassium sorbate 0.27% as preservative.

Uses *Mode of Action:* Fucidin H Ointment, H Gel and H Cream combine the potent topical antibacterial action of fusidic acid with the anti-inflammatory and antipruritic effects of hydrocortisone. Concentrations of 0.03–0.12 microgram fusidic acid per ml inhibit nearly all strains of *Staphylococcus aureus*. Topical application of fusidic acid is also effective against Streptococci, Corynebacteria, Neisseria and certain Clostridia.

Indications: Fucidin H Ointment, H Gel and H Cream are indicated in eczema and dermatitis with secondary bacterial infections, including atopic eczema, primary irritant dermatitis, allergic and seborrhoeic dermatitis and acne vulgaris.

Dosage and administration *Adults and children:* Uncovered lesions – apply gently, three or four times daily. Covered lesions – less frequent applications may be adequate.

Contra-indications, warnings, etc
Contra-indications: As with other topical corticosteroid preparations, Fucidin H Ointment, H Gel and H Cream are contra-indicated in primary bacterial, viral and fungal skin infections.

Fucidin H Ointment, H Gel and H Cream are contra-indicated in patients with hypersensitivity to fusidic acid and its salts.

Precautions: Fucidin H Ointment should not be used in or near the eye, as sodium fusidate causes conjunctival irritation.

Fusidic acid does not appear to cause conjunctival irritation in experimental animals. Caution should still be exercised, however, when Fucidin H Gel or Fucidin H Cream is used near the eye.

Steroid-antibiotic combinations should not be continued for more than 7 days in the absence of any clinical improvement since in this situation occult extension of the infection may occur due to the masking of the steroid. Similarly, steroids may also mask hypersensitivity reactions.

Bacterial resistance has been reported to occur with the use of fusidic acid applied topically. As with all topical antibiotics, extended or recurrent application may increase the risk of contact sensitisation and the development of antibiotic resistance.

Pregnancy and lactation: There is inadequate evidence of safety in human pregnancy.

Topical administration of corticosteroids to pregnant animals can cause abnormalities of foetal development including cleft palate and intra-uterine growth retardation. There may, therefore, be a very small risk of such effects in the human foetus.

Animal studies and many years of clinical experience have suggested that fusidic acid is devoid of teratogenic effects. There is evidence to suggest that when given systemically, fusidic acid can penetrate the placental barrier. The use of topical Fucidin in pregnancy requires that the potential benefits be weighed against the possible hazards to the foetus.

Safety in nursing mothers has not been established.

When fusidic acid (as the sodium salt) has been given systemically, levels have been detected in breast milk, but with topical use the possible amount of drug present is unlikely to affect the infant.

In infants, long-term continuous topical therapy with corticosteroids should be avoided. Adrenal suppression can occur even without occlusion.

Adverse reactions: Hypersensitivity reactions to the active ingredient in the form of skin rashes and mild stinging and irritation on application, have been reported rarely.

Overdosage: Not applicable.

Pharmaceutical precautions *Fucidin H Gel:* Store below 25°C but do not freeze.

Fucidin H Ointment and H Cream: Nil.

Legal category POM.

Package quantities Tubes of 15 g (OP) and 30 g (OP).

Further information Fusidic acid and its salts exhibit no cross hypersensitivity with other antibiotics in clinical use.

Despite many years of clinical use, resistance to fusidic acid amongst *Staphylococcus aureus*, remains low.

The ointment base contains lanolin.

The gel base is non-staining and contains no lanolin or other fatty constituents.

The cream base is a vanishing base and contains no lanolin.

Product licence numbers

Fucidin H Cream	0043/0093
Fucidin H Gel	0043/0024R
Fucidin H Ointment	0043/5012R

FUCIBET* CREAM

Presentation FuciBet cream contains betamethasone 0.1% (as the valerate ester) and Fusidic Acid BP 2% in a smooth white to off-white water miscible base; chlorocresol 0.1% as preservative.

Uses FuciBet combines the well-known anti-inflammatory and antipruritic effects of betamethasone with the potent topical antibacterial action of fusidic acid.

Betamethasone valerate is a topical steroid rapidly effective in those inflammatory dermatoses which normally respond to this form of therapy. More refractory conditions can often be treated successfully.

When applied topically, fusidic acid is effective against *Staphylococcus aureus*, Streptococci, Corynebacteria, Neisseria and certain Clostridia and Bacteroides. Concentrations of 0.03 to 0.12 microgram per ml inhibit nearly all strains of *S. aureus.* The antibacterial activity of fusidic acid is not diminished in the presence of betamethasone.

Indications: FuciBet is indicated for the treatment of eczematous dermatoses including atopic eczema, infantile eczema, discoid eczema, stasis eczema, contact eczema and seborrhoeic eczema when secondary bacterial infection is confirmed or suspected.

Dosage and administration A small quantity should be applied to the affected area two or three times daily until a satisfactory response is obtained. It may then be possible to maintain improvement by less frequent application or by the use of a less potent topical steroid/antibacterial preparation such as Fucidin H Ointment or Fucidin H Gel.

In the more resistant lesions the effect of FuciBet can be enhanced by occlusion with polythene film. Overnight occlusion is usually adequate.

Contra-indications, warnings, etc

Contra-indications: Acne rosacea and peri-oral dermatitis. Skin lesions of viral, fungal or bacterial origin. Hypersensitivity to the preparation.

Precautions: Long-term continuous topical therapy should be avoided, particularly in infants and children. Adrenal suppression can occur even without occlusion. Atrophic changes may occur on the face and to a lesser degree in other parts of the body, after prolonged treatment with potent topical steroids.

Caution should be exercised if FuciBet is used near the eye. Glaucoma might result if the preparation enters the eye. Systemic chemotherapy is required if bacterial infection persists.

Pregnancy: Topical administration of any corticosteroid to pregnant animals can cause abnormalities of foetal development. The relevance of this finding to human beings has not been established; however, topical steroids should not be used extensively in pregnancy, i.e. in large amounts or for prolonged periods.

Adverse reactions: Prolonged and intensive treatment with potent corticosteroids may cause local atrophic changes in the skin, including striae, thinning and dilation of superficial blood vessels, particularly when applied to the flexures or when occlusion is employed.

As with other topical corticosteroids sufficient systemic absorption to produce hypercorticism can occur with prolonged or extensive use. Infants and children are at particular risk, more so if occlusive dressings are used. A napkin may act as an occlusive dressing in infants.

Hypersensitivity reactions to fusidic acid are rare and FuciBet does not contain lanolin. However, if signs of hypersensitivity occur, treatment should be withdrawn.

Overdosage: Not applicable.

Pharmaceutical precautions Nil.

Legal category POM.

Package quantities Tubes of 15 g (OP) and 30 g (OP).

Further information The least potent corticosteroid, which controls the disease, should be used.

Product licence number 0043/0091.

FUCITHALMIC*

Presentation Sterile viscous drops of a 1% aqueous sustained release formulation of Fusidic Acid BP preserved with benzalkonium chloride.

Uses

Mode of action: Fucithalmic is active against a wide range of Gram-positive organisms, particularly *Staphylococcus aureus.* Other species against which Fucithalmic has been shown to have *in-vitro* activity include *Streptococcus, Neisseria, Haemophilus, Moraxella* and *Corynebacteria.*

The sustained release formulation of Fucithalmic ensures a prolonged contact with the conjunctival sac. Twice daily application provides sufficient fusidic acid concentrations in all relevant tissues of the eye. Fusidic acid penetrates well into the aqueous humour.

Indications: Fucithalmic is indicated for the topical treatment of bacterial conjunctivitis where the organism is known to be sensitive to the antibiotic.

Dosage and administration For all ages: One Fucithalmic drop to be instilled into the eye twice daily. Treatment should be continued for at least 48 hours after the eye returns to normal.

Contra-indications, warnings, etc

Contra-indications: Hypersensitivity to any of its components.

Precautions: Should not be used when contact lenses are being worn.

Side-effects: Transient stinging after application has been encountered. Hypersensitivity may occur.

Overdosage: Not applicable.

Pharmaceutical precautions Store below 25°C.

Keep the tube tightly closed. The tube should be discarded one month after opening.

Legal category POM.

Package quantities Available in 5 g tubes (OP).

Further information Nil.

Product licence number 0043/0137.

HEPARIN (MUCOUS) INJECTION BP

Presentation Heparin (Mucous) Injection BP 1,000 units per ml: each ml contains 1,000 units sodium heparin. (Presented in 5 ml ampoules without preservative, and 5 ml vials with 0.5% chlorbutol as preservative.)

Heparin (Mucous) Injection BP 5,000 units per ml: each ml contains 5,000 units sodium heparin (with 0.5% chlorbutol as preservative). Presented in 5 ml vials.

Heparin (Mucous) Injection BP 25,000 units per ml: each ml contains 25,000 units sodium heparin (with 0.4% chlorbutol as preservative). Presented in 5 ml vials.

Uses *Mode of Action:* Heparin is a naturally occurring anticoagulant which prevents the coagulation of blood *in-vivo* and *in-vitro.* It potentiates the inhibition of several activated coagulation factors, including thrombin and factor X.

Indications: Treatment of thrombo-embolic disorders such as deep vein thrombosis, acute arterial embolism or thrombosis, thrombophlebitis, pulmonary embolism, fat embolism.

Prophylaxis against deep vein thrombosis and thromboembolic events in susceptible patients.

Dosage and administration
Treatment dosage

Intravenous administration: 5,000–10,000 units every 4 hours or 500 units/kg bodyweight daily as a continuous infusion in sodium chloride injection or dextrose injection. The dose should be individually adjusted according to coagulation tests.

Subcutaneous administration: The initial dose is 250 units/kg bodyweight. Further doses should be given every 12 hours and individually adjusted according to coagulation tests.

Dosage adjustment: It is recommended that dosages be adjusted to maintain a thrombin clotting time, whole blood clotting time or activated partial thromboplastin time 1.5–2 times that of control on blood withdrawn 4–6 hours after the first injection or commencement of infusion and at similar intervals until the patient is stabilised.

Prophylactic dosage
Administration is by subcutaneous injection.

Patients undergoing major elective surgery: 5000 units should be given 2 hours pre-operatively and then every 8–12 hours post-operatively for 10–14 days or until the patient is ambulant whichever is the longer.

Following myocardial infarction: 5000 units should be given twice daily for 10 days or until the patient is mobile.

Other patients: 5000 units should be given every 8–12 hours.

These standard prophylactic regimens do not require routine control.

Dosage in children

Treatment dosage: Standard treatment dosages should be given initially. Subsequent dosages and/or dosage intervals should be individually adjusted according to changes in thrombin clotting time, whole blood clotting time and/or activated partial thromboplastin time.

Dosage in the elderly

Treatment dosage: Lower treatment dosages may be required, however, standard treatment dosages should be given initially and then subsequent dosages and/or dosage intervals should be individually adjusted according to changes in thrombin clotting time, whole blood clotting time and/or activated partial thromboplastin time.

Prophylactic dosage: Dosage alterations are unnecessary for prophylaxis in the elderly.

Pregnancy

Treatment dosage: Standard treatment dosages should be given initially by continuous intravenous infusion or every 12 hours by subcutaneous injection. Intermittent intravenous injections are not advised. Subsequent dosages and/or dosage intervals should be individually adjusted according to changes in thrombin clotting time, whole blood clotting time and/or activated partial thromboplastin time.

Prophylactic dosage: It is recommended that plasma heparin levels be maintained below 0.4 units/ml, as determined by specific anti-Xa assay. A suggested dosage is 5,000 units every 12 hours in early pregnancy, increasing to 10,000 units every 12 hours in the last trimester. The dosage should be reduced during labour and the standard prophylactic dosage is suitable in the puerperium.

Contra-indications, warnings, etc
Contra-indications: Haemorrhagic disorders and patients with an actual or potential bleeding site e.g. peptic ulcer.

Precautions: Heparin therapy should be given with caution to patients about to undergo surgery, and those with impaired renal or hepatic function.

Oral anticoagulants or drugs which interfere with platelet function, eg aspirin and dextran solutions should be administered with caution.

Pregnancy and lactation: Although animal studies have not been performed, epidemiological studies indicate that if drug therapy is needed in pregnancy, the use of heparin in the recommended dosage is acceptable. Heparin does not cross the placenta or appear in breast milk.

Adverse reactions: Hypersensitivity and acute reversible thrombocytopenia may occur rarely. Osteoporosis and alopecia have been reported after prolonged therapy.

Overdosage: The effect of heparin can be reversed immediately by intravenous administration of a 1% protamine sulphate solution. The dose of protamine sulphate required for neutralisation should be determined accurately by titrating the patient's plasma. It is important to avoid overdosage of protamine sulphate because protamine itself has anticoagulant properties. A single dose of protamine sulphate should never exceed 50 mg. Intravenous injection of protamine may cause a sudden fall in blood pressure, bradycardia, dyspnoea and transitory flushing, but these may be avoided or diminished by slow and careful administration.

Pharmaceutical precautions Store below 25°C. Heparin has been reported to be incompatible in aqueous solutions with certain substances, eg, some antibiotics, hydrocortisone and phenothiazines, narcotic analgesics and some antihistamines.

Legal category POM.

Package quantities *Heparin 1,000 units per ml:* 5 ml ampoules (without preservative), 5 ml vials (with preservative): Packs of 5.
Heparin 5,000 units per ml: 5 ml vials. Packs of 5 vials.
Heparin 25,000 units per ml: 5 ml vials. Packs of 1.

Further information Nil.

Product licence numbers

1,000 units (with preservative)	0043/0041R
1,000 units (without preservative)	0043/0085
5,000 units (with preservative)	0043/0038R
25,000 units (with preservative)	0043/0039R

HEP-FLUSH*

Presentation Heparin flush solution; 2 ml ampoule, each ml containing 100 units sodium heparin in saline with 0.5% chlorbutol as preservative. (i.e. 200 units per ampoule).

Uses
Mode of action: Heparin is a naturally occurring anticoagulant which prevents the coagulation of blood in-vivo and in-vitro. It potentiates the inhibition of several activated coagulation factors, including thrombin and factor X.

Indications: To maintain the patency of in-dwelling intravenous lines. It is not recommended for therapeutic use.

Dosage and administration For routine use, 2 ml containing 200 units of heparin should be administered into the catheter/cannula every 4 to 8 hours or as required.

Contra-indications, warnings, etc When used as recommended the low dose of heparin reaching the blood should have no systemic effects.

Pharmaceutical precautions Store below 25°C.
Hep-flush is compatible with normal saline. Heparin has been reported to be incompatible in aqueous solution with certain substances, e.g. some antibiotics, hydrocortisone, phenothiazines, narcotic analgesics and antihistamines.

Legal category POM.

Package quantities Packs of 10 × 2 ml ampoules.

Further information Nil.

Product licence number 0043/0057

HEPLOK*

Presentation Heparin flush solution; 5 ml ampoule, each ml containing 10 units sodium heparin in saline (no preservative), (i.e. 50 units per ampoule).

Uses
Mode of action: Heparin is a naturally occurring anticoagulant which prevents the coagulation of blood in-vivo and in-vitro. It potentiates the inhibition of several activated coagulation factors, including thrombin and factor X.

Indications: To maintain the patency of in-dwelling intravenous lines. It is not recommended for therapeutic use.

Dosage and administration For routine use 1–5 ml (10–50 units heparin) should be administered into the catheter/cannula every 4 to 8 hours or as required.

Contra-indications, warnings, etc When used as recommended the low dose of heparin reaching the blood should have no systemic effects.

Pharmaceutical precautions Store below 25°C. Heplok is compatible with normal saline. Heparin has been reported to be incompatible in aqueous solutions with certain substances, e.g. some antibiotics, hydrocortisone, phenothiazines, narcotic analgesics and antihistamines.

Legal category POM.

Package quantities Packs of 10 × 5 ml ampoules.

Further information Nil.

Product licence number 0043/0092.

IMUNOVIR*

Presentation White, ovoid tablets with the number 148 on one side and the letters IMV on the other. Each tablet contains 500 mg inosine pranobex.

Uses Imunovir is an agent demonstrating anti-viral activity and possessing immunopotentiating action in viral diseases.

Indications: Imunovir is indicated in the management of:
(a) Mucocutaneous infections due to herpes simplex virus (type I and/or type II).
(b) Genital warts as adjunctive therapy to podophyllin or carbon dioxide laser.
(c) Subacute sclerosing panencephalitis.

Dosage and administration
Mucocutaneous herpes simplex: 1 g q.d.s. (4 g daily) for 7–14 days.
Genital warts: 1 g t.d.s. (3 g daily) for 14–28 days as adjunctive therapy to podophyllin or carbon dioxide laser.
Subacute sclerosing panencephalitis: 50–100 mg/kg daily in divided doses every 4 hours.

Dosage in the elderly: No dosage alterations are necessary in the elderly.

Children: No information is available in children.

Contra-indications, warnings, etc
Contra-indications: None known.

Warnings: As the inosine component of Imunovir is metabolised to uric acid, it should be used with caution in patients with renal impairment, a history of gout or hyperuricaemia.

Pregnancy: Although animal tests have shown no teratogenic effect, the use of Imunovir in women where pregnancy is suspected or confirmed, should be avoided.

Adverse reactions: Side-effects are rare and usually of a mild and transitory nature. The only commonly associated adverse effects occurring during treatment with Imunovir are elevated serum and urinary concentrations of uric acid. These return to normal once treatment is withdrawn.

Symptoms and treatment of overdosage: There has been no experience of overdosage with Imunovir. However, serious adverse effects, apart from increased levels of uric acid in the body, seem unlikely in view of the animal toxicity studies. Treatment should be restricted to symptomatic and supportive measures.

Pharmaceutical precautions Store below 25°C.

Legal category POM.

Package quantities Available in bottles of 100 tablets.

Further information Nil.

Product licence number 0043/0153.

LEO* K TABLETS

Presentation Potassium Chloride BP 600 mg (8 mmol potassium in a slow-release wax core). White film-coated, ovoid tablets with no superficial markings.

Uses *Mode of Action:* Potassium depletion can occur insidiously, as the symptoms often resemble those of the underlying condition and may be easily overlooked. It is difficult to assess potassium depletion from serum potassium levels because there is no correlation between intracellular and extracellular potassium concentrations.

Intake of dietary potassium may not be adequate to restore normal levels in patients who already have low cellular potassium. These patients require potassium supplements.

Because of the risk of localised high concentrations of potassium salts in the small bowel, the potassium of Leo K is included in an inert wax core, from which it is released slowly over at least six hours.

Indications: As a potassium supplement, to reduce the risk of potassium depletion which may be associated with prolonged use of diuretics, and corticosteroids;

congestive heart failure; primary or secondary aldosteronism; renal tubular acidosis; malabsorption syndrome, ulcerative colitis, liver cirrhosis and other conditions where potassium loss may be severe.

Dosage and administration 3–5 tablets daily in divided doses (24–40 mmol potassium) are often adequate. A smaller dose may be adequate in those patients with a more satisfactory dietary intake of potassium, but some patients, particularly those with hepatic or renal insufficiency, may require considerably more potassium chloride.

The tablets should be swallowed whole with at least 100 mls water.

Dosage in the elderly: Serum potassium levels should be monitored and dosage adjusted according to response.

Contra-indications, warnings, etc

Contra-indications: All solid forms of potassium medication are contra-indicated in the presence of obstructions in the digestive tract (e.g. resulting from compression of the oesophagus due to dilation of the left atrium or from stenosis of the gut).

Precautions: To avoid hyperkalaemia, a potassium supplement should be used with great caution in renal insufficiency or with the potassium-sparing diuretics like spironolactone, triamterene or amiloride. Some patients may develop potassium depletion despite the use of potassium supplements. This is a particular danger to digitalised patients or those with hepatic ascites.

Non-specific small bowel lesions, characterised by stenosis and possibly accompanied by ulceration have been associated with the oral administration of tablets and capsules containing potassium salts. Symptoms and signs which might indicate ulceration or obstruction of the small bowel in patients taking tablets or capsules containing potassium salts are indications for stopping treatment with such a preparation immediately.

Overdosage: Symptoms of overdosage include asthenia, hypotension, mental confusion, parasthesia, and cardiac arrhythmias.

Characteristic ECG changes also occur. Hyperkalaemia should be treated with an intravenous infusion of sodium bicarbonate or by intravenous injection of calcium chloride or calcium gluconate (10–20 ml of a 1% solution).

Pharmaceutical precautions Nil.

Legal category GSL.

Package quantities Packs of 100 and 1,000 tablets.

Further information Nil.

Product licence number 0043/5006R.

MINIHEP* MINIHEP* CALCIUM

Presentation *Minihep:* Heparin (Mucous) Injection BP. Single dose ampoules containing sodium heparin 5,000 units in 0.2 ml (no preservative).

Minihep Calcium: Heparin (Mucous) Injection BP. Single dose ampoules containing calcium heparin 5,000 units in 0.2 ml (no preservative).

Uses

Mode of Action: Heparin is a naturally occurring anticoagulant which prevents the coagulation of blood in-vivo and in-vitro. It potentiates the inhibition of several activated coagulation factors, including thrombin and factor X.

Indications: Prophylaxis against deep vein thrombosis and thromboembolic events in susceptible patients.

Dosage and administration Administration is by subcutaneous injection.

Patients undergoing major elective surgery: 5,000 units in 0.2 ml should be given two hours pre-operatively and then every 8–12 hours post-operatively for 10–14 days, or until the patient is ambulant, whichever is the longer.

Following myocardial infarction: 5,000 units in 0.2 ml should be given twice daily for 10 days, or until the patient is mobile.

Other patients: 5,000 units in 0.2 ml should be given every 8–12 hours.

These standard dosage regimens do not require routine control.

Dosage in the elderly: Dosage alterations are unnecessary for prophylaxis in the elderly.

Pregnancy: It is recommended that plasma heparin levels be maintained below 0.4 units/ml as determined by specific anti-Xa assay. A suggested dosage is 5,000 units every 12 hours in early pregnancy increasing to 10,000 units every 12 hours in the last trimester. The dosage should be reduced during labour and the standard prophylactic dosage is suitable in the puerperium.

Contra-indications, warnings, etc

Contra-indications: Haemorrhagic disorders and patients with an actual or potential bleeding site, e.g. peptic ulcer.

Precautions: Heparin therapy should be given with caution to patients with impaired renal or hepatic function.

Oral anticoagulants or drugs which interfere with platelet function, e.g. aspirin and dextran solutions, should be administered with caution.

Pregnancy and lactation: Although animal studies have not been performed, epidemiological studies indicate that if drug therapy is needed in pregnancy, the use of heparin in the recommended dosage is acceptable. Heparin does not cross the placenta or appear in breast milk.

Adverse reactions: Hypersensitivity and acute reversible thrombocytopenia may occur rarely. Osteoporosis and alopecia have been reported after prolonged therapy.

Overdosage: The effect of heparin can be reversed immediately by intravenous administration of a 1% protamine sulphate solution. The dose of protamine sulphate required for neutralisation should be determined accurately by titrating with the patient's plasma.

It is important to avoid over-dosage of protamine sulphate because protamine itself has anticoagulant properties. A single dose of protamine sulphate should never exceed 50 mg. Intravenous injection of protamine may cause a sudden fall in blood pressure, bradycardia, dyspnoea and transitory flushing, but these may be avoided or diminished by slow and careful administration.

Pharmaceutical precautions Store below 25°C.

Legal category POM.

Package quantities Packs of 10 × 0.2 ml ampoules.

Further information Nil.

Product licence numbers

Minihep	0043/0088
Minihep Calcium	0043/0051

ONE-ALPHA* CAPSULES ONE-ALPHA* SOLUTION

Presentation *One-Alpha Capsules:* Capsules contain alfacalcidol (1α hydroxy-vitamin D) in two strengths: Brown capsule – contains 1 microgram alfacalcidol; white capsule – contains 0.25 microgram alfacalcidol.

One-Alpha Solution: A clear or slightly opalescent solution, one ml contains 0.2 microgram alfacalcidol.

Uses

Action: Alfacalcidol (One-Alpha) is converted rapidly in the liver to 1,25 dihydroxyvitamin D. This is the metabolite of vitamin D which acts as a regulator of calcium and phosphate metabolism. Since this conversion is rapid, the clinical effects of One-Alpha and 1,25 dihydroxyvitamin D are very similar.

Impaired 1α hydroxylation by the kidneys reduces endogenous 1,25 dihydroxyvitamin D production. This contributes to the disturbances in mineral metabolism found in several disorders, including renal bone disease, hypoparathyroidism, neonatal hypocalcaemia and vitamin D dependent rickets. These disorders, which require high doses of parent vitamin D for their correction, will respond to small doses of One-Alpha.

The delay in response and high dosage required in treating these disorders with parent vitamin D makes dosage adjustment difficult. This can result in unpredictable hypercalcaemia which may take weeks or months to reverse. The major advantage of One-Alpha is the more rapid onset of response, which allows a more accurate titration of dosage. Should inadvertent hypercalcaemia occur it can be reversed within days of stopping treatment.

Indications: One-Alpha is indicated in all conditions, where there is disturbance of calcium metabolism due to impaired 1α hydroxylation such as when there is reduced renal function.

The main indications are:

(a) Renal osteodystrophy
(b) Hyperparathyroidism (with bone disease)
(c) Hypoparathyroidism
(d) Neonatal hypocalcaemia
(e) Nutritional and malabsorptive rickets and osteomalacia
(f) Pseudo-deficiency (D dependent) rickets and osteomalacia
(g) Hypophosphataemic Vitamin D resistant rickets and osteomalacia

Dosage and administration One-Alpha may be administered as capsules or solution. One-Alpha Solution should be administered using the enclosed oral dispenser. Initial dosage for all indications is:

Adults	1 microgram/day
Dosage in the elderly	0.5 microgram/day
Neonates and premature infants	0.05–0.1 microgram/kg/day
Children under 20 kg bodyweight	0.05 microgram/kg/day
Children over 20 kg bodyweight	1 microgram/day

The dose of One-Alpha should be adjusted thereafter to avoid hypercalcaemia according to the biochemical response.

Indices of response include plasma levels of calcium (ideally corrected for protein binding), alkaline phosphatase, parathyroid hormone, as well as radiographic and histological investigations.

Plasma levels should initially be measured at weekly intervals. The daily dose of One-Alpha may be increased by increments of 0.25–0.5 microgram. When the dose is stabilised, measurements may be taken every 2–4 weeks.

Most adult patients respond to doses between 1 and 3 micrograms per day. When there is biochemical or radiographic evidence of bone healing (and in hypoparathyroid patients when normal plasma calcium levels have been attained), the dose generally decreases. Maintenance doses are generally in the range of 0.25 to 1 microgram per day. If hypercalcaemia occurs, One-Alpha should be stopped until plasma calcium returns to normal (approximately 1 week) then restarted at half the previous dose.

(a) Renal bone disease: Patients with relatively high initial plasma calcium levels may have autonomous hyperparathyroidism, often unresponsive to One-Alpha. Other therapeutic measures may be indicated.

Before and during treatment with One-Alpha, phosphate binding agents should be considered to prevent hyperphosphataemia. It is particularly important to make frequent plasma calcium measurements in patients with chronic renal failure because prolonged hypercalcaemia may aggravate the decline of renal function.

(b) Hyperparathyroidism: In patients with primary or tertiary hyperparathyroidism about to undergo parathyroidectomy, pre-operative treatment with One-Alpha for 2–3 weeks alleviates bone pain and myopathy without aggravating pre-operative hypercalcaemia. In order to decrease post-operative hypocalcaemia, One-Alpha should be continued until plasma alkaline phosphatase levels fall to normal or hypercalcaemia occurs.

(c) Hypoparathyroidism: In contrast to the response to parent vitamin D, low plasma calcium levels are restored to normal relatively quickly with One-Alpha. Severe hypocalcaemia is corrected more rapidly with higher doses of One-Alpha (e.g. 3–5 micrograms) together with calcium supplements.

(d) Neonatal hypocalcaemia: Although the normal starting dose of One-Alpha is 0.05–0.1 microgram/kg/day (followed by careful titration) in severe cases doses of up to 2 microgram/kg/day may be required. Whilst ionised serum calcium levels may provide a guide to response, measurement of plasma alkaline phosphatase activity may be more useful. Levels of alkaline phosphatase approximately 7.5 times above the adult range indicates active disease.

A dose of 0.1 microgram/kg/day of One-Alpha has proven effective as prophylaxis against early neonatal hypocalcaemia in premature infants.

(e) Nutritional and malabsorptive rickets and osteomalacia: Nutritional rickets and osteomalacia can be cured rapidly with One-Alpha. Malabsorptive osteomalacia (responding to large doses of IM or IV parent vitamin D) will respond to small oral doses of One-Alpha.

(f) Pseudo-deficiency (D-dependent) rickets and osteomalacia: Although large doses of parent vitamin D would be required, effective doses of One-Alpha are similar to those required to heal nutritional Vitamin D deficiency rickets and osteomalacia.

(g) Hypophosphataemic vitamin D-resistant rickets and osteomalacia: Neither large doses of parent vitamin D nor phosphate supplements are entirely satisfactory. Treatment with One-Alpha at normal dosage rapidly relieves myopathy when present and increases calcium and phosphate retention. Phosphate supplements may also be required in some patients.

Contra-indications, warnings, etc

Precautions and side-effects: If hypercalcaemia occurs during treatment with One-Alpha this can be rapidly corrected by stopping treatment until plasma calcium levels return to normal (about 1 week). One-Alpha may then be restarted at half the previous dose.

Patients taking barbiturates or anticonvulsants may require larger doses of One-Alpha to produce the desired effect.

Pregnancy and lactation: There is inadequate evidence of safety of One-Alpha in human pregnancy but it has been in wide use for many years without apparent ill consequence. Animal studies have shown no hazard. If drug therapy is needed in pregnancy, One-Alpha can be used if there is no alternative.

Although it has not been established, it is likely that increased amounts of 1,25 dihydroxyvitamin D will be found in the milk of lactating mothers treated with One-Alpha. This may influence calcium metabolism in the infant.

Overdosage: Hypercalcaemia is treated by stopping One-Alpha. Severe hypercalcaemia may be additionally treated with a 'loop' diuretic and intravenous fluids, or with corticosteroids.

Pharmaceutical precautions One-Alpha capsules: Protect from direct sunlight.

One-Alpha solution: Protect from direct sunlight and store in a cool place (below 15°C).

Legal category POM.

Package quantities Capsules: Bottles of 100 capsules. Solution: Amber glass bottle of 60 ml (OP); an oral dispenser is enclosed.

Further information One-Alpha Solution is sugar free and contains no colouring agents.

Product licence numbers

Capsules 1 microgram	0043/0050
Capsules 0.25 microgram	0043/0052
Solution	0043/0133

PONDOCILLIN* TABLETS
PONDOCILLIN* SUSPENSION
PONDOCILLIN* SACHETS

Presentation *Tablets:* Each tablet contains 500mg pivampicillin – a white film-coated ovoid tablet with the number 128 printed on one side and an Assyrian lion on the other.

Suspension: Bottles containing powder for the preparation of 50 ml and 100ml suspension. When reconstituted each 5 ml contains 175 mg pivampicillin.

Sachets: Each unit dose sachet contains 175 mg pivampicillin as off-white granules.

Uses Pondocillin (pivampicillin) is the pivaloyloxymethyl ester of ampicillin, and is rapidly hydrolysed in the body to ampicillin by non-specific enzymes present in serum, gastro-intestinal mucosa and other tissues.

After oral administration of Pondocillin, the plasma levels of ampicillin are 2–3 times higher than those obtained with equimolar doses of oral ampicillin. The tablets are formulated to disintegrate readily and produce rapid therapeutic plasma levels. A peak level generally occurs after 1 hour compared to approximately 2 hours with oral ampicillin. These levels are comparable to those obtained with an equimolar dose of intramuscular ampicillin.

Concentrations achieved in the urine are similarly raised. Generally, twice the amount of antibiotic can be recovered after treatment with Pondocillin when compared with equimolar doses of oral ampicillin. Whereas between 30–40% of the administered dose appears in the urine in the first 6 hours after oral administration of ampicillin, 70% can be recovered after an equimolar dose of Pondocillin.

Pondocillin is stable in the presence of gastric acid, and, unlike oral ampicillin, absorption is not affected by the presence of food. Plasma concentrations achieved in the post-prandial state do not differ significantly when compared with the fasting state. Like ampicillin, Pondocillin is destroyed by penicillinase-producing bacteria.

Indications: Like ampicillin, Pondocillin has a broad spectrum of activity against both gram-negative and gram-positive organisms. It is particularly indicated for the treatment of infections caused by susceptible strains *of Shigella, Salmonella, N. gonorrhoea, Esch. coli, H. influenzae, Pr. mirabilis* and is also indicated for pneumococcal, streptococcal and non-penicillinase-producing staphylococcal infections.

Specific infections include:

(a) Acute and chronic bronchitis
(b) Pneumonia
(c) Ear, nose and throat infections
(d) Gynaecological infections
(e) Urinary tract infections
(f) Skin and soft tissue infections
(g) Gonorrhoea

Dosage and administration *Tablets:* Usual dosage for adults: 500 mg pivampicillin to be administered twice daily. Dosage may be doubled in cases of severe infection. Gonorrhoea: 1.5–2 g pivampicillin as a single dose. 1 g probenecid can be given concurrently as desired. The medication may be taken with food or fluids.

Suspension (in bottle): Infants under 1 yr: 40–60 mg/Kg bodyweight per day.

Children aged 1–5 yrs: 10–15 ml per day

Children aged 6–10 yrs: 15–20 ml per day

Adults and children over 10 yrs: 30ml per day.

Sachets (for suspension): Children aged 1–5 years: 2–3 sachets per day.

Children aged 6–10 yrs: 3–4 sachets per day

Adults and children over 10 yrs: 6 sachets per day.

The daily dosage may be given either as 2 or 3 equal divided doses.

Dosage may be doubled where appropriate.

Dosage in the elderly: Renal excretion of ampicillin is delayed in the elderly but significant accumulation of the drug is not likely at the recommended adult dosage of Pondocillin.

Contra-indications, warnings, etc
Contra-indications: Pondocillin is contra-indicated in any patient with a history of hypersensitivity to any of the penicillins or cephalosporins. Because of the high frequency of exanthemata associated with ampicillin therapy in infectious mononucleosis, treatment with Pondocillin is contra-indicated in this disease.

Pondocillin is also contra-indicated in infections caused by penicillinase-producing bacteria.

Precautions: Care should be exercised when treating patients with a history of sensitivity to a variety of allergens, since serious hypersensitivity (anaphylactic) reactions are more likely to occur. If lymphatic leukaemia is treated with Pondocillin then caution is urged because of the frequency of exanthemata associated with ampicillin therapy.

The use of concurrent antacid therapy with Pondocillin is not recommended, since it reduces absorption of the antibiotic, and may cause underdosing.

During long-term therapy and in patients with severe renal or hepatic impairment it is advisable to carry out routine liver and kidney function tests.

Pregnancy: In keeping with current practice use during the first trimester of pregnancy should be avoided. Ampicillin crosses the placenta and small amounts have been detected in breast milk.

Adverse Reactions: Pondocillin is a compound of low toxicity. Like ampicillin, skin rashes of two types have been noted: a non-specific erythema which usually disappears during treatment, and urticaria which may cause withdrawal of the drug. As with other penicillins, fever, joint pains, angioedema and anaphylactic shock in hypersensitive patients may occur.

Upper gastro-intestinal disturbances, such as nausea, vomiting, retrosternal pain and flatulence have occurred more frequently when a dose has been given on an empty stomach. Diarrhoea has been reported, but less frequently than with ampicillin. This observation underlines the importance of giving Pondocillin with or just after a meal. None of these effects appear to be dose-related. Other side effects reported are dizziness and pruritis.

Warning: Pondocillin suspension is not recommended for the treatment of *severe* infections in infancy.

Overdosage: There is no experience of overdosage with Pondocillin. However, excessive doses of Pondocillin are likely to induce nausea, vomiting and gastritis. Treatment should be restricted to symptomatic and supportive measures.

Pharmaceutical precautions *Tablets:* Nil.
Suspension: Pondocillin suspension when reconstituted, is stable for 14 days at room temperature or for 4 weeks when kept in a refrigerator.

Sachets: Contain a single dose and when reconstituted, use suspension immediately.

Legal category POM.

Package quantities *Tablets:* Bottles of 500 and 100 tablets.

Suspension: Available in amber bottles making 50 ml (OP) or 100 ml (OP) suspension when dispensed.

Sachets: Boxes of 10 sachets (OP).

Further information Nil.

Product licence numbers

Tablets	0043/0067
Suspension	0043/0031R
Sachets	0043/0152

PONDOCILLIN* PLUS

Presentation White, film coated tablets, marked with an Assyrian lion on one side and 139 on the other. Each tablet contains pivampicillin 250 mg and pivmecillinam hydrochloride 200 mg.

Uses Pondocillin Plus contains the orally active derivatives of mecillinam and ampicillin – pivmecillinam hydrochloride and pivampicillin respectively. Following oral administration, there is rapid absorption and pivmecillinam and pivampicillin are hydrolysed in the body by non-specific enzymes present in blood and other tissues liberating mecillinam and ampicillin. Both drugs produce maximum plasma levels at $\frac{1}{4}$–1 hour after administration. Mecillinam and ampicillin are both mainly excreted unchanged in the urine within the first 8 hours of administration. Smaller amounts of both compounds are excreted with the bile. Pondocillin Plus shows high antibacterial activity against most commonly occurring Gram-negative and Gram-positive pathogens. Sensitive organisms include: Gram-positive: penicillin-sensitive *Staph. aureus, Strep. pyogenes, Strep. faecalis, Strep. viridans, Strep. pneumoniae* and Clostridia species. Gram-negative: *Neisseria meningitidis, Neisseria gonorrhoeae, Haemophilus influenzae, Escherichia coli, Proteus mirabilis, Proteus vulgaris, Klebsiella pneumoniae*, Enterobacter and Citrobacter species, *Salmonella typhi, Salmonella paratyphi*, other Salmonella species and species of Serratia, Shigella and Yersinia.

The anti-bacterial effect of Pondocillin Plus is further enhanced by the synergistic action of mecillinam and ampicillin which has been demonstrated with many of the Gram-negative organisms.

Penicillinase-producing Staphylococci and *Pseudomonas aeruginosa* are resistant to Pondocillin Plus.

Indications: The treatment of acute bronchitis, pneumonia, acute exacerbations of chronic bronchitis, otitis media, sinusitis, tonsillitis, tracheitis, laryngitis, pharyngitis and urinary tract infections due to organisms sensitive to the combination.

Dosage and administration The tablets must be taken with at least half a glass of water and preferably with or immediately after a meal.

For acute uncomplicated infections: Adults and children over 10 years: One Pondocillin Plus tablet twice daily.

For severe infections: Adults and children over 10 years: Dosages of up to 2 Pondocillin Plus tablets twice daily, have been given to adults.

Dosage in the elderly: Renal excretion of mecillinam and ampicillin is delayed in the elderly but significant accumulation of the drug is not likely at the recommended adult dosage.

Contra-indications, warnings, etc

Contra-indications: Penicillin and cephalosporin hypersensitivity. Because of the high frequency of exanthemata associated with ampicillin therapy in infectious mononucleosis, treatment with Pondocillin Plus is contra-indicated in this disease.

Precautions: During long term usage, it is advisable to carry out routine liver and kidney function tests. As with other antibiotics which are excreted mainly by the kidneys, raised blood levels of mecillinam and ampicillin may occur if repeated doses are given to patients with impaired renal function.

Caution is urged if patients with lymphatic leukaemia are treated with Pondocillin Plus because of the frequency of exanthemata associated with ampicillin therapy.

Pregnancy: Although tests in two animal species have shown no teratogenic effect, in keeping with current practice, use during the first trimester of pregnancy should be avoided. The drug, as mecillinam and ampicillin, crosses the placenta. Ampicillin has been detected in breast milk.

Adverse reactions: Side-effects are rare and usually of a mild and transitory nature. Urticaria, erythematous rash and pruritis may occur. Upper gastrointestinal disturbances in the form of dyspepsia, nausea and vomiting have been observed but can generally be avoided by administration with meals. Diarrhoea has been reported infrequently. Anaphylactic reactions, though not yet reported, may occur.

Overdosage: There has been no experience of overdosage with Pondocillin Plus. However, excessive doses are likely to induce nausea, vomiting and gastritis. Treatment should be restricted to symptomatic and supportive measures.

Pharmaceutical precautions Nil.

Legal category POM.

Package quantities Bottles of 100 tablets.

Further information Nil.

Product licence number 0748/0033.
Product licence held by Edwin Burgess Limited

PRESTIM* TABLETS
PRESTIM* FORTE TABLETS

Presentation *Prestim:* White, flat, petal-shaped tablets engraved with 132 on the scored face and with an Assyrian lion on the reverse. Each tablet contains Timolol Maleate BP 10 mg and Bendrofluazide BP 2.5 mg.

Prestim Forte: White, flat, petal-shaped tablets engraved with 146 on the scored face and with an Assyrian lion on the reverse. Each tablet contains Timolol Maleate BP 20 mg and Bendrofluazide BP 5 mg.

Uses *Mode of Action:* Bendrofluazide, a thiazide diuretic, has an established action in the treatment of hypertension.

Timolol maleate is a beta-adrenergic receptor blocking agent with marked hypotensive activity lasting up to 24 hours.

It has been shown that the combination of a beta-blocking agent with a thiazide diuretic gives an enhanced antihypertensive effect. This means that a relatively lower dose of the beta-blocker is required.

Indications: For the treatment of mild to moderate hypertension.

Dosage and administration The recommended dosage range is:

For Prestim Tablets: 1–4 tablets daily. Most patients are controlled on 1 or 2 tablets.

For Prestim Forte Tablets: $\frac{1}{2}$–2 tablets daily.

The dosage can be taken in the morning or in two divided doses, morning and evening.

If blood pressure control is not achieved on 4 tablets Prestim daily or 2 tablets Prestim Forte daily, consideration should be given to titrating timolol and bendrofluazide separately or adding another agent with hypotensive activity.

Dosage in the elderly: Initiate treatment with 1 tablet Prestim or $\frac{1}{2}$ tablet Prestim Forte daily and thereafter adjust according to response.

Contra-indications, warnings, etc

Contra-indications: Anuria. Prestim should not be used in patients with renal failure or with a history of hypersensitivity to the thiazides.

Uncontrolled heart failure, bradycardia, cardiogenic shock, bronchial asthma, chronic obstructive pulmonary disease, patients receiving adrenergic augmenting drugs (monoamine oxidase inhibitors and tricyclic antidepressants).

Anaesthesia with agents that produce myocardial depression, such as chloroform and ether.

Pregnancy.

As with other diuretics, Prestim should not be administered concurrently with lithium salts. Diuretics can reduce lithium clearance resulting in high serum levels of lithium.

Precautions: The continued depression of sympathetic drive through beta blockade may lead to cardiac failure, and, if it occurs, digitalisation should be considered.

Caution should be exercised in patients with diabetes mellitus, spontaneous hypoglycaemia, impaired renal or hepatic function and in patients receiving catecholamine depleting drugs, such as reserpine or guanethidine.

Adverse Reactions: Side-effects associated with beta blockade, e.g. gastro-intestinal symptoms, dizziness, insomnia, sedation, depression, weakness, dyspnoea, bradycardia, heart block, bronchospasm and heart failure.

Thiazide diuretics may cause excessive depletion of fluid and electrolytes during prolonged or intense use. Symptoms are muscle pain or fatigue, thirst and oliguria. With thiazide diuretics hypokalaemia is more severe in patients already depleted of potassium, as in renal or hepatic insufficiency. Coma may be precipitated in hepatic cirrhosis.

The thiazides may induce hyperglycaemia and glycosuria in diabetic and other susceptible patients. The thiazides increase blood urea, which is most pronounced in patients with renal disease and pre-existing retention of nitrogen. Hyperuricaemia sometimes can occur.

Reports of other adverse reactions to the thiazides include skin rashes with associated photosensitivity, necrotising vasculitis, acute pancreatitis, blood dyscrasias and aggravation of pre-existing myopia.

Warning: There have been reports of skin rashes and/or dry eyes associated with the use of beta-adrenergic blocking drugs. The reported incidence is small and in most cases the symptoms have cleared when treatment was withdrawn. Discontinuance of the drug should be considered if any such reaction is not otherwise explicable. Cessation of therapy with the beta-blocker should be gradual.

Overdosage: The most common signs of overdosage are bradycardia, hypotension, bronchospasm and acute cardiac failure. Suggested treatments are as follows:

Severe bradycardia: I.V. atropine sulphate 0.25–2 mg. If bradycardia persists, I.V. isoprenaline 25 micrograms may be given.

Severe hypotension: I.V. noradrenaline or adrenaline.

Bronchospasm: Isoprenaline hydrochloride, orciprenaline or salbutamol.

Acute cardiac failure: Digitalis, diuretics and oxygen. In refractory cases I.V. aminophylline and I.V. glucagon 0.5–1 mg have been reported useful.

General measures should be taken to restore blood volume, maintain blood pressure and correct electrolyte imbalance.

Pharmaceutical precautions Nil.

Legal category POM.

Package quantities Prestim: Glass bottles of 100 and 500 tablets.

Prestim Forte: Glass bottles of 100 tablets.

Further information Both constituents cross the placenta and appear in breast milk.

Product licence numbers

Prestim	0043/0047
Prestim Forte	0043/0084

PUMP-HEP*
Heparin for Continuous Infusion

Presentation Heparin (Mucous) Injection BP 1000 units/ml. Single dose ampoules of 20 ml, 10 ml or 5 ml containing 1,000 units sodium heparin per ml, in saline, without preservative (i.e. 20,000, 10,000 or 5,000 units per ampoule respectively).

Uses

Mode of action: Heparin is a naturally occurring anticoagulant which prevents the coagulation of blood in vivo and in vitro. It potentiates the inhibition of several activated coagulation factors, including thrombin and factor X.

Indications: Treatment of thrombo-embolic disorders such as: deep vein thrombosis, acute arterial embolism or thrombosis, thrombophlebitis, pulmonary embolism, fat embolism.

Dosage and administration Pump-Hep may be used when heparin is being administered intravenously as an alternative to diluting heparin taken from multidose vials.

500 units/kg bodyweight daily or 5,000–10,000 units every 4 hours as a continuous infusion in sodium chloride injection or dextrose injection. The dose should be individually adjusted according to coagulation tests.

Dosage adjustment: It is recommended that the dosages be adjusted to maintain a thrombin clotting time, whole blood clotting time or activated partial thromboplastin time 1.5 to 2 times that of control on blood withdrawn 4–6 hours after commencement of infusion and at similar intervals until the patient is stabilised.

Dosage in the elderly: Lower dosages may be required, however, standard dosages should be given initially and then subsequent dosages and/or dosage intervals should be individually adjusted according to changes in thrombin clotting time, whole blood clotting time and/or activated partial thromboplastin time.

Pregnancy: Standard dosages should be given initially. Intermittent intravenous injections are not advised. Subsequent dosages and/or dosage intervals should be individually adjusted according to changes in thrombin clotting time, whole blood clotting time and/or activated partial thromboplastin time.

Contra-indications, warnings, etc

Contra-indications: Haemorrhagic disorders and patients with an actual or potential bleeding site, eg, peptic ulcer.

Precautions: Heparin therapy should be given with caution to patients with impaired renal or hepatic functions.

Oral anticoagulants or drugs which interfere with platelet function, eg aspirin and dextran solutions should be administered with caution.

Pregnancy and lactation: Although animal studies have not been performed, epidemiological studies indicate that if drug therapy is needed in pregnancy, the use of heparin in the recommended dosage is acceptable. Heparin does not cross the placenta or appear in breast milk.

Adverse reactions: Hypersensitivity and acute thrombocytopenia may occur rarely. Osteoporosis and alopecia have been reported after prolonged therapy.

Overdosage: The effect of heparin can be reversed immediately by intravenous administration of a 1% protamine sulphate solution. The dose of protamine sulphate required for neutralisation should be determined accurately by titrating the patient's plasma.

It is important to avoid overdosage of protamine sulphate because protamine itself has anticoagulant properties. A single dose of protamine should never exceed 50 mg. Intravenous injection of protamine may cause a sudden fall in blood pressure, bradycardia, dyspnoea and transitory flushing, but these may be avoided or diminished by slow and careful administration.

Pharmaceutical precautions Store below 25°C.

Heparin has been reported to be incompatible in aqueous solutions with certain substances, eg some antibiotics, hydrocortisone, phenothiazines, narcotic analgesics and some antihistamines.

Legal category POM.

Package quantities Packs of 10 × 20 ml ampoules; 10 × 10 ml ampoules; 10 × 5 ml ampoules.

Further information Nil.

Product licence number 0748/0047.

Product licence held by: Edwin Burgess Limited.

SELEXID* TABLETS
SELEXID* SUSPENSION

Presentation *Tablets:* Each tablet contains 200 mg pivmecillinam hydrochloride – a white film-coated tablet with convex surfaces, an Assyrian lion printed on one side and the number 137 on the other.

Suspension: Unit-dose foil sachets, each containing 100 mg of pivmecillinam as white granules.

Uses Selexid is an orally active antibiotic. Chemically it is the pivaloyloxymethyl ester of the amidino-penicillanic acid, mecillinam. On oral administration, it is well absorbed and subsequently hydrolysed in the body to mecillinam, the active antibacterial agent, by non-specific esterases present in blood, gastro-intestinal mucosa and other tissues. Peak serum levels of mecillinam averaging 5 microgram/ml are reached after one hour following a dose of 10 mg/kg body weight in children and 400 mg in adults.

The serum half-life is 1.2 hours. The protein binding amounts to 5–10%. Approximately 50% of the administered dose is excreted as mecillinam in the urine within the first six hours. Mecillinam is partly excreted with the bile giving rise to biliary concentrations about three times the serum levels. Concurrent administration of probenecid delays the renal excretion of mecillinam, producing more sustained serum levels. The absorption of Selexid is practically unaffected by taking the tablets or suspension with food.

Selexid is highly active against most Enterobacteriaceae, including E. coli, Klebsiella, Proteus, Enterobacter, Serratia, Salmonella, Shigella, and Yersinia.

Selexid is less active against gram-positive bacteria, and organisms such as *Pseudomonas aeruginosa* and *Streptococcus faecalis* are practically resistant to mecillinam.

Whilst Selexid, like the penicillins and cephalosporins, interferes with the biosynthesis of the bacterial cell wall, the target of the inhibition is different. This different mode of action is probably responsible for the synergistic action which has been found, both *in-vitro* and *in-vivo*, between Selexid and various penicillins and cephalosporins.

Indications: Selexid is indicated in the treatment of infections due to mecillinam sensitive organisms, including:

(a) Urinary tract infections.
(b) Salmonellosis.

Preliminary experience in a small number of patients suggests Selexid may be a useful alternative antibiotic in the treatment of acute typhoid fever, and in some carriers of salmonellae when antibiotic treatment is considered essential.

Dosage and administration The tablets must be taken with at least half a glass of water and preferably taken with or immediately after a meal. Similarly the suspension should preferably be taken with or immediately after a meal or with bland fluids such as water or milk.

Suspension: Mix the contents of the sachet in a little water (5–10 mls) and stir before taking. The suspension should be taken immediately.

Dosage for adults and children weighing more than 40 kg:

Urinary tract infections:
Tablets:

(a) Acute uncomplicated cystitis: 2 tablets stat then 1 tablet 3 times daily to a total of 10 tablets.

(b) Chronic or recurrent bacteriuria: 2 tablets three to four times daily.

Sachets:

(a) Acute uncomplicated cystitis: 4 sachets stat then 2 sachets 3 times daily to a total of 20 sachets.

(b) Chronic or recurrent bacteriuria: 4 sachets three to four times daily.

Salmonellosis:

1. Enteric fever: 1.2–2.4 g daily for 14 days.
2. Salmonella carriers: 1.2–2.4 g daily for 2–4 weeks.

Dosage for children weighing less than 40 kg:

Urinary tract infections: 20–40 mg/kg body weight, daily, in three to four divided doses.

Salmonellosis: 30–60 mg/kg body weight, daily, in three to four divided doses.

Dosage in the elderly: Renal excretion of mecillinam is delayed in the elderly, but significant accumulation of the drug is not likely at the recommended adult dosage of Selexid.

Contra-indications, warnings, etc
Contra-indications: Penicillin and cephalosporin hypersensitivity.

Precautions: During long term usage, it is advisable to carry out routine liver and kidney function tests.

As with other antibiotics which are excreted mainly by the kidneys, raised blood levels of mecillinam may occur if repeated doses are given to patients with impaired renal function.

Pregnancy: Although tests in two animal species have shown no teratogenic effects, in keeping with current practice, use during the first trimester of pregnancy should be avoided. The drug, as mecillinam, crosses the placenta.

Adverse Reactions: Anaphylactic reactions, though not yet reported, may occur. Upper gastro-intestinal disturbances such as nausea, vomiting and indigestion have occurred, more frequently when a dose has been given on an empty stomach. Other side effects reported are diarrhoea and urticarial rash.

Overdosage: There has been no experience of overdosage with Selexid. However, excessive doses are likely to induce nausea, vomiting and gastritis. Treatment should be restricted to symptomatic and supportive measures.

Pharmaceutical precautions *Tablets:* Store below 25°C in a dry place. *Suspension:* Store below 15°C. Once reconstituted use the suspension immediately.

Legal category POM.

Package quantities *Tablets:* Bottles of 100 tablets. *Suspension:* Boxes of 20 sachets (OP).

Further information Nil.

Product licence numbers

Tablets	0043/0048
Suspension	0043/0053

SELEXIDIN* INJECTION

Presentation Each vial contains 400 mg mecillinam, a white crystalline powder.

Uses Selexidin is the amidino-penicillanic acid, mecillinam. It may be administered by both intravenous and intramuscular injection.

Peak serum levels averaging 6 microgram/ml and 12 microgram/ml are obtained following intramuscular doses of 200 mg and 400 mg respectively. Intravenous injection produces initially very high concentrations, which rapidly decline as the compound is excreted. The serum half life is 1.2 hours, and the protein binding amounts to 5–10%. Approximately 50–60% of the dose may be recovered in the urine within the first six hours. Mecillinam is partly excreted with the bile giving rise to biliary concentrations about three times the serum level. Concurrent administration of probenecid delays the renal excretion of mecillinam.

Selexidin is highly active against most Enterobacteriaceae, including *E. coli*, Klebsiella, Proteus, Enterobacter, Serratia, Salmonella, Shigella and Yersinia.

Selexidin is less active against gram-positive bacteria. *Streptococcus faecalis* and *Pseudomonas aeruginosa* are practically resistant to mecillinam.

Whilst Selexidin, like the penicillins and cephalosporins, interferes with the biosynthesis of the bacterial cell wall, the target of the inhibition is different. This different mode of action is probably responsible for the synergistic action which has been found, both *in-vivo* and *in-vitro*, between Selexidin and various penicillins and cephalosporins.

Indications: Selexidin injection is indicated in the treatment of serious infections due to mecillinam-sensitive organisms, and in those patients where oral therapy, with Selexid, is considered inappropriate.

Dosage and administration Selexidin should be dissolved in Water for Injections and administered either intramuscularly or by slow intravenous injection (three to four minutes) in the following concentrations:

Intravenous: Dissolve the mecillinam, in sterile water, as a 10% w/v solution, e.g. 400 mg in 4 ml.

Intramuscular: Dissolve 400 or 800 mg in 2 ml sterile water.

Alternatively, mecillinam, following dissolution in Water for Injections BP, may be added to either Sodium Chloride Injection or 5% dextrose and infused over 15–30 minutes. Such solutions should be made immediately before use and not stored. It is not recommended to store aqueous solutions of mecillinam. Mecillinam should not be added to infusion fluids containing other antibiotics.

Dosage: Adults and children.

1. *Urinary tract infections:* 5 mg/kg body weight every six to eight hours.
2. *Severe gram-negative infections due to susceptible organisms:* 10 mg/kg body weight every six hours.
3. *Enteric fever:* 12.5–15.0 mg/kg body weight every six hours. (Probenecid may also be administered.)

In some instances, for example where there was reason to expect a synergistic interaction, mecillinam has been given in combination with a broad-spectrum penicillin or cephalosporin. When combination therapy has been employed, normal dosages of both compounds were given.

Dosage in the elderly: Renal excretion of mecillinam is delayed in the elderly, but significant accumulation of the drug is not likely at the recommended adult dosage of Selexidin.

Contra-indications, warnings, etc
Contra-indications: Penicillin and cephalosporin hypersensitivity.

Precautions: During long-term usage, it is advisable to carry out routine liver and kidney function tests.

As with other antibiotics which are excreted mainly by the kidneys, raised blood levels of mecillinam may occur if repeated doses are given to patients with impaired renal function.

Pregnancy: Although tests in two animal species have shown no teratogenic effects, in keeping with current practice, use during the first trimester of pregnancy should be avoided. The drug, as mecillinam, crosses the placenta.

Adverse reactions: Reported side-effects include urticarial rash, and suspected drug fever in a few patients with enteric fever. Anaphylactic reactions, though not yet reported, may occur. Preliminary experience indicates that intramuscular injections of mecillinam are well tolerated.

Overdosage: There has been no experience of overdosage with Selexidin. Treatment should be restricted to symptomatic and supportive measures.

Pharmaceutical precautions Store below 25°C.

Legal category POM.

Package quantities Boxes of 10 vials.

Further information Nil.

Product licence number 0043/0055

TREOSULFAN* CAPSULES TREOSULFAN* INJECTION

Presentation *Capsules:* White opaque capsules each containing 250 mg Treosulfan (L-threitol 1,4 dimethane sulfonate).

Injection: Infusion bottles containing 5 g Treosulfan (L-threitol 1,4 dimethane sulfonate), a white crystalline powder.

Uses Treosulfan is a bifunctional alkylating agent which has been shown to possess anti-neoplastic activity in the animal tumour screen and in clinical trials. The activity of Treosulfan is due to the formation of epoxide compounds in vivo.

Indications: For the treatment of all types of ovarian cancer, either supplementary to surgery or palliatively. Some uncontrolled studies have suggested activity in a wider range of neoplasms.

Because of a lack of cross-resistance reported between Treosulfan and other cytotoxic agents Treosulfan may be useful in any neoplasm refractive to conventional therapy.

Treosulfan has been used in combination regimens in conjunction with vincristine, methotrexate, 5-FU and procarbazine.

Dosage and administration *Capsules:* The following dosage regimens have been indicated. All regimens indicate that a total dose of 21–28 g of Treosulfan should be given in the initial 8 weeks of treatment.

Regimen A: 1 g daily, given in four divided doses for four weeks followed by four weeks off therapy.

Regimen B: 1 g daily, given in four divided doses for two weeks, followed by two weeks off therapy.

Regimen C: 1.5 g daily, given in three divided doses for one week only, followed by three weeks off therapy. If no evidence of haematological toxicity at this dose in Regimen C, increase to 2 g daily in four divided doses for one week for the second and subsequent courses.

These cycles should be repeated with the dose being adjusted if necessary, as outlined below, according to the effect on the peripheral blood counts.

The capsules should be swallowed whole and not allowed to disintegrate within the mouth.

Dose modification (All regimens): For excessive haematological toxicity (white blood cell count less than 3,000/microlitre or thrombocyte count less than 100,000/microlitre) a repeat blood count should be made after 1–2 weeks interval and treatment restarted if haematological parameters are satisfactory, reducing dose as follows:

Regimen A: 1 g daily × 28 to 0.75 g daily × 28 (and to 0.5 g daily × 28 if necessary).

Regimen B: 1 g daily × 14 to 0.75 g daily × 14 (and to 0.5 g daily × 14 if necessary).

Regimen C: 2 g daily × 7 to 1.5 g daily × 7 (and to 1 g daily × 7 if necessary).

Present evidence, whilst not definitive, suggests that Regimens B and C are less myelosuppressive than Regimen A, whilst retaining maximum cytotoxic efficacy.

Injection: 5–15 g i.v. every 1–3 weeks depending on blood count and concurrent chemotherapy. Single injections of up to 15 g have been given with no serious adverse effects. Doses of up to 3 g have been given intraperitoneally. Doses up to 5 g Treosulfan may be given as a bolus injection. Larger doses should be administered as an i.v. infusion at a rate of 5 g every 5–10 minutes. The contents of each infusion bottle should be dissolved in 100 mls Water for Injection, a transfer needle may be used for this purpose. The resulting solution should be used immediately and any contents not used at once should be discarded.

Treatment should not be given if the white blood cell count is less than 3,000/microlitre or the thrombocyte count less than 100,000/microlitre. A repeat blood count should be made after a weeks interval, when treatment may be restarted if haematological parameters are satisfactory. Lower doses of Treosulfan should be used if other cytotoxic drugs or radiotherapy are being given concurrently. Treatment is initiated as soon as possible after diagnosis.

Care should be taken in administration of the injection to avoid extravasation into tissues since this will cause local pain and tissue damage. If extravasation occurs, the injection should be discontinued immediately and any remaining portion of the dose should be introduced into another vein.

Dosage in the elderly: Treosulfan is renally excreted. Blood counts should be carefully monitored in the elderly and dosage adjusted accordingly.

Children: Not recommended.

Contra-indications, warnings, etc
Warning: This product should not normally be administered to patients who are pregnant or to mothers who are breast feeding.

Adverse reactions: The major side-effect of Treosulfan is one of bone marrow depression and, in common with other alkylating agents, there have been reports of patients who have developed acute myeloid leukaemia. Reduction in white blood cell and thrombocyte counts occur during treatment and minimal levels may not occur until two or three weeks after discontinuing treatment. These counts usually return to normal within four weeks of cessation of therapy.

Patients showing marked bone marrow depression in the first course of treatment often respond similarly during subsequent courses. In all cases blood cell counts should be monitored regularly. Other adverse reactions include gastro-intestinal complaints such as nausea, vomiting and abdominal pain, mild allergic reactions in the form of exanthema and skin pigmentation. Alopecia may occur. Stomatitis may occur if the capsules are chewed; the capsules should be swallowed whole. Parenteral therapy has shown no local side-effects (unless extravasation is allowed to occur) and no systemic side-effects apart from the expected bone marrow depression.

Overdosage: Although there is no experience of acute overdosage with Treosulfan, nausea, vomiting and gastritis may occur.

Prolonged or excessive therapeutic doses may result in bone marrow depression which has occasionally been irreversible. The drug should be withdrawn, a blood transfusion given and general supportive measures given.

Pharmaceutical precautions Once brought into solution the injection should be used immediately.

Guidelines for the safe handling of antineoplastic agents:
1. Trained personnel should reconstitute the drug.
2. This should be performed in a designated area.
3. Adequate protective gloves, masks and clothing should be worn.
4. Precautions should be taken to avoid the drug accidentally coming into contact with the eyes.
5. Cytotoxic preparations should not be handled by staff who may be pregnant.
6. Adequate care and precautions should be taken in the disposal of items (syringes, needles, etc.) used to reconstitute cytotoxic drugs.
7. The work surface should be covered with disposable plastic-backed absorbent paper.
8. Use Luer-lock fittings on all syringes and sets. Large bore needles are recommended to minimize pressure and the possible formation of aerosols. The latter may also be reduced by the use of a venting needle.

Legal category POM.

Package quantities *Capsules:* Amber glass bottles of 100 capsules.
Injection: Boxes of 5 × 100 ml infusion bottles, each containing 5 g Treosulfan, complete with 5 transfer needles and 5 plastic bottle holders.

Further information All centres using Treosulfan have reported noteworthy improvements in the general condition of patients responding to treatment, particularly in regard to reduction or disappearance of ascites. Treosulfan is remarkably well tolerated allowing many patients to become fully ambulatory and return to their normal day to day work.

Product licence numbers
Capsules 0043/0040R
Injection 0043/0072.

UNIHEP LEO* 1,000
UNIHEP LEO* 5,000
UNIHEP LEO* 10,000
UNIHEP LEO* 25,000

Presentation
Unihep Leo 1,000: Heparin (Mucous) Injection BP 1,000 units per ml. Single dose ampoules containing Sodium Heparin 1,000 units in 1 ml (no preservative).

Unihep Leo 5,000: Heparin (Mucous) Injection BP 5,000 units per ml. Single dose ampoules containing Sodium Heparin 5,000 units in 1 ml (no preservative).

Unihep Leo 10,000: Heparin (Mucous) Injection BP 10,000 units per ml. Single dose ampoules containing Sodium Heparin 10,000 units in 1 ml (no preservative).

Unihep Leo 25,000: Heparin (Mucous) Injection BP 25,000 units per ml. Single dose ampoules containing Sodium Heparin 25,000 units in 1 ml (no preservative).

Uses
Mode of action: Heparin is a naturally occurring anticoagulant which prevents the coagulation of blood in-vivo and in-vitro. It potentiates the inhibition of several activated coagulation factors, including thrombin and factor X.

Indications: Treatment of thromboembolic disorders such as: deep vein thrombosis, acute arterial embolism or thrombosis, thrombophlebitis, pulmonary embolism, fat embolism.

Prophylaxis against deep vein thrombosis and thromboembolic events in susceptible patients.

Dosage and administration
Treatment dosage
Intravenous administration: 5,000–10,000 units every 4 hours or 500 units/kg bodyweight daily as a continuous infusion in sodium chloride injection or dextrose injection. Doses should be individually adjusted according to coagulation tests.

Subcutaneous administration: The initial dose is 250 units/kg bodyweight. Further doses should be given every 12 hours and individually adjusted according to coagulation tests.

Dosage adjustment: It is recommended that dosages be adjusted to maintain a thrombin clotting time, whole blood clotting time or activated partial thromboplastin time 1.5 to 2 times that of control on blood withdrawn 4–6 hours after the first injection or commencement of infusion, and at similar intervals until the patient is stabilised.

Prophylactic dosage
Administration is by subcutaneous injection.

Patients undergoing major elective surgery: 5,000 units should be given 2 hours pre-operatively and then every 8–12 hours post-operatively for 10–14 days or until the patient is ambulant whichever is the longer.

Following myocardial infarction: 5,000 units should be given twice daily for 10 days or until the patient is mobile.

Other patients: 5,000 units should be given every 8–12 hours.

These standard prophylactic regimens do not require routine control.

Dosage in children
Treatment dosage: Standard treatment dosages should be given initially. Subsequent dosages and/or dosage intervals should be individually adjusted according to changes in thrombin clotting time, whole blood clotting time and/or activated partial thromboplastin time.

Dosage in the elderly
Treatment dosage: Lower treatment dosages may be required, however, standard treatment dosages should be given initially and then subsequent dosages and/or dosage intervals should be individually adjusted accord-

ing to changes in thrombin clotting time, whole blood clotting time and/or activated partial thromboplastin time.

Prophylactic dosage: Dosage alterations are unnecessary for prophylaxis in the elderly.

Pregnancy
Treatment dosage: Standard treatment dosages should be given initially by continuous intravenous infusion or every 12 hours by subcutaneous injection. Intermittent intravenous injections are not advised. Subsequent dosages and/or dosage intervals should be individually adjusted according to changes in thrombin clotting time, whole blood clotting time and/or activated partial thromboplastin time.

Prophylactic dosage: It is recommended that plasma heparin levels be maintained below 0.4 units/ml, as determined by specific anti-Xa assay. A suggested dosage is 5,000 units every 12 hours in early pregnancy increasing to 10,000 units every 12 hours in the last trimester. The dosage should be reduced during labour and the standard prophylactic dosage is suitable in the puerperium.

Contra-indications, warnings, etc
Contra-indications: Haemorrhagic disorders and patients with an actual or potential bleeding site, e.g. peptic ulcer.

Precautions: Heparin therapy should be given with caution to patients with impaired renal or hepatic function.

Oral anticoagulants or drugs which interfere with platelet function, e.g. aspirin and dextran solutions should be administered with caution.

Pregnancy and lactation: Although studies have not been performed, epidemiological studies indicate that if drug therapy is needed in pregnancy, the use of heparin in the recommended dosage is acceptable. Heparin does not cross the placenta or appear in breast milk.

Adverse reactions: Hypersensitivity and acute reversible thrombocytopenia may occur rarely. Osteoporosis and alopecia have been reported after prolonged therapy.

Overdosage: The effect of heparin can be reversed immediately by intravenous administration of a 1% protamine sulphate solution. The dose of protamine sulphate required for neutralisation should be determined accurately by titrating with the patient's plasma.

It is important to avoid overdosage of protamine sulphate because protamine itself has anticoagulant properties. A single dose of protamine sulphate should never exceed 50 mg. Intravenous injection of protamine may cause a sudden fall in blood pressure, bradycardia, dyspnoea and transitory flushing but these may be avoided or diminished by slow and careful administration.

Pharmaceutical precautions Store below 25°C.
Heparin has been reported to be incompatible in aqueous solutions with certain substances, e.g. some antibiotics, hydrocortisone, phenothiazines, narcotic analgesics and some antihistamines.

Legal category POM.

Package quantities

Unihep Leo 1,000:	Packs of 5 × 10 ampoules
Unihep Leo 5,000:	Packs of 5 × 10 ampoules
Unihep Leo 10,000:	Packs of 10 ampoules
Unihep Leo 25,000:	Packs of 10 ampoules

Further information Nil.

Product licence numbers

Unihep Leo 1,000	0043/0085
Unihep Leo 5,000	0043/0086
Unihep Leo 10,000	0043/0064
Unihep Leo 25,000	0043/0087

**Trade Mark*

Eli Lilly & Company Limited
Kingsclere Road
Basingstoke
Hants RG21 2XA

AMYTAL*

Presentation Tablets (white, coded T56) each containing 30 mg Amylobarbitone BP.

Tablets (white, coded T37) each containing 50 mg Amylobarbitone BP.

Tablets (white, coded T32) each containing 100 mg Amylobarbitone BP.

Tablets (white, coded U13) each containing 200 mg Amylobarbitone BP.

Uses For the treatment of severe, intractable insomnia.

Dosage and administration For oral administration to adults only. Normal dosage is 100–200 mg at bedtime. Occasionally a larger dose may be necessary.

The effects should become apparent between 30 and 60 minutes after administration.

The elderly: Amytal is not recommended for use in elderly or debilitated patients.

Contra-indications, warnings, etc
Contra-indications: Hypersensitivity to barbiturates, a history of manifest or latent porphyria, marked impairment of liver function, or respiratory disease in which dyspnoea or obstruction is evident. Oral barbiturates should not be administered in the presence of uncontrolled acute or chronic pain, because paradoxical excitement may be induced or important symptoms may be masked.

Barbiturates should not be administered to children, young adults, patients with a history of drug or alcohol abuse, the elderly and the debilitated.

Usage in pregnancy: Barbiturates are contra-indicated during pregnancy.

Labour and delivery: Respiratory depression has been noted in infants born following the use of barbiturates during labour.

Nursing mothers: Small amounts of barbiturates are excreted in the milk and they are therefore contra-indicated for the nursing mother.

Warnings
Addiction potential: Barbiturates have a high addiction potential. Long-term use, or use of high dosage for short periods, may lead to tolerance and subsequently to physical and psychological dependence.

Signs of acute intoxication with barbiturates include unsteady gait, slurred speech and sustained nystagmus. Symptoms of dependence or chronic intoxication include confusion, defective judgement, loss of emotional control, insomnia and somatic complaints.

To minimise the possibility of overdosage or development of dependence, the amount prescribed should be limited to that required for the interval until the next appointment.

Withdrawal symptoms occur after long-term normal use (and particularly after abuse) on rapid cessation of barbiturate treatment. Symptoms include nightmares, irritability and insomnia, and in severe cases, tremors, delirium, convulsions and death.

Barbiturates should be withdrawn gradually from any patient known to be taking excessive doses over long periods.

Information for patients: The following information should be given to patients receiving amylobarbitone:

1. The use of amylobarbitone carries with it an associated risk of psychological and/or physical dependence. The patient should be warned against increasing the dose of the drug without consulting a physician.

2. Amylobarbitone may impair the mental and/or physical abilities required for the performance of potentially hazardous tasks, such as driving a car or operating machinery. The patient should be cautioned accordingly.

3. Alcohol should not be consumed while taking amylobarbitone. The concurrent use of amylobarbitone with other CNS depressants (e.g. alcohol, narcotics, tranquillisers and antihistamines) may result in additional CNS depressant effects.

Drug interactions: Amylobarbitone in combination with alcohol, tranquillisers and other CNS depressants, has additive depressant effects, and the patient should be so advised. Toxic effects and fatalities have occurred following overdoses of amylobarbitone alone and in combination with other CNS depressants. Caution should be exercised in prescribing unnecessarily large amounts of amylobarbitone for patients who have a history of emotional disturbances or suicidal ideation or who have misused alcohol or other CNS drugs.

Barbiturates cause induction of the liver enzymes responsible for metabolising many other drugs; in particular they should not be administered concurrently with coumarin-type anticoagulants. They may also affect the metabolism of systemic steroids (including oral contraceptives), phenytoin, griseofulvin, rifampicin, tricyclic antidepressants, and phenothiazines such as chlorpromazine.

Monoamine oxidase inhibitors prolong the effects of barbiturates, probably because the metabolism of the barbiturate is inhibited.

Precautions: Barbiturates should be administered with caution, if at all, to patients who are mentally depressed or have suicidal tendencies. They should also be used with great caution and at reduced dosage in those with marked renal dysfunction, shock or respiratory depression.

Prolonged therapy with barbiturates should be accompanied by periodic evaluation of haematopoietic, renal and hepatic systems (but see 'Uses').

Elderly or debilitated patients may react to barbiturates with marked excitement, depression or confusion (see 'Contra-indications'). In some persons, barbiturates repeatedly produce excitement rather than depression.

A cumulative effect may occur with the barbiturates leading to features of chronic poisoning including headache, depression and slurred speech.

Automatism may follow the use of an hypnotic dose of a barbiturate.

The systemic effects of exogenous hydrocortisone and endogenous hydrocortisone (cortisol) may be diminished by amylobarbitone. This product should therefore be administered with caution to patients with borderline hypoadrenal function, regardless of whether it is of pituitary or of primary adrenal origin.

Side-effects: Common adverse reactions include drowsiness, sedation, ataxia and vertigo.

Hypersensitive skin reactions may occur in some patients, especially those with asthma, urticaria or angioneurotic oedema.

Other idiosyncratic reactions include a hangover effect, paradoxical excitement, pain, confusion and memory defects.

Overdosage: The toxic dose of barbiturates varies considerably. In general, an oral dose of 1 g of most barbiturates produces serious poisoning in an adult. Death commonly occurs after 2 to 10 g of ingested barbiturate. Barbiturate intoxication may be confused with alcoholism, bromide intoxication, and various neurological disorders.

Symptoms: The manifestations of overdosage are early hypothermia followed by fever, sluggish or absent reflexes, respiratory depression, gradual appearance of circulatory collapse, pulmonary oedema and coma.

In extreme overdose, all electrical activity in the brain may cease, in which case a 'flat' EEG normally equated with clinical death cannot be accepted. This effect is fully reversible unless hypoxic damage occurs. Consideration should be given to the possibility of barbiturate intoxication even in situations that appear to involve trauma.

Treatment: General management should consist of symptomatic and supportive therapy, including gastric lavage, administration of intravenous fluids, and maintenance of blood pressure, body temperature and adequate respiratory exchange. Haemodialysis will increase the rate of removal of barbiturates from the body fluids. Antibiotics may be required to control pulmonary complications.

Pharmaceutical precautions Nil.

Legal category CD (Sch 3) POM.

Package quantities
Tablets 30 mg: Bottles of 500.
Tablets 50 mg: Bottles of 500.
Tablets 100 mg: Bottles of 100.
Tablets 200 mg: Bottles of 100.

Further information Nil.

Product licence numbers

Tablets 30 mg	0006/5058
Tablets 50 mg	0006/5059
Tablets 100 mg	0006/5060
Tablets 200 mg	0006/5061

AVENTYL*

Presentation Capsules (yellow and white, coded H17) each containing Nortriptyline Hydrochloride BP equivalent to 10 mg nortriptyline.

Capsules (yellow and white, coded H19) each containing Nortriptyline Hydrochloride BP equivalent to 25 mg nortriptyline.

Uses Aventyl is indicated for the relief of symptoms of depression. It may also be used for the treatment of some cases of nocturnal enuresis.

Dosage and administration For oral administration.

Adults: The usual adult dose is 25 mg three or four times daily. Dosage should begin at a low level and be increased as required. Alternatively, the total daily dose may be given once a day. When doses above 100 mg daily are administered, plasma levels of nortriptyline should be monitored and maintained in the optimum range of 50 to 150 ng/ml. Doses above 150 mg per day are not recommended.

Lower than usual dosages are recommended for elderly patients and adolescents. Lower dosages are also recommended for outpatients than for hospitalised patients who will be under close supervision. The physician should initiate dosage at a low level and increase it gradually, noting carefully the clinical response and any evidence of intolerance. Following remission, maintenance medication may be required for a longer period of time at the lowest dose that will maintain remission.

If a patient develops minor side-effects, the dosage should be reduced. The drug should be discontinued promptly if adverse effects of a serious nature or allergic manifestations occur.

The elderly: 30 to 50 mg/day in divided doses.

Adolescent patients: 30 to 50 mg/day in divided doses.

Plasma levels: Optimal responses to nortriptyline have been associated with plasma concentrations of 50 to 150 ng/ml. Higher concentrations may be associated with more adverse experiences. Plasma concentrations are difficult to measure, and physicians should consult the laboratory professional staff. Larger plasma concentrations of the active nortriptyline metabolite 10-hydroxy-nortriptyline have been reported in older patients. In one case, such a condition was associated with apparent cardiotoxicity, despite the fact that nortriptyline concentrations were within the 'therapeutic range'. Clinical findings should predominate over plasma concentrations as primary determinants of dosage changes.

Children: (for nocturnal enuresis only).

Age (years)	*Weight*		*Dose (mg)*
	kg	*lbs*	
6–7	20–25	44–55	10
8–11	25–35	55–77	10–20
>11	35–54	77–119	25–35

The dose should be administered thirty minutes before bedtime.

The maximum period of treatment should not exceed three months. A further course of treatment should not be started until a full physical examination has been made and an ECG performed.

Contra-indications, warnings, etc

Contra-indications: Hypersensitivity to nortriptyline. Recent myocardial infarction, any degree of heart block or other cardiac arrhythmia. Severe liver disease. Mania. Nortriptyline is contra-indicated for the nursing mother and for children under the age of six years. (Please also refer to 'Drug interactions' section.)

Warnings: As improvement may not occur during the initial weeks of therapy, patients, especially those posing a high suicidal risk, should be closely monitored during this period.

Withdrawal symptoms, including insomnia, irritability and excessive perspiration may occur on abrupt cessation of therapy.

The use of nortriptyline in schizophrenic patients may result in an exacerbation of the psychosis or may activate latent schizophrenic symptoms. If administered to overactive or agitated patients, increased anxiety and agitation may occur. In manic-depressive patients, nortriptyline may cause symptoms of the manic phase to emerge.

Cross-sensitivity between nortriptyline and other tricyclic antidepressants is a possibility.

Patients with cardiovascular disease should be given nortriptyline only under close supervision because of the tendency of the drug to produce sinus tachycardia and to prolong the conduction time. Myocardial infarction, arrhythmia and strokes have occurred. Great care is necessary if nortriptyline is administered to hyperthyroid patients or patients receiving thyroid medication, since cardiac arrhythmia may develop.

The use of nortriptyline should be avoided, if possible, in patients with a history of epilepsy. If it is used, however, the patients should be observed carefully at the beginning of treatment, for nortriptyline is known to lower the convulsive threshold.

Nortriptyline may impair the mental and/or physical abilities required for the performance of hazardous tasks, such as operating machinery or driving a car; therefore the patient should be warned accordingly.

Drug interactions: Under no circumstances should nortriptyline be given concurrently with, or within two weeks of cessation of, therapy with monoamine oxidase inhibitors. Hyperpyretic crises, severe convulsions and fatalities have occurred when similar tricyclic antidepressants were used in such combinations.

Nortriptyline should not be given with sympathomimetic agents such as adrenaline, ephedrine, isoprenaline, noradrenaline, phenylephrine and phenylpropanolamine.

Nortriptyline may decrease the antihypertensive effect of guanethidine, debrisoquine, bethanidine and possibly clonidine. Concurrent administration of reserpine has been shown to produce a 'stimulating' effect in some depressed patients. It would be advisable to review all antihypertensive therapy during treatment with tricyclic antidepressants.

Barbiturates may increase the rate of metabolism of nortriptyline.

Anaesthetics given during tricyclic antidepressant therapy may increase the risk of arrhythmias and hypotension. If surgery is necessary, the drug should be discontinued, if possible, for several days prior to the procedure, or the anaesthetist should be informed if the patient is still receiving therapy.

Tricyclic antidepressants may potentiate the CNS depressant effect of alcohol.

The potentiating effect of excessive consumption of alcohol may lead to increased suicidal attempts or overdosage, especially in patients with histories of emotional disturbances or suicidal ideation.

Steady-state serum concentrations of the tricyclic antidepressants are reported to fluctuate significantly as cimetidine is either added to or deleted from the drug regimen. Higher than expected steady-state serum concentrations of the tricyclic antidepressant have been observed when therapy is initiated in patients already taking cimetidine. A decrease may occur when cimetidine therapy is discontinued.

Greater than two-fold increases in previously stable plasma levels of nortriptyline have occurred when fluoxetine was administered concomitantly. Fluoxetine and its active metabolite, norfluoxetine, have long half-lives (7–9 days for norfluoxetine).

Supervision and adjustment of dosage may be required when nortriptyline is used with other anticholinergic drugs.

Usage in pregnancy: The safety of nortriptyline for use during pregnancy has not been established, nor is there evidence from animal studies that it is free from hazard. Aventyl should not, therefore, be administered to pregnant women or women of childbearing age unless the potential benefits clearly outweigh any potential risk.

Usage in nursing mothers: See 'Contra-indications'.

Precautions: The elderly are particularly liable to experience adverse reactions, especially agitation, confusion and postural hypotension.

Troublesome hostility in a patient may be aroused by the use of nortriptyline.

Behavioural changes may occur in children receiving therapy for nocturnal enuresis.

If possible, the use of nortriptyline should be avoided in patients with narrow angle glaucoma or symptoms suggesting prostatic hypertrophy.

The possibility of a suicide attempt by a depressed patient remains after the initiation of treatment. This possibility should be considered in relation to the quantity of drug to be dispensed at any one time.

When it is essential, nortriptyline may be administered with electro-convulsive therapy, although the hazards may be increased.

Both elevation and lowering of blood sugar levels have been reported. Significant hypoglycaemia was reported in a Type II diabetic patient maintained on chlorpropamide (250 mg/day), after the addition of nortriptyline (125 mg/day).

Side-effects: Included in the following list are a few adverse reactions that have not been reported with this specific drug. However, the pharmacological similarities among the tricyclic antidepressant drugs require that each of the reactions be considered when nortriptyline is administered.

Cardiovascular: Hypotension, hypertension, tachycardia, palpitation, myocardial infarction, arrhythmias, heart block, stroke.

Psychiatric: Confusional states (especially in the elderly) with hallucinations, disorientation, delusions; anxiety, restlessness, agitation; insomnia, panic, nightmares; hypomania; exacerbation of psychosis.

Neurological: Numbness, tingling, paraesthesia of extremities; incoordination, ataxia, tremors; peripheral neuropathy; extrapyramidal symptoms; seizures, alteration of EEG patterns; tinnitus.

Anticholinergic: Dry mouth and, rarely, associated sublingual adenitis or gingivitis; blurred vision, disturbance of accommodation, mydriasis; constipation, paralytic ileus; urinary retention, delayed micturition, dilation of the urinary tract.

Allergic: Rash, petechiae, urticaria, itching, photosensitisation (avoid excessive exposure to sunlight); oedema (general or of face and tongue), drug fever, cross-sensitivity with other tricyclic drugs.

Haematological: Bone-marrow depression, including agranulocytosis; aplastic anaemia; eosinophilia; purpura; thrombocytopenia.

Gastro-intestinal: Nausea and vomiting, anorexia, epigastric distress, diarrhoea; peculiar taste, stomatitis, abdominal cramps, black tongue, constipation, paralytic ileus.

Endocrine: Gynaecomastia in the male; breast enlargement and galactorrhoea in the female; increased or decreased libido, impotence; testicular swelling; elevation or depression of blood sugar levels; syndrome of inappropriate secretion of antidiuretic hormone.

Other: Jaundice (simulating obstructive); altered liver function, hepatitis and liver necrosis; weight gain or loss; sweating; flushing; urinary frequency, nocturia; drowsiness, dizziness, weakness, fatigue; headache; parotid swelling; alopecia.

Withdrawal symptoms: Though these are not indicative of addiction, abrupt cessation of treatment after prolonged therapy may produce nausea, headache and malaise.

Overdose

Signs and symptoms: 50 mg of a tricyclic antidepressant can be an overdose in a child. Of patients who are alive at presentation, mortality of 0–15% has been reported. Symptoms may begin within several hours and may include blurred vision, confusion, restlessness, dizziness, hypothermia, hyperthermia, agitation, vomiting, hyperactive reflexes, dilated pupils, fever, rapid heart rate, decreased bowel sounds, dry mouth, inability to void, myoclonic jerks, seizures, respiratory depression, myoglobinuric renal failure, nystagmus, ataxia, dysarthria, choreoathetosis, coma, hypotension and cardiac arrhythmias. Cardiac conduction may be slowed, with prolongation of QRS complex and QT intervals, right bundle branch and AV block, ventricular tachyarrhythmias (including Torsade de pointes and fibrillation) and death. Prolongation of QRS duration to more than 100 msec is predictive of more severe toxicity. The absence of sinus tachycardia does not ensure a benign course. Hypotension may be caused by vasodilatation, central and peripheral alpha-adrenergic blockade and cardiac depression. In a healthy young person, prolonged resuscitation may be effective; one patient survived 5 hours of cardiac massage.

Treatment: Symptomatic and supportive therapy is recommended. Activated charcoal may be more effective than emesis or lavage to reduce absorption.

Ventricular arrhythmias, especially when accompanied by lengthened QRS intervals, may respond to alkalinisation by hyperventilation or administration of sodium bicarbonate. Serum electrolytes should be monitored and managed. Refractory arrhythmias may respond to propranolol, bretylium or lignocaine. Quinidine and procainamide usually should not be used because they may exacerbate arrhythmias and conduction already slowed by the overdose.

Seizures may respond to diazepam. Phenytoin may treat seizures and cardiac rhythm disturbances. Physostigmine may antagonise atrial tachycardia, gut immotility, myoclonic jerks and somnolence. The effects of physostigmine may be short-lived.

Diuresis and dialysis have little effect. Haemoperfusion is unproven. Monitoring should continue, at least until the QRS duration is normal.

Pharmaceutical precautions Keep containers tightly closed and protect from light. Store below 25°C.

Legal category POM.

Package quantities
Capsules 10 mg: Bottles of 100.
Capsules 25 mg: Bottles of 100.

Further information Nil.

Product licence numbers

Capsules 10 mg	0006/5054
Capsules 25 mg	0006/5055

AXID*

Presentation Capsules (pale yellow and dark yellow, coded 3144) containing 150 mg nizatidine INN.

Capsules (pale yellow and brown, coded 3145) containing 300 mg nizatidine INN.

Uses For the treatment of the following diseases where reduction of gastric acid is indicated: Duodenal ulcer; benign gastric ulcer; prevention of duodenal ulcer recurrence; gastric oesophageal reflux disease (including erosions, ulcerations and associated heartburn).

Dosage and administration Axid is administered orally.

Adults: For treatment of duodenal ulcer, the recommended daily dose is 300 mg in the evening. Treatment should continue for four weeks, although this period may be reduced if healing is confirmed earlier by endoscopy. Most ulcers will heal within four weeks, but if complete ulcer healing has not occurred after four weeks therapy, patients should continue therapy for a further four weeks.

For the treatment of benign gastric ulcer, the recommended daily dose is 300 mg in the evening for four or, if necessary, eight weeks. Prior to treatment with nizatidine, care should be taken to exclude the possibility of gastric cancer.

If preferred, the 300 mg daily dose for the treatment of duodenal or benign gastric ulcer may be given as two divided doses of 150 mg in the morning and evening.

For the prevention of duodenal ulcer recurrence (prophylactic maintenance therapy) the recommended daily dose is 150 mg in the evening. Treatment may continue for up to one year.

For the treatment of gastric oesophageal reflux disease, the recommended dosage is from 150 mg twice daily, up to 300 mg twice daily. Therapy for up to 12 weeks is indicated for erosions and ulcerations.

The elderly: Age does not significantly influence efficacy or safety. Normally dosage modification is not required except in patients who have moderate to severe renal impairment (creatinine clearance less than 50 ml/min).

Children: Not recommended, as safety and efficacy have not been established.

Patients with impaired renal function: Nizatidine is principally excreted via the kidneys. For patients on 300 mg daily and who have moderate renal impairment (creatinine clearance less than 50 ml/min), the dose should be reduced by 50% to 150 mg in the evening. For patients on 300 mg daily and who have severe renal impairment (creatinine clearance less than 20 ml/min), the dose should be reduced by 75%, to 150 mg on alternate days.

For gastric oesophageal reflux disease patients receiving the higher dose of 600 mg daily and who have moderate renal impairment (creatinine clearance less than 50 ml/min), the dose should be reduced by 50% to 150 mg twice daily. For such patients with severe renal impairment (creatinine clearance less than 20 ml/min), the dose should be reduced by 75% to 150 mg daily.

For prevention of duodenal ulcer recurrence in patients with moderate renal impairment (creatinine clearance less than 50 ml/min), the dose may be reduced to 150 mg on alternate days. If renal impairment is severe (creatinine clearance less than 20 ml/min), the dose may be reduced to 150 mg every third day.

Contra-indications, warnings, etc

Contra-indication: Known hypersensitivity to H_2-receptor antagonists.

Warnings

Usage in pregnancy: The safety of nizatidine for use during pregnancy has not been established. Animal studies have shown no evidence of impaired fertility or teratogenicity attributable to nizatidine. In one species, however, (Dutch Belted rabbits) at a dose equivalent to 300 times the human dose, effects on fetal development have been observed. Nizatidine should only be used in pregnant women, or in those planning pregnancy, if considered absolutely necessary, and then with caution.

Usage in lactation: Studies conducted in lactating women have shown that 0.1% of the administered oral dose of nizatidine is secreted in human milk in proportion to plasma concentrations. Because of the growth depression in pups reared by lactating rats treated with nizatidine, Axid should be administered to nursing mothers only if considered absolutely necessary.

Drug interactions: There is evidence that nizatidine does not affect the serum levels of concomitantly administered aminophylline, theophylline, chlordiazepoxide, diazepam, lignocaine, phenytoin, ibuprofen, metoprolol, warfarin or lorazepam. Nizatidine does not inhibit the hepatic cytochrome P450-linked drug metabolising enzyme system, but may increase absorption of salicylates when they are used in very high dosage. Approximately 35 per cent of nizatidine is bound to plasma protein. Warfarin, diazepam, paracetamol, propantheline, phenobarbitone and propranolol did not effect plasma protein binding of nizatidine *in vitro*.

Absorption of nizatidine is not clinically significantly affected by food intake, anticholinergic agents or antacids.

Precautions: As nizatidine is partially metabolised by the liver and principally excreted by the kidneys, patients with impaired liver or kidney function should be treated with caution. (See 'Dosage and Administration' section.)

Symptomatic response to nizatidine therapy does not preclude the presence of gastric malignancy.

Side-effects: In large scale clinical trials, sweating, urticaria and somnolence were significantly more common in nizatidine treated patients when compared with placebo.

In the same trials, patients treated with both nizatidine and placebo had mild, transient, asymptomatic elevations of transaminases or alkaline phosphatase; rare instances of marked elevations (>500 iu/l) occurred in nizatidine treated patients. The overall rate of occurrences of elevated liver enzymes and elevations to 3 times the upper limit of normal, however, did not differ significantly from placebo. All abnormalities were reversible after discontinuation of nizatidine. Since introduction hepatitis and jaundice have been reported. Rare cases of cholestatic or mixed hepatocellular and cholestatic injury with jaundice have been reported, with reversal of the abnormalities after discontinuation.

The following effects have also been rarely reported, although a causal relationship has not always been established: thrombocytopenic purpura, fatal thrombocytopenia, exfoliative dermatitis, gynaecomastia, hyperuricaemia, fever, nausea and reversible mental confusion. Rare episodes of hypersensitivity reactions (eg, bronchospasm, laryngeal oedema, rash and eosinophilia) have been reported.

Overdosage: There is little experience of overdose in humans. Tested at very high doses in animals, nizatidine has been shown to be relatively non-toxic. Animal studies suggest that cholinergic-type effects, including lacrimation, salivation, emesis, miosis and diarrhoea, may occur following very large oral doses.

Treatment: Symptomatic and supportive therapy is recommended. Activated charcoal, emesis or lavage may reduce nizatidine absorption. Renal dialysis does not substantially increase clearance of nizatidine due to its large volume of distribution.

Pharmaceutical precautions Store below 25°C.

Legal category POM.

Package quantities
Capsules 150 mg: Blister packs of 28 (4 strips of 7 capsules).
Capsules 300 mg: Blister packs of 28 (4 strips of 7 capsules).

Further information Nizatidine is a potent, selective, competitive and fully reversible histamine H_2-receptor antagonist with a rapid onset of action. It significantly decreases acid concentration together with the volume of basal and stimulated gastric secretion. In clinical trials, nizatidine usually abolished ulcer pain within the first week of therapy. Nizatidine 300 mg at bedtime significantly reduced overnight gastric secretion, but did not increase subsequent basal or meal stimulated gastrin production. Intrinsic factor is not decreased in subjects administered nizatidine.

Nizatidine has no significant effect on the serum concentrations of gonadotrophins, prolactin, growth hormone, antidiuretic hormone, cortisol, tri-iodothyronine, thyroxine, testosterone, 5α-dihydrotestosterone, androstenedione or oestradiol.

Experience in clinical trials indicates that nizatidine has no greater potential than placebo for antiandrogenic effects.

Product licence numbers
Capsules 150 mg 0006/0230
Capsules 300 mg 0006/0231

BRIETAL* Sodium

Presentation Brietal Sodium (methohexitone sodium for injection), in crystalline form, is supplied as follows:

100 mg (with anhydrous Sodium Carbonate BP 6 mg) in 10 ml rubber-stoppered vials.

500 mg (with anhydrous Sodium Carbonate BP 30 mg) in 50 ml rubber-stoppered vials.

Uses
Action: Methohexitone sodium is a rapid, ultrashort-acting barbiturate anaesthetic agent.

Indications: Brietal Sodium is an intravenous anaesthetic agent for the induction of anaesthesia. It is used alone for short surgical procedures, or in combination with other agents for more prolonged anaesthesia.

Dosage and administration Pre-anaesthetic medication is generally advisable. Brietal Sodium may be used with any recognised pre-anaesthetic medications, but the phenothiazines are less satisfactory than the combination of an opiate and a belladonna derivative.

Facilities for assisting respiration and administering oxygen are necessary adjuncts for intravenous anaesthesia. Since cardiorespiratory arrest may occur, patients should be observed carefully during and after use of Brietal Sodium. Resuscitative equipment (i.e. intubation and cardioversion equipment, oxygen, suction and a secure intravenous line) and personnel qualified in its use must be immediately available.

Brietal Sodium is administered by intravenous injection (not infusion), usually in a 1% solution (10 mg per ml). Higher concentrations markedly increase the incidence of muscular movements and irregularities in respiration and blood pressure.

Adults: As an initial guide, an injection rate of 1 ml of a 1% solution (10 mg) in five seconds may be used – although a faster rate than this is preferred by some anaesthetists. The dose usually ranges between 5 and 12 ml (50–120 mg, with an average of about 70 mg), but it must be adjusted to the needs of the individual patient. The induction dose maintains unconsciousness for about five to seven minutes.

The elderly: Onset of anaesthesia may be slow due to sluggish circulation, therefore methohexitone should be injected slowly.

Children: The dose should be adjusted for age and/or weight. Doses of approximately 1 mg/kg are usually satisfactory.

Maintenance: Brietal Sodium is best used simply as an induction agent. If further injection for maintenance is needed the dose must be individualised; but, as a guide, 2–4 ml of a 1% solution every four to seven minutes may be used.

Preparation of solutions: The recommended diluent for Brietal Sodium is Water for Injections PhEur. Solutions may also be prepared in Sodium Chloride Intravenous Infusion BP or 5% Dextrose Intravenous Infusion BP. These solutions are not stable for more than twenty-four hours. Brietal Sodium is not compatible with Compound Sodium Lactate Intravenous Infusion BP or diluents containing bacteriostats.

For a 1% solution (10 mg per ml) vial contents should be diluted as follows:

100 mg: add 10 ml diluent.
500 mg: add 50 ml diluent.

Contra-indications, warnings, etc
Contra-indications: Hypersensitivity to barbiturates. When general anaesthesia is contra-indicated, Brietal Sodium should not be used. Patients with latent or manifest porphyria should not receive barbiturates in any form.

Warnings: Because the liver is involved in demethylation and oxidation of methohexitone and because barbiturates may enhance pre-existing circulatory depression, severe hepatic dysfunction, severe cardiovascular instability, or a shock-like condition, may be reason for selecting another induction agent.

Methohexitone is not recommended for use in patients in status asthmaticus or in individuals with a history of epilepsy. Psychomotor seizures may be elicited in susceptible individuals.

Unintended intra-arterial injection of barbiturate solutions may be followed by the production of platelet aggregates and thrombosis, starting in arterioles distal to the site of injection. The resulting necrosis may lead to gangrene, which may require amputation.

Drug interactions: Barbiturates may stimulate the enzymes responsible for metabolising many other drugs; in particular, they should not be administered concurrently with coumarin-type anticoagulants. They may also affect the metabolism of endogenous steroids.

Prolonged administration may result in cumulative effects, including extended somnolence, protracted unconsciousness and respiratory and cardiovascular depression.

The central nervous system depressant effect of methohexitone may be additive with that of other CNS depressants, including alcohol and antihistamines.

Cyclizine and some phenothiazines, especially promethazine, have been reported to increase the incidence of abnormal muscle movements.

Usage in pregnancy: The safety of methohexitone sodium for use during pregnancy has not been established. Brietal Sodium should not be used in the pregnant patient unless, in the opinion of the clinician, the expected benefit outweighs the possible risk. Animal studies have shown no evidence of teratogenicity.

Labour and delivery: Methohexitone sodium has been used in caesarean section delivery but, because of its solubility, it readily and rapidly traverses the placenta and may therefore cause respiratory depression in the newly delivered baby. The obstetrician and paediatrician should be aware of this fact.

Nursing mothers: Caution should be exercised when methohexitone is administered to a nursing woman.

Precautions: Brietal Sodium should be administered only by persons who are experienced in anaesthesia and who have appropriate equipment on hand for the prevention and treatment of anaesthetic emergencies. Respiratory depression, apnoea, hypotension or cardiorespiratory arrest may occur owing to individual variations in tolerance or to the physical status of the patient. Caution should be exercised in debilitated patients or in those with impaired function of respiratory, circulatory, renal, hepatic or endocrine systems. It is essential that a free airway be maintained at all times. As with any potent anaesthetic agent, pulmonary ventilation should be maintained if prolonged apnoea occurs.

The patient's stomach should be empty. The usual pre-anaesthetic medications may be administered for the production of sedation and inhibition of secretions. If increased muscular relaxation is required for the performance of certain surgical procedures, it may be accomplished by the concomitant use of Brietal Sodium and skeletal muscle relaxants.

Extravasation of the solution may cause pain, swelling, ulceration and necrosis. Should it occur, moist heat may be applied to the infiltrated area.

When appropriate, patients should be instructed as to the hazards of drowsiness that may follow use of methohexitone sodium. Outpatients should be released in the company of another individual, and no skilled activities, such as operating machinery or driving a motor vehicle, should be engaged in for at least 24 hours.

Liver function studies may be influenced by administration of a single dose of barbiturates.

Side-effects: During the induction, especially if it is too rapid, transitory apnoea may occur. This is easily treated by maintaining pulmonary ventilation for a short time until spontaneous respiration is resumed. Following induction, temporary hypotension and tachycardia may occur.

Too rapid induction, inadequate dosage, or insufficient or unsuitable pre-anaesthetic medication may result in skeletal muscle hyperactivity, laryngospasm, cough, sneezing or hiccups. Postanaesthetic shivering may also occur.

Pain at the site of injection and a burning sensation along the course of the vein have occasionally been reported.

Other reported side-effects include: circulatory or respiratory depression, cardiorespiratory arrest, injury to nerves adjacent to injection site, headache, salivation, nausea, emesis, thrombophlebitis, bronchospasm and emergence delirium.

Acute allergic reactions, such as rash, erythema, urticaria, pruritus, rhinitis, dyspnoea, hypotension, restlessness, anxiety, abdominal pain, peripheral vascular collapse and convulsions in association with cardiorespiratory arrest have been reported with the use of Brietal Sodium.

Overdose: The onset of toxicity following an overdose of intravenously administered methohexitone will be within seconds. If methohexitone is administered rectally or is ingested, the onset of toxicity may be delayed. The manifestations include central nervous system depression, respiratory depression, hypotension, loss of peripheral vascular resistance, and muscular hyperactivity ranging from twitching to convulsive-like movements or actual convulsions. Other findings may include allergic reactions. Following massive exposure to any barbiturate, pulmonary oedema, circulatory collapse with loss of peripheral vascular tone, and cardiac arrest may occur.

Management: No specific antidote is known. Treatment consists of the usual life supporting measures.

Pharmaceutical precautions Owing to differences in pH, solutions of Brietal Sodium should not be mixed with acid solutions such as atropine sulphate, tubocurarine and succinylcholine chloride.

Do not use solvents containing bacteriostats, as these may cause precipitation.

Solutions of Brietal Sodium are incompatible with silicone and should not be allowed to come in contact with rubber stoppers or parts of disposable syringes that have been treated with silicone.

Vials of Brietal Sodium should be stored below 25°C.

After reconstitution: Solutions should be used within 24 hours.

Legal category POM.

Package quantities
100 mg in 10 ml vial: Pack of 10 vials.
500 mg in 50 ml vial: Single vials.

Further information Nil.

Product licence numbers

100 mg	0006/5050
500 mg	0006/5051

CELANCE* ▼

Presentation Tablets (ivory, modified rectangle shaped, scored, marked Lilly 4131) containing 50 micrograms pergolide base.

Tablets (green, modified rectangle shaped, scored, marked Lilly 4133) containing 250 micrograms pergolide base.

Tablets (pink, modified rectangle shaped, scored, marked Lilly 4135) containing 1000 micrograms pergolide base.

Uses Pergolide mesylate is indicated as adjunctive treatment to levodopa in the management of the signs and symptoms of Parkinson's disease. Pergolide mesylate is a dopamine receptor agonist at both D1 and D2 receptor sites.

Dosage and administration For oral administration to adults only.

Administration of pergolide mesylate should be initiated with a daily dosage of 50 micrograms for the first 2 days. The dosage should then be gradually increased by 100 or 150 micrograms/day every third day over the next 12 days of therapy. The dosage may then be increased by 250 micrograms/day every third day until an optimal therapeutic dosage is achieved.

Pergolide mesylate is usually administered in divided doses 3 times per day. During dosage titration, the dosage of concurrent *l*-dopa may be cautiously decreased.

In clinical studies, the mean therapeutic daily dosage of pergolide mesylate was 3 mg/day (3000 micrograms/day). The average concurrent daily dosage of *l*-dopa/carbidopa (expressed as *l*-dopa) was approximately 650 mg/day. The efficacy of pergolide mesylate at doses above 5 mg/day (5000 micrograms/day) has not been systematically evaluated.

Children: Safety and effectiveness have not been established.

The major route of excretion is via the kidney.

Contra-indications, warnings, etc

Contra-indication: Hypersensitivity to this drug or other ergot derivatives.

Warnings: Patients should be warned to begin therapy with low doses and to increase dosage in carefully adjusted increments over a period of 3 to 4 weeks (see 'Dosage and administration') to minimise the risk of symptomatic postural and/or sustained hypotension. With gradual dosage titration, tolerance to the hypotension usually develops, (but see 'Drug interactions').

In controlled trials, pergolide mesylate with *l*-dopa caused hallucinosis in about 14 per cent of patients, as opposed to 3 per cent taking placebo with *l*-dopa. This was of sufficient severity to cause discontinuation of treatment in about 3 per cent of those enrolled. Tolerance to this untoward effect was not observed.

In the placebo-controlled trial, 2 of 187 patients treated with placebo died, as compared with 1 of 189 patients treated with pergolide mesylate. Of the 2299 patients treated with pergolide mesylate in pre-marketing studies evaluated in October 1988, 6.2 per cent died while on the drug or shortly after discontinuation. The patient population under evaluation was elderly, ill and at high risk for death. A case-by-case review of the patients who died failed to disclose any unique set of signs, symptoms, or laboratory results that would suggest that treatment with pergolide caused these deaths.

Caution should be exercised when administering to patients prone to cardiac dysrhythmias or with significant underlying cardiac disease.

In a placebo-controlled study, patients taking pergolide mesylate had significantly more episodes of atrial premature contractions (APC's) and sinus tachycardia.

Precautions: Use in patients on *l*-dopa may cause and/or exacerbate pre-existing states of confusion and hallucinations (see 'Warnings'). Abrupt discontinuation of pergolide mesylate, in patients receiving it chronically as an adjunct to *l*-dopa, may precipitate the onset of hallucinations and confusion; these may occur within a span of several days. Discontinuation of pergolide should be undertaken gradually, even if the patient is to remain on *l*-dopa.

Administration to patients receiving *l*-dopa may cause and/or exacerbate pre-existing dyskinesia.

Patients and their families should be informed of the common adverse consequences of the use of pergolide mesylate and the risk of hypotension.

Patients should be advised to tell their doctor if they become pregnant or intend to become pregnant during therapy. They should also tell their doctor if they are breast feeding.

No specific laboratory tests are essential for the management of patients. Periodic routine evaluation is appropriate.

Drug interactions: Dopamine antagonists, such as the neuroleptics (phenothiazines, butyrophenones, thioxanthines) or metoclopramide, ordinarily should not be administered concurrently with pergolide mesylate (a dopamine agonist); these agents may diminish the effectiveness of pergolide mesylate.

Because pergolide mesylate is approximately 90 per cent associated with plasma proteins, caution should be exercised if it is co-administered with other drugs known to affect protein binding.

There are no studies involving the concomitant administration of pergolide and warfarin. When these two drugs are co-prescribed, careful monitoring of anticoagulation should be performed, with adjustments of dosage as necessary.

Because of the risk of postural and/or sustained hypotension in patients taking pergolide, caution should be exercised if it is co-administered with antihypertensive agents.

Carcinogenesis, mutagenesis and impairment of fertility: Two year carcinogenicity studies in mice and rats used doses up to 340 and 12 times the maximum human oral dose (6 mg or 6000 micrograms/day equivalent to 120 micrograms/kg/day). A low incidence of uterine neoplasms occurred in both rats and mice. Endometrial adenomas and carcinomas were observed in rats. Endometrial sarcomas were observed in mice. These occurrences are probably attributable to the high oestrogen/progesterone ratio, which would occur in rodents as a result of the prolactin-inhibiting action of pergolide mesylate. These endocrine mechanisms are not present in humans. However, there are no human data with pergolide to substantiate this conclusion concerning the lack of potential for human risk.

Mutagenic potential was evaluated in a battery of tests. A weak response was noted in one test but the other three tests were negative. The relevance to humans is unknown.

Impaired fertility was observed in mice at the highest dose (5.6 mg or 5600 micrograms/kg/day). This may be related to depressed prolactin levels.

Pregnancy: In animal studies there was no evidence of harm to the fetus due to pergolide mesylate. There are, however, no adequate and well-controlled studies in pregnant women. In pre-marketing studies there were 33 pregnancies that resulted in healthy babies and 5 pregnancies that resulted in congenital abnormalities, although a causal relationship has not been established. This drug should be used during pregnancy only if clearly needed.

Nursing mothers: It is not known whether pergolide is excreted in human milk. The pharmacological action of pergolide mesylate suggests it may interfere with lactation. A decision should be made whether to discontinue nursing or the drug, taking into account the importance of the drug to the mother.

Side-effects: The following adverse events, which are listed in decreasing order of frequency under body system, were observed during placebo-controlled clinical trials at a frequency of one per cent or greater and at a significantly higher incidence than placebo (P value $\leq$ 0.05):

Body as a whole: Pain, abdominal pain.

Digestive system: Nausea, dyspepsia.

Nervous system: Dyskinesia, hallucinations, somnolence.

Respiratory system: Rhinitis, dyspnoea.

Special senses: Diplopia.

Other events that have been reported include insomnia, confusion, constipation, diarrhoea, hypotension, atrial premature contractions and sinus tachycardia.

The more common events that caused discontinuation were related to the nervous system, primarily hallucinations and confusion.

Overdosage: There is no clinical experience with massive overdosage. Overdoses of 60 mg on one day, 19 mg/day for 3 days, or 14 mg/day for 23 days have occurred. Symptoms and signs included vomiting, hypotension, agitation, severe hallucinations, severe involuntary movements and tingling sensations. Another patient who inadvertently received 7 mg, instead of the prescribed 0.7 mg (700 micrograms), experienced palpitations, hypotension and ventricular extrasystoles. The highest daily dose (prescribed for several patients with refractory Parkinson's disease) has exceeded 30 mg.

In animals, manifestations of overdosage include nausea, vomiting, convulsions, decreased blood pressure and CNS stimulation.

Treatment: Symptomatic supportive therapy and cardiac monitoring is recommended.

Arterial blood pressure should be maintained. An antiarrhythmic agent may be necessary. If signs of CNS stimulation are present, a phenothiazine, or other butyrophenone neuroleptic agent, may be indicated.

Activated charcoal may be considered instead of, or in addition to, gastric emptying.

Dialysis or haemoperfusion are unlikely to be of benefit.

Pharmaceutical precautions Store at room temperature.

Legal category POM.

Package quantities

Tablets 50 micrograms:	Bottles of 30.
Tablets 250 micrograms:	Bottles of 100.
Tablets 1000 micrograms:	Bottles of 100.

Further information Nil.

Product licence numbers

Tablets 50 micrograms:	0006/0250
Tablets 250 micrograms:	0006/0251
Tablets 1000 micrograms:	0006/0252

CESAMET*

Presentation Capsules (blue and white, coded Lilly 3101) containing 1 mg nabilone.

Uses Nabilone is indicated for the control of nausea and vomiting, caused by chemotherapeutic agents used in the treatment of cancer, in patients who have failed to respond adequately to conventional antiemetic treatments.

Dosage and administration Nabilone is for oral administration to adults only. It is not recommended for use in children younger than 18 years of age as safety and efficacy have not been established.

The usual adult dosage is 1 mg or 2 mg twice a day. To minimise side-effects, it is recommended that the lower starting dose is used and that the dose is increased as necessary. The first dose should be administered the night before initiation of chemotherapy, and the second dose should be given one to three hours before the first dose of the oncolytic agent is administered.

The maximum daily dose should not exceed 6 mg, given in three divided doses.

Nabilone may be administered throughout each cycle of chemotherapy and, if necessary, for 48 hours after the last dose of each cycle. Data on the chronic use of nabilone are not available.

The elderly: As for adults (see 'Precautions').

Contra-indications, warnings, etc
Contra-indication: Nabilone is contra-indicated in patients with a known allergy to cannabinoid agents and when the nausea and vomiting arises from any cause other than cancer chemotherapy.

Warnings: As nabilone is excreted primarily by the biliary route, the drug is not recommended for use in patients with severe liver dysfunction.

Nabilone may impair the mental and/or physical abilities required for the performance of potentially hazardous tasks such as operating machinery or driving a car; therefore the patient should be advised accordingly. The effects of nabilone may persist for a variable and unpredictable period of time following its oral administration. Adverse psychiatric reactions can persist for 48 to 72 hours following cessation of treatment.

Patients receiving nabilone should be closely observed, if possible, within an inpatient setting. This is especially important during the treatment of naive patients. However, even patients experienced with cannabinoid agents may have serious untoward responses not predicted by prior uneventful exposure. Patients should be made aware of possible changes of mood and other adverse behavioural effects of the drug.

Usage in pregnancy: Laboratory studies have so far shown no evidence of teratogenicity. There are no adequate and well controlled studies in pregnant women. Nabilone should be used during pregnancy only if clearly needed.

Reproduction studies performed in rats at 150 times the human dose and rabbits at 40 times the human dose revealed a dose-related reduction in litter size, an increase in the incidence of fetal resorptions, and an increase in the incidence of stillborn pups. The number of implantations was unaffected by treatment. These effects appear related to the dose-dependent reduction in maternal food intake and gain in body weight induced by nabilone. At 150 times the maximum recommended human dose, nabilone produced a reduction in neonatal survival that may be related to reduced milk production by mothers. Nabilone is known to have an inhibitory effect on prolactin release, which could contribute to the observed reduction in milk production. Hypothermia was also reported in the offspring of high-dose groups of female rats, which may have also contributed to reduced neonatal survival.

Nursing mothers: It is not known whether this drug is excreted in breast milk. It is not recommended that nabilone be given to nursing mothers.

Precautions: Since nabilone can elevate supine and standing heart rates and cause postural hypotension, it should be used with caution in the elderly and in patients with hypertension and heart disease.

Nabilone should be administered with caution to patients who are taking other psychoactive drugs or CNS depressants, including alcohol, barbiturates and narcotic analgesics, or to those with a history of psychiatric disorder (including manic-depressive illness and schizophrenia). Nabilone has been shown to have an additive CNS depressant effect when given with either diazepam, secobarbitone sodium, alcohol, or codeine.

Side-effects: During controlled clinical trials of nabilone, virtually all patients experienced at least one adverse reaction. These included psychotomimetic reactions.

In these trials, the commonest statistically significant adverse events (in decreasing order of incidence) were: drowsiness, vertigo/dizziness, euphoria (high), dry mouth, ataxia, visual disturbance, concentration difficulties, sleep disturbance, dysphoria, hypotension, headache and nausea.

Other reported events include confusion, disorientation, hallucinations, psychosis, depression, decreased co-ordination, tremors, tachycardia, decreased appetite and abdominal pain.

Tolerance to such CNS effects as relaxation, drowsiness and euphoria develops rapidly and is readily reversible.

Drug abuse and dependence: Nabilone is an abusable substance, capable of producing side-effects, such as euphoria or 'high', at therapeutic doses. Prescriptions should be limited to the amount necessary for a single cycle of chemotherapy (ie, a few days). The physical dependence capability of nabilone is unknown. Patients who participated in clinical trials, up to 5 days duration, showed no withdrawal symptoms on cessation of dosing.

Overdosage: Signs and symptoms are an extension of the psychotomimetic and physiological effects of nabilone. Overdosage may be considered to have occurred, even at prescribed dosages, if disturbing psychiatric symptoms are present. Subsequent doses should be withheld until patients have returned to their baseline mental status; routine dosing, possibly at a lower dose, may then be resumed if clinically indicated. In controlled clinical trials, alterations in mental status, related to the use of nabilone, resolved within 72 hours without specific medical therapy. Vital signs should be monitored, since hypertension, hypotension, and tachycardia have occurred.

No cases of overdosage with more than 10 mg/day of nabilone have been reported during clinical trials. Signs and symptoms to be anticipated in large overdose situations are psychotic episodes, including hallucinations and anxiety reactions, respiratory depression and coma.

Treatment: Conservative management, if possible (ie, verbal support and comfort). In more severe cases, antipsychotic drugs may be useful, although they have not been systematically evaluated. Such patients should be closely monitored because of the potential for drug interactions (eg, additive CNS depressant effects due to nabilone and chlorpromazine).

General supportive care is recommended. Consider giving activated charcoal to decrease absorption from the gastro-intestinal tract. The use of forced diuresis, peritoneal dialysis, haemodialysis, charcoal haemoperfusion, or cholestyramine, has not been reported. Most of a dose of nabilone is eliminated through the biliary system.

Treatment for respiratory depression and comatose state consists of symptomatic and supportive therapy. Attention should be paid to the occurrence of hypothermia. Consider fluids, inotropes and/or vasopressors for hypotension.

Pharmaceutical precautions Keep containers tightly closed. Store at room temperature (15°–25°C).

Legal category POM.

Package quantities Bottles of 20.

Further information Nil.

Product licence number 0006/0155.

CINOBAC*

Presentation Capsules (green and orange, coded 3056) containing 500 mg cinoxacin.

Uses Cinoxacin is indicated for acute, recurrent and chronic upper and lower urinary tract infections (including cystitis, pyelonephritis or pyelitis and asymptomatic bacteriuria) caused by susceptible micro-organisms.

A single dose of 500 mg taken at bedtime has been shown to be effective as preventive therapy in reducing the number of episodes of infection in patients subject to recurrent urinary tract infections.

Cinoxacin is active against most strains of the following organisms: *Enterobacter* spp. (including *Ent. aerogenes, Ent. cloacae* and *Ent. hafniae), Escherichia coli, Klebsiella* spp., *Proteus mirabilis*, and *Pr. vulgaris*.

Cinoxacin is also active against approximately 50 per

cent of strains of *Pr. rettgeri, Providencia* and *Serratia* species.

Dosage and administration The usual adult dose is 1 g daily administered orally as 500 mg b.d. for seven to fourteen days.

For prophylactic use, a single dose of 500 mg daily, taken at bedtime.

Not recommended for use in children.

The elderly: As for adults, unless renal function is impaired (see 'Precautions').

Contra-indications, warnings, etc
Contra-indication: Hypersensitivity to cinoxacin.

Warnings: Since cinoxacin, like other drugs in its class, causes arthropathy in immature animals, its use during pregnancy or for pre-pubertal children is not recommended.

Usage in pregnancy or lactation: Cinoxacin should not be administered during pregnancy or to the nursing mother as safety has not been established. Animal studies showed no evidence of teratogenicity or toxicity. It is not known whether cinoxacin is excreted in human milk.

Convulsions have been reported with cinoxacin, although no causal relationship has been established. Convulsions, increased intracranial pressure, toxic psychoses and CNS stimulation (tremors, restlessness, lightheadedness, confusion and hallucinations) have been reported with other quinolones. Cinoxacin should be used with caution in patients with CNS disorders, such as cerebral arteriosclerosis, epilepsy, or other factors predisposed to seizures. If such reactions occur discontinue treatment.

Serious and, occasionally, fatal hypersensitivity (anaphylactoid) reactions, some following the first dose, have been reported in patients during quinolone therapy. Some reactions were accompanied by cardiovascular collapse, loss of consciousness, tingling, pharyngeal and face oedema, dyspnoea, urticaria and itching. Only a few patients had a history of hypersensitivity reactions.

Precautions: Since cinoxacin is eliminated primarily by the kidney, dosage should be reduced or time between doses increased in patients with reduced renal function. Administration of cinoxacin is not recommended for patients with severely impaired renal function.

Cinoxacin should be used with caution in patients with a history of hepatic disease.

Drug interactions: Cinoxacin may enhance the effects of oral anticoagulants, such as warfarin. When concomitant administration cannot be avoided, daily coagulation tests are essential.

Elevated plasma levels of theophylline and theophylline-related side-effects have been reported with concomitant quinolone use. Therefore, the monitoring of theophylline plasma levels should be considered.

Side-effects: The most frequently reported adverse events in postmarketing surveillance have been nausea/vomiting and rash.

Gastro-intestinal: Nausea, anorexia, vomiting, abdominal cramps, and diarrhoea have been reported.

Hypersensitivity: Rash, pruritus, urticaria, oedema, angio-oedema and eosinophilia. Anaphylaxis, anaphylactoid reactions and toxic epidermal necrolysis have been reported rarely. Erythema multiforme has been reported with cinoxacin, and Stevens-Johnson syndrome with other quinolones.

Haematological: Thrombocytopenia has been reported rarely.

Nervous system: Dizziness, headache, insomnia, tingling sensation, perineal burning, photophobia and tinnitus.

Laboratory values: Transient changes in AST, ALT, blood urea, ALP, and creatinine clearance have been observed occasionally.

Overdosage

Signs and symptoms: May include anorexia, nausea, vomiting, epigastric distress and diarrhoea. The severity of epigastric distress and diarrhoea are dose related. Headache, dizziness, insomnia, photophobia, tinnitus and tingling sensation have also been reported.

Treatment: Patients should be kept well hydrated to prevent crystalluria. Symptomatic and supportive therapy is recommended. Activated charcoal should be considered instead of, or in addition to, gastric emptying. Forced diuresis, peritoneal dialysis, haemodialysis, or charcoal haemoperfusion have not been established as beneficial.

Pharmaceutical precautions Store at room temperature (15°–25°C).

Legal category POM.

Package quantity Blister pack of 14.

Further information Nil.

Product licence number 0006/0124.

COLOGEL*

Presentation An aromatised solution each 100 ml containing 9 g methylcellulose in a lemon-flavoured vehicle, with alcohol 5%.

Uses Cologel is a liquid bulk laxative, which does not irritate the intestinal mucosa or interfere with the absorption of foods or vitamins. It is indicated for the treatment of chronic or acute constipation.

Dosage and administration For oral administration.

Adults: 5–15 ml (1–3 teaspoonfuls) with a full glass of water three times daily after meals.

Maintenance dosage: 5–15 ml with a full glass of water once daily. In severe cases, up to 30 ml with a full glass of water may be administered once daily.

Children: The dosage should be scaled down in proportion to size.

The elderly: As for adults.

Contra-indications, warnings, etc
Contra-indications: Cologel should not be given to children who are dehydrated. It should not be used in patients with intestinal obstruction or faecal impaction.

Warnings: Intestinal obstruction has been reported after the administration of bulk laxatives, therefore it is essential that an adequate quantity of water be taken with each dose.

Usage in pregnancy: This product is not absorbed from the gastro-intestinal tract and is therefore considered to be safe for use during pregnancy.

Pharmaceutical precautions Exposure to high temperatures may cause this product to gel. If this occurs, place in a refrigerator. Cologel should not be frozen.

Legal category GSL.

Package quantities Bottles of 500 ml.

Further information Nil.

Product licence number 0006/5047.

CYCLOSERINE

Presentation Capsules (red and grey, coded F04) each containing 250 mg Cycloserine BP.

Uses
Actions: Cycloserine inhibits cell wall synthesis in susceptible strains of Gram-positive and Gram-negative bacteria and in *Mycobacterium tuberculosis.*

Indications: Cycloserine is indicated in the treatment of active pulmonary and extra-pulmonary tuberculosis (including renal disease) when the organisms are susceptible to this drug and after failure of adequate treatment with the primary medications (streptomycin, isoniazid, rifampicin and ethambutol). Like all anti-tuberculous drugs, cycloserine should be administered in conjunction with other effective chemotherapy and not as the sole therapeutic agent.

Cycloserine may be effective in the treatment of acute urinary tract infections caused by susceptible strains of Gram-positive and Gram-negative bacteria, especially *Klebsiella/Enterobacter* species and *Escherichia coli*. It is generally no more and may be less effective than other antimicrobial agents in the treatment of urinary tract infections caused by bacteria other than mycobacteria. Use of cycloserine in these infections should be considered only when the more conventional therapy has failed and when the organism has been demonstrated to be sensitive to the drug.

Dosage and administration Cycloserine is administered orally.

Adults: The usual dosage is 500 mg to 1 g daily in divided doses, monitored by blood level determinations. The initial adult dosage most frequently given is 250 mg twice daily at 12-hour intervals for the first two weeks. A daily dosage of 1 g should not be exceeded.

Children: The usual starting dose is 10 mg/kg/day, then adjusted according to blood levels obtained and therapeutic response.

The elderly: As for adults but reduce dosage if renal function is impaired.

Contra-indications, warnings, etc
Contra-indications: Cycloserine is contra-indicated in the presence of any of the following: hypersensitivity to cycloserine; epilepsy; depression, severe anxiety or psychosis; severe renal insufficiency; alcohol abuse.

Warnings: Administration of cycloserine should be discontinued or the dosage reduced if the patient develops allergic dermatitis or symptoms of central nervous system toxicity such as convulsions, psychosis, somnolence, depression, confusion, hyper-reflexia, headache, tremor, vertigo, paresis or dysarthria.

Toxicity is usually associated with blood levels of greater than 30 mg/l, which may be the result of high dosage or inadequate renal clearance. The therapeutic index for this drug is low. The risk of convulsions is increased in chronic alcoholics (see 'Precautions' section).

Patients should be monitored by haematological, renal excretion, blood level and liver function studies.

Drug interactions: Concurrent administration of ethionamide has been reported to potentiate neurotoxic side-effects. Alcohol and cycloserine are incompatible, especially during a regimen calling for large doses of the latter. Alcohol increases the possibility and risk of epileptic episodes. Patients receiving cycloserine and isoniazid should be monitored for signs of CNS toxicity, such as dizziness and drowsiness, as these drugs have a combined toxic action on the CNS. Dosage adjustments may be necessary.

Usage in pregnancy: Concentrations in fetal blood approach those found in the serum. A study in 2 generations of rats given doses up to 100 mg/kg/day demonstrated no teratogenic effect in offspring. It is not known whether cycloserine can cause fetal harm when administered to a pregnant woman or can affect reproduction capacity. Cycloserine should be given to a pregnant woman only if clearly needed.

Usage in nursing mothers: Concentrations in the mother's milk approach those found in the serum. A decision should be made whether to discontinue nursing or to discontinue the drug, taking into account the importance of the drug to the mother.

Precautions: Before treatment with cycloserine is begun, cultures should be taken and the susceptibility of the organism to the drug should be established. In tuberculous infections, sensitivity to the other anti-tuberculous agents in the regimen should also be demonstrated.

Blood levels should be determined at least weekly for patients having reduced renal function, for individuals receiving a daily dosage of more than 500 mg, and for those showing signs and symptoms suggestive of toxicity. The dosage should be adjusted to keep the blood level below 30 mg/l.

Anticonvulsant drugs or sedatives may be effective in controlling symptoms of central nervous system toxicity, such as convulsions, anxiety or tremor. Patients receiving more than 500 mg of cycloserine daily should be closely observed for such symptoms. The value of pyridoxine in preventing CNS toxicity from cycloserine has not been proved.

Administration of cycloserine and other anti-tuberculous drugs has been associated in a few instances with vitamin B_{12} and/or folic acid deficiency, megaloblastic anaemia and sideroblastic anaemia. If evidence of anaemia develops during treatment, appropriate investigations and treatment should be carried out.

Side-effects: Most side-effects occurring during treatment with cycloserine involve the nervous system or are manifestations of drug hypersensitivity. The following side-effects have been observed: nervous system manifestations, which appear to be related to higher dosages of drug, i.e. more than 500 mg daily, can be convulsions, drowsiness, somnolence, headache, tremor, dysarthria, vertigo, confusion and disorientation with loss of memory, psychosis, possibly with suicidal tendencies, character changes, hyperirritability, aggression, paresis, hyper-reflexia, paraesthesiae, major and minor localised clonic seizures and coma.

Other reported side-effects include allergy, rash, megaloblastic anaemia and elevated serum aminotransferases, especially in patients with pre-existing liver disease.

Sudden development of congestive heart failure, in patients receiving 1 to 1.5 g of cycloserine daily, has been reported.

Overdosage
Signs and symptoms: Acute toxicity can occur if more than 1 g is ingested by an adult. Chronic toxicity is dose related and can occur if more than 500 mg is administered daily. For patients with renal impairment see 'Contra-indications' and 'Warnings'. Toxicity commonly affects the central nervous system. Effects may include headache, vertigo, confusion, drowsiness, hyperirritability, paraesthesias, dysarthria and psychosis. Following larger ingestions, paresis, convulsions and coma often occur. Ethanol may increase the risk of seizures.

Treatment: Symptomatic and supportive therapy is recommended. Activated charcoal may be more effective in reducing absorption than emesis or lavage. In adults, many neurotoxic effects can be both treated and prevented with 200–300 mg of pyridoxine daily. Haemodialysis removes cycloserine from the bloodstream but should be reserved for life-threatening toxicity.

Pharmaceutical precautions Keep containers tightly closed. Store below 25°C. Protect from moisture.

Legal category POM.

Package quantities Capsules 250 mg: Bottles of 100.

Further information Nil.

Product licence number 0006/5045.

DIMELOR*

Presentation Tablets (yellow, scored, coded U07) each containing 500 mg Acetohexamide BP.

Uses For the treatment of non-insulin-dependent diabetes mellitus (Type II, maturity onset) where dietary treatment has proved inadequate and there is no evidence of ketosis or acidosis.

Dosage and administration The daily dose may range from 250 mg to 1.5 g. No loading dose is required.

Patients who do not respond to 1.5 g daily are unlikely to benefit from a higher dose and for this reason doses exceeding 1.5 g daily are not recommended. The majority of patients receiving 1 g or less daily can be controlled on a once-daily dosage. Patients requiring 1.5 g daily usually benefit from twice-daily dosage, given before the morning and evening meals.

Previously untreated patients: In mild stable diabetes (after dietary regulation) treatment can be started with

250 mg daily before breakfast. The dose can be increased by 250–500 mg every five to seven days as necessary.

Elderly patients: Because some elderly patients are unusually responsive, patients in this group should be started with a single daily dose of one-half tablet (250 mg) before breakfast, and their blood and urine sugars should be monitored during the first 24 hours of treatment. If control is satisfactory, this dose may be continued on a daily basis or, if necessary, gradually increased. Any tendency towards hypoglycaemia is an indication for reduction of dosage or even discontinuation.

Children: Use in children is not recommended.

Transfer from other oral agents: Patients who have been maintained on other oral agents may be transferred directly to Dimelor. It should be remembered that Dimelor is intermediate in potency between tolbutamide and chlorpropamide, and the first dose of Dimelor should be only half the previous tolbutamide dose. When the transfer is from chlorpropamide, it is likely that Dimelor will be required at double the previous chlorpropamide dose. A transition period is usually required because of the long half-life of chlorpropamide. Adjustment of dosage should be made according to clinical response, bearing in mind the maximum recommended dose of 1.5 g.

Transfer from insulin: In general, patients who were previously maintained on small doses of insulin of up to 20 units daily may be transferred directly to Dimelor with discontinuation of the insulin. Some older patients may need to be observed in hospital during the transition period, because of the potential hazards of hypoglycaemia in the elderly.

Contra-indications, warnings, etc

Contra-indications: Acetohexamide is contra-indicated in patients known to be intolerant of sulphonylureas or sulphonamides, as sole therapy in insulin-dependent Type I diabetes mellitus, in patients with diabetic ketoacidosis with or without coma, patients with hyperglycaemia and glycosuria associated with primary renal disease (in whom blood sugar reduction should also be effected by insulin), and diabetes when complicated by pregnancy.

Warnings: In stress situations such as fever, trauma, infection or surgical intervention, it may be necessary to add insulin to the Dimelor treatment or to switch entirely to insulin treatment to achieve control until the stress is over.

In patients with impaired hepatic and/or renal function or with adrenal and pituitary insufficiency and in debilitated or malnourished individuals, there is a possibility that hypoglycaemia may occur. Careful observation and appropriate adjustment of dosage are therefore necessary in such patients.

Hypoglycaemia may also appear in patients who eat irregularly or who exercise without caloric supplementation and this is most likely to occur during a period of transition from insulin. Hypoglycaemia may also occur in association with alcohol ingestion or when more than one hypoglycaemic agent is in use.

Special warning on increased risk of cardiovascular mortality: In 1970, a publication from the University Group Diabetes Program reported that patients treated for 5 to 8 years with diet plus a fixed dose of tolbutamide (1.5 g/day) had a rate of cardiovascular mortality approximately 2.5 times that of patients treated with diet alone. A significant increase in total mortality was not observed, but the use of tolbutamide was discontinued based on the increase in cardiovascular mortality, thus limiting the opportunity for the study to show an increase in overall mortality. Despite controversy regarding the interpretation of these results, the findings of the UGDP study provide an adequate basis for this warning. The patient should be informed of the potential risks and advantages of Dimelor and of alternative modes of therapy.

Although only one drug in the sulphonylurea class (tolbutamide) was included in this study, it is prudent from a safety standpoint to consider that this warning may also apply to other oral hypoglycaemic drugs in this class, in view of their close similarities in mode of action and chemical structure.

Drug interactions: The hypoglycaemic action of sulphonylurea drugs may be potentiated by various drugs including non-steroidal anti-inflammatory agents and other drugs that are highly protein bound, namely, salicylates, sulphonamides, chloramphenicol, probenecid, coumarins, monoamine oxidase inhibitors and beta-adrenergic blocking agents. When such drugs are administered to a patient receiving Dimelor, the patient should be observed closely in case hypoglycaemia should occur. Also, when such drugs are withdrawn, the patient should be observed in case diabetic control should be lost.

Certain drugs that tend to have a hyperglycaemic action may also induce loss of control. Such drugs include thiazide and other diuretics, corticosteroids, phenothiazines, thyroid products, oestrogens, oral contraceptives, phenytoin, nicotinic acid, sympathomimetics, calcium channel blockers and isoniazid. When such drugs are administered to a patient receiving Dimelor, the patient should be observed lest control be lost and conversely, when such drugs are withdrawn from a patient also receiving Dimelor, the possibility of the occurrence of hypoglycaemia should be remembered.

Patients receiving sulphonylureas may experience a disulfiram-type reaction following the ingestion of alcohol. Symptoms may include flushing, nausea and vomiting, headache and hypotension.

Usage in pregnancy: Acetohexamide has not been shown to be teratogenic in animals. However, teratogenesis in animals has been observed following administration of high doses of other sulphonylureas. There are no adequate and well-controlled studies in pregnant women. Therefore, acetohexamide is not recommended for the management of diabetes when complicated by pregnancy. Many experts recommend that insulin be used during pregnancy to maintain blood glucose levels as close to normal as possible.

In addition, prolonged severe hypoglycaemia (4 to 10 days) has been reported in neonates whose mothers were receiving a sulphonylurea drug at the time of delivery. This has been reported more frequently with the use of drugs with prolonged half-lives.

Usage in nursing mothers: Acetohexamide is not recommended for mothers who are breast-feeding. It is not known whether acetohexamide is excreted in human breast milk.

Precautions: Secondary failures and the tendency for the severity of diabetes mellitus to fluctuate spontaneously may result in loss of control. Patients should therefore be re-evaluated regularly.

Side-effects

Gastro-intestinal: The most common side-effects are gastro-intestinal disturbances, e.g. nausea, epigastric fullness and heartburn, and occur in 1 in 40 patients. These reactions tend to be dose-related and may disappear when dosage is reduced.

Hepatic: Cholestatic jaundice may occur rarely; if it does, Dimelor should be discontinued.

Dermatological: Allergic skin reactions, e.g. pruritus, erythema, urticaria, and morbilliform or maculopapular eruptions, occur in less than 1 in 100 patients. These may be transient and may disappear despite continued use of Dimelor. If skin reactions persist, the drug should be discontinued.

Porphyria cutanea tarda and photosensitivity reactions have been reported with sulphonylurea agents.

Endocrine: There have been reports of hyponatraemia and the syndrome of inappropriate antidiuretic hormone (SIADH) secretion with acetohexamide and other sulphonylurea agents.

Haematological: As with other sulphonylurea drugs, leucopenia, thrombocytopenia, pancytopenia, agranulocytosis, aplastic anaemia and haemolytic anaemia have been reported.

Metabolic: Hepatic porphyria and disulfiram-like reactions have been reported with sulphonylurea agents.

Overdosage

Signs and symptoms: Hypoglycaemia may be preceded by nausea, vomiting and mild epigastric pain. Symptoms of hypoglycaemia may include headache, weakness, confusion, dizziness, lethargy, convulsions, coma and death. Patients may be especially susceptible to hypoglycaemia if they are elderly, if they have had restricted carbohydrate intake (especially during periods of exercise), or if they have kidney or liver dysfunction.

Treatment: Mild hypoglycaemic symptoms, without loss of consciousness or neurological findings, should be treated with oral glucose and adjustments in drug dosage and/or meal patterns. Severe hypoglycaemic reactions, with coma, seizure, or other neurological impairment, occur infrequently but constitute medical emergencies. If hypoglycaemic coma is diagnosed or suspected, the patient should be given a rapid intravenous injection of concentrated (50%) glucose solution. This should be followed by a continuous infusion of a more dilute (10%) glucose solution at a rate that will maintain the blood glucose at a level of about 100 mg/dl (5.6 mmol/l). Patients should be closely monitored for a minimum of 24 to 48 hours, since hypoglycaemia may recur after apparent clinical recovery.

General symptomatic and supportive therapy is recommended. Activated charcoal should be considered instead of, or in addition to, gastric emptying.

Pharmaceutical precautions Keep containers tightly closed.

Legal category POM.

Package quantities Bottles of 100.

Further information Nil.

Product licence number 0006/5069.

DISTACLOR*

Presentation Capsules (violet and white, printed Distaclor 250) containing 250 mg cefaclor.

Capsules (violet and grey, printed Distaclor 500) containing 500 mg cefaclor.

Granules (pink) for suspension containing 125 mg cefaclor/5 ml.

Granules (pink) for suspension containing 250 mg cefaclor/5 ml.

Uses Distaclor is indicated for the treatment of the following infections due to susceptible micro-organisms:

Respiratory tract infections, including pneumonia, bronchitis, exacerbations of chronic bronchitis, pharyngitis and tonsillitis, and as part of the management of sinusitis
Otitis media
Skin and soft tissue infections
Urinary tract infections, including pyelonephritis and cystitis
Distaclor has been found to be effective in both acute and chronic urinary tract infections.

Cefaclor is active against the following organisms *in vitro:*

Alpha- and beta-haemolytic streptococci
Staphylococci; including coagulase-positive, coagulase-negative and penicillinase-producing strains
Streptococcus pneumoniae
Streptococcus pyogenes (group A beta-haemolytic streptococci)
Branhamella catarrhalis
Escherichia coli
Proteus mirabilis
Klebsiella species
Haemophilus influenzae, including ampicillin-resistant strains.

Cefaclor has no activity against *Pseudomonas* species, *Acinetobacter calcoaceticus,* or against most strains of enterococci (*Str. faecalis*), *Enterobacter,* indole-positive *Proteus* and *Serratia* species. Some rare strains of staphylococci are resistant to cefaclor.

Dosage and administration Distaclor is administered orally.

Adults: The usual adult dosage is 250 mg every eight hours. For more severe infections or those caused by less susceptible organisms, doses may be doubled. Doses of 4 g per day have been administered safely to normal subjects for 28 days, but the total daily dosage should not exceed this amount.

Distaclor may be administered in the presence of impaired renal function. Under such conditions dosage is usually unchanged (see 'Precautions').

Patients undergoing haemodialysis: Haemodialysis shortens serum half-life by 25–30%. In patients undergoing regular haemodialysis, a loading dose of 250 mg–1 g administered prior to dialysis and a therapeutic dose of 250–500 mg every six to eight hours maintained during interdialytic periods is recommended.

The elderly: As for adults.

Children: The usual recommended daily dosage for children is 20 mg/kg/day in divided doses every eight hours, as indicated. Safety and efficacy have not been established for use in infants aged less than one month.

Distaclor suspension

	125 mg/5 ml	250 mg/5 ml
<1 year (9 kg)	2.5 ml tid	
1–5 years (9–18 kg)	5.0 ml tid	
Over 5 years		5.0 ml tid

In more serious infections, otitis media, sinusitis and infections caused by less susceptible organisms, 40 mg/kg/day in divided doses is recommended, up to a daily maximum of 1 g.

In the treatment of beta-haemolytic streptococcal infections, therapy should be continued for at least 10 days.

Contra-indications, warnings, etc

Contra-indication: Hypersensitivity to cephalosporins.

Warnings: Before instituting therapy with cefaclor, every effort should be made to determine whether the patient has had previous hypersensitivity reactions to the cephalosporins, penicillins or other drugs. Cefaclor should be given cautiously to penicillin-sensitive patients. There is some clinical and laboratory evidence of partial cross-allergenicity of the penicillins and cephalosporins. Patients have had severe reactions (including anaphylaxis) to both types of drugs.

Pseudomembranous colitis has been reported with virtually all broad-spectrum antibiotics, including macrolides, semi-synthetic penicillins and cephalosporins. It is important, therefore, to consider its diagnosis in patients who develop diarrhoea in association with the use of antibiotics. Such colitis may range in severity from mild to life-threatening. Mild cases usually respond to drug discontinuance alone. In moderate to severe cases, appropriate measures should be taken.

Usage in pregnancy: Although laboratory studies and clinical experience have shown no evidence of teratogenicity, caution should be exercised when prescribing for the pregnant patient.

Usage in nursing mothers: Small amounts of cefaclor have been detected in breast milk following administration of single 500 mg doses. Average levels of about 0.2 micrograms/ml or less were detected up to 5 hours later. Trace amounts were detected at one hour. As the effect on nursing infants is not known, caution should be exercised when cefaclor is administered to a nursing woman.

Precautions: If an allergic reaction to cefaclor occurs, the drug should be discontinued and the patient treated with the appropriate agents.

Cefaclor should be administered with caution in the presence of markedly impaired renal function. Since the half-life of cefaclor in anuric patients is 2.3 to 2.8 hours, dosage adjustments for patients with moderate or severe renal impairment are not usually required. Clinical experience with cefaclor under such conditions is limited; therefore, careful clinical observation and laboratory studies should be made.

Broad-spectrum antibiotics should be prescribed with caution in individuals with a history of gastro-intestinal disease, particularly colitis.

Prolonged use of cefaclor may result in the overgrowth of non-susceptible organisms. If superinfection occurs during therapy, appropriate measures should be taken.

Positive direct Coombs' tests have been reported during treatment with the cephalosporin antibiotics. In haematological studies or in transfusion cross-matching procedures, when anti-globulin tests are performed on the minor side, or in Coombs' testing of newborns whose mothers have received cephalosporin antibiotics before parturition, it should be recognised that a positive Coombs' test may be due to the drug.

A false-positive reaction for glucose in the urine may occur with Benedict's or Fehling's solutions or with copper sulphate test tablets.

Drug interactions: There have been rare reports of increased prothrombin time, with or without clinical bleeding, in patients receiving cefaclor and warfarin concomitantly. It is recommended that in such patients, regular monitoring of prothrombin time should be considered, with adjustment of dosage if necessary.

Side-effects

Gastro-intestinal: The most frequent side-effect has been diarrhoea. It is rarely severe enough to warrant cessation of therapy. Colitis, including rare instances of pseudomembranous colitis, has been reported. Nausea and vomiting have also occurred.

Hypersensitivity: Allergic reactions such as morbilliform eruptions, pruritus and urticaria have been observed. These reactions usually subside upon discontinuation of therapy. Serum sickness-like reactions (erythema multiforme minor, rashes or other skin manifestations accompanied by arthritis/arthralgia, with or without fever) have been reported. Lymphadenopathy and proteinuria are infrequent, there are no circulating immune complexes and no evidence of sequelae. Serum sickness-like reactions are apparently due to hypersensitivity and have usually occurred during or following a second (or subsequent) course of therapy with cefaclor. Such reactions have been reported more frequently in children than in adults. Signs and symptoms usually occur a few days after initiation of therapy and usually subside within a few days of cessation of therapy. Antihistamines and corticosteroids appear to enhance resolution of the syndrome. No serious sequelae have been reported.

There are rare reports of erythema multiforme major (Stevens-Johnson syndrome), toxic epidermal necrolysis, and anaphylaxis. Anaphylaxis may be more common in patients with a history of penicillin allergy.

Haematological: Eosinophilia; positive Coombs' tests; and, rarely, thrombocytopenia. Transient lymphocytosis, leucopenia and, rarely, haemolytic anaemia and reversible neutropenia of possible clinical significance.

Hepatic: Transient hepatitis and cholestatic jaundice have been reported rarely; slight elevations in AST, ALT or alkaline phosphatase values.

Renal: Reversible interstitial nephritis has occurred rarely; also slight elevations in blood urea or serum creatinine or abnormal urinalysis.

Central Nervous System: Reversible hyperactivity, nervousness, insomnia, confusion, hypertonia, dizziness and somnolence have been reported rarely.

Miscellaneous: Genital pruritus and vaginitis.

Overdosage: Symptoms of nausea, vomiting, epigastric distress and diarrhoea would be anticipated.

Treatment: Unless 5 times the normal total daily dose has been ingested, gastrointestinal decontamination will not be necessary.

General management may consist of supportive therapy.

Pharmaceutical precautions Store at room temperature (15°–25°C). Keep containers tightly closed and protect from light. After reconstitution, the suspension should be stored in a refrigerator (2°–8°C) and be used within 14 days. When dilution is unavoidable, Syrup BP should be used after the suspension has been prepared according to the manufacturer's instructions.

Legal category POM.

Package quantities
Capsules 250 mg: Bottles of 20 and 100.
Capsules 500 mg: Bottles of 50.
Suspension 125 mg/5 ml: Bottles of 100 ml.
Suspension 250 mg/5 ml: Bottles of 100 ml.

Further information Nil.

Product licence numbers

Capsules 250 mg	0006/0118
Capsules 500 mg	0006/0119
Suspension 125 mg/5 ml	0006/0120
Suspension 250 mg/5 ml	0006/0121

DOBUTREX*

Presentation Dobutrex (dobutamine hydrochloride for injection) is available as:— Dobutrex Solution: Vials containing 20 ml of sterile solution, for intravenous use only. Each ml contains 12.5 mg dobutamine, 0.24 mg sodium bisulphite and water for injection.

Uses *Actions:* The primary action of dobutamine is to augment cardiac contractility by stimulating the β_1 receptors of the heart. It is a direct-acting agent.

Indications: Dobutrex is indicated for adults who require inotropic support in the treatment of low output cardiac failure associated with myocardial infarction, open heart surgery, cardiomyopathies, septic shock and cardiogenic shock. Dobutrex can also increase or maintain cardiac output during positive end expiratory pressure (PEEP) ventilation.

Dobutrex may also be used for cardiac stress testing as an alternative to exercise in patients for whom routine exercise testing cannot be satisfactorily performed. This use of dobutamine should only be undertaken in units which already perform exercise stress testing and all normal care and precautions required for such testing are also required when using dobutamine for this purpose.

Dosage and administration For intravenous administration only.

Dobutrex Solution must be further diluted to at least 50 ml prior to administration in an i.v. container with one of the intravenous solutions listed below:

Sodium Chloride Intravenous Infusion BP
5% Dextrose Intravenous Infusion BP
5% Dextrose + 0.9% Sodium Chloride Intravenous Infusion BP
5% Dextrose + 0.45% Sodium Chloride Intravenous Infusion BP
Sodium Lactate Intravenous Infusion BP

If diluting to 250 ml or 500 ml, dilution will give a concentration for administration as follows:

250 ml contains 1,000 micrograms/ml of dobutamine
500 ml contains 500 micrograms/ml of dobutamine

The prepared solution should be used within 24 hours.

Administration: Due to its short half-life, Dobutrex must be administered as a continuous intravenous infusion. After dilution, Dobutrex should be administered intravenously through an intravenous needle or catheter. An i.v. drip chamber or other suitable metering device is essential for controlling the rate of flow in drops per minute.

Recommended dosage for adults and the elderly: Most patients will respond satisfactorily to doses ranging from 2.5 to 10 micrograms/kg/minute. Occasionally, however, a dose as low as 0.5 micrograms/kg/minute will elicit a response. Rarely, a dose as high as 40 micrograms/kg/minute is required.

The rate of administration and the duration of therapy should be adjusted according to the patient's response as determined by heart rate, blood pressure, urine flow, and, if possible, measurement of cardiac output.

Rather than abruptly discontinuing therapy with Dobutrex, it is often advisable to decrease the dosage gradually.

Side-effects, which are dose-related, are infrequent when Dobutrex is administered at rates below 10 micrograms/kg/minute. Rates as high as 40 micrograms/kg/minute have been used occasionally without significant adverse effects.

The final volume administered should be determined by the fluid requirements of the patient. Concentrations as high as 5,000 micrograms/ml have been used in patients on a restricted fluid intake. High concentrations of dobutamine should only be given with an infusion pump, to ensure accurate dosage.

Cardiac stress testing: When used as an alternative to exercise for cardiac stress testing the recommended dose is an incremental increase of 5 micrograms/kg/min from 5 up to 20 micrograms/kg/min, each dose being infused for 8 minutes. Continuous ECG monitoring is essential and the infusion terminated in the event of >3 mm ST segment depression or any ventricular arrhythmia. The infusion should also be terminated if heart rate reaches the age/sex maximum, systolic blood pressure rises above 220 mm Hg or any side-effects occur – see 'Side-effects'.

Paediatric use: The safety and efficacy of dobutamine for use in children have not been established.

Contra-indications, warnings, etc

Contra-indication: Previous hypersensitivity to dobutamine.

Warnings: If an undue increase in heart rate or systolic blood pressure occurs or if an arrhythmia is precipitated, the dose of dobutamine should be reduced or the drug should be discontinued temporarily.

Dobutamine may precipitate or exacerbate ventricular ectopic activity; rarely has it caused ventricular tachycardia or fibrillation. Because dobutamine facilitates atrioventricular conduction, patients with atrial flutter or fibrillation may develop rapid ventricular responses.

Particular care should be exercised when dobutamine is used in patients with acute myocardial infarction because any significant increase in heart rate or excessive increases in arterial pressure that occur may intensify ischaemia and cause anginal pain and ST segment elevation.

Inotropic agents, including dobutamine, do not improve haemodynamics in most patients with mechanical obstruction that hinders either ventricular filling or outflow, or both. Inotropic response may be inadequate in patients with markedly reduced ventricular compliance. Such conditions are present in cardiac tamponade, valvular aortic stenosis, and idiopathic hypertrophic subaortic stenosis.

Minimal vasoconstriction has occasionally been observed, most notably in patients recently treated with a β-blocking drug. As the inotropic effect of dobutamine stems from stimulation of cardiac β_1 receptors, this effect is prevented by β-blocking drugs. However, dobutamine has been shown to counteract the cardiodepressive effects of β-blocking drugs. Conversely, α-adrenergic blockade may make the β_1 and β_2 effects apparent, resulting in tachycardia and vasodilatation.

The use of dobutamine as an alternative to exercise for cardiac stress testing is not recommended for patients with unstable angina, bundle branch block, valvular heart disease, aortic outflow obstruction or any cardiac condition that could make them unsuitable for exercise stress testing.

Usage in pregnancy: Reproduction studies performed in rats and rabbits have revealed no evidence of impaired fertility, harm to the fetus, or teratogenic effects due to dobutamine. As there are no adequate and well-controlled studies in pregnant women, and as animal reproduction studies are not always predictive of human response, dobutamine should not be used during pregnancy unless the potential benefits outweigh the potential risks to the fetus.

Precautions: During the administration of dobutamine, as with any parenteral catecholamine, heart rate and rhythm, arterial blood pressure, and infusion rate should be monitored closely. When initiating therapy, electrocardiographic monitoring is advisable until a stable response is achieved.

Precipitous decreases in blood pressure have occasionally been described in association with dobutamine therapy. Decreasing the dose or discontinuing the infusion typically results in rapid return of blood pressure to base-line values, but rarely intervention may be required and reversibility may not be immediate.

Dobutamine should be used with caution in the presence of severe hypotension complicating cardiogenic shock (mean arterial pressure less than 70 mm Hg).

Hypovolaemia should be corrected when necessary with whole blood or plasma before dobutamine is administered.

If arterial blood pressure remains low or decreases progressively during administration of dobutamine despite adequate ventricular filling pressure and cardiac output, consideration may be given to the concomitant use of a peripheral vasoconstrictor agent, such as dopamine or noradrenaline.

Dobutrex contains sodium bisulphite. Sulphites may cause allergic-type reactions, including anaphylactic symptoms and life-threatening or less severe asthmatic episodes in certain susceptible people. Sulphite sensitivity is seen more frequently in asthmatic than in non-asthmatic people.

Side-effects: For cardiovascular effects, see 'Warnings' and 'Precautions' sections.

Reactions at site of intravenous infusion: Phlebitis has occasionally been reported. Local inflammatory changes have been described following inadvertent infiltration.

The following side-effects have been reported rarely: nausea, headache, anginal pain, nonspecific chest pain, palpitations, shortness of breath, and reactions suggestive of hypersensitivity, including rash, fever, eosinophilia and bronchospasm.

As with other catecholamines, decreases in serum potassium concentrations have occurred, rarely to hypokalaemic values.

Long-term safety: Infusions for up to 72 hours have revealed no adverse effects other than those seen with shorter infusions. There is evidence that partial tolerance develops with continuous infusions of dobutamine for 72 hours or more; therefore, higher doses may be required to maintain the same effects.

Overdosage: Overdoses of dobutamine have been reported rarely. The symptoms of toxicity may include anorexia, nausea, vomiting, tremor, anxiety, palpitations, headache, shortness of breath and anginal and non-specific chest pain. The positive inotropic and chronotropic effects of dobutamine may cause hypertension, tachyarrhythmias, myocardial ischaemia and ventricular fibrillation. Hypotension may result from vasodilatation.

The duration of action of dobutamine hydrochloride is generally short (half-life, approximately 2 minutes).

Temporarily discontinue dobutamine until the patient's condition stabilises. The patient should be monitored and any appropriate resuscitative measures initiated promptly.

Forced diuresis, peritoneal dialysis, haemodialysis, or charcoal haemoperfusion have not been established as beneficial.

If the product is ingested, unpredictable absorption may occur from the mouth and gastrointestinal tract.

Pharmaceutical precautions

Undiluted vials of Dobutrex Solution: Store below 25°C.

Prepared intravenous solutions are stable for 24 hours at room temperature.

Do not add Dobutrex to 5% Sodium Bicarbonate Intravenous Infusion BP or to any other strongly alkaline solutions. Because of potential physical incompatibilities, it is recommended that dobutamine hydrochloride not be mixed with other drugs in the same solution.

Dobutamine hydrochloride should not be used with other agents or diluents containing both sodium bisulphite and ethanol.

Solutions containing Dobutrex may turn pink; the colour may intensify with time. This colour change is due to slight oxidation of the drug, but there is no significant loss of potency during the recommended storage period.

Legal category POM.

Package quantity
Dobutrex Solution: Single 20 ml vials containing 250 mg dobutamine hydrochloride.

Further information Nil.

Product licence number 0006/0180

DOLOXENE*

Presentation Capsules (opaque orange, coded H64) containing 100 mg Dextropropoxyphene Napsylate BP (approximately equivalent to 65 mg dextropropoxyphene hydrochloride or 60 mg dextropropoxyphene base).

Uses
Actions: Dextropropoxyphene is a mild narcotic analgesic structurally related to methadone.

Indication: For the relief of mild to moderate pain.

Dosage and administration For oral administration to adults only. The usual dose is one capsule three or four times daily, and should not normally be exceeded. Consideration should be given to a reduced total daily dosage in patients with hepatic or renal impairment.

The elderly: There is evidence of prolonged half-life in the elderly, so reduction in dosage should be considered.

Children: Dextropropoxyphene is not recommended for use in children.

Contra-indications, warnings, etc
Contra-indications: Hypersensitivity to dextropropoxyphene.

Use in patients who are suicidal or addiction prone.

Warnings: PATIENTS SHOULD BE ADVISED NOT TO EXCEED THE RECOMMENDED DOSE AND TO AVOID ALCOHOL.

Dextropropoxyphene products in excessive doses, either alone or in combination with other CNS depressants, including alcohol, are a major cause of drug-related deaths. Fatalities within the first hour of overdosage are not uncommon and can occur within 15 minutes. Some deaths have occurred as a consequence of the accidental ingestion of excessive quantities of dextropropoxyphene alone, or in combination with other drugs.

Dextropropoxyphene should be prescribed with caution for those patients whose medical condition requires the concomitant administration of sedatives, tranquillisers, muscle relaxants, antidepressants or other CNS-depressant drugs. Patients should be advised of the additive depressant effects of these combinations. Doloxene should also be prescribed with caution in patients who use alcohol in excess.

Drug dependence: Dextropropoxyphene, when taken in higher than recommended doses over long periods of time, can produce drug dependence.

Ambulatory patients: Dextropropoxyphene may impair abilities required for tasks such as driving a car or operating machinery. The patient should be cautioned accordingly.

Pregnancy: Safety in pregnancy has not been established relative to possible adverse effects on fetal development. Withdrawal symptoms in neonates have been reported following use during pregnancy. Therefore, dextropropoxyphene should not be used in pregnant women unless, in the judgement of the physician, the potential benefits outweigh the possible hazards.

Nursing mothers: Low levels of dextropropoxyphene have been detected in human milk. In postpartum studies involving nursing mothers who were given dextropropoxyphene, no adverse effects were noted in the infants.

Precautions: Dextropropoxyphene should be administered with caution to patients with hepatic or renal impairment since higher serum concentrations or delayed elimination may occur.

Drug interactions: The CNS-depressant effect of dextropropoxyphene is additive with that of other CNS depressants, including alcohol.

Dextropropoxyphene may interfere with the metabolism of antidepressants, anticonvulsants and warfarin-like drugs. Severe neurological signs, including coma, have occurred with concomitant use of carbamazepine.

Side-effects: The most frequently reported have been dizziness, sedation, nausea and vomiting. Some of these side-effects may be alleviated if the patient lies down.

Other side-effects include constipation, abdominal pain, rashes, light-headedness, headache, weakness, euphoria, dysphoria, hallucinations and minor visual disturbances.

Dextropropoxyphene therapy has been associated with abnormal liver function tests and, more rarely, with instances of reversible jaundice.

Subacute painful myopathy has occurred following chronic dextropropoxyphene overdosage.

Chronic ingestion of dextropropoxyphene in doses exceeding 720 mg per day has caused toxic psychoses and convulsions.

Overdosage: Initial consideration should be given to the management of the CNS effects of dextropropoxyphene overdosage. Resuscitative measures should be initiated promptly.

In the acute phase dextropropoxyphene produces symptoms typical of narcosis, with somnolence or coma and respiratory depression, sometimes with convulsions. Blood pressure falls and cardiac performance deteriorates. Cardiac arrhythmias and conduction delay may be present. A combined respiratory-metabolic acidosis occurs, which may be severe if large amounts of salicylates have also been ingested. Death may occur.

Naloxone will reduce the respiratory depression and 0.4–2 mg iv should be administered promptly. (This may be repeated at 2–3 minute intervals, but if there is no response after 10 mg of naloxone the diagnosis should be questioned.) The duration of antagonism may be brief and need repeating for up to 24 hours. Mechanical ventilation, with oxygen may be required, and PEEP ventilation is desirable if pulmonary oedema is present.

Blood gases, pH and electrolytes should be monitored and electrocardiographic monitoring is essential. Ventricular fibrillation or cardiac arrest may occur. Respiratory acidosis rapidly subsides as ventilation is restored and hypercapnoea eliminated, but lactic acidosis may require iv bicarbonate for prompt correction. In addition to the use of a narcotic antagonist, the patient may require titration with an anti-convulsant to control convulsions. Gastric lavage may be useful and activated charcoal can absorb a significant amount of ingested dextropropoxyphene.

Treatment of dextropropoxyphene overdose in children: See general comments above. Naloxone at 0.01 mg/kg body weight iv should be administered promptly. If there is no response a dose of 0.1 mg/kg iv may be used.

Pharmaceutical precautions Store below 25°C.

Legal category CD (Sch 5), POM.

Package quantity Blister packs of 100 (10 strips of 10 capsules).

Further information Animal toxicology studies indicate that, on a molar basis, the napsylate salt of dextropropoxyphene is less toxic than the hydrochloride. This may be due to its relative insolubility and retarded absorption.

Product licence number 0006/5068.

DOLOXENE* Compound

Presentation Hard gelatin capsules (light grey opaque cap, red opaque body, coded H91) each containing: Dextropropoxyphene Napsylate BP 100 mg (approximately equivalent to 65 mg dextropropoxyphene hydrochloride or 60 mg dextropropoxyphene base)

Aspirin PhEur	375 mg
Caffeine PhEur	30 mg

Uses

Actions: Dextropropoxyphene is a mild narcotic analgesic structurally related to methadone.

Indication: For the relief of mild to moderate pain.

Dosage and administration For oral administration to adults only. The usual dose is one capsule three or four times daily, and should not normally be exceeded. Consideration should be given to a reduced total daily dosage in patients with hepatic or renal impairment.

The elderly: There is evidence of prolonged half-life in the elderly, so reduction in dosage should be considered. The elderly are more likely to experience gastric side-effects and tinnitus with aspirin.

Children: Doloxene Compound is not recommended for use in children.

Contra-indications, warnings, etc

Contra-indications

Hypersensitivity to any of the constituents, hypoprothrombinaemia, haemophilia and active peptic ulceration.

Use in patients who are suicidal or addiction-prone.

Warnings: PATIENTS SHOULD BE ADVISED NOT TO EXCEED THE RECOMMENDED DOSE AND TO AVOID ALCOHOL.

Dextropropoxyphene products in excessive doses, either alone or in combination with other CNS depressants, including alcohol, are a major cause of drug-related deaths. Fatalities within the first hour of overdosage are not uncommon and can occur within 15 minutes. Some deaths have occurred as a consequence of the accidental ingestion of excessive quantities alone, or in combination with other drugs.

Doloxene Compound should be prescribed with caution for those patients whose medical condition requires the concomitant administration of sedatives, tranquillisers, muscle relaxants, antidepressants or other CNS-depressant drugs; patients should be advised of the additive depressant effects of these combinations. Doloxene Compound should also be prescribed with caution in patients who use alcohol in excess.

Salicylates should be used with caution in patients with a history of peptic ulceration or coagulation abnormalities. They may also induce gastro-intestinal haemorrhage, occasionally major.

In large doses, salicylates may also decrease insulin requirements.

High doses of caffeine may cause tremors and palpitations.

Drug dependence: Dextropropoxyphene, when taken in higher than recommended doses over long periods of time, can produce drug dependence.

Ambulatory patients: Dextropropoxyphene may impair abilities required for tasks such as driving a car or operating machinery. The patient should be cautioned accordingly.

Pregnancy: Safety in pregnancy has not been established relative to possible adverse effects on fetal development. Instances of withdrawal symptoms in the neonate have been reported following usage of dextropropoxyphene. Aspirin may prolong labour and contribute to maternal and neonatal bleeding and it is best avoided at term. Therefore, Doloxene Compound should not be used in pregnant women unless, in the judgement of the physician, the potential benefits outweigh the possible hazards.

Nursing mothers: Low levels of dextropropoxyphene have been detected in human milk. In postpartum studies involving nursing mothers who were given dextropropoxyphene, no adverse effects were noted in the infants. Aspirin is also excreted in breast milk.

Precautions: Dextropropoxyphene should be administered with caution to patients with hepatic or renal impairment since higher serum concentrations or delayed elimination may occur.

Drug interactions: The CNS-depressant effect of dextropropoxyphene is additive with that of other CNS depressants, including alcohol.

Dextropropoxyphene may interfere with the metabolism of antidepressants, anticonvulsants and warfarin-like drugs. Severe neurological signs, including coma, have occurred with concurrent use of carbamazepine.

Aspirin may enhance the effect of anticoagulants, inhibit uricosuric agents, precipitate bronchospasm or induce asthma in susceptible individuals.

Side-effects: The most frequently reported have been dizziness, sedation, nausea and vomiting. Some of these side-effects may be alleviated if the patient lies down.

Other side-effects include constipation, abdominal pain, rashes, light-headedness, headache, weakness, euphoria, dysphoria, hallucinations and minor visual disturbances.

Dextropropoxyphene therapy has been associated with abnormal liver function tests and, more rarely, with instances of reversible jaundice.

Subacute painful myopathy has occurred following chronic dextropropoxyphene overdosage.

Chronic ingestion of dextropropoxyphene in doses exceeding 720 mg per day has caused toxic psychoses and convulsions.

Salicylates may induce hypersensitivity, asthma, urate kidney stones, chronic gastro-intestinal blood loss, tinnitus, nausea and vomiting.

Overdosage: Initial consideration should be given to the management of the CNS effects of dextropropoxyphene overdosage. Resuscitative measures should be initiated promptly.

Dextropropoxyphene: In the acute phase dextropropoxyphene produces symptoms typical of narcosis, with somnolence or coma and respiratory depression, sometimes with convulsions. Blood pressure falls and cardiac performance deteriorates. Cardiac arrhythmias and conduction delay may be present. A combined respiratory-metabolic acidosis occurs, which may be severe if large amounts of salicylates have also been ingested. Death may occur.

Naloxone will reduce the respiratory depression and 0.4–2 mg iv should be administered promptly. (This may be repeated at 2–3 minute intervals, but if there is no response after 10 mg of naloxone the diagnosis should be questioned.) The duration of antagonism may be brief and need repeating for up to 24 hours. Mechanical ventilation, with oxygen may be required, and PEEP ventilation is desirable if pulmonary oedema is present.

Blood gases, pH and electrolytes should be monitored and electrocardiographic monitoring is essential. Ventricular fibrillation or cardiac arrest may occur. Respiratory acidosis rapidly subsides as ventilation is restored and hypercapnoea eliminated, but lactic acidosis may require iv bicarbonate for prompt correction. In addition to the use of a narcotic antagonist, the patient may require titration with an anticonvulsant to control convulsions. Gastric lavage may be useful and activated charcoal can absorb a significant amount of ingested dextropropoxyphene.

Treatment of dextropropoxyphene overdose in children: See general comments above. Naloxone at 0.01 mg/kg body weight iv should be administered promptly. If there is no response a dose of 0.1 mg/kg iv may be used.

Aspirin: Overdosage produces dizziness, tinnitus, sweating, nausea and vomiting, confusion and hyperventilation. Gross overdosage may lead to CNS depression with coma, cardiovascular collapse and respiratory depression. If overdosage is suspected, the patient should be kept under observation for at least 24 hours, as symptoms and salicylate blood levels may not become apparent for several hours. Treatment of overdosage consists of gastric lavage and forced alkaline diuresis. Haemodialysis may be necessary in severe cases.

Pharmaceutical precautions Store below 25°C.

Legal category CD (Sch 5), POM.

Package quantity Blister packs of 100 (10 strips of 10 capsules).

Further information Nil.

Product licence number 0006/0091.

ELDISINE*

Presentation Vials containing 5 mg Eldisine (vindesine sulphate for injection) and 25 mg Mannitol BP. (Supplied in a combination package with an accompanying vial of diluting solution, 5 ml containing 45 mg Sodium Chloride PhEur with 2% Benzyl Alcohol BP as a preservative.)

Uses Eldisine is an anti-neoplastic drug for intravenous use which can be used alone or in combination with other oncolytic drugs. Information available at present suggests that Eldisine as a single agent may be useful for the treatment of: acute lymphoblastic leukaemia of childhood resistant to other drugs; blastic crises of chronic myeloid leukaemia; malignant melanoma unresponsive to other forms of therapy; advanced carcinoma of the breast, unresponsive to appropriate endocrine surgery and/or hormonal therapy.

Dosage and administration This preparation is for intravenous use only. Intrathecal administration has resulted in death (see 'Warnings' for treatment).

Extreme care must be used in calculating and administering the dose of vindesine, since overdosage may have a very serious or fatal outcome.

It is recommended that the drug be administered intravenously in a single rapid bolus injection at weekly intervals. The size of the dose is determined by body surface area. In adults and the elderly, the recommended starting dose is 3 mg/m^2, and children may be started at 4 mg/m^2. Thereafter, granulocyte counts should be made prior to each subsequent dose to determine the patient's sensitivity to the drug. Provided there is no granulocytopenia or other toxicity (see 'Adverse Reactions') the dosage may be increased in 0.5 mg/m^2 steps at weekly intervals.

In adults, the maximum total weekly dosage for which data exists is 4 mg/m^2. The optimum dose of vindesine is that which produces mild to modest granulocytopenia. Sustained granulocyte counts lower than 2,500 cells/mm^3 are to be avoided.

Those with decreased marrow function from leukaemia infiltration or replacement will require full doses to attempt to restore marrow function. This must be done under close supervision.

The dose should not be increased after that dose which: (i) reduces the granulocyte count to below 1500 cells/mm^3 or, on rare occasions, (ii) reduces the platelet count to below 100,000/mm^3; (iii) causes acute abdominal pain (see under 'Precautions').

On each of the above occasions there should be full recovery before administering the next dose, which should be reduced from the one causing the adverse reaction. For most patients, however, the weekly dosage will prove to be in the range of 3.0 to 4.0 mg/m^2 in adults and 4.0 to 5.0 mg/m^2 in children.

The use of small amounts of vindesine daily for long periods is not advised, even though the resulting total weekly dosage may be similar to that recommended. Little or no added therapeutic advantage has been demonstrated when such regimens have been used, and side-effects are increased. Strict adherence to the recommended dosage schedule is very important.

To prepare a solution containing 1 mg/ml add the 5 ml of accompanying diluting solution to the 5 mg of Eldisine in the sterile vial. The drug dissolves rapidly to give a clear solution.

The dose of Eldisine solution (calculated to provide the desired number of milligrams per square metre of the patient's surface area) may be injected either into the tubing of a running intravenous infusion (*compatible infusions are 5% Dextrose Intravenous Infusion BP, Sodium Chloride Intravenous Infusion BP and dextrose/saline infusions)* or directly into a vein.

The latter procedure is readily adaptable to outpatient therapy. In either case, the injection should be completed in 1 to 3 minutes. If care is taken to ensure that the needle is securely within the vein and that no solution containing vindesine is spilled extravascularly, cellulitis and/or phlebitis is unlikely to occur.

Because of the enhanced possibility of thrombosis, it is considered inadvisable to inject a solution into an extremity in which the circulation is impaired, or potentially impaired, by such conditions as compressing or invading neoplasm, phlebitis or varicosity.

Caution: It is extremely important to choose the largest accessible vein and to be certain that the needle is properly positioned in the vein before any vindesine is injected. If leakage into surrounding tissue should occur during intravenous administration, it may cause considerable irritation. The injection should be discontinued as soon as leakage occurs, and any remaining portion of the dose should then be introduced into another vein. Local injection of hyaluronidase and the application of moderate heat to the area of leakage help disperse the drug and are thought to minimise discomfort and the possibility of cellulitis.

Contra-indications, warnings, etc
Contra-indications
Intrathecal administration: Intrathecal administration has resulted in death (see 'Warnings' for treatment).

Use in patients who have drug-induced severe granulocytopenia (less than 1,500 granulocytes per mm^3) or severe thrombocytopenia. Vindesine should not be used in the presence of bacterial infection. Such infections must be brought under control with antiseptics or antibiotics before using vindesine.

Patients with the demyelinating form of Charcot-Marie-Tooth syndrome should not be given vindesine.

Warning

Syringes containing this product should be labelled 'WARNING – VINDESINE SULPHATE FOR INTRAVENOUS USE ONLY'.

The following treatment successfully arrested progressive paralysis in a single patient mistakenly given the related vinca alkaloid, vincristine sulphate, intrathecally. This treatment should be initiated immediately:

1. Removal of as much CSF as is safely possible.
2. Flushing with Lactated Ringer's solution by continuous infusion at 150 ml/h, through a catheter in a cerebral lateral ventricle and removed through lumbar access, until fresh frozen plasma became available.
3. Fresh frozen plasma, 25 ml, diluted with 1 l of Lactated Ringer's was then infused similarly at 75 ml/h. The rate of infusion should be adjusted to maintain a spinal fluid protein level of 150 mg/dl.
4. Glutamic acid, 10 gm, was given iv over 24 hours, followed by 500 mg tds by mouth for 1 month. Glutamic acid may not be essential.

Usage in pregnancy or lactation: The safety of this product for use during pregnancy has not been established. Animal studies with vindesine suggest that teratogenic effects may occur. The benefit-to-risk ratio must be carefully considered before use in pregnant patients. Eldisine should not normally be given to mothers who are breast feeding.

Precautions: Clinically, the dose-limiting toxicity of vindesine is granulocytopenia, although in general oncolytic activity is obtained at doses causing little or no effect on the granulocytes. Individual patient variation has been observed with respect to the severity of side-effects, including neurotoxicity, granulocytopenia, alopecia, and decrease in bowel motility.

When granulocytopenia occurs, the nadir in the granulocyte count may be expected to occur 3–5 days after the last day of drug administration. Recovery of the granulocyte count is rapid thereafter and is usually complete within 7–10 days after the last dose.

The thrombocyte count is usually either unaffected or increased by weekly therapy with vindesine. However, significant thrombocytopenia has occurred occasionally, particularly when doses are given more frequently than once a week. It is probably more likely to occur when patients are thrombocytopenic (less than 100,000 cells/mm^3) prior to therapy with vindesine.

The effect of vindesine upon the red blood cell count and haemoglobin concentration is usually insignificant when other treatment does not complicate the picture. It should be remembered, however, that patients with malignant disease may exhibit anaemia even in the absence of any treatment.

If granulocytopenia with less than 1,000 granulocytes/mm^3 occurs following a dose of vindesine, the patient should be watched carefully for evidence of infection until the granulocyte count has returned to a safe level.

While neurotoxicity is not usually dose-limiting, there have been instances in which neurotoxicity has made it necessary to reduce the dosage or temporarily discontinue use of vindesine. Neurotoxicity induced by vindesine is believed to be generally less severe and less progressive in nature than the effects observed with vincristine.

Particular attention should be given to dosage and neurological side-effects if vindesine is administered to patients with pre-existing neuromuscular disease, and also when other drugs with neurotoxic potential are being used. The neurotoxicity associated with vindesine therapy may be additive.

Care should be exercised when vindesine has been the cause of acute abdominal pain, as paralytic ileus may be a significant risk if further doses of vindesine are given, particularly if the dose is increased. Prophylactic measures should be taken to prevent obstipation that may result from a decrease in bowel motility.

As vindesine is excreted principally by the liver, it may be necessary to reduce initial doses in the presence of significantly impaired hepatic or biliary function.

When chemotherapy is being given in conjunction with radiation therapy through portals which include the liver, the use of vindesine should be delayed until radiation therapy has been completed.

Acute shortness of breath and severe bronchospasm have been reported following the administration of vindesine. These reactions have been encountered most frequently when vindesine was used in combination with mitomycin-C and may be serious when there is pre-existing pulmonary dysfunction. The onset may be within minutes, or several hours after the drug is injected and may occur up to 2 weeks after a dose of mitomycin-C.

The simultaneous oral or intravenous administration of phenytoin and antineoplastic chemotherapy combinations have been reported to have reduced blood levels of the anticonvulsant and to have increased seizure activity. Although the contribution of the vinca alkaloids has not been established, dosage adjustment of phenytoin may need to be made when used in combination with vindesine.

Extreme care should be exercised to prevent injection outside the vein. Extravasation during intravenous injection will cause cellulitis and phlebitis. If the amount of extravasation is great, sloughing will occur. Healing of such wounds may require several weeks and be attended by severe pain. The discomfort may persist after healing of the ulcer.

Care must be taken to avoid contamination of the eye with concentrations of vindesine used clinically. If accidental contamination occurs, severe irritation and/or corneal ulceration may result. The eye should be washed immediately and thoroughly with water or saline.

Adverse reactions: Prior to the use of the drug, patients and/or their parents/guardians should be advised of the possibility of untoward symptoms. Acute toxicity appears to be dose related and is more likely to occur if doses above 4 mg/m^2 are employed. Granulocytopenia is usually the dose-limiting factor. Neurotoxicity is common and appears to be related to the cumulative total dose given.

The following side-effects have been reported:

Gastrointestinal: Nausea, vomiting, constipation, vesiculation of the mouth, ileus, diarrhoea, anorexia, abdominal pain, dysphagia, dyspepsia, perforated duodenal ulcer (nausea and vomiting usually may be controlled by antiemetic agents).

Neurological: Numbness and tingling of digits, peripheral neuritis, jaw pain, mental depression, loss of deep-tendon reflexes, foot drop, headache, convulsions. Cortical blindness has been reported in patients treated with multiple-agent chemotherapy that has included vindesine. The contribution of vindesine to this reaction is unknown.

Haematological: Granulocytopenia, thrombocytopenia, thrombocytosis, mild anaemia.

Pulmonary: See under 'Precautions'.

Cutaneous: Alopecia from mild to total is the commonest side-effect. Regrowth of hair may occur while still on therapy. Maculopapular rashes, cellulitis with extravasation.

Miscellaneous: Generalised musculoskeletal pain, malaise, chills and fevers, asthenia.

Overdosage: Side-effects following the use of vindesine are dose related. Therefore, following administration of more than the recommended dose, patients can be expected to experience these effects in an exaggerated fashion.

Supportive care should include: (a) daily blood counts for guidance in transfusion requirement; (b) prevention of the side-effects that result from the syndrome of inappropriate secretion of antidiuretic hormone. This includes restriction of fluid intake and, perhaps, the use of a diuretic drug acting on the loop of Henle and distal tubule function; (c) use of cathartics to prevent ileus; (d) administration of an anticonvulsant; (e) monitoring the patient's cardiovascular system.

The use of folinic acid in addition to the other supportive measures recommended may be considered although, unlike vincristine, studies have not been conducted to confirm its protective action. Clinical experience of vindesine overdosage is extremely limited, with only one published case.

Pharmaceutical precautions

Guidelines for the safe handling of antineoplastic agents: Cytotoxic preparations should not be handled by pregnant staff.

Trained personnel should reconstitute the drug. This should be performed in a designated area. The work surface should be covered with disposable plastic-backed absorbent paper.

Adequate protective gloves, masks and clothing should be worn. Precautions should be taken to avoid the drug accidentally coming into contact with the eyes. If accidental contamination occurs, the eye should be washed with water or saline thoroughly and immediately.

Use Luer-lock fittings on all syringes and sets. Large bore needles are recommended to minimise pressure and the possible formation of aerosols. The latter may also be reduced by the use of a venting needle.

Adequate care and precaution should be taken in the disposal of items (syringes, needles, etc.) used to reconstitute cytotoxic drugs.

Vials of Eldisine should be stored in a refrigerator between 2° and 8°C.

After reconstitution: After a portion of the solution has been removed from a vial, the remainder of the contents of the vial may be stored in a refrigerator for future use for 30 days without significant loss of potency. When the reconstituted vial of Eldisine is to be stored for more than 48 hours, it is essential to use the accompanying diluting solution or a diluent which contains a preservative.

Eldisine should never be mixed with any other drug.

Legal category POM.

Package quantities Vials 5 mg: Single vials.

Further information Nil.

Product licence numbers
Vials 5 mg 0006/0137
Diluent 0006/5174

GLUCAGON

Presentation The product is in lyophilised form and is supplied with an accompanying diluting solution.

Vials containing 1 unit (1.09 mg) of glucagon as the hydrochloride with 49 mg of Lactose PhEur. (Diluting solution, 1 ml, containing Glycerol PhEur, 1.6%, with phenol, 0.2%, as a preservative. Sodium hydroxide and/or hydrochloric acid may have been added during manufacture to adjust the pH.)

Crystalline glucagon is a white powder containing less than 0.05% zinc. It is relatively insoluble in water but is soluble at a pH of less than 3 or more than 9.5. Glucagon is stable in lyophilised form at room temperatures.

Uses *Actions:* Glucagon causes an increase in blood glucose concentrations and is used in the treatment of hypoglycaemic states. It is effective in small doses. Glucagon acts only on liver glycogen, converting it to glucose, and is therefore helpful only if liver glycogen is available. It is of little or no help in states of starvation, adrenal insufficiency or chronic hypoglycaemia. The patient with Type I diabetes does not have as great a response in blood glucose levels as does the Type II stable diabetic, therefore supplementary carbohydrate should be given as soon as possible, especially to juvenile patients.

Parenteral administration of glucagon produces relaxation of the smooth muscle of the stomach, duodenum, small bowel and colon.

Indications: Glucagon is useful in counteracting severe hypoglycaemic reactions.

Glucagon is indicated as a diagnostic aid in the radiological examination of the stomach, duodenum, small bowel and colon, when a hypotonic state would be advantageous.

Glucagon is as effective for this examination as the anti-cholinergic drugs, but it has fewer side-effects. When glucagon is administered concomitantly with an anticholinergic agent, the response is not significantly greater than when either drug is used alone. However, the addition of the anticholinergic agent results in increased side-effects.

Dosage and administration The diluent is provided for use only in the preparation of glucagon for *intermittent* parenteral injection and for no other use.

Glucagon should not be used at concentrations greater than 1 unit/ml (1 mg/ml).

Glucagon may be given by subcutaneous, intramuscular or intravenous injection. Administration as a continuous intravenous infusion for long periods is not recommended.

Dosage in the elderly: As for adults.

Directions for the use of glucagon in hypoglycaemia:

1. Dissolve the lyophilised glucagon in the accompanying diluent.
2. Give 0.5–1 unit (0.5–1 mg) of glucagon by subcutaneous, intramuscular or intravenous injection. These doses are equally suitable for adults and children.
3. The patient will normally awaken in 15 minutes. If the response is delayed, there is no contra-indication to the administration of 1 or 2 additional doses of glucagon: however, in view of the deleterious effects of cerebral hypoglycaemia and depending on the duration and depth of coma, the use of parenteral glucose must be considered.
4. Intravenous glucose *must* be given if the patient fails to respond to glucagon.
5. When the patient responds, give supplementary carbohydrate to restore the liver glycogen and prevent secondary hypoglycaemia.

It is important that the patient be aroused as quickly as possible, because prolonged hypoglycaemic reactions may result in cortical damage. Glucagon or intravenous glucose will awaken the patient sufficiently so that oral carbohydrates may be taken.

Although the patient or family members may use glucagon for the treatment of hypoglycaemia during an emergency, a doctor must still be notified when hypoglycaemic reactions occur so that the treatment regimen may be adjusted if necessary.

For use as a diagnostic aid: Dissolve the lyophilised glucagon in the accompanying diluting solution. Glucagon should not be used at concentrations greater than 1 unit/ml (1 mg/ml).

The following doses may be administered for relaxation of the stomach, duodenum, and small bowel, depending on the time of onset of action and the duration of effect required for the examination. Since the stomach is less sensitive to the effect of glucagon, 0.5 unit (0.5 mg) i.v. or 2 units (2 mg) i.m. are recommended.

Dose† (units)	*Route of administration*	*Time of onset of action (min)*	*Approximate duration of effect (min)*
0.25–0.5	i.v.	1	9–17
1	i.m.	8–10	12–27
2*	i.v.	1	22–25
2*	i.m.	4–7	21–32

*2-unit (2 mg) doses are associated with a higher incidence of nausea and vomiting than lower doses.
†1 unit equals 1 mg.

For examination of the colon, it is recommended that a 2-unit dose be administered intramuscularly approximately 10 minutes prior to initiation of the procedure. Relaxation of the colon and reduction of discomfort to the patient will allow the radiologist to perform a more satisfactory examination.

Contra-indications, warnings, etc
Contra-indications: Hypersensitivity to glucagon. Patients with phaeochromocytoma, where glucagon can cause the tumour to release catecholamines, which result in sudden and marked hypertension.

Warnings: Glucagon should be administered cautiously to patients with known or suspected insulinoma. In these patients intravenous administration of glucagon will produce an initial increase in blood glucose but, because of its insulin-releasing effect, may subsequently cause severe hypoglycaemia. A patient developing symptoms of hypoglycaemia after a dose of glucagon should be given glucose orally, intravenously, or by gavage, whichever is more appropriate.

Exogenous glucagon also stimulates the release of catecholamines. In the presence of phaeochromocytoma, glucagon can cause the tumour to release catecholamines, which results in a sudden and marked increase in blood pressure. Five to 10 mg of phentolamine mesylate may be administered i.v. in an attempt to control the blood pressure.

Glucagon may enhance the anticoagulant effect of warfarin.

Usage in pregnancy: Animal reproduction studies have revealed no evidence of impaired fertility or fetal harm due to glucagon. However, in the absence of adequate human studies, glucagon should be used during pregnancy only if clearly needed.

Usage in nursing mothers: It is not known whether this drug is excreted in human milk. Although the plasma half-life is only 3 to 6 minutes and it is not active when taken orally, caution should be exercised when glucagon is administered to a nursing woman.

Precautions: Glucagon is helpful in hypoglycaemia only if liver glycogen is available. Because glucagon is of little or no help in states of starvation, adrenal insufficiency, or chronic hypoglycaemia, glucose should be considered for the treatment of hypoglycaemia.

Blood glucose determinations may be obtained to follow the patient in hypoglycaemic shock until he is asymptomatic.

Glucagon should be used with caution as a diagnostic aid in diabetic patients.

Side-effects: Glucagon is relatively free of adverse reactions, except for occasional nausea and vomiting, which may also occur with hypoglycaemia. Diarrhoea and hypokalaemia have rarely been reported as well as generalised allergic reactions, including urticaria, respiratory distress and hypotension.

Overdosage

Signs and symptoms: Although there is a lack of human experience and glucagon is generally well tolerated, nausea, vomiting, gastric hypotonicity and diarrhoea would be expected. Intravenous glucagon has positive inotropic and chronotropic effects. Increases in blood pressure and pulse might be more severe in patients taking beta-blockers and might require therapy in patients with phaeochromocytoma, insulinomas or coronary artery disease. When large doses (0.5–16 mg/hour by continuous infusion for periods of 5–166 hours) were given to cardiac patients, positive inotropy occurred and side-effects included nausea, vomiting and decreasing serum potassium.

As a polypeptide, glucagon would be rapidly destroyed if ingested.

Treatment: The plasma half-life of glucagon is approximately 3–6 minutes. Symptomatic and supportive therapy might include supplemental potassium for hypokalaemia, or phentolamine if a dramatic increase in blood pressure occurs. Forced diuresis, peritoneal dialysis, haemodialysis, or charcoal haemoperfusion have not been established as beneficial.

Pharmaceutical precautions *Prior to reconstitution:* Store below 25°C. Use accompanying diluting fluid for reconstitution.

After reconstitution: Solutions should be used immediately. Glucagon solutions should not be used unless they are clear and of a water-like consistency.

If glucagon is to be given at doses higher than 2 units (2 mg), it should be reconstituted with Sterile Water for Injection, instead of the diluting solution supplied, and used immediately.

Legal category POM.

Package quantities Vials No. 666, 1 unit (1.09 mg) glucagon as the hydrochloride accompanied by Vials No. 667 containing 1 ml of diluent.

Further information Nil.

Product licence numbers

Vials 1 unit	0006/5110
Vials Diluting Solution	0006/5112

HUMATROPE* ▼

Presentation Vials containing 4 iu (1.48 mg) of somatropin as a sterile, white, lyophilised powder. The vial also contains mannitol, glycine and dibasic sodium phosphate. pH may have been adjusted with phosphoric acid and/or sodium hydroxide. Each vial is supplied in a combination package with an accompanying 2 ml vial of sterile Diluent containing 0.3% m-cresol as a preservative, and 1.7% glycerol.

Reconstituted solutions have a pH of approximately 7.5.

Uses Growth failure in children due to deficiency of endogenous growth hormone, as verified by appropriate tests of pituitary function. Growth failure in children associated with Turner's syndrome, as confirmed by chromosomal analysis. At present the effect on final height has not been determined.

Dosage and administration Humatrope is administered either as a subcutaneous or intramuscular injection. If injected subcutaneously, the injection sites should be rotated to minimise the risk of lipo-atrophy.

Growth hormone deficiency: The dosage and administration schedule should be individualised for each patient. Humatrope may be given either daily or three times a week. Treatment should stop at the time of epiphyseal fusion.

Daily: Dosage should be calculated according to body weight up to a maximum of 0.07 iu/kg (0.026 mg/kg) per day.

OR

Three times weekly: Dosage should be calculated according to body weight up to a maximum of 0.16 iu/kg (0.06 mg/kg) per dose.

Turner's syndrome: a dosage of 0.8–0.9 iu/kg (24–28 iu/m^2 or 0.3–0.33 mg/kg) of body weight, per week, is recommended. This weekly dose should be divided in 6–7 subcutaneous injections, to be administered in the evening.

To reconstitute, add the accompanying 2 ml of sterile Diluent. The Diluent should be injected into the vial of Humatrope by aiming the stream of liquid against the glass wall. The vial should then be swirled GENTLY until the contents are completely dissolved. DO NOT SHAKE. The resulting solution should be clear, without particulate matter. If the solution is cloudy or contains particulate matter, it must not be injected.

Before and after injection, the septum of the vial should be wiped with rubbing alcohol or another alcoholic antiseptic solution to prevent contamination of the contents by repeated needle insertions. Sterile disposable syringes and needles should be used for administration of Humatrope.

The volume of the syringe should be small enough so that the prescribed dose can be withdrawn from the vial with reasonable accuracy. The needle should be of sufficient length (usually 1 inch or more) to ensure that the injection reaches the muscle layer.

Contra-indications, warnings, etc

Contra-indications: Use in patients in whom epiphyseal fusion has occurred.

It should not be used when there is any evidence of activity of a tumour. Intracranial lesions must be inactive and antitumour therapy complete prior to starting Humatrope therapy. Humatrope should be discontinued if there is evidence of tumour growth.

Known hypersensitivity to m-cresol (but see 'Further information' section).

Warnings:

Usage in pregnancy and lactation: In the event of a pregnancy occurring during therapy with Humatrope, treatment should be discontinued as there is no evidence from either human or animal studies of the safety of growth hormone treatment during pregnancy.

No information is available as to whether peptide hormones pass into breast milk.

Precautions: Therapy with Humatrope should be directed by physicians who are experienced in the diagnosis and management of patients with growth hormone deficiency, and there should be appropriate monitoring of clinical, biochemical and radiological response.

Patients with growth hormone deficiency secondary to an intracranial lesion should be examined frequently for progression or recurrence of the underlying disease process.

In children who are both growth hormone deficient and diabetic, glycaemic control and insulin needs should be carefully monitored during somatropin therapy. An increased dose of insulin may be required. Also, as somatropin may induce a state of insulin resistance, patients should be observed for evidence of glucose intolerance.

Excessive glucocorticoid therapy will inhibit the growth promoting effect of somatropin. Thus, patients with coexisting ACTH deficiency should have their glucocorticoid replacement dose carefully adjusted to avoid an inhibitory effect on growth.

Hypothyroidism may develop during treatment with somatropin, and inadequate treatment of hypothyroidism may prevent optimal response to somatropin. Therefore, patients should have periodic thyroid function tests and be treated with thyroid hormone when indicated.

Patients with endocrine disorders, including growth

hormone deficiency, may develop slipped capital epiphyses more frequently. Any child with the onset of a limp during growth hormone therapy should be reviewed by a clinician.

Side-effects: A very small number of patients have developed antibodies to somatropin during clinical trials of Humatrope, but there is no evidence of growth attenuation associated with these antibodies. The long-term implications of antibody development are uncertain at present. Any patient who fails to respond to therapy should be tested for antibodies to human growth hormone.

In trials in Turner's syndrome, where higher doses of Humatrope are used, up to 8% of patients developed antibodies to growth hormone.

Other side-effects may include hypothyroidism (see 'Precautions'), oedema, and injection site reactions including pain.

Leukaemia has been reported in a small number of children who have been treated with growth hormone, including growth hormone of pituitary origin and recombinant somatropin. The relationship, if any, between leukaemia and growth hormone therapy is uncertain.

Overdosage: Acute overdosage could lead initially to hypoglycaemia and subsequently to hyperglycaemia. Long-term overdosage could result in signs and symptoms consistent with the known effects of human growth hormone excess.

Pharmaceutical precautions Both before and after reconstitution, Humatrope and Diluent should be stored in a refrigerator between 2° and 8°C. Avoid freezing the Diluent and reconstituted vial. If kept under these conditions, Humatrope is stable for up to 14 days after reconstitution.

The storage of reconstituted Humatrope solutions in plastic syringes should be avoided.

Legal category POM.

Package quantities Vials 4 iu (1.48 mg) accompanied by vials containing 2 ml of Diluent.

Further information Pharmacologically, somatropin behaves like endogenous growth hormone. After administration of Humatrope, somatomedin C (IGF-1) levels are seen to rise, cellular and organ growth increase as well as linear skeletal growth. Protein metabolism is altered as reflected by improved nitrogen balance and lipid metabolism altered as measured by increased lipid mobilisation. Mineral and connective tissue metabolism are also influenced.

If sensitivity to the Diluent should occur, Humatrope may be reconstituted with Water for Injection but only 1 reconstituted dose may be used per vial. The solution should be refrigerated between 2° and 8°C if not used immediately and must be used within 24 hours. Discard the unused portion.

Product licence numbers
Vials 4 iu 0006/0237
Diluent 0006/0254

HUMULIN VIALS AND CARTRIDGES
HUMULIN* S
HUMULIN* I
HUMULIN* Lente
HUMULIN* Zn
HUMULIN* M1
HUMULIN* M2
HUMULIN* M3
HUMULIN* M4

Presentation *Humulin S (Soluble):* A sterile, clear, colourless, aqueous solution of human insulin (prb) adjusted to a pH of 6.6–8.0.

Humulin I (Isophane): A sterile suspension of a white, crystalline precipitate of isophane human insulin (prb) in an isotonic phosphate buffer adjusted to a pH of 6.9–7.5.

Humulin Lente (Zinc suspension): A sterile suspension of 30% amorphous and 70% crystalline human insulin (prb) zinc suspension, adjusted to a pH of 6.9–7.5 (vials only).

Humulin Zn (Zinc suspension): A sterile, white suspension of crystalline human insulin (prb) zinc suspension, adjusted to a pH of 6.9–7.5 (vials only).

Humulin M1: A sterile suspension of human insulin (prb) in the proportion of 10% soluble insulin and 90% isophane insulin.

Humulin M2: A sterile suspension of human insulin (prb) in the proportion of 20% soluble insulin and 80% isophane insulin.

Humulin M3: A sterile suspension of human insulin (prb) in the proportion of 30% soluble insulin and 70% isophane insulin.

Humulin M4: A sterile suspension of human insulin (prb) in the proportion of 40% soluble insulin and 60% isophane insulin.

Each presentation contains 100 iu/ml.

Humulin S contains m-cresol as a preservative. Humulin I and the M mixtures contain m-cresol and phenol. Humulin Zn and Humulin Lente contain methyl parahydroxybenzoate as a preservative.

Humulin I and the M mixtures contain protamine. Humulin Lente and Humulin Zn contain zinc oxide.

Uses For the treatment of insulin-dependent diabetes mellitus.

Humulin S may also be of value during preparation of a diabetic patient for surgery, or in hyperglycaemic coma, trauma or severe infection.

Dosage and administration The dosage or type of insulin should be determined and adjusted only under medical supervision, according to the requirements of the patient.

All Humulin preparations may be given by subcutaneous or intramuscular injection, but only Humulin S in vials may be given intravenously.

Subcutaneous administration, preferably by the patient, should be in the upper arms, thighs, buttocks or abdomen. Use of injection sites should be rotated so that the same site is not used more than approximately once a month.

Care should be taken to ensure that a blood vessel has not been entered. The injection site should not be massaged.

Humulin cartridges are for use in Becton Dickinson pen injection devices only. The pen manufacturer's directions should be followed carefully for loading the pen and for priming it. Patients should be advised to always keep a spare syringe and vial of Humulin in case the pen injection device or cartridges get lost or damaged.

Single agent therapy: Humulin S may be administered alone, using multiple daily injections. Humulin I, Lente or Zn may also be administered alone once or twice daily.

Combination therapy: For some patients, the addition of Humulin S to Humulin I, Lente or Zn may be considered necessary to intensify the initial effect (see 'Pharmaceutical Precautions' section).

The effects of mixing with insulins of animal origin, or insulin preparations of other manufacturers, have not been studied and this practice is not recommended.

Mixtures: The Humulin M preparations are ready-made mixtures designed to avoid the need for combination therapy. They should normally be administered twice daily, usually with two thirds of the daily requirement being given in the morning and the remainder in the evening. For any one injection, the dose should not exceed 50 iu.

Usage in pregnancy: It is essential to maintain good control of the insulin-treated (insulin-dependent or gestational) diabetic patient throughout pregnancy. Insulin requirements usually fall during the first trimester and increase during the second and third trimesters.

Time-action profiles are given in the following table:

Humulin presentation	*S*	*I*	*Lente*	*Zn*	*M1*	*M2*	*M3*	*M4*
Onset of action (Hours after administration)	½	1	2½	3	½	½	½	½
Duration of action (Hours after administration)	5–7	18–20	Up to 24	20–24	16–18	14–16	14–15	14–15
Peak activity (Hours after administration)	1–3	2–8	4–16	6–14	1½–9	1–9½	1–8½	1–8

Patients should be advised to inform their doctors if they are pregnant or are contemplating pregnancy.

Usage in nursing mothers: Diabetic patients who are nursing may require adjustments in insulin dose and/or diet.

Contra-indications, warnings, etc

Contra-indications: Hypoglycaemia.

Under no circumstances should any Humulin preparation, except Humulin S in vials, be given intravenously.

Precautions

Transferring from other insulins: A small number of patients transferring from insulins of animal origin may require a reduced dosage and/or a change in the ratio of soluble to intermediate preparations, especially if they are very tightly controlled and bordering on hypoglycaemia. The dosage reduction may occur immediately after transfer or be a gradual process lasting for several weeks. There is a risk of hypoglycaemia if insulin requirement is decreased, and both the physician and the patient should be aware of this possibility. The risk can be considered minimal if the daily dosage is less than 40 iu. Insulin-resistant patients receiving more than 100 iu daily should be referred to hospital for transfer.

A few patients who experienced hypoglycaemic reactions after transfer to human insulin have reported that the early warning symptoms were less pronounced or different from those experienced with their previous insulin. Patients whose blood glucose control is greatly improved, e.g. by intensified insulin therapy, may lose some or all of the warning symptoms of hypoglycaemia and should be advised accordingly. Uncorrected hypoglycaemic and hyperglycaemic reactions can cause loss of consciousness, coma or death.

Insulin requirements may be increased during illness or emotional disturbances, or by concurrent administration of drugs with hyperglycaemic activity, e.g. oral contraceptives, corticosteroids or thyroid hormone replacement therapy.

Insulin requirements may be reduced in the presence of renal or hepatic impairment, or by the concurrent administration of drugs with hypoglycaemic activity e.g. monoamine oxidase inhibitors and beta-adrenergic blockers.

Adjustment of insulin dosage may also be necessary if patients undertake increased physical activity or change their usual diet.

Side-effects: Lipodystrophy, insulin resistance and hypersensitivity reactions are among the side-effects associated with insulins of animal origin. However, the incidence of such side-effects with Humulin is minimal. In the rare event of a severe allergy to Humulin, treatment is required immediately. A change of insulin or desensitisation may be required.

Overdosage: Overdosage causes hypoglycaemia, with accompanying symptoms which may include listlessness, confusion, headache, palpitations, sweating and vomiting.

Treatment: Mild hypoglycaemic episodes will respond to oral administration of glucose or sugar, and rest.

Correction of moderately severe hypoglycaemia can be accomplished by intramuscular or subcutaneous administration of glucagon, followed by oral carbohydrate when the patient recovers sufficiently.

If the patient is comatose or has failed to respond to glucagon injection, Strong Dextrose Injection BPC should be given intravenously.

Pharmaceutical precautions Humulin preparations should be stored in a refrigerator between 2° and 8°C. They should not be frozen or exposed to excessive heat or sunlight.

Vials or cartridges in use

Vials: If refrigeration is not possible, the vial in use may be kept at room temperature (up to 25°C) for 1 month.

Cartridges: When in use, the cartridge should be kept at room temperature (15°–25°C) and should not be refrigerated. The maximum storage period for a cartridge in use is 21 days for all Humulins, *except* Humulin S, for which it is 28 days.

Resuspension

Vials of Humulin I, Lente, Zn, M1, M2, M3 and M4: The vial should be rotated in palms of hands immediately before use to re-suspend. Do not shake vigorously as this may cause frothing which may interfere with the correct measurement of the dose.

Cartridges of Humulin I, M1, M2, M3 or M4: A cartridge of Humulin must be rolled between the palms 10 times and inverted 180° 10 times (see Patient Leaflet). Before insertion into the Becton Dickinson pen, the cartridge should be inspected for uniform resuspension and the above repeated as necessary. Humulin I or M should look uniformly cloudy or milky after resuspension. Do not use if the insulin substance remains at the bottom of the cartridge after resuspension. *A cartridge of Humulin I or M should not be used if there are clumps floating in the insulin after resuspension, or if solid white particles stick to the bottom or wall of the cartridge, giving it a frosted appearance.*

Mixing of insulins (vials only): The shorter-acting insulin should be drawn into the syringe first, to prevent contamination of the vial by the longer-acting preparation. It is advisable to inject immediately after mixing, especially with Humulin Lente or Zn. However, if a delay is necessary, a consistent routine must be followed.

Humulin cartridges are not designed to allow any other insulin to be mixed in the cartridge. The cartridges are not designed to be refilled.

Legal category P.

Package quantities 10 ml glass vials in packs of 5. 1.5 ml glass cartridges in packs of 5.

Further information Nil.

Product licence numbers

Humulin S	100 iu/ml	0006/0216 (vial) 0006/0242 (cartridge)
Humulin I	100 iu/ml	0006/0228 (vial) 0006/0257 (cartridge)
Humulin Lente	100 iu/ml	0006/0224 (vial)
Humulin Zn	100 iu/ml	0006/0226 (vial)
Humulin M1	100 iu/ml	0006/0220 (vial) 0006/0258 (cartridge)
Humulin M2	100 iu/ml	0006/0222 (vial) 0006/0259 (cartridge)

Humulin M3	100 iu/ml	0006/0233 (vial) 0006/0260 (cartridge)
Humulin M4	100 iu/ml	0006/0235 (vial) 0006/0261 (cartridge)

KEFLEX*

Presentation Tablets (pillow shaped, 16 mm long, scored, peach, marked Lilly U49) containing 500 mg Cephalexin BP.

Tablets (9.5 mm diameter, peach, marked Lilly U57) containing 250 mg Cephalexin BP.

Capsules (pale green and dark green, coded H71) containing 500 mg Cephalexin BP.

Capsules (green and white, coded H69) containing 250 mg Cephalexin BP.

Suspension (pink granules) containing 125 mg Cephalexin BP per 5 ml.

Suspension (orange granules) containing 250 mg Cephalexin BP per 5 ml.

Uses Cephalexin is indicated in the treatment of the following infections due to susceptible micro-organisms: respiratory tract infections; otitis media; skin and soft tissue infections; bone and joint infections; genito-urinary tract infections, including acute prostatitis; dental infections.

Cephalexin is active against the following organisms *in vitro*: Beta-haemolytic streptococci; staphylococci, including coagulase-positive, coagulase-negative and penicillinase-producing strains; *Streptococcus pneumoniae*; *Escherichia coli*; *Proteus mirabilis*; *Klebsiella* species; *Haemophilus influenzae*; *Branhamella catarrhalis*.

Most strains of enterococci (*Streptococcus faecalis*) and a few strains of staphylococci are resistant to cephalexin. It is not active against most strains of *Enterobacter* species, *Morganella morganii* and *Pr. vulgaris*. It has no activity against *Pseudomonas* or *Herellea* species. When tested by *in vitro* methods, staphylococci exhibit cross-resistance between cephalexin and methicillin-type antibiotics.

Dosage and administration Keflex is administered orally.

Adults: The adult dosage ranges from 1–4 g daily in divided doses; most infections will respond to a dosage of 500 mg every 8 hours. For skin and soft tissue infections, streptococcal pharyngitis and mild, uncomplicated urinary tract infections, the usual dosage is 250 mg every 6 hours, or 500 mg every 12 hours.

For more severe infections or those caused by less susceptible organisms, larger doses may be needed. If daily doses of Keflex greater than 4 g are required, parenteral cephalosporins, in appropriate doses, should be considered.

The elderly and patients with impaired renal function: As for adults. Reduce dosage if renal function is markedly impaired (see 'Precautions').

Children: The usual recommended daily dosage for children is 25–50 mg/kg (10–20 mg/lb) in divided doses. For skin and soft tissue infections, streptococcal pharyngitis and mild, uncomplicated urinary tract infections, the total daily dose may be divided and administered every 12 hours. For most infections the following schedule is suggested:

Children under 5 years: 125 mg every 8 hours.

Children 5 years and over: 250 mg every 8 hours.

In severe infections, the dosage may be doubled. In the therapy of otitis media, clinical studies have shown that a dosage of 75 to 100 mg/kg/day in 4 divided doses is required.

In the treatment of beta-haemolytic streptococcal infections, a therapeutic dose should be administered for at least 10 days.

Contra-indications, warnings, etc

Contra-indication: Cephalexin is contra-indicated in patients with known allergy to the cephalosporin group of antibiotics.

Warnings: Before instituting therapy with cephalexin, every effort should be made to determine whether the patient has had previous hypersensitivity reactions to the cephalosporins, penicillins or other drugs. Cephalexin should be given cautiously to penicillin-sensitive patients. There is some clinical and laboratory evidence of partial cross-allergenicity of the penicillins and cephalosporins. Patients have had severe reactions (including anaphylaxis) to both drugs.

Pseudomembranous colitis has been reported with virtually all broad-spectrum antibiotics, including macrolides, semisynthetic penicillins and cephalosporins. It is important, therefore, to consider its diagnosis in patients who develop diarrhoea in association with the use of antibiotics. Such colitis may range in severity from mild to life-threatening. Mild cases of pseudomembranous colitis usually respond to drug discontinuance alone. In moderate to severe cases, appropriate measures should be taken.

Usage in pregnancy: Although laboratory and clinical studies have shown no evidence of teratogenicity, caution should be exercised when prescribing for the pregnant patient.

Usage in nursing mothers: The excretion of cephalexin in human breast milk increased up to 4 hours following a 500 mg dose. The drug reached a maximum level of 4 micrograms/ml, then decreased gradually and had disappeared 8 hours after administration. Caution should be exercised when cephalexin is administered to a nursing woman.

Precautions: If an allergic reaction to cephalexin occurs, the drug should be discontinued and the patient treated with the appropriate agents.

Prolonged use of cephalexin may result in the overgrowth of non-susceptible organisms. Careful observation of the patient is essential. If superinfection occurs during therapy, appropriate measures should be taken.

Cephalexin should be administered with caution in the presence of markedly impaired renal function. Careful clinical and laboratory studies should be made because safe dosage may be lower than that usually recommended.

Positive direct Coombs' tests have been reported during treatment with the cephalosporin antibiotics. In haematological studies, or in transfusion cross-matching procedures when antiglobulin tests are performed on the minor side, or in Coombs' testing of newborns whose mothers have received cephalosporin antibiotics before parturition, it should be recognised that a positive Coombs' test may be due to the drug.

A false positive reaction for glucose in the urine may occur with Benedict's or Fehling's solutions or with copper sulphate test tablets.

Side-effects

Gastro-intestinal: Symptoms of pseudomembranous colitis may appear either during or after antibiotic treatment. Nausea and vomiting have been reported rarely. The most frequent side-effect has been diarrhoea. It was very rarely severe enough to warrant cessation of therapy. Dyspepsia and abdominal pain have also occurred. As with some penicillins and some other cephalosporins, transient hepatitis and cholestatic jaundice have been reported rarely.

Hypersensitivity: Allergic reactions have been observed in the form of rash, urticaria, angioedema, and rarely erythema multiforme, Stevens-Johnson syndrome and toxic epidermal necrolysis. These reactions usually subsided upon discontinuation of the drug, although in some cases supportive therapy may be necessary. Anaphylaxis has also been reported.

Other: These have included genital and anal pruritus, genital candidiasis, vaginitis and vaginal discharge, dizziness, fatigue, headache, agitation, confusion, hallucinations, arthralgia, arthritis and joint disorder. Reversible interstitial nephritis has been reported rarely.

Eosinophilia, neutropenia, thrombocytopenia, and slight elevations in AST and ALT have been reported.

Treatment of overdosage: Symptoms of oral overdose may include nausea, vomiting, epigastric distress, diarrhoea and haematuria.

In the event of severe overdosage, general supportive care is recommended, including close clinical and laboratory monitoring of haematological, renal and hepatic functions, and coagulation status until the patient is stable. Forced diuresis, peritoneal dialysis, haemodialysis, or charcoal haemoperfusion have not been established as beneficial for an overdose of cephalexin. It would be extremely unlikely that one of these procedures would be indicated.

Unless 5 to 10 times the normal total daily dose has been ingested, gastrointestinal decontamination should not be necessary.

There have been reports of haematuria without impairment of renal function in children accidentally ingesting more than 3.5 g of cephalexin in a day. Treatment has been supportive (fluids) and no sequelae have been reported.

Pharmaceutical precautions
Capsules and tablets: Keep containers tightly closed.

Suspensions: After mixing, Keflex suspensions should be stored in a cool place (6°–15°C) or in a refrigerator (2°–8°C) and be used within 10 days. Where dilution is unavoidable, Syrup BP should be used after the suspension has been prepared according to the manufacturer's instructions.

Legal category POM.

Package quantities
Tablets 500 mg: Bottles of 20, 100 and 500.
Tablets 250 mg: Bottles of 20, 100 and 500.
Capsules 500 mg: Bottles of 20, 100 and 500.
Capsules 250 mg: Bottles of 20, 100 and 500.
Suspension 125 mg/5 ml: Bottles of 100 ml.
Suspension 250 mg/5 ml: Bottles of 100 ml.

Further information Nil.

Product licence numbers

Tablets 500 mg	0006/5096
Tablets 250 mg	0006/0073
Capsules 500 mg	0006/0076
Capsules 250 mg	0006/5103
Suspension 125 mg/5 ml	0006/5097
Suspension 250 mg/5 ml	0006/5098

KEFLIN*

Presentation Vials containing the equivalent of 1 g cephalothin as the sodium salt.

30 mg/g of sodium bicarbonate has been added to give a pH of the reconstituted solution between 6 and 8.5. The total sodium content is approximately 63 mg per g of cephalothin.

Uses Keflin is indicated in the treatment of serious infections of the respiratory tract, genito-urinary tract, soft tissue and skin, gastro-intestinal tract, bones and joints, blood stream and cardiovascular system when due to susceptible organisms. It has also been effective in cases of peritonitis and septic abortion.

Cases of staphylococcal and pneumococcal meningitis have also responded to treatment. However, as only low levels of cephalothin are found in the cerebrospinal fluid, the drug is not reliable for the treatment of this condition and should only be considered when other more reliably effective antibiotics cannot be used.

Prophylactic use: Perioperative administration has been beneficial in reducing the incidence of postoperative infection in patients undergoing contaminated or potentially contaminated surgical procedures associated with a high risk of infection, in surgical patients with reduced host resistance to bacterial infection, or when the occurrence of a postoperative infection could be especially serious. The best results are observed if cephalothin is administered immediately prior to the operative procedure, thus providing adequate antibiotic concentration in the tissues before bacterial contamination occurs.

Cephalothin is usually active against the following organisms *in vitro:*

Staphylococci, including coagulase-positive, coagulase-negative and penicillinase-producing strains
Clostridia
Streptococcus pneumoniae
Haemophilus influenzae
Escherichia coli and other coliform bacteria
Klebsiella species
Proteus mirabilis
Salmonella species
Shigella species
Beta-haemolytic and other streptococci (many strains of enterococci e.g. *Streptococcus faecalis,* are relatively resistant).

Pseudomonas species are resistant to cephalothin, as are most indole-positive *Proteus* and motile *Enterobacter* species.

Dosage and administration
Adults and the elderly: The usual dosage range is 500 mg to 1 g every 4 to 6 hours. In milder infections a dose of 500 mg every six hours may be indicated. In severe infections, 500 mg–1 g every 4 hours may be used. In life-threatening infections, doses up to 2 g every 4 hours may be required. Limit the dose to a maximum of 6 g daily in patients with oliguria or blood urea elevation above 17.8 mmol/l (107 mg/100 ml).

Infants and children: The dosage should be proportionately less in accordance with age, weight and severity of infection. Daily administration of 100 mg/kg (80–160 mg/kg) in divided doses has been found effective for most infections.

Antibiotic therapy for beta-haemolytic streptococcal infections should continue for at least 10 days.

Prophylactic use: The following dosages are recommended for perioperative use:

1 to 2 g iv prior to surgical incision, followed by 1 to 2 g during surgery and 1 to 2 g every 6 hours for 24 hours postoperatively. In children, 20 to 30 mg/kg may be given at the times designated above.

Since cephalothin has a serum half-life of 30–50 minutes, it is important that 1) the preoperative dose be given just prior to the start of surgery and 2) during surgery, administration is made at appropriate intervals to provide sufficient levels of the antibiotic.

Postoperative administration of cephalothin should be discontinued after twenty-four hours unless signs of infection are present, in which case cultures should be performed and appropriate therapy instituted. Longer courses of preventive antibiotic therapy may be considered necessary when surgical procedures involve implantation of prosthetic devices.

Dosage in renal impairment: When renal function is reduced, an intravenous loading dose of 1–2 g may be given. Continued dosage schedule should be determined by degree of renal impairment, severity of infection and susceptibility of the causative organism. The maximum doses administered should be based on the following recommendations.

Dosage of Keflin when renal function is impaired

Status of renal function	*Maximum adult dosage (maintenance)*
Mild impairment (C_{cr}=80–50 ml/min)	2 g q 6 h
Moderate impairment (C_{cr}=50–25 ml/min)	1.5 g q 6 h
Severe impairment (C_{cr}=25–10 ml/min)	1 g q 6 h
Marked impairment (C_{cr}=10–2 ml/min)	0.5 g q 6 h
Essentially no function (C_{cr}= <2 ml/min)	0.5 g q 8 h

Cephalothin is best given intravenously but the intramuscular route may also be used (see below).

For direct intravenous administration: A solution containing 1 g cephalothin in 10 ml of diluent may be slowly injected directly into the vein over a period of three to five minutes, or may be given through the tubing when the patient is receiving parenteral solutions. The cephalothin solution may be further diluted to a larger volume if desired to facilitate measurement of the rate of injection.

Cephalothin may be administered in one of the following intravenous fluids:
Water for Injections PhEur
Sodium Chloride Intravenous Infusion BP
Dextrose Intravenous Infusion BP
Sodium Lactate Intravenous Infusion BP
Compound Sodium Lactate Intravenous Infusion BP
Sodium Chloride and Dextrose Intravenous Infusion BP.

Intra-peritoneal administration: In peritoneal dialysis procedures, cephalothin has been added to dialysis fluid in concentrations up to 6 mg/100 ml and instilled into the peritoneal space throughout an entire dialysis (16–30 hours). Careful assay procedures have shown that 44% of the administered drug was absorbed into the blood stream. Serum levels of 10 mg/l were reported, with no evidence of accumulation and no untoward or systemic reaction.

The intraperitoneal administration of solutions containing 0.1 to 4% Keflin in saline has been used in treating patients with peritonitis or contaminated peritoneal cavities. (The total daily dosage of Keflin should take into account the amount given by the intraperitoneal route.)

Intramuscular injection deep into a large muscle mass such as the gluteus or lateral aspect of the thigh may be used to minimise pain and induration.

Each g of cephalothin should be diluted in 4 ml of Sterile Water for Injection. If the vial contents do not completely dissolve, an additional small amount of diluent (eg, 0.2 to 0.4 ml) may be added and the contents warmed slightly.

Contra-indications, warnings, etc
Contra-indication: Hypersensitivity to cephalosporin antibiotics.

Warnings: Before cephalothin therapy is instituted, careful enquiry should be made concerning previous hypersensitivity reactions to cephalosporins and penicillin. Cephalosporin C derivatives should be given cautiously to penicillin-sensitive patients.

Serious acute hypersensitivity reactions may require adrenaline and other emergency measures.

There is some clinical and laboratory evidence of partial cross-allergenicity of the penicillins and the cephalosporins. Patients have been reported to have had severe reactions (including anaphylaxis) to both drugs.

Antibiotics should be administered with caution to any patient who has demonstrated some form of allergy, particularly to drugs.

Pseudomembranous colitis has been reported with virtually all broad-spectrum antibiotics, including macrolides, semisynthetic penicillins and cephalosporins. Therefore it is important to consider its diagnosis in patients who develop diarrhoea in association with the use of antibiotics. Such colitis may range in severity from mild to life-threatening. Mild cases of pseudomembranous colitis usually respond to drug discontinuance alone. In moderate to severe cases, appropriate measures should be taken.

Usage in pregnancy: Animal studies have shown no evidence of teratogenicity or impaired fertility. There are, however, no adequate and well-controlled studies in pregnant women. Cephalothin should not be administered during pregnancy unless considered essential by the physician.

Usage in nursing mothers: As small amounts are excreted in breast milk, this drug should be used with caution in nursing mothers.

Precautions: If an allergic reaction to cephalothin occurs, the drug should be discontinued and the patient treated with the appropriate agents.

Although cephalothin rarely produces alteration in kidney function, evaluation of renal status is recommended, especially in seriously ill patients receiving maximum doses. Patients with impaired renal function should be placed on the dosage schedule recommended under 'Dosage and Administration'. Usual doses in such individuals may result in excessive serum concentrations.

An increased incidence of nephrotoxicity has been reported following concomitant administration of cephalosporins and aminoglycoside antibiotics.

When intravenous doses of cephalothin larger than 6 g daily are given by infusion for periods longer than 3 days, they may be associated with thrombophlebitis, and the veins may have to be alternated. The addition of 10 to 25 mg of hydrocortisone to intravenous solutions containing 4 to 6 g of cephalothin may reduce the incidence of thrombophlebitis. The use of small iv needles in the larger available veins may be preferred.

Broad-spectrum antibiotics should be prescribed with caution in individuals with a history of gastro-intestinal disease, particularly colitis.

Prolonged use of cephalothin may result in the overgrowth of non-susceptible organisms. Careful observation of the patient is essential. If superinfection occurs, appropriate measures should be taken.

A false-positive reaction for glucose in the urine may occur with Benedict's or Fehling's solutions or with copper sulphate test tablets.

Side-effects:
Hypersensitivity: Maculopapular rash, urticaria, reactions resembling serum sickness and anaphylaxis have been reported. Eosinophilia and drug fever have been observed to be associated with other allergic reactions. These reactions are most likely to occur in patients with a history of allergy, particularly to penicillin.

Haematological: Neutropenia, leucopenia, granulocytopenia, thrombocytopenia and haemolytic anaemia have been reported. Some individuals, particularly those with uraemia, have developed positive direct Coombs' tests during cephalothin therapy.

Hepatic: Transient rise in AST and alkaline phosphatase has been noted. Toxic intrahepatic cholestasis has been reported.

Renal: Rises in blood urea and decreased creatinine clearances have been reported, particularly in patients with prior renal impairment. Proteinuria has been observed.

Gastro-intestinal: Symptoms of pseudomembranous colitis may appear either during or after antibiotic treatment. Diarrhoea, nausea and vomiting have been reported rarely.

Injection site reactions: Pain, induration, tenderness and elevation of temperature have been reported following repeated intramuscular injections. Thrombophlebitis has occurred, and is usually associated with daily doses of over 6 g given by infusion for more than three days.

Overdosage: The administration of inappropriately large doses of parenteral cephalosporins may cause seizures, particularly in patients with renal impairment. Dosage reduction is necessary when renal function is impaired (see 'Dosage and Administration'). If seizures occur, the drug should be promptly discontinued; anticonvulsant therapy may be administered if clinically indicated.

In the event of serious overdosage, general supportive care is recommended. Haemodialysis may be considered in cases of overwhelming overdosage.

Pharmaceutical precautions *Unreconstituted vials:* Store below 25°C.

After reconstitution: When stored under refrigeration (2°–8°C), the solution has a satisfactory potency for 48 hours. Solutions may precipitate; they can be redissolved by being warmed.

Kept at *room temperature,* solutions for intramuscular injection should be given within 12 hours after being mixed. Intravenous infusions should be started within 12 hours and completed within 24 hours. For prolonged infusions, replace with a freshly prepared solution at least every 24 hours.

The concentrated solution will darken, especially at room temperature.

Legal category POM.

Package quantities 1 g vials: Single vials in packs of 10.

Further information Nil.

Product licence number 0006/5099.

KEFZOL*

Presentation Kefzol is supplied in rubber-stoppered vials containing the equivalent of 500 mg and 1 g cephazolin as the sodium salt. The sodium content is 48.3 mg per g of cephazolin sodium. The pH of the reconstituted solution is between 4.5 and 6.

Uses Kefzol is indicated in the treatment of the following infections due to susceptible micro-organisms:

Respiratory tract infections
Genito-urinary tract infections
Skin and soft tissue infections
Bone and joint infections
Septicaemia
Endocarditis
Biliary tract infections

Prophylactic use: Perioperative administration of cephazolin may reduce the incidence of postoperative infections in patients undergoing contaminated or potentially contaminated surgical procedures associated with a high risk of infection, or where the occurrence of a postoperative infection could be especially serious.

Cephazolin is active against the following organisms *in vitro:*

Staphylococcus aureus (penicillin-sensitive and penicillin-resistant)

Staphylococcus epidermidis, Group A beta-haemolytic streptococci and other strains of streptococci (many strains of enterococci are resistant) – *Streptococcus pneumoniae, Escherichia coli, Klebsiella* species, *Proteus mirabilis, Haemophilus influenzae, Enterobacter aerogenes.*

Most strains of *Enterobacter cloacae, Morganella morganii* and indole-positive Proteus *(Pr. vulgaris, Pr. rettgeri)* are resistant. Methicillin-resistant staphylococci, *Serratia, Pseudomonas* and *Acinetobacter calcoaceticus* are almost uniformly resistant to cephazolin.

Dosage and administration After reconstitution, Kefzol may be administered intramuscularly or intravenously.

Intramuscular administration: Reconstitute with Water for Injections PhEur 0.9% Sodium Chloride Intravenous Infusion BP, or 5% Dextrose Intravenous Infusion BP according to Table 1. Shake well until dissolved. Kefzol should be injected into a large muscle mass.

Table 1. Dilution table

Vial size	*Diluent to be added*	*Approximate available volume*	*Approximate average concentration*
500 mg	4.0 ml	4.1 ml	125 mg/ml
500 mg	2.0 ml	2.2 ml	225 mg/ml
1 g†	2.5 ml	3.0 ml	330 mg/ml

†The 1 g vial should be reconstituted only with Water for Injections PhEur.

Intravenous administration: Kefzol may be administered by intravenous injection or by continuous or intermittent infusion. Total daily dosages are the same as for intramuscular injection.

Intermittent intravenous infusion: Kefzol may be administered along with primary intravenous fluid management programmes in a volume control set or in a separate secondary i.v. bottle. Reconstituted 500 mg or 1 g of Kefzol may be diluted in 50 to 100 ml of Water for Injections PhEur or one of the following intravenous solutions:

0.9% Sodium Chloride Intravenous Infusion BP.
5% or 10% Dextrose Intravenous Infusion BP.
5% Dextrose in Compound Sodium Lactate Intravenous Infusion BP.
0.9% Sodium Chloride and 5% Dextrose Intravenous Infusion BP.
0.45% Sodium Chloride and 5% Dextrose Intravenous Infusion BP.
Compound Sodium Lactate Intravenous Infusion BP.
5% or 10% Invert Sugar in Water for Injections PhEur.

Direct intravenous injection: Dilute 500 mg or 1 g of reconstituted Kefzol in a minimum of 10 ml of Water for Injections PhEur and inject solution slowly over a period of three to five minutes. Do not inject in less than 3 minutes. The injection may be made directly into a vein or, for patients receiving the above parenteral fluids, through the tubing.

Dosage: The usual adult dosages are given in Table 2.

In adults with renal impairment, cephazolin is not readily excreted. After a loading dose appropriate to the severity of the infection, the following recommendations (Table 3) may be used as a guide.

Table 2. Usual adult dosage

Type of infection	*Dose*	*Frequency*
Pneumococcal pneumonia	500 mg	q 12 h
Mild infections caused by susceptible Gram-positive cocci	250 mg to 500 mg	q 8 h
Acute uncomplicated urinary tract infections	1 g	q 12 h
Moderate to severe infections	500 mg to 1 g	q 6 to 8 h
Severe, life-threatening infections (eg, endocarditis and septicaemia)*	1 g to 1.5 g	q 6 h

*In rare instances, doses up to 12 g cephazolin per day have been used.

In patients undergoing peritoneal dialysis (2 l/h), mean serum levels of cephazolin were approximately 10 and 30 micrograms/ml after 24 hours' instillation of a dialysing solution containing 50 mg/l and 150 mg/l respectively.

The elderly: As for adults.

Table 3. Dosage of Kefzol in adults with reduced renal function

Creatinine clearance (ml/min)	*Serum creatinine (mg %)*	*Dosage reduction*
≥55	≤1.5	None
35–54	1.6 to 3.0	None q 8+ hrs
11–34	3.1–4.5	50% q 12 hrs
≤10	≥4.6	50% q 18–24 hrs

Paediatric dosage: In children, a total daily dosage of 25 to 50 mg/kg of body weight, divided into three or four equal doses, is effective for most mild to moderately severe infections (Table 4). Total daily dosage may be increased to 100 mg/kg of body weight for severe infections.

In children with mild to moderate renal impairment (creatinine clearance of 70–40 ml/min), 60% of the normal daily dose given in divided doses q 12 h should be sufficient. In children with moderate impairment (creatinine clearance of 40–20 ml/min), 25% of the normal daily dose in divided doses q 12 h should be adequate. In children with marked impairment (creatinine clearance of 20–5 ml/min), 10% of the normal daily dose given q 24 h should be sufficient. All dosage recommendations apply after an initial loading dose.

Table 4. Paediatric dosage guide

Weight kg	*25 mg/kg/day divided into 3 doses*		*25 mg/kg/day divided into 4 doses*	
	Approximate single dose (q 8 h)	*Vol. needed with dilution of 125 mg/ml*	*Approximate single dose (q 6 h)*	*Vol. needed with dilution of 125 mg/ml*
4.5	40 mg	0.35 ml	30 mg	0.25 ml
9.0	75 mg	0.6 ml	55 mg	0.45 ml
13.5	115 mg	0.9 ml	85 mg	0.7 ml
18.0	150 mg	1.2 ml	115 mg	0.9 ml
22.5	190 mg	1.5 ml	140 mg	1.1 ml

Weight kg	*50 mg/kg/day divided into 3 doses*		*50 mg/kg/day divided into 4 doses*	
	Approximate single dose (q 8 h)	*Vol. needed with dilution of 225 mg/ml*	*Approximate single dose (q 6 h)*	*Vol. needed with dilution of 225 mg/ml*
4.5	75 mg	0.35 ml	55 mg	0.25 ml
9.0	150 mg	0.7 ml	110 mg	0.5 ml
13.5	225 mg	1.0 ml	170 mg	0.75 ml
18.0	300 mg	1.35 ml	225 mg	1.0 ml
22.5	375 mg	1.7 ml	285 mg	1.25 ml

Since safety for use in premature infants and in infants under 1 month of age has not been established, the use of cephazolin in these patients is not recommended.

Prophylactic use: The following doses are recommended for perioperative use:

Adults: 1 g intravenously or intramuscularly one-half to one hour prior to surgical incision, followed by 0.5 to 1 g intravenously or intramuscularly every six to eight hours for 24 hours postoperatively. Additionally, for lengthy operative procedures (e.g. two hours or more), 0.5 to 1 g intravenously or intramuscularly during surgery.

The prophylactic administration of cephazolin should usually be discontinued within a 24 hour period after the surgical procedure. For patients undergoing open-heart surgery or implantation of prosthetic devices, administration may be continued for three to five days.

Contra-indications, warnings, etc

Contra-indication: Cephazolin is contra-indicated in patients with known allergy to the cephalosporin group of antibiotics.

Warnings: Before instituting therapy with cephazolin, every attempt should be made to determine if the patient has had previous hypersensitivity reactions to the cephalosporins, penicillins, or other drugs, in which case this product should be given cautiously. Serious acute hypersensitivity reactions may require adrenaline and other emergency measures.

There is some evidence of partial cross-allergenicity between the penicillins and the cephalosporins. Patients have been reported to have had severe reactions (including anaphylaxis) to both drugs.

Antibiotics should be administered cautiously to any patient who has demonstrated some form of allergy, particularly to drugs.

The results of experimental studies in animals given cephalosporins suggest that the concurrent use of potent diuretics, such as frusemide or ethacrynic acid, may increase the risk of renal toxicity.

Pseudomembranous colitis has been reported with virtually all broad-spectrum antibiotics, so it is important to consider this diagnosis in patients who develop diarrhoea in association with the use of antibiotics. Severity ranges from mild to life-threatening; mild cases usually respond to drug discontinuance alone. In moderate to severe cases, appropriate measures should be taken.

Usage in pregnancy: Although animal studies have shown no evidence of impaired fertility or teratogenicity, there are no adequate and well-controlled studies in pregnant women. Therefore, caution should be exercised when prescribing for the pregnant patient. When cephazolin has been administered prior to caesarean section, drug levels in cord blood have been approximately one fourth to one third of maternal drug levels. The drug appeared to have no adverse effect on the fetus.

Usage in nursing mothers: Caution is required when cephazolin is administered to a nursing woman, as very low concentrations of cephazolin have been found in breast milk.

Usage in neonates: The safety of this product for use in prematures and infants under one month of age has not been established.

Precautions: If an allergic reaction to cephazolin occurs, the drug should be discontinued and the patient treated with the usual agents (e.g. adrenaline or other pressor amines, antihistamines, or corticosteroids).

Broad-spectrum antibiotics should be prescribed with caution in individuals with a history of gastro-intestinal disease, particularly colitis.

Prolonged use of cephazolin may result in the overgrowth of non-susceptible organisms. Careful observation of the patient is essential. If superinfection occurs during therapy, appropriate measures should be taken.

When cephazolin is administered to patients with impaired renal function, the daily dosage should be reduced to avoid toxicity (see 'Dosage and administration').

A false positive reaction for glucose in the urine may occur with Benedict's or Fehling's solutions or with copper sulphate test tablets.

Positive direct and indirect antiglobulin (Coombs') tests have occurred; these may also occur in neonates whose mothers received cephalosporins before delivery.

Drug interactions: Probenecid may decrease renal tubular secretion of cephalosporins when used concurrently, which results in increased and more prolonged cephalosporin blood levels.

Side-effects: The following side-effects have been reported:

Gastro-intestinal: Symptoms of pseudomembranous colitis may appear either during or after treatment. Nausea, anorexia, vomiting, diarrhoea and oral candidiasis have been reported.

Hypersensitivity: Drug fever, rash, vulvar pruritus, eosinophilia and anaphylaxis.

Haematological: Neutropenia, leucopenia, thrombocythaemia, and positive direct and indirect Coombs' tests.

Neurological: Convulsions have occasionally been reported, especially after administration of high doses to patients with marked renal impairment.

Renal: Transient rise in blood urea nitrogen levels has been observed without clinical evidence of renal impairment. Interstitial nephritis and other renal disorders have been reported rarely. Most patients experiencing these reactions have been seriously ill and were receiving multiple drug therapies. The role of cephazolin has not been determined.

Hepatic: Transient rises in AST, ALT and ALP levels have been observed rarely. As with some penicillins and some other cephalosporins, transient hepatitis and cholestatic jaundice have been reported rarely.

Other: Pain on intramuscular injection, sometimes with induration has occurred infrequently. Phlebitis at the site of intravenous injection has been noted. Other side-effects have included genital and anal pruritus, genital candidiasis and vaginitis.

Overdosage

Signs and symptoms: May include pain, inflammation and phlebitis at the injection site.

The administration of inappropriately large doses of parenteral cephalosporins may cause dizziness, paraesthesiae and headaches. Seizures may occur with some cephalosporins, particularly in patients with renal impairment in whom accumulation is likely to occur.

Laboratory abnormalities may include elevations in creatinine, BUN, liver enzymes and bilirubin, a positive Coombs' test, thrombocytosis, thrombocytopenia, eosinophilia, leucopenia and prolongation of prothrombin time.

Treatment: In the event of serious overdosage, general supportive care is recommended, with monitoring of haematological, renal and hepatic functions and coagulation status until the patient is stable. If seizures occur, the drug should be discontinued promptly. Anticonvulsant therapy may be clinically indicated. General supportive therapy is recommended.

In cases of severe overdosage, especially in a patient with renal failure, combined haemodialysis and haemoperfusion may be considered, although supporting data are not available.

Pharmaceutical precautions Extemporaneous mixtures with other antibiotics (including aminoglycosides) are not recommended.

Unreconstituted vials: Protect from light.

After reconstitution: If stored below 25°C, use within 24 hours. If kept in a refrigerator (2°–8°C), use within 96 hours.

Prior to administration, parenteral drug products should be inspected visually for particulate matter and discolouration, whenever solution and container permit.

Legal category POM.

Package quantities
500 mg vials: Single vials in packs of 10.
1 g vials: Single vials in packs of 10.

Further information Nil.

Product licence number 0006/0078.

NEBCIN*

Presentation Nebcin is presented in vials in the following strengths: 1 ml vials containing tobramycin sulphate equivalent to 40 mg tobramycin base.

2 ml vials containing tobramycin sulphate equivalent to 80 mg tobramycin base.

2 ml vials containing tobramycin sulphate equivalent to 20 mg tobramycin base.

Also containing 0.5% w/v Phenol BP with sodium bisulphite and Disodium Edetate BP.

Uses Nebcin is indicated for the treatment of the following infections caused by susceptible micro-organisms:

Central nervous system infections, including meningitis, septicaemia and neonatal sepsis
Gastro-intestinal infections, including peritonitis and other significant infections such as:
Complicated and recurrent urinary tract infections, including pyelonephritis and cystitis
Lower respiratory tract infections, including pneumonia, bronchopneumonia and acute bronchitis
Skin, bone and soft tissue infections, including burns.

Nebcin may be considered in serious staphylococcal infections for which penicillin or other less potentially toxic drugs are contra-indicated and when bacterial susceptibility testing and clinical judgement indicate its use.

Tobramycin is usually active against most strains of the following organisms:

Pseudomonas aeruginosa
Proteus species (indole-positive and indole-negative), including *Pr. mirabilis, Pr. rettgeri* and *Pr. vulgaris; Morganella morganii, Escherichia coli, Klebsiella-Enterobacter-Serratia* species, *Citrobacter* species, *Providencia* species, Staphylococci including *Staphylococcus aureus* (coagulase-positive and coagulase-negative).

Most strains of enterococci demonstrate *in vitro* resistance. The combination of penicillin G and tobramycin results in a synergistic bactericidal effect *in vitro* against certain strains of *Enterococcus faecalis* (formerly *Streptococcus faecalis*). However, this combination is not synergistic against other closely related organisms, e.g. *E. faecium (formerly S. faecium)*. Speciation of enterococci alone cannot be used to predict susceptibility. Susceptibility testing and tests for antibiotic synergism are emphasised.

Cross-resistance between aminoglycosides occurs and depends largely on inactivation by bacterial enzymes.

The combination of tobramycin and carbenicillin is synergistic *in vitro* against most strains of *Ps. aeruginosa.* Other Gram-negative organisms may be affected synergistically by the combination of tobramycin and a cephalosporin.

Dosage and administration Nebcin may be given intramuscularly or intravenously. The patient's pretreatment body weight should be obtained for calculation of correct dosage.

The intramuscular dose is the same as the intravenous dose.

It is recommended that both peak and trough serum levels should be determined whenever possible to ensure the correct dosage is given. Blood levels should always be determined in patients with chronic infections such as cystic fibrosis, or where longer duration of treatment may be necessary, or in patients with decreased renal function.

Patients with normal renal function:

Adults: The usual recommended dosage for adults with serious infections is 3 mg/kg/day, administered in three equal doses every eight hours (see Table 1). For life-threatening infections, dosages up to 5 mg/kg/day may be administered in three or four equal doses. The dosage should be reduced to 3 mg/kg/day as soon as clinically indicated. To prevent increased toxicity due to excessive blood levels, dosage should not exceed 5 mg/kg/day unless serum levels are monitored (see 'Warnings' and 'Precautions').

Table 1. Dosage schedule guide for adults with normal renal function
(Dosage at 8–hour intervals)

Patient weight kg	*Usual dose for serious infections 1 mg/kg q 8 h (total 3 mg/kg/day)*		*Maximum dose for life-threatening infections (reduce as soon as possible) 1.66 mg/kg q 8 h (total 5 mg/kg/day unless monitored)*	
	mg/dose	ml/dose†	mg/dose	ml/dose†
120	120	3.0	200	5.0
100	100	2.5	166	4.0
80	80	2.0	133	3.0
60	60	1.5	100	2.5
40	40	1.0	66	1.6

† Applicable to 40 mg/ml product forms.

To achieve therapeutic serum levels in patients with cystic fibrosis, it may be necessary to administer up to 8 to 10 mg/kg/day in equally divided doses. Because serum concentrations of tobramycin vary from one patient to another, serum levels should be monitored.

In adults with normal renal function, mild to moderate infections of the urinary tract have responded to a dosage of 2–3 mg/kg/day administered as a single intramuscular injection.

The elderly: As for adults, but see recommendations for patients with impaired renal function.

Children: The recommended dosage is 6–7.5 mg/kg/day, administered in three or four equally divided doses. In some patients it may be necessary to administer higher doses.

Premature or full-term neonates: Dosages of up to 4 mg/kg/day may be administered in two equal doses every 12 hours, for those between 1.5 and 2.5 kg body weight.

The usual duration of treatment is 7 to 10 days. A longer course of therapy may be necessary in difficult and complicated infections. In such cases, monitoring of renal, auditory and vestibular functions is advised, because neurotoxicity is more likely to occur when treatment is extended for longer than 10 days.

Obese patients: The appropriate dose may be calculated using the patient's estimated lean body weight, plus 40% of the excess, as the weight on which to determine mg/kg.

Patients with impaired renal function: Following a loading dose of 1 mg/kg, subsequent dosage in these patients must be adjusted, either with lower doses administered at eight-hour intervals or with normal doses at prolonged intervals (see Table 2). Both of these regimens are suggested as guides to be used when serum levels of tobramycin cannot be measured directly. They are based on either the creatinine clearance or the serum creatinine of the patient, because these values correlate with the half-life of tobramycin. Neither regimen should be used when dialysis is being performed.

Reduced dosage at eight-hour intervals (Regimen I): An appropriately reduced dosage range can be found in the accompanying table (Table 2) for any patient for whom the blood urea, creatinine clearance or serum creatinine values are known. The choice of dose within the indicated range should be based on the severity of the infection, the sensitivity of the pathogen, and individual patient considerations, especially renal function. An alternative rough guide for determining reduced dosage at eight-hour intervals (for patients whose steady-state serum creatinine values are known) is to divide the normally recommended dose by the patient's serum creatinine value (mg/100 ml).

Normal dosage at prolonged intervals (Regimen II): Recommended intervals between doses are given in the accompanying table (Table 2). As a general rule, the dosage frequency in hours can be determined by multiplying the patient's serum creatinine level (mg/100 ml) by six.

The dosage schedules derived from either method should be used in conjunction with careful clinical and laboratory observations of the patient and should be modified as necessary (see 'Warnings').

Intramuscular administration: Nebcin may be administered by withdrawing the appropriate dose directly from the vial.

Intravenous administration: For intravenous administration, the usual volume of diluent (0.9% Sodium Chloride Intravenous Infusion BP or 5% Dextrose Intravenous Infusion BP) for adult doses is 50–100 ml. For children, the volume of diluent should be proportionately less than for adults. The diluted solution should be infused over a period of 20–60 minutes avoiding admixture with any other drug. Nebcin may be administered slowly by direct intravenous injection or into the tubing of a drip set. When given in this way, serum levels may exceed 12 mg/l for a short time (see 'Contra-indications, warnings, etc.').

Contra-indications, warnings, etc

Contra-indications: Intrathecal administration. Hypersensitivity to any aminoglycoside is a contra-indication to the use of tobramycin because of the known cross-allergenicity of drugs in this class.

Warnings: Nebcin contains sodium bisulphite which may cause allergic-type reactions, including anaphylactic symptoms and life-threatening or less severe asthmatic episodes, in certain susceptible people. The overall prevalence of sulphite sensitivity in the general population is unknown and probably low, but it occurs more frequently in asthmatic patients.

Patients treated with tobramycin should be under close observation because tobramycin and other aminoglycoside antibiotics have an inherent potential for causing nephrotoxicity and ototoxicity.

Both vestibular and auditory ototoxicity can occur. Eighth cranial nerve impairment may develop in patients with pre-existing renal damage and if tobramycin is administered for longer periods or in higher doses than those recommended. Other manifestations of neurotoxicity may include numbness, skin tingling, muscle twitching and convulsions. The risk of aminoglycoside-induced hearing loss increases with the degree of exposure to either high peak or high trough serum concentrations. Patients who develop cochlea damage may not have symptoms during therapy to warn them of eighth-nerve toxicity, and partial or total irreversible bilateral deafness may continue to develop after the drug has been discontinued. Rarely, nephrotoxicity may not become manifest until the first few days after cessation of therapy. Aminoglycoside-induced nephrotoxicity is usually reversible.

Therefore, renal and eighth cranial nerve function should be closely monitored in patients with known or suspected renal impairment and also in those whose renal function is initially normal but who develop signs of renal dysfunction during therapy. Evidence of impairment in renal, vestibular and/or auditory function requires discontinuation of the drug or dosage adjustment.

Monitoring of renal function is particularly important in elderly patients who may have reduced renal function that may not be evident in the results of routine screening tests, such as blood urea or serum creatinine. A creatinine clearance determination may be more useful.

Serum concentrations should be monitored when feasible, and prolonged concentrations above 12 mg/l should be avoided. Rising trough levels (above 2 mg/l) may indicate tissue accumulation. A useful guideline would be to perform serum level assays after two or three doses, so that the dosage could be adjusted if necessary,

Table 2. Two maintenance regimens based on renal function and body weight following an initial dose of 1 mg/kg†

Renal function‡					*Regimen I* or		*Regimen II*
					Adjusted doses at 8-hour intervals		*Normal dosage at prolonged intervals*
Blood urea		*Serum creatinine*		*Creatinine clearance*	*Weight*		*Weight/Dose 50–60 kg:60 mg 60–80 kg:80 mg*
mg/100 ml	*mmol/l*	*mg/100 ml*	*micromoles/l*	*ml/min*	*50–60 kg*	*60–80 kg*	
Normal:							
<42	<7.0	<1.3	<114.9	>70	60 mg	80 mg	q 8 h
42–74	7.0–12.3	1.4–1.9	123.8–168	69–40	30–60 mg	50–80 mg	q 12 h
75–105	12.5–17.5	2.0–3.3	176.8–291.7	39–20	20–25 mg	30–45 mg	q 18 h
106–140	17.7–23.3	3.4–5.3	300.6–468.5	19–10	10–18 mg	15–24 mg	q 24 h
141–160	23.5–26.7	5.4–7.5	477.4–663	9–5	5–9 mg	7–12 mg	q 36 h
>160	>26.7	>7.6	>671.8	<4	2.5–4.5 mg	3.5–6 mg	q 48 h§

†For life-threatening infections, dosages 50% above those normally recommended may be used. The dosages should be reduced as soon as possible when improvement is noted.

‡If used to estimate degree of renal impairment, blood urea and serum creatinine concentrations should reflect a steady state of renal uraemia.

§When dialysis is not being performed.

and also at three to four day intervals during therapy. In the event of changing renal function, more frequent serum levels should be obtained and the dosage or dosage intervals adjusted according to the guidelines provided in the 'Dosage and Administration' section. In order to measure the peak level, a serum sample should be drawn about 30 minutes following intravenous infusion or at one hour after intramuscular injection. Trough levels are measured by obtaining serum samples at eight hours or just prior to the next dose of tobramycin.

Urine should be examined for increased excretion of protein, cells and casts. Serum creatinine or creatinine clearance (preferred over blood urea) should be measured periodically. When feasible, it is recommended that serial audiograms be obtained in patients old enough to be tested, particularly high-risk patients.

The risk of toxic reactions is low in patients with normal renal function who do not receive tobramycin in higher doses or for longer periods of time than those recommended.

Patients with reduced renal function, however, are particularly prone to the potential ototoxic and nephrotoxic effects of this drug, so dosage should be adjusted carefully on the basis of regular monitoring of serum drug concentrations and of renal function.

Concurrent and/or sequential use of other potentially neurotoxic and/or nephrotoxic drugs, particularly other aminoglycosides (eg. amikacin, streptomycin, neomycin, kanamycin, gentamicin and paromomycin), amphotericin B, cephaloridine, viomycin, polymyxin B, colistin, cisplatin and vancomycin, requires careful monitoring. Other factors that may increase patient risk are advanced age and dehydration.

Tobramycin should not be given concurrently with potent diuretics. Some diuretics themselves cause ototoxicity, and intravenously administered diuretics enhance aminoglycoside toxicity by altering antibiotic concentrations in serum and tissue.

Usage in pregnancy: Aminoglycosides can cause fetal harm when administered to a pregnant woman. Aminoglycoside antibiotics cross the placenta, and there have been several reports of total irreversible bilateral congenital deafness in children whose mothers received streptomycin during pregnancy. Serious side-effects to mother, fetus, or newborn have not been reported in the treatment of pregnant women with other aminoglycosides, but tobramycin should not be administered to the pregnant patient unless the potential benefits clearly outweigh any potential risk. If tobramycin is used during pregnancy or if the patient becomes pregnant whilst taking tobramycin, she should be informed of the potential hazard to the fetus.

Usage in nursing mothers: Tobramycin is excreted in the breast milk and should be avoided in nursing women.

Precautions: Use in neonates: Tobramycin should be used with caution in premature and neonatal infants because of their renal immaturity and the resulting prolongation of serum half-life of the drug.

General: Serum calcium, magnesium, and sodium should be monitored. It is particularly important to monitor serum levels closely in patients with known renal impairment.

In patients with extensive burns, altered pharmacokinetics may result in reduced serum concentrations of aminoglycosides. In such patients treated with tobramycin, measurement of serum concentration is especially recommended as a basis for determination of appropriate dosage.

Aminoglycosides may be absorbed in significant quantities from body surfaces for local irrigation or application and may cause neurotoxicity and nephrotoxicity.

Aminoglycosides should be used with caution in patients with muscular disorders, such as myasthenia gravis or parkinsonism, since these drugs may aggravate muscle weakness because of their potential curare-like effect on neuromuscular function.

Neuromuscular blockade or respiratory paralysis may occur following rapid intravenous administration of many aminoglycosides and have been reported in cats receiving very high doses of tobramycin (40 mg/kg). The possibility of prolonged secondary apnoea should be considered if tobramycin is administered to anaesthetised patients who are also receiving neuromuscular blocking agents such as succinylcholine, tubocurarine or decamethonium, or to patients receiving massive transfusions of citrated blood. If neuromuscular blockade occurs, it may be reversed by the administration of calcium salts.

The inactivation of tobramycin by beta-lactam antibiotics (penicillins or cephalosporins) has been demonstrated *in vitro* and in patients with severe renal impairment. Such inactivation has not been found in patients with normal renal function if the drugs are administered by separate routes.

If overgrowth of non-susceptible organisms occurs, appropriate therapy should be initiated.

Side-effects: Renal function changes, as shown by rising blood urea and serum creatinine and by oliguria, cylindruria and increased proteinuria, have been reported, especially in patients with a history of renal impairment who are treated for longer periods or with higher doses than those recommended. These changes can occur in patients with initially normal renal function.

Side-effects on both vestibular and auditory branches of the eighth cranial nerve have been reported, especially in patients receiving high doses or prolonged therapy, in those given previous courses of therapy with an ototoxin, and in cases of dehydration. Symptoms include dizziness, vertigo, tinnitus, roaring in the ears and hearing loss. Hearing loss is usually irreversible and is manifested initially by diminution of high-tone acuity.

Other reported side-effects, possibly related to tobramycin, include increased AST, ALT, and serum bilirubin; decreased serum calcium, magnesium, sodium and potassium; anaemia, granulocytopenia, thrombocytopenia, leucopenia, leucocytosis and eosinophilia; and fever, rash, itching, urticaria, nausea, vomiting, diarrhoea, headache, lethargy, pain at the injection site, mental confusion and disorientation.

Overdosage: Severity of the manifestations of a tobramycin overdose depend on the dose, the patient's renal function, state of hydration, age and whether concurrent medication with similar toxicities is being given.

Nephrotoxicity following the parenteral administration of an aminoglycoside is most closely related to the AUC of serum concentration versus time. Nephrotoxicity is more likely if trough levels fail to fall below 2 mg/l and is also proportional to the average blood concentration. Patients who are elderly, have renal impairment, are receiving other nephrotoxic or ototoxic drugs, or are volume depleted, are at greater risk for developing acute tubular necrosis or auditory and vestibular toxicity. These patients often experience dizziness, tinnitus, vertigo and a loss of high-tone acuity. Neuromuscular blockade or respiratory failure may occur following rapid intravenous administration of many aminoglycosides. These reactions and prolonged respiratory paralysis may occur more commonly in patients with myasthenia gravis or Parkinson's disease, or those receiving decamethonium, tubocurarine or succinylcholine.

Toxicity from ingested tobramycin is unlikely because aminoglycosides are poorly absorbed from an intact gastro-intestinal tract.

Treatment: Resuscitative measures should be initiated promptly if respiratory paralysis occurs. Neuromuscular blockade may be reversed by giving calcium salts. Fluid balance, creatinine clearance and tobramycin plasma levels should be carefully monitored until the tobramycin level falls below 2 mg/l. Haemodialysis or peritoneal dialysis will help remove tobramycin from the blood. Between 25% and 70% of the administered dose may be removed, depending on the duration and type of dialysis employed; haemodialysis is the more effective method.

Pharmaceutical precautions *Undiluted vials:* Store below 25°C. Nebcin should not be physically premixed with other drugs but should be administered separately according to the recommended dose and route.

Prior to administration, parenteral drug products should be inspected visually for particulate matter and discolouration whenever solution and container permit.

Legal category POM.

Package quantity Boxes of 10 rubber-stoppered injection vials.

Further information Nil.

Product licence numbers
40 mg per 1 ml 0006/0084
10 mg per 1 ml 0006/0085

NU-SEALS* Aspirin

Presentation Enteric sealed tablets of aspirin. Nu-Seals Aspirin is available in two sizes containing 300 mg (coded B01) and 600 mg (coded B06) Acetylsalicylic Acid PhEur covered in a special coating, red in colour.

Uses Aspirin has analgesic, antipyretic and anti-inflammatory actions. It also has an anti-thrombotic action, mediated through inhibition of platelet activation, which has been shown to be useful in secondary prophylaxis following myocardial infarction, and in patients with unstable angina or cerebral transient ischaemic attacks.

Nu-Seals Aspirin is indicated wherever high and prolonged dosage of aspirin is required. The special coating resists dissolution in gastric juice, but will dissolve readily in the relatively less acid environment of the duodenum. Owing to the delay that the coating imposes on the release of the active ingredient, Nu-Seals Aspirin is unsuitable for the short-term relief of pain.

Dosage and administration Nu-Seals Aspirin is for oral administration to adults only.

Analgesic, antipyretic and anti-inflammatory actions: The usual dose of aspirin is 300–900 mg repeated three to four times daily according to clinical needs. In acute rheumatic disorders the dose is in the range of 4–8 g daily, taken in divided doses.

Antithrombotic action: For its antithrombotic effect following myocardial infarction, transient ischaemic attack, or in patients with unstable angina, the recommended dose is 300 mg daily.

The elderly: Analgesic, antipyretic and anti-inflammatory actions: As for adults. The elderly are more likely to experience gastric side-effects and tinnitus. *Antithrombotic action:* The risk-benefit ratio has not been fully established.

Contra-indications, warnings, etc
Contra-indications: Hypersensitivity to aspirin. Hypoprothrombinaemia, haemophilia and active peptic ulceration.

Warnings: Aspirin should not be given to children, particularly those under 12 years, unless the expected benefits outweigh the possible risks. Aspirin may be a contributory factor in the causation of Reye's syndrome in some children.

Salicylates should be used with caution in patients with a history of peptic ulceration or coagulation abnormalities. They may also induce gastro-intestinal haemorrhage, occasionally major.

In large doses, salicylates may also decrease insulin requirements.

Usage in pregnancy: Although clinical and epidemiological evidence would suggest the safety of aspirin for use during pregnancy, caution should be exercised when prescribing for pregnant patients. Aspirin may prolong labour and contribute to maternal and neonatal bleeding, and it is best avoided at term.

Usage in nursing mothers: As aspirin is excreted in breast milk, Nu-Seals should not be taken by patients who are breast-feeding.

Precautions: Salicylates may enhance the effect of anticoagulants and inhibit the uricosuric effect of probenecid. They may also precipitate bronchospasm or induce attacks of asthma in susceptible subjects.

Patients with hypertension should be carefully monitored.

Side-effects: Salicylates may induce hypersensitivity, asthma, urate kidney stones, chronic gastro-intestinal blood loss, tinnitus, nausea and vomiting. The special coating of Nu-Seals Aspirin helps to reduce the incidence of side-effects resulting from gastric irritation.

Overdosage: Overdosage produces dizziness, tinnitus, sweating, nausea and vomiting, confusion and hyperventilation. Gross overdosage may lead to CNS depression with coma, cardiovascular collapse and respiratory depression. If overdosage is suspected, the patient should be kept under observation for at least 24 hours, as symptoms and salicylate blood levels may not become apparent for several hours. Treatment of overdosage consists of gastric lavage and forced alkaline diuresis. Haemodialysis may be necessary in severe cases.

Pharmaceutical precautions Keep containers tightly closed.

Legal category P.

Package quantities
Tablets 300 mg: Bottles of 100 and 500.
Tablets 600 mg: Bottles of 100.

Further information Nil.

Product licence numbers
Tablets 300 mg 0006/5093R
Tablets 600 mg 0006/5094R

ONCOVIN*

Presentation Vials containing 1 mg Oncovin (Vincristine Sulphate BP) and 10 mg Lactose PhEur.

Oncovin is supplied in a combination package with an accompanying vial of diluting solution, 10 ml containing 90 mg Sodium Chloride PhEur with 2% Benzyl Alcohol BP as a preservative.

Oncovin Solution: 1 ml vials containing 1 mg Oncovin (Vincristine Sulphate BP) and 100 mg Mannitol BP.

2 ml vials containing 2 mg Oncovin (Vincristine Sulphate BP) and 200 mg Mannitol BP.

The vials also contain 1.8 mg per 1 ml Methyl Hydroxybenzoate PhEur and 0.2 mg per 1 ml Propyl Hydroxybenzoate PhEur as preservatives. Acetic acid and sodium acetate have been added for pH control.

Uses Oncovin is an anti-neoplastic drug for intravenous use.

Information available at present suggests that Oncovin may be useful either alone or in conjunction with other oncolytic drugs for the treatment of:

1. Leukaemias, including acute lymphocytic leukaemia, chronic lymphocytic leukaemia, acute myelogenous leukaemia and blastic crisis of chronic myelogenous leukaemia.
2. Malignant lymphomas, including Hodgkin's disease and non-Hodgkin's lymphomas.
3. Multiple myeloma.
4. Solid tumours, including breast carcinoma, small cell bronchogenic carcinoma, head and neck carcinoma and soft tissue sarcomas.
5. Paediatric solid tumours, including Ewing's sarcoma, embryonal rhabdomyosarcoma, neuroblastoma, Wilms' tumour, retinoblastoma and medulloblastoma.
6. Idiopathic thrombocytopenic purpura.

Dosage and administration This preparation is for intravenous use only. Intrathecal administration usually results in death (see 'Warnings' for treatment).

Extreme care must be used in calculating and administering the dose of vincristine since overdosage may have a very serious or fatal outcome.

The drug is administered intravenously at weekly intervals. The recommended dose is 1.4 to 1.5 mg/m^2, up to a maximum weekly dose of 2 mg.

The dosage must always be adjusted individually because of the narrow range between therapeutic and toxic levels, and individual variations in response.

The elderly: As for adults.

Solutions of Oncovin ranging from 0.01 mg to 1 mg/ml have been administered with equally satisfactory results. With these concentrations, there have been no reports of phlebitis or cellulitis at the site of injection unless extravasation occurred. Various solvents have been employed for the drug, including Water for Injections PhEur and Sodium Chloride Intravenous Infusion BP. Both of the latter appear to be equally satisfactory.

To prepare a solution containing 1 mg/ml add 1 ml of the accompanying diluting solution to the 1 mg vial. The drug dissolves rapidly to give a clear solution.

The calculated dose of the resulting solution or of the solution for injection is drawn up into a syringe and injected either directly into a vein or into the tubing of a running intravenous infusion, whichever is more suitable for the patient.

Oncovin solution: The concentration of vincristine is 1 mg/ml. Do not add extra fluid to the vial prior to removal of the dose. Withdraw the solution of Oncovin into an accurate dry syringe, measuring the dose carefully. Do not add extra fluid to the vial in an attempt to empty it completely.

Care should be taken to avoid infiltration of subcutaneous tissues. Injection may be completed in about one minute.

Caution: If leakage into surrounding tissue should occur during intravenous administration of vincristine, it may cause considerable irritation. The injection should be discontinued immediately and any remaining portion of the dose should then be introduced into another vein. Local injection of hyaluronidase and the application of moderate heat to the area of leakage help to disperse the drug and are thought to minimise discomfort and the possibility of cellulitis.

Contra-indications, warnings, etc

Contra-indications: Intrathecal administration usually results in death (see 'Warnings' for treatment).

Patients with the demyelinating form of Charcot–Marie–Tooth syndrome should not be given vincristine.

Warnings: Syringes containing this product should be labelled 'WARNING – VINCRISTINE FOR INTRAVENOUS USE ONLY'.

After intrathecal administration, removal of cerebrospinal fluid, and flushing with Lactated Ringer's and other solutions, has not prevented ascending paralysis leading to death. In one adult paralysis was arrested, with some recovery, by the following treatment initiated immediately:

1. Removal of as much CSF as is safely possible.
2. Flushing with Lactated Ringer's solution by continuous infusion at 150 ml/h, through a catheter in a cerebral lateral ventricle and removed through lumbar access, until fresh frozen plasma became available.
3. Fresh frozen plasma, 25 ml, diluted with 1 l of Lactated Ringer's was then infused similarly at 75 ml/h. The rate of infusion was adjusted to maintain a spinal fluid protein level of 150 mg/dl.
4. Glutamic acid, 10 gm, was given iv over 24 hours, followed by 500 mg tds by mouth for 1 month. Glutamic acid may not be essential.

Usage in pregnancy: Caution is necessary with the use of all oncolytic drugs during pregnancy.

Vincristine can cause fetal harm when administered to a pregnant woman, although there are no adequate and well controlled studies. In several animal species, vincristine can induce teratogenic effects as well as embryolethality with doses that are nontoxic to the pregnant animal. Women of childbearing potential should be advised to avoid becoming pregnant while receiving vincristine. If vincristine is used during pregnancy or if the patient becomes pregnant while receiving this drug she should be informed of the potential hazard to the fetus.

Usage in nursing mothers: It is not known whether Oncovin is excreted in human breast milk. Because of the potential for serious adverse reactions due to Oncovin in nursing infants, a decision should be made whether to discontinue nursing or the drug, taking into account the importance of the drug to the mother.

Precautions: Effective therapy with Oncovin is less likely to be followed by granulocytopenia than is the case with Velbe (vinblastine sulphate) and other oncolytic agents. A study of the side-effects of Oncovin in all age groups reveals that it is usually neuromuscular rather than bone marrow toxicity that limits dosage. However, because of the possibility of granulocytopenia, both clinician and patient should remain alert for signs of any complicating infection. Although pre-existing granulocytopenia does not necessarily contra-indicate the administration of Oncovin, the appearance of granulocytopenia during treatment warrants careful consideration before giving the next dose.

Acute uric acid nephropathy, which may occur after the administration of oncolytic agents, has also been reported with Oncovin.

If central-nervous-system leukaemia is diagnosed, additional agents may be required, since vincristine does not appear to cross the blood-brain barrier in adequate amounts.

Particular attention should be given to dosage and neurological side effects if Oncovin is administered to patients with pre-existing neuromuscular disease and also when other drugs with neurotoxic potential are being used.

Acute shortness of breath and severe bronchospasm have been reported following the administration of vinca alkaloids. These reactions have been encountered most frequently when the vinca alkaloid was used in combination with mitomycin-C and may be serious when there is pre-existing pulmonary dysfunction. The onset may be within minutes or several hours after the vinca is injected and may occur up to 2 weeks following the dose of mitomycin. Progressive dyspnoea, requiring chronic therapy, may occur. Vincristine should not be readministered.

The simultaneous oral or intravenous administration of phenytoin and antineoplastic chemotherapy combinations, that included vincristine sulphate, have been reported to reduce blood levels of the anticonvulsant and to increase seizure activity. Although the contribution of the vinca alkaloids has not been established, dosage adjustment of phenytoin, based on serial blood level monitoring, may need to be made when it is used in combination with vincristine.

An increase in the severity of side effects may be experienced by patients with liver disease sufficient to decrease biliary excretion. A 50 per cent reduction in the dose of vincristine is recommended for patients having a direct serum bilirubin value above 3 mg/100 ml.

When Oncovin is used in combination with L-asparaginase, it should be given 12 to 24 hours before administration of the enzyme in order to minimise toxicity, since administering L-asparaginase first may reduce hepatic clearance of vincristine.

When chemotherapy is being given in conjunction with radiation therapy through portals which include the liver, the use of vincristine should be delayed until radiation therapy has been completed.

Both *in vivo* and *in vitro* laboratory tests have failed to demonstrate conclusively that this product is mutagenic. Fertility following treatment with vincristine alone for malignant disease has not been studied in humans. Clinical reports of both male and female patients who received multiple-agent chemotherapy that included vincristine indicate that azoospermia and amenorrhoea can occur in postpubertal patients. Recovery occurred many months after completion of chemotherapy in some but not all patients. When the same treatment is administered to prepubertal patients, it is much less likely to cause permanent azoospermia and amenorrhoea.

Patients who received vincristine chemotherapy in combination with anticancer drugs known to be carcinogenic have developed second malignancies. The contributing role of vincristine in this development has not been determined. No evidence of carcinogenicity was found following intraperitoneal administration in rats and mice, although this study was limited.

Care must be taken to avoid contamination of the eye with concentrations of Oncovin used clinically. If accidental contamination occurs, severe irritation (or, if the drug was delivered under pressure, even corneal ulceration) may result. The eye should be washed immediately and thoroughly.

Adverse reactions: Prior to the use of this drug, patients and/or their parents/guardians should be advised of the possibility of untoward symptoms.

In general, adverse reactions are reversible and are related to dosage size and cumulative dosage. The use of small amounts of vincristine daily for long periods is not advised. The most common adverse reaction is alopecia; the most troublesome adverse reactions are neuromuscular in origin.

When single weekly doses of the drug are employed, the adverse reactions of granulocytopenia, neuritic pain, and constipation are usually of short duration (i.e. less than 7 days). When the dosage is reduced, these reactions may lessen or disappear. They seem to be increased when the calculated amount of drug is given in divided doses. Other adverse reactions, such as alopecia, sensory loss, paraesthesia, difficulty in walking, slapping gait, loss of deep-tendon reflexes and muscle wasting may persist for at least as long as therapy is continued. Generalised sensorimotor dysfunction may become progressively more severe with continued treatment. In most instances, they have disappeared by about the sixth week after discontinuance of treatment, but the neuromuscular difficulties may persist for prolonged periods in some patients. Regrowth of hair may occur while maintenance therapy continues.

The following adverse reactions have been reported:

Neuromuscular (often dose limiting): Neuritic pain, sensory loss, paraesthesiae, difficulty in walking, slapping gait, loss of deep tendon reflexes, muscle wasting, ataxia, paralysis, foot drop and cranial nerve palsies, especially affecting the extraocular and laryngeal muscles. Jaw pain, pharyngeal pain, parotid gland pain, bone pain, back pain, limb pain, and myalgias have been reported; pain in these areas may be severe. Convulsions, frequently with hypertension, have been reported in a few patients receiving vincristine. Several instances of convulsions followed by coma have been reported in children. Transient cortical blindness and optic atrophy with blindness have been reported. Frequently, there appears to be a sequence in the development of neuromuscular side-effects. Initially, one may encounter only sensory impairment and paraesthesiae. With continued treatment, neuritic pain may appear and later, motor difficulties. No reports have yet been made of any agent that can reverse the neuromuscular manifestations of Oncovin.

Haematological: Granulocytopenia; vincristine does not appear to have any constant or significant effect upon the platelets or the red blood cells, however, anaemia and thrombocytopenia have been reported. If thrombocytopenia is present when treatment with Oncovin is begun, it may actually improve before the appearance of marrow remission.

Gastro-intestinal: Constipation, abdominal cramps, paralytic ileus, diarrhoea, weight loss, nausea, vomiting, oral ulceration, intestinal necrosis and/or perforation, and anorexia have occurred. The constipation which may be encountered responds well to such usual measures as enemas and laxatives. Constipation may take the form of upper colon impaction and the rectum may be found to be empty on physical examination. Colicky abdominal pain, coupled with an empty rectum, may mislead the clinician. A flat film of the abdomen is useful in demonstrating this condition. A routine prophylactic regimen against constipation is recommended for all patients receiving Oncovin. Paralytic ileus may occur, particularly in young children. The ileus will reverse itself upon temporary discontinuance of vincristine and with symptomatic care.

Pulmonary: See under 'Precautions'.

Endocrine: Rare occurrences of a syndrome attributable to inappropriate antidiuretic hormone secretion have been observed in patients treated with vincristine. There is a high urinary sodium excretion in the presence of hyponatraemia; renal or adrenal disease, hypotension, dehydration, azotaemia and clinical oedema are absent. With fluid deprivation, improvement occurs in the hyponatraemia and in the renal loss of sodium.

Genitourinary: Polyuria, dysuria and urinary retention due to bladder atony have occurred. Other drugs known to cause urinary retention (particularly in the elderly) should, if possible, be discontinued for the first few days following administration of vincristine.

Cardiovascular: Hypertension and hypotension have occurred. Chemotherapy combinations which have included vincristine, when given to patients previously treated with mediastinal radiation, have been associated with coronary artery disease and myocardial infarction. Causality has not been established.

Hypersensitivity: Rare cases of allergic-type reactions, such as anaphylaxis, rash and oedema, temporally related to vincristine therapy have been reported in patients receiving vincristine as a part of multi-drug chemotherapy regimens.

Cutaneous: Alopecia, rash.

Other: Fever, headache.

Overdosage: Side-effects following the use of vincristine are dose related. In children under 13 years of age, death has occurred following doses of vincristine that were 10 times those recommended for therapy. Severe symptoms may occur in this patient group following dosages of 3 to 4 mg/m^2. Adults can be expected to experience severe symptoms after single doses of 3 mg/m^2 or more. Therefore, following administration of doses higher than those recommended, patients can be expected to experience side-effects in an exaggerated fashion. Supportive care should include the following: (a) prevention of side-effects resulting from the syndrome of inappropriate antidiuretic hormone secretion (this would include restriction of fluid intake and perhaps the administration of a diuretic affecting the function of Henle's loop and the distal tubule); (b) administration of anticonvulsants; (c) use of enemas or cathartics to prevent ileus (in some instances, decompression of the gastrointestinal tract may be necessary); (d) monitoring the cardiovascular system; (e) determining daily blood counts for guidance in transfusion requirements.

Folinic acid has been observed to have a protective effect in normal mice which were administered lethal doses of vincristine. Isolated case reports suggest that folinic acid may be helpful in treating humans who have received an overdose. A suggested schedule is to administer 100 mg of folinic acid intravenously every 3 hours for 24 hours and then every 6 hours for at least 48 hours. Theoretical tissue levels of vincristine derived from pharmacokinetic data are predicted to remain significantly elevated for at least 72 hours. Treatment with folinic acid does not eliminate the need for the above-mentioned supportive measures.

Most of an intravenous dose of vincristine is excreted into the bile after rapid tissue binding. Because only very small amounts of the drug appear in dialysate, haemodialysis is not likely to be helpful in cases of overdosage.

Enhanced fecal excretion of parenterally administered vincristine has been demonstrated in dogs pretreated with cholestyramine. There are no published clinical data on the use of cholestyramine as an antidote in humans.

There are no published clinical data on the consequences of oral ingestion of vincristine. Should oral ingestion occur, the stomach should be evacuated followed by oral administration of activated charcoal and a cathartic.

Pharmaceutical precautions

Guidelines for the safe handling of antineoplastic agents: Cytotoxic preparations should not be handled by pregnant staff.

Trained personnel should reconstitute the drug. This should be performed in a designated area. The work surface should be covered with disposable plastic-backed absorbent paper.

Adequate protective gloves, masks and clothing should be worn. Precautions should be taken to avoid the drug accidentally coming into contact with the eyes.

If accidental contamination occurs, the eye should be washed with water thoroughly and immediately.

Use Luer-lock fittings on all syringes and sets. Large bore needles are recommended to minimise pressure and the possible formation of aerosols. The latter may also be reduced by the use of a venting needle.

Adequate care and precaution should be taken in the disposal of items (syringes, needles, etc.) used to reconstitute cytotoxic drugs.

Vials of Oncovin should be stored in a refrigerator between 2° and 8°C.

After reconstitution: After a portion of the solution has been removed from a vial, the remainder of the contents of the vial may be stored in a refrigerator for further use for 14 days without significant loss of potency. When the reconstituted vial of Oncovin is to be stored for more than 48 hours, it is essential to use the accompanying diluting solution or a diluent which contains a preservative.

Oncovin Solution: Store in a refrigerator between 2° and 8°C. Protect from light.

Oncovin should never be mixed with any other drug and should not be diluted in solutions that raise or lower the pH outside the range of 3.5 to 5.5.

Legal category POM.

Package quantities
Vials 1 mg: Single vials.
Vials 1 mg/1 ml: Single vials.
Vials 2 mg/2 ml: Single vials.

Further information Nil.

Product licence numbers

Vials 1 mg	0006/5070
Diluent	0006/5174
Vials 1 mg/1 ml	0006/0169
Vials 2 mg/2 ml	0006/0169

PROGESIC*

Presentation Tablets each containing fenoprofen calcium equivalent to 200 mg of fenoprofen. The tablets are round, yellow, 9.5 mm in diameter and marked Lilly 4015.

Uses For the treatment of osteoarthritis, rheumatoid arthritis and ankylosing spondylitis. For the relief of mild/moderate pain. Pyrexia.

Dosage and administration For oral administration to adults only, and not recommended for administration to children.

Dosage: 200–600 mg three or four times a day. The maximum daily dose should not exceed 3 g.

If fenoprofen is administered with meals the total amount absorbed is not affected, although peak blood levels are delayed and diminished.

The elderly: There is no difference in the metabolism or pharmacokinetics of fenoprofen in the elderly. However, it may be advisable to start therapy with a low dose, as side-effects of non-steroidal anti-inflammatory drugs are more pronounced in this patient population.

Contra-indications, warnings, etc

Contra-indications: Hypersensitivity to the drug. Active, or a history of, peptic or intestinal ulceration.

Fenoprofen should not be given to patients in whom aspirin and other non-steroidal anti-inflammatory drugs induce the symptoms of asthma, rhinitis, or urticaria, because cross-sensitivity to these drugs occurs in a high proportion of patients.

Patients with a history of significantly impaired renal function.

Warnings

Gastro-intestinal: Serious toxicity, such as bleeding, ulceration and perforation, can occur at any time, without warning symptoms, in patients treated chronically. Elderly or debilitated patients tolerate ulceration or bleeding less well than other individuals and most spontaneous reports of fatal gastro-intestinal events are in this population. Minor upper gastro-intestinal problems, such as dyspepsia, are common, usually developing early in therapy.

Fenoprofen should only be given under close supervision to patients with a history of upper gastro-intestinal disease or peptic ulcer risk factors.

Genito-urinary: The most frequently reported problems have been episodes of dysuria, cystitis, haematuria, interstitial nephritis and nephrotic syndrome. This syndrome may be preceded by the appearance of fever, rash, arthralgia, oliguria and uraemia, and may progress to anuria. Early recognition of the syndrome and withdrawal of the drug have been followed by rapid recovery. Patients who have had similar reactions with other non-steroidal anti-inflammatory drugs should not be given fenoprofen. Patients likely to have compromised renal function should be monitored periodically.

Bronchospasm may be precipitated in patients suffering from, or with a previous history of, bronchial asthma or allergic disease.

Usage in pregnancy: The safety of fenoprofen for use during pregnancy has not been established; therefore it should not be used during pregnancy unless considered essential by the physician. Animal studies showed prolongation of parturition, but no evidence of teratogenicity.

Usage in nursing mothers: Safety has not been established, therefore administration to nursing mothers is not recommended.

Precautions: In patients with conditions leading to reduction in renal blood flow or blood volume, administration of non-steroidal anti-inflammatory drugs may precipitate overt renal decompensation. Patients at greatest risk of this reaction are those with impaired renal function, heart failure, liver dysfunction, those taking diuretics, and the elderly. Discontinuation of therapy is typically followed by recovery to the pre-treatment state.

Since fenoprofen is eliminated primarily by the kidneys, patients with possibly compromised renal function (such as the elderly) should be closely monitored; a lower daily dosage should be anticipated to avoid excessive drug accumulation.

Some patients have developed elevation of serum transaminase, LDH and alkaline phosphatase and it is recommended that fenoprofen be discontinued if any significant liver abnormalities occur. Borderline elevations of one or more liver function tests may occur in up to 15% of patients. Severe hepatic reactions, including jaundice and cases of fatal hepatitis, have been reported.

Patients with initial low haemoglobin values who are receiving long-term therapy with fenoprofen should have a haemoglobin determination at reasonable intervals.

Peripheral oedema has been observed in some patients taking fenoprofen, therefore it should be used with caution in patients with compromised cardiac function or hypertension. The possibility of renal involvement should be considered.

Studies to date have not shown changes in the eyes attributable to the administration of fenoprofen. However, adverse ocular effects have been observed with other anti-inflammatory drugs, so eye examinations should be performed if visual disturbances occur in patients taking fenoprofen.

Caution should be exercised by patients whose activities require alertness if they experience central nervous system side-effects.

Since the safety of fenoprofen has not been established in patients with impaired hearing, these patients should have periodic tests of auditory function during chronic therapy.

Fenoprofen decreases platelet aggregation and may prolong bleeding time.

Laboratory test interactions: Values of total and free triiodothyronine in patients receiving fenoprofen have been reported as falsely elevated. Thyroid stimulating hormone, total thyroxine and thyrotropin releasing hormone response are not affected.

Drug interactions: The concurrent use of fenoprofen and salicylates is not recommended.

Chronic administration of phenobarbitone may be associated with a decrease in the plasma half-life of fenoprofen. Dosage adjustment of fenoprofen may be required.

Patients treated with fenoprofen may be resistant to the effects of loop diuretics.

In vitro studies have shown that fenoprofen may displace other drugs, for example hydantoins, sulphonamides, or sulphonylureas, from their binding sites and this may lead to drug interaction. Theoretically, fenoprofen could likewise be displaced. In patients receiving coumarin-type anti-coagulants, the addition of fenoprofen could prolong the prothrombin time.

Side-effects

Gastro-intestinal: These are the most commonly observed side-effects and include dyspepsia, constipation, diarrhoea, nausea, vomiting, anorexia, ulceration of the buccal mucosa, abdominal pain, flatulence, dry mouth, gastritis, metallic taste, pancreatitis and occult blood in the stool. Cases of peptic ulceration, including some complicated by bleeding or perforation have occurred.

Renal: Cases of acute renal insufficiency, in association with interstitial nephritis, nephrotic syndrome or papillary necrosis, have been reported. Episodes of dysuria, cystitis and haematuria, oliguria, azotaemia and anuria have occurred.

Hepatic: Severe hepatic reactions, including jaundice and fatal hepatitis, have been reported rarely. Increases in alkaline phosphatase, LDH and AST have been observed.

Haematological: Various syndromes involving the bone marrow have been reported rarely; thrombocytopenia, pancytopenia and aplastic anaemia have occurred. Purpura, bruising, haemorrhage, haemolytic anaemia and agranulocytosis have also been reported.

Allergic/skin: Pruritus, rash, urticaria, anaphylaxis, Stevens-Johnson syndrome, angioneurotic oedema, increased sweating, exfoliative dermatitis, toxic epidermal necrolysis and alopecia have been reported.

Neurological: Reactions reported include headache, somnolence, dizziness, tremor, confusion and insomnia, depression, disorientation, seizures and trigeminal neuralgia.

Cardiovascular: Palpitations, tachycardia, atrial fibrillation, pulmonary oedema, ECG changes and supraventricular tachycardia have been reported.

Miscellaneous: Tinnitus, hearing decrease, amblyopia, blurred vision, diplopia, optic neuritis, nervousness, peripheral oedema, asthenia, dyspnoea, fatigue, malaise, burning tongue, personality change, lymphadenopathy, mastodynia, fever, upper respiratory infection and nasopharyngitis have been reported.

Overdosage: Symptoms of overdose appear within several hours and generally involve the gastro-intestinal and central nervous systems. They include dyspepsia, nausea, vomiting, abdominal pain, dizziness, headache, ataxia, tinnitus, tremor, drowsiness and confusion. Hyperpyrexia, tachycardia, hypotension and acute renal failure may occur rarely following overdose. Respiratory depression and metabolic acidosis have also been reported following overdose with certain non-steroidal anti-inflammatory drugs.

Treatment: Standard therapy to evacuate gastric contents and to support vital functions should be employed. Alkalinisation of the urine, forced diuresis, peritoneal dialysis, haemodialysis and charcoal haemoperfusion do not enhance systemic drug elimination.

Pharmaceutical precautions Store at room temperature (15°–25°C).

Legal category POM.

Package quantities Tablets 200 mg. Blister packs of 100 tablets.

Further information Nil.

Product licence number 0006/0141.

SECONAL* SODIUM

Presentation Capsules (orange, coded F42) containing 50 mg Secobarbitone Sodium PhEur.

Capsules (orange, coded F40) containing 100 mg Secobarbitone Sodium PhEur. (The British Approved Name is quinalbarbitone sodium.)

Uses For the short-term treatment of severe, intractable insomnia.

Dosage and administration For oral administration to adults only. Normal dosage is 100 mg at bedtime.

The onset of action is 10 to 15 minutes and the duration ranges from 3 to 4 hours. The rate of absorption is increased if taken on an empty stomach. The plasma half-life in adults ranges between 15 to 40 hours, with a mean of 28 hours.

The elderly: Seconal is not recommended for use in elderly or debilitated patients.

In studies, secobarbitone sodium has been found to lose most of its effectiveness for both inducing and maintaining sleep by the end of 2 weeks of continued drug administration, even with the use of multiple doses.

Contra-indications, warnings, etc

Contra-indications: Hypersensitivity to barbiturates, a history of manifest or latent porphyria, marked impairment of liver function, or respiratory disease in which dyspnoea or obstruction is evident. Oral barbiturates should not be administered in the presence of acute or chronic pain, because paradoxical excitement may be induced or important symptoms may be masked.

Barbiturates should not be administered to children, young adults, patients with a history of drug or alcohol addiction or abuse, the elderly and the debilitated.

Usage in pregnancy: Barbiturates are contra-indicated during pregnancy since they can cause fetal harm. A higher than expected incidence of fetal abnormalities may be connected with maternal consumption of barbiturates. Barbiturates readily cross the placental barrier and are distributed throughout fetal tissues, with highest concentrations in placenta, fetal liver and brain. Withdrawal symptoms occur in infants born to women who receive barbiturates during the last trimester of pregnancy. If a patient becomes pregnant whilst taking this drug, she should be told of the potential hazard to the fetus.

Reports of infants suffering from long-term barbiturate exposure *in utero* included the acute withdrawal syndrome of seizures and hyperirritability, from birth to a delayed onset of up to 14 days.

Labour and delivery: Respiratory depression has been noted in infants born following the use of barbiturates during labour. Premature infants are particularly susceptible. Resuscitation equipment should be available.

Nursing mothers: Small amounts of barbiturates are excreted in the milk, and they are therefore contra-indicated for the nursing mother.

Warnings: Addiction potential: Secobarbitone sodium may be habit forming. Tolerance and psychological and physical dependence may occur with continued use. Patients who have psychological dependence on barbiturates may increase the dosage or decrease the dosage interval without consulting a doctor, and subsequently may develop a physical dependence on barbiturates.

To minimise the possibility of overdosage or development of dependence, the amount prescribed should be limited to that required for the interval until the next appointment.

Withdrawal symptoms occur after long-term normal use (and particularly after abuse) on rapid cessation of barbiturate treatment. Symptoms include nightmares, irritability and insomnia, and in severe cases, tremors, delirium, convulsions and death.

Barbiturates should be withdrawn gradually from any patient known to be taking excessive doses over long periods.

Information for patients: The following information should be given to patients receiving secobarbitone:

1. The use of secobarbitone carries with it an associated

risk of psychological and/or physical dependence. The patient should be warned against increasing the dose of the drug without consulting a doctor.

2. Secobarbitone may impair the mental and/or physical abilities required for the performance of potentially hazardous tasks, such as driving a car or operating machinery. The patient should be cautioned accordingly.

3. Alcohol should not be consumed while taking secobarbitone. The concurrent use of secobarbitone with other CNS depressants (e.g. alcohol, narcotics, tranquillisers and antihistamines) may result in additional CNS depressant effects.

Precautions: Barbiturates should be administered with caution, if at all, to patients who are mentally depressed or have suicidal tendencies. They should also be used with great caution and at reduced dosage in those with hepatic disease, marked renal dysfunction, shock or respiratory depression.

Elderly or debilitated patients may react to barbiturates with marked excitement, depression or confusion (see 'Contra-indications'). In some persons, barbiturates repeatedly produce excitement rather than depression.

Barbiturates should not be administered to patients showing the premonitory signs of hepatic coma (see 'Contra-indications').

A cumulative effect may occur with the barbiturates leading to features of chronic poisoning including headache, depression and slurred speech.

Automatism may follow the use of an hypnotic dose of barbiturate.

The systemic effects of exogenous and endogenous corticosteroids may be diminished by secobarbitone. This product should therefore be administered with caution to patients with borderline hypoadrenal function, regardless of whether it is of pituitary or of primary adrenal origin.

Laboratory tests: Prolonged therapy with barbiturates should be accompanied by periodic evaluation of eg, the haematopoietic, renal and hepatic systems (but see 'Uses').

Drug interactions: Toxic effects and fatalities have occurred following overdoses of secobarbitone alone and in combination with other CNS depressants. Caution should be exercised in prescribing unnecessarily large amounts of secobarbitone for patients who have a history of emotional disturbances or suicidal ideation or who have misused alcohol or other CNS drugs.

Anticoagulants: Barbiturates cause induction of the liver microsomal enzymes responsible for metabolising many other drugs; in particular they may result in increased metabolism and decreased anticoagulant response of oral anticoagulants (eg, warfarin). Patients stabilised on anticoagulant therapy may require dosage adjustments if barbiturates are added to or withdrawn from their regimen.

Corticosteroids: Barbiturates appear to enhance the metabolism of exogenous corticosteroids, and steroid dosage may also need adjustment.

Griseofulvin: Barbiturates may interfere with the absorption of oral griseofulvin, thus decreasing its blood level. Concomitant administration should be avoided if possible.

Doxycycline: Barbiturates may shorten the half-life of doxycycline for as long as 2 weeks after the barbiturate is discontinued. If administered concomitantly, the clinical reponse to doxycycline should be monitored closely.

Phenytoin, sodium valproate, valproic acid: The effect of barbiturates on phenytoin metabolism is variable. Phenytoin and barbiturate blood levels should be monitored more frequently if administered concomitantly. Sodium valproate and valproic acid increase secobarbitone serum levels. Therefore, these levels should be monitored and dosage adjustments made as clinically indicated.

CNS depressants: Concomitant use of other CNS depressants, including other sedatives or hypnotics, antihistamines, tranquillisers or alcohol, may produce additive depressant effects.

Monoamine oxidase inhibitors (MAOIs): Prolong the effects of barbiturates.

Oestradiol, oestrone, progesterone and other steroidal hormones: There have been reports of patients treated with antiepileptic drugs (eg, phenobarbitone) who became pregnant while taking oral contraceptives. Barbiturates may decrease the effect of oestradiol. An alternative contraceptive method might be suggested to women taking barbiturates.

Carcinogenesis: Animal data show that phenobarbitone can be carcinogenic after lifetime administration.

Human data: In a 29 year epidemiological study of 9,136 patients who were treated on an anticonvulsant protocol that included phenobarbitone, results indicated a higher than normal incidence of hepatic carcinoma. Previously, some of these patients had been treated with thorotrast, a drug that is known to produce hepatic carcinomas. Thus, this study did not provide sufficient evidence that phenobarbitone is carcinogenic in humans.

A retrospective study of 84 children with brain tumours, matched to 73 normal controls and 78 cancer controls (malignant disease other than brain tumours), suggested an association between exposure to barbiturates prenatally and an increased incidence of brain tumours.

Side-effects: The following adverse reactions and their incidences were compiled from surveillance of thousands of hospitalised patients who received barbiturates. As such patients may be less aware of certain of the milder adverse effects of barbiturates, the incidence of these reactions may be somewhat higher in fully ambulatory patients:

More than 1 in 100 patients: The most common adverse reaction, estimated to occur at a rate of 1 to 3 patients per 100, is the following:

Nervous System: Somnolence.

Less than 1 in 100 patients: Adverse reactions estimated to occur at a rate of less than 1 in 100 patients are listed below, grouped by organ system and by decreasing frequency:

Neurological: Agitation, confusion, hyperkinesia, ataxia, CNS depression, nightmares, nervousness, psychiatric disturbance, hallucinations, insomnia, anxiety, dizziness, abnormal thinking.

Respiratory: Hypoventilation, apnoea.

Cardiovascular: Bradycardia, hypotension, syncope.

Digestive: Nausea, vomiting, constipation.

Other: Headache, hypersensitivity reactions (angioneurotic oedema, rashes, exfoliative dermatitis), fever, liver damage. Hypersensitivity is more likely to occur in patients with asthma, urticaria or angioneurotic oedema.

Drug abuse and dependence: Barbiturates may be habit forming; tolerance, psychological and physical dependence may occur, especially following prolonged use of high doses. Daily administration in excess of 400 mg secobarbitone, for approximately 90 days, is likely to produce some degree of physical dependence. A dosage of 600–800 mg, for at least 35 days, is sufficient to produce withdrawal seizures. The average daily dose for the barbiturate addict is usually about 1.5 g.

As tolerance to barbiturates develops, the amount needed to maintain the same level of intoxication increases; tolerance to a fatal dosage, however, does not increase more than twofold. As this occurs, the margin between intoxicating dosage and fatal dosage becomes smaller. The lethal dose of a barbiturate is far less if alcohol is also ingested.

Symptoms of acute intoxication include unsteady gait, slurred speech, and sustained nystagmus, Mental signs of chronic intoxication include confusion, poor judgement, irritability, insomnia and somatic complaints.

The symptoms of barbiturate withdrawal can be severe and may cause death. Minor withdrawal symptoms may appear 8 to 12 hours after the last dose of a barbiturate. These symptoms usually appear in the following order: anxiety, muscle twitching, tremor of hands and fingers, progressive weakness, dizziness, distortion in visual perception, nausea, vomiting, insomnia, and orthostatic hypotension. Major withdrawal symptoms (convulsions and delirium) may occur within 16 hours and last up to 5 days after abrupt cessation of barbiturates. Intensity of withdrawal symptoms gradually declines over a period of approximately 15 days. Individuals susceptible to barbiturate abuse and dependence include alcoholics and opiate abusers, as well as other sedative-hypnotic and amphetamine abusers.

Dependence on barbiturates arises from repeated administration on a continuous basis, generally in amounts exceeding therapeutic dose levels. Treatment of dependence consists of cautious and gradual withdrawal of the drug. Barbiturate-dependent patients can be withdrawn by using a number of withdrawal regimens. In all cases, withdrawal takes an extended period. One method involves substituting a 30 mg dose of phenobarbitone for each 100–200 mg dose of barbiturate that the patient has been taking. The total daily amount of phenobarbitone is then administered in 3 or 4 divided doses, not to exceed 600 mg daily. Should signs of withdrawal occur on the first day of treatment, a loading dose of 100 to 200 mg of phenobarbitone may be administered intramuscularly in addition to the oral dose. After stabilisation on phenobarbitone, the total daily dose is decreased by 30 mg a day as long as withdrawal is proceeding smoothly. A modification of this regimen involves initiating treatment at the patient's regular dosage level and decreasing the daily dosage by 10% as tolerated by the patient.

Infants that are physically dependent on barbiturates may be given phenobarbitone, 3 to 10 mg/kg/day. After withdrawal symptoms (hyperactivity, disturbed sleep, tremors, and hyperreflexia) are relieved, the dosage of phenobarbitone should be gradually decreased and completely withdrawn over a 2 week period.

Overdosage: The toxic dose of barbiturates varies considerably. In general, an oral dose of 1 g of most barbiturates produces serious poisoning in an adult. Death commonly occurs after 2 to 10 g of ingested barbiturate. The sedated, therapeutic blood levels of secobarbitone range between 0.5 and 5 mg/l; the usual lethal blood level ranges from 15 to 40 mg/l. Barbiturate intoxication may be confused with alcoholism, bromide intoxication, and various neurological disorders. Potential tolerance must be considered when evaluating significance of dose and plasma concentration.

Signs and symptoms: Symptoms of oral overdose may occur within 15 minutes and begin with CNS depression, absent or sluggish reflexes, underventilation, hypotension and hypothermia, which may progress to pulmonary oedema and death. Haemorrhagic blisters may develop, especially at pressure points.

In extreme overdose, all electrical activity in the brain may cease, in which case a 'flat' EEG normally equated with clinical death cannot be accepted. This effect is fully reversible unless hypoxic damage occurs. Consideration should be given to the possibility of barbiturate intoxication even in situations that appear to involve trauma.

Complications such as pneumonia, pulmonary oedema, cardiac arrhythmias, congestive heart failure and renal failure may occur. Uraemia may increase CNS sensitivity to barbiturates if renal function is impaired. Differential diagnosis should include hypoglycaemia, head trauma, cerebrovascular accidents, convulsive states and diabetic coma.

Treatment: General management should consist of symptomatic and supportive therapy. Activated charcoal may be more effective than emesis or lavage. Diuresis and peritoneal dialysis are of little value. Haemodialysis and haemoperfusion enhance drug clearance and should be considered in serious poisoning. If the patient has chronically abused sedatives, withdrawal reactions may be manifest following acute overdose.

Pharmaceutical precautions Keep containers tightly closed. Store below 25°C.

Legal category CD (Sch 2) POM.

Package quantities Capsules 50 mg and 100 mg: Bottles of 100.

Further information Nil.

Product licence numbers
Capsules 50 mg 0006/5065
Capsules 100 mg 0006/5066

SODIUM AMYTAL* CAPSULES
SODIUM AMYTAL* TABLETS

Presentation Capsules (blue, coded F23) each containing 60 mg Amylobarbitone Sodium PhEur.

Capsules (blue, coded F33) each containing 200 mg Amylobarbitone Sodium PhEur.

Tablets (uncoated, white, coded U43) each containing 60 mg Amylobarbitone Sodium PhEur.

Tablets (uncoated, white, coded U16) each containing 200 mg Amylobarbitone Sodium PhEur.

Uses For the treatment of severe, intractable insomnia.

Dosage and administration For oral administration to adults only. Normal dosage is 60–200 mg at bedtime. Occasionally a larger dose may be necessary.

The effects should become apparent between 30 and 45 minutes after administration.

The elderly: Sodium Amytal is not recommended for use in elderly or debilitated patients.

Contra-indications, warnings, etc
Contra-indications: Hypersensitivity to barbiturates, a history of manifest or latent porphyria, marked impairment of liver function, or respiratory disease in which dyspnoea or obstruction is evident. Oral barbiturates should not be administered in the presence of uncontrolled acute or chronic pain, because paradoxical excitement may be induced or important symptoms may be masked.

Barbiturates should not be administered to children, young adults, patients with a history of drug or alcohol abuse, the elderly and the debilitated.

Usage in pregnancy: Barbiturates are contra-indicated during pregnancy.

Labour and delivery: Respiratory depression has been noted in infants born following the use of barbiturates during labour.

Nursing mothers: Small amounts of barbiturates are excreted in the milk, and they are therefore contra-indicated for the nursing mother.

Warnings
Addiction potential: Barbiturates have a high addiction potential. Long-term use, or use of high dosage for short periods, may lead to tolerance and subsequently to physical and psychological dependence.

Signs of acute intoxication with barbiturates include unsteady gait, slurred speech and sustained nystagmus. Symptoms of dependence or chronic intoxication include confusion, defective judgement, loss of emotional control, insomnia and somatic complaints.

To minimise the possibility of overdosage or development of dependence, the amount prescribed should be limited to that required for the interval until the next appointment.

Withdrawal symptoms occur after long-term normal use (and particularly after abuse) on rapid cessation of barbiturate treatment. Symptoms include nightmares, irritability and insomnia, and in severe cases, tremors, delirium, convulsions and death.

Barbiturates should be withdrawn gradually from any patient known to be taking excessive doses over long periods.

Information for patients: The following information should be given to patients receiving amylobarbitone:

1. The use of amylobarbitone carries with it an associated risk of psychological and/or physical dependence. The patient should be warned against increasing the dose of the drug without consulting a physician.

2. Amylobarbitone may impair the mental and/or

physical abilities required for the performance of potentially hazardous tasks, such as driving a car or operating machinery. The patient should be cautioned accordingly.

3. Alcohol should not be consumed while taking amylobarbitone. The concurrent use of amylobarbitone with other CNS depressants (e.g. alcohol, narcotics, tranquillisers and antihistamines) may result in additional CNS depressant effects.

Drug interactions: Amylobarbitone in combination with alcohol, tranquillisers, and other CNS depressants, has additive depressant effects, and the patient should be so advised. Toxic effects and fatalities have occurred following overdoses of amylobarbitone alone and in combination with other CNS depressants. Caution should be exercised in prescribing unnecessarily large amounts of amylobarbitone for patients who have a history of emotional disturbances or suicidal ideation or who have misused alcohol or other CNS drugs.

Barbiturates cause induction of the liver enzymes responsible for metabolising many other drugs; in particular they should not be administered concurrently with coumarin-type anticoagulants. They may also affect the metabolism of systemic steroids (including oral contraceptives), phenytoin, griseofulvin, rifampicin, tricyclic antidepressants, and phenothiazines such as chlorpromazine.

Monoamine oxidase inhibitors prolong the effects of barbiturates, probably because the metabolism of the barbiturate is inhibited.

Precautions: Barbiturates should be administered with caution, if at all, to patients who are mentally depressed or have suicidal tendencies. They should also be used with great caution and at reduced dosage in those with marked renal dysfunction, shock or respiratory depression.

Prolonged therapy with barbiturates should be accompanied by periodic evaluation of haematopoietic, renal and hepatic systems (but see 'Uses').

Elderly or debilitated patients may react to barbiturates with marked excitement, depression or confusion (see 'Contra-indications'). In some persons, barbiturates repeatedly produce excitement rather than depression.

A cumulative effect may occur with the barbiturates leading to features of chronic poisoning including headache, depression and slurred speech.

Automatism may follow the use of an hypnotic dose of a barbiturate.

The systemic effects of exogenous hydrocortisone and endogenous hydrocortisone (cortisol) may be diminished by amylobarbitone. This product should therefore be administered with caution to patients with borderline hypoadrenal function, regardless of whether it is of pituitary or of primary adrenal origin.

Side-effects: The following adverse reactions have been reported:

Neurological: Residual sedation or 'hangover'; drowsiness, lethargy, ataxia, paradoxical excitement, confusion, pain, memory defects, vertigo.

Respiratory/circulatory: Respiratory depression, apnoea and circulatory collapse.

Hypersensitivity: Allergic reactions, especially in individuals with asthma, urticaria, angioneurotic oedema or similar conditions; skin eruptions.

Other: Nausea and vomiting; headache.

Overdosage: The toxic dose of barbiturates varies considerably. In general, an oral dose of 1 g of most barbiturates produces serious poisoning in an adult. Death commonly occurs after 2 to 10 g of ingested barbiturate. Barbiturate intoxication may be confused with alcoholism, bromide intoxication, and various neurological disorders.

Symptoms: The manifestations of overdosage are early hypothermia followed by fever, sluggish or absent reflexes, respiratory depression, gradual appearance of circulatory collapse, pulmonary oedema and coma.

In extreme overdose, all electrical activity in the brain may cease, in which case a 'flat' EEG normally equated with clinical death cannot be accepted. This effect is fully reversible unless hypoxic damage occurs. Consideration should be given to the possibility of barbiturate intoxication even in situations that appear to involve trauma.

Treatment: General management should consist of symptomatic and supportive therapy, including gastric lavage, administration of intravenous fluids, and maintenance of blood pressure, body temperature and adequate respiratory exchange. Haemodialysis will increase the rate of removal of barbiturates from the body fluids. Antibiotics may be required to control pulmonary complications.

Pharmaceutical precautions *Capsules and tablets:* Keep containers tightly closed. Store below 25°C.

Legal category CD (Sch 3) POM.

Package quantities
Capsules 60 mg: Bottles of 100.
Capsules 200 mg: Bottles of 100.
Tablets 60 mg: Bottles of 100.
Tablets 200 mg: Bottles of 100.

Further information Nil.

Product licence numbers

Capsules 60 mg	0006/5084
Capsules 200 mg	0006/5085
Tablets 60 mg	0006/5080
Tablets 200 mg	0006/5082

SODIUM AMYTAL* INJECTION

Presentation Vials containing 250 mg Amylobarbitone Sodium PhEur for injection.

Uses Sodium Amytal may be used parenterally to control status epilepticus, but it is not the barbiturate of choice in the routine treatment of grand mal epilepsy.

Dosage and administration
Adults: The usual adult dose is in the range of 250 mg–1 g. The maximum single dose should not exceed 1 g and the maximum intramuscular dose at any one site should not exceed 500 mg. The final dosage is largely determined by the patient's reaction to the slow administration of the drug.

The elderly: Dosage should be reduced in the elderly, since they may be more sensitive to barbiturates. Dosage reduction is also necessary if renal or hepatic function is impaired (see 'Precautions').

Children: The final dosage is determined to a great extent by the patient's reaction to the slow administration of the drug. Usually, 65 mg to 500 mg may be given to a child 6 to 12 years of age. Safety and efficacy have not been established in children below the age of 6 years. In neonates, the half-life is significantly prolonged.

Solutions should be made up aseptically with Sterilised Water for Injections PhEur. The accompanying table will aid in preparing solutions of various concentrations; ordinarily, a 10% solution is used. After Sterilised Water for Injections PhEur is added, the vial should be rotated to facilitate solution of the powder. Do not shake the vial.

Several minutes may be required for the drug to dissolve completely, but under no circumstances should a solution be injected if it has not become absolutely clear within five minutes. Also, a solution that forms a precipitate after clearing should not be used. Amylobarbitone sodium hydrolyses in solution or upon exposure to air. Not more than 30 minutes should elapse from the time the vial is opened until its contents are injected. Prior to administration, parenteral drug products should be inspected visually for particulate matter and discolouration, whenever containers permit.

Quantity of Sterilised Water for Injections PhEur to be added to the vial contents to obtain a solution of a desired percentage. Solutions derived will be in Weight/Volume.

Vial Content	1%	2.5%	5%	10%	20%
250 mg	25 ml	10 ml	5 ml	2.5 ml	1.25 ml

Intramuscular use: No more than 5 ml (irrespective of concentration) should be injected at any one site. Injections should be made deeply into large muscles, such as the gluteus maximus. Superficial intramuscular or subcutaneous injections may be painful and may produce sterile abscesses or sloughing.

If it is desirable to reduce the dosage volume, a 20% solution may be used.

Intravenous use: For intravenous use, the contents of the vial should be diluted.

Slow intravenous injection is essential, with vital signs observed, to maintain blood pressure, respiratory and cardiac function. The rate of iv injection, for adults, should not exceed 50 mg/min, to prevent sleep or sudden respiratory depression.

Parenteral solutions of barbiturates are highly alkaline. Therefore, extreme care should be taken to avoid perivascular extravasation or intra-arterial injection. Extravascular injection may cause local tissue damage, with subsequent necrosis. Consequences of intra-arterial injection may vary from transient pain to gangrene of the limb. Any complaint of pain in the limb warrants stopping the injection.

Caution: The intravenous administration of Sodium Amytal carries with it the potential dangers inherent in the intravenous use of any potent hypnotic.

Contra-indications, warnings, etc

Contra-indications: Hypersensitivity to barbiturates, a history of manifest or latent porphyria, marked impairment of liver function, or respiratory disease in which dyspnoea or obstruction is evident.

Sodium Amytal should not be administered in the presence of uncontrolled acute or chronic pain, because paradoxical excitement may be induced or important symptoms may be masked.

Warnings

Intravenous administration: Too rapid administration may cause respiratory depression, apnoea, laryngospasm, or vasodilatation with fall in blood pressure.

Addiction potential: Amylobarbitone sodium may be habit forming. Tolerance and psychological and physical dependence may occur with continued use. Patients who have psychological dependence on barbiturates may increase the dosage or decrease the dosage interval without consulting a doctor, and subsequently may develop a physical dependence on barbiturates.

Withdrawal symptoms occur after long-term normal use (and particularly after abuse) on rapid cessation of barbiturate treatment. Symptoms include nightmares, irritability and insomnia, and in severe cases, tremors, delirium, convulsions and death.

Barbiturates should be withdrawn gradually from any patient known to be taking excessive doses over long periods.

Information for patients: The following information should be given to patients receiving barbiturates:

1. The use of barbiturates carries with it an associated risk of psychological and/or physical dependence. The patient should be warned against increasing the dose of the drug without consulting a doctor.
2. Barbiturates may impair the mental and/or physical abilities required for the performance of potentially hazardous tasks, such as driving a car or operating machinery. The patient should be cautioned accordingly.
3. Alcohol should not be consumed while taking barbiturates. The concurrent use of amylobarbitone with other CNS depressants (eg. alcohol, narcotics, tranquillisers and antihistamines) may result in additional CNS depressant effects.

Usage in pregnancy: Barbiturates can cause fetal damage when administered to a pregnant woman. If amylobarbitone sodium is used during pregnancy, or if the patient becomes pregnant while taking this drug, she should be told of the potential hazard to the fetus.

A higher than expected incidence of fetal abnormalities may be connected with maternal consumption of barbiturates. Barbiturates readily cross the placental barrier and are distributed throughout fetal tissues, with highest concentrations in placenta, fetal liver and brain. Fetal blood levels approach maternal blood levels following parenteral administration. Withdrawal symptoms occur in infants born to women who receive barbiturates during the last trimester of pregnancy.

Reports of infants suffering from long-term barbiturate exposure *in utero* included the acute withdrawal syndrome of seizures and hyperirritability, from birth to a delayed onset of up to 14 days.

Labour and delivery: Respiratory depression has been noted in infants born following the use of barbiturates during labour. Premature infants are particularly susceptible. Resuscitation equipment should be available.

Nursing mothers: Small amounts of barbiturates are excreted in the milk, and this product should not be administered to nursing mothers unless considered to be essential by the doctor.

Precautions: Amylobarbitone sodium should be used with caution in patients with decreased liver function, since a prolongation of effect may occur. A reduced dosage may be required in patients with decreased hepatic or renal function. Barbiturates should not be administered to patients showing the premonitory signs of hepatic coma.

Barbiturates should be administered with caution, if at all, to patients who are mentally depressed, have suicidal tendencies, or have a history of drug abuse.

Elderly or debilitated patients may react to barbiturates with marked excitement, depression, or confusion.

The systemic effects of exogenous and endogenous corticosteroids may be diminished by amylobarbitone sodium. This product should therefore be administered with caution to patients with borderline hypoadrenal function, regardless of whether it is of pituitary or of primary adrenal origin.

Dosage and rate of administration should be selected with great care in patients with hypertension, hypotension or pulmonary or cardiovascular diseases.

Amylobarbitone sodium is not recommended as an anaesthetic agent but, if a patient develops physical signs of severe depression, he should be treated as though he is deeply anaesthetised. Pulmonary oedema may complicate long periods of unconsciousness.

Laboratory tests: Prolonged therapy with barbiturates should be accompanied by periodic evaluation of e.g., the haematopoietic, renal and hepatic symptoms.

Drug interactions: Toxic effects and fatalities have occurred following overdoses of amylobarbitone alone and in combination with other CNS depressants. Caution should be exercised in prescribing unnecessarily large amounts of amylobarbitone for patients who have a history of emotional disturbances or suicidal ideation, or who have misused alcohol or other CNS drugs.

Anticoagulants: Barbiturates cause induction of the liver microsomal enzymes responsible for metabolising many other drugs; in particular they may result in increased metabolism and decreased anticoagulant response of oral anticoagulants (eg, warfarin). Patients stabilised on anticoagulant therapy may require dosage adjustments if barbiturates are added to or withdrawn from their regimen.

Corticosteroids: Barbiturates appear to enhance the metabolism of exogenous corticosteroids, and steroid dosage may also need adjustment.

Griseofulvin: Barbiturates may interfere with the absorption of oral griseofulvin, thus decreasing its blood level. Concomitant administration should be avoided if possible.

Doxycycline: Barbiturates may shorten the half-life of

doxycycline for as long as 2 weeks after the barbiturate is discontinued. If administered concomitantly, the clinical response to doxycycline should be monitored closely.

Phenytoin, sodium valproate, valproic acid: The effect of barbiturates on phenytoin metabolism is variable. Phenytoin and barbiturate blood levels should be monitored more frequently if administered concomitantly. Sodium valproate and valproic acid increase amylobarbitone serum levels. Therefore, these levels should be monitored and dosage adjustments made as clinically indicated.

CNS depressants: Concomitant use of other CNS depressants, including other sedatives or hypnotics, antihistamines, tranquillisers or alcohol, may produce additive depressant effects.

Monoamine oxidase inhibitors (MAOIs): Prolong the effects of barbiturates.

Oestradiol, oestrone, progesterone and other steroidal hormones: There have been reports of patients treated with antiepileptic drugs (e.g., phenobarbitone) who became pregnant while taking oral contraceptives. Barbiturates may decrease the effect of oestradiol. An alternative contraceptive method might be suggested to women taking barbiturates.

Carcinogenesis: Animal data show that phenobarbitone can be carcinogenic after lifetime administration.

Human data: In a 29 year epidemiological study of 9,136 patients who were treated on an anticonvulsant protocol that included phenobarbitone, results indicated a higher than normal incidence of hepatic carcinoma. Previously, some of these patients had been treated with thorotrast, a drug that is known to produce hepatic carcinomas. Thus, this study did not provide sufficient evidence that phenobarbitone is carcinogenic in humans.

A retrospective study of 84 children with brain tumours, matched to 73 normal controls and 78 cancer controls (malignant disease other than brain tumours), suggested an association between exposure to barbiturates prenatally and an increased incidence of brain tumours.

Side-effects: In the general use of barbiturates by the intravenous route, respiratory depression is the most serious side-effect. Laryngospasm may develop during normal induction or as a result of improper dosage. Rapid intravenous administration may also induce apnoea, vasodilatation, and some fall in blood pressure.

The following adverse reactions and their incidences were compiled from surveillance of thousands of hospitalised patients who received barbiturates. As such patients may be less aware of certain of the milder adverse effects of barbiturates, the incidence of these reactions may be somewhat higher in fully ambulatory patients:

More than 1 in 100 patients: The most common adverse reaction, estimated to occur at a rate of 1 to 3 patients per 100, is the following:

Nervous system: Somnolence.

Less than 1 in 100 patients: Adverse reactions estimated to occur at a rate of less than 1 in 100 patients are listed below, grouped by organ system and by decreasing frequency:

Neurological: Agitation, confusion, hyperkinesia, ataxia, CNS depression, nightmares, nervousness, psychiatric disturbance, hallucinations, insomnia, anxiety, dizziness, abnormal thinking.

Respiratory: Hypoventilation, apnoea, postoperative atelectasis.

Cardiovascular: Bradycardia, hypotension, syncope.

Digestive: Nausea, vomiting, constipation.

Other: Headache, injection site reactions, hypersensitivity reactions, (angioneurotic oedema, rashes, exfoliative dermatitis), fever, liver damage. Hypersensitivity is more likely to occur in patients with asthma, urticaria or angioneurotic oedema.

Drug abuse and dependence: Barbiturates may be habit forming; tolerance, psychological and physical dependence may occur, especially following prolonged use of high doses. Daily administration in excess of 400 mg pentobarbitone or secobarbitone, for approximately 90 days, is likely to produce some degree of physical dependence. A dosage of 600–800 mg, for at least 35 days, is sufficient to produce withdrawal seizures. The average daily dose for the barbiturate addict is usually about 1.5 g.

As tolerance to barbiturates develops, the amount needed to maintain the same level of intoxication increases; tolerance to a fatal dosage, however, does not increase more than twofold. As this occurs, the margin between intoxicating dosage and fatal dosage becomes smaller. The lethal dose of a barbiturate is far less if alcohol is also ingested.

Symptoms of acute intoxication include unsteady gait, slurred speech, and sustained nystagmus. Mental signs of chronic intoxication include confusion, poor judgement, irritability, insomnia, and somatic complaints.

The symptoms of barbiturate withdrawal can be severe and may cause death. Minor withdrawal symptoms may appear 8 to 12 hours after the last dose of a barbiturate. These symptoms usually appear in the following order: anxiety, muscle twitching, tremor of hands and fingers, progressive weakness, dizziness, distortion in visual perception, nausea, vomiting, insomnia, and orthostatic hypotension. Major withdrawal symptoms (convulsions and delirium) may occur within 16 hours and last up to 5 days after abrupt cessation of barbiturates. Intensity of withdrawal symptoms gradually declines over a period of approximately 15 days. Individuals susceptible to barbiturate abuse and dependence include alcoholics and opiate abusers, as well as other sedative-hypnotic and amphetamine abusers.

Dependence on barbiturates arises from repeated administration on a continuous basis, generally in amounts exceeding therapeutic dose levels. Treatment of dependence consists of cautious and gradual withdrawal of the drug. Barbiturate-dependent patients can be withdrawn by using a number of withdrawal regimes. In all cases, withdrawal takes an extended period. One method involves substituting a 30 mg dose of phenobarbitone for each 100–200 mg dose of barbiturate that the patient has been taking. The total daily amount of phenobarbitone is then administered in 3 or 4 divided doses, not to exceed 600 mg daily. Should signs of withdrawal occur on the first day of treatment, a loading dose of 100 to 200 mg of phenobarbitone may be administered intramuscularly in addition to the oral dose. After stabilisation on phenobarbitone, the total daily dose is decreased by 30 mg a day as long as withdrawal is proceeding smoothly. A modification of this regimen involves initiating treatment at the patient's regular dosage level and decreasing the daily dosage by 10% as tolerated by the patient.

Infants that are physically dependent on barbiturates may be given phenobarbitone, 3 to 10 mg/kg/day. After withdrawal symptoms (hyperactivity, disturbed sleep, tremors, and hyperreflexia) are relieved, the dosage of phenobarbitone should be gradually decreased and completely withdrawn over a 2 week period.

Overdosage: The toxic dose of barbiturates varies considerably. In general, an oral dose of 1 g of most barbiturates produces serious poisoning in an adult. Death commonly occurs after 2 to 10 g of ingested barbiturate. The sedated therapeutic blood levels of amylobarbitone range between 2 to 10 mg/l; the usual lethal blood level ranges from 40 to 80 mg/l. Barbiturate intoxication may be confused with alcoholism, bromide intoxication, and various neurological disorders. Potential tolerance must be considered when evaluating significance of dose and plasma concentration.

Signs and symptoms: The manifestations of overdosage are early hypothermia followed by CNS depression, sluggish or absent reflexes, underventilation, hypotension, and may progress to pulmonary oedema and death. Haemorrhagic blisters may develop, especially at pressure points.

In extreme overdose, all electrical activity in the brain may cease, in which case a 'flat' EEG normally equated with clinical death cannot be accepted. This effect is fully reversible unless hypoxic damage occurs. Consideration should be given to the possibility of barbiturate intoxication even in situations that appear to involve trauma.

Complications, such as pneumonia, pulmonary oedema, cardiac arrhythmias, congestive heart failure and renal failure, may occur. Uraemia may increase CNS sensitivity to barbiturates if renal function is impaired. Differential diagnosis should include hypoglycaemia, head trauma, cerebrovascular accidents, convulsive states, and diabetic coma.

Treatment: General management should consist of symptomatic and supportive therapy. Diuresis and peritoneal dialysis are of little value. Haemodialysis and haemoperfusion enhance drug clearance and should be considered in serious poisoning. If the patient has chronically abused sedatives, withdrawal reactions may be manifest following acute overdose.

Pharmaceutical precautions *Unreconstituted vials:* Store at room temperature (15°–25°C).

Legal category CD (Sch 3), POM.

Package quantity
Vials 250 mg: Packs of 25.

Further information Nil.

Product licence number 0006/5086

TUINAL*

Presentation Capsules (orange and blue, coded F65) containing 100 mg Tuinal (50 mg Secobarbitone Sodium PhEur and 50 mg Amylobarbitone Sodium PhEur). (The British Approved Name for Secobarbitone is quinalbarbitone.)

Uses For the treatment of severe, intractable insomnia, for those patients already habituated to barbiturates. It is not advised to start new patients with this preparation.

Dosage and administration *For adults only:* 100–200 mg at bedtime.

The elderly: Oral barbiturates are contra-indicated in the elderly.

The effects should become apparent between 15 and 30 minutes after administration.

Attempts should be made to wean patients off this preparation, but this should be done gradually (see 'Warnings').

Contra-indications, warnings, etc
Contra-indications: Hypersensitivity to barbiturates, a history of manifest or latent porphyria, marked impairment of liver function, or respiratory disease in which dyspnoea or obstruction is evident. Oral barbiturates should not be administered in the presence of uncontrolled acute or chronic pain, because paradoxical excitement may be induced or important symptoms may be masked.

Barbiturates should not be administered to children, young adults, patients with a history of drug or alcohol abuse, the elderly and the debilitated.

Usage in pregnancy: Barbiturates are contra-indicated during pregnancy.

Labour and delivery: Respiratory depression has been noted in infants born following the use of barbiturates during labour.

Nursing mothers: Small amounts of barbiturates are excreted in the milk, and they are therefore contra-indicated for the nursing mother.

Warnings
Addiction potential: Barbiturates have a high addiction potential. Long-term use, or use of high dosage for short periods, may lead to tolerance and subsequently to physical and psychological dependence.

Signs of acute intoxication with barbiturates include unsteady gait, slurred speech and sustained nystagmus. Symptoms of dependence or chronic intoxication include confusion, defective judgement, loss of emotional control, insomnia and somatic complaints.

To minimise the possibility of overdosage or development of dependence, the amount prescribed should be limited to that required for the interval until the next appointment.

Withdrawal symptoms occur after long-term normal use (and particularly after abuse) on rapid cessation of barbiturate treatment. Symptoms include nightmares, irritability and insomnia, and in severe cases, tremors, delirium, convulsions and death.

Barbiturates should be withdrawn gradually from any patient known to be taking excessive doses over long periods.

Information for patients: The following information should be given to patients receiving Tuinal:

1. The use of Tuinal carries with it an associated risk of psychological and/or physical dependence. The patient should be warned against increasing the dose of the drug without consulting a physician.

2. Tuinal may impair the mental and/or physical abilities required for the performance of potentially hazardous tasks, such as driving a car or operating machinery. The patient should be cautioned accordingly.

3. Alcohol should not be consumed while taking Tuinal. The concurrent use of Tuinal with other CNS depressants (e.g. alcohol, narcotics, tranquillisers and antihistamines) may result in additional CNS depressant effects.

Drug interactions: Tuinal in combination with alcohol, tranquillisers, and other CNS depressants, has additive depressant effects, and the patient should be so advised. Toxic effects and fatalities have occurred following overdoses of Tuinal alone and in combination with other CNS depressants. Caution should be exercised in prescribing unnecessarily large amounts of Tuinal for patients who have a history of emotional disturbances or suicidal ideation or who have misused alcohol or other CNS drugs.

Barbiturates cause induction of the liver enzymes responsible for metabolising many other drugs; in particular they should not be administered concurrently with coumarin-type anticoagulants. They may also affect the metabolism of systemic steroids (including oral contraceptives), phenytoin, griseofulvin, rifampicin, tricyclic antidepressants, and phenothiazines such as chlorpromazine.

Monoamine oxidase inhibitors prolong the effects of barbiturates, probably because the metabolism of the barbiturate is inhibited.

Precautions: Barbiturates should be administered with caution, if at all, to patients who are mentally depressed or have suicidal tendencies. They should also be used with great caution and at reduced dosage in those with marked renal dysfunction, shock or respiratory depression.

Prolonged therapy with barbiturates should be accompanied by periodic evaluation of haematopoietic, renal and hepatic systems (but see 'Uses').

Elderly or debilitated patients may react to barbiturates with marked excitement, depression or confusion (see 'Contra-indications'). In some persons, barbiturates repeatedly produce excitement rather than depression.

A cumulative effect may occur with the barbiturates leading to features of chronic poisoning including headache, depression and slurred speech.

Automatism may follow the use of an hypnotic dose of a barbiturate.

The systemic effects of exogenous hydrocortisone and endogenous hydrocortisone (cortisol) may be diminished by Tuinal. This product should therefore be administered with caution to patients with borderline hypoadrenal function, regardless of whether it is of pituitary or of primary adrenal origin.

Side-effects: The following adverse reactions have been reported:

Neurological: Residual sedation or 'hangover'; drowsiness, lethargy, ataxia, paradoxical excitement, confusion, pain, memory defects, vertigo.

Respiratory/circulatory: Respiratory depression, apnoea and circulatory collapse.

Hypersensitivity: Allergic reactions, especially in individuals with asthma, urticaria, angioneurotic oedema or similar conditions; skin eruptions.

Other: Nausea and vomiting; headache.

Overdosage: The toxic dose of barbiturates varies considerably. In general, an oral dose of 1 g of most barbiturates produces serious poisoning in an adult. Death commonly occurs after 2 to 10 g of ingested barbiturate. Barbiturate intoxication may be confused with alcoholism, bromide intoxication, and various neurological disorders. Potential tolerance must be considered when evaluating significance of dose and plasma concentration.

Signs and symptoms: Symptoms of oral overdose may occur within 15 minutes and begin with CNS depression, underventilation, hypotension and hypothermia, which may progress to pulmonary oedema and death. Haemorrhagic blisters may develop, especially at pressure points.

In extreme overdose, all electrical activity in the brain may cease, in which case a 'flat' EEG normally equated with clinical death cannot be accepted. This effect is fully reversible unless hypoxic damage occurs. Consideration should be given to the possibility of barbiturate intoxication even in situations that appear to involve trauma.

Complications such as pneumonia, pulmonary oedema, cardiac arrhythmias, congestive heart failure and renal failure may occur. Uraemia may increase CNS sensitivity to barbiturates if renal function is impaired. Differential diagnosis should include hypoglycaemia, head trauma, cerebrovascular accidents, convulsive states and diabetic coma.

Treatment: General management should consist of symptomatic and supportive therapy. Activated charcoal may be more effective than emesis or lavage. Diuresis and peritoneal dialysis are of little value. Haemodialysis and haemoperfusion enhance drug clearance and should be considered in serious poisoning. If the patient has chronically abused sedatives, withdrawal reactions may be manifest following acute overdose.

Pharmaceutical precautions Keep containers tightly closed. Store below 25°C.

Legal category CD (Sch 2), POM.

Package quantities
Capsules 100 mg: Bottles of 100.

Further information Nil.

Product licence number
Capsules 100 mg 0006/5077R

V-CIL-K*

Presentation

1. Phenoxymethylpenicillin Potassium Capsules BP (pink, coded H37) containing the equivalent of 250 mg phenoxymethylpenicillin (400,000 units).

2. Phenoxymethylpenicillin Potassium Tablets BP (white, coded C29) containing the equivalent of 250 mg phenoxymethylpenicillin (400,000 units).

3. Paediatric syrup: orange/pink granules for the preparation of Phenoxymethylpenicillin Elixir BP. Each 5 ml contains the equivalent of 125 mg Phenoxymethylpenicillin PhEur (200,000 units).

The potassium content is 14.03 mg (0.36 m Eq) in 125 mg, and 28.06 mg (0.72 m Eq) in 250 mg.

Uses Penicillin exerts high activity *in vitro* against staphylococci (except penicillinase-producing strains), streptococci (groups A, C, G, H, L, and M), pneumococci, *Corynebacterium diphtheriae, Bacillus anthracis, Actinomyces bovis, Streptobacillus moniliformis, Listeria monocytogenes, Neisseria gonorrhoeae, Treponema pallidum, Clostridium* species and Leptospira.

Phenoxymethylpenicillin and potassium phenoxymethylpenicillin are indicated in the treatment of mild to moderately severe infections associated with microorganisms whose susceptibility to penicillin is within the range of serum levels attained with these dosage forms.

Note: Severe empyema, bacteraemia, pericarditis, meningitis and arthritis should not be treated with penicillin V during the acute phase.

The following infections will usually respond to adequate doses:

Streptococcal infections (without bacteraemia) – Mild to moderate infections of the upper respiratory tract, scarlet fever and mild erysipelas.

Pneumococcal infections – Mild to moderately severe infections of the respiratory tract.

Staphylococcal infections sensitive to penicillin – Mild infections of the skin and soft tissues.

Fusospirochaetosis (Vincent's gingivitis and pharyngitis) – Mild to moderately severe infections of the oropharynx usually respond to therapy with oral penicillin.

Prophylactic use: Prophylaxis with oral penicillin has proved effective in preventing recurrence of rheumatic fever and chorea.

Patients with a past history of rheumatic fever receiving continuous prophylaxis may harbour penicillin-resistant organisms. In these patients, the use of another prophylactic agent should be considered.

Note: Oral penicillin should not be used as adjunctive prophylaxis for genito-urinary instrumentation or surgery, lower intestinal tract surgery, sigmoidoscopy and childbirth.

Dosage and administration For oral administration.

Adults: 125 or 250 mg every four to six hours, depending on the severity of the condition.

The elderly: As for adults. Reduce dosage if renal function is markedly impaired.
Children over 5 years: The adult dose.
Children 5 years or less: 125 mg every six hours.
Infants (up to 1 year): 62.5 mg every six hours.

In all but the most serious cases, the last dose of the day may be doubled to avoid disturbing sleep. Ideally, each dose should be given half an hour before (or at least three hours after) a meal.

Prophylactic use: 125 mg twice daily is recommended for long term prophylaxis of rheumatic fever.

Contra-indications, warnings, etc
Contra-indication: A previous hypersensitivity reaction to any penicillin.

Warning: All degrees of hypersensitivity, including fatal anaphylaxis, have been observed with oral penicillin. These reactions are more likely to occur in individuals with a history of sensitivity to penicillins, cephalosporins and other allergens. Enquiry should be made for such a history before therapy with a penicillin is begun. If an allergic reaction occurs, the drug should be discontinued and the patient treated with the usual agents (eg, adrenaline and other pressor amines, antihistamines and corticosteroids).

Usage in pregnancy: Although laboratory and clinical studies have shown no evidence of teratogenicity, caution should be exercised when prescribing for the pregnant patient.

Precautions: Penicillin should be used with caution in individuals with histories of significant allergies and/or asthma.

Oral therapy should not be relied upon in patients with severe illness, or with nausea, vomiting, gastric dilatation, cardiospasm or intestinal hypermotility. Occasionally, patients do not absorb therapeutic amounts of orally administered penicillin.

Administer with caution in the presence of markedly impaired renal function, as safe dosage may be lower than that usually recommended.

Streptococcal infections should be treated for a minimum of 10 days, and post-therapy cultures should be performed to confirm the eradication of the organisms.

Prolonged use of antibiotics may promote the overgrowth of non-susceptible organisms, including fungi. If super-infection occurs, appropriate measures should be taken.

Side-effects: Although reactions have been reported

much less frequently after oral than after parenteral therapy, it should be remembered that all degrees of hypersensitivity, including fatal anaphylaxis, have been observed with oral penicillin.

The most common reactions to oral penicillin are nausea, vomiting, epigastric distress, diarrhoea and black, hairy tongue. The hypersensitivity reactions noted are skin eruptions (ranging from maculopapular to exfoliative dermatitis); urticaria; reactions resembling serum sickness, including chills, fever, oedema, arthralgia and prostration; laryngeal oedema; and anaphylaxis. Fever and eosinophilia may frequently be the only reactions observed. Haemolytic anaemia, leucopenia, thrombocytopenia, neuropathy and nephropathy are infrequent reactions and are usually associated with high doses of parenteral penicillin.

Overdosage

Signs and symptoms: A large oral overdose of penicillin may cause nausea, vomiting, stomach pain, diarrhoea and, rarely, major motor seizures. If other symptoms are present consider the possibility of an allergic reaction.

Hyperkalaemia may result from overdosage, particularly in patients with renal insufficiency.

Treatment: No specific antidote is known. Symptomatic and supportive therapy is recommended. Activated charcoal with a cathartic, such as sorbitol, may hasten drug elimination. Penicillin may be removed by haemodialysis.

Pharmaceutical precautions Keep containers tightly closed.

Capsules: Store below 25°C.

Syrup: Reconstituted preparations may be stored for seven days at room temperature (15°–25°C) or fourteen days in a refrigerator (2°–8°C).

Legal category POM.

Package quantities
Capsules 250 mg: Bottles of 100.
Tablets 250 mg: Bottles of 100, 500 and 1,000.
Paediatric syrup 125 mg/5 ml: Bottles of 100 ml.

Further information Nil.

Product licence numbers

Capsules 250 mg	0006/5126
Tablets 250 mg	0006/5164
Paediatric syrup 125 mg/5 ml	0006/5128

VANCOCIN* CP INJECTION

Presentation Rubber-stoppered 10 ml vials each containing chromatographically purified vancomycin hydrochloride, 250,000 iu or 500,000 iu, equivalent to 250 mg or 500 mg vancomycin respectively, as an off-white lyophilised plug. Rubber-stoppered 20 ml vials containing chromatographically purified vancomycin hydrochloride, 1,000,000 iu, equivalent to 1 g vancomycin, as an off-white lyophilised plug. When reconstituted in water, it forms a clear solution with a pH range of 2.8 to 4.5.

Uses Vancomycin is a glycopeptide antibiotic derived from *Nocardia orientalis* (formerly *Streptomyces orientalis*), and is active against many Gram-positive bacteria including *Staphylococcus aureus*, *Staph. epidermidis*, α and β haemolytic streptococci, group D streptococci, corynebacteria and clostridia.

Vancomycin is indicated in potentially life-threatening infections which cannot be treated with other effective, less toxic antimicrobial drugs, including the penicillins and cephalosporins.

Vancomycin is useful in the therapy of severe staphylococcal infections in patients who cannot receive or who have failed to respond to the penicillins and cephalosporins, or who have infections with staphylococci resistant to other antibiotics.

Vancomycin is used in the treatment of endocarditis and as prophylaxis against endocarditis in patients at risk from dental or surgical procedures.

Its effectiveness has been documented in other infections due to staphylococci, including osteomyelitis, pneumonia, septicaemia and soft tissue infections.

Vancomycin may be used orally for the treatment of staphylococcal enterocolitis and pseudomembranous colitis due to *Clostridium difficile*.

Vancomycin is not significantly absorbed from the normal gastro-intestinal tract and is therefore not effective by the oral route for other types of infection. Intravenous administration may be used concomitantly if required.

Dosage and administration For intravenous infusion and oral use only and not for intramuscular administration.

Infusion-related adverse events are related to both concentration and rate of administration of vancomycin. Concentrations of no more than 5 mg/ml are recommended. In selected patients in need of fluid restriction, a concentration up to 10 mg/ml may be used; use of such higher concentrations may increase the risk of infusion-related events. Infusions should be given over at least 60 minutes. In adults, if doses exceeding 500 mg are used, a rate of infusion of no more than 10 mg/min is recommended. Infusion-related events may occur, however, at any rate or concentration.

Intravenous Infusion in patients with normal renal function

Adults: The usual intravenous dose is 500 mg every six hours or 1 g every 12 hours, in Sodium Chloride Intravenous Infusion BP or 5% Dextrose Intravenous Infusion BP. Each dose should be administered at no more than 10 mg/min. Other patient factors, such as age, obesity or pregnancy, may call for modification of the usual daily dose. The majority of patients with infections caused by organisms sensitive to the antibiotic show a therapeutic response within 48–72 hours. The total duration of therapy is determined by the type and severity of the infection and the clinical response of the patient. In staphylococcal endocarditis, treatment for three weeks or longer is recommended.

Pregnancy: It has been reported that significantly increased doses may be required to achieve therapeutic serum concentrations in pregnant patients, but see 'Warnings'.

The elderly: Dosage reduction may be necessary to a greater extent than expected because of decreasing renal function (see below). Monitor auditory function – see 'Warnings' and 'Precautions'.

Children: The usual intravenous dosage is 10 mg/kg per dose given every 6 hours (total daily dosage 40 mg/kg of body weight). Each dose should be administered over a period of at least 60 minutes.

In neonates and young infants, the total daily dosage may be lower. An initial dose of 15 mg/kg is suggested, followed by 10 mg/kg every 12 hours in the first week of life and every 8 hours thereafter until one month of age. Each dose should be administered over 60 minutes. Close monitoring of serum vancomycin concentrations may be warranted in these patients.

Patients with impaired renal function: Dosage adjustments must be made to avoid toxic serum levels. In premature infants and the elderly, greater dosage reductions than expected may be necessary because of decreased renal function. Regular monitoring of serum levels is advised in such patients, as accumulation has been reported, especially after prolonged therapy. Vancomycin serum concentrations may be determined by use of a microbiological assay, radioimmunoassay, fluorescence polarisation immunoassay, fluorescence immunoassay or high-pressure liquid chromatography. The following nomogram, based on creatinine clearance values, is provided.

The nomogram is not valid for functionally anephric patients on dialysis. For such patients, a loading dose of 15 mg/kg body weight should be given to achieve therapeutic serum levels promptly, and the dose required to maintain stable levels is 1.9 mg/kg/24 hours. Since individual maintenance doses of 250 mg to 1 g are convenient, in patients with marked renal impairment a dose may be given every several days rather than on a

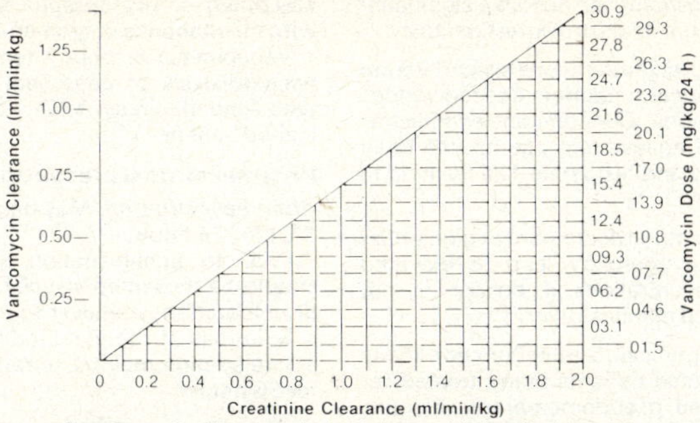

Dosage Nomogram for Vancomycin in Patients with Impaired Renal Function

daily basis. In anuria a dose of 1 g every 7 to 10 days has been recommended.

Measurement of serum concentrations:
Following multiple intravenous doses, peak serum concentrations, measured 2 hours after infusion is complete, range from 18–26 mg/l. Trough levels measured immediately prior to the next dose should be 5–10 mg/l. Ototoxicity has been associated with serum drug levels of 80–100 mg/l, but this is rarely seen when serum levels are kept at or below 30 mg/l.

Preparation of solution: At the time of use, add 10 ml of Water for Injections PhEur to the vial. Vials reconstituted in this manner will give a solution of 50 mg/ml.

FURTHER DILUTION IS REQUIRED. Read instructions which follow:

1. *Intermittent infusion* is the preferred method of administration. The above solution (containing 500 mg vancomycin) can be added to 100–200 ml Sodium Chloride Intravenous Infusion BP or 5% Dextrose Intravenous Infusion BP. The desired dose should be given by intravenous infusion over a period of at least 60 minutes. If administered over a shorter period of time or in higher concentrations, there is the possibility of inducing marked hypotension in addition to thrombophlebitis. Rapid administration may also produce flushing and a transient rash over the neck and shoulders.

2. *Continuous infusion* (should be used only when intermittent infusion is not feasible). Two to four vials (1–2 g) can be added to a sufficiently large volume of Sodium Chloride Intravenous Infusion BP or 5% Dextrose Intravenous Infusion BP to permit the desired daily dose to be administered slowly by intravenous drip over a 24-hour period.

Oral administration: The contents of the 500 mg vial for parenteral administration may be used.

Adults and the elderly: The usual daily dose given is 500 mg in divided doses for 7 to 10 days, although up to 2 g/day have been used in severe cases. The total daily dosage should not exceed 2 g. Each dose may be reconstituted in 30 ml water and either given to the patient to drink, or administered by nasogastric tube.

Children: The usual daily dose is 40 mg/kg in three or four divided doses for 7 to 10 days. The total daily dosage should not exceed 2 g.

Common flavouring syrups may be added to the solution at the time of administration to improve the taste.

Capsules are also available.

Contra-indications, warnings, etc
Contra-indication: Hypersensitivity to vancomycin.

Warnings: Rapid bolus administration (e.g. over several minutes) may be associated with exaggerated hypotension, including shock, and, rarely, cardiac arrest. Vancomycin should be infused in a dilute solution over a period of not less than 60 minutes to avoid rapid infusion-related reactions. Stopping the infusion usually results in a prompt cessation of these reactions (see 'Dosage and administration' and 'Side-effects' sections).

Since vancomycin is not usually significantly absorbed from the gastro-intestinal tract, the toxicity encountered with parenteral therapy is unlikely to occur after oral administration.

Due to its potential ototoxicity and nephrotoxicity, vancomycin should be used with care in patients with renal insufficiency and the dose should be reduced according to the degree of renal impairment. The risk of toxicity is appreciably increased by high blood concentrations or prolonged therapy. Blood levels should be monitored and renal function tests should be performed regularly.

Vancomycin should also be avoided in patients with previous hearing loss. If it is used in such patients, the dose should be regulated, if possible, by periodic determination of the drug level in the blood. Deafness may be preceded by tinnitus. The elderly are more susceptible to auditory damage. Experience with other antibiotics suggests that deafness may be progressive despite cessation of treatment.

There have been reports that the frequency of infusion-related events increases with the concomitant administration of anaesthetic agents. Infusion-related events may be minimised by the administration of vancomycin as a 60-minute infusion prior to anaesthetic induction.

Concurrent or sequential systemic or topical use of other potentially neurotoxic or nephrotoxic drugs, such as amphotericin B, aminoglycosides, bacitracin, polymixin B, colistin, viomycin or cisplatin, when indicated, requires careful monitoring.

Drug interaction: Concomitant administration of vancomycin and anaesthetic agents has been associated with erythema, histamine-like flushing and anaphylactoid reactions.

Vancomycin solution has a low pH that may cause chemical or physical instability when it is mixed with other compounds.

Usage in pregnancy: Teratology studies have been performed at 5 times the human dose in rats and 3 times the human dose in rabbits, and have revealed no evidence of harm to the fetus due to vancomycin. In a controlled clinical study, the potential ototoxic and nephrotoxic effects of vancomycin hydrochloride on infants were evaluated when the drug was administered to pregnant women for serious staphylococcal infections complicating intravenous drug abuse. Vancomycin hydrochloride was found in cord blood. No sensorineural hearing loss or nephrotoxicity attributable to vancomycin was noted. One infant, whose mother received vancomycin in the third trimester, experienced conductive hearing loss that was not attributable to vancomycin. Because vancomycin was administered only in the second and third trimesters, it is not known whether it causes fetal harm. Vancomycin should be given in pregnancy only if clearly needed and blood levels should be monitored carefully to minimise the risk of fetal toxicity. It has been reported, however, that pregnant patients may require significantly increased doses of vancomycin to achieve therapeutic serum concentrations.

Usage in nursing mothers: Vancomycin hydrochloride is excreted in human milk. Caution should be exercised when vancomycin is administered to a nursing woman.

It is unlikely that a nursing infant can absorb a significant amount of vancomycin from its gastro-intestinal tract.

Usage in paediatrics: In premature neonates and young infants, it may be appropriate to confirm desired vancomycin serum concentrations. Concomitant administration of vancomycin and anaesthetic agents has been associated with erythema and histamine-like flushing in children.

Usage in the elderly: The natural decrement of glomerular filtration with increasing age may lead to elevated vancomycin serum concentrations if dosage is not adjusted (see 'Dosage and administration').

Precautions: Clinically significant serum concentrations have been reported in some patients being treated for active *C. difficile*-induced pseudomembranous colitis after multiple oral doses of vancomycin.

Patients with borderline renal function and individuals over the age of 60 should be given serial tests of auditory function and of vancomycin blood levels. All patients receiving the drug should have periodic haematological studies, urine analysis and renal function tests.

Vancomycin is very irritating to tissue, and causes necrosis when injected intramuscularly; it must be infused intravenously. Pain and thrombophlebitis occur in many patients receiving vancomycin and are occasionally severe.

The frequency and severity of thrombophlebitis can be minimised by administering the drug slowly as a dilute solution (2.5 to 5.0 g/l) and by rotating the sites of infusion.

Prolonged use of vancomycin may result in the overgrowth of non-susceptible organisms. Careful observation of the patient is essential. If super-infection occurs during therapy, appropriate measures should be taken. In rare instances, there have been reports of pseudomembranous colitis, due to *C. difficile*, developing in patients who received intravenous vancomycin.

Side-effects

Infusion-related events: During or soon after rapid infusion of vancomycin, patients may develop anaphylactoid reactions including hypotension, wheezing, dyspnoea, urticaria or pruritus. Rapid infusion may also cause flushing of the upper-body ('red-neck') or pain and muscle spasm of the chest and back. These reactions usually resolve within 20 minutes but may persist for several hours. In animal studies, hypotension and bradycardia occurred in animals given large doses of vancomycin at high concentrations and rates. Such events are infrequent if vancomycin is given by slow infusion over 60 minutes. In studies of normal volunteers, infusion-related events did not occur when vancomycin was administered at a rate of 10 mg/min or less.

Nephrotoxicity: Rarely, renal failure, principally manifested by increased serum creatinine or blood urea concentrations, have been observed, especially in patients given large doses of intravenously administered vancomycin. Rare cases of interstitial nephritis have been reported. Most occurred in patients who were given aminoglycosides concomitantly or who had pre-existing kidney dysfunction. When vancomycin was discontinued, azotaemia resolved in most patients.

Ototoxicity: Hearing loss associated with intravenously administered vancomycin has been reported. Most of these patients had kidney dysfunction, pre-existing hearing loss, or concomitant treatment with an ototoxic drug. Vertigo, dizziness and tinnitus have been reported rarely.

Haematological: Reversible neutropenia, usually starting one week or more after onset of intravenous therapy or after a total dose of more than 25 g. Neutropenia appears to be promptly reversible when vancomycin is discontinued. Thrombocytopenia has rarely been reported.

Miscellaneous: Phlebitis, anaphylaxis, nausea, chills, fever, eosinophilia and rashes, including exfoliative dermatitis, Stevens-Johnson syndrome, and rare cases of vasculitis.

Treatment of overdosage: Supportive care is advised with maintenance of glomerular filtration.

Vancomycin is poorly removed from the blood by haemodialysis or peritoneal dialysis. Haemoperfusion with Amberlite resin XAD-4 has been reported to be of limited benefit.

Pharmaceutical precautions Store below 25°C.

After reconstitution: May be stored in a refrigerator (2°–8°C) for 24 hours.

Prior to administration, parenteral drug products should be inspected visually for particulate matter and discolouration whenever solution or container permits.

Solutions of the parenteral powder intended for oral administration may be stored in a refrigerator (2°–8°C) for 96 hours.

Legal category POM.

Package quantities
Vials 250 mg (250,000 iu vancomycin). Single vials.
Vials 500 mg (500,000 iu vancomycin). Single vials.
Vials 1 g (1,000,000 iu vancomycin). Single vials.

Further information Nil.

Product licence number 0006/5076.

VANCOCIN* MATRIGEL CAPSULES

Presentation Matrigel capsules (dark blue and grey, coded Lilly 3126) containing chromatographically purified vancomycin hydrochloride, equivalent to 250 mg vancomycin base. Matrigel capsules (dark blue and peach, coded Lilly 3125) containing chromatographically purified vancomycin hydrochloride, equivalent to 125 mg vancomycin base.

This preparation is for oral use only. If parenteral vancomycin therapy is desired, use Vancocin CP Injection (Sterile Vancomycin Hydrochloride BP) and consult literature accompanying that preparation.

Uses Vancomycin may be used orally for the treatment of staphylococcal enterocolitis and pseudomembranous colitis due to *Clostridium difficile*.

Vancomycin is not significantly absorbed from the normal gastro-intestinal tract and is therefore not effective by the oral route for other types of infection. Intravenous administration may be used concomitantly if required.

Dosage and administration For oral administration. Either the Matrigel capsules or the contents of the 500 mg vial for parenteral administration may be used.

Adults and the elderly: The usual daily dose is 500 mg in divided doses for 7 to 10 days, although up to 2 g/day have been used in severe cases. The total daily dosage should not exceed 2 g.

Children: The usual daily dose is 40 mg/kg in three or four divided doses for 7 to 10 days. The total daily dosage should not exceed 2 g.

Oral solution: The contents of the 500 mg vial for parenteral administration may be used and either given to the patient to drink, or administered by nasogastric tube. Mix thoroughly to dissolve. Common flavouring syrups may be added to the solution at the time of administration to improve the taste.

Contra-indications, warnings, etc
Contra-indication: Hypersensitivity to vancomycin.

Warnings

Usage in pregnancy: Animal reproduction studies have not been conducted with vancomycin. It is not known whether vancomycin can affect reproduction capacity. In a controlled clinical study, the potential ototoxic and nephrotoxic effects of vancomycin hydrochloride on infants were evaluated when the drug was administered to pregnant women for serious staphylococcal infections complicating intravenous drug abuse. Vancomycin hydrochloride was found in cord blood. No sensorineural hearing loss or nephrotoxicity attributable to vancomycin was noted. One infant, whose mother received vancomycin in the third trimester, experienced conductive hearing loss that was not attributable to vancomycin. Because vancomycin was administered only in the second and third trimesters, it is not known whether it causes fetal harm. Therefore vancomycin should be given to a pregnant woman only if clearly needed.

Usage in nursing mothers: Vancomycin hydrochloride is excreted in human milk. Caution should be exercised when vancomycin is administered to a nursing woman.

Precautions: Clinically significant serum concentrations have been reported in some patients who have taken multiple oral doses of vancomycin for acute *C. difficile*-induced pseudomembranous colitis.

Some patients with inflammatory disorders of the intestinal mucosa may have significant systemic absorption of vancomycin and, therefore, may be at risk for the development of adverse reactions associated with the parenteral administration of vancomycin (see package insert accompanying the intravenous preparation). The risk is greater in patients with renal impairment. It should be noted that the total systemic and renal clearances of vancomycin are reduced in the elderly.

Ototoxicity has occurred in patients receiving vancomycin. It may be transient or permanent. It has been reported mostly in patients who have been given excessive intravenous doses, have an underlying hearing loss, or are receiving concomitant therapy with an ototoxic agent such as an aminoglycoside. Serial tests of auditory function may be helpful in order to minimise the risk of ototoxicity.

When treating patients with underlying renal dysfunction or patients receiving concomitant therapy with an aminoglycoside, serial monitoring of renal function should be performed.

Side-effects: Since vancomycin is not usually significantly absorbed from the gastro-intestinal tract, the toxicity encountered with parenteral therapy is unlikely to occur after oral administration (but see 'Precautions').

Nephrotoxicity: Rarely, renal failure, principally manifested by increased serum creatinine or blood urea concentrations, have been observed, especially in patients given large doses of intravenously administered vancomycin. Rare cases of interstitial nephritis have been reported. Most occurred in patients who were given aminoglycosides concomitantly or who had pre-existing kidney dysfunction. When vancomycin was discontinued, azotaemia resolved in most patients.

Ototoxicity: Hearing loss associated with *intravenously* administered vancomycin has been reported. Most of these patients had kidney dysfunction, pre-existing hearing loss, or concomitant treatment with an ototoxic drug. Vertigo, dizziness and tinnitus have been reported rarely.

Haematological: Reversible neutropenia, usually starting one week or more after onset of *intravenous* therapy or after a total dose of more than 25 g. Neutropenia appears to be promptly reversible when vancomycin is discontinued. Thrombocytopenia has been reported rarely.

Miscellaneous: Anaphylaxis, chills, fever, eosinophilia, nausea and rashes, including exfoliative dermatitis, Stevens-Johnson syndrome and rare cases of vasculitis.

Treatment of overdosage: Supportive care is advised, with maintenance of glomerular filtration. Vancomycin is poorly removed by dialysis. Haemofiltration and haemoperfusion with Amberlite resin XAD-4 have been reported to be of limited benefit.

Pharmaceutical precautions Protect from moisture. Store below 25°C.

After reconstitution, solutions of the parenteral powder intended for oral administration may be stored in a refrigerator (2°–8°C) for 96 hours.

Legal category POM.

Package quantity Blister packs of 20 (2 strips of 10 capsules).

Further information The bitter taste of vancomycin can be avoided by the use of the matrigel capsules. Vancomycin powder should be used when the patient is unable to swallow the capsules.

Product licence numbers
Matrigel Capsules 125 mg 0006/0193
Matrigel Capsules 250 mg 0006/0194

VELBE*

Presentation Vials containing 10 mg Velbe (Vinblastine Sulphate BP) in the form of a lyophilised plug.

Velbe is supplied in a combination package with an accompanying vial of diluting solution, 10 ml containing 90 mg Sodium Chloride PhEur, with 2% Benzyl Alcohol BP as a preservative.

Uses Velbe is an anti-neoplastic drug for intravenous use.

Information available at present suggests that Velbe may be useful, either alone or in combination with other oncolytic drugs for the treatment of: Hodgkin's disease; non-Hodgkin's lymphoma; carcinoma of the breast; methotrexate-resistant choriocarcinoma; renal cell carcinoma; testicular teratoma and seminoma; histiocytosis-X.

Other neoplasms occasionally show a marked response to Velbe, but less frequently than the more susceptible conditions listed above.

Dosage and administration This preparation is for intravenous use only. Intrathecal administration has resulted in death (see 'Warnings' for treatment).

The recommended dose for adults, the elderly and children is 6 mg/m^2 usually administered no more frequently than once every seven days. For testicular tumours, the dosage may be increased to 0.2 mg/kg administered on each of two consecutive days every three weeks.

To prepare a solution containing 1 mg/ml, add 10 ml of the accompanying diluting solution to the 10 mg vial. The drug dissolves rapidly to give a clear solution.

The dose of Velbe solution may be injected either into the tubing of a running intravenous infusion of sodium chloride 0.9% or directly into a vein. In either case, the injection should be completed in about one minute. If care is taken to ensure that the needle is securely within the vein and that no solution containing vinblastine is spilled extravascularly, cellulitis and/or phlebitis will not occur.

To minimise further the possibility of extravascular spillage, it is suggested that the syringe and needle be rinsed with venous blood before withdrawal. The dose should not be diluted in large volumes of diluent (i.e. 100 to 250 ml) or given intravenously for prolonged periods (ranging from 30 to 60 minutes or more), since this frequently results in irritation of the vein and increases the chance of extravasation.

Because of the enhanced possibility of thrombosis, it is considered inadvisable to inject a solution of Velbe into an extremity in which the circulation is impaired, or potentially impaired, by such conditions as compressing or invading neoplasm, phlebitis or varicosity.

Caution: If leakage into surrounding tissue should occur during intravenous administration of vinblastine, it may cause considerable irritation. The injection should be discontinued immediately, and any remaining portion of the dose should then be introduced into another vein. Local injection of hyaluronidase and the application of moderate heat to the area of leakage help disperse the drug and are thought to minimise discomfort and the possibility of cellulitis.

Contra-indications, warnings, etc
Contra-indications
Intrathecal administration has resulted in death (see 'Warnings' for treatment).

Vinblastine is contra-indicated in patients who are granulocytopenic unless this is the result of the disease being treated. It should not be used in the presence of bacterial infection. Such infections must be brought under control with antiseptics or antibiotics before using vinblastine.

Warnings
Syringes containing this product should be labelled 'WARNING – VINBLASTINE FOR INTRAVENOUS USE ONLY'.

The following treatment successfully arrested progressive paralysis in a single patient mistakenly given the related vinca alkaloid, vincristine sulphate, intrathecally. This treatment should be initiated immediately:

1. Removal of as much CSF as is safely possible.
2. Flushing with Lactated Ringer's solution by continuous infusion at 150 ml/h, through a catheter in a cerebral lateral ventricle and removed through lumbar access, until fresh frozen plasma became available.
3. Fresh frozen plasma, 25 ml, diluted with 1 l of Lactated Ringer's was then infused similarly at 75 ml/h. The rate of infusion should be adjusted to maintain a spinal fluid protein level of 150 mg/dl.
4. Glutamic acid, 10 gm, was given iv over 24 hours, followed by 500 mg tds by mouth for 1 month. Glutamic acid may not be essential.

Usage in pregnancy: Caution is necessary with the use of all oncolytic drugs during pregnancy. Information on the use of vinblastine during human pregnancy is very limited but vinblastine can cause fetal harm when administered to a pregnant woman. There are no adequate and well-controlled studies in pregnant women. Animal studies with vinblastine suggest that teratogenic effects may occur. Laboratory animals given this drug early in pregnancy suffer resorption of the conceptus; surviving fetuses demonstrate gross deformities.

Women of childbearing potential should be advised to avoid becoming pregnant while receiving vinblastine. If Velbe is used during pregnancy or if the patient becomes pregnant while receiving this drug she should be informed of the potential hazard to the fetus.

Usage in nursing mothers: It is not known whether vinblastine is excreted in human milk. Because of the potential for serious adverse reactions due to Velbe in nursing infants, a decision should be made whether to discontinue nursing or the drug taking into account the importance of the drug to the mother.

Aspermia has been reported in men. Animal studies show metaphase arrest and degenerative changes in germ cells. Amenorrhea has occurred in some patients treated with vinblastine in combination with other drugs. Recovery of menses was frequent.

Stomatitis and neurological toxicity, although not common or permanent, can be disabling.

Precautions: The dose-limiting factor is bone marrow toxicity. Effective therapy with vinblastine is more likely to be followed by granulocytopenia than is the case with Oncovin (vincristine sulphate).

In general, the larger the dose employed, the more profound and longer lasting the granulocytopenia will be. The fact that the granulocyte count returns to normal levels after drug-induced granulocytopenia is an indication that the granulocyte-producing mechanism is not permanently depressed.

Following therapy with vinblastine, the nadir in the granulocyte count may be expected to occur five to ten days after the last day of drug administration. Recovery of the granulocyte count is fairly rapid thereafter and is usually complete within another seven to fourteen days.

If granulocytopenia with less than 1,000 granulocytes/mm^3 occurs following a dose of vinblastine, the patient should be watched carefully for evidence of infection until the granulocyte count has returned to a safe level. Any infection must be brought under control immediately.

When cachexia or ulcerated areas of the skin surface are present, there may be a more profound granulocytopenic response to the drug; therefore, its use should be avoided in older persons suffering from either of these conditions.

Although the thrombocyte count is not usually significantly lowered by therapy with vinblastine, patients whose bone marrow has been recently impaired by prior therapy with radiation or with other oncolytic drugs may show thrombocytopenia (less than 150,000 platelets/mm^3). When other chemotherapy or radiation has not been employed previously, thrombocyte reduction below the level of 150,000/mm^3 is rarely encountered, even when vinblastine may be causing significant granulocytopenia. Rapid recovery from thrombocytopenia within a few days is the rule.

The effect of vinblastine upon the red blood cell count and haemoglobin is usually insignificant when other treatment does not complicate the picture.

In patients with malignant-cell infiltration of the bone marrow, the granulocyte and platelet counts have sometimes fallen drastically after moderate doses of vinblastine. Further use of the drug in such patients is inadvisable.

As vinblastine is excreted principally by the liver, toxicity may be increased when there is hepatic insufficiency and it may be necessary to reduce initial doses in the presence of significantly impaired hepatic or biliary function. A reduction of 50% in the dose is recommended for patients having a direct serum bilirubin value above 3 mg/100 ml. Since metabolism and excretion are primarily hepatic, no modification is recommended for patients with impaired renal function.

When chemotherapy is being given in conjunction with radiation therapy through portals which include the liver, the use of vinblastine should be delayed until radiation therapy has been completed.

Acute shortness of breath and severe bronchospasm have been reported following the administration of the vinca alkaloids. These reactions have been encountered most frequently when the vinca alkaloid was used in combination with mitomycin-C and may be serious when there is pre-existing pulmonary dysfunction. The onset may be within minutes, or several hours after the vinca is injected, and may occur up to 2 weeks following a dose of mitomycin.

Progressive dyspnoea, requiring chronic therapy, may occur. Vinblastine should not be readministered.

The simultaneous oral or intravenous administration of phenytoin and antineoplastic chemotherapy combinations, that included vinblastine sulphate, have been reported to reduce blood levels of the anticonvulsant and to increase seizure activity. Although the contribution of the vinca alkaloids has not been established, dosage adjustment of phenytoin, based on serial blood level monitoring, may need to be made when it is used in combination with vinblastine.

Care must be taken to avoid contamination of the eye with concentrations of Velbe used clinically. If accidental contamination occurs, severe irritation (or, if the drug was delivered under pressure, even corneal ulceration) may result. The eye should be washed with water immediately and thoroughly.

Sperm abnormalities have been noted in mice. Additional studies in mice demonstrated no reduction in fertility of males. Breaks and aberrations were not observed on chromosome analysis of marrow cells from patients treated with vinblastine although chromosomal changes have been noted in some hamster lung cell *in vitro* tests.

There is no currently available evidence to indicate that vinblastine itself has been carcinogenic in humans although some patients have developed leukaemia following radiation therapy and the administration of vinblastine in combination with alkylating agents.

Adverse reactions: Granulocytopenia is the most common adverse reaction and is usually the dose-limiting factor.

In general, the incidence of side-effects attending the use of Velbe appears to be related to the size of dosage employed. Symptoms commonly encountered when high doses are employed include constipation, abdominal pain, ileus and myalgia.

The use of small amounts of vinblastine daily for long periods is not advisable, even though the resulting total dosage may be similar to the recommended dosage. Little or no therapeutic advantage has been demonstrated when such regimens have been used and side effects are increased.

The constipation which may be encountered responds well to such usual measures as enemas and laxatives. Constipation may take the form of upper colon impaction and the rectum may be found to be empty on physical examination. A flat film of the abdomen is useful in demonstrating this condition. A routine prophylactic regimen against constipation is recommended for patients receiving high doses of vinblastine.

The following symptoms may occur after usual doses of vinblastine:

Haematological: Granulocytopenia, thrombocytopenia, anaemia.

Gastro-intestinal: Nausea, vomiting, constipation, ileus, diarrhoea, anorexia, abdominal pain, rectal bleeding, pharyngitis, haemorrhagic enterocolitis, bleeding from an old peptic ulcer.

Neurological: Numbness, paraesthesiae, peripheral neuritis, mental depression, loss of deep tendon reflexes, headache, convulsions.

Pulmonary: See under 'Precautions'.

Cutaneous: Ulceration of the mouth and skin, and alopecia. When alopecia develops it is frequently not total and, in some cases, hair regrows while maintenance therapy continues.

Cardiovascular: Hypertension. Cases of unexpected myocardial infarction and cerebrovascular accidents have occurred in patients undergoing combination chemotherapy with vinblastine, bleomycin and cisplatin.

Miscellaneous: malaise, weakness, dizziness, bone pain, jaw pain, and pain in tumour site. Inappropriate ADH secretion has been reported with higher than recommended doses. Raynaud's phenomenon has occurred when patients are being treated with vinblastine in combination with bleomycin and cisplatin for testicular cancer.

Overdosage: Side-effects following the use of vinblastine are dose related. Therefore, following administration of more than the recommended dose, patients can be expected to experience these effects in an exaggerated fashion. Any dose that results in elimination of platelets and neutrophils from blood and marrow and their precursors from marrow is life-threatening.

Overdoses occurring during prolonged, consecutive day infusions may be more toxic than the same total dose given by rapid iv injection.

In addition, neurotoxicity similar to that seen with Oncovin (vincristine sulphate) may be observed.

Supportive care should include: (a) prevention of the side-effects that result from the syndrome of inappropriate secretion of antidiuretic hormone. This includes restriction of fluid intake and perhaps the use of a diuretic acting on the loop of Henle and distal tubule function; (b) administration of an anticonvulsant; (c) prevention and treatment of ileus; (d) monitoring the patient's cardiovascular system; (e) daily blood counts for guidance in transfusion requirement and assessing the risk of infection.

The major effect of excessive doses of vinblastine will be on granulocytopoiesis, and this may be life-threatening.

There is no specific antidote. The use of folinic acid in addition to the other supportive measures recommended may be considered although, unlike vincristine, studies have not been conducted to confirm its protective action.

There is no information regarding the effectiveness of dialysis nor of cholestyramine for the treatment of overdosage.

Vinblastine in the dry state is irregularly and unpredictably absorbed from the gastro-intestinal tract following oral administration. Absorption of the solution has not been studied. If vinblastine is swallowed, activated charcoal in a water slurry may be given by mouth along with a cathartic. The use of cholestyramine in this situation has not been reported.

Pharmaceutical precautions
Guidelines for the safe handling of antineoplastic agents: Cytotoxic preparations should not be handled by pregnant staff.

Trained personnel should reconstitute and administer the drug. This should be performed in a designated area. The work surface should be covered with disposable plastic-backed absorbent paper.

Adequate protective gloves, masks and clothing should be worn. Precautions should be taken to avoid the drug accidentally coming into contact with the eyes. If accidental contamination occurs, the eye should be washed with water thoroughly and immediately.

Use Luer-lock fittings on all syringes and sets. Large bore needles are recommended to minimise pressure and the possible formation of aerosols. The latter may also be reduced by the use of a venting needle.

Adequate care and precaution should be taken in the disposal of items (syringes, needles, etc.) used to reconstitute cytotoxic drugs.

Vials of Velbe should be stored in a refrigerator between 2° and 8°C.

After reconstitution: After a portion of the solution has been removed from a vial, the remainder of the contents of the vial may be stored in a refrigerator for further use for 30 days without significant loss of potency. When the reconstituted vial of Velbe is to be stored for more than 48 hours, it is essential to use the accompanying diluting solution or a diluent which contains a preservative.

Velbe should never be mixed with any other drug and should not be diluted with solvents that raise or lower the pH from between 3.5 and 5.0.

Legal category POM.

Package quantity Vials 10 mg: Single vials.

Further information The presence of this drug or its metabolites in blood or body tissues is not known to interfere with clinical laboratory tests.

Product licence numbers

Vials 10 mg:	0006/5073
Diluent:	0006/5174

**Trade Mark*

Lipha Pharmaceuticals Limited
Harrier House, High Street
Yiewsley
West Drayton
Middlesex UB7 7QG

GLUCOPHAGE*

Presentation White, film-coated tablets containing Metformin Hydrochloride BP. 500 mg marked GL500; 850 mg marked GL850.

Uses *Indications:* Non-insulin dependent diabetes when diet has failed and especially if the patient is overweight. Glucophage can be given alone as initial therapy, or can be administered in combination with a sulphonylurea.

In insulin-dependent diabetes, Glucophage may be given as an adjuvant to patients whose symptoms are poorly controlled.

Pharmacology: Glucophage is a biguanide oral anti-hyperglycaemic agent. Its mode of action is thought to be multifactorial and includes delayed uptake of glucose from the gastro-intestinal tract, increased peripheral glucose utilisation mediated by increased insulin sensitivity and inhibition of increased hepatic and renal gluconeogenesis.

Dosage and administration
Adults: Initially, one 850 mg tablet twice a day or one 500 mg tablet three times a day, with or after food. Good diabetic control may be achieved within a few days, but it is not unusual for the full effect to be delayed for up to two weeks. If control is incomplete a cautious increase in dosage to a maximum of 3 g daily is justified. Once control has been obtained it may be possible to reduce the dosage of Glucophage.

Children: Glucophage is not recommended for use.

Elderly: Glucophage is indicated in the elderly, but not when renal function is impaired.

Contra-indications, warnings, etc
Contra-indications: Hypersensitivity to the drug. Diabetic coma and ketoacidosis, impairment of renal function, chronic liver disease, cardiac failure and recent myocardial infarction. History of, or states associated with, lactic acidosis such as shock or pulmonary insufficiency, alcoholism (acute or chronic), and conditions associated with hypoxaemia.

Precautions: Glucophage is excreted by the kidney and regular monitoring of renal function is advised in all diabetics. Glucophage therapy should be stopped 2–3 days before surgery and clinical investigations such as intravenous urography and intravenous angiography, and reinstated only after control of renal function has been regained. The use of Glucophage is not advised in conditions which may cause dehydration or in patients suffering from serious infections or trauma.

Patients receiving continuous Glucophage therapy should have an annual estimation of Vitamin B_{12} levels because of reports of decreased Vitamin B_{12} absorption.

During concomitant therapy with a sulphonylurea, blood glucose should be monitored because combined therapy may cause hypoglycaemia. Stabilisation of diabetic patients with Glucophage and insulin should be carried out in hospital because of the possibility of hypoglycaemia until the correct ratio of the two drugs has been obtained.

Reduced renal clearance of Glucophage has been reported during cimetidine therapy, so a dose reduction should be considered. As with a number of drugs, an interaction between Glucophage and anticoagulants is a possibility and dosage of the latter may need adjustment.

Use in pregnancy and lactation: Pregnancy: The use of Glucophage is not advised. Lactation: No information is available.

Adverse reactions: Glucophage is normally well tolerated but gastro-intestinal disturbances sometimes occur. These are usually minor and can often be avoided by taking Glucophage with or after food. Occasionally a temporary lowering of the dose may be needed. It is important that Glucophage treatment is not abandoned at the first sign of intolerance, since this has been found to resolve spontaneously.

Lactic acidosis has been associated with Glucophage but, in the few cases reported, has occurred in patients with contra-indications to therapy. In patients with a metabolic acidosis lacking evidence of ketoacidosis (ketonuria and ketonaemia), lactic acidosis should be suspected and Glucophage therapy stopped. Lactic acidosis is a medical emergency which must be treated in hospital.

Overdosage – Signs and Symptoms: Hypoglycaemia does not occur with Glucophage monotherapy (fifty tablets have been ingested with no untoward effects on blood glucose levels). However, it can occur when Glucophage is given concomitantly with a sulphonylurea, insulin or alcohol.

In excessive dosage, and particularly if there is a possibility of accumulation, lactic acidosis may develop.

Overdosage – Treatment: Intensive supportive therapy is recommended which should be particularly directed at correcting fluid loss and metabolic disturbance.

Pharmaceutical precautions Store below 25°C in a dry place. The shelf-life is 5 years.

Legal category POM.

Package quantities 500 mg: 84 tablets (28 days' supply as an original dispensing pack). 850 mg: 56 tablets (28 days' supply as an original dispensing pack).

Further information Glucophage does not lower blood glucose levels in non-diabetics, and does not cause hypoglycaemia in diabetics when used as mono-therapy. Weight loss often occurs during therapy and levels of plasma cholesterol, triglycerides and prebeta-lipoproteins may be lowered. Glucophage has been shown to improve peripheral glucose metabolism.

Product licence numbers
Glucophage 500 mg 3759/0012
Glucophage 850 mg 3759/0013

IONAMIN*

Presentation Capsules marked 'IONAMIN' and with the capsule strength, containing Phentermine INN in a sustained-release formulation. 15 mg: Opaque grey and yellow capsule. 30 mg: Opaque yellow capsule.

Ionamin also contains lactose and sunset yellow (E110).

Uses Ionamin is an anorectic agent intended for short term use as an adjunct to the treatment of patients with moderate to severe obesity for whom close support and supervision are also to be provided.

Dosage and administration
Adults: 15 or 30 mg daily before breakfast or 10 to 14 hours before retiring. The recommended dose should not be exceeded in an attempt to increase the anorectic effect and the drug should be discontinued in non-responsive cases.

Several clinical studies have indicated that an intermittent dosage regime consisting of treatment for up to 4 weeks followed by a similar period without medication may be as effective as continuous treatment.

The efficacy and safety of Ionamin in intermittent use for more than 6 months have not been established. The possibility of dependence with continuous use should be considered.

Children and the Elderly: Ionamin is not recommended for use.

Contra-indications, warnings, etc
Contra-indications: Hypersensitivity to sympathomimetic amines. Severe hypertension, thyrotoxicosis, a history of psychiatric illness, or drug or alcohol abuse. Emotional instability or vulnerable personalities. Concurrent or recent use of monoamine oxidase inhibitors (MAOIs). Concurrent administration of other anorectic agents.

Warnings: Phentermine is structurally and pharmacologically related to the amphetamines, drugs which have been extensively abused for euphoriant effect, and are capable of inducing physical dependence. Experience has shown that generally neither of these are problems, although dependence has been reported in a few cases.

Phentermine may produce mild CNS excitation and there is a theoretical risk of sedation on withdrawal of the drug: if the patient is affected, his ability to drive or operate machinery may be impaired. Phentermine may enhance the response to alcohol.

Precautions: Caution should be exercised when Ionamin is administered with anti-hypertensive, psychotropic and sympathomimetic drugs. The use of Ionamin in combination with dietary regimes may alter the insulin requirements of patients receiving anti-diabetic medication.

Use in pregnancy and lactation: Pregnancy: There is inadequate evidence of safety of Ionamin in human pregnancy; there is evidence of harmful effects in animals with amphetamines. As with amphetamines, treatment should cease during pregnancy.

Lactation: No information is available.

Adverse reactions: Dry mouth, restlessness, nervousness, insomnia, palpitations, constipation, nausea, vomiting, rashes, euphoria and agitation have been reported. There is a theoretical possibility of raised blood pressure.

Overdosage – Signs and Symptoms: CNS stimulation such as restlessness, agitation and hallucinations may occur, usually followed by fatigue and depression. Cardiovascular effects include arrhythmias, hypertension and circulatory collapse. Gastrointestinal effects include nausea, vomiting, diarrhoea and abdominal cramps. Since Ionamin is a sustained release product, effects may be slow in onset and prolonged.

Overdosage – Treatment: Management includes emesis or gastric lavage (depending on the clinical state of the patient), and activated charcoal. The patient should be kept quiet and chlorpromazine used if necessary for sedation. Cardiovascular function should be monitored and treated symptomatically. In serious cases, forced acid diuresis may be indicated but only after discussion with a poisons centre.

Pharmaceutical precautions Store below 25°C in a dry place. The shelf-life is 3 years.

Legal category CD (Sch 3), POM.

Package quantities 100 capsules.

Further information Nil.

Product licence numbers
Ionamin 15 mg 3759/0007R
Ionamin 30 mg 3759/0008R

KELOCYANOR*

Presentation Clear 20 ml ampoules filled with a rose-coloured solution and each containing 300 mg Dicobalt Edetate INN (15 mg/ml).

Excipients: Dextrose, water for injections.

Uses
Indications: Kelocyanor is a specific antidote for acute cyanide poisoning. In view of the difficulty of certain diagnosis in emergency situations, it is recommended that Kelocyanor only be given when the patient is tending to lose, or has lost, consciousness. The product should not be used as a precautionary measure (see warnings section).

Pharmacology: Cyanide blocks intracellular respiration by binding to cytochrome oxidase. Kelocyanor forms a stable complex with the cyanide thereby acting as an antidote.

Dosage and administration
Adults: One 300 mg ampoule intravenously over approximately one minute. If the patient shows inadequate response, a second ampoule may be given. If there is no response after a further five minutes, a third ampoule may be administered.

Each ampoule of Kelocyanor may be followed immediately by 50 ml Dextrose Intravenous Infusion BP 500 g/l.

When the patient's condition is less severe but, in the physician's judgement, still warrants the use of Kelocyanor, the period over which the injection is given should be extended to 5 minutes.

Children: There is no clinical experience of the use of Kelocyanor in children. As with adults, the dose required will be related to the quantity of cyanide ingested.

Elderly: There is no clinical experience of the use of Kelocyanor in the elderly, but there is no reason to believe that the dosage schedule should be different from that for adults.

Cyanide poisoning must be treated as quickly as possible and intensive supportive measures must be instituted: clear airways and adequate ventilation are essential. 100% oxygen should be administered concurrently with Kelocyanor.

Expert advice on the treatment of poisoning is available from the local Poisons Centre.

Contra-indications, warnings, etc
Warnings: There is a reciprocal antidote action between cyanide and cobalt. Thus in the absence of cyanide, Kelocyanor is itself toxic. It is therefore essential that the product only be used in cases of cyanide poisoning. When the patient is fully conscious, it is unlikely that the extent of poisoning warrants the use of Kelocyanor.

Adverse reactions: The initial effects of Kelocyanor are vomiting, a fall in blood pressure, and compensatory tachycardia. After this the patient should recover.

Overdosage – Signs and Symptoms: These may be due to cobalt toxicity or to an anaphylactic type reaction, which may be dramatic. Oedema (particularly of the face and neck), vomiting, chest pain, sweating, hypotension, cardiac irregularities and rashes may occur.

Overdosage – Treatment: Intensive supportive therapy is required.

Pharmaceutical precautions Store below 25°C. The shelf-life is 3 years.

Legal category POM.

Package quantities 6 ampoules.

Further information Nil.

Product licence number 3759/5901R.

NITROLINGUAL* SPRAY

Presentation Metered-dose aerosol which delivers 400 micrograms glyceryl trinitrate per spray emission. This presentation provides for very rapid buccal absorption from the spray droplets producing an almost immediate effect.

Uses *Indications:* For the treatment and prophylaxis of angina pectoris and the treatment of variant angina.

For emergency treatment of pulmonary oedema secondary to acute left ventricular failure until such time as appropriate intravenous therapy can be instituted.

Pharmacology: Glyceryl trinitrate relieves angina pectoris by reduction of cardiac work and dilation of the coronary arteries. In this way, not only is there a lessening in arterial oxygen requirement, but the amount of oxygenated blood reaching the ischaemic heart is increased.

In heart failure glyceryl trinitrate acts primarily by relaxing venous smooth muscle, and this leads to a decrease in venous return and lower ventricular filling pressure thus relieving pulmonary congestion.

Dosage and administration
Dosage: Adults and the Elderly: At the onset of an attack: one or two 400 microgram metered-doses sprayed under the tongue. No more than three metered-doses are generally recommended at any one time. For the prevention of exercise-induced angina or in other precipitating conditions: one or two 400 microgram metered-doses sprayed under the tongue immediately prior to the event.

In the emergency treatment of pulmonary oedema secondary to acute left ventricular failure, two 400 microgram metered doses should be sprayed under the tongue as quickly as possible. This dose may be repeated as necessary.

Children: Nitrolingual spray is not recommended for use.

Administration: In angina: During application the patient should rest, ideally in the sitting position. The canister should be held vertically with the valve head uppermost and the spray orifice as close to the mouth as possible. The dose should be sprayed under the tongue and the mouth should be closed immediately after each dose. The spray should not be inhaled. Patients should be instructed to familiarize themselves with the position of the spray orifice, which can be identified by the finger rest on top of the valve, in order to facilitate orientation for administration at night.

In acute left ventricular failure: When used for the emergency treatment of acute left ventricular failure, the patient should be maintained as nearly as possible in an upright sitting position and the canister held upright whilst two metered dose sprays are directed under the tongue.

Contra-indications, warnings, etc These are common to all nitrates.

Contra-indications: Hypersensitivity to nitrates. Hypotensive shock, severe anaemia, cerebral haemorrhage and brain trauma, mitral stenosis, arterial hypoxaemia, uncorrected hypovolaemia and angina caused by hypertrophic obstructive cardiomyopathy.

Precautions: Tolerance to this drug and cross tolerance to other nitrates may occur. Alcohol may potentiate the hypotensive effect.

Use in pregnancy and lactation: No information is available.

Adverse reactions: Headache, postural hypotension, flushing, tachycardia and paradoxical bradycardia have been reported.

Overdosage – Signs and Symptoms: Flushing, severe headache, a feeling of suffocation, hypotension, fainting and rarely cyanosis and methaemoglobinaemia may occur. In a few patients there may be a reaction comparable to shock with nausea, vomiting, weakness, sweating and syncope.

Overdosage – Treatment: Recovery often occurs without special treatment. Hypotension may be corrected by elevation of the legs to promote venous return. Methaemoglobinaemia should be treated by intravenous methylene blue. Symptomatic treatment should be given for respiratory and circulatory defects in more serious cases.

Pharmaceutical precautions Store below 25°C. Pressurised container. Protect from sunlight and do not expose to temperatures exceeding 50°C. Do not pierce or burn, even after use. Do not spray on a naked flame or any incandescent material. The shelf-life is 3 years.

Legal category P.

Package quantities Single canisters.

Further information Unlike glyceryl trinitrate sublingual tablets, Nitrolingual Spray does not deteriorate on storage. No loss of potency occurs throughout the 3 year shelf-life of the product.
Glyceryl trinitrate is also known as nitroglycerin, trinitroglycerin and trinitrin.

Product licence number 3759/0035.

NITRONAL*

Presentation Amber glass 5 ml ampoules and 50 ml clear glass vials filled with a colourless isotonic solution containing 1 mg/ml glyceryl trinitrate.

Excipients: Dextrose, polyethylene glycol 400, water for injections.

Uses
Indications:

1. Unresponsive congestive heart failure, including that secondary to acute myocardial infarction.
2. Refractory unstable angina pectoris and coronary insufficiency, including Prinzmetal's angina.
3. Control of hypertensive episodes and/or myocardial ischaemia during and after cardiac surgery. For the induction of controlled hypotension for surgery.

Pharmacology: Glyceryl trinitrate exerts a spasmolytic action on smooth muscle, particularly in the vascular system. The predominant effect is an increase in venous capacitance resulting in marked diminution of both the left ventricular filling pressure and volume (preload). There is also a reduction in afterload due to moderate dilation of the arteriolar resistance vessels. These haemodynamic changes lower the myocardial oxygen demand. By direct action and through the reduction of myocardial wall tension, glyceryl trinitrate also lowers the resistance to flow in the coronary collateral channels and allows re-distribution of blood flow to ischaemic areas of the myocardium.

Administration of Nitronal by intravenous infusion to patients with congestive heart failure results in a marked improvement in haemodynamics, reduction of elevated left ventricular filling pressure and systolic wall tension, and an increase in the depressed cardiac output. It reduces the imbalance that exists between myocardial oxygen demand and delivery, thereby diminishing myocardial ischaemia and controlling ischaemia-induced ventricular arrhythmias.

Dosage and administration
Dosage: Adults and the Elderly – The dose should be titrated against the individual clinical response.

1. Unresponsive congestive heart failure. The normal dose range is 10–100 micrograms/minute administered as a continuous intravenous infusion with frequent monitoring of blood pressure and heart rate. The infusion should be started at the lower rate and increased cautiously until the desired clinical response is achieved. Other haemodynamic measurements are extremely important in monitoring response to the drug: these may include pulmonary capillary wedge pressure, cardiac output and precordial electrocardiogram depending on the clinical picture.
2. Refractory unstable angina pectoris. An initial infusion rate of 10–15 micrograms/minute is recommended; this may be increased cautiously in increments of 5–10 micrograms until either relief of

angina is achieved, headache prevents further increase in dose, or the mean arterial pressure falls by more than 20 mm Hg.

3. Use in surgery. An initial infusion rate of 25 micrograms/minute is recommended; this should be increased gradually until the desired systolic arterial pressure is attained. The usual dose is 25–200 micrograms/minute.

Children: Nitronal is not recommended for use.

Administration: Nitronal need not be diluted before use but can be diluted with Dextrose Injection BP, Sodium Chloride and Dextrose Injection BP, 0.9% Sodium Chloride Injection BP or other protein-free infusion solution, if required.

The solution, whether or not diluted, should be infused *slowly* (see dosage section) and *not* given by bolus injection.

To ensure a constant infusion rate of glyceryl trinitrate, it is recommended that Nitronal be administered by means of a syringe pump or polyethylene infusion bag with a counter, with a glass or rigid polyethylene syringe and polyethylene tubing. Systems made of polyvinylchloride may adsorb up to 50% of the glyceryl trinitrate from the solution, thus reducing the efficacy of the infusion. If the recommended type of system is unavailable, a 1:10 dilution of Nitronal should be used and the infusion rate modified according to the haemodynamic response of the patient, until the required parameters are attained.

Contra-indications, warnings, etc These are common to all nitrates.

Contra-indications: Hypersensitivity to nitrates. Hypotensive shock, severe anaemia, cerebral haemorrhage, arterial hypoxaemia, uncorrected hypovolaemia and angina caused by hypertrophic obstructive cardiomyopathy.

Precautions: Caution should be exercised in patients with severe liver or renal disease, hypothermia or hypothyroidism. Glyceryl trinitrate may potentiate the action of other hypotensive drugs and the hypotensive and anticholinergic effects of tricyclic anti-depressants; it may also slow the metabolism of morphine-like analgesics.

Pregnancy and lactation: No information is available.

Adverse reactions: Nitronal is generally well tolerated because a minimum dose is administered in unit time. Headache, dizziness, flushing, hypotension and tachycardia may be encountered, particularly if the infusion is administered too rapidly. Nausea, diaphoresis, restlessness, retrosternal discomfort, abdominal pain and paradoxical bradycardia have been reported. These symptoms should be readily reversible on reducing the rate of infusion or, if necessary, discontinuing treatment.

Overdosage – Signs and Symptoms: Vomiting, restlessness, hypotension, syncope, cyanosis, coldness of the skin, impairment of respiration, bradycardia, psychosis and methaemoglobinaemia may occur.

Overdosage – Treatment: The symptoms may be readily reversed by discontinuing treatment; if hypotension persists, raising the foot of the bed and the use of vasoconstrictors such as intravenous methoxamine or phenylephrine is recommended. Methaemaglobinaemia should be treated by intravenous methylene blue. Oxygen and assisted respiration may be required.

Pharmaceutical precautions Store in a cool place away from light. The vial is for single dose use only, and should be stored in the carton until ready for use. The shelf life is 2 years.

The diluted solution should be administered as soon as possible; it is stable for up to 24 hours in the recommended infusion system.

Legal category POM.

Package quantities 10 ampoules; single vials.

Further information Nitronal is free of alcohol, propylene glycol and potassium. See package insert for further details on administration sets, etc. Glyceryl trinitrate is also known as nitroglycerin, trinitroglycerin and trinitrin.

Product licence number 3759/0025.

PRAXILENE*

Presentation Pale pink capsules marked PRAXILENE and LIPHA, each containing 100 mg of naftidrofuryl oxalate.

Uses *Indications:* Peripheral vascular disorders – intermittent claudication, night cramps, rest pain, incipient gangrene, trophic ulcers, Raynaud's syndrome, diabetic arteriopathy and acrocyanosis.

Cerebral vascular disorders – cerebral insufficiency and cerebral atherosclerosis, particularly where these manifest themselves as mental deterioration and confusion in the elderly.

Pharmacology: Praxilene has been shown to exert a direct effect on intracellular metabolism. Thus it has been demonstrated in man and animals that it produces an increase of ATP levels and a decrease of lactic acid levels in ischaemic conditions, evidence for an enhancement of cellular oxidative capacity. Furthermore Praxilene is a powerful spasmolytic agent.

Dosage and administration
Adults and the Elderly: Peripheral vascular disorders: one or two 100 mg capsules three times daily for a minimum of three months, or at the discretion of the Physician.

Cerebral vascular disorders: one 100 mg capsule three times daily for a minimum of three months, or at the discretion of the Physician.

Children: There is no recommended dose.

Contra-indications, warnings, etc
Contra-indications: Hypersensitivity to the drug.

Use in pregnancy and lactation: Pregnancy: There is no, or inadequate, evidence of safety of Praxilene in human pregnancy, but it has been in wide use for many years without apparent ill consequence, animal studies having shown no hazard. If drug therapy is needed in pregnancy, this drug can be used if there is no safer alternative.

Lactation: No information is available.

Adverse reactions: Praxilene is normally well tolerated in the dosage recommended. Occasionally nausea, epigastric pain and rashes have been noted.

Overdosage – Signs and symptoms: Depression of cardiac conduction and convulsions may occur.

Overdosage – Treatment: The stomach should be emptied by gastric lavage and emesis. Activated charcoal may be employed if necessary. Cardiovascular function and respiration should be monitored and, in severe cases, electrical pacemaking or the use of isoprenaline should be considered. Convulsions may be managed by diazepam.

Pharmaceutical precautions Store below 20°C in a dry place away from light. The shelf-life is 3 years.

Legal category POM.

Package quantities Blister pack of 84 capsules (OP); Securitainers of 100 and 500 capsules.

Further information For the treatment of peripheral vascular disorders when symptoms of gross ischaemia, rest pain or incipient gangrene are present, parenteral treatment with Praxilene Forte should be given in conjunction with oral therapy. The recommended dosing schedule is one 200 mg Praxilene Forte ampoule twice daily, given by infusion, for 7 to 10 days, together with one or two 100 mg capsules three times daily.

Product licence number 3759/0002.

PRAXILENE FORTE*

Presentation Clear, 10 ml ampoules filled with a colourless solution, each containing 200 mg of naftidrofuryl oxalate (20 mg/ml).

Excipients: Sorbitol, water for injections.

Uses *Indications:* For the treatment of peripheral vascular disease when symptoms of gross ischaemia, rest pain or incipient gangrene are present.

Pharmacology: Praxilene has been shown to exert a direct effect on intracellular metabolism. Thus, it has been demonstrated in man and animals that it produces an increase of ATP levels and a decrease of lactic acid levels in ischaemic conditions, evidence for an enhancement of cellular oxidative capacity. Furthermore, Praxilene is a powerful spasmolytic agent.

Dosage and administration
Adults and the Elderly: One 200 mg ampoule twice daily administered by intravenous or intra-arterial infusion in 250 to 500 ml of saline or dextrose over a minimum of 90 minutes, for a period of 7 to 10 days. Praxilene Forte may be administered in low molecular weight dextran provided the data sheet recommendations on dosage and administration for the appropriate product are observed. Praxilene Forte must NOT be given by bolus injection.

Children: There is no recommended dose.

Contra-indications, warnings, etc
Contra-indications: Hypersensitivity to the drug. Atrio-ventricular block.

Precautions: Caution should be exercised in patients with severe cardiac insufficiency, conduction disorders and renal or hepatic insufficiency. The possibility of an additive effect occurring between Praxilene Forte and antiarrhythmic and beta-adrenergic blocking drugs should be considered.

Warning: Praxilene Forte must not be given by bolus injection.

Use in pregnancy and lactation: Pregnancy: There is no, or inadequate, evidence of safety of Praxilene in human pregnancy, but it has been in wide use for many years without apparent ill consequence, animal studies having shown no hazard. If drug therapy is needed in pregnancy, this drug can be used if there is no safer alternative.

Lactation: No information is available.

Adverse reactions: Praxilene Forte is normally well tolerated in the dosage recommended. Occasionally nausea has been noted.

Overdosage – Signs and symptoms: Depression of cardiac conduction and convulsions may occur.

Overdosage – Treatment: In severe cases, treatment with isoprenaline injection or electrical pace-making should be considered. Convulsions may be managed by diazepam.

Pharmaceutical precautions Store below 25°C away from light. The shelf-life is 3 years.

The diluted solution is chemically stable for up to 72 hours in the recommended diluents. However, from a microbiological viewpoint, it is recommended that the diluted solution be administered as soon as possible and any solution not used within 24 hours discarded.

Praxilene Forte should not be given in solutions containing calcium ions.

Legal category POM.

Package quantities 10 ampoules.

Further information One or two 100 mg Praxilene capsules three times daily should be given with the infusion therapy. On completion of the infusion therapy, the patient should continue on oral treatment, 1 or 2 100 mg capsules three times daily for a minimum of three months, or at the discretion of the Physician.

Product licence number 3759/0004.

SLO-PHYLLIN*

Presentation Capsules marked SLO-PHYLLIN, LIPHA and with the capsule strength, containing Theophylline BP (anhydrous) in a timed release formulation which provides a prolonged therapeutic effect over 12 hours.

60 mg: Opaque white capsule with a clear colourless cap, filled with white pellets.

125 mg: Opaque dark brown capsule with a clear colourless cap, filled with white pellets.

250 mg: Opaque blue capsule with a clear colourless cap, filled with white pellets.

Slo-Phyllin also contains sucrose.

Uses As a bronchodilator in the symptomatic and prophylactic treatment of asthma and for reversible bronchoconstriction associated with chronic bronchitis, bronchial asthma and emphysema.

Dosage and administration
Children:

2–6 years (10–20 kg)	60–120 mg twice daily
6–12 years (20–35 kg)	125–250 mg twice daily
Over 12 years	250–500 mg twice daily

Adults: 250–500 mg twice daily.

Elderly: There is a tendency for theophylline clearance to decrease with age leading to higher serum levels. A reduction of the adult dosage may therefore be necessary, and close monitoring is advised.

Each patient should be titrated to a suitable dosage regimen by clinical assessment. It may also be necessary to measure plasma theophylline levels.

Initially the lowest dosage for each group is recommended. This may be increased gradually if optimal bronchodilator effects are not achieved. The total dosage should not normally exceed 24 mg/kg bodyweight for children and 13 mg/kg for adults. However the plasma theophylline level measured 4–8 hours after dosing and at least 3 days after any dosage adjustment, provides a more accurate assessment of the patient's dosage need, especially as significant variations in the rate of drug elimination can occur between individuals. The following table provides a guide:

Plasma level (microgram/ml)	*Result*	*Directions (if clinically indicated)*
Below 10	Too low	Increase dose by 25%
10–20	Correct	Maintain dose
20–25	Too high	Decrease dose by 10%
25–30		Miss next dose and decrease subsequent doses by 25%
Over 30		Miss next 2 doses and decrease subsequent doses by 50%

It is advisable to recheck the plasma level after dose adjustment and every 6–12 months.

It is not possible to ensure bioequivalence between different sustained release theophylline products. Once titrated to an effective dose, patients should not be changed from Slo-Phyllin to another sustained release xanthine preparation without re-titration and clinical assessment.

Patients should be instructed not to chew or suck the capsules or pellets as this destroys the timed release properties. However, for those who experience difficulty in swallowing capsules, the contents of a capsule may be sprinkled on to a spoonful of soft food, e.g. yoghurt.

Contra-indications, warnings, etc
Contra-indications: Hypersensitivity to theophylline or other xanthines. Concomitant use with ephedrine in children.

Precautions: Smoking and alcohol consumption can increase the clearance of theophylline and a higher dosage may be necessary.

Careful monitoring is recommended for patients with

congestive heart failure, chronic alcoholism, hepatic dysfunction or viral infections as they may have lower total clearance of theophylline which could lead to higher than normal plasma levels.

Caution should be exercised in patients with peptic ulcers, cardiac arrhythmias, other cardiovascular diseases, hyperthyroidism or hypertension.

Slo-Phyllin should not be used concurrently with other preparations containing xanthine derivatives. If it is necessary to administer aminophylline to a patient who is already receiving Slo-Phyllin, plasma theophylline concentrations should be monitored.

Use in pregnancy and lactation: Pregnancy: Slo-Phyllin is not recommended since theophylline is known to cross the placenta and its safety in pregnancy has not been established.

Lactation: Theophylline is distributed in breast milk and therefore Slo-Phyllin should be used with caution in nursing mothers.

Adverse reactions: These usually occur when theophylline blood levels exceed 20 micrograms/ml and include gastric irritation, nausea, vomiting, abdominal discomfort, palpitations, a fall in blood pressure, headache, occasional diarrhoea and insomnia. CNS stimulation and diuresis may also occur, especially in children.

Overdosage – Signs and Symptoms: Headache, nausea, vomiting, restlessness, hypotension, tachycardia, arrhythmias (usually supraventricular tachyarrhythmias), hypokalaemia, CNS depression, convulsions, dehydration and coma may occur. Massive overdosage may result in cardiac inhibition, circulatory and respiratory failure.

Overdosage – Treatment: The stomach should be emptied by gastric lavage and emesis. Repeated doses of activated charcoal should be considered. Blood glucose, electrolytes, arterial gases and pH should be monitored. Serum theophylline should be measured 4 h after ingestion and at 4 to 12 hourly intervals thereafter if symptoms are severe.

Intensive supportive therapy may be required to maintain respiration and cardiovascular function. Convulsions may be controlled by diazepam. Haemoperfusion may be necessary.

Slo-Phyllin is a timed-release capsule and effects may be slow in onset and prolonged.

Drug interactions: Theophylline has been reported to interact with a number of drugs.

The following increase clearance and it may therefore be necessary to increase dosage to ensure a therapeutic effect: barbiturates, carbamazepine, lithium, phenytoin, rifampicin, and sulphinpyrazone.

The following reduce clearance and a reduced dosage may therefore be necessary to avoid side-effects: allopurinol, cimetidine, ciprofloxacin, corticosteroids, erythromycin, frusemide, isoprenaline, oral contraceptives and thiabendazole.

There is some evidence of an interaction between theophylline and influenza vaccine.

Xanthines can potentiate hypokalaemia resulting from $beta_2$ agonist therapy, steroids, diuretics and hypoxia. Particular caution is advised in severe asthma. It is recommended that serum potassium levels are monitored in such situations.

Pharmaceutical precautions Store below 25°C in a dry place. The shelf-life is 3 years.

Legal category P.

Package quantities Blister pack of 56 capsules (OP); Securitainer of 100 capsules (250 mg strength only).

Further information The active pellets in each strength of Slo-Phyllin capsule are identical and the three presentations are therefore equally bioavailable. The three strengths thus allow optimum dose titration.

Product licence numbers
Slo-Phyllin 60 mg 0161/0021
Slo-Phyllin 125 mg 0161/0019
Slo-Phyllin 250 mg 0161/0020

SONI-SLO*

Presentation Capsules containing Isosorbide Dinitrate INN in a timed release formulation which provides a prolonged therapeutic effect.

20 mg: Size 3 transparent pink capsules with a clear colourless cap, filled with off-white pellets.

40 mg: Size 2 transparent red capsule with a clear colourless cap, filled with off-white pellets.

Soni-Slo also contains sucrose.

Uses For the prophylactic treatment of angina pectoris.

Dosage and administration
Adults and the Elderly: 40–120 mg daily in divided doses, generally morning and evening but eight hourly administration may be found necessary in severe cases.

Initially the lowest dosage is recommended. This may be increased gradually until the maximum therapeutic effect is achieved. Gradual reduction of dosage after long-term therapy is recommended whenever possible.

Children: Soni-Slo is not recommended for use.

Patients should be instructed not to chew or suck the capsules or pellets as this destroys the timed release properties.

Contra-indications, warnings, etc These are common to all nitrates.

Contra-indications: Hypersensitivity to nitrates. Hypotensive shock, severe anaemia, and angina caused by hypertrophic obstructive cardiomyopathy.

Precautions: Tolerance to this drug and cross tolerance to other nitrates may occur. Alcohol may potentiate the hypotensive effect.

Use in pregnancy and lactation: No information is available.

Adverse reactions: Headache, postural hypotension, flushing, tachycardia and paradoxical bradycardia have been reported.

Overdosage – Signs and Symptoms: Flushing, severe headache, a feeling of suffocation, hypotension and fainting and rarely, cyanosis and methaemoglobinaemia may occur. In a few patients there may be a reaction comparable to shock, with nausea, vomiting, weakness, sweating and syncope.

Overdosage – Treatment: Recovery often occurs without special treatment. Hypotension may be corrected by elevation of the legs to promote venous return. Methaemoglobinaemia should be treated by intravenous methylene blue. Symptomatic treatment should be given for respiratory and circulatory defects in more serious cases. Gastric lavage should be considered after careful assessment of the patient's condition, in particular the level of consciousness.

Pharmaceutical precautions Store in a cool dry place protected from light. Keep tightly closed. The shelf-life is 3 years.

Legal category P.

Package quantities 100 capsules.

Further information Nil.

Product licence numbers
Soni-Slo 20 mg 3759/0020
Soni-Slo 40 mg 3759/0021.

**Trade Mark*

Lorex Pharmaceuticals Ltd
PO Box 293
Lane End Road
High Wycombe
Buckinghamshire HP12 4HL

KERLONE*

Presentation White, biconvex, film-coated tablets engraved KE20 on one side with breakline on reverse. Each tablet contains betaxolol hydrochloride 20 mg.

Uses

Actions: Kerlone (betaxolol hydrochloride) is a beta-adrenoceptor blocking agent which is cardio-selective, i.e. acts preferentially on $beta_1$-adrenergic receptors in the heart. It has prolonged activity, permitting once-daily administration which aids patient compliance. Its principal effects are to lower heart rate, especially on exercise, and to lower systolic and diastolic blood pressure in hypertensive subjects. It is devoid of intrinsic sympathomimetic activity and has little membrane stabilising activity. As with other beta-blockers, its mechanism of action in the treatment of hypertension is unclear. Absorption from the gastro-intestinal tract is complete and not affected by food. There is little first-pass extraction in the liver. This results in blood levels which vary little within and between subjects and a reproducible bioavailability of 80–90%.

Its long elimination half-life of 16–20 hours results in protection from excessive or inappropriate sympathetic activity throughout the 24 hours after administration of a once daily dose.

Indications: Management of hypertension.

Dosage and administration

Adults: The usual adult dose is one tablet (20 mg) daily. The single daily dose may be increased to two tablets (40 mg) if response is inadequate.

Elderly patients or those with a history of bronchospasm: A starting dose of half tablet (10 mg) daily is recommended.

Impaired renal function: An adjustment of dose is usually unnecessary in patients with renal insufficiency where creatinine clearance is greater than 20 ml/min. However, clinical surveillance is recommended at the start of treatment until steady state blood levels are attained (4 days on average).

For patients on haemo- or peritoneal dialysis the initial recommended dose is 10 mg daily independent of the dialysis schedule.

Hepatic insufficiency: Adjustment of dosage is usually unnecessary in patients with hepatic insufficiency. However, clinical surveillance is recommended at the start of treatment.

Children: Paediatric experience with Kerlone is limited and for this reason it is not currently recommended for use in children.

Most of the reduction of blood pressure is seen during the first 3 hours following the initial dose, permitting an early evaluation of the anti-hypertensive effect. Little further reduction is seen after seven days of treatment and the response is undiminished in subsequent months. Should an inadequate response be obtained, a further decrease may be achieved by combining Kerlone with another antihypertensive agent such as a diuretic. However, in a large series of controlled clinical trials, 70–80% of patients responded to betaxolol alone.

Patients can be transferred to Kerlone from other antihypertensive treatments with the exception of clonidine (see precautions below).

Contra-indications, warnings, etc

Contra-indications: Kerlone is contra-indicated in cardiogenic shock, in patients with uncontrolled congestive cardiac failure and in second or third degree AV block if no pacemaker is present and in patients with marked bradycardia (heart rate less than 50 beats per minute).

Warnings: Concomitant administration of Kerlone and a myocardial depressant or inhibitor of AV conduction, such as the calcium antagonists of the verapamil type, should be carried out only under close supervision, especially in the case of intravenous administration.

Although cardio-selective beta-blockers may have less effect on lung function than non-selective beta-blockers, as with all beta-blockers these should be avoided in patients with reversible obstructive airways disease unless there are compelling clinical reasons for their use.

It is recommended that Kerlone treatment is started at the dose of 10 mg daily in such patients. If any increase in airway resistance is provoked, it can be relieved by $beta_2$-mimetics whose effect is not inhibited.

Precautions: Secondary sympathetic hyperactivity has sometimes been reported following discontinuation of treatment with other beta-blockers. Even though Kerlone blood levels decrease slowly, care should be exercised if treatment is withdrawn, especially in patients with ischaemic heart disease.

Patients with a history of cardiac failure, cardiomyopathy, or cardiomegaly should be monitored carefully during treatment with a beta-blocker as sympathetic stimulation may be essential to their circulatory function.

Use with caution where the PR conduction interval is prolonged.

Studies in normal subjects have shown that, unlike non-selective beta-blockers, Kerlone does not inhibit the recovery from insulin-induced hypoglycaemia, nor does it mask the cardiovascular response. Due to its $beta_1$ selectivity, Kerlone is unlikely to interfere with glucose metabolism in insulin-treated diabetics. However, caution is advised when treating such patients.

Anaesthesia: In the event of surgical intervention, the anaesthetist should be advised in advance that the patient is receiving Kerlone. In patients with severe ischaemic heart disease the risk/benefits of continuation of treatment have to be evaluated. If treatment is continued care should be taken when using anaesthetic agents such as ether, cyclopropane and trichloroethylene.

Drug interactions: As with other beta-blockers, use with care in combination with myocardial depressants or drugs which depress AV conduction. If Kerlone and clonidine are given concurrently, clonidine should not be discontinued until several days after withdrawal of the beta-blocker.

Pregnancy: No teratogenic effects have been demonstrated in animal studies but the safety of Kerlone during human pregnancy has not been established. Like other beta-blockers, Kerlone crosses the placental barrier and its use in pregnant women requires that the anticipated benefit be weighed against the possible hazards to the mother and foetus.

Nursing mothers: Kerlone is excreted in human breast milk and the possibility of bradycardic and hypotensive effects on the new-born should therefore be considered if Kerlone is given to nursing mothers.

Side effects: Kerlone is generally well tolerated. The side effects are usually those due to its pharmacological actions and rarely require discontinuation of treatment. Minor side effects include lassitude at the start of treatment, exacerbation of Raynaud's disease or intermittent claudication, and paraesthesia of the extremities. Possible side effects include marked bradycardia and hypotension, AV block, cardiac insufficiency and bronchospasm. There have been reports of rashes and dry eyes associated with the use of all beta-blockers but in most cases the signs and symptoms have cleared when treatment was withdrawn. Nevertheless, the drug should be discontinued if any such reaction is suspected.

Overdosage: Excessive bradycardia can usually be corrected with atropine. If there is no response isoprenaline may be administered with caution. Cardiac failure should be managed with digitalisation and diuretics. Hypotension may be managed with vasopressors such as adrenaline.

Pharmaceutical precautions No special precautions are indicated for Kerlone.

Legal category POM.

Package quantities Calendar pack of 28 tablets (2 × 14).

Further information Kerlone is unique in having high bioavailability, long blood half-life and high selectivity for cardiac $beta_1$-receptors. Unlike most other cardioselective beta-blockers it has high lipid solubility. This may facilitate rapid arrival of the drug at the receptor, but does not induce an increased incidence of side effects.

These characteristics and the rapidity of response increase patient compliance by virtue of the drug's acceptability, the simple dose regimen and narrow dose range.

The only active metabolite is cardio-selective and does not contribute to the clinical effect. Kerlone does not modify the hypoglycaemic response to insulin nor mask the cardiovascular response. It can be used in patients with respiratory disease, and is compatible with most other hypotensive agents.

Product licence number 4969/0001.

TILDIEM*

Presentation Off-white biconvex tablets, engraved Tildiem 60. Each tablet contains 60 mg of diltiazem hydrochloride in a modified release formulation.

Uses

Actions: Tildiem (diltiazem hydrochloride) is a calcium antagonist. It selectively reduces calcium entry through voltage-dependent calcium channels into vascular smooth muscle cells and myocardial cells. This lowers the concentration of intracellular calcium which is available to activate contractile proteins. This action of diltiazem results in dilation of coronary arteries causing an increase in myocardial oxygen supply. It reduces cardiac work by moderating the heart rate and reducing systemic vascular resistance thus reducing oxygen demand.

When Tildiem is given alone or with a beta-blocking agent only slight negative inotropic effects have been reported in patients with preserved ventricular function.

Indications: Angina pectoris.

Dosage and administration

Adults: The usual dose is one tablet (60 mg) three times daily. However, patient responses may vary and dosage requirements can differ significantly between individual patients. If necessary the dosage may be increased to 360 mg/day. Higher doses up to 480 mg/day have been used with benefit in some patients especially in unstable angina. There is no evidence of any decrease in efficacy at these high doses.

Children: Safety and efficacy in children have not been established.

Elderly and patients with impaired hepatic or renal function: The recommended starting dose is one tablet (60 mg) twice daily. The heart rate should be measured regularly in these groups of patients and the dose should not be increased if the heart rate falls below 50 beats per minute.

Contra-indications, warnings, etc

Contra-indications: Tildiem is contra-indicated in pregnancy and in women of child-bearing potential.

Tildiem depresses atrioventricular node conduction and is therefore contra-indicated in patients with marked bradycardia, sick sinus syndrome, left ventricular failure with stasis, or second or third degree AV block except in the presence of a functioning pacemaker.

Tildiem, like any calcium antagonist, should not be administered concurrently with dantrolene infusion because of the risk of ventricular fibrillation.

Warnings and precautions: Tildiem should be used with caution in patients with reduced left ventricular function. Patients with mild bradycardia, first degree AV block or prolonged PR interval should be observed closely.

Drug interactions: In common with other calcium antagonists, when Tildiem is used with drugs which may induce bradycardia or with other antiarrhythmic drugs the possibility of an additive effect should be borne in mind.

Case reports have suggested that blood levels of carbamazepine, cyclosporin, and theophylline may be increased when given concurrently with diltiazem hydrochloride. Care should be exercised in patients taking these drugs. In common with other calcium antagonists Tildiem may cause small increases in plasma levels of digoxin.

In patients taking H2 antagonists concurrently with Tildiem there may be increased levels of diltiazem.

Tildiem has been used safely in combination with beta-blockers, diuretics, ACE inhibitors and other antihypertensive agents. It is recommended that patients receiving these combinations should be regularly monitored. Concomitant use of Tildiem with alpha blockers such as prazosin should be strictly monitored because of the possible synergistic hypotensive effect of this combination.

Diltiazem hydrochloride treatment has been continued without problem during anaesthesia, but the anaesthetist should be informed that the patient is receiving a calcium antagonist.

Pregnancy: Diltiazem hydrochloride is teratogenic in some animal species. In the absence of adequate evidence of safety in human pregnancy, Tildiem should not be used in pregnancy or in women of child bearing potential.

Nursing mothers: Diltiazem hydrochloride is excreted in breast milk. One report suggests that concentrations in breast milk reach similar levels to those in serum. If use of Tildiem is considered essential, an alternative method of infant feeding should be instituted.

Side-effects: The following have been reported: ankle oedema, malaise, headache, hot flushes, gastro-intestinal disturbances and very rarely symptomatic bradycardia, sino-atrial block and atrio-ventricular block. Rash has been reported in association with diltiazem. These reactions are generally mild and resolve on cessation of therapy, however, severe vascular skin reactions have been reported occasionally. Isolated cases of moderate and transient elevation of liver transaminases have been observed at the start of treatment. Isolated cases of clinical hepatitis have been reported which resolved on cessation of therapy.

The current literature suggests that the effects of vasodilation, particularly ankle oedema, are dose dependent and are more frequent in the elderly.

Overdosage: The clinical consequences of overdose can be severe hypotension leading to collapse, and sinus bradycardia which may be accompanied by isorhythmic dissociation and atrioventricular conduction disturbances. Observation in a coronary care unit is advisable. Vasopressors such as adrenaline may be indicated in patients exhibiting profound hypotension. Calcium gluconate may help reverse the effects of calcium entry blockade. Atropine administration and temporary cardiac pacing may be required to manage bradycardia and/or conduction disturbances.

Pharmaceutical precautions Store in a dry place below 30°C (86°F).

Legal category POM.

Package quantities Blister strips of 10 tablets in packs of 100 tablets.

Further information Diltiazem hydrochloride is effective in angina, protecting the heart against ischaemia, vasodilating coronary arteries and reducing myocardial oxygen requirements. It is well tolerated and does not generally give rise to side effects associated with peripheral vasodilators, nor cause significant myocardial depression.

In pharmacokinetic studies in healthy volunteers, diltiazem was well absorbed. Peak plasma concentrations were reached 3 to 4 hours after dosing. Due to a first pass effect the bioavailability of the Tildiem tablet is about 50%. Mean apparent plasma half life is 5 hours. Diltiazem in plasma is 80–85% protein bound and is poorly dialysed. Diltiazem is extensively metabolised by the liver. The two major active circulating metabolites, desacetyl-diltiazem and N-monodemethyl diltiazem possess pharmacological activity equivalent to about 50% of that of diltiazem. Only 0.2 to 4% of diltiazem is found unchanged in the urine.

There is a linear relationship between dose and plasma concentration. During long-term administration in any one patient plasma concentrations of diltiazem remained constant.

Product licence number 4969/0005.

TILDIEM* RETARD 90
TILDIEM* RETARD 120

Presentation Off white biconvex sustained release tablets containing 90 mg and 120 mg diltiazem hydrochloride.

Uses

Mode of action: Tildiem Retard (diltiazem hydrochloride) is a calcium antagonist. It selectively reduces calcium entry through voltage-dependent calcium channels into vascular smooth muscle cells and myocardial cells. This lowers the concentration of intracellular calcium which is available to activate contractile proteins. This action of diltiazem results in dilation of coronary arteries causing an increase in myocardial oxygen supply. It reduces cardiac work by moderating the heart rate and by reducing the systemic vascular resistance thus reducing oxygen demand.

It also consequently exerts an antihypertensive effect which appears principally related to a lowering of peripheral resistance without producing reflex tachycardia.

Indications: Angina pectoris and mild to moderate hypertension.

Dosage and administration

Adults

Adults and hypertension: The usual starting dose is one tablet (120 mg) twice daily. The tablets should be swallowed with a little water and not chewed. Patient responses may vary and dosage requirements can differ significantly between individual patients. Higher divided doses up to 480 mg/day have been used with benefit in some angina patients especially in unstable angina. Doses of 360 mg/day may be required to provide adequate BP control in hypertensive patients. The heart rate should be monitored in groups of patients requiring dose reduction (e.g., elderly, patients with impaired hepatic or renal function) and the dose should not be increased if the heart rate falls below 50 beats per minute.

Elderly and patients with impaired hepatic or renal function

Angina: The recommended starting dose is one 60 mg tablet twice daily. This dose may be increased to one 90 mg or one 120 mg Tildiem Retard tablet twice daily.

Hypertension: The starting dose should be one 120 mg Tildiem Retard tablet daily. Dose adjustment is one 90 mg or one 120 mg Tildiem Retard tablet twice daily may be required.

Tildiem Retard tablets should be swallowed with a little water and not chewed.

Children

Safety and efficacy in children have not been established.

Contra-indications, warnings, etc

Contra-indications: Tildiem Retard is contra-indicated in pregnancy and in women of childbearing potential.

Tildiem Retard depresses atrioventricular node conduction and is therefore contraindicated in patients with marked bradycardia, sick sinus syndrome, left ventricular failure with stasis, or second or third degree AV block except in the presence of functioning pacemaker.

Tildiem Retard, like any calcium antagonist, should not be administered concurrently with dantrolene infusion because of the risk of ventricular fibrillation.

Warnings and precautions: Tildiem Retard should be used with caution in patients with reduced left ventricular function. Patients with mild bradycardia, first degree AV block or prolonged PR interval should be observed closely.

Unlike some other calcium antagonists, diltiazem does not affect the glucose or endogenous insulin responses to hypoglycaemia.

It does not have a significant myocardial depressant action in man.

Drug interactions: In common with other calcium antagonists, when Tildiem Retard is used with drugs which may induce bradycardia or with other antihypertensive drugs the possibility of an additive effect should be borne in mind.

Case reports have suggested that blood levels of carbamazepine, cyclosporin, and theophylline may be increased when given concurrently with diltiazem hydrochloride. Care should be exercised in patients taking these drugs. In common with other calcium antagonists Tildiem Retard may cause small increases in plasma levels of digoxin.

In patients taking H_2 antagonists concurrently with Tildiem Retard there may be increased levels of diltiazem.

Tildiem Retard has been used safely in combination with betablockers, diuretics, ACE inhibitors and other antihypertensive agents. It is recommended that patients receiving these combinations should be regularly monitored. Concomitant use of Tildiem Retard with alpha blockers such as prazosin should be strictly monitored because of the possible synergistic hypotensive effect of this combination.

Diltiazem hydrochloride treatment has been continued without problem during anaesthesia, but the anaesthetist should be informed that the patient is a receiving a calcium antagonist.

Pregnancy: Diltiazem hydrochloride is teratogenic in some animal species. In the absence of adequate evidence of safety in human pregnancy, Tildiem Retard should not be used in pregnancy or in women of child bearing potential.

Nursing mothers: Diltiazem hydrochloride is excreted in breast milk. One report suggest that concentrations in breast milk reach similar levels to those in serum. If use of Tildiem Retard is considered essential, an alternative method of infant feeding should be instituted.

Adverse effects: The following have been reported: ankle oedema, malaise, headache, hot flushes, gastro-intestinal disturbances and very rarely symptomatic bradycardia, sino-atrial block and atrio-ventricular block. Rash has been reported in association with diltiazem. These reactions are generally mild and resolve on cessation of therapy; however, severe vascular skin reactions have been reported occasionally. Isolated cases of moderate and transient elevation of liver transaminases have been observed at the start of treatment. Isolated cases of clinical hepatitis have been reported which resolved on cessation of therapy.

The current literature suggests that the effects of vasodilatation, particularly ankle oedema, are dose dependent and are more frequent in the elderly.

Overdosage: The clinical consequences of overdose can be severe hypotension leading to collapse, and sinus bradycardia which may be accompanied by isorhythmic dissociation and atrioventricular conduction disturbances. Observation in a coronary care unit is advisable. Vasopressors such as adrenaline may be indicated in patients exhibiting profound hypotension. Calcium gluconate may help reverse the effects of calcium entry blockade. Atropine administration and temporary cardiac pacing may be required to manage bradycardia and/or conduction disturbances.

Pharmaceutical precautions Store in a dry place below 30°C (86°F).

Legal category POM.

Package quantities Blister strip packs of 56 tablets.

Further information In pharmacokinetic studies in healthy volunteers, diltiazem was well absorbed (>90%). Peak plasma concentrations are reached 4 to 8 hours after dosing. Due to a first pass effect the bioavailability of Tildiem Retard is about 40%. The apparent plasma half life is on average 7–8 hours. After repeated administration there is an increase of 30% with respect to the theoretical value, in the following parameters: C_{max}, AUC, C_{min}. This increase is due to the partial saturation of hepatic first pass. Diltiazem in plasma is 80–85% protein bound and is poorly dialysed. Diltiazem is extensively metabolised by the liver. The two major active circulating metabolites, desacetyl-diltiazem and N-monodemethyl diltiazem possess pharmacological activity in angina equivalent to about 50% of that of diltiazem. Only 0.2 to 4% of diltiazem is found unchanged in the urine.

During long term administration in any one patient plasma concentrations of diltiazem remained constant. Plasma concentrations in elderly patients and in hepatic failure are in general higher than in young subjects, due to an increase in bioavailability. In renal failure, a reduction in dosage is only necessary as a function of the clinical response.

Product licence number
Tildiem Retard 90 4969/0012
Tildiem Retard 120 4969/0013

**Trade Mark*

LRC Products Limited
North Circular Road
London E4 8QA

durex®

DURAGEL*
DURACREME*

Presentation
Duragel: A colourless unscented gel containing Nonoxynol 9 USP, 2% w/w.
Duracreme: A white unscented cream containing Nonoxynol 9 USP, 2% w/w.
Other constituents:
Duracreme: Docusate Sodium BP, Isopropyl Alcohol BP, Propylene Glycol EP, Sodium Hydroxide BP, Carbomer 934P USP, Zinc Stearate EP, Benzoic Acid EP, Purified Water EP.
Duragel: Docusate Sodium BP, Isopropyl Alcohol BP, Propylene Glycol EP, Sodium Hydroxide BP, Carbomer 934P USP, Benzoic Acid EP, Purified Water EP.

Uses Duragel and Duracreme are for use as spermicidal contraceptives in conjunction with barrier methods of contraception.

Dosage and administration For use only by adult females of child bearing age.
Vaginal diaphragm
At insertion: Two strips (5 cm each) on each side of the diaphragm.
At topping up: 1 applicator full (approximately 22 cm strip).
Cervical Cap
At insertion: One 5 ml teaspoonful inside the cap.
At topping up: 1 applicator full (approximately 22 cm strip).
All uses:
Apply or top up not more than 3 hours before intercourse. Top up between repeated acts of intercourse. Leave in place for at least 6 hours after last intercourse. Do not leave in place for longer than 24 hours.

Contra-indications, warnings, etc
Contra-indications: Hypersensitivity to Nonoxynol 9 or to any component of the preparation. Patients with absent vaginal sensation e.g. paraplegics and quadriplegics.
Undesirable effects: May cause irritation of the vagina or penis.
Use in pregnancy and lactation: there is no evidence from animal and human studies that Nonoxynol 9 is teratogenic. Human epidemiological studies have not shown any firm evidence of adverse effects on the foetus, however some studies have shown that Nonoxynol 9 may be embryotoxic in animals. This product should not be used if pregnancy is suspected or confirmed. Animal studies have detected Nonoxynol 9 in milk after intravaginal administration. Use by lactating women has not been studied.
Other special warnings and precautions: Spermicidal intravaginal preparations are intended for use in conjunction with barrier methods of contraception such as condoms, diaphragms and caps.
Where avoidance of pregnancy is important the choice of contraceptive method should be made in consultation with a doctor or a family planning clinic.
If vaginal or penile irritation occurs discontinue use. If symptoms worsen or continue for more than 48 hours medical advice should be sought.
Overdose: If taken orally the surfactant properties of this preparation may cause gastric irritation. General supportive therapy should be carried out. Hepatic and renal function should be monitored if medically indicated.

Pharmaceutical precautions Store below 30°C. Do not freeze.

Legal category GSL.

Package quantities The products are presented in collapsible tubes containing 100 g. The tubes are supplied in packs of four.

Further information Duragel and Duracreme are suitable for patients requiring extra lubrication in addition to spermicidal action.
Durex spermicide applicators are available from chemists. Other makes of applicator should not be used.

Product licence numbers

Duragel	2156/5001R
Duracreme	2156/5002R

**Trade Mark*

Lundbeck Limited
Lundbeck House
Hastings Street
Luton Bedfordshire LU1 5BE

ACLACIN* ▼

Presentation Aclacin is a yellow or orange-yellow freeze-dried powder containing aclarubicin hydrochloride equivalent to 20 mg aclarubicin.

Uses
Pharmacology: Aclarubicin is a cytotoxic antibiotic of the anthracycline group (Class II). The precise mode of action is uncertain, although aclarubicin has been shown to preferentially inhibit RNA synthesis.

Indications: Acute non-lymphocytic leukaemia in patients who have relapsed or are resistant or refractory to first line chemotherapy.

Dosage and administration Aclarubicin should be administered by intravenous infusion over 30 to 60 minutes.

Adults, including the elderly: The usual initial dosage is 175–300 mg/m^2 body surface over 3 to 7 consecutive days, e.g. 80–100 mg/m^2 on 3 consecutive days or 25 mg/m^2 daily for 7 consecutive days. Repetition of treatment schedules will be dependent on the patient's haematological profile and the response of the primary disease.

Maintenance dosage should be treatments of 25–100 mg/m^2 of body surface given as a single infusion every 3 to 4 weeks.

This is a guide to dosage using the drug alone. In combination with other cytotoxic drugs dosage may need to be reduced.

The maximum total dosage given to any individual patient should be decided according to their cardiological status. Most patients treated have received a maximum of 400 mg/m^2, however, larger dosages in some patients have been used without ill consequence.

Children: Experience suggests that aclarubicin is well tolerated by children at the standard dosage level.

Preparation of solutions: The vial contents should be reconstituted with 10 ml of 0.9% sodium chloride injection or water for injections. The concentration of this reconstituted solution is 2 mg/ml.

To prepare an infusion solution dilute the required volume of reconstituted solution with 200 to 500 ml 0.9% sodium chloride intravenous infusion or, if necessary, 5% glucose intravenous infusion (of pH value between 5 and 6). The final concentration should be 0.2–0.5 mg/ml.

Administration: Either (i) in a freely flowing iv peripheral line or (ii) in a patent central venous line.

Contra-indications, warnings, etc
Contra-indications: Severe bone marrow depression.

Use in pregnancy and lactation: There is no evidence of the drug's safety in human pregnancy. There is evidence from animal work that it is foetotoxic but not teratogenic. Avoid in pregnancy unless there is no safer alternative. If used in pregnancy patients should be warned of the potential risk to the foetus.

Women of childbearing age should take adequate contraceptive precautions.

If the use of Aclarubicin is considered essential, nursing mothers should be advised to stop breast-feeding.

Precautions: Patients receiving aclarubicin require close observation and frequent laboratory monitoring therefore, treatment should be carried out by doctors experienced in the use of cytotoxic drugs. Treatment should be carried out at centres where there are adequate laboratory facilities, supportive treatment and facilities for monitoring heart disease readily available. Therapy should be initiated cautiously in patients with compromised hepatic, renal or cardiac function.

The patient's haematological profile should be taken into account when instituting therapy and monitored during the recovery phase post treatment. Anaemia and thrombocytopenia should be treated with appropriate blood product replacement.

Hyperuricaemia should be avoided (fluid and xanthine oxidase inhibitors) and infections should be treated.

Cardiac function should be monitored by ECG.

There have been reports of increased toxicity consequent upon irradiation treatment shortly before the administration of anthracyclines. No such reactions have been observed following treatment with aclarubicin but the theoretical risk should be borne in mind.

Interactions with other medication: Aclarubicin is a powerful myelosuppressive agent. The concurrent use of other chemotherapeutic drugs with similar actions may be expected to lead to additive myelosuppression and dosage reduction should be considered.

Aclarubicin has caused higher than expected myelosuppression in patients previously treated with nitrosourea or mitomycin.

Warnings and adverse effects
Haematological: The dose-limiting toxicity of aclarubicin is haematological with myelosuppression seen as leucopenia and thrombocytopenia. The platelet nadir precedes the leucocyte nadir. Myelosuppression is severe at total dosages greater than 300 mg/m^2. Higher total dosages should be administered in a cyclic schedule including rest periods for recovery of the bone marrow. Myelosuppression is not reduced by dividing a single dose over 2 to 5 days. Thrombocytopenia is at a maximum 1 to 2 weeks after the start of drug administration with recovery within 2 to 4 weeks. Leucopenia is greatest 2 to 3 weeks after drug administration with recovery within 3 to 4 weeks.

Gastrointestinal: Nausea and vomiting have been observed in 20–100% (average 60%) of patients depending on dosage and dose schedule used. Single dosages greater than 120 mg/m^2 given by iv infusion caused nausea and vomiting in all patients.

The same dosage divided over 5 days is better tolerated. A daily dose of up to 30 mg/m^2 for 7 consecutive days caused nausea and vomiting, (controllable with antiemetics) in about 50% of patients. Bolus injections of more than 50 mg/m^2 should not be given due to severe gastrointestinal side-effects. Diarrhoea, occasionally haemorrhagic, has been observed in 10–35% (average 26%) of patients. Diarrhoea has been most pronounced after high single dosages or consecutive use of low dosages for more than 10 days. Mucositis/stomatitis has been observed in 15–55% (average 30%) of patients and is also more pronounced at high dosages.

Cardiac: Acute cardiotoxicity during and after drug administration has been associated with ECG changes (including arrhythmia, atrial flutter, flattening or inversion of T waves, sinus tachycardia, ST depression and premature beats) in 10–40% (average 17%) of patients. The frequency of ECG changes is greater with high single doses of aclarubicin. The ECG changes are generally reversible, transient and frequently without clinical signs of cardiotoxicity. ECG QTc prolongation may herald a clinical risk of ventricular fibrillation.

Chronic cardiotoxicity has been observed rarely: in a follow-up study of about 1,600 patients congestive heart failure occurred in 5 patients and in 2 patients clinical signs of cardiomyopathy were seen. The risk of cardiotoxicity may be increased in patients previously treated with other cytotoxic agents or irradiation to the thorax.

Alopecia: Mild alopecia has been observed in 1–5% of patients.

Hepatic: Transient and reversible serum transaminase elevation and hepatic dysfunction have been reported in 4–6% of patients.

Other: Phlebitis is rare, occurring in up to 7% of patients. It may be eliminated by dilution of infusion solutions. Allergic reactions (angioedema, urticaria, skin rash, conjunctivitis) have occurred in isolated cases.

After accidental extravasation, aclarubicin caused inflammation and induration, but no tissue necrosis.

Results from some mutagenicity studies with aclarubicin were positive and it showed the capacity to induce chromosomal aberrations. The carcinogenic potential of aclarubicin in man is unknown. The possibility of a carcinogenic effect should be kept in mind when planning long-term therapy.

Aclarubicin is a novel anthracycline, any unexpected side-effect or unusual response should be reported immediately.

Effect on ability to drive or operate machinery: The patient's general condition is likely to be more significant in this consideration than any drug-induced effects.

Overdosage: The haematologic profile should be monitored and, in the event of dangerously low haemoglobin, white cell or platelet counts, treatment with appropriate blood products should be carried out as clinically required. Fevers should be investigated and treated properly.

Cardiac function should be monitored and arrhythmias or congestive cardiac failure treated as they appear.

Pharmaceutical precautions Aclarubicin should only be reconstituted using 0.9% sodium chloride injection or water for injections. Reconstituted aclarubicin should only be added to 0.9% intravenous sodium chloride infusion or to glucose infusion solutions having pH values between 5 and 6.

Aclarubicin is not stable at pH of less than 4. Exposure of very dilute solutions to light promotes degradation.

Infusion solutions should be used immediately, and protected from sunlight during administration.

Water and saline solutions should be stored, protected from light, below 4°C and used within 24 hours of preparation or within 6 hours at room temperature.

In the dry state, the product has a shelf-life of 3 years when stored at room temperature and protected from light.

Guidelines for the safe handling of antineoplastic agents
(a) Trained personnel should reconstitute the drug.
(b) This should be performed in a designated area. The safety cabinet should be used when preparing solutions of aclarubicin.
(c) Adequate protective gloves, goggles and mask should be worn.
(d) Precautions should be taken to avoid the drug accidentally coming into contact with the eyes, skin or mucous membranes. In case of contamination of the eyes, skin or mucous membranes rinse thoroughly with water.
(e) The cytotoxic preparation should not be handled by pregnant staff.
(f) Adequate care and precautions should be taken in the disposal of items (syringes, needles, etc) used to reconstitute cytotoxic drugs. All items used for reconstitution, administration or cleaning should be placed in high-risk, waste-disposal bags and incinerated at a temperature of 1000°C.
(g) The work surface should be covered with disposable plastic backed absorbent paper.
(h) Use Luer-lock fittings on all syringes and sets. Large bore needles are recommended to minimise pressure and the possible formation of aerosols. The latter may also be reduced by the use of a venting needle.

Legal category POM.

Package quantities Boxes of 10 × 20 mg vials.

Further information Nil.

Product licence number 0458/0062.

BLEOMYCIN INJECTION

Presentation Bleomycin Lundbeck Injection is a whitish-yellow freeze-dried plug of bleomycin sulphate equivalent to 15 I.U. bleomycin in a clear glass ampoule.

Active ingredients: 15 I.U. bleomycin per ampoule, as the sulphate.

Uses *Pharmacology:* Bleomycin is a basic water-soluble glycopeptide with cytotoxic activity. The mechanism of action of bleomycin is believed to involve single-strand scission of DNA, leading to inhibition of cell division, of growth and of DNA synthesis in tumour cells.

Apart from its antibacterial and antitumour properties, bleomycin is relatively free from biological activity. When injected intravenously it may have a histamine-like effect on blood pressure and may cause a rise in body temperature. Blood concentrations of bleomycin in patients indicate that the drug is excreted more rapidly after intravenous than after intramuscular injection and that up to one third of the dose is excreted unchanged in the urine within 24 hours.

Indications:

1. Squamous cell carcinoma affecting the mouth, nasopharynx and paranasal sinuses, larynx, oesophagus, external genitalia, cervix or skin. Well-differentiated tumours usually respond better than anaplastic ones.
2. Hodgkin's disease and other malignant lymphomas, including mycosis fungoides.
3. Testicular teratoma.
4. Malignant effusions of serous cavities.
5. Secondary indications in which bleomycin has been shown to be of some value (alone or in combination with other drugs) include metastatic malignant melanoma, carcinoma of the thyroid, lung and bladder.

Dosage and administration *Adults:* Bleomycin is usually administered intramuscularly but may be given intravenously (bolus or drip), intra-arterially, intrapleurally or intraperitoneally as a solution in physiological saline. Local injection directly into the tumour may occasionally be indicated.

1. *Squamous cell carcinoma and testicular teratoma:* The following dosage schedules are recommended for adults:

Age in years	*Total dose (I.U.)*	*Dose per week (I.U.)*
80 and over	100	15
70–79	150–200	30
60–69	200–300	30–60
Under 60	500	30–60

These doses may need to be adjusted when bleomycin is used in combination therapy.

A total dose of 500 I.U. should not normally be exceeded, but young men with testicular tumours have frequently tolerated twice this amount.

Used alone normal dose frequency is 15 I.U. three times a week or 30 I.U. twice a week, either intramuscularly or intravenously until the total dose indicated in the above table is administered. Continuous intravenous infusion at a rate of 15 I.U./24 hours for up to 10 days, or 30 I.U./24 hours for up to five days may produce a therapeutic effect more rapidly. The development of stomatitis is the most useful guide to the determination of individual tolerance of maximum therapeutic dose.

2. *Malignant lymphomas:* Used alone the recommended dosage regimen is 15 I.U. once or twice a week, intramuscularly, to a total dose of 225 I.U. For patients 60 years and over, 75% of the dosage recommended in 1 above should be used. These doses may need to be adjusted when bleomycin is used in combination chemotherapy.

3. *Malignant effusions (particularly those associated with carcinoma of breast):* After drainage of the serous cavity affected 60 I.U. bleomycin dissolved in 100 ml physiological saline is introduced via the drainage needle or cannula, which is then withdrawn.

Bleomycin is commonly used in conjunction with radiotherapy, particularly in the treatment of cancer of the head and neck region. Such a combination may enhance mucosal reactions if full doses of both forms of treatment are used and bleomycin dosage may require reduction, e.g. to 5 I.U. at the time of each radiotherapy fraction five days a week. Bleomycin is frequently used as one of the drugs in multiple chemotherapy regimens (e.g. in squamous cell carcinoma, testicular teratoma, lymphoma). The mucosal toxicity of bleomycin should be borne in mind in the selection and dosage of drugs with similar toxic potential used in such combinations.

Children: Until further data are available, administration of bleomycin to children should take place only under exceptional circumstances and in special centres. The dosage should be based on that recommended for adults and adjusted to body surface area or body weight.

Reduced kidney function: With serum creatinine values of 2–4 mg%, half the above individual dosage is recommended. With serum creatinine above 4 mg%, a further reduction in dose is indicated.

Preparation of solutions: For intramuscular injections the required dose is dissolved in up to 5 ml of a suitable solvent such as physiological saline. If pain occurs at the site of injection a 1% solution of lignocaine may be used as a solvent.

For intravenous injections the dose required is dissolved in 5–200 ml of physiological saline and injected slowly or added to the reservoir of a running intravenous infusion. For intra-arterial administration a slow infusion in physiological saline is used. For intra-cavitary injection 60 I.U. is dissolved in 100 ml normal saline.

For local injections bleomycin is dissolved in physiological saline to make a 1–3 I.U./ml solution.

Contra-indications, warnings, etc This product should not normally be administered to patients who are pregnant or to mothers who are breast feeding. It is also contra-indicated in patients with acute pulmonary infection or greatly reduced lung function.

Adverse reactions: Like most cytotoxic agents bleomycin can give rise both to immediate and to delayed toxic effects. The most immediate effect is fever on the day of injection. Anorexia, tiredness or nausea also may occur. Local pain may occur after intravenous or intracavitary injection, and other rare adverse effects are hypotension and local thrombophlebitis after intravenous administration. Acute anaphylactoid reactions with hyperpyrexia and cardiorespiratory collapse have been reported after intravenous injections of doses higher than those recommended. The incidence of such reactions is minimised if the dosing schedule recommended above is adhered to. Hypotension, hyperpyrexia and drug related deaths have been reported rarely following intracavitary injection.

The most serious delayed effect is interstitial pneumonia, which may develop during, or occasionally after, a course of treatment. This condition may sometimes develop into fatal pulmonary fibrosis, although such an occurrence is rare on recommended doses. Previous or concurrent radiotherapy to the chest is an important factor in increasing the incidence and severity of lung toxicity. It has been suggested that those patients who have received bleomycin preoperatively are at a greater risk of developing pulmonary toxicity, and a reduction in inspired oxygen concentration during the operation and post-operatively is recommended.

The majority of patients who receive a full course of bleomycin develop lesions of the skin or oral mucosa. Induration, hyperkeratosis, reddening, tenderness, and swelling of the tips of the fingers, ridging of the nails, bulla formation over pressure points such as elbows, loss of hair and stomatitis are rarely serious and usually disappear soon after completion of the course.

Precautions: Patients undergoing treatment with bleomycin should have chest X-rays weekly. These should continue to be taken for up to four weeks after completion of the course. If breathlessness or infiltrates, not obviously attributable to tumour or to co-existent lung disease, appear, administration of the drug must be stopped immediately and patients should be treated with a corticosteroid (e.g. hydrocortisone 100 mg i.m. as the sodium succinate daily for five days, followed by oral prednisolone 10 mg twice daily) and a broad-spectrum antibiotic. No specific clinical incompatibilities with other drugs or food have been encountered.

Overdosage: No specific antidote. The acute reaction to an overdosage with bleomycin would probably include hypotension, fever, rapid pulse and general symptoms of shock. Treatment is purely symptomatic. In the event of respiratory complications, the patient should be treated with a corticosteroid and a broad-spectrum antibiotic.

Pharmaceutical precautions Freeze-dried bleomycin has a shelf life of three years from the date of manufacture when stored at room temperature. Bleomycin should be administered as a freshly prepared solution.

Because of possible skin changes, direct contact of bleomycin with the skin should be avoided.

Pharmaceutical incompatibilities: Bleomycin solutions should not be mixed with solutions of essential amino acids, riboflavine, ascorbic acid, dexamethasone, aminophylline or frusemide. Loss of bleomycin activity may occur when it is mixed with solutions of carbenicillin, cephazolin, cephalothin, nafcillin, benzylpenicillin, methotrexate, mitomycin, hydrocortisone, sodium succinate, aminophylline, ascorbic acid or terbutaline.

Legal category POM.

The supply of bleomycin is restricted to centres with special experience in the chemotherapy of malignant diseases and is available on prescription only.

Package quantities Boxes of 10 × 15 I.U. ampoules.

Further information Bleomycin has little or no toxic effect on the bone marrow, and has no immunosuppressive action.

Product licence number 0458/0009.

CCNU LUNDBECK CAPSULES

Presentation Blue/white gelatin capsules containing 10 mg lomustine, and blue gelatin capsules containing 40 mg lomustine.

Active ingredient: 10 mg and 40 mg lomustine (CCNU; 1-(2-chloroethyl)-3-cyclohexyl-1-nitrosourea).

Uses The mechanism of action is believed to be partly as an alkylating agent and partly by inhibition of several other vital enzymatic processes. Cross-resistance with other nitrosoureas is usual but cross-resistance with conventional alkylating agents is unusual.

Indications: As palliative or supplementary treatment, usually in combination with radiotherapy and/or surgery or as part of multiple drug regimens in:

brain tumours (primary or metastatic);
lung tumours (especially oat-cell carcinoma);
Hodgkin's disease (resistant to conventional combination chemotherapy);
malignant melanoma (metastatic).

CCNU may also be of value as second-line treatment in non-Hodgkin's lymphoma, myelomatosis, gastrointestinal tumours, carcinoma of the kidney, the testis, the ovary, the cervix uteri and the breast.

Dosage and administration *Adults:* CCNU is given

by mouth. The recommended dose in patients with normally functioning bone marrow receiving CCNU as their only chemotherapy is 120–130 mg/m^2 as a single dose every six to eight weeks (or as a divided dose over three days, e.g. 40 mg/m^2/day).

Dosage is reduced if:

(a) CCNU is being given as part of a drug regimen which includes other marrow-depressant drugs, and
(b) in the presence of leucopenia below 3,000/mm^3 or thrombocytopenia below 75,000/mm^3.

Marrow depression after CCNU is longer sustained than after nitrogen mustards and recovery of white cell and platelet counts may not occur for six weeks or more. Blood elements depressed below the above levels should be allowed to recover to 4,000/mm^3 (WBC) and 100,000/mm^3 (platelets) before repeating CCNU dosage.

Administration to children: Until further data are available administration of CCNU to children with malignancies other than brain tumours should be restricted to specialised centres and exceptional situations. Dosage in children, like that in adults, is based on body surface area (120–130 mg/m^2 every six to eight weeks, with the same qualifications as apply to adults).

Contra-indications, warnings, etc This product should not normally be administered to patients who are pregnant or to mothers who are breast feeding. Other contra-indications are: 1. Previous hypersensitivity to nitrosoureas; 2. Previous failure of the tumour to respond to other nitrosoureas; 3. Severe bone marrow depression.

Precautions: Patients receiving CCNU chemotherapy should be under the care of doctors experienced in cancer treatment. Blood counts should be carried out before starting the drug and at frequent intervals (preferably weekly) during treatment. Treatment and dosage is governed principally by the haemoglobin, white cell count and platelet count. Liver function should also be assessed periodically.

Adverse effects: Haematological: The principal adverse effect is marrow toxicity of a delayed or prolonged nature. Thrombocytopenia appears about four weeks after a dose of CCNU and lasts one to two weeks at a level around 80–100,000/mm^3; leucopenia appears after six weeks and persists for one to two weeks at about 4–5,000/mm^3. The haematological toxicity may be cumulative, leading to successively lower white cell and platelet counts with successive doses of the drug.

Gastrointestinal: Nausea and vomiting usually occur four to six hours after a full single dose of CCNU and last for 24–48 hours, followed by anorexia for two to three days. The effects are less troublesome if the six-weekly dose is divided into three doses and given on each of the first three days of the six-week period. Gastrointestinal tolerance is usually good, however, if prophylactic antinauseants are given (e.g. metoclopramide or chlorpromazine). Transient elevation of liver enzymes (SGOT, SGPT, LDH or alkaline phosphatase) are occasionally observed. More rarely patients are troubled by stomatitis.

Other side-effects: Loss of scalp hair has been reported infrequently.

Overdosage: There is no specific antidote. In the event of dangerously low red cell, white cell or platelet counts, cross-matched whole blood should be given as necessary.

Pharmaceutical precautions The capsules should be stored in the original container and protected from light and moisture. The preparation has a shelf life of two years from the date of manufacture, when stored at room temperature.

Legal category POM.

The supply of CCNU capsules is restricted to centres with special experience in the chemotherapy of malignant disease. CCNU capsules are available on prescription only.

Package quantities Bottles of 20 capsules each containing 10 mg or 40 mg lomustine.

Further information Nil.

Product licence number 0458/0018.
0458/0024

CLOPIXOL *ACUPHASE* INJECTION

Presentation Clopixol Acuphase Injection is a sterile, yellowish, clear solution of 5% zuclopenthixol acetate in thin vegetable oil (Viscoleo®). It is presented in clear glass ampoules of 1 ml and 2 ml capacity (1 ml = 50 mg).

Uses

Pharmacology: Zuclopenthixol is a neuroleptic of the thioxanthene series. The antipsychotic effect of neuroleptics is believed to be related to their dopamine receptor blocking effect. Thioxanthenes have a high affinity for D1 and D2 receptors.

Indications: Initial treatment for acute psychoses, including mania and exacerbation of chronic psychoses, particularly where a rapid onset of action, and a duration of effect of two to three days is desirable.

Dosage and administration

Note: As with all oil based injections it is important to ensure, by aspiration before injection, that inadvertent intravascular entry does not occur.

Adults: Dosage should be adjusted according to the severity of the patient's illness. Clopixol Acuphase is administered by deep intramuscular injection, into the upper outer buttock or lateral thigh.

The usual dosage is 50–150 mg (1–3 ml), repeated if necessary after 2 or 3 days. Some patients may need an additional injection between 1 and 2 days after the *first* injection.

Clopixol Acuphase is not intended for long-term use and duration of treatment should not be more than two weeks. The maximum accumulated dosage in a course should not exceed 400 mg and the number of injections should not exceed four.

Patients with compromised hepatic function should receive half the recommended dosages for normal patients. Where there is reduced renal function, it is not necessary to reduce the dosage but where there is renal failure dosage should be reduced to half the normal dosage.

Maintenance treatment where required can be continued with Clopixol tablets or Clopixol injection, according to the following guidelines:

(1) Introduce Clopixol tablets at a dosage of 20–60 mg/day in divided doses, 2 to 3 days after the last injection of Clopixol Acuphase. If necessary increase the tablet dosage by 10–20 mg each day up to a maximum of 150 mg/day.

or

(2) Concomitantly with the last injection of Clopixol Acuphase, administer 200–400 mg (1–2 ml) of Clopixol injection by deep intramuscular injection and repeat the Clopixol injection at intervals of 2 to 4 weeks. Higher dosages or a shorter interval may be necessary.

Elderly: The dosage may need to be reduced in the elderly owing to reduced rates of metabolism and elimination. Maximum dosage per injection should be 100 mg.

Children: Not recommended for children.

Contra-indications, warnings, etc

Contra-indications: Comatose states, including acute alcohol, barbiturate, and opiate intoxication.

Use in pregnancy, lactation and puerperium: Animal tests have not revealed any evidence that zuclopenthixol causes an increased incidence of foetal damage. Nevertheless, zuclopenthixol acetate should not be administered during pregnancy or to women of childbearing potential, unless they are taking adequate contraceptive precautions or unless the expected benefit to the patient outweighs the potential risk to the foetus.

Zuclopenthixol is found in very low concentrations in the breast milk of mothers receiving Clopixol treatment.

It is recommended that mothers treated with Clopixol Acuphase should not breast feed.

Precautions: Caution should be exercised in patients having convulsive disorders, or advanced hepatic, renal or cardiovascular disease.

Interaction with other medication: Zuclopenthixol enhances the response to alcohol and the effects of barbiturates and other CNS depressants. Potentiation of the effects of general anaesthetics may occur. Zuclopenthixol acetate should not be given concomitantly with guanethidine or similarly acting compounds, since neuroleptics may block the antihypertensive effect of these compounds. Tricyclic antidepressants and neuroleptics mutually inhibit the metabolism of each other. Zuclopenthixol may reduce the effect of levodopa and the effect of adrenergic drugs. Concomitant use of metoclopramide and piperazine increases the risk of extrapyramidal symptoms.

The possibility of interaction with lithium salts should be borne in mind.

Warnings and adverse effects: Zuclopenthixol is not suitable for patients who do not tolerate oral neuroleptic drugs or for patients suffering from Parkinson's disease.

Drowsiness, sedation, dry mouth and nasal stuffiness may occur, particularly with high dosage and at the start of treatment. Postural hypotension may occur, particularly in the elderly. Other anticholinergic type side-effects that should be borne in mind include blurring of vision, tachycardia, constipation and urinary hesitancy or retention.

Extrapyramidal reactions in the form of acute dystonias (including oculogyric crisis), Parkinsonian rigidity, tremor, akinesia and akathisia may occur in susceptible patients. Antiparkinson agents should not be prescribed routinely because of the possible risk of causing anticholinergic side-effects, precipitating toxic-confusional states or impairing therapeutic efficacy. They should only be given if required and their requirement reassessed at regular intervals.

Confusional states or epileptic fits can occur. The hormonal effects of antipsychotic neuroleptic drugs include hyperprolactinaemia, which may be associated with galactorrhoea, gynaecomastia, oligomenorrhoea or amenorrhoea.

Neuroleptics have been reported to affect cardiac conduction, but no specific reports have been received relating to patients receiving zuclopenthixol.

Body temperature regulation, especially in the elderly, may be compromised. Hypothermia has been reported rarely.

Jaundice and other liver abnormalities have been reported rarely.

The ability to drive a car or operate machinery may be affected and patients should be warned of this risk.

Overdosage: Overdosage may cause somnolence, or even coma, extrapyramidal symptoms, convulsions, hypotension, shock, hyper- or hypothermia. Treatment is symptomatic and supportive. Measures to support the respiratory and cardiovascular systems should be instituted. Adrenaline should not be given. There is no specific antidote.

Pharmaceutical precautions Clopixol Acuphase should be stored at room temperature and protected from light. Under these conditions, the product has a shelf-life of 2 years.

Clopixol Acuphase should not be mixed in the same syringe with other injection fluids.

Legal category POM. Clopixol Acuphase is available on prescription only.

Package quantities Boxes of 5 × 50 mg (1 ml). Boxes of 5 × 100 mg (2 ml).

Further information Zuclopenthixol is a potent neuroleptic of the thioxanthene series with a piperazine side-chain. Clopixol Acuphase injection contains the acetic ester of zuclopenthixol in a vegetable oil (Viscoleo®). The acetic ester is slowly released from the oil depot and is rapidly hydrolysed to release zuclopenthixol. A single injection of Clopixol Acuphase has an onset of sedative action shortly after injection and an antipsychotic action persisting for 2 to 3 days. In this period, maintenance treatment with tablets or a longer acting depot neuroleptic can be initiated.

Product licence number 0458/0063.

CLOPIXOL* INJECTION
CLOPIXOL*-CONC. INJECTION

Presentation Clopixol Injection is a 20% (200 mg/ml) sterile, straw-coloured solution of zuclopenthixol decanoate in thin vegetable oil. It is presented in clear glass ampoules (1 ml) and vials (10 ml).

Clopixol-Conc. Injection is a sterile, straw-coloured solution of 50% (500 mg/ml) zuclopenthixol decanoate in thin vegetable oil. It is presented in clear glass ampoules (1 ml).

Uses

Pharmacology: Zuclopenthixol is a neuroleptic of the thioxanthene series. The antipsychotic effect of neuroleptics is believed to be related to their dopamine receptor blocking effect. Thioxanthenes have a high affinity for D1 and D2 receptors. Zuclopenthixol possesses a marked specific calming effect and a non-specific sedative action.

Indications: Clopixol Injection and Clopixol-Conc. Injection are depot neuroleptic preparations for maintenance treatment of schizophrenia and paranoid psychoses, especially where compliance with oral medication is a problem. They are especially suitable for patients who are agitated or aggressive.

Dosage and administration

Adults: Clopixol Injection and Clopixol-Conc. Injection are administered by deep intramuscular injection into the upper, outer buttock or lateral thigh. The usual dosage range for Clopixol Injection is 200–400 mg (1–2 ml) every two to four weeks, and for Clopixol-Conc. Injection 250–500 mg ($\frac{1}{2}$ ml–1 ml) every 1–4 weeks, depending on response. A few patients may need higher doses or shorter intervals between doses. The maximum recommended dose of either strength is 600 mg a week. Injection volumes greater than 2 ml should be distributed between two injection sites. Treatment is usually started with 100 mg. One week later, or when symptoms recur (but not more than four weeks later) a second injection of 100–200 mg or more is given.

Elderly: In accordance with standard medical practice the dose may need to be reduced in the frail and elderly. The use of Clopixol Injection (20%) will usually be most appropriate.

Children: Clopixol Injection and Clopixol Conc. Injection should not be administered to children.

Contra-indications, warnings, etc

Contra-indications: Comatose states.

Use in pregnancy, lactation and puerperium: Animal tests have not revealed any evidence that zuclopenthixol causes an increased incidence of foetal damage. Nevertheless, zuclopenthixol decanoate should not be administered during pregnancy or to women of childbearing potential, unless they are taking adequate contraceptive precautions or unless the expected benefit to the patient outweighs the potential risk to the foetus.

Zuclopenthixol is found in low concentrations in the breast milk of mothers receiving Clopixol treatment. Mothers treated with Clopixol should not breast feed.

Precautions: Clopixol Injection and Clopixol-Conc. Injection are unsuitable for patients whose psychoses are accompanied by features of apathy or withdrawal.

Caution should be exercised in patients having: liver disease; cardiac disease or arrhythmias; severe respiratory disease; renal failure; epilepsy (and conditions predisposing to epilepsy, eg alcohol withdrawal or brain damage); Parkinson's disease; patients who have shown hypersensitivity to other neuroleptics. The general caution for the use of neuroleptics in hypothyroidism, thyrotoxicosis, myasthenia gravis, phaeochromocytoma or prostatic hypertrophy should be observed, but there is no evidence to suggest that Clopixol gives rise to any particular problem in such conditions. Care should also be taken in the elderly, particularly if frail or at risk of hypothermia, and in patients with personal or family history of narrow angle glaucoma.

Drug interactions: Zuclopenthixol enhances the response to alcohol and the effects of barbiturates and other CNS depressants. Potentiation of the effects of general anaesthetics may occur. Zuclopenthixol should not be given concomitantly with guanethidine or similarly acting compounds, since neuroleptics may block the antihypertensive effect of these compounds. Tricyclic antidepressants and neuroleptics inhibit the metabolism of each other. Zuclopenthixol may reduce the effect of levodopa, adrenergic drugs and anticonvulsants. Concomitant use of metoclopramide and piperazine increases the risk of extrapyramidal symptoms.

The possibility of interaction with lithium salts should be borne in mind.

Warnings: Zuclopenthixol decanoate is unsuitable for patients who do not tolerate oral neuroleptic drugs or for patients suffering from Parkinson's disease.

The ability to drive a car or operate machinery may be affected and patients should be warned of this risk.

Adverse effects: Drowsiness, sedation, dry mouth and nasal stuffiness may occur, particularly with high dosage and at the start of treatment. Postural hypotension may occur, particularly in the elderly. Other anticholinergic type side-effects that should be borne in mind include blurring of vision, tachycardia, constipation and urinary hesitancy or retention.

Extrapyramidal reactions in the form of acute dystonias (including oculogyric crisis), parkinsonian rigidity, tremor, akinesia and akathisia may occur in susceptible patients. Antiparkinson agents should not be prescribed routinely because of the possible risk of causing anticholinergic side-effects, precipitating toxic-confusional states or impairing therapeutic efficacy. They should only be given if required and their requirement reassessed at regular intervals.

Sexual function including erection and ejaculation may rarely be impaired. Weight gain and less commonly weight loss has been reported. Oedema has occasionally been reported and is considered to be allergic in origin. Blood dyscrasias have occasionally been reported.

Confusional states or epileptic fits can occur. The hormonal effects of antipsychotic neuroleptic drugs include hyperprolactinaemia, which may be associated with galactorrhoea, gynaecomastia, oligomenorrhoea or amenorrhoea.

Neuroleptics have been reported to affect cardiac conduction, but no specific reports have been received relating to patients receiving zuclopenthixol.

Body temperature regulation, especially in the elderly, may be compromised. Hypothermia has been reported rarely.

Jaundice and other liver abnormalities have been reported rarely.

Tardive dyskinesia is more common with phenothiazines at high doses for prolonged periods and has been reported at lower dosage for short periods. It has been observed occasionally in patients receiving Clopixol. The concurrent use of anticholinergic antiparkinson drugs may exacerbate this effect. The potential irreversibility and seriousness, as well as the unpredictability of the syndrome, requires especially careful assessment of the risk versus the benefit, and the lowest possible dosage and duration of treatment consistent with therapeutic efficacy. Short-lived dyskinesia may occur after abrupt withdrawal of the drug.

The neuroleptic malignant syndrome has been reported rarely in patients receiving neuroleptics. The syndrome is characterised by hyperthermia, a fluctuating level of consciousness, muscular rigidity and autonomic dysfunction with pallor, tachycardia, labile blood pressure, sweating and urinary incontinence. Neuroleptic therapy should be discontinued immediately and vigorous symptomatic treatment implemented. The administration of bromocriptine and dantrolene has been reported to aid recovery.

Overdosage: Overdosage may cause somnolence, or even coma, extrapyramidal symptoms, convulsions, hypotension, shock, hyper or hypothermia. Treatment is symptomatic and supportive. Measures to support the respiratory and cardiovascular systems should be instituted. Adrenaline should not be given. There is no specific antidote.

Pharmaceutical precautions Store at room temperature and protect from light. Under these conditions the preparations have a shelf life of 2 years from the date of manufacture.

Legal category POM.

Clopixol Injection and Clopixol-Conc. Injection are available through hospitals, clinics and on prescription only through registered pharmacies for patients whose treatment has been initiated by a psychiatrist.

Package quantities
Clopixol injection
Boxes of 10 × 200 mg (1 ml ampoules).
Boxes of 1 × 2000 mg (10 ml vials).
Clopixol-Conc. Injection
Boxes of 5 × 500 mg (1 ml ampoules).

Further information Zuclopenthixol is a potent neuroleptic of the thioxanthene series with a piperazine side-chain. Clopixol Injection and Clopixol Conc. Injection contain the decanoic ester of zuclopenthixol in a vegetable oil (Viscoleo*). The decanoic ester is slowly released from the oil depot and is rapidly hydrolysed to release zuclopenthixol. Whereas zuclopenthixol itself is relatively short acting, the decanoic ester in oil provides a predictable slow release depot preparation of the active constituent.

Product licence numbers
Clopixol Injection: 0458/0017
Clopixol-Conc. Injection: 0458/0060

CLOPIXOL* TABLETS

Presentation Clopixol tablets contain zuclopenthixol 2 mg, 10 mg and 25 mg as the dihydrochloride. The tablets are round, biconvex and film coated. The 2 mg tablets are pink with a diameter of 5 mm, the 10 mg tablets are light brown with a diameter of 6 mm and the 25 mg tablets are brown with a diameter of 7 mm.

Uses
Pharmacology: Zuclopenthixol is a neuroleptic of the thioxanthene series. The antipsychotic effect of neuroleptics is believed to be related to their dopamine receptor blocking effect. Thioxanthenes have a high affinity for D1 and D2 receptors. Zuclopenthixol possesses a marked specific calming effect and a non-specific sedative action.

Indications: Clopixol Tablets are indicated in the treatment of schizophrenia and other psychoses, particularly in patients who are agitated or aggressive.

Dosage and administration
Adults: The usual initial dose is 20–30 mg/day, increasing as necessary to a maximum of 150 mg/day, in divided doses. The usual maintenance dose in chronic schizophrenia is 20–50 mg/day in divided doses. Lower doses may be appropriate depending on individual patient response.

Elderly: The dosage may need to be reduced in the elderly owing to reduced rates of metabolism and elimination.

Children: Not recommended.

Contra-indications, warnings, etc
Contra-indications: Comatose states.

Use in pregnancy, lactation and puerperium: Animal tests have not revealed any evidence that zuclopenthixol causes an increased incidence of foetal damage. Nevertheless, zuclopenthixol should not be administered during pregnancy or to women of childbearing potential, unless they are taking adequate contraceptive precautions or unless the expected benefit to the patient outweighs the potential risk to the foetus.

Zuclopenthixol is found in very low concentrations in the breast milk of mothers receiving Clopixol treatment. Mothers treated with Clopixol should not breast feed.

Precautions: Clopixol tablets are unsuitable for patients whose psychoses are accompanied by features of apathy or withdrawal.

Caution should be exercised in patients having: liver disease; cardiac disease or arrhythmias; severe respiratory disease; renal failure; epilepsy (and conditions predisposing to epilepsy, e.g. alcohol withdrawal or brain damage); Parkinson's disease; patients who have shown hypersensitivity to other neuroleptics. The general caution for the use of neuroleptics in hypothyroidism, thyrotoxicosis, myasthenia gravis, phaeochromocytoma or prostatic hypertrophy should be observed, but there is no evidence to suggest that Clopixol gives rise to any particular problem in such conditions. Care should also be taken in the elderly, particularly if frail or at risk of hypothermia, and in patients with personal or family history of narrow angle glaucoma.

Drug interactions: Zuclopenthixol enhances the response to alcohol and the effects of barbiturates and other CNS depressants. Potentiation of the effects of general anaesthetics may occur. Zuclopenthixol should not be given concomitantly with guanethidine or similarly acting compounds, since neuroleptics may block the antihypertensive effect of these compounds. Tricyclic antidepressants and neuroleptics inhibit the metabolism of each other. Zuclopenthixol may reduce the effect of levodopa, adrenergic drugs and anticonvulsants. Concomitant use of metoclopramide and piperazine increases the risk of extrapyramidal symptoms.

The possibility of interaction with lithium salts should be borne in mind.

Warnings: The ability to drive a car or operate machinery may be affected and patients should be warned of this risk.

Adverse effects: Drowsiness, sedation, dry mouth and nasal stuffiness may occur, particularly with high dosage and at the start of treatment. Postural hypotension may occur, particularly in the elderly. Other anticholinergic type side-effects that should be borne in mind include blurring of vision, tachycardia, constipation and urinary hesitancy or retention.

Extrapyramidal reactions in the form of acute dystonias (including oculogyric crisis), parkinsonian rigidity, tremor, akinesia and akathisia may occur in susceptible patients. Antiparkinson agents should not be prescribed routinely because of the possible risk of causing anticholinergic side-effects, precipitating toxic-confusional states or impairing therapeutic efficacy. They should only be given if required and their requirement reassessed at regular intervals.

Sexual function including erection and ejaculation may rarely be impaired. Weight gain and less commonly weight loss has been reported. Oedema has occasionally been reported and is considered to be allergic in origin. Blood dycrasias have occasionally been reported.

Confusional states or epileptic fits can occur. The hormonal effects of antipsychotic neuroleptic drugs include hyperprolactinaemia, which may be associated with galactorrhoea, gynaecomastia, oligomenorrhoea or amenorrhoea.

Neuroleptics have been reported to affect cardiac conduction, but no specific reports have been received relating to patients receiving zuclopenthixol.

Body temperature regulation, especially in the elderly, may be compromised. Hypothermia has been reported rarely.

Jaundice and other liver abnormalities have been reported rarely.

Tardive dyskinesia is more common with phenothiazines at high dosages for prolonged periods and has been reported at lower dosage for short periods. It has been observed occasionally in patients receiving Clopixol. The concurrent use of anticholinergic antiparkinson drugs may exacerbate this effect. The potential irreversibility and seriousness, as well as the unpredictability of the syndrome, requires especially careful assessment of the risk versus benefit, and the lowest possible dosage and duration of treatment consistent with therapeutic efficacy. Short-lived dyskinesia may occur after abrupt withdrawal of the drug.

The neuroleptic malignant syndrome has been reported rarely in patients receiving neuroleptics. The syndrome is characterised by hyperthermia, a fluctuating level of consciousness, muscular rigidity and autonomic dysfunction with pallor, tachycardia, labile blood pressure, sweating and urinary incontinence. Neuroleptic therapy should be discontinued immediately and vigorous symptomatic treatment implemented. The administration of bromocriptine and dantrolene has been reported to aid recovery.

Overdosage: Overdosage may cause somnolence, or even coma, extrapyramidal symptoms, convulsions, hypotension, shock, hyper or hypothermia. Measures to support the respiratory and cardiovascular systems should be instituted. Adrenaline should not be given. There is no specific antidote.

Pharmaceutical precautions The tablets should be stored at room temperature in their original containers, protected from light and moisture. Under these conditions the preparation has a shelf life of three years from the date of manufacture.

Legal category POM.

Package quantities Clopixol tablets 2 mg, 10 mg and 25 mg are packed in bottles containing 100 tablets.

Further information Nil.

Product licence numbers

2 mg	0458/0027
10 mg	0458/0028
25 mg	0458/0029

DEPIXOL* INJECTION
DEPIXOL*-CONC INJECTION

Presentation Depixol Injection is a 2% sterile, straw-coloured solution of cis(Z)-flupenthixol decanoate in thin vegetable oil. It is presented as 20 mg (1 ml) and 40 mg (2 ml) doses in clear glass ampoules, syringes (1 ml and 2 ml) and a vial (10 ml).

Depixol-Conc. Injection is a 10% sterile, straw-coloured solution of cis(Z)-flupenthixol decanoate in thin vegetable oil. It is presented as 50 mg (0.5 ml) and 100 mg (1 ml) doses in glass ampoules and a 500 mg (5 ml) vial.

Uses

Pharmacology: Cis-(Z)-flupenthixol is a neuroleptic of the thioxanthene series. The antipsychotic effect of neuroleptics is believed to be related to their dopamine receptor blocking effect. Thioxanthenes have a high affinity for D1 and D2 receptors.

Indications: Depixol Injection and Depixol-Conc. Injection are depot neuroleptic preparations, indicated in the treatment of schizophrenia and paranoid psychoses, especially where compliance with oral medication is a problem. Depixol is unsuitable for patients in whom sedation is required.

Dosage and administration Note: As with all oily injections it is important to ensure, by aspiration before injection, that inadvertent intravascular entry does not occur.

Adults: Depixol Injection is administered by deep intramuscular injection into the upper, outer buttock or lateral thigh in doses of 20 to 40 mg (1 to 2 ml) at intervals of 2 to 4 weeks depending on the response. Those not previously treated with long-acting antipsychotic injections should continue with oral neuroleptic drugs but in diminishing dosage.

Some patients may need larger doses or need them at

shorter intervals. Injection volumes exceeding 2 ml should be distributed between two injection sites. The dosage range of Depixol-Conc. lies between 50 mg every 4 weeks and 300 mg every two weeks but some patients may require up to 400 mg weekly. Adequate control of severe psychotic symptoms by Depixol-Conc. Injection is usually achieved within 4 to 6 months and this may justify a return to lower dose maintenance treatment with standard Depixol 2% Injection.

Elderly: In accordance with standard medical practice initial dosage may need to be reduced to a quarter or half the normal starting dose in the frail and elderly.

Children: Depixol Injection and Depixol-Conc. Injection are not indicated for children.

Contra-indications, warnings, etc
Contra-indications: Comatose states. Depixol Injection and Depixol-Conc. Injection are not recommended for excitable or agitated patients.

Use in pregnancy, lactation and puerperium: There is insufficient evidence of safety in human pregnancy, nor is there evidence from animal studies that it is free from hazard. Do not use Depixol during pregnancy, especially the first and last trimesters.

The newborn of mothers treated with *phenothiazines* in late pregnancy, or labour, may show signs of intoxication such as lethargy, tremor and hyperexcitability, and have a low apgar score.

Flupenthixol is excreted into breast milk. If the use of Depixol is considered essential, nursing mothers should be advised to stop breast-feeding.

Precautions: Caution should be exercised in patients having: liver disease; cardiac disease, or arrhythmias; severe respiratory disease; renal failure; epilepsy (and conditions predisposing to epilepsy, e.g. alcohol withdrawal or brain damage); Parkinson's disease; patients who have shown hypersensitivity to other neuroleptics; myasthenia gravis; phaeochromocytoma.

The elderly require close supervision because they are specially prone to experience such adverse effects as sedation, hypotension, confusion and temperature changes (see also under 'Warnings').

Care should be taken when Depixol is used in patients with narrow angle glaucoma, prostatic hypertrophy and hypothyroidism.

Drug interactions: The anticholinergic effects of atropine and tricyclic antidepressants may be increased, and undesirable anticholinergic effects can be enhanced by antiparkinson drugs, and tardive dyskinesia precipitated.

Depixol *weakly* antagonises the action of adrenaline and other sympathomimetic agents, and may reverse the blood pressure lowering effects of adrenergic blocking agents, such as guanethidine, possibly also clonidine.

It may possibly affect the control of diabetes or the action of anticoagulants.

Phenothiazines may enhance the cardiac depressant effect of quinidine, the absorption of corticosteroids and digoxin, the effect of diazoxide and of neuromuscular blocking agents.

Warnings and adverse effects: Drowsiness and sedation are unusual. Sedation, if it occurs, is more often seen with high dosage and at the start of treatment, particularly in the elderly. Other adverse effects include blurring of vision, tachycardia and urinary incontinence and frequency. Dose-related postural hypotension may occur, particularly in the elderly.

Because Depixol may impair alertness, especially at the start of treatment or following the consumption of alcohol, patients should be warned of this risk and advised not to drive or operate machinery, until their susceptibility is known.

Extrapyramidal reactions in the form of acute dystonias (including oculogyric crisis), parkinsonian rigidity, tremor, akinesia and akathisia have been reported and may occur even at lower dosage in susceptible patients. Such effects would usually be encountered early in treatment, but delayed reactions may also occur. Antiparkinson agents should not be prescribed routinely because of the possible risk of precipitating toxic-confusional states, impairing therapeutic efficacy or causing anticholinergic side-effects. They should only be given if required and their requirement reassessed at regular intervals.

Tardive dyskinesia is more common with *phenothiazines* at high doses for prolonged periods and has been reported at lower dosage for short periods. The risk seems to be greater in the elderly, especially females. It has been reported that fine vermicular movements of the tongue are an early sign. It has been observed occasionally in patients receiving Depixol. The concurrent use of anticholinergic antiparkinson drugs may exacerbate this effect. The potential irreversibility and seriousness, as well as the unpredictability of the syndrome, requires especially careful assessment of the risk versus benefit, and the lowest possible dosage and duration of treatment consistent with therapeutic efficacy. Short-lived dyskinesia may occur after abrupt withdrawal of the drug.

In schizophrenia, the response to antipsychotic treatment may be delayed. If drugs are withdrawn, recurrence of symptoms may not become apparent for several weeks or months.

Flupenthixol, even in low doses, in susceptible (especially non-psychotic) individuals may unusually, cause nausea, dizziness or headache, excitement, agitation, insomnia or unpleasant subjective feelings of being mentally dulled or slowed down.

Epileptic fits have occasionally been reported. Confusional states can occur. The hormonal effects of antipsychotic drugs include hyperprolactinaemia, which may be associated with galactorrhoea, gynaecomastia, oligomenorrhoea or amenorrhoea. Sexual function, including erection and ejaculation may be impaired; but increased libido has also been reported. Weight gain and less commonly weight loss have been reported; oedema has occasionally been reported and has been considered to be allergic in origin. Rashes have occurred rarely. Although less likely than with *phenothiazines*, flupenthixol can rarely cause increased susceptibility to sunburn.

ECG changes with prolongation of the QT interval and T-wave changes may occur with moderate to high doses; they are reversible on reducing the dose.

Flupenthixol may impair body temperature control, and cases of hyperthermia have occurred rarely. The possible development of hypothermia, particularly in the elderly and hypothyroid, should be borne in mind.

The neuroleptic malignant syndrome has rarely been reported in patients receiving neuroleptics. The syndrome is characterised by hyperthermia, a fluctuating level of consciousness, muscular rigidity and autonomic dysfunction with pallor, tachycardia, labile blood pressure, sweating and urinary incontinence. Neuroleptic therapy should be discontinued immediately and vigorous symptomatic treatment implemented. The administration of bromocriptine and dantrolene has been reported to aid recovery.

Because acute withdrawal symptoms, including nausea, vomiting and insomnia have rarely been described after abrupt cessation of high doses of *phenothiazines*, gradual withdrawal of Depixol is advisable.

Blood dyscrasias have occasionally been reported. Blood counts should be carried out if a patient develops signs of persistent infection. Jaundice and other liver abnormalities have been reported rarely, but have never been confirmed to be Depixol-induced.

Overdosage: Overdosage should be treated:
(a) By anticholinergic antiparkinson drugs if extrapyramidal symptoms occur.
(b) By sedation (with benzodiazepines) in the unlikely event of agitation or excitement.
(c) By noradrenaline in saline intravenous drip if the patient is in shock.

Otherwise, observation and symptomatic management should be adequate.

Pharmaceutical precautions Store at room temperature and protect from light. Under these conditions the preparations have a shelf life of two years from date of manufacture.

Legal category POM.

For use in hospitals and hospital clinics and in registered pharmacies for dispensing prescriptions in respect of patients stabilised on Depixol. Depixol is available on prescription only.

Package quantities
Depixol Injection:
Boxes of 10 × 20 mg (1 ml) ampoules and 5 × 20 mg (1 ml) syringes
Boxes of 10 × 40 mg (2 ml) ampoules and 5 × 40 mg (2 ml) syringes
Boxes of 1 × 200 mg (10 ml) vial
Depixol-Conc. Injection:
Boxes of 10 × 50 mg (0.5 ml) ampoules
Boxes of 10 × 100 mg (1 ml) ampoules
Boxes of 1 × 500 mg (5 ml) vial

Further information Flupenthixol is a potent neuroleptic drug with antipsychotic and anxiolytic effects. It is particularly beneficial in patients who are withdrawn, apathetic, anergic or depressed in mood, or in whom neuroleptics with a marked sedative effect cause fatigue or drowsiness. Depixol Injection and Depixol-Conc. Injection, contain the decanoic ester of flupenthixol in a vegetable oil (Viscoleo*). The decanoic ester is slowly released from the oil depot and is rapidly hydrolysed to release flupenthixol. Whereas flupenthixol itself is relatively short acting, the decanoic ester in oil provides a predictable slow-release depot preparation. Pharmacokinetic studies have shown that a maximal blood concentration of flupenthixol is reached 4 to 7 days after injection. The characteristics of the serum concentration curve indicate that dosage intervals of 2 to 4 weeks are appropriate. Studies in patients have confirmed the pharmacokinetic similarity between Depixol Injection (2%) and Depixol-Conc. Injection (10%).

Product licence numbers

Depixol Injection	0458/0007
Depixol-Conc. Injection	0458/0015

DEPIXOL* TABLETS 3 mg

Presentation Depixol tablets 3 mg contain flupenthixol 3 mg as the dihydrochloride. The tablets are round, biconvex, yellow, sugar coated and have a diameter of about 9 mm. The Lundbeck logo is printed in black on one face.

Uses
Pharmacology: Flupenthixol is a neuroleptic of the thioxanthene series. The antipsychotic effect of neuroleptics is believed to be related to their dopamine receptor blocking effect. Thioxanthenes have a high affinity for D1 and D2 receptors.

Indications: Depixol tablets 3 mg are indicated in the treatment of schizophrenia and other psychoses.
Depixol is unsuitable for patients in whom sedation is desirable.

Dosage and administration
Adults: 1–3 tablets twice daily, to a maximum of 18 mg (6 tablets) per day. It is recommended that commencement of treatment and increase in dosage should be carried out under close supervision. As with all neuroleptic drugs, the dose of Depixol should be titrated to the needs of each patient.

Elderly: In accordance with standard medical practice initial dosage may need to be reduced to a quarter or half the normal starting dose in the frail and elderly.

Children: Depixol tablets are not indicated for children.

Contra-indications, warnings, etc
Contra-indications: Comatose states. Depixol tablets 3 mg are not recommended for excitable or agitated patients.

Use in pregnancy, lactation and puerperium: There is insufficient evidence of safety in human pregnancy, nor is there evidence from animal studies that it is free from hazard. Do not use Depixol during pregnancy, especially the first and last trimesters.

The newborn of mothers treated with *phenothiazines* in late pregnancy, or labour, may show signs of intoxication such as lethargy, tremor and hyperexcitability, and have a low apgar score.

Flupenthixol is excreted into the breast milk. If the use of Depixol is considered essential, nursing mothers should be advised to stop breast-feeding.

Precautions: Caution should be exercised in patients having: liver disease; cardiac disease or arrhythmias; severe respiratory disease; renal failure; epilepsy (and conditions predisposing to epilepsy, e.g. alcohol withdrawal or brain damage); Parkinson's disease; patients who have shown hypersensitivity to other neuroleptics; myasthenia gravis; phaeochromocytoma.

The elderly require close supervision because they are specially prone to experience such adverse effects as sedation, hypotensiion, confusion and temperature changes (see also under 'Warnings'). Care should be taken when Depixol is used in patients with narrow angle glaucoma, prostatic hypertrophy and hypothyroidism.

Drug interactions: The anticholinergic effects of atropine and tricyclic antidepressants may be increased, and undesirable anticholinergic effects can be enhanced by antiparkinson drugs, and tardive dyskinesia precipitated.

Depixol *weakly* antagonises the action of adrenaline and other sympathomimetic agents, and may reverse the blood pressure lowering effects of adrenergic blocking agents, such as guanethidine, possibly also clonidine.

It may possibly affect the control of diabetes or the action of anticoagulants.

Antacids can impair absorption of *phenothiazines* and tea and coffee may prevent absorption by causing insoluble precipitates.

Phenothiazines may enhance the cardiac depressant effect of quinidine, the absorption of corticosteroids and digoxin, the effect of diazoxide and of neuromuscular blocking agents.

Warnings and adverse effects: Drowsiness and sedation are unusual. Sedation, if it occurs, is more often seen with high dosage and at the start of treatment, particularly in the elderly. Other adverse effects include blurring of vision, tachycardia and urinary incontinence and frequency. Dose-related postural hypotension may occur, particularly in the elderly.

Because Depixol may impair alertness, especially at the start of treatment or following the consumption of alcohol, patients should be warned of this risk and advised not to drive or operate machinery, until their susceptibility is known.

Extrapyramidal reactions in the form of acute dystonias (including oculogyric crisis), parkinsonian rigidity, tremor, akinesia and akathisia have been reported and may occur even at low dosage in susceptible patients. Such effects would usually be encountered early in treatment, but delayed reactions may also occur. Antiparkinson agents should not be prescribed routinely because of the possible risk of precipitating toxic-confusional states, impairing therapeutic efficacy or causing anticholinergic side-effects. They should only be given if required and their requirement reassessed at regular intervals.

Tardive dyskinesia is more common with *phenothiazines* at high doses for prolonged periods and has been reported at lower dosage for short periods. The risk seems to be greater in the elderly, especially females. It has been reported that fine vermicular movements of the tongue are an early sign. It has been observed occasionally in patients receiving Depixol. The concurrent use of anticholinergic antiparkinson drugs may exacerbate this effect. The potential irreversibility and seriousness, as well as the unpredictability of the syndrome, requires especially careful assessment of risk versus benefit, and the lowest possible dosage and duration of treatment consistent with therapeutic efficacy. Short-lived dyskinesia may occur after abrupt withdrawal of the drug.

In schizophrenia, the response to antipsychotic treatment may be delayed. If drugs are withdrawn, recurrence of symptoms may not become apparent for several weeks or months.

Flupenthixol, even in low doses, in susceptible (especially non-psychotic) individuals may unusually cause nausea, dizziness or headache, excitement, agitation, insomnia or unpleasant subjective feelings of being mentally dulled or slowed down.

Epileptic fits have occasionally been reported. Confusional states can occur. The hormonal effects of antipsychotic neuroleptic drugs include hyperprolactinaemia, which may be associated with galactorrhoea, gynaecomastia, oligomenorrhoea or amenorrhoea. Sexual function, including erection and ejaculation may be impaired, but increased libido has also been reported. Weight gain and less commonly weight loss have been reported; oedema has occasionally been reported and has been considered to be allergic in origin. Rashes have occurred rarely. Although less likely than with *phenothiazines*, flupenthixol can rarely cause increased susceptibility to sunburn.

ECG changes with prolongation of the QT interval and T-wave changes may occur with moderate to high doses; they are reversible on reducing the dose.

Flupenthixol may impair body temperature control, and cases of hyperthermia have occurred rarely. The possible development of hypothermia, particularly in the elderly and hypothyroid, should be borne in mind.

The neuroleptic malignant syndrome has rarely been reported in patients receiving neuroleptics. The syndrome is characterised by hyperthermia, a fluctuating level of consciousness, muscular rigidity and autonomic dysfunction with pallor, tachycardia, labile blood pressure, sweating and urinary incontinence. Neuroleptic therapy should be discontinued immediately and vigorous symptomatic treatment implemented. The administration of bromocriptine and dantrolene has been reported to aid recovery.

Because acute withdrawal symptoms, including nausea, vomiting and insomnia have rarely been described after abrupt cessation of high doses of *phenothiazines*, gradual withdrawal of Depixol is advisable.

Blood dyscrasias have occasionally been reported. Blood counts should be carried out if a patient develops signs of persistent infection. Jaundice and other liver abnormalities have been reported rarely, but have never been confirmed to be Depixol-induced.

Overdosage: Overdosage should be treated by gastric lavage, and by parenteral antiparkinson drugs if severe extrapyramidal symptoms occur. Cardiac monitoring is advisable for at least 48 hours and longer if required.

Pharmaceutical precautions The tablets should be stored in their original container protected from light and moisture. Under these conditions the preparation has a shelf life of 5 years from the date of manufacture.

Legal category POM.

Package quantities Bottles of 100 tablets of 3 mg.

Further information Flupenthixol is a potent neuroleptic with antipsychotic and anxiolytic effects. It is particularly useful in patients who are withdrawn, apathetic, anergic or depressed, or in whom neuroleptics with a marked sedative effect cause fatigue or drowsiness.

Product licence number 0458/0013.

FLUANXOL* TABLETS

Presentation Fluanxol tablets contain flupenthixol as the dihydrochloride. The tablets are red, round, biconvex and sugar-coated, with 'Lundbeck' printed on one face. The 0.5 mg tablet has a diameter of 6 mm and 'Lundbeck' printed in black on one face. The 1 mg tablet has a diameter of 8 mm and 'Lundbeck' printed in white on one face.

Uses Fluanxol tablets are indicated in the short-term symptomatic treatment of depression of mild to moderate severity (with or without anxiety) or where treatment with other antidepressants has failed.

Dosage and administration *Adults:* Standard initial dosage is 1 mg as a single morning dose. After one week the dose may be increased to 2 mg if there is inadequate clinical response. Daily dosage of more than 2 mg should be in divided doses up to a maximum 3 mg. In view of the activating properties of Fluanxol it is advisable to give the last dose of the day no later than 4.00 p.m.

Patients often respond to Fluanxol within two or three days. If no effect has been observed within one week at maximum dosage the drug should be withdrawn.

Elderly: Standard initial dosage is 0.5 mg as a single morning dose. After one week, if response is inadequate, dosage may be increased to 1 mg once a day. Caution should be exercised in further increasing the dosage but occasional patients may require up to a maximum of 2 mg a day which should be given in divided doses (1 mg at breakfast time and 1 mg at about 4.00 pm).

Children: Not recommended for children.

Contra-indications, warnings, etc Fluanxol is not recommended for the treatment of severe depression requiring ECT and/or hospitalisation. It is not recommended in states of excitement or overactivity (including mania).

Precautions: Fluanxol should be used with caution in patients with Parkinson's disease, severe arteriosclerosis, senile confusional state or severe hepatic, renal or cardiovascular disease.

Warnings and adverse effects: precipitation of hypomania has been occasionally reported. Restlessness or insomnia are occasional side-effects. Others more rarely reported include, dizziness, tremor, visual disturbances, headache, migraine and hyperprolactinaemia. Extrapyramidal symptoms, such as akinesia, may occur rarely at the recommended dose and if they do occur treatment with Fluanxol should be withdrawn. Late onset movement disorders, including tardive dyskinesia, have occasionally been reported in patients receiving flupenthixol but no cases have been reported in patients treated with Fluanxol within the data sheet recommendations. Fluanxol may initially cause drowsiness. Patients should be warned of this possibility if driving or operating machinery. Alcohol may potentiate this effect.

Recurrence of depressive symptoms on abrupt withdrawal is rare. However gradual reduction of dosage is advisable. Dependence has not been reported.

Pregnancy: As there is no unequivocal evidence as to the safety of Fluanxol in human pregnancy, use during pregnancy, especially the first and last trimesters, should be avoided.

Treatment of overdose: Overdosage should be treated by gastric lavage and supportive therapy. The toxic hazard is less than with overdosage of tricyclic antidepressants.

Further information Clinical trials have shown that symptoms of apathy, lowered mood, asthenia, despondency, lack of initiative, or inertia are likely to respond well to Fluanxol. Its high therapeutic index is an advantage in view of the suicide risk associated with depressive illness.

No adverse interactions have been reported between Fluanxol and benzodiazepines or tricyclic antidepressants.

Flupenthixol is available in higher doses as Depixol tablets. These are indicated only in the treatment of functional psychotic disorders.

Pharmaceutical precautions The tablets should be stored in their original container, protected from light and moisture. Under these conditions the 0.5 mg tablet and 1.0 mg tablet have a shelf life of five and three years respectively.

Legal category POM.

Package quantities 0.5 mg tablets in bottles of 100 tablets.
1.0 mg tablets in packs of 60, as 6 × 10 blister strips.

Product licence numbers 0458/0011
0458/0037

NICORETTE*

Presentation Square pieces of chewing gum containing 2 mg or 4 mg nicotine.

Active ingredient: 2 mg or 4 mg nicotine as the resin in a chewing gum base.

Uses Nicotine replacement. When Nicorette is chewed, nicotine is slowly released into the mouth and is absorbed through the buccal mucosa. A proportion, by the swallowing of nicotine-containing saliva, reaches the stomach and intestine and any nicotine absorbed by this route is inactivated.

Indications: Nicorette is intended to help smokers who want to give up smoking, but experience great difficulty in doing so because of their nicotine dependence.

Dosage and administration *Adults:* The strength of gum to be used depends upon the smoking habits of the individual. It is recommended that patients beginning treatment should always start with Nicorette 2 mg to determine its acceptability. If more than 15 × 2 mg Nicorette per day are required, transfer to the 4 mg gum may be considered.

Nicorette should be chewed slowly, when there is an urge to smoke, up to a maximum of 15 × 4 mg pieces per day; however the patient's individual need may be considerably less than this number. Most patients require about 10 pieces of 2 mg per day initially.

All available nicotine is released from a piece of gum after about 30 minutes chewing. Since effective absorption is through the buccal mucosa, the rate of chewing should be adjusted to minimise the swallowing and inactivation of nicotine contained in saliva.

After 3 months ad libitum dosage Nicorette should be gradually withdrawn.

Children: Not to be administered to children.

Contra-indications, warnings, etc Nicotine in any form is contra-indicated in pregnancy. Smokers who wear dentures may experience difficulty in chewing Nicorette. Dependence is a rare side-effect and is both less harmful and easier to break than smoking dependence.

Precautions:

1. Swallowed nicotine may exacerbate symptoms in patients suffering from gastritis or peptic ulcer.
2. Nicotine's cardiovascular effects may be deleterious to patients with angina or a history of coronary artery disease. Nicorette presents a lesser hazard, however, than smoking which introduces carbon monoxide as an additional toxic factor.

Adverse effects: Nicorette in the recommended dose has not been found to cause any serious adverse effects. Nicotine from the gum may sometimes cause a slight irritation of the throat at the start of treatment, and may also cause increased salivation. Excessive swallowing of dissolved nicotine may, at first, cause hiccupping. Those with a tendency to indigestion may suffer initially from minor degrees of indigestion or heartburn if the 4 mg gum is used; slower chewing and the use of the 2 mg gum (if necessary more frequently) will usually overcome this problem.

Excessive consumption of Nicorette by patients who have not been in the habit of inhaling tobacco smoke could possibly lead to nausea, faintness or headaches (as may be experienced by such patients if tobacco smoke is inhaled).

Overdosage: Overdosage of Nicorette can occur only if many pieces are chewed simultaneously. The fatal acute dose of nicotine in man is probably about 60 mg. Risk of overdosage with Nicorette is, however, small since nausea or vomiting usually occurs at an early stage.

Risk of poisoning by swallowing the gum is also small, since the release of nicotine from the gum is slow. Therefore very little nicotine is absorbed from the stomach or intestine and any that is will be inactivated in the liver. Nicotine is excreted in acid urine four times as rapidly as in alkaline urine.

Treatment of overdosage: In the event of overdosage vomiting should be induced with syrup of ipecacuanha or gastric lavage carried out (wide bore tube). A suspension of activated charcoal should then be passed through the tube and left in the stomach. Artificial respiration with oxygen should be instituted if needed and continued for as long as necessary. Other therapy, including treatment of shock, is purely symptomatic.

Pharmaceutical precautions No special storage conditions are necessary. The preparation has a shelf life at room temperature of 30 months from the date of manufacture.

Legal category POM.

Package quantities Package of 105 pieces, in the form of 7 blister-packed strips each containing 15 pieces (2 mg or 4 mg).

Further information Nicorette should be chewed slowly. Sufficient nicotine may be released from the gum by chewing intermittently and leaving the gum under the lip or in the corner of the mouth between chews.

Nicorette is sugar-free.

Product licence numbers
2 mg: 0458/0020
4 mg: 0458/0021

NYCOPREN*

Presentation Nycopren (naproxen) is a non-steroidal anti-inflammatory agent. It is presented as:

(i) An oblong white enteric coated tablet containing 250 mg of naproxen.
(ii) An oblong white enteric coated tablet containing 500 mg of naproxen.

Uses
Indications: Nycopren is indicated for the treatment of rheumatoid arthritis, juvenile rheumatoid arthritis, osteoarthrosis (degenerative arthritis), ankylosing spondylitis, acute gout and acute inflammatory musculoskeletal disorders.

Pharmacology: Nycopren is covered with an acid resistant film coating and will pass through the stomach without disintegrating. It is broken down and absorbed in the intestinal tract. Direct, local damaging effects on the gastric mucosa may thus be prevented.

Naproxen is a non-steroidal anti-inflammatory agent with analgesic and antipyretic properties. It inhibits prostaglandin synthetase, as do other non-steroidal anti-inflammatory agents. As with other agents however, the exact mechanism of its anti-inflammatory action is not known.

Dosage and administration Enteric coated tablets should be swallowed whole preferably with sufficient to drink. It is recommended not to take the tablets in connection with heavy meals to prevent further delay in absorption.

Adults: For rheumatoid arthritis, osteoarthrosis and ankylosing spondylitis, the usual dose is 500 mg to 1 g per day taken in two doses at 12 hour intervals.

Where 1 g per day is needed, the suggested regimen is one Nycopren 500 mg tablet twice daily.

In the following cases a loading dose of 750 mg or 1 g per day for the acute phase is recommended:

(a) In patients reporting severe night-time pain and/or morning stiffness.
(b) In patients being switched to Nycopren from a high dose of another anti-rheumatic compound.
(c) In osteoarthrosis where pain is the predominant symptom.

For the patient who requires 750 mg per day, the size of the morning and evening doses can be adjusted on the basis of the predominant symptoms, i.e. night-time pain or morning stiffness.

In acute gout, the recommended dosage is 750 mg at once, then 250 mg every eight hours until the attack has passed.

For the treatment of acute musculoskeletal disorders, the recommended dose is 500 mg initially followed by

250 mg at 8 hour intervals as needed, with a maximum daily dose after the first day of 1250 mg.

Elderly: One study indicates that although total plasma concentration of naproxen is unchanged, the unbound plasma fraction of naproxen is increased in the elderly. The implication of this finding for naproxen dosing is unknown, but caution is advised when high doses are required. For the effect of reduced elimination in the elderly refer to the section 'Use in patients with impaired renal function.'

Children: For the treatment of juvenile rheumatoid arthritis in children over 50 kg: Adult dosage.

Contra-indications, warnings, etc *Contra-indications:* Active peptic ulceration. Hypersensitivity to naproxen or naproxen sodium formulations. Since the potential exists for cross-sensitivity reactions, Nycopren should not be given to patients in whom aspirin or other non-steroidal anti-inflammatory/analgesic drugs induce the syndrome of asthma, rhinitis or urticaria.

Special precautions and warnings: Episodes of gastrointestinal bleeding have been reported in patients with naproxen therapy. Nycopren should be given under close supervision to patients with a history of gastrointestinal disease.

Bronchospasm may be precipitated in patients suffering from, or with a history of, bronchial asthma or allergic disease.

Sporadic abnormalities in laboratory tests (e.g. liver function tests) have occurred in patients on naproxen therapy, but no definite trend was seen in any test indicating toxicity. Naproxen decreases platelet aggregation and prolongs bleeding time. This effect should be kept in mind when bleeding times are determined.

Mild peripheral oedema has been observed in a few patients receiving naproxen. Although sodium retention has not been reported in metabolic studies, it is possible that patients with questionable or compromised cardiac function may be at a greater risk when taking Nycopren.

Use in patients with impaired renal function: As naproxen is eliminated to a large extent (95%) by urinary excretion via glomerular filtration it should be used with great caution in patients with impaired renal function and the monitoring of serum creatinine and/or creatinine clearance is advised in these patients. Naproxen is not recommended to patients having baseline creatinine clearance less than 20 ml/minute.

Certain patients, specifically those where renal blood flow is compromised, such as in extracellular volume depletion, cirrhosis of the liver, sodium retention, congestive heart failure, and pre-existing renal disease, should have renal function assessed before and during naproxen therapy. Some elderly patients in whom impaired renal function may be expected could also fall within this category. A reduction in daily dosage should be considered to avoid the possibility of excessive accumulation of naproxen metabolites in these patients.

Use in patients with impaired liver function: Chronic alcoholic liver disease and probably also other forms of cirrhosis reduce the total plasma concentration of naproxen but the plasma concentration of unbound naproxen is increased. The implication of this finding for Nycopren therapy is unknown, but caution is advised when high doses are required.

Interactions with other drugs: Due to the high plasma protein binding of naproxen, patients simultaneously receiving hydantoins, anti-coagulants or a highly protein-bound sulphonamide should be observed for signs of overdosage of these drugs. No interactions have been observed in clinical studies with naproxen and anticoagulants or sulphonylureas, but caution is nevertheless advised since interaction has been seen with other non-steroidal agents of this class.

The natriuretic effect of frusemide has been reported to be inhibited by some drugs of this class.

Inhibition of renal lithium clearance leading to increases in plasma lithium concentrations has also been reported.

Nycopren and other non-steroidal anti-inflammatory drugs can reduce the anti-hypertensive effect of propranolol and other beta-blockers.

Probenecid given concurrently increases Nycopren plasma levels and extends its plasma half-life considerably.

Caution is advised where methotrexate is administered concurrently because of possible enhancement of its toxicity, since Nycopren, among other non-steroidal anti-inflammatory drugs, has been reported to reduce the tubular secretion of methotrexate in an animal model.

It is suggested that Nycopren therapy be temporarily discontinued 48 hours before adrenal function tests are performed because Nycopren may artifactually interfere with some tests for 17 ketogenic steroids. Similarly, Nycopren may interfere with some assays of urinary 5-hydroxyindoleacetic acid and colitis.

Side effects:
Gastro-intestinal: The more frequent reactions are nausea, vomiting, abdominal discomfort and epigastric distress. More serious reactions which may occur occasionally are gastro-intestinal bleeding and peptic ulceration (sometimes with haemorrhage and perforation).

Dermatological/hypersensitivity: Skin rashes, urticaria, angio-oedema. Anaphylactic reactions to naproxen and naproxen sodium formulations and eosinophilic pneumonitis, alopecia, erythema multiforme, Stevens Johnson Syndrome, epidermal necrolysis and photosensitivity reactions may occur rarely.

CNS: Headache, insomnia, inability to concentrate and cognitive dysfunction have been reported.

Haematological: Thrombocytopenia, granulocytopenia, aplastic anaemia and haemolytic anaemia may occur rarely.

Other: Tinnitus, hearing impairment, vertigo, mild peripheral oedema. Jaundice, fatal hepatitis, nephropathy, haematuria, visual disturbances, vasculitis, aseptic meningitis and ulcerative stomatitis have been reported rarely.

Use in pregnancy and breast feeding: Teratology studies in rats and rabbits, at dose levels equivalent on a human multiple basis to those which have produced foetal abnormality with certain other non-steroidal anti-inflammatory agents e.g. aspirin, have not produced evidence of foetal damage with naproxen. As with other drugs of this type, naproxen produces delay in parturition in animals (the relevance of this finding to human patients is unknown) and also affects the human foetal cardiovascular system (closure of the ductus arteriosus).

Good medical practice indicates minimal drug usage in pregnancy, and use of this class of therapeutic agent requires cautious balancing of possible benefit against potential risk to the mother and foetus especially in the first and third trimesters.

The use of Nycopren should be avoided in patients who are breast feeding.

Overdosage: Few reports of poisoning with naproxen have been published in the literature. It is not known what dose of the drug would be life-threatening. One patient who was reported to have ingested 25 g of naproxen developed only mild transient nausea and indigestion. Hypoprothrombinemia was observed in a patient who ingested 10 g naproxen. In a pharmacokinetic study no side-effects were reported other than mild epigastric pain in one volunteer after receiving 3 g naproxen. (All the reports concern plain naproxen tablets).

Significant overdosage of naproxen may be characterised by: headache, tinnitus, drowsiness, indigestion, nausea, vomiting, tachycardia, hypoprothrombinemia or renal dysfunction.

Management: Supportive and symptomatic. The stomach may be emptied by lavage or inducing emesis. Activated charcoal may be given with the intention of reducing the absorption of naproxen. Further treatment is symptomatic.

Pharmaceutical precautions No special precautions are required. The tablets should be stored in their original container (rheuma-container) at room temperature. Under these conditions the product has a shelf-life of 4 years.

Legal category POM.

Package quantities Nycopren enteric-coated tablets are supplied in rheuma-containers in the following quantities:
Nycopren 250 mg: 250 tablets.
Nycopren 500 mg: 60 tablets. 100 tablets.

Further information Due to the fact that Nycopren is broken down and absorbed in the intestinal tract, the absorption is delayed compared with plain tablets. An evening dosage will thus normally give a higher plasma concentration in the morning.

Product licence numbers
250 mg 4517/0009
500 mg 4517/0010

Product licence holder: Nycomed UK Limited, Nycomed House, 2111, Coventry Road, Sheldon, Birmingham B26 3EA.
Distributed by Lundbeck Ltd.

**Trade Mark*

3M Health Care Limited
Morley Street
Loughborough
Leics LE11 1EP

3M Health Care

ACUPAN*

Presentation *Acupan Tablets:* White, film-coated, circular, biconvex tablets, 7 mm in diameter, marked APN on one side. Each tablet contains nefopam hydrochloride 30 mg.

Acupan Injection: Each 2 ml ampoule contains 1 ml of a solution of nefopam hydrochloride 20 mg/ml.

It also contains the following inactive ingredients: Sodium Acid Phosphate BP; Sodium Phosphate PhEur.

Uses Acupan is indicated for the relief of acute and chronic pain, including: post-operative pain; dental pain; musculo-skeletal pain; acute traumatic pain and cancer pain.

Acupan is a potent and rapidly-acting analgesic. It is totally distinct from other centrally-acting analgesics such as morphine, codeine, pentazocine and propoxyphene.

Unlike the narcotic agents, Acupan has been shown not to cause respiratory depression. There is no evidence of habituation occurring with Acupan.

Dosage and administration *Adults: Acupan Tablets:* Dosage may range from 1 to 3 tablets three times daily depending on response. The recommended starting dosage is 2 tablets three times daily.

Acupan Injection: 20 mg (1 ml) intramuscularly repeated if necessary every six hours (see instructions for administration). Onset of effect after intramuscular injection is within 15–20 minutes and peak effect is reached at one to one-and-a-half hours after administration.

Treatment started with Acupan injection may be continued with Acupan Tablets. 60 mg Acupan (2 tablets) is approximately bioequivalent to 20 mg (1 ampoule) given by injection.

Instructions for administration of Acupan Injection: Acupan Injection should always be given with the patient lying down and after injection the patient should remain lying down for 15–20 minutes. The patient should then get up slowly.

Elderly: Elderly patients may require reduced dosage due to slower metabolism. It is strongly recommended that the starting dose does not exceed one tablet three times daily as the elderly appear more susceptible to, in particular, the CNS side-effects of Acupan and some cases of hallucination and confusion have been reported in this age group.

Children: Since Acupan has not been evaluated in children no dosage recommendation can be given for patients under 12 years.

Contra-indications, warnings, etc *Side-effects:* Nausea, nervousness, dry mouth, lightheadedness and urinary retention may occur. Less frequently, vomiting, blurred vision, drowsiness, sweating, insomnia, headache and tachycardia have been reported.

Caution: The side-effects of Acupan may be additive to those of other agents with anticholinergic or sympathomimetic activity.

It should not be used in the treatment of myocardial infarction since there is no clinical experience in this indication.

Hepatic and renal insufficiency may interfere with the metabolism and excretion of nefopam.

Caution should be exercised when nefopam is administered concurrently with tricyclic antidepressants.

Acupan should be used with caution in patients with, or at risk of, urinary retention. Rarely a temporary, harmless pink discolouration has occurred.

Use in pregnancy: There is no evidence as to the drug safety in human pregnancy nor is there evidence from animal work that it is free from hazard. Avoid in pregnancy unless there is no safer treatment.

Contra-indications: Acupan is contra-indicated in patients with a history of convulsive disorders and should not be given to patients taking mono-amine-oxidase (MAO) inhibitors.

Overdosage: The clinical pattern of nefopam toxicity in overdose is on the neurological (convulsions, hallucinations and agitation) and cardiovascular systems (tachycardia with a hyperdynamic circulation). Routine supportive measures should be taken and prompt removal of ingested drug by gastric lavage or induced vomiting with Syrup of Ipecacuanha should be carried out. Oral administration of activated charcoal may help prevent absorption. Convulsions and hallucinations should be controlled (e.g. with intravenously or rectally administered diazepam). Beta-adrenergic blockers may help control the cardiovascular complications.

Pharmaceutical precautions Store in a cool, dry place.

Package quantities *Acupan Tablets;* Packs of 90 tablets (OP).
Acupan Injection; Boxes containing 5 × 2 ml ampoules filled with 1 ml of solution.

Legal category POM.

Further information Nil.

Product licence numbers

Acupan Tablets	0068/0061
Acupan Injection	0068/0069

AEROLIN* AUTOHALER*

Presentation Aerolin Autohaler is a breath-actuated pressurised aerosol for bronchodilator inhalation therapy. Each actuation delivers Salbutamol Sulphate BP equivalent to Salbutamol 100 micrograms. It also delivers the following inactive ingredients: sorbitan trioleate; propellants 11, 12 and 114.

Uses Aerolin is indicated for the treatment and prophylaxis of bronchial asthma and for the treatment of reversible airways obstruction associated with bronchitis and emphysema. It is also suitable for routine maintenance therapy in chronic asthma and chronic bronchitis, because of its prolonged action. Aerolin may be used to relieve attacks of acute dyspnoea and may also be taken prophylactically before exertion or to prevent exercise-induced asthma. It is suitable for treating bronchospasm in patients with co-existing heart disease or hypertension, including those taking beta-blocking drugs, because of its selective action on the bronchial receptors and lack of effects on the cardiovascular system. Salbutamol is a sympathomimetic agent which has a highly selective action on beta-adrenergic receptors in bronchial muscle. At therapeutic levels it has little activity on cardiac receptors.

Dosage and administration
Adults: For the relief of acute bronchospasm and for

managing intermittent episodes of asthma: one or two inhalations as a single dose; for chronic maintenance or prophylactic therapy: two inhalations, three or four times daily; for prevention of exercise-induced bronchospasm: two inhalations before exertion.

Children: For the relief of acute bronchospasm, management of episodic asthma or before exercise: one inhalation; for routine maintenance or prophylaxis: one inhalation three or four times a day, increasing if necessary to two inhalations three or four times daily.

Elderly: The dosage is the same as for other adults.

Contra-indications, warnings, etc
Contra-indications: There are no contra-indications to inhaled Aerolin therapy.

Warnings: Potentially serious hypokalaemia has been reported in patients taking B_2-agonist therapy.

Hypokalaemia may also occur in hypoxic patients and those treated with xanthine derivatives, steroids, diuretics and long-term laxatives. Extra care should therefore be taken if B_2-agonists are used in these groups of patients and serum potassium levels should be monitored.

Precautions: Administer cautiously to patients with thyrotoxicosis. The patient should be advised to seek medical advice if the treatment ceases to be effective.

Side-effects: Mild tremor, headache and transient muscle cramps may rarely occur. Potentially serious hypokalaemia has been reported in patients taking B_2-agonist therapy.

Overdosage: Treatment: A cardioselective beta-blocking agent should be administered, but these should be used with caution in patients with a history of bronchospasm.

Use in pregnancy: The use of inhaled salbutamol during the first trimester of pregnancy is not recommended unless the clinical need outweighs the risk.

Pharmaceutical precautions Aerolin should be stored in a cool place, protected from frost and direct sunlight. As the vial is pressurised, no attempt should be made to puncture or dispose of it by burning.

Legal category POM.

Package quantities Aerolin Autohaler is supplied as a complete unit delivering 200 inhalations (OP).

Further information Aerolin is not contra-indicated in patients under treatment with MAOIs (monoamine oxidase inhibitors). It does not cause difficulty in micturition as salbutamol does not stimulate alpha-adrenoceptors.

Product licence number 0068/0117

ALU-CAP*

Presentation Opaque green/red hard gelatin capsule, size 0, marked 'RIKER'. Each capsule contains 475 mg Dried Aluminium Hydroxide Gel BP as a white powder.

It also contains the following inactive ingredients: E104; E110; E127; E131.

Uses Alu-Cap is recommended for use as a phosphate-binding agent in the management of renal failure. It may also be used as an antacid.

In the gut, aluminium hydroxide adsorbs phosphate ions. This reduces absorption of phosphate into the body, and thereby reduces serum phosphate levels. In patients with renal failure, the problem of high serum phosphate levels may be partially solved by a diet low in phosphorus. However, a more liberal diet is feasible when a phosphate-binding agent, such as aluminium hydroxide, is used.

Aluminium hydroxide gel is a slow-acting antacid. It is used to provide symptomatic relief in gastric hyperacidity. In addition, the antipeptic and demulcent activity of aluminium hydroxide helps to protect inflamed gastric mucosa against further irritation by gastric secretions.

Dosage and administration *For phosphate-binding: Adults and children:* The dosage must be selected in accordance with individual patient requirements, and may range from 4 to 20 capsules of Alu-Cap daily (approximately 2–10 g dried aluminium hydroxide gel), taken with meals.

As an antacid: Adults: One Alu-Cap four times daily and on retiring. Alu-Cap is not suitable for antacid therapy in children.

Elderly: No special dosage recommendations are made for elderly patients.

Contra-indications, warnings, etc
Side-effects: Aluminium hydroxide is astringent and may cause constipation.

Precautions: Serum phosphate levels should be monitored in all patients receiving phosphate binders, to prevent the development of a phosphate depletion syndrome.

Aluminium hydroxide may form complexes with certain antibiotics (tetracyclines); concomitant administration may result in reduced absorption of the antibiotic.

Pregnancy: There is no evidence of safety of the drug in human pregnancy but it has been in wide use for many years without apparent ill consequence – animal studies having shown no hazard.

Contra-indications: Patients with hypophosphataemia.

Overdosage: Symptoms and treatment: A single massive dose of aluminium hydroxide is unlikely to have harmful sequelae, as aluminium is not absorbed systemically to any great extent. Gastric lavage should be administered, followed by a mild aperient if required.

Pharmaceutical precautions Store in a cool, dry place.

Legal category P.

Package quantities Bottles of 120 capsules (OP).

Further information Nil.

Product licence number 0068/0052.

CALCISORB*

Presentation Creamy-white to beige fibrous powder. The active ingredient is the sodium salt of the phosphate ester of cellulose. Each dose of 5 g is supplied in sachet form and contains approximately 4.7 g of the active ingredient and 0.3 g of moisture.

Uses Sodium cellulose phosphate is an ion-exchange compound with a particular affinity for divalent cations. The product binds calcium ions in the lumen of the stomach and intestine and thus prevents hyperabsorption of dietary calcium. Calcium bound by cellulose phosphate is no longer available for absorption and is therefore excreted in the faeces.

Each 5 g dose will bind approximately 350 mg of calcium.

Calcisorb is used to diminish calcium absorption from the diet: 1) in the treatment of hypercalciuria and recurrent formation of renal stones: 2) in osteopetrosis; 3) as a basis of a test for calcium absorption.

Other possible uses are: 1) treatment of idiopathic hypercalcaemia of infancy; 2) treatment of hypercalcaemic sarcoidosis; 3) treatment of vitamin D intoxication.

Dosage and administration
Adults: 15 g daily, divided as three 5 g doses with meals.

Children: 10 g daily, divided as three doses with meals.

The required dose should be dispersed in water and taken orally. Alternatively the powder may be sprinkled onto food.

Elderly: No special dosage recommendations are made for elderly patients.

Contra-indications, warnings, etc
Contra-indications: Renal failure. Congestive heart failure and other conditions in which a low sodium intake is essential.

Interactions: May occur with oral preparations containing calcium or magnesium salts such as some antacids and laxatives.

Side-effects: Side-effects are rare. Isolated cases of diarrhoea have been reported. One patient with mild renal disease developed a moderate magnesium deficiency. This was readily corrected by halving the dose.

No signs of calcium deficiency have been reported during the continuous use of cellulose phosphate for up to 11 years. This theoretical hazard is particularly relevant to pregnancy, but in view of the absence of data on the effect of cellulose phosphate on calcium levels in pregnant women it is recommended that treatment is discontinued during pregnancy and lactation. Likewise growing children should be prescribed Calcisorb only at the discretion of a senior physician and under his direct supervision.

Pharmaceutical precautions Since cellulose phosphate is an ester, some hydrolysis occurs on storage, the rate increasing with temperature. Calcisorb should therefore be kept in a refrigerator for long-term storage.

For short-term storage by the patient, i.e. of the order of one month, refrigeration is unnecessary. The product is supplied with a minimum expiry date of two years from manufacture.

Legal category P.

Package quantities Supplied in packs of 90 sachets (OP).

Further information Calcisorb should be used in conjunction with a low calcium diet in which dairy products in particular are severely restricted.

During treatment with Calcisorb restriction of oxalate-rich foods, such as spinach, rhubarb, peanuts, beetroot and chocolate, may be beneficial. An oral magnesium supplement of 58–87 mg elemental magnesium, twice daily, in patients receiving 10 and 15 g sodium cellulose phosphate daily, respectively, is also recommended. This supplement should be administered at least 1 hour before or 1 hour after Calcisorb.

Product licence number 0068/5900R

DIFFLAM* CREAM

Presentation Difflam is a white, pleasant-smelling cream, containing benzydamine hydrochloride 3% w/w.

It also contains the following inactive ingredients: Cutina* MD; Cetyl Alcohol USNF; Cetiol* V; Eumulgin* B1; Propylene Glycol PhEur; Perfume, Crematest*; Methyl Hydroxybenzoate PhEur; Propyl Hydroxybenzoate PhEur.

Uses Difflam cream is a topical analgesic and non-steroidal anti-inflammatory agent. It is recommended as a short-term treatment for the relief of symptoms associated with painful inflammatory conditions of the musculo-skeletal system, including:

Acute inflammatory disorders such as myalgia and bursitis.

Traumatic conditions such as sprains, strains, contusions and the after-effects of fractures.

Difflam cream is well absorbed through the skin and it has been shown to have anti-inflammatory and local anaesthetic actions.

Dosage and administration Difflam cream should be massaged lightly into the affected area. Depending on the size of the site to be treated, 35–85 mm (1–2 g) should be applied three times daily and at the discretion of the doctor, up to six times daily in more severe conditions. It is recommended that treatment be limited to not more than 10 days.

Elderly: No special dosage recommendations are made for elderly patients.

Contra-indications, warnings, etc *Side-effects:* Photosensitivity reactions have been reported and local skin reactions which have varied from erythema to papular eruption. The skin returned to normal on stopping treatment.

Use in pregnancy: There is inadequate evidence of safety of the drug in human pregnancy but it has been in wide use for many years without apparent ill consequence.

Caution: To avoid possible irritation, Difflam cream should be kept away from eyes and mucosal surfaces.

Overdosage: Difflam is unlikely to cause adverse systemic effects, even if accidental ingestion should occur. No special measures are required.

Pharmaceutical precautions Avoid extremes of temperature. Store in a cool dry place.

Legal category P.

Package quantities Tubes containing 50 g and 100 g (OP).

Further information Nil.

Product licence number 0068/0088.

DIFFLAM* ORAL RINSE

Presentation Difflam Oral Rinse is a pleasant tasting, clear, green solution, containing benzydamine hydrochloride 0.15% w/v. It also contains the following inactive ingredients: Methylhydroxybenzoate PhEur; E104; E131.

Uses Difflam Oral Rinse is a locally acting analgesic and anti-inflammatory treatment for the relief of painful inflammatory conditions of the mouth and throat including:

Traumatic conditions: Pharyngitis following tonsillectomy or the use of a naso-gastric tube.

Inflammatory conditions: Pharyngitis, aphthous ulcers and oral ulceration due to radiation therapy.

Dentistry: For use after dental operations.

Benzydamine exerts an anti-inflammatory and analgesic action by stabilising the cellular membrane and inhibiting prostaglandin synthesis.

Dosage and administration Rinse or gargle with 15 ml (approximately 1 tablespoonful) every 1½ to 3 hours as required for pain relief. Not suitable for children aged 12 years or under. The solution should be expelled from the mouth after use. Difflam Oral Rinse should generally be used undiluted, but if 'stinging' occurs the rinse may be diluted with water. Uninterrupted treatment should not exceed seven days, unless under medical supervision.

Elderly: No special dosage recommendations are made for elderly patients.

Contra-indications, warnings, etc *Side-effects:* Side-effects are minor. Occasionally, oral tissue numbness or 'stinging' sensations may occur.

Overdosage: Difflam is unlikely to cause adverse systemic effects, even if accidental ingestion should occur. No special measures are required.

Use in pregnancy: There is inadequate evidence of safety of the drug in human pregnancy, but it has been in wide use for many years without apparent ill consequence.

Pharmaceutical precautions Do not leave the uncartonned bottle in direct sunlight.

Legal category P.

Package quantities Bottle containing 200 ml (OP).

Further information Nil.

Product licence number 0068/0096.

DIFFLAM* SPRAY

Presentation Difflam Spray is a metered-dose pump spray which delivers a pleasant tasting, clear, green solution, containing benzydamine hydrochloride 0.15% w/v, 150 μl per puff. It also contains the following inactive ingredient: Methylhydroxybenzoate PhEur.

Uses Difflam Spray is a locally acting analgesic and anti-inflammatory treatment for the throat and mouth.

It is especially useful for the relief of pain in traumatic conditions such as following tonsillectomy or the use of a naso-gastric tube; dental surgery.

Benzydamine exerts an anti-inflammatory and analgesic action by stabilising the cellular membrane and inhibiting prostaglandin synthesis.

Dosage and administration
Adults and elderly: 4 to 8 puffs, 1½ to 3 hourly.

Children (6 to 12): 4 puffs, 1½ to 3 hourly.

Children under 6: 1 Puff to be administered per 4 kg body weight, up to a maximum of 4 puffs, 1½–3 hourly.

Because of the small amount of drug applied, elderly patients can receive the same dose as adults.

The spray should be directed on to the affected area.

Contra-indications, warnings, etc
Side-effects: Side-effects are minor. Occasionally, oral tissue numbness or 'stinging' sensations may occur. The stinging has been reported to disappear upon continuation of the treatment, however, if it persists, it is recommended that treatment be discontinued.

Overdosage: Difflam is unlikely to cause adverse systemic effects, even if accidental ingestion should occur. No special measures are required.

Use in pregnancy: There is inadequate evidence of safety of the drug in human pregnancy, but it has been in wide use for many years without apparent ill consequence.

Pharmaceutical precautions After use the nozzle should be wiped with a tissue to prevent blockage.

It is important that the unit be used and stored upright.

Legal category P.

Package quantities Bottle containing 30 ml (OP).

Further information Nil.

Product licence number 0068/0112.

DISALCID*

Presentation Grey and orange hard gelatin capsule, size 0, marked DS on one half and RIKER on the other.

Each 'Disalcid' capsule contains Salsalate BP 500 mg.

It also contains the following inactive ingredients: E104; E127.

Uses Disalcid is indicated in the treatment of chronic inflammatory conditions of joints, tendons, muscles and connective tissue – for example, osteoarthritis, rheumatoid arthritis, tendinitis, bursitis, fibrositis and polymyalgia.

Salsalate is an ester which after absorption is slowly hydrolysed to two molecules of free salicylic acid. Its insolubility in gastric juice renders it very unlikely to cause the gastric irritation, erosion and haemorrhage associated with acetylsalicylic acid. Moreover, its prolonged biological half-life is a real therapeutic advantage at night and in the relief of morning stiffness.

Dosage and administration *Adults:* 4 capsules daily in divided doses. Where a greater anti-inflammatory effect is required dosage may be increased to 2 capsules three or four times daily.

The last dose should be taken at bedtime. Disalcid should be taken immediately before or with food.

Disalcid should not be given to children under 12 years.

Elderly: Use with caution in elderly patients at a reduced dosage.

Contra-indications, warnings, etc
Side-effects: Allergic reactions may occur rarely with salsalate, as with other salicylates. If tinnitus and deafness occur they are usually signs of overdosage and are reversible by reducing dosage.

Caution: Although Disalcid is relatively free from the risk of gastric erosion usually associated with anti-inflammatory agents, caution should be observed in patients with active peptic ulcer.

Disalcid should be used with caution in patients with renal impairment.

Disalcid may enhance the activity of anticoagulants and hypoglycaemic agents.

Patients should be warned not to take aspirin or any other salicylate-containing medication whilst they are receiving treatment with Disalcid as this will increase the likelihood of overdosage.

Pregnancy: There is no evidence of safety of the drug in human pregnancy; it has been in wide use for many years without apparent ill consequence; there is evidence of harmful effects of salicylates in pregnancy in animals. It is recommended that Disalcid Capsules should not be taken by breast feeding mothers.

Contra-indications: Disalcid is contra-indicated in patients with known hypersensitivity to salicylic acid or its derivatives.

Overdosage: Symptoms: Overdosage with Disalcid produces the usual symptoms of salicylism: tinnitus and deafness, vertigo, headache, sweating, hyperventilation and confusion are likely to occur.

Treatment: The stomach should be emptied by lavage with sodium bicarbonate or water.

Patients suffering from severe intoxication should in addition have forced alkaline diuresis by intravenous infusions of sodium bicarbonate solution. Haemodialysis or peritioneal dialysis may be needed in extreme cases, especially in the presence of cardiac or renal impairment.

Pharmaceutical precautions Disalcid should be stored in a cool, dry place. The container should be kept tightly closed.

Legal category POM.

Package quantities *Disalcid Capsules:* Bottles of 120 (OP).

Further information Nil.

Product licence number 0068/0089.

DUROMINE*

Presentation *Duromine* is available in two strengths. Each capsule contains phentermine 15 mg or 30 mg as an ion-exchange resin complex. It also contains the following inactive ingredients: lactose; E104; E123; E131.

Duromine 15 mg: Opaque green/grey size number three capsules printed *Duromine* 15.

Duromine 30 mg: Opaque maroon/grey size number three capsules printed *Duromine* 30.

Uses Duromine is an appetite-depressant for short-term use as an adjunct to the treatment of some patients with moderate to severe obesity, for whom close control and supervision should be provided.

After ingestion, the active constituent phentermine is gradually released from the ion-exchange resin complex over a period of 10–14 hours.

The prolonged release of phentermine gives sustained plasma levels devoid of absorption peaks, thus minimising the risk of adverse CNS reactions.

Dosage and administration *Adults:* One 15 mg or 30 mg capsule daily at breakfast time. Duromine is not recommended for the elderly or children.

Intermittent dosage: Treatment for 4 to 8 weeks followed by a similar period without medication may be as effective as continuous treatment, and reduces the risk of dependence.

Efficacy in use for more than 3–6 months and safety in long-term use has not been established and may carry an increased risk of dependence.

The stated dose should not be exceeded.

Treatment should be discontinued if weight loss does not occur or ceases.

Contra-indications, warnings, etc
Contra-indications: Duromine is contra-indicated in patients under treatment with monoamine-oxidase (MAO) inhibitors, and should not be given within 2 weeks of stopping such treatment. It is also contra-indicated in thyrotoxicosis, severe hypertension, and in patients sensitive to sympathomimetic agents.

Duromine should not be given to patients with a history of psychiatric illness, emotionally unstable or vulnerable personalities, or those with previous drug or alcohol abuse. It should not be used concurrently with other appetite depressant drugs or by women during lactation.

Use in pregnancy: Do not use in pregnancy. There is inadequate evidence of safety in human pregnancy, and there is no information from animal studies.

Caution: Duromine should be used with caution in patients under treatment with antihypertensive agents, since it may cause some loss of blood pressure control, and in patients receiving psychotropic drugs, including sedatives and sympathomimetic agents.

Side-effects: Patients have been withdrawn from trials due to the following adverse reactions: insomnia, CNS stimulation, vomiting, dry mouth, facial oedema, rash and headache. Other side-effects which were well tolerated included constipation, urinary frequency, nausea, dizziness, nervousness and depression.

Palpitations, tachycardia, high blood pressure, psychosis and hallucinations may also occur.

Patients may be at risk whilst driving or operating machinery, and there may be an interaction with alcohol. There is also a possibility of dependence.

Overdosage
Symptoms: Initially irritability, agitation, disorientation and tremor may occur, followed by cardiac arrhythmias, convulsions, hallucinations and coma.

Treatment: The stomach should be emptied by emesis or stomach tube and washed out with water if the preparation has been ingested within the last three or four hours. Diazepam, preferably by mouth (cautiously by intravenous injection) should be used to control marked excitement and convulsions. Provided renal function is adequate, elimination of phentermine may be assisted by acidification of the urine by agents such as lysine hydrochloride or arginine hydrochloride.

Pharmaceutical precautions Store in a cool, dry place.

Legal category CD (Sch 3), POM.

Package quantities
Duromine 15 mg: Bottles of 30 capsules.
Duromine 30 mg: Bottles of 30 capsules.

Further information There is a possibility that amphetamine-type dependence may occur and Duromine may be socially abused for euphoriant effect.

Product licence numbers
Duromine 15 mg: 0068/5055R
Duromine 30 mg: 0068/5056R

EXIREL* CAPSULES

Presentation Exirel is available as capsules containing 10 mg or 15 mg of pirbuterol as the hydrochloride. Each capsule also contains the following inactive ingredient: lactose.

The 10 mg capsule has a turquoise body and an olive cap printed 'MXR 10' and '3M'. The 15 mg capsule has a turquoise body and a beige cap printed 'MXR 15' and '3M'.

Pirbuterol hydrochloride is a white crystalline powder which is very soluble in water.

Uses *Actions:* Exirel is a beta-adrenergic receptor agonist, which has been shown *in vitro* and in *in vivo* animal studies to exert a more selective action on beta$_2$-adrenergic receptors located in the lung than on beta$_1$ receptors in the heart muscle. No data exist to confirm this in man.

Indications: Exirel capsules are indicated for the treatment and prophylaxis of bronchial asthma and the reversible bronchospasm which may be associated with bronchitis and emphysema.

Dosage and administration For adults, and children 12 years and above, the effective dosage of Exirel capsules is 10 mg or 15 mg administered three or four times daily.

The maximum total daily recommended dose is 60 mg.

Contra-indications, warnings, etc
Contra-indications: Exirel capsules are contra-indicated in patients known to be sensitive to sympathomimetic agents, and in patients who are receiving non-selective beta-adrenergic blocking agents.

Warnings: If the recommended dose of Exirel capsules fails to maintain effective relief, patients should be advised to seek immediate medical attention.

Potentially serious hypokalaemia has been reported in patients taking B_2-agonist therapy. Hypokalaemia may also occur in hypoxic patients and those treated with xanthine derivatives, steroids, diuretics and long term laxatives. Extra care should therefore be taken if B_2-agonists are used in these groups of patients and serum potassium levels should be monitored.

Use in pregnancy: Animal tests show no teratogenic effects, but the safety of Exirel capsules for use during pregnancy or lactation has not yet been established. The expected therapeutic effects of the drug should be weighed against the possible hazard to the mother or child in these situations.

Use in children: Exirel capsules are not recommended for children below the age of 12 years.

Use in the elderly: No additional recommendations are made for elderly patients. Use of the lowest dose giving adequate clinical efficacy is advised.

Precautions: As with other sympathomimetic agents, Exirel capsules should be used with caution in patients with thyrotoxicosis, coronary artery disease or cardiac dysrhythmias.

Side-effects: Side-effects such as tremors, headache, nervousness, insomnia, palpitations have been reported infrequently and are similar to those reactions recorded with other beta$_2$-adrenergic agonists.

Overdosage: In the event of overdosage with Exirel, supportive and symptomatic treatment is indicated. Cardioselective beta-blocking drugs may be useful but should be used with caution in patients with a history of bronchospasm.

Pharmaceutical precautions Exirel capsules should be stored below 30°C.

Legal category POM.

Package quantities Exirel capsules, 10 mg or 15 mg are supplied in packs of 90.

Further information Following administration of Exirel capsules a clinically significant improvement in pulmonary function is usually observed within one hour with maximum effect within 1–2 hours. Following oral administration the duration of action of Exirel is six hours or more. The efficacy of Exirel is not diminished on chronic administration.

In man maximum levels of drug appear in plasma 1–3 hours after oral dosing. The half-life is approximately two hours. The drug is extensively metabolised with the sulphate conjugate being the chief urinary excretion product.

Product licence numbers
Exirel Capsules 10 mg 0068/0136
Exirel Capsules 15 mg 0068/0137

EXIREL* METERED INHALER

Presentation Exirel is presented as a metered dose inhaler, delivering 200 micrograms pirbuterol as the acetate per actuation. It also delivers the following inactive ingredients: sorbitan trioleate, freon 11 and freon 12. Each canister is capable of delivering at least 200 individual doses. Pirbuterol acetate is a white crystalline powder which is very soluble in water.

Uses *Actions:* Exirel is a beta-adrenergic receptor agonist, which has been shown *in vitro* and in *in vivo* animal studies to exert a more selective action on $beta_2$-adrenergic receptors located in the lung than on $beta_1$-receptors in the heart muscle. No data exist to confirm this in man.

Indications: Exirel inhaler is indicated for the treatment or prophylaxis of bronchial asthma and the reversible bronchospasm which may be associated with bronchitis and emphysema.

Dosage and administration The dose of Exirel for adults and children over 12 years is 1 or 2 inhalations (200 microgram or 400 microgram). For maintenance or prophylactic therapy the recommended dosage is 2 inhalations (400 microgram) three or four times daily which can be increased, but the total should not exceed 12 inhalations (2400 microgram) daily. With repetitive dosing, inhalation should usually not be repeated more often than every four hours. To use the Exirel inhaler, patients should actuate the valve shortly after the beginning of a slow inhalation which should be followed by at least 10 second breath holding.

Contra-indications, warnings, etc
Contra-indications: Exirel inhaler is contra-indicated in patients known to be sensitive to sympathomimetic agents, and in patients who are receiving non-selective beta-adrenergic blocking agents.

Warnings: If the recommended dose of Exirel inhaler fails to maintain effective relief, patients should be advised to seek immediate medical attention.

Excessive use of sympathomimetic inhalants has been associated with an increased incidence of adverse reactions including life-threatening dysrhythmias.

Potentially serious hypokalaemia has been reported in patients taking B_2-agonist therapy. Hypokalaemia may also occur in hypoxic patients and those treated with xanthine derivatives, steroids, diuretics and long-term laxatives. Extra care should therefore be taken if B_2-agonists are used in these groups of patients and serum potassium levels should be monitored.

Use in pregnancy: Animal tests show no teratogenic effects, but the safety of Exirel inhaler during pregnancy or lactation has not yet been established. The expected therapeutic effects of the drug should be weighed against the possible hazard to the mother or child in these situations.

Use in children: Exirel inhaler is not presently recommended for children below the age of 12 due to lack of clinical data in this age group.

Use in the elderly: No additional recommendations are made for elderly patients. Use of the lowest dose giving adequate clinical efficacy is advised.

Precautions: As with other sympathomimetic agents, Exirel inhaler should be used with caution in patients with thyrotoxicosis.

Side-effects: Side-effects such as tremors, headache, nervousness, insomnia, palpitations have been reported infrequently and are similar to those reactions recorded with other $beta_2$-adrenergic agonists. Potentially serious hypokalaemia has been reported in patients taking B_2-agonist therapy.

Overdosage: In the event of overdosage with Exirel inhaler, supportive and symptomatic treatment is indicated. Cardioselective beta-blocking drugs may be useful but should be used with caution in patients with a history of bronchospasm.

Pharmaceutical precautions The Exirel inhaler should be stored below 30°C. It must not be exposed to heat or punctured.

Legal category POM.

Package quantities Each canister of Exirel inhaler contains sufficient material to give at least 200 metered doses of pirbuterol as pirbuterol acetate.

Further information Following administration of Exirel inhaler a clinically significant improvement in pulmonary function is usually observed within 5–10 minutes with maximum effect within 15–30 minutes. The duration of action of Exirel is at least five hours. The efficacy of Exirel is not diminished on chronic administration.

In man plasma levels of drug following inhaler administration were undetectable. However urine contained approximately 15% of the dose as unchanged drug and approximately 36% as the sulphate conjugate after oral dosing.

Product licence number Exirel inhaler 0068/0135.

HIPREX*

Presentation White, oblong tablet with breakline, marked HX on one side and RIKER on the other. Each Hiprex tablet contains methenamine hippurate 1 g.

Uses
Hiprex is indicated in the prophylaxis and treatment of urinary tract infections:

1. As maintenance therapy after successful initial treatment of acute infections with antibiotics.
2. As long-term therapy in the prevention of recurrent cystitis.
3. To suppress urinary infection in patients with indwelling catheters and to reduce the incidence of catheter blockage.
4. To provide prophylaxis against the introduction of infection into the urinary tract during instrumental procedures.
5. Asymptomatic bacteriuria.

Methenamine hippurate is readily absorbed from the gastro-intestinal tract and excreted via the kidney.

With Hiprex, as with other specific urinary antibacterial agents of this type, antibacterial activity is confined to the urinary tract.

The antibacterial action is achieved by the slow release of the bactericidal formaldehyde, from the methenamine part, in the urine; acid pH less than pH 5.5 is necessary for this reaction to occur. It is obtained and maintained there by the presence of hippuric acid.

Hiprex has a wide antibacterial spectrum covering both gram-positive and gram-negative organisms. It is active against the bacteria which most commonly cause urinary tract infection – *Escherichia coli, Aerobacter aerogenes*, Pseudomonas and some strains of Proteus. Urinary antibacterial activity can be shown within 30 minutes of administration.

Hiprex is particularly useful for long-term treatment because neither tolerance to its effect nor bacterial resistance occurs. The incidence of side-effects is extremely low.

Dosage and administration *Adults:* 1 g twice daily.

In patients with catheters the dosage may be increased to 1 g three times daily.

Children: 6–12 years: 500 mg twice daily.

The tablets may be halved, or they can be crushed and taken with a drink of milk or fruit juice if the patient prefers.

Contra-indications, warnings, etc *Side-effects:* Occasionally rashes, gastric irritation or irritation of the bladder may occur.

All side-effects are reversible on withdrawal of the drug.

Contra-indications: Severe dehydration, metabolic acidosis, or severe renal failure (creatinine clearance or GFR < 10 ml/min.). Hiprex may be used where mild (20–50 ml/min.) to moderate (10–20 ml/min.) renal insufficiency is present. (If the GFR is not available, the serum creatinine concentration can be used as a guide).

Hiprex should not be administered concurrently with sulphonamides because of the possibility of crystalluria, or with alkalising agents, such as mixture of potassium citrate.

Use in pregnancy: There is inadequate evidence of safety of the drug in human pregnancy but it has been in wide use for many years without apparent ill consequence, animal studies having shown no hazard.

Methenamine is excreted in breast milk but the quantities will be insignificant to the infant.

Overdosage: Vomiting and haematuria may occur. These can be treated by the use of an anti-emetic and drinking copious quantities of water respectively. Bladder symptoms can be treated by the consumption of copious quantities of water and 2–3 teaspoonfuls of bicarbonate of soda.

Pharmaceutical precautions The container should be kept tightly closed.

Legal category P.

Package quantities Bottles of 60 tablets (OP).

Further information Nil.

Product licence number 0068/5003R.

INTRALGIN*

Presentation Intralgin contains Benzocaine BP 2 per cent w/w and salicylamide 5 per cent w/w in an alcoholic vehicle. It contains the following inactive ingredients: Carbopol*; Brij*; Isopropyl Alcohol BP; Strong Ammonia Solution BP. Intralgin is a clear, pleasant-smelling preparation – non-greasy and non-staining.

Uses Intralgin is indicated for the relief of muscle pain from strains, sprains and injuries, and pain associated with fibrositis, lumbago and non-articular rheumatism.

The use of isopropyl alcohol as a vehicle for the medicaments contributes significantly to the action of Intralgin. Isopropyl alcohol because of its penetrative properties facilitates the percutaneous absorption of benzocaine and salicylamide so that they reach underlying tissue to relieve pain rapidly. Vigorous massage is not needed with Intralgin, unlike traditional rubs which rely for effect on erythema or counter-irritation.

Dosage and administration Intralgin Gel should be applied liberally and rubbed gently into the skin until penetration is complete. Vigorous massage is unnecessary.

For more rapid absorption the painful area should be warmed before applying Intralgin.

Children and the elderly: There are no special dosage recommendations for children and elderly patients.

Contra-indications, warnings, etc
Contra-indications: None.

Precautions: If irritation or itching occurs due to hypersensitivity, Intralgin should be discontinued and a soothing cream applied.

Interactions: There are no known interactions with Intralgin therapy.

Side-effects: Local sensitivity reactions to the benzocaine constituent have occasionally been reported.

Overdosage: Not applicable.

Use in pregnancy: There is inadequate evidence of the safety of Intralgin in human pregnancy but it has been in wide use for many years without apparent ill consequence. Excretion in breast milk, if any, is expected to be too low to affect the infant.

Pharmaceutical precautions The tube should be kept tightly closed and kept away from direct heat.

Legal category P.

Package quantities Tubes of 50 g (OP).

Further information Nil.

Product licence number 0068/5076R.

LERGOBAN*

Presentation Creamy-white, circular, bi-convex tablets, 0.25 inch (6.4 mm) in diameter. The markings are 'LB' on one side and 'RIKER' on the other. Each Lergoban Tablet contains Diphenylpyraline Hydrochloride BP 5 mg.

Uses Lergoban is indicated in: allergic rhinitis, allergic conjunctivitis, angioneurotic oedema, hay fever, urticaria, allergic skin conditions and associated irritation.

Diphenylpyraline is an antihistamine with the general properties of antihistamine compounds, but with a low incidence of side-effects. In Lergoban its therapeutic usefulness is greatly increased by the long-acting presentation. Lergoban Tablets consist of a porous plastic matrix in which the diphenylpyraline is dispersed. In the gastro-intestinal tract, the active ingredient is gradually leached from the pores of the matrix and absorbed systemically. The release rate is not affected by changes in pH, digestive enzymes, viscosity, surface tension or electrolyte concentration. The small plastic skeleton is insoluble and is excreted unchanged in the faeces.

The duration of effect from each dose of Lergoban is about 10 hours, so that only two doses every 24 hours are required.

Dosage and administration *Adults:* One or two 5 mg tablets every 12 hours, or as directed by the physician.

Children: Older children may be given one 5 mg tablet every 12 hours.

Lergoban is not recommended for children under 10 years.

Elderly: Elderly patients may require a reduced dosage due to slower metabolism.

Contra-indications, warnings, etc
Side-effects: Slight drowsiness and dizziness, flushing, headache and anorexia may occur. Possible anticholinergic effects include urinary retention, blurred vision, dry mouth and gastro-intestinal disturbance.

Pregnancy: There is inadequate evidence of safety of Lergoban in human pregnancy but it has been in wide use for many years without apparent ill consequence, animal studies having shown no hazard. If drug therapy is needed in pregnancy, this drug can be used if there is no safer alternative.

Contra-indications: None.

Caution: Doses greater than those recommended may cause sedation and drowsiness. Patients undergoing treatment with an antihistamine should be warned of this possibility if they are in control of vehicles or machinery, where loss of attention may lead to accidents.

In some patients, the action of antihistamines may be potentiated by alcohol or other CNS depressants.

Antihistamines should be used with caution in patients with epilepsy, prostatic hypertrophy, glaucoma and hepatic disease.

Interactions: Antihistamines potentiate the effect of hypnotics and anxiolytics, and show antagonism when used concurrently with betahistine (a histamine analogue). When used with anticholinergic drugs such as benzhexol, increased side-effects may occur.

Overdosage: In adults, overdosage of antihistamines usually causes sedation, varying from drowsiness to deep sleep. Conversely in children, antihistamines often act as cerebral stimulants and may cause convulsions and hyperpyrexia. Stimulation may also occur in some adults.

Treatment: If the drug has recently been taken, the stomach should be emptied by gastric lavage, using a tube greater than 7 mm in diameter. Excitement may be controlled with diazepam given by mouth; the ECG should be monitored.

Pharmaceutical precautions Store in a cool, dry place.

Legal category P.

Package quantities Bottles of 60 tablets (OP).

Further information Nil.

Product licence number 0068/5002R.

MEDIHALER-EPI*

Presentation Medihaler-Epi is a pressurised aerosol for inhalation therapy. The vial contains a creamy-white suspension of Adrenaline Acid Tartrate BP 14 mg/ml in aerosol propellent, and delivers 400 measured doses, each containing 280 micrograms Adrenaline Acid Tartrate BP. The vial contains the following inactive ingredients: sorbitan trioleate; propellants 11, 12 and 114.

Uses Medihaler-Epi may be used as an adjunct to the standard therapy in anaphylactic reactions due to drug sensitivity or insect stings.

Adrenaline is a sympathomimetic amine which activates both alpha- and beta-adrenergic receptors. As a result, it causes vasoconstriction, bronchodilatation, relieves mucosal congestion and is a cardiac stimulant.

By inhalation, adrenaline relaxes bronchial smooth muscle and constricts bronchial mucosal vessels, relieving congestion and oedema. However, tolerance to adrenaline can develop after repeated use and the action of adrenaline in reducing bronchial secretion may make mucus more viscid.

Dosage and administration Each puff from Medihaler-epi delivers a measured dose of 280 micrograms adrenaline acid tartrate.

Correct technique is essential if the patient is to obtain full benefit from each treatment. It is important that the doctor shows the patient how to use Medihaler-epi by personal demonstration, as patients may not be familiar with the use of inhalers. A Demonstration Unit containing no active medicament can be obtained for this purpose, on request.

Adults: In the adjunctive treatment of anaphylactic reactions, a minimum dose of 20 puffs is recommended.

Children: Medihaler-epi has not been evaluated in children but, should the need arise, it may be used as an adjunct to standard anaphylactic therapy. A dose of 10 to 15 puffs is recommended. Medihaler-epi should be administered to children only under the supervision of a responsible adult.

Elderly: No special dosage recommendations are made for elderly patients.

Contra-indications, warnings, etc
Side-effects: Gastric pain has been reported, probably as a result of swallowed adrenaline. Overdosage may cause dry mouth, palpitations or nervousness.

Contra-indications: Medihaler-epi should be used with caution in the presence of cardiac disease, hypertension and hyperthyroidism.

Prolonged use of adrenaline may lead to the development of tolerance (adrenaline 'fastness'). When this occurs, isoprenaline is a most effective alternative.

Theoretically, no interaction with monoamine oxidase inhibitors (MAOI) would be expected, but some enhancement of the cardiovascular effects of adrenaline is seen especially if the MAOI induces hypotension.

Pregnancy: There is inadequate evidence of safety of the drug in human pregnancy but it has been in wide use for many years without apparent ill consequence, animal studies having shown no hazard. If drug therapy is needed in pregnancy, this drug can be used if there is no safer alternative.

Overdosage
Acute poisoning: No cases have been reported. The following guidance is based on acute adrenaline poisoning following parenteral administration.

Symptoms: Restlessness, palpitations, rapid pulse, tremor, weakness, dizziness, headache, coldness of extremities, elevated blood pressure, tachycardia. The symptoms are rapid in onset and of short duration.

Treatment: It is essential to administer immediately intravenous injections of quick-acting sympatholytics, e.g. phentolamine or piperoxan.

Chronic poisoning: Some cases have been reported, but no details of treatment have been given, other than withdrawal of the aerosol.

Pharmaceutical precautions Medihaler-epi shold be stored in a cool place, protected from frost and sunlight.

As the Medihaler vial is pressurised, no attempt should be made to puncture it or to dispose of it by burning.

Legal category POM.

Package quantities Standard pack (complete unit): vial contains 400 doses (OP).

Further information Nil.

Product licence number 0068/5060R.

MEDIHALER* ERGOTAMINE

Presentation Creamy-white suspension in pressurised container. Medihaler Ergotamine contains a suspension of Ergotamine Tartrate BP 9 mg/ml in aerosol propellant, and delivers to the patient 75 measured doses, each containing 360 micrograms ergotamine tartrate.

Medihaler Ergotamine contains the following inactive ingredients: sorbitan trioleate; propellants 11, 12 and 114.

Uses Medihaler Ergotamine is indicated for rapid relief of migraine.

Micronised ergotamine tartrate taken by inhalation is rapidly absorbed from the highly vascular epithelium of the respiratory tract into the systemic circulation. Two factors make this route of administration particularly effective: speed of absorption and lack of interference with the drug's action by either the digestive tract or the liver. Another advantage is that the dose is retained in spite of vomiting.

One or two inhalations from Medihaler Ergotamine can abort the migraine attack before cephalic vasodilatation becomes fixed and before oedema of the vascular wall and perivascular tissues has developed. In the majority of patients, full therapeutic effect is achieved within 15 minutes.

Dosage and administration
Adults and children aged 10 or over: One inhalation should be taken at the first sign of attack and should be repeated if necessary after five minutes.

Caution: No more than 6 inhalations should be taken in any 24-hour period. Maximum dosage in one week should not exceed 15 inhalations.

Elderly: No special dosage recommendations are made for elderly patients.

Children: Medihaler Ergotamine is not recommended for children younger than 10 years of age.

To obtain full benefit from treatment, the patient should follow these simple steps:
Remove the dust-cap and shake the unit.
Place the mouthpiece well into the mouth with lips closed firmly around it.
Breathe out fully.
Start to breathe in and then press the vial firmly down into the adapter with the forefinger. This operates Medihaler Ergotamine and the dose is released.
Release pressure on the vial. Remove the unit from the mouth and hold the breath as long as possible before breathing out.
After use, replace the dust cap.

Contra-indications, warnings, etc
Side-effects: Ergotamine tartrate may cause nausea and vomiting in some patients. As these symptoms can occur in migraine attacks, it may be difficult to determine whether the illness or the medication is responsible.

Muscular pain may occasionally be experienced. This can be controlled by reduction of dosage.

Contra-indications: Septic conditions, coronary disease, peripheral vascular disease, renal or hepatic dysfunction, hypertension or pregnancy.

Overdosage: Symptoms: Acute poisoning is rare. Symptoms are nausea, vomiting, diarrhoea, thirst, coldness of the skin, pruritus, rapid and weak pulse, numbness and tingling of the extremities, confusion and unconsciousness.

Treatment: Treatment of poisoning is symptomatic. Vasodilators such as choline esters, nitrites or papaverine may be used, together with mechanical procedures to restore the circulation. Nausea and vomiting may be relieved by atropine.

Pharmaceutical precautions Medihaler Ergotamine has a shelf-life of 2 years and should be stored at 5°C until dispensed.

Once dispensed the shelf life is 6 months.

As the Medihaler Ergotamine vial is pressurised no attempt should be made to puncture it or to dispose of it by burning.

Legal category POM.

Package quantities Standard pack (complete unit): pressurised vial containing 75 doses (OP).

Further information Nil.

Product licence number 0068/5014R

MEDIHALER-ISO* MEDIHALER-ISO* FORTE

Presentation *Medihaler-iso* and *Medihaler-iso Forte* are pressurised aerosols for inhalation therapy.

The *Medihaler-iso* vial contains a creamy-white suspension of Isoprenaline Sulphate BP 4 mg/ml in aerosol propellent, and delivers 400 measured doses, each containing 80 micrograms Isoprenaline Sulphate BP. The vial contains the following inactive ingredients: Sorbitan trioleate; propellants 11, 12 and 114.

The *Medihaler-iso Forte* vial contains a creamy-white suspension of Isoprenaline Sulphate BP 20 mg/ml in aerosol propellent, and delivers 400 measured doses, each containing 400 micrograms Isoprenaline Sulphate BP. The vial contains the same inactive ingredients as Medihaler-Iso.

Uses Isoprenaline is a bronchodilator, and Medihaler-iso and Medihaler-iso Forte are indicated for the relief of bronchospasm in bronchial asthma and chronic bronchitis. It is recommended that these products be used only in patients responsive to bronchodilators, and that this be determined by measurement of respiratory parameters before and after inhalation of isoprenaline.

Isoprenaline is a directly acting sympathomimetic amine which activates both β_1 and β_2 adrenergic receptors. It has virtually no affinity for α-receptors. As a result it is a bronchodilator which also produces vasodilatation in all blood vessels, including those of the pulmonary system. Pulse rate and cardiac output are increased, the degree of cardiac stimulation being proportional to the blood level. Isoprenaline is quickly eliminated from the blood and therefore has no cumulative effect. It inhibits histamine release in the lungs and has a beneficial effect on cilia and mucus flow.

By inhalation, isoprenaline has a rapid onset of bronchodilatation. It has a duration of action of 1–2 hours. Cardiac stimulation does not usually occur and the maximum possible bronchodilatation is produced at doses below those which result in significant tachycardia. Appreciable cardiac stimulation occurs only at the upper end of the therapeutic dose range.

Dosage and administration Each puff from Medihaler-iso delivers a measured dose of 80 micrograms isoprenaline sulphate and from Medihaler-iso Forte, 400 micrograms isoprenaline sulphate. One, two or at the most three puffs should be sufficient to provide relief in most cases. Before taking a further inhalation, the patient should wait at least one minute to allow the full effect of the previous puff to become apparent. It should not be necessary for the patient to take further treatment for at least 30 minutes, or more than eight treatments in any 24-hour period.

Children: Medihaler-iso should be administered to children who are responsive to bronchodilators only under the supervision of a responsible adult. Medihaler-iso Forte is not recommended for children.

Elderly: No special dosage recommendations are made for elderly patients.

Contra-indications, warnings, etc
Side-effects: Overdosage may cause dry mouth, palpitations or nervousness. Rebound bronchospasm has been reported, but this is rare. Elderly patients are more susceptible to side-effects.

Contra-indications: Medihaler-iso and Medihaler-iso Forte should not be used in the presence of severe cardiac disease, pre-existing ventricular arrhythmias, severe hypertension and hyperthyroidism.

Precautions: Use with care in patients with heart disease and hypertension, and those taking other sympathomimetic agents. There is a theoretical possibility that isoprenaline could trigger or aggravate cardiac arrhythmias.

Theoretically, no interaction with monoamine oxidase inhibitors (MAOI) would be expected, but some enhancement of the cardiovascular effects of isoprenaline is seen, particularly if the MAOI induces hypotension.

Interactions: Concurrent administration of cardiac glycosides, antidepressants, xanthine derivatives, thyroxine and anaesthetics may result in the myocardium being sensitised. This is also seen in patients with abnormalities of electrolytes and blood gases.

Pregnancy: There is inadequate evidence of the safety of the drug in human pregnancy but it has been in wide use for many years without apparent ill consequence, animal studies having shown no hazard. If drug therapy is needed in pregnancy, this drug can be used if there is no safer alternative.

Medihaler-iso Forte: It is recognised that even following topical use, significant systemic absorption of isoprenaline could occur following the use of Medihaler-iso Forte, and give rise to systemic effects. Excessive use near the term could delay the onset of labour. There is no information on the excretion of the drug in breast milk.

Overdosage: Acute poisoning in non-asthmatics: No cases have been reported. In the absence of details of such practical experience, the following guidance is based on theoretical considerations.

Symptoms of acute isoprenaline poisoning are likely to be mainly cardiovascular effects, e.g. tachycardia, palpitations, peripheral vasodilatation and fall in blood pressure.

Treatment: General symptomatic therapy.

Chronic poisoning in asthmatics: Some cases have been reported, but no details of treatment have been given, other than withdrawal of the aerosol.

Excessive use during an attack of asthma indicates lack of response. This is a grave sign suggestive of status asthmaticus, or that the patient is ill. Patients should therefore be advised to seek urgent medical attention. It is recommended that 100 mg hydrocortisone be given immediately by intravenous injection, and the patient admitted to hospital without delay. Beta-blocking drugs should not be used.

Pharmaceutical precautions *Medihaler-iso* and *Medihaler-iso Forte* should be stored in a cool place, protected from frost and sunlight. The shelf-life of *Medihaler-iso* and *Medihaler-iso Forte* is three years.

As the *Medihaler* vial is pressurised, no attempt should be made to puncture it or to dispose of it by burning.

Legal category POM.

Package quantities *Medihaler-iso, Medihaler-iso Forte:* are both supplied as complete units containing 400 doses (OP).

Further information Nil.

Product licence numbers
Medihaler-iso 0068/5082R
Medihaler-iso Forte 0068/5072R

NORFLEX* INJECTION

Presentation Each 2 ml ampoule contains Orphenadrine Citrate BP 30 mg/ml. It also contains the following inactive ingredients: Sodium Chloride PhEur; Sodium Hydroxide BP.

Uses Norflex injection is indicated for the short term symptomatic relief of painful conditions of the musculoskeletal system such as low back pain and lumbago.

Orphenadrine acts centrally by blocking reticular facilitation, i.e. it blocks preferentially those pathways whose hyperactivity leads to an exaggeration of motor function such as spasticity, rigidity or muscle spasm.

Dosage and administration *Adults:* 60 mg (one 2 ml ampoule) administered intramuscularly or intravenously.

Note: An intravenous injection should be administered over a period of about five minutes.

Elderly: The cautions and contra-indications apply particularly to elderly patients. It is recommended that these patients receive a reduced dose. Orphenadrine may cause confusion (delirium) in the elderly.

Norflex is not recommended for children under 12 years.

Contra-indications, warnings, etc *Contra-indications:* Contra-indications to Norflex result from the parasympatholytic action of orphenadrine. Norflex should not be given to patients with glaucoma, urinary retention (e.g. due to prostatic hypertrophy or obstruction of the bladder neck) and myasthenia gravis. It should not be given to lactating mothers.

Side-effects: Blurring of vision, dry mouth, nausea, dizziness, confusion and tremor may occur in some patients susceptible to the parasympatholytic action of orphenadrine. These symptoms rapidly disappear following reduction of dosage or cessation of treatment. Some patients may experience a transient feeling of lightheadedness or dizziness following an injection of Norflex.

Caution: Norflex should be used with caution in patients with tachycardia.

Pregnancy: There is no evidence as to drug safety in human pregnancy nor is there evidence from animal work that it is free from hazard. Avoid in pregnancy unless there is no safer treatment.

Orphenadrine is excreted into breast milk and 'Norflex' is contra-indicated in lactating mothers.

Overdosage: Symptoms of orphenadrine citrate overdosage: Excitement, confusion and delirium leading to coma, convulsions, tachycardia. Dilated pupils and urinary retention may occur.

Treatment: Convulsions and delirium respond to relatively large doses of diazepam, preferably by mouth. Adequate hydration of the patient is important.

Pharmaceutical precautions Store in a cool, dry place.

Legal category POM.

Package quantities *Ampoules (30 mg/ml):* 3 × 2 ml.

Further information Nil.

Product licence number 0068/5078R.

NUELIN*

Presentation White, circular, biconvex tablet with breakline, 9 mm in diameter, marked NL/125 on one side and 'RIKER' on the other.

Each Nuelin tablet contains Theophylline BP 125 mg in microcrystalline form. It also contains the following inactive ingredient: lactose.

Uses Nuelin is indicated for the prophylaxis and treatment of reversible broncho-spasm in asthma, bronchitis and emphysema.

Theophylline is well established in the treatment of bronchospasm. In Nuelin, the theophylline is present as microfine particles to give a very high rate of dissolution which results in rapid and predictable absorption.

Dosage and administration *Adults:* One tablet three or four times daily, preferably after food; this can be increased to two tablets three or four times daily depending on response.

Elderly: Elderly patients may require lower doses due to reduced theophylline clearance.

Children: 7–12 years (20–35 kg): Half or 1 tablet three or four times daily, preferably after food.

The difficulty of dividing the tablet accurately makes Nuelin unsuitable for use in children under the age of seven.

Nuelin tablets are soluble in water.

Contra-indications, warnings, etc
Contra-indications: Hypersensitivity to theophylline or other xanthines.

Warnings: Xanthines can potentiate hypokalaemia resulting from B_2-agonist therapy, steroids, diuretics and hypoxia. Particular caution is advised in severe asthma. It is recommended that serum potassium levels are monitored in such situations.

Precautions: Use with caution in patients with cardiac arrythmias, peptic ulcer, hyperthyroidism and severe hypertension.

Smoking and alcohol consumption may increase theophylline clearance and increased doses of theophylline are therefore required. In patients with cardiac failure, hepatic dysfunction/disease and fever the reverse is true and these patients may require a reduced dosage.

Epilepsy may become uncontrolled.

It is not recommended that the product be used concurrently with other preparations containing xanthine derivatives.

Interactions: Cimetidine, allopurinol, corticosteroids, frusemide, isoprenaline, oral contraceptives, thiobendazole, ciprofloxacin, erythromycin or other macrolide antibiotics delay the elimination of theophylline. A reduction of the theophylline dosage is recommended. Phenytoin, carbamazepine, barbiturates, lithium, rifampicin, sulphin pyrazone increase theophylline clearance and therefore the theophylline dosage may need to be increased.

Also see 'Warnings'.

Side-effects: Nausea or other gastric disturbances may occur rarely. Palpitations, headache, CNS stimulation and insomnia have been reported occasionally.

Overdosage

Symptoms: Characterised by nausea, vomiting and gastro-intestinal irritation. Tachycardia, convulsions and hypotension may also occur.

Treatment: Gastric lavage and general supportive measures (e.g. to maintain circulation, respiration and fluid and electrolyte balance) are recommended. Oral activated charcoal may reduce serum theophylline levels, whilst in severe cases charcoal haemoperfusion may be required.

Use in pregnancy: There is inadequate evidence of safety of the drug in human pregnancy but it has been in wide use for many years without apparent ill consequences; there is evidence of harmful effects in pregnancy in animals. Use in pregnancy only when there is no safer alternative and when the condition itself carries risks for the mother.

Theophylline is excreted in breast milk and has been shown to cause irritability in infants. It is therefore recommended that the mother nurse her infant just prior to taking her next dose, when plasma theophylline levels are expected to be low.

Pharmaceutical precautions Store in a cool, dry place.

Legal category P.

Package quantities Packs of 90 tablets (OP).

Further information Nil.

Product licence number 0068/0064R.

NUELIN* LIQUID

Presentation Clear, light brown, pleasantly flavoured liquid. Each 5 ml dose of Nuelin Liquid contains the equivalent of 60 mg Theophylline Hydrate BP as the sodium glycinate salt. It also contains the following inactive ingredients: sucrose; Sodium Butyl Hydroxybenzoate BP.

Uses Nuelin Liquid is indicated for the prophylaxis and treatment of reversible bronchospasm in asthma, bronchitis and emphysema. Nuelin in tablet form (microcrystalline theophylline 125 mg) is established as a highly effective bronchodilator. Nuelin Liquid is designed to offer comparable relief of bronchospasm with the same low incidence of side-effects, for patients who prefer a liquid presentation. Each 10 ml of Nuelin Liquid approximates to one 125 mg Nuelin tablet.

Dosage and administration *Adults:* 10–20 ml (two to four 5 ml spoonfuls) three or four times daily, preferably after food.

Children: 7–12 years: One-and-a-half or two 5 ml spoonfuls three or four times daily, preferably after food.

2–6 years: One or one-and-a-half 5 ml spoonfuls three or four times daily, preferably after food.

Under 2 years: Nuelin liquid is not recommended for children under 2 years of age.

Elderly: Elderly patients may require lower doses due to reduced theophylline clearance.

Contra-indications, warnings, etc
Contra-indications: Hypersensitivity to theophylline or other xanthines.

Warnings: Xanthines can potentiate hypokalaemia resulting from B_2-agonist therapy, steroids, diuretics and hypoxia. Particular caution is advised in severe asthma. It is recommended that serum potassium levels are monitored in such situations.

Precautions: Use with caution in patients with cardiac arrhythmias, peptic ulcer, and severe hypertension.

Smoking and alcohol consumption may increase theophylline clearance and increased doses of theophylline are therefore required. In patients with cardiac failure, hepatic dysfunction/disease and fever the reverse is true and these patients may require a reduced dosage.

Epilepsy may become uncontrolled.

It is not recommended that the product be used concurrently with other preparations containing xanthine derivatives.

Interactions: Cimetidine, allopurinol, corticosteroids, frusemide, isoprenaline, oral contraceptives, thiobendazole, ciprofloxacin, erythromycin or other macrolide antibiotics delay the elimination of theophylline. A reduction of the theophylline dosage is recommended. Phenytoin, carbamazepine, barbiturates, lithium, rifampicin, sulphin pyrazone increase theophylline clearance and therefore the theophylline dosage may need to be increased.

Also see 'Warnings'.

Side-effects: Nausea or other gastric disturbances may occur rarely. Palpitations, headache, CNS stimulation and insomnia have been reported occasionally.

Overdosage

Symptoms: Characterised by nausea, vomiting and gastro-intestinal irritation. Tachycardia, convulsions and hypotension may also occur.

Treatment: Gastric lavage and general supportive measures (e.g. to maintain circulation, respiration and fluid and electrolyte balance) are recommended. Oral activated charcoal may reduce serum theophylline levels, whilst in severe cases charcoal haemoperfusion may be required.

Use in pregnancy: There is inadequate evidence of safety of the drug in human pregnancy but it has been in wide use for many years without apparent ill consequences; there is evidence of harmful effects in pregnancy in animals. Use in pregnancy only when there is no safer alternative and when the condition itself carries risks for the mother.

Theophylline is excreted in breast milk and has been shown to cause irritability in infants. It is therefore recommended that the mother nurse her infant just prior to taking her next dose, when plasma theophylline levels are expected to be low.

Pharmaceutical precautions Store in a cool, dry place.

Legal category P.

Package quantities Bottles of 200 ml (OP).

Further information Each 5 ml spoonful of Nuelin Liquid contains 0.38 mEq sodium (8.7 mg Na).

Product licence number 0068/0084.

NUELIN* SA

Presentation *Nuelin SA:* White, biconvex, round tablets, 9 mm in diameter and marked NLS 175 on one side and RIKER on the other.

Each Nuelin SA tablet contains 175 mg anhydrous theophylline in a slow release formulation which gives a particularly smooth release of medicament over a prolonged period. It also contains the following inactive ingredient: lactose.

Nuelin SA-250: White, biconvex, round tablets with breakline, 11 mm in diameter and marked NLS 250 on one side and 3M RIKER on the other. Each Nuelin SA-250 tablet contains 250 mg anhydrous theophylline in a slow release formulation. It contains the same inactive ingredients as Nuelin SA.

Uses Nuelin SA and Nuelin SA-250 tablets are indicated for the prophylaxis and treatment of reversible bronchospasm in asthma, bronchitis and emphysema.

Because effective plasma levels are maintained for up to twelve hours from a single dose, less frequent dosing is required than with conventional theophylline preparations.

Dosage and administration *Nuelin SA: Adults:* One tablet twice daily, preferably after food, increasing to two tablets twice daily if necessary.

Children: 6 to 12 years: one tablet twice daily, preferably after food.

Nuelin SA-250: Adults: One tablet twice daily, preferably after food, increasing to two tablets twice daily if necessary.

Children: 6 to 12 years: Half or one tablet twice daily, preferably after food.

Nuelin SA and Nuelin SA-250 tablets are not recommended for children under six years.

Elderly: Elderly patients may require lower dosage due to reduced theophylline clearance.

Nuelin SA tablets should be swallowed whole and not crushed or chewed.

Nuelin SA-250 tablets are scored and may be halved but should not be crushed or chewed.

Contra-indications, warnings, etc
Contra-indications: Hypersensitivity to theophylline or other xanthines.

Warnings: Xanthines can potentiate hypokalaemia resulting from B_2-agonist therapy, steroids, diuretics and hypoxia. Particular caution is advised in severe asthma. It is recommended that serum potassium levels are monitored in such situations.

Precautions: In the case of an acute asthmatic attack in a patient receiving a sustained action theophylline preparation, great caution should be taken when administering intravenous aminophylline. Half the recommended loading dose of aminophylline (generally 6 mg/kg) should be given, i.e. 3 mg/kg, cautiously.

Use with caution in patients with cardiac arrhythmias, peptic ulcer and severe hypertension.

Smoking and alcohol consumption may increase theophylline clearance and increased doses of theophylline are therefore required. In patients with cardiac failure, hepatic dysfunction/disease and fever the reverse is true and these patients may require a reduced dosage.

Epilepsy may become uncontrolled.

It is not recommended that the product be used concurrently with other preparations containing xanthine derivatives.

Interactions: Cimetidine, allopurinol, corticosteroids, frusemide, isoprenaline, oral contraceptives, thiobendazole, ciprofloxacin, erythromycin or other macrolide antibiotics delay the elimination of theophylline. A reduction of the theophylline dosage is recommended. Phenytoin, carbamazepine, barbiturates, lithium, rifampicin, sulphin pyrazone increase theophylline clearance and therefore the theophylline dosage may need to be increased.

Also see 'Warnings'.

Side-effects: The side-effects commonly associated with xanthine derivatives such as nausea, gastric irritation, palpitations, headache, CNS stimulation and insomnia are much diminished when a sustained action preparation such as Nuelin SA is used. These side-effects are mild and infrequent when the plasma concentration is maintained at less than 20 microgrammes/ml.

Overdosage

Symptoms: Characterised by nausea, vomiting and gastro-intestinal irritation. Tachycardia, convulsions and hypotension may also occur.

Treatment: Gastric lavage and general supportive measures (e.g. to maintain circulation, respiration and fluid and electrolyte balance) are recommended. Oral activated charcoal may reduce serum theophylline levels, whilst in severe cases charcoal haemoperfusion may be required.

Use in pregnancy: There is inadequate evidence of safety of the drug in human pregnancy but it has been in wide use for many years without apparent ill consequence; there is evidence of harmful effects in animals. Use in pregnancy only when there is no safer alternative and when the condition itself carries risks for the mother.

Theophylline is excreted in breast milk and has been shown to cause irritability in infants. As it is recommended that the mother nurse her infant just prior to taking her next dose when theophylline levels are expected to be low, a non-sustained release form such as Nuelin is therefore preferable for nursing mothers.

Pharmaceutical precautions Store in a cool, dry place.

Legal category P.

Package quantities *Nuelin SA:* Packs of 60 tablets (OP).
Nuelin SA-250: Packs of 60 tablets (OP).

Further information Nil.

Product licence numbers

Nuelin SA	0068/0092
Nuelin SA-250	0068/0093

NUMOTAC*

Presentation White to creamy-white, circular biconvex tablets 7.14 mm diameter, marked 'NT' on one side and RIKER on the other. Each tablet contains Isoetharine Hydrochloride USP 10 mg in a porous plastic matrix. It also contains the following inactive ingredient: Sodium Metabisulphite BP.

Uses Numotac is indicated for the relief of bronchospasm in chronic bronchitis, bronchial asthma and pulmonary emphysema.

Isoetharine is a sympathomimetic amine with a marked bronchodilator action. It is rapidly absorbed from the gastro-intestinal tract and has a relatively fast onset of action.

A notable feature of isoetharine is that at normal dosage levels it acts selectively on the β_2-receptors of bronchial muscle and has little effect on the β_1 cardiac receptors. Cardiac side-effects are therefore reduced to negligible levels, and occur only at higher doses or in hypersensitive patients.

Numotac contains isoetharine hydrochloride embedded in a porous plastic matrix. By this means, the release of isoetharine is controlled, giving Numotac a duration of action of between four and six hours. This formulation reduces the possibility of side-effects associated with uneven blood levels.

Dosage and administration *Adults:* One or two tablets three or four times daily.

For patients who have not previously been prescribed oral bronchodilator therapy or who are known to be sensitive to the action of sympathomimetic amines, treatment should be started on the lower dosages (3 or 4 tablets daily). Dosage may then be gradually adjusted upwards, if necessary, to achieve optimum response. At high doses, cardiac and CNS effects begin to occur.

Clinical and pharmacological studies have shown that 'Numotac' acts for between four and six hours. In susceptible patients administration at shorter intervals may give rise to side-effects. When this occurs dosage should be adjusted accordingly.

Children: The 10 mg tablet should not be broken, and this dose is not recommended for children aged 12 years or under.

Elderly: Elderly patients may require a reduced dosage due to slower metabolism and their greater sensitivity to sympathomimetic agents.

Patients with diabetes, hepatic or renal dysfunction: Diabetic patients using isoetharine should be closely monitored to ensure that the control of diabetes is re-established. Formal studies on the use of isoetharine in patients with hepatic or renal dysfunction are not available.

Contra-indications, warnings, etc

Side-effects: Cardiovascular effects include vasodilatation, tachycardia, palpitation and lightheadedness whilst CNS effects are fine tremor, nervousness, headache and insomnia. Susceptibility to these reactions is increased by hypoxia and in patients receiving other concurrent sympathomimentic drugs.

Rebound (paradoxical) bronchoconstriction has been reported following repeated or excessive use, although this is rare. One of the excipients is sodium metabisulphite which can give rise to nausea, diarrhoea, acute asthma, anaphylaxis and loss of consciousness in asthmatic patients.

Contra-indications: The use of Numotac is contra-indicated in thyrotoxicosis.

Cautions: Numotac should be used with great caution in the presence of caridiac disease, or hypertension.

Interactions: Except in patients with ischaemic heart disease, no interactions of significance have been reported with anaesthetic agents and isoetharine is therefore suitable for use before and after surgery. However, its use with digoxin is contra-indicated as it may provoke or worsen ventricular arrhythmias, and it should not be used with other sympathomimetic aerosols. Interactions have been reported with beta-blockers which cause a risk of hypertension and with nitrates and antihypertensive agents where there is a risk of hypotension. The effects of isoetharine may be enhanced by the concomitant administration of xanthines.

Pregnancy: There is no evidence as to the drug safety in human pregnancy nor is there evidence from animal work that it is free from hazard. Avoid in pregnancy unless there is no safer treatment. The use of the drug near the term could delay the onset of labour. There is no information on whether isoetharine is excreted in breast milk.

Overdosage: Symptoms: Chest pain, palpitation, nausea, hypotension, dizziness, headache, restlessness, tremor and weakness.

Treatment: General symptomatic treatment. If the drug

has recently been taken, the stomach should be emptied by gastric lavage, using a tube greater than 8 mm in diameter. Cautious use of sedatives should be considered if potential benefits exceed their risk.

Pharmaceutical precautions Store in a cool, dry place.

Legal category POM.

Package quantities Bottles of 90 tablets (OP).

Further information Nil.

Product licence number 0068/5054R.

PULMADIL* INHALER
PULMADIL* AUTO

Presentation Pulmadil Inhaler is a pressurised aerosol for bronchodilator inhalation therapy. The vial contains a suspension of rimiterol hydrobromide 10 mg/ml in aerosol propellant and delivers to the patient 300 measured doses each containing 200 micrograms rimiterol hydrobromide. The vial contains the following inactive ingredients: sorbitan trioleate; propellants 11, 12 and 114.

Pulmadil Auto is a breath-actuated, pressurised aerosol for bronchodilator inhalation therapy. The vial contains a suspension of rimiterol hydrobromide 10 mg/ml in aerosol propellent and delivers to the patient 300 measured doses each containing 200 micrograms rimiterol hydrobromide. The vial contains the same inactive ingredients as Pulmadil Inhaler.

Uses Pulmadil is indicated for the relief of bronchospasm in bronchial asthma and chronic bronchitis.

Rimiterol hydrobromide is a sympathomimetic agent which has a rapid and highly selective action on β_2-adrenergic receptors in bronchial muscle. At therapeutic dose levels it has virtually no effect on β_1-adrenergic receptors. Cardiac stimulation is therefore reduced to negligible levels and occurs only at high doses or in hypersensitive patients. The plasma half life of rimiterol in man is less than five minutes.

Dosage and administration One to three puffs should provide relief in most cases. This treatment dose should not be repeated in less than thirty minutes. No more than eight treatments should be taken in any 24-hour period.

Children: Pulmadil Inhaler and Pulmadil Auto should be administered to children only under the supervision of a responsible adult.

Elderly: No special dosage recommendations are made for elderly patients.

Instructions for use: Pulmadil Inhaler: With the dust cap removed, Pulmadil Inhaler should be shaken to disperse the particles of medicament in the propellent.

The patient shold breathe out gently and then place the mouthpiece in the mouth with the lips closed firmly around it.

As soon as the patient starts to breathe in, the vial should be pressed firmly down into the adapter. This releases a dose. The adapter should now be taken from the mouth and the breath held for as long as possible to avoid exhalation of particles of medicament.

Before taking a further inhalation, the patient should wait at least one minute to allow the full effect of the first to become apparent.

Pulmadil Auto: To obtain full benefit from Pulmadil Auto the patient should follow these simple steps:

1. Shake the unit with the mouthpiece cover closed. Then open the mouthpiece cover downwards.
2. Breathe out as much as possible, then close the lips tightly round the mouthpiece. Keep the teeth apart and the tongue flat (to allow the flow of medicament into the lungs).
3. Suck in air through the mouthpiece as rapidly and deeply as possible. When the unit operates a click will be heard. *Continue to breathe in after the click* until the lungs are full. Hold the breath for a few seconds. Then take the inhaler away from the mouth and breathe out slowly through pursed lips. If no click is heard, repeat step 3, making sure that the lips are well sealed round the mouthpiece.
4. *The unit must be reset before another dose can be taken,* by closing the mouthpiece cover upwards. It is important to keep the cover closed when it is not in use.

Contra-indications, warnings, etc
Contra-indications: There are no contra-indications to inhaled Pulmadil therapy.

Warnings: Potentially serious hypokalaemia has been reported in patients taking B_2-agonist therapy. Hypokalaemia may also occur in hypoxic patients and those treated with xanthine derivatives, steroids, diuretics and long-term laxatives. Extra care should therefore be taken if B_2-agonists are used in these groups of patients and serum potassium levels should be monitored.

Precautions: Administer cautiously to patients with thyrotoxicosis. The patient should be advised to seek medical advice if the treatment ceases to be effective.

Interactions: See 'Warnings'.

Side-effects: Side-effects such as headache and rash have been reported infrequently and are similar to those reactions recorded with other B_2-agonists. Potentially serious hypokalaemia has been reported in patients taking B_2-agonist therapy.

Overdosage: As rimiterol is rapidly eliminated from the blood, it carries little risk of accumulation even if used excessively. No cases of overdosage have been reported and the following guidance is based on theoretical considerations.

Symptoms: The blood pressure may fall and cause dizziness and fainting. Anxiety, tremor and tachycardia may be present.

Treatment: A cardioselective beta-blocking agent should be administered, but these should be used with caution in patients with a history of bronchospasm.

Use in pregnancy: There is inadequate evidence of safety of the drug in human pregnancy but it has been in wide use for many years without apparent ill consequence, animal studies having shown no hazard.

It is very unlikely that sufficient drug will be excreted in the breast milk to affect the infant.

Pharmaceutical precautions Pulmadil Inhaler and Pulmadil Auto should be stored in a cool place, protected from frost and direct sunlight.

As the Pulmadil vial is pressurised, no attempt should be made to puncture or dispose of it by burning.

The shelf-life of both Pulmadil preparations is three years.

Legal category POM.

Package quantities Pulmadil Inhaler is supplied as a complete standard pack, comprising a vial delivering 300 doses and an adapter (OP).

Pulmadil Auto is supplied as a complete unit for which replacement cartridges are available. Each cartridge delivers 300 doses (OP).

Further information
Excessive use in asthmatics: Excessive use of any bronchodilator aerosol can indicate lack of response. This is a grave sign suggestive of status asthmaticus. It is recommended that 100 mg of hydrocortisone be given intravenously immediately and the patient admitted to hospital without delay.

Product licence number 0068/0030R.

RIKOSPRAY* BALSAM

Presentation Brown solution in a pressurised glass bottle. Pressurised bottle contains:

Dissolved solids of Benzoin BP (equivalent to Sumatra Benzoin BP 12.5% w/w)	9% w/w
Prepared Storax BP	2.5% w/w

It also contains the following inactive ingredients:

Solvent and aerosol propellants 11 and 12 to 100% w/w.

Uses Rikospray Balsam is indicated in all conditions where tincture of benzoin is, or would be, applied topically, e.g. under adhesive plaster dressings; in colostomy and ileostomy hygiene.

Rikospray Balsam delivers benzoin and storax to the skin in a thin transparent film which is protective and non-irritant.

Benzoin and storax are naturally occurring balsamic oleoresins containing mixtures of resins and benzoic and cinnamic acids. The natural resins provide protection against the physical and chemical irritation of adhesive plaster; against skin maceration in ileostomy and colostomy.

The benzoin and cinnamic acid compounds are mild antiseptics.

Administration *Directions for use:* Shake the bottle. The affected part should be sprayed sparingly, keeping the nozzle about 15 to 20 cm from the skin. To obtain an adequate and evenly distributed film, the bottle should be kept moving during application.

Contra-indications, warnings, etc
Contra-indications: Rikospray Balsam should not be applied over areas of obvious infection. It is not intended for use by inhalation.

Precautions: None.

Interactions: There are no known interactions with Rikospray Balsam therapy.

Side-effects: Skin sensitisation may occur.

Overdosage: Not applicable.

Use in pregnancy: There is inadequate evidence of the safety of Rikospray Balsam in human pregnancy but it has been in wide use for many years without apparent ill consequence. Excretion in breast milk, if any, is expected to be low to affect the infant.

Pharmaceutical precautions As the Rikospray Balsam bottle is pressurised, it should not be punctured, incinerated or exposed to heat, including the sun, even when empty.

Rikospray Balsam is inflammable and should not be used near a fire or flame.

To clear a blocked valve, invert bottle and spray in this position for 2–3 seconds.

Legal category GSL.

Package quantities Bottles of 50 g (OP).

Further information For external use only.

Product licence number 0068/5028R.

RIKOSPRAY* SILICONE

Presentation White suspension in a pressurised aerosol container. The application of Rikospray Silicone delivered to the skin contains:

Aluminium dihydroxyallantoinate	0.5% w/w
Dimethicone 1,000 BP to	100%

It also contains the following inactive ingredients: Cetylpyridinium Chloride BP, propellants 11 and 12.

Uses Rikospray Silicone is indicated in: the prevention and treatment of bedsores, particularly in incontinent patients; the prevention and treatment of napkin rash; colostomy hygiene.

Rikospray Silicone delivers a spray which coats the skin with a film of virtually 100% silicone. The silicone compounds are well known for their water-repellent and protective properties. The protective film is instantly impervious to water, urine or faeces.

Aluminium dihydroxyallantoinate has astringent and healing properties and is also a mild antiperspirant. No irritant or sensitising properties have been reported from its use.

Administration *Directions for use:* Before applying Rikospray Silicone, the affected area should be washed thoroughly and the skin dried carefully.

The canister should be shaken before use, and then held about 15 to 20 cm from the skin. Rikospray Silicone should be applied sparingly to cover the entire area. This should be done twice daily for at least one week, then application once daily will often be sufficient.

Contra-indications, warnings, etc
Contra-indications: None.

Precautions: None.

Interactions: There are no known interactions with Rikospray Silicone therapy.

Side-effects: Skin irritation or sensitisation, although theoretically possible, have not been reported.

Overdosage: Not applicable.

Use in pregnancy: There is inadequate evidence of the safety of Rikospray Silicone in human pregnancy but it has been in wide use for many years without apparent ill consequence. Excretion in breast milk, if any, is expected to be too low to affect the infant.

Pharmaceutical precautions The shelf life of Rikospray Silicone is five years.

As the Rikospray Silicone canister is pressurised, it should not be punctured, incinerated or exposed to heat, including the sun, even when empty.

Legal category GSL.

Package quantities Canisters of 200 g (OP).

Further information As Silicone can make some surfaces slippery, care should be taken to avoid the spray coming into contact with the floor. For external use only.

Product licence number 0068/5080R.

SALBULIN* INHALER

Presentation Salbulin Inhaler is a pressurised aerosol for bronchodilator inhalation therapy. It delivers to the patient 200 measured doses each containing 100 micrograms Salbutamol BP. Each dose contains the following inactive ingredients: Sorbitan trioleate; propellants 11 and 12.

Uses Salbulin Inhaler is indicated for the treatment and prophylaxis of bronchial asthma and for the treatment of reversible airways obstruction associated with bronchitis and emphysema. It is also suitable for routine maintenance therapy in chronic asthma and chronic bronchitis, because of its prolonged action. Salbulin Inhaler may be used to relieve attacks of acute dyspnoea and may also be taken prophylactically before exertion or to prevent exercise-induced asthma. It is suitable for treating bronchospasm in patients with co-existing heart disease or hypertension, including those taking beta-blocking drugs, because of its selective action on the bronchial receptors and lack of effects on the cardiovascular system. Salbutamol is a sympathomimetic agent which has a highly selective action on beta-adrenergic receptors in bronchial muscle. At therapeutic levels it has little activity on cardiac receptors.

Dosage and administration
Adults: For the relief of acute bronchospasm and for managing intermittent episodes of asthma: one or two inhalations as a single dose; for chronic maintenance or prophylactic therapy: two inhalations, three or four times daily; for prevention of exercise-induced bronchospasm: two inhalations before exertion.

Children: For the relief of acute bronchospasm, management of episodic asthma or before exercise: one inhalation; for routine maintenance or prophylaxis: one inhalation three or four times a day, increasing if necessary to two inhalations three or four times daily.

Elderly: The dosage is the same as for other adults.

Contra-indications, warnings, etc
Contra-indications: There are no contra-indications to *Salbulin* Inhaler therapy.

Warnings: Potentially serious hypokalaemia has been reported in patients taking B_2-agonist therapy. Hypokalaemia may also occur in hypoxic patients and those treated with xanthine derivatives, steroids, diuretics and long-term laxatives. Extra care should therefore be taken if B_2-agonists are used in these groups of patients and serum potassium levels should be monitored.

Precautions: Administer cautiously to patients with thyrotoxicosis. The patient should be advised to seek medical advice if the treatment ceases to be effective.

Side-effects: Mild tremor, headache and transient muscle cramps may rarely occur. Potentially serious hypokalaemia has been reported in patients taking B_2-agonist therapy.

Overdosage: Treatment: A cardioselective beta-blocking agent should be administered, but these should be used with caution in patients with a history of bronchospasm.

Use in pregnancy: The use of inhaled salbutamol during the first trimester of pregnancy is not recommended unless the clinical need outweighs the risk.

Pharmaceutical precautions Salbulin Inhaler should be stored in a cool place, protected from frost and direct sunlight. As the vial is pressurised, no attempt should be made to puncture or dispose of it by burning.

Legal category POM.

Package quantities Each canister provides 200 inhalations (OP).

Further information Salbulin Inhaler is not contra-indicated in patients under treatment with MAOIs (monoamine oxidase inhibitors). It does not cause difficulty in micturition as salbutamol does not stimulate alpha-adrenoceptors.

Product licence number 68/0108.

TAMBOCOR*

Presentation *Tambocor tablets:* White, circular, biconvex tablets, 8.5 mm in diameter marked RIKER on one side and TR 100 with a break-line on the other. Each tablet contains flecainide acetate 100 mg.

Tambocor injection: Each ampoule contains 15 ml of a solution of flecainide acetate 10 mg/ml, for intravenous use only. It also contains the following inactive ingredients: Sodium Acetate PhEur; Glacial Acetic Acid BP.

Uses Tambocor is a Class I anti-arrhythmic (local anaesthetic) agent for the treatment of the conditions listed below. It is recommended that treatment with Tambocor should be initiated in hospitals.

Tambocor slows conduction through the heart. Its actions may be reflected in the ECG by prolongation of the PR interval and widening of the QRS complex. The effect on the JT interval is insignificant.

Indications

Tablets: Tambocor tablets are indicated for:

(a) AV nodal reciprocating tachycardia; Wolff-Parkinson-White Syndrome and similar conditions with accessory pathway and anterograde or retrograde conduction.
(b) Symptomatic sustained ventricular tachycardia.
(c) Premature ventricular contractions and/or non-sustained ventricular tachycardia which are causing disabling symptoms, where these are resistant to other therapy or when other treatment has not been tolerated.

Tambocor tablets can be used for the maintenance of normal rhythm following conversion by other means.

Injection: Tambocor injection is indicated when rapid control or short term prophylaxis of the following arrhythmias is the main clinical requirement:

(a) Ventricular tachyarrhythmias where these are resistant to other treatment.
(b) AV nodal reciprocating tachycardia; Wolff-Parkinson-White Syndrome and similar conditions with accessory pathway and anterograde or retrograde conduction.

Dosage and administration *Tablets: Adults:* The recommended starting dosage is one tablet twice daily (200 mg). The maximum daily dose is 400 mg. This is normally reserved for patients of large build or where rapid control of the arrhythmia is required. After 3–5 days it is recommended that the dosage be progressively adjusted to the lowest level which maintains control of the arrhythmia. It may be possible to reduce dosage during long-term treatment.

Children: Tambocor is not recommended in children under 12, as there is insufficient evidence of its use in this age group.

Elderly patients: The rate of flecainide elimination from plasma may be reduced in elderly people. An initial dose of one tablet twice daily will usually be adequate, and it may well be possible to reduce this dose for maintenance therapy after one week.

Injection:

a) *Bolus injection:* Tambocor can be given in an emergency or for rapid effect by a slow injection of 2 mg/kg over not less than ten minutes, or in divided doses. If preferred the dose may be diluted with 5% dextrose and given as a mini-infusion.
Continuous ECG monitoring is recommended in all patients receiving the bolus dose. The injection should be stopped when there is control of the arrythmia.
It is recommended that Tambocor should be administered more slowly to patients in sustained ventricular tachycardia with careful monitoring of the electrocardiogram. Similar caution should apply to patients with a history of cardiac failure, who may become decompensated during the administration. For such patients it is recommended that the initial dose is given over 30 minutes.
The maximum recommended bolus dose is 150 mg.

b) *Intravenous infusion:* When prolonged parenteral administration is required, it is recommended that therapy is initiated by slow injection of 2 mg/kg over 30 minutes as above and continued by intravenous infusion at the following rates:
First hour: 1.5 mg/kg per hour. *Second and later hours:* 0.1–0.25 mg/kg per hour.
It is recommended that the infusion duration should not exceed 24 hours. However, where this is considered necessary, or for patients receiving the upper end of the dose range, plasma level monitoring is strongly recommended. The maximum cumulative dose given in the first 24 hours should not exceed 600 mg.
In patients with severe renal impairment (creatinine clearance of less than 35 ml/min/1.73 sq m), each of the above dosage recommendations should be reduced by half.
Transition to oral dosing should be accomplished as soon as possible by stopping the infusion and administering the first required oral dose.
Oral maintenance is then continued as indicated in the relevant oral dosage instructions.

Plasma levels: Based on PVC suppression, it appears that plasma levels of 200–1000 ng/ml may be needed to obtain the maximum therapeutic effect. Plasma levels above 700–1000 ng/ml are associated with increased likelihood of adverse experiences.

Dosage in impaired renal function: In patients with significant renal impairment (creatinine clearance of 35 ml/min/1.73 sq. m. or less) the maximum initial dosage should be 100 mg daily (or 50 mg twice daily). When used in such patients, frequent plasma level monitoring is strongly recommended.

Contra-indications, warnings, etc

Contra-indications: Tambocor is contra-indicated in cardiac failure, and in patients with a history of myocardial infarction who have either asymptomatic ventricular ectopics or asymptomatic non-sustained ventricular tachycardia.

Unless pacing rescue is available, Tambocor should not be given to patients with sinus node dysfunction, atrial conduction defects, second degree or greater atrioventricular block, bundle branch block or distal block.

Precautions: Electrolyte disturbances should be corrected before using Tambocor.

Since flecainide elimination from the plasma can be markedly slower in patients with significant hepatic impairment, flecainide should not be used in such patients unless the potential benefits clearly outweigh the risks. Plasma level monitoring is strongly recommended in these circumstances.

Tambocor is known to increase endocardial pacing thresholds – ie. to decrease endocardial pacing sensitivity. This effect is reversible and is more marked on the acute pacing threshold than on the chronic. Tambocor should thus be used with caution in all patients with permanent pacemakers or temporary pacing electrodes, and should not be administered to patients with existing poor thresholds or non-programmable pacemakers unless suitable pacing rescue is available.

Generally, a doubling of either pulse width or current is sufficient to regain capture, but it may be difficult to obtain ventricular thresholds less than 1 Volt at initial implantation in the presence of Tambocor.

The minor negative inotropic effect of flecainide may assume importance in patients predisposed to cardiac failure. Difficulty has been experienced in defibrillating some patients. Most of the cases reported had pre-existing heart disease with cardiac enlargement, a history of myocardial infarction, arterio-sclerotic heart disease and cardiac failure.

In a large scale, placebo-controlled clinical trial in post-myocardial infarction patients with asymptomatic ventricular arrhythmia, oral flecainide was associated with a 2.2 fold higher incidence of mortality or non-fatal cardiac arrest as compared with its matching placebo. In that same study, an even higher incidence of mortality was observed in flecainide-treated patients with more than one myocardial infarction. Comparable placebo-controlled clinical trials have not been done to determine if flecainide is associated with higher risk of mortality in other patient groups.

Use in Pregnancy and Lactation: There is no evidence as to drug safety in human pregnancy.

In New Zealand White rabbits high doses of flecainide caused some foetal abnormalities, but these effects were not seen in Dutch Belted rabbits or rats. The relevance of these findings to humans has not been established.

The possibility of flecainide being excreted in milk should be considered.

Drug interactions: Use of flecainide with other Class I antiarrhythmics is not recommended. Treatment with Tambocor is compatible with use of oral anticoagulants. Flecainide can cause the plasma digoxin level to rise by about 15%, which is unlikely to be of clinical significance for patients with plasma levels in the therapeutic range. It is recommended that the digoxin plasma level in digitalised patients should be measured not less than six hours after any digoxin dose, before or after administration of flecainide. The possibility of additive negative inotropic effects of beta-blockers and other cardiac depressants with flecainide should be recognised.

Limited data in patients receiving known enzyme inducers (phenytoin, phenobarbital, carbamazepine) indicate only a 30% increase in the rate of flecainide elimination. In healthy subjects receiving cimetidine (1 g daily) for one week, plasma flecainide levels increased by about 30% and the half-life by about 10%.

When flecainide is given in the presence of amiodarone, the usual flecainide dosage should be reduced by 50% and the patient monitored closely for adverse effects. Plasma level monitoring is strongly recommended in these circumstances.

Side-effects: Most commonly giddiness, dizziness and lightheadedness. Visual disturbances, such as double vision and blurring of vision, may occur. More rarely nausea and vomiting have been reported. These effects are usually transient and disappear upon continuing or reducing the dosage.

Pro-arrhythmic effects occur but are most likely in patients with structural heart disease and/or significant left ventricular impairment.

A number of cases of elevated liver enzymes and jaundice have been reported in association with Tambocor treatment. So far this has always been reversible on stopping treatment.

Overdosage: No specific antidote is known. There is no known way of rapidly removing flecainide from the system, but forced acid diuresis may theoretically be helpful. Neither dialysis nor haemoperfusion are helpful and injections of anticholinergics are not recommended. Treatment may include therapy with an inotropic agent, intravenous calcium, giving circulatory assistance (e.g. balloon pumping) mechanically assisting respiration, or temporarily inserting a transvenous pacemaker if there are severe conduction disturbances or the patient's left ventricular function is otherwise compromised.

Pharmaceutical precautions

Storage: Tambocor tablets should be stored in a cool, dry place. Tambocor injection should be protected from light.

Dilution: When necessary Tambocor injection should be diluted with, or injected into, sterile solutions of 5% dextrose. If chloride containing solutions, such as sodium chloride or Ringer's lactate are used, the injection should be added to a volume of not less than 500 ml, otherwise a precipitate will form.

Legal category POM.

Package quantities *Tablets* – packs of 60 tablets (OP).
Injection – 5 × 15 ml ampoules.

Further information Nil.

Product licence numbers
Tablets 0068/0102
Injection 0068/0101

THEODROX*

Presentation White to creamy-white, circular, biconvex tablets, 12.0 mm diameter, marked TX on one side and RIKER on the other. Each tablet contains Dried Aluminium Hydroxide Gel BP 260 mg and Aminophylline BP 195 mg.

Uses Theodrox is indicated in the prophylaxis of reversible bronchospasm in asthma and chronic bronchitis.

Aminophylline is a combination of theophylline and ethylenediamine. It has properties very similar to those of theophylline but is more soluble. It relaxes smooth muscle and relieves bronchial spasm. In common with other xanthine compounds, aminophylline has a diuretic action.

Administered orally, aminophylline can cause gastric irritation. However, in Theodrox this possibility is reduced by the simultaneous administration of aluminium hydroxide gel, which counteracts gastric acidity and retards the breakdown of aminophylline to theophylline in the stomach. By this means, larger doses of aminophylline can be given with less risk of side-effects such as nausea and vomiting.

Dosage and administration

Adults: Dosage optimisation should be achieved by step-wise increments starting with 1 tablet every 8 hours and increasing to a maximum of 1–2 tablets every 6–8 hours.

Children: Theodrox is not recommended for children.

Elderly: Elderly patients may require a reduced dosage due to slower drug clearance.

Plasma level monitoring is recommended in all patients to achieve optimum plasma concentrations in the therapeutic range of 10–20 micrograms/ml (22–44 μmol/l).

Contra-indications, warnings, etc

Contra-indications: There are no contra-indications to Theodrox therapy.

Warnings: Xanthines can potentiate hypokalaemia resulting from B_2-agonist therapy, steroids, diuretics and hypoxia. Particular caution is advised in severe asthma. It is recommended that serum potassium levels are monitored in such situations.

Precautions: Theodrox should be administered with caution to patients with peptic ulcer, hepatic and cardiac disease.

Interactions: Cimetidine, erythromycin or other macrolide antibiotics delay the elimination of aminophylline. A reduction of aminophylline dosage is recommended. Phenytoin increases aminophylline clearance. It is not recommended that the product be used concurrently with sympathomimetic agents or with other preparations containing xanthine derivatives.

Aluminium hydroxide may form complexes with certain antibiotics (tetracyclines); concurrent administration may result in reduced absorption of the antibiotic.

Also see 'Warnings'.

Side-effects: Occasionally, nausea or vomiting or dyspepsia may occur in some patients. In addition, dizziness, lightheadedness, headache, insomnia, tremor and/or agitation are possible side-effects, as well as palpitation, tachycardia, flushing and arrhythmia.

Overdosage: Symptoms: Epigastric pain, vomiting, diarrhoea, haematemesis, hyper-reflexia, fasciculations, convulsions, hypertension, shock, tachypnoea, hyperthermia and collapse.

Pregnancy and breastfeeding: There is inadequate evidence of safety of aminophylline and aluminium hydroxide in human pregnancy but both have been in wide use for many years without apparent ill consequence. There is evidence of harmful effects of aminophylline in pregnancy in animals. Use in pregnancy only when there is no safer alternative.

Aminophylline is excreted in breast milk and has been shown to cause irritability in infants. It is recommended that the mother nurse her infant immediately prior to taking her next dose when plasma levels are expected to be low.

Treatment: If necessary, the stomach should be emptied by aspiration and lavage. The patient shold be sedated and plasma levels monitored. The use of iv fluids is recommended.

Oral activated charcoal may reduce serum theophylline levels, whilst in severe cases charcoal haemoperfusion may be required. The use of sympathomimetic agents is not recommended.

Pharmaceutical precautions Store in a cool, dry place.

Legal category P.

Package quantities Bottles of 120 tablets (OP).

Further information Nil.

Product licence number 0068/5011R.

TITRALAC*

Presentation White, circular, bi-convex tablets, 11.2 mm in diameter, marked 'TC' on one side and 'RIKER' on the other. Each tablet contains Calcium Carbonate BP 420 mg and Glycine BP 180 mg.

Uses Titralac is indicated as a calcium supplement or phosphate binding agent in the management of renal failure.

Dosage and administration As calcium supplement: According to the requirements of the patient. Each Titralac tablet contains 4.2 mmol (168 mg) calcium.

As phosphate binding agent: According to the requirements of the patient. Each Titralac tablet binds, in vitro, about 340 mg phosphate.

These dosage instructions apply to adults, elderly and children.

Titralac tablets may be chewed, allowed to dissolve in the mouth or swallowed whole as desired.

Contra-indications, warnings, etc

Side-effects: Hypercalcaemia and hypophosphataemia are possible complications of vigorous therapy.

Symptoms of hypercalcaemia include anorexia, nausea, vomiting, constipation, abdominal pain, muscle weakness, thirst, polyuria, drowsiness, confusion, and cardiac arrhythmias leading to cardiac arrest.

Symptoms of hypophosphataemia include weakness, paraesthesia, seizures and coma.

Hypophosphataemic red cell dysfunction impairs effective oxygen delivery to the periphery.

Precautions: Serum phosphate levels should be monitored in all patients receiving phosphate binders, to prevent the development of a phosphate depletion syndrome.

In long-term treatment, serum and urinary calcium levels should be monitored to prevent hypercalcaemia occurring. Serum albumin, magnesium and potassisum levels should also be monitored to ensure Ca++/PO4--- homeostasis, particularly following dialysis.

Sarcoidosis may increase the risk of hypercalcaemia.

Pregnancy and lactation: Epidemiological studies have shown no increase in the teratogenic hazard to the foetus if used in the usual doses recommended for calcium supplementation. The safety of high doses of calcium, however, is not established.

Although some supplemental calcium may be excreted in breast milk, the concentration is not sufficient to produce an adverse effect on the neonate and problems in humans have not been documented.

Contra-indications: Patients with hypophosphataemia, hypercalcaemia or hypercalciuria.

Interactions: Concurrent administration of 1,25-dihydroxycholecalciferol or thiazides increases the risk of hypercalcaemia. There is a risk of digoxin toxicity if hypercalcaemia develops in well-digitalised patients. Corticosteroids may interfere with calcium absorption while calcium interferes with absorption of tetracyclines.

Overdosage: Acute hypercalcaemia may result and this may be aggravated by dehydration. Management of acute hypercalcaemia should be along standard recommendations and should include full hydration, monitoring of other electrolytes, judicious use of frusemide and other symptomatic and supportive measures. ECG monitoring of cardiac rhythm is particularly advisable in patients with renal failure.

Pharmaceutical precautions Store in a cool, dry place.

Legal category GSL.

Package quantities Bottles of 180 tablets (OP).

Further information Nil.

Product licence number 0068/5004R.

TRIBIOTIC* SPRAY

Presentation Pressurised aerosol canister contains creamy-white suspension of:

Neomycin Sulphate BP	500,000 units
Bacitracin Zinc BP	10,000 units
Polymyxin B Sulphate BP	150,000 units

It contains the following inactive ingredients: sorbitan trioleate; propellants 11, 12 and 114 to 110 g.

The contents of the canister are sterile.

Uses Tribiotic Spray is indicated for the prevention and control of bacterial infection in surgery, at any stage of surgical procedures.

Because neomycin is well absorbed from broken or inflamed skin, the spray should not be used on large denuded areas, including those due to burns, sunburn, chronic ulcers and chronic inflammatory dermatoses.

Also, it is not indicated for pruritis and minor skin disorders.

The combination of neomycin, bacitracin and polymyxin B in Tribiotic Spray provides an almost complete spectrum of activity against the common pathogenic organisms likely to occur in wounds and infected skin conditions. It provides a quick non-touch application; the antibiotic powders are micronised during manufacture to produce a fine dry spray which is evenly distributed over the skin.

Neomycin is a broad-spectrum antibiotic, primarily bactericidal rather than bacteriostatic. It is not inactivated by pus, exudates, gastro-intestinal secretions, bacterial growth products or enzymes. Hypersensitivity reactions are uncommon.

Bacitracin is effective against most Gram-positive organisms. However, it is not destroyed by Gram-negative bacteria and can be of value in the control of mixed infections.

Polymyxin B is selectively bactericidal to Gram-negative bacteria (particularly *Pseudomonas aeruginosa, Escherichia coli, Aerobacter aerogenes, Haemophilus influenzae*, Friedlander's bacillus and the dysentery group) but exerts no action on *Proteus*. Topical applications of polymyxin B have been found effective in the prophylaxis and treatment of infection in granulating surfaces.

Dosage and administration *Directions for use:* The canister should be shaken before and between applications, and held 15 to 25 cm from the skin.

The spray should be applied sparingly to cover the affected area and should be kept clear of the eyes.

Important: During use, the canister should not be inverted or inclined at an angle greater than 45°.

Application of Tribiotic Spray should be limited in adults to a maximum of one canister per day for no more than seven days. Patients with renal impairment are particularly vulnerable to neomycin ototoxicity and the dose should be appropriately reduced.

Dosage should not exceed 15 mg neomycin/kg body weight/day in children. Each 1 second spray contains approximately 15 mg neomycin.

Greater caution should be exercised when treating infants.

Occasionally, blockage may occur from agglomeration of the powder in the outlet of the actuating button. This can easily be cleared with a sterile hypodermic needle (No. 15–17).

Elderly: Use with caution in the elderly as they are more susceptible to ototoxicity, particularly if renal insufficiency is present.

Use in pregnancy: Due to lack of sufficient information, the product should not be administered during the first trimester of pregnancy or during lactation unless the clinical need outweighs the possible risk.

Contra-indications, warnings, etc
Contra-indications: Because of the risk of systemic absorption Tribiotic Spray is not recommended for the treatment of burns. The only other contra-indication is allergic sensitivity to one or more of the constituents.

Precautions: The quantity of neomycin absorbed after topical administration is usually small. However, if high doses are applied, sufficient absorption can occur to cause permanent loss of hearing; the maximum recommended dose should not therefore be exceeded. Nephrotoxicity, resulting in ototoxicity may also occur. Care should be taken in patients with a hearing loss.

The concurrent use with other aminoglycoside antibiotics is not recommended and caution should be exercised in case of cross hypersensitivity to other aminoglycoside antibiotics.

The possibility of resistant organisms should be considered.

Neomycin has inherent neuromuscular blocking activity and may potentiate the action of similar agents, causing respiratory depression.

Overdosage: Overdosage only occurs with chronic use rather than acute.

Pharmaceutical precautions
Storage: Store in a cool place. The shelf-life of Tribiotic Spray is three years.

Container: As the Tribiotic Spray canister is pressurised, it should not be punctured, incinerated or exposed to heat, including the sun, even when empty.

Legal category POM.

Package quantities Canister of 110 g (OP).

Further information Nil.

Product licence number 0068/5075R.

VIDENE* POWDER

Presentation Videne Powder is a cream coloured powder containing red/brown particles, presented in a translucent polythene squeeze bottle. Contains Povidone-Iodine USP 5% w/w.

It also contains the following inactive ingredient: lactose.

Uses Videne powder is a wide spectrum antiseptic for topical use. It presents all the bactericidal, fungicidal and virucidal properties of iodine, normally without the risk of skin sensitisation encountered with elemental iodine.

Videne powder is indicated for topical application to superficial wounds and minor burns, in the treatment and prevention of infection.

Dosage and administration Apply a light dusting of powder to the affected area. When dry this forms a protective antiseptic layer over the area treated.

There are no special dosage recommendations for children or elderly patients.

Contra-indications, warnings, etc
Precautions: Care must be taken when used on known iodine sensitive subjects, although they do not normally react to povidone iodine.

Excess powder can be washed off readily with warm water.

Contra-indications: Not to be administered internally.

Pregnancy: Videne powder is not recommended for use during pregnancy because of the possibility of absorption through broken skin and subsequent interference with tests of thyroid function.

Overdosage:

Symptoms: Symptoms of overdosage include metabolic acidosis, hypernatraemia and renal impairment.

Treatment: In cases where Videne powder has been taken orally, gastric lavage with dilute starch mucilage or a 1% solution of sodium thiosulphate should be administered. The electrolyte balance must be corrected and any lost fluids replaced.

Pharmaceutical precautions Videne powder should be stored away from heat, and direct sunlight. It should be used directly from the container. Videne powder is sterile until open.

Legal category GSL.

Package quantities Videne powder is supplied as 15 g polythene squeeze bottles (OP).

Further information Nil.

Product licence number 0068/0116.

**Trade Mark*

Macfarlan Smith Limited
Wheatfield Road
Edinburgh EH11 2QA

DF118*

Presentation
DF118 Tablets: White tablets engraved DF118. Each tablet contains Dihydrocodeine Tartrate BP 30 mg.

Elixir DF118: A brown syrup. Each 5 ml contains Dihydrocodeine Tartrate BP 10 mg.

DF118 Injection: A colourless solution. Each ampoule contains in 1 ml Dihydrocodeine Tartrate BP 50 mg.

Uses Relief of moderate to severe pain. 30 mg given parenterally has been shown to have an analgesic potency equivalent to that of 10 mg of morphine; in a study of oral analgesics for the relief of chronic pain, the same dose was found to be equivalent to 100 mg of pethidine. In both these trials dihydrocodeine was found to have a lower incidence of side effects than either morphine or pethidine.

In the recommended doses sedative or hypnotic effects are rare and it causes little or no respiratory depression; in addition to being a potent analgesic the compound also exhibits well-defined antitussive activity.

DF118 is indicated in all painful conditions where an alert patient is desired, viz, sciatica, osteo-arthritis, chronic rheumatoid arthritis, arthritis of the spine, peripheral vascular disease, post-herpetic neuralgia, Paget's disease, malignant disease, post-operative pain. Because DF118, in the recommended doses, causes little or no respiratory depression, its use in the treatment of post-operative pain may reduce the risk of chest complications.

Dosage and administration The oral route is to be preferred whenever possible. The analgesic effect of DF118 is not materially enhanced by increasing the dose above that recommended below; in severe cases the interval between doses should be reduced to obtain the requisite analgesic cover.

DF118 is best administered with or after food. It is not recommended for administration to children under 4 years.

Elixir DF118 is a pleasant tasting liquid suitable for administration to patients who may have difficulty swallowing the tablets.

Dosage – Analgesia
Adults: DF118 Tablets: 1 Tablet (30 mg) every four to six hours or at the discretion of the physician.

Elixir DF118: One to three 5 ml spoonfuls (10 to 30 mg) every four to six hours or at the discretion of the physician.

DF118 Injection: Patients who, for one reason or another are unable to be treated with the tablets or elixir may be given up to 50 mg by intramuscular or deep subcutaneous injection.

Children aged 4 to 12 years: 0.5 to 1 mg/kg bodyweight every four to six hours. The Elixir is to be preferred.

Dosage – Antitussive
Adults: Elixir DF118: One 5 ml spoonful (10 mg) every four to six hours or at the discretion of the physician.

Children aged 4 to 12 years: 200 micrograms/kg bodyweight every four to six hours. The Elixir is to be preferred.

Contra-indications, warnings, etc Respiratory depression; obstructive airways disease.

Precautions: As Dihydrocodeine may bring about histamine-release, DF118 should not be given during an attack of asthma and it should be administered with due care to persons liable to such attacks.

Dosage should be reduced in the elderly, in hypothyroidism, in chronic hepatic disease and in renal insufficiency. Alcohol should be avoided whilst under treatment with DF118.

Pregnancy: There is no, or inadequate evidence of safety in human pregnancy but the drug has been used for many years without apparent ill consequence.

Side-effects: Constipation, nausea, vomiting, headache and vertigo occur and are relatively more common when the dose is increased above 30 mg. If constipation occurs, it can be treated with a gentle laxative.

Overdosage: Conservative management is recommended; gastric lavage should be carried out. Severe respiratory depression can be treated with naloxone hydrochloride 0.4 to 2 mg subcutaneously, repeated as required at 2 or 3 minute intervals.

Pharmaceutical precautions The recommended diluent of the Elixir is Unpreserved Syrup BP, or syrup preserved with p-hydroxybenzoic acid. The resulting dilution with keep for 14 days at room temperature. DF118 preparations should be protected from light.

Legal category
DF118 Tablets CD (Sch 5), POM.
Elixir DF118 CD (Sch 5), POM.
DF118 Injection CD (Sch 2), POM.

Package quantities DF118 Tablets are available in packs of 100 and 500. Elixir DF118 is available in bottles of 150 ml. DF118 Injection is available in boxes of 5 ampoules of 1.1 ml.

Further information In patients already habituated to a drug such as pethidine, the substitution of dihydrocodeine in equi-analgesic doses has led to the appearance of abstinence symptoms. This suggests that dihydrocodeine, despite its effectiveness as an analgesic, has a low addiction potential. Nevertheless, when dihydrocodeine is prescribed for chronic use the physician should take care to avoid any unnecessary increase in dosage, especially where there is a previous history of drug dependence or abuse.

Product licence numbers

DF118 Tablets	0021/5063R
Elixir DF118	0021/0053R
DF118 Injection	0021/5028R

Product licence holder Duncan Flockhart & Co Ltd, 700 Oldfield Lane North, Greenford, Middlesex, UB6 0HD.

PARAMOL TABLETS*
(Co-dydramol – Dihydrocodeine and Paracetamol Tablets)

Presentation
A white tablet engraved Paramol, each tablet containing:

Paracetamol BP	500 mg
Dihydrocodeine Tartrate BP	10 mg

Uses Paracetamol is an effective analgesic possessing a remarkably low level of side-effects. Its broad clinical utility has been extensively reported, and it now largely replaces aspirin for routine use. Paracetamol is well tolerated; having a bland effect on gastric mucosa, unlike aspirin, it neither exacerbates symptoms of peptic ulcer nor precipitates bleeding. Dihydrocodeine tartrate has been widely used for a number of years as a powerful analgesic; 30 mg of dihydrocodeine has been reported to have analgesic potency equal to 60 to 120 mg codeine.

In addition the compound exhibits well-defined antitussive activity.

By fortifying paracetamol with 10 mg dihydrocodeine, Paramol provides an effective combination of drugs for the treatment of mild to moderate pain and as an antipyretic.

Dosage and administration Paramol Tablets should, if possible, be taken during or after meals.

Adults and children over 12 years: Analgesia: 1 tablet every four hours. This may be increased to 2 tablets four times a day if necessary.

Antitussive: 1 tablet every four hours.

Paramol is not recommended for children under 12 years.

Contra-indications, warnings, etc Respiratory depression, obstructive airways disease.

Precautions: Additive CNS depression may occur with alcohol.

Paramol should be given with caution to patients with allergic disorders and should not be given during an attack of asthma. Caution should also be observed if there is marked impairment of liver function or advanced kidney disease.

Dosage should be reduced in the elderly, in hypothyroidism and in chronic hepatic disease. An overdose can cause hepatic necrosis.

Pregnancy: There is no, or inadequate evidence of safety in human pregnancy but the drug has been used for many years without apparent ill consequence.

Side-effects: Constipation, if it occurs, is readily treated with a mild laxative. Nausea, headache, vertigo and giddiness may occur in a few patients.

Overdosage: Conservative management is recommended : gastric lavage should be carried out. Severe respiratory depression can be treated with naloxone hydrochloride 0.4 to 2 mg subcutaneously, repeated as required at 2 or 3 minute intervals. Treatment for paracetamol overdosage should be commenced as soon as possible after ingestion using preferably acetylcysteine or cysteamine or methionine.

Pharmaceutical precautions No special requirements or precautions.

Legal category CD (Sch 5), POM.

Package quantities Paramol Tablets are available in containers of 100 and 500.

Further information Nil.

Product licence number 0021/5056R.

**Trade Mark*

Martindale Pharmaceuticals Limited
Bampton Road
Harold Hill
Romford, Essex RM3 8UG

GTN 300 micrograms

Presentation Plain white uncoated tablets each containing Glyceryl Trinitrate BP 300 micrograms.

Uses As a short acting vasodilator in the prophylaxis and treatment of attacks of angina pectoris.

Dosage and administration One tablet is allowed to dissolve slowly under the tongue; the treatment may be repeated as required.

Contra-indications, warnings, etc As with all glyceryl trinitrate preparations the tablets should not be used in patients with marked anaemia, incipient glaucoma or those with head trauma or cerebral haemorrhage.

Side effects reported include headaches and facial flushing.

Toxic effects include vomiting, restlessness, hypotension, syncope, cyanosis and methaemoglobinaemia. Severe poisoning may result in bradycardia, respiratory depression and psychosis.

Treatment of toxic effects: To minimise the effects of hypotension, the patient is treated in the recumbent position with the head lowered. The stomach should be emptied to prevent further absorption and general supportive measures such as oxygen, assisted respiration, plasma expanders, employed as necessary. Methaemoglobinaemia may be treated with methylene blue intravenously 1–4 mg/kg.

Pharmaceutical precautions Store in a cool dry place with cap tightly closed.

Legal category P.

Package quantities Bottles of 100 tablets.

Further information Nil.

Product licence number 1883/5958.

MEDILAVE* GEL

Presentation Pale buff-coloured gel. Contains Benzocaine PhEur 1.0% and Cetylpyridinium Chloride BP 0.01% in a specially formulated water-immiscible protective base.

Uses For the relief of pain from abrasions and ulcers of the gums, palate, cheek, tongue and lips.

Dosage and administration Cover the affected area 3 to 4 times daily with a thin film as required, filling the depression in the ulcer, particularly before meals. Do not rub in.

Contra-indications, warnings, etc Not recommended for children under 12 years of age. In cases of dental abrasion, care should be taken to remove the underlying cause of the lesion. Consult doctor or dentist if symptoms persist. Some individuals may be hypersensitive to Benzocaine. If so, cease treatment immediately.

Pharmaceutical precautions No special precautions required.

Legal category P.

Package quantities Tube of 10 g.

Further information Nil.

Product licence number 0156/0014.

MITOMYCIN-C KYOWA*

Presentation Purple crystalline powder for intravenous injection containing Mitomycin C Kyowa 2 mg with 48 mg sodium chloride, 10 mg with 240 mg sodium chloride, 20 mg with 480 mg sodium chloride for dissolving in water for injections using the volume recommended for each strength.

Uses *Action:* Mitomycin C Kyowa is an antitumour antibiotic that is activated in the tissues to an alkylating agent which disrupts deoxyribonucleic acid (DNA) in cancer cells by forming a complex with DNA and also acts by inhibiting division of cancer cells by interfering with the biosynthesis of DNA. In vivo, Mitomycin C Kyowa is rapidly cleared from the serum after intravenous administration. The time required to reduce the serum concentration by 50% after a 30 mg bolus injection is 17 minutes. After injection of 30 mg, 20 mg, or 10 mg I.V., the maximal serum concentrations were 2.4 mcg/ml, 1.7 mcg/ml and 0.52 mcg/ml respectively. Clearance is effected primarily by metabolism in the liver, but metabolism occurs in other tissues as well. The rate of clearance is inversely proportional to the maximal serum concentration because, it is thought, of saturation of the degradative pathways. Approximately 10% of a dose of Mitomycin C Kyowa is excreted unchanged in the urine. Since metabolic pathways are saturated at relatively low doses, the percentage dose excreted in the urine increases with increasing the dose. In children, excretion of intravenously administered Mitomycin C Kyowa is similar to that in adults.

Indications: Antimitotic and Cytotoxic. Mitomycin C Kyowa is recommended for certain types of cancer, either in combination with other drugs or after primary therapy has failed. In particular, Mitomycin C Kyowa has been successfully used to improve subjective and objective symptoms in a wide range of neoplastic conditions including carcinomas of the stomach, pancreas, breast and uterus; adenocarcinoma of the lung; peritonitis carcinomatosa; colonic, bladder, rectal and skin cancer. In addition, Mitomycin C Kyowa may also be of some value in sarcomas, hepatic cancer, acute and chronic leukaemias and Hodgkin's disease.

Dosage and administration For systemic administration, Mitomycin C Kyowa should be given intravenously using great care to avoid extravasation. The usual dosage is in the range 4–10 mg (0.06–0.15 mg/kg) at 1–6 weekly intervals, depending on whether other drugs are given in combination and on bone marrow recovery. In a number of combination schedules, the dose of Mitomycin C Kyowa per treatment course is 10 mg/m^2 of body surface area, the course being repeated at intervals for as long as required. A dosage course ranging from 40–80 mg (0.58–1.2 mg/kg) is often required for a satisfactory response both when Mitomycin C Kyowa is used alone or as part of a combination. A higher dosage course may be given when Mitomycin C Kyowa is used alone or as part of particular combination schedules and total cumulative doses exceeding 2 mg/kg have been given.

For reconstitution, the contents of the 2 mg vial should be dissolved in 5 ml water for injections, or 20% dextrose solution. The 10 mg vial should be dissolved in at least 10 ml and the 20 mg vial in at least 20 ml of the same solvents and administered by intravenous injection.

The dose should be adjusted according to the age and condition of the patient.

For administration to specific tissues, Mitomycin C Kyowa can be given also into the pleural and peritoneal cavities and, by the arterial route, directly into tumours.

Because of cumulative myelosuppression, patients should be fully re-evaluated after each course of Mitomycin C Kyowa and the dose reduced if the patient has experienced any toxic effects. Doses greater than 0.6 mg/kg have not been shown to be more effective and are more toxic than lower doses.

Treatment of superficial urinary bladder tumours: In the prevention of recurrent bladder tumours, the usual dose is the equivalent of 4–10 mg (0.06–0.15 mg/kg) potency of Mitomycin C Kyowa instilled into the bladder through a urethral catheter once or three times a week. In the treatment of bladder tumours, the usual dose is the equivalent of 10–40 mg (0.15–0.6 mg/kg) potency of Mitomycin C Kyowa instilled into the bladder either weekly or three times a week for a total of 20 doses. In either case, it should be dissolved in 20 ml–40 ml of water for injections before use. The dose should be adjusted in accordance with the age and condition of the patient.

Contra-indications, warnings, etc Mitomycin C Kyowa should be administered under the supervision of a physician experienced in cytotoxic cancer chemotherapy. Patients should be monitored closely during each course of treatment, paying particular attention to peripheral blood count including platelet count.

The principal toxicity of Mitomycin C Kyowa is bone marrow suppression, particularly thrombocytopenia and leucopenia. The nadir is usually around four weeks after treatment and toxicity is cumulative, with increasing risk after each course of treatment.

No repeat dosage should be given until leucocyte count has returned to 3.0×10^9/l and platelet count to 90.0×10^9/l. If disease progression continues after two courses of treatment, the drug should be stopped since the chances of response are then minimal.

Severe renal toxicity has occasionally been reported after treatment and renal function should be monitored before starting treatment and again after each course.

Nausea and vomiting are sometimes experienced immediately after treatment but these are usually mild and of short duration. Local ulceration and cellulitis may be caused by tissue extravasation during intravenous injection and utmost care should be taken in administration. In the event of extravasation following an intravenous injection of Mitomycin C Kyowa, it is recommended that 5 ml of Sodium Bicarbonate 8.4% solution is immediately infiltrated into the area where extravasation has occurred followed by an injection of 4 mg Dexamethasone. In addition, a systemic injection of 200 mg Vitamin B6 may be of some value in promoting the regrowth of tissues that have been damaged.

Mitomycin C Kyowa should not normally be administered to patients who are pregnant or to mothers who are breast feeding. Teratological changes have been noted in animal studies. The effect of Mitomycin C Kyowa on fertility is unknown. Mitomycin C Kyowa is contraindicated in patients who have demonstrated a hypersensitive or idiosyncratic reaction to it in the past.

The person administering the injection of Mitomycin C Kyowa should not allow the solution to come into contact with his or her skin.

Treatment of skin or eye contact: Any Mitomycin C Kyowa substance or solution in contact with the skin should be washed several times with 8.4% sodium bicarbonate solution, followed by washing with soap and water. Use of handcreams or other emollient preparations is inappropriate as this may assist the penetration of any traces of Mitomycin C Kyowa into the epidermal tissue.

Contact with the eye: The eye should be rinsed several times with sodium bicarbonate eye lotion and the eye examined for several days after contact for evidence of corneal damage. If this occurs, appropriate treatment should be instituted.

Pharmaceutical precautions Unreconstituted Mitomycin C Kyowa remains stable for four years after manufacture when stored at room temperature. Reconstitution, as directed, should be accomplished using aseptic technique and the resulting solutions are best used immediately. If reconstituted Mitomycin C Kyowa must be stored prior to use, it should be protected from light and kept in a cool place – it should not be refrigerated. Solutions stored in this way should be discarded if unused after 12 hours.

When reconstituted solution is added to infusion fluids, especially where these contain dextrose, the resulting solution should be used immediately.

Legal category POM.

Package quantities 2 mg, 10 mg and 20 mg vials for intravenous injection.

Further information Mitomycin C Kyowa vials are available through hospital pharmacies for use in hospitals and hospital clinics and can be supplied to retail chemists for dispensing prescriptions for patients whose treatment has been initiated in hospital practice.

Product licence number 0156/5903.

PAMERGAN P100*

Presentation Pamergan P100 is a colourless solution for injection containing the following ingredients in each 2 ml ampoule:

Pethidine Hydrochloride BP	100 mg
Promethazine Hydrochloride BP	50 mg

Uses Promethazine hydrochloride is a powerful antihistamine agent possessing additional sedative, antiemetic and anticholinergic actions as well as a potentiating effect on central nervous system depressants.

Pethidine hydrochloride is a major analgesic which causes less respiratory depression than morphine.

Pamergan P100 is indicated for pre-anaesthetic medication, obstetrical analgesia and amnesia, and the management of severe pain.

Dosage and administration Pamergan P100 is usually injected intramuscularly; it may be given by the intravenous route after dilution to at least 10 ml with water for injections.

Pre-anaesthetic medication, obstetrical analgesia, severe pain: Administered by intramuscular injection.

Pre-anaesthetic medication: Adults: 2 ml (children: 8–12 years 0.75 ml; 12–16 years 1 ml). Administered 60–90 minutes before anaesthesia.

Obstetrical analgesia and amnesia: 1–2 ml when labour is well established, repeated at four-hourly intervals as required.

Severe pain: 1–2 ml every four to six hours in adults.

Contra-indications, warnings, etc The administration of Pamergan P100 solution to a patient who is or has recently been under treatment with a monoamine oxidase inhibitor may be followed by cerebral excitement, confusion and collapse, or by severe respiratory depression. It is important therefore that Pamergan P100 should not be given to patients receiving such treatment or within two weeks of its discontinuation.

Because of its pethidine content Pamergan P100 should not be given to patients with severe liver disease or for pain following cholecystectomy, biliary colic or increased intracranial pressure.

Because this preparation may cause or exacerbate respiratory depression, its use is contra-indicated in patients suffering from respiratory depression or obstructive airways disease.

Although no embryopathic effects have been reported with Pamergan P100 as with all drugs, it should only be used in pregnancy when the physician considers that the benefits outweigh the potential risks.

Precautions: This preparation may cause drowsiness: patients should not be allowed to drive or operate machinery until any such effects have worn off. Avoid the intake of alcohol during use. Administration during labour may cause some respiratory depression in the new born infant. In elderly patients, those with hypothyroidism or with chronic hepatic disease, a reduced dosage regime should be contemplated.

Warnings and adverse effects: Dryness of the mouth, blurring of vision, slight disorientation and dizziness occur in some patients and an occasional patient may develop a feeling of weakness or syncope accompanied by profuse perspiration.

Prolonged treatment with this preparation may give rise to tolérance and dependance to the pethidine component.

Overdosage: Accidental overdose may give rise to respiratory depression, hypotension, convulsions and circulatory collapse.

Treatment: Establish and maintain a patent airway, assisting respiration if necessary. If respiration is severely depressed give a small intravenous dose of naloxone (adults: 0.4 mg, children: 0.005–0.01 mg/kg, neonates: 0.01 mg/kg) repeated if necessary at intervals of 2–3 minutes. Hypotension may improve with improved oxygenation but may require treatment with an infusion of plasma or suitable electrolyte solution. Convulsions may be treated with a short acting muscle relaxant, intubation and controlled respiration.

Pharmaceutical precautions Protect from light. Pamergan P100 has a pH of 5.0–6.0 and is incompatible with alkaline preparations including thiopentone sodium injection.

Legal category CD (Sch 2) POM.

Package quantities Box of 10 × 2 ml ampoules.

Further information Nil.

Product licence number 0156/0020R.

**Trade Mark*

May & Baker Pharmaceuticals
A Division of Rhône-Poulenc U.K. Ltd
Dagenham
Essex RM10 7XS

Please refer to the entry under Rhône-Poulenc Rorer Limited for products previously distributed by this company.

Medo Pharmaceuticals Limited
East Street
Chesham
Bucks HP5 1DG

DIOCTYL*

Presentation
Dioctyl Tablets: Yellow, biconvex tablets containing 100 mg docusate sodium.

Dioctyl 1% Solution: Clear solution with a minty odour, containing 50 mg docusate sodium per 5 ml.

Dioctyl Paediatric Solution: Clear solution with an orange odour, containing 12.5 mg docusate sodium per 5 ml.

Uses
1. To prevent and treat chronic constipation.
2. As an adjunct in abdominal radiological procedures.

Dosage and administration
Adults and elderly: Up to 500 mg daily in divided doses Dioctyl tablets or Dioctyl 1% solution should be used.

Children (2–12 years): 12.5 to 25 mg three times a day.

Infants (over 6 months): 12.5 mg three times a day. Dioctyl tablets and Dioctyl 1% solution are not recommended for children or infants. Dioctyl paediatric should be used.

Tablets and solution should be taken with a glass of water.

Dioctyl tablets should be swallowed whole.

For use with barium meals – 400 mg should be taken with the barium meal.

Contra-indications, warnings, etc
Contra-indications: Docusate sodium should not be administered when abdominal pain, nausea, vomiting or intestinal obstruction is present. Docusate sodium should not be given to infants under six months old.

Interactions: Concurrent administration with mineral oil is contra-indicated. Anthraquinone derivatives should be taken in reduced dose when administered with docusate sodium as it increases their absorption.

Pregnancy and lactation: There is inadequate evidence of safety of the drug in human pregnancy, nor is there evidence from animal work that it is free from hazard. However, it has been in wide use for many years without apparent ill consequence. Therefore Dioctyl should only be used in pregnancy if the benefits outweigh the potential risk.

Docusate sodium is excreted in breast milk and should therefore be used with caution in breastfeeding mothers.

Overdose: In rare cases of overdose, excessive loss of water and electrolytes may occur. This should be treated by encouraging the patient to drink plenty of fluid.

Pharmaceutical precautions None.

Legal category P.

Package quantities Dioctyl Tablets are available in packs of 30, 100 and 250 tablets. Dioctyl 1% Solution is available in bottles of 300 ml. Dioctyl Paediatric Solution is available in bottles of 125 ml, 300 ml.

Further information Docusate sodium exerts its clinical effect in the gastro-intestinal tract by means of its physical surfactant properties, by allowing penetration of water and fats into hard, dry faeces. There is some evidence to suggest that Docusate sodium is absorbed from the gastro-intestinal tract and that it may enhance absorption of compounds administered concomitantly.

Product licence numbers

Dioctyl Tablets	4147/5910R
Dioctyl 1% Solution	4147/5909R
Dioctyl Paediatric Solution	4147/5908R

DIOCTYL* EAR DROPS

Presentation A clear liquid containing docusate sodium 5% w/w in polyethylene glycol in a 10 ml glass amber dropper bottle.

Uses For the softening of ear wax to facilitate its removal.

Dosage and administration
Adults and Elderly: Four drops should be instilled into the ear twice daily for 2–3 days. The head should be inclined to one side and the ear plugged with cotton wool soaked in Dioctyl Ear Drops if necessary. After 2–3 days the wax should be easy to remove. Patients prone to persistent problems with ear wax should use Dioctyl Ear Drops every two weeks.

Children: The number of drops instilled may be reduced to the level required to fill ear with solution.

Contra-indications, warnings, etc
Contra-indication: Not to be used if the ear drum is known or suspected to be perforated, or if there is inflammation of the ear.

Warnings: Slight stinging or irritation may occur. If pain or inflammation occurs, treatment should be stopped.

Pharmaceutical precautions None.

Legal category GSL.

Package quantities Dioctyl Ear Drops are available in a 10 ml amber glass bottle with a removable glass dropper unit.

Further information Dioctyl Ear Drops are for use only in the ear. Docusate sodium is the British Approved Name for dioctyl sodium sulphosuccinate.

Product licence number 4147/0045.

PHOLCOMED* D LINCTUS PHOLCOMED DIABETIC FORTE LINCTUS

Presentation
Pholcomed D: A red, blackcurrant flavoured, sugar-free linctus. Each 5 ml contains pholcodine BP 5 mg.

Pholcomed Diabetic Forte: A red, blackcurrant flavoured, sugar-free linctus. Each 5 ml contains pholcodine BP 10 mg.

Uses Pholcomed is used for the relief of irritating, unproductive coughs. Pholcodine exerts an inhibitory action on the cough centre and has a less constipating effect than codeine.

Dosage and administration
Pholcomed D
Adults and Elderly: One or two 5 ml spoonfuls, three to four times a day.
Children (2–12 years): One 5 ml spoonful three times a day.

Children (1–2 years): Half a 5 ml spoonful three times a day.
Children under 1 year: Not recommended.

Pholcomed Diabetic Forte
Adults and Elderly: One 5 ml spoonful three times a day.
Children: Not recommended.

Contra-indications, warnings, etc
Contra-indications: Pholcomed is contra-indicated in patients who suffer from liver disease, ventilatory failure, or asthma. This product is not advised for use by patients with bronchitis and bronchiectasis. It should also not be used in patients who are hypersensitive to pholcodine or any other ingredient.

Precautions: The CNS depressant effects may be potentiated by concurrent use of other CNS depressants and alcohol.

If pholcodine is taken within two weeks of monoamine oxidase inhibitor therapy, CNS excitation may occur.

Constipation and nausea may occur. Drowsiness occassionally occurs, if affected do not drive or operate machinery.

Pholcodine may delay absorption of some drugs, e.g. mexiletine.

Pholcomed contains parabens which may cause hypersensitivity reactions in some susceptible individuals.

Pregnancy and lactation: The safety of pholcodine during pregnancy or lactation has yet to be established. Therefore this product should not be used unless the possible benefit is thought to outweigh any possible risk.

Overdosage: Symptoms of overdosage are nausea, drowsiness and respiratory depression. Symptomatic treatment and/or gastric lavage is indicated. In severe cases, use of an opioid antagonist such as naloxone may be considered.

Pharmaceutical precautions None.

Legal category CD (Sch 5), P.

Package quantities Pholcomed D is available in bottles of 125 ml and 300 ml. Pholcomed Diabetic Forte is available in bottles of 125 ml.

Further information Pholcomed D Linctus and Pholcomed Diabetic Forte Linctus contains no sugar, have negligible calorific value, and are therefore suitable for both diabetic and non-diabetic patients.

Both Pholcomed D Linctus, and Pholcomed Diabetic Forte Linctus are tartrazine free but do contain amaranth (E123).

Product licence numbers

Pholcomed D Linctus	4147/5902R
Pholcomed Diabetic Forte Linctus	4147/5904R

PHOLCOMED* PASTILLES

Presentation Blackcurrant flavoured, sugar coated disc shaped pastilles containing Pholcodine BP 4 mg

Uses Pholcomed Pastilles are used for the relief of irritating unproductive coughs.

Dosage and administration
Adults: One to two pastilles every hour.

Children (over 6 years): One pastille every hour.

Maximum adult dose: Fifteen pastilles daily.
Maximum children's dose: Seven pastilles daily.

Contra-indications, warnings, etc Pholcomed pastilles should not be given to patients with liver disease, ventilatory failure, or asthma.

This product is not advised for use by patients with bronchitis and bronchiectasis.

These pastilles should not be used by patients who are hypersensitive to pholcodine or other ingredients.

Precautions: The CNS depressant effects may be potentiated by concurrent use of other CNS depressants and alcohol.

If Pholcodine is taken within two weeks of monoamine oxidase inhibitor therapy, CNS excitation may occur.

Constipation and nausea may occur, drowsiness occasionally occurs. If affected do not drive or operate machinery.

Pholcodine may delay the absorption of some drugs, e.g. mexiletine.

Pregnancy and lactation: The safety of pholcodine during pregnancy or lactation has yet to be established.

The product should not be used unless the possible benefit is thought to outweigh any possible risks.

Overdosage: Symptoms of overdosage are nausea, drowsiness and respiratory depression. Symptomatic treatment and/or gastric lavage is indicated.

In severe cases, use of an opioid antagonist such as naloxone may be considered.

Pharmaceutical precautions Store in a cool, dry place.

Legal category CD (Sch 5), P.

Package quantities Cartons containing 20 pastilles.

Further information Nil.

Product licence number 4147/5905R.

**Trade Mark*

E. Merck Pharmaceuticals
(A Division of Merck Ltd)
Four Marks
Alton
Hampshire GU34 5HB

MERCK

BALNEUM*

Presentation A liquid preparation for external use.

Active ingredient: Soya oil 84.75% w/w.

Inactive ingredients: Laureth 4, oleic acid diethanolamide, perfume oil, antioxidant (containing propylene glycol and butylated hydroxytoluene).

Uses Balneum has emollient properties and is recommended for the treatment of dry skin conditions including those associated with dermatitis and eczema.

Dosage and administration For full bath (~100 L)–20 ml = 1 measure.

For bath for children (~25 L)–5 ml = ¼ measure.

For partial bath (~5L)–2.5 ml = ⅛ measure.

For particularly dry skin, 2–3 times the above quantities can be used.

Add Balneum to the bath water and mix well. The frequency and duration of bathing will depend on the type and severity of the condition. Generally 2–3 baths should be taken weekly. For babies and infants a daily bath is recommended.

Contra-indications, warnings, etc Balneum is contra-indicated in patients with a known hypersensitivity to any of the ingredients.

No side-effects have been observed.

Pharmaceutical precautions None.

Legal category P.

Package quantities Bottles of 200 ml, 500 ml and 1000 ml.

Further information Balneum contains vegetable oil well tolerated by the skin. Since the product contains no wool alcohols or lanolin it can be safely used by patients sensitive to these materials. The bath can easily be cleaned after use.

Product licence number 0493/0064.

BALNEUM PLUS*

Presentation an oily liquid for external use.

Active ingredients: soya oil 82.95% w/w and mixed lauromacrogols 15% w/w.

Inactive ingredients: liquid paraffin, stabiliser, perfume oil, antioxidant (containing butylated hydroxytoluene and propylene glycol)

Uses Balneum Plus is a bath oil which has emollient and local anaesthetic properties and provides relief of pruritus. It is recommended for the treatment of dry skin conditions including those associated with dermatitis and eczema where pruritus is also experienced.

Dosage and administration After shaking the bottle Balneum Plus is added to the bath water and mixed well. Frequency and duration of the application depends on the type and severity of the condition. Balneum Plus should be used when bathing.

For babies and infants a daily application is recommended.

For full bath (~100 L) – 20 ml = 1 measure.

For bath for children (~25 L) – 5 ml = ¼ measure.

For partial bath (~5 L) – 2.5 ml = ⅛ measure.

A partial bath may be required when the condition is localised eg the arm.

Balneum Plus can also be used in the shower. In this case the preparation should first be evenly applied over the body without dilution. Subsequently the excess is removed under the shower. Soap, which would remove the desired oil film on the skin, should not be used.

If the skin requires considerable moisturising, 2–3 times the above quantities can be used.

Excessive rinsing with water after the bath counteracts the therapeutic action of Balneum Plus.

After the bath the skin should only be lightly dabbed with a towel. Strong wiping and rubbing decreases the therapeutic effect.

The bath can be easily cleaned after use.

Contra-indications, warnings, etc Balneum Plus should not be used for the treatment of patients sensitive to any of the ingredients.

As Balneum Plus deposits a film of oil over the skin, care should be taken to guard against slipping, especially in the bath or shower.

Legal category P.

Package quantities Bottles of 500 ml.

Further information Balneum Plus contains a vegetable oil that is well tolerated by the skin. Since the product contains no wool alcohols or lanolin it can be used safely by patients sensitive to these materials. Cooler bath temperatures (circa 30°C) will enhance the anti-pruritic effect of the lauromacrogols.

The lauromacrogols contained in the product exert their local anaesthetic action directly to the skin surface, where it is required, thus optimising their efficacy.

Product licence number 0493/0137.

BALNEUM* WITH TAR

Presentation Balneum with Tar is a clear, brownish-black medicinal bath oil.

Active ingredients: Soya oil 55% w/w, coal tar distillate 30% w/w.

Inactive ingredient: Laureth 4.

Uses Balneum with Tar is particularly recommended in the treatment of eczema, psoriasis, pruritic dermatoses and ichthyosis.

Dosage and administration Balneum with Tar is added to the bath water and well mixed. Frequency and duration of bathing depends on the type and severity of the condition. Unless otherwise prescribed by a physician, 2 to 3 baths weekly for up to 20 minutes each are recommended.

Adults: One measure (20 ml) of Balneum with Tar should be added to the usual bath of ~100 litres.

Children over 2 years: In small baths (~50 litres), up to half a measure (10 ml) will be sufficient.

Contra-indications, warnings, etc
Contra-indications: Do not apply the preparation to moist and weeping dermatoses, or severely broken skin. Not recommended for use in children under 2 years old, or in children over 2 years old for longer than 6 weeks at a time.

Warnings: Avoid contact with the eyes and prolonged exposure to sunlight after bathing.

Side-effects: Very rarely sensitisation of normal skin may occur.

Pharmaceutical precautions No special requirements.

Legal category P.

Package quantities Bottles of 225 ml.

Further information Balneum with Tar combines the emollient properties of the medicinal bath oil Balneum with the therapeutic properties of coal tar distillate.

Product licence number 0493/0113.

BALTAR* SHAMPOO

Presentation Baltar Shampoo is a clear, light brown liquid for scalp application.

Active ingredient: Coal tar distillate 1.5% w/w.

Inactive ingredients: Coconut fatty acid derivatives, sodium laureth sulphate, perfume oil, sodium chloride, purified water.

Uses For the treatment of scalp disorders such as psoriasis, eczema, dandruff, seborrhoeic and pruritic dermatoses.

Dosage and administration Wet hair and scalp. Apply sufficient Baltar shampoo to make a rich lather and massage well into the scalp. Wait one minute. Rinse and repeat. Finally rinse hair thoroughly.

Baltar shampoo should be used as above once to three times weekly, depending on the severity of the condition, or as directed by the physician.

Contra-indications, warnings, etc
Contra-indications: Do not apply the preparation to moist and weeping dermatoses, or severely broken skin.

Not recommended for use in children under 2 years old.

Warnings: Avoid contact with the eyes.

Side-effects: Very rarely, sensitisation of normal skin may occur.

Pharmaceutical precautions No special requirements.

Legal category GSL.

Package quantities Bottles of 225 ml or 500 ml.

Further information Baltar Shampoo combines the properties of a soap-free skin cleansing agent with the therapeutic effects of tar in a formulation designed to encourage patient compliance.

Product licence number 0493/0123.

EMCOR*
EMCOR LS

Presentation Emcor LS tablets, containing 5 mg bisoprolol fumarate (2:1) are heart-shaped, pale yellow and film-coated. Emcor tablets, containing 10 mg bisoprolol fumarate (2:1) are heart-shaped, pale orange and film-coated. Both tablets are scored.

Uses
(i) Management of hypertension
(ii) Management of angina pectoris

Mode of action: Bisoprolol is a potent, highly β_1-selective-adrenoreceptor blocking agent devoid of intrinsic sympathomimetic activity and without relevant membrane stabilising activity.

As with other β_1-blocking agents, the mode of action in hypertension is not clear but it is known that bisoprolol markedly depresses plasma renin activity.

In patients with angina, the blockade of β_1-receptors reduces heart action and thus reduces oxygen demand. Hence bisoprolol is effective in eliminating or reducing the symptoms.

Pharmacokinetics: Bisoprolol is absorbed almost completely from the gastrointestinal tract. Together with the very small first pass effect in the liver, this results in a high bioavailability of approximately 90%. The drug is cleared equally by the liver and kidney.

The plasma elimination half-life (10–12 hours) provides 24 hours efficacy following a once daily dosage. About 95% of the drug substance is excreted through the kidney, half of this is as unchanged bisoprolol. There are no active metabolites in man.

Dosage and administration
Adults: The usual dose is 10 mg once daily with a maximum recommended dose of 20 mg per day. In some patients 5 mg per day may be adequate. In patients with final stage impairment of renal (creatinine clearance <20 ml/min) or liver function, the dose should not exceed 10 mg bisoprolol once daily.

Experience of the use of bisoprolol in renal dialysis patients is limited, however, there is no evidence that the dosage regimen needs to be altered.

Elderly: No dosage adjustment is normally required but 5 mg per day may be adequate in some patients; as for other adults, dosage may have to be reduced in cases of severe renal or hepatic dysfunction.

Children: There is no paediatric experience with bisoprolol, therefore its use cannot be recommended for children.

Contra-indications, warnings, etc
Contra-indications: As with other β_1-adrenoceptor antagonists, bisoprolol should not be used in cases of untreated cardiac failure, cardiogenic shock, sinoatrial block, second or third degree AV block, marked bradycardia (heart rate less than 50 beats/min), extreme hypotension, or severe asthma.

Precautions: Use with care in patients with a prolonged PR conduction interval, poor cardiac reserve and peripheral circulatory disturbances, such as Raynaud's phenomenon.

In patients with ischaemic heart disease, treatment should not be withdrawn abruptly.

Although bisoprolol is a highly selective β_1-adrenoceptor blocking agent, it should be used with caution in patients with chronic obstructive airways diseases or a family history of asthma. In some asthmatic patients some increase in airways resistance may occur, this may be regarded as a signal to discontinue therapy. This bronchospasm can usually be reversed by commonly used bronchodilators such as salbutamol.

Due to the low affinity of bisoprolol for β_2-receptors, the drug does not appear to have a hypoglycaemic effect. However, it should be used with caution in diabetic patients since the symptoms of hypoglycaemia (in particular, tachycardia) may be masked.

Pregnancy: No teratogenic effects have been demonstrated in animal studies, but the safety of bisoprolol during human pregnancy has not been established. Like other β-blockers, the benefits of use during pregnancy should be weighed against the possible hazard to mother and foetus. Studies in animals suggest that no clinically relevant levels of bisoprolol reach the milk. However, as in pregnancy, caution should be exercised for use during lactation.

Drug interactions: Bisoprolol may potentiate the effect of other concurrently administered antihypertensive drugs. Concomitant treatment with reserpine, α-methyldopa and clonidine may cause an exaggerated decrease in heart rate. In particular, if clonidine is to be discontinued, this should not be done until bisoprolol treatment has been discontinued for several days.

Bisoprolol should also be used with care when myocardial depressants, inhibitors of AV conduction such as calcium antagonists of the verapamil and diltiazem type, or class I antidysrhythmic agents such as disopyramide are used concurrently.

The intravenous administration of calcium antagonists and antiarrythmic agents is not recommended during bisoprolol therapy.

The concurrent use of rifampicin can reduce the elimination half-life of bisoprolol, although an increase in dose is generally not necessary. The effects of insulin or oral hypoglycaemic agents may be potentiated when used concurrently with bisoprolol.

Anaesthesia: Prior to anaesthesia, the anaesthetist should be informed if the patient is taking bisoprolol. In cases of severe ischaemic heart disease the risk/benefit of continuing treatment should be evaluated. Care should be taken when using either cyclopropane or trichloroethylene.

Side-effects: Bisoprolol is well tolerated. The reported side effects are generally attributable to its pharmacological actions and include lassitude, dizziness, mild headache, perspiration, aggravation of intermittent claudication or Raynaud's disease and parasthaesia of the extremities. Occasionally a marked decrease in blood pressure, and pulse rate or a disturbance of AV conduction, skin rashes and dry eyes may be observed. Sleep disturbances of the type noted with other β-blockers have rarely been reported.

Overdosage: In the case of overdosage or a precipitous drop in pulse rate and/or blood pressure, treatment with bisoprolol must be discontinued. If necessary, the following antidotes should be administered alone or consecutively: intravenous atropine 0.5–2.0 mg, intravenous orciprenaline 0.5 mg by slow intravenous injection; also glucagon may be given at a dose level of 1 to 5 mg.

Pharmaceutical precautions No special requirement.

Legal category POM.

Package quantities Calendar blister packs of 28 tablets OP. Strips of 14 tablets, two strips in each carton.

Further information Bisoprolol is effective in hypertension and angina pectoris for at least 24 hours following a single oral dose. Since it is β_1-selective even in the higher therapeutic dose range, bisoprolol may, with care, be used successfully in the treatment of patients with concurrent respiratory disease who cannot tolerate a less selective β_1-blocker. The high bioavailability and the dual pathway of clearance lead to predictable blood levels. Patient compliance is increased by the reliable and simple administration regimen.

Product licence numbers
Emcor LS 0493/0126
Emcor 0493/0127

EMFLEX* ▼

Presentation Yellow/orange capsules containing 60 mg acemetacin.

Inactive ingredients: gelatin capsule (colourings erythrosine red E104, quinoline yellow E127 and titanium dioxide E171), lactose, magnesium stearate, silicon dioxide, talc.

Uses Emflex is a non-steroidal anti-inflammatory drug (NSAID) indicated for rheumatoid arthritis and post-operative pain and inflammation.

Mode of action: Acemetacin is a glycolic acid ester of indomethacin and the pharmacological activity resulting from acemetacin administration in man is derived from the presence of both therapeutic agents. The precise pharmacological mode of action of acemetacin is not known, however, unlike other NSAIDs, acemetacin is only a relatively weak inhibitor of prostaglandin synthetase. Prostaglandins are known to have an antisecretory and cytoprotective effect on the gastric mucosa. Acemetacin does show activity in many of the established in vitro tests of anti-inflammatory activity including inhibition of the release of a number of mediators of inflammation.

Pharmacokinetics: Acemetacin is well absorbed after oral administration. Its major metabolite is indomethacin, which, after repeated administration is present at levels in excess of those of acemetacin. Acemetacin is bound to plasma protein to a slightly lesser extent than indomethacin and has a relatively short plasma elimination half life. It is eliminated by both hepatic and renal mechanisms. The pharmacokinetics appear to be linear at recommended therapeutic doses, unaffected by moderate renal or hepatic impairment and unchanged in the elderly.

Dosage and administration The recommended starting dose is 120 mg/day in divided doses, increasing to 180 mg/day in divided doses depending upon patient response. Emflex should be taken with food, milk or an antacid to reduce the possibility of any gastrointestinal disturbance.

Use in the elderly: No dosage adjustment is usually required, however, non-steroidal anti-inflammatory drugs should be used with caution in older patients who may be more prone to adverse reactions.

Contra-indications, warnings, etc Active peptic ulceration or history of recurrent ulceration. Emflex should not be used in patients with nasal polyps associated with angioneurotic oedema, previous hypersensitivity to the drug or indomethacin or in asthmatic patients in whom attacks of asthma, urticaria or acute rhinitis are precipitated by aspirin or non-steroidal anti-inflammatory drugs. The safety of use in children is not established.

Pregnancy: The safety of this product for use in human pregnancy or lactation has not been established. Animal reproduction studies do not provide reassurance regarding the lack of reproductive toxicity/teratogenicity. Due to maternal toxicity, the studies were conducted at doses below the therapeutic dose or a very low multiple of the therapeutic dose. It should not therefore be used in pregnancy or lactation or in women of childbearing age unless they are taking adequate contraceptive precautions.

Precautions: Rare instances of peptic ulceration have been reported in patients receiving Emflex and drug administration should be closely supervised in patients with a history of upper gastro-intestinal disease. Emflex should be discontinued if peptic ulceration or gastro-intestinal bleeding occurs.

In common with other non-steroidal anti-inflammatory drugs, Emflex may inhibit platelet aggregation and this should be taken into account in treating patients receiving concurrent anti-coagulant therapy. Ability to drive a car or operate machinery may be affected. Caution should be exercised initially until individual reaction to treatment is known.

Emflex should be used with caution in patients with a psychiatric disorder, epilepsy or parkinsonism, as it may aggravate these conditions. Non-steroidal anti-inflammatory drugs may mask the signs and symptoms of infection. For patients with reduced renal blood flow, prostaglandins may play an important part in maintaining renal perfusion. Emflex should therefore be used with caution in such patients. In patients at particular risk – such as those with renal or hepatic dysfunction, congestive heart failure, electrolyte or fluid imbalance, sepsis, concomitant use of nephrotoxic drugs – renal function should be monitored. As with other non-steroidal anti-inflammatory drugs patients on long-term treatment should be periodically screened as a precautionary measure for renal and hepatic function and blood counts.

Chronic rheumatoid disease can result in eye changes which may be the result of the disease or therapy. It is recommended that patients receive periodic ophthalmological examinations and therapy is discontinued if eye changes occur.

Borderline elevation of liver and renal function test parameters have occasionally occurred. If these persist or worsen, Emflex therapy should be stopped.

Hyperkalaemia has been reported with the use of indomethacin and this should be considered when administration with potassium sparing diuretics is proposed.

Drug interactions: Emflex is highly protein bound and it may therefore be necessary to modify the dosage of other highly protein bound drugs eg anti-coagulants. As there is a possibility of either pharmacokinetic or pharmacodynamic interaction with aspirin or other salicylates, diflusinal, probenecid, lithium, triamterene, ACE inhibitors, haloperidol and methotrexate, patients receiving such combinations should be carefully monitored and dosages adjusted as necessary. Non-steroidal anti-inflammatory drugs may reduce the anti-hypertensive effects of beta-blockers, although clinical studies showed no propensity for Emflex to antagonise the effects of propranolol. Likewise the reduction of diuretic and anti-hypertensive effects of thiazides and frusemide may occur with non-steroidal anti-inflammatory drugs and this should be borne in mind when treating patients with compromised cardiac function or hypertension.

Side-effects: The following side-effects have been either reported with Emflex or could possibly occur as they are common to a number of NSAIDs:

Gastro-intestinal – Gastro-intestinal discomfort/pain, anorexia, nausea, vomiting, indigestion, diarrhoea and constipation, peptic ulceration, gastrointestinal perforation and haemorrhage.

Central nervous system – Symptoms most frequently encountered are headache, dizziness, vertigo and insomnia. Rarely, confusion, depressed mood, irritability.

Hepatic – Occasional elevation of liver function test parameters without overt clinical symptomology. Very rarely, symptoms of cholestasis.

Cardiovascular/renal – Rarely, oedema, chest pain, palpitations, blood urea elevation.

Dermatological/hypersensitivity – Pruritus, urticaria, erythema, skin rash, alopecia, angio-neurotic oedema and excessive sweating have been reported.

Haematological – Rarely, thrombocytopenia, leucopenia and reduced haemoglobin levels. Very rarely, reversible agranulocytosis, bone marrow depression.

Ocular/auditory – Infrequently, tinnitus, blurred vision and rarely, eye pain.

Treatment of overdose: Symptomatic and supportive therapy is indicated. If ingestion is recent, vomiting should be induced or gastric lavage should be performed. Progress should be followed for several days as gastro-intestinal ulceration and haemorrhage have been reported with overdosage of other NSAIDs. Antacids may be helpful.

Pharmaceutical precautions Store below 25°C.

Legal category POM.

Package quantities Containers of 90 capsules OP.

Further information Emflex is an NSAID which has been available in other European countries for a number of years and has been entered into extensive long term and post marketing studies.

Emflex is presented in plastic containers with specially designed 'easy to open' screw caps which should help patients with limited grip strength.

Product licence number 0493/0141.

ENDOBIL*

Presentation Endobil 100 ml bottle contains a 9.91% w/v concentration of the meglumine salt of iodoxamic acid for intravenous infusion, equivalent to an iodine content of 45 mg/ml.

Uses Intravenous cholecystography and cholangiography.

Dosage and administration
Adults: The recommended duration of intravenous infusion is between fifteen and thirty minutes.

Patients undergoing cholegraphic procedures with Endobil should be adequately prepared with only a light meal on the night before examination and an enema. Endobil should be warmed to body temperature and administered intravenously with the patient lying down.

Elderly: Dosage as for adults.

Children: The use of Endobil in children is not recommended until further evidence has been accumulated and reviewed.

Contra-indications, warnings, etc
Contra-indications: Proven or suspected hypersensitivity to iodine-containing preparations.

Warnings, side-effects: Endobil should be used with caution in patients with severe functional impairment of the liver, kidneys or myocardium, severe hyperthyroidism and macroglobulinaemia (Waldenströms disease).

X-ray examination of women should if possible be conducted during the pre-ovulation phase of the menstrual cycle and should be avoided during pregnancy; also since it has not been demonstrated that Endobil is safe for use in pregnant women, it should be administered only if the procedure is considered essential by the physician.

Side-effects following the administration of Endobil are generally mild and relatively rare, the most common being facial flushing and nausea.

As with any contrast medium, injection solutions of adrenaline, a vasopressor, a corticosteroid and an antihistamine should be immediately available in case of hypersensitivity. To cover the remote possibility of delayed hypersensitivity the patient should be attended for 20 minutes following injection.

Pharmaceutical precautions Store away from light.

Legal category POM.

Package quantities Box containing 10 × 100 ml bottles for intravenous infusion (4.5 g iodine).

Further information Nil.

Product licence number 0493/0074.

GAMANIL*

Presentation Round, film-coated, brownish violet tablets with a spindle shaped scoring on one side, containing lofepramine hydrochloride equivalent to 70 mg lofepramine base.

Use The treatment of symptoms of depressive illness.

Dosage and administration
Adults: The usual dose 70 mg twice daily (140 mg) or three times daily (210 mg) depending upon patient response.

Elderly: Elderly patients may respond to lower doses in some cases.

Children: Not recommended.

Contra-indications, warnings, etc
Contra-indications: Lofepramine should not be used in patients hypersensitive to dibenzazepines, in mania, severe liver impairment and/or severe renal impairment, heart block, cardiac arrythmias, or during the recovery phase following a myocardial infarction.

Precautions and warnings: Lofepramine should be used with caution in patients with cardiovascular disease, impaired liver or renal function, narrow angle glaucoma, symptoms suggestive of prostatic hypertrophy, a history of epilepsy or recent convulsions, hyperthyroidism, blood dyscrasias or porphyria.

Ability to drive a car and operate machinery may be affected. Therefore caution should be exercised initially until the individual reaction to treatment is known.

Use in pregnancy: The safety of lofepramine for use during pregnancy has not been established and there is evidence of harmful effects in pregnancy in animals when high doses are given. Lofepramine has been shown to be excreted in breast milk. The administraton of lofepramine in pregnancy and during breast feeding therefore, is not advised unless there are compelling medical reasons.

Side-effects: Lofepramine has been shown to be well tolerated and side-effects when they occur tend to be mild.

Comparative clinical trials have shown that lofepramine is associated with a low incidence of anticholinergic side-effects.

The following side-effects have been reported with lofepramine:

Cardiovascular: hypotension, tachycardia.

CNS and neuromuscular: dizziness, drowsiness, agitation, confusion, headache, malaise, paraesthesia and rarely hypomania and convulsions.

Anticholinergic: dryness of mouth, constipation, disturbances of accommodation, urinary hesitancy, urinary retention, sweating and tremor.

Allergic: skin rash, allergic skin reactions.

Gastrointestinal: nausea, vomiting.

Endocrine: rarely, inappropriate secretion of antidiuretic hormone, interference with sexual function.

Haematological/biochemical: rarely, bone marrow depression including isolated reports of: agranulocytosis, eosinophilia, granulocytopenia, leucopenia, pancytopenia, thrombocytopenia.

Rises in liver enzymes have been observed in some patients, usually occurring within the first three months of starting therapy. There have been a small number of reports of jaundice. These reactions are reversible on cessation of therapy.

The following adverse effects have been encountered in patients under treatment with tricyclic antidepressants and should therefore be considered as theoretical hazards of lofepramine even in the absence of substantiation: psychotic manifestations, including mania and paranoid delusions may be exacerbated during treatment with tricyclic antidepressants; withdrawal symptoms may occur on abrupt cessation of therapy and include insomnia, irritability and excessive perspiration; adverse effects such as withdrawal symptoms, respiratory depression and agitation have been reported in neonates whose mothers have taken tricyclic antidepressants during the last trimester of pregnancy.

Drug interactions: Lofepramine should not be administered concurrently with or within 2 weeks of cessation of therapy with monoamine oxidase inhibitors. It should then be introduced cautiously using a low initial dosage.

Lofepramine should not be given with sympathomimetic agents, central nervous depressants including alcohol or thyroid hormone therapy since its effects may be potentiated.

Lofepramine may decrease the antihypertensive effect of adrenergic neurone-blocking drugs; it is therefore advisable to review this form of antihypertensive therapy during treatment.

Anaesthetics given during tricyclic antidepressant therapy may increase the risk of arrhythmias and hypotension. If surgery is necessary, the anaesthetist should be informed that a patient is being so treated. Barbiturates may increase the rate of metabolism.

Overdosage: Treatment of overdosage is symptomatic and supportive. It should include immediate gastric lavage and routine close monitoring of cardiac function.

Reports of overdosage with lofepramine, with quantities ranging from 0.7 g up to 6.72 g, have shown no serious sequelae directly attributable to the drug.

Pharmaceutical precautions The tablets should be stored at room temperature, in their original container, protected from light and moisture.

Legal category POM.

Package quantities Containers of 250 tablets 70 mg. Blister calendar packs of 4 × 14 tablets 70 mg(OP).

Further information Nil.

Product licence number 0493/0060.

GASTROMIRO*

Presentation Gastrimiro contains 61.2% w/v iopamidol as an orange flavoured sugar free aqueous solution. The iodine content is 300 mgI/ml.

Uses Gastromiro is an X-ray contrast medium specifically formulated for radiological investigation of the gastro-intestinal tract. It may be used either orally or as an enema and is indicated especially in those cases in which the use of other contrast media is unsatisfactory, undesirable or contra-indicated.

Gastromiro is of particular value in the following indications:

1. Paediatric radiology of the gastro-intestinal tract (GIT) where there is the possibility of:
   (i) Spill into the respiratory tract, for example in:
      (a) Swallowing disorders.
      (b) Oesophageal obstruction as with foreign body, atresia or stricture.
      (c) Tracheo-oesophageal fistula.
   (ii) Spill into the mediastinum, pleura, peritoneum or retroperitoneal tissues, for example due to perforation of the GIT.
   (iii) Inspissation of fluid, for example in:
      (a) Meconium ileus equivalent.
      (b) Intussusception.
      (c) Colonic obstruction.
      (d) Hirschsprung's disease.
2. Adult radiology of the gastro-intestinal tract, such as:
   (i) Suspected upper gastro-intestinal perforation for example in: oesophagogastrectomy, endoscopy, partial gastrectomy, pneumonectomy, ingestion of foreign body, duodenal ulceration, small bowel resection, Whipples procedure and blunt abdominal trauma.
   (ii) Computer Tomography (CT) of the abdominal and pelvic regions, for example:
      (a) Suspicion of expanding lesions of pancreas, liver and gall bladder.
      (b) Space occupying metastatic lesions originating from prostate or recto-sigmoidal region in post-surgical staging of cancer.

Dosage and administration
Adults

Radiology of gastro-intestinal tract
Oral: 40–100 ml undiluted
Rectal: 200 ml of a 50% dilution, up to 1000 ml of a 2% dilution

Computer tomography
Oral:
Abdominal CT: 100 ml of a 17% dilution, up to 600 ml of a 3% dilution.
Rectal – pelvic CT: 500–700 ml of a 3% dilution

Infants and children

Radiology of gastro-intestinal tract
Oral: 10–100 ml undiluted or, for use in infants 20–200 ml of up to a 50% dilution to provide isotonic contrast medium
Rectal: 200 ml of 50–60% dilution

Elderly: Dosage as for adults.

Dilution of Gastromiro should be carried out using sterile water. Any unused solution should be discarded after 6 hours.

Contra-indications, warnings, etc
Contra-indications: Proven or suspected hypersensitivity to iodine containing preparations of this type. It must not be used for parenteral administration.

Warnings: Disturbances in water or electrolyte balance must first be corrected. This product is formulated for gastro-intestinal use only and should not be used parenterally.

Care should also be exercised in patients with severe functional impairment of the liver, kidney or myocardium, severe systemic disease and in myelomatosis. In such patients adequate hydration should be maintained and parameters of hepatic and renal function, especially urinary output should be monitored after the procedure.

Patients with hepato-renal insufficiency should not be examined unless benefits clearly outweigh risks and re-examination should be delayed for 5–7 days.

In patients with a history of adverse reactions during similar investigations additional caution should be exercised and the procedure only carried out if benefits clearly outweigh any risks.

X-ray examination of women should be conducted as far as possible during the pre-ovulation phase of the menstrual cycle. This product may interfere with tests of thyroid function.

Side-effects: Systemic effects are rare since Gastromiro is only poorly absorbed from the alimentary tract. Owing to slight hypertonicity Gastromiro may occasionally cause vomiting and diarrhoea particularly in infants and children.

Pregnancy and lactation: The safety of iopamidol during pregnancy and lactation has not been demonstrated clinically. Due, however, to the extremely low absorption of iopamidol from the gastro-intestinal tract it is unlikely that a foetus could be exposed to significant levels. In animal experiments iopamidol is neither teratogenic nor foetotoxic. Similarly, during lactation breast fed infants are unlikely to be exposed to significant levels of iopamidol. However, the product should not be used during pregnancy or when breast feeding unless it is considered essential.

Pharmaceutical precautions Protect from light.

Legal category POM.

Package quantities 10 × 20 ml bottles
10 × 50 ml bottles
10 × 100 ml bottles

Further information This new class of iodinated, non-ionic, low osmolality contrast medium for use in the gastro-intestinal tract offers a dramatic improvement in terms of general and local toxicity, imaging and ease of use. After oral or rectal administration of Gastromiro only about 1% of the dose is absorbed and available systemically.

Gastromiro does not damage the bowel mucosa and is less irritating to body tissues, such as the peritoneal cavity and lungs, than other diagnostic radiographic material and hypertonic water soluble iodinated agents.

Inactive ingredients: Citric acid, disodium edetate dihydrate, flavouring, saccharin, sodium cyclamate, sodium hydroxide, water.

Product licence number 0493/0139.

MULTIBIONTA* for INFUSION

Presentation A 10 ml ampoule of an aqueous solution containing:

Active ingredients:

Vitamin A palmitate (corresponding to 10,000 Units of Vitamin A)	5.5 mg
Vitamin B_1 hydrochloride	50 mg
Vitamin B_2-5 phosphate sodium salt	10 mg
Nicotinamide	100 mg
Pantothenyl alcohol	25 mg
Vitamin B_6 hydrochloride	15 mg
Vitamin C	500 mg
Vitamin E acetate	5 mg

Inactive ingredients: Polysorbate 80, propylene glycol, glycerol 85%, benzyl alcohol, DL-α-tocopherol, trometamol.

Uses Intravenous infusions of vitamins should only be considered when oral intake is impossible or inadequate.

Infants: Multibionta for infusion is indicated as part of a total parenteral feeding regimen in young children in the following conditions.

1. Protracted diarrhoea unresponsive to dietary treatment.
2. Renal failure.

In older children and adults:

1. Obstructing lesions of the gastro-intestinal tract.
2. Massive bowel resection.
3. Extensive burns.
4. Major trauma and severe infections.
5. Acute states of inflammatory bowel disease.
6. Severe uncontrolled malabsorptive states with undernutrition.
7. Disorders of swallowing as might occur in poliomyelitis, tetanus or following severe trauma.
8. Prolonged coma.

Dosage and administration The exact requirements of intravenously administered vitamins (particularly in sick infants) are not known. For adults 10 ml of Multibionta in an average daily dose should be added to a full infusion bottle containing not less than 250 ml of the infusion. For small children 2 ml per litre of the infusion fluid is adequate; alternatively the dose can be calculated as 0.15 ml/kilogram/24 hours. However, if preferred, the adult dose may be used with complete safety.

There is no preparation which contains all the essential vitamins in recommended amounts. It is, therefore, suggested that the following are given during prolonged intravenous nutrition in the dosage indicated.

Folic acid	0.1–0.5 mg/day
Vitamin B_{12}	100 micrograms/month
Vitamin D	300 Units/day (administered IM as calciferol. 1 ml contains 300,000 Units)
Vitamin K	3 mg twice weekly
Choline chloride	500 mg/day (normally present in adequate amounts as cholinephosphatides in fat emulsions)

Their compatibility with the carrier intravenous infusion should always be checked with the pharmacy before addition.

Additional information: The miscibility of 10 ml of Multibionta has been tested and it was found to be compatible with amino-acid solutions, carbohydrate solutions such as glucose at various concentrations, and fat solutions.

Although Multibionta is compatible with many infusion fluids, it is best introduced into separate normal saline or dextrose-saline mixtures.

Contra-indications, warnings, etc Rarely, intravenous B_1 may act as an allergen.

Multibionta must not be used in neonates, especially in immature preterm babies, because of the benzyl alcohol content.

Multibionta should only be given in pregnancy if there are compelling reasons because of the possible embryotoxic effect of propylene glycol.

In order to minimise possible loss of active substance in a mixture (masked incompatibility), it is recommended that solutions to which Multibionta is added should not be kept for longer than six hours. Amino-acid solutions or dextran solutions containing Multibionta should not be kept longer than one hour.

A mixture should be discarded if visible turbidity or crystallisation appear in the infusion solution.

Especial care should be taken to avoid exposure of a plastic bag or giving set containing Multibionta to direct sunlight.

Pharmaceutical precautions Should be stored at a temperature not exceeding 8°C.

Legal category POM.

Package quantities 10 ml ampoules in packs of 3.

Further information Nil.

Product licence number 0493/0076.

NIOPAM*

Presentation Ampoules or bottles containing sterile aqueous solutions of varying strengths of iopamidol.

Niopam 150: contains a 30.62% w/v concentration of the active constituent equivalent to 15% iodine or 150 mg iodine/ml.

Niopam 200: contains a 40.8% w/v concentration of the active constituent equivalent to 20% iodine or 200 mg iodine/ml.

Niopam 300: contains a 61.2% w/v concentration of the active constituent equivalent to 30% iodine or 300 mg iodine/ml.

Niopam 340: contains a 69.4% w/v concentration of the active constituent equivalent to 34% iodine or 340 mg iodine/ml.

Niopam 370: contains a 75.5% w/v concentration of the active constituent equivalent to 37% iodine or 370 mg iodine/ml.

Uses X-ray contrast media for lumbar and thoraco-cervical myelography, cerebral angiography, peripheral arteriography and venography, angiocardiography, digital subtraction angiography, left ventriculography and coronary arteriography, aortography, selective visceral angiography, computer tomography enhancement, urography, arthrography.

NIOPAM – Recommended Dosage Schedule

Procedure	*Niopam product and dosage*	
Lumbar Myelography	Niopam 200 Niopam 300	Adults 10–15 ml Adults 5–10 ml
Thoraco-Cervical Myelography	Niopam 200 Niopam 300	Adults 5–15 ml Adults 5–10 ml
Cerebral Angiography	Niopam 300	Adults 5–10 ml* Children 5–7 ml**
Peripheral Arteriography	Niopam 300 Niopam 340 Niopam 370	Adults 20–50 ml* Children **
Venography	Niopam 300	Adults 20–50 ml Children **
Angiocardiography & Left Ventriculography	Niopam 340 Niopam 370	Adults 30–80 ml Children **
Coronary Arteriography	Niopam 340 Niopam 370	Adults 4–8 ml per artery*
Aortography —retrograde	Niopam 340 Niopam 370	Adults 30–80 ml
Selective Renal Arteriography	Niopam 340 Niopam 370	Adults 5–10 ml Children **
Selective Visceral Angiography: Hepatic Coeliac Superior Mesenteric Inferior Mesenteric	Niopam 340 Niopam 370	Adults 30–70 ml 40–70 ml 25–70 ml 5–30 ml
Digital Subtraction Angiography Intra-arterial injection	Niopam 150	Adults 1–40 ml Children 0.5–0.75 ml/kg
Intra-venous injection	Niopam 340 Niopam 370	Adults 30–50 ml Children 0.5–0.75 ml/kg**
Left ventriculography	Niopam 340 Niopam 370 Niopam 150	Adults 25 ml Children 1.0–1.5 ml/kg
Selective coronary arteriography by intra-arterial DSA	Niopam 340 Niopam 370	Adults 2–5 ml
Computer Tomography Enhancement	Niopam 200 Niopam 300 Niopam 340	Adults *Brain Scanning* 50–100 ml *Whole Body Scanning* 40–100 ml
Intravenous Urography	Niopam 300 Niopam 340 Niopam 370	Adults 40–80 ml In severe renal failure the usual high dose methods should be employed (up to 1.5 ml/kg) Children 1–2.5 ml/kg or**
Arthrography	Niopam 300 Niopam 340	Adults 1–10 ml According to joint being examined.

* Repeat as necessary.
** According to body size and age.

Dosage and administration See table on previous page.

Elderly: There are no special dosage requirements for elderly patients, but as with all medicines, the lowest effective dose should be used.

Contra-indications, warnings, etc
Contra-indications: Proven or suspected hypersensitivity to iodine containing preparations of this type.

Warnings: As with all other contrast media this product may provoke anaphylaxis or other manifestations of allergy with nausea, vomiting, dyspnoea, erythema, urticaria and hypotension. A positive history of allergy, asthma or untoward reaction during previous similar investigations indicates a need for extra caution; the benefit should clearly outweigh the risk in such patients. Appropriate resuscitative measures should be immediately available.

Care should be exercised in carrying out radiographic procedures with contrast media in patients with severe functional impairment of the liver or myocardium, severe systemic disease and in myelomatosis. In the latter condition patients should not be exposed to dehydration; similarly abnormalities of fluid or electrolyte balance should be corrected prior to use.

Care should also be exercised in patients with moderate to severe impairment of renal function (as reflected by a raised blood urea) or in diabetes. Substantial deterioration in renal function is minimised if the patient is well hydrated. Renal function parameters should be monitored after the procedure in these patients.

Patients with severe hepato-renal insufficiency should not be examined unless absolutely indicated. Re-examination should be delayed for 5–7 days.

Special care should be exercised when this product is injected into the right heart or pulmonary artery in patients with pulmonary hypertension. Right heart angiography should be carried out only when absolutely indicated.

During intracardiac and/or coronary arteriography, ventricular arrhythmias may infrequently occur.

In patients who are known epileptics or have a history of epilepsy, anticonvulsant therapy should be maintained before and following myelographic procedures. In some instances, anticonvulsant therapy may be increased for 48 hours before the examination.

Use of this product may interfere with tests for thyroid function.

Niopam should be used with caution in patients with hyperthyroidism. It is possible that hyperthyroidism may recur in patients previously treated for Graves' disease.

Non-ionic contrast media have less anti-coagulant activity in-vitro than ionic media. Meticulous attention should therefore be paid to angiographic technique. Non-ionic media should not be allowed to remain in contact with blood in the syringe and intravascular catheters should be flushed frequently, to minimise the risk of clotting, which rarely has led to serious thromboembolic complications after procedures.

X-ray examination of women should if possibe be conducted during the pre-ovulation phase of the menstrual cycle and should be avoided during pregnancy; also since it has not been demonstrated that Niopam is safe for use in pregnant women, it should be administered only if the procedure is considered essential by the physician.

Side Effects: Side effects are infrequent and normally mild and may consist of headache, nausea, vomiting, heat sensation, dyspnoea and hypotension. Skin rashes may occur in some patients.

Following use in myelography, headaches, dizziness, nausea and vomiting may occasionally occur.

More severe reactions involving the cardiovascular system may call for emergency treatment; appropriate resuscitative measures should be immediately available.

No other drugs should be mixed with the contrast medium.

Pharmaceutical precautions Protect the solution from light. Store at room temperature.

Discard if solution is not clear of particulate matter.

Legal category POM.

Package quantities

Niopam 150:	Box containing 10 × 50 ml bottles
	Box containing 10 × 100 ml bottles
	Box containing 10 × 200 ml bottles
Niopam 200:	Box containing 5 × 10 ml ampoules
	Box containing 5 × 20 ml ampoules
	Box containing 10 × 50 ml bottles
Niopam 300:	Box containing 5 × 10 ml ampoules
	Box containing 5 × 20 ml ampoules
	Box containing 10 × 50 ml bottles
	Box containing 10 × 70 ml bottles
	Box containing 10 × 100 ml bottles
Niopam 340:	Box containing 10 × 50 ml bottles
	Box containing 10 × 100 ml bottles
Niopam 370:	Box containing 5 × 10 ml ampoules
	Box containing 5 × 20 ml ampoules
	Box containing 10 × 50 ml bottles
	Box containing 10 × 70 ml bottles
	Box containing 10 × 100 ml bottles
	Box containing 10 × 200 ml bottles

Further information Niopam is one of the new generation of water soluble non-ionic contrast media. The development of this compound has led to considerable reduction in general toxicity particularly with regard to vascular endothelium and nervous tissues.

Product licence numbers

Niopam 150	0493/0119
Niopam 200	0493/0065
Niopam 300	0493/0066
Niopam 340	0493/0131
Niopam 370	0493/0067

NUTRIZYM* GR

Presentation Hard gelatin capsules with opaque olive green cap and orange body each containing: Pancreatin BP 300 mg with not less than the following activities:

Lipase	10,000 BPU
Protease	650 BPU
Amylase	10,000 BPU

Use Fibrocystic disease of the pancreas, chronic pancreatitis, steatorrhoea and other pancreatic deficiency states.

Dosage and administration
Adults: 1–2 capsules with meals. In severe cases dosage may be increased.

Children: 1–2 capsules to be taken with meals and further capsules may be taken according to the degree of exocrine insufficiency.

Capsules should be swallowed whole with water. Where swallowing of capsules proves difficult, the capsule may be opened and the pellets sprinkled on soft foods which do not require chewing. When Nutrizym GR is mixed with foods in this way, the resulting mixture should not be allowed to stand for more than one hour prior to use.

Contra-indications, warnings, etc
Contra-indications: Known hypersensitivity to active ingredient (porcine pancreatin).

Precautions: Hyperuricaemia and hyperuricosuria have been reported to occur in cystic fibrosis patients; pancreatin extracts contain a very small amount of purine which might, in high doses, contribute to this condition.

Use in pregnancy: Safety in pregnancy has not been established.

Side-effects: Very rarely hypersensitivity reactions may occur. As with any pancreatin extract, high doses may cause buccal and perianal irritation, in rare cases amounting to inflammation.

Pharmaceutical precautions Store below 25° C in tightly closed containers.

Legal category P.

Package quantities Containers of 100 capsules OP.

Further information Each Nutrizym GR capsule contains enteric coated pellets of pancreatin extract thus giving maximum enzymatic activity in the gastrointestinal tract.

Product licence number 0493/0121.

OPTIMAX*

Presentation Optimax Tablets: Yellow capsule shaped film coated tablets each containing 500 mg L-tryptophan, 5 mg pyridoxine hydrochloride, 10 mg ascorbic acid, bearing the name OPTIMAX on one side and a break line on the other.

Optimax tablets are available without vitamins; they are of similar appearance and are marked OPTIMAX WV.

Optimax Powder: A chocolate-flavoured powder for mixing into a drink with warm milk or water. Each 6 g of powder contains 1 g L-tryptophan, 10 mg pyridoxine hydrochloride, 20 mg ascorbic acid.

Uses Optimax is indicated for the relief of symptoms of mild to moderate depressive illness. Long term efficacy and safety of L-tryptophan have not been established; therefore, it is recommended that L-tryptophan be used for short term therapy with a review at three monthly intervals. For the treatment of more severe depressive illness Optimax may be administered with other antidepressant drugs.

Dosage and administration
Adults: The usual dose is two tablets, three times daily or one sachet three times daily (equivalent to 3 g L-tryptophan daily); for some patients up to 6 g L-tryptophan may be required. There is no evidence to suggest that dosage in the elderly should be different.

Children: Not recommended.

When used in combination with other antidepressants it may be necessary to adjust the dosage of either component.

Contra-indications, warnings, etc
Contra-indications: No absolute contra-indications known.

Precautions and Drug Interactions: Where Optimax is combined with an MAO Inhibitor the side effects of the latter may be enhanced.

In patients taking Optimax in conjunction with phenothiazines or benzodiazepines there have been isolated reports of sexual disinhibition.

Pyridoxine should not be administered to patients undergoing treatment with L-Dopa.

L-tryptophan is not advised, except for relatively short periods, in patients with active bladder disease or known bladder lesions.

Warnings and Adverse Effects: L-tryptophan may produce drowsiness. Patients should be warned of the possible hazard when driving or operating machinery.

In some patients Optimax may cause a slight feeling of nausea which usually disappears within 2 or 3 days. Such nausea can be minimised by giving Optimax after food. Other adverse reactions include headache and lightheadedness.

Safety in pregnancy has not been established.

Overdosage: Drowsiness and vomiting may occur; supportive measures should be employed.

Pharmaceutical precautions Store in a cool dry place.

Legal category POM.

Package quantities *Optimax Tablets:* Containers of 100 tablets (OP) and of 500 tablets.

Optimax Powder: Cartons of 100 sachets OP.

Further information L-tryptophan, one of the essential amino acids, is the major precursor of the brain amine 5-hydroxytryptamine (5-HT). There is convincing evidence that levels of 5-HT are depleted in the CNS of depressed patients.

Abnormal tryptophan metabolism may occur in patients who are pyridoxine deficient. Such deficiency may occur in women taking oral contraceptives.

For some patients it may be beneficial to prescribe tablets for the morning and midday dose and powder for the night time dose.

Product licence numbers
Optimax Tablets 0493/5903
Optimax WV Tablets 0493/5900
Optimax Powder 0493/5902

SEPTOPAL* CHAINS

Presentation Methylmethacrylate-methylacrylate copolymer (PMMA) beads (7 mm in diameter) each containing gentamicin sulphate 7.5 mg (corresponding to 4.5 mg of gentamicin base) and 20 mg of zirconium dioxide as X-ray medium.

Chains consisting of 10 or 30 beads threaded on multiple-thread surgical wire.

Uses Gentamicin is a proven broad spectrum antibiotic active against both gram-positive and gram-negative organisms. Following insertion of the Chains, gentamicin is released gradually from the PMMA beads over a prolonged period and the high bactericidal concentrations of the antibiotic reached at the site of infection enable the infection to be controlled, or provide protection against infection when used prophylactically.

Septopal Chains are indicated for:

Short term and longer term therapy in bone infection, e.g. osteomyelitis, infected pseudoarthroses, infected osteosyntheses.

Short term preventive treatment of potentially infected bone injuries.

Short term prevention and therapy of soft tissue infections associated with abdominoperineal resections; operations on the small or large bowel. Other therapeutic indications for use include bacterial peritonitis, infection associated with cholecystectomies, infective fistulae, infected vascular grafts, soft tissue abscesses.

Dosage and administration
Administration: Septopal Chains are implanted in the cavity resulting from thorough surgical removal of infected tissue and/or sequestrated bone or that remaining after operation in the sacral cavity. The chains are laid in the cavity in such a way as to facilitate easy removal.

Septopal Chains may be used as follows:

1. Bone Infection
(a) *Short term application:* For the implantation of Chains, it is recommended to take into account the direction in which the Chain will later be pulled out and to let the last bead anchored by a loose suture, project above skin level through a separate stab incision in order that the Chain may be removed by careful, steady traction a few beads at a time daily. The Chains are in general removed within 10–14 days following insertion and preferably not more than 10 days after the operation.

Where there is evidence of persisting local infection beyond 5 days post-operatively, it is recommended that the Chain be removed and the cause of infection determined prior to recommending further antibacterial therapy.

The less the Chains are fixed to connective tissue, the easier it is to remove them; this procedure is thus also less painful and more comfortable for the patient.

If the beads become fixed to connective tissue to an advanced extent, or if the traction on the beads is not adapted to the tissue conditions, one or several beads may rarely detach themselves from the multistranded wire or, in exceptional circumstances the wire may break on the removal of the Chain. In such an event one should generally try to remove the single beads (together with the remaining wire). Should, however, extensive surgical procedures be necessary, the single beads may be left in the body, taking into consideration the comparative risk of reoperation. For the above reasons the surgeons should count the beads on their removal as a check.

(b) Longer Term Application: This may be as above or if circumstances require it, the Chains may be implanted completely, and removed by reoperation up to 3 months later. The length of time the Chains are left in situ prior to secondary intervention will depend on the orthopaedic procedure. Inserted Chains will be completely enclosed by primary wound closure. Control of local infection allows subsequent surgical procedures, e.g. cancellous bone grafting.

2. Soft tissue infections (Short term applications only): The insertion of chains is carried out as described under 1a above. In this indication, the chains are best removed by the sixth and the very latest by the tenth day after the operation. In most cases it is advised that the chains are withdrawn gradually a few beads at a time daily from about the second post insertion day.

In considering wound closure/drainage it should be remembered that excess drainage will dilute the gentamicin concentration at the site of infection so, if possible, primary wound closure should always be employed. Local circumstances and degree of inflammation however should be considered.

An overflow drain may be employed only when considered necessary. Suction drainage is not employed but may be temporarily used in cases of obstructed wound secretion flow.

Toxic effects due to the antibiotics are not anticipated since after use of Septopal Chains, barely detectable systemic gentamicin concentrations (no more than 0.5 micrograms/ml) are found in the serum for up to 4 days postoperatively following insertion of the Chains.

Dosage: The number of Chains used will depend upon the size of the cavity. Usually 1–3 Chains are inserted but up to 5 have been used.

Contra-indications, warnings, etc There is no absolute contra-indication other than established intolerance of gentamicin.

Septopal Chains should not be used concurrently in apposition to metal-containing implants because of the theoretical possibility of surgical wire and implant corrosion. Septopal Chains should be removed prior to implant of a metal prosthesis.

Since the beads are strung on surgical wire containing chrome and nickel, there is a potential for local sensitivity reactions to these metals.

Gentamicin crosses the placenta barrier and may cause ototoxicity in the foetus although no problems in clinical use have been positively identified. Implantation of Septopal Chains results in only a transient, barely detectable plasma concentration of gentamicin which is well below toxic levels therefore, no ototoxic effects on the foetus are to be expected. Nevertheless, it is recommended that the product should not be used in pregnancy.

Septopal Chains should not be used alone in those situations where culture of wound secretion reveals the presence of anaerobic bacteria, or organisms which could be insensitive to gentamicin therapy. In these instances, additional systemic therapy with an appropriate antibiotic should be used.

Septopal may be used in all orthopaedic surgical procedures where gentamicin sensitive organisms are found to be present from routine bacteriological screening. Where resistant organisms are encountered to the standard 10 microgram disc test, a MIC determination is recommended. In view of the high bactericidal gentamicin concentration at the infection site, organisms found resistant to the standard 10 microgram sensitivity disc screen may in fact be sensitive and therefore results of such screening may not give a true reflection of clinical effectiveness.

In soft tissue, the chains should not be implanted intraperitoneally.

Young and elderly: There is no evidence to suggest that use of Septopal Chains is either nephrotoxic or ototoxic. Nevertheless, for those patients who have moderate to severe impairment of renal function and when Septopal therapy is desirable, monitoring of renal state is advised.

Pharmaceutical precautions Store at room temperature – do not freeze.

Resterilisation of Septopal Chains should not be attempted under any circumstances.

Legal category POM.

Package quantities One Chain consists of 10 or 30 beads threaded on surgical wire in a sterile inner sachet (peel-off pack). Packs of 1 chain of 10 beads. Packs of 1 Chain of 30 beads. Packs of 5 Chains of 30 beads.

Further information Septopal Chains have been sterilised in ethylene oxide. They are contained in a triple sachet. The two outer sachets are opened (aluminium covering followed by the non-sterile peel-off pack) and the chain in the inner, sterile sachet is then removed under aseptic conditions.

Gentamicin is released in bactericidal concentrations at the site of infection with negligible systemic spread. Granulation tissue grows into the hollow spaces between the beads during the healing process, the flow of secretion is not inhibited and the bio-mechanics of the bone are not changed. Local control of infection lessens the risk of secondary infection developing with subsequent bone grafting.

Product licence number 0493/0091.

TUTOPLAST* DURA

Presentation Tutoplast Dura is solvent dehydrated human dura mater in the form of absorbable collagen for homotransplantation. It is highly purified, free from antigens and enzymes, and sterilised by gamma irradiation.

Uses Tutoplast Dura may be used to effect a repair or closure in the following areas: Thoracic surgery, abdominal surgery, neurosurgery and urology.

It should be used in procedures in which the use of human dura is essential, consideration having been given to the use of autologous tissue or synthetic materials.

Dosage and administration Tutoplast Dura, of suitable size for the area under transplantation, should be soaked in a sterile solution of 0.9% saline at room temperature for several minutes prior to use. This makes the Dura softer and easier to work with during surgery.

Contra-indications, warnings, etc

Contra-indication: Dura implantation is contra-indicated if local infection is present.

Warning: As with all biological products, it is not possible to give an absolute guarantee of freedom from Human Immunodeficiency Virus (HIV) or Creutzfeldt–Jakob Disease (CJD) agent although treatments shown to be capable of reducing the risk of any transmission are used in the processing of Tutoplast Dura.

Pharmaceutical precautions Opened and unused material should be discarded.

Legal category POM.

Package quantities

1/1 calotte: pack containing 1 piece
1/2 calotte: pack containing 1 piece
4 × 5 cm: pack containing 2 pieces
1.5 × 3 cm: pack containing 5 pieces
2 × 10 cm: pack containing 2 pieces
4 × 10 cm: pack containing 1 piece
2 × 30 cm: pack containing 1 piece

Other sizes available on request from E Merck Ltd.

Further information Transplanted Tutoplast Dura provides the basis for the formation of endogenous connective tissue. Within a period of 3–4 months, about 85% of the transplant is absorbed and replaced by collagenous connective tissue. This endogenous tissue formation is contingent on the size of the transplant and the tissue reactivity in the surrounding transplant area.

Product licence number 0493/0090.

UNGUENTUM MERCK*

Presentation Unguentum Merck is a stable emulsion system with a uniform distribution of fat and water (ambiphilic); thus it combines the properties of a) an oil in water emulsion (cream) and b) a water in oil emulsion (ointment), for use on dry or weeping conditions of the skin.

Composition: Dispersed silicic acid; liquid paraffin; white soft paraffin; cetostearyl alcohol; polysorbate-40; glyceryl monostearate; saturated neutral oils; sorbic acid; propylene glycol; purified water, sodium hydroxide. Fat content: about 60%. Water content: about 40%.

Uses Unguentum Merck is to be used as a diluent for various topical corticosteroid formulations in those instances where a lower strength preparation is considered desirable by the physician and as a general base for extemporaneous dispensing.

Unguentum Merck has emollient properties and is recommended for the symptomatic treatment of dermatitis, nappy rash, ichthyosis, eczema, protection of raw and abraded skin areas, pruritus and related conditions where dry scaly skin is a problem, and as a pre-bathing emollient for dry/eczematous skin, to alleviate drying effects.

Dosage and administration *Administration:* A thin application of the cream should be gently massaged into the skin three times daily or at appropriate intervals.

When used as a protective cream Unguentum Merck should be applied sparingly to the affected areas of the skin before, or immediately after, exposure to a potentially harmful factor.

Contra-indications, warnings, etc Unguentum Merck should not be used for the treatment of patients sensitive to any of the ingredients.

Pharmaceutical precautions No special requirements.

Legal category P.

Package quantities Tubes of 50 g, 100 g. Jar of 500 g. 200 ml dispenser.

Further information Unguentum Merck contains no common allergens such as lanolin or parabens.

Product licence number 0493/0013.

UROMIRO* 300, 340, 380, 420 SODIUM UROMIRO* 300

Presentation Ampoules or bottles containing sterile aqueous solutions of varying strengths of meglumine and sodium iodamide.

Uromiro 300: Contains a 65% w/v concentration of the meglumine salt of iodamide equivalent to 30% iodine or 300 mg/ml.

Uromiro 340: Contains a concentration of 18.3% w/v meglumine iodamide and 43.4% w/v of sodium iodamide equivalent to 34% iodine or 340 mg/ml.

Uromiro 380: Contains a concentration of 70% w/v meglumine iodamide and 9.7% w/v sodium iodamide equivalent to 38% iodine or 380 mg/ml.

Uromiro 420: Contains a concentration of 40.8% w/v meglumine iodamide and 39.4% w/v sodium iodamide equivalent to 42% iodine or 420 mg/ml.

Sodium Uromiro 300: Contains a concentration of 52.66% w/v sodium iodamide equivalent to 30% iodine or 300 mg/ml.

Uses X-ray contrast media for the opacification of the vascular and renal systems, e.g. urography, cerebral angiography, peripheral arteriography, venography, operative and T-tube cholangiography, angiocardiography, coronary arteriography and aortography.

Dosage and administration See Table.

Elderly: Dosage as for adults.

Contra-indications, warnings, etc

Contra-indications: Proven or suspected hypersensitivity to iodine-containing preparations of this type.

Warnings, side-effects: Care should be exercised in patients with severe systemic disease, in hyperthyroidism, in allergic subjects and in myelomatosis; patients with this condition should not be exposed to dehydration.

X-ray examination of women should if possible be conducted during the pre-ovulation phase of the menstrual cycle and should be avoided during pregnancy;

Intravenous Urography	Sodium Uromiro 300 Uromiro 300 Uromiro 340 Uromiro 380 Uromiro 420	Adults 40–80 ml Children 1 ml/kg	In severe renal failure the usual high dose methods of Urography should be applied (up to 1.5 ml/kg)
Cerebral Angiography	Uromiro 300	Adults 8 ml Children 5–7 ml according to body size and age	
Angiocardiography	Uromiro 380 Uromiro 420	Adults 20–50 ml Children 1 ml/kg In both adults and children requiring frequent multiple injections, a total of 3–5 ml per kg should seldom be exceeded. Inject rapidly within 1–2 sec.	
Coronary Arteriography	Uromiro 380	Adults 5–8 ml per artery	
Peripheral Arteriography	Uromiro 300 Uromiro 340 Uromiro 380	Adults 20–30 ml Children according to body size and age	
Venography	Uromiro 300 Uromiro 340	Adults 20–30 ml Children according to body size and age	
Operative and T-tube Cholangiography	Uromiro 300	During the period of operation 10–15 ml of contrast medium are injected into the cystic duct or its stump by means of a fine needle. In the postoperative period this may be done through a T-tube left in situ at operation	
Aortography retrograde	Uromiro 380 Uromiro 420	Adults 20–40 ml Children according to body size and age	
Selective renal arteriography	Uromiro 380 Uromiro 420	Adults 8 ml Children according to body size and age	

also since it has not been demonstrated that Uromiro is safe for use in pregnant women, it should be administered only if the procedure is considered essential by the physician.

Use of the product may give rise to side-effects including anaphylactoid or shock-like manifestations with nausea, vomiting, widespread reddening of the skin and heat sensation, headache, and sometimes coryza; oedema of the larynx, fever, sweating, asthenia, dizziness, pallor, dyspnoea, and moderate hypotension. Skin rashes of various description may occur in some patients.

More severe reactions involving the cardiovascular system may call for emergency treatment. Appropriate resuscitative measures should be immediately available. No other drugs should be mixed with the contrast medium.

Fluid intake should not be limited in neonates and small children.

Before using hypertonic contrast media any abnormalities of water and electrolyte balance should be corrected.

Pharmaceutical precautions Store away from light.

Legal category POM.

Package quantities
Uromiro 300:
Box containing 10 × 50 ml bottles.

Uromiro 340:
Box containing 5 × 20 ml ampoules.
Box containing 10 × 50 ml bottles.

Uromiro 380:
Box containing 10 × 50 ml bottles.

Uromiro 420:
Box containing 10 × 50 ml bottles.

Sodium Uromiro 300:
Box containing 10 × 50 ml bottles.

Further information Nil.

Product licence numbers
Uromiro 300 0493/0086
Uromiro 340 0493/0087
Uromiro 380 0493/0088
Uromiro 420 0493/0089
Sodium Uromiro 300 0493/0085

**Trade Mark*

Merck Sharp & Dohme Limited
Hertford Road
Hoddesdon
Hertfordshire EN11 9BU

MSD
MERCK SHARP & DOHME

ALDOMET*

Presentation Yellow, film-coated tablets containing Methyldopa BP equivalent to the following amounts of anhydrous methyldopa: 125 mg (marked 'ALDOMET MSD 135'), 250 mg (marked 'ALDOMET MSD 401'), or 500 mg (marked 'ALDOMET MSD 516').

Fruit-flavoured, oral suspension containing 250 mg of methyldopa per 5 ml. The oral suspension contains sodium metabisulphite as preservative

Injection, ampoules containing 50 mg Methyldopate Hydrochloride BP per millilitre, as a colourless solution. The injection contains sodium metabisulphite as preservative.

Uses Hypertension. Aldomet Injection is indicated for hypertension when parenteral medication is required. Treatment of acute hypertensive crises may be initiated with Aldomet Injection when an immediate effect is not necessary.

Mode of action: The antihypertensive effect of methyldopa is probably due to its metabolism to alphamethylnoradrenaline, which lowers arterial pressure by stimulation of central inhibitory alpha-adrenergic receptors, false neurotransmission, and/or reduction of plasma renin activity.

Dosage and administration *Oral therapy – Adults: Initial dosage:* Usually 250 mg two or three times a day, for two days.

Adjustment: Usually adjusted at intervals of not less than two days, until an adequate response is obtained. The maximum recommended daily dosage is 3 g.

Many patients experience sedation for two or three days when therapy with Aldomet is started or when the dose is increased. When increasing the dosage, therefore, it may be desirable to increase the evening dose first.

General considerations: Methyldopa is largely excreted by the kidney, and patients with impaired renal function may respond to smaller doses.

Withdrawal of Aldomet is followed by return of hypertension, usually within 48 hours. This is not complicated generally by an overshoot of blood pressure.

Therapy with Aldomet may be initiated in most patients already on treatment with other antihypertensive agents by terminating these antihypertensive medications gradually if required (see manufacturer's recommendations on stopping these drugs). Following such previous antihypertensive therapy, Aldomet should be limited to an initial dose of not more than 500 mg daily and increased as required at intervals of not less than two days.

A thiazide may be added at any time during methyldopa therapy and is recommended if therapy has not been started with a thiazide or if effective control of blood pressure cannot be maintained on 2.0 g of methyldopa daily.

Aldomet may also be used concomitantly with the combination of amiloride hydrochloride and hydrochlorothiazide (such as Moduretic*) or beta-blocking agents, such as timolol maleate (Blocadren*).

When methyldopa is given to patients on other antihypertensives the dose of these agents may need to be adjusted to effect a smooth transition.

Oral therapy – Children: Initial dosage is based on 10 mg/kg of body weight daily in 2–4 oral doses. The daily dosage then is increased or decreased until an adequate response is achieved. The maximum dosage is 65 mg/kg or 3.0 g daily, whichever is less.

Intravenous therapy: Aldomet Injection is for intravenous use only, it must not be given intramuscularly or subcutaneously. An effective dose will produce a fall in blood pressure that may begin in 4 to 6 hours and be maintained for 10 to 16 hours.

The required dose of Aldomet Injection should be added to 100 ml of 5% Dextrose Injection BP. Alternatively, Aldomet may be given with 5% dextrose infusion solution BP at a concentration of 100 mg to each 10 ml solution. This intravenous infusion should be given slowly over a period of 30 to 60 minutes.

When practicable, oral therapy with Aldomet may be substituted, starting with the same dosage as that being used by the parenteral route.

Usual adult dosage: 250–500 mg (5–10 ml) six-hourly. In severe cases, up to 1 g (20 ml) six-hourly may be needed, and this is the maximum recommended dosage. If there is renal impairment, lower dosages should suffice.

Children's dosage: The recommended intravenous dosage for children is 20–40 mg/kg of body weight daily in divided doses every six hours. The maximum dosage is 65 mg/kg or 3.0 g daily, whichever is less. If there is renal impairment, lower dosages should suffice.

Use in the elderly: The initial dose in elderly patients should be kept as low as possible, not exceeding 250 mg daily; an appropriate starting dose in the elderly would be 125 mg b.d. increasing slowly as required, but not to exceed a maximum daily dosage of 2 g.

Contra-indications, warnings, etc
Contra-indications: Active hepatic disease, such as acute hepatitis and active cirrhosis; hypersensitivity (including hepatic disorders associated with previous methyldopa therapy), depression.

Aldomet is not recommended for the treatment of phaeochromocytoma (see 'Precautions').

Precautions: Acquired haemolytic anaemia has occurred rarely; should symptoms suggest anaemia, haemoglobin and/or haematocrit determinations should be made. If anaemia is confirmed, tests should be done for haemolysis. If haemolytic anaemia is present, Aldomet should be discontinued. Stopping therapy, with or without giving a corticosteroid, has usually brought prompt remission. Rarely, however, deaths have occurred.

Some patients on continued therapy with methyldopa develop a positive direct Coombs test. From the reports of different investigators, the incidence averages between 10% and 20%. A positive Coombs test rarely develops in the first six months of therapy, and if it has not developed within 12 months, it is unlikely to do so later on continuing therapy. Development is also dose-related, the lowest incidence occurring in patients receiving 1 g or less of methyldopa per day. The test becomes negative usually within weeks or months of stopping methyldopa.

Prior knowledge of a positive Coombs reaction will aid in evaluating a cross-match for transfusion. If a patient with a positive Coombs reaction shows an incompatible minor cross-match, an indirect Coombs test should be performed. If this is negative, transfusion with blood compatible in the major cross-match may be carried out. If positive, the advisability of transfusion should be determined by a haematologist.

Reversible leucopenia, with primary effect on granulocytes has been reported rarely. The granulocyte count returned to normal on discontinuing therapy. Reversible thrombocytopenia has occurred rarely.

Occasionally, fever has occurred within the first three weeks of therapy, sometimes associated with eosinophilia or abnormalities in liver function tests. Jaundice, with or without fever, also may occur. Its onset is usually within the first two or three months of therapy. In some patients the findings are consistent with those of cholestasis. Rare cases of fatal hepatic necrosis have been reported. Liver biopsy, performed in several patients with liver dysfunction, showed a microscopic focal necrosis compatible with drug hypersensitivity. Liver function tests and a total and differential white blood cell count are advisable before therapy and at intervals during the first six weeks to twelve weeks of therapy, or whenever an unexplained fever occurs. Should fever, abnormality in liver function, or jaundice occur, therapy should be withdrawn. If related to methyldopa, the temperature and abnormalities in liver function will then return to normal. Methyldopa should not be used again in these patients. Methyldopa should be used with caution in patients with a history of previous liver disease or dysfunction.

When methyldopa and lithium are given concomitantly the patient should be monitored carefully for symptoms of lithium toxicity.

When methyldopa is used with other antihypertensive drugs, potentiation of antihypertensive action may occur. The progress of patients should be carefully followed to detect side reactions or manifestations of drug idiosyncrasy.

The antihypertensive effect of Aldomet may be diminished by sympathomimetics, phenothiazines, tricyclic antidepressants and MAOIs.

A paradoxical pressor response has been reported with Aldomet Injection.

Patients may require reduced doses of anaesthetics when on methyldopa. If hypotension does occur during anaesthesia, it can usually be controlled by vasopressors. The adrenergic receptors remain sensitive during treatment with methyldopa.

Dialysis removes methyldopa; therefore, hypertension may recur after this procedure.

Rarely, involuntary choreoathetotic movements have been observed during therapy with methyldopa in patients with severe bilateral cerebrovascular disease. Should these movements occur, therapy should be discontinued.

Aldomet should be used with extreme caution in patients, or in near relatives of patients, with hepatic porphyria.

The preservatives in both Aldomet Injection and Suspension have been reported to cause hypersensitivity. Sodium metabisulphite in particular is associated with circulatory collapse, and depression of the central nervous system in certain susceptible individuals with allergic tendencies.

Interference with laboratory tests: Methyldopa may interfere with the measurement of urinary uric acid by the phosphotungstate method, serum creatinine by the alkaline picrate method, and AST (SGOT) by colorimetric method. Interference with spectrophotometric methods for AST (SGOT) analysis has not been reported.

As methyldopa fluoresces at the same wavelengths as catecholamines, spuriously high amounts of urinary catecholamines may be reported interfering with a diagnosis of phaeochromocytoma.

It is important to recognise this phenomenon before a patient with a possible phaeochromocytoma is subjected to surgery. Methyldopa does not interfere with measurements of VMA (vanillylmandelic acid) by those methods which convert VMA to vanillin.

Rarely, when urine is exposed to air after voiding, it may darken because of breakdown of methyldopa or its metabolites.

Pregnancy and breast-feeding mothers: Aldomet has been used under close medical supervision for the treatment of hypertension during pregnancy. There was no clinical evidence that Aldomet caused fetal abnormalities or affected the neonate.

Methyldopa crosses the placental barrier and appears in cord blood and breast milk.

Although no obvious teratogenic effects have been reported, the possibility of fetal injury cannot be excluded and the use of the drug in women who are, or may become, pregnant or who are breast-feeding their newborn infant requires that anticipated benefits be weighed against possible risks.

Side-effects: Sedation, usually transient, may occur during the initial period of therapy or whenever the dose is increased. If affected, patients should not attempt to drive, or operate machinery. Headache, asthenia or weakness may be noted as early and transient symptoms.

Significant side-effects due to Aldomet have been infrequent and this agent usually is well tolerated.

The following reactions have been reported:

Central nervous system: Sedation (usually transient), headache, asthenia or weakness, paraesthesiae, parkinsonism, Bell's palsy, involuntary choreoathetotic movements. Psychic disturbances including nightmares, impaired mental acuity and reversible mild psychoses or depression. Dizziness, light-headedness, and symptoms of cerebrovascular insufficiency (may be due to lowering of blood pressure).

Cardiovascular: Bradycardia, prolonged carotid sinus hypersensitivity, aggravation of angina pectoris. Orthostatic hypotension (decrease daily dosage). Oedema (and weight gain) usually relieved by use of a diuretic. (Discontinue methyldopa if oedema progresses or signs of heart failure appear.)

Gastro-intestinal: Nausea, vomiting, distension, constipation, flatus, diarrhoea, colitis, mild dryness of mouth, sore or 'black' tongue, pancreatitis, sialadenitis.

Hepatic: Liver disorders including hepatitis, jaundice, abnormal liver function tests.

Haematological: Positive Coombs test, haemolytic anaemia, bone marrow depression, leucopenia, granulocytopenia, thrombocytopenia. Positive tests for antinuclear antibody, LE cells, and rheumatoid factor.

Allergic: Drug-related fever and lupus-like syndrome, myocarditis, pericarditis.

Dermatological: Rash as in eczema or lichenoid eruption, toxic epidermal necrolysis.

Other: Nasal stuffiness, rise in blood urea, breast enlargement, gynaecomastia, hyperprolactinaemia, amenorrhoea, lactation, impotence, decreased libido, failure of ejaculation, mild arthralgia with or without joint swelling, myalgia.

Overdosage: Acute overdosage may produce acute hypotension with other responses attributable to brain and gastro-intestinal malfunction (excessive sedation, weakness, bradycardia, dizziness, light-headedness, constipation, distension, flatus, diarrhoea, nausea, and vomiting). If ingestion is recent, emesis may be induced or gastric lavage performed. There is no specific antidote. Methyldopa is dialysable. Treatment is symptomatic. Infusions may be helpful to promote urinary excretion. Special attention should be directed towards cardiac rate and output, blood volume, electrolyte balance, paralytic ileus, urinary function and cerebral activity. Administration of sympathomimetic agents may be indicated. When chronic overdosage is suspected, Aldomet should be discontinued.

The plasma half-life of methyldopa is 105 minutes. Peak plasma levels were reached about two hours after oral ingestion.

Pharmaceutical precautions Keep containers well closed and store the tablets and suspension below 25°C, protected from light. The injection should also be protected from freezing. Only 5% dextrose should be used as diluent for the injection.

Aldomet Suspension should not be diluted.

Legal category POM.

Package quantities *Tablets 125 mg:* Bottles of 100.

Tablets 250 mg: Bottles of 100 and 500.
Tablets 500 mg: Bottles of 100 and 500.
Oral Suspension 250 mg/5 ml: Bottles of 200 ml.
Injection: Ampoules of 5 ml.

Further information Aldomet reduces both supine and standing blood pressure. Symptomatic postural hypotension, exercise hypotension and diurnal blood pressure variations rarely occur. By adjustment of dosage, morning hypotension can be prevented without sacrificing control of afternoon blood pressure.

Methyldopa has no direct effect on cardiac function and usually does not reduce glomerular filtration rate, renal blood flow or filtration fraction. Cardiac output usually is maintained without cardiac acceleration. In some patients, the heart rate is slowed.

Because of its relative freedom from adverse effects on kidney function, methyldopa can be of benefit in the control of high blood pressure, even in the presence of renal impairment. It may help arrest or retard the progression of renal function impairment and damage due to sustained elevation of blood pressure.

Normal or elevated plasma renin activity may decrease in course of methyldopa therapy.

Product licence numbers

Tablets 125 mg	0025/0098
Tablets 250 mg	0025/0099
Tablets 500 mg	0025/0100
Oral Suspension 250 mg/5 ml	0025/0154
Injection	0025/5003

ARAMINE*

Presentation A clear, colourless solution containing, in each millilitre, Metaraminol Tartrate BP equivalent to 10 mg metaraminol. Aramine also contains methylparaben, propylparaben and sodium bisulphite as preservatives; with the solution made isotonic by the inclusion of sodium chloride.

Uses Sympathomimetic amine (vasopressor agent). For the treatment of acute hypotension due to loss of vasoconstrictor tone as may occur during spinal anaesthesia, and as an adjunct to accepted remedial procedures (e.g. tilting of patient and attention to fluid volumes). (See 'Precautions'.)

The pressor effect of a single dose of Aramine lasts from about twenty minutes up to one hour. Its onset is around one or two minutes after direct intravenous injection.

Dosage and administration Aramine Injection may be given intravenously either directly or by infusion. Because the maximum effect is not immediately apparent, allow at least ten minutes before increasing the dose. Since the vasopressor effect tapers off when therapy is stopped, be prepared to restart promptly if the blood pressure falls too rapidly. Patients with coexistent shock and acidosis may show poor response.

Direct intravenous injection is recommended only in grave emergencies. *Particular care should be taken to use the correct dose.*

Intravenous infusion (for adjunctive treatment of hypotension): 15–100 mg (1.5–10 ml) in 500 ml of Sodium Chloride Injection BP or 5% Dextrose Injection BP, adjusting the rate of infusion to maintain the blood pressure at the desired level. Higher concentrations of Aramine 150–500 mg per 500 ml of infusion fluid, have been used. If the patient needs additional saline or dextrose at a rate of flow that would provide an excessive dose of Aramine when used as recommended, the volume of infusion fluid should be increased accordingly. Aramine may also be added to *less* than 500 ml of infusion fluid if a smaller volume is desired.

Aramine is physically and chemically compatible with Injection Sodium Chloride BP, 5% Injection Dextrose BP, Ringer's Injection USP, Lactated Ringer's Injection USP, Dextran 70 Injection.

When Aramine is mixed with an infusion solution, sterile precautions should be observed. Mixtures should be used within 24 hours since infusion solutions do not contain preservatives.

Direct intravenous injection (to be employed only in grave emergencies, when immediate action is necessary to save life): 0.5–5 mg (0.05–0.5 ml), followed by an infusion of 15–100 mg (1.5–10 ml) in 500 ml of infusion liquid. *Particular care should be taken to use the correct dose when injecting undiluted Aramine.*

Children: Aramine should not be used in children.

Use in the elderly: The dosage may not require modification for elderly patients; however geriatric patients may be more sensitive to sympathomimetic agents, therefore particular caution should be taken in this age group.

Contra-indications, warnings, etc
Contra-indications: Concurrent use with cyclopropane or halothane anaesthesia, unless clinical circumstances demand it. Hypersensitivity to any component of Aramine. Children.

Precautions and side-effects: Caution should be exercised to avoid excessive blood pressure changes since response to treatment with Aramine is very variable and the ensuing control of the blood pressure may prove difficult.

In choosing the site for injection, it is important to avoid those areas generally recognised as being unsuitable for the use of any pressor agent and to discontinue the infusion immediately if infiltration or thrombosis occurs. Although the urgent nature of the patient's condition may force the choice of an unsuitable injection site, the preferred areas of injection should be used when possible. The larger veins of the antecubital fossa or thigh are preferred to the veins in the ankle or dorsum of the hand, particularly in patients with peripheral vascular disease, diabetes mellitus, Buerger's disease or conditions with coexistent hypercoagulability.

Monoamine oxidase inhibitors have been reported to potentiate the action of sympathomimetic amines. The pressor effect of Aramine is decreased but not reversed by alpha-adrenergic blocking agents.

Aramine should be used with caution in cases of heart disease, hypertension, thyroid disease or diabetes mellitus because of its vasoconstrictor action.

Sympathomimetic amines may provoke a relapse in patients with a history of malaria.

Sympathomimetic amines, including Aramine, may cause sinus or ventricular tachycardia, or other arrhythmias, especially in patients with myocardial infarction.

Each preservative in Aramine has been reported to cause hypersensitivity. Sodium bisulphite in particular is associated with circulatory or respiratory collapse, and depression of the CNS in certain susceptible individuals, particularly in those with asthma.

Abscess formation, tissue necrosis, and sloughing rarely may follow the use of Aramine.

Rapidly induced hypertensive responses have been reported to cause acute pulmonary oedema, cardiac arrhythmias and arrest. Aramine should be used with caution in patients with cirrhosis; electrolyte levels should be adequately restored if a diuresis ensues. A fatal ventricular arrhythmia was reported in a patient with Laënnec's cirrhosis while receiving metaraminol tartrate. In several instances, ventricular extrasystoles that appeared during infusion of Aramine promptly subsided when the rate of flow was reduced. Aramine should be used with caution in digitalised patients since the combination of digitalis and sympathomimetic amines is capable of causing ectopic arrhythmic activity.

With the prolonged action of Aramine, a cumulative effect is possible. An excessive vasopressor response may cause a prolonged elevation of blood pressure, even after discontinuation of therapy.

When vasopressor amines are used for long periods, the resulting vasoconstriction may prevent adequate expansion of circulating volume and may cause perpetuation of the shock state. There is evidence that plasma volume may be reduced in all types of shock, and that the measurement of central venous pressure is useful in assessing the adequacy of the circulating blood volume.

Blood, or plasma-volume expanders, should therefore be employed when the principal reason for hypotension or shock is decreased circulating volume.

Overdosage: Aramine acts rapidly. Its major therapeutic effects are complete within an hour of parenteral administration.

If the drug has been ingested, induce emesis or perform gastric lavage. If Aramine has been administered by subcutaneous or intramuscular injection, local ice packs may be applied to delay absorption. Intravenous infusion should be stopped immediately, but reinstated if hypotension occurs. If needed, an alpha-adrenergic blocking agent such as phenoxybenzamine may be used to reduce hypertension. Intravenous beta-adrenergic blocking agents may also be useful for reducing hypertension and may have a beneficial effect on cardiac arrhythmia, if present. Parenteral diazepam may be given for convulsions.

Accidental spillage of Aramine on the skin can cause dermatitic reactions linked to the presence of the agent's preservatives.

Pharmaceutical precautions Store below 25°C, protected from light and from freezing. Aramine is physically and chemically compatible with Injection Sodium Chloride BP, 5% Injection Dextrose BP, Ringer's Injection USP, Lactated Ringer's Injection USP, Dextran 70 Injection. The ampoule may be autoclaved.

Legal category POM.

Package quantities Ampoules of 1 ml.

Further information Aramine is a potent sympathomimetic amine which increases the force of myocardial contractions as well as having a peripheral vasoconstrictor action. It increases both systolic and diastolic blood pressures.

Renal, coronary, and cerebral blood flow are a function of perfusion pressure and regional resistance. In most instances of cardiogenic shock, the beneficial effect of sympathomimetic amines is attributable to their positive inotropic effect. In patients with insufficient or failing vasoconstriction, there is additional advantage to the peripheral action of Aramine, but in most patients with shock, vasoconstriction is adequate and any further increase is unnecessary. Therefore, blood flow to vital organs may decrease with Aramine if the regional resistance increases excessively.

The pressor effect of Aramine is decreased but not reversed by alpha-adrenergic blocking agents. Primary or secondary fall in blood pressure and tachyphylactic response to repeated use are uncommon.

Product licence number 10 mg/ml injection 0025/5020.

BENEMID*

Presentation White, half-scored tablets, marked 'MSD 501', containing 500 mg Probenecid BP.

Uses Benemid is a uricosuric and renal tubular blocking agent designed for maintenance treatment of gout and gouty arthritis. It inhibits the reabsorption of urate ions in the renal tubules, thus increasing urinary excretion of uric acid and decreasing serum uric acid levels. This action is reversible upon withdrawal of the drug and is demonstrable in normal individuals as well as in patients under treatment. Effective uricosuria reduces the miscible urate pool, retards the deposition of urates, and promotes reabsorption of urate deposits. Also selectively inhibits the urinary excretion of β-lactam antibiotics (other than cephaloridine) and p-aminosalicyclic acid.

Gout and other forms of hyperuricaemia: Benemid is an effective uricosuric agent for the treatment of hyperuricaemia in gout and gouty arthritis. Time is required to achieve clinical results with Benemid despite its marked uricosuric activity. Although acute attacks may occur in the early stages of therapy, as therapy is continued, these attacks should become less frequent and less intense.

Benemid may also be given prophylactically to treat the asymptomatic hyperuricaemia that often occurs in 'gouty' families, in an attempt to forestall the development of acute gouty attacks and urate deposition in tissues.

Benemid may be used to control the hyperuricaemia induced or aggravated by diuretics employed in oedema and hypertension.

β-lactam antibiotic therapy: Benemid is indicated as an adjunctive therapy with β-lactam antibiotics (other than cephaloridine). Benemid interferes with the renal tubular excretion of these substances and thus elevates and prolongs the plasma levels by whatever route the antibiotics are given. A twofold to fourfold increase in plasma concentration has been demonstrated for penicillin G, or V, the synthetic penicillins, ampicillin, methicillin, oxacillin, cloxacillin, and carbenicillin, and for the cephamycin, cefoxitin sodium, and the cephalosporins, cephalothin, cephalexin and cephaloglycin.

Adjunctive therapy of this type is particularly useful when treating severe or resistant infections, such as gonorrhoea, subacute bacterial endocarditis, staphylococcal osteomyelitis, staphylococcal septicaemia, and meningitis due to Gram-positive organisms.

Dosage and administration *Uricosuric therapy: Usual adult dosage:* ½ tablet (250 mg) twice a day for one week, followed thereafter by 1 tablet (500 mg) twice a day.

Some degree of renal impairment is common in patients with gout, therefore, a daily dosage of 2 tablets (1 g) may be adequate in many patients. If, however, symptoms of gouty arthritis remain uncontrolled or the 24-hour urate excretion is not above 700 mg, the daily dosage may be increased by 1 tablet (500 mg) every four weeks within tolerance [usually not more than 4 tablets (2 g) a day]. Benemid may not be effective in chronic renal insufficiency, particularly when the glomerular filtration rate is 30 ml/min or less.

Gastric intolerance may be indicative of overdosage, and may be corrected by reducing the dosage without losing the therapeutic response.

Beremid should be continued at a dosage that will maintain a normal serum uric acid level. When acute attacks have been absent for at least six months and serum uric acid levels remain within normal limits, dosage may be reduced by 1 tablet (500 mg) every 6 months to the minimum effective dosage. The dosage should not be reduced to the point where serum uric acid levels tend to rise.

β-lactam antibiotic therapy (general): Adults: 4 tablets (2 g) a day in divided doses. Elderly patients with suspected renal impairment should be given a reduced dosage. Benemid should not be given concurrently with a β-lactam antibiotic in known cases of renal impairment.

Children over 2 years: 25 mg per kg body weight (or 700 mg/m^2 body surface) initially, followed by 40 mg per kg (or 1,200 mg/m^2) a day in divided doses every six hours. For children weighing more than 50 kg, the adult dosage is recommended.

Gonorrhoea: For uncomplicated gonorrhoea in men or women: a single dose of 2 tablets (1 g) with adequate doses of either oral ampicillin or intramuscular aqueous procaine penicillin or cefoxitin. If oral ampicillin is used, Benemid should be given simultaneously; if a parenteral antibiotic is administered, Benemid should be given at least 30 minutes beforehand.

Use in the elderly: As with all drugs which are primarily renally excreted, care should be taken in the elderly whose renal function may be impaired.

Contra-indications, warnings, etc

Contra-indications: Known hypersensitivity to any component of this product. History of blood dyscrasias. Uric acid kidney stones. Children under two years old. Therapy with Benemid should not be started until an acute gouty attack has subsided. Salicylates are contra-indicated in patients taking Benemid.

Precautions: Benemid should be used with caution in patients with a history of peptic ulcer.

If hypersensitivity reactions appear during therapy, the drug should be withdrawn.

Haematuria, renal colic, costovertebral pain and the formation of urate stones associated with the use of probenecid in gouty patients may be prevented by a liberal fluid intake and enough sodium bicarbonate (3–7.5 g daily) or potassium citrate (7.5 g daily) to keep the urine alkaline. When alkali is given, the acid-base balance of the patient should be carefully monitored.

Exacerbation of gout during therapy with Benemid may occur; if so, a full therapeutic dosage of colchicine, indomethacin or other appropriate therapy should be given.

Use in pregnancy: Probenecid crosses the placental barrier and appears in cord blood. Its use in women of childbearing age requires that the anticipated benefit be weighed against possible hazards.

Drug interactions: The use of acetylsalicylic acid is contraindicated because it antagonises the uricosuric action of probenecid. If patients on 'Benemid' need a mild analgesic, paracetamol is preferred.

Since probenecid decreases the renal excretion of conjugated sulphonamides, plasma concentrations of the latter should be determined from time to time when a sulphonamide and probenecid are given together for prolonged periods. Probenecid may prolong or enhance the action of oral sulphonylureas and thereby increase the risk of hypoglycaemia.

Benemid increases the mean plasma elimination half-life of a number of other drugs, which can lead to increased peak plasma concentrations. These drugs include paracetamol, naproxen, indomethacin, ketoprofen, meclofenamate, lorazepam, and rifampicin. The clinical significance of this is not known; however, adjustment in the usual dosage of these drugs may be required.

Caution should be used if 'Benemid' is administered simultaneously with methotrexate. Benemid has been reported to decrease the tubular secretion of methotrexate and to potentiate toxicity.

If Benemid is given with methotrexate, the dosage of methotrexate should be reduced and serum levels may need to be monitored.

The uricosuric action of Benemid is antagonised by pyrazinamide.

Because of the mechanism of action, Benemid is not recommended in conjunction with a beta-lactam antibiotic in the presence of known renal impairment.

In addition to its effects on the excretion of uric acid and the β-lactam antibiotics (other than cephaloridine). Benemid decreases the urinary excretion of ρ-aminosalicylic acid (PAS), ρ-aminohippuric acid (PAH), phenolsulphonylphthalein (PSP), pantothenic acid, 17-ketosteroids, sodium iodomethamate and related iodinated organic acids. Benemid decreases both hepatic and renal excretion of sulphabromophthalein (BSP). The renal tubular reabsorption of phosphorus is inhibited in hypoparathyroid but not in euparathyroid individuals.

Benemid does not affect the excretion of streptomycin, chloramphenicol, chlortetracycline, oxytetracycline, or neomycin. The effects on the excretion of cephaloridine are not clinically significant.

Side-effects: Headache, gastro-intestinal symptoms (e.g. anorexia, nausea, vomiting), frequency of micturition, hypersensitivity reactions (including anaphylaxis, dermatitis, pruritus, urticaria and fever), sore gums, flushing, alopecia and dizziness, anaemia and haemolytic anaemia (in some cases associated with genetic deficiency of glucose-6-phosphate dehydrogenase in red blood cells) have occurred. The nephrotic syndrome, leucopenia, hepatic necrosis, and aplastic anaemia occur rarely. In gouty patients, exacerbation of gout, and uric acid stones with or without haematuria, renal colic, or costovertebral pain, has been seen.

Laboratory Tests: A reducing substance may appear in the urine of patients receiving Benemid. This may give a false-positive Benedict's test, but the substance disappears when therapy is discontinued.

Falsely high readings for theophylline have been reported in an in vitro study using the Schack and Waxler technique, when therapeutic concentrations of theophylline and Benemid were added to human plasma.

Overdosage: Limited data are available on overdosage in humans. A case of massive overdosage (ninety five 500 mg tablets) was admitted to hospital in status epilepticus. Within an hour of admission, the patient vomited copiously, became progressively stuporous and lapsed into a coma. He then had 2 successive grand mal seizures and his serum urate fell to very low levels. The patient's condition improved steadily but on the third day he had a temperature of 102°F, visual hallucinations, and generalised mild tremors. After recovery, the patient was discharged.

No specific antidote is available. Treatment of overdosage should be symptomatic and supportive. If ingestion is recent, emesis should be induced or gastric lavage performed. If signs of CNS excitation are present, a short-acting barbiturate or intravenous diazepam should be given parenterally. Adrenaline should be given for anaphylactoid reactions. For less severe hypersensitivity reactions, antihistamines or corticosteroids may be given.

The plasma half-life of probenecid is between six to 12 hours; between 85 to 95% of the drug is bound to plasma proteins.

Pharmaceutical precautions Keep container tightly closed. Store in a cool place, protected from light.

Legal category POM.

Package quantities Bottles of 100.

Further information Benemid has been in use since 1952. It can generally be given indefinitely because of its low toxicity.

Product licence number 0025/5021.

BLOCADREN*

Presentation Blue, half-scored tablets, marked 'MSD 136' on one side with 'BLOCADREN' on the other, containing 10 mg Timolol Maleate BP.

Uses Beta-adrenergic-receptor blocking agent. For the treatment of essential hypertension and in angina pectoris due to ischaemic heart disease.

Blocadren is also indicated for the long-term prevention of myocardial infarction and cardiac death (including sudden death) in those who have survived the acute phase of a myocardial infarction.

Prophylactic treatment of common and classic migraine.

Dosage and administration

Hypertension: The initial dosage is 10 mg a day in a single or divided dosage. Depending on the response of the patient, increases in dosage may be made gradually to a maximum of 60 mg daily. Daily dosages above 20 mg should be given on a divided dose schedule.

Use with Moduretic (amiloride hydrochloride and hydrochlorothiazide, MSD):* Studies have shown that Blocadren can be administered once daily when used concomitantly with Moduretic. The majority of patients will respond to a regimen of 10 or 20 mg of Blocadren once a day and 1 tablet of Moduretic.

Use with other antihypertensives: Blocadren may be used with thiazides, hydralazine, or methyldopa. Dosage adjustments are usually required.

For concomitant use with catecholamine-depleting drugs such as reserpine or guanethidine, see 'Precautions'.

Angina: Therapy should be initiated with 5 mg two or three times a day. Dosage increases may be necessary, depending on the symptomatic response, pulse rate, and blood pressure. The first increase should not exceed 10 mg a day in divided doses, and subsequent increases should not exceed 15 mg a day in divided doses. There should be an interval of at least three days between increases in dosage.

The usual dosage range is 15 to 45 mg a day. The majority of patients respond to a dosage in the range of 35 to 45 mg a day.

Preventive use in ischaemic heart disease: For long-term preventive use in patients who have survived the acute phase of myocardial infarction, the maintenance dose is 10 mg twice daily. Therapy should be initiated with 5 mg twice daily and the patient observed carefully. If no adverse reaction occurs, the dosage should then be increased after 2 days to 10 mg twice daily. In the studies evaluating Blocadren following myocardial infarction, treatment was begun 7 to 28 days after the acute phase.

Migraine: The recommended dosage in the prophylactic treatment of common and classic migraine is 10 to 20 mg administered once-a-day.

Paediatric use: not established (see 'Precautions').

Use in the elderly: Initial dosage should be 5 mg b.d. Dosage may be increased cautiously depending on clinical response. *For the preventive use in ischaemic heart disease:* The dosage should be increased to 10 mg b.d. after the second day of treatment.

Contra-indications, warnings, etc

Contra-indications: Bronchospasm (including bronchial asthma), history of bronchospasm, severe chronic obstructive pulmonary disease; sinus bradycardia; atrioventricular block; overt heart failure (see 'Precautions'); right ventricular failure secondary to pulmonary hypertension; significant cardiomegaly; cardiogenic shock; hypersensitivity to this product.

See also 'Use in pregnancy and breast-feeding mothers', under 'Precautions'.

Precautions: Congestive heart failure: Blocadren may be given cautiously to patients with a history of cardiac failure who are well compensated, usually with digitalis or diuretics. Both digitalis and timolol maleate slow AV conduction. If cardiac failure persists, Blocadren should be withdrawn.

In patients without history of cardiac failure: At the first sign or symptom of cardiac failure, patients receiving Blocadren should be digitalised and/or given a diuretic, and the response closely observed. If cardiac failure still continues, Blocadren should be withdrawn.

Thyrotoxicosis: Beta-adrenergic blockade may mask certain clinical signs (e.g. tachycardia) of hyperthyroidism. Patients suspected of developing thyrotoxicosis should be managed carefully to avoid abrupt withdrawal of Blocadren which might precipitate a thyroid storm.

Exacerbation of ischaemic heart disease following abrupt withdrawal: Hypersensitivity to catecholamines has been seen in patients withdrawn from beta-blocker therapy; exacerbation of angina and, in some cases, myocardial infarction has occurred after *abrupt* withdrawal of such therapy.When discontinuing chronically administered Blocadren, particularly in patients with ischaemic heart disease, the dosage should be gradually reduced over one to two weeks and the patient carefully monitored. If angina markedly worsens or acute coronary insufficiency develops, Blocadren should be reinstated promptly, at least temporarily, and other appropriate measures taken. Patients should be warned against interruption or discontinuation of Blocadren without the physicians advice. Because coronary artery disease is both common and may be unrecognised, it may be prudent not to discontinue Blocadren abruptly, even when only treating hypertension.

Major surgery: Because beta-adrenergic-receptor blockade impairs the heart's response to beta-adrenergic mediated reflex stimuli, some patients on beta-adrenergic receptor blocking agents have shown protracted severe hypotension during anaesthesia. Difficulty in restarting and maintaining the heartbeat has also been reported.

Some authorities now recommend gradual withdrawal of beta-adrenergic-receptor blocking agents from anginal patients before elective surgery. If necessary during surgery, the effects of Blocadren may be reversed by sufficient doses of such agonists as isoprenaline, dopamine, dobutamine or noradrenaline (see 'Overdosage').

Diabetes mellitus: Blocadren should be administered with caution to patients liable to spontaneous hypoglycaemia, or to diabetic patients (especially those with labile diabetes) who are receiving insulin or oral hypoglycaemic agents. Beta-adrenergic receptor blocking agents may mask the premonitory signs and symptoms of acute hypoglycaemia.

Impaired hepatic or renal function: Since Blocadren is partially metabolised in the liver and excreted mainly by the kidney, dosage reduction may be necessary when hepatic and/or renal insufficiency is present.

In the presence of marked renal failure: Although the pharmacokinetics of Blocadren are not greatly altered by renal impairment, marked hypotensive responses have been seen in patients with marked renal impairment undergoing dialysis after 20 mg doses. Dosing in such patients should, therefore, be especially cautious.

Musculoskeletal: Beta-blockers have been reported to induce myasthenic symptoms such as diplopia, ptosis and generalised weakness. Timolol has been reported rarely to increase muscle weakness in some patients with myasthenic symptoms.

Cerebrovascular insufficiency: As an agent affecting both pulse and blood pressure, Blocadren should be used cautiously in patients with cerebrovascular insufficiency. Signs or symptoms suggesting reduced cerebral blood flow should prompt consideration of withdrawing therapy with Blocadren.

General: There have been reports of skin rashes and/or dry eyes associated with the use of beta-adrenoceptor-blocking drugs. The reported incidence is small and in most cases the symptoms have cleared when treatment was withdrawn. Discontinuation of the drug should be considered if any such reaction is not otherwise explicable. Cessation of therapy involving beta-blockade should be gradual.

Paediatric use: Safety and efficacy in children has not been established.

Use in pregnancy and breast-feeding mothers: There are no adequate and well-controlled studies in pregnant women. Blocadren should only be used if the potential benefit justifies the risk to the fetus.

Because of the potential for serious adverse reactions in breast-feeding babies, a decision to discontinue breast-feeding, or Blocadren, should be made taking into account the importance of the drug to the mother.

Drug interactions: Close observation of the patient is recommended when Blocadren is administered to patients on catecholamine-depleting drugs such as reserpine, because of possible additive effects and the production of hypotension and/or marked bradycardia, which may produce vertigo, syncope, or postural hypotension.

Attenuation of the antihypertensive effect of beta-blockers by NSAIDs has been reported. Patients treated with both agents should be monitored to confirm that the desired therapeutic effect has been obtained.

Oral calcium antagonists may be combined with Blocadren only when heart function is normal. The potential exists for hypotension, AV conduction disturbances, and left ventricular failure to occur in patients receiving a beta-blocking agent when an oral calcium antagonist is added to the treatment regimen. The nature of any cardiovascular adverse effect tends to depend on the type of calcium antagonist used. Dihydropyridine derivatives, such as nifedipine, may lead to hypotension, whereas verapamil or diltiazem have a greater propensity to lead to AV conduction disturbances or left ventricular failure when used with a beta-blocker. Intravenous calcium antagonists and Blocadren should only be used together with caution.

Concomitant use of beta-blockers and digitalis with either diltiazem or verapamil may further prolong the AV conduction time.

Side-effects: Blocadren is usually well tolerated. Most adverse reactions have been mild and transient. *General:* Asthenia, fatigue, headache, chest pain, extremity pain, decreased exercise tolerance, weight loss. *Cardiovascular:* Bradycardia, cardiac arrest, cerebral vascular accident, palpitation, arrhythmia, sino-atrial block, AV block (2nd or 3rd degree), syncope, hypotension, oedema, pulmonary oedema, cardiac failure, Raynaud's phenomenon, cold extremities, claudication, worsening of arterial insufficiency or angina pectoris, vasodilatation. *Digestive:* Dyspepsia, nausea, vomiting, diarrhoea, hepatomegaly. *Endocrine:* Hyperglycaemia, hypoglycaemia. *Integumentary:* Rash, pruritus, skin irritation, increased pigmentation, sweating, exfoliative dermatitis (one case). *Musculoskeletal:* Arthralgia. *Nervous system:* Dizziness, vertigo, paraesthesiae, local weakness. *Psychiatric:* Nervousness, diminished concentration, hallucinations, nightmares, increased dreaming, insomnia, depression, somnolence, decreased libido. *Haematological:* Non-thrombocytopenic purpura. *Respiratory:* Dyspnoea, bronchial spasm, rales, cough. *Special senses:* Tinnitus, visual disturbances, diplopia, ptosis, eye irritation, dry eyes. *Urogenital:* Impotence, micturition difficulties. *Clinical laboratory tests:* Changes in clinical laboratory tests are rare. Slight increases in blood urea, serum potassium and serum uric acid, and slight decreases in haemoglobin and haematocrit occurred, but were not progressive or associated with clinical manifestations.

Overdosage: No specific data are available in humans. A study in patients with renal failure suggests that Blocadren does not readily dialyse.

The most common signs and symptoms to be expected following overdosage with a beta-adrenergic-receptor blocking agent are symptomatic bradycardia, hypotension, bronchospasm, acute cardiac failure, and heart block. If overdosage occurs, the following measures are suggested. In all cases therapy with Blocadren should be stopped, and the patient closely observed.

1. Gastric lavage.
2. Symptomatic bradycardia: atropine sulphate, 0.25 to 2 mg intravenously, should be used to induce vagal blockade. If bradycardia persists, intravenous isoprenaline hydrochloride should be administered cautiously. In refractory cases, the use of a cardiac pacemaker may be considered.
3. Hypotension: a sympathomimetic pressor agent such as dopamine, dobutamine or noradrenaline should be used. In refractory cases, the use of glucagon has been reported to be useful.
4. Bronchospasm: isoprenaline hydrochloride should be used. Additional therapy with aminophylline may be considered.
5. Acute cardiac failure: conventional therapy with digitalis, diuretics, and oxygen should be instituted immediately. In refractory cases, the use of intravenous aminophylline is suggested. This may be followed, if necessary, by glucagon which has been reported useful.
6. Heart block: isoprenaline hydrochloride or a pacemaker should be used.

Timolol is rapidly and nearly completely absorbed following ingestion. Plasma half-life is approximately four hours.

Pharmaceutical precautions Keep container well closed; store in a cool place, protected from light.

Legal category POM.

Package quantities Bottles of 100.

Further information Blocadren reduces blood pressure without acute hypotensive episodes in most patients with essential hypertension. The exact mechanism of action is still unknown. Blocadren does not usually affect normal blood pressure.

Blocadren effectively delays or prevents the development of anginal pain in most patients. It acts by modifying the cardiac response to stress or exercise.

Blocadren has been shown to be highly effective in reducing the incidence of cardiac death, including sudden death, and of reinfarction in patients who have survived the acute phase of a myocardial infarction.

Product licence number 0025/0091.

CLINORIL*
CLINORIL* 200

Presentation Brilliant yellow, scored, hexagonal tablets, biconvex in shape, containing 200 mg and 100 mg Sulindac BP. The 200 mg tablets are marked 'MSD 942' and the 100 mg tablets are marked 'MSD 943'.

Uses Non-steroidal, analgesic/anti-inflammatory agent with antipyretic properties.

Indicated in osteoarthritis, rheumatoid arthritis, ankylosing spondylitis, acute gouty arthritis, peri-articular disorders such as bursitis, tendinitis, and tenosynovitis.

Mode of action: Clinoril is a prodrug. Following absorption, sulindac undergoes two major biotransformations: reversible reduction to the sulphide metabolite, and irreversible oxidation to the inactive sulphone metabolite. The sulphide metabolite is a potent inhibitor of prostaglandin synthesis.

Dosage and administration The dosage should be taken twice a day and adjusted to the severity of the disease.

The usual dose is 400 mg a day. However, the dosage may be lowered depending on the response. Doses above 400 mg per day are not recommended.

In the treatment of acute gouty arthritis, therapy for seven days is usually adequate.

In peri-articular disorders, treatment should be limited to seven to ten days.

Clinoril should be adminstered with fluids or food.

Children: The use of Clinoril in children is contra-indicated.

Use in the elderly: The dosage does not require modification for the elderly patient.

Contra-indications, warnings, etc
Contra-indications: Hypersensitivity to any component of this product.

Clinoril should not be used in patients in whom acute asthmatic attacks, urticaria, or rhinitis have been precipitated by aspirin or other non-steroidal anti-inflammatory agents.

The drug should not be administered to patients with active gastro-intestinal bleeding.

The use of Clinoril should be avoided in patients with active peptic ulcer.

Since paediatric indications and dosage have not yet been established, Clinoril should not be given to children.

Clinoril should not be given to pregnant or lactating women, since safety for its use has not been established.

Precautions: Clinoril should be used with caution in patients having a history of gastro-intestinal haemorrhage or ulcers. In patients with renal functional impairment, since the major route of excretion of the drug is via the kidney, the dosage may need to be reduced.

A potentially life-threatening, apparent hypersensitivity syndrome has been reported. In cases where the syndrome is suspected, therapy should be discontinued immediately, and not recontinued. This syndrome may include constitutional symptoms (fever, chills), cutaneous findings (rash or other dermatological reactions), involvement of major organs (changes in liver function tests, jaundice, pancreatitis, pneumonitis with or without pleural effusion, leucopenia, eosinophilia, disseminated intravascular coagulation, anaemia, renal impairment, including renal failure), and other less specific findings (adenitis, arthralgia, myalgia, fatigue, malaise, hypotension, chest pain, tachycardia).

While Clinoril has less effect on platelet function and bleeding time than aspirin, it is a moderate to weak inhibitor of platelet function and, therefore, patients who may be adversely affected by these actions should be carefully observed when Clinoril is administered.

A patient with signs and/or symptoms suggesting liver dysfunction, or in whom an abnormal liver function test has occurred, should be evaluated for evidence of a more severe hepatic reaction while on therapy. Significant elevations of AST(SGOT) and ALT(SGPT) (three times higher than normal) were seen in less than 1% of patients in controlled clinical trials.

Poor liver function may alter the blood levels of circulating metabolites of Clinoril. Patients with liver dysfunction on Clinoril should be monitored closely; daily dosage reduction may be required.

Cases of hepatitis, jaundice, or both, with or without

fever, may occur within the first three months of therapy. In some patients, the findings are consistent with those of cholestatic hepatitis.

Fever or other evidence of hypersensitivity including abnormalities in one or more liver function tests and skin reactions have occurred during therapy. Some fatalities have occurred.

Whenever a patient develops unexplained fever, rash or other dermatological reaction, or constitutional symptoms, Clinoril should be permanently stopped and liver function investigated. Fever and abnormal liver function are reversible.

Sulindac metabolites have been reported rarely as the major or a minor component in renal stones in association with other calculus components. Clinoril should be used with caution in patients with a history of renal lithiasis and they should be kept well hydrated while receiving Clinoril.

Drug interactions: Dimethyl sulphoxide should not be used with Clinoril. Concomitant use has been reported to reduce plasma levels of the active metabolite of Clinoril, and also cause peripheral neuropathy.

Although sulindac and its sulphide metabolite are highly bound to protein, studies (in which Clinoril was given at a dose of 400 mg daily) have shown no clinically significant interaction with oral anticoagulants or oral hypoglycaemic agents. However, patients should be monitored carefully until it is certain that no change in their anticoagulant or hypoglycaemic dose is required.

Concomitant administration with aspirin in normal volunteers significantly depressed plasma levels of the active sulphide metabolite. Clinical study of the combination showed an increase in GI side effects with no improvement in the therapeutic response to Clinoril. The combination is not recommended.

Concomitant administration with diflunisal in normal volunteers reduced the plasma level of active sulphide metabolite by approximately one-third.

Probenecid given concomitantly with sulindac had only a slight effect on plasma sulphide levels, while plasma levels of sulindac and sulphone were increased. Sulindac was shown to produce a modest reduction in the uricosuric action of probenecid which probably is not usually significant.

Neither dextropropoxyphene hydrochloride nor paracetamol had any effect on the plasma levels of sulindac or its sulphide metabolite.

In a drug interaction study, an antacid, (magnesium and aluminium hydroxides in suspension) was administered with Clinoril with no significant difference in absorbance.

In contrast to most other non-steroidal anti-inflammatory drugs, Clinoril does not reduce the antihypertensive effect of thiazides and a variety of other agents used to treat mild-to-moderate hypertension. However, the blood pressure of patients taking Clinoril with antihypertensive agents should be closely monitored.

Side-effects: Clinoril is generally well tolerated. Those side-effects experienced are usually mild and may often respond to a reduction in dosage.

Gastro-intestinal: The most frequent types of side-effects occurring with Clinoril are gastro-intestinal; these include gastro-intestinal pain, dyspepsia, nausea with or without vomiting, diarrhoea, constipation, flatulence, anorexia, and gastro-intestinal cramps.

Dermatological: Rash, pruritus.

Central nervous system: Dizziness, headache, nervousness.

Special senses: Tinnitus.

Miscellaneous: Oedema.

The following side-effects were reported less frequently. The probability exists of a causal relationship between Clinoril and these side-effects:

Gastro-intestinal: Stomatitis, gastritis or gastro-enteritis. Peptic ulcer, colitis, as well as gastro-intestinal bleeding and perforations have been reported rarely. Fatalities have occurred. Liver function abnormalities, jaundice sometimes with fever, cholestasis, hepatitis, pancreatitis, ageusia and glossitis. It has also been reported that a probable sulindac metabolite has been found in biliary sludge in patients with symptoms of cholecystitis who underwent a cholecystectomy.

Dermatological: Sore or dry mucous membranes, alopecia, photosensitivity. Erythema multiforme, toxic epidermal necrolysis, Stevens-Johnson syndrome, exfoliative dermatitis.

Cardiovascular: Congestive heart failure, especially in patients with marginal cardiac function, palpitation, hypertension.

Haematological: Thrombocytopenia, ecchymosis, purpura, leucopenia, agranulocytosis, neutropenia, bone marrow depression including aplastic anaemia, haemolytic anaemia, increased prothrombin time in patients on oral anticoagulants.

Genito-urinary: Urine discoloration, vaginal bleeding, haematuria, proteinuria, crystalluria, renal impairment, interstitial nephritis, nephrotic syndrome.

Nervous system: Vertigo, somnolence, insomnia, sweating, asthenia, paraesthesiae, convulsions, syncope, depression, psychic disturbances including acute psychosis, aseptic meningitis.

Metabolic: hyperkaelemia.

Special senses: Visual disturbances including blurred vision, decreased hearing, metallic or bitter taste.

Respiratory: Epistaxis.

Hypersensitivity reactions: Anaphylaxis and angioneurotic oedema. Bronchial spasm, dyspnoea, hypersensitivity vasculitis, hypersensitivity syndrome.

Causal relationship unknown: Other reactions have been reported in clinical trials or since the drug was marketed, but occurred under circumstances where a causal relationship could not be established. However, in these rarely reported events, that possibility cannot be excluded. Therefore, these observations are listed to serve as alerting information to physicians.

Nervous system: Neuritis.

Cardiovascular: Arrhythmia.

Miscellaneous: Gynaecomastia.

Metabolic: Hyperglycaemia.

Overdosage: Cases of overdosage have been reported and, rarely, fatalities have occurred. Stupor, coma, diminished urine output and hypotension have been seen.

In the event of acute overdosage, if ingestion is recent, the stomach should be emptied by inducing vomiting or by gastric lavage, and the patient carefully observed and given symptomatic and supportive treatment.

Animal studies show that absorption is decreased by the prompt administration of activated charcoal and excretion is enhanced by alkalinisation of the urine.

The readiness of sulindac and its metabolites to dialyse is unknown at present. But because they are highly bound to plasma proteins, dialysis is not likely to be effective.

The mean half-life of sulindac is 7.8 hours while the mean half-life of the active sulphide metabolite is 16.4 hours.

Pharmaceutical precautions Keep container well closed; store in a cool place, protected from light.

Legal category POM.

Package quantities *200 mg:* Bottles of 100 and 500. *100 mg:* Bottles of 100.

Further information Clinoril usually provides symptomatic relief of inflammation, pain and tenderness and promotes early improvement in joint mobility. Clinoril has a prolonged duration of activity, which permits a twice-a-day dose schedule. Based on extensive studies, Clinoril has been shown to be suitable for the long-term relief of pain and inflammation.

Prostaglandin synthetase inhibition is hypothesised as the basis by which non-steroidal anti-inflammatory agents act. Following absorption, sulindac undergoes two major biotransformations: reversible reduction to the sulphide metabolite; and irreversible oxidation to the inactive sulphone metabolite. The sulphide metabolite is a potent inhibitor of prostaglandin synthesis and accounts for the activity of sulindac (Clinoril). Sulindac is thus a prodrug.

Product licence numbers
100 mg 0025/0121
200 mg 0025/0122

COGENTIN*

Presentation White, quarter-scored tablets, marked 'MSD 60', containing 2 mg Benztropine Mesylate BP.

An injection containing in each millilitre 1 mg Benztropine Mesylate BP, as a colourless solution.

Uses Anti-parkinsonian agent with powerful anticholinergic effects.

For symptomatic treatment of all types of 'classical' parkinsonism including arteriosclerotic, post-encephalitic, and idiopathic parkinsonism, and of extrapyramidal reactions induced by phenothiazines or reserpine.

Cogentin is particularly effective in the relief of rigidity and tremor. Among other symptoms which it can ameliorate are: sialorrhoea, drooling, mask-like facies, oculogyric crises, speech and writing difficulties, gait disturbances, dysphagia, and pain and insomnia due to muscle spasm and cramps.

Cogentin often is helpful in patients who have become unresponsive to other agents. Therapy is directed toward control of disturbing symptoms to permit the patient maximum integration of function with minimum discomfort. In non-drug-induced parkinsonism, partial control of symptoms is usually achieved.

Dosage and administration As Cogentin is cumulative in action, treatment should begin with a low dosage, which can be increased by amounts of 0.5 mg at intervals of five to six days, to the smallest dosage necessary for optimal relief without excessive side-effects. Maximum dosage, 6 mg a day.

Cogentin Injection may be used intramuscularly or intravenously in emergencies, or for patients unable to swallow tablets. (As there is no significant difference in time of onset of effect between intramuscular and intravenous administration, the intravenous route is not usually necessary.)

In emergencies, 1–2 ml (1–2 mg) of Cogentin Injection will normally provide quick relief. If signs of parkinsonism begin to return, the dose can be repeated.

'Classical' parkinsonism: Usual dosage: 1–2 mg a day, with a range of 0.5–6 mg a day, orally or parenterally. Dosage must be adjusted on an individual basis, taking into consideration the age and weight of the patient, and the type of parkinsonism. Older patients, thin patients and those with arteriosclerotic parkinsonism usually cannot tolerate large dosages. Most patients with post-encephalitic parkinsonism need and indeed tolerate fairly large dosages. Patients with a poor mental outlook may respond poorly. In arteriosclerotic and idiopathic parkinsonism, therapy may be initiated with a single daily dose of 0.5–1 mg at bedtime. This dosage will be adequate in some patients, whereas 4–6 mg a day may be required by others. In post-encephalitic parkinsonism, therapy may be initiated in most patients with 2 mg a day in one or more doses. In highly sensitive individuals, therapy may be initiated with 0.5 mg at bedtime, and increased as necessary.

Some patients obtain greatest relief by taking the entire dose at bedtime; others react more favourably to divided dosage, two to four times a day. One dose a day frequently is sufficient; divided doses may be unnecessary or even undesirable.

See also 'Further information'.

Drug-induced parkinsonism: Usual dosage range: 1–4 mg once or twice a day.

Acute dystonic reactions: 1–2 ml (1–2 mg) by intravenous injection followed usually by 1–2 mg orally twice a day.

Extrapyramidal reactions appearing soon after starting phenothiazine or reserpine therapy are likely to be temporary, and are usually controlled in one or two days by 1–2 mg of Cogentin orally two or three times a day. Cogentin should be withdrawn after one or two weeks to determine if it is still needed. It can be reinstated if necessary.

Certain extrapyramidal reactions which develop slowly (e.g. tardive dyskinesia) do not usually respond to Cogentin.

Paediatric use: Use with caution in children over 3 years old (see 'Contra-indications').

Use in the elderly: As with younger patients, dosage should be the smallest possible for optimum relief of symptoms. Initial dosage should be 0.5–1 mg preferably at night, increasing until optimum effect is seen. Older patients usually cannot tolerate large doses.

Contra-indications, warnings, etc

Contra-indications: Because of the atropine-like side-effects, Cogentin is contra-indicated in children under 3 years old and should be used with caution in older children. Cogentin is contra-indicated in patients who are hypersensitive to this product.

Precautions: Cogentin may impair the mental alertness and physical ability required for the performance of such hazardous tasks as driving a car or operating machinery.

Continued supervision of patients is recommended as Cogentin has a cumulative action. Patients with a tendency towards tachycardia and those with prostatic hypertrophy, should be closely observed.

Patients with mental disorders should be carefully supervised when Cogentin is used to control drug-induced extrapyramidal reactions, especially when therapy is started or the dosage of Cogentin is increased. Intensification of mental symptoms may occasionally occur. Cogentin should be temporarily withdrawn if the reactions are severe.

Drug interactions: Extra care should be taken when Cogentin is given concomitantly with phenothiazines or other drugs with anticholinergic or antihistaminic activity. Patients should be advised to report gastro-intestinal complaints promptly. Paralytic ileus, sometimes fatal, has occurred in patients taking anticholinergic-type anti-parkinsonian drugs, including Cogentin, in combination with phenothiazines and/or tricyclic antidepressants.

Tardive dyskinesia may appear in some patients on long-term therapy with phenothiazines or related agents, or after discontinuation of such therapy. Anti-parkinsonian agents do not usually alleviate symptoms of tardive dyskinesia, and in some cases may aggravate or unmask them. Cogentin is not recommended in tardive dyskinesia.

Cogentin has anticholinergic effects, and glaucoma is a possibility. Although Cogentin does not appear to have any adverse effect on simple glaucoma, its use is probably not advisable in narrow-angle glaucoma. It may cause anhidrosis; this should be borne in mind, particularly in hot weather, especially when given concomitantly with other atropine-like drugs to the chronically ill, alcoholics, or patients with a central nervous system disease and those who do manual labour in a hot environment. Cogentin should be used cautiously in patients with or prone to abnormalities of sweating. If there is evidence of anhidrosis, the possibility of hyperthermia should be considered. Dosage should be decreased as necessary to maintain body heat equilibrium by the action of perspiration. Severe anhidrosis and fatal hyperthermia have occurred.

Use in pregnancy: It is not known whether Cogentin can cause fetal harm when administered to a pregnant woman or can affect reproductive capacity. Cogentin should be given to a pregnant woman only if clearly needed.

Breast-feeding mothers: It is not known whether this drug is excreted in human milk. Because many drugs are excreted in human milk, caution should be exercised when Cogentin is administered to a breast-feeding mother.

Side-effects: Side effects, most of which are anticholinergic or antihistaminic in nature are listed below by body system in order of decreasing severity.

Cardiovascular: Tachycardia.

Digestive: Constipation, dry mouth, nausea, vomiting.

If dry mouth is so severe that there is difficulty in swallowing or speaking, or loss of appetite and weight occur, reduce dosage, or discontinue the drug temporarily.

Slight reduction in dosage may control nausea and still give sufficient relief of symptoms. Vomiting may be controlled by temporary discontinuation, followed by resumption at a lower dosage.

Nervous system: Toxic psychosis, including confusion, disorientation, memory impairment, visual hallucinations; exacerbation of pre-existing psychotic symptoms; nervousness; depression; listlessness; numbness of fingers.

Special senses: Blured vision, dilated pupils.

Urogenital: Urinary retention, dysuria.

Metabolic/Immune and Skin: Occasionally, an allergic reaction, e.g. skin rash, develops. If this cannot be controlled by dosage reduction, the medication should be discontinued.

Overdosage: Symptoms may be any of those seen in atropine poisoning or antihistamine overdosage: CNS depression, preceded or followed by stimulation; confusion; nervousness; listlessness; intensification of mental symptoms or toxic psychosis in patients with mental illness being treated with neuroleptic drugs (e.g. phenothiazines); hallucinations (especially visual); dizziness; muscle weakness; ataxia; dry mouth; mydriasis; blurred vision; palpitations; tachycardia; nausea; vomiting; dysuria; numbness of fingers; dysphagia, allergic reactions, e.g. skin rash; headache; hot, dry, flushed skin; delirium; coma; shock; convulsions; respiratory arrest; anhidrosis; hyperthermia; glaucoma; constipation.

Physostigmine salicylate (1–2 mg, subcutaneously or intravenously) is reported to reverse symptoms of anticholinergic intoxication. A second injection may be given after two hours if needed. Otherwise, treatment is symptomatic and supportive.

If ingestion is recent, emesis should be induced or gastric lavage performed. A short-acting barbiturate may be used for CNS excitement, but with caution to avoid subsequent depression. Supportive care for CNS depression may be required (such convulsant stimulants as picrotoxin, leptazol or bemegride should be avoided). In severe respiratory depression, artificial respiration may be required. Also needed may be a local miotic for mydriasis and cycloplegia, ice bags or other cold applications and alcohol sponges for hyperpyrexia, a vasopressor and fluids for circulatory collapse, and a darkened room for photophobia.

Data on the metabolism of benztropine maleate are not available at present; but a death was recorded $1\frac{1}{2}$ hours after ingestion.

Pharmaceutical precautions *Tablets:* Keep container tightly closed; store in a cool place, protected from light.

Injection: Store in a cool place, protected from light and freezing.

Legal category POM.

Package quantities *Tablets:* Bottles of 500.
Injection: Ampoules of 2 ml.

Further information Cogentin may be used in combination with other agents employed in the treatment of parkinsonism; the dosage of such agents may be reduced or they may be gradually discontinued. Many patients obtain greatest relief with a combination of Cogentin and other agents.

Cogentin may be used concomitantly with levodopa, in which case the usual dosage of each may need to be reduced. However, if it is continued when Sinemet* (carbidopa and levodopa, MSD) is introduced the dosage of Cogentin may need to be adjusted.

The oral LD_{50} in the mouse is 94 mg/kg. The intravenous LD_{50} in the mouse is 24 mg/kg.

Product licence numbers

Tablets	0025/5023
Injection	0025/5024

CONCORDIN*

Presentation Concordin-5, salmon-red, film-coated tablets, marked 'MSD 26', containing 5 mg Protriptyline Hydrochloride BP.

Concordin-10, white, film-coated tablets, marked 'MSD 47', containing 10 mg Protriptyline Hydrochloride BP.

Uses Symptoms of depressive illness.

Concordin may be used successfully in depression that is a manifestation of psychosis or neurosis, whether endogenous or reactive. Endogenous depression is more likely to respond. Concordin is especially recommended in apathetic, withdrawn patients, because it promptly relieves anergia, and it lacks sedative activity.

The following 'target' symptoms of depression may be expected to respond well to Concordin: depressed mood; excessive crying; apathy; withdrawal; psychomotor retardation; loss of interest; fatigue; lassitude; feelings of guilt; anorexia; headache; functional somatic complaints (e.g. gastro-intestinal symptoms).

Dosage and administration Dosage should be adjusted for each patient, bearing in mind the cyclic nature and variable severity of depression, the danger of relapse, and the possibility of spontaneous remission.

Adults: Dosage range, 15–60 mg. Usual starting dosage, 30–40 mg a day, divided into 3 or 4 doses. Any increase in dosage should be made gradually, and added to the morning dose first. If insomnia is present, the last dose should be given no later than mid-afternoon. When a satisfactory response is noted, the dosage should be reduced to the smallest amount necessary to maintain relief. Maintenance therapy should be continued for at least three months after satisfactory improvement. If relapse occurs, Concordin may be reinstated.

If the dosage required for adequate antidepressant effect produces overstimulation, concurrent use of a tranquilliser will provide effective control. Overstimulation is unlikely if the dosage of Concordin is kept below 20 mg a day.

Therapy may be usefully initiated with a tranquilliser and preventive supervision in suicidal patients, because these patients usually have a high level of anxiety, and Concordin may relieve anergia before recovery from depression is complete.

Children: Concordin is not recommended for children under 16 years old.

Elderly patients: Initially 5 mg three times a day. These patients may not tolerate higher doses as well as other patients. If the elderly receive more than 20 mg a day, they should be observed for effects on the cardiovascular system.

Contra-indications, warnings, etc
Contra-indications: Hypersensitivity to any component of this product. Concurrent use with a monoamine oxidase inhibitor. Hyperpyretic crises, severe convulsions, and deaths have occurred when tricyclic antidepressants and MAOIs have been given simultaneously (see also 'Precautions'); the acute recovery phase after recent myocardial infarction; known sensitivity to protriptyline. Any degree of heart block or other cardiac arrhythmias, mania, marked agitation, severe liver disease, during breast feeding. For 'Use in pregnancy', see 'Precautions'.

Precautions: Protriptyline should be used with caution in patients with a history of epilepsy, impaired liver function, a tendency to urinary retention, prostatic hypertrophy, or increased intra-ocular pressure.

Concordin should be used cautiously in elderly patients and patients with cardiovascular disorders. Such patients should be closely observed because of the tendency of protriptyline to produce tachycardia, hypotension, arrhythmias, and prolongation of the conduction time. The elderly are particularly liable to experience agitation and confusion. Myocardial infarction and stroke have occurred with drugs of this class.

Protriptyline may impair abilities needed for performing hazardous tasks, such as driving a vehicle or operating machinery.

In patients who may use alcohol excessively, potentiation may increase the danger inherent in any suicide attempt or overdosage.

Psychotic symtoms may be aggravated when Concodin is used in schizophrenic patients. Manic depressive patients may shift towards the manic phase. Paranoid delusions, with or without hostility, may be exaggerated. In any of these circumstances, it may be advisable to reduce the dosage, or to use a major tranquilliser concurrently.

Concordin may aggravate anxiety or agitation in overactive or agitated patients.

The possibility of suicide in depressed patients remains during treatment until significant remission has occurred; suicidal patients should not have access to large quantities of Concordin tablets and should be carefully supervised.

The natural course of depression often is of many months' duration. It is appropriate, therefore, to continue maintenance therapy for three months or longer to lessen the possibility of relapse.

Discontinue the drug several days before elective surgery if possible.

Drug interactions: A minimum of 14 days should elapse between discontinuing a monoamine oxidase inhibitor and introducing Concordin, which should then be started cautiously, with gradual increases in dosage until optimum response is achieved.

Protriptyline may block the antihypertensive effect of guanethidine, debrisoquine, bethanidine, and possibly clonidine or similar compounds. Review all antihypertensive therapy during treatment.

Protriptyline should not be given with sympathomimetic agents such as ephedrine, isoprenaline, noradrenaline, phenylephrine, and phenylpropanolamine.

Protriptyline may enhance the response to alcohol and the effects of barbiturates and other CNS depressants.

Cimetidine is reported to reduce hepatic metabolism of certain tricyclic antidepressants.

Concurrent administration of Concordin may increase the hazards of electroconvulsive therapy. Such combined treatment should be limited to those for whom it is essential.

Anaesthetics given during tricyclic antidepressant therapy may increase the risk of arrhythmias and hypotension. If surgery is necessary, the anaesthetist should be informed that the patient is receiving protriptyline.

On rare occasions, hyperthyroid patients or those receiving thyroid medication may develop arrhythmias when protriptyline is given.

Use in pregnancy and lactation: Safe use in pregnancy and lactation has not been established. Avoid during pregnancy, especially during the first and last trimesters. Use in pregnant women, breast-feeding mothers or women who may become pregnant requires that possible benefits be weighed against possible hazards to the mother and child.

There is no evidence as to drug safety in human pregnancy, nor is there evidence from animal work that it is free from hazard.

Side-effects: Some of the adverse reactions below have not been specifically reported for Concordin, but are included because of the similar pharmacological properties of the tricyclic group of antidepressants. Concordin is more likely to aggravate anxiety and agitation and to produce such cardiovascular reactions as tachycardia and hypotension.

As improvement may not occur during the first two to four weeks of treatment, patients should be closely monitored during this period.

Cardiovascular: Hypotension (particularly orthostatic hypotension), hypertension, tachycardia, palpitation, myocardial infarction, arrhythmias, heart block, stroke.

Psychiatric: Confusional states (especially in the elderly) with hallucinations, disorientation, delusions, anxiety, restlessness, agitation; insomnia, panic, and nightmares; hypomania; exacerbation of psychosis.

Neurological: Numbness, tingling and paraesthesiae of extremities; incoordination, ataxia, tremors, peripheral neuropathy; extrapyramidal symptoms; seizures; alteration in EEG patterns, tinnitus, drowsiness, dizziness, weakness and fatigue; headache.

Anticholinergic: Dry mouth and rarely associated sublingual adenitis; blurred vision, disturbance of accommodation, mydriasis; constipation, paralytic ileus; hyperpyrexia; urinary retention, delayed micturition, dilatation of the urinary tract.

Allergic: Skin rash, petechiae, urticaria, itching, oedema (generally, or of face and tongue), drug fever. Some rashes have been associated with photosensitisation. In view of this, patients should avoid excessive exposure to sunlight, including sunbathing.

Haematological: Bone-marrow depression; agranulocytosis; leucopenia; eosinophilia; purpura; thrombocytopenia.

Gastro-intestinal: Nausea and vomiting, anorexia, epigastric distress, diarrhoea, peculiar taste, stomatitis, abdominal cramps, black tongue.

Endocrine: Gynaecomastia in the male; breast enlargement and galactorrhoea in the female; increased or decreased libido, impotence; testicular swelling; elevation or depression of blood sugar levels; syndrome of inappropriate ADH secretion.

Other: Jaundice (simulating obstructive); altered liver function; weight gain or loss; perspiration; flushing; urinary frequency; nocturia; parotid swelling; alopecia.

Withdrawal symptoms: Though not indicative of addiction, abrupt cessation of treatment after prolonged therapy may produce nausea, insomnia, irritability, excessive perspiration, headache and malaise.

Gradual dosage reduction has been reported to produce, within two weeks, transient symptoms including irritability, restlessness, and dream and sleep disturbance. These symptoms are not indicative of addiction. Rare instances have been reported of mania or hypomania occurring within 2–7 days following cessation of chronic therapy with tricyclic antidepressants.

Withdrawal symptoms in neonates whose mothers receive tricyclic antidepressants during the third trimester have also been reported.

Overdosage: High doses may cause temporary confusion, disturbed concentration, or transient visual hallucinations. Overdosage may cause drowsiness; hypothermia; tachycardia and other arrhythmic abnormalities, for example bundle branch block; ECG evidence of impaired conduction; congestive heart failure; dilated pupils; convulsions; severe hypotension; stupor; and coma. Other symptoms may be agitation, hyperactive reflexes, muscle rigidity, vomiting, and hyperpyrexia, or any of those listed under 'Side-effects'.

Experience in the management of overdosage with protriptyline is limited. All patients suspected of having taken an overdosage should be admitted to a hospital as soon as possible. Treatment is symptomatic and supportive. If ingestion is recent, empty the stomach as quickly as possible by emesis followed by gastric lavage upon arrival at the hospital. Following gastric lavage, activated charcoal may be administered; 20 to 30 g of activated charcoal may be given every four to six hours during the first 24 to 48 hours after ingestion. An ECG should be taken and close monitoring of cardiac function instituted if there is any sign of abnormality. Maintain an open airway and adequate fluid intake; regulate body temperature.

Anticonvulsants may be given to control convulsions.

Dialysis is of no value because of low plasma concentrations of the drug.

The intravenous administration of 1–3 mg of physostigmine salicylate is reported to reverse the symptoms of tricyclic antidepressant poisoning in humans. Because physostigmine is rapidly metabolised, the dosage of physostigmine should be repeated as required, particularly if life-threatening signs such as arrhythmias, convulsions, and deep coma recur or persist after the initial dosage of physostigmine. Because physostigmine itself may be toxic, it is not recommended for routine use.

Standard measures should be used to manage circulatory shock and metabolic acidosis. Cardiac arrhythmias may be treated with neostigmine, pyridostigmine, or propranolol. Should cardiac failure occur, the use of digitalis should be considered. Close monitoring of cardiac function for not less than five days is advisable.

Protriptyline has been estimated to have a very prolonged half-life ranging from 55 to 198 hours, which may be further prolonged in overdosage.

Pharmaceutical precautions Keep container well closed; store in a cool place, protected from light.

Legal category POM.

Package quantities
5 mg: Bottles of 100.
10 mg: Bottles of 100.

Further information Concordin is a member of the tricyclic group of antidepressants. Concordin is not a monoamine oxidase inhibitor, and dietary restrictions are not necessary. Concordin has not produced addiction or habituation.

Concordin has a rapid onset of effect, which can be of particular importance where there is a risk of suicide. It is advisable, however, to administer a tranquilliser and to ensure preventative supervision when starting Concordin in suicidal patients since they usually have a high level of anxiety, and especially because Concordin may relieve the anergia before there is complete recovery from the depressed state.

When Concordin has to be used in conjunction with ECT, the total number of shock treatments required may be reduced.

Product licence numbers
5 mg 0025/5004
10 mg 0025/5005

COSMEGEN,* LYOVAC*

Presentation Yellow, lyophilised powder, in a vial containing 500 micrograms dactinomycin with 20 mg of mannitol.

Uses Cytotoxic, antineoplastic antibiotic with immunosuppressant properties.

Mode of action: Cosmegen inhibits the proliferation of cells by forming a stable complex with DNA and interfering with DNA-dependent RNA synthesis.

Recommended only in the treatment, under appropriate supervision, of hospitalised patients with Wilms' tumour, rhabdomyosarcoma, and carcinoma of the testis or uterus. All other indications for dactinomycin are as yet experimental (e.g. Ewing's sarcoma, osteogenic sarcoma).

Wilms' tumour: The neoplasm responding most frequently to Cosmegen is Wilms' tumour. With low doses of both dactinomycin and radiotherapy, temporary objective improvement may be as good as, and may last longer than, that obtained with higher doses of each given alone.

Rhabdomyosarcoma: Temporary regression of the tumour and beneficial subjective results have occurred with dactinomycin in rhabdomyosarcoma, which, like most soft-tissue sarcomas, is comparatively radio-resistant.

Carcinoma of testis and uterus: The sequential use of dactinomycin and methotrexate, along with meticulous monitoring of human chorionic gonadotrophin levels until normal, has resulted in survival in the majority of women with metastatic choriocarcinoma.

Sequential therapy is used if there is:

1. Stability in gonadotrophin titres following two successive courses of an agent.
2. Rising gonadotrophin titres during treatment.
3. Severe toxicity preventing adequate therapy.

In patients with non-metastatic choriocarcinoma, dactinomycin or methotrexate or both, have been used successfully, with or without surgery.

Cosmegen has been beneficial as a single agent in the treatment of metastatic non-seminomatous testicular carcinoma.

Other neoplasms: Dactinomycin has been given intravenously or by regional perfusion, alone or with other antineoplastic compounds or with X-ray therapy, in the palliative treatment of Ewing's sarcoma and sarcoma botryoides. For non-metastatic Ewing's sarcoma, promising results were obtained when dactinomycin (45 micrograms/m^2) and cyclophosphamide (1,200 mg/m^2) were given sequentially and with radiotherapy, over an eighteen-month period. Those with metastatic disease remain the subject of continued investigation with a more aggressive chemotherapeutic regimen employed initially.

Temporary objective improvement and relief of pain and discomfort have followed the use of dactinomycin, usually in conjunction with radiotherapy for sarcoma botryoides. This palliative effect ranges from transitory inhibition of tumour growth to a considerable but temporary regression in tumour size.

Cosmegen and radiation therapy: Much evidence suggests that Cosmegen potentiates the effects of X-ray therapy. The converse also appears likely; that Cosmegen may be more effective when radiation therapy is given concurrently.

With combined Cosmegen and radiation therapy, the normal skin, as well as the buccal and pharyngeal mucosa, shows early erythema. When given with dactinomycin, a smaller than usual X-ray dose causes erythema and vesiculation, which progresses more rapidly through the stages of tanning and desquamation. Healing may occur in four to six weeks rather than in two to three months. Erythema from previous X-ray therapy may be reactivated by the administration of Cosmegen alone, especially when the interval between the two forms of therapy is brief. This potentiation of radiation effects represents a special problem when the irradiation treatment area includes the mucous membrane. When irradiation is directed towards the nasopharynx, the combination may produce severe oropharyngeal mucositis.

Severe reactions may ensue if high doses of both Cosmegen and radiation therapy are used, or if the patient is particularly sensitive to such combined therapy.

Because of this potentiating effect, Cosmegen may be tried in radio-sensitive tumours not responding to doses of X-ray therapy that can be tolerated. Objective improvement in tumour size and activity may be observed when lower, better tolerated doses of both types of therapy are employed.

Isolation-perfusion technique: Cosmegen, alone or with other antineoplastic agents, has also been given by the isolation-perfusion technique, either as palliative treatment or as an adjunct to resection of a tumour. Some tumours that are considered resistant to chemotherapy and radiation therapy may respond when the drug is given by the perfusion technique. Neoplasms in which dactinomycin has been tried by this technique include various types of sarcoma, carcinoma and adenocarcinoma.

In some instances, tumours regressed, pain was relieved for variable periods, and surgery made possible. On other occasions, however, the outcome has been less favourable. Nevertheless, in selected cases, Cosmegen given by the perfusion technique may provide more effective palliation than when given systemically.

Dosage and administration Toxic reactions due to Cosmegen are frequent and may be severe, thus limiting the amount that may be given in many cases. However, the severity of toxicity varies markedly and is only partly dependent on the dosage used. Cosmegen must only be given in short courses.

Intravenous use: The dosage of Cosmegen will vary with the tolerance of the patient, the size and location of the neoplasm, and the use of other forms of therapy. It may be necessary to reduce the usual dosage suggested below when other chemotherapy or X-ray therapy is used concurrently, or has been employed previously.

The dosage of Cosmegen is calculated in micrograms. The dosage for adults or children should not exceed 15 mcg/kg or 400–600 mcg/square meter of body surface daily intravenously for five days. Calculation of the dosage for obese or oedematous patients should be on the basis of surface area in an effort to relate dosage to lean body mass.

Adults: Usually 500 micrograms a day for a maximum of five days, given intravenously.

Children: 15 micrograms per kg body weight a day for a maximum of five days, given intravenously. Alternatively, a total dosage of 2500 micrograms/m^2 body surface is given intravenously over a one-week period.

Cosmegen should not normally be given to infants under the age of 12 months.

In both adults and children, a second course may be given, but not until at least three weeks have elapsed, and all evidence of toxicity has disappeared.

Isolation-perfusion technique: Administration by the isolation-perfusion technique offers certain advantages, provided leakage of the drug through the general circulation into other areas of the body is minimal. By this technique, dactinomycin is in continuous contact with the tumour for the duration of treatment. The dose may be increased well above that used by the systemic route, usually without adding to the danger of toxic effects. If the agent is confined to an isolated part, it should not interfere with the patient's defence mechanisms. Systemic absorption of toxic products from neoplastic tissue can be minimised by removing the perfusate when the procedure is finished.

The dosage schedules and the technique itself vary from one investigator to another; the published literature should, therefore, be consulted for details. In general, the following doses are suggested:

For a lower extremity or pelvis – 50 micrograms per kg body weight.

For an upper extremity – 35 micrograms per kg body weight.

It may be advisable to use lower doses in obese patients, or when previous chemotherapy or radiation therapy has been employed.

Use in the elderly: The general considerations already outlined also apply to elderly patients.

Reconstitution and administration: Cosmegen is reconstituted by adding 1.1 ml of Water for Injections BP without preservative to the vial. For injection, 1.0 ml of the reconstituted solution, which will contain 500 micrograms of dactinomycin, is withdrawn into the syringe. Only Water for Injections BP (which does not contain preservatives) should be used. Other injection fluids may cause precipitation.

Cosmegen should be inspected for particulate matter and discoloration, whenever possible. The reconstituted solution is clear and gold-coloured.

When reconstituted, the solution of dactinomycin can be added to an infusion solution of 5% dextrose injection or sodium chloride injection, either directly or into the tubing of a running intravenous infusion.

Since dactinomycin is extremely corrosive to soft tissue, precautions for materials of this nature should be observed. To avoid extravasation, the calculated dose of Cosmegen should be given through the tubing of a running intravenous infusion, so that when administration is completed, the tubing can be flushed immediately to avoid damage to the vein. If extravasation occurs, stop the infusion and disconnect the IV administration set, but leave the cannula or needle in situ. Attempt to aspirate the extravasated drug via the cannula or needle, inject antidote if desired, and remove the cannula or needle. Elevate the limb and apply a cold compress for 45 minutes. There is no generally-accepted antidote for local use, but the following have been used with some success: Sodium thiosulphate 25% (1.6 ml+3 ml of water for injection), Sodium thiosulphate 10% (4 ml+6 ml of water for injection), ascorbic acid injection (50 mg/ml) (1 ml). In severe cases, debridement may become necessary.

Partial removal of dactinomycin from intravenous solutions by cellulose ester membrane filters used in some intravenous in-line filters has been reported.

If Cosmegen is to be injected directly into the vein without the use of an infusion, the 'two-needle' technique should be used. The calculated dose should be reconstituted and withdrawn from the vial with one sterile needle; direct injection into the vein should then be performed with another sterile needle.

Although reconstituted Cosmegen is chemically stable, the product does not contain a preservative and accidental microbial contamination might result. Any unused portion of the solution should be discarded. Use of water-containing preservatives (benzyl alcohol or parabens) to reconstitute cosmegen for injection, results in the formation of a precipitate.

Contra-indications, warnings, etc

Contra-indications: If Cosmegen is given at or about the time of infection with chickenpox or herpes zoster, a severe generalised disease, which may be fatal, can occur.

Warning: Cosmegen should be administered only under the supervision of a physician who is experienced in the use of a cancer chemotherapeutic agent.

Precautions: Cosmegen is highly toxic and both powder and solution must be handled and administered with care. This drug is extremely corrosive to soft tissue. If extravasation occurs during intravenous use, severe damage to soft tissues will occur.

Cosmegen, like all antineoplastic agents, is a toxic drug, and very careful and frequent observation of the patient for adverse reactions is necessary. These reactions may involve any tissue of the body. The possibility of an anaphylactoid reaction should be borne in mind.

Dactinomycin can affect male fertility adversely.

An increased incidence of gastro-intestinal toxicity and bone-marrow depression has been reported when dactinomycin was given with X-ray therapy.

Particular caution is necessary when administering dactinomycin within two months of irradiation for the treatment of right-sided Wilms' tumour, since hepatomegaly and elevated AST (SGOT) levels have been seen.

Nausea and vomiting due to dactinomycin make it necessary to give Cosmegen intermittently. It is extremely important to observe the patient daily for toxic side-effects when combined therapy is employed, since a full course of therapy is occasionally not tolerated. If stomatitis, diarrhoea, or severe haemopoietic depression appear during therapy, these drugs should be discontinued until the patient has recovered.

Recent reports indicate an increased incidence of second primary tumours following treatment with radiation and anti-neoplastic agents, such as dactinomycin. Multi-modal therapy creates the need for careful, long-term observation of cancer survivors.

Drug/laboratory test interactions: A variety of abnormalities of renal, hepatic and bone-marrow function have been reported in patients with neoplastic disease receiving dactinomycin. It is advisable to make frequent checks of renal, hepatic, and bone-marrow function.

It has been reported that dactinomycin may interfere with bioassay procedures for the determination of antibacterial drug levels.

Use in pregnancy and nursing mothers: This product has been shown to be teratogenic in animals and should not normally be given to pregnant women.

Dactinomycin should not be administered to mothers who are breast feeding.

Use in children: As there is a greater frequency of toxic effects of dactinomycin in infants, Cosmegen should not normally be given to children less than 12 months old.

Side-effects: Toxic effects (except nausea and vomiting) do not usually become apparent until two to four days after a course of therapy is stopped, and may not reach a maximum before one to two weeks have elapsed. Deaths have been reported. However, side-effects are usually reversible on discontinuing therapy. They include the following:

General: Malaise, fatigue, lethargy, fever, myalgia, proctitis, hypocalcaemia.

Oral: Cheilitis, dysphagia, oesophagitis, ulcerative stomatitis, pharyngitis.

Gastro-intestinal: Anorexia, nausea, vomiting, abdominal pain, diarrhoea, gastro-intestinal ulceration, liver toxicity including ascites, hepatomegaly, hepatitis, and liver function test abnormalities. Nausea and vomiting, which occur early during the first few hours after administration, may be alleviated by giving anti-emetics.

Haematological: Anaemia (even to the point of aplastic anaemia, agranulocytosis, leucopenia, thrombocytopenia, pancytopenia, reticulocytopenia). Platelet and white blood cell counts should be done daily to detect severe haemopoietic depression. If either count shows a marked decrease, dactinomycin should be withheld to allow marrow recovery. This often takes up to three weeks.

Dermatological: Alopecia, skin eruptions, acne, flare-up of erythema or increased pigmentation of previously irradiated skin.

Soft tissues: Dactinomycin is extremely corrosive to soft tissues. If extravasation occurs during intravenous use, severe damage to soft tissues will occur. In at least one instance, this has led to contracture of the arms.

Side-effects relating especially to the isolation-perfusion technique: Complications of the perfusion technique are related mainly to the amount of drug that escapes into the systemic circulation and may consist of haemopoietic depression, increased susceptibility to infection, absorption of toxic products from massive destruction of neoplastic tissue, impaired wound healing, and superficial ulceration of the gastric mucosa. Other side-effects may include oedema of the extremity involved, damage to the soft tissues of the perfused area, and potentially venous thrombosis.

Overdosage: Dactinomycin is extremely corrosive to soft tissue. Extravasation in at least one instance has lead to contracture of the arms.

In the event of overdosage, dactinomycin therapy should be withdrawn immediately. Many abnormalities of renal, hepatic and bone marrow function can be expected. Treatment should be symptomatic and supportive. There is no known antidote.

Study has indicated that the terminal plasma half-life was approximately 36 hours. Some 30% of the dose of dactinomycin was recovered in the urine and faeces in one week.

Pharmaceutical precautions Store below 25°C protected from light. Avoid freezing.

It is recommended that Cosmegen is reconstituted only by trained personnel wearing protective gloves. A designated area should be set aside for this purpose and the work surface covered with disposable plastic-backed absorbent paper.

Luer-lock fittings on all syringes and sets are recommended, and use of large-bore needles or a venting needle will help to minimise back pressure and the possible formation of aerosols. Accidental splashing on to the skin or eye should be treated immediately with copious irrigation of isotonic saline or water. Pregnant staff should not handle Cosmegen.

Adequate care should be taken in the disposal of equipment after contact with Cosmegen.

Legal category POM.

Package quantities Vials containing 500 micrograms dactinomycin with 20 mg mannitol.

Further information Generally, the actinomycins inhibit Gram-positive and Gram-negative bacteria and some fungi. However, the toxic properties of the actinomycins (including dactinomycin) in relation to antibacterial activity preclude their use as antibiotics in the treatment of infectious diseases.

Because the actinomycins are cytotoxic, they have an antineoplastic effect which has been demonstrated in experimental animals with various types of tumour implant. This cytotoxic action is the basis for their use in the palliative treatment of certain types of cancer.

Dactinomycin is minimally metabolised. It tends to concentrate in nucleated cells and does not cross the blood-brain barrier.

Product licence number 0025/5075.

DARANIDE*

Presentation Yellow, half-scored tablets, marked 'MSD 49', containing 50 mg Dichlorphenamide BP.

Uses Carbonic anhydrase inhibitor.

For chronic simple (open-angle) glaucoma and secondary glaucoma. May be useful for pre-operative control of intra-ocular tension in acute angle-closure glaucoma.

Dosage and administration Although Daranide can be used alone, it is usually more effective when given concurrently with miotics.

Initial adult dosage: Usually 2–4 tablets followed by 2 tablets every 12 hours.

Maintenance dosage: ½–1 tablet one to three times a day.

Dosage must be carefully adjusted to the individual requirements of each patient. In acute angle-closure glaucoma, Daranide may be administered with miotics and osmotic agents. If this does not reduce the intra-ocular tension rapidly, surgery may be mandatory.

Use in the elderly: The dosage above also applies to the elderly, but use with particular caution in this age group (see 'Precautions' and 'Side-effects').

Paediatric use is not recommended.

Contra-indications, warnings, etc

Contra-indications: Hepatic insufficiency, renal failure, adrenocortical insufficiency, hyperchloraemic acidosis, depressed sodium or potassium levels or chronic non-congestive closed-angle glaucoma. Should not be used in patients with severe pulmonary obstruction who are unable to increase their alveolar ventilation, since acidosis may be increased. Hypersensitivity to dichlorphenamide.

See also 'Use in pregnancy' under 'Precautions'.

Precautions: Daranide increases potassium excretion, and hypokalaemia may develop under the following circumstances: when diuresis is brisk; in the presence of severe cirrhosis; during concomitant therapy with steroids or ACTH; interference with adequate oral electrolyte intake. Digitalised patients are particularly sensitive to the effects of potassium depletion. Hypokalaemia may be treated by administration of potassium chloride or giving foods with a high potassium content.

Like all carbonic anhydrase inhibitors, high doses of Daranide cause some decrease in renal blood flow and glomerular filtration rate.

Daranide should be used with caution in the presence of severe degrees of respiratory acidosis.

Carbonic anhydrase inhibitors may potentiate the effects of folic acid antagonists, hypoglycaemic agents, oral anticoagulants and local anaesthetics, and may increase the risk of salicylate toxicity in patients taking salicylates. Instances of severe osteomalacia have been reported in patients taking carbonic anhydrase inhibitors with anticonvulsants.

Use in pregnancy: Studies with dichlorphenamide in rats have demonstrated teratogenic effects (skeletal anomalies) at high dosages. There is no evidence of these effects in humans; however, dichlorphenamide is not recommended for use in women of child bearing age or in pregnant patients, especially during the first trimester. If pregnancy is present or suspected, the benefits of using Daranide should be weighed against possible hazards to the fetus.

Side-effects: The side-effects characteristic of carbonic anhydrase inhibitors may occur. These include: gastro-intestinal disturbances (anorexia, nausea, and vomiting); loss of weight; constipation; urinary frequency; renal colic; renal calculi; skin eruptions; pruritus; leucopenia; agranulocytosis; thrombocytopenia; headache; weakness; nervousness; globus hystericus; sedation; lassitude; depression; confusion; disorientation; dizziness; ataxia; tremor; tinnitus; paraesthesiae of hands, feet and tongue.

Overdosage: Symptoms of overdosage or toxicity may include drowsiness, anorexia, nausea, vomiting, dizziness, paraesthesiae, ataxia, tremor and tinnitus.

In the event of recent overdosage, induce emesis or perform gastric lavage. Fluids and electrolytes should, if necessary, be replenished. The electrolyte disturbance most likely to be encountered from overdosage is hyperchloraemic acidosis that may respond to bicarbonate administration. Potassium supplementation may be required. The patient should be carefully observed and given supportive treatment.

Data on the metabolism of dichlorphenamide are not available. Onset of therapeutic action begins within an hour and reaches maximal effect in two to four hours. Activity of a single dose is maintained for approximately six to twelve hours.

Pharmaceutical precautions Keep container well closed; store in a cool place, protected from light.

Legal category POM.

Package quantities Bottles of 100.

Further information Nil.

Product licence number 0025/5025.

DECADRON* INJECTION

Presentation A clear, colourless solution containing, in each millilitre, Dexamethasone Sodium Phosphate BP equivalent to 4 mg dexamethasone phosphate or approximately 3.33 mg dexamethasone.

Uses Corticosteroid.

For use in certain endocrine and non-endocrine disorders responsive to corticosteroid therapy.

Systemic administration: Decadron Injection is recommended for systemic administration by intravenous or intramuscular injection when oral therapy is not feasible or desirable in the following conditions.

Endocrine disorders:
Primary or secondary adrenocortical insufficiency: (Hydrocortisone or cortisone is the first choice, but synthetic analogues may be used with mineralocorticoids where applicable and, in infancy, mineralocorticoid supplementation is particularly important.)

Non-endocrine disorders: Decadron Injection may be used in the treatment of non-endocrine corticosteroid responsive conditions including:

Allergy and anaphylaxis: Angioneurotic oedema and anaphylaxis.

Gastro-intestinal: Crohn's disease and ulcerative colitis.

Infection (with appropriate chemotherapy): Miliary tuberculosis and endotoxic shock.

Neurological disorders: Raised intracranial pressure secondary to cerebral tumours and infantile spasms.

Respiratory: Bronchial asthma and aspiration pneumonitis.

Skin disorders: Toxic epidermal necrolysis.

Shock: Adjunctive treatment where high pharmacological doses are needed. Treatment is an adjunct to, and not a substitute for specific and supportive measures the patient may require. Dexamethasone has been shown to be beneficial when used in the early treatment of shock, but it may not influence overall survival.

Local administration
Decadron Injection is suitable for intra-articular or soft-tissue injection as adjunctive therapy for short-term administration in:

Soft-tissue disorders such as carpal tunnel syndrome and tenosynovitis.

Intra-articular disorders such as rheumatoid arthritis and osteoarthritis with an inflammatory component.

Decadron Injection may be injected intralesionally in selected skin disorders such as cystic acne vulgaris, localised lichen simplex, and keloids.

Dosage and administration Decadron Injection can be given without mixing or dilution, but if preferred, can be added without loss of potency to sodium chloride injection or dextrose injection or compatible blood for transfusion, and given by intravenous drip. The infusion mixture must be used within 24 hours, and the usual aseptic techniques for injections should be observed.

All dosage recommendations are given in units of dexamethasone phosphate.

Intravenous and intramuscular injection:
General considerations: Generally, initial and maintenance dosages must be determined individually according to the disease under treatment and to the response of the patient. The lowest possible dosage adequate to control the disease process should be used.

Usually the parenteral dosage ranges are one-third to one-half the oral dose, given every 12 hours.

The usual initial dosage is 0.5–20 mg (0.125–5 ml) a day. In situations of less severity, lower doses will generally suffice. However, in certain overwhelming, acute, life-threatening situations, administration in dosages exceeding the usual dosages may be justified. In these circumstances, the slower rate of absorption by intramuscular administration should be recognised.

The initial dosage should be maintained or adjusted until a satisfactory response is noted.

Both the dose in the evening, which is useful in alleviating morning stiffness, and the divided dosage regimen are associated with greater suppression of the hypothalamo-pituitary-adrenal axis. (If, after a reasonable time, there is a lack of satisfactory clinical response, Decadron Injection should be discontinued and the patient transferred to other appropriate therapy.) After a favourable response is noted, the proper maintenance dosage should be determined by decreasing the initial dosage by small amounts at appropriate intervals to the lowest dosage which will maintain an adequate clinical response. Chronic dosage should preferably not exceed 500 micrograms dexamethasone daily. Close monitoring of drug dosage is needed.

If Decadron is to be stopped after it has been given for more than a few days, it should be withdrawn gradually rather than stopped abruptly.

Whenever possible, the intravenous route should be used for the initial dose and for as many subsequent doses as are given while the patient is in shock (because of the irregular rate of absorption of any medicament administered by any other route in such patients). When the blood pressure responds, use the intramuscular route until oral therapy can be substituted. For the comfort of the patient, not more than 2 ml should be injected intramuscularly at any one site.

In emergencies, the usual dose of Decadron Injection by intravenous or intramuscular injection is 4–20 mg (1–5 ml), depending on the severity of the condition (see also 'Shock'). This dose may be repeated until adequate response is discernible.

After initial improvement, single doses of 2–4 mg (0.5–1 ml) repeated as necessary, may be sufficient. The total daily dosage usually need not exceed 80 mg (20 ml), even in severe conditions.

When constant maximal effect is desired, dosage must be repeated at three-hour or four-hour intervals, or maintained by slow intravenous drip.

Intravenous and intramuscular injections are advised in acute illness. When the acute stage has passed, oral steroid therapy should be substituted as soon as feasible.

Shock (of haemorrhagic, traumatic, surgical or septic

origin): Usually 2 to 6 mg/kg body weight as a single intravenous injection. This may be repeated in two to six hours if shock persists. Alternatively, this may be followed immediately by the same dose in an intravenous infusion. Therapy with Decadron Injection is an adjunct to, and not a replacement for conventional therapy.

Administration of these high doses should be continued only until the patient's condition has stabilised and usually no longer than 48–72 hours.

Cerebral oedema: Associated with primary or metastatic brain tumour, pre-operative preparation of patients with increased intracranial pressure secondary to brain tumour: initially 10 mg (2.5 ml) intravenously, followed by 4 mg (1 ml) intramuscularly every six hours until symptoms of cerebral oedema subside. Response is usually noted within 12–24 hours; dosage may be reduced after two to four days and gradually discontinued over five to seven days.

High doses of Decadron Injection are recommended for initiating short-term intensive therapy for acute life-threatening cerebral oedema. Following the high loading dose schedule of the first day of therapy, the dose is scaled down over the seven- to ten-day period of intensive therapy and subsequently reduced to zero over the next seven to ten days. When maintenance therapy is required, substitute oral Decadron as soon as possible. (See table below.)

Palliative management of recurrent or inoperable brain tumours: Maintenance therapy should be determined for each patient; 2 mg (0.5 ml) two or three times a day may be effective.

The smallest dosage necessary to control cerebral oedema should be used.

Suggested high dose schedule in cerebral oedema:

Adults:	
Initial Dose	50 mg IV
1st day	8 mg IV every 2 hours
2nd day	8 mg IV every 2 hours
3rd day	8 mg IV every 2 hours
4th day	4 mg IV every 2 hours
5th–8th day	4 mg IV every 4 hours
Thereafter	decrease by daily reduction of 4 mg
Children (35 kg and over):	
Initial Dose	25 mg IV
1st day	4 mg IV every 2 hours
2nd day	4 mg IV every 2 hours
3rd day	4 mg IV every 2 hours
4th day	4 mg IV every 4 hours
5th–8th day	4 mg IV every 6 hours
Thereafter	decrease by daily reduction of 2 mg
Children (below 35 kg):	
Initial Dose	20 mg IV
1st day	4 mg IV every 3 hours
2nd day	4 mg IV every 3 hours
3rd day	4 mg IV every 3 hours
4th day	4 mg IV every 6 hours
5th–8th day	2 mg IV every 6 hours
Thereafter	decrease by daily reduction of 1 mg

Dual therapy: In acute self-limiting allergic disorders or acute exacerbations of chronic allergic disorders, the following schedule combining oral and parenteral therapy is suggested:

First day	Decadron Injection, 4 mg–8 mg (1 ml–2 ml) intramuscularly
Second day	Two 500 microgram Decadron Tablets twice a day
Third day	Two 500 microgram Decadron Tablets twice a day
Fourth day	One 500 microgram Decadron Tablet twice a day
Fifth day	One 500 microgram Decadron Tablet twice a day
Sixth day	One 500 microgram Decadron Tablet
Seventh day	One 500 microgram Decadron Tablet
Eighth day	Reassessment day

(For information on Decadron Tablets, see separate entry.)

Intrasynovial, intralesional, and soft-tissue injection: In general, these injections are employed when only one or two joints or areas are affected.

Some of the usual single doses are:

Site of injection	*Amount of dexamethasone phosphate*
Large joints (e.g. knee)	2–4 mg (0.5–1 ml)
Small joints (e.g. interphalangeal, temporomandibular)	0.8–1 mg (0.2–0.25 ml)
Bursae	2–3 mg (0.5–0.75 ml)
Tendon sheaths*	0.4–1 mg (0.1–0.25 ml)
Soft-tissue infiltration	2–6 mg (0.5–1.5 ml)
Ganglia	1–2 mg (0.25–0.5 ml)

* Injection should be made into the tendon sheath, and not directly into the tendon.

Frequency of injection: once every three to five days to once every two to three weeks, depending on response.

Use in children: Dosage should be limited to a single dose on alternate days to lessen retardation of growth and minimise suppression of the hypothalamo-pituitary-adrenal axis.

Use in the elderly: Treatment of elderly patients, particularly if long term, should be planned bearing in mind the more serious consequences of the common side effects of corticosteroids in old age, especially osteoporosis, diabetes, hypertension, susceptibility to infection and thinning of the skin.

Contra-indications, warnings, etc

Contra-indications: Systemic fungal infection; hypersensitivity to any component.

Warnings: Frequent intra-articular injections over a prolonged period may lead to joint destruction with bone necrosis. Intra-articular injection of corticosteroid may produce systemic adverse reactions including adrenal suppression.

Precautions: Corticosteroids may exacerbate systemic fungal infections and, therefore, should not be used in the presence of such infections unless they are needed to control drug reactions due to amphotericin. Moreover, there have been cases reported in which concomitant use of amphotericin and hydrocortisone was followed by cardiac enlargement and congestive failure.

The dosage of corticosteroid should be reduced gradually.

Average and large doses of hydrocortisone or cortisone can cause elevation of blood pressure, retention of salt and water, and increased excretion of potassium, but these effects are less likely to occur with synthetic derivatives, except when used in large doses. Dietary salt restriction and potassium supplementation may be necessary. All corticosteroids increase calcium excretion.

The slower rate of absorption by intramuscular administration should be recognised.

In patients on corticosteroid therapy subjected to unusual stress, dosage should be increased before, during and after the stressful situation.

Drug-induced secondary adrenocortical insufficiency may be minimised by gradual dosage reduction, but may persist for months after discontinuation of therapy. In any stressful situation during that period, therefore, corticosteroid therapy should be reinstated. If the patient is already receiving corticosteroids, the dosage may have to be increased. Salt and/or a mineralocorticoid should be given concurrently, since mineralocorticoid secretion may be impaired.

Stopping corticosteroids after prolonged therapy may cause withdrawal symptoms including fever, myalgia, arthralgia, and malaise. This may occur in patients even without evidence of adrenal insufficiency.

Because anaphylactoid reactions have occurred, rarely, in patients receiving parenteral corticosteroid therapy, appropriate precautions should be taken prior to administration, especially when the patient has a history of allergy to any drug.

Administration of live virus vaccines is contraindicated in individuals receiving immunosuppressive doses of corticosteroids. If inactivated viral or bacterial vaccines are administered to individuals receiving immunosuppressive doses of corticosteroids, the expected serum antibody response may not be obtained. However, immunisation procedures may be undertaken in patients who are receiving corticosteroids as replacement therapy, e.g. for Addison's disease.

Aspirin should be used cautiously in conjunction with corticosteroids in hypoprothrombinaemia.

The use of Decadron Injection in active tuberculosis should be restricted to those cases of fulminating or disseminated tuberculosis in which the corticosteroid is used for the management of the disease in conjunction with an appropriate antituberculosis regimen. If the corticosteroids are indicated in patients with latent tuberculosis or tuberculin reactivity, close observation is necessary as reactivation may occur. During prolonged corticosteroid therapy, these patients should receive prophylactic chemotherapy.

Corticosteroids should be used with caution in renal insufficiency, hypertension, diabetes or in those with a family history of diabetes, congestive heart failure, osteoporosis, previous steroid myopathy, glaucoma (or previous history), myasthenia gravis, non-specific ulcerative colitis, diverticulitis, fresh intestinal anastomoses, active or latent peptic ulcer. Signs of peritoneal irritation following gastro-intestinal perforation in patients receiving large doses of corticosteroids may be minimal or absent. Fat embolism has been reported as a possible complication of hypercortisonism.

Corticosteroids should be used cautiously in patients with ocular herpes simplex because of possible corneal perforation.

There is an enhanced effect of corticosteroids in patients with hypothyroidism and in those with cirrhosis. Corticosteroids may increase or decrease motility and number of spermatozoa.

As phenytoin, barbiturates, ephedrine and rifampicin may enhance the metabolic clearance of corticosteroids, resulting in decreased blood levels and reduced physiological activity, the dosage may have to be adjusted. These interactions may interfere with dexamethasone suppression tests which should be interpreted with caution during administration of these drugs.

The prothrombin time should be checked frequently in patients who are receiving corticosteroids and coumarin anticoagulants at the same time.

When corticosteroids are administered concomitantly with potassium-depleting diuretics, patients should be observed closely for development of hypokalaemia.

Corticosteroids may mask some signs of infection, and new infections may appear during their use. There may be decreased resistance, and inability to localise infection.

A report shows that the use of corticosteroids in cerebral malaria is associated with a prolonged coma and an increased incidence of pneumonia and gastro-intestinal bleeding.

Corticosteroids may activate latent amoebiasis. Therefore, it is recommended that latent or active amoebiasis be excluded before initiating corticosteroid therapy in any patient who has either spent time in the tropics, or has unexplained diarrhoea.

Alterations in the patient's mental state may appear when corticosteroids are used, ranging from psychological dependence, euphoria, insomnia, mood swings, personality changes and severe depression, to frank psychotic manifestations.

Prolonged use of corticosteroids may produce posterior subcapsular cataracts, glaucoma with possible damage to the optic nerves, and may enhance the establishment of secondary infections.

Local steroid injection should be undertaken in an aseptic environment to reduce the particular risk of bacterial infection. Injection of a steroid into an infected site should be avoided.

Appropriate examination of joint fluid is necessary to exclude a septic process.

A marked increase in pain accompanied by local swelling, further restriction of joint motion, fever, and malaise are suggestive of septic arthritis. If this complication occurs and the diagnosis of sepsis is confirmed, appropriate antimicrobial therapy should be instituted.

Patients should understand the great importance of not over-using joints that are still diseased despite symptomatic improvement.

Corticosteroids should not be injected into unstable joints.

Frequent intra-articular injections have been reported to cause development of Charcot-like arthropathies.

Children: Corticosteroids cause growth retardation in infancy, childhood and adolescence. Treatment should be limited to the minimum dosage for the shortest possible time. In order to minimise suppression of the hypothalamo-pituitary-adrenal axis and growth retardation, treatment should be limited, where possible, to a single dose on alternate days.

Growth and development of infants and children on prolonged corticosteroid therapy should be carefully monitored.

Use in pregnancy and the nursing mother: There is inadequate evidence of safety in human pregnancy and there may be a very small risk of cleft palate and intrauterine growth retardation in the fetus; there is evidence of harmful effects on pregnancy in animals.

Corticosteroids appear in breast milk and could suppress growth, interfere with endogenous corticosteroid production, or cause other unwanted effects. Mothers taking pharmacological doses of corticosteroids should be advised not to nurse.

Side-effects: Fluid and electrolyte disturbances: Sodium retention, fluid retention, congestive heart failure in susceptible patients, potassium loss, hypokalaemic alkalosis, hypertension, increased calcium excretion.

Musculoskeletal: Muscle weakness, steroid myopathy, loss of muscle mass, osteoporosis (especially in post-menopausal females), vertebral compression fractures, aseptic necrosis of femoral and humeral heads, pathological fracture of long bones, tendon rupture, and post-injection flare (following intra-articular use).

Gastro-intestinal: Peptic ulcer with possible perforation and haemorrhage, perforation of the small and large bowel, particularly in patients with inflammatory bowel disease, pancreatitis, abdominal distension, ulcerative oesophagitis, dyspepsia, oesophageal candidiasis.

Dermatological: Impaired wound healing, thin fragile skin, petechiae and ecchymoses, erythema, striae, telangiectasia, acne, increased sweating, possible suppression of skin tests, burning or tingling especially in the perineal area (after intravenous injection), other cutaneous reactions such as allergic dermatitis, urticaria, angioneurotic oedema, and hypo- or hyper-pigmentation.

Neurological: Convulsions, increased intracranial pressure with papilloedema (pseudotumour cerebri) usually after treatment, vertigo, headache, and rare instances of blindness associated with intra-lesional therapy around the face and head.

Endocrine: Menstrual irregularities, amenorrhoea, development of Cushingoid state, suppression of growth in children, secondary adrenocortical and pituitary unresponsiveness, particularly in times of stress, as in trauma, surgery or illness, decreased carbohydrate tolerance, manifestations of latent diabetes mellitus, increased requirements for insulin or oral hypoglycaemic agents in diabetes.

Ophthalmic: Posterior subcapsular cataracts, increased intra-ocular pressure, papilloedema, corneal or scleral thinning, exacerbation of ophthalmic viral disease, glaucoma, exophthalmos.

Metabolic: Negative nitrogen balance due to protein catabolism.

Other: Anaphylactoid or hypersensitivity reactions, leucocytosis, thrombo-embolism, weight gain, increased appetite, nausea, malaise, and sterile abscess.

Teratogenicity: See pregnancy warning under 'Use in pregnancy and the nursing mother'.

Overdosage: Reports of acute toxicity and/or deaths following overdosage with glucocorticoids are rare. No antidote is available. Treatment is probably not indicated for reactions due to chronic poisoning unless the patient has a condition that would render him unusually susceptible to ill effects from corticosteroids. In this case, symptomatic treatment should be instituted as necessary.

Anaphylactic and hypersensitivity reactions may be treated with adrenaline, positive-pressure artificial respiration and aminophylline. The patient should be kept warm and quiet.

The biological half-life of dexamethasone in plasma is about 190 minutes.

Pharmaceutical precautions Decadron Injection is sensitive to heat and should not be autoclaved to sterilise the outside of the vial. Store below 25°C, protected from light and freezing. Only sodium chloride injection or dextrose injection should be used as diluent. Any infusion mixture must be used within 24 hours.

Legal category POM.

Package quantities Vials of 2 ml.

Further information Also available is Injection Decadron Shock-Pak containing, per millilitre, dexamethasone sodium phosphate equivalent to 20 mg dexamethasone, indicated exclusively for intravenous use as adjunctive therapy in severe shock. For information about this special high-dose form of Decadron Injection, see separate entry.

Decadron Injection is ready for immediate use. An adequate dose is contained in a small volume of vehicle, and small-bore needles can be used wherever appropriate.

Product licence number 0025/5045.

INJECTION DECADRON* SHOCK-PAK

Presentation An injection containing, per millilitre, dexamethasone sodium phosphate equivalent to 20 mg dexamethasone, as a colourless solution.

Uses Corticosteroid.

Only for the adjunctive treatment of shock where massive doses of corticosteroids are needed. It is an adjunct to, and not a substitute for, specific or supportive measures that the patient may require, e.g. restoration of circulating blood volume, correction of fluid and electrolyte balance, oxygen, surgical measures and antibiotics. Dexamethasone has been shown to be beneficial when used early in the treatment of septic shock, but it may not influence overall survival.

Dosage and administration Injection Decadron Shock-Pak is for administration by the intravenous route only.

Intravenous injection in shock: Injection Decadron Shock-Pak can be used without mixing or diluting. Injection should be made slowly.

The usual dosage by intravenous injection is 2–6 mg/kg body weight given as a single intravenous injection. This may be repeated in two to six hours, if shock persists. As an alternative, the initial intravenous injection may be followed immediately by an intravenous infusion containing the same dose. (Although Injection Decadron Shock-Pak was not primarily designed for intravenous infusion, it can be added to sodium chloride injection, or to dextrose injection, and administered by intravenous drip without loss of potency. When the Shock-Pak is added to an infusion solution, the mixture must be used within 24 hours as infusion solutions do not contain preservatives.)

These dosages are large in comparison with the usual recommended dosages of dexamethasone sodium phosphate. They are, however, for emergency use in acute conditions needing massive doses of corticosteroid, and reflect the tendency in current medical practice to use such high doses in the treatment of shock.

Therapy with Injection Decadron Shock-Pak is an adjunct to, and not a replacement for, conventional therapy. Administration of high doses of corticosteroids should be continued only until the patient's condition has stabilised, and usually no longer than 48–72 hours. Prolonged therapy at such high doses should be avoided to prevent possible complications, such as adrenal suppression or gastro-intestinal ulceration.

Use in the elderly: These dosage recommendations apply to all adults, including the elderly.

Contra-indications, warnings, etc

Contra-indications: Systemic fungal infections; hypersensitivity to any component.

Precautions: Injection Decadron Shock-Pak is for adjunctive use in the treatment of shock, and therapy must be accompanied by the usual standard measures employed in its management. In shock of septic origin, appropriate antibiotic therapy must be continued for as long as required.

The pronounced hormonal effects associated with prolonged corticosteroid therapy will probably not be seen when this injection is used for short-term adjunctive therapy in shock.

Use in pregnancy: There is inadequate evidence of safety in human pregnancy and there may be a very small risk of cleft palate and intra-uterine growth retardation in the fetus; there is evidence of harmful effects on pregnancy in animals.

Side-effects: Although adverse reactions associated with short-term corticosteroid therapy in high doses are uncommon, peptic ulceration may occur. However, for details of side-effects seen with prolonged dexamethasone therapy, please see previous entry on Decadron Injection. Some patients have reported transitory burning or tingling sensations, often in the perineal area, when intravenous injections of large doses of dexamethasone sodium phosphate were given. The usual aseptic techniques governing injections should be observed.

Overdosage: Reports of acute toxicity and/or deaths following overdosage with glucocorticoids are rare. No antidote is available. Treatment is probably not indicated for reactions due to chronic poisoning unless the patient has a condition that would render him unusually susceptible to ill effects from corticosteroids. In this case, symptomatic treatment should be instituted as necessary.

Anaphylactic and hypersensitivity reactions may be treated with adrenaline, positive-pressure artificial respiration and aminophylline. The patient should be kept warm and quiet.

The biological half-life of dexamethasone in plasma is about 190 minutes.

Pharmaceutical precautions Injection Decadron Shock-Pak is sensitive to heat, and should not be autoclaved to sterilise the outside of the vial. It should be stored in a cool place and protected from freezing.

Only sodium chloride injection or dextrose injection should be used as diluents for infusion. Any infusion mixture must be used within 24 hours.

Legal category POM.

Package quantities Vials of 5 ml.

Further information Injection Decadron Shock-Pak is a special dosage form of dexamethasone sodium phosphate designed exclusively for intravenous use as adjunctive therapy in the treatment of severe shock. For other indications requiring an injectable steroid, Decadron Injection, a formulation containing, per millilitre, dexamethasone sodium phosphate equivalent to 4 mg dexamethasone phosphate (approximately 3.33 mg dexamethasone), is available.

Product licence number 0025/0077.

DECADRON* TABLETS

Presentation White, half-scored tablets, marked 'MSD 41', containing 500 micrograms Dexamethasone BP.

Uses Corticosteroid.

For use in certain endocrine and non-endocrine disorders, in certain cases of cerebral oedema, and for diagnostic testing of adrenocortical hyperfunction.

Endocrine disorders: Primary or secondary adrenocortical insufficiency (the first choice is hydrocortisone or cortisone, but synthetic analogues may be used with mineralocorticoids where applicable; in infancy, mineralocorticoid supplementation is particularly important), congenital adrenal hyperplasia.

Non-endocrine disorders: Dexamethasone may be used in the treatment of non-endocrine corticosteroid responsive conditions including:

Allergy and anaphylaxis: Angioneurotic oedema, anaphylaxis.

Arteritis collagenosis: Polymyalgia rheumatica, polyarteritis nodosa.

Blood disorders: Haemolytic anaemia, leukaemia, myeloma.

Cardiovascular disorders: Post-myocardial infarction syndrome.

Gastro-intestinal: Crohn's disease, ulcerative colitis.

Hypercalcaemia: Sarcoidosis.

Infections (with appropriate chemotherapy): Miliary tuberculosis.

Muscular disorders: Polymyositis.

Neurological disorders: Raised intra-cranial pressure secondary to cerebral tumours.

Ocular disorders: Anterior and posterior uveitis, optic neuritis.

Renal disorders: Lupus nephritis.

Respiratory disease: Bronchial asthma, aspiration pneumonitis.

Rheumatic disorders: Rheumatoid arthritis.

Skin disorders: Pemphigus vulgaris.

Dosage and administration *General considerations:* Dosage must be individualised on the basis of the disease and the response of the patient. The lowest possible dosage adequate to control the disease process should be used.

The initial dosage varies from 0.5–9 mg a day depending on the disease being treated. In more severe diseases, doses higher than 9 mg may be required. The initial dosage should be maintained or adjusted until the patient's response is satisfactory. Both the dose in the evening, which is useful in alleviating morning stiffness, and the divided dosage regimen are associated with greater suppression of the hypothalamo-pituitary-adrenal axis. If satisfactory clinical response does not occur after a reasonable period of time, discontinue Decadron Tablets and transfer the patient to other therapy.

After a favourable initial response, the proper maintenance dosage should be determined by decreasing the initial dosage in small amounts to the lowest dosage that maintains an adequate clinical response. Chronic dosage should preferably not exceed 1.5 mg dexamethasone daily.

Patients should be monitored for signs that might require dosage adjustment, including changes in clinical status resulting from remissions or exacerbations of the disease, individual drug responsiveness, and the effect of stress (e.g. surgery, infection, trauma). During stress it may be necessary to increase dosage temporarily.

If the drug is to be stopped after more than a few days of treatment, it should be withdrawn gradually.

The following equivalents facilitate changing to Decadron from other glucocorticoids.

Milligram for milligram, dexamethasone is approximately equivalent to bethamethasone, 4 to 6 times more potent than methylprednisolone and triamcinolone, 6 to 8 times more potent than prednisone and prednisolone, 25 to 30 times more potent than hydrocortisone, and about 35 times more potent than cortisone.

In acute, self-limiting allergic disorders or acute exacerbations of chronic allergic disorders, the following dosage schedule combining parenteral and oral therapy is suggested.

First day	Decadron Injection, 4 mg or 8 mg (1 ml or 2 ml) intramuscularly
Second day	Two 500 microgram Decadron Tablets twice a day
Third day	Two 500 microgram Decadron Tablets twice a day
Fourth day	One 500 microgram Decadron Tablet twice a day
Fifth day	One 500 microgram Decadron Tablet twice a day
Sixth day	One 500 microgram Decadron Tablet
Seventh day	One 500 microgram Decadron Tablet
Eighth day	Reassessment day

This schedule is designed to ensure adequate therapy during acute episodes while minimising the risk of overdosage in chronic cases.

Dexamethasone suppression tests:

1. *Tests for Cushing's syndrome:* Two milligrams of Decadron is given orally at 11 p.m., then blood is drawn for plasma cortisol determination at 8 a.m. the following morning.

For greater accuracy, 500 microgram Decadron is given orally every 6 hours for 48 hours. Plasma cortisol is measured at 8 a.m. on the third morning. Twenty-four-hour urine collections are made for determination of 17-hydroxycorticosteroid excretion.

2. *Test to distinguish Cushing's syndrome caused by pituitary ACTH excess from the syndrome induced by other causes:* Two milligrams of Decadron is given orally every 6 hours for 48 hours. Plasma cortisol is measured at 8 a.m. on the morning following the last dose. Twenty-four-hour urine collections are made for determination of 17-hydroxycorticosteroid excretion.

Use in children: Dosage should be limited to a single dose on alternate days to lessen retardation of growth and minimise suppression of hypothalamo-pituitary-adrenal axis.

Use in the elderly: Treatment of elderly patients, particularly if long term, should be planned bearing in mind the more serious consequences of the common side effects of corticosteroids in old age, especially osteoporosis, diabetes, hypertension, susceptibility to infection and thinning of the skin.

Contra-indications, warnings, etc

Contra-indications: Systemic fungal infections; hypersensitivity to the drug.

Precautions: The dosage of corticosteroid should be reduced gradually.

Corticosteroids may exacerbate systemic fungal infections and should not be used unless they are needed to control drug reactions due to amphotericin.

Cases have been reported in which concomitant use of amphotericin and hydrocortisone was followed by cardiac enlargement and heart failure.

A report shows that the use of corticosteroids in cerebral malaria is associated with a prolonged coma and an increased incidence of pneumonia and gastro-intestinal bleeding.

Average and large doses of hydrocortisone or cortisone can cause elevation of blood pressure, retention of salt and water, and increased excretion of potassium, but these effects are less likely to occur with synthetic derivatives, except when used in large doses. Dietary salt restriction and potassium supplementation may be necessary. All corticosteroids increase calcium excretion.

In patients on corticosteroid therapy subjected to unusual stress, dosage should be increased before, during and after the stressful situation. Drug-induced secondary adrenocortical insufficiency may result from too rapid withdrawal of corticosteroids and may be minimised by gradual dosage reduction, but may persist for months after discontinuation of therapy. In any stressful situation during that period, therefore, corticosteroid therapy should be reinstated. If the patient is already receiving corticosteroids, the dose may have to be increased. Salt and/or a mineralocorticoid should be given concurrently, since mineralocorticoid secretion may be impaired.

Stopping corticosteroids after prolonged therapy may cause withdrawal symptoms including fever, myalgia, arthralgia, and malaise. This may occur in patients even without evidence of adrenal insufficiency.

Administration of live virus vaccines is contra-indicated in individuals receiving immunosuppressive doses of corticosteroids. If inactivated viral or bacterial vaccines are administered to individuals receiving immunosuppressive doses of corticosteroids, the expected serum antibody response may not be obtained. However, patients who are receiving corticosteroids as replacement therapy, e.g. for Addison's disease, may be immunised.

Aspirin should be used cautiously in conjunction with corticosteroids in hypoprothrombinaemia.

The use of Decadron Tablets in active tuberculosis should be restricted to those cases of fulminating or disseminated tuberculosis in which the corticosteroid is used for the management of the disease in conjunction with an appropriate antituberculous regimen. If corticosteroids are indicated in patients with latent tuberculosis or tuberculin reactivity, close observation of the disease is necessary as reactivation may occur. During prolonged corticosteroid therapy, these patients should receive prophylactic chemotherapy.

Corticosteroids should be used with caution in renal insufficiency, hypertension, diabetes or in those with a family history of diabetes, congestive heart failure, osteoporosis, previous steroid myopathy, glaucoma (or previous history), myasthenia gravis, non-specific ulcerative colitis, diverticulitis, fresh intestinal anastomosis, active or latent peptic ulcer. Signs of peritoneal irritation following gastro-intestinal perforation in patients receiving large doses of corticosteroids may be minimal or absent. Fat embolism has been reported as a possible complication of hypercortisonism.

Corticosteroids should be used cautiously in patients with ocular herpes simplex, because of possible corneal perforation.

There is an enhanced effect of corticosteroids in patients with hypothyroidism and in those with cirrhosis.

Corticosteroids may mask some signs of infection, and new infections may appear during their use. There may be decreased resistance and inability to localise infection in patients on corticosteroids.

Corticosteroids may activate latent amoebiasis. Therefore, it is recommended that latent or active amoebiasis be excluded before initiating corticosteroid therapy in any patient who has either spent time in the tropics, or has unexplained diarrhoea.

Alterations in the patient's mental state may appear when corticosteroids are used, ranging from psychological dependence, euphoria, insomnia, mood swings, personality changes and severe depression, to frank psychotic manifestations.

Prolonged use of corticosteroids may produce subcapsular cataracts, glaucoma with possible damage to the optic nerves, and may enhance the establishment of secondary infections.

Steroids may increase or decrease the motility and number of spermatozoa.

As phenytoin, barbiturates, ephedrine and rifampicin may enhance the metabolic clearance of corticosteroids, resulting in decreased blood levels and reduced physiological activity, the dosage of Decadron may have to be adjusted. These interactions may interfere with dexamethasone suppression tests which should be interpreted with caution during administration of these drugs.

The prothrombin time should be checked frequently in patients who are receiving corticosteroids and coumarin anticoagulants at the same time.

When corticosteroids are administered concomitantly with potassium-depleting diuretics, patients should be observed closely for development of hypokalaemia.

Children: Corticosteroids cause growth retardation in infancy, childhood and adolescence. Treatment should be limited to the minimum dosage for the shortest possible time. In order to minimise suppression of the hypothalamo-pituitary-adrenal axis and growth retardation, treatment should be limited, where possible, to a single dose on alternate days.

Growth and development of infants and children on prolonged corticosteroid therapy should be carefully monitored.

Use in pregnancy and the nursing mother: There is inadequate evidence of safety in human pregnancy and there may be a very small risk of cleft palate and intra-uterine growth retardation in the fetus; there is evidence of harmful effects on pregnancy in animals.

Corticosteroids appear in breast milk and could suppress growth, interfere with endogenous corticosteroid production, or cause other unwanted effects. Mothers taking pharmacological doses of corticosteroids should be advised not to nurse.

Side-effects: Fluid and electrolyte disturbances: Sodium retention, fluid retention, congestive heart failure in susceptible patients, potassium loss, hypokalaemic alkalosis, hypertension, increased calcium excretion.

Musculoskeletal effects: Muscle weakness, steroid myopathy, loss of muscle mass, osteoporosis (especially in post-menopausal females), vertebral compression fractures, aseptic necrosis of femoral and humeral heads, pathological fracture of long bones, tendon rupture.

Gastro-intestinal: Peptic ulcer with possible perforation and haemorrhage, perforation of the small and large bowel particularly in patients with inflammatory bowel disease, pancreatitis, abdominal distension, ulcerative oesophagitis, dyspepsia, oesophageal candidiasis.

Dermatological: Impaired wound healing, thin fragile skin, petechiae and ecchymoses, erythema, striae, telangiectasia, acne, increased sweating, suppressed reaction to skin tests, other cutaneous reactions such as allergic dermatitis, urticaria, angioneurotic oedema.

Neurological: Convulsions, vertigo, headache. Increased intracranial pressure with papilloedema (pseudotumour cerebri) may occur usually after treatment.

Endocrine: Menstrual irregularities, amenorrhoea, development of Cushingoid state, suppression of growth in children, secondary adrenocortical and pituitary unresponsiveness (particularly in times of stress as in trauma, surgery or illness), decreased carbohydrate tolerance, manifestations of latent diabetes mellitus, increased need for insulin or oral hypoglycaemic agents in diabetics.

Ophthalmic: Posterior subcapsular cataracts, increased intra-ocular pressure, papilloedema, corneal or scleral thinning, exacerbation of ophthalmic viral disease, glaucoma, exophthalmos.

Metabolic: Negative nitrogen balance due to protein catabolism.

Other: Hypersensitivity, leucocytosis, thrombo-embolism, weight gain, increased appetite, nausea, malaise.

Teratogenicity: See pregnancy warning under 'Use in pregnancy and the nursing mother'.

Overdosage: Reports of acute toxicity and/or deaths following overdosage with glucocorticoids are rare. No antidote is available. Treatment is probably not indicated for reactions due to chronic poisoning unless the patient has a condition that would render him unusually susceptible to ill effects from corticosteroids. In this case, the stomach should be emptied and symptomatic treatment should be instituted as necessary.

Anaphylactic and hypersensitivity reactions may be treated with adrenaline, positive-pressure artificial respiration and aminophylline. The patient should be kept warm and quiet.

The biological half-life of dexamethasone in plasma is about 190 minutes.

Pharmaceutical precautions Keep container well closed; store in a cool place, protected from light.

Legal category POM.

Package quantities *0.5 mg:* Bottles of 100.

Further information Decadron is a potent glucocorticoid with little mineralocorticoid activity. It has considerable anti-inflammatory properties, but its effect on electrolyte metabolism is slight, and thus, electrolyte imbalance is not normally a problem with Decadron. In low or average doses, Decadron does not usually cause elevation of blood pressure, salt and water retention, or excessive potassium excretion.

Product licence number
500 microgram tablet 0025/5046

DEMSER*

Presentation Available as, two-tone blue, opaque capsules, marked 'MSD 690', and 'DEMSER', containing 250 mg metirosine.

Uses The treatment of phaeochromocytoma during: pre-operative preparation of patients for surgery; management of patients when surgery is contra-indicated; prolonged treatment of patients with phaeochromocytoma.

Demser is not recommended for the control of essential hypertension.

Dosage and administration *Adults and children over 12 years of age:* Initially, 1 capsule (250 mg) four times a day. This may be increased by 1 or 2 capsules (250 or 500 mg) daily to a maximum of 4 g daily in divided doses. When used pre-operatively, the optimum dosage should be given for at least five to seven days before surgery.

The optimum dosage range is usually between 8 and 12 capsules (2 to 3 g) a day, titrated by monitoring clinical symptoms and catecholamine excretion. In patients who are hypertensive, dosage should be adjusted to lower blood pressure and control symptoms; in patients whose blood pressure is normal, adjust dosage until the urinary excretion of catecholamines and/or vanillylmandelic acid is reduced by 50% or more.

It is recommended that an alpha-adrenergic blocking agent such as phenoxybenzamine be added if control with Demser is not adequate.

The use of Demser in children under twelve years of age has been limited, and a dosage recommendation cannot be made.

Use in the elderly: These dosage recommendations apply to all adults, including the elderly.

Contra-indications, warnings, etc
Contra-indications: Hypersensitivity.

Warnings: When Demser is used pre-operatively, especially in combination with alpha-adrenoceptor blocking agents, blood volume must be maintained during and after surgery to avoid hypotension and decreased perfusion of vital organs. During surgery, life-threatening arrhythmias may occur requiring treatment with a beta-blocker or lignocaine. Blood pressure and ECG should be monitored continuously throughout surgery.

Demser does not eliminate the danger of arrhythmias or hypertensive crises occurring during manipulation of the tumour and additional alpha-blockade may be necessary.

Precautions: Crystalluria and urolithiasis have occurred in dogs; and crystalluria has been seen in a few patients. To minimise the risk, fluid intake should be sufficient to maintain a urine volume of 2,000 ml or more daily. Urine should be examined routinely, and if metirosine crystals (needles or rods) are seen, fluid intake should be increased. If crystalluria persists, the dosage of Demser should be reduced or discontinued.

Caution should be observed in administering Demser to patients receiving phenothiazines or haloperidol because the extrapyramidal effects of these drugs can be expected to be potentiated by inhibition of catecholamine synthesis; this has been documented to date only for haloperidol.

No evidence of adverse effects on hepatic, haematological or other functions (except for a few instances of increased AST) has been seen during clinical trials. However, total experience in man is limited to approximately 300 patients, and few patients have been studied long-term. Therefore, suitable laboratory tests should be carried out periodically in patients on prolonged therapy, particularly those with impaired hepatic or renal function.

Demser may cause spurious increases in urinary catecholamine measurements.

Breast-feeding mothers: It is not known whether Demser is excreted in human milk. Mothers who need Demser should stop breast-feeding.

Pregnancy: Demser is not recommended for use in pregnant patients. Complete reproduction studies have not been performed in animals to determine whether Demser affects fertility in males or females, has teratogenic potential, or has other adverse effects on the fetus. There are no well-controlled studies of Demser in pregnant women. The use of Demser in pregnant women should be avoided, if possible, but may be appropriate when anticipated benefits outweigh the potential risks.

Adverse reactions: The most common adverse reaction to Demser is moderate to severe sedation, which has been observed in almost all patients. It occurs at both low and high dosages. Sedative effects begin within the first 24 hours of therapy, are maximal after two to three days, and tend to wane during the next few days. Sedation usually is not obvious after one week unless the dosage is increased, but at dosages greater than 2,000 mg/day some degree of sedation or fatigue may persist.

When receiving Demser, patients should be warned about engaging in activities requiring mental alertness and motor co-ordination, such as driving a motor vehicle or operating machinery. Demser may have additive effects with alcohol and other CNS depressants, e.g. hypnotics, sedatives, tranquillisers, anti-anxiety agents.

In most patients who experience sedation, temporary changes in sleep pattern occur following withdrawal of the drug. Changes consist of insomnia that may last for two or three days and feelings of increased alertness and ambition. Even patients who do not experience sedation while on Demser may report symptoms of psychic stimulation when the drug is discontinued.

Extrapyramidal signs such as drooling, speech difficulty and tremor have been reported in approximately 10% of patients, occasionally with trismus and frank parkinsonism.

Anxiety, depression, hallucinations, disorientation and confusion have occurred but may disappear on reduction of the dosage.

Diarrhoea occurs in about 10% of patients, and may be severe. Infrequently, slight swelling of the breast, galactorrhoea, nasal stuffiness, decreased salivation, dry mouth, headache, nausea, vomiting, abdominal pain, and impotence or failure of ejaculation may occur. Crystalluria transient dysuria and haematuria have been seen in a few patients. Eosinophilia, increased AST levels, peripheral oedema, and hypersensitivity such as urticaria and pharyngeal oedema has been reported rarely.

Overdosage: Signs of metirosine overdosage include the CNS effects seen at therapeutic dosages such as fatigue, anxiety or agitated depression, neuromuscular effects, diarrhoea, and decreased salivation. At therapeutic levels, reduction of dose or cessation of treatment usually results in the disappearance of these symptoms.

Since there is little clinical experience, the treatment of overdosage has not been identified. There is no antidote.

Metirosine is well-absorbed from the gastro-intestinal tract. Maximal biochemical effect is usually seen within two or three days.

Pharmaceutical precautions Store in a cool place, protected from light.

Legal category POM.

Package quantities Bottles of 100.

Further information Nil.

Product licence number 0025/0132.

EDECRIN*

Presentation White, half-scored tablets, marked 'MSD 90', containing 50 mg Ethacrynic Acid BP.

Injection, vials containing sodium ethacrynate equivalent to 50 mg ethacrynic acid, as a dry, lyophilised powder.

Uses Diuretic. Edecrin is indicated when urgent and potent diuresis is essential. It is particularly recommended in oedema associated with: Congestive heart failure; pulmonary oedema; renal oedema; hepatic cirrhosis with ascites; ascites due to malignancy; oedema due to other causes, including idiopathic oedema and lymphoedema.

In children over 2 years old: Edecrin Tablets are indicated for the treatment of oedema due to the nephrotic syndrome or to congenital heart disease. (Edecrin Injection is not recommended for children.)

Dosage and administration Dosage should be carefully regulated to prevent a more rapid or substantial diuresis than necessary. Daily weighing of the patient and, where possible, serum electrolyte determinations will greatly contribute to the success of treatment.

Oral therapy: Usual initial adult dosage: 50 mg (1 tablet) a day given immediately after breakfast.

Adjustment: Increase, as necessary, by amounts of 25–50 mg ($\frac{1}{2}$–1 tablet) a day, to the lowest dosage which will produce a gradual weight loss (about $\frac{1}{2}$–1 kg a day).

Effective dosage range: Usually 50–150 mg (1–3 tablets) a day. Patients with severe refractory oedema may need a higher dosage. This should be achieved gradually, and in no case should exceed 400 mg (8 tablets) a day. When the total daily requirement is higher than 50 mg, it should be divided into 2 doses after meals.

Maintenance dosage: Treatment may be maintained by continuous or intermittent therapy. Intermittent therapy can usually be used without loss of therapeutic response. Edecrin may be administered on alternate days, or preferably for two- to three-day periods alternating with two or three days' rest.

Children: Initially 25 mg ($\frac{1}{2}$ tablet) taken immediately after breakfast. If necessary, this should be carefully increased by 25 mg ($\frac{1}{2}$ tablet) a day until an effective dosage is achieved. Do not use in children under two years of age.

Parenteral therapy: Edecrin Injection is intended for intravenous injection when oral treatment is impractical or when urgent diuresis is essential, as in acute pulmonary oedema.

Usual adult intravenous dose: 0.5–1 mg/kg of bodyweight. The dosage for an average-sized adult is 50 mg. Usually only one dose is necessary; however, if a second dose is required, it should be given at a new injection site to avoid thrombophlebitis.

Single intravenous doses of up to 100 mg have been used in critical situations.

The solution may be given slowly through the tubing of a running infusion, or by direct intravenous injection over several minutes.

Edecrin Injection should not be mixed with whole blood or blood derivatives. If it is desired to administer it at the same time as a blood transfusion, it should be given independently.

Children: As paediatric experience with Edecrin Injection is limited, it is not recommended for children.

Use in the elderly: The general considerations on adjustment of dosage to meet individual needs apply equally to elderly patients (see 'Precautions').

Contra-indications, warnings, etc

Contra-indications: Anuria, infants (under 2 years). For 'Use in pregnancy' and 'Use in breast-feeding mothers', see 'Precautions'. Hypersensitivity to this product.

Precautions: The effects of Edecrin on electrolytes are based on its renal pharmacology and are usually dose related.

To minimise the possibility of profound electrolyte and water loss, therapy should be initiated with a low dosage and this carefully adjusted as necessary; intermittent dosage should be used where possible and the patient weighed regularly throughout treatment. If diuresis is excessive, Edecrin should be withdrawn until homeostasis is restored.

Frequent serum electrolyte, alkali reserve and blood urea determinations should be made early in therapy, and periodically thereafter while active diuresis is taking place. Any electrolyte abnormality should be corrected or the drug temporarily withdrawn. If increasing electrolyte imbalance, azotaemia and/or oliguria occur during treatment of severe progressive renal disease, the diuretic should be discontinued.

Inclusion of potassium supplements or potassium-sparing agents is often advisable, especially during the treatment of cirrhotic or nephrotic patients and patients receiving digitalis.

Although treatment with Edecrin generally allows patients greater freedom with their salt intake, cirrhotic patients should usually have their salt moderately restricted while on therapy.

Edecrin should be given with caution to patients with advanced cirrhosis of the liver, particularly those with a history of episodes of electrolyte imbalance or hepatic encephalopathy. Edecrin may precipitate hepatic coma and death.

When metabolic alkalosis may be anticipated (e.g. in cirrhosis with ascites), a potassium-conserving agent or potassium chloride may mitigate or prevent hypokalaemia.

Loop diuretics may cause hypomagnesaemia.

Too vigorous a diuresis may induce an acute hypotensive episode. In elderly cardiac patients, severe diuresis may cause a rapid contraction of plasma volume, which should be avoided to prevent possible thrombo-embolic episodes.

Weakness, muscle cramps, paraesthesiae, thirst, anorexia, and signs of hyponatraemia, hypokalaemia and/or hypochloraemic alkalosis may follow vigorous or excessive diuresis or be accentuated by rigid salt restriction. Rarely, tetany has been reported following vigorous diuresis. Adequate salt intake and potassium chloride supplements are often necessary.

A few patients have had a sudden onset of profuse watery diarrhoea. If this occurs and other causes are eliminated, Edecrin should be discontinued and not re-administered.

Edecrin should be used cautiously in critically ill patients, particularly (1) those patients with severe myocardial disease who have been receiving digitalis; they may develop acute hypokalaemia with fatal arrhythmias. (2) Patients with severely decompensated hepatic cirrhosis with ascites (with or without accompanying encephalopathy) who are in electrolyte imbalance may undergo further deterioration of the electrolyte defect. A number of possible drug-related deaths have occurred among such patients.

Edecrin has little or no effect on glomerular filtration rate or renal blood flow, except immediately after a pronounced reduction in plasma volume following rapid diuresis. An increase in blood urea may occur, although transient it may usually be readily reversed by discontinuing Edecrin.

Edecrin may potentiate the effect of carbonic anhydrase inhibitors, increasing sodium and potassium excretion. If Edecrin is given to patients already receiving a carbonic anhydrase inhibitor, the initial dose and increments should be only 25 mg ($\frac{1}{2}$ tablet).

Drug interactions

Antihypertensive agents may require adjustment of dosage with concurrent use. Orthostatic hypotension may occur in patients on antihypertensive agents when given Edecrin.

Antibiotics: The concurrent use of such drugs as aminoglycosides with Edecrin should be avoided because of the risk of increasing their ototoxic potential.

Warfarin: Several drugs, including Edecrin, have been shown to displace warfarin from plasma protein. In patients receiving both types of drug, a reduction in the dosage of the anticoagulant may therefore be required.

Lithium: Lithium should generally not be given to patients receiving diuretics, since the risk of lithium toxicity is very high in such patients.

Corticosteroids: Edecrin may increase the risk of gastric haemorrhage associated with corticosteroid treatment.

Use in pregnancy: As clinical experience is limited, Edecrin is not recommended in pregnant patients. The routine use of diuretics in otherwise healthy pregnant women with or without mild oedema is not indicated because they may be associated with hypovolaemia, increased blood viscosity and decreased placental perfusion. If administration in confirmed or suspected pregnancy is considered, the benefits of therapy should be weighed against the possible hazard to the fetus.

Use in breast-feeding mothers: Edecrin is contra-indicated in breast-feeding mothers. If its use is deemed essential, the patient should stop breast-feeding.

Side-effects
Gastro-intestinal: Anorexia, malaise, abdominal discomfort or pain, dysphagia, nausea, vomiting and diarrhoea. A few patients have had profuse, watery diarrhoea, gastro-intestinal bleeding, and acute pancreatitis.

Metabolic: Reversible hyperuricaemia, decreased urinary urate excretion and hyperglycaemia may occur. Acute gout may be precipitated. Rarely, acute symptomatic hypoglycaemia with convulsions, jaundice and abnormal liver-function tests have been reported.

Haematological: Agranulocytosis, severe neutropenia, thrombocytopenia and Henoch-Schönlein purpura have been reported rarely.

Special senses: Deafness, tinnitus and vertigo with a sense of fullness in the ears, and blurred vision have occurred.

Central nervous system: Fatigue, apprehension and confusion.

Other: Skin rash, headache, fever, rigors, and haematuria. Edecrin Injection has occasionally caused local irritation and pain due to extravasation of injected fluid.

Overdosage: Ethacrynic acid, especially as a dust, is irritant to the eyes, mucous membranes and skin. Treatment should be symptomatic and supportive; no specific antidote is available. Dehydration, electrolyte imbalance, hepatic coma and hypotension should be corrected by standard methods. If respiration is impaired, oxygen or artificial respiration should be given.

The drug is fairly rapidly absorbed after ingestion with a plasma half-life of 30 minutes to one hour. Ethacrynic acid is bound to plasma proteins: haemodialysis is unlikely to be effective.

Pharmaceutical precautions Keep tablet container well closed. Store tablets and injection in a cool place, protected from light. Injection: to reconstitute the lyophilised material, add 50 ml of 5% dextrose injection or of isotonic saline to the vial. (Some 5% dextrose injection solutions have a pH below 5. If such a preparation is used as diluent, the resulting solution may be cloudy. The use of such a solution is not recommended.) Any unused reconstituted solution should be discarded after 24 hours.

Legal category POM.

Package quantities
Tablets: Bottles of 100.
Injection: Vials containing sodium ethacrynate equivalent to 50 mg ethacrynic acid.

Further information Nil.

Product licence numbers

Tablets	0025/5006
Injection	0025/5007

HYDROCORTONE* TABLETS

Presentation White, quarter-scored tablets, marked 'MSD 619', containing 10 mg hydrocortisone. White, half-scored tablets, marked 'MSD 625', containing 20 mg hydrocortisone.

Uses Corticosteroid.

For use as replacement therapy in primary, secondary, or acute adrenocortical insufficiency.

Pre-operatively, and during serious trauma or illness in patients with known adrenal insufficiency or doubtful adrenocortical reserve.

Dosage and administration Dosage must be individualised according to the response of the individual patient. The lowest possible dosage should be used.

Patients should be observed closely for signs that might require dosage adjustment, including changes in clinical status resulting from remissions or exacerbations of the disease, individual drug responsiveness, and the effect of stress (e.g. surgery, infection, trauma). During stress it may be necessary to increase the dosage temporarily.

If the drug is to be stopped after more than a few days of treatment, it should be withdrawn gradually.

In chronic adrenocortical insufficiency, a dosage of 10–20 mg a day or occasionally more is recommended, together with 4–6 g of sodium chloride or 1–3 mg of desoxycorticosterone acetate. When immediate support is mandatory, one of the soluble adrenocortical hormone preparations (e.g. Decadron* Injection, dexamethasone sodium phosphate, MSD), which may be effective within minutes after parenteral administration, can be life-saving.

Use in children: In chronic adrenocortical insufficiency, the dosage should be approximately 0.4 to 0.8 mg/kg/day in two or three divided doses, adjusted to the needs of the individual child.

Use in the elderly: Treatment of elderly patients, particularly if long term, should be planned bearing in mind the more serious consequences of the common side effects of corticosteroids in old age, especially osteoporosis, diabetes, hypertension, susceptibility to infection and thinning of the skin.

Contra-indications, warnings, etc
Contra-indications: Systemic fungal infections. Hypersensitivity to the drug.

Precautions: The lowest possible dosage of corticosteroid should be used and when reduction in dosage is possible, the reduction should be gradual.

Average and large dosages of hydrocortisone or cortisone can cause elevation of blood pressure, salt and water retention, and increase excretion of potassium. These effects are less likely to occur with the synthetic derivatives except when used in large doses. Dietary salt restriction and potassium supplementation may be necessary. All corticosteroids increase calcium excretion.

Corticosteroids may exacerbate systemic fungal infections and should not be used unless they are needed to control drug reactions due to amphotericin.

Cases have been reported in which concomitant use of amphotericin and hydrocortisone was followed by cardiac enlargement and congestive heart failure.

A report shows that the use of corticosteroids in cerebral malaise is associated with a prolonged coma and an increased incidence of pneumonia and gastro-intestinal bleeding.

In patients on corticosteroid therapy subjected to unusual stress, increased dosage of rapidly acting corticosteroids before, during and after the stressful situation is indicated.

Drug-induced secondary adrenocortical insufficiency may result from too rapid a withdrawal of corticosteroids and may be minimised by gradual reduction of dosage. This type of relative insufficiency may persist for months after discontinuation of therapy; therefore, in any situation of stress occurring during that period, corticosteroid therapy should be reinstated. If the patient is receiving steroids already, the dosage may have to be increased. Since mineralocorticoid secretion may be impaired, salt and/or a mineralocorticoid should be administered concurrently.

Stopping corticosteroids after prolonged therapy may cause withdrawal symptoms including fever, myalgia, arthralgia, and malaise. This may occur in patients even without evidence of adrenal insufficiency.

Aspirin should be used cautiously in conjunction with corticosteroids in hypoprothrombinaemia.

If corticosteroids are indicated in patients with latent tuberculosis or tuberculin reactivity, close observation is necessary as reactivation may occur. During prolonged corticosteroid therapy, these patients should receive prophylactic chemotherapy.

The use of Hydrocortone Tablets in active tuberculosis should be restricted to those cases of fulminating or disseminated tuberculosis.

Corticosteroids should be used with caution in renal insufficiency, hypertension, diabetes or in those with a family history of diabetes, congestive heart failure, osteoporosis, previous steroid myopathy, glaucoma (or previous history), myasthenia gravis, non-specific ulcerative colitis, diverticulitis, fresh intestinal anastomoses, active or latent peptic ulcer. Signs of peritoneal irritation following gastro-intestinal perforation in patients receiving large doses of corticosteroids may be minimal or absent. Fat embolism has been reported as a possible complication of hypercortisonism.

Corticosteroids should be used cautiously in patients with ocular herpes simplex because of possible corneal perforation.

There is an enhanced effect of corticosteroids in patients with hypothyroidism and in those with cirrhosis.

Corticosteroids may mask some signs of infection, and new infections may appear during their use. There may be decreased resistance and inability to localise infection in patients on corticosteroids.

Corticosteroids may activate latent amoebiasis. Therefore, it is recommended that latent or active amoebiasis be excluded before initiating corticosteroid therapy in any patient who has either spent time in the tropics, or has unexplained diarrhoea.

Alterations in the patient's mental state may appear when corticosteroids are used, ranging from psychological dependence, euphoria, insomnia, mood swings, personality changes and severe depression, to frank psychotic manifestations.

Prolonged use of corticosteroids may produce posterior subcapsular cataracts, glaucoma with possible damage to the optic nerves, and may enhance the establishment of secondary ocular infections.

Corticosteroids may increase or decrease motility and number of spermatozoa.

Phenytoin, ephedrine, barbiturates and rifampicin may enhance the metabolic clearance of corticosteroids, resulting in decreased blood levels and lessened physiological activity, thus requiring adjustment in corticosteroid dosage.

The prothrombin time should be checked frequently in patients who are receiving corticosteroids and coumarin anticoagulants at the same time.

When corticosteroids are administered concomitantly with potassium-depleting diuretics, patients should be observed closely for development of hypokalaemia.

Children: Corticosteroids cause growth retardation in infancy, childhood and adolescence. Treatment should be limited to the minimum dosage in order to minimise suppression of the hypothalamo-pituitary-adrenal axis and growth retardation.

Growth and development of infants and children on prolonged corticosteroid therapy should be carefully monitored.

Use in pregnancy and the nursing mother: There is inadequate evidence of safety in human pregnancy and there may be a very small risk of cleft palate and intrauterine growth retardation in the fetus; there is evidence of harmful effects on pregnancy in animals.

Corticosteroids appear in breast milk and could suppress growth, interfere with endogenous corticosteroid production, or cause other unwanted effects. Mothers taking pharmacological doses of corticosteroids should be advised not to nurse.

Side-effects: Fluid and electrolyte disturbances: Sodium retention, fluid retention, congestive heart failure in susceptible patients, potassium loss, hypokalaemic alkalosis, hypertension, increased calcium excretion.

Musculoskeletal effects: Muscle weakness, steroid myopathy, loss of muscle mass, osteoporosis (especially in post-menopausal females), vertebral compression fractures, aseptic necrosis of femoral and humeral heads, pathological fracture of long bones, tendon rupture.

Gastro-intestinal: Peptic ulcer with possible perforation and haemorrhage, perforation of the small and large bowel particularly in patients with inflammatory bowel disease, pancreatitis, abdominal distension, ulcerative oesophagitis, dyspepsia, oesophageal candidiasis.

Dermatological: Impaired wound healing, thin fragile skin, petechiae, and ecchymoses, erythema, striae, telangiectasia, acne, increased sweating, may suppress reactions to skin tests, other cutaneous reactions such as allergic dermatitis, urticaria, angioneurotic oedema.

Neurological: Convulsions, increased intracranial pressure with papilloedema (pseudotumour cerebri) usually after treatment, vertigo, headache.

Endocrine: Menstrual irregularities, amenorrhoea, development of Cushingoid state, suppression of growth in children, secondary adrenocortical and pituitary unresponsiveness (particularly in times of stress, as in trauma, surgery, or illness), decreased carbohydrate tolerance, manifestations of latent diabetes mellitus, increased requirements for insulin or oral hypoglycaemic agents in diabetics, hirsutism.

Ophthalmic: Posterior subcapsular cataracts, increased intra-ocular pressure, papilloedema, corneal or scleral thinning, exacerbation of ophthalmic viral disease, glaucoma, exophthalmos.

Metabolic: Negative nitrogen balance due to protein catabolism.

Other: Hypersensitivity, leucocytosis, thrombo-embolism, weight gain, increased appetite, nausea, malaise.

Teratogenicity: See pregnancy warning under 'Use in pregnancy and the nursing mother'.

Overdosage: Reports of acute toxicity and/or deaths following overdosage with glucocorticoids are rare. No antidote is available. Treatment is probably not indicated for reactions due to chronic poisoning unless the patient has a condition that would render him unusually susceptible to ill effects from corticosteroids. In this case, symptomatic treatment should be instituted as necessary.

Anaphylactic and hypersensitivity reactions may be treated with adrenaline, positive-pressure artificial respiration and aminophylline. The patient should be kept warm and quiet.

The biological half-life of hydrocortisone is about 100 minutes.

Pharmaceutical precautions Keep container well closed, store in a cool place, protected from light.

Legal category POM.

Package quantities *10 mg:* Bottles of 100. *20 mg:* Bottles of 100.

Further information Nil.

Product licence numbers
10 mg 0025/5053
20 mg 0025/5054

HYDROMET*

Presentation Salmon-pink, film-coated tablets, marked 'MSD 423', containing Methyldopa BP, equivalent to 250 mg anhydrous methyldopa, and 15 mg Hydrochlorothiazide BP.

Uses Antihypertensive.

A highly effective combination of methyldopa and hydrochlorothiazide, two antihypertensive agents with complementary properties for the treatment of hypertension.

Mode of action: The antihypertensive effect of methyldopa is probably due to its metabolism to alpha-methylnoradrenaline, which lowers arterial pressure by stimulation of central inhibitory alpha-adrenergic receptors, false neurotransmission, and/or reduction of plasma renin activity.

It is not known how hydrochlorothiazide controls hypertension. While it does not usually affect normal blood pressure, it is particularly effective when used in conjunction with other antihypertensive agents.

Dosage and administration *Initial dosage:* Usually 1 tablet twice a day for two days.

Adjustment: Upwards or downwards. Preferably at intervals of at least two days, until an adequate response is obtained.

The maximum recommended daily dosage of the components is 3 g of methyldopa and 100 mg hydrochlorothiazide.

Many patients experience sedation for two or three days when therapy with Hydromet is started or when the dose is increased. When increasing the dosage, therefore, it may be desirable to increase the evening dose first.

General considerations: Methyldopa is largely excreted by the kidney and patients with impaired kidney function may respond to smaller doses of Hydromet.

Withdrawal of Hydromet is followed by return of hypertension usually within 48 hours. This is not complicated by an overshoot of blood pressure.

Therapy with Hydromet may be initiated in most patients already on treatment with other antihypertensive agents by terminating these antihypertensive medications, gradually if required (see manufacturer's recommendations on stopping these drugs). Following such previous antihypertensive therapy, Hydromet should be limited to an initial dose of 1 tablet daily and increased as required at intervals of not less than two days.

When Hydromet is given to patients on other antihypertensives, the dose of these agents may need to be adjusted to effect a smooth transition.

Paediatric use of Hydromet is not usually recommended.

Use in the elderly: The initial dose should not exceed 1 tablet daily. Particular caution is needed in the elderly because of their susceptibility to electrolyte imbalance: the dosage may be increased slowly as required by the initial response.

Contra-indications, warnings, etc

Contra-indications: Severe liver disease (such as acute hepatitis and active cirrhosis); severe renal failure; anuria; Addison's disease; hypercalcaemia; concurrent lithium therapy, and depression. Known sensitivity to methyldopa, hydrochlorothiazide or sulphonamides, including hepatic disorders associated with previous methyldopa therapy. Hydromet is not recommended for the treatment of phaeochromocytoma (see 'Precautions'). See also 'Precautions' for 'Use in pregnancy' and 'Use in the breast-feeding mother'.

Precautions: The precautions relating to the use of Hydromet are generally those of its components.

Methyldopa: Acquired haemolytic anaemia has occurred rarely. Should symptoms suggest anaemia, haemoglobin and/or haematocrit determinations should be made. If anaemia is confirmed, tests should be done for haemolysis. If haemolytic anaemia is present, Hydromet should be discontinued. Stopping therapy, with or without corticosteroids, has usually brought prompt remission. Rarely, however, deaths have occurred.

Some patients on continued therapy with methyldopa develop a positive direct Coombs test. From the reports of different investigators, the incidence averages between 10% and 20%. A positive Coombs reaction rarely develops in the first six months of therapy, and if it has not developed within 12 months, it is unlikely to do so later on continuing therapy. Development is also dose-related, the lowest incidence occurring in patients receiving 1 g or less of methyldopa per day. The test becomes negative usually within weeks to months after methyldopa is discontinued.

Prior knowledge of a positive Coombs reaction will aid in evaluation of cross-matching for transfusions. If a patient with a positive Coombs reaction shows an incompatible minor cross-match, an indirect Coombs test should be performed. If this is negative, transfusion with blood otherwise compatible in the major cross-match may be carried out. If positive, the advisability of transfusion should be determined by a haematologist.

Reversible leucopenia, with primary effect on granulocytes, has been reported rarely. The granulocyte count returned promptly to normal on discontinuing therapy. Reversible thrombocytopenia has occurred rarely.

Occasionally, fever has occurred within the first three weeks of therapy, sometimes associated with eosinophilia or abnormalities in liver function tests. Jaundice, with or without fever, also may occur. Its onset is usually within the first two or three months of therapy. In some patients the findings are consistent with those of cholestasis. Rare cases of fatal hepatic necrosis have been reported. Liver biopsy performed in several patients with liver dysfunction showed a microscopic focal necrosis compatible with drug hypersensitivity.

Liver function tests, and a total and differential white blood cell count, are advisable at intervals during the first six to twelve weeks of therapy, or whenever an unexplained fever occurs. Should fever, abnormality in liver function, or jaundice occur, therapy should be withdrawn. If related to methyldopa, the temperature and abnormalities in liver function have characteristically reverted to normal when methyldopa has been discontinued. Methyldopa should not be reinstated in these patients. Methyldopa should be used with caution in patients with a history of previous liver disease or dysfunction.

When methyldopa is used with other antihypertensive drugs, potentiation of antihypertensive action may occur. The progress of patients should be carefully followed to detect side reactions or unusual manifestations of drug idiosyncrasy.

Patients may require reduced doses of anaesthetics when on methyldopa. If hypotension does occur during anaesthesia, it can usually be controlled by vasopressors. The adrenergic receptors remain sensitive during treatment with methyldopa.

Dialysis removes methyldopa; therefore, hypertension may recur after this procedure.

Rarely, involuntary choreoathetotic movements have been observed during therapy with methyldopa in patients with severe bilateral cerebrovascular disease. Should these movements occur, therapy should be discontinued.

Hydromet should be used with extreme caution in patients, or in near relatives of patients, with hepatic porphyria.

Interference with laboratory tests: Methyldopa may interfere with the measurement of urinary uric acid by the phosphotungstate method, serum creatinine by the alkaline picrate method, and AST (SGOT) by colorimetric method. Interference with spectrophotometric methods for AST analysis has not been reported.

As methyldopa fluoresces at the same wavelengths as catecholamines, spuriously high amounts of urinary catecholamines may be reported, giving rise to a false-positive diagnosis of phaeochromocytoma.

It is important to recognise this phenomenon before a patient with a possible phaeochromocytoma is subjected to surgery. Methyldopa does not interfere with measurement of VMA (vanillylmandelic acid) by those methods which convert VMA to vanillin.

Rarely, when urine is exposed to air after voiding, it may darken because of breakdown of methyldopa or its metabolites.

Hydrochlorothiazide:

Electrolyte imbalance: Patients should be carefully monitored for signs of fluid and electrolyte imbalance (hyponatraemia, hypomagnesaemia, hypochloraemic alkalosis and hypokalaemia). It is particularly important to make serum and urine electrolyte determinations if the patient is vomiting excessively or receiving parenteral fluids. Warning signs are dryness of the mouth, thirst, weakness, lethargy, drowsiness, restlessness, muscle pains or cramps, muscular fatigue, hypotension, oliguria, tachycardia and gastro-intestinal disturbance such as nausea and vomiting.

Hypokalaemia may develop, especially with brisk diuresis, after prolonged therapy or when severe cirrhosis is present. Hypokalaemia can sensitise or exaggerate the response of the heart to the toxic effects of digitalis (e.g. increased ventricular irritability).

Diuretic-induced hyponatraemia is usually mild and asymptomatic. However, hyponatraemia may become severe and symptomatic in a few patients who will require immediate attention and appropriate treatment.

Thiazides may decrease urinary calcium excretion with intermittent and slight elevation of serum calcium in the absence of known disorders of calcium metabolism. Thiazides should be discontinued before testing for parathyroid function.

Impaired renal function and/or azotaemia: When creatinine clearance falls below 30 ml/min, thiazides become ineffective.

Azotaemia may be precipitated or increased by hydrochlorothiazide. Cumulative effects of hydrochlorothiazide may develop in patients with impaired renal function. Renal function should be monitored. If increasing azotaemia and oliguria occur during treatment of severe progressive renal disease, Hydromet should be discontinued.

Hepatic disease: Thiazides should be used with caution in patients with impaired hepatic function or progressive liver disease, since minor alterations of fluid and electrolyte balance or of serum ammonia may precipitate hepatic coma.

Metabolic: Hyperuricaemia may occur, or gout may be precipitated or aggravated in certain patients receiving thiazide therapy.

Thiazide therapy may impair glucose tolerance. Dosage adjustment of antidiabetic agents, including insulin, may be required.

Other: The possibility of exacerbation or activation of systemic lupus erythematosus has been reported.

The occurrence of pancreatitis as an adverse reaction to thiazide therapy suggests a cautious use of 'Hydromet' in patients with hyperlipidaemia. Diabetes mellitus which has been latent may become manifest during thiazide administration.

Drug interactions:

Alcohol, barbiturates or narcotics: Co-administration may potentiate orthostatic hypotension.

Sympathomimetics, tricyclic antidepressants, phenothiazines, and MAOIs reduce the antihypertensive effect of 'Hydromet'. *Oral and parenteral antidiabetic drugs* may require adjustment of dosage with concurrent use. *Other antihypertensive drugs* may be potentiated by 'Hydromet'. Discontinuation of diuretic therapy 2–3 days before the initiation of treatment with an ACE-inhibitor may reduce the likelihood of first-dose hypotension. The antihypertensive effect of the drug may be enhanced in the post-sympathectomy patient. *Corticosteroids or ACTH* may intensify any thiazide-induced electrolyte depletion, particularly hypokalaemia. *Pressor amines such as adrenaline* may show decreased arterial responsiveness when used with 'Hydromet', but this reaction is not enough to preclude their therapeutic usefulness. *Non-polarising muscle relaxants such as tubocurarine* may possibly interact with 'Hydromet' to increase muscle relaxation. *Non-steroidal anti-inflammatory drugs* may attenuate the diuretic and antihypertensive effect of diuretics.

Drug/laboratory tests: Because thiazides may affect calcium metabolism, Hydromet may interfere with tests for parathyroid function.

Use in pregnancy: The routine use of diuretics in otherwise healthy, pregnant women with or without mild oedema is not indicated because their use may be associated with hypovolaemia, increased blood viscosity and decreased placental perfusion. Thiazides do not prevent the development of toxaemia of pregnancy, and there is no satisfactory evidence to support their use in its treatment.

Methyldopa and thiazides cross the placental barrier and appear in the cord blood. The use of 'Hydromet' when pregnancy is present or suspected, requires that the benefits of the drug be weighed against the possible hazards to the fetus. These hazards include neonatal jaundice, thrombocytopenia, hypoglycaemia, electrolyte imbalance and possibly other adverse reactions which have occurred in the adult.

Use in the breast-feeding mother: Thiazides also appear in breast milk. If use of Hydromet is deemed essential, the patient should stop breast-feeding.

Side-effects: The side-effects of Hydromet are generally those of its components; combination of methyldopa and hydrochlorothiazide has not produced any additional side-effects.

Methyldopa: Significant side-effects due to methyldopa have been infrequent and this agent is usually well tolerated.

Sedation, usually transient, may occur initially or when the dosage is increased. If affected, patients should not attempt to drive, or operate machinery. Other early transient effects which may occur are headache, asthenia and weakness.

Central nervous system: Sedation (usually transient) headache, asthenia or weakness, paraesthesiae, parkinsonism, Bell's palsy, involuntary choreoathetotic movements. Psychic disturbances including nightmares, impaired mental activity and reversible mild psychoses or depression. Dizziness, light-headedness, and symptoms of cerebrovascular insufficiency (may be due to lowering of blood pressure).

Cardiovascular: Bradycardia, prolonged carotid sinus hypersensitivity, aggravation of angina pectoris. Orthostatic hypotension (decrease daily dosage). Oedema (and weight gain) usually relieved by use of a diuretic. (Discontinue methyldopa if oedema progresses or signs of heart failure appear.)

Gastro-intestinal: Nausea, vomiting, distension, constipation, flatus, diarrhoea, colitis, mild dryness of the mouth, sore or 'black' tongue, pancreatitis, salivary gland inflammation.

Hepatic: Liver disorders including hepatitis, jaundice, abnormal liver function tests.

Haematological: Positive Coombs test, haemolytic anaemia, bone-marrow depression, leucopenia, granulocytopenia, thrombocytopenia. Positive tests for antinuclear antibody, LE cells, and rheumatoid factor.

Allergic: Drug-related fever, lupus-like syndrome, myocarditis, pericarditis.

Dermatological: Rash as in eczema or lichenoid eruption, toxic epidermal necrolysis.

Other: Nasal stuffiness, rise in blood urea, breast enlargement, gynaecomastia, hyperprolactinaemia, amenorrhoea, lactation, impotence, decreased libido, failure of ejaculation, mild arthralgia with or without joint swelling, myalgia.

Hydrochlorothiazide: Gastro-intestinal system: Anorexia, gastric irritation, nausea, vomiting, cramps, diarrhoea, constipation, jaundice (intrahepatic cholestatic jaundice), pancreatitis, salivary gland inflammation.

Central nervous system: Dizziness, vertigo, paraesthesiae, headache, yellow vision.

Haematological: Leucopenia, agranulocytosis, thrombocytopenia, aplastic anaemia, haemolytic anaemia.

Cardiovascular: Orthostatic hypotension (may be aggravated by alcohol, barbiturates or narcotics).

Hypersensitivity: Purpura, photosensitivity, rash, urticaria, necrotising angiitis (vasculitis, cutaneous vasculitis), fever, respiratory distress including pneumonitis and pulmonary oedema, anaphylactic reactions.

Metabolic: Hyperglycaemia, glycosuria, hyperuricaemia, electrolyte imbalance.

Other: Muscle spasm, weakness, restlessness, transient blurred vision, loss of libido, impotence.

Overdosage: The most common signs and symptoms observed are those caused by electrolyte depletion (hypokalaemia, hypochloraemia, hyponatraemia) and dehydration resulting from excessive diuresis. Dizziness, sedation, weakness, nausea and vomiting due to methyldopa, as well as lethargy and dizziness due to hydrochlorothiazide can be regarded as early symptoms of overdosage. If digitalis has also been administered, hypokalaemia may accentuate cardiac arrhythmias.

In the event of overdosage, symptomatic and supportive measures should be employed with special attention to signs of depressed cerebral activity. If ingestion is recent, emesis should be induced or gastric lavage performed. Dehydration, electrolyte imbalance, hepatic coma and hypotension should be corrected by established procedures. Signs of cardiac depression with AV conduction defects and hypovolaemia may occur. If required, give oxygen or artificial respiration for respiratory impairment.

The plasma half-life of methyldopa is 105 minutes; that of hydrochlorothiazide is 5.6 hours with a subsequent longer terminal phase.

Pharmaceutical precautions Keep container well closed; store in a cool place, protected from light.

Legal category POM.

Package quantities Bottles of 100 and 500.

Further information Hydromet reduces both supine and standing blood pressure. Symptomatic postural hypotension, exercise hypotension and diurnal blood pressure variations rarely occur. By adjustment of dosage, morning hypotension can be prevented without sacrificing control of afternoon blood pressure.

Product licence number 0025/5008.

HYDROSALURIC*

Presentation White, half-scored tablets, marked 'MSD 42', containing 25 mg Hydrochlorothiazide BP.

White, half-scored tablets, marked 'MSD 105', containing 50 mg Hydrochlorothiazide BP.

Uses Thiazide diuretic and antihypertensive.

Oedema associated with congestive heart failure, hepatic cirrhosis, premenstrual tension and oedema due to various forms of renal dysfunction (i.e. the nephrotic syndrome, acute glomerulonephritis, chronic renal failure). Hypertension, either alone or as an adjunct to other antihypertensive drugs.

Dosage and administration Dosage should be determined on an individual basis, and the lowest dosage necessary to achieve the desired result should be used.

Adults – for oedema: Usually 25–100 mg once or twice a day. Many patients respond to intermittent therapy; for example, every other day, or three to five days a week. Intermittent therapy is less likely to produce excessive diuretic response with resulting undesirable electrolyte imbalance. The maximum recommended daily dose is 200 mg.

In oedema accompanying premenstrual tension: 25–50 mg once or twice a day, from the first morning of symptoms until the onset of the menses.

Adults – for control of hypertension: Usual starting dosage, 25 mg or 50 mg a day as a single or divided dose. In some patients, a starting dose of 12.5 mg, alone or with another antihypertensive, may be sufficient. Dosage should be adjusted to response, but should not exceed 100 mg.

Thiazides may add to the action of other antihypertensives. If HydroSaluric is used with other antihypertensive agents, it may be necessary to reduce the dosage of such agents so as to prevent an excessive drop in blood pressure.

Infants and children: Usually 2.5 mg per kg bodyweight a day, given in two doses. Infants under 6 months may need up to 3.5 mg per kg a day, in two doses. Infants up to 2 years of age may be given 12.5–37.5 mg of HydroSaluric a day in two doses. Children from 2 to 12 years of age may be given 37.5–100 mg a day in two doses. Dosage should be based on bodyweight.

Uses in the elderly: Particular caution is needed in the elderly because of their susceptibility to electrolyte imbalance; the dosage should be carefully adjusted according to renal function and clinical response. If lower dosage is required, 25 mg tablets are available.

Contra-indications, warnings, etc

Contra-indications: Anuria, known hypersensitivity to this product or to other sulphonamide-derived drugs, severe renal or hepatic failure, Addison's disease, hypercalcaemia, concurrent lithium therapy. See 'Use in pregnancy' and 'Use in breast-feeding mothers', under 'Precautions'.

Precautions: Patients should be carefully monitored for signs of fluid and electrolyte imbalance (hyponatraemia, hypochloraemic alkalosis, hypokalaemia and hypomagnesaemia). It is particularly important to make serum and urine electrolyte determinations when the patient is vomiting excessively or receiving parenteral fluids. Warning signs or symptoms of fluid and electrolyte imbalance include: dryness of mouth, thirst, weakness, lethargy, drowsiness, restlessness, seizures, muscle pains or cramps, muscle fatigue, hypotension, oliguria, tachycardia, and gastro-intestinal disturbances such as nausea and vomiting.

Hypokalaemia may develop, especially with brisk diuresis, when severe cirrhosis is present, or after prolonged therapy. Hypokalaemia can sensitise or exaggerate the response of the heart to the toxic effects of digitalis (e.g. increased ventricular irritability).

Sensitivity reactions may occur in patients with or without history of allergy or bronchial asthma.

Hypokalaemia may be avoided or treated in the adult by concurrent use of amiloride hydrochloride (Midamor*), a potassium-conserving agent. It may also be avoided by giving potassium chloride or foods with a high potassium content. (Note that symptoms and signs which might indicate ulceration or obstruction of the small bowel in patients taking tablets or capsules containing potassium salts are indications for stopping treatment with such preparations immediately.)

Diuretic-induced hyponatraemia is usually mild and asymptomatic. Dilutional hyponatraemia may occur in oedematous patients in hot weather; and, except in rare instances when hyponatraemia is life-threatening, appropriate therapy is water restriction rather than administration of salt.

Thiazides may decrease serum PBI levels without signs of thyroid disturbances.

Thiazides may decrease urinary calcium excretion, and may also cause intermittent and slight elevation of serum calcium in the absence of known disorders of calcium metabolism. Thiazides should be discontinued before carrying out tests for parathyroid function.

When creatinine clearance falls below 30 ml/min, thiazide diuretics become ineffective.

Azotaemia may be precipitated or increased by chlorothiazide. Cumulative effects of the drug may develop in patients with impaired renal function. If increasing azotaemia and oliguria occur during treatment of renal disease, HydroSaluric should be discontinued.

Thiazides should be used with caution in patients with impaired hepatic function or progressive liver disease, since minor alterations of fluid and electrolyte balance may precipitate hepatic coma.

Hyperuricaemia may occur, or gout may be precipitated, in certain patients receiving thiazide therapy.

Thiazide therapy may impair glucose tolerance.

Increases in cholesterol and triglyceride levels may be associated with thiazide diuretic therapy.

The possibility of exacerbation or activation of systemic lupus erythematosus has been reported.

Latent diabetes may become manifest during thiazide administration.

Use in pregnancy: Thiazides cross the placental barrier and appear in cord blood. The use of HydroSaluric when pregnancy is present or suspected requires, therefore, that the benefits of the drug be weighed against possible hazards to the fetus. These hazards include fetal or neonatal jaundice, thrombocytopenia, and possibly other adverse reactions which have occurred in the adult. The routine use of diuretics in otherwise healthy pregnant women with or without mild oedema is not indicated because their use may be associated with hypovolaemia, increased blood viscosity and decreased placental perfusion.

Use in breast-feeding mothers: Thiazides appear in breast milk. If use of the drug is deemed essential, the patient should stop breast-feeding.

Drug interactions: Alcohol, barbiturates or narcotics: Co-administration may potentiate orthostatic hypotension. *Oral and parenteral antidiabetic drugs* may require adjustment of dosage with concurrent use. *Other antihypertensive drugs* may have an additive effect. Discontinuation of diuretic therapy 2–3 days before the initiation of treatment with an ACE inhibitor may reduce the likelihood of first-dose hypotension. The antihypertensive effect of the drug may be enhanced in the post-sympathectomy patient. *Corticosteroids or ACTH* may intensify any thiazide-induced electrolyte depletion, particularly hypokalaemia. *Pressor amines such as adrenaline* may show decreased arterial responsiveness when used with HydroSaluric, but this reaction is not enough to preclude their therapeutic usefulness. *Non-depolarising muscle relaxants such as tubocurarine* may possibly interact with HydroSaluric to increase muscle relaxation. *Non-steroidal anti-inflammatory drugs* may attenuate the diuretic and antihypertensive effect of diuretics.

Drug/laboratory tests: Because thiazides may affect calcium metabolism, HydroSaluric may interfere with tests for parathyroid function.

Side-effects

Gastro-intestinal system: Anorexia, gastric irritation, nausea, vomiting, cramps, diarrhoea, constipation, jaundice (intrahepatic cholestatic jaundice), pancreatitis, salivary gland inflammation.

Central nervous system: Dizziness, vertigo, paraesthesiae, headache, yellow vision.

Haematological: Leucopenia, agranulocytosis, thrombocytopenia, aplastic anaemia, haemolytic anaemia.

Cardiovascular: Hypotension, including orthostatic hypotension (may be aggravated by alcohol, barbiturates, narcotics or antihypertensive drugs).

Hypersensitivity: Purpura, photosensitivity, rash, urticaria, necrotising angiitis (vasculitis, cutaneous vasculitis), fever, respiratory distress including pneumonitis and pulmonary oedema, anaphylactic reactions.

Metabolic: Hyperglycaemia, glycosuria, hyperuricaemia, electrolyte imbalance.

Renal: Renal dysfunction, interstitial nephritis, renal failure.

Other: Muscle spasm, weakness, restlessness, transient blurred vision, impotence.

Whenever side-effects are moderate to severe, thiazide dosage should be reduced or therapy withdrawn.

Overdosage: The most common signs and symptoms observed are those caused by electrolyte depletion (hypokalaemia, hypochloraemia, hyponatraemia) and dehydration resulting from excessive diuresis. If digitalis has also been administered, hypokalaemia may accentuate cardiac arrhythmias.

In the event of overdosage, treatment should be symptomatic and supportive. No specific antidote is known. If ingestion is recent, the stomach should be emptied by emesis or gastric lavage. Dehydration, electrolyte imbalance, hepatic coma and hypotension should be corrected by standard methods. For impaired respiration, oxygen or artificial respiration should be given.

The plasma half-life of hydrochlorothiazide is 5.6 hours with a subsequent longer terminal phase. The biological half-life is 14.8 hours when the plasma level can be followed for at least 24 hours.

Pharmaceutical precautions Keep container tightly closed; store in a cool place, protected from light.

Legal category POM.

Package quantities 25 mg: Bottles of 500.
50 mg: Bottles of 500.

Further information Diuresis begins within two hours following administration, is at a peak after four hours and persists for six to twelve hours. No rigid dietary salt restriction required.

Product licence numbers
25 mg tablet 0025/5009
50 mg tablet 0025/5010

INNOVACE

Presentation Peach-coloured, triangular tablets, marked 'INNOVACE', containing 20 mg enalapril maleate, MSD.

Red, triangular tablets, marked 'INNOVACE', containing 10 mg enalapril maleate, MSD.

White, half-scored, triangular tablets, marked 'INNOVACE', containing 5 mg enalapril maleate, MSD.

White, round tablets, marked 'INNOVACE', containing 2.5 mg enalapril maleate, MSD.

Uses

Indications:

Hypertension: All grades of essential hypertension and renovascular hypertension.

Congestive heart failure: In congestive heart failure, Innovace should be used as an adjunctive therapy with digitalis and/or diuretics. Treatment with Innovace should always be initiated in hospital under close supervision.

Mode of action: Following oral administration, Innovace is rapidly absorbed and hydrolysed to enalaprilat, a highly specific, long-acting, non-sulphydryl angiotensin-converting enzyme inhibitor.

Innovace modulates a specific physiological mechanism, the renin-angiotensin-aldosterone system, which plays a major role in the regulation of blood pressure. Its onset of action begins smoothly and gradually within one hour and its effects continue usually for 24 hours after a single daily dose. Data indicate no loss of effect during long-term therapy. Rebound hypertension does not occur following abrupt cessation of therapy.

Congestive heart failure patients benefit particularly from reduction in pre-load and after-load of the heart, with an increase in cardiac output, without reflex tachycardia.

Dosage and administration The maximum daily dose is 40 mg.

The absorption of Innovace is not affected by food.

Essential and renovascular hypertension:

Treatment should be initiated with 5 mg once a day. Where concomitant therapy is a diuretic, the recommended initial dose of Innovace is 2.5 mg (see 'With concomitant diuretic therapy' section). The dose should be titrated to give optimum control of blood pressure. The usual maintenance dose is 10–20 mg given once daily. In severe hypertension, the dosage may be increased incrementally to a maximum of 40 mg once daily.

The dosage of other antihypertensive agents being used together with Innovace may need to be adjusted. Where Innovace replaces a beta-blocking drug in the therapeutic regime, the beta-blocking agent should not be discontinued abruptly; the dosage should be titrated down after commencing therapy with Innovace (see manufacturer's recommendations).

With concomitant diuretic therapy: The recommended initial dose of Innovace is 2.5 mg. Symptomatic hypotension can occur following the initial dose of Innovace; this is more likely when Innovace is added to previous diuretic therapy. Caution is recommended, therefore, since these patients may be volume or salt depleted. If possible, the diuretic therapy should be discontinued for 2–3 days prior to initiation of therapy with Innovace.

Innovace minimises the development of thiazide-induced hypokalaemia and hyperuricaemia.

Use in the elderly (*over 65 years*)*:* The starting dose should be 2.5 mg. Innovace is effective in the treatment of hypertension in the elderly. Some elderly patients may be more responsive to Innovace than younger patients.

The dose should be titrated according to need for the control of blood pressure.

Congestive heart failure: Innovace can be used as adjunctive therapy with digitalis and/or diuretics in congestive heart failure. Therapy with Innovace should be initiated under close supervision in hospital, with a recommended starting dose of 2.5 mg. If possible, the dose of diuretic should be reduced before beginning treatment. Blood pressure and renal function should be monitored closely both before and during treatment with Innovace because severe hypotension and, more rarely, consequent renal failure have been reported (see 'Precautions').

In the absence of, or after effective management of, symptomatic hypotension following initiation of therapy with Innovace in congestive heart failure, the dose should be gradually increased, depending on the patient's response, to the usual maintenance dose (10–20 mg) given in a single or divided dose. This dose titration may be performed over a two- to four-week period, or more rapidly if indicated by the presence of residual signs and symptoms of heart failure.

The appearance of hypotension after the initial dose of Innovace does not preclude subsequent careful dose titration with the drug, following effective treatment of the hypotension.

Use in impaired renal function: (See 'Precautions') Innovace is excreted by the kidney. It should be used with caution in patients with renal impairment. The recommended starting dose is 2.5 mg. The dose should be titrated against the response, and should be kept as low as possible to maintain adequate control of blood pressure or heart failure.

Innovace is dialysable. Dialysis patients may be given the usual dose of Innovace on dialysis days. On the days when patients are not on dialysis the dosage should be tailored to the blood pressure response.

Children: The paediatric use of Innovace has not been studied.

Contra-indications, warnings, etc

Contra-indications

Pregnancy: Innovace has been shown to be fetotoxic in rabbits during middle and late pregnancy.

Effects of exposure of the fetus to ACE inhibitors during the first trimester of human pregnancy are unknown. Fetal exposure during the second and third trimesters of pregnancy has been associated with fetal and neonatal morbidity and mortality.

ACE inhibitors in human pregnancy have been associated with oligohydramnios. Hypotension and renal failure have occurred in the newborn.

Because of these findings Innovace is contra-indicated in pregnancy.

Hypersensitivity to the product or any of its components, and in patients with a history of angioneurotic oedema relating to previous treatment with an ACE inhibitor.

Precautions

Pretreatment assessment of renal function: Evaluation of the patient should include assessment of renal function prior to initiation of therapy, and during treatment where appropriate.

Symptomatic hypotension was seen rarely in uncomplicated hypertensive patients. It has been reported mainly in patients with severe heart failure. It is more likely to occur in patients who have been volume-depleted by diuretic therapy, dietary salt restriction, dialysis, diarrhoea or vomiting.

In these patients, by discontinuing diuretic therapy or significantly reducing the diuretic dose for two to three days prior to initiating Innovace, the possibility of this occurrence is reduced. By initiating therapy with a small dose (2.5 mg Innovace) the duration of any hypotensive effect may be lessened.

Similar considerations in terms of initiating therapy with a small dose may apply also to patients with ischaemic heart or cerebrovascular disease in whom severe hypotension could result in a myocardial infarct or cerebrovascular accident.

Severe hypotension has been reported, mainly in patients with severe heart failure with or without associated renal insufficiency. This is most likely in those patients on high doses of loop diuretics, or with hyponatraemia or functional renal impairment.

If hypotension develops, the patient should be placed in a supine position. Volume repletion with oral fluids or intravenous normal saline may be required. Intravenous atropine may be necessary if there is associated bradycardia. A transient hypotensive response is not a contra-indication to further doses, which can usually be given without difficulty once the blood pressure has increased after volume expansion.

In some patients with congestive heart failure who have normal or low blood pressure, additional lowering of systemic blood pressure may occur with Innovace. If such hypotension becomes symptomatic, a reduction of dose or discontinuation of Innovace may become necessary.

The appearance of hypotension after the initial dose of Innovace does not preclude subsequent careful dose titration with the drug after effective management of the hypotension.

Impaired renal function: Innovace should be used with caution in patients with renal insufficiency as they may require reduced or less frequent doses (see 'Dosage'). Close monitoring of renal function before and during therapy should be performed as deemed appropriate in those with renal insufficiency. In the majority, renal function will not alter, or may improve.

Renal failure has been reported in association with Innovace and has been mainly in patients with severe congestive heart failure or underlying renal disease, including renal artery stenosis. If recognised promptly and treated appropriately, renal failure when associated with therapy with Innovace is usually reversible.

Some hypertensive patients, with no apparent pre-existing renal disease have developed increases in blood urea and creatinine when Innovace has been given concurrently with a diuretic. Dosage reduction of Innovace and/or discontinuation of the diuretic may be required. This situation should raise the possibility of underlying renal artery stenosis (see 'Renovascular hypertension').

As with all antihypertensive agents, renal function should be assessed in patients with hypertension or congestive heart failure before initiating therapy.

Renovascular hypertension: Innovace can be used when surgery is not indicated, or prior to surgery. In some patients with bilateral renal artery stenosis or stenosis of the artery to a solitary kidney, increases of blood urea and creatinine, reversible upon discontinuation of therapy, have been seen. This is especially likely in patients treated with diuretics and/or those with renal insufficiency.

Surgery/anaesthesia: In patients undergoing major surgery or during anaesthesia with agents that produce hypotension, Innovace blocks angiotensin II formation secondary to compensatory renin release. This may lead to hypotension which can be corrected by volume expansion.

General: Where Innovace has been used as a single agent in hypertension, Afro-Caribbean patients may show a reduced therapeutic response.

Innovace should not be used in patients with aortic stenosis or outflow obstruction.

Drug interactions: Combination with other antihypertensive agents such as beta-blockers, methyldopa, calcium antagonists, and diuretics may increase the antihypertensive efficacy. Adrenergic-blocking drugs should only be combined with Innovace under careful supervision. Concomitant propranolol may reduce the bioavailability of Innovace, but this does not appear to be of any clinical significance.

Concomitant therapy with lithium may increase the serum lithium concentration.

Plasma potassium usually remains within normal limits,

although cases of hyperkalaemia have been reported. If Innovace is given with a potassium-losing diuretic, the likelihood of diuretic-induced hypokalaemia may be lessened. Innovace may elevate plasma potassium levels in patients with renal failure. Potassium supplements, potassium-sparing diuretics and potassium-containing salt substitutes are not recommended, particularly in patients with impaired renal function, since they may lead to significant increases in plasma potassium.

However, if the concomitant use of these agents is deemed appropriate, they should be used with caution and with frequent monitoring of plasma potassium.

Breast-feeding mothers: Because it is not known whether Innovace is excreted in human milk, caution should be exercised if Innovace is given to breast-feeding mothers.

Side-effects

Severe hypotension and renal failure have occurred in association with therapy with Innovace. These appear to occur in certain specific sub-groups (see 'Precautions').

Angioneurotic oedema has been reported with angiotensin-converting enzyme inhibitors, including Innovace. In such cases, Innovace should be discontinued immediately and the patient observed. Where swelling is confined to the face, lips and mouth the condition will usually resolve without further treatment, although antihistamines may be useful in relieving symptoms. These patients should be followed carefully until the swelling has resolved. However, where there is involvement of the tongue, glottis or larynx, likely to cause airways obstruction, subcutaneous adrenaline (0.5 ml 1:1,000) should be administered promptly when indicated.

Other hypersensitivity reactions, including urticaria, have been reported.

Other adverse reactions: Dizziness and headaches are the more commonly reported side effects. Fatigue and asthenia were reported in 2–3% of patients. Other side-effects occurred in less than 2% of patients, and included hypotension, orthostatic hypotension, syncope, nausea, diarrhoea, muscle cramps, rash and cough. Less frequently renal dysfunction, renal failure, and oliguria have been reported. Less common side-effects include:

Cardiovascular: Myocardial infarction or cerebrovascular accident, possibly secondary to severe hypotension in high-risk patients (see 'Precautions'), chest pain, palpitations, rhythm disturbances, angina pectoris.

Gastro-intestinal: Ileus, pancreatitis, hepatitis or cholestatic jaundice, abdominal pain, vomiting, dyspepsia, constipation, anorexia, stomatitis.

Nervous system/Psychiatric: Depression, confusion, somnolence, insomnia, nervousness, paraesthesiae, vertigo.

Respiratory: Bronchospasm, asthma, dyspnoea, rhinorrhoea, sore throat and hoarseness.

Other: Hyperhidrosis, impotence, pruritus, alopecia, flushing, taste alteration, tinnitus, glossitis, blurred vision.

A complex of symptoms has been reported which may include fever, serositis, vasculitis, myalgia, arthralgia/arthritis, a positive ANA, elevated ESR, eosinophilia, and leucocytosis. Rash, photosensitivity or other dermatological manifestations may occur.

Laboratory test findings: Increases in blood urea and plasma creatinine, reversible on discontinuation of Innovace, are most likely in the presence of severe heart failure or bilateral renal artery stenosis, especially in patients with renal insufficiency (see 'Precautions'). However, increases in blood urea and plasma creatinine may occur without evidence of pre-existing renal impairment, especially in patients taking diuretics. In this event undiagnosed renal artery stenosis should be suspected. Dosage reduction of Innovace and/or discontinuation of the diuretic should be considered.

Hyperkalaemia and hyponatraemia have also been reported in a few cases (see 'Plasma potassium' for further information).

Decreases in haemoglobin and haematocrit as well as elevation of liver enzymes and/or serum bilirubin have been reported in a few patients, and are usually reversible upon discontinuation of Innovace.

Decreases in platelets and white cell count, and rare cases of neutropenia, thrombocytopenia, bone marrow depression, and agranulocytosis have been reported, but a causal relationship to Innovace has not been established.

Overdosage: Limited data are available for overdosage in humans. The most prominent features of overdosage reported to date are marked hypotension, beginning some six hours after ingestion of tablets, concomitant with blockade of the renin-angiotensin system, and stupor.

Serum enalaprilat levels 100 times and 200 times higher than usually seen after therapeutic doses have been reported after ingestion of 300 mg and 400 mg of enalapril, respectively.

The recommended treatment of overdosage is intravenous infusion of normal saline solution. If ingestion is recent, induce emesis. Innovace can be removed from the general circulation by haemodialysis.

Pharmaceutical precautions Store in a dry place below 25°C, protected from light.

Legal category POM.

Package quantities
Tablets 20 mg: Calendar packs of 28 tablets, bottles of 50 tablets
Tablets 10 mg: Calendar packs of 28 tablets, bottles of 50 tablets
Tablets 5 mg: Calendar packs of 28 tablets, bottles of 50 tablets
Tablets 2.5 mg: Bottles of 50 tablets

Further information Nil.

Product licence numbers

2.5 mg tablet	0025/0220
5 mg tablet	0025/0194
10 mg tablet	0025/0195
20 mg tablet	0025/0196

INNOZIDE*

Presentation Round, fluted, yellow tablets with MSD 718 on one side and scored. Each tablet contains 20 mg enalapril maleate and 12.5 mg hydrochlorothiazide.

Uses For the treatment of mild to moderate hypertension in patients who have been stabilised on the individual components given in the same proportions.

Mode of action: Innozide is a combination of an angiotensin-converting enzyme inhibitor (enalapril maleate) and a diuretic (hydrochlorothiazide).

Innozide is highly effective in the treatment of hypertension. The antihypertensive effects of the two components are additive and are sustained for at least 24 hours. A higher percentage of patients with hypertension respond satisfactorily to Innozide than to either component administered alone.

Enalaprilat, the active metabolite of enalapril maleate, is a highly specific, long-acting, non-sulphydryl angiotensin-converting enzyme inhibitor. Enalapril maleate modulates a specific physiological mechanism, the renin-angiotensin-aldosterone system, which plays a major role in the regulation of blood pressure.

Hydrochlorothiazide is a diuretic and antihypertensive agent. Use of this agent alone results in increased renin secretion. Although enalapril maleate alone is antihypertensive, concomitant administration with hydrochlorothiazide results in a greater reduction in blood pressure. Enalapril maleate attenuates the potassium loss associated with hydrochlorothiazide.

Dosage and administration The dosage of Innozide should be determined primarily by the experience with the enalapril maleate component.

Adults

Essential hypertension: The usual dosage is one tablet,

taken once daily. If necessary, the dosage may be increased to two tablets, taken once daily.

Prior diuretic therapy: Symptomatic hypotension may occur following the initial dose of enalapril; this is more likely in patients who are volume and/or salt depleted as a result of prior diuretic therapy. The diuretic therapy should be discontinued for 2–3 days prior to initiation of therapy with enalapril.

Dosage in renal insufficiency: Thiazides may not be appropriate diuretics for use in patients with renal impairment and are ineffective at creatinine clearance values of 30 ml/min or below (i.e. moderate or severe renal insufficiency).

In patients with creatinine clearance of >30 and <80 ml/min, Innozide should be used only after titration of the individual components.

Use in the elderly: In clinical studies the efficacy and tolerability of enalapril maleate and hydrochlorothiazide, administered concomitantly, were similar in both elderly and younger hypertensive patients.

Paediatric use: Safety and effectiveness in children have not been established.

Contra-indications, warnings, etc

Contra-indications: Innozide is contra-indicated in patients with anuria.

Innozide is contra-indicated in patients who are hypersensitive to any component of the product and in patients with a history of angioneurotic oedema relating to previous treatment with an angiotensin-converting enzyme inhibitor.

Innozide is contra-indicated in patients who are hypersensitive to other sulphonamide-derived drugs.

Innozide is contra-indicated in pregnancy. ACE inhibitors have been shown to be fetotoxic in rabbits during middle and late pregnancy. Effects of exposure of the fetus to ACE inhibitors during the first trimester of human pregnancy are unknown. Fetal exposure during the second and third trimesters of pregnancy has been associated with fetal and neonatal morbidity and mortality. ACE inhibitors in human pregnancy have been associated with oligohydramnios. Hypotension and renal failure have occurred in the newborn.

See also 'Breast-feeding mothers' under 'Precautions'.

Precautions

Hypotension and electrolyte/fluid imbalance: As with all antihypertensive therapy, symptomatic hypotension may occur in some patients. This was rarely seen in uncomplicated hypertensive patients but is more likely in the presence of fluid or electrolyte imbalance, e.g. volume depletion, hyponatraemia, hypochloraemic alkalosis, hypomagnesaemia or hypokalaemia which may occur from prior diuretic therapy, dietary salt restriction, dialysis, or during intercurrent diarrhoea or vomiting. Periodic determination of serum electrolytes should be performed at appropriate intervals in such patients.

Particular consideration should be given when therapy is administered to patients with ischaemic heart or cerebrovascular disease because an excessive fall in blood pressure could result in a myocardial infarction or cerebrovascular accident.

If hypotension occurs, the patient should be placed in the supine position and, if necessary, should receive an intravenous infusion of normal saline. A transient hypotensive response is not a contra-indication to further doses. Following restoration of effective blood volume and pressure, reinstitution of therapy at reduced dosage may be possible; or either of the components may be used appropriately alone.

Renal function impairment: Thiazides may not be appropriate diuretics for use in patients with renal impairment and are ineffective at creatinine clearance values of 30 ml/min or below (i.e. moderate or severe renal insufficiency).

Innozide should not be administered to patients with renal insufficiency (creatinine clearance ≤80 ml/min) until titration of the individual components has shown the need for the doses present in the combination tablet.

Some hypertensive patients with no apparent pre-existing renal disease have developed usually minor and transient increases in blood urea and serum creatinine when enalapril maleate has been given concomitantly with a diuretic. If this occurs during therapy with Innozide, the combination should be discontinued. Reinstitution of therapy at reduced dosage may be possible, or either of the components may be used appropriately alone.

In some patients, with bilateral renal artery stenosis or stenosis in the artery to a solitary kidney, increases in blood urea and serum creatinine, reversible upon discontinuation of therapy, have been seen with angiotensin-converting enzyme (ACE) inhibitors.

Hepatic disease: Thiazides should be used with caution in patients with impaired hepatic function or progressive liver disease, since minor alterations of fluid and electrolyte balance may precipitate hepatic coma.

Surgery/anaesthesia: In patients undergoing major surgery or during anaesthesia with agents that produce hypotension, enalaprilat blocks angiotensin-II formation secondary to compensatory renin release. If hypotension occurs and is considered to be due to this mechanism, it can be corrected by volume expansion.

Metabolic and endocrine effects: Thiazide therapy may impair glucose tolerance. Dosage adjustment of antidiabetic agents, including insulin, may be required.

Thiazides may decrease urinary calcium excretion and may cause intermittent and slight elevation of serum calcium. Marked hypercalcaemia may be evidence of hidden hyperparathyroidism. Thiazides should be discontinued before carrying out tests for parathyroid function.

Increases in cholesterol and triglyceride levels may be associated with thiazide diuretic therapy.

Thiazide therapy may precipitate hyperuricaemia and/or gout in certain patients. However, enalapril may increase urinary uric acid and thus may attenuate the hyperuricaemic effect of hydrochlorothiazide.

Hypersensitivity/angioneurotic oedema: Angioneurotic oedema of the face, extremities, lips, tongue, glottis and/or larynx has been reported rarely in patients treated with angiotensin-converting enzyme inhibitors, including enalapril maleate. In such cases, enalapril maleate should be discontinued promptly and appropriate monitoring should be carried out to ensure complete resolution of symptoms before dismissing the patient.

In those instance where swelling has been confined to the face and lips the condition generally resolved without treatment, although antihistamines have been useful in relieving symptoms.

Angioneurotic oedema associated with laryngeal oedema may be fatal. Where there is involvement of the tongue, glottis or larynx, likely to cause airway obstruction, appropriate therapy such as subcutaneous adrenalin solution 1:1000 (0.3 ml to 0.5 ml) should be administered promptly.

Patients with a history of angioedema unrelated to ACE-inhibitor therapy may be at increased risk of angioedema while receiving an ACE inhibitor. (See also: 'Contra-indications').

In patients receiving thiazides, sensitivity reactions may occur with or without a history of allergy or bronchial asthma. Exacerbation or activation of systemic lupus erythematosus has been reported with the use of thiazides.

Cough: Cough has been reported with the use of ACE inhibitors. Characteristically, the cough is non-productive, persistent and resolves after discontinuation of therapy. ACE inhibitor-induced cough should be considered as part of the differential diagnosis of cough.

Breast-feeding mothers: Both enalapril and thiazides appear in human milk. If use of Innozide is deemed essential, breast-feeding should stop.

Drug Interactions

Serum potassium: The potassium-losing effect of thiazide diuretics is usually attenuated by the effect of enalapril maleate. Serum potassium usually remains within normal limits, although in clinical trials with enalapril maleate hyperkalaemia did occur in a few cases.

The use of potassium supplements, potassium-sparing agents or potassium-containing salt substitutes, particularly in patients with impaired renal function, may lead to a significant increase in serum potassium. If concomitant use of 'Innozide' and any of these agents is deemed appropriate, they should be used with caution and with frequent monitoring of serum potassium.

Lithium: Lithium generally should not be given with diuretics or ACE inhibitors (ACE-I). Diuretic agents and ACE-I reduce the renal clearance of lithium and add a high risk of lithium toxicity. Refer to the prescribing information for lithium preparations before use of such preparations.

Non-depolarising muscle relaxants: Thiazides may increase the responsiveness to tubocurarine.

Other agents: The combination of enalapril maleate with beta-adrenergic blocking agents, methyldopa, or calcium entry blockers has been shown to improve the efficacy of lowering the blood pressure.

Ganglionic-blocking agents or adrenergic-blocking agents, combined with enalapril, should only be administered under careful observation of the patient.

When administered concurrently, the following drugs may interact with thiazide diuretics:

Alcohol, barbiturates, narcotics or phenothiazines: Potentiation of orthostatic hypotension may occur.

Antidiabetic drugs (oral agents and insulin): Dosage adjustment of the antidiabetic drug may be required.

Corticosteroids, ACTH: Intensified electrolyte depletion, particularly hypokalaemia.

Pressor amines (e.g. adrenalin): Possible decreased response to pressor amines but not sufficient to preclude their use.

Non-steroidal anti-inflammatory drugs: In some patients, the administration of non-steroidal anti-inflammatory agent can reduce the diuretic, natriuretic, and antihypertensive effects of diuretics.

Side-effects: Innozide is usually well tolerated. In clinical studies, side effects have usually been mild and transient, and in most instances have not required interruption of therapy.

The most common clinical side-effects were dizziness and fatigue, which generally responded to dosage reduction and seldom required discontinuation of therapy.

Other side-effects (1–2%) were: Muscle cramps, nausea, asthenia, orthostatic effects including hypotension, headache, cough, and impotence.

Less common side-effects which occurred either during controlled trials or during marketed use include:

Cardiovascular: Syncope, non-orthostatic hypotension, palpitation, tachycardia, chest pain.

Gastro-intestinal: Diarrhoea, vomiting, dyspepsia, abdominal pain, flatulence, constipation.

Nervous system/psychiatric: Insomnia, somnolence, paraesthesia, vertigo, nervousness.

Respiratory: Dyspnoea.

Skin: Stevens–Johnson syndrome, rash, pruritis, diaphoresis.

Other: Renal dysfunction, renal failure, decreased libido, dry mouth, gout, tinnitus, arthralgia.

A symptom complex has been reported which may include fever, serositis, vasculitis, myalgia, arthralgia/arthritis, a positive ANA, elevated ESR, eosinophilia and leucocytosis. Rash, photosensitivity or other dermatological manifestations may occur.

Hypersensitivity/angioneurotic oedema: Angioneurotic oedema of the face, extremities, lips, tongue, glottis and/or larynx has been reported rarely (see 'Precautions').

Side-effects due to individual components: Additional side-effects that have been seen with one of the individual components and may be potential side-effects with Innozide are the following:

Enalapril maleate: Ileus, pancreatitis, either hepatocellular or cholestatic jaundice, depression, confusion, bronchospasm/asthma, rhythm disturbances, angina pectoris, myocardial infarction or cerebrovascular accident, rhinorrhoea, photosensitivity, alopecia, flushing, taste alteration, anorexia, blurred vision, urticaria, stomatitis, glossitis, oliguria, toxic epidermal necrolysis, erythema multiforme, exfoliative dermatitis.

Hydrochlorothiazide: Anorexia, gastric irritation, constipation, jaundice (intrahepatic cholestatic jaundice), pancreatitis, sialoadenitis, vertigo, xanthopsia, leucopenia, agranulocytosis, thrombocytopenia, aplastic anaemia, haemolytic anaemia, purpura, photosensitivity, fever, urticaria, necrotising angiitis (vasculitis), respiratory distress (including pneumonitis and pulmonary oedema), anaphylactic reaction, glycosuria, electrolyte imbalance including hyponatraemia, restlessness, muscle spasm, transient blurred vision.

Laboratory test findings: Clinically important changes in standard laboratory parameters were rarely associated with administration of 'Innozide'. Occasional hyperglycaemia, hyperuricaemia and hyper- or hypokalaemia have been noted. Increases in blood urea and serum creatinine, and elevations of liver enzymes and/or serum bilirubin have been seen. Decreases in haemoglobin and haematocrit have been reported in hypertensive patients treated with Innozide. These are usually reversible upon discontinuation of Innozide.

Decreases in platelets and white cell count, and rare cases of neutropenia, thrombocytopenia and bone marrow depression have been reported, but a causal relationship to 'Innozide' has not been established.

Hyponatraemia has occurred with enalapril and may be a potential finding with 'Innozide'.

Overdosage: No specific information is available on the treatment of overdosage with 'Innozide'. Treatment is symptomatic and supportive. Therapy with 'Innozide' should be discontinued and the patient observed closely. Suggested measures include induction of emesis and/or gastric lavage, and correction of dehydration, electrolyte imbalance and hypotension by established procedures.

Enalapril maleate: The most prominent feature of overdosage reported to date is marked hypotension, beginning some six hours after ingestion of tablets, concomitant with blockade of the renin-angiotensin system, and stupor. Serum enelaprilat levels 100 times and 200 times higher than usually seen after therapeutic doses have been reported after ingestion of 300 mg and 440 mg of enalapril maleate respectively.

Enalaprilat may be removed from the general circulation by haemodialysis.

Hydrochlorothiazide: The most common signs and symptoms observed are those caused by electrolyte depletion (hypokalaemia, hypochloraemia, hyponatraemia) and dehydration resulting from excessive diuresis. If digitalis has also been administered, hypokalaemia may accentuate cardiac arrhythmias.

Pharmaceutical precautions Store in a dry place below 25°C, protected from light.

Legal category POM.

Package quantities Calendar pack of 28 tablets.

Further information Nil.

Product licence number 0025/0249.

MEFOXIN* INJECTION

Presentation In vials containing 1 g or 2 g of cefoxitin as the sodium salt. Each gram of cefoxitin contains approximately 2.3 mEq sodium.

Uses Mefoxin is indicated for the treatment of the following infections caused by sensitive bacteria: peritonitis and other intra-abdominal and intrapelvic infections; gonorrhoea; female genital tract infections; septicaemia; urinary tract infections; respiratory tract infections; bone and joint infections; and skin and soft-tissue infections.

Mefoxin is a broad-spectrum bactericidal antibiotic indicated for the treatment of infections caused by susceptible strains of Gram-positive and Gram-negative pathogens both aerobic and anaerobic.

Mefoxin has been clinically effective not only in infections due to antibiotic-sensitive organisms, but also in infections due to organisms resistant to one or more of the following antibacterial agents: penicillin, ampicillin, carbenicillin, tetracyclines, erythromycin, chloramphenicol, cephalosporins, kanamycin, gentamicin, tobramycin, and sulphamethoxazole-trimethoprim.

Many Gram-negative pathogens are resistant to penicillins and cephalosporins through the action of the beta-lactamases which are produced by these pathogens. Mefoxin is remarkably stable in the presence of these bacterial beta-lactamases, both penicillinases and cephalosporinases. Hence, the clinical efficacy of Mefoxin extends to many infections caused by such pathogens.

Mefoxin is indicated for the treatment of mixed infections caused by susceptible strains of aerobic and anaerobic bacteria. The majority of these mixed infections are associated with contamination by faecal flora as well as flora originating from the vagina, skin, and mouth. In these mixed infections, *Bacteroides fragilis* is the most commonly encountered anaerobic pathogen and is usually resistant to aminoglycosides, cephalosporins, and virtually all penicillins. However, *Bacteroides fragilis* is usually susceptible to Mefoxin.

Mefoxin is indicated for adjunctive therapy in the surgical treatment of infections, including abscesses, infection complicating hollow visceral perforations, cutaneous infections, and infections of serous surfaces, whether caused by aerobes, mixed aerobes and anaerobes, or anaerobes.

Clinical experience has demonstrated that Mefoxin can be administered to patients who are also receiving carbenicillin, kanamycin, gentamicin, tobramycin, or amikacin (see 'Precautions' and 'Dosage and administration').

Prophylaxis: Mefoxin is indicated for the prevention of certain post-operative infections in patients undergoing contaminated or potentially contaminated surgical procedures or where the occurrence of post-operative infection could be especially serious.

Microbiology: Mefoxin is active in vitro *against:* Aerobic bacteria: *Gram-positive cocci* including: *Staphylococci:* (including coagulase-positive, coagulase-negative, and penicillinase-producing strains); Group A beta-haemolytic streptococci (*Streptococcus pyogenes*); Group B beta-haemolytic streptococci (*Streptococcus agalactiae*); *Streptococcus pneumoniae* (*Diplococcus pneumoniae*); other streptococci (except group D streptococci including enterococci, most strains of which are resistant, e.g. *Streptococcus faecalis*), *Gram-negative cocci* including: *Neisseria gonorrhoeae* (including penicillinase-producing strains); *Neisseria meningitidis. Gram-negative rods* (*facultative anaerobes*) including: *Escherichia coli*; *Klebsiella pneumoniae*; Klebsiella spp.; *Proteus mirabilis. Proteus* (indole-positive): *Morganella morganii* (formerly *Proteus* morganii); *Proteus vulgaris; Haemophilus influenzae; Serratia marcescens*; Providencia spp.; *Providencia rettgeri* (formerly *Proteus rettgeri*); Salmonella and Shigella spp.

Anaerobic bacteria: *Gram-positive cocci* including: Peptococcus spp.; Peptostreptococcus spp.; Microaerophilic streptococcus. *Gram-positive rods* including: *Clostridium perfringens*; Clostridium spp.; Eubacterium spp.; *Propionibacterium acnes. Gram-negative cocci* including: Veillonella spp. *Gram-negative rods* including: *Bacteroides fragilis; Bacteroides melaninogenicus*; Bacteroides spp. (including both penicillin-susceptible and penicillin-resistant strains); Fusobacterium spp.

Mefoxin is active against some strains of the following bacteria: *Acinetobacter calcoaceticus* var. *anitratum* (*Herellea vaginicola*); *Acinetobacter calcoaceticus* var. *lwoffi* (*Mima polymorpha*); *Alcaligenes faecalis*; Citrobacter spp. and Flavo-bacterium spp.; Enterobacter spp.

Mefoxin is not active against Pseudomonas spp., most strains of enterococci, many strains of *Enterobacter cloacae*, methicillin-resistant staphylococci, and *Listeria monocytogenes*.

Human pharmacology: Mefoxin administered parenterally, produces high serum and urine concentrations. It is excreted virtually unchanged as active Mefoxin by the kidneys, and has a mean terminal serum half-life of approximately one hour. Mefoxin passes rapidly into body fluids such as pleural, bile, and ascitic fluids. Probenecid slows tubular excretion and increases and prolongs blood levels.

Intravenous: Peak serum concentrations of Mefoxin following 1 g infused intravenously over 3 minutes was 125 micrograms/ml, infused over 30 minutes was 72 micrograms/ml, and infused over 120 minutes was 25 micrograms/ml. Following 2 g infused intravenously over 3 minutes, peak serum concentration was 221 micrograms/ml.

In a number of studies using 0.5 g, 1 g, or 2 g intravenous doses of Mefoxin mean total urinary recovery ranged from 77% to 99% of the cefoxitin dose.

Intramuscular: When Mefoxin was reconstituted for intramuscular injection with 0.5% or 1% lignocaine hydrochloride, the lignocaine had no effect on the absorption or elimination of Mefoxin.

Intramuscular injections of 1 g of Mefoxin in 0.5% lignocaine hydrochloride solution produced a peak serum concentration of 30 micrograms/ml at 20 minutes. Approximately 85% of an intramuscular dose is excreted by the kidneys in the first six hours; this results in high urine levels (e.g. >3,000 micrograms/ml between one and two hours after a 1 g dose).

Dosage and administration Mefoxin may be administered intravenously or intramuscularly. (See reconstitution directions for each route.) Dosage and route of administration should be determined by severity of infection, susceptibility of the causative organisms, and condition of the patient.

Therapy may be started while awaiting the results of susceptibility testing.

Usual adult dosage

Type of infection	*Dose (g)*	*Frequency (hrs)*	*Total daily dosage*
Uncomplicated	1	Every 8 (occasionally every 6)	3 g (4 g)
Moderately severe or severe	2	Every 8 (occasionally every 6)	6 g (8 g)
Infections generally needing antibiotics in higher dosage	3 (2)	Every 6 (every 4)	12 g

Maintenance dosage of Mefoxin in adults with reduced renal function

Renal function	Creatinine clearance (ml/min)	Dose (g)	Frequency (hrs)
Mild impairment	50–30	1–2	Every 8–12
Moderate impairment	29–10	1–2	Every 12–24
Severe impairment	9–5	0.5–1	Every 12–24
Essentially no function	<5	0.5–1	Every 24–48

Adults Dosage: The usual dosage is 1 g or 2 g of Mefoxin every eight hours. (See 'Usual adult dosage' chart.)

In adults with renal insufficiency, an initial loading dose of 1 g to 2 g may be given. After a loading dose, the following recommendations for *maintenance dosage* may be used as a guide.

In the patients undergoing haemodialysis, the loading dose of 1–2 g should be given after each haemodialysis, and the maintenance dose should be given as indicated in the chart giving 'Maintenance dosage of Mefoxin in adults with reduced renal function'.

Uncomplicated urinary tract infections: In uncomplicated urinary tract infections due to susceptible organisms, 1 g intramuscularly twice a day has been shown to be effective.

Uncomplicated gonorrhoea: For single dose therapy of uncomplicated gonorrhoea, including that caused by penicillinase-producing strains, the recommended dose is 2 g of Mefoxin intramuscularly given with 1 g of probenecid by mouth (at the same time or up to one hour before).

Neonates, infants and children:

Neonates	
0–1 week of age	20–40 mg/kg every 12 hours
1–4 weeks of age	20–40 mg/kg every 8 hours
Infants	20–40 mg/kg every 6 hours or every 8 hours
Children	20–40 mg/kg every 6 hours or every 8 hours

In severe infections, the total daily dosage may be increased to 200 mg/kg, but not to exceed 12 g per day.

Mefoxin is not recommended for the therapy of meningitis. If meningitis is suspected an appropriate antibiotic should be used.

In children with renal insufficiency dosage frequency should be reduced as indicated for adults.

Prophylactic administration to adults: 2 g administered intramuscularly or intravenously just prior to surgery (½–1 hour before incision), then 2 g every 6 hours. Prophylactic therapy should not usually be given for more than 24 hours.

Prophylactic administration for neonates, infants and children: In infants and children, 30–40 mg/kg doses may be given at the same times as designated for adults. However, in neonates, 30–40 mg/kg doses may be given ½ to 1 hour before initial incision and the second and third dose may be given every 8–12 hours.

Obstetric and gynaecological surgery: For patients undergoing caesarean section, a single 2 g dose is administered intravenously as soon as the cord is clamped.

In gynaecological surgical procedures, a single prophylactic dose of 2 g intravenously or intramuscularly has been effective given ½ to 1 hour before surgery.

In prolonged or heavily contaminated cases, additional 2 g doses may be given at 6-hour intervals. Prophylactic therapy does not ordinarily extend beyond 24 hours.

Intravenous administration: Reconstitute Mefoxin with Water for Injections BP: 1 g is soluble in 2 ml. Although Mefoxin is very soluble, for intravenous use it is preferable to add 10 ml of Water for Injections BP to the 1 g vial or to the 2 g vial. Shake to dissolve and then withdraw entire contents of vial into syringe.

Solutions of Mefoxin range from clear to light amber in colour. The pH of freshly reconstituted solutions usually ranges from 4.2 to 7.0.

For direct intravenous injection, Mefoxin may be slowly injected into the vein over a period of three to five minutes or may be given through the tubing when the patient is receiving parenteral solutions.

An intermittent intravenous infusion of Mefoxin may be employed when large amounts of fluid are to be given. However, during infusion of the solution containing Mefoxin, it may be advisable temporarily to discontinue administration of any other infusion solution at the same site (by using an appropriate IV infusion set).

A solution of Mefoxin may also be given by continuous intravenous infusion (see opposite for compatibility and stability).

Intramuscular administration ONLY: Reconstitute Mefoxin 1 g with 2 ml of Water for Injections BP, or 0.5% or 1% lignocaine hydrochloride (without adrenaline) solution. Mefoxin is given by deep injection into a large muscle mass. Avoid injection into a blood vessel.

Note: Some patients may be hypersensitive to lignocaine.

Preparation of solution: The following table is provided for convenience in reconstituting Mefoxin for both intravenous and intramuscular administration.

Strength	*Amount of diluent to be added (ml*)*	*Approximate final volume (ml)*	*Approximate average concentration (mg/ml)*
1 gram vial	2 (Intramuscular)	2.5	400
1 gram vial	10 (IV)	10.5	95
2 gram vial	10 or 20 (IV)	11 or 21	180 or 95

* Shake to dissolve and let stand until clear.

Compatibility and stability: A solution of Mefoxin in Water for Injections BP may be added to the following solutions: 0.9% Sodium Chloride Injection BP, 5% or 10% Dextrose Injection BP, Dextrose and Sodium Chloride Injection BP (5%/0.9%, 5%/0.45%, or 5%/0.2%). Lactated Ringer's Injection USP, 5% Dextrose Injection in 0.02% sodium bicarbonate solution, 5% Dextrose in Lactated Ringer's Injection, 5% or 10% invert sugar in water, 10% invert sugar in saline solution, 5% Sodium Bicarbonate Injection BP, M/6 Sodium Lactate Injection BP, insulin (in normal saline or 10% invert sugar), heparin (100 units/ml and 0.1 units/ml), mannitol (2.5%, 5% and 10%).

Mefoxin has been shown to be chemically and visually compatible with aminoglycosides such as amikacin, gentamicin, kanamycin, and tobramycin mixed in 200 ml of 0.9% sodium chloride or 5% dextrose in water.

Use in the elderly: The dosage should be determined by the severity of the infection, the susceptibility of the causative organisms, the patient's clinical condition and renal function.

Contra-indications, warnings, etc

Contra-indications: Mefoxin is contra-indicated in persons who have shown hypersensitivity to cefoxitin. In the absence of clinical experience, Mefoxin should not be administered to patients who have shown hypersensitivity to cephalosporins.

Precautions: There is some clinical and laboratory evidence of partial cross-allergenicity between cephamycins and other beta-lactam antibiotics, penicillins, and cephalosporins. Severe reactions (including anaphylaxis) have been reported with most beta-lactam antibiotics.

Before therapy with Mefoxin, careful inquiry should be made concerning previous hypersensitivity reactions to beta-lactam antibiotics. Mefoxin should be given cautiously to penicillin-allergic patients.

Any patient who has demonstrated some form of allergy, particularly to drugs, should receive antibiotics cautiously. If an allergic reaction to Mefoxin occurs, the drug should be discontinued.

Pseudomembranous colitis, reported with virtually all antibiotics, can range from mild to life threatening in severity. Antibiotics should be prescribed with caution in patients with a history of gastro-intestinal disease, particularly colitis. Treatment-related diarrhoea should always be considered as a pointer to this diagnosis. While studies indicate that a toxin of *Clostridium difficile* is one of the primary causes of antibiotic-related colitis, other causes should be considered.

The total daily dosage should be reduced when Mefoxin is administered to patients with transient or persistent reduction of urinary output due to renal insufficiency (see 'Dosage and administration') because high and prolonged serum antibiotic concentrations can occur from usual doses.

Interference with laboratory tests: A false-positive reaction to glucose in the urine may occur with reducing substances but not with the use of specific glucose oxidase methods.

Using the Jaffe technique, falsely high creatinine values in serum may occur if Mefoxin serum concentrations exceed 100 mcg/ml. Serum samples from patients treated with Mefoxin should not be analysed for creatinine if withdrawn within two hours of drug administration.

High concentration of cefoxitin in the urine may interfere with the measurement of 17-hydroxy-corticosteroids by the Porter-Silber reaction to give slight, falsely increased results.

Use in pregnancy: Use of the drug in women of childbearing potential requires that the anticipated benefits be weighed against possible hazards. Reproductive and teratogenic studies have been performed in mice and rats and have revealed no evidence of impaired fertility or harm to the fetus due to Mefoxin. There are no controlled studies with Mefoxin in pregnant women.

Nursing mothers: Mefoxin is excreted in human milk. Caution should be exercised if use is indicated.

Side-effects: Mefoxin is generally well tolerated. Side-effects have usually been mild and transient and treatment rarely needs to be stopped. The most common side effects have been local reactions following intravenous or intramuscular injection.

Local reactions: Thrombophlebitis has occurred with intravenous administration. Pain, induration and tenderness after intramuscular injections have been reported.

Allergic: Rash including exfoliative dermatitis, urticaria, pruritus, eosinophilia, fever and other allergic reactions (including anaphylaxis) have been noted.

Cardiovascular: Hypotension.

Gastro-intestinal: Symptoms of pseudomembraneous colitis can appear during or after antibiotic treatment. Nausea and vomiting have been reported rarely.

Blood: Eosinophilia, leucopenia including granulocytopenia, neutropenia, anaemia including haemolytic anaemia, thrombocytopenia and bone-marrow depression have been reported. Some individuals, particularly those with azotaemia, may develop positive direct Coombs tests during therapy with Mefoxin.

Liver function: Transient elevations in AST (SGOT), ALT (SGPT), serum LDH, serum alkaline phosphatase and jaundice have been reported.

Kidney function: Elevations in serum creatinine and/or blood urea levels have been observed. Acute renal failure has been reported rarely. The role of Mefoxin in changes in renal function tests is difficult to assess, since factors predisposing to pre-renal azotaemia or to impaired renal function usually have been present.

Overdosage: Cefoxitin is not absorbed from the GI tract and so reaction on accidental ingestion is unlikely.

After injection, cefoxitin has a half-life between 45 and 60 minutes with a 70% binding to plasma proteins.

The parenteral dose of Mefoxin is carefully controlled by the physician and no case of overdosage has been recorded. No known antidote is available.

Pharmaceutical precautions Mefoxin, as reconstituted below, maintains satisfactory potency for 24 hours at room temperature, for one week under refrigeration (below 5°C) and for at least 30 weeks in the frozen state and will maintain potency after thawing for at least 24 hours at room temperature.

Mefoxin may be reconstituted with Water for Injections BP, Water for Injections BP preserved with parabens or benzyl alcohol, 0.9% Sodium Chloride Injection BP, 5% Dextrose Injection BP, or 0.5% and 1.0% lignocaine hydrochloride (preserved in parabens).

When reconstituting Mefoxin for neonates, Water for Injections must be preservative free.

After reconstitution with Water for Injections BP and subsequent storage in disposable plastic syringes, 'Mefoxin' is stable for 24 hours at room temperature and 48 hours under refrigeration.

After the periods mentioned above, any unused solutions or frozen material should be discarded. Do not refreeze.

Note: Mefoxin in the dry state should be stored below 30°C. Avoid exposure to temperatures above 50°C. The dry material as well as solutions tend to darken, depending on storage conditions; product potency, however, is not adversely affected.

Legal category POM.

Package quantities Sterile Mefoxin is supplied in vials containing 1 g or 2 g of cefoxitin as the sodium salt, both strengths available in packs of 5 vials.

Further information Nil.

Product licence numbers
1 g 0025/0130
2 g 0025/0131

MINTEZOL*

Presentation Orange-coloured chewable tablets, marked 'MSD 907', containing 500 mg Thiabendazole BP.

Uses Anthelmintic.

Mintezol is indicated as primary treatment against Strongyloidiasis; Cutaneous larva migrans (creeping eruption); Dracunculiasis (guinea worm); Visceral larva migrans.

Mintezol is indicated as secondary treatment against Enterobiasis (threadworm) when the infestation is mixed with a primary indication.

Mintezol can relieve the symptoms and fever of trichinosis during the invasion stage.

Mintezol is indicated (a) when specific therapy is unavailable, (b) when other therapy cannot be used or (c) as additive therapy against *Necator americanus* and *Ancylostoma duodenale* (hookworm); *Trichuriasis* (whipworm); *Ascariasis* (large roundworm).

Dosage and administration Dosage depends on the body weight of the patient and is independent of the condition being treated. Usually, 2 doses are given each day. For patients weighing less than 60 kg (132 lb), each dose is based on 25 mg thiabendazole per kg body weight. For patients weighing 60 kg or more, each dose is 1.5 g thiabendazole. The maximum daily dosage for adults weighing 60 kg or more is 3 g.

Mintezol should be taken with meals and chewed before swallowing. Dietary restrictions, complementary medications and cleansing enemas are not necessary.

The table below relates dosage to body weight:

Patient's weight		*Dose (twice daily)*
kg	*lb*	*Tablets (500 mg thiabendazole)*
10	22	½
20	44	1
30	66	1½
40	88	2
50	110	2½
60 (or more)	132 (or more)	3

Clinical experience, as well as safety experience in children weighing less than 15 kg has been limited. Duration of therapy depends on the particular nematode infestation, and is as follows:

Strongyloidiasis, ascariasis, uncinariasis and trichuriasis: 2 doses a day for two successive days. Alternatively, a single dose of 50 mg/kg may be given, but a higher incidence of side-effects would be expected.

Cutaneous larva migrans: 2 doses a day for two successive days. If active lesions are still present two days after completion of this therapy, a second similar course is recommended.

Visceral larva migrans: 2 doses a day for 7 successive days. (Safety and efficacy data on this duration of treatment are limited.)

Trichinosis: 2 doses a day for two to four successive days, according to the response of the patient. The optimum dosage in trichinosis has not yet been established.

Dracunculiasis: 50–100 mg/kg in two equally divided doses for one day. The lower dosage for patients with 1 or 2 visible worms; the higher dosage for patients with multiple infection (3 or more worms). In massive infections (10 worms or more), a second dose of 50 mg/

kg can be given five to eight days after treatment, if required.

Further considerations: In certain patients, 2 doses a day may lead to a higher incidence of side-effects. In these circumstances, 25 mg per kg body weight may be given after the largest meal on the first day and repeated 24 hours later after a similar meal on the second day.

For mass treatment, a single dose of 50 mg/kg after the evening meal is highly effective and most convenient, though a higher incidence of side-effects may be expected.

Use in the elderly: Since CNS and hepatic side effects have been reported to occur and since excretion is primarily renal, use with caution in elderly patients who have renal, hepatic or CNS dysfunction. As with younger patients, the dosage should be calculated on the basis of body weight.

Use in children: Clinical experience, as well as safety experience with thiabendazole treatment in children weighing less than 15 kg has been limited.

Contra-indications, warnings, etc

Contra-indication: Hypersensitivity to any component of this product.

Precautions: If any hypersensitivity reactions occur, therapy should be discontinued immediately and not resumed. Erythema multiforme, including fatal cases of Stevens-Johnson syndrome, has been associated with thiabendazole therapy.

Mintezol may impair alertness in some patients, who should avoid driving, operating machinery, or other activities made hazardous by diminished alertness.

Ideally, anaemic, dehydrated or malnourished patients should be given supportive therapy before starting treatment with Mintezol. Liver and renal function should be carefully monitored in patients with disorders of these organs.

Mintezol should not be used prophylactically.

Pregnancy and the nursing mother: Mintezol should not be used during pregnancy or lactation. Reports have suggested that thiabendazole is teratogenic in mice, although reproduction studies in generations of rabbits, rats, sheep, cattle and pigs have shown no fetal abnormalities attributable to the drug. Nevertheless, Mintezol should not be used in women of childbearing potential unless pregnancy has been excluded.

Drug interactions: Thiabendazole may compete with other drugs, such as theophylline, for sites of metabolism in the liver and thus elevate the serum levels of such drugs to potentially toxic levels. Therefore, when the concomitant use of thiabendazole and xanthine derivatives is anticipated, it may be necessary to monitor blood levels and/or reduce the dosage of such compounds. Such concomitant use should only be made under careful medical supervision.

Side-effects: The most common are anorexia, nausea, vomiting and dizziness. Diarrhoea, epigastric distress, pruritus, weariness, giddiness, headache and drowsiness occur less often.

Rare side-effects are tinnitus, collapse, abnormal sensation in the eyes, blurring of vision, hyperirritability, numbness, hyperglycaemia, yellow vision, enuresis, hypotension, jaundice, transient leucopenia, perianal rash, crystalluria, haematuria, convulsions, psychic disturbances, drying of mucous membranes (mouth, eyes etc.), intrahepatic cholestasis and parenchymal liver damage. The appearance of live ascaris in the mouth and nose has been reported on rare occasions.

Hypersensitivity reactions include fever, facial flush, rigor, conjunctival injection, angioneurotic oedema, anaphylaxis, skin rashes, erythema multiforme including Stevens-Johnson syndrome, and lymphadenopathy.

Some patients excrete a metabolite which imparts a characteristic odour to their urine, similar to that which occurs after eating asparagus.

Laboratory test findings: Rarely a transient rise in cephalin flocculation and SGOT has occurred in patients receiving Mintezol.

Overdosage: The stomach should be emptied promptly either by inducing emesis, if necessary, or by gastric lavage. Toxic disturbances of the GI and CNS systems can be expected and these should be treated symptomatically and supportively. There is no known antidote.

Thiabendazole is readily absorbed from the GI tract with a peak plasma level reached in 1 to 2 hours.

Pharmaceutical precautions Store in a dry place below 25°C.

Legal category POM.

Package quantities *Tablets:* Packs of 6.

Further information Nil.

Product licence number 0025/5031.

PERIACTIN*

Presentation White, half-scored tablets, marked 'MSD 62', containing Cyproheptadine Hydrochloride BP equivalent to 4 mg anhydrous cyproheptadine hydrochloride.

A yellow syrup containing, in each 5 ml, Cyproheptadine Hydrochloride BP equivalent to 2 mg anhydrous cyproheptadine hydrochloride.

Uses Periactin is a serotonin and histamine antagonist with anticholinergic and sedative properties.

In allergy and pruritus: Periactin has a wide range of anti-allergic and antipruritic activity, and can be used successfully in treatment of acute and chronic allergic and pruritic conditions, such as: dermatitis, including neurodermatitis and neurodermatitis circumscripta; eczema; eczematoid dermatitis; dermatographism; mild, local allergic reactions to insect bites; hay fever and other seasonal rhinitis; perennial allergic and vasomotor rhinitis; allergic conjunctivitis due to inhalant allergies and foods; urticaria; angioneurotic oedema; drug and serum reactions; anogenital pruritus; pruritus of chickenpox.

Periactin is indicated as adjunctive therapy to adrenaline and other standard measures for the relief of anaphylactic reactions after the acute manifestations have been controlled.

In migraine headache: Periactin has been reported to have beneficial effects in a significant number of patients having vascular types of headache. Many patients who have responded inadequately to all other agents have reported amelioration of symptoms with Periactin. The characteristic headache and feeling of malaise may disappear within an hour or two of the first dose.

As an appetite stimulant: Periactin is recommended for those patients with decreased appetite where, in the opinion of the physician, stimulation of the appetite and consequent weight gain is desirable. Periactin is not a substitute for food: an adequate diet is essential for successful therapy. The physician should treat any underlying disease or condition which may be responsible for the weight loss.

Dosage and administration There is no recommended dosage for children under 2 years old. Periactin is not recommended for elderly debilitated patients.

In allergy and pruritus: Dosage must be determined on an individual basis. The effect of a single dose usually lasts for four to six hours. For continuous effective relief, the daily requirement should be given in divided doses, three or four times a day, or as often as necessary.

Adults: 4–20 mg a day, most patients requiring 12–16 mg a day.

Maximum: 32 mg a day.

Children aged 7–14 years: Usually 4 mg two or three times a day, according to the patient's weight and response. Any additional dosage should be given at bedtime. Maximum 16 mg a day.

Children aged 2–6 years: Initially 2 mg two or three times a day, adjusted according to the patient's weight and response. Any additional dosage should be given at bedtime. Maximum 12 mg a day.

In vascular headache and migraine: For both prophylactic and therapeutic use at an initial dose of 4 mg repeated if necessary after half an hour. Patients who respond usually obtain relief with 8 mg, and this dose should not be exceeded within a 4- to 6-hour period.

Maintenance: 4 mg every four to six hours.

As an appetite stimulant: Daily dosage may be given as a single dose once a day in the evening or alternatively in divided doses. Dosage should be individualised according to the needs and response of the patient.

Adults and adolescents: The dosage of 12 mg (3 tablets or six 5 ml spoonfuls) a day is usually satisfactory. Larger doses are neither required nor recommended for appetite stimulation.

Children aged 7–14 years: The dosage should not exceed 12 mg (3 tablets or six 5 ml spoonfuls) a day.

Children aged 2–6 years: The dosage should not exceed 8 mg (2 tablets or four 5 ml spoonfuls) a day.

The effect of Periactin on appetite and weight gain only occurs during the period of its administration. After therapy is stopped, there may be some weight loss, but usually not to pre-treatment levels.

Use in the elderly: Periactin should not be used in elderly, debilitated patients. Elderly patients are more likely to experience dizziness, sedation, and hypotension.

Contra-indications, warnings, etc
Contra-indications: Therapy of an acute asthmatic attack; newborn or premature infants; nursing mothers; known sensitivity to cyproheptadine hydrochloride or drugs with similar chemical structure; concurrent use with monoamine oxidase inhibitors; glaucoma; stenosing peptic ulcer; symptomatic prostatic hypertrophy; bladder neck obstruction; pyloroduodenal obstruction; elderly, debilitated patients; predisposition to urinary retention.

Precautions: Antihistamines should not be used to treat lower respiratory tract symptoms including those of acute asthma.

The safety and efficacy of Periactin is not established in children under 2 years old.

Antihistamines may diminish mental alertness; conversely, particularly in the young child, they may occasionally produce excitation.

Patients should be warned against engaging in activities requiring motor co-ordination and mental alertness such as driving a car or operating machinery.

Patients with severe appetite loss should be carefully assessed to exclude serious underlying pathology.

Rarely, prolonged therapy with antihistamines may cause blood dyscrasias.

Because Periactin has an atropine-like action, it should be used cautiously in patients with a history of bronchial asthma, increased intra-ocular pressure, hyperthyroidism, cardiovascular disease, or hypertension.

Periactin Syrup contains sucrose which may produce dental caries and destabilise otherwise well-controlled diabetes.

Drug interactions: MAO inhibitors prolong and intensify the anticholinergic effects of antihistamines.

Antihistamines may have additive effects with alcohol and other CNS depressants, e.g. hypnotics, sedatives, tranquillisers and anti-anxiety agents.

Pregnancy and nursing mothers: The use of any drug in pregnancy or in women of child-bearing age requires that the potential benefit of the drug should be weighed against possible hazards to the embryo or fetus. It is not known whether Periactin is excreted in human milk. Because many drugs are excreted in human milk, and because of the potential for serious adverse reactions in nursing infants from Periactin, a decision should be made whether to discontinue nursing or to discontinue the drug, taking into account the importance of the drug to the mother (see 'Contra-indications').

Side-effects: Side-effects reported with antihistamines are:

Central nervous system: Sedation, sleepiness (often transient), dizziness, disturbed co-ordination, confusion, restlessness, excitation, nervousness, tremor, irritability, insomnia, parasthesiae, neuritis, convulsions, euphoria, hallucinations, hysteria, faintness.

Integumentary: Allergic manifestations of rash and oedema, excessive perspiration, urticaria, photosensitivity.

Special senses: Acute labyrinthitis, blurred vision, diplopia, vertigo, tinnitus.

Cardiovascular: Hypotension, palpitation, tachycardia, extrasystoles, anaphylactic shock.

Haematological: Haemolytic anaemia, leucopenia, agranulocytosis, thrombocytopenia.

Digestive system: Dryness of mouth, epigastric distress, anorexia, nausea, vomiting, diarrhoea, constipation, jaundice.

Genito-urinary: Frequency and difficulty of micturition, urinary retention, early menses.

Respiratory: Dryness of the nose and throat, thickening of bronchial secretions, tightness of chest and wheezing, nasal stuffiness.

Miscellaneous: Fatigue, rigors, headache.

Overdosage: Antihistamine overdosage may vary from CNS depression or stimulation to convulsions and death, especially in infants and children. Atropine-like and GI symptoms may occur.

If vomiting has not occurred spontaneously, it should be induced in the conscious patient with syrup of ipecac. If the patient cannot vomit, gastric lavage with isotonic or half isotonic saline is indicated followed by activated charcoal.

Precautions against aspiration must be taken, especially in infants and children.

Life-threatening CNS signs and symptoms should be treated appropriately.

Saline cathartics usefully draw water into the bowel by osmosis to dilute bowel content rapidly.

Central stimulants must not be used, but vasopressors may be used to counteract hypotension.

Pharmaceutical precautions Periactin should be stored in a dry place below 25°C; the syrup should also be protected from freezing. Periactin Syrup may be diluted with Syrup BP; the mixture should be used within 14 days.

Legal category P.

Package quantities *Tablets:* Bottles of 100. *Syrup:* Bottles of 200 ml.

Further information Nil.

Product licence numbers
Tablets 0025/5017
Syrup 0025/5018

PRIMAXIN*▾

Presentation
For intravenous infusion: Vials containing sterile powders of:

250 mg imipenem (as the monohydrate) with 250 mg cilastatin (as the sodium salt) named Primaxin IV 250 mg.

500 mg imipenem (as the monohydrate) with 500 mg cilastatin (as the sodium salt) named Primaxin IV 500 mg.

For intramuscular administration: Vials containing sterile powders of:

500 mg imipenem (as the monohydrate) with 500 mg cilastatin (as the sodium salt), named Primaxin IM 500 mg.

Uses Broad-spectrum beta-lactam antibiotic.

Primaxin contains imipenem, a member of a new class of beta-lactam antibiotics – the thienamycins; and cilastatin sodium, a specific enzyme-inhibitor, that blocks the metabolism of imipenem in the kidney and substantially increases the concentration of unchanged imipenem in the urinary tract.

Primaxin is bactericidal against an unusually wide-spectrum of Gram-positive, Gram-negative, aerobic and anaerobic pathogens. Primaxin is useful for treating single, and polymicrobic infections, and initiating therapy prior to identification of the causative organisms.

Primaxin is indicated for the treatment of the following infections due to susceptible organisms:

Primaxin IV	*Primaxin IM*
Lower respiratory tract infections	Lower respiratory tract infections (except those caused by *Pseudomonas aeruginosa)*
Intra-abdominal infections	Intra-abdominal infections
Genito-urinary infections	Genito-urinary infections
Gynaecological infections	Gynaecological infections
Septicaemia	Not indicated
Bone and joint infections	Bone and joint infections (there is limited experience in patients with these infections)
Skin and soft tissue infections	Skin and soft tissue infections

Note: Primaxin is not indicated against central nervous system infections.

Because of lack of data, the use of Primaxin alone in the treatment of infections in patients with neutropenia is not recommended.

Primaxin is indicated against mixed infections caused by susceptible aerobic and anaerobic bacteria. The majority of these infections are associated with contamination by faecal flora, or flora originating from the vagina, skin, and mouth.

In these mixed infections, Primaxin is usually effective against *Bacteroides fragilis* sp., the most commonly encountered anaerobic pathogen that is usually resistant to the aminoglycosides, cephalosporins and penicillins.

Prophylaxis: Primaxin IV is also indicated for the prevention of certain post-operative infections in patients undergoing contaminated or potentially contaminated surgical procedures or where the occurrence of post-operative infection could be especially serious.

Mode of action: Imipenem is a potent inhibitor of bacterial cell wall synthesis and is highly reactive towards penicillin-binding protein. Imipenem is more potent in its bactericidal effect than other antibiotics studied. Imipenem also provides extraordinary stability to degradative bacterial beta-lactamases. Imipenem is therefore active against a high percentage of organisms resistant to other beta-lactam antibiotics.

Cilastatin sodium is a competitive, reversible, and specific inhibitor of dehydropeptidase-I, the renal enzyme which metabolises and inactivates imipenem. Cilastatin sodium is devoid of intrinsic antibacterial activity itself and does not affect the antibacterial activity of imipenem.

Bacteriology: Primaxin has a unique anti-bacterial spectrum. Against Gram-negative species, it shares the spectrum of the newer cephalosporins and penicillins; against Gram-positive species Primaxin exerts the high bacterial potency previously only associated with narrow-spectrum beta-lactam antibiotics and the first-generation cephalosporins.

The antibiotic spectrum of Primaxin is broader than other antibiotics studied and includes virtually all clinically significant pathogenic genera.

Organisms against which Primaxin is usually active *in vitro* include:

Gram-negative aerobes: *Escherichia coli*; *Proteus mirabilis*; *Proteus vulgaris*; *Proteus* spp.; *Morganella morganii* (formerly *Proteus morganii*); *Providencia rettgeri* (formerly *Proteus rettgeri*); *Providencia stuartii*; *Providencia* spp; *Hafnia alvei*; *Serratia marcescens*; *Serratia liquefaciens*; *Serratia* spp.; *Klebsiella oxytoca*; *Klebsiella pneumoniae*; *Klebsiella* spp.; *Enterobacter aerogenes*; *Enterobacter agglomerans*; *Enterobacter cloacae*; *Enterobacter* spp.; *Citrobacter freundii*; *Citrobacter diversus*; *Citrobacter* spp.; *Campylobacter* spp.; *Salmonella typhi*; *Salmonella* spp.; *Shigella* spp.; *Pseudomonas aeruginosa*; *Pseudomonas fluorescens*; *Pseudomonas* spp.†; *Acinetobacter* spp. (formerly *Mima-Herellea*); *Haemophilus influenzae* (including beta-lactamase-producing strains); *Haemophilus parainfluenzae*; *Neisseria gonorrhoeae* (including penicillinase-producing strains); *Moraxella* spp.; *Pasteurella multocida*; *Aeromonas hydrophila*; *Yersinia* spp. (formerly *Pasteurella); Yersinia enterocolitica*; *Achromobacter* spp.; *Gardnerella* spp.

†*Xanthomonas maltophilia* and some strains of *Pseudomonas cepacia* are generally not sensitive to Primaxin.

Gram-positive aerobes: Streptococcus Group A (*S. pyogenes*); Streptococcus Group B (*S. agalactiae*); Streptococcus Group C; Enterococcus including *Enterococcus faecalis*; Streptococcus Group D; Streptococcus Group G; *Streptococcus pneumoniae*; *Viridans streptococci* (including alpha and gamma haemolytic strains); *Staphylococcus aureus* (including penicillinase-producing strains); *Staphylococcus epidermidis* (including penicillinase-producing strains); *Erysipelothrix rhusiopathiae.*

Some methicillin-resistant staphylococci and some group D streptococci are not sensitive to Primaxin.

Microaerophilic streptococcus

Gram-negative anaerobes: *Bacteroides fragilis*; *Bacteroides vulgatus*; *Bacteroides melaninogenicus*; *Bacteroides asaccharolyticus*; *Bacteroides distasonis*; *Bacteroides ovatus*; *Bacteroides thetaiotaomicron*; *Bacteroides* spp.; *Fusobacterium nucleatum*; *Fusobacterium necrophorum*; *Fusobacterium* spp.; *Veillonella* spp.

Gram-positive anaerobes: *Actinomyces* spp.; *Clostridium perfringens*; *Clostridium* spp.; *Eubacterium* spp.; *Peptococcus* spp.; *Peptostreptococcus* spp.; *Propionibacterium* spp. including *P. acnes*.

In vitro tests show that imipenem acts synergistically with aminoglycoside antibiotics against some isolates of *Pseudomonas aeruginosa*.

Dosage and administration The total daily dosage and route of administration of Primaxin should be based on the type or severity of infection, consideration of degree of susceptibility of the pathogen(s), renal function and bodyweight. Doses cited are based on a bodyweight of 70 kg. The total daily requirement should be given in equally divided doses.

The dosage recommendations that follow specify the amounts of imipenem to be given. An equivalent amount of cilastatin is provided with this. One vial of Primaxin IV 250 mg therefore provides the equivalents of 250 mg anhydrous imipenem and 250 mg cilastatin; similarly one vial of Primaxin IV or IM 500 mg provides the equivalents of 500 mg anhydrous imipenem and 500 mg cilastatin.

Use in the elderly: Age does not affect the safety and efficacy of Primaxin. The dosage should be determined by the severity of the infection, the susceptibility of the causative organism(s), the patient's clinical condition, and renal function.

INTRAVENOUS ADMINISTRATION: This formulation should not be used intramuscularly. The dosage of Primaxin IV should be determined by the severity of the infection, the antibiotic susceptibility of the causative organism(s) and the condition of the patient.

Note: All recommended doses refer to the imipenem fraction of Primaxin.

Adults (based on 70 kg bodyweight): The usual adult daily dosage is 1–2 g of Primaxin administered in 3–4 equally divided doses (see chart below). In infections due to less sensitive organisms, the daily dose of Primaxin may be increased to a maximum dose of 50 mg/kg/day (or not exceeding 4 g daily).

Usual adult intravenous dosage

Severity of infection	I.V. administration Dose	Dosage interval	Total daily dose
Mild	250 mg	6 hours	1.0 g
Moderate	500 mg	8 hours	1.5 g
Severe – fully susceptible	500 mg	6 hours	2.0 g
Severe and/or life-threatening infections due to less sensitive organisms (primarily some strains of *P. aeruginosa*)	1000 mg 1000 mg	8 hours 6 hours	3.0 g 4.0 g

Each 250 mg or 500 mg dose should be given by intravenous infusion over 20–30 minutes. Each 1000 mg dose should be infused over 40–60 minutes. In patients who develop nausea during infusion, the infusion rate may be slowed.

Prophylactic use: For prophylaxis against post-surgical infections in adults, 1 g Primaxin should be given intravenously on induction of anaesthesia and 1 g three hours later. For high-risk (i.e. colorectal) surgery, two additional 0.5 g doses can be given at 8 and 16 hours after induction.

In patients with renal insufficiency: As in patients with normal renal function, dosing is based on the severity of the infection. The maximum dosage for patients with various degrees of renal functional impairment is shown in the following Table. Doses cited are based on a bodyweight of 70 kg. Proportionate reduction in dose administered should be made for patients with lower bodyweight.

Maximum dosage in relation to renal function

Renal function	*Creatinine clearance (ml/min)*	*Dose (mg)*	*Dosage interval (hrs)*	*Maximum total daily dose† (g)*
Mild impairment	31–70	500	6–8	1.5–2
Moderate impairment	21–30	500	8–12	1–1.5
Severe‡ impairment	0–20	250–500	12	0.5–1.0

†The higher dose should be reserved for infections caused by less susceptible organisms.

‡Patients with creatinine clearance of 6–20 ml/min should be treated with 250 mg (or 3.5 mg/kg, whichever is lower) every 12 hours for most pathogens. When the 500 mg dose is used in these patients, there may be an increased risk of convulsions.

Patients with a creatinine clearance of ≤ 5 ml/min should not receive Primaxin IV unless haemodialysis is started within 48 hours.

Primaxin is cleared by haemodialysis. The patient should receive Primaxin IV immediately after haemodialysis and at 12-hourly intervals thereafter. Dialysis patients, especially those with background CNS disease, should be carefully monitored; patients on haemodialysis should only receive Primaxin IV when the benefit outweighs the potential risk of convulsions (see 'Precautions').

There are currently inadequate data to recommend the use of Primaxin IV for patients on peritoneal dialysis.

Paediatric dosage

Age	*Dose*	*Dosage interval*	*Total daily dose*
3 months of age and older (less than 40 kg bodyweight)	15 mg/kg	6 hours	60 mg/kg

Children over 40 kg bodyweight should receive adult doses.

The maximum daily dose should not exceed 2 g.

Clinical data are insufficient to recommend an optimal dose for children under 3 months of age or infants and children with impaired renal function.

Primaxin IV is not recommended for the therapy of meningitis. If meningitis is suspected an appropriate antibiotic should be used.

Primaxin IV may be used in children with sepsis as long as they are not suspected of having meningitis.

Preparation of solution: The following table is provided for convenience in reconstituting Primaxin IV for intravenous infusion.

Amount of Primaxin (mg)	*Volume of diluent added (ml)†*	*Approximate average concentration (mg/ml)*
Primaxin IV 500 mg	100	5
Primaxin IV 250 mg	50	5

†Shake to dissolve to a colourless or yellow solution. Variation of colour within this range does not affect potency.

Compatibility and stability: In keeping with good clinical and pharmaceutical practice, Primaxin IV should be administered as a freshly prepared solution. On the few occasions where changing circumstances make this impracticable, reconstituted Primaxin IV retains satisfactory potency for 3 hours at room temperature (up to 25°C) or 24 hours in a refrigerator (below 4°C) when prepared in any of the following diluents: 0.9% Sodium Chloride Injection; 5% Dextrose and 0.9% Sodium Chloride; 5% Dextrose and 0.225% Sodium Chloride; 5% Mannitol; 2.5% Mannitol.

Primaxin IV is chemically incompatible with lactate and should not be reconstituted with diluents containing lactate. Primaxin IV can, however, be administered into an IV tubing through which a lactate solution is being infused.

Primaxin IV should not be mixed with, or physically added to, other antibiotics.

INTRAMUSCULAR ADMINISTRATION: This formulation is for intramuscular use only and should not be administered intravenously.

Note: All recommended doses refer to the imipenem fraction of Primaxin.

Adults: A single 500 mg dose of the intramuscular formulation may be used for the treatment of urethritis or cervicitis due to non-penicillinase-producing *Neisseria gonorrhoea.*

The intramuscular formulation may be used as an alternative to the intravenous formulation in the treatment of mild and moderate infections.

Primaxin IM should be given by deep intramuscular injection into a large muscle mass (such as the gluteal or lateral part of the thigh).

Usual adult intramuscular dose

Type or severity of infection	*IM administration* Dose of imipenem	*Dosage interval*	*Total daily dose*
Gonococcal urethritis/cervicitis	500 mg	single dose	0.5 g
Mild infections	500 mg	12 hours	1.0 g
Moderate infections	750 mg	12 hours	1.5 g

In infants and children: The safety and efficacy of the intramuscular formulation have not been studied in the paediatric group.

In patients with renal insufficiency: The safety and efficacy of the intramuscular formulation have not been studied in patients with renal insufficiency.

Preparation of intramuscular suspension: The following table is provided for convenience in reconstituting Primaxin IM with 1% lignocaine solution for intramuscular use.

Strength	*Volume of 1% lignocaine solution to be added (ml†)*	*Final volume (ml)*
Primaxin IM 500 mg	2	2.8

† Shake to prepare a white to light-tan-coloured suspension. Variation of colour within this range does not affect potency. Use immediately after making up.

Contra-indications, warnings, etc

Contra-indication: Hypersensitivity to this product.

Warning: There is some clinical and laboratory evidence of partial cross-allergenicity between Primaxin and the other beta-lactam antibiotics, penicillins and cephalosporins. Severe reactions (including anaphylaxis) have been reported with most beta-lactam antibiotics. Before initiating therapy with Primaxin, careful inquiry should be made concerning previous hypersensitivity reactions to beta-lactam antibiotics. If an allergic reaction to Primaxin occurs, the drug should be discontinued and appropriate measures undertaken.

Precautions: Pseudomembranous colitis, reported with virtually all antibiotics, can range from mild to life-threatening in severity. Primaxin should be prescribed with caution in patients with a history of gastro-intestinal disease, particularly colitis. Treatment-related diarrhoea should always be considered as a pointer to this diagnosis. While studies indicate that a toxin of *Clostridium difficile* is one of the primary causes of antibiotic-associated colitis, other causes should be considered.

Use in pregnancy and lactation: Pregnant monkeys showed evidence of maternal and fetal toxicity with bolus injections at doses equivalent to twice the human dose.

The use of Primaxin in pregnant women has not been studied and Primaxin should therefore not be given in pregnancy unless the anticipated benefit to the mother outweighs the possible risk to the fetus.

It is not known whether Primaxin is excreted in human milk. Because many drugs are excreted by this route, the breast feeding mother should not receive Primaxin. If the use of Primaxin is deemed essential, the mother should stop breast feeding.

Paediatric use: Primaxin IV: Efficacy and tolerability in infants under three months of age have yet to be established; therefore, Primaxin is not recommended for use below this age.

Primaxin IM: Safety and efficacy of 'Primaxin' IM have not yet been studied in the paediatric group; therefore, at present, Primaxin IM is not recommended for use in this group.

Drug interactions: There are no data on adverse drug interactions. However, concomitant probenecid has been shown to double the plasma level and half-life of cilastatin, but with no effect on its urinary recovery.

Concomitant probenecid showed only minimal increases in plasma level and half-life of imipenem, with urinary recovery of active imipenem decreased to approximately 60% of the administered dose.

Central nervous system: Patients with CNS disorders and/or compromised renal function (accumulation of Primaxin may occur) have shown CNS side effects, especially when recommended dosages based on body weight and renal function were exceeded. Hence it is recommended that the dosage schedules of Primaxin should be strictly adhered to, and established anticonvulsant therapy continued.

If focal tremors, myoclonus or convulsions occur, the patient should be evaluated neurologically and placed on anticonvulsant therapy if not already instituted. If these symptoms still continue, the dosage should be reduced, or Primaxin withdrawn completely.

Use in patients with renal insufficiency: Primaxin IV: Patients with creatinine clearances of ≤5 ml/min should not receive Primaxin IV unless haemodialysis is instituted within 48 hours. For patients on haemodialysis, Primaxin IV is only recommended when the benefit outweighs the potential risk of convulsions.

Primaxin IM: Safety and efficacy of Primaxin IM have not yet been studied in patients with renal insufficiency, therefore, at present, Primaxin IM is not recommended for use in this group.

Side-effects: Primaxin is generally well tolerated. Side-effects rarely require cessation of therapy and are generally mild and transient; serious side-effects are rare.

Local reactions: Erythema, local pain and induration, thrombophlebitis.

Allergic: Rash, pruritus, urticaria, toxic epidermal necrolysis (rarely), fever, anaphylactic reactions.

Gastro-intestinal: Nausea, vomiting, diarrhoea. Pseudomembranous colitis has been reported.

Blood: Eosinophilia, leucopenia, neutropenia including agranulocytosis, thrombocytopenia, thrombocytosis decreased haemoglobin, and hepatitis (rarely). A positive direct Coombs test may develop.

Liver function: Mild increases in serum transaminases, bilirubin and/or serum alkaline phosphatase have been reported.

Renal function: Oliguria anuria, polyuria, acute renal failure (rarely). The role of Primaxin in changes in renal function is difficult to assess, since factors predisposing to pre-renal azotemia or to impaired renal function usually have been present. Elevated serum creatinine and blood urea have been seen. A harmless reddish urine discoloration, not to be confused with haematuria, has been seen in children.

Central nervous system: Myoclonic activity, psychic disturbances, confusional states or convulsions have been reported.

Special senses: Taste perversion.

Other reported reactions with an unknown causal relationship

Gastro-intestinal: Haemorrhagic colitis, gastro-enteritis, abdominal pain, glossitis, tongue papillar hypertrophy, heartburn, pharyngeal pain, increased salivation.

Central nervous system: Dizziness, somnolence, encephalopathy, paraesthesiae, vertigo, headache.

Special senses: Transient hearing loss in patients with impaired hearing, tinnitus.

Respiratory: Chest discomfort, dyspnoea, hyperventilation, thoracic spine pain.

Cardiovascular: Hypotension, palpitations, tachycardia.

Skin: Erythema multiforme, facial oedema, flushing, cyanosis hyperhidrosis, skin texture changes, candidiasis, pruritus vulvae.

Body as a whole: Polyarthralgia, asthenia/weakness.

Treatment of overdosage: No information is available at present.

Pharmaceutical precautions Vials of dry Primaxin should be stored below 25°C protected from light until immediately before use. They should not be frozen, or exposed to temperatures above 50°C.

Legal category POM.

Package quantities *For intravenous use:* Single 60-ml vial containing sterile powders of 250 mg imipenem (as the monohydrate) with 250 mg cilastatin (as the sodium salt).

Single 120-ml vial containing sterile powders of 500 mg imipenem (as the monohydrate) with 500 mg cilastatin (as the sodium salt).

For intramuscular use: Single 15-ml vial containing sterile powders of 500 mg imipenem (as the monohydrate) with 500 mg cilastatin (as the sodium salt).

Further information *The differences between intramuscular and intravenous administration should be recognised.*

Intramuscular use has a 75% bioavailability of intravenous infusion. Effective absorption from the intramuscular site is longer; plasma levels of a single 500 mg or 750 mg dose of imipenem remained above 2 mcg/ml for at least six to eight hours. This is above the MIC_{90} of such pathogens as *Serratia* spp., *Acinetobacter* spp.,

Bacteroides fragilis and all Gram-positive cocci except enterococci. Alternatively, intravenous infusion offers peak plasma levels from single 250, 500 and 1000 mg doses of 17, 39 and 66 mcg/ml, respectively. The plasma levels of these doses decline below 1 microgram/ml or less in four to six hours.

Approximately 70% of the antibiotic administered intravenously was recovered intact from the urine in 10 hours. Concentrations exceeded 10 micrograms/ml for up to eight hours after a single intravenous dose of 500 mg Primaxin.

However, intramuscular administration of a single dose of 500 mg or 750 mg of the antibiotic gave urine levels above 10 micrograms/ml for 12 hours with a total urinary recovery of 50% of the dose.

No accumulation of imipenem is seen in patients with normal kidney function in either plasma or urine at any of the dosage regimens recommended.

Product licence numbers
Primaxin for intravenous administration:
250 mg 0025/0228
500 mg 0025/0229

Primaxin for intramuscular administration: 500 mg 0025/0230.

SALURIC*

Presentation White, half-scored tablets, marked 'MSD 432', containing 500 mg Chlorothiazide BP.

Uses Thiazide diuretic and antihypertensive.

Oedema associated with congestive heart failure, hepatic cirrhosis, premenstrual tension, and in oedema due to various forms of renal dysfunction (i.e. nephrotic syndrome, acute glomerulonephritis and chronic renal failure). Hypertension, either alone or as an adjunct to other antihypertensive drugs.

Dosage and administration Dosage should be determined on an individual basis, and the lowest dosage necessary to achieve the desired result should be used.

Adults–for oedema: Usually ½–2 tablets (250–1,000 mg) once or twice a day. Many patients respond to intermittent therapy: every other day, or three to five consecutive days a week. Intermittent therapy is less likely to produce excessive diuretic response with resulting electrolyte imbalance. The maximum recommended daily dose is 4 tablets (2,000 mg).

In oedema accompanying premenstrual tension: ½–1 tablet (250–500 mg) once or twice a day, from the first morning of symptoms until the onset of the menses.

Adults – for control of hypertension: The usual starting dose is ½–1 tablet (250–500 mg) a day as a single or divided dose.

In some patients, a ¼ tablet (125 mg), alone or with another antihypertensive, may be sufficient to initiate therapy. Dosage should be adjusted to response, but should not exceed 2 tablets (1,000 mg) a day.

Thiazides may add to the action of other antihypertensives. If Saluric is added to therapy with other antihypertensive agents, dosage reduction of such agents may be necessary to prevent an excessive drop in blood pressure.

Infants and children: Usually 25 mg per kg bodyweight a day, given in two doses. Infants under six months may need up to 35 mg per kg a day, in two doses.

On this basis, infants up to two years of age may be given 125–375 mg of Saluric daily in two doses. Children from 2 to 12 years of age may be given 375 mg to 1.0 g daily in two doses. Dosage in both age groups should be based on bodyweight.

Use in the elderly: Particular caution is needed in the elderly because of their susceptibility to electrolyte imbalance; the dosage should be carefully adjusted according to renal function and clinical response.

Contra-indications, warnings, etc
Contra-indications: Anuria, known hypersensitivity to this product or to other sulphonamide-derived drugs, severe renal or hepatic failure, Addison's disease, hypercalcaemia, concurrent lithium therapy. See 'Use in pregnancy' and 'Use in breast-feeding mothers', under 'Precautions'.

Precautions: Patients should be carefully monitored for signs of fluid and electrolyte imbalance (hyponatraemia, hypochloraemic alkalosis, hypokalaemia and hypomagnesaemia). It is particularly important to make serum and urine electrolyte determinations when the patient is vomiting excessively or receiving parenteral fluids. Warning signs or symptoms of fluid and electrolyte imbalance include: dryness of mouth, thirst, weakness, lethargy, drowsiness, restlessness, seizures, muscle pains or cramps, muscular fatigue, hypotension, oliguria, tachycardia, and gastro-intestinal disturbances such as nausea and vomiting.

Hypokalaemia may develop, especially with brisk diuresis, when severe cirrhosis is present, or after prolonged therapy. Hypokalaemia can sensitise or exaggerate the response of the heart to the toxic effects of digitalis (e.g. increased ventricular irritability).

Sensitivity reactions may occur in patients with or without history of allergy or bronchial asthma.

Hypokalaemia may be avoided or treated in the adult by concurrent use of amiloride hydrochloride (Midamor*), a potassium-conserving agent. It may also be avoided by giving potassium chloride or foods with a high potassium content. (Note that symptoms and signs which might indicate ulceration or obstruction of the small bowel in patients taking tablets or capsules containing potassium salts are indications for stopping treatment with such preparations immediately.)

Diuretic-induced hyponatraemia is usually mild and asymptomatic. Dilutional hyponatraemia may occur in oedematous patients in hot weather; and, except in rare instances when hyponatraemia is life-threatening, appropriate therapy is water restriction rather than administration of salt.

Thiazides may decrease serum PBI levels without signs of thyroid disturbances.

Thiazides may decrease urinary calcium excretion, and may also cause intermittent and slight elevation of serum calcium in the absence of known disorders of calcium metabolism. Thiazides should be discontinued before carrying out tests for parathyroid function.

When creatinine clearance falls below 30 ml/min, thiazide diuretics become ineffective.

Azotaemia may be precipitated or increased by Saluric. Cumulative effects of chlorothiazide may develop in patients with impaired renal function. If increasing azotaemia and oliguria occur during treatment of renal disease, Saluric should be discontinued.

Thiazides should be used with caution in patients with impaired hepatic function or progressive liver disease, since minor alterations of fluid and electrolyte balance may precipitate hepatic coma.

Hyperuricaemia may occur, or gout may be precipitated, in certain patients receiving thiazide therapy.

Thiazide therapy may impair glucose tolerance.

Increases in cholesterol and triglyceride levels may be associated with thiazide diuretic therapy.

The possibility of exacerbation or activation of systemic lupus erythematosus has been reported.

Latent diabetes may become manifest during thiazide administration.

Use in pregnancy: Thiazides cross the placental barrier and appear in the cord blood. The use of Saluric when pregnancy is present or suspected, requires that the benefits of the drug be weighed against the possible hazards to the fetus. These hazards include fetal or neonatal jaundice, thrombocytopenia, and possibly other adverse reactions which have occurred in the adult. The routine use of diuretics in otherwise healthy, pregnant women with or without mild oedema is not indicated, because their use may be associated with hypovolaemia, increased blood viscosity and decreased placental perfusion.

Use in breast-feeding mothers: Thiazides appear in breast milk. If use of the drug is deemed essential, the patient should stop breast-feeding.

Drug interactions: Alcohol, barbiturates or narcotics: Co-administration may potentiate orthostatic hypotension. *Oral and parenteral antidiabetic drugs* may require adjustment of dosage with concurrent use. *Other anti-hypertensive drugs* may have an additive effect. Discontinuation of diuretic therapy 2–3 days before the initiation of treatment with an ACE-inhibitor may reduce the likelihood of first-dose hypotension. The antihypertensive effect of the drug may be enhanced in the post-sympathectomy patient. *Corticosteroids or ACTH* may intensify any thiazide-induced electrolyte depletion, particularly hypokalaemia. *Pressor amines such as adrenaline* may show decreased arterial responsiveness when used with Saluric, but this reaction is not enough to preclude their therapeutic usefulness. *Non-depolarising muscle relaxants such as tubocurarine* may possibly interact with Saluric to increase muscle relaxation. *Non-steroidal anti-inflammatory drugs* may attenuate the diuretic and antihypertensive effect of diuretics.

Drug/laboratory tests: Because thiazides may affect calcium metabolism, Saluric may interfere with tests for parathyroid function.

Side-effects

Gastro-intestinal system: Anorexia, gastric irritation, nausea, vomiting, cramps, diarrhoea, constipation, jaundice (intrahepatic cholestatic jaundice), pancreatitis, salivary gland inflammation.

Central nervous system: Dizziness, vertigo, paraesthesiae, headache, yellow vision.

Haematological: Leucopenia, agranulocytosis, thrombocytopenia, aplastic anaemia, haemolytic anaemia.

Cardiovascular: Hypotension, including orthostatic hypotension (may be aggravated by alcohol, barbiturates, narcotics or antihypertensive drugs).

Hypersensitivity: Purpura, photosensitivity, rash, urticaria, necrotising angiitis (vasculitis, cutaneous vasculitis), fever, respiratory distress including pneumonitis and pulmonary oedema, anaphylactic reactions.

Metabolic: Hyperglycaemia, glycosuria, hyperuricaemia, electrolyte imbalance.

Renal: renal dysfunction, interstitial nephritis, renal failure.

Other: Muscle spasm, weakness, restlessness, transient blurred vision, impotence.

Whenever side-effects are moderate or severe, thiazide dosage should be reduced or therapy withdrawn.

Overdosage: The most common signs and symptoms observed are those caused by electrolyte depletion (hypokalaemia, hypochloraemia, hyponatraemia) and dehydration resulting from excessive diuresis. If digitalis has also been administered, hypokalaemia may accentuate cardiac arrhythmias.

In the event of overdosage, treatment should be symptomatic and supportive; no specific antidote is known. If ingestion is recent, the stomach should be emptied by emesis or gastric lavage. Dehydration, electrolyte imbalance, hepatic coma, and hypotension should be corrected by standard methods. For impaired respiration, oxygen or artificial respiration should be given.

The plasma half-life of chlorothiazide is 45–120 minutes.

Pharmaceutical precautions Keep container tightly closed; store in a cool place, protected from light.

Legal category POM.

Package quantities Bottles of 100.

Further information Diuresis usually begins within two hours, is at a peak after four hours and persists for six to twelve hours. No rigid dietary salt restriction required.

Product licence number 0025/5019.

SODIUM PARA-AMINOHIPPURATE

Presentation A clear, colourless to slightly yellow solution for intravenous injection, containing in each 10 ml of sterile solution 2 g sodium para-aminohippurate. Inactive ingredient: Sodium Hydroxide BP.

Uses As a diagnostic agent for the estimation of effective renal plasma flow (RPF). In research procedures, for the measurement of the functional capacity of the renal tubular secretory mechanism (Tm_{PAH}).

Dosage and administration For intravenous use only.

For the measurement of RPF, the concentration of sodium para-aminohippurate in the plasma is maintained at 2 mg per 100 ml. As a research procedure for the measurement of Tm_{PAH}, the plasma level of sodium para-aminohippurate must be sufficient to saturate the capacity of the tubular secretory cells. Concentrations of from 40 to 60 mg per 100 ml are necessary.

Contra-indications, warnings, etc

Precautions: Intravenous solutions must be administered with caution in patients with low cardiac reserve, since a rapid increase in plasma volume can precipitate congestive heart failure.

For measurement of RPF, small doses of sodium para-aminohippurate are used. However, in research procedures for Tm_{PAH} determinations high plasma levels are required to saturate the capacity of the tubular cells. During these procedures the intravenous administration of sodium para-aminohippurate solutions should be carried out slowly and with caution. The patient should be continuously observed for any adverse reactions.

Renal clearance measurement of sodium para-aminohippurate cannot be made with any significant accuracy in patients receiving sulphonamides, procaine or thiazolesulphone. These compounds interfere with chemical colour development essential to the analytical procedures.

Probenecid depresses tubular secretion of certain weak acids such as sodium para-aminohippurate. Therefore, patients receiving probenecid will have erroneously low RPF and Tm_{PAH} values. Clearance is also affected by penicillins and salicylates.

Side-effects: Vasomotor disturbances, flushing, tingling, nausea, vomiting, cramps. Patients may have a sensation of warmth or the desire to defaecate or urinate during or shortly after the administration of a primary dose.

Overdosage: The dose is carefully controlled by experiment; no data are available on the symptoms of overdosage. No antidote is available.

The biological half-life of sodium para-aminohippurate is 10.2 minutes.

Pharmaceutical precautions No special requirements.

Legal category POM.

Package quantities Vials of 10 ml.

Further information Methods of calculating renal function are to be found in the package leaflet.

Product licence number 0025/5080.

TIMOPTOL*

Presentation Clear, colourless to light yellow, sterile eye drops containing Timolol Maleate BP equivalent to 0.25% and 0.5% w/v solution of timolol.

Uses Timoptol Ophthalmic Solution is a beta-adrenergic receptor blocking agent used topically in the reduction of elevated intra-ocular pressure in various conditions including the following: patients with ocular hypertension; patients with chronic open-angle glaucoma including aphakic patients; some patients with secondary glaucoma.

Dosage and administration Recommended therapy

is one drop 0.25% solution in the affected eye twice a day.

If clinical response is not adequate, dosage may be changed to one drop 0.5% solution in each affected eye twice a day. If needed, Timoptol may be used with miotics, adrenaline or systemically-administered carbonic anhydrase inhibitors.

Intra-ocular pressure should be reassessed approximately four weeks after starting treatment because response to Timoptol may take a few weeks to stabilise.

Provided that the intra-ocular pressure is maintained at satisfactory levels, many patients can then be placed on once-a-day therapy.

Transfer from other agents: When another topical beta-blocking agent is being used, discontinue its use after a full day of therapy and start treatment with 'Timoptol' the next day with one drop of 0.25% Timoptol in each affected eye twice a day. The dosage may be increased to one drop of 0.5% solution in each affected eye twice a day if the response is not adequate.

When transferring a patient from a single anti-glaucoma agent other than a topical beta-blocking agent, continue the agent and add one drop of 0.25% Timoptol in each affected eye twice a day. On the following day, discontinue the previous agent completely, and continue with Timoptol. If a higher dosage of Timoptol is required, substitute one drop of 0.5% solution in each affected eye twice a day (see 'Further information').

Paediatric use is not currently recommended.

Use in the elderly: There has been wide experience with the usage of timolol maleate in elderly patients. The dosage recommendations above reflect the clinical data derived from this experience.

Contra-indications, warnings, etc

Contra-indications: Bronchial asthma, history of bronchial asthma, or severe chronic obstructive pulmonary disease; sinus bradycardia, second and third degree AV block, overt cardiac failure, cardiogenic shock; and hypersensitivity to this product or other beta-blocking agents.

Precautions: Like other topically applied ophthalmic drugs, Timoptol may be absorbed systemically and adverse reactions seen with oral beta-blockers may occur.

Cardiac failure should be adequately controlled before beginning therapy with Timoptol. Patients with a history of severe cardiac disease should be watched for signs of cardiac failure and have their pulse rates checked.

Respiratory and cardiac reactions, including death due to bronchospasm in patients with asthma and, rarely, death associated with cardiac failure have been reported.

The effect on intra-ocular pressure or the known effects of systemic beta-blockade may be exaggerated when Timoptol is given to patients already receiving an oral beta-blocking agent. The response of these patients should be closely observed.

There have been reports of skin rashes and/or dry eyes associated with the use of beta-adrenergic receptor blocking drugs. The reported incidence is small and in most cases the symptoms have cleared when treatment was withdrawn. Discontinuation of the drug should be considered if any such reaction is not otherwise explicable. Cessation of therapy involving beta-blockade should be gradual.

Timoptol contains benzalkonium chloride as a preservative and, therefore, should not be used in patients who continue to wear hydrophilic (soft) contact lenses.

In patients with open angle glaucoma, the immediate objective of treatment is to reopen the angle. This requires constricting the pupil with a miotic. Timoptol has little or no effect on the pupil. When Timoptol is used to reduce elevated intraocular pressure in angle closure glaucoma it should be used with a miotic and not alone.

Drug interactions: Although Timoptol alone has little or no effect on pupil size, mydriasis has occasionally been reported when Timoptol is given with adrenaline.

Timoptol may potentially add to the effects of oral calcium antagonists, rauwolfia alkaloids or beta-blockers to induce hypotension and/or marked bradycardia.

Breast-feeding: A decision for breast-feeding mothers either to stop taking Timoptol or stop nursing should be based on the importance of the drug to the mother.

Use in pregnancy: Timoptol has not been studied in human pregnancy. The use of Timoptol requires that the anticipated benefit be weighed against possible hazards.

Side-effects: Timoptol is usually well tolerated.

Special senses: Signs and symptoms of ocular irritation, including conjunctivitis, blepharitis, keratitis, and decreased corneal sensitivity. Visual disturbances, including refractive changes (due to withdrawal of miotic therapy in some cases), diplopia, and ptosis.

Cardiovascular: Bradycardia, arrhythmia, hypotension, syncope, heart block, cerebrovascular accident, cerebral ischaemia, congestive heart failure, palpitation, cardiac arrest.

Respiratory: Bronchospasm (predominantly in patients with pre-existing bronchospastic disease), respiratory failure, dyspnoea.

Body as a whole: Headache, asthenia, nausea, dizziness, depression, fatigue.

Integumentary: Hypersensitivity reactions including localised and generalised rash and urticaria.

Causal relationship unknown: The following adverse effects have been reported, but a causal relationship to Timoptol has not been established; aphakic cystoid macular oedema, dry mouth, nasal congestion, anorexia, dyspepsia, CNS effects (e.g. behavioural change including confusion, hallucinations, anxiety, disorientation, nervousness, somnolence, and other psychiatric disturbances), hypertension, and retroperitoneal fibrosis. The adverse reactions seen with oral timolol maleate may occur with Timoptol.

Overdosage: No specific data are available. The most common signs and symptoms to be expected following overdosage with a beta-adrenoreceptor blocking agent are symptomatic bradycardia, hypotension, bronchospasm, and acute cardiac failure. If overdosage occurs, the following measures should be considered.

1. Gastric lavage, if ingested. Studies have shown that timolol does not dialyse readily.
2. Symptomatic bradycardia: Atropine sulphate, 0.25 to 2 mg intravenously, should be used to induce vagal blockade. If bradycardia persists, intravenous isoprenaline hydrochloride should be administered cautiously. In refractory cases, the use of a cardiac pacemaker may be considered.
3. Hypotension: A sympathomimetic pressor agent such as dopamine, dobutamine or noradrenaline should be used. In refractory cases, the use of glucagon has been reported to be useful.
4. Bronchospasm: Isoprenaline hydrochloride should be used. Additional therapy with aminophylline may be considered.
5. Acute cardiac failure: Conventional therapy with digitalis, diuretics, and oxygen should be instituted immediately. In refractory cases, the use of intravenous aminophylline is suggested. This may be followed, if necessary, by glucagon which has been reported useful.
6. Heart block (second or third degree): Isoprenaline hydrochloride or a pacemaker should be used.

Pharmaceutical precautions Timoptol is stable at room temperature. Protect from light.

Legal category POM.

Package quantities Both the 0.25% and 0.5% w/v solution are presented in special metered-dose Ocumeter* Dispensers, each containing 5 ml.

Further information Unlike miotics, Timoptol reduces IOP with little or no effect on accommodation or pupil size. In patients with cataracts, the inability to see around lenticular opacities when the pupil is constricted is avoided. When changing patients from miotics to Timoptol a refraction might be necessary when these effects of the miotic have passed.

Diminished response after prolonged therapy with Timoptol has been reported in some patients.

Timoptol has been generally well tolerated in glaucoma patients wearing conventional hard contact lenses. Timoptol has not been studied in patients wearing lenses made with material other than polymethylmethacrylate (PMMA).

Product licence numbers

0.25%	Ophthalmic Solution	0025/0134
0.5%	Ophthalmic Solution	0025/0135

TYROZETS*

Presentation Pink, aniseed-flavoured lozenges, marked 'MSD' one side and Tyrozets the other, containing 1 mg tyrothricin and 5 mg Benzocaine BP.

Uses Antibiotic and local analgesic-anaesthetic.

For minor mouth and throat irritations; secondary irritation following tonsillectomy and other mouth and throat surgery.

Dosage and administration *Adults:* 1 lozenge every three hours; maximum, 8 lozenges in 24 hours.

Children: Dosage of Tyrozets should be reduced in children. Tyrozets are not recommended for children under the age of three years.

If an adequate response is not evident within two days, consider stopping Tyrozets. Do not use for longer than five consecutive days.

To allow maximum contact with inflamed tissues, Tyrozets should not be chewed or swallowed whole, but allowed to dissolve slowly in the mouth.

Contra-indications, warnings, etc

Contra-indications: Hypersensitivity to tyrothricin or to benzocaine. If evidence of sensitivity occurs during therapy. Tyrozets should be discontinued.

Precautions: The use of antibiotics may cause overgrowth of non-susceptible organisms. If new infections due to bacteria or fungi appear during therapy, Tyrozets should be stopped and appropriate measures taken.

Topical use of Tyrozets as an aid to prevention of local infection in no way alters the need for adequate systemic therapy if an infection should develop.

Tyrozets contain sucrose, which may produce dental caries and destabilise otherwise well-controlled diabetes.

Due to the local anaesthetic property of Tyrozets, it may be necessary either to avoid food when anaesthesia is at its maximum, or to rinse the mouth with water after eating, to prevent any further trauma to the mucous membranes.

Side-effects: Blackness or soreness of the tongue may occur, but usually disappears when therapy is stopped.

Skin rashes have been reported to occur after benzocaine administration.

Methaemoglobinaemia has been reported to occur rarely in infants and children after benzocaine absorption.

Overdosage: Tyrozets should only be sucked in the mouth. Insertion into the nasal cavity can damage the sensory epithelium with risk of prolonged loss of smell. Parenteral use may result in haemolysis, liver, and kidney damage.

No antidote to either tyrothricin or benzocaine is available. Treatment of overdosage should be symptomatic and supportive; emesis should be induced or gastric lavage performed.

Pharmaceutical precautions Store in a cool, dry place.

Legal category P.

Package quantities Twin vials of 12 lozenges.

Further information Since tyrothricin is used only locally and has a low index of sensitisation and toxicity, cross-sensitisation with antibiotics used systemically in more serious infections is unlikely.

Product licence number 0025/5072.

UTINOR* ▼

Presentation White, oval tablets marked Utinor containing 400 mg norfloxacin.

Uses Broad spectrum, bactericidal agent indicated for the treatment of upper and lower, complicated and uncomplicated, acute and chronic urinary tract infections. These infections include cystitis, pyelitis, pyelonephritis, chronic prostatitis and those urinary infections associated with urological surgery, neurogenic bladder or nephrolithiasis caused by bacteria susceptible to Utinor.

Mode of action: Utinor inhibits bacterial deoxyribonucleic acid synthesis and is bactericidal. At the molecular level, three specific events were attributed to Utinor in *Escherichia coli* cells:

(1) inhibition of the ATP-dependent DNA supercoiling reaction catalysed by DNA gyrase;
(2) inhibition of the relaxation of supercoiled DNA;
(3) promotion of double-stranded DNA breakage.

Spontaneous mutation resistance to norfloxacin has occurred rarely and resistance of the organism during therapy has developed in less than 1% of patients treated.

Bacteriology: Utinor has a broad spectrum of antibacterial activity against Gram-positive and Gram-negative aerobic pathogens. The fluorine atom at the 6 position provides increased potency against Gram-negative organisms and the piperazine moiety at the 7 position is responsible for the anti-pseudomonal activity.

Utinor is active *in vitro* against the following bacteria:

Bacteria found in urinary tract infections:

Enterobacteriaceae – Citrobacter spp; *Citrobacter diversus*; *Citrobacter freundii*; *Edwardsiella tarda*; *Enterobacter* spp; *Enterobacter agglomerans*; *Enterobacter aerogenes*; *Enterobacter cloacae*; *Escherichia coli*; *Hafnia* spp; *Klebsiella* spp; *Klebsiella oxytoca*; *Klebsiella pneumoniae*; *Morganella morganii*; *Proteus* spp. (indole positive); *Proteus mirabilis*; *Proteus vulgaris*; *Providencia* spp; *Providencia rettgeri*; *Providencia stuartii*; *Serratia* spp; *Serratia marcescens*.

Pseudomonadaceae – Pseudomonas aeruginosa; *Pseudomonas cepacia*; *Pseudomonas fluorescens*.

Other – Alcaligenes spp; *Flavobacterium* spp.

Gram-positive cocci – Enterococci; *Staphyloccus* spp; *Staphylococcus* Coag. negative; *Staphylococcus aureus*; *Staphylococcus epidermidis*; *Staphylococcus saprophyticus*; *Streptococcus* Group B, Group D, Group G; *Streptococcus viridans*.

In addition, Utinor is active against *Bacillus cereus*, *Neisseria gonorrhoea*, *Ureaplasma urealyticum*, and *Haemophilus influenzae*.

Utinor is not active against anaerobes, including *Actinomyces* spp, *Fusobacterium* spp., *Bacteroides* spp, and *Clostridium* spp, other than *C. perfringens*.

There is no cross-resistance between norfloxacin and structurally unrelated antibacterial agents such as penicillins, cephalosporins, tetracyclines, macrolides, aminocyclitols and sulphonamides, 2,4 diaminopyrimidines, or combinations thereof (e.g. co-trimoxazole).

Dosage and administration Susceptibility of the causative organism to Utinor should be tested. However, therapy may be initiated before obtaining the results of these tests.

Diagnosis	*Dosage*	*Therapy duration*
Uncomplicated lower urinary tract infections (e.g. cystitis)†	400 mg twice daily	3 days
Urinary tract infections	400 mg twice daily	7–10 days
Chronic relapsing urinary tract infection††	400 mg twice daily	up to 12 wks

†Trials in over 600 patients have demonstrated the efficacy and tolerability of Utinor in the three-day treatment of uncomplicated urinary tract infections.
††If adequate suppression is obtained within the first four weeks of therapy, the dose of Utinor may be reduced to 400 mg daily.

Patients with renal impairment: Utinor is suitable for the treatment of patients with impaired renal function. In patients with a creatinine clearance of less than 30 ml/min, the plasma half-life is increased from 3–4 hours to 6.5 hours and the recommended dose is one 400 mg tablet once daily. At this dosage, concentrations in appropriate body tissues or fluids exceed the MICs for most pathogens sensitive to Utinor, even when the glomerular filtration rate is as low as 10 ml/min. There are insufficient data to recommend treatment in patients whose creatinine clearance is less than 10 ml/min.

Use in the elderly: Pharmacokinetic studies have shown no appreciable changes, when compared to younger patients, apart from a slight prolongation of half-life. In the absence of renal impairment no adjustment of dosage is necessary. Limited clinical studies have shown Utinor to be well tolerated.

Contra-indications, warnings, etc
Contra-indications: Hypersensitivity to any component of this product or any chemically related quinolone antibacterials.

Utinor is contra-indicated in prepubertal children and growing adolescents.

Precautions: Convulsions have been reported rarely with norfloxacin although a causal relationship has not been established.

As with other drugs in this class, Utinor should not be used in patients with a history of convulsions unless there is an overwhelming clinical need.

Use in pregnancy and lactation: There is no evidence from animal studies that norfloxacin has any teratogenic or mutagenic effects. Embryotoxicity secondary to maternotoxicity was observed after large doses in rabbits. Embryonic losses were observed in cynomolgus monkeys without any teratogenic effects. The relevance of these findings for humans is uncertain.

The safe use of Utinor in pregnant women has not been established; however, as with other quinolones, norfloxacin has been shown to cause arthropathy in immature animals and therefore its use during pregnancy is not recommended.

It is not known whether Utinor is excreted in human milk; administration to breast-feeding mothers is thus not recommended.

Use in children: As with other quinolones, Utinor has been shown to cause arthropathy in immature animals. The safety of Utinor in children has not been adequately explored and therefore the use of Utinor in prepubertal children or growing adolescents is contra-indicated.

Drug interactions: Co-administration of probenecid does not affect serum concentrations of norfloxacin, but urinary excretion of the drug diminishes.

As with other organic acid antibacterials, antagonism has been demonstrated *in vitro* between Utinor and nitrofurantoin.

Elevated plasma levels of theophylline have been reported with concomitant quinolone use. There have been rare reports of theophylline-related side effects in patients on concomitant therapy with norfloxacin and theophylline. Therefore, monitoring of theophylline plasma levels should be considered and dosage of theophylline adjusted as required.

Elevated serum levels of cyclosporin have been reported with concomitant use of norfloxacin. Cyclosporin serum levels should be monitored and appropriate cyclosporin dosage adjustments made when these drugs are used concomitantly.

Sucralfate or antacids should not be administered concomitantly with norfloxacin or within two hours of administration of norfloxacin.

Quinolones, including norfloxacin, may enhance the effects of the anticoagulant warfarin, or its derivatives, by displacing significant amounts from serum albumin-binding sites. When concomitant administration of these products cannot be avoided, measurements of prothrombin time or other suitable coagulation tests should be carried out.

Side-effects: The overall incidence of drug-related side-effects reported during clinical trials was approximately 3%.

The most common side-effects have been gastrointestinal, neuropsychiatric and skin reactions, and include nausea, headache, dizziness, rash, heartburn, abdominal pain/cramps and diarrhoea.

Less commonly, other events such as anorexia, sleep disturbances, depression, anxiety/nervousness, irritability, euphoria, disorientation, hallucination, tinnitus and epiphora have been reported.

Abnormal laboratory values observed during clinical trials included: leucopenia, elevation of ALAT (SGPT), ASAT (SGOT), eosinophilia, neutropenia, thrombocytopenia.

With more widespread use the following additional side-effects have been reported:

Hypersensitivity reactions: Hypersensitivity reactions including angioedema and urticaria; arthritis, myalgia, arthralgia.

Skin – Photosensitivity; Stevens-Johnson syndrome; toxic epidermal necrolysis, exfoliative dermatitis.

Gastro-intestinal – Pseudomembranous colitis.

Treatment of overdosage: No information is available at present.

In the event of acute overdosage, the stomach should be emptied by induced vomiting or by gastric lavage and the patient carefully observed and given symptomatic and supportive treatment. Adequate hydration must be maintained.

Pharmaceutical precautions Store in a cool, dry place protected from light.

Legal category POM.

Package quantities Utinor is available as blister packs of 6 and 14 tablets.

Further information Nil.

Product licence numbers 0025/0254.

ZINAMIDE*

Presentation White, half-scored tablets, marked 'MSD 504', containing 500 mg Pyrazinamide BP.

Uses Antituberculous agent.

Zinamide is indicated in patients with active tuberculosis caused by *Mycobacterium tuberculosis*. Zinamide is not active against the atypical mycobacteria. Zinamide should only be given in combination with other antituberculous agents.

Dosage and administration *Usual adult dosage:* 20–35 mg/kg a day divided into three or four doses; the maximum daily dosage is 3 g regardless of body weight. Zinamide should be administered with at least one other effective antituberculous drug. The use of Zinamide in combination therapy does not modify the accepted dosages of other antituberculous agents.

Paediatric use has not been established (see 'Precautions').

Use in the elderly: The general considerations outlined above should also apply to elderly patients.

Contra-indications, warnings, etc
Contra-indications: Zinamide is contra-indicated in patients hypersensitive to it; in patients with hepatic disease; and in those with hyperuricaemia and/or gouty arthritis.

Zinamide is contra-indicated in breast-feeding mothers. If its use is deemed essential, the patient should stop breast-feeding.

Precautions: Zinamide should only be used when close daily observation of the patient is possible, and when laboratory facilities are available for performing frequent liver function tests and blood uric acid determinations. Pre-treatment examinations should include *in vitro* sensitivity tests of recent cultures of *M. tuberculosis* from the patient as measured against the usual antituberculous drugs.

Liver function tests, especially aspartate transferase (AST) and alanine transferase (ALT) determinations, should be carried out prior to therapy, and then every two to four weeks during therapy. Therapy with Zinamide should be withdrawn and not reinstated if signs of hepatocellular damage occur.

If hyperuricaemia accompanied by an acute gouty arthritis occurs, therapy should be discontinued and not reinstated. Close monitoring is advised to detect any increasing difficulty in the management of patients with a history of gout or diabetes mellitus.

Reduction in the size and/or frequency of dose is recommended for patients with renal insufficiency.

Children: The safety of Zinamide for use in children has not been established. Because of its potential toxicity, the use of Zinamide in children should be avoided unless it is considered crucial.

Pregnancy: There have been no well-controlled studies in pregnant women. Zinamide should only be used if the potential benefit justifies the risk to the fetus.

Side-effects: A hepatic reaction is the most common side-effect of Zinamide. This varies from a symptomless abnormality of hepatic cell function, detectable only by laboratory tests, through a mild syndrome of fever, anorexia, malaise, liver tenderness, hepatomegaly and splenomegaly, to more serious reactions such as clinical jaundice, and rare cases of progressive fulminating acute yellow atrophy and death.

Other side-effects – active gout, sideroblastic anaemia, arthralgias, anorexia, nausea and vomiting, dysuria, malaise, fever, urticaria, aggravation of peptic ulcer.

Overdosage: There has been no experience reported with pyrazinamide poisoning. Liver toxicity and hyperuricaemia may occur with overdosage.

The stomach should be emptied by gastric lavage if necessary.

There is no specific antidote. General supportive measures should be employed. Liver function should be monitored closely, and a high-carbohydrate, low-fat diet employed. Care should be taken to avoid exposure of the patient to other potential hepatotoxic agents, including alcohol. Benzodiazepines may be given if there is evidence of central nervous system stimulation. Probenecid may be given for hyperuricaemia.

The plasma half-life of pyrazinamide is about nine to ten hours.

Pharmaceutical precautions Keep container tightly closed; store in a cool place, protected from light.

Legal category POM.

Package quantities Bottles of 100. Pure pyrazinamide powder, for sensitivity tests, is available on request.

Further information Zinamide has been used with other agents, notably rifampicin, isoniazid or streptomycin. The use of such combinations has produced sputum conversion in a high proportion of patients able to continue therapy for at least six months.

Product licence number 0025/5038.

ZOCOR*▼

Presentation Peach, oval-shaped, film-coated tablets, marked 'ZOCOR 10' on one side, containing 10 mg simvastatin, MSD.

Tan, oval-shaped, film-coated tablets, marked 'ZOCOR 20' on one side, containing 20 mg simvastatin, MSD.

Uses For use in patients with primary hypercholesterolaemia, intolerant or not responsive to other forms of therapy, with a cholesterol level in excess of 7.8 mmol/l.

Mode of action: Zocor is metabolised after oral ingestion to a substance which inhibits 3-hydroxy-3 methylglutaryl coenzyme A (HMG-CoA) reductase, an enzyme which catalyses an early and rate-limiting step in the biosynthesis of cholesterol. As a result, Zocor, in clinical studies reduced total serum cholesterol, low-density lipoprotein (LDL) and very-low-density lipoprotein (VLDL) cholesterol concentrations. It also moderately increased HDL cholesterol and reduced plasma-triglycerides.

In animal studies, after oral dosing, simvastatin had high selectivity for the liver, where it achieved substantially higher concentrations than in non-target tissues. Simvastatin undergoes extensive first-pass extraction in the liver, the primary site of action, with subsequent excretion of drug in the bile. Systemic exposure of the active form of simvastatin in man has been found to be less than 5% of the oral dose. Of this, 95% is bound to human plasma proteins.

Dosage and administration
Adults: The recommended starting dose is 10 mg once daily taken in the evening. The dose range is 10 to 40 mg a day in single doses taken at night.

A marked response to Zocor is seen within two weeks and the maximum therapeutic response occurs within four to six weeks. The response is maintained during continuation of therapy.

Adjustments of dosage, if required, should be made at intervals of not less than four weeks depending on the patient's individual response. If total serum cholesterol levels fall below 3.6 mmol/litre or if LDL cholesterol falls below 1.94 mmol/litre, consideration should be given to reducing the dose of Zocor. The patient should be placed on a standard cholesterol-lowering diet before receiving Zocor and should continue on this diet during treatment with Zocor.

Concomitant therapy: Zocor is effective alone or in combination with the bile-acid sequestrants.

Dosage in renal insufficiency: Because Zocor does not undergo significant renal excretion, modification of dosage should not be necessary in patients with renal insufficiency.

Elderly: Although experience in elderly patients is limited, efficacy using standard doses appears similar to that seen in the population as a whole. There is no apparent increase in the frequency of clinical or laboratory adverse findings.

Children: Studies to show the safety and effectiveness in children have not been carried out.

Contra-indications, warnings, etc
Contra-indications: Hypersensitivity to this product; active liver disease or unexplained persistent elevations of serum transaminases; pregnancy and breast-feeding (see also 'Precautions'); women of childbearing potential unless adequately protected by non-hormonal methods.

Precautions
Homozygous familial hypercholesterolaemia: In patients with the homozygous form of familial hypercholesterolaemia, in whom there is a complete absence of LDL receptors, thereapy with Zocor is unlikely to result in clinical benefit.

Hypertriglyceridaemia: Zocor has only a moderate triglyceride-lowering effect and is not indicated where hypertriglyceridaemia is the abnormality of most concern (i.e. hyperlipidaemia types I, IV and V).

Hepatic effects: Minor asymptomatic transient rises in

serum transaminases may occur soon after initiation of treatment which do not require the drug to be discontinued. There is no evidence that these changes are due to hypersensitivity to Zocor.

It is recommended that liver-function tests be performed before treatment begins and periodically thereafter in all patients. Special attention should be paid to patients who develop elevated serum transaminase levels, and in these patients measurements should be repeated promptly and then performed more frequently. If the transaminase levels show evidence of progression, particularly if they rise to three times the upper limit of normal and are persistent, the drug should be discontinued.

The drug should be used with caution in patients who consume substantial quantities of alcohol and/or have a past history of liver disease. Active liver diseases or unexplained transaminase elevations are contraindications to the use of simvastatin.

Muscle effects: Therapy with HMG-COA reductase inhibitors has rarely been associated with myopathy. Myopathy should be considered in any patient with marked elevations of creatine phosphokinase (CPK) levels ($\geq$10 times the upper limit of normal), or with diffuse myalgias, muscle tenderness and such marked elevations of CPK levels. The patient should be asked to report promptly unexplained muscle pain, tenderness or weakness. Therapy with Zocor should be discontinued if markedly elevated CPK levels occur or if myopathy is diagnosed. These CPK elevations should be considered in the differential diagnosis of chest pain in a patient on therapy with Zocor.

Transient mild elevations of creatine phosphokinase (CPK) levels (from skeletal muscle) have been seen commonly in patients receiving Zocor, but these have been usually of no clinical significance. Myopathy, as defined above, has occasionally been reported (incidence of $<$0.1%).

Myopathy has been reported in patients receiving lovastatin (another closely related HMG-COA reductase inhibitor) concomitantly with lipid lowering doses of nicotinic acid, or a fibric acid derivative, and with immunosuppressant drugs (including cyclosporin). There have been reports of severe rhabdomyolysis with secondary acute renal failure.

Therapy with Zocor should be temporarily withheld or discontinued in any patient with an acute, serious condition suggestive of a myopathy or having a risk factor predisposing to the development of renal failure secondary to rhabdomyolysis.

Ophthalmic evaluations: In the absence of any drug therapy, an increase in the prevalence of lens opacities with time is expected as a result of ageing. Current long-term data from clinical trials do not indicate an adverse effect of simvastatin on the human lens.

Pregnancy: The active metabolite of simvastatin was shown to produce fetal malformations in the offspring of pregnant rats. There are no data available for the use of Zocor in pregnant women. Therefore Zocor is contraindicated for use in pregnancy and women of childbearing potential unless adequately protected by non-hormonal methods.

An interval of one month should elapse between the end of therapy with Zocor and planned conception.

Breast-feeding mothers: It is not known whether simvastatin or its metabolites are excreted in human milk. Zocor should be avoided during lactation.

Drug interactions

Phenazone is a model for drugs metabolised by the microsomal hepatic enzyme system (cytochrome P-450 system). Because Zocor had little or no detectable effect on the pharmacokinetics of phenazone in hypercholesterolaemic patients, the potential for significant interactions with other drugs metabolised via this mechanism is negligible.

Propranolol: In normal volunteers, there was no clinically significant pharmacokinetic or pharmacodynamic interaction with concomitant administration of single doses of Zocor and propranolol.

Digoxin: Concomitant administration of Zocor and digoxin in normal volunteers resulted in a slight elevation (less than 0.3 ng/ml) in drug concentrations (as measured by a digoxin radio-immuno-assay) in plasma compared to concomitant administration of placebo and digoxin.

Coumarin derivatives: The administration of Zocor appeared to enhance slightly the anticoagulant effect of warfarin (mean changes in prothrombin time less than two seconds) in normal volunteers maintained in a state of low therapeutic anticoagulation. The clinical importance of these findings for fully anticoagulated patients receiving concomitant chronic therapy with Zocor is unkown.

In patients taking coumarin anticoagulants, prothrombin time should be determined prior to starting therapy with simvastatin and, thereafter, monitored at the intervals usually recommended for patients on coumarin anticoagulants.

Fibric acid derivatives: (see 'Muscle effects')

Other concomitant therapy: Caution should be exercised in the concomitant use of Zocor with immunosuppressant therapy or nicotinic acid (see 'Precautions'). In clinical studies, Zocor was used concomitantly with beta-blockers, calcium antagonists, diuretics and non-steroidal anti-inflammatory drugs (NSAIDs) without evidence of clinically significant adverse interactions.

Side effects: Zocor is generally well tolerated; for the most part, side-effects have been usually mild and transient in nature. Less than 2% of patients on Zocor were discontinued from controlled clinical studies due to side-effects attributable to Zocor.

In all clinical studies, controlled and uncontrolled, adverse effects occurring with a frequency of 1% or more and considered by the investigator as possibly, probably or definitely drug-related were: abdominal pain, constipation, flatulence and nausea. Other side effects occurring in 0.5–0.9% of patients were: asthenia, acid regurgitation, dyspepsia, headache, insomnia, diarrhoea, and rash.

Myopathy has been reported rarely.

Laboratory test findings: Marked and persistent increases of serum transaminases have been reported infrequently. Liver-function test abnormalities have generally been mild and transient. Increases in serum creatine phosphokinase (CPK) levels derived from skeletal muscle have been reported (see 'Precautions').

Overdosage: There are no data on overdosage available. No antidote is available. General measures should be adopted in the event of overdosage and liver function should be closely monitored.

The maximum plasma concentration of inhibitors occurred within 1.3 to 2.4 hours of administration.

Pharmaceutical precautions Store in a cool place below 25°C, protected from light.

Legal category POM.

Package quantities
Tablets 10 mg: Calendar packs of 28.
Tablets 20 mg: Calendar packs of 28.

Further information Nil.

Product licence numbers
10 mg Tablet 0025/0241
20 mg Tablet 0025/0242

**Trade Mark*

Merieux UK Ltd
Clivemont House
Clivemont Road
Maidenhead
Berkshire
SL6 7BU

MERIEUX UK LTD
A PASTEUR MERIEUX COMPANY

IMMRAVAX*
Measles, Mumps and Rubella Vaccine, Live, Attenuated

Presentation Immravax is a lyophilized vaccine containing 3 hyperattenuated live viruses. Each 0.5 ml dose of the reconstituted vaccine contains:

Measles virus (Schwarz strain, not less than 1000 $TCID_{50}$).
Mumps virus (Urabe Am 9 strain, not less than 5000 $TCID_{50}$).
Rubella virus (RA 27/3 strain, not less than 1000 $TCID_{50}$).

The measles and mumps viruses are both cultured in chick embryo tissue; the rubella virus is grown in human diploid cells.

The vaccine also contains albumin, traces of kanamycin, not more than 25 μg of neomycin per dose and no preservative.

Uses Immravax is indicated for active immunisation of children and susceptible adults against measles, mumps and rubella.

Dosage and administration
Adults and children: 0.5 ml of the reconstituted vaccine is given deep subcutaneously or intramuscularly. The vaccine is reconstituted using the sterile diluent provided. Any vaccine remaining one hour after reconstitution should be discarded.

The vaccine is rapidly inactivated by ether, alcohol and detergents and therefore care must be taken with any skin cleaning technique to avoid contact with these substances.

Contra-indications, warnings, etc Immravax must not be given to any woman who is pregnant or suspected to be pregnant. Following its administration, pregnancy must be avoided for at least three months.

Immravax should not be given in the presence of acute infectious disease, or currently evolving acute or chronic disease (particularly tuberculosis or respiratory tract infection).

It is contra-indicated in states of altered immunity including malignancy, leukaemia, lymphoma or in those receiving corticosteroids, cytotoxic drugs or irradiation.

The vaccine contains small traces of egg protein and is therefore contra-indicated in those who have a known serious allergy to egg protein (documented anaphylactic reaction to egg protein).

It also contains traces of neomycin and kanamycin and should not be given to those known to be hypersensitive to these antibiotics.

Although anaphylaxis is extremely rare, remedial facilities such as a solution of 1:1000 adrenaline should always be available during immunisation.

Immravax must not be given to those who previously have had severe reactions to measles, mumps or rubella vaccines.

Precautions: Children with a personal or close family history of convulsions may be immunised with Immravax, provided their parents understand that there may be a febrile response 5–10 days following immunisation. Advice should be given in such cases about measures such as removal of clothing, tepid sponging and the administration of paracetamol which may be indicated.

Because of the potential interference from passive antibodies, Immravax should not normally be given to infants below the age of one year. Immunisation should be deferred for at least 3 months following a blood or plasma transfusion or the administration of human immunoglobulin. If the vaccine is inadvertently given in these circumstances, serum antibody levels should be checked subsequently.

Other live vaccines may be given simultaneously at different sites or with an interval of three weeks between vaccines. A three week interval should be allowed before BCG vaccine is given. Tuberculin testing should be deferred for 8 weeks after immunisation with Immravax since false-negative results may occur.

Adverse reactions: A moderate fever is not uncommon, usually between 5–10 days after immunisation, and high fever associated with febrile convulsions has been reported. Malaise, sore throat, headache, fever, rash, local erythema, induration and tenderness, lymphadenopathy, orchitis, thrombocytopenia and purpura, arthritis, arthralgia and polyneuritis have all been reported with measles, mumps or rubella vaccines. Rarely parotitis may occur, usually at about 21 days following immunisation. Allergic reactions occur very rarely. Encephalitis has been reported very rarely in the period following measles, mumps and rubella immunisation. No causal relationship has been established between isolated reports of ocular palsies and Guillain-Barré syndrome and measles vaccines.

Pharmaceutical precautions Protect from light. Immravax should be stored at +2°C to +8°C and should not be frozen (lower temperatures will not harm the vaccine but may damage the diluent).

The vaccine should be reconstituted using the sterile diluent provided (Water for Injections with no added preservatives). The colour of the reconstituted vaccine is pale yellow, pinkish yellow, or orange yellow. Once reconstituted Immravax should be used immediately. Any vaccine remaining one hour after reconstitution should be discarded.

Legal category POM.

Package quantities Single dose vial of vaccine with syringe of diluent.

Further information Nil.

Product licence numbers

Vaccine	6745/0020
Diluent	6745/0024

MEASAVAX*
Measles Vaccine, Live, BP

Presentation Measavax is a lyophilized vaccine containing hyperattenuated live measles virus. Each 0.5 ml dose of reconstituted vaccine contains not less than 1000 $TCID_{50}$ of Schwarz strain virus cultured in chick embryo tissue.

The vaccine also contains albumin, not more than 25 μg of neomycin per dose and no preservative.

Use Measavax is indicated for active immunisation of children and susceptible adults against measles. The vaccine, if given to contacts within 3 days of exposure to measles, can suppress the full clinical disease.

Dosage and administration
Adults and children over 1 year of age: 0.5 ml of the reconstituted vaccine is given deep subcutaneously or intramuscularly. The vaccine is reconstituted using the sterile diluent provided. Any vaccine remaining one hour after reconstitution should be discarded.

The vaccine is rapidly inactivated by ether, alcohol and detergents and therefore care must be taken with any skin cleaning technique to avoid contact with these substances.

Contra-indications, warnings, etc Measavax should not be given in the presence of acute infectious disease, or currently evolving acute or chronic disease (particularly tuberculosis or respiratory tract infection).

It is contra-indicated in states of altered immunity including malignancy, leukaemia, lymphoma or in those receiving corticosteroids, cytotoxic drugs or irradiation. Children with compromised immunity who come into contact with measles should be given normal immunoglobulin as soon as possible after exposure.

The vaccine contains small traces of egg protein and is therefore contra-indicated in those who have a known serious allergy to egg protein (documented anaphylactic reaction to egg protein).

It also contains traces of neomycin and should not be given to those known to be hypersensitive to this antibiotic.

Although anaphylaxis is extremely rare, remedial facilities such as a solution of 1:1000 adrenaline should always be available during immunisation.

Measavax must not be given to those who previously have had severe reactions to measles vaccine. There is inadequate data on the theoretical risk from the use of the vaccine in pregnancy. Measles vaccine is therefore contraindicated in pregnant women.

Precautions: Children with a personal history of convulsions or whose parents or siblings have a history of idiopathic epilepsy should be immunised with Measavax, provided their parents understand that there may be a febrile response 5–10 days following immunisation. Advice should be given in such cases about measures such as removal of clothing, tepid sponging and the administration of paracetamol which may be indicated.

Because of the potential interference from passive antibodies, Measavax should not normally be given to infants below the age of one year. Immunisation should be deferred for at least 3 months following a blood or plasma transfusion or the administration of human immunoglobulin. If the vaccine is given within 3 months of human immunoglobulin, revaccination should be considered.

Other live vaccines may be given simultaneously at different sites or with an interval of three weeks between vaccines. A three week interval should be allowed before BCG vaccine is given. Tuberculin testing should be deferred for 8 weeks after immunisation with Measavax since false-negative results may occur.

Adverse reactions: A moderate fever is not uncommon, usually between 5–10 days after immunisation, and high fever associated with febrile convulsions has been reported. Malaise, pharyngitis, headache, cough, conjunctivitis, coryza, fever, rash, local erythema, induration and tenderness, lymphadenopathy and neuropathies have all been reported with measles vaccines. Allergic reactions occur very rarely. Encephalitis and thrombocytopenic purpura have been reported very rarely in the period following measles immunisation. No causal relationship has been established between isolated reports of ocular palsies and Guillain-Barré syndrome and measles vaccines.

Pharmaceutical precautions Protect from light. Measavax should be stored at +2°C to +8°C and should not be frozen (lower temperatures will not harm the vaccine but may damage the diluent).

The vaccine should be reconstituted using the sterile diluent provided (Water for Injections with no added preservatives). The colour of the reconstituted vaccine is pale yellow to pinkish yellow. Once reconstituted Measavax should be used immediately. Any vaccine remaining one hour after reconstitution should be discarded.

Legal category POM.

Package quantities Single dose vial of vaccine with syringe of diluent.

Further information Nil.

Product licence numbers
Vaccine 6745/0017
Diluent 6745/0024

MENGIVAC (A+C)* Meningococcal Polysaccharide Vaccine PhEur

Presentation An inactivated polysaccharide vaccine against meningococcal serogroups A and C. It is purified, heat stable and lyophilised. It is obtained by culturing bacterial A2 Branham strain of group A and No. 11 Gotschlich strain of group C Neisseria meningitidis. Surface polysaccharides are extracted by precipitation with cetrimide, followed by centrifugation. The vaccine is lyophilised and stabilised with lactose. It is prepared to World Health Organisation accepted standards.

Each dose of 0.5 ml contains a minimum of 50 μg of Neisseria meningitidis serogroup A polysaccharide, a minimum of 50 μg of Neisseria meningitidis serogroup C polysaccharide and 2 mg of lactose.

Isotonic buffered diluent is supplied with each dose.

Uses Prophylaxis against meningococcal meningitis of serogroups A and C. Vaccination is recommended for unprotected people travelling to endemic regions. It is also recommended for use during an epidemic.

Post-vaccination immunity lasts approximately 3 years.

Dosage and administration
Adults and children over 18 months: A single dose of 0.5 ml of reconstituted vaccine given deep subcutaneously or intramuscularly. For children aged under 18 months see 'Precautions'.

Use in elderly: No special comment.

For reconstitution the diluent provided should be used. This is carefully injected into the vial containing lyophilised vaccine and gently agitated prior to withdrawal into the syringe.

Multidose vials are best reconstituted by first adding a small amount of diluent then gently agitating prior to the addition of the remaining diluent. The vial should be agitated prior to each dose being withdrawn.

Contra-indications, warnings, etc
Contra-indication: The vaccine must not be given to those who have previously experienced a serious reaction to the vaccine or its components.

Vaccination should be delayed if an acute infection is present.

Precautions: A+C meningococcal vaccines should not generally be given to children under 18 months except during epidemics. Clinical data has confirmed the efficacy of the serogroup A component over 3 months of age. The response to the serogroup C component is only transitory but can be of limited value during a severe epidemic. Transient side effects are more commonly reported below the age of 18 months.

Meningococcal A+C polysaccharide vaccine protects against meningitis caused by meningococci of serogroups A and C. It does not protect against meningitis caused by meningococci of serogroup B, Haemophilus influenzae, Streptococcus pneumoniae, etc.

Although anaphylaxis is extremely rare, facilities for its

management should always be available when vaccination is carried out.

Side and adverse effects: Reactions to this vaccine are rare and are seen less often in adults than in children. Local reactions at the site of vaccination have been reported and are transitory. Low grade fever, irritability and fatigue may occasionally occur in the first 72 hours following vaccination.

Use in pregnancy and lactation: There is no animal data and insufficient data in humans to recommend routinely the use of the vaccine in pregnancy and lactation. However, vaccination may be considered if the benefit outweighs the risk e.g in the event of an epidemic.

Treatment of overdose: Not applicable.

Pharmaceutical precautions Store at +2°C to + 8°C. The diluent must not be frozen. The diluent is a sterile, isotonic buffered solution. After reconstitution, the vaccine must be used within 1 hour.

Legal category POM.

Package quantities Carton of 1 single dose vial of lyophilised vaccine with syringe of diluent (0.5 ml).

Carton of 1 × 10 dose vial of lyophilisd vaccine + vial of diluent (5 ml).

Carton of 25 × 50 dose vials of lyophilised vaccine.

Carton of 25 vials of diluent for reconstitution of 50 dose vials of lyophilised vaccine.

Product licence numbers

Diluent	6745/0029
Lyophilised vaccine	6745/0030

MERIEUX* INACTIVATED RABIES VACCINE

Human Diploid Cell Rabies Vaccine

Presentation The vaccine is a lyophilised, stabilised suspension of inactivated Wistar rabies virus strain PM/ WI38 1503–3M, cultured on human diploid cells (MRC_5) and inactivated by beta-propiolactone. The dry vaccine is coloured off-white but, after reconstitution with the diluent supplied, it turns a pinkish colour due to the presence of phenol red. The potency of the reconstituted vaccine is not less than 2.5 International Units per dose (1 ml).

Uses

(a) Prophylactic immunisation against rabies.

(b) Treatment of patients following suspected rabies contact.

Dosage and administration The dose of reconstituted vaccine in all cases is 1 ml given by deep subcutaneous or intramuscular injection. The vaccine should be administered into the deltoid region but not the gluteal region. Reconstitution: Inject the diluent from the syringe into the vial, agitate to ensure complete reconstitution and withdraw the contents back into the syringe.

(a) Prophylaxis: Give one dose of vaccine (1 ml) followed by a second dose 28 days later. A booster dose should be given a further 6–12 months later. To maintain high antibody titres, a further booster should be given every two to three years if risk of infection continues. For treatment after contact with a suspected rabid animal see section (b) below.

(b) Treatment:

(i) *In persons known to have adequate prophylaxis.* In the event of contact with a suspected rabid animal, two further boosters should be given on day 0 and on day 3 to 7.

(ii) *In persons with no, or possibly inadequate, prophylaxis.* The first injection of MIRV should be given as soon as possible after the suspected contact (day 0) and followed by five further doses on days 3, 7, 14, 30 and 90. The use of Human Rabies Immunoglobulin on day 0 should be considered but only in persons with no adequate prophylaxis. The treatment schedule may be stopped if the animal concerned is found conclusively to be free of rabies.

Contra-indications, warnings, etc There are no absolute contra-indications to inactivated rabies vaccine cultured on human diploid cells. Redness, swelling or tenderness at the site of injection may occur during the first 48 hours. A mild fever, malaise and influenza-like symptoms have been reported.

Although anaphylaxis is extremely rare remedial facilities such as adrenaline should always be available during vaccination.

The vaccine contains traces of neomycin.

Pharmaceutical precautions Store at +2°C to + 8°C. Do not freeze. Use immediately after reconstituting the vaccine. Discard any vaccine unused one hour after reconstitution.

Legal category POM.

Package quantities A vial of lyophilised vaccine containing one dose together with a disposable syringe containing 1 ml of diluent. The diluent is Water for Injections with no added preservatives.

Further information The British National Formulary and DHSS Memorandum on Rabies (HMSO) both contain reference to rabies.

Product licence number 6745/0007

MFV-JECT*

Presentation MFV-Ject is Inactivated Influenza Vaccine (Split Virion) BP, purified by zonal ultra-centrifugation and extraction with ether. Merieux Flu Vaccine contains the strains of influenza virus currently recommended by the WHO. Each dose contains not more than 0.05 mg of thiomersal as preservative.

Uses Prophylaxis against influenza. Particularly recommended in at risk groups, especially the elderly, which include those suffering from the following:

Chronic pulmonary disease.
Chronic heart disease.
Chronic renal disease.
Diabetes and other less common endocrine disorders.
Patients receiving immunosuppressive therapy.

Immunisation against influenza is also recommended in:

School children over 4 years of age and elderly persons in residential establishments.

Doctors, nurses and others at special risk of infection by contact with influenza sufferers.

Dosage and administration By deep subcutaneous or intramuscular injection.

Adults, elderly and children (over 13 years): single dose, 0.5 ml.

Children (4–13 years): 0.5 ml. A second dose of 0.5 ml should be given after an interval of 4–6 weeks unless the child is known to have been previously infected or has received trivalent influenza vaccine in the past 4 years.

Contra-indications, warnings, etc

Contra-indications: Merieux Flu Vaccine is contra-indicated in persons hypersensitive to egg, chicken or influenza viral proteins.

Immunisation should be postponed in patients with febrile illness.

Warnings, side-effects: Local effects such as transient erythema, tenderness or pain at the site of injection, or rarely systemic effects such as mild fever, may appear within the first 48 hours.

Precautions: The vaccine should be used with caution in patients with a history of allergy.

Although anaphylaxis is extremely rare, facilities for its management should always be available during vaccination.

Use in pregnancy: Not recommended.

Overdosage: Not applicable.

Pharmaceutical precautions Store protected from light at +2°C to +8°C. Do not freeze.

Legal category POM.

Package quantities Single dose prefilled syringe (unit pack and pack of 10).

Further information Nil.

Product licence number 6745/0038.

RUBAVAX*
Rubella Vaccine, Live, BP

Presentation Rubavax is a lyophilised vaccine containing hyperattenuated live rubella virus. Each 0.5 ml dose of the reconstituted vaccine contains not less than 1000 $TCID_{50}$ of the Wistar RA 27/3 strain rubella virus cultured in human diploid cells.

The vaccine also contains albumin, not more than 25 µg of neomycin per dose and no preservative.

Uses Rubavax is indicated for active immunisation against rubella in girls of 10–14 years and *non-pregnant* women of child-bearing age who are seronegative.

Dosage and administration
Adults and children: 0.5 ml of the reconstituted vaccine is given deep subcutaneously or intramuscularly. The vaccine is reconstituted using the sterile diluent provided. Any vaccine remaining one hour after reconstitution should be discarded.

The vaccine is rapidly inactivated by ether, alcohol and detergents and therefore care must be taken with any skin cleaning technique to avoid contact with these substances.

Contra-indications, warnings, etc Rubavax must not be given to any woman who is pregnant or suspected to be pregnant. Following its administration, pregnancy must be avoided for at least three months.

Rubavax should not be given in the presence of acute infectious disease, or currently evolving acute or chronic disease.

It is contra-indicated in states of altered immunity including malignancy, leukaemia, lymphoma or in those receiving corticosteroids, cytotoxic drugs or irradiation.

The vaccine contains traces of neomycin and should not be given to those known to be hypersensitive to this antibiotic.

Although anaphylaxis is extremely rare, remedial facilities such as a solution of 1:1000 adrenaline should always be available during immunisation.

Rubavax must not be given to those who previously have had severe reactions to rubella vaccine.

Precautions: Immunisation should be deferred for at least 3 months following a blood or plasma transfusion or the administration of human immunoglobulin. If the vaccine is given within 3 months of human immunoglobulin, revaccination should be considered. Other live vaccines may be given simultaneously at different sites or with an interval of three weeks between vaccines.

Adverse reactions: These are usually mild and transient; slight fever, malaise, sore throat, erythema, induration or pain at site of injection. Regional lymphadenopathy, rubella-like rash, pharyngitis, arthralgia, and arthritis have been reported. Transient joint symptoms are more common in women than young girls. Neurological symptoms have been reported rarely following the administration of rubella vaccine.

Pharmaceutical precautions Protect from light. Rubavax should be stored at +2°C to +8°C and should not be frozen (lower temperatures will not harm the vaccine but may damage the diluent).

The vaccine should be reconstituted using the sterile diluent provided (Water for Injections with no added preservatives). The colour of the reconstituted vaccine may be yellow to purplish red in colour. Once reconstituted Rubavax should be used immediately. Any vaccine remaining one hour after reconstitution should be discarded.

Legal category POM.

Package quantities Single dose vial of vaccine with syringe of diluent.

Further information Nil.

Product licence numbers
Vaccine 6745/0014
Diluent 6745/0024

TETAVAX*
Adsorbed Tetanus Vaccine BP (Tet/Vac/Ads)

Presentation Tetavax is a sterile aqueous suspension of purified tetanus toxoid. The toxoid is adsorbed onto aluminium hydroxide with thiomersal added as preservative.

Each 0.5 ml dose contains not less than 40 International Units (IU) of tetanus toxoid.

Uses Active immunisation against tetanus. Reinforcement of immunity to tetanus.

Dosage and administration By deep subcutaneous or intramuscular injection. Shake before use.

Primary immunisation: 3 injections each of 0.5 ml with an interval of 4 weeks between the first and second doses and 4 weeks between the second and third doses.

Reinforcing doses: Following primary immunisation, a reinforcing dose of 0.5 ml is recommended after 10 years and a further 0.5 ml dose 10 years later.

Management of tetanus prone wounds: Following a tetanus prone injury, a single dose of the vaccine should be administered to persons who have not received a booster dose nor completed a primary course during the preceding 10 years. Persons who have never received a primary course or in whom the immunisation history is not known, should commence or complete a primary course in addition to tetanus immunoglobulin, as appropriate.

Adsorbed tetanus vaccine may be administered simultaneously with tetanus immunoglobulin but must be given at a separate site.

Contra-indications, warnings, etc
Contra-indications: Acute infectious illness except when used in the management of tetanus prone injuries. The vaccine should not be given to persons who have had a severe reaction to a previous dose.

Warnings: Not for intradermal injection.

In immunised adults, booster doses at less than 10 year intervals are unnecessary and may cause excess reactions.

Side effects: General reactions are uncommon but may include transient pyrexia, headache, malaise, local swelling, redness and tenderness (especially in adults), acute allergic reactions, pallor, dyspnoea, urticaria, angioneurotic oedema, acute anaphylactic reactions and rarely, peripheral neuropathy. A small painless nodule may form at the injection site especially if administered into the superficial layers of subcutaneous tissue.

Precautions: Although anaphylaxis is extremely rare, facilities for its management should always be available during vaccination.

Pharmaceutical precautions Store at +2° to +8°C. Do not freeze.

Multidose containers which are partly used should be discarded at the end of the vaccination session.

Legal category POM.

Package quantities Single dose pre-filled syringe (unit pack and pack of 10); single dose ampoule (pack of 5) or 10 dose (5 ml) vial.

Further information Active immunisation against tetanus is recommended for everybody. Adsorbed tetanus vaccine may be administered to persons of any age.

Product licence numbers
Single dose 6745/0002
Multi dose 6745/0003

**Trade Mark*

Merrell Dow Pharmaceuticals Limited
Lakeside House
Stockley Park
Uxbridge
Middlesex UB11 1BE

Merrell Dow

CLOMID*

Presentation Pale yellow, round, flat, bevelled tablet. A scored bisect line on one side and the other engraved 'M' within two circles. Each tablet contains 50 mg Clomiphene Citrate BP.

Uses
Action: The ovulatory response to cyclic Clomid therapy appears to be mediated through increased output of pituitary gonadotrophins, which in turn stimulates the maturation and endocrine activity of the ovarian follicle and the subsequent development and function of the corpus luteum. The role of the pituitary is indicated by increased urinary excretion of gonadotrophins and the response of the ovary is manifested by increased urinary oestrogen excretion.

Indications: Clomid is indicated for the treatment of ovulatory failure in women desiring pregnancy.

Clomid is indicated only for patients in whom ovulatory dysfunction is demonstrated, who meet the conditions described in this data sheet. Other causes of infertility must be excluded or adequately treated before giving Clomid.

Good levels of endogenous oestrogen (as estimated from vaginal smears, endometrial biopsy, assay of urinary oestrogen, or endometrial bleeding in response to progesterone) provide a favourable prognosis for ovulatory response induced by Clomid. A low level of oestrogen, although clinically less favourable, does not preclude successful outcome of therapy.

Clomid therapy is ineffective in patients with primary pituitary or primary ovarian failure. Clomid therapy cannot substitute for specific treatment of other causes of ovulatory failure, such as thyroid or adrenal disorders. For hyperprolactinaemia there is other preferred treatment.

Clomid is not first line treatment for low-weight related amenorrhoea, with infertility, and has no value if a high FSH blood level is observed following an early menopause.

Dosage and administration
General considerations: The work-up and treatment should be supervised by physicians experienced in management of gynaecological or endocrine disorders. Patients should be chosen for therapy with Clomid only after careful diagnostic evaluation. The plan of therapy should be outlined in advance. Other causes of infertility should be excluded or adequately treated before giving Clomid.

Many patients will respond to 50 mg daily for 5 days. In the determination of a starting dose efficacy must be balanced against potential adverse effects. For example, the data available suggest that ovulation and pregnancy are slightly more attainable on 100 mg/day for 5 days than on 50 mg/day for 5 days. As the dosage is increased, however, ovarian hyperstimulation and other adverse effects may increase. Furthermore, although the data do not yet establish a relationship between dosage and multiple births, it would seem reasonable on pharmacological grounds that such a relationship does exist.

For these reasons it would seem prudent to begin treatment with the lower dose, 50 mg daily for 5 days, and to increase the dose only in patients who do not respond to the first course. Special care with lower dosage or duration of treatment for the first course is particularly recommended if unusual sensitivity to pituitary gonadotrophin is suspected, such as in patients with polycystic ovary syndrome.

Recommended dosage: The recommended dose for the first course of Clomid is 50 mg (1 tablet) daily for 5 days. Therapy may be started at any time in the patient who has had no recent uterine bleeding. If progestin-induced bleeding is planned, or if spontaneous uterine bleeding occurs before therapy, the regimen of 50 mg daily for 5 days should be started on or about the fifth day of the cycle. When ovulation occurs at this dosage, there is no advantage to increasing the dose in subsequent cycles of treatment.

If ovulation appears not to have occurred after the first course of therapy, a second course of 100 mg daily (two 50 mg tablets given as a single daily dose) for five days should be given. This course may be started as early as 30 days after the previous one. *Increase of the dosage or duration of therapy beyond 100 mg/day for 5 days should not be undertaken.*

The majority of patients who are going to respond will respond to the first course of therapy, and 3 courses should constitute an adequate therapeutic trial. If ovulatory menses have not yet occurred, the diagnosis should be re-evaluated. Treatment beyond this is not recommended in the patient who does not exhibit evidence of ovulation.

Pregnancy: The importance of properly timed coitus cannot be over-emphasised (i.e. at about the time of ovulation). For regularity of cyclic ovulatory response it is also important that each course of Clomid be started on or about the fifth cycle day, once ovulation has been established. Clomid therapy follows the rule of diminishing returns, such that likelihood of conception diminishes with each succeeding course of therapy. Before starting treatment, patients and their male partners should be advised of the possibility of multiple pregnancy and its potential hazards if conception occurs in relationship to Clomid therapy.

Long-term cyclic therapy: Not recommended.

The relative safety of long-term cyclic therapy has not been conclusively demonstrated, and since the majority of patients will ovulate following 3 courses, long-term cyclic therapy is not recommended.

Contra-indications, warnings, etc
Contra-indications
Use in pregnancy: Clomid is not indicated during pregnancy. Although there is no evidence that Clomid has a harmful effect on the human foetus, there is evidence that Clomid has a deleterious effect on rat and rabbit foetuses when given in high doses to the pregnant animal. To help avoid inadvertent Clomid administration during early pregnancy, the basal body temperature should be recorded throughout all treatment cycles and the patient carefully observed to determine whether ovulation occurs. If the basal temperature following Clomid is biphasic and not followed by menses, the patient should be examined carefully and have a pregnancy test.

Liver disease: Clomid therapy is contra-indicated in patients with liver disease or a history of liver dysfunction.

Abnormal uterine bleeding: Clomid is contra-indicated

in patients with abnormal bleeding of undetermined origin.

Ovarian cyst: See 'Precautions'.

Precautions

Ovarian cyst: Pelvic examination is necessary prior to start of and before each subsequent course of Clomid treatment. Clomid should not be given in the presence of an ovarian cyst (including endometriosis involving the ovary), except polycystic ovary since further enlargement of the cyst may occur.

To minimise the hazard of the abnormal ovarian enlargement associated with Clomid therapy, the lowest dose consistent with expectation of good results should be used. The patient should be instructed to inform the physician of any abdominal or pelvic pain, discomfort or distension after taking Clomid. Maximal enlargement of the ovary may not occur until several days after discontinuation of the course of Clomid.

The patient who complains of abdominal or pelvic pain, discomfort, or distension after taking Clomid should be examined because of the possible presence of an ovarian cyst or other cause. If abnormal enlargement occurs, Clomid should not be given until the ovaries have returned to pre-treatment size. The ovarian enlargement and cyst formation associated with Clomid therapy usually regress spontaneously within a few days or weeks after discontinuing treatment. Most of these patients should be managed conservatively. The dosage and/or duration of the next dose should be reduced.

Multiple pregnancy: There is an increased chance of multiple pregnancy when conception occurs in relationship to Clomid therapy. During the clinical investigation studies, the incidence of multiple pregnancy was 7.9% (186 of 2369 Clomid associated pregnancies on which outcome was reported). Among these 2369 pregnancies, 2183 (92.1%) were single, 165 (6.9%) twin, 11 (0.5%) triplet, 7 (0.3%) quadruplet, and 3 (0.13%) quintuplet.

Pregnancy wastage and birth anomalies: The overall incidence of reported birth anomalies from pregnancies associated with maternal Clomid ingestion (before or after conception) during the investigational studies was within the range of that reported in published references for the general population. Among the birth anomalies spontaneously reported in the published literature as individual cases, the proportion of neural tube defects has been high among pregnancies associated with ovulation induced by Clomid, but this has not been supported by data from population-based studies.

The physician should explain so that the patient understands the assumed risk of any pregnancy whether the ovulation was induced with the aid of Clomid or occurred naturally.

The patient should be informed of the greater pregnancy risks associated with certain characteristics or conditions of any pregnant woman: e.g. age of female and male partner, history of spontaneous abortions, Rh genotype, abnormal menstrual history, infertility history (regardless of cause), organic heart disease, diabetes, exposure to infectious agents such as rubella, familial history of birth anomaly, and other risk factors that may be pertinent to the patient for whom Clomid is being considered. Based upon the evaluation of the patient, genetic counselling may be indicated.

Population-based reports have been published on possible elevation of risk of Down's Syndrome in ovulation induction cases and of increase in trisomy defects among spontaneously aborted foetuses from subfertile women receiving ovulation inducing drugs (no women with Clomid alone without additional inducing drugs). However, as yet, the reported observations are too few to confirm or not confirm the presence of an increased risk that would justify amniocentesis, other than for the usual indications because of age and family history.

The experience from patients of all diagnoses during clinical investigation of Clomid shows a pregnancy wastage or foetal loss rate of 21.4% (abortion rate of 19.0% and other loss rate of 2.4%).

Clomid therapy after conception was reported for 158 of the 2369 delivered and reported pregnancies in the clinical investigations. Of these 158 pregnancies 8 infants (born of 7 pregnancies) were reported to have birth defects.

There was no difference in reported incidence of birth defects whether Clomid was given before the 19th day after conception or between the 20th and 35th day after conception. This incidence is within the anticipated range of general population.

Warnings

Visual symptoms: Patients should be advised that blurring or other visual symptoms may occasionally occur during or shortly after therapy with Clomid. Patients should be warned that visual symptoms may render such activities as driving a car or operating machinery more hazardous than usual, particularly under conditions of variable lighting. The significance of these visual symptoms is not understood. If the patient has any visual symptoms, treatment should be discontinued and ophthalmological evaluation performed.

Side-effects

Symptoms/signs/conditions: Adverse effects appeared to be dose related, occurring more frequently at higher dose and with the longer courses of treatment used in investigational studies. At recommended dosage, adverse effects are not prominent and infrequently interfere with treatment.

During investigational studies, the more common reported adverse effects included ovarian enlargement (13.6%), vasomotor flushes (10.4%), abdominal-pelvic discomfort (distension, bloating) (5.5%). The vasomotor symptoms resembling menopausal 'hot flushes' were rarely severe and disappeared promptly after treatment was discontinued. Abdominal symptoms were most often related to ovulatory (mittelschmerz) or premenstrual phenomena, or to ovarian enlargement.

Ovarian enlargement: At recommended dosage, abnormal ovarian enlargement is infrequent, although the usual cyclic variation in ovarian size may be exaggerated. Similarly, cyclic ovarian pain (mittelschmerz) may be accentuated. With higher or prolonged dosage, more frequent ovarian enlargement and cyst formation may occur, and the luteal phase of the cycle may be prolonged.

Rare instances of massive ovarian enlargement are recorded. Such an instance has been described in a patient with polycystic ovary syndrome whose Clomid therapy consisted of 100 mg daily for 14 days. Abnormal ovarian enlargement usually regresses spontaneously; most of the patients with this condition should be treated conservatively.

Eye/visual symptoms: Symptoms described usually as 'blurring' or spots or flashes (scintillating scotomata), increase in incidence with increasing total dose and usually disappear within periods ranging from a few days to a few weeks after Clomid is discontinued.

These symptoms appear to be due to intensification and prolongation of after-images. Symptoms often first appear or are accentuated with exposure to bright-lit environment. While measured visual acuity has not generally been affected, one investigational patient (not anovulatory) taking Clomid 200 mg daily developed visual blurring on the seventh day of treatment, which progressed to severe diminution of visual acuity by the tenth treatment day. No other abnormality was found and the visual acuity returned to normal on the third day after treatment was stopped.

Ophthalmologically definable scotomata and retinal cell function (electroretinographic) changes have been reported. A patient treated during clinical studies developed phosphenes and scotomata during prolonged Clomid administration, but they disappeared by the 32nd day after stopping therapy.

There are rare reports of cataracts. In a 34-year-old patient who had taken 3 courses of Clomid, slit-lamp microscopic examination showed a mild amount of posterior cortical subcapsular opacity in each eye. Ophthalmoscopic examination revealed normal findings. The diagnosis was reported as 'posterior cortical senile cataracts'. In another patient previously treated with

Clomid posterior vitreous detachment was the reported diagnosis. Other isolated reports include conditions such as: optic neuritis, retinal haemorrhage/thrombosis/vascular spasm, temporary loss of vision, and macular oedema.

Dermatoses: Dermatitis and rash were reported by investigational patients. Conditions such as rash and urticaria were the most common ones reported after prescription availability but also reported were conditions such as allergic reaction, erythema multiforme, ecchymosis and angioneurotic oedema. Hair thinning has been reported very rarely.

CNS symptoms: In investigational patients, CNS symptoms/signs/conditions of dizziness, light-headedness/vertigo (0.9%), nervous tension/insomnia (0.8%), and fatigue/depression (0.7%) were reported. After prescription availability, there were isolated additional reports of these conditions and also reports of other conditions such as syncope/fainting, cerebrovascular accident, cerebral thrombosis, psychotic reactions including paranoid psychosis, neurologic impairment, disorientation and speech disturbance.

Liver function: Bromsulphalein (BSP) retention of greater than 5% was reported in 32 of 141 patients in whom it was measured, including 5 of 43 patients who took approximately the dose of Clomid now recommended. Retention was usually minimal unless associated with prolonged continuous Clomid administration or with apparently unrelated liver disease. Other liver function tests were usually normal. In a later study in which patients were given 6 consecutive monthly courses of Clomid (50 or 100 mg daily for 3 days) or matching placebo, BSP tests were done on 94 patients. Values in excess of 5% retention were recorded in 11 patients, 6 of whom had taken drug and 5 placebo.

In a separate report, one patient taking 50 mg of Clomid daily developed jaundice on the 19th day of treatment; liver biopsy revealed bile stasis without evidence of hepatitis.

Overdosage: There is no experience of acute overdosage with Clomid.

Pharmaceutical precautions Clomid tablets should be protected from light, moisture and excessive heat.

Legal category POM.

Package quantities Clomid is obtainable in packs of 30 and 100 tablets in blister packs.

Further information Clomid is prescribable under the supervision of an appropriate specialist.

Orally administered 14C labelled clomiphene citrate was readily absorbed when administered to humans. Cumulative excretion of the 14C label by way of the urine and faeces averaged about 50% of the oral dose after 5 days in 6 subjects, with mean urinary excretion of 7.8% and mean faecal excretion of 42.4%. A mean rate of excretion of 0.73% per day of the 14C dose after 31 days to 35 days and 0.45% per day of the 14C dose after 42 days to 45 days was seen in faecal and urine samples collected from 6 subjects for 14 to 53 days after clomiphene citrate 14C administration. The remaining drug/metabolites may be slowly excreted from a sequestered enterohepatic recirculation pool.

Product licence number 4425/5900.

DESTOLIT*

Presentation White half-scored tablet containing 150 mg ursodeoxycholic acid marked Destolit.

Uses Destolit is indicated for the dissolution of radiolucent (i.e. non-radio opaque) cholesterol gallstones in patients with a functioning gallbladder.

Dosage and administration The daily dose for most patients is 3 or 4 tablets of 150 mg according to body weight. This dose should be divided into 2 administrations after meals, with one administration always to be taken after the evening meal.

A *daily dose* of about 8 to 10 mg/kg will produce cholesterol desaturation of bile in the majority of cases. The measurement of the lithogenic index on bile-rich duodenal drainage fluid after 4–6 weeks of therapy may be useful for determining the minimal effective dose. The lowest effective dose has been found to be 4 mg/kg.

The *duration of treatment* required to achieve gallstone dissolution will usually not be extended beyond 2 years and should be monitored by regular cholecystograms. Treatment should be continued for 3–4 months after the radiological disappearance of the gallstones.

Any temporary discontinuation of treatment, if prolonged for 3–4 weeks, will allow the bile to return to a state of supersaturation and will extend the total time required for litholysis. In some cases stones may recur after successful treatment.

Contra-indications, warnings, etc *Use in pregnancy and lactation:* In common with all drugs, it is advised that ursodeoxycholic acid should not be given during the first trimester of pregnancy. (In the rabbit, embryotoxicity has been observed, but this has not been seen in the rat.) Treatment in women of child-bearing age should only be undertaken if measures to prevent pregnancy are used. Non-hormonal contraceptive measures are recommended. In cases of conception during treatment, therapy should be discontinued.

Contra-indications: Active gastric or duodenal ulcers are contra-indications, as are hepatic and intestinal conditions interfering with the enterohepatic circulation of bile acids (ileal resection and stoma, regional ileitis, extra and intra-hepatic cholestasis, severe, acute, and chronic liver diseases). A product of this class has been found to be carcinogenic in animals. The relevance of these findings to the clinical use of ursodeoxycholic acid has not been established.

Precautions: Excessive dietary intake of calories and cholesterol should be avoided; a low cholesterol diet will probably improve the effectiveness of Destolit tablets.

Drug Interactions: It is also recommended that drugs known to increase cholesterol elimination in bile, such as oestrogenic hormones, oral contraceptive agents and certain blood cholesterol lowering agents should also not be prescribed concomitantly.

Side-effects: Destolit is normally well tolerated. Diarrhoea has been found to occur only occasionally. No significant alterations have so far been observed in liver function.

Overdosage: It is unlikely that overdosage will cause serious adverse effects. Diarrhoea may occur and it is recommended that liver function tests be monitored. Ion-exchange resins may be useful to bind bile acids in the intestines.

Pharmaceutical precautions None.

Legal category POM.

Package quantities Blister packs of 60 tablets.

Further information Nil.

Product licence number 4425/0045.

KOLANTICON* GEL

Presentation Kolanticon Gel is a white, viscous, peppermint-flavoured suspension, each 5 ml containing:

Dicyclomine Hydrochloride BP	2.5 mg
Dried Aluminium Hydroxide Gel BP	200 mg
Light Magnesium Oxide BP	100 mg
Simethicone USP	20 mg

Uses Kolanticon is an antacid-antiflatulent-anti-spasmodic-demulcent indicated for the treatment and prophylaxis of symptoms of peptic ulcer and functional dyspepsia especially in patients in whom gastric distress results from hyperacidity, smooth muscle spasm and flatulence. Also indicated for symptomatic relief in oesophagitis, hiatus hernia, gastritis and iatrogenic gastritis.

Dosage and administration Two to four 5 ml spoonfuls every four hours as required.

Contra-indications, warnings, etc
Contra-indications: Known idiosyncrasy to any of the ingredients. Should not be used in patients with obstructive uropathy, obstructive disease of the gastro-intestinal tract, paralytic ileus and intestinal atony, severe ulcerative colitis, and myasthenia gravis.

Precautions: In the presence of renal insufficiency magnesium salts may cause central nervous system depression. Aluminium hydroxide in the presence of low phosphorous diets may cause phosphorous deficiency. Aluminium hydroxide may reduce absorption of tetracyclines when given concomitantly. Products containing dicyclomine hydrochloride should be used with caution in any patient with or suspected of having glaucoma or prostatic hypertrophy. Use with care in patients with hiatus hernia associated with reflux oesophagitis because anticholinergic drugs may aggravate this condition.

Use in pregnancy and lactation: Epidemiological studies in pregnant women with products containing dicyclomine hydrochloride (at doses up to 40 mg/day) have not shown that dicyclomine increases the risk of foetal abnormalities if administered during the first trimester of pregnancy. Reproduction studies have been performed in rats and rabbits at doses of up to 100 times the maximum recommended dose (based on 60 mg per day for an adult person) and have revealed no evidence of impaired fertility or harm to the foetus due to dicyclomine.

Since risk of teratogenicity cannot be excluded with absolute certainty for any product, the drug should be used during pregnancy only if clearly needed.

It is not known whether dicyclomine is secreted into human milk. Because many drugs are excreted in human milk, caution should be exercised when dicyclomine is administered to a nursing woman.

Side-effects: In particularly sensitive patients dicyclomine hydrochloride may cause atropine-like side-effects such as dry mouth, blurred vision, urinary retention or constipation.

Overdosage: Signs and symptoms of dicyclomine hydrochloride overdose include: headache, nausea and vomiting, blurred vision, dilated pupils, hot dry skin, dizziness, vertigo, dryness of mouth, difficulty in swallowing and CNS stimulation.

Treatment may include emetics, gastric lavage and symptomatic therapy if indicated.

Pharmaceutical precautions Store in a cool place. Shake well before use.

Legal category P.

Package quantities Amber glass bottles of 200 ml and 500 ml (original pack).

Further information Nil.

Product licence number 4425/0032.

LURSELLE*

Presentation White, non-coated tablets imprinted on one face with the name 'Lurselle' and a bisect line on the other, containing 250 mg probucol [4-4' (iso-propylidenedithio) bis (2,6-di-t-butylphenol)].

Uses Lurselle is indicated as ancillary therapy to diet for the reduction of elevated serum cholesterol in patients with hypercholesterolaemia, or in patients with combined hypercholesterolaemia and hypertriglyceridaemia where levels of cholesterol are a cause of concern.

Dosage and administration The recommended dose for adults is two tablets of 250 mg twice a day with the morning and evening meals.

Paediatric dosage has not been established.

Contra-indications, warnings, etc
Use in pregnancy and lactation: Reproduction studies in animals have not demonstrated any impairment of fertility or any harm to the foetus or offspring due to Lurselle. As yet there are no adequate studies in pregnant women, and the use of Lurselle during pregnancy is therefore not recommended. If a patient wishes to become pregnant, it is recommended that the drug be withdrawn and birth control procedures should be continued for at least six months, due to the persistence of the drug in the fatty tissues of the body.

In animals it has been shown that some of the drug is excreted in the milk. It is recommended that nursing mothers should not be treated with Lurselle.

Precautions: Before starting Lurselle, an attempt should be made to control elevated serum cholesterol by appropriate dietary regimens, weight reduction, and the treatment of any underlying disorder which might be the cause of the hypercholesterolaemia. Serum cholesterol and triglyceride levels should be monitored during the first months of treatment with Lurselle and periodically thereafter.

A favourable trend in cholesterol reduction should be evident during the first two months of Lurselle administration. An assessment should be made by the sixth month whether adequate reduction is being attained. A discontinuation in Lurselle treatment is usually followed by a gradual return of cholesterol to pre-treatment values.

If a marked sustained rise in serum triglycerides occurs during Lurselle therapy, consideration should be given to improving dietary compliance, alcohol abstinence, further restriction of calories, or adjustment of carbohydrate intake. If hypertriglyceridaemia persists, Lurselle should be discontinued.

Because probucol may cause prolongation of the QT interval (QTc), caution should be exercised in administering probucol to patients with evidence of recent or progressive myocardial damage or findings suggestive of serious ventricular arrhythmias or cardiovascular associated syncope. Caution should also be exercised in patients with QT prolongation due to other underlying conditions or to concomitant treatment. An ECG should be recorded before starting treatment.

Side-effects: The side-effects associated with Lurselle are generally mild to moderate and of short duration. They include diarrhoea, which occurs in about 1 in 10 patients, flatulence, abdominal pain, nausea and vomiting. These reactions are usually transient and seldom require the drug to be discontinued.

During the clinical studies in which patients have been treated for as long as 9 years, Lurselle had to be discontinued in less than 3 percent of the patients because of adverse gastrointestinal reactions.

Hypersensitivity reactions including angioneurotic oedema have been reported. Ventricular arrhythmias have also been reported.

Overdosage: In cases of overdosage symptomatic treatment and supportive measures should be instituted according to the individual symptoms.

Concomitant Therapy
The dosage of hypoglycaemic agents and oral anticoagulants need not usually be modified when given with Lurselle and these drugs do not alter the effect of Lurselle on serum cholesterol.

Administration of Lurselle with a second lipid lowering drug has been shown to produce further significant reductions in serum cholesterol. The most effective combinations were Lurselle with either ion exchange resins or nicotinic acid.

Pharmaceutical precautions Lurselle tablets should be stored in a well closed container, protected from light, heat and moisture.

Legal category POM.

Package quantities Original pack of 120 tablets.

Further information Absorption of Lurselle from the gastrointestinal tract is limited; food intake improves absorption and consequently induces higher and less variable peak blood levels. Lurselle is eliminated slowly from the body; the major pathway of excretion is the biliary tract.

Studies in man on the mode of action of Lurselle are

still underway but they have shown that Lurselle lowers serum cholesterol by increasing the excretion of bile acids and by inhibiting an early stage of cholesterol biosynthesis. In addition there may be a slight decrease in absorption of dietary cholesterol.

Studies with Lurselle have shown no evidence of biliary tract pathology or related gallstone formation.

Product licence number 4425/0043.

MERBENTYL* SYRUP

Presentation Merbentyl Syrup is colourless, and raspberry flavoured. Each 5 ml contains 10 mg Dicyclomine Hydrochloride BP.

Uses Merbentyl is a smooth muscle antispasmodic primarily indicated for the treatment of functional conditions involving smooth muscle spasm of the gastro-intestinal tract. The commonest of these is irritable colon (mucous colitis, spastic colon).

Dosage and administration *Adults:* One to two 5 ml spoonfuls (10–20 mg) three times daily before or after meals.

Children (2–12 years): One 5 ml spoonful (10 mg) three times daily.

Children (6 months–2 years): 5–10 mg three or four times daily, 15 minutes before feeds. Do not exceed a daily dose of 40 mg. If it is necessary to dilute Merbentyl Syrup this may be done using Syrup BP or, if diluted immediately prior to use, with water.

Contra-indications, warnings, etc
Contra-indications: Known idiosyncrasy to dicyclomine hydrochloride. Infants under 6 months of age.

Precautions: Products containing dicyclomine hydrochloride should be used with caution in any patient with, or suspected of having, glaucoma or prostatic hypertrophy. Use with care in patients with hiatus hernia associated with reflux oesophagitis because anticholinergic drugs may aggravate the condition.

There are rare reports of infants, 3 months of age and under, administered dicyclomine hydrochloride syrup, who have evidenced respiratory symptoms (breathing difficulty, shortness of breath, breathlessness, respiratory collapse, apnoea), as well as seizures, syncope, asphyxia, pulse rate fluctuations, muscular hypotonia and coma. The above symptoms have occurred within minutes of ingestion and lasted 20–30 minutes. The symptoms were reported in association with dicyclomine hydrochloride syrup therapy but the cause and effect relationship has neither been disproved nor proved. The timing and nature of the reactions suggest that they were a consequence of local irritation and/or aspiration, rather than to a direct pharmacological effect. Although no causal relationship between these effects, observed in infants, and dicyclomine administration has been established, dicyclomine hydrochloride is contra-indicated in infants under 6 months of age. See 'Contra-indications' above.

Use in pregnancy and lactation: Epidemiological studies in pregnant women with products containing dicyclomine hydrochloride (at doses up to 40 mg/day) have not shown that dicyclomine hydrochloride increases the risk of foetal abnormalities if administered during the first trimester of pregnancy. Reproduction studies have been performed in rats and rabbits at doses of up to 100 times the maximum recommended dose (based on 60 mg per day for an adult person) and have revealed no evidence of impaired fertility or harm to the foetus due to dicyclomine.

Since the risk of teratogenicity cannot be excluded with absolute certainty for any product, the drug should be used during pregnancy only if clearly needed.

It is not known whether dicyclomine is secreted in human milk. Because many drugs are excreted in human milk, caution should be exercised when dicyclomine is administered to a nursing woman.

Side-effects: Side-effects seldom occur with Merbentyl. However, in susceptible individuals, dry mouth, thirst and dizziness may occur. On rare occasions, fatigue, sedation, blurred vision, rash, constiptation, anorexia, nausea and vomiting, headache, and dysuria have also been reported.

Overdosage: Symptoms of Merbentyl overdosage are headache, dizziness, nausea, dry mouth, difficulty in swallowing, dilated pupils and hot dry skin. Treatment may include emetics, gastric lavage and symptomatic therapy if indicated.

Pharmaceutical precautions Should be stored and dispensed in amber glass bottles.

Legal category POM.
P – Preparations of Dicyclomine Hydrochloride for internal use with a maximum dose of 10 mg and a maximum daily dose of 60 mg.

Package quantities Amber glass bottles of 125 ml (original pack) and 500 ml.

Further information Nil.

Product licence number 4425/0047.

MERBENTYL* AND MERBENTYL 20* TABLETS

Presentation
Merbentyl Tablets: White, round, plain biconvex tablets, stamped 'M' in two concentric circles, containing Dicyclomine Hydrochloride BP 10 mg.

Merbentyl 20 Tablets: White, biconvex, oval tablets stamped MERBENTYL 20 containing Dicyclomine Hydrochloride BP 20 mg.

Uses Merbentyl is a smooth muscle antispasmodic primarily indicated for the treatment of functional conditions involving smooth muscle spasm of the gastro-intestinal tract.

Dosage and administration *Adults:* 10–20 mg three times daily before or after meals.

Children: (2–12 years): 10 mg three times daily.

Contra-indications, warnings, etc Known idiosyncrasy to dicyclomine hydrochloride.

Precautions: Products containing dicyclomine hydrochloride should be used with caution in any patient with, or suspected of having glaucoma or prostatic hypertrophy. Use with care in patients with hiatus hernia associated with reflux oesophagitis because anticholinergic drugs may aggravate the condition.

Use in pregnancy and lactation: Epidemiological studies in pregnant women with products containing dicyclomine hydrochloride (at doses up to 40 mg/day) have not shown that dicyclomine hydrochloride increases the risk of foetal abnormalities if administered during the first trimester of pregnancy. Reproduction studies have been performed in rats and rabbits at doses of up to 100 times the maximum recommended dose (based on 60 mg per day for an adult person) and have revealed no evidence of impaired fertility or harm to the foetus due to dicyclomine.

Since the risk of teratogenicity cannot be excluded with absolute certainty for any product, the drug should be used during pregnancy only if clearly needed.

It is not known whether dicyclomine is secreted in human milk. Because many drugs are excreted in human milk, caution should be exercised when dicyclomine is administered to a nursing woman.

Side-effects: Side-effects seldom occur with Merbentyl. However, in susceptible individuals, dry mouth, thirst and dizziness may occur. On rare occasions, fatigue, sedation, blurred vision, rash, constipation, anorexia, nausea and vomiting, headache and dysuria have also been reported.

Overdosage: Symptoms of Merbentyl overdosage are headache, dizziness, nausea, dry mouth, difficulty in swallowing, dilated pupils and hot dry skin. Treatment may include emetics, gastric lavage and symptomatic therapy if indicated.

Pharmaceutical precautions None.

Legal category POM.
P – Preparations of Dicyclomine Hydrochloride for internal use with a maximum dose of 10 mg and a maximum daily dose of 60 mg.

Package quantities
Merbentyl Tablets: blister pack of 100 tablets.
Merbentyl 20 Tablets: original pack of 84 tablets.

Further information Nil.

Product licence numbers

Merbentyl Tablets	4425/0035
Merbentyl 20 Tablets	4425/0081

PERFAN* INJECTION

Presentation Perfan Injection is a 5 mg/ml solution of enoximone presented in ampoules containing 20 ml.

Other ingredients are alcohol (95%), sodium hydroxide, propylene glycol and Water for Injections.

Perfan Injection is a sterile, clear yellow solution (pH approximately 12.0) for intravenous administration, which must be diluted before use. Containers of diluted product are intended for single use only.

Uses
Actions: Perfan has positive inotropic and vasodilator properties.

Indications: Perfan Injection is indicated for the treatment of congestive heart failure, typically where cardiac output is reduced and filling pressures increased, in patients who require intravenous therapy and who can be closely monitored. The duration of therapy should depend on the patient's continued positive and beneficial response. Sustained haemodynamic and clinical effects have been observed in patients treated for up to 48 hours.

Dosage and administration Perfan Injection must be diluted before use. Dilutions should be used immediately and any unused portion discarded.

Dilution: The pH of Perfan Injection is approximately 12.0. Perfan Injection must be diluted with an equal volume of 0.9% Sodium Chloride Injection or Water for Injections before administration.

Do not use more dilute solutions or other diluents, particularly dextrose injection, as crystal formation may occur.

Since crystal formation has been observed within approximately 1 hour after mixing Perfan Injection in glass containers or syringes, only plastic containers or syringes should be used for dilutions.

Administration: The following procedure is recommended for the administration of the diluted Perfan Injection.

Initial therapy: Therapy should be initiated with a dose of 0.5–1.0 mg/kg given as a slow injection (not faster than 12.5 mg/min); further doses of 0.5 mg/kg may be given similarly every 30 minutes until a satisfactory response is achieved or a total initial dose of 3.0 mg/kg is reached. Alternatively, treatment may be initiated as an infusion at a rate of 90 micrograms/kg/minute administered over 10 to 30 minutes until the required haemodynamic response is achieved.

Maintenance therapy: To maintain the effects of Perfan Injection the initial dose (not more than 3.0 mg/kg) may be repeated as required every 3–6 hours and adjusted according to the response of the patient. Alternatively, a continuous or intermittent infusion at a rate of 5 to 20 micrograms/kg/minute may be instituted. Total dose over 24 hours should not normally exceed 24.0 mg/kg. In patients with renal impairment the dosage or dosage frequency may need to be reduced.

Precautions should be taken to avoid venous extravasation during administration.

This dosing regimen will produce, in the majority of patients, a 30% or greater increase in cardiac output and/or decreases in pulmonary capillary wedge pressure of about 30% and right atrial pressure of about 40%. It should be noted that the initial haemodynamic response determines the subsequent rate of administration as well as the duration of treatment.

Use in children: Safety and effectiveness in children have not been established.

Contra-indications, warnings, etc
Contra-indications: Perfan Injection is contra-indicated in patients with a known hypersensitivity to Perfan or its components.

Use in pregnancy and lactation: There is no evidence of animal teratogenicity with oral therapy. Reproduction studies performed in rats at doses up to 300 mg/kg/day and 100 mg/kg/day have revealed reductions in maternal food consumption, maternal body weight gain and in pup weight at weaning and sexual maturity when enoximone was administered throughout pregnancy and lactation. Sexual behaviour and reproductive capability were unaltered by enoximone treatment. There are no adequate and well-controlled studies in pregnant women. Perfan Injection should be used during pregnancy only if the potential benefit justifies the potential risk. It is not known whether this drug is excreted in human milk. Because many drugs are excreted in human milk, caution should be exercised when Perfan Injection is administered to a nursing mother.

Precautions: Perfan Injection should be used cautiously when heart failure is associated with hypertrophic cardiomyopathy, stenotic or obstructive valvular disease or other outlet obstruction.

During treatment with Perfan Injection the following parameters should be monitored: blood pressure, heart rate, ECG, central venous pressure and fluid and electrolyte status; monitoring of platelet counts and hepatic enzyme levels is recommended.

Drug/laboratory interactions: No clinical manifestations of untoward drug interaction were observed in patients receiving Perfan Injection most of whom concomitantly received one or more of the following: diuretics (amiloride, triamterene, frusemide and spironolactone), digitalis glycosides (digoxin), potassium supplements, antiarrhythmics (diltiazem, propranolol, lignocaine, nifedipine, procainamide and quinidine), vasodilators (captopril, hydralazine, nitroprusside and nitrates), anticoagulants (warfarin and heparin), analgesics (acetylsalicylic acid, paracetamol and codeine), sedatives (chloral hydrate, diazepam and lorazepam) and positive inotropic agents (dobutamine and dopamine).

In general, administration of Perfan Injection has not been associated with clinically significant alterations in laboratory tests. However, some changes have been noted in platelet counts (reduction in a small percentage of patients) and hepatic enzyme levels (a few patients with minor abnormalities). Monitoring of these parameters is recommended.

Side-effects: Whilst Perfan Injection has not been shown to be arrhythmogenic in electrophysiological studies, ectopic beats have been observed in some patients during or after Perfan Injection administration. Ventricular tachycardias or supraventricular arrhythmias have been reported less frequently and are more likely to occur in patients with pre-existing arrhythmias. Perfan Injection may induce hypotension as a consequence of its vasodilator activity. Temporary discontinuation of treatment or a reduction in dosage will usually reverse these conditions.

Other side-effects reported include headache, insomnia, nausea and/or vomiting, and diarrhoea.

Isolated cases of chills, oliguria, fever, urinary retention and upper and lower extremity pain have also been reported.

Overdosage: Intravenous administration of Perfan Injection has been shown to produce reductions in blood pressure with occasional instances of hypotensive symptoms. If symptomatic hypotension is observed, administration of Perfan Injection should be reduced or discontinued. No specific antidote is known, but general measures for circulatory support should be taken.

Pharmaceutical precautions Store ampoules in a cold place (36°–46°F, 2°–8°C). Use only 0.9% Sodium Chloride Injection or Water for Injections as diluents.

After dilution, use immediately and discard unused portion. If immediate administration is not possible, do not refrigerate dilutions as crystal formation may occur.

Do not administer unless diluted product is a clear yellow solution.

Other drugs should not be mixed in the same container as Perfan Injection.

Legal category POM.

Package quantities Ampoules of 20 ml in cartons of 10 ampoules.

Further information Nil.

Product licence number 4425/0086.

RIFADIN*

Presentation
Rifadin capsules 150 mg: Blue and red marked 'Lepetit' containing 150 mg Rifampicin BP.
Rifadin capsules 300 mg: Red marked 'Lepetit' containing 300 mg Rifampicin BP.
Rifadin syrup: Raspberry colour and flavour, containing 100 mg Rifampicin BP in each 5 ml.

Uses
Mode of action: Rifadin is a semi-synthetic antibiotic with bactericidal activity against most Mycobacteria and Gram-positive organisms. Rifadin is also active against Gram-negative organisms at higher concentrations.

Indications:
Tuberculosis: Rifadin, used in combination with other active anti-tuberculosis drugs, is indicated in the treatment of all forms of tuberculosis, including fresh, advanced, chronic and drug-resistant cases. Rifadin is also effective against most atypical strains of Mycobacteria.

Leprosy: Rifadin, used in combination with at least one other active anti-leprosy drug, is indicated in the management of multibacillary and paucibacillary leprosy to effect conversion of the infectious state to a non-infectious state.

Other Infections: Rifadin is indicated in the treatment of Brucellosis, Legionnaires Disease, and serious staphylococcal infections. To prevent emergence of resistant strains of the infecting organisms, Rifadin should be used in combination with another antibiotic appropriate for the infection.

Prophylaxis of meningococcal meningitis: Rifadin is indicated for the treatment of asymptomatic carriers of *N. meningitidis* to eliminate meningococci from the nasopharynx.

Haemophilus influenzae: Rifadin is indicated for the treatment of asymptomatic carriers of *H. influenzae* and as chemoprophylaxis of exposed children, 4 years of age or younger.

Dosage and administration The daily dose of Rifadin, calculated from the patient's body weight, should preferably be taken at least 30 minutes before a meal or 2 hours after a meal to ensure rapid and complete absorption.

Tuberculosis: Rifadin should be given with other effective anti-tuberculosis drugs to prevent the possible emergence of rifampicin-resistant strains of Mycobacteria.

Adults: The recommended single daily dose in tuberculosis is 8–12 mg/kg.

Usual daily dose: Patients weighing less than 50 kg – 450 mg. Patients weighing 50 kg or more – 600 mg.

Children: In children, oral doses of 10–20 mg/kg body weight daily are recommended, although a total daily dose should not usually exceed 600 mg.

Leprosy: 600 mg doses of rifampicin should be given once per month. Alternatively, a daily regimen may be used. The recommended single daily dose is 10 mg/kg.

Usual daily dose: Patients weighing less than 50 kg – 450 mg. Patients weighing 50 kg or more – 600 mg.

In the treatment of leprosy, rifampicin should always be used in conjunction with at least one other antileprosy drug.

Brucellosis, Legionnaires Disease or serious staphylococcal infections
Adults: The recommended daily dose is 600 – 1200 mg given in 2 to 4 divided doses, together with another appropriate antibiotic to prevent the emergence of resistant strains of the infecting organisms.

Prophylaxis of meningococcal meningitis
Adults: 600 mg twice daily for 2 days.
Children (1–12 years): 10 mg/kg twice daily for 2 days.
Children (3 months–1 year): 5 mg/kg twice daily for 2 days.

Prophylaxis of Haemophilus influenzae
Adults and children: For members of households exposed to H. influenzae B disease when the household contains a child 4 years of age or younger, it is recommended that all members (including the child) receive rifampicin 20 mg/kg once daily (maximum daily dose 600 mg) for 4 days.

Index cases should be treated prior to discharge from hospital.

Neonates (1 month): 10 mg/kg daily for 4 days.

Impaired liver function: A daily dose of 8 mg/kg should not be exceeded in patients with impaired liver function.

Use in the elderly: In elderly patients, the renal excretion of rifampicin is decreased proportionally with physiological decrease of renal function; due to compensatory increase of liver excretion, the terminal half-life in serum is similar to that of younger patients. However, as increased blood levels have been noted in one study of rifampicin in elderly patients, caution should be exercised in using rifampicin in such patients, especially if there is evidence of impaired liver function.

Contra-indications, warnings, etc
Contra-indications: Rifadin is contra-indicated in the presence of jaundice, and in patients who are hypersensitive to the rifamycins.

Use in pregnancy and lactation: At very high doses in animals rifampicin has been shown to have teratogenic effects. There are no well controlled studies with rifampicin in pregnant women. Therefore, Rifadin should be used in pregnant women or in women of child bearing potential only if the potential benefit justifies the potential risk to the foetus. When Rifadin is administered during the last few weeks of pregnancy it may cause post-natal haemorrhages in the mother and infant for which treatment with Vitamin K1 may be indicated.

Rifampicin is excreted in breast milk, patients receiving rifampicin should not breast feed unless in the physician's judgement the potential benefit to the patient outweighs the potential risk to the infant.

Precautions: Patients with impaired liver function should only be given rifampicin in cases of necessity, and then with caution and under close medical supervision. In these patients, lower doses of rifampicin are recommended and careful monitoring of liver function, especially serum glutamic pyruvic transaminase (SGPT) and serum glutamic oxaloacetic transaminase (SGOT) should be carried out prior to therapy and then every two to four weeks during therapy. If signs of hepatocellular damage occur, rifampicin should be withdrawn. In patients with impaired liver function, elderly patients, malnourished patients, and possibly, children under two years of age, caution is particularly recommended when instituting therapeutic regimens in which isoniazid is to be used concurrently with Rifadin. It is rarely necessary, in the absence of clinical findings, to increase the frequency of performing routine liver function tests in patients with normal pretreatment liver function.

In some patients hyperbilirubinaemia can occur in the early days of treatment. This results from competition between rifampicin and bilirubin for hepatic excretion.

An isolated report showing a moderate rise in bilirubin and/or transaminase level is not in itself an indication for interrupting treatment; rather the decision should be made after repeating the tests, noting trends in the levels and considering them in conjunction with the patient's clinical condition.

Because of the possibility of immunological reaction (see Side-effects) occurring with intermittent therapy (less than 2 to 3 times per week) patients should be closely monitored. Patients should be cautioned against interrupting treatment.

Rifampicin has enzyme-inducing properties including induction of delta amino levulinic acid synthetase. Isolated reports have associated porphyria exacerbation with rifampicin administration.

Drug/laboratory interactions: Rifampicin has been shown in animals and man to have liver enzyme inducing properties and may reduce the activity of anticoagulants, corticosteroids, cyclosporin, digitalis preparations, oral contraceptives, oral hypoglycaemic agents, dapsone, phenytoin, quinidine, narcotics and analgesics. It may be necessary to adjust the dosage of these drugs if they are given concurrently with Rifadin, particularly when it is initiated or withdrawn.

Patients on oral contraceptives should be advised to use alternative, non-hormonal methods of birth control during Rifadin therapy. Also diabetes may become more difficult to control.

If *p*-aminosalicylic acid and rifampicin are both included in the treatment regimen, they should be given not less than eight hours apart to ensure satisfactory blood levels.

Therapeutic levels of rifampicin have been shown to inhibit standard microbiological assays for serum folate and Vitamin B12. Thus alternative assay methods should be considered. Transient elevation of BSP and serum bilirubin have been reported. Therefore, these tests should be performed before the morning dose of rifampicin.

Side-effects: Reactions occurring with either daily or intermittent dosage regimens include:

Cutaneous reactions which are mild and self-limiting and do not appear to be hypersensitivity reactions. Typically they consist of flushing and itching with or without a rash.

Gastrointestinal reactions consist of anorexia, nausea, vomiting, abdominal discomfort, and diarrhoea. Pseudomembranous colitis has been reported with rifampicin therapy.

Hepatitis can be caused by rifampicin and liver function tests should be monitored (see Precautions).

Thrombocytopenia with or without purpura may occur, usually associated with intermittent therapy, but is reversible if drug is discontinued as soon as purpura occurs. Cerebral haemorrhage and fatalities have been reported when rifampicin administration has been continued or resumed after the appearance of purpura.

Eosinophilia, leucopenia, oedema, muscle weakness and myopathy have been reported to occur in a small percentage of patients treated with rifampicin.

Reactions usually occurring with intermittent dosage regimens and probably of immunological origin include:

- 'Flu Syndrome' consisting of episodes of fever, chills, headache, dizziness, and bone pain appearing most commonly during the 3rd to the 6th month of therapy. The frequency of the syndrome varies but may occur in up to 50% of patients given once-weekly regimens with a dose of rifampicin of 25 mg/kg or more.
- Shortness of breath and wheezing.
- Decrease in blood pressure and shock.
- Acute haemolytic anaemia.
- Acute renal failure usually due to acute tubular necrosis or acute interstitial nephritis.

If serious complications arise, e.g. renal failure, thrombocytopenia or haemolytic anaemia, rifampicin should be stopped and never restarted.

Occasional disturbances of the menstrual cycle have been reported in women receiving long term anti-tuberculosis therapy with regimens containing rifampicin.

Rifampicin may produce a reddish discolouration of the urine, sputum and tears. The patient should be forewarned of this. Soft contact lenses may be permanently stained.

Overdosage: In cases of overdosage with Rifadin, gastric lavage should be performed as soon as possible. Intensive supportive measures should be instituted and individual symptoms treated as they arise.

Pharmaceutical precautions Rifadin syrup should not be diluted. It should be dispensed in clear or amber glass bottles.

Rifadin capsules should be protected from light and moisture and stored below 25°C.

Legal category POM.

Package quantities
Rifadin capsules 150 mg: Blister packs of 100 capsules.
Rifadin capsules 300 mg: Blister packs of 100 capsules.
Rifadin syrup 100 mg/5 ml: Bottles of 120 ml.

Further information An oral dose of 450–600 mg Rifadin produces therapeutically effective levels in the blood, with the peak concentrations being observed approximately 2 hours after administration. There is a good distribution of rifampicin into body tissues and fluids including lung, bone, lymph nodes and inflammatory exudates. Rifampicin is excreted mainly in the bile and urine, and high concentrations are reached in both these fluids. No cross resistance has been shown between Rifadin and other anti-Mycobacteria agents.

Product licence numbers

Rifadin capsules 150 mg	4425/5915
Rifadin capsules 300 mg	4425/5916
Rifadin syrup	4425/5917

RIFADIN* FOR INFUSION

Presentation 20 ml vial containing 600 mg Rifampicin BP (red lyophilised powder) and 10 ml ampoule of clear colourless solvent solution (pyrogen free water plus polysorbate 81).

Uses
Mode of action: Rifadin is a semi-synthetic antibiotic with bactericidal activity against most Mycobacteria and Gram-positive organisms. Rifadin is also active against Gram-negative organisms at higher concentrations.

Indications: Rifadin for Infusion is indicated for acutely ill patients who are unable to tolerate oral therapy e.g. post operative or comatose patients or patients in whom gastrointestinal absorption is impaired.

Oral therapy should be used where possible. As soon as patients are able to accept oral medication, they should be transferred to Rifadin Capsules or Syrup.

Tuberculosis: Rifadin, used in combination with other active anti-tuberculosis drugs, is indicated in the treatment of all forms of tuberculosis, including fresh, advanced, chronic and drug-resistant cases. Rifadin is also effective against most atypical strains of Mycobacteria.

Other infections: Rifadin is indicated in the treatment of Legionnaires Disease, and serious staphylococcal infections. To prevent emergence of resistant strains of the infecting organisms. Rifadin should be used in combination with another antibiotic appropriate for the infection.

Preparation of infusion: Rifadin for Infusion is prepared by aseptically adding the solvent to the vial of rifampicin powder and shaking vigorously and continuously for about 30 seconds. When the powder has completely dissolved, the solution should be immediately diluted in 500 ml 5% glucose solution, or other suitable infusion fluid (see 'Pharmaceutical precautions'). It is suggested that the infusion is administered over a period of 2–3 hours. Rifadin solution should be used within 6 hours of preparation.

Dosage and administration Treatment with Rifadin for Infusion should include concomitant use of other appropriate antibacterials to prevent the emergence of resistant strains of the causative organism.

Tuberculosis

Adults: A single daily administration of 600 mg given by intravenous infusion over 2 to 3 hours has been found to be effective and well tolerated for adult patients. Serum concentrations following this dosage regimen are similar to those obtained after 600 mg by mouth.

Children: The usual paediatric regimen is a single daily dose of up to 20 mg/kg bodyweight; the total daily dose should not normally exceed 600 mg.

Legionnaires Disease or serious staphylococcal infections:

Adults: The recommended daily dose is 600 – 1200 mg given in 2 to 4 divided doses, together with another antibacterial agent with similar properties to prevent the emergence of resistant strains.

Impaired liver function: A daily dose of 8 mg/kg should not be exceeded in patients with impaired liver function.

Use in the elderly: In elderly patients, the renal excretion of rifampicin is decreased proportionally with physiological decrease of renal function; due to compensatory increase of liver excretion, the serum terminal half-life is similar to that of younger patients. However, as increased blood levels have been noted in one study of rifampicin in elderly patients, caution should be exercised in using rifampicin in such patients, especially if there is evidence of liver function impairment.

Contra-indications, warnings, etc

Contra-indications: Rifadin for Infusion is contra-indicated in patients who are hypersensitive to rifamycins.

Although not recommended for use in patients with jaundice, the therapeutic benefit of Rifadin for Infusion should be weighed against the possible risks.

Use in pregnancy and lactation: At very high doses in animals rifampicin has been shown to have teratogenic effects. There are no well controlled studies with rifampicin in pregnant women. Therefore, Rifadin for Infusion should be used in pregnant women or in women of child bearing potential only if the potential benefit justifies the potential risk to the foetus. When rifampicin is administered during the last few weeks of pregnancy it may cause post-natal haemorrhages in the mother and infant for which treatment with Vitamin K1 may be indicated.

Rifampicin is excreted in breast milk and patients receiving rifampicin should not breast feed unless in the physician's judgement the potential benefit to the patient outweighs the potential risk to the infant.

Precautions: Patients with impaired liver function should only be given rifampicin in cases of necessity, and then with caution and under close medical supervision. In these patients, lower doses of rifampicin are recommended and careful monitoring of liver function, especially serum glutamic pyruvic transaminase (SGPT) and serum glutamic oxaloacetic transaminase (SGOT) should be carried out. If signs of hepatocellular damage occur, rifampicin should be withdrawn. In patients with impaired liver function, elderly patients, malnourished patients, and possibly, children under two years of age, caution is particularly recommended when instituting therapeutic regimens in which isoniazid is to be used concurrently with rifampicin.

It is rarely necessary, in the absence of clinical findings, to increase the frequency of performing routine liver function tests in patients with normal pretreatment liver function. In the presence of complete renal failure, rifampicin is excreted entirely in the bile: provided hepatic function is not impaired the dosage of rifampicin need not be adjusted.

In some patients hyperbilirubinaemia resulting from competition between rifampicin and bilirubin for excretory pathways of the liver at the cell level can occur in the early days of treatment. An isolated report showing a moderate rise in bilirubin and/or transaminase level is not in itself an indication for interrupting treatment; rather the decision should be made after repeating the tests, noting trends in the levels and considering them in conjunction with the patient's clinical condition.

Rifampicin has enzyme-inducing properties including induction of delta amino levulinic acid synthetase. Isolated reports have associated porphyria exacerbation with rifampicin administration.

Drug/laboratory interactions: Rifampicin has been shown in animals and man to have liver enzyme inducing properties and may reduce the activity of anticoagulants, corticosteroids, cyclosporin, digitalis preparations, oral contraceptives, oral hypoglycaemic agents, dapsone, phenytoin, quinidine, narcotics and analgesics. It may be necessary to adjust the dosage of these drugs if they are given concurrently with Rifadin, particularly when it is initiated or withdrawn.

Therapeutic levels of rifampicin have been shown to inhibit standard microbiological assays for serum folate and Vitamin B12. Thus alternative assay methods should be considered. Transient elevation of BSP and serum bilirubin have been reported. Therefore, these tests should be performed before the daily administration of Rifadin for Infusion.

Side-effects: Rifadin for Infusion is generally well tolerated and accepted by patients, although hypersensitivity reactions have been described and occasionally patients have experienced fever, skin rashes and nausea/vomiting.

Occasional instances of phlebitis and pain at the infusion site have been reported.

Reactions occurring with either daily or intermittent dosage regimens include:

Cutaneous reactions which are mild and self-limiting may occur and do not appear to be hypersensitivity reactions. Typically they consist of flushing and itching with or without a rash.

Gastro-intestinal reactions consist of anorexia, nausea, vomiting, abdominal discomfort, and diarrhoea. Pseudomembranous colitis has been reported with rifampicin therapy.

Hepatitis can be caused by rifampicin and liver function tests should be monitored (see Precautions).

Thrombocytopenia with or without purpura may occur, usually associated with intermittent therapy, but is reversible if drug is discontinued as soon as purpura occurs. Cerebral haemorrhage and fatalities have been reported when rifampicin administration has been continued or resumed after the appearance of purpura.

Eosinophilia, leucopenia, oedema, muscle weakness and myopathy have been reported to occur in a small percentage of patients treated with rifampicin.

Reactions usually occurring with intermittent dosage regimens and probably of immunological origin include:

- 'Flu Syndrome' consisting of episodes of fever, chills, headache, dizziness, and bone pain appearing most commonly during the 3rd to the 6th month of therapy. The frequency of the syndrome varies but may occur in up to 50% of patients given once-weekly regimens with a dose of rifampicin of 25 mg/kg or more.
- Shortness of breath and wheezing.
- Decrease in blood pressure and shock.
- Acute haemolytic anaemia.
- Acute renal failure usually due to acute tubular necrosis or acute interstitial nephritis.

If serious complications arise, (renal failure, thrombocytopenia or haemolytic anaemia), rifampicin should be stopped and never restarted.

Occasional disturbances of the menstrual cycle have been reported in women receiving long term anti-tuberculosis therapy with regimens containing rifampicin.

Rifampicin may produce a reddish discolouration of the urine, sputum and tears. The patient should be forewarned of this. Soft contact lenses may be permanently stained.

Pharmaceutical precautions Rifadin for Infusion should be freshly prepared.

Compatibilities: Rifadin for Infusion is compatible with the following infusion solutions for up to 6 hours: Mannitol 10% and 20%, Macrodex with Saline Solution,

Macrodex with Glucose Solution, Rheomacrodex, Sodium Bicarbonate 1.4%, Laevulose 5% and 10%, Ringer Lactate, Ringer Acetate, Dextrose 5% and 10%, Saline Solution.

Incompatibilities: Rifadin for Infusion is incompatible with the following: Perfudex, Sodium Bicarbonate 5%, Sodium Lactate 0.167M, Ringer Acetate with Dextrose.

Legal category POM.

Package quantities Combined pack of one vial containing 600 mg Rifampicin BP, and one ampoule containing 10 ml solvent.

Further information Nil.

Product licence number 4425/0051.

RIFATER*

Presentation Smooth, round, shiny, pink-beige, sugar coated tablets containing Isoniazid BP 50 mg, Pyrazinamide BP 300 mg and Rifampicin BP 120 mg.

Uses Rifater is indicated in the treatment of pulmonary tuberculosis.

Dosage and administration Rifater is recommended in the initial intensive phase of the short-course treatment of pulmonary tuberculosis. During this phase, which lasts for 2 months, Rifater should be administered on a daily continuous basis. The concomitant administration of ethambutol or intramuscular streptomycin over the same period of time is advised.

Each Rifater tablet contains isoniazid (INH), pyrazinamide (Z) and rifampicin (RAMP) in such a ratio that the administration of 9–12 mg/kg RAMP, 4–5 mg/kg INH and 23–30 mg/kg Z can be achieved by giving 3 tablets daily to patients weighing less than 40 kg, 4 tablets to patients weighing 40–49 kg, 5 tablets to patients weighing 50–64 kg and 6 tablets to patients weighing 65 kg or more.

Rifater should be given as a single dose and preferably on an empty stomach at least 30 minutes before a meal or 2 hours after a meal to ensure rapid and complete absorption.

Once the initial intensive phase of treatment has been completed treatment can be continued with the combination rifampicin-isoniazid (Rifinah*) always on a daily basis.

This regimen, if correctly applied, is 100% effective with very few, if any, relapses. The clinical evidence indicates that these occur generally in the first 6 months after stopping treatment with bacilli fully sensitive to the drugs employed, so that changes in the drugs to be utilised for further treatment are not required. The regimen has been found to be fully effective also in the presence of a bacillary population resistant to isoniazid, to streptomycin or to both drugs.

Children: The ratio of the three drugs in Rifater may not be appropriate in children (e.g. higher mg/kg doses of INH are usually given in children than in adults). Rifater can be used only in special cases, after careful consideration of the mg/kg dose of each component.

Use in the elderly: Caution should be exercised in such patients, in view of the possible decrease of the excretory function of the kidney and of the liver.

Contra-indications, warnings, etc
Contra-indications: Rifater is contra-indicated in patients who are hypersensitive to any one of the components of the combination. Rifater is contra-indicated in the presence of jaundice.

Use in pregnancy and lactation: At very high doses in animals rifampicin has been shown to have teratogenic effects. There are no well controlled studies with Rifater in pregnant women. Therefore, Rifater should be used in pregnant women or in women of child-bearing potential only if the potential benefit justifies the potential risk to the foetus. When administered during the last few weeks of pregnancy, Rifater may cause post-natal haemorrhages in the mother and infant, for which treatment with Vitamin K1 may be indicated.

Rifampicin and isoniazid are excreted in breast milk and patients receiving Rifater should not breast feed unless in the physician's judgement the potential benefit to the patient outweighs the potential risk to the infant.

Precautions: The precautions for the use of Rifater are the same as those considered when a triple individual administration of rifampicin, isoniazid and pyrazinamide is required. Each of these drugs has been associated with liver dysfunction. Patients with impaired liver function should only be given Rifater in cases of necessity and then with caution and under strict medical supervision. In these patients, careful monitoring of liver function, especially serum glutamic pyruvic transaminase (SGPT) and serum glutamic oxaloacetic transaminase (SGOT) should be carried out prior to therapy and then every two to four weeks during therapy. If signs of hepatocellular damage occur, Rifater should be withdrawn. Care should be exercised in the treatment of elderly or malnourished patients who may also require Vitamin B6 supplementation with the isoniazid therapy.

In some cases hyperbilirubinaemia resulting from competition between rifampicin and bilirubin for excretory pathways of the liver at the cell level can occur in the early days of treatment. An isolated report showing a moderate rise in bilirubin and/or transaminase level is not in itself an indication for interrupting treatment; rather, the decision should be made after repeating the tests, noting trends in the levels and considering them in conjunction with the patient's clinical condition.

Rifater should be used with caution in patients with a history of gout. If hyperuricaemia accompanied by an acute gouty arthritis occurs, the patient should be transferred to a regimen not containing pyrazinamide (e.g. Rifinah 150 or 300).

The possibility of pyrazinamide having an adverse effect on blood clotting time or vascular integrity should be borne in mind in patients with haemoptysis.

Because of the possibility of immunological reaction (see 'Side-effects') occurring with intermittent rifampicin therapy (less than 2 to 3 per week) patients should be closely monitored. Patients should be cautioned against interruption of dosage regimens since these reactions may occur.

Drug/laboratory interactions: Rifampicin has liver enzyme-inducing properties and may reduce the activity of a number of drugs including anticoagulants, corticosteroids, cyclosporin, digitalis preparations, quinidine, oral contraceptives, oral hypoglycaemic agents, dapsone, narcotics and analgesics. It may be necessary to adjust the dosage of these drugs if they are given concurrently with Rifater.

Patients using oral contraceptives should be advised to change to non-hormonal methods of birth control during Rifater therapy. Also diabetes may become more difficult to control.

If p-aminosalicylic acid and rifampicin are both included in the treatment regimen, they should be given not less than eight hours apart to ensure satisfactory blood levels.

Therapeutic levels of rifampicin have been shown to inhibit standard microbiological assays for serum folate and Vitamin B12. Thus alternative assay methods should be considered. Transient elevation of BSP and serum bilirubin have been reported. Therefore, these tests should be performed before the morning dose of rifampicin. Isoniazid may decrease the excretion of phenytoin or may enhance its effects. Appropriate adjustment of the anti-convulsant dose should be made.

Side-effects: Rifampicin: Reactions occurring with either daily or intermittent dosage regimens include:

Cutaneous reactions which are mild and self-limiting and do not appear to be hypersensitivity reactions. Typically they consist of flushing and itching with or without a rash.

Gastro-intestinal reactions consist of anorexia, nausea, vomiting, abdominal discomfort, and diarrhoea. Pseudomembranous colitis has been reported with rifampicin therapy.

Hepatitis can be caused by rifampicin and liver function tests should be monitored. (See 'Precautions').

Thrombocytopenia with or without purpura may occur, usually associated with intermittent therapy, but is reversible if drug is discontinued as soon as purpura occurs. Cerebral haemorrhage and fatalities have been reported when rifampicin administration has been continued or resumed after the appearance of purpura.

Eosinophilia, leucopenia, oedema, muscle weakness and myopathy have been reported to occur in a small percentage of patients treated with rifampicin.

Reactions usually occurring with intermittent dosage regimens and probably of immunological origin include:

- 'Flu Syndrome' consisting of episodes of fever, chills, headache, dizziness, and bone pain appearing most commonly during the 3rd to the 6th month of therapy. The frequency of the syndrome varies but may occur in up to 50% of patients given once-weekly regimens with a dose of rifampicin of 25 mg/kg or more.
- Shortness of breath and wheezing.
- Decrease in blood pressure and shock.
- Acute haemolytic anaemia.
- Acute renal failure usually due to acute tubular necrosis or to acute interstitial nephritis.

If serious complications arise, (renal failure, thrombocytopenia or haemolytic anaemia), Rifater should be stopped and never restarted.

Occasional disturbances of the menstrual cycle have been reported in women receiving long term anti-tuberculosis therapy with regimens containing rifampicin.

Rifampicin may produce a reddish discolouration of the urine, sputum and tears. The patient should be forewarned of this. Soft contact lenses may be permanently stained.

Isoniazid: Severe and sometimes fatal hepatitis may occur with isoniazid therapy. Polyneuritis associated with isoniazid, presenting as paraesthesia, muscle weakness, loss of tendon reflexes, is unlikely to occur with the recommended daily dose of Rifater. Various haematological disturbances have been identified during treatment with isoniazid, including eosinophilia, agranulocytosis, and anaemia. High doses of isoniazid can cause convulsions. The possibility that the frequency of seizures may be increased in patients with epilepsy should be borne in mind.

Pyrazinamide: Adverse reactions, other than hepatic reactions, which have been attributed to pyrazinamide are active gout (pyrazinamide has been reported to reduce urate excretion), sideroblastic anaemia, arthralgia, anorexia, nausea and vomiting, dysuria, malaise, fever, urticaria and aggravation of peptic ulcer. The hepatic reaction is the most common adverse reaction and varies from a symptomless abnormality of hepatic cell function detected only through laboratory liver function tests, through a mild syndrome of fever, malaise and liver tenderness, to more serious reactions such as clinical jaundice and rare cases of acute yellow atrophy and death.

Overdosage: In cases of overdosage with Rifater, gastric lavage should be performed as soon as possible. Intensive supportive measures should be instituted and individual symptoms treated as they arise. Parenteral pyridoxine (Vitamin B6) should be given. Symptoms are more likely to be related to isoniazid, including coma, respiratory distress, hyperglycaemia and metabolic ketoacidosis.

Pharmaceutical precautions None.

Legal category POM.

Package quantities Blister strips of 20's in packs of 100's.

Further information Nil.

Product licence number 4425/0060.

RIFINAH*

Presentation *Rifinah 300:* orange, capsule-shaped tablets marked RH300 containing 300 mg Rifampicin BP and 150 mg Isoniazid BP.

Rifinah 150: cyclamen, round biconvex tablets marked RH150 containing 150 mg Rifampicin BP and 100 mg Isoniazid BP.

Uses Rifinah 300 and Rifinah 150 are indicated in the treatment of all forms of tuberculosis, including fresh, advanced and chronic cases.

Dosage and administration Another anti-tuberculosis drug may be given concurrently with Rifinah until the susceptibility of the infecting organism to rifampicin and isoniazid has been confirmed.

Adults: Patients should be given the following single daily dose preferably on an empty stomach at least 30 minutes before a meal or 2 hours after a meal:

Rifinah 150: Patients weighing less than 50 kg – 3 tablets.

Rifinah 300: Patients weighing 50 kg or more – 2 tablets.

Use in the elderly: Caution should be exercised in such patients especially if there is evidence of liver impairment.

Contra-indications, warnings, etc

Contra-indications: Rifinah 300 and Rifinah 150 are contra-indicated in the presence of jaundice. Rifinah 300 and Rifinah 150 are contra-indicated in patients who are hypersensitive to rifamycins or isoniazid.

Use in pregnancy and lactation: Rifampicin has been shown to be teratogenic in rodents when given in large doses. There are no well controlled studies with Rifinah in pregnant women. Therefore, Rifinah should be used in pregnant women or in women of child bearing potential only if the potential benefit justifies the potential risk to the foetus.

When administered during the last few weeks of pregnancy, rifampicin can cause post-natal haemorrhages in the mother and infant, for which treatment with Vitamin K1 may be indicated.

Rifampicin and isoniazid are excreted in breast milk and patients receiving Rifinah should not breast feed unless in the physician's judgement the potential benefit to the patient outweighs the potential risk to the infant.

Precautions: Rifinah is a combination of 2 drugs, each of which has been associated with liver dysfunction.

Patients with impaired liver function should only be given Rifinah in cases of necessity, and then with caution and under close medical supervision. In these patients, careful monitoring of liver function, especially serum glutamic pyruvic transaminase (SGPT) and serum glutamic oxaloacetic transaminase (SGOT) should be carried out prior to therapy and then every two to four weeks during therapy. Similar care should be exercised in elderly patients, malnourished patients and children under two years of age. If signs of hepatocellular damage occur, Rifinah should be withdrawn. Care should be exercised in the treatment of elderly or malnourished patients who may also require Vitamin B_6 supplementation with the isoniazid therapy.

In some cases hyperbilirubinaemia resulting from competition between rifampicin and bilirubin for excretory pathways of the liver at the cell level can occur in the early days of treatment. An isolated report showing a moderate rise in bilirubin and/or transaminase level is not in itself an indication for interrupting treatment; rather the decision should be made after repeating the tests, noting trends in the levels and considering them in conjunction with the patient's clinical condition.

Because of the possibility of immunological reaction (see 'Side-effects') occurring with intermittent rifampicin therapy (less than 2 to 3 times per week) patients should be closely monitored. Patients should be cautioned against interruption of dosage regimens since these reactions may occur.

Drug/laboratory interactions: Rifampicin has liver-enzyme inducing properties and may reduce the activity of a number of drugs including anticoagulants, corticosteroids, cyclosporin, digitalis preparations, quinidine, oral contraceptives, oral hypoglycaemic agents, dapsone, narcotics and analgesics. It may be necessary to adjust the dosage of these drugs if they are given concurrently with Rifinah. Patients using oral contraceptives should be advised to change to non-hormonal methods of birth control during Rifinah therapy. Also, diabetes may become more difficult to control. When rifampicin is taken with para-aminosalicylic acid (P.A.S.), rifampicin levels in the serum may decrease. Therefore the drugs should be taken at least eight hours apart. Therapeutic levels of rifampicin have been shown to inhibit standard microbiological assays for serum folate and Vitamin B_{12}. Thus, alternative assay methods should be considered. Transient elevation of BSP and serum bilirubin have been reported. Therefore, these tests should be performed before the morning dose of rifampicin. Isoniazid may decrease the excretion of phenytoin or may enhance its effects. Appropriate adjustments of the anticonvulsant dose should be made.

Side-effects:
Rifampicin: Reactions to rifampicin occurring with either daily or intermittent dosage regimens include:

Cutaneous reactions which are mild and self-limiting and do not appear to be hypersensitivity reactions. Typically they consist of flushing and itching with or without a rash. More serious hypersensitivity cutaneous reactions occur but are uncommon.

Gastro-intestinal reactions consist of anorexia, nausea, vomiting, abdominal discomfort, and diarrhoea. Pseudomembranous colitis has been reported with rifampicin therapy.

Hepatitis can be caused by rifampicin and liver function tests should be monitored. (See 'Precautions').

Thrombocytopenia with or without purpura may occur, usually associated with intermittent therapy, but is reversible if drug is discontinued as soon as purpura occurs. Cerebral haemorrhage and fatalities have been reported when rifampicin administration has been continued or resumed after the appearance of purpura.

Eosinophilia, leucopenia, oedema, muscle weakness and myopathy have been reported to occur in a small percentage of patients treated with rifampicin.

Reactions usually occurring with intermittent dosage regimens and probably of immunological origin include:

- 'Flu Syndrome' consisting of episodes of fever, chills, headache, dizziness, and bone pain appearing most commonly during the 3rd to the 6th month of therapy. The frequency of the syndrome varies but may occur in up to 50% of patients given once-weekly regimens with a dose of rifampicin of 25 mg/kg or more.
- Shortness of breath and wheezing.
- Decrease in blood pressure and shock.
- Acute haemolytic anaemia.
- Acute renal failure usually due to acute tubular necrosis or to acute interstitial nephritis.

If serious complications arise, e.g. renal failure, thrombocytopenia or haemolytic anaemia, rifampicin should be stopped and never restarted.

Occasional disturbances of the menstrual cycle have been reported in women receiving long term antituberculosis therapy with regimens containing rifampicin.

Rifampicin may produce a reddish discolouration of the urine, sputum and tears. The patient should be forewarned of this. Soft contact lenses may be permanently stained.

Isoniazid: Severe and sometimes fatal hepatitis may occur with isoniazid therapy. Polyneuritis associated with isoniazid, presenting as paraesthesia, muscle weakness, loss of tendon reflexes, is unlikely to occur with the recommended daily dose of Rifinah. Various haematological disturbances have been identified during treatment with isoniazid, including eosinophilia, agranulocytosis, and anaemia. High doses of isoniazid can cause convulsions. The possibility that the frequency of seizures may be increased in patients with epilepsy should be borne in mind.

Overdosage: In cases of overdosage with Rifinah 300 or Rifinah 150, gastric lavage should be performed as soon as possible. Intensive supportive measures should be instituted and individual symptoms treated as they arise. Parenteral pyridoxine (Vitamin B_6) should be given. Symptoms are more likely to be related to isoniazid, including coma, respiratory distress, hyperglycaemia and metabolic ketoacidosis.

Pharmaceutical precautions Store below 25°C.

If it proves necessary to open a blister pack, Rifinah 300 and Rifinah 150 should be dispensed in amber glass or plastic containers. Protect from moisture.

Legal category POM.

Package quantities *Rifinah 300:* Original packs of 56 tablets (4-weeks calendar packs); Blister packs of 100 tablets.
Rifinah 150: Original packs of 84 tablets (4-weeks calendar packs); Blister packs of 100 tablets.

Further information The recommended daily dose of Rifinah 300 or Rifinah 150 produces therapeutically effective blood levels of rifampicin and isoniazid, two of the most powerful antituberculosis drugs. Serum concentrations and the biological half-life of the two component drugs do not differ significantly from values obtained when the drugs are given alone.

Product licence numbers
Rifinah 150 4425/0041
Rifinah 300 4425/0042

SABRIL* TABLETS ▼

Presentation White, oval, biconvex tablets with a breakline on one side and 'SABRIL' on the other. Each tablet contains 500 mg vigabatrin.

Uses
Mode of action: Vigabatrin is a selective, irreversible inhibitor of GABA-transaminase. Treatment with Sabril leads to an increase in brain levels of GABA (gamma aminobutyric acid), the major inhibitory neurotransmitter in the brain.

Indications: Sabril is indicated for the treatment of epilepsy which is not satisfactorily controlled by other antiepileptic drugs.

Dosage and administration Sabril is for oral administration once or twice daily and may be taken before or after meals. It should be added to the patient's current therapeutic regimen.

Adults: The recommended daily starting dose is 2 g (4 tablets).

If necessary the dose may be increased or decreased in 0.5 g or 1.0 g increments depending upon clinical response and tolerability.

Increasing the dose above 4 g/day does not usually result in improved efficacy. There is no direct correlation between plasma concentration and efficacy. The duration of the effects of the drug are dependent on the rate of enzyme resynthesis rather than the concentration of drug in the plasma.
Children: The recommended daily starting dose is 1 g (2 tablets) in children aged 3–9 years and 2 g (4 tablets) in older children.

Elderly: Dosage reduction may be necessary in patients with impaired renal function, particularly patients with creatinine clearance less than 60 ml/min. See 'Precautions'.

Contra-indications, warnings, etc
Use in pregnancy and lactation: There is inadequate evidence of safety in human pregnancy. In animal studies vigabatrin was not teratogenic in the rat, but in the rabbit a slight increase in the incidence of cleft palate was seen at high doses. The use of Sabril during pregnancy is therefore contra-indicated.

There is no evidence of the safety of Sabril treatment whilst breast-feeding and so it is not recommended.

Precautions: As with other antiepileptic drugs abrupt withdrawal may lead to rebound seizures. If treatment is to be discontinued it is recommended that this is done by gradually reducing the dose over 2–4 weeks.

Sabril should be used with caution in patients with a history of psychosis or behavioural problems (see 'Side-effects').

Sabril is eliminated via the kidney and therefore caution should be exercised when administering the product to elderly patients and more particularly patients with creatinine clearance of less than 60 ml/min. Reduced doses should be used and patients monitored closely for adverse events such as sedation and confusion.

Warning: Animal safety studies indicate that vigabatrin causes intramyelinic oedema in the brain white matter tracts. Currently there is no evidence to suggest that this effect occurs in man. However, it is recommended that patients treated with Sabril are closely observed for adverse effects on neurological function. Details of animal findings are given under 'Further Information'.

Effects on driving ability: Drowsiness has been observed in clinical trials and patients should be warned of this possibility before treatment. Special care should be taken by patients driving, operating machinery or performing any hazardous task.

Side-effects: Adverse events are mainly CNS related and probably a secondary consequence of the increase in GABA caused by Sabril. Aggression and psychosis have been reported and a previous history of psychosis or a behavioural problem appears to be a predisposing factor to such reactions. Other reported events are drowsiness and fatigue, dizziness, nervousness, irritability, depression, headache and less commonly confusion, memory disturbance and vision complaints such as diplopia.

Other adverse events reported include weight gain and minor gastrointestinal side-effects.

In children excitation and agitation have been seen.

The sedative effect of vigabatrin decreases with continuing treatment.

As with other antiepileptic drugs, some patients may experience an increase in seizure frequency with vigabatrin. Patients with myoclonic seizures may be particularly liable to this effect.

There is no evidence of neurotoxicity in humans. Tests done to confirm lack of significant adverse effect on neurological function include evoked potentials, CAT scans, magnetic resonance imaging, CSF analyses and in a small number of cases, neuropathological examinations of brain specimens.

Laboratory data indicate that Sabril treatment does not lead to renal or hepatic toxicity. Decreases in SGOT and SGPT have been observed and may be a result of inhibition of these transaminases by Sabril. Chronic treatment with Sabril may be associated with a slight decrease in haemoglobin which rarely attains clinical significance.

Drug interactions: Sabril is not metabolised, or protein bound and does not induce hepatic cytochrome P450 or drug metabolising enzymes so interactions with other drugs are unlikely. In clinical studies a gradual reduction of about 20% in plasma phenytoin concentration has been observed. The mechanism is not understood but this is unlikely to be of therapeutic significance. No clinically significant interactions have been seen with carbamazepine, phenobarbitone or sodium valproate in clinical trials.

Overdose: There is no specific antidote and the usual supportive measures should be employed. Overdoses of 14 and 30 g of Sabril have been reported without any sequelae.

Pharmaceutical precautions None.

Legal category POM.

Package quantities Blister strips of 10 in cartons of 100.

Further information Animal safety studies carried out in rat, mouse, dog and monkey have indicated that vigabatrin has no significant adverse effects on the liver, kidney, lung, heart or gastrointestinal tract. In the brain, microvacuolation has been observed in white matter tracts of rat, mouse and dog at doses of 30–50 mg/kg/day. In the monkey these lesions are minimal or equivocal. This effect is caused by a separation of the outer lamellar sheath of myelinated fibres, a change characteristic of intramyelinic oedema. In both rat and dog the intramyelinic oedema was reversible on stopping vigabatrin treatment and even with continued treatment histologic regression was observed. However, in rodents, minor residual changes consisting of swollen axons (eosinophilic spheroids) and mineralised microbodies have been observed. In the dog, the results of an electrophysiological study indicate that intramyelinic oedema is associated with an increase in the latency of the somatosensory evoked potential which is reversible when the drug is withdrawn.

In man, however, no tendency towards increased evoked potential latencies has been observed even on prolonged treatment. Similarly, in rats treated with high doses of vigabatrin, changes in brain proteins have been observed in the CSF, but in man no similar changes have been detected.

Product licence number 4425/0098.

TARGOCID* ▼

Presentation For intravenous or intramuscular injection or intravenous infusion.

Targocid 200 mg: Each vial provides 200 mg teicoplanin presented as a lyophilisate for reconstitution. Each pack contains an ampoule of diluent (Water for Injections PhEur).

Targocid 400 mg: Each vial provides 400 mg teicoplanin presented as a lyophilisate for reconstitution. Each pack contains an ampoule of diluent (Water for Injections PhEur).

The vials do not contain any preservative.

Uses

Properties: Teicoplanin is a bactericidal, glycopeptide antibiotic, produced by fermentation of *Actinoplanes teicomyceticus.* It is active against both aerobic and anaerobic Gram-positive bacteria.

Species usually sensitive: *Staphylococcus aureus* and coagulase negative staphylococci (sensitive or resistant to methicillin), streptococci, enterococci, *Listeria monocytogenes*, micrococci, group *JK corynebacteria* and Gram-positive anaerobes including *Clostridium difficile*, and peptococci.

Species usually resistant: *Nocardia asteroides*, lactobacillus sp, leuconostoc and all Gram-negative bacteria. Bactericidal synergy has been demonstrated *in vitro* with aminoglycosides against group D streptococci and staphylococci. *In vitro* combinations of teicoplanin with rifampicin or fluorinated quinolones show primarily additive effects and sometimes synergy.

One-step resistance to teicoplanin could not be obtained *in vitro* and multi-step resistance was only reached *in vitro* after 11–14 passages.

Teicoplanin does not show cross-resistance with other classes of antibiotics.

Susceptibility testing: Sensidiscs are charged with 30 micrograms of teicoplanin. Strains showing an inhibition zone diameter of 14 mm or more are susceptible, and those of 10 mm or less are resistant.

Indications: Targocid is indicated in potentially serious Gram-positive infections including those which cannot be treated with other antimicrobial drugs, e.g. penicillins and cephalosporins.

Targocid is useful in the therapy of serious staphylococcal infections in patients who cannot receive or who have failed to respond to the penicillins and cephalosporins, or who have infections with staphylococci resistant to other antibiotics.

The effectiveness of teicoplanin has been documented in the following infections: Skin and soft tissue infections, urinary tract infections, lower respiratory tract infections, joint and bone infections, septicaemia, endocarditis and peritonitis related to continuous ambulatory peritoneal dialysis.

Dosage and administration

Preparation of injection: The entire contents of the water ampoule should be slowly added to the vial of Targocid and the vial rolled gently until the powder is completely dissolved, taking care to avoid formation of foam. If the solution does become foamy then allow to stand for about 15 minutes for the foam to subside.

A calculated excess is included in each vial of Targocid so that, when prepared as described above, a full dose of 200 mg or 400 mg will be obtained if all the reconstituted solution is withdrawn from the vial by a syringe.

Administration: The reconstituted Targocid injection may be administered directly either intravenously or intramuscularly. The intravenous injection may be administered either as a bolus or as a 30 minute infusion. Dosage is usually once daily but, in cases of severe infection, a second injection should be administered on the first day in order to reach more rapidly the required serum concentrations. The majority of patients with infections caused by organisms sensitive to the antibiotic show a therapeutic response within 48–72 hours. The total duration of therapy is determined by the type and severity of the infection and the clinical response of the patient. In endocarditis and osteomyelitis, treatment for three weeks or longer is recommended.

Determination of teicoplanin serum concentrations may optimise therapy. In severe infections, trough serum concentrations should not be less than 10 mg/l. Peak concentrations measured one hour after a 400 mg intravenous dose are usually in the range of 20–50 mg/l; peak serum concentrations of up to 250 mg/l have been reported after intravenous doses of 25 mg/kg. A relationship between serum concentration and toxicity has not been established.

Therapeutic dosage

Adult or elderly patients with normal renal function:

Moderate infections: skin and soft tissue infection, urinary tract infection, lower respiratory tract infection.

Loading dose: one single i.v. injection of 400 mg on the first day.

Maintenance dose: a single i.v. or i.m. injection of 200 mg daily.

Severe infections: joint and bone infection, septicaemia, endocarditis.

Loading dose: 400 mg i.v. injection every 12 hours for the first 3 doses.

Maintenance dose: a single i.v. or i.m. injection of 400 mg daily.

NB:

1. Standard doses of 200 and 400 mg equate respectively to mean doses of 3 and 6 mg/kg. In patients weighing more than 85 kg it is recommended to adapt the dosage to the weight following the same therapeutic schedule: moderate infection 3 mg/kg, severe infection 6 mg/kg.
2. In some clinical situations, such as infected, severely burned patients or *Staphylococcus aureus* endocarditis, unit maintenance doses of up to 12 mg/kg have been administered intravenously.

Children: In patients under 14 years doses of 6 mg/kg of Targocid should be given every 12 hours for the first 3 doses followed by 3 mg/kg daily; this will provide adequate cover for most infections caused by susceptible organisms. In severe infections a daily dose of 6 mg/kg is recommended.

Adults and elderly patients with renal insufficiency: For patients with impaired renal function, reduction of dosage is not required until the fourth day of Targocid treatment. Measurement of the serum concentration of teicoplanin may optimise therapy (see section 'Administration').

From the fourth day of treatment:

In mild renal insufficiency: Creatinine clearance between 40 and 60 ml/min, Targocid dose should be halved, either by administering the initial unit dose every two days, or by administering half of this dose once a day.

In severe renal insufficiency: Creatinine clearance less than 40 ml/min, and in haemodialysed patients, Targocid dose should be one third of the normal either by administering the initial unit dose every third day, or by administering one third of this dose once a day. Teicoplanin is not removed by dialysis.

In continuous ambulatory peritoneal dialysis: After a single loading IV dose of 400 mg if the patient is febrile, the recommended dosage is 20 mg/l per bag in the first week, 20 mg/l in alternate bags in the second week, and 20 mg/l in the overnight dwell bag only during the third week.

Contra-indications, warnings, etc

Contra-indications: Hypersensitivity to teicoplanin.

Warnings: Targocid should be administered with caution in patients known to be hypersensitive to vancomycin since cross hypersensitivity may occur. However, a history of the 'Red Man Syndrome' that can occur with vancomycin is not a contra-indication to Targocid.

Thrombocytopenia has been reported with teicoplanin, especially at higher doses than those usually recommended. It is advisable for periodic haematological studies to be performed during treatment. Liver and renal function tests are advised during treatment.

Serial renal and auditory function tests should be undertaken in the following circumstances:

- prolonged treatment in patients with renal insufficiency.
- concurrent and sequential use of other drugs which may have neurotoxic and/or nephrotoxic properties. These include aminoglycosides, colistin, amphotericin B, cyclosporin, cisplatin, frusemide and ethacrynic acid.

However, there is no evidence of synergistic toxicity with combinations with Targocid.

Dosage must be adapted in patients with renal impairment (see 'Dosage').

The use of Targocid may result in overgrowth of non-susceptible organisms. If new infections due to bacteria or fungi appear during treatment appropriate measures should be taken.

Use in pregnancy: Animal reproduction studies have not shown evidence of impairment of fertility or teratogenic effects. At high doses in rats there was an increased incidence of stillbirths and neonatal mortality. It is recommended that Targocid should not be used during confirmed or presumed pregnancy or during lactation unless a physician considers that the potential benefits outweigh any possible risk. There is no information about the excretion of teicoplanin in milk or placental transfer of the drug.

Interactions: In clinical trials teicoplanin has been administered to many patients already receiving various medications including other antibiotics, antihypertensives, anaesthetic agents, cardiac drugs, and antidiabetic agents without evidence of adverse interaction. In particular, in patients treated with concomitant aminoglycosides there was no evidence of synergistic oto- or nephro-toxicity. Animal studies have shown lack of interaction with diazepam, thiopentone, morphine, neuromuscular blocking agents or halothane.

Side-effects: Targocid is generally well tolerated. Side-effects rarely require cessation of therapy and are generally mild and transient; serious side-effects are rare. The following adverse events have been reported:

Local reactions: erythema, local pain, thrombophlebitis.

Allergic: rash, pruritus, fever, bronchospasm, anaphylactic reactions.

Gastro-intestinal: nausea, vomiting, diarrhoea.

Blood: eosinophilia, leucopenia, neutropenia, thrombocytopenia, thrombocytosis.

Liver function: increases in serum transaminases and/or serum alkaline phosphatase.

Renal function: transient elevations of serum creatinine.

Central nervous system: dizziness and headache.

Other reported events with an unknown causal

relationship: Mild hearing loss, tinnitus and vestibular disorder.

Overdosage: Targocid is not removed by haemodialysis. Treatment of overdosage should be symptomatic. Several overdoses of 100 mg/kg day have been administered in error to two neutropenic paediatric patients, aged 4 and 8 years. Despite high plasma concentrations of teicoplanin up to 300 mg/l, there were no symptoms or laboratory abnormalities.

Pharmaceutical precautions In keeping with good clinical and pharmaceutical practice reconstituted vials of Targocid should be used immediately and any unused portion discarded. On the few occasions when changing circumstances make this impracticable reconstituted solutions should be kept at 4°C and discarded within 24 hours.

The reconstituted solution may be injected directly, or alternatively diluted with: 0.9% Sodium Chloride Injection; Compound Sodium Lactate Injection (Ringer-Lactate Solution, Hartmanns Solution); 5% Dextrose Injection; 0.18% Sodium Chloride and 4% Dextrose Injection; Peritoneal dialysis solution containing 1.36% or 3.86% Dextrose.

Vials of dry Targocid should be stored below 25°C and protected from heat.

Legal category POM.

Package quantities
Targocid 200 mg: Combined pack of one vial providing 200 mg teicoplanin and one ampoule containing Water for Injections.
Targocid 400 mg: Combined pack of one vial providing 400 mg teicoplanin and one ampoule containing Water for Injections.

Further information
Pharmacokinetics: Following injection teicoplanin rapidly penetrates into tissues, including skin, fat and bone, and reaches the highest concentrations in the kidney, trachea, lungs and adrenals. Teicoplanin does not readily penetrate into the cerebrospinal fluid.

In man the plasma level profile after intravenous administration indicates a biphasic distribution (with a rapid distribution phase having a half life of about 0.3 hour, followed by a more prolonged distribution phase having a half life of about 3 hours), followed by slow elimination (with an elimination half life of 70–100 hours). The apparent volume of distribution at steady state is similar to total body water, i.e. 0.6 l/kg. The volume of distribution in children is not substantially different from that in adults.

Approximately 90–95% teicoplanin is bound with weak affinity to plasma proteins. Teicoplanin penetrates readily into blister exudates and into joint fluid; it penetrates neutrophils and enhances their bactericidal activity; it does not penetrate red blood cells.

No metabolites of teicoplanin have been identified; more than 97% of the administered teicoplanin is excreted unchanged.

The elimination of teicoplanin from the plasma is prolonged with a terminal half life of elimination in man of 70–100 hours. Teicoplanin is excreted mainly in the urine.

Product licence numbers

Targocid 200 mg vial	4425/0088
400 mg vial	4425/0089
Water for Injections	4425/0090

TENUATE DOSPAN*

Presentation White, flat, bevelled, oblong tablets, scored on one side and stamped "Merrell" on the other. Each contains Diethylpropion Hydrochloride BP 75 mg in a hydrophilic colloid gum designed to release the ingredient over a 10-hour period.

Uses An anorectic agent for short term use as an adjunct to the treatment of some patients with moderate or severe obesity when close support and supervision are also provided.

Dosage and administration *Adults:* One 75 mg tablet swallowed whole in mid-morning.

Not recommended for children or the elderly.

Current medical opinion supports intermittent use of an appetite suppressant. Courses of Tenuate Dospan may be given over periods of six to eight weeks with intervening periods of similar length without treatment and this may reduce the risk of dependence. The stated dose should not be exceeded. Efficacy in use for more than 3 to 6 months, and safety in long term use have not been established. Tenuate Dospan should be discontinued if weight loss does not occur or when patients stop losing weight.

Contra-indications, warnings, etc Tenuate Dospan should not be given concurrently with monoamine oxidase inhibitors (MAOI's) or other appetite suppressant drugs. It should not be given to patients hypersensitive to sympathomimetic agents, patients with uncontrolled thyrotoxicosis, emotionally unstable individuals or those with a history of psychiatric illness nor to patients known to be susceptible to drug or alcohol abuse. Although diethylpropion has less marked peripheral effects than the amphetamines, it should not be used in moderate/severe hypertension and severe cardivascular disease.

Use in pregnancy: There is inadequate evidence of safety in human pregnancy. The use of diethylpropion during any stage of pregnancy or lactation is not recommended. There is evidence from animal studies that the drug may be harmful to the foetus.

Isolated spontaneous reports of congenital malformations have been recorded in humans, but no causal relationship to diethylpropion has been established.

Precautions and drug interactions: Tenuate Dospan should be used with caution when administered concurrently with antihypertensive medication, antidiabetic medication, psychotropic drugs (including sedatives) and sympathomimetic agents.

Warnings and adverse effects: Rarely severe enough to require discontinuation of therapy, side-effects associated with diethylpropion hydrochloride have been reported to occur in relatively low incidence. These have included dry mouth, restlessness, nervousness, euphoria, agitation, insomnia, palpitations, tachycardia, raised blood pressure, depression, psychosis, hallucinations, dependence, constipation and rashes. Gynaecomastia has been reported rarely. Infrequent occurrences of nausea and vomiting have been noted, but diarrhoea is exceedingly rare. Hypertensive crises may result from the administration during treatment with, or within 14 days of, monoamine oxidase inhibitors. Patients should be warned against driving or operating machinery until it is established that they are not over-stimulated or suffer from rebound sedation while taking, or after discontinuing, Tenuate Dospan. Alcoholic drink should be avoided.

Overdosage: Manifestations of acute overdosage include restlessness, tremor, hyper-reflexia, rapid respiration, confusion, assaultiveness, hallucinations, panic states. Fatigue and depression usually follow the central stimulation.

Cardiovascular effects include arrhythmias, hypertension or hypotension and circulatory collapse. Gastrointestinal symptoms include nausea, vomiting, diarrhoea and abdominal cramps. Overdose of pharmacologically similar compounds has resulted in fatal poisoning, usually terminating in convulsions and coma. Management of acute diethylpropion hydrochloride intoxication is largely symptomatic and includes lavage and sedation with a barbiturate. Experience with haemodialysis or peritoneal dialysis is inadequate to permit recommendation. Intravenous phentolamine has been suggested on pharmacological grounds for possible acute, severe hypertension, if this complicates overdosage.

Pharmaceutical precautions Store in a cool dry place.

Legal category CD (Sch 3), POM.

Package quantities Original packs of 30 tablets.

Further information Prolonged use of diethylpropion may induce dependence with withdrawal syndrome on cessation of therapy. Hallucinations have occurred rarely following high doses of the drug. Several cases of toxic psychosis have been reported following the excessive use of the drug and a very small number have been reported in which the recommended dose appears not to have been exceeded. The psychosis was temporary and cleared up after the drug was discontinued.

Product licence number 4425/0015.

TRILUDAN* TABLETS
TRILUDAN* FORTE TABLETS
TRILUDAN* SUSPENSION

Presentation
Triludan Tablets: White, round, flat faced, bevel edged tablets with 'M' in two concentric circles on one side and a scored bisect line on the other. Each tablet contains 60 mg terfenadine.

Triludan Forte Tablets: White, convex, capsule shaped tablets with inscribed 'T' on one face. Each tablet contains 120 mg terfenadine.

Triludan Suspension: A white, oral, sugar-free suspension with a banana flavour containing 30 mg terfenadine in 5 ml.

Uses Triludan is an antihistamine, indicated for the symptomatic relief of hay fever, allergic rhinitis and allergic skin conditions.

Dosage and administration
Adults and children over 12 years: 60 mg twice daily or 120 mg once daily in the morning.

Children 6–12 years: 30 mg twice daily.

Children 3–6 years: 15 mg twice daily.

Contra-indications, warnings, etc
Contra-indications: Patients with known hypersensitivity to the drug.

Precautions: Terfenadine undergoes extensive metabolism in the liver. Caution is required when treating patients with impaired hepatic function or those receiving treatment with potent inhibitors of hepatic oxidation (See 'Drug Interactions') or with conditions leading to QT prolongation, as reports of QT prolongation and/or ventricular tachycardia have been recorded. The events may be related to altered metabolism of the drug, to electrolyte imbalance or both.

Use in pregnancy and lactation: Although animal studies have not indicated adverse effects, Triludan, like most medications, should not be used during pregnancy nor during lactation unless, in the opinion of the physician, the potential benefits outweigh any potential risk.

Drug interactions: Ketoconazole significantly alters the metabolism of terfenadine and therefore their concurrent use is not recommended. Concurrent use of other potent inhibitors of hepatic oxidation (e.g. certain macrolides) with terfenadine should be approached with caution (see 'Precautions').

Side-effects: The following side-effects have been reported: abdominal pain and dyspepsia, alopecia (hair loss and thinning), anaphylaxis, angioedema, arrhythmias, bronchospasm, confusion, convulsions, depression, dizziness, headache, insomnia, jaundice, liver dysfunction including transaminase elevations, menstrual disorders, musculoskeletal pain, nightmares, palpitations, paraesthesia, photosensitivity reactions, skin rash, sweating, tremor, visual disturbances.

In objective tests Triludan has been shown to be free from central nervous system side-effects. Reports of drowsiness are extremely rare. This means that patients usually may drive or perform tasks requiring concentration. However, in order to identify sensitive people who have unusual reaction to drugs, it is advisable to check the individual response before driving or performing complicated tasks.

Overdosage: Several cases of overdosage have been reported. Generally signs and symptoms were absent or mild. However, arrhythmias including ventricular tachycardia or fibrillation or torsade de pointes have been reported at overdoses of 900–3360 mg and have occurred up to 15 hours after the dose. In a clinical pharmacology study of terfenadine, 300 mg twice a day for 7 days, ECG's showed changes in T wave morphology and development of U waves in some patients; the mean corrected QT interval increased 43 msec without clinical symptoms, or signs of arrhythmia. Therefore, in cases of overdosage, cardiac monitoring for at least 24 hours is recommended along with standard measures to remove any unabsorbed drug. Haemodialysis does not effectively remove the major metabolite of terfenadine from blood.

Pharmaceutical precautions None.

Legal category P.

Package quantities
Triludan Tablets: Original packs of 60 tablets.
Triludan Forte Tablets: Original packs of 30 tablets.
Triludan Suspension: Amber glass bottles of 200 ml.

Further information In actual driving tests, Triludan does not impair performance, nor is there a change in mood.

Product licence numbers

Triludan Tablets	4425/0024
Triludan Forte Tablets	4425/0091
Triludan Suspension	4425/0057

**Trade Mark*

Thomas Morson Pharmaceuticals
Division of Merck Sharp & Dohme Limited
Hertford Road, Hoddesdon
Hertfordshire EN11 9BU

CARACE

Presentation Blue, oval tablets, marked 'MSD 15', containing 2.5 mg lisinopril, MSD.

White, half-scored, oval tablets, marked 'CARACE' and '5', containing 5 mg lisinopril, MSD.

Yellow, half-scored, oval tablets, marked 'CARACE' and '10', containing 10 mg lisinopril, MSD.

Orange, half-scored, oval tablets, marked 'CARACE' and '20', containing 20 mg lisinopril, MSD.

Uses

Indications

Hypertension: All grades of essential hypertension and renovascular hypertension. Carace may be used alone or with other antihypertensive agents.

Congestive heart failure: In the treatment of congestive heart failure as adjunctive therapy with non-potassium-sparing diuretics and, where appropriate, digitalis. Treatment with Carace should always be initiated in hospital under close medical supervision.

Mode of action: Carace is an orally active specific inhibitor of angiotensin I converting enzyme, a membrane bound enzyme which catalyses the conversion of the inactive decapeptide angiotensin I to the active octapeptide angiotensin II. Carace thus reduces levels of angiotensin II, a very powerful vasoconstrictor substance. As a consequence, blood pressure may be reduced in hypertensive patients and cardiac workload may be reduced in patients with congestive heart failure. The onset of action begins gradually, with the maximum effect usually occurring four to six hours after the first dose, with effects persisting for 24 hours after a single daily dose.

Dosage and administration The absorption of Carace is not affected by food.

Hypertension: The need for dosage titration should be determined by measurement of the blood pressure just before the next dose.

Essential and renovascular hypertension: Treatment should be started with 2.5 mg once daily, and titrated upwards to achieve optimal blood pressure control. A 2.5 mg dose seldom achieves a therapeutic response.

The usual effective dose range is 10–20 mg once daily.

The maximum recommended dose is 40 mg daily.

Diuretic-treated patients: If possible, the diuretic should be discontinued or the dose reduced, two to three days before beginning therapy with Carace (see 'Precautions') and may be resumed later if required.

Use in the elderly: Age alone does not appear to affect the efficacy or safety profile of Carace. Thus, elderly patients should start treatment with Carace as directed above.

Congestive heart failure: Carace may be used as adjunctive therapy with non-potassium-sparing diuretics with or without digitalis.

Initial dosage: Treatment should be initiated in hospital under close medical supervision, with a recommended starting dose of 2.5 mg with subsequent dose titration. If possible, the dose of diuretic should be reduced before beginning treatment.

Blood pressure and renal function should be monitored closely both before and during treatment because severe hypotension and, more rarely, consequent renal failure have been reported with angiotensin-converting enzyme (ACE) inhibitors (see 'Precautions').

The appearance of hypotension after the initial dose of Carace does not preclude subsequent careful dose adjustment with the drug, following effective treatment of the hypotension.

Maintenance dosage: The dose should be gradually increased, depending on the patient's response, to the usual maintenance dose (5–20 mg). This dose adjustment may be performed over a two- to four-week period, or more rapidly if clinically indicated.

Impaired renal function: Carace is excreted by the kidney, and should be used with caution in patients with renal insufficiency.

Carace is dialysable. Dialysis patients may be given the usual dose of 'Carace' on dialysis days. On the days when patients are not on dialysis the dosage should be tailored to the blood pressure response.

Paediatric use: Carace has not been studied for use in children.

Contra-indications, warnings, etc

Contra-indications

Pregnancy: Carace has been shown to be fetotoxic in rabbits during middle and late pregnancy.

Effects of exposure of the fetus to ACE inhibitors during the first trimester of human pregnancy are unknown. Fetal exposure during the second and third trimesters of pregnancy has been associated with fetal and neonatal morbidity and mortality.

ACE inhibitors in human pregnancy have been associated with oligohydramnios. Hypotension and renal failure have occurred in the newborn.

Because of these findings Carace is contra-indicated in pregnancy.

Hypersensitivity to Carace, and in patients with a history of angioneurotic oedema relating to previous treatment with an ACE inhibitor.

Precautions

Assessment of renal function: Evaluation of the patient should include assessment of renal function prior to initiation of therapy, and during treatment.

Impaired renal function: Carace should be used with caution in patients with renal insufficiency, as they may require reduced or less frequent doses (see 'Dosage'). Close monitoring of renal function during therapy should be performed as deemed appropriate in those with renal insufficiency. In the majority, renal function will not alter, or may improve.

Renal failure has been reported in association with ACE inhibitors and has been mainly in patients with severe congestive heart failure or underlying renal disease, including renal artery stenosis. If recognised promptly and treated appropriately, renal failure is usually reversible.

Some hypertensive patients, with no apparent pre-existing renal disease, have developed increases in blood urea and creatinine when Carace has been given concurrently with a diuretic. Dosage reduction of Carace and/or discontinuation of the diuretic may be required. This situation should raise the possibility of underlying renal artery stenosis (see 'Renovascular hypertension').

Symptomatic hypotension was seen rarely in uncomplicated hypertensive patients. It is more likely to occur in patients who have been volume-depleted by diuretic therapy, dietary salt restriction, dialysis, diarrhoea, or vomiting. In these patients, by discontinuing diuretic therapy or significantly reducing the diuretic dose for two to three days prior to initiating Carace, the possibility of this occurrence is reduced.

Similar caution and close supervision may apply also to patients with ischaemic heart or cerebrovascular disease in whom severe hypotension could result in a myocardial infarct or cerebrovascular accident.

Severe hypotension has been reported with ACE inhibitors, mainly in patients with severe heart failure. Many of these patients were on high doses of loop diuretics, and some had hyponatraemia or functional renal impairment. If hypotension develops, the patient should be placed in a supine position. Volume repletion with oral fluids or intravenous normal saline may be required. Intravenous atropine may be necessary if there is associated bradycardia. Treatment with Carace may be restarted with careful dose titration following restoration of effective blood volume and pressure.

In some patients with congestive heart failure who have normal or low blood pressure, additional lowering of systemic blood pressure may occur with Carace. If such hypotension becomes symptomatic, a reduction of dose or discontinuation of Carace may become necessary.

The appearance of hypotension after the initial dose of Carace does not preclude subsequent careful dose titration with the drug after effective management of hypotension.

Renovascular hypertension: Carace can be used when surgery is not indicated, or prior to surgery. In some patients with bilateral renal artery stenosis or stenosis of the artery to a solitary kidney, increases of blood urea and creatinine, reversible upon discontinuation of therapy, have been seen. This is especially likely in patients treated with diuretics and/or those with renal insufficiency.

Surgery/anaesthesia: In patients undergoing major surgery or during anaesthesia with agents that produce hypotension, Carace blocks angiotensin II formation secondary to compensatory renin release. This may lead to hypotension which can be corrected by volume expansion.

General: Carace should not be used in patients with aortic stenosis, cor pulmonale or outflow tract obstruction.

Where Carace is used as a single agent in hypertension, Afro-Caribbean patients may show a reduced therapeutic response.

Drug interactions: Combination with other antihypertensive agents such as beta-blockers and diuretics may increase the antihypertensive efficacy.

Carace has been used with nitrates without significant clinical interaction.

Carace minimises the development of thiazide-induced hypokalaemia and hyperuricaemia.

Indomethacin may reduce the antihypertensive efficacy of Carace.

As Carace may reduce the elimination of lithium, serum levels of lithium should be monitored if lithium salts are administered.

Plasma potassium usually remains within normal limits, although a few cases of hyperkalaemia have occurred. If Carace is given with a diuretic, the likelihood of diuretic-induced hypokalaemia may be lessened. Carace may elevate plasma potassium levels in patients with renal failure. Potassium supplements, potassium-sparing diuretics and potassium-containing salt substitutes are not recommended.

Breast-feeding mothers: Because it is not known whether Carace is excreted in human milk, caution should be exercised if Carace is given to breast-feeding mothers.

Side-effects: Hypotension has occurred in association with therapy with Carace. This appears to occur in certain specific sub-groups (see 'Precautions').

Angioneurotic oedema: It has been reported with angiotensin-converting enzyme inhibitors, including Carace. In such cases, Carace should be discontinued immediately and the patient observed. Where swelling is confined to the face, lips and mouth, the condition will usually resolve without further treatment, although antihistamines may be useful in relieving symptoms. These patients should be followed carefully until the swelling has resolved. However, where there is involvement of the tongue, glottis or larynx likely to cause airways obstruction, subcutaneous adrenaline (0.5 ml 1:1,000) should be administered promptly when indicated.

Other hypersensitivity reactions have been reported.

Other adverse reactions: Dizziness, headache, diarrhoea, cough, nausea and fatigue are the most frequent. Other less frequent side effects include rash, and asthenia. Palpitation and impotence have been observed rarely.

Laboratory test findings: Increases in blood urea and creatinine, reversible on discontinuation of Carace, are most likely in the presence of bilateral renal artery stenosis, especially in patients with renal insufficiency (see 'Precautions'). However, increases in blood urea and creatinine may occur without evidence of pre-existing renal impairment, especially in patients taking diuretics. In this event, undiagnosed renal artery stenosis should be suspected. Dosage reduction of Carace and/or discontinuation of the diuretic should be considered.

Increases in liver enzymes and serum bilirubin have occurred which are usually reversible on discontinuation of Carace.

Decreases in haemoglobin and haematocrit have been reported in a few patients, but a causal relationship to Carace has not been established.

Hyperkalaemia has occurred in a few cases (see also 'Plasma potassium').

Overdosage: Available data are limited. The most likely manifestation of overdosage would be hypotension, which can be treated, if necessary, by intravenous infusion of normal saline solution. Carace can be removed by haemodialysis.

Pharmaceutical precautions Store in a dry place below 25°C.

Legal category POM.

Package quantities
Tablets 20 mg: Calendar packs of 28 tablets, bottles of 50 tablets.
Tablets 10 mg: Calendar packs of 28 tablets, bottles of 50 tablets.
Tablets 5 mg: Calendar packs of 28 tablets, bottles of 50 tablets.
Tablets 2.5 mg: Bottles of 50 tablets.

Further information Nil.

Product licence numbers

2.5 mg tablet	0025/0239
5 mg tablet	0025/0233
10 mg tablet	0025/0234
20 mg tablet	0025/0235

CARACE* PLUS

Presentation Hexagonal, yellow tablets marked MSD 140 on one side and scored. Each tablet contains 20 mg lisinopril and 12.5 mg hydrochlorothiazide.

Uses For the treatment of mild to moderate hypertension in patients who have been stabilised on the individual components given in the same proportions.

Mode of action: Carace Plus is a combination of an angiotensin-converting enzyme inhibitor (lisinopril) and a diuretic (hydrochlorothiazide). Carace Plus is highly effective in the treatment of hypertension. Hydrochlorothiazide stimulates the renin-angiotensin-aldosterone system which produces an additive effect with lisinopril.

Lisinopril is an inhibitor of the angiotensin-converting enzyme (ACE). Inhibition of the formation of angiotensin II results in vasodilatation and a fall in blood pressure.

Hydrochlorothiazide is a diuretic and antihypertensive agent. Use of this agent alone results in increased renin secretion. Although lisinopril alone is antihypertensive, even in patients with low renin hypertension, concomitant administration with hydrochlorothiazide results in a greater reduction in blood pressure. Lisinopril attenuates the potassium loss associated with hydrochlorothiazide.

Dosage and administration

Adults

Essential hypertension: The usual dosage is 1 tablet, administered once daily. If necessary, the dosage may be increased to 2 tablets, administered once daily.

Dosage in renal insufficiency: Thiazides may not be appropriate diuretics for use in patients with renal impairment and are ineffective at creatinine clearance values of 30 ml/min or below (i.e. moderate or severe renal insufficiency).

Carace Plus is not to be used as initial therapy in any patient with renal insufficiency.

In patients with creatinine clearance of >30 and <80 ml/min, Carace Plus may be used, but only after titration of the individual components.

Prior diuretic therapy: Symptomatic hypotension may occur following the initial dose of lisinopril: this is more likely in patients who are volume and/or salt depleted as a result of prior diuretic therapy. If possible, the diuretic therapy should be discontinued for 2–3 days prior to initiation of therapy with lisinopril alone, in a 2.5 mg dose.

Use in the elderly: Lisinopril was equally effective in elderly (65 years or older) and non-elderly hypertensive patients. In elderly hypertensive patients, monotherapy with lisinopril was as effective in reducing diastolic blood pressure as monotherapy with either hydrochlorothiazide or atenolol. In clinical studies, age did not affect the tolerability of lisinopril.

In clinical studies the efficacy and tolerability of lisinopril and hydrochlorothiazide, administered concomitantly, were similar in both elderly and younger hypertensive patients.

Paediatric use: Safety and effectiveness in children have not been established.

Contra-indications, warnings, etc

Contra-indications: Carace Plus is contra-indicated in patients with anuria.

Carace Plus is contra-indicated in patients who are hypersensitive to any component of the product and in patients with a history of angioneurotic oedema relating to previous treatment with an angiotensin-converting-enzyme inhibitor.

Carace Plus is contra-indicated in patients who are hypersensitive to other sulphonamide-derived drugs.

Carace Plus is contra-indicated in pregnancy, and treatment should be stopped if pregnancy is suspected because lisinopril has been shown to be fetotoxic in rabbits.

See also 'Breast-feeding mothers' under 'Precautions'.

Precautions

Hypotension and electrolyte/fluid imbalance: As with all antihypertensive therapy, symptomatic hypotension may occur in some patients. This was rarely seen in uncomplicated hypertensive patients but is more likely in the presence of fluid or electrolyte imbalance, e.g. volume depletion, hyponatraemia, hypochloraemic alkalosis, hypomagnesaemia or hypokalaemia which may occur from prior diuretic therapy, dietary salt restriction, dialysis, or during intercurrent diarrhoea or vomiting. Periodic determination of serum electrolytes should be performed at appropriate intervals in such patients.

Particular consideration should be given when therapy is administered to patients with ischaemic heart or cerebrovascular disease, because an excessive fall in blood pressure could result in myocardial infarction or cerebrovascular accident.

If hypotension occurs, the patient should be placed in the supine position and, if necessary, should receive an intravenous infusion of normal saline. A transient hypotensive response is not a contra-indication to further doses. Following restoration of effective blood volume and pressure, reinstitution of therapy at reduced dosage may be possible; or either of the components may be used appropriately alone.

Renal function impairment: Thiazides may not be appropriate diuretics for use in patients with renal impairment and are ineffective at creatinine clearance values of 30 ml/min or below (i.e. moderate or severe renal insufficiency). Carace Plus should not be administered to patients with renal insufficiency (creatinine clearance ≤80 ml/min) until titration of the individual components has shown the need for the doses present in the combination tablet.

Some hypertensive patients, with no apparent pre-existing renal disease, have developed usually minor and transient increases in blood urea and serum creatinine when lisinopril has been given concomitantly with a diuretic. If this occurs during therapy with Carace Plus, the combination should be discontinued. Reinstitution of therapy at reduced dosage may be possible, or either of the components may be used appropriately alone.

In some patients, with bilateral renal artery stenosis or stenosis of the single artery to a solitary kidney, increases in blood urea and serum creatinine, reversible upon discontinuation of therapy, have been seen with angiotensin-converting enzyme (ACE) inhibitors.

Hepatic disease: Thiazides should be used with caution in patients with impaired hepatic function or progressive liver disease, since minor alterations of fluid and electrolyte balance may precipitate hepatic coma.

Surgery/anaesthesia: In patients undergoing major surgery or during anaesthesia with agents that produce hypotension, lisinopril may block angiotensin II formation secondary to compensatory renin release. If hypotension occurs and is considered to be due to this mechanism, it can be corrected by volume expansion.

Metabolic and endocrine effects: Thiazide therapy may impair glucose tolerance. Dosage adjustment of antidiabetic agents, including insulin, may be required.

Thiazides may decrease urinary calcium excretion and may cause intermittent and slight elevation of serum calcium. Marked hypercalcaemia may be evidence of hidden hyperparathyroidism. Thiazides should be discontinued before carrying out tests for parathyroid function.

Increases in cholesterol and triglyceride levels may be associated with thiazide diuretic therapy.

Thiazide therapy may precipitate hyperuricaemia and/or gout in certain patients. However, lisinopril may increase urinary uric acid and thus may attenuate the hyperuricaemic effect of hydrochlorothiazide.

Hypersensitivity/angioneurotic oedema: Angioneurotic oedema of the face, extremities, lips, tongue, glottis, and/or larynx has been reported rarely in patients treated with angiotensin-converting enzyme inhibitors, including lisinopril. In such cases, Carace Plus should be discontinued promptly, and appropriate monitoring should be instituted to ensure complete resolution of symptoms prior to dismissing the patient.

In those instances where swelling has been confined to the face and lips, the condition generally resolved without treatment, although antihistamines have been useful in relieving symptoms. Angioneurotic oedema associated with laryngeal oedema may be fatal. Where there is involvement of the tongue, glottis or larynx, likely to cause airway obstruction, appropriate therapy such as subcutaneous adrenaline solution 1:1,000 (0.3 ml to 0.5 ml) should be administered promptly. Patients with a history of angioedema unrelated to ACE-inhibitor therapy may be at increased risk of angioedema while receiving an ACE inhibitor. (See also 'Contra-indications').

In patients receiving thiazides, sensitivity reactions may occur with or without a history of allergy or bronchial asthma. Exacerbation or activation of systemic lupus erythematosus has been reported with the use of thiazides.

Cough: Cough has been reported with the use of ACE inhibitors. Characteristically, the cough is non-productive, persistent, and resolves after discontinuation of therapy. ACE inhibitor-induced cough should be considered as part of the differential diagnosis of cough.

Breast-feeding mothers: It is not known whether lisinopril is secreted in human milk; however, thiazides do appear in human milk. Because of the potential for serious reactions in nursing infants, a decision should be made whether to discontinue breast-feeding or to discontinue Carace Plus, taking into account the importance of the drug to the mother.

Serum potassium: The potassium-losing effect of thiazide diuretics is usually attenuated by the potassium-conserving effect of lisinopril.

The use of potassium supplements, potassium-sparing agents or potassium-containing salt substitutes, particularly in patients with impaired renal function, may lead to a significant increase in serum potassium. If concomitant use of Carace Plus and any of these agents is deemed appropriate, they should be used with caution and with frequent monitoring of serum potassium.

Lithium: Lithium generally should not be given with diuretics or ACE inhibitors. Diuretic agents and ACE inhibitors reduce the renal clearance of lithium and add a high risk of lithium toxicity. Refer to prescribing information for lithium preparations before use of such preparations.

Other agents: Indomethacin may diminish the hypertensive effect of concomitantly administered Carace Plus. The antihypertensive effect of Carace Plus may be potentiated when given concomitantly with other agents likely to cause postural hypotension.

Thiazides may increase the responsiveness to tubocurarine.

Side-effects: Carace Plus is usually well tolerated. In clinical studies, side effects have usually been mild and transient, and in most instances have not required interruption of therapy. The side-effects that have been observed have been limited to those reported previously with lisinopril or hydrochlorothiazide.

The most common clinical side-effect was dizziness, which generally responded to dosage reduction and seldom required discontinuation of therapy.

Other, less frequent side-effects were headache, dry cough, fatigue, and hypotension including orthostatic hypotension.

Still less common were diarrhoea, nausea, vomiting, dry mouth, rash, gout, palpitation, chest discomfort, muscle cramps and weakness, paraesthesia, asthenia, and impotence.

Hypersensitivity/angioneurotic oedema: Angioneurotic oedema of the face, extremities, lips, tongue, glottis and/or larynx has been reported rarely (see 'Precautions').

A symptom complex has been reported which may include fever, vasculitis, myalgia, arthralgia/arthritis, a positive ANA, elevated ESR, eosinophilia, and leucocytosis. Rash photosensitivity, or other dermatological manifestations may occur.

Laboratory test findings: Laboratory side-effects have rarely been of clinical importance. Occasional hyperglycaemia, hyperuricaemia and hyperkalaemia or hypokalaemia have been noted. Usually minor and transient increases in blood urea nitrogen and serum creatinine have been seen in patients without evidence of pre-existing renal impairment. If such increases persist, they are usually reversible upon discontinuation of Carace Plus. Small decreases in haemoglobin and haematocrit have been reported frequently in hypertensive patients treated with Carace Plus but were rarely of clinical importance unless another cause of anaemia co-existed. Rarely, elevation of liver enzymes and/or serum bilirubin have occurred, but a causal relationship to Carace Plus has not been established.

Other side-effects reported with the individual components alone, and which may be potential side-effects with Carace Plus, are:

Hydrochlorothiazide: anorexia, gastric irritation, constipation, jaundice (intrahepatic cholestatic jaundice), pancreatitis, sialoadenitis, vertigo, xanthopsia, leucopenia, agranulocytosis, thrombocytopenia, aplastic anaemia, haemolytic anaemia, purpura, photosensitivity, urticaria, necrotising angiitis (vasculitis, cutaneous vasculitis), fever, respiratory distress including pneumonitis and pulmonary oedema, anaphylactic reactions, hyperglycaemia, glycosuria, hyperuricaemia, electrolyte imbalance including hyponatraemia, muscle spasm, restlessness, transient blurred vision, renal failure, renal dysfunction, and interstitial nephritis.

Lisinopril: myocardial infarction or cerebrovascular accident possibly secondary to excessive hypotension in high-risk patients, tachycardia, abdominal pain, mood alterations, urticaria, diaphoresis, uraemia, oliguria/anuria, renal dysfunction, acute renal failure, hepatitis (hepatocellular or cholestatic) and jaundice.

Overdosage: No specific information is available on the treatment of overdosage with Carace Plus. Treatment is symptomatic and supportive. Therapy with Carace Plus should be discontinued and the patient observed closely. Suggested measures include induction of emesis and/or gastric lavage, if ingestion is recent, and correction of dehydration, electrolyte imbalance and hypotension by established procedures.

Lisinopril: The most likely features of overdosage would be hypotension, for which the usual treatment would be intravenous infusion of normal saline solution.

Lisinopril may be removed from the general circulation by haemodialysis.

Hydrochlorothiazide: The most common signs and symptoms observed are those caused by electrolyte depletion (hypokalaemia, hypochloraemia, hyponatraemia) and dehydration resulting from excessive diuresis. If digitalis has also been administered, hypokalaemia may accentuate cardiac arrhythmias.

Pharmaceutical precautions Store at room temperature.

Legal category POM.

Package quantities Bottles and/or calendar packs of 28 tablets. Bottles of 56 tablets.

Further information Nil.

Product licence number 0025/0251.

DOLOBID*
DOLOBID* 500

Presentation Peach-coloured, capsule-shaped, film-coated tablets, marked 'DOLOBID', containing 250 mg Diflunisal BP; and orange-coloured, film-coated tablets, marked 'DOLOBID', containing 500 mg Diflunisal BP.

Uses Dolobid is indicated for the relief of pain.

Dolobid is also indicated in the relief of pain and inflammation associated with osteoarthritis and rheumatoid arthritis.

Dolobid is indicated in the relief of pain and associated symptoms of primary dysmenorrhoea.

Dosage and administration Tablets should be swallowed whole, not crushed or chewed.

For relief of pain: An initial dose of 1000 mg, followed by 500 mg every 12 hours, is recommended for most patients. Following the initial dose some patients may require 500 mg every eight hours. Maintenance doses higher than 1500 mg a day are not recommended.

For osteoarthritis and rheumatoid arthritis: The recommended dosage range is 500 mg to 1000 mg per day. Dolobid may be administered once or twice a day.

Dosage should be adjusted to the nature and intensity of the pain being treated.

For dysmenorrhoea: The recommended dosage is 1000 mg at the onset of cramps or bleeding, followed by 500 mg every 12 hours for as long as symptoms last, usually a maximum of five days.

Dolobid is not recommended for children.

Use in the elderly: The dosage does not require modification for elderly patients.

Contra-indications, warnings, etc

Contra-indications: Hypersensitivity.

In patients who have previously experienced acute asthmatic attacks, urticaria, or rhinitis precipitated by aspirin or non-steroidal anti-inflammatory agents.

The drug should not be administered to patients with active gastro-intestinal bleeding.

The use of Dolobid should be avoided in patients with active peptic ulcer.

Dolobid should not be given to pregnant women, since the safety for this use has not been established. Breast-feeding mothers should not take Dolobid, or should stop breast-feeding.

Precautions: Although Dolobid has less effect on platelet function and bleeding time than aspirin, it does inhibit platelet function at higher doses; patients who may be adversely affected should be carefully observed.

Because of reports of adverse eye findings with agents of this class, eye complaints developing during treatment with Dolobid should be fully examined.

Dolobid should be used with caution in patients having a history of gastro-intestinal haemorrhage or ulcers. Fatalities have occurred, rarely.

Although there have been no known reports associated with the use of Dolobid to date, acetylsalicylic acid has been associated with Reye's syndrome. Because diflunisal is a compound related to salicylic acid, the possibility of an association with Reye's syndrome cannot be excluded.

As with other NSAIDs, Dolobid should be used with caution in patients with reduced renal blood flow since renal prostaglandins play a supportive role in the maintenance of renal perfusion.

The dosage of Dolobid may need to be reduced in patients with renal functional impairment since the major route of excretion is via the kidney. In patients with severe renal impairment, the drug should not be used.

In rats and dogs, high oral doses of diflunisal (50–200 mg/kg/day) as with aspirin, produced similar pathological changes (gastro-intestinal ulceration and renal papillary oedema). These dosages are approximately 3 to 12 times the maximum dosages recommended in man.

Peripheral oedema has been observed in some patients taking Dolobid. Therefore, as with other drugs in this class, Dolobid should be used with caution in patients with compromised cardiac function, hypertension, or other conditions predisposing to fluid retention.

A potentially fatal apparent hypersensitivity syndrome has been reported which may include constitutional symptoms, (fever, rigors); dermatological findings listed above, involvement of major organs (changes in liver function, jaundice leucopenia, thrombocytopenia, eosinophilia, renal impairment including renal failure); and less specific findings such as adenitis, arthralgia, malaise, anorexia, and disorientation.

Laboratory tests: AST (SGOT) and ALT (SGPT) rose significantly by three times the upper limit of normal in less than 1% of patients in controlled clinical trials of non-steroidal anti-inflammatory drugs. A patient on Dolobid with signs or symptoms suggesting liver disease or in whom abnormal liver function tests have occurred should be evaluated for evidence of a more severe hepatic reaction. If abnormal liver tests persist or worsen, if signs or symptoms of liver disease develop or if systemic manifestations such as eosinophilia or rash occur, Dolobid should be discontinued.

Drug interactions: Indomethacin: The combined use of indomethacin and Dolobid has been associated with fatal gastro-intestinal haemorrhage. The combination should not be used. Co-administration of Dolobid with indomethacin increases the plasma level of indomethacin by about 30 to 35% with a concomitant decrease in renal clearance of indomethacin and its conjugate. *Aspirin:* Co-administration of aspirin causes approximately a 15% decrease in plasma levels of Dolobid. *Codeine:* Co-administration with Dolobid improves the analgesic efficacy of either drug taken alone. *Methotrexate:* Caution should be used if Dolobid is administered concomitantly with methotrexate. Non-steroidal anti-inflammatory drugs have been reported to decrease the tubular secretion of methotrexate and potentiate the toxicity. *Oral anticoagulant drugs:* The concomitant administration of Dolobid and warfarin or nicoumalone resulted in prolongation of prothrombin time in normal volunteers. This may occur because diflunisal competitively displaces coumarins from protein binding sites. Accordingly, prothrombin time should be monitored during and for several days after the concomitant drug administration of Dolobid and oral anticoagulants. The dosage of oral anticoagulants may require adjustment. *Tolbutamide:* No significant changes occurred in the plasma levels of tolbutamide or in the fasting blood sugar levels of diabetic patients who also took Dolobid. *Hydrochlorothiazide:* Co-administration increases the plasma levels of hydrochlorothiazide by 25 to 35% with a concomitant decrease in renal clearance. This change is not clinically important. Dolobid counteracts the hyperuricaemic effect of hydrochlorothiazide. *Frusemide:* Co-administration did not affect the diuretic activity of frusemide in normal volunteers, but its hyperuricaemic activity was decreased by Dolobid. *Antacids:* The clinical effect of occasional doses of antacid is insignificant, but this becomes significant when antacids are used continuously. Co-administration of aluminium hydroxide suspension significantly decreases the absorption of Dolobid by approximately 40%. *Paracetamol:* Co-administration significantly increased the plasma levels of paracetamol by 50%, but the plasma levels of Dolobid were unaffected. *Other non-steroidal, anti-inflammatory agents:* No clinical data on the safety and efficacy of concomitant administration are available. No recommendations can be made. However, normal volunteers given sulindac and Dolobid showed significantly lower levels of the active sulphide metabolite of sulindac. Normal volunteers given naproxen and Dolobid showed no changes in plasma levels of either drug, but a significant decrease in urinary excretion of naproxen and its glucuronide metabolite. *Gold salts:* In clinical studies of patients with rheumatoid arthritis Dolobid added to the regimen of gold salts usually resulted in additional symptomatic relief.

Side effects: 3% to 9% incidence: Gastro-intestinal: gastro-intestinal pain, dyspepsia, diarrhoea, nausea. *Dermatological:* rash. *Central nervous system:* headache.

1% to 3% incidence: Gastro-intestinal: vomiting, constipation, flatulence. *Central nervous system/Psychiatric:* dizziness, somnolence, insomnia. *Special senses:* tinnitus. *Miscellaneous:* fatigue.

Less than 1% incidence: Gastro-intestinal: peptic ulcer, gastro-intestinal perforation and bleeding, anorexia, jaundice, cholestasis, liver function abnormality, hepatitis, gastitis. *Dermatological:* pruritus, sweating, dry mucous membranes, stomatitis, photosensitivity, urticaria, erythema multiforme and Stevens-Johnson syndrome, toxic epidermal necrolysis, exfoliative dermatitis. *Genito-urinary:* dysuria, renal impairment including renal failure, interstitial nephritis, haematuria. *Central nervous system/Psychiatric:* vertigo, light-headedness, paraesthesiae, nervousness, depression, hallucinations, confusion. *Haematological:* thrombocytopenia, granulocytosis, haemolytic anaemia. *Special senses:* transient visual disturbances including blurred vision. *Miscellaneous:* asthenia, oedema. *Hypersensitivity reactions:* acute anaphylactic reaction with bronchospasm, angioedema, hypersensitivity vasculitis, hypersensitivity syndrome.

A potentially fatal apparent hypersensitivity syndrome has been reported which may include constitutional symptoms (fever, rigors); dermatological findings listed above; involvement of major organs (changes in liver function, jaundice, leucopenia, thrombocytopenia, eosinophilia, renal impairment including renal failure); and less specific findings such as adenitis, arthralgia, arthritis, malaise, anorexia, and disorientation.

Other reported reactions with an unknown causal relationship: Respiratory: Dyspnoea. *Cardiovascular:* Palpitation, syncope. *Musculoskeletal:* Muscle cramps. *Miscellaneous:* Chest pain. *Genitourinary:* Nephrotic syndrome.

Treatment of overdosage:

Cases of overdosage have occurred and fatalities have been reported. The most common signs and symptoms observed with overdosage were drowsiness, vomiting, nausea, diarrhoea, hyperventilation, tachycardia, sweating, tinnitus, disorientation, stupor, and coma. Diminished urine output and cardiorespiratory arrest have also been reported. The lowest dose of Dolobid alone at which death was reported was 15 g; death has been reported from a mixed drug overdose that included 7.5 g Dolobid.

In the event of recent overdosage, the stomach should be emptied by inducing vomiting or gastric lavage, and the patient observed carefully and given symptomatic and supportive treatment.

To facilitate urinary elimination of the drug, attempt to maintain renal function. Because of the high degree of protein binding, haemodialysis is not recommended.

The initial plasma half-life following single oral doses of diflunisal seems to be dose dependent, ranging from approximately 7.5 hours for a 250 mg dose to 11 hours for a 500 mg dose.

Pharmaceutical precautions Store in a cool place, protected from light.

Legal category POM.

Package quantities Dolobid 250 mg tablets are supplied in packs of 50, 100 and 1,000 tablets; the 500 mg tablets in packs of 100.

Further information Following a single therapeutic dose, significant relief of pain usually occurs within the first hour, reaches a maximum in 2–3 hours and lasts for up to 12 hours or more.

Dolobid has a dose-related effect on platelet function. In normal volunteers given Dolobid over eight days, 250 mg twice daily had no effect on platelet function and 500 mg twice daily affected platelet function only slightly. However, at 1,000 mg twice daily, which exceeds the maximum recommended dose, platelet function was inhibited. In contrast to aspirin, these effects were reversible.

Bleeding time was unaffected by 250 mg twice daily, slightly increased at 500 mg twice daily, and the greater increase at 1,000 mg twice daily was not statistically significant from placebo.

Faecal blood loss is significantly less following treatment with Dolobid (250 mg b.d.) than that associated with aspirin (600 mg q.i.d.).

Product licence numbers
250 mg tablet 0025/0128
500 mg tablet 0025/0146

INDOCID*

Presentation Ivory, opaque capsules containing 25 mg or 50 mg Indomethacin BP, marked 'INDOCID 25' and 'INDOCID 50' respectively.

Opaque ivory headed, transparent blue based, sustained release capsules carrying white and blue pellets containing 75 mg indomethacin, marked 'INDOCID R 693'. The 75 mg of indomethacin provides 25 mg of free indomethacin for immediate dissolution, and 50 mg of time-release coated pellets.

A fruit-flavoured suspension containing in each 5 ml, 25 mg indomethacin.

Polyethylene glycol suppositories containing 100 mg Indomethacin BP.

Uses Non-steroidal anti-inflammatory agent indicated for the active stages of rheumatoid arthritis, osteoarthritis, ankylosing spondylitis, degenerative joint disease of the hip, acute musculoskeletal disorders, low-back pain, and acute gout.

Also indicated in inflammation, pain and oedema following orthopaedic procedures; and the treatment of pain and associated symptoms of primary dysmenorrhoea.

Indocid Suppositories may be used where night pain and morning stiffness are prominent. One suppository at bedtime will frequently give relief from pain and stiffness for 13 to 16 hours after administration.

Indocid-R: Indocid-R may be substituted for all the indications of Indocid except acute gout, as clinical evidence is not currently available for this dosage form in this condition.

Dosage and administration The dosage of Indocid should be carefully adjusted to suit the needs of the individual patient.

Oral therapy: In order to reduce the possibility of gastro-intestinal disturbances, *Indocid/Indocid-R Capsules and Suspension should always be taken with food, milk or an antacid.* (Note, however, that Indocid Suspension should not be mixed with an antacid, but should be taken separately, because indomethacin is unstable in an alkaline medium.) Indocid Suspension should not be diluted.

In chronic conditions, starting therapy with a low dosage, increasing this gradually as necessary, and continuing a trial of therapy for an adequate period (in some cases, up to one month) will give the best results with a minimum of unwanted reactions.

The recommended oral dosage range is 50–200 mg daily in divided doses. Paediatric dosage not established.

Dosage in acute gouty arthritis: 150–200 mg daily in divided doses until all symptoms and signs subside.

Dosage in dysmenorrhoea: Up to 75 mg a day, starting with onset of cramps or bleeding, and continuing for as long as the symptoms usually last.

Adult dosage for suppositories: 1 suppository to be inserted once or twice a day. One should be used at bedtime. If another is necessary, it should be used in the morning.

Dosage for Indocid-R: The sustained-release capsule may be given once or, where necessary, twice a day depending on patient needs and response.

Use in the elderly: Indocid should be used with particular care in older patients who are more prone to adverse reactions.

Contra-indications, warnings, etc
Contra-indications: Active peptic ulcer; a recurrent history of gastro-intestinal lesions; in patients who have nasal polyps associated with angioneurotic oedema, who show sensitivity to Indocid, or who have experienced acute asthmatic attacks, urticaria or rhinitis as a result of therapy with aspirin or other non-steroidal anti-inflammatory drugs. Safety for use in children has not been established. Indocid Suppositories are contra-indicated in patients with a history of proctitis or recent rectal bleeding.

Indocid should not be used during pregnancy or lactation (it is secreted in breast milk).

Precautions: Headache, sometimes accompanied by dizziness and lightheadedness, may occur, usually early in treatment. Starting therapy with a low dosage and increasing it gradually will usually minimise the incidence of headache. These symptoms frequently disappear on continuing therapy or reducing the dosage, but if headache persists despite dosage reduction, Indocid should be withdrawn. Patients should be warned that they may experience dizziness and, if they do, should not drive a car or undertake potentially dangerous activities needing alertness.

Indocid should be used cautiously in patients with psychiatric disorders, epilepsy, or parkinsonism, as it may tend to aggravate these disorders.

Gastro-intestinal disturbances may be minimised by giving Indocid orally with food, milk or an antacid. They usually disappear on reducing the dosage; if not, the risks of continuing therapy should be weighed against the possible benefits. If gastro-intestinal bleeding does occur, Indocid should immediately be discontinued.

Single or multiple ulcerations, including perforation and haemorrhage of the oesophagus, stomach, duodenum or small or large intestine have been reported to occur with Indocid. Fatalities have been reported in some instances. Rarely, intestinal ulceration has been associated with stenosis and obstruction.

Gastro-intestinal bleeding without obvious ulcer formation and perforation of pre-existing sigmoid lesions (diverticulum, carcinoma, etc.) have occurred. Increased abdominal pain in ulcerative colitis patients or the development of ulcerative colitis and regional ileitis have been reported to occur rarely.

Fluid retention and peripheral oedema have been observed in some patients taking Indocid. It should therefore be used with caution in patients with cardiac dysfunction, hypertension or other conditions predisposing to fluid retention.

Tenesmus and irritation of the rectal mucosa have been reported occasionally with Indocid Suppositories.

Indocid may mask the signs and symptoms of infection. Indocid should be used with caution in patients with existing, but controlled infection.

In patients with rheumatoid arthritis, eye changes may occur which may be related to the underlying disease or to the therapy. Therefore, in chronic rheumatoid disease, ophthalmological examinations at periodic intervals are recommended. Discontinue therapy if eye changes are observed.

Patients should be periodically observed to allow early detection of any unwanted effects on peripheral blood (anaemia), liver function or gastro-intestinal tract.

Indocid can inhibit platelet aggregation. The effect usually disappears within 24 hours of discontinuing Indocid. Bleeding time is prolonged (but within normal range) in normal adults. Because this effect may be exaggerated in patients with underlying haemostatic defects, Indocid should be used cautiously in patients with coagulation defects.

As with other non-steroidal anti-inflammatory drugs, there have been reports of acute interstitial nephritis with haematuria, proteinuria, and occasionally nephrotic syndrome, in patients receiving long-term administration of indomethacin.

In patients with reduced renal blood flow where renal prostaglandins play a major role in maintaining renal perfusion, administration of a non-steroidal anti-inflammatory agent may precipitate overt renal decompensation. Patients at greatest risk of this reaction are those with renal or hepatic dysfunction, diabetes mellitus, advanced age, extracellular volume depletion, congestive heart failure, sepsis, or concomitant use of any nephrotoxic drug. A non-steroidal anti-inflammatory drug should be given with caution and renal function should be monitored in any patient who may have reduced renal reserve. Discontinuation of non-steroidal anti-inflammatory therapy is usually followed by recovery to the pretreatment state.

Increases in plasma potassium concentration, including hyperkalaemia, have been reported, even in some patients without renal impairment. In patients with normal renal function, these effects have been attributed to a hyporeninaemic-hypoaldosteronism state (see 'Drug interactions').

Since Indocid is eliminated primarily by the kidneys, patients with significantly impaired renal function should be closely monitored; a lower daily dosage should be used to avoid excessive drug accumulation.

Laboratory tests: Borderline elevations of one or more liver tests may occur, and significant elevations of ALT (SGPT) or AST (SGOT) have been seen in less than 1% of patients receiving therapy with non-steroidal anti-inflammatory drugs in controlled clinical trials. If abnormal liver tests persist or worsen, if clinical signs and symptoms consistent with liver disease develop or if systemic manifestations such as rash or eosinophilia occur, Indocid should be stopped.

False negative results in the dexamethasone suppression test (DST) in patients being treated with Indocid have been reported. Thus, results of this test should be used with caution in these patients.

Drug interactions: The use of Indocid with aspirin or other salicylates is not recommended. Controlled clinical studies have shown no enhanced therapeutic effect, and one study showed a significant increase in the incidence of gastro-intestinal side effects. A study in normal volunteers showed that chronic administration of 3.6 g aspirin with indomethacin lowered the indomethacin blood levels by approximately 20%.

Co-administration of diflunisal with Indocid increases the plasma level of indomethacin by about a third with a concomitant decrease in renal clearance. Fatal gastro-intestinal haemorrhage has occurred. The combination should not be used.

Although clinical studies suggest that Indocid does not influence the hypoprothrombinaemia induced by anticoagulants, patients also receiving anticoagulants should be closely observed for alterations of the prothrombin time.

Co-administration of probenecid may increase plasma levels of indomethacin.

Caution should be exercised with simultaneous use of Indocid with methotrexate. Indocid has been reported to decrease the tubular secretion of methotrexate and to potentiate toxicity.

Indomethacin 50 mg three times a day produced a clinically relevant elevation of plasma lithium and reduction in renal lithium clearance in psychiatric patients and normal subjects with steady state plasma lithium concentrations. This effect has been attributed to inhibition of prostaglandin synthesis. As a consequence, when indomethacin and lithium are given concomitantly, the patient should be observed carefully for signs of lithium toxicity.

In addition, the frequency of monitoring serum lithium concentrations should be increased at the outset of such combination drug treatment.

In some patients, the administration of Indocid can reduce the diuretic and antihypertensive effects of loop, potassium-sparing, and thiazide diuretics. Therefore, when Indocid and diuretics are used concomitantly, the patient shoud be observed closely to determine if the desired effect of the diuretic is obtained.

Indocid reduces basal plasma renin activity (PRA), as well as those elevations of PRA induced by frusemide administration, or salt or volume depletion. These facts should be considered when evaluating plasma renin activity in hypertensive patients.

It has been reported that the addition of triamterene to a maintenance schedule of Indocid resulted in reversible acute renal failure in two of four healthy volunteers. Indocid and triamterene should not be administered together.

Indocid and potassium-sparing diuretics each may be associated with increased plasma potassium levels. The potential effects of Indocid and potassium-sparing diuretics on potassium kinetics and renal function should be considered when these agents are administered concurrently.

Most of the above effects concerning diuretics have been attributed, at least in part, to mechanisms involving inhibition of prostaglandin synthesis by Indocid.

Because Indocid may reduce the antihypertensive effect of beta-blockers, patients receiving dual therapy should have the antihypertensive effect of their therapy reassessed.

Warnings and adverse reactions: CNS reactions – headaches, dizziness, lightheadedness, depression, vertigo, and fatigue (including malaise and listlessness). Reactions reported infrequently include mental confusion, anxiety, syncope, drowsiness, convulsions, coma, peripheral neuropathy, muscle weakness, involuntary muscle movements, insomnia, psychiatric disturbances such as depersonalisation; and, rarely, paraesthesiae, aggravation of epilepsy and parkinsonism. These are often transient and disappear frequently with continued or reduced dosage. However, occasionally, severe reactions require stopping therapy.

Gastro-intestinal – the more frequent reactions are nausea, anorexia, vomiting, epigastric distress, abdominal pain, constipation, and diarrhoea. Others are ulceration (single or multiple) of oesophagus, stomach, duodenum or elsewhere in the small or large intestine, sometimes with haemorrhage and perforation (a few fatalities have been reported); gastro-intestinal tract bleeding without obvious ulcer formation; increased abdominal pain in patients with pre-existing ulcerative colitis. Rarely, intestinal ulceration followed by stenosis and obstruction has been reported. Reactions occurring infrequently are stomatitis; gastritis; flatulence; bleeding from the sigmoid colon (occult or from a diverticulum); perforation of pre-existing sigmoid lesions such as diverticulae and carcinomata; ulcerative colitis and regional ileitis (causal relationship not established). With suppositories, tenesmus and irritation of the rectal mucosa have occasionally been reported.

Hepatic – rarely, hepatitis and jaundice (some fatalities reported).

Cardiovascular/renal – oedema, increased blood pressure, tachycardia, chest pain, arrhythmia, palpitation, hypotension, congestive heart failure, blood urea elevation and haematuria (all infrequent).

Dermatological/hypersensitivity – pruritus, urticaria, angioneurotic oedema, angiitis, erythema nodosum, skin rash, exfoliative dermatitis, Stevens-Johnson syndrome, erythema multiforme, toxic epidermal necrolysis, loss of hair, rapid fall in blood pressure resembling a shock-like state, acute anaphylaxis, acute respiratory distress including sudden dyspnoea, asthma and pulmonary oedema (all infrequent). Bronchospasm may be precipitated in patients suffering from or with a history of bronchial asthma or allergic disease.

Haematological – infrequently, blood dyscrasias may occur including leucopenia, petechiae or ecchymosis, purpura, aplastic or haemolytic anaemia, agranulocytosis, bone-marrow depression, disseminated intravascular coagulation, and particularly thrombocytopenia. Because some patients may develop anaemia secondary to obvious or occult gastro-intestinal bleeding, appropriate blood determinations are recommended.

Ocular – infrequently, blurred vision, diplopia, and orbital and peri-orbital pain. Corneal deposits and retinal disturbances including those of the macula have been reported in patients with rheumatoid arthritis on prolonged therapy, but similar changes may also be expected in patients with rheumatoid arthritis who have not received Indocid.

Aural – tinnitus, hearing disturbances (rarely deafness).

Genito-urinary – proteinuria, nephrotic syndrome, interstitial nephritis and renal insufficiency including renal failure (all rare).

Miscellaneous – vaginal bleeding, hyperglycaemia, glycosuria, hyperkalaemia, flushing and sweating, epistaxis, breast changes including enlargement and tenderness, gynaecomastia, and ulcerative stomatitis (all rare).

The following adverse reactions have been associated with use of Indocid Suppositories: tenesmus; proctitis; rectal bleeding, burning, pain, discomfort, and itching.

Overdosage: The following symptoms may be observed following overdosage: nausea, vomiting, intense headache, dizziness, mental confusion, disorientation, or lethargy. There have been reports of paraesthesiae, numbness, and convulsions. Treatment is symptomatic and supportive. The stomach should be emptied as quickly as possible if the ingestion is recent. If vomiting has not occurred spontaneously, the patient should be induced to vomit with syrup of ipecac. If the patient is unable to vomit, gastric lavage should be performed. Once the stomach has been emptied, 25 or 50 g of activated charcoal may be given. Depending on the condition of the patient, close medical observation and nursing care may be required. The patient should be followed for several days because gastro-intestinal ulceration and haemorrhage have been reported as adverse reactions of indomethacin. Use of antacids may be helpful.

The plasma elimination of indomethacin is biphasic with the half-life of the terminal plasma half-life phase between 2.6 and 11.2 hours.

Pharmaceutical precautions Keep container well closed; store in a dry place below 25°C, protected from light. Indocid Suspension should also be protected from freezing.

Indocid/Indocid-R Capsules and Suspension should always be taken with food, milk or an antacid. (Note, however, that Indocid Suspension should not be mixed with an antacid but should be taken separately because indomethacin is unstable in an alkaline medium.) Indocid Suspension should not be diluted.

Legal category POM.

Package quantities *Capsules:* 25 mg, bottles of 100 and 500; 50 mg, bottles of 100; 75 mg, bottles of 100. *Suppositories:* Boxes of 10. *Suspension:* Bottles of 200 ml.

Further information Nil.

Product licence numbers

25 mg	0025/0111
50 mg	0025/0112
75 mg	0025/0125
Suppositories	0025/0062
Suspension	0025/0120

INDOCID* PDA

Presentation Available in vials containing a sterile, off-white to yellow lyophilised mass of indomethacin sodium trihydrate equivalent to 1.0 mg indomethacin.

Uses The closure of patent ductus arteriosus in premature babies.

Mode of action: Although the exact mechanism of action is not known, it is believed that indomethacin closes a patent ductus arteriosus by inhibiting prostaglandin synthesis. In the newborn with certain congenital heart malformations, PGE1 dilates the ductus arteriosus; indomethacin causes its constriction.

Dosage and administration *For intravenous use only.*

A course of therapy is defined as three intravenous doses of Indocid PDA given at 12- to 24-hour intervals, with careful attention to urinary output.

If anuria or marked oliguria (urinary output of 0.6 ml/kg/hr) is evident at the time of the scheduled second or third dose, Indocid PDA must not be given until laboratory studies indicate that renal function has returned to normal.

Dosage recommendations depend closely on the age of the infant:

	Dosage (mg/kg)		
Age at first dose	*1st*	*2nd*	*3rd*
Less than 48 hours	0.2	0.1	0.1
2–7 days	0.2	0.2	0.2
Over 7 days	0.2	0.25	0.25

If the ductus arteriosus is closed or significantly reduced in size 48 hours after the first course of therapy, no further treatment is necessary. If the ductus arteriosus reopens, a second course of therapy may be given.

If the condition is unchanged after the second course of therapy, surgery may then be necessary. If severe adverse reactions occur, stop the treatment.

Directions for use: The solution should be prepared only with 1 to 2 ml 0.9% Sodium Chloride Injection BP or Water for Injections PhEur. Preparations containing dextrose must not be used.

Preservatives should be carefully avoided at every stage because of the risk of toxicity in the newborn; any unused portion remaining in the opened vial should be discarded.

A fresh solution should be prepared just prior to each administration according to the dilution table below:

Amount of diluent used for each vial	*Concentration achieved*
1 ml	0.1 mg/0.1 ml
2 ml	0.05 mg/0.1 ml

The indomethacin solution may be injected intravenously over 5 to 10 seconds.

Further dilution with intravenous infusion solutions is not recommended.

Contra-indications, warnings, etc

Contra-indications: Indocid PDA is contra-indicated in infants with established or suspected untreated infection; infants who are bleeding, especially with active intracranial haemorrhage or gastro-intestinal bleeding; infants with congenital heart disease in whom patency of the ductus arteriosus is necessary for satisfactory pulmonary or systemic blood flow (e.g. pulmonary atresia, severe tetralogy of Fallot, severe coarctation of the aorta); infants with thrombocytopenia; infants with coagulation defects; infants with known or suspected necrotising enterocolitis; infants with significant impairment of renal function.

Precautions
General: Indocid may mask the usual signs and symptoms of infection. The drug must therefore be used cautiously in the presence of existing controlled infection.

Because severe hepatic reactions have been reported in adults on prolonged therapy with oral indomethacin, Indocid PDA should be discontinued if signs and symptoms consistent with liver disease develop in the neonate.

Indocid PDA should be administered carefully to avoid extravasation and resultant irritation to tissues.

Gastro-intestinal effects: Clinical results indicate that major gastro-intestinal bleeding was no more common in those babies receiving indomethacin than those receiving placebo. However, minor gastro-intestinal bleeding (i.e. chemical detection of blood in the stool) was more common in infants treated with indomethacin. Severe gastro-intestinal effects have been reported in adults treated for prolonged periods with oral indomethacin.

CNS reactions: Prematurity *per se* is associated with an increased incidence of spontaneous intraventricular haemorrhage. Because indomethacin may inhibit platelet aggregation, the potential for intraventricular bleeding may be increased.

Renal effects: Indocid PDA may cause significant reduction in urine output (50% or more) with elevated blood urea and creatinine, and reduced GFR and creatinine clearance. In most babies, these effects are transient and disappear when therapy with Indocid PDA is stopped. However, because adequate renal function can depend on renal prostaglandin synthesis, Indocid PDA may precipitate renal insufficiency. This is most likely in babies with conditions such as CHF, sepsis, or hepatic dysfunction or who are undergoing therapy with nephrotoxic drugs which may affect renal function. Whenever a significant suppression of urine volume occurs with treatment, treatment with Indocid PDA must stop until urine output returns to normal.

Indocid PDA may suppress water excretion in premature babies to a greater extent than the excretion of sodium. This may result in hyponatraemia. Renal function and plasma electrolytes should be monitored.

Drug interactions: The half-life of digitalis in premature babies with patent ductus arteriosus and with cardiac failure is often prolonged by indomethacin. When both drugs are used concomitantly, frequent monitoring of ECG and serum digitalis may help to prevent or detect digitalis toxicity early.

In a study of premature infants treated with Indocid PDA and also receiving gentamicin and amikacin, both peak and trough levels of these amino-glycosides were significantly elevated.

Indocid may reduce the diuretic effect of frusemide.

Side-effects
Haemorrhagic: Gross or microscopic bleeding into the gastro-intestinal tract; oozing from the skin after needle puncture; pulmonary haemorrhage; and disseminated intravascular coagulopathy.

Renal: Renal dysfunction including one or more of the following: reduced urinary output; reduced urine sodium, chloride or potassium, urine osmolality, free water clearance, or glomerular filtration rate; uraemia; transient oliguria; and hypercreatininaemia.

Gastro-intestinal: Vomiting; abdominal distension; melaena; and transient ileus, and localised perforations of the small and/or large intestine.

Metabolic: Hypersensitivity; hyponatraemia; elevated plasma potassium; elevated blood urea; hypoglycaemia.

Cardiovascular: Pulmonary hypertension.

Coagulation: Decreased platelet aggregation.

General: Weight gain (fluid retention); and exacerbation of infection.

Causal relationship unknown: Although the following reactions have been reported in babies, a definite causal relationship has not been established.

Cardiovascular: intracranial bleeding; bradycardia.

Respiratory: apnoea; exacerbation of pre-existing pulmonary infection.

Haematological: Disseminated intravascular coagulation.

Metabolic: acidosis, alkalosis.

Gastro-intestinal: necrotising enterocolitis.

Ophthalmic: Retrolental fibroplasia.

See data sheet for Indocid (indomethacin) for additional information concerning side-effects and other cautionary statements.

Overdosage: It is recommended that Indocid PDA should only be administered in a neonatal intensive-care unit. No antidote is available. Dosage is critical, and any complications occurring in the gastro-intestinal, renal and central nervous systems should be treated symptomatically and supportively.

Plasma half-life of intravenous indomethacin was inversely variable to the post-natal age and weight of the baby. In one study, a mean plasma half-life in babies less than a week old averaged 20 hours, while older babies showed a 12-hour average. Grouping the same babies by weight, the mean plasma half-life seen in babies under 1000 g was 21 hours, in heavier babies the half-life was reduced to an average of 15 hours.

Pharmaceutical precautions The vial may be shipped and stored at room temperature. Intravenous solution should be prepared just prior to use and any unused portion remaining in the opened vial should be discarded.

When reconstituted, Indocid PDA is acceptable for use only when clear and free from particulate matter.

Further dilution with intravenous infusion solutions is not recommended. Indocid PDA is not buffered and reconstitution at pH levels below 6 may cause precipitation of insoluble indomethacin.

Legal category POM.

Package quantities Available in cartons of three 1 ml vials containing sterile, lyophilised indomethacin sodium trihydrate equivalent to 1.0 mg indomethacin.

Further information Nil.

Product licence number 0025/0201.

MIDAMOR*

Presentation Yellow, diamond-shaped tablets, marked 'MSD 92', containing Amiloride Hydrochloride BP equivalent to 5 mg anhydrous amiloride hydrochloride.

Uses Potassium-conserving agent; diuretic.

Although Midamor may be used alone, its principal indication is as concurrent therapy with thiazides or more potent diuretics to conserve potassium during periods of vigorous diuresis and during long-term maintenance therapy.

In *hypertension*, it is used as an adjunct to prolonged therapy with thiazides and similar agents to prevent potassium depletion.

In *congestive heart failure*, Midamor may be effective alone, but its principal indication is for concomitant use in patients receiving thiazides or more potent diuretic agents.

In *hepatic cirrhosis with ascites*, Midamor usually provides adequate diuresis, with diminished potassium loss and less risk of metabolic alkalosis, when used alone. It may be used with more potent diuretics when a greater diuresis is required while maintaining a more balanced serum electrolyte pattern.

Dosage and administration *Midamor alone:* The usual initial dosage is 10 mg (as a single dose or 5 mg twice a day). The total daily dose should not exceed 20 mg (4 tablets) a day. After diuresis has been achieved, the dosage may be reduced by 5 mg increments to the least amount required.

Midamor with other diuretic therapy: When Midamor is used with a diuretic which is given on an intermittent basis, it should be given at the same time as the diuretic.

Hypertension: 5 or 10 mg (1 or 2 tablets) a day, together with the usual antihypertensive dosage of the thiazide concurrently employed. It is not usually necessary to exceed 10 mg of Midamor a day; in any event, not more than 20 mg (4 tablets) of Midamor a day should be given.

Congestive heart failure: Initially, 5 or 10 mg (1 or 2 tablets) a day, together with the usual dosage of the diuretic concurrently employed. If diuresis is not achieved with minimal dosage of both agents, the dosage of both may be gradually increased, but that of Midamor should not exceed 20 mg (4 tablets) a day. Once diuresis has been achieved, reduction in dosage of both agents may be attempted for maintenance therapy. The dosage of both drugs is determined by the diuresis and the level of plasma potassium.

Hepatic cirrhosis with ascites: Treatment should be started with a small dose of Midamor, i.e. 5 mg (1 tablet), plus a low dosage of the other diuretic agent. If necessary, dosage of both agents may be increased gradually.

The dosage of Midamor should not exceed 20 mg (4 tablets) a day. Maintenance doses may be lower than those required to initiate diuresis; reduction in the daily dosage should therefore be attempted when the patient's weight is stabilised.

Children: The use of Midamor in children is contra-indicated.

Use in the elderly: The elderly are more susceptible to electrolyte imbalance, and more likely to experience hyperkalaemia since renal reserve may be reduced. The dosage should be carefully adjusted according to renal function, blood electrolytes and diuretic response.

Contra-indications, warnings, etc
Contra-indications: Hyperkalaemia (plasma potassium over 5.5 mmol/l); other potassium-conserving agents or potassium supplements (see 'Precautions'); anuria, acute renal failure, severe progressive renal disease, diabetic nephropathy (see 'Precautions'); prior sensitivity to this product. Safety for use in children is not established. See also 'Use in pregnancy' and 'Use in the breast-feeding mother' under 'Precautions'.

Precautions – Diabetes mellitus: To minimise the risk of hyperkalaemia in known or suspected diabetic patients, the status of renal function should be determined before initiating therapy. Midamor should be discontinued for at least three days before a glucose-tolerance test.

Metabolic or respiratory acidosis: Potassium-conserving therapy should be initiated only with caution in severely ill patients in whom metabolic or respiratory acidosis may occur, e.g. patients with cardiopulmonary disease of decompensated diabetes. Shifts in acid-base balance alter the balance of extracellular-intracellular potassium, and the development of acidosis may be associated with rapid increases in plasma potassium.

Hyperkalaemia: This has been observed in patients receiving amiloride hydrochloride, alone or with other diuretics. These patients should be observed carefully for clinical, laboratory, and ECG evidence of hyperkalaemia.

Some deaths have been reported in this group of patients. Hyperkalaemia has been noted particularly in the elderly and in hospital patients with hepatic cirrhosis or cardiac oedema who have known renal involvement, who were seriously ill, or were undergoing vigorous diuretic therapy.

Neither potassium-conserving agents nor a diet rich in potassium should be used with Midamor except in severe and/or refractory cases of hypokalaemia. If the combination is used, plasma potassium levels must be continuously monitored.

Impaired renal function: Patients with increases in blood urea over 10 mmol/l, serum creatinine over 130 µmol/l, or with diabetes mellitus, should not receive amiloride hydrochloride without careful, frequent monitoring of serum electrolytes and blood urea levels. In renal impairment, use of a potassium-conserving agent may result in rapid development of hyperkalaemia.

Treatment of hyperkalaemia: If hyperkalaemia occurs, Midamor should be discontinued immediately and, if necessary, active measures taken to reduce the plasma potassium level.

Electrolyte imbalance and reversible blood urea increases: Hyponatraemia and hypochloraemia may occur when amiloride hydrochloride is used with other diuretics. Reversible increases in blood urea levels have been reported accompanying vigorous diuresis, especially when diuretics were used in seriously ill patients, such as those with hepatic cirrhosis with ascites and metabolic alkalosis, or those with resistant oedema. Careful monitoring of serum electrolytes and blood urea levels should therefore be carried out when Midamor is given with other diuretics to such patients.

Cirrhotic patients: Oral diuretic therapy is more frequently accompanied by side effects in patients with hepatic cirrhosis with or without ascites, because these patients are intolerant of acute shifts in electrolyte balance, and because they often already have hypokalaemia as a result of associated aldosteronism.

In patients with pre-existing severe liver disease, hepatic encephalopathy, manifested by tremors, confusion, and coma, and increased jaundice, have been reported in association with diuretics, including amiloride hydrochloride.

Use in pregnancy: Because clinical experience is limited, Midamor is not recommended for use during pregnancy. The routine use of diuretics in otherwise healthy pregnant women with or without mild oedema is not indicated because they may be associated with hypovolaemia, increased blood viscosity and decreased placental perfusion. Fetal and neonatal jaundice, fetal bone marrow depression and thrombocytopenia have also been described. The potential benefits of the drug must be weighed against possible hazards to the fetus if it is administered to a woman of childbearing age.

Use in the breast-feeding mother: It is not known whether Midamor is excreted in human milk. Because many drugs are excreted by this route, and because there is risk that it might take this route of excretion, and that it might then cause serious side effects in the breast-feeding infant, the mother should either stop breast-feeding or stop taking the drug. The decision depends on the importance of the drug to the mother.

Drug interactions: Lithium should not be given with diuretics because they reduce its renal clearance and add a high risk of lithium toxicity.

When combined with thiazide diuretics, amiloride can act synergistically with chlorpropamide to increase the risk of hyponatraemia.

When amiloride hydrochloride is administered concomitantly with an angiotensin-converting enzyme inhibitor, the risk of hyperkalaemia may be increased. Therefore, if concomitant use of these agents is indicated because of demonstrated hypokalaemia, they should be used with caution and with frequent monitoring of serum potassium.

Side effects: Midamor is usually well tolerated, although minor side effects are reported relatively frequently. Except for hyperkalaemia, significant side-effects are infrequent. Nausea/anorexia, abdominal pain, flatulence, and mild skin rash are probably due to amiloride; but other side-effects are generally associated with diuresis or with the underlying disease being treated.

Body as a whole: Headache, weakness, fatigue, back pain, chest pain, neck/shoulder ache, pain in the extremities.

Cardiovascular: Angina pectoris, orthostatic hypotension, arrhythmias, palpitation, one patient with partial heart block developed complete heart block.

Digestive: Anorexia, nausea, vomiting, diarrhoea, constipation, abdominal pain, GI bleeding, jaundice, thirst, dyspepsia, flatulence.

Metabolic: Elevated plasma potassium levels above 5.5 mmol/l, hyponatraemia.

Integumentary: Pruritus, rash, dryness of mouth, alopecia.

Musculoskeletal: Muscle cramps, joint pain.

Nervous: Dizziness, vertigo, paraesthesiae, tremors, encephalopathy.

Psychiatric: Nervousness, mental confusion, insomnia, decreased libido, depression, somnolence.

Respiratory: Cough, dyspnoea.

Special senses: Nasal congestion, visual disturbances, increased intra-ocular pressure, tinnitus.

Urogenital: Impotence, polyuria, dysuria, bladder spasms, frequency of micturition.

Reactions in which no causal relationship could be established were activation of probable pre-existing peptic ulcer, aplastic anaemia, neutropenia and abnormal liver function tests. In a few cirrhotic patients, jaundice associated with the underlying disease has deepened, but the drug relationship is uncertain.

Overdosage: No data are available; and it is not known whether the drug is dialysable.

The most likely signs and symptoms are dehydration and electrolyte imbalance which should be treated by established methods. Therapy should be discontinued and the patient observed closely. No specific antidote is available. If ingestion is recent, emesis should be induced or gastric lavage performed. Treatment is symptomatic and supportive. If hyperkalaemia occurs, active measures should be taken to reduce plasma potassium levels.

The plasma half-life of amiloride is about six hours.

Pharmaceutical precautions Keep container well closed; store in a cool place, protected from light.

Legal category POM.

Package quantities Bottles of 100.

Further information Combined with hydrochlorothiazide, Midamor causes less magnesium excretion than either the thiazides or loop diuretics when used alone.

Product licence number 0025/5015.

MODUCREN*

Presentation Blue, square, half-scored tablets, marked 'MODUCREN', containing 25 mg hydrochlorothiazide, 2.5 mg amiloride hydrochloride, and 10 mg timolol maleate.

Uses Mild to moderate hypertension.

Dosage and administration 1 to 2 tablets once a day.

Use in the elderly: Moducren has been shown to be as well tolerated in the elderly as in younger patients. The recommended starting dose is one tablet daily.

Children: Because the safety and efficacy of Moducren has not been established in children, it is not recommended for paediatric use.

Contra-indications, warnings, etc

Contra-indications: Patients with bronchial asthma or with a history of bronchial asthma, severe chronic obstructive pulmonary disease, sinus bradycardia, second- or third-degree AV block, overt cardiac failure, right ventricular failure secondary to pulmonary hypertension, significant cardiomegaly, and cardiogenic shock. Hyperkalaemia (plasma potassium over 5.5 mmol/l). Anuria, acute and chronic renal insufficiency, severe progressive renal disease and diabetic nephropathy. Patients with blood urea over 10 mmol/l or serum creatinine over 130 μmol/l or diabetes mellitus should not receive Moducren without careful and frequent serum urea and serum electrolyte monitoring.

Anaesthetic agents causing myocardial depression, hypersensitivity to any component of Moducren or to sulphonamide-derived drugs. Use with other potassium-conserving agents. Use with potassium supplements or potassium-rich food except in severe and/or refractory cases of hypokalaemia when careful monitoring of the serum potassium level is necessary.

See also 'Pregnancy', 'Breast-feeding mothers' and 'Children'.

Precautions:

Congestive cardiac failure: care should be exercised before and during treatment of patients with cardiomegaly or history of cardiac failure. *Cardiac arrhythmias:* patients at risk of congestive heart failure should be carefully observed for bradycardia, AV block and respiratory distress. If congestive cardiac failure persists, Moducren should be withdrawn. Beta-adrenergic blocking agents should be used with caution in patients with cerebrovascular insufficiency. If signs or symptoms suggesting reduced cerebral blood flow are observed, consideration should be given to discontinuing these agents. *Exacerbation of ischaemic heart disease following abrupt withdrawal:* Exacerbation of angina and, in some cases, myocardial infarction have occurred after abrupt withdrawal of beta-blocker therapy. Therefore, it is recommended that if Moducren is to be withdrawn, dosage should be gradually reduced. *Elective or emergency surgery:* Moducren should also be gradually withdrawn prior to elective surgery of anginal patients. Agonists such as isoprenaline, dopamine, dobutamine or noradrenaline may be used to counter the effects of beta-blockade in emergency surgery. *Renal and hepatic disease and electrolyte disturbances:* Moducren should be used with caution in patients with renal or hepatic disease and in those patients in whom fluid and electrolyte balance is critical. When creatinine clearance falls below 30 ml/min, thiazide diuretics are ineffective. Azotemia may be precipitated or increased by hydrochlorothiazide. Cumulative effects of the drug may develop in patients with impaired renal function. If increasing azotemia and oliguria occur during treatment of renal disease, the diuretic should be discontinued. *Metabolic or respiratory acidosis:* acid-base balance should be monitored frequently in severely ill patients at risk of respiratory or metabolic acidosis. *Electrolyte and fluid balance:* serum and urine electrolyte determinations should be made in patients vomiting excessively or receiving parenteral fluids. Dilutional hyponatraemia may occur in patients with oedema in hot weather which calls for appropriate therapy; hypochloraemia requires specific treatment only under exceptional circumstances. Hyponatraemia, hypochloraemic alkalosis, hypokalaemia, hyperkalaemia or hypomagnesaemia may occur. If hyperkalaemia occurs, Moducren should be discontinued immediately and, if necessary, active measures taken to reduce the plasma potassium level. The degree of thiazide-induced hypomagnesaemia is reduced. *Diabetes mellitus, hypoglycaemia:* Moducren should be given with caution to diabetic patients and to patients subject to spontaneous hypoglycaemia as the symptoms and signs of acute hypoglycaemia may be masked. To minimise the risk of hyperkalaemia in diabetic or suspected diabetic patients, the status of renal function should be known before initiating therapy with Moducren. Therapy should be discontinued for at least three days prior to glucose tolerance testing. Thiazide therapy may impair glucose tolerance. Dosage adjustment of antidiabetic agents, including insulin, may be required. *Skin and sensitivity reactions:* there have been reports of skin rashes and/or dry eyes associated with the use of beta-adrenergic blocking drugs. The reported incidence is small and in most cases the symptoms have cleared when treatment was withdrawn. Discontinuation of the drug should be considered if any such reaction is not otherwise explicable. Withdrawal should be gradual. Sensitivity reactions to Moducren may occur with or without a history of allergy or bronchial asthma. Possible exacerbation or activation of systemic lupus erythematosus reactions have been reported with thiazide diuretics. *Metabolic and endocrine:* beta-adrenergic blocking agents may mask the signs of hyperthyroidism. Patients suspected of developing thyrotoxicosis should be managed carefully to avoid abrupt withdrawal of beta blockade which might precipitate a thyroid storm. Hypercalcaemia and hypophosphataemia have also been reported with thiazide diuretics. Moducren should be discontinued in patients prior to testing for parathyroid function. Increases in cholesterol and triglyceride levels may be associated with thiazide diuretic therapy. Hyperuricaemia or acute gout may be precipitated in some patients. *Musculoskeletal:* beta-blockers have been reported to induce myasthenic symptoms such as diplopia, ptosis, and generalised weakness.

Drug interactions: Moducren may potentiate other antihypertensive agents, such as reserpine or guanethidine. The antihypertensive effect of beta-blockers may be reduced by NSAIDs. NSAIDs may reduce the diuretic, natriuretic and antihypertensive effects of diuretics. Its effect may be enhanced in the post-sympathectomy patient.

Oral calcium antagonists may be combined with Moducren only when heart function is normal. When the heart function is impaired, combination of beta-blockers with dihydropyridine derivatives such as nifedipine may lead to hypotension; and combination with verapamil or diltiazem may cause AV conduction disturbances or left ventricular failure.

Intravenous calcium antagonists and Moducren should only be used together with caution.

Concomitant beta-blockers and digitalis with either diltiazem or verapamil may further prolong the AV conduction time.

Alcohol, barbiturates, or narcotics: Co-administration may potentiate orthostatic hypotension. *Oral and parenteral antidiabetic drugs* may require adjustment of dosage with concurrent use.

Corticosteroids or ACTH may intensify any thiazide-induced electrolyte depletion, particularly hypokalaemia. *Pressor amines such as adrenaline* may show decreased arterial responsiveness when used with Moducren, but this reaction is not enough to preclude their therapeutic usefulness. *Non-depolarising muscle relaxants such as tubocurarine* may possibly interact with Moducren to increase muscle relaxation. *Lithium* should not generally be given with diuretics, because they reduce its renal clearance and add a high risk of lithium toxicity. *Drug laboratory tests:* because thiazides may affect calcium metabolism, Moducren may interfere with tests for parathyroid function (see 'Precautions').

Breast-feeding mothers: Thiazides appear in breast milk, but it is not known whether timolol maleate or amiloride are also excreted. If the use of Moducren is deemed essential, the mother should stop breast-feeding.

Pregnancy: Moducren is not recommended for use during pregnancy. The use of any drug in women of child-bearing age requires that the anticipated benefit be weighed against possible hazards, which include fetal or neonatal jaundice, thrombocytopenia, and possibly other adverse reactions which have occurred in the adult.

Side effects: Moducren is usually well tolerated with significant side effects only infrequently reported.

Most common side-effects are dizziness, asthenia, fatigue, and bradycardia. Other clinical adverse reactions are: *Body as a whole:* Asthenia, fatigue, headache. *Cardiovascular:* Bradycardia, peripheral vascular disorder (cold extremities), hypotension, syncope, arrhythmia, angina pectoris. *Respiratory:* Dyspnoea, wheezing. *Digestive:* Nausea, dyspepsia, constipation, diarrhoea, vomiting, GI pain, anorexia, thirst, dry mouth, stomatitis. *Urogenital:* Impotence. *Nervous:* Dizziness, vertigo, paraesthesiae, tremors. *Integumentary:* Sweating. *Musculoskeletal:* Muscle cramps. *Psychiatric:* Insomnia, nervousness, depression, somnolence, abnormal dreaming, sleep disturbance. *Special senses:* Visual disturbances.

Side-effects that have been reported with the individual components may be considered as potential side-effects of Moducren.

Amiloride-related effects
Digestive: abnormal liver function, activation of probable pre-existing peptic ulcer, dyspepsia, jaundice. *Integumentary:* dry mouth, alopecia, diaphoresis. *Haematological:* aplastic anaemia, neutropenia. *Cardiovascular:* one patient with partial heart block developed complete heart block, palpitation. *Psychiatric:* decreased libido. *Respiratory:* cough. *Special senses:* tinnitus, increased intraocular pressure. *Urogenital:* polyuria, urinary frequency, bladder spasm.

Hydrochlorothiazide-related effects
Body as a whole: Anaphylactic reaction, fever. *Cardiovascular:* Necrotising angiitis (vasculitis, cutaneous vasculitis). *Digestive:* Jaundice (intrahepatic cholestatic jaundice), pancreatitis, cramping, gastric irritation. *Integumentary:* Photosensitivity. *Endocrine/metabolic:* Glycosuria, hyperglycaemia, hyperuricaemia, sialadenitis, urticaria. *Psychiatric:* Restlessness. *Respiratory:* respiratory distresses including pneumonitis, pulmonary oedema. *Special senses:* Transient blurred vision, xanthopsia. *Haematological:* Agranulocytosis, aplastic anaemia, haemolytic anaemia, leucopenia, purpura, thrombocytopenia.

Timolol maleate-related effects.
Body as a whole: Asthenia, fatigue, headache, chest pain, extremity pain, decreased exercise tolerance, weight loss. *Cardiovascular:* bradycardia, cardiac arrest, cerebral vascular accident, palpitation, arrhythmia, second- or third-degree AV block, sino-atrial block, syncope, hypotension, oedema and pulmonary oedema, cardiac failure, Raynaud's phenomenon, cold extremities, claudication, worsening of arterial insufficiency and angina pectoris, vasodilatation. *Digestive:* Dyspepsia, nausea, vomiting, diarrhoea, hepatomegaly. *Endocrine:* Hyperglycaemia, hypoglycaemia. *Integumentary:* Rash, Pruritus, skin irritation, increased pigmentation, sweating, exfoliative dermatitis (one case). *Musculoskeletal:* arthralgia. *Nervous system:* Dizziness, vertigo, paraesthesiae, local weakness. *Psychiatric:* Nervousness, diminished concentration, hallucinations, nightmares, increased dreaming, insomnia, depression, somnolence, decreased libido. *Haematological:* Non-thrombocytopenic purpura. *Respiratory:* Dyspnoea, bronchial spasm, rales, cough. *Special senses:* Tinnitus, visual disturbances, diplopia, ptosis, eye irritation, dry eyes. *Urogenital:* Impotence, micturition difficulties.

Clinical laboratory tests: Changes in clinically important laboratory tests associated with timolol maleate are rare. Slight increases in blood urea, serum potassium and serum uric acid, and slight decreases in haemoglobin and haematocrit occurred but were not progressive or associated with clinical manifestations.

Overdosage: No specific data are available in humans. Little is known about dialysability of its components: a study of patients with renal failure showed that timolol did not readily dialyse. No antidote is available. Treatment is symptomatic and supportive.

Therapy with Moducren should be stopped and emesis and/or gastric lavage induced.

Hydrochlorothiazide and amiloride hydrochloride: The signs and symptoms most likely are dehydration and electrolyte imbalance. If hyperkalaemia occurs, active measures should be taken to reduce plasma potassium levels.

Timolol maleate: The most common signs and symptoms to be expected following overdosage with a beta-blocker are symptomatic bradycardia, hypotension, bronchospasm, acute cardiac failure, and heart block.

If overdosage occurs, the following measures are recommended:

1. *Gastric lavage*

2. *For symptomatic bradycardia:* Atropine sulphate, 0.25 to 2 mg intravenously, should be used to induce vagal blockade. If bradycardia persists, intravenous isoprenaline hydrochloride should be administered cau-

tiously. In refractory cases, the use of a transvenous cardiac pacemaker may be considered.

3. *For hypotension:* A sympathomimetic pressor agent such as dopamine, dobutamine or noradrenaline should be used. In refractory cases, the use of glucagon has been reported useful.

4. *For bronchospasm:* Isoprenaline hydrochloride should be used. Additional therapy with aminophylline may be considered.

5. *For acute cardiac failure:* Conventional therapy with digitalis, diuretics, and oxygen should be instituted immediately. In refractory cases, the use of intravenous aminophylline is suggested. This may be followed, if necessary, by glucagon which has been reported useful.

6. *For heart block:* Isoprenaline hydrochloride or a transvenous cardiac pacemaker should be used.

The components of Moducren have, respectively, plasma half-lives of: Hydrochlorothiazide at 5.6 hours with a longer terminal phase; amiloride at about six hours; and timolol at about four hours.

Pharmaceutical precautions Store in a dry place below 25°C, protected from light.

Legal category POM.

Package quantities Calendar packs of 28 tablets.

Further information The combination of amiloride with hydrochlorothiazide has been shown to cause less magnesium excretion than either the thiazides or loop diuretics alone.

Similar dosage schedules and similar bioavailability rationalise the combination of hydrochlorothiazide (a saluretic), timolol maleate (a beta-adrenergic receptor blocking agent), and amiloride hydrochloride (a potassium-conserving agent) for the treatment of hypertension.

Product licence number 0025/0141.

MUMPSVAX*

Presentation Lyophilised powder which, when reconstituted, contains in each dose not less than 5,000 $TCID_{50}$ (tissue culture infectious doses) of mumps virus vaccine expressed in terms of the assigned titre of the FDA (USA) Reference Mumps Virus. It is prepared from the Jeryl Lynn (B Level) strain, named after the patient from whom the virus was initially recovered.

Uses Mumps virus vaccine.

Mumpsvax induces a modified, non-communicable mumps infection in susceptible persons. Clinical trials have shown Mumpsvax to be highly immunogenic and well tolerated. A single injection has been shown to induce antibody response in approximately 97% of susceptible children and 93% of susceptible adults.

The vaccine is indicated for immunisation against mumps in children over 12 months of age, or adults. A booster is not needed. It is not recommended for children younger than this because they may retain maternal mumps-neutralising antibodies which may interfere with the immune response.

Evidence indicates that the vaccine will not offer protection when given after exposure to natural mumps.

Revaccination: Based on available evidence, there is no need to revaccinate children who were originally vaccinated when 12 months or older. However, patients should be revaccinated if there is evidence that initial immunisation was ineffective.

Use with other vaccines: Routine administration of diphtheria, tetanus and pertussis vaccine and/or oral poliomyelitis vaccine with Mumpsvax is not recommended because of insufficient data. However, if circumstances do dictate concurrent vaccination, separate syringes and separate sites for injection should be used.

Mumpsvax should not be given less than one month before or after immunisation with other virus vaccines.

Dosage and administration *Adults and children:* After suitably cleansing the immunisation site, the total volume of reconstituted vaccine should be injected subcutaneously, preferably into the outer aspect of the upper arm. Mumpsvax must not be injected intravenously.

The dosage of vaccine is the same for all patients. *Do not give serum globulin (ISG) concurrently with Mumpsvax.*

Reconstitution: To reconstitute the vaccine, all the diluent provided should be injected into the vial of lyophilised vaccine, and agitated to ensure thorough mixing. The entire contents of the vial should then be drawn back into the syringe for subcutaneous injection.

Contra-indications, warnings, etc
Contra-indications: Do not give Mumpsvax to pregnant women, since the possible effects of the vaccine on fetal development are not known at this time. If vaccination of post-pubertal females is undertaken, pregnancy should be avoided for three months following vaccination (see 'Pregnancy').

Mumpsvax should not be given to children less than one year of age.

Anaphylactoid reaction to neomycin (each dose of reconstituted vaccine contains approximately 25 micrograms of neomycin).

Patients with active untreated tuberculosis should not be given Mumpsvax.

Malignant disease. Those with impaired immune responsiveness, whether occurring naturally or as a result of treatment with steroids, radiotherapy, cytotoxic drugs or other therapy. This contra-indication does not apply to patients who are receiving corticosteroids as replacement therapy, e.g. for Addison's disease.

Any active or suspected infection is reason for delaying vaccination.

Those with a family history of congenital or hereditary immunodeficiency should not be vaccinated until their immune competence is demonstrated.

Hypersensitivity to eggs, chicken, or chicken feathers: Live mumps vaccine is produced in cell cultures of chick embryo.

Patients with a history of anaphylactoid or other immediate reactions to eating eggs (e.g. hives, swelling of the mouth and throat, difficult breathing, hypotension and shock) should not be vaccinated. Evidence indicates, however, that patients with egg allergies that are not anaphylactoid may be vaccinated in the usual way. There is also no evidence to suggest that allergy to chicken or feathers increases the risk of reaction.

Pregnancy: Animal reproduction studies have not been conducted with Mumpsvax. It is also not known whether Mumpsvax can damage the fetus or affect the mother's reproductive capacity.

Although mumps virus is capable of infecting the placenta and fetus, there is no good evidence that it causes congenital malformation in humans. Mumps vaccine virus has also been shown to affect the placenta, but the virus has not been isolated from fetal tissues taken from susceptible women who were vaccinated and underwent elective abortions.

Precautions: A sterile syringe and Adrenaline Injection BP (1 : 1,000) should be ready for immediate use should an anaphylactoid reaction occur.

Vaccination should be deferred for at least three months following blood or plasma transfusions, or administration of human immune serum globulin. If any of these substances have been used near to the time of vaccination, a test for the presence of mumps antibody should be made at a later date.

It has been reported that live mumps virus vaccine may temporarily depress tuberculin skin sensitivity. Therefore, if a tuberculin test is to be done, it should be scheduled before or simultaneously with mumps vaccine.

As with any vaccine, Mumpsvax does not provide seroconversion in 100% of susceptible vaccinees.

Nursing mothers: Because it is not known whether Mumpsvax is secreted in human milk, caution should be exercised when considering the use of the vaccine in nursing mothers.

Adverse reactions: Because of the slight acidity of the vaccine (pH 6.2–6.6) patients may complain of burning and/or stinging at the injection site for a short time.

Mild fever occurs occasionally. Fever above 103°F (39.4°C) is uncommon.

Parotitis has been reported to occur in very low incidence, and orchitis rarely, in persons who were vaccinated. In most instances investigated, prior exposure to natural mumps was established. In other instances, whether or not this was due to vaccine, to prior natural mumps exposure or to other causes has not been established.

Reports of purpura and allergic reactions such as wheal and flare at the injection site, or urticaria have been extremely rare.

Forms of optic neuritis, including retrobulbar neuritis and papillitis, may infrequently follow viral infections and have been reported to occur one to three weeks following vaccination with some live virus vaccines.

Very rarely, encephalitis, febrile seizures, nerve deafness, and other nervous system reactions have occurred in recipients of the vaccine. A cause-effect relationship has not been established.

Overdosage: Poisoning is unlikely. Swallowing Mumpsvax would render the live vaccine benign, and the content of neomycin (25 micrograms/ml) is not likely to cause toxicity. No case of overdosage has been reported.

Anaphylactoid reaction should be treated immediately with Adrenaline Injection BP (1:1,000).

Pharmaceutical precautions During shipment, the vaccine should be maintained at a temperature below 10°C to insure that there is no loss of potency.

Prior to reconstitution, the vaccine should be stored between 2°C–8°C. *Protect from light.*

A separate sterile disposable needle and syringe should be used on each occasion, free from preservatives, antiseptics and detergents which may inactivate the vaccine.

The vaccine should be reconstituted using only the diluent provided, and used immediately after reconstitution.

When reconstituted, the vaccine is yellow. It is acceptable for use only when clear and free from particulate matter.

Legal category POM.

Package quantities One 0.5 ml single-dose vial of lyophilised vaccine with an ampoule containing diluent.

Further information Mumpsvax is grown in cell cultures of chick embryos free of avian leucosis and other adventitious agents.

Vaccine-induced antibody levels have persisted for at least 15 years without substantial decline. The pattern of antibody closely resembles that observed for natural mumps, although the antibody level is significantly lower than that following the natural infection. If this pattern continues, it will provide a basis for expectation that immunity following the vaccine will be permanent. However, continued observation will be required to demonstrate this point.

No reports have been received of transmission of mumps from vaccinees to susceptible contacts.

Product licence number 0025/0072.

PEPCID* PM

Presentation Brown, round-cornered square tablets, marked 'PEPCID PM' on one face with '40' on the other, containing 40 mg famotidine.

Beige, round-cornered square tablets, marked 'PEPCID PM' on one face with '20' on the other, containing 20 mg famotidine.

Uses
Indications: Duodenal ulcer.

Prevention of relapses of duodenal ulceration.

Benign gastric ulcer.

Hypersecretory conditions such as Zollinger-Ellison syndrome.

Mode of action: Pepcid PM is a novel, highly specific and potent competitive H_2-receptor antagonist. It has a rapid onset of action. Although the plasma half-life of famotidine in patients is approximately 3.0 hours, Pepcid PM has a long duration of action, and a single 40 mg dose has been shown to reduce gastric acid secretion for at least 10 hours.

Pepcid PM reduces the acid and pepsin content, as well as the volume of basal, nocturnal and stimulated gastric secretion.

Dosage and administration In benign gastric and duodenal ulceration, the dose of Pepcid PM is one 40 mg tablet at night.

It is unnecessary to time the dose in relation to meals; bioavailability is not clinically affected by food in the stomach. In all cases the clinical response of the patient should be taken into consideration

Duodenal ulcer: The recommended initial dose is one 40 mg tablet of Pepcid PM at night. Treatment should continue for four to eight weeks. In most patients, healing occurs on this regimen within four weeks. In those patients whose ulcers have not healed completely after four weeks, a further four-week period of treatment is recommended.

Maintenance therapy: For preventing the recurrence of duodenal ulceration, the reduced dose of 20 mg of Pepcid PM at night is recommended. This 20 mg maintenance dose has been continued effectively in clinical studies of 12 months duration.

Benign gastric ulcer: The recommended dose is one 40 mg tablet of Pepcid PM at night. Treatment should continue for four to eight weeks unless endoscopy reveals earlier healing.

Zollinger-Ellison syndrome: Patients without prior antisecretory therapy should be started on 20 mg of Pepcid PM every six hours. Dosage should then be adjusted to individual response: doses up to 800 mg daily have been used up to one year without the development of significant adverse effects or tachyphylaxis. Patients who have been receiving another H_2 antagonist may be switched directly to Pepcid PM at a dose higher than that recommended for new cases. This starting dose will depend on the severity of the condition and the last dose of H_2 antagonist previously used.

Use in the elderly: The recommended dosage in most elderly patients is the same as in younger patients for all indications (see above). No change in the incidence or type of side effects were seen in treated elderly patients.

Use in impaired renal function: Since Pepcid PM is excreted primarily by the kidney, caution should be observed in patients with impaired renal function. The dose should be reduced to 20 mg *nocte* if creatinine clearance falls below 10 ml/min.

Paediatric use: The efficacy and safety of Pepcid PM in children have not been established.

Contra-indications, warnings, etc
Contra-indications: Hypersensitivity to any component of this product.

Precautions
Gastric carcinoma: Gastric malignancy should be excluded prior to initiation of therapy of gastric ulcer with Pepcid PM. Symptomatic response of gastric ulcer to therapy with Pepcid PM does not preclude the presence of gastric malignancy.

Impaired renal function: Since Pepcid PM is primarily excreted via the kidney, caution should be exercised when treating patients with impaired renal function.
The dose should be reduced to 20 mg *nocte* when creatinine clearance falls below 10 ml/min.

Pregnancy: Pepcid PM is not recommended for use in pregnancy, and should be prescribed only if clearly needed. Before a decision is made to use Pepcid PM during pregnancy, the physician should weigh the potential benefits from the drug against the possible risks involved.

Breast-feeding mothers: Pepcid PM is secreted in human milk, therefore breast-feeding mothers should either stop breast-feeding or stop taking the drug.

Drug interactions: No clinically important drug interactions have been identified. Pepcid PM does not interact with the cytochrome P450-linked drug metabolising enzyme system. Compounds metabolised by this system which have been tested in man have included warfarin, theophylline, phenytoin, diazepam, propranolol, aminopyrine and phenazone. Indocyanine green as an index of hepatic blood flow and/or hepatic drug extraction has been tested and no significant effects have been found.

Side-effects: In controlled studies, Pepcid PM has been shown to be generally well tolerated.

Headache, dizziness, constipation, and diarrhoea have been reported rarely. Other side effects reported even less frequently included dry mouth, nausea and/or vomiting, abdominal discomfort or distension, anorexia, fatigue, rash, pruritis and urticaria, liver enzyme abnormalities, cholestatic jaundice, anaphylaxis, angioedema, arthralgia. Pancytopenia and leukopenia have been reported, however, a causal relationship to therapy with Pepcid PM has not been established.

Overdosage: There is no experience to date with overdosage.

The usual measures to remove unabsorbed material from the gastro-intestinal tract, clinical monitoring, and supportive therapy should be employed.

Patients with Zollinger-Ellison syndrome have tolerated a dosage of 800 mg daily for up to a year without significant adverse effects.

Pharmaceutical precautions Store in a dry place below 25°C.

Legal category POM.

Package quantities Calendar packs of 28 tablets; bottles of 50 tablets.

Further information Pepcid PM is a chemically novel competitive H_2-receptor antagonist with a guanidinothiazole ring. Pepcid PM is rapidly absorbed, with dose-related peak plasma concentrations reached in one to three hours. When used as recommended, there was no accumulation effect with repeated doses.

In clinical studies, a single dose of Pepcid PM at night relieved the pain associated with peptic ulcer, usually within a week, and suppressed gastric secretion.

Studies in animals and human volunteers have not shown anti-androgenic effects.

Product licence numbers
20 mg tablets 0025/0215
40 mg tablets 0025/0216

PNEUMOVAX* II

Presentation Single-dose vial containing, in 0.5 ml, 25 micrograms of each polysaccharide type derived from capsules of the 23 most prevalent pneumococci dissolved in isotonic saline containing 0.25% phenol.

Uses A pneumococcal vaccine.

Pneumovax II is a sterile liquid vaccine consisting of a mixture of highly purified capsular polysaccharides from the 23 most prevalent or invasive pneumococcal types accounting for at least 90% of pneumococcal blood isolates and at least 85% of all pneumococcal isolates from usually sterile sites determined by ongoing surveillance (see chart).

23 pneumococcal capsular types included in Pneumovax II

Nomenclature	Pneumococcal types							
Danish	1	2	3	4	5	6B	7F	8
U.S.	1	2	3	4	5	26	51	8
Danish	9N	9V	10A	11A	12F	14	15B	17F
U.S.	9	68	34	43	12	14	54	17
Danish	18C	19F	19A	20	22F	23F	33F	
U.S.	56	19	57	20	22	23	70	

Protective capsular type-specific antibody levels usually develop by the third week following vaccination.

Pneumovax II is indicated for immunisation against pneumococcal disease caused by those pneumococcal types included in the vaccine. Pneumovax II will not immunise against capsular types of pneumococcus other than those contained in the vaccine. It should be considered for all persons 2 years of age or older in whom there is an increased risk of morbidity and mortality from pneumococcal pneumonia.

Pneumovax II may not be effective in preventing infection resulting from basilar skull fracture or from external communication with cerebrospinal fluid.

Dosage and administration *Do not inject intravenously; avoid intradermal administration.*

Administer a single 0.5 ml dose of Pneumovax II subcutaneously or intramuscularly (preferably in the deltoid muscle or lateral mid-thigh) with appropriate precautions to avoid intravascular administration.

Revaccination: Revaccination of adults is not recommended. Adults previously immunised with any polyvalent pneumococcal vaccine should not receive Pneumovax II, since an increased, incidence and severity of adverse reactions among healthy adults receiving such re-injections have been noted, most likely due to sustained high antibody levels.

Certain groups of children at very high risk of pneumococcal disease (e.g. children with sickle cell disease or nephrotic syndrome) may have lower peak levels of antibody response and/or more rapid rates of decline in antibody levels than do healthy adults. However, insufficient data are currently available to formulate guidelines for the reimmunisation of high-risk children. Such children should not, however be revaccinated within three years.

Contra-indications, warnings, etc

Contra-indications: Hypersensitivity to any component of the vaccine. Adrenaline injection BP (1:1,000) must be immediately available should an acute anaphylactoid reaction occur.

Revaccination of adults is contra-indicated. Adults previously immunised with any polyvalent pneumococcal vaccine should not receive Pneumovax II.

Do not use Pneumovax II less than ten days prior to or during immunosuppressive therapy.

Patients with Hodgkin's disease who have received extensive chemotherapy and/or nodal irradiation.

Pneumovax II should not be given to pregnant women, since it is not known whether the vaccine can cause fetal harm, or affect the outcome of pregnancy.

Breast-feeding mothers should not be given Pneumovax II.

Warnings: The expected serum antibody response may not be obtained in patients receiving immunosuppressive therapy.

Intradermal administration may cause severe local reactions.

Precautions; Caution and appropriate care should be exercised in administering Pneumovax II to individuals with severely compromised cardiac and/or pulmonary function in whom a systemic reaction would pose a significant risk.

Delay the use of Pneumovax II in any febrile respiratory illness or other active infection except when this delay may involve even greater risk.

Required prophylactic antibiotic therapy against pneumococcal infection should not be stopped after immunisation with Pneumovax II.

It is recommended that a clear note of vaccination with Pneumovax II be kept in the patient's hospital and general practitioner records.

Children under 2 years of age: Pneumovax II is not recommended because antibody response to capsular types that most often cause pneumococcal disease in this age group may be poor.

Adverse reactions: Local erythema and soreness at the injection site, usually of less than 48 hours' duration, commonly occur; local induration occurs less frequently. Rarely, rash and arthralgia have been reported.

Low-grade fever (less than 38.3°C) occurs occasionally, usually within 24 hours of vaccination. Rarely, fever over 38.9°C has been reported.

On rare occasions, patients with otherwise stabilised idiopathic thrombocytopenic purpura have relapsed with a thrombocytopenia that has recurred 2–14 days after vaccination, and lasted for up to 2 weeks.

Reactions of greater severity, duration, or extent are unusual. Neurological disorders such as paraesthesiae and acute radiculoneuropathy, including the Guillain-Barre syndrome, have rarely been reported at the time of vaccination, but with no established cause and effect relationship.

Rarely, anaphylactoid reactions have been reported.

Pharmaceutical precautions Store at 2° to 8°C. The vaccine is used directly as supplied. No dilution or reconstitution is necessary. Phenol 0.25% is present as preservative. All vaccine must be discarded after the expiration date.

Pneumovax II should be inspected before injection to see that it a clear, colourless liquid without suspended particles.

Legal category POM.

Package quantities A single-dose vial.

Further information Invasive pneumococcal disease causes high morbidity and mortality in spite of effective antimicrobial control by antibiotics. These effects of pneumococcal disease appear to be due to irreversible pathological damage caused by bacteria during the first five days following onset of illness, irrespective of antimicrobial therapy.

Although the duration of the protective effect of Pneumovax II is presently unknown, previous studies with other pneumococcal vaccines suggest that induced antibodies may persist for five years. Type-specific antibody levels induced by 14-valent Pneumovax decline over a 42-month period of observation, but remain significantly higher than prevaccination levels in almost all recipients who responded initially.

Product licence number 0025/0213.

TRYPTIZOL*

Presentation Tryptizol 75, clear orange, slow-release capsules, marked 'MSD 649', containing 75 mg amitriptyline hydrochloride as a pelleted formulation.

Blue, film-coated tablets, marked 'MSD 23', containing 10 mg Amitriptyline Hydrochloride BP; yellow, film-coated tablets, marked 'MSD 45', containing 25 mg; and brown, film-coated tablets, marked 'MSD 102', containing 50 mg.

Injection, a colourless solution containing per ml 10 mg amitriptyline hydrochloride.

Syrup, a pink suspension containing, in each 5 ml, Amitriptyline Embonate BP equivalent to 10 mg amitriptyline.

Uses Symptoms of depression (especially where sedation is required); also effective in nocturnal enuresis where organic pathology is excluded.

Dosage and administration *Depression.*

Oral therapy: Therapy should be started with a low dosage and increased gradually, according to the clinical response and any evidence of intolerance.

Adults – initial dosage: Usually 75 mg a day in divided doses (or a single dose at night). If necessary, this may be increased to a total of 150 mg a day, the additional doses being given in the late afternoon and/or at bedtime.

The sedative effect is usually rapidly apparent. The antidepressant activity may be seen within three or four days or may take up to 30 days to develop adequately.

Adults – maintenance dosage: Usually 50–100 mg a day. For maintenance therapy, the total dosage may be given in a single dose preferably in the evening or at bedtime. When satisfactory improvement has been reached, dosage should be reduced to the lowest amount that will maintain relief of symptoms. Maintenance therapy should be continued for three months or longer to lessen the chances of relapse.

Parenteral therapy: Parenteral use of amitriptyline should be restricted to patients for whom oral therapy is inappropriate or difficult. Substitute oral therapy as soon as possible: 10–20 mg (1–2 ml) four times a day. The dosage should not exceed that for oral therapy and should always be given in divided doses, intramuscularly or intravenously.

Children: Due to lack of clinical experience, Tryptizol is not recommended for the treatment of *depression* in children under 16 years of age.

Enuresis: Children aged 6–10 years may receive 10–20 mg a day, while those aged 11–16 years may need 25–50 mg a day. The recommended dosage must not be exceeded, and therefore Tryptizol 75 is not suitable for the treatment of enuresis. Treatment should not exceed three months.

This medication should be kept out of the reach of children. Tryptizol Syrup can be diluted with Syrup BP.

Plasma levels: Because of the wide variation in the absorption and distribution of tricyclic antidepressants in body fluids, dosage should be adjusted to clinical response and not based on plasma levels. However, plasma levels may be used as a guide to toxicity or to non-compliance.

Elderly patients: In general, lower dosages are recommended for these patients and an initial dosage of 10–25 mg t.d.s. is recommended, which should be increased slowly. A daily dosage of 50 mg may be satisfactory in elderly patients who may not tolerate higher dosages. The required dosage may be administered either as divided doses or as a single dose preferably in the evening or at bedtime.

Contra-indications, warnings, etc
Contra-indications: Co-administration with monoamine oxidase inhibitors; prior sensitisation to amitriptyline; during the recovery phase after myocardial infarction; arrhythmias, particularly heartblock of any degree; mania; severe liver disease; lactation; children under 6 years of age. See also 'Use in pregnancy' under 'Precautions'.

Precautions: Tryptizol should be used with caution in patients with a history of epilepsy, in patients with impaired liver function and, because of its atropine-like action, in patients with a history of urinary retention, prostatic hypertrophy, narrow-angle glaucoma, or increased intra-ocular pressure. In patients with narrow-angle glaucoma, even average doses may precipitate an attack of glaucoma.

Patients with cardiovascular disorders, hyperthyroid patients, and those receiving thyroid medication or anticholinergic agents should be closely supervised and the dosage of all medications carefully adjusted.

Elderly patients are particularly liable to experience adverse reactions: especially agitation, confusion, and postural hypotension.

Tryptizol may impair alertness in some patients and

activities made hazardous by diminished alertness (e.g. driving a car) should be avoided.

When Tryptizol is used for the depressive component of schizophrenia, psychotic symptoms may be aggravated. In manic-depressives, a shift towards the manic phase may occur; paranoid delusions, with or without associated hostility, may be aggravated. In such cases, a major tranquilliser should be given concurrently, or the dosage of Tryptizol reduced.

The risk of suicide remains during treatment of depressed patients and until significant remission occurs. Such patients require careful supervision.

Concurrent administration with ECT may increase the hazards of treatment, and should be limited to patients for whom it is deemed essential.

If possible, discontinue Tryptizol several days before surgery. But if emergency surgery is unavoidable, the anaesthetist should be informed that the patient is being treated with Tryptizol, because anaesthesia may increase the risk of hypotension and arrhythmias.

Behavioural changes have been observed in children receiving tricyclics for the treatment of enuresis.

Use in pregnancy: The safety of Tryptizol for use during pregnancy has not been established. Tryptizol is not recommended during pregnancy, especially during the first and third trimesters unless there are compelling reasons, and in these patients the benefits should be weighed against possible hazards to the fetus, child, or mother. Clinical experience of the use of Tryptizol in pregnancy has been limited. Animal studies have shown harmful effects at exceptionally high doses.

Breast-feeding mothers: Amitriptyline is detectable in breast milk. Because of the potential for serious adverse reactions in infants from amitriptyline, a decision should be made whether to discontinue breast-feeding or discontinue the drug.

Drug interactions: The concurrent use of antidepressants having varying modes of action should be made only with due recognition of their possible potentiation and with a thorough knowledge of their respective pharmacologies. Monoamine oxidase inhibitors can potentiate the effects of tricyclic antidepressants such as Tryptizol, and hyperpyretic crises, severe convulsions, and fatalities have occurred. A minimum of 14 days should elapse between discontinuing an MAOI and starting Tryptizol, which should be introduced cautiously and dosage increased gradually.

Tryptizol may block the antihypertensive action of guanethidine, debrisoquine, bethanidine, and possibly clonidine. It would be advisable to review all antihypertensive therapy during treatment with tricyclic antidepressants.

Amitriptyline should not be given with sympathomimetic agents such as adrenaline, ephedrine, isoprenaline, noradrenaline, phenylephrine, and phenylpropanolamine.

Tryptizol may enhance the response to alcohol, barbiturates, and other CNS depressants. In turn, barbiturates may decrease, and methylphenidate may increase, the antidepressant action of amitriptyline. Delirium has been reported in patients taking amitriptyline with disulfiram.

Paralytic ileus may occur in patients taking tricyclic antidepressants in combination with drugs having an anticholinergic action.

Cimetidine is reported to reduce hepatic metabolism of certain tricyclic antidepressants. Caution is advised if patients receive large doses of ethchlorvynol concurrently. Transient delirium has been reported in patients treated with 1 g ethchlorvynol and 75 mg to 150 mg of Tryptizol.

Warnings and adverse effects: In general, Tryptizol is well tolerated. The side effects given below are essentially a combined list of all those of the tricyclic group of antidepressants. Some of them have not been reported with Tryptizol, but are included because of the similar pharmacologies of the group members. As the antidepressant effects of Tryptizol may not become apparent for the first 2–4 weeks of therapy, patients should be closely monitored during this period.

Cardiovascular reactions: hypotension, syncope, postural hypotension, hypertension, tachycardia, palpitations, myocardial infarction, arrhythmias, heart block, stroke, non-specific ECG changes and changes in AV conduction. Arrhythmias and severe hypotension are likely to occur with high dosage or overdosage.

CNS and neuromuscular: confusional states, disturbed concentration, disorientation, delusions, hallucinations, hypomania, excitement, anxiety, restlessness, insomnia, nightmares, numbness, tingling, and paraesthesiae of the extremities, peripheral neuropathy, incoordination, ataxia, tremors, coma, convulsions, alteration of the EEG, extrapyramidal symptoms, including abnormal involuntary movements and tardive dyskinesia, dysarthria, tinnitus.

Anticholinergic: dry mouth, blurred vision, disturbance of accommodation, increased intra-ocular pressure, constipation, paralytic ileus, hyperpyrexia, urinary retention, urinary tract dilatation.

Allergic: skin rash, urticaria, photosensitisation, oedema of face and tongue.

Haematological: bone-marrow depression including agranulocytosis, leucopenia, eosinophilia, purpura, thrombocytopenia.

Gastro-intestinal: nausea, epigastric distress, vomiting, anorexia, stomatitis, unpleasant taste, diarrhoea, parotid swelling, black tongue, rarely hepatitis (including altered liver function and jaundice).

Endocrine: testicular swelling, gynaecomastia; breast enlargement, galactorrhoea, increased or decreased libido, impotence, interference with sexual function, elevation or lowering of blood sugar levels, syndrome of inappropriate ADH (antidiuretic hormone) secretion.

Other reactions: dizziness, weakness, fatigue, headache, weight loss, increased perspiration, urinary frequency, mydriasis, alopecia, drowsiness, increased appetite and weight gain (may be a drug reaction or due to relief of the depression). Abrupt withdrawal after prolonged administration has caused nausea, headache and malaise. Reports have associated gradual withdrawal with transient symptoms including irritability, restlessness, as well as dream and sleep disturbances during the first two weeks of dosage reduction. These symptoms are not indicative of addiction.

Adverse reactions such as withdrawal symptoms, respiratory depression and agitation have been reported in neonates whose mothers had taken tricyclic antidepressants in the last trimester of pregnancy.

Mania or hypomania has been reported rarely within 2–7 days of stopping chronic therapy with tricyclic antidepressants.

Side effects in enuresis: Dosages used in enuresis are low compared with those used in depression, and side effects are therefore less frequent. The most common are drowsiness and anticholinergic effects. The only other side effects, reported infrequently at these dosages, have been mild sweating and itching.

The recommended dosage must not be exceeded.

Overdosage: High dosage may cause temporary confusion, disturbed concentration, or transient visual hallucinations. Overdosage may cause drowsiness; hypothermia; tachycardia and other arrhythmic abnormalities such as bundle branch block; ECG evidence of impaired conduction; congestive heart failure; dilated pupils; convulsions; severe hypotension; stupor, coma and polyradiculoneuropathy. Other symptoms may be agitation, hyperactive reflexes, muscle rigidity, vomiting, hyperpyrexia, or any of those listed as adverse effects.

All persons suspected of having taken an overdosage should be admitted to hospital as soon as possible. Treatment is symptomatic and supportive. The stomach should be emptied as quickly as possible by emesis, followed by gastric lavage upon arrival at hospital. Following lavage, activated charcoal may be given during the first 24–48 hours at a dosage of 20–30 g every four to six hours. An ECG should be taken and close monitoring of cardiac function instituted if there is any sign of abnormality. An open airway and an adequate fluid intake should be maintained, and body temperature regulated.

Intravenous physostigmine salicylate, 1–3 mg, has been reported to reverse the symptoms of tricyclic antidepressant poisoning. Because physostigmine is rapidly metabolised, the dosage of physostigmine should be repeated as required, particularly if life-threatening signs such as arrhythmias, convulsions, and deep coma recur or persist after the initial dose of physostigmine. Because physostigmine itself may be toxic, it is not recommended for routine use.

Standard measures should be used to manage circulatory shock and metabolic acidosis. Cardiac arrhythmias may be treated with neostigmine, pyridostigmine or propanolol. Should cardiac failure occur, use of digitalis should be considered. Close monitoring of cardiac function for not less than five days is advisable.

If convulsions occur, they should be treated with paraldehyde, diazepam or an inhalation anaesthetic. Barbiturates should not be used because Tryptizol increases their CNS-depressant action.

Dialysis is of no value because of low plasma concentrations of amitriptyline. Since overdosage is often deliberate, patients may attempt suicide by other means during the recovery phase. Deaths by deliberate or accidental overdosage have occurred with this class of medicament.

Pharmaceutical precautions Keep containers well closed and store below 25°C, protected from light. The injection and the syrup should also be protected from freezing. Tryptizol Syrup may be diluted with Syrup BP; the mixture should be used within 14 days.

Legal category POM.

Package quantities *Capsules 75 mg:* Bottles of 100.
Tablets 10 mg: Bottles of 100 and 500.
Tablets 25 mg: Bottles of 100 and 500.
Tablets 50 mg: Bottles of 100.
Injection: Vials of 10 ml.
Syrup: Bottles of 200 ml and 1,000 ml.

Further information Tryptizol is a member of the tricyclic group of antidepressants. Its mode of action in man is not known, but it is not a monoamine oxidase inhibitor (special dietary restrictions are not necessary), and it does not act primarily by stimulating the CNS.

Product licence numbers

Capsules 75 mg	0025/0116
Tablets 10 mg	0025/0093
Tablets 25 mg	0025/0094
Tablets 50 mg	0025/0095
Injection	0025/5036
Syrup	0025/5037

**Trade Mark*

Napp Laboratories Limited
Cambridge Science Park
Milton Road
Cambridge CB4 4GW

ADIZEM*-60 TABLETS

Presentation White, film coated, capsule shaped tablets marked with 60/DL on one side. Each tablet contains 60 mg of diltiazem hydrochloride in a modified release formulation.

Uses
Actions: Diltiazem is a calcium antagonist. It restricts the slow channel entry of calcium ions into the cell and so reduces the liberation of calcium from stores in the sarcoplasmic reticulum. This results in a reduction in the amount of available intra-cellular calcium and consequently a (1) reduction of myocardial oxygen consumption (2) dilation of small and large coronary arteries (3) mild peripheral vasodilation (4) negative dromotropic effects (5) reflex positive chronotropic and inotropic effects due to reflex sympathetic activity are partially inhibited and result in a slight reduction or no change in heart rate.

The antianginal effect is due to reduction in cardiac oxygen demand with maintenance of coronary blood flow. Cardiac contractility and ventricular ejection fraction are unchanged. Diltiazem increases exercise capacity and improves indices of myocardial ischaemia in the angina patient. Diltiazem relieves the spasm of vasospastic (Prinzmetal) angina.

Indications: Management of angina pectoris.

Dosage and administration The tablets should be swallowed whole and not chewed.

Adults: The usual dose is one tablet (60 mg) three times a day, however, patients' responses may vary and dosage requirements can differ significantly between individual patients. There is no evidence of any decrease in efficacy at high doses. If necessary the dose may be increased to 480 mg/day.

Elderly (over 65 years) and patients with renal or hepatic impairment: The recommended starting dose is one tablet (60 mg) twice daily. The heart rate should be measured regularly in these groups of patients and the dosage should not be increased if the heart rate falls below 50 beats per minute.

Children: Adizem-60 tablets are not recommended for children.

Contra-indications, warnings, etc
Contra-indications: Sick sinus syndrome not requiring pacemaker, second or third degree AV-block, bradycardia (less than 40 beats per minute). Pregnant women or those of child bearing potential.

Warnings and precautions: Patients with either mild bradycardia or a prolonged PR interval should be observed closely. Diltiazem does not have a significant myocardial depressant effect and is well tolerated in patients with poor left ventricular function.

Drug interactions: If a beta-blocker is given together with Adizem-60 Tablets then the heart rate should be observed closely at the start of treatment and the doses adjusted as required. Patients with pre-existing conduction defects should not receive this combination. The blood levels of beta-blockers with a low bioavailability (e.g. propranolol) may be increased and small increases in the plasma levels of digitalis glycosides have been observed. The absorption of diltiazem is not affected by antacids or aspirin. Diltiazem causes elevation of carbamazepine levels and, in patients with renal failure, elevated cyclosporin levels occur. Diltiazem metabolism is inhibited by cimetidine and to a lesser extent by ranitidine. Drugs that increase hepatic microsomal activity (e.g. phenobarbitone and phenytoin) lead to decreased plasma diltiazem levels. Diltiazem has been used during anaesthesia without problems, but the anaesthetist should be made aware of the treatment regimen.

Side-effects: Diltiazem is generally well tolerated. Occasional undesirable effects are nausea, finger swelling, headache, skin rashes and oedema. Bradycardia and first degree heart block may also be encountered.

Overdosage: Empty stomach contents; symptomatic treatment and observation in a coronary care unit is advisable. Corrective measures for possible hypotension and conduction disturbances should be available.

Pharmaceutical precautions Store in a dry place at less than 30°C.

Legal category POM.

Package quantities Securitainers of 100 tablets.

Further information Adizem-60 tablets are effective in angina, protecting the heart against ischaemia and reducing myocardial oxygen requirements. Diltiazem is well tolerated and does not normally give rise to the side effects associated with peripheral vasodilators, nor cause significant myocardial depression. It protects against excessive catecholamine stimulation but is free of the side effects seen with beta-blockade. Although Diltiazem tends to lower blood pressure in hypertensive patients, Adizem-60 tablets are not currently recommended for this indication. Adizem-60 tablets do not interfere with glucose metabolism.

Product licence number 0337/0163.

ADIZEM*-SR TABLETS 120 mg

Presentation White, film coated, capsule shaped tablets marked with 120/DL on one side. Each tablet contains 120 mg of diltiazem hydrochloride in a controlled release formulation.

Uses
Actions: Diltiazem is a calcium antagonist. It restricts the slow channel entry of calcium ions into the cell and so reduces the liberation of calcium from stores in the sarcoplasmic reticulum. This results in a reduction in the amount of available intra-cellular calcium and consequently a (1) reduction of myocardial oxygen consumption (2) dilation of small and large coronary arteries (3) mild peripheral vasodilation (4) negative dromotropic effects (5) reflex positive chronotropic and inotropic effects due to reflex sympathetic activity are partially inhibited and result in a slight reduction or no change in heart rate.

The antianginal effect is due to reduction in cardiac oxygen demand with maintenance of coronary blood flow. Cardiac contractility and ventricular ejection fraction are unchanged. Diltiazem increases exercise capacity and improves indices of myocardial ischaemia in the angina patient. Diltiazem relieves the spasm of vasospastic (Prinzmetal) angina.

Indications: Management of angina pectoris.

Dosage and administration The tablets should be swallowed whole and not chewed.

Adults: The usual dose is one tablet (120 mg) twice a day. However, patients' responses may vary and dosage requirements can differ significantly between individual patients. There is no evidence of any decrease in efficacy at high doses. If necessary the dose may be increased to 480 mg/day.

Elderly (over 65 years) and patients with renal or hepatic impairment: Adizem-SR Tablets 120 mg are contra-indicated in these patients. Adizem-SR Tablets 120 mg are not suitable for use in such patients where the patients should be initiated with 60 mg twice daily dosage.

Children: Adizem-SR tablets 120 mg are not recommended for children.

Contra-indications, warnings, etc
Contra-indications: Sick sinus syndrome not requiring pacemaker, second or third degree AV-block, bradycardia (less than 40 beats per minute). Pregnant women or those of child bearing potential. The elderly and patients with impaired renal or hepatic function.

Warnings and precautions: Patients with either mild bradycardia or a prolonged PR interval should be observed closely. Diltiazem does not have a significant myocardial depressant effect and is well tolerated in patients with poor left ventricular function.

Drug interactions: If a beta-blocker is given together with Adizem-SR Tablets 120 mg then the heart rate should be observed closely at the start of treatment and the doses adjusted as required. Patients with pre-existing conduction defects should not receive this combination. The blood levels of beta-blockers with a low bioavailability (e.g. propranolol) may be increased and small increases in the plasma levels of digitalis glycosides have been observed. The absorption of diltiazem is not affected by antacids or aspirin. Diltiazem causes elevation of carbamazepine levels and, in patients with renal failure, elevated cyclosporin levels occur. Diltiazem metabolism is inhibited by cimetidine and to a lesser extent by ranitidine. Drugs that increase hepatic microsomal activity (e.g. phenobarbitone and phenytoin) lead to decreased plasma diltiazem levels. Diltiazem has been used during anaesthesia without problems, but the anaesthetist should be made aware of the treatment regimen.

Side-effects: Diltiazem is generally well tolerated. Occasional undesirable effects are nausea, finger swelling, headache, skin rashes and oedema. Bradycardia and first degree heart block may also be encountered.

Overdosage: Empty stomach contents; symptomatic treatment and observation in a coronary care unit is advisable. Corrective measures for possible hypotension and conduction disturbances should be available. The formulation is a controlled release matrix which will continue to release diltiazem for some hours.

Pharmaceutical precautions Store in a dry place at less than 30°C.

Legal category POM.

Package quantities Blister packs containing 56 tablets (OP).

Further information Nil.

Product licence number 0337/0137.

AUDAX* EAR DROPS

Presentation Ear drops containing the Mundicylat* brand of choline salicylate 20.0% w/w and Glycerol BP 12.6% w/v.

Uses For the symptomatic relief of ear pain in acute and chronic otitis media and externa. Patients with ear pain should always seek medical advice.

For softening of ear wax as an aid to ear wax removal.

Dosage and administration
For pain relief: With the head tilted to one side, the external ear canal is filled completely with Audax Ear Drops using the dropper provided. The ear should be plugged with cotton wool soaked with the ear drops. A wick may be inserted if preferred, using the ear drops to keep it moist. Audax Ear Drops should be instilled every 3–4 hours but should the pain persist for longer than 24 hours the patient must seek medical advice.

For softening of ear wax: Apply as described above, twice daily for four days.

Contra-indications, warnings, etc Not to be used in children under 1 year of age without medical advice being sought. Salicylate sensitivity. Perforated ear drum.

Where infection of the ear necessitates topical and/or systemic antibiotics, the Audax Ear Drops are designed as an adjuvant therapy.

Overdosage: Each bottle of Audax Ear Drops contains 1.6 g of choline salicylate equivalent to 1.2 g of aspirin. Accidental or deliberate ingestion of the contents of a bottle of Audax Ear Drops is therefore only of concern in small infants. In such cases signs of intoxication may include dizziness, tinnitus, sweating, vomiting, confusion and hyperventilation. Gross overdosage may lead to CNS depression. Management should include, as appropriate, induced vomiting, correction of fluid and electrolyte balance and measurement of plasma salicylate levels. At concentrations in excess of 300 mg l^{-1} measures such as forced alkaline diuresis and haemodialysis to enhance clearance may be appropriate.

Pharmaceutical precautions Store at or below 20°C.

Legal category P.

Package quantities Bottle containing 8 ml with dropper.

Further information The low surface tension of Audax Ear Drops ensures rapid penetration to the site of action. Choline salicylate gives quick and prolonged analgesia. The pH of Audax Ear Drops is adjusted to approximate closely that normally found in the external auditory meatus.

Audax Ear Drops contain no irritants or sensitising local anaesthetics. Audax Ear Drops eliminate the need to resort to oral salicylates and other systemic analgesics. In addition, Audax Ear Drops exert local anti-inflammatory and anti-pruritic effects in the ear and have their own spectrum of anti-microbial activity.

Product licence number 0337/5004R.

BETADINE* ALCOHOLIC SOLUTION

Presentation A golden brown alcoholic solution containing the Mundidone* brand of Povidone Iodine USP 10% w/v.

Uses For use as an antiseptic skin cleanser for major and minor surgical procedures where a quick drying effect is desired.

For topical administration.

Dosage and administration
Adults: Apply full strength as an antiseptic skin cleanser.

Children and the elderly: As for adults.

Povidone iodine is not recommended for regular use in neonates and is contra-indicated in very low birth weight infants (below 1500 grams).

Contra-indications, warnings, etc
Contra-indications: Known or suspected iodine hypersensitivity.

Regular use is contra-indicated in patients and users with thyroid disorders (in particular nodular colloid goitre, endemic goitre and Hashimoto's thyroiditis).

Interactions with other medicaments and other forms of interaction: Absorption of iodine from povidone iodine through either intact or damaged skin may interfere with thyroid function tests.

Contamination with povidone iodine of several types of tests for the detection of occult blood in faeces or blood in urine may produce false-positive results.

Effects on ability to drive and use machines: None known.

Other undesirable effects: Povidone iodine may produce local skin reactions although it is less irritant than iodine.

The application of povidone iodine to large wounds or severe burns may produce systemic adverse effects such as metabolic acidosis, hypernatraemia and impairment of renal function.

Use in pregnancy and lactation: Regular use of povidone iodine should be avoided in pregnant or lactating women as absorbed iodine can cross the placental barrier and can be secreted into breast milk. Although no adverse effects have been reported from limited use, caution should be recommended and therapeutic benefit must be balanced against possible effects of the absorption of iodine on foetal thyroid function and development.

Other special warnings and precautions: Special caution is needed when regular applications to broken skin are made to patients with pre-existing renal insufficiency.

Regular use should be avoided in patients on concurrent lithium therapy.

This preparation is flammable and caution is advised during surgical procedures involving hot wire cautery or diathermy.

Overdosage: Excess iodine can produce goitre and hypothyroidism or hyperthyroidism. Systemic absorption of iodine after repeated application of povidone iodine to large areas of wounds or burns may lead to a number of adverse effects:

Metallic taste in mouth, increased salivation, burning or pain in the throat or mouth, irritation and swelling of the eyes, pulmonary oedema, skin reactions, gastrointestinal upset and diarrhoea, metabolic acidosis, hypernatraemia and renal impairment.

In the case of accidental ingestion of large quantities of Betadine symptomatic and supportive treatment should be provided with special attention to electrolyte balance and renal and thyroid function.

Pharmaceutical precautions Store in a dry place at or below 20°C and protected from light.

Legal category P.

Package quantities Containers of 500 ml and 5 litres.

Further information Betadine Alcoholic Solution has a rapid and prolonged germicidal action and with repeated use, a cumulative germicidal action. It is active against a wide range of organisms including Gram positive and Gram negative bacteria, fungi, protozoa, viruses and bacterial spores. In the presence of blood, serum, purulent exudate and necrotic tissue, its activcity persists whilst the colour remains.

Product licence number 0337/5902.

BETADINE* ANTISEPTIC PAINT

Presentation A golden brown alcoholic solution containing the Mundidone* brand of Povidone Iodine USP 10% w/v.

Uses Betadine Antiseptic Paint is a broad spectrum, quick drying antiseptic for the treatment and prevention of infection. It is ideal for herpes simplex, herpes zoster, grazes, abrasions, cuts and wounds or any break in the skin which requires protection from infection. Betadine Antiseptic Paint is effective in the treatment of dermal infections caused by bacteria, fungi, yeasts and viruses (e.g. herpes virus types I and II).

Dosage and administration Apply Betadine Antiseptic Paint undiluted as necessary to affected area and allow to dry. Use twice daily and cover with a dressing if desired. Rinse the brush thoroughly after use.

Contra-indications, warnings, etc

Contra-indications: Hypersensitivity to iodine. History of abnormal thyroid function or goitre.

Warnings: If local irritation or sensitivity develop, then discontinue treatment.

Interactions: None known.

Precautions: Use in pregnancy and lactation should be limited to minor lesions only and although no adverse effects are anticipated from such limited usage, caution is recommended and the therapeutic benefit must be balanced against the possible effect of the absorption of iodine on foetal thyroid development and function.

Overdosage: In the case of deliberate or accidental ingestion of large quantities, symptomatic and supportive treatment should be provided with special attention to electrolyte balance and thyroid and renal function.

Pharmaceutical precautions Store in a dry place at or below 20°C and protected from light.

Legal category GSL.

Package quantities Glass bottles containing 8 ml with an applicator brush.

Further information Betadine Antiseptic Paint has a rapid and prolonged germicidal action against a wide spectrum of organisms including Gram positive and Gram negative bacteria, fungi, protozoa and viruses. It is also active against bacterial spores. In the presence of soap, blood, serum, purulent exudate and necrotic tissue, its activity persists whilst the golden brown colour remains.

Product licence number 0337/0047.

STANDARDISED BETADINE* ANTISEPTIC SOLUTION

Presentation A golden brown solution containing the Mundidone* brand of Povidone Iodine USP 10% w/v.

Uses For use as a pre-operative and post-operative antiseptic skin cleanser for major and minor surgical procedures.

For topical application.

Dosage and administration

Adults: Apply full strength as a pre-operative and post-operative antiseptic skin cleanser. Avoid pooling both under the patients and in the skin folds. Wash off excess solution before using occlusive dressings.

Children and the elderly: As for adults.

Povidone iodine is not recommended for regular use in neonates and is contra-indicated in very low birth weight infants (below 1500 grams).

Contra-indications, warnings, etc

Contra-indications: Known or suspected iodine hypersensitivity.

Regular use is contra-indicated in patients and users with thyroid disorders (in particular nodular colloid goitre, endemic goitre and Hashimoto's thyroiditis).

Interactions with other medicaments and other forms of interaction: Absorption of iodine from povidone iodine through either intact or damaged skin may interfere with thyroid function tests.

Contamination with povidone iodine of several types of tests for the detection of occult blood in faeces or blood in urine may produce false-positive results.

Effects on ability to drive and use machines: None known.

Other undesirable effects: Povidone iodine may produce local skin reactions although it is less irritant than iodine.

The application of povidone iodine to large wounds or severe burns may produce systemic adverse effects such as metabolic acidosis, hypernatraemia and impairment of renal function.

Use in pregnancy and lactation: Regular use of povidone iodine should be avoided in pregnant or lactating women as absorbed iodine can cross the placental barrier and can be secreted into breast milk. Although no adverse effects have been reported from limited use, caution should be recommended and therapeutic benefit must be balanced against possible effects of the absorption of iodine on foetal thyroid function and development.

Other special warnings and precautions: Special caution is needed when regular applications to broken skin are made to patients with pre-existing renal insufficiency.

Regular use should be avoided in patients on concurrent lithium therapy.

Overdosage: Excess iodine can produce goitre and hypothyroidism or hyperthyroidism. Systemic absorption of iodine after repeated application of povidone iodine to large areas of wounds or burns may lead to a number of adverse effects:

Metallic taste in mouth, increased salivation, burning or pain in the throat or mouth, irritation and swelling of the eyes, pulmonary oedema, skin reactions, gastrointestinal upset and diarrhoea, metabolic acidosis, hypernatraemia and renal impairment.

In the case of accidental ingestion of large quantities of Betadine symptomatic and supportive treatment should be provided with special attention to electrolyte balance and renal and thyroid function.

Pharmaceutical precautions Store in a dry place at or below 20°C and protected from light.

Legal category P.

Package quantities Containers of 500 ml and 5 litres.

Further information Standardised Betadine Antiseptic Solution has a rapid and prolonged germicidal action and with repeated use, a cumulative germicidal action. It is active against a wide range of organisms including Gram positive and Gram negative bacteria, fungi, protozoa, viruses and bacterial spores. In the presence of blood, serum, purulent exudate and necrotic tissue, its activity persists whilst the colour remains.

Product licence number 0337/5901.

BETADINE* DRY POWDER SPRAY

Presentation Pressurised aerosol can containing a brown powder consisting of the Mundidone* brand of Povidone Iodine USP 2.5% w/v.

Uses As a skin antiseptic for treatment and prevention of infection in wounds including ulcers, burns, cuts and other minor injuries.

Dosage and administration
Adults and children: Shake the can well, spray the required area from a distance of 6–10 inches until coated with powder.

Contra-indications, warnings, etc
Contra-indications: Not for use in infants under 2 years. Hypersensitivity to iodine. History of abnormal thyroid function or goitre.

Warnings: Avoid inhalation or spraying into the eyes. If local irritation or sensitivity develops, then discontinue treatment. Iodine is absorbed through burns and broken skin and to a lesser extent, through intact skin. Following prolonged application of Betadine Dry Powder Spray to severe burns or large areas of denuded skin, systemic effects such as metabolic acidosis, hypernatraemia, renal impairment and thyroid dysfunction may occur.

Interactions: None known.

Precautions: Use in pregnancy and lactation should be limited and although no adverse effects are anticipated from such limited usage, caution is recommended and the therapeutic benefit must be balanced against the possible effects of the absorption of iodine on foetal thyroid development and function.

Overdosage: In the case of deliberate or accidental ingestion of large quantities, symptomatic and supportive treatment should be provided with special attention to electrolyte balance, thyroid and renal function.

Pharmaceutical precautions Store in a dry place at or below 20°C, away from direct heat and sunlight. The can must not be autoclaved or punctured or destroyed by burning even when empty.

Legal category GSL.

Package quantities Aerosol cans containing 150 g.

Further information Betadine Dry Powder Spray has a rapid and prolonged germicidal action against a wide spectrum of organisms including Gram positive and Gram negative bacteria, fungi, protozoa and viruses. It is also active against bacterial spores. In the presence of soap, blood, serum, purulent exudate and necrotic tissue, its activity persists whilst the golden brown colour remains.

Product licence number 0337/0114.

BETADINE* GARGLE AND MOUTHWASH

Presentation A pleasantly flavoured amber coloured solution containing the Mundidone* brand of Povidone Iodine USP 1% w/v.

Uses For the treatment of acute mucosal infections of the mouth and pharnyx.

For oral hygiene, prior to, during and after dental and oral surgery.

Dosage and administration
Adults, the elderly and children over six years: Use undiluted or diluted with an equal volume of warm water. Gargle or rinse with up to 10 mls for up to 30 seconds without swallowing. Repeat up to four times daily, for up to 14 consecutive days, or as directed.

Contra-indications, warnings, etc
Contra-indications: Not for use in children under six years of age.

Known or suspected iodine hypersensitivity.

Regular use is contra-indicated in patients and users with thyroid disorders (in particular nodular colloid goitre, endemic goitre and Hashimoto's thyroiditis).

Regular use is contra-indicated in pregnant or lactating women.

Interactions with other medicaments and other forms of interaction: Absorption of iodine from povidone iodine may interfere with thyroid function tests.

Contamination with povidone iodine of several types of tests for the detection of occult blood in faeces or blood in urine may produce false-positive results.

Effects on ability to drive and use machines: None known.

Other undesirable effects: Idiosyncratic mucosal irritation and hypersensitivity reactions may occur.
Excessive absorption of iodine may produce systemic adverse effects such as metabolic acidosis, hypernatraemia and impairment of renal function.

Use in pregnancy and lactation: Regular use of povidone iodine should be avoided in pregnant or lactating women as absorbed iodine can cross the placental barrier and can be secreted into breast milk. Although no adverse effects have been reported from limited use, caution should be recommended and therapeutic benefit must be balanced against possible effects of the absorption of iodine on foetal thyroid function and development. The use of Betadine Gargle and Mouthwash in pregnant and lactating women should be limited to a single treatment session only.

Other special warnings and precautions: Regular use must be avoided as prolonged use may lead to the absorption of a significant amount of iodine. Do not use for more than 14 days.

If sores or ulcers in the mouth do not heal within 14 days seek medical or dental advice.

Regular use should be avoided in patients on concurrent lithium therapy.

Overdosage: Excess iodine can produce goitre and hypothyroidism or hyperthyroidism. Acute overdose may result in symptoms of metallic taste in the mouth, increased salivation, burning or pain in the throat or mouth, irritation and swelling in the eyes, skin reactions, gastrointestinal upset and diarrhoea, and difficulty in breathing due to pulmonary oedema.

Metabolic acidosis, hypernatraemia and renal impairment may occur.

In the case of accidental ingestion of large quantities

of Betadine, symptomatic and supportive treatment should be provided with special attention to electrolyte balance and renal and thyroid function.

Pharmaceutical precautions Store in a dry place at or below 20°C and protected from light.

Legal category GSL.

Package quantities Bottles containing 250 ml.

Further information Betadine Gargle and Mouthwash does not stain the skin, mucous membranes or teeth despite its powerful germicidal action. It is effective against a wide spectrum of organisms including Gram positive and Gram negative bacteria, fungi, protozoa and viruses. It is also active against bacterial spores. In the presence of soap, blood, serum, purulent exudate and necrotic tissue, its activity persists whilst the colour remains.

Product licence number 0337/0009.

BETADINE* OINTMENT

Presentation A golden brown water soluble ointment containing the Mundidone* brand of Povidone Iodine USP 10% w/w.

Uses Betadine Ointment is a broad spectrum antiseptic for the topical treatment or prevention of infection in minor cuts and abrasions, minor surgical procedures and small areas of burns. Treatment of mycotic and bacterial skin infections and pyodermas.

Treatment of infections in decubitus and stasis ulcers.

Dosage and administration

For the treatment of infection: Apply once or twice daily for a maximum of 14 days.

For the prevention of infection: Apply once or twice a week, for as long as necessary.

The affected skin should be cleaned and dried. Apply Betadine Ointment to the affected area. May be covered with a dressing or bandage.

Contra-indications, warnings, etc

Contra-indications: Known or suspected iodine hypersensitivity.

Regular use is contra-indicated in patients and users with thyroid disorders (in particular nodular colloid goitre, endemic goitre and Hashimoto's thyroiditis).

Not for use in children under two years of age.

Interactions with other medicaments and other forms of interaction: Absorption of iodine from povidone iodine through either intact or damaged skin may interfere with thyroid function tests.

Contamination with povidone iodine of several types of tests for the detection of occult blood in faeces or blood in urine may produce false-positive results.

Effects on ability to drive and use machines: None known.

Other undesirable effects: Povidone iodine may produce local skin reactions although it is less irritant than iodine.

The application of povidone iodine to large wounds or severe burns may produce systemic adverse effects such as metabolic acidosis, hypernatraemia and impairment of renal function.

Use in pregnancy and lactation: Regular use of povidone iodine should be avoided in pregnant or lactating women as absorbed iodine can cross the placental barrier and can be secreted into breast milk. Although no adverse effects have been reported from limited use, caution should be recommended and therapeutic benefit must be balanced against possible effects of the absorption of iodine on foetal thyroid function and development.

Other special warnings and precautions: Special caution is needed when regular applications to broken skin are made to patients with pre-existing renal insufficiency.

Regular use should be avoided in patients on concurrent lithium therapy.

Thyroid function tests should be performed during prolonged use.

Overdosage: Excess iodine can produce goitre and hypothyroidism or hyperthyroidism. Systemic absorption of iodine after repeated application of povidone iodine to large areas of wounds or burns may lead to a number of adverse effects:

Metallic taste in mouth, increased salivation, burning or pain in the throat or mouth, irritation and swelling of the eyes, pulmonary oedema, skin reactions, gastrointestinal upset and diarrhoea, metabolic acidosis, hypernatraemia and renal impairment.

In the case of accidental ingestion of large quantities of Betadine symptomatic and supportive treatment should be provided with special attention to electrolyte balance and renal and thyroid function.

Incompatibilities (major): None.

Pharmaceutical precautions Store in a dry place at or below 20°C and protected from light.

Legal category GSL.

Package quantities Tubes of 20 gm and 80 gm.

Further information Betadine Ointment has a rapid and prolonged germicidal action against a wide range of organisms including Gram positive and Gram negative bacteria, fungi, protozoa and viruses. It is also active against bacterial spores. In the presence of soap, blood, serum, purulent exudate and necrotic tissue, its activcity persists whilst the colour remains.

Product licence number 0337/5005.

BETADINE* SCALP AND SKIN CLEANSER

Presentation A golden brown cleansing and sudsing surfactant solution containing Mundidone* brand of Povidone Iodine USP 7.5% w/v.

Uses For seborrhoeic conditions of the scalp and acne vulgaris of the face and neck.

Dosage and administration

Adults, children and the elderly

For the treatment of seborrhoeic conditions of the scalp: Use as a shampoo. Allow to remain on the hair for at least five minutes. Rinse hair with warm water. Repeat application and rinse again.

Repeat twice weekly until improvement is noted. Afterwards use once weekly.

For the treatment of acne vulgaris of the face and neck: Apply directly or with a moistened sponge. Cleanse area thoroughly. Repeat application. Rinse with warm water and dry with a clean or sterile towel or gauze.

Repeat daily (morning and evenings) until improvement is noted. Afterwards use once daily.

Contra-indications, warnings, etc

Contra-indications: Not for use in infants under 2 years. Hypersensitivity to iodine. History of abnormal thyroid function or goitre.

Warnings: If local irritation or sensitivity develops, then discontinue treatment. Do not use on broken skin.

Interactions: None known.

Precautions: Use in pregnancy and lactation should be limited and although no adverse effects are anticipated from such limited usage, caution is recommended and the therapeutic benefit must be balanced against the possible effects of the absorption of iodine on foetal thyroid function.

Overdosage: In the case of deliberate or accidental ingestion of large quantities, symptomatic and supportive treatment should be provided with special attention to electrolyte balance, thyroid and renal function.

Pharmaceutical precautions Store in a dry place at or below 20°C and protected from light.

Legal category GSL.

Package quantities Plastic bottle containing 250 ml.

Further information Betadine Scalp and Skin

Cleanser has a highly effective germicidal activity. This activity is maintained in the presence of exfoliative debris and infected scalp lesions whilst the colour persists. It does not stain the skin.

Product licence number 0337/5023R.

BETADINE* SHAMPOO

Presentation A golden brown cleansing and sudsing surfactant solution containing Mundidone* brand of Povidone Iodine USP 4% w/v.

Uses Seborrhoeic conditions of the scalp associated with excessive dandruff, pruritus, scaling, exudation and erythema of the scalp; Pityriasis capitis; Infected lesions of the scalp – pyodermas (recurrent furunculosis, infective folliculitis and impetigo).

Dosage and administration
Adults and children over 12:
1. Having first wetted the hair, apply 2 or 3 capfuls of Betadine Shampoo, use warm water to lather. Rinse.
2. Again apply 2 or 3 capfuls of Betadine Shampoo and massage into the scalp with the tips of the fingers.
3. Work up to a golden lather using warm water.
4. Repeat treatment twice weekly until improvement is noted. Afterwards, use Betadine Shampoo once a week.

Children 2–12: As for children over 12, substituting 1 or 2 capfuls of Betadine Shampoo.

Contra-indications, warnings, etc
Contra-indications: Known or suspected iodine hypersensitivity.

Regular use is contra-indicated in patients and users with thyroid disorders (in particular nodular colloid goitre, endemic goitre and Hashimoto's thyroiditis).

Not for use in children under 2 years.

Interactions with other medicaments and other forms of interaction: Absorption of idodine from povidone iodine through either intact or damaged skin may interfere with thyroid function tests.

Contamination with povidone iodine of several types of tests for the detection of occult blood in faeces or blood in urine may produce false-positive results.

Effect on ability to drive and use machines: None known.

Other undesirable effects: Povidone iodine may produce local skin reactions although it is less irritant than iodine.

Use in pregnancy and lactation: Regular use of povidone iodine should be avoided in pregnant or lactating women as absorbed iodine can cross the placental barrier and can be secreted into breast milk. Although no adverse effects have been reported from limited use, caution should be recommended and therapeutic benefit must be balanced against possible effects of the absorption of iodine on foetal thyroid function and development.

Other special warnings and precautions: Special caution is needed when regular applications to broken skin are made to patients with pre-existing renal insufficiency.

Regular use should be avoided in patients on concurrent lithium therapy.

Overdosage: Excess iodine can produce goitre and hypothyroidism or hyperthyroidism.

In the case of accidental ingestion of large quantities of Betadine symptomatic and supportive treatment should be provided with special attention to electrolyte balance and renal and thyroid function.

Incompatibilities (major): None.

Pharmaceutical precautions Store in a dry place at or below 20°C and protected from light.

Legal category GSL.

Package quantities Plastic bottle containing 250 ml.

Further information Betadine Shampoo has a highly effective germicidal activity. This activity is maintained in the presence of exfoliative debris and infected scalp lesions whilst the colour persists. It does not stain the skin.

Product licence number 0337/5033.

BETADINE* SKIN CLEANSER

Presentation A penetrating golden brown sudsing surfactant solution containing Mundidone* brand of Povidone Iodine USP 4% w/v.

Uses Acne vulgaris of the face and neck. For general disinfection of the skin (as a liquid soap).

Dosage and administration
Adults, elderly and children over 2 years: Apply directly or with moistened sponge to the affected areas and work up a rich lather. Allow to remain on the skin for 3 to 5 minutes then rinse off thoroughly with warm water and dry with a clean or sterile towel or gauze. Repeat twice daily.

Contra-indications, warnings, etc
Contra-indications: Not for use in infants under 2 years. Hypersensitivity to iodine. History of abnormal thyroid function or goitre.

Warnings: If local irritation or sensitivity develops, then discontinue treatment. Do not use on broken skin. Iodine is absorbed through burns and broken skin and to a lesser extent, through intact skin.

Interactions: None known.

Precautions: Use in pregnancy and lactation should be limited and although no adverse effects are anticipated from such limited usage, caution is recommended and the therapeutic benefit must be balanced against the possible effect of the absorption of iodine on foetal thyroid function.

Overdosage: In cases of deliberate or accidental ingestion of large quantities, symptomatic and supportive treatment should be provided with special attention to electrolyte balance, thyroid and renal function.

Pharmaceutical precautions Store in a dry place at or below 20°C, and protected from light.

Legal category GSL.

Package quantities Plastic bottle containing 250 ml.

Further information Betadine Skin Cleanser has a highly effective germicidal activity. This activity is maintained in the presence of exfoliative debris and infected scalp lesions whilst the colour persists. It does not stain the skin.

Product licence number 0337/5034R.

BETADINE* SURGICAL SCRUB

Presentation A golden brown surfactant solution containing Mundidone* brand of Povidone Iodine USP 7.5% w/v with non-ionic surfactants.

Uses For use as an antiseptic skin cleanser for pre-operative scrubbing and washing by surgeons and theatre staff; and pre-operative preparation of patients' skin.

Dosage and administration
Adults: Apply full strength as a pre-operative antiseptic skin cleanser.

Children and the elderly: As for adults.

Povidone iodine is not recommended for regular use in neonates and is contra-indicated in very low birth weight infants (below 1500 grams).

Contra-indications, warnings, etc
Contra-indications: Known or suspected iodine hypersensitivity.

Regular use is contra-indicated in patients and users with thyroid disorders (in particular nodular colloid goitre, endemic goitre and Hashimoto's thyroiditis).

Interactions with other medicaments and other forms of interaction: Absorption of iodine from povidone iodine through either intact or damaged skin may interfere with thyroid function tests.

Contamination with povidone iodine of several types of tests for the detection of occult blood in faeces or blood in urine may produce false-positive results.

Effects on ability to drive and use machines: None known.

Other undesirable effects: Povidone iodine may produce local skin reactions although it is considered to be less irritant than iodine.

The application of povidone iodine to large wounds or severe burns may produce systemic adverse effects such as metabolic acidosis, hypernatraemia and impairment of renal function.

Use in pregnancy and lactation: Regular use of povidone iodine should be avoided in pregnant or lactating women as absorbed iodine can cross the placental barrier and can be secreted into breast milk. Although no adverse effects have been reported from limited use, caution should be recommended and therapeutic benefit must be balanced against possible effects of the absorption of iodine on foetal thyroid function and development.

Other special warnings and precautions: Special caution is needed when regular applications to broken skin are made to patients with pre-existing renal insufficiency.

Regular use should be avoided in patients on concurrent lithium therapy.

Betadine Surgical Scrub can permanently discolour white gold jewellery and it is recommended that this type of jewellery should be removed before using Betadine Surgical Scrub.

Overdosage: Excess iodine can produce goitre and hypothyroidism or hyperthyroidism. Systemic absorption of iodine after repeated application of povidone iodine to large areas of wounds or burns may lead to a number of adverse effects:

Metallic taste in mouth, increased salivation, burning or pain in the throat or mouth, irritation and swelling of the eyes, pulmonary oedema, skin reactions, gastrointestinal upset and diarrhoea, metabolic acidosis, hypernatraemia and renal impairment.

In the case of accidental ingestion of large quantities of Betadine symptomatic and supportive treatment should be provided with special attention to electrolyte balance and renal and thyroid function.

Pharmaceutical precautions Store at or below 20°C and protected from light.

Legal category P.

Package quantities Containers of 500 ml and 5 litres.

Further information Betadine Surgical Scrub has a rapid and prolonged germicidal action and with repeated use, a cumulative germicidal action. It is active against a wide range of organisms including Gram positive and Gram negative bacteria, fungi, protozoa, viruses and bacterial spores. In the presence of blood, serum, purulent exudate and necrotic tissue, its activity persists whilst the colour remains.

Product licence number 0337/5903.

BETADINE* VAGINAL CLEANSING KIT

Presentation The Betadine V.C. Kit consists of Betadine V.C. Concentrate, containing 250 ml of Mundidone* brand of Povidone Iodine USP 10% w/v with an applicator squeeze bottle and a plastic vaginal applicator.

Uses Vaginitis due to candidal, trichomonal, non-specific or mixed infections, and pre-operative preparation of the vagina.

Dosage and administration
In adults and the elderly: Once a day (preferably in the morning) for a 14-day period, including days of menstruation.

The Betadine V.C. Concentrate should be diluted 1:10 using the measuring cap, and used according to the patient instruction leaflet provided.

The applicators should only be used for the administration of the diluted V.C. concentrate.

May be used in combination with Betadine Vaginal Pessaries or Betadine Vaginal Gel.

In children: Contra-indicated for use in pre-pubertal children.

Contra-indications, warnings, etc
Contra-indications: Known or suspected iodine hypersensitivity.

Regular use is contra-indicated in patients and users with thyroid disorders (in particular nodular colloid goitre, endemic goitre and Hashimoto's thyroiditis).

Interactions with other medicaments and other forms of interaction: Absorption of iodine from povidone iodine through either intact or damaged skin may interfere with thyroid function tests.

Contamination with povidone iodine of several types of tests for the detection of occult blood in faeces or blood in urine may produce false-positive results.

Effects on ability to drive and use machines: None known.

Other undesirable effects: If local irritation, redness or swelling develops discontinue treatment. Iodine is absorbed from the vagina and following prolonged use, thyroid dysfunction may develop. The product may be spermicidal and should not be used when conception is desired.

Use in pregnancy and lactation: Regular use of povidone iodine should be avoided in pregnant or lactating women as absorbed iodine can cross the placental barrier and can be secreted into breast milk. Although no adverse effects have been reported from limited use, caution should be recommended and therapeutic benefit must be balanced against possible effects of the absorption of iodine on foetal thyroid function and development.

Other special warnings and precautions: Special caution is needed when regular applications to broken skin are made to patients with pre-existing renal insufficiency.

Regular use should be avoided in patients on concurrent lithium therapy.

Overdosage: Excess iodine can produce goitre and hypothyroidism or hyperthyroidism.

In the case of accidental ingestion of large quantities of Betadine symptomatic and supportive treatment should be provided with special attention to electrolyte balance and renal and thyroid function.

Incompatibilities (major): Compatibility with barrier contraceptives has not been established. Therefore this product should not be used with such methods of contraception as their reliability may be affected.

Pharmaceutical precautions Store in a dry place at or below 20°C.

Legal category GSL.

Package quantities Carton containing plastic bottle of 250 ml Betadine V.C. Concentrate, an empty applicator squeeze bottle and a plastic vaginal applicator.

Further information Betadine V.C. Concentrate is fungicidal, trichomonacidal and bactericidal to the pathogenic organisms that cause vaginitis. In the presence of blood, serum and necrotic tissue, its activity persists whilst the colour remains. The preparation is water soluble and does not stain the skin.

Product licence number 0337/5021.

BETADINE* VAGINAL GEL

Presentation A golden brown gel containing Mundidone* brand of Povidone Iodine USP 10% w/w.

Uses Vaginitis due to candidal, trichomonal, non-specific or mixed infections, and pre-operative preparation of the vagina.

Dosage and administration
In adults and the elderly: Insert an applicator full of gel (5 g) every night for up to 14 days. The regimen may be varied to combine the use of Betadine Vaginal Gel and Betadine Vaginal Pessaries or in combination with the Betadine V.C. Kit using one in the morning and one at night for up to 14 days.

If menstruation occurs during treatment, it is important to continue treatment during the days of the period.

In children: Contra-indicated for use in pre-pubertal children.

Contra-indications, warnings, etc
Contra-indications: Known or suspected iodine hypersensitivity.

Regular use is contra-indicated in patients and users with thyroid disorders (in particular nodular colloid goitre, endemic goitre and Hashimoto's thyroiditis).

Interactions with other medicaments and other forms of interaction: Absorption of iodine from povidone iodine through either intact or damaged skin may interfere with thyroid function tests.

Contamination with povidone iodine of several types of tests for the detection of occult blood in faeces or blood in urine may produce false-positive results.

Effects on ability to drive and use machines: None known.

Other undesirable effects: If local irritation, redness or swelling develops discontinue treatment. Iodine is absorbed from the vagina and following prolonged use, thyroid dysfunction may develop. The product may be spermicidal and should not be used when conception is desired.

Use in pregnancy and lactation: Regular use of povidone iodine should be avoided in pregnant or lactating women as absorbed iodine can cross the placental barrier and can be secreted into breast milk. Although no adverse effects have been reported from limited use, caution should be recommended and therapeutic benefit must be balanced against possible effects of the absorption of iodine on foetal thyroid function and development.

Other special warnings and precautions: Special caution is needed when regular applications to broken skin are made to patients with pre-existing renal insufficiency.

Regular use should be avoided in patients on concurrent lithium therapy.

Overdosage: Excess iodine can produce goitre and hypothyroidism or hyperthyroidism.

In the case of accidental ingestion of large quantities of Betadine symptomatic and supportive treatment should be provided with special attention to electrolyte balance and renal and thyroid function.

Incompatibilities (major): Compatibility with barrier contraceptives has not been established. Therefore this product should not be used with such methods of contraception as their reliability may be affected.

Pharmaceutical precautions Store in a dry place at or below 20°C.

Legal category GSL.

Package quantities 80 g with applicator.

Further information Betadine Vaginal Gel is fungicidal, trichomonacidal and bactericidal to the pathogenic organisms that cause vaginitis. In the presence of blood, serum and necrotic tissue, its activity persists whilst the colour remains. The preparation is water soluble and does not stain the skin.

Product licence number 0337/5020.

BETADINE* VAGINAL PESSARIES

Presentation Vaginal pessaries, golden brown in colour, each contain Mundidone* brand of Povidone Iodine USP 200 mg in a water-soluble base.

Uses Vaginitis due to candidal, trichomonal, non-specific or mixed infections, and pre-operative preparation of the vagina.

Dosage and administration
In adults and the elderly: Using the applicator, insert one pessary night and morning for up to 14 days. Each pessary should be wetted with water immediately prior to insertion, thus ensuring maximum dispersion of the active constituent and avoiding risk of local irritation.

If menstruation occurs during treatment, it is important to continue treatment during the days of the period.

In children: Contra-indicated for use in pre-pubertal children

Contra-indications, warnings, etc
Contra-indications: Known or suspected iodine hypersensitivity.

Regular use is contra-indicated in patients and users with thyroid disorders (in particular nodular colloid goitre, endemic goitre and Hashimoto's thyroiditis).

Interactions with other medicaments and other forms of interaction: Absorption of iodine from povidone iodine through either intact or damaged skin may interfere with thyroid function tests.

Contamination with povidone iodine of several types of tests for the detection of occult blood in faeces or blood in urine may produce false-positive results.

Effects on ability to drive and use machines: None known.

Other undesirable effects: If local irritation, redness or swelling develops discontinue treatment. Iodine is absorbed from the vagina and following prolonged use, thyroid dysfunction may develop. The product may be spermicidal and should not be used when conception is desired.

Use in pregnancy and lactation: Regular use of povidone iodine should be avoided in pregnant or lactating women as absorbed iodine can cross the placental barrier and can be secreted into breast milk. Although no adverse effects have been reported from limited use, caution should be recommended and therapeutic benefit must be balanced against possible effects of the absorption of iodine on foetal thyroid function and development.

Other special warnings and precautions: Special caution is needed when regular applications to broken skin are made to patients with pre-existing renal insufficiency.

Regular use should be avoided in patients on concurrent lithium therapy.

Overdosage: Excess iodine can produce goitre and hypothyroidism or hyperthyroidism.

In the case of accidental ingestion of large quantities of Betadine symptomatic and supportive treatment should be provided with special attention to electrolyte balance and renal and thyroid function.

Incompatibilities (major): Compatibility with barrier contraceptives has not been established. Therefore this product should not be used with such methods of contraception as their reliability may be affected.

Pharmaceutical precautions Store in a dry place at or below 20°C.

Legal category GSL.

Package quantities 28 with applicator (OP).

Further information Betadine Vaginal Pessaries are fungicidal, trichomonacidal and bactericidal to the pathogenic organisms that cause vaginitis. In the presence of blood, serum and necrotic tissue, their activity persists whilst the colour remains. The preparation is water soluble and does not stain the skin.

Product licence number 0337/5019.

BRADILAN* TABLETS

Presentation Enteric and white sugar coated tablets each containing tetranicotinoylfructose (nicofuranose) 250 mg.

Uses In peripheral vascular disease including primary

and secondary Raynaud's disease, intermittent claudication, night cramps, perniosis and cerebrovascular disease.

In hyperlipidaemia, i.e. hypertriglyceridaemia, hypercholesterolaemia, and lipid abnormalities associated with atherosclerosis.

Dosage and administration Dosage needs to be adjusted to the individual. An average dose of 2 tablets three times a day is often sufficient, but doses of 3–4 tablets three times a day may be indicated in some patients. It is better to start therapy with 2 tablets three times a day and increase this dosage over a period of days until the effects of vasodilation are appreciated by the patient and noticed by the doctor. If minimal facial flushing is well tolerated by the patient, the dosage should be maintained at this level. However, the beneficial effects of therapy are not lost by reducing the dosage slightly until flushing disappears.

Contra-indications, warnings, etc Adjust daily dosage to suit each patient individually to ambient temperature.

Patients entering an overheated room or going into a warm bed should not take Bradilan tablets immediately before doing so or they may experience increased vasodilator effects.

The vasodilator effect of Bradilan tablets is enhanced by alcoholic beverages, but their concomitant consumption is not contra-indicated.

Because of the special structure of Bradilan tablets they should not be chewed or broken, but swallowed whole.

Bradilan tablets should not be given in the 24 hours before a surgical operation.

Overdosage: In the event of accidental or deliberate overdosage, facial flushing, vasodilation and possibly hypotension, headaches, gastric irritation, nausea, diarrhoea, hyperglycaemia and hyperthermia may occur. Gastric lavage should be performed and symptomatic treatment given in patients with diabetes, a history of gastro-intestinal ulceration and those susceptible to hyperthermia.

Pharmaceutical precautions Store in a well-closed container, in a cool dry place protected from light.

Legal category P.

Package quantities 50 and 250 tablets.

Further information With Bradilan tablet therapy a clinical response is observed within days.

Correct Bradilan tablet dosage and continued therapy do not result in continued facial flushing, headache, gastric irritation and nausea which are commonly associated with nicotinic acid and its salts. Because of its sustained therapeutic activity Bradilan tablets need be given only three to four times a day.

Product licence number 0337/5006.

CARYLDERM* LOTION

Presentation A clear, colourless, alcohol-based lotion containing carbaryl 0.5% w/v.

Uses For the treatment of head and pubic lice infestations.

Dosage and administration The source of infestation should be sought and treated.

For head lice:

1. Sprinkle the lotion on the hair and rub gently on to the head until the entire scalp is moistened. Pay special attention to the back of the neck and area behind the ears. Take care to avoid the eyes.
2. Allow the hair to dry naturally – use NO heat.
3. As all lice and eggs will have been killed, the hair may shampooed after 2 hours. If a residual effect is desired, however, it is recommended that shampooing be carried out after 12 hours.
4. While still wet, comb the hair with an ordinary comb. The fine-toothed Napp Comb can then be used to remove the dead lice and eggs.

For pubic lice: Application and dosage etc. are as for the head. Apply the lotion to the pubic hair and the hair between the legs and around the anus. Allow to dry naturally using NO heat. Transient, mild stinging may be experienced due to the alcohol content.

Contra-indications, warnings, etc Contains flammable alcohol. Apply and dry with care. Avoid naked flames or lighted objects. Do not use artificial heat (e.g. electric dryers). Dry in a well-ventilated room. Do not cover the head before the lotion has dried completely. The alcohol content may cause wheezing in asthmatic patients and stinging or inflammation of the skin in people with severe eczema.

Children under the age of six months should be treated under medical supervision.

When Carylderm Lotion is used by a school nurse or other health officer in the mass treatment of large numbers of children, it is advisable that protective plastic or rubber gloves be worn.

Treatment of overdosage: In the event of deliberate or accidental ingestion, as for ethyl alcohol, empty stomach contents and keep patient warm. In the event of massive ingestion, atropine, in doses of 1 or 2 mg may be required to counteract cholinesterase inhibition.

Pharmaceutical precautions Store in a cool place protected from light.

Legal category P.

Package quantities Sprinkler-top bottles of 55 ml and 110 ml.

Further information The volatile alcoholic base used in Carylderm Lotion evaporates quickly leaving a high concentration of Carbaryl on the hair. This is rapidly lethal to both lice and their eggs and may give several weeks' protection from reinfestation. For this protective effect to be optimal Carylderm Lotion should be left on the scalp for 12 hours before shampooing and no artifical heat used to dry the hair after shampooing.

Product licence number 0337/0038.

CARYLDERM* SHAMPOO

Presentation A pleasantly perfumed, clear yellow liquid shampoo containing carbaryl 1% w/v.

Uses For the treatment of head and pubic lice infestation.

Dosage and administration The source of infestation should be sought and treated.

For head lice:

1. Wet the hair thoroughly with warm water and apply sufficient shampoo to work up a rich lather and ensure that no part of the scalp is left uncovered. Pay special attention to the back of the neck and area behind the ears. Take care to avoid the eyes.
2. Leave for at least five minutes.
3. Rinse thoroughly with clean, warm water and repeat procedure.
4. While the hair is still wet, comb with an ordinary comb. The fine-toothed Napp Comb can then be used to remove the dead lice and eggs.
5. This treatment should be carried out a total of three times at three day intervals.

For pubic lice:

1. Wet area and apply shampoo directly to the pubic hair and the hair between the legs and around the anus.
2. Cover the skin and hair completely with the shampoo.
3. Work up a lather and leave for at least five minutes.
4. Rinse thoroughly.
5. Repeat procedure. The fine-toothed Napp Comb can then be used to remove the dead lice and eggs.

Contra-indications, warnings, etc Children under

the age of six months should be treated under medical supervision.

As with all shampoos, avoid contact with the eyes. When Carylderm Shampoo is used by a school nurse or other health officer in the mass treatment of large numbers of children, it is advisable that protective plastic or rubber gloves be worn.

Treatment of overdosage: In the event of deliberate or accidental ingestion, empty stomach contents and keep patient warm. In the event of massive ingestion, atropine, in doses of 1 or 2 mg may be required to counteract cholinesterase inhibition.

Pharmaceutical precautions None.

Legal category P.

Package quantities Bottle of 100 ml.

Further information Carylderm Shampoo contains an insecticide of the carbamate group, which is rapidly lethal to both lice and their eggs.

Product licence number 0337/0044.

CO-DANTHRAMER SUSPENSION (Codalax)
STRONG CO-DANTHRAMER SUSPENSION (Codalax Forte)

Presentation Co-Danthramer Suspension is a peach flavoured, viscous, orange coloured liquid. Each 5 ml spoonful contains: Poloxamer 188 200 mg and Danthron BP 25 mg.

Strong Co-Danthramer Suspension is also a peach flavoured, viscous, orange coloured liquid. Each 5 ml spoonful contains: Poloxamer 188 1000 mg and Danthron BP 75 mg.

Uses

Action: As a lubricant, faecal softener and laxative for oral administration. Danthron is a hydroquinone compound which acts on the nerve endings of the myenteric plexus to stimulate the muscle of the large intestine. It acts between 6 and 12 hours after administration.

Poloxamer 188 increases the penetration of water into faecal material thus preventing the faecal mass from drying and hardening excessively. The surface activity of poloxamer improves the penetration of water and the total effect is one of useful lubrication of the distal colonic contents.

Indications:

(a) Constipation in geriatric practice.

(b) In analgesic induced constipation in the terminally ill, in all age groups.

(c) For the prophylaxis of analgesic induced constipation in terminally ill cancer patients.

(d) Constipation in cardiac failure and coronary thrombosis, conditions in which defaecation must be free of strain.

Both products are noted for their effectiveness and in particular, their freedom from griping which can be caused by other preparations.

Dosage and administration

Co-Danthramer Suspension:

Adults: one or two 5 ml spoonfuls at bedtime.

Children: half to one 5 ml spoonful at bedtime.

Strong Co-Danthramer Suspension: Half to one 5 ml spoonful at bedtime or as directed. Not recommended for children under 12 years. Danthron acts between 6 and 12 hours after administration.

Contra-indications, warnings, etc

Contra-indications: In common with other gastrointestinal evacuants Co-Danthramer and Strong Co-Danthramer Suspensions should not be given when acute or painful conditions of the abdomen are present, or the cause of constipation is suspected to be intestinal inflammation or obstruction.

Caution: Co-Danthramer suspensions may cause staining of the buttocks in incontinent and/or bedridden patients. This may lead to superficial sloughing of the skin. Therefore, Co-Danthramer preparations should not be given to infants in nappies and be used with caution in all incontinent patients.

Use in pregnancy: There is inadequate evidence of the safety of Co-Danthramer preparations in pregnancy and therefore its use is not recommended.

Special warning: Oral administration of Danthron has been reported to cause intestinal tumours in rats and mice. It has also been reported to be hepatocarcinogenic in rats as well as in mice. There is no sound evidence to conclude a no effect dose and therefore there may be a risk of such effects in humans.

Side-effects: Danthron may cause temporary harmless pink or red colouring of the urine and perianal skin. With prolonged high dosage the mucosa of the large intestine may become coloured.

Overdosage: Patients should be given plenty of fluids. An anticholinergic preparation such as atropine methonitrate may be given to offset the excessive intestinal motility.

Pharmaceutical precautions Store in a cool place, away from stong light.

Diluents: Tragacanth Mucilage BP or Syrup BP should be used if diluents are required.

N.B. It is not possible to diluted Strong Co-Danthramer Suspension to obtain Suspension of Co-Danthramer since the proportions of the two active ingredients are different.

Legal category POM.

Package quantities Bottles of 100 ml, 300 ml and 1 litre.

Further information Nil.

Product licence numbers

Co-Danthramer Suspension	0549/0062
Strong Co-Danthramer Suspension	0549/0063

COMPLOMENT* CONTINUS* TABLETS

Presentation Bi-convex, yellow tablets, marked C on one side and the logo NAPP on the other. Each tablet contains 100 mg Vitamin B_6 (pyridoxine hydrochloride) in the patented Continus controlled release system.

Uses For the treatment of Pyridoxine (Vitamin B_6) deficiency, including that induced by usage of the oral contraceptive pill.

Dosage and administration One tablet to be taken daily, or as directed by the physician.

Contra-indications, warnings, etc None known.

Treatment of overdosage: Ingestion of twenty to thirty tablets may cause headache and will alter the kinetics of levodopa. No treatment is necessary.

Pharmaceutical precautions Comploment Continus tablets should be stored in a cool place, protected from light.

Legal category P.

Package quantities Blister packs containing 28 tablets (OP).

Further information Fifty per cent of women who have symptoms of pessimism, anxiety, dissatisfaction, lethargy and loss of libido associated with the taking of the oral contraceptive pill have been reported to have an absolute deficiency of vitamin B_6 (pyridoxine hydrochloride) (Lancet i, 897, 1973).

Comploment Continus tablets will effectively correct such pyridoxine deficiency. The controlled release system ensures adequate supplementation of the pyridoxine from a single tablet taken daily.

Product licence number 0337/0045.

DHC CONTINUS* TABLETS

Presentation
DHC Continus Tablets 60 mg are white capsule-shaped, biconvex tablets with DHC 60 on one side. Each tablet contains 60 mg Dihydrocodeine Tartrate BP in a patented controlled release system.
DHC Continus Tablets 90 mg are white to off-white, capsule-shaped, biconvex tablets with DHC 90 on one side. Each tablet contains 90 mg of Dihydrocodeine Tartrate BP in a patented controlled release system.
DHC Continus Tablets 120 mg are white to off-white, capsule-shaped, biconvex tablets with DHC 120 on one side. Each tablet contains 120 mg of Dihydrocodeine Tartrate BP in a patented controlled release system.

Uses For the relief of chronic severe pain.

Dosage and administration
Adults and children over 12 years: For DHC Continus Tablets 60 mg the dosage is one or two tablets 12 hourly. For DHC Continus Tablets 90 and 120 mg the dosage is one tablet 12 hourly. Tablets should be swallowed whole and not chewed.

Elderly: Dosage should be reduced.

Children 12 years or under: Not recommended.

Contra-indications, warnings, etc
Contra-indications: Respiratory depression and obstructive airways disease. As dihydrocodeine may cause the release of histamine it should not be given during an attack of asthma and should be given with caution to asthmatics.

Precautions: Dosage should be reduced in the elderly, in hypothyroidism, chronic hepatic disease and renal insufficiency. Alcohol should be avoided whilst under treatment with dihydrocodeine. Dihydrocodeine should be used with caution in patients taking mono-amine oxidase inhibitors. Opioid analgesics should be avoided in those patients with raised intracranial pressure or head injury. Dihydrocodeine may cause drowsiness and, if affected, patients should not drive or operate machinery.

Pregnancy: There is little published data on safety in human pregnancy but dihydrocodeine has been used for many years without apparent ill effects. Dihydrocodeine has not been reported to be excreted in breast milk, however it is advisable that dihydrocodeine only be administered to breast-feeding mothers if considered esssential.

Side-effects: Constipation, nausea, vomiting, headache, vertigo and urinary retention can occur. Constipation can be treated with a gentle laxative.

Overdosage: Conservative management is recommended and should include gastric lavage. Severe respiratory depression can be treated with naloxone hydrochloride 0.4 mg intravenously, repeated as required or at 2–3 minute intervals.

Pharmaceutical precautions DHC Continus Tablets should be stored at or below 20°C.

Legal category POM.

Package quantities Packs of 56 tablets.

Further information The risk of dependence with dihydrocodeine is very low.

Product licence numbers
60 mg 0337/0115
90 mg 0337/0140
120 mg 0337/0141

FLEXIN* CONTINUS* TABLETS

Presentation Yellow capsule-shaped tablets with 75 IC embossed on one side. Each tablet contains 75 mg Indomethacin BP in a patented controlled release system.

Uses Non-steroidal anti-inflammatory agent indicated in rheumatoid arthritis; osteoarthritis; ankylosing spondylitis; gout; degenerative joint disease of the hip; painful musculoskeletal disorders; low-back pain; and any periarticular disorders such as bursitis, tendinitis, synovitis, tenosynovitis and capsulitis. Also indicated in inflammation, pain and oedema following orthopaedic procedures and treatment of dysmenorrhoea.

Dosage and administration In order to reduce the possibility of gastro-intestinal disturbance, Flexin Continus Tablets should always be given with food, milk or an antacid.

Adults: One tablet once or twice daily, depending on patient needs and response. In dysmenorrhoea one tablet daily, starting with the onset of cramps or bleeding and continuing for as long as the symptoms usually last.

Elderly: Indomethacin should be used with particular care in older patients who are more prone to adverse reactions.

Children: A paediatric dose has not been established.

Contra-indications, warnings, etc
Contra-indications: Since safety of indomethacin has not been established in children, pregnant and lactating women, Flexin Continus Tablets should not be given to such patients.

Also contra-indicated in active peptic ulcer, a history of recurrent gastro-intestinal lesions. Sensitivity to indomethacin, aspirin or other non-steroidal anti-inflammatory drugs.

Precautions: Flexin Continus Tablets should be used with caution in patients with hepatic or renal dysfunction. Hepatitis and jaundice have been reported rarely with indomethacin treatment.

Patients should be warned not to drive or operate machinery if they become dizzy or light-headed.

In common with other anti-inflammatory analgesic anti-pyretic agents, indomethacin may mask the signs and symptoms of infection.

Flexin Continus Tablets should be used with caution in patients with psychiatric disorders, epilepsy or Parkinsonism as indomethacin may tend to aggravate these disorders.

Flexin Continus Tablets should be used with caution in patients with coagulation defects. Indomethacin can inhibit platelet aggregation. The effect usually disappears within 24 hours of discontinuing therapy.

Drug interactions: Co-administration of aspirin may decrease blood levels of indomethacin. Diflunisal and probenecid may increase plasma levels of indomethacin.

Indomethacin and triamterine should not be administered together.

Flexin Continus Tablets may reduce the anti-hypertensive effect of beta-blockers and the diuretic and anti-hypertensive effect of thiazides and frusemide in some patients.

When Flexin Continus Tablets are used in patients receiving anti-coagulant therapy, they should be closely observed for changes in prothrombin time.

Flexin Continus Tablets may reduce the tubular secretion and therefore potentiate the toxicity of methotrexate.

Co-administration to patients with steady state lithium concentrations may reduce clearance of lithium and raise plasma lithium levels.

Warnings and adverse effects: Starting treatment with one Flexin Continus Tablet per day and increasing to two per day, if necessary for symptomatic relief will minimise the incidence of side effects.

Headache, dizziness and dyspepsia may occur. If headache persists, even after dosage reduction, indomethacin should be withdrawn.

Other CNS side-effects which may occur include mental confusion, depression, convulsions, depersonalisation and tinnitus. These are often transient and disappear with time or on reduction of dosage. Coma has also been reported.

Gastro-intestinal side-effects which may occur with indomethacin therapy are anorexia, nausea, vomiting, epigastric distress, abdominal pain and diarrhoea. Giving indomethacin with food, milk or antacids lowers the incidence of these side-effects. Ulceration of the oesophagus, stomach or duodenum, which may be accompanied by either haemorrhage or perforation has been reported with indomethacin preparations. Use of Flexin Continus Tablets will minimise these gastro-intestinal effects. Gastro-intestinal bleeding without obvious ulceration may also occur. If this happens indomethacin treatment should be discontinued.

Blood dyscrasias, particularly thrombocytopenia, have been reported with indomethacin therapy.

Blurred vision and orbital and peri-orbital pain are seen infrequently with indomethacin therapy. Corneal deposits and retinal disturbances have been reported in some patients with rheumatoid arthritis on prolonged therapy with indomethacin, and ophthalmic examinations are desirable in patients given prolonged treatment.

Oedema and increased blood pressure and haematuria have been reported with indomethacin therapy.

Reported hypersensitivity reactions to indomethacin include pruritus, urticaria, angiitis, erythema nodosum. Hair loss may also occur.

Acute respiratory distress including sudden dyspnoea and asthma, have been reported on rare occasions with indomethacin therapy. Bronchospasm may be precipitated in patients suffering from, or with a previous history of bronchial asthma or allergic disease.

Treatment of overdosage: Empty stomach contents. Supportive therapy should be initiated and a watch should be kept for gastro-intestinal bleeding for several days. Antacids may be useful.

Pharmaceutical precautions Store at or below 20°C.

Legal category POM.

Package quantities Containers of 28 tablets (OP).

Product licence number 0337/0128.

FULL MARKS* LOTION

Presentation A clear, colourless, alcohol-based lotion containing phenothrin 0.2% w/v.

Uses For the treatment of head and pubic lice infestations.

Dosage and administration The source of infestation should be sought and treated.

For head lice:

1. Ensure the hair is dry before commencing treatment.
2. Sprinkle the lotion on the hair and rub gently onto the head until the entire scalp is moistened. Pay special attention to the back of the neck and area behind the ears. Take care to avoid the eyes.
3. Allow to dry naturally – use NO heat. Ensure the hair is dry before going to bed.
4. As all lice and eggs will have been killed, the hair may be shampooed after 2 hours.
5. While still wet, comb the hair with an ordinary comb. A fine-toothed Napp* Comb can then be used to remove the dead lice and eggs.

For pubic lice: Application and dosage are as for the head. Apply the lotion to the pubic hair and the hair between the legs and around the anus. Allow to dry naturally using NO heat. Transient, mild stinging may be experienced due to the alcohol content.

Contra-indications, warnings, etc Contains flammable alcohol. Apply and dry with care. Avoid naked flames or lighted objects. Do not use artificial heat (e.g. electric dryers). Dry in a well-ventilated room. Do not cover the head before the lotion has dried completely. Do not use if sensitive to pyrethroid insecticides.

The alcohol content may cause wheezing in asthmatic patients and stinging or inflammation of the skin in people with severe eczema.

Children under the age of six months should be treated under medical supervision.

Nursing staff using Full Marks Lotion in the treatment of a large number of children are advised to wear protective plastic or rubber gloves.

Treatment of overdosage: In the event of deliberate or accidental ingestion, as for ethyl alcohol, empty stomach contents and keep patient warm.

Pharmaceutical precautions Store bottle in the carton at or below 30°C.

Legal category P.

Package quantities Sprinkler-top bottles of 55 ml and 110 ml.

Further information The volatile alcoholic base used in Full Marks Lotion evaporates quickly leaving a high concentration of phenothrin in the hair. This is rapidly lethal to both lice and their eggs.

Product licence number 0337/0153.

FULL MARKS* SHAMPOO

Presentation A pleasantly perfumed clear orange liquid shampoo containing phenothrin 0.2% w/w.

Uses Pediculicide for the treatment of head lice infestations.

Dosage and administration The source of infestation should be sought and treated.

For all age groups:

1. Wet the hair thoroughly with warm water. Apply sufficient shampoo to work up a rich lather and ensure that no part of the scalp is left uncovered. Particular attention should be paid to the nape of the neck and behind the ears.
2. Leave for at least five minutes.
3. Rinse thoroughly with clean, warm water and repeat procedure.
4. While hair is still wet, comb with an ordinary comb. The fine toothed Napp Comb can now be used to remove all dead lice and eggs.

Contra-indications, warnings, etc

Contra-indications: Full Marks Shampoo should not be used on patients with a history of sensitivity to pyrethroid insecticides or commercially available shampoos.

Warnings: Children under the age of six months should be treated under medical supervision. As with all shampoos, avoid contact with the eyes. When Full Marks Shampoo is used by a school nurse or other health officer in the mass treatment of large numbers of children, it is advisable that gloves be worn.

Overdosage: In the event of accidental or deliberate ingestion of a large quantity of Full Marks Shampoo, empty stomach contents and provide symptomatic treatment.

Pharmaceutical precautions None.

Legal category P.

Package quantities Bottles of 125 ml.

Further information Full Marks Shampoo contains a pyrethroid insecticide which is highly effective against lice and their eggs whilst having an extremely low toxicity to mammals compared with other insecticides.

Product licence number 0337/0104.

GASTROBID* CONTINUS* TABLETS

Presentation White biconvex tablets with (NAPP) on one side and 15 mg on the other. Each tablet contains 15 mg Metoclopramide Hydrochloride BP equivalent to 15 mg of the anhydrous substance in a patented controlled release system.

Uses Gastrobid Continus Tablets restore normal coordination and tone to the upper digestive tract and relieve symptoms of gastro-duodenal dysfunction including heartburn, dyspepsia, nausea and vomiting associated with such conditions as reflux oesophagitis, gastritis, duodenitis and hiatus hernia.

Gastrobid Continus Tablets are also indicated as an

anti-emetic for the treatment of nausea and vomiting associated with cytostatic and cytotoxic drugs.

Dosage and administration
20 years and over: 1 tablet (15 mg) twice daily.
Under 20 years: Contra-indicated.
Elderly patients: As for adults.

To avoid adverse reactions adhere strictly to dosage recommendations and where prolonged therapy is considered necessary patients should be regularly reviewed.

Contra-indications, warnings, etc
Contra-indications: Gastrobid Continus Tablets are contra-indicated in patients under 20 years, since dosage titration is not possible.

Precautions: Gastrobid Continus Tablets should not be given during, or within 15 days of completing treatment with monoamine oxidase inhibitors, nor with tricyclic antidepressants or sympathomimetic drugs. It is also recommended that combination with neuroleptics (synergy of central effect) and derivatives of anticholinergic drugs (neutralisation of effect) be avoided.

Special care should be taken if Gastrobid Continus Tablets are administered concomitantly with other medicines. For example, the presence of metoclopramide may decrease gastric absorption of digoxin and increase the intestinal absorption of paracetamol.

Although animal tests in several mammalian species have shown no teratogenic effects, treatment with Gastrobid Continus Tablets is not advised during the first trimester of pregnancy.

Following operations such as pyloroplasty or gut anastomosis, therapy with Gastrobid Continus Tablets should be withheld for three or four days as vigorous muscular contractions may impair healing.

Side-effects: The following side-effects have occasionally been reported with metoclopramide therapy: drowsiness, lethargy, dizziness and headache. More rarely, various extrapyramidal reactions, usually of the dystonic type, have been reported. These include spasm of the facial muscles, trismus, rhythmic protrusion of the tongue, a bulbar type of speech, spasm of extra-ocular muscles including oculogyric crises, unnatural positioning of the head and shoulders and opisthotonos. These have been shown to be more common in young adults, particularly females aged 12–19. Parkinsonian reactions are significantly more common in the elderly. Tardive dyskinesia has been reported during prolonged treatment with metoclopramide in a small number of mainly elderly patients. Insomnia, diarrhoea and flatulence have also been reported.

The majority of reactions occur within 36 hours of starting treatment and the effects are reversible, usually disappearing within 24 hours of stopping treatment.

Raised serum prolactin levels have been observed during metoclopramide therapy; this effect is similar to that noted with many other compounds. Metoclopramide may induce an acute hypertensive response in patients with phaeochromocytoma.

Overdosage: Gastric lavage and intensive supportive therapy should be initiated. Should treatment of a dystonic reaction be required, an anticholinergic antiparkinsonian drug, or a benzodiazepine may be used. The physician should be aware that tablets remaining in the intestine will continue to release metoclopramide hydrochloride for a period of hours.

Pharmaceutical precautions Store in a cool, dry place, protected from light.

Legal category POM.

Package quantities Blister packs of 56 tablets.

Further information The action of Gastrobid Continus Tablets is closely associated with parasympathetic nervous control of the upper gastro-intestinal tract, where it has the effect of encouraging normal peristaltic action. This provides a fundamental approach to the treatment of those conditions where disturbed gastro-intestinal motility is a common underlying factor. The controlled release formulation allows Gastrobid Continus Tablets to be administered twice daily.

Product licence number 0337/0106.

MST* CONTINUS* TABLETS

Presentation
MST Continus Tablets 10 mg are golden brown, film-coated and bi-convex. Each tablet contains 10 mg of morphine sulphate incorporated within a patented controlled release system. The tablets are marked with the NAPP logo on one side and 10/mg on the other.

MST Continus Tablets 30 mg are dark purple, film coated and bi-convex. Each tablet contains 30 mg of morphine sulphate BP incorporated within a patented controlled release system. The tablets are marked with the NAPP logo on one side and 30/mg on the other.

MST Continus Tablets 60 mg are orange, film-coated and bi-convex. Each tablet contains 60 mg of morphine sulphate BP incorporated within a patented controlled release system. The tablets are marked with the NAPP logo on one side and 60/mg on the other.

MST Continus Tablets 100 mg are grey, film-coated and bi-convex. Each tablet contains 100 mg of morphine sulphate BP incorporated within a patented controlled release system. The tablets are marked with the NAPP logo on one side and 100/mg on the other.

MST Continus Tablets 200 mg are teal-green, film-coated and bi-convex. Each tablet contains 200 mg of morphine sulphate BP incorporated within a patented controlled release system. The tablets are marked with the NAPP logo on one side and 200/mg on the other.

Uses MST Continus Tablets are indicated for the prolonged relief of severe and intractable pain.

MST Continus Tablets up to 30 mg 12 hourly are indicated for the relief of post-operative pain.

Dosage and administration MST Continus Tablets must be swallowed whole and not chewed.

For the prolonged relief of severe and intractable pain
Adults: MST Continus Tablets should be used at 12-hourly intervals. The dosage is dependent upon the severity of the pain, the patient's age and previous history of analgesic requirements.

Increasing severity of pain will require an increased dosage of MST Continus Tablets using 10 mg, 30 mg, 60 mg, 100 mg and 200 mg alone or in combination to achieve pain relief. The correct dosage for any individual patient is that which controls the pain for a full 12 hours.

A patient presenting with severe pain uncontrolled by weaker opioids should normally be started on 30 mg MST Continus Tablets 12 hourly increasing to 60 mg 12 hourly when required. If higher doses are necessary they should be made in 25%–50% increments.

In debilitated and underweight patients a reduction in starting dose is advisable.

Patients previously on normal release oral morphine or diamorphine should be given the same total daily dose as MST Continus Tablets but in divided doses at 12 hourly intervals.

Patients receiving MST Continus tablets in place of parenteral morphine should be given a sufficiently increased dosage to compensate for any reduction in analgesic effects associated with oral administration. Usually such increased requirement is of the order of 50%–100%. In such patients individual dose adjustments are required.

Children: For severe and intractable pain in cancer a starting dose in the range of 0.2 to 0.8 mg/kg 12 hourly is recommended. Doses should be titrated in the normal way as for adults.

Elderly: As with all narcotics, a reduction in dosage may be advisable in the elderly.

Post-operative pain

Adults and elderly: MST Continus tablets are not recommended in the first 24 hours post-operatively; thereafter it is suggested that the following dosage schedule be observed at the physician's discretion:

(a) MST Continus tablets 20 mg 12 hourly to patients under 70 kilograms.

(b) MST Continus tablets 30 mg 12 hourly to patients over 70 kilograms.

Supplemental parenteral morphine may be given if required but with careful attention to the total dosage of morphine, and bearing in mind the prolonged effects of morphine in the MST Continus formulation.

As with all oral morphine preparations, MST Continus Tablets should be used with caution post-operatively, and particularly in 'acute abdomen' and following abdominal surgery.

Children: MST Continus Tablets are not recommended for treatment of post-operative pain in children.

Contra-indications, warnings, etc Respiratory depression, paralytic ileus, delayed gastric emptying, obstructive airways disease, known morphine sensitivity, acute hepatic disease, concurrent administration of monoamine oxidase inhibitors (MAOIs) or within two weeks of discontinuation of their use. MAOIs have been reported to interact with narcotic analgesics, producing CNS excitation or depression with hyper or hypotensive crisis.

MST Continus Tablets are not recommended for use in pregnancy or for the treatment of post-operative pain in children.

Pre-operative administration of MST Continus Tablets is not recommended and is not an approved indication.

Precautions: As with all narcotics a reduction in dosage may be advisable in the elderly, in hypothyroidism, in renal and chronic hepatic disease.

Morphine may modify the patients reactions when driving to a varying extent depending on the dosage and individual susceptibility.

Use with caution in patients with raised intracranial pressure.

Warnings and adverse effects: MST Continus Tablets should not be used where there is a possibility of paralytic ileus occurring. Should paralytic ileus be suspected or occur during use, MST Continus Tablets should be discontinued immediately. As with all morphine preparations, patients who are to undergo cordotomy or other pain relieving surgical procedures should not receive MST Continus Tablets for 24 hours prior to surgery. If further treatment with MST Continus Tablets is then indicated the dosage should be adjusted to the new post-operative requirement.

Tolerance and dependence may occur. When nausea and vomiting are troublesome, MST Continus Tablets can be readily combined with phenothiazine antiemetics. It should be noted however, that morphine potentiates the effects of tranquillisers, anaesthetics, hypnotics and sedatives. As with all morphine preparations, constipation may occur, which may be treated with appropriate laxatives.

Overdosage: Signs of morphine toxicity and overdosage:

These are likely to consist of pin-point pupils, respiratory depression and hypotension. Circulatory failure and deepening coma may occur in more severe cases.

Treatment of morphine overdosage:

Administer naloxone 0.4 mg intravenously. Repeat at 2–3 minute intervals as necessary, or by an infusion of 2 mg in 500 ml of normal saline or 5% dextrose (0.004 mg/ml).

The infusion should be run at a rate related to the previous bolus doses administered and should be in accordance with the patient's response. Empty the stomach. A 0.02% aqueous solution of potassium permanganate may be used for lavage. Assist respiration if necessary. Maintain fluid and electrolyte levels.

In the case of MST Continus Tablets, the physician should be aware that tablets remaining in the intestine will continue to release morphine sulphate for a period of hours.

Pharmaceutical precautions MST Continus Tablets should be stored at or below 25°C.

Legal category CD (Sch 2) POM.

Package quantities Blister packs of 60 tablets.

Further information Morphine Sulphate BP is readily absorbed from the gastro-intestinal tract following oral administration. The patented controlled release system maintains plasma levels of morphine over a period of up to 12 hours and reduces the likelihood of morphine associated side-effects.

Transferability: It is not possible to ensure bioequivalence between different controlled release morphine products. Therefore, it should be emphasised that patients, once titrated to an effective dose, should not be changed from MST Continus Tablet preparations to other slow, sustained or controlled release morphine preparations without retitration and clinical assessment.

Product licence numbers

10 mg	0337/0055
30 mg	0337/0059
60 mg	0337/0087
100 mg	0337/0088
200 mg	0337/0149

PHYLLOCONTIN* CONTINUS* TABLETS 225 mg PHYLLOCONTIN FORTE CONTINUS TABLETS 350 mg PHYLLOCONTIN PAEDIATRIC CONTINUS TABLETS 100 mg

Presentation

Phyllocontin Continus tablets are pale yellow, film-coated tablets with the logo (NAPP) on one side and SA on the other. Each tablet contains Aminophylline BP 225 mg in a patented controlled release system.

Phyllocontin Forte Continus tablets are pale yellow, film-coated, capsule-shaped tablets with the logo (NAPP) on one side and SA/350 on the other. Each tablet contains Aminophylline BP 350 mg in a patented controlled release system.

Phyllocontin Paediatric Continus tablets are pale mottled peach, bi-convex tablets with the logo (NAPP) on one side and SA/2 on the other. Each tablet contains Aminophylline BP 100 mg in a patented controlled release system.

Uses Aminophylline is a bronchodilator. In addition it affects the function of a number of cells involved in the inflammatory processes associated with asthma and chronic obstructive airways disease. Of most importance may be enhanced suppressor T-lymphocyte activity and reduction of eosinophil and neutrophil function. These actions may contribute to anti-inflammatory prophylactic activity in asthma and chronic obstructive airways disease.

For the treatment and prophylaxis of bronchospasm associated with asthma, emphysema and chronic bronchitis. Also indicated in adults for the treatment of cardiac asthma and left ventricular or congestive cardiac failure.

Dosage and administration

N.B. Tablets should be swallowed whole and not chewed.

Children: Not recommended for children under 3 years of age. The maintenance dose (expressed as mg aminophylline) is 12 mg/kg twice daily adjusted to the nearest 100 mg. It is recommended that half the maintenance dose be given for the first week of therapy if the patient has not previously been receiving xanthine preparations.

Some children with chronic asthma require and tolerate much higher doses (13–20 mg/kg twice daily). Lower doses (based on the usual adult dose) may be required by adolescents.

Adults: The usual daily dose is two Phyllocontin Continus tablets 225 mg twice-daily following an initial week of therapy on one tablet twice-daily.

The elderly: The dose should be adjusted following the response to the initial week of therapy on one tablet twice-daily.

Dose titration: Patients vary in their response to xanthines and it may be necessary to titrate dosage individually. Steady state theophylline levels are generally attained 3–4 days after dose adjustment. If a satisfactory clinical response is not achieved, serum theophylline should be measured 4–6 hours after the last dose. Based on serum theophylline assay results dosage should be titrated using the following as a guide:

Peak serum theopylline level	*Dosage adjustment to nearest 120 mg*
< 10 micrograms/ml	Increase total daily dose by half.
10–15 micrograms/ml	Increase total daily dose by one quarter if symptoms persist.
16–20 micrograms/ml	No adjustment required.
21–25 micrograms/ml	Decrease dose by one quarter.
26–30 micrograms/ml	Miss next dose and decrease maintenance dose by one half.

It is advisable to re-check serum theophylline concentration after dose adjustment, when steady state is attained.

Pharmacokinetics: In-vivo and *in-vitro* bioavailability/dissolution studies have shown that the three strengths of Phyllocontin Continus tablets are equally bioavailable. It has also been demonstrated that twice-daily dosing produces minimal peak to trough variation and with appropriate dose titration plasma theophylline levels can be maintained within the therapeutic range of 10–20 micrograms/ml throughout the 12-hour dosing interval.

Transferability: It is not possible to ensure bioequivalence between different sustained release theophylline products. Therefore, it should be emphasised that patients, once titrated to an effective dose, should not be changed from Phyllocontin Continus tablet preparations to other slow or sustained release xanthine preparations without re-titration and clinical assessment.

Contra-indications, warnings, etc
Contra-indications: Should not be given concomitantly with ephedrine in children.

Warnings: Theophylline has been reported to interact with a number of drugs.

The following increase clearance and it may therefore be necessary to increase dosage to ensure a therapeutic effect: phenytoin, carbamazepine, rifampicin, sulphinpyrazone and barbiturates. Smoking and alcohol consumption can also increase clearance of theophylline.

The following reduce clearance and a reduced dosage may therefore be necessary to avoid side-effects: ciprofloxacin, allopurinol, cimetidine, erythromycin, thiabendazole, isoprenaline and oral contraceptives. Factors such as viral infections, liver disease and heart failure also reduce theophylline clearance. There are conflicting reports concerning the potentiation of theophylline by influenza vaccine and physicians should be aware that interaction may occur. A reduction of dosage may also be necessary in the elderly patient.

The hypokalaemia resulting from $Beta_2$ agonist therapy, steroids, diuretics and hypoxia may be potentiated by xanthines. Particular care is advised in patients suffering from severe asthma who require hospitalisation. It is recommended that serum potassium levels are monitored in such situations.

The following should also be used with caution in patients taking Phyllocontin Continus tablet preparations: halothane, lomustine and lithium.

Phyllocontin Continus Tablets should be used with caution in pregnancy and lactation. Safety in human pregnancy has not been established, however, use during human pregnancy has been reported without attributable adverse foetal effects. Theophylline crosses the placental barrier and is secreted in breast milk. Control of severe asthma during pregnancy and lactation is of importance to maternal and foetal wellbeing and the physician should balance the potential therapeutic gain against any risk to the foetus or neonate. During pregnancy, the pharmacokinetics of theophylline may change and it is therefore advised that plasma levels be monitored during and after pregnancy.

Side-effects: The risk of side-effects usually associated with aminophylline and xanthine derivatives such as nausea, gastric irritation, headache, palpitations and CNS stimulation are only frequent above 20 micrograms/ml theophylline plasma concentrations. Phyllocontin Continus tablets reduce the risk of such effects by minimising peak/trough variations in plasma levels.

Overdosage: Empty stomach contents. Monitor electrocardiogram and maintain fluid balance. Oral activated medical charcoal has been found to reduce high theophylline blood levels. In severe poisoning employ charcoal-column haemoperfusion. Treat symptoms on appearance. The physician should be aware that tablets in the intestine will continue to release aminophylline for a period of hours.

In the event of hypokalaemia, potassium chloride should be given by slow intravenous infusion. Repeated measurements of plasma potassium should be made.

Pharmaceutical precautions Store at room temperature in a dry place protected from light.

Legal category P.

Package quantities
Phyllocontin Continus tablets 225 mg: Blister packs of 60 tablets (OP), containers of 250 and 1000 tablets.
Phyllocontin Forte Continus tablets 350 mg: Containers of 60 tablets (OP).
Phyllocontin Paediatric Continus tablets 100 mg: Containers of 50 (OP) and 250 tablets.

Further information By incorporating aminophylline in the patented Continus controlled release system, therapeutic blood levels of theophylline between 10 and 20 micrograms/ml can be maintained over a full 24-hour period on a simple twice daily dosage. The availability of three strengths of Phyllocontin Continus tablets permits ideal dosage flexibility. The Continus tablet formulation shows minimal tablet to tablet variation in aminophylline release.

Product licence numbers
Phyllocontin Continus tablets 225 mg 0337/0026
Phyllocontin Forte Continus tablets 350 mg 0337/0090
Phyllocontin Paediatric Continus tablets 100 mg 0337/0040

PLESMET* SYRUP

Presentation Blackcurrant flavoured syrup containing the equivalent of 25 mg ferrous iron per 5 ml dose in the chelated form as ferrous glycine sulphate.

Uses Treatment and prophylaxis of iron deficiency anaemia.

Dosage and administration
Treatment of iron deficiency anaemia
Adults and children > 30 kg: 10 ml three times a day
Children 15–30 kg: 5 ml three times a day
7.5–14.9 kg: 2.5 ml three times a day
5.0–7.4 kg: 2.5 ml twice a day
2.5–4.9 kg: 2.5 ml daily

Prophylaxis of iron deficiency anaemia
Adults and children >30 kg: 5 ml three times a day
Children 15–30 kg: 2.5 ml three times a day
7.5–14.9 kg: 2.5 ml daily
<7.4 kg: Not recommended

Plesmet Syrup may be diluted with Syrup BP.

Contra-indications, warnings, etc
Precautions: Absorption of iron salts may be reduced by tetracyclines, magnesium trisilicate, trientine and zinc salts.

Absorption of tetracyclines may be reduced by iron salts.

Side-effects: Side-effects due to chelated iron are uncommon. However, dose-related nausea and epigastric pain may occur. Administration of Plesmet Syrup with food may alleviate these symptoms if they do arise but iron absorption may be diminished. Diarrhoea and constipation (in the elderly in particular) may occur.

Overdosage: Initial symptoms of overdosage include nausea, vomiting, diarrhoea, abdominal pain, haematemesis, rectal bleeding, lethargy and circulatory collapse. Hyperglycaemia and metabolic acidosis may occur.

Treatment of overdosage:
1. Administer an emetic.
2. Emesis should be followed by gastric lavage with desferrioxamine solution (2 g/l). Desferrioxamine 5 g in 50–100 ml water should be introduced into the stomach following gastric emptying.
3. Keep the patient under constant surveillance to detect possible aspiration of vomitus. Maintain suction apparatus and standby emergency oxygen in case of need.
4. In adults, a drink of mannitol or sorbitol should be given to induce small bowel emptying. Inducing diarrhoea in children may be dangerous and should not be undertaken in young children.
5. Severe poisoning: in the presence of shock and/or coma with high serum iron levels (Adults >142 umol/l, children >90 umol/l), immediate supportive measures should be introduced. Desferrioxamine should be given by slow i.v. infusion (Adults 5 mg/kg/h, children 15 mg/kg/h). The maximum dose is 80 mg/kg/24 h. Warning: hypotension may occur if the infusion rate is too rapid.
6. Less severe poisoning: i.m. desferrioxamine should be administered (Adults 50 mg/kg to a maximum of 4 g, children 1 g 4–6 hourly).
7. Serum iron levels should be monitored throughout.

Pharmaceutical precautions Store at or below 20°C.

Legal category P.

Package quantities Bottles of 100 ml and 1 litre.

Further information Chelated iron is more rapidly absorbed and utilised than the more conventional forms of iron.

Product licence number 0337/5904

PRIODERM* CREAM SHAMPOO

Presentation A light-orange pearlescent cream shampoo containing malathion 1.0% w/w.

Uses For the treatment of head and pubic lice infestation.

Dosage and administration The source of infestation should be sought and treated.

For head lice:
1. Wet the hair thoroughly with warm water and apply sufficient shampoo to work up a rich lather and ensure that no part of the scalp is left uncovered. Pay special attention to the back of the neck and area behind the ears. Take care to avoid the eyes.
2. Leave for at least five minutes.
3. Rinse thoroughly with clean, warm water and repeat procedure.
4. While the hair is still wet, comb with an ordinary comb. The fine-toothed Napp comb can then be used to remove the dead lice and eggs.
5. This treatment should be carried out a total of three times at three day intervals.

For pubic lice:
1. Wet area and apply shampoo directly to the pubic hair and the hair between the legs and around the anus.
2. Cover the skin and hair completely with the shampoo.
3. Work up a lather and leave for at least five minutes.
4. Rinse thoroughly.
5. Repeat procedure. The fine-toothed Napp comb can then be used to remove the dead lice and eggs.

Contra-indications, warnings, etc Children under the age of six months should be treated under medical supervision.

As with all shampoos, avoid contact with the eyes. When Prioderm Cream Shampoo is used by a school nurse or other health officer in the mass treatment of large numbers of children, it is advisable that protective plastic or rubber gloves be worn.

Treatment of overdosage: In the event of deliberate or accidental ingestion, empty stomach contents and keep patient warm. In the event of massive ingestion atropine and pralidoxime may be required to counteract cholinesterase inhibition.

Pharmaceutical precautions None.

Legal category P.

Package quantities Tube of 40 g.

Further information Prioderm Cream Shampoo contains the insecticide malathion which is rapidly lethal to both lice and their eggs.

Product licence number 0337/0036.

PRIODERM* LOTION

Presentation A clear, colourless, alcohol-based lotion containing malathion 0.5% w/v.

Uses For the treatment of head and pubic lice infestations and scabies.

Dosage and administration The source of infestation should be sought and treated.

For head lice:
1. Sprinkle the lotion on the hair and rub gently on to the head until the entire scalp is moistened. Pay special attention to the back of the neck and area behind the ears. Take care to avoid the eyes.
2. Allow the hair to dry naturally – use NO heat.
3. As all lice and eggs will have been killed the hair may be shampooed after 2 hours. If a residual effect is desired, however, it is recommended that shampooing be carried out after 12 hours.
4. While still wet, comb the hair with an ordinary comb. The fine-toothed Napp comb can then be used to remove the dead lice and eggs.

For pubic lice: Application and dosage etc. are as for the head. Apply the lotion to the pubic hair and the hair between the legs and around the anus. Allow to dry naturally using NO heat. Transient, mild stinging may be experienced due to the alcohol content.

For scabies:
1. Use cotton wool to apply lotion to all parts of the body except face and scalp.
2. Rub in well and allow to dry naturally. Do not bathe until 12 hours after treatment.

Contra-indications, warnings, etc Contains flammable alcohol. Apply and dry with care. Avoid naked flames or lighted objects. Do not use artificial heat (e.g. electric dryers). Dry in a well-ventilated room. Do not cover the head before the lotion has dried completely.

The alcohol content may cause wheezing in asthmatic patients and stinging or inflammation of the skin in people with severe eczema.

Children under the age of six months should be treated under medical supervision.

When Prioderm Lotion is used by a school nurse or other health officer in the mass treatment of large numbers of children, it is advisable that protective plastic or rubber gloves be worn.

Treatment of overdosage: In the event of deliberate or accidental ingestion, as for ethyl alcohol, empty stomach contents and keep patient warm. In the event of massive ingestion atropine and pralidoxime may be required to counteract cholinesterase inhibition.

Pharmaceutical precautions Store in a cool place protected from light.

Legal category P.

Package quantities Sprinkler-top bottle of 55 ml and 110 ml.

Further information The volatile alcoholic base used in Prioderm Lotion evaporates quickly leaving a high concentration of malathion on the hair. This is rapidly lethal to both lice and their eggs and may give several weeks' protection from reinfestation. For this protective effect to be optimal Prioderm Lotion should be left on the scalp for 12 hours before shampooing and no artificial heat used to dry the hair after shampooing.

Product licence number 0199/5002.

SEVREDOL* TABLETS 10 mg and 20 mg

Presentation
Sevredol Tablets 10 mg are blue, film coated, capsule shaped, biconvex tablets with a score line on one side. 'IR' is marked on the left side and '10' on the right. Each tablet contains 10 mg of Morphine Sulphate BP.
Sevredol Tablets 20 mg are pink, film coated, capsule shaped, biconvex tablets with a score line on one side. 'IR' is marked on the left side and '20' on the right. Each tablet contains 20 mg of Morphine Sulphate BP.

Uses Sevredol Tablets 10 mg and 20 mg are indicated for the relief of both acute and chronic, severe pain.

Dosage and administration
Adults and children over 12 years: Sevredol Tablets 10 mg and 20 mg should be used at 4-hourly intervals. The dosage is dependent upon the severity of the pain and the patients' previous history of analgesic requirements. A patient presenting with severe pain should normally be started on a dosage of one Sevredol Tablet 10 mg 4-hourly. Increasing severity of pain or tolerance to morphine will require increased dosage of Sevredol using 10 mg and 20 mg tablets alone or in combination to achieve the desired relief.

Patients receiving Sevredol Tablets in place of parenteral morphine should be given a sufficiently increased dosage to compensate for any reduction in analgesic effects associated with oral administration. Usually such increased requirement is of the order of 50% to 100%. In such patients individual dose adjustments are required.

When changing to MST Continus* Tablets the total daily (24 hours) mg dosage of Sevredol should be divided by 2 to give the 12 hourly dose.

Elderly: A reduction in adult dosage may be advisable.

Children: 3–5 years – 5 mg 4-hourly.
6–12 years – 5–10 mg 4-hourly.

Contra-indications, warnings, etc
Contra-indications: Respiratory depression, coma, obstructive airways disease, acute abdomen, known morphine sensitivity, acute hepatic disease, concurrent administration of mono-amine oxidase inhibitors or within two weeks of discontinuation of their use. Sevredol Tablets are not recommended for children under 3 years of age. Sevredol Tablets should be avoided in patients with raised intracranial pressure or head injury and also in patients with convulsive disorders or acute alcoholism.

Precautions: As with all narcotics, a reduction in dosage may be advised in the elderly, in hypothyroidism, in renal and chronic hepatic disease, adrenocortical insufficiency, prostatic hypertrophy, shock or reduced respiratory reserve. Sevredol Tablets are not recommended in the first 24 hours post-operatively. After this time, they should be used with caution particularly following abdominal surgery.

Pregnancy and lactation: Sevredol Tablets are not recommended in pregnancy or in the breast-feeding mother.

Warnings and adverse effects: Sevredol Tablets should not be used where there is the possibility of paralytic ileus occurring. Should paralytic ileus be suspected or occur during use, Sevredol Tablets should be discontinued immediately.

As with all morphine preparations, patients about to undergo cordotomy or other pain relieving surgical procedures should not receive Sevredol Tablets for 4 hours prior to surgery. If further treatment with Sevredol Tablets is indicated then dosage should be adjusted to the new post-operative requirement. Tolerance may occur with Sevredol Tablets. Urinary retention may also occur. When nausea and vomiting are troublesome, Sevredol Tablets can be readily combined with anti-emetics. It should be noted however, that morphine potentiates the effects of tranquillisers, anaesthetics, hypnotics and sedatives. As with all morphine preparations, constipation may occur which may be treated with appropriate laxatives.

Morphine may cause drowsiness and patients should not drive or operate machinery if so affected.

Overdosage: Signs of morphine toxicity and overdosage include pinpoint pupils, respiratory depression, and hypotension. Circulatory failure and deepening coma may occur in more severe cases.

Treatment of morphine overdosage: Administer naloxone 0.4 mg intravenously. Repeat at 2–3 minute intervals as necessary, or by an infusion of 2 mg in 500 ml of normal saline or 5% dextrose (0.004 mg/ml). The infusion should be run at a rate relative to the previous bolus doses administered and should be in accordance with the patient's response. The stomach should be emptied. A 0.02% aqueous solution of potassium permanganate may be used for lavage. Respiration should be assisted if necessary. Fluid and electrolyte levels should be maintained.

Pharmaceutical precautions Store at or below 30°C.

Legal category CD (Sch 2), POM.

Package quantities
Sevredol Tablets 10 mg: blister packs of 56 tablets (OP).
Sevredol Tablets 20 mg: blister packs of 56 tablets (OP).

Product licence numbers
Sevredol Tablets 10 mg 0337/0142
Sevredol Tablets 20 mg 0337/0143

TRILISATE* TABLETS

Presentation Pale orange, capsule shaped, scored tablets containing 500 mg salicylate as choline magnesium trisalicylate. The tablets embossed (NAPP) and '500' on one side and 'TRILISATE' on the reverse.

Uses Trilisate tablets are indicated for relief of the signs and symptoms of rheumatoid arthritis, osteoarthritis and other arthroses.

Dosage and administration (a) One or two tablets twice a day for osteoarthritis and mild to moderate arthroses.

(b) Two or three tablets twice a day for rheumatoid arthritis and the more severe arthroses.

For maintenance therapy the total daily dosage may be given as a single daily dosage.

Contra-indications, warnings, etc *Contra-indications:* Hypersensitivity to aspirin. Active peptic ulceration. Haemophilia.

Precautions; Concurrent administration with other analgesics containing aspirin. As with other salicylates, Trilisate tablets should be used with caution in patients with chronic renal insufficiency, or with erosive gastritis or peptic ulcer.

Trilisate tablets should be used with caution in pregnancy.

Warnings and adverse effects: May induce gastrointestinal haemorrhage. Reports indicate that when salicylates are given with steroids, the butazones or alcohol, the risk of gastrointestinal ulceration is increased.

Trilisate tablets are not recommended for children under twelve years of age. As with all medicines, Trilisate tablets should be kept out of reach of children.

Overdosage: Empty stomach contents and lavage stomach with 5% sodium bicarbonate solution. Severe overdosage should be treated by diuresis induced by intravenous saline with sodium bicarbonate, or dextrose solution. Electrolyte levels and acid base balance should be monitored and corrected as necessary.

Pharmaceutical precautions Trilisate tablets should be stored in a cool, dry place, protected from light.

Legal category P.

Package quantities Containers of 60 tablets.

Further information When Trilisate tablets are administered, the salicylate is absorbed rapidly and reaches peak blood levels within two hours. At recommended doses, the therapeutic range of 5 to 30 mg/100 ml is achieved, and a steady state condition is normally reached after 4–5 doses.

Trilisate tablets do not cause any significant faecal blood loss nor do they affect platelet aggregation.

Trilisate tablets do not cause any observable stomach mucosal irritation as determined by endoscopic examination.

Product licence number 0337/0053.

UNIPHYLLIN* CONTINUS* TABLETS 400 mg
UNIPHYLLIN* CONTINUS* TABLETS 300 mg
UNIPHYLLIN* PAEDIATRIC CONTINUS* TABLETS 200 mg

Presentation *Uniphyllin Continus tablets 400 mg* are white, capsule-shaped scored tablets with the logo (NAPP) U400 embossed on one side and 'UNIPHYLLIN' on the other. Each tablet contains Theophylline BP 400 mg in a patented controlled release system.

Uniphyllin Continus tablets 300 mg are white, capsule-shaped, scored tablets with U300 embossed on one side. Each tablet contains Theophylline BP 300 mg in a patented controlled release system.

Uniphyllin Paediatric Continus tablets 200 mg are white, capsule-shaped, scored tablets with U200 embossed on one side. Each tablet contains Theophylline BP 200 mg in a patented controlled release system.

Uses Theophylline is a bronchodilator. In addition it affects the function of a number of cells involved in the inflammatory processes associated with asthma and chronic obstructive airways disease. Of most importance may be enhanced suppressor T-lymphocyte activity and reduction of eosinophil and neutrophil function. These actions may contribute to anti-inflammatory prophylactic activity in asthma and chronic obstructive airways disease.

For the treatment and prophylaxis of bronchospasm associated with asthma, emphysema and chronic bronchitis. Also indicated in adults for the treatment of cardiac asthma and left ventricular or congestive cardiac failure.

Dosage and administration

N.B. Tablets should be swallowed whole and not chewed.

Children: Not recommended for children under 5 years of age. The maintenance dose is 9 mg/kg twice daily. Some children with chronic asthma require and tolerate much higher doses (10–16 mg/kg twice daily). Lower dosages (based on usual adult dose) may be required by adolescents.

Adults: The usual maintenance dose for elderly patients or those less than 70 kg body weight is 300 mg 12-hourly following an initial week of therapy on 200 mg 12-hourly.

The usual maintenance dose for patients of 70 kg body weight or over is 400 mg 12-hourly following an initial week of therapy on 300 mg 12-hourly.

It may be appropriate to administer a larger evening or morning dose in some patients, in order to achieve optimum therapeutic effect when symptoms are most severe, e.g. at the time of the 'morning dip' in lung function.

In patients whose night time or day time symptoms persist despite other therapy and who are not currently receiving theophylline, then the total daily requirement of Uniphyllin Continus tablets (as specified above) may be added to their treatment regimen as either a single evening or morning dose.

Elderly: The dose should be 200 mg 12-hourly increasing to 300 mg 12-hourly.

Dose titration: Patients vary in their response to xanthines and it may be necessary to titrate dosage individually. Steady state theophylline levels with 12-hourly dosing are generally attained 3–4 days after dose adjustment. If a satisfactory clinical response is not achieved, serum theophylline should be measured 6–8 hours after the last dose. Based on serum theophylline assay results, dosage should be titrated using the following as a guide:

Peak serum theophylline level	*Dosage adjustment to nearest 100 mg*
< 10 micrograms/ml	Increase total daily dose by half.
10–15 micrograms/ml	Increase total daily dose by one quarter if symptoms persist.
16–20 micrograms/ml	No adjustment required.
21–25 micrograms/ml	Decrease dose by one quarter.
26–30 micrograms/ml	Miss next dose and decrease maintenance dose by one half.

It is advisable to re-check serum theophylline concentration after dose adjustment, when steady state is attained.

Pharmacokinetics: In-vivo bioavailability studies have shown that the three strengths of Uniphyllin Continus tablets are equally bioavailable. It has also been demonstrated that twice-daily dosing produces minimal peak to trough variation and plasma theophylline levels can be maintained within the therapeutic range of 10–20 micrograms/ml throughout the 12-hour dosing interval.

Transferability: It is not possible to ensure bioequivalence between different sustained release theophylline products. Therefore, it should be emphasised that patients, once titrated to an effective dose, should not be changed from Uniphyllin Continus tablet preparations to other slow or sustained release xanthine preparations without re-titration and clinical assessment.

After an effective therapeutic regimen is attained, it is important that practitioners, pharmacists and patients be aware of the possible dangers of inefficacy or toxicity if an alternative sustained release theophylline preparation is substituted. This may be a particular hazard because the products are available without prescription. Likewise there may be a hazard if the doctor prescribes 'generically' or if the preparation used in hospital is unknown by the general practitioner.

Contra-indications, warnings, etc

Contra-indications: Should not be given concomitantly with ephedrine in children.

Warnings: Theophylline has been reported to interact with a number of drugs.

The following increase clearance and it may therefore be necessary to increase dosage to ensure a therapeutic effect: phenytoin, carbamazepine, rifampicin, sulphinpyrazone and barbiturates. Smoking and alcohol consumption can also increase clearance of theophylline.

The following reduce clearance and a reduced dosage may therefore be necessary to avoid side-effects: allupurinol, cimetidine, ciprofloxacin, erythromycin, thiabendazole, isoprenaline and oral contraceptives. Factors such as viral infections, liver disease and heart failure also reduce theophylline clearance. There are conflicting reports concerning the potentiation of theophylline by influenza vaccine and physicians should be aware that interaction may occur. A reduction of dosage may also be necessary in the elderly patient.

The hypokalaemia resulting from $Beta_2$ agonist therapy, steroids, diuretics and hypoxia may be potentiated by xanthines. Particular care is advised in patients suffering from severe asthma who require hospitalisation. It is recommended that serum potassium levels are monitored in such circumstances.

The following should also be used with caution in patients taking Uniphyllin Continus tablet preparations: halothane, lomustine and lithium.

Safety in human pregnancy has not been established. However, use during human pregnancy has been reported without teratogenicity or other adverse foetal effect. Theophylline crosses the placental barrier and is secreted in breast milk.

Side-effects: The risk of side-effects usually associated with theophylline and xanthine derivatives such as nausea, gastric irritation, headache and CNS stimulation is significantly reduced when Uniphyllin Continus tablet preparations are given. Furthermore, the side-effects can be minimised by dose titration downwards.

Overdosage: Empty stomach contents. Monitor electrocardiogram and maintain fluid balance. Oral activated medical charcoal has been found to reduce high theophylline blood levels. In severe poisoning employ charcoal-column haemoperfusion. Treat symptoms on appearance. The physician should be aware that tablets in the intestine will continue to release theophylline for a period of hours.

In the event of hypokalaemia, potassium chloride should be given by slow intravenous infusion. Repeated measurements of plasma potassium should be made.

Pharmaceutical precautions Store at room temperature in a dry place protected from light.

Legal category P.

Package quantities Uniphyllin Continus tablets 400 mg: Blister packs of 56 tablets (OP), containers of 250 and 1000 tablets.

Uniphyllin Continus tablets 300 mg: Blister packs of 56 tablets (OP) and containers of 250 tablets.

Uniphyllin Paediatric Continus tablets 200 mg: Blister packs of 56 tablets (OP).

Further information By incorporating theophylline in the patented Continus controlled release system, therapeutic blood levels of theophylline between 10 and 20 micrograms/ml can be maintained over a full 24 hour period on a simple twice daily dosage. The availability of 3 strengths of Uniphyllin Continus tablets permits ideal dosage flexibility. The Continus tablet formulation shows minimal tablet to tablet variation in theophylline release.

Product licence numbers
Uniphyllin Continus tablets 400 mg 0337/0074
Uniphyllin Continus tablets 300 mg 0337/0129
Uniphyllin Paediatric Continus tablets 200 mg 0337/0057

X-PREP* LIQUID

Presentation A chocolate-flavoured, brown liquid containing the Primolax* brand of purified, standardised extract of senna fruit equivalent to 72 mg total Sennosides in each 72 ml dose.

Uses A single-dose pre-radiographic purgative given the day prior to radiographic examination, particularly in gastro-intestinal and urological procedures.

Dosage and administration The following doses apply to all age groups:

Patients with bodyweight of 72 kgs or more – complete bottle, 72 ml (72 mg sennosides), should be taken between 2.00 and 4.00 pm on the day before the X-ray examination.

Patients with bodyweight of less than 72 kgs – dosage is 1 ml (1 mg sennosides) per kg bodyweight taken between 2.00 and 4.00 pm on the day before the X-ray examination.

In either case the dosage may be split into two equal volumes with one hour between each administration. Each administration should be followed by at least half a pint of water and the patient should drink a further half a pint of water every hour throughout the afternoon and evening.

Patients should be advised to expect a strong thorough bowel action to begin approximately six to eight hours later.

Contra-indications, warnings, etc
Contra-indications: The usual clinical contra-indications for purgatives apply to X-Prep Liquid. X-Prep Liquid should not be used in patients with bowel obstruction.

Warnings: Caution should be exercised in the elderly and in patients with inflammatory bowel disease or suspected diverticular disease.

As with all purgatives mild to severe griping and some nausea occasionally occur; however, these are generally less of a problem with X-Prep Liquid and are minimised by drinking at least the recommended volume of water.

A light, bland, fat-free meal should precede administration. No solid food should be taken after administration and nothing at all after 10.00 pm on the day before the X-ray examination.

In diabetic patients the doctor should be aware of the sugar content of X-Prep Liquid (47.52 g per 72 ml dose).

Overdosage: In the event of deliberate or accidental ingestion of large amounts where diarrhoea is severe, excessive loss of water and electrolytes may occur. Treatment is supportive with generous amounts of fluid. Electrolytes, especially potassium, should be monitored.

Pharmaceutical precautions Store in a cool, dry place protected from light.

Legal category P.

Package quantities Bottles containing 72 ml (OP).

Further information Nil.

Product licence number 0337/5017.

**Trade Mark*

Nicholas Laboratories Limited
PO Box 17
Slough
Berkshire SL1 4AU

ALBUCID* EYE DROPS 10%

Presentation Albucid Eye Drops 10% is a sterile solution containing 10% w/v Sulphacetamide Sodium PhEur. Cetrimide BP (0.01% w/v) is included as a preservative.

Uses Mild infections of the conjunctiva and eyelids. Industrial eye injuries. Prophylaxis against infection.

Dosage and administration All ages: 2–4 drops two to six hourly.

Contra-indications, warnings, etc
Contra-indications: Known sensitivity to sulphonamides.

Side-effects: Some transient irritation may occur.

Use in pregnancy: No special precautions required.

Overdosage: Not applicable.

Pharmaceutical precautions Store at room temperature (15–25°C). Do not freeze.

Legal Category POM.

Package quantities Opaque white polythene bottle with green cap, containing 10 ml of sterile solution.

Further information Nil.

Product licence number 0188/5912

ELECTROLADE* Banana
ELECTROLADE* Melon

Presentation Paper/aluminium foil sachet containing white free flowing powder, flavoured with banana or melon.
Each sachet contains:

Sodium chloride Ph.Eur	0.236 g
Potassium chloride Ph.Eur	0.300 g
Sodium bicarbonate Ph.Eur	0.500 g
Glucose Ph.Eur	4.000 g

Also contains: Saccharin sodium, flavourings.

Uses Oral replacement therapy of electrolyte and fluid loss in children and adults arising from dehydration associated with diarrhoea of various origins (including viral). Also a corrective treatment of dehydration associated with other feverish illnesses.

Dosage and administration
Reconstitution: Only with water and at the volume stated.

Adults and children: The contents of each sachet should be dissolved in approximately 200 ml of cool, fresh, clean drinking water. The resulting solution is both clear and colourless with an aroma of banana or melon.

Infants: The water should be boiled then cooled before reconstitution as above.

The reconstituted cooled solution should be used immediately and the unused remainder discarded, or stored in a refrigerator for no longer than 24 hours. Do not boil after reconstitution. The product must only be used at the recommended dilution.

Dosage: Oral fluid replacement and maintenance therapy must be tailored by the physician to individual patients needs. The volume of solution used will depend on the weight and age of the patient, using the basic principle of firstly rehydrating the patient by replacing lost fluid and thereafter maintaining fluid replacement in line with the volume of fluid lost from stools or vomiting plus normal daily requirements. As a basic guide, a daily intake of 150 ml/kg bodyweight for infants (under 2 years of age) or 100–120 ml/kg for adults and children is needed.

Replacement of fluid losses with Electrolade solution:
Infants (under 2 years of age): Reconstitute sachets according to directions and administer at 1–1½ times usual feed volume. No milk (other than breast milk) or solids should be given during the first 24 hours. In breast-fed infants, Electrolade should be given before the feed. The re-introduction of normal feeding should only take place when symptoms of diarrhoea are abating and should be added gradually to make up the total daily fluid requirements.

Children: One sachet after every loose motion, up to 12 sachets in 24 hours.

Adults: 1–2 sachets after every loose motion, up to 16 sachets in 24 hours.

Elderly persons: As for adults but care must be taken not to over-hydrate.

In adults and children Electrolade can be given in amounts necessary to satisfy thirst. As with infants, solids should be avoided during the first day, but may be gradually resumed as necessary during day 2.

It is extremely difficult to over-hydrate by mouth, thus when there is normal renal function it is better to give more Electrolade than less.

Pregnancy and lactation: The dose is the above adult dose. Breast feeding can be continued as normal.

If vomiting is a problem then Electrolade solution should be taken in frequent small volumes.

Contra-indications, warnings, etc There are no absolute contra-indications to using Electrolade. However, it would be unwise to give the solution where there is renal failure with oliguria or anuria, in acute abdominal patients prior to surgery or where parenteral therapy should be given.

The solution must be made up without adding extra sugar or salt. In treating diabetics with gastroenteritis, the sugar content must be noted.

Solutions of greater concentration may result in hypernatraemia. Those of greater dilution may result in inadequate replacement.

Overdosage: In oral electrolyte replacement therapy toxicity is rare in previously healthy people. In subjects with renal impairment, hypernatraemia and hyperkalaemia might occur. If these conditions occur, full biochemical profile under hospital conditions will be needed and the physician should take the appropriate measures.

Pharmaceutical precautions Electrolade should be stored in a dry place at 15–25°C.

Legal category P.

Package quantities Boxes of 4 and 20 sachets containing a patient information leaflet.

Further information A reconstituted solution of Electrolade (1 sachet/200 ml) has the following composition:

	mmol/l
Sodium	50
Potassium	20
Chloride	40
Bicarbonate	30
Dextrose	111

Because of Electrolade's palatability, there is a greater chance, particularly in younger children, of achieving a treatment success.

The sodium and glucose concentration should give optimum water replacement; solutions with higher concentrations reverse this process.

Potassium and bicarbonate included in the formula will replace the large amounts lost in diarrhoea and will combat metabolic acidosis.

Product licence numbers
Electrolade Banana 0188/0077
Electrolade Melon 0188/0101

GENTICIN* CREAM
GENTICIN* OINTMENT

Presentation Genticin Cream is a white, sterile cream which contains Gentamicin Sulphate PhEur≡0.3% w/w gentamicin base in a water-miscible base. Methylhydroxybenzoate PhEur and Butylhydroxybenzoate BP are included as preservatives.

Genticin Ointment is a colourless, sterile ointment which contains Gentamicin Sulphate PhEur≡0.3% w/w gentamicin base in a greasy base.

Uses For the topical treatment of primary bacterial skin infections.

Genticin Cream and Ointment are indicated in the treatment of gentamicin-sensitive bacterial skin infections, including impetigo, sycosis barbae, folliculitus, and infected wounds and ulcers. Dermatological use of gentamicin in the hospital environment should be restricted to treatment of bacteriologically proven pseudomonas or proteus infection.

Dosage and administration For all ages: Genticin Cream and Ointment are intended for topical use only and should be applied three to four times daily to the infected area, covering with a gauze dressing if necessary. Cream preparations are recommended for moist lesions and ointment for dry conditions.

Contra-indications, warnings, etc
Contra-indications: None, except in cases of known sensitisation to aminoglycoside antibiotics.

Other undesirable effects: Extended or recurrent application may increase the risk of contact sensitisation. The risk of inducing bacterial resistance should be borne in mind when gentamicin is used in a closed hospital environment.

Use in pregnancy: When gentamicin is administered systemically in pregnancy, the risk of foetal ototoxicity should be considered. Consideration should therefore also be given to the possibility of foetal ototoxicity when gentamicin is applied topically to lage denuded areas of skin.

Other special warnings and precautions: When gentamicin is applied topically to large denuded areas of skin, the small risk of ototoxicity from systemic absorption should be considered, especially in the elderly and in those with impaired renal function.

If irritation, sensitisation or super-infection develop, treatment with Gentamicin should be discontinued and appropriate therapy instituted.

Overdosage: Not applicable.

Pharmaceutical precautions Store at room temperature. Do not freeze.

In order to preserve the therapeutic activity of these products they should not be diluted.

Legal category POM.

Package quantities Genticin Cream and Ointment are each available in 15 g and 100 g tubes.

Further information Nil.

Product licence numbers
Genticin Cream 0188/5926R
Genticin Ointment 0188/5927R

GENTICIN* EYE/EAR DROPS

Presentation Gentamicin Sulphate PhEur≡0.3% w/v gentamicin base in a sterile, aqueous, isotonic solution in a 10 ml dropper bottle. Benzalkonium Chloride BP is included as preservative.

Uses Genticin (gentamicin) is a proven bactericidal antibiotic active against an extremely broad spectrum of Gram-positive and Gram-negative bacteria. Genticin Eye/Ear Drops are therefore particularly useful in superficial infections of the eye or ear caused by organisms sensitive to gentamicin, and for prophylaxis against infection in trauma of the eye or ear.

Dosage and administration For all ages:
Eyes: 1–2 drops instilled in affected eye up to six times a day or more frequently if required. (Severe infections may require one or two drops every fifteen to twenty minutes initially, reducing the frequency of instillation gradually as the infection is controlled.)

Ears: The area should be cleaned and 2–3 drops instilled three to four times a day and at night, or more frequently if required.

Contra-indications, warnings, etc
Contra-indications: Hypersensitivity to Gentamicin or to any of the ingredients. (Cross sensitivity with other aminoglycoside antibiotics may occur.)

Interactions with other medicaments: None relevant to topical use.

Effects on ability to drive and use machines: May cause transient blurring of vision. If affected do not drive or operate machinery.

Other undesirable effects: Hypersensitivity reactions, usually of the delayed type may occur with local treatment with gentamicin. Irritation, burning, stinging, itching and dermatitis may occur.

Use in pregnancy: Safety for use in pregnancy and lactation has not been established. Use only when considered essential by the physician.

Other special warnings and precautions: In severe infections topical use of gentamicin should be supplemented with appropriate systemic treatment.

Prolonged use should be avoided as it may lead to skin sensitisation and the emergence of resistant organisms.

Gentamicin may cause irreversible partial or total deafness when given systemically or when applied topically to open wounds or damaged skin. This effect is dose-related and is enhanced by renal or hepatic impairment. Although this effect has not been reported following topical ocular use the possibility should be considered when high dose topical treatment is given to small children or infants.

Topical application of aminoglycoside antibiotics into the middle ear carries a theoretical risk of causing hearing loss due to ototoxicity. The benefits of gentamicin therapy should be considered against the risk of infection itself causing hearing loss.

Contact lenses should be removed during the period of treatment.

Overdose: Not applicable. The oral ingestion of the contents of one bottle is unlikely to cause any significant adverse effect.

Pharmaceutical precautions Store at room temperature. Do not freeze.

Legal category POM.

Package quantities Genticin Eye/Ear Drops are available in 10 ml opaque, white, polythene dropper bottles with white plastic caps.

Further information Gentisone HC Ear Drops are also available where a mild steroid (Hydrocortisone Acetate

1.0% w/v) is required in addition to Genticin (gentamicin 0.3% w/v) to treat ear infections complicated by an inflammatory condition.

Product licence number 0188/5924R.

GENTICIN* EYE OINTMENT

Presentation Genticin Eye Ointment is a sterile, colourless ointment which contains Gentamicin Sulphate PhEur≡0.3% w/w gentamicin base in a greasy base.

Uses Genticin (gentamicin) is a proven bactericidal antibiotic active against an extremely broad spectrum of Gram-positive and Gram-negative bacteria. Genticin Eye Ointment is therefore particularly useful in external bacterial infections of the eye, where the bacterial organisms are often very varied.

In particular Genticin Eye Ointment is indicated in conjunctivitis, blepharitis, styes, corneal ulcers, and prophylaxis in trauma.

Dosage and administration For all ages: Genticin Eye Ointment should be applied three to four times daily to the infected eye.

Contra-indications, warnings, etc
Contra-indications: There are no specific contra-indications except in cases of true sensitivity to one of the ingredients.

Precautions: If irritation, sensitization or super-infection develop, treatment with Genticin should be discontinued and appropriate therapy instituted.

Overdosage: Not applicable.

Use in pregnancy: No additional precautions required.

Pharmaceutical precautions Store at room temperature. Do not freeze.

Legal category POM.

Package quantities Genticin Eye Ointment is available in 3g tubes.

Further information The wide range and degree of antibacterial activity of Genticin coupled with freedom from troublesome side effects make it particularly suitable for bacterial eye conditions where the pathogens involved or their sensitivity to antibiotics are unknown.

Product licence number 0188/0057.

GENTICIN* INJECTABLE

Presentation Each 2 ml multidose vial and snap-off ampoule contains a 2 ml solution of Gentamicin Sulphate PhEur≡80 mg gentamicin base. Methylhydroxybenzoate PhEur and Propylhydroxybenzoate PhEur are included as preservatives.

Uses Genticin (gentamicin) is a proven bactericidal antibiotic active against an extremely broad spectrum of Gram-positive and Gram-negative pathogens including *E. coli,* Klebsiella, Proteus, *Pseudomonas aeruginosa* and penicillin-resistant strains of *Staph. aureus.*

Indications for the use of Genticin are bacteraemia, septicaemia, urinary-tract infections, severe chest infections, severe neonatal infections and other systemic infections due to susceptible bacteria.

Dosage and administration Genticin is normally administered intramuscularly, but may be given intravenously if required.

If intravenous administration is necessary the normal intramuscular dose should be given as a bolus injection into the tubing of the giving set or directly into the venous system over a period of two to three minutes. Genticin should not be given as a slow infusion or mixed with other drugs before use (see below for incompatibilities).

With either intramuscular or intravenous administration the following dosage applies for normal renal function:

Adults: 3–4 mg/kg body weight daily in divided doses.
Typical doses:
Over 60 kg: 80 mg eight-hourly
Less than 60 kg: 60 mg eight-hourly

In cases of impaired renal function a reduction in dosage frequency is recommended. The following table is a guide to recommended dosage schedule.

Blood urea (mg/100 ml)	*Creatinine clearance (GFR) (ml/min)*	*Dose and frequency of administration*
<40	>70	80 mg† 8-hourly
40–100	30–70	80 mg† 12-hourly
100–200	10–30	80 mg† daily
>200	5–10	80 mg† every 48 hours
Twice-weekly intermittent haemodialysis	<5	80 mg† after dialysis

† 60 mg if body weight <60 kg.

Urinary-tract infections: As above.

Alternatively, if renal function is not impaired, 160 mg once daily may be used.

In life-threatening infections the frequency of dosage may need to be increased to six-hourly and the quantity of each dose may also be increased at the discretion of the clinician up to a total dosage of 5 mg/kg in 24 hours. In such cases it is advisable to monitor gentamicin serum levels.

Elderly persons: Adjust dosage according to weight and renal function. Periodic serum monitoring is desirable.

Children: In children and in neonates, it can be expected that serum levels will be lower than those found in adults at equivalent dosage per body weight.

The recommended paediatric dosage is therefore as follows:

Up to 12 years: 6.0 mg/kg in 24 hours in 3 equally divided doses (i.e. 2.0 mg/kg eight-hourly).

In infants up to two weeks this dosage should be given in 2 equally divided doses (i.e. 3.0 mg/kg 12-hourly).

Serum levels should preferably be monitored daily.

In neonates, infants and children, subsequent dosage will often need to be increased to achieve therapeutic serum levels. Peak levels should be measured about one hour after intramuscular or intravenous injection and should reach 4 micrograms/ml, but not exceed 10 micrograms/ml.

Contra-indications, warnings, etc
Contra-indications: There are no absolute contra-indications other than sensitivity to one of the ingredients, allergy to gentamicin and myasthenia gravis.

Interactions: The potential nephrotoxicity of cephalosporins may be increased in the presence of gentamicin and kidney monitoring is therefore recommended with this combination.

Frusemide and piretanide may potentiate the ototoxicity of gentamicin, and ethacrynic acid, which is ototoxic in its own right, should be avoided with gentamicin.

Neuromuscular blockade and respiratory paralysis have occasionally been reported from administration of aminoglycosides to patients who have received curare-type muscle relaxants during anaesthesia.

Bacteriostatic antibiotics may give an antagonistic interaction, but in some cases (e.g. with clindamycin and lincomycin) the disadvantage of antagonism may be outweighed by the addition of activity against anaerobic organisms.

Other undesirable effects: As with all aminoglycosides, at critical levels gentamicin exhibits toxicity. Nephrotoxicity may occur, resulting in a gradual reduction in creatinine clearance after about two weeks of treatment. This is rapidly reversed if the drug is withdrawn. Most cases have pre-existing renal disease or have received other nephrotoxic agents. With gentamicin the vestibular mechanism may be affected when serum levels of 10 micrograms/ml or when a trough level of 2 micrograms/

ml are exceeded. This is usually reversible if observed promptly and the dose adjusted. In the patient with normal renal function it is virtually impossible to achieve these levels at standard dosage.

Use in pregnancy and lactation: Although there is no animal evidence of teratogenicity, gentamicin crosses the placenta and there is a risk of ototoxicity in the foetus and gentamicin should only be used where the seriousness of the mother's condition justifies the risk.

Other special warnings and precautions: Where renal function is impaired through disease or old age the frequency, but not the amount, of each dose should be reduced according to the degree of impairment. Gentamicin is excreted by simple glomerular filtration, and dosage frequency may be predicted by assessing creatinine clearance rates or blood urea and reducing the frequency accordingly.

It is also advisable to check serum levels to confirm that peak (one hour) levels do not exceed 10 micrograms/ml and that trough levels (before next injection) do not exceed 2 micrograms/ml.

Overdose: Symptoms: dizziness, vertigo and hearing loss if overdose accidentally given parenterally. Treatment: if reaction severe consider haemodialysis.

Incompatibilities: In general mixing Genticin Injectable with other drugs prior to administration is not advised. In particular the following are incompatible in mixed solution: penicillins, cephalosporins, erythromycin, lipiphysan, heparins and sodium bicarbonate†.

Dilution in the body will obviate the danger of physical and chemical incompatibility and enable Genticin Injectable to be given concurrently with the drugs listed above either as a bolus injection into the drip tubing with adequate flushing, or at separate sites. However, in the case of carbenicillin and gentamicin they should only be given at separate sites.

Pharmaceutical precautions Genticin is a remarkably stable antibiotic and does not require to be kept under refrigerated conditions. Store at room temperature.

Legal category POM.

Package quantities Ampoules and vials are packed in boxes of 5.

Further information Nil.

Product licence number 0188/5905R.

† Carbon dioxide may be liberated on addition of the two solutions. Normally this will dissolve in the solution, but under some circumstances small bubbles may form.

GENTICIN* PURE POWDER

Approved name: Gentamicin Sulphate

Presentation Available as a sterile hygroscopic powder. The weight of powder will vary according to potency but will be approximately 1.8 g Gentamicin Sulphate PhEur ≡ 1 g gentamicin base (1 million units). Genticin Pure Powder is sterilised by irradiation.

Uses Genticin Pure Powder is supplied for the preparation of preservative-free solutions of gentamicin for intrathecal and intraventricular administration in meningitis and ventriculitis and other indications where a preservative free solution, or different concentrations are required.

Dosage and administration The recommended daily dose is 1 mg gentamicin base intrathecally or intraventricularly plus 2–4 mg/kg/day intramuscularly in three equally divided doses at eight hourly intervals in adult patients.

In children the supportive dosage is: Up to 12 years: 6.0 mg/kg in 24 hours in three equally divided doses (i.e. 2.0 mg/kg eight hourly). In infants up to two weeks this doage should be given in two equally divided doses (i.e. 3.0 mg/kg 12 hourly).

Elderly persons: No special dosage regimen required.

The intraventricular/inthrathecal dose may need to be increased at the discretion of the clinician to obtain adequate CSF levels which can be controlled by assay, particularly if a severe degree of hydrocephalus is present. Treatment should continue until the CSF is shown to be bacteriologically clear.

Contra-indications, warnings, etc

Contra-indications: There are no absolute contra-indications other than sensitivity to one of the ingredients, allergy to gentamicin and myasthenia gravis.

Interactions: The potential nephrotoxicity of cephalosporins may be increased in the presence of gentamicin and kidney monitoring is therefore recommended with this combination.

Frusemide and piretanide may potentiate the ototoxicity of gentamicin, and ethacrynic acid, which is ototoxic in its own right, should be avoided with gentamicin.

Neuromuscular blockade and respiratory paralysis have occasionally been reported from administration of aminoglycosides to patients who have received curare-type muscle relaxants during anaesthesia.

Bacteriostatic antibiotics may give an antagonistic interaction, but in some cases (e.g. with clindamycin and lincomycin) the disadvantage of antagonism may be outweighed by the addition of activity against anaerobic organisms.

Other undesirable effects: As with all aminoglycosides, at critical levels gentamicin exhibits toxicity. Nephrotoxicity may occur, resulting in a gradual reduction in creatinine clearance after about two weeks of treatment. This is rapidly reversed if the drug is withdrawn. Most cases have pre-existing renal disease or have received other nephrotoxic agents. With systemic gentamicin the vestibular mechanism may be affected when serum levels of 10 micrograms/ml or when a trough level of 2 micrograms/ml are exceeded. This is usually reversible if observed promptly and the dose adjusted. In the patient with normal renal function it is virtually impossible to achieve these levels at standard dosage. Local ventricular inflammation may give rise to radiculitis.

Use in pregnancy and lactation: Although there is no animal evidence of teratogenicity, gentamicin crosses the placenta and there is a risk of ototoxicity in the foetus and gentamicin should only be used where the seriousness of the mother's condition justifies the risk.

Other special warnings and precautions: Where renal function is impaired through disease or old age the frequency, but not the amount, of each dose by the systemic route should be reduced according to the degree of impairment. Gentamicin is excreted by simple glomerular filtration, and dosage frequency may be predicted by assessing creatinine clearance rates or blood urea and reducing the frequency accordingly.

It is also advisable to check serum levels to confirm that peak (one hour) levels do not exceed 10 micrograms/ml and that trough levels (before next injection) do not exceed 2 micrograms/ml.

Overdose: Symptoms: dizziness, vertigo and hearing loss if overdose accidentally given parenterally. Treatment: if reaction severe consider haemodialysis.

Incompatibilities: In general mixing genticin with other drugs prior to systemic administration is not advised. In particular the following are incompatible in mixed solution: penicillins, cephalosporins, erythromycin, lipiphysan, heparins and sodium bicarbonate.

Dilution in the body will obviate the danger of physical and chemical incompatibility and enable systemic genticin to be given concurrently with the drugs listed above either as a bolus injection into the drip tubing with adequate flushing, or at separate sites. However, in the case of carbenicillin and gentamicin they should only be given at separate sites.

Pharmaceutical precautions Genticin Pure Powder should be stored at room temperature.

Care should be taken after the container has been opened to replace the stopper immediately.

Genticin Pure Powder may be dissolved in water or in normal saline for injection purposes in order to obtain a preservative-free solution. This should be sterilised before use, preferably by membrane filtration.

Legal category POM.

Package quantities Genticin Pure Powder is available in vials containing 1 g or 0.5 g sterile gentamicin base.

Further information The package leaflet contained in every pack gives a suggested method for the preparation of intrathecal injection based on 1 mg of gentamicin base per 1 ml.

Product licence number 0188/5906R.

GENTISONE* HC CREAM
GENTISONE* HC OINTMENT

Presentation Gentisone HC Cream is a sterile, white cream which contains Hydrocortisone Acetate PhEur 1.0% w/w, and Gentamicin Sulphate PhEur≡0.3% w/w gentamicin base in a water-miscible base. Methylhydroxybenzoate PhEur and Butylhydroxybenzoate BP are included as preservatives.

Gentisone HC Ointment is a colourless, sterile ointment which contains Hydrocortisone Acetate PhEur 1.0% w/w and Gentamicin Sulphate PhEur≡0.3% w/w gentamicin base in a greasy base.

Uses Genticin has been combined with 1.0% w/w hydrocortisone for the topical treatment of those inflammatory skin conditions where gentamicin-sensitive secondary bacterial infections may be involved.

Gentisone HC Cream and Ointment are indicated particularly in infective eczemas (infantile, atopic, allergic, seborrhoeic, etc), infective contact dermatitis, otitis externa, and infected pruritus.

Dermatological use of gentamicin in the hospital environment should be restricted to treatment of bacteriologically proven pseudomonas or proteus infection.

Dosage and administration For all ages: Gentisone HC Cream and Ointment are intended for topical use only and should be applied three to four times daily to the infected area, covering with a gauze dressing if necessary. Cream preparations are recommended for moist lesions and ointment for dry conditions.

Contra-indications, warnings, etc
Contra-indications: Primary bacterial infections. Known sensitisation to aminoglycoside antibiotics.

Other undesirable effects: In infants, adrenal suppression can occur even without occlusion. In the closed hospital environment, inducing bacterial resistance is a risk.

Use in pregnancy and lactation: Foetal ototoxicity could occur when gentamicin is applied topically to large denuded areas of skin. Topical administration of corticosteroids to pregnant animals can cause abnormalities of foetal development and there is therefore a very small risk of such effects in the human foetus.

Other special warnings and precautions: If irritation, sensitisation or super-infection develop treatment with Gentisone HC Cream or Ointment should be discontinued and appropriate therapy instituted. Long term continuous topical therapy should be avoided. In the elderly or those with impaired renal function there is a small risk of ototoxicity from systemic absorption when gentamicin is administered topically to large denuded areas of skin.

Overdosage: Not applicable.

Pharmaceutical precautions Store at room temperature. Do not freeze.

In order to preserve the therapeutic activity of these products they should not be diluted.

Legal category POM.

Package quantities Gentisone HC Cream and Ointment are available in tubes of 15 g.

Further information Nil.

Product licence numbers

Gentisone HC Cream	0188/5922R
Gentisone HC Ointment	0188/5928R

GENTISONE* HC EAR DROPS

Presentation Gentamicin Sulphate PhEur≡0.3% w/v gentamicin base plus Hydrocortisone Acetate PhEur 1.0% w/v in a sterile aqueous suspension in a 10 ml polythene dropper bottle. Benzalkonium Chloride BP is included as preservative.

Uses Genticin (gentamicin) is a proven bactericidal antibiotic active against an extremely broad spectrum of Gram-positive and Gram-negative bacteria. Gentisone HC Ear Drops are therefore particularly useful in combating bacterial infections of the ear where the offending organisms are often varied and difficult to identify.

Gentisone HC Ear Drops are indicated for the treatment of eczema and infection of the outer ear (otitis externa), for prophylaxis against otitis externa following trauma, for post-operative local use in surgery to infected mastoid cavities, and in chronic suppurative otitis media.

Dosage and administration For all ages: The area should be cleaned and 2–4 drops instilled three to four times a day and at night. In middle ear infections the cavity may be filled with drops.

Contra-indications, warnings, etc
Contra-indications: The topical application of gentamicin as with other aminoglycosides in chronic suppurative otitis media carries a theoretical risk of causing a decrease in hearing perception; however the benefits of treating with gentamicin should be weighed against the risk of the chronic infection itself causing hearing loss. There are no other specific contra-indications except in cases of true sensitivity to one of the ingredients.

Other undesirable effects: Prolonged use of an anti-infective may result in the development of super-infection due to organisms becoming resistant to the anti-infective. In infants, adrenal suppression can occur even without occlusion.

Use in pregnancy and lactation: Topical administration of any corticosteroid to pregnant animals can cause abnormalities of foetal development. The relevance of this finding to human beings has not been established. However, topical steroids should not be used extensively in pregnancy, i.e. in large amounts or for prolonged periods.

Other special warnings and precautions: If irritation, sensitisation or super-infection develop treatment with Gentisone HC should be discontinued and appropriate therapy instituted. Long term continuous topical therapy should be avoided.

Overdosage: Not applicable.

Pharmaceutical precautions Store at room temperature. Do not freeze.

Legal category POM.

Package quantities Gentisone HC Ear Drops are available in 10 ml opaque white polythene dropper bottles with orange plastic caps.

Further information Genticin Eye/Ear Drops are also available where a plain antibiotic solution is required for topical application, for example, in the treatment of simple infections of the eye and ear.

Product licence number 0188/5925R.

HAMARIN* 100 TABLETS
HAMARIN* 300 TABLETS

Presentation Hamarin 100 – White biconvex tablets, engraved on one side with a break-line and 'Hamarin' and '100', and with a triangle logo on the other side. Each tablet contains Allopurinol BP 100 mg.

Hamarin 300 – White biconvex tablets, engraved on one side with a break-line and 'Hamarin' and '300', and with a triangle logo on the other side. Each tablet contains Allopurinol BP 300 mg.

Uses Gout: Primary hyperuricaemia.

Secondary hyperuricaemia: Prophylaxis of uric acid and calcium oxalate stones.

Dosage and administration *Adults:* The initial dose should be in the range 100–300 mg per day, as a single daily dose. The dose should be adjusted by monitoring serum uric acid levels at appropriate intervals, until the desired effect is achieved, which may take one to three weeks.

The maintenance dose is normally 200–600 mg per day. It is rarely found necessary to exceed 900 mg per day. Doses in excess of 300 mg should be administered in divided doses.

Dosage in impaired renal function, and renal dialysis: Allopurinol and its metabolites are excreted via the kidney. Impairment of kidney function may lead to retention of the drug and its metabolites, with consequent prolongation of action. The amount and frequency of dosage may need to be reduced, as indicated by monitoring serum uric acid levels.

Allopurinol and metabolites are removed by dialysis. The table below gives recommended doses for adults.

Creatinine clearance	*Dose*
>20 ml/minute	Standard dose
10–20 ml/minute	100–200 mg/day
<10 ml/minute	100 mg/day, or at longer intervals.
Renal dialysis	300–400 mg after each dialysis (none in the interim).

Children: Dosage should be in the range 10–20 mg/kg/day. Use in children is indicated largely in leukaemia and other malignant conditions, and enzyme disorders such as Lesch-Nyhan syndrome.

Elderly persons: Use of allopurinol in elderly persons should take full cognizance of the increased risk of renal or hepatic impairment in such patients, and the dose should be reduced accordingly.

Contra-indications, warnings, etc

Contra-indications: Acute gout. Known intolerance of allopurinol.

Precautions: Treatment with allopurinol should not be started during an acute attack of gout. Prophylactic therapy with allopurinol may be started when the acute attack has completely subsided; anti-inflammatory agents should be given concurrently.

Dosage should be reduced in patients with renal or hepatic disorders.

Fluid intake should ensure adequate urinary output.

Use in pregnancy and lactation: There is no evidence that allopurinol taken orally in humans causes foetal abnormalities. However, allopurinol should be used with caution in pregnancy. Allopurinol has been associated with foetal abnormalities in mice after intraperitoneal administration, but oral administration in animals has shown no such effects.

There is no data on the excretion of allopurinol and metabolites in breast milk.

Drug interactions: When administered concurrently with allopurinol the dose of 6-mercaptopurine and azathioprine should be reduced to one quarter of the usual dose. The activity of these drugs is prolonged by inhibition of xanthine oxidase.

The possibility of interaction with anti-coagulants whose activity may be enhanced should be borne in mind when allopurinol is concurrently administered. Prothrombin times should be checked.

There may be an increased risk of prolonged hypoglycaemic activity when allopurinol is administered with chlorpropamide, in patients with impaired renal function.

Allopurinol may interact with uricosuric agents.

Adverse effects: Adverse effects are usually rare and mainly of a minor nature. They are more common in patients with renal impairment.

An acute attack of gouty arthritis may be precipitated during the early stages of treatment with allopurinol. (See initiation of therapy).

Skin reactions: Skin reactions are the most common adverse effect, and may occur at any time during treatment. They may be pruritic, maculopapular, sometimes scaly or purpuric and, rarely, exfoliative.

Allopurinol should be withdrawn immediately should such reactions occur.

After recovery from mild skin reactions, allopurinol may be re-introduced at low dose (e.g. 50 mg/day); this may be gradually increased.

If the rash recurs, allopurinol should be withdrawn immediately and permanently.

General hypersensitivity: Skin reactions may rarely be associated with exfoliation, fever, lymphadenopathy, arthralgia and eosinophilia.

In such cases, allopurinol should be withdrawn immediately and permanently.

Corticosteroids may be beneficial in treating such reactions, which occur usually in patients with pre-existing hepatic or renal disorders.

Gastro-intestinal disorders: Nausea and vomiting can be avoided by taking allopurinol after meals.

Blood and lymphatic system: Transient reduction in the numbers of blood cells and platelets have been occasionally reported, usually in association with hepatic and/or renal disorder. The clinical significance has yet to be demonstrated.

Miscellaneous: In conditions which give rise to an increased miscible urate pool (e.g. malignant disease and its treatment, Lesch-Nyhan syndrome), allopurinol rarely leads to tissue deposition of xanthine. High fluid intake and alkalinisation should ensure adequate urinary output. Xanthine crystals seen in muscle tissue of patients receiving allopurinol appear to have no clinical significance.

The following have been reported, but do not have a clear cause and effect relationship with administration of allopurinol: nausea, vomiting, abdominal pain, diarrhoea, alopecia, headache, drowsiness, general malaise, granulomatous hepatitis, hepatic necrosis, cataracts, visual disorders, macular changes, impotence, diabetes, furunculosis, hypertension, haematuria, oedema.

Initiation of therapy: In common with uricosuric agents, allopurinol may precipitate an acute attack of gouty arthritis during the early stages of treatment. It is therefore advisable to give concurrently a suitable anti-inflammatory agent, or colchicine, for at least one month.

Use with uricosuric agents: Allopurinol may be given concurrently with uricosuric agents; this may be useful in patients with large tophaceous deposits. The possibility of interactions between allopurinol and uricosuric agents, perhaps necessitating dosage adjustment of one or both drugs, should be borne in mind.

When changing from uricosuric therapy to allopurinol, one to three weeks overlap of treatments is advisable, to ensure continuous hypouricaemic effect.

Use with cytotoxic drugs: When used to prevent uric acid nephropathy in neoplastic conditions, allopurinol treatment should be started before cytotoxic therapy.

When allopurinol is administered concurrently with 6-mercaptopurine or azathioprine, only one quarter of the usual dose of cytotoxic agent should be given. There is no unequivocal evidence that allopurinol potentiates the action of other cytotoxic drugs.

Interference with tests: Allopurinol has been reported to interfere with liver function tests.

Toxicity and treatment of overdosage: The most likely effect of overdosage is gastro-intestinal disturbance.

Massive absorption of allopurinol may lead to marked xanthine oxidase inhibition. This should have no untoward effect, unless 6-mercaptopurine and/or azathioprine is being taken concurrently, when the activity of these drugs may be increased.

Adequate hydration to maintain diuresis facilitates excretion of allopurinol and its metabolites.

Dialysis may rarely be needed if clinically appropriate.

Pharmaceutical precautions Store in a cool dry place.

Legal category POM.

Package quantities Hamarin 100: Containers of 100 tablets.
Hamarin 300: Containers of 30 tablets.

Further information Hamarin may also be used in the treatment of hyperuricaemia that may be associated with neoplastic disease or its treatment, enzyme disorders, especially the Lesch-Nyhan syndrome, diuretic therapy and psoriasis.

Product licence numbers Hamarin 100: 0188/0068.
Hamarin 300: 0188/0069.

MICROPAQUE* HD

Presentation A fine white powder which, when reconstituted with water, produces a suspension with a bland taste of vanilla, containing 96% w/w Barium Sulphate PhEur.

Uses Double contrast radiological investigations of the gastrointestinal tract.

Dosage and administration Micropaque HD Powder must be reconstituted before use by adding water.

A table of dilutions is provided to enable the user to select the concentration most suited to their technique.

% w/v Barium sulphate	*Water (mls)*	*Final volume (mls)*
200	93	168
210	85	160
220	78	153
230	71	146
240	65	140

As a guide, findings indicate that a concentration of between 230 and 240% will give optimum results.

Optimum dispersion is obtained by shaking for approximately one minute.

Although the volume of suspension used will depend on the patient, the procedure and technique involved, the following dosages of Micropaque HD represent a basic guide to the quantities suitable for routine examinations of the upper gastrointestinal tract.

Barium swallow	40–60 ml
Double contrast stomach and duodenum examination	100–150 ml
Follow-through examination of the small bowel	150–250 ml

Elderly persons: No special dosage regimen is required, but care should be taken to observe the contra-indications and warnings below.

Contra-indications, warnings, etc Perforation of any region of the gastrointestinal tract and intestinal obstruction. Pyloric stenosis might be considered as a contra-indication to the use of barium sulphate. Administration of a barium enema should proceed with particular care in patients with existing intestinal disease, in children, the elderly or the debilitated. In choosing the route of administration, the possibility of actual or incipient bowel obstruction should be borne in mind.

Overdosage: Not applicable.

Use in pregnancy: Micropaque is not absorbed.

Pharmaceutical precautions Store at room temperature in a dry place. Micropaque HD should be used as soon as possible after reconstitution and in any event within two hours of adding water.

Legal category P.

Package quantities 500 ml polypropylene beaker containing 350 g barium sulphate (96% w/w).

Further information Micropaque HD produces a high density, low viscosity suspension on reconstitution that is especially designed for double contrast examinations of the upper gastrointestinal tract. It should be used in conjunction with a compatible gas producing agent such as Nicholas CO_2 Granules.

Product licence number 0188/0055.

MICROPAQUE* STANDARD

Presentation A creamy-white suspension with a bland characteristic taste of butterscotch/vanilla, containing 100% w/v Barium Sulphate PhEur.

Uses Radiological investigations of the gastro-intestinal tract.

Dosage and administration *Adults: Oesophagus:* Use 40–60 mls of undiluted Micropaque Standard orally as required. For prolonged adhesion use Microtrast Oesophageal Paste.

Stomach and duodenum: To demonstrate the mucosal pattern use up to 50 ml of undiluted Micropaque Standard orally. Follow this with a further 100 ml of Micropaque Standard diluted with 100 ml of water for demonstration of stomach distension and emptying function. If this biphased technique is not used, 150 ml of Micropaque Standard diluted with 50 ml of water may be given.

Small intestine: Use 100 ml of Micropaque Standard diluted with 150 ml of water or follow through from stomach examination.

Colon: For examination by barium enema using the filled colon technique, use 1 volume of Micropaque Standard to 2 volumes of water made up to the required quantity. For double contrast studies use 1–2 volumes of Micropaque Standard to 1 volume of water. 400 ml total volume is usually sufficient. An important pre-requisite is a thorough cleansing preparation of the colon and an examination time of preferably not greater than 15 minutes.

Children: No children's dosage is recommended as such investigations in children are rare and specialised. The dosage will therefore be tailored by the radiologist to suit the special requirements in each case.

Elderly persons: No special dosage regimen required, but care should be taken to observe the contra-indications and warnings below.

Contra-indications, warnings, etc Perforation of any region of the gastro-intestinal tract. Intestinal obstruction. Pyloric stenosis might be considered as a contra-indication to the use of barium sulphate preparations. Administration of a barium enema should proceed with particular care in patients with existing intestinal disease, in children, the elderly or the debilitated. In choosing the route of administration, the possibility of actual or incipient bowel obstruction should be borne in mind.

Overdosage: Not applicable.

Use in pregnancy: Micropaque is not absorbed.

Pharmaceutical precautions Shake before use.

Store at room temperature. Do not freeze. A light brown supernatant layer may appear and is quite normal. It will disappear when the bottle is shaken.

Legal category P.

Package quantities Plastic bottles containing 250 ml and 2 litres.

Further information Nil.

Product licence number 0188/5903R.

NEO MERCAZOLE* 5
NEO MERCAZOLE* 20

Presentation *Neo Mercazole 5:* Pale pink, circular shallow convex compression-coated tablets, containing a white core. The tablets are impressed with a tear-drop symbol enclosing the letters "BS" on one side, and a figure "5" on the other side. Neo Mercazole 5 contains 5 mg Carbimazole BP.

Neo Mercazole 20: Pink, circular shallow convex compression-coated tablets, containing a white core. The tablets are impressed with a tear-drop symbol enclosing the letters "BS" on one side, and a figure "20" on the other side. Neo Mercazole 20 contains 20 mg Carbimazole BP.

Uses Neo Mercazole is an anti-thyroid agent. It is indicated in all conditions where reduction of thyroid function is required.

1. Hyperthyroidism.
2. Preparation for thyroidectomy in hyperthyroidism.
3. Preparation for, and as concomitant therapy with, radio-iodine treatment.

Dosage and administration
Adults: The initial dose is in the range 20–60 mg, taken as two-three divided doses. This is continued until the patient is euthyroid. Subsequent therapy may then be administered in one of two ways.

(i) *Maintenance regime:* Dosage is gradually reduced so as to maintain a euthyroid state. Final dosage is usually in the range 5–15 mg per day, which may be taken as a single daily dose. Therapy should be continued for at least six, and up to eighteen months.

(ii) *Blocking-replacement regime:* Dosage is maintained at the initial level i.e. 20–60 mg per day, and supplemental l-thyroxine, 50–150 micrograms per day, is administered concomitantly, in order to prevent hypothyroidism. Therapy should be continued for at least six months, and up to eighteen months.

Children: The usual initial daily dose is 15 mg per day.

Elderly persons: No special dosage regime is required, but care should be taken to observe the contra-indications and warnings below.

Contra-indications, warnings, etc
Contra-indications: Previous history of adverse reactions to carbimazole.

Warnings: Patients should be warned about the onset of sore throats, mouth ulcers or other manifestations which might suggest the early development of bone marrow depression. In such cases it is important that drug treatment is stopped and medical advice sought immediately. Early withdrawal of the drug will increase the chance of complete recovery. Carbimazole should be stopped temporarily at the time of administration of radio-iodine.

Pregnancy: Carbimazole crosses the placenta, but provided that the mother's dose is within the standard range, and her thyroid status is monitored, there is no evidence of neo-natal thyroid abnormalities. Studies have shown that the incidence of congenital malformations is greater in the children of mothers whose hyperthyroidism has remained untreated than in those to whom treatment with carbimazole has been given. However, treatment with carbimazole has been associated very rarely with aplasia cutis in the neonate. The dose of Neo Mercazole must be regulated by the patient's clinical condition. The lowest dose possible should be used, and this should not exceed 15 mg per day in the last trimester. Neo Mercazole can often be discontinued three to four weeks before term, in order to reduce the risk of neo-natal complications. The blocking-replacement regime should not be used during pregnancy since very little thyroxine crosses the placenta in the last trimester. Carbimazole is secreted in breast milk, and the patient should not breast feed her baby whilst taking the drug.

Adverse effects: Adverse reactions usually occur in the first eight weeks of treatment. The most common minor reactions are nausea, headache, arthralgia, mild gastric distress, skin rashes and pruritis. Hair loss has been occasionally reported. These reactions are usually self-limiting, and may not require withdrawal of the drug.

Bone marrow depression has been reported and can lead to agranulocytosis. Patients should always be instructed to recognise symptoms which may suggest bone marrow depression, to stop the drug and to seek immediate medical advice.

Overdosage: No symptoms are likely from a single large dose, and so no specific treatment is indicated.

Pharmaceutical precautions Store at room temperature.

Legal category POM.

Package quantities
Neo Mercazole 5: Containers of 100 and 500 tablets.
Neo Mercazole 20: Containers of 100 tablets.

Further information Nil.

Product licence numbers
Neo Mercazole 5: 0188/5907R
Neo Mercazole 20: 0188/0081

NICHOLAS CO_2 GRANULES

Presentation Sachet containing:

Betaine hydrochloride	1830.0 mg
Sodium Bicarbonate PhEur	1000.0 mg
Dimethicone BPC	75.0 mg

Uses Gas producing agent for double contrast radiography of the gastro-intestinal tract.

Each sachet generates approximately 267 ml CO_2.

Dosage and administration 1–2 sachets as required per examination. Each sachet should be administered with a little water or barium suspension at the beginning of the examination.

The films should be taken as rapidly as possible after coating of the stomach wall with barium suspension, and the patient should be instructed to suppress eructation for as long as possible.

Elderly persons: No special dosage regimen required.

Contra-indications, warnings, etc There are no specific contra-indications.

Use in pregnancy: No special precautions.

Overdosage: not applicable.

Pharmaceutical precautions Store in a cool, dry place.

Legal category P.

Package quantities Supplied in boxes of 10 sachets.

Further information Nicholas CO_2 Granules contain a defoaming agent which reduces excessive bubbling during formation of gas and enhances the visualisation of mucosal detail.

Product licence number 0188/0007.

PALAPRIN FORTE*

Presentation Pale orange, oval tablets, with the letter 'P' impressed on one face. The other face has a break-line across the short axis. Each tablet contains Aloxiprin BP 600 mg, equivalent to aspirin 500 mg.

Uses As an analgesic/anti-inflammatory agent in rheumatoid arthritis, osteo-arthritis, various forms of spondylitis and other 'rheumatic' conditions where high dosage salicylate therapy is indicated.

Dosage and administration *Adults:* Usual dose 300–1200 mg, up to four times a day (max 4.8 g per day). In acute rheumatic conditions, up to 9.6 g per day, in divided doses.

In order to ensure the maintenance of plasma salicylate levels adequate for anti-inflammatory, as well as analgesic effect, dosage may be calculated on a body-weight basis, at the rate of one tablet (600 mg) per 6 kg body weight per day, in divided doses.

Dosage should be carefully controlled, and in conditions where high dosage therapy is used, e.g. Still's disease, plasma salicylate levels should be monitored.

The tablets should preferably be dispersed in water

before administration, but can be chewed, sucked or swallowed whole with a draught of water.

Children up to age 12: Not to be given to children under 12, except on medical advice. In acute rheumatic conditions, dosage is calculated on a body weight basis, at the rate of 100 mg/kg per day, in divided doses.

Elderly persons: No special dosage regimen required but exercise caution where renal function is impaired.

Contra-indications, warnings, etc
Contra-indications: Palaprin Forte, as other aspirin products, is contra-indicated in patients with active peptic ulceration, haemophilia, or who have hypersensitivity to aspirin. High doses of Palaprin Forte are contra-indicated during breast-feeding, because of the theoretical risk of affecting clotting mechanisms.

Precautions and warnings: Aspirin may precipitate bronchospasm, and induce asthmatic attacks in susceptible subjects; it may induce gastro-intestinal haemorrhage, occasionally major, and may cause constipation and tinnitus at high doses. Should tinnitus occur, dosage should be reduced.

Drug interactions: Aspirin may enhance the effects of anti-coagulants, and may inhibit the action of uricosuric agents.

Use in pregnancy: There is clinical and epidemiological evidence of safety of aspirin in pregnancy, but it may prolong labour and contribute to maternal and neo-natal bleeding, and so is best avoided during the week prior to anticipated onset of labour.

Overdosage: Gastric lavage, forced alkaline diuresis and supportive therapy may be employed. Restoration of acid-base balance may be necessary.

Pharmaceutical precautions Store at room temperature.

Legal category P.

Package quantities Containers of 250 tablets.

Further information In high dosage aspirin has a uricosuric effect, and may reduce plasma bicarbonate, and prolong prothrombin time.
Aloxiprin releases salicylate largely in the small intestine, thereby reducing the likelihood of salicylate induced dyspepsia.

Product licence number 0188/5011R.

PLATET* 100

Presentation Round, white bevelled edge tablets. Each tablet contains Aspirin PhEur 100 mg in an effervescent base.

Uses Platet 100 inhibits platelet aggregation and is indicated for use in patients following aorto-coronary bypass surgery to prevent graft occlusion.

Dosage and administration Platet 100 tablets should be dissolved in water before administration. Following aortocoronary bypass surgery, treatment should commence within 36 hours.

Adults: One tablet to be taken daily, at the same time each day.

Elderly persons: No special dosage regimen required.

Children: Contra-indicated in children under 12 because of a possible association between Reye's syndrome and use of aspirin in feverish children.

Contra-indications, warnings, etc
Contra-indications: Platet 100, as other aspirin products, is contra-indicated in patients with active peptic ulceration, haemophilia and other bleeding disorders, or who have hypersensitivity to aspirin.

Precautions and warnings: Aspirin may precipitate bronchospasm, and induce asthmatic attacks in susceptible subjects; it may induce gastro-intestinal haemorrhage, occasionally major. It should be used with caution in subjects with gout.

Drug interactions: Aspirin may enhance the effects of anti-coagulants.

Use in pregnancy: There is clinical and epidemiological evidence of safety of aspirin in pregnancy, but it may prolong labour and contribute to maternal and neo-natal bleeding, therefore discontinue use one week before planned delivery or onset of labour.

Overdosage: Overdosage is unlikely, owing to the low dose of aspirin in Platet 100. If necessary gastric lavage, forced alkaline diuresis and supportive therapy may be employed. Restoration of acid-base balance may be necessary.

Pharmaceutical precautions Store in a dry place, at room temperature.

Legal category P.

Package quantities Platet 100 tablets are individually packed in aluminium foil, in cartons of 30 tablets.

Further information Nil.

Product licence number 0188/0092.

PLATET* 300

Presentation Round, white bevelled edge tablets. Each tablet contains Aspirin PhEur 300 mg in an effervescent base.

Uses To reduce the risk of myocardial infarction in patients with unstable angina or who have had a previous myocardial infarction. To reduce the risk of occlusive stroke and recurrent transient cerebral ischaemic attacks in patients with a history of such thrombotic events.

Dosage and administration Platet 300 tablets should be dissolved in water before administration. Following a primary myocardial infarction, treatment should commence as soon as possible.

Adults: One tablet to be taken daily, at the same time each day.

Elderly persons: No special dosage regimen required.

Children: Contra-indicated in children under 12 because of a possible association between Reye's syndrome and use of aspirin in feverish children.

Contra-indications, warnings, etc
Contra-indications: Platet 300, as other aspirin products, is contra-indicated in patients with active peptic ulceration, hypertension, haemophilia and other bleeding disorders, or who have a hypersensitivity to aspirin.

Precautions and warnings: Aspirin may precipitate bronchospasm, and induce asthmatic attacks in susceptible subjects; it may induce gastro-intestinal haemorrhage, occasionally major. It should be used with caution in subjects with gout. Risk/benefit ratios in the elderly have not been fully established.

Drug interactions: Aspirin may enhance the effects of anti-coagulants.

Use in pregnancy: There is clinical and epidemiological evidence of safety of aspirin in pregnancy, but it may prolong labour and contribute to maternal and neo-natal bleeding, therefore discontinue use one week before planned delivery or onset of labour.

Overdosage: Gastric lavage, forced alkaline diuresis and supportive therapy may be employed. Restoration of acid-base balance may be necessary.

Pharmaceutical precautions Store in a dry place, at room temperature.

Legal category: P.

Package quantities: Platet 300 tablets are individually packed in aluminium foil, in cartons of 30 tablets.

Further information Nil.

Product licence number 0188/0104.

POLYCROL* GEL

Presentation A white peppermint-flavoured suspension containing in each 5 ml:

Activated dimethicone	25 mg
Magnesium Hydroxide PhEur	100 mg
Aluminium hydroxide gel≡Al_2O_3	201.5 mg

Uses Disorders of the upper gastrointestinal tract, including dyspepsia, peptic ulcer, gastritis, flatulence, heartburn, oesophagitis and hiatus hernia. Polycrol Gel rapidly relieves acid pain, disperses gastric foam and assists eructation of gas and air.

Dosage and administration *Adults:* One or two 5 ml spoonfuls of gel between meals and at bedtime.

Children: Under 5 years: Half 5 ml spoonful with food, up to 4 doses per day.

5–12 years: One 5 ml spoonful with food, up to 4 doses per day.

Elderly persons: No special dosage regimen required but care should be taken to observe the contra-indications below which may be particularly applicable to elderly persons.

Contra-indications, warnings, etc
Contra-indications: Polycrol Gel should not be administered to patients with renal failure, or who are severely debilitated.

Warnings: Polycrol Gel may rarely give rise to nausea.

Drug interactions: As with other antacids, Polycrol Gel may inhibit the absorption of other drugs, e.g. tetracyclines, digoxin and vitamins. This may be avoided if such drugs are not administered within two hours of taking Polycrol.

Use in pregnancy: There is no evidence to contra-indicate the use of Polycrol Gel in pregnancy.

Overdosage: Not applicable.

Pharmaceutical precautions Store at room temperature (15–25°C).

Legal category P.

Package quantities Plastic bottle containing 300 ml.

Further information Polycrol contains a balanced mixture of antacids (aluminium and magnesium hydroxides) together with a deflatulent (activated dimethicone).

The antacids are balanced to reduce the risk of any bowel reaction and with Polycrol Gel neither constipation nor diarrhoea should occur.

Polycrol Gel contains 0.075 mmol sodium per 5 ml.

Product licence number 0188/5930R.

POLYCROL* TABLETS

Presentation Circular, flat bevelled-edge tablet consisting of two layers, green and white. The green face is impressed with the letter 'N'. Each tablet contains:

Activated dimethicone	25 mg
Aluminium hydroxide/magnesium carbonate co-dried gel	275 mg
Magnesium Hydroxide PhEur	100 mg

Uses Disorders of the upper gastrointestinal tract including dyspepsia, peptic ulcer, gastritis, flatulence, heartburn, oesophagitis and hiatus hernia. Polycrol Tablets rapidly relieve acid pain, disperse gastric foam and assist eructation of gas and air.

Dosage and administration *Adults:* 1 or 2 tablets to be chewed between meals and at bedtime.

Children: Under 5 years: Half a tablet to be chewed two or three times a day.

5–12 years: 1 tablet to be chewed two to three times a day.

Elderly persons: No special dosage regimen required, but care should be taken to observe the contra-indications below, which may be particularly applicable to elderly persons.

Contra-indications, warnings, etc
Contra-indications: Polycrol Tablets should not be administered to patients with renal failure, or who are severely debilitated.

Warnings: Polycrol Tablets may rarely give rise to nausea.

Drug interactions: As with other antacids, Polycrol Tablets may inhibit the absorption of other drugs, e.g. tetracyclines, digoxin and vitamins. This may be avoided if such drugs are not administered within two hours of taking Polycrol.

Use in pregnancy: There is no evidence to contra-indicate the use of Polycrol Tablets in pregnancy.

Overdosage: Not applicable.

Pharmaceutical precautions Store at room temperature (15–25°C).

Legal category P.

Package quantities Box of 200 tablets.

Further information Polycrol Tablets contain a balanced mixture of antacids (aluminium and magnesium hydroxides) together with a deflatulent (activated dimethicone).

The antacids are balanced to reduce the risk of any bowel reaction and with Polycrol Tablets neither constipation nor diarrhoea should occur.

Product licence number 0188/5919R.

POLYCROL* FORTE GEL

Presentation A white, viscous, peppermint-flavoured gel containing in 5 ml:

Activated dimethicone	125 mg
Magnesium Hydroxide PhEur	100 mg
Aluminium hydroxide gel≡Al_2O_3	201.5 mg

Uses In antacid/deflatulent therapy in conditions such as dyspepsia of functional or organic origin, heartburn, hiatus hernia, flatulence and abdominal distension, oesophagitis, gastritis, symptomatic treatment of peptic ulcer and other conditions where flatulence and hyperacidity may be present.

Polycrol Forte Gel rapidly relieves acid pain, disperses gastric foam and assists eructation of gas and air.

Dosage and administration *Adults:* One to two 5 ml spoonfuls of gel between meals and at bedtime.

Children: Under 5 years: Half 5 ml spoonful with food up to 4 doses per day.

5–12 years: One 5 ml spoonful with food up to 4 doses per day.

Elderly persons: No special dosage regimen required, but care should be taken to observe the contra-indications below, which may be particularly applicable to elderly persons.

Contra-indications, warnings, etc
Contra-indications: Polycrol Forte Gel should not be administered to patients with renal failure, or who are severely debilitated.

Warnings: Polycrol Forte Gel may rarely give rise to nausea.

Drug interactions: As with other antacids, Polycrol Forte Gel may inhibit the absorption of other drugs, e.g. tetracyclines, digoxin and vitamins. This may be avoided if such drugs are not administered within two hours of taking Polycrol.

Use in pregnancy: There is no evidence to contra-indicate the use of Polycrol Forte Gel in pregnancy.

Overdosage: Not applicable.

Pharmaceutical precautions Store at room temperature (15–25°C).

Legal category P.

Package quantities Plastic bottle containing 300 ml.

Further information Polycrol Forte Gel contains a balanced mixture of antacids (aluminium and magnesium hydroxides) together with a deflatulent (activated dimethicone).

The antacids are balanced to reduce the risk of any bowel reaction and with Polycrol Forte Gel, neither constipation nor diarrhoea should occur.

Polycrol Forte Gel contains 0.075 mmol sodium per 5 ml.

Product licence number 0188/5929R.

POLYCROL* FORTE TABLETS

Presentation White, circular, flat-faced tablets. One face is plain and the other is impressed with a triangle and the words 'POLYCROL FORTE' round the periphery. Each tablet contains:

Activated dimethicone	250 mg
Aluminium hydroxide/magnesium carbonate co-dried gel	275 mg
Magnesium Hydroxide PhEur	100 mg

Uses In antacid/deflatulent therapy in conditions such as dyspepsia of functional or organic origin, heartburn, hiatus hernia, flatulence and abdominal distension, oesophagitis, gastritis, symptomatic treatment of peptic ulcer and other conditions where flatulence and hyperacidity may be present.

Polycrol Forte Tablets rapidly relieve acid pain, disperse gastric foam and assist eructation of gas and air.

Dosage and administration *Adults:* One or two tablets to be chewed between meals and at bedtime.

Children: Not recommended for children under 12 years.

Elderly persons: No special dosage regimen required, but care should be taken to observe the contra-indications below, which may be particularly applicable to elderly persons.

Contra-indications, warnings, etc
Contra-indications: Polycrol Forte Tablets should not be administered to patients with renal failure, or who are severely debilitated.

Warnings: Polycrol Forte Tablets may rarely give rise to nausea.

Drug interactions; As with other antacids, Polycrol Forte Tablets may inhibit the absorption of other drugs, e.g. tetracyclines, digoxin and vitamins. This may be avoided if such drugs are not administered within two hours of taking Polycrol.

Use in pregnancy: There is no evidence to contra-indicate the use of Polycrol Forte Tablets in pregnancy.

Overdosage: Not applicable.

Pharmaceutical precautions Store at room temperature (15–25°C).

Legal category P.

Package quantities Box of 120 tablets.

Further information Polycrol Forte Tablets contain a balanced mixture of antacids (aluminium and magnesium hydroxides) together with a deflatulent (activated dimethicone).

The antacids are balanced to reduce the risk of any bowel reaction and with Polycrol Forte Tablets, neither constipation nor diarrhoea should occur.

Product licence number 0188/5918R.

VASCARDIN* 10 mg

Presentation Vascardin 10 mg tablets are circular, white, flat-faced, bevelled edge tablets with a break-line on one side and '10' within a triangle impressed on the reverse. Each tablet contains Diluted Isosorbide Dinitrate BP ≡ 10 mg isosorbide dinitrate.

Uses Angina pectoris – reduction of frequency and severity of attacks. Reduction of cardiac workload and oxygen consumption. Used alone or in combination with β-blockade in certain patients.

Congestive cardiac failure as adjunctive therapy.

Dosage and administration For adults only.

Angina: Treatment: As directed, ½–1 10 mg tablet sublingually at the onset, or for prevention of acute anginal attacks.

Prophylaxis: 30–120 mg orally in divided doses daily, or as required. Dosage should be increased gradually to minimise the possibility of nitrate headache and achieve tolerance. If the headache does occur it can be relieved by simple analgesics.

Congestive cardiac failure: 10–30 mg orally four times daily, according to patient requirements. The dose should be increased gradually to an optimum, using continuous haemodynamic monitoring to determine the level. Vascardin should be used as adjunctive therapy to other standard drugs (cardiac glycosides and diuretics) in cases of severe congestive cardiac failure.

Elderly persons: No special dosage regimen required.

Contra-indications, warnings, etc
Contra-indications: A known sensitivity to nitrates. Obstructive and restrictive cardiac conditions such as valvular stenosis and pericarditis. Severe anaemia, head trauma and cerebral haemorrhage.

Interactions: If used concurrently with anticoagulant therapy, aspirin and other salicylates should not be taken. This product may reduce or abolish the effects of sympathomimetics; there may be a synergistic effect with beta-blockers. If used concurrently with other vasodilators, effects are likely to be additive.

Other undesirable effects: During the first few days of treatment some patients may experience 'nitrate headache' (see under Dosage and Administration). Postural hypotension may occur if the dose is increased too rapidly. Facial flushing and/or tachycardia may be experienced by some patients.

Pregnancy and lactation: Isosorbide Dinitrate should not be used during pregnancy unless considered essential by the physician. There is no evidence that Isosorbide Dinitrate is excreted in breast milk, however, treatment of nursing mothers must be at the discretion of the physician.

Other special warnings and precautions: Use with caution in patients with glaucoma. Pulmonary capillary pressure should not usually be allowed to fall below 15 mmHg or the systolic blood pressure below the physiological range in normal and hypertensive patients. There should be no fall at all in patients with hypotension in the range of 90–110 mmHg of systolic pressure. In certain sensitive patients vasodilators, including Vascardin may cause excessive hypotension leading to increased ischaemia, extension of myocardial damage and progressive congestive heart failure. Tolerance to isosorbide dinitrate may develop but this can be reversed by an overnight washout period.

Overdosage: Although isosorbide dinitrate is quickly absorbed, gastric lavage is advised. The main effect of overdosage is hypotension, which should be treated by raising the patient's legs. Other symptoms are vomiting, syncope, cyanosis and, rarely, methaemaglobinaemia. Treatment should include support of cardiovascular and respiratory functions. In cases of methaemaglobinaemia, treatment is by a 1% solution of methylene blue, intravenously, at a dose of 1–4 mg/kg body weight.

Pharmaceutical precautions Store at room temperature (15–25°C).

Legal category P.

Package quantities Containers of 100 or 250 tablets.

Further information Nil.

Product licence number 0188/5931R.

**Trade Mark*

Norgine Limited
116–120 London Road
Headington
Oxford OX3 9BA

ALVERCOL*

Presentation Beige, coated granules containing:

Sterculia BP	62%
Alverine Citrate USNF XIII	0.5%

Uses Treatment of hypertonic disorders of the colon. Irritable bowel syndrome.

Dosage and administration Granules for oral administration.

Adults (including the elderly): 1–2 heaped 5 ml spoonfuls once or twice after meals.

Children (6–12 years): One half the above amount.

The granules should be placed dry on the tongue and, without chewing or crushing, swallowed immediately with plenty of water.

Contra-indications, warnings, etc

Contra-indications: Intestinal obstruction, faecal impaction, and total atony of the colon.

Precautions: Not to be taken immediately before retiring to bed, especially in the elderly. Adequate fluid intake should be maintained.

Use in pregnancy: No teratogenic effects have been reported but caution should be exercised during the first trimester of pregnancy.

Side-effects: Abdominal distension. Intestinal obstruction is possible if the product is taken in overdosage or is not adequately washed down with fluid.

Overdosage: Intestinal obstruction is possible, particularly in combination with inadequate fluid intake. Management is as for intestinal obstruction from other causes. Alverine in overdosage can produce hypotension and atropine-like toxic effects, which should be treated as for atropine poisoning.

Pharmaceutical precautions Store in a cool, dry place.

Legal category P.

Package quantities Packs of 500 g.

Further information Nil.

Product licence number 0322/5009.

CAMCOLIT*

Presentation *Camcolit 250:* White film coated tablets with 'Camcolit' engraved on one side and a break line on the reverse, each containing 250 mg Lithium Carbonate BP (equivalent to 6.8 millimoles).

Camcolit 400: White film coated controlled release tablets, with 'Camcolit S' engraved on one side and a break line on the reverse, each containing 400 mg Lithium Carbonate BP (equivalent to 10.8 millimoles).

Uses Treatment and prophylaxis of mania, manic-depressive illness and recurrent depression. Treatment of aggressive or self mutilating behaviour.

Dosage and administration Tablets for oral administration. Camcolit 400 may be given in divided or single daily doses, whereas Camcolit 250 should be given in divided dosage.

Acute mania: Treatment of mania should be initiated in hospital where regular monitoring of serum lithium levels can be conducted.

The dosage of Camcolit should be adjusted to produce a serum lithium level between 0.6 and 1.2 mmol/l 12 hours after the last dose. The required serum lithium level may be achieved in one of two ways but, whichever is adopted, regular estimations must be carried out to ensure maintenance of levels within the therapeutic range. For consistent results it is essential that the blood samples for serum lithium estimations are taken 12 hours after the last dose of lithium.

1. 1,500–2,000 mg of lithium carbonate are administered daily for the first five or seven days. A blood sample for serum lithium estimation is taken 12 hours after the last dose on the fifth or seventh day, and the dosage of Camcolit is adjusted to keep the serum lithium level within the therapeutic range.

Subsequently, regular serum lithium estimations must be carried out and, where necessary, the dosage of Camcolit adjusted accordingly.

The precise initial dose of lithium should be decided in the light of the age and weight of the patient; young patients often require a dose higher than average and older patients a lower dose.

2. A lithium clearance test is carried out and the initial dosage calculated from the results. Even when the initial dosage is calculated in this way, it is still desirable that serum lithium levels should be determined at weekly intervals during the first three weeks of treatment, and any necessary adjustments to dosage made as a result of the levels actually obtained.

Most of the above applies in the treatment of hypomania as well as mania, but the patient (if not too ill) can be started on treatment as an outpatient provided that facilities for periodic serum lithium monitoring are available.

Prophylaxis of recurrent affective disorders (including unipolar mania, unipolar depressions and bipolar manic-depressive illness): A dosage of 500–1,200 mg of lithium carbonate can be administered daily for the first seven days. A blood sample for serum lithium estimation is then taken 12 hours after the last dose, and the dosage of Camcolit is adjusted to keep the plasma lithium level within the effective range. Clinical improvement is usually associated with serum concentrations of 0.5 mmol/l or above. Toxic symptoms are usually associated with concentrations exceeding 1.5 mmol/l.

Use in elderly: Usually 500–1,000 mg/day.

Toxic symptoms are likely with serum concentrations above 1.0 mmol/l.

Use in children: Not recommended.

Measurement of serum lithium concentrations: Lithium therapy should not be initiated unless adequate facilities for routine monitoring of serum concentrations are available. On initiation of therapy serum concentrations should be measured weekly until stabilisation is achieved, then weekly for one month and at monthly intervals thereafter. Additional measurements should be made if signs of lithium toxicity occur (see below), on dosage alteration, development of significant intercurrent disease, signs of manic or depressive relapse and if significant change in sodium or fluid intake occurs. More frequent monitoring is required if patients are receiving diuretics.

As bioavailability may vary between formulations, should a change of preparation be made, blood levels should be monitored weekly until re-stabilisation is achieved.

Contra-indications, warnings, etc The first consideration in lithium therapy is the selection of proper candidates. The second is the physical state of the patient, which must be adequate to handle the lithium ion when it is introduced into the body.

Contra-indications: Patients with renal disease, cardiovascular disease, Addison's disease or those breast feeding.

Precautions: Pre-treatment and periodic routine clinical monitoring is essential. This should include assessment of renal function, urine analysis, assessment of thyroid function and cardiac function, especially in patients with cardiovascular disease.

Patients should be euthyroid before the initiation of lithium therapy.

Clear instructions regarding the symptoms of impending toxicity should be given by the doctor to all patients receiving long-term lithium therapy (see Warnings and Adverse Effects). Patients should also be warned to report if polyuria or polydipsia develop. Episodes of nausea and vomiting or other conditions leading to salt/water depletion (including severe dieting) should also be reported. Patients should be advised to maintain their usual salt and fluid intake.

Elderly patients are particularly liable to lithium toxicity.

Lower doses of lithium may be needed during diuretic therapy as lithium clearance is reduced.

Raised plasma levels of ADH may occur during treatment.

Symptoms of nephrogenic diabetes are particularly prevalent in patients receiving concurrent treatment with tri/tetracyclic antidepressants.

Serum lithium concentrations may increase during concomitant therapy with indomethacin or tetracycline.

Warnings: Long-term treatment with lithium may result in permanent changes in the kidney and impairment of renal function. High serum concentrations of lithium, including episodes of acute lithium toxicity may enhance these changes. The minimum clinically effective dose of lithium should always be used. Patients should be maintained on lithium after 3–5 years only if, on assessment, benefit persists.

Renal function should be routinely monitored in patients with polyuria and polydipsia.

Use in pregnancy: There is epidemiological evidence that the drug may be harmful in human pregnancy. Should the use of lithium be unavoidable, close monitoring of serum concentrations should be made throughout the pregnancy and during parturition.

Side-effects: Side effects are usually related to serum lithium concentrations and are infrequent at levels below 1.0 mmol/l.

Mild gastro-intestinal effects, nausea, vertigo, muscle weakness and a dazed feeling may occur, but frequently disappear after stabilisation. Fine hand tremors, polyuria and mild thirst may persist. Some studies suggest that the tremor can be controlled by relatively small doses of propranolol.

Long term treatment with lithium is frequently associated with disturbances of thyroid function including goitre and hypothyroidism. These can be controlled by administration of small doses of thyroxine (0.05–0.2 mg daily) concomitantly with lithium. Thyrotoxicosis has also been reported.

Mild cognitive impairment may occur during long term use.

Hypercalcaemia, hypermagnesaemia, hyperparathyroidism and an increase in antinuclear antibodies have also been reported.

Exacerbation of psoriasis may occur.

Signs of impending toxicity: Appearance or aggravation of gastro-intestinal symptoms, muscle weakness, lack of co-ordination, drowsiness or lethargy may be early signs of intoxication. With increasing toxicity there is ataxia, giddiness, tinnitus, blurred vision, coarse tremor, muscle twitching and a large output of dilute urine. At blood levels above 2–3 mmol/l, there is increasing disorientation, seizures, coma and death.

Overdosage: There is no antidote to lithium poisoning. In the event, lithium treatment should be stopped immediately and serum lithium levels estimated every 6 hours. When ingestion is recent, gastric lavage should be carried out, together with general supportive measures. Special attention must be given to the maintenance of fluid and electrolyte balance, also of adequate renal function. Sodium-depleting diuretics should not be used in any circumstances. Forced alkaline diuresis may be used or, if the serum lithium level is above 4.0 mmol/l, if there is a deterioration in the patient's condition, or if the serum lithium concentration is not falling at a rate equivalent to a half-life of less than 30 hours, peritoneal dialysis or haemodialysis should be instituted promptly. This should be continued until the serum and dialysis fluid are free of lithium. Serum lithium levels should be monitored for at least another 7 days, as a rebound rise is possible as a result of delayed diffusion from tissues.

Pharmaceutical precautions Store in a cool, dry place.

Legal category POM.

Package quantities *Camcolit 250:* Packs of 100 and 1,000 tablets.
Camcolit 400: Packs of 100 and 500 tablets.

Further information Several studies have confirmed that patients who had been receiving their daily dose of lithium carbonate in the form of another 'controlled-release' preparation can be changed to the same daily dose of lithium carbonate in the form of Camcolit 400 without significant change in plasma lithium levels.

Product licence numbers
Camcolit 250 0322/5900R.
Camcolit 400 0322/0015.

CYCLOBRAL*

Presentation Pink/brown hard gelatin capsules imprinted CYCLOBRAL. Each capsule contains 400 mg cyclandelate.

Uses As an adjunct to the management of elderly patients with arterio-sclerotic dementia, and for peripheral vascular disorders such as intermittent claudication, Raynaud's syndrome, night cramps, acrocyanosis, cold extremities, chilblains and 'restless legs'.

Dosage and administration Capsules for oral administration.

Adults (including the elderly): 1 capsule three or four times daily.

Children: Not recommended.

Contra-indications, warnings, etc
Contra-indications: Acute phase of cerebrovascular accidents or recent myocardial infarction. Actual or incipient peripheral gangrene or frostbite.

Precautions: Glaucoma.

Use in pregnancy: No teratogenic effects have been reported, but caution should be exercised during the first trimester of pregnancy.

Side-effects: Nausea, gastro-intestinal distress or flushing may occasionally occur.

Overdosage: Gastric lavage, followed, if necessary, by administration of vasopressors.

Pharmaceutical precautions Store in a cool, dry place.

Legal category P.

Package quantities Packs of 250 capsules.

Further information Cyclandelate has a low order of toxicity and for maximum therapeutic effect it is recommended that four capsules daily should be given.

Product licence number 0322/0036.

FYBRANTA*

Presentation Mottled, light brown tablets containing bran 2 g.

Uses The treatment of all colonic and other gastroenterological diseases where administration of bran is indicated, including the treatment of constipation, symptomatic relief in diverticular disease and the irritable bowel syndrome. Treatment of conditions requiring a high-fibre regimen.

Dosage and administration *Adults (including the elderly):* Usually 1–3 tablets three or four times daily, preferably with meals.

At the discretion of the physician, larger quantities may be prescribed in individual cases.

Children (5–12 years): A lower dose, at the discretion of the physician.

Children (below 5 years): Only on the direction of a physician.

Fybranta tablets should be chewed, part of a tablet at a time if necessary, and swallowed with a drink.

No attempt should be made to swallow the tablets whole.

Contra-indications, warnings, etc
Contra-indications: Intestinal obstruction, gluten enteropathies.

Precautions: None known.

Use in pregnancy: There is no evidence to suggest that Fybranta should not be taken during pregnancy.

Side-effects: None reported.

Overdosage: Has not been reported but if taken without fluid, intestinal obstruction is theoretically possible, and should be managed as intestinal obstruction from other causes.

Pharmaceutical precautions Store in a cool, dry place.

Legal category GSL.

Package quantities Packs of 100 tablets.

Further information Fybranta tablets contain calcium phosphate which ensures neutralisation of the phytic acid in bran, which may otherwise interfere with calcium absorption.

Product licence number 0322/0016R.

GUARINA*

Presentation A fine off-white dispersible granulate in unit dose sachets. Each sachet contains 5 g of guar gum (USNF).

Uses As an adjunct in the treatment of diabetes mellitus.

Dosage and administration
Dosage: Adults: Initially, one sachet daily, increasing if necessary to a maximum of three sachets daily from the third week of therapy. It is important that all doses should be taken before or with meals.

Children: No specific recommendations can be made for children.

To be taken immediately before or with meals. The contents of one sachet should be added to 150 ml ($\frac{1}{4}$ pint) of a cold drink (sugar-free squash, juice or water), stirred briskly and taken straight away. Alternatively the contents may be sprinkled on, or mixed with, suitable foods, which must be accompanied by a drink of 150 ml.

Contra-indications, warnings, etc
Contra-indications: 1. Oesophageal disease or dysfunction. 2. Intestinal obstruction.

Precautions: Careful monitoring is required during the initial stages of treatment, to minimise the dangers of hypoglycaemia.

Side-effects: Flatulence, some alteration in bowel habit or nausea may occur in a few patients, but these effects are usually transient.

Pharmaceutical precautions Store in a cool, dry place, below 25°C.

Legal category P.

Package quantities Cartons of 60 sachets.

Further information Guar is used to slow the rate of glucose absorption, thereby reducing the post-prandial peak in the blood-glucose level. This may allow a reduction in dosage of insulin or oral hypoglycaemic agents.

Product licence number 0322/0053.

KAMILLOSAN*

Presentation Light brown ointment containing Chamomile extracts 10.5% (standardised to provide 0.01% L-α bisabolol) in a base containing lanolin.

Uses Prophylaxis and treatment of sore nipples in nursing mothers, nappy rash, nappy chafe and chapped hands.

Dosage and administration Ointment for topical application.

Sore nipples: Apply after breastfeeding.

Nappy rash: Apply at every nappy change.

Other conditions: Apply twice daily as necessary.

Contra-indications, warnings, etc
Contra-indications: None known.

Precautions: None known.

Use in pregnancy: There is no evidence to suggest that Kamillosan should not be used during pregnancy.

Side-effects: None reported.

Pharmaceutical precautions Store in a cool, dry place.

Legal category GSL.

Package quantities Tubes of 24 g and 5 g.

Further information Nil.

Product licence number 0322/5914R.

KLEAN-PREP*

Presentation An off-white powder, packed in 4 sachets. Each sachet contains:

Polyethylene Glycol 3350 USNF	59.00 g
Anhydrous Sodium Sulphate PhEur	5.685 g
Sodium Bicarbonate PhEur	1.685 g
Sodium Chloride PhEur	1.465 g
Potassium Chloride PhEur	0.7425 g

The contents of each sachet to be reconstituted with 1 litre of water. When the contents of a sachet are reconstituted with one litre of water the resulting solution contains:

Sodium	125 mmol/L
Potassium	10 mmol/L
Sulphate	40 mmol/L
Chloride	35 mmol/L
Bicarbonate	20 mmol/L

The solution also contains aspartame.

Uses Bowel preparation before colonoscopy, colonic surgery, radiological examination and other related procedures.

Dosage and administration Reconstituted solution for oral administration.

Adults (including the elderly): The contents of one sachet to be dissolved in 1 litre of water. 250 ml to be drunk rapidly every 10–15 minutes until all the solution has been consumed.

The procedure to be repeated with all four sachets or until the rectal effluent is clear. The solution from all 4 sachets should be drunk within 4–6 hours. No dosage changes need be made for patients with renal insufficiency. If administered by nasogastric tube the rate of administration should be 20–30 ml/minute.

Children: Not recommended.

Contra-indications, warnings, etc
Contra-indications: Gastro-intestinal obstruction or perforation, ileus, gastric retention, acute intestinal or gastric ulceration, toxic colitis or megacolon. Patients with body weight less than 20 kg.

Warnings: Extra care should be taken in patients with impaired gag reflex, reflux oesophagitis, those with diminished levels of consciousness and in ulcerative colitis. It should be noted that any oral medication administered within 1 hour of administration of Klean-Prep may be flushed from the gastro-intestinal tract and not absorbed.

Side-effects: Nausea, abdominal fullness, bloating may be experienced. Abdominal cramps, vomiting and anal irritation occur less frequently. These effects normally subside rapidly. Urticaria and allergic reactions have been reported rarely. Should distension or pain arise the rate of administration should be slowed or temporarily stopped until symptoms subside. There is no effect on the ability to drive or to use machines.

In case of gross accidental overdose, where diarrhoea is severe, conservative measures are usually sufficient; generous amounts of fluid, especially fruit juices, should be given.

Use in pregnancy: Klean-Prep should only be used during pregnancy if considered essential by the physician. There is no experience of use during pregnancy. The purpose and mechanism of use should be borne in mind if the physician is considering administration.

Overdosage: In cases of gross accidental overdosage, where diarrhoea is severe, conservative measures are usually sufficient; generous amounts of fluid, especially fruit juices, should be given.

Pharmaceutical precautions Store in a cool, dry place below 25 C. The reconstituted solution should be refrigerated and used within 24 hours. Any unused portion should be discarded.

Legal category P.

Package quantity Unit dose pack of 4 sachets.

Further information Flavouring, such as fruit cordials, may be added if required. Metoclopramide or domperidone may be given, 30 minutes before starting to take Klean-Prep, to facilitate gastric emptying.

Product licence number 5628/0003.

Product licence holder: Birex Pharmaceuticals Ltd.

MURIPSIN*

Presentation Orange, film-coated tablets, each containing:

Glutamic Acid Hydrochloride USNF XIII 500 mg

Uses The symptomatic treatment of gastric hydrochloric acid deficiency.

Dosage and administration Tablets for oral administration. *Adults (including the elderly):* 1 or 2 tablets with each meal.

Children: No specific dosage can be recommended.

Contra-indications, warnings, etc
Contra-indications: Gastric or duodenal ulcer.

Precautions: None known.

Use in pregnancy: No teratogenic effects have been reported, but caution should be exercised during the first trimester of pregnancy.

Side-effects: None reported.

Overdosage: Can cause gastric ulceration and metabolic acidosis. Management is as for the ingestion of mineral acid.

Pharmaceutical precautions Store in a cool, dry place.

Legal category GSL.

Package quantities Packs of 50 tablets.

Further information Each Muripsin tablet is approximately equivalent to the oral administration of 1 ml Dilute Hydrochloric Acid BP.

Product licence number 0322/5005R.

NORMACOL*

Presentation White, coated granules containing Sterculia BP 62%.

Uses Treatment of constipation, particularly simple or idiopathic constipation, and constipation arising in pregnancy.

Management of colostomies and ileostomies.

The 'high residue diet' management of diverticular disease of the colon and other conditions requiring a high fibre regime.

The initiation and maintenance of bowel action after rectal and anal surgery.

Administration after ingestion of sharp foreign bodies to provide a coating and reduce the possibility of intestinal damage during transit.

Dosage and administration Granules for oral administration.

Adults: (including the elderly): 1 or 2 sachets or 1–2 heaped 5 ml spoonfuls, once or twice daily after meals.

Children (6–12 years): One half of the above amount.
Children (under 6 years): Only on the direction of the doctor.

The granules should be placed dry on the tongue and, without chewing or crushing, swallowed immediately with plenty of liquid (water or a cool drink).

Contra-indications, warnings, etc
Contra-indications: Intestinal obstruction, faecal impaction, and total atony of the colon.

Precautions: Not to be taken immediately before retiring to bed, especially in the elderly. Adequate fluid intake should be maintained. Caution should be exercised in cases of ulcerative colitis.

Use in pregnancy and lactation: Normacol is recommended for use during pregnancy or lactation.

Side-effects: Abdominal distension. Intestinal obstruction is possible if the product is taken in overdosage or if it is not adequately washed down with fluid.

Pharmaceutical precautions Store in a cool, dry place.

Legal category GSL.

Package quantities Packs of 60 sachets (2 × 30), each sachet containing 7 g of granules, or packs of 500 g.

Further information Each 7 g sachet of granules contains 1.72 g of available carbohydrate, equivalent to 6.75 kcal.

Product licence number 0322/5010R.

NORMACOL* PLUS

Presentation Brown, coated granules containing:

Sterculia BP	62%
Frangula BPC 1949	8%

Uses Treatment of constipation, particularly hypotonic or slow transit constipation resistant to bulk alone.

The initiation and maintenance of bowel action after rectal surgery and after haemorrhoidectomy.

Dosage and administration Granules for oral administration.

Adults (including the elderly): 1 or 2 sachets or 1–2 heaped 5 ml spoonfuls once or twice daily after meals.

Children (6–12 years): A reduced amount may be given at the discretion of the physician.

The granules should be placed dry on the tongue and, without chewing or crushing, swallowed immediately with plenty of liquid (water or a cool drink).

Contra-indications, warnings, etc
Contra-indications: Intestinal obstruction, faecal impaction, and total atony of the colon.

Precautions: Not to be taken immediately before retiring to bed, especially in the elderly. Adequate fluid intake should be maintained. Caution should be exercised in cases of ulcerative colitis.

Use in pregnancy: No teratogenic effects have been reported, but caution should be exercised during the first trimester of pregnancy.

Use during lactation: There is no evidence to suggest that Normacol Plus is unsuitable for use during lactation, though Normacol (sterculia alone) is available, if preferred.

Side-effects: Abdominal distension. Intestinal obstruction is possible if the product is taken in overdosage or is not adequately washed down with fluid.

Pharmaceutical precautions Store in a cool, dry place.

Legal category GSL.

Package quantities Packs of 60 sachets (2×30), each sachet containing 7 g of granules, or packs of 200 g and 500 g.

Further information Each 7 g sachet of granules contains 1.72 g of available carbohydrate, equivalent to 6.75 kcal.

Product licence number 0322/5011R.

POSALFILIN*

Presentation Dark brown ointment containing:

Podophyllum Resin BP	20%
Salicylic Acid BP	25%

Uses Treatment of plantar warts (verrucae plantaris).

Dosage and administration Ointment for topical administration. *Adults (including the elderly) and children:*

1. Place a felt corn ring around the wart, if necessary adjusting the size of the hole by snipping, allowing the wart to protrude through the hole.
2. Apply the ointment (using a minimum amount) to exposed wart only. Cover with a piece of plaster.
3. The dressing may be renewed two or three times weekly. When wart appears soft and spongy leave exposed to the air for a day or two when it will usually drop off. If not, repeat the above procedure.
4. Wash hands thoroughly after applying the ointment, and if a waterproof plaster is used normal washing will not affect the efficacy of the treatment.

Contra-indications, warnings, etc
Contra-indications: Pregnancy.

Precautions: The patient should be warned that Posalfilin is caustic to healthy skin. Posalfilin should not be applied to sensitive areas of the face, armpits or ano-genital region.

Use in pregnancy: Contra-indicated. Posalfilin should not be used during pregnancy or when there is a possibility of pregnancy.

Side-effects: Inflammation of the surrounding skin may occur, in which case treatment should be suspended.

Pharmaceutical precautions Store in a cool, dry place.

Legal category P.

Package quantities Tubes of 10 g.

Further information Nil.

Product licence number 0322/5901.

PREFIL*

Presentation Brown, coated granules containing Sterculia BP 55%.

Uses Treatment of obesity, in conjunction with a calorie-controlled diet.

Dosage and administration Granules for oral administration. *Adults (including the elderly):* Two rounded 5 ml spoonfuls, ½ to 1 hour before each meal. The granules should be placed dry on the tongue, in small quantities if necessary, and without chewing or crushing, swallowed with ½ pint of low-calorie drink.

Children: At the discretion of the physician, when a reduced dosage may be given.

Contra-indications, warnings, etc
Contra-indications: Intestinal obstruction.

Precautions: None known.

Use in pregnancy: There is no evidence to suggest that Prefil should not be used during pregnancy.

Side-effects: Some patients who have become accustomed to an unusually low residue diet may experience slight abdominal discomfort from the increase in bulk which follows the administration of full doses of Prefil. These patients may be advised to take a smaller dose initially, increasing to the full dose over a period of one week. In these circumstances, the full clinical effect may not be experienced until the end of the first week.

Pharmaceutical precautions Store in a cool, dry place.

Legal category GSL.

Package quantities Packs of 200 g and 500 g.

Further information Available carbohydrate content approx. 1.6 g per spoonful (as sucrose) equivalent to 6 Cals.

Product licence number 0322/0035.

SOMNITE*

Presentation An off-white, translucent, thixotropic suspension with a cherry flavour. Each 5 ml spoonful contains Nitrazepam BP 2.5 mg.

Uses Short term treatment of insomnia where daytime sedation is acceptable. Benzodiazepines should be used to treat insomnia only when it is severe, disabling, or subjecting the individual to extreme distress. An underlying cause for insomnia should be sought before deciding upon the use of benzodiazepines for symptomatic relief.

Dosage and administration Suspension for oral administration. *Adults:* 5 mg (two 5 ml spoonfuls) before retiring. This dose may, if necessary, be increased to 10 mg.

Elderly patients: 2.5 mg before retiring. This dose may, if necessary, be increased to 5 mg.

Children: Not recommended.

The lowest dose which can control the symptoms should be used. It should not be continued beyond four weeks. Long term chronic use is not recommended. Treatment should always be tapered off gradually. Patients who have taken benzodiazepines for a long time may require a longer period during which doses are reduced. When a benzodiazepine is used as a hypnotic, treatment should, if possible, be intermittent.

Contra-indications, warnings, etc
Contra-indications: Known sensitivity to benzodiazepines. Acute pulmonary insufficiency.

Precautions: Chronic pulmonary insufficiency. In chronic renal or hepatic disease. In labour. High single doses or repeated low doses have been reported to produce hypotonia, poor sucking and hypothermia in the neonate and irregularities in the foetal heart. Avoid if possible in lactation. The concurrent use of other CNS depressant drugs should be avoided. Benzodiazepines should not be used alone to treat depression or anxiety associated with depression. Suicide may be precipitated in such patients. They should not be used for phobic or obsessional states. They should not be used for the treatment of chronic psychosis. In cases of loss or bereavement, psychological adjustment may be inhibited by benzodiazepines. Disinhibiting effects may be manifested in various ways. Suicide may be precipitated in patients who are depressed, and aggressive behaviour towards self and others may be precipitated. Extreme caution should therefore be used in prescribing benzodiazepines in patients with personality disorders.

Use in pregnancy: There is no evidence as to drug safety in human pregnancy nor is there evidence from animal work that it is free from hazard. Do not use during pregnancy, especially during the first and last trimesters, unless there are compelling reasons.

Side-effects: Common adverse effects include drowsiness, sedation, blurring of vision, unsteadiness and ataxia. These effects occur following single as well as repeated dosage and may persist well into the following day. Performance at skilled tasks and alertness may be impaired. Patients should be warned of this hazard and advised not to drive or operate machinery during treatment. These effects are potentiated by alcohol. The elderly are particularly liable to experience these symptoms together with confusion especially if organic brain symptoms are present. See also Dependence Potential and Withdrawal Symptoms below.

Abnormal psychological reactions to benzodiazepines have been reported. Rare behavioural adverse effects include paradoxical aggressive outbursts, excitement, confusion, and the uncovering of depression with suicidal tendencies.

Other rare adverse effects including hypotension, gastro-intestinal and visual disturbances, skin rashes, urinary retention, headache, vertigo, changes in libido; blood dyscrasias and jaundice have also been reported.

Dependence potential and withdrawal symptoms: In general the dependence potential of benzodiazepines is low but this increases when high dosages are attained, especially when given over long periods. This is particularly so in patients with a history of alcoholism, drug abuse or in patients with marked personality disorders. Regular monitoring of treatment in such patients is essential and routine repeat prescriptions should be avoided.

Treatment in all patients should be withdrawn gradually. Withdrawal from benzodiazepines may be associated with physiological and psychological symptoms of withdrawal including depression, nervousness, rebound insomnia, irritability, sweating and diarrhoea. Withdrawal symptoms occur with benzodiazepines following normal therapeutic doses given for short periods of time.

Abrupt withdrawal following excessive dosage may produce confusion, toxic psychosis, convulsions or a condition resembling delirium tremens.

Overdosage: The primary symptoms of overdosage are drowsiness, dizziness, ataxia and slurred speech. Treatment is symptomatic but gastric lavage may be useful if performed soon after ingestion.

Pharmaceutical precautions Somnite suspension should be stored in a cool place, protected from light.

Somnite suspension may be diluted to a maximum of 1 in 5 with Syrup BP (preserved). The shelf life of the diluted suspension is not more than 14 days.

Legal category CD (Sch 4) POM.

Package quantities Bottles of 150 ml

Further information Nil.

Product licence number 0322/0039.

SPASMONAL*

Presentation Blue/grey, opaque, hard gelatin capsules, marked '78' on one half and with a sailing boat design on the other. Each capsule contains 60 mg Alverine Citrate USNF XIII.

Uses Smooth muscle spasmolytic effective on smooth muscle of the alimentary tract and uterus. Spasmonal is indicated for use in the relief of smooth muscle spasm, in conditions such as irritable bowel syndrome, painful diverticular disease of the colon, primary dysmenorrhoea.

Dosage and administration Capsules for oral administration.

Adults (including the elderly): 1 or 2 capsules one to three times daily.

Children (8–12 years): 1 capsule 3 times daily.

Contra-indications, warnings, etc
Contra-indications: Paralytic ileus.

Precautions: None known.

Use in pregnancy: No teratogenic effects have been reported, but caution should be exercised during the first trimester of pregnancy.

Side-effects: None reported at normal therapeutic doses.

Overdosage: Can produce hypotension and atropine-like toxic effects. Management is as for atropine poisoning with supportive therapy for hypotension.

Pharmaceutical precautions Store in a cool, dry place.

Legal category P.

Package quantities Containers of 100 capsules.

Further information Alverine citrate is a synthetic, non-narcotic, non-habit-forming spasmolytic of a low order of toxicity in comparison with other anti-spasmodics. It has a specific effect on the smooth muscle of the intestine and uterus, but not on those of the respiratory or cardiovascular system.

Product licence number 0322/5014.

WAXSOL*

Presentation Colourless liquid containing:

Docusate Sodium BP 0.5% in a water-miscible base.

Uses Cerumenolytic.

Dosage and administration For aural use only.
Adults (including the elderly) and children: The patient should be directed to fill the ear with Waxsol on not more than two consecutive nights, before attending for syringing.

Contra-indications, warnings, etc
Contra-indications: Perforation of the ear drum; inflammation of the ear.

Precautions: If pain or inflammation is experienced, treatment should be discontinued.

Use in pregnancy: There is no evidence to suggest that Waxsol should not be used during pregnancy.

Side-effects: Rarely, transient stinging or irritation may occur.

Pharmaceutical precautions Store in a cool place.

Legal category GSL.

Package quantities 10 ml bottle with dropper.

Further information Waxsol, because of its low surface tension and its water-miscibility, rapidly penetrates the dry matrix of the ceruminous mass, reducing the solid material to a semi-solid debris which can be syringed away readily or, in less severe and in chronic cases, is ejected by normal physiological processes.

Product licence number 0322/5016R.

**Trade Mark*

Norwich Eaton Limited
New Sandgate House
City Road
Newcastle Upon Tyne NE99 1YD

Norwich Eaton

ALPHADERM*

Presentation Alphaderm contains Hydrocortisone PhEur 1% w/w and Urea BP 10% w/w in a specially formulated base which assists the percutaneous transportation of the active ingredients to the site of action. Due to this formulation Alphaderm acts as a moderately potent topical corticosteroid. The base is self-occlusive and fulfils the functions of both an ointment and a cream. Alphaderm does not contain lanolin and is preservative free.

Uses Alphaderm is indicated for the treatment of all dry ichthyotic, eczematous conditons of the skin, including atopic, infantile, chronic allergic and irritant eczema, asteatotic, hyperkeratotic and lichenified eczema, neurodermatitis and prurigo.

Dosage and administration Adults, children and the elderly: a small amount should be applied topically to the preferably dry affected areas twice daily. In resistant lesions occlusive dressings may be used but this is usually unnecessary because of the self-occlusive nature of the special base.

Contra-indications, warnings, etc Alphaderm is contra-indicated in primary bacterial, viral and fungal diseases of the skin and secondarily infected eczemas or intertrigo and, in general, should not be used on weeping surfaces.

Known hypersensitivity.

Precautions: Caution should be exercised when using in children. In infants and children, long term continuous therapy should be avoided, as adrenal suppression can occur even without occlusion. Excessive absorption may occur when applied under napkins.

Application to moist or fissured skin may cause temporary irritation. Urea may also enhance the absorption of the corticosteroid and this possibility should be borne in mind, especially when long term treatment is contemplated.

As with corticosteroids in general, prolonged application to the face and eyelids is undesirable.

Use in pregnancy and lactation: There is inadequate evidence for safety in human pregnancy. Topical administration of corticosteroids to pregnant animals can cause abnormalities of foetal development including cleft palate and intra-uterine growth retardation. There may, therefore, be a very small risk of such effects in the human foetus.

Overdosage: Chronically, grossly excessive over-use on large areas of skin in, for example, children, could result in adrenal suppression of the hypothalamic-pituitary axis (HPA) as well as topical and systemic signs and symptoms of high corticosteroid dosage. In such cases, treatment should not stop abruptly. Adenal insufficiency may require treatment with systemic hydrocortisone. Ingestion of a large amount of Alphaderm would be expected to result in gastrointestinal irritation, nausea, and possibly vomiting. Symptomatic and supportive care should be given. Liberal oral administration of milk or water may be helpful.

Pharmaceutical precautions Store at a temperature not exceeding 25°C.

Legal category POM.

Package quantities Alphaderm is available in tubes of 30 g and 100 g.

Further information Optimum rehydration of dry skin is achieved without the use of occlusive dressings.

Product licence number 0364/0019R.

AQUADRATE*

Presentation Aquadrate contains urea 10% w/w in a specially formulated base. It has keratolytic action and helps to hydrate the skin. The base is self-occlusive and it fulfils the functions of both an ointment and a cream. Aquadrate does not contain lanolin and is preservative free.

Uses Aquadrate is indicated in atopic eczema, ichthyosis, xeroderma, hyperkeratosis and other chronic dry skin conditions.

Dosage and administration Aquadrate is applied topically. Wash affected areas well, rinse off all traces of soap, dry, and apply sparingly twice daily. Occlusive dressings may be used but are usually unnecessary because of the self-occlusive nature of the base.

Contra-indications, warnings, etc In some instances, Aquadrate may cause irritation when applied to sensitive skin.

Pharmaceutical precautions Store at a temperature not exceeding 30°C.

Legal category P.

Package quantities Aquadrate is available in tubes of 30 g and 100 g.

Further information Nil.

Product licence number 0364/0018.

CACIT* TABLETS

Presentation Cacit Tablets 500 mg: Pink, slightly speckled, circular, orange flavoured, effervescent calcium tablets. Each effervescent tablet contains 1.25 g calcium carbonate PhEur which, when dispersed in water, provides 500 mg calcium as calcium citrate.

Uses Treatment of calcium deficiency states including osteomalacia, rickets and malabsorption syndromes affecting the upper gastrointestinal tract.

An adjunct to conventional therapy in the arrest or slowing down of bone demineralisation in osteoporosis.

In the arrest or slowing down of bone demineralisation in osteoporosis, where other effective treatment is contra-indicated.

As a therapeutic supplement during times when intake may be inadequate, particularly those associated with the increased demand of childhood, old age, pregnancy and lactation.

Dosage and administration The tablets must be dissolved in a glass of water and the solution should then be drunk immediately after complete dissolution of the tablets.

Adults: For simple calcium deficiency states and malabsorption, dosage should be tailored to the individual patient's needs. In osteomalacia 1–3 g per day is recommended.

For the treatment of osteoporosis a dose of up to 1.5 g per day is normally required. In women with adequate dietary calcium intake (at least 1 g/day), 500 mg daily may be sufficient.

Up to 1.5 g of calcium per day is the recommended dosage for therapeutic supplementation.

Children: For calcium deficiency states, malabsorption and rickets, the recommendation given under adult dosage should be followed.

For therapeutic supplementation a dose of up to 1 g per day is recommended.

Elderly: No evidence exists that tolerance of Cacit is directly affected by advanced age; however, elderly patients should be supervised as factors sometimes associated with aging, such as poor diet or impaired renal function, may indirectly affect tolerance and may require dosage reduction.

Contra-indications, warnings, etc
Contra-indications: Patients with hypercalcaemia or hypercalciuria. Cacit Tablets are also contra-indicated in patients where prolonged immobilisation is accompanied by hypercalciuria and/or hypercalcaemia. In these cases calcium treatment should only be resumed when the patient becomes mobile.

Precautions: Cacit Tablets should be used with caution in patients suffering from impaired renal function or a history of renal stone formation. In patients with renal insufficiency, serum and urinary calcium levels should be monitored regularly to prevent hypercalcaemia occurring.

Vitamin D causes an increase in calcium absorption and plasma calcium levels may continue to rise after stopping Vitamin D therapy. Concomitant administration of Cacit Tablets and Vitamin D should therefore be carried out with caution. Patients treated with high doses of Vitamin D or who are receiving prolonged calcium treatment, should undergo regular measurements of plasma calcium levels which should be interpreted in conjunction with measurements of plasma protein levels.

Calcium salts reduce the absorption of some drugs, in particular tetracyclines. It is, therefore, suggested that administration of Cacit Tablets be separated from these products by at least 3 hours.

Use in pregnancy: Calcium supplements have been in wide use for many years without apparent ill consequence.

Side-effects: Mild gastro-intestinal disturbances have occurred rarely (e.g. constipation, diarrhoea). Although hypercalcaemia would not be expected in patients unless their renal function were impaired, the following symptoms could indicate the possibility of hypercalcaemia: nausea, vomiting, anorexia, constipation, abdominal pain, bone pain, thirst, polyuria, muscle weakness, drowsiness or confusion.

Overdosage: The amount of calcium absorbed following overdosage with Cacit Tablets will depend on the individual's calcium status. Deliberate overdosage is unlikely with effervescent preparations and acute overdosage has not been reported. It might cause gastro-intestinal disturbances but would not be expected to cause hypercalcaemia except in patients treated with excessive doses of Vitamin D. Treatment should be aimed at lowering serum calcium levels e.g. administration of oral phosphates.

Pharmaceutical precautions Cacit Tablets are hygroscopic and should be dispensed in the original container. Store at room temperature in a dry place.

Legal category P.

Package quantities Boxes of 76 (4 tubes of 19).

Further information Cacit Tablets contain no sugar and have a low sodium content.

Product licence number 0364/0045.

DANTRIUM*

Presentation Dantrium capsules are available in two strengths, containing either 25 mg or 100 mg dantrolene sodium per capsule.

Dantrium is presented in orange/light brown capsules. The 25 mg capsule carries the monogram Dantrium 25 mg on the cap and 0149, 0030 and a single coding bar on the body. The 100 mg capsule carries the monogram Dantrium 100 mg on the cap and 0149, 0033 and triple coding bars on the body.

Uses Dantrium produces relaxation of contracted skeletal muscle by affecting the contractile response at a site beyond the myoneural junction. Dantrium produces a dissociation of excitation-contraction coupling, probably interfering with the release of Ca^{++} from the sarcoplasmic reticulum. The effect is seen in both fast and slow fibres but is more pronounced in the former.

Dantrium is indicated for the treatment of chronic, severe spasticity in adults resulting from such disorders as stroke, multiple sclerosis, spinal cord injury and cerebral palsy. It is useful in these conditions whenever spasticity is so severe that increased muscular resistance to stretch, clonus or exaggerated reflex posturing interfere with the activity of daily living such as exercise, posture, equilibrium, walking, transfer manoeuvres or the use of braces.

Occasionally, only a subtle but perceptible improvement in spasticity may occur with Dantrium therapy. In such instances information regarding improvement should be sought from the patient and those who are in constant daily contact and attendance on him. Brief withdrawal of Dantrium for a period of two to four days will frequently demonstrate exacerbation of the spasticity and may help to reinforce a previously indefinable clinical impression.

Dosage and administration Before commencing Dantrium therapy, it is important to set an attainable therapeutic goal for the individual patient. Such a goal would be a reduction in spasticity which allows the patient or his attendants to carry out a function which could not previously be performed, or one that he or his attendants consider important.

The need for patience and attention to the individual patient's needs in titrating Dantrium dosage is of paramount importance.

Dosage should be increased until the maximum benefit compatible with the patient's neurological deficit is achieved.

Dosage for use in spasticity for adults: For the individual patient, the lowest dose compatible with optimal response is recommended. Dosage in excess of 400 mg/day is not recommended.

A recommended dosage increment scale is shown below:

Week	*Recommended dosage*
First	One 25 mg capsule daily
Second	One 25 mg capsule twice daily
Third	Two 25 mg capsules twice daily
Fourth	Two 25 mg capsules three times daily
Fifth	Three 25 mg capsules three times daily
Sixth	Three 25 mg capsules four times daily
Seventh	One 100 mg capsule four times daily

Each dose level should be maintained for seven days, in order to determine the patient's response. Therapy with a dose four times daily may offer maximum benefit to some patients. Maximum daily doses should not exceed 400 mg.

In view of the potential for hepatotoxicity in long term use, if no observable benefit is derived from the administration of Dantrium after a total of 45 days, therapy should be discontinued.

Many patients experience side-effects such as weakness and fatigue during the first four weeks of therapy whilst the patient adjusts to the changes in muscle tone induced by the drug. They are usually transient and mild in nature. Patients should be warned of them and encouraged to persevere with treatment. Should it be necessary, the dosage of Dantrium may be reduced and then gradually increased according to the patient's tolerance.

A similar titration schedule should be used with the elderly, where assessment of therapeutic aims and effect is equally important to any other age group.

Contra-indications, warnings, etc
Contra-indications: Dantrium is contra-indicated where spasticity is utilised to sustain upright posture and balance in locomotion, or whenever spasticity is utilised to obtain or maintain increased function.

Dantrium is contra-indicated in patients with evidence of hepatic dysfunction. Dantrium is not indicated for the treatment of acute skeletal muscle spasm.

Dantrium should not be administered to children.

Warnings
Use in pregnancy: Although teratological studies in animals have proved satisfactory, use of Dantrium is not advised in pregnancy and nursing mothers.

Dantrolene sodium showed some evidence of tumourgenicity at high dose levels in Sprague-Dawley female rats. However, these effects were not seen in other studies in Fischer 344 rats or HaM/ICR mice. There is no clinical evidence of carcinogenicity in humans, however, this possibility cannot be absolutely excluded.

Precautions: It is important to recognise that fatal and non-fatal liver disorders of an idiosyncratic or hypersensitivity type may occur with Dantrium therapy.

At the start of Dantrium therapy, it is desirable to do liver function studies (SGOT/ALT, SGPT/AST, alkaline phosphatase, total bilirubin) for a baseline or to establish whether there is pre-existing liver disease. If baseline liver abnormalities exist and are confirmed, there is a clear possibility that the potential for Dantrium hepatotoxicity could be enhanced, although such a possibility has not yet been established.

Liver function studies (e.g. serum, SGOT/AST, SGPT/ALT) should be performed at appropriate intervals during Dantrium therapy. If such studies reveal abnormal values, therapy should generally be discontinued. Only where benefits of the drug have been of major importance to the patient, should re-introduction or continuation of therapy be considered. Some patients have revealed a return to normal laboratory values in the face of continued therapy while others have not.

If symptoms compatible with hepatitis, accompanied by abnormalities in liver function tests or jaundice appear, Dantrium should be discontinued. If caused by Dantrium and detected early, the abnormalities in liver function have reverted to normal when the drug was discontinued.

Dantrium has been re-introduced in a few patients who have developed clinical signs, or elevated serum enzymes, of hepatocellular injury.

Re-introduction of Dantrium therapy should only be contemplated in patients who clearly need the drug, and only after complete reversal of the signs of hepatotoxicity and liver function tests. Patients being re-challenged with Dantrium should be hospital in-patients, and small, gradually increasing doses should be used. Laboratory test monitoring should be frequent, and the drug should be withdrawn immediately if there is any indication of recurrent liver abnormality. Some patients have reacted with unmistakeable signs of liver abnormality upon administration of an initial test dose, whilst others have not.

The use of Dantrium with other potentially hepatotoxic drugs should be avoided.

There are isolated cases of possibly significant effects of Dantrium on the cardiovascular and respiratory systems. These cases also have other features suggesting a pre-disposition to cardiovascular disease, and impaired respiratory function, particularly obstructive pulmonary disease. Dantrium should be used with caution in such patients.

Patients should be advised not to drive a motor vehicle or to undertake potentially dangerous work until Dantrium therapy has been stabilised, because some patients experience drowsiness and dizziness. Caution should be exercised in the simultaneous administration of tranquillising agents and alcohol.

Action in event of overdosage: For acute overdosage, general supportive measures and gastric lavage should be employed as well as measures to reduce the absorption of Dantrium. The theoretical possibility of crystalluria in overdose has not been reported for Dantrium, but would be treated according to general principles, including administration of fluids.

Side-effects and adverse reactions: The most frequently reported unwanted effects associated with the use of Dantrium have been drowsiness, dizziness, weakness, general malaise, fatigue and diarrhoea. These effects are generally transient, occur early in treatment, and can often be obviated by careful determination and regulation of the dosage. Diarrhoea may be severe, and may necessitate temporary withdrawal of Dantrium. If diarrhoea recurs upon re-introduction of Dantrium, then Dantrium therapy should probably be withdrawn permanently. Other frequent side effects include anorexia, nausea, headache, and skin rash. Less frequent side-effects include: constipation, dysphagia, speech disturbance, visual disturbance, confusion, nervousness, depression, seizures, increased urinary frequency, and insomnia. Rare reports include tachycardia, erratic blood pressure, dyspnoea, haematuria, crystalluria (unconfirmed reports), urinary incontinence, and urinary retention. Pleural effusion and/or pericarditis in patients using Dantrium have been rarely reported. Chills and fever have occasionally been reported.

Dantrium has a potential for hepatotoxicity. Symptomatic hepatitis (fatal and non-fatal) has been reported at various dose levels although the incidence is greater in patients taking more than 400 mg/day. Liver dysfunction as evidenced by blood chemical abnormalities alone (liver enzyme elevation) has been observed in patients exposed to Dantrium for varying periods of time. Overt hepatitis has occurred at varying intervals after initiation of therapy, but has most frequently been observed between the second and twelfth month of treatment. *The risk of hepatic injury appears to be greater in females, in patients over 30 years old and in patients taking concomitant medication.* There is some evidence that hepatic injury is more likely in patients using concomitant oral oestrogens.

An idiosyncratic interaction between verapamil and intravenous Dantrium, involving hypotension, hyperkalaemia, and myocardial depression, has been reported as a single case. This interaction has been replicated in dogs and pigs.

Pharmaceutical precautions Dantrium capsules should be stored at a temperature not exceeding 30°C.

Legal category POM.

Package quantities Dantrium capsules 25 mg and Dantrium capsules 100 mg are supplied in containers of 100 capsules.

Further information The duration and intensity of skeletal muscle relaxation in patients on Dantrium is related to the dosage and blood levels. The mean biological half-life of Dantrium is about nine hours after a 100 mg dose.

Studies specifically designed to determine compatibility with diazepam and phenobarbitone revealed that neither of these drugs appears to affect Dantrium metabolism.

Product licence numbers

Dantrium capsules 25 mg	0364/0015R
Dantrium capsules 100 mg	0364/0016R

DANTRIUM* INTRAVENOUS

Presentation Dantrium Intravenous is supplied as a sterile, lyophilized powder. Each vial contains a mixture of 20 mg dantrolene sodium, 3 g mannitol and sufficient sodium hydroxide to yield a pH of approximately 9.5 when reconstituted with 60 ml of Water for Injections PhEur.

Uses Dantrium Intravenous is indicated for the treatment of malignant hyperthermia. It is for intravenous use only.

Mode of action: In isolated muscle preparations, dantrolene sodium uncouples the excitation and contraction of skeletal muscle, probably by interfering with the release of calcium from the sarcoplasmic reticulum.

In the malignant hyperthermia syndrome, evidence points to an intrinsic abnormality of muscle tissue. It has been postulated that 'triggering agents' (i.e. skeletal muscle relaxants and inhalation anaesthetics) induce a sudden rise in myoplasmic calcium, either by preventing the sarcoplasmic reticulum from accumulating calcium adequately, or by accelerating its release. This rise in myoplasmic calcium activates the acute catabolic processes involved in the malignant hyperthermia crisis.

Dantrolene sodium may prevent the increases in myoplasmic calcium and the acute catabolism within the muscle cell by interfering with the release of calcium from the sarcoplasmic reticulum to the myoplasm. Thus the physiological, metabolic and biochemical changes associated with the crisis may be reversed or attenuated.

Dosage and administration As soon as the malignant hyperthermia syndrome is recognised all anaesthetic agents should be discontinued. An initial Dantrium Intravenous dose of 1 mg/kg should be given rapidly into the vein. It must not be mixed with other intravenous infusions. If the physiological and metabolic abnormalities persist or reappear, this dose may be repeated up to a cumulative dose of 10 mg/kg. Clinical experience to date has shown that the average dose of Dantrium Intravenous required to reverse the manifestations of malignant hyperthermia has been 2.5 mg/kg. If a relapse or recurrence occurs, Dantrium Intravenous should be readministered at the last effective dose.

Mixing instructions: Each vial of Dantrium Intravenous should be reconstituted by adding 60 ml of Water for Injections PhEur, and shaking until the solution is clear. Use within six hours of reconstitution, protecting from light and temperatures above 30°C and below 15°C.

Contra-indications, warnings, etc
Precautions: 1. In some subjects as much as 10 mg/kg of Dantrium Intravenous has been needed to reverse the crisis. In a 70 kg man this dose would require approximately 36 vials. Such a volume has been administered in approximately one and a half hours.

2. Because of the high pH of the intravenous formulation of Dantrium, care must be taken to prevent extravasation of the intravenous solution into the surrounding tissues.

3. *Pregnancy:* The safety of Dantrium Intravenous in pregnant women has not been established; it should be given only when the potential benefits have been weighed against the possible risk to mother and child.

4. *Drug interactions:* The combination of therapeutic doses of intravenous dantrolene sodium and verapamil in halothane/alpha-chloralose anaesthetized swine has resulted in ventricular fibrillation and cardiovascular collapse in association with marked hyperkalaemia. It is recommended that the combination of intravenous dantrolene sodium and calcium channel blockers, such as verapamil, not be used during the reversal of a malignant hyperthermia crisis until the relevance of these findings to humans is established.

Warnings: The use of Dantrium Intravenous in the management of malignant hyperthermia is not a substitute for previously known supportive measures. It will be necessary to discontinue the suspect triggering agents, attend to increased oxygen requirements and manage the metabolic acidosis. When necessary institute cooling, attend to urinary output and monitor for electrolyte imbalance.

Side-effects and adverse reactions: No side-effects have been attributed to Dantrium Intravenous in patients treated with short-term therapy for malignant hyperthermia. The nature of the emergency and the complexity of concomitant therapy will make it extremely difficult to isolate cause and effect relationships for any of the drugs used. Hepatotoxic reactions have been noted in a small number of subjects given long term oral dantrolene therapy.

Pharmaceutical precautions Unreconstituted product should be protected from light and stored below 30°C.

Legal category POM.

Package quantities Dantrium Intravenous is available in packs of twelve vials each containing 20 mg dantrolene sodium.

Further information Because of the nature of the freeze-drying process used in the manufacture of Dantrium Intravenous, the freeze-dried cake of Dantrium Intravenous may have a mottled orange/white appearance or be in the form of loose aggregates. This is an entirely normal artefact and in no way compromises the stability of the product.

Product licence number 0364/0030.

DIDRONEL* I.V.

Presentation Didronel I.V. is a clear colourless sterile solution of Etidronate Disodium USP. Each ampoule contains 300 mg Etidronate Disodium USP in 6 ml Water for Injections PhEur.

Uses Didronel I.V., together with achievement and maintenance of adequate hydration, is indicated in the initial intravenous therapy for hypercalcaemia of malignancy. Patients with and without metastasis to bone have been responsive to treatment with Didronel I.V.

Didronel I.V. is also indicated for the treatment of hypercalcaemia of malignancy when other modes of therapy, such as hydration, have inadequately reduced elevated serum calcium.

Dosage and administration The recommended daily dose of Didronel I.V. is 7.5 mg/kg/day for three successive days. This daily dose should be diluted in at least 250 ml of 0.9% w/v Sodium Chloride Intravenous Infusion BP, but can be added to volumes of fluid greater than 250 ml when convenient. Diluted Didronel I.V. should be administered intravenously over a period of at least 2 hours. Regardless of the volume of solution in which Didronel I.V. is diluted slow infusion is important to safety. The minimum infusion time of 2 hours at the recommended dose, or at smaller doses, should be observed.

Retreatment with Didronel I.V. may be appropriate if hypercalcaemia recurs. There should be at least a 7 day interval between courses of treatment with Didronel I.V. The dose and manner of treatment is the same as that for the initial treatment. The safety and efficacy of more than two courses of therapy has not been established.

In the presence of impaired renal function reduction of the dose may be advisable.

It is recommended that in addition to Didronel I.V., oral or intravenous fluids should be given in amounts adequate to establish or maintain normal hydration.

Safety and efficacy in children have not been established.

Contra-indications, warnings, etc
Contra-indications: Known hypersensitivity to etidronate disodium. Didronel I.V. therapy should be withheld from patients with impaired renal function where serum creatinine is greater than 440 μmol/litre.

Warnings: Occasional mild to moderate abnormalities in renal function (elevated blood urea nitrogen and/or serum creatinine) have been observed when Didronel I.V. was given as directed to patients with hypercalcaemia of malignancy. These changes were reversible or remained stable, without worsening, after completion of the course of Didronel I.V. In some patients with pre-existing renal impairment or in those who had received potentially nephrotoxic drugs, further depression of renal function was sometimes seen. This suggests that Didronel I.V. may produce or aggravate the depression of renal function in approximately 8 out of 203 treatment courses when used to treat hypercalcaemia of malignancy. Therefore, it is recommended that appropriate monitoring of renal function with serum creatinine and/or blood urea nitrogen be carried out with Didronel I.V. treatment.

Since Didronel is excreted by the kidney, it is important to know that renal function is adequate to handle not only the increased fluid load but also the excretion of the drug itself.

The effect of Didronel I.V. administration on renal function in patients with serum creatinine greater than 220 μmol/l has not been systematically examined in controlled trials. Reduction of the dose of Didronel I.V. may be advisable in patients with renal functional impairment, with serum creatinine levels of 220–440 μmol/l and Didronel I.V. should be used only if the potential benefit of hypercalcaemia correction will substantially exceed the potential for worsening of renal function. In patients with serum creatinine levels greater than 440 μmol/l Didronel I.V. should be withheld.

Precautions: Hypercalcaemia may cause or exacerbate impaired renal function. In clinical trials, while elevations of serum creatinine or blood urea nitrogen were seen in patients with hypercalcaemia of malignancy prior to treatment with Didronel I.V., these measurements improved or remained unchanged in most patients. Nevertheless elevations in serum creatinine during treatment with Didronel I.V. have been observed in approximately 10% of patients.

In the principal clinical trial of Didronel I.V., 18% of patients treated one or more times with Didronel I.V. had serum calcium values below the lower limits of normal. When adjusted for levels of reduced serum albumin, less than 1% of patients are estimated to have hypocalcaemic ionised serum calcium levels. No adverse effects have been traced to hypocalcaemia.

The hypercalcaemia of hyperparathyroidism is usually refractory to Didronel I.V. It is possible for this disease to coexist in patients with malignancy. Didronel I.V. is not contra-indicated in patients with hyperparathyroidism; however, it may be ineffective if increased renal tubular reabsorption of calcium is an important mechanism contributing to the hypercalcaemia. This contribution is usual in patients with hyperparathyroidism.

In clinical studies there have been no reports of adverse effects attributed to the concurrent use of Didronel I.V. with corticosteroids, phosphate, calcitonin or frusemide therapies and the effects may be additive. Concurrent use with plicamycin has not been investigated.

Pregnancy and lactation: No adequate well controlled reproduction or teratology studies have been carried out with intravenous etidronate disodium. Reproduction/teratology studies performed in rats and rabbits at perioral doses up to five times the maximum oral human dose have revealed no evidence of impaired fertility or harm to the foetus due to Didronel. At oral doses of 22 times the maximum oral human dose, a decrease in live foetuses were observed in rats. The only incidence of malformations occurred in rats at exaggerated doses following subcutaneous administration and was skeletal in nature. These malformations were deemed the result of the pharmacological action of the drug. There are no adequate, well controlled studies in pregnant women. Because animal reproduction studies are not always predictive of human response, this drug should be used during pregnancy only if clearly needed.

Nursing mothers: It is not known whether this drug is excreted in human milk. Because many drugs are excreted in human milk, caution should be exercised when Didronel IV is administered to a nursing woman.

Side-effects and adverse reactions: Metallic or altered taste, or loss of taste during and/or after infusion, which disappears within a few hours.

Hypercalcaemia of malignancy is frequently associated with abnormal elevations of serum creatinine and blood urea nitrogen. However, a causal relationship between increases in serum creatinine and the administration of Didronel I.V. cannot be ruled out.

Action in event of an overdose: Rapid intravenous administration of Didronel I.V. at doses above 27 mg/kg has produced ECG changes and bleeding problems in animals. These abnormalities are probably related to marked and/or rapid decreases in ionised calcium levels in blood and tissue fluids. They are thought to be due to the chelation of calcium by massive amounts of the diphosphonate. These abnormalities have been shown to be reversible in animal studies by the administration of ionisable calcium salts.

Overdose would be clinically manifested as the signs and symptoms of hypocalcaemia, such as paraesthesia and carpopedal spasm. The chelation effects of etidronate disodium should be reversible with the intravenous administration of calcium gluconate.

Pharmaceutical precautions Didronel I.V. should be stored at a temperature not exceeding 30°C. Protect the diluted solution from temperatures below 15°C and above 30°C. Use within 24 hours of dilution.

Legal category POM.

Package quantities Didronel I.V. is available in packs containing six ampoules. Each ampoule contains a solution of 300 mg Etidronate Disodium USP in 6 ml of Water for Injections Ph. Eur.

Further information Didronel is also known as EHDP (the disodium salt of ethane-1-hydroxy-1, 1-diphosphonate).

Product licence number 0364/0041.

DIDRONEL* TABLETS

Presentation White, rectangular tablets, marked with 'P&G' on one face and '402' on the other. Each tablet contains Etidronate Disodium USP 200 mg.

Uses

Indications:

(a) Paget's disease of bone: Didronel is indicated for the treatment of Paget's disease of bone (osteitis deformans). Effectiveness has been demonstrated primarily in patients with polyostotic Paget's disease with symptoms of pain and with clinically significant elevations of urinary hydroxyproline and serum alkaline phosphatase. In other circumstances in which there is extensive involvement of the skull or the spine with the prospect of irreversible neurological damage, or when a weight-bearing bone may be involved, the use of Didronel may be considered.

(b) Hypercalcaemia of malignancy: Oral Didronel treatment is indicated in hypercalcaemia of malignancy to help maintain clinically acceptable serum calcium levels following successful initial intravenous treatment with Didronel I.V.

Dosage and administration 5 mg/kg/day to 20 mg/kg/day as detailed below.

(a) Paget's disease:

Adults: The recommended initial dose of Didronel for most patients is 5 mg/kg body weight/day, for a period not exceeding six months. Doses above 10 mg/kg should be reserved for use when there is an overriding requirement for suppression of increased bone turnover associated with Paget's disease or when the patient requires more prompt reduction of elevated cardiac output. Treatment with doses above 10 mg/kg/day should be approached cautiously and should not exceed three months duration. Doses in excess of 20 mg/kg/day are not recommended.

Retreatment should be undertaken only after a drug-free period of at least three months and after it is evident that reactivation of the disease has occurred and biochemical indices of the disease have become substantially re-elevated or approach pre-treatment values (approximately twice the upper limit of normal or 75% of pre-treatment value). In no case should duration of retreatment exceed the maximum duration of the initial treatment. Premature retreatment should be avoided. In clinical trials the biochemical improvements obtained during drug therapy have generally persisted for a period of three months to, in some cases, up to two years after drug withdrawal.

Children: Disorders of bone in children, referred to as

juvenile Paget's disease, have been reported rarely. The relationship to adult Paget's disease has not been established. Didronel has not been studied in children for Paget's disease.

(b) Hypercalcaemia of malignancy:
Adults: Didronel tablets may be administered on the day following the last intravenous dose of Didronel I.V. in order to help maintain clinically acceptable serum calcium levels. The recommended dose for patients who have had hypercalcaemia is 20 mg/kg/day for 30 days. If serum calcium levels remain normal or at clinically acceptable levels, treatment may be extended. Treatment for more than 90 days has not been adequately studied and is not recommended.

Children: Safety and efficacy have not been established in children.

Directions for use: Didronel should be administered as a single, oral dose, two hours before a meal. It may be given with fruit juice or water. Food in the stomach or upper portions of the small intestine, particularly materials with a high calcium content such as milk and vitamins with mineral supplements or antacids, may reduce absorption. Therefore, eating should be avoided for two hours before and after drug administration.

Daily dosage guide

Body weight		Required daily regimen of 200 mg tablets		
Kilograms	Stones	5 mg/kg*	10 mg/kg*	20 mg/kg†
50	8	1	3	5
60	9.5	2	3	6
70	11	2	4	7
80	12.5	2	4	8
90	14	2	5	9

* Course of therapy – 6 months
† Course of therapy – 3 months

Contra-indications, warnings, etc Known hypersensitivity to etidronate disodium.

Precautions:

1. *General:* Didronel retards mineralisation of osteoid laid down during the bone accretion process. This effect is dose and time dependent. There may be an overlap of beneficial and mineralisation inhibition effects in some patients at higher doses. Extended periods of medication should be approached cautiously. When administered at doses of 20 mg/kg/day Didronel suppresses bone turnover and essentially greatly reduces mineralisation of new bone in Pagetic lesions and, to a lesser extent, in the uninvolved skeleton. Mineralisation of Pagetic lesions has been demonstrated to occur normally after discontinuation of the drug.

At lower doses (5 mg/kg/day), mineralisation inhibition is uncommon and when it occurs it is focal in nature. This does not usually present a clinical problem. However, should a patient present with significant osteolysis in a weight-bearing bone, special efforts should be taken to prevent the possibility of a combination of mineralisation inhibition and a failure of the drug to inhibit resorption leading to an adverse effect on bone.

It is recommended that serum phosphate, serum alkaline phosphatase and if possible urinary hydroxyproline be measured before commencing medication and at three month intervals during treatment. If after three months of medication the pretreatment levels of serum alkaline phosphatase and/or urinary hydroxyproline have not been reduced by at least 25%, the patient may be relatively resistant to therapy. If the serum phosphate level is essentially unchanged in the "resistant" patient, consideration should be given to increasing the dose since the absorption of pharmacologically active amounts of Didronel is typically accompanied by a rise in serum phosphate. This rise usually correlates with reductions in the biochemical indices of disease activity. If after three or more months of medication elevations of serum phosphate above the upper limit of normal are not accompanied by clinical or biochemical evidence of reduced activity, resistance of the disease to the action of Didronel is probable and termination of Didronel medication should be considered. Patients in whom serum phosphate elevations are high and reductions of disease activity are low may be particularly prone to retarded mineralisation of new osteoid. In those cases where 200 mg per day (a single tablet) may be excessive, doses may be administered less frequently.

Patients with Paget's disease of bone should maintain an adequate nutritional status, and particularly, an adequate intake of calcium and vitamin D. Patients with restricted vitamin D and calcium intake may be particularly sensitive to drugs that affect calcium homeostasis and should be closely monitored during Didronel therapy.

Didronel is not metabolised but excreted unchanged via the kidney; therefore, treatment of patients with impaired renal function should be approached very cautiously, if at all.

Hyperphosphataemia may occur in patients taking 10 mg/kg or more of Didronel daily. No adverse effects of drug induced hyperphosphataemia have been observed and hyperphosphataemia is not a contraindication for therapy. It is apparently due to drug-related increased tubular re-absorption of phospate by the kidney. Serum phosphate levels generally return to normal 2–4 weeks post-therapy.

Didronel therapy has been withheld from patients with enterocolitis because increased frequency of bowel movements and diarrhoea are seen in some patients when Didronel is administered at a dose of 20 mg/kg/day and may be increased occasionally at lower doses.

2. *Pregnancy: Teratogenic effects:* Reproduction/teratology studies performed in rats and rabbits at oral doses up to five times the maximum human oral dose by the intended route of administration have revealed no evidence of impaired fertility or harm to the foetus due to Didronel. At oral doses of 22 times the maximum human dose, a decrease in live foetuses was observed in rats. The only incidence of malformations occurred in rats at exaggerated doses following subcutaneous administration and were skeletal in nature. These malformations were deemed the result of the pharmacological action of the drug. There are no adequate well controlled studies in pregnant women. Because animal reproduction studies are not always predictive of human response, this drug should be used during pregnancy only if clearly needed.

3. *Nursing mothers:* It is not known whether this drug is excreted in human milk. Because many drugs are excreted in human milk, caution should be exercised when Didronel is administered to a nursing woman.

Warnings: In Pagetic patients the physician should adhere to the recommended dose regimen in order to avoid overtreatment with Didronel. The response to therapy may be of slow onset and may continue even for months after treatment when the drug has been discontinued. Dosage should not be increased prematurely nor should treatment be resumed before there is clear evidence of reactivation of the disease process. Retreatment should not be initiated until the patient has had at least a three-month drug-free interval.

Increased or recurrent bone pain at existing Pagetic sites and/or the appearance of pain at sites previously asymptomatic has been reported. At a dose of 5 mg/kg/day 1 out of 10 patients reported the phenomenon; at higher doses the figure rose to 2 out of 10. In placebo-treated patients, the occurrence was 1 out of 15. In Didronel treated patients, the pain resolved while therapy was continued in some patients but persisted for several months in others.

Fractures are recognised as a common feature in patients with Paget's disease. There has been no evidence of increased risk at the recommended dose of 5 mg/kg/day for six months. The risk of fracture may be increased when Didronel is taken at a dose level of 20 mg/kg/day in excess of three months. This risk may be greater in patients with extensive and severe disease, a history of multiple fractures, and/or rapidly advancing osteolytic lesions. It is recommended that the drug be discontinued when fractures occur and that the therapy not be reinstated until fracture healing is complete.

The incidence of osteogenic sarcoma is known to be increased in Paget's disease. Pagetic lesions, with or without therapy, may appear by X-ray to progress markedly, possibly with some loss of definition of periosteal margins. Such lesions should be evaluated carefully to differentiate these from osteogenic sarcoma.

Side-effects: Gastro-intestinal complaints such as diarrhoea and nausea are increased in some patients when Didronel is administered at doses greater than 5 mg/kg/day. The incidence is about 1 out of 15 in both placebo-treated patients and in patients on Didronel, 5 mg/kg/day. The incidence rises to approximately 2 out of 10 patients with Didronel at the dose of 20 mg/kg/day.

At oral doses of 20 mg/kg/day, mineralisation of newly formed osteoid may be impaired. At lower doses, occasionally, focal but not universal mineralisation inhibition has been reported. Adverse reactions associated with such changes have not been reported in patients treated for hypercalcaemia at this dose. Mineralisation occurs normally after discontinuation of the drug.

Hypersensitivity reactions, including angioneurotic oedema/urticaria, rash and/or pruritus, have been reported rarely.

Overdosage: Overdose would be manifested as the signs and symptoms of hypocalcaemia. Treatment should be by cessation of therapy, correction of hypocalcaemia with intravenous calcium gluconate and maintenance of an adequate nutritional status, artificially supplemented if necessary.

Pharmaceutical precautions Normal pharmaceutical storage and handling are indicated. Store below 30°C.

Legal category POM.

Package quantities 60 × 200 mg tablets.

Further information Didronel is also known as EHDP (the disodium salt of ethane-1-hydroxy-1, 1-diphosphonate).

Product licence number 0364/0039.

FURADANTIN*

Presentation Furadantin Tablets are yellow in colour and have a pentagonal shape. Each tablet has a break line on one face and the tablet strength is shown on the opposite face. Furadantin Tablets are available in two strengths, containing 100 mg or 50 mg Nitrofurantoin PhEur. Furadantin Suspension is a yellow suspension containing 25 mg Nitrofurantoin PhEur per 5 ml.

Uses Furadantin is indicated for the treatment of and prophylaxis against acute or recurrent, uncomplicated lower urinary tract infections or pyelitis either spontaneous or following surgical procedures.

Nitrofurantoin is specifically indicated for the treatment of infections when due to susceptible strains of *Escherichia coli*, enterococci, staphylococci, *Citrobacter*, *Klebsiella* and *Enterobacter*.

Most strains of *Proteus* and *Serratia* are resistant. All *Pseudomonas* strains are resistant.

Furadantin is not indicated for the treatment of associated renal cortical or perinephric abscesses.

Dosage and administration
Adults: Furadantin is administered orally. The dose should be taken with each meal and at bedtime, with food or milk. In the event of severe nausea the dose may be reduced, but not below the adult equivalent of 200 mg in 24 hours. Should it persist the drug should be withdrawn.

For acute uncomplicated urinary tract infections: 50 mg four times daily for 7 days.

For severe chronic recurrent infections: 100 mg four times daily for 7 days.

For long-term suppressive therapy: When such therapy is desirable 50 mg–100 mg once a day at bedtime is suggested. See 'Precautions and warnings' regarding risks associated with long-term therapy.

For prophylaxis: 50 mg four times daily on the day of the procedure and for 3 days thereafter is recommended.

Children: Furadantin Suspension or Furadantin Tablets 50 mg may be used:

For acute urinary tract infections: 3 mg/kg/day in four divided doses for seven days.

For suppressive therapy: 1 mg/kg/day once a day.

Elderly patients: Provided there is no significant renal impairment, in which nitrofurantoin is contra-indicated, the dosage should be that for any normal adult. See 'Precautions' for risks to elderly patients associated with long-term therapy.

Contra-indications, warnings, etc
Contra-indications: Furadantin is contra-indicated in patients suffering from renal dysfunction with a creatinine clearance of less than 60 ml/minute or elevated serum creatinine.

Furadantin is contra-indicated in infants under one month of age as well as pregnant patients at term (during labour and delivery) because of the theoretical possibility of haemolytic anaemia in the foetus or in the newborn infant due to immature erythrocyte enzyme systems.

Furadantin is also contra-indicated in those patients with known hypersensitivity to nitrofurantoin or other nitrofurans.

Precautions: Nitrofurantoin is not effective for the treatment of parenchymal infections of unilaterally functioning kidney. A surgical cause for infections should be excluded in recurrent or severe cases.

Peripheral neuropathy which may become severe or irreversible has occurred and may be life threatening. Nitrofurantoin should be used with caution in patients with anaemia, diabetes mellitus, electrolyte imbalance, debilitating conditions, vitamin B (particularly folate) deficiency. Therefore, treatment should be stopped at the first signs of neural involvement (paraesthesiae).

Since pre-existing conditions may mask hepatic or pulmonary adverse reactions, nitrofurantoin should be used with caution in patients with pulmonary disease, hepatic dysfunction, neurological disorders and allergic diathesis.

Acute, subacute or chronic pulmonary reactions have been observed in patients treated with nitrofurantoin. If these reactions occur, Furadantin should be discontinued and appropriate measures taken. Reports have cited pulmonary reactions as a contributing cause of death.

Chronic pulmonary reactions (diffuse interstitial pneumonitis or pulmonary fibrosis or both) can develop insidiously. These reactions occur rarely and generally in patients receiving therapy for six months or longer. Chronic pulmonary reactions may occur more commonly in elderly patients. Close monitoring of the pulmonary condition of patients receiving long term therapy is warranted and requires that the benefits of therapy be weighed against potential risks.

Hepatic reactions, including cholestatic jaundice and chronic active hepatitis, occur rarely. Fatalities have been reported. Cholestatic jaundice is generally associated with short-term therapy (usually up to two weeks). Chronic active hepatitis is generally associated with long-term therapy (usually after six months); the onset may be insidious, and patients should be monitored periodically for changes in liver function. If hepatitis occurs, the drug should be withdrawn immediately and appropriate measures taken.

Ten percent of black patients and a variable percentage of ethnic groups of Mediterranean, Near Eastern and Asian origin, suffer from a deficiency of glucose-6-phosphate dehydrogenase in their blood cells. In such people, nitrofurantoin in common with many other therapeutic agents may cause haemolysis. This enzyme deficiency is extremely rare in Caucasians. Any sign of haemolysis is an indication to discontinue the drug. Haemolysis ceases when the drug is withdrawn.

Discontinue treatment with nitrofurantoin if otherwise unexplained pulmonary, hepatotoxic, haematological or neurologic syndromes occur.

For long-term treatment monitor patient closely for appearance of hepatic or pulmonary symptoms and other evidence of toxicity.

Pregnancy and lactation: Based on animal reproduction

studies and clinical experience in humans over many years, there is no evidence of any teratogenic effects of nitrofurantoin on the foetus. When antibiotic therapy is required during pregnancy, nitrofurantoin may be considered appropriate. However, caution should be exercised while breast feeding an infant known or suspected to have any erythrocyte enzyme deficiency as nitrofurantoin is detected in trace amounts in breast milk.

However, as with all drugs, the maternal side effects may adversely affect the course of the pregnancy. The drug should be used at the lowest effective dose as appropriate for the specific indication only after careful assessment of benefits against potential risks.

Action in event of overdosage: Symptoms and signs of overdosage include gastric irritation, nausea and vomiting. There is no known specific antidote. Nitrofurantoin can be haemodialysed. Standard treatment is by induction of emesis or by gastric lavage in cases of recent ingestion. Standard monitoring procedures for drug overdose, e.g. full blood count, liver function tests and pulmonary function, are recommended. A high fluid intake should be maintained to promote urinary excretion of the drug.

Adverse effects: Respiratory: Actue, subacute or chronic pulmonary reactions may occur.

Acute pulmonary reactions are commonly manifested by fever, chills, cough, chest pain, dyspnoea, pulmonary infiltration with consolidation or pleural effusion on X-ray and eosinophilia. Acute reactions usually occur within the first week of treatment and are reversible with cessation of therapy. Resolution often is dramatic.

In subacute pulmonary reactions, fever and eosinophilia occur less often than in the acute form. Upon cessation of therapy, recovery may require several months. If the symptoms are not recognised as being drug-related and therapy is not stopped, they may become more severe.

Chronic pulmonary reactions may occur in patients who have received continuous therapy for six months or more. Chronic pulmonary reactions may occur more commonly in elderly patients. Malaise, dyspnoea on exertion, cough and altered pulmonary function are common manifestations which can occur insidiously. Radiological and histological findings of diffuse interstitial pneumonitis or fibrosis, or both, are also common manifestations of the chronic pulmonary reactions. Fever is rarely prominent. The severity of chronic pulmonary reactions and their degree of resolution appear to be related to the duration of therapy after the first clinical signs appear. Pulmonary function may be impaired permanently, even after cessation of therapy. The risk is greater when chronic pulmonary reactions are not recognised early.

Gastro-intestinal: Nausea and anorexia have been reported. Emesis, abdominal pain and diarrhoea are less common gastro-intestinal reactions. These reactions may be minimised by taking the drug with food or milk or by adjustment of dosage.

Hepatic reactions including cholestatic jaundice and chronic active hepatitis occur rarely.

Hypersensitivity: Exfoliative dermatitis and erythema multiforme (including Stevens-Johnson syndrome) have been reported rarely.

Allergic skin reactions manifesting as angioneurotic oedema, maculopapular, erythematous or eczematous eruptions, urticaria, rash, and pruritus have occurred. Lupus-like syndrome associated with pulmonary reaction to nitrofurantoin has been reported.

Other hypersensitivity reactions include anaphylaxis, sialadenitis, pancreatitis, drug fever, and arthralgia.

Haematological: Agranulocytosis, leucopenia, granulocytopenia, haemolytic anaemia, thrombocytopenia, glucose-6-phosphate dehydrogenase deficiency anaemia, megaloblastic anaemia and eosinophilia have occurred. Cessation of therapy has generally returned the blood picture to normal. Aplastic anaemia has been reported rarely.

Neurological: Peripheral neuropathy, which may become severe or irreversible, has occurred. Less frequent reactions, of unknown causal relationship are nystagmus, vertigo, dizziness, asthenia, headache and drowsiness.

Miscellaneous: Transient alopecia has been reported.

As with other antimicrobial agents superinfections by fungi or resistant organisms such as *Pseudomonas* may occur. However, these are limited to the genito-urinary tract because suppression of normal bacterial flora does not occur elsewhere in the body.

Interactions: Concomitant administration of magnesium trisilicate with nitrofurantoin reduces both the rate and extent of absorption.

Uricosuric drugs such as probenecid and sulphinpyrazone may inhibit renal tubular secretion of nitrofurantoin. The resulting increase in serum levels may increase toxicity and the decreased urinary levels could lessen its efficacy as a urinary tract antibacterial.

Nitrofurantoin may antagonise the antibacterial efficacy of the quinolones. Concurrent use is not recommended.

Unlike many drugs, the presence of food or agents delaying gastric emptying can increase the bioavailability of nitrofurantoin presumably by allowing better dissolution in gastric juices.

There may be decreased antibacterial activity for nitrofurantoin in the presence of carbonic anhydrase inhibitors and urine alkalinising agents.

Pharmaceutical precautions Furadantin Tablets are supplied in polypropylene containers with polythene pilfer-proof caps. The tablets should be stored in light-proof and preferably moisture-resistant containers. Storage temperature must not exceed 30°C.

Furadantin Suspension is supplied in amber bottles and should be protected from light as exposure will cause darkening of the active principle. Because of this, amber bottles should be used in dispensing. The glass should preferably be neutral since discoloration will occur on contact with alkaline materials. Furadantin Suspension should be stored at a temperature not exceeding 30°C and should be protected from freezing.

It is not recommended to dilute Furadantin Suspension.

Legal category POM.

Package quantities Furadantin Tablets 100 mg and 50 mg are supplied in packs of 100.

Furadantin suspension is supplied in bottles of 300 ml.

Further information The urine of patients receiving Furadantin may be coloured a dark yellow or brown. This results from the presence of drug and/or metabolite(s) and is quite harmless. Furadantin can interfere with certain laboratory tests. False positive or spuriously high readings may be produced with urine glucose tests utilising the copper sulphate reduction method, e.g. Benedict's reagent, Clinitest (Ames). However, there is no interference with the Clinistix test.

Product licence numbers

Furadantin Tablets 50 mg	0364/0008R
Furadantin Tablets 100 mg	0364/0009R
Furadantin Suspension	0364/0010R

MACRODANTIN*

Presentation Macrodantin is presented in hard gelatin capsules and is available in two strengths, containing 100 mg or 50 mg Nitrofurantoin PhEur macrocrystals.

The 100 mg capsule has an opaque yellow body and cap and bears the monogram 'Macrodantin 100'.

The 50 mg capsule has an opaque yellow cap and opaque white body and bears the monogram 'Macrodantin 50'.

Uses Macrodantin is indicated for the treatment of and prophylaxis against acute or recurrent, uncomplicated lower urinary tract infections or pyelitis either spontaneous or following surgical procedures.

Nitrofurantoin is specifically indicated for the treatment of infections when due to susceptible strains of *Escherichia coli*, enterococci, staphylococci, *Citrobacter*, *Klebsiella* and *Enterobacter*.

Most strains of *Proteus* and *Serratia* are resistant. All *Pseudomonas* strains are resistant.

Macrodantin is not indicated for the treatment of associated renal cortical or perinephric abscesses.

The nitrofurantoin macrocrystals of Macrodantin are specially formulated. The crystal size is designed to control the rate of absorption and thus reduce the incidence of nausea. Clinical and animal studies indicate that Macrodantin therapy decreases the likelihood of nausea in patients who might experience these symptoms on nitrofurantoin therapy. This special reformulation of nitrofurantoin has not caused any decrease in antibacterial efficacy.

Dosage and administration

Adults: Macrodantin is administered orally. The dose should be taken with each meal and at bedtime, with food or milk. In the event of severe nausea the dose may be reduced, but not below the adult equivalent of 200 mg in 24 hours. Should it persist the drug should be withdrawn.

For acute uncomplicated urinary tract infections: 50 mg four times daily for 7 days.

For severe chronic recurrent infections: 100 mg four times daily for 7 days.

For long-term suppressive therapy: When such therapy is desirable 50 mg–100 mg once a day at bedtime is suggested. See 'Precautions and warnings' regarding risks associated with long-term therapy.

For prophylaxis: 50 mg four times daily on the day of the procedure and for 3 days after is recommended.

Children: For acute urinary tract infections: 3 mg/kg/day in four divided doses for seven days.

For suppressive therapy: 1 mg/kg/day once a day.

For children under 25 kg bodyweight consideration should be given to the use of Furadantin Suspension.

Elderly patients: Provided there is no significant renal impairment, in which nitrofurantoin is contra-indicated, the dosage should be that for any normal adult. See 'Precautions' for risks to elderly patients associated with long-term therapy.

Contra-indications, warnings, etc

Contra-indications: Macrodantin is contra-indicated in patients suffering from renal dysfunction with a creatinine clearance of less than 60 ml/minute or elevated serum creatinine.

Macrodantin is contra-indicated in infants under one month of age as well as pregnant patients at term (during labour and delivery) because of the theoretical possibility of haemolytic anaemia in the foetus or in the newborn infant due to immature erythrocyte enzyme systems.

Macrodantin is also contra-indicated in those patients with known hypersensitivity to nitrofurantoin or other nitrofurans.

Precautions: Nitrofurantoin is not effective for the treatment of parenchymal infections of unilaterally functioning kidney. A surgical cause for infections should be excluded in recurrent or severe cases.

Peripheral neuropathy which may become severe or irreversible has occurred and may be life threatening. Nitrofurantoin should be used with caution in patients with anaemia, diabetes mellitus, electrolyte imbalance, debilitating conditions, vitamin B (particularly folate) deficiency. Therefore, treatment should be stopped at the first signs of neural involvement (paraesthesiae).

Since pre-existing conditions may mask hepatic or pulmonary adverse reactions, nitrofurantoin should be used with caution in patients with pulmonary disease, hepatic dysfunction, neurological disorders and allergic diathesis.

Acute, subacute or chronic pulmonary reactions have been observed in patients treated with nitrofurantoin. If these reactions occur, Macrodantin should be discontinued and appropriate measures taken. Reports have cited pulmonary reactions as a contributing cause of death.

Chronic pulmonary reactions (diffuse interstitial pneumonitis or pulmonary fibrosis or both) can develop insidiously. These reactions occur rarely and generally in patients receiving therapy for six months or longer. Chronic pulmonary reactions may occur more commonly in elderly patients. Close monitoring of the pulmonary condition of patients receiving long term therapy is warranted and requires that the benefits of therapy be weighed against potential risks.

Hepatic reactions, including cholestatic jaundice and chronic active hepatitis, occur rarely. Fatalities have been reported. Cholestatic jaundice is generally associated with short-term therapy (usually up to two weeks). Chronic active hepatitis is generally associated with long-term therapy (usually after six months); the onset may be insidious, and patients should be monitored periodically for changes in liver function. If hepatitis occurs, the drug should be withdrawn immediately and appropriate measures taken.

Ten percent of black patients and a variable percentage of ethnic groups of Mediterranean, Near Eastern and Asian origin, suffer from a deficiency of glucose-6-phosphate dehydrogenase in their blood cells. In such people, nitrofurantoin in common with many other therapeutic agents may cause haemolysis. This enzyme deficiency is extremely rare in Caucasians. Any sign of haemolysis is an indication to discontinue the drug. Haemolysis ceases when the drug is withdrawn.

Discontinue treatment with nitrofurantoin if otherwise unexplained pulmonary, hepatotoxic, haemotological or neurologic syndromes occur.

For long-term treatment monitor patient closely for appearance of hepatic or pulmonary symptoms and other evidence of toxicity.

Pregnancy and lactation: Based on animal reproduction studies and clinical experience in humans over many years, there is no evidence of any teratogenic effects of nitrofurantoin on the foetus. When antibiotic therapy is required during pregnancy, nitrofurantoin may be considered appropriate. However, caution should be exercised while breast feeding an infant known or suspected to have any erythrocyte enzyme deficiency as nitrofurantoin is detected in trace amounts in breast milk.

However, as with all drugs, the maternal side effects may adversely affect the course of the pregnancy. The drug should be used at the lowest effective dose as appropriate for the specific indication only after careful assessment of benefits against potential risks.

Action in event of overdosage: Symptoms and signs of overdosage include gastric irritation, nausea and vomiting. There is no known specific antidote. Nitrofurantoin can be haemodialysed. Standard treatment is by induction of emesis or by gastric lavage in cases of recent ingestion. Standard monitoring procedures for drug overdose, e.g. full blood count, liver function tests and pulmonary function, are recommended. A high fluid intake should be maintained to promote urinary excretion of the drug.

Adverse effects: Respiratory: Actue, subacute or chronic pulmonary reactions may occur.

Acute pulmonary reactions are commonly manifested by fever, chills, cough, chest pain, dyspnoea, pulmonary infiltration with consolidation or pleural effusion on X-ray and eosinophilia. Acute reactions usually occur within the first week of treatment and are reversible with cessation of therapy. Resolution often is dramatic.

In subacute pulmonary reactions, fever and eosinophilia occur less often than in the acute form. Upon cessation of therapy, recovery may require several months. If the symptoms are not recognised as being drug-related and therapy is not stopped, they may become more severe.

Chronic pulmonary reactions may occur in patients who have received continuous therapy for six months or more. Chronic pulmonary reactions may occur more commonly in elderly patients. Malaise, dyspnoea on exertion, cough and altered pulmonary function are common manifestations which can occur insidiously. Radiological and histological findings of diffuse interstitial pneumonitis or fibrosis, or both, are also common manifestations of the chronic pulmonary reactions. Fever is rarely prominent. The severity of chronic pulmonary reactions and their degree of resolution appear to be related to the duration of therapy after the first clinical signs appear. Pulmonary function may be impaired permanently, even after cessation of therapy. The risk is greater when chronic pulmonary reactions are not recognised early.

Gastro-intestinal: Nausea and anorexia have been reported. Emesis, abdominal pain and diarrhoea are less common gastro-intestinal reactions. These reactions may be minimised by taking the drug with food or milk or by adjustment of dosage.

Hepatic reactions including cholestatic jaundice and chronic active hepatitis occur rarely.

Hypersensitivity: Exfoliative dermatitis and erythema multiforme (including Stevens-Johnson syndrome) have been reported rarely.

Allergic skin reactions manifesting as angioneurotic oedema, maculopapular, erythematous or eczematous eruptions, urticaria, rash, and pruritus have occurred. Lupus-like syndrome associated with pulmonary reaction to nitrofurantoin has been reported.

Other hypersensitivity reactions include anaphylaxis, sialadenitis, pancreatitis, drug fever, and arthralgia.

Haematological: Agranulocytosis, leucopenia, granulocytopenia, haemolytic anaemia, thrombocytopenia, glucose-6-phosphate dehydrogenase deficiency anaemia, megaloblastic anaemia and eosinophilia have occurred. Cessation of therapy has generally returned the blood picture to normal. Aplastic anaemia has been reported rarely.

Neurological: Peripheral neuropathy, which may become severe or irreversible, has occurred. Less frequent reactions, of unknown causal relationship are nystagmus, vertigo, dizziness, asthenia, headache and drowsiness.

Miscellaneous: Transient alopecia has been reported.

As with other antimicrobial agents superinfections by fungi or resistant organisms such as *Pseudomonas* may occur. However, these are limited to the genito-urinary tract because suppression of normal bacterial flora does not occur elsewhere in the body.

Interactions: Concomitant administration of magnesium trisilicate with nitrofurantoin reduces both the rate and extent of absorption.

Uricosuric drugs such as probenecid and sulphinpyrazone may inhibit renal tubular secretion of nitrofurantoin. The resulting increase in serum levels may increase toxicity and the decreased urinary levels could lessen its efficacy as a urinary tract antibacterial.

Nitrofurantoin may antagonise the antibacterial efficacy of the quinolones. Concurrent use is not recommended.

Unlike many drugs, the presence of food or agents delaying gastric emptying can increase the bioavailability of nitrofurantoin presumably by allowing better dissolution in gastric juices.

There may be decreased antibacterial activity for nitrofurantoin in the presence of carbonic anhydrase inhibitors and urine alkalinising agents.

Pharmaceutical precautions Both Macrodantin 50 and 100 mg Capsules should be stored at temperatures not exceeding 30°C. Macrodantin 100 mg Capsules should be stored in light-proof and preferably moisture-resistant containers.

Legal category POM.

Package quantities Macrodantin 50 mg Capsules are supplied in blister packs of 28. Each pack comprises 7 blister cards containing 4 capsules on each card. Macrodantin Capsules 100 mg are supplied in polypropylene containers with polythene pilfer-proof caps. Each container holds 100 tablets.

Further information The urine of patients receiving Macrodantin may be coloured a dark yellow or brown. This results from the presence of drug and/or metabolite(s) and is quite harmless. Macrodantin can interfere with certain laboratory tests. False positive or spuriously high readings may be produced with urine glucose tests utilising the copper sulphate reduction method, e.g. Benedict's reagent, Clinitest (Ames). However, there is no interference with the Clinistix test.

Product licence numbers

Macrodantin Capsules 50 mg	0364/0005R
Macrodantin Capsules 100 mg	0364/0006R

PSORADRATE CREAM*

Presentation Psoradrate cream is a smooth textured, unperfumed, bland, yellow cream containing 0.1% w/w Dithranol BP; 0.2% w/w Dithranol BP or 0.4% w/w Dithranol BP in a specially formulated powder-in-cream base which includes stabilised, hypermolar urea to assist percutaneous transportation of the active ingredient. Psoradrate cream does not contain lanolin parabens or preservatives.

Uses Psoradrate cream is indicated for the treatment of subacute and chronic psoriasis. In addition, Psoradrate 0.1% is indicated for the treatment of psoriasis of the scalp.

Dosage and administration Wash affected areas well, dry thoroughly and apply directly to the lesions twice daily. Treatment should be continued until the raised lesions have disappeared and the skin is smooth. Occlusive dressings should not be used because they may increase the incidence of staining and stinging on normal skin. For use on the scalp, shampoo and dry hair, then rub Psoradrate 0.1% into the lesions, preferably at night. Remove the next morning with shampoo.

Before using creams containing high concentrations of dithranol it is advisable to establish the patient's tolerance. In cases in which tolerance has not been established, treatment of psoriatic lesions should be commenced with a low concentration of dithranol, namely Psoradrate 0.1%. If the patient's skin can tolerate Psoradrate 0.1% cream, but the lesions appear resistant, then treatment should be changed to increased strength Psoradrate creams to aid the clearance of the lesions. If, however, the patient is known to have a high tolerance to dithranol then therapy can be commenced using Psoradrate 0.2% cream, or Psoradrate 0.4% cream.

Contra-indications, warnings, etc Psoradrate cream is contra-indicated in pustular psoriasis.

The active ingredient of Psoradrate cream, dithranol, may cause a tingling or stinging sensation when applied to skin or lesions. It is irritant to the eyes and mucosa. If eye contact occurs, wash out immediately with a neutral solution. If mucosal contact occurs, wash with plenty of water. Exercise care when applying to the face and intertrigenous areas. Skin staining may occur and clothing may occasionally be discoloured. For external use only.

Pharmaceutical precautions Store in a cool place.

Legal category P.

Package quantities Psoradrate 0.1% and 0.2% are available in tubes of 30 g and 100 g. Psoradrate 0.4% is available in 100 g tubes.

Further information Use of a descaling agent such as salicylic acid is not necessary with Psoradrate creams. The creams are absorbed into the skin and the inconvenience of removing the application is avoided. Relapse rate with dithranol therapy has been reported as being less than that seen with steroids. Stains on clothes can be removed with a solvent such as trichloroethylene.

Product licence numbers

Psoradrate Cream 0.1%	0364/0027
Psoradrate Cream 0.2%	0364/0031
Psoradrate Cream 0.4%	0364/0037

TOPICYCLINE*

Presentation Topicycline is presented in two separate bottles as a yellow powder and a solvent which must be combined prior to use.

The powder contains 154 mg of Tetracycline Hydrochloride PhEur as the active ingredient, as well as 230 mg

4-epitetracycline hydrochloride and 70 mg sodium bisulphite.

The solvent contains 1.25 mg per ml of n-decyl methyl sulphoxide (DecMSO) and citric acid in a 40% ethanol solution.

Once reconstituted, Topicycline contains 2.2 mg per ml of tetracycline hydrochloride. The n-decyl methyl sulphoxide enhances penetration of tetracycline into the skin.

Uses Topicycline is indicated in the treatment of acne vulgaris.

Dosage and administration Topicycline is first prepared according to the manufacturer's instructions.

Topicycline is applied topically, twice daily. It should be applied generously, to the entire affected area, not just to individual lesions, until the skin is thoroughly wet.

The average amount of Topicycline delivered to the skin by application to the face and neck twice a day is approximately 1.3 ml/day. This quantity of the medication contains approximately 2.9 mg of tetracycline hydrochloride. Twice-daily use of Topicycline on other acne-involved areas, in addition to the face and neck, has resulted in an average application of about 2.2 ml/day, or 4.8 mg of tetracycline hydrochloride.

Contra-indications, warnings, etc Topicycline is contra-indicated in patients who have shown hypersensitivity to any of its ingredients or to any of the other tetracyclines.

Topicycline is for external use only, and care should be taken to keep it out of the eyes, nose and mouth.

Because the serum level of tetracycline resulting from the use of Topicycline (less than 0.1 microgram/ml) is less than 7% of that associated with a therapeutic dose of 500 mg/day of tetracycline administered orally, liver damage from the use of Topicycline is highly unlikely, even in patients with renal impairment. Nevertheless, the warnings associated with the use of tetracycline orally should be considered before prescribing Topicycline for patients with renal impairment.

Reproduction studies in rats and rabbits have revealed no evidence of impaired fertility or harm to the foetus from Topicycline. There are no data, however, on the use of this product in pregnant women.

It is not known whether tetracycline or any other component of Topicycline administered in this topical form, is secreted in human milk. Because many drugs are secreted in human milk, caution should be exercised if Topicycline is administered to nursing mothers.

Safety and effectiveness in children below the age of eleven have not been established.

Side-effects: Some patients may experience a stinging or burning sensation upon application of Topicycline. The sensation normally lasts no more than a few minutes, and does not occur at every application and often diminishes with continued use of the product.

Pharmaceutical precautions Unreconstituted product should be stored at a temperature not exceeding 25°C.

Reconstituted Topicycline should be used within 8 weeks of reconstitution, and should be stored at room temperature or below.

Any unused material should be discarded.

Legal category POM.

Package quantities Topicycline is supplied in a single carton containing one plastic bottle of powder (454 mg) and one of liquid (70 ml); these two phases must be combined prior to use. At the time of dispensing, the liquid is poured into the powder-containing bottle and the powder contents are dissolved by shaking the bottle. An applicator and overcap are supplied. Reconstituted Topicycline contains 154 mg of tetracycline hydrochloride/70 ml of medication as dispensed.

Further information Reconstituted Topicycline provides about an eight-week supply for treating the face and neck, or about a four week supply for treating the face, neck and additional acne-involved areas.

Product licence number 0522/0010.

Product licence holder: Procter & Gamble Ltd., Newcastle upon Tyne.

**Trade Mark*

Novex Pharma
A Division of Innovex Medical Products Ltd
Innovex House
Reading Road
Henley-on-Thames
Oxon RG9 1EL

MINTEC* CAPSULES

Presentation Green and ivory enteric-coated, soft gelatin capsules (size 4), each containing 0.2 ml Peppermint Oil BP.

Uses Peppermint oil is an aromatic carminative, which acts locally to relax gastro-intestinal smooth muscle and relieve gastro-intestinal flatulence and colic. The enteric coating of the capsule is designed to delay release of the peppermint oil beyond the stomach and upper small bowel.

Mintec is indicated for the treatment of discomfort, pain and distension associated with the irritable bowel or spastic colon syndrome.

Dosage and administration
Adults (including the elderly) only: One capsule orally three times a day, preferably before meals and taken with a small quantity of water, but **not** immediately after food. The capsules must not be broken or chewed.

When symptoms are more severe, the dosage may be increased to two capsules three times a day.

Mintec should be taken until symptoms resolve, but may be continued for up to 2 to 3 months.

Contra-indications, warnings, etc
Caution: In patients with pre-existing heartburn, symptoms may be exacerbated.

Use in pregnancy and lactation: The usual precautions concerning the administration of any drug during pregnancy should be observed.

Adverse reactions: Heartburn, rarely allergic reactions including erythematous skin rash, headache, bradycardia, muscle tremor and ataxia.

Overdosage: Treatment consists of gastric lavage, together with symptomatic and supportive measures.

Pharmaceutical precautions Store capsules at a temperature not exceeding 25°C and protect from light.

Legal category P.

Package quantities Packs of 100 capsules.

Further information Nil.

Product licence number 0002/0142.

Product licence holder: Smith Kline and French Laboratories Ltd, Welwyn Garden City, Hertfordshire AL7 1EY.

TROSYL* NAIL SOLUTION

Presentation Trosyl Nail Solution is a clear, slightly yellow solution containing 28% w/w tioconazole. Each ml of solution contains 280 mg tioconazole.

Uses Tioconazole is a broad spectrum imidazole antifungal agent. Trosyl Nail Solution is indicated for the topical treatment of nail infections due to susceptible fungi (dermatophytes and yeasts).

Dosage and administration
Adults: The solution should be applied to the affected nails and immediately surrounding skin every twelve hours using the applicator brush supplied.

The duration of treatment is up to six months but may be extended to twelve months.

Use in the elderly: No special precautions are required. Use the adult dose.

Use in children: No special precautions are required. Use the adult dose.

Contra-indications, warnings, etc
Contra-indications: Trosyl Nail Solution is contra-indicated in individuals who have been shown to be hypersensitive to imidazole antifungal agents, or to any of the components of the solution.

Use in pregnancy: In animal studies tioconazole was not teratogenic. At high doses it increased the incidence of renal abnormalities in rat embryos, but this effect was minor and transient and was not evident in weaned animals. There is insufficient evidence as to the drug's safety in human pregnancy, although absorption after topical administration is negligible. Because of the extensive duration of treatment required for nail infections, the use of Trosyl Nail Solution is contra-indicated throughout pregnancy.

Precautions: Trosyl Nail Solution is not for ophthalmic use.

Side-effects: Trosyl Nail Solution is well tolerated following local application and no systemic adverse reactions have been observed. Symptoms of local irritation have been reported by some patients, but are usually seen during the first week of treatment and are transient and mild.

However, if a sensitivity reaction develops with the use of Trosyl Nail Solution, treatment should be discontinued and appropriate therapy instituted.

Overdosage: No cases of overdosage with Trosyl Nail Solution have been reported. In the event of excessive oral ingestion, gastrointestinal symptoms may occur. Appropriate means of gastric lavage should be considered.

Pharmaceutical precautions Store between 4°C and 30°C. Avoid flame and heat.

Legal category POM.

Package quantities Amber glass bottles containing 12 ml of solution.

Further information Nil.

Product licence number 0057/0236.

Product licence holder: Pfizer Limited, Sandwich, Kent.

**Trade Mark*

Novo Nordisk Pharmaceuticals Limited

Novo Nordisk House, Broadfield Park
Brighton Road, Pease Pottage
Crawley, West Sussex, RH11 9RT

HUMAN ACTRAPID* PENFILL* PENMIX* 30/70 PENFILL* HUMAN PROTAPHANE* PENFILL*

Presentation *Human Actrapid Penfill* (Neutral Insulin Injection BP) is a clear neutral solution of human insulin (pyr), containing glycerol, and m-cresol as added preservative.

PenMix 30/70 Penfill (Biphasic Isophane Insulin Injection) is a neutral suspension of human insulin (pyr), consisting of soluble human insulin and isophane human insulin in the ratio 3:7.

Human Protaphane Penfill (Isophane Insulin Injection BP) is a neutral suspension of isophane human insulin (pyr).

PenMix 30/70 Penfill and Human Protaphane Penfill contain glycerol, sodium phosphate, protamine sulphate as retarding agent, and m-cresol and phenol as added preservative.

The Penfill preparations are contained in 1.5 ml cartridges; when agitated up and down the suspensions appear white and cloudy. Each preparation is available in a strength of 100 iu/ml.

Uses The treatment of insulin requiring diabetics.

Dosage and administration *Adults and children:* The dosage is determined by the physician according to the needs of the patient. The Penfill preparations are intended for use only in the NovoPen® and NovoPen®II injection devices; when used in these devices they are given by subcutaneous injection. Instructions for use of these preparations in NovoPen and NovoPen II are included with the devices and must be carefully followed. Prior to injection the suspensions should be agitated up and down until the insulin appears white and cloudy; a glass ball is included in the cartridge to facilitate resuspension.

When injected subcutaneously, Human Actrapid Penfill has a duration of action of some $\frac{1}{2}$ to 8 hours and its maximum effect is exerted between $2\frac{1}{2}$ and 5 hours after injection. When used alone it is usually given three or more times daily; it is most commonly used in regimens where an intermediate or long acting insulin is given in addition. When injected subcutaneously, PenMix 30/70 Penfill has a duration of action of some $\frac{1}{2}$ to 24 hours and its maximum effect is exerted between 2 and 12 hours after injection, and Human Protaphane Penfill has a duration of action of some $1\frac{1}{2}$ to 24 hours and its maximum effect is exerted between 4 and 12 hours after injection. PenMix 30/70 Penfill and Human Protaphane Penfill may be given once, or more commonly, twice daily. PenMix 30/70 Penfill is used especially when a strong initial effect is desired. Human Protaphane Penfill may also be supplemented with shorter acting insulin.

The Penfill preparations must not be used or refilled with conventional syringes.

Use in the elderly: There are no precautions concerning the use of insulin which are specific to the elderly diabetic. However, injection procedures may be difficult for the infirm, the poorly sighted, or the confused patient, and the simplest regimen consistent with keeping the patient symptom-free should be considered.

Contra-indications, warnings, etc
Contra-indications: Insulin is contra-indicated in hypoglycaemia.

Precautions: Owing to their strong early effect, injections of Human Actrapid Penfill or PenMix 30/70 Penfill should be followed by a meal within 30 minutes of administration.

When patients are transferred from other insulins to Human Monocomponent insulin the change should be made according to the following general guidelines:

For patients currently controlled on Human Monocomponent, porcine monocomponent or other highly purified human or porcine insulin preparations, no dosage change is anticipated other than the routine adjustments made in order to maintain stable diabetic control.

Patients currently stabilised on mixed species or bovine insulin may require a dosage adjustment dependent upon dosage, purity, species and formulation of the insulin preparation(s) currently administered. Variations in glycaemic control may occur and adjustments in therapy should be made under the guidance of a physician.

A few patients have reported that after being transferred to human insulin, the early warning symptoms for hypoglycaemia were less pronounced than they were with animal source insulin.

Patients whose blood glucose control is greatly improved, e.g. by intensified insulin therapy, may experience a change in their usual warning symptoms of hypoglycaemia, and possibly lose some or all of the symptoms, and should be advised accordingly.

Use in pregnancy: Intensified control in the treatment of pregnant insulin-dependent diabetics is recommended. Insulin requirements usually fall in the first trimester and increase during the second and third trimester. Insulin does not pass the placental barrier.

Concomitant use of other drugs may influence insulin requirements. The following substances may enhance the hypoglycaemic effect of insulin: monoamine oxidase inhibitors (MAOI), alcohol, beta-adrenergic blocking agents. Other drugs may increase insulin requirements: corticosteroids, thyroid hormones, oral contraceptives. Beta-adrenergic blocking agents may blur the symptoms of hypoglycaemia.

Side-effects: Allergies to human insulin are very rare, and are mostly due to cross-reacting antibodies to animal insulins. Lipodystrophy at injection sites is also rare and should be prevented by constantly changing injection sites.

Overdosage: Overdosage causes hypoglycaemia, symptoms are variable but may include confusion, palpitations, sweating, malaise, and loss of consciousness.

In the event of an overdose, glucose should be given orally if the patient is conscious. Where the patient is unconscious an intra-muscular, subcutaneous or intravenous injection of glucagon should be given and oral carbohydrate administered when the patient responds. Alternatively intravenous glucose may be administered; it must be given if there is no response to glucagon.

Pharmaceutical precautions The Penfill cartridge preparations should be stored between 2 and 8°C, and should not be allowed to freeze. Cartridges in use or carried as a spare may be kept at ambient temperature (e.g. in the pocket or handbag) for up to one month, but should not be exposed to excessive heat or sunlight. Cartridges in use must not be stored in a refrigerator.

Legal category P.

Package quantities Pack of 5 × 1.5 ml cartridges.

Further information Sole Distributor: Farillon Limited, Ashton Road, Harold Hill, Romford, Essex RM3 8UE. Tel: Ingrebourne 71136.

Product licence numbers

Human Actrapid Penfill	4668/0024
PenMix 30/70 Penfill	4668/0020
Human Protaphane Penfill	4668/0019

Product licence holder: Novo Nordisk A/S.

HUMAN ACTRAPID* HUMAN MONOTARD* HUMAN PROTAPHANE* HUMAN ACTRAPHANE* 30/70 HUMAN ULTRATARD*

Presentation *Human Actrapid* (Neutral Insulin Injection BP) is a clear neutral solution of human insulin (pyr), containing glycerol, and m-cresol as added preservative.

Human Monotard (Insulin Zinc Suspension BP) is a neutral suspension of amorphous (30%) and crystalline (70%) human insulin (pyr).

Human Protaphane (Isophane Insulin Injection BP) is a neutral suspension of isophane human insulin (pyr).

Human Actraphane 30/70 (Biphasic Isophane Insulin Injection) is a neutral suspension of human insulin (pyr), consisting of soluble human insulin and isophane human insulin in the ratio 3:7.

Human Ultratard (Insulin Zinc Suspension Crystalline BP) is a neutral suspension of crystalline human insulin (pyr).

Human Monotard and Human Ultratard contain sodium chloride, sodium acetate, zinc as retarding agent and methyl parahydroxybenzoate as added preservative. Human Protaphane and Human Actraphane 30/70 contain glycerol, sodium phosphate, protamine sulphate as retarding agent, and m-cresol and phenol as added preservative. When shaken, the suspensions appear white and cloudy.

Each preparation is available in a strength of 100 iu/ml.

Uses The treatment of insulin requiring diabetics.

Dosage and administration
Adults and children: The dosage is determined by the physician according to the needs of the patient.

Human Actrapid may be given by subcutaneous, intramuscular or intravenous injection. When injected subcutaneously it has a duration of action of some ½ to 8 hours and its maximum effect is exerted between 2½ and 5 hours after injection.

The suspensions may be given by subcutaneous or intramuscular injection. The vial should be gently shaken before use to ensure that the insulin is uniformly distributed throughout the liquid. The dose should then be immediately drawn into the syringe and injected.

Human Monotard and Human Protaphane may be used in once, or more commonly, twice daily injection regimens. When injected subcutaneously, Human Monotard has a duration of action of some 2½ to 24 hours and its maximum effect is exerted between 7 and 15 hours after injection, and Human Protophane has a duration of action of some 1½ to 24 hours and its maximum effect is exerted between 4 and 12 hours after injection.

Human Actraphane 30/70 may be given once, or more commonly, twice daily, especially when a strong initial effect is desired. When injected subcutaneously it has a duration of action of some ½ to 24 hours and its maximum effect is exerted between 2 and 12 hours after injection.

Human Ultratard is usually given as a once daily insulin but may also be given twice daily if required. It is often used as a basal insulin in multiple injection regimens. Human Ultratard may be used as a once daily injection (if necessary with the addition of rapid acting insulin) in maturity onset diabetes when diet or oral hypoglycaemic drugs fail to produce good control. When injected subcutaneously Human Ultratard has a duration of action of some 4 to 28 hours and its maximum effect is exerted between 8 and 24 hours after injection.

The suspensions may be mixed in the syringe with Human Actrapid to intensify the initial effect. The Human Actrapid should be drawn into the syringe first and the injection given immediately after mixing.

Infusion pumps: Due to the risk of precipitation in some pump catheters, Human Actrapid is not recommended for use in insulin infusion pumps.

The suspensions must not be used in insulin infusion pumps.

Use in the elderly: There are no precautions concerning the use of insulin which are specific to the elderly diabetic. However the injection procedure may be difficult for the infirm, the poorly sighted, or the confused patient, and the simplest regimen consistent with keeping the patient symptom-free should be considered.

Contra-indications, warnings, etc
Contra-indications: Insulin is contra-indicated in hypoglycaemia.

Precautions: Owing to their strong early effect, injections of Human Actrapid or Human Actraphane 30/70 should be followed by a meal within 30 minutes of administration.

When patients are transferred from other insulins to Human Monocomponent insulin the change should be made according to the following general guidelines:

For patients currently controlled on Human Monocomponent, porcine monocomponent, or other highly purified human or porcine insulin preparation, no dosage change is anticipated other than the routine adjustments made in order to maintain stable diabetic control.

Patients currently stabilised on mixed species or bovine insulin may require a dosage adjustment dependent upon dosage, purity, species, and formulation of the insulin preparation(s) currently administered. Variations in glycaemic control may occur and adjustment in therapy should be made under the guidance of a physician.

A few patients have reported that after being transferred to human insulin, the early warning symptoms for hypoglycaemia were less pronounced than they were with animal source insulin.

Patients whose blood glucose control is greatly improved, e.g. by intensified insulin therapy, may experience a change in their usual warning symptoms of hypoglycaemia, and possibly lose some or all of the symptoms, and should be advised accordingly.

Use in pregnancy: Intensified control in the treatment of pregnant insulin dependent diabetics is recommended. Insulin requirements usually fall in the first trimester and increase during the second and third trimester. Insulin does not pass the placental barrier.

Concomitant use of other drugs may influence insulin requirements. The following substances may enhance the hypoglycaemic effect of insulin: monoamine oxidase inhibitors (MAOI), alcohol, beta-adrenergic blocking agents. Other drugs may increase insulin requirements: corticosteroids, thyroid hormones, oral contraceptives. Beta-adrenergic blocking agents may blur the symptoms of hypoglycaemia.

Side-effects: Allergies to human insulin are very rare, and are mostly due to cross-reacting antibodies to animal insulins. Lipodystrophy at injection sites is also rare and should be prevented by constantly changing injection sites.

Overdosage: Overdosage causes hypoglycaemia, symptoms are variable but may include confusion, palpitations, sweating, malaise, and loss of consciousness.

In the event of an overdose, glucose should be given orally if the patient is conscious. Where the patient is unconscious an intra-muscular, subcutaneous or intravenous injection of glucagon should be given and oral carbohydrate administered when the patient responds. Alternatively intravenous glucose may be administered; it must be given if there is no response to glucagon.

Pharmaceutical precautions The human insulin preparations should be stored between 2° and 8°C. They should not be exposed to excessive heat or sunlight and should not be allowed to freeze. The vial in use may be kept at room temperature (max. 25°C) for up to four weeks.

Legal category P.

Package quantities 10 ml glass vials.

Further information Sole distributor: Farillon Limited, Ashton Road, Harold Hill, Romford, Essex RM3 8UE. Tel: Ingrebourne 71136.

Product licence numbers

Human Actrapid	4668/0025
Human Monotard	4668/0021
Human Protaphane	4668/0018
Human Actraphane	4668/0023
Human Ultratard	4668/0022

Product licence holder: Novo Nordisk A/S.

HUMAN VELOSULIN* HUMAN INSULATARD* HUMAN MIXTARD* 30/70 HUMAN INITARD* 50/50

Presentation

Human Velosulin (Neutral Insulin Injection) is a clear neutral solution of highly purified human insulin (emp).

Human Insulatard (Isophane Insulin Injection, NPH) is a cloudy neutral suspension of highly purified microcrystalline human insulin (emp).

Human Mixtard 30/70 is a cloudy neutral suspension of highly purified human insulin (emp) comprising 30% Neutral Insulin in solution and 70% Isophane Insulin in microcrystalline form.

Human Initard 50/50 is a cloudy neutral suspension of highly purified human insulin (emp) comprising 50% Neutral Insulin in solution and 50% Isophane Insulin in microcrystalline form.

All the above insulins are available in 10 ml vials containing 100 iu/ml and are buffered with Sodium Phosphate PhEur 2.4 mg/ml. Human Velosulin is preserved with m-Cresol BP 3.0 mg/ml; and Human Insulatard, Human Mixtard 30/70 and Human Initard 50/50 are preserved with m-Cresol BP 1.5 mg/ml and Phenol BP 0.6 mg/ml

The vials are fitted with tamper evident orange-coloured disposable plastic caps as a security safeguard. No attempt should be made to refit the caps after removal. Additionally, to aid identification by those with visual impairment, Human Velosulin has one, Human Insulatard two, Human Mixtard 30/70 three and Human Initard 50/50 four raised tactile marks on the aluminium closure ring.

Uses For the treatment of insulin-requiring diabetic patients.

Human Velosulin has a rapid onset and a short duration of action, making it particularly suitable for the treatment of diabetic coma and pre-coma.

Human Mixtard 30/70 contains 30% soluble insulin and 70% isophane insulin designed to avoid the necessity for self titration in the majority of patients requiring a combination of quick and intermediate acting insulin.

Human Initard 50/50 contains a higher ratio of neutral insulin in solution and should be used when a more intense initial effect is required.

Dosage and administration The dosage of insulin is determined by the physician according to the needs of the patient.

Human Velosulin may be given by subcutaneous, intramuscular or intravenous injection or infusion.

Human Insulatard, Human Mixtard 30/70 and Human Initard 50/50 may be given by subcutaneous or intramuscular injection. The suspension should be well mixed by gently inverting the vial several times prior to drawing up the insulin. The patient should then check that the insulin suspension appears a uniform cloudy grey/white which indicates that the isophane crystals have been completely resuspended. Care should be taken to avoid accidental intravascular injection.

Human Velosulin and Human Insulatard may be mixed together, or with Human Mixtard 30/70 and Human Initard 50/50 in all proportions without changing the characteristic effect of any of the types of insulin.

The injection site should be changed regularly according to a set routine.

Subcutaneous injection: Human Velosulin has an onset of action of approximately half an hour after subcutaneous injection with a duration of about 8 hours, the maximum effect being exerted between 1 and 3 hours after injection.

Human Insulatard has an onset of action of approximately 1½ hours with a duration of action of up to 24 hours, the maximum effect being exerted 4 to 12 hours after injection.

Human Mixtard 30/70 and Human Initard 50/50 have an onset of action of about half an hour with a duration of action of up to 24 hours. A maximum effect is exerted 4–8 hours after injection, Human Initard 50/50 having a stronger initial effect than Human Mixtard 30/70.

Intramuscular injection: Following intramuscular injection, the onset of action is more rapid, while the overall duration of action is shorter, provided the injection site is well perfused muscle.

Use in pregnancy and lactation: It is important to maintain continuous good glycaemic control during conception and throughout pregnancy. In insulin-requiring pregnant diabetic patients, insulin requirements generally fall during the first trimester and increase during the second and third trimesters.

Use in the elderly: Clearance rates may be reduced in the elderly due to declining renal function. Insulin may therefore have a more prolonged action. Dose requirements should be regularly reviewed.

Contra-indications, warnings, etc

Contra-indications: Insulin is contra-indicated in hypoglycaemia.

Precautions: Variations in lifestyle and other factors, e.g. infection and pregnancy, can affect insulin requirements.

Some patients previously treated with insulin of beef or pork origin may require a dosage adjustment on transfer to highly purified human insulin (emp). This is more likely in patients previously treated with beef or mixed beef/pork insulin.

Hypoglycaemia may be precipitated by some drugs including the following: asprin; sulphonylureas and agents affecting them; and certain steroids. Hypoglycaemia may also occur following excessive physical activity, alcohol intake or reduced food intake.

Hyperglycaemia can be enhanced by drugs including the following: triiodothyronine; thyroxine; various natural and synthetic steroids, including some oral contraceptives; diuretics including thiazides; and cyclophosphamide.

Certain beta-blockers, especially propranolol, may affect insulin requirements and mask the signs of hypoglycaemia mediated by the sympathetic nervous system. Monoamine oxidase inhibitors (MAOI) may potentiate the action of insulin.

A few patients have reported that after being transferred to human insulin, their early warning symptoms for hypoglycaemia were less pronounced than they had been with beef or porcine insulin. Patients should be alerted to this possibility on being transferred to human insulin.

Patients whose blood glucose control is greatly improved, e.g. by intensified insulin therapy, may experience a change in their usual warning symptoms of hypoglycaemia, and possibly lose some or all of the symptoms, and should be advised accordingly.

Side- and adverse effects: The most important side-effect is hypoglycaemia. Reduction of hyperglycaemia in newly diagnosed diabetic patients may alter visual refraction.

Insulin and protamine, like any other injected proteins are potentially immunogenic. This may or may not have clinical implications. Local reactions at the injection site may include transient erythema, induration, urticaria and oedema. The incidence is minimal with highly purified human insulin (emp) and these usually resolve with continuing insulin usage. True generalised hypersensitivity reactions approaching anaphylaxis are very rare.

Clinical evidence suggests that highly purified human insulin (emp) is unlikely to cause localised lipodystrophy. However, at present, this possibility cannot be totally excluded.

Toxicity and treatment of overdosage: The symptoms and signs of hypoglycaemia depend on the patient's clinical state and on the rate and extent of the fall in blood glucose levels.

If possible, glucose, sucrose, or rapidly absorbable carbohydrate should be taken by mouth. Failing this, hypoglycaemia should be reversed as rapidly as possible by intravenous injection of glucose 50% solution. Alternative emergency treatments include the subcutaneous injection of up to 1 ml of adrenaline solution 1:1000 or the subcutaneous, intramuscular or intravenous injection of lyophilised glucagon 0.5–1.0 mg (1 unit = 1.0 mg). Both adrenaline and glucagon injections mobilise hepatic glycogen, but this effect is short lived and must be supplemented by freely available carbohydrate as soon as possible.

Pharmaceutical precautions Store at a temperature between 2 and 8°C, protected from sunlight. The shelf life is 3 years from the date of manufacture. Insulin which has been frozen should not be used.

Legal category P.

Package quantities 10 ml glass vials in individual cartons.

Further information Sole distributor: The Wellcome Foundation Ltd., Crewe Hall, Crewe, Cheshire, CW1 1UB. Tel: Crewe (0270) 583151.

Product licence numbers

Human Velosulin	3132/0031
Human Insulatard	3132/0034
Human Mixtard 30/70	3132/0037
Human Initard 30/50	3132/0040

VELOSULIN* INSULATARD* MIXTARD* 30/70 INITARD* 50/50

Presentation Velosulin (Neutral Insulin Injection BP) is a clear neutral solution of highly purified pork insulin.

Insulatard (Isophane Insulin Injection BP [NPH]) is a cloudy neutral suspension of highly purified microcrystalline pork insulin.

Mixtard 30/70 is a cloudy neutral suspension of highly purified pork insulin comprising 30% Neutral Insulin in solution and 70% Isophane Insulin in microcrystalline form.

Initard 50/50 is a cloudy neutral suspension of highly purified pork insulin comprising 50% Neutral Insulin in solution and 50% Isophane Insulin in microcrystalline form.

All the above insulins are available in 100 units/ml strength and are buffered with Sodium Phosphate PhEur 2.4 mg/ml. Velosulin is preserved with m-Cresol BP 3 mg/ml and Insulatard, Mixtard 30/70 and Initard 50/50 are preserved with m-Cresol BP 1.5 mg/ml and Phenol BP 0.6 mg/ml.

The vials are fitted with orange coloured disposable plastic caps as a security safeguard. No attempt should be made to refit the caps after removal. Additionally, to aid identification, Velosulin has one, Insulatard two, Mixtard 30/70 three and Initard 50/50 four raised tactile marks on the aluminium closure ring.

Uses The treatment of insulin-requiring diabetic patients. Velosulin has a rapid onset and a short duration of action making it particularly suitable for the treatment of diabetic coma and pre-coma.

Dosage and administration The dosage of insulin is determined by the physician according to the needs of the patient. Velosulin, Insulatard, Mixtard 30/70 and Initard 50/50 may be mixed in all proportions without changing the characteristic effect of any of the types of insulin.

Velosulin may be given by subcutaneous, intramuscular or intravenous injection or infusion. It has an onset of action of approximately 30 minutes after subcutaneous injection with duration of about 8 hours, the maximum effect being 1 to 3 hours after injection.

Insulatard, Mixtard 30/70 and Initard 50/50 should be well mixed by gently inverting the vial several times before being given by subcutaneous or intramuscular injection. Insulatard, Mixtard 30/70 and Initard 50/50 should not be given intravenously.

Insulatard has an onset of action of approximately 1½ hours after subcutaneous injection with an overall duration of action which may extend to 24 hours, the maximum effect occurring 4 to 12 hours after injection.

Mixtard 30/70 and Initard 50/50 each have a duration of action of some ½ to 24 hours after subcutaneous injection, the maximum effect occurring 4 to 8 hours after injection. Initard 50/50 has a stronger initial effect than Mixtard 30/70.

Onset of action is more rapid and overall duration of action shorter following intramuscular injection than with the subcutaneous route assuming adequate vascular perfusion.

Use in pregnancy and lactation: It is essential to maintain continuous good glycaemic control throughout pregnancy. In the insulin-treated (gestational or insulin-dependent) pregnant diabetic patient, the insulin requirements fall during the first trimester and increase during the second and third trimesters.

Use in the elderly: Clearance rates may be reduced in the elderly due to falling renal function. Insulin may therefore have a more prolonged action. Dose requirements should be regularly reviewed.

Contra-indications, warnings, etc

Contra-indications: Insulin is contra-indicated in hypoglycaemia.

Precautions: Variations in lifestyle and other factors, eg. infection and pregnancy, can affect insulin requirements.

Some patients previously treated with insulin of beef or mixed beef/pork origin may require a dosage adjustment on transfer to highly purified pork insulin.

Hypoglycaemia can be enhanced by drugs including the following: aspirin; sulphonylureas and agents affecting them; certain steroids.

Hyperglycaemia can be enhanced by drugs including the following: triiodothyronine; thyroxine; various natural and synthetic steroids, including some oral contraceptives; diuretics, including thiazides; cyclophosphamide.

Certain beta-blockers, especially propranolol, may affect insulin requirements and mask the signs of hypoglycaemia mediated by the sympathetic nervous system.

Monoamine oxidase inhibitors (MAOI) may potentiate the action of insulin.

Patients whose blood glucose control is greatly improved, e.g. by intensified insulin therapy, may experience a change in their usual warning symptoms of hypoglycaemia, and possibly lose some or all of the symptoms, and should be advised accordingly.

Side-and adverse effects: The most important side-effect is hypoglycaemia. Reduction of hyperglycaemia in newly diagnosed diabetics may alter visual refraction.

Insulin and protamine, like any other injected proteins, are potentially immunogenic. This may or may not have clinical implications. Local reactions at the injection site may include transient erythema, induration, urticaria and oedema. The incidence is minimal with highly purified pork insulin. These usually resolve with continuing usage of insulin. True generalised hypersensitivity reactions approaching anaphylaxis are very rare.

Clinical evidence suggests that highly purified pork insulins are unlikely to cause localised lipodystrophies, however, at present, this possibility cannot be totally excluded.

Toxicity and treatment of overdosage: The symptoms and signs of hypoglycaemia depend on the patient's clinical state and on the rate and extent of the fall in blood glucose levels.

If possible, glucose, sucrose, or rapidly absorbable carbohydrate should be taken by mouth. Failing this, hypoglycaemia should be reversed as rapidly as possible by intravenous injection of glucose 50% solution. Alternative emergency treatments include the subcutaneous injection of up to 1 ml of adrenaline solution 1:1000 or the subcutaneous, intramuscular or intravenous injection of lyophilised glucagon 0.5–1.0 mg (1 unit = 1.0 mg). Both adrenaline and glucagon injections mobilise hepatic glycogen, but the effect is short lived and must be supplemented by freely available carbohydrate as soon as possible.

Pharmaceutical precautions The highly purified pork insulin preparations should be stored between 2 and 8°C, protected from sunlight. Under these storage conditions they have a shelf life of 3 years from date of manufacture. Insulin which has been frozen should not be used.

Legal category P.

Package quantities 10 ml glass vials.

Further information Sole distributor: The Wellcome Foundation Ltd., Crewe Hall, Crewe, Cheshire, CW1 1UB. Tel: Crewe (0270) 583151.

Product licence numbers

Velosulin	3132/0019
Insulatard	3132/0018
Mixtard 30/70	3132/0021
Initard 50/50	3132/0020

SEMITARD* MC
RAPITARD* MC
LENTARD* MC

Presentation Semitard MC (Insulin Zinc Suspension Amorphous BP) is a neutral suspension of amorphous porcine MC insulin, containing sodium chloride, sodium acetate, zinc as retarding agent and methyl parahydroxybenzoate as added preservative.

Rapitard MC (Biphasic Insulin Injection BP) is a neutral suspension comprising porcine MC insulin (25%) in solution and crystalline bovine MC insulin (75%), and containing sodium chloride, sodium acetate, and methyl parahydroxybenzoate as added preservative.

Lentard MC (Insulin Zinc Suspension BP) is a neutral suspension of amorphous porcine MC insulin (30%) and crystalline bovine MC insulin (70%), containing sodium chloride, sodium acetate, zinc as retarding agent, and methyl parahydroxybenzoate as added preservative.

When shaken the suspensions appear white and cloudy.

The MC insulin preparations are available in a strength of 100 iu/ml.

Uses The treatment of insulin requiring diabetic patients.

Dosage and administration *Adults and children:* The dosage of insulin is determined by the physician according to the needs of the patient.

Suspensions may be given by subcutaneous or intramuscular injection. The vial should be gently shaken before use to ensure that the insulin is uniformly distributed throughout the liquid. The dose should then be immediately drawn into the syringe and injected.

Semitard MC is usually given twice daily. It has a duration of action of some 1½ to 16 hours and its maximum effect is exerted between 5 and 10 hours after injection.

Rapitard MC has a duration of action of some ½ to 22 hours and its maximum effect is exerted between 4 and 12 hours after injection. Rapitard MC may be used once or twice daily.

Lentard MC has a duration of action of some 2½ to 24 hours and its maximum effect is exerted between 7 and 15 hours after injection. It may be given once or twice daily.

The MC insulin suspensions may be mixed in the syringe with Human Actrapid to intensify the initial effect. The insulin mixture should be injected immediately. When longer acting insulins are mixed with short acting soluble insulins, the short acting insulin should be drawn into the syringe first.

100 iu/ml insulin must only be used with syringes specifically designed for this strength of insulin.

Infusion pumps: Insulin suspensions must not be used in insulin infusion pumps.

Use in pregnancy: It is essential to maintain continuous good control of the insulin requiring diabetic patient throughout pregnancy. In the insulin treated (gestational or insulin dependent) pregnant diabetic patient the insulin requirements usually fall in the first trimester and increase during the second and third trimester.

Use in the elderly: There are no precautions concerning the use of insulin which are specific to the elderly diabetic. However the injection procedure may be difficult for the infirm, the poorly sighted, or the confused patient, and the simplest regimen consistent with keeping the patient symptom-free should be considered.

Contra-indications, warnings, etc

Contra-indications: Insulin is contra-indicated in hypoglycaemia.

Precautions: Owing to its strong early effect, the injection of Rapitard MC should be followed by a meal within 30 minutes of administration.

Patients transferred from conventional (predominantly bovine) insulins may require a smaller dosage. The dosage reduction may occur immediately after transfer or gradually over a period of weeks or months. In order to reduce the risk of hypoglycaemia, the patient and the physician should be aware of the possibility that the insulin requirement may be reduced.

If the daily insulin dosage is below 40 iu the risk is considered minimal. However, when higher dosages are required, stricter supervision of the patient is necessary and possibly a dosage reduction should be made initially on transfer. Insulin resistant patients receiving over 100 units daily should be referred to hospital for transfer.

Patients whose blood glucose control is greatly improved, e.g. by intensified insulin therapy, may experience a change in their usual warning symptoms of hypoglycaemia, and possibly lose some or all of the symptoms, and should be advised accordingly.

The addition of corticosteroids, oral contraceptives or thyroid hormone replacement therapy may lead to an increase in insulin requirements. The addition of a beta-adrenergic blocking agent or a monoamine oxidase inhibitor (MAOI), may also necessitate an adjustment of insulin dosage.

Side-effects: Lipodystrophy, insulin resistance and hypersensitivity reactions have been associated with insulin therapy, but the incidence and severity of these unwanted effects is minimal with the MC insulins.

Severe local or generalised allergic reactions require immediate treatment and, in some cases, desensitisation may be necessary.

Overdosage: In the event of an overdose, glucose should be given orally if the patient is conscious. Where the patient is unconscious, an intramuscular, subcutaneous or intravenous injection of glucagon should be given and oral carbohydrate administered when the patient responds. Alternatively, intravenous glucose may be administered; it must be given if there is no response to glucagon.

Pharmaceutical precautions The mixing of phosphate containing insulin preparations with insulin zinc suspensions should be avoided.

The MC insulin preparations should be stored between 2°C and 8°C. They should not be exposed to excessive heat or sunlight, neither should they be frozen. The vial in use may be kept at room temperature (max. 25°C) for one month.

Legal category P.

Package quantities 10 ml glass vials.

Further information Sole distributor: Farillon Limited, Ashton Road, Harold Hill, Romford, Essex RM3 8UE. Tel: Ingrebourne 71136.

Product licence numbers

Semitard MC	100 iu/ml	0542/0027
Rapitard MC	100 iu/ml	0542/0029
Lentard MC	100 iu/ml	0542/0030

Product licence holder: Farillon Limited.

VELOSULIN* CARTRIDGE
Neutral Insulin Injection BP, highly purified pork

Presentation Velosulin Cartridge is a clear neutral solution of highly purified pork insulin available in 5.7 ml glass cartridge vials containing 100 iu/ml for use only in the Nordisk Infuser*. Other ingredients include: buffer Sodium Phosphate PhEur 2.4 mg/ml and preservative Phenol BP 0.6 mg/ml.

Uses The treatment of insulin-requiring diabetic patients. To be used only with the Nordisk Infuser.

Dosage and administration Velosulin Cartridge is intended to be administered as subcutaneous infusion using the Nordisk Wellcome Infuser System.

Basal rate and prandial doses are to be determined by the physician according to the needs of the patient.

Velosulin Cartridge should only be used with the infusion set supplied with the Nordisk Infuser. No attempt should be made to refill the cartridges. When empty, they should be discarded and a fresh cartridge inserted. In order to minimise the risk of infusion site irritation or infection, it is recommended that the infusion set is changed every 2–3 days. The infusion site should be cleansed thoroughly and the needle taped securely in place. The infusion site should be changed according to a suitable routine and should be cleansed regularly. The procedure (given in the User's Manual) should be followed when the cartridge or infusion set is changed. The maximum in-use life of Velosulin Cartridge used in the Nordisk Infuser is 14 days.

Velosulin Cartridge is stable at normal Infuser operating temperatures (30–37°C if worn under outdoor clothing), although care must be taken to avoid extremes of temperature, eg. when sunbathing, winter sports, etc.

Use in pregnancy and lactation: It is essential to maintain continuous good glycaemic control throughout pregnancy. In the insulin-treated (gestational or insulin-dependent) pregnant diabetic patient, the insulin requirements fall in the first trimester and increase during the second and third trimesters.

Use in the elderly: No specific studies regarding continuous subcutaneous insulin infusion (CSII) in the elderly have yet been conducted. Clearance rates may be reduced in the elderly due to falling renal function. Insulin may therefore have a more prolonged action. Dose requirements should be regularly reviewed.

Contra-indications, warnings, etc

Contra-indications: Insulin is contra-indicated in hypoglycaemia.

Precautions: Variations in lifestyle and other factors, eg. infection and pregnancy, can affect insulin requirements.

Patients previously treated by subcutaneous insulin injection may require a dosage adjustment when transferred to subcutaneous infusion.

Hypoglycaemia can be enhanced by drugs including the following: aspirin; sulphonylureas, and agents affecting them; certain steroids.

Hyperglycaemia can be enhanced by drugs including the following: triiodothyronine; thyroxine; various natural and synthetic steroids, including some oral contraceptives; diuretics, including thiazides; cyclophosphamide.

Certain beta-blockers, especially propranolol, may affect insulin requirements and mask the signs of hypoglycaemia mediated by the sympathetic nervous system.

Monoamine oxidase inhibitors (MAOI) may potentiate the action of insulin.

Patients whose blood glucose control is greatly improved, e.g. by intensified insulin therapy, may experience a change in their usual warning symptoms of hypoglycaemia, and possibly lose some or all of the symptoms, and should be advised accordingly.

Side-and adverse effects: The most important side-effect is hypoglycaemia. Reduction of hyperglycaemia in newly diagnosed diabetics may alter visual refraction.

Insulin, like many other injected substances, is potentially immunogenic. This may or may not have clinical implications. Local reactions at the infusion site may include transient erythema, induration, urticaria and oedema. The incidence is minimal with highly purified pork insulin. These usually resolve with continuing usage of insulin. True generalised hypersensitivity reactions approaching anaphylaxis are very rare.

Clinical evidence suggests that highly purified pork insulins are unlikely to cause localised lipodystrophies, however, at present, this possibility cannot be totally excluded.

Toxicity and treatment of overdosage: The symptoms and signs of hypoglycaemia depend on the patient's clinical state and on the rate and extent of the fall in blood glucose levels.

Infusion with Velosulin Cartridge should be reduced or suspended until normal blood glucose levels are restored.

If possible, glucose, sucrose, or rapidly absorbable carbohydrate should be taken by mouth. Failing this, hypoglycaemia should be reversed as rapidly as possible by intravenous injection of glucose 50% solution. Alternative emergency treatments include the subcutaneous injection of up to 1 ml of adrenaline solution 1:1000 or the subcutaneous, intramuscular or intravenous injection of lyophilised glucagon 0.5–1.0 mg (1 unit = 1.0 mg). Both adrenaline and glucagon injections mobilise hepatic glycogen, but the effect is short lived and must be supplemented by freely available carbohydrate as soon as possible.

Pharmaceutical precautions Velosulin Cartridge should be stored between 2 and 8°C, protected from sunlight. Insulin which has been frozen should not be used. Velosulin Cartridge insulin which appears turbid (cloudy) should not be used.

Legal category P.

Package quantities 1 × 5.7 ml glass cartridge vials.

Further information Sole distributor: The Wellcome Foundation Ltd., Crewe Hall, Crewe, Cheshire, CW1 1UB. Tel: Crewe (0270) 583151.

Product licence number 3132/0043

GLUCAGON NOVO

Presentation Glucagon Novo is available as the hydrochloride in lyophilised form with accompanying diluent in two pack sizes:

1 mg – a vial containing 1 mg (1 i.u.) glucagon (as hydrochloride) and lactose 107 mg; a vial containing 1.1 ml Water for Injections, and a sterile plastic disposable syringe.

10 mg – a vial containing 10 mg (10 i.u.) glucagon (as hydrochloride) and lactose 140 mg, and a vial containing 10 ml of diluent (comprising glycerol 200 mg, methyl hydroxybenzoate 10 mg and propyl hydroxy-benzoate 1.5 mg as added preservatives, Water for Injections to 10 ml).

Uses

Indications: Treatment of severe hypoglycaemic reactions which may occur in the management of diabetic patients receiving insulin or oral hypoglycaemic agents.

Termination of insulin coma during insulin shock therapy in psychiatric patients.

As an adjunct for examinations of the gastro-intestinal tract by radiography or endoscopy.

Actions: Glucagon is a hyperglycaemic agent that mobilises hepatic glycogen which is released into the blood as glucose.

Independent of its hyperglycaemic effect glucagon also has an inhibitory action on the motility of the gastro-intestinal tract.

Dosage and administration *Adults and children:*

1. Treatment of severe hypoglycaemic reactions. Dissolve the lyophilised glucagon in the accompanying diluent. Give 0.5 to 1 mg (0.5 to 1 i.u.) of Glucagon Novo by subcutaneous, intramuscular or intravenous injection. If the patient does not awaken within 10 minutes, intravenous glucose must be given. When the patient responds, administer oral carbohydrate to restore the liver glycogen and prevent secondary hypoglycaemia.

2. Termination of insulin shock therapy. Dissolve the lyophilised glucagon in the accompanying diluent. 1–2 mg (1–2 iu) of Glucagon Novo is administered by subcutaneous, intramuscular or intravenous injection. If the patient does not awaken within 10 minutes, intravenous glucose must be given. When the patient responds, administer oral carbohydrate to restore the liver glycogen and prevent secondary hypoglycaemia.

In very deep states of coma, intravenous glucose may be given concurrently with Glucagon Novo.

3. Radiography and endoscopy of the gastro-intestinal tract. Doses range from 0.2–2 mg depending on the diagnostic technique used and the route of administration. The usual diagnostic dose for relaxation of the stomach, duodenal bulb, duodenum and small bowel is 0.2–0.5 mg given intravenously or 1 mg given intramuscularly; the usual dose to relax the colon is 0.5–0.75 mg intravenously or 1–2 mg intramuscularly.

Onset of action after an intravenous injection of 0.2–0.5 mg occurs within one minute and the duration of the effect is between 5 and 20 minutes depending on the organ under examination. The onset of action after an intramuscular injection of 1–2 mg occurs after 4–14 minutes and lasts approximately 10–40 minutes depending on the organ.

Contra-indications, warnings, etc *Contra-indications:* Glucagon Novo is contra-indicated in phaeochromocytoma, insulinoma and glucagonoma.

The presence of fibril formation or solid particles in the solution is a contra-indication to its use at any time.

Warnings: Glucagon reacts antagonistically towards insulin.

Precautions: Caution must be observed if Glucagon Novo is used in diabetic patients as an adjunct in radiography or endoscopy of the gastro-intestinal tract. Since glucagon is a protein, there is a theoretical possibility of hypersensitivity.

Side-effects: Nausea and vomiting may occur occasionally especially with doses above 1 mg, or if the injection is given too fast. No evidence of toxicity has been reported.

Pharmaceutical precautions Glucagon as the dry substance should be stored below 25°C.

1 mg pack: The solution should be prepared immediately prior to use.

10 mg pack: The solution should be prepared immediately prior to use but can be stored at 4°C for up to one week. Do not use solution unless clear.

Legal category POM.

Package quantities A single dose pack consisting of a vial containing 1 mg (1 i.u.) glucagon (as hydrochloride), a vial containing 1.1 ml Water for Injection, and a sterile plastic disposable syringe. A multiple dose pack consisting of a vial containing 10 mg (10 i.u.) glucagon (as hydrochloride) and a vial containing 10 ml diluent.

Further information *Sole distributors:* Farillon Limited, Ashton Road, Harold Hill, Romford, Essex RM3 8UE. Tel: Ingrebourne 71136.

Product licence numbers
1 mg 0542/0016
10 mg 0542/0017

Product licence holder: Farillon Limited.

NORDITROPIN* ▼

Presentation Pack comprising two vials, one vial containing somatropin (epr) 12 iu powder for injection, the second vial containing 3 ml sterile diluent for reconstituting the injection.

Ingredients: Vial 1 – Norditropin 12 iu, Glycine, Sodium Hydrogen Carbonate, Mannitol; Vial 2 – benzyl alcohol 9 mg/ml, Water for Injections.

Uses Treatment of short stature prior to epiphyseal fusion due to an inadequate secretion of growth hormone (growth hormone deficiency) or Turner's Syndrome. The diagnosis should be verified by an investigation of pituitary function before the preparation is administered. Data on long term efficacy of human growth hormone in Turner's Syndrome are currently not available.

Dosage and administration The dosage is individually determined for each patient.

Growth hormone deficiency: Generally 2–3 iu/m^2 body surface area or 0.07–0.1 iu/kg body weight, administered subcutaneously 6 to 7 times per week is recommended.

Turner's Syndrome: Generally 0.1 iu/kg body weight, 6 to 7 times per week is recommended.

Administration: The injection site should be varied to prevent lipoatrophy.

The injection is reconstituted by adding 3 ml of solvent to the dry powder for injection.

Prior to administration, the rubber seals of the vials should be wiped with antiseptic solution. The solvent is then drawn into a syringe and injected into the vial containing the dry powder whilst directing the stream against the glass wall of the vial. The powder is dissolved by inverting the vial several times; vigorous shaking should be avoided. The final Norditropin concentration of the reconstituted solution is 4 iu/ml.

Contra-indications, warnings, etc
Contra-indications: Norditropin should not be used where there is evidence of active tumour. Anti-tumour therapy should be completed prior to the institution of therapy. Norditropin should be discontinued if there is any evidence of recurrent tumour growth.

Pregnancy and lactation: There is currently insufficient evidence of safety of human growth hormone therapy during pregnancy, Norditropin is, therefore, contraindicated during pregnancy. In the event of pregnancy occurring during treatment, Norditropin therapy should be discontinued.

The possibility that human growth hormone is secreted in breast milk cannot be discounted.

Precautions: Patients treated with Norditropin should be regularly assessed by a specialist in child growth.

Growth hormone has a diabetogenic action which includes the induction of hyperglycaemia and ketosis. Norditropin should be used with caution in patients with diabetes mellitus or who have a family history of diabetes mellitus. Regular urine testing for evidence of glycosuria should be carried out in all patients.

A state of hypothyroidism may develop during growth hormone treatment. Since untreated hypothyroidism may interfere with the response to Norditropin, patients should have a periodic thyroid function test and should be treated with thyroid hormone when indicated.

Patients with growth hormone deficiency secondary to an intracranial lesion should be examined frequently for progression or recurrence of the underlying disease process.

Concomitant glucocorticoid therapy may inhibit the growth promoting effect of Norditropin. Patients with coexisting ACTH deficiency should have their glucocorticoid replacement dose carefully adjusted to avoid an inhibiting effect on growth.

Side-effects: Formation of antibodies directed against somatropin has rarely been observed during Norditropin therapy. The titres and binding capacities of these antibodies have been very low and have not interfered with the growth response to Norditropin. Patients failing to respond to treatment should, however, be tested for antibodies.

Local discomfort at the injection site has been reported occasionally.

Overdosage: Acute overdosage could lead initially to hypoglycaemia and subsequently to hyperglycaemia. Long-term overdosage could result in signs and symptoms consistent with the known effects of human growth hormone excess.

Pharmaceutical precautions The dry powder and reconstituted solution should be stored at 2–8°C and protected from direct sunlight. The dry powder has a shelf life of 3 years, expiry dates are stated on the label.

After reconstitution with Norditropin solvent the solution may be stored for up to 14 days at 2–8°C. The solution should not be frozen and should be protected from direct sunlight.

Legal category POM.

Package quantities Package containing one vial of Norditropin 12 iu and one vial of 3 ml sterile diluent.

Further information Norditropin is a registered trademark for highly purified biosynthetic somatropin of recombinant DNA origin, synthesised by a strain of E. coli carrying the gene for human growth hormone. Norditropin contains a sequence of 191 amino acids, identical to naturally occurring pituitary human growth hormone (molecular weight of about 22,000 daltons). The biological potency is approximately 3 iu/mg somatropin as determined by the tibia test and the weight gain test.

Sole distributor: The Wellcome Foundation Ltd., Crewe Hall, Crewe, Cheshire, CW1 1UB. Tel: Crewe (0270) 583151.

Product licence numbers

Norditropin 12 iu	3132/0046
Diluent	3132/0065

TRISEQUENS*

Presentation Trisequens is supplied in a calendar dial-pack of 28 sequential tablets:

12 blue biconvex tablets marked 'NOVO 270' on one side, blank on the other side, each containing 2 mg oestradiol and 1 mg oestriol.

10 white biconvex tablets marked 'NOVO 271' on one side, blank on the other side, each containing 2 mg oestradiol, 1 mg oestriol and 1 mg Norethisterone Acetate BP.

6 red biconvex tablets marked 'NOVO 272' on one side, blank on the other side, each containing 1 mg oestradiol, and 0.5 mg oestriol.

Uses Trisequens is indicated for the treatment of symptoms due to oestrogenic deficiency and for the prophylaxis of postmenopausal osteoporosis in women at risk of developing fractures.

The oestrogen components of Trisequens counteract falling oestrogen levels during the menopause, whilst the progestogen component counteracts hyper-stimulation of the endometrium. A regular shedding of the endometrium is normally induced by Trisequens during the red tablet phase or at the end of the white tablet phase.

Studies based on measurement of bone mineral content have shown that Trisequens is effective in the prevention of progressive bone loss following the menopause.

Dosage and administration Trisequens is administered orally without chewing, one tablet daily without interruption, starting with the blue tablets. In menstruating women the first tablet should be taken on the fifth day of menstrual bleeding. If menstruation has stopped altogether or is infrequent and sporadic (2–4 monthly intervals) the first tablet can be taken at any time.

Menopausal symptoms: Treatment may be stopped at approximately 6–12 monthly intervals to establish whether continued therapy for relief of menopausal symptoms is still required.

Postmenopausal oesteoporosis: Epidemiological studies which have examined risk factors for osteoporotic fractures (hip, lower forearm and spine) indicate that a useful reduction in fracture frequency is achieved with continuous long-term oestrogen therapy. In these studies, treatment for 5–6 years gave a reduction in fracture frequency of about 50%. Ideally, prophylactic therapy should commence during the perimenopausal period or as soon as possible thereafter. At present there is no diagnostic test for determining women at risk of developing osteoporotic fractures. Epidemiological studies give some indication of those women at risk. White women are more at risk than black women; other risk factors for fracture include: low body weight, tallness, early menopause, surgical menopause, cigarette smoking and high alcohol intake. A dietary intake of calcium ⩾1000 mg/day is probably also important in maintaining bone mass and supplementation should be considered if the diet is deficient.

Not intended for children or males.

Contra-indications, warnings, etc

Contra-indications: Known or suspected mammary or genital carcinoma. Known or suspected oestrogen-dependent tumours. Thrombophlebitis, thromboembolic disorders or patients with a past history of these conditions.

Undiagnosed irregular vaginal bleeding. Acute or chronic liver disease or history of liver disease where the liver function tests have failed to return to normal. Jaundice or history of jaundice in pregnancy. Rotor syndrome or Dubin-Johnson syndrome. Hyperlipoproteinaemia, especially in the presence of other risk factors which may indicate a predisposition to cardiovascular or cerebrovascular disorders. Patients with existing cerebrovascular or cardiovascular disease. A history during pregnancy of severe pruritus, herpes gestationis, or a deterioration of otosclerosis. Pregnancy or suspected pregnancy.

Precautions and warnings: Before initiation of therapy with Trisequens it is advisable to undertake a thorough examination to exclude any possibility of genital or mammary tumours. Women receiving long-term therapy with Trisequens should be given a similar examination every 6 months. Special attention should be paid to body weight, blood pressure, heart, breasts, pelvic organs, legs and skin.

It has been established that treatment of women with an intact uterus with oestrogens unopposed by progestogens increases the risk of endometrial cancer. Endometrial hyperplasia (atypical or adenomatous) often precedes endometrial cancer. Recent prospective studies, however, suggest that endometrial hyperplasia can virtually be avoided if the endometrium is protected by administration of a sufficient dose of progestogen for at least 10 days each cycle.

Long-term use of oestrogen replacement therapy in high doses shows an increase in breast cancer risk. Use of small doses for short periods show no measurable increase in risk. The effects of smaller doses of oestrogens for long periods are not adequately studied but appear unlikely to be associated with any substantially increased risk of breast cancer.

Patients with epilepsy, migraine, diabetes, asthma ocardiac dysfunction should be carefully controlled, as oestrogens may worsen these conditions.

Thromboembolism has been reported in connection with oestrogen replacement therapy but there is no background to believe that the overall incidence is increased.

The indications for immediate withdrawal of therapy

are as follows: thrombophlebitis; thromboembolic disorders; the appearance of jaundice; the occurrence of migraine-like headaches; sudden visual disturbances or a significant increase in blood pressure.

It is also advisable to withdraw treatment 6 weeks before elective surgery and during prolonged periods of immobilisation.

Trisequens may potentiate the side-effects of phenothiazines. Drugs such as barbiturates, phenytoin, and rifampicin, which induce the activity of hepatic microsomal drug-metabolizing enzymes, may decrease the effectiveness of Trisequens. Mineral oil may decrease the intestinal absorption of Trisequens.

Trisequens has no contraceptive effect.

Pre-existing uterine fibromyomata may increase in size under the influence of oestrogens and if this is observed administration of the preparation should be discontinued.

Side-effects: During the first few months of treatment, tension in the breasts, spotting or break-through bleeding can occur. These side-effects are usually of a temporary character and normally disappear after continued treatment. Other side-effects such as headache, oedema or nausea seldom occur.

Pharmaceutical precautions Protect from light.

Legal category POM.

Package quantities Trisequens is supplied in a calendar dial-pack of 28 tablets.

Further information *Sole distributor:* Farillon Limited, Ashton Road, Harold Hill, Romford, Essex RM3 8UE. Tel: Ingrebourne 71136.

Product licence number 4668/0015.

Product licence holder: Novo Nordisk A/S.

TRISEQUENS* FORTE

Presentation Trisequens forte is supplied in a calendar dial pack of 28 sequential tablets.

12 yellow biconvex tablets marked NOVO 273 on one side, blank on the other side, each containing 4 mg oestradiol and 2 mg oestriol.

10 white biconvex tablets marked NOVO 274 on one side, blank on the other side, each containing 4 mg oestradiol, 2 mg oestriol and 1 mg norethisterone acetate BP.

6 red biconvex tablets marked NOVO 272 on one side, blank on the other side, each containing 1 mg oestradiol and 0.5 mg oestriol.

Uses Trisequens forte is indicated for the treatment of symptoms due to oestrogenic deficiency. The oestrogen components of Trisequens forte counteract falling oestrogen levels during the menopause, whilst the progestogen component counteracts hyperstimulation of the endometrium. A regular shedding of the endometrium is normally induced by Trisequens forte during the red tablet phase or at the end of the white tablet phase.

Dosage and administration Trisequens forte is administered orally without chewing, one tablet daily without interruption, starting with the yellow tablets. In menstruating women, the first tablet should be taken on the fifth day of menstrual bleeding. If menstruation has stopped altogether, or is infrequent and sporadic (2–4 monthly intervals), the first tablet can be taken at any time. Treatment may be stopped at approximately 6–12 monthly intervals to establish whether continued therapy for relief of menopausal symptoms is still required.

Not intended for children or males.

Contra-indications, warnings, etc

Contra-indications: Known or suspected mammary or genital carcinoma. Known or suspected oestrogen-dependent tumours. Thrombophlebitis, thromboembolic disorders or patients with a past history of these conditions.

Undiagnosed irregular vaginal bleeding. Acute or chronic liver disease or history of liver disease where the liver function tests have failed to return to normal. Jaundice or history of jaundice in pregnancy. Rotor syndrome or Dubin-Johnson syndrome. Hyperlipoproteinaemia, especially in the presence of other risk factors which may indicate a predisposition to cardiovascular or cerebrovascular disorders. Patients with existing cerebrovascular or cardiovascular disease. A history during pregnancy or severe pruritus, herpes gestationis, or a deterioration of otosclerosis. Pregnancy or suspected pregnancy.

Precautions and warnings: Before initiation of therapy with Trisequens forte, it is advisable to undertake a thorough examination to exclude any possibility of genital or mammary tumours. Women receiving long-term therapy should be given a similar examination every 6 months. Special attention should be paid to body weight, blood pressure, heart, breasts, pelvic organs, legs and skin.

It has been established that treatment of women with an intact uterus with oestrogens unopposed by progestogens increases the risk of endometrial cancer. Endometrial hyperplasia (atypical or adenomatous) often precedes endometrial cancer. Recent prospective studies, however, suggest that endometrial hyperplasia can virtually be avoided if the endometrium is protected by administration of a sufficient dose of progestogen for at least 10 days each cycle.

Long-term use of oestrogen replacement therapy in high doses shows an increase in breast cancer risk. Use of small doses for short periods show no measurable increase in risk. The effects of smaller doses of oestrogens for long periods are not adequately studied but appear unlikely to be associated with any substantially increased risk of breast cancer.

Patients with epilepsy, migraine, diabetes, asthma or cardiac dysfunction should be carefully controlled, as oestrogens may worsen these conditions.

Thromboembolism has been reported in connection with oestrogen replacement therapy but there is no background to believe that the overall incidence is increased.

The indications for immediate withdrawal of therapy are as follows: thrombophlebitis, thromboembolic disorders, the appearance of jaundice, the occurrence of migraine-like headaches, sudden visual disturbances or a significant increase in blood pressure.

It is also advisable to withdraw treatment 6 weeks before elective surgery and during prolonged periods of immobilisation.

Trisequens forte may potentiate the side effects of phenothiazines. Drugs such as barbiturates, phenytoin, and rifampicin, which induce the activity of hepatic microsomal drug-metabolising enzymes, may decrease the effectiveness of Trisequens forte. Mineral oil may decrease the intestinal absorption of Trisequens forte.

Trisequens forte has no contraceptive effect.

Pre-existing uterine fibromyomata may increase in size under the influence of oestrogens and if this is observed administration of the preparation should be discontinued.

Side-effects: During the first few months of treatment, tension in the breasts, spotting or break-through bleeding can occur. These side effects are usually of a temporary character and normally disappear after continued treatment. Other side-effects such as headache, oedema or nausea seldom occur.

Pharmaceutical precautions Protect from light.

Legal category POM.

Package quantities Trisequens forte is supplied in a calendar dial pack of 28 tablets.

Further information Sole distributor: Farillon Limited, Ashton Road, Harold Hill, Romford, Essex RM3 8UE. Tel: Ingrebourne 71136.

Product licence number
Trisequens forte 0542/0021.

Product licence holder: Farillon Limited.

VAGIFEM*

Presentation White shallow concave, film-coated vaginal tablet, diam. 6 mm, containing 25 micrograms Oestradiol USP. The tablet formulation is based on a hydrophillic cellulose-derived matrix which gives a controlled release of the oestradiol.

Each tablet is inset in a polypropylene/polyethylene applicator. Each applicator with inset vaginal tablet is packed in a laminated bubble pack.

Uses
Indications: The treatment of atrophic vaginitis due to oestrogen deficiency.

Actions: Oestradiol is readily absorbed by the vagina and increases maturation of the vaginal epithelial cells, and cervical secretory activity.

Dosage and administration Vagifem is administered intravaginally using the applicator. An initial dose of 1 tablet daily for two weeks will usually improve vaginal atrophy and associated symptoms; a maintenance dose of 2 tablets per week may then be instituted. Treatment should be discontinued after about 3 months to assess whether further therapy is necessary.

Method of use: The applicator is inserted into the vagina up to the end of the smooth part of the applicator (approx. 9 cm). The tablet is released by pressing the plunger. The applicator is then withdrawn and disposed of.

Vagifem is not intended for children or males.

Contra-indications, warnings, etc
Contra-indications: Known, suspected, or past history of carcinoma of the breast. Known or suspected oestrogen dependent neoplasia, e.g. endometrial carcinoma or other hormone dependent tumours. Abnormal genital bleeding of unknown aetiology. Known or suspected pregnancy. Acute thrombophlebitis or thromboembolic disorders or a past history of these conditions, associated with previous oestrogen use.

Precautions and warnings: Although the dose of oestradiol is low and the treatment is local, a minor degree of systemic absorption may occur. Because of this the increased risk of endometrial cancer after treatment with unopposed oestrogens should be kept in mind. Endometrial hyperplasia (atypical or adenomatous) often precedes endometrial cancer.

Patients with the following conditions who are treated with Vagifem should be monitored more frequently and if any of the conditions worsen Vagifem treatment should be withdrawn: Thrombophlebitis, thromboembolic disorders or cerebrovascular accident or a past history of these disorders.

Acute or chronic liver disease or history of liver disease where the liver function tests have failed to return to normal.

Haemoglobinopathies or sickle cell anaemia.
Porphyria.
Epilepsy.
Migraine.
Diabetes.
Asthma.
Cardiac dysfunction.
Hypertension requiring treatment.

Before initiation of therapy with Vagifem it is advisable to undertake a thorough examination to exclude any possibility of genital or mammary tumours. Vaginal infections should be treated before initiation of Vagifem therapy.

Persistent or recurring vaginal bleeding should be investigated.

The present bulk of evidence shows that oestrogens given to post-menopausal women do not increase the risk of breast cancer.

Side-effects: Few side-effects have been observed. Slight vaginal bleeding, vaginal discharge and skin rash have rarely been reported.

Overdosage: Vagifem is intended for intravaginal use. The dose of oestradiol is so low that a considerable number of tablets would have to be ingested to approach a significant oral dose.

Pharmaceutical precautions Store at room temperature. Each applicator with inset tablet is intended for use only once.

Legal category POM.

Package quantities Laminated bubble strips containing 5 applicators with inset tablet. Packed in cartons containing 3 strips (15 tablets and applicators).

Further information Sole distributor: Farillon Limited, Ashton Road, Harold Hill, Romford, Essex RM3 8UE. Tel: Ingrebourne 71136.

Product licence number 4668/0026.

Product licence holder: Novo Nordisk A/S.

**Trade Mark*

Organon Laboratories Limited

Cambridge Science Park
Milton Road
Cambridge CB4 4FL

BOLVIDON*

Presentation White, film-coated, bi-convex tablets 6 mm in diameter, coded CT4 on one side and 'Organon' on the reverse side, each containing *10 mg* Mianserin Hydrochloride BP.

White, film-coated, bi-convex tablets 7 mm in diameter, coded CT6 on one side and 'Organon' on the reverse side, each containing *20 mg* Mianserin Hydrochloride BP.

White, film-coated, bi-convex tablets 8 mm in diameter, coded CT7 on one side and 'Organon' on the reverse side, each containing *30 mg* Mianserin Hydrochloride BP.

Other ingredients: Starch, aerosil, magnesium stearate, methyl cellulose tylopur MHB 50 and calcium hydrogen phosphate $2H_2O$.

Uses Symptoms of depressive illness.

Dosage and administration The daily dose can be taken either in divided doses or preferably (in view of the favourable effect on sleep) as a single dose at night.

It is often advantageous to maintain antidepressant treatment for several months after initial clinical improvement has occurred.

The tablets should be swallowed whole without chewing.

Adults: Treatment should usually commence with 30 mg or 40 mg per day for the first few days. The effective daily dosage usually lies between 30 mg and 90 mg.

Elderly: Not more than 30 mg a day initially. The dose should be slowly increased under close supervision. A lower than the normal maintenance dose may be sufficient to produce a satisfactory clinical response.

Children: Not recommended.

Contra-indications, warnings, etc

Contra-indications: Mania. Severe liver disease.

Use during pregnancy and breast feeding: Bolvidon is contraindicated during breast feeding. Breast feeding should be discontinued if treatment with Bolvidon is considered essential.

Do not use during pregnancy unless there are compelling reasons. There is no evidence of safety in human pregnancy. Animal studies have not shown hazard.

Precautions and warnings: Care should always be taken in patients with recent myocardial infarction or heart block. Serious cardiotoxic effects appear to be rare at therapeutic dosage, even in patients with pre-existing cardiac disease, recent myocardial infarction or cardiac insufficiency.

The elderly are less liable to experience adverse reactions such as agitation, confusion and postural hypotension with Bolvidon than with tricyclics or bridged tricyclics, but all anti-depressant therapy should be used with caution in this group of patients.

Patients posing a high suicidal risk require close initial supervision.

Avoid if possible in patients with epilepsy. When treating patients with diabetes, hepatic or renal insufficiency, normal precautions should be exercised and the dosages of any concurrent therapy kept under review. Patients with narrow angle glaucoma or symptoms suggestive of prostatic hypertrophy should also be monitored even though anticholinergic side-effects are not anticipated with Bolvidon therapy.

There are indications that Bolvidon, like other antidepressants, may precipitate hypomania in susceptible subjects with bipolar affective illness. In such a case treatment with Bolvidon should be withdrawn.

If surgery is necessary during Bolvidon therapy the anaesthetist should be informed of the treatment being given.

Drug interactions: Bolvidon may potentiate the central nervous depressant action of alcohol. Bolvidon should not be given concurrently with, or within two weeks of cessation of therapy with monoamine oxidase inhibitors.

Phenytoin plasma levels should be monitored in patients treated concurrently with Bolvidon.

Interactions with sympathomimetic agents have not been reported, and are unlikely.

Clinical experience has shown that Bolvidon does not interact with the anti-hypertensives bethanidine, clonidine, hydralazine, guanethidine or propranolol (either alone or in combination with hydralazine). Nevertheless, the monitoring of blood pressure is recommended for those patients receiving concurrent anti-hypertensive therapy.

Concurrent anticoagulant therapy of the coumarin type (e.g. warfarin) is also permissible, but close additional monitoring procedures should be carried out.

Warnings and adverse effects: As an improvement may not occur during the first 2–4 weeks of treatment, patients should be closely monitored during this period.

It is advisable to maintain treatment with Bolvidon for several months after initial clinical improvement.

The most commonly occurring side effect is drowsiness, particularly during the first few days of treatment. Patients should be warned of the possible hazard in driving or operating machinery. Any drowsiness may be potentiated by alcohol.

In order to ensure an optimal antidepressant effect, the dosage of Bolvidon should not be reduced.

The frequency and severity of depression-related symptoms such as blurred vision, dry mouth and constipation do not usually increase during treatment with Bolvidon; in fact an actual decrease has been observed in many cases.

Bone marrow depression, usually presenting as granulocytopenia or agranulocytosis, has been reported during treatment with Bolvidon. These reactions have occurred most commonly after 4–6 weeks of treatment and were generally reversible on stopping treatment. A full blood count is recommended every four weeks during the first three months of treatment. In addition, monitoring of the patient's clinical condition should continue and if a patient develops fever, sore throat, stomatitis or other signs of infection, treatment should be stopped and a full blood count obtained. These adverse reactions have been observed in all age groups but appear to be more common in the elderly.

Jaundice, usually mild, hypomania and convulsions have also been reported at therapeutic dosage and under such circumstances treatment should be withdrawn.

Additional adverse effects that may occur include breast disorders (gynaecomastia, nipple tenderness and non-puerperal lactation), disturbances of liver function, arthralgia, dizziness, postural hypotension, oedema, polyarthropathy, skin rash, sweating and tremor.

Psychotic manifestations, including mania and paranoid delusions, may be exacerbated during antidepressant therapy.

The following adverse effects although not reported with Bolvidon can occur with tricyclics and bridged tricyclics: interference with sexual function; withdrawal symptoms in adults; withdrawal symptoms (e.g. neuromuscular irritability) in neonates whose mothers received tricyclic or bridged tricyclic antidepressants during pregnancy.

Overdosage: Symptoms of overdosage are normally confined to prolonged sedation. Cardiac arrhythmias, convulsions, severe hypotension and respiratory depression are unlikely to occur. There is no specific antidote. Treatment is by gastric lavage with appropriate symptomatic and supportive therapy for vital functions.

Pharmaceutical precautions Protect from light.

Legal category POM.

Package quantities

All strengths are available in Securitainers of 100 and 500 tablets.

Further information Bolvidon is an antidepressant. Its active substance belongs to the piperazino-azepine group of compounds which are chemically not related to the tricyclic antidepressants (TADs). Its structure lacks the basic side-chain which is considered to be responsible for the anticholinergic activity of the TADs. The overall antidepressant efficacy of Bolvidon is comparable with that of other currently used antidepressants. Moreover, it possesses anxiolytic properties which are of value in treating patients with anxiety associated with depressive illness.

Bolvidon is well tolerated, in particular by the elderly and by patients with cardiovascular disease. At therapeutically effective dosages Bolvidon is devoid of anticholinergic action and does not produce significant effects on the cardiovascular system. As compared to the TADs, it causes less cardiotoxic effects on overdosage.

Elderly: Pharmacokinetic studies of Bolvidon in the elderly patient suggest a longer half-life and slower metabolic clearance. This information implies that a single night-time dose of Bolvidon should be preferable to divided doses in the elderly patient; in addition, a lower than the normal maintenance dose may be sufficient to produce a satisfactory clinical response.

Product licence numbers
10 mg tablets – 0065/0031R
20 mg tablets – 0065/0057R
30 mg tablets – 0065/0061R

COTAZYM*

Presentation Dark green gelatine capsules, containing pancreatic enzymes in powder form.

Each capsule contains Pancreatin EP with not less than 14,000 BP-Units lipase.

Uses As an adjunct in the treatment of pancreatic exocrine deficiency.

Dosage and administration The usual dose is 6 capsules daily in divided doses. The capsules should be opened and the contents sprinkled on to the food.

Dosage can easily be adjusted according to the requirements of the individual patient. In severe cases of pancreatic insufficiency, much higher dosages have been used with good results. In patients with severe gastric hyperacidity the concurrent use of an antacid or an H_2-receptor antagonist may be considered.

Contra-indications, warnings, etc
Contra-indications: Patients with a known allergy to the active ingredients (porcine protein).

Precautions and warnings: Buccal and perianal irritation may occur, and rarely inflammation, when large doses are used.

This product contains lactose and this should be taken into account when treating patients with lactose intolerance.

Use during pregnancy: There is no evidence of safety in use during pregnancy and animal reproduction-toxicological studies are lacking. Therefore, during pregnancy the benefits of the use of Cotazym capsules should be weighed against the possible hazards to the foetus.

Adverse reactions: As with any pancreatic extract, Cotazym capsules may have adverse effects in high dosages. These may include hyperuricosuria or hyperuricaemia (due to the purine content of the product), and buccal or perianal irritation, rarely amounting to frank inflammation.

Pharmaceutical precautions Store in a cool, dry place between 2 and 15°C and protect the capsules from light.

Legal category P.

Package quantities Securitainer of 56 capsules.

Further information Nil.

Product licence number 0065/5054R.

DECA-DURABOLIN*

Presentation Deca Durabolin is a clear, sterile, oily, solution for injection containing Nandrolone Decanoate BP, 25 mg or 50 mg per ml.

Other constituents: Benzyl Alcohol PhEur 0.1 ml and Arachis Oil PhEur to 1.0 ml.

Uses For use in osteoporosis in post-menopausal women.

Established osteoporosis should have been diagnosed by the following parameters:
i) crush or wedge fractures of the vertebrae
ii) other osteoporotic fractures
iii) established reduction in bone mineral content as measured by accepted BMC measurements.

Dosage and administration
Dosage: Post-menopausal women – 50 mg every three weeks.

Administration: The duration of treatment depends on the clinical response and the possible occurrence of side-effects.

The continuation of therapy as well as its discontinuation in case of side effects is at the clinicians discretion. It is recommended that all patients are informed about the possible side effects of Deca-Durabolin therapy in conjunction with its benefits.

Deca-Durabolin should be administered by deep intramuscular injection.

Contra-indications, warnings, etc
Contra-indications: Pregnancy. Known or suspected carcinoma of prostate or mammary carcinoma in the male.

Precautions and warnings: If signs of virilisation develop, discontinuation of the treatment should be considered.

Patients, especially the elderly, with the following conditions should be monitored: Latent or overt cardiac failure, renal dysfunction, hypertension, epilepsy or migraine (or a history of these conditions), since anabolic steroids may occasionally induce sodium and water retention;

Diabetes, or latent diabetes, since anabolic steroids may improve the glucose tolerance and decrease the need for insulin or other antidiabetic drugs;

Incomplete statural growth, since anabolic steroids in high dosages may accelerate epiphyseal closure;

Skeletal metastases, since anabolic steroids may induce hypercalcaemia and hypercalciuria in these patients;

Liver dysfunction.

Adverse reactions: Deca-Durabolin at the *recommended* dosages is unlikely to produce virilising effects.

High dosages, prolonged treatment and/or too frequent administration may cause:

Virilisation which appears in sensitive women as hoarseness, acne, hirsutism and increase of libido; in prepubertal boys as an increased frequency of erections and phallic enlargement, and in girls as an increase of pubic hair and clitoral hypertrophy. Hoarseness may be the first symptom of vocal change which may end in

long-lasting, sometimes irreversible deepening of the voice;
Amenorrhoea and inhibition of spermatogenesis;
Premature epiphyseal closure;
Sodium and water retention.

Pharmaceutical precautions Protect from light. Store at room temperature (15° to 25°C).

After storage at lower temperatures precipitation of the arachis oil vehicle may occur. By heating the ampoules at 100°C for a few minutes or at 40°C for one hour the solution becomes clear. The precipitation and rewarming does not affect the activity of the injection.

Legal category POM.

Package quantities
25 mg per ml: 1 ml ampoules in boxes of 3 and 1 ml Orgaject Disposable Syringes singly.
50 mg per ml: 1 ml ampoules in boxes of 3 and 1 ml Orgaject Disposable Syringes singly.

Further information In controlled trials periods of 6 months to 2 years have been used. The average duration of therapy was 9–12 months. The effect on bone continued for a considerable time period after therapy ended; in most cases for a period equalling the duration for which therapy was given.

Product licence numbers
25 mg/ml 0065/5005R
50 mg/ml 0065/5063R.

DECA-DURABOLIN* 100

Presentation Deca Durabolin 100 is a clear, sterile, oily, solution for injection containing Nandrolone Decanoate EP, 100 mg per ml.

Other ingredients: Benzyl Alcohol EP 0.1 ml and Arachis Oil EP to 1.0 ml.

Uses Deca Durabolin 100 is a higher dosage form of nandrolone decanoate intended for adjuvant therapy in the treatment of certain blood disorders.

Indicated in such conditions as: Anaemia of chronic renal failure; aplastic anaemia; anaemia due to cytotoxic therapy.

Dosage and administration Deca Durabolin 100 should be administered by deep intramuscular injection.

Adults: Anaemia of chronic renal failure – males 200 mg weekly; females 100 mg weekly.

Aplastic anaemia – 50–150 mg weekly.

Anaemia due to cytotoxic therapy – 200 mg weekly, starting 2 weeks prior to the course of cytotoxic therapy. This treatment should be continued throughout cytotoxic therapy and thereafter during the recovery period until the blood count has returned to normal.

Children: A dosage scheme for children cannot be given because of insufficient clinical experience.

Treatment with Deca-Durabolin 100 does not substitute for other therapeutic measures.

The onset of a therapeutic effect may vary widely among patients. If no satisfactory response occurs after 3–6 months of treatment, administration should be discontinued.

After a satisfactory improvement or a normalisation of the red blood picture has been obtained, treatment should be withdrawn gradually on the basis of regular monitoring of the haematological parameters.

Should a relapse occur at any time whilst the dose is being reduced or after stopping the treatment, re-institution of therapy should be considered.

Contra-indications, warnings, etc
Contra-indications: Pregnancy.

Known or suspected carcinoma of prostate or breast carcinoma in the male.

Use in pregnancy and lactation: This medicine is contra-indicated in pregnancy because of possible masculinisation of the foetus. There are insufficient data on the use of this medicine during breast-feeding to assess potential harm to the infant or a possible influence on milk production.

The recommended doses should not be exceeded.

If signs of virilisation develop, discontinuation of the treatment should be considered, preferably in consultation with the patient.

It is recommended that patients, with any of the following conditions should be monitored: latent or overt cardiac failure, renal dysfunction, hypertension, or migraine (or a history of these conditions), since anabolic steroids may occasionally induce sodium and water retention; incomplete statural growth, since anabolic steroids in high dosages may accelerate epiphyseal closure; skeletal metastases of breast carcinoma. In these patients hypercalcaemia may develop both spontaneously and as a result of anabolic steroid therapy. The latter can be indicative of a positive tumour response to the treatment. Nevertheless, the hypercalcaemia should first be treated appropriately and after restoration of normal calcium levels the therapy can be resumed; liver dysfunction.

Adverse reactions: The high dosages which are required to obtain a therapeutic effect in the indications mentioned may cause: virilisation which appears in sensitive women as hoarseness, acne, hirsutism and increase of libido; in prepubertal boys as an increased frequency of erections and phallic enlargement, and in girls as an increase of pubic hair and clitoral hypertrophy. Hoarseness may be the first symptom of vocal change which may end in long-lasting, sometimes irreversible deepening of the voice; amenorrhoea; inhibition of spermatogenesis; premature epiphyseal closure; fluid retention. Occasionally, abnormal values in some liver function tests. These changes appear to be reversible after completion of the treatment course.

Interactions: Although only one possible case of interaction with an oral anticoagulant has been observed, it is advisable to check the prothrombin time regularly when Deca Durabolin 100 is used in conjunction with such an agent.

Anabolic steroids may improve the glucose tolerance and decrease the need for insulin or other antidiabetic medicines in diabetes.

Overdose: The acute toxicity of nandrolone decanoate in animals is very low. There are no reports of acute overdosage with Deca-Durabolin 100 in the human.

Pharmaceutical precautions Protect from light.

Store at room temperature (15° to 25°C).

After storage at lower temperatures precipitation of the arachis oil vehicle may occur. By heating the ampoules at 100°C for a few minutes or at 40°C for one hour the solution becomes clear. The precipitation and rewarming does not affect the activity of the injection.

Legal category POM.

Package quantities 100 mg per ml: 1 ml ampoules in boxes of 3.

Further information In the human, Deca-Durabolin 100 stimulates erythropoiesis as demonstrated by rises in the red blood cell mass, and in the haemoglobin and haematocrit values. This effect is utilised therapeutically in the treatment of anaemia due to a decreased production of erythropoietin, bone marrow depression induced by chemotherapy, or hypoplasia of the stem cells in the bone marrow. In the latter condition (e.g. aplastic anaemia) the erythropoietic response is frequently accompanied by a positive effect on leucopoiesis and thrombopoiesis.

Product licence number 0065/0036R.

DEXAMETHASONE INJECTION

Presentation Each ml aqueous solution contains 5 mg Dexamethasone Sodium Phosphate BP, equivalent to approximately 4 mg dexamethasone.

Other ingredients: 1 ml ampoule – Glycerol EP 22.5 mg, Disodium Edetate EP 100 micrograms, Water for Injections EP to 1 ml. 2 ml vials – Glycerol EP 45.0 mg, Disodium Edetate EP 200 micrograms, Methylparaben BP 1.7 mg, Propylparaben BP 300 micrograms and Water for injections EP to 2 ml.

Uses Dexamethasone injection can be used for all forms of general and local glucocorticoid injection therapy and all acute conditions in which intravenous glucocorticoids may be life-saving.

Dosage and administration

Dosage: N.B. All dosages are expressed as mg dexamethasone sodium phosphate.

In general, glucocorticoid dosage depends on the severity of the condition and response of the patient. Under certain circumstances, for instance in stress, extra dosage adjustments may be necessary. If no favourable response is noted within a couple of days, glucocorticoid therapy should be discontinued.

Adults: Once the disease is under control the dosage should be reduced or tapered off to the lowest suitable level under continuous monitoring and observation of the patient. This should be done by administering one early morning dose, daily (or preferably every other morning), of an oral glucocorticoid with a shorter biological half-life than dexamethasone e.g. prednisolone.

For acute life-threatening situations (e.g. anaphylaxis, acute severe asthma) substantially higher dosages may be needed. Cerebral oedema (adults): initial dose 10–20 mg i.v. followed by 6 mg i.v. or i.m. every 6 hours, until a satisfactory result has been obtained. In brain surgery these dosages may be necessary until several days after the operation. Thereafter, the dosage has to be tapered off gradually. Increase of intracranial pressure associated with brain tumours can be counteracted by continuous treatment.

For local treatment, the following dosages can be recommended:

intra-articularly:	2–4 mg large joints
	0.8–1 mg small joints;
intrabursally:	2–4 mg;
in tendon sheaths:	0.4–1 mg.

The frequency of these injections may vary from every 3–5 days to every 2–3 weeks.

For rectal drip in cases of ulcerative colitis: 5 mg diluted in 120 ml saline.

Suggested doses for children: Dosage requirements are variable and may have to be changed according to individual needs. Usually 0.25 mg/kg to 0.50 mg/kg of body weight daily.

Administration: Dexamethasone may be administered intravenously, subcutaneously, intramuscularly, by local injection or as a rectal drip. For administration by intravenous infusion: see section on compatibility with infusion fluids. With intravenous administration high plasma levels can be obtained rapidly.

Rapid intravenous injection of massive doses of glucocorticoids may sometimes cause cardiovascular collapse; the injection should therefore be given slowly over a period of several minutes.

Intra-articular injections should be given under strictly aseptic conditions.

Discontinuation of prolonged therapy should be carried out by gradual reduction of dosage and under strict medical supervision, since withdrawal may result in acute exacerbation of the disease, acute adrenocortical insuffiency and polyarteritis.

Use with infusion fluids: Dexamethasone has been shown to retain its potency for at least 24 hours at room temperature, and in daylight conditions, when diluted with one of the following infusion fluids:

sodium chloride 0.9%
anhydrous glucose 5%
invert sugar 10%
sorbitol 5%
Ringer's solution
Hartmann's solution (Ringer-lactate)
Rheomacrodex
Haemaccel

Using these infusion fluids, Dexamethasone can also be injected directly into the infusion line without causing precipitation of the ingredients. Direct injection into the infusion line is also possible with the following infusion fluids:

mannitol 10%
Vamin N

Use during pregnancy and breast-feeding: During pregnancy, the benefits of the use of glucocorticoids should be weighed against the possible hazards to the mother or foetus. Infants whose mothers received substantial doses of glucocorticoids during pregnancy should be carefully observed for signs of adrenal insufficiency.

Glucocorticoids appear in breast milk in very small quantities. Mothers taking high doses of glucocorticoids should be advised not to breast-feed.

Contra-indications, warnings, etc

Contra-indications: No contra-indications exist when glucocorticoids, in a large single dose, are used in conditions where life is endangered.

Systemic glucocorticoids are generally contra-indicated in patients with Cushing's Syndrome, gastro-intestinal ulcers, glaucoma, hypersensitivity to glucocorticoids, systemic fungal infections or certain viral infections, e.g. varicella and herpes genitalis and ocular herpes infections, active tuberculosis and acute psychosis.

Local injection of a glucocorticoid is contra-indicated in bacteraemia, and systemic fungal infections, unstable joints, hypersensitivity to glucocorticoids, and infections at the injection site e.g. septic arthritis resulting from gonorrhoea or tuberculosis.

Precautions and warnings: Patients, especially the elderly, with the following conditions should be monitored:

latent or overt cardiac failure, renal dysfunction, hypertension, epilepsy or migraine, since glucocorticoids may induce fluid retention;
osteoporosis, since glucocorticoids have a negative effect on the calcium balance;
a history of psychotic illness;
latent tuberculosis, since glucocorticoids, may induce reactivation;
certain parasitic infestations, in particular amoebiasis;
incomplete statural growth, since glucocorticoids on prolonged administration may accelerate epiphyseal closure.

Glucocorticoid therapy is non-specific, suppresses the symptoms and signs of disease and decreases the resistance to infections. Appropriate antimicrobial therapy should accompany glucocorticoid therapy when necessary, e.g. in tuberculosis, and viral and fungal infections of the eye.

If a live vaccine is to be administered it should be borne in mind that glucocorticoids exert an immunosuppressive effect.

Patients on long-term glucocorticoid therapy should be regularly examined for increased intra-ocular pressure and posterior subcapsular cataracts.

Patients on long-term glucocorticoid therapy should be regularly examined with respect to their glucose metabolism.

Before, during and after stressful situations, dosage may need to be increased in patients who have undergone prolonged glucocorticoid treatment in the previous year.

Local injection of a glucocorticoid may produce systemic effects.

After parenteral administration of glucocorticoids serious anaphylactoid reactions, such as glottis oedema, urticaria and bronchospasm, have occasionally occurred, particularly in patients with a history of allergy. If such an anaphylactoid reaction occurs, the following measures are recommended: immediate slow intravenous injection of 0.1–0.5 ml of adrenaline (solution of 1:1000: 0.1–0.5 mg adrenaline dependent on body weight), intravenous administration of aminophylline and artificial respiration if necessary.

Cases of ruptured tendon have been reported following

the injection of glucocorticoids directly into a tendon. In the treatment of conditions such as tendinitis or tenosynovitis care should be taken to inject into the space between the tendon sheath and the tendon.

Adverse reactions: Adverse reactions associated with prolonged systemic glucocorticoid therapy are unlikely when high doses are administered over a short period of time. Nevertheless, gastric and duodenal ulceration, with possible perforation and haemorrhage, may occasionally occur.

The following adverse reactions have been associated with prolonged systemic glucocorticoid therapy:

Endocrine and metabolic disturbances: Cushing-like syndrome, hirsutism, menstrual irregularities, premature epiphyseal closure, secondary adrenocortical and pituitary unresponsiveness, decreased glucose tolerance, negative nitrogen and calcium balance.

Fluid and electrolyte disturbances: sodium and water retention, abdominal distension, hypertension, potassium loss, hypokalaemic alkalosis.

Muscular-skeletal effects: myopathy, osteoporosis, aseptic necrosis of femoral and humeral heads.

Gastro-intestinal effects: gastric and duodenal ulceration, perforation and haemorrhage.

Dermatologic effects: impaired wound healing, skin atrophy, striae, petechiae and ecchymoses, bruising, facial erythema, increased sweating, acne.

C.N.S. effects: psychic disturbances ranging from euphoria to frank psychotic manifestations, convulsions, in children pseudotumor cerebri (benign intracranial hypertension) with vomiting and papilloedema.

Opthalmic effects: glaucoma, increased intra-ocular pressure, posterior subcapsular cataracts.

Immunosuppressive effects: diminished lymphoid tissue and immune response, increased susceptibility to infections, decreased responsiveness to vaccination and skin tests, diminished inflammatory response.

Hypersensitivity reactions may occasionally occur.

A transient burning or tingling sensation, mainly in the perineal area, following intravenous injection of large doses of corticosteroid phosphates.

Local adverse reactions include post-injection flare, and a painless destruction of the joint reminiscent of Charcots arthropathy, especially with repeated intra-articular injections.

Interactions: Patients concomitantly using glucocorticoids and one of the following drugs should be monitored:

diuretics and/or cardiac glycosides, since potassium loss may be enhanced. This is a particular risk in patients using cardiac glycosides, since hypokalaemia increases the toxicity of these drugs.

antidiabetics, since glucocorticoids may impair glucose tolerance, thereby increasing the need for antidiabetic drugs.

non-steroidal anti-inflammatory drugs, since the incidence and/or severity of gastro-intestinal ulceration may increase.

oral anticoagulants, since glucocorticoids increase blood coagulability and therefore alter the need for these drugs.

Glucocorticoids may be less effective when used concomitantly with liver enzyme-inducing drugs, such as rifampicin, ephedrine, barbiturates, phenytoin, primidone, and phenylbutazone.

If patients undergoing long-term therapy with glucocorticoids are concomitantly given salicylates, any reduction in glucocorticoid dosage should be made with caution, since salicylate intoxication has been reported in such cases. Additionally, there may be interaction with salicylates, in patients with hypoprothrombinaemia.

Pharmaceutical precautions Store below 25°C, protected from light.

Legal category POM.

Package quantities Boxes of 10 × 2 ml vials containing Dexamethasone Sodium Phosphate BP 5 mg/ml equivalent to Dexamethasone (4 mg/ml).
Boxes of 10 × 1 ml ampoules. Each ampoule containing 5 mg/ml Dexamethasone Sodium Phosphate BP.

Further information After administration of Dexamethasone injection, dexamethasone sodium phosphate is rapidly converted into dexamethasone. This is a synthetic glucocorticoid whose anti-inflammatory potency is 7 times greater than prednisolone and 30 times that of the natural glucocorticoid, hydrocortisone. Like other glucocorticoids, dexamethasone also has anti-allergic, antipyretic and immunosuppressive properties. Dexamethasone has practically no sodium and water-retaining properties and is, therefore, particularly suitable for use in patients with cardiac failure or hypertension.

Because of its long biological half-life (36–54 hours), dexamethasone is especially suitable in conditions where continuous glucocorticoid action is desired.

Product licence numbers

2 ml/vial	0065/5013R
1 ml ampoule	0065/0106R

DEXAMETHASONE TABLETS BP

Presentation Round, flat white tablets in two strengths. 500 micrograms Dexamethasone BP code marked XC/4 with Organon and a star on the reverse side and 2 mg Dexamethasone BP code marked XC/8 with Organon and a star on the reverse side.

Uses Indicated in a wide variety of disorders amenable to glucocorticoid therapy, as well as an adjunct in the control of cerebral oedema.

Dosage and administration In general, glucocorticoid dosage depends on the severity of the condition and response of the patient. Under certain circumstances, for instance in stress, extra dosage adjustments may be necessary. If no favourable response is noted within a couple of days, glucocorticoid therapy should be discontinued.

Adults: Usually, daily oral dosages of 0.5–10 mg are sufficient. In some patients higher dosages may be temporarily required to control the disease. Once the disease is under control the dosage should be reduced or tapered off to the lowest suitable level under continuous monitoring and observation of the patient. This should be done by administering one early morning dose, daily (or preferably every other morning), of an oral glucocorticoid with a shorter biological half-life than dexamethasone e.g. prednisolone.

For a short dexamethasone suppression test, 1 mg dexamethasone is given at 11 p.m. and plasma cortisol measured the next morning. Patients who do not show a decrease in cortisol can be exposed to a longer test: 500 micrograms dexamethasone is given at 6 hourly intervals for 48 hours followed by 2 mg every 6 hours for a further 48 hours. 24 hour-urine collections are made before, during and at the end of the test for determination of 17-hydroxycorticosteroids.

Discontinuation of prolonged therapy should be carried out by gradual reduction of dosage and under strict medical supervision, since withdrawal may result in acute exacerbation of the disease and acute adrenocortical insufficiency.

Children: 0.01–0.1 mg/kg of body weight daily.

Dosage of glucocorticoids should be adjusted on the basis of the individual patient's response.

Use during pregnancy and breast-feeding During pregnancy, the benefits of the use of glucocorticoids should be weighed against the possible hazards to the mother or foetus. Infants whose mothers received substantial doses of glucocorticoids during pregnancy should be carefully observed for signs of adrenal insufficiency.

Glucocorticoids appear in breast milk in very small quantities. Mothers taking high doses of glucocorticoids should be advised not to breast-feed.

Contra-indications, warnings, etc

Contra-indications: No contra-indications exist when glucocorticoids, in a large single dose, are used in conditions where life is endangered.

Glucocorticoids are generally contra-indicated in

patients with Cushing's Syndrome, gastro-intestinal ulcers, glaucoma, hypersensitivity to glucocorticoids, systemic fungal infections or certain viral infections, e.g. varicella and herpes genitalis.

Precautions and warnings: Patients, especially the elderly, with the following conditions should be monitored:

latent or overt cardiac failure, renal dysfunction, hypertension, epilepsy or migraine, since glucocorticoids may induce fluid retention;
osteoporosis, since glucocorticoids have a negative effect on the calcium balance;
a history of psychotic illness;
latent tuberculosis, since glucocorticoids may induce reactivation;
certain parasitic infestations, in particular amoebiasis;
incomplete statural growth, since glucocorticoids on prolonged administration may accelerate epiphyseal closure.

Glucocorticoid therapy is non-specific, suppresses the symptoms and signs of disease and decreases the resistance to infections. Appropriate antimicrobial therapy should accompany glucocorticoid therapy when necessary, e.g. in tuberculosis, and viral and fungal infections of the eye.

If a live vaccine is to be administered it should be borne in mind that glucocorticoids exert an immunosuppressive effect.

Patients on long-term glucocorticoid therapy should be regularly examined for increased intra-ocular pressure and posterior subcapsular cataracts.

Patients on long-term glucocorticoid therapy should be regularly examined with respect to their glucose metabolism.

Before, during and after stressful situations, dosage may need to be increased in patients currently on glucocorticoids or resumed in patients who have undergone glucocorticoid treatment in the previous year.

Adverse reactions: Adverse reactions associated with prolonged systemic glucocorticoid therapy are unlikely when high doses are administered over a short period of time. Nevertheless, gastric and duodenal ulceration, with possible perforation and haemorrhage, may occasionally occur.

The following adverse reactions have been associated with prolonged systemic glucocorticoid therapy:

Endocrine and metabolic disturbances: Cushing-like syndrome, hirsutism, menstrual irregularities, premature epiphyseal closure, secondary adrenocortical and pituitary unresponsiveness, decreased glucose tolerance, negative nitrogen and calcium balance.

Fluid and electrolyte disturbances: sodium and water retention, abdominal distention, hypertension, potassium loss, hypokalaemic alkalosis.

Muscular-skeletal effects: myopathy, osteoporosis, aseptic necrosis of femoral and humeral heads.

Gastro-intestinal effects: gastric and duodenal ulceration, perforation and haemorrhage.

Dermatologic effects: impaired wound healing, skin atrophy, striae, petechiae and ecchymoses, bruising, facial erythema, increased sweating, acne.

C.N.S. effects: psychic disturbances ranging from euphoria to frank psychotic manifestations, convulsions, in children pseudotumor cerebri (benign intracranial hypertension) with vomiting and papilloedema.

Ophthalmic effects: glaucoma, increased intraocular pressure, posterior subcapsular cataracts.

Immunosuppressive effects: increased susceptibility to infections, decreased responsiveness to vaccination and skin tests, diminished inflammatory response.

Hypersensitivity reactions may occasionally occur.

Interactions: Patients treated concomitantly with glucocorticoids and one of the following drugs should be monitored:

diuretics and/or cardiac glycosides, since potassium loss may be enhanced. This is a particular risk in patients using cardiac glycosides, since hypokalaemia increases the toxicity of these drugs.
antidiabetics, since glucocorticoids may impair glucose tolerance, thereby increasing the need for antidiabetic drugs.
non-steroidal anti-inflammatory drugs since the incidence and/or severity of gastro-intestinal ulceration may increase.
oral anticoagulants, since glucocorticoids may alter the need for these drugs.

Glucocorticoids may be less effective when used concomitantly with liver enzyme-inducing drugs, such as rifampicin, ephedrine, barbiturates, phenytoin, primidone.

If patients undergoing long-term therapy with glucocorticoids are concomitantly given salicylates, any reduction in glucocorticoid dosage should be made with caution, since salicylate intoxication has been reported in such cases.

Antacids, especially those containing magnesium trisilicate, have been reported to impair the gastro-intestinal absorption of glucocorticoids. Therefore doses of one agent should be spaced as far as possible from the other.

Pharmaceutical precautions Protect from light.

Legal category POM.

Package quantities Dexamethasone tablets BP 500 micrograms: pack of 500 tablets. Dexamethasone tablets BP 2 mg: pack of 100 or 500 tablets.

Further information Dexamethasone is a synthetic glucocorticoid whose anti-inflammatory potency is 7 times greater than prednisolone. Like other glucocorticoids, dexamethasone also has anti-allergic, antipyretic and immunosuppressive properties.

Dexamethasone has practically no water and salt-retaining properties and is, therefore, particularly suitable for the use in patients with cardiac failure or hypertension. Because of its long biological half-life (36–54 hours), dexamethasone is especially suitable in conditions when continuous glucocorticoid action is desired.

Product licence numbers

500 microgram	0065/5044R
2 mg	0065/5045R

DURABOLIN*

Presentation Durabolin is a clear, sterile, oily, solution for injection containing nandrolone phenylpropionate, 25 mg or 50 mg per ml.

Other constituents: Benzyl Alcohol PhEur 0.1 ml and Arachis Oil PhEur to 1.0 ml.

Uses For use in osteoporosis in post-menopausal women.

Established osteoporosis should have been diagnosed by the following parameters:

i) crush or wedge fractures of the vertebrae
ii) other osteoporotic fractures
iii) established reduction in bone mineral content as measured by accepted BMC measurements.

Dosage and administration
Dosage: Post-menopausal women – 50 mg every week.

Administration: The duration of treatment depends on the clinical response and the possible occurrence of side-effects.

The continuation of therapy as well as its discontinuation in case of side effects is at the clinicians discretion. It is recommended that all patients are informed about the possible side effects of Deca-Durabolin therapy in conjunction with its benefits.

Durabolin should be administered by deep intramuscular injection.

Contra-indications, warnings, etc
Contra-indications: Pregnancy. Known or suspected carcinoma of prostate or mammary carcinoma in the male.

Precautions and warnings: If signs of virilisation develop, discontinuation of the treatment should be considered.

Patients, especially the elderly, with the following conditions should be monitored:

Latent or overt cardiac failure, renal dysfunction, hypertension, epilepsy or migraine (or a history of these conditions), since anabolic steroids may occasionally induce sodium and water retention.

Diabetes, or latent diabetes, since anabolic steroids may improve the glucose tolerance and decrease the need for insulin or other antidiabetic drugs;

Incomplete statural growth, since anabolic steroids in high dosages may accelerate epiphyseal closure.

Skeletal metastases, since anabolic steroids may induce hypercalcaemia and hypercalciuria in these patients.

Liver dysfunction.

Adverse reactions: Durabolin at the *recommended* dosages is unlikely to produce virilising effects.

High dosages, prolonged treatment and/or too frequent administration may cause: Virilisation which appears in sensitive women as hoarseness, acne, hirsutism and increase of libido; in prepubertal boys as an increased frequency of erections and phallic enlargement, and in girls as an increase of pubic hair and clitoral hypertrophy. Hoarseness may be the first symptom of vocal change which may end in long-lasting, sometimes irreversible deepening of the voice;

Amenorrhoea and inhibition of spermatogenesis;
Premature epiphyseal closure;
Sodium and water retention.

Pharmaceutical precautions Protect from light. Store at room temperature (15° to 25°C).

After storage at lower temperatures precipitation of the arachis oil vehicle may occur. By heating the ampoules at 100°C for a few minutes or at 40°C for one hour the solution becomes clear. The precipitation and rewarming does not affect the activity of the injection.

Legal category POM.

Package quantities
25 mg per ml: 1 ml ampoules in boxes of 3 and 1 ml Orgaject Disposable Syringes singly.
50 mg per ml: 1 ml Orgaject Disposable Syringes singly.

Further information In controlled trials periods of 6 months to 2 years have been used. The average duration of therapy was 9–12 months. The effect on bone continued for a considerable time period after therapy ended; in most cases for a period equalling the duration for which therapy was given.

Product licence numbers

25 mg/ml: 1 ml ampoules and 1 ml Orgajects	0065/5007R
50 mg/ml: 1 ml Orgajects	0065/5091R

GESTANIN*

Presentation Round, flat, white tablets with bevelled edges, diameter 9.00 mm, code-marked 'GK' above, and 4 below a single breakline on one side, with 'Organon' and a star on the reverse side. Each tablet contains 5 mg of allylestrenol.

Other constituents: dl-alpha-tocopherol, lactose, potato starch, disodium edetate, talc, glycerol and magnesium stearate.

Uses Threatened abortion, habitual abortion and threatened premature labour.

Dosage and administration
Dosage: Adults.

In threatened abortion: 1 tablet three times daily for 5–7 days. If necessary, the treatment period may be extended. After disappearance of the symptoms the dosage should be gradually reduced unless symptoms return.

In habitual abortion: 1–2 tablets daily as soon as pregnancy has been diagnosed. The administration should be continued until at least one month after the end of the critical period.

In threatened premature labour: The dosage must be determined individually. High dosages (up to 40 mg daily) have been used.

Elderly: Not applicable.

Children: Not applicable.

Administration: Gestanin tablets are for oral administration.

Contra-indications, warnings, etc
Contra-indications: Abnormal liver function.

Precautions and warnings: No precautions and warnings are applicable.

Side-effects: Gastrointestinal complaints (nausea, vomiting) have been occasionally reported.

Pharmaceutical precautions Store between 2 and 25°C, protected from moisture and light.

Legal category POM.

Package quantities Polypropylene containers of 100 tablets.

Further information Administration of Gestanin, in combination with bedrest, can remove or prevent the threat of abortion in early pregnancy or stop threatened premature labour. Gestanin is generally well tolerated. Serious adverse reactions have neither been reported in the mother nor in the offspring.

Product licence number 0065/5030R.

HUMEGON*

Presentation Human menopausal gonadotrophins (HMG) containing human follicle stimulating hormone (hFSH) and human luteinizing hormone (hLH) activities in a ratio of approximately 1, in a freeze-dried sterile preparation.

Ampoules containing 75 or 150 I.U. HMG i.e. 75 or 150 I.U. of hFSH and 75 I.U. or 150 I.U. hLH activities each. Human chorionic gonadotrophin (hCG) is added to achieve the labelled activity of LH i.e. 3.7–10.2 I.U. hCG to achieve an LH activity of 75 I.U. and 7.4–20.4 I.U. hCG to achieve an activity of 150 I.U. LH.

Other ingredients: Humegon 75 I.U. – mannitol 5 mg, disodium hydrogen phosphate (anhydrous) 250 micrograms, sodium dihydrogen phosphate (anhydrous) 250 micrograms. Humegon 150 I.U. – mannitol 10 mg, disodium hydrogen phosphate (anhydrous) 500 micrograms, sodium dihydrogen phosphate (anhydrous) 500 micrograms.

Ampoules containing one ml solvent (0.9% saline).

Uses For the treatment of female and male fertility disorders due to inadequate gonadotrophin stimulation of the gonads, and for controlled superovulation in medically assisted reproduction programmes.

In the female
Infertility caused by anovulation: HMG can be used to promote the development of a single follicle in the following categories of anovulatory women:
– Amenorrhoeic patients with no evidence of endogenous oestrogen production, non-elevated prolactin levels, normal or low gonadotrophins.
– Amenorrhoeic patients with evidence of endogenous oestrogen production, normal prolactin, and normal gonadotrophin levels.
– Patients with a variety of menstrual cycle disturbances, e.g., luteal phase insufficiency and anovulatory cycles with normal prolactin.

Patients belonging to the latter 2 categories should preferentially be treated with other ovulation – inducing agents influencing the steroid feed-back mechanisms, such as clomiphene. Patients who have not reacted to such agents, may be selected for gonadotrophin therapy.

Controlled superovulation in medically assisted reproduction programmes: The objective is to increase the number of oocytes available for collection in medically assisted reproduction programmes. In vitro fertilization followed by embryo transfer (IVF/ET) may be indicated in cases of infertility due to disorders, such as total obstruction, endometriosis, male factors, absent or non-functional ovaries, immunological and idiopathic causes. Another alternative in the treatment of infertility, mainly in andrological and idiopathic infertility, is gamete intra-fallopian transfer (GIFT). A prerequisite in this case, is that at least one adequately functioning fallopian tube is present.

In the male

Deficient spermatogenesis: In hypogonadotrophic hypogonadal men HMG is given primarily to augment hFSH for the stimulation of the Sertoli cells. The much higher hLH activity needed to stimulate the Leydig cells is mainly provided by additional therapy with hCG (Pregnyl). Cases of idiopathic dysspermias have also been reported to respond to combined HMG-hCG treatment.

Dosage and administration After addition of the solvent to the freeze-dried substance, the reconstituted Humegon solution should be administered intramuscularly.

Since an opened ampoule cannot be resealed in such a way to further guarantee the sterility of the contents, the solution should be used immediately after reconstitution.

Anovulatory infertility: There are large inter- and intra-individual variations in the response of the ovaries to exogenous gonadotrophins. This makes it impossible to set a uniform dosage scheme. Since the objective of therapy is the development of a single mature follicle the dosage should be adjusted individually depending on the ovarian response. This requires monitoring of oestrogen levels, ultrasonography and/or clinical evaluation of oestrogen activity. In general, a sequential treatment scheme is recommended. This starts with daily administration of 75 or 150 I.U. HMG. Administration on alternate days may also be considered. The dose is gradually increased until oestrogen levels start to rise. The effective dose is then maintained until adequate pre-ovulatory oestrogen levels are reached. If oestrogen levels rise too rapidly, the dose should be decreased.

As a measure of follicle maturity the following values can be taken:

- total urinary oestrogen: 75–150 microgram (270–540 nmol)/24 hours:
- plasma 17beta-oestradiol: 400–800 picogram/ml (1500–3000 pmol/L).

When adequate pre-ovulatory oestrogen levels have been reached, Humegon is witheld. Ovulation may then be induced by administering hCG (Pregnyl) in a dose of 5000–10000 I.U.

Up to three repeat injections of up to 5000 I.U. hCG (Pregnyl) each may be given within the following 9 days to prevent insufficiency of the corpus luteum. In women with polycystic ovarian disease, induction of a hypogonadotrophic state by a GnRH agonist before treatment with HMG may result in better pregnancy rates than without the use of an agonist.

Controlled superovulation in medically assisted reproduction programmes: The objective of therapy is to stimulate multiple follicular growth, thereby increasing the number of oocytes available for fertilisation or replacement in IVF and GIFT respectively.

Various stimulation protocols are applied. Stimulation of follicular growth is generally achieved by daily administration of 75–300 I.U. HMG alone or in combination with clomiphene citrate or a GnRH agonist. When using HMG alone, treatment may be started between days 1–5 of the menstrual cycle and continued until maturation of the follicles. Maturation of follicles is monitored by measurement of oestrogen levels, ultrasonography and/or clinical evaluation of oestrogen activity. It is recommended there should be at least 3 follicles greater than 17 mm in diameter with 17-beta oestradiol levels of at least 3,500 pmol/L, (920 picogram/ml). Follicles are prepared for punction by administration of hCG (Pregnyl) in a dose of 5000–10000 I.U. 30–40 hours after the last Humegon injection. Pregnyl should not be administered if these criteria have not been met. Oocyte collection is carried out 32–36 hours after the hCG injection.

Male infertility: 75 I.U. HMG are given daily or 2–3 times a week. These injections are generally combined with 1000–2000 I.U. hCG (Pregnyl) 2–3 times a week to achieve the necessary hLH effect. This treatment should be continued for at least 3 months before any improvement in spermatogenesis can be expected. During this treatment testosterone replacement therapy should be suspended. Once achieved, the improvement may in some cases be maintained by hCG alone.

Contra-indications, warnings, etc

Contra-indications: Ovarian, testicular and pituitary tumours.

Precautions and warnings: Prior to treating patients for inadequate endogenous stimulation of the gonads, an examination should be performed to exclude anatomical abnormalities of the genital organs or nongonadal endocrinopathies (e.g. thyroid or adrenal disorders, diabetes). Primary ovarian failure should be excluded by the determination of gonadotrophin levels.

In pregnancies occurring after induction of ovulation with gonadotrophic preparations, there is an increased risk of miscarriage and multiplets.

Unwanted hyperstimulation: During treatment of female patients, determinations of oestrogen levels and assessment of ovarian size and, if possible, ultrasonography should be performed prior to treatment and at regular intervals during treatment. High dosages may cause oestrogen levels to rise excessively rapidly, e.g. more than doubling on 2 or 3 consecutive days, and possibly reaching excessively high pre-ovulatory values.

If unwanted hyperstimulation occurs (i.e. not as part of a treatment preparing for IVF/ET or GIFT), the administration of HMG should be discontinued immediately. hCG must not be given, because the administration of an hLH-active gonadotrophin at this stage may induce, in addition to multiple ovulations, the ovarian hyperstimulation syndrome. This warning is particularly important with respect to patients with polycystic ovarian disease.

The severe form of ovarian hyperstimulation syndrome may be life-threatening and is characterized by large ovarian cysts (prone to rupture), ascites, very often hydrothorax and occasionally thrombo-embolic phenomena.

Adverse reactions: Skin rashes have rarely been reported.

Overdosage: The acute toxicity of HMG has been shown to be very low. However, too high a dosage for more than one day may lead to hyperstimulation of the ovaries (see Unwanted hyperstimulation).

Pharmaceutical precautions The product has a shelf-life of 3 years when stored in the dark at a temperature between 2 and 25°C.

Legal category POM.

Package quantities Humegon 75 I.U. – packs of 1 or 10 ampoules plus solvent (0.9% saline).

Humegon 150 I.U. – packs of 1 or 10 ampoules plus solvent (0.9% saline).

Product licence numbers

Humegon 75 I.U.	0065/0112
Humegon 150 I.U.	0065/0113
Solvent (0.9% saline)	0065/0114

HYDROCORTISONE SODIUM SUCCINATE

Presentation A white, freeze-dried, sterile powder which on reconstitution with water for injections forms a solution of hydrocortisone sodium succinate. There are two concentrations available equivalent to 100 mg or 500 mg hydrocortisone base.

Uses Injectable glucorticoids may be indicated in the following conditions, especially if oral therapy is impossible or undesirable.

Immuno-allergology: in some cases, especially in exacerbation, of systemic lupus erythematosus, nephrotic syndrome with minimal change lesions, periarteritis nodosa, mixed connective tissue disease, arteritis temporalis; usually in combination with adrenaline in anaphylaxis; hypersensitivity reactions to drugs or chemicals, serum sickness, transfusion reactions, angioneurotic oedema, Stevens-Johnson syndrome.

Rheumatology: in general as adjunctive therapy for short-term administration (either systemically or locally) in serious cases of rheumatoid arthritis and rheumatic osteoarthritis, synovitis, ankylosing spondylitis, polymyalgia rheumatica, acute rheumatic carditis: for local administration in cases of acute and subacute bursitis, synovitis, epicondylitis, tendinitis.

Endocrinology: primary or secondary adrenocortical insufficiency, adrenogenital syndromes, polycystic ovary syndrome, non suppurative thyroiditis, thyrotoxic crisis; in surgery, severe stress or trauma in cases of decreased or doubtful adrenocortical function.

Dermatology: severe cases of pemphigus and pemphigoid, exfoliative and other serious cases of dermatitis, mycosis fungoides, erythema multiforme; locally in keloids and some cases of alopecia areata.

Ophthalmology: severe acute or chronic allergic inflammatory processes of the eye and its adnexa (subconjunctivally, retrobulbarly or systemically) such as allergic conjunctivitis, iritis, iridocyclitis, choroiditis, optic neuritis, sympathetic ophthalmia; scar-prevention in eye surgery and eye injuries.

Gastro-enterology: to induce remission of ulcerative colitis and regional enteritis; in some cases of chronic hepatitis, especially the aggressive form with hyperimmunity; oesophagitis corrosiva, in some cases of coeliac disease eosinophylic (gastro) enteritis.

Cardiology: in some cases of pericarditis (idiopathic, postmyocardial infarction and postcommissurotomic syndrome).

Pulmonology: asthmatic pulmonary eosinophilia and allergic alveolitis, aspiration pneumonitis, severe bronchial asthma and other chronic non-specific obstructive lung diseases; diffuse interstitial pulmonary processes; as part of the treatment of laryngotracheobronchitis and the respiratory distress syndrome in adults; in combination with tuberculostatic therapy in fulminating tuberculosis.

Haematology and oncology: idiopathic and secondary thrombocytopenic purpura (i.v. only), auto-immune haemolytic anaemia, idiopathic immuno-granulocytopenia (agranulocytosis), acute and chronic lymphocytic leukaemia, acute myelocytic leukaemia (blastemic crisis), Hodgkin's disease, other malignancies of the lymphoid and histiocytic tissue, multiple myeloma, macroglobulinaemia; as an anti-emetic in antineoplastic regimens; for palliative treatment in terminal stages of neoplastic disease.

Neurology: cerebral oedema, particularly those forms resulting from brain tumours, brain abscesses and neurosurgical interventions (in the latter case also for prevention of brain oedema); myoclonic seizures in epilepsy, pseudotumor cerebri, severe myasthenia gravis resistant to anticholinesterase therapy and thymectomy, in some cases of acute multiple sclerosis and peripheral neuritis.

Other indications: in the prevention of inflammatory oedema and adhesions in surgery; in most cases of tuberculous meningitis, pericarditis, peritonitis and pleuritis (in combination with tuberculostatic therapy); antenatal, for prophylaxis only in pre-term labour, of neonatal respiratory distress syndrome; severe trichinosis, hypercalcaemia such as associated with neoplastic diseases, hypervitaminosis-D, idiopathic infantile hypercalcaemia.

Dosage and administration

Route of administration: After addition of the solvent to the freeze-dried substance, the reconstituted solution can be administered by intravenous, subcutaneous, intramuscular and local injection as well as by rectal drip.

Dosage: In general, glucocorticoid dosage depends on the severity of the condition and the response of the patient. Under certain circumstances, for instance in stress and changed clinical picture, extra dosage adjustments may be necessary. If no favourable response is noted within a couple of days, continuation of glucocorticoid therapy is undesirable.

For systemic therapy, one injection of 50–200 mg daily is usually sufficient. As soon as symptoms diminish, dosage should be reduced under continuous observation of the clinical picture to the lowest possible level, or tapered off completely. This should be done by giving one daily dose in the early morning, preferably every other day, of an oral glucorticoid.

For acute life-endangering situations (e.g. anaphylaxis, acute severe asthma) higher intravenous dosages, up to 500 mg, may be needed. Cerebral oedema (adults): initial dose 250–500 mg i.v. followed by 150 mg i.v. or i.m. every 6 hours, until a satisfactory result has been obtained. In brain surgery these dosages may be necessary until several days after the operation. Thereafter, the dosage has to be tapered off gradually. Increase of intracranial pressure associated with brain tumours can be counteracted by continuous treatment.

For local therapy, one injection of 100 mg is usually sufficient; if necessary the injection may be repeated. Sometimes one or more injections of 40–60 mg will be an adequate dosage.

For rectal drip in cases of ulcerative colitis: 100 mg diluted in 120 ml saline.

Use in children: Corticosteroids cause growth retardation in infancy, childhood and adolescence. Treatment should be limited to the minimum dosage for the shortest possible time. In order to minimise suppression of the hypothalomo-pituitary adrenal axis and growth retardation, treatment should be administered where possible as a single dose on alternate days.

Use in elderly: Treatment of elderly patients, particularly if long term, should be planned bearing in mind the more serious consequences of the common side-effects of corticosteroids in old age, especially osteoporosis, diabetes, hypertension, susceptibility to infection and thinning of the skin.

Contra-indications, warnings, etc

Contra-indications

For systemic therapy: Gastric and duodenal ulcers; systemic fungal infections; certain viral infections, e.g. varicella and herpes genitalis infections; glaucoma; hypersensitivity to glucocorticoids.

For local therapy: Infection at the affected site, e.g. septic arthritis resulting from gonorrhoea or tuberculosis; bacteraemia and systemic fungal infections; instability of the joint; hypersensitivity to glucocorticoids

In general no contra-indications apply in conditions where the use of glucocorticoids may be life-saving.

Use in pregnancy and lactation: There is inadequate evidence of safety in human pregnancy and there may be a very small risk of cleft palate and intra-uterine growth retardation in the foetus. There are indications for a harmful effect in animal experiments. Infants whose mothers received substantial doses of glucocorticoids during pregnancy should be carefully observed for signs of adrenal insufficiency. Glucocorticoids appear in breast milk in very small quantities, but it is unknown whether this can adversely affect the infant.

Precautions and warnings: Patients with any of the following conditions should be monitored:

latent or overt cardiac failure, renal dysfunction, hypertension or migraine since glucocorticoids may induce fluid retention;
osteoporosis, since glucocorticoids have a negative effect on the calcium balance;
a history of psychotic illness;
latent tuberculosis, since glucocorticoids may induce reactivation;
certain parasitic infestations, in particular amoebiasis;
incomplete statural growth, since glucocorticoids on prolonged administration may accelerate epiphyseal closure.

Glucocorticoid therapy is non-specific, suppresses the symptoms and signs of disease and decreases the resistance to infections. Appropriate antimicrobial therapy should accompany glucocorticoid therapy when necessary, e.g. in tuberculosis, and viral and fungal infections of the eye.

Patients on long-term glucocorticoid therapy should be regularly examined for increased intra-ocular pressure and posterior subcapsular cataracts.

Patients on long-term glucocorticoid therapy should be regularly examined with respect to their glucose metabolism.

Before, during and after stressful situations, dosage may need to be increased in patients currently on glucocorticoids or resumed in patients who have undergone prolonged glucocorticoid treatment in the previous year.

Discontinuation of prolonged therapy should be carried out by gradual reduction of dosage and under strict medical supervision, since withdrawal may result in acute exacerbation of the disease and acute adrenocortical insufficiency.

Local injection of a glucocorticoid may produce systemic effects.

After parenteral administration of glucocorticoids serious anaphylactoid reactions, such as glottis oedema and bronchospasm, have occasionally occurred, particularly in patients with a history of allergy. If such an anaphylactoid reaction occurs, the following measures are recommended:

immediate slow intravenous injection of 0.1–0.5 ml of adrenaline 1:1000 (0.1–0.5 mg), intravenous administration of aminophylline and artificial respiration.

The use of corticosteroids may influence the results of certain laboratory tests.

Adverse effects: Adverse reactions, associated with prolonged systemic glucocorticoid therapy, are unlikely when high doses are administered over a short period of time. Nevertheless, gastric and duodenal ulceration, with possible perforation and haemorrhage, may occasionally occur.

The following adverse reactions have been associated with prolonged systemic glucocorticoid therapy:

Endocrine and metabolic disturbances: Cushing-like syndrome, hirsutism, menstrual irregularities, premature epiphyseal closure, secondary adrenocortical and pituitary unresponsiveness, decreased glucose tolerance, negative nitrogen and calcium balance.

Fluid and electrolyte disturbances: sodium and fluid retention, hypertension, potassium loss, hypokalaemic alkalosis.

Musculo-skeletal effects: myopathy, abdominal distention, osteoporosis, aseptic necrosis of femoral and humeral heads.

Gastro-intestinal effects: gastric and duodenal ulceration, perforation and haemorrhage.

Dermatologic effects: impaired wound healing, skin atrophy, striae, petechiae and ecchymoses, bruising, facial erythema, increased sweating and acne.

C.N.S. effects: psychic disturbances ranging from euphoria to frank psychotic manifestations, convulsions, in children pseudotumour cerebri (benign intracranial hypertension) with vomiting and papilloedema.

Ophthalmic effects: glaucoma, increased intraocular pressure, posterior subcapsular cataracts.

Immunosuppressive effects: increased susceptibility to infections, decreased responsiveness to vaccination and skin tests.

Hypersensitivity reactions may occasionally occur.

Local adverse reactions include post-injection flare and a painless destruction of the joint reminiscent of Charcot's arthropathy, especially with repeated intra-articular injections.

Interactions: Concomitant use of glucocorticoids with any of the following drugs or substances may lead to the occurrence of clinically relevant interactions:

diuretics and/or cardiac glycosides
(potassium loss may be enhanced which is a particular risk in patients using cardiac glycosides, since hypokalaemia increases the toxicity of these drugs).

antidiabetics
(glucocorticoids may impair glucose tolerance, thereby increasing the need for antidiabetic drugs).

non-steroidal anti-inflammatory drugs
(the incidence and/or severity of gastro-intestinal ulceration may increase).

oral anticoagulants
(glucocorticoids may alter the need for these drugs).

active vaccines
(glucocorticoids may suppress the immune response of the body; extra caution should be exercised with live vaccines).

Glucocorticoids may be less effective when used concomitantly with liver enzyme-inducing drugs, such as rifampicin, ephedrine, barbiturates, phenytoin and primidone.

If patients undergoing long-term therapy with glucocorticoids are concomitantly given salicylates, any reduction in glucocorticoid dosage should be made with caution, since salicylate intoxication has been reported in such cases.

Incompatibilities: Hydrocortisone sodium succinate has been shown not to lose its potency for at least 24 hours (at room temperature and in daylight conditions) when diluted with any of the following infusion fluids:

sodium chloride 0.9%
anhydrous glucose 5%
sorbitol 5%
Ringer's solution

Using these fluids, Hydrocortisone Sodium Succinate can also be injected directly into the infusion line without causing precipitation of the ingredients. Direct injection into the infusion line is also possible with the following infusion fluids but the 24-hours stability has not been established:

Rheomacrodex
mannitol 10%
Vamin N

Overdosage: In animal experiments the acute toxicity of hydrocortisone has been shown to be very low. There are no symptoms of an acute parenteral overdosage known.

Pharmaceutical precautions Shelf-life 2 years, stored at room temperature and protected from light.

Legal category POM.

Package quantities 10 × 10 ml vials of 500 mg hydrocortisone sodium succinate.
10 × 2 ml vials of 100 mg hydrocortisone sodium succinate and 2 ml ampoules of water for injections BP.
10 × 2 ml ampoules of 100 mg hydrocortisone sodium succinate and 2 ml ampoules of water for injections.

Product licence numbers

10 ml vial 500 mg	0065/5071
2 ml vial 100 mg	0065/0110
2 ml ampoule 100 mg	0065/5009

LIVIAL*▼

Presentation Round, flat, white tablets with 'Organon' and a star on one side and a code 'MK2' on the other side, packed in press-through strips of 28 tablets.

Each tablet contains 2.5 mg of tibolone.

Other ingredients: potato starch, magnesium stearate, ascorbyl palmitate and lactose.

Uses In the treatment of vasomotor symptoms, such as hot flushes, sweating, depressed mood, decreased libido, resulting from the natural or surgical menopause. At present there is insufficient evidence to recommend the use of Livial in post-menopausal osteoporosis.

Dosage and administration The dosage is one tablet per day. Improvement of symptoms generally occurs within a few weeks, but optimal results are obtained when therapy is continued for at least 3 months.

At the recommended dosage, Livial may be used uninterrupted for longer periods.

The tablets should be swallowed without chewing, preferably at the same time of day.

Use in children: Not applicable.

Contra-indications, warnings, etc
Contra-indications: Pregnancy or lactation; known or suspected hormone-dependent tumours; cardiovascular or cerebrovascular disorders, e.g. thrombophlebitis, thrombo-embolic processes or a history of these conditions; vaginal bleeding of unknown etiology; severe liver disorders.

Precautions and warnings: Livial is not intended for contraceptive use.

During prolonged treatment with steroids with hormonal activity, periodic medical examination is advisable.

Livial should not be prescribed in the premenopause because in view of the ovulation inhibition, cycle regularity may be disturbed.

In postmenopausal women Livial does not stimulate the endometrium; the incidence of vaginal bleeding is no higher than that with placebo use. In women in whom some endogenous estrogen is still produced, vaginal bleeding may occur during Livial therapy because of an apparently stimulated endometrium. Normally such a bleeding is of short duration. Bleeding of longer duration should be investigated.

In women changing from another form of hormonal substitution therapy to Livial therapy, it is always advisable to induce a withdrawal bleed with a progestogen, because the endometrium may already be stimulated in these women.

Treatment should be discontinued if signs of thrombo-embolic processes occur, if results of liver function tests become abnormal, or if cholestatic jaundice appears.

Patients with any of the following conditions should be monitored:
renal dysfunction, epilepsy or migraine or a history of these conditions, since the use of steroids with hormonal activity may occasionally induce fluid retention;
hypercholesterolaemia, since during Livial treatment changes in the serum lipid profile have been observed;
impaired carbohydrate metabolism, since Livial may diminish glucose tolerance and increase the need for insulin or other antidiabetic drugs;
The sensitivity of patients to anticoagulants may be enhanced during Livial therapy because of enhanced blood fibrinolytic activity (lower fibrinogen levels, higher antithrombin III, plasminogen and fibrin plate fibrinolytic activity values).

N.B. The changes in biochemical parameters mentioned above are known to be induced by steroids with hormonal activity. Values mentioned above return to pretreatment values after cessation of therapy.

Use in pregnancy and lactation: Contra-indicated.

Adverse reactions: Livial is well tolerated and the incidence of adverse reactions during treatment is low. The following adverse reactions have been occasionally observed: change in body weight, dizziness, seborrhoeic dermatosis, vaginal bleeding, headache, gastrointestinal upset, changes in liver function parameters, increased facial hair growth and pretibial oedema.

Interactions: Enzyme-inducing compounds such as phenytoin, carbamazepine and rifampicin can accelerate the metabolism of tibolone and thus decrease its activity.

Overdosage: The acute oral toxicity of Livial is very low. Therefore toxic symptoms will not occur when several tablets are taken simultaneously. If several tablets are taken simultaneously gastric disturbances may occur. Specific treatment is not required.

Pharmaceutical precautions Store in the dark under dry conditions at 2–25°C.

Legal category POM.

Package quantities Calendar pack of 1 press-through strip of 28 tablets. Pack of 3 strips.

Further information Livial stabilizes the hypothalmic-pituitary system after failure of the ovarian function in the climacteric. This central effect results from a favourable combination of hormonal properties, e.g. estrogenic, progestogenic and weak androgenic activities, which are demonstrated by the following effects: Livial, in a daily oral dose of 2.5 mg, suppresses the gonadotrophin levels in postmenopausal women and inhibits ovulation in fertile women. In this same dosage, Livial does not stimulate the endometrium in postmenopausal women. Only a few patients showed slight proliferation; the degree of proliferation did not increase with the duration of treatment. A stimulatory effect on vaginal mucosa was also seen.

Like other steroidal compounds, tibolone is metabolized in the liver and converted to metabolites which are excreted in urine and faeces. Some of the metabolites may contribute to the biological effects of the drug.

Product licence number 0065/0086.

MARVELON*

Presentation White, round, biconvex tablets, diameter 6 mm, coded TR5 on one side and ORGANON* on the reverse side.

Each tablet contains 150 micrograms of Desogestrel and 30 micrograms Ethinyloestradiol BP.

Other ingredients: dl-alpha-tocopherol, potato starch, povidone, stearic acid, magnesium stearate, aerosil and lactose.

Uses Oral contraception.

Dosage and administration It is preferable that tablet intake from the first pack is started on the first day of menstruation in which case no extra contraceptive precautions are necessary.

If menstruation has already begun, (that is 2, 3, or 4 days previously), tablet taking should commence on day 5 of the menstrual period. In this case additional contraceptive precautions must be taken for the first 7 days of tablet taking.

If menstruation began more than 5 days previously then the patient should be advised to wait until her next menstrual period before starting to take Marvelon.

How to take Marvelon: One tablet is taken daily at the same time, (preferably in the evening) without interruption for 21 days, followed by a break of 7 tablet-free days. Each subsequent pack is started after the 7 tablet-free days have elapsed.

Additional contraceptive precautions are not then required.

Use during pregnancy and breast feeding: Marvelon is contra-indicated for use during pregnancy or suspected pregnancy and in mothers who are breast-feeding.

Post-partum administration: Following childbirth oral contraceptive administration to non-breast feeding mothers can be started 21–28 days post-partum in which case no additional contraceptive precautions are required.

If intercourse has taken place post-partum, oral contraceptive use should be delayed until the first day of the first menstrual period.

If post-partum administration of Marvelon begins more than 28 days after delivery then additional contraceptive precautions are required for the first 7 days.

N.B. Mothers who are breast feeding should be advised not to use the pill since this may reduce the amount of breast-milk, but may be advised instead to use a progestogen-only pill (POP).

After miscarriage or abortion administration should start immediately in which case no additional contraceptive precautions are required.

Changing from a 21 day pill or another 22 day pill to Marvelon: All tablets in the old pack should be finished. The first Marvelon tablet is taken the next day i.e. no gap is left between taking tablets nor does the patient need to wait for her period to begin. Tablets should be taken as instructed in 'How to take Marvelon'. Additional contraceptive precautions are not required. The patient will not have a period until the end of the first Marvelon pack, but this is not harmful, nor does it matter if she experiences some bleeding on tablet-taking days.

Changing from a combined Every Day Pill (28 day tablets) to Marvelon: Marvelon should be started after taking the last **active** tablet from the 'Every Day Pill' pack (i.e. after taking 21 or 22 tablets). The first Marvelon tablet is taken the next day i.e. no gap is left between taking tablets nor does the patient need to wait for her period to begin. Tablets should be taken as instructed in 'How to take Marvelon'. Additional contraceptive precautions are not required. Remaining tablets from the Every Day (ED) pack should be discarded. The patient will not have a period until the end of the first Marvelon pack, but this is not harmful, nor does it matter if she experiences some bleeding on tablet-taking days.

Changing from a Progestogen-only Pill (POP or Mini Pill) to Marvelon: The first Marvelon tablet should be taken on the first day of the period, even if the patient has already taken a mini pill on that day. Tablets should be taken as instructed in 'How to take Marvelon'. Additional contraceptive precautions are not required. All the remaining progestogen-only pills in the mini pack should be discarded.

If the patient is taking a (mini) pill, then she may not always have a period, especially when she is breast feeding. The first Marvelon tablet should be taken on the day *after* stopping the mini pill. All remaining pills in the mini pill packet must be discarded. Additional contraceptive precautions must be taken for the first 7 days.

Additional contraceptive precautions: When additional contraceptive precautions are required the patient should be advised either not to have sex, or to use a cap plus spermicide, or for her partner to use a condom. Rhythm methods should not be advised as the pill disrupts the usual cyclical changes associated with the natural menstrual cycle e.g. changes in temperature and cervical mucus.

To skip a period: To skip a period, a new pack of Marvelon should be started on the day after finishing the current pack (the patient skips the tablet-free days). Tablet-taking should be continued in the usual way. During the use of the second pack she may experience slight spotting or break-through bleeding but contraceptive protection will not be diminished provided there are no tablet omissions. The next pack of Marvelon is started after the usual 7 tablet-free days, regardless of whether the period has completely finished or not.

Reduced reliability: The reliability of Marvelon may be reduced under the following circumstances:

Forgotten tablets: If the forgotten tablet is taken *within 12 hours*, no further precautions are necessary.

If a tablet is forgotten for *more than 12 hours*, the forgotten tablet should be skipped, and the patient should take additional contraceptive precautions and follow the '7-day rule'.

If more than one tablet is forgotten, the patient should be advised to stop tablet taking, and to use additional contraceptive precautions until the next menstrual period. If the next period fails to occur, a pregnancy test should be performed, and the patient advised to use additional contraceptive precautions before considering resuming use of Marvelon.

(See 'Precautions and Warnings' for further advice.)

Vomiting or diarrhoea: If symptoms persist for more than 12 hours the patient should follow the '7-day rule'. (See 'Precautions and Warnings' for further advice.)

Interactions: The doctor should consider the possibility of interactions between oral contraceptives and other drugs commonly prescribed such as antibiotics, anticonvulsants and barbiturates. (See 'Interactions' for further advice.)

Surgery, varicose veins or immobilisation: It is advisable to discontinue oral contraceptive use at least 4 to 6 weeks prior to these procedures, and to (re)start not less than 2 weeks after full ambulation. (See 'Precautions and Warnings' for further advice.)

Contra-indications, warnings, etc

Absolute contra-indications: Pregnancy or suspected pregnancy (that cannot yet be excluded) or breast feeding.

Circulatory disorders (cardiovascular or cerebrovascular) such as thrombophlebitis and thromboembolic processes (or a history of these conditions), moderate to severe hypertension, hyperlipoproteinaemia.

In addition the presence of more than one of the risk factors for arterial disease which are discussed under 'Serious Adverse Reactions'.

Severe liver disease, cholestatic jaundice or hepatitis (viral or non-viral), or a history of these conditions if the results of liver function tests have failed to return to normal, and for 3 months after liver function tests have been found to be normal; a history of jaundice of pregnancy or jaundice due to the use of steroids, Rotor syndrome and Dubin-Johnson syndrome, hepatic cell tumours and porphyria.

Cholelithiasis.

Known or suspected oestrogen-dependent tumours, (see 'Serious Adverse Reactions'); endometrial hyperplasia; undiagnosed vaginal bleeding.

Systemic lupus erythematosus or a history of this condition.

A history during pregnancy or previous use of steroids of: severe pruritis, herpes gestationis, a manifestation or deterioration of otosclerosis.

Relative contra-indications: If any of the relative contra-indications listed below is present, the benefits of oestrogen/progestogen-containing preparations must be weighed against the possible risks for each individual case and the patient kept under close supervision. In case of aggravation or appearance of any of these conditions whilst the patient is taking the pill, its use should be discontinued.

– Conditions implicating an increasing risk of developing venous thrombo-embolic complications, e.g. severe varicose veins or prolonged immobilisation or major surgery (see 'Precautions and Warnings'). Disorders of coagulation.
– Presence of any risk factor for arterial disease e.g. smoking, hyperlipidaemia or hypertension (see 'Serious Adverse Reactions').
– Other conditions associated with an increased risk of circulatory disease such as latent or overt cardiac failure, renal dysfunction, or a history of these conditions.
– Epilepsy or a history of this condition.
– Migraine or a history of this condition.
– A history of cholelithiasis.
– Presence of any risk factor for oestrogen-dependent tumours; oestrogen-sensitive gynaecological disorders such as uterine fibromyomata and endometriosis (see also under 'Serious Adverse Reactions').
– Diabetes mellitus.
– Severe depression or a history of this condition. If this is accompanied by a disturbance in tryptophan metabolism, administration of vitamin B_6 might be of therapeutic value.
– Sickle cell haemoglobinopathy, since under certain circumstances, e.g. during infections or anoxia, oestrogen-containing preparations may induce thromboembolic processes in patients with this condition.
– If the result of liver function tests become abnormal, use should be discontinued.

Precautions and warnings

Reduced reliability: When Marvelon is taken according to the directions for use the occurrence of pregnancy is highly unlikely. However, the reliability of oral contraceptives may be reduced under the following circumstances.

Forgotten tablets: Provided she is *less than 12 hours late* in taking her tablet the patient should take it as soon as she remembers. Marvelon will still give contraceptive protection during this cycle.

If she is *more than 12 hours late* in taking any tablet then she will *not* be protected for the next 7 days. The forgotten tablet should be skipped and the patient should take additional contraceptive precautions and follow the '7-day rule'.

If the patient has forgotten to take more than one

tablet, she should stop taking the tablets, and use additional contraceptive precautions until the next menstrual period. If the next period fails to occur, a pregnancy test should be performed, and she should be advised to use additional contraceptive precautions before considering resuming use of Marvelon.

Vomiting or diarrhoea: If after tablet intake vomiting or diarrhoea occurs, a tablet may not be absorbed properly by the body. If the symptoms disappear within 12 hours of tablet-taking, the patient should take an extra tablet from a spare pack and continue with the rest of the pack as usual. However, if the symptoms continue beyond those 12 hours, additional contraceptive precautions are necessary for any sexual intercourse during the stomach or bowel upset and for the following 7 days (the patient must be advised to follow '7-day rule').

If the patient is taking certain other medicines: If the patient is taking any of the medicines given in the 'Interactions' section she should be advised to follow the '7-day rule':

The 7-day rule.

If any one tablet is forgotten for more than 12 hours:

If the patient has vomiting or diarrhoea for more than 12 hours:

If the patient is taking any of the drugs listed under 'Interactions':

The patient should continue to take her tablets as usual and:

- Additional contraceptive precautions must be taken for the next 7 days.
- *BUT – if these 7 days run beyond the end of the current pack*, the next pack must be started as soon as the current one is finished, i.e. no gap should be left between packs. (This prevents an extended break in tablet taking which may increase the risk of the ovaries releasing an egg and thus reducing contraceptive protection). The patient will not have a period until the end of 2 packs but this is not harmful nor does it matter if she experiences some bleeding on tablet taking days.

If after taking Marvelon for several months there is a sudden occurrence of spotting or breakthrough bleeding (not observed in previous cycles) or the absence of withdrawal bleeding, contraceptive effectiveness may be reduced. If withdrawal bleeding fails to occur and none of the above mentioned events has taken place, pregnancy is highly unlikely and oral contraceptive use can be continued until the end of the next pack. (If withdrawal bleeding fails to occur at the end of the second cycle, tablet intake should be discontinued and pregnancy excluded before oral contraceptive use can be resumed.) However, if withdrawal bleeding is absent and any of the above mentioned events has occurred, tablet intake should be discontinued and pregnancy excluded before oral contraceptive use can be resumed.

Medical examination/consultation: A complete medical history and physical examination should be taken prior to the initiation or reinstitution of oral contraceptives and should be repeated periodically.

These physical examinations should include special reference to blood pressure, breasts, abdomen and pelvic organs, including cervical cytology and, where indicated by the medical or family history, relevant laboratory tests.

Caution should be observed when prescribing oral contraceptives to young women whose cycles are not yet stabilised.

Surgery, varicose veins or immobilisation: In patients using oestrogen-containing preparations, the risk of deep-vein thrombosis may be temporarily increased when undergoing a major operation (e.g. abdominal, orthopaedic), any surgery to the legs, medical treatment for varicose veins or prolonged immobilisation. Therefore, it is advisable to discontinue oral contraceptive use at least 4 to 6 weeks after prior to these procedures if performed electively and to (re)start not less than 2 weeks after full ambulation. The latter is also valid with regard to immobilisation after an accident or emergency surgery. In case of emergency surgery, thrombotic prophylaxis is usually indicated e.g. with subcutaneous heparin.

Chloasma: Chloasma may occasionally occur, especially in women with a history of chloasma gravidarum. Women with a tendency to chloasma should avoid exposure to the sun or ultraviolet radiation whilst taking this preparation.

Laboratory tests: The use of steroids may influence the results of certain laboratory tests. In the literature, at least a hundred different parameters have been reported to possibly be influenced by oral contraceptive use, predominantly by the oestrogenic component. Among these are: biochemical parameters of the liver, thyroid, adrenal and renal function, plasma levels of (carrier) proteins and lipid/lipoprotein fractions and parameters of coagulation and fibrinolysis.

Adverse reactions: Various adverse reactions have been associated with oral contraceptive use. The serious reactions are dealt with in more detail. The first appearance of symptoms indicative of any one of these reactions necessitates immediate cessation of oral contraceptive use while appropriate diagnostic and therapeutic measures are undertaken.

Serious adverse reactions: Various reports have associated oral contraceptive use with the occurrence of deep venous thrombosis, pulmonary embolism and other embolisms.

Other investigations involving oral contraceptives have suggested an increased risk of oestrogen and/or progestogen dose-dependent coronary thromboses and cerebrovascular accidents, predominantly in heavy smokers. Thrombosis has very rarely been reported to occur in other veins or arteries, e.g. hepatic, mesenteric, renal or retinal. It should be noted that there is no consensus about the often contradictory findings obtained in early studies. The physician should bear in mind, the possibility of vascular events occurring and take into account the presence of risk factors for arterial disease and deep venous thrombosis when prescribing oral contraceptives. Risk factors for arterial disease include smoking, the presence of hyperlipidaemia, hypertension, or diabetes mellitus. Signs and symptoms of a thromboembolic event may include: sudden severe pain in the chest, whether or not reaching to the left arm; sudden breathlessness; any unusual severe, prolonged headache, especially if it occurs for the first time or gets progressively worse, or is associated with any of the following symptoms: sudden partial or complete loss of vision or diplopia, aphasia, vertigo, a bad fainting attack or collapse with or without focal epilepsy, weakness or very marked numbness suddenly affecting one side or one part of the body, motor disturbances; severe pain in the calf of one leg; acute abdomen.

Cigarette smoking increases the risk of serious cardiovascular adverse reactions to oral contraceptive use. This risk increases with age and with heavy smoking and is more marked in women over 35 years of age. Women who use oral contraceptives should be strongly advised not to smoke.

The use of oestrogen-containing oral contraceptives may promote growth of existing sex steroid dependent tumours. For this reason, the use of these oral contraceptives in patients with such tumours is contra-indicated.

Numerous epidemiological studies have been reported on the risk of ovarian, endometrial, cervical and breast cancer in women using combined oral contraceptives. The evidence is clear that combined oral contraceptives offer substantial protection against both ovarian and endometrial cancer.

An increased risk of cervical cancer in long term users of combined oral contraceptives has been reported in some studies, but there continues to be controversy about the extent to which this is attributable to the confounding effects of sexual behaviour and other factors.

The evidence linking combined oral contraceptive use and breast cancer remains inconclusive. The results of some studies suggest an increased risk of breast cancer presenting below the age of about 35, the risk rising with duration of use. Any possible increased risk of breast cancer with combined oral contraceptives is however likely to be small, and may be expected to be less with low dose pills. This possible risk should be weighed against the many benefits of combined oral contraceptives, including their protective effects against ovarian and endometrial cancers.

Malignant hepatic tumours have been reported on rare occasions in long-term users of oral contraceptives. Benign hepatic tumours have also been associated with oral contraceptive usage. A hepatic tumour should be considered in the differential diagnosis when upper abdominal pain, enlarged liver or signs of intra-abdominal haemorrhage occur.

The use of oral contraceptives may sometimes lead to the development of cholestatic jaundice or cholelithiasis.

On rare occasions the use of oral contraceptives may trigger or reactivate systemic lupus erythematosus.

A further rare complication of oral contraceptive use is the occurrence of Sydenhams' chorea which can be reversed by discontinuing the pill. The majority of cases of oral-contraceptive-induced chorea show a pre-existing predisposition which often relates to acute rheumatism.

Other adverse reactions

Cardiovascular system: rise of blood pressure. If hypertension develops, treatment should be discontinued.

Genital tract: intermenstrual bleeding, post-medication amenorrhoea, changes in cervical secretion, increase in size of uterine fibromyomata, aggravation of endometriosis and certain vaginal infections, e.g. candidiasis.

Breast: tenderness, pain, enlargement, secretion.

Gastro-intestinal tract: nausea, vomiting, cholelithiasis, cholestatic jaundice.

Skin: erythema nodosum, rash, chloasma.

Eyes: discomfort of the cornea if contact lenses are used.

CNS: headache, migraine, mood changes, depression.

Metabolic: fluid retention, change in body weight, reduced glucose tolerance.

Interactions: Irregular cycles and reduced reliability of oral contraceptives may occur when these preparations are used concomitantly with drugs such as anticonvulsants, barbiturates, antibiotics, (e.g. tetracyclines, ampicillin, rifampicin, etc), griseofulvin, activated charcoal and certain laxatives.

Special consideration should be given to patients being treated with antibiotics for acne.

They should be advised to use a non-hormonal method of contraception, or to use an oral contraceptive containing a progestogen showing minimal androgenicity, which have been reported as helping to improve acne without using an antibiotic.

Oral contraceptives may diminish glucose tolerance and increase the need for insulin or other antidiabetic drugs in diabetics.

Overdosage: There have been no reports of serious ill-effects from overdosage even when a considerable number of tablets have been taken by a small child. In general, it is therefore unnecessary to treat overdosage. However, if overdosage is discovered within two or three hours and is large, then gastric lavage can be safely used. There are no antidotes and further treatment should be symptomatic.

Pharmaceutical precautions Store in a cool, dry place and protect from light.

Legal category POM.

Package quantities Plastic/aluminium foil blister strips containing 21 tablets, overwrapped with a sealed aluminium laminated sachet. Pack of 1 or 3 strips.

Product licence number 0065/0071.

MERCILON*

Presentation White, round, biconvex tablets, 6 mm in diameter, engraved with Organon motif on one side and T_4R on the other. Each pack of Mercilon consists of 21 tablets.

Each tablet contains:

Desogestrel (a progestogen) 150 micrograms
Ethinyloestradiol (an oestrogen) BP 20 micrograms.

Other ingredients: dl-alpha-tocopherol, potato starch, povidone, stearic acid, magnesium stearate, aerosil and lactose.

Uses Oral contraception.

Dosage and administration It is preferable that tablet intake from the first pack is started on the first day of menstruation in which case no extra contraceptive precautions are necessary.

If menstruation has already begun, (that is 2, 3, or 4 days previously), tablet taking should commence on day 5 of the menstrual period. In this case additional contraceptive precautions must be taken for the first 7 days of tablet taking.

If menstruation began more than 5 days previously then the patient should be advised to wait until her next menstrual period before starting to take Mercilon.

How to take Mercilon: One tablet is taken daily at the same time, (preferably in the evening) without interruption for 21 days, followed by a break of 7 tablet-free days. Each subsequent pack is started after the 7 tablet-free days have elapsed.

Additional contraceptive precautions are not then required.

Use during pregnancy and breast feeding: Mercilon is contra-indicated for use during pregnancy or suspected pregnancy and in mothers who are breast-feeding.

Post-partum administration: Following childbirth oral contraceptive administration to non-breast feeding mothers can be started 21–28 days post-partum in which case no additional contraceptive precautions are required.

If intercourse has taken place post-partum, oral contraceptive use should be delayed until the first day of the first menstrual period.

If post-partum administration of Mercilon begins more than 28 days after delivery then additional contraceptive precautions are required for the first 7 days.

N.B. Mothers who are breast feeding should be advised not to use the pill since this may reduce the amount of breast-milk, but may be advised instead to use a progestogen-only pill (POP).

After miscarriage or abortion administration should start immediately in which case no additional contraceptive precautions are required.

Changing from a 21 day pill or another 22 day pill to Mercilon: All tablets in the old pack should be finished. The first Mercilon tablet is taken the next day i.e. no gap is left between taking tablets nor does the patient need to wait for her period to begin. Tablets should be taken as instructed in 'How to take Mercilon'. Additional contraceptive precautions are not required. The patient will not have a period until the end of the first Mercilon pack, but this is not harmful, nor does it matter if she experiences some bleeding on tablet-taking days.

Changing from a combined Every Day Pill (28 day tablets) to Mercilon: Mercilon should be started after taking the last **active** tablet from the 'Every Day Pill' pack (i.e. after taking 21 or 22 tablets). The first Mercilon tablet is taken the next day i.e. no gap is left between taking tablets nor does the patient need to wait for her period to begin. Tablets should be taken as instructed in 'How to take Mercilon'. Additional contraceptive precautions are not required. Remaining tablets from the Every Day (ED) pack should be discarded. The patient will not have a period until the end of the first Mercilon pack, but this is not harmful, nor does it matter if she experiences some bleeding on tablet-taking days.

Changing from a Progestogen-only Pill (POP or Mini Pill) to Mercilon: The first Mercilon tablet should be taken on the first day of the period, even if the patient has already taken a mini pill on that day. Tablets should be taken as instructed in 'How to take Mercilon'. Additional contraceptive precautions are not required. All the remaining progestogen-only pills in the mini pack should be discarded.

If the patient is taking a (mini) pill, then she may not

always have a period, especially when she is breast feeding. The first Mercilon tablet should be taken on the day *after* stopping the mini pill. All remaining pills in the mini pill packet must be discarded. Additional contraceptive precautions must be taken for the first 7 days.

Additional contraceptive precautions: When additional contraceptive precautions are required the patient should be advised either not to have sex, or to use a cap plus spermicide, or for her partner to use a condom. Rhythm methods should not be advised as the pill disrupts the usual cyclical changes associated with the natural menstrual cycle e.g. changes in temperature and cervical mucus.

To skip a period: To skip a period, a new pack of Mercilon should be started on the day after finishing the current pack (the patient skips the tablet-free days). Tablet-taking should be continued in the usual way. During the use of the second pack she may experience slight spotting or break-through bleeding but contraceptive protection will not be diminished provided there are no tablet omissions. The next pack of Mercilon is started after the usual 7 tablet-free days, regardless of whether the period has completely finished or not.

Reduced reliability: The reliability of Mercilon may be reduced under the following circumstances:

Forgotten tablets: If the forgotten tablet is taken *within 12 hours*, no further precautions are necessary.

If a tablet is forgotten for *more than 12 hours*, the forgotten tablet should be skipped, and the patient should take additional contraceptive precautions and follow the '7-day rule'.

If more than one tablet is forgotten, the patient should be advised to stop tablet taking, and to use additional contraceptive precautions until the next menstrual period. If the next period fails to occur, a pregnancy test should be performed, and the patient advised to use additional contraceptive precautions before considering resuming use of Mercilon. (See 'Precautions and Warnings' for further advice.)

Vomiting or diarrhoea: If symptoms persist for more than 12 hours the patient should follow the '7-day rule'. (See 'Precautions and Warnings' for further advice.)

Interactions: The doctor should consider the possibility of interactions between oral contraceptives and other drugs commonly prescribed such as antibiotics, anticonvulsants and barbiturates. (See 'Interactions' for further advice.)

Surgery, varicose veins or immobilisation: It is advisable to discontinue oral contraceptive use at least 4 to 6 weeks prior to these procedures, and to (re)start not less than 2 weeks after full ambulation. (See 'Precautions and Warnings' for further advice.)

Contra-indications, warnings, etc

Absolute contra-indications: Pregnancy or suspected pregnancy (that cannot yet be excluded) or breast feeding.

Circulatory disorders (cardiovascular or cerebrovascular) such as thrombophlebitis and thromboembolic processes (or a history of these conditions), moderate to severe hypertension, hyperlipoproteinaemia.

In addition the presence of more than one of the risk factors for arterial disease which are discussed under 'Serious Adverse Reactions'.

Severe liver disease, cholestatic jaundice or hepatitis (viral or non-viral), or a history of these conditions if the results of liver function tests have failed to return to normal, and for 3 months after liver function tests have been found to be normal; a history of jaundice of pregnancy or jaundice due to the use of steroids, Rotor syndrome and Dubin-Johnson syndrome, hepatic cell tumours and porphyria.

Cholelithiasis.

Known or suspected oestrogen-dependent tumours, (see 'Serious Adverse Reactions'); endometrial hyperplasia; undiagnosed vaginal bleeding.

Systemic lupus erythematosus or a history of this condition.

A history during pregnancy or previous use of steroids of: severe pruritis, herpes gestationis, a manifestation or deterioration of otosclerosis.

Relative contra-indications: If any of the relative contra-indications listed below is present, the benefits of oestrogen/progestogen-containing preparations must be weighed against the possible risks for each individual case and the patient kept under close supervision. In case of aggravation or appearance of any of these conditions whilst the patient is taking the pill, its use should be discontinued.

- Conditions implicating an increasing risk of developing venous thrombo-embolic complications, e.g. severe varicose veins or prolonged immobilisation or major surgery (see 'Precautions and Warnings'). Disorders of coagulation.
- Presence of any risk factor for arterial disease e.g. smoking, hyperlipidaemia or hypertension (see 'Serious Adverse Reactions').
- Other conditions associated with an increased risk of circulatory disease such as latent or overt cardiac failure, renal dysfunction, or a history of these conditions.
- Epilepsy or a history of this condition.
- Migraine or a history of this condition.
- A history of cholelithiasis.
- Presence of any risk factor for oestrogen-dependent tumours; oestrogen-sensitive gynaecological disorders such as uterine fibromyomata and endometriosis (see also under 'Serious Adverse Reactions').
- Diabetes mellitus.
- Severe depression or a history of this condition. If this is accompanied by a disturbance in tryptophan metabolism, administration of vitamin B_6 might be of therapeutic value.
- Sickle cell haemoglobinopathy, since under certain circumstances, e.g. during infections or anoxia, oestrogen-containing preparations may induce thromboembolic processes in patients with this condition.
- If the result of liver function tests become abnormal, use should be discontinued.

Precautions and warnings

Reduced reliability: When Mercilon is taken according to the directions for use the occurrence of pregnancy is highly unlikely. However, the reliability of oral contraceptives may be reduced under the following circumstances.

Forgotten tablets: Provided she is *less than 12 hours late* in taking her tablet the patient should take it as soon as she remembers. Mercilon will still give contraceptive protection during this cycle.

If she is *more than 12 hours late* in taking any tablet then she will *not* be protected for the next 7 days. The forgotten tablet should be skipped and the patient should take additional contraceptive precautions and follow the '7-day rule'.

If the patient has forgotten to take more than one tablet, she should stop taking the tablets, and use additional contraceptive precautions until the next menstrual period. If the next period fails to occur, a pregnancy test should be performed, and she should be advised to use additional contraceptive precautions before considering resuming use of Mercilon.

Vomiting or diarrhoea: If after tablet intake vomiting or diarrhoea occurs, a tablet may not be absorbed properly by the body. If the symptoms disappear within 12 hours of tablet-taking, the patient should take an extra tablet from a spare pack and continue with the rest of the pack as usual. However, if the symptoms continue beyond those 12 hours, additional contraceptive precautions are necessary for any sexual intercourse during the stomach or bowel upset and for the following 7 days (the patient must be advised to follow '7-day rule').

If the patient is taking certain other medicines: If the patient is taking any of the medicines given in the 'Interactions' section she should be advised to follow the '7-day rule':

The 7-day rule.

If any one tablet is forgotten for more than 12 hours:

If the patient has vomiting or diarrhoea for more than 12 hours:

If the patient is taking any of the drugs listed under 'Interactions':

The patient should continue to take her tablets as usual and:

- Additional contraceptive precautions must be taken for the next 7 days.
- *BUT – if these 7 days run beyond the end of the current pack*, the next pack must be started as soon as the current one is finished, i.e. no gap should be left between packs. (This prevents an extended break in tablet taking which may increase the risk of the ovaries releasing an egg and thus reducing contraceptive protection). The patient will not have a period until the end of 2 packs but this is not harmful nor does it matter if she experiences some bleeding on tablet taking days.

If after taking Mercilon for several months there is a sudden occurrence of spotting or breakthrough bleeding (not observed in previous cycles) or the absence of withdrawal bleeding, contraceptive effectiveness may be reduced. If withdrawal bleeding fails to occur and none of the above mentioned events has taken place, pregnancy is highly unlikely and oral contraceptive use can be continued until the end of the next pack. (If withdrawal bleeding fails to occur at the end of the second cycle, tablet intake should be discontinued and pregnancy excluded before oral contraceptive use can be resumed.) However, if withdrawal bleeding is absent and any of the above mentioned events has occurred, tablet intake should be discontinued and pregnancy excluded before oral contraceptive use can be resumed.

Medical examination/consultation: A complete medical history and physical examination should be taken prior to the initiation or reinstitution of oral contraceptives and should be repeated periodically.

These physical examinations should include reference to blood pressure, breasts, abdomen and pelvic organs, including cervical cytology and, where indicated by the medical or family history, relevant laboratory tests.

Caution should be observed when prescribing oral contraceptives to young women whose cycles are not yet stabilised.

Surgery, varicose veins or immobilisation: In patients using oestrogen-containing preparations, the risk of deep-vein thrombosis may be temporarily increased when undergoing a major operation (e.g. abdominal, orthopaedic), any surgery to the legs, medical treatment for varicose veins or prolonged immobilisation. Therefore, it is advisable to discontinue oral contraceptive use at least 4 to 6 weeks prior to these procedures if performed electively and to (re)start not less than 2 weeks after full ambulation. The latter is also valid with regard to immobilisation after an accident or emergency surgery. In case of emergency surgery, thrombotic prophylaxis is usually indicated e.g. with subcutaneous heparin.

Chloasma: Chloasma may occasionally occur, especially in women with a history of chloasma gravidarum. Women with a tendency to chloasma should avoid exposure to the sun or ultraviolet radiation whilst taking this preparation.

Laboratory tests: The use of steroids may influence the results of certain laboratory tests. In the literature, at least a hundred different parameters have been reported to possibly be influenced by oral contraceptive use, predominantly by the oestrogenic component. Among these are: biochemical parameters of the liver, thyroid, adrenal and renal function, plasma levels of (carrier) proteins and lipid/lipoprotein fractions and parameters of coagulation and fibrinolysis.

Adverse reactions: Various adverse reactions have been associated with oral contraceptive use. The serious reactions are dealt with in more detail. The first appearance of symptoms indicative of any one of these reactions necessitates immediate cessation of oral contraceptive use while appropriate diagnostic and therapeutic measures are undertaken.

Serious adverse reactions: Various reports have associated oral contraceptive use with the occurrence of deep venous thrombosis, pulmonary embolism and other embolisms.

Other investigations involving oral contraceptives have suggested an increased risk of oestrogen and/or progestogen dose-dependent coronary thromboses and cerebrovascular accidents, predominantly in heavy smokers. Thrombosis has very rarely been reported to occur in other veins or arteries, e.g. hepatic, mesenteric, renal or retinal. It should be noted that there is no consensus about the often contradictory findings obtained in early studies. The physician should bear in mind, the possibility of vascular events occurring and take into account the presence of risk factors for arterial disease and deep venous thrombosis when prescribing oral contraceptives. Risk factors for arterial disease include smoking, the presence of hyperlipidaemia, hypertension, or diabetes mellitus. Signs and symptoms of a thromboembolic event may include: sudden severe pain in the chest, whether or not reaching to the left arm; sudden breathlessness; any unusual severe, prolonged headache, especially if it occurs for the first time or gets progressively worse, or is associated with any of the following symptoms: sudden partial or complete loss of vision or diplopia, aphasia, vertigo, a bad fainting attack or collapse with or without focal epilepsy, weakness or very marked numbness suddenly affecting one side or one part of the body, motor disturbances; severe pain in the calf of one leg; acute abdomen.

Cigarette smoking increases the risk of serious cardiovascular adverse reactions to oral contraceptive use. This risk increases with age and with heavy smoking and is more marked in women over 35 years of age. Women who use oral contraceptives should be strongly advised not to smoke.

The use of oestrogen-containing oral contraceptives may promote growth of existing sex steroid dependent tumours. For this reason, the use of these oral contraceptives in patients with such tumours is contra-indicated.

Numerous epidemiological studies have been reported on the risk of ovarian, endometrial, cervical and breast cancer in women using combined oral contraceptives. The evidence is clear that combined oral contraceptives offer substantial protection against both ovarian and endometrial cancer.

An increased risk of cervical cancer in long term users of combined oral contraceptives has been reported in some studies, but there continues to be controversy about the extent to which this is attributable to the confounding effects of sexual behaviour and other factors.

The evidence linking combined oral contraceptive use and breast cancer remains inconclusive. The results of some studies suggest an increased risk of breast cancer presenting below the age of about 35, the risk rising with duration of use. Any possible increased risk of breast cancer with combined oral contraceptives is however likely to be small, and may be expected to be less with low dose pills. This possible risk should be weighed against the many benefits of combined oral contraceptives, including their protective effects against ovarian and endometrial cancers.

Malignant hepatic tumours have been reported on rare occasions in long-term users of oral contraceptives. Benign hepatic tumours have also been associated with oral contraceptive usage. A hepatic tumour should be considered in the differential diagnosis when upper abdominal pain, enlarged liver or signs of intra-abdominal haemorrhage occur.

The use of oral contraceptives may sometimes lead to the development of cholestatic jaundice or cholelithiasis.

On rare occasions the use of oral contraceptives may trigger or reactivate systemic lupus erythematosus.

A further rare complication of oral contraceptive use is the occurrence of Sydenhams' chorea which can be reversed by discontinuing the pill. The majority of cases of oral-contraceptive-induced chorea show a pre-existing predisposition which often relates to acute rheumatism.

Other adverse reactions

Cardiovascular system: rise of blood pressure. If

hypertension develops, treatment should be discontinued.

Genital tract: intermenstrual bleeding, post-medication amenorrhoea, changes in cervical secretion, increase in size of uterine fibromyomata, aggravation of endometriosis and certain vaginal infections, e.g. candidiasis.

Breast: tenderness, pain, enlargement, secretion.

Gastro-intestinal tract: nausea, vomiting, cholelithiasis, cholestatic jaundice.

Skin: erythema nodosum, rash, chloasma.

Eyes: discomfort of the corneal if contact lenses are used.

CNS: headache, migraine, mood changes, depression.

Metabolic: fluid retention, change in body weight, reduced glucose tolerance.

Interactions: Irregular cycles and reduced reliability of oral contraceptives may occur when these preparations are used concomitantly with drugs such as anticonvulsants, barbiturates, antibiotics, (e.g. tetracyclines, ampicillin, rifampicin, etc), griseofulvin, activated charcoal and certain laxatives.

Special consideration should be given to patients being treated with antibiotics for acne.

They should be advised to use a non-hormonal method of contraception, or to use an oral contraceptive containing a progestogen showing minimal androgenicity, which have been reported as helping to improve acne without using an antibiotic.

Oral contraceptives may diminish glucose tolerance and increase the need for insulin or other antidiabetic drugs in diabetics.

Overdosage: There have been no reports of serious ill-effects from overdosage even when a considerable number of tablets have been taken by a small child. In general, it is therefore unnecessary to treat overdosage. However, if overdosage is discovered within two or three hours and is large, then gastric lavage can be safely used. There are no antidotes and further treatment should be symptomatic.

Pharmaceutical precautions Store in a cool, dry place and protect from light.

Legal category POM.

Package quantities Plastic/aluminium foil blister strips containing 21 tablets, overwrapped with a sealed aluminium laminated sachet. Pack of 1 or 3 strips.

Product licence number 0065/0085.

MULTILOAD* Cu250 MULTILOAD Cu250 SHORT and MULTILOAD Cu375

Presentation Multiload Cu250, Multiload Cu250 Short and Multiload Cu375 are intrauterine devices made of polyethylene with a copper wire wound round the stem, giving a total copper surface area of 250 mm^2 for Multiload Cu250 and Multiload Cu250 Short and 375 mm^2 for Multiload Cu375. The flexible side arms ensure that Multiload remains in position as high as possible against the fundus, without the uterine cavity being stretched at all. A monofilament nylon thread is attached to the stem. The contraceptive action of the device is probably due to a number of foreign body reactions with the uterine endometrium and the presence of metallic copper. The latter not only improves contraceptive efficacy, but also makes the stem radio-opaque. The plastic body itself is not radio-opaque.

Uses Intrauterine contraception.

Recommendations for the type of Multiload to be fitted

Adults: The Multiload Cu250 and Multiload Cu375 are suitable for insertion in uteri with a sound length between 6 and 9 cm.

Multiload Cu250 Short is suitable for insertion in uteri with a sound length between 5 and 7 cm.

Elderly patients: Not applicable.

Children: Not applicable.

Contra-indications, warnings, etc

Contra-indications:

Absolute: Malignant disease of the corpus uteri or cervix. Pregnancy (established or suspected). History of ectopic pregnancy or the presence of predisposing factors for this condition such as, salpingitis, endometritis or pelvic peritonitis in the medical history. Active pelvic inflammatory disease (PID) or a history of recurrent PID. Presence of, or a history of veneral disease excluding bacterial vaginitis, candidiasis, recurrent herpes virus infection, hepatitis B or cytomegalovirus infection. Infected abortion in the past 3 months. Active genital infection (with the exception of candidiasis). Congenital or acquired malformations or distortions of the uterus or the cervix, large or multiple uterine fibromyomata in the presence of excessively heavy menstrual periods, endometrial hyperplasia, cervical dysplasia. Postpartum subinvolution of the uterus or uterine depth over 9 cm. Undiagnosed vaginal bleeding. Established or suspected allergy to copper. Severe anaemia.

Relative contra-indications: Valvular heart disease. Use of an IUD in these cases may increase the risk of subacute bacterial endocarditis. Antibiotic prophylaxis should be given when inserting or removing the IUD. Anaemia, or a history of excessive uterine bleeding. Severe dysmenorrhoea. Uterine scars from previous surgery other than caesarean section or previous perforation of the uterus. Small uterine fibromyomata, endometrial polyps, or endometriosis. Regular pelvic examination of a patient with fibroids is advised to assess any change in size. Treatment with corticosteroids or non-steroidal anti-inflammatory drugs. Immunosuppressive therapy. Any disorder of copper metabolism, e.g. Wilson's disease. Multiple sexual partners (Absolute for nulliparous women in areas of high known or suspected prevalence of sexually transmitted disease). Coagulopathy or current administration of anti-coagulants. Nulliparity.

Use in pregnancy and lactation: The use of Multiload is contra-indicated in established or suspected pregnancy, and in patients with a history of ectopic pregnancy, or the presence of predisposing factors for this condition such as, salpingitis, endometritis or pelvic peritonitis in the medical history.

Multiload may be inserted in breast-feeding women. However, in view of the increased risk of uterine perforation during lactation, particular care should be taken.

Precautions and warnings

Medical examination: Prior to insertion of an IUD the medical contraindications for IUD use should be excluded on the basis of both the medical history and the physical examination of the woman. Physical examination should include a pelvic examination, cervical smear, and if possible, appropriate tests for sexually transmitted disease.

IUD users should be re-examined shortly after the first postinsertion period or within a month after immediate postabortion or postpartum insertion. Thereafter, appropriate examination should be carried out at regular intervals e.g. every six months.

If Multiload strings cannot be felt in a woman who has not noticed expulsion, examination is necessary to exclude perforation. Ultrasound or X-ray may be used to locate the device. The copper wire is radio-opaque whereas the plastic body and the threads of the IUD are not.

Nulliparity: In nulliparous women the risks and benefits of intrauterine contraception should be assessed with special consideration of their future fertility.

Pain during and after insertion is more likely to occur in nulliparous than in multiparous women.

Pelvic inflammatory disease (PID): During the first few months of IUD use there is an increased risk of PID which is attributed to contamination of the uterine cavity during insertion. PID that develops more than 4 months after insertion appears to be due to other factors, such as acquisition of a sexually transmitted disease.

PID may lead to tubal occlusion resulting in impairment of future fertility, increase the risk of subsequent ectopic pregnancy and, if a tubo-ovarian abscess develops, may necessitate hysterectomy and oophorectomy. Therefore, in nulliparous women and in women with a recent history of treated pelvic infection, contraceptive benefits of IUD use have to be weighed against potential risks. The following clinical symptoms may be indicative of PID: pyrexia, lower abdominal tenderness or pain, abnormal vaginal discharge, deep dyspareunia, prolonged or heavy menstrual bleeding, pain on manipulation of the cervix, tenderness or pain on bimanual examination of the uterus and uterine adnexae. If women fitted with an IUD are suspected of PID, the following is advised:

- In mild cases the diagnosis should be established and treatment with antibiotics started. If there is no response after 24 hours the IUD should be removed.
- In moderate cases with more definite clinical signs the IUD should be removed before starting antibiotic therapy and the patient referred for a gynaecological opinion.
- In severe cases associated with marked lower abdominal pain and fever the IUD should be removed and the patient should be admitted to hospital.

Reasons for removal:

- Pregnancy (see below).
- PID (see above).
- Excessive and persistent bleeding or cramping.
- Perforation of the cervical or uterine wall. This is extremely rare with Multiload but if it should happen, the device should be removed. If X-ray is used to locate the device note that only the Multiload copper wire is radio-opaque.
- Partial downward displacement of Multiload into the cervical canal.
- Translocation of stemmed IUDs may occur after immediate postpartum insertion. If translocation occurs, the IUD should be removed.
- It is advised that the Multiload Cu250 and Multiload Cu250 Short are replaced every 3 years and the Multiload Cu375 is replaced every 5 years.

N.B. For the removal procedure and the possible complications encountered therewith see the relevant section elsewhere.

Additional warnings: Insertion of an IUD may precipitate a seizure in women suffering from epilepsy. Special care is therefore recommended during insertion.

Medical diathermy (shortwave and microwave) of the abdominal and sacral areas should be used cautiously as it may induce heat injuries because of the presence of metallic copper on the IUD.

In women fitted with an IUD blood loss due to heavier periods may lead to iron deficiency anaemia.

Pregnancy despite IUD use: IUDs protect against pregnancy but should a pregnancy occur with an IUD in situ the clinician should consider the possible risk of this being an ectopic pregnancy. There is no convincing evidence of a cause-and-effect relationship between IUD use and ectopic pregnancy.

Should a pregnancy occur with an IUD in situ, it is necessary to determine e.g. by ultrasonography, whether this pregnancy is intrauterine or ectopic.

1. *Intrauterine pregnancy:* If intrauterine pregnancy occurs with an IUD in situ the following is strongly recommended:

- up to 12 weeks gestation, the device should be removed if the threads are visible.
- beyond 12 weeks, or if no threads are visible, termination of pregnancy should be considered and offered to the woman as an option, bearing in mind that the risks associated with elective abortion increase with gestational age.

If the woman insists on continuing the pregnancy with the IUD in situ, refer early for antenatal care. Some reports indicate an increased incidence of septic abortion in patients becoming pregnant with an IUD in situ. In some instances septic abortion has been complicated by septicaemia, sometimes with fatal outcome. The onset of septicaemia may be insidious. If pregnancy is continued with the IUD in situ, the woman must be closely observed and advised to report immediately all abnormal symptoms such as flu-like syndrome, fever, abdominal cramping and pain, dyspareunia, bleeding or vaginal discharge.

If left in situ throughout pregnancy the device is usually expelled before or with placenta and membranes. If not, X-ray or ultrasound should be used early in the puerperium to locate it. So far, there is no evidence that, when a pregnancy continues to term with an IUD in situ, this will lead to birth defects.

2. *Ectopic pregnancy:* IUDs are more protective against intrauterine rather than extrauterine pregnancy. IUD-related pelvic infection may cause tubal damage which predisposes to ectopic implantation. If ectopic pregnancy is suspected early diagnosis is vital. If ectopic pregnancy is established immediate gynaecological intervention is required. Clinical features include amenorrhoea for 6–8 weeks accompanied by symptoms of pregnancy and (severe) unilateral pelvic pain with or without vaginal bleeding which is often scanty and black. However, these symptoms are not always present. The period may not even be late. In addition shouldertip pain or the recent onset of dizziness or fainting may be present.

Patient counselling: The patient should always be given a copy of the leaflet contained in the pack which explains the importance of seeking medical advice in the very unlikely event of pregnancy or if complications occur.

The physician should inform the user about:

The necessity to read the 'Information for the user' very carefully and to follow the instructions to the letter. This is particularly relevant with regard to the paragraph in the section 'Medical advice' covering the early symptoms of genito-urinary infection and the possibility of device failure and pregnancy. Women desiring future pregnancy should be made aware of the slightly increased risk of PID and its possible interference with future fertility.

How to feel each month after the end of her period for the thread(s) of Multiload coming through the cervical os.

How to feel the cervix each month after the end of her period and to ensure that no firm plastic is protruding.

The necessity to contact a doctor:

- if she can not feel the thread(s) of Multiload.
- if she feels the plastic end of Multiload protruding.
- if she experiences heavy menstrual bleeding or troublesome intermenstrual bleeding or spotting as a new complaint occurring after the first few months after insertion, or postcoital bleeding.
- if she experiences dysmenorrhoea or dyspareunia.
- if she misses a period.
- if signs or symptoms of a genito-urinary infection or of an extrauterine pregnancy appear, i.e. prolonged or heavy menstrual bleeding, (persistent) lower abdominal pain or shouldertip pain, deep dyspareunia, fever in excess of 38°C and/or flu-like syndrome, abnormal vaginal discharge, dizziness or fainting.

Adverse reactions: After insertion uterine cramps and/or abdominal pain may occur. In addition some women, particularly nulliparous women, are more prone to syncope, bradycardia and other neuro-vascular episodes during or immediately after insertion or removal of IUDs. Following insertion of an IUD breakthrough bleeding and/or spotting, often occurs during the first cycle. In some women this may recur for several subsequent cycles. Prolongation of menstruation and an increase in menstrual blood loss may occur, especially during the first two or three cycles. Dysmenorrhoea may occur or be aggravated.

In addition the following adverse reactions have rarely been reported: backpain, pains in the legs, dyspareunia, genito-urinary infections (e.g. PID), abnormal vaginal discharge, perforation of uterus or cervix, increased risk of spontaneous abortion and septicaemia, ectopic pregnancy and urticarial allergic skin reactions.

Time of insertion: The optimum time of insertion of an IUD is the last days of the menstrual flow or in the first days afterwards (so-called interval insertion). This is to reduce the possibility of insertion in the presence of an existing undiagnosed pregnancy.

An IUD may also be inserted immediately (no later than 15 minutes) postabortion or postpartum, although in these cases the chances of pregnancy, PID, perforation and expulsion are higher.

If a postabortion or postpartum insertion is not done immediately, it should be delayed until involution is complete i.e. at least 6 weeks after delivery or abortion (so-called delayed post-partum insertion). After caesarian section, insertion should not be attempted until 12 weeks after delivery.

Recommended insertion procedure: It is imperative that a no-touch technique is employed throughout the insertion procedure to ensure sterile handling.

A. Interval insertion

Preparation

1. Perform a careful bimanual examination to determine the version, flexion axis and other aspects of the uterus.
2. Insert a bivalve speculum to expose the cervix. Cleanse the cervix and vaginal walls with sterile cotton wool dipped in antiseptic solution. Wipe all secretion away from the external os.
3. Grasp the anterior lip of the cervix with a single-tooth tenaculum taking a good bite through the cervical lip so that *steady downward traction to straighten the uterine axis* can be maintained without risk of cervical laceration.

   Reflex contraction, which causes cramp of the uterus when the tenaculum is applied, can be prevented by injection of a local anaesthetic into the anterior lip or a paracervical block.
4. Carefully sound the uterus to determine its depth and to confirm the direction of its axis. If the sound meets more than normal resistance at the internal os, it may be advisable to gently dilate the cervical canal to 4–5 mm, using sterile, tapered rather than cylindrical dilators. In the absence of other instruments for measurement of the internal dimensions of the uterine cavity, the sound may be used to obtain an idea of its configuration.

Inserting the Multiload

1. Lay the Multiload pack on a flat surface. Strip the wrapping from the Multiload by lifting the transparent front sheet of the pack from the distal end.
2. The vertical stem of the Multiload is already preloaded in the introducer tube. The side-arms do not require loading into the tube. They are sufficiently flexible to adapt to the shape of the cervical canal.
3. Pick up the introducer tube (with pre-loaded IUD) grasping the tube at the indentation near its distal end and move the cervical stop to the numbered mark corresponding to the sounded length in cm.
4. The distal end of the introducer tube may be held without risk of contaminating the device. Hold the introducer tube and pre-loaded IUD upwards, so that the IUD does not fall from the tube.
5. Carefully insert the Multiload into the uterus until it touches the fundus and the cervical stop rests against the external os whilst *maintaining steady downward traction with the tenaculum to straighten the uterine axis.* No attempt should be made to force insertion.

   Insufficient axial straightening may, on occasion, result in a sub-endometrial insertion. This risk may be reduced by exerting an adequate downward pulling force on the external os, thereby fully straightening the axis of the uterus against its ligamentous frame.
6. When the Multiload touches the fundus, it is released into the uterine cavity by simply withdrawing the introducer tube. During this procedure continue to apply downward traction with the tenaculum. No push-rod is required to insert the Multiload. Check the cervical canal with the sound to ensure that the tail of the Multiload is entirely within the uterine cavity. Trim the threads of the Multiload to 2 to 3 cm measured from the external os.

We must emphasise the importance of precisely following the recommended insertion procedure in order to minimise the risk of a sub-endometrial insertion, which may, in turn, lead to full or partial endometrial embedding of the IUD. Should this occur, an excessive force may need to be applied to remove the IUD from this incorrect location, which may increase the risk of side-arm breakages. Furthermore, it may be clinically difficult to confirm the IUD's sub-endometrial location, since this is usually not obvious to the doctor during insertion of the device and the patient probably experiences no pain. It is anticipated that correctly inserting the device may reduce the incidence of both side-arm breakages and perforations.

B. Immediate post-partum insertion

1. Insert a bivalve speculum to expose the cervix after delivery of the placenta and membranes (no later than 15 minutes). Cleanse the cervix and vaginal walls with sterile cotton wool dipped in antiseptic solution.
2. Grasp both the anterior and the posterior lips with one or two ring forceps and draw the cervix down for close inspection.
3. Take the introducer tube (with pre-loaded IUD) and insert the Multiload along the palmar aspect of two fingers into the uterine cavity until it touches the fundus. Check the position of the Multiload with the flat hand on the abdominal wall covering the fundal region.
4. When the Multiload touches the fundus, it is released into the uterine cavity by very gentle withdrawal of the inserter tube. Take care not to pull on the threads which are left uncut until the first follow-up visit.

Removal procedure: Prepare the vulva, insert the speculum, cleanse the cervix and *straighten the uterine axis* with the tenaculum as for insertion.

When removing the device, we recommend that the doctor always uses a tenaculum to straighten out the uterine axis, thereby possibly reducing the risk of side-arm breakages.

Use a forceps to grasp both threads of the Multiload as near to the exit from the external os as possible. Steady downward traction with the tenaculum to straighten the uterine axis should facilitate removal and also minimise the likelihood of side-arm breakages. *No excessive force must be used.*

Difficult removal and breakage during removal: Sometimes difficulties are encountered when removing the IUD. In the event of a more than usual force being required for removal, consideration should be given to the probability that the Multiload is embedded. There have been reports of part of an embedded device (in particular an embedded side-arm) breaking off within the uterine cavity, when a greater than normal force needs to be applied for removal. Retained fragments may be expelled painlessly with the menstrual period and embedded side-arms may be freed by uterine contractions. There have also been some rare reports of breakage not associated with embedding.

If the device cannot be withdrawn by normal force or if a fragment has remained behind, diagnostic steps should be taken to exclude perforation or embedding. Remember that only the copper wire of the Multiload is visible by X-rays and the plastic frame is radiotranslucent. Plastic fragments, such as the side-arms, may be located using ultrasound or hysteroscopy. The latter technique allows removal at the same time. However, reports indicate that curettage for removal of a fragment, whether or not located in advance, is successful in many cases.

Pharmaceutical precautions Multiloads are supplied sterile in a peel-open pouch, which should not be opened until required for insertion. When handling the device aseptic technique should be used. Care should be taken to ensure that the sterile package is not damaged; it should be stored in cool, dry conditions.

Legal category POM.

Package quantities Single packs containing one Multiload ready for immediate use fitted in a disposable inserter.

Product licence numbers

Multiload Cu250 0065/0062

Multiload Cu250 Short	0065/0075
Multiload Cu375	0065/0092

OESTRADIOL IMPLANTS (ORGANON)

Presentation Pellets of fused, crystalline oestradiol for implantation. Each pellet contains either 25 mg, 50 mg, or 100 mg of Oestradiol.

The 25 mg weight has a diameter of 2.2 mm and the 50 mg and 100 mg weights have a diameter of 4.5 mm.

Uses Indicated in females for:

Major post-menopausal symptoms due to oestrogen deficiency, including prevention of post-menopausal osteoporosis in hysterectomised patients.

Should women with an intact uterus be prescribed Oestradiol implants then the lowest effective dose should be used and it must be co-administered with a progestogen for 10–13 days in each cycle.

Dosage and administration 25–100 mg.

Frequency of replacement depends on the duration of activity of the implants administered and the severity of the symptoms. Patients require a further implant when symptoms return, usually every 4 to 8 months.

Because of the sustained absorption of oestradiol, the endometrium of post-menopausal or ovariectomised women is liable to progressive hypertrophy. Therefore, in women with an intact uterus, additional administration of a progestogen is essential, for 10–13 days in each cycle, to prevent endometrial hyperplasia.

When the patient no longer requires or seeks re-implantation with oestradiol pellets, it is recommended that, in those women with an intact uterus, cyclical administration of an oral progestogen should be continued until there is a cessation of withdrawal bleeding, in order to prevent the possibility of continued endometrial stimulation.

Since the rate of release of the active substance depends on the surface area of the pellet, the dosage is not only determined by the total implanted dose, but also by the number of separate pellets, sited on separate tracks.

Oestradiol Implants should be inserted subcutaneously, (either by means of a trocar and cannula or in the wound at the time of laparotomy), into an area where there is relatively little movement or blood supply, such as the lower abdominal wall or the buttock. Insertion is made under local anaesthesia and the wound is closed either with an adhesive dressing or a fine suture. The implants must be placed subcutaneously to facilitate removal if necessary.

Full aseptic 'no touch' technique should be adopted.

Use during pregnancy and breast-feeding: Oestradiol implants are contraindicated during pregnancy. This is based on epidemiological evidence that use during pregnancy is harmful to the foetus.

Oestradiol implants are not recommended in lactating women. It is known that oestradiol is excreted in breast milk and may decrease milk production.

Contra-indications, warnings, etc

Contra-indications: Pregnancy.

Cardiovascular or cerebrovascular disorders, e.g. thrombophlebitis, thrombo-embolic processes or a history of these conditions.

Moderate to severe hypertension.

Severe liver disease or history of this condition if results of liver function tests have failed to return to normal; cholestatic jaundice, a history of jaundice in pregnancy or jaundice due to the use of steroids; Rotor syndrome and Dubin-Johnson syndrome.

Known or suspected oestrogen-dependent tumours.

Endometrial hyperplasia.

Undiagnosed vaginal bleeding.

Prophyria.

Hyperlipoproteinaemia, especially in the presence of other risk factors predisposing to cardiovascular disorders.

A history during pregnancy or previous steroid use of severe pruritus or herpes gestationis.

Precautions and warnings: If any signs of thrombo-embolic processes occur, the implants must be removed immediately.

In the presence of severe varicose veins the benefits of oestrogen-containing preparations must be weighed against the possible risks.

In patients using oestrogen-containing preparations, the risk of deep-vein thrombosis may be temporarily increased when undergoing major surgery or prolonged immobilization.

Prolonged exposure to unopposed oestrogens is not recommended because it increases the risk of endometrial carcinoma in non-hysterectomised women.

The implant(s) should be removed if liver function tests become abnormal.

Chloasma is occasionally seen during the use of oestrogen- and/or progestogen-containing preparations, especially in women with a history of chloasma gravidarum. Women with a tendency to chloasma should avoid exposure to the sun while taking this preparation.

Pain in the breasts or excessive production of cervical mucus may be indicative of too high a dosage.

The use of steroids may influence the results of certain laboratory tests e.g. thyroid function tests.

During prolonged treatment with oestrogen-containing preparations periodical medical examinations are advisable.

Patients, especially the elderly, with any of the following conditions should be monitored;

- latent or overt cardiac failure, renal dysfunction, epilepsy or migraine (or a history of these conditions), since the use of steroids may occasionally induce fluid retention.
- hypertension (or a history of this condition); if hypertension develops, the implant should be removed.
- sickle cell haemoglobinopathy, since under certain circumstances, e.g. during infections or anoxia, oestrogen-containing preparations may induce thromboembolic processes in patients with this condition.
- oestrogen-sensitive gynaecological disorders, e.g. uterine fibromyomata which may increase in size and endometriosis which may become aggravated during oestrogen treatment.

Adverse reactions: The following adverse reactions have been associated with oestrogen therapy:

Genito-urinary tract: Intermenstrual bleeding, increase in the size of the uterine fibromyomata, endometrial proliferation, excessive production of cervical mucus, aggravation of endometriosis.

Breast: Tenderness, pain, enlargement, secretion.

Gastro-intestinal tract: Nausea, vomiting, cholelithiasis, cholestatic jaundice.

Cardiovascular system: Thrombosis, rise of blood pressure.

Skin: Chloasma, erythema nodosum, rash.

Eyes: Discomfort of the cornea if contact lenses are used.

CNS: Headache, migraine, mood changes.

Metabolic: Sodium and water retention, reduced glucose tolerance, and change in body weight.

High dosages and/or prolonged use of oestrogens may cause psychotic disturbances.

Interactions: Oestrogen and/or progestogen-containing preparations may diminish glucose tolerance and increase the need for insulin or other antidiabetic drugs in diabetics.

Overdosage: The acute toxicity of oestradiol in animals is very low. In the event of overdosage the pellets should be removed.

Pharmaceutical precautions Protect from light.

Legal category POM.

Package quantities Each sterile implant is supplied singly, in a sealed glass tube, available in the following weights: 25 mg, 50 mg, and 100 mg.

Further information Oestradiol implants, when inserted subcutaneously, provide a very slow release of the natural oestrogen, oestradiol. Oestradiol implants can be used in conditions requiring a uniform and sustained oestrogenic activity for a prolonged period of time.

A 2.2 mm diameter trocar and cannula should be used to introduce the 25 mg Oestradiol Implant and a 4.5 mm trocar and cannula should be used to introduce either a 50 mg or 100 mg Oestradiol implant. On each occasion before reuse it is important to sterilise the trocar and cannula set by washing and subsequent heat sterilisation. This may be carried out by boiling in water for 30 minutes or through the use of an autoclave.

Product licence numbers	25 mg	0065/5074R
	50 mg	0065/5075R
	100 mg	0065/5076R

OVESTIN* CREAM

Presentation An intravaginal cream containing 1 mg oestriol in 1 g of cream

Other ingredients: 2 octyl-dodecanol; cetaceum; glycerin; cetyl alcohol; Stearyl alcohol; Polysorbate 60; sorbitan monostearate; Chlorhexidine hydrochloride; lactic acid; sodium hydroxide to pH 4, purified water.

Uses Vulvo-vaginal complaints due to oestrogen deficiency associated with the climacteric and the post-menopause or after oophorectomy: Atrophic vaginitis; kraurosis vulvae; pruritus vulvae; dyspareunia due to an atrophic vaginal mucosa; as pre-surgery therapy for vaginal operations and during subsequent convalescence.

Dosage and administration Ovestin Cream should be given at the lowest dose to control the symptoms and for as short a time as is found necessary.

Ovestin Cream is administered intravaginally by means of a calibrated applicator before retiring at night.

One applicator-dose (applicator filled to the red mark) is 500 mg Ovestin Cream containing 500 micrograms oestriol.

Usual dose for vulvo-vaginal complaints associated with the menopause: One application per day for 2 to 3 weeks.

As maintenance dosage, one application twice a week is recommended.

Medication should be discontinued every 2 to 3 months for a period of 4 weeks to assess the necessity for further treatment.

Pre-surgery therapy (one application per day) should begin 2 weeks before the operation. Following surgery a period of at least 2 weeks should be allowed before resuming therapy.

The following 'Instructions for use' should be given to the patient and are included in the package interior leaflet:

Instructions for use

Apply the cream before retiring at night.

Remove the cap from the tube, invert it, and use the sharp point to open the tube.

Withdraw the plunger to the red mark and screw the nozzle end of the applicator on to the tube.

Squeeze the tube to force sufficient cream into the applicator to fill it to the red mark.

Unscrew the applicator from the tube and replace the cap on the tube.

To apply cream, lie down, insert the end of the applicator deeply into the vagina and slowly push the plunger all the way in.

After use, pull the plunger out of the barrel and wash both in warm, soapy water. Rinse well afterwards. Do not use detergent.

DO NOT PUT THE APPLICATOR IN HOT OR BOILING WATER.

Contra-indications, warnings, etc

Use during pregnancy and breast feeding: Ovestin Cream is contraindicated during pregnancy.

There are insufficient data on the use of Ovestin Cream during breast-feeding to assess potential harm to the infant. It is known, however, that oestriol is excreted in breast milk and may decrease milk production.

Contra-indications: Pregnancy or suspected pregnancy and during lactation.

Thrombophlebitis, thrombo-embolic processes, or a history of these conditions.

Known or suspected oestrogen-dependent tumours, e.g. mammary, genital carcinoma.

Undiagnosed vaginal bleeding.

Acute or chronic liver disease or history of liver disease where the liver function tests have failed to return to normal. Jaundice or history of jaundice in pregnancy. Rotor syndrome or Dubin-Johnson syndrome.

Porphyria.

Cerebrovascular or cardiovascular disease.

Hyperlipoproteinaemia, especially in the presence of other risk factors which may indicate a predisposition to cerebrovascular or cardiovascular disorders.

A history during pregnancy or previous use of steroids of severe pruritus, herpes gestationis or a deterioration of otosclerosis.

Precautions and warnings: In the event of persistent or recurring vaginal bleeding, appropriate diagnostic measures should be taken to rule out malignancy. In case of vaginal infections these should be treated before therapy with Ovestin Cream is started.

Prolonged exposure to unopposed oestrogens may increase the risk of the development of endometrial carcinoma.

Pain in the breasts or excessive production of cervical mucus may be indicative of too high a dosage.

During prolonged treatment with oestrogens, periodic medical examinations are advisable.

A cervical smear should be taken at regular intervals.

Oestrogen preparations may increase the risk of thrombosis and this should be taken into account when surgery is to be performed in patients using these preparations. Where possible, oestrogens should be discontinued approximately six weeks prior to elective surgery and not recommenced until the patient has recovered and is mobile.

Patients, especially the elderly, with any of the following conditions should be monitored: Latent or overt cardiac failure; renal or hepatic dysfunction; hypertension; epilepsy or migraine or a history of these conditions; a history of thromboembolic disorders (since oestrogens may cause sodium and water retention and exacerbate the above conditions); endometriosis; fibrocystic mastopathy; diabetes mellitus.

Adverse reactions: As with any preparation that is to be applied to mucosal surfaces, Ovestin Cream may cause local irritation or itching at the beginning of treatment. During the first weeks of therapy, occasional mastodynia may occur. In general, these complaints are transient in nature.

Interactions: There is insufficient evidence to support the occurrence of clinically relevant interactions.

Overdosage: The acute toxicity of oestriol in animals is very low. Symptoms that may occur in the case of an acute oral overdosage are nausea, vomiting and possibly withdrawal bleeding in females. No specific antidote is known. If necessary a symptomatic treatment should be instituted.

Pharmaceutical precautions The preparation should be stored at room temperature (15–25°C).

Legal category POM.

Package quantities Tube (+applicator) containing 15 g cream.

Further information Ovestin Cream contains the natural female hormone, oestriol. In comparison to other oestrogens, oestriol is short-acting.

The atrophic changes, developing in the lower female genito-urinary tract in conditions of oestrogen deficiency, may cause symptoms and complaints which can be alleviated by local application of oestriol. Oestriol induces the normalisation of the vaginal epithelium and thus helps to restore the physiological pH in the vagina. As a result, it increases the resistance of the vaginal epithelial cells to infection and inflammation.

During the use of Ovestin Cream, systemic absorption of oestriol occurs. As a rule, however, this will not result in endometrial proliferation provided that the recommended dosage is adhered to.

Product licence number 0065/0074.

OVESTIN* TABLETS

Presentation Round, flat, white tablets, diameter 8 mm, code-marked 'DG4' on one side, with 'Organon' and a star on the reverse side.

Each tablet contains 250 micrograms of Oestriol.

Other constituents: propylene glycol, lactose, potato starch and magnesium stearate.

Uses In oestrogen deficiency states for genito-urinary complaints due to recurrent urogenital infections.

Infertility due to poor cervical penetration.

Dosage and administration The tablets should be swallowed without chewing. It is important that the total daily dose is taken at one time.

Genito-urinary infections: 0.5–3 mg daily for up to 1 month. Maintenance dose 0.5–1 mg daily until restoration of the epithelial integrity and normal balance of vaginal flora is established.

Infertility due to poor cervix penetration: 0.25–1 mg per day on days 6–15 of cycle.

NB. Oestrogen therapy should be reviewed according to the individual patient's requirements and clinical picture. Long-term therapy requires regular monitoring procedures.

Use during pregnancy and breast feeding: Ovestin tablets are contra-indicated during pregnancy. This is based on observations in the human which have indicated that the use of oestrogens may be harmful in pregnancy.

There is insufficient data on the use of Ovestin tablets at recommended dosages during breast-feeding to assess potential harm to the child. It is known, however, that oestriol is excreted in breast milk and may inhibit lactation.

Contra-indications, warnings, etc

Contra-indications: Pregnancy; Thrombosis; known or suspected oestrogen-dependent tumours; undiagnosed vaginal bleeding; porphyria; severe hypertension; hepatic diseases.

Precautions and warnings: Prolonged exposure to unopposed oestrogens may increase the risk of the development of endometrial carcinoma.

Pain in the breasts or excessive production of cervical mucus may be indicative of too high a dosage.

During prolonged treatment with oestrogens, periodic medical examinations are advisable.

With vaginal infections, a concomitant specific treatment is recommended.

Patients, with the following conditions should be monitored: a history of thromboembolic disorders; latent or overt cardiac failure; fluid retention due to renal dysfunction; hypertension; epilepsy or migraine (or a history of these conditions); endometriosis; fibrocystic mastopathy; hyperlipoproteinaemia; diabetes mellitus; a history during pregnancy or previous use of steroids of severe pruritus or herpes gestationis.

Adverse reactions: the following adverse reactions, associated with oestrogen treatment may occur during oestriol therapy: Nausea and vomiting; breast tenderness or pain in the breasts; spotting during or on withdrawal of therapy; excessive production of cervical mucus; headache.

Interactions: There is insufficient evidence to support the potential occurrence of clinically relevant interactions.

Overdosage: The acute toxicity of the natural hormone oestriol is very low. Symptoms that may possibly occur in the case of an acute overdosage are nausea and vomiting. No specific antidote is known. If necessary a symptomatic treatment will probably be sufficient.

Pharmaceutical precautions Protect from light.

Legal category POM.

Package quantities Bottles of 100 tablets.

Further information Ovestin tablets contain the natural female hormone, oestriol. In comparison to other oestrogens, oestriol is short-acting. This is due to its short nuclear retention time in the target tissues, its low affinity for plasma proteins and its rapid metabolic clearance. As a result, Ovestin tablets are capable of regenerating oestrogen-dependent tissues without causing proliferation of the endometrium, provided that the preparation is administered as an undivided daily dose.

Product licence number 0065/5049R.

PREGNYL*

Presentation Pregnyl contains purified human chorionic gonadotrophin (hCG) prepared from the urine of pregnant women. Ampoules containing a white, freeze-dried plug, with 1 ml ampoules of solvent. Active ingredient: Chorionic Gonadotrophin BP 500 Units, 1500 Units or 5000 Units.

Other ingredients: sodium carboxymethylcellulose USP 50 micrograms, mannitol USP 5 mg, disodium hydrogen phosphate EP 250 micrograms (calculated as anhydrous), sodium dihydrogen phosphate EP 250 micrograms (calculated as anhydrous).

Uses

In the male: Hypogonadotrophic hypogonadism. Delayed puberty associated with insufficient gonadotrophic pituitary function. Sterility in selected cases of deficient spermatogenesis.

In the female: Sterility due to the absence of follicle-ripening or ovulation. In conjunction with human menopausal gonadotrophins (HMG), in the promotion of controlled superovulation in medically assisted reproduction programs.

Dosage and administration

In the male

Hypogonadotrophic hypogonadism: 500–1000 Units 2–3 times weekly.

Delayed puberty associated with insufficient gonadotrophic pituitary function: 1500 Units twice weekly for at least 6 months.

Sterility in selected cases of deficient spermatogenesis: Usually, 3000 Units per week in combination with a Human Menopausal Gonadotrophins (HMG) preparation.

In the female

Sterility due to the absence of follicle-ripening or ovulation: Usually, 5,000–10,000 Units hCG to induce ovulation, following treatment with an HMG (human menopausal gonadotrophin) preparation. Up to 3 repeat injections of up to 5,000 Units hCG each, may be given within the following 9 days to prevent insufficiency of the corpus luteum.

In conjunction with HMG, in the promotion of controlled superovulation in medically assisted reproduction programs: 5000–10 000 units hCG 30–40 hours after the last HMG injection.

Pregnyl should not be administered if the following criteria have not been met: It is recommended that at least 3 follicles greater than 17 mm in diameter are present with 17B oestradiol levels of at least 3500 pmol/L (920 picogram/ml).

Oocyte collection is carried out 32–36 hours after the hCG injection.

After addition of the solvent to the freeze-dried substance, the solution should be used immediately by intramuscular injection.

Contra-indications, warnings, etc
Contra-indications: Known or suspected androgen-dependent tumours, carcinoma of the prostate or mammary carcinoma in males.

Precautions and warnings:
Treatment of male patients with Pregnyl leads to increased androgen production. Therefore: Pregnyl should be used cautiously in prepubertal boys to avoid premature epiphyseal closure or precocious sexual development.

Patients with latent or overt cardiac failure, renal dysfunction, hypertension, epilepsy or migraine (or a history of these conditions) should be monitored, since sodium and fluid retention have been observed after administration of high dosages of hCG.

Prior to treating patients for inadequate endogenous stimulation of the gonads, an examination should be performed to exclude anatomical abnormalities of the genital organs or nongonadal endocrinopathies (e.g. thyroid or adrenal disorders, diabetes). Primary ovarian failure should be excluded by the determination of gonadotrophin levels.

In the pregnancies occurring after induction of ovulation with gonadotrophic preparations, there is an increased risk of abortion and multiplets.

Unwanted hyperstimulation: During treatment of female patients, determinations of oestrogen levels and assessment of ovarian size and if possible, ultrasonography should be performed prior to treatment and at regular intervals during treatment. High dosages may cause oestrogen levels to rise excessively rapidly, e.g. more than doubling on 2 or 3 consecutive days, and possibly reaching excessively high pre-ovulatory values.

If unwanted hyperstimulation occurs (i.e. not as part of a treatment preparing for IVF/ET or GIFT or other assisted reproduction techniques), the administration of HMG should be discontinued immediately, hCG must not be given, because the administration of an hLH-active gonadotrophin at this stage may induce, in addition to multiple ovulations, the ovarian hyperstimulation syndrome. This warning is particularly important with respect to patients with polycystic ovarian disease.

The severe form of ovarian hyperstimulation syndrome may be life-threatening and is characterised by large ovarian cysts (prone to rupture), ascites, very often hydrothorax and occasionally thrombo-embolic phenomena.

Adverse reactions: Skin rashes have occasionally been reported.

Sodium and water retention is occasionally seen in males after administration of high dosages; this is regarded as a result of excessive androgen production.

Overdose: The toxicity of human chorionic gonadotrophic hormone is very low. However, too high a dose may lead to hyperstimulation of the ovaries (see 'Unwanted Hyperstimulation').

Pharmaceutical precautions Protect from light and store at a temperature between 2 and 15°C. In the dry state, in sealed containers, Pregnyl will retain its full activity for three years from the date of manufacture. Solutions are unstable and should be used freshly prepared.

Legal category POM.

Package quantities Single ampoules of Pregnyl 500 Units, 1,500 Units or 5,000 Units with solvent. Boxes of 10 ampoules of Pregnyl 5,000 Units with solvent.

Further information Pregnyl stimulates the steroidogenesis in the gonads by virtue of a biological effect similar to that of LH (luteinizing hormone, which is the same as interstitial cell stimulating hormone). In the male it promotes the production of testosterone and in the female the production of oestrogens and particularly of progesterone after ovulation. In certain cases, this preparation is used in combination with human menopausal gonadotrophin (HMG). Because hCG is of human origin, no antibody formation is to be expected.

Product licence numbers

Pregnyl 500 Units	0065/5077
Pregnyl 1500 Units	0065/5078
Pregnyl 5000 Units	0065/5079
Solvent	0065/0114 (Sodium Chloride solution for injection 0.9% w/v)

RESTANDOL*

Presentation Soft, oval, reddish-brown gelatin capsules each containing 40 mg of testosterone undecanoate in oleic acid. Code marked D_3V and ORG.

Uses Restandol is an orally active testosterone preparation.

Indications:

Testosterone replacement therapy in male hypogonadal disorders, for example: After castration; eunuchoidism; hypopituitarism; endocrine impotence; male climacteric symptoms like decreased libido and decreased mental and physical activity; certain types of infertility due to disorders of spermatogenesis.

Testosterone therapy may also be indicated in osteoporosis due to androgenic deficiency.

Dosage and administration
Adults: The initial dosage required will usually be 120–160 mg daily for 2–3 weeks. Subsequent dosage (40–120 mg daily) should be based on the clinical effect obtained during the first weeks of therapy.

Elderly: It should be noted that smaller and less frequent doses may achieve the same response.

The capsules should be taken after meals, if necessary with a little water, and be swallowed whole without chewing. It is preferable that half of the daily dose be taken in the morning and the other half in the evening. If an uneven number of capsules is taken daily, the greater part should be taken in the morning.

Contra-indications, warnings, etc
Contra-indications: Known or suspected prostatic or mammary carcinoma; hypercalciuria, hypercalcaemia, nephrotic syndrome, ischaemic heart disease or untreated congestive heart failure.

Precautions and warnings:
Patients, especially the elderly, with the following conditions should be monitored: Latent or overt cardiac failure, renal or hepatic dysfunction, hypertension, epilepsy or migraine (or a history of these conditions), since androgens may occasionally induce sodium and water retention.

Mammary carcinoma, hypernephroma, bronchial carcinoma, and skeletal metastases, since these conditions may produce hypercalcaemia or hypercalciuria which may in turn be exacerbated by androgen therapy. If hypercalcaemia or hypercalciuria develops treatment should be discontinued.

A decrease in protein-bound iodine (PBI) may occur, but this has no clinical significance.

Androgens should be used cautiously in prepubertal boys to avoid premature epiphyseal closure or precocious sexual development.

Androgen therapy should only be used in male hypogonadism in which testosterone levels have been demonstrated to be low.

In treating males, stimulation to the point of increasing nervous, mental and physical activities beyond the patient's cardiovascular capacity should be avoided.

Tumours and other histological abnormalities and disturbances of liver function have been reported in patients subjected to prolonged treatment with some testosterone derivatives. Most of these compounds were 17-alpha alkyl derivatives but a smaller number of cases has occurred with certain 17-beta esters of testosterone. The possibility that such changes result from the use of Restandol has not been excluded.

Adverse reactions: Restandol, like any other androgen therapy, may give rise to the following adverse reactions:

Priapism and other signs of excessive sexual stimulation.

Precocious sexual development, an increased frequency of erections, phallic enlargement and premature epiphyseal closure in pre-pubertal males.

Sodium and water retention.

Oligospermia and a decreased ejaculatory volume.

Treatment should be interrupted until these symptoms have disappeared after which it should be continued at a lower dosage.

Hoarseness of the voice may be the first symptom of vocal change which may lead to irreversible lowering of the voice. If signs of virilisation, particularly lowering of the voice, develop, treatment should be discontinued.

Interactions: Concurrent administration of liver enzyme inducing drugs such as rifampicin, barbiturates, carbamazepine, dichloralphenazone, phenylbutazone, phenytoin or primidone may decrease the effect of Restandol.

Overdosage: Treatment of overdosage is by gastric lavage with appropriate supportive therapy. Standard resuscitative measures should be given as required.

Pharmaceutical precautions Store in a cool (6–15°C) dry place. Protect from light.

Legal category POM.

Package quantities 60 capsules.

Further information Restandol is an orally effective testosterone preparation. The therapeutic substance is tesosterone undecanoate, a fatty acid ester of the natural androgen testosterone. Testosterone is inactive on oral administration because it is prematurely inactivated by the liver. Testosterone undecanoate is able to by-pass the liver via the lymphatic system and is therefore orally active.

Product licence number 0065/0059.

SUSTANON* 100

Presentation Sustanon 100 is a clear, sterile, oily solution containing in each millilitre 20 mg Testosterone Propionate BP, 40 mg Testosterone Phenylpropionate BP and 40 mg Testostrone Isocaproate BP.

Other constituents: Benzyl Alcohol PhEur 0.1 ml and Arachis Oil PhEur to 1.0 ml.

Uses Sustanon 100 is an androgenic preparation for intramuscular administration containing three different esters of the natural hormone testosterone.

Indications: Testosterone replacement therapy in male hypogonadal disorders, for example: After castration; eunuchoidism; hypopituitarism; endocrine impotence; male climacteric symptoms like decreased libido; certain types of infertility due to disorders of spermatogenesis.

Testosterone therapy may also be indicated for the prevention and treatment of osteoporosis in hypogonodal males.

Dosage and administration In general, dosage should be adjusted to the individual response of the patient.

Adults: Usually, one injection of 1 ml per two weeks will be adequate.

Elderly: It should be noted that smaller and less frequent doses may achieve the same response.

Children: It should be noted that smaller and less frequent doses may achieve the same response.

Sustanon 100 should be administered by deep intramuscular injection.

Contra-indications, warnings, etc

Contra-indications: Known or suspected prostatic or mammary carcinoma.

Precautions and warnings: Patients, especially the elderly, with the following conditions should be monitored: ischaemic heart disease, since androgens may produce hypercholesterolaemia; latent or overt cardiac failure, renal dysfunction, hypertension, epilepsy or migraine (or a history of these conditions), since this may occasionally induce salt and fluid retention; skeletal metastases, since androgens may induce hypercalcaemia or hypercalciuria in these patients.

A decrease in protein-bound iodine (PBI) may occur, but this has no clinical significance.

Androgens should be used cautiously in prepubertal boys to avoid premature epiphyseal closure or precocious sexual development.

Adverse reactions: Sustanon 100 like any other androgen therapy, may give rise to the following adverse reactions: Priapism and other signs of excessive sexual stimulation.

Precocious sexual development, an increased frequency of erections, phallic enlargement and premature epipyseal closure in pre-pubertal males.

Oligospermia and a decreased ejaculatory volume.

Water and salt retention.

Treatment should be interrupted until these symptoms have disappeared, after which it should be continued at a lower dosage.

Hoarseness of the voice may be the first symptom of vocal change which may lead to irreversible lowering of the voice. If signs of virilisation, particularly lowering of the voice, develop, treatment should be discontinued.

Pharmaceutical precautions Protect from light.

Store at room temperature (15 to 25°C).

After storage at lower temperatures precipitation of the arachis oil vehicle may occur. By heating the ampoules at 100°C for a few minutes or at 40°C for one hour, the solution will become clear. The precipitation and rewarming does not affect the activity of the injection.

Legal category POM.

Package quantities 1 ml ampoules in boxes of 3.

Further information Testosterone propionate has a rapid onset and short duration of action. Testosterone phenylpropionate and isocaproate have a less rapid onset and a long duration of action. By combining these testosterone esters the action of Sustanon 100 starts shortly after injection and is maintained for about two weeks.

Sustanon 100 is generally well tolerated and has no adverse effect on the liver.

Product licence number 0065/5019.

SUSTANON* 250

Presentation Sustanon 250 is a clear, sterile, oily solution containing in each millilitre 30 mg Testosterone Propionate BP, 60 mg Testosterone Phenylpropionate BP, 60 mg Testosterone Isocaproate BP, and 100 mg Testosterone Decanoate BP.

Other constituents: Benzyl Alcohol PhEur 0.1 ml and Arachis Oil PhEur to 1.0 ml.

Uses Sustanon 250 is an androgenic preparation for intramuscular administration containing four different esters of the natural hormone testosterone.

Indications: Testosterone replacement therapy in male hypogonadal disorders, for example: after castration; eunuchoidism; hypopituitarism; endocrine impotence; male climacteric symptoms like decreased libido; certain types of infertility due to disorders of spermatogenesis.

Testosterone therapy may also be indicated for the prevention and treatment of osteoporosis in hypogonadal males.

Dosage and administration In general, dosage should be adjusted to the individual response of the patient.

Adults: Usually, one injection of 1 ml per three weeks will be adequate.

Elderly: It should be noted that smaller and less frequent doses may achieve the same response.

Children: It should be noted that smaller and less frequent doses may achieve the same response.

Sustanon 250 should be administered by deep intramuscular injection.

Contra-indications, warnings, etc
Contra-indications: Known or suspected prostatic or mammary carcinoma.

Precautions and warnings: Patients, especially the elderly, with the following conditions should be monitored: ischaemic heart disease, since androgens may produce hypercholesterolaemia; latent or overt cardiac failure, renal dysfunction, hypertension, epilepsy or migraine (or a history of these conditions), since androgens may occasionally induce fluid and sodium retention; skeletal metastases, since androgens may induce hypercalcaemia or hypercalciuria in these patients.

A decrease in protein-bound iodine (PBI) may occur, but this has no clinical significance.

Androgens should be used cautiously in prepubertal boys to avoid premature epiphyseal closure or precocious sexual development.

Adverse reactions: Sustanon 250 like any other androgen therapy, may give rise to the following adverse reactions: Priapism and other signs of excessive sexual stimulation.

Precocious sexual development, an increased frequency of erections, phallic enlargement and premature epiphyseal closure in pre-pubertal males.

Sodium and water retention.

Oligospermia and a decreased ejaculatory volume.

Treatment should be interrupted until these symptoms have disappeared, after which it should be continued at a lower dosage.

Hoarseness of the voice may be the first symptom of vocal change which may lead to irreversible lowering of the voice. If signs of virilisation, particularly lowering of the voice, develop, treatment should be discontinued.

Pharmaceutical precautions Protect from light. Store at room temperature (15 to 25°C).

After storage at lower temperatures precipitation of the arachis oil vehicle may occur. By heating the ampoules at 100°C for a few minutes or at 40°C for one hour, the solution will become clear. The precipitation and rewarming does not affect the activity of the injection.

Legal category POM.

Package quantities 1 ml ampoules in boxes of 3.

Further information Testosterone propionate has a rapid onset and short duration of action. Testosterone phenylpropionate and isocaproate have a less rapid onset and long duration of action. Testosterone decanoate has a slow onset and long duration of action. By combining these testosterone esters the action of Sustanon 250 starts shortly after injection and is maintained for about three weeks.

Sustanon 250 is generally well tolerated and has no adverse effect on the liver.

Product licence number 0065/5086.

TETRABID-ORGANON*

Presentation Hard gelatin capsules (purple cap/ yellow body).

Each capsule contains 250 mg Tetracycline Hydrochloride PhEur.

Other ingredients: Aerosil, fumaric acid, purified talc, povidone and shellac.

Uses Treatment of infections caused by organisms sensitive to tetracycline, including bronchitis and non-specific urethritis.

Treatment and prophylaxis against acute exacerbations of chronic bronchitis caused by organisms sensitive to tetracycline.

In the treatment of acne vulgaris.

Dosage and administration
Adults and children over 12 years: Two capsules initially, followed by one capsule every 12 hours. For more severe infections, dosage may be increased at the discretion of the physician. The daily dose should be divided over a 24-hour period.

Apart from the initial dose, no more than one capsule should be taken at any one time.

Treatment should continue for at least two or three days after achievement of the desired clinical response.

In prophylaxis: half the usual daily dosage.

In treatment of acne vulgaris: One capsule daily for at least three months.

Capsules should be swallowed whole with a sufficient amount of fluid in the upright or sitting position. They should not be taken with milk products (see 'Interactions'). They should preferably be taken one hour before, or two hours after meals.

Contra-indications, warnings, etc
Contra-indications: Pregnancy or suspected pregnancy (unless specifically indicated by bacterial sensitivity tests and where the risk involved is justified) and during lactation.

Severe renal impairment.

Hypersensitivity to tetracyclines.

Children under 8 years of age, because tetracycline is selectively taken up in developing bones and teeth of foetuses and children, causing dental staining and enamel hypoplasia.

Use during pregnancy and breast feeding: Since Tetrabid-Organon contains tetracycline it should not be used during pregnancy, unless bacterial sensitivity tests leave no other choice and the risk involved is justified.

Tetracyclines are excreted in breastmilk. Because tetracyclines may form nonabsorbable complexes with calcium in breastmilk, use is contraindicated during lactation.

Precautions and warnings: Tetracyclines should be administered with caution in patients with renal or hepatic impairment or those receiving potentially hepatotoxic drugs; this may be of particular relevance to the elderly group of patients in whom such impairment is relatively more common; a reduction of the dosage or a longer time interval between doses is indicated.

Broad-spectrum antibiotic therapy may result in overgrowth of non-susceptible organisms. If such superinfection should occur, resulting in the development of oral thrush, pruritis ani or gastrointestinal side-effects, the antibiotic therapy should be discontinued and appropriate measures taken.

If long-term therapy is intended, then laboratory monitoring of certain functions (including haemopoietic, renal and hepatic tests) should be performed.

In some patients, treatment with tetracyclines may induce hypersensitivity reactions ranging from rashes to drug fever or anaphylactic shock. If a serious anaphylactic reaction occurs, appropriate therapy should be instituted which may include immediate slow intravenous injection of 0.1–0.5 ml of adrenaline 1:1000 (0.1–0.5 mg) as well as high doses of water-soluble glucorticoids (e.g. dexamethasone).

Adverse reactions: Bulging fontanelles in infants and benign intracranial hypertension in adults has been reported. Treatment should cease if evidence of raised intracranial pressure develops.

Skin photosensitivity reactions are occasionally observed in patients on tetracycline therapy. Treatment should be discontinued at the first sign of skin erythema.

Nausea, vomiting, diarrhoea.

A Fanconi-type syndrome may occasionally occur.

Interactions: Concomitant use with any of the following drugs or substances may lead to the occurrence of clinically relevant interactions:

— Antacids, urinary alkalinizers, zinc and bismuth salts, haematinics and milk products (since these products may impair the intestinal absorption of tetracycline. Therefore doses of one drug should be spaced as far as possible from the other).

— Oral anticoagulants (since tetracyclines may reduce plasma prothrombin activity, the dosage of oral anticoagulant may have to be reduced).

— Bactericidal antibiotics, such as penicillins (since bacteriostatic drugs may antagonise the bactericidal effect of penicillins).

— Methoxyflurane (since tetracyclines may increase its potential nephrotoxicity).
— Digoxin (since tetracyclines may increase the bioavailability of digoxin).
— Oral contraceptives: their reliability may be reduced.

Overdosage: After oral ingestion the toxicity of tetracyclines is generally low. Symptoms and signs that may occur after an acute overdosage include: transient fever, vomiting, melaena, jaundice and haematoma formation; transaminases may be elevated and prothrombin time prolonged.

In cases of overdosage, treatment should be instituted as soon as possible, especially in young children. The stomach should be washed out by gastric lavage, followed by appropriate symptomatic and supportive measures. Antacids may be used to reduce tetracycline absorption. In severe cases of poisoning, peritoneal or haemodialysis should be performed.

Pharmaceutical precautions Store at a temperature below 30°C and in dry conditions.

Legal category POM.

Package quantities Securitainer of 100 or 500 capsules.

Further information Tetrabid-Organon is a sustained-action tetracycline formulation which requires only half the daily dose and half the frequency of administration of conventional tetracycline.

Twice-daily Tetrabid-Organon provides tetracycline therapy with a reduced incidence of side-effects. The formulation allows sustained release of tetracycline throughout the gastro-intestinal tract and fumaric acid (33 mg) provides a localised low pH environment at the point of release which favours increased absorption.

Product licence number 0065/0028.

**Trade Mark*

Organon Teknika Limited
Science Park
Milton Road
Cambridge

NORCURON*

Presentation Vial containing 10 mg vecuronium bromide in a buffered freeze-dried form, with a 5 ml ampoule of Water for Injections PhEur as solvent.

Other ingredients: Citric Acid Monohydrate PhEur, Disodium Hydrogen Phosphate Dihydrate and Mannitol USP.

Uses Norcuron is a non-depolarising neuromuscular blocking agent with a short to medium duration of action. It is used as an adjunct in surgical anaesthesia to obtain relaxation of the skeletal muscles in a wide range of surgical procedures. Norcuron has no ganglion blocking properties, lacks vagolytic action and histamine release is not expected to occur.

Norcuron has no cumulative effects. Several maintenance doses can therefore be given in succession. These properties make Norcuron highly suitable for short as well as for long-lasting operations. The relatively low renal elimination and the transient liver storage of Norcuron suggest that biliary excretion is the major excretion route. The elimination half-life ranges from 30–70 minutes. Norcuron is well tolerated by the patient.

Dosage and administration Norcuron is administered intravenously.

When calculating the dose of neuromuscular blocking agents the following factors must be taken into account: the anaesthetic technique used, potential interactions with the drugs used during and before anaesthesia, and the condition of the individual patient.

The following may be used as a general guide to dosage for adults, children and infants.

For intubation and subsequent surgical procedures.

Initial dose: 80–100 micrograms/kg (good to excellent intubation conditions within 90–120 seconds).
Incremental doses: 30–50 micrograms/kg.
Infusion dose: 50–80 micrograms/kg/hr

The onset of action of Norcuron is more rapid in infants and children than in adults.

At the initial dose of 80–100 micrograms/kg, skeletal muscle relaxation can be expected to have the following duration:

Adults	20–30 minutes
Children	15–20 minutes
Infants	30–40 minutes

Supplemental doses will be required at longer intervals for infants, and shorter intervals for children.

Should there be any reason for the selection of larger doses, initial doses ranging from 150–250 micrograms/kg may be administered. In these cases duration of action will be increased to 50 minutes at doses of 150 micrograms/kg and 80 minutes at doses of 250 micrograms/kg. Recovery index (time from 25–75% recovery) increases from 14 minutes at 100 micrograms/kg to 30 minutes at 250 micrograms/kg.

In the elderly the recovery index may be even more prolonged.

In obese patients a reduction of the dose is recommended.

The use of a peripheral nerve stimulator is recommended for monitoring neuromuscular block and recovery.

In general it is not recommended that Norcuron should be mixed with other agents in the same syringe or with solutions for intravenous infusion, except for the following intravenous infusion fluids which have been shown to be compatible with Norcuron: 0.9% Sodium Chloride solution; 5.0% Glucose solution; Ringer's solution; Ringer-glucose solution.

When administered by intravenous infusion the Norcuron freeze-dried substance should first be dissolved in the 5 ml of solvent (Water for Injections) provided and the resultant solution added to the infusion fluid. The diluted solution will remain stable for 24 hours at room temperature and in daylight. In practice the infusion containing Norcuron will only be used as long as muscle relaxation is required, at maximum for a few hours. Afterwards the solution should be discarded.

Use in pregnancy: Since there is no experience with the use of Norcuron in pregnant women, it cannot be recommended during pregnancy.

Norcuron can be used in childbirth by Caesarean section without effect on the newly born child.

Contra-indications, warnings, etc

Contra-indications: There are no known contra-indications for the use of Norcuron.

Precautions and warnings: Norcuron should be administered only by anaesthetists familiar with its use, and only when facilities for controlled ventilation, insufflation with oxygen and endotracheal intubation are available for immediate use. Since Norcuron causes relaxation of the respiratory muscles, respiration must be assisted in all patients. It is essential to ensure that the patient is breathing spontaneously, deeply and regularly before leaving the theatre after anaesthesia. The neuromuscular blockade achieved with Norcuron can be reversed with a cholinesterase inhibiting agent (e.g. neostigmine) in an adequate dose, together with atropine as an anticholinergic agent.

Administration of a depolarising drug (e.g. suxamethonium) following a non-depolarising agent (e.g. Norcuron) is dangerous (see 'Interactions' section).

Before the administration of Norcuron, conditions such as electrolyte disturbance, altered pH and dehydration should if possible be corrected.

Care should be exercised if there is a danger of regurgitation when intubating the patient.

Like pancuronium bromide, d-tubocurarine or other non-depolarising neuromuscular blocking agents, Norcuron may cause a reduction in the partial thromboplastin time and the prothrombin time.

The following disease states may influence the pharmacokinetics and/or pharmacodynamics of Norcuron:

Renal failure: In patients with renal insufficiency a slight prolongation of the neuromuscular blockade can be expected after the use of Norcuron.

Hepatic and/or biliary tract disease: Patients with liver disease or liver insufficiency do not usually require a reduction of the initial dose. In some patients the required dose may even be higher.

Neuromuscular disease: Extreme caution should be exercised, and very small doses used in patients with myasthenia gravis or myasthenic syndrome, unless it is intended to administer prolonged post-operative respiratory assistance. In cases of myopathy, neuromuscular disease and poliomyelitis Norcuron should be used with caution.

Hypothermia: In operations requiring hypothermia the neuromuscular blockade of non-depolarising drugs is decreased and increases when re-warming the patient.

Other conditions which may increase the effect of

Norcuron: Hypokalaemia (e.g. after severe vomiting, diarrhoea, digitalisation and diuretic therapy), hypermagnesaemia, hypocalcaemia (after massive transfusion), hypoproteinaemia, dehydration, acidosis, hypercapnoea, cachexia.

Interactions: The following drugs have been shown to influence the magnitude and/or duration of action of non-depolarising neuromuscular blocking agents:

Increased effect:

Anaesthetics: Halothane, ether, enflurane, isoflurane, methoxyflurane, cyclopropane, thiopentone, methohexital, ketamine, fentanyl, gammahydroxybutyrate, etomidate, propanidid.

Other drugs: Other non-depolarising muscle relaxants, prior administration of suxamethonium, aminoglycoside and polypeptide antibiotics, diuretics, beta-adrenergic blocking agents, thiamine, M.A.O. inhibiting agents, quinidine, protamine, alpha-adrenergic blocking agents, imidazole, metronidazole and calcium antagonists.

Decreased effect: Neostigmine, edrophonium, prior chronic administration of corticosteroids, noradrenaline, azathioprine, theophylline, KCl, NaCl, $CaCl_2$.

Variable effect: Depolarising muscle relaxants given after the administration of vecuronium bromide may produce potentiation or attenuation of the neuromuscular blocking effect. The non-depolarising drug increases resistance towards the neuromuscular blocking effect of the depolarising drug. Therefore high doses of a depolarising drug are necessary before muscular relaxation can be obtained. These high doses of a depolarising drug may cause endplate desensitisation and prolonged postoperative apnoea. Unlike a non-depolarising block, a depolarising block cannot be overcome by an anticholinesterase agent and may even be worsened.

Recent evidence suggests that alkylating drugs (nitrogen mustards) should be considered a possible hazard when given to patients during anaesthesia involving the use of muscle relaxants.

Side-effects: On rare occasions unwanted effects have been reported in association with Norcuron; e.g. reactions at the site of injection, bronchospasm and in rare instances, anaphylactoid reactions. However, in all instances Norcuron had been administered concomitantly with other drugs and causality is difficult to establish.

Overdosage: The spontaneous reversal of the neuromuscular blockade caused by Norcuron is rapid.

In the event of an overdosage i.e. a failure of neostigmine to reverse the neuromuscular block, the patient must continue to be ventilated. When administration of a cholinesterase inhibiting agent fails to reverse the neuromuscular blocking effects of Norcuron, ventilation must be continued until spontaneous breathing is restored. Repeated dosage of a cholinesterase inhibitor can be dangerous.

Pharmaceutical precautions Store in the dark at a temperature below 25°C.

Legal category POM.

Package quantities 20 vials each containing 10 mg vecuronium bromide.

20 ampoules each containing 5 ml solvent (Water for Injections PhEur.)

Further information Norcuron is an amino-steroidal derivative which is a highly active non-depolarising neuromuscular blocking agent. The drug is highly selective in its action at the neuromuscular junction and therefore much larger doses would be required to produce ganglion block, vagal block, histamine release and noradrenaline uptake block. Overall a highly significant lack of cardiovascular side-effects has been observed even with doses much higher than those producing neuromuscular block. Norcuron offers a shorter time to intubation, a shorter duration of action and a consistently more rapid rate of recovery in comparison to standard non-depolarisers.

Norcuron has no cumulative effects, even in renal failure patients. Norcuron induced block is readily reversed by standard agents and the predictability of duration of action relative to dose employed, in addition to rapid rate of recovery, promise that an antagonist will on occasion be unnecessary at the end of surgery.

Extensive clinical studies show Norcuron to cause little or no change in cardiovascular parameters and that it is even less active than pancuronium in causing histamine release. Hence Norcuron should be most useful where little change in cardiovascular or pulmonary systems is desirable. This stability, in conjunction with the predictability of its action, allows Norcuron to be used safely and reliably over prolonged periods by infusion where this is desirable as well as in short surgical procedures where a fast time to intubation and short duration of action are required of a non-depolarising neuromuscular blocking agent.

Product licence number 3524/0013.

PAVULON*

Presentation Pancuronium Bromide BP 2 ml ampoules. A clear, aqueous solution. Active ingredient: Each 2 ml ampoule contains Pancuronium Bromide BP 4 mg. Other ingredients: Sodium Chloride PhEur, Sodium Acetate PhEur, Acetic Acid Glacial BP to pH 4.

Uses Pavulon is a non-depolarising neuromuscular blocking agent with a medium duration of action. It is used as an adjunct in surgical anaesthesia to obtain relaxation of the skeletal muscles in a wide range of surgical procedures.

Pavulon is also used for neuromuscular blockade during intensive care therapy for a variety of pathologies, including intractable status asthmaticus and tetanus.

Dosage and administration Pavulon is administered intravenously.

When determining the dose, the method of anaesthesia, expected duration of surgery, potential interaction with other drugs that are administered before or during anaesthesia and the condition of the patient should be taken into account. The use of a peripheral nerve stimulator is recommended for monitoring neuromuscular block and recovery.

The following may be used as a general guide to dosage:

Adult surgery: Initial dose: 50–80 micrograms/kg (intubation accomplished within 150–120 seconds) or 80–100 micrograms/kg (intubation accomplished within 120–090 seconds). Incremental doses: 10–20 micrograms/kg.

Child surgery: Initial dose: 60–100 micrograms/kg. Incremental doses: 10–20 micrograms/kg.

Neonatal surgery: 30–40 micrograms/kg. Incremental doses: As neonates are sensitive this dose should be adjusted according to the initial response but generally incremental doses lie in the range 10–20 micrograms/kg body weight.

Following the administration of suxamethonium the dosage of Pavulon may be considerably reduced.

Adults: Initial dose: 20–60 micrograms/kg. Incremental doses: 10–20 micrograms/kg.

Children: Initial dose: 20–60 micrograms/kg. Incremental doses: 10–20 micrograms/kg.

In obese patients all of these doses should be reduced.

The duration of action depends upon the clinical condition of the patient and the dose administered, but in normal subjects receiving perioperative muscle relaxant doses the duration of action is usually 45–60 minutes.

Pavulon is longer-acting in the intensive-care patient, and an intravenous dose of 60 micrograms/kg every one to one and a half hours, or even less frequently, is usually adequate.

The neuromuscular blocking activity of Pavulon is prolonged in the elderly.

In the control of tetanus, duration of Pavulon relaxation probably depends on the severity of the spasm: duration of effect can therefore be variable.

Pavulon should not be mixed with other agents in the

same syringe, or with solutions for intravenous infusion, as a change in pH may induce precipitation.

Any unused solution should be discarded.

Use in pregnancy: There are insufficient data on the use of Pavulon during animal or human pregnancy to assess potential harm to the foetus. The drug should only be administered to a pregnant woman when the attending physician decides that the benefits outweigh the risks.

Caesarean section: Studies with Pavulon have shown its safety for use in Caesarean section. Pavulon does not affect Apgar score, foetal muscle tonus nor cardiorespiratory adaptation of the newborn. From assays of the Pavulon concentration in umbilical blood samples it is apparent that only very limited placental transfer of Pavulon occurs.

Warning: Reversal of neuromuscular block induced by Pavulon may be unsatisfactory in patients receiving magnesium sulphate for toxaemia of pregnancy because magnesium salts enhance neuromuscular blockade.

Dosages should be reduced in such cases.

Contra-indications, warnings, etc

Contra-indications: Patients with a known hypersensitivity to Pavulon injection.

Use before or concurrently with a depolarising neuromuscular blocking drug e.g. suxamethonium.

Precautions and warnings: Pavulon should be administered only by anaesthetists familiar with its use, and only when facilities for controlled ventilation, insufflation with oxygen and endotracheal intubation are available for immediate use.

Since Pavulon causes relaxation of the respiratory muscles, respiration must be assisted in all patients. It is essential to ensure that the patient is breathing spontaneously, deeply and regularly before leaving the theatre after anaesthesia. The neuromuscular blockade achieved with Pavulon can be reversed with a cholinesterase inhibiting agent (e.g. neostigmine) in an adequate dose, together with atropine as an anticholinergic agent.

Care should be exercised if there is a danger of regurgitation when intubating the patient, for example during crash induction.

Pavulon (like d-tubocurarine) causes a reduction in the partial thromboplastin time and the prothrombin time.

The following disease states may influence the pharmacokinetics and/or pharmacodynamics of Pavulon:

Renal failure: Since renal excretion is the major elimination route of Pavulon, the elimination half-life is prolonged and the plasma clearance is reduced in patients with renal failure. Pavulon should be used with caution in patients with severe renal impairment as the duration of action can be prolonged.

The prolongation of half-life in patients with renal failure is often but not always associated with an extended duration of neuromuscular blockade. In these patients the recovery from neuromuscular block may also be prolonged.

Hyperdiuresis may result in a decreased neuromuscular blocking effect.

Hepatic and/or biliary tract disease: Despite the modest role of the liver in the elimination of Pavulon, major pharmacokinetic changes have been observed in patients with liver disease.

Resistance to the neuromuscular blocking activity of Pavulon may occur, because these conditions are characterised by a considerable increase (up to 50%) in the volume of distribution of the drug.

At the same time hepatic and/or biliary tract disease can prolong the elimination half-life of Pavulon and prolong the recovery from neuromuscular block.

The possibility of slower onset, higher total dosage requirements and prolongation of neuromuscular blockade and recovery time must be taken in consideration when Pavulon is used in these patients.

Altered circulation time: Conditions associated with slower circulation time, such as cardiovascular disease, old age, oedematous states resulting in an increased volume of distribution, may contribute to an increase of onset time.

Neuromuscular disease: As is the case with other curariform agents, in cases of neuromuscular disease or after poliomyelitis, Pavulon should be used with extreme caution since the response to neuromuscular blocking agents may be considerably altered in these patients. The magnitude and direction of this alteration may vary widely. In patients with myasthenia gravis or the myasthenic (Eaton Lambert) syndrome, small doses of Pavulon may have profound effects and only very small doses of Pavulon should be used initially.

Hypothermia: In operations requiring hypothermia the neuromuscular blockade of non-depolarising drugs is decreased and increases when re-warming the patient. Hypothermia in neonates therefore, requires a reduced dosage of Pavulon.

Other conditions which may increase the effect of Pavulon are: hypokalaemia (e.g. after severe vomiting, diarrhoea, digitalisation and diuretic therapy), hypermagnesaemia, hypocalcaemia (after massive transfusions), hypoproteinaemia, dehydration, acidosis, hypercapnoea, cachexia.

Severe electrolyte disturbances, altered blood pH or dehydration should therefore be corrected when possible.

Patients with carcinomatosis especially when associated with bronchial carcinoma, may exhibit a marked sensitivity to this agent, and the neuromuscular block produced may respond poorly to neostigmine.

Interactions: The following drugs have been shown to influence the magnitude and/or duration of action of non-depolarising neuromuscular blocking agents:

Increased effect:

Anaesthetics: Halothane, ether, enflurane, isoflurane, methoxyflurane, cyclopropane, thiopentone, methohexital, ketamine, fentanyl, gammahydroxybutyrate, etomidate.

Other drugs: Other non-depolarising muscle relaxants, prior administration of succinylcholine, aminoglycoside and polypeptide antibiotics, diuretics, beta-adrenergic blocking agents, thiamine, M.A.O. inhibiting agents, quinidine, protamine, phenytoin, alpha-adrenergic, blocking agents, imidazoles, metronidazole, nitroglycerin, diazepam, magnesium sulphate, narcotic analgesics.

Decreased effect:

Anaesthetics: Neurolept analgesia, propanidid

Other drugs: Neostigmine, edrophonium, pyridostigmine, prior chronic administration of corticosteroids, noradrenaline, adrenalin, azathioprine, theophylline, KCl, NaCl, $CaCl_2$ heparin (temporary decrease).

Variable effect: Depolarising muscle relaxants given after the administration of Pavulon may produce potentiation or attenuation of the neuromuscular blocking effect.

The non-depolarising drug increases resistance towards the neuromuscular blocking effect of the depolarising drug. Therefore high doses of a depolarising drug are necessary before muscular relaxation can be obtained. These high doses of a depolarising drug may cause endplate desensitisation and prolong post-operative apnoea.

Unlike a non-depolarising block, a depolarising block cannot be overcome by, and may even by worsened by an anticholinesterase agent.

Influence on the cardiovascular system: Pavulon does not intensify the hypotension induced by halothane; in addition the cardiac depression is partly restored. The excessive bradycardia induced by neurolept analgesia and some of the cholinergic effects of morphine derivatives are counteracted by Pavulon.

Pavulon should be given with caution to a patient receiving chronic tricyclic antidepressant therapy who is anaesthetised with halothane or any inhalation anaesthetic, since this enhances the predisposition to the development of cardiac arrhythmias associated with tricyclic antidepressants.

Recent evidence suggests that alkylating drugs (nitrogen mustards) should be considered a possible hazard when given to patients during anaesthesia involving the use of muscle relaxants.

Side-effects: After Pavulon a slight to moderate rise in arterial pressure may occur. Increased pulse rate and cardiac output are frequently reported, showing Pavulon to have weak vagolytic activity. In general this is considered to be a favourable effect. Pavulon decreases intra-ocular pressure and induces miosis, both effects being favourable in ophthalmic surgery. A few cases of localised reactions at the site of injection have been reported. Although rare instances of bronchospasm have been reported, Pavulon has in general a lack of associated bronchospasm.

Overdosage: In the event of an overdosage i.e. a failure of neostigmine to reverse the neuromuscular block, the patient must continue to be ventilated. When administration of a cholinesterase inhibiting agent fails to reverse the neuromuscular blocking effects of Pavulon, ventilation must be continued until spontaneous breathing is restored. Repeated dosage of a cholinesterase inhibitor can be dangerous.

Pharmaceutical precautions In the pharmacy, Pavulon should be stored at 2–8°C and protected from light, when it will retain its stability for two years. Pavulon is stable for six weeks at 25°C.

Opened ampoules of Pavulon should be discarded if the contents are not used within a few hours.

Legal category POM.

Package quantities Boxes of 25 ampoules 2 ml.

Further information The active substance of Pavulon is pancuronium bromide, an amino steroid which effectively blocks transmission of motor nerve impulses to the striated muscle receptors. Endplate depolarisation does not occur. Pancuronium bromide has no hormonal activity. An initial dose of Pavulon of 80 micrograms/kg i.v. has a mean onset of action of 45 seconds, a maximum effect after 90–120 seconds, and a mean duration of action of 60 minutes (these data are approximations since, as is well-known, all muscle relaxants display dose-response variability). The potency ratio of Pavulon: d-tubocurarine is approximately 6–7 : 1.

Pavulon is accepted as one of the standard preparations in anaesthesia, and is widely used in all fields of surgery. It has a smooth onset of action, extremely low toxicity and the virtual absence of such side-effects as histamine release, and although rare instances of bronchospasm have been reported Pavulon has, in general, a lack of associated bronchospasm. There is a lack of ganglion blockade and thus no hypotensive effect, unlike some other muscle relaxants.

Pavulon is of considerable value when used in conjunction with halothane, since it helps to counteract the cardiovascular depression normally induced by halothane. Pavulon is particularly suitable for use in poor risk patients and in intensive-care units. Pavulon is used widely with good results in Caesarean section.

Product licence number 0065/5014R.

**Trade Mark*

Ortho Division of Cilag Limited
PO Box 79, Saunderton
High Wycombe
Buckinghamshire HP14 4HJ.

BINOVUM*

Presentation ¼-inch diameter, circular tablets with flat faces and bevelled edges. The 7 white tablets are engraved C over 535 on both faces and contain 500 micrograms Norethisterone PhEur and 35 micrograms Ethinyloestradiol PhEur. The 14 peach tablets are engraved C over 135 on both faces and contain 1 mg Norethisterone PhEur and 35 micrograms Ethinyloestradiol PhEur.

Uses Contraception and the recognised indications for such oestrogen/progestogen combinations.

Action: Through the mechanism of gonadotrophin suppression by the oestrogenic and progestational actions of the ingredients. Although the primary mechanism of action is inhibition of ovulation, alterations to the cervical mucus and to the endometrium may also contribute to the efficacy of the product.

Dosage and administration The basic dosage regimen is a 28 day cycle, of 1 tablet daily for 21 days, followed by 7 tablet-free days. A white tablet is taken every day for 7 days, then a peach coloured tablet is taken every day for 14 days. For initial therapy, the first white tablet is taken on the first day of bleeding of the menstrual cycle. If Binovum* Tablets are first taken later than the first day of bleeding of the first menstrual cycle of medication, contraceptive reliance should be not placed on this product until after the first 14 consecutive days of administration.

Subsequent cycles: Each subsequent course is started after 7 tablet-free days have followed the preceding course.

Changing from another combined oral contraceptive: The first white tablet should be taken on the first day of the withdrawal bleed after the completion of the previous course of tablets.

Changing from a progestogen-only contraceptive: The first white tablet should be taken on the first day of bleeding that occurs either during the last course of tablets or following completion of the tablet course.

Post-partum use: After pregnancy, oral contraception may be initiated immediately post-partum in the non-nursing patient or as soon as spontaneous menstruation has been resumed. Another method of contraception should be used in the interval between delivery and the first course of tablets, unless it is started within seven days of delivery. After a miscarriage or first-trimester abortion, oral contraception may be started immediately.

If the patient forgets more than one tablet, she should recommence the course as soon as she remembers, taking the appropriate tablet for that day and omitting any tablets delayed more than 12 hours. She should then use an additional method of contraception until the next withdrawal bleed. To obtain maximum contraceptive effectiveness, all contraceptive tablets should be taken exactly as directed and at approximately the same time each day.

If the patient has vomiting or diarrhoea, absorption of the hormones will be impaired, making it advisable to use an additional reliable method of contraception until her next menstrual period. Should a bleeding fail to occur at the usual time, the possibility of pregnancy should be excluded before starting the next pack.

Contra-indications, warnings, etc
Contraindications: Existing thrombophlebitis, thromboembolic disorders, cerebrovascular disease, myocardial infarction, or a past history of these conditions. Sickle-cell anaemia. Markedly impaired liver function. Congenital or existing disorders of lipid metabolism. Known or suspected carcinoma of the breast. Known or suspected oestrogen-dependent neoplasia. History during pregnancy of idiopathic jaundice, severe pruritus, shingles or deterioration of otosclerosis. Dubin-Johnson syndrome. Rotor syndrome. Undiagnosed abnormal genital tract bleeding. Known or suspected pregnancy.

Warnings: An increased risk of thrombophlebitis, cerebrovascular disorders, myocardial infarction and pulmonary embolism associated with the use of oral contraceptives has been reported in several retrospective case control studies. The increased risk has been estimated in these studies to be approximately 4 to 11 times higher (for cerebral haemorrhage two times higher) for users when compared to non users. This reported risk according to two of the studies is not related to duration of use nor does it persist after discontinuance according to one of the studies. An interim report of a large scale continuing prospective study has tended to confirm these retrospective studies for thrombophlebitis and possible cerebrovascular disorders. This study also reported that the risk of superficial and deep vein thrombosis was lower in women using preparations containing 50 micrograms of oestrogen or less. There may not be full recovery from such disorders and it should be realised that in a few cases they are fatal.

Because of a possible increased risk of post surgical thromboembolic complications in oral contraceptive users, therapy should be discontinued at least six weeks prior to elective surgery. Caution should be exercised in administering oestrogen/progestogen combinations to women with a history of hypertension. An increased risk of surgically confirmed gall bladder disease associated with the use of oral contraceptives has been reported in a retrospective case control study.

Malignant hepatic tumours have been reported on rare occasions in long-term users of oral contraceptives. Benign hepatic tumours have also been associated with oral contraceptive usage. A hepatic tumour should be considered in the differential diagnosis when upper abdominal pain, enlarged liver or signs of intra-abdominal haemorrhage occur.

A small fraction of the active ingredients in oral contraceptives has been identified in the milk of mothers receiving these drugs. The effects, if any, on the breast-fed child have not been determined. If possible the use of oral contraceptives should be deferred until the infant is weaned.

When women have taken hormones during pregnancy there have been some reports of the possibility of adverse effects on the developing child. A direct relationship between such effects and oral contraceptives has not been confirmed, but as with any other drug, avoidance of continuing oral contraception in early pregnancy is desirable. Therefore pregnancy should be ruled out before initiating or continuing the administration of oral contraceptives to patients who have missed one menstrual period.

Certain factors may entail some risk of thrombosis, e.g. smoking, obesity, varicose veins, cardiovascular diseases, diabetes, and migraine. The suitability of a combined oral contraceptive should be judged according to the severity of such conditions in the individual case, and should be discussed with the patient before she decides to take it. The risk of arterial thrombosis associated with combined oral contraceptives increases with age and this risk is aggravated by cigarette smoking. The use of combined oral contraceptives in women in the older age group, especially those who are cigarette smokers, should therefore be discouraged and alternative methods advised.

Reduced efficacy and increased incidence of breakthrough bleeding have been associated with concomitant use of oral contraceptives and rifampicin. A similar association has been suggested with oral contraceptives and barbiturates, phenytoin sodium, ampicillin, tetracycline and griseofulvin.

Numerous epidemiological studies have been reported on the risk of ovarian, endometrial, cervical and breast cancer in women using combined oral contraceptives. The evidence is clear that combined oral contraceptives offer substantial protection against ovarian and endometrial cancer.

An increased risk of cervical cancer in long-term users of combined oral contraceptives has been reported in some studies, but there continues to be controversy about the extent to which this is attributable to the confounding effects of sexual behaviour and other factors.

The evidence linking combined oral contraceptive use and breast cancer remains inconclusive. The results of some studies suggest an increased risk of breast cancer presenting below the age of about 35, the risk rising with duration of use. Any possible increased risk of breast cancer with combined oral contraceptives is, however, likely to be small, and may be expected to be less with low dosage pills. This possible risk should be weighed against the many benefits of combined oral contraceptives, including their protective effects against ovarian and endometrial cancers.

Reasons for stopping oral contraceptives immediately: Early manifestations of thrombotic or thromboembolic disorders, thrombophlebitis, cerebrovascular disorders (including haemorrhage), myocardial infarction, pulmonary embolism or retinal thrombosis. Hypertension. Gradual or sudden, partial or complete loss of vision. Proptosis or diplopia. Onset or aggravation of migraine or development of headaches of a new pattern which are recurrent, persistent or severe. Papilloedema or any evidence of retinal vascular lesions. During periods of immobility (e.g. after accidents). Pregnancy. Manifestations of liver tumours.

Precautions: Examination of the pelvic organs, breasts and blood pressure should precede the prescribing of any oral contraceptive, and should be repeated regularly.

The following are some of the conditions reported to be influenced by oral contraceptive therapy, and where the physician will have to exercise medical judgement to commence, continue or discontinue therapy as appropriate.

(a) Pre-existing uterine fibromyomata may increase in size.
(b) A decrease in glucose tolerance in a significant number of women.
(c) An increase in blood pressure in a small but significant number of women.
(d) Cholestatic jaundice. Patients with a history of cholestatic jaundice of pregnancy are more likely to develop cholestatic jaundice during oral contraceptive therapy.
(e) Amenorrhoea during and after oral contraceptive therapy. Women with a past history of oligomenorrhoea or secondary amenorrhoea or women with irregular cycles may be more likely to remain anovulatory or to become amenorrhoeic post oral contraceptive therapy.
(f) Depression.
(g) Fluid retention. Conditions which might be influenced by this factor include epilepsy, migraine, asthma, cardiac or renal dysfunction.
(h) Varicose veins.
(i) Multiple sclerosis.
(j) Porphyria.
(k) Tetany.
(l) Wearing of contact lenses.

or any condition that is prone to worsen during pregnancy.

The following laboratory determinations may be altered in patients using oral contraceptives:

Hepatic: Increased BSP retention and other tests.
Coagulation: Increased prothrombin, Factors VII, VIII, IX and X, decreased antithrombin III, increased platelet aggregability.
Endocrine: Increased PBI and butanol extractable protein bound iodine and decreased T3 uptake, increased glucose blood levels.
Other: Increased phospholipids and tri-glycerides, decreased serum folate values and disturbance in tryptophan metabolism, decreased pregnanediol excretion, reduced response to metyrapone test.

These tests usually return to pre-therapy values after discontinuing oral contraceptive use. However, the physician should be aware that these altered determinations may mask an underlying disease.

Side effects: Those most commonly reported in early cycles of oral contraceptive therapy include breakthrough bleeding, spotting, nausea, vomiting and other gastrointestinal disturbances. These frequently decrease with continued use. Other common side-effects include: change in menstrual flow, change in weight, oedema, chloasma (which may persist post therapy), amenorrhoea, breast changes (tenderness, enlargement and secretion).

In addition to the conditions and disorders discussed above, the following have been reported as adverse reactions in patients using combined oral contraceptives:

Neuro-ocular lesions	Haemorrhagic eruptions
Rash	Cystitis-like syndrome
Cervical erosion and secretions	Headache
Suppression of lactation	Nervousness
Pre-menstrual like syndrome	Fatigue
Changes in libido	Hirsutism
Leg cramp	Loss of scalp hair
Relative pyridoxine deficiency	Erythema multiforme
	Erythema nodosum
	Itching
	Vaginal candidiasis
	Porphyria

Overdosage: Serious ill effects have not been reported following acute ingestion of large doses of oral contraceptives by young children. Overdosage may cause nausea, and withdrawal bleeding may occur in females. An appropriate method of gastric emptying may be used if considered desirable.

Pharmaceutical precautions Protect from light.

Legal category POM.

Package quantities Carton containing 3 pushpaks each of 21 tablets – sufficient for 3 cycles.

Further information Nil.

Product licence number 0076/0090.

CILEST* 250/35 ORAL CONTRACEPTIVE TABLETS ▼

Presentation Cilest Oral Contraceptive tablets are dark blue $\frac{1}{4}$ inch diameter, circular tablets with flat faces and bevelled edges engraved C 250 on each face. Each tablet contains 0.25 mg Norgestimate and 35 micrograms Ethinyloestradiol EP.

Uses Contraception and the recognised indications for such oestrogen/progestogen combinations.

Action: Through the mechanism of gonadotrophin suppression by the oestrogenic and progestational actions of the ingredients.

Although the primary mechanism of action is inhibition of ovulation, alterations to the cervical mucus and to the endometrium may also contribute to the efficacy of the product.

Dosage and administration It is preferable that tablet intake from the first pack is started on the first day of menstruation in which case no extra contraceptive precautions are necessary.

If menstruation has already begun (that is 2, 3 or 4 days previously), tablet taking should commence on day 5 of the menstrual period. In this case additional contraceptive precautions must be taken for the first 7 days of tablet taking. (See further information for additional contraceptive precautions).

If menstruation began more than 5 days previously then the patient should be advised to wait until her next menstrual period before starting to take Cilest.

How to take Cilest: One tablet is taken daily at the same time (preferably in the evening) without interruption for 21 days, followed by a break of 7 tablet-free days. Each subsequent pack is started after the 7 tablet-free days have elapsed. Additional contraceptive precautions are not then required.

Use during pregnancy and breast feeding: Cilest is contra-indicated for use during pregnancy or suspected pregnancy and in mothers who are breast feeding.

Post-partum administration: Following childbirth, oral contraceptive administration to non-breast feeding mothers can be started 21–28 days post-partum, in which case no additional contraceptive precautions are required.

If intercourse has taken place post-partum, oral contraceptive use should be delayed until the first day of the first menstrual period. If post-partum administration of Cilest begins more than 28 days after delivery then additional contraceptive precautions are required for the first 7 days.

N.B. Mothers who are breast feeding should be advised not to use the pill since this may reduce the amount of breast-milk, but may be advised instead to use a progestogen-only pill (POP).

After miscarriage or abortion administration should start immediately in which case no additional contraceptive precautions are required.

Changing from a 21 day pill or another 22 day pill to Cilest: All tablets in the old pack should be finished. The first Cilest tablet is taken the next day i.e. no gap is left between taking tablets nor does the patient need to wait for her period to begin. Tablets should be taken as instructed in 'How to take Cilest'. Additional contraceptive precautions are not required. The patient will not have a period until the end of the first Cilest pack, but this is not harmful, nor does it matter if she experiences some bleeding on tablet-taking days.

Changing from a combined Every Day Pill (28 day tablets) to Cilest: Cilest should be started after taking the last active tablet from the 'Every Day Pill' pack (i.e. after taking 21 or 22 tablets). The first Cilest tablet is taken the next day i.e. no gap is left between taking tablets nor does the patient need to wait for her period to begin. Tablets should be taken as instructed in 'How to take Cilest'. Additional contraceptive precautions are not required. Remaining tablets from the Every Day (ED) pack should be discarded. The patient will not have a period until the end of the first Cilest pack, but this is not harmful, nor does it matter if she experiences some bleeding on tablet-taking days.

Changing from a Progestogen-only Pill (POP or Mini Pill) to Cilest: The first Cilest tablet should be taken on the first day of the period, even if the patient has already taken a mini pill on that day. Tablets should be taken as instructed in 'How to take Cilest'. Additional contraceptive precautions are not required. All the remaining progestogen-only pills in the mini pill pack should be discarded.

If the patient is taking a (mini) pill, then she may not always have a period, especially when she is breast feeding. The first Cilest tablet should be taken on the day *after* stopping the mini pill. All remaining pills in the mini pill packet must be discarded. Additional contraceptive precautions must be taken for the first 7 days.

To skip a period: To skip a period, a new pack of Cilest should be started on the day after finishing the current pack (the patient skips the tablet-free days). Tablet-taking should be continued in the usual way. During the use of the second pack she may experience slight spotting or break-through bleeding but contraceptive protection will not be diminished provided there are no tablet omissions.

The next pack of Cilest is started after the usual 7 tablet-free days, regardless of whether the period has completely finished or not.

Reduced reliability: The reliability of Cilest may be reduced under the following circumstances.

Forgotten tablets: For further advice on the above please see precautions and warnings.

Vomiting or diarrhoea: For further advice on the above, please see precautions and warnings.

Interactions: For further advice on the above, please see precautions and warnings.

Contra-indications, warnings, etc

Absolute contra-indications: Pregnancy or suspected pregnancy (that cannot yet be excluded) or breast feeding.

Circulatory disorders (cardiovascular or cerebrovascular) such as thrombophlebitis and thromboembolic processes (or a history of these conditions), moderate to severe hypertension, hyperlipoproteinaemia. In addition the presence of more than one of the risk factors for arterial disease which are discussed under 'Serious adverse reactions'.

Severe liver disease, cholestatic jaundice or hepatitis (viral or non-viral) or a history of these conditions if the results of liver function tests have failed to return to normal, and for 3 months after liver function tests have been found to be normal; a history of jaundice or pregnancy or jaundice due to the use of steroids, Rotor syndrome and Dubin-Johnson syndrome, hepatic cell tumours and porphyria.

Cholelithiasis.

Known or suspected oestrogen-dependent tumours, (see 'Serious Adverse Reactions'); endometrial hyperplasia; undiagnosed vaginal bleeding.

Systemic lupus erythematosus or a history of this condition.

A history during pregnancy or previous use of steroids for: severe pruritus; herpes gestationis; a manifestation or deterioration of otosclerosis.

Relative contra-indications: If any of the relative contra-indications listed below is present, the benefits of oestrogen/progestogen-containing preparations must be weighed against the possible risk for each individual case and the patient kept under close supervision. In case of aggravation or appearance of any of these conditions whilst the patient is taking the pill, its use should be discontinued.

- Conditions implicating an increasing risk of developing venous thrombo-embolic complications, e.g. severe varicose veins or prolonged immobilisation or major surgery (see Precautions and Warnings). Disorders of coagulation.
- Presence of any risk factor for arterial disease e.g. smoking, hyperlipidaemia or hypertension (see 'Serious Adverse Reactions').
- Other conditions associated with an increased risk of circulatory disease such as latent or overt cardiac failure, renal dysfunction, or a history of these conditions.
- Epilepsy or a history of this condition.
- Migraine or a history of this condition.
- A history of cholelithiasis.
- Presence of any risk factor for oestrogen-dependent tumours; oestrogen-sensitive gynaecological disorders such as uterine fibromyomota and endometriosis (see also under 'Serious Adverse Reactions').
- Diabetes mellitus.
- Severe depression or a history of this condition. If this

is accompanied by a disturbance in tryptophan metabolism, administration of vitamin B6 might be of therapeutic value.
- Sickle cell haemoglobinopathy, since under certain circumstances, e.g. during infections or anoxia, oestrogen-containing preparations may induce thromboembolic process in patients with this condition.
- If the results of liver function tests become abnormal, use should be discontinued.

Precautions and warnings
Reduced reliability: When Cilest is taken according to the directions for use the occurrence of pregnancy is highly unlikely. However, the reliability of oral contraceptives may be reduced under the following circumstances:

Forgotten tablets: If the patient forgets to take a tablet, she should take it as soon as she remembers and take the next one at the normal time. This may mean that 2 tablets are taken in one day. The rest of the pack should be taken as usual.

Provided she is *less than 12 hours late* in taking her tablet, Cilest will still give contraceptive protection during this cycle.

If she is *more than 12 hours late* in taking any tablet then she will not be protected for the next 7 days, the forgotten tablet should be skipped, and then she should take additional contraceptive precautions and follow the '7-day rule'. (See further information on 7 day rule).

If the patient has forgotten to take more than one tablet, she should stop taking the tablets, and use additional contraceptive precautions until the next menstrual period. If the next period fails to occur, a pregnancy test should be performed, and she should be advised to use additional contraceptive precautions before considering resuming use of Cilest.

Vomiting or diarrhoea: If after tablet intake vomiting or diarrhoea occurs, a tablet may not be absorbed properly by the body. If the symptoms disappear within 12 hours of tablet-taking, the patient should take an extra tablet from a spare pack and continue with the rest of the pack as usual.

However, if the symptoms continue beyond those 12 hours, additional contraceptive precautions are necessary for any sexual intercourse during the stomach or bowel upset and for the following 7 days (the patient must be advised to follow '7-day rule').

Change in bleeding pattern: If after taking Cilest for several months there is a sudden occurrence of spotting or break-through bleeding (not observed in previous cycles) or the absence of withdrawal bleeding, contraceptive effectiveness may be reduced. If withdrawal bleeding fails to occur and none of the above mentioned events has taken place, pregnancy is highly unlikely and oral contraceptive use can be continued until the end of the next pack.

(If withdrawal bleeding fails to occur at the end of the second cycle, tablet intake should be discontinued and pregnancy excluded before oral contraceptive use can be resumed.) However, if withdrawal bleeding is absent and any of the above mentioned events has occurred, tablet intake should be discontinued and pregnancy excluded before oral contraceptive use can be resumed.

Interactions: Irregular cycles and reduced reliability of oral contraceptives may occur when these preparations are used concomitantly with drugs such as anticonvulsants, barbiturates, antibiotics, (e.g. tetracyclines, ampicillin, rifampicin, etc.), griseofulvin, activated charcoal and certain laxatives. Special consideration should be given to patients being treated with antibiotics for acne. They should be advised to use a non-hormonal method of contraception, or to use an oral contraceptive containing a progestogen showing minimal androgenicity, which have been reported as helping to improve acne without using an antibiotic. Oral contraceptives may diminish glucose tolerance and increase the need for insulin or other antidiabetic drugs in diabetics.

Medical examination/consultation: A complete medical history and physical examination should be taken prior to the initiation or reinstitution of oral contraceptives and should be repeated periodically.

These physical examinations should include special reference to blood pressure, breasts, abdomen and pelvic organs, including cervical cytology and, where indicated by the medical or family history, relevant laboratory tests. Caution, should be observed when prescribing oral contraceptives to young women whose cycles are not yet stabilised.

Surgery, varicose veins or immobilisation: In patients using oestrogen-containing preparations the risk of deep vein thrombosis may be temporarily increased when undergoing a major operation (e.g. abdominal, orthopaedic), any surgery to the legs, medical treatment for varicose veins or prolonged immobilisation. Therefore, it is advisable to discontinue oral contraceptive use at least 4 to 6 weeks prior to these procedures if performed electively and to (re)start not less than 2 weeks after full ambulation. The latter is also valid with regard to immobilisation after an accident or emergency surgery. In case of emergency surgery, thrombotic prophylaxis is usually indicated e.g. with subcutaneous heparin.

Chloasma: Chloasma may occasionally occur, especially in women with a history of chloasma gravidarum. Women with a tendency to chloasma should avoid exposure to the sun or ultraviolet radiation whilst taking this preparation.

Laboratory tests: The use of steroids may influence the results of certain laboratory tests. In the literature, at least a hundred different parameters have been reported to possibly be influenced by oral contraceptive use, predominantly by the oestrogenic component. Among these are: biochemical parameters of the liver, thyroid, adrenal and renal function, plasma levels of (carrier) proteins and lipid/lipoprotein fractions and parameters of coagulation and fibrinolysis.

Adverse reactions: Various adverse reactions have been associated with oral contraceptive use. The serious reactions are dealt with in more detail. The first appearance of symptoms indicative of any one of these reactions necessitates immediate cessation of oral contraceptive use while appropriate diagnostic and therapeutic measures are undertaken.

Serious adverse reactions: Various reports have associated oral contraceptive use with the occurrence of deep venous thrombosis, pulmonary embolism and other embolisms. Other investigations of these oral contraceptives have suggested an increased risk of oestrogen and/ or progestogen dose-dependent coronary and cerebrovascular accidents, predominately in heavy smokers. Thrombosis has very rarely been reported to occur in other veins or arteries, e.g. hepatic, mesenteric, renal or retinal.

It should be noted that there is no consensus about the often contradictory findings obtained in early studies. The physician should bear in mind, the possibility of vascular accidents occurring and take into account the presence of risk factors for arterial disease and deep venous thrombosis when prescribing oral contraceptives. Risk factors for arterial disease include smoking, the presence of hyperlipidaemia, hypertension, or diabetes.

Signs and symptoms of a thrombotic event may include: sudden severe pain in the chest, whether or not reaching to the left arm; sudden breathlessness; any unusual severe, prolonged headache, especially if it occurs for the first time or gets progressively worse, or is associated with any of the following symptoms: sudden partial or complete loss of vision or diplopia, aphasia, vertigo, a bad fainting attack or collapse with or without focal epilepsy, weakness or very marked numbness suddenly affecting one side or one part of the body, motor disturbances; severe pain in the calf of one leg; acute abdomen.

Cigarette smoking increases the risk of serious cardiovascular adverse reactions to oral contraceptive use. The risk increases with age and with heavy smoking and is more marked in women over 35 years of age. Women who use oral contraceptives should be strongly advised not to smoke.

The use of oestrogen-containing oral contraceptives may promote growth of existing sex steroid dependent tumours. For this reason, the use of these oral contraceptives in patients with such tumours is contra-indicated. Numerous epidemiological studies have been reported on the risk of ovarian, endometrial, cervical and breast cancer in women using combined oral contraceptives.

The evidence is clear that combined oral contraceptives offer substantial protection against both ovarian and endometrial cancer. An increased risk of cervical cancer in long term users of combined oral contraceptives has been reported in some studies, but there continues to be controversy about the extent to which this is attributable to the confounding effects of sexual behaviour and other factors.

The evidence linking combined oral contraceptive use and breast cancer remains inconclusive. The results of some studies suggest an increased risk of breast cancer presenting below the age of about 35, the risk rising with duration of use. Any possible increased risk of breast cancer with combined oral contraceptives is however likely to be small, and may be expected to be less with low dose pills. This possible risk should be weighed against the many benefits of combined oral contraceptives, including their protective effects against ovarian and endometrial cancers.

Malignant hepatic tumours have been reported on rare occasions in long-term users of oral contraceptives. Benign hepatic tumours have also been associated with oral contraceptive usage. A hepatic tumour should be considered in the differential diagnosis when upper abdominal pain, enlarged liver or signs of intra-abdominal haemorrhage occur.

The use of oral contraceptives may sometimes lead to the development of cholestatic jaundice or cholelithiasis.

On rare occasions the use of oral contraceptives may trigger or reactivate systemic lupus erythematosus.

A further rare complication of oral contraceptive use is the occurrence of chorea which can be reversed by discontinuing the pill. The majority of cases of oral-contraceptive-induced chorea show a pre-existing predisposition which often relates to acute rheumatism.

Other adverse reactions: Cardiovascular system – rise of blood pressure. If hypertension develops, treatment should be discontinued.

Genital tract – intermenstrual bleeding, post-medication amenorrhoea, changes in cervical secretion, increase in size of uterine fibromyomata, aggravation of endometriosis, certain vaginal infections, e.g. candidiasis.

Breast – tenderness, pain, enlargement, secretion.

Gastro-intestinal tract – nausea, vomiting, cholelithiasis, cholestatic jaundice.

Skin – erythema nodosum, rash, chloasma.

Eyes – discomfort of the cornea if contact lenses are used.

CNS – headache, migraine, mood changes, depression.

Metabolic – fluid retention, change in body weight, reduced glucose tolerance.

Overdosage: There have been no reports of serious ill-health from overdosage even when a considerable number of tablets have been taken by a small child. In general, it is therefore unnecessary to treat overdosage. However, if overdosage is discovered within two or three hours and is large, then gastric lavage can be safely used. There are no antidotes and further treatment should be symptomatic.

Further information
Additional contraceptive precautions: When additional contraceptive precautions are required the patient should be advised either not to have sex, or to use a cap plus spermicide or for her partner to use a condom. Rhythm methods should not be advised as the pill disrupts the usual cyclical changes associated with the natural menstrual cycle e.g. changes in temperature and cervical mucus.

The 7-day rule
If any one tablet is forgotten for more than 12 hours:
If the patient has vomiting or diarrhoea for more than 12 hours:
If the patient is taking any of the drugs listed under 'Interactions':
The patient should continue to take her tablets as usual and additional contraceptive precautions must be taken for the next 7 days.

BUT – if these 7 days run beyond the end of the current pack, the next pack must be started as soon as the current one is finished, i.e. no gap should be left between packs. (This prevents an extended break in tablet taking which may increase the risk of the ovaries releasing an egg and thus reducing contraceptive protection.) The patient will not have a period until the end of 2 packs but this is not harmful nor does it matter if she experiences some bleeding on tablet taking days.

Pharmaceutical precautions Store in a cool, dry place and protect from light.

Legal category POM.

Package quantities Carton containing 3 push packs of 21 tablets – sufficient for 3 cycles.

Product licence number 0076/0134.

DELFEN* CONTRACEPTIVE FOAM

Presentation Delfen Contraceptive Foam is a white, non-staining aerosol foam which contains nonoxynol-9 12.5% w/w and buffered to normal vaginal pH of 4.5.

Uses Delfen Contraceptive Foam is a spermicidal foam for the control of conception. It provides rapid dispersion and extensive, uniform coverage of the cervix. A higher degree of protection against pregnancy will be afforded by using another method of contraception in addition to a spermicidal contraceptive. It is suitable for use with an occlusive device.

Dosage and administration One applicatorful intravaginally prior to coitus. A fresh application must be made if intercourse is repeated or delayed by more than one hour. If a douche is desired, it should be deferred for at least six hours after intercourse.

Contra-indications, warnings, etc Hypersensitivity to the product.

Warnings: Where avoidance of pregnancy is essential, the choice of contraceptive should be made in consultation with a doctor or a family planning clinic.

Side-effects: Irritation of the vagina or penis has been reported. In such cases the medication should be discontinued.

Overdosage: Delfen Contraceptive Foam is intended for intravaginal use only, and if taken orally by mistake is likely to taste unpleasant. If excess quantities are swallowed this may give rise to gastric irritation as the product contains a surfactant, and general supportive therapy should be carried out if necessary.

Pharmaceutical precautions Contents are under pressure. Do not burn or puncture container. Store at room temperature, not over 49°C (120°F).

Legal category GSL.

Package quantities 20 g aerosol container with the Delfen* Contraceptive Foam Applicator.

Further information Nil.

Product licence number 0076/5003.

GYNOL* II CONTRACEPTIVE JELLY

Presentation Gynol II Contraceptive Jelly is a clear, unscented, unflavoured water-dispersible spermicidal jelly which contains nonoxynol-9 2% w/w buffered to normal vaginal pH.

Uses Gynol II Contraceptive Jelly is a spermicidal jelly for use in conjunction with an occlusive vaginal diaphragm, whenever the control of conception is desirable.

A higher degree of protection against pregnancy will

be afforded by using another method of contraception in addition to a spermicidal contraceptive.

Dosage and administration The jelly should be spread over the surface of the diaphragm which will be in contact with the cervix and on the rim. The diaphragm must be allowed to remain in situ for at least six to eight hours after coitus. A fresh application of jelly or other spermicides, e.g. Orthoforms* Contraceptive Pessaries, must be made prior to any subsequent act of coitus within this period of time, without removing the diaphragm. (A vaginal applicator should be used for inserting more cream or jelly.)

Contra-indications, warnings, etc
Contra-indications: Hypersensitivity to the product.

Warnings: Where avoidance of pregnancy is essential, the choice of contraceptive should be made in consultation with a doctor or family planning clinic.

Occasional irritation of the vagina or penis has been reported. In such cases the medication should be discontinued.

The diaphragm should not remain in position for longer than 24 hours.

Overdosage: Gynol II Contraceptive Jelly is intended for intravaginal use only. If excess quantities are taken orally by mistake this may give rise to gastric irritation as the product contains a surfactant, and general supportive therapy should be carried out if necessary.

Pharmaceutical precautions None known.

Legal category GSL.

Package quantities Tube containing 81 g. Also tube containing 30 g with applicator. Ortho* Vaginal Applicator available separately.

Further information Nil.

Product licence number 0076/0127.

MICRONOR* ORAL CONTRACEPTIVE TABLETS

Presentation White, $\frac{1}{4}$ inch diameter, circular tablets with flat faces and bevelled edges, bearing on each face the engraving C over 035. Micronor Oral Contraceptive Tablets each contain 350 micrograms Norethisterone PhEur.

Uses Contraception.

Action: Micronor has a progestational effect on the endometrium and on the cervical mucus. The exact mechanism of how it prevents conception has not been confirmed.

Dosage and administration Micronor is administered orally on a continuous daily dosage regimen starting on the first day of menstruation. One tablet is taken at the same time each day, every day of the year, whether menstruation occurs or not. When starting Micronor therapy the patient should be instructed to use an additional reliable non-hormonal method of contraception during the first 14 days of the first cycle.

The non-nursing patient may be prescribed Micronor in the post partum period whether or not menstruation has resumed provided the possibility of pregnancy has been excluded.

The possibility of ovulation and conception prior to initiation of medication should be considered.

Strict adherence to the dosage regimen is important. If the patient should fail to take 1 tablet at the usual time protection is reduced. She should take the missed tablet as soon as she remembers and take the next tablet on the day it is due. When a tablet is missed an additional reliable means of contraception should be used in addition to taking Micronor until her next period occurs.

If the patient does not have a period within 45 days of her last period, pregnancy should be excluded.

If the patient has vomiting or diarrhoea, absorption of the hormone will be impaired, making it advisable to use an additional reliable method of contraception until the next menstrual period.

Contra-indications, warnings, etc Any of the following conditions should be regarded as contra-indications for the use of Micronor. Existing thrombophlebitis, thromboembolic disorders, cerebral vascular disease, myocardial infarction, or a past history of these conditions. Markedly impaired liver function. Known or suspected hormone dependent neoplasia. Known or suspected carcinoma of the breast. Undiagnosed abnormal genital tract bleeding. Known or suspected pregnancy.

Warnings: Because of a possible increased risk of post surgery thromboembolic complications in oral contraceptive users, therapy should be discontinued six weeks prior to elective surgery.

Masculinisation of the female foetus has occurred when progestogens have been used in pregnant women, although this has been observed at doses much higher than that contained in Micronor. Pregnancy should be ruled out before continuing administration of Micronor to patients who have gone 45 days without a menstrual period.

A small fraction of the active ingredients in oral contraceptives has been identified in the milk of mothers receiving these drugs. The effects, if any, on the breast-fed child have not been determined. If possible the use of oral contraceptives should be deferred until the infant is weaned.

Malignant hepatic tumours have been reported on rare occasions in long-term users of oral contraceptives. Benign hepatic tumours have also been associated with oral contraceptive usage. A hepatic tumour should be considered in the differential diagnosis when upper abdominal pain, enlarged liver or signs of intra-abdominal haemorrhage occur.

Reduced efficacy and increased incidence of breakthrough bleeding have been associated with concomitant use of oral contraceptives and rifampicin. A similar association has been suggested with oral contraceptives and barbiturates, phenytoin sodium, ampicillin, tetracycline and griseofulvin.

Reasons for stopping oral contraceptives immediately: Early manifestations of thrombotic or thromboembolic disorders, thrombophlebitis, cerebrovascular disorders (including haemorrhage), myocardial infarction, pulmonary embolism. Gradual or sudden, partial or complete loss of vision. Proptosis or diplopia. Onset or aggravation of migraine or development of headaches of a new pattern which are recurrent, persistent or severe. Papilloedema or any evidence of retinal vascular lesions. During periods of immobility (e.g. after accidents). Pregnancy. Manifestations of liver tumours.

Precautions: Examination of the pelvic organs, breasts and blood pressure should precede the prescribing of any oral contraceptive, and should be repeated regularly. The following are some of the medical conditions reported to be influenced by the combined pill, and may be affected by Micronor. The physician will have to exercise medical judgement to commence, continue or discontinue therapy as appropriate.

a) Pre-existing uterine fibromyomata may increase in size.

b) A decrease in glucose tolerance in a significant number of women.

c) An increase in blood pressure in a small but significant number of women.

d) Cholestatic jaundice. Patients with a history of cholestatic jaundice of pregnancy are more likely to develop cholestatic jaundice during oral contraceptive therapy.

e) Amenorrhoea during and after oral contraceptive therapy. Women with a past history of oligomenorrhoea or secondary amenorrhoea or women with irregular cycles may be more likely to remain anovulatory or to become amenorrhoeic post oral contraceptive therapy.

f) Depression.

g) Fluid retention. Conditions which might be influenced by this factor include epilepsy, migraine, asthma, cardiac or renal dysfunction.

h) Varicose veins.
i) Multiple sclerosis.
j) Porphyria.
k) Tetany.
l) Wearing of contact lenses.

or any condition that is prone to worsen during pregnancy.

The following laboratory determinations may be altered in patients using oral contraceptives.

Hepatic: Increased BSP retention and other tests.

Coagulation: Increased prothrombin, Factors VII, VIII, IX and X, decreased antithrombin III, increased platelet aggregability.

Endocrine: Increased PBI and butanol extractable protein bound iodine and decreased T3 uptake, increased glucose blood levels.

Other: Increased phospholipids and tri-glycerides, decreased serum folate values and disturbance in tryptophan metabolism, decreased pregnanediol excretion, reduced response to metyrapone test.

These tests usually return to pre-therapy values after discontinuing oral contraceptive use. However, the physician should be aware that these altered determinations may mask an underlying disease.

Side-effects: Micronor has been found to be a well tolerated drug. Side-effects are usually self-limiting and of relatively short duration. Amongst the symptoms reported are headaches, nausea, vomiting, breast changes, change in weight, chloasma, break-through bleeding and spotting. Particularly in the early cycles of therapy the menstrual pattern becomes irregular, some cycles being short and others long. It is important that patients should be advised that whilst on Micronor therapy they will experience that variation in cycle length.

Overdosage: Serious ill effects have not been reported following acute ingestion of large doses of oral contraceptives by young children. Overdosage may cause nausea, and withdrawal bleeding may occur in females. An appropriate method of gastric emptying may be used if considered desirable.

Pharmaceutical precautions Protect from light.

Legal category POM.

Package quantities Carton containing 3 pushpaks each of 28 tablets – sufficient for 3 cycles.

Further information Nil.

Product licence number 0076/0017.

NEOCON* 1/35 ORAL CONTRACEPTIVE TABLETS

Presentation Peach coloured $\frac{1}{4}$ inch diameter, circular tablets with flat faces and bevelled edges, bearing the engraving C over 135 on each face. Each tablet contains 1 mg Norethisterone PhEur and 35 micrograms Ethinyloestradiol PhEur.

Uses Contraception and the recognised indications for such oestrogen/progestogen combinations.

Action: Through the mechanism of gonadotrophin suppression by the oestrogenic and progestational actions of the ingredients. Although the primary mechanism of action is inhibition of ovulation, alteration to the cervical mucus and to the endometrium may also contribute to the efficacy of the product.

Dosage and administration The basic dosage regimen is a 28-day cycle of 1 tablet daily for 21 days followed by seven tablet-free days. For initial therapy the first tablet is taken on the fifth day of the menstrual cycle, counting the first day of bleeding as Day 1. Each subsequent course is started after seven tablet-free days have followed the preceding course. To obtain maximal contraceptive effectiveness, all contraceptive tablets should be taken exactly as directed and at approximately the same time each day. Contraception can be initiated immediately post partum in the non-nursing patient. The possibility of ovulation and conception prior to initiation of medication should be considered.

The patient should be advised that during the first 14 days of the first course an additional reliable non-hormonal form of contraception should be used. If the patient misses more than 1 tablet, she should begin taking tablets again as soon as remembered and an additional reliable method of contraception used until the next withdrawal bleed. If the patient has vomiting or diarrhoea, absorption of the hormones will be impaired, making it advisable to use an additional reliable method of contraception until her next menstrual period. Should a bleeding fail to occur at the usual time, the possibility of pregnancy should be excluded before starting the next pack.

Contra-indications, warnings, etc Existing thrombophlebitis, thromboembolic disorders, cerebral vascular disease, myocardial infarction, or a past history of these conditions. Sickle-cell anaemia. Markedly impaired liver function. Congenital or existing disorders of lipid metabolism. Known or suspected carcinoma of the breast. Known or suspected oestrogen-dependent neoplasia. History during pregnancy of idiopathic jaundice, severe pruritus, shingles or deterioration of otosclerosis. Dubin-Johnson syndrome. Rotor Syndrome. Undiagnosed abnormal genital tract bleeding. Known or suspected pregnancy.

Warnings: An increased risk of thrombophlebitis, cerebrovascular disorders, myocardial infarction and pulmonary embolism associated with the use of oral contraceptives has been reported in several retrospective case control studies. The increased risk has been estimated in these studies to be approximately 4 to 11 times higher (for cerebral haemorrhage two times higher) for users when compared to non users. This reported risk according to two of the studies is not related to duration of use nor does it persist after discontinuance according to one of the studies. An interim report of a large scale continuing prospective study has tended to confirm these retrospective studies for thrombophlebitis and possible cerebrovascular disorders. This study also reported that the risk of superficial and deep vein thrombosis was lower in women using preparations containing 50 micrograms of oestrogen or less. There may not be full recovery from such disorders and it should be realised that in a few cases they are fatal.

Because of a possible increased risk of post surgery thromboembolic complications in oral contraceptive users, therapy should be discontinued at least six weeks prior to elective surgery. Caution should be exercised in administering oestrogen/progestogen combinations to women with a history of hypertension. An increased risk of surgically confirmed gall bladder disease associated with the use of oral contraceptives has been reported in a retrospective case control study.

Malignant hepatic tumours have been reported on rare occasions in long-term users of oral contraceptives. Benign hepatic tumours have also been associated with oral contraceptive usage. A hepatic tumour should be considered in the differential diagnosis when upper abdominal pain, enlarged liver or signs of intra-abdominal haemorrhage occur.

A small fraction of the active ingredients in oral contraceptives has been identified in the milk of mothers receiving these drugs. The effects, if any, on the breast-fed child have not been determined. If possible the use of oral contraceptives should be deferred until the infant is weaned.

When women have taken hormones during pregnancy there have been some reports of the possibility of adverse effects on the developing child. A direct relationship between such effects and oral contraceptives has not been confirmed, but as with any other drug, avoidance of continuing oral contraception in early pregnancy is desirable. Therefore pregnancy should be ruled out before initiating or continuing the administration of oral contraceptives to patients who have missed one menstrual period.

Certain factors may entail some risk of thrombosis, eg

smoking, obesity, varicose veins, caridovascular diseases, diabetes, and migraine. The suitability of a combined oral contraceptive should be judged according to the severity of such conditions in the individual case, and should be discussed with the patient before she decides to take it. The risk of arterial thrombosis associated with combined oral contraceptives increases with age and this risk is aggravated by cigarette smoking. The use of combined oral contraceptives in women in the older age group, especially those who are cigarette smokers, should therefore be discouraged and alternative methods advised.

Reduced efficacy and increased incidence of breakthrough bleeding have been associated with concomitant use of oral contraceptives and rifampicin. A similar association has been suggested with oral contraceptives and barbiturates, phenytoin sodium, ampicillin, tetracycline and griseofulvin.

Numerous epidemiological studies have been reported on the risk of ovarian, endometrial, cervical and breast cancer in women using combined oral contraceptives. The evidence is clear that combined oral contraceptives offer substantial protection against ovarian and endometrial cancer.

An increased risk of cervical cancer in long-term users of combined oral contraceptives has been reported in some studies, but there continues to be controversy about the extent to which this is attributable to the confounding effects of sexual behaviour and other factors.

The evidence linking combined oral contraceptive use and breast cancer remains inconclusive. The results of some studies suggest an increased risk of breast cancer presenting below the age of about 35, the risk rising with duration of use. Any possible increased risk of breast cancer with combined oral contraceptives is, however, likely to be small, and may be expected to be less with low dosage pills. This possible risk should be weighed against the many benefits of combined oral contraceptives, including their protective effects against ovarian and endometrial cancers.

Reasons for stopping oral contraception immediately: Early manifestation of thrombotic or thromboembolic disorders, thrombophlebitis, cerebrovascular disorders (including haemorrhage), myocardial infarction, pulmonary embolism or retinal thrombosis. Hypertension. Gradual or sudden, partial or complete loss of vision. Proptosis or diplopia. Onset or aggravation of migraine or development of headaches of a new pattern which are recurrent, persistent or severe. Papilloedema or any evidence of retinal vascular lesions. During periods of immobility (eg. after accidents). Pregnancy. Manifestations of liver tumours.

Precautions: Examination of the pelvic organs, breasts and blood pressure should precede the prescribing of any oral contraceptive, and should be repeated regularly. The following are some of the conditions reported to be influenced by oral contraceptive therapy, and where the physician will have to exercise medical judgement to commence, continue or discontinue therapy as appropriate.

a) Pre-existing uterine fibromyomata may increase in size.
b) A decrease in glucose tolerance in a significant number of women.
c) An increase in blood pressure in a small but significant number of women.
d) Cholestatic jaundice. Patients with a history of cholestatic jaundice of pregnancy are more likely to develop cholestatic jaundice during oral contraceptive therapy.
e) Amenorrhoea during and after oral contraceptive therapy. Women with a past history of oligomenorrhoea or secondary amenorrhoea or women with irregular cycles may be more likely to remain anovulatory or to become amenorrhoeic post oral contraceptive therapy.
f) Depression.
g) Fluid retention. Conditions which might be influenced by this factor including epilepsy, migraine, asthma, cardiac or renal dysfunction.
h) Varicose veins.
i) Multiple sclerosis.
j) Porphyria.
k) Tetany.
l) Wearing of contact lenses

or any condition that is prone to worsen during pregnancy.

The following laboratory determinations may be altered in patients using oral contraceptives:

Hepatic: Increased BSP retention and other tests.
Coagulation: Increased prothrombin, Factors VII, VIII, IX and X; decreased antithrombin III; increased platelet aggregability.
Endocrine: Increased PBI and butanol extractable protein bound iodine and decreased T3 uptake, increased glucose blood levels.
Other: Increased phospholipids and tri-glycerides, decreased serum folate values and disturbance in tryptophan metabolism. Decreased pregnanediol excretion, reduced response to metyrapone test.

These tests usually return to pre-therapy values after discontinuing oral contraceptive use. However, the physician should be aware that these altered determinations may mask an underlying disease.

Side-effects: Side-effects most commonly reported in early cycles of oral contraceptive therapy include breakthrough bleeding, spotting, nausea, vomiting and other gastrointestinal disturbances. These frequently decrease with continued use. Other common side-effects include: change in menstrual flow, change in weight, oedema, chloasma (which may persist post therapy), amenorrhoea, breast changes (tenderness, enlargement and secretion).

In addition to the conditions and disorders discussed above, the following have been reported as adverse reactions in patients using combined oral contraceptives:

Neuro-ocular lesions	Haemorrhagic eruptions
Rash	Cystitis-like syndrome
Cervical erosion and secretions	Headache
Suppression of lactation	Nervousness
Pre-menstrual like syndrome	Fatigue
Changes in libido	Hirsutism
Leg cramp	Loss of scalp hair
Relative pyridoxine deficiency	Erythema multiforme
	Erythema nodosum
	Itching
	Vaginal candidiasis
	Porphyria

Overdosage: Serious ill effects have not been reported following acute ingestion of large doses of oral contraceptives by young children. Overdosage may cause nausea, and withdrawal bleeding may occur in females. An appropriate method of gastric emptying may be used if considered desirable.

Pharmaceutical precautions Protect from light.

Legal category POM.

Package quantities Carton containing 3 pushpaks each of 21 tablets – sufficient for 3 cycles.

Further information Nil.

Product licence number 0076/0054.

ORTHO-CREME* CONTRACEPTIVE CREAM

Presentation Ortho-Creme Contraceptive Cream is a white spermicidal cream which contains nonoxynol-9 2.0% w/w, buffered to normal vaginal pH.

Uses Ortho-Creme Contraceptive Cream is a spermicidal cream for use in conjunction with an occlusive vaginal diaphragm, whenever the control of conception is desirable. A higher degree of protection against pregnancy will be afforded by using another method of contraception in addition to a spermicidal contraceptive.

Dosage and administration The cream should be spread over the surface of the diaphragm which will be in contact with the cervix, and on the rim. The diaphragm, and spermicide must be allowed to remain undisturbed for at least six to eight hours after coitus. A fresh application of cream or other spermicides, e.g. Orthoforms Contraceptive Pessaries, must be made prior to any subsequent act of coitus within this period of time, without removing the diaphragm. (A vaginal applicator should be used for inserting more cream or jelly.)

Douching is not recommended; but if it is desired it should be deferred for at least six hours after intercourse.

Contra-indications, warnings, etc Hypersensitivity to the product.

Warning: Where avoidance of pregnancy is essential, the choice of contraceptive should be made in consultation with a doctor or a family planning clinic.

Occasional irritation of the vagina or penis has been reported. In such cases the medication should be discontinued.

The diaphragm should not remain in position for longer than 24 hours.

Overdosage: Ortho-Creme Contraceptive Cream is intended for intravaginal use only, and if taken orally by mistake is likely to taste unpleasant. If excess quantities are swallowed, this may give rise to gastric irritation as the product contains a surfactant, and general supportive therapy should be carried out if necessary.

Pharmaceutical precautions None known.

Legal category GSL.

Package quantities Tubes containing 70 g.
Ortho Plastic Vaginal Applicator available separately.

Further information Nil.

Product licence number 0076/5008.

ORTHO* DIENOESTROL CREAM

Presentation A white non-staining cream containing 0.01% w/w Dienoestrol PhEur.

Uses For intravaginal use only. Indicated in the treatment of atrophic vaginitis and kraurosis vulvae in post menopausal women, and for the treatment of pruritus vulvae and dyspareunia when associated with the atrophic vaginal epithelium.

Dosage and administration Given for short term use only. The lowest dose that will control symptoms should be chosen and medication should be discontinued as promptly as possible.

Attempts to discontinue or taper medication should be made at three to six month intervals, following physical examination. The usual dosage range is one or two applicatorfuls per day for one or two weeks, then gradually reduced to one half initial dosage for a similar period. A maintenance dose of one applicatorful, one to three times a week, may be used after restoration of the vaginal mucosa has been achieved. If the treatment is continued, treated patients with an intact uterus should be monitored closely for signs of endometrial cancer and appropriate diagnostic measures should be taken to rule out malignancy in the event of persistent or recurring abnormal vaginal bleeding.

Studies of the addition of a progestin for seven or more days of a cycle of oestrogen administration have reported a lowered incidence of endometrial hyperplasia. Morphological and biochemical studies of endometrium suggest that 10 to 13 days of progestin are needed to provide maximal maturation of the endometrium and to eliminate any hyperplastic changes. In women with an intact uterus the addition of a progestogen is essential. There are possible additional risks which may be associated with the inclusion of progestin in oestrogen replacement regimens. The potential risks include adverse effects on carbohydrate and lipid metabolism.

As a general rule it is advisable that patients receiving any form of oestrogen replacement therapy should have a complete physical examination at least once a year.

Contra-indications, warnings, etc Pregnancy is an absolute contra-indication to the use of Dienoestrol cream since it may be harmful to the developing foetus.

Oestrogens should not be used in women with any of the other following conditions: known or suspected oestrogen-dependent neoplasia; endometrial hyperplasia; uterine fibromyomata; undiagnosed abnormal genital bleeding; cardiovascular disorders, e.g., thrombophlebitis, thrombosis or thromboembolic disorders; severe liver disease; porphyria.

Thromboembolic disorders: While an increased rate of thromboembolic and thrombotic disease in post-menopausal users of oestrogen has not been found this does not rule out the possibility that such an increase may be present or that subgroups of women who have underlying risk factors or who are receiving relatively large doses of oestrogen may have increased risk. Therefore oestrogens should not be used in persons with active thrombophlebitis or thromboembolic disorders, and they should not be used (except in treatment of malignancy) in persons with a history of such disorders. If any signs of thrombosis develop, whether cardiovascular or cerebrovascular, in patients receiving oestrogen, discontinue treatment. Oestrogen treatment should be stopped before surgery in order to decrease the risk of deep vein thrombosis.

Prolonged exposure to unopposed oestrogen may increase the risk of development of endometrial carcinoma, induction of other malignant neoplasms, and the risk of cancer of the breast: long term continuous administration of natural and synthetic oestrogens in certain animal species increases the frequency of carcinomas of the breast, cervix, vagina and liver. There is now evidence that oestrogens increase the risk of carcinoma of the endometrium in humans. At the present time there is no satisfactory evidence that oestrogens given to post-menopausal women increase the risk of cancer of the breast, although a recent long-term follow up of a single physician has raised this possibility. However, because of animal data there is a need for caution in prescribing oestrogens for women with a strong family history of breast cancer or who have breast nodules, fibrocystic disease, or abnormal mammograms.

Gall bladder disease: A recent study has reported a two to three-fold increase in the risk of surgically confirmed gall bladder disease in women receiving post-menopausal oestrogens, similar to the two-fold increase previously noted in users of oral contraceptives.

Hepatic adenoma: Benign hepatic adenomas appear to be associated with the use of oral contraceptives. Although benign, and rare, these may rupture and may cause death through intra-abdominal haemorrhage. Such lesions have not yet been reported in association with other oestrogen or progestogen preparations but should be considered in oestrogen users having abdominal pain and tenderness, abdominal mass, or hypovolemic shock.

Elevated blood pressure: It has been reported that this may occur with the use of oestrogens in the menopause and blood pressure should be monitored with oestrogen use, especially if high doses are used. Treatment should be discontinued with emergent or increasing hypertension.

Precautions: A complete medical and family history should be taken prior to the initiation of any oestrogen therapy. The pretreatment and periodic physical examinations should include special reference to blood pressure, breasts, abdomen, and pelvic organs, and should include a Papanicolaou smear.

A pathologist should be advised of oestrogen therapy when relevant specimens are submitted. Certain endocrine and liver function tests may be affected by oestrogen containing products. These are:

Increased B.S.P. retention
Increased prothrombin and factors VII, VIII, IX, and X; decreased antithrombin 3, increased norepinephrine-induced platelet aggregability

Impaired glucose tolerance.
Increased thyroid binding globulin (TBG) leading to increased circulating total thyroid hormone, as measured by PBI, T4 by column or T4 by RIA. Free T3 resin uptake is decreased, reflecting the elevated TRG; free T4 is unaltered
Decreased pregnanediol excretion
Reduced response to metyrapone
Reduced serum folate concentration
Increased serum triglyceride and phospholipid concentration

Certain patients may develop undesirable manifestations of excessive oestrogenic stimulations, such as abnormal or excessive uterine bleeding, mastodynia, etc. Pre-existing uterine fibroids may increase in size during oestrogen use.

Patients with a past history of jaundice during pregnancy have an increased risk of recurrence of jaundice while receiving oestrogen. The medication should be discontinued while the cause is investigated.

Oestrogens may cause fluid retention. Conditions possibly affected by this factor such as epilepsy, migraine and cardiac or renal dysfunction require careful monitoring.

Oestrogens should be used with caution in patients with:

Metabolic bone diseases that are associated with hypercalcaemia
Impaired liver function
A history of mental depression
Diabetes
Contact lenses.

Oestrogens should be used judiciously in patients in whom bone growth is not complete.

Ortho Dienoestrol is generally well tolerated. There have been occasional reports of burning, itching and irritation. The doctor should also be aware of those adverse reactions reported to occur with systemic administration of oestrogens.

Genito-urinary tract: intermenstrual bleeding, increase in the size of uterine fibromyomata, change in amount of cervical secretion.

Breast: tenderness, enlargement, secretion.

Gastrointestinal tract: nausea, vomiting, cholestatic jaundice.

Skin: erythema nodosum, rash, chloasma.

Eyes: corneal discomfort if contact lenses are used.

CNS: headache, migraine, mood changes.

Metabolic: reduced glucose tolerance and changes in body weight.

Other events normally associated with the use of oral contraceptives may result from prolonged use of unopposed oestrogens.

Overdosage: Ortho Dienoestrol Cream is intended for intravaginal use. If accidental ingestion of large quantities of the product occurs, an appropriate method of gastric emptying may be used if considered desirable. Overdosage may cause nausea, and in females withdrawal bleeding may occur.

Pharmaceutical precautions Store at room temperature.

Legal category POM.

Package quantities Tube containing 78 g with the Ortho* Plastic Vaginal Applicator.

Further information Nil.

Product licence number 0076/5010R.

ORTHOFORMS* CONTRACEPTIVE PESSARIES

Presentation White, opaque pessaries. Each pessary contains nonoxynol-9 5% w/w.

Uses Whenever the control of conception is desired. Placed in the vagina, the pessary melts and rapidly forms a smooth emollient cream which spreads, mixing intimately with secretions and seminal fluid. Orthoforms Contraceptive Pessaries melt rapidly between 34°C and 37°C – the normal vaginal temperature range.

Orthoforms Contraceptive Pessaries are intended to add reliability to the use of other methods, such as the diaphragm, the sheath, the cervical cap, the IUCD, or when intercourse is repeated without removing the appliance.

A higher degree of protection against pregnancy will be afforded by using another method of contraception in addition to a spermicidal contraceptive.

Dosage and administration The Orthoforms Contraceptive Pessary should be inserted as high as possible into the vagina approximately 5 minutes before intercourse to permit the pessary to melt. It retains its spermicidal activity for approximately 1 hour. Any subsequent acts of intercourse should not be undertaken before the insertion of an additional pessary.

Contra-indications, warnings, etc Hypersensitivity to the product.

Side-effects: Irritation of the vagina or penis has been reported. In such cases the medication should be discontinued.

Warnings: Where avoidance of pregnancy is essential the choice of contraceptive should be made in consultation with a doctor or a family planning clinic.

Overdosage: Orthoforms Contraceptive Pessaries are intended for intravaginal use only, and if taken orally by mistake are likely to taste unpleasant. If excess quantities are swallowed this may give rise to gastric irritation as the product contains a surfactant, and general supportive therapy should be carried out if necessary.

Pharmaceutical precautions Orthoforms Contraceptive Pessaries should be stored in a cool place.

Legal category GSL.

Package quantities Pack of 15 pessaries.

Further information Nil.

Product licence number 0076/5006.

ORTHO-GYNEST* CREAM AND PESSARIES

Presentation Cream: White to faint yellowish cream with fat like odour containing 0.01% w/w oestriol. Pessaries: White pessaries each containing 0.5 mg oestriol and melting at 37°C.

Uses Oestriol is a naturally occurring oestrogen which exerts specific actions on the vulva, vagina and cervix.

Ortho-Gynest Cream and Pessaries are indicated for the treatment of atrophic vaginitis and kraurosis vulvae in post menopausal women, and for the treatment of pruritus vulvae and dyspareunia when associated with atrophic vaginal epithelium.

For intravaginal use only.

Dosage and administration The lowest dose that will control symptoms should be chosen and medication should be discontinued as promptly as possible. Attempts to taper and discontinue medication should be made at three to six month intervals following initiation of therapy and in conjunction with physical examination.

The recommended initial daily dose is one applicatorful or one pessary inserted high into the vagina, preferably in the evening.

A maintenance dose of one applicatorful or one pessary twice a week may be used after restoration of the vaginal mucosa has been achieved.

Contra-indications, warnings, etc Prolonged exposure to unopposed oestrogens may increase the risk of development of endometrial carcinoma. Although publications indicate that oestriol may occupy a somewhat different position with respect to mammary and endometrial carcinomas than other oestrogens, contra-indications for treatment with Ortho-Gynest Cream and

Pessaries should be the same as for other oestrogen products.

Oestrogens should not be used in women with any of the following conditions: known or suspected cancer of the breast, known or suspected oestrogen-dependent neoplasia, undiagnosed abnormal genital bleeding, active thrombophlebitis or thromboembolic disorders, a past history of thrombophlebitis, thrombosis or thromboembolic disorders. Markedly impaired liver function. Congenital or existing disorders of lipid metabolism. History during pregnancy of idiopathic jaundice, severe pruritus, herpes gestationis or otosclerosis. Dubin-Johnson syndrome. Rotor syndrome.

Ortho-Gynest Cream and Pessaries are contra-indicated in pregnancy; therapy should be discontinued immediately pregnancy is suspected.

An increased risk of gall-bladder disease has been reported in women receiving post-menopausal oestrogens, similar to the increase noted in users of oral contraceptives.

Benign hepatic adenomas appear to be associated with the use of oral contraceptives and although rare, these may rupture and cause death, through intra-abdominal haemorrhage. Such lesions have not yet been reported in association with other oestrogen or progestogen preparations but should be considered in oestrogen users having abdominal pain and tenderness, abdominal mass or hypovolemic shock.

It has been reported that elevated blood pressure may occur with the use of oestrogens in menopausal women and blood pressure should be monitored with oestrogen use.

Precautions: A complete medical and family history should be taken prior to the initiation of any oestrogen therapy. The pre-treatment and periodic physical examinations should include special reference to blood pressure, breasts, abdomen, and pelvic organs and should include a Papanicolaou smear.

A pathologist should be advised of oestrogen therapy when relevant specimens are submitted.

Certain patients may develop undesirable manifestations of excessive oestrogenic stimulation such as abnormal or excessive uterine bleeding, mastodynia etc. Bleeding occurring during therapy should be investigated to exclude serious concomitant pathology. Pre-existing uterine fibroids may increase in size during oestrogen use.

Oestrogen may aggravate cases of porphyria.

Patients with a past history of jaundice during pregnancy have an increased risk of recurrence of jaundice while receiving oestrogen therapy. If jaundice develops in any patient receiving oestrogen, the medication should be discontinued while the cause is investigated.

Overdosage: Ortho-Gynest Cream and Pessaries are intended for intravaginal use. If accidental ingestion of large quantities of the product occurs, an appropriate method of gastric emptying may be used if considered desirable.

Pharmaceutical precautions Store at room temperature.

Legal category POM.

Package quantities Cream: Tube containing 78 g with the Ortho Plastic Vaginal Applicator.

Pessaries: Pack of 15 individually sealed pessaries.

Further information Nil.

Product licence numbers

Cream	0076/0082
Pessaries	0076/0081

ORTHO* GYNE-T* INTRAUTERINE COPPER CONTRACEPTIVE DEVICE

Presentation Each device consists of a polyethylene 'T' shaped support with 120 mg pure copper wire (providing a surface area of 200 sq. mm) wound around the vertical section of the 'T'.

The support is impregnated with a radiopaque substance and has a polyethylene suture attached to the base of the 'T'.

Uses Contraception.

Dosage and administration Ortho Gyne-T Intrauterine Copper Contraceptive Device may be used in any woman of child-bearing age.

One device is inserted by its introducer into the uterus. The device should be removed after three years of use. If continued contraception is required a new device should be inserted. The device should be placed as high as possible within the uterine cavity and the patient should check periodically, particularly after menstruation, to ensure that the threads still protrude from the cervix. She should return to her doctor if she becomes aware that the device has been expelled. When the threads cannot be felt by the patient and cannot be seen by her doctor further investigation is necessary.

Contra-indications, warnings, etc

Contra-indications: The use of the device is contraindicated in the following conditions:

1. Pregnancy or suspicion of pregnancy. History of ectopic pregnancy.
2. Abnormalities of the uterus resulting in distortion of the uterine cavity, including developmental abnormalities.
3. Pelvic inflammatory disease or a history of repeated pelvic inflammatory disease.
4. Post-partum endometritis or infected abortion in the last three months.
5. Known or suspected uterine or cervical malignancy including unresolved abnormal cervical smear or endometrial disease.
6. Uterine bleeding of unknown aetiology.
7. Severe dysmenorrhoea.
8. Cervicitis until the infection is controlled.
9. Significant anaemia.
10. Valvular heart disease.
11. Leukaemia.
12. Use of chronic corticosteroid therapy because of increased susceptibility to infection.
13. Wilsons disease or a hypersensitivity to copper.
14. Medical diathermic or ultrasonic therapy to the abdominal or sacral regions is contra-indicated because of the possibility of heat injury to surrounding tissues.

The device should be removed for the following reasons:

1. Excessive and persistent bleeding or cramping.
2. Perforation of the uterus and location of the device outside the uterine cavity. In this case hospital investigation and surgical removal will be required.
3. Partial downward displacement of the device within the cervical canal.
4. Development of either a Papanicolaou smear Class III or higher or treatment resistant cervical erosions or suspected dysplasia or neoplasia of the genital tract.
5. Pelvic infection resistant to treatment.
6. Menorrhagia producing significant anaemia or intractable pain.

Warnings: An increased incidence of pelvic inflammatory disease and menorrhagia associated with the use of IUCD's has been reported. Pelvic infection may result in future infertility. This risk appears to be greatest for nulliparous women who have a multiplicity of sexual partners.

Syncope or bradycardia may occur in some women during insertion or removal of an IUCD. In the event of early signs of vasovagal attack, insertion may need to be abandoned or the device removed. The woman should be kept supine, the head lowered and the legs elevated to the vertical position if necessary in order to restore cerebral blood flow. A clear airway must be maintained. persistent bradycardia may be controlled with intravenous atropine. If oxygen is available it may be administered.

Post-insertion cramps are usually of only a few minutes duration, but some women may experience cramps for several hours or days. Spotting, intermenstrual bleeding or increased menstrual flow may occur. Expulsion rate may be increased when insertions are made before normal uterine involution occurs following delivery.

Pregnancy/ectopic pregnancy: The risk of ectopic pregnancy is reported to be greater in women who conceive with an IUCD 'in situ' than those without an IUCD. Therefore, if a woman becomes pregnant with an IUCD 'in situ', she should be carefully evaluated for possible ectopic pregnancy.

If a patient is found to be pregnant with an Ortho Gyne-T *in situ* and the thread is visible it is recommended that, in the absence of reasons to the contrary, the device be removed as soon as possible. It is possible that should a second trimester abortion occur, sepsis will supervene, and hence the desirability of removing the device as soon as possible. If the thread is not visible then it is recommended that the device is left *in situ* until the pregnancy goes to term or a decision is made to terminate the pregnancy.

There have been reports of an increased incidence of septic abortion, associated in some instances with septicaemia, septic shock and death, in women who become pregnant with an IUCD 'in situ'. Women who are pregnant with an IUCD 'in situ' should be closely observed and told to report immediately all abnormal symptoms such as 'flu-like symptoms, fever, cramp-like pain, bleeding or excessive discharge, as the onset of septicaemia associated with septic abortion may be insidious with general symptoms rather than initial signs of spontaneous abortion.

If the women elects to continue the pregnancy, careful observation is required. The long term effects of intrauterine copper on the foetus are not known.

Precautions: Prior to insertion of an IUCD a thorough history and physical examination, including a pelvic examination and Papanicolaou smear, should be performed. Pregnancy should be ruled out. Insertion of an IUCD into a uterine cavity measuring less than 6.5 cm by sounding may increase the incidence of expulsion, bleeding, pain and perforation. The patient should be re-examined within three months after insertion and thereafter at yearly intervals to ensure the device is still in place. The patient should be advised to contact her doctor immediately if she misses a menstrual period or has any other reason to think she may be pregnant.

IUCD's should be used with caution in patients with: anaemia, menorrhagia, hypermenorrhoea, a history of previous uterine incision or perforation of the uterus and those receiving anticoagulant steroid therapy or having a coagulopathy.

The possibility of a seizure being precipitated in an epileptic, at or shortly after insertion of an IUCD should be borne in mind.

It has been reported that IUCD's may be less effective in insulin-dependent diabetics.

Patients with known or suspected cardiac abnormalities should receive appropriate antibiotic cover during insertion of the device. No method of contraception is 100% effective. In some cases it may be appropriate to recommend the use of an additional reliable method of contraception at mid-cycle.

Adverse reactions

1. Perforation of the body of the uterus, with or without translocation of the device into the abdominal cavity.
2. Perforation of the cervix.
3. Copper allergy.
4. Pelvic infection including salpingitis with tubal damage or occlusion, which may result in future infertility.
5. The following complaints have also been reported in IUCD users: amenorrhoea or delayed menses, backaches, cervical erosion, cystic masses in the pelvis, vaginitis, urticarial allergic skin reactions, leg pain or soreness, weight loss or gain, nervousness, dyspareunia, cystitis, endometritis, septic abortion, septicemia, leukorrhea, infection of reproductive organs with actinomycosis, ectopic pregnancy, difficult removal, uterine embedment, anaemia, pain, neurovascular episodes including bradycardia and syncope associated with insertion or removal, dysmenorrhoea, fragmentation of the copper wire on the IUD and breakage of the string.

Lost threads: When the threads cannot be felt by the patient or cannot be seen by the doctor further investigation is necessary. A uterine sound should be introduced into the endometrial cavity following the same technique as for insertion. In most instances the IUCD can be detected by the sound. If the threads have retracted into the uterine cavity, they may be brought back down through the cervix and into the vagina. If such is the case there is usually no need to replace the device providing there is no evidence of infection.

If the device cannot be detected in the uterine cavity by the sound, a soft tissue x-ray should be taken of the pelvis and lower abdomen. A positive roentgenogram should be followed by appropriate radiological techniques for localising the device. If the device is extra-uterine, surgical removal is recommended.

Overdosage: Not applicable.

Pharmaceutical precautions If the seal of the sterile pack is broken the device inside should not be used.

Legal category POM. Also available through family planning clinics.

Package quantities Each sterile Ortho Gyne-T Intrauterine Copper Contraceptive Device unit is supplied in a sealed transparent envelope.

Full fitting instructions and advice for the patient are supplied with each device.

Further information Nil.

Product licence number 0076/0046.

ORTHO*GYNE-T* 380 SLIMLINE INTRAUTERINE COPPER CONTRACEPTIVE DEVICE

Presentation Each device consists of a polyethylene 'T' shaped support with 180 mg pure copper wire (providing a surface area of 320 mm^2) wound around the vertical section of the 'T' and one collar with 70 mg pure copper providing an exposed surface area of 30 mm^2 on the distal portion of each transverse arm. The support is impregnated with a radiopaque substance and has a polyethylene suture attached to the base of the 'T'.

Uses Contraception.

Dosage and administration Ortho Gyne-T 380 Slimline Intrauterine Copper Contraceptive Device may be used in any woman of child bearing age.

One device is inserted by its introducer into the uterus preferably at the end of the menstrual period. The device should be removed after four years of use. If continued contraception is required a new device should be inserted. The device should be place as high as possible within the uterine cavity and the patient should check periodically, particularly after menstruation, to ensure that the threads still protrude from the cervix. She should return to her doctor if she becomes aware that the device has been expelled. When the threads cannot be felt by the patient and cannot be seen by her doctor further investigation is necessary.

Contra-indications, warnings, etc

Contra-indications: The use of the device is contra-indicated in the following conditions:

1. Pregnancy or suspicion of pregnancy. History of ectopic pregnancy.
2. Abnormalities of the uterus resulting in distortion of the uterine cavity, including developmental abnormalities.
3. Pelvic inflammatory disease or a history of repeated pelvic inflammatory disease.
4. Post-partum endometritis or infected abortion in the last three months.
5. Known or suspected uterine or cervical malignancy including unresolved cervical smear or endometrial disease.

6. Uterine bleeding of unknown aetiology.
7. Severe dysmenorrhoea.
8. Cervicitis, until the infection is controlled.
9. Significant anaemia.
10. Valvular heart disease.
11. Leukaemia.
12. Use of chronic corticosteroid therapy because of increased susceptibility to infection.
13. Wilsons disease or a hypersensitivity to copper.
14. Medical diathermic or ultrasonic therapy to the abdominal or sacral regions is contra-indicated because of the possibility of heat injury to surrounding tissues.

The device should be removed for the following reasons:

1. Excessive and persistent bleeding or cramping.
2. Perforation of the uterus and location of the device outside the uterine cavity. In this case hospital investigation and surgical removal will be required.
3. Partial downward displacement of the device within the cervical canal.
4. Development of either a Papanicolaou smear Class III or higher or treatment resistant cervical erosions or suspected dysplasia or neoplasia of the genital tract.
5. Pelvic infection resistant to treatment.
6. Menorrhagia producing significant anaemia or intractable pain.

Warnings: An increased incidence of pelvic inflammatory disease and menorrhagia associated with the use of IUCD's has been reported. Pelvic infection may result in future infertility. This risk appears to be greatest for nulliparous women who have a multiplicity of sexual partners.

Syncope or bradycardia may occur in some women during insertion or removal of an IUCD. In the event of early signs of vasovagal attack, insertion may need to be abandoned or the device removed. The woman should be kept supine, the head lowered and the legs elevated to the vertical position if necessary in order to restore cerebral blood flow. A clear airway must be maintained. Persistent bradycardia may be controlled with intravenous atropine. If oxygen is available it may be administered.

Post insertion cramps are usually of only a few minutes duration, but some women may experience cramps for several hours or days. Spotting, intermenstrual bleeding or increased menstrual flow may occur. Expulsion rate may be increased when insertions are made before normal uterine involution occurs following delivery.

Pregnancy/ectoptic pregnancy: The risk of ectopic pregnancy is reported to be greater in women who conceive with an IUCD 'in situ' than those without an IUCD. Therefore, if a woman becomes pregnant with an IUCD 'in situ', she should be carefully evaluated for possible ectopic pregnancy.

If a patient is found to be pregnant with an Ortho Gyne-T 380 Slimline 'in situ' and the thread is visible, it is recommended that, in the absence of reasons to the contrary, the device be removed as soon as possible. It is possible that should a second trimester abortion occur, sepsis will supervene and hence the desirability of removing the device as soon as possible. If the thread is not visible, then it is recommended that the device is left 'in situ' until the pregnancy goes to term or a decision is made to terminate the pregnancy.

There have been reports of an increased incidence of septic abortion, associated in some instances with septicaemia, septic shock and death, in women who became pregnant with an IUCD 'in situ'. Women who are pregnant with an IUCD 'in situ' should be closely observed and told to report immediately all abnormal symptoms such as 'flu-like symptoms, fever, cramp-like pain, bleeding or excessive discharge, as the onset of septicaemia associated with septic abortion may be insidious with general symptoms rather than initial signs of spontaneous abortion.

If the women elects to continue the pregnancy, careful observation is required. The long-term effects of intrauterine copper on the foetus are not known.

Precautions: Prior to insertion of an IUCD a thorough history and physical examination, including a pelvic examination and Papanicolaou smear should be performed. Pregnancy should be ruled out. Insertion of an IUCD into a uterine cavity measuring less than 6.5 cm by sounding may increase the incidence of expulsion, bleeding, pain and perforation. The patient should be re-examined within three months after insertion and thereafter at yearly intervals to ensure the device is still in place. The patient should be advised to contact her doctor immediately if she misses a menstrual period or has any other reason to think she may be pregnant.

IUCD's should be used with caution in patients with anaemia, menorrhagia, hypermenorrhoea, a history of previous uterine incision or perforation of the uterus and those receiving anticoagulant steroid therapy or having a coagulopathy.

The possibility of a seizure being precipitated in an epileptic, at or shortly after insertion of an IUCD should be born in mind.

It has not been reported that IUCD's may be less effective in insulin-dependent diabetics.

Patients with known or suspected cardiac abnormalities should receive appropriate antibiotic cover during insertion of the device. No method of contraception is 100% effective. In some cases it may be appropriate to recommend the use of an additional reliable method of contraception at mid-cycle.

Adverse reactions

1. Perforation of the body of the uterus, with or without translocation of the device into the abdominal cavity.
2. Perforation of the cervix.
3. Copper allergy.
4. Pelvic infection including salpingitis with tubal damage or occlusion, which may result in future infertility.
5. The following complaints have also been reported in IUCD users: amenorrhoea or delayed menses, backaches, cervical erosion, cystic masses in the pelvis, vaginitis, urticarial allergic skin reactions, leg pain or soreness, weight loss or gain, nervousness, dyspareunia, cystitis, endometritis, septic abortion, septicemia, leukorrhea, infection of reproductive organs with actinomycosis, ectopic pregnancy, difficult removal, uterine embedment, anaemia, pain, neurovascular episodes including bradycardia and syncope associated with insertion or removal, dysmenorrhoea, fragmentation of the copper wire on the IUD and breakage of the string.

Lost threads: When the threads cannot be felt by the patient or cannot be seen by the doctor further investigation is necessary. A uterine sound should be introduced into the endometrial cavity following the same technique as for insertion. In most instances the IUCD can be detected by the sound. If the threads have retracted into the uterine cavity, they may be brought back down through the cervix and into the vagina. If such is the case there is usually no need to replace the device providing there is no evidence of infection.

If the device cannot be detected in the uterine cavity by the sound, a soft tissue x-ray should be taken of the pelvis and lower abdomen. A positive roentgenogram should be followed by appropriate radiological techniques for localising the device. If the device is extra-uterine, surgical removal is recommended.

Overdosage: Not applicable.

Pharmaceutical precautions If the seal of the sterile pack is broken the device inside should not be used.

Legal category POM. (Also available through family planning clinics.)

Package quantities Each sterile Ortho Gyne-T 380 Slimline Intrauterine Copper Contraceptive Device unit is supplied in a sealed transport envelope. Full fitting instructions and advice for the patient are supplied with each device.

Further information Nil.

Product licence number 0076/0093.

ORTHO-GYNOL* CONTRACEPTIVE JELLY

Presentation Ortho-Gynol Contraceptive Jelly is a water-dispersible spermicidal jelly having a pH of 4.5, which contains *p*-diisobutylphenoxypolyethoxyethanol 1.0% w/w.

Uses Ortho-Gynol Contraceptive Jelly is a spermicidal jelly for use in conjunction with an occlusive vaginal diaphragm, whenever the control of conception is desirable.

A higher degree of protection against pregnancy will be afforded by using another method of contraception in addition to a spermicidal contraceptive.

Dosage and administration The jelly should be spread over the surface of the diaphragm which will be in contact with the cervix and on the rim. The diaphragm and spermicide must be allowed to remain undisturbed for at least six to eight hours after coitus. A fresh application of jelly or other spermicides, e.g. Orthoforms Contraceptive Pessaries, must be made prior to any subsequent act of coitus within this period of time, without removing the diaphragm. (A vaginal applicator should be used for inserting more cream or jelly.)

Douching is not recommended; but if desired it should be deferred for at least six hours after intercourse.

Contra-indications, warnings, etc Hypersensitivity to the product.

Warning: Where avoidance of pregnancy is essential, the choice of contraceptive should be made in consultation with a doctor or family planning clinic.

Occasional irritation of the vagina or penis has been reported. In such cases the medication should be discontinued.

The diaphragm should not remain in position for longer than 24 hours.

Overdosage: Ortho-Gynol Contraceptive Jelly is intended for intravaginal use only, and if taken orally by mistake is likely to taste unpleasant. If excess quantities are swallowed this may give rise to gastric irritation as the product contains a surfactant, and general supportive therapy should be carried out if necessary.

Pharmaceutical precautions None known.

Legal category GSL.

Package quantities Tube containing 81 g.

Ortho* Plastic Vaginal Applicator available separately.

Further information Nil.

Product licence number 0076/5007

ORTHO-NOVIN* 1/50 ORAL CONTRACEPTIVE TABLETS

Presentation White $\frac{1}{4}$ inch diameter, circular tablets with flat faces and bevelled edges, bearing on each face the engraving C over 150. Each tablet contains 1 mg Norethisterone PhEur and 50 micrograms Mestranol PhEur.

Uses Oral contraception and menstrual disorders such as heavy, irregular or painful periods.

Action: Through the mechanism of gonadotrophin suppression by the oestrogenic and progestational actions of the ingredients. Although the primary mechanism of action is inhibition of ovulation, alterations to the cervical mucus and to the endometrium may also contribute to the efficacy of the product.

Dosage and administration The basic dosage regimen is a 28-day cycle of 1 tablet daily for 21 days followed by seven tablet-free days. For initial therapy the first tablet is taken on the fifth day of the menstrual cycle, counting the first day of bleeding as Day 1. Each subsequent course is started after seven tablet-free days have followed the preceding course. To obtain maximal contraceptive effectiveness all contraceptive tablets should be taken exactly as directed and at approximately the same time each day. Contraception can be initiated immediately post partum in the non-nursing patient. The possibility of ovulation and conception prior to the initiation of medication should be considered. The patient should be advised that during the first 14 days of the first course an additional reliable non-hormonal form of contraception should be used. If the patient misses more than one tablet she should begin taking tablets again as soon as remembered and an additional reliable method of contraception used until the next withdrawal bleed.

If the patient has vomiting or diarrhoea, absorption of the hormones will be impaired, making it advisable to use an additional reliable method of contraception until her next menstrual period. Should a bleeding fail to occur at the usual time, the possibility of pregnancy should be excluded before starting the next pack.

Contra-indications, warnings, etc

Contra-indications: Existing thrombophlebitis, thromboembolic disorders, cerebral vascular disease, myocardial infarction, or a past history of these conditions. Sickle-cell anaemia. Markedly impaired liver function. Congenital or existing disorders of lipid metabolism. Known or suspected carcinoma of the breast. Known or suspected oestrogen-dependent neoplasia. History during pregnancy of idiopathic jaundice, severe pruritus, shingles or deterioration of otosclerosis. Dubin-Johnson syndrome. Rotor syndrome. Undiagnosed abnormal genital tract bleeding. Known or suspected pregnancy.

Warnings: An increased risk of thrombophlebitis, cerebrovascular disorders, myocardial infarction and pulmonary embolism associated with the use of oral contraceptives has been reported in several retrospective case control studies. The increased risk has been estimated in these studies to be approximately 4 to 11 times higher (for cerebral haemorrhage two times higher) for users when compared to non users. This reported risk according to two of the studies is not related to duration of use nor does it persist after discontinuance according to one of the studies. An interim report of a large scale continuing prospective study has tended to confirm these retrospective studies for thrombophlebitis and possible cerebrovascular disorders. This study also reported that the risk of superficial and deep vein thrombosis was lower in women using preparations containing 50 micrograms of oestrogen or less. There may not be full recovery from such disorders and it should be realised that in a few cases they are fatal.

Because of a possible increased risk of post surgery thromboembolic complications in oral contraceptive users, therapy should be discontinued at least six weeks prior to elective surgery. Caution should be exercised in administering oestrogen/progestogen combinations to women with a history of hypertension. An increased risk of surgically confirmed gall bladder disease associated with the use of oral contraceptives has been reported in a retrospective case control study.

Malignant hepatic tumours have been reported on rare occasions in long-term users of oral contraceptives. Benign hepatic tumours have also been associated with oral contraceptive usage. A hepatic tumour should be considered in the differential diagnosis when upper abdominal pain, enlarged liver or signs of intra-abdominal haemorrhage occur.

A small fraction of the active ingredients in oral contraceptives has been identified in the milk of mothers receiving these drugs. The effects, if any, on the breast-fed child have not been determined. If possible the use of oral contraceptives should be deferred until the infant is weaned.

When women have taken hormones during pregnancy there have been some reports of the possibility of adverse effects on the developing child. A direct relationship between such effects and oral contraceptives has not been confirmed, but as with any other drug, avoidance of continuing oral contraception in early pregnancy is desirable. Therefore pregnancy should be ruled out before initiating or continuing the administration of oral contraceptives to patients who have missed one menstrual period.

Certain factors may entail some risk of thrombosis, e.g.

smoking, obesity, varicose veins, cardiovascular diseases, diabetes, and migraine. The suitability of a combined oral contraceptive should be judged according to the severity of such conditions in the individual case, and should be discussed with the patient before she decides to take it. The risk of arterial thrombosis associated with combined oral contraceptives increases with age and this risk is aggravated by cigarette smoking. The use of combined oral contraceptives in women in the older age group, especially those who are cigarette smokers, should therefore be discouraged and alternative methods advised.

Reduced efficacy and increased incidence of breakthrough bleeding have been associated with concomitant use of oral contraceptives and rifampicin. A similar association has been suggested with oral contraceptives and barbiturates, phenytoin sodium, ampicillin, tetracycline and griseofulvin.

Numerous epidemiological studies have been reported on the risk of ovarian, endometrial, cervical and breast cancer in women using combined oral contraceptives. The evidence is clear that combined oral contraceptives offer substantial protection against ovarian and endometrial cancer.

An increased risk of cervical cancer in long-term users of combined oral contraceptives has been reported in some studies, but there continues to be controversy about the extent to which this is attributable to the confounding effects of sexual behaviour and other factors.

The evidence linking combined oral contraceptive use and breast cancer remains inconclusive. The results of some studies suggest an increased risk of breast cancer presenting below the age of about 35, the risk rising with duration of use. Any possible increased risk of breast cancer with combined oral contraceptives is, however, likely to be small, and may be expected to be less with low dosage pills. This possible risk should be weighed against the many benefits of combined oral contraceptives, including their protective effects against ovarian and endometrial cancers.

Reasons for stopping oral contraceptives immediately: Early manifestations of thrombotic or thromboembolic disorders, thrombophlebitis, cerebrovascular disorders (including haemorrhage), myocardial infarction, pulmonary embolism or retinal thrombosis. Hypertension. Gradual or sudden, partial or complete loss of vision. Proptosis or diplopia. Onset or aggravation of migraine or development of headaches of a new pattern which are recurrent, persistent or severe. Papilloedema or any evidence of retinal vascular lesions. During periods of immobility (e.g. after accidents). Pregnancy. Manifestations of liver tumours.

Precautions: Examination of the pelvic organs, breasts and blood pressure should precede the prescribing of any oral contraceptive, and should be repeated regularly. The following are some of the medical conditions reported to be influenced by oral contraceptive therapy, and where the physician will have to exercise medical judgement to commence, continue or discontinue therapy as appropriate:

1. Pre-existing uterine fibromyomata may increase in size.
2. A decrease in glucose tolerance in a significant number of women.
3. An increase in blood pressure in a small but significant number of women.
4. Cholestatic jaundice. Patients with a history of cholestatic jaundice of pregnancy are more likely to develop cholestatic jaundice during oral contraceptive therapy.
5. Amenorrhoea during and after oral contraceptive therapy. Women with a past history of oligomenorrhoea or secondary amenorrhoea or women with irregular cycles may be more likely to remain anovulatory or to become amenorrhoeic post oral contraceptive therapy.
6. Depression.
7. Fluid retention. Conditions which might be influenced by this factor include epilepsy, migraine, asthma, cardiac or renal dysfunction.
8. Varicose veins.
9. Multiple sclerosis.
10. Porphyria.
11. Tetany.
12. Wearing of contact lenses

or any condition that is prone to worsen during pregnancy.

The following laboratory determinations may be altered in patients using oral contraceptives:

Hepatic: Increased BSP retention and other tests.

Coagulation: Increased prothrombin, Factors VII, VIII, IX and X; decreased antithrombin III; increased platelet aggregability.

Endocrine: Increased PBI and butanol extractable protein bound iodine and decreased T3 uptake; increased glucose blood levels.

Other: Increased phospholipids and tri-glycerides, decreased serum folate values and disturbance in tryptophan metabolism. Decreased pregnanediol excretion, reduced response to metyrapone test.

These tests usually return to pre-therapy values after discontinuing oral contraceptive use. However, the physician should be aware that these altered determinations may mask an underlying disease.

Side-effects: Side-effects most commonly reported in early cycles of oral contraceptive therapy include breakthrough bleeding, spotting, nausea, vomiting and other gastro-intestinal disturbances. These frequently decrease with continued use. Other common side-effects include: change in menstrual flow, change in weight, oedema, chloasma (which may persist post therapy), amenorrhoea, breast changes (tenderness, enlargement and secretion).

In addition to the conditions and disorders discussed above, the following have been reported as adverse reactions in patients using combined oral contraceptives:

Neuro-ocular lesions
Rash
Cervical erosion and secretions
Suppression of lactation
Pre-menstrual-like syndrome
Changes in libido
Leg cramp
Relative pyridoxine deficiency
Haemorrhagic eruptions
Cystitis like syndrome
Headache
Nervousness
Fatigue
Hirsutism
Loss of scalp hair
Erythema multiforme
Erythema nodosum
Itching
Vaginal candidiasis
Porphyria

Overdosage: Serious ill effects have not been reported following acute ingestion of large doses of oral contraceptives by young children. Overdosage may cause nausea, and withdrawal bleeding may occur in females. An appropriate method of gastric emptying may be used if considered desirable.

Pharmaceutical precautions Protect from light.

Legal category POM.

Package quantities Carton containing 3 pushpaks each of 21 tablets – sufficient for 3 cycles.

Further information Nil.

Product licence number 0076/5000.

OVYSMEN* 0.5/35 ORAL CONTRACEPTIVE TABLETS

Presentation White $\frac{1}{4}$ inch diameter, circular tablets with flat faces and bevelled edges, bearing the engraving

C over 535 on each face. Each tablet contains 500 micrograms Norethisterone PhEur and 35 micrograms Ethinyloestradiol PhEur.

Uses Contraception and the recognised indications for such oestrogen/progestogen combinations.

Action: Through the mechanism of gonadotrophin suppression by the oestrogenic and progestational actions of the ingredients. Although the primary mechanism of action is inhibition of ovulation, alterations to the cervical mucus and to the endometrium may also contribute to the efficacy of the product.

Dosage and administration The basic dosage regimen is a 28-day cycle of 1 tablet daily for 21 days followed by seven tablet-free days. For initial therapy the first tablet is taken on the fifth day of the menstrual cycle, counting the first day of bleeding as Day 1. Each subsequent course is started after seven tablet-free days have followed the preceding course. To obtain maximal contraceptive effectiveness, all contraceptive tablets should be taken exactly as directed and at approximately the same time each day. Contraception can be initiated immediately post partum in the non-nursing patient. The possibility of ovulation and conception prior to initiation of medication should be considered. The patient should be advised that during the first 14 days of the first course an additional reliable non-hormonal form of contraception should be used. If the patient misses more than 1 tablet, she should begin taking tablets again as soon as remembered and an additional reliable method of contraception used until the next withdrawal bleed.

If the patient has vomiting or diarrhoea, absorption of the hormones will be impaired, making it advisable to use an additional reliable method of contraception until her next menstrual period. Should a bleeding fail to occur at the usual time, the possibility of pregnancy should be excluded before starting the next pack.

Contra-indications, warnings, etc

Contra-indications: Existing thrombophlebitis, thromboembolic disorders, cerebral vascular disease, myocardial infarction, or a past history of these conditions. Sickle-cell anaemia. Markedly impaired liver function. Congenital or existing disorders of lipid metabolism. Known or suspected carcinoma of the breast. Known or suspected oestrogen-dependent neoplasia. History during pregnancy of idiopathic jaundice, severe pruritus, shingles or deterioration of otosclerosis. Dubin-Johnson syndrome. Rotor syndrome. Undiagnosed abnormal genital tract bleeding. Known or suspected pregnancy.

Warnings: An increased risk of thrombophlebitis, cerebrovascular disorders, myocardial infarction and pulmonary embolism associated with the use of oral contraceptives has been reported in several retrospective case control studies. The increased risk has been estimated in these studies to be approximately 4 to 11 times higher (for cerebral haemorrhage two times higher) for users when compared to non users. This reported risk according to two of the studies is not related to duration of use nor does it persist after discontinuance according to one of the studies. An interim report of a large scale continuing prospective study has tended to confirm these retrospective studies for thrombophlebitis and possible cerebrovascular disorders. This study also reported that the risk of superficial and deep vein thrombosis was lower in women using preparations containing 50 micrograms of oestrogen or less. There may not be full recovery from such disorders and it should be realised that in a few cases they are fatal.

Because of a possible increased risk of post surgery thromboembolic complications in oral contraceptive users, therapy should be discontinued at least six weeks prior to elective surgery. Caution should be exercised in administering oestrogen/progestogen combinations to women with a history of hypertension. An increased risk of surgically confirmed gall bladder disease associated with the use of oral contraceptives has been reported in a retrospective case control study.

Malignant hepatic tumours have been reported on rare occasions in long-term users of oral contraceptives. Benign hepatic tumours have also been associated with oral contraceptive usage. A hepatic tumour should be considered in the differential diagnosis when upper abdominal pain, enlarged liver or signs of intra-abdominal haemorrhage occur.

A small fraction of the active ingredients in oral contraceptives has been identified in the milk of mothers receiving these drugs. The effects, if any, on the breast-fed child have not been determined. If possible the use of oral contraceptives should be deferred until the infant is weaned.

When women have taken hormones during pregnancy there have been some reports of the possibility of adverse effects on the developing child. A direct relationship between such effects and oral contraceptives has not been confirmed, but as with any other drug, avoidance of continuing oral contraception in early pregnancy is desirable. Therefore pregnancy should be ruled out before initiating or continuing the administration of oral contraceptives to patients who have missed one menstrual period.

Certain factors may entail some risk of thrombosis, e.g. smoking, obesity, varicose veins, cardiovascular diseases, diabetes, and migraine. The suitability of a combined oral contraceptive should be judged according to the severity of such conditions in the individual case, and should be discussed with the patient before she decides to take it. The risk of arterial thrombosis associated with combined oral contraceptives increases with age and this risk is aggravated by cigarette smoking. The use of combined oral contraceptives in women in the older age group, especially those who are cigarette smokers, should therefore be discouraged and alternative methods advised.

Reduced efficacy and increased incidence of breakthrough bleeding have been associated with concomitant use of oral contraceptives and rifampicin. A similar association has been suggested with oral contraceptives and barbiturates, phenytoin sodium, ampicillin, tetracycline and griseofulvin.

Numerous epidemiological studies have been reported on the risk of ovarian, endometrial, cervical and breast cancer in women using combined oral contraceptives. The evidence is clear that combined oral contraceptives offer substantial protection against ovarian and endometrial cancer.

An increased risk of cervical cancer in long-term users of combined oral contraceptives has been reported in some studies, but there continues to be controversy about the extent to which this is attributable to the confounding effects of sexual behaviour and other factors.

The evidence linking combined oral contraceptive use and breast cancer remains inconclusive. The results of some studies suggest an increased risk of breast cancer presenting below the age of about 35, the risk rising with duration of use. Any possible increased risk of breast cancer with combined oral contraceptives is, however, likely to be small, and may be expected to be less with low dosage pills. This possible risk should be weighed against the many benefits of combined oral contraceptives, including their protective effects against ovarian and endometrial cancers.

Reasons for stopping oral contraceptives immediately: Early manifestations of thrombotic or thromboembolic disorders, thrombophlebitis, cerebrovascular disorders (including haemorrhage), myocardial infarction, pulmonary embolism or retinal thrombosis. Hypertension. Gradual or sudden, partial or complete loss of vision. Proptosis or diplopia. Onset or aggravation of migraine or development of headaches of a new pattern which are recurrent, persistent or severe. Papilloedema or any evidence of retinal vascular lesions. During periods of immobility (e.g. after accidents). Pregnancy. Manifestations of liver tumours.

Precautions: Examination of the pelvic organs, breasts and blood pressure should precede the prescribing of any oral contraceptive, and should be repeated regularly. The following are some of the conditions reported to be influenced by oral contraceptive therapy, and where the physician will have to exercise medical judgement to commence, continue or discontinue therapy as appropriate.

a) Pre-existing uterine fibromyomata may increase in size.

b) A decrease in glucose tolerance in a significant number of women.

c) An increase in blood pressure in a small but significant number of women.

d) Cholestatic jaundice. Patients with a history of cholestatic jaundice of pregnancy are more likely to develop cholestatic jaundice during oral contraceptive therapy.

e) Amenorrhoea during and after oral contraceptive therapy. Women with a past history of oligomenorrhoea or secondary amenorrhoea or women with irregular cycles may be more likely to remain anovulatory or to become amenorrhoeic post oral contraceptive therapy.

f) Depression.

g) Fluid retention. Conditions which might be influenced by this factor including epilepsy, migraine, asthma, cardiac or renal dysfunction.

h) Varicose veins.

i) Multiple sclerosis.

j) Porphyria.

k) Tetany.

l) Wearing of contact lenses.

or any condition that is prone to worsen during pregnancy.

The following laboratory determinations may be altered in patients using oral contraceptives:

Hepatic: Increased BSP retention and other tests.

Coagulation: Increased prothrombin, Factors VII, VIII, IX and X; decreased antithrombin III; increased platelet aggregability.

Endocrine: Increased PBI and butanol extractable protein bound iodine and decreased T3 uptake, increased glucose blood levels.

Other: Increased phospholipids and tri-glycerides, decreased serum folate values and disturbance in tryptophan metabolism. Decreased pregnanediol excretion, reduced response to metyrapone test.

These tests usually return to pre-therapy values after discontinuing oral contraceptive use. However, the physician should be aware that these altered determinations may mask an underlying disease.

Side-effects: Side-effects most commonly reported in early cycles of oral contraceptive therapy include breakthrough bleeding, spotting, nausea, vomiting and other gastro-intestinal disturbances. These frequently decrease with continued use. Other common side-effects include: change in menstrual flow, change in weight, oedema, chloasma (which may persist post therapy), amenorrhoea, breast changes (tenderness, enlargement and secretion).

In addition to the conditions and disorders discussed above, the following have been reported as adverse reactions in patients using combined oral contraceptives:

Neuro-ocular lesions
Rash
Cervical erosion and secretions
Suppression of lactation
Pre-menstrual like syndrome
Changes in libido
Leg cramp
Relative pyridoxine deficiency
Haemorrhagic eruptions
Cystitis-like syndrome
Headache
Nervousness
Fatigue
Hirsutism
Loss of scalp hair
Erythema multiforme
Erythema nodosum
Itching
Vaginal candidiasis
Porphyria

Overdosage: Serious ill effects have not been reported following acute ingestion of large doses of oral contraceptives by young children. Overdosage may cause nausea, and withdrawal bleeding may occur in females. An appropriate method of gastric emptying may be used if considered desirable.

Pharmaceutical precautions Protect from light.

Legal category POM.

Package quantities Carton containing 3 pushpaks each of 21 tablets – sufficient for 3 cycles

Further information Nil.

Product licence number 0076/0047.

TRINOVUM*

Presentation $\frac{1}{4}$ inch diameter, circular tablets with flat faces and bevelled edges engraved on each face as follows: the seven white tablets each contain 500 micrograms Norethisterone PhEur and 35 micrograms Ethinyloestradiol PhEur and are engraved C535; the seven light peach coloured tablets each contain 750 micrograms Norethisterone PhEur and 35 micrograms Ethinyloestradiol PhEur and are engraved C735; the seven peach coloured tablets each contain 1 mg Norethisterone PhEur and 35 micrograms Ethinyloestradiol PhEur and are engraved C135.

Uses Contraception and the recognised indications for such oestrogen/progestogen combinations.

Action: Through the mechanism of gonadotrophin suppression by the oestrogenic and progestational actions of the ingredients. Although the primary mechanism of action is inhibition of ovulation, alterations to the cervical mucus and to the endometrium may also contribute to the efficacy of the product.

Dosage and administration The basic dosage regimen is a 28-day cycle of one tablet daily for 21 days followed by seven tablet-free days. A white tablet is taken on every day for 7 days, a light peach coloured tablet is taken every day for 7 days, followed by a peach coloured tablet every day for 7 days. For initial therapy, the first white tablet is taken on the first day of bleeding of the menstrual cycle. If Trinovum* tablets are first taken later than the first day of bleeding of the first menstrual cycle of medication, contraceptive reliance should be not placed on the product until after the first 14 consecutive days of administration.

Subsequent cycles: Each subsequent course is started after 7 tablet-free days have followed the preceding course.

Changing from another combined oral contraceptive: The first white tablet should be taken on the first day of the withdrawal bleed after the completion of the previous course of tablets.

Changing from a progestogen-only contraceptive: The first white tablet should be taken on the first day of bleeding that occurs either during the last course of tablets or following completion of the tablet course.

Post-partum use: After pregnancy, oral contraception may be initiated immediately post-partum in the non-nursing patient or as soon as spontaneous menstruation has been resumed. Another method of contraception should be used in the interval between delivery and the first course of tablets, unless it is started within seven days of delivery. After a miscarriage or first-trimester abortion, oral contraception may be started immediately.

If the patient forgets more than one tablet, she should recommence the course as soon as she remembers, taking the appropriate tablet for that day and omitting any tablets delayed more than 12 hours. She should then use an additional method of contraception until the next withdrawal bleed. To obtain maximum contraceptive effectiveness, all contraceptive tablets should be taken exactly as directed and at approximately the same time each day.

If a patient has vomiting or diarrhoea, absorption of the hormones will be impaired, making it advisable to use an additional method of contraception until her next menstrual period. Should a bleeding fail to occur at the usual time, the possibility of pregnancy should be excluded before starting the next pack.

Contra-indications, warnings, etc

Contra-indications: Existing thrombophlebitis, thromboembolic disorders, cerebral vascular disease, myocardial infarction, or a past history of these conditions. Sickle-cell anaemia. Markedly impaired liver function. Congenital or existing disorders of lipid metabolism. Known or suspected carcinoma of the breast. Known or suspected oestrogen-dependent neoplasia. History during pregnancy of idiopathic jaundice, severe pruritus, shingles or deterioration of otosclerosis. Dubin-Johnson syndrome. Rotor syndrome. Undiagnosed abnormal genital tract bleeding. Known or suspected pregnancy.

Warnings: An increased risk of thrombophlebitis, cerebrovascular disorders, myocardial infarction and pulmonary embolism associated with the use of oral contraceptives has been reported in several retrospective case control studies. The increased risk has been estimated in these studies to be approximately 4 to 11 times higher (for cerebral haemorrhage two times higher) for users when compared to non users. This reported risk according to two of the studies is not related to duration of use nor does it persist after discontinuance according to one of the studies. An interim report of a large scale continuing prospective study has tended to confirm these retrospective studies for thrombophlebitis and possible cerebrovascular disorders. This study also reported that the risk of superficial and deep vein thrombosis was lower in women using preparations containing 50 micrograms of oestrogen or less. There may not be full recovery from such disorders and it should be realised that in a few cases they are fatal.

Because of a possible increased risk of post surgery thromboembolic complications in oral contraceptive users, therapy should be discontinued at least six weeks prior to elective surgery. Caution should be exercised in administering oestrogen/progestogen combinations to women with a history of hypertension. An increased risk of surgically confirmed gall bladder disease associated with the use of oral contraceptives has been reported in a retrospective case control study.

Malignant hepatic tumours have been reported on rare occasions in long-term users of oral contraceptives. Benign hepatic tumours have also been associated with oral contraceptive usage. A hepatic tumour should be considered in the differential diagnosis when upper abdominal pain, enlarged liver or signs of intra-abdominal haemorrhage occur.

A small fraction of the active ingredients in oral contraceptives has been identified in the milk of mothers receiving these drugs. The effects, if any, on the breast-fed child have not been determined. If possible the use of oral contraceptives should be deferred until the infant is weaned.

When women have taken hormones during pregnancy there have been some reports of the possibility of adverse effects on the developing child. A direct relationship between such effects and oral contraceptives has not been confirmed, but as with any other drug, avoidance of continuing oral contraception in early pregnancy is desirable. Therefore pregnancy should be ruled out before initiating or continuing the administration of oral contraceptives to patients who have missed one menstrual period.

Certain factors may entail some risk of thrombosis e.g. smoking, obesity, varicose veins, cardiovascular diseases, diabetes, and migraine. The suitability of a combined oral contraceptive should be judged according to the severity of such conditions in the individual case, and should be discussed with the patient before she decides to take it. The risk of arterial thrombosis associated with combined oral contraceptives increases with age and this risk is aggravated by cigarette smoking. The use of combined oral contraceptives in women in the older age group, especially those who are cigarette smokers, should therefore be discouraged and alternative methods advised.

Reduced efficacy and increased incidence of breakthrough bleeding have been associated with concomitant use of oral contraceptives and rifampicin. A similar association has been suggested with oral contraceptives and barbiturates, phenytoin sodium, ampicillin, tetracycline and griseofulvin.

Numerous epidemiological studies have been reported on the risk of ovarian, endometrial, cervical and breast cancer in women using combined oral contraceptives. The evidence is clear that combined oral contraceptives offer substantial protection against ovarian and endometrial cancer.

An increased risk of cervical cancer in long-term users of combined oral contraceptives has been reported in some studies, but there continues to be controversy about the extent to which this is attributable to the confounding effects of sexual behaviour and other factors.

The evidence linking combined oral contraceptive use and breast cancer remains inconclusive. The results of some studies suggest an increased risk of breast cancer presenting below the age of about 35, the risk rising with duration of use. Any possible increased risk of breast cancer with combined oral contraceptives is, however, likely to be small, and may be expected to be less with low dosage pills. This possible risk should be weighed against the many benefits of combined oral contraceptives, including their protective effects against ovarian and endometrial cancers.

Reasons for stopping oral contraceptives immediately: Early manifestations of thrombotic or thromboembolic disorders, thrombophlebitis, cerebrovascular disorders (including haemorrhage), myocardial infarction, pulmonary embolism or retinal thrombosis. Hypertension. Gradual or sudden, partial or complete loss of vision. Proptosis or diplopia. Onset or aggravation of migraine or development of headaches of a new pattern which are recurrent, persistent or severe. Papilloedema or any evidence of retinal vascular lesions. During periods of immobility (e.g. after accidents). Pregnancy. Manifestations of liver tumours.

Precautions: Examination of the pelvic organs, breasts and blood pressure should precede the prescribing of any oral contraceptive, and should be repeated regularly.

The following are some of the conditions reported to be influenced by oral contraceptive therapy, and where the physician will have to exercise medical judgement to commence, continue or discontinue therapy as appropriate.

a) Pre-existing uterine fibromyomata may increase in size.
b) A decrease in glucose tolerance in a significant number of women.
c) An increase in blood pressure in a small but significant number of women.
d) Cholestatic jaundice. Patients with a history of cholestatic jaundice of pregnancy are more likely to develop cholestatic jaundice during oral contraceptive therapy.
e) Amenorrhoea during and after oral contraceptive therapy. Women with a past history of oligomenorrhoea or secondary amenorrhoea or women with irregular cycles may be more likely to remain anovulatory or to become amenorrhoeic post oral contraceptive therapy.
f) Depression.
g) Fluid retention. Conditions which might be influenced by this factor include epilepsy, migraine, asthma, cardiac or renal dysfunction.
h) Varicose veins.
i) Multiple sclerosis.
j) Porphyria.
k) Tetany.
l) Wearing of contact lenses.

or any condition that is prone to worsen during pregnancy.

The following laboratory determinations may be altered in patients using oral contraceptives:

Hepatic: Increased BSP retention and other tests.

Coagulation: Increased prothrombin, Factors VII, VIII, IX and X: decreased antithrombin III, increased platelet aggregability.
Endocrine: Increased PBI and butanol extractable protein bound iodine and decreased T3 uptake, increased glucose blood levels.
Other: Increased phospholipids and tri-glycerides, decreased serum folate values and disturbance in tryptophan metabolism, decreased pregnanediol excretion, reduced response to metyrapone test.

These tests usually return to pre-therapy values after discontinuing oral contraceptive use. However, the physician should be aware that these altered determinations may mask an underlying disease.

Side-effects: Most commonly reported in early cycles of oral contraceptive therapy include breakthrough bleeding, spotting, nausea, vomiting and other gastrointestinal disturbances. These frequently decrease with continued use. Other common side-effects include: change in menstrual flow, change in weight, oedema, chloasma (which may persist post therapy), amenorrhoea, breast changes (tenderness, enlargement and secretion).

In addition to the conditions and disorders discussed above, the following have been reported as adverse reactions in patients using combined oral contraceptives:

Neuro-ocular lesions	Haemorrhagic eruptions
Rash	Cystitis-like syndrome
Cervical erosion and secretions	Headache
	Nervousness
Suppression of lactation	Fatigue
Pre-menstrual like syndrome	Hirsutism
	Loss of scalp hair
Changes in libido	Erythema multiforme
Leg cramp	Erythema nodosum
Relative pyridoxine deficiency	Itching
	Vaginal candidiasis
	Porphyria

Overdosage: Serious ill effects have not been reported following acute ingestion of large doses of oral contraceptives by young children. Overdosage may cause nausea, and withdrawal bleeding may occur in females. An appropriate method of gastric emptying may be used if considered desirable.

Pharmaceutical precautions Protect from light.

Legal category POM.

Package quantities Carton containing 3 pushpaks each of 21 tablets – sufficient for 3 cycles.

Further information Nil.

Product licence number 0076/0095.

TRINOVUM* ED

Presentation $\frac{1}{4}$-inch diameter, circular tablets with flat faces and bevelled edges engraved on each face as follows: the seven white tablets each contain 500 micrograms Norethisterone PhEur and 35 micrograms Ethinyloestradiol PhEur and are engraved C535; the seven light peach coloured tablets each contain 750 micrograms Norethisterone PhEur and 35 micrograms Ethinyloestradiol PhEur and are engraved C735; the seven peach coloured tablets each contain 1.0 mg Norethisterone PhEur and 35 micrograms Ethinyloestradiol PhEur and are engraved C135; the seven green tablets are placebo tablets and are engraved C-C in a diamond.

Uses Contraception and the treatment of menstrual disorders such as heavy, irregular or painful periods.

Action: Through the mechanism of gonadotrophin suppression by the oestrogenic and progestational actions of the ingredients. Although the primary mechanism of action is inhibition of ovulation, alterations to the cervical mucus and to the endometrium may also contribute to the efficacy of the product.

Dosage and administration The dosage regimen is a 28-day cycle of one tablet daily. There are no tablet-free days. A white tablet is taken on every day for seven days, a light peach coloured tablet is taken every day for seven days, a peach coloured tablet every day for seven days, followed by a green tablet every day for seven days. For initial therapy, the first white tablet is taken on the first day of bleeding of the menstrual cycle. If TriNovum ED tablets are first taken later than the first day of bleeding of the menstrual cycle, contraceptive reliance should be not placed on the product until after the first 14 consecutive days of administration.

Subsequent cycles: Each subsequent course is started immediately after completing the preceding course. There is no tablet-free interval.

Changing from another combined oral contraceptive: The first white tablet should be taken on the first day of the withdrawal bleed after the completion of the previous course of tablets.

Changing from a progestogen-only contraceptive: The first white tablet should be taken on the first day of bleeding that occurs either during the last course of tablets or following completion of the tablet course.

Post-partum use: After pregnancy, oral contraception may be initiated immediately post-partum in the non-nursing patient or as soon as spontaneous menstruation has been resumed. Another method of contraception should be used in the interval between delivery and the first course of tablets, unless it is started within seven days of delivery. After a miscarriage or first-trimester abortion, oral contraception may be started immediately.

If the patient forgets more than one tablet, she should recommence the course as soon as she remembers, taking the appropriate tablet for that day and omitting any tablets delayed more than 12 hours. She should then use an additional method of contraception until the next withdrawal bleed. To obtain maximum contraceptive effectiveness, all contraceptive tablets should be taken exactly as directed and at approximately the same time each day.

If a patient has vomiting or diarrhoea, absorption of the hormones will be impaired, making it advisable to use an additional method of contraception until her next menstrual period. Should a bleeding fail to occur at the usual time, the possibility of pregnancy should be excluded before starting the next pack.

Contra-indications, warnings, etc
Contra-indications: Existing thrombophlebitis, thromboembolic disorders, cerebrovascular disease, myocardial infarction, or a past history of these conditions. Sickle-cell anaemia. Markedly impaired liver function. Congenital or existing disorders of lipid metabolism. Known or suspected carcinoma of the breast. Known or suspected oestrogen-dependent neoplasia. History during pregnancy of idiopathic jaundice, severe pruritus, shingles or deterioration of otosclerosis. Dubin-Johnson syndrome. Rotor syndrome. Undiagnosed abnormal genital tract bleeding. Known or suspected pregnancy.

Warnings: An increased risk of thrombophlebitis, cerebrovascular disorders, myocardial infarction and pulmonary embolism associated with the use of oral contraceptives has been reported in several retrospective case control studies. The increased risk has been estimated in these studies to be approximately 4 to 11 times higher (for cerebral haemorrhage two times higher) for users when compared to non-users. This reported risk according to two of the studies is not related to duration of use nor does it persist after discontinuance according to one of the studies. An interim report of a large-scale continuing prospective study has tended to confirm these retrospective studies for thrombophlebitis and possible cerebrovascular disorders. This study also reported that the risk of superficial and deep vein thrombosis was lower in women using preparations containing 50 micrograms of oestrogen or less. There may not be full recovery from such disorders and it should be realised that in a few cases they are fatal.

Because of a possible increased risk of post-surgical thromboembolic complications in oral contraceptive users, therapy should be discontinued at least six weeks prior to elective surgery. Caution should be exercised in administering oestrogen/progestogen combinations to women with a history of hypertension. An increased risk of surgically confirmed gall bladder disease associated with the use of oral contraceptives has been reported in a retrospective case control study.

Malignant hepatic tumours have been reported on rare occasions in long-term users of oral contraceptives. Benign hepatic tumours have also been associated with oral contraceptive usage. A hepatic tumour should be considered in the differential diagnosis when upper abdominal pain, enlarged liver or signs of intra-abdominal haemorrhage occur.

A small fraction of the active ingredients in oral contraceptives has been identified in the milk of mothers receiving these drugs. The effects, if any, on the breast-fed child have not been determined. If possible the use of oral contraceptives should be deferred until the infant is weaned.

When women have taken hormones during pregnancy there have been some reports of the possibility of adverse effects on the developing child. A direct relationship between such effects and oral contraceptives has not been confirmed but, as with any other drug, avoidance of continuing oral contraception in early pregnancy is desirable. Therefore pregnancy should be ruled out before initiating or continuing the administration of oral contraceptives to patients who have missed one menstrual period.

Certain factors may entail some risk of thrombosis e.g. smoking, obesity, varicose veins, cardiovascular disease, diabetes, and migraine.

The suitability of a combined oral contraceptive should be judged according to the severity of such conditions in the individual case, and should be discussed with the patient before she decides to take it. The risk of arterial thrombosis associated with combined oral contraceptives increases with age and this risk is aggravated by cigarette smoking. The use of combined oral contraceptives in women in the older age group, especially those who are cigarette smokers, should therefore be discouraged and alternative methods advised.

Reduced efficacy and increased incidence of breakthrough bleeding have been associated with concomitant use of oral contraceptives and rifampicin. A similar association has been suggested with oral contraceptives and barbiturates, phenytoin sodium, ampicillin, tetracycline and griseofulvin.

Numerous epidemiological studies have been reported on the risk of ovarian, endometrial, cervical and breast cancer in women using combined oral contraceptives. The evidence is clear that combined oral contraceptives offer substantial protection against ovarian and endometrial cancer.

An increased risk of cervical cancer in long-term users of combined oral contraceptives has been reported in some studies, but there continues to be controversy about the extent to which this is attributable to the confounding effects of sexual behaviour and other factors.

The evidence linking combined oral contraceptive use and breast cancer remains inconclusive. The results of some studies suggest an increased risk of breast cancer presenting below the age of about 35, the risk rising with duration of use. Any possible increased risk of breast cancer with combined oral contraceptives is, however, likely to be small, and may be expected to be less with low dosage pills. This possible risk should be weighed against the many benefits of combined oral contraceptives, including their protective effects against ovarian and endometrial cancers.

Reasons for stopping oral contraceptives immediately: Early manifestations of thrombotic or thromboembolic disorders, thrombophlebitis, cerebrovascular disorders (including haemorrhage), myocardial infarction, pulmonary embolism or retinal thrombosis. Hypertension. Gradual or sudden, partial or complete loss of vision. Proptosis or diplopia. Onset or aggravation of migraine or development of headaches of a new pattern which is recurrent, persistent or severe. Papilloedema or any evidence of retinal vascular lesions. During periods of immobility (e.g. after accidents). Pregnancy. Manifestations of liver tumours.

Precautions: Examination of the pelvic organs, breasts and blood pressure should precede the prescribing of any oral contraceptive, and should be repeated regularly.

The following are some of the conditions reported to be influenced by oral contraceptive therapy, and where the physician will have to exercise medical judgement to commence, continue or discontinue therapy as appropriate.

a) Pre-existing uterine fibromyomata may increase in size.
b) A decrease in glucose tolerance in a significant number of women.
c) An increase in blood pressure in a small but significant number of women.
d) Cholestatic jaundice. Patients with a history of cholestatic jaundice of pregnancy are more likely to develop cholestatic jaundice during oral contraceptive therapy.
e) Amenorrhoea during and after oral contraceptive therapy. Women with a past history of oligomenorrhoea or secondary amenorrhoea or women with irregular cycles may be more likely to remain anovulatory or to become amenorrhoeic post-oral contraceptive therapy.
f) Depression.
g) Fluid retention. Conditions which might be influenced by this factor include epilepsy, migraine, asthma, cardiac or renal dysfunction.
h) Varicose veins.
i) Multiple sclerosis.
j) Porphyria.
k) Tetany.
l) Wearing of contact lenses.

or any condition that is prone to worsen during pregnancy.

The following laboratory determinations may be altered in patients using oral contraceptives:

Hepatic: Increased BSP retention and other tests.
Coagulation: Increased prothrombin, Factors VII, VIII, IX and X: decreased antithrombin III, increased platelet aggregability.
Endocrine: Increased PBI and butanol extractable protein bound iodine and decreased T3 uptake, increased glucose blood levels.
Other: Increased phospholipids and tri-glycerides, decreased serum folate values and disturbance in tryptophan metabolism, decreased pregnanediol excretion, reduced response to metyrapone test.

These tests usually return to pre-therapy values after discontinuing oral contraceptive use. However, the physician should be aware that these altered determinations may mask an underlying disease.

Side-effects: Those most commonly reported in early cycles of oral contraceptive therapy include breakthrough bleeding, spotting, nausea, vomiting and other gastro-intestinal disturbances. These frequently decrease with continued use. Other common side-effects include: change in menstrual flow, change in weight, oedema, chloasma (which may persist post-therapy), amenorrhoea, breast changes (tenderness, enlargement and secretion).

In addition to the conditions and disorders discussed above, the following have been reported as adverse reactions in patients using combined oral contraceptives:

Neuro-ocular lesions
Rash
Cervical erosion and secretions
Suppression of lactation
Pre-menstrual like syndrome
Changes in libido
Leg cramp
Relative pyridoxine deficiency
Haemorrhagic eruptions
Cystitis-like syndrome
Headache
Nervousness
Fatigue
Hirsutism
Loss of scalp hair
Erythema multiforme
Erythema nodosum
Itching
Vaginal candidiasis
Porphyria

Overdosage: Serious ill effects have not been reported following acute ingestion of large doses of oral contraceptives by young children. Overdosage may cause nausea, and withdrawal bleeding may occur in females. An appropriate method of gastric emptying may be used if considered desirable.

Pharmaceutical precautions Protect from light.

Legal category POM.

Package quantities Cartons containing 3 pushpacks each of 28 tablets – sufficient for 3 cycles.

Further information Nil.

Product licence number 0076/0140.

**Trade Mark*

Paines & Byrne Limited
Greenford
Middlesex UB6 7HG

APROTININ INJECTION BP

Presentation A sterile, pyrogen-free, clear, colourless solution of Aprotinin 5.56 BP/EP Units per ml/ 10,000 KIU (Kallikrein Inactivator Units) per ml in 0.9% sodium chloride solution presented in 50 ml vials containing 70 mg aprotinin (500,000 KIU) and 5 ml ampoules containing 7 mg aprotinin (50,000 KIU).

Uses Aprotinin is a polyvalent protease inhibitor, isolated from animal tissue. It is active against certain proteolytic enzymes such as kallikrein, kinin, trypsin, chymotrypsin, plasmin, plasmin-activator, fibrin enzymes and tissue proteases. Aprotinin may be used therapeutically or prophylactically when these enzyme systems fail.

Aprotinin is a haemostatic. High doses offer major reductions in peri-operative blood loss and the need for donor blood transfusions. It is indicated for the treatment of life-threatening haemorrhage due to hyperplasminaemia.

Dosage and administration Intravenously by slow injection or infusion.

Dosage in adults: 500,000 to 1,000,000 KIU (277.8–555.6 EP Units) given by slow IV infusion (maximum rate 5 ml/min), followed by 200,000 KIU (111.1 EP Units) hourly until bleeding stops.

Dosage in the elderly: The dosage given above applies to persons of average bodyweight. Reductions of these doses should be considered in patients of below average weight.

Dosage in children: It is recommended that a dose proportional to the adult dose is calculated.

Contra-indications, warnings, etc
Contra-indications: Known hypersensitivity to aprotinin.

Interactions: None known.

Effects on ability to drive/use machines: None known; unlikely to be applicable as indications are for hospitalised patients.

Side-effects: Aprotinin is usually well tolerated but local thrombophlebitis, nausea and vomiting, diarrhoea, muscle pains, and blood-pressure changes can occur.

Allergic reactions such as erythema, urticaria, and bronchospasm have occasionally been reported and can occur on first administration. On repeated dosage, a reddening may occur at the point of injection, but this disappears after 1 or 2 hours. Anaphylaxis, tachycardia, pallor or cyanosis and dyspnoea have also occurred.

Use in pregnancy/lactation: There is no evidence that aprotinin has teratogenic or embryotoxic effects in animals. Experience in human pregnancy and lactation is limited and inadequate to assess safety. As the use of aprotinin is in life-threatening situations it may be used in pregnancy and lactation when the benefit is considered to outweigh the risk.

Warnings/precautions: Rapid IV injection of large doses should be avoided for the high basicity of aprotinin may cause liberation of histamine and lead to an anaphylactic reaction. Aprotinin should be administered slowly (maximum 5 ml/min) with the patient lying down. Care shold be taken in treating patients intermittently and in those who have received Aprotinin previously. If hypersensitivity reactions are observed, the injection/infusion must be stopped immediately and the appropriate therapeutic measures initiated (administration of adrenaline, antihistamines, intravenous corticosteroids). Intra-ocular or intra-dermal testing may be useful for detecting allergic patients.

Overdose: There is no specific antidote and symptomatic treatment is advised. The use of more than 6×10^6 KIU (equivalent to 12×50 ml vials) per day is not recommended.

Incompatibilities: Antibiotics which react with proteins, corticosteroid and nutrient solutions containing amino-acids or fat emulsions.

Pharmaceutical precautions Store at a temperature not exceeding 25°C and protect from light. Both 5 ml ampoules and 50 ml vials should be considered as single dose containers and any contents not used in a single administration should be discarded.

Legal category POM.

Package quantities 5 ml ampoules each containing 50,000 KIU in boxes of 10 ampoules; 50 ml vials containing 500,000 KIU.

Further information Nil.

Product licence numbers

5 ml ampoule	0051/0027
50 ml vial	0051/0028

COBALIN-H*

Presentation 1 ml ampoules containing a sterile, clear, red solution providing 1000 micrograms hydroxocobalamin per millilitre for injection. Cobalin-H complies with the specification for Hydroxocobalamin Injection BP.

Uses Addisonian pernicious anaemia. Prophylaxis and treatment of other macrocytic anaemias due to B_{12} deficiency. Tobacco amblyopia and Leber's atrophy.

Dosage and administration The following dosages are suitable for children and adults. Addisonian pernicious anaemia and other macrocytic anaemias *without* neurological involvement: *Initially* – 250 micrograms to 1000 micrograms intramuscularly on alternate days for one or two weeks then 250 micrograms weekly until blood count is normal. *Maintenance* – 1000 micrograms every two or three months.

Addisonian pernicious anaemia and other macrocytic anaemias *with* neurological involvement: *Initially* – 1000 micrograms on alternate days as long as improvement continues. *Maintenance* – 1000 micrograms every two months.

Prophylaxis of macrocytic anaemias associated with Vitamin B_{12} deficiency resulting from gastrectomy, ileal resection, certain malabsorption states and vegetarianism: 1000 micrograms every two or three months.

Tobacco amblyopia and Leber's optic atrophy: *Initially* – 1000 micrograms daily by intramuscular injection for two weeks then twice weekly as long as improvement is maintained. *Maintenance* – 1000 micrograms every three months or as required.

Contra-indications, warnings, etc
Contra-indications: Sensitivity to hydroxocobalamin.

Precautions: Should not be given before a megaloblastic marrow has been demonstrated.

Pharmaceutical precautions Store in a cool place protected from light.

Legal category POM.

Package quantities Boxes of 5 ampoules.

Further information Hydroxocobalamin injection has completely replaced Cyanocobalamin injection and is now the form of Vitamin B_{12} therapy of choice.

Product licence number 0051/5041R

DALIVIT* CAPSULES

Presentation Oval red, soft gelatin capsule containing an oily yellow suspension of the following formula:

	per capsule
Vitamin A (as palmitate)	7,500 Units
Vitamin D_2 (ergocalciferol)	1,000 Units
Vitamin B_1 (thiamine mononitrate)	3 mg
Vitamin B_2 (riboflavine)	3 mg
Vitamin B_6 (pyridoxine hydrochloride)	1 mg
Vitamin C (ascorbic acid)	75 mg
Nicotinamide	25 mg
Calcium pantothenate	5 mg

Uses For the prevention of vitamin deficiency in older children, adults, and the elderly.

Dosage and administration
Adults, children more than 12 years, and the elderly: One Dalivit Capsule daily by mouth or as directed by physician.

Contra-indications, warnings, etc
Contra-indications: Hypersensitivity to any of the active ingredients. Hypercalcaemia.

Interactions: The absorption of Vitamins A and D may be reduced in conditions of fat malabsorption as well as with the concurrent administration of neomycin, cholestyramine and liquid paraffin.

Effects on ability to drive and use machines: None known.

Other undesirable effects: Excessive doses of Vitamins A and D can lead to hypervitaminosis.

Use in pregnancy and lactation: During first trimester of pregnancy large doses of Vitamin A may be teratogenic. Patients should be warned not to take Vitamin A supplements if pregnant or likely to become pregnant, except on the advice of a doctor or antenatal clinic. Large doses of Vitamin D in lactating mothers may cause hypercalcaemia in infants.

Other warnings and precautions: When multivitamin preparations are prescribed allowance must be made for vitamins from other sources e.g. cod-liver oil and fortified foods.

Overdose: Symptoms of overdosage may include anorexia, nausea, vomiting, rough dry skin, polyuria, thirst, loss of hair, painful bones and joints as well as raised plasma and urine calcium and phosphate concentration. No emergency procedure or antidote is applicable and symptoms are rapidly reduced upon withdrawal of the preparation.

Incompatibilities: None known.

Pharmaceutical precautions Store in a cool dry place and protect from light.

Legal category P.

Package quantities 30 capsules.

Further information Nil.

Product licence number 0051/5018R

DALIVIT* DROPS

Presentation Deep yellow liquid with a characteristic taste and odour in a 15 ml amber glass bottle with integral dropper.

Each 0.6 ml contains:

Vitamin A Palmitate	5000 Units
Ergocalciferol (Vitamin D_2)	400 Units
Thiamine Hydrochloride	1 mg
Riboflavine	400 micrograms
Pyridoxine Hydrochloride	500 micrograms
Ascorbic Acid	50 mg
Nicotinamide	5 mg

Uses As a supplement for the prevention of vitamin deficiency states and as an aid to the maintenance of normal health and growth in infants and young children.

Dosage and administration Dalivit Drops are administered orally.

Infants from 6 weeks up to one year: 0.3 ml daily (7 drops).

Older children, adults: 0.6 ml daily (14 drops). Or as directed by the physician.

Contra-indications, warnings, etc
Contra-indications: Hypersensitivity to any of the ingredients. Hypercalcaemia.

Interactions: None known.

Effects on ability to drive and use machines: None known.

Other undesirable effects: Excessive doses of Vitamins A and D can lead to hypervitaminosis.

Use in pregnancy and lactation: During first trimester of pregnancy large doses of Vitamin A may be teratogenic. Patients should be warned not to take Vitamin A supplements if pregnant or likely to become pregnant, except on the advice of a doctor or antenatal clinic. Vitamin D is secreted in breast milk and may cause hypercalcaemia in infants.

Other special warnings and precautions: When multivitamin preparations are prescribed allowance must be made for vitamins from other sources.

Overdose: Symptoms of vitamin overdosage may include anorexia, nausea, vomiting, rough dry skin, polyuria, thirst, loss of hair, painful bones and joints as well as raised plasma and urine calcium and phosphate concentration.

Incompatibilities: None known.

Pharmaceutical precautions Store in a cool place protected from light.

Legal category GSL.

Package quantities 2 × 15 ml dropper bottles.

Further information Dalivit Drops are prescribable on the NHS. A daily dose of 14 drops is useful for preventing vitamin deficiency in the elderly who may find drops easier to take than other forms of vitamin supplementation.

Product licence number 0051/5016R

FOLICIN*

Presentation White sugar-coated tablets each containing: Dried Ferrous Sulphate BP 200 mg (Approx. 60 mg of iron), Copper Sulphate BPC 2.5 mg, Manganese Sulphate BP 2.5 mg, Folic Acid BP 2.5 mg.

Uses For the prophylaxis and treatment of pregnancy anaemia.

Dosage and administration 1–2 tablets daily throughout the ante-natal period.

This product is not suitable for administration to children.

Contra-indications, warnings, etc Diagnosis of pernicious anaemia should be excluded before folic acid therapy is instituted. Folicin may cause gastro-intestinal discomfort, diarrhoea or vomiting in some patients. Constipation may follow long term use.

Overdosage with iron: Induce emesis and follow by gastric lavage with sodium bicarbonate 1% solution. Dissolve 2 g of desferrioxamine in Water for Injections and inject intramuscularly. Also give orally or by stomach tube 5 g of desferrioxamine dissolved in 50 ml of water.

Pharmaceutical precautions Store in a cool dry place.

Legal category POM.

Package quantities 100.

Further information Folicin is prescribable under the NHS.

Product licence number 0051/5030R

GESTONE*

Presentation Ampoules of a sterile straw-coloured solution of Progesterone BP 25 or 50 mg per ml in ethyl oleate for injection containing 10% v/v benzyl alcohol.

Uses Gestone is indicated for the treatment of dysfunctional uterine bleeding.

It is also indicated for the maintenance of early pregnancy in cases of documented history of repeated miscarriages due to luteal phase defect and in selected cases as an adjunct to successful treatment of infertility with techniques such as in-vitro fertilisation (IVF) or gamete intra-fallopian transfer (GIFT) in order to facilitate uterine implantation of the fertilised ovum.

Dosage and administration Gestone is given by intramuscular injection. It should be injected deep into the buttock, rather than the thigh or deltoid, using a 1.5 inch (3.8 cm) needle. This site has ample fat cells where a depot of progesterone can be formed for slow release.

Dysfunctional uterine bleeding: 5–10 mg daily for 5–10 days until 2 days before anticipated onset of menstruation.

Maintenance of pregnancy: Twice weekly or more frequent (maximum: daily) injections of 25–100 mg from approximately day 15, or day of transfer of embryo or gametes usually until 8–16 weeks of pregnancy when secretion of progesterone from the placenta should be established.

Daily dosage can be increased to 200 mg at the discretion of the physician.

As the indications for Gestone are restricted to women of child-bearing age, dosage recommendations for children and the elderly are not appropriate.

Contra-indications, warnings, etc

Contra-indications: Hypersensitivity to progestins, undiagnosed vaginal bleeding, missed or incomplete abortion, history of thrombo-embolism, mammary or genital tract carcinoma, thrombo-phlebitis, cerebral haemorrhage, marked hepatic dysfunction. Contraindicated as a diagnostic test for pregnancy.

Interactions: Gestone may interfere with the effects of bromocriptine. Gestone may affect the results of laboratory tests of hepatic and/or endocrine functions. Gestone may raise the plasma concentration of cyclosporin.

Effects on ability to drive and use machinery: No known effect.

Other undesirable effects: Breakthrough bleeding, change in menstrual flow, amenorrhoea, changes in cervical erosion and secretions, breast changes, oedema, weight gain, catabolism, cholestatic jaundice, allergic reactions and rashes, acne, chloasma, mental depression, pyrexia, insomnia, somnolence, nausea, alopecia, hirsutism, local reactions at site of injection.

Use in pregnancy and lactation: Gestone may be used to maintain pregnancy where there is deficient production of endogenous progesterone from the corpus luteum. It should not be necessary to administer Gestone once there is adequate secretion of placental progesterone. Gestone contains progesterone itself, the same as the naturally secreted hormone, and is not associated with masculinization of a female foetus as are synthetic progestins.

Detectable amounts of progesterone enter the breast milk. As the effect on the suckling infant has not been determined, the use of Gestone during lactation is not recommended.

Other special warnings and precautions: Gestone should be used cautiously in patients with conditions that might be aggravated by fluid retention (e.g. hypertension, cardiac disease, renal disease, epilepsy), with a history of mental depression, diabetes, mild to moderate hepatic dysfunction, acute intermittent porphyria, migraine or photosensitivity.

If unexplained, sudden or gradual, partial or complete loss of vision, proptosis or diplopia, papilloedema, retinal vascular lesions or migraine occur during therapy, the drug should be discontinued and appropriate diagnostic and therapeutic measures instituted.

Overdosage: This is unlikely and is not expected to produce any adverse effects. Treatment is observation and, if necessary, symptomatic and supportive measures should be provided.

Pharmaceutical precautions Protect from light. On storage, solid matter may separate and this should be redissolved by warming before use.

Legal category POM.

Package quantities Ampoules containing: 25 mg in 1 ml; 50 mg in 1 ml; 100 mg in 2 ml. Boxes of 10.

Further information Nil.

Product licence numbers

25 mg	0051/5036R
50 mg	0051/5037R
100 mg	0051/5038R

GONADOTRAPHON LH*

Presentation Gonadotraphon LH is presented in ampoules containing a white, sterile, freeze-dried plug of 1000 or 5000 Units of Chorionic Gonadotrophin BP (HCG) in a lactose base, for injection. Both strengths are supplied with 2 ml ampoules of solvent for reconstitution of the powder.

Uses Human chorionic gonadotrophin (HCG) is obtained from the urine of pregnant women. The action of HCG is predominantly that of the pituitary luteinising hormone.

In the female: In the management of anovulatory infertility, Gonadotraphon LH can be given to induce ovulation after follicular development has been stimulated with follicle stimulating hormone.

In the male: HCG stimulates the interstitial cells to secrete testosterone. Gonadotraphon LH can therefore be used in the management of delayed puberty, undescended testes and oligospermia.

Dosage and administration Gonadotraphon LH is given by intramuscular injection. Treatment should only commence after expert assessment.

In the female: Induction of ovulation: 10,000 units mid-cycle if plasma oestrogen levels are favourable following follicular stimulation.

In the male: Delayed puberty: Dose should be titrated against plasma testosterone, starting with 500 units twice weekly. Treatment should be continued for 4–6 weeks.

Undescended testes: Treatment should begin before puberty, the optimum age range being 7–10 years. 500 units three times weekly is a suitable starting dose, but this may be increased up to 4000 units thrice weekly if necessary. Treatment should continue for 6–10 weeks. In males over 17 years of age a commencing dose of 1000 units twice weekly can be given. Treatment should be continued for one or two months after testicular descent.

Oligospermia: Dose should be titrated against seminal analysis starting with 500 units two or three times weekly. Treatment should be continued for 16 weeks.

Contra-indications, warnings, etc

Contra-indications: HCG should not be given to patients with disorders that might be exacerbated by androgen release.

Warnings: HCG should be given with care to patients in

whom fluid retention might be a hazard, as in asthma, epilepsy, migraine, or cardiac or renal disorders.

Allergic reactions may occur and patients thought to be susceptible should be given skin tests before treatment.

HCG preparations should only be used under the supervision of a specialist having available adequate facilities for appropriate laboratory monitoring.

In the female: Use in induction of ovulation may result in ovarian enlargement or cysts, acute abdominal pain, superovulation, or multiple pregnancies, particularly if endocrine monitoring is inadequate.

In the male: Treatment for undescended testes may produce precocious puberty; use should cease immediately. Gynaecomastia has been reported. A growth spurt may also be associated with use and this should be kept in mind particularly where epiphyseal growth is still potentially active.

Side-effects: Headache, tiredness and mood changes have been described.

Pharmaceutical precautions In the dry state, in sealed ampoules, Gonadotraphon LH will remain stable if protected from light and stored at a temperature not exceeding 20°C. Solutions are unstable and should be freshly prepared.

Legal category POM.

Package quantities
1000 units: Boxes of 5
5000 units: Boxes of 1 or 5

Further information The solvent contains 0.5% Phenol BP in Water for Injections BP. This has been found to reduce the pain of injections.

Product licence numbers
1000 Units 0051/5027
5000 Units 0051/5028

KETOVITE* LIQUID

Presentation A pink to yellow liquid containing the following active constituents in a formulation which does not include sucrose, glucose, fructose, lactose, starch, sodium or artificial colouring.

	per 5 ml
Vitamin A	2,500 Units
Ergocalciferol BP	400 Units
Choline chloride	150 mg
Cyanocobalamin BP	12.5 micrograms

Uses As a therapeutic supplement for the prevention of vitamin deficiency in conditions such as galactosaemia, disaccharide intolerance, phenylketonuria and other disorders of carbohydrate or amino acid metabolism, as well as in patients who are on restricted, specialised or synthetic diets.

Dosage and administration Ketovite Liquid should be administered orally. The dose for adults, children and the elderly is 5 ml daily.

Contra-indications, warnings, etc
Contra-indications: Hypersensitivity to the product. Hypercalcaemia.

Interactions: Absorption of some vitamins in the preparation may be reduced in conditions of fat malabsorption or with the concurrent use of neomycin, cholestyramine, liquid paraffin, aminoglycosides, aminosalicylic acid, anticonvulsants, biguanides, chloramphenicol, cimetidine, colchicine, potassium salts and methyl-dopa. Serum B_{12} concentrations may be decreased by concurrent administration of oral contraceptives.

Effects on ability to drive and to use machines: None known.

Other undesirable effects: None in the absence of overdosage.

Use in pregnancy and lactation: Caution should be used in pregnancy as excessive doses of Vitamin A may be teratogenic, especially when taken in the first trimester. Large doses of Vitamin D in lactating mothers may cause hypercalcaemia in infants.

Other special warnings and precautions: The recommended dose should not be exceeded without medical advice. No other vitamin supplement containing Vitamins A and D should be taken with Ketovite Liquid except under medical supervision.

Overdose: Symptoms of overdosage may include anorexia, nausea, vomiting, rough dry skin, polyuria, thirst, loss of hair, painful bones and joints as well as raised plasma and urine calcium and phosphate concentration.

No emergency procedure or antidote is applicable and symptoms are rapidly reduced upon withdrawal of the preparation.

Incompatibilities (major): None known.

Pharmaceutical precautions Store at a temperature between 5° and 15°C.

Legal category P.

Package quantities 150 ml.

Further information For complete vitamin supplementation, Ketovite Liquid should be used in conjunction with Ketovite Tablets. Ketovite Liquid is available on NHS prescription.

Product licence number 0051/5080R

KETOVITE* TABLETS

Presentation Yellow biconvex tablets. Each tablet contains the following vitamins in a formulation which does not contain sucrose, glucose, fructose, lactose, starch, sodium, artificial colouring or preservatives:

Thiamine Hydrochloride BP	1.0 mg
Riboflavine BP	1.0 mg
Pyridoxine Hydrochloride BP	330 micrograms
Nicotinamide BP	3.3 mg
Calcium Pantothenate PhEur	1.16 mg
Ascorbic Acid BP	16.6 mg
Alpha Tocopheryl Acetate BP	5.0 mg
Inositol	50.0 mg
Biotin	170 micrograms
Folic Acid BP	250 micrograms
Acetomenaphthone 1973 BP	500 micrograms

Uses As a therapeutic supplement for the prevention of vitamin deficiency in conditions such as galactosaemia, disaccharide intolerance, phenylketonuria and other disorders of carbohydrate or amino acid metabolism, as well as in patients who are on restricted, specialised or synthetic diets.

Dosage and administration Ketovite Tablets should be administered orally. The dose for adults, children and the elderly is one tablet three times a day.

Contra-indications, warnings, etc
Contra-indications: Hypersensitivity to the product.

Interactions: Pyridoxine may increase the peripheral metabolism of levodopa reducing therapeutic efficacy in patients with Parkinson's disease.

Effects on ability to drive and to use machines: None known.

Other undesirable effects: None known.

Use in pregnancy and lactation: The recommended dose should not be exceeded without medical advice.

Overdose: Large overdosages of water-soluble vitamins are readily excreted in the urine.

No emergency procedure or antidote is applicable and any symptoms are rapidly reduced upon withdrawal of the preparation.

Incompatibilities (major): None known.

Pharmaceutical precautions Store in a cool dry place.

Legal category POM.

Package quantities 100.

Further information For complete vitamin supplementation, Ketovite Tablets should be used in conjunction with Ketovite Liquid. Ketovite Tablets are available on NHS prescription.

Product licence number 0051/5079R.

PANCREX* GRANULES

Presentation Pancrex Granules (Pancreatin Granules BP) – Coated granules of pancreatin with not less than the following BP Units of activity in each gram: Free protease 300, lipase 5,000, amylase 4,000.

Uses To compensate for reduced intestinal enzyme activity in pancreatic deficiency states.

Indications: Fibrocystic disease of the pancreas (cystic fibrosis), chronic pancreatitis and pancreatic steatorrhoea following pancreatectomy, vagotomy or gastrectomy.

Dosage and administration Oral. Dosage may vary considerably according to the needs of the individual patient and should be determined by the physician.

An average dose for adults and children who are able to take granules satisfactorily is: 5–10 g four times daily to be swallowed dry or mixed with a little water or milk just before meals.

Contra-indications, warnings, etc
Contra-indications: None stated.

Interactions: None stated.

Effects on ability to drive and use machines: None stated.

Other undesirable effects: There are no known major adverse effects. Rare cases of hyperuricosuria and hyperuricaemia have been reported when extremely high doses of pancreatin have been taken.

Use in pregnancy and lactation: Safety in pregnancy has not been established. However no teratogenic effects have been observed in clinical cases.

Other special warnings and precautions: Chewing the granules and retaining them in the mouth may cause irritation of the mucosa of the mouth. Skin around the anus may suffer irritation. A barrier cream may prevent this.

Overdose: None stated.

Incompatibilities: None stated.

Pharmaceutical precautions Store at a temperature not exceeding 15°C.

Further information Pancrex is prepared from Pancreatin of porcine origin. Three level 5 ml spoonfuls provide aproximately 10 g of Pancrex Granules. Palatability may be improved by mixing with fruit juice or puree.

Legal category GSL.

Package quantities 500 g.

Product licence number 0051/5003R.

PANCREX* V CAPSULES
PANCREX* V CAPSULES 125 mg

Presentation
Pancrex V Capsules: Ivory coloured opaque hard gelatin capsules imprinted 'Pancrex V' and company logo containing Pancreatin BP and providing not less than the following BP Units of activity per capsule: Free protease 430, lipase 8,000, amylase 9,000.

Pancrex V Capsules '125': Clear hard gelatin capsules containing Pancreatin BP and providing not less than the following BP Units of activity: Free protease 160, lipase 2,950, amylase 3,300.

Uses To compensate for reduced intestinal enzyme activity in pancreatic deficiency states.

Indications: Fibrocystic disease of the pancreas (cystic fibrosis), chronic pancreatitis and pancreatic steatorrhoea following pancreatectomy. May also be indicated following gastrectomy as an aid to digestion.

Dosage and administration Oral. Dosage should be adjusted according to the needs of the individual patient and the amount and type of food consumed.

The following dosage ranges provide a suitable basis for adjustment.

Pancrex V Capsules
Infants: The contents of 1–2 capsules mixed with feeds.
Older children and adults: The contents of 2–6 capsules with each snack or meal. The capsules may be swallowed.

The capsules may provide a suitable alternative to the enteric coated presentations in cases where the pH of the duodenum is not sufficiently alkaline to dissolve the enteric coat.

Capsules provide a simple and convenient method of dose measurement of pancreatin for administration to younger children reequiring a low dose.

Pancrex V Capsules 125 mg: These low dose capsules may be used when small amounts of Pancrex are required, for example for neonates.

Neonates: The contents of 1–2 capsules mixed with feeds.

Contra-indications, warnings, etc
Contra-indications: None stated.

Interactions: None stated.

Effects on ability to drive and use machines: None stated.

Other undesirable effects: Rare cases of hyperuricosuria and hyperuricaemia have been reported when extremely high doses of pancreatin have been taken.

Use in pregnancy and lactation: Safety in pregnancy has not been established. However no teratogenic effects have been observed in clinical cases.

Other special warnings and precautions: It is possible that some irritation of the skin of the mouth may occur if capsules are chewed or the contents retained in the mouth. Irritation of the anus may also occur. A barrier cream may prevent this local irritation.

Allergic/asthmatic reactions have occasionally occurred on handling the capsule contents.

If the capsule contents are mixed with liquids or feeds, the resulting mixture should not be allowed to stand for more than one hour prior to use.

Overdose: None stated.

Incompatibilities: None stated.

Pharmaceutical precautions Store at a temperature not exceeding 15°C.

Further information Pancrex is prepared from Pancreatin of porcine origin. Palatability of capsule contents may be improved by mixing with fruit juice or puree.

Some of the activity is destroyed by the acidity of the stomach. Dosage recommendations reflect this. Cimetidine given 30–45 minutes before meals has been found to potentiate the enzyme activity by reducing gastric acid secretion.

Legal category GSL.

Package quantities 500 Pancrex V Capsules.
300 Pancrex V Capsules 125 mg.

Product licence numbers
0051/5043R
0051/5104R (125 mg)

PANCREX* V POWDER

Presentation Pancrex V Powder (Pancreatin BP): A white or buff coloured powder having not less than the following BP Units of activity in each gram: Free Protease 1,400, Lipase 25,000, Amylase 30,000.

Uses To compensate for reduced intestinal enzyme activity in pancreatic deficiency states.

Indications: Fibrocystic disease of the pancreas (cystic fibrosis), chronic pancreatitis and pancreatic steatorrhoea following pancreatectomy. May also be indicated following gastrectomy as an aid to digestion.

Dosage and administration Oral. Dosage should be adjusted according to the needs of the individual patient and the amount and type of food consumed.

The following dosage ranges provide a suitable basis for adjustment:

Adults and children: 0.5–2 g. Swallowed dry or mixed with a little water or milk with each snack or meal.

Newborn infants: 0.25–0.5 g with each feed.

Contra-indications, warnings, etc
Contra-indications: None stated.

Interactions: None stated.

Effects on ability to drive and use machines: None stated.

Other undesirable effects: Rare cases of hyperuricosuria and hyperuricaemia have been reported when extremely high doses of pancreatin have been taken.

Use in pregnancy and lactation: Safety in pregnancy has not been established. However no teratogenic effects have been observed in clinical cases.

Other special warnings and precautions: It is possible that some irritation of the skin of the mouth may occur if the powder is retained in the mouth. Irritation of the anus may also occur. A barrier cream may prevent this local irritation.

Allergic/asthmatic reactions have occasionally occurred on handling the powder.

If Pancrex is mixed with liquids or feeds, the resulting mixture should not be allowed to stand for more than one hour prior to use.

Overdose: None stated.

Incompatibilities: None stated.

Pharmaceutical precautions Store at a temperature not exceeding 15°C.

Further information Pancrex is prepared from Pancreatin of porcine origin. One level 5 ml spoonful will provide approximately 2 g of Pancrex V Powder.

Palatability may be improved by mixing with fruit juice or puree. Some of the activity is destroyed by the acidity of the stomach. Dosage recommendations reflect this. Cimetidine given 30–45 minutes before meals has been found to potentiate the enzyme activity by reducing gastric acid secretion.

Legal category GSL.

Package quantities 300 g.

Product licence number 0051/5004R.

PANCREX* V FORTE TABLETS

Presentation
Pancrex V Forte Tablets (Pancreatin Tablets BP) (Pancreatin BP/Pancreas Powder EP 222 mg): White sugar and enteric coated tablets each containing not less than the following BP Units of activity: Free protease 330, lipase 5,600, amylase 5,000.

Uses To compensate for reduced intestinal enzyme activity in pancreatic deficiency states.

Indications: Fibrocystic disease of the pancreas (cystic fibrosis), chronic pancreatitis and pancreatic steatorrhoea following pancreatectomy. May also be indicated following gastrectomy as an aid to digestion.

Dosage and administration Oral. Dosage should be adjusted according to the needs of the individual patient and the amount and type of food consumed.

The following dosage range provides a suitable basis for adjustment.

Adults and children: 6–10 tablets before each snack or meal swallowed whole.

Contra-indications, warnings, etc
Contra-indications: None stated.

Interactions: None stated.

Effects on ability to drive and use machines: None stated.

Other undesirable effects: Rare cases of hyperuricosuria and hyperuricaemia have been reported when extremely high doses of pancreatin have been taken.

Use in pregnancy and lactation: Safety in pregnancy has not been established. However no teratogenic effects have been observed in clinical cases.

Other special warnings and precautions: Variations in response to treatment may be due to enteric coating. It is possible that some irritation of the skin of the mouth may occur if tablets are chewed. Irritation of the anus may also occur. A barrier cream may prevent this local irritation.

Overdose: None stated.

Incompatibilities: None stated.

Pharmaceutical precautions Store at a temperature not exceeding 15°C.

Further information Pancrex is prepared from Pancreatin of porcine origin.

Legal category GSL.

Package quantities 250.

Product licence number 0051/5000R

VIRORMONE*

Presentation Ampoules of 100 mg of Testosterone Propionate BP in ethyl oleate for intramuscular injection.

Uses Testosterone is the androgenic hormone of male testis. It is used as replacement therapy in castrated adults and in those who are hypogonadal due to either pituitary or testicular disease.

May also be used for control of carcinoma of the breast in post-menopausal women.

Dosage and administration
In the male: Hypogonadism (adults), delayed puberty, cryptorchidism.

In the female: Carcinoma of the breast in post-menopausal women.

Hypogonadism	50 mg 2–3 times weekly
Delayed puberty cryptorchidism	50 mg weekly
Carcinoma of the breast	100 mg 2–3 times weekly

Contra-indications, warnings, etc
Cautions: Do not use before puberty in males, unless for treatment of delayed puberty. In any case caution is advised since the fusion of the epiphyses is hastened and may lead to short stature.

Use with care in patients with cardiac, renal or hepatic impairment, circulatory failure, hypertension or epilepsy. A reduced dosage may be advisable in elderly male patients since hyperstimulation can occur.

Virilism may occur in female patients on high doses.

Contra-indications: Breast cancer in men, prostatic carcinoma, pregnancy, breast feeding and nephrosis.

Warning: Tumours of the liver have been reported occasionally in patients subjected to prolonged treatment with androgenic-anabolic steroids. The possibility that these compounds may induce or enhance the development of hepatic tumours cannot at present be excluded and this should be considered when the use of this product is proposed, especially in young people who are not suffering with life threatening disorders.

Pharmaceutical precautions Protect from light.

Legal category POM.

Package quantities 100 mg in 2 ml ampoules. Boxes of 10.

Further information Nil.

Product licence number 0051/5059R

**Trade Mark*

Panpharma Limited
Hayes Gate House
27 Uxbridge Road
Hayes, Middlesex UB4 0JN

ANACAL* SUPPOSITORIES
ANACAL* RECTAL OINTMENT

Presentation

	Anacal Suppository (a smooth white suppository) (g%)	*Anacal Rectal Ointment (a white translucent ointment) (g%)*
Mucopolysaccharide polysulphuric acid ester (Heparinoid)	0.2	0.2
Oxypolyethoxydodecane (Lauromacrogol-400)	2.5	5.0

Uses For the relief of symptoms associated with haemorrhoids (including perianal haematomas), perianal eczema, pruritus, anal fissure, proctitis, periproctitis, and after-care of haemorrhoids treated by surgery or injection.

Dosage and administration Adults, the elderly and children over the age of five years.
Anacal Suppositories: One suppository to be inserted once or twice daily.

Anacal Rectal Ointment: To be applied one to four times daily, as required. (Nozzle supplied for internal application.)

Contra-indications, warnings, etc
Contra-indications: Not intended for administration to children below the age of 7 years.

Pregnancy and lactation: There is no evidence to suggest that Anacal should not be used during pregnancy and lactation.

Pharmaceutical precautions Store suppositories in a cool place.

Legal category P.

Package quantities *Anacal Suppositories:* Packs of 10 (2 g ea.).
Anacal Rectal Ointment: Tubes of 30 g.

Further information Nil.

Product licence numbers
Anacal Suppositories 0542/5004R
Anacal Rectal Ointment 0542/5005R

Product licence holder: Farillon Ltd, Romford, Essex RM3 8UE.

HIRUDOID* CREAM
HIRUDOID* GEL

Presentation Hirudoid Cream contains organo-heparinoid 'Luitpold' 0.3 g (25,000 units) in 100 g of a white vanishing-cream base.
Hirudoid Gel contains the same active constituent in a colourless gel base.

Uses For the treatment of superficial thrombophlebitis and the soothing relief of superficial bruising and haematoma.

Dosage and administration Adults, the elderly and children over the age of 5 years.
Hirudoid Cream: Two to six inches (5–15 cm) to be applied up to four times daily to the affected area and gently massaged into the skin. If the area is tender to touch or if there is evidence of thrombosis, Hirudoid Cream should be applied thickly to the skin and covered with gauze or lint. In such cases it may be massaged very gently into the skin surrounding the affected area.

Hirudoid Gel: To be applied as a thin layer up to four times daily. Recommended when its cooling effect and rapid action are especially required.

Contra-indications, warnings, etc
Contra-indications: Not to be used on large areas of skin, broken skin, sensitive areas of skin or mucous membranes.

Precautions: Should not be used on children under the age of 5 years. For external use only.

Pregnancy and lactation: There is no evidence to suggest that Hirudoid should not be used during pregnancy and lactation.

Pharmaceutical precautions Nil.

Legal category P.

Package quantities *Hirudoid Cream or Gel:* Tubes of 40 g.

Further information Nil.

Product licence numbers
Hirudoid Cream 0542/5000R
Hirudoid Gel 0542/0005R

Product licence holder: Farillon Ltd, Romford, Essex RM3 8EU.

MOVELAT* CREAM
MOVELAT* GEL

Presentation Movelat Cream contains mucopolysaccharide polysulphate (MPS) 0.2 g and salicylic acid 2.0 g in 100 g of a white vanishing-cream base. Movelat Gel contains the same active constituents in a colourless gel base.

Uses For the relief of symptoms associated with painful inflammatory conditions of the musculo-skeletal system, including traumatic conditions such as sprains and strains.

Dosage and administration
Movelat Cream: Two to six inches (5–15 cm) to be massaged into the affected area up to four times daily. The cream may also be used with a dressing, when it should be applied thickly.

Movelat Gel: Two to six inches (5–15 cm) to be applied to the affected area up to four times daily.

Contra-indications, warnings, etc
Contra-indications: Should not be used on large areas of skin. Should not be used on broken skin, sensitive areas of skin or on mucous membranes. Should not be used on children under the age of 12 years.

Precautions: In cases of sensitivity to salicylates, allergic skin reactions may occur. For external use only.

Pregnancy and lactation: There is no evidence to suggest

that Movelat should not be used during pregnancy and lactation.

Pharmaceutical precautions Nil.

Legal category P.

Package quantities *Movelat Cream or Gel:* Tubes of 100 g.

Further information Nil.

Product licence numbers
Cream 0542/5001R
Gel 0542/0006R

Product licence holder: Farillon Limited, Romford, Essex, RM3 8UE.

NORDOX*

Presentation Green capsules containing 100 mg doxycycline, as the hydrochloride, coded NORDOX 100.

Uses
Actions: Nordox is postulated to exert its antimicrobial effect by the inhibition of protein synthesis and can thus be considered to be primarily bacteriostatic. Nordox is clinically effective in the treatment of a variety of infections caused by a wide range of Gram-negative and Gram-positive bacteria, as well as certain other micro-organisms. After oral administration, Nordox is almost completely absorbed in the gastro-intestinal tract and, unlike several other tetracyclines, the absorption is not unduly altered by the ingestion of milk or food.

Genito-urinary tract infections: Cystitis, urethritis, pyelonephritis, caused by susceptible strains of *Escherichia coli, Neisseria gonorrhoeae*, the *Klebsiella-Enterobacter* group, *Staphylococcus* species and *Chlamydia trachomatis*. A single large dose of doxycycline has effectively treated acute gonococcal anterior urethritis in the adult male. However, a more extended therapy elicited the highest cure rates.

Soft tissue infections: Infected traumatic and postoperative wounds, furunculosis, impetigo, cellulitis, abscess and paronychia, caused by susceptible strains of the *Klebsiella-Enterobacter* group, as well as susceptible strains of *Staphylococcus aureus, Streptococcus* species, *E. coli* and *Staphylococcus albus*. Nordox treatment of soft tissue infections should always be carried out in conjunction with any necessary indicated surgical procedures.

Pneumonia: Nordox is effective against single and multilobe pneumonia and broncho-pneumonia caused by susceptible strains of *H. influenzae, Klebsiella pneumoniae, pneumococci* and other *streptococcus* species, *Staphylococcus* and *Mycoplasma pneumoniae*. Other respiratory tract infections: Bronchitis, tonsillitis, pharyngitis, otitis media and sinusitis, due to susceptible strains of *pneumococci, H. influenzae, staphylococcus* species and beta-haemolytic streptococci.

As Nordox is one of the tetracycline group of antibiotics, it may be expected to be useful in the treatment of infections which respond to other tetracyclines such as:

Gastro-intestinal infections: Caused by susceptible strains of such organisms as *Shigella* species, *Salmonella* species, *Entamoeba histolytica* and enteropathogenic *E. coli*.

Ophthalmic infections: Caused by susceptible strains of staphylococci, gonococci and *H. influenzae*. Nordox is indicated for the treatment of inclusion conjunctivitis either alone or in combination with topical agents. Nordox is also suitable in the treatment of trachoma. However, the infectious agent is not eliminated on all occasions, as tested by immunofluorescence techniques.

Miscellaneous: Trigonitis and Prostatitis caused by *Proteus* species. *Psittacosis*. Certain other infections caused by susceptible strains of *Bacteroides* species, *Listeria* species, *Rickettsia* species, *Yersinia* species, *Brucella* species (in combination with streptomycin) and *Bordatella pertussis, Calymmato-bacterium granulomatis*, spirochaetes (*Treponema* species), *Bacillus anthracis, Neisseria meningitis* and *Clostridium welchii*.

Nordox may be a useful adjunct to amoebicides in the treatment of acute intestinal amoebiasis.

Further, Nordox may be useful in the treatment of acne vulgaris and acne conglobata.

Dosage and administration
Adults: The recommended dose of Nordox is 200 mg on the first day of treatment—which can be given as a single dose or it can be divided into two 100 mg doses with a 12 hour interval—followed by a 100 mg/day maintenance dose. For more severe infections, especially chronic urinary tract infections, a daily dose of 200 mg should be administered during the period of treatment.

Elderly: In elderly patients over 70 years of age, a liquid or dispersible form of doxycycline would be more appropriate.

Children: Nordox is not recommended for children under 12 years of age.

As doxycycline is liable to cause oesophageal irritation and ulceration, it is recommended that Nordox should be taken with an adequate volume of fluid (at least half a glass) preferably taken in the upright position and not immediately prior to going to bed. It is further recommended that Nordox be taken with food or milk if gastric irritation occurs. The absorption of Nordox is not markedly influenced by the simultaneous ingestion of food or milk.

Dosage restriction is not normally required in cases of renal impairment.

If the recommended dosage is exceeded, an increase in the incidence of side-effects may ensue. Treatment should be continued for at least 24 to 48 hours beyond the period when symptoms and fever have abated. In the specific case of streptococcal infections, treatment should be continued for 10 days in order that the development of glomerulonephritis or rheumatic fever is prevented.

Primary and secondary syphilis: A recommended daily dosage of 300 mg in divided doses to be administered for at least 10 days.

Acute gonococcal infections in the adult female: A dosage schedule of 100 mg twice a day to be continued until cure is effected.

Acute gonococcal anterior urethritis in males: A dosage schedule of 100 mg twice a day for two to four days or a single dose of 300 mg. The dose should preferably be taken with food, including milk or carbonated drink, as necessary.

Uncomplicated urethral, endocervical, or rectal infection in adults, caused by Chlamydia trachomatis: 100 mg by mouth, twice daily for at least 7 days.

Typhus of the louse-borne variety has been successfully treated with a single dose of 100 to 200 mg depending on the severity of infection.

Concurrent treatment: Patients taking Nordox should not be simultaneously ingesting antacids containing magnesium, aluminium or calcium salts as these impair absorption. Studies indicate that doxycycline at usual dosage in patients with renal impairment does not lead to excessive accumulation of the antibiotic within the body.

Concurrent use of doxycycline with bactericidal antibiotics, e.g. penicillin, is not recommended.

Contra-indications, warnings, etc
Contra-indications: Known hypersensitivity to tetracyclines.

Warnings: Tetracyclines may cause a yellow to brown discolouration of the teeth and enamel hypoplasia in the developing foetus or child and, therefore, Nordox should only be administered if considered essential, to pregnant or lactating women and to children under twelve years of age.

As with other tetracyclines, Nordox forms a stable calcium complex in any bone-forming tissue. A decrease in the fibula growth rate has been observed in prematures given oral tetracycline in doses of 25 mg/kg every 6 hours. This reaction was shown to be reversible when the drug was discontinued.

The antianabolic action of tetracyclines may cause an increase in BUN. Studies indicate that this does not occur with the use of Nordox in patients with renal impairment.

Tetracyclines have been reported as causing photo-sensitivity and allergic skin reactions. Patients should be advised to avoid direct exposure to natural or artificial sunlights and that treatment should be discontinued at the first signs of skin discomfort.

Pregnancy and lactation: (See Warnings above about using during tooth development).

Nordox has not been studied in pregnant patients. It should not be used in pregnant women unless, in the judgement of the physician, it is essential for the welfare of the patient.

Results of animal studies indicate that tetracyclines cross the placenta, are found in foetal tissues and can have toxic effects on the developing foetus (often related to retardation of the skeletal development). Evidence of embryotoxicity has also been noted in animals treated early in pregnancy.

Tetracyclines are present in the milk of lactating women who are taking a drug of this class and should therefore be avoided in nursing mothers.

Precautions: Where syphilis is suspected as co-existing with gonorrhoea, proper diagnostic procedures should be utilised, including darkfield examinations. Monthly serological tests in such cases should be performed for at least four months.

As with all antibiotics, overgrowth of resistant organisms may cause glossitis, stomatitis, vaginitis or staphylococcal enteritis. Should any of these occur, treatment should cease and the appropriate therapy be instituted.

Infections due to group A beta-haemolytic streptococci should be treated for at least 10 days.

Drug interactions: Tetracyclines depress plasma prothrombin activity, therefore reduced dosages of concurrent anti-coagulants may be required.

Barbiturates, carbamazepine and phenytoin decrease the half-life of doxycycline.

The concurrent use of tetracycline and methoxyflurane has been reported to result in fatal renal toxicity.

Adverse reactions: Due to the fact that Nordox is virtually completely absorbed, gastro-intestinal side-effects are infrequent. Patients receiving doxycycline are known, however, to exhibit the following adverse reactions.

Oesophagitis and oesophageal ulceration.

Gastro-intestinal: Diarrhoea, nausea, vomiting and anorexia may occur.

Skin: Maculopapular and erythematous rashes. Exfoliative dermatitis has been reported but is uncommon. Photo-sensitivity is discussed in the 'Warnings' section.

Hypersensitivity reactions: Anaphylaxis, anaphylactoid purpura, angioneurotic oedema, urticaria, pericarditis and exacerbation of systemic lupus erythematosis.

Bulging fontanelles in infants and benign intracranial hypertension in adults have been reported. Treatment should cease if evidence of raised intracranial pressure develops.

Blood: Thrombocytopenia, haemolytic anaemia, eosinophilia and neutropenia have all been reported with tetracyclines.

Tetracyclines given over prolonged periods have been reported to produce a brown/black microscopic discolouration of thyroid tissue. No abnormalities of thyroid function are known to occur.

Overdose and toxic effects: No specific antidote. Gastric lavage plus appropriate supportive treatment.

Toxic effects are usually due to hypersensitivity reactions and should be treated as such.

Pharmaceutical precautions Store in a cool dry place. Protect from light.

Legal category POM.

Package quantities Packs of 10 capsules.

Further information Nil.

Product licence number 8265/0001.

**Trade Mark*

Parke-Davis Research Laboratories
Chestnut Avenue
Eastleigh
Hampshire SO5 3ZQ

PARKE-DAVIS
RESEARCH LABORATORIES

ABIDEC*

Presentation Oral drops: A clear yellow liquid, with a characteristic odour and taste.

Composition: Each 0.6 ml contains:

Vitamin A PhEur	4000 units
Vitamin B_1 (Thiamine Hydrochloride PhEur)	1 mg
Vitamin B_2 (Riboflavine PhEur)	400 micrograms
Vitamin B_6 (Pyridoxine Hydrochloride PhEur)	500 micrograms
Vitamin C (Ascorbic Acid PhEur)	50 mg
Vitamin D_2 (Calciferol PhEur)	400 units
Nicotinamide PhEur	5 mg

Uses The prevention of vitamin deficiencies and for the maintenance of normal growth and health during the early years of infancy and childhood; multivitamin supplement.

Dosage and administration Oral.
Infants less than one year old: 0.3 ml daily.

Older children and adults: 0.6 ml daily.

Elderly (over 65 years): As for adults.

Contra-indications, warnings, etc Hypersensitivity to any of the active constituents. Excessive dosage of vitamins A and D can lead to hypervitaminosis. When prescribing Abidec, as with other multivitamin preparations, allowance should be made for vitamins obtained from other sources.

Treatment of overdosage: Not applicable.

Pharmaceutical precautions Product has an expiry date of 2 years. Store below 25°C.

Legal category GSL.

Package quantities 50 ml pack (2×25 ml+2 droppers graduated at 0.3 ml and 0.6 ml). 25 ml pack.

Further information Nil.

Product licence number 0018/5021.

ACCUPRO*

Presentation Brown, film coated, tablets imprinted with the dosage strength. The 5 mg tablet is elliptical. The 10 mg tablet is triangular. The 20 mg tablet is round.

Composition: Tablets containing 5 mg, 10 mg or 20 mg, of quinapril.

Uses
Action: Quinapril is rapidly de-esterified to quinaprilat (quinapril diacid, the principal metabolite), which is a potent angiotensin-converting enzyme (ACE) inhibitor.

Indications: For the treatment of all grades of essential hypertension where standard therapy is ineffective or inappropriate because of adverse effects. Accupro is effective as monotherapy or concomitantly administered with diuretics in patients with hypertension.

For the treatment of congestive heart failure when given concomitantly with a diuretic and/or cardiac glycoside. Treatment of congestive heart failure with Accupro should always be initiated in hospital.

Dosage and administration Oral.
Adults
Hypertension: The recommended initial dosage is 5 mg once daily. A 5 mg dose seldom achieves a therapeutic response. Depending upon clinical response, patient's dosage may be titrated (by doubling the dose allowing adequate time for dosage adjustment) to a maintenance dosage of 20 to 40 mg/day given as a single dose or divided into 2 doses. Long-term control is maintained in most patients with a single daily dosage regimen. Patients have been treated with dosages up to 80 mg/day.

Concomitant diuretics: In order to determine if excess hypotension will occur, an initial dosage of 2.5 mg of Accupro is recommended in patients who are also being treated with a diuretic. After this the dosage of Accupro should be titrated (by doubling the dose allowing adequate time for dosage adjustment) to the optimal response.

Congestive heart failure: In order to closely monitor patients for symptomatic hypotension, a single 2.5 mg initial dose is recommended. After this, patients should be titrated to an effective dose (up to 40 mg/day) given in 2 doses with concomitant diuretic and/or cardiac glycoside therapy. Patients are usually maintained effectively on doses of 10–20 mg/day given in 2 doses with concomitant therapy.

Elderly/renal impairment: In elderly patients and in patients with a creatinine clearance of less than 40 ml/min, an initial dosage in essential hypertension of 2.5 mg once daily is recommended followed by titration to the optimal response.

Children: Not recommended. Safety and efficacy in children has not been established.

Contra-indications, warnings, etc Hypersensitivity to any of the ingredients.

Pregnancy: Accupro is contra-indicated throughout pregnancy. Accupro has been shown to be foetotoxic in rabbits. Use of ACE inhibitors in the second and third trimesters of human pregnancy has been associated with oligohydramnios. Hypotension and renal failure have occurred in the newborn.

Precautions: In patients with renal insufficiency, monitoring of renal function during therapy should be performed as deemed appropriate, although in the majority renal function will not alter or may improve.

Renal failure has been reported in association with ACE inhibitors and has occurred mainly in patients with severe congestive heart failure or underlying renal disease, including renal artery stenosis. If recognised promptly and treated appropriately, renal failure is usually reversible.

Drug interactions
Tetracycline: Because of the presence of magnesium carbonate in the formulation Accupro has been shown in healthy volunteers to reduce the absorption of tetracycline in concomitant administration. It is recommended that concomitant administration with tetracycline be avoided.

Concomitant diuretic therapy: Patients treated with diuretics may occasionally experience an excessive reduction of blood pressure after initiation of therapy with Accupro. This hypotensive effect may be effectively minimised by either discontinuing the diuretic or increasing the salt intake prior to the initial dose of Accupro. If discontinuation of the diuretic is not possible, medical supervision should be provided for up to two hours following administration of the initial dose.

Agents increasing serum potassium: Concomitant treatments with potassium sparing diuretics, potassium supplements or potassium salts should be used with caution and with appropriate monitoring of serum potassium.

Surgery/anaesthesia: Although no data are available to indicate there is an interaction between Accupro and anaesthetic agents that produces hypotension, caution should be exercised when patients undergo major surgery or anaesthesia since angiotensin converting enzyme inhibitors have been shown to block angiotensin II formation secondary to compensatory renin release. This may lead to hypotension which can be corrected by volume expansion.

Side-effects: The most frequent clinical adverse reactions in hypertension and congestive heart failure are headache, dizziness, rhinitis, coughing, upper respiratory tract infection, fatigue, nausea and vomiting. Other less frequent side effects are dyspepsia, myalgia, chest pain, abdominal pain, diarrhoea, back pain, sinusitis, insomnia, paraesthesia, nervousness, asthenia, pharyngitis, hypotension.

Increases ($>$1.25 times the upper limit of normal) in serum creatinine and blood urea nitrogen were observed in 3% and 4% respectively of the patients on monotherapy. Such increases are more likely to occur in patients receiving concomitant diuretic therapy than those on monotherapy with Accupro. These observed increases will often reverse on continued therapy.

Angioedema: Angioedema has been reported in patients treated with angiotensin-converting enzyme inhibitors. If laryngeal stridor or angioedema of the face, tongue, or glottis occur, treatment should be discontinued immediately, the patient treated appropriately in accordance with accepted medical care, and carefully observed until the swelling disappears. In instances where swelling is confined to the face and lips, the condition generally resolves without treatment; antihistamines may be useful in relieving symptoms. Angioedema associated with laryngeal involvement may be fatal. Where there is involvement of the tongue, glottis, or larynx likely to cause airway obstruction, appropriate therapy eg, subcutaneous adrenaline solution 1:1000 (0.3 to 0.5 ml) should be promptly administered.

Hypotension: Symptomatic hypotension was rarely seen in hypertensive patients treated with Accupro but is a possible consequence of ACE inhibition therapy particularly in salt/volume depleted patients such as those previously treated with diuretics.

Neutropenia/agranulocytosis: ACE inhibitors have been rarely associated with agranulocytosis and bone marrow depression in patients with uncomplicated hypertension but more frequently in patients with renal impairment, especially if they also have collagen vascular disease. As with other ACE inhibitors, monitoring of white blood cell counts in patients with collagen vascular disease and/or renal diseases should be considered.

Use in nursing mothers: Since it is not known if this drug is secreted in human milk caution should be exercised when the product is given to a nursing mother.

Overdosage: No data are available with respect to overdosage in humans. The most likely clinical manifestation would be symptoms attributable to severe hypotension, which should normally be treated by intravenous volume expansion. It is not known if quinapril or its metabolites are removed by haemodialysis.

Pharmaceutical precautions Store at a temperature not exceeding 30°C.

Legal category POM.

Package quantities: 5 mg, 10 mg and 20 mg strength are packed in blister strips of 7 tablets, 4 strips in a carton (28 tablets) (OP).

Further information: Nil.

Product licence numbers 0018/0148–0150.

AGAROL*

Presentation A stable, white emulsion containing the following active constituents per 5 ml:

Phenolphthalein BP	66 mg
Liquid Paraffin PhEur	1.6 ml
Agar PhEur	10 mg

Inactive ingredients: Benzoic Acid PhEur; Sodium Benzoate PhEur.

Uses Agarol provides balanced cathartic and laxative properties. For the temporary relief of constipation. Agarol may be especially required when straining at stool is a hazard e.g. in patients with hernia, cardiac or hypertensive conditions, during convalescence after surgery, pre and post operatively in the surgical treatment of haemorrhoids and other allied ano-rectal conditions, obstetric patients and patients confined to bed.

Dosage and administration Oral
Adults: One to three 5 ml spoonfuls to be taken at bedtime. If necessary the dose may be repeated 2 hours after breakfast. This product is for temporary use only.

Elderly (over 65 years): As for adults. Long term over-indulgence in laxatives has been reported. This is of particular importance in the elderly where a degree of dehydration may already exist. This product is for temporary use only.

Children (5–12 years) One 5 ml spoonful to be taken at bedtime or 2 hours after breakfast. Agarol may be mixed with water, milk or fruit juices. This product is for temporary use only.

Contra-indications, warnings, etc
Contra-indications: Sensitivity to phenolphthalein. Use is contra-indicated in children under 5 years.

Warnings: Caution is required in patients with swallowing difficulties. Repeated use is not recommended. Patients should be advised to consult their Doctor if laxatives are needed every day, if they have persistent abdominal pain or have a condition which makes swallowing difficult. This product should not be used repeatedly.

Precautions: Agarol should not be taken within 2 hours of a meal since there is a theoretical risk that the liquid paraffin content could interfere with absorption of fat soluble vitamins.

Side-effects: Rarely, sensitivity to phenolphthalein.

Overdosage: Overdosage may cause excessive purgation and may produce skin eruptions or rash in sensitive persons. Gastric lavage is unnecessary, but fluid (and electrolyte) replacement may be required. Skin rash should be treated symptomatically.

Pharmaceutical precautions Store below 25°C. Keep container tightly closed.

Legal category P.

Package quantities Bottles containing 200 ml.

Further information Nil.

Product licence number 0018/0160.

ALOPHEN*

Presentation Brown film-coated pills.

Composition: Each pill contains:

Aloin BP	15 mg
Belladonna dry extract PhEur	5 mg
Prepared Ipecacuanha PhEur	4 mg
Phenolphthalein BP	30 mg

Inactive ingredients: Lactose.

Uses Alophen Pills are for the relief of constipation due to torpidity of the lower bowel. They act promptly, evacuation normally occurring within 8–10 hours.

Dosage and administration Oral.
Adults: 1 to 3 pills at bedtime.

Elderly (over 65 years): As for adults. Long term over-indulgence in laxatives has been reported. This is of particular importance in the elderly where a degree of dehydration may already exist.

Children: Not recommended.

Contra-indications, warnings, etc Should not be used without the advice of a physician when nausea, vomiting or abdominal pain are present. Should not be given to patients with inflammatory bowel diseases or with glaucoma. Use with caution in patients with prostatic enlargement.

Prolonged continuous use is not recommended.

Treatment of overdosage: Treatment should be supportive together with fluid replacement.

Pharmaceutical precautions Store below 30°C.

Legal category P.

Package quantities Packs of 50.

Further information Nil.

Product licence number 0018/0062.

AMSIDINE* CONCENTRATE FOR INFUSION

Presentation Amsidine is formulated as two sterile liquids that are combined prior to use: *Drug ampoule* – a 2 ml clear, neutral glass printed ampoule containing a clear bright orange/red coloured solution; *Diluent vial* – a 20 ml amber glass vial containing a clear colourless solution.

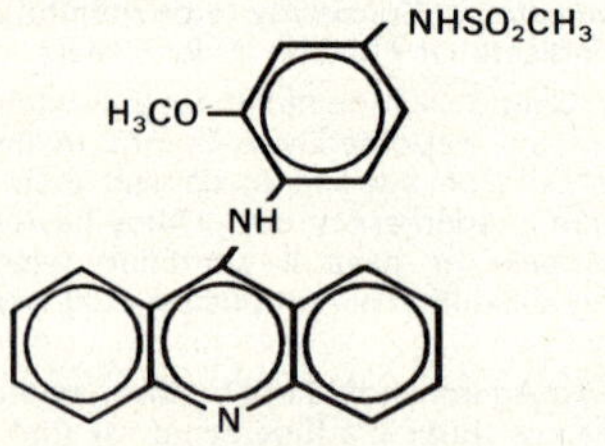

Each 2 ml ampoule contains 1.5 ml of amsacrine solution in anhydrous N,N-dimethylacetamide in a strength of 50 mg amsacrine per ml. That is, each ampoule contains 75 mg amsacrine. Each 20 ml amber vial contains 13.5 ml of 0.0353M L-lactic acid. Exactly 1.5 ml of the solution from the ampoule is removed by the aid of a graduated glass syringe and immediately added to the vial with L-lactic acid and the contents are mixed thoroughly by shaking. The resulting red solution contains 5 mg/ml Amsidine.

Uses

Action: Amsidine is a sterile antitumour chemotherapeutic agent for intravenous infusion. Although not completely clarified, the mode of action of amsacrine is related to its property of binding the DNA through intercalation and external (electrostatic) forces. Amsacrine inhibits the synthesis of DNA while the RNA may not be directly affected. An additional mode of action, involving modification of cell membrane function, has been suggested.

Indications: Amsidine is indicated for the induction and maintenance of remission in acute leukaemia of adults. It is effective in patients refractory to the anthracycline antibiotics used singly or in combination with other chemotherapeutic agents, and in patients who were formerly treated with maximum cumulative doses of these antibiotics.

Dosage and administration Amsidine must be diluted in 500 ml 5% Dextrose Injection BP and infused over 60 to 90 minutes. Phlebitis or pain at the injection site may occur at doses greater than 70 mg/m^2. (*Note: do not use other diluents. Amsidine is incompatible with saline.*) Care must be taken that no extravasation occurs which might produce severe irritation or necrosis. Caution in the handling and preparation of the solution should be exercised, and the use of polyethylene gloves is recommended. If the solution of Amsidine contacts the skin or mucosae, immediately wash thoroughly with soap and water. (See enclosure leaflet.)

Adults

Induction of remission phase: The usual dosage of Amsidine in the induction phase is 90 mg/m^2 every day for five consecutive days (total dose 450 mg/m^2 per course of treatment). If bone marrow biopsy performed on day six displays over 50% cellularity and the blasts count is over 30%, the treatment may be extended for an additional three days, bringing the total dose per course of treatment to 720 mg/m^2.

More than one course of treatment may be required to achieve induction. Depending on the effectiveness of the first course in producing myelosuppression, the subsequent courses are given at two-week (if not effective) to four-week (if effective) intervals. In cases where a hypocellular marrow has not been achieved after the first course of treatment, the daily dose of Amsidine may be escalated to 120 mg/m^2 per day for the subsequent courses, provided that this is not contra-indicated for reasons of non-myelosuppressive toxicity.

For patients with impaired liver function or impaired renal function, the dose of Amsidine should be decreased by 20–30% (to 60–75 mg/m^2 per day).

Maintenance phase: The maintenance dose is about one third the induction dose, given either as a single IV infusion or divided in three daily doses, e.g. 150 mg/m^2 given once every 3–4 weeks or 50 mg/m^2 per day for three consecutive days, repeated every 3–4 weeks. Each maintenance course should bring down the granulocyte count to 1,000–1,500/mm^3 and the platelet count to 50,000–100,000/mm^3. If this is not accomplished the maintenance dose may be escalated by 20% every second course. The granulocyte and platelet counts should be allowed to recover between the courses to over 1,500/mm^3 and 100,000/mm^3 respectively; otherwise the subsequent course should be delayed.

Children under 12 years: None.

Contra-indications, warnings, etc

Contra-indications: Treatment with Amsidine should not be started in patients who have pre-existing marked bone marrow suppression induced by other chemotherapeutic agents or radiotherapy.

Precautions: Patients should be hospitalised during the induction phase of treatment for close observation and extensive laboratory monitoring. Amsidine should be used only by physicians experienced in cancer chemotherapy. The drug may cause severe myelosuppression, and complete blood counts must be performed frequently. Leucocyte, red cell and platelet transfusions should be available.

With recommended dose schedules, leucopenia is usually transient, reaching its nadir at 10–13 days after treatment, with recovery usually following by the 17th to 25th day. White blood cell counts of 1,000/mm^3 or lower are to be expected during treatment with appropriate doses of Amsidine. Doses higher than recommended may produce more severe or more prolonged marrow suppression. The potential for cardiotoxicity may be increased particularly by hypokalaemia, also concurrent use of diuretics, aminoglycosides or other nephrotoxic drugs and previous exposure to other anthracycline therapy. Periodic monitoring of bone marrow, cardiac, liver, kidney and CNS functions should be carried out in patients receiving Amsidine and particularly in those with pre-existing disorders of these systems. In the case of an exceedingly large fall in white cell count and excessive depression of bone marrow, suspension of treatment or reduction of dosage may be necessary.

Studies have demonstrated a mutagenic potential. No carcinogenic studies have been carried out. As with other antineoplastic agents there is a possibility that prolonged use may lead to a carcinogenic effect. This should be borne in mind when undertaking long-term treatment.

Use in pregnancy: Animal studies have indicated that amsacrine has foetotoxic and teratogenic properties. In addition there may be an effect on fertility. There is no information on use in human pregnancy, therefore, the benefit/risk considerations should be carefully weighed when administering Amsidine.

Adverse reactions
Haematopoietic system: The dose-limiting toxicity associated with Amsidine is myelosuppression and pancytopenia, requiring supportive treatment with white and red blood cells and platelets. Major complications during therapy were infections and haemorrhages treated respectively, with antibiotics and platelet transfusions.

Gastro-intestinal: Nausea with or without vomiting occurred frequently, but these symptoms were usually mild to moderate. Mucositis (stomatitis and oesophagitis) was almost as frequent and ranged in severity from mild to life-threatening; its frequency and severity were not strictly dose-related.

Central nervous system: A few cases of grand mal seizures in acute leukaemia patients have occurred during treatment with Amsidine. These patients were suffering, however, from a number of conditions related to far-advanced disease and were heavily pretreated; and it is unclear whether the seizures were attributable to Amsidine. The seizures generally were responsive to standard treatment, such as phenytoin.

Hepatic: Liver function tests showed occasional transient elevations of serum bilirubin and alkaline phosphatase, sometimes accompanied by jaundice, which required lowering the dose of Amsidine.

Renal: Occasional occurrence of haematuria, anuria, and rarely acute renal failure have been reported.

Cardiac: Cardiotoxicity occurred in several patients. It ranged from grand mal seizures followed by ventricular tachycardia to congestive heart failure or cardiac arrest.

Cutaneous: Local tissue irritation, necrosis and phlebitis have been reported. This problem is related to the concentration of drug infused per unit time; it is ameliorated by diluting the drug in a large volume of 5% Dextrose Injection BP and infusing over a longer period of time (1 to 2 hours).

Alopecia occurred in about 1 in 7 patients, sometimes precipitously. Since most patients were previously treated with other chemotherapeutic agents and/or radiation, it is not clear whether this was a cumulative effect of all treatments.

Treatment of overdosage: Treatment of overdosage should be supportive and the blood picture should be closely monitored with appropriate blood transfusions being given if necessary.

Pharmaceutical precautions Store below 25°C. Protect from light. Caution in handling and preparation of solution should be exercised, and the use of polyethylene gloves is recommended (see enclosure leaflet). If the solution of Amsidine contacts the skin or mucosae, immediately wash thoroughly with soap and water.

Amsidine must be diluted in 500 ml 5% Dextrose Injection BP and infused over 60 to 90 minutes. (*Note: do not use other diluents. Amsidine is incompatible with saline*).

The solution when diluted for infusion is stable for eight hours at room temperature. It should be protected from exposure to sunlight, and any unused solution should be discarded (see enclosure leaflet). *Glass syringes must be used. Amsidine in solution reacts with plastic syringes.*

Legal category POM.

Package quantities Each carton contains six 2 ml ampoules containing amsacrine solution and six 20 ml vials of diluent.

Further information Nil.

Product licence number 0018/0124.

ANUGESIC*-HC CREAM

Presentation Buff-coloured cream with the characteristic odour of Balsam Peru. Each 100 g of cream contains:

Pramoxine Hydrochloride USP	1.00 g
Hydrocortisone Acetate PhEur	0.50 g
Benzyl Benzoate BP	1.20 g
Bismuth Oxide	0.875 g
Balsam Peru BPC 1973	1.85 g
Zinc Oxide PhEur	12.35 g

Inactive ingredients: Glyceryl Monostearate PhEur; Propylene Glycol PhEur; Methyl p-Hydroxybenzoate PhEur; Propyl p-Hydroxybenzoate PhEur; Polysorbate 60 PhEur; Sorbitan Monostearate BP; Liquid Paraffin BP; Titanium Dioxide PhEur; Water, Purified PhEur.

Uses Anugesic-HC Cream provides antiseptic, astringent, emollient and decongestant properties. In addition hydrocortisone exerts an anti-inflammatory effect. Pramoxine is a rapidly acting local anaesthetic. The cream may be used to provide lubrication for suppositories.

Anugesic-HC Cream is indicated for the comprehensive symptomatic treatment of severe and acute discomfort or pain associated with internal and external haemorrhoids and pruritus.

Dosage and administration Topical.
Adults: Apply cream to the affected area at night, in the morning and after each evacuation.

Thoroughly cleanse the affected area, dry and apply cream by gently smoothing onto the affected area. For internal conditions use rectal nozzle provided and clean it after each use.

Not to be taken orally.

Elderly (over 65 years): As for adults.

Children: Not recommended.

Contra-indications, warnings, etc
Contra-indications: Tubercular, fungal and most viral lesions including herpes simplex, vaccinia and varicella. History of sensitivity to any of the constituents.

Warnings: As with all products containing topical steroids the possibility of systemic absorption should be borne in mind.

Prolonged or excessive use may produce systemic corticosteroid effects, and use for periods longer than seven days is not recommended.

Use in pregnancy: There is inadequate evidence of safety in human pregnancy and there may be a very small risk of cleft palate and intrauterine growth retardation as well as suppression of the neonatal HPA axis. There is evidence of harmful effects in animals. Use in pregnancy only when there is no safer alternative and when the disease itself carries risks for the mother or child.

Precautions: Following symptomatic relief definite diagnosis should be established.

Side-effects: Rarely, sensitivity reactions.

Patients may occasionally experience transient burning on application, especially if the anoderm is not intact.

Overdosage: If swallowed, fever, nausea, vomiting, stomach cramps and diarrhoea may develop 3–12 hours after ingestion.

Pramoxine is relatively non-toxic and less sensitising than other local anaesthetics.

Hydrocortisone normally does not produce toxic effects in an acute single overdose.

Treatment of a large acute overdosage should include gastric lavage, purgation with magnesium sulphate and complete bed rest. If necessary, give oxygen, and general supportive measures. Methaemoglobinaemia should be treated by intravenous methylene blue.

Pharmaceutical precautions Store at a temperature not exceeding 25°C.

Legal category POM.

Package quantity Tubes containing 30 g.

Further information Anugesic-HC Cream is prepared in a water-miscible base which provides intimate contact with the area to be treated without having to cross an anhydrous barrier. A cream is also more convenient to use being aesthetically more acceptable than ointments.

Product licence number 0018/0161.

ANUGESIC*-HC SUPPOSITORIES

Presentation Buff-coloured suppositories. Each 2.8 g suppository contains:

Pramoxine Hydrochloride USP	27 mg
Hydrocortisone Acetate PhEur	5 mg
Benzyl Benzoate BP	33 mg
Bismuth Oxide	24 mg
Bismuth Subgallate BP	59 mg
Balsam Peru BPC 1973	49 mg
Zinc Oxide PhEur	296 mg

Inactive ingredients: Calcium Hydrogen Phosphate PhEur; Cocoa Butter BP.

Uses Anugesic-HC Suppositories provide antiseptic, astringent, emollient and decongestant properties. In addition hydrocortisone exerts an anti-inflammatory effect. Pramoxine is a rapidly acting local anaesthetic.

Anugesic-HC Suppositories are indicated for the comprehensive symptomatic treatment of severe and acute discomfort or pain associated with internal haemorrhoids, and pruritus ani.

Dosage and administration *Adults:* Remove plastic cover and insert one suppository into the anus at night, in the morning and after each evacuation.

Not to be taken orally.

Elderly (over 65 years): As for adults.

Children: Not recommended.

Contra-indications, warnings, etc
Contra-indications: Tubercular, fungal and most viral lesions including herpes simplex, vaccinia and varicella. History of sensitivity to any of the constituents.

Warnings: As with all products containing topical steroids the possibility of systemic absorption should be borne in mind.

Prolonged or excessive use may produce systemic corticosteroid effects, and use for periods longer than seven days is not recommended.

Use in pregnancy: There is inadequate evidence of safety in human pregnancy and there may be a very small risk of cleft palate and intrauterine growth retardation as well as suppression of the neonatal HPA axis. There is evidence of harmful effects in animals. Use in pregnancy only when there is no safer alternative and when the disease itself carries risks for the mother or child.

Precautions: Following symptomatic relief definite diagnosis should be established.

Side-effects: Rarely, sensitivity reactions.

Patients may occasionally experience transient burning on application, especially if the anoderm is not intact.

Overdosage: If swallowed, fever, nausea, vomiting, stomach cramps and diarrhoea may develop 3–12 hours after ingestion.

Pramoxine is relatively non-toxic and less sensitising than other local anaesthetics.

Hydrocortisone normally does not produce toxic effects in an acute single overdose.

Treatment of a large acute overdosage should include gastric lavage, purgation with magnesium sulphate and complete bed rest. If necessary, give oxygen, and general supportive measures. Methaemoglobinaemia should be treated by intravenous methylene blue.

Pharmaceutical precautions Store in a dry place, at a temperature not exceeding 25°C.

Legal category POM.

Package quantity Box of 12 suppositories.

Further information Nil.

Product licence number 0018/0162.

ANUSOL* CREAM & OINTMENT

Presentation *Anusol Cream:* A buff-coloured cream having the characteristic odour of Balsam Peru. Each 100 g of cream contains:

Bismuth Oxide	2.14 g
Balsam Peru BPC 1973	1.80 g
Zinc Oxide PhEur	10.75 g.

Inactive ingredients: Glycerol Monostearate PhEur; Propylene Glycol PhEur; Methyl p-Hydroxybenzoate PhEur; Propyl p-Hydroxybenzoate PhEur; Sorbitan Monostearate BP; Paraffin Liquid PhEur; Titanium Dioxide PhEur; Polysorbate 60 PhEur; Water, Purified PhEur.

Anusol Ointment: A light buff coloured ointment having the characteristic odour of Balsam Peru. Each 100 g of ointment contains:

Bismuth Subgallate BP	2.25 g
Bismuth Oxide	0.875 g
Balsam Peru BPC 1973	1.875 g
Zinc Oxide PhEur	10.75 g.

Inactive ingredients: Magnesium Stearate PhEur; Cocoa Butter BP; Lanolin Anhydrous PhEur; Castor Oil PhEur; Kaolin Light BP; Petroleum Jelly White BP; Calcium Hydrogen Phosphate.

Uses Anusol Cream and Anusol Ointment provide antiseptic, astringent and emollient properties which help to relieve discomfort associated with minor ano-rectal conditions. Anusol Cream also provides lubricating properties for use with suppositories. Indicated for the symptomatic relief of uncomplicated internal and external haemorrhoids, pruritus ani, proctitis and fissures. Also indicated post-operatively in ano-rectal surgical procedures and after excision of thrombosed or sclerosed ano-rectal veins.

Dosage and administration Topical
Adults: Apply to the affected area at night, in the morning and after each evacuation until the condition is controlled. Thoroughly cleanse the affected area, dry and apply cream or ointment. Anusol Ointment should be applied on a gauze dressing. Anusol Cream is prepared in a vanishing cream base and may be gently smoothed onto the affected area without the need to apply a gauze dressing. For internal conditions use rectal nozzle provided, and clean it after each use.

Not to be taken orally.

Elderly (over 65 years): As for adults.

Children: Not recommended.

Contra-indications, warnings, etc
Contra-indications: History of sensitivity to any of the constituents.

Warnings: None applicable.

Precautions: None applicable.

Pregnancy: Whilst formal studies on the effect of this product during human pregnancy have not been conducted, there is no epidemiological evidence of adverse effect, either to the pregnant mother or the foetus.

Side-effects: Rarely, sensitivity reactions. Patients may occasionally experience transient burning on application, especially if the anoderm is not intact.

Overdosage: Treatment of a large acute overdose should include gastric lavage, purgation with magnesium sulphate and complete bed rest. If necessary, apply oxygen, and give general supportive measures.

Pharmaceutical precautions Store at a temperature not exceeding 25°C.

Legal category GSL.

Package quantities Anusol Cream: Tubes containing 23 g., Anusol Ointment: Tubes containing 25 g.

Further information The formula of Anusol Cream is similar to that of Anusol Ointment. The advantage of the cream preparation is that the water-miscible base gives intimate contact with the area to be treated and the medicaments do not have to cross an anhydrous barrier. A cream is also more convenient to use, being aesthetically more acceptable than ointments.

Product licence numbers

Anusol Cream	0018/0163.
Anusol Ointment	0018/0164.

ANUSOL* SUPPOSITORIES

Presentation White suppositories. Each 2.8 g suppository contains:

Bismuth Subgallate BP	59 mg
Bismuth Oxide	24 mg
Balsam Peru BPC 1973	49 mg
Zinc Oxide PhEur	296 mg

Inactive ingredients: Kaolin Light BP; Titanium Dioxide PhEur; Miglyol 812; Glycerol; vegetable oils.

Uses The relief of discomfort associated with internal haemorrhoids (piles) and other related ano-rectal conditions.

Dosage and administration *Adults:* Remove wrapper and insert one suppository into the anus at night, in the morning and after each evacuation.

Not to be taken orally.

Elderly (over 65 years): As for adults.

Children: Not recommended.

Contra-indications, warnings, etc
Contra-indications: History of sensitivity to any of the constituents.

Warnings: None applicable.

Precautions: None applicable.

Pregnancy: Whilst formal studies on the effect of this product during human pregnancy have not been conducted, there is no epidemiological evidence of adverse effect, either to the pregnant mother or the foetus.

Side-effects: Rarely, sensitivity reactions. Patients may occasionally experience transient burning on application, especially if the anoderm is not intact.

Overdosage: Treatment of a large acute overdose should include gastric lavage, purgation with magnesium sulphate and complete bed rest. If necessary, give oxygen and general supportive measures.

Pharmaceutical precautions Store at a temperature not exceeding 25°C.

Legal category GSL.

Package quantities Box of 12 or 24 suppositories.

Further information Nil.

Product licence number 0018/0165.

ANUSOL*-HC OINTMENT

Presentation A buff-coloured ointment having a characteristic odour of Balsam Peru. Each 100 g of ointment contains:

Hydrocortisone Acetate PhEur	0.25 g
Benzyl Benzoate BP	1.25 g
Bismuth Subgallate BP	2.25 g
Bismuth Oxide	0.875 g
Balsam Peru BPC 1973	1.875 g
Zinc Oxide PhEur	10.75 g

Inactive ingredients: Kaolin Light BP; Magnesium Stearate PhEur; Castor Oil PhEur; Cocoa Butter BP; Lanolin Anhydrous PhEur; Petroleum Jelly White BP; Calcium Hydrogen Phosphate PhEur.

Uses Anusol-HC Ointment provides antiseptic, astringent, emollient and decongestant properties. In addition hydrocortisone exerts an anti-inflammatory effect.

Indicated for the comprehensive symptomatic treatment of external and internal haemorrhoids and pruritus ani.

Dosage and administration Topical
Adults: Apply ointment to the affected area at night, in the morning and after each evacuation.

Thoroughly cleanse the affected area, dry and apply ointment on a gauze dressing. For internal conditions use rectal nozzle provided and clean it after each use.

Not to be taken orally.

Elderly (over 65 years): As for adults.

Children: Not recommended.

Contra-indications, warnings, etc
Contra-indications: Tubercular, fungal and most viral lesions including herpes simplex, vaccinia and varicella. History of sensitivity to any of the constituents.

Warnings: As with all products containing topical steroids the possibility of systemic absorption should be borne in mind.

Prolonged or excessive use may produce systemic corticosteroid effects, and use for periods longer than seven days is not recommended.

Use in pregnancy: There is inadequate evidence of safety in human pregnancy and there may be a very small risk of cleft palate and intrauterine growth retardation as well as suppression of the neonatal HPA axis. There is evidence of harmful effects in animals. Use in pregnancy only when there is no safer alternative and when the disease itself carries risks for the mother or child.

Precautions: Following symptomatic relief definite diagnosis should be established.

Side-effects: Rarely, sensitivity reactions.

Patients may occasionally experience transient burning on application, especially if the anoderm is not intact.

Overdosage: If swallowed, fever, nausea, vomiting, stomach cramps and diarrhoea may develop 3–12 hours after ingestion.

Hydrocortisone normally does not produce toxic effects in an acute single overdose.

Treatment of a large acute overdose should include gastric lavage, purgation with magnesium sulphate and complete bed rest. If necessary, give oxygen, and general supportive measures. Methaemoglobinaemia should be treated by intravenous methylene blue.

Pharmaceutical precautions Store at a temperature not exceeding 25°C.

Legal category POM.

Package quantities Tubes containing 30 g.

Further information Nil

Product licence number 0018/0166.

ANUSOL*-HC SUPPOSITORIES

Presentation Olive green suppositories. Each 2.8 g suppository contains:

Hydrocortisone Acetate PhEur	10 mg
Benzyl Benzoate BP	33 mg
Bismuth Subgallate BP	59 mg
Bismuth Oxide	24 mg
Balsam Peru BPC 1973	49 mg
Zinc Oxide PhEur	296 mg

Inactive ingredients: Tartrazine Lake 397; Indigo Carmine A1 Lake 34%; Cocoa Butter BP; Calcium Hydrogen Phosphate PhEur.

Uses Anusol-HC Suppositories provide antiseptic, astringent, emollient and decongestant properties which help to relieve discomforts associated with minor ano-rectal conditions. In addition hydrocortisone exerts an anti-inflammatory effect.

Anusol-HC Suppositories are indicated for the symptomatic relief of internal haemorrhoids and pruritus ani.

Dosage and administration *Adults:* Remove wrapper and insert one suppository into the anus at night, in the morning and after each evacuation.

Not to be taken orally.

Elderly (over 65 years): As for adults.

Children: Not recommended.

Contra-indications, warnings, etc
Contra-indications: Tubercular, fungal and most viral lesions including herpes simplex, vaccinia and varicella. History of sensitivity to any of the constituents.

Warnings: As with all products containing topical steroids the possibility of systemic absorption should be borne in mind. Prolonged or excessive use may produce systemic corticosteroid effects and use for periods longer than seven days is not recommended.

Use in pregnancy: There is inadequate evidence of safety in human pregnancy and there may be a very small risk of cleft palate and intrauterine growth retardation as well as suppression of the neonatal HPA axis. There is evidence of harmful effects in animals. Use in pregnancy only when there is no safer alternative and when the disease itself carries risks for the mother or child.

Precautions: Following symptomatic relief definite diagnosis should be established.

Side-effects: Rarely, sensitivity reactions.

Patients may occasionally experience transient burning on application, especially if the anoderm is not intact.

Overdosage: If swallowed, fever, nausea, vomiting, stomach cramps and diarrhoea may develop 3–12 hours after ingestion.

Hydrocortisone normally does not produce toxic effects in an acute single overdose.

Treatment of a large acute overdose should include gastric lavage, purgation with magnesium sulphate and complete bed rest. If necessary, give oxygen, and general supportive measures. Methaemoglobinaemia should be treated by intravenous methylene blue.

Pharmaceutical precautions Store at a temperature not exceeding 25°C.

Legal category POM.

Package quantities Box of 12 suppositories.

Further information Nil.

Product licence number 0018/0167.

CHLOROMYCETIN* CAPSULES 250 mg and PALMITATE SUSPENSION

Presentation
Chloromycetin Capsules 250 mg: Hard gelatin capsule with white opaque body/light grey opaque cap imprinted 'PARKE-DAVIS'.

Inactive ingredient: Lactose.

Chloromycetin Palmitate Suspension: A white suspension with no bitter taste.

Inactive ingredients: Sodium Benzoate PhEur; Sucrose; Ethanol BP; Propylene Glycol PhEur.

Composition: Each capsule contains:
Chloramphenicol PhEur 250 mg.
Each 5 ml suspension contains:
Chloramphenicol Palmitate BP equivalent to Chloramphenicol PhEur 125 mg.

Action: Chloramphenicol palmitate which contains the effective polymorph is hydrolysed to the free antibiotic before absorption. Resulting blood concentrations are similar to those produced by the administration of other oral forms of chloramphenicol.

Chloramphenicol exerts mainly a bacteriostatic effect on a wide range of gram-negative and gram-positive bacteria, and is particularly active against *Salmonella typhi* and *Haemophilus influenzae*. The mode of action is through interference with or inhibition of protein synthesis in intact cells. Development of resistance to chloramphenicol, both experimentally and in man, appears to be low in contrast to other antibiotics.

Chloramphenicol administered orally is absorbed rapidly from the gastro-intestinal tract producing detectable concentrations in the blood within one half hour after administration. Average peak serum levels of free chloramphenicol after the first dose generally occur within one or two hours.

The principal route of excretion of chloramphenicol is through the kidneys, total urinary excretion ranging from 68 to over 90 per cent. Small amounts of active drug are found in the bile and faeces. Chloramphenicol diffuses rapidly throughout tissues and body fluids. Chloramphenicol enters cerebrospinal fluid even in the absence of meningeal inflammation. Measurable levels are also detectable in pleural and ascitic fluids, saliva and milk. It diffuses readily into the aqueous and vitreous humours of the eye. Transport across the placental barrier occurs with somewhat lower concentration in cord blood than in maternal blood.

Uses Chloramphenicol is a potent therapeutic agent and should not be used for trivial infections. It should be administered according to the instructions of a medical practitioner. It is recommended that chloramphenicol should be reserved for use in typhoid fever, *Haemophilus influenzae* meningitis, serious chest infections and situations where clinical assessment usually supplemented by laboratory studies indicates that no other antibiotic would suffice.

Dosage and administration
Adults and children over 2 weeks old: The conventional dosage of chloramphenicol of 50 mg/kg of bodyweight per day in divided doses at six-hour intervals is recommended for the average patient. In exceptional cases, such as with patients having infections due to moderately resistant organisms or suffering from infections such as septicaemia or meningitis, dosage schedules up to 100 mg/kg/day may be prescribed. However, these higher doses should be decreased as soon as clinically indicated. To prevent relapses, treatment should be continued after the temperature has returned to normal for 4 days in rickettsial diseases and for 8–10 days in typhoid fever.

In instances of impaired hepatic or renal function, the ability to metabolise or excrete chloramphenicol may be reduced and the medical practitioner should adjust the dose accordingly.

Elderly (over 65 years): As for adults.

Chloramphenicol has been used successfully at normal dosage in elderly patients. The pattern and incidence of adverse effects does not appear to differ from younger adults. Chloramphenicol is mainly conjugated in the liver to form an inactive glucuronide. Mildly decreased renal function in the elderly will not therefore significantly affect levels of chloramphenicol.

Premature and newborn infants and children with immature metabolic processes: (see gray syndrome under Adverse reactions).

A total of 25 mg/kg/day divided into four doses at six-hour intervals usually produces and maintains a concentration of chloramphenicol in blood and tissues adequate to control most infections in premature and new born infants and children with immature metabolic processes. After the first two weeks of life, full term infants ordinarily may receive up to a total of 50 mg/kg/day equally divided into four doses at six-hour intervals. Precise control of serum chloramphenicol levels should be achieved through analytical methods, wherever this is feasible.

Contra-indications, warnings, etc Chloramphenicol is contra-indicated in individuals with a history of previous hypersensitivity and/or toxic reaction to the drug.

Blood dyscrasias including aplastic anaemia may be associated with the administration of chloramphenicol. If facilities are available, it is well to determine the routine blood profile before therapy, and blood studies should be repeated at appropriate intervals especially during prolonged or intermittent therapy. The intervals at which such studies should be performed depends on the circumstances of each individual case. Consideration should be given to discontinuing the drug if evidence of depression of any of the blood elements appears attributable to chloramphenicol, weighing these effects against the seriousness and course of the disease under treatment. Repeated courses of chloramphenicol and concurrent therapy with other drugs known to cause bone marrow depression or even aplastic anaemia should be avoided. Chloramphenicol should be administered according to the direction of a medical practitioner, and it should not be used for the treatment of trivial infections. Excessive blood levels, as with other antibiotics may result from administration of the recommended dose to patients with impaired liver or kidney function, including those due to immature metabolic processes in the premature and full-term infant. Chloramphenicol should not be administered intravenously during labour. The medical practitioner should also remember that chloramphenicol is excreted in the milk of the lactating mother. Therefore mothers taking this drug should not breast-feed their infants.

Chloramphenicol should not be used during pregnancy unless considered essential by the physician.

As with other antibiotics, the use of chloramphenicol may result in an overgrowth of non-susceptible organisms including fungi.

Chloramphenicol is not alone in the phenomenon of drug interaction and when patients are concurrently receiving anti-coagulants or anti-convulsants, dosage adjustment of these agents may be necessary. The half-life of chloramphenicol is considerably prolonged in patients receiving paracetamol (acetaminophen). Concurrent administration of these drugs should be avoided.

Adverse reactions: Haematological reactions: Blood dyscrasias including aplastic anaemia have been attributed to the administration of chloramphenicol. Two types of bone marrow depression have been observed. One type may occur during therapy, is reversible on cessation of treatment and is dose related. The second type which may occur weeks to months after therapy is rare; it may be genetically related, and is not dose related. In more than half the cases, it is irreversible. It may lead to aplastic anaemia which may be fatal. The reported incidence of aplastic anaemia varies throughout the world. There have been reports of aplastic anaemia, attributed to chloramphenicol, which terminated in leukaemia.

Paroxysmal nocturnal haemoglobinuria has also been reported.

Hypoplastic anaemia, thrombocytopenia and agranulocytosis have also been described following administration of chloramphenicol.

Gastro-intestinal reactions: Nausea, vomiting, glossitis and stomatitis, diarrhoea and enterocolitis may occur; incidence is low.

Neurological reactions: Optic and peripheral neuritis have been reported usually following long-term dosage.

Hypersensitivity reactions: Sensitivity reactions are sometimes encountered.

Gray syndrome: Toxic reactions including fatalities have occurred in the premature and newborn infant; the signs and symptoms associated with these reactions are known as the 'gray syndrome'. Single reports have appeared in an infant as old as three months, and in an infant born of a mother receiving chloramphenicol intravenously during labour. The following points summarise the studies of the 'gray syndrome'.

1. In most instances therapy has been instituted within the first 48 hours of life.
2. Symptoms first appeared after 3 to 4 days of continued treatment with conventional adult dosage of chloramphenicol not tolerated by and incorrect for this age group.
3. The symptoms appeared in the following order.
   (a) Abdominal distension with or without vomiting.
   (b) Progressive pallid cyanosis.
   (c) Vasomotor collapse, frequently accompanied by irregular respiration.
   (d) Death within a few hours of onset of symptoms.
4. Progression of symptoms from onset to exitus was accelerated with higher dosage schedules.
5. In some cases upon early recognition of the associated symptomatology, termination of therapy frequently reversed the process with complete recovery.

Treatment of overdosage: If more than 120 ml suspension or 12 capsules are swallowed, the stomach should be emptied and any symptoms treated accordingly.

Pharmaceutical precautions Store at a temperature not exceeding 30°C; protect from light.

Chloromycetin Palmitate Suspension: Suitable diluent Syrup BP. When diluted use within 14 days of preparation.

Legal category POM.

Package quantities Chloromycetin Capsules 250 mg: Available in packs of 100 capsules.

Chloromycetin Palmitate Suspension: Available in packs of 100 ml.

Further information Nil.

Product licence numbers

Chloromycetin Capsules 250 mg	0018/5097
Chloromycetin Palmitate Suspension	0018/5076.

CHLOROMYCETIN* HYDROCORTISONE OPHTHALMIC OINTMENT

Presentation Chloromycetin Hydrocortisone Ophthalmic Ointment 1%.

White translucent sterile ointment.

Composition

Chloromycetin Hydrocortisone Ophthalmic Ointment 1% contains:

Chloramphenicol PhEur	1%
Hydrocortisone Acetate PhEur	0.5%

Inactive ingredients: Heavy liquid paraffin; White Soft Paraffin BP.

Action: Chloromycetin (chloramphenicol PhEur) has a wide range of antibacterial activity and is effective against virtually all bacterial pathogens known to cause diseases of the eye. Chloromycetin does not provide adequate coverage against *Pseudomonas aeruginosa* and *Serratia marcescens*. It penetrates the non-inflamed eye better than any other antibiotic regardless of the mode of administration and resistance is slow to develop, moderate in degree and not necessarily permanent.

Indications Ocular inflammation due to allergy when this is coexistent with a bacterial infection sensitive to chloramphenicol.

Dosage and administration Topical to the eye. *Adults:* The frequency of administration of the ointment depends on the type and severity of the disease and varies from every hour to once or twice a day. Treatment should not be stopped abruptly.

Elderly (over 65 years): As for adults.

Children and infants: All age groups: as for adults.

Contra-indications, warnings, etc Chloromycetin Hydrocortisone Ophthalmic Ointment should not be administered to patients hypersensitive to chloramphenicol. Transient burning or stinging sensations may occur with the use of Chloromycetin. The prolonged use of antibiotics may occasionally result in overgrowth of non-susceptible organisms including fungi. If any new infection appears during treatment the antibiotic should be discontinued and appropriate measures taken. Chloramphenicol should be reserved for use only in infections for which it is specifically indicated. Bone marrow hypoplasia, including aplastic anaemia has been reported following topical use of chloramphenicol. Whilst the hazard is a rare one, it should be borne in mind when assessing the benefits expected from the use of this compound.

In treating bacterial diseases of the eye it is considered that the use of steroids is dangerous unless the organism is already under antibiotic control, for although the external appearance improves, the progress of the disease may be concealed.

Prolonged use of steroids may result in raised intraocular pressure with possible development of glaucoma and infrequent optic nerve damage; defects in visual acuity and fields of vision; posterior subcapsular cataract formation; and delayed wound healing.

Pharmaceutical precautions Store at a temperature not exceeding 30°C.

Legal category POM.

Package quantities Available in 4 g Tube.

Further information Nil.

Product licence number 0018/5050R.

CHLOROMYCETIN* OPHTHALMIC PREPARATIONS

Presentation Eye drops, eye ointment.

Composition: Chloromycetin Redidrops* (Ophthalmic) 0.5% (Chloramphenicol Eye Drops BP):

Chloromycetin Redidrops conform to the requirements of the BP 1980 for chloramphenicol eye drops containing 0.5% w/v Chloramphenicol PhEur in a sterile solution of purified water containing suitable buffering agents (Borax BP; Boric Acid BP) and 0.002% w/v phenyl mercuric acetate as a preservative.

Chloromycetin Ophthalmic Ointment (Chloramphenicol Eye Ointment BP) contains 1% Chloramphenicol Ph Eur in a petrolatum base.

Action Chloromycetin (Chloramphenicol Ph Eur) has a wide range of antibacterial activity and is effective against virtually all bacterial pathogens known to cause diseases of the eye. Chloromycetin does not provide adequate coverage against *Pseudomonas aeruginosa* and *Serratia marcescens.* It penetrates the non-inflamed eye better than any other antibiotic regardless of the mode of administration, and resistance to it is slow to develop, moderate in degree and not necessarily permanent. Clinical studies have shown that preparations of Chloromycetin for local treatment of ocular conditions are well tolerated.

Indications Treatment of bacterial conjunctivitis caused by the organisms *Escherichia coli, Haemophilus influenzae, Staphylococcus aureus, Streptococcus haemolyticus,* Morax-Axenfeld and others.

Dosage and administration The recommended dosage for adults, children and infants of all age groups is 2 drops, or a small amount of ointment to be applied to the affected eye every three hours or more frequently if required: treatment should be continued for at least 48 hours after the eye appears normal.

Elderly (over 65 years): As for adults.

Chloramphenicol has been used successfully at normal dosage in elderly patients. The pattern and incidence of adverse effects does not appear to differ from younger adults.

Contra-indications, warnings, etc Chloromycetin Ophthalmic Preparations should not be administered to patients hypersensitive to chloramphenicol. Transient burning or stinging sensations may occur with the use of Chloromycetin.

In severe infections the topical use of chloramphenicol should be supplemented by appropriate systemic treatment. The prolonged use of antibiotics may occasionally result in overgrowth of non-susceptible organisms, including fungi. If any new infection appears during treatment the antibiotic should be discontinued and appropriate measures taken. Chloramphenicol should be reserved for use only in infections for which it is specifically indicated.

Bone marrow hypoplasia, including aplastic anaemia has been reported following topical use of chloramphenicol. Whilst the hazard is a rare one, it should be borne in mind when assessing the benefits expected from the use of this compound.

Treatment of overdosage: Not applicable.

Pharmaceutical precautions *Chloromycetin Redidrops:* Store between 2 and 8°C. Protect from light. Contents must be used within four weeks of being dispensed.

Chloromycetin Ophthalmic Ointment 1%: Store at a temperature not exceeding 30°C. Use within one month of opening.

Legal category POM.

Package quantities *Chloromycetin Redidrops:* 5 ml and 10 ml in polythene dropper bottle.

Chloromycetin Ophthalmic Ointment 1%: Tube of 4 g.

Further information Nil

Product licence numbers

Chloromycetin Redidrops	0018/0065R
Chloromycetin Ophthalmic Ointment 1%	0018/5074R

CHLOROMYCETIN* SUCCINATE

Presentation A plug of freeze-dried sterile powder which when reconstituted with Water for Injection makes a clear solution for injection.

Composition: Each 1.2 g vial contains: Chloramphenicol Sodium Succinate BP equivalent to Chloramphenicol PhEur 1.2 g.

Each 300 mg vial contains: Chloramphenicol Sodium Succinate BP equivalent to Chloramphenicol PhEur 300 mg.

Inactive ingredient: Sodium Hydroxide BP.

Action: Chloramphenicol sodium succinate when administered intravenously is hydrolysed to the free antibiotic within the body. Part of the parenterally administered chloramphenicol sodium succinate is excreted by the kidneys prior to hydrolysis and although serum levels of free chloramphenicol are lower than when a comparable dose of chloramphenicol is given orally, they are clinically effective.

Chloramphenicol exerts mainly a bacteriostatic effect on a wide range of gram-negative and gram-positive bacteria and is also active against rickettsial organisms and the lymphogranuloma-psittacosis group. It is particularly active against *Salmonella typhi* and *Haemophilus influenzae.* The mode of action is through interference with or inhibition of protein synthesis in intact cells. Development of resistance to chloramphenicol both experimentally and in man, appears to be low in contrast to other antibiotics. The principal route of excretion of chloramphenicol is through the kidneys, total urinary excretion ranging from 68 to over 90 per cent. Small amounts of active drug are found in the bile and faeces. Chloramphenicol diffuses rapidly throughout the tissues and body fluids. Chloramphenicol enters cerebrospinal fluid even in the absence of meningeal inflammation. Measurable levels are also detectable in pleural and ascitic fluids, saliva, and in milk. It diffuses readily into the aqueous and vitreous humours of the eye. Transport across the placental barrier occurs with somewhat lower concentration in cord blood than in maternal blood.

Uses Chloramphenicol is a potent therapeutic agent and should not be used for trivial infections. It should be administered according to the instructions of a medical practitioner. It is recommended that chloramphenicol should be reserved for use in typhoid fever, *Haemophilus influenzae* meningitis, serious chest infections and situations where clinical assessment usually supplemented by laboratory studies indicates that no other antibiotic would suffice.

Dosage and administration

Adults and children over 2 weeks old: The conventional dosage of chloramphenicol of 50 mg/kg of bodyweight per day in divided doses at six-hour intervals is recommended for the average patient. In exceptional cases, such as with patients having infections due to moderately resistant organisms or suffering from infections such as septicaemia or meningitis, dosage schedules up to 100 mg/kg/day may be prescribed. However, these high dosages should be decreased as soon as clinically indicated. To prevent relapses treatment should be continued after the temperature has returned to normal for 4 days in rickettsial diseases and for 8–10 days in typhoid fever. Chloramphenicol in the form of chloramphenicol succinate should be administered intravenously in seriously ill patients or under conditions in which the patient is not able to take the drug by mouth. In such instances, it is highly desirable that the physician change over to orally administered chloramphenicol as soon as is practicable. In instances of impaired hepatic or renal function, the ability to metabolise or excrete chloramphenicol may be reduced and the medical practitioner should adjust the dose accordingly.

Elderly (over 65 years): As for adults.

Chloramphenicol has been used successfully at normal dosage in elderly patients. The pattern and incidence of adverse effects does not appear to differ from younger adults.

Premature and newborn infants and children with immature metabolic processes: (see Gray syndrome under Adverse reactions).

25 mg/kg/day divided into four doses at six-hour intervals usually produces and maintains a concentration of chloramphenicol in blood and tissues adequate to control most infections in premature and newborn infants and children with immature metabolic processes. After the first two weeks of life, full term infants ordinarily may receive up to a total of 50 mg/kg/day equally divided into four doses at six hour intervals. Precise control of serum chloramphenicol levels should be achieved through analytical methods, wherever this is feasible.

For administration to young children, infants, and neonates in particular, the Chloromycetin Succinate 300 mg vial is recommended for preparation of the solution. The Chloromycetin Succinate 1.2 g vial is more suitable for preparation of the solution for older children and adults. See above for actual dosage to be given.

Method of preparation.

Chloromycetin 300 mg vial: Prepare a solution of 25 mg/ml (2.5%) by the addition of 11.75 ml of aqueous diluent. This solution should be injected intravenously over at least a one minute period, the amount administered depending on the bodyweight of the patient.

Chloromycetin 1.2 g vial: Prepare a solution of 100 mg/ml (10%) by the addition of 11 ml of aqueous diluent. This solution should be injected intravenously over at least a one minute period, the amount administered depending on the bodyweight of the patient.

Further information is contained in the package insert, which should be consulted before preparation and administration.

Contra-indications, warnings, etc Chloramphenicol succinate is contra-indicated in persons with a history of previous hypersensitivity and/or toxic reaction to the drug.

Blood dyscrasias including aplastic anaemia may be associated with the administration of chloramphenicol succinate. If facilities are available, it is well to determine the routine blood profile before therapy, and blood studies should be repeated at appropriate intervals especially during prolonged or intermittent therapy.

The intervals at which such studies should be performed depends on the circumstances of each individual case. Consideration should be given to discontinuing the drug if evidence of depression of any of the blood elements appear attributable to chloramphenicol, weighing these effects against the seriousness and course of the disease under treatment. Repeated courses of chloramphenicol succinate and concurrent therapy with other drugs known to cause bone marrow depression or even aplastic anaemia should be avoided. Chloramphenicol succinate should be administered according to the direction of a medical practitioner, and it should not be used for the treatment of trivial infections. Excessive blood levels, as with other antibiotics, may result from administration of the recommended dose to patients with impaired liver or kidney function, including those due to immature metabolic processes in the premature and full-term infant. Chloramphenicol succinate should not be administered intravenously during labour. The medical practitioner should also remember that chloramphenicol is excreted in the milk of the lactating mother. Therefore mothers taking this drug should not breastfeed their infants. Chloramphenicol should not be used during pregnancy unless considered essential by the physician.

As with other antibiotics, the use of chloramphenicol succinate may result in an overgrowth of non-susceptible organisms including fungi.

Chloramphenicol succinate is not alone in the phenomenon of drug interaction and when patients are concurrently receiving anti-coagulants or anti-convulsants, dosage adjustment of these agents may be necessary. The half-life of chloramphenicol is considerably prolonged in patients receiving paracetamol (acetaminophen). Concurrent administration of these drugs should be avoided.

Adverse reactions:

Haematological reactions: Blood dyscrasias including aplastic anaemia have been attributed to the administration of chloramphenicol. Two types of bone marrow depression have been observed. One type may occur during therapy, is reversible on cessation of treatment, and is dose related.

The second type which may occur weeks to months after therapy is rare; it may be genetically related and is not dose related. In more than half of the cases, it is irreversible. It may lead to aplastic anaemia which may be fatal. The reported incidence of aplastic anaemia varies throughout the world.

There have been reports of aplastic anaemia, attributed to chloramphenicol, which terminated in leukaemia.

Paroxysmal nocturnal haemoglobinuria has also been reported.

Hypoplastic anaemia, thrombocytopenia and agranulocytosis have also been described following the administration of chloramphenicol.

Gastro-intestinal reactions: Nausea, vomiting, glossitis and stomatitis, diarrhoea and enterocolitis may occur; incidence is low.

Neurological reactions: Optic and peripheral neuritis have been reported usually following long-term dosage.

Hypersensitivity reactions: Sensitivity reactions are sometimes encountered.

Gray syndrome: Toxic reactions including fatalities have occurred in the premature and newborn infant; the signs and symptoms associated with these reactions are known as the 'gray syndrome'. Single reports have appeared in an infant as old as three months, and in an infant born of a mother receiving chloramphenicol intravenously during labour. The following points summarise the studies of the 'gray syndrome'.

1. In most instances therapy has been instituted within the first 48 hours of life.
2. Symptoms first appeared after 3 to 4 days of continued treatment with conventional adult dosage of chloramphenicol not tolerated by and incorrect for this age group.
3. The symptoms appeared in the following order.
   (a) Abdominal distension with or without vomiting.
   (b) Progressive pallid cyanosis.
   (c) Vasomotor collapse, frequently accompanied by irregular respiration.
   (d) Death within a few hours of onset of symptoms.
4. Progression of symptoms from onset to exitus was accelerated with higher dosage schedules.
5. In some cases upon early recognition of the associated symptomatology, termination of therapy frequently reversed the process with complete recovery.

Treatment of overdose: There is no known antidote. General supportive therapy to prevent cardiovascular collapse.

Pharmaceutical precautions Protect from light.

Store at a temperature not exceeding 30°C.

To reduce the risk of microbial and particulate contamination the reconstituted solution should be used on one occasion only, immediately after preparation.

Legal category POM.

Further information Chloramphenicol sodium succinate is generally compatible with infusion fluids when the pH range is 5.5 to 7.0. For further information contact the manufacturer.

Package quantities Vials of 1.2 mg and 300 mg.

Product licence numbers

Chloromycetin Succinate 1.2 g	0018/5078
Chloromycetin Succinate 300 mg	0018/5077

CHOLEDYL*

Presentation Coated pink, bi-convex tablets with a debossed 'Choledyl 100' on one side, containing 100 mg Choline Theophyllinate BP.

Coated yellow, bi-convex tablets with a debossed 'Choledyl 200' on one side, containing 200 mg Choline Theophyllinate BP.

An amber-coloured, chocolate-flavoured, clear syrup. Each 5 ml spoonful contains Choline Theophyllinate BP 62.5 mg.

Uses For the relief and prophylaxis of bronchospasm in chronic bronchitis and asthma.

Dosage and administration
Tablets: Oral administration.

Adults: 400–1,600 mg daily in divided doses. The usual adult dose is 100–400 mg four times daily.

An initial dose of 5 mg/kg may be increased slowly over three-day periods until an optimum clinical response is achieved. The peak serum theophylline levels should not reach values greater than 20 micrograms/ml.

There is considerable individual variation in the rate of drug clearance, therefore the dosage should be titrated to individual needs and monitoring of serum drug levels is recommended.

Smokers: Theophylline clearance tends to increase with smoking and therefore, smokers may tend to have lower serum theophylline levels. Consequently they may require up to 40% greater doses than non-smokers to obtain a therapeutic response.

Elderly (over 65 years): As for adults. Theophylline clearance tends to decrease slightly with age and elderly patients will, therefore, tend to have higher serum theophylline levels. They should, therefore, be monitored closely for signs of toxicity during dosage adjustment.

Adults over 75 years may require doses 15–20% lower than the normal adult dose.

Children (over 6 years): 3 or 4 × 100 mg tablets daily in divided doses. The 200 mg tablet should not be administered to children.

Syrup: Oral administration.

Children: (3–6 years): One to two 5 ml spoonfuls three times daily. Use in children at more than six hourly intervals.

Contra-indications, warnings, etc
Contra-indications: Use in patients with a known hypersensitivity to the xanthine group of drugs is contra-indicated.

Precautions and warnings: Caution should be exercised in patients suffering from cardiac or liver disease as such individuals may show marked reductions in theophylline clearance, with consequent high serum levels at normal therapeutic doses. Great caution should especially be used in patients with congestive heart failure. It is particularly important that careful serum level monitoring is carried out in these patients and doses of choline theophyllinate adjusted accordingly. Half life may be prolonged in patients with chronic obstructive airways disease or cor pulmonale and in neonates. Care should be taken in its use in patients suffering from insomnia.

Xanthines can potentiate hypokalaemia resulting from $beta_2$ agonist therapy, steroids, diuretics and hypoxia. Particular caution is advised in severe asthma. It is recommended that serum potassium levels are monitored in such situations.

Theophylline clearance may be decreased in patients receiving troleandomycin, erythromycin, cimetidine, high-dose allopurinol, propranolol, oral contraceptives, or influenza vaccine. Plasma concentrations of theophylline may be reduced when aminoglutethimide, carbamazepine, phenytoin, rifampicin and sulphinpyrazone are administered concurrently.

Smoking increases theophylline metabolism and this effect persists for 3–24 months after cessation of smoking. Care should be taken in its concomitant use with beta adrenergic agonists, glucagon and the other xanthine drugs as these will potentiate the effect of theophylline. The incidence of toxic effects may be enhanced by the concomitant use of ephedrine. Choledyl syrup contains invert sugar syrup (3.7 ml/5 ml) and due care should be taken where it is prescribed for patients with diabetes mellitus.

Use in pregnancy and lactation: There is no conclusive evidence of safety in pregnancy, but choline theophyllinate has been widely used for many years and only one case of irritability and apnoea has been reported in a newborn infant exposed to theophylline during the third trimester of pregnancy. In view of this it is recommended that Choledyl should only be administered during the last trimester of pregnancy if no safer alternative is available. Methylxanthines are excreted in breast milk and irritability has been reported in breast-fed infants. It is therefore recommended that mothers taking Choledyl should not breast feed.

Side-effects: Gastro-intestinal upsets, palpitations and CNS stimulation may occur occasionally.

Overdosage: Characterised by nausea, vomiting, gastro-intestinal irritation, hypokalaemia, unusual thirst, CNS stimulation including convulsions in severe cases, tachycardia, arrhythmias, fall in BP and collapse.

Treatment: Gastric lavage. For fall in blood pressure, nurse in head-down position and treat with fluid replacement if necessary. Use general supportive measures and treat symptoms accordingly. Diazepam i.v. may be given to control convulsions. Charcoal haemoperfusion can be considered in severely intoxicated patients. Supportive treatment is indicated for hypokalaemia.

Pharmaceutical precautions Choledyl Syrup and Tablets should be stored in a dry place at a temperature not exceeding 25°C, and protected from light.

Legal category P.

Package quantities *Tablets 100 mg:* Bottles containing 100 tablets.
Tablets 200 mg: Bottles containing 100 tablets.
Choledyl Syrup: Bottles containing 200 ml.

Further information Nil.

Product licence numbers

Tablets 100 mg	0018/0170
Tablets 200 mg	0018/0171
Syrup	0018/0169

COMPRECIN* TABLETS

Presentation Comprecin tablets 200 mg: light blue, oval, film-coated tablets each containing enoxacin 200 mg.

Uses Comprecin is a broad spectrum fluoroquinolone antibacterial agent for oral administration.

Comprecin is indicated for the treatment of the following infections caused by susceptible organisms: Genito-urinary tract infections (simple and complicated); skin and skin structure infections (infected eczema, folliculitis, cellulitis, impetigo, superficial wounds and chancroid); genital tract infections (simple urethral and endocervical gonorrhoea); and shigellosis.

The organisms normally susceptible to Comprecin include:

Gram-positive: *Staphylococcus aureus* and coagulase negative species (e.g. *S. epidermidis*) including methicillin- and penicillin-resistant strains.

Enterobacteriaceae: *Escherichia coli*, Klebsiella species (including *K. pneumoniae*, *K. oxytoca*, and *K. ozaneae*), Enterobacter species (including *E. aerogenes*, *E. agglomerans*, and *E. cloacae*), *Citrobacter diversus*, *Citrobacter freundii*, *Citrobacter koseri*, *Morganella morganii*, Proteus species (including *P. mirabilis* and *P. vulgaris*), *Providencia alcalifaciens*, *Providencia rettgeri*, *Providencia stuartii*, Salmonella species (including *S. enteritidis*, *S. typhi*, and *S. typhimurium*), Serratia species (including *S. liquifaciens* and *S. marcescens*), Shigella species, *Yersinia enterocolitica*.

Gram-negative (non-Enterobacteriaceae): *Pseudomonas aeruginosa*, Campylobacter species (including *C. jejuni* and *C. fetus*), *Haemophilus influenzae*, *Haemophilus ducreyi*, *Acinetobacter calcoaceticus*, *Alcaligenes faecalis*, Aeromonas species (including *A. hydrophila*).

Miscellaneous organisms: *Neisseria gonorrhoeae* and *N. meningitidis* (including penicillinase producing strains), *Bordetella pertussis*, *Branhamella catarrhalis*, *Listeria monocytogenes*, *Ureaplasma urealyticum*.

Many strains of Streptococcus species and anaerobes exhibit resistance to Comprecin.

Dosage and administration Oral.

Adults: Comprecin tablets are for oral administration. Comprecin is usually taken twice a day (see specific dosage instructions below) and may be taken with or without food.

Elderly (over 65 years): Higher enoxacin serum concentrations (15–30%) are found in the elderly. These patients should receive 200 mg Comprecin taken twice daily; or 400 mg as a single dose for the treatment of genital tract infection.

Children (up to the age of puberty and growing adolescents): Not recommended.

Impaired renal function: Patients with moderate-to-severe renal impairment (creatinine clearance ≤30 ml/min) should receive 200 mg Comprecin taken twice daily; or 400 mg as a single dose for the treatment of genital tract infection.

Urinary tract infections: The usual dose for acute infections is 200 mg Comprecin taken twice a day for three days. The dose for complicated infections is 400 mg Comprecin taken twice a day for 7 to 14 days.

Skin and skin structure infections: The dose is 400 mg Comprecin taken twice a day for 7 to 14 days. For chancroid the usual dose is 400 mg taken 12 hourly for 3 doses.

Genital tract infections: For simple, urethral or endocervical gonorrhoea including infections caused by penicillinase-producing *N. gonorrhoeae*, the usual dose of Comprecin is a single 400 mg dose.

Shigellosis: The dose is 400 mg Comprecin taken twice a day for five days.

Contra-indications, warnings, etc

Contra-indications: Comprecin should not be administered to patients with a known sensitivity to the quinolone class of antibacterials.

Since Comprecin and other quinolones cause arthropathy in immature animals, it should not be administered to prepubertal children or growing adolescents.

Warnings: Patients with moderate-to-severe renal impairment require dosage adjustment (see 'Dosage and administration' above).

Bacteriological studies to determine the causative organisms and their susceptibility to Comprecin should be performed. Therapy may be initiated prior to obtaining the results from bacteriological and susceptibility studies when there is reason to believe the infection may involve any of the organisms listed above. Once the results of bacteriological testing are known, therapy should be adjusted if appropriate. As with other quinolones, Comprecin may cause central nervous system (CNS) stimulation which may lead to tremor, restlessness, lightheadedness, confusion, very rarely to hallucinations, and rarely to seizures.

Comprecin has been associated with a higher risk of seizures in patients with predisposing conditions such as a history of epilepsy, structural CNS lesions, or severe cerebral arteriosclerosis. Comprecin should not be used in these patients unless there is an overwhelming clinical need. Caution should also be exercised in the elderly, where there is an increased prevalence of these conditions.

Use in pregnancy and lactation: There is no evidence from mutagenicity or animal studies that Comprecin has any mutagenic, embryotoxic or teratogenic effect.

There are, however, no adequate and well-controlled studies in pregnant women. Since enoxacin, like other drugs in its class, causes arthropathy in immature animals, it should not be used in pregnant women.

Although enoxacin is excreted in the milk of lactating rats it is not known whether enoxacin is excreted in human milk. Other drugs of this class, however, are excreted in human milk. Therefore, Comprecin should not be administered to nursing mothers unless the benefits clearly outweigh the risks.

Drug interactions: Comprecin, as with some other quinolones, interferes with the metabolism of theophylline thereby raising the serum theophylline concentrations. Adverse effects such as nausea, vomiting, or central nervous system effects, which may be related to the higher concentration of theophylline, have occurred in patients receiving concomitant therapy with Comprecin. If concomitant use cannot be avoided, patients receiving theophylline should be instructed to decrease their normal maintenance dose by 50–75% when Comprecin is started. Plasma levels of theophylline should be monitored and further dose adjustments made as appropriate.

Enoxacin markedly inhibits caffeine metabolism. Thus, patients receiving enoxacin and caffeine are likely to have increased plasma caffeine concentrations which may result in adverse events. Therefore, patients should avoid or minimise caffeine intake during Comprecin therapy.

Enoxacin does not affect the pharmacokinetics of the S-isomer of warfarin, but it decreases the metabolic clearance of the less pharmacologically active R-isomer. In a small study of healthy subjects, this pharmacokinetic change was not accompanied by any changes in prothrombin time. Because of this pharmacokinetic interaction, prothrombin times should be monitored when Comprecin and warfarin are co-administered.

Seizures have been reported rarely in patients taking Comprecin and fenbufen concurrently (in Japan only). Animal studies also suggest a potential for seizures when these two drugs are given together. Therefore, co-administration of Comprecin and fenbufen should be avoided.

No clinically significant interactions were observed when Comprecin was co-administered with either phenytoin or chlorpropamide.

Adverse effects: Of those adverse reactions reported as possibly, probably, or definitely related to Comprecin the most frequent were nausea or vomiting, dizziness, altered taste, dyspepsia, headache, abdominal pain, and rash.

Less-frequently reported enoxacin-related adverse reactions were oedema, fatigue, palpitation, tachycardia, diarrhoea, dry mouth/throat, stomatitis, insomnia, seizures, tremor, nervousness, pruritus, photosensitivity, amblyopia and tinnitus.

Overdosage: No cases of overdosage with Comprecin have been reported to date. No specific antidote is currently known. The usual supportive measures for overdosage should be taken.

Pharmaceutical precautions Store in a cool place at a temperature not exceeding 30°C.

Legal category POM.

Package quantities Blisterpacks of 6 tablets (OP).

Further information Comprecin is an inhibitor of the bacterial enzyme DNA gyrase. It is bactericidal at or near the MIC. Due to its mechanism of action, Comprecin is usually active against pathogens resistant to other drug classes, including beta-lactams and aminoglycosides.

Comprecin administered in single or multiple doses is rapidly absorbed, achieving peak plasma concentrations at 1–2 hours after drug administration in healthy subjects. Plasma concentrations are sustained after dosing with a half-life of 4–6 hours. Steady state is achieved within 2–3 days with a twice daily dosing schedule which may be due to a 30% reduction in steady state plasma clearance as compared to clearance after a single dose.

Enoxacin penetrates sputum, bronchial mucosa, bile, blister fluid, kidney, prostate, pelvic tissue, and muscle, often at levels exceeding serum concentrations. Concentrations in these tissues and fluids exceed the MICs of susceptible organisms. Enoxacin is approximately 30% bound to plasma proteins.

Product licence number 0018/0143.

EPANUTIN* CAPSULES, SUSPENSION AND INFATABS*

Presentation

Epanutin Capsules 25 mg: A white powder in a No 4 hard gelatin capsule with a white opaque body and purple cap, radially printed 'EPANUTIN 25'.

Epanutin Capsules 50 mg: A white powder in a No 4 hard gelatin capsule with a white opaque body and a pale pink opaque cap, radially printed 'EPANUTIN 50'.

Epanutin Capsules 100 mg: A white powder in a No 3 hard gelatin capsule with a white opaque body and orange cap, radially printed 'EPANUTIN 100'.

Epanutin Suspension: Cherry red suspension.

Epanutin Infatabs: A yellow triangular flat chewable tablet with a breaking line on one side and with a spearmint flavour.

Composition:
Epanutin Capsules (Phenytoin Capsules BP): Capsules containing 25 mg, 50 mg or 100 mg phenytoin sodium Ph Eur.

Epanutin Suspension (Phenytoin Mixture BP): Suspension containing 30 mg phenytoin BP in 5 ml.

Epanutin Infatabs: Each Infatab contains 50 mg Phenytoin BP.

Uses

Pharmacology: Anticonvulsant which appears to stabilise rather than raise the seizure threshold and prevent spread of seizure activity rather than abolish the primary focus of seizure discharge.

A small percentage of individuals who have been treated with phenytoin have been shown to metabolise the drug more slowly than normal and this appears to be genetically determined.

Phenytoin is hydroxylated in the liver by an enzyme system which is saturable. Small incremental doses may produce very substantial increases in serum levels when these are in the upper range of therapeutic concentrations.

Indications: Control of tonic-clonic seizures (grand mal epilepsy), partial (focal including temporal lobe) seizures or a combination of these and the prevention and treatment of seizures occurring during or following neurosurgery and/or severe head injury. Epanutin has also been employed in the treatment of trigeminal neuralgia but it should only be used as second line therapy if carbamazepine is ineffective or patients are intolerant to carbamazepine.

Dosage and administration

Dosage: Dosage should be individualised as there may be wide interpatient variability in phenytoin serum levels with equivalent dosage. Epanutin should be introduced in small dosages with gradual increments until control is achieved or until toxic effects appear. In some cases serum level determinations may be necessary for optimal dosage adjustments – the clinically effective level is usually 10–20 mg/l (40–80 micromoles/l) although some cases of tonic-clonic seizures may be controlled with lower serum levels of phenytoin. With recommended dosage a period of seven to ten days may be required to achieve steady state serum levels with Epanutin and changes in dosage should not be carried out at intervals shorter than seven to ten days. Maintenance of treatment should be the lowest dose of anticonvulsant consistent with control of seizures.

Epanutin Capsules, Suspension and Infatabs: Epanutin Capsules contain phenytoin sodium whereas Epanutin Suspension and Epanutin Infatabs contain phenytoin. Although 100 mg of phenytoin sodium is equivalent to 92 mg of phenytoin on a molecular weight basis; these molecular equivalents are not necessarily biologically equivalent. Physicians should therefore exercise care in those situations where it is necessary to change the dosage form and serum level monitoring is advised.

Adults: Initially 3 to 4 mg/kg/day with subsequent dosage adjustment if necessary. For most adults a satisfactory maintenance dose will be 200 to 500 mg daily in single or divided doses. Exceptionally, a daily dose outside this range may be indicated. Dosage should normally be adjusted according to serum levels where assay facilities exist.

Elderly: (over 65 years): As with adults the dosage of Epanutin should be titrated to the patient's individual requirements using the same guidelines. As elderly patients tend to receive multiple drug therapies, the possibility of drug interactions should be borne in mind.

Infants and children: Initially, 5 mg/kg/day in two divided doses, with subsequent dosage individualised to a maximum of 300 mg daily. A recommended daily maintenance dosage is usually 4–8 mg/kg. Epanutin Infatabs may be chewed.

Neonates: The absorption of phenytoin following oral administration in neonates is unpredictable. Furthermore, the metabolism of phenytoin may be depressed. It is therefore especially important to monitor serum levels in the neonate.

Contra-indications, warnings, etc

Use in pregnancy: Anticonvulsants including phenytoin may produce congenital abnormalities in the offspring of a small number of epileptic patients. The exact role of drug therapy in these abnormalities is unclear and genetic factors, in some studies, have also been shown to be important. Epanutin should only be used during pregnancy, especially early pregnancy, if in the judgement of the physician the potential benefits clearly outweigh the risk.

In addition to the reports of increased incidence of congenital malformations, such as cleft lip/palate and heart malformations in children of women receiving phenytoin and other antiepileptic drugs, there have more recently been reports of a foetal hydantoin syndrome. This consists of prenatal growth deficiency, microencephaly and mental deficiency in children born to mothers who have received phenytoin, barbiturates, alcohol, or trimethadione. However, these features are all interrelated and are frequently associated with intrauterine growth retardation from other causes.

There have been isolated reports of malignancies, including neuroblastoma, in children whose mothers received phenytoin during pregnancy.

An increase in seizure frequency during pregnancy occurs in a proportion of patients, and this may be due to altered phenytoin absorption or metabolism. Periodic measurement of serum phenytoin levels is particularly valuable in the management of a pregnant epileptic patient as a guide to an appropriate adjustment of dosage. However, postpartum restoration of the original dosage will probably be indicated.

Neonatal coagulation defects have been reported within the first 24 hours in babies born to epileptic mothers receiving phenytoin. Vitamin K_1 has been shown to prevent or correct this defect and may be given to the mother before delivery and to the neonate after birth.

Lactation: Small quantities of phenytoin are excreted in breast milk.

Contra-indications: Hypersensitivity to hydantoins.

Warnings: Abrupt withdrawal of phenytoin in epileptic patients may precipitate status epilepticus. When, in the judgement of the clinician, the need for dosage reduction, discontinuation, or substitution of alternative antiepileptic medication arises, this should be done gradually. However, in the event of an allergic or hypersensitivity reaction, rapid substitution of alternative therapy may be necessary. In this case, alternative therapy should be an anti-epileptic drug not belonging to the hydantoin chemical class.

Precautions: Phenytoin is highly protein bound and extensively metabolised by the liver. Reduced dosage to prevent accumulation and toxicity may therefore be required in patients with impaired liver function. Where protein binding is reduced, as in uraemia, total serum phenytoin levels will be reduced accordingly. However, the pharmacologically active free drug concentration is unlikely to be altered. Therefore, under these circumstances therapeutic control may be achieved with total phenytoin levels below the normal range of 10–20 mg/l (40–80 micromoles/l).

Phenytoin should be discontinued if a skin rash appears. If the rash is exfoliative, purpuric, or bullous or if lupus erythematosus or Stevens-Johnson syndrome or toxic epidermal necrolysis is suspected, use of the drug should not be resumed (see Adverse Reactions). If the rash is of a milder type (measles-like or scarlatiniform), therapy may be resumed after the rash has completely disappeared. If the rash occurs upon reinstitution of therapy, further phenytoin medication is contraindicated.

Phenytoin may affect glucose metabolism and hyperglycaemia has been reported in association with toxic levels.

Phenytoin therapy may interfere with Vitamin D metabolism. In the absence of an adequate dietary intake of Vitamin D or exposure to sunlight, osteomalacia or rickets may develop.

Adverse reactions: Acute alcohol intake may increase phenytoin serum levels while chronic alcoholism may decrease serum levels.

Central nervous system: The most common manifestations encountered with phenytoin therapy are referable to this system and are usually dose-related. These include nystagmus, ataxia, slurred speech, and mental confusion. Dizziness, insomnia, transient nervousness, motor twitchings, and headaches have also been observed. There have also been rare reports of phenytoin induced dyskinesias, including chorea, dystonia, tremor and asterixis, similar to those induced by phenothiazine and other neuroleptic drugs. There are occasional reports of irreversible cerebellar dysfunction associated with severe phenytoin overdosage. Peripheral neuropathy has also been reported on rare occasions.

Gastrointestinal: Nausea, vomiting and constipation.

Dermatological: Dermatological manifestations sometimes accompanied by fever have included scarlatiniform or morbilliform rashes. A moribilliform rash is the most common; dermatitis is seen more rarely. Other more serious and rare forms have included bullous, exfoliative or purpuric dermatitis, lupus erythematosus, Stevens-Johnson syndrome and toxic epidermal necrolysis (see 'Precautions').

Connective tissue: Coarsening of the facial features, enlargement of the lips, gingival hyperplasia, hirsutism, and Peyronie's Disease.

Haemopoietic: Haemopoietic complications have occasionally been reported in association with administration of phenytoin. These have included thrombocytopenia, leucopenia, granulocytopenia, agranulocytosis, pancytopenia and aplastic anaemia. While macrocytosis and megaloblastic anaemia have occurred, these conditions usually respond to folic acid therapy.

There have been a number of reports suggesting a relationship between phenytoin and the development of lymphadenopathy (local and generalised) including benign lymph node hyperplasia, pseudolymphoma, lymphoma, and Hodgkin's Disease. Although a cause and effect relationship has not been established, the occurrence of lymphadenopathy indicates the need to differentiate such a condition from other types of lymph node pathology. Lymph node involvement may occur with or without symptoms and signs resembling serum sickness, eg fever, rash and liver involvement. In all cases of lymphadenopathy, follow-up observation for an extended period is indicated and every effort should be made to achieve seizure control using alternative antiepileptic drugs.

Other: Systemic lupus erythematosus, polyarteritis nodosa, toxic hepatitis, liver damage, polyarthropathy and immuno-globulin abnormalities may occur rarely.

Drug interactions:

1. Drugs which may *increase* phenytoin serum levels include: chloramphenicol, certain sulphonamides, dicoumarol, disulfiram, isoniazid, cimetidine, and phenylbutazone.
2. Drugs which may *decrease* phenytoin serum levels include: carbamazapine and chronic alcohol abuse.
3. Drugs which may either *increase* or *decrease* phenytoin serum levels include: Phenobarbitone, sodium valproate and certain antacids. Similarly, the effect of phenytoin on phenobarbitone and valproic acid serum levels is unpredictable.
4. Although not a true pharmacokinetic interaction, tricylic antidepressants and phenothiazines may precipitate seizures in susceptible patients and phenytoin dosage may need to be adjusted.
5. Drugs whose effect is *decreased* by phenytoin include: corticosteroids, dicourmarol, oral contraceptives, quinidine, and Vitamin D.
6. Drugs whose effect is *increased* or *decreased* by phenytoin include: warfarin. The effect of phenytoin on warfarin is variable and prothrombin times should be determined when these agents are combined.

Serum level determinations are especially helpful when possible drug interactions are suspected.

Drug/laboratory test interactions: Phenytoin may cause a slight decrease in serum levels of total and free thyroxine, possibly as a result of enhanced peripheral metabolism. These changes do not lead to clinical hypothyroidism and do not affect the levels of circulating TSH. The latter can therefore be used for diagnosing hypothyroidism in the patient on phenytoin. Phenytoin does not interfere with uptake and suppression tests used in the diagnosis of hypothyroidism. It may, however, produce lower than normal values for dexamethasone or metyrapone tests. Phenytoin may cause raised serum levels of glucose, alkaline phosphatase, and gamma glutamyl transpeptidase and lowered serum levels of calcium and folic acid.

Overdosage: The mean lethal dose for adults is estimated to be 2 to 5 g. The initial symptoms are nystagmus, ataxia and dysarthria. The patient then becomes comatose, the pupils are unresponsive and hypotension occurs followed by respiratory depression and apnoea. There are marked variations among individuals with respect to phenytoin serum levels where toxicity may occur. As much as 25 times therapeutic dose has been taken to result in serum concentrations over 100 mg/l (400 micromoles/l) with complete recovery.

Treatment: Treatment is non-specific since there is no known antidote. If ingested within the previous 4 hours the stomach should be emptied. If the gag reflex is absent, the airway should be supported. Oxygen, and assisted ventilation may be necessary for central nervous system, respiratory and cardiovascular depression. The total exchange transfusion has been utilised in the treatment of severe intoxication in children.

Pharmaceutical precautions Store at a temperature not exceeding 30°C. Epanutin Suspension – Suitable diluent Syrup BP. When diluted use within 14 days of preparation.

Legal category POM.

Package quantities Epanutin Capsules 25 mg are available in containers of 500.

Epanutin Capsules 50 mg are available in containers of 500.

Epanutin Capsules 100 mg are available in containers of 500 and 1000.

Epanutin Suspension (30 mg per 5 ml) is available in bottles of 500 ml.

Epanutin Infatabs 50 mg are available in containers of 100.

Further information The 25 mg Epanutin Capsule has been introduced because incremental doses of the drug should become progressively smaller as the serum concentration increases, since there is no linear relationship between dose and serum level – for example, an incremental dose of 50 mg may be enough to increase a serum level in a particular patient from 10 mg/l (40 micromoles/l) to a toxic level.

Product licence numbers

Epanutin Capsules	25 mg	0018/0112
Epanutin Capsules	50 mg	0018/5079
Epanutin Capsules	100 mg	0018/5080
Epanutin Suspension		0018/5106
Epanutin Infatabs		0018/0069

EPANUTIN* READY MIXED PARENTERAL

(Phenytoin Injection BP)

Presentation Ampoule containing clear sterile solution for parenteral administration. Each 5 ml ampoule contains 250 mg Phenytoin Sodium PhEur. *Inactive ingredients:* Sodium Hydroxide PhEur; Propylene Glycol PhEur; Ethanol.

Uses

Pharmacology: Anticonvulsant which appears to stabilise rather than raise the seizure threshold and prevent spread of seizure activity rather than abolish the primary focus of seizure discharge.

A small percentage of individuals who have been treated with phenytoin have been shown to metabolise the drug more slowly than normal and this appears to be genetically determined.

Phenytoin is hydroxylated in the liver by an enzyme system which is saturable. Small incremental doses may produce very substantial increases in serum levels when these are in the upper range.

Indications: Parenteral Epanutin is indicated for the control of status epilepticus of the tonic-clonic (grand mal) type and prevention and treatment of seizures occurring during or following neurosurgery and/or severe head injury.

It is of use in the treatment of cardiac arrhythmias where first line therapy is not effective. It is of particular value when these are digitalis induced.

Dosage and administration Parenteral Epanutin is suitable for use as long as it remains free of haziness and precipitate. Upon refrigeration or freezing a precipitate might form; this will dissolve again after the solution is allowed to stand at room temperature. The product is still suitable for use. Only a clear solution should be used. A faint yellow coloration may develop, however, this has no effect on the potency of this solution.

Parenteral Epanutin should be injected *slowly* directly into a large vein through a large-gauge needle or intravenous catheter.

Each injection of intravenous Epanutin should be followed by an injection of sterile saline through the same needle or catheter to avoid local venous irritation due to alkalinity of the solution.

Continuous infusion should be avoided; the addition of Parenteral Epanutin to intravenous infusion fluids is not recommended because of the likelihood of crystallization.

Continuous monitoring of the electrocardiogram and blood pressure is essential. Cardiac resuscitative equipment should be available. The patient should be observed for signs of respiratory depression. If administration of intravenous Epanutin does not terminate seizures, the use of other measures, including general anaesthesia, should be considered.

Status epilepticus: In a patient having continuous seizure activity, as compared to the more common rapidly recurring seizures, i.e. serial epilepsy, because of its rapid onset of action, intravenous diazepam is recommended prior to administration of Epanutin.

Following the use of diazepam in patients having continuous seizures and in the initial management of serial epilepsy a loading dose of Epanutin 10–15 mg/kg should be injected *slowly* intravenously, at a rate not exceeding 50 mg per minute (this will require approximately 20 minutes in a 70-kg patient). The loading dose should be followed by maintenance doses of 100 mg orally or intravenously every 6 to 8 hours.

Recent work in neonates has shown that absorption of phenytoin is unreliable after oral administration, but a loading dose of 15–20 mg/kg of Epanutin intravenously will usually produce serum concentrations of phenytoin within the generally accepted therapeutic range (10–20 mg/l). The drug should be injected slowly intravenously at a rate of 1–3 mg/kg/min.

Determination of phenytoin serum levels is advised when using Epanutin in the management of status epilepticus and in the subsequent establishing of maintenance dosage. The clinically effective level is usually 10–20 mg/l although some cases of tonic-clonic seizures may be controlled with lower serum levels of phenytoin.

Intramuscular administration should not be used in the treatment of status epilepticus because the attainment of peak plasma levels may require up to 24 hours.

Use in cardiac arrhythmias: 3.5–5 mg per kg of bodyweight intravenously initially, repeated once if necessary.

Other clinical conditions: It is not possible to set forth a universally applicable dosage schedule. *The intravenous route of administration is preferred.* Dosage and dosing interval will, of necessity, be determined by the needs of the individual patient. Factors such as previous antiepileptic therapy, seizure control, age and general medical condition must be considered. Notwithstanding the slow absorption of Epanutin when given intramuscularly its use in certain conditions may be appropriate.

When short term intramuscular administration is necessary for a patient previously stabilised orally, compensating dosage adjustments are essential to maintain therapeutic serum levels. An intramuscular dose 50% greater than the oral dose is necessary to maintain these levels. When returned to oral administration, the dose should be reduced by 50% of the original oral dose to prevent excessive serum levels due to continued release from intramuscular tissue sites.

In a patient who has not previously received the drug, Parenteral Epanutin 100–200 mg (2–4 ml) may be given intramuscularly at approximately 4-hour intervals prophylactically during neurosurgery and continued during the postoperative period for 48–72 hrs. The dosage should then be reduced to a maintenance dose of 300 mg and adjusted according to serum level estimations.

If the patient requires more than a week of intramuscular Epanutin alternative routes should be explored such as gastric intubation. For time periods less than one week, the patient switched from intramuscular administration should receive one half the original oral dose for the same period of time the patient received Epanutin intramuscularly. Measurement of serum levels is of value as a guide to an appropriate adjustment of dosage.

Elderly: Elderly (over 65 years): As for adults. However, complications may occur more readily in elderly patients.

Neonates: Recent work in neonates has shown that absorption of phenytoin is unreliable after oral administration, but a loading dose of 15–20 mg/kg of Epanutin intravenously will usually produce serum concentrations of phenytoin within the generally accepted therapeutic range (10–20 mg/l). The drug should be injected slowly intravenously at a rate of 1–3 mg/kg/min.

Infants and children: As for adults. However, it has been shown that children tend to metabolise phenytoin more rapidly than adults. This should be borne in mind when determining dosage regimens. The use of serum level monitoring being particularly beneficial in such cases.

Use in pregnancy and lactation: In considering the use

of Epanutin intravenously in the management of status epilepticus in pregnancy, the following information should be weighed in assessing the risks and the benefits. The potential adverse effects upon the foetus of status epilepticus, specifically hypoxia, make it imperative to control the condition in the shortest possible time.

There is some evidence that phenytoin may produce congenital abnormalities in the offspring of a small number of epileptic patients, therefore it should not be used as first drug during pregnancy, especially early pregnancy, unless in the judgement of the physician the potential benefits outweigh the risk.

In addition to the reports of increased incidence of congenital malformations, such as cleft lip/palate and heart malformations in children of women receiving phenytoin and other antiepileptic drugs, there have more recently been reports of a foetal hydantoin syndrome. This consists of prenatal growth deficiency, microencephaly and mental deficiency in children born to mothers who have received phenytoin, barbiturates, alcohol, or trimethadione. However, these features are all interrelated and are frequently associated with intrauterine growth retardation from other causes.

There have been isolated reports of malignancies, including neuroblastoma, in children whose mothers received phenytoin during pregnancy.

An increase in seizure frequency during pregnancy occurs in a proportion of patients, because of altered phenytoin absorption or metabolism. Periodic measurement of serum phenytoin levels is particularly valuable in the management of a pregnant epileptic patient as a guide to an appropriate adjustment of dosage. However, post partum restoration of the original dosage will probably be indicated. Neonatal coagulation defects have been reported within the first 24 hours in babies born to epileptic mothers receiving phenytoin. Vitamin K has been shown to prevent or correct this defect and may be given to the mother before delivery and to the neonate after birth.

Small quantities of phenytoin are excreted in breast milk.

Contra-indications, warnings, etc

Contra-indications: Phenytoin is contra-indicated in patients who are hypersensitive to phenytoin or other hydantoins.

Intra-arterial administration must be avoided in view of the high pH of the preparation.

Because of its effect on ventricular automaticity, phenytoin is contraindicated in sinus bradycardia, sino-atrial block, and second and third degree A-V block, and patients with Adams-Stokes syndrome.

Warnings: In adults, intravenous administration should not exceed 50 mg per minute. In neonates, the drug should be administered at a rate of 1–3 mg/kg/min.

The most notable signs of toxicity associated with the intravenous use of this drug are cardiovascular collapse and/or central nervous system depression. Severe cardiotoxic reactions and fatalities due to depression of atrial and ventricular conduction and ventricular fibrillation, respiratory arrest and tonic seizures have been reported particularly in elderly or gravely ill patients, if the preparation is given too rapidly or in excess.

Hypotension usually occurs when the drug is administered rapidly by the intravenous route.

Subcutaneous or perivascular injection should be avoided because of the highly alkaline nature of the solution. Such injection may cause irritation of the tissues varying from slight tenderness to extensive necrosis, sloughing and in rare instances has led to amputation.

The intramuscular route is not recommended for the treatment of status epilepticus because of slow absorption. Serum levels of phenytoin in the therapeutic range cannot be rapidly achieved by this method.

Precautions

General: Intravenous Epanutin should be used with caution in patients with hypotension and severe myocardial insufficiency.

Phenytoin is highly protein bound and extensively metabolised by the liver. Reduced maintenance dosage to prevent accumulation and toxicity may therefore be required in patients with impaired liver function. Where protein binding is reduced, as in uraemia, total serum phenytoin levels will be reduced accordingly. However, the pharmacologically active free drug concentration is unlikely to be altered. Therefore, under these circumstances therapeutic control may be achieved with total phenytoin levels below the normal range 10–20 mg/l.

Phenytoin may affect glucose metabolism and hyperglycaemia has been reported. Caution is advised when treating diabetic patients.

Laboratory tests: Phenytoin serum level determinations may be necessary to achieve optimal dosage adjustments.

Adverse reactions: Signs of toxicity are associated with cardiovascular and central nervous system depression.

Cardiovascular: Atrial and ventricular arrhythmias, hypotension which may lead to cardiovascular collapse in severe cases.

Respiratory: Alterations in respiratory function including respiratory arrest may occur.

Central nervous system: Drowsiness, nystagmus, vertigo, paraesthesia. These symptoms are usually transient. Tonic seizures have also been reported.

Injection site: Local irritation, inflammation and tenderness. Necrosis and sloughing have been reported after subcutaneous or perivascular injection. Subcutaneous or perivascular injection should be avoided. Soft tissue irritation and inflammation have occurred at the site of injection with and without extravasation of intravenous phenytoin.

Dermatological system: Dermatological manifestations sometimes accompanied by fever have included scarlatiniform or moribilliform rashes. A moribilliform rash (measles-like) is the most common. Other types of dermatitis are seen more rarely. Other more serious forms which may be fatal have included bullous, exfoliative or purpuric dermatitis, lupus erythematosus, Stevens-Johnson syndrome, and toxic epidermal necrolysis.

Haemopoietic system: There have been a number of reports suggesting a relationship between phenytoin and the development of lymphadenopathy (local or generalized) including benign lymph node hyperplasia, pseudolymphoma, lymphoma, and Hodgkin's Disease. Although a cause and effect relationship has not been established, the occurrence of lymphadenopathy indicates the need to differentiate such a condition from other types of lymph node pathology. Lymph node involvement may occur with or without symptoms and signs resembling serum sickness, e.g. fever, rash and liver involvement.

In all cases of lymphadenopathy, follow-up observation for an extended period is indicated and every effort should be made to achieve seizure control using alternative antiepileptic drugs.

Drug interactions:

1. Drugs which may *increase* phenytoin serum levels include: chloramphenicol, certain sulphonamides, dicoumarol, disulfiram, isoniazid, cimetidine, sulthiame and phenylbutazone.

2. Drugs which may *decrease* phenytoin serum levels include: carbamazepine and chronic alcohol abuse and folic acid.

3. Drugs which may either *increase* or *decrease* phenytoin serum levels include: Phenobarbitone, sodium valproate and certain antacids. Similarly the effect of phenytoin on phenobarbitone, valproic acid and sodium valproate serum levels is unpredictable.

4. Although not a true drug – drug interaction, tricyclic antidepressants and phenothiazines may precipitate seizures in susceptible patients and phenytoin dosage may need to be adjusted.

5. Drugs whose effect is impaired by phenytoin include: corticosteroids, dicoumarol, doxycycline, oral contraceptives, quinidine, and vitamin D.

6. Drugs whose effects are enhanced by phenytoin include warfarin.

Serum level determinations are especially helpful when possible drug interactions are suspected.

Drug/laboratory test interactions: Phenytoin may cause decreased serum levels of protein-bound iodine (PBI). It may also produce lower than normal values for dexamethasone or metyrapone tests. Phenytoin may cause raised serum levels of glucose, alkaline phosphatase, gamma glutamyl transpepidase and lowered serum levels of calcium and folic acid.

Overdosage: The lethal dose in children is not known. The mean lethal dose in adults is estimated to be 2 to 5 grams. The initial symptoms are nystagmus, ataxia, and dysarthria. Other signs are tremor, hyperflexia, lethargy, nausea, vomiting. The patient may become comatose and hypotensive. Death is due to respiratory and circulatory depression.

Attempts to relate serum levels of the drug to toxic effects have shown wide interpatient variation. As much as 25 times the therapeutic dose, which resulted in a serum concentration of 100 mg/l was taken with complete recovery.

Treatment: Treatment is non-specific since there is no known antidote.

The adequacy of the respiratory and circulatory systems should be carefully observed and appropriate supportive measures employed. Total exchange transfusion has been used in the treatment of severe intoxication in children.

In acute overdosage the possibility of other CNS depressants, including alcohol, should be borne in mind.

Pharmaceutical precautions Store at room temperature not exceeding 25°C. Protect from light.

The product should not be used if a precipitate or haziness develops in the solution in the ampoule.

Epanutin Ready Mixed Parenteral should not be added to intravenous infusion fluids because of precipitation of the acid.

Legal category POM.

Package quantities 10 × 5 ml ampoules.

Further information There may be wide interpatient variability in phenytoin serum levels with equivalent dosages. Serum level determinations in such patients may be particularly helpful. Optimum control without clinical signs of toxicity occurs more often with serum levels between 10 and 20 micrograms/ml although some cases of tonic-clonic seizures may be controlled with lower serum levels of phenytoin. Phenytoin is hydroxylated in the liver by an enzyme system which is saturable. Small incremental doses may produce very substantial increases in serum levels, when these are in the upper range.

Product licence number 0018/0070R.

ERYMAX*

Presentation Capsules containing 250 mg erythromycin activity as enteric coated pellets of Erythromycin PhEur; orange and white enteric coated pellets in a size 0 capsule with an opaque orange cap and a clear orange body, radially imprinted Erymax 250 mg on each capsule half. *Inactive ingredients:* lactose; sunset yellow.

Uses Erythromycin is an antibiotic effective in the treatment of bacterial disease caused by susceptible organisms.

Examples of its use are in the treatment of upper and lower respiratory tract infections of mild to moderate severity; skin and soft tissue infections including pustular acne. Erythromycin is usually active against the following organisms *in vitro* and in clinical infection: *Streptococcus pyogenes; Alpha haemolytic streptococci; Staphylococcus aureus; Streptococcus pneumoniae; Mycoplasma pneumoniae; Treponema pallidum; Corynebacterium diphtheriae; Corynebacterium minutissimum; Entamoeba histolytica; Listeria monocytogenes; Neisseria gonorrhoeae; Bordetella pertussis; Legionella pneumophila; Haemophilus influenzae; Chlamydia trachomatis, Propionibacterium acnes.*

Dosage and administration Oral.

Adults: 250 mg every six hours – before or with meals. 500 mg every twelve hours may be given if desired; b.i.d. dosage should not be used if dosage exceeds one gram.

Elderly (over 65 years): As for adults.

Children: 30–50 mg/kg/day in divided doses given every six hours or twice daily. For the treatment of more severe infections, this dose may be doubled; elevated doses should be given every six hours. The drug should be given before or with meals. This product may be given to children of any age group who can swallow the intact capsules.

Streptococcal infections

For active infection – a full therapeutic dose is given for at least ten days.

For continuous prophylaxis against recurrences of streptococcal infections in patients with evidence of rheumatic fever heart disease, the dose is 250 mg b.i.d.

For the prevention of bacterial endocarditis in patients with valvular disease scheduled for dental or surgical procedures of the upper respiratory tract, adult dose is 1.0 gram (children 20 mg/kg) 2 hours before surgery. Following surgery, 500 mg for adults (children 10 mg/kg) orally every six hours for 8 doses.

Primary syphilis: 30–40 grams given in divided doses over a period of 10–15 days.

Intestinal amoebiasis: 250 mg four times daily for 10 to 14 days for adults: 30 to 50 mg/kg/day in divided doses for 10 to 14 days for children.

Legionnaires' disease: 1–4 g daily until clinical signs and symptoms indicate a clinical cure. Treatment may be prolonged.

Pertussis: 30–50 mg/kg/day given in divided doses for 5–14 days, depending upon eradication of a positive culture.

Acne: Initially, 250 mg twice daily, which may be reduced to a maintenance dose of 250 mg once daily after one month according to response.

Contra-indications, warnings, etc

Contra-indications: Erymax is contra-indicated in patients with known hypersensitivity to erythromycin.

Use in pregnancy: Like all drugs, erythromycin should be used in pregnancy only when clearly indicated.

Nursing mothers: Erythromycin is excreted in human milk.

Precautions: In patients with impaired hepatic function, liver function should be monitored, since a few reports of hepatic dysfunction have been received in patients taking erythromycin as the estolate, base or stearate.

Prolonged use of erythromycin has caused overgrowth of nonsusceptible bacteria or fungi; this is a rare occurrence.

In a few patients receiving high doses of theophylline, concomitant use of erythromycin has caused increase of serum theophylline levels and signs of toxicity. Erythromycin administration in patients receiving carbamazepine has been reported to cause increased serum levels of carbamazepine with subsequent development of signs of carbamazepine toxicity.

Concomitant administration of erythromycin and digoxin has been reported to result in elevated digoxin serum levels.

There have been reports of increased anticoagulant effects when erythromycin and oral anticoagulants were used concomitantly.

Serious allergic reaction, including anaphylaxis, has been reported.

Side effects: Rarely, hypersensitivity and superinfections. Nausea and abdominal discomfort can occur at elevated doses; diarrhoea and vomiting are less common.

Overdosage: Nausea, vomiting and diarrhoea have been reported.

Treatment: Gastric lavage and general supportive therapy.

Pharmaceutical precautions Store below 25°C. Protect from moisture and light.

Legal category POM.

Package quantities Securitainers containing 100 capsules.

Further information Nil.

Product licence number 0018/0133.

GELUSIL* TABLETS

Presentation A white bevel-edge tablet marked GELUSIL on one side containing:

Magnesium Trisilicate Ph Eur	500 mg
Dried Aluminium Hydroxide Gel BP	250 mg

Inactive ingredient: Sucrose.

Uses Gelusil is an antacid indicated for the relief of gastric hyperacidity, indigestion and heartburn when occurring alone or in association with peptic ulcer.

Dosage and administration Oral.
Adults: One or two tablets to be chewed or sucked after meals or whenever symptoms arise.

Elderly (over 65 years): As for adults. No clinical or pharmacokinetic data specific to this age group is available. However, at normal dosage no problems have been reported.

Children (6–12 years): Half the adult dose or as directed by the physician.

Contra-indications, warnings, etc
Contra-indications: None known.

Warnings: None applicable.

Precautions: Prolonged or intensive therapy in patients with severe renal insufficiency may lead to hypermagnesaemia.

Antacids are known to interfere with the absorption of certain drugs including cimetidine, mexiletine, chlorpromazine, diflunisal, ketaconazole, penicillamine, pivampicillin and the tetracyclines.

Gelusil tablets contain 561 mg sugar per tablet and due care should be taken when they are prescribed for patients with diabetes mellitus.

Side-effects: None is observed at the therapeutic dosage.

Overdosage: Symptoms are unlikely and treatment is rarely required.

Pharmaceutical precautions No special precautions.

Legal category GSL.

Package quantities 2 blister packs of 10 tablets in a carton.
5 blister packs of 10 tablets in a carton.

Further information Nil.

Product licence number 0018/0172.

KETALAR*

Presentation Parenteral general anaesthetic.

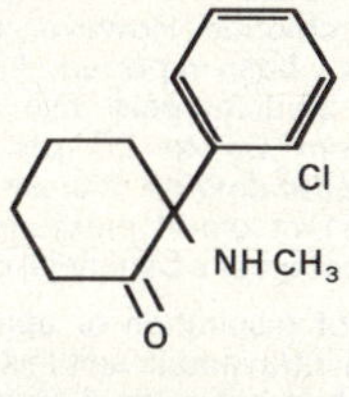

HCl

Ketalar: (ketamine hydrochloride) dl 2-(o-chlorophenyl)-2-(methylamino) cyclohexanone hydrochloride, is a white crystalline solid, soluble in water to 20% clear and colourless solution.

The base component is 86.7% of the salt. It is supplied as a slightly acid (pH 3.5–5.5) solution for intravenous or intramuscular injection in concentrations containing the equivalent of either 10, 50 or 100 mg ketamine base per ml. The latter two concentrations contain 1:10,000 Phemeride* (benzethonium chloride) as a preservative. The 10 mg per ml solution has been made isotonic with sodium chloride.

Uses Ketalar *is recommended:*

1. As the sole anaesthetic agent for diagnostic and surgical procedures. Although best suited for short procedures, Ketalar can be used, with additional doses, for longer procedures. If skeletal muscle relaxation is desired, a muscle relaxant should be used and respiration should be supported.
2. For the induction of anaesthesia prior to the administration of other general anaesthetic agents.
3. To supplement other anaesthetic agents.

Specific areas of application or types of procedures:

1. When the intramuscular route of administration is preferred.
2. Debridement, painful dressings, and skin grafting in burned patients, as well as other superficial surgical procedures.
3. Neurodiagnostic procedures such as pneumoencephalograms, ventriculograms, myelograms, and lumbar punctures.
4. Diagnostic and operative procedures of the eye, ear, nose, and mouth, including dental extractions. *Note:* Eye movements may persist during ophthalmological procedures.
5. Anaesthesia in poor-risk patients with depression of vital functions or where depression of vital functions must be avoided, if at all possible.
6. Orthopaedic procedures such as closed reductions, manipulations, femoral pinning, amputations, and biopsies.
7. Sigmoidoscopy and minor surgery of the anus and rectum, circumcision and pilonidal sinus.
8. Cardiac catheterization procedures.
9. Caesarian section; as an induction agent in the absence of elevated blood pressure.
10. Anaesthesia in the asthmatic patient, either to minimise the risks of an attack of bronchospasm developing, or in the presence of bronchospasm where anaesthesia cannot be delayed.

Dosage and administration
Adults, elderly (over 65 years) and children: For surgery in elderly patients ketamine has been shown to be suitable either alone or supplemented with other anaesthetic agents.

Preoperative preparations:

1. Ketalar has been safely used alone when the stomach was not empty.

However, since the need for supplemental agents and muscle relaxants cannot be predicted, when preparing for elective surgery it is advisable that nothing be given by mouth for at least six hours prior to anaesthesia.

2. Atropine, scopolamine, or another drying agent should be given at an appropriate interval prior to induction.
3. Midazolam, diazepam, lorazepam, or flunitrazepam used as a premedicant or as an adjunct to ketamine, have been effective in reducing the incidence of emergence reactions.

Onset and duration: As with other general anaesthetic agents, the individual response to Ketalar is somewhat varied depending on the dose, route of administration, age of patient, and concomitant use of other agents, so that dosage recommendation cannot be absolutely fixed. The dose should be titrated against the patient's requirements.

Because of rapid induction following intravenous injection, the patient should be in a supported position during administration. An intravenous dose of 2 mg/kg of body-weight usually produces surgical anaesthesia within 30 seconds after injection and the anaesthetic effect usually lasts 5 to 10 minutes. An intramuscular dose of 10 mg/kg of body-weight usually produces surgical anaesthesia within 3 to 4 minutes following injection and the anaesthetic effect usually lasts 12 to 25 minutes. Return to consciousness is gradual.

A. Ketalar as the sole anaesthetic agent:

Intravenous Infusion: The use of Ketalar by continuous infusion enables the dose to be titrated more closely, thereby reducing the amount of drug administered compared with intermittent administration. This results in a shorter recovery time and better stability of vital signs.

A solution containing 1 mg/ml of ketamine in dextrose 5% or sodium chloride 0.9% is suitable for administration by infusion.

Induction: An infusion corresponding to 0.5–2 mg/kg† as total induction dose.

Maintenance of anaesthesia: Anaesthesia may be maintained using a microdrip infusion of 10–45 microgram/kg/min (1–3 mg/min). The rate of infusion will depend on the patient's reaction and response to anaesthesia. The dosage required may be reduced when a long acting neuromuscular blocking agent is used.

Intermittent Injection

Induction

Intravenous route: The initial dose of Ketalar administered intravenously may range from 1 mg/kg to 4.5 mg/kg.† The average amount required to produce 5 to 10 minutes of surgical anaesthesia has been 2 mg/kg. It is recommended that intravenous administration be accomplished slowly (over a period of 60 seconds). More rapid administration may result in respiratory depression.

Intramuscular route: The initial dose of Ketalar administered intramuscularly may range from 6.5 to 13 mg/kg.† A low initial intramuscular dose of 4 mg/kg has been used in diagnostic manoeuvres and procedures not involving intensely painful stimuli. A dose of 10 mg/kg will usually produce 12 to 25 minutes of surgical anaesthesia.

Maintenance of anaesthesia: Lightening of anaesthesia may be indicated by nystagmus, movements in response to stimulation, and vocalization. Anaesthesia is maintained by the administration of additional doses of Ketalar by either the intravenous or intramuscular route.

Each additional dose is from ½ to the full induction dose recommended above for the route selected for maintenance, regardless of the route used for induction.

The larger the total amount of Ketalar administered, the longer will be the time to complete recovery.

Purposeless and tonic-clonic movements of extremities may occur during the course of anaesthesia. These movements do not imply a light plane and are not indicative of the need for additional doses of the anaesthetic.

B. Ketalar as induction agent prior to the use of other general anaesthetics: Induction is accomplished by a full intravenous or intramuscular dose of Ketalar as defined above. If Ketalar has been administered intravenously and the principal anaesthetic is slow-acting, a second dose of Ketalar may be required 5 to 8 minutes following the initial dose. If Ketalar has been administered intramuscularly and the principal anaesthestic is rapid-acting, administration of the principal anaesthetic may be delayed up to 15 minutes following the injection of Ketalar.

C. Ketalar as supplement to anaesthetic agents: Ketalar is clinically compatible with the commonly used general and local anaesthetic agents when an adequate respiratory exchange is maintained. The dose of Ketalar for use in conjunction with other anaesthetic agents is usually in the same range as the dosage stated above; however, the use of another anaesthetic agent may allow a reduction in the dose of Ketalar.

Management of patients in recovery: Following the procedure the patient should be observed but left undisturbed. This does not preclude the monitoring of vital signs. If, during the recovery, the patient shows any indication of emergence delirium, consideration may be given to the use of one of the following agents: diazepam (5 to 10 mg IV in an adult). A hypnotic dose of a thiobarbiturate (50 to 100 mg IV) may be used to terminate severe emergence reactions. If any one of these agents is employed, the patient may experience a longer recovery period.

† *In terms of ketamine base.*

Contra-indications, warnings, etc

Contra-indications: Ketalar is contra-indicated in persons in whom an elevation of blood pressure would constitute a serious hazard (see Adverse Reactions section). Ketalar should not be used in patients with eclampsia or pre-eclampsia.

Precautions:

1. To be used only in hospitals by or under the supervision of experienced medically qualified anaesthetists except under emergency conditions.
2. As with any general anaesthetic agent, resuscitative equipment should be available and ready for use.
3. Barbiturates and Ketalar, being chemically incompatible because of precipitate formation, should not be injected from the same syringe.
4. Prolonged recovery time may occur if barbiturates and/or narcotics are used concurrently with Ketalar.
5. Emergence delirium phenomena may occur during the recovery period.

The incidence of these reactions may be reduced if verbal and tactile stimulation of the patient is minimised during the recovery period. This does not preclude the monitoring of vital signs.

6. Because pharyngeal and laryngeal reflexes usually remain active, mechanical stimulation of the pharynx should be avoided unless muscle relaxants, with proper attention to respiration, are used.
7. Although aspiration of contrast medium has been reported during Ketalar anaesthesia under experimental conditions (Taylor, P. A., and Towey, R. M., *Brit. med. J.* 1971, **2**: 688) in clinical practice aspiration is seldom a problem.
8. Cardiac function should be continually monitored during the procedure in patients found to have hypertension or cardiac decompensation.
9. Since an increase in cerebrospinal fluid pressure has been reported during Ketalar anaesthesia, Ketalar should be used with special caution in patients with preanaesthetic elevated cerebrospinal fluid pressure.
10. Respiratory depression may occur with overdosage of Ketalar, in which case supportive ventilation should be employed. Mechanical support of respiration is preferred to the administration of analeptics.
11. The intravenous dose should be administered over a period of 60 seconds. More rapid administration may result in transient respiratory depression or apnoea.
12. In surgical procedures involving visceral pain pathways, Ketalar should be supplemented with an agent which obtunds visceral pain.
13. Use with caution in the chronic alcoholic and the acutely alcohol-intoxicated patient.
14. When Ketalar is used on an outpatient basis, the patient should not be released until recovery from anaesthesia is complete and then should be accompanied by a responsible adult.

Adverse reactions:

Cardiovascular: Temporary elevation of blood pressure and pulse rate is frequently observed following administration of ketamine hydrochloride. However, hypotension and bradycardia have been reported. Arrhythmia has also occurred. The medium peak rise of blood pressure has ranged from 20 to 25 per cent of preanaesthetic values. Depending on the condition of the patient, this elevation of blood pressure may be considered an adverse reaction or a beneficial effect.

Respiratory: Depression of respiration or apnoea may occur following too rapid intravenous administration or high doses of ketamine hydrochloride. Laryngospasm and other forms of airway obstruction have occurred during ketamine hydrochloride anaesthesia.

Ocular: Diplopia and nystagmus may occur following ketamine hydrochloride administration. A slight elevation in intraocular pressure may also occur.

Psychological: During recovery from anaesthesia the patient may experience emergence delirium, characterised by vivid dreams (pleasant or unpleasant), with or without psychomotor activity, manifested by confusion and irrational behaviour. The fact that these reactions are observed less often in the young (15 years of age or less) makes Ketalar especially useful in paediatric anaesthesia. These reactions are also less frequent in the elderly (over 65 years of age) patient. The incidence of emergence reactions is reduced as experience with the drug is gained. No residual psychological effects are known to have resulted from the use of Ketalar.

Neurological: In some patients, enhanced skeletal muscle tone may be manifested by tonic and clonic movements sometimes resembling seizures. These movements do not imply a light plane of anaesthesia and are not indicative of a need for additional doses of the anaesthetic.

Gastro-intestinal: Anorexia, nausea, and vomiting have been observed, however, these are minimal and are not usually severe. The great majority of patients are able to take liquids by mouth shortly after regaining consciousness.

Other: Local pain and exanthema at the injection site have infrequently been reported. Transient erythema and/or morbilliform rash have also been reported. Increased salivation leading to respiratory difficulties may occur unless an antisialogogue is used.

Symptoms and treatment of overdosage: Respiratory depression can result from an overdosage of ketamine hydrochloride. Supportive ventilation should be employed. Mechanical support of respiration that will maintain adequate blood oxygen saturation and carbon dioxide elimination is preferred to administration of analeptics.

Ketalar has a wide margin of safety; several instances of unintentional administration of overdoses of Ketalar (up to 10 times that usually required) have been followed by prolonged but complete recovery.

Pharmaceutical precautions Barbiturates and Ketalar, being chemically incompatible because of precipitation formation, should not be injected from the same syringe. Protect from light. Store at a temperature not exceeding 30°C.

A 1 mg/ml solution of Ketamine in dextrose 5% or sodium chloride 0.9% is stable for 24 hours.

Legal category POM.

Ketamine hydrochloride is to be used only in hospitals by or under the supervision of experienced medically qualified anaesthetists.

Package quantities Vials of 20 ml containing 10 mg ketamine base per ml.
Vials of 10 ml containing 50 mg ketamine base per ml.
Vials of 5 ml containing 100 mg ketamine base per ml.

Further information Nil.

Product licence numbers

Ketalar 10 mg per ml	0018/5117
Ketalar 50 mg per ml	0018/5118
Ketalar 100 mg per ml	0018/0015

LENTIZOL*

Presentation Capsules containing 50 mg Amitriptyline Hydrochloride BP – white pellets in a size 2 capsule with a pink body and a red cap radially marked 'LENTIZOL 50'. *Inactive ingredient:* Sucrose.

Capsules containing 25 mg Amitriptyline Hydrochloride BP – white pellets in a size 3 all-pink capsule radially marked 'LENTIZOL 25'. *Inactive ingredient:* Sucrose.

The pellets are prepared in a special sustained-release presentation which allows the active constituent to be released over a period of up to 12 hours.

Uses Symptoms of depressive illness especially where sedation is required.

Dosage and administration Oral administration:

Adults and adolescents over 16 years old: Initially 50–100 mg as a single dose at night, increasing to 200 mg/day according to clinical response. Maintenance dose 50–100 mg at night.

Elderly (over 65 years): 25–75 mg a day initially. The initial dose should be increased with caution under close supervision. Half the normal maintenance dose may be sufficient to produce a satisfactory clinical response.

The elderly are particularly liable to experience adverse reactions especially agitation, confusion and postural hypotension.

Children (under 16 years): Not recommended.

Use in pregnancy: Do not use during pregnancy, especially during the first and last trimesters, unless there are compelling reasons. There is no, or inadequate, evidence of safety of the drug in human pregnancy; although it has been in wide use for many years without apparent ill-consequence. There is evidence of harmful effects in pregnancy in animals, when given in exceptionally high doses.

Contra-indications, warnings, etc

Contra-indications: Recent cardiac infarction and patients with any degree of heart block or disorders of cardiac rhythm, and those suffering from coronary artery insufficiency. Patients with mania, severe liver disease, or known hypersensitivity to dibenzazepines. Lentizol should not be given to mothers during breast feeding.

Precautions: Unless essential it is inadvisable to combine Lentizol with ECT.

Avoid if possible in patients with narrow angle glaucoma, symptoms suggestive of prostatic hypertrophy and a history of epilepsy. Lentizol should be used with caution in hyperthyroid patients.

Patients posing a high suicidal risk require close initial supervision.

Tricyclic anti-depressants potentiate the central nervous depressant action of alcohol.

Anaesthetics given during tri/tetracyclic anti-depressant therapy may increase the risk of arrhythmias and hypotension. If surgery is necessary, the anaesthetist should be informed that a patient is being so treated.

Drug interactions: Lentizol should not be administered concurrently or within 14 days of termination of treatment with MAO inhibitors. It should not be given with directly acting sympathomimetic agents such as adrenaline, ephedrine, isoprenaline, noradrenaline, phenylephrine, and phenylpropanolamine, and should be used with caution when administered concurrently with anticholinergic drugs.

Lentizol may counteract the effect of adrenergic neurone blocking agents, and possibly clonidine, and therefore it would be advisable to review all antihypertensive therapy during treatment.

The action of Lentizol may be decreased by barbiturates, and potentiated by methyl phenidate.

Warnings: As improvement may not occur during the first 2–4 weeks of treatment, patients should be closely monitored during this period.

Amitriptyline may initially impair alertness. Patients should be warned of the possible hazard when driving or operating machinery.

Cardiac arrhythmias and severe hypotension are likely to occur with high dosage or in deliberate overdosage. They may also occur in patients with pre-existing heart disease taking normal dosage.

Adverse effects: The following adverse effects, although not necessarily all reported with amitriptyline, have occurred with other tricyclic anti-depressants.

Amitriptyline may produce excessive perspiration and has some anticholinergic activity which may cause dryness of mouth, blurred vision, constipation, tachycardia and urinary retention. These symptoms are common but usually lessen on continuing therapy.

Other common adverse effects include postural hypotension, tremor and skin rashes. Interference with sexual function, nausea, anorexia and dizziness may also occur. Drowsiness may occur in some patients but this can usually be controlled by reducing the dose. If necessary the dose may subsequently be gradually increased.

Serious adverse effects are rare; those reported include:

depression of the bone marrow, including agranulocytosis, cholestatic jaundice, hypomania, convulsions and peripheral neuropathy, paralytic ileus.

Psychotic manifestations, including mania and paranoid delusions, may be exacerbated during treatment with tricyclic anti-depressants.

Withdrawal symptoms may occur on abrupt cessation of therapy and include insomnia, irritability and excessive perspiration.

Adverse effects such as withdrawal symptoms, respiratory depression and agitation have been reported in neonates whose mothers had taken amitriptyline during the last trimester of pregnancy.

Overdosage: Amitriptyline exerts an anticholinergic effect as well as antihistamine and adrenaline blocking actions. Large doses produce convulsions, coma, apnoea and cardiac irregularities, with intestinal stasis.

Treatment: Gastric lavage and emesis if appropriate. Vital signs should be continuously monitored and patients should be treated in ICUs wherever possible. General supportive measures with careful attention to electrolyte balance. Cardiac irregularities may need controlling with antiarrhythmic drugs and physostigmine salicylate is also indicated. Forced diuresis and haemodialysis have no place in treatment.

Pharmaceutical precautions Store in a dry place at a temperature not exceeding 25°C.

Legal category POM.

Package quantities *50 mg:* Bottles containing 50 and 250 capsules.
25 mg: Bottles containing 50 and 250 capsules.

Further information Nil.

Product licence numbers
50 mg 0018/0174R
25 mg 0018/0173R

LOESTRIN*

Presentation Loestrin 20: A pale blue-grey film-coated tablet. Each tablet contains Norethisterone Acetate BP 1 mg and Ethinyloestradiol PhEur 20 micrograms. *Inactive ingredients:* Lactose.

Loestrin 30: A green film-coated tablet. Each tablet contains Norethisterone acetate BP 1.5 mg and Ethinyloestradiol PhEur 30 micrograms. *Inactive ingredients:* Lactose; Sunset Yellow.

Action Loestrin achieves contraceptive effect primarily by inhibition of ovulation through gonadotrophin suppression. It is possible that other sites of action such as changes in cervical mucus and in the endometrium may contribute to the efficacy of combined oral contraceptives.

Indications Control of conception.

Dosage and administration *Oral:* One Loestrin 20 tablet or one Loestrin 30 tablet should be taken daily for three weeks, starting on the first day of menstrual bleeding, and then an interval of one week allowed before commencing the second course of tablets. If the starting day was not the first day of menstrual bleeding, it is advisable to use another method of contraception for the first 7 days of the first cycle in addition to taking the tablets. Second and subsequent courses should be taken for three weeks with one week without tablets between courses. Thus each new course of tablets is always started on the same day of the week. It is important that the tablets are taken as directed. Tablets should be taken without regard to menstrual bleeding except in the initial cycle.

If a tablet is not taken at the usual time, it must be taken as soon as possible and the next tablet taken at the normal time. If the delay exceeds 12 hours additional contraception (barriers and spermicides) should be used for the next 7 days, while the next 7 tablets are being taken. Additionally, therefore, if pills have been missed during the last 7 days of a pack, there should be no break before the next pack is started.

Gastro-intestinal upset: Vomiting or diarrhoea may reduce efficacy by preventing full absorption. Barriers and spermicides should be used until 7 days after the upset, and, if those 7 days overrun the end of a pack, the next pack should be started without a break. It has been suggested that certain drugs may produce increased metabolism of oral contraceptive steroids. Patients receiving additional drugs, including phenobarbitone, phenytoin and some antibiotics, might be advised to use non-hormonal additional methods of contraception whilst taking the drug and for 7 days after. If those 7 days overrun the end of the pack, the next pack should be started without a break.

Post-partum: Oral contraception is usually started as soon as spontaneous menstruation has resumed after childbirth. However, oral contraception can be started within 7–12 days of a vaginal delivery, provided that the patient is ambulant and there are no puerperal complications. If medication is started within 12 days of delivery, additional contraceptive precautions are unnecessary. After a first trimester abortion, oral contraceptives can normally be started immediately.

Children: None.

Contra-indications, warnings, etc
Contra-indications: Thromboembolic disorders, or a past history of these conditions; sickle cell anaemia; known or suspected disorders of lipid metabolism; markedly impaired liver function; known or suspected carcinoma of the breast; known or suspected oestrogen dependent neoplasms; undiagnosed abnormal vaginal bleeding. Loestrin should not be given during pregnancy, or to patients with a history of severe pruritus during pregnancy or of herpes of pregnancy. Loestrin should not be given to patients with a history of otosclerosis, idiopathic jaundice; Dubin-Johnson or Rotor syndromes or any significant liver disease.

Warnings: The use of oral contraceptives has been shown to be associated with an increased risk of thromboembolic disorders. The physician should be alert to the earliest manifestations of these disorders, (thrombophlebitis, cerebrovascular disorders, pulmonary embolism, and retinal thrombosis). Should any of these occur or be suspected, Loestrin should be discontinued immediately.

Certain factors may predispose to the development of thrombosis, e.g. smoking, obesity, age, the presence of varicose veins, cardiovascular disease, diabetes and migraine. The suitability of combined oral contraceptives for patients with any of these conditions should be discussed with the patient before a final decision is taken.

The risk of arterial thrombosis associated with combined oral contraceptives increases with age, and the risk is aggravated by cigarette smoking. The use of combined oral contraceptives by women in the older age group, especially those who are cigarette smokers, should therefore be discouraged, and alternative methods advised.

Benign hepatic tumours have been associated with oral contraceptive usage. Malignant hepatic tumours have also been reported on rare occasions in long term users of oral contraceptives. A hepatic tumour should be considered in the differential diagnosis when upper abdominal pain, enlarged liver or signs of intra-abdominal haemorrhage occur.

Numerous epidemiological studies have been reported on the risks of ovarian, endometrial, cervical and breast cancer in women using combined oral contraceptives. The evidence is clear that combined oral contraceptives offer substantial protection against both ovarian and endometrial cancer.

An increased risk of cervical cancer in long-term users of combined oral contraceptives has been reported in some studies, but there continues to be controversy about the extent to which this is attributable to the confounding effects of sexual behaviour and other factors.

The evidence linking combined oral contraceptive use and breast cancer remains inconclusive. The results of some studies suggest an increased risk of breast cancer presenting below the age of about 35, the risk rising with duration of use. Any possible increased risk of breast cancer with combined oral contraceptives is however likely to be small, and may be expected to be less with low dosage pills. This possible risk should be weighed against the many benefits of combined oral contraceptives, including their protective effects against ovarian and endometrial cancers.

Medication should be discontinued pending examination if there is a sudden onset of proptosis, diplopia or migraine.

Patients with a history of depression should be carefully observed and the drug discontinued if the depression recurs to a serious degree.

Since the safety of Loestrin in pregnancy has not been demonstrated, it is recommended that for any patient who has missed a period, the absence of pregnancy should be established before continuing the contraceptive regimen.

Combined oral contraceptives should be stopped at least six weeks before elective surgery and during immobilisation, e.g. after accidents etc.

Loestrin should be discontinued if the patient becomes jaundiced or has a significant rise in blood pressure.

Precautions: The pre-treatment and periodic physical examination should include special reference to breast and pelvic organs, including Papanicolaou smear since oestrogens have been known to produce tumours, some of them malignant in five species of subprimate animals.

Oestrogen-progestogen preparations should be used with caution in patients with a history of hypertension. Some women experience an increase in blood pressure following administration of contraceptive steroids. Pregnancy should be excluded before starting treatment.

Because these agents may cause some degree of fluid retention, patients with conditions which might be influenced by this such as epilepsy, migraine, asthma and cardiac or renal dysfunction, should be carefully observed.

A decrease in glucose tolerance has been observed in a significant percentage of patients on oral contraceptives. The mechanism of this decrease is obscure. For this reason, diabetic patients should be carefully observed while receiving Loestrin.

Under the influence of oestrogen-progestogen preparations, pre-existing uterine fibroleiomyomata may increase in size.

The following conditions also require careful consideration: multiple sclerosis, porphyria, tetany, disturbed liver function, gallstones, cardiovascular disease, renal disease, chloasma, the wearing of contact lenses or any disease that is prone to worsen during pregnancy. The deterioration or first appearance of any of these conditions may indicate that the oral contraceptive should be stopped.

Loestrin may mask the onset of the climacteric.

The following laboratory results may be altered by the use of oral contraceptives: hepatic function (increased sulphobromophthalein retention and other tests); thyroid function (thyroid-binding globulin, T3, T4 serum levels); haematological tests (increase in prothrombin factors VII, VIII, IX, and X; decreased antithrombin; increased adrenalin-induced platelet aggregation); measurement of pregnanediol excretion (reduced). Therefore, if such tests are abnormal in a patient taking Loestrin, it is recommended that they be repeated after Loestrin has been withdrawn for two months.

The pathologist should be advised of the administration of Loestrin when relevant specimens are submitted.

Any possible influence of prolonged administration of Loestrin on pituitary, ovarian, adrenal, hepatic and uterine functions is unknown at present.

A small fraction of the hormonal agents in oral contraceptives have been identified in the milk of mothers receiving these drugs. The long range effect to the nursing infant is at present unknown.

Adverse effects: The following adverse effects which have been reported in patients receiving oral contraceptives are believed to be drug-related.

Nausea, vomiting, gastro-intestinal symptoms (such as abdominal cramps and bloating), breakthrough bleeding, spotting, change in menstrual flow, amenorrhoea during and after treatment, oedema, chloasma or melasma, breast changes (tenderness, enlargement and secretion), change in weight, cervical erosion and changes in cervical secretion, suppression of lactation when given immediately post-partum, cholestatic jaundice, migraine, rash (allergic), rise in blood pressure, depression, and thromboembolic disorders.

Although the following adverse effects have been reported in women taking oral contraceptives, an association has been neither confirmed nor refuted: prolonged amenorrhoea after discontinuing oral contraceptives, pre-menstrual like syndrome, headache, nervousness, dizziness, fatigue, cataract, backache, hirsutism, loss of scalp hair, erythema multiforme, erythema nodosum, haemorrhagic eruption and itching.

In most women the menstrual flow is reduced and occasionally may be missed altogether. This reduced flow is not normally indicative of pregnancy, particularly if the tablets have been taken correctly, but pregnancy should be ruled out before a new course of tablets is started.

Breakthrough bleeding happens more often in the first two or three cycles after starting the tablets. The patient should continue taking the tablets according to the schedule if breakthrough bleeding occurs. Probably it will amount to no more than spotting and will not last more than a day or two. If breakthrough bleeding is experienced after the third cycle, the patient should consult her physician.

Treatment of overdosage: The usual effects in children are nausea, and drowsiness. Slight vaginal bleeding occasionally occurs in girls. In view of the low toxicity following overdosage with oral contraceptives, it is suggested that treatment should be conservative.

Pharmaceutical precautions Store below 30°C in a dry place.

Legal category POM.

Package quantities Available in packs of 21 tablets (OP).

Further information Nil.

Product licence numbers
Loestrin 20: 0018/0086
Loestrin 30: 0018/0087

LOPID*

Presentation *Lopid 300 capsules:* A white powder in a No 0 hard gelatin capsule with a white body and maroon cap, overprinted "LOPID 300". Each capsule contains gemfibrozil 300 mg. Other ingredients: polysorbate 80 PhEur.

Lopid 600 tablets: A white, elliptical, film-coated tablet debossed with "LOPID" on one side. Each tablet contains gemfibrozil 600 mg. Other ingredients Polysorbate 80 PhEur.

Uses

Action: Lopid is a lipid-regulating agent which decreases total serum cholesterol and serum triglycerides. These decreases occur in the low density lipoprotein (LDL) fraction and in the very low density lipoprotein (VLDL) fraction. In addition, Lopid increases high density lipoprotein (HDL) cholesterol.

Indications: Lopid is indicated for the primary prevention of coronary heart disease in men between 40–55 years of age and with hyperlipidaemias who have not responded to diet and other appropriate measures.

Lopid is also indicated for the treatment of patients with hyperlipidaemias of Fredrickson Type IIa (hypercholesterolaemia), Fredrickson Type IIb (mixed hyperlipidaemia), Fredrickson Type III (familial dysbetalipoproteinaemia), Fredrickson Type IV (hypertriglyceridaemia) and Type V (hypertriglyceridaemia).

Lopid should be prescribed only for patients with lipid or lipoprotein abnormalities demonstrated by laboratory tests and where diet alone is insufficient to correct the condition.

Dosage and administration
Adult: 1200 mg daily in divided doses usually twice daily. 900 mg as a total daily dose may be given in cases of intolerance at normal dosage. When maximum triglyceride reduction is desired as in Type V patients, up to 1500 mg daily may be needed.

Elderly: As for adults.

Patients 60 years or older with lipid levels consistent with increased risk of coronary heart disease should be treated with diet for at least three months. If diet therapy is not effective, treatment with gemfibrozil in this age group should be considered. The incidence of side-effects associated with gemfibrozil therapy has not been shown to be different in elderly subjects compared with younger ones.

Children: Not recommended.

Contra-indications, warnings, etc
Contra-indications: Hypersensitivity to gemfibrozil, alcoholism, hepatic dysfunction, pre-existing gallstones.

Use in pregnancy: Safe use in human pregnancy has not been established. It is not known whether gemfibrozil is secreted in human milk. Like most drugs, gemfibrozil should normally be avoided during pregnancy and lactation.

Precautions: Before instituting Lopid therapy, attempts should be made to control serum lipids with appropriate diet, exercise, cessation of smoking, limitation of alcohol intake, weight loss in obese patients, and treatment of the causes of secondary hyperlipidaemias such as hypothyroidism and diabetes mellitus. Since long-term administration of Lopid is recommended, all baseline values including lipid profile, blood count and liver function tests, should be measured before treatment and periodic determinations of serum lipids should be obtained. The drug should be withdrawn or additional therapy instituted if the lipid response is inadequate after 3 months. In addition, Lopid should be withdrawn if after 3 months the response is paradoxical. Paradoxical response has been occasionally observed, usually in patients with alcoholic hepatic disease. The blood level of LDL cholesterol occasionally rises on treatment with Lopid. A further estimation of LDL cholesterol should therefore be made during treatment to confirm that the desired therapeutic effect has been achieved.

Adverse effects have not been reported in patients with renal disease, but such patients should start treatment at 900 mg daily, which may be increased after careful assessment of response and renal function.

Concomitant anticoagulant dosage may need to be reduced and frequent determinations of prothrombin carried out to confirm that the desired prothrombin level has been re-established. There have been reports of severe myositis with marked elevation of creatine kinase and myoglobinuria (rhabdomyolysis) when Lopid and lovastatin were used concomitantly. In most subjects who have had an unsatisfactory lipid response to either drug alone, the possible benefit of combined therapy with lovastatin and Lopid does not outweigh the risks of severe myopathy, rhabdomyolysis and acute renal failure.

Long-term toxicity studies in rats and mice were carried out at one and ten times the human dose on a weight for weight basis. In male rats receiving ten times the human dose, there was a significant increase in incidence of benign liver nodules and liver carcinomas. Male rats receiving a dose equivalent to the human dose had no statistically significant increase in the incidence of liver carcinomas. At all dose levels, there were no statistically significant differences from controls in the incidence of liver tumours in female rats, or in mice of either sex.

Electron microscopy demonstrated a marked hepatic peroxisome proliferation following Lopid administration to the male rat. Similar changes have been sought but not found in the human liver at up to 27 months continuous gemfibrozil therapy.

Male rats had a dose-related increase of benign Leydig cell tumours. Subcapsular bilateral cataracts occurred in 10%, and unilateral cataracts in 6.3% of the high dose males.

Lopid may increase cholesterol excretion into the bile, raising the potential for gallstone formation. If cholelithiasis is suspected, gallbladder studies are indicated. Lopid therapy should be discontinued if gallstones are found.

Elevated liver function tests (SGOT, and SGPT) increased alkaline phosphatase, LDH, and bilirubin have occasionally been reported with Lopid administration. These are usually reversible when Lopid is discontinued. Therefore liver function tests are recommended during the first year of therapy – and treatment with Lopid should be terminated if abnormalities persist.

Significant mild haemoglobin, haematocrit and white cell decreases have been observed, unrelated to dosage and not progressive beyond six months' treatment. Eosinophilia has been occasionally reported. Rarely, severe anaemia, leucopenia, thrombocytopenia and bone marrow hypoplasia have been reported. Therefore periodic blood counts are recommended during the first 12 months of treatment.

Serial ophthalmological examinations have not provided evidence of drug-related abnormalities, though a non-significantly greater, but still small, number of participants on Lopid underwent cataract surgery in the Helsinki Heart Study. Nevertheless, an annual eye examination with an ophthalmoscope is recommended.

Warnings and adverse effects: Significant side-effects in decreasing order of frequency were abdominal pain, diarrhoea, nausea, epigastric pain, vomiting and flatulence; occasionally and possibly attributable to Lopid were rash, dermatitis, pruritus, urticaria, impotence, headache, dizziness, blurred vision, painful extremities; rarely, myalgia accompanied by increases in creatine kinase.

Other reactions where a causal relationship is difficult to establish to which the physician should be alert: Dry mouth, constipation, anorexia, dyspepsia, back pain, arthralgia, muscle cramps, swollen joints, vertigo, insomnia, paraesthesia, tinnitus, leucopenia, hypokalaemia, fatigue, malaise and syncope. Viral and bacterial infections (common cold, cough and urinary tract infections) were more common in Lopid than in placebo-treated patients.

Treatment of overdosage: While there has been no reported case of overdosage, symptomatic supportive measures should be taken should it occur.

Pharmaceutical precautions Store in a dry place at a temperature not exceeding 30°C.

Legal category POM.

Package quantities Lopid 300 capsules: Securitainers containing 100 capsules. Lopid 600 tablets: Blister packs containing 56 tablets.

Further information Nil.

Product licence numbers

Lopid 300 capsules	0018/0153
Lopid 600 tablets	0018/0157

NARDIL*

Presentation Orange, film-coated tablets each containing 15 mg phenelzine (as the sulphate BP).

Inactive ingredient: Sunset yellow.

Uses Phenelzine is a monoamine oxidase inhibitor. Nardil is indicated as follows:

Symptoms of depressive illness, especially where phobic symptoms are present or where treatment with other anti-depressants has failed.

Dosage and administration Oral.

Adults: One 15 mg tablet three times a day. A response is usually seen within the first week. If no response is evident after two weeks, the dosage may be increased to a maximum of one 15 mg tablet four times a day. Doses of up to two 15 mg tablets three times a day may be used in hospitals. The effectiveness of the drug may not become apparent in less than four weeks' therapy. After a satisfactory response has been achieved, the dosage may be reduced very gradually to a suitable maintenance level. This may be as low as one 15 mg tablet every other day.

Elderly (over 65 years): As for adults.

Postural hypotension may be an unwanted effect of MAOIs in the elderly. Elderly patients as a group tend to receive multiple drug therapies and the possibility of increased risk of drug interactions should be borne in mind. Nardil should only be used with great caution in elderly patients. Despite these problems, MAOIs (including Nardil) have been found to be useful in the treatment of depression in the elderly.

Children: Nardil is not indicated for children.

Contra-indications, warnings, etc

Contra-indications: Nardil should not be given where there is any history of hepatic damage or insufficiency. Toxic hepatitis due to Nardil, as well as other monoamine oxidase inhibitors, has been reported. Incidence is low, occurring no more than once in every 37,500 courses of treatment with Nardil. Contra-indicated in cerebrovascular disease. In general tricyclic anti-depressants, e.g. clomipramine, imipramine, desipramine, butriptyline, nortriptyline, protriptyline, should not be given with, or within 14 days of treatment with MAOI therapy, although it is recognised that there is some division of consultant opinion on this matter.

Use in pregnancy: Do not use during pregnancy, especially during the first and last trimesters, unless there are compelling reasons. There is no evidence as to drug safety in human pregnancy nor is there evidence from animal work that it is free from hazard.

Precautions: Nardil may potentiate the action of pethidine, morphine, adrenaline, amphetamines and other sympathomimetic amines such as fenfluramine, ephedrine, phenylpropanolamine, dopamine and levodopa. Many patients on Nardil react quite normally to therapeutic doses of pethidine or morphine. However, if it is necessary to administer either of these drugs to a patient on Nardil, a trial dose of one-tenth to one-fifth of the normal dose should be given initially. If this is without adverse effect the dosage may be built up to the normal over a further period of two to three hours. Nardil may also potentiate the effects of anti-hypertensives, hypoglycaemic agents, sympathomimetics, anti-parkinson drugs, local anaesthetics and CNS depressants including barbiturates.

Nardil should be withdrawn two weeks before elective surgery/dentistry.

Patients under treatment with Nardil should avoid cheese, cooked or plain, and foods containing a high proportion of degraded protein – Oxo, Bovril, Marmite, etc – during treatment, and up to 14 days after ceasing treatment. Flavoured textured vegetable protein, hung game, pickled herrings or broad bean pods may also present a hazard. Patients should not consume alcoholic drinks or non-alcoholic beers, lagers or wines. Patients should be warned against self-medication, particularly cold cures. Where a reaction between Nardil and certain foodstuffs occurs the intensity of the reaction is usually related to the tyramine content of the food. The reaction is now well recognised and serious hypertensive episodes are extremely rare. Should such a reaction occur, the hypertension should promptly be controlled by slow administration of phentolamine 5–10 mg i.v., repeated if necessary. Care should be taken in administering Nardil with trimipramine or amitriptyline.

Nardil should only be used with great caution in elderly or agitated patients, or those who have cardiovascular disease, epilepsy, blood dyscrasias, phaeochromocytoma or patients with liver toxicity, or diabetes; patients taking diuretics. Nardil may also potentiate the effects of alcohol.

Warnings and adverse effects: Minor side-effects are: dizziness, drowsiness, weakness and fatigue, oedema and gastro-intestinal disturbances (nausea, vomiting, dryness of the mouth, constipation), insomnia, blurred vision, adverse effects on driving ability and postural hypotension. Less common side-effects are: headache, nervousness, euphoria, paraesthesia, sweating, increased appetite and weight, rash, difficulty in micturition, muscle tremor, peripheral neuritis, behavioural changes, arrhythmias, convulsions, impotence and delayed ejaculation, purpura and blood dyscrasias.

Overdosage: Large doses may produce hypomania, euphoria, followed by coma with hypotension, or acute hypertension with sometimes sub-arachnoid haemorrhage. In a few cases, extra-pyramidal symptoms have been recorded.

Treatment: Gastric lavage (tablets dissolve slowly in stomach). Absolute bed rest: raise feet in hypotension. Vasopressors are best avoided. Hypertension should be urgently controlled with phentolamine i.v. Avoid hypnotics, such as morphine, pethidine, barbiturates. Use phenothiazine derivates (chlorpromazine) to control restlessness and intravenous therapy to maintain fluid and electrolyte balance. In deep coma and severe hypotension hydrocortisone by injection may be tried. There is no specific antidote for Nardil.

Pharmaceutical precautions Store in a dry place at a temperature not exceeding 25°C.

Legal category POM.

Package quantity Tampertainers of 100 tablets.

Further information Nil.

Product licence number 0018/0177.

OPILON* TABLETS

Presentation Opilon 40 mg: Pale yellow film-coated tablets. Each tablet contains: Thymoxamine hydrochloride BP (Moxisylyte Hydrochloride INN) equivalent to thymoxamine base 40 mg. *Inactive ingredients:* Lactose, Propylene Glycol PhEur, sunset yellow.

Opilon 80 mg: Orange film-coated tablets. Each tablet contains: Thymoxamine hydrochloride BP (Moxisylyte Hydrochloride INN) equivalent to thymoxamine base 80 mg. *Inactive ingredients:* Lactose, Polyethylene Glycol BP, Quinoline Yellow and Sunset Yellow.

Uses Thymoxamine is an alpha adrenergic blocking agent. Opilon is indicated in the short term control of the symptoms of primary Raynaud's phenomenon.

Dosage and administration

Adults: Oral administration. Initially one tablet to be taken four times a day. This may be increased to two tablets four times a day if initial response is poor. For patients exposed to the cold during the daytime, one tablet should be administered every three hours during the period when symptoms are most likely to occur. In the event that a response is not evident within 2 weeks, the drug should be discontinued.

Elderly (over 65 years): As for adults. No clinical or pharmacokinetic data specific to this age group is available. Whilst at normal dosage no problems have been reported, caution nevertheless is advised when Opilon is prescribed in the elderly.

Children: Opilon tablets are not indicated for use in children.

Contra-indications, warnings, etc

Contra-indications: Hypersensitivity to any of the ingredients.

Warnings: The alpha-adrenergic blocking action of Opilon will produce a vasodilatating effect which may theoretically potentiate the effect of a number of drugs used in the management of hypertension. In practice, with the recommended dosage of Opilon, this has not been reported.

Precautions: Opilon should be used with caution in diabetes as, theoretically, insulin requirements may be reduced. Tricyclic antidepressants may increase any hypotensive effect produced by alpha blockade.

Pregnancy and lactation: The safety of Opilon for use during pregnancy and lactation has not been established. It should not therefore be used by women who are pregnant or breast feeding.

Side-effects: Occasionally mild nausea, diarrhoea, vertigo, headache and facial flushing may be encountered. These are, however, rare and transient.

Overdosage: In excessive overdosage, a fall in blood pressure is the main symptom. The patient should be nursed in the supine position until the blood pressure has been restored to normal.

Pharmaceutical precautions Store in a cool dry place at a temperature not exceeding 30°C.

Legal category POM.

Package quantities Opilon 40 mg and Opilon 80 mg: Blister strips of 30 tablets, four strips in a carton (120 tablets) (OP).

Further information Nil.

Product licence numbers
Opilon 40 mg 0018/0179
Opilon 80 mg 0018/0190

PITRESSIN*

Presentation A clear, sterile, colourless solution for injection.

Composition: Each ml contains Argipressin 20 units. *Inactive ingredients:* Glacial Acetic Acid.

Action: Pitressin has a direct antidiuretic action on the kidney. It also constricts peripheral vessels and causes contraction of the smooth muscle of the intestine, gall bladder and urinary bladder.

Uses For use in diabetes insipidus and control of bleeding from oesophageal varices.

Dosage and administration
Adults
Diabetes insipidus: 0.25 ml to 1 ml (5 to 20 units) by subcutaneous or intramuscular injection every four hours.

Oesophageal varices: For the initial control of variceal bleeding Pitressin should be given intravenously. Pitressin, 20 units diluted in 100 ml Dextrose 5% w/v may be infused over a 15 minute period (Shields R, Brit J Hosp Med, p. 126, February 1977).

Elderly (over 65 years): As for adults. No clinical or pharmacokinetic data specific to this age group is available. However, at normal dosage no problems have been reported.

Children and infants: No dose recommended.

Contra-indications, warnings, etc Anaphylaxis or hypersensitivity to the drug or its components.

Warnings: This drug should not be used in patients with vascular disease, especially disease of the coronary arteries, except with extreme caution. In such patients, even small doses may precipitate anginal pain, and with larger doses, the possibility of myocardial infarction should be considered.

Pitressin may produce water intoxication. The early signs of drowsiness, listlessness, and headaches should be recognized to prevent terminal coma and convulsions.

Precautions: Pitressin should be used cautiously in the presence of epilepsy, migraine, asthma, heart failure, or any state in which a rapid addition to extracellular water may produce hazard for an already overburdened system.

Chronic nephritis with nitrogen retention contraindicates the use of Pitressin until reasonable nitrogen blood levels have been attained.

Adverse effects: Local or systemic allergic reactions may occur in hypersensitive individuals. The following side-effects have been reported following the administration of Pitressin: tremor, sweating, vertigo, circumoral pallor, 'pounding' in head, abdominal cramps, passage of gas, nausea, vomiting, urticaria, bronchial constriction. Anaphylaxis (cardiac arrest and/or shock) has been observed shortly after injection of Pitressin.

Treatment of overdosage: If water intoxication occurs, no fluids should be given. In severe cases, small amounts of hypertonic saline may be administered. Urea and mannitol infusions may be helpful in cases of cerebral oedema. If a patient should experience anginal pain after administration of Pitressin, amyl nitrate by inhalation, or glyceryl trinitrate sublingually, may be given.

Pharmaceutical precautions Store between 2°C and 8°C. Do not freeze.

Legal category POM.

Package quantities Available in packs of 10 × 1 ml ampoules.

Further information Nil.

Product licence number 0018/5056.

PONSTAN* Capsules
(Mefenamic Acid Capsules BP)

PONSTAN* Paediatric Suspension
(Mefenamic Acid Suspension 50 mg/5 ml)

Presentation *Capsules:* An off-white powder in a No. 1 hard gelatin capsule with an ivory opaque body and aqua-blue opaque cap, radially printed PONSTAN 250. Each capsule contains Mefenamic Acid BP 250 mg. *Inactive ingredients:* Lactose.

Paediatric Suspension: An off-white suspension, with a typical aroma and taste. Each 5 ml suspension contains Mefenamic Acid BP 50 mg. *Inactive ingredients:* Sodium benzoate; sucrose; ethanol.

Action Mefenamic acid is a non-steroidal anti-inflammatory agent with analgesic properties and a demonstrable antipyretic effect. It has also been shown to inhibit prostaglandin activity.

Indications 1. As an anti-inflammatory analgesic for the symptomatic relief of rheumatoid arthritis (including Still's Disease), osteoarthritis, and pain including muscular, traumatic and dental pain, headaches of most aetiology, post-operative and post-partum pain; pyrexia in children.

2. Primary dysmenorrhoea.

3. Menorrhagia due to dysfunctional causes and presence of an IUD when other pelvic pathology has been ruled out.

Dosage and administration Oral.
Adults: 2 capsules (500 mg) three times daily.

In menorrhagia to be administered on the first day of excessive bleeding and continued according to the judgement of the physician.

In dysmenorrhoea to be administered at the onset of menstrual pain and continued according to the judgement of the physician.

Elderly (over 65 years): As for adults. Whilst no pharmacokinetic or clinical studies specific to the elderly have been undertaken with Ponstan, it has been used at normal dosage in trials which included many elderly patients.

Ponstan should be used with caution in elderly patients suffering from dehydration and renal disease.

Non oliguric renal failure and proctocolitis have been reported mainly in elderly patients who have not discontinued Ponstan after the development of diarrhoea.

Children: It is recommended that children under 12 years

of age should be given Ponstan Paediatric Suspension (50 mg/5 ml) in the following dosage regime.
Infants over 6 months – 25 mg/kg of body weight daily in divided doses, or
6 months to 1 year – one 5 ml spoonful.
2 years to 4 years – two 5 ml spoonfuls.
5 years to 8 years – three 5 ml spoonfuls.
9 years to 12 years – four 5 ml spoonfuls.
Dose may be repeated as necessary, up to three times daily.

Apart from the treatment of Still's Disease, therapy should not be continued for longer than seven days in children.

Contra-indications, warnings, etc Patients hypersensitive to Mefenamic acid. Mefenamic acid is contra-indicated in inflammatory bowel disease and in patients suffering from peptic and/or intestinal ulceration, and in patients with renal or hepatic impairment.

Precautions: Safety in pregnancy has not been established. In patients suffering from dehydration and renal disease, particularly the elderly. Concurrent therapy with other plasma protein binding drugs may necessitate a modification in dosage. In the case of anticoagulants the dose of the anticoagulant may need to be reduced.

In dysmenorrhoea and menorrhagia lack of response should alert the physician to investigate other causes.

Warnings and adverse effects: Diarrhoea occasionally occurs following the use of mefenamic acid. Although this may occur soon after starting treatment, it may also occur after several months of continuous use. The diarrhoea has been investigated in some patients who have continued this drug in spite of its continued presence. These patients were found to have associated proctocolitis.

If diarrhoea does develop, the drug should be withdrawn immediately and this patient should not receive mefenamic acid again.

Skin rashes have been observed following the administration of mefenamic acid and occurrence of a rash is a definite indication to withdraw medication.

As with other prostaglandin inhibitors allergic glomerulonephritis has occurred occasionally: non-oliguric renal failure has been reported on a few occasions in elderly patients with dehydration usually from diarrhoea. It has been suggested that the recovery is more rapid and complete than with other forms of analgesic induced renal impairment.

Rarely, thrombocytopenia has been reported with mefenamic acid.

In some cases reversible haemolytic anaemia has occurred. Temporary lowering of the white blood cell count, which may have been due to mefenamic acid, has been reported. Blood studies should therefore be carried out during long-term administration.

Bronchospasm may be precipitated in patients suffering from, or with a previous history of, bronchial asthma or allergic disease. Patients on prolonged therapy should also be kept under surveillance with particular attention to liver dysfunction. Should this appear it is an indication to discontinue therapy.

Drowsiness and dizziness have rarely been reported.

Note: A positive reaction in certain tests for bile in the urine of patients receiving mefenamic acid has been demonstrated to be due to the presence of the drug and its metabolites and not to the presence of bile.

Treatment of overdosage: Gastric lavage in the conscious patient and intensive supportive therapy where necessary. Activated charcoal has been shown to be a powerful adsorbent for mefenamic acid and its metabolites. Studies in experimental animals and humans showed that a 5 to 1 ratio of charcoal to mefenamic acid resulted in considerable suppression of absorption of the drug.

Pharmaceutical precautions Store at a temperature not exceeding 30°C. Recommended diluent for Suspension – Syrup BP. When diluted use within 14 days of preparation.

Legal category POM.

Package quantities *Capsules:* Blister strips of 28 capsules, 6 strips in a carton (168 capsules) (OP).

Suspension: Available in packs of 125 ml.

Further information Nil.

Product licence numbers

Ponstan Capsules	0018/0094R
Ponstan Paediatric Suspension	0018/5025R

PONSTAN* DISPERSIBLE TABLETS

Presentation A blue, flat, bevel-edged tablet with 'Ponstan D' debossed on one side. Each tablet contains mefenamic acid BP 250 mg.

Uses
Action: Mefenamic acid is a non-steroidal anti-inflammatory agent with analgesic properties, and a demonstrable antipyretic effect. It has also been shown to inhibit prostaglandin activity.

Indications:
1. As an anti-inflammatory analgesic for the symptomatic relief of rheumatoid arthritis (including Still's Disease), osteoarthritis and pain, including muscular, traumatic and dental pain, headaches of most aetiology, post-operative and post-partum pain; pyrexia in children.
2. Primary dysmenorrhoea.
3. Menorrhagia due to dysfunctional causes and presence of an IUD when other pelvic pathology has been ruled out.

Dosage and administration Oral.

Adults: 2 tablets (500 mg) dissolved in half a tumbler of water three times daily. In menorrhagia, to be administered on the first day of excessive bleeding and continued according to the judgement of the physician. In dysmenorrhoea to be administered at the onset of menstrual pain and continued according to the judgement of the physician.

Elderly (over 65 years): As for adults.

Whilst no pharmacokinetic or clinical studies specific to the elderly have been undertaken with Ponstan, it has been used at normal dosage in trials which included many elderly patients.

Ponstan should be used with caution in elderly patients suffering from dehydration and renal disease.

Non oliguric renal failure and proctocolitis have been reported mainly in elderly patients who have not discontinued Ponstan after the development of diarrhoea.

Children: It is recommended that children under 12 years of age should be given Ponstan Paediatric Suspension.

Contra-indications, warnings, etc
Contra-indications: Patients hypersensitive to Mefenamic acid. Mefenamic acid is contra-indicated in inflammatory bowel disease and in patients suffering from peptic and/or intestinal ulceration, and in patients with renal or hepatic impairment.

Precautions: Safety in pregnancy has not been established.

In patients suffering from dehydration and renal disease, particularly the elderly.

Concurrent therapy with other plasma protein binding drugs may necessitate a modification in dosage. In the case of anticoagulants the dose of the anticoagulant may need to be reduced.

In dysmenorrhoea and menorrhagia lack of response should alert the physician to investigate other causes.

Warnings and adverse effects: Diarrhoea occasionally occurs following the use of mefenamic acid. Although this may occur soon after starting treatment, it may also occur after several months of continuous use. The diarrhoea has been investigated in some patients who have continued this drug in spite of its continued presence; these patients were found to have associated proctocolitis.

If diarrhoea does develop, the drug should be withdrawn immediately and this patient should not receive mefenamic acid again.

Skin rashes have been observed following the administration of mefenamic acid and the occurrence of a rash is a definite indication to withdraw medication.

As with other prostaglandin inhibitors allergic glomerulonephritis has occurred occasionally: non-oliguric renal failure has been reported on a few occasions in elderly patients with dehydration usually from diarrhoea. It has been suggested that the recovery is more rapid and complete than with other forms of analgesic induced renal impairment. Rarely, thrombocytopenia has been reported with mefenamic acid. In some cases reversible haemolytic anaemia has occurred. Temporary lowering of white blood cell count, which may have been due to mefenamic acid, has been reported. Blood studies should therefore be carried out during long term administration.

Bronchospasm may be precipitated in patients suffering from, or with a previous history of, bronchial asthma or allergic disease. Patients on prolonged therapy should also be kept under surveillance with particular attention to liver dysfunction. Should this appear it is an indication to discontinue therapy.

Drowsiness and dizziness have rarely been reported.

Note: A positive reaction in certain tests for bile in the urine of patients receiving mefenamic acid has been demonstrated to be due to the presence of the drug and its metabolites and not to the presence of bile.

Treatment of overdosage: Gastric lavage in the conscious patient and intensive supportive therapy where necessary. Activated charcoal has been shown to be a powerful adsorbent for mefenamic acid and its metabolites. Studies in experimental animals and humans showed that a 5 to 1 ratio of charcoal to mefenamic acid resulted in considerable suppression of absorption of the drug.

Pharmaceutical precautions Store in a dry place at a temperature not exceeding 25°C.

Legal category POM.

Package quantities Available in packs of 100.

Further information Nil.

Product licence number 0018/0129.

PONSTAN FORTE*

Presentation Yellow film-coated ovoid tablet inscribed PONSTAN FORTE on one side.

Composition: Each tablet contains Mefenamic Acid BP 500 mg. *Inactive ingredient:* Sunset Yellow.

Action Mefenamic acid is a non-steroidal anti-inflammatory agent with analgesic properties and a demonstrable antipyretic effect. It has also been shown to inhibit prostaglandin activity.

Indications

1. As an anti-inflammatory analgesic for the symptomatic relief of rheumatoid arthritis (including Still's Disease) osteoarthritis, and pain including muscular, traumatic and dental pain, headaches of most aetiology, post-operative and post-partum pain.
2. Primary dysmenorrhoea.
3. Menorrhagia due to dysfunctional causes and presence of an IUD when other pelvic pathology has been ruled out.

Dosage and administration Oral.

Adults: 1 tablet (500 mg) three times daily.

In menorrhagia to be administered on the first day of excessive bleeding and continued according to the judgement of the physician. In dysmenorrhoea to be administered at the onset of menstrual pain and continued according to the judgement of the physician.

Elderly (over 65 years): As for adults. Whilst no pharmacokinetic or clinical studies specific to the elderly have been undertaken with Ponstan, it has been used at normal dosage in trials which included many elderly patients.

Ponstan should be used with caution in elderly patients suffering from dehydration and renal disease.

Non oliguric renal failure and proctocolitis have been reported mainly in elderly patients who have not discontinued Ponstan after the development of diarrhoea.

Children: It is recommended that children under 12 years of age should be given Ponstan Paediatric Suspension (see Ponstan data sheet).

Contra-indications, warnings, etc Patients hypersensitive to mefenamic acid. Mefenamic acid is contra-indicated in inflammatory bowel disease and in patients suffering from peptic and/or intestinal ulceration, and in patients with renal or hepatic impairment.

Precautions: Safety in pregnancy has not been established. In patients suffering from dehydration and renal disease, particularly the elderly. Concurrent therapy with other plasma protein binding drugs may necessitate a modification in dosage. In the case of anticoagulants the dose of the anticoagulant may need to be reduced. In dysmenorrhoea and menorrhagia, lack of response should alert the physician to investigate other causes.

Warnings and adverse effects: Diarrhoea occasionally occurs following the use of mefenamic acid. Although this may occur soon after starting treatment, it may also occur after several months of continuous use. The diarrhoea has been investigated in some patients who have continued this drug in spite of its continued presence. These patients were found to have associated proctocolitis.

If diarrhoea does develop, the drug should be withdrawn immediately and this patient should not receive mefenamic acid again.

Skin rashes have been observed following the administration of mefenamic acid and the occurrence of a rash is a definite indication to withdraw medication.

As with other prostaglandin inhibitors allergic glomerulonephritis has occurred occasionally: non-oliguric renal failure has been reported on a few occasions in elderly patients with dehydration usually from diarrhoea. It has been suggested that the recovery is more rapid and complete than with other forms of analgesic induced renal impairment.

Rarely, thrombocytopenia has been reported with mefenamic acid.

In some cases reversible haemolytic anaemia has occurred. Temporary lowering of the white blood cell count, which may have been due to mefenamic acid, has been reported. Blood studies should therefore be carried out during long-term administration.

Bronchospasm may be precipitated in patients suffering from, or with a previous history of, bronchial asthma or allergic disease.

Patients on prolonged therapy should also be kept under surveillance with particular attention to liver dysfunction. Should this appear it is an indication to discontinue therapy.

Drowsiness and dizziness have rarely been reported.

Note: A positive reaction in certain tests for bile in the urine of patients receiving mefenamic acid has been demonstrated to be due to the presence of the drug and its metabolites and not to the presence of bile.

Treatment of overdosage: Gastric lavage in the conscious patient and intensive supportive therapy where necessary. Activated charcoal has been shown to be a powerful adsorbent for mefenamic acid and its metabolites. Studies in experimental animals and humans showed that a 5 to 1 ratio of charcoal to mefenamic acid resulted in considerable suppression of absorption of the drug.

Pharmaceutical precautions Store at a temperature not exceeding 30°C.

Legal category POM.

Package quantities Available in packs of 100.

Further information Nil.

Product licence number 0018/0095R.

SYTRON*

Presentation A clear red mixture with a cherry taste.

Composition: Each 5 ml contains:
Sodium Ironedetate 190 mg
(Equivalent to 27.5 mg of Iron)

Inactive ingredients: Ethanol; Ponceau 4R; Methyl Hydroxybenzoate PhEur; Propyl p-Hydroxybenzoate PhEur.

Action: Sodium ironedetate is not an iron salt as it contains iron in an un-ionised form. In this compound the iron is 'insulated' or 'sequestered' with the sodium salt of ethylenediamine tetra-acetic acid to form a chelate. This accounts for the fact that Sytron is not astringent and does not discolour teeth. Studies using radio-active tracers, have shown that iron chelate is split within the gastro-intestinal tract, releasing elemental iron which is absorbed and rendered available for haemoglobin regeneration.

Uses Iron deficiency anaemia, in paediatrics, in anaemias complicating rheumatoid arthritis. It is especially suitable in pregnancy when other forms of oral iron are not well tolerated.

Dosage and administration *Oral: Adults:* 5 ml increasing gradually to 10 ml three times daily.

Elderly (over 65 years): As for adults.

Children: (including premature infants) up to 1 year: 2.5 ml twice daily; somewhat smaller doses should be used initially. 1 to 5 years: 2.5 ml three times daily. 6 to 12 years: 5 ml three times daily.

Contra-indications, warnings, etc Patients have occasionally complained of nausea or mild diarrhoea in the early stages of treatment. In such cases it has been found that if treatment is withdrawn for a short time, these symptoms quickly disappear and subsequently the patient will tolerate further doses, which should be on a somewhat reduced scale. Normal individuals have taken Sytron in twice the recommended dosage and some of these have experienced mild diarrhoea. This should be taken into account if dosage is increased much higher than the recommended scale.

Treatment of overdosage: Probably not required but if indicated, treatment should be according to any symptoms that may arise.

Pharmaceutical precautions Store below 30°C. Recommended diluent: Water. When diluted use within 14 days of preparation.

Legal category P.

Package quantities Containers of 500 ml and 2.25 litre.

Further information Nil.

Product licence number 0018/5029.

ZARONTIN*

Presentation Zarontin Syrup (Ethosuximide Elixir BP) is a clear red, raspberry-flavoured syrup. Each 5 ml contains Ethosuximide BP 250 mg. *Inactive ingredients:* Sodium benzoate; sucrose; carmoisine; Sunset yellow.

Zarontin Capsules (Ethosuximide Capsules BP) are amber, oblong soft gelatin capsules containing a clear liquid and imprinted 'P-D' in ivory ink. Each capsule contains Ethosuximide BP 250 mg. *Inactive ingredients:* Ponceau 4R; polyethylene glycol USP; quinolone yellow.

Action Ethosuximide suppresses the paroxysmal spike and wave pattern common to petit mal seizures. The frequency of epileptiform attacks is reduced, apparently by depression of the motor cortex and elevation of the threshold of the central nervous system to convulsive stimuli. Compared with other succinimide anticonvulsants, ethosuximide is more specific for pure petit mal.

Indications Primarily useful in petit mal epilepsy. When grand mal and other forms of epilepsy co-exist with petit mal, Zarontin may be administered in combination with other anticonvulsants such as phenobarbitone, Epanutin* (Phenytoin Sodium Ph Eur) and primidone.

Dosage and administration Oral.

Adults and children over 6 years: initially 2 capsules or two 5 ml spoonfuls daily and adjusted thereafter to the patient's needs; daily dosage should be increased by small increments, for example, by 1 capsule or 5 ml every four to seven days, until control is achieved with minimal side-effects; although 4–6 capsules or 20–30 ml daily in divided doses often produce control of seizures, 7–8 capsules or 35–40 ml daily is not an unusual requirement.

Children and infants under 6 years: The initial dose is 5 ml daily which is adjusted by small increments until control is achieved with minimal side-effects.

Contra-indications, warnings, etc Hypersensitivity to succinimides.

There is some evidence that the succinimides may produce congenital abnormalities in the offspring of a small number of epileptic patients, and therefore they should only be used in pregnancy if in the judgement of the physician the potential benefits outweigh the risk. Ethosuximide may be excreted in breast milk. Zarontin should be used with caution in patients with impaired hepatic or renal function.

Mild side-effects, which are usually transient, may occur initially. These include apathy, drowsiness, depression, mild euphoria, headache, ataxia, dizziness, anorexia, gastric upset, nausea and vomiting. Psychotic states thought to be induced or exacerbated by anticonvulsant therapy have been reported. Skin rashes have been seen in a few patients. Systemic lupus erythematosus has occasionally been associated with the use of ethosuximide. Haematological reactions to ethosuximide appear to be uncommon. Cases of leucopenia, agranulocytosis and aplastic anaemia have been reported. The extent to which ethosuximide is implicated in these reactions is yet to be determined. Monocytosis, leucocytosis and transitory mild eosinophilia have also been noted. In most cases of leucopenia, the blood picture has been restored to normal on reduction of the dosage or discontinuation of the drug. Where leucopenia has occurred with other drugs, the polymorph count has in some cases increased steadily after starting treatment with ethosuximide and discontinuing previous medication. If the patient has been receiving other anticonvulsants the sudden withdrawal of the drugs may precipitate a series of attacks before Zarontin has been given in sufficient amounts to exercise control. This may be avoided by gradually replacing with Zarontin the anticonvulsant previously used.

Treatment of overdosage: If less than 2 g have been taken, fluids should be given by mouth. If a larger dose has been taken the stomach should be emptied, respiration maintained and any other symptoms treated accordingly.

Pharmaceutical precautions *Capsules:* Store at a temperature not exceeding 30°C.

Syrup: Store at a temperature not exceeding 25°C.

Recommended diluent – Syrup BP. When diluted use within 14 days of preparation.

Legal category POM.

Package quantities *Capsules 250 mg:* 50 and 500. *Syrup:* 250 ml.

Further information Nil.

Product licence numbers
Zarontin Syrup 0018/5040R
Zarontin Capsules 0018/0078R

**Trade Mark*

Perstorp Pharma Limited
Wound Care Division
Studio 1
Intec 2
Wade Road
Basingstoke
Hampshire RG24 0NE

IODOSORB* OINTMENT

Presentation Tubes of sterile cadexomer iodine (INN) ointment containing Iodine PhEur at a concentration of 0.9% w/w for topical application. The cadexomer iodine, a modified starch gel microbead, is formulated in an inert ointment base. Each tube is for a single application only.

The formulation includes polyethylene glycol 400, 40.8%; polyethylene glycol 4000, 7.2%; pluronic L64 2.0%.

Uses For the treatment of chronic leg ulcers. When applied to the wound, Iodosorb Ointment absorbs pus and exudate, cleans the wound surface and reduces bacterial count. In chronic ulcers it stimulates granulation, reduces pain and accelerates healing.

The ointment formulation improves the ease of application on awkward wound sites.

Dosage and administration Iodosorb Ointment is applied topically to the wound surface to a depth of approximately 3 mm ($\frac{1}{8}$"). A single application should not exceed 50 g (5 × 10 g tubes). The total amount of Iodosorb Ointment used in one week must not exceed 15 tubes. The preparation should be changed approximately three times per week or when the Iodosorb Ointment has become saturated with wound exudate, indicated by a loss of colour. Each time the dressing is changed and at the end of treatment, the remaining Iodosorb should be gently removed from the ulcer surface either with a stream of sterile water or saline, or with a sterile wet swab. The duration of treatment should not exceed 3 months in any single course of treatment. When venous insufficiency is a contributory factor, support bandages or stockings can be applied in conjunction with the use of Iodosorb Ointment.

Contra-indications, warnings, etc
Contra-indications: As Iodosorb Ointment contains 0.9% w/w iodine it should not be used in patients with known or suspected iodine sensitivity. Iodosorb Ointment is contra-indicated in Hashimoto's thyroiditis.

In patients with a prior history of Graves Disease it is not recommended to use iodine containing products, which includes Iodosorb Ointment.

The ointment should not be used in the case of non-toxic nodular goitre.

Warnings: Patients with a past history of any thyroid disorder are more susceptible to alteration in thyroid metabolism with chronic Iodosorb therapy.

Iodine is absorbed systemically especially when large wounds are treated.

In endemic goitre there have been isolated reports of hyperthyroidism associated with Iodosorb.

There is a potential for interaction of iodine with the following drugs and therefore co-administration is not recommended, lithium, sulphafurazoles and sulphonylureas.

It has been observed occasionally that an adherent crust can form when the dressing is not changed with significant frequency.

Pregnancy: Iodine can cross the placental barrier and is secreted into milk. Do not use Iodosorb in pregnant or lactating women.

Pharmaceutical precautions Store at room temperature or below.

Legal category POM.

Package quantities Four unit dose tubes containing 10 g of ointment per pack (OP).

Further information On contact with wound exudate, the ointment absorbs fluid, removing exudate, pus and debris from the wound surface. Iodine is physically immobilised within the matrix of the ointment and is slowly released in an active form during uptake of wound fluid. This mechanism of release provides antibacterial activity both at the wound surface and within the formed gel. The gel can be removed with a stream of water without damaging the fragile new epithelium.

Product licence number 3863/0004.

IODOSORB* POWDER

Presentation Sterile sachets of cadexomer iodine, a dry yellow-brown powder of modified starch gel microbeads containing Iodine PhEur at a concentration of 0.9% w/w for topical application.

Uses Treatment of moist wounds including decubitus ulcers and chronic leg ulcers associated with venous disease. When applied to the wound cadexomer iodine absorbs pus and exudate, cleans the wound surface and reduces bacterial counts. In chronic venous ulcers and decubitus ulcers it stimulates granulation, reduces pain and accelerates healing.

Dosage and administration Cadexomer iodine is applied to the wound surface to form a layer approximately 3 mm deep and then covered with a dry dressing of gauze. The dressing should be changed daily, or when all applied cadexomer iodine has become saturated with wound exudate. Each time the dressing is changed and at the end of treatment, the remaining cadexomer iodine gel should be gently washed from the surface either with a gentle stream of sterile water or saline or with a sterile wet swab.

To avoid the risk of cross-contamination, it is recommended that the use of a single sachet of cadexomer iodine be confined to one patient.

Cadexomer iodine is a dressing for the wound and has no influence on the underlying cause of the chronic wound.

Contra-indications, warnings, etc Iodine is absorbed systemically, especially when large wounds are treated. This should be taken into consideration in patients in whom thyroid function is under investigation. Cadexomer iodine contains 0.9% iodine and must not be used in patients with known or suspected iodine sensitivity. Iodine can cross the placental barrier and is secreted into milk. Use of cadexomer iodine should therefore be avoided in pregnant or lactating women.

It has been observed occasionally that an adherent crust can form when the dressing is not changed with sufficient frequency.

Pharmaceutical precautions Iodosorb should be stored protected from heat and moisture.

Legal category POM.

Package quantities Unit dose sachet of 3 g in boxes of 7 sachets (OP).

Further information One gram of cadexomer iodine can absorb up to 6 ml of fluid. Iodine is physically immobilised within the matrix of the dry cadexomer iodine and is slowly released in an active form during uptake of wound fluid. This mechanism of release provides antibacterial activity at the wound surface and within the formed gel. The gel can be removed with a stream of water without damaging the fragile new epithelium beneath.

Product licence number 3863/0001.

**Trade Mark*

Pfizer Limited
Sandwich
Kent CT13 9NJ

ALEXAN* AND ALEXAN 100

Presentation Alexan (cytarabine) is available as either an isotonic solution (Alexan) or as a hypertonic solution (Alexan 100) in ampoules ready for injection.

Alexan ampoules contain either 2 ml or 5 ml of a solution of 20 mg/ml cytarabine. Inactive excipients: These are sodium chloride, sodium lactate solution, sodium hydroxide and water.

Alexan 100 ampoules contain 1 ml or 10 ml of a solution of 100 mg/ml cytarabine. Inactive excipients: These are sodium lactate solution, lactic acid and water.

Uses Cytarabine is a cytostatic agent for induction of clinical remission and/or maintenance therapy in patients with: acute myeloid leukaemia, acute non-lymphoblastic leukaemias, acute lymphoblastic leukaemias, blast crises of chronic myeloid leukaemia, diffuse histiocytic lymphomas (non-Hodgkin's lymphomas of high malignancy).

Dosage and administration

Alexan ampoules: Alexan is administered by continuous intravenous infusion, intravenous injection, intrathecal injection, intramuscular or subcutaneous injection.

To prepare an infusion solution, Alexan can be added to sodium chloride intravenous infusion or dextrose intravenous infusion. Alexan is incompatible with 5-fluorouracil and methotrexate.

Continuous infusions have ranged from 8–12 hours to 120–168 hours. In comparison with the single i.v. injections, continuous infusions of the same dosage show more pronounced gastrointestinal side-effects. Intrathecal, lumbar or intraventricular administration of Alexan can be carried out with the original solution. It is recommended that 5–8 ml of cerebrospinal fluid (CSF) be drawn up, mixed with the injection solution in the syringe and slowly re-injected. Systemic toxicity is not to be expected using this route of administration.

Intramuscular and subcutaneous injections are usually used only in maintenance therapy. Intracutaneous injections should be avoided, due to the risk of oedema.

Alexan 100: In high dose schedules, Alexan 100 should be administered by continuous intravenous infusion in either sodium chloride intravenous infusion or dextrose intravenous infusion. Alexan 100 is incompatible with 5-fluorouracil and methotrexate. Infusion times of less than one hour appear to increase the toxicity of this regimen. To reduce the toxicity of Alexan 100 in high dose schedules, the duration of infusion should be not less than 1 hour.

Subcutaneous injection of Alexan 100 is not recommended at present due to lack of clinical data.

Intrathecal/intramuscular use of Alexan 100 is contra-indicated due to slight hypertonicity of this formulation.

The dosage required should be as exact as possible for each patient and is best calculated according to body surface area. Unless otherwise indicated in special combinations, Alexan should be used in the following doses:

Alexan

Remission Induction Therapy:

Acute leukaemias: 100–200 mg/m^2/day or 3–6 mg/kg/day.

Administer 100 mg/m^2 twice daily when rapid intravenous injection is used. However, when continuous infusion is employed, 100 mg/m^2/day is recommended as a starting dose. The duration will depend on clinical and morphological (bone marrow) findings.

Either: Treat the patient with Alexan for up to seven days and then allow 7–14 days treatment free to allow the bone marrow to recover before applying consolidation cycles (often of reduced duration of treatment) until remission or toxicity occurs.

Or: Continue to treat the patient with Alexan until the appearance of bone marrow hypoplasia, which may be considered a tolerance limit. Before repeating the therapy cycle (often of reduced duration) there should be a treatment free period of at least 14 days or until the bone marrow has recovered. For remission induction therapy, patients should be supervised in a centre with laboratory and supportive resources sufficient to monitor drug tolerance and protect and maintain a patient compromised by drug toxicity.

Remission Maintenance:

Leukaemias: 75–100 mg/m^2/day or 1.5–3 mg/kg/day for five consecutive days once a month or for one day each week.

CNS leukaemias: 10–30 mg/m^2 three times weekly, intrathecally.

Lymphomas: These conditions are usually treated with a suitable combination of agents.

Alexan 100

High dose therapy should be reserved for treatment of resistant or refractory cases. The evidence suggests that the maximum tolerated dose is 3 g/m^2 every 12 hours for 6 days. The dosage should be based on the schedules employed in clinical practice, and it is strongly recommended that current literature be consulted before initiating therapy with high dose Alexan 100.

Use in children: Children show greater tolerance than adults to Alexan. Upper dosage levels of Alexan and Alexan 100 may be administered to children.

Use in the elderly: Elderly patients may tolerate side-effects less well and such patients should be carefully monitored.

Contra-indications, warnings, etc

Contra-indications: Patients who already have bone marrow suppression should be excluded from treatment with Alexan or Alexan 100 unless the clinician considers that the benefit of such treatment outweighs its risk for the individual patient. Hypersensitivity to cytarabine.

Warnings: Hyperuricaemic prophylaxis is an absolute requirement, particularly in patients with acute monoblastic leukaemia, with large tumour masses or with high blast counts. The clinician should monitor the patient's blood uric acid level and use such supportive and pharmacological measures as might be necessary to control this. Because of the possible teratogenic effect of cytarabine on male and female germ cells, adequate conception control should be established during and for a sufficient period after treatment.

To minimise the risks associated with remission induction therapy (granulocytopenia and associated infection, haemorrhage secondary to thrombocytopenia), Alexan and Alexan 100 should be used only in centres where adequate supportive therapy is available.

Cytarabine has also been reported to cause chromosome breaks in human leucocytes in vitro. Cytarabine inhibits DNA synthesis in mammalian cell cultures. These factors should be considered in long term administration.

Use in pregnancy and lactation: Cytarabine has been shown to be teratogenic in some animal species. Alexan and Alexan 100 should not be used in pregnancy or lactation unless considered absolutely essential by the physician.

Precautions: Cytarabine is a potent bone marrow suppressant. During induction therapy patients should be closely supervised and leucocyte and platelet counts performed daily. Remission maintenance may be carried out under out-patient conditions, but effects on blood and bone marrow must be carefully monitored. If the platelet count falls below $50{,}000/mm^3$ or the leucocyte count falls below $1{,}000/mm^3$ suspension or modification of therapy should be considered. The blood count may continue to fall following discontinuation of Alexan or Alexan 100. Treatment may be recommenced if indicated, when bone marrow recovery is confirmed by bone marrow biopsy.

Haematopoietic, renal and liver function should be regularly monitored.

Drug interaction: 5-flurocytosine should not be administered together with Alexan or Alexan 100. The therapeutic efficacy of 5-flurocytosine has been shown to be abolished during such therapy.

Side-effects: In standard doses, Alexan has been associated with bone marrow suppression, thrombocytopenia, leukopenia, anaemia, megaloblastosis, immunosuppression, nausea and vomiting, diarrhoea, oral inflammation or ulceration, fever, pneumonia, anorexia and hepatic dysfunction. Rash, thrombophlebitis and bleeding may also occur.

In high-dose schedules, all conventional side-effects are likely to be increased, and, in addition, several side-effects not normally reported may become obvious:

Haematological: Cytarabine is a potent myelosuppressant associated with depression of all bone marrow constituents. Leucopenia may be of 28 days duration (range 22–40 days), and thrombocytopenia 25 days duration (range 16–41 days). Leucopenia can be associated with fever and with fatal infective episodes. Thrombocytopenia has a potential for mortality due to haemorrhage.

Gastrointestinal: The most frequent side-effects are nausea and vomiting which tend to be mild and transient. Diarrhoea may also occur and whilst usually mild and transient, can be so severe on occasions as to produce a clinical syndrome of diarrhoea, ileus, pain and fever, which can mimic an "acute abdomen".

Central nervous system (CNS): CNS toxicity has only been reported with high dosage regimens, but, because of its importance, is described more fully.

CNS toxicity is a dose limiting phenomenon and does not appear to be related to CNS leukaemia, previous intrathecal therapy, cranial irradiation, or infection. The symptoms are predominantly cerebellar with dysarthria, dysdiadochokinesia and ataxia. In some patients this is associated with mild cognitive dysfunction, manifesting as personality changes and somnolence. The symtomatology usually begins 6–8 days after initiation of therapy, lasting for 3–7 days, and can be fatal, even when the leukaemia is in complete remission. CNS toxicity may be alleviated by the use of pyridoxine. The occurrence of CNS toxicity should probably be considered sufficient grounds for immediate discontinuation of therapy.

Dermatological: Usually presents as a generalised erythematous maculo-papular rash, often accompanied by an intense painful erythema of the palms and soles, which in most cases is accompanied by bulla formation and desquamation. Alopecia is often associated with this therapy and when it occurs tends to be severe.

Ocular: May present as ocular pain, excessive lacrimation, foreign-body sensation, photophobia and blurred vision. The use of hydrocortisone eye drops before the first dose of Alexan or Alexan 100 may either prevent or ameliorate this complication.

The Cytarabine (Ara-C) Syndrome: A "cytarabine syndrome" has been described. It is characterised by fever, myalgia, bone pain, occasionally chest pain, maculopapular rash, conjunctivitis, and malaise usually occurring 6 to 12 hours following cytarabine administration. Treatment with corticosteroids should be considered while continuing therapy with Alexan or Alexan 100. The "cytarabine syndrome" may be found to be more a complication of high dose than of conventional therapy.

Respiratory: Respiratory failure has been reported with pulmonary infiltrates followed by severe respiratory distress, especially in patients with pre-existing respiratory disease.

Other reported side-effects include mucosal ulceration, hepatic dysfunction, fever, psychiatric disturbance, oesophagitis, tinnitus, tachycardia, fatigue, myalgia and bone pain.

Pharmaceutical precautions Store below 15°C.

Alexan and Alexan 100 do not contain any preservatives. An opened ampoule should be used or discarded within 24 hours.

Alexan and Alexan 100 are stable for at least 24 hours following dilution with sodium chloride intravenous infusion or dextrose intravenous infusion.

The increasing use of cytotoxic drugs and the potential hazards associated with them, requires special precautions to be taken in their handling, preparation and administration. These recommendations provide a basis for the safe handling of Alexan/Alexan 100.

1. All staff working with Alexan/Alexan 100 should receive special training.

2. Dilution of Alexan/Alexan 100 should be performed in a designated aseptic area which gives maximum protection to the surrounding environment.

3. Adequate protective clothing including gloves and safety spectacles should be worn.

Should spillage on the skin occur, the affected area should be washed with copious quantities of water.

Should spillage into the eye occur, immediately cleanse thoroughly using copious quantities of sodium chloride eye wash. (If sodium chloride eye wash is not available, water can be used as an alternative.) Should eye irritation continue medical help should be sought.

4. Alexan/Alexan 100 should not be handled by pregnant staff.

5. Adequate care and precautions should be taken in the disposal of items used to dilute Alexan/Alexan 100.

Disposal procedure:
Unopened ampoules: Place in a suitable closed container† and incinerate at 1000°C.

Diluted solution: Inactivate with hydrochloric acid adjusting to pH2. Absorb diluted liquid on to paper, ash or sawdust. Place in a high risk waste disposal bag† and incinerate at 1000°C.

Disposal of swabs, etc: Swabs, etc, should be placed in a high risk waste disposal bag† and incinerated at 1000°C.

Accidental spillage: Should spillage on the floor or breakage of an ampoule occur, adequate protective clothing, including gloves and safety spectacles should be worn. The area should be cleaned with absorbent paper and the floor wiped with cloths soaked in hydrochloric acid solution at pH2, then the floor should be washed with copious quantities of water. The absorbent paper, cloths, gloves and other materials used in the management of the spillage should be placed in a high risk waste disposal bag† and incinerated at 1000°C.

Care should be taken in disposing of broken glass from ampoules, which should go into a closed container† for incineration.

Legal category POM.

Package quantities
Alexan
2 ml ampoule (40 mg cytarabine) in packs of 10.
5 ml ampoule (100 mg cytarabine) in packs of 10.
Alexan 100
1 ml ampoule (100 mg cytarabine) in packs of 10.
10 ml ampoule (1000 mg cytarabine) in packs of 5.

Further information There is extensive literature available on the effectiveness of cytarabine both alone and in combination with other agents in the treatment of conditions for which it is indicated.

Product licence numbers

Alexan	0057/0190
Alexan 100	0057/0259

† The containers and bags should be those specified in the 'Safe disposal of clinical waste'. Health & Safety Advisory Committee HMSO 1982.

ATARAX*

Presentation Atarax (hydroxyzine hydrochloride) is available as:

10 mg sugar-coated tablets, coloured orange and coded on one side with 'Pfizer'.

25 mg sugar-coated tablets, coloured green and coded on one side with 'Pfizer'.

Inactive excipients: Atarax tablets include lactose, sucrose, butyl parahydroxybenzoate and an azo dye sunset yellow. In addition, Atarax 10 mg tablets contain erythrosine and Atarax 25 mg tablets contain quinoline yellow and patent blue V.

Syrup 10 mg/5 ml clear, flavoured with sucrose, peppermint, spearmint and caramel flavour and also containing sodium benzoate and ethanol.

Atarax preparations are gluten free.

Uses *Actions:* Atarax is unrelated chemically to phenothiazine, reserpine, and meprobamate.

Atarax has been shown clinically to be a rapid-acting anxiolytic with a wide margin of safety. It induces a calming effect in anxious, tense adults. It is not a cortical depressant, but its action may be due to a suppression of activity in certain key regions of the subcortical area of the central nervous system.

Antihistamine effects have been demonstrated experimentally and confirmed clinically; it is highly effective in alleviating pruritus.

Atarax is rapidly absorbed from the gastro-intestinal tract and effects are usually noted within 15 to 30 minutes after oral administration.

Indications: Atarax is indicated to assist in the management of anxiety in adults.

Atarax is indicated for the management of pruritus associated with acute and chronic urticaria, including cholinergic and physical types, and atopic and contact dermatoses in adults and children.

Dosage and administration Anxiety: Adults, 50–100 mg four times daily.

Pruritus: Adults, starting dose of 25 mg at night increasing as necessary to 25 mg three or four times daily; children from 6 months to 6 years 5–15 mg rising to 50 mg daily in divided doses and for children over 6 years, 15–25 mg rising to 50–100 mg daily in divided doses.

As with all medications, the dosage should be adjusted according to the patient's response to therapy.

Use in elderly patients: Atarax may be used in elderly patients with no special precautions other than the care always necessary in this age group. The lowest effective maintenance dose and careful observation for side effects are important.

Contra-indications, warnings, etc
Contra-indications: Atarax is contra-indicated in patients who have shown a previous hypersensitivity to it.

Use in pregnancy: Atarax is contra-indicated in early pregnancy. Hydroxyzine, when administered to the pregnant mouse, rat and rabbit, induced foetal abnormalities at doses substantially above the human therapeutic range. Clinical data in humans are inadequate to establish safety in early pregnancy. There is inadequate evidence of safety in the later stages of pregnancy. Use in later pregnancy only when there is no safer alternative or when the disease itself carries risks for the mother or child.

Warnings: Use in nursing mothers: It is not known whether Atarax is excreted in human milk. Since many drugs are so excreted, Atarax should not be given to nursing mothers.

Use in renal insufficiency: Atarax should be used with caution in patients with impaired renal function. It is uncertain whether the drug may accumulate or have other adverse effects in such patients.

Patients should be warned that Atarax may impair their ability to perform activities requiring mental alertness or physical co-ordination such as operating machinery or driving a vehicle.

Patients should be warned that Atarax may enhance their response to alcohol, barbiturates and other CNS depressants.

Side-effects: Therapeutic doses of Atarax seldom produce marked impairment of mental alertness. Drowsiness may occur; if so, it is usually transitory and may disappear after a few days of continued therapy or upon reduction of the dose. Dryness of the mouth may be encountered at higher doses. Dizziness, weakness, headache and confusion have been reported.

Extensive clinical use has substantiated the absence of toxic effects on the liver or bone marrow when administered in the recommended doses for over four years of uninterrupted therapy. The absence of side-effects has been further demonstrated in experimental studies in which excessively high doses were administered.

Involuntary motor activity, including rare instances of tremor and convulsions, have been reported, usually with doses considerably higher than those recommended. Continuous therapy with over 1 g/day has been employed in some patients without these effects having been encountered.

Overdosage: The most common manifestation of Atarax overdosage is hypersedation. As in the management of overdosage with any drug, it should be borne in mind that multiple agents may have been taken.

If vomiting has not occurred spontaneously in conscious patients, it should be induced. Immediate gastric lavage is also recommended. General supportive care, including frequent monitoring of the vital signs and close observation of the patient is indicated. Hypotension, though unlikely, may be controlled with intravenous fluids and noradrenaline, or metaraminol. Adrenaline should not be used in this situation as Atarax counteracts its pressor action.

There is no specific antidote. It is doubtful that haemodialysis would be of any value in the treatment of overdosage with Atarax. However, if other agents such as barbiturates have been ingested concomitantly, haemodialysis may be indicated.

Pharmaceutical precautions Store below 25°C.

Legal category POM.

Package quantities
Tablets 10 mg: Original packs of 84 tablets (in blister strips of 6 × 14 tablets).
Tablets 25 mg: Original packs of 28 tablets (in blister strips of 2 × 14 tablets).
Syrup: Bottle of 150 ml.

Further information Nil.

Product licence numbers

Tablets 10 mg	0057/5003R
Tablets 25 mg	0057/5004R
Syrup	0057/5005R.

COMBANTRIN*

Presentation Combantrin is available as orange tablets containing 125 mg pyrantel as pyrantel pamoate.

Inactive excipients: These include an azo dye sunset yellow FCF. The product is free of gluten, lactose and other sugars.

Uses *Actions:* Combantrin is an anthelmintic agent highly effective against infections due to pinworm (*Enterobius vermicularis*), roundworm (*Ascaris lumbricoides*), hookworm (*Ancylostoma duodenale* and *Necator americanus*), and *Trichostrongylus colubriformis* and *orientalis*. Combantrin has some activity against whipworm (*Trichuris trichiura*).

Combantrin exercises a neuromuscular blocking effect on susceptible helminths. By virtue of its action, Combantrin immobilises ascarides and brings about their expulsion without producing excitation, or stimulating migration of the affected worms. Within the intestinal tract Combantrin is effective against mature and immature forms of susceptible helminths. The normal migratory stages of worms are unaffected. Combantrin is poorly absorbed from the gastro-intestinal tract. More than 50% is excreted unchanged in the faeces following oral administration; less than 7% is found in the urine unchanged and in the form of metabolites.

Indications: Combantrin is specifically indicated for the treatment of infection with any of the following gastro-intestinal parasites when these are present either alone or as a mixed infection.

1. *Enterobius vermicularis* (threadworm, pinworm)
2. *Ascaris lumbricoides* (roundworm)
3. *Ancylostoma duodenale* (hookworm)
4. *Necator americanus* (hookworm)
5. *Trichostrongylus colubriformis* and *orientalis*.

Combantrin should be used for the treatment of infection with one or more of these parasites in both adults and children. It is well tolerated and will not stain the oral mucosa upon ingestion or the clothing by faecal contamination. The presence of an infection with any of the five parasites in one member of a family or group of persons in close proximity may indicate unidentified infection in other members. In these circumstances, Combantrin administration to all the family or group members is recommended. (Rigorous cleaning of living quarters and clothing to destroy helminthic ova will help prevent reinfection.)

Dosage and administration The recommended dose of Combantrin for the treatment of infections with *Enterobius vermicularis, Ascaris lumbricoides, Ancylostoma duodenale, Necator americanus, Trichostrongylus colubriformis* and *orientalis* is 10 mg/kg of patient body weight, administered orally as a single dose. A simplified dosage schedule, based on the above and on estimated weights at various ages follows:

Age of patient	*Weight*	*Tablets of 125 mg*
6 months to 2 years	less than 12 kg	1
2 to 6 years	12 to 22 kg	2
6 to 12 years	22 to 41 kg	4
over 12 years	41 to 75 kg	6
	Adults over 75 kg	8

For more severe infections of *Necator americanus*, the recommended dosage is 20 mg/kg bodyweight administered as a single dose on each of two consecutive days, or 10 mg/kg bodyweight administered as a single dose on each of three consecutive days.

Infection due to *Ascaris lumbricoides* alone can be successfully treated with a dose of 5 mg/kg bodyweight administered as a single dose.

A simplified dosage schedule for ascariasis based on the above and on estimated weights at various ages follows:

Age of patient	*Weight*	*Tablets of 125 mg*
6 months to 2 years	less than 12 kg	½
2 to 6 years	12 to 22 kg	1
6 to 12 years	22 to 41 kg	2
over 12 years	41 to 75 kg	3
	adults over 75 kg	4

In mass treatment programmes directed against *Ascaris lumbricoides* infestation alone, a single dose of 2.5 mg/kg bodyweight can be used. A simplified dosage schedule based on the preceding and on estimated weight at various ages follows:

Age of patient	*Weight*	*Tablets of 125 mg*
6 months to 2 years	less than 12 kg	¼
2 to 6 years	12 to 22 kg	½
6 to 12 years	22 to 41 kg	1
over 12 years	41 to 75 kg	1½
	adults over 75 kg	2

Use in the elderly: No additional precautions.

Contra-indications, warnings, etc

Use in pregnancy: Although animal reproductive studies have not demonstrated any teratogenic effects, Combantrin has not been studied in the pregnant patient. Accordingly, it should not be used during pregnancy unless in the judgement of the physician it is essential for the welfare of the patient.

Precautions: Combantrin should be used with caution in patients with pre-existing hepatic dysfunction, as minor transient elevations of the SGOT have occurred in a small percentage of patients.

Side-effects: Clinical experience has shown Combantrin to be extremely well tolerated. Side-effects, if encountered, usually relate to the gastro-intestinal tract – anorexia, abdominal cramps, nausea, vomiting and diarrhoea. Other side effects that may occur are: headache, dizziness, drowsiness, insomnia and rash.

Overdosage: No cases of overdose with Combantrin have been reported. In the event of overdosage, gastric lavage plus supportive treatment is indicated.

Pharmaceutical precautions Store below 25°C.

Legal category POM.

Package quantities Pack of 6 tablets (Original pack).

Further information Nil.

Product licence number 0057/0057.

DELTACORTRIL* ENTERIC

Presentation Deltacortril Enteric tablets 2.5 mg uniformly brown in colour and coded 'Pfizer'.

Deltacortril Enteric tablets 5 mg uniformly red in colour and coded 'Pfizer'.

Deltacortril is the synthetic crystalline steroid prednisolone.

Inactive excipients: These include lactose, sucrose and methyl parahydroxybenzoate. In addition, the 2.5 mg tablet contains red/brown oxide, and the 5 mg tablet an azo dye ponceau 4R. The tablets are gluten free.

Uses *Actions:* Naturally occurring glucocorticoids (hydrocortisone and cortisone), which also have salt-retaining properties, are used as replacement therapy in adrenocortical deficiency states. Their synthetic analogues such as prednisolone are primarily used for their potent anti-inflammatory effect in disorders of many organ systems. Prednisolone is about four times as active as hydrocortisone on a weight for weight basis.

Deltacortril Enteric is one of the highly potent glucocorticoid steroids having anti-inflammatory, hormonal, and metabolic effects qualitatively similar to those of hydrocortisone.

Glucocorticoids cause profound and varied metabolic effects. In addition, they modify the body's immune responses to diverse stimuli.

Indications

Allergy and anaphylaxis: Bronchial asthma, drug hypersensitivity reactions, serum sickness, angioneurotic oedema, anaphylaxis.

Arteritis/collagenosis: Giant cell arteritis/polymyalgia rheumatica, mixed connective tissue disease, polyarteritis nodosa, polymyositis.

Blood disorders: Haemolytic anaemia (autoimmune), leukaemia (acute and lymphatic), malignant lymphoma, multiple myeloma, idiopathic thrombocytopenic purpura.

Cardiovascular disorders: Post myocardial infarction syndrome, rheumatic fever with severe carditis.

Endocrine disorders: Primary and secondary adrenal insufficiency, congenital adrenal hyperplasia.

Gastro-intestinal disorders: Crohn's disease, ulcerative colitis, persistent coeliac syndrome (coeliac disease unresponsive to gluten withdrawal), auto-immune chronic active hepatitis, multisystem disease affecting liver, biliary peritonitis.

Hypercalcaemia: Sarcoidosis, vitamin D excess.

Infections (with appropriate chemotherapy): Helminthic infestations, Herxheimer reaction, infectious mononucleosis, miliary tuberculosis, mumps orchitis (adult), tuberculous meningitis, rickettsial disease.

Muscular disorders: Polymyositis, dermatomyositis.

Neurological disorders: Infantile spasms, Shy-Drager syndrome, sub-acute demyelinating polyneuropathy.

Ocular disease: Scleritis, posterior uveitis, retinal vasculitis, pseudo tumours of the orbit, giant cell arteritis, malignant ophthalmic Graves disease.

Renal disorders: Lupus nephritis, acute interstitial nephritis, minimal change nephrotic syndrome.

Respiratory disease: Allergic pneumonitis, bronchial asthma, occupational asthma, pulmonary aspergillosis, pulmonary fibrosis, pulmonary alveolitis, aspiration of foreign body, aspiration of stomach contents, pulmonary sarcoid, drug induced lung disease, adult respiratory distress syndrome, spasmodic croup.

Rheumatic disorders: Rheumatoid arthritis, polymyalgia rheumatica, juvenile chronic arthritis, systemic lupus erythematosus, dermatomyositis, mixed connective tissues disease.

Skin disorders: Pemphigus vulgaris, bullous pemphigoid, systemic lupus erythematosus, pyoderma gangrenosum.

Miscellaneous: Sarcoidosis, hyperpyrexia, Behcets disease, immuno-suppression in organ transplantation.

Dosage and administration The initial dosage of Deltacortril Enteric may vary from 5 mg to 60 mg daily depending on the disorder being treated. Divided daily dosage is usually used.

The following therapeutic guidelines should be kept in mind for all therapy with corticosteroids:

Corticosteroids are palliative symptomatic treatment by virtue of their anti-inflammatory effects; they are never curative.

The appropriate individual dose must be determined by trial and error and must be re-evaluated regularly according to activity of the disease.

As corticosteroid therapy becomes prolonged and as the dose is increased, the incidence of disabling side-effects increases.

Abrupt cessation of prolonged, high dosage corticosteroid therapy is associated with a significant risk of potentially life-threatening adrenal insufficiency.

In general, initial dosage should be maintained or adjusted until the anticipated response is observed. The dose should then be gradually reduced until the lowest dose which will maintain an adequate clinical response is reached.

During prolonged therapy, dosage may need to be temporarily increased during periods of stress or during exacerbations of the disease.

When the drug is to be stopped, it must be withdrawn gradually and not abruptly.

If there is lack of a satisfactory clinical response to Deltacortril Enteric, the drug should be gradually discontinued and the patient transferred to alternative therapy.

Intermittent dosage regimen: A single dose of Deltacortril on alternate days or at longer intervals is acceptable therapy for some patients. When this regimen is practical, the degree of pituitary-adrenal suppression can be minimised.

Specific dosage guidelines: The following recommendations for some corticosteroid-responsive disorders are for guidance only. Acute or severe disease may require initial high dose therapy with reduction to the lowest effective maintenance dose as soon as possible. Dosage reductions should not exceed 5–7.5 mg daily during chronic treatment.

Allergic and skin disorders: Initial doses of 5–15 mg daily are commonly adequate.

Collagenosis: Initial doses of 20–30 mg daily are frequently effective. Those with more severe symptoms may require higher doses.

Rheumatoid arthritis: The usual initial dose is 10–15 mg daily. The lowest daily maintenance dose compatible with tolerable symptomatic relief is recommended.

Blood disorders and lymphoma: An initial daily dose of 15–60 mg is often necessary with reduction after an adequate clinical or haematological response.

Higher doses may be necessary to induce remission in acute leukaemia.

Use in children: Although appropriate fractions of the actual dose may be used, dosage will usually be determined by clinical response as in adults. Corticosteroids cause growth retardation in infancy, childhood and adolescence. Treatment should be limited to the minimum dosage for the shortest possible time. In order to minimise suppression of the hypothalamo-pituitary adrenal axis and growth retardation, treatment should be administered where possible as a single dose on alternate days.

Use in the elderly: Treatment of elderly patients, particularly if long term, should be planned bearing in mind the more serious consequences of the common side-effects of corticosteroids in old age, especially osteoporosis, diabetes, hypertension, susceptibility to infection and thinning of the skin.

Contra-indications, warnings, etc

Contra-indications: Systemic infections unless specific anti-infective therapy is employed.

Warnings

Use in pregnancy: There is inadequate evidence of safety in human pregnancy and there may be a very small risk of cleft palate and intra-uterine growth retardation in the foetus; there is evidence of harmful effects on pregnancy in animals. The use of corticosteroids in pregnancy, nursing mothers or women of childbearing potential requires that possible benefits be weighed against potential hazards to mother and foetus.

Precautions: Caution is necessary when oral corticosteroids, including Deltacortril Enteric, are prescribed in patients with the following conditions:

Tuberculosis: Those with a previous history of or X-ray changes characteristic of tuberculosis. The emergence of active tuberculosis can, however, be prevented by the prophylactic use of antituberculous therapy.

Hypertension.

Diabetes mellitus or in those with a family history of diabetes.

Osteoporosis: This is of special importance in post-menopausal females who are at particular risk.

Glaucoma or in those with a family history of glaucoma.

Patients with a history of severe affective disorders and particularly those with a previous history of steroid induced psychoses.

Epilepsy.

Peptic ulceration.

Previous steroid myopathy.

Corticosteroid treatment is likely to reduce the response of the pituitary-adrenal axis to stress and relative adrenal insufficiency may persist for up to a year after discontinuation of therapy. Therapy may need to be reintroduced during a period of stress.

The effect of corticosteroids may be enhanced in patients with hypothyroidism and in those with chronic liver disease with impaired hepatic function. Corticosteroids should be used cautiously in patients with ocular herpes simplex because of possible perforation.

Side-effects:

Gastro-intestinal: Dyspepsia, peptic ulceration with perforation and haemorrhage, abdominal distension, oesophageal ulceration, oesophageal candidiasis, acute pancreatitis.

Musculo-skeletal: Proximal myopathy, osteoporosis, vertebral and long bone fractures, avascular osteonecrosis, tendon rupture.

Fluid and electrolyte disturbance: Sodium and water retention, hypertension, hypokalaemic alkalosis.

Dermatological: Impaired healing, skin atrophy, bruising, striae, telangiectasia, acne.

Endocrine/metabolic: Suppression of the hypothalamo-pituitary adrenal axis, growth suppression in childhood and adolescence, menstrual irregularity and amenorrhoea. Cushingoid facies, hirsutism, weight gain, impaired carbohydrate tolerance with increased requirement for antidiabetic therapy, negative nitrogen balance.

Neuropsychiatric: Euphoria, psychological dependence, depression, insomnia. Intracranial hypertension in children. Aggravation of schizophrenia.

Ophthalmic: Increased intra-ocular pressure, glaucoma, papilloedema, cataracts, corneal or scleral thinning, exacerbation of ophthalmic viral disease.

General: Opportunistic infection, recurrence of dormant tuberculosis, leucocytosis, hypersensitivity, thromboembolism, increased appetite, nausea, malaise.

Withdrawal symptoms: Fever, myalgia, arthralgia, adrenal insufficiency.

Teratogenicity: See 'Warnings'.

Drug interactions: Drugs which can cause liver enzyme induction such as phenobarbitone, phenytoin and rifampicin may reduce the therapeutic efficacy of corticosteroids by increasing the rate of metabolism. Lack of expected response may be observed and dosage of corticosteroid may need to be increased.

Response to anticoagulants may be reduced or, less often, enhanced by corticosteroids.

Concurrent administration of corticosteroids and diuretics may cause excessive potassium loss.

Overdosage: Treatment is unlikely to be needed. Serum electrolytes should be monitored.

Pharmaceutical precautions Store below 25°C.

Legal category POM.

Package quantities Deltacortril Enteric Tablets 2.5 mg and 5 mg: Original packs of 56 tablets. Hospital packs of 500 tablets are only available direct from Pfizer Ltd.

Further information Nil.

Product licence numbers
2.5 mg tablets 0057/5012R
5 mg tablets 0057/0128.

DIABINESE*

Presentation Diabinese (chlorpropamide) is available as a white scored tablet in two different strengths:

Diabinese 100 mg tablet coded DIA/100 on one side and 'Pfizer' on the other.

Diabinese 250 mg tablet coded DIA/250 on one side and 'Pfizer' on the other.

Diabinese is classified as an arylsulphonylurea.

The tablets are free of gluten, lactose and other sugars.

Uses Diabinese is a potent, orally active sulphonylurea which effectively reduces blood glucose in selected patients with mild to moderately severe, maturity-onset, stable diabetes (Type II diabetes).

The mode of action of Diabinese is believed to be that of stimulation of synthesis and release of endogenous insulin from the beta-cells of pancreatic islet tissue. Extra pancreatic effects may play a part in the mechanism of action of oral sulphonylureas.

Diabinese is rapidly absorbed from the gastrointestinal tract. Within one hour after a single oral dose, it is readily detectable in the blood, and reaches a maximum within two to four hours. It is metabolised and excreted in the urine as unchanged drug and as hydroxylated or hydrolyzed metabolites. The biological half-life of chlorpropamide averages about 36 hours. Within 96 hours, 80 to 90% of a single oral dose is excreted in the urine. However, long-term administration of therapeutic doses does not result in undue accumulation in the blood, since absorption and excretion rates become stabilized in about 5 to 7 days after the initiation of therapy.

Diabinese exerts a hypoglycaemic effect in normal humans within one hour, becoming maximal at 3 to 6 hours and persisting for at least 24 hours.

There is now evidence that improvement in pancreatic beta cell function, with consequent improvement in glucose tolerance, may occur with prolonged administration of Diabinese. Accordingly, in individuals with asymptomatic diabetes mellitus, principally manifested by an abnormal glucose tolerance, continuous use of Diabinese may result in 'normalization' of their tolerance to glucose.

Indications:

Diabetes mellitus: Diabinese is indicated as an adjunct to diet to lower the blood glucose in patients with non-insulin-dependent diabetes mellitus (NIDDM/Type II), whose hyperglycaemia cannot be controlled by diet alone.

The use of Diabinese in asymptomatic patients has not been definitely established to be effective in preventing the long-term cardiovascular or neurological complications of diabetes.

Diabinese may prove effective in patients who have not responded or have ceased to respond to other sulphonylureas (primary or secondary failures).

Concurrent Diabinese – biguanide therapy: Concurrent treatment with a biguanide is indicated in stable, nonketotic, NIDDM which cannot be controlled by diet alone, by diet and insulin, or by diet and sulphonylurea agents. The appropriate biguanide data sheet should be consulted for complete details of patient selection, indications, warnings and dose.

Diabetes insipidus: Limited studies have shown that Diabinese has an antidiuretic action which is useful in the treatment of diabetes insipidus.

It is essential that physicians considering Diabinese for the treatment of diabetes insipidus read this data sheet completely and particularly those paragraphs relating to Precautions and Adverse Reactions.

Dosage and administration The total daily dose of Diabinese should be taken as a single dose each morning with breakfast. The occasional case of gastrointestinal intolerance may be relieved by dividing the daily dosage. A loading or primary dose is not necessary.

Initial therapy in diabetes mellitus: Patients should be given a 7 day therapeutic trial with Diabinese and if there is no ketonuria and satisfactory control of glycosuria and hyperglycaemia, this indicates that their diabetes can be controlled by Diabinese.

The recommended starting dose is 250 mg daily.

Use in children: Safety and effectiveness in children have not been established.

Use in the elderly: Elderly patients should be started on 100–125 mg daily as some are more sensitive to the hypoglycaemic effect of sulphonylureas.

Initial therapy in diabetes insipidus: Because of the risk of hypoglycaemia in this group of patients, the initial dose should be low, for example 100 mg.

Titration: Five to seven days after initial therapy Diabinese blood levels reach a plateau. Dosage may then be adjusted up or down by increments of not more than 50–125 mg at intervals of 3 to 5 days to obtain optimal control.

Maintenance therapy: Most moderately severe, middle-aged stable diabetic patients are controlled by approximately 250 mg daily. Milder diabetics may do well on daily doses of 100–125 mg or less. Some severe diabetics may require doses of 500 mg daily. The maximum recommended maintenance daily dose is 500 mg.

In elderly patients, debilitated or malnourished patients, and patients with impaired renal or hepatic function, the initial and maintenance dosing should be conservative to avoid hypoglycaemic reactions (see Precautions section).

Transfer from other oral agents: No transition period is necessary when transferring patients from other oral hypoglycaemic agents. However due consideration must be given to the greater potency of Diabinese.

Patients receiving insulin: The large majority of patients receiving insulin can have their insulin abruptly discontinued and be placed directly on the oral drug. For patients needing more than 40 units of insulin daily, therapy with Diabinese may be started with a 50% reduction in insulin for the first few days, with further reduction dependent upon the response. During insulin withdrawal the patient should test his urine for sugar and ketone bodies at least 3 times daily. If they are abnormal the doctor should be notified. In some instances hospitalisation during the transition period should be considered.

Diabinese/Metformin dosage: The dosage of Diabinese should be maintained at or increased to 500 mg. If control is still inadequate, metformin may be added at a dosage of 500 mg twice daily, increasing by 500 mg to 1.0 gram every one to two weeks to a maximum of 3 grams daily.

If adequate control is obtained without side-effects, reduction in dosage of both Diabinese and metformin should be undertaken slowly (reducing the dosage of one drug at a time) in an attempt to maintain control with the least possible medication.

Contra-indications, warnings, etc

Contra-indications: Hypersensitivity to Diabinese: Insulin dependent (juvenile) diabetes mellitus; diabetic ketoacidosis, with or without coma, major surgery, severe infection, or severe trauma; patients with serious impairment of hepatic, renal or thyroid function.

Use in pregnancy: Diabinese is contra-indicated during pregnancy. Serious consideration should be given to the potential hazard of using Diabinese in women of childbearing age who may become pregnant.

Nursing mothers: Diabinese is excreted in breast milk and it is not recommended that a woman breast feed while taking this medication.

Precautions

General: Hypoglycaemia: Severe hypoglycaemia may occur with all sulphonylureas. Proper patient selection, dosage and instructions are important to avoid hypoglycaemic episodes. Renal or hepatic insufficiency may cause elevated blood levels of Diabinese and the latter may also diminish gluconeogenic capacity, both of which increase the risk of serious hypoglycaemic reactions. Elderly, debilitated or malnourished patients, and those with adrenal or pituitary insufficiency are particularly susceptible to the hypoglycaemic action of glucose-lowering drugs. Hypoglycaemia may be difficult to recognise in the elderly, and in people who are taking beta-adrenergic blocking drugs. Hypoglycaemia is more likely to occur when caloric intake is deficient, after severe or prolonged exercise, when alcohol is ingested, or when more than one glucose-lowering drug is used.

Because of the long half-life of Diabinese, patients who become hypoglycaemic during therapy require careful supervision of the dose and frequent meals for at least 3 to 5 days. Hospitalisation and intravenous glucose may be necessary.

Loss of control of blood glucose: When a patient stabilised on any diabetic regimen is exposed to stress such as fever, trauma, infection, or surgery, a loss of control may occur. At such times, it may be necessary to discontinue Diabinese and administer insulin. (See Contra-indications.)

The effectiveness of any oral hypoglycaemic drug, like Diabinese, in lowering blood glucose to a desired level, decreases in many patients over a period of time. This may be due to progression of the severity of the diabetes or to diminished responsiveness to the drug. This phenomenon is known as secondary failure, to distinguish it from primary failure in which the drug is ineffective in an individual patient when first given.

Information for patients: Patients should be informed of the potential risks and advantages of Diabinese and of alternative modes of therapy. They should also be informed about the importance of adherence to dietary instructions, of a regular exercise programme, and of regular testing of urine and/or blood glucose.

The risks of hypoglycaemia, its symptoms and treatment, and conditions that predispose to its development should be explained to patients and responsible family members. Primary and secondary failure should also be explained.

Patients should be instructed to contact their physician promptly if they experience symptoms of hypoglycaemia or other adverse reactions.

Laboratory tests: Blood and urine glucose should be monitored periodically. Measurement of glycosylated haemoglobin may be useful.

Use in diabetes insipidus: Patients and the parents of young patients suffering from diabetes insipidus should be warned of the possibility and management of hypoglycaemic reactions especially during intercurrent infections or other periods of impaired food intake. In such cases treatment should be discontinued and the patient's physician informed.

Drug interactions: The following drugs may prolong or potentiate the effect of sulphonylureas, including Diabinese, so increasing the risk of hypoglycaemia. Drugs that are highly protein bound such as nonsteroidal anti-inflammatory agents, salicylates, sulphonamides, chloramphenicol, probenecid, coumarins, monoamine oxidase inhibitors and beta-adrenergic blocking agents.

A disulfiram-like reaction may be produced by the ingestion of alcohol.

Certain drugs tend to produce hyperglycaemia and may lead to loss of control. These include the thiazides and other diuretics, corticosteroids, phenothiazines, thyroid products, oestrogens, oral contraceptives, phenytoin, nicotinic acid, sympathomimetics, calcium channel blocking drugs and isoniazid. Diabetic control may be altered in patients also treated with cyclophosphamide.

Use in the elderly: Elderly diabetic patients appear to be more sensitive to the hypoglycaemic effect of sulphonylurea drugs, so should be started on doses of 100–125 mg daily. The elderly are also particularly susceptible to the effects of hypoglycaemia.

Use in renal insufficiency: Diabinese should be used with caution in patients with renal insufficiency and, like other sulphonylureas, is generally contra-indicated in patients with an elevated blood urea or serum creatinine. Serum half-life may be prolonged and drug accumulation may occur thereby enhancing the hypoglycaemic effect of Diabinese and the possibiity of adverse effects.

Side-effects: The majority of side-effects have been dose-related, transient, and have responded to dose reduction or withdrawal of the medication. However, as with other sulphonylureas, some side-effects associated with hypersensitivity may be severe and some deaths have been reported.

Hypoglycaemia: See 'Precautions' and 'Overdosage' sections.

Gastrointestinal reactions: Cholestatic jaundice may occur rarely; Diabinese should be discontinued if this occurs. Gastrointestinal disturbances are the most common reactions; nausea has been reported in less than 5% of patients and diarrhoea, vomiting, anorexia, and hunger in less than 2%. Other gastrointestinal disturbances have occurred in less than 1% of patients.

Dermatological reactions: Pruritus has been reported in less than 3% of patients. Other allergic skin reactions, e.g., urticaria and maculopapular eruptions have been reported in 1% or less of patients. If skin reactions persist, Diabinese should be discontinued.

Porphyria cutanea tarda and photosensitivity reactions.

Skin eruptions progressing to erythema multiforme and exfoliative dermatitis.

Haematological reactions: Leucopenia, agranulocytosis, thrombocytopenia, haemolytic anaemia, aplastic anaemia, and pancytopenia.

Metabolic reactions: Hepatic porphyria and disulfiram-like reactions occur rarely. See 'Drug interactions' section.

Endocrine reactions: A reaction identical to the syndrome of inappropriate antidiuretic hormone (ADH) secretion occurs rarely. The features of this syndrome result from excessive water retention and include hyponatraemia, low serum osmolality, and high urine osmolality.

Overdosage: Overdosage of sulphonylureas including Diabinese can produce hypoglycaemia. Mild hypoglycaemic symptoms without loss of consciousness or neurological findings should be treated aggressively with oral glucose and adjustments in drug dosage and/or meal patterns. Close monitoring should continue until the physician is assured that the patient is out of danger. Severe hypoglycaemic reactions with coma, seizure, or other neurological impairment occur infrequently, but constitute medical emergencies requiring immediate hospitalisation. If hypoglycaemic coma is diagnosed or suspected, the patient should be given a rapid intravenous injection of concentrated (50%) glucose solution. This should be followed by a continuous infusion of a more dilute (10%) glucose solution at a rate that will maintain the blood glucose at a level above 5.6 mmol/l (100 mg/dl). Patients should be closely monitored for a minimum of 24 to 48 hours since hypoglycaemia may recur after apparent clinical recovery.

Pharmaceutical precautions Store below 25°C.

Legal category POM.

Package quantities Diabinese 100 mg and 250 mg tablets are packed in original packs of 28 tablets (in blister strips of 2 × 14 tablets).

Further information Diabinese does not interfere with the usual tests to detect albumin in the urine.

Product licence numbers
100 mg Tablets 0057/5015R
250 mg Tablets 0057/5016R

DIFLUCAN*

Presentation Diflucan 50 mg capsules are light turquoise blue and white, coded 'FLU 50' and 'PFIZER', containing 50 mg fluconazole.

Diflucan 150 mg capsules are light turquoise blue, coded 'FLU 150' and 'PFIZER', containing 150 mg fluconazole.

Diflucan 200 mg capsules are purple and white, coded 'FLU 200' and 'PFIZER', containing 200 mg fluconazole.

Diflucan Intravenous Infusion contains fluconazole 2 mg/ml in a 0.9% sodium chloride solution.

Inactive excipients: All the capsule strengths include lactose and titanium dioxide, in addition the 50 mg and 150 mg capsules contain patent blue V, and the 200 mg capsule contains erythrosine and indigotine.

Diflucan preparations are free of other sugars, gluten and azo dyes.

Uses Fluconazole, a member of a new triazole class of antifungal agents, is a potent and selective inhibitor of fungal enzymes necessary for the synthesis of ergosterol.

Diflucan is indicated for:

1. Vaginal candidiasis, acute or recurrent.
2. Mucosal candidiasis. These include oropharyngeal, oesophageal, non-invasive bronchopulmonary infections, candiduria, mucocutaneous and chronic oral atrophic candidiasis (denture sore mouth). Normal hosts and patients with compromised immune function may be treated.
3. Systemic candidiasis including candidaemia, disseminated candidiasis and other forms of invasive candidal infection. These include infections of the peritoneum, endocardium and pulmonary and urinary tracts. Candidal infections in patients with malignancy, in intensive care units or those receiving cytotoxic or immunosuppressive therapy, may be treated.
4. Cryptococcosis, including cryptococcal meningitis and infections of other sites (e.g. pulmonary, cutaneous). Normal hosts and patients with acquired immune deficiency syndrome (AIDS), organ transplants or other causes of immunosuppression may be treated. Diflucan can be used as maintenance therapy to prevent relapse of cryptococcal disease in patients with AIDS.

Dosage and administration Diflucan may be administered either orally, or by intravenous infusion at a rate of approximately 5–10 ml/min, the route being dependent on the clinical state of the patient. On transferring from the intravenous to the oral route or vice versa, there is no need to change the daily dose. Diflucan intravenous infusion is formulated in 0.9% sodium chloride solution, each 200 mg (100 ml bottle) containing 15 mmol each of Na^+ and Cl^-.

Adults:

1. *Vaginal candidiasis:* 150 mg single oral dose.
2. *Mucosal candidiasis:* Oropharyngeal candidiasis: the recommended dose is 50 mg once daily for 7 to 14 days. Treatment should not normally exceed 14 days except in severely immunocompromised patients.

Atrophic oral candidiasis associated with dentures: the recommended dose is 50 mg once daily for 14 days administered concurrently with local antiseptic measures to the denture.

For other candidal infections of the mucosa, (except vaginal candidiasis see above), e.g. oesophagitis, non-invasive bronchopulmonary infections, candiduria, mucocutaneous candidiasis etc.: the recommended dose is 50 mg daily, given for 14 to 30 days.

In unusually difficult cases of mucosal candidal infections the dose may be increased to 100 mg daily.

3. *For candidaemia, disseminated candidiasis and other invasive candidal infections:* the recommended dose is 400 mg on the first day followed by 200 mg once daily. Depending on the clinical response the dose may be increased to 400 mg once daily. Duration of treatment is based upon the clinical response.

4a. *For cryptococcal meningitis and cryptococcal infections at other sites:* the recommended dose is 400 mg on the first day followed by 200 mg–400 mg once daily. Duration of treatment for cryptococcal infections will depend on the clinical and mycological response, but is usually at least 6 to 8 weeks for cryptococcal meningitis.

4b. *For the prevention of relapse of cryptococcal meningitis in patients with AIDS:* after the patient receives a full course of primary therapy, Diflucan may be administered indefinitely at a daily dose of at least 100 mg.

Use in children: Limited data are available on the use of Diflucan in children below the age of 16 years; therefore use at present is not recommended in these patients unless antifungal treatment is imperative and no suitable alternative exists.

For children aged > 1 year with normal renal function the suggested daily dose is 1 to 2 mg/kg for superficial candidal infections, and 3 to 6 mg/kg for systemic candidal/cryptococcal infections.

For children with impaired renal function the daily dose should be reduced in accordance with the guidelines given for adults.

There are no available data on the use of Diflucan in infants and its use in children below the age of 1 year is therefore not recommended.

Use in the elderly: The normal dose should be used if there is no evidence of renal impairment. In patients with renal impairment (creatinine clearance less than 40 ml/min) the dosage schedule should be adjusted as described below.

Use in renal impairment: Fluconazole is excreted predominantly in the urine as unchanged drug. No adjustments in single dose therapy are required. In multiple dose therapy of patients with renal impairment, normal doses should be given on days 1 and 2 of treatment and thereafter the dosage intervals or daily dose should be modified in accordance with creatinine clearance as follows:

Creatinine clearance (ml/min)	*Dosage interval/daily dose*
>40	24 hours (normal dosage regimen)
21–40	48 hours *or* half normal daily dose
10–20	72 hours *or* one-third normal daily dose
Patients receiving regular haemodialysis	One dose after every dialysis session

Compatibility of intravenous infusion: Although further dilution is unnecessary Diflucan intravenous infusion is compatible with the following administration fluids:
Dextrose 20%
Ringer's solution
Hartmann's solution
Potassium chloride in dextrose
Sodium bicarbonate 4.2%
Normal saline (0.9%)

Diflucan may be infused through an existing line with one of the above listed fluids. No specific incompatibilities have been noted, although mixing with any other drug prior to infusion is not recommended.

Contra-indications, warnings, etc Contra-indications: Diflucan should not be used in patients with known hypersensitivity to fluconazole or to related triazole compounds.

Use in pregnancy: Adverse foetal effects have been seen in animals only at dose levels associated with maternal toxicity. These levels are many times in excess of those recommended for therapeutic use. There has been little use during human pregnancy. Accordingly, Diflucan should not be used in pregnancy or in women of child-bearing potential unless adequate contraception is employed.

Warnings: In some patients, particularly those with serious underlying diseases such as AIDS and cancer, abnormalities of hepatic, renal, haematological and other biochemical function tests have been observed during treatment with Diflucan but the clinical significance and relationship to treatment is uncertain.

Very rarely patients, who died with severe underlying disease and who had received multiple dose Diflucan, had post-mortem findings which included hepatic necrosis. These patients were receiving multiple concomitant medications, some known to be potentially hepatotoxic, and/or had underlying diseases which could have caused the hepatic necrosis. Consequently, because a causal relationship with Diflucan cannot be excluded, the risk-benefit ratio of continued Diflucan treatment should be asssessed in those patients in whom a significant rise of liver enzymes occurs.

Patients with AIDS are more prone to the development of severe cutaneous reactions to many drugs. A small number of AIDS patients have developed such reactions usually while receiving Diflucan concomitantly with other agents known to be associated with severe exfoliation. If a rash develops in a patient treated for oral candidiasis which is considered attributable to Diflucan, further therapy with this agent should be discontinued. In patients with invasive/systemic fungal infections who develop rashes, they should be monitored closely and Diflucan discontinued if bullous lesions or erythema multiforme develop.

Use during lactation: No data on fluconazole levels in breast milk are available and the use of Diflucan in nursing mothers is not recommended.

Use in children: As stated in the Dosage section the use in children below the age of 16 years is not recommended unless the treating physician considers Diflucan therapy imperative.

There are no available data on the use of Diflucan in infants and its use in children below the age of 1 year is therefore not recommended.

Driving/use of machinery: Experience with Diflucan indicates that therapy is unlikely to impair a patient's ability to drive or use machinery.

Drug interactions: In an interaction study, Diflucan increased the prothombin time after warfarin administration in healthy males. Though the magnitude of change was small (12%), careful monitoring of prothrombin time in patients receiving coumarin-type anticoagulants is recommended.

Diflucan has been shown to prolong the serum half-life of concomitantly administered oral sulphonylureas (chlorpropamide, glibenclamide, glipizide and tolbutamide) in healthy volunteers. Diflucan and oral sulphonylureas may be co-administered to diabetic patients, but the possibility of a hypoglycaemic episode should be borne in mind.

In a kinetic interaction study, co-administration of multiple-dose hydrochlorothiazide to healthy volunteers receiving Diflucan increased plasma concentrations of fluconazole by 40%. An effect of this magnitude should not necessitate a change in the Diflucan dose regimen in subjects receiving concomitant diuretics, although the prescriber should bear it in mind.

Concomitant administration of Diflucan and phenytoin may increase the levels of phenytoin to a clinically significant degree. If it is necessary to administer both drugs concomitantly, phenytoin levels should be monitored and the phenytoin dose adjusted to maintain therapeutic levels.

Concomitant administration of Diflucan and rifampicin has resulted in a 25% decrease in the AUC and 20% shorter half-life of fluconazole. In patients receiving concomitant rifampicin, an increase in the Diflucan dose should be considered.

Kinetic interaction studies with multiple-dose Diflucan have shown the following: 50 mg daily does not affect endogenous steroid levels or the kinetics of the oral contraceptive in females; 100 mg daily does not affect cyclosporin levels in patients with bone marrow transplants; 200–400 mg daily has no clinically significant effect on endogenous steroid levels or on ACTH stimulated response in healthy male volunteers. These conclusions are also applicable to a 150 mg single dose.

Interaction studies have shown that when oral Diflucan is co-administered with food, cimetidine, antacids or following total body irradiation for bone marrow transplantation, no clinically significant impairment of fluconazole absorption occurs.

Side-effects: Diflucan is generally well tolerated. The commonest side-effects associated with Diflucan are symptoms associated with the gastro-intestinal tract; these include nausea, abdominal discomfort, diarrhoea and flatulence. Other adverse events such as rash are rarely encountered (incidences less than 1%).

Overdosage: In the event of overdosage, supportive measures and symptomatic treatment, with gastric lavage if necessary, may be adequate.

As fluconazole is excreted largely in the urine, forced volume diuresis would probably increase the elimination rate. A three hour session of haemodialysis decreases plasma levels by approximately 50%.

Pharmaceutical precautions Store below 30°C.

Intravenous infusion: Do not freeze. The infusion does not contain any preservatives. It is for single use only. Discard any remaining solution.

Legal category POM.

Package quantities Single dose therapy (vaginal candidiasis): Blister pack containing 1 × 150 mg Diflucan capsule.
Multiple dose therapy: Calendar blister packs containing 7 × 50 mg or 7 × 200 mg Diflucan capsules.
Diflucan Intravenous Infusion 2 mg/ml: Bottle of 25 ml (50 mg); Bottle of 100 ml (200 mg).

Further information Nil.

Product licence numbers

Diflucan Capsules 50 mg	0057/0289
Diflucan Capsules 150 mg	0057/0290
Diflucan Capsules 200 mg	0057/0317
Diflucan Intravenous Infusion 2 mg/ml	0057/0315

FASIGYN*

Presentation Fasigyn (tinidazole) is available as 500 mg film coated white tablets.

Inactive excipients: These include titanium dioxide. The product is free of gluten, lactose and other sugars.

Uses *Actions:* Fasigyn is rapidly and completely absorbed after oral therapy. Peak serum levels usually occur within two hours after administration and decline slowly, with an elimination half-life of 12 to 14 hours.

In healthy volunteers, peak plasma concentrations at 2 hours after a single oral 2 g dose vary between 40–51 micrograms/ml. At 24 hours the values are between 11–19 micrograms/ml. Detectable levels of approximately 1 microgram/ml are still observed up to 72 hours.

Studies with labelled Fasigyn in humans show that Fasigyn is excreted mainly in the urine and to a lesser extent in faeces in a proportion of 5 to 1 measured as radioactivity excreted after 5 days. The urinary recovery of unchanged Fasigyn is around 25% of administered drug while metabolites account for approximately 12%.

In patients with moderate to severe renal impairment the pharmacokinetic characteristics are not markedly changed in comparison with those in normal volunteers. Thus modification of the dosage in patients with impaired renal function is not necessary.

The plasma protein binding is approximately 12%.

Following dosing with Fasigyn the compound is well distributed into body tissues in clinically effective concentrations and effectively passes the blood brain barrier.

Fasigyn is active against both protozoa and obligate anaerobic bacteria. The activity against protozoa involves *Trichomonas vaginalis*, *Entamoeba histolytica* and *Giardia lamblia*.

The mode of action of Fasigyn against anaerobic bacteria and protozoa involves penetration of the drug into the cell of the micro-organism and subsequent damage of DNA strands or inhibition of their synthesis.

Fasigyn is active against *Gardnerella vaginalis* and most anaerobic bacteria including *Bacteroides fragilis*, *Bacteroides melaninogenicus*, *Bacteroides* spp., *Clostridium* spp., *Eubacterium* spp., *Fusobacterium* spp., *Peptococcus* spp., *Peptostreptococcus* spp., and *Veillonella* spp.

Indications: 1. *Prophylaxis:* The prevention of post-operative infections caused by anaerobic bacteria, especially those associated with colonic, gastro-intestinal and gynaecological surgery.

2. *Treatment of anaerobic infections such as:*

Intraperitoneal infections: peritonitis, abscess.

Gynaecological infections: endometritis, endomyometritis, tubo-ovarian abscess.

Bacterial septicaemia.

Post-operative wound infections.

Skin and soft tissue infections.

Upper and lower respiratory tract infections: pneumonia, empyema, lung abscess.

3. Non-specific vaginitis.
4. Acute ulcerative gingivitis.
5. Urogenital trichomoniasis in both male and female patients.
6. Giardiasis.
7. Intestinal amoebiasis.
8. Amoebic involvement of the liver.

Dosage and administration

1. *Prevention of post-operative infections: Adults: Oral:* A single oral dose of 2 g approximately 12 hours before surgery.

Children less than 12 years: Data are not available to allow dosage recommendations for children below the age of 12 years in the prophylaxis of post-operative infections.

2. *Treatment of anaerobic infections: Adults: Oral:* An initial dose of 2 g the first day followed by 1 g daily given as a single dose or as 500 mg twice daily.

Treatment for 5 to 6 days will generally be adequate but clinical judgement must determine the duration of therapy, particularly when eradication of infection from certain sites may be difficult.

Regular clinical and laboratory observation is advised if it is considered necessary to continue therapy for more than 7 days.

Children less than 12 years: Data are not available to allow dosage recommendations for children below the age of 12 years in the treatment of anaerobic infections.

3. *Non-specific vaginitis: Adults:* Non-specific vaginitis is treated with a single oral dose of 2 g. Higher cure rates have been achieved with 2 g single daily doses on two consecutive days (total dosage 4 g).

4. *Acute ulcerative gingivitis: Adults:* A single oral dose of 2 g.

5. *Urogenital trichomoniasis:* When infection with *Trichomonas vaginalis* is confirmed, simultaneous treatment of the consort is recommended.

Adult preferred regimen: A single oral dose of 2 g.

Children: A single oral dose of 50 to 75 mg/kg of body weight.

In adults and children, it may be necessary to repeat this dose once in some cases.

6. *Giardiasis: Adults:* A single oral dose of 2 g.

Children: A single oral dose of 50 to 75 mg/kg of body weight.

In adults and children, it may be necessary to repeat this dose once in some cases.

7. *Intestinal amoebiasis: Adults:* A single oral daily dose of 2 g for two or three days.

Children: A single oral daily dose of 50 to 60 mg/kg of body weight on each of three successive days.

8. *Amoebic involvement of the liver: Adults:* Total dosage varies from 4.5 to 12g, depending on the virulence of the *Entamoeba histolytica*.

Treatment should be initiated with 1.5 to 2 g as a single oral daily dose for 3 days. In the occasional instance where a three-day course is ineffective, treatment may be continued for up to a total of five days.

Children: A single oral daily dose of 50 to 60 mg/kg of body weight on each of five successive days.

In amoebic involvement of the liver, the aspiration of pus may be required in addition to therapy with Fasigyn.

Oral administration: It is recommended that oral Fasigyn be taken during or after a meal.

Use in the elderly: There are no special recommendations for this age group.

Contra-indications, warnings, etc

Contra-indications: As with other drugs of similar structure, Fasigyn is contra-indicated in patients having, or with a history of blood dyscrasia although no persistent haematological abnormalities have been noted in clinical or animal studies.

Fasigyn should be avoided in patients with organic neurological disorders.

Fasigyn should not be administered to patients with known hypersensitivity to the drug.

Use in pregnancy: Fasigyn crosses the placental barrier and is present in the breast milk when administered to nursing mothers. Since the effects of compounds of this class on foetal development and in the newborn are not definitely known, Fasigyn is contra-indicated during the first trimester of pregnancy and in nursing mothers during the neo-natal period. While there is no evidence that Fasigyn is harmful during the later stages of pregnancy, its use during the last two trimesters of pregnancy requires that the potential benefits be weighed against possible hazards to mother and foetus.

Precautions: Fasigyn and related compounds when

taken together with alcoholic beverages have caused abdominal cramps, flushing, and vomiting.

Drugs of similar chemical structure have also produced various neurological disturbances such as dizziness, vertigo, inco-ordination, and ataxia. If, during therapy with Fasigyn, abnormal neurological signs develop, therapy should be discontinued.

Side-effects: Reported side-effects have generally been infrequent, mild and self-limiting.

Gastro-intestinal side-effects include nausea, vomiting, anorexia, diarrhoea and metallic taste.

Hypersensitivity reactions, occasionally severe, may occur in rare cases in the form of skin rash, pruritus, urticaria and angioneurotic oedema.

As with related compounds, Fasigyn may produce transient leucopenia. Other rarely reported side-effects are headache, tiredness, furry tongue and dark urine.

Overdosage: There is no specific treatment for gross overdosage of Fasigyn, but early gastric lavage is recommended following overdosage by mouth.

Pharmaceutical precautions Tablets – Store below 25°C in a dry place, away from light.

Legal category POM.

Package quantities 20 × 500 mg tablets.

Further information Nil.

Product licence number
500 mg tablet 0057/0150.

FELDENE* CAPSULES
FELDENE* 20 CAPSULES
FELDENE* DISPERSIBLE TABLETS
FELDENE* SUPPOSITORIES

Presentation Feldene capsules are maroon and blue capsules, coded 'Pfizer' and 'FEL 10' containing 10 mg piroxicam. Feldene 20 capsules are maroon capsules coded 'Pfizer' and 'FEL 20' containing 20 mg piroxicam.

Feldene dispersible tablets are available in two strengths: 10 mg – white to off-white flat round tablets coded 'FEL' and '10' on one side, with an incised line between, and 'Pfizer' on the other. 20 mg – white to off-white capsular tablets coded 'FEL 20' on one side and lettered 'PFIZER' on the other.

Feldene suppositories (white to off-white) containing 20 mg piroxicam.

Inactive excipients: Feldene capsules and tablets contain lactose. Feldene capsules also contain erythrosine, indigotin and titanium dioxide. Feldene preparations are free of other sugars, gluten and azo dyes.

Uses Feldene is a non-steroidal anti-inflammatory drug indicated for a variety of conditions requiring anti-inflammatory and/or analgesic activity, such as rheumatoid arthritis, oesteoarthritis (arthrosis, degenerative joint disease) ankylosing spondylitis, acute musculoskeletal disorders and acute gout. Children with definitely diagnosed juvenile chronic arthritis (Still's disease).

Dosage and administration
Rheumatoid arthritis, osteoarthritis, ankylosing spondylitis: The recommended starting dose is 20 mg given as a single daily dose. The majority of patients will be maintained on 20 mg daily. A relatively small group of patients may be maintained on 10 mg daily. Some patients may require up to 30 mg daily given in single or divided doses. Long-term administration of doses 30 mg or higher carries an increased risk of gastro-intestinal side-effects.

Acute gout: Therapy should be initiated by a single dose of 40 mg, followed on the next four to six days with 40 mg daily, given in single or divided dosage. Feldene is not indicated for the long-term management of gout.

Acute musculoskeletal disorders: Therapy should be initiated with 40 mg daily for the first two days, given in single or divided doses. For the remainder of the seven to fourteen day treatment period, the dose should be reduced to 20 mg daily.

Juvenile chronic arthritis (Still's disease): As little data are available in very young children, it is recommended that only children aged 6 years and older are treated with Feldene dispersible tablets according to the following dosage schedule:

Body weight (kg)	*Once-daily dose*
less than 15	5 mg
16–25	10 mg
26–45	15 mg
46 and above	20 mg

Dosage recommendations and indications for use in children other than in juvenile chronic arthritis have not been established.

Feldene dispersible tablets: These can be swallowed whole with a fluid, or may be dispersed in a minimum of 50 ml of water and then swallowed.

Rectal: For each indication (not for use in juvenile chronic arthritis), the dosage of Feldene suppositories when used alone, is identical with the dosage of Feldene capsules or dispersible tablets.

Combined administration: The total daily dosage of Feldene administered as capsules, dispersible tablets and suppositories should not exceed the maximal recommended daily dosage as indicated above.

Use in the elderly: Elderly, frail or debilitated patients may tolerate side-effects less well and such patients should be carefully supervised.

As with other non-steroidal anti-inflammatory drugs, caution should be used in the treatment of elderly patients who are more likely to be suffering from impaired renal, hepatic or cardiac function.

Contra-indications, warnings, etc
Contra-indications:

1. Active peptic ulceration or a history of recurrent ulceration.
2. Feldene should not be used in those patients who have previously shown a hypersensitivity to the drug. The potential exists for cross sensitivity to aspirin and other non-steroidal anti-inflammatory drugs. Feldene should not be given to patients in whom aspirin and other non-steroidal anti-inflammatory drugs induce the symptoms of asthma, nasal polyps, angioedema or urticaria.
3. Feldene suppositories should not be used in patients with any inflammatory lesions of the rectum or anus, or in patients with a recent history of rectal or anal bleeding.

Warnings
Use in pregnancy: Although no teratogenic effects were seen in animal testing, the safety of Feldene during pregnancy or during lactation has not yet been established. Feldene inhibits prostaglandin synthesis and release through a reversible inhibition of the cyclo-oxygenase enzyme. This effect, as with other non-steroidal anti-inflammatory drugs has been associated with an increased incidence of dystocia and delayed parturition in pregnant animals when drug administration was continued into late pregnancy. Non-steroidal anti-inflammatory drugs are also known to induce closure of the ductus arteriosus in infants.

Nursing mothers: A study indicates that piroxicam appears in breast milk at about 1% to 3% of the maternal plasma concentrations. No accumulation of piroxicam occurred in milk relative to that in plasma during treatment for up to 52 days. Feldene is not recommended for use in nursing mothers as clinical safety in neonates has not been established.

Precautions: Drug administration should be closely supervised in patients with a history of upper gastro-intestinal disease. Feldene should be withdrawn if peptic ulceration or gastro-intestinal bleeding occurs.

In rare cases, non-steroidal anti-inflammatory drugs may cause interstitial nephritis, glomerulonephritis, papillary necrosis and the nephrotic syndrome. Such agents inhibit the synthesis of renal prostaglandin which plays a supportive role in the maintenance of renal perfusion in patients whose renal blood flow and blood volume are decreased. In these patients, administration of a non-steroidal anti-inflammatory drug may precipitate overt renal decompensation which is typically followed by recovery to pretreatment state upon discontinuation of non-steroidal anti-inflammatory therapy. Patients at greatest risk of such a reaction are those with congestive heart failure, liver cirrhosis, nephrotic syndrome and overt renal disease. Such patients should be carefully monitored whilst receiving non-steroidal anti-inflammatory drug therapy.

Because of reports of adverse eye findings with non-steroidal anti-inflammatory drugs, it is recommended that patients who develop visual complaints during treatment with Feldene have ophthalmic evaluation.

Drug interactions: Non-steroidal anti-inflammatory drugs may cause sodium, potassium and fluid retention, and may interfere with the natriuretic action of diuretic agents. These properties should be kept in mind when treating patients with compromised cardiac function or hypertension since they may be responsible for a worsening of those conditions.

As with other non steroidal anti-inflammatory drugs, bleeding has been reported rarely when Feldene has been administered to patients on coumarin-type anticoagulants. Patients should be monitored closely if Feldene and oral anticoagulants are administered together.

Feldene, like other non-steroidal anti-inflammatory drugs, decreases platelet aggregation and prolongs bleeding time. This effect should be kept in mind when bleeding times are determined.

As with other non-steroidal anti-inflammatory drugs, the use of Feldene in conjunction with aspirin or the concomitant use of two non-steroidal anti-inflammatory drugs is not recommended because data are inadequate to demonstrate that the combination produces greater improvement than that achieved with the drug alone and the potential for adverse reactions is increased.

Studies in man have shown that the concomitant administration of Feldene and aspirin resulted in a reduction of plasma levels of piroxicam to about 80% of the normal values. Concomitant administration of antacids had no effect on piroxicam plasma levels. Neither did concurrent therapy with Feldene and digoxin, or Feldene and digitoxin, affect the plasma levels of either drug.

Feldene is highly protein-bound, and therefore might be expected to displace other protein-bound drugs. The physician should closely monitor patients for change in dosage requirements when administering Feldene to patients on highly protein-bound drugs. Non-steroidal anti-inflammatory drugs, including Feldene, have been reported to increase steady state plasma lithium levels. It is recommended that these levels are monitored when initiating, adjusting and discontinuing Feldene.

Results of two separate studies indicate a slight but significant increase in absorption of piroxicam following cimetidine administration but no significant changes in elimination rate constants or half-life. The small increase in absorption is unlikely to be clinically significant.

Side-effects: Gastro-intestinal: These are the most commonly encountered side-effects but in most instances do not interfere with the course of therapy. They include stomatitis, anorexia, epigastric distress, nausea, constipation, abdominal discomfort, flatulence, diarrhoea, abdominal pain and indigestion. Objective evaluations of gastric mucosal appearances and intestinal blood loss show that 20 mg/day of Feldene administered either in single or divided daily doses is significantly less irritating to the gastro-intestinal tract than aspirin. Peptic ulceration, perforation and gastro-intestinal bleeding, in rare cases fatal, have been reported with Feldene.

Long-term administration of doses of 30 mg or higher carries an increased risk of gastro-intestinal side-effects.

Ano-rectal reactions to suppositories have presented as local pain, burning, pruritus and tenesmus. Rare instances of rectal bleeding have occurred.

Oedema: As with other non-steroidal anti-inflammatory drugs, oedema, mainly of the ankle, has been reported in a small percentage of patients and the possibility of precipitating congestive cardiac failure in elderly patients or those with compromised cardiac function should therefore be borne in mind.

CNS: Dizziness, headache, somnolence, insomnia, depression, nervousness, hallucinations, mood alterations, dream abnormalities, mental confusion, paraesthesias and vertigo have been reported rarely.

Dermal hypersensitivity: Rash and pruritus. Onycholysis and alopecia have rarely been reported. Photosensitivity reactions occur infrequently. As with other non-steroidal anti-inflammatory drugs, toxic epidermal necrolysis (Lyell's disease) and Stevens-Johnson syndrome may develop in rare cases. Vesiculo bullous reactions have been reported rarely.

Hypersensitivity reactions: Hypersensitivity reactions such as anaphylaxis, bronchospasm, urticaria/angiodema, vasculitis and serum sickness have been reported rarely.

Renal function: Reversible elevations of BUN and creatinine have been reported (see Precautions).

Haematological: Decreases in haemoglobin and haematocrit, unassociated with obvious gastro-intestinal bleeding, have occurred. Anaemia. Thrombocytopenia and non-thrombocytopenic purpura (Henoch-Schoenlein), leucopenia and eosinophilia. Rare cases of aplastic anaemia and haemolytic anaemia. Epistaxis has rarely been reported.

Liver function: Changes in various liver function parameters have been observed. As with most other non-steroidal anti-inflammatory drugs, some patients may develop increased serum transaminase levels during treatment with Feldene. Severe hepatic reactions, including jaundice and cases of fatal hepatitis have been reported. Although such reactions are rare, if abnormal liver function tests persist or worsen, if clinical signs and symptoms consistent with liver disease develop, or if systemic manifestations occur (e.g. eosinophilia, rash), Feldene should be discontinued.

Other: The following have been reported rarely: Palpitations and dyspnoea, anecdotal cases of positive ANA, anecdotal cases of hearing impairment, metabolic abnormalities such as hypoglycaemia, hyperglycaemia, weight increase or decrease.

Swollen eyes, blurred vision, and eye irritations have been reported. Routine ophthalmoscopy and slit-lamp examination have revealed no evidence of ocular changes. Malaise and tinnitus may occur.

Overdosage: In the event of overdosage with Feldene, supportive and symptomatic therapy is indicated. Studies indicate that administration of activated charcoal may result in reduced absorption and re-absorption of piroxicam thus reducing the total amount of active drug available.

Pharmaceutical precautions
Capsules and Dispersible Tablets: Store below 30°C.
Suppositories: Store below 25°C. Do not refrigerate.

Legal category POM.

Package quantities
Feldene Capsules 10 mg: Original packs of 56.
Feldene 20 Capsules 20 mg: Original packs of 28.
Feldene Dispersible Tablets 10 mg: Original packs of 56.
Feldene Dispersible Tablets 20 mg: Original packs of 28.
Feldene Suppositories 20 mg: Original packs of 10.

Further information Feldene pharmacokinetics are similar following oral or rectal administration. Following oral administration with food there is a slight delay in the rate but not the extent of absorption. The plasma half-life is approximately 50 hours in man and stable plasma concentrations are maintained throughout the day on once-daily dosage. Continuous treatment with 20 mg/day for periods of one year produces similar blood levels to those seen once steady state is first achieved.

Feldene is extensively metabolised and less than 5% of the daily dose is excreted unchanged in urine and faeces. One important metabolic pathway is hydroxylation of the pyridyl ring of the piroxicam side chain, followed by conjugation with glucuronic acid and urinary elimination.

Product licence numbers

Feldene Capsules 10 mg	0057/0145
Feldene 20 Capsules 20 mg	0057/0146
Feldene Dispersible Tablets 10 mg	0057/0240
Feldene Dispersible Tablets 20 mg	0057/0242
Feldene Suppositories 20 mg	0057/0219

FELDENE* GEL
FELDENE* SPORTS GEL

Presentation Topical Feldene is available as a clear pale yellow gel containing 5 mg piroxicam in each gram. Topical Feldene is available in two tube sizes: 30 g Feldene Sports Gel and 60 g Feldene Gel.

Inactive excipients: These are benzyl alcohol, propylene glycol, ethanol, carbopol 940, di-isopropanolamine, hydroxyethyl cellulose and water.

Uses Feldene Gel and Feldene Sports Gel contain piroxicam, a non-steroidal anti-inflammatory agent indicated for a variety of conditions characterised by pain and inflammation, or stiffness.

Feldene Gel is effective in the treatment of osteoarthritis of superficial joints such as the knee, acute musculoskeletal injuries, periarthritis, epicondylitis, tendinitis, and tenosynovitis.

Feldene Sports Gel is in a 30 g tube which is specifically designed for the short-term treatment of acute musculoskeletal injuries, providing treatment for approximately 7–10 days.

Feldene Gel and Feldene Sports Gel are for topical use only.

Dosage and administration Feldene Gel and Feldene Sports Gel are for external use only. No occlusive dressings should be employed. Apply 1 g of the Gel, corresponding to 3 cms, (approximately $1\frac{1}{4}$ inches) and rub into the affected site three to four times daily leaving no residual material on the skin. Therapy should be reviewed after four weeks.

Use in children: Dosage recommendations and indications for the use of Feldene Gel and Feldene Sports Gel in children have not been established.

Use in the elderly: No special precautions are required.

Contra-indications, warnings, etc

Contra-indications: Feldene Gel and Feldene Sports Gel should not be used in those patients who have previously shown a hypersensitivity to the Gel or piroxicam in any of its forms. The potential exists for cross sensitivity to aspirin and other non-steroidal anti-inflammatory agents.

Feldene Gel and Feldene Sports Gel should not be given to patients in whom aspirin and other non-steroidal anti-inflammatory agents induce the symptoms of asthma, nasal polyps, angioedema or urticaria.

Precautions: If local irritation develops, the use of the Gel should be discontinued and appropriate therapy instituted as necessary.

Keep away from the eyes and mucosal surfaces. Do not apply to any sites affected by open skin lesions, dermatoses or infection.

Use in Pregnancy: Although no teratogenic effects were seen when Feldene was orally administered in animal testing, the safety of the Gel during pregnancy or during lactation has not yet been established. Feldene inhibits prostaglandin synthesis and release through a reversible inhibition of the cyclo-oxygenase enzyme. This effect, as with other non-steroidal anti-inflammatory agents, has been associated with an increased incidence of dystocia and delayed parturition in pregnant animals when drug administration was continued into late pregnancy. Non-steroidal anti-inflammatory agents are also known to induce closure of the ductus arteriosus in infants.

Nursing mothers: A study indicates that following oral administration piroxicam is found in breast milk at about 1% to 3% of the maternal plasma concentrations. No accumulation of piroxicam occurred in milk relative to that in plasma during treatment for up to 52 days. Feldene Gel and Feldene Sports Gel are not recommended for use in nursing mothers as clinical safety has not been established.

Side-effects: Mild or moderate local irritation, erythema, rash, pityroid desquamation, pruritus, and related local reactions at the application site have been reported. Mild but transient skin discolouration and staining of clothing have been noted when the Gel is not rubbed in completely.

The systemic side-effects associated with oral or rectal administration of Feldene are listed below. Some of these effects of a minor nature have been reported with the Gel.

Gastro-intestinal: These are the most commonly encountered side-effects but in most instances do not interfere with the course of therapy. They include stomatitis, anorexia, epigastric distress, nausea, constipation, abdominal discomfort, flatulence, diarrhoea, abdominal pain and indigestion. Objective evaluations of gastric mucosal appearances and intestinal blood loss show that 20 mg/day of Feldene administered either in single or divided daily doses is significantly less irritating to the gastro-intestinal tract than aspirin. Peptic ulceration, perforation and gastro-intestinal bleeding, in rare cases fatal, have been reported with Feldene.

Long-term administration of doses of 30 mg per day or higher carries an increased risk of gastro-intestinal side-effects.

Oedema: As with other non-steroidal anti-inflammatory drugs, oedema, mainly of the ankle, has been reported in a small percentage of patients and the possibility of precipitating congestive cardiac failure in elderly patients or those with compromised cardiac function should therefore be borne in mind.

CNS: Dizziness, headache, somnolence, insomnia, depression, nervousness, hallucinations, mood alteration, dream abnormalities, mental confusion, paraesthesia and vertigo have been reported rarely.

Dermal hypersensitivity: Rash and pruritus. Onycholysis and alopecia have rarely been reported. Photosensitivity reactions occur infrequently. As with other non-steroidal anti-inflammatory drugs, toxic epidermal necrolysis (Lyell's disease), and Stevens-Johnson syndrome may develop in rare cases. Vesiculo-bullous reactions have been reported rarely.

Hypersensitivity reactions: Hypersensitivity reactions such as anaphylaxis, bronchospasm, urticaria/angiodema, vasculitis and serum sickness have been reported rarely.

Renal function: Reversible elevations of BUN and creatinine have been reported.

Haematological: Decreases in haemoglobin and haematocrit, unassociated with obvious gastro-intestinal bleeding, have occured. Anaemia. Thrombocytopenia and non-thrombocytopenic purpura (Henoch-Schoenlein), leucopenia and eosinophilia. Rare cases of aplastic anaemia and haemolytic anaemia. Epistaxis has rarely been reported.

Liver function: Changes in various liver function parameters have been observed. As with most other non-steroidal anti-inflammatory drugs, some patients may develop increased serum transaminase levels during treatment with Feldene. Severe hepatic reactions, including jaundice and cases of fatal hepatitis have been reported. Although such reactions are rare, if abnormal liver function tests persist or worsen, if clinical signs and symptoms consistent with liver disease develop, or if systemic manifestations occur (e.g. eosinophilia, rash) Feldene should be discontinued.

Other: The following have been reported rarely, palpitations and dyspnoea, anecdotal cases of positive ANA, anecdotal cases of hearing impairment, metabolic abnormalities such as hypoglycaemia, hyperglycaemia, weight increase or decrease.

Swollen eyes, blurred vision, and eye irritations have

been reported. Routine ophthalmoscopy and slit-lamp examination have revealed no evidence of ocular changes. Malaise and tinnitus may occur.

Overdosage: Overdosage is unlikely to occur with this topical preparation.

Pharmaceutical precautions Store below 30°C.

Legal category POM.

Package quantities
Feldene Gel: 60 g tube.
Feldene Sports Gel: 30 g tube.

Further information On the basis of various pharmacokinetic and tissue distribution studies in animals, with the Gel, the highest concentrations of piroxicam were achieved in the tissues below the site of application with low concentrations being reached in the plasma. The Gel was continuously and gradually released from the skin to underlying tissues, equilibrium between skin, and muscle or synovial fluid appeared to be reached rapidly, within a few hours of application.

From a pharmacokinetic study in man, 2 g of the Gel was applied to the shoulders of normal volunteers twice daily (corresponding to 20 mg piroxicam/day) for 14 days, plasma levels of piroxicam rose slowly, reaching steady state after about 11 days. The plasma levels at this time were between 300–400 ng/ml, or one-twentieth of those observed in subjects receiving 20 mg orally.

The Gel was well tolerated in volunteers with a history of contact allergy.

Product licence number 0057/0284.

GLIBENESE*

Presentation Glibenese (glipizide) is available as white oblong tablets marked GBS/5 on the scored side and 'Pfizer' on the other. Each tablet contains 5 mg glipizide.

Inactive excipients: These include lactose. The product is free of gluten, sucrose and invert sugar.

Uses *Actions:* Glibenese is an orally active sulphonylurea which effectively reduces blood glucose to the normal range in properly selected patients with non-insulin-dependent diabetes mellitus (NIDDM). It eliminates or diminishes glycosuria and ameliorates symptoms such as polyuria, polydipsia and pruritus.

The primary mode of action of Glibenese in experimental animals is the stimulation of insulin secretion from the beta-cells of pancreatic islet tissue. In man, stimulation of insulin secretion by Glibenese in response to a meal is undoubtedly of major importance. Fasting insulin levels are not elevated even on long-term Glibenese administration, but the post-prandial insulin response continues to be enhanced after at least 6 months of treatment. The insulinotropic response to a meal occurs within 30 minutes after an oral dose of Glibenese in diabetic patients, but elevated insulin levels do not persist beyond the time of the meal challenge. There is also increasing evidence that extrapancreatic effects involving potentiation of insulin action form a significant component of the activity of Glibenese.

Blood sugar control persists for up to 24 hours after a single dose of Glibenese even though plasma levels have declined to a small fraction of peak levels by that time. Once-daily administration of doses up to 15 mg has been shown to be safe and effective maintenance therapy in selected patients.

Some patients fail to respond initially, or gradually lose their responsiveness to sulphonylurea drugs, including Glibenese. Alternatively, Glibenese, may be effective in some patients who have not responded or have ceased to respond to other sulphonylureas.

Gastrointestinal absorption of Glibenese in man is uniform, rapid and essentially complete. Peak plasma concentrations occur 1–3 hours after a single oral dose. The half-life of elimination ranges from 2–4 hours in normal subjects, whether given intravenously or orally. The metabolic and excretory patterns are similar with the two routes of administration, indicating that first-pass metabolism is not significant. Glibenese does not accumulate in plasma on repeated oral administration. Total absorption and disposition of an oral dose was unaffected by food in normal volunteers, but absorption was delayed by about 40 minutes. Thus, Glibenese was more effective when administered about 30 minutes before, rather than with a test meal in diabetic patients. Protein binding was studied in serum from volunteers who received either oral or intravenous Glibenese and found to be 98–99% one hour after either route of administration. The apparent volume of distribution of Glibenese after intravenous administration was 11 litres, indicative of localisation within the extracellular fluid compartment.

The metabolism of Glibenese is extensive and occurs mainly in the liver. The primary metabolites are inactive hydroxylation products and polar conjugates and are excreted mainly in the urine. Less than 10% unchanged Glibenese is found in the urine.

In a placebo-controlled, crossover study in normal volunteers, Glibenese showed no antidiuretic activity, and, in fact, led to a slight increase in free water clearance.

Indications: Glibenese is indicated as an adjunct to diet to lower the blood glucose in patients with non-insulin-dependent diabetes mellitus (type II, NIDDM), formerly known as maturity onset diabetes, whose hyperglycaemia cannot be controlled by diet alone.

In initiating treatment for non-insulin dependent diabetes, diet should be emphasised as the primary form of treatment. Caloric restriction and weight loss are essential in the obese diabetic patient. Proper dietary management alone may be effective in controlling the blood glucose and symptoms of hyperglycaemia. The importance of regular physical activity should also be stressed, cardiovascular risk factors should be identified and corrective measures taken where possible.

Use of Glibenese must be viewed by both the physician and patient as a treatment in addition to diet, and not as a substitute for diet or as a convenient mechanism for avoiding dietary restraint. Furthermore, loss of blood glucose control on diet alone also may be transient, thus requiring only short-term administration of Glibenese.

During maintenance programmes, Glibenese should be discontinued if satisfactory lowering of blood glucose is no longer achieved. Judgments should be based on regular clinical and laboratory evaluation.

In considering the use of Glibenese in asymptomatic patients, it should be recognised that controlling the blood glucose in non-insulin-dependent diabetes, has not been definitely established to be effective in preventing the long-term cardiovascular or neurological complications of diabetes.

Patient selection: The most likely patient for therapy is one in whom diabetes is of the NIDDM type, stable, and not controlled by dietary regulation alone. A past history of diabetic coma does not necessarily preclude successful therapeutic control with Glibenese. A trial period may be indicated in certain patients who might be expected to respond to this type of medication, but who failed in initial trials with, or after having been on other oral sulphonylurea agents, or in patients whose diabetic control on such agents has not been satisfactory. Glibenese may prove effective and provide improved control of the diabetes. The final evaluation of response in patients who qualify as candidates for Glibenese is a therapeutic trial for a period of at least seven days. During the trial period, the absence of ketonuria together with a satisfactory control, indicates that the patient is responsive and amenable to control with the drug. However, the development of ketonuria within 24 hours after withdrawal of insulin usually will be indicative of a poor response. The patient is considered unresponsive if he fails to achieve satisfactory lowering of blood sugar levels or fails to obtain objective or subjective clinical improvement and if he develops ketonuria or glycosuria. Insulin is indicated for the therapy of such patients.

Dosage and administration There is no fixed dosage

regimen for the management of diabetes mellitus with Glibenese or any other hypoglycaemic agent. In addition to the usual monitoring of urinary glucose, the patient's blood glucose must also be monitored periodically to determine the minimum effective dose for the patient, to detect primary failure: i.e. inadequate lowering of blood glucose at the maximum recommended dose of medication, and to detect secondary failure, i.e. loss of adequate blood-glucose-lowering response after an initial period of effectiveness. Glycosylated haemoglobin levels may also be of value in monitoring the patient's response to therapy.

Short term administration of Glibenese may be sufficient during periods of transient loss of control in patients usually controlled well on diet.

In general, Glibenese should be given approximately 30 minutes before a meal to achieve the greatest reduction in post-prandial hyperglycaemia.

Initial dose: The recommended starting dose is 5 mg, given before breakfast or the midday meal. Mild diabetics, elderly patients or those with liver disease may be started on 2.5 mg.

Titration: Dosage adjustments should ordinarily be in increments of 2.5 to 5 mg, as determined by blood glucose response. At least several days should elapse between titration steps. The maximum recommended single dose is 15 mg. Doses above 15 mg should ordinarily be divided.

Maintenance: Some patients may be effectively controlled on a once-a-day regimen. Total daily dosage above 15 mg should ordinarily be divided. Total daily dosage above 30 mg has been given safely on a twice daily basis to long term patients. Patients can usually be stabilised on a dosage ranging from 2.5 to 30 mg daily. The maximum recommended daily dosage is 40 mg.

Use in the elderly: Elderly diabetics are more sensitive to the hypoglycaemic effect of sulphonylurea drugs and should therefore be prescribed a low starting dose of 2.5 mg daily. The elderly are also particularly susceptible to the effects of hypoglycaemia. Hypoglycaemia may be difficult to recognise in the elderly.

In elderly, debilitated or malnourished patients, and patients with an impaired renal or hepatic function, the initial and maintenance dosing should be conservative to avoid hypoglycaemic reactions (see Precautions section).

Use in children: Safety and effectiveness in children have not been established.

Patients receiving insulin: As with other sulphonylurea class hypoglycaemics, many stable non-insulin-dependent diabetic patients receiving insulin may be safely placed on Glibenese. When transferring patients from insulin to Glibenese, the following general guidelines should be considered.

For patients whose daily insulin requirement is 20 units or less, insulin may be discontinued and Glibenese therapy begun at usual dosages. Several days should elapse between Glibenese titration steps.

For patients whose daily insulin requirement is greater than 20 units, the insulin dose should be reduced by 50% and Glibenese therapy initiated at usual dosages. Subsequent reductions in insulin dosage should depend on individual patient response. Several days should elapse between Glibenese steps.

During the insulin withdrawal period, the patient should test urine samples for sugar and ketone bodies at least three times daily. Patients should be instructed to contact the prescriber immediately if these tests are abnormal. In some cases, especially when the patient has been receiving greater than 40 units of insulin daily, it may be advisable to consider hospitalisation during the transition period.

Patients receiving other oral hypoglycaemic agents: As with other sulphonylurea class hypoglycaemics, no transition period is necessary when transferring patients to Glibenese. Patients should be observed carefully (1–2 weeks) for hypoglycaemia when being transferred from longer half-life sulphonylureas (e.g. chlorpropamide) to Glibenese due to potential overlapping of drug effect.

Concurrent biguanide therapy: As with other sulphonylureas, a proportion of patients who do not achieve optimal control with Glibenese alone, or who experience secondary failure, may be expected to have their control improved or restored by the addition of a biguanide.

For such patients, it is suggested that the dosage of Glibenese should be maintained and the biguanide chosen should be added using low doses initially and increasing the dosage of the biguanide progressively until adequate control is achieved or restored. Should gastrointestinal side-effects appear, an attempt should be made to reduce the dosage of the biguanide.

Contra-indications, warnings, etc

Contra-indications: Glibenese is contra-indicated in the following conditions:

1. Known hypersensitivity to Glibenese.
2. Diabetic ketoacidosis, with or without coma. This condition should be treated with insulin.
3. Insulin dependent (juvenile-onset) diabetes.
4. Severe renal, hepatic or thyroid impairment, coexistent renal and hepatic disease.

Warnings: The metabolism and excretion of Glibenese may be slowed in patients with impaired renal and/or hepatic function. If hypoglycaemia should occur in such patients, it may be prolonged.

Precautions

General: Hypoglycaemia: All sulphonylurea drugs are capable of producing severe hypoglycaemia. Proper patient selection, dosage, and instructions are important to avoid hypoglycaemic episodes. Renal or hepatic insufficiency may cause elevated blood levels of Glibenese and the latter may also diminish gluconeogenic capacity, both of which increase the risk of serious hypoglycaemic reactions. Elderly, debilitated or malnourished patients, and those with adrenal or pituitary insufficiency are particularly susceptible to the hypoglycaemic action of glucose-lowering drugs. Hypoglycaemia may be difficult to recognise in the elderly, and in people who are taking beta-adrenergic blocking drugs. Hypoglycaemia is more likely to occur when caloric intake is deficient, after severe or prolonged exercise, when alcohol is ingested, or when more than one glucose-lowering drug is used.

Loss of control of blood glucose: When a patient stabilised on any diabetic regimen is exposed to stress such as fever, trauma, infection, or surgery, a loss of control may occur. At such times, it may be necessary to discontinue Glibenese and administer insulin.

The effectiveness of any oral hypoglycaemic drug, including Glibenese, in lowering blood glucose to a desired level decreases in many patients over a period of time, which may be due to progression of the severity of the diabetes or to diminished responsiveness to the drug. This phenomenon is known as secondary failure, to distinguish it from primary failure in which the drug is ineffective in an individual patient when first given.

Information for patients: Patients should be informed of the potential risks and advantages of Glibenese and of alternative modes of therapy. They should also be informed about the importance of adherence to dietary instructions, of a regular exercise programme, and of regular testing of urine and/or blood glucose.

The risk of hypoglycaemia, its symptoms and treatment, and conditions that predispose to its development should be explained to patients and responsible family members. Primary and secondary failure should also be explained.

Laboratory tests: Blood and urine glucose should be monitored periodically. Measurement of glycosylated haemoglobin may be useful.

Driving/use of machinery: Clinical experience with Glibenese indicates that it is unlikely to impair a patient's ability to drive or use machinery.

Use in pregnancy: Glibenese is contra-indicated during pregnancy. Diabetes in pregnancy should be treated with insulin and not with sulphonylureas. Recent evidence suggests that hyperglycaemia in pregnancy is associated with a higher incidence of congenital abnormalities.

Nursing mothers: Although it is not known whether Glibenese is excreted in human milk, some sulphonylurea drugs are known to be excreted in human milk. Caution is therefore necessary if a sulphonylurea drug is prescribed because of the possibility of hypoglycaemia in the infant.

Use in renal insufficiency: Glibenese is not recommended in patients with renal insufficiency.

Drug interactions: The hypoglycaemic action of sulphonylureas may be potentiated by certain drugs including nonsteroidal anti-inflammatory agents and other drugs that are highly protein bound, salicylates, sulphonamides, chloramphenicol, probenecid, coumarins, monoamine oxidase inhibitors and beta-adrenergic blocking agents. When such drugs are administered to a patient receiving Glibenese, the patient should be observed closely for hypoglycaemia. When such drugs are withdrawn from a patient receiving Glibenese, the patient should be observed closely for loss of control.

Certain drugs tend to produce hyperglycaemia and may lead to loss of control. These drugs include the thiazides and other diuretics, corticosteroids, phenothiazines, thyroid products, oestrogens, oral contraceptives, phenytoin, nicotinic acid, sympathomimetics, calcium antagonists and isoniazid. When such drugs are administered to or withdrawn from a patient receiving Glibenese, the patient should be closely observed for loss of control.

In the mouse, Glibenese pre-treatment did not cause an accumulation of acetaldehyde after ethanol administration. Clinical experience has confirmed the virtual absence of an alcohol interaction in man.

Side-effects: The majority of side-effects have been dose related, transient, and have responded to dose reduction or withdrawal of the medication. However, clinical experience thus far has shown that, as with other sulphonylureas some side-effects associated with hypersensitivity may be severe and deaths have been reported in some instances.

Hypoglycaemia: See 'Precautions' and 'Overdosage' sections.

Gastrointestinal: Gastrointestinal complaints include nausea, diarrhoea, constipation and gastralgia. They appear to be dose related and usually disappear on division or reduction of dosage.

Dermatological: Allergic skin reactions including erythema, morbilliform or maculopapular reactions, urticaria, pruritis and eczema have been reported. They frequently disappear with continued therapy. However, if they persist, the drug should be discontinued.

Miscellaneous: Dizziness, drowsiness and headache have each been reported in patients treated with Glibenese. They are usually transient and seldom require discontinuance of therapy.

Laboratory tests: The pattern of laboratory test abnormalities observed with Glibenese is similar to that for other sulphonylureas. Occasional mild to moderate elevations of AST (SGOT), LDH, alkaline phosphatase, BUN and creatinine were noted. One case of jaundice was reported. The relationship of these abnormalities to Glibenese is uncertain, and they have rarely been associated with clinical symptoms.

Overdosage: There is no well documented experience with Glibenese overdosage. The acute oral toxicity was extremely low in all species tested (LD_{50} greater than 4g/kg).

Overdosage of sulphonylureas including Glibenese can produce hypoglycaemia. Mild hypoglycaemic symptoms without loss of consciousness or neurological findings should be treated aggressively with oral glucose and adjustments in drug dosage and/or meal patterns. Close monitoring should continue until the physician is assured that the patient is out of danger. Severe hypoglycaemic reactions with coma, seizure, or other neurological impairment occur infrequently, but constitute medical emergencies requiring immediate hospitalisation. If hypoglycaemic coma is diagnosed or suspected, the patient should be given a rapid intravenous injection of concentrated (50%) glucose solution. This should be followed by continuous infusion of a more dilute (10%) glucose solution at a rate that will maintain the blood glucose at a level above 5.6 mmol/l (100 mg/dl). Patients should be closely monitored for a minimum of 24 to 48 hours since hypoglycaemia may recur after apparent clinical recovery. Clearance of Glibenese from plasma would be prolonged in persons with liver disease. Because of the extensive protein binding of Glibenese, dialysis is unlikely to be of benefit.

Pharmaceutical precautions Store below 25°C.

Legal category POM.

Package quantities Glibenese tablets 5 mg: Original packs of 56 tablets (in blister strips of 4 × 14 tablets).

Further information Nil.

Product licence number 0057/0113R.

ISTIN* ▼

Presentation Istin is available in two strengths as white, round, normal convex tablets containing 5 mg and 10 mg amlodipine as the besylate salt:

5 mg tablets coded 'ITN5' on one side and 'PFIZER' on the other.

10 mg tablets coded 'ITN 10' on one side and 'PFIZER' on the other.

The product is free of gluten, lactose and other sugars.

Uses

Actions: Istin is a calcium antagonist (calcium blocker, calcium slow channel blocker) of the dihydropyridine group, and inhibits the transmembrane influx of calcium ions into cardiac and smooth muscle.

The mechanism of the antihypertensive action of Istin is due to a direct relaxant effect on vascular smooth muscle. The precise mechanism by which Istin relieves angina has not been fully determined but Istin reduces total ischaemic burden by the following two actions:

1. Istin dilates peripheral arterioles and thus reduces the total peripheral resistance (afterload) against which the heart works. Since there is no associated reflex tachycardia, this unloading of the heart reduces myocardial energy consumption and oxygen requirements and probably accounts for the effectiveness of Istin in myocardial ischaemia.

2. The mechanism of action of Istin probably involves dilation of the main coronary arteries and coronary arterioles, both in normal and ischaemic regions.

After oral administration of therapeutic doses, amlodipine is well absorbed with peak blood levels between 6–12 hours post-dose. The terminal plasma elimination half-life is about 35–50 hours and is consistent with once-daily administration. Steady state plasma levels are reached after 7–8 days. Amlodipine is predominantly cleared by metabolism to inactive metabolites with most metabolites excreted in the urine. Amlodipine is approximately 97.5% plasma protein bound.

In patients with hypertension, once daily dosing provides clinically significant reductions of blood pressure in both the supine and standing positions throughout the 24 hour interval. Due to the slow onset of action, acute hypotension is not a feature of Istin administration.

In patients with angina, once daily administration of Istin increases total exercise time and decreases both angina attack frequency and glyceryl trinitrate tablet consumption.

Istin has not been associated with any adverse metabolic effects or changes in plasma lipids and is suitable for use in patients with asthma, diabetes, and gout.

Indications: Istin is indicated for the first-line treatment of hypertension and can be used as the sole agent to control blood pressure in the majority of patients. Patients not adequately controlled on a single antihypertensive agent may benefit from the addition of Istin, which has been used in combination with a thiazide diuretic, beta-adrenoceptor blocking agent, or an angiotensin-converting enzyme inhibitor.

Istin is indicated for the first-line treatment of myocardial ischaemia, due to fixed obstruction of the coronary vasculature (stable angina). Istin may be used as monotherapy, or in combination with other antianginal drugs in patients with angina that is refractory to nitrates and/or adequate doses of beta-adrenoceptor blocking agents.

Dosage and administration
Adults: For both hypertension and angina, the recommended initial dose is 5 mg Istin orally once daily which may be increased to a maximum dose of 10 mg depending on the individual patient's response.

The dose does not need adjusting when Istin is given concurrently with thiazide diuretics, beta-adrenoceptor blocking agents or angiotensin-converting enzyme inhibitors. Istin can be administered with or without food.

Use in children: Since there is no clinical experience in patients of less than 18 years, use in children is not currently recommended.

Use in the elderly: Although elderly patients may have higher plasma concentrations of amlodipine than younger patients, the terminal elimination half-lives are similar. Istin is similarly well-tolerated in elderly or younger patients. Therefore the normal dosage is recommended.

Use with renal impairment: Amlodipine is extensively metabolised to inactive metabolites with 10% excreted as unchanged drug in the urine. Changes in amlodipine plasma concentration are not correlated with the degree of renal impairment, therefore the normal dosage is recommended. Amlodipine is not dialysable.

Use in patients with impaired hepatic function: The half-life of amlodipine is prolonged in patients with impaired liver function and dosage recommendations have not been established. Istin should therefore be administered with caution in these patients.

Contra-indications, warnings, etc
Contra-indications: Istin is contra-indicated in patients with a known sensitivity to dihydropyridines (e.g. nifedipine, nicardipine, isradipine).

Warnings and precautions
Use during pregnancy and lactation: Although some dihydropyridine compounds have been found to be teratogenic in animals, data in the rat and rabbit for amlodipine provide no evidence for a teratogenic effect. There is, however, no clinical experience with Istin in pregnancy or lactation. Accordingly, Istin should not be administered during pregnancy, or lactation, or to women of child-bearing potential unless effective contraception is used.

Driving/use of machinery: Clinical experience with Istin indicates that it is unlikely to impair a patient's ability to drive or use machinery.

Drug interactions: Istin has been safely administered with thiazide diuretics, beta-adrenoceptor blocking drugs, angiotensin-converting enzyme inhibitors, long-acting nitrates, sublingual glyceryl trinitrate, non-steroidal anti-inflammatory drugs, antibiotics, and oral hypoglycaemic agents.

Co-administration of Istin with digoxin did not change serum digoxin levels or digoxin renal clearance in normal volunteers. Co-administration of cimetidine did not alter the pharmacokinetics of amlodipine.

In healthy volunteers, co-administration of Istin did not significantly alter the effect of warfarin on prothrombin time. The introduction of Istin is not likely to result in the need for modification of an established warfarin regimen.

In vitro data from studies with human plasma indicate that amlodipine has no effect on protein binding of digoxin, phenytoin, warfarin, or indomethacin.

Side-effects: Istin is well tolerated. In placebo controlled clinical trials involving patients with hypertension or angina, the most commonly observed side-effects were headache, oedema, fatigue, nausea, flushing and dizziness. No clinically significant pattern of laboratory test abnormalities related to Istin has been observed.

Overdosage: There is no well documented experience with Istin overdosage. Since amlodipine absorption is slow, gastric lavage may be worthwhile in some cases. Available data suggest that gross overdosage could result in excessive peripheral vasodilation with subsequent marked and probably prolonged systemic hypotension. Clinically significant hypotension due to Istin overdosage calls for active cardiovascular support including monitoring of cardiac and respiratory function, elevation of extremities, and attention to circulating fluid volume and urine output. A vasoconstrictor agent may be helpful in restoring vascular tone and blood pressure, provided that there is no contra-indication to its use. Since amlodipine is highly protein-bound, dialysis is unlikely to be of benefit.

Pharmaceutical precautions Store below 30°C.

Legal category POM.

Package quantities
5 mg: Calendar pack of 28 tablets
10 mg: Calendar pack of 28 tablets

Further information Nil.

Product licence numbers
Istin Tablets 5 mg 0057/0297
Istin Tablets 10 mg 0057/0298

MITHRACIN*

Presentation Mithracin (plicamycin) is available in vials as a freeze-dried preparation for intravenous administration. Each vial contains 2500 micrograms of plicamycin with 100 mg of mannitol and sufficient disodium phosphate to maintain pH 7.

Uses
Indications: Mithracin is indicated for the treatment of refractory hypercalcaemia associated with a variety of neoplasms, specifically where standard therapeutic methods have failed. The use of Mithracin in other types of neoplastic disease is not recommended.

Actions: Mithracin lowers serum calcium levels. The exact mechanism (or mechanisms) by which the drug exerts this effect is unknown. It appears that Mithracin may block the hypercalcaemic action of pharmacologic doses of vitamin D. It has also been suggested that Mithracin may lower calcium serum levels by inhibiting the effect of parathyroid hormone upon osteoclasts. Mithracin inhibition of DNA-dependent RNA synthesis appears to render osteoclasts unable to fully respond to parathyroid hormone with the biosynthesis necessary for osteolysis. Decreases in serum phosphate levels and urinary calcium excretion accompany the lowering of serum calcium concentrations.

Dosage and administration (please see *Warnings* section). The daily dose of Mithracin is based on the patient's body weight. If a patient has abnormal fluid retention, the patient's ideal weight rather than actual body weight should be used to calculate the dose.

In hypercalcaemia associated with advanced malignancy the recommended course of treatment with Mithracin is 25 micrograms/kg body weight/day for 3 to 4 days.

If the desired degree of reversal of hypercalcaemia is not achieved with the initial course of therapy, additional courses of therapy may then be administered at intervals of one week or more to achieve the desired result or to maintain serum calcium at normal levels. It may be possible to maintain normal calcium balance with single weekly doses or with a schedule of 2 or 3 doses per week.

Dosage recommendations have not been established in patients with impaired liver or renal function. The drug should therefore be administered with caution in these patients.

Mithracin should be administered intravenously only. The appropriate daily dose of Mithracin should be diluted in one litre of either 5% dextrose intravenous infusion or sodium chloride intravenous infusion in water and administered by slow intravenous infusion over a period of 4 to 6 hours. Rapid direct intravenous injection of Mithracin should be avoided as it may be associated with a higher incidence and greater severity of gastro-intestinal side-effects. Extravasation of solutions of Mithracin may cause local irritation and cellulitis. Should thrombophlebitis or perivascular cellulitis occur, the infusion should be terminated and reinstituted at another site. The application of moderate heat to the site of extravasation may help to disperse the compound and minimise discomfort and local tissue irritation. The use of anti-emetic compounds prior to and during treatment with Mithracin may be helpful in relieving nausea and vomiting.

To reconstitute, add aseptically 4.9 ml of Water for Injections PhEur to the contents of the vial and shake to dissolve. Each ml of the resulting solution will then contain 500 micrograms of Mithracin. After removal of the appropriate dose, the remaining unused solution must be discarded. Fresh solution must be prepared in the above manner each day of therapy.

Contra-indications, warnings, etc

Contra-indications: Mithracin is contra-indicated in patients with thrombocytopenia, thrombocytopathy, co-agulation disorder or an increased susceptibility to bleeding due to other causes. Mithracin should not be administered to any patient with impairment of bone marrow function.

Mithracin should not be used in the treatment of patients who are not hospitalised and who cannot be observed carefully and frequently during and after therapy, or whenever appropriate laboratory facilities are unavailable.

Use in pregnancy: Mithracin may cause foetal harm when administered to a pregnant woman. This drug is contra-indicated in women who are or may become pregnant. If used during pregnancy, or if the patient becomes pregnant while taking this drug, the patient should be apprised of the potential hazard to the foetus.

Warnings: The information contained in this Data Sheet should be thoroughly reviewed before administering the preparation: In the treatment of each patient, the physician must weigh carefully the possibility of achieving therapeutic benefit versus the risk of toxicity which may occur with Mithracin therapy.

It is recommended that Mithracin be administered only to hospitalised patients by or under the supervision of a qualified physician who is experienced in the use of cytotoxic agents, because of the possibility of severe reactions. Facilities for the determination of necessary laboratory studies must be available.

Severe thrombocytopenia, a haemorrhagic tendency and even death, may result from the use of Mithracin. Although severe toxicity is more apt to occur in patients who have far-advanced disease or are otherwise considered poor risks for therapy, serious toxicity may also occasionally occur even in patients who are in relatively good condition.

Antineoplastic and cytotoxic agents have been shown to be mutagenic and carcinogenic in animals and possibly man. Only limited animal and *in vitro* mutagenicity studies have been carried out with plicamycin; the possibility that plicamycin has similar effects to other antineoplastic and cytotoxic agents should be borne in mind.

Use in lactation: It is not known whether this drug is excreted in human milk. Because many drugs are excreted in human milk and because of the potential for serious adverse reactions in nursing infants from Mithracin, a decision should be made whether to discontinue nursing or to discontinue the drug, taking into account the importance of the drug to the mother.

Precautions: Mithracin should be administered only to patients who are hospitalised and who can be observed frequently and carefully during and after therapy.

Electrolyte imbalance, especially hypokalaemia and hypophosphataemia should be corrected with appropriate electrolyte therapy prior to treatment with Mithracin.

Mithracin should be used with extreme caution in patients with significant impairment of renal or hepatic function.

Renal function should be carefully monitored before, during and after treatment.

In the treatment of each patient, the physician must weigh carefully the possibility of achieving therapeutic benefit versus the risk of toxicity which may occur with Mithracin therapy.

The following laboratory studies should be obtained frequently during therapy and for several days following the last dose: platelet count, prothrombin time, bleeding time. The occurrence of thrombocytopenia or a significant prolongation of prothrombin time or bleeding time is an indication for the termination of therapy.

Side-effects: The most important form of toxicity associated with the use of Mithracin consists of a bleeding syndrome which usually begins with an episode of epistaxis. This bleeding tendency may consist of a single or several episodes of epistaxis only and progress no further. However, in some cases, this haemorrhagic syndrome can start with an episode of haematemesis which may progress to more widespread haemorrhage in the gastrointestinal tract or to a more generalised bleeding tendency. This haemorrhagic diathesis is most likely due to abnormalities in multiple clotting factors.

Other haematological abnormalities include depression of platelet count, white blood cell count, haemoglobin and prothrombin content, elevation of clotting time and bleeding time, abnormal clot retraction.

Thrombocytopenia may be rapid in onset and may occur at any time during the therapy or within several days following the last dose. With the occurrence of severe thrombocytopenia, the infusion of platelet concentrates or platelet-rich plasma may be helpful in elevating the platelet count.

The occurrence of leucopenia with the use of Mithracin is relatively uncommon, occurring only in approximately 6% of patients.

It has been uncommon for abnormalities in clotting time or clot retraction to be demonstrated prior to the onset of an overt bleeding episode noted in some patients treated with Mithracin. Nevertheless, the performance of these tests periodically is recommended because in a few instances an abnormality in one of these studies may have served as a warning to terminate therapy because of impending serious toxicity.

The most common side-effects reported with the use of Mithracin consist of gastro-intestinal symptoms: anorexia, nausea, vomiting, diarrhoea, and stomatitis. Other less frequently reported side-effects include fever, drowsiness, weakness, lethargy, malaise, headache, depression, phlebitis, facial flushing, and skin rash.

The following laboratory abnormalities have been reported during therapy with Mithracin and in most instances were reversible following cessation of treatment.

Abnormal liver function tests: Increased levels of serum glutamic oxalacetic transaminase, serum glutamic pyruvic transaminase, lactic dehydrogenase, alkaline phosphatase, serum bilirubin, ornithine carbamyl transferase, isocitric dehydrogenase, and increased retention of bromsulphalein.

Abnormal renal function: Increased blood urea nitrogen and serum creatinine; proteinuria.

Abnormalities in electrolyte concentrations: Depression of serum phosphorus and potassium.

Overdosage: Generally, adverse effects following the use of Mithracin, especially the haemorrhagic syndrome, are dose related. Therefore, following administration of an overdose, patients can be expected to experience an exaggeration of the usual adverse effects. Close monitoring of the haematologic picture, including factors involved in the clotting mechanism, hepatic and renal functions, and serum electrolytes, is necessary. No specific antidote for Mithracin is known. Management of overdosage would include general supportive measures to sustain the patient through the period of toxicity.

Pharmaceutical precautions Store at 2°C to 8°C.

The increasing use of cytotoxic drugs and the potential hazards associated with them, requires special precautions to be taken in their handling, preparation and administration. These recommendations provide a basis for the safe handling of Mithracin.

1. All staff working with Mithracin should receive special training.
2. Reconstitution of Mithracin should be performed in a designated aseptic area which gives maximum protection to the surrounding environment.
3. Adequate protective clothing including gloves and safety spectacles should be worn.

Should spillage on the skin occur, the affected area should be washed with copious quantities of water.

Should spillage into the eye occur, immediately cleanse thoroughly using copious quantities of sodium chloride eye wash. (If sodium chloride eye wash is not available water can be used as an alternative). Should eye irritation continue medical help should be sought.

4. Mithracin should not be handled by pregnant staff.
5. Adequate care and precautions should be taken in the disposal of items used to reconstitute Mithracin.

Disposal procedure
Unopened vials: Place in a suitable closed container† and incinerate at 1000°C.

Reconstituted solution: Dilute small volumes with larger volumes of 10% w/v trisodium phosphate solution. Absorb diluted liquid on to paper, ash or sawdust. Place in high risk waste disposal bag† and incinerate at 1000°C.

Disposal of swabs, etc: Swabs etc. should be placed in a high risk waste disposal bag† and incinerated at 1000°C.

Accidental spillage: Should spillage on the floor or breakage of a vial of reconstituted solution occur, adequate protective clothing, including gloves and safety spectacles should be worn. The area should be cleaned with absorbent paper and the floor wiped with cloths soaked in 10% w/v trisodium phosphate solution or 0.1N sodium hydroxide solution, then washed with copious quantities of water. The absorbent paper, cloths, gloves and other materials used in the management of the spillage should be placed in a high risk waste disposal bag† and incinerated at 1000°C.

If Mithracin is still as the freeze dried powder, damp down quickly to avoid dispersion and proceed as above.

Care should be taken in disposing of broken glass from vials, which should go into a closed container† for incineration.

Legal category POM.

Package quantities Vial containing 2500 micrograms.

Further information Nil.

Product licence number 0057/5022R.

†The containers and bags should be those specified in 'Safe disposal of clinical waste'. Health and Safety Advisory Committee HMSO 1982.

NEPHRIL*

Presentation Nephril is available as white scored tablets coded NEP/1 on one side and 'Pfizer' on the other, each containing 1 mg polythiazide.

Inactive excipients: These include lactose. The product is free of gluten, sucrose and invert sugar.

Uses *Actions:* The mechanism of action results in an interference with the renal tubular mechanism of electrolyte reabsorption. At maximal therapeutic dosage, all thiazides are approximately equal in their diuretic potency. The mechanism whereby thiazides function in the control of hypertension is unknown.

Indications: Nephril is an orally effective, non-mercurial diuretic, saluretic and antihypertensive agent. Nephril is indicated as adjunctive therapy in oedema associated with congestive cardiac failure, hepatic cirrhosis and corticosteroid and oestrogen therapy.

Nephril has also been found useful in oedema due to certain forms of renal dysfunction, such as nephrotic syndrome, acute glomerulonephritis and chronic renal failure (see Warnings).

Nephril is indicated in the management of hypertension either as the sole therapeutic agent or to enhance the effectiveness of other antihypertensive drugs in the more severe forms of hypertension.

Dosage and administration The usual dosage of Nephril for diuretic therapy is 1 to 4 mg once daily. For antihypertensive therapy the usual maintenance dose is between 2 and 4 mg daily although some patients may be optimally controlled on doses of 500 micrograms or 1 mg daily. However, few patients will require doses as high as 4 mg daily and at such a dose level serum electrolytes should be monitored frequently. Dosage should be individualised according to response and should be titrated to gain the maximum therapeutic effect with the minimum dose required to maintain that therapeutic response.

Use in children: Nephril is not recommended for use in children.

Use in the elderly: Elderly patients are especially liable to the adverse effects of diuretics. It is therefore particularly important that the dose should be the lowest possible consistent with adequate effect. The possibility of drug interactions should also be considered in view of the frequency of multiple drug therapy in this age group.

Contra-indications, warnings, etc
Contra-indications: Anuria, hypersensitivity to polythiazide and other thiazide diuretics and other sulphonamide derived drugs.

Warnings:

Use in renal insufficiency: Thiazides should be used with caution in severe renal disease. In patients with renal disease, thiazides may precipitate azotaemia. Cumulative effects of the drug may develop in patients with impaired renal function. If progressive renal impairment becomes evident, as indicated by a rising nonprotein nitrogen or blood urea nitrogen, a careful reappraisal of therapy is necessary with probable cessation of treatment.

Use in hepatic disease: Thiazides should be used with caution in patients with impaired hepatic function or progressive liver disease, since minor alterations of fluid and electrolyte balance may precipitate hepatic coma.

Thiazides may add to or potentiate the action of other antihypertensive drugs. Potentiation occurs with ganglionic or peripheral adrenergic blocking drugs.

Sensitivity reactions may occur in patients with a history of allergy or bronchial asthma. The possibility of exacerbation or activation of systemic lupus erythematosus has been reported.

Use in pregnancy: The routine use of diuretics in healthy pregnant women is inappropriate and may expose mother and foetus to unnecessary hazard. Diuretics do not prevent development of toxaemia of pregnancy and there is no satisfactory evidence that they are useful in the treatment of established toxaemia.

Oedema during pregnancy may arise from pathological causes or from physiological and mechanical consequences of pregnancy. Physiological hypervolaemia during pregnancy may be associated with generalised oedema including dependent oedema. This oedema is properly treated by recumbency and support hose. Thiazides may be indicated in pregnancy when oedema is due to pathological causes other than toxaemia. Rarely short courses of thiazides are indicated where physiological oedema is unrelieved by rest and where the oedema causes extreme discomfort.

Thiazides cross the placental barrier and appear in cord blood. The use of thiazides in pregnant women requires that the anticipated benefit be weighed against possible hazards to the foetus. These hazards include foetal or neonatal jaundice, thrombocytopenia and other side-effects which have occurred in the adult.

Use in nursing mothers: Thiazides appear in breast milk.

If use of Nephril is deemed essential, breast feeding should be discontinued.

Precautions: All patients receiving thiazide therapy should have periodic determinations of serum electrolytes at appropriate intervals to detect possible electrolyte imbalance. Such patients should also be observed for clinical signs of fluid or electrolyte imbalance; namely hyponatraemia, hypochloraemic alkalosis and hypokalaemia. Serum and urine electrolyte determinations are particularly important when the patient is vomiting or receiving parenteral fluids. Warning signs of possible electrolyte imbalance, irrespective of cause, are: dryness of mouth, thirst, weakness, lethargy, drowsiness, restlessness, muscle pains or cramps, muscular fatigue, hypotension, oliguria, tachycardia and gastro-intestinal disturbances such as nausea and vomiting.

Hypokalaemia may develop with thiazides as with any other potent diuretic, especially with brisk diuresis, when severe cirrhosis is present, or during concomitant use of corticosteroids or ACTH.

Interference with adequate oral electrolyte intake will also contribute to hypokalaemia. Hypokalaemia may exaggerate metabolic effects of digitalis therapy especially with reference to myocardial activity.

Any chloride deficit is generally mild and usually does not require specific treatment except under extraordinary circumstances (as in liver disease or renal disease). Dilutional hyponatraemia may occur in oedematous patients in hot weather; appropriate therapy is water restriction, rather than administration of salt except in rare instances, when the hyponatraemia is life threatening. In actual salt depletion, appropriate replacement is the therapy of choice. Hyperuricaemia may occur or frank gout may be precipitated in certain patients receiving thiazide therapy.

Insulin requirements in diabetic patients may be increased, decreased or unchanged. Latent diabetes mellitus may become manifest during thiazide administration.

Thiazide drugs may increase the responsiveness to tubocurarine.

The antihypertensive effects of thiazides may be enhanced in the post-sympathectomy patient. Thiazides may decrease arterial responsiveness to noradrenaline. This diminution is not sufficient to preclude effectiveness of the pressor agent for therapeutic use.

If progressive renal impairment becomes evident, as indicated by a rising non-protein nitrogen or blood urea nitrogen a careful reappraisal of therapy is necessary with probable discontinuation of therapy with Nephril.

Thiazides may decrease serum protein-bound iodine levels without signs of thyroid disturbance.

Side-effects:

Gastro-intestinal – anorexia, gastric irritation, nausea, vomiting, cramping, diarrhoea, constipation, jaundice (intrahepatic cholestatic jaundice), pancreatitis.

Central nervous system – dizziness, vertigo, paraesthesia, headache, xanthopsia.

Haematological – leucopenia, agranulocytosis, thrombocytopenia, aplastic anaemia.

Dermatological – purpura, photosensitivity, rash, urticaria, necrotising angiitis (vasculitis) (cutaneous vasculitis).

Cardiovascular – orthostatic hypotension may occur and be aggravated by alcohol, barbiturates or narcotics.

Other – hyperglycaemia, glycosuria, hyperuricaemia, muscle spasm, weakness, restlessness.

Whenever adverse reactions are moderate or severe, thiazide dosage should be reduced or therapy withdrawn.

Overdosage: Gastric lavage and supportive therapy. Treatment of acute renal failure if present. Potassium supplements.

Pharmaceutical precautions Store below 25°C.

Legal category POM.

Package quantities Nephril 1 mg: Original packs of 28 tablets.

Further information Nil.

Product licence number 0057/5024R.

SINEQUAN*

Presentation Sinequan (doxepin hydrochloride) is available in capsules of four strengths. All capsules bear the name 'Pfizer'.

The four sizes of capsules are distinguished by their colour and coding as follows:

Sinequan 10 mg capsule coded 'SQN 10' (opaque red).

Sinequan 25 mg capsule coded 'SQN 25' (opaque blue cap/opaque red body).

Sinequan 50 mg capsule coded 'SQN 50' (opaque blue).

Sinequan 75 mg capsule coded 'SQN 75' (opaque blue cap/opaque rich yellow body).

Inactive excipients: Sinequan 10, 25 mg and 50 mg tablets contain lactose.

Sinequan 10 mg and 25 mg contain two azo dyes sunset yellow and amaranth, also erythrosine and titanium dioxide. Sinequan 25 mg also contains patent blue V.

Sinequan 50 mg and 75 mg contain erythrosine, patent blue V and titanium dioxide. Sinequan 75 mg also contains quinoline yellow. Sinequan preparations are free of gluten, sucrose and invert sugar.

Uses *Actions:* Sinequan is a tricyclic antidepressant. The mechanism of action of Sinequan is not definitely known. It is not a central nervous stimulant nor a monoamine oxidase inhibitor. The current hypothesis is that the clinical effects are due, at least in part, to influences on the adrenergic activity at the synapses so that deactivation of noradrenaline by reuptake into the nerve terminals is prevented. In animal studies anticholinergic, antiserotonin and antihistamine effects on smooth muscle have been demonstrated. At higher than usual clinical doses, adrenaline response was potentiated in animals. This effect was not demonstrated in humans.

Indications: Symptoms of depressive illness, especially where sedation is required.

Sinequan may be used with benefit where symptoms are of short or long duration prior to treatment and in patients with a wide range of intensity of illness.

As with other psychotherapeutic agents, the degree of response varies with each patient. In patients exhibiting a beneficial response, this may be seen within a few days of commencing therapy, while others may not respond for two weeks or longer.

Due to its excellent toleration, Sinequan is particularly useful in ambulatory patients seen in general practice as well as in the treatment of hospitalised patients.

Dosage and administration The optimum oral dose depends on the severity of the condition and the individual patient's response. The dose varies from 30–300 mg daily, and is usually administered in three divided doses daily.

For the majority of patients with moderate or severe symptoms, it is recommended that treatment commences with an initial dose of 75 mg daily. Many of these patients will respond satisfactorily at this dose level. For patients who do not, the dosage may be adjusted according to individual response. In more severely ill patients, it may be necessary to administer a dose of up to 300 mg a day to obtain a clinical response.

The total daily dosage of Sinequan may be given on a divided or once daily schedule. If the once daily schedule is employed, the maximum recommended dose is 100 mg/day. This dose may be given at bedtime.

In patients where insomnia is a troublesome symptom, it is recommended that the total daily dose be divided so that a higher proportion is given for the evening dose; similarly, if drowsiness is experienced as a side effect of treatment, Sinequan may be administered by this regimen, or the dosage may be reduced.

It is often possible, having once obtained a satisfactory

therapeutic response, to reduce the dose for maintenance therapy.

The optimal antidepressant effect may not be evident for two to three weeks.

Use in children: The use of Sinequan in children under 12 years is not recommended, because safe conditions for its use have not been established.

Use in the elderly: In general, lower dosages are recommended. Where the presenting symptoms are mild in nature, it is advisable to initiate treatment at a dose of 10–50 mg daily. A satisfactory clinical response is obtained in many of these patients at a daily dose of 30–50 mg. The dosage may be adjusted according to the individual response.

Contra-indications, warnings, etc

Contra-indications: Hypersensitivity, mania, severe liver disease, lactation, glaucoma, tendency to urinary retention.

Precautions: The once-a-day dosage regimen of Sinequan in patients with intercurrent illness or patients taking other medications should be carefully adjusted. This is especially important in patients receiving other medications with anticholinergic effects.

The use of Sinequan on a once-a-day dosage regimen in geriatric patients should be adjusted carefully on the basis of the patient's condition. The elderly are particularly liable to experience toxic effects, especially agitation, confusion and postural hypotension. The initial dose should be increased with caution under close supervision. Half the normal maintenance dose may be sufficient to produce a satisfactory clinical response.

Use with caution in patients who have experienced a recent myocardial infarction.

Since suicide is an inherent risk in any depressed patient until significant improvement has occurred, patients should be closely supervised during early therapy.

Drug interactions: Combined use with other antidepressants, alcohol or antianxiety agents should be undertaken with due recognition of the possibility of potentiation. It is known, for example, that monoamine oxidase inhibitors may potentiate other drug effects, therefore Sinequan should not be given concurrently, or within two weeks of cessation of therapy, with monoamine oxidase inhibitors.

Cimetidine has been reported to produce clinically significant fluctuations in steady-state serum concentrations of various tricylic antidepressants.

Anaesthetics given during tricyclic or tetracyclic antidepressant therapy may increase the risk of arrhythmias and hypotension. If surgery is necessary, the anaesthetist should be informed that a patient is being so treated.

Use with caution in patients with a history of epilepsy.

Sinequan may decrease the antihypertensive effect of agents such as debrisoquine, bethanidine, guanethidine and possibly clonidine. It usually requires daily doses of Sinequan in excess of 150 mg before any effect on the action of guanethidine is seen. It would be advisable to review all antihypertensive therapy during treatment with tricyclic antidepressants.

Sinequan should not be given with sympathomimetic agents, such as ephedrine, isoprenaline, noradrenaline, phenylephrine and phenylpropanolamine.

Barbiturates may increase the rate of metabolism of Sinequan.

The dose of thyroid hormone medication may need reducing if Sinequan is being given concurrently.

Driving/use of machinery: Since drowsiness may occur with the use of Sinequan, patients should be warned of the possibility and cautioned against driving a car or operating machinery while taking this drug.

Use in pregnancy: There is inadequate evidence of safety in human pregnancy but the drug has been widely used for many years without apparent ill consequences and animal studies have not shown any hazard.

Side-effects: Note: Some of the side-effects noted below have not been specifically reported with Sinequan. However, due to the close pharmacological similarities amongst the tricyclics, the reactions should be considered when prescribing Sinequan.

Anticholinergic effects: Dry mouth, blurred vision, constipation and urinary retention have been reported. If they do not subside with continued therapy, or if they become severe, it may be necessary to reduce the dosage.

Central nervous system effects: Drowsiness is the most commonly noticed side-effect. This tends to disappear as therapy is continued. Other infrequently reported CNS side-effects are confusion, disorientation, hallucinations, paraesthesiae, ataxia and extrapyramidal symptoms, tremor and convulsions.

Psychotic manifestations, including mania and paranoid delusions may be exacerbated during treatment with tricyclic antidepressants.

Cardiovascular: Although Sinequan carries less risk than other tricyclic antidepressants, caution should be observed in the treatment of patients with heart block or cardiac arrhythmias. Cardiovascular effects including hypotension and tachycardia have been reported occasionally.

Allergic: Skin rash, facial oedema, photosensitisation and pruritus have occasionally occurred.

Haematological: Eosinophilia has been reported in a few patients. There have been occasional reports of bone marrow depression manifesting as agranulocytosis, leucopenia, thrombocytopenia and purpura.

Gastro-intestinal: Nausea, vomiting, indigestion, taste disturbances, diarrhoea and anorexia have been reported. (See Anticholinergic effects).

Endocrine: Raised or lowered libido, testicular swelling, gynaecomastia, enlargement of breasts and galactorrhoea in the female, raising or lowering of blood sugar levels and inappropriate antidiuretic hormone secretion have been reported following the administration of tricyclics.

Other: Dizziness, tinnitus, weight gain, sweating, chills, fatigue, weakness, flushing, jaundice and alopecia have been occasionally observed as adverse effects.

Withdrawal: Withdrawal symptoms may occur on abrupt cessation of tricyclic antidepressant therapy and include insomnia, irritability, and excessive perspiration. Withdrawal symptoms in neonates whose mothers received tricyclic antidepressants during the third trimester have also been reported and include respiratory depression, convulsions and 'jitteriness' (hyper-reflexia).

Overdosage:

A. *Signs and Symptoms:*

1. Mild: Drowsiness, stupor, blurred vision, excessive dryness of mouth.

2. Severe: Respiratory depression, hypotension, coma, convulsions, cardiac arrhythmias and tachycardias.

Also: urinary retention (bladder atony), decreased gastro-intestinal motility (paralytic ileus), hyperthermia (or hypothermia), hypertension, dilated pupils, hyperactive reflexes.

B. *Management and Treatment:*

1. Mild: Observation and supportive therapy is all that is usually necessary.

2. Severe: Medical management of severe Sinequan overdosage consists of aggressive supportive therapy. If the patient is conscious, gastric lavage, with appropriate precautions to prevent pulmonary aspiration, should be performed even though Sinequan is rapidly absorbed. The use of activated charcoal has been recommended, as has been continuous gastric lavage with saline for 24 hours or more. An adequate airway should be established in comatose patients and assisted ventilation used if necessary. ECG monitoring may be required for several days, since relapse after apparent recovery has been reported. Arrhythmias should be treated with the appropriate anti-arrhythmic agent. It has been reported that many of the cardiovascular and CNS symptoms of tricyclic antidepressant poisoning in adults may be

reversed by the slow intravenous administration of 1 mg to 3 mg of physostigmine salicylate. Because physostigmine is rapidly metabolised, the dosage should be repeated as required. Convulsions may respond to standard anticonvulsant therapy. However, barbiturates may potentiate any respiratory depression. Dialysis and forced diuresis generally are not of value in the management of overdosage due to high tissue and protein binding of Sinequan.

Pharmaceutical precautions Store below 25°C.

Legal category POM.

Package quantities
Capsules 10 mg: Original packs of 56 capsules (in blister strips of 4 × 14 capsules).
Capsules 25 mg: Original packs of 28 capsules (in blister strips of 2 × 14 capsules).
Capsules 50 mg: Original packs of 28 capsules (in blister strips of 2 × 14 capsules).
Capsules 75 mg: Original packs of 28 capsules (in blister strips of 2 × 14 capsules).

Further information Nil.

Product licence numbers

10 mg capsules	0057/5032R
25 mg capsules	0057/5033R
50 mg capsules	0057/5034R
75 mg capsules	0057/0133

TERRAMYCIN*

Presentation Terramycin (oxytetracycline) is available as:

Tablets 250 mg: Each sugar-coated yellow tablet contains 250 mg Oxytetracycline Dihydrate PhEur and coded 'Pfizer'.

Capsules 250 mg: Hard gelatin capsules, opaque yellow cap and body printed TER250 and 'Pfizer', each containing 250 mg Oxytetracycline as the Hydrochloride PhEur.

Inactive excipients: The tablet excipients include sucrose, methyl hydroxybenzoate, sunset yellow, quinoline yellow and titanium dioxide. The capsule excipients include erythrosine, quinoline yellow and titanium dioxide. Both formulations are free of gluten and lactose.

Uses *Actions:* Oxytetracycline is primarily bacteriostatic and is thought to exert its antimicrobial effect by the inhibition of protein synthesis. Terramycin is active against a wide range of Gram-negative and Gram-positive organisms.

The drugs in the tetracycline class have closely similar antimicrobial spectra and cross resistance among them is common.

Oxytetracycline and its salts are readily absorbed orally and are 10–40% bound to plasma proteins. Between 40 and 70% is excreted unchanged in the urine via glomerular filtration. A serum half-life of 6–10 hours has been reported for Terramycin in patients with normal renal function.

Oxytetracycline diffuses readily through the placenta into the foetal circulation, into the pleural fluid and, under some circumstances, into the cerebrospinal fluid. It appears to be well concentrated in the hepatic system and excreted in the bile, so that it appears in the faeces, as well as in the urine, in a biologically active form.

Indications: Terramycin is indicated in infections caused by the following micro-organisms:
Rickettsiae (Rocky Mountain spotted fever, typhus fever and the typhus group, Q fever, rickettsialpox and tick fevers),
Mycoplasma pneumoniae (PPLO, Eaton Agent),
Chlamydia psittaci (formerly agents of psittacosis and ornithosis),
Chlamydia trachomatis (formerly agents of lymphogranuloma venereum),
Calymmatobacterium (Donovania) *granulomatis* (formerly agents of granuloma inguinale),
The spirochaetal agent of relapsing fever (*Borrelia recurrentis*).

The following Gram-negative micro-organisms:
Neisseria gonorrhoea,
Haemophilus ducreyi (chancroid),
Yersinia pestis (formerly *Pasteurella pestis*),
Francisella tularensis (formerly *Pasteurella tularensis*),
Bartonella bacilliformis,
Bacteroides species.
Vibrio cholerae (formerly *Vibrio comma*),
Campylobacter foetus (formerly *Vibrio foetus*),
Brucella species (in conjunction with streptomycin).

Because many strains of the following groups of micro-organisms have been shown to be resistant to tetracyclines, culture and susceptibility testing are recommended.

Terramycin is indicated for treatment of infections caused by the following Gram-negative micro-organisms, when bacteriological testing indicates appropriate susceptibility to the drug:
Escherichia coli,
Enterobacter aerogenes (formerly *Aerobacter aerogenes*),
Shigella species,
Acinetobacter species (formerly *Mima* species and *Herellea* species),
Haemophilus influenzae (respiratory infections),
Klebsiella species (respiratory and urinary infections).

Terramycin is indicated for treatment of infections caused by the following Gram-positive micro-organisms when bacteriological testing indicates appropriate susceptibility to the drug:
Streptococcus pneumoniae (formerly *Diplococcus pneumoniae*),
Staphylococcus aureus (skin and soft-tissue infections).

When penicillin is contra-indicated, tetracyclines are alternative drugs in the treatment of infections due to:
Treponema pallidum and *Treponema pertenue* (syphilis and yaws),
Listeria monocytogenes,
Clostridium species,
Bacillus anthracis,
Leptotrichia buccalis (formerly *Fusobacterium fusiforme*) (Vincent's infection),
Actinomyces species.

In acute intestinal amoebiasis, the tetracyclines may be a useful adjunct to amoebicides.

In severe acne vulgaris and rosacea, Terramycin is useful in long-term treatment.

Tetracyclines are indicated in the treatment of trachoma, although the infectious agent is not always eliminated, as judged by immunofluorescence.

Inclusion conjunctivitis may be treated with oral tetracyclines or with a combination of oral and topical agents.

Dosage and administration Oral administration.
Adults: The usual daily dosage of Terramycin is 1–2 g divided in four equal doses, depending on the severity of the infection.

Children above 8 years of age: The usual daily dose is 25–50 mg/kg of body weight divided in four equal doses (see 'Warnings' Section).

Use in the elderly: Terramycin may be given at the usual adult dosage. The possibility of sub-clinical renal insufficiency should be kept in mind, as it may lead to drug accumulation.

Total daily dosage should be administered in equally divided doses, given every 6 hours. Therapy should be continued for at least 24–48 hours after symptoms and fever have subsided.

For the treatment of brucellosis: 500 mg of Terramycin four times daily for 3 weeks should be accompanied by streptomycin, 1 g intramuscularly twice daily the first week, and once daily the second week.

For the treatment of uncomplicated gonorrhoea and non-gonococcal urethritis: Terramycin 500 mg four times daily for seven days for a total dose of 14 g.

For the treatment of early syphilis (primary, secondary, latent syphilis of less than 1 year's duration) Terramycin 500 mg four times a day for 15 days.

Syphilis of more than 1 year's duration (latent syphilis of indeterminate or more than 1 year's duration, cardiovascular or late benign syphilis), except neurosyphilis, should be treated with Terramycin 500 mg, by mouth, 4 times a day for 30 days. Patient compliance with this regimen may be difficult, so care should be taken to encourage optimal compliance. Close follow-up, including laboratory tests, is recommended.

For treatment of uncomplicated urethral, endocervical, or rectal chlamydia infections in adults, Terramycin 500 mg, by mouth, 4 times a day for at least 7 days.

For treatment of sexually transmitted epididymo-orchitis, Terramycin 500 mg, by mouth, 4 times a day for at least 10 days after initial treatment with an appropriate beta-lactam antibiotic.

Food and some dairy products also interfere with absorption. Oral forms of Terramycin should be given 1 hour before or 2 hours after meals.

In patients with renal impairment (See Warnings), total dosage should be decreased by reduction of recommended individual doses and/or by extending time intervals between doses.

Contra-indications, warnings, etc Terramycin is contra-indicated in persons who have shown hypersensitivity to any of the tetracyclines.

Use in pregnancy: Terramycin is contra-indicated in pregnancy. If this drug is used during pregnancy, or if the patient becomes pregnant while taking this drug, the patient should be appraised of the potential hazard to the foetus.

Results of animal studies with the tetracycline family of antimicrobials indicate that tetracyclines cross the placenta, are found in foetal tissues and can have toxic effects on the developing foetus (often related to retardation of skeletal development). Evidence of embryotoxicity has also been noted in animals treated early in pregnancy.

Warnings: Use in newborns, infants and children: The use of drugs of the tetracycline class during tooth development (last half of pregnancy, infancy and childhood to the age of 8 years) may cause permanent discoloration of the teeth (yellow-grey-brown). This adverse reaction is more common during long term use of the drugs but has been observed, following repeated short-term courses. Enamel hypoplasia has also been reported. Tetracycline drugs, therefore, should not be used in this age group unless other drugs are not likely to be effective or are contra-indicated.

All tetracyclines form a stable calcium complex in any bone-forming tissue. A decrease in the fibular growth rate has been observed in premature infants given oral tetracyclines in dosages of 25 mg/kg every 6 hours. This reaction was shown to be reversible when the drug was discontinued.

If renal impairment exists, even usual oral or parenteral doses may lead to excessive systemic accumulation of the drug and possible liver toxicity. Under such circumstances, lower than usual total doses are indicated and, if therapy is prolonged, serum level determinations of the drug may be advisable. The antianabolic action of the tetracyclines may cause an increase in BUN. While this in not a problem in those with normal renal function, in patients with significantly impaired renal function, higher serum levels of Terramycin may lead to azotaemia, hyperphosphataemia and acidosis.

Photosensitivity manifested by an exaggerated sunburn reaction has been observed in some individuals taking tetracyclines. Persons apt to be exposed to direct sunlight or ultraviolet light should be advised that this reaction can occur with tetracycline drugs.

Precautions: As with other antibiotic preparations, Terramycin may result in overgrowth of nonsusceptible organisms, including fungi. If superinfection occurs, the antibiotic should be discontinued and appropriate therapy instituted.

In venereal diseases when coexistent syphilis is suspected, a dark field examination should be performed before treatment is started and the blood serology repeated monthly for at least four months.

In long-term therapy, periodic laboratory evaluation of organ systems, including heamatopoietic, renal and hepatic studies should be performed.

All infections due to Group A beta-haemolytic streptococci should be treated for at least 10 days.

Nursing mothers: Tetracyclines are excreted in human milk. Because of the potential for serious adverse reactions in breastfeeding infants, Terramycin should be used only when in the opinion of the physician, potential benefit outweighs potential risk.

Drug interactions: Because tetracyclines have been shown to depress plasma prothrombin activity, patients who are on anticoagulant therapy may require downward adjustment to their anticoagulant dosage.

Since bacteriostatic drugs may interfere with the bactericidal action of penicillin, it is advisable to avoid giving Terramycin in conjunction with penicillin.

Absorption of tetracyclines is impaired by antacids containing aluminium, calcium, or magnesium, and iron-containing preparations.

The concurrent use of tetracyclines and methoxyflurane has been reported to result in fatal renal toxicity.

Side-effects: Gastro-intestinal: anorexia, nausea, vomiting, diarrhoea, glossitis, dysphagia, enterocolitis, and inflammatory lesions (with monilial overgrowth) in the anogenital region. These reactions have been caused by both the oral and parenteral administration of tetracyclines.

Skin: Maculopapular and erythematous rashes. Exfoliative dermatitis has been reported but is uncommon. Photosensitivity.

Renal toxicity: Rise in BUN has been reported and is apparently dose related. (See Warnings.)

Hypersensitivity reactions: Urticaria, angioneurotic oedema, anaphylaxis, anaphylactoid purpura, pericarditis and exacerbation of systemic lupus erythematosis.

Bulging fontanelles in infants and benign intracranial hypertension in adults have been reported in individuals receiving full therapeutic dosages. These conditions disappeared rapidly when the drug was discontinued.

Blood: Haemolytic anaemia, thrombocytopenia, neutropenia and eosinophilia have been reported.

When given over prolonged periods, tetracyclines have been reported to produce brown-black microscopic discoloration of thyroid glands. No abnormalities of thyroid function are known to occur.

Overdosage: Acute overdosage with antibiotics is rare. In the event of overdosage, gastric lavage plus appropriate supportive treatment is indicated.

Pharmaceutical precautions Store below 25°C. Protect from light.

Legal category POM.

Package quantities
Tablets 250 mg: Original packs of 28 tablets.
Capsules 250 mg: Original packs of 28 capsules.

Further information Nil.

Product licence numbers

Tablets 250 mg	0057/5080
Capsules 250 mg	0057/5036

TERRA-CORTRIL* EAR SUSPENSION

Presentation Terra-Cortril Ear Suspension contains 5 mg of Oxytetracycline as the Hydrochloride PhEur, 15 mg of Hydrocortisone Acetate PhEur and 10,000 units of Polymyxin B Sulphate PhEur in each millilitre of a mineral oil suspension.

Inactive excipients: Aluminium tristearate and liquid paraffin.

Uses
Actions: Terra-Cortril Ear Suspension combines the anti-infective activity of oxytetracycline and polymyxin B with the anti-inflammatory activity of hydrocortisone.

Oxytetracycline is a broad-spectrum antibiotic active against both Gram-positive and Gram-negative organisms. Polymyxin B has antimicrobial activity against a wide variety of Gram-negative micro-organisms. It is particularly effective against infections caused by *Pseudomonas aeruginosa*.

Indications: Terra-Cortril Ear Suspension is recommended for the topical treatment of ear conditions in which hydrocortisone is indicated and where there is the possibility of the presence of infection by organisms sensitive to the tetracyclines or polymyxin B. The preliminary identification of the infecting organism and determination of antibiotic sensitivity is essential.

Terra-Cortril Ear Suspension may be used in allergic external otitis of mixed origin, atopic external otitis, excessive inflammatory reactions, pruritus and chronic eczema of the external ear canal.

If the infection is found to be deep-seated or spreading, systemic antibiotic therapy should be considered.

Dosage and administration

Adults: For the treatment of infections of the external ear canal, it is recommended that two to four drops be instilled three times daily for a maximum of 5–7 days, or as prescribed by the physician. The patient should be instructed to avoid contamination of the dropper with exudate from the infected site.

Use in the elderly: No special precautions. The possibility of sub-clinical renal insufficiency should be considered.

Use in children: Not recommended. See 'Contra-indications'.

Contra-indications, warnings, etc

Contra-indications:

1. Hypersensitivity to any of the components of the preparation.
2. Acute herpes simplex, vaccinia, varicella.
3. Fungal diseases of the skin.
4. Tuberculosis of the skin.
5. Primary bacterial infections, e.g. impetigo, pyoderma, furunculosis.
6. Patients with perforation of the eardrum.
7. Patients with existing loss of hearing.
8. Pregnancy, and in infants and small children because of the theoretical risk of damage to permanent dentition.

Acute purulent infections may be masked or enhanced by the presence of the steroid.

Warnings: Specific antimicrobial therapy by the systemic route is indicated for the treatment of deep infections of the ear.

Precautions: Terra-Cortril Ear Suspension should not be continued for more than seven days in the absence of any clinical improvement, since in this situation occult extension of infection may occur due to the masking effect of the steroid.

The use of oxytetracycline and other antibiotics may result in an overgrowth of resistant organisms – particularly Candida and staphylococci. Constant observation of the patient for this possibility is essential. If new infections due to non-susceptible bacteria or fungi appear during therapy, Terra-Cortril Ear Suspension should be withdrawn.

If irritation develops, the product should be discontinued and appropriate therapy instituted.

Use in renal insufficiency: Terra-Cortril Ear Suspension should be used with caution because polymyxin B is potentially nephrotoxic.

Side-effects: Oxytetracycline, hydrocortisone, and polymyxin B are well tolerated by the epithelial tissues and may be used topically with minimal untoward effects. Allergic reactions may occur occasionally, but are rare. The use of Terra-Cortril Ear Suspension should be discontinued if such reactions occur.

Overdosage: No cases of overdosage with Terra-Cortril Ear Suspension have been reported. No special antidotes are required following accidental ingestion.

Pharmaceutical precautions Store below 25°C.

Legal category POM.

Package quantities 5 ml Tube with specially designed narrow nozzle.

Further information Nil.

Product licence number 0057/5073R.

TERRA-CORTRIL* SPRAY

Presentation Terra-Cortril Spray contains Oxytetracycline Hydrochloride PhEur and Hydrocortisone PhEur in finely divided form as a pressure packed presentation for topical application.

Terra-Cortril Spray is available as an aerosol in:

42 g (30 ml) container (50 mg Hydrocortisone PhEur and 150 mg Oxytetracycline as the Hydrochloride PhEur);

84 g (60 ml) container (100 mg Hydrocortisone PhEur and 300 mg Oxytetracycline as the Hydrochloride PhEur).

Inactive excipients: Lecithin, sorbitan trioleate, isopropyl myristate and Arcton 12/11.

Uses

Actions: Terra-Cortril Spray possesses both the anti-inflammatory activity of hydrocortisone and the broad spectrum antibacterial activity of oxytetracycline, which is active against a wide variety of Gram-positive and Gram-negative organisms.

Where topical therapy with hydrocortisone is of value, the concurrent use of oxytetracycline may help to eradicate secondary bacterial infection.

Indications: Terra-Cortril Spray is indicated in exudative and secondarily infected eczema including atopic eczema, primary irritant dermatitis, allergic and seborrhoeic dermatitis. Secondarily infected insect bite reactions.

In exudative flexural intertrigo Terra-Cortril Spray can be used for up to seven days.

Like other tetracyclines, oxytetracycline is generally ineffective against Pseudomonas and Proteus species. Because these are recognised secondary infecting organisms in exudative dermatoses, preliminary identification of the organism and determination of antibiotic sensitivity is important.

Terra-Cortril Spray is for topical administration only.

Dosage and administration

Adults: After thorough cleansing of the affected skin areas, a small amount of the spray should be applied covering the whole surface and keeping the container at a proper distance (approximately 20–25 cm). Applications should be made two to four times daily.

Use in the elderly: No special precautions.

Use in children: Not recommended. See 'Contra-indications'.

Contra-indications, warnings, etc

Contra-indications:

1. Hypersensitivity to any of the components of the preparation.
2. Primary bacterial infections, e.g. impetigo, pyoderma, furunculosis.
3. Acute herpes simplex, vaccinia and varicella.
4. Tuberculosis of the skin.
5. Fungal diseases of the skin.
6. Pregnancy, and in infants and small children because of the theoretical risk of damage to permanent dentition.

Warnings: When used on the face, the eyes should be closed and protected. Inhalation of the spray should be avoided.

Precautions: If irritation develops, the product should be discontinued and appropriate therapy instituted.

Terra-Cortril Spray should not be continued for more than seven days in the absence of any clinical improvement, since in this situation occult extension of infection may occur due to the masking effect of the steroid.

Extended or recurrent applications may increase the risk of contact sensitization and should be avoided.

The use of oxytetracycline and other antibiotics may result in an overgrowth of resistant organisms – particularly Candida and staphylococci. Careful observation of the patient for this possibility is essential. If new infections due to nonsusceptible bacteria or fungi appear during therapy, Terra-Cortril Spray should be discontinued.

If extensive areas are treated, there may be increased systemic absorption of the corticosteroid and suitable precautions should be taken.

Terra-Cortril Spray is not recommended for ophthalmic use.

Side-effects: Hydrocortisone and oxytetracycline are well tolerated by the epithelial tissues and may be used topically with minimal untoward effects. Allergic reactions may occur occasionally, but are rare.

The following local side-effects have been reported with topical corticosteroids, especially under occlusive dressings: burning, itching, irritation, dryness, folliculitis, hypertrichosis, acneiform eruptions, hypopigmentation, perioral dermatitis, allergic contact dermatitis, maceration of the skin, secondary infection, skin atrophy, striae, miliaria.

The use of Terra-Cortril Spray should be discontinued if such reactions occur.

Overdosage: No cases of overdosage with Terra-Cortril Spray have been reported.

Pharmaceutical precautions Store below 25°C.

Legal category POM.

Package quantities 42 g (30 ml) aerosol; 84 g (60 ml) aerosol.

Further information Nil.

Product licence number 0057/5074R.

TERRA-CORTRIL* TOPICAL OINTMENT

Presentation Terra-Cortril Topical Ointment contains 30 mg Oxytetracycline as the Hydrochloride PhEur and 10 mg Hydrocortisone PhEur in each gram of paraffin base, comprising white soft and liquid paraffin.

Uses

Actions: Terra-Cortril Topical Ointment possesses both the anti-inflammatory activity of hydrocortisone and the broad-spectrum antibacterial activity of oxytetracycline, which is active against a wide variety of Gram-positive and Gram-negative organisms.

Where topical therapy with hydrocortisone is of value the concurrent use of oxytetracycline may help eradicate secondary bacterial infection.

Indications: Terra-Cortril Topical Ointment is indicated in the following disorders: exudative and secondarily infected eczema including atopic eczema, primary irritant dermatitis, allergic and seborrhoeic dermatitis. Secondarily infected insect bite reactions.

In exudative flexural intertrigo Terra-Cortril Topical Ointment can be used for up to seven days.

Like other tetracyclines, oxytetracycline is generally ineffective against Pseudomonas and Proteus species. Because these are recognised secondary infecting organisms in exudative dermatoses, preliminary identification of the organism and determination of antibiotic sensitivity is important.

Terra-Cortril Topical Ointment is for topical administration only.

Dosage and administration

Adults: After thorough cleansing of the affected skin areas, a small amount of the ointment should be applied gently two to four times daily.

Use in the elderly: No special precautions.

Use in children: Not recommended. See 'Contra-indications'.

Contra-indications, warnings, etc

Contra-indications:

1. Hypersensitivity to any of the components of the preparation.
2. Primary bacterial infections, e.g. impetigo, pyoderma, furunculosis.
3. Acute herpes simplex, vaccinia and varicella.
4. Tuberculosis of the skin.
5. Fungal diseases of the skin.
6. Pregnancy, and in infants and small children because of the theoretical risk of damage to permanent dentition.

Precautions: If irritation develops, the product should be discontinued.

Terra-Cortril Topical Ointment should not be continued for more than seven days in the absence of any clinical improvement, since in this situation occult extension of infection may occur due to the masking effect of the steroid.

Extended or recurrent application may increase the risk of contact sensitization and should be avoided.

The use of oxytetracycline and other antibiotics may result in an overgrowth of resistant organisms – particularly Candida and staphylococci. Careful observation of the patient for this possibility is essential. If new infections due to nonsusceptible bacteria or fungi appear during therapy, Terra-Cortril Topical Ointment should be discontinued.

If extensive areas are treated or if the occlusive technique is used, there may be increased systemic absorption of the corticosteroid and suitable precautions should be taken.

Terra-Cortril Topical Ointment is not recommended for ophthalmic use.

Side-effects: Hydrocortisone and oxytetracycline are well tolerated by the epithelial tissues and may be used topically with minimal untoward effects. Allergic reactions may occur occasionally, but are rare.

The following local side-effects have been reported with topical corticosteroids, especially under occlusive dressings: burning, itching, irritation, dryness, folliculitis, hypertrichosis, acneiform eruptions, hypopigmentation, perioral dermatitis, allergic contact dermatitis, maceration of the skin, secondary infection, skin atrophy, striae, miliaria.

The use of Terra-Cortril Topical Ointment should be discontinued if such reactions occur.

Overdosage: No cases of overdosage with Terra-Cortril Topical Ointment have been reported. No special antidotes are required following accidental ingestion.

Pharmaceutical precautions Store below 25°C.

Legal category POM.

Package quantities 15 g tube; 30 g tube.

Further information Nil.

Product licence number 0057/5076R.

TERRA-CORTRIL* NYSTATIN CREAM

Presentation Terra-Cortril Nystatin Cream contains 30 mg oxytetracycline as Oxytetracycline Calcium BP., 10 mg Hydrocortisone PhEur and 100,000 units nystatin BP in each gram of perfumed homogeneous yellow cream.

Inactive excipients: These are sodium metabisulphite, polysorbate 80, soft white paraffin, liquid paraffin, stearyl alcohol, stearic acid, cetomacrogol 1000, di-sodium hydrogen ortho-phosphate, sodium hydroxide, propyl and methyl hydroxybenzoates, propylene glycol, fragrance lavender-citrus and water.

Uses *Actions:* Terra-Cortril Nystatin Cream is ideal for use in conditions where topical, nonsystemic action is desired. The oxytetracycline present will prevent or overcome superficial infections caused by organisms susceptible to it. Concomitantly, the concentration of hydrocortisone supplied is ample for inflammatory reactions resulting from allergy, infection or trauma. Nystatin is an antifungal antibiotic which is both fungistatic and fungicidal *in vitro* against a wide variety of yeasts and yeast-like fungi. It is effective for the treatment of cutaneous infections caused by *Candida albicans* and other Candida as well as other yeasts.

Thus this product provides the combined broad-spectrum activity of oxytetracycline against the primarily causative or secondarily infecting organisms, and the effectiveness of hydrocortisone, an anti-allergic, anti-inflammatory hormone, which controls excessive tissue reaction to infections, allergens, and trauma along with nystatin which prevents or eradicates secondary fungal infections.

Indications: The use of Terra-Cortril Nystatin Cream is indicated in the treatment of steroid-responsive dermatoses. The added presence of oxytetracycline and nystatin will serve to prevent or eradicate secondary bacterial and fungal complications. Since varying degrees of bacterial and/or fungal infection frequently complicate those skin conditions for which hydrocortisone topical therapy is indicated, this combined preparation may offer therapeutic advantages over the use of hydrocortisone alone.

Among these conditions are: Atopic dermatitis: including allergic eczema, both disseminated and circumscribed neurodermatitis, pruritus with lichenification, eczematoid dermatitis and food eczema.

Cutaneous infections: including superficial pyogenic infections, pyoderma, pustular dermatitis, and infections associated with minor burns or wounds.

Contact dermatitis: due to plants, drugs, cosmetics, clothing material and miscellaneous substances.

Non-specific pruritus: of the anus, vulva or scrotum.

Dosage and administration
Adults: After thorough cleansing of the affected skin areas, a small amount of the cream should be applied gently. Applications should be made two to four times daily. When actual infection is present, the cream may be applied on sterile gauze and, by this means, kept in contiguous contact with the affected area. Care should be taken not to discontinue therapy too soon after the initial response has been obtained.

Supplementary therapy with oral antibiotics is advisable in the treatment of severe infections or those which may become systemic.

Use in the elderly: No special precautions.

Use in children: Not recommended. See 'Contra-indications'.

Contra-indications, warnings, etc
Contra-indications:
1. Acute herpes simplex, vaccinia and varicella.
2. Tuberculosis of the skin.
3. Hypersensitivity to any of the components of the cream.
4. Acute purulent infections.
5. Pregnancy, and in infants and small children because of the theoretical risk of damage to permanent dentition.

Precautions: The use of oxytetracycline and other antibiotics may result in an overgrowth of resistant organisms. Observation of the patient for this possibility is required.

If irritation develops, the product should be discontinued and appropriate therapy instituted.

If a favourable response does not occur promptly, the corticosteroid should be discontinued until the infection has been adequately controlled.

If extensive areas are treated or if the occlusive technique is used there will be increased systemic absorption of the corticosteroid and suitable precautions should be taken.

Terra-Cortril Nystatin Cream is not for ophthalmic use.

Side-effects: Oxytetracycline, hydrocortisone and nystatin are well tolerated by the epithelial tissues and may be used topically with minimal untoward effects. Allergic reactions may occur occasionally, but are rare.

The following local side-effects have been reported with topical corticosteroids, especially under occlusive dressings: burning, itching, irritation, dryness, folliculitis, hypertrichosis, acneiform eruptions, hypopigmentation, perioral dermatitis, allergic contact dermatitis, maceration of the skin, secondary infection, skin atrophy, striae, miliaria.

The use of Terra-Cortril Nystatin Cream should be discontinued if such reactions occur.

Overdosage: No cases of overdosage with Terra-Cortril Nystatin Cream have been reported. No special antidotes are required following accidental ingestion.

Pharmaceutical precautions Store below 25°C.

Legal category POM.

Package quantities 30 g tube.

Further information Nil.

Product licence number 0057/0099.

TROSYL* NAIL SOLUTION

Presentation Trosyl Nail Solution is a clear, slightly yellow solution containing 28% w/w tioconazole. Each ml of solution contains 280 mg tioconazole.

Inactive excipients: These are undecylenic acid and ethyl acetate.

Uses Tioconazole is a broad spectrum imidazole antifungal agent. Trosyl Nail Solution is indicated for the topical treatment of nail infections due to susceptible fungi (dermatophytes and yeasts).

Dosage and administration
Adults: The solution should be applied to the affected nails and immediately surrounding skin every twelve hours using the applicator brush supplied.

The duration of treatment is up to six months but may be extended to twelve months.

Use in the elderly: No special precautions are required. Use the adult dose.

Use in children: No special precautions are required. Use the adult dose.

Contra-indications, warnings, etc
Contra-indications: Trosyl Nail Solution is contra-indicated in individuals who have been shown to be hypersensitive to imidazole antifungal agents, or to any of the components of the solution.

Use in pregnancy: In animal studies tioconazole was not teratogenic. At high doses it increased the incidence of renal abnormalities in rat embryos, but this effect was minor and transient and was not evident in weaned animals. There is insufficient evidence as to the drug's safety in human pregnancy, although absorption after topical administration is negligible. Because of the extensive duration of treatment required for nail infections, the use of Trosyl Nail Solution is contra-indicated throughout pregnancy.

Precautions: Trosyl Nail Solution is not for ophthalmic use.

Side-effects: Trosyl Nail Solution is well tolerated following local application and no systemic adverse reactions have been observed. Symptoms of local irritation have been reported by some patients, but are usually seen during the first week of treatment and are transient and mild.

However, if a sensitivity reaction develops with the use of Trosyl Nail Solution, treatment should be discontinued and appropriate therapy instituted.

Overdosage: No cases of overdosage with Trosyl Nail Solution have been reported. In the event of excessive oral ingestion, gastrointestinal symptoms may occur. Appropriate means of gastric lavage should be considered.

Pharmaceutical precautions Store between 4°C and 30°C. Avoid flame and heat.

Legal category POM.

Package quantities Amber glass bottles containing 12 ml of solution.

Further information Nil.

Product licence number 0057/0236.

**Trade Mark*

Pharbita Limited
33 Liberty Close
Woolsbridge Industrial Park
Three Legged Cross
Wimborne, Dorset BH21 6SY

pharbita φβ

SALBUTAMOL CYCLOCAPS*

Presentation Salbutamol Cyclocaps are intended only for use in the Cyclohaler* and together present an alternative system for administering salbutamol as a breath actuated dry powder inhalation that is effective at relatively low inspiratory flow rates.

Salbutamol Cyclocaps are available in capsules containing the equivalent of either 200 micrograms or 400 micrograms of micronised salbutamol together with suitable excipients. The 200 micrograms Cyclocap has a light green opaque cap and a clear transparent body and is imprinted φβ 935. The 400 micrograms Cyclocap has a dark green opaque cap and a clear transparent body and is imprinted φβ 945. The contents of the Cyclocaps have been specifically designed to give optimum results using the Cyclohaler and they are not suitable for use with other inhalers. Neither are other types of inhalation cartridges suitable for use with the Cyclohaler.

Cyclocaps are blister packed enabling patients to hygienically carry a small supply together with the Cyclohaler in the specially designed Cyclohaler box.

Uses Salbutamol is a β-adrenergic stimulant which when inhaled in therapeutic doses has a selective action on bronchial β_2-adrenoceptors with almost no effect on cardiac β_1-receptors. Salbutamol Cyclocaps are therefore indicated in the management, (treatment and prevention), of bronchial asthma in which reversible bronchial obstruction is present. Salbutamol Cyclocaps can also be used in the treatment of (acute) reversible airway obstructions and as maintenance treatment in chronic asthma and bronchitis.

Salbutamol Cyclocaps have a rapid beneficial effect when inhaled and are thus suitable for treatment of acute attacks, whilst their relatively long duration of action makes them suitable for maintenance and prophylactic therapy.

Dosage and administration

Adults: For the treatment of acute bronchospasms or periodic episodes of asthma 200 micrograms or 400 micrograms to be inhaled as a single dose. For maintenance therapy in chronic obstructive lung disease a dosage regime of 400 micrograms three or four times daily is recommended.

Children: For the treatment of acute bronchospasms or periodic episodes of asthma 200 micrograms to be inhaled as a single dose. For maintenance therapy in chronic obstructive lung disease a dosage regime of 200 micrograms three or four times daily is recommended.

Salbutamol Cyclocaps are for inhalation only and may only be inhaled using the Cyclohaler in accordance with the instructions for use included in the Cyclohaler box. For optimum results in most patients Salbutamol Cyclocaps should be used on a regular basis.

Contra-indications, warnings, etc

Contra-indications: Hypersensitivity to salbutamol, lactose or gelatine. Inhaled salbutamol preparations are not suitable for managing premature labour and should not be used for threatened abortion during the first and second trimester of pregnancy.

Precautions: Avoid using combinations of salbutamol with beta-blocking agents if possible, particularly non-selective beta-blocking drugs such as propranolol. Salbutamol should be used carefully in patients with thyrotoxicosis, hypertension, myocardial insufficiency or cardiac arrhythmias. The duration of action of Salbutamol Cyclocaps is about 6 hours, patients should be advised that if the effects of a single inhalation persist for less than three hours they should seek medical advice as a change in their treatment regime may be advisable.

Pregnancy: There is insufficient data to evaluate any possible harmful effects of salbutamol when used during pregnancy in humans, animal studies have indicated some evidence of harmful effects on the foetus. If possible the use of salbutamol during pregnancy should therefore be avoided.

Side-effects: At normal therapeutic doses side effects are usually rare, transient and mild. They are due to the pharmacological properties of the drug and are the result of over-stimulation of the adrenergic receptors leading to muscle tremors, peripheral vasodilation, headache and a positive inotropic and chronotropic effect. At very high doses tachycardias and arrhythmias have been reported. As with other inhalation therapy the potential for paradoxical bronchospasm and muscle cramps should be borne in mind and if they occur therapy with salbutamol should be discontinued.

Overdosage: Patients should be warned of the risks of exceeding the prescribed dose. If beta-adrenergic stimulation is so great as to require treatment one may have recourse to cardioselective beta blocking agents, but these must be used with caution in patients with a history of bronchospasm.

Pharmaceutical precautions To keep the Cyclocaps in the best condition it is important that they are stored in a dry place and are not exposed to extremes of heat or cold. Storage under adverse conditions for sustained periods can adversely affect the operation of the Cyclohaler/Cyclocap system.

Legal category POM.

Package quantities Salbutamol Cyclocaps 200 µg and 400 µg are supplied in blister strips in packs containing 100 Cyclocaps each. Up to 1 blister strip of 10 Cyclocaps can be stored in the special Cyclohaler carrying case for patient convenience and to assist compliance.

Further information Salbutamol Cyclocaps have not been shown to be incompatible with other pharmaceutical products, but possible adverse effects of beta-blocking agents should be considered.

Product licence numbers

Salbutamol Cyclocaps 200 micrograms	5322/0001
Salbutamol Cyclocaps 400 micrograms	5322/0002

**Trade Mark*

Pharmax Limited
Bourne Road
Bexley
Kent DA5 1NX

COLOMYCIN* INJECTION

Presentation Colomycin Injection is Colistin Sulphomethate Injection BP presented as a neutral glass vial containing a creamy-white crystalline powder (before reconstitution). Available as:
Colistin Sulphomethate Sodium BP 500,000 units;
Colistin Sulphomethate Sodium BP 1,000,000 units.

Uses By aerosol inhalation, as adjunct therapy in patients already receiving standard antibiotic therapy.

Parenterally or via other routes where routine antibiotic therapy has been unsuccessful.

Colomycin injection should only be used to treat severe systemic or localised infections caused by sensitive gram negative organisms, e.g. respiratory infection and septicaemia.

Dosage and administration Colomycin Injection is administered by aerosol, intramuscularly or intravenously following reconstitution with sterile water or saline, but when indicated can be introduced via other routes such as subconjunctivally (used with 0.5% lidocaine) and by local instillation.

Normal recommendations for systemic treatment are:

Children (up to 60 kg): 50,000 units/kg body weight in 24 hours, divided into three eight-hourly doses. Serum levels should be measured if used in the newborn.

Adults (including elderly) (over 60 kg): 6,000,000 units in 24 hours (i.e. 2 × 1,000,000 unit vials every eight hours).

Infusion therapy: Daily dosage as above. Infusion should preferably be completed within six hours.

Aerosol therapy: Daily dosage as above, concomitant with parenteral administration. For the aerosol, colistin is dissolved in water or saline for use in a suitable nebuliser attached to an air/oxygen supply.

Bladder irrigation: 1,000,000 units are dissolved in 50 ml water or saline and instilled during catheterisation. In the presence of infection, administration is carried out twice daily.

The above are expressed as average doses. Should clinical or bacteriological response be slow, dosage may be increased as indicated by the patient's condition. Minimum of five days treatment is recommended.

Where there is moderate or severe renal impairment excretion of the antibiotic is delayed. Therefore, size of dose and dosage interval should be adjusted in relation to renal function. The table below is a guide to dosage modifications in order to prevent accumulation of Colomycin. It is stressed that adjustments may still have to be made on evaluation of the individual patient. Blood level estimations are recommended: 10–15 microgram/ml should be adequate.

Contra-indications, warnings, etc Colomycin injection is contra-indicated in patients with known sensitivity to colistin. With appropriate dosage modifications, Colomycin need not be withheld in cases of renal impairment. Curariform muscle relaxants should be used with extreme caution in patients receiving Colomycin injection.

Adverse effects on renal function have been reported, usually following use of higher than recommended doses in patients with normal renal function, or failure to reduce the dosage in patients with renal impairment or during concomitant use of other nephrotoxic antibiotics. The effects are usually reversible on discontinuation of therapy.

Other reversible adverse effects may include transient sensory disturbances such as facial paraesthesia and vertigo, and rarely, vasomotor instability, slurred speech, visual disturbance, confusion or psychosis. Neurotoxicity has been reported in association with overdosage, failure to reduce dosage in patients with renal insufficiency and the concomitant use of either curariform agents or antibiotics with similar neurotoxic effects. Therapy need not be discontinued and reduction of dosage may alleviate symptoms.

Bronchospasm may occur on antibiotic inhalation; this may be treated with $beta_2$ agonists.

Permanent nerve damage such as deafness or vestibular damage has not been reported. Local irritation at the site of injection is minimal.

Overdosage: Overdose can result in renal insufficiency, muscle weakness and apnoea.

There is no specific antidote; management is supportive treatment plus attempts to increase the rate of elimination of colistin, e.g. mannitol diuresis, prolonged haemodialysis or peritoneal dialysis.

Use in pregnancy and lactation: Safety in human pregnancy has not been established. Animal studies do not indicate teratogenic properties; however, single dose studies in human pregnancy show that Colomycin crosses the placental barrier, and there is a risk of foetal toxicity if repeated doses are given to pregnant patients. Colomycin is secreted in breast milk and patients to whom the drug is administered should not breast feed an infant.

Pharmaceutical precautions Vials should be stored in a cool, dry place, protected from light. Solutions of colomycin for parenteral administration should preferably be freshly prepared. Compatible infusion solutions are normal saline; 5% dextrose; 5% fructose; Ringer's solution. Infusions should be completed within six hours.

Mixed infusions or injections involving Colomycin should be avoided.

Legal category POM.

Package quantities Boxes of 10 × 500,000 unit vials and 10 × 1,000,000 unit vials.

Further information Colistin is a polypeptide antibiotic which possesses bactericidal activity against most Gram-negative organisms. Clinically it is of particular

Creatinine clearance (ml/min)	*B.U.N. (mg/100 ml)*	*(mmol/l)*	*Adult dosage*	*Childrens' dosage*
20–72	>60	>10	1–2 million units every 8 hr	12,500–16,000 units/kg every 8 hr
10–20	>100	>16.5	1 million units every 12–18 hr	12,500 units/kg every 12–18 hr
<10	>200	>33	1 million units every 18–24 hr	8,000 units/kg every 18–24 hr

value in serious infections caused by pathogens such as Pseudomonas aeruginosa, Escherichia coli, Klebsiella spp. It cannot be recommended for Proteus spp.

Susceptible organisms do not readily develop or acquire resistance and R factor mediated resistance has not been encountered.

(1 mg of colistin sulphomethate sodium is approx. 12,500 units).

Product licence numbers
500,000 units 0108/5005
1,000,000 units 0108/5006.

COLOMYCIN* STERILE POWDER

Presentation White crystalline powder in neutral glass vial containing Colistin Sulphate BP 1 g. (1 mg of colistin sulphate is approx. 19,500 units.)

Uses Colistin is a polypeptide antibiotic which possesses bactericidal activity against most Gram-negative organisms. Clinically it is of particular value in serious infections caused by pathogens such as *Pseudomonas aeruginosa, Escherichia coli*, Klebsiella spp. It cannot be recommended for Proteus spp.

Colomycin Sterile Powder is used for the treatment of topical infections caused by sensitive gram-negative organisms.

Dosage and administration Colomycin sterile powder is applied topically as a 1% solution, powder, or ointment according to the site of infection, as follows:

1% solution in water or saline – for use as eye and ear drops, wound irrigation, application to dressings.

1% dispersed powder in lactose or Biosorb – for application to infected leg ulcers and in other skin infections.

The undiluted powder should NOT be applied topically.

1% ointment in Simple Cream BP, simple cream plus hydrous lanolin (90:10), Hydrous Ointment BP; Macrogol Ointment BPC for use in skin infections.

COLOMYCIN STERILE POWDER MUST NOT BE USED FOR THE PREPARATION OF INJECTABLE SOLUTIONS.

Contra-indications, warnings, etc
Contra-indications: Colomycin preparations are contra-indicated in patients with known sensitivity to colistin. Colomycin powder should not be used for the treatment of otitis externa if the tympanic membrane is perforated.

Precautions and warnings: Colistin absorption has not been detected following limited topical application. Absorption may however increase with prolonged use and in the case of topical treatment absorption may be enhanced if applied to large areas of broken skin. Nevertheless, caution should be applied in the use of Colomycin Powder in patients with renal failure, and in patients receiving curariform muscle relaxants.

Use in pregnancy and lactation: Safety in human pregnancy has not been established. Animal studies do not indicate teratogenic properties; however parenteral single dose studies in human pregnancy show that Colomycin crosses the placental barrier, and there is a risk of foetal toxicity if repeated doses are given to pregnant patients. Colomycin is secreted in breast milk and patients to whom the drug is administered should not breast feed an infant.

Side-effects: Topical therapy is well tolerated; transient irritation at the site of application has been reported infrequently. Allergic sensitisation has not occurred.

Systemic side-effects have not been reported following topical administration, however following systemic therapy with colistin adverse effects on renal function have been reported, usually following use of higher than recommended doses in patients with normal renal function, or failure to reduce the dosage in patients with renal impairment, or during concomitant use of other nephrotoxic antibiotics. The effects are usually reversible on discontinuation of therapy.

Adverse effects following systemic administration may include transient sensory disturbances such as perioral paraesthesia and vertigo. Neurotoxicity has been reported in association with overdosage, failure to reduce dosage in patients with renal insufficiency and the concomitant use of either curariform agents or antibiotics with similar neurotoxic effects. Therapy need not be discontinued and reduction of dosage may alleviate symptoms.

Permanent nerve damage such as deafness or vestibular damage has not been reported.

Overdosage: No symptoms of overdosage have been reported following topical use of Colistin. However, use of the undiluted powder causes stinging and is not recommended. Following systemic administration overdosage can result in renal insufficiency, muscle weakness and apnoea.

There is no specific antidote; management is supportive treatment plus attempts to increase the rate of elimination of colistin e.g. mannitol diuresis, prolonged haemodialysis or peritoneal dialysis.

Pharmaceutical precautions All Colomycin preparations should be stored in a cool, dry place, protected from light.

Colymycin Powder Solutions should be freshly prepared and stored between 2–8°C. Any unused solution should be discarded within 24 hours. Ointments or dispersed powders prepared from Colomycin Sterile Powder (See Dosage and Administration) may be stored for up to one month at room temperature, as may preserved solutions.

Eye and ear drop solutions may be preserved using 0.002% phenylmercuric nitrate.

Legal category POM.

Package quantities Vials of 1 g.

Further information A solution of Colomycin Sterile Powder in water may be used as an alternative to Colomycin Syrup where a sugar free solution for oral treatment is required. (See data sheet for Colomycin Syrup and Tablets.)

Product licence number 0108/5010.

COLOMYCIN* SYRUP

Presentation Pale pink powder for reconstitution, containing Colistin Sulphate BP 4,000,000 units per bottle (i.e. 250,000 units/5 ml, when dispensed). This product also contains sucrose, benzoic acid and methyl parabens.

Uses The treatment of gastro-intestinal infections caused by sensitive Gram-negative organisms. Also bowel preparation. Colistin Sulphate is not absorbed from the gastro-intestinal tract, and must *not therefore be used for systemic infections.*

Dosage and administration Oral
Children up to 15 kg: 250,000–500,000 units (i.e. 5–10 ml syrup) every eight hours.

Children of 15–30 kg: 750,000–1,500,000 units every eight hours.

Adults, elderly and children over 30 kg: 1,500,000–3,000,000 units every eight hours.

A minimum of five days treatment is recommended. Should clinical or bacteriological response be slow, dosage may be increased.

Bowel preparation: A 24-hour course of Colistin Sulphate at the normal dosage above. Treatment should preferably finish 12 hours before surgery.

Contra-indications, warnings, etc There are no absolute contra-indications to oral therapy, and side-effects are rare. The syrup base contains sucrose. In cases of intolerance a solution of Colomycin Sterile Powder can be used.

Pharmaceutical precautions Colomycin preparations should be stored in a cool dry place, protected from light.

After reconstitution with water, Colomycin Syrup is stable for two weeks at room temperature.

Legal category POM.

Package quantities Bottle for reconstitution to 80 ml.

Further information 1 mg Colistin Sulphate is approx. 19,500 units.

Product licence number 0108/5009.

COLOMYCIN* TABLETS

Presentation White tablet with 'P' in a hexagon on one face and two crossed score-marks on reverse, each containing Colistin Sulphate BP 1,500 units. (1 mg of Colistin Sulphate is approx. 19,500 units.)

Uses Colistin is a polypeptide antibiotic which possesses bactericidal activity against most Gram-negative organisms. Clinically it is of particular value in serious infections caused by pathogens such as *Pseudomonas aeruginosa, Escherichia coli,* Klebsiella spp. It cannot be recommended for Proteus spp.

Colomycin Tablets may be used for the treatment of gastro-intestinal infections caused by sensitive Gram-negative organisms. Also for bowel preparation.

Colistin sulphate is not absorbed from the gastro-intestinal tract, except in infants under the age of 6 months, and must not be given orally for the treatment of systemic infections in any age group.

Dosage and administration *Oral:* Children up to 15 kg: 250,000–500,000 units (i.e. 5–10 ml syrup) every 8 hours. Children 15–30 kg: 750,000–1,500,000 units every 8 hours. Adults (including the elderly) (over 30 kg): 1,500,000–3,000,000 units every 8 hours.

A minimum of 5 days' treatment is recommended. Dosage may be increased when clinical or bacteriological response is slow.

For bowel preparation, a 24-hour course at the normal dosage above is given. Treatment should preferably finish 12 hours before surgery.

Contra-indications, warnings, etc
Contra-indications: Colomycin preparations are contra-indicated in patients with known sensitivity to colistin.

Precautions and warnings: Colistin is subject to limited and unpredictable absorption from the GI tract in infants under 6 months. Studies in older children and in adults have demonstrated no systemic absorption of Colistin following oral administration.

Nevertheless, caution should be employed in the use of Colomycin Tablets in patients with renal failure, and in patients, receiving curariform muscle relaxants.

Use in pregnancy and lactation: Safety in human pregnancy has not been established. Animal studies do not indicate teratogenic properties; however parenteral single dose studies in human pregnancy show that Colomycin crosses the placental barrier, and there is a risk of foetal toxicity if repeated doses are given to pregnant patients. Colomycin is secreted in breast milk and patients to whom the drug is administered should not breast feed an infant.

Side-effects: Systemic side-effects have not been reported following oral administration; however following systemic therapy with colistin adverse effects on renal function have been reported, usually following use of higher than recommended doses in patients with normal renal function, or failure to reduce the dosage in patients with renal impairment, or during concomitant use of other nephrotoxic antibiotics. The effects are usually reversible on discontinuation of therapy.

Adverse effects following systemic administration may include transient sensory disturbances such as perioral paraesthesia and vertigo. Neurotoxicity has been reported in association with overdosage, failure to reduce dosage in patients with renal insufficiency and the concomitant use of either curariform agents or antibiotics with similar neurotoxic effects. Therapy need not be discontinued and reduction of dosage may alleviate symptoms.

Permanent nerve damage such as deafness or vestibular damage has not been reported.

Overdosage: No symptoms of overdosage have been reported following oral use of Colistin. However, following systemic administration, overdosage can result in renal insufficiency, muscle weakness and apnoea.

There is no specific antidote; management is supportive treatment plus attempts to increase the rate of elimination of colistin e.g. mannitol diuresis, prolonged haemodynamics or peritoneal dialysis.

Pharmaceutical precautions All Colomycin preparations should be stored in a cool, dry place, protected from light.

Legal category POM.

Package quantities Securitainers of 50 tablets.

Further information Nil.

Product licence number 0108/5008.

FLETCHERS'* ARACHIS OIL RETENTION ENEMA

Presentation Ready-to-use, self-contained single-dose, disposable enema containing Arachis Oil BP 130 ml.

Uses To soften impacted faeces.

Dosage and administration For rectal administration only.
Adults and elderly patients: 1 enema as required.

Children: In proportion, according to bodyweight.

The enema should be warmed before use by placing in warm water.

Contra-indications, warnings, etc Not for use in children unless under medical supervision. Use with caution in patients with intestinal obstruction.

Care should be taken not to use undue force in administration of the enema especially in elderly or debilitated patients or those with neurological disorders.

Pharmaceutical precautions Store at room temperature.

Legal category P.

Package quantities Box of 10 enemas.

Further information Nil.

Product licence number 0108/5016.

FLETCHERS' ENEMETTE*

Presentation Ready-to-use, self-contained single-dose, disposable microenema of 5 ml liquid containing: Docusate Sodium BP 90 mg, Glycerol PhEur 3780 mg.

This product also contains sorbic acid.

Uses Routine treatment of constipation. Pre- and post-operative cleansing of the bowel, in obstetrics and prior to proctoscopy, sigmoidoscopy or X-ray examination.

Dosage and administration For rectal administration only.
Adults, elderly and children over 3 years: 1 enema as required.
Children under 3 years: Not recommended.

Contra-indications, warnings, etc
Contra-indications: Nil

Precautions: Use with caution in patients with intestinal obstruction.

Care should be taken not to use undue force in administration of the enema especially in elderly or debilitated patients or those with neurological disorders.

Pharmaceutical precautions Store in a cool place. Protect from heat.

Legal category P.

Package quantities Box of 12 microenemas.

Further information The formulation of docusate sodium, a faecal softening agent, in glycerol (which when administered rectally promotes peristalsis and evacuation of the lower bowel) and polyethylene glycol, provides an easy-to-use, efficacious, low-volume enema.

Product licence number 0108/0078.

FLETCHERS'* PHOSPHATE ENEMA

Presentation Fletchers' Phosphate Enema is Phosphate Enema BPC, Formula B, in a ready-to-use, self-contained, disposable, single-dose enema of 128 ml aqueous solution containing:

Sodium Acid Phosphate BP	10.0% w/v
Sodium Phosphate PhEur	8.0% w/v

This product also contains disodium edetate.

Available with standard or long rectal tube.

Uses Routine treatment of constipation. Pre- and post-operative cleansing of the bowel, in obstetrics and prior to proctoscopy, sigmoidoscopy or X-ray examination.

Dosage and administration For rectal administration only.
Adults and elderly patients: 1 enema, as required.

Children: Under 3 years, contra-indicated. Over 3 years, in proportion, according to bodyweight.

The enema may be administered at room temperature, or warmed in warm water before use. The long-tube variety will provide better operating distance for staff and easier control for self-administration.

Contra-indications, warnings, etc
Contra-indications: Contra-indicated in patients with inflammatory or ulcerative conditions of the large bowel, in those with increased colonic absorptive capacity e.g. Hirschsprung's disease, and in those with acute gastrointestinal conditions.

This product should not be used in children under three years old.

Precautions: There have been occasional reports of apparent vasovagal attacks occurring in elderly patients following the administration of phosphate enemata.

Prolonged use may lead to irritation of the anal canal. This product should be used with caution in patients requiring a reduced sodium intake and electrolyte balance should be maintained during extended use.

Use with caution in patients with intestinal obstruction.

Care should be taken not to use undue force in administration of the enema especially in elderly or debilitated patients or those with neurological disorders.

Pharmaceutical precautions Store in a cool place.

Legal category P.

Package quantities Box of 50 enemas.

Further information Nil.

Product licence number 0108/5015.

INFACOL*

Presentation A white opaque liquid, containing activated dimethicone 40 mg/ml (as Simethicone Emulsion USP). This product also contains methyl and propyl parabens.

Uses An antiflatulent for the relief of griping pain, colic or wind due to swallowed air.

Dosage and administration Oral.
Infants: 20 or 40 mg (0.5 or 1.0 ml) administered before feeds.

Adults and elderly: not applicable.

Contra-indications, warnings, etc
Contra-indications: None known.

Warning: If symptoms persist, seek medical advice.

Side-effects: None known.

Use in pregnancy and lactation: Not applicable.

Overdosage: In the event of deliberate or accidental overdosage, treat symptoms on appearance.

Pharmaceutical precautions Store at room temperature (25°C).

Legal category GSL.

Package quantities Bottle of 50 ml.

Further information Treatment with Infacol will provide a progressive improvement in symptoms over several days.

Product licence number 0108/0100.

LASMA*

Presentation White capsule shaped tablets, imprinted 'PHARMAX' on one side and single scored on the reverse. Lasma is a sustained release tablet containing Theophylline PhEur 300 mg.

Uses Lasma tablets are indicated for the treatment and prophylaxis of bronchospasm associated with asthma (including nocturnal asthma), emphysema and bronchitis.

Dosage and administration Oral.
Adults: Therapy should commence with 2 tablets (600 mg daily), preferably after food. In patients of 70 kg body weight or over the dosage should be increased after 1 week to 3 tablets (900 mg) daily.

The daily dosage is administered as one Lasma tablet every 12 hours, preferably after food. The dosage may be increased, as necessary, by half tablet increments.

Nocturnal asthma: In patients where nocturnal symptoms predominate, therapeutic benefit of up to 12 hours duration may be achieved by administration of Lasma tablets as a single dose in the late evening to prevent the characteristic 'early-morning dip' in peak expiratory flow rate, thus allowing patients an uninterrupted nights sleep. Any day-time symptoms may then be controlled by inhaled bronchodilators.

Contra-indications, warnings, etc
Contra-indications: There are no absolute contra-indications to theophylline, however caution should be exercised in the treatment of patients with cardiac arrhythmias, peptic ulcers or severe hypertension. Cardiac failure or hepatic dysfunction decreases theophylline clearance and patients with such conditions should be carefully monitored.

Precautions: Lasma tablets should be swallowed whole and not chewed. It is recommended, as with all xanthine preparations, that patients are individually titrated to their correct daily dosage by blood level estimations. Once a patient is stabilised on an effective dosage regime of Lasma tablets this should not be changed, nor should an alternative product be substituted without re-titration of the dosage by clinical assessment and blood-level estimations.

Side-effects: Side-effects (particularly tremor) are rare at plasma theophylline concentrations of less than 20 microgram/ml but may include gastro-intestinal disturbances, headache, CNS stimulation and tremor.

Use in pregnancy and lactation: Safety in human pregnancy has not been established. Theophylline crosses the placental barrier and is secreted in breast milk.

Interactions: Lasma should not be used concurrently with other preparations containing xanthine derivatives. Theophylline has been reported to interact with a number of drugs.

The following increase clearance and it may therefore be necessary to increase dosage to ensure a therapeutic effect: phenytoin, carbamazepine, rifampicin, sulphinpyrazone and barbiturates. Smoking and alcohol consumption can also increase clearance of theophylline. The following reduce clearance and a reduced dosage may therefore be necessary to avoid side-effects: allopurinol, cimetidine, erythromycin, thiabendazole, ciprofloxacin, isoprenaline and oral contraceptives. Factors such as viral infections, liver disease and heart failure also reduce theophylline clearance. There are conflicting reports concerning the potentiation of theophylline by influenza vaccine and physicians should be aware that interaction may occur. A reduction of dosage may also be necessary in the elderly patient.

The following should also be used with caution in patients taking theophylline preparations: halothane, lomustine and lithium.

Xanthines can potentiate hypokalaemia resulting from $beta_2$ agonist therapy, steroids, diuretics and hypoxia.

Particular caution is advised in severe asthma. It is recommended that serum potassium levels are monitored in such situations.

Overdosage: Symptoms may include nausea, vomiting, gastro-intestinal irritation, cramps, convulsions, tachycardia and hypotension.

The stomach contents should be emptied and supportive measures employed to maintain circulation, respiration and fluid and electrolyte balance. Electrocardiographic monitoring should be carried out and in severe poisoning charcoal haemoperfusion should be used.

Pharmaceutical precautions None.

Legal category P.

Package quantities Bottles of 100 tablets.

Further information Lasma is a sustained release formulation of theophylline designed to facilitate the control of plasma theophylline levels within the optimum range. This reduced diurnal variation in plasma levels provides for:

(i) Reduced risk of rapid and excessive absorption of theophylline and hence improved safety.

(ii) Maintenance of the desired plasma levels, so providing continuous protection.

(iii) Improved convenience of dosing for the patient.

Product licence number 0108/0075.

MUCOGEL* SUSPENSION AND TABLETS

Presentation
Suspension: A white mint flavoured suspension. Each 5 ml contains:

Aluminium Hydroxide equivalent to dried gel BP	220 mg
Magnesium Hydroxide BP	195 mg

This product also contains methyl and propyl parabens.

Tablets: White mint flavoured tablet containing

Dried Aluminium Hydroxide Gel BP	400 mg
Magnesium Hydroxide BP	400 mg

This product also contains sucrose.

Uses Antacid therapy in gastric and duodenal ulcer, gastritis, heartburn, gastric hyperacidity. Treatment of indigestion.

Suspension only: Relief of symptoms of heartburn and dyspepsia associated with gastric reflux in hiatus hernia, reflux oesophagitis and similar conditions.

Dosage and administration Oral.
Suspension: Adults, elderly and children over 12 years old: 10–20 ml three times daily 20 minutes to one hour after meals, and at bedtime, or as required.
Children under 12 years: Not recommended.

Tablets: Adults, elderly and children over 12 years old: One or two tablets, well chewed, should be taken 20 minutes to one hour after meals and at bedtime or as required.
Children under 12 years: Not recommended.

Contra-indications, warnings, etc
Contra-indications: Mucogel should not be used in patients who are severely debilitated or suffering from kidney failure. Antacids inhibit the absorption of tetracyclines and vitamins and should not be taken concomitantly.

Adverse effects: Gastrointestinal side-effects are uncommon. This formulation minimises the problems of diarrhoea and constipation.

Use in pregnancy and lactation: Unnecessary drug therapy should be avoided in the first trimester of pregnancy.

Overdosage: Serious symptoms are unlikely to follow overdosage.

Pharmaceutical precautions Suspension; Do not freeze. Tablets: No special precautions.

Legal category GSL.

Package quantities Suspension: Bottles of 500 ml. Tablets: Packs of 100.

Further information Mucogel is a pleasant-tasting, well tolerated antacid containing balanced quantities of aluminium and magnesium.

Product licence numbers
Suspension: 0108/0074
Tablets: 0108/0079.

PREDENEMA*

Presentation Ready-to-use, self-contained, single-dose, disposable enema of 100 ml aqueous solution containing Prednisolone Metasulphobenzoate Sodium, equivalent to Prednisolone 20 mg. This product also contains disodium edetate and methyl, propyl and ethyl parabens.

Uses Local treatment of ulcerative colitis.

Dosage and administration For rectal administration only.
Adults only: 1 enema nightly for two to four weeks, extending the course when a good response is being obtained. The long tube presentation facilitates self-administration.

The enema may be administered at room temperature or warmed in warm water before use.

Contra-indications, warnings, etc Administration of prednisolone via this route for this indication is seldom associated with adverse effects. It is contra-indicated in local conditions such as peritonitis, fistulae, intestinal obstruction, perforation of the bowel where it might mask infection or impair healing.

Precautions: Symptoms of adrenal insufficiency have not been reported, but prolonged therapy should be carefully monitored. Use with caution in patients with intestinal obstruction.

Use in pregnancy: Topical administration of corticosteroids to pregnant animals can cause abnormalities of foetal development. The relevance of this finding to human beings has not been established. However, physicians should be aware of the possibility of teratogenic effects, and also of potential suppression of the HPA axis, and should weigh up the risk/benefit ratio before using Predenema in pregnancy. If treatment is instituted with Predenema, the minimum dosage and frequency of administration required for clinical control should be employed, and prolonged usage should be avoided.

Pharmaceutical precautions Store below 25°C, protected from light.

Legal category POM.

Package quantities Long tube box of 7 enemas
Standard tube box of 10 enemas.

Further information Nil

Product licence number 0108/5018.

PREDFOAM*

Presentation A white, mucoadherent aerosol foam containing prednisolone metasulphobenzoate sodium equivalent to 20 mg prednisolone per metered dose.

This product also contains disodium edetate and Phenonip (phenoxyethanol and 4-hydroxybenzoate acid esters).

Uses Treatment of proctitis and ulcerative colitis.

Dosage and administration
Adults and elderly patients: One metered dose inserted rectally once or twice daily for two weeks, extending treatment for a further two weeks when a good response is obtained. Use should be discontinued at the discretion of the physician once the disease is stable and under control.

Children: Not recommended.

Contra-indications, warnings, etc
Contra-indications: Local conditions where infection might be masked or healing impaired e.g. peritonitis, fistulae, intestinal obstruction, perforation of the bowel.

Precautions: This product should be used with extreme caution in the presence of severe ulcerative colitis. The possible occurrence of masking of local or systemic infection should be borne in mind when using this product. For rectal use only.

Side-effects: The consequences of systemic absorption should be considered with extensive use over prolonged periods. As with all rectal corticosteroids, prolonged continuous use is undesirable.

Use in pregnancy and lactation: There is inadequate evidence of safety in human pregnancy. Topical administration of corticosteroids to pregnant animals can cause abnormalities of foetal development including cleft palate and intra-uterine growth retardation. There may therefore be a very small risk of such effects in the human foetus.

Overdosage: Overdosage by this route is unlikely.

Pharmaceutical precautions Pressurised container. Protect from sunlight and do not expose to temperatures above 50°C. Do not pierce or burn even after use. Shake before use.

Legal category POM.

Package quantities Box consisting of an aerosol canister containing 25 g (approximately 14 applications) plus 14 disposable applicators.

Further information Nil.

Product licence number 0108/0101.

SAVENTRINE* TABLETS

Presentation White tablet with grey/brown surface speckling and 'P' in hexagon embossed on one face. Each tablet contains Isoprenaline Hydrochloride BP 30 mg.

This product also contains sucrose.

Uses As a second-line treatment in chronic atrioventricular dissociation as a temporary measure where pacing is not available or has been declined.

Dosage and administration Oral.
Adults and elderly patients: Dosage must be tailored to the requirements of the individual patient. Treatment is best initiated under observation in hospital with facilities available for monitoring ECG and for cardiac resuscitation.

The usual initial dosage is 1 tablet (30 mg) six-hourly and this can be increased quite rapidly if required. Daily dosage may range from 90 mg in some patients to 840 mg in others, with frequency of administration varying from eight-hourly to two-hourly. Optimum dosage is that which satisfactorily controls the heart rate with minimum side-effects.

Tablets must be swallowed whole, they are not for sublingual administration.

Children: Contra-indicated.

Contra-indications, warnings, etc
Contra-indications: Saventrine is contra-indicated in acute coronary disease and in patients prone to episodes of ventricular fibrillation or tachycardia.

Side-effects: Include palpitations, tremor, tachycardia, precordial pain. Sweats, facial flushing, headache and diarrhoea have also been reported. Incidence of side-effects with this presentation is less than with sublingual isoprenaline, and side-effects usually respond to dosage adjustment.

Use in pregnancy and lactation: Not recommended unless considered essential by the physician.

Overdosage: Symptoms of overdosage are as listed in the 'Side-effects' section above. Fatality may also occur in cases of serious overdosage. In the event of overdosage, toxic effects may be diminished by a beta-adrenergic blocking drug and should be accompanied by monitoring of heart rhythm.

Pharmaceutical precautions Store below 25°C.

Legal category POM.

Package quantities Securitainers of 30 and 250 tablets.

Further information Saventrine contains granules of Isoprenaline Hydrochloride coated with varying numbers of layers of ethylcellulose.

Isoprenaline is a potent sympathomimetic amine acting almost exclusively via beta-adrenergic receptors, and exerts positive chronotropic and inotropic effects on the heart.

Product licence number 0108/5028.

SAVENTRINE* i.v.

Presentation Glass ampoules containing a stabilised solution of Isoprenaline Hydrochloride BP for injection. Each ampoule contains 2 ml of 1 mg/ml solution (pH 2.5–2.8).

This product also contains ascorbic acid, disodium edetate and Water for Injections PhEur.

Uses
1. Cardiogenic or endotoxic shock states.
2. Acute Stokes-Adams attacks and other cardiac emergencies.
3. Severe bradycardia precipitated by beta-adrenergic antagonists and disopyramide.
4. Evaluation of congenital heart defects.

Dosage and administration The usual route is by intravenous infusion, in 5% dextrose solution or Water for Injections PhEur. Widely varying doses have been used with success.

Adults and elderly patients:
1. Shock states: 0.5–10 microgram/min or alternatively intracardiac injection of 0.1 mg in 10 ml water.
2. Acute Stokes-Adams attack: 4–8 microgram/min or alternatively, intracardiac injection of 0.1 mg in 10 ml water.
3. Severe bradycardia: 1–4 microgram/min.
4. Evaluation of congenital cardiac defects: 1.5–4 microgram/min.

Children: Adjust above dosage in proportion to weight.

Contra-indications, warnings, etc Saventrine i.v. is contra-indicated in acute coronary disease and in patients prone to episodes of ventricular fibrillation or tachycardia secondary to their slow rate.

Isoprenaline may precipitate ventricular extrasystoles and arrhythmias, especially in patients who may be hypersensitive to the drug. In such cases the infusion rate should be reduced or possibly discontinued.

Precautions: Use with caution in patients with hyperthyroidism or diabetes. This product is not recommended for oral administration.

Side-effects: These may include palpitations, tremor, precordial pain, sweats, facial flushing, headache.

Interactions: Isoprenaline may induce arrhythmias when administered with halothane, cyclopropane and trichloroethylene.

Pregnancy and lactation: Safety during pregnancy and lactation has not been established. The risk to benefit ratio should be assessed in individual circumstances.

Overdosage: Symptoms of overdosage are as listed in the 'Side-effects' section above. Fatality may also occur in cases of serious overdosage. A beta-adrenergic blocking drug may diminish toxic effects and should be accompanied by monitoring of heart rhythm.

Pharmaceutical precautions Store in a cool place protected from light.

Legal category POM.

Package quantities Carton of 6 ampoules.

Further information Isoprenaline Hydrochloride is a sympathomimetic amine with potent activity at beta-adrenergic receptors.

Product licence number 0108/5030.

SUSCARD* BUCCAL TABLETS

Presentation White biconvex tablets, marked with the dosage strength on one face. Suscard is a controlled release presentation of glyceryl trinitrate in four strengths, 1 mg, 2 mg, 3 mg and 5 mg, for buccal administration (see below).

Uses The management and treatment of angina pectoris. This product may also be of benefit in the in-patient management of unstable angina. Acute and congestive cardiac failure.

Dosage and administration
Administration Buccal.
The Suscard tablet is placed high up between the upper lip and the gum to either side of the front teeth.

The diagrams below show the correct placement of the tablet.

The onset of action of Suscard tablets is extremely rapid, and the tablets may be substituted for sublingual glyceryl trinitrate tablets in the treatment of acute angina pectoris. The duration of action of the Suscard tablet, once in place, as shown above, correlates with the dissolution time of the tablet. This is normally 3–5 hours. However, the first few doses may dissolve more rapidly until the patient is used to the presence of the tablet.

During the dissolution period the tablet will soften and adhere to the gum; in practice the presence of the tablet is not noticeable to the patient after a short time.

Patients should be instructed as to the correct placement of the tablet and should note the following points:

(a) The tablet should not be moved about the mouth with the tongue, as this will cause it to dissolve more rapidly.
(b) A slight stinging sensation (as for sublingual glyceryl trinitrate) may be felt for a few minutes after placement of the tablet.
(c) If a tablet is **accidentally** swallowed it may be replaced by a further tablet.
(d) In patients who wear dentures, the tablet may be placed in any comfortable position between the lip and the gum.
(e) The patient may alternate the placement of successive tablets on the right and left sides of the front teeth.

Suscard tablets do not interfere with the ingestion of food or liquids.

Dosage: Adults and elderly patients
Angina: administration of Suscard tablets should start with the 2 mg strength. If angina occurs while the tablet is in place, the dosage strength used should be increased to 3 mg where necessary. The 5 mg dosage strength should be reserved for patients with severe angina

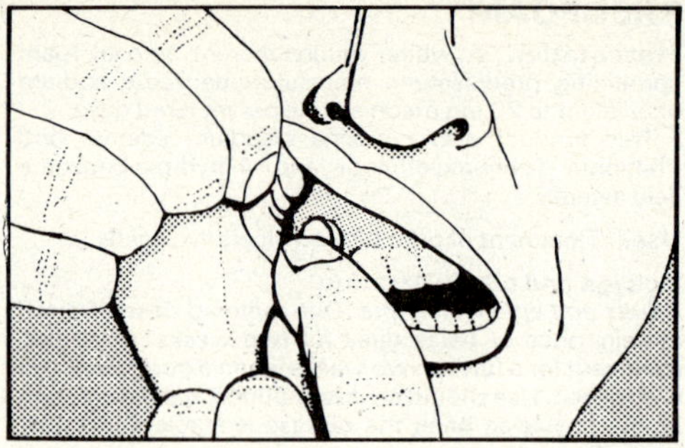

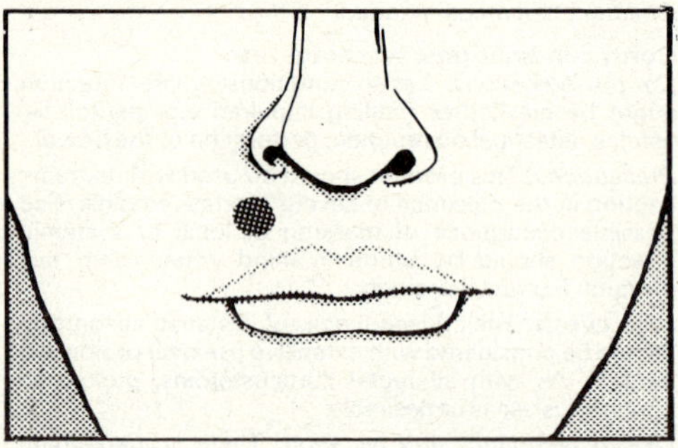

THE TABLETS SHOULD *NOT* BE PLACED UNDER THE TONGUE, CHEWED OR INTENTIONALLY SWALLOWED.

pectoris refractory to treatment with the lower dosage strengths. A 1 mg dosage strength is also available and may be considered for the small number of patients who initially show intolerance to the 2 mg strength as a starting dose.

Suggested dosage frequency in angina:

(a) For patients suffering only occasional angina pectoris – The tablets may be administered on a p.r.n. basis, to relieve the acute attack.
(b) For patients suffering angina pectoris in response to known stimuli – The tablet may be administered a few minutes prior to encountering the angina-precipitating stimulus.
(c) For patients in whom chronic therapy is indicated – The tablet should be administered on a thrice daily basis or as dictated by the dissolution rate of the tablet in an individual patient. If angina occurs during the period between the disappearance of one tablet and the time the next tablet is due to be put in place, dosage frequency should be increased.

Note that if an acute attack of angina pectoris is suffered while a tablet is in place, an additional tablet may be positioned on the opposite side of the mouth.

Acute heart failure: Administer 5 mg repeated as indicated by patient response until symptoms abate.

Unstable angina: Dosage should be rapidly titrated upwards in order to relieve and prevent symptoms. Suscard Tablets may be used in addition to pre-existing anti-anginal therapy, where considered appropriate.

As indicated in the section above the higher 5 mg dosage strength may be required to achieve a satisfactory therapeutic response in patients exhibiting severe symptoms.

Unstable angina is a serious condition managed under hospitalised conditions and involving continuous monitoring of ECG changes with frequent monitoring of appropriate haemodynamic variables. In common with other nitrate therapy a fall in systolic blood pressure of 10–15 mm Hg may occur.

Congestive cardiac failure: Dosage should commence with the 5 mg strength, administered three times daily. In moderately severe or severe cases, particularly where patients have not responded to standard therapy (digitalis/diuretics), the dosage may need to be increased to 10 mg (2 × 5 mg tablets) t.i.d. over a period of three or four days. In such instances one tablet should be placed between the upper lip and the gum, on each side of the front teeth.

Contra-indications, warnings, etc Contra-indications are as for glyceryl trinitrate. Suscard tablets should not be used in patients with marked anaemia, head trauma, cerebral haemorrhage or closed angle glaucoma nor in patients with known hypersensitivity to nitrates.

Precautions: Rarely, prolonged use in susceptible individuals with poor dental hygiene and associated plaque may lead to an increased risk of dental caries. Patients should therefore be instructed to alternate the site of application and careful attention should be paid to dental hygiene, particularly in those areas where the tablet is applied.

Use in pregnancy and lactation: There is no information on the safety of nitrates in pregnancy and lactation; nitrates should not be administered to pregnant women and nursing mothers unless considered essential by the physician.

Side-effects: Side-effects are predominantly headache, dizziness, facial flushing and postural hypotension. In the unlikely event of severe side-effects, the tablet may simply be removed from the mouth.

Overdosage: Toxic effects of glyceryl trinitrate include vomiting, restlessness, cyanosis, methaemoglobinaemia and syncope. Overdosage (i.e. if large numbers of tablets have been swallowed) should be treated with gastric aspiration and lavage, plus attention to respiratory and circulatory symptoms.

Pharmaceutical precautions Store at room temperature.

Legal category P.

Package quantities Blister strips of 10 tablets in packs of 100 tablets (OP).

Further information Nil.

Product licence numbers
1 mg 0108/0067
2 mg 0108/0069
3 mg 0108/0073
5 mg 0108/0071.

SUSTAC*

Presentation Pink tablets with surface speckling and 'P' in hexagon embossed on one face. Sustac is a prolonged release presentation of glyceryl trinitrate in three strengths; 2.6 mg, 6.4 mg and 10.0 mg. These products also contain lactose and sucrose.

Uses Prophylactic therapy of angina pectoris.

Dosage and administration
Adults and elderly patients: Sustac tablets must be swallowed whole and not chewed. They are not for sublingual administration. Dosage should be tailored to the requirements of the individual patient, but it is usually 1 or 2 tablets of the 2.6 mg or 6.4 mg strength taken three times daily, or 1 tablet of the 10 mg strength two or three times daily. Tablets should be taken between meals.

Contra-indications, warnings, etc
Contra-indications: Contra-indications are as for glyceryl trinitrate. Sustac should not be used in patients with marked anaemia, head trauma, cerebral haemorrhage, incipient glaucoma.

Use in pregnancy and lactation: There is no evidence relating to the safety of nitrates in pregnancy and lactation; nitrates should not be administered to pregnant women and nursing mothers unless considered essential by the physician.

Side-effects: Include facial flushing and headache, hypotension and coldness of the skin.

Withdrawal from therapy: As with other drugs for the treatment of angina pectoris, abrupt discontinuation of therapy may lead to an exacerbation of symptoms. When discontinuing long-term treatment, the dosage should be reduced gradually over several days, and the patient carefully monitored.

Overdosage: In the event of accidental or deliberate overdosage toxic effects of glyceryl trinitrate include vomiting restlessness, cyanosis, methaemoglobinaemia tachycardia and syncope. Patients should receive gastric aspiration and lavage and be given respiratory and circulatory support. The physician should be aware that tablets in the intestine will release their content over several hours.

Pharmaceutical precautions Can be stored at room temperature.

Legal category P.

Package quantities 2.6 mg and 6.4 mg: Securitainers of 250 tablets. 10 mg: Bottles of 100 tablets.

Further information Sustac can be used in combination with reduced beta-blockade dosage to give a patient full anti-anginal support, and at the same time reduce the likelihood of beta-blockade side-effects.

Product licence numbers
2.6 mg 0108/5031
6.4 mg 0108/5032
10 mg 0108/0064

**Trade Mark*

Porton Products Ltd
Porton House
Vanwall Road
Maidenhead
Berkshire SL6 4UB

PORTON

DYSPORT* ▼

Presentation Dysport is supplied as a white freeze-dried pellet containing 500 units of *Clostridium botulinum* type A toxin-haemagglutinin complex in a clear glass vial, for use in a single patient. One unit is defined as the median lethal intraperitoneal dose in mice.

Uses Dysport is used for the treatment of blepharospasm and hemifacial spasm.

Dosage and administration The exposed central portion of the rubber stopper should be cleaned with alcohol immediately prior to piercing the septum. Using a sterile 23 or 25 gauge needle, 2.5 ml of Sodium Chloride Injection BP (0.9%) at room temperature should be injected into the vial and mixed gently to dissolve the contents. This will yield a clear solution containing 200 units per ml of Dysport.

In the treatment of bilateral blepharospasm the recommended initial dose is 120 units per eye.

After the skin around each eye has been cleaned, the following injections should be made subcutaneously using a 2 ml syringe with a 23 or 25 gauge needle. A dose of 0.1 ml (20 units) should be made medially and of 0.2 ml (40 units) should be made laterally into the junction between the preseptal and orbital parts of both the upper and lower orbicularis oculi muscles of each eye. For injections into the upper lid, the needle should be directed away from its centre to avoid the levator muscle. A diagram to aid placement of these injections is provided in the package insert.

The relief of symptoms may be expected to begin within two to four days with maximal effect within two weeks.

Injections should be repeated approximately every eight weeks or as required to prevent recurrence of symptoms.

On such subsequent administrations the dose may need to be reduced to 80 units per eye – viz: 0.1 ml (20 units) medially and 0.1 ml (20 units) laterally above and below each eye in the manner previously described. The dose may be further reduced to 60 units per eye by omitting the medial lower lid injection.

In cases of unilateral blepharospasm, the injections should be confined to the affected eye.

Patients with hemifacial spasm should be treated as for unilateral blepharospasm.

The doses recommended are applicable to adults of all ages including the elderly.

The safety and effectiveness of Dysport in children has not been demonstrated.

Contra-indications, warnings, etc Teratological and other reproductive studies have not been performed with Dysport. The safety of its use in pregnant or lactating women, or women of child-bearing age has not been demonstrated.

Side-effects may occur from deep or misplaced injections of Dysport temporarily paralysing other nearby muscle groups. They may also occur from exacerbation of pre-existing eyelid abnormalities or from an initial over-correction. Ptosis is the most common unwanted effect and will be experienced from time to time by the majority of patients. A few patients may also experience diplopia or symptoms from spread of the paralytic effect to mid-facial muscles. These side-effects may be expected to resolve within two to four weeks. Keratitis and dry eyes due to reduced blinking have also been reported. The use of artificial tears could be considered for such patients. Minor bruising and lid swelling may occur but are short lived. Reversible external ophthalmoplegia has been reported after excessive dosing. In conformity with normal clinical practice, all patients should be alerted to possible side effects.

There are no reports of any immune response after the local administration of *Clostridium botulinum* type A toxin-haemagglutinin complex in accordance with these dosage recommendations.

Excessive doses may produce distant and profound neuromuscular paralysis. There is no specific antidote; antitoxin should not be expected to be beneficial. General supportive care is advised with artificial respiratory support, if necessary, until symptoms resolve.

Pharmaceutical precautions Unopened vials must be maintained at temperatures between 2°C and 8°C. After reconstitution, Dysport should be used within one hour and should not be frozen.

Immediately after treatment of the patient, any residual Dysport which may be present in either vial or syringe, should be inactivated with dilute hypochlorite solution (1% available chlorine). Thereafter all items should be disposed of in accordance with standard hospital practice.

Spillage of Dysport should be wiped up with an absorbent cloth soaked in dilute hypochlorite solution.

Legal category POM.

Package quantities Each pack contains two vials.

Further information Botulinum type A toxin blocks the release of acetylcholine from motor nerve terminals. It binds specifically and permanently to the motor end plate. Repeat injections are necessary as new nerve end plates usually form within two to three months.

Product licence number 6958/0003.

ERWINASE*

Crisantaspase (asparaginase from *Erwinia chrysanthemi*)

Presentation Erwinase is supplied as a white freeze-dried powder in clear glass vials containing 10,000 International Units (I.U.) of Erwinia L-asparaginase.

Uses Erwinase is used in combination with other antineoplastic agents to treat acute lymphoblastic leukaemia. It may also be used in other neoplastic conditions where depletion of asparagine might be expected to have a useful effect. Patients receiving treatment with L-asparaginase from *Escherichia coli* and who develop hypersensitivity to that enzyme may be able to continue treatment with Erwinase since the enzymes are antigenically different.

Dosage and administration The usual dose is 200 I.U./kg bodyweight (5,000–6,000 I.U./m^2 body surface area) but reference to recent MRC leukaemia trials should be made for current information on dose, route and frequency of treatment. Erwinase solution should be given by intramuscular or subcutaneous injection; infusion or intravenous route may also be used.

Contra-indications, warnings, etc Erwinase is a bacterial protein and it may be considered necessary to test patients for hypersensitivity before starting treatment. For this purpose an intradermal injection of 50 I.U. in 0.1–0.2 ml should be given and the site observed for 3 hours. Erwinase should not be given if there is a severe reaction. It should also preferably be given without interruption. If, however, an interruption cannot be avoided, treatment should be resumed with a low dose, 10 I.U./kg/day, and increased to the full dose over 5 days if tolerated. Anaphylaxis is rare but facilities should be made available for its management during administration.

Erwinase should not be given to women who are, or are likely to become pregnant.

Adverse reactions are generally reversible. The following side-effects have been reported: fever, nausea, vomiting, CNS depression, hypersensitivity. Various plasma biochemical changes have been seen including increased BSP retention, increased bilirubin, AspAT, alkaline phosphatase and cholesterol levels. Decreased fibrinogen and some other clotting factors have also been noted.

Overdosage is unlikely to occur because of the method of presentation and the need to establish each patient's dose after testing for hypersensitivity.

Pharmaceutical precautions Store at 2 to 8°C. Shelf life is three years.

Erwinase is not a typical cytotoxic drug and so does not require the special precautions needed for handling cytotoxic drugs. It should be handled in the same way as other therapeutic enzymes such as hyaluronidase.

The contents of each vial should be reconstituted in 1 to 2 ml of Sodium Chloride for Injection BP and dissolved by gentle mixing with minimal contact with the cap. The solution should be administered without delay since contact with the rubber stopper denatures the reconstituted drug producing a few minute filaments of insoluble material. The effect is not progressive and does not affect the potency but the solution should be administered without delay.

Legal category POM.

Package quantities Each pack contains 20 vials.

Further information Erwinase is now well established as an effective agent, when used in conjunction with other anti-neoplastic drugs for induction of remission in patients with acute lymphoblastic leukaemia. The incidence of side-effects is less with Erwinia asparaginase than with *E. coli* asparaginase. Intramuscular injection appears to minimise the risk of hypersensitivity and is the preferred route of administration.

Product licence number 4073/0003.

HYATE*:C ▼

Presentation Hyate:C is a highly purified freeze dried concentrate of porcine antihaemophilic factor (Factor VIII:C). Hyate:C is in the form of a white lyophilised powder for reconstitution with 20 ml Water for Injections BP per vial. Each vial contains between 400–700 units of Factor VIII:C. The assayed amount of activity is stated on the label.

Uses Hyate:C is intended for the treatment or prevention of bleeding in patients with haemophilia A who have inhibitors to Human Factor VIII:C.

Dosage and administration The dosage of Hyate:C required for control of bleeding varies for individual patients. The required dose is dependent upon:

1. The weight of the patient.
2. The activity of the antibody against Hyate:C.
3. The type of haemorrhage and desired plasma Factor VIII:C level.

The required dose is determined by administering a preliminary dose of Hyate:C and assaying the post-infusion level of Factor VIII:C in the patient's plasma. According to the response, dosage can then be increased or decreased for subsequent infusions. It is commonly observed that recovery of Factor VIII:C increases during a course of treatment, possibly as a result of saturation of circulating antibody. It is therefore desirable to monitor pre and post infusion levels of Factor VIII:C for each dose.

An estimate of the preliminary dose of Hyate:C required for the initial infusion can be made in the following ways:

1. If the patient's antibody titre against Hyate:C is not known, but the anti-human Factor VIII:C titre is less than 50 Bethesda Units/ml, an initial dose of 25–50 units/Kg body weight for a moderately severe joint or muscle bleed, or 100 units/Kg body weight, for a major life threatening bleed is recommended.[1]

2. If the patient's antibody titre against Hyate:C is known or can be determined, a prediction of the dose of Hyate:C required to neutralise the antibody can be made using the formula:

Neutralising dose =
Plasma volume (ml) × antibody titre (Bethesda Units/ml).

The incremental dose must then be added to this neutralising dose to increase the Plasma Factor VIII level by the desired amount. This increment can be calculated by assuming that 1 unit of Hyate:C per Kg body weight will give rise to a 1.5 units/decilitre increase in plasma Factor VIII:C activity.[2]

Example:
Patient body weight: 55 Kg
Haematocrit: 0.5 litre/litre
Antibody titre: 3 Bethesda units
Desired Factor VIII:C Level: 40% of normal i.e. 40 units Factor VIII/dl of Plasma.
Dose-response relationship: 1 unit of Hyate:C per Kg body weight will give rise to a 1.5 units/decilitre increase in plasma factor VIII:C activity.
Average blood volume: 80 ml/Kg

(i) *Plasma volume*
Patient's body weight × Average Blood Volume × (1 minus Haematocrit)
i.e. Plasma Volume: 55 × 80 × (1–0.5) = 2,200 ml.

(ii) *Neutralising dose*
Plasma Volume × Antibody Titre
i.e. Neutralising Dose: 2,200 × 3 = 6,600 units

(iii) *Incremental dose*

$$\frac{\text{Desired plasma Factor VIII:C level} \times \text{Patient's body weight}}{\text{Dose-response relationship}}$$

i.e. Incremental dose: $\frac{40 \times 55}{1.5} = 1466$ units

(iv) *Total dose:* Neutralising Dose + Incremental Dose
i.e. Total Dose: 6,600 × 1466 = 8066 units.

3. If the patient's antibody titre against Hyate:C is not known, but the anti-human Factor VIII:C level is greater than 50 Bethesda units/ml, an initial dose of 100–250 units/Kg body weight is suggested, followed by determination of the Plasma Factor VIII:C level.[1]

4. If a patient has previously been treated with Hyate:C, this may provide a guide to his likely response, and therefore assist in estimation of the preliminary dose.

Subsequent dose administration: Following administration of the preliminary dose, if the recovery of Factor VIII:C in the patient's plasma is not sufficient, a further dose should be administered. If the recovery after the second dose is still insufficient a third and higher dose may prove effective.

Determination of the activity of the inhibitor against Hyate:C: A modification of the Bethesda assay[3] is recommended. Hyate:C should be diluted to 1 unit per ml in haemophilic plasma and used as a substrate in the Bethesda assay.

Reconstitution and administration:

1. Warm the unopened vials of Hyate:C to between 20°C and 37°C.
2. Clean the exposed central portion of the rubber stopper with antiseptic immediately prior to piercing.
3. Using a sterile needle and syringe slowly inject 20 ml of Water for Injections BP into the vial.
4. Withdraw the needle and shake the vial gently, avoiding frothing, until the powder is completely dissolved. This usually takes less than 5 minutes.
5. Withdraw the solution into a syringe using a filter needle.
6. Replace the filter needle with a sterile injection needle and administer intravenously at a rate of not more than 2–5 ml per minute.

Contra-indications, warnings, etc There are no known contra-indications to Hyate:C.

Acute infusion reactions: On rare occasions Hyate:C may give rise to acute infusion reactions, such as anaphylactic shock.

Adrenaline, hydrocortisone and facilities for resuscitation should be available in case these reactions occur.

Mild infusion reactions: Hyate:C may give rise to reactions such as fever, chills, headache, nausea, vomiting and skin rashes. These reactions are more common after the first infusion of a course of treatment, and tend to lessen in frequency and severity as further infusions are given. Hydrocortisone and/or antihistamine may alleviate these effects and may be prescribed as a precautionary measure.

Immune response to Hyate:C: Infusion of Hyate:C may be followed by a rise in plasma levels of inhibitor to both human and porcine Factor VIII:C. Inhibitor levels to both porcine and human Factor VIII:C should therefore be monitored after treatment.

Effect on the platelet count: A significant fall in the patient's platelet count occurs on rare occasions after infusion of Hyate:C. However, monitoring of the platelet count during the treatment period is recommended.

Pharmaceutical precautions Hyate:C should be stored at a temperature of −15°C to −20°C and should be used before the expiry date stated on the package. Reconstituted Hyate:C must not be stored and should be used within 3 hours.

Legal category POM.

Package quantities Vials contain not less than 400 units of Porcine Factor VIII:C Hyate:C.

Further information The ease of reconstitution of Hyate:C in 20 ml Water for Injections BP makes it suitable for syringe administration facilitating high dose therapy.

References

[1] Kernoff P. B. A. et al. Blood *63*: 31–41, 1984.
[2] Gatti L. and Manucci P. H. Thromb. & Haemostas *51*: 379–384, 1984.
[3] Kasper C. K. et al. Thrombos. Diathes. Hamorrh. *34*: 869–872, 1975.

Product licence number 3070/0007.

**Trade Mark*

Quinoderm Limited
Manchester Road
Oldham OL8 4PB

CEANEL* CONCENTRATE

Presentation
Active ingredients:

Phenylethyl Alcohol BPC	7.5%
Cetrimide BP	10%
Undecenoic Acid BP	1%

Other ingredients: Lauric diethanolamide, diethanolamine, fragrance, poly oxy propylene stearyl ether.

Appearance: Ceanel Concentrate is a clear, viscous, amber-coloured liquid.

Uses *Main pharmacological action:* Cetrimide is particularly active against Gram-positive organisms. This feature combined with the bactericidal action of phenylethyl alcohol and the fungicidal properties of undecenoic acid makes Ceanel Concentrate particularly effective in the treatment of dermatological conditions. Ceanel Concentrate is effective in removing debris and scale in seborrhoea capitis, and psoriasis of the scalp.

Indications: As an adjunct in the management of psoriasis of the scalp, seborrhoeic dermatitis, dandruff, psoriasis of the trunk and limbs.

Dosage and administration
Adults, children and the elderly: Scalp conditions: Wet the scalp and hair with warm water. Protect the eyes with a towel to avoid discomfort. Apply $\frac{1}{2}$–1 teaspoonful of Ceanel to the wetted scalp. Then apply a small amount of water and work up into a lather. Rinse and repeat. Finally rinse the hair and scalp *thoroughly*. Use three times in the first week and twice weekly thereafter.

Other areas of the body: Wet the area to be treated with warm water; apply sufficient Ceanel Concentrate by gentle massage to cover the wetted area. Allow to remain in contact for two minutes. Remove the Ceanel by thorough rinsing with warm water. Use as required.

Contra-indications, warnings, etc *Precaution:* The eyes should be protected during treatment. A simple way to do this is with a towel.

Overdosage: Ceanel Concentrate is for external use only. Following accidental ingestion, nausea and vomiting may occur as well as respiratory problems and hypotension. Treatment is supportive and symptomatic avoiding gastric lavage.

Warning: There is inadequate evidence of safety in human pregnancy, but it has been in wide use for many years without apparent ill consequence. As with other medicaments it may be used during pregnancy if the anticipated benefits outweigh the risks. No problems are anticipated during lactation.

Pharmaceutical precautions *Storage:* No special precaution required.

Diluents: Ceanel Concentrate is easily removed by warm water.

Legal category P.

Package quantities Available in packs of 50 ml, 150 ml and 500 ml.

Further information In clinical trials Ceanel Concentrate was used on 31 patients suffering from psoriasis, seborrhoeic eczema, atopic eczema or infected eczema of the scalp. A complete clearing of scaling was obtained in 24 of the 25 patients with psoriasis, and in all six patients with eczema.

Greasiness of the scalp was eliminated in 20 of the 21 patients with psoriasis who showed this feature.

Product licence number 0291/5002R.

ECZEDERM* CREAM

Presentation
Active ingredients:

Calamine BP	20.88%
Arachis Oil BP	12.5%

Other ingredients: Fragrance, pentaerythritol dioleate, Isopropyl Myristate BP, Sorbitan Mono Oleate BP, White Soft Paraffin BP, Maize Starch BP, Dehymuls F (high molecular weight fatty acids and salts), triethylene glycol (trace), 1,2 propylene glycol (trace), 5 chloro-2-methyl-4-isothiazoline-3-one (trace), benzyl alcohol (trace), 2 methyl-4-isothiazoline-3-one (trace).

Appearance: Eczederm is a pink-coloured cream.

Uses *Main pharmacological action:* The soothing and healing properties of calamine have been combined with the bland cooling effect from the special emollient base. This has produced a unique blend of useful therapeutic properties.

Indications: Mild dermatoses including both wet and dry eczemas especially where steroid-containing preparations should be avoided.

Dosage and administration *Adults and children:* Spread thinly over the affected area up to three times a day. The use of occlusive dressings may be considered in dry scaly dermatoses.

Contra-indications, warnings, etc Eczederm Cream is for topical use only. There are no known contra-indications except true hypersensitivity to one of the ingredients. Ingestion should be avoided.

Pharmaceutical precautions *Storage:* Eczederm should be stored in a cool place and extremes of temperature avoided.

Diluents etc: Eczederm is not suitable for dilution or reformulation.

Legal category GSL.

Package quantities Eczederm is supplied in tubes of 30 g and 60 g. Also available in plastic containers of 500 g.

Further information This preparation does not contain parabens-type compounds or lanolin. It is of special use where steroid-containing preparations are contra-indicated.

Product licence number 0291/0003.

GELCOSAL*

Presentation
Active ingredients:

Strong Coal Tar Solution BPC	5%
Tar BP (Pine Tar)	5%
Salicylic Acid BP	2%

Other ingredients: Poly oxy propylene stearyl ether, Hydroxy Propyl Methyl Cellulose BPC.

Appearance: Gelcosal is a light-brown thixotropic gel which spreads easily and cleanly on the skin. It is non-sticky, non-greasy and being water-miscible is easily removed and does not permanently stain the skin.

Uses
Main pharmacological action: The combination of two different tars in Gelcosal provides a preparation with antipruritic, keratolytic and antiseptic properties. The combination also provides the usual therapeutic activity of tars.

Salicylic acid provides a keratolytic action.

The salicylic acid constituent of Gelcosal allows removal of scale and thus access of the tar components to the underlying diseased areas.

The base has been developed with the objective of providing a cosmetically acceptable thixotropic formulation at the same time as retaining the therapeutic efficacy of crude tar.

Indications: Treatment of psoriasis in the chronic scaling phase. Treatment of dermatitis in the chronic scaling phase.

Dosage and administration
Adults and Children: By gentle massage over all the affected area twice daily. Unless hands are being treated, rinse hands thoroughly following application.

Contra-indications, warnings, etc
Contra-indications: Known sensitivity or intolerance to any of the ingredients.

Precautions: For external use only. Keep away from eyes and other muscosal surfaces.

Overdosage: Not applicable.

Main side-effects/adverse reactions: N.B. Prolonged use over large areas of topical preparations containing salicylic acid may result in symptoms of salicylism e.g. tinnitus. In view of this extra caution should be exercised when treating children.

Pharmaceutical precautions *Storage:* Store in a cool place.

Legal category P.

Package quantities 50 g.

Further information If sensitivity occurs or infection appears, discontinue use and institute appropriate therapy. Some patients may not be able to tolerate salicylic acid in which case Gelcotar may be a suitable alternative.

Gelcosal is water-miscible and does not permanently stain the skin.

Product licence number 0291/0019.

GELCOTAR*

Presentation
Active ingredients:

Strong Coal Tar Solution BPC	5%
Tar BP (Pine tar)	5%

Other ingredients: Poly oxy propylene stearyl ether, Hydroxy Propyl Methyl Cellulose BPC.

Appearance: Gelcotar is a light-brown thixotropic gel which spreads easily and cleanly on the skin. It is non-sticky, non-greasy and being water-miscible is easily removed and does not permanently stain the skin.

Uses *Main pharmacological action:* The combination of two different tars in Gelcotar provides a preparation with antipruritic, keratolytic and antiseptic properties. The combination also provides the usual therapeutic activity of tars.

The base has been developed with the objective of providing a cosmetically acceptable thixotropic formulation at the same time as retaining the efficacy of crude tar.

Indications: Treatment of psoriasis.

Treatment of dermatitis in the chronic phase.

Dosage and administration *Adults and children:* By gentle massage over all the affected area twice daily.

Contra-indications, warnings, etc
Contra-indications: Known sensitivity or intolerance to any of the ingredients.

Precautions: For external use only. Keep away from the eyes and other mucosal surfaces.

Overdosage: Not applicable.

Main side-effects/adverse reactions: None reported.

Pharmaceutical precautions *Storage:* Store in a cool place.

Legal category P.

Package quantities 50 g and 500 g.

Further information If sensitivity occurs or infection appears discontinue use and institute appropriate therapy.

Gelcotar is water-miscible and does not permanently stain the skin.

Product licence number 0291/0011.

GELCOTAR* LIQUID

Presentation
Active ingredients:

Strong Coal Tar Solution BP	1.25%
Cade Oil BPC	0.5%

Other ingredients: Lauric diethanolamide, triethylene glycol (trace), 1,2 propylene glycol (trace), 5 chloro-2-methyl-4-isothiazoline-3-one (trace), benzyl alcohol (trace), 2-methyl-4-isothiazoline-3-one (trace), poly ethylene mono tallowate, di sodium fatty acid monoethanolamide sulpho succinate, ricinoleic propyl amido trimethyl ammonium metho sulphate, triethanolamine lauryl sulphate, lecithin, fragrance.

Appearance: Gelcotar Liquid is a completely clear deep red/brown viscous liquid.

Uses *Main pharmacological action:* The combination of strong coal tar solution and cade oil provides a preparation with antiseptic and keratolytic properties to be used as a medicated scalp cleanser.

Indications: Psoriasis of the scalp, seborrhoeic dermatitis and dandruff.

Dosage and administration *Adults and children:* Wet the scalp and hair with warm water. Sufficient Gelcotar Liquid should be applied to produce a generous lather. Massage the scalp and surrounding area with the fingertips. Rinse and repeat. Finally rinse the hair and scalp thoroughly.

Use twice weekly or as directed by the medical practitioner.

Contra-indications, warnings, etc
Contra-indications: Patients with known sensitivity or intolerance to strong coal tar solution or cade oil should not use Gelcotar liquid.

Precautions: Contact with eyes and other mucosal surfaces should be avoided. All medicines should be kept out of reach of children.

Pharmaceutical precautions *Storage:* No special precaution required.

Diluents: Gelcotar Liquid can be easily removed by warm water.

Legal category GSL.

Package quantities Gelcotar Liquid is available in bottles of 150 ml and 350 ml.

Further information Gelcotar Liquid is of value in removing pastes and pomades used to treat psoriasis.

Product licence number 0291/0018.

HIOXYL* CREAM

Presentation
Active ingredients:

Stabilised Hydrogen Peroxide BP	1.5%

Other ingredients: Lactic Acid BP, White Soft Paraffin BP, Sodium Acid Phosphate BP, Maize Starch BP, cetyl stearyl alcohol, sodium cetyl stearyl sulphate, PEG 40 castor oil.

Appearance: A smooth, white, non-greasy cream with virtually no odour.

Uses *Main pharmacological action:* The antiseptic effect of hydrogen peroxide is a result of its ready release of oxygen when applied to tissues. The effect only lasts as long as oxygen is being released, and for solutions of hydrogen peroxide, this is only of short duration.

Hioxyl Cream is a unique formulation in which hydrogen peroxide has been stabilised in a soothing, easy to apply, cream to give prolonged antiseptic action.

Indications: The treatment of leg ulcers, pressure sores, minor wounds and infections.

Dosage and administration *Adults and children:* Hioxyl Cream is applied freely using a piece of lint or gauze. If necessary it may be covered with a dressing. The application can be repeated as required.

Contra-indications, warnings, etc There are no known contra-indications or warnings to the use of Hioxyl Cream.

Pharmaceutical precautions Store in a cool place.

Legal category P.

Package quantities Tubes of 25 g and 100 g.

Further information Care should be taken to avoid usage with other topical medicaments due to possible chemical interaction negating the active principle.

Product licence number 0291/0008.

HYDROMOL* CREAM

Presentation

Active ingredients:

Arachis Oil BP	10.0%
Isopropyl Myristate BP	5.0%
Liquid Paraffin BP	10.0%
Sodium pyrrolidone carboxylate	2.5%
Sodium Lactate	1.0%
Emollient base to	100%

Other ingredients: Cetomacrogol Emulsifying Wax BP, myristyl myristate, Cetomacrogol 1000 BP, triethylene glycol (trace), 1,2 propylene glycol (trace), 5 chloro-2-methyl-4-isothiazoline-3-one (trace), benzyl alcohol (trace), 2 methy-4-isothiazoline-3-one (trace).

Appearance: Hydromol Cream is a soft, white, oil in water cream which can be massaged easily into the skin.

Uses

Main pharmacological action: The combination of oils in Hydromol Cream helps to lubricate and hydrate the skin. Moisture loss from the stratum corneum is reduced by the formation of an occlusive film by arachis oil and liquid paraffin on the surface of the skin. Isopropyl myristate, a fatty acid ester, is easily absorbed into the skin and helps to improve skin softness.

The combination of sodium pyrrolidone carboxylate and sodium lactate positively aids the hydration of the skin.

Indications: Any condition in which 'dry skin' is a feature, including all forms of dermatitis/eczema – all degrees of ichthyosis and senile pruritus.

Dosage and administration

Adults and children: Apply liberally to the affected area and massage well into the skin. Hydromol Cream may be used as often as required.

Hydromol Cream is especially beneficial when used immediately after washing or bathing, when the resultant warmth of the skin enhances absorption.

Contra-indications, warnings, etc

Contra-indications: There are no contra-indications except true hypersensitivity to any of the ingredients.

Pharmaceutical precautions The formulation is not designed for use as a diluent.

Legal category GSL.

Package quantities 50 g, 100 g tubes and 500 g pump dispenser.

Further information Hydromol Cream provides soothing, antipruritic symptomatic relief in addition to the longer term therapeutic activity outlined above.

Hydromol Cream does not contain lanolin or fragrance and may thus be used on patients sensitive to these substances.

Product licence number 0291/0023.

HYDROMOL* EMOLLIENT

Presentation

Active ingredients:

Light Liquid Paraffin BP	37.8%
Isopropyl Myristate BP	13.0%

Other ingredients: C12-C14 alcohol with 3 molecules of ethylene oxide, polyol fatty acid ester; iso-octyl stearate.

Appearance: Hydromol Emollient is a clear colourless water-dispersible bath additive resulting in an emulsion of dispersed oils together with an homogenised film on the surface.

Main pharmacological action: The combination of oils used in Hydromol Emollient are deposited on the skin surface during bathing and thus reduce moisture loss, provide antipruritic action, lubricate and soften the skin.

Hydromol Emollient is particularly suitable for infant bathing. The preparations can also be used as a cleanser where soaps etc. are best avoided.

Indications: For the treatment of dry skin conditions such as eczema, icthyosis and senile pruritus.

Dosage and administration Hydromol Emollient should always be either added to water or applied to wet skin.

1. For use in the bath

(a) Adults/Children: Add 1–3 capfuls to an 8 inch bath of water. Soak for 10–15 minutes.

(b) Infants: Add ½–2 capfuls to a small bath of water.

2. For application to the skin as a sponge bath or in the shower

Adults and Children: Pour a small quantity on to a wet sponge or flannel and rub onto wet skin. Rinse and pat dry.

Contra-indications, warnings, etc Keep away from eyes. Take care to avoid slipping in the bath/shower.

Pharmaceutical precautions Nil.

Legal category P.

Package quantities Polyethylene bottles of 150 ml, 350 ml and 1 litre.

Further information In order to ensure a complete coverage of the emulsion in patients with large areas of body involvement, Hydromol Emollient should be used as a bath additive. The bath can be easily cleansed after use.

Hydromol Emollient does not contain lanolin or fragrance and may thus be used on patients sensitive to these substances.

Product licence number 0291/0022.

QUINOCORT* CREAM

Presentation

Active ingredients:

Potassium Hydroxyquinoline Sulphate BP	0.5%
Hydrocortisone BP	1.0%

Other ingredients: Lactic Acid BP, White Soft Paraffin BP, EDTA, Sodium Acid Phosphate BP, Maize Starch BP, cetyl stearyl alcohol, sodium cetyl stearyl sulphate,

PEG 40 castor oil, triethylene glycol (trace), 1,2 propylene glycol (trace), 5 chloro-2-methyl-4-isothiazoline-3-one (trace), benzyl alcohol (trace), 2-methyl-4-isothiazoline-3-one (trace).

Appearance: The active ingredients are formulated in a vanishing cream base and the preparation is faintly yellow in appearance.

Uses *Main pharmacological action:* Hydrocortisone provides anti-inflammatory action yet is the least potent topical corticosteroid available. Potassium hydroxyquinoline sulphate provides broad spectrum antibacterial and anticandidal activity. The combination facilitates treatment of steroid-responsive dermatoses where complication by infection with bacteria or yeast is evident, suspected, or a possibility.

Indications: The treatment of infected eczema, intertrigo and other steroid-responsive dermatoses where anti-infective cover is appropriate.

Dosage and administration *Adults and children:* By gentle massage over all the affected area two to three times daily.

Contra-indications, warnings, etc
Precautions: Caution should be exercised when using this preparation in infants.

Avoid contact with eyes and other mucosal surfaces.

Warning: In pregnant animals administration of corticosteroids can cause abnormalities of foetal development. The relevance of this finding in human beings has not been established. However topical steroids should not be used extensively in pregnancy i.e. in large amounts or for long periods.

In infants long term continuous topical therapy should be avoided. Adrenal suppression can occur even without occlusion.

Contra-indications: Known sensitivity or intolerance to any of the ingredients.

Pharmaceutical precautions *Storage:* Store in a cool place avoiding extremes of temperature.

Legal category POM.

Package quantities Tubes of 30 g.

Further information Nil.

Product licence number 0291/0014.

QUINODERM* CREAM

Presentation

Active ingredients:

Benzoyl Peroxide BP	10.0%
Potassium Hydroxyquinoline Sulphate BP	0.5%

Other ingredients: Lactic Acid BP, White Soft Paraffin BP, EDTA, Sodium Acid Phosphate BP, Maize Starch BP, cetyl stearyl alcohol, sodium cetyl stearyl sulphate, PEG 40 castor oil.

Appearance: Quinoderm Cream is a creamy white astringent vanishing cream.

Uses The combination of the mild keratolytic properties of benzoyl peroxide and the antibacterial and antifungal properties of potassium hydroxyquinoline sulphate in a specially formulated bland water-miscible base makes this preparation valuable in the treatment of acne vulgaris, acneform eruptions and folliculitis.

Dosage and administration
Adults, children and the elderly: By gentle massage over all the affected area two or three times daily.

Contra-indications, warnings, etc
Contra-indications: Quinoderm Cream is contra-indicated in acne rosacea. Patients with known sensitivity to either of the active ingredients should not use Quinoderm Cream. Quinoderm Cream is for topical use only.

Warning: Benzoyl peroxide is an oxidising agent. Hence Quinoderm Cream should not be used at the same time as other topical agents which would react with an oxidising agent.

Precautions: In a few isolated cases overreaction to Quinoderm Cream may occur. To minimise this possibility, select a small area of skin behind the ear, apply the cream and leave for twelve hours. If severe irritation or pronounced redness occurs, do not proceed. Contact with mouth and eyes should be avoided. Care should be taken to avoid contact with dyed fabrics as this preparation may adversely affect dye fastness.

Pharmaceutical precautions
Storage: Quinoderm Cream should be stored in a cool place avoiding extremes of temperature.

Diluents, etc: Quinoderm Cream can be easily removed by warm water and soap.

Legal category P.

Package quantities Quinoderm Cream is supplied in tubes of 25 g and 50 g.

Product licence number 0291/5000R.

QUINODERM* CREAM 5

Presentation

Active ingredients:

Benzoyl Peroxide BP	5.0%
Potassium Hydroxyquinoline Sulphate BP	0.5%

Other ingredients: Lactic Acid BP, White Soft Paraffin BP, EDTA, Sodium Acid Phosphate BP, Maize Starch BP, cetyl stearyl alcohol, sodium cetyl stearyl sulphate, PEG 40 castor oil.

Appearance: Quinoderm Cream 5 is a creamy white astringent vanishing cream.

Uses *Main pharmacological action:* The combination of the mild keratolytic properties of benzoyl peroxide and the antibacterial, antifungal and deodorant properties of potassium hydroxyquinoline sulphate in a specially formulated bland water-miscible base make this preparation valuable in the treatment of pustular affections of the skin particularly when associated with staphylococcal infection.

Indications: Acne vulgaris, acneform eruptions, folliculitis.

Dosage and administration *Adults and children:* By gentle massage over all the affected area, two or three times daily.

Contra-indications, warnings, etc Quinoderm Cream 5 is contra-indicated in acne rosacea. Patients with known sensitivity to either of the active ingredients should not use Quinoderm Cream 5. Quinoderm Cream 5 is used topically.

Precaution: In a few isolated cases overreaction to Quinoderm Cream 5 may occur. To minimise this possibility, select a small area of skin behind the ear, apply the cream and leave for 12 hours. If severe irritation or pronounced redness occurs do not proceed.

All medicines should be kept out of the reach of children.

Pharmaceutical precautions *Storage:* Quinoderm Cream 5 should be stored in a cool place, avoiding extremes of temperature.

Diluents, etc: Quinoderm Cream 5 can be easily removed by warm water and soap.

Legal category P.

Package quantities Quinoderm Cream 5 is supplied in tubes of 50 g.

Further information Contact with mouth and eyes should be avoided. Care should be taken to avoid contact with dyed fabrics as this preparation may adversely affect dye fastness.

Product licence number 0291/0012.

QUINODERM* CREAM WITH 1% HYDROCORTISONE

Presentation
Active ingredients:

Benzoyl Peroxide BP	10.0%
Potassium Hydroxyquinoline Sulphate BP	0.5%
Hydrocortisone BP	1.0%

Other ingredients: Lactic Acid BP, White Soft Paraffin BP, EDTA, Sodium Acid Phosphate BP, Maize Starch BP, cetyl stearyl alcohol, sodium cetyl stearyl sulphate, PEG 40 castor oil.

Appearance: Quinoderm Cream with 1% Hydrocortisone is a creamy white astringent vanishing cream.

Uses The combination of the anti-inflammatory properties of hydrocortisone, the keratolytic action of benzoyl peroxide, the antibacterial and antifungal properties of potassium hydroxyquinoline sulphate in a specially formulated bland water-miscible base, make this preparation valuable in the treatment of acne vulgaris, acneform eruptions and folliculitis especially where inflamed lesions are present.

Dosage and administration
Adults, children and the elderly: Spread thinly over the affected area and then gently massage until no trace of the cream can be seen on the skin surface. Apply two or three times daily. It is important that the whole area be treated not just individual spots or blemishes.

Contra-indications, warnings, etc
Contra-indications: Quinoderm Cream with 1% Hydrocortisone is contra-indicated in acne rosacea, primary bacterial infections, viral and fungal infections. Patients with known sensitivity to any of the active ingredients should not use Quinoderm Cream with 1% Hydrocortisone. Quinoderm Cream with 1% Hydrocortisone is for topical use only.

Warnings: As the preparation contains a corticosteroid, long term continuous topical therapy should be avoided in infants. Adrenal suppression can occur even without occlusion. Benzoyl peroxide is an oxidising agent. Hence Quinoderm Cream with 1% Hydrocortisone should not be used at the same time as other agents which would react with an oxidising agent.

Precautions: Contact with mouth and eyes should be avoided. Care should be taken to avoid contact with dyed fabrics as this preparation may adversely affect dye fastness.

Use in pregnancy: In pregnant animals, administration of corticosteroids can cause abnormalities of foetal development. The relevance of this finding to human beings has not been established. However, topical steroids should not be used extensively in pregnancy, i.e. large amounts or for long periods.

Pharmaceutical precautions
Storage: Quinoderm Cream with 1% Hydrocortisone should be stored in a cool place avoiding extremes of temperature.

Diluents: The cream is easily removed by warm water and soap.

Legal category POM.

Package quantities Quinoderm Cream with 1% Hydrocortisone is available in tubes of 30 g.

Product licence number 0291/5001R.

QUINODERM* LOTIO-GEL 5%

Presentation
Active ingredients:

Benzoyl Peroxide BP	5%
Potassium Hydroxyquinoline Sulphate BP	0.5%

Other ingredients: Lactic Acid BP, EDTA, Sodium Acid Phosphate BP, Maize Starch BP, Cetomacrogol 1000 BP, cetyl stearyl alcohol, sodium cetyl stearyl sulphate, PEG 40 castor oil, Light Liquid Paraffin BP.

Appearance: A homogeneous astringent gel formulated to give the colour and consistency of a creamy white lotion.

Uses
Main pharmacological action: The main pharmacological action of benzoyl peroxide is considered to be keratolytic and comedolytic. Potassium hydroxyquinoline sulphate has broad spectrum antibacterial activity. This combination is formulated in a specifically researched and developed base and is designed to aid the resolution of the polymorphic lesions of acne.

The base has been developed with the objective of providing a stable pharmaceutical form which maximises the advantages of a gel and lotion in a system which does not employ organic solvents and therefore has a correspondingly lower irritancy, toxicity and abuse potential.

Indications: Quinoderm Lotio-gel 5% is indicated in the treatment of acne.

Dosage and administration *Adults and children:* The preparation should be applied by gentle massage over all the affected area, one to three times daily.

Contra-indications, warnings, etc
Contra-indications: Patients with known sensitivity to either of the active constituents should not use Quinoderm Lotio-Gel 5%.

Precautions: In a few isolated cases overreaction to Quinoderm Lotio-Gel 5% may occur. To minimise this possibility, select a small area of skin behind the ear, apply the Lotio-Gel 5% and leave for twelve hours. If severe irritation or pronounced redness occurs, do not proceed.

All medicines should be kept out of the reach of children.

Contact with mouth and eyes should be avoided.

Care should be taken to avoid contact with dyed fabrics as this preparation may adversely affect dye fastness.

Pharmaceutical precautions *Storage:* Quinoderm Lotio-Gel 5% should be stored in a cool place avoiding extremes of temperature.

Legal category P.

Package quantities Quinoderm Lotio-Gel 5% is available in plastic bottles of 30 ml.

Further information Patients may vary in their response to benzoyl peroxide preparations. The stability of benzoyl peroxide in Quinoderm Lotio-Gel 5% is enhanced to minimise any variation in response which may be attributable to variations in the concentration of this active constituent.

Product licence number 0291/0009.

QUINOPED* CREAM

Presentation
Active ingredients:

Benzoyl Peroxide BP	5%
Potassium Hydroxyquinoline Sulphate BP	0.5%

Other ingredients: Lactic Acid BP, White Soft Paraffin BP, EDTA, Sodium Acid Phosphate BP, Maize Starch BP, cetyl stearyl alcohol, sodium cetyl stearyl sulphate, PEG 40 castor oil.

Appearance: Quinoped Cream is a cream-coloured astringent cream.

Uses *Main pharmacological action:* Benzoyl peroxide functions as a keratolytic and facilitates the removal of macerated tissue and associated debris. Potassium hydroxyquinoline sulphate has antifungal and deodorant properties.

Indications: Athlete's foot (tinea pedis) and related fungal infections.

Dosage and administration *Adults and children:* Spread thinly over all the affected area and gently massage until no trace of the cream can be seen on the skin surface. Apply morning and night.

Contra-indications, warnings, etc Not applicable.

Pharmaceutical precautions *Storage:* Quinoped Cream should be stored in a cool place, avoiding extremes of temperature.

Diluents: The cream is easily removed with warm water and soap.

Legal category P.

Package quantities Quinoped Cream is available in tubes of 25 g.

Further information Quinoped Cream is a balanced formulation to counteract the effect of *T. rubrum, T. interdigitale* and *E. floccosum.*

Product licence number 0291/0002.

**Trade Mark*

Reckitt & Colman Products

Dansom Lane
Hull HU8 7DS

Associated companies:
Lloyd-Hamol Ltd
Westminster Laboratories Ltd

BONJELA* ORAL PAIN RELIEVING GEL

Presentation Bonjela is a clear, almost colourless gel containing choline salicylate 8.7% w/w and cetalkonium chloride 0.01% w/w, in a sugar free base. This product contains ethanol.

Uses For the relief of pain and discomfort of common mouth ulcers, cold sores, denture sore spots and infant teething.

Dosage and administration By topical application to the oral mucosa..

Adults: Using a clean finger, massage aproximately half an inch of the gel onto the sore area, not more than once every three hours.

Children: (from 4 months): using a clean finger, massage approximately one quarter inch of gel onto the sore area, not more than once every three hours and not more than six doses in any twenty-four hour period.

Elderly: There is no evidence that dosage need be modified for the elderly.

Denture sore spots: Apply Bonjela to the gums and leave at least 30 minutes before reinsertion of the dentures. Do not apply this product directly to the dentures.

Contra-indications, warnings, etc Preparations containing aspirin should not be given to children under 12 during Bonjela treatment. Unwanted effects are those of salicylates. Bonjela should not be given to patients suffering from active peptic ulceration or known to be allergic to salicylates. Not to be used in infants under four months.

Salicylates may precipitate bronchospasm, and induce attacks of asthma in susceptible subjects.

Use in pregnancy: There is clinical evidence of the safety of salicylates in pregnancy but they may prolong bleeding and contribute to maternal and neonatal bleeding and are best avoided at term.

Use in lactation: Salicylates are excreted in low concentrations in breast milk but are unlikely to adversely affect the breast fed infant.

Drug interactions: Salicylates may enhance the effect of anticoagulants and inhibit the action of uricosurics.

Interferences with laboratory tests: Salicylates may produce falsely increased results for blood creatinine, urate (low dose aspirin) and urea. Falsely decreased results may be obtained for blood thyroxine and urate (>4 g/day aspirin) and for urinary 5-HIAA (with nitrosonaphthol method). Urinary VMA (HMMA) levels may be falsely increased or decreased depending on the method of analysis.

Treatment of overdosage: The usual procedure for salicylate overdosage should be followed, including general supportive measures and gastric lavage if necessary.

Pharmaceutical precautions None.

Legal category GSL.

Package quantities Tubes of 15 g.

Product licence number 0107/5002.

Product licence holder: Lloyd's Pharmaceuticals.

BUCCASTEM*

Presentation Buccastem tablets are circular, biconvex, pale yellow and uncoated with J1 engraved on the face; the reverse is plain. They contain 3 mg prochlorperazine maleate. This product contains sucrose.

Uses Buccastem is a potent phenothiazine neuroleptic. It is indicated in the symptomatic treatment of vertigo due to Meniere's disease, labyrinthitis and other causes; for nausea and vomiting from whatever cause and in the treatment of migraine.

Dosage and administration
Dosage: Adults and children aged 12 years and over: One or two 3 mg Buccastem tablets twice a day.

Elderly patients: For the indications shown above, there is no evidence that the dosage needs to be modified but the lower dosage is recommended for initial use.

Administration: The tablet should be placed high up between the upper lip and the gums to either side of the front teeth, where it will soften and adhere to the gum.

Patients should be instructed as to the correct placement of the tablet and should note the following points:

(a) The tablet should be left undisturbed.
(b) Slight numbness of the gum and tongue may be observed but this is transient.
(c) If a tablet is accidentally swallowed during insertion, it may be replaced by a further tablet.
(d) In patients who wear dentures, the tablet may be placed in any comfortable position between the lip and the gum.

Contra-indications, warnings, etc
Contra-indications: Buccastem is contra-indicated in patients with impaired renal or liver function, existing blood dyscrasias, known hypersensitivity to the active ingredient, epilepsy, Parkinson's disease, prostatic hypertrophy, and narrow angle glaucoma.

Use in pregnancy and lactation: There is inadequate evidence of safety in human pregnancy, although prochlorperazine has been used widely for many years without apparent ill effects. However, as with other drugs, use of Buccastem in the first trimester of pregnancy should be avoided unless absolutely necessary. Since data from animal studies show that prochlorperazine may be found in breast milk, Buccastem should not be used during lactation.

Warnings: Hypotension, usually postural, may occur, particularly in elderly or volume depleted subjects.

Parkinsonism or tardive dyskinesia may occur occasionally, although are normally associated with higher doses than are recommended for Buccastem.

Alcohol and other CNS depressants should be used with caution, as should α-adrenoreceptor blocking antihypertensives.

Patients who drive or operate machinery should be warned of the possibility of drowsiness.

Adverse reactions: Drowsiness, dizziness, dry mouth, insomnia, agitation and mild skin reactions may occur. Extrapyramidal reactions are very unlikely at the recommended dosage.

Other adverse effects which have occurred rarely with prochlorperazine and other phenothiazine neuroleptics include jaundice, blood dyscrasias and, very rarely, hyperprolactinaemic effects. Neuroleptic malignant syndrome (hyperthermia, rigidity, autonomic dysfunction and altered consciousness) may occur with any neuroleptic.

Overdosage: The signs and symptoms will be predominantly extrapyramidal and may be accompanied by either restlessness and agitation or central nervous depression. Hypotension may also occur. Treatment is essentially symptomatic and supportive. There is no specific antidote. Gastric lavage is helpful, particularly when carried out within 6 hours of ingestion. Do not induce vomiting. Particular attention must be directed to maintaining a clear airway, since this may be threatened by the extrapyramidal muscle dystonias. Severe dystonic reactions usually respond to procyclidine (5–10 mg) or orphenadrine (20–40 mg) given i.m. or i.v. If convulsions occur they should be treated using i.v. diazepam. If hypotension is present strict attention to ventilation and posturing of the patient will often secure the desired effect but failing this, consideration should be given to volume expansion by i.v. fluids. If this is insufficient, positive inotropic agents such as dopamine may be tried, but peripheral vasoconstrictor agents are not generally recommended. Adrenaline should *not* be used.

Pharmaceutical precautions Protect from light.

Legal category POM.

Package quantities Packs of 60 tablets, in blister foils of 15 tablets each.

Further information Pharmacokinetic studies have shown that prochlorperazine is absorbed via the buccal mucosa. One Buccastem tablet administered twice daily produces steady state plasma levels equivalent to those achieved after oral administration of 5 mg three times daily.

Product licence number 0044/0089

COLVEN*

Presentation Colven is presented as grapefruit flavoured granules of yellowish-brown colour contained in a sachet.

Active ingredients: Each sachet contains Ispaghula Husk BP 3.5 g and mebeverine hydrochloride 135 mg. This product contains aspartame.

Uses Colven is indicated for the treatment of conditions where abdominal pain and bowel dysfunction occur, such as irritable bowel syndrome, or where these symptoms occur in patients with gastrointestinal diseases such as colitis, Crohn's disease, ulcerative colitis or gastritis.

Dosage and administration
Adults, children over 12: One sachet morning and evening, half an hour before meals. An additional sachet may be taken before the midday meal if symptoms are not controlled at this time.

The contents of one sachet of Colven should be stirred into a glass of cold water and taken immediately.

There is no indication that dosage need be modified for the elderly.

Contra-indications, warnings, etc Colven is contra-indicated in cases of intestinal obstruction and colonic atony such as senile megacolon. As this product contains 6.1 mmol of sodium per sachet, its use is contra-indicated where strict control of salt intake is required, for example, in severe renal and cardiovascular conditions. The product is not at present recommended for children under 12 and, in common with most drugs, care should be taken in prescribing during pregnancy.

In the event of overdosage, conservative measures should be taken. The patient may notice abdominal discomfort and flatulence and attention should be paid to maintaining an adequate fluid intake, particularly if the granules have been taken without water, contrary to the administration instructions.

Pharmaceutical precautions Store in a cool dry place.

Legal category POM.

Package quantities Carton of 60 (6 × 10) sachets.

Further information Studies by Ritchie and Truelove (1979, 1980) have demonstrated that a combination of ispaghula and mebeverine gave better overall relief of the symptoms of irritable bowel syndrome when compared to bran or another antispasmodic agent. Ispaghula with mebeverine is presented as effervescent granules which disperse readily in water. References: Ritchie, J.A. & Truelove, S.C. (1979) *Br.Med.J.*, **1**, 376. Ritchie, J.A. & Truelove, S.C. (1980) *Br.Med.J.*, **281**, 1317.

Colven has no known effects on diagnostic laboratory tests.

Product licence number 0044/0075.

DISPROL* PAEDIATRIC

Presentation A sugar-free suspension of Paracetamol PhEur in a pale yellow banana-flavoured liquid. Each 5 ml dose contains 120 mg of paracetamol.

This product contains methyl and propyl hydroxybenzoates.

Uses For the treatment of mild to moderate pain, including headache, migraine, neuralgia, toothache, pain in teething, sore throat, aches and pains. Symptomatic relief of rheumatic aches and pains. Symptomatic relief of influenza, feverishness and feverish colds. Symptomatic relief of reactions due to vaccination or immunisation.

Dosage and administration
Children 3–12 months: Half to one 5 ml spoonful every four hours.

1 year to under 6 years: One to two 5 ml spoonfuls every four hours.

6 to 12 years: Two to four 5 ml spoonfuls every four hours.

Dosage for children under 3 months is at a physician's discretion.

Disprol Paediatric may be diluted with an equal volume of boiled then cooled water to produce a 12 mg/ml solution (60 mg/5 ml spoonful) with a 14 day shelf life.

For a 2 month old weighing 4.4 kg or above, prescribe one 2.5 ml spoonful of undiluted Disprol or one 5 ml spoonful of diluted Disprol every six hours.

For a 2 month old weighing less than 4.4 kg, prescribe 1 ml/kg (12 mg/kg) of diluted Disprol every six hours, to be administered via an oral measuring syring to ensure an accurate dose.

Not more than 4 doses should be administered in any 24-hour period.

Contra-indications, warnings, etc Disprol Paediatric should not be given to patients with a history of hypersensitivity to paracetamol. It should be used with caution in patients with hepatic or renal dysfunction.

Each 5 ml dose of suspension contains approximately 3.25 g of hydrogenated glucose syrup (up to 12 Kcal). This should be borne in mind when treating diabetic children.

Side-effects from paracetamol administered in normal doses are rare. There have been isolated reports of agranulocytosis, methaemoglobinaemia and thrombocytopenic purpura, and after overdosage or prolonged administration, isolated cases of chronic hepatic necrosis, acute pancreatitis and nephrotoxicity.

Drug interactions: Drugs which induce hepatic microsomal enzymes, such as alcohol, barbiturates and tricyclic antidepressants, may increase the hepatotoxicity of paracetamol particularly after overdosage.

Interferences with laboratory tests: In paracetamol overdosage, the following tests for blood glucose may be distorted:

Reduction methods and YSI analyser – falsely increased results.

Glucose oxidase method – falsely decreased results.

There is no interference with the hexokinase method.

There may be analytical interference with catecholamine estimations.

Treatment of overdosage: Overdosage should be treated promptly by gastric lavage followed by I.V. N-acetylcysteine or oral methionine since liver damage following overdosage does not become apparent for 1–6 days after ingestion. Initial mild symptoms consist of nausea, vomiting and pallor. Measurement of the blood paracetamol level and the time elapsed since ingestion is important in order to determine whether further therapy with N-acetylcysteine is necessary.

Pharmaceutical precautions Store below 25°C and protect from light, avoid freezing.

Legal category P.

Package quantities 100 ml bottles and 500 ml bottles, 5 ml sachets.

Product licence number 0044/0085.

FYBOGEL* and FYBOGEL* ORANGE

Presentation Flaky granules of a pale buff colour. Fybogel Orange has an orange flavouring. One sachet of granules contains Ispaghula Husk BP 3.5 g in a base containing 7 mmol potassium, beta-carotene colour and saccharin. Fybogel and Fybogel Orange are gluten free and contain no mono or disaccharides.

Uses Fybogel is recommended for the treatment of patients requiring a high-fibre regimen. It is effective in relieving constipation and restoring regular bowel function. Ispaghula husk is capable of absorbing up to forty times its own weight of water in vitro, and part of its activity can be attributed to its action as a simple bulking agent. In addition, colonic bacteria are believed to use the hydrated material as a metabolic substrate. This results in an increase in the bacterial cell mass which softens the faeces to allow easy evacuation and avoiding episodes of straining. Fybogel effervescent granules disperse readily to form a palatable drink in water. The unflavoured form of Fybogel may be mixed with fruit squash to vary the flavour.

Dosage and administration
Adults: children over 12: One sachet morning and evening.

Children 6–12: Half to one level 5 ml spoonful depending on age and size, morning and evening.

Children under 6: To be taken only on medical advice: Dose: half to one level 5 ml spoonful, depending on age and size, morning and evening.

Elderly: There is no indication that dosage need be modified for the elderly.

Fybogel should be stirred into approximately $\frac{1}{4}$ pint (150 ml) water and taken as quickly as possible, preferably after meals.

Contra-indications, warnings, etc Fybogel is contra-indicated in cases of intestinal obstruction and colonic atony such as senile megacolon.

Use in pregnancy and lactation: May be used during pregnancy and lactation since the ispaghula is not absorbed from the gastrointestinal tract.

Drug interactions: There have been no interactions reported when Fybogel granules have been used with other drugs.

Interference with laboratory tests: Fybogel has no known effects on diagnostic laboratory tests.

Treatment of overdosage: In the event of overdosage, conservative measures should be taken. The patient may notice abdominal discomfort and flatulence and attention should be paid to maintaining an adequate fluid intake, particularly if the granules have been taken without water, contrary to the administration instructions.

Pharmaceutical precautions Store below 30°C in a dry place.

Legal category GSL.

Package quantities Carton of 60 (6 × 10) sachets.

Product licence numbers
Fybogel 0044/0041
Fybogel Orange 0044/0068.

LIQUID GAVISCON*

Presentation A pink suspension with a flavour of fennel (similar to aniseed).

10 ml of Liquid Gaviscon contains Sodium Alginate BPC 500 mg, Sodium Bicarbonate PhEur 267 mg, Calcium Carbonate PhEur 160 mg.

This product contains parabens and erythrosine.

Uses Gaviscon alleviates the painful conditions resulting from the reflux of gastric acid and bile into the oesophagus by suppressing the reflux itself. It is indicated in heartburn, including heartburn of pregnancy, dyspepsia associated with gastric reflux, hiatus hernia, reflux oesophagitis, regurgitation and all cases of epigastric and retrosternal distress where the underlying cause is gastric reflux.

Dosage and administration *Adults, children over 12:* 10–20 ml after meals and at bedtime.

Children under 12: 5–10 ml after meals and at bedtime. Not recommended for Infants, see Infant Gaviscon. If desired, the standard dose of Liquid Gaviscon may be taken diluted with not more than an equal quantity of water, well stirred.

There is no indication that dosage need be modified for the elderly.

Contra-indications, warnings, etc There are no specific contra-indications.

As Gaviscon's mode of action is physical, overdosage in terms of the alginate content presents virtually no hazard. The only likely consequence is abdominal distension, which is best treated conservatively.

Pharmaceutical precautions Store below 30°C; avoid freezing.

Legal category GSL.

Package quantities Amber bottles of 200 ml and 500 ml.

Further information On ingestion Gaviscon reacts with gastric acid to produce in the stomach a floating viscous gel of near neutral pH which effectively impedes reflux. In severe cases the gel itself may be refluxed into the oesophagus, where it protects the inflamed mucosa, thus allowing healing to take place and preventing further inflammation.

The sodium content of a dose of 10 ml liquid is 141 mg (6.2 mmol). This may be of importance when a highly restricted salt diet is required as in some renal and cardiovascular conditions.

May be used during lactation since the alginate is not absorbed from the gastrointestinal tract.

Liquid Gaviscon has no known effects on diagnostic laboratory tests.

Product licence number 0044/0058.

GAVISCON* TABLETS

Presentation White, mint-flavoured tablet engraved on both sides with the word 'Gaviscon' and a sword symbol. Each tablet contains:

Alginic Acid BPC 500 mg
Magnesium Trisilicate PhEur 25 mg
Dried Aluminium Hydroxide Gel BP 100 mg
Sodium Bicarbonate PhEur 170 mg

in a sugar free peppermint flavoured base containing calcium carbonate (40 mg) and saccharin.

Uses Gaviscon alleviates the painful conditions resulting from the reflux of gastric acid and bile into the oesophagus by suppressing the reflux itself.

On ingestion, Gaviscon reacts with gastric acid to produce in the stomach a floating viscous gel of near neutral pH which effectively impedes reflux. In severe cases the gel itself may be refluxed into the oesophagus, where it protects the inflamed mucosa, thus allowing the healing to take place and preventing further inflammation. Gaviscon is indicated for heartburn, including heartburn of pregnancy, dyspepsia associated with gastric reflux, hiatus hernia, reflux oesophagitis, regurgitation and all cases of epigastric and retrosternal distress where the underlying cause is gastric reflux.

Dosage and administration
Adults and children over 12: 1 or 2 tablets after meals and at bedtime.

Children under 12: 1 tablet after meals and at bedtime. Not recommended for infants, see Infant Gaviscon.

Elderly: There is no indication that dosage need be modified for the elderly.

Tablets should be thoroughly chewed. It is recommended they be broken in half and chewed a little at a time. This may be followed by a drink of water.

Contra-indications, warnings, etc There are no specific contra-indications.

Aluminium hydroxide containing products should be used with caution in patients with renal dysfunction or hypophosphataemia. The sodium content of a tablet is 47 mg (2.04 mmol).

Use in pregnancy: Gaviscon is indicated for heartburn, including heartburn of pregnancy.

Use in lactation: May be used during lactation since the alginate is not absorbed from the gastrointestinal tract.

Drug interactions: There have been no interactions reported when Gaviscon Tablets have been used with other drugs. Although large doses of antacids interfere with the absorption of some drugs, the amount of antacid in two Gaviscon tablets is unlikely to interact with other drugs.

Interference with laboratory tests: Gaviscon Tablets have no known effects on diagnostic laboratory tests.

Treatment of overdosage: As Gaviscon's mode of action is physical, overdosage in terms of the alginate presents virtually no hazard. The only likely consequence is abdominal distension which is best treated conservatively.

Pharmaceutical precautions Store below 30°C in a dry place.

Legal category GSL.

Package quantities Carton containing 3 tubes of 20 tablets.

Product licence number 0044/0021.

INFANT GAVISCON*

Presentation Infant Gaviscon is a fine, white powder packed in a sachet and sterilised. Each sachet contains sodium alginate 225 mg, magnesium alginate 87.5 mg and dried Aluminium Hydroxide BP 112.5 mg in a base containing colloidal silica (Aerosil) and Mannitol BP.

Uses Infant Gaviscon reacts with gastric acid to form a viscous gel which when mixed with stomach contents thickens them and helps prevent reflux into the oesophagus.

It is indicated for gastric regurgitation, including that seen when the competence of the cardiac sphincter has not been fully established, gastro-oesophageal reflux and reflux associated with hiatus hernia in infants and young children.

Dosage and administration Not to be used except on a doctor's recommendation, or in infants under 1 year except under medical supervision. Mix immediately before use as directed below.

Breast-fed infants: Under 10 lb (4.5 kg), one dose. Over 10 lb (4.5 kg), two doses. Add 1 teaspoon (5 ml) of boiled, cooled water to the powder in a glass, mix to a smooth paste, add two more teaspoons of the water and mix. Give after each feed using a spoon or feeding bottle.

Bottle-fed infants: Under 10 lb (4.5 kg), one dose to be mixed into not less than 4 fluid oz (115 ml) of each feed in the bottle and shaken well. Over 10 lb (4.5 kg), two doses to be mixed into not less than 8 fluid oz (225 ml) of each feed in the bottle and shaken well.

Young children: Two doses, prepared as for breast-fed infants, to be drunk after each meal.

Contra-indications, warnings, etc Contra-indicated in cases of intestinal obstruction and in cases of established diarrhoea.

Attention should be paid to the dosage instructions to avoid an excessive amount of product per feed and the possible risk of hypernatraemia.

Infant Gaviscon's mode of action is physical resulting in a thickening of the gastric contents. An excessive concentration of Infant Gaviscon may lead to gastric distension.

Not to be used in premature infants or in situations where excessive water loss is likely, e.g. fever, diarrhoea, vomiting or high room temperature. Not to be used in gastroenteritis, where the appropriate treatment is rehydration with fluid replacement.

Not to be used when treating infants with known or suspected impairment of renal function as the sodium content (approximately 21 mg or 0.92 mmol per dose) may add to the risk of hypernatraemia. A medical review of the patient's condition should be undertaken seven days after initiating treatment or before if symptoms worsen.

Drug interactions: There have been no interactions reported when Infant Gaviscon was used with other drugs.

Interference with laboratory tests: Infant Gaviscon has no known effects on diagnostic laboratory tests.

Treatment of overdosage: Rare instances have occurred in which an intragastric mass has developed, comprising Gaviscon and milk proteins. Overdosage may have contributed to the development of such masses. The majority resolved spontaneously when the child was admitted, Infant Gaviscon was discontinued and a regime of adequate fluid intake and monitoring of fluid and electrolyte balance was installed. If spontaneous resolution of the mass does not occur, removal by surgical or endoscopic means may be required.

If hypernatraemia occurs it should be treated with oral fluids and monitoring of the infant's electrolytes. Severe cases should be treated by the cautious use of hypo-osmotic solutions.

Pharmaceutical precautions Nil.

Legal category P.

Package quantities Carton of 15 dual sachets (30 doses).

Product licence number 0044/5007.

PRIPSEN*

Presentation Pripsen is a cream-coloured powder presented in a dual sachet pack. The powder forms a fine red suspension in milk or water. Each individual sachet contains 4 g Piperazine Phosphate BP and standardised senna equivalent to 15.3 mg total sennosides calculated as sennoside B. Pripsen is sweetened with saccharin and coloured with natural carmine.

Uses Pripsen is a potent anthelmintic recommended for the eradication of enterobiasis (pinworm, threadworm) and ascariasis (roundworm).

Dosage and administration Pripsen should be stirred into a small glass of milk or water and drunk immediately.

1. Threadworms:

Age (yrs)	*First dose*	*Second dose*
Adult and children over 6	1 sachet	Repeat after 14 days.
Children aged 1–6	2/3 sachet (1 level 5 ml spoonful)	Repeat after 14 days.
Infants 3 months to one year. To be taken only when prescribed by a doctor	1/3 sachet (1 level 2.5 ml spoonful)	Repeat after 14 days.

2. Roundworms: The initial dose relative to age is as for threadworms. Additional single prophylactic doses at monthly intervals up to three months, may be necessary to eliminate the risk of reinfestation.

Elderly: There is no indication that dosage needs to be modified for the elderly.

The piperazine in Pripsen paralyses the worms which are then evacuated by the laxative action of the standardised senna. The life cycle of the threadworm is approximately thirty days. Since some worms may still be in the larval stage when the first dose of Pripsen is administered, a follow up dose should be taken after 14 days to eliminate the possibility of reinfestation.

Contra-indications, warnings, etc Pripsen is contra-indicated in patients with epilepsy, severe bilateral renal dysfunction, hepatic dysfunction or with a known sensitivity to piperazine.

Unwanted effects resulting from Pripsen therapy are rare. When such reactions do occur the most frequent are allergic in nature such as rash, urticaria, itching or, rarely, bronchospasm. Isolated cases of Stevens Johnson syndrome and angio-neurotic oedema have also been reported. Secondly, mild gastrointestinal disturbances such as nausea, vomiting, colic or diarrhoea. A few cases of neurotoxic reactions have been reported such as drowsiness, confusion or clonic contractions if administered to patients with neurological or renal abnormalities.

A few cases of neurotoxic reactions such as ataxia and vertigo have been reported in normal subjects.

Use in pregnancy: Although no causal relationship has been established, isolated instances of foetal malformation have been reported when piperazine was part of the patient's therapy. Use in the first trimester of pregnancy is therefore not advised. Unless symptoms warrant immediate treatment the administration of Pripsen should be postponed until after parturition.

Use in lactation: Piperazine is excreted in breast milk but no unwanted effects in the infant have been reported. To minimise the amount of piperazine ingested by the baby it is recommended that the infant be fed immediately before the mother takes Pripsen then allow eight hours before breast feeding is resumed. During this eight hour period, milk should be expressed and discarded at the usual feeding interval.

Drug interactions: Pyrantel pamoate antagonises the mode of action of piperazine and therefore should not be co-administered. Although caution should be exercised when co-administering phenothiazines or tricyclic antidepressants, due to a possible interaction, this has not been shown to be a problem in clinical practice.

Interference with laboratory tests: Pripsen has no known effects on diagnostic laboratory tests.

Treatment of overdosage: Mild symptoms would be expected from overdosage of Pripsen being either gastrointestinal (diarrhoea, nausea, vomiting) or neurological (muscular hypotonia, ataxia and vertigo). General supportive measures including maintenance of an adequate fluid intake should be adopted, and if necessary anticonvulsant therapy administered.

Pharmaceutical precautions Store below 25°C in a dry place. Any unused powder should be discarded.

Legal category P.

Package quantities Outers containing dual dose sachets.

Product licence number 0063/5004.

Product licence holder: Westminster Laboratories Ltd.

SENOKOT*

Presentation *Tablets:* Small brown tablets engraved on one side only with the word Senokot and a sword symbol. One tablet contains standardised senna equivalent to 7.5 mg total sennosides calculated as sennoside B. Senokot tablets contain lactose and parabens.

Granules: Brown chocolate-flavoured granules. One 5 ml level spoonful (2.73 g) contains standardised senna equivalent to 15 mg total sennosides calculated as sennoside B. Senokot granules contain sucrose.

Syrup: Brown, fruit-flavoured syrup. One 5 ml spoonful contains standardised senna extract equivalent to 7.5 mg total sennosides calculated as sennoside B. Senokot syrup contains sucrose and ethanol.

Uses In the management of constipation, including:
Simple constipation, whether self-induced or environmental, e.g. neglect of the call to stool or poor sanitary conditions.
Constipation in old age, especially where maintenance treatment is required.
Constipation in pregnancy and the puerperium.
Idiopathic slow-transit constipation.
Constipation in the irritable bowel syndrome.
Conservative treatment of haemorrhoids.
Avoidance of straining after surgery and in cerebral and cardiovascular disease.

The physiological action of the anthrone glycoside in Senokot is virtually colon specific. The anthroquinones are protected by a natural sugar moiety which safeguards their transport to the large bowel, where bacterial action breaks the sugar-anthrone bond and releases the active fraction. Peristalsis is then stimulated via the submucosal and myenteric plexuses.

Being colon specific, Senokot does not affect the vital nutritional functions of the upper gastro-intestinal tract.

Dosage and administration The correct dose of Senokot is the smallest required to produce a comfortable soft-formed motion. It varies between individuals, but is generally found within the following ranges:

Adults: 2 tablets (up to 4 on medical advice) or one 5 ml spoonful of granules (up to 10 ml on medical advice) or 10 ml of syrup (up to 20 ml on medical advice) at bedtime.

Children over 6 years: Half the adult dosages, taken in the morning.

Children 2–6 years: Senokot syrup ½ to one 5 ml spoonful for preference.

There is no indication that dosage need be modified for the elderly.

New users should start with the lowest dose of the preferred formulation. These are available from a range of general sales packs advising only the lowest dose and available for self medication as described above. Alternatively the product may be dispensed to allow, if necessary, an increase by half the initial dose each day until a comfortable formed motion is produced. If no bowel action has occurred after three days' progressively increased dosage a medical examination should be considered.

Senokot is best taken as a single dose, at bedtime by adults and in the morning by children. The tablets can be taken with a drink, the granules can be stirred into hot milk, sprinkled on food, or eaten as they are.

Once regularity has been achieved, dosage should be reduced and can usually be stopped.

Contra-indications, warnings, etc Senokot like all laxatives, should not be given when any undiagnosed acute or persistent abdominal symptoms are present. Temporary mild griping may occur during adjustment of dosage.

Diabetic patients should use the tablets as these have a negligible sugar content.

Use in lactation: Clinical studies have shown that breast fed infants of mothers taking Senokot did not show any side effects of the drug.

Interference with laboratory tests: Senokot has no known effects on diagnostic laboratory tests.

Treatment of overdosage: In cases of accidental overdosage, where diarrhoea is severe, conservative measures are usually sufficient: generous amounts of fluid especially fruit drinks should be given.

Pharmaceutical precautions The tablets and granules should be kept in closed airtight containers, and the syrup in amber bottles as supplied. Store in a cool place.

Legal category GSL, sales restricted to pharmacies.

Package quantities
Tablets: 24 in foil: 50, 100, and 500 in Securitainers.
Granules: 100 and 500 g in Securitainers.
Syrup: Bottles of 100 ml and 500 ml.

Further information Nil.

Product licence numbers

Tablets	0063/5000R
Granules	0063/5002
Syrup	0063/5003

Product licences held by Westminster Laboratories Ltd.

SOLPRIN* 75 MG

Presentation White tablets engraved on one side with the code H sword motif 3, the other side being plain. Each tablet contains Aspirin PhEur 75 mg, and when dissolved in water provides a solution of calcium acetylsalicylate.

Uses For the relief of pain.

Dosage and administration
Adults (including elderly) and children aged 12 years and over: As considered necessary by the physician. Each tablet to be dissolved in water.

Children under 12 years: Not to be given to children under 12 unless under strict medical supervision.

Contra-indications, warnings, etc Not to be given to patients known to be allergic to aspirin or suffering from peptic ulceration or haemophilia.

Aspirin may enhance the effects of anticoagulants and inhibit the effects of uricosurics. Aspirin may precipitate bronchospasm and induce attacks of asthma or hypersensitivity in susceptible subjects. May also induce gastrointestinal haemorrhage, occasionally major.

There is clinical and epidemiological evidence of the safety of aspirin in human pregnancy, but it may prolong labour and contribute to maternal and neonatal bleeding and is best avoided at term.

The usual procedure for aspirin overdosage should be followed including general supportive measures and gastric lavage if necessary.

Pharmaceutical precautions Keep in a dry place below 30°C.

Legal category GSL (available only through pharmacies)

Package quantities Carton containing 24 tablets in strips of alumininium foil.

Further information Solprin is aspirin in a soluble form. Because the aspirin is taken in solution, effective blood levels and the relief of pain may be achieved more rapidly than with ordinary aspirin; further, it is less likely to cause gastric upsets. Aspirin has been shown to inhibit the aggregation of blood platelets. (Hanley S. P. et al., (1981), Lancet, **I**, 969. Weksley B. B. et al., (1983), N Engl J Med, **308**, 800).

Solprin has no known effects on diagnostic laboratory tests.

Product licence number 0044/5002R.

TEMGESIC* INJECTION

Presentation Temgesic Injection is a colourless liquid containing 300 micrograms/ml buprenorphine, as the hydrochloride, in a 5% dextrose solution, adjusted to pH range 3.5–5.5 with hydrochloric acid. Clear glass snap ampoules of 1 ml (300 micrograms) or 2 ml (600 micrograms).

Temgesic Injection contains 50 mg dextrose per ml, but no sodium, potassium or preservative.

Uses As a strong analgesic for the relief of moderate to severe pain.

Dosage and administration *Adults and children over 12 years old:* The recommended dosage is 1 to 2 ml (300–600 micrograms buprenorphine), by IM or slow IV injection, every six to eight hours or as required. Temgesic Injection may be employed in balanced anaesthetic techniques as a premedication at a dose of 300 micrograms intramuscularly or as an analgesic supplement at doses of 300–450 micrograms intravenously.

Children under 12 years: Temgesic is suitable for children under 12 at a dose of 3–6 micrograms/kg body weight every 6–8 hours. In refractory cases up to 9 micrograms/kg may be administered. There is no clinical experience in infants below the age of six months.

Elderly: There is no evidence that dosage need be modified for the elderly though they may be more susceptible to hallucinations and other psychotomimetic effects.

Contra-indications, warnings, etc Controlled human and animal studies indicate that buprenorphine has a substantially lower dependence liability than pure agonist analgesics. In patients abusing opioids in moderate doses substitution with buprenorphine may prevent withdrawal symptoms. In man limited euphorigenic effects have been observed. This has resulted in some abuse of the product and caution should be exercised when prescribing it to patients known to have, or suspected of having, problems with drug abuse.

There is evidence to indicate that therapeutic doses of buprenorphine do not reduce the analgesic efficacy of standard doses of an opioid agonist, and that when buprenorphine is employed within the normal range, standard doses of opioid agonist may be administered before the effects of the former have ended without compromising analgesia. However, in individuals on high doses of opioids, buprenorphine may precipitate abstinence effects due to its properties as a partial agonist.

Temgesic may cause some drowsiness which may be potentiated by other centrally-acting agents, including alcohol, tranquillisers, sedatives and hypnotics. Ambulant patients should be warned not to drive or operate machinery if affected by drowsiness.

Temgesic occasionally causes significant respiratory depression and, as with other strong centrally acting analgesics, care should be taken when treating patients with impaired respiratory function or patients who are receiving drugs which can cause respiratory depression. Although volunteer studies have indicated that opioid antagonists may not fully reverse the effects of Temgesic, clinical experience has shown that naloxone may be of benefit in reversing a reduced respiratory rate. Respiratory stimulants such as doxapram are also effective.

Since buprenorphine is metabolised in the liver, the intensity and duration of its action may be affected in patients with impaired liver function.

Temgesic should be used with caution in patients receiving monoamine oxidase inhibitors, although animal studies have given no indication of interactions.

Temgesic has no known effects on diagnostic laboratory tests.

Temgesic is not recommended for use during pregnancy. Animal studies indicate that the amounts of buprenorphine excreted in milk are very low and in human use are unlikely to be of clinical significance to the baby. There is indirect evidence in animal studies to suggest that Temgesic may cause a reduction in milk flow during lactation. Although this occurred only at doses well in excess of the human dose, it should be borne in mind when treating lactating women.

Overdosage: Temgesic has a wide safety margin, and in clinical practice doses well in excess of those recommended have been used without untoward effect. Supportive measures should be instituted and, if appropriate, naloxone or respiratory stimulants can be used.

The expected symptoms of overdosage would be drowsiness, nausea and vomiting; marked miosis may occur.

Side-effects: Drowsiness, or sleep from which the patient can be easily aroused, may occur particularly in the postoperative period. In common with other strong analgesics, nausea, vomiting, dizziness, sweating and drowsiness have been reported which may be more frequent in ambulant patients. Should nausea and vomiting occur, concurrent administration of an anti-emetic is advised. Hallucinations and other psychotomimetic effects have occurred although more rarely than with other agonist-antagonists.

Pharmaceutical precautions Temgesic Injection, though stable, should be kept cool and protected from light. It may be diluted with 5% Injection Dextrose BP or Injection Sodium Chloride BP.

Legal category CD (Sch 3), POM.

Package quantities Packs of 5 ampoules (1 ml or 2 ml).

Product licence numbers
Temgesic Injection 1 ml 0044/0056
Temgesic Injection 2 ml 0044/0057

TEMGESIC* SUBLINGUAL

Presentation Temgesic Sublingual is presented as white, biconvex tablets containing 200 micrograms (0.2 mg) or 400 micrograms (0.4 mg) of buprenorphine as the hydrochloride, engraved on one side with a 2 or a 4 respectively and on the other with a sword symbol. This product contains lactose.

Uses As a strong analgesic for the relief of moderate to severe pain.

Dosage and administration
Adults and children over 12: 200–400 micrograms (0.2–0.4 mg) buprenorphine to be dissolved under the tongue every 6–8 hours or as required. The recommended starting dose for moderate to severe pain of the type typically presenting in general practice is 200–400 micrograms (0.2–0.4 mg) every eight hours. The tablet should not be chewed or swallowed as this will reduce efficacy.

Temgesic Sublingual may be employed in balanced anaesthetic techniques as a premedication at a dose of 400 micrograms.

Children under 12 years: Temgesic Sublingual 0.2 mg is suitable for use in children as follows:

16–25 kg (35–55 lb), 100 micrograms (half a tablet).
25–37.5 kg (55–82.5 lb), 100–200 micrograms (half to one tablet).
37.5–50 kg (82.5–110 lb), 200–300 micrograms (one to one and a half tablets).

There is no clinical experience in infants below the age of six months.

Elderly: There is no evidence that dosage need be modified for the elderly though they may be more susceptible to hallucinations and other psychotomimetic effects.

Contra-indications, warnings, etc Controlled human and animal studies indicate that buprenorphine has a substantially lower dependence liability than pure agonist analgesics. In patients abusing opioids in moderate doses substitution with buprenorphine may prevent withdrawal symptoms. In man limited euphorigenic effects have been observed. This has resulted in some abuse of the product and caution should be exercised when prescribing it to patients known to have, or suspected of having, problems with drug abuse.

There is evidence to indicate that therapeutic doses of buprenorphine do not reduce the analgesic efficacy of standard doses of an opioid agonist, and clinical studies have shown that when buprenorphine is employed within the normal therapeutic range, standard doses of narcotic agonist may be administerd before the effects of the former have ended without compromising analgesia. However, in individuals on high doses of narcotics, buprenorphine may precipitate withdrawal effects due to its properties as a partial agonist.

Temgesic may cause some drowsiness which may be potentiated by other centrally-acting agents, including alcohol, tranquillisers, sedatives and hypnotics. Ambulant patients should be warned not to drive or operate machinery if affected by drowsiness.

Temgesic occasionally causes significant respiratory depression and, as with other strong centrally acting analgesics, care should be taken when treating patients with impaired respiratory function or patients who are receiving drugs which can cause respiratory depression. Although volunteer studies have indicated that opioid antagonists may not fully reverse the effects of Temgesic, clinical experience has shown that naloxone may be of benefit in reversing a reduced respiratory rate. Respiratory stimulants such as doxapram are also effective.

Since buprenorphine is metabolised in the liver, the intensity and duration of its action may be affected in patients with impaired liver function.

Temgesic should be used with caution in patients who are receiving monoamine oxidase inhibitors, although animal studies have given no indication of interactions.

Temgesic has no known effects on diagnostic laboratory tests.

Temgesic is not recommended for use during pregnancy. Animal studies indicate that the amounts of buprenorphine excreted in milk are very low and in human use are unlikely to be of clinical significance to the baby. There is indirect evidence in animal studies to suggest that Temgesic may cause a reduction in milk flow during lactation. Although this occurred only at doses well in excess of the human dose, it should be borne in mind when treating lactating women.

Overdosage: Temgesic Sublingual has a wide safety margin and in clinical practice doses of buprenorphine well in excess of those recommended have been used without untoward effect. Supportive measures should be instituted and, if appropriate, naloxone or respiratory stimulants can be used. The expected symptoms of overdosage would be drowsiness, nausea and vomiting; marked miosis may occur.

Side-effects: Drowsiness, or sleep from which the patient can easily be aroused, may occur particularly in the postoperative period. In common with other strong analgesics, nausea, vomiting, dizziness, sweating and drowsiness have been reported and may be more frequent in ambulant patients. Should nausea and vomiting occur, concurrent administration of an anti-emetic is advised. Hallucinations and other psychotomimetic effects have occurred although more rarely than with other agonist-antagonists.

Pharmaceutical precautions Store in a cool place.

Legal category CD (Sch 3), POM.

Package quantities Cartons of 50 tablets as blister-packs of 10 each.

Further information Nil.

Product licence numbers
Temgesic sublingual 0.2 mg 0044/0063
Temgesic sublingual 0.4 mg 0044/0109

TIMODINE*

Presentation Pale yellow cream containing (w/w):

Nystatin BP	100,000 i.u./g
Hydrocortisone PhEur	0.5%

Benzalkonium Chloride Solution BP	0.2%
Dimethicone 350 BP	10.0%

The cream contains nitrocellulose, dibutylphthalate, glycerylmonostearate, stearic acid, cetostearyl alcohol, parabens, sorbic acid, sodium metabisulphite and butylated hydroxyanisole.

Uses For the treatment of dermatoses, including intertrigo, eczema, seborrhoeic dermatitis, "housewife's eczema" and pruritus ani and vulvae, in which infection with *Candida albicans* is a factor. For the treatment of severe napkin rash in which *Candida albicans* is a factor.

Dosage and administration
Dermatoses: Sufficient Timodine should be applied to cover the lesion in a thin layer. It should then be massaged into the skin until the cream disappears. The treatment should be repeated three times a day until the lesion has healed.

There is no indication that dosage need be modified for the elderly.

Napkin Rash: After removal of the soiled napkin, the affected area should be cleaned and dried and a thin layer of Timodine applied. The treatment should be repeated after every napkin change. In infants, long term continuous topical steroid therapy should be avoided and a course of treatment should not normally exceed seven days.

Contra-indications, warnings, etc
Contra-indications: Sensitivity to benzalkonium chloride or nystatin.

Precaution: Keep away from the eyes.

Topical administration of corticosteroids to pregnant animals can cause abnormalities of foetal development. The relevance of this finding to human beings has not been established; however, topical steroids should not be used extensively in pregnancy, i.e. in large amounts or for prolonged periods.

Side-effects: None have been reported.

Pharmaceutical precautions Store below 15°C.

Legal category POM.

Package quantities Tubes of 30 g.

Further information Timodine is particularly indicated in the treatment of dermatoses occurring in sites, such as the skin folds, in which the special environmental conditions present predispose to maceration and chafing, leading to secondary infection with *Candida albicans* and bacteria, and causing additional inflammation and persistent pruritus.

Timodine has no known effects on diagnostic laboratory tests.

Product licence number 1839/0001.

Product licence held by Lloyd-Hamol Ltd.

**Trade Mark*

Rhône-Poulenc Rorer Limited

Dagenham
Essex RM10 7XS

RHÔNE-POULENC RORER

AAA* MOUTH AND THROAT SPRAY

Presentation The can contains 10.92 g with a valve providing 60 metered doses.

Each metered dose contains:

Benzocaine PhEur 1.5 mg

Other ingredients: ethanol, glycerin, sodium saccharin, cetalkonium chloride and an inert, flavoured propellant.

Uses Analgesic oral spray for the temporary relief of soreness or pain associated with sore throats and minor mouth infections.

Dosage and administration Shake can before use. *Adults (including elderly):* 2 shots every two to three hours if required (not more than 16 shots in 24 hours) or as directed by the physician.

Children aged 6–12: 1 shot every two to three hours if required (not more than 8 shots in 24 hours) or as directed by the physician. Not for use in children under 6 years.

Contra-indications, warnings, etc
Contra-indications: Known hypersensitivity to benzocaine.

Side-effects: Hypersensitivity reactions to benzocaine have been reported.

Interactions: As benzocaine may hydrolyse to p-aminobenzoic acid it should not be used with sulphonamides.

Precautions: This preparation should not be administered to children under 6 or used for more than three consecutive days unless directed by a physician.

If a sore throat is severe, persistent or accompanied by fever or headache, a physician should be consulted before use of this product.

Avoid spraying into eyes. Avoid inhalation of the product.

Contents under pressure – do not puncture.

Keep away from heat and flames – do not throw finished container into fire.

Use in pregnancy: There is no current evidence of hazard from benzocaine although only limited information is available. The product should not be used in pregnancy unless considered essential by a doctor.

Pharmaceutical precautions Store in a cool place. Shake can before use.

Legal category P.

Package quantities Single can containing 10.92 g with a valve providing 60 × 133 mg metered doses (shots) (OP).

Further information Nil.

Product licence number 0231/5026.

ASCABIOL*

Presentation Ascabiol is a mildly perfumed white emulsion containing 25% benzyl benzoate.

Uses Ascabiol is an efficient acaricide and is used in the treatment of scabies. It is also indicated in the treatment of pediculosis.

Benzyl benzoate is lethal to Sarcoptes scabei and to the adult and larval forms of head lice.

Dosage and administration *Scabies:* After a hot bath and drying, Ascabiol is applied to the whole body except the head and face. If the application is thorough, one treatment should suffice, but the possibility of failure is lessened if a second application is made within five days of the first.

Alternatively, Ascabiol can be applied to the whole body, except the head and face, on three occasions at 12-hourly intervals. The patient has a hot bath 12 hours after the last application and changes to clean clothes and sheets.

Pediculosis: The affected region is coated with Ascabiol followed by a wash 24 hours later with soap and water. In severe cases this procedure may need to be repeated two or three times. An examination should always be made a week after the last treatment to confirm disinfestation.

Elderly patients: No specific recommendations.

Children: Ascabiol can be diluted with an equal quantity of water for older children and with three parts of water for babies.

Contra-indications, warnings, etc Ascabiol causes little skin irritation, but may cause a transient burning sensation. This is usually mild but can occasionally be severe in sensitive individuals. In the event of a severe skin reaction, the preparation should be washed off using soap and warm water. Ascabiol is also irritating to the eyes, therefore these should be protected if it is applied to the scalp.

Pregnancy: There is inadequate evidence of the safety of Ascabiol in human pregnancy, but it has been widely used without apparent ill consequence. Nevertheless, Ascabiol should not be used during pregnancy unless considered essential.

Lactation: Breast feeding should be suspended during treatment with Ascabiol. Feeding may be restarted after the emulsion has been washed off the body.

If this preparation is accidentally taken by mouth, treatment should consist of gastric lavage or the administration of an emetic. An anticonvulsant should be given if necessary, otherwise treatment is symptomatic. Urinary retention in adults and convulsions in infants, have been reported following excessive use of topical benzyl benzoate. The body should be washed to remove excess benzyl benzoate, otherwise treatment is symptomatic.

Pharmaceutical precautions Store below 25°C.

Legal category P.

Package quantities Bottles of 100 ml.

Further information Patients should be warned that undiluted Ascabiol may adversely affect acrylic/plastic bathroom furniture.

Product licence number 0012/5104.

AVOMINE*

Presentation Avomine is presented as white tablets, each containing 25 mg promethazine theoclate, indented 'Avomine' on one face and with a break line on the reverse. The tablets also contain lactose, sodium metabisulphite and other ingredients.

Uses Long-acting anti-emetic, indicated for prevention and treatment of nausea and vomiting arising from various causes including motion sickness and postoperative vomiting. Vertigo due to Ménière's syndrome, labyrinthitis and other causes. Promethazine theoclate has central sedative, antihistamine and anticholinergic properties.

Kinetics: Promethazine is well absorbed after oral administration, peak plasma concentrations occurring in 2–3 hours. It is distributed widely in the body, metabolised in the liver and slowly excreted in the urine. The drug is highly plasma protein bound. It enters the brain and crosses the placenta. Phenothiazines pass into the milk in low concentrations.

Dosage and administration *Motion sickness: Adults:* For prevention on long journeys: one 25 mg tablet each evening at bedtime, starting the day before setting out. The duration of action is such that a second dose in 24 hours is not often necessary.

For prevention of motion sickness on short journeys: one 25 mg tablet one or two hours before travelling or as soon after as possible.

Treatment of motion sickness: One 25 mg tablet as soon as possible and repeated the same evening followed by a third tablet on the following evening.

Nausea and vomiting due to other causes: Adults: One 25 mg tablet at night is often sufficient, but two or three tablets are sometimes necessary. Alternatively, more frequent administration such as 25 mg two or three times a day may be required for some patients. It is not often necessary to give more than four of the 25 mg Avomine tablets in 24 hours.

Children: In the above indications children over 10 years of age may be given the lower adult doses described above. Children between 5 and 10 years may be given half the adult dose.

Elderly: No specific dosage recommendations.

Contra-indications, warnings, etc Avomine should not be used in patients who are in a coma or suffering from CNS depression of any cause. It must not be given to neonates, premature infants or patients hypersensitive to phenothiazines. Avomine should be avoided in patients who have been taking monoamine oxidase inhibitors within the previous 14 days.

Avomine may thicken or dry lung secretions and impair expectoration, it should therefore be used with caution in patients with asthma, bronchitis or bronchiectesis. Use with care in patients with severe coronary artery disease, narrow angle glaucoma, epilepsy or hepatic and renal insufficiency. Caution should be exercised in patients with bladder neck or pyloro-duodenal obstruction. Promethazine may mask the warning signs of ototoxicity caused by ototoxic drugs e.g. salicylates.

It may also delay the early diagnosis of intestinal obstruction or raised intracranial pressure through the suppression of vomiting.

Use in pregnancy: There is epidemiological evidence for the safety of promethazine in pregnancy, and animal studies have shown no hazard, nevertheless it should not be used in pregnancy unless the physician considers it essential. The use of Avomine tablets is not recommended in the two weeks prior to delivery in view of the risk of irritability and excitement in the neonate.

Use in lactation: Available evidence suggests that the amount excreted in milk is insignificant. However there are risks of neonatal irritability and excitement.

Ambulant patients receiving Avomine for the first time should not be in control of vehicles or machinery for the first few days until it is established that they are not hypersensitive to the central nervous effects of the drug and do not suffer from disorientation, confusion or dizziness.

Interactions: Avomine may enhance the action of any anticholinergic agent, tricyclic antidepressant, sedative or hypnotic. Alcohol should be avoided during treatment.

Avomine may interfere with immunologic urine pregnancy tests to produce false-positive or false-negative results. Avomine should be discontinued at least 72 hours before the start of skin tests using allergen extracts as it may inhibit the cutaneous histamine response thus producing false-negative results.

In nausea and vomiting of unknown origin, it is essential to establish the diagnosis before giving an anti-emetic, to ensure that a serious underlying condition is not masked.

Side-effects: Side-effects may be seen in a few patients: drowsiness, dizziness, restlessness, headaches, nightmares, tiredness, and disorientation. Anticholinergic side-effects such as blurred vision, dry mouth and urinary retention occur occasionally. Newborn and premature infants are susceptible to the anticholinergic effects of promethazine while other children may display paradoxical hyperexcitability. The elderly are particularly susceptible to the anticholinergic effects and confusion due to promethazine. Other side-effects include anorexia, gastric irritation, palpitations, hypotension, arrhythmias, extrapyramidal effects, muscle spasms and tic-like movements of the head and face. Anaphylaxis, jaundice and blood dyscrasias including haemolytic anaemia rarely occur. Photosensitive skin reactions have been reported; strong sunlight should be avoided during treatment.

Treatment of overdosage: Symptoms of severe overdosage are variable. They are characterised in children by various combinations of excitation, ataxia, inco-ordination, athetosis and hallucinations, while adults may become drowsy and lapse into coma. Convulsions may occur in both adults and children; coma or excitement may precede their occurrence. Cardiorespiratory depression is uncommon. If the patient is seen soon enough after ingestion, it should be possible to induce vomiting despite the anti-emetic effect of promethazine; alternatively, gastric lavage may be used.

Treatment is otherwise supportive with attention to maintenance of adequate respiratory and circulatory status. Convulsions should be treated with diazepam or other suitable anticonvulsant.

Pharmaceutical precautions Protect from light.

Legal category P.

Package quantities Containers of 30 × 25 mg tablets (OP).

Further information Nil.

Product licence number 0012/5253.

CALCITARE*

Presentation *For intramuscular or subcutaneous use only.* Each vial contains 160 international units Calcitonin (Pork) BP.

Uses For short term treatment in
i) *Paget's disease of bone*

ii) *Hypercalcaemia:* The calcium lowering effect of calcitonin is usually rapid. Treatment should be regarded as an adjunct to more specific long-term measures. The fall in serum calcium is more pronounced in hypercalcaemic patients with a raised bone turnover, e.g. Paget's disease and thyrotoxicosis. Treatment may also be beneficial in patients with hypercalcaemia due to immobilisation in Paget's disease, malignancy, vitamin D intoxication and hyperparathyroidism. Calcitonin is of particular value when such patients have concurrent renal or cardiac failure.

Dosage and administration Calcitare can be given subcutaneously or intramuscularly.

1. *Paget's disease of bone:* Clinical and biochemical improvement has been observed with dosage regimens ranging from 80 international units three times a week to 160 international units daily in single or divided doses.

Daily injections of 80 international units or 160 international units are recommended for three to six months in patients with bone pain or nerve compression syndromes.

Clinical improvement is usually seen within three months but may occasionally be delayed for as long as a year. When clinical improvement occurs, an attempt to reduce the dose and/or frequency of injection may be made, consistent with maintaining a remission. Alternatively, treatment can be stopped and restarted at a later date when necessary. Duration of dosage should be a maximum of two six month courses.

Biochemical improvement is shown by a reduction in serum alkaline phosphatase and urinary hydroxyproline excretion, the fall in urinary hydroxyproline often occurring in a matter of days. The fall in serum alkaline phosphatase occurs in a matter of weeks. Serum alkaline phosphatase and urinary hydroxyproline levels return slowly towards pre-treatment values (at different rates) on withdrawal of calcitonin therapy.

When changing from synthetic salmon calcitonin (Calsynar) to porcine calcitonin (Calcitare), 80 international units of Calcitare may be conveniently substituted for 50 international units of Calsynar and 160 international units for 100 international units respectively.

2. *Hypercalcaemia:* The optimum dosage pattern must essentially be gauged by the magnitude of the hypocalcaemic response obtained in a particular patient. In general the greatest response will be observed in cases of rapid bone turnover. Four international units per kg per day of Calcitare may produce a fall in serum calcium. However, larger doses of calcitonin may be necessary, but are inconvenient to administer as Calcitare, in which case treatment with Calsynar is advised.

Elderly: No special precautions.

Children: Calcitare should not be given to children for more than a few weeks unless the physician considers that longer treatment is indicated on compelling medical grounds; careful surveillance of bone growth is recommended.

Contra-indications, warnings and side-effects A species and strain-specific dose-related increase of pituitary adenomas has been observed in long term toxicity studies in the rat. As the significance of these findings to man is uncertain, long term use is not recommended.

Calcitonin may cause nausea, vomiting, facial flushing and tingling of the hands. An unpleasant taste and inflammatory reactions at the injection site have been reported. The nausea and flushing are usually transient and rarely necessitate withdrawal of treatment. If necessary, the injections can be administered at night with an antiemetic.

In any patient with a history of allergy, a scratch (or intradermal) test should be conducted prior to administration of Calcitare using a 1:100 dilution in Sodium Chloride Injection BP. To detect gelatin sensitivity a similar test should be carried out using gelatin diluent in the same dilution.

Some patients will develop porcine calcitonin binding antibodies after several months of treatment. The antibodies are generally of low titre and are more likely to occur in patients on the higher doses. The development of these antibodies is not usually related to loss of clinical efficacy. It is possible that this may be analogous to treated diabetic patients in whom insulin binding antibodies frequently develop, but who rarely manifest clinical resistance to insulin. The presence of these antibodies appears to bear no relationship to allergic reactions which are very rare. Secondary hyperparathyroidism is not thought to occur following calcitonin therapy.

There are several reports of the value of calcitonin in the acute treatment of severe hypercalcaemia in patients with concurrent renal or cardiac failure; however, care should be exercised when treating such patients. Trace amounts of T_3/T_4 are present in Calcitare. Experience over a number of years has not revealed any significant metabolic effects due to T_3 and T_4, when Calcitare has been given at the maximum recommended dose for Paget's disease of 160 international units daily. At higher doses (e.g. 4 international units/kg) used in the treatment of hypercalcaemia, the amounts of T_3/T_4 normally detected in the product are most unlikely to have any adverse effect, except in highly susceptible patients such as those with significant ischaemic heart disease.

Use in pregnancy and lactation: Studies have not been carried out in pregnant patients. Animal studies have suggested a possible relationship between calcitonin and retardation of foetal growth and inhibition of lactation. Unless considered essential, calcitonin should not be used in women of child bearing potential or nursing mothers.

Treatment of overdosage: No specific antidote. Following overdosage, e.g., 600 international units as a single injection one might experience flushing of the face and/or extremities or gastrointestinal disturbance. Acute hypocalcaemia is unlikely to occur.

Pharmaceutical precautions Calcitare is presented as a sterile, lyophilised powder providing 160 international units porcine calcitonin per vial. Calcitare should normally be used immediately after aseptic reconstitution. The reconstituted product will, however, maintain its potency for up to 24 hours at room temperature or 7 days in a refrigerator (2°–8°C). Typically, however, the reconstituted product should be stored at 2°–8°C and used within 48 hours.

The lyophilised powder when stored at less than 25°C will retain its potency for three years.

Legal category POM.

Package quantities *For intramuscular or subcutaneous use:* Boxes of 5 vials Calcitare 160 international units per vial sterile, lyophilised, with 5 ampoules gelatin diluent, sterile.

Boxes of 10 vials Calcitare 160 international units per vial sterile, lyophilised, with 10 ampoules gelatin diluent, sterile.

Further information The calcium lowering ability of the calcitonins is measured in international units. The international unit is based on a rat bioassay in which one fortieth of the weight of salmon calcitonin, as compared with weights of porcine and human calcitonin, produces the same fall in serum calcium. The weights of pure calcitonin equivalent to 100 international units in this assay are: human calcitonin, 1 mg. porcine calcitonin, 1 mg, and salmon calcitonin, 0.025 mg.

Product licence number 0231/0011.

CALSYNAR*

Presentation

Multidose vials: An aqueous solution containing 400 international units of synthetic Salmon Calcitonin in 2 mls. The solution also contains Sodium Chloride, Sodium Acetate, Acetic Acid and Phenol.

Ampoule: An aqueous solution containing 100 international units of Synthetic Salmon Calcitonin in 1 ml of solution. The injection also contains Sodium Chloride, Sodium Acetate and Acetic Acid.

Uses For the short term treatment of:

(a) Paget's disease of bone.
(b) Advancing osteolytic hypercalcaemia of malignancy.
(c) Pain associated with advanced metastatic bone cancer: The use of Calsynar has been reported to be beneficial in the relief of pain in some patients with advanced metastatic bone cancer.
(d) Postmenopausal osteoporosis: Studies based on total body calcium determinators have indicated that Calsynar may be effective in the prevention of progressive loss of bone mass in the treatment of postmenopausal osteoporosis.

Dosage and administration For subcutaneous or intramuscular use only.

(a) Paget's disease of bone: Clinical and biochemical improvement has been observed with dosage regimens ranging from 50 international units three times a week to 100 international units daily in single or divided doses.

When clinical improvement occurs, a dosage reduction may maintain a remission in some patients. Alternatively, treatment can be stopped and restarted at a later date when necessary.

Biochemical improvement is shown by a reduction in serum alkaline phosphatase and urinary hydroxyproline excretion, the fall in urinary hydroxyproline often occurring in a matter of days, the fall in serum alkaline phosphatase and urinary hydroxyproline levels return slowly towards pretreatment values (at different rates) on withdrawal of calcitonin therapy.

When changing from porcine calcitonin (Calcitare) to synthetic salmon calcitonin (Calsynar) 50 international units of Calsynar may be conveniently substituted for 80 international units of Calcitare and 100 international units for 160 international units of Calcitare.

(b) Advancing osteolytic hypercalcaemia of malignancy: Treatment should be adjusted to the patient's clinical and biochemical response.

Severe hypercalcaemia may require high doses of Calsynar and initially 400 international units may be given every 6 or 8 hours. Lower doses may be satisfactory in some patients and dosage may be adjusted according to the patient's clinical and biochemical response. There is no additional benefit to be gained from doses in excess of 8 international units per kg given every 6 hours.

(c) Pain associated with metastatic bone cancer: The usual dose is 200 international units, 6-hourly or 400 international units 12-hourly for 48 hours. Concomitant analgesic medication may be reduced as appropriate. The treatment course may be repeated at the discretion of the physician.

Many patients with advanced malignant disease already suffer from anorexia and nausea. In these cases, prior administration of anti-emetic therapy may reduce the incidence of nausea and vomiting sometimes associated with calcitonin therapy.

(d) Post menopausal osteoporosis: The recommended dose of Calsynar is 100 international units per day. Patients should also receive supplementary calcium (equivalent to 600 mg elemental calcium daily) and vitamin D (400 units daily). An adequate diet is also essential. (See also 'Further Information').

Elderly: No special precautions.

Children: Calsynar should not be given to children for periods of more than a few weeks unless the physician considers that longer treatment is indicated on compelling medical grounds. Careful surveillance of bone growth is recommended.

Contra-indications, warnings, etc
Precautions: Rat carcinogenicity studies have shown a dose related excess of pituitary tumours. As the significance of this finding is uncertain, long term use is not recommended.

There are several reports of the value of Calcitonin in the acute treatment of severe hypercalcaemia in patients with concurrent renal or cardiac failure, however, care should be exercised when treating such patients.

Following injections of calcitonin serum calcium levels may be transiently lowered to below normal values. This effect is noted most frequently on initiation of therapy where bone turnover is abnormally high, but diminishes as osteoclastic activity is reduced with Calsynar. Whilst this phenomenon does not usually give rise to complications, care should be exercised in patients who are receiving concurrent cardiac glycosides as dosage adjustments of these drugs may be necessary in view of the fact that their effect may be modified by changes in cellular electrolyte concentrations.

Prior to treatment with Calsynar any patients who have a history of allergy should undergo a scratch (or intradermal) test using a 1:100 dilution of Calsynar in Sodium Chloride injection BP.

Side-effects: Calcitonin may cause nausea, vomiting, facial flushing, tingling of the hands and an unpleasant taste. Inflammatory reactions at the injection site have been reported. The nausea and flushing are usually transient and rarely necessitate withdrawal of treatment. If necessary, the injections can be administered at night with an antiemetic.

Some patients will develop salmon calcitonin binding antibodies after several months of treatment. The antibodies are generally of low titre and are more likely to occur in patients on the higher doses. The development of these antibodies is not usually related to loss of clinical efficacy. It is possible that this may be analogous to treated diabetic patients in whom insulin binding antibodies frequently develop, but who rarely manifest clinical resistance to insulin. The presence of antibodies appears to bear no relationship to allergic reactions which are very rare. Secondary hyperparathyroidism is not thought to occur following calcitonin therapy.

Administration of salmon calcitonin has been reported in a few cases to cause serious allergic type reactions (e.g. bronchospasm, swelling of the tongue or throat and anaphylactic shock). Allergic reactions should be differentiated from generalised flushing and hypotension.

Use in pregnancy and lactation: Studies have not been carried out in pregnant women. Animal studies have suggested a possible relationship between Calcitonin and retardation of foetal growth and inhibition of lactation. Hence unless considered essential, Calcitonin should not be used in women of child bearing potential or nursing mothers.

Treatment of overdosage: Symptoms following overdosage, e.g. 400 international units administered as a single injection, may include flushing of the face and or extremities, and gastrointestinal disturbance. Acute hypocalcaemia is unlikely to occur. There is no specific antidote.

Pharmaceutical precautions
Calsynar multidose vials: Store between 2–8°C. Do not freeze.
Calsynar Ampoules: Store between 2–8°C. Do not freeze.

Legal category POM.

Package quantities Multidose vial: Box of 1 and cartons of 4 vials.
Ampoules: Cartons of 5.

Further information
Postmenopausal osteoporosis: There is evidence from published literature on postmenopausal osteoporosis that cyclical therapy may be useful in some patients.

Units and potency: The calcium lowering ability of the calcitonins is measured in international units. The international unit is based on a rat bioassay in which one fortieth of the weight of salmon calcitonin, as compared with weights of porcine and human calcitonin, produces the same fall in serum calcium. The weights of pure calcitonin equivalent to 100 international units in this assay are approximately: human calcitonin 1 mg; porcine calcitonin 1 mg and salmon calcitonin 0.025 mg.

Product licence numbers

Multidose vials:	0231/0027
Ampoules:	0231/0055

CEPLAC

Presentation Rose coloured tablets engraved CEPLAC on one face and plain on the reverse face. Each tablet contains 6 mg erythrosine (E127).

Uses As an aid to the efficient teaching of oral hygiene.

Dosage and administration *Adults (including elderly) and children:* The patient should be given a Ceplac Tablet in the surgery. This will at once demonstrate the shortcomings of his current oral hygiene techniques and make it easier to gain his co-operation.

When he has been shown the correct method of brushing his teeth, he should be sent home with a supply of Ceplac Tablets and instructions on how to use them. Ceplac will play a central role in helping him to acquire the habit of regular and correct tooth brushing.

Initially use once a day. The patient should crush one Ceplac Tablet between his teeth before cleaning them, and distribute saliva to all tooth and gum surfaces with the aid of the tongue for at least half a minute. He should then spit out into a bowl of running water, and rinse his mouth once or twice with water.

He should then brush his teeth in the way he has been shown until all red stain has been removed.

Once a sound brushing technique has been established the patient can use Ceplac from time to time after brushing, as a check on continuing proficiency.

In the same way, patients should be given Ceplac on visits to the surgery, to assess their progress.

Contra-indications, warnings, etc There are no known contra-indications or adverse reactions.

Use in pregnancy: No known contra-indications to use in pregnancy. Do not use, however, unless recommended by your doctor.

Treatment of overdosage: Gastric lavage.

Pharmaceutical precautions No special precautions.

Legal category GSL.

Package quantities Pack of 14 (OP).

Further information Ceplac stains bacterial plaque and food debris a brilliant red. The stain is non-persistent and is easily removed from lips or clothing with soap and water.

Product licence number 0152/5032.

CLEXANE* ▼

Presentation Clexane is available in single dose prefilled syringes.

Clexane 20 mg contains 20 mg enoxaparin in 0.2 ml of clear, colourless to pale yellow solution and has an anti-Factor Xa activity of 2000 iu (with reference to the WHO First International Low Molecular Weight Heparin Reference Standard).

Clexane 40 mg contains 40 mg enoxaparin in 0.4 ml of clear, colourless to pale yellow solution and has an anti-Factor Xa activity of 4000 iu.

Uses
Indications: Clexane is indicated for:

(1) The prophylaxis of thromboembolic disorders of venous origin, in particular those which may be associated with orthopaedic or general surgery.

(2) The prevention of thrombus formation in the extracorporeal circulation during haemodialysis.

Properties: Enoxaparin is a low molecular weight heparin which has antithrombotic properties. It is characterised by a higher ratio of anti-Factor Xa to anticoagulant activity than unfractionated heparin. At the recommended doses, it does not significantly influence platelet aggregation or binding of fibrinogen to platelets, nor does it affect global blood clotting tests. (i.e. prothrombin time or Activated Partial Thromboplastin Time (APTT)). It is, therefore, unnecessary to monitor treatment with these tests. However, biological and chromogenic assays can be used to measure anti-Factor Xa activity, if considered necessary.

Pharmacokinetics: Enoxaparin is rapidly and completely absorbed after subcutaneous injection. Maximum plasma anti-Factor Xa activity occurs 1 to 4 hours after injection; the peak activities are approximately 0.16 iu/ml after injection of 20 mg (2000 iu) and 0.38 iu/ml after injection of 40 mg (4000 iu). The anti-Factor Xa activity generated by enoxaparin is localised within the vascular compartment and elimination is characterised by a half-life of approximately 4–5 hours; for a dose of 40 mg (4000 iu) anti-Factor Xa activity may persist in the plasma for up to 24 hours after injection.

Enoxaparin is excreted renally, in the intact or slightly degraded form, although the overall elimination rate remains unchanged in patients with renal insufficiency. Hepatic metabolism of enoxaparin occurs mainly by desulphation and depolymerisation. The half-life is prolonged in the elderly to between 6 and 7 hours, although no alteration of the dosage is necessary.

Enoxaparin, as detected by anti-Factor Xa activity, does not cross the placental barrier during the second trimester of pregnancy.

Dosage and administration
Administration: Clexane may be administered by subcutaneous injection, or through the arterial line of a dialysis circuit. It must not, however, be administered by intramuscular injection.

Subcutaneous injection technique: Patients should be lying down and Clexane administered by deep subcutaneous injection. Administration should be alternated between the left and the right anterolateral and left and right posterolateral abdominal wall. The whole length of the needle should be introduced vertically into a skin fold held between the thumb and forefinger; the skin fold should be held throughout the injection. Do not purge the syringes of air before use.

Adult dosage: In patients with a low to moderate risk of venous thromboembolism, such as in general surgery, the recommended dose of Clexane is 20 mg (2000 iu) once daily by subcutaneous injection. Treatment should be continued for 7 to 10 days or until the risk of thromboembolism has diminished. In patients undergoing surgery, the initial dose should be given approximately 2 hours preoperatively.

In patients with a higher risk of venous thromboembolism, such as in orthopaedic surgery, the dose should be increased to 40 mg (4000 iu) administered once daily by subcutaneous injection with the initial dose being given approximately 12 hours preoperatively.

In extracorporeal circulation during haemodialysis, 1 mg/kg (100 iu/kg) enoxaparin is introduced into the arterial line of the circuit at the beginning of the dialysis session. The effect of this dose is usually sufficient for a 4 hour session although, if fibrin rings are found, such as after a longer than normal session, a further dose of 500 to 1000 micrograms/kg (50 to 100 iu/kg) may be given. For patients with a high risk of haemorrhage the dose should be reduced to 500 micrograms/kg for double vascular access or 750 micrograms/kg for single vascular access.

Elderly: No dosage adjustment is necessary in the elderly.

Children: Dosage not established.

Contra-indications, warnings, etc
Contra-indications: Clexane is contra-indicated in patients with acute bacterial endocarditis, major bleeding disorders, thrombocytopenia in patients with a positive 'in-vitro' aggregation test in the presence of enoxaparin, active peptic ulcer, hypersensitivity to enoxaparin, stroke (except if due to systemic emboli) and in other patients with increased risk of haemorrhage.

Warning: Clexane must not be administered by the intramuscular route.

Precautions: Clexane should be used with care in patients with hepatic insufficiency, uncontrolled arterial hypertension or a history of gastrointestinal ulceration.

As different low molecular weight heparins may not be equivalent, alternative products should not be introduced during a course of treatment.

Use in pregnancy: There is inadequate evidence of the safety of enoxaparin in human pregnancy, although animal studies have shown no hazard. Clexane does not cross the placental barrier in animals or during the second trimester of human pregnancy. As a precaution, Clexane should not be used during pregnancy unless no safer alternative can be found.

Use in lactation: There is no experience of the use of enoxaparin during human lactation, although it is poorly absorbed orally and fertility studies in rodents were free of any effect on lactation. As a precaution, lactating mothers receiving Clexane should be advised to avoid breast-feeding.

Interactions: Clexane should be used with care in patients receiving oral anticoagulants, platelet aggregation inhibitors, non-steroidal anti-inflammatory drugs, aspirin or dextran.

Adverse reactions: Thrombocytopenia may occur rarely and liver abnormalities, such as changes in transaminase and alkaline phosphatase, are possible during treatment with Clexane. Ecchymosis and other haemorrhagic, manifestations may occur occasionally.

Overdosage: Orally administered Clexane is poorly absorbed and so even large oral doses should not lead to any serious consequences. This may be checked by plasma assays of the anti-Factor Xa and anti-Factor IIa activities.

Accidental overdosage following subcutaneous administration of Clexane may lead to haemorrhagic complications. This may be largely neutralised by the slow intravenous injection of protamine (sulphate or hydrochloride). The dose of protamine should be equal to the dose of Clexane injected: 100 anti-heparin units of protamine should neutralise the anti-Factor IIa activity generated by 1 mg (100 iu) of Clexane. Under these conditions, the thrombin time and anti-Factor Xa activity are corrected in a manner comparable to unfractionated heparin. However, even with higher doses of protamine, the APTT may remain more prolonged than under normal conditions found following administration of conventional heparin. In all these cases the anti-Factor Xa activity is never completely neutralised (maximum about 60%). Particular care should be taken to avoid overdosage with protamine.

Pharmaceutical precautions Do not mix Clexane with other injections or infusions. Clexane should be stored at room temperature (22° ± 4°C).

Legal category POM.

Package quantities Clexane is available in packs of 10 prefilled syringes.

Further information Nil.

Product licence numbers
Clexane 20 mg 0012/0196.
Clexane 40 mg 0012/0197.

CONRAY*

Presentation Ampoules or vials containing colourless sterile solutions of varying strengths of meglumine or sodium iothalamate. The aqueous solutions also contain sodium calciumedetate and sodium dihydrogen phosphate.

Conray 280: Meglumine iothalamate injection 60% w/v containing 280 mg iodine in combined form per ml.

Conray 325: Sodium iothalamate injection 54% w/v containing 325 mg iodine in combined form per ml.

Conray 420: Sodium iothalamate injection 70% w/v containing 420 mg iodine in combined form per ml.

Uses X-ray contrast media are used for the opacification of the vascular and renal systems and the female genital tract and do not normally possess any pharmacological action. See the table below for detailed uses of each product.

Kinetics: If renal function is not impaired Conray is rapidly excreted unchanged by glomerular filtration.

Dosage and administration See table below.

There are no specific dosage recommendations for the elderly.

Contra-indications, warnings, etc *Pregnancy:* There is inadequate evidence as to the safety of Conray in human pregnancy. The pregnant female should not be submitted to X-rays unless the radiologist considers it essential.

Conray preparations must NEVER be injected into the subarachnoid space.

For cerebral arteriography, Conray 280 should be used; Conray 325 and 420 should not be employed in this procedure and are not recommended in any peripheral arteriography.

Precautions: Following the use of any contrast medium of this type, there is the remote possibility of severe sensitivity reactions occurring. When they do, they tend to occur in the first few minutes following injection and the patient should be kept under observation during this period. It is essential to have immediately available emergency resuscitation equipment, including appropriate drugs, oxygen and means of administration.

Subjects with a history of allergy or previous reactions to drugs or severe cardiovascular disease are more at risk than others.

Side-effects: Side-effects which may occur are nausea, vomiting, metallic taste, sensation of heat, weakness, headache, dizziness, thirst, coughing, sneezing, itching, urticaria, pallor, tachycardia and hypotension. Rarely: convulsions, circulatory failure and cardiac arrest. Pain may be felt at the site of injection.

Overdosage: Overdosage is unlikely in clinical practice. In the event of accidental overdosage it is important to keep the patient well hydrated. Other treatment should be symptomatic, with particular reference to the cardiovascular system.

Pharmaceutical precautions Protect from light.

Apart from Water for Injections and Dextrose Saline, Conray should not be mixed with any other substance.

Legal category POM.

Package quantities *Conray 280:* Box of 10 × 20 ml ampoules. Box of 10 × 50 ml bottles.
Conray 325: Box of 10 × 50 ml bottles.
Conray 420: Box of 10 × 20 ml ampoules. Box of 10 × 50 ml bottles.

Further information Nil.

Product licence numbers
Conray 280: 0012/5033R
Conray 325: 0012/5034R
Conray 420: 0012/5035R

Procedure	Conray 280	Conray 325	Conray 420
Intravenous urography	*Adults:* 40–80 ml. In the absence of preliminary dehydration 40–100 ml may be used. *Infants and children:* Under 12 kg: 2 ml/kg body weight. Over 12 kg: 1.5 ml/kg body weight (with a minimum of 24 ml). Over 10 years of age: Lower range of adult dosage.	As for Conray 280.	40 ml is usually adequate but the schedule for Conray 280 can be used with safety.
Femoral and other peripheral arteriography.	15–20 ml injected into the femoral or iliac artery will provide excellent visualisation of the arterial tree of the leg. A similar or smaller dose is indicated for smaller arteries.	**Do not use**	**Do not use**
Cerebral arteriography (carotid and vertebral)	Average adult dose is 6–10 ml for each injection. Exceptionally, up to 10 injections of 8 ml each have been made into the carotid artery.	**Do not use**	**Do not use**
Abdominal aortography (direct puncture or retrograde catheterisation)	*Adults:* 20–30 ml.	*Adults:* 20–30 ml.	*Adults:* 20–30 ml.
Thoracic aortography (including arch aortography)	Often adequate in children: 0.5–1 ml per kg body weight. May be used as a test dose in positioning catheter tip.	*Adults and children:* 0.5–1 ml per kg body weight. The usual volume employed in the adult is 20–40 ml.	
Intravenous aortography	**Do not use**	**Do not use**	*Adults and children:* 1 ml per kg body weight. In adults 80–100 ml or more per injection is often used. Frequently this amount is subdivided equally and given by rapid simultaneous bilateral injection.
Angiocardiography	May be used as test dose in positioning catheter tip. Volumes of up to 40 ml have been used for this purpose prior to the diagnostic dose of more concentrated medium.	**Do not use**	*Adults and children over 14 years of age:* 20 to 50 ml per injection. *Small children and infants:* 0.5–1.0 ml per kg body weight with a minimum of 3 ml. Multiple injections may be required and the above doses may be repeated with confidence but 3 ml per kg body weight should not be exceeded.
Splenography, portal venography	*Adults;* 20–40 ml.	*Adults;* 20–40 ml.	*Adults:* 20–40 ml.
Femoral venography and/or inferior vena cavography	*Adults:* 20–60 ml.	*Adults:* 20–60 ml.	*Adults:* 20–60 ml.
Hysterosalpingography	About 10 ml are usually required, administered by slow injection into the uterine cervical canal via a syringe and suitable canula.	**Do not use**	**Do not use**

CREMALGIN* BALM

Presentation Pink balm containing methyl nicotinate 1.0% w/w, capsicin 0.1% w/w, glycol salicylate 10.0% w/w. Other ingredients: lannette wax, stearic acid, white soft paraffin, triethanolamine, Ponceau 4R (E124).

Uses Rubefacient balm. For the symptomatic relief of rheumatism, sciatica, lumbago, fibrositis and muscular stiffness.

Dosage and administration Two or three times daily or as required. Place a sufficient quantity on the skin over the affected area and massage gently. To be applied to the unbroken skin only.

Contra-indications, warnings, etc Cremalgin is contra-indicated in those patients with salicylate hypersensitivity. Erythematous reactions may occur in sensitive patients.

Use in pregnancy: No information available on use in pregnancy. Do not use unless recommended by a doctor.

Pharmaceutical precautions No special precautions.

Legal category GSL.

Package quantities Tubes of 30 g (OP).

Further information Nil.

Product licence number 5272/0031.

FLAGYL* & FLAGYL-S* SUSPENSION

Presentation Tablets containing 200 mg and 400 mg metronidazole. The 200 mg tablets are off white to cream, film coated, engraved 'Flagyl 200' around the outer margin. The 400 mg tablets are capsule shaped, off white to cream, film coated, engraved 'Flagyl 400' on one side.

Flagyl-S Suspension: White to cream yellow, each 5 ml containing 320 mg metronidazole benzoate, equivalent to 200 mg metronidazole.

Flagyl-S suspension contains 68% w/v sugars, ethanol, methyl and propyl hydroxybenzoate.

Suppositories containing 500 mg and 1.0 gram metronidazole.

Injection (for intravenous infusion) metronidazole 0.5 per cent w/v in 100 ml bottles or 100 ml Viaflex containers or 20 ml ampoules. The injection also contains sodium phosphate, citric acid and sodium chloride.

Uses Flagyl is indicated in the prophylaxis and treatment of infections in which anaerobic bacteria have been identified or are suspected to be the cause.

Flagyl is active against a wide range of pathogenic micro-organisms notably species of Bacteroides, Fusobacteria, Clostridia, Eubacteria, anaerobic cocci and Gardnerella vaginalis.

It is also active against Trichomonas, Entamoeba histolytica, Giardia lamblia and Balantidium coli.

It is indicated in:

1. The prevention of postoperative infections due to anaerobic bacteria, particularly species of bacteroides and anaerobic streptococci.
2. The treatment of septicaemia, bacteraemia, peritonitis, brain abscess, necrotising pneumonia, osteomyelitis, puerperal sepsis, pelvic abscess, pelvic cellulitis, and post-operative wound infections from which susceptible pathogenic anaerobes have been isolated.
3. Urogenital trichomoniasis in the female (trichomonal vaginitis) and in the male.
4. Bacterial vaginosis (also known as non-specific vaginitis, anaerobic vaginosis or Gardnerella vaginitis).
5. All forms of amoebiasis (intestinal and extra-intestinal disease and that of symptomless cyst passers).
6. Giardiasis.
7. Acute ulcerative gingivitis.
8. Anaerobically-infected leg ulcers and pressure sores.
9. Acute dental infections (e.g. acute pericoronitis and acute apical infections).

Kinetics: Metronidazole is rapidly and almost completely absorbed on administration of Flagyl Tablets; peak plasma concentrations occur after 20 min to 3 hours.

The bioavailability of metronidazole in Flagyl suppositories is 60–80%. Effective blood concentrations are achieved 5–12 hours after the first suppository and are maintained by the recommended 8 hourly regimen.

Metronidazole is widely distributed in body tissues after injection. At least half the dose is excreted in urine as metronidazole and metabolites. The elimination half-life of metronidazole is approximately 8.5 ± 2.9 hours.

Metronidazole can be used in chronic renal failure; it is rapidly removed from the plasma by dialysis.

Metronidazole is excreted in milk but the intake of a suckling infant of a mother receiving normal dosage would be considerably less than the therapeutic dosage for infants.

Dosage and administration *Flagyl tablets* should be swallowed with water (NOT CHEWED). It is recommended that the tablets be taken during or after a meal.

Flagyl S suspension should be taken at least one hour before a meal.

Flagyl suppositories are unsuitable for initiating treatment of serious conditions owing to slower absorption and lower plasma concentrations of metronidazole.

Flagyl injection should be infused intravenously at an approximate rate of 5 ml/minute. Oral medication should be substituted as soon as feasible.

Only those substances and diluents listed under 'Pharmaceutical Precautions' should be mixed with Flagyl Injection. For intravenous administration, on no account should substances other than those specified be administered concurrently by the same route.

Anaerobic infections: Treatment for 7 days should be satisfactory for most patients but, depending on clinical and bacteriological assessments, the physician may decide to prolong treatment, for example, for the eradication of infection from sites which cannot be drained or are liable to endogenous recontamination by anaerobic pathogens from the gut, oropharynx or genital tract.

A. *Prophylaxis:* against anaerobic infection – chiefly in the context of abdominal (especially colorectal) and gynaecological surgery.

Intravenous: 500 mg shortly before operation, repeated 8 hourly, oral doses of 400 mg 8 hourly to be started as soon as feasible.

Children: 7.5 mg/kg (1.5 ml) 8 hourly.

Oral: 400 mg at 8 hourly intervals during the 24 hours preceding operation followed by postoperative intravenous or rectal administration until patient is able to take tablets.

Children 7.5 mg/kg 8 hourly.

Rectal: 1 g 8 hourly.

Children: one half or a quarter of a 500 mg suppository 8 hourly.

Elderly: Caution is advised in the elderly, particularly at high doses, although there is limited information available on modification of dosage.

B. *Treatment of established anaerobic infection:*

Intravenous: to be used initially if patient's condition or symptoms preclude oral therapy: 500 mg 8 hourly.

Children: 7.5 mg/kg 8 hourly.

Oral: 800 mg followed by 400 mg 8 hourly.

Children: 7.5 mg/kg 8 hourly.

Rectal: 1 g 8 hourly. Substitute oral medication as early as possible. If rectal administration is prolonged beyond 3 days reduce dose to 1 g 12 hourly for remainder of course.

Children: 7.5 mg/kg 8 hourly.

C. *Treatment of Protozoal and other infections:* See table.

Contra-indications, warnings, etc

Use in pregnancy: There is inadequate evidence of the safety of metronidazole in pregnancy. Flagyl should not therefore be given during pregnancy or during lactation unless the physician considers it essential; in these circumstances the short, high-dosage regimens are not recommended.

Contra-indication: Known hypersensitivity to metronidazole.

Precautions: Regular clinical and laboratory monitoring are advised if administration of Flagyl for more than 10 days is considered to be necessary.

There is a possibility that after Trichomonas vaginalis has been eliminated a gonococcal infection might persist.

The elimination half-life of metronidazole remains unchanged in the presence of renal failure. The dosage of metronidazole therefore needs no reduction. Such patients however retain the metabolites of metronidazole. The clinical significance of this is not known at present. In patients undergoing haemodialysis metronidazole and metabolites are efficiently removed during an eight-hour period of dialysis. Metronidazole should therefore be re-administered immediately after haemodialysis.

No routine adjustment in the dosage of 'Flagyl' need be made in patients with renal failure undergoing intermittent peritoneal dialysis (IPD) or continuous ambulatory peritoneal dialysis (CAPD).

Dosage is given in terms of metronidazole or metronidazole equivalent

	Duration of dosage in days	*Adults and children over 10 years‡*	*Children†*		
			7 to 10 years	*3 to 7 years*	*1 to 3 years*
Urogenital trichomoniasis Where re-infection is likely, in adults the consort should receive a similar course of treatment concurrently.	7	200 mg three times daily or 400 mg twice daily	100 mg three times daily	100 mg twice daily	50 mg three times daily
	or 2	800 mg in the morning and 1,200 mg in the evening			
	or 1	2.0 g as a single dose			
Bacterial vaginosis	7	400 mg twice daily			
	1	2·0 g as a single dose			
Amoebiasis (a) Invasive intestinal disease in susceptible subjects	5	800 mg three times daily	400 mg three times daily	200 mg four times daily	200 mg three times daily
(b) Intestinal disease in less susceptible subjects and chronic amoebic hepatitis	5–10				
(c) Amoebic liver abscess also other forms of extra-intestinal amoebiasis	5	400 mg three times daily	200 mg three times daily	100 mg four times daily	100 mg three times daily
(d) Symptomless cyst passers	5–10	400–800 mg three times daily	200–400 mg three times daily	100–200 mg four times daily	100–200 mg three times daily
Giardiasis	3	2.0 g once daily	1.0 g once daily	600–800 mg once daily	500 mg once daily
Acute ulcerative gingivitis	3	200 mg three times daily	100 mg three times daily	100 mg twice daily	50 mg three times daily
Acute dental infections	3–7	200 mg three times daily			
Leg ulcers and pressure sores	7	400 mg three times daily			
Anaerobic infections (general)			See data sheet text		

† Children and babies weighing less than 10 kg should receive proportionately smaller dosages.
‡ *Elderly:* Flagyl is well tolerated by the elderly, but a pharmacokinetic study suggests cautious use of high dosage regimens in this age group.

Metronidazole is mainly metabolised by hepatic oxidation. Substantial impairment of metronidazole clearance may occur in the presence of advanced hepatic insufficiency. Significant cumulation may occur in patients with hepatic encephalopathy and the resulting high plasma concentrations of metronidazole may contribute to the symptoms of the encephalopathy. Flagyl should, therefore, be administered with caution to patients with hepatic encephalopathy. The daily dosage should be reduced to one-third and may be administered once daily.

Caution is advised in patients with active disease of the central nervous system other than brain abscess.

Patients should be advised not to take alcohol during metronidazole therapy because of the possibility of a disulfiram-like reaction.

Some potentiation of anticoagulant therapy has been reported when metronidazole has been used with the warfarin type oral anticoagulants. Dosage of the latter may require reducing. Prothrombin times should be monitored. No interactions have been reported with anticoagulants of the heparin type. However, anticoagulant activity should be routinely monitored with these products. Lithium retention accompanied by evidence of possible renal damage has been reported in patients treated simultaneously with lithium and metronidazole. Lithium treatment should be tapered or withdrawn before administering metronidazole. Plasma concentration of lithium, creatinine and electrolytes should be monitored in patients under treatment with lithium while they receive metronidazole.

Patients receiving phenobarbitone metabolise metronidazole at a much greater rate than normally, reducing the half life to approximately 3 hours.

Aspartate amino transferase assays may give spuriously low values in patients taking metronidazole, depending on the method used.

Clinicians who contemplate continuous therapy for the relief of chronic conditions, for periods longer than those recommended, are advised to consider the possible therapeutic benefit against the risk of peripheral neuropathy.

Warnings and adverse effects: Serious adverse reactions occur very rarely with standard recommended regimens. Unpleasant taste in the mouth, furred tongue, nausea, vomiting gastro-intestinal disturbance, and urticaria and angioedema occur occasionally. Anaphylaxis may occur rarely.

Drowsiness, dizziness, headache, ataxia, skin rashes, pruritus, incoordination of movement, darkening of the urine (due to metronidazole metabolite) have been reported but very rarely.

During intensive and/or prolonged metronidazole therapy, a few instances of peripheral neuropathy or transient epileptiform seizures have been reported. In most cases neuropathy disappeared after treatment was stopped or when dosage was reduced. A moderate leucopenia has been reported in some patients but the white cell count has always returned to normal before or after treatment has been completed.

Treatment of overdosage: Uneventful recovery has followed attempts at suicide with quantities of 30 and 60 × 200 mg tablets.

There is no specific treatment for gross overdosage of Flagyl.

Pharmaceutical precautions Protect from light. Suppositories – store below 20°C. Flagyl-S suspension and Viaflex containers 100 mls – store below 25°C. Protect from light. 20 ml ampoules and 100 ml bottles of injection solution. Protect from light.

Cefuroxime sodium is physically and chemically compatible with Flagyl Injection. The following drugs have been shown to be physically compatible in terms of pH and appearance over the normal period of administration, although there is no information on chemical stability: amikacin sulphate, ampicillin sodium, carbenicillin sodium, cephazolin sodium, cefotaxime sodium, cephalothin sodium, chloramphenicol sodium succinate, clindamycin phosphate, gentamicin sulphate, hydrocortisone sodium succinate, latamoxef disodium, netilmicin sulphate and tobramycin sulphate.

In patients maintained on intravenous fluids, Flagyl Injection may be diluted with appropriate volumes of sodium chloride solution 0.9% w/v, dextrose and sodium chloride, dextrose 5% w/v or potassium chloride (20 or 40 mmol/litre) intravenous infusions.

Flagyl Injection must not be mixed with cefamandole nafate, cefoxitin sodium, dextrose 10% w/v infusion, compound sodium lactate injection, penicillin G potassium or any other substance unless specified above.

Legal category POM.

Package quantities Blister packs of 21 × 200 mg (OP) and 14 × 400 mg (OP) tablets.

Bottles of 100 ml (OP) suspension (metronidazole benzoate).

Containers of 10 × 500 mg (OP) and 10 × 1.0 gram (OP) suppositories.

Boxes of 10 × 100 ml bottles injection 0.5 per cent w/v.

Cartons of 20 × 100 ml injection 0.5 per cent w/v in Viaflex containers.

Carton of 10 × 20 ml ampoules 0.5 per cent w/v.

Further information Metronidazole has no useful direct activity against aerobic and facultatively anaerobic bacteria.

Flagyl injection does not contain a preservative; the 100 ml bottle is not, therefore, intended as a 'multi-dose'.

Dilution of Flagyl-S suspension, if necessary, should be carried out with syrup BP. The diluted suspension has a shelf life of 14 days.

Viaflex is a registered trade mark of Baxter Healthcare Ltd.

Product licence numbers

Tablets 200 mg	0012/5256
Tablets 400 mg	0012/0084
Suppositories 500 mg	0012/0113
Suppositories 1.0 g	0012/0114
Injection 100 ml	0012/0107
Injection 20 ml	0012/0125
Suspension	0012/0131

FLAGYL* COMPAK

Presentation Flagyl Compak is a combined treatment pack containing: 14 × 400 mg Flagyl (metronidazole)

Tablets, 14 × 100,000 units nystatin vaginal inserts, 1 vaginal insert, applicator.

The 400 mg metronidazole tablets are capsule-shaped, off-white to cream, film coated, engraved 'Flagyl 400' on one face.

The 100,000 units nystatin vaginal inserts are yellowish-cream, almond shaped, indented 'M&B' on one face. The inserts also contain lactose.

Uses Flagyl is a potent trichomonacide. It is also active against other protozoa and anaerobic bacteria.

Nystatin is a fungistatic and fungicidal antibiotic which is active topically against Candida albicans.

Flagyl Compak is indicated in the treatment of vaginitis where a mixed trichomonal/candidal infection is diagnosed or suspected. Presenting symptoms may include vaginal discharge, pruritus vulvae and dyspareunia.

Kinetics: Metronidazole is rapidly and almost completely absorbed from the tablets leading to peak plasma concentrations after 20 min to 3 hours. Metronidazole is excreted in milk but the intake of a suckling infant of a mother receiving normal dosage would be considerably less than the therapeutic dosage for infants.

Nystatin is not absorbed through the skin or mucous membranes when applied topically.

Dosage and administration One Flagyl Tablet to be swallowed whole, with half a glassful of water during or after meals, twice daily for seven days.

Concurrently, one nystatin vaginal insert to be moistened and introduced high into the vagina night and morning for seven days. Some physicians may prefer to instruct patients to use one insert nightly, before retiring, for fourteen nights. Full patient instructions for use of the applicator are included in each Compak.

This product is not recommended for girls under 10 years of age.

Elderly: No specific dosage recommendations.

Where cross infection with Trichomonas vaginalis is confirmed or suspected the male consort should be treated concurrently with one Flagyl 400 tablet by mouth twice daily for seven days.

Contra-indications, warnings, etc

Use in pregnancy: There is inadequate evidence of the safety of metronidazole in pregnancy. Flagyl Compak should not therefore be given during pregnancy or during lactation unless the physician considers it essential.

Contra-indications: Known hypersensitivity to metronidazole.

Precautions: Regular clinical and laboratory monitoring are advised if administration of Flagyl for more than 10 days is considered to be necessary.

There is a possibility that after *Trichomonas vaginalis* has been eliminated a gonococcal infection might persist.

The elimination half-life of metronidazole remains unchanged in the presence of renal failure. The dosage of metronidazole therefore needs no reduction. Such patients however retain the metabolites of metronidazole. The clinical significance of this is not known at present. Metronidazole is mainly metabolised by hepatic oxidation. Substantial impairment of metronidazole clearance may occur in the presence of advanced hepatic insufficiency. Significant cumulation may occur in patients with hepatic encephalopathy and the resulting high plasma concentrations of metronidazole may contribute to the symptoms of the encephalopathy. Flagyl should, therefore, be administered with caution to patients with hepatic encephalopathy. The daily dosage should be reduced to one-third and may be administered once daily.

Patients should be advised not to take alcohol during metronidazole therapy because of the possibility of a disulfiram-like reaction.

Some potentiation of anticoagulant therapy has been reported when metronidazole has been used with the warfarin type oral anticoagulants. Dosage of the latter may require reducing. Prothrombin times should be monitored. There is no interaction with heparin. Lithium retention accompanied by evidence of possible renal damage has been reported in patients treated simultaneously with lithium and metronidazole. Lithium treatment should be tapered or withdrawn before administering metronidazole. Plasma concentration of lithium creatinine and electrolytes should be monitored in patients under treatment with lithium while they receive metronidazole.

Patients receiving phenobarbitone metabolise metronidazole at a much greater rate than normally, reducing the half life to approximately 3 hours.

Aspartate amino transferase assays may give spuriously low values in patients taking metronidazole, depending on the method used.

Warnings and adverse effects: Serious adverse reactions occur very rarely with standard recommended regimens. There have been reports of an unpleasant taste in the mouth, furred tongue, nausea, vomiting, gastro-intestinal disturbance, and of urticaria and angioedema. Anaphylaxis may occur rarely.

Drowsiness, dizziness, headache, ataxia, skin rashes, pruritus, inco-ordination of movements and darkening of the urine (due to metronidazole metabolite) have been reported but very rarely.

No adverse effects due to the use of nystatin vaginal inserts have been reported.

Pharmaceutical precautions Protect from light. Flagyl Compak should be stored in a cool place.

Legal category POM.

Package quantities Combined treatment pack containing 14 × 400 mg Flagyl Tablets, 14 × 100,000 units nystatin vaginal inserts, 1 vaginal insert applicator, full instructions for the patient (OP).

Further information There is no evidence of resistant organisms developing to either Flagyl or nystatin.

Product licence number 0012/5091.

FLAXEDIL*

Presentation Colourless injection solution containing gallamine triethiodide 4% w/v. The injection solution also contains sodium sulphite.

Uses Non-depolarising (competitive-blocking) muscle relaxant having a duration of action of 20–30 minutes. Flaxedil is used as an adjunct to induce skeletal muscle relaxation and also to manage patients undergoing mechanical ventilation.

Pharmacokinetics: Gallamine acts 1–2 minutes after intravenous administration with a duration of action of 20–30 minutes. It is excreted unchanged in urine with negligible amounts in bile.

Dosage and administration Flaxedil is administered intravenously after the patient has been anaesthetised. Dosage must be adjusted to individual requirements, the nature of the general anaesthetic used, and the duration of the operation. Some anaesthetists recommend that a test dose of 20 mg should be given before anaesthesia is induced to exclude sensitivity.

As a guide the average adult requires 80–120 mg of Flaxedil given intravenously for the provision of adequate muscular relaxation. Supplementary doses of 20–40 mg are given as required. Where no suitable vein is available, Flaxedil may be given intramuscularly with or without hyaluronidase.

Elderly: No specific dosage recommendations.

For children a dosage of 1.5 mg per kg should be given intravenously.

Neonates: As neonates are more sensitive to gallamine a dose of 600 micrograms/kg is recommended.

Contra-indications, warnings, etc
Contra-indications: Flaxedil is contra-indicated in patients suffering from myasthenia gravis, shock, severe renal impairment and hypersensitivity to gallamine, iodine or sulphite.

Since gallamine is excreted by the kidneys it should not be used in patients with renal dysfunction (G.F.R. less than 50 mls per minute).

Pregnancy: In early pregnancy, there is inadequate evidence of safety. Flaxedil has however been widely used for many years without apparent ill consequence. Avoid unless there is no safer alternative available.

In operative obstetrics, because gallamine passes rapidly through the placental barrier, it should be used with care until after delivery of the foetus.

Lactation: Gallamine is inactive orally and should therefore cause no problems in infants of breastfeeding mothers.

Precautions: Since gallamine is excreted by the kidneys extra care is necessary in its use in patients with renal dysfunction (GFR below 50 mls/min). Flaxedil should only be used when facilities for securing an effective airway and providing controlled respiration with adequate oxygen are available.

Care is advised in the use of gallamine in patients with cardiac disorders, hypertension and pulmonary dysfunction.

The action of gallamine may be affected by body temperature, hydration status, electrolyte imbalance and the presence of bronchogenic carcinoma.

Flaxedil contains sulphite as a preservative and a reaction to sulphite, characterised by cardiorespiratory collapse, can occur in some susceptible individuals.

Interactions: The action of muscle relaxants is enhanced by the antibiotics amikacin, gentamicin, kanamycin, neomycin, streptomycin, polymixin, tobramycin and by potent anaesthetics such as halothane, ether and methoxyflurane. Diazepam has been reported to delay recovery from gallamine. Quinidine enhances the action of neuromuscular blocking agents and may lead to recurarisation if given after surgery. Azathioprine can reverse or decrease neuromuscular blockade by gallamine.

Muscular relaxation with Flaxedil is normally free from side-effects, other than tachycardia which occurs in the majority of patients and which is associated with its vagolytic action. Care is advised in its use in patients with heart conditions. Anaphylactic and anaphylactoid reactions have been reported occasionally.

Overdosage with Flaxedil is an unlikely event. If it is necessary to reverse the effects of Flaxedil rapidly, the antagonist neostigmine methylsulphate should be injected intravenously in a dosage of 1 mg initially followed by increments of 0.5 mg until the respiratory exchange is adequate. The use of neostigmine must always be preceded by the intravenous injection of atropine sulphate 0.5–1 mg. No patient who has received neostigmine should be left alone until all risk of excessive bradycardia and of recrudescence of muscular paralysis has passed.

Pharmaceutical precautions Protect from light.

Flaxedil is compatible with solutions of thiopentone sodium, but it is important to add the Flaxedil to the thiopentone solution, not vice versa. Flaxedil is incompatible with pethidine hydrochloride solutions.

Legal category POM.

Package quantities Boxes of 10 × 2 ml ampoules.

Further information Nil.

Product licence number 0012/5077R.

FRUMIL*

Presentation
Frumil: Orange tablets with a breakline, marked Frumil each containing 40 mg Frusemide BP and Amiloride Hydrochloride BP equivalent to amiloride hydrochloride anhydrous 5 mg. Other ingredients include lactose, sunset yellow (E110).

Frumil LS (low strength): Orange tablets marked 'LS' containing 20 mg Frusemide BP and Amiloride Hydrochloride BP equivalent to amiloride hydrochloride anhydrous 2.5 mg.

Frumil Forte: Orange tablets with a breakline, marked 'DS', and containing 80 mg Frusemide BP and Amiloride Hydrochloride BP equivalent to amiloride hydrochloride anhydrous 10 mg.

Uses Frumil is indicated where a prompt diuresis is required. It is of particular value in conditions where potassium conservation is important: congestive cardiac failure, nephrosis, corticosteroid therapy, oestrogen therapy. Ascites associated with cirrhosis.

Dosage and administration The tablets should be taken in the morning.

Frumil: The normal adult dose is one tablet although this may be increased to two tablets.

Frumil LS: When weaker diuresis is required one Frumil LS tablet (equivalent to half a Frumil tablet) should be taken.

Frumil Forte: When more powerful diuresis is required, i.e., necessitating two Frumil tablets, a single Frumil Forte tablet may be given as an alternative.

Elderly: The dosage should be adjusted according to diuretic response: serum electrolytes and urea should be carefully monitored.

Contra-indications, warnings, etc
Contra-indications: Hyperkalaemia (serum potassium >5.3 mmol/litre), Addison's disease, acute renal failure, anuria, severe progressive renal disease, electrolyte imbalance, precomatose states associated with cirrhosis, concomitant potassium supplements or potassium-sparing diuretics, known sensitivity to frusemide or amiloride.

Frumil is contra-indicated in children as safety in this age group has not been established.

Warnings: Hyperkalaemia has been observed in patients receiving amiloride hydrochloride. As ACE inhibitors may elevate serum potassium levels, especially in the presence of renal impairment, combination with Frumil is best avoided in elderly patients or in any others in whom renal function may be compromised. If use of the combination is deemed essential, clinical condition and serum electrolytes must be carefully and continuously monitored.

Frusemide may cause latent diabetes to become manifest. It may be necessary to increase the dose of hypoglycaemic agents in diabetic patients.

Patients with prostatic hypertrophy or impairment of micturition have an increased risk of developing acute urinary retention during diuretic therapy.

Serum uric acid levels may rise during treatment with Frumil and acute attacks of gout may be precipitated.

Cephaloridine nephrotoxicity may be increased by concomitant administration of potent diuretics such as Frumil.

Precautions: Patients who are being treated with this preparation require regular supervision, with monitoring of fluid and electrolyte states to avoid excessive loss of fluid.

Frumil should be used with particular caution in elderly patients or those with potential obstruction of the urinary tract or disorders rendering electrolyte balance precarious.

Hyponatraemia, hypochloraemia and raised blood urea nitrogen may occur during vigorous diuresis, especially in seriously ill patients. Careful monitoring of serum electrolytes and urea should therefore be undertaken in these patients.

The dosage of concurrently administered cardiac glycosides, lithium, non-depolarising muscle relaxants or antihypertensive agents may require adjustment.

Frumil should be discontinued before a glucose tolerance test.

Pregnancy and lactation: The safety of Frumil use during pregnancy and lactation has not been established.

Side effects: Malaise, gastric upset, nausea, vomiting, diarrhoea, and constipation may occur.

If skin rashes or pruritus occur, treatment should be withdrawn.

Rare complications may include minor psychiatric disturbances, disturbances in liver function tests and ototoxicity.

Bone marrow depression occasionally complicates treatment, necessitating withdrawal of the product. The haematopoietic state should be regularly monitored during treatment.

Treatment of overdosage: Treatment of overdosage should be aimed at reversing dehydration and correcting electrolyte imbalance, particularly hyperkalaemia. Emesis should be induced or gastric lavage performed. Treatment is symptomatic and supportive. If hyperkalaemia is seen, appropriate measures to reduce serum potassium must be instituted.

Pharmaceutical precautions Store in a cool, dry place, protect from light.

Legal category POM.

Package quantities Frumil: Cartons of 28 tablets consisting of 2 calendar foils of 14 tablets (OP).

Cartons of 56 tablets consisting of 4 calendar foils of 14 tablets (OP).

Frumil LS: Cartons of 28 tablets consisting of 2 calendar foils of 14 tablets (OP).

Cartons of 56 tablets consisting of 4 calendar foils of 14 tablets (OP).

Frumil Forte: Cartons of 28 tablets consisting of 2 calendar foils of 14 tablets (OP).

Cartons of 56 tablets consisting of 4 calendar foils of 14 tablets (OP).

Further information Frumil is particularly suitable for patients at risk from hypokalaemia and causes significantly less potassium excretion than frusemide during the 12 hours after administration. The daily loss of potassium with Frumil is equivalent to normal potassium excretion.

Product licence number

Frumil	5272/0017
Frumil LS	5272/0024
Frumil Forte	5272/0026

GARDENAL* SODIUM

Presentation A clear, very slightly yellow injection solution containing 200 mg phenobarbitone sodium per ml in a propylene glycol/water mixture.

Uses Gardenal Sodium is a long-acting barbiturate with anticonvulsant properties. It may be used to control seizures in epilepsy and similar conditions.

Kinetics: Barbiturates are rapidly absorbed and widely distributed in the body. They diffuse across the placenta and appear in the milk. Phenobarbitone is excreted mainly unchanged in the urine. The plasma half life is shorter in children than adults but longer in neonates.

Dosage and administration May be injected undiluted by the intramuscular route. Before intravenous administration Gardenal Sodium injection should be diluted to 10 times its own volume with Water for Injections immediately before use.

For the emergency control of convulsions:

Adults: 200 mg i.m. repeated if necessary after 6 hours.

Elderly: No specific dosage recommendations, but see 'Precautions' below.

Children: 15 mg/kg i.m. is required as a loading dose to achieve adequate blood levels. This may be followed by 5 mg/kg daily by mouth (divided if appropriate).

In status epilepticus Gardenal Sodium is preferably

given i.v. 400–800 mg in the adult, small doses being relatively ineffective.

Contra-indications, warnings, etc
Pregnancy and lactation: There is evidence of harmful effects in animals, therefore avoid its use during first trimester pregnancy unless there is no safer alternative. Hypo-prothrombinaemia and withdrawal symptoms have been seen in neonates whose mothers have been treated during late pregnancy. Barbiturates should be used with caution in the nursing mother.

Contra-indication: Acute intermittent porphyria is an absolute contra-indication.

Precautions: Gardenal Sodium should be used with care in infants, elderly or frail patients.

Dosage should be reduced in the presence of marked renal or hepatic failure.

Interactions: Gardenal Sodium should not be administered to patients known to have taken alcohol or other CNS depressants. In patients stabilized on phenytoin phenobarbitone may lead to lower serum concentrations of phenytoin. Sodium valproate could enhance the action of phenobarbitone. The following drugs may become less effective on administration of phenobarbitone: Warfarin, chloramphenicol, corticosteroids and oral contraceptives.

Warnings and adverse effects: Idiosyncratic reactions have occasionally occurred in the form of a hangover, followed by vertigo or gastro-intestinal upset or excitement or localised or diffuse pain. Hypersensitivity reactions appearing as localised swellings, particularly about the face have also been reported.

Toxicity and treatment of overdosage: Overdosage produces severe, persistent respiratory depression.

Treatment includes general measures for the support of the respiratory and cardiovascular systems.

Pharmaceutical precautions Protect from light. Store below 25°C.

Legal category POM.

Package quantities Box of 10 × 1 ml ampoules.

Further information Nil.

Product licence number 0012/5076.

HALOTHANE – M&B*

Presentation Halothane is an almost colourless liquid with a distinctive, pleasant odour. It contains thymol as an inactive ingredient.

Uses Halothane is a general anaesthetic used in inhalation anaesthesia. It is of particular value:

1. When cautery or diathermy is to be used.
2. In giving a pleasant and rapid induction particularly in children.
3. As it suppresses secretions from the salivary, bronchial and gastric glands.
4. In maintaining the required plane of anaesthesia which is easily reversed.
5. Since relaxation is adequate for most operations and respiration is readily controlled.
6. Since recovery is rapid and nausea and vomiting are rare.
7. As it is suitable for most types of surgery.
8. As it can be given with a very high percentage of oxygen when this is indicated.

Dosage and administration *The technique of Halothane anaesthesia:*

1. *Pre-medication:* A small dose of pethidine with or without the addition of promethazine will produce satisfactory sedation in most patients and will reduce the tendency to tachypnoea. Atropine in an appropriate dose should be administered to all patients.

2. *Induction:* This is most conveniently carried out with a sleep dose of thiopentone sodium, to allow the application of a face mask. A gas flow of 8 litres/minute should be administered, of which at least 30% should be oxygen, and then the Halothane should slowly be introduced. Administration should start at 0.5% and be increased by a further 0.5% every few breaths until the inspired gases contain 3% Halothane. Intubation can be carried out after five minutes' inhalation of 3% Halothane in a carrier gas flow of 8 litres/minute or before exposure to Halothane if an intubating dose of suxamethonium is given. If intubation is performed before exposing the patient to Halothane, the introduction of Halothane must still be stepwise.

3. *Maintenance:* At a gas flow of 8 litres/minute, Halothane concentrations of between 0.5% and 1.5% are usually adequate. At a 2 litres/minute gas flow with the vaporiser out of circuit (VOC) a concentration of 2–2.5% fed into the absorber circuit will suffice. A low resistance vaporiser may be placed within the circuit (VIC), but in this case controlled or assisted ventilation must not be used. A vaporiser for VIC use must not be capable of delivering a concentration greater than 3%.

4. *Recovery:* This is usually rapid and uneventful. If the Halothane is withdrawn as skin closure starts, reflexes will have returned by the time the dressings are in place. Shivering is occasionally seen during recovery if there is a marked temperature differential between the theatre and the ward. This is readily controlled by the administration of a small dose of chlorpromazine, but supplementary oxygen may be required for a few minutes.

Methods of administration: Halothane is a potent anaesthetic and should, wherever possible, be administered via a specially calibrated and temperature-compensated vaporiser. A number of such vaporisers are now available.

Halothane can also be administered from the ordinary bottle vaporiser of a Boyle's machine, but the scale should be extended to allow fine adjustment in the concentration of Halothane delivered.

Open-drop anaesthesia with Halothane is not generally recommended; however, a few drops carefully applied to the mask may smooth the subsequent administration of ether.

Draw-over machines and inhalers can be satisfactorily used with Halothane, but if air is the carrier gas, supplementary oxygen or assisted respiration may be necessary to maintain full oxygenation.

Contra-indications, warnings, etc Halothane can induce liver damage. Minor changes in serum aminotransferase activity have been reported to occur in about 20% of patients. The incidence of severe liver damage (jaundice, which may lead to hepatic failure as a consequence of massive hepatic cell necrosis) is not known. However the risk of developing hepatic failure appears to be greatly increased by repeated exposure to Halothane. Although short intervals of time between exposures are likely to increase the risk of hepatotoxicity, even long intervals between exposure may not reduce the risks, since some patients have developed severe reactions to Halothane given many years after the previous exposure. On the information which is available at the present time, it is advised that the following precautions be taken:

(i) A careful anaesthetic history is to be taken from patients due to undergo anaesthesia in order to determine whether exposure to Halothane took place and the nature of any adverse reaction to this agent.

(ii) History of unexplained jaundice or pyrexia after a previous exposure to Halothane is an absolute contra-indication to its future use in that patient.

(iii) Further exposure to Halothane within three months is to be avoided unless there are overriding reasons for its re-use.

(iv) Patients who have exhibited adverse reactions to Halothane should be informed and strictly instructed to alert their physician. Details of the reaction should be entered on the patient's medical records.

Particular care should be exercised in the following conditions:

1. In obstetrics – uterine relaxation and post-partum haemorrhage may result.
2. In neurosurgery – a rise in CSF pressure has been

recorded, the effects of which may be mitigated by the use of moderate hyperventilation.

3. When injection of Adrenaline is used concurrently – cardiac arrhythmias may occur.

The use of beta-adrenergic blocking agents during Halothane anaesthesia is at the discretion of the anaesthetist.

Muscle relaxants: All commonly used muscle relaxants may be used in conjunction with Halothane, but, as Halothane potentiates the actions of gallamine and *d*-tubocurarine, the doses of these muscle relaxants must be reduced. The association of *d*-tubocurarine with Halothane may lead to a marked fall in blood pressure.

Ganglion blocking agents: Potentiation occurs between Halothane and the standard hypotensive agents such as pentolinium, pempidine and trimetaphan. These drugs must be used in reduced dosage when administered in conjunction with Halothane.

Vaporiser: Halothane must not be used in the EMO ether vaporiser as it attacks the metal; a vaporiser specially constructed for Halothane should be used.

Pharmaceutical precautions Store in a dark place below 25°C. Keep well closed. The vaporiser should be drained at regular intervals. Any discoloured Halothane should be discarded.

Legal category P.

Package quantities Bottle of 250 ml.

Further information Nil.

Product licence number 0012/0095.

HEXABRIX*

Presentation
Hexabrix 320: Ampoules and bottles of a sterile, light yellow solution of meglumine ioxaglate 39.30% w/v and sodium ioxaglate 19.65% w/v containing 320 mg iodine in combined form per ml.

Hexabrix 200: Bottles of a sterile, light yellow solution of meglumine ioxaglate 24.56% w/v and sodium ioxaglate 12.28% w/v containing 200 mg iodine in combined form per ml.

Hexabrix 200 and Hexabrix 320 also contain sodium calciumedetate.

Uses Low osmolar X-ray contrast medium for the opacification of the vascular system, urinary tract, joints and female genital tract, the indications for which are given in the table on the next page.

Kinetics: Hexabrix is rapidly eliminated by the kidneys with a half-life of about 90 minutes. 99% of the dose is eliminated in 24 hours. Some biliary excretion also occurs and opacification of the gall bladder may be observed 24 hours after administration. Biliary excretion may be of some importance in kidney impairment. The compound is not metabolised.

Dosage and administration See table on next page. For ease of injection it may be found helpful to warm Hexabrix to near body temperature.

Elderly: No specific dosage recommendations.

Contra-indications, warnings, etc Hexabrix must never be injected by the subarachnoid or epidural route. It is definitely contra-indicated for myelography.

Pregnancy: There is no evidence that this product is safe during pregnancy, nor is there evidence in animal work that it is free from hazard. The product should not be used during pregnancy unless benefit outweighs the risk and is considered essential by the physician. The ten day rule in women of childbearing age should be observed.

Precautions: Since the causes of severe reactions to iodinated water-soluble contrast media are unknown and preliminary testing is unreliable as an indication that a patient will react unfavourably, the only other safeguards are physical examination and a careful evaluation of the patient's history to screen out subjects known to suffer from allergy, asthma, or severe cardiovascular disease. The provision of facilities for resuscitation and the training of staff members in their prompt use is mandatory.

A positive history of allergy, asthma or of untoward reactions during previous similar investigations does not necessarily contra-indicate the use of the contrast agent, but it emphasises the need for extra caution, for a sensitivity-test dose before the definitive injection, possibly steroid cover, and for even greater than usual preparedness to deal promptly with any reaction that might occur.

Extra caution should be exercised in carrying out radiographic procedures with contrast media in patients with severe systemic disease, asthma, and in allergic subjects. In patients with advanced renal disease and inadequate renal function as reflected by a raised blood urea, and in diabetics, the normally rapid excretion of the contrast medium may be markedly impaired. Even in patients with kidney disease substantial deterioration of renal function is minimised if the patient is well hydrated. Urine output must be carefully checked in these patients after the procedure.

Patients with hepatorenal insufficiency should not be examined unless the possibility of benefit clearly outweighs the additional risk. Re-examination should be delayed for five to seven days.

Special care should be exercised when Hexabrix is injected into the right heart or pulmonary artery in patients with pulmonary arterial hypertension. Right heart angiography is probably best avoided in patients with pulmonary arterial hypertension.

Patients with MYELOMATOSIS, and to a lesser degree, DIABETES, show poor tolerance of all intravenous radio-diagnostic compounds, the use of which should be avoided unless the possibility of benefit clearly outweighs the risk. These patients must be particularly well hydrated should intravascular iodinated injections be necessary and urine output must be carefully monitored.

All organic iodine contrast media interfere with tests of thyroid function. If required, such diagnostic tests should be undertaken before procedures with Hexabrix or a few weeks after the procedures.

Sensitivity testing: Hypersensitivity to Hexabrix has been very rare but may be tested for by any of the standard techniques. It is doubtful, however, whether routine sensitivity testing is justified, providing careful enquiry has been made concerning a history of allergy or of untoward reactions on any previous occasion. A 'negative' sensitivity test-dose does not imply that the patient will tolerate a larger volume.

Resuscitation: It is essential to have at hand injections of adrenaline, a vasopressor, an anti-histaminic and hydrocortisone, together with appropriate sterile syringes, needles etc. Means for administering oxygen under positive pressure and maintaining an adequate air-way should always be available.

Because of the possibility, remote though it may be, of a delayed reaction to the contrast agent, the patient should never be left unsupervised for the thirty minutes immediately after the injection.

Warnings and adverse effects: In cerebral arteriography, the only frequent side-effect is facial heat, usually of mild degree. In femoral and iliac arteriography a warm feeling is usually experienced and very rarely slight pain may be felt but leg movement and/or vocal protests are unusual.

After the rapid injection of Hexabrix for angiocardiography or aortography, patients may experience a wave of mild warmth, associated with flushing passing over the body. Slight coughing may occur after right heart or pulmonary artery injections. Other transient reactions reported rarely are nausea, vomiting, hypotension, headache and a metallic taste.

A few ventricular extrasystoles are common after any rapid intraventricular injection and the injection flow should not exceed 12 ml/sec in the adult ventricle. Ventricular fibrillation may occur very infrequently after intra-cardiac or intra-coronary injection and a DC

Procedure	*Product*	*Dosage and administration*
Femoral and other peripheral arteriographies	Hexabrix 320	15–20 ml injected into the femoral or iliac artery will provide excellent visualisation of the arterial tree of the leg. A similar or smaller dose is indicated for smaller arteries.
Cerebral angiography (carotid and vertebral)	Hexabrix 320	Average adult dose: 6–8 ml for each injection. Up to 10 injections each of 8 ml may be required.
Angio-cardiography	Hexabrix 320	Multiple small test injections may be used for positioning catheter tip. Adults and children over 14 years: 30–50 ml per injection. Children (14 years and under) and infants: 1–1.5 ml per kg bodyweight. Multiple injections may be required. Total dosage should not normally exceed 4 ml per kg bodyweight. In exceptional circumstances, this total dose may be exceeded according to the clinical condition.
Abdominal aortography (direct puncture or catheterization)	Hexabrix 320	Adults: 20–30 ml. Up to 50 ml may be used particularly if films of the legs are also taken following the same injection.
Thoracic aortography (including arch aortography)	Hexabrix 320	Adults and children: 0.5–1 ml per kg bodyweight up to 40 ml per injection. This may be repeated if necessary. Total dosage should not normally exceed 4 ml per kg bodyweight.
Pulmonary angiography	Hexabrix 320	Adults: 20–40 ml. Children: 0.5–1 ml per kg bodyweight. Special care should be exercised in patients with pulmonary arterial hypertension.
Coronary arteriography	Hexabrix 320	Adults: 3–8 ml per injection, depending on size of artery. Several injections are usually given for complete demonstration, particularly in the left coronary artery.
Digital subtraction angiography	Hexabrix 320 to be diluted 50% with Water for Injection BP or Sodium Chloride and Dextrose Injection BP to produce a solution containing 160 mg of Iodine per ml	The appropriate volume of diluted medium (depending on the part of the body to be visualised) should be injected into a suitable artery.
Intravenous aortography	Hexabrix 320	Adults and children: 1–1.5 ml per kg bodyweight. In adults 100 ml is often used; frequently this amount is sub-divided equally and given by simultaneous rapid bilateral injection.
Femoral venography and/or inferior vena cavography	Hexabrix 320	Adults: 20–50 ml.
Leg phlebography	Hexabrix 200 Hexabrix 320	50–150 ml injected into a vein in the foot. 20–50 ml injected into a vein in the foot.
Intravenous urography	Hexabrix 320	Adults: 20–80 ml. 60–100 ml may be used provided that the patient is not dehydrated. Children: Under 12 kg–2 ml per kg bodyweight. Over 12 kg–1.5 ml per kg bodyweight (with a minimum of 24 ml). Over 10 years of age—lower range of adult dosage. Patients with severe renal disease or diabetes should be well hydrated. Particular care is necessary in these patients as temporary deterioration in renal function has been reported.
Splenography portal venography	Hexabrix 320	Adults: 20–40 ml by splenic puncture.
Knee arthrography (double contrast)	Hexabrix 320	By injection into the knee joint. Adults: 4.5 ml together with injections of air before and after the positive contrast medium.
Hysterosalpingography	Hexabrix 320	About 10 ml is usually required, administered by slow injection into the uterine cervical canal via a syringe and suitable cannula.

defibrillator and other equipment necessary for defibrillation must always be available during these studies.

Following intracardiac, ascending aortic or coronary artery injection, the QRST complex of the ECG may be altered briefly. After prolonged cardiac catheterisation (with or without injection of a contrast medium), 5 to 10 per cent of patients may develop some degree of shivering or shock.

In intravenous urography, nausea, vomiting, dizziness and urticaria have been reported occasionally but have been of little consequence.

Interactions: Special care should be exercised in patients being treated with a calcium ion antagonist (eg verapamil) and who are to undergo coronary angiography; in such circumstances, a few instances of serious arrhythmias have been reported.

Toxicity and treatment of overdosage: In laboratory animals, the main signs of toxicity are convulsions, pulmonary congestion and oedema, respiratory depression, prostration, darkening of the eyes and hypersalivation; it is most unlikely that such toxic signs would occur in man, as it would be necessary to inject far greater doses than the maximum of those recommended. In man, overdosage as such should not arise but, since the causes of severe reactions to iodinated water-soluble contrast media are unknown, the information detailed causes of severe reactions to iodinated water-soluble contrast media are unknown, the information detailed under *Precautions and resuscitation* should be carefully studied.

Pharmaceutical precautions Protect from light.

Apart from Water for Injections and Dextrose Saline, Hexabrix should not be mixed with any other substance.

Legal category POM.

Package quantities

Hexabrix 320: Box of 10 × 20 ml ampoules.
Box of 10 × 50 ml bottles.
Box of 10 × 100 ml bottles.

Hexabrix 200: Box of 10 × 50 ml bottles.

Further information Nil.

Product licence numbers

Hexabrix 320: 0012/0135
Hexabrix 200: 0012/0167

INTRAVAL* SODIUM

Presentation Vials or bottles of thiopentone sodium.

It is supplied in vials of 0.5 g and bottles of 2.5 g for extemporaneous preparation of 2.5% solutions. A sterile transfer device, with instructions for use, is supplied with each 2.5 g bottle.

Uses Administered intravenously Intraval Sodium produces general anaesthesia of short duration.

Intraval Sodium is indicated for the induction of general anaesthesia; for general anaesthesia of short duration with or without the addition of a muscle relaxant; for the control of convulsive states. It is administered rectally for the induction of basal anaesthesia.

Other information: Although bound to plasma proteins it rapidly crosses the blood-brain barrier and reaches maximum concentration in the brain within 30 seconds of injection. It is slowly metabolised by the liver. Only a small proportion of the active drug is excreted in the urine.

Dosage and administration Intraval Sodium is administered usually as a 2.5% solution, but a 5% solution is sometimes used. A 2.5% solution is advised for all elderly and bad-risk patients. The injection may be given through any superficial vein.

Definite dosage cannot be stated for every case. The response of each patient must be observed and the dose regulated according to the onset of unconsciousness. Fractional administration is advised rather than the single-dose method, as this gives close control and greater flexibility of the anaesthetic and helps to prevent overdosage.

Most patients will require not more than 0.5 g otherwise recovery will be prolonged and possibly complicated. The patient should in all cases be premedicated with atropine and if necessary with an analgesic or tranquiliser, although the latter will increase the recovery time. If chlorpromazine or promethazine are used for pre-medication the amount of Intraval Sodium required for induction should be reduced.

Solutions are prepared by adding Water for Injections (BP). They must be used within 24 hours or discarded.

For induction: Inject 2–3 ml of the 5% solution or twice this volume of the 2.5% solution in 10–15 seconds, then pause for 30 seconds to 1 minute to observe the effect of the drug, depending on the state of the patient's circulation. Usually there is loss of consciousness and some relaxation. A further quantity of the solution may then be given if indicated, otherwise anaesthesia should be maintained by an appropriate inhalation agent.

For minor operations: Induction is as described above with additional quantities of the anaesthetic solution being given as required to maintain anaesthesia at a level adequate to obtund pain reflexes. The level of anaesthesia is best judged by the depth of respiration; surgical anaesthesia is usually present when respiration is depressed. It cannot be too strongly emphasised that the airway must be kept open with the patient breathing an adequate concentration of oxygen. In these circumstances the depressed respiration is not dangerous and the patient should remain a good colour with the skin warm and dry.

Intravenous anaesthesia is not recommended for the maintenance of unconsciousness in lengthy procedures, so that for these, after induction, it should always be supplemented by the chosen inhalation agent.

Children: Intraval Sodium is suitable for use in children as well as adults. The dosage is 2–7 mg/kg intravenously.

Contra-indications, warnings, etc

Use in pregnancy: There is epidemiological and clinical evidence of the safety of barbiturates in pregnancy including thiopentone. This drug readily crosses the placenta and appears in human milk. Dosage in the pregnant female should not exceed 250 mg.

Contra-indications: A history of acute intermittent porphyria is an absolute contra-indication to any barbiturate. Special care is required in patients with the following conditions: hypovolaemia; severe haemorrhage; burns; dehydration; severe anaemia; cardiovascular disease; status asthmaticus; severe liver disease; myasthenia gravis and muscular dystrophies; adrenocortical insufficiency even when controlled by cortisone; cachexia and severe toxaemia; raised intracranial pressure; raised blood urea; raised plasma potassium; metabolic disorders, e.g. thyrotoxicosis, myxoedema, diabetes.

Precautions: Reduced doses are required in the elderly and in patients heavily pre-medicated with narcotics and other central depressants. On the other hand, those addicted to drugs are difficult subjects to anaesthetise with normal thiopentone dosage and it is advised that supplementary analgesic agents and relaxants be given as necessary.

The jaw drops rapidly after starting the injection and must be supported, since it is imperative to keep the airway open. The patient should always be in a recumbent position to avoid cerebral ischaemia.

If Intraval Sodium is used in dental work a mouth prop is inserted before injection is commenced. The throat must be properly packed to prevent access of blood, etc. to the larynx and the dose employed should not exceed 0.25 g otherwise recovery will be delayed. Facilities for intubation and administration of oxygen under positive pressure must always be available.

To prevent accidental intra-arterial injection the site of administration must be palpated carefully and after insertion of the needle a little blood should be drawn into the syringe to observe its colour. Intra-arterial injection produces severe arterial spasm with intense burning pain in the hand and fingers. The patient can sometimes warn the anaesthetist of this before losing consciousness. In the event of such accident, inject procaine hydrochloride directly into the artery and perform a stellate ganglion block. Early anticoagulant therapy is advisable.

Side-effects: Adverse effects: Coughing, sneezing or laryngeal spasm may occur during induction. Extravasation causes pain and possible tissue necrosis. Thrombophlebitis may result from the use of 5% solution. Skin rashes, fever, arthralgia and weakness are rare side-effects. Allergic reactions and hypersensitivity have been documented.

Toxicity and treatment of overdosage: Respiratory depression during thiopentone anaesthesia must be treated by artificial ventilation with oxygen, as should cardiac arrhythmia associated with anoxia or hypercarbia. A fall in blood pressure is often noted initially, while overdose may lead to circulatory failure.

Apnoea or serious respiratory depression must be treated by controlled respiration with oxygen. Cardiovascular collapse requires immediate lowering of the head of the table; if the blood pressure fails to rise a pressor agent such as mephentermine or a plasma expander should be given. If the heart stops immediate cardiac massage should be given.

Pharmaceutical precautions Aqueous solutions of thiopentone sodium are strongly alkaline; a 2.5% solution has a pH about 10.5. The solution is incompatible with acids, acidic salts and oxidising agents. Solutions decompose on standing giving cloudiness, precipitation or crystallisation; any such solution must not be used.

Solutions should be freshly prepared and used within 24 hours or discarded.

Legal category POM.

Package quantities
For the preparation of 2.5% solution:

Boxes of 10 × 2.5 g.
Boxes of 10 × 2.5 g + 10 × 100 ml Water for Injection.
Boxes of 25 × 0.5 g.
Boxes of 25 × 0.5 g + 25 × 20 ml Water for Injection.

Further information Nil.

Product licence number 0012/5043.

LARGACTIL*

Presentation White to off-white film coated tablets containing 10 mg, 25 mg, 50 mg, or 100 mg chlorpromazine hydrochloride. The tablets also contain lactose.

The tablets are impressed LG/10, LG/25, LG/50 and LG/100 respectively on one face, reverse plain.

Pale straw coloured injection solution containing 2.5% w/v chlorpromazine hydrochloride in ampoules of 2 ml.

The injection solution also contains sodium sulphite, sodium metabisulphite, sodium chloride and sodium citrate.

Syrup: A clear bright golden-brown syrupy liquid, each 5 ml containing 25 mg chlorpromazine hydrochloride. The syrup also contains sodium sulphite, sodium metabisulphite, sodium benzoate and 68% w/v sugars.

Forte suspension coloured orange, each 5 ml containing 145 mg chlorpromazine embonate equivalent to 100 mg chlorpromazine hydrochloride. The suspension also contains sodium benzoate and Sunset Yellow.

Uses Largactil is a phenothiazine neuroleptic. It is indicated in the following conditions:

- Schizophrenia and other psychoses (especially paranoid), mania and hypomania.
- In anxiety psychomotor agitation excitement, violent or dangerously impulsive behaviour. Largactil is used as an adjunct in the short term management of these conditions.
- Intractable hiccup.
- Nausea and vomiting of terminal illness (where other drugs have failed or are not available).
- Induction of hypothermia is facilitated by Largactil which prevents shivering and causes vasodilatation.
- Childhood schizophrenia and autism.

Kinetics: Chlorpromazine is rapidly absorbed and widely distributed in the body. It is metabolised in the liver and excreted in the urine and bile. Whilst plasma concentration of chlorpromazine itself rapidly declines excretion of chlorpromazine metabolites is very slow. The drug is highly bound to plasma protein. It readily diffuses across the placenta. Small quantities have been detected in milk from treated women. Children require smaller dosages per kg than adults.

Dosage and administration See the general remarks below and Tables 1, 2 and 3.

Oral administration should be used whenever possible. Patients unwilling to swallow tablets may be treated with suspension or syrup. Dosages should be low to begin with and gradually increased under close supervision until the optimum dosage within the recommended range for the individual is reached. Individuals vary considerably and the optimum dose may be affected by the formulation used.

Parenteral formulations may be used in emergencies. They may only be administered by *deep* intramuscular injection. Largactil is too irritant to give subcutaneously. Repeated injections should be avoided if possible.

Contra-indications, warnings, etc
Pregnancy: There is inadequate evidence of the safety of Largactil in human pregnancy but it has been widely used for many years without apparent ill consequence. There is evidence of harmful effects in animals. Like other drugs it should be avoided in pregnancy unless the physician considers it essential. It may occasionally prolong labour and at such a time should be withheld until the cervix is dilated 3–4 cm. Possible adverse effects on the neonate include lethargy or paradoxical hyperexcitability, tremor and low Apgar score. Largactil being excreted in milk, breastfeeding should be suspended during treatment.

Precautions: Largactil should be avoided in patients with liver or renal dysfunction, epilepsy, Parkinson's disease, hypothyroidism, cardiac failure, phaeochromocytoma, myasthenia gravis, prostate hypertrophy. It should be avoided in patients known to be hypersensitive to phenothiazines or with a history of narrow angle glaucoma. It should be used with caution in the elderly, particularly during very hot or very cold weather (risk of hyper-, hypothermia).

Patients should be warned about drowsiness during the early days of treatment, and advised not to drive or operate machinery.

Postural hypotension with tachycardia as well as local pain or nodule formation may occur after i.m. administration. The patient should be kept supine and B.P. monitored when receiving parenteral chlorpromazine.

The elderly are particularly susceptible to postural hypotension.

Interactions of phenothiazine neuroleptics:

The CNS depressant actions of Largactil and other neuroleptic agents may be intensified (additively) by alcohol, barbiturates and other sedatives. Respiratory depression may occur.

The hypotensive effect of most antihypertensive drugs especially alpha-adrenoceptor blocking agents may be exaggerated by Largactil.

The mild anticholinergic effect of Largactil may be enhanced by other anticholinergic drugs possibly leading to constipation, heat stroke, etc.

The action of some drugs may be opposed by Largactil; these include amphetamine, levodopa, clonidine, guanethidine, adrenaline.

Anticholinergic agents may reduce the antipsychotic effect of Largactil.

Some drugs interfere with absorption of neuroleptic agents: antacids, anti-Parkinson, lithium. Increases or decreases in the plasma concentrations of a number of drugs, e.g. propranolol, phenobarbitone have been observed but were not of clinical significance.

High doses of Largactil reduce the response to hypoglycaemic agents the dosage of which might have to be raised.

Documented adverse clinically significant interactions occur with alcohol, guanethidine and hypoglycaemic agents. Adrenaline must not be used in patients overdosed with Largactil. Other interactions are of a theoretical nature and not serious.

Simultaneous administration of desferrioxamine and prochlorperazine has been observed to induce a transient metabolic encephalopathy characterised by loss of consciousness for 48–72 hours. It is possible that this may occur with Largactil since it shares many of the pharmacological activities of prochlorperazine.

Minor side effects are nasal stuffiness, dry mouth, insomnia, agitation.

Adverse effects: Liver function: Jaundice, usually transient, occurs in a very small percentage of patients taking chlorpromazine. A premonitory sign may be a sudden onset of fever after one to three weeks of treatment followed by the development of jaundice. Chlorpromazine jaundice has the biochemical and other characteristics of obstructive jaundice and is associated with obstructions of the canaliculi by bile thrombi; the frequent presence of an accompanying eosinophilia indicates the allergic nature of this phenomenon. Treatment should be withheld on the development of jaundice.

Table 1: Dosage of chlorpromazine in schizophrenia, other psychoses, anxiety and agitation etc.

Route	*Adult*	*Children under 1 year*	*Children 1–5 years*	*Children 6–12 years*	*Elderly or debilitated patients*
Oral	Initially 25 mg t.d.s. or 75 mg at bedtime increasing by daily amounts of 25 mg to an effective maintenance dose. This is usually in the range 75 to 300 mg daily, but some patients may require up to 1 g daily.	Do not use unless need is life saving.	0.5 mg/kg bodyweight every 4–6 hours to a maximum recommended dose of 40 mg daily.	$\frac{1}{3}$ to $\frac{1}{2}$ the adult dose to a maximum recommended dose of 75 mg daily.	Start with $\frac{1}{3}$ to $\frac{1}{2}$ the usual adult dose with a more gradual increase in dosage.
i.m.	For acute relief of symptoms 25–50 mg every 6–8 hours.	As above.	0.5 mg/kg bodyweight every 6–8 hours. Dosage is not advised to exceed 40 mg daily.	0.5 mg/kg bodyweight every 6–8 hours. Dosage is not advised to exceed 75 mg daily.	Doses in the lower range for adults should be sufficient to control symptoms i.e. 25 mg 8 hourly.

Table 2: Hiccup. Induction of hypothermia

Indication	*Route*	*Adult dose*	*Children under 1 year*	*Children 1–5 years*	*Children 6–12 years*	*Elderly or debilitated patients*
Hiccups	Oral	25–50 mg t.d.s. or q.d.s.	No information available			
	i.m.	25–50 mg and if this fails 25–50 mg in 500–1000 ml sodium chloride injection infused slowly.				
Induction of hypothermia to prevent shivering.	i.m.	25–50 mg every 6–8 hours.	Do not use.	Initial dose 0.5 mg to 1 mg/kg. Maintenance 0.5 mg/kg every 4–6 hours.	Initial dose 0.5 mg to 1 mg/kg. Maintenance 0.5 mg/kg every 4–6 hours.	No data available.

Table 3: Nausea and vomiting of terminal illness

Form	*Adults*	*Children under 1 year*	*Children 1–5 years*	*Children 6–12 years*	*Elderly or debilitated patients*
Oral	10–25 mg every 4–6 hours.	Do not use unless need is life saving.	0.5 mg/kg every 4–6 hours. Maximum daily dosage should not exceed 40 mg.	0.5 mg/kg every 4–6 hours. Maximum daily dosage should not exceed 75 mg.	Initially $\frac{1}{3}$ to $\frac{1}{2}$ the adult dose. The physician should then use his clinical judgment to obtain control.
i.m.	25 mg initially then 25–50 mg every 3–4 hours until vomiting stops then drug to be taken orally.	Do not use unless need is life saving.	0.5 mg/kg 6–8 hourly. It is advised that maximum daily dosage should not exceed 40 mg.	0.5 mg/kg every 6–8 hours. It is advised that maximum daily dosage should not exceed 75 mg.	For oral use only.

Cardiorespiratory: Hypotension, usually postural, commonly occurs. Elderly or volume depleted subjects are particularly susceptible; it is more likely to occur after intramuscular administration.

Cardiac arrhythmias, including atrial arrhythmia, A-V block, ventricular tachycardia and fibrillation have been reported during neuroleptic therapy, possibly related to dosage. Pre-existing cardiac disease, old age, hypokalaemia and concurrent tricyclic antidepressants may predispose. ECG changes, usually benign, include widened QT interval, ST depression, U-waves and T-wave changes.

Respiratory depression is possible in susceptible patients.

Blood picture: A mild leucopenia occurs in up to 30% of patients on prolonged high dosage. Agranulocytosis may occur rarely; it is not dose related. The occurrence of unexplained infections or fever requires immediate haematological investigation.

Extrapyramidal: Acute dystonias or dyskinesias, usually transitory are commoner in children and young adults, and usually occur within the first 4 days of treatment or after dosage increases.

Akathisia characteristically occurs after large initial doses.

Parkinsonism is commoner in adults and the elderly. It usually develops after weeks or months of treatment. One or more of the following may be seen: tremor, rigidity, akinesia or other features of Parkinsonism. Commonly just tremor.

Tardive dyskinesia: If this occurs it is usually, but not necessarily, after prolonged or high dosage. It can even occur after treatment has been stopped. Dosage should therefore be kept low whenever possible.

Skin and eyes: Contact skin sensitisation is a serious but rare complication in those frequently handling preparations of chlorpromazine; the greatest care must be taken to avoid contact of the drug with the skin. Skin rashes of various kinds may also be seen in patients treated with the drug. Patients on high dosage should be warned that they may develop photosensitivity in sunny weather and should avoid exposure to direct sunlight.

Ocular changes and the development of a metallic greyish-mauve colouration of exposed skin have been noted in some individuals mainly females, who have received chlorpromazine continuously for long periods (four to eight years).

Endocrine: Hyperprolactinaemia which may result in galactorrhoea, gynaecomastia, amenorrhoea; impotence.

Neuroleptic malignant syndrome (hyperthermia, rigidity autonomic dysfunction and altered consciousness) may occur with any neuroleptic.

Toxicity and treatment of overdosage: Symptoms of chlorpromazine overdosage include drowsiness or loss of consciousness, hypotension, tachycardia, E.C.G. changes, ventricular arrhythmias and hypothermia. Severe extra-pyramidal dyskinesias may occur.

If the patient is seen sufficiently soon (up to 6 hours) after ingestion of a toxic dose, gastric lavage may be attempted. Pharmacological induction of emesis is unlikely to be of any use. Activated charcoal should be given. There is no specific antidote. Treatment is supportive.

Generalised vasodilatation may result in circulatory collapse; raising the patient's legs may suffice, in severe cases, volume expansion by intravenous fluids may be needed; infusion fluids should be warmed before administration in order not to aggravate hypothermia.

Positive inotropic agents such as dopamine may be tried if fluid replacement is insufficient to correct the circulatory collapse. Peripheral vasoconstrictor agents are not generally recommended; avoid the use of adrenaline.

Ventricular or supraventricular tachy-arrhythmias usually respond to restoration of normal body temperature and correction of circulatory or metabolic disturbances. If persistent or life threatening, appropriate anti-arrhythmic therapy may be considered. Avoid lignocaine and, as far as possible, long acting anti-arrhythmic drugs.

Pronounced central nervous system depression requires airway maintenance or, in extreme circumstances, assisted respiration. Severe dystonic reactions usually respond to procyclidine (5–10 mg) or orphenadrine (20–40 mg) administered intramuscularly or intravenously. Convulsions should be treated with intravenous diazepam.

Neuroleptic malignant syndrome should be treated with cooling. Dantrolene sodium may be tried.

Pharmaceutical precautions Protect from light. Largactil Injection Solutions, on exposure to light, rapidly develop a pink or yellow coloration; any such solution should be discarded. Largactil Injection Solutions have a pH of 5.0–6.5; they are incompatible with benzylpenicillin potassium, pentobarbitone sodium and phenobarbitone sodium.

Largactil Forte Suspension: The contents of the bottle should be used within six months of opening.

Largactil Forte Suspension and Syrup may be diluted with Syrup BP without preservative. Dilutions of Largactil Forte Suspension should be used within one week and dilutions of Largactil Syrup within two weeks of preparation.

Tablets should not be crushed and solutions should be handled with care because of the risk of contact dermatitis.

Store tablets below 30°C and other products below 25°C.

Legal category POM.

Package quantities *Tablets 10 mg and 25 mg:* Containers of 56 (OP); *50 mg and 100 mg:* Containers of 56 (OP).

Injection Solution 2.5%; Boxes of 10 × 2 ml ampoules.

Syrup: Bottles of 100 ml (OP).

Forte Suspension: Bottle of 100 ml (OP).

Further information Nil.

Product licence numbers

Tablets 10 mg	0012/5108R
Tablets 25 mg	0012/5109R
Tablets 50 mg	0012/5110R
Tablets 100 mg	0012/5111R
Injection Solution 2.5%	0012/5308R
Syrup	0012/5083R
Forte Suspension	0012/5001R

LIPIODOL ULTRA FLUID*

Presentation Lipiodol Ultra Fluid is a pale-yellow oil which is a sterile iodine addition product of the ethyl esters of the fatty acids of poppyseed oil, containing approximately 38% w/v organically combined iodine.

Uses An X-ray contrast medium for use in certain radiological investigations where it is desirable to outline a viscous or other structure with directly instilled radio-opaque material. It is used in lymphography, hysterosalpingography and sialography. From most sites in the body it is slowly absorbed, but from the peritoneal cavity (after hysterosalpingography) absorption is relatively rapid.

On account of its low viscosity Lipiodol Ultra Fluid is suitable for introduction into narrow channels and may therefore be used in ducts and sinuses.

Kinetics: Following intralymphatic administration, Lipiodol is transported in blood to the liver, to the lungs where the lipid droplets are rapidly dispersed in the pulmonary alveoli, to the spleen and to the adipose tissue. Disappearance of droplets in the lungs or other tissues proceeds slowly. During metabolism, iodine is released which is eliminated in urine as iodide. Lipiodol can remain in the body for several weeks or months after lymphography.

Dosage and administration The medium should be administered via a suitable syringe and cannula, the volume to be administered depending on the technique being carried out and the size of the patient.

Lipiodol Ultra Fluid may be used for children or elderly patients at the surgeon's discretion.

Contra-indications, warnings, etc
Contra-indications: Lipiodol Ultra Fluid is unsuitable for bronchography as it would rapidly fill the bronchioles and the alveoli. The medium is contra-indicated in cases of recent haemorrhage.

Precautions: Care should be taken in those subjects presenting a history of previous allergic manifestations or of thyroid dysfunction. The injection of the medium into certain fistulae should be conducted with great care in order to avoid penetration of vascular channels and the possibility of oil embolism.

Iodism occurs more frequently with Lipiodol than with water-soluble organic iodine derivatives.

Lipidiol Ultra Fluid should be used with care in patients with impaired lung function.

The administration of iodine-containing contrast media may interfere with thyroid function tests for periods of 3 months or more.

The product should only be used in patients with iodine hypersensitivity if the benefits likely to be derived outweigh the risks entailed, and if adequate facilities are available for control of immediate and delayed reactions.

Use in pregnancy: There is no evidence that this product is safe during pregnancy nor is there evidence in animal work that it is free from hazard. The product should not be used during pregnancy unless benefit outweighs the risk and is considered essential by the physician. The ten day rule in women of child bearing age should be observed.

Treatment of overdosage: Gross overdosage is most unlikely to occur in lymphography. Complications and adverse reactions are more frequent with the higher doses. Treatment of adverse effects is symptomatic.

Pharmaceutical precautions Store below 25°C. Protect from light. If the product becomes opaque or dark amber in colour it should not be used.

Legal category POM.

Package quantities 5 × 10 ml ampoules.

Further information Lipiodol Ultra Fluid has been shown to dissolve polystyrene; for this reason disposable syringes made from this material must not be used to administer this preparation.

Product licence number 0012/5061R.

MAALOX* SUSPENSION AND TABLETS

Presentation White peppermint-flavoured suspension. Each 5 ml contains:

Dried Aluminium Hydroxide Gel BP	220 mg
Magnesium Hydroxide BP	195 mg

Other ingredients include parabens.

White peppermint-flavoured tablet containing:

Dried Aluminium Hydroxide Gel BP	400 mg
Magnesium Hydroxide BP	400 mg

Other ingredients include sucrose.

Uses Antacid therapy for the relief of gastritis, dyspepsia and gastric hyperacidity.

Dosage and administration Maalox is administered orally and can be taken with milk or water if required.

Adult (including elderly): 5–10 ml four times daily, taken 20 minutes to one hour after meals and at bedtime, or as required. One or two tablets well chewed, 20 minutes to one hour after meals and at bedtime, or as required.

Not recommended for children under 14 years.

Contra-indications, warnings, etc Maalox should not be used in patients who are severely debilitated or suffering from kidney failure or if there is severe abdominal pain and/or the possibility of bowel obstruction.

Maalox will inhibit absorption of tetracyclines and vitamins if taken concurrently. Gastro-intestinal side-effects are uncommon. Occasional diarrhoea or constipation may occur if use is excessive.

Use in pregnancy: It is wise to avoid taking preparations containing antacids in the first trimester of pregnancy and during lactation.

Treatment of overdosage: Serious symptoms are unlikely following overdosage. Discontinue medication and correct fluid deficiency if necessary.

Pharmaceutical precautions The suspension must be kept from freezing and the bottle kept tightly closed.

Legal category GSL

Package quantities Suspension: Plastic bottle containing 500 ml. Carton containing 20 sachets of 10 ml.

Tablets: Carton containing 100 strip-packed tablets.

Further information Maalox is a highly palatable balanced combination of two reliable antacids and has minimal gastro-intestinal side-effects. It is therefore especially suitable when prolonged therapy is necessary.

Product licence numbers
Suspension 0050/5002
Tablets 0050/5003

MAALOX* TC SUSPENSION AND TABLETS

Presentation
Suspension: White, peppermint flavoured suspension. Each 5 ml contains:

Dried Aluminium Hydroxide BP	600 mg
Magnesium Hydroxide BP	300 mg

Other ingredients include parabens.

Tablets: White, peppermint flavoured tablets marked 'Maalox TC' on one face and 'Rorer' on the other face. Each tablet contains:

Dried Aluminium Hydroxide BP	600 mg
Magnesium Hydroxide BP	300 mg

Other ingredients include sucrose.

Uses
Properties: Maalox TC is a concentrated antacid formulation providing a high acid neutralising capacity per unit dose.

Indications: The management of the symptoms of heartburn, gastric hyperacidity and gastritis.

The treatment of duodenal ulcer.

The management of the symptoms of peptic ulceration.

The prevention of duodenal ulcer recurrence.

Dosage and administration Maalox TC is administered orally and can be taken with milk or water if required.

Adult doses (including elderly):
Management of heartburn, gastric hyperacidity, gastritis and peptic ulceration:

Suspension: 5–10 ml four times daily taken 20 minutes to 1 hour after meals and at bedtime.

Tablets: 1–2 tablets four times daily taken 20 minutes to 1 hour after meals and at bedtime.

Treatment of duodenal ulcer:

Suspension: 15 ml four times daily taken 1 hour after meals and at bedtime.

Tablets: 3 tablets four times daily taken 1 hour after meals and at bedtime.

Prevention of duodenal ulcer recurrence:

Suspension: 15 ml in the morning, after food, and 15 ml at bedtime.

Tablets: 3 tablets in the morning, after food, and 3 tablets at bedtime.

Contra-indications, warnings, etc Contra-indicated in alkalosis and hypermagnesaemia, where abdominal distension may be due to partial or complete intestinal obstruction. Not recommended for severely debilitated patients or those with impaired renal function.

Precautions: Magnesium salts, in the presence of renal insufficiency may cause CNS depression. Aluminium hydroxide, in the presence of low phosphorus diets, may cause phosphorus deficiency.

Maalox TC is a balanced formulation of antacids which will minimise bowel reaction, however, mild diarrhoea may be experienced at high doses.

Do not administer concomitantly with tetracycline antibiotics or iron preparations as antacids may interfere with the absorption of these drugs.

Use in pregnancy: The safety of Maalox TC in pregnancy has not been established and it is wise to avoid taking preparations containing antacids in the first trimester of pregnancy and during lactation.

Treatment of overdosage: Serious symptoms are unlikely following overdosage and specific therapy is rarely required.

Pharmaceutical precautions The suspension must be kept from freezing and the bottle tightly closed.

Legal category GSL.

Package quantities
Suspension: Plastic bottle containing 500 ml.
Tablets: Carton containing 100 strip-packed tablets.

Further information Nil.

Product licence numbers
Suspension 5272/0021
Tablets 5272/0019.

MUCODYNE*

Presentation
Mucodyne Capsules: Opaque yellow capsules marked 'MUCODYNE 375', each containing carbocisteine 375 mg. Other ingredients include lactose, tartrazine (E102).

Mucodyne Syrup: Clear amber syrup containing carbocisteine 250 mg in each 5 ml. Other ingredients include parabens, sucrose, tartrazine (E102).

Mucodyne Paediatric Syrup: Clear red syrup containing carbocisteine 125 mg in each 5 ml. Other ingredients include parabens, sucrose, Ponceau 4R (E124).

Uses Mucolytic agent for the adjunctive therapy of respiratory tract disorders, characterised by excessive or viscous mucus, including Glue Ear in children.

Mucodyne reduces the viscosity of bronchial secretions and facilitates expectoration. There is also evidence that during treatment with Mucodyne, the physical and chemical characteristics of the mucin components of sputum return to a more normal pattern, with reduction of fucose and sulphate content and an increase in the proportions of sialomucins.

Dosage and administration *Adults (including elderly):* (Syrup and Capsules.) Dosage is based upon an initial daily dosage of 2250 mg carbocisteine in divided doses reducing to 1500 mg daily in divided doses when a satisfactory response has been obtained, e.g. for normal syrup 15 ml tds reducing to 10 ml tds.

Children: The normal daily dose is 20 mg/kg body weight in divided doses. The following dosage is recommended for the Mucodyne Paediatric syrup: 2 to 5 years: 2.5–5 ml four times a day; 5 to 12 years: 10 ml three times a day. Dosage in younger children and infants has not been established.

Contra-indications, warnings, etc There have been rare reports of skin rashes or gastro-intestinal bleeding occurring during treatment with Mucodyne. Contra-indicated in active peptic ulceration.

Use in pregnancy: Although tests in mammalian species have revealed no teratogenic effects, Mucodyne is not recommended during the first trimester of pregnancy.

Use in lactation: Effects not known.

Treatment of overdosage: Gastric lavage may be beneficial, followed by observation. Gastro-intestinal disturbance is the most likely symptom of Mucodyne overdosage.

Pharmaceutical precautions The syrups should be stored in a cool place. Mixture with linctus of pholcodeine causes precipitation of carbocisteine from solution. Dilution of Mucodyne Syrup may be effected with unpreserved Syrup BP but diluted preparations should not be kept for more than 14 days.

Legal category POM.

Package quantities *Mucodyne Capsules:* Containers of 30.
Mucodyne Syrup: Bottles of 300 ml with dosage cap.
Mucodyne Paediatric Syrup: Bottles of 300 ml with dosage cap.

Further information Nil.

Product licence numbers

Capsules	0152/0098R
Syrup	0152/0042R
Paediatric Syrup	0152/0166

NEULACTIL*

Presentation Tablets, uncoated, yellow, containing 2.5, 10 or 25 mg pericyazine, embossed 'Neulactil', 'Neulactil' 10 or 'Neulactil' 25 respectively on one face, with a break-line on the reverse. Neulactil tablets contain lactose and methylhydroxybenzoate.

Forte Syrup, clear orange brown syrupy liquid, each 5 ml containing 10 mg pericyazine. The content of sugars is about 68% w/v, and it also contains sodium sulphite, sodium metabisulphite and sodium benzoate.

Uses Pericyazine is a neuroleptic with cardiovascular and antihistamine effects similar to those of chlorpromazine, but it has a stronger antiserotonin effect and a powerful central sedative effect.

Neulactil Tablets are indicated for use:

(a) In adults with schizophrenia or other psychoses, for the treatment of symptoms or prevention of relapse.

(b) In adults with anxiety, psychomotor agitation, violent or dangerously impulsive behaviour. Neulactil is used as an adjunct to the short-term management of these conditions.

Neulactil Tablets are not recommended for children.

Neulactil Forte Syrup is indicated for use:

(c) In children with schizophrenia or other psychoses; for the treatment of symptoms or prevention of relapse.

(d) In children with behavioural disorders.

Kinetics: There is little information about plasma concentrations, distribution and excretion in humans. The rate of metabolism and excretion of phenothiazines decreases in old age.

Dosage and administration Dosage requirement varies with the individual and the severity of the condition being treated. Initial dosage should be low with progressive increases until the desired response is obtained, after which dosage should be adjusted to maintain control of symptoms.

Severe conditions Indication (a)	*Mild or moderate conditions Indication (b)*
Adults	
Initially 75 mg per day in divided doses. Dosage should be increased by 25 mg per day at weekly intervals until the optimum effect is achieved. Maintenance therapy would not normally be expected to exceed 300 mg per day.	Initially 15–30 mg daily, divided into two portions, with a larger dose being given in the evening.
Elderly	
Initially 15–30 mg per day in divided doses. If this is well tolerated the dosage may be increased if necessary for optimum control of behaviour.	5 to 10 mg per day is suggested as a starting dose. It may be divided so that a larger portion is given in the evening. Half or quarter the normal adult dose may be sufficient for maintenance therapy.

Children: The initial daily dose should be calculated on bodyweight. A child weighing 10 kg should receive 0.5 milligram and this initial dose should be increased by 1 mg for each additional 5 kg of bodyweight up to a total daily dose of 10 mg daily. This dosage may be gradually increased until the desired effect is achieved but the daily maintenance dose should not exceed twice the initial amount. Neulactil is not recommended for use in children below 1 year of age.

Contra-indications, warnings, etc

Pregnancy: There is inadequate evidence of the safety of Neulactil in human pregnancy but it has been widely used for many years without apparent ill consequence. There is evidence with some neuroleptics of harmful effects in animals. Like other drugs Neulactil should be avoided in pregnancy unless the physician considers it essential. It may occasionally prolong labour and at such a time should be withheld until the cervix is dilated 3–4 cm. Possible adverse effects on the neonate include lethargy or paradoxical hyperexcitability, tremor and low Apgar score. Phenothiazines may be excreted in milk therefore breastfeeding should be suspended during treatment.

Precautions: Neuroleptics should be avoided in patients with liver or renal dysfunction, epilepsy, Parkinson's disease, hypothyroidism, cardiac failure, phaeochromocytoma, myasthenia gravis, prostate hypertrophy. It should be avoided in patients known to be hypersensitive to phenothiazines or with a history of narrow angle glaucoma. It should be used with caution in the elderly, particularly during very hot or very cold weather (risk of hyper-, hypothermia).

Patients should be warned about drowsiness during the early days of treatment, and advised not to drive or operate machinery.

The elderly are particularly susceptible to postural hypotension.

Interactions of phenothiazine neuroleptics. The CNS depressant actions of neuroleptic agents may be intensified (additively) by alcohol, barbiturates and other sedatives. Respiratory depression may occur.

The hypotensive effect of most antihypertensive drugs especially alpha adrenoceptor blocking agents may be exaggerated by neuroleptics.

The mild anticholinergic effect of neuroleptics may be enhanced by other anticholinergic drugs possibly leading to constipation, heat stroke, etc.

The action of some drugs may be opposed by neuroleptics; these include amphetamine, laevodopa clonidine, guanethidine, adrenaline.

Anticholinergic agents may reduce the antipsychotic effect of neuroleptics.

Some drugs interfere with absorption of neuroleptic agents: antacids, anti-Parkinson, lithium. Increases or decreases in the plasma concentrations of a number of drugs, e.g. propranolol, phenobarbitone have been observed but were not of clinical significance.

High doses of neuroleptics may reduce the response

to hypoglycaemic agents the dosage of which might have to be raised.

Adrenaline must *not* be used in patients overdosed with neuroleptics. Most of the above interactions are of a theoretical nature and not serious.

Simultaneous administration of desferrioxamine and prochlorperazine has been observed to induce a transient metabolic encephalopathy characterised by loss of consciousness for 48–72 hours.

It is possible that this may occur with Neulactil since it shares many of the pharmacological activities of prochlorperazine.

Minor side-effects are nasal stuffiness, dry mouth, insomnia, agitation.

Adverse effects: Liver function: Jaundice, occurs in a very small percentage of patients taking neuroleptics. A premonitory sign may be a sudden onset of fever after one to three weeks of treatment followed by the development of jaundice. Neuroleptic jaundice has the biochemical and other characteristics of obstructive jaundice and is associated with obstruction of the canaliculi by bile thrombi; the frequent presence of an accompanying eosinophilia indicates the allergic nature of this phenomenon. Treatment should be withheld on the development of jaundice.

Cardiorespiratory: Hypotension, usually postural, commonly occurs. Elderly or volume depleted subjects are particularly susceptible.

Cardiac arrhythmias, including atrial arrhythmia, A-V block, ventricular tachycardia and fibrillation have been reported during neuroleptic therapy, possibly related to dosage. Pre-existing cardiac disease, old age, hypokalaemia and concurrent tricyclic antidepressants may predispose. ECG changes, usually benign, include widened QT interval, ST depression, U-waves and T-wave changes.

Respiratory depression is possible in susceptible patients.

Blood picture: A mild leukopaenia occurs in up to 30% of patients on prolonged high dosage of neuroleptics. Agranulocytosis may occur rarely; it is not dose related. The occurrence of unexplained infections or fever requires immediate haematological investigation.

Extrapyramidal: Acute dystonias or dyskinesias, usually transitory are commoner in children and young adults, and usually occur within the first 4 days of treatment or after dosage increases.

Akathisia characteristically occurs after large initial doses.

Parkinsonism is commoner in adults and the elderly. It usually develops after weeks or months of treatment. One or more of the following may be seen: tremor, rigidity, akinesia or other features of Parkinsonism. Commonly just tremor.

Tardive dyskinesia: If this occurs it is usually, but not necessarily, after prolonged or high dosage. It can even occur after treatment has been stopped. Dosage should therefore be kept low whenever possible.

Skin and eyes: Contact skin sensitisation is a serious but rare complication in those frequently handling preparations of phenothiazines; the greatest care must be taken to avoid contact of the drug with the skin. Skin rashes of various kinds may also be seen in patients treated with the drug. Patients on high dosage should be warned that they may develop photosensitivity in sunny weather and should avoid exposure to direct sunlight.

Endocrine: hyperprolactinaemia which may result in galactorrhoea, gynaecomastia, amenorrhoea; impotence.

Neuroleptic malignant syndrome (hyperthermia, rigidity autonomic dysfunction and altered consciousness) may occur with any neuroleptic.

Toxicity and treatment of overdosage: Symptoms of neuroleptic overdosage include drowsiness or loss of consciousness, hypotension, tachycardia, E.C.G. changes, ventricular arrhythmias and hypothermia. Severe extra-pyramidal dyskinesias may occur.

If the patient is seen sufficiently soon (up to 6 hours) after ingestion of a toxic dose, gastric lavage may be attempted. Pharmacological induction of emesis is unlikely to be of any use. Activated charcoal should be given. There is no specific antidote. Treatment is supportive.

Generalised vasodilatation may result in circulatory collapse; raising the patient's legs may suffice, in severe cases, volume expansion by intravenous fluids may be needed; infusion fluids should be warmed before administration in order not to aggravate hypothermia.

Positive inotropic agents such as dopamine may be tried if fluid replacement is insufficient to correct the circulatory collapse. Peripheral vasoconstrictor agents are not generally recommended; avoid the use of adrenaline.

Ventricular or supraventricular tachy-arrhythmias usually respond to restoration of normal body temperature and correction of circulatory or metabolic disturbances. If persistent or life threatening, appropriate antiarrhythmic therapy may be considered. Avoid lignocaine and, as far as possible, long acting anti-arrhythmic drugs.

Pronounced central nervous system depression requires airway maintenance or, in extreme circumstances, assisted respiration. Severe dystonic reactions usually respond to procyclidine (5–10 mg) or orphenadrine (20–40 mg) administered intramuscularly or intravenously. Convulsions should be treated with intravenous diazepam.

Neuroleptic malignant syndrome should be treated with cooling. Dantrolene sodium may be tried.

Pharmaceutical precautions Protect from light. Neulactil Forte Syrup can be diluted with Syrup BP without preservative. Such dilutions have a shelf-life of 14 days.

Legal category POM.

Package quantities Containers of 84 × 2.5 mg (OP) and 10 mg tablets and of 50 × 25 mg tablets.

Bottles of 100 ml (OP) Neulactil Forte Syrup.

Further information Nil.

Product licence numbers

Tablets 2.5 mg	0012/5276
Tablets 10 mg	0012/5277
Tablets 25 mg	0012/5278
Forte Syrup	0012/5016

NIVAQUINE*

Presentation

Tablets: Yellowish buff film-coated tablets containing 200 mg chloroquine sulphate (equivalent to 150 mg chloroquine base) impressed 'Nivaquine 200' on one face, reverse plain. The tablets also contain glucose.

Syrup: A bright, golden syrup containing 68 mg chloroquine sulphate (equivalent to 50 mg chloroquine base) in each 5 ml. Nivaquine syrup also contains saccharin sodium, sugars, sodium L-glutamate, methyl hydroxybenzoate and propyl hydroxybenzoate.

Injection: A colourless injection solution of chloroquine sulphate 5.45% w/v equivalent to 40 mg chloroquine base per ml in ampoules of 5 ml.

Uses Chloroquine is a 4-aminoquinoline derivative, which has a high degree of activity against the asexual erythrocytic forms of all species of malaria parasites. It is indicated for the suppression and clinical cure of all forms of malaria and, in addition, produces radical cure of falciparum malaria.

Nivaquine exerts a beneficial effect in certain collagen diseases and protects against the effects of solar radiation. It is also indicated in the treatment of rheumatoid arthritis, juvenile rheumatoid arthritis, discoid and systemic lupus erythematosus and skin conditions aggravated by sunlight.

Nivaquine is also active against Entamoeba histolytica and Giardia lamblia and when metronidazole is not available it may be used in hepatic amoebiasis and giardiasis.

Dosage and administration

Suppression of malaria: It is advisable to start taking Nivaquine 2 weeks before entering an endemic area and to continue for 4 weeks after leaving.

Age group	*Dose to be taken once a week on the same day each week*
Adults	Two Nivaquine tablets (300 mg chloroquine base)
Infants and children up to twelve years	5 mg chloroquine base per kg bodyweight

These dosages are those recommended by the World Health Organisation.

Treatment of malaria
(1) Non-immune subjects

(a) Oral route

Adults

Day of treatment	*Dosage*
Day 1	Four Nivaquine tablets (600 mg chloroquine base) in one dose followed by a further two tablets (300 mg chloroquine base) six hours later.
Day 2	Two Nivaquine tablets (300 mg chloroquine base).
Day 3	Two Nivaquine tablets (300 mg chloroquine base).

The above dosage is intended as a guide in the treatment of Plasmodium falciparum malaria. However, due to variation in the strain sensitivity, it may sometimes be necessary to increase the duration of treatment by administering two Nivaquine tablets (300 mg chloroquine base) daily on days 4 to 7.

Infants and children: Nivaquine syrup can be conveniently used in this age group to permit flexibility of dosage.

Day of treatment	*Dosage*
Day 1	10 mg chloroquine base/kg bodyweight (maximum 600 mg base) followed by 5 mg chloroquine base/kg bodyweight (maximum 300 mg base) six hours later.
Day 2	5 mg chloroquine base/kg bodyweight (maximum 300 mg base).
Day 3	5 mg chloroquine base/kg bodyweight (maximum 300 mg base).

(b) Injection

Adults and children: Slow intravenous infusion: 10 mg/kg bodyweight chloroquine base to be administered in sodium chloride 0.9% injection by slow intravenous infusion over eight hours followed by three further 8 hour infusions containing 5 mg base/kg (total dose 25 mg base/kg over 32 hours). The dose should not be modified in renal or hepatic disease.

Exceptionally, where intravenous administration is not possible, Nivaquine may be given by intramuscular or subcutaneous injection in small divided doses of 3.5 mg chloroquine base/kg bodyweight every 6 hours or 2.5 mg base/kg every 4 hours.

(2) Partially immune subjects
Adults: A single dose of four Nivaquine tablets (600 mg chloroquine base) will provide an effective course of treatment.

Infants and children: Repeated infection with many species and strains of malaria parasite prevalent in highly endemic malarial areas eventually produces a high degree of immune response frequently resulting in modification of the symptoms of clinical attack. This is particularly obvious in adults but less so in adolescents and children. Immunity is uncommon in very young age groups with the exception of infants up to the age of about 6 months who are partly protected by trans-placentally derived maternal antibodies. It is therefore advisable to treat previously exposed children in the same way as non-immune children.

Other indications:

Indication	*Age group*	*Dose*
Rheumatoid arthritis	Adults	One Nivaquine tablet (150 mg chloroquine base) daily.
	Children	3 mg/kg bodyweight as base per day
Systemic lupus erythematosus	Adults	One Nivaquine tablet (150 mg chloroquine base) daily until maximum improvement is obtained followed by a smaller maintenance dosage.
	Children	3 mg/kg bodyweight as base per day.
Light-senstive skin eruptions	Adults	One or two Nivaquine tablets (150 mg to 300 mg chloroquine base) daily during the period of maximum light exposure.
	Children	3 mg/kg bodyweight as base per day during the period of maximum light exposure.

Treatment should be discontinued if no improvement has occurred after 6 months.

Dosage in the elderly: No specific dosage recommendations.

Contra-indications, warnings, etc

Precautions: Caution is advised in cases of porphyria,

severe gastrointestinal, neurological and blood disorders. Nivaquine should be used with care in patients with a history of epilepsy as it has been reported to provoke seizures. Caution should be exercised in patients with hepatic or renal disease. Retinopathy: Irreversible retinal damage may occur with prolonged treatment. Ophthalmological examination should always be carried out before and regularly (3–6 monthly intervals) during treatment. Retinal damage is particularly likely to occur if treatment has been given for longer than one year or if the total dosage has exceeded 1.6 g/kg bodyweight. These precautions also apply to patients receiving chloroquine continuously at weekly intervals as a prophylactic against malarial attack for more than three years.

Nivaquine has a temporary effect on visual accommodation and patients should be warned regarding driving or operating machinery.

Use in pregnancy: Nivaquine is generally contra-indicated in pregnancy. However, clinicians may decide to administer Nivaquine to pregnant women for the prevention or treatment of malaria. Ocular or inner ear damage may occur in infants born of mothers who receive high doses of chloroquine throughout pregnancy.

Side-effects: The more common side-effects include gastro-intestinal disturbances, headache and skin eruptions. Psoriasis may be exacerbated. Retinal damage and depigmentation or loss of hair may also occur. These effects usually disappear on cessation of treatment. Convulsions have been reported rarely (these may result from cerebral malaria, such patients should receive an injection of phenobarbitone to prevent seizures in a dose of 3.5 mg/kg in addition to intravenous administration of Nivaquine). Bone marrow depression, including aplastic anaemia, occurs rarely. Full blood counts should therefore be carried out regularly during extended treatment. Allergic and anaphylactic reactions have occurred rarely.

Treatment of overdosage: Chloroquine is highly toxic in overdose; children are particularly susceptible to toxic doses of chloroquine. The chief symptoms of overdosage include circulatory collapse due to a potent cardiotoxic effect, respiratory arrest and coma. Symptoms may progress rapidly after initial nausea and vomiting.

Death may result from circulatory or respiratory failure or cardiac dysrhythmia.

Gastric lavage should be carried out urgently, first protecting the airway and instituting artificial ventilation where necessary. There is a risk of cardiac arrest following aspiration of gastric contents in more serious cases. Activated charcoal left in the stomach may reduce the absorption of any remaining chloroquine from the gut. Circulatory status (with central venous pressure measurement), respiration, plasma electrolytes and blood gases should be monitored, with correction of hypokalaemia and acidosis if indicated. Cardiac arrhythmias should not be treated unless life threatening; drugs with quinidine-like effect should be avoided.

Early administration of the following has been shown to improve survival in cases of serious poisoning:

1. Adrenaline infusion 0.25 micrograms/kg/min initially with increments of 0.25 micrograms/kg/min until adequate systolic blood pressure (more than 100 mm Hg) is restored; adrenaline reduces the effects of chloroquine on the heart through its inotropic and vasoconstrictor effects.

2. Diazepam infusion (2 mg/kg over 30 minutes as a loading dose, followed by 1–2 mg/kg/day for up to 2–4 days). Diazepam may minimise cardiotoxicity.

Acidification of the urine, haemodialysis, peritoneal dialysis or exchange transfusion have not been shown to be of value in treating chloroquine poisoning. Chloroquine is excreted very slowly, therefore symptomatic cases merit observation for several days.

Pharmaceutical precautions
Tablets: Protect from light.
Syrup: Store below 25°C and protect from light.
Injection: Protect from light.

Legal category Nivaquine Tablets and Syrup POM, but when supplied for prevention of malaria in a container specifically labelled for that purpose, P.

Nivaquine Injection POM.

Package quantities 30 × 200 mg Tablets. 100 ml bottles of syrup. Injection: 10 ampoules of 5 ml per carton.

Further information Nil.

Product licence numbers
Injection 0012/5048R
Tablets 0012/5260R
Syrup 0012/5020R

NOZINAN*

Presentation
Injection: Colourless isotonic solution containing 2.5% w/v methotrimeprazine hydrochloride in ampoules of 1 ml. The injection also contains ascorbic acid, sodium sulphite and sodium chloride.

Tablets: Greyish white or cream tablets containing 25 mg methotrimeprazine maleate impressed NOZINAN '25' on one face, with a break line on the reverse.

Uses Methotrimeprazine resembles chlorpromazine and promethazine in the pattern of its pharmacology. It possesses anti-emetic, anti-histamine and anti-adrenaline activity and exhibits a strong sedative effect.

Nozinan potentiates the action of other central nervous system depressants but may be given in conjunction with appropriately modified doses of narcotic analgesics in the management of severe pain. Nozinan does not significantly depress respiration and is particularly useful where pulmonary reserve is low.

Nozinan is indicated in the management of severe pain and accompanying anxiety and distress.

Nozinan is also indicated in psychiatry as an alternative to Largactil in schizophrenia especially when it is desirable to reduce psychomotor activity.

Kinetics: Maximum serum concentrations are achieved in 2–3 hours depending on route of administration. Excretion is slow, with a half-life of about 30 hours. It is eliminated via urine and faeces.

Dosage and administration Dosage varies with the condition and individual response of the patient.

1. *Terminal illness:* The usual dose for adults is 12.5–25 mg (0.5–1 ml) by intramuscular injection, or by the intravenous route after dilution with an equal volume of normal saline immediately before use. In cases of severe agitation up to 50 mg (2 ml) may be used, repeated every six to eight hours.

Continuous subcutaneous infusion: Nozinan may be administered over a 24 hour period via a syringe driver. The required dose of Nozinan (25–200 mg per day) should be diluted with the calculated volume of normal saline. Diamorphine hydrochloride is compatible with this solution and may be added if greater analgesia is required.

Nozinan tablets 25 mg may be substituted for the injection if oral therapy is more convenient the dosage being 12.5–50 mg 4–8 hourly.

Elderly: No specific dosage recommendations.

2. *Psychiatric conditions*
Adults: Ambulant patients: initially the total daily oral dose should not exceed 25–50 mg, usually divided into 3 doses; a larger portion of the dosage may be taken at bedtime to minimise diurnal sedation. The dosage is then gradually increased to the most effective level compatible with sedation and other side-effects.

Bed patients: Initially the total daily oral dosage may be 100–200 mg, usually divided into 3 doses, gradually increased to 1 g daily if necessary. When the patient is stable attempts should be made to reduce the dosage to an adequate maintenance level.

Children: Children are very susceptible to the hypotensive and soporific effects of methotrimeprazine. It is advised that a total daily oral dosage of 40 mg should not be exceeded. The average effective daily intake for a 10-year-old is 15–20 mg.

Elderly patients: It is not advised to give methotrimeprazine to ambulant patients over 50 years of age unless the risk of a hypotensive reaction has been assessed.

Contra-indications, warnings, etc Safety in pregnancy has not been established.

There are no absolute contra-indications to the use of Nozinan in terminal care.

The drug should be avoided or used with caution in patients with liver dysfunction or cardiac disease.

Precautions: The hypotensive effects of Nozinan should be taken into account when it is administered to patients with cardiac disease and the elderly or debilitated. Patients receiving large initial doses should be kept in bed.

Nozinan may cause drowsiness, disorientation, confusion or excessive hypotension, which may affect patient's ability to drive or operate machinery. Avoid alcoholic drinks.

Side-effects: Somnolence and asthenia are frequent side effects. Dry mouth is encountered occasionally. Hypotension may occur, especially in elderly patients. A raised ESR may occasionally be encountered. Agranulocytosis has been reported, as have photosensitivity and allergic skin reactions.

Parkinsonian-like reactions may occur in patients receiving prolonged high dosage. Jaundice is a rare side effect. Other adverse effects common to phenothiazine neuroleptics may be seen.

Interactions: Simultaneous administration of desferrioxamine and prochlorperazine has been observed to induce a transient metabolic encephalopathy characterised by loss of consciousness for 48–72 hours. It is possible that this may occur with Nozinan since it shares many of the pharmacological activities of prochlorperazine. Adrenaline must not be used in patients overdosed with neuroleptics.

Toxicity and treatment of overdosage: Symptoms of methotrimeprazine overdosage include drowsiness or loss of consciousness, hypotension, tachycardia, E.C.G. changes, ventricular arrhythmias and hypothermia. Severe extra-pyramidal dyskinesias may occur.

If the patient is seen sufficiently soon (up to 6 hours) after ingestion of a toxic dose, gastric lavage may be attempted. Pharmacological induction of emesis is unlikely to be of any use. Activated charcoal should be given. There is no specific antidote. Treatment is supportive.

Generalised vasodilatation may result in circulatory collapse; raising the patient's legs may suffice, in severe cases, volume expansion by intravenous fluids may be needed; infusion fluids should be warmed before administration in order not to aggravate hypothermia.

Positive inotropic agents such as dopamine may be tried if fluid replacement is insufficient to correct the circulatory collapse. Peripheral vasoconstrictor agents are not generally recommended; avoid the use of adrenaline.

Ventricular or supraventricular tachy-arrhythmias usually respond to restoration of normal body temperature and correction of circulatory or metabolic disturbances. If persistent or life threatening, appropriate anti-arrhythmic therapy may be considered. Avoid lignocaine and, as far as possible, long acting anti-arrhythmic drugs.

Pronounced central nervous system depression requires airway maintenance or, in extreme circumstances, assisted respiration. Severe dystonic reactions usually respond to procyclidine (5–10 mg) or orphenadrine (20–40 mg) administered intramuscularly or intravenously. Convulsions should be treated with intravenous diazepam.

Neuroleptic malignant syndrome should be treated with cooling. Dantrolene sodium may be tried.

Pharmaceutical precautions Protect from light. Nozinan Injection Solution, on exposure to light, rapidly develops a pink or yellow colouration and any such solution should be discarded. Nozinan Injection Solution is incompatible with alkaline solutions.

Legal category POM.

Package quantities Injection Solution 2.5% Box of 10 × 1 ml ampoules.

Tablets container of 500 × 25 mg.

Further information Dilutions of Nozinan injection in normal saline, with or without the addition of diamorphine hydrochloride, are stable for 24 hours and may be used in syringe drivers.

Product licence numbers

Injection Solution 2.5%	0012/5007
Tablets 25 mg	0012/5305

OCUSERT*

Presentation Ocusert Pilocarpine therapeutic systems are elliptically-shaped units designed to release pilocarpine continuously following placement into the upper or lower conjunctival sac. The systems consist of a core reservoir of pilocarpine surrounded by a membrane which controls the drug's diffusion from the system into the tear fluid. Two systems are available, Pilo-20 and Pilo-40, which release 20 and 40 microgram per hour, respectively, for one week. The Pilo-20 system is 5.7 × 13.4 mm across its axis, 0.3 mm thick, and contains 5 mg pilocarpine, the Pilo-40 system is 5.5 × 13 mm on its axis, 0.5 mm thick, and contains 11 mg pilocarpine. Except for the opaque white margin, the systems are clear.

Uses The Ocusert pilocarpine system is indicated for control of elevated intra-ocular pressure in glaucoma in pilocarpine-responsive patients.

Dosage and administration *Initiation of therapy:* The Ocusert Pilo-20 system will usually control a patient previously controlled by 1 per cent or 2 per cent pilocarpine eye drops; a patient who has used higher strengths of pilocarpine eye drops may require the Pilo-40. However, there is no direct correlation between the two strengths of Ocusert and the strength of pilocarpine eye drops necessary to achieve the required reduction of pressure. The Ocusert systems reduce the amount of pilocarpine necessary to achieve adequate reduction of intra-ocular pressure; therapy may be started therefore with the Ocusert Pilo-20 system irrespective of the strength of pilocarpine eye drops used previously by the patient. If the pressure is satisfactorily reduced with the Ocusert Pilo-20 system the patient should continue its use, replacing each unit every seven days; if greater reduction of intra-ocular pressure is required, the patient should be transferred to the Pilo-40 system. Depending on the patient's age, family history, and disease status, the ophthalmologist may elect to begin therapy with the Pilo-40 system.

Concomitant therapy: Where necessary, adrenaline or timolol eye drops or a diuretic of the carbonic anhydrase inhibitor type may be used concurrently with Ocusert systems. The release rate of pilocarpine from the Ocusert systems is not influenced by the beta adrenoceptor antagonist, by carbonic anhydrase inhibitors, adrenaline eye drops, fluorescein, or local anaesthetics, antibiotics or anti-inflammatory steroid eye drops.

Placement and removal of the Ocusert systems: Patient instructions for the placement of the Ocusert systems in the eye and their removal are included in each package. It is strongly recommended that the patient's ability to manage the placement and removal of the system be reviewed at the first patient visit after initiation of therapy.

Since pilocarpine-induced myopia from the Ocusert systems may occur during the first few hours of therapy, the patient should be advised to place the system into the conjunctival sac at bedtime. By morning the induced myopia is at a stable level.

Handling precautions: Patients should be instructed to wash their hands thoroughly with soap and water before touching or manipulating the Ocusert systems. If a displaced unit contacts unclean surfaces, rinsing with cool tap water before replacing is advisable. Biologically contaminated units should be discarded and replaced with fresh ones.

Retention in the eye: During the initial adaptation period, the Ocusert unit may slip out of the conjuctival sac on to the cheek. The patient is usually aware of such movement and can replace the unit without difficulty.

In those patients in whom retention of the Ocusert unit is a problem, placement in the upper conjuctival sac is often more acceptable. The Ocusert unit can be manipulated from the lower to the upper conjunctival sac by a gentle digital massage through the lid, a technique readily learned by the patient. For best retention, the unit should be moved before sleep to the upper conjunctival sac. Should the unit slip out of the conjunctival sac during sleep, its ocular hypotensive effect continues for a period of time comparable to that following instillation of eye drops. The patient should be instructed to check for the presence of the Ocusert unit before sleep and on rising.

Contra-indications, warnings, etc Ocusert systems are contra-indicated where pupillary constriction is undesirable, such as glaucomas associated with acute inflammatory disease of the anterior segment of the eye, and glaucomas occurring or persisting after extracapsular cataract extraction where posterior synechiae may occur.

Ocusert systems should not be used in patients with acute infectious conjuctivitis or keratitis except on specialist advice. Damaged or deformed systems should not be placed or retained in the eye. Systems believed to be associated with an unexpected increase in drug action should be removed and replaced with new systems. The effect of pilocarpine on visual accommodation may affect the patient's ability to drive and use machinery.

The safety of Ocusert systems in patients with retinal detachment or with filtration blebs has not been established. Although eye drops have been used effectively in conjunction with the Ocusert systems, systemic reactions consistent with an increased rate of absorption from the eye of an autonomic drug, such as adrenaline, have been observed. In rare instances, reactions of this type can be severe. The conjunctival erythema and oedema associated with adrenaline eye drops are not substantially altered by concomitant use of an Ocusert system. The use of pilocarpine eye drops should be considered when intense miosis is desired in certain ocular conditions.

Ciliary spasm is encountered with pilocarpine usage but is not a contra-indication to continued therapy unless the induced myopia is debilitating to the patient. Irritation from pilocarpine has been frequently encountered and may require cessation of therapy depending on the judgement of the doctor. True allergic reactions are uncommon but require discontinuation of therapy if they occur.

Although withdrawal of the peripheral iris from the anterior chamber angle by miosis may reduce the tendency for narrow angle closure, miotics can occasionally precipitate angle closure by increasing the resistance to aqueous flow from posterior to anterior chamber. Miotic agents may also cause retinal detachment; thus, care should be exercised with all miotic therapy especially in young myopic patients.

Some patients may notice signs of conjuctival irritation, including mild erythema with or without a slight increase in mucous secretion when they first use Ocusert systems. These signs tend to lessen or disappear after the first week of therapy. In rare instances a sudden increase in pilocarpine effects has been reported.

Pharmaceutical precautions Store in a refrigerator at 2° to 8°C, i.e. not in the freezer compartment.

Legal category POM.

Package quantities Ocusert Pilo-20 (OP) or Ocusert Pilo-40 systems (OP) are available in containers of eight individual sterile systems.

Further information The decrease in intra-ocular pressure obtained with both the Pilo-20 and Pilo-40 systems is fully established within 1½ or 2 hours after placement in the conjunctival sac and is maintained for 24 hours a day for seven days. Intra-ocular pressure reduction with Ocusert systems for an entire week is achieved with either 3.4 mg or 6.7 mg pilocarpine (20 mcg or 40 mcg times 24×7, respectively), as compared with 28 mg of pilocarpine administered as a 2 per cent ophthalmic solution four times a day.

Ocusert systems may be used in association with contact lenses.

Product licence numbers
Pilo-20 0012/0118
Pilo-40 0012/0119

ORUDIS*

Presentation Capsules each containing 50 mg ketoprofen, bicoloured (opaque green/opaque purple) with each half printed 'Orudis 50' in white. Capsules each containing 100 mg ketoprofen (flesh opaque) printed 'Orudis 100' in black. The capsules also contain lactose.

Cream coloured suppositories each containing 100 mg ketoprofen.

Uses Orudis is recommended in the management of rheumatoid arthritis, osteoarthritis, ankylosing spondylitis, acute articular and periarticular disorders (bursitis, capsulitis, synovitis, tendonitis), fibrositis, cervical spondylitis, low back pain (strain, lumbago, sciatica, fibrositis), painful musculo-skeletal conditions, dysmenorrhoea, acute gout and control of pain and inflammation following orthopaedic surgery. Orudis suppositories are *not* recommended for treatment of dysmenorrhoea.

Orudis is a potent non-steroidal anti-inflammatory analgesic agent and a strong inhibitor of prostaglandin synthetase.

Orudis reduces joint pain and inflammation, and facilitates increase in mobility and functional independence. As with other non-steroidal anti-inflammatory agents, it does not cure the underlying disease.

Kinetics: Ketoprofen is completely absorbed from Orudis capsules and maximum plasma concentration occurs after ½–1 hour. It declines thereafter with an elimination half-life of about 2–3 hours. There is no accumulation on continued daily dosing. Ketoprofen is rapidly absorbed from the suppository dosage form with maximum plasma concentrations at 1–2 hours with an elimination half-life of 2–3 hours. Plasma levels obtained are comparable to those obtained from equal oral doses. Ketoprofen is very highly bound to plasma protein.

Dosage and administration Orudis is administered orally and/or rectally; to limit occurrence of gastrointestinal disturbance, capsules should always be taken with food (milk, meals).

Oral dosage is 50–100 mg twice daily, depending on patient weight and on severity of symptoms; medication should be taken early in the morning and late at night.

Rectal dosage is one suppository (100 mg) late at night supplemented as required with Orudis capsules during the daytime.

Orudis suppositories are especially appropriate for controlling overnight symptoms (severity of night and morning pain; duration and severity of morning stiffness). Suppositories administered late at night provide more consistent effective control of overnight symptoms than oral medication.

Best results are obtained by titrating dosage to suit each patient; start with a low dosage in mild chronic disease and a high dosage in acute or severe disease. Some patients derive greater benefit by treatment with capsules only; some with a combined capsule/suppository regimen; and others with a higher dosage at night-time than at early morning. Where patients require a maximum oral dosage initially, an attempt should be made to reduce this dosage for maintenance, since lower dosage might be better tolerated for purposes of long-term treatment.

Elderly: As with other medications, it is generally advisable to begin ketoprofen therapy at the lower end of the dose range and to maintain such patients on the lowest effective dosage.

Paediatric: Dosage is not established.

Contra-indications, warnings, etc Active peptic ulceration; a history of recurrent peptic ulceration or chronic dyspepsia; severe renal dysfunction; disease in children (safety/dosage during long-term treatment has not been established).

Suppositories should not be used following recent proctitis or in association with haemorrhoids.

Ketoprofen should not be given to patients with a known hypersensitivity to ketoprofen or to aspirin or other non-steroidal anti-inflammatory agents. Severe bronchospasm might be precipitated in these subjects, and in patients suffering from, or with a history of, bronchial asthma or allergic disease.

Precautions
Use in pregnancy: No embryopathic effects have been demonstrated in animals and there is epidemiological evidence of the safety of ketoprofen in human pregnancy. Nevertheless, it is recommended to avoid ketoprofen unless considered essential in which case it should be discontinued within one week of expected confinement when NSAIDs might cause premature closure of the ductus arteriosus or persistent pulmonary hypertension in the neonate. They also may delay labour. Trace amounts of ketoprofen are also excreted in breast milk; avoid use of ketoprofen unless considered essential.

Warnings: Inhibition of renal prostaglandin synthesis by non-steroidal anti-inflammatory agents may interfere with renal function especially in the presence of existing renal disease. Ketoprofen should therefore be used with caution in patients with renal impairment.

Orudis capsules should always be prescribed 'To be taken with food' to minimise gastric intolerance.

Interactions: Ketoprofen is highly protein-bound. Concomitant use of other protein-binding drugs, e.g. anticoagulants, sulphonamides, hydantoins, might necessitate modification of dosage in order to avoid increased levels of such drugs resulting from competition for plasma protein-binding sites. Similar acting drugs such as aspirin or other non-steroidal anti-inflammatory agents should not be administered concomitantly with ketoprofen as the potential for adverse reactions is increased.

Serious interactions have been recorded after the use of high dose methotrexate with non-steroidal anti-inflammatory agents including ketoprofen.

Adverse effects: Minor adverse effects, frequently transient, consist for the most part of gastrointestinal effects such as indigestion, dyspepsia, nausea, constipation, diarrhoea, heartburn and various types of abdominal discomfort. Other minor effects such as headache, dizziness, mild confusion, vertigo, drowsiness, oedema, mood change and insomnia may occur less commonly.

Major gastrointestinal adverse effects such as peptic ulceration, haemorrhage or perforation may rarely occur.

Major adverse effects involving other organ systems such as haematological reactions including thrombocytopenia, hepatic or renal damage, dermatological reactions, bronchospasm and anaphylaxis are exceedingly rare.

In all cases of major adverse effects Orudis should be withdrawn at once.

Use of suppositories is sometimes associated with change in stool consistency mostly of mild softening. In a study of 64 patients treated for up to six months with one suppository each night (supplemented during daytime with Orudis capsules), local intolerance to suppositories sufficiently severe to discontinue treatment occurred in only four subjects.

Overdosage: Like other propionic acid derivatives, ketoprofen is of low toxicity in overdosage; symptoms after acute ketoprofen intoxication are largely limited to drowsiness, abdominal pain and vomiting, but adverse effects seen after overdosage with propionic acid derivatives such as hypotension, bronchospasm and gastrointestinal haemorrhage should be anticipated. Treatment is otherwise supportive and symptomatic.

Pharmaceutical precautions Store in a dry place, below 25°C.

Legal category POM.

Package quantities Orudis 50: Containers of 112 × 50 mg (OP).
Orudis 100: Containers of 56 × 100 mg (OP) capsules.
Blister pack of 7 × 100 mg (OP) suppositories.

Further information Nil.

Product licence numbers

50 mg capsules	0012/0122
100 mg capsules	0012/0133
100 mg suppositories	0012/0109

ORUVAIL* and ORUVAIL* I.M. INJECTION

Presentation
Oruvail 100: Transparent pink capsules with opaque purple cap (each half printed 'Oruvail 100' in white), holding white pellets. Each capsule contains 100 mg ketoprofen in a pH sensitive controlled release delivery system.

Oruvail 200: Transparent pink capsules with opaque white cap (each half printed 'Oruvail' 200 in blue), holding white pellets. Each capsule contains 200 mg ketoprofen in a pH sensitive controlled release delivery system. Oruvail 100 and Oruvail 200 both contain sucrose.

Oruvail I.M. Injection: Brown glass ampoules containing 100 mg ketoprofen in 2 ml colourless aqueous solution. Also contains arginine, benzyl alcohol and citric acid.

Uses Oruvail Capsules are recommended for management of rheumatoid arthritis, osteoarthritis, ankylosing spondylitis, acute articular and periarticular disorders (bursitis, capsulitis, synovitis, tendinitis), cervical spondylitis, low back pain (strain, lumbago, sciatica, fibrositis), painful musculoskeletal conditions, acute gout, dysmenorrhoea and control of pain and inflammation following orthopaedic surgery.

Oruvail I.M. Injection is recommended for management of acute exacerbations of rheumatoid arthritis, osteoarthritis, ankylosing spondylitis, periarticular conditions such as fibrositis, bursitis, capsulitis, tendinitis and tenosynovitis, low back pain of musculoskeletal origin, sciatica, other musculoskeletal conditions, acute gout and control of pain and inflammation following orthopaedic surgery.

Oruvail is a potent non-steroidal anti-inflammatory analgesic agent and a stong inhibitor of prostaglandin synthetase.

Oruvail reduces joint pain and inflammation, and facilitates increase in mobility and functional independence. As with other non-steroidal anti-inflammatory agents, it does not cure the underlying disease.

Kinetics: Ketoprofen is slowly but completely absorbed from Oruvail capsules. Maximum plasma concentration occurs after 6–8 hours. It declines thereafter with a half-life of about 8 hours. There is no accumulation on continued daily dosing. Ketoprofen is rapidly and completely absorbed after I.M. injection reaching maximum plasma concentration in 20–30 minutes. Elimination half life is 1.8 hours. Ketoprofen is very highly bound to plasma protein.

Dosage and administration
Adults: Oruvail capsules: 100–200 mg once daily, depending on patient weight and on severity of symptoms. The capsules should be taken orally, usually with food.

I.M. Injection: 50–100 mg every 4 hours, repeated up to a maximum of 200 mg in 24 hours. Administer by deep intramuscular injection into the upper, outer quadrant of the buttock. Following a satisfactory response, oral therapy should be instituted with capsules.

It is recommended that the injection should not be used for longer than 3 days. The injection must not be given by the intravenous route.

Elderly: There is no evidence of an excess of adverse reactions in the elderly. However, as with other medications, it is generally advisable to begin ketoprofen therapy at the lower end of the dose range and to maintain such patients on the lowest effective dosage.

Paediatric dosage is not established.

Contra-indications, warnings, etc Active peptic ulceration; a history of recurrent peptic ulceration or chronic dyspepsia. Severe renal dysfunction.

Ketoprofen should not be given to patients with a known hypersensitivity to ketoprofen or sensitive to aspirin or other non-steroidal anti-inflammatory agents. Severe bronchospasm might be precipitated in these patients and in those suffering from, or with a history of bronchial asthma or allergic disease. The injection must not be given by the intravenous route.

Pregnancy and lactation: No embryopathic effects have been demonstrated in animals and there is epidemiological evidence of the safety of ketoprofen in human pregnancy. Nevertheless, it is recommended to avoid ketoprofen unless considered essential in which case it should be discontinued within one week of expected confinement when NSAIDs might cause premature closure of the ductus arteriosus or persistent pulmonary hypertension in the neonate. They may also delay labour. Trace amounts of ketoprofen are excreted in breast milk, avoid use of ketoprofen unless considered essential.

Warnings: Inhibition of renal prostaglandin synthesis by non-steroidal anti-inflammatory agents may interfere with renal function especially in the presence of existing renal disease. Ketoprofen should therefore be used with caution in patients with renal impairment.

Oruvail capsules should always be prescribed 'To be taken with food' to minimise gastric intolerance.

Interactions: Ketoprofen is highly protein-bound. Concomitant use of other protein-binding drugs, e.g. anticoagulants, sulphonamides, hydantoins, might necessitate modification of dosage in order to avoid increased levels of such drugs resulting from competition for plasma protein-binding sites. Similar acting drugs such as aspirin or other non-steroidal anti-inflammatory agents should not be administered concomitantly with ketoprofen as the potential for adverse reactions is increased.

Serious interactions have been recorded after the use of high dose methotrexate with non-steroidal anti-inflammatory agents including ketoprofen.

Adverse effects: Minor adverse effects, frequently transient, consist for the most part of gastrointestinal effects such as indigestion, dyspepsia, nausea, constipation, diarrhoea, heartburn and various types of abdominal discomfort. Other minor effects such as headache, dizziness, mild confusion, vertigo, drowsiness, oedema, mood change and insomnia may occur less commonly.

Major gastrointestinal adverse effects such as peptic ulceration, haemorrhage or perforation may rarely occur.

Major adverse effects involving other organ systems such as haematological reactions including thrombocytopenia, hepatic or renal damage, dermatological reactions, bronchospasm and anaphylaxis are exceedingly rare.

In all cases of major adverse effects Oruvail should be withdrawn at once.

Local reactions at the injection site can occur and may include pain or a burning sensation.

Overdosage: Like other propionic acid derivatives, ketoprofen is of low toxicity in overdosage; symptoms after acute ketoprofen intoxication are largely limited to drowsiness, abdominal pain and vomiting, but adverse effects seen after overdosage with propionic acid derivatives such as hypotension, bronchospasm and gastrointestinal haemorrhage should be anticipated.

Owing to the slow release characteristics of Oruvail, it should be expected that ketoprofen will continue to be absorbed for up to 16 hours after ingestion.

Gastric lavage, aimed at recovering pellets that may still be in the stomach, should be performed if the patient is seen soon after ingestion. It should be possible to identify the pellets in the gastric contents. Treatment is otherwise supportive and symptomatic.

Administration of activated charcoal in an attempt to reduce absorption of slowly-released ketoprofen should be considered.

Pharmaceutical precautions Store in a dry place, below 25°C.

Legal category POM.

Package quantities
Oruvail 100: Containers of 56 capsules (OP).
Oruvail 200: Calendar blister pack of 28 capsules (OP).
Oruvail I.M. Injection: Boxes of 10 × 2 ml ampoules.

Further information The above mentioned blister pack is a convenient calendar pack containing 28 capsules to aid administration and compliance.

Product licence numbers

Oruvail 100:	0012/0143
Oruvail 200:	0012/0158
Oruvail I.M. Injection:	0012/0186

PACITRON*

Presentation Film-coated oblong orange-yellow tablets marked 'PCT 500', each containing L-tryptophan 500 mg. Other ingredients include sunset yellow (E110).

Uses L-tryptophan is a metabolic precursor of 5-hydroxytryptamine (serotonin) which acts as a neurotransmitter in the central nervous system. L-tryptophan is indicated for the short-term relief of mild to moderate depressive illness. It is recommended that therapy be reviewed at 3-monthly intervals. L-tryptophan may enhance the action of amitriptyline and other antidepressant drugs.

Dosage and administration
Adults: The usual adult dosage is 3 g daily in divided doses. Some patients may require up to 6 g daily. L-tryptophan may also be given to patients responding inadequately to monoamine oxidase inhibitors (MAOI) but when the two are given together the side-effects of both may be increased. Pacitron should therefore be introduced more slowly, beginning at 500 mg daily for the first week, 1 g daily for the second. Normal dosage may be given from the third week onwards, but Pacitron should be discontinued at once if headache or blurring of vision occurs.

Children: L-tryptophan is not recommended in children.

Elderly: No special precaution.

Contra-indications, warnings, etc
Contra-indications: The use of Pacitron should not replace standard management in patients with severe depression and/or a risk of suicide. There is no absolute contra-indication to the use of Pacitron.

Precautions: Concurrent use of MAOI may potentiate the adverse reactions of both drugs.

In patients taking Pacitron together with or after phenothiazines or benzodiazepines, there have been rare reports of sexual disinhibition and of reversible Parkinsonian-like rigidity and dyskinesias. Since these other drugs may reduce plasma binding of tryptophan it is recommended that initial dosage of Pacitron should not exceed one tablet three times daily if the patient is taking or has just finished treatment with a major tranquilliser.

Pacitron should be used with caution in patients with overt nutritional deficiency.

Pacitron is not advised, except for relatively short periods in patients with active bladder disease or known bladder lesions.

Warnings, Side-effects etc.: L-tryptophan may produce drowsiness. Patients should be warned of the possible hazard when driving or operating machinery.

Other reported side-effects include nausea, headache and light-headedness.

There is at present no information on safety and efficacy after long-term administration of Pacitron.

Abnormal tryptophan metabolism may occur in patients who are pyridoxine deficient, such deficiency may occur in women taking oral contraceptives or in elderly or undernourished patients who have an inadequate vitamin intake. Pyridoxine supplements may be advisable in patients suspected of deficiency.

Use in Pregnancy: Evidence from animal studies is insufficient to establish safety in pregnancy. Use in pregnant and nursing mothers is not advised.

Treatment of overdosage: No serious consequences are known to result from overdosage. Gastric lavage might be helpful followed by observation and general supportive measures.

Pharmaceutical precautions No special precautions.

Legal category POM.

Package quantities Containers of 100 tablets.

Further information As with other antidepressant drugs the full therapeutic effect may not be seen for two or three weeks and patients should be told this.

Product licence number 0152/0117.

PENTACARINAT*

Presentation A sterile white powder supplied in single dose vials containing 300 mg pentamidine isethionate.

Uses Pentamidine isethionate is indicated in the treatment of the following conditions:

- pneumonia due to *Pneumocystis carinii* occurring in debilitated or immunocompromised patients e.g. in the acquired immune deficiency syndrome (AIDS). *P. carinii* pneumonia (PCP) is the commonest lethal opportunistic infection in patients with AIDS.
- Leishmaniasis: (visceral and cutaneous).
- early phase African sleeping sickness caused by *Trypanosoma gambiense*.

All the above indications may be treated parenterally. *P. carinii* pneumonia can also be treated by the inhalation route in view of the presence of these organisms in the alveolar space.

Pentacarinat is also indicated for the prevention of *P. carinii* pneumonia in patients infected by the human immunodeficiency virus (HIV) who have experienced a previous episode of PCP. Administration is by the inhalation route.

Kinetics: After intravenous infusion, plasma levels of pentamidine fall rapidly during the first two hours to one twentieth of peak levels, followed by a much slower decline thereafter. After intramuscular administration, the apparent volume of distribution of pentamidine is significantly greater (>3 times) than that observed following intravenous administration.

Elimination half-lives after parenteral administration were estimated to be about 6 hours after intravenous infusion in patients with a normal renal function. The elimination half-life following intramuscular injection was found to be about 9 hours.

Following parenteral administration pentamidine appears to be widely distributed in the body and probably accumulates in tissue, particularly the liver and kidney. Only a small amount is excreted unchanged in the urine. When administered by use of a nebuliser, human kinetic studies revealed significant differences when compared to parenteral administration. Aerosol administration resulted in a 10-fold increase in bronchial alveolar lavage (BAL) supernatant fluid and an 80-fold increase in BAL sediment concentrations in comparison with those seen with equivalent intravenous doses.

Limited data suggest that the half-life of pentamidine in BAL fluid is greater than 10 to 14 days. Peak plasma concentrations after inhalation therapy were found to be approximately 10% of those observed with equivalent intramuscular doses and less than 5% of those observed following intravenous administration. This suggests that systemic effects by the inhalation route are less likely.

Long-term pulmonary parenchymal effects of aerosolised pentamidine are not known. Lung volume and alveolar capillary diffusion, however, have not been shown to be affected by high doses of pentamidine administered by inhalation to AIDS patients.

Dosage and administration

Dosage by the inhalation route: For the treatment of *P. carinii* pneumonia the recommended dosage is 600 mg pentamidine isethionate (2 × 300 mg Pentacarinat vials) daily for three weeks.

For the secondary prevention of *P. carinii* pneumonia the dosage is 300 mg pentamidine isethionate administered as a single inhalation every 4 weeks.

Dosage by intramuscular or intravenous administration: The following dosage regimes relate to both intramuscular and intravenous administration and are recommended for adults, children and infants.

Treatment of *P. carinii* pneumonia; pentamidine isethionate 4 mg/kg bodyweight daily for at least 14 days, preferably by slow intravenous infusion.

Leishmaniasis: Visceral (Kala-azar): pentamidine isethionate 3 to 4 mg/kg bodyweight on alternate days to a maximum of 10 injections, preferably by the intramuscular route. A repeat course may be needed.

Cutaneous: pentamidine isethionate 3 to 4 mg/kg bodyweight once or twice weekly by intramuscular injection until the condition resolves.

Trypanosomiasis: Pentamidine isethionate 4 mg/kg bodyweight daily or on alternate days to a total of 7 to 10 injections using either of the parenteral routes.

Dosage in the elderly: No specific dosage recommendations.

Dosage in renal failure: (creatinine clearance <10 ml/minute): In life-threatening cases of *P. carinii* pneumonia the recommended dosage of pentamidine isethionate is 4 mg/kg bodyweight, by either parenteral route, once daily for 7 to 10 days. Treatment should then continue at the same dosage on alternate days to complete the course of at least 14 doses. In less severe cases pentamidine isethionate 4 mg/kg bodyweight should be administered on alternate days to complete the course of at least 14 doses.

No dosage reduction is necessary in renally impaired patients with leishmaniasis or trypanosomiasis.

Dosage in hepatic failure: No information available.

Administration by inhalation: Solutions for inhalation should be prepared as described below and then used immediately.

Treatment for P. carinii pneumonia: Dissolve the contents of two Pentacarinat vials (2 × 300 mg pentamidine isethionate) in 6 ml of Water for Injections BP.

Prevention of P. carinii pneumonia: Dissolve the contents of one Pentacarinat vial (300 mg pentamidine isethionate) in 4–6 mls of Water for Injections BP.

The freshly prepared solution should be administered by inhalation using a suitable nebuliser such as a 'Respirgard II', modified 'Acorn System 22' or an equivalent device. This should be fitted with either a portable compressor or piped oxygen at a flow rate of 6 to 10 litres/minute.

The optimal particle size for alveolar deposition is between 1 and 2 microns.

A suitable, well-fitted one-way system should be employed such that the nebuliser stores the aerosolised drug during exhalations and disperses exhaled pentamidine into a reservoir. A filter should be fitted to the exhaust line to reduce atmospheric pollution. It is advisable to use a suitable exhaust tube which vents directly through a window to the external atmosphere. Care should be taken to ensure that passers-by will not be exposed to the exhaust.

Parenteral administration: In order to reduce the incidence of sudden, severe hypotension Pentacarinat should be administered parenterally only by deep intramuscular injection or by slow intravenous infusion with the patient lying down. Bolus intravenous injections should be avoided if possible and never be given rapidly.

Pentacarinat must be reconstituted only with Water

for Injections BP. The reconstituted solution may be further diluted for intravenous infusion using either Glucose Intravenous Infusion 5% BP or 0.9% Sodium Chloride Injection BP. It must not be mixed or diluted with any other injection solutions.

For deep intramuscular administration the contents of one vial of Pentacarinat (300 mg pentamidine isethionate) should be dissolved in 3 ml Water for Injections BP. The dose calculated for the individual patient then should be administered by deep intramuscular injection, preferably into the buttock.

For slow intravenous infusion, the contents of one Pentacarinat vial (300 mg pentamidine isethionate) should be dissolved in a known volume (3 to 5 ml) of Water for Injections BP. The dose calculated for an individual patient may then be diluted further in 50 to 250 ml of Glucose Intravenous Infusion 5% BP or in 0.9% Sodium Chloride Injection BP. The resulting solution of pentamidine isethionate should be infused over a period of at least 60 minutes with the patient remaining supine and under close medical supervision.

Contra-indications, warnings, etc The drug should not be administered to patients with a known hypersensitivity to pentamidine.

Pregnancy: There is no evidence of the safety of pentamidine isethionate in human pregnancy. Pentamidine isethionate should not be administered to pregnant patients unless considered essential.

Lactation: The use of pentamidine isethionate is contra-indicated in breast-feeding mothers unless considered essential by the physician.

Precautions: Pentacarinat should be used with particular caution in patients with hepatic and/or renal dysfunction, hypertension or hypotension, hyperglycaemia or hypoglycaemia, leucopenia, thrombocytopenia or anaemia.

Sudden, severe hypotension may occur in patients after a single dose of Pentacarinat has been given either intramuscularly or by intravenous infusion. Baseline blood pressure should be established and patients should receive the drug lying down. Blood pressure should be closely monitored during administration and at regular intervals until treatment is concluded.

Laboratory monitoring: The following tests should be carried out before, during and after treatment by the parenteral route.

(i) Blood urea nitrogen and serum creatinine daily during therapy.
(ii) Complete blood and platelet counts daily during therapy.
(iii) Fasting blood glucose measurements daily during therapy, and at regular intervals after completion of therapy. Hyperglycaemia and diabetes mellitus, with or without preceding hypoglycaemia have occurred up to several months after cessation of therapy.
(iv) Liver function tests (LFTs) including bilirubin, alkaline phosphatase, aspartate aminotransferase (AST/SGOT), and alanine aminotransferase (ALT/SGPT). If baseline measurements are normal and remain so during therapy, test weekly thereafter. When there is baseline elevation in LFTs and/or LFTs increase during therapy, continue monitoring weekly unless the patient is on other hepatotoxic agents, when monitoring every 3–5 days is appropriate.
(v) Serum calcium, test weekly.
(vi) Urine analysis and serum electrolytes daily during therapy.
(vii) Electrocardiograms at regular intervals.

Interactions: None known.

Adverse effects

(a) Parenteral route. Severe reactions, sometimes fatal due to hypotension, hypoglycaemia, pancreatitis, and cardiac arrhythmias have been reported. Other life-threatening reactions requiring immediate corrective measures and withdrawal of Pentacarinat have included leucopenia (<1000 per cubic millimetre), thrombocytopenia (<20,000 per cubic millimetre), acute renal failure (serum creatinine >6 mg/dL), hypocalcaemia, and ventricular tachycardia. A possible case of Stevens-Johnson syndrome has been reported.

Less severe reactions may be observed consisting of azotemia (elevated serum creatinine levels 2.4 to 6 mg/dL), abnormal liver function tests, leucopenia, anaemia, thrombocytopenia, hyperkalaemia, hyperglycaemia, hypoglycaemia, nausea and vomiting, hypotension, dizziness, syncope, flushing, rash and taste disturbances.

Local reactions can occur ranging in severity from discomfort and pain to induration, abscess formation and muscle necrosis. Raised serum creatinine phosphokinase (CPK) and lactic dehydrogenase levels have also been observed.

Side-effects including metabolic disturbances, hepatic impairment, haematological disorders or hypotension have been reported in 5–10% of patients.

(b) Inhalation route: Bronchospasm has been reported to occur following use of the nebuliser. This has been particularly noted in patients who have a history of smoking or asthma. This can usually be controlled by prior use of bronchodilators. The occurrence of cases of pneumothorax has been reported in patients presenting a history of PCP. Although the aetiology of the pneumothorax was not linked primarily to the aerosolised administration of pentamidine in the majority of cases, a causal relationship to pentamidine cannot be ruled out.

Local reactions involving the upper respiratory tract can occur ranging in severity from cough, shortness of breath and wheezing to bronchospasms.

Other side-effects reported were hypoglycaemia, pancreatitis and renal insufficiency, rash, fever, decrease in appetite, bad taste, fatigue, lightheadedness and nausea.

A miscarriage has been reported following prophylactic aerosolised administration.

Treatment of overdosage: Treatment is symptomatic. However, no cases of overdosage have been recorded with Pentacarinat.

Pharmaceutical precautions This product should be reconstituted in a laminar flow cabinet. Store the dry product below 30°C. Store dilute reconstituted drug solutions between 2–8°C, and discard all unused portions within 24 hours of preparation. Concentrated solutions for administration by the inhalation or intramuscular routes should be used immediately.

After reconstitution with Water for Injections BP, Pentacarinat should not be mixed with any injection solutions other than Glucose Intravenous Infusion 5% BP and 0.9% (Normal) Sodium Chloride Injection BP.

Legal category POM.

Package quantities Box of 5 × 300 mg vials.

Further information Pentamidine isethionate is an aromatic diamidine. It is an antiprotozoal agent which acts by interfering with DNA and folate transformation, and by inhibition of RNA and protein synthesis. Dosage equivalence: 4 mg of pentamidine isethionate contains 2.3 mg pentamidine base: 1 mg of pentamidine base is equivalent to 1.74 mg pentamidine isethionate.

Displacement value: 300 mg of pentamidine isethionate displaces approximately 0.15 ml of water.

All bystanders including medical personnel are advised to minimise exposure to atmospheric pentamidine from nebulisers.

Product licence number 0012/0193.

Trade marks: Acorn System 22 is a Trade Mark of Medic-Aid and Respirgard II is a Trade Mark of Marquest, Medical Products Inc.

PENTACARINAT* READY-TO-USE SOLUTION

Presentation A clear colourless, solution, supplied in a 10 ml unit-dose container, containing 300 mg pentamidine isethionate. The solution also contains glucose and sodium acetate buffer.

Uses Pentacarinat Ready-to-Use Solution is indicated

in the treatment of *Pneumocystis carinii* pneumonia (PCP)in the patients infected by the human immunodeficiency virus (HIV).

Pentacarinat Ready-to-Use Solution is also indicated for the prevention of Pneumocystis carinii pneumonia in patients infected by the human immunodeficiency virus who have experienced a previous episode of PCP.

Kinetics: When administered by the use of a nebuliser, human kinetic studies revealed significant differences compared to parenteral administration. Aerosol administration resulted in a 10-fold increase in bronchial alveolar lavage (BAL) supernatant fluid, and an 80-fold increase in BAL sediment concentrations in comparison with those seen with equivalent parenteral doses.

Limited data suggest that the half-life of pentamidine in BAL fluid is greater than 10 to 14 days.

Long-term pulmonary parenchymal effects of aerosolised pentamidine are not known. Lung volume and alveolar capillary diffusion, however, have not been shown to be affected by high doses of pentamidine administered by inhalation to AIDS patients.

Dosage and administration
Treatment: For the treatment of P. carinii pneumonia, the dosage is 600 mg (two bottles of solution), given once daily for 3 weeks.

Prophylaxis: For prevention of P. carinii pneumonia, the dosage is 300 mg once a month or 150 mg every two weeks.

The solution containing the required dosage should be administered by inhalation using a suitable nebuliser such as a Respirgard II*, modified Acorn System 22* or an equivalent device with either a compressor or piped oxygen at a flow rate of 6 to 10 litres/minute.

The optimal particle size for alveolar deposition is between 1 and 2 microns.

A suitable, well fitted one-way system should be employed such that the nebuliser stores the aerosolised drug during exhalations and disperses exhaled pentamidine into a reservoir. A filter should be fitted to the exhaust line to reduce atmospheric pollution. It is advisable to use a suitable exhaust tube which vents directly through a window to the external atmosphere. Care should be taken to ensure that passers-by will not be exposed to the exhaust.

Elderly: No specific dosage recommendations.

Hepatic failure: No information available.

Contra-indications, warnings, etc The drug should not be administered to patients with a known hypersensitivity to pentamidine.

Pregnancy: There is no evidence of the safety of aerosolised pentamidine in human pregnancy. Pentamidine isethionate should not be administered to pregnant patients unless considered essential.

Lactation: The use of pentamidine isethionate is contraindicated in breast-feeding mothers unless considered essential by the physician.

Precautions: Pentamidine isethionate should be used with particular caution in patients with hepatic or renal dysfunction, hypertension or hypotension, hyperglycaemia or hypoglycaemia, leucopenia, thrombocytopenia or anaemia.

Bronchospasm has been reported to occur following use of nebulised pentamidine. This has been noted particularly in patients who have a history of smoking or asthma and can usually be controlled by prior use of bronchodilators.

The benefit of aerosolised pentamidine therapy in patients at high risk of a pneumothorax should be weighed against the clinical consequences of such an occurrence.

Interactions: None known.

Adverse effects: Cases of pneumothorax have been reported in patients with a history of PCP. Although the aetiology of the pneumothorax was not linked primarily to the aerosolised administration of pentamidine in the majority of cases, a causal relationship to pentamidine cannot be ruled out.

Local reactions involving the upper respiratory tract can occur ranging in severity from cough, shortness of breath and wheezing to bronchospasms.

Other adverse effects reported with the use of aerosolised pentamidine include hypoglycaemia, pancreatitis, renal insufficiency, rash, fever, decrease in appetite, bad taste, fatigue, lightheadedness and nausea.

A miscarriage within the first trimester of pregnancy has been reported following prophylactic administration of aerosolised pentamidine.

Treatment of overdosage: No cases of overdosage have been recorded with pentamidine. Should overdosage occur treatment should be symptomatic.

Pharmaceutical precautions Store between 15°C–25°C. Any solid material should be redissolved by gentle warming before use.

Legal category POM.

Package quantities 10 × 300 mg bottles.

Further information Pentamidine isethionate is an aromatic diamidine. It is an antiprotozoal agent which acts by interfering with DNA and folate transformation, and by inhibition of RNA and protein synthesis. Dosage equivalence: 4 mg of pentamidine isethionate contains 2.3 mg pentamidine base; 1 mg of pentamidine base is equivalent to 1.74 mg pentamidine isethionate.

All bystanders including medical personnel, and especially pregnant women, are advised to minimise exposure to atmospheric pentamidine resulting from nebuliser usage.

Product licence number 0012/0221.

Trade marks: "Acorn System 22" is a Trade Mark of Medic-Aid and "Respirgard II" is a Trade Mark of Marquest Medical Products Inc.

PHENERGAN*

Presentation
Tablets: Pale blue, film-coated tablets containing 10 mg promethazine hydrochloride, impressed 'PN10' on one side.

Pale blue, film-coated tablets containing 25 mg promethazine hydrochloride, impressed 'PN 25' on one side.

Phenergan 10 mg and 25 mg tablets contain lactose.

Elixir: Promethazine oral solution BP (sugar-free). A clear bright golden syrupy liquid containing 5 mg promethazine hydrochloride per 5 ml. The elixir contains sodium sulphite, sodium metabisulphite, hydrogenated glucose and sodium benzoate.

Injection: A colourless injection solution containing 2.5% w/v promethazine hydrochloride. The injection also contains sodium sulphite and sodium metabisulphite.

Uses As an adjunct in preoperative sedation in surgery and obstetrics.

Potent long-acting antihistamine with additional, antiemetic anticholinergic and sedative/calming effects.

Indicated in symptomatic treatment of allergic conditions of the upper respiratory tract and skin: sensitisation reactions to drug or foreign proteins; anaphylactic reactions.

For sedation and treatment of insomnia in adults.

As a paediatric sedative.

As an antiemetic.

Kinetics: Promethazine is well absorbed after oral dosing and slowly excreted via urine and bile. It is distributed widely in the body. It enters the brain and crosses the placenta. Phenothiazines pass into the milk at low concentrations.

Dosage and administration
Adults: Oral administration: Initial dose one 25 mg tablet at night; may be increased to two or three 25 mg tablets at night if necessary. In allergic conditions more frequent administration, twice or three times daily, may be necessary, starting with one or two 10 mg tablets and increasing as required. For travel sickness, 25 mg on the night before the journey. This dose may be repeated after 6–8 hours.

Parenteral administration: The usual adult dose is 25–

50 mg by deep intramuscular injection or, in emergency, by slow intravenous injection after dilution of 2.5% solution to 10 times its volume with Water for Injections immediately before use. Maximum parenteral dose 100 mg.

Elderly: No specific dosage recommendations.

Children: They may be treated more conveniently by the elixir containing 5 mg per 5 ml.

As an antihistamine in allergy:

Below 1 year:	Not recommended
1–2 years:	Use as recommended by a doctor
2–5 years:	5–15 mg
5–10 years:	10–25 mg

In cases where two doses in 24 hours are required the lower amount stated should be given.

As a sedative:

Below 1 year:	Not recommended
1–2 years:	Use as recommended by a doctor
2–5 years:	15–20 mg
5–10 years:	20–25 mg

Given as a single night-time dose.

As an anti-emetic:

Below 1 year:	Not recommended
1–2 years:	Use as recommended by a doctor
2–5 years:	5 mg
5–10 years:	10 mg
Over 10 years:	25 mg

To be taken the night before the journey and repeated after 6–8 hours if required.

Parenteral: Half the oral dose, i.e. 6.25–12.5 mg for children from 5 to 10 years may be given by deep intramuscular injection.

Contra-indications, warnings, etc Phenergan should not be used in patients who are in a coma or suffering from CNS depression of any cause. It must not be given to neonates, premature infants or patients hypersensitive to phenothiazines. Phenergan should be avoided in patients who have been taking monoamine oxidase inhibitors within the previous 14 days.

The Elixir contains hydrogenated glucose and is not suitable for diabetics.

Use in pregnancy: There is epidemiological evidence for the safety of promethazine in pregnancy, and animal studies have shown no hazard, nevertheless it should not be used in pregnancy unless the physician considers it essential. The use of Phenergan is not recommended in the two weeks prior to delivery in view of the risk of irritability and excitement in the neonate.

Use in lactation: Available evidence suggests that the amount excreted in milk is insignificant. However there are risks of neonatal irritability and excitement.

Ambulant patients receiving Phenergan for the first time should not be in control of vehicles or machinery for the first few days until it is established that they are not hypersensitive to the central nervous effects of the drug and do not suffer from disorientation, confusion or dizziness.

Phenergan may thicken or dry lung secretions and impair expectoration, it should therefore be used with caution in patients with asthma, bronchitis or bronchiectesis. Use with care in patients with severe coronary artery disease, narrow angle glaucoma, epilepsy or hepatic and renal insufficiency. Caution should be exercised in patients with bladder neck or pyloroduodenal obstruction. Promethazine may mask the warning signs of ototoxicity caused by ototoxic drugs e.g. salicylates. It may also delay the early diagnosis of intestinal obstruction or raised intracranial pressure through the suppression of vomiting.

Accidental intraarterial injection may lead to peripheral gangrene and necrosis while subcutaneous injections may lead to local necrosis.

Interactions: Phenergan may enhance the action of any anticholinergic agent, tricyclic antidepressant, sedative or hypnotic. Alcohol should be avoided during treatment.

Phenergan may interfere with immunologic urine pregnancy tests to produce false-positive or false-negative results.

Phenergan should be discontinued at least 72 hours before the start of skin tests using allergen extracts as it may inhibit the cutaneous histamine response thus producing false-negative results.

Phenergan injection has been known to increase glucose tolerance.

Side-effects may be seen in a few patients: drowsiness, dizziness, restlessness, headaches, nightmares, tiredness, and disorientation. Anticholinergic side-effects such as blurred vision, dry mouth and urinary retention occur occasionally. Newborn and premature infants are susceptible to the anticholinergic effects of promethazine while other children may display paradoxical hyperexcitability. The elderly are particularly susceptible to the anticholinergic effects and confusion due to promethazine. Other side-effects include anorexia, gastric irritation, palpitations, hypotension, arrhythmias, extrapyramidal effects, muscle spasms and tic-like movements of the head and face. Anaphylaxis, jaundice and blood dyscrasias including haemolytic anaemia rarely occur. Photosensitive skin reactions have been reported; strong sunlight should be avoided during treatment. The preservatives used in Phenergan injection have been reported to cause hypersensitivity reactions, characterised by circulatory collapse with CNS depression, in certain susceptible individuals with allergic tendencies.

The preservatives used in Phenergan elixir have been reported to cause hypersensitivity reactions.

Treatment of overdosage: Symptoms of severe overdosage are variable. They are characterised in children by various combinations of excitation, ataxia, inco-ordination, athetosis and hallucinations, while adults may become drowsy and lapse into coma. Convulsions may occur in both adults and children; coma or excitement may precede their occurrence. Cardiorespiratory depression is uncommon. If the patient is seen soon enough after ingestion, it should be possible to induce vomiting with ipecacuanha despite the anti-emetic effect of promethazine; alternatively, gastric lavage may be used.

Treatment is otherwise supportive with attention to maintenance of adequate respiratory and circulatory status. Convulsions should be treated with diazepam or other suitable anticonvulsant.

Pharmaceutical precautions Protect from light. Solutions of Phenergan are incompatible with alkaline substances, which precipitate the insoluble promethazine base. Store the tablets below 30°C and the elixir below 25°C.

Legal category Tablets and Elixir P.
Injection Solution POM.

Package quantities Containers of 56 tablets of both strengths (OP). Injection Solution 2.5%: Boxes of 10 × 1 ml. Elixir: Bottles of 100 ml (OP).

Further information Nil.

Product licence numbers

Tablets 10 mg	0012/5285
Tablets 25 mg	0012/5286
Elixir	0012/5025
Injection	0012/5054

PIPORTIL* DEPOT INJECTION

Presentation Straw coloured viscous liquid containing pipothiazine palmitate 5.0% w/v (50 mg per ml) in sesame oil.

Uses Piportil Depot is a long-acting phenothiazine neuroleptic indicated for the maintenance treatment of schizophrenia and paranoid psychoses, and prevention of relapse, especially where compliance with oral medication is a problem.

Kinetics: There is little information about blood levels, distribution and excretion in humans. The rate of metabolism and excretion of phenothiazines decreases in old age.

Dosage and administration Patients should be stabilised on Piportil Depot under psychiatric supervision. Administration should be by deep intramuscular injection into the gluteal region.

Adults: Initially 25 mg (0.5 ml) should be given to assess the response of the patient to the drug. Further doses should be administered at appropriate intervals, increasing by increments of 25 or 50 mg until a satisfactory response is obtained. In clinical practice Piportil Depot has been shown to have a long duration of action, allowing intervals of 4 weeks between injections for maintenance therapy. Dosage should be adjusted under close supervision to suit each individual patient in order to obtain the best therapeutic response compatible with tolerance.

The duration of action depends on the dose administered, allowing dosage intervals to be varied to suit individual circumstances.

Most patients respond favourably to a dose of 50–100 mg (1–2 ml) every 4 weeks. The maximum recommended dose is 200 mg (4 ml) every four weeks.

Elderly: Neuroleptics should be used cautiously in the elderly; a reduced starting dose is recommended, i.e. 5–10 mg might be considered.

Children: Not recommended for use in children.

Contra-indications, warnings, etc Piportil Depot should not be administered to patients in comatose states or with marked cerebral atherosclerosis, phaeochromocytoma, renal or liver failure, severe cardiac insufficiency or hypersensitivity to other phenothiazine derivatives.

Precautions: Piportil Depot should be used with caution in patients suffering from or who have a history of, the following conditions: severe respiratory disease, epilepsy, alcohol withdrawal symptoms, brain damage, Parkinson's disease or marked extrapyramidal symptoms with previously used neuroleptics, personal or family history of narrow angle glaucoma, hypothyroidism, myaesthenia gravis, prostatic hypertrophy, thyrotoxicosis. Care is required in very hot or very cold weather particularly in elderly frail patients.

Pregnancy: There is inadequate evidence of safety of Piportil Depot in human pregnancy, although animal studies have shown no hazard. The drug should not be used during pregnancy or lactation unless the physician considers it essential.

Interactions of phenothiazine neuroleptics: The CNS depressant actions of neuroleptic agents may be intensified (additively) by alcohol, barbiturates and other sedatives. Respiratory depression may occur.

The hypotensive effect of most antihypertensive drugs especially alpha adrenoceptor blocking agents may be exaggerated by neuroleptics.

The mild anticholinergic effect of neuroleptics may be enhanced by other anticholinergic drugs possibly leading to constipation, heat stroke, etc.

The action of some drugs may be opposed by phenothiazine neuroleptics; these include amphetamine, levodopa, clonidine, guanethidine, adrenaline.

Anticholinergic agents may reduce the antipsychotic effect of neuroleptics.

Some drugs interfere with absorption of neuroleptic agents: antacids, anti-Parkinson, lithium. Increases or decreases in the plasma concentrations of a number of drugs, e.g. propranolol, phenobarbitone have been observed but were not of clinical significance.

High doses of neuroleptics reduce the response to hypoglycaemic agents the dosage of which might have to be raised.

Adrenaline must *not* be used in patients overdosed with phenothiazine neuroleptics. Most of the above interactions are of a theoretical nature and not dangerous.

Simultaneous administration of desferrioxamine and prochlorperazine has been observed to induce a transient metabolic encephalopathy characterised by loss of consciousness for 48–72 hours.

It is possible that this may occur with Piportil since it shares many of the pharmacological activities of prochlorperazine.

Adverse effects of neuroleptics: Minor side effects of neuroleptics are nasal stuffiness, dry mouth, insomnia, agitation and weight gain. Other possible adverse effects are listed below.

Liver function: jaundice, usually transient, occurs in a very small percentage of patients taking neuroleptics. A premonitory sign may be a sudden onset of fever after one to three weeks of treatment followed by the development of jaundice. Neuroleptic jaundice has the biochemical and other characteristics of obstructive jaundice and is associated with obstructions of the canaliculi by bile thrombi; the frequent presence of an accompanying eosinophilia indicates the allergic nature of this phenomenon. Treatment should be withheld on the development of jaundice.

Cardiorespiratory: Hypotension, usually postural, commonly occurs. Elderly or volume depleted subjects are particularly susceptible; it is more likely to occur after intramuscular administration.

Cardiac arrhythmias, including atrial arrhythmia, A-V block, ventricular tachycardia and fibrillation have been reported during neuroleptic therapy, possibly related to dosage. Pre-existing cardiac disease, old age, hypokalaemia and concurrent tricyclic antidepressants may predispose. ECG changes, usually benign, include widened QT interval, ST depression, U-waves and T-wave changes.

Respiratory depression is possible in susceptible patients.

Blood picture: A mild leukopaenia occurs in up to 30% of patients on prolonged high dosage of neuroleptics. Agranulocytosis may occur rarely; it is not dose related. The occurrence of unexplained infections or fever requires immediate haematological investigation.

Extrapyramidal: Acute dystonias or dyskinesias, usually transitory, are commoner in children and young adults, and usually occur within the first 4 days of treatment or after dosage increases.

Akathisia characteristically occurs after large initial doses.

Parkinsonism is commoner in adults and the elderly. It usually develops after weeks or months of treatment. One or more of the following may be seen: tremor, rigidity, akinesia or other features of Parkinsonism. Commonly just tremor.

Tardive dyskinesia: If this occurs it is usually, but not necessarily, after prolonged or high dosage. It can even occur after treatment has been stopped. Dosage should therefore be kept low whenever possible.

Skin and eyes: Contact skin sensitisation is a serious but rare complication in those frequently handling preparations of phenothiazines; the greatest care must be taken to avoid contact of the drug with the skin. Skin rashes of various kinds may also be seen in patients treated with these drugs. Patients on high dosage should be warned that they may develop photosensitivity in sunny weather and should avoid exposure to direct sunlight.

Ocular changes and the development of a metallic greyish-mauve coloration of exposed skin have been noted in some individuals mainly females, who have received chlorpromazine continuously for long periods (four to eight years). Other neuroleptics have been implicated but less frequently.

Endocrine: hyperprolactinaemia which may result in galactorrhoea, gynaecomastia, amenorrhoea; impotence.

Neuroleptic malignant syndrome (hyperthermia, rigidity, autonomic dysfunction and altered consciousness) may occur with any neuroleptic.

Toxicity and treatment of neuroleptic overdosage: Symptoms of phenothiazine overdosage include drowsiness or loss of consciousness, hypotension, tachycardia, E.C.G. changes, ventricular arrhythmias and hypothermia. Severe extra-pyramidal dyskinesias may occur.

Generalised vasodilatation may result in circulatory collapse; raising the patient's legs may suffice, in severe cases, volume expansion by intravenous fluids may be needed; infusion fluids should be warmed before administration in order not to aggravate hypothermia.

Positive inotropic agents such as dopamine may be tried if fluid replacement is insufficient to correct the circulatory collapse. Peripheral vasoconstrictor agents are not generally recommended; avoid the use of adrenaline.

Ventricular or supraventricular tachy-arrhythmias usually respond to restoration of normal body temperature and correction of circulatory or metabolic disturbances. If they are persistent or life threatening, appropriate anti-arrhythmic therapy may be considered. Avoid lignocaine and, as far as possible, long acting anti-arrhythmic drugs.

Pronounced central nervous system depression requires airway maintenance or, in extreme circumstances, assisted respiration. Severe dystonic reactions usually respond to procyclidine (5–10 mg) or orphenadrine (20–40 mg) administered intramuscularly or intravenously. Convulsions should be treated with intravenous diazepam.

Neuroleptic malignant syndrome should be treated with cooling. Dantrolene sodium may be tried.

Pharmaceutical precautions Piportil Depot should be protected from light. It can be stored at room temperature. Piportil Depot should not be mixed with any other substance.

Legal category POM.

Package quantities Boxes of 10 × 1 ml (50 mg) and 10 × 2 ml (100 mg) ampoules.

Further information Nil.

Product licence number
Injection 5.0% w/v 0012/0117.

PRIMALAN*

Presentation White bi-convex tablets embossed Primalan on one side, unmarked on reverse. Each tablet contains 5 mg mequitazine. The tablets also contain lactose.

Uses Antihistamine for the symptomatic treatment of allergic conditions such as hay fever, perennial rhinitis, urticaria, pruritus of allergic origin and allergic reactions associated with insect bites and stings.

Dosage and administration

Adults: One 5 mg tablet to be taken orally twice a day.

Elderly: There is no information on specific dosage recommendation in the elderly. Caution should therefore be exercised in this group of patients.

Children: Primalan is not recommended for children under the age of 12.

Contra-indications, warnings, etc Primalan should not be given to patients sensitive to phenothiazines or given concurrently with monoamine oxidase inhibitors. As with all antihistamines, it should be used with caution in epilepsy, prostatic hypertrophy, glaucoma and hepatic disease. Primalan should not be administered during pregnancy.

In objective tests, Primalan has been shown to have no significant effect on alertness, performance or reaction time. As drowsiness can occur in some patients, it is advisable to check individual responses prior to driving or operating machinery.

Potentiation of the sedative effects of alcohol may occur in individual patients. Primalan may potentiate sympathomimetic amines.

Side-effects: Anticholinergic effects such as dryness of the mouth and disturbance of visual accommodation may occasionally occur, particularly in the early days of treatment.

Treatment of overdosage: Gastric lavage and supportive therapy. Avoid sedation with other phenothiazine derivatives.

Pharmaceutical precautions Store in a cool dry place and protect from light.

Legal category POM.

Package quantities Blister pack of 56 tablets (OP).

Further information Primalan has a prolonged action, allowing adequate control of symptoms with twice daily dosage.

Product licence numbers 0012/0161.

SECADREX*

Presentation Secadrex tablets are white, round, slightly biconvex, and film-coated, imprinted 'SECADREX' on one face; each contains the equivalent of 200 mg acebutolol (in the form of the hydrochloride) and 12.5 mg hydrochlorothiazide. The tablets also contain lactose.

Uses Mild and moderate hypertension. Secadrex has been shown to be particularly suitable for elderly patients.

Dosage and administration One Secadrex tablet once daily, usually in the morning, is sufficient in most patients. If response is inadequate, the dosage may be increased to two Secadrex tablets once daily. Two Secadrex tablets may be particularly suitable in moderately severe hypertension when satisfactory control of arterial blood pressure cannot be obtained with either a beta-blocker or a diuretic used alone. Secadrex is not intended for use in children.

Contra-indications, warnings, etc

(a) Cardiogenic shock is an absolute contra-indication to beta-blockade and caution is required in patients with blood pressures of the order of 100/60 or below.
(b) Heart block. Administration of any beta-adrenoceptor blocking agent is considered inadvisable (except perhaps in first degree block).
(c) Severe kidney and liver failure.
(d) Hypersensitivity to hydrochlorothiazide.
(e) Secadrex tablets should not be used with verapamil or within several days of verapamil therapy (and vice-versa).
(f) Insulin-dependent diabetes. Use in non-insulin dependent diabetics may be inadvisable since thiazide diuretics may cause further impairment of glucose tolerance.
(g) Gout or hyperuricaemia.
(h) Reversible obstructive airways disease. Although cardioselective betablockers may have less effect on lung function than non-selective betablockers, as with all betablockers these should be avoided in patients with reversible obstructive airways disease unless there are compelling reasons for their use.
(i) *Pregnancy:* Secadrex should not be administered to female patients during the first trimester of pregnancy unless the physician considers it essential. Animal studies with acebutolol have shown no teratogenic hazard.

Thiazides are not generally recommended in the treatment of pregnancy hypertension; it may be preferable to use monotherapy with Sectral* or another suitable anti-hypertensive drug in pregnant patients.

Precautions:
Caution should be exercised:

(a) If Secadrex tablets are administered in the presence of bradycardia (depending on the circumstances).
(b) If Secadrex tablets are to be prescribed with a catecholamine-depleting drug, such as reserpine.
(c) In the presence of signs of heart failure, since acebutolol has a slight but acceptable cardio-depressant action.
(d) In anaesthesia: some anaesthetists prefer to discontinue therapy 48 hours before anaesthesia, others do not consider this essential. Withdrawal should be made gradually. Thiazides may increase responsiveness to tubocurarine.

If Secadrex tablets and clonidine are given concurrently, the clonidine should not be discontinued until several days after the withdrawal of the beta-blocker (see also prescribing information on clonidine).

All patients receiving hydrochlorothiazide therapy (as in Secadrex tablets) should be monitored periodically for clinical signs of fluid or electrolyte imbalance, hypokalaemia, hyponatraemia and hypochloraemic alkalosis. Hypokalaemia can sensitise or exaggerate the response of the heart to the toxic effects of digitalis (eg increased ventricular irritability).

With the low dose of hydrochlorothiazide present in Secadrex tablets the possibility of significant imbalance becomes less likely.

Side effects: No serious side-effects have been reported with Secadrex treatment. The most common, ie those related to beta-blockade – hypotension, bradycardia, gastro-intestinal effects and depression have been met with infrequently, and usually do not require interruption or withdrawal of therapy.

There have been reports of skin rashes and/or dry eyes associated with the use of beta-adrenoceptor antagonists. The reported incidence is small and in most cases the symptoms have cleared when treatment was withdrawn. Discontinuation of the drug should be considered if any such reaction is not explicable. Cessation of treatment with a beta-blocker should be gradual. Bronchospasm has occurred rarely with use of acebutolol.

Skin rashes and photosensitivity due to hydrochlorothiazide have been reported as have blood dyscrasias including thrombocytopenia but these are rare.

Drug interactions: Tricyclic antidepressants and MAO inhibitors should not be used concurrently with Secadrex tablets. Lithium should generally not be given to patients receiving diuretics since the risk of lithium toxicity is very high in such patients.

Treatment of overdosage: In the rare event of excessive bradycardia or hypotension, 1 mg atropine sulphate administered intravenously should be given without delay. If this proves insufficient, it should be followed by a slow intravenous injection of isoprenaline (5 mcg per minute) with constant monitoring until a response occurs. In cases of severe poisoning with beta-adrenoceptor antagonists the injection of 10 mg glucagon intravenously has produced rapid improvement. If bradycardia becomes severe electrical pacing may be necessary.

Pharmaceutical precautions Store in a dry place below 30°C.

Legal category POM.

Package quantities Calendar (blister) pack of 28 tablets (OP).

Further information Secadrex is an effective antihypertensive agent, which combines Sectral, a cardioselective beta-adrenoceptor antagonist with partial agonist activity and hydrochlorothiazide, an effective and acceptable diuretic/antihypertensive agent. The combination of these two medicaments in a single tablet may facilitate the management of hypertension and improve patient compliance.

Product licence number 0012/0137.

SECTRAL*

Presentation Sectral capsules each containing the equivalent of 100 mg acebutolol (in the form of the hydrochloride). The capsules are bi-coloured (opaque buff/opaque white) each half printed 'SECTRAL 100' in black.

Sectral 200 capsules each containing the equivalent of 200 mg acebutolol (in the form of the hydrochloride). The capsules are bi-coloured (opaque buff/opaque pink) each half printed 'SECTRAL 200' in black.

Sectral 400 tablets each containing the equivalent of 400 mg acebutolol (in the form of the hydrochloride). The tablets are off white and film coated with one face impressed 'Sectral 400' and the reverse side plain. The tablets also contain lactose.

Uses *Mode of action:* Sectral is a beta adrenoceptor antagonist which is cardioselective, ie acts preferentially on beta-l adrenergic receptors in the heart. Its principal effects are to reduce heart rate especially on exercise and to lower blood pressure in hypertensive subjects. Sectral and its equally active metabolite, diacetolol have anti-arrhythmic activity, the combined plasma half-life of the active drug and metabolite being 7–10 hours. Both have partial agonist activity (PAA) also known as intrinsic sympathomimetic activity (ISA). This property ensures that some degree of stimulation of beta receptors is maintained. Under conditions of rest this tends to balance the negative chronotropic and negative inotropic effects. Sectral blocks the effects of excessive catecholamine stimulation resulting from stress.

Sectral is indicated in the following conditions:

1. The management of all grades of hypertension.
2. The management of angina pectoris.
3. The control of tachyarrhythmias.

Nifedipine may be usefully combined with acebutolol for hypertension.

Dosage and administration
Elderly: There are no specific dosage recommendations for the elderly with normal glomerular filtration rate. Dosage reduction is necessary if moderate to severe renal impairment is present. Withdrawal of treatment by beta-blockers should be achieved by gradual dosage reduction. Beta-blockers may mask signs of thyrotoxicosis.

1. *Hypertension:* Initial dosage of 400 mg orally once daily at breakfast or 200 mg orally twice daily. If response is not adequate within two weeks, dosage may be increased up to 400 mg orally twice daily. If the hypertension is not adequately controlled consideration should be given to adding a second antihypertensive agent such as a compatible calcium antagonist or a small dose of a thiazide diuretic.

2. *Angina pectoris:* Initial dosage of 400 mg orally once daily at breakfast or 200 mg twice daily. In severe forms up to 300 mg three times daily may be required; up to 1,200 mg daily has been used.

3. *Cardiac arrhythmias:* Maximal anti-arrhythmic effect may not be achieved until up to 3 hours after oral administration.

The daily dose requirement for long term anti-arrhythmic activity should lie between 400 and 1200 mg daily. The dose can be gauged by response. Since the presence of more consistent beta-blockade may be necessary for the control of arrhythmias, better control may be achieved by divided doses rather than single daily doses.

Contra-indications, warnings, etc Cardiogenic shock is an absolute contra-indication and caution is required in patients with blood pressures of the order of 100/60 mm Hg or below. Sectral is also contra-indicated in patients with atrioventricular block, hypersensitivity to acebutolol or beta-blockers, marked bradycardia and uncontrolled heart failure. Although cardioselective betablockers may have less effect on lung function than non-selective agents, as with all betablockers these should be avoided in patients with reversible obstructive airways disease unless there are compelling clinical reasons for their use. (Drug-induced bronchospasm is usually at least partially reversible by the use of a suitable agonist).

Pregnancy: Sectral should not be administered to female patients during the 1st trimester of pregnancy unless the physician considers it essential. Animal studies have shown no teratogenic hazard. Beta-blockers administered in late pregnancy may give rise to bradycardia, hypotension and hypoglycaemia in the foetus/neonate.

Lactation: Acebutolol and its active metabolites are excreted in breast milk and the half life of acebutolol in the neonate is double that in adults. In view of this the use of Sectral in nursing mothers requires careful assessment of the risk to the suckling infant.

Renal impairment is not a contraindication to the use of Sectral which has both renal and non-renal excretory pathways. Some caution should be exercised when administering high doses to patients with severe renal failure as cumulation could possibly occur in these circumstances. As a guide, the dose of Sectral should be reduced by 50% and 75% when glomerular filtration rates are between 25–50 ml/min and below 25 ml/min respectively. Caution should be exercised in patients with obstructive airways disease and asthmatic subjects. Bronchospasm is usually at least partially reversible by the use of a suitable agonist.

Interactions: Sectral should not be used with verapamil or within several days of verapamil therapy (and vice-versa). In patients with labile and insulin-dependent diabetes the dosage of the hypoglycaemic agent may need to be reduced. However, beta-blockers have also been known to blunt the effect of glibenclamide. Concurrent use of digoxin and beta-blockers may occasionally induce serious bradycardia. The antihypertensive effects of beta-blockers may be attenuated by non-steroidal anti-inflammatory agents. Cross reactions due to displacement of other drugs from plasma protein binding sites are unlikely due to the low degree of plasma protein binding exhibited by acebutolol and diacetolol. If a beta-adrenoceptor antagonist is used concurrently with clonidine the latter should not be withdrawn until several days after the former is discontinued. Acebutolol is a cardioselective beta-blocker and it may antagonise the effect of sympathomimetic and xanthine bronchodilators but to a lesser extent than non-cardioselective beta-blockers.

There is a theoretical risk that concurrent administration of monoamine oxidase inhibitors and high doses of beta-blockers, even if they are cardioselective, can produce hypertension. Sectral therapy should be brought to the attention of the anaesthetist prior to general anaesthesia. If treatment is continued, special care should be taken when using anaesthetic agents such as ether, cyclopropane and trichlorethylene.

Side-effects: Sectral possesses antihypertensive effects but these are unlikely to be noted in normotensive subjects. Those common to beta-blockade, bradycardia, gastrointestinal effects, cold extremities, dizziness, headache, shortness of breath, nightmares, loss of libido and lethargy have been met with infrequently. The low lipid solubility and lack of cumulation in CNS tissues of acebutolol and its active metabolite reduces the likelihood of sleep disturbances, depression or other central effects and such occurrences are rare.

There have been reports of skin rashes and/or dry eyes associated with the use of beta adrenoceptor blocking drugs. The reported incidence is small and in most cases the symptoms have cleared when treatment was withdrawn. Discontinuation of the drug should be considered if any such reaction is not otherwise explicable. Cessation of therapy with a beta blocker should be gradual. Although some patients have developed antinuclear factor titres, the incidence of associated clinical symptoms is rare and when present these clear promptly upon discontinuation of treatment. Bronchospasm has occurred rarely with usage of acebutolol (see contra-indications).

Treatment of overdosage: Excessive bradycardia or chypotension are the main features of overdosage with Sectral and 1 mg atropine sulphate administered intravenously should be given without delay. If this is insufficient it should be followed by a slow intravenous injection of isoprenaline (5 mcg per minute) with constant monitoring until a response occurs. In severe cases of self poisoning with circulatory collapse unresponsive to atropine and catecholamines the intravenous injection of glucagon 10–20 mg may produce a dramatic improvement. Cardiac pacing may be employed if bradycardia becomes severe. Judicious use of vasopressors, diazepam, phenytoin, lidocaine, digoxin and bronchodilators should be considered depending on the presentation of the patient. Acebutolol can be removed from the blood by haemodialysis. Other symptoms and signs of overdosage include cardiogenic shock, AV block, conduction defects, pulmonary oedema, depressed level of consciousness, bronchospasm, hypoglycaemia and rarely hyperkalaemia.

Pharmaceutical precautions Sectral capsules should be stored in a dry place below 25°C. Protect from light.

Legal category POM.

Package quantities *Capsules 100 mg:* containers of 84 (OP).
Capsules 200 mg ('Sectral 200'): containers of 56 (OP).
Tablets 400 mg ('Sectral 400'): foil pack of 28 (2 × 14) (OP).

Further information Sectral 400 tablets are available as a calendar pack containing 28 tablets for ease of use in once daily therapy for hypertension.

Product licence numbers

100 mg Capsules	0012/0100
200 mg Capsules ('Sectral 200')	0012/0101
400 mg Tablets ('Sectral 400')	0012/0124

SONERYL*

Presentation Pink tablets each containing 100 mg butobarbitone, with the name 'Soneryl' indented on one face and a break line on the reverse.

Uses Soneryl is a barbiturate with a medium duration of action. It is a powerful hypnotic and is indicated for severe, intractable insomnia. Sleep is usually induced within 30–40 minutes and lasts for six to ten hours.

Dosage and administration One or two tablets at bedtime; may be increased to 3 or 4 in obstinate cases. These doses may be modified at the physician's discretion, but it is advisable not to exceed 6 tablets in 24 hours.

Elderly: Do not use.

Children: Do not use.

Contra-indications, warnings, etc
Contra-indications: Porphyria is an absolute contra-indication to the use of Soneryl. Patients with uncontrolled pain, or those with a history of alcohol or drug abuse should not be given Soneryl.

Soneryl should not be used in children, young adults, the elderly and the debilitated.

Pregnancy. Soneryl should not be administered during pregnancy or breast feeding.

Precautions: Reduced dosage should be used in patients with renal or hepatic failure.

Drug interactions: Barbiturates cause the induction of liver enzymes and this may affect the availability and blood concentrations of drugs given concurrently that are metabolised in the liver. These include the following: coumarin-type anticoagulants, synthetic steroids (including oral contraceptives), phenytoin, griseofulvin, rifampicin, phenothiazines such as chlorpromazine and tricyclic antidepressants.

Warnings and adverse effects: Drowsiness, sedation. Unsteadiness, vertigo and inco-ordination are common adverse effects.

Performance and alertness may be impaired during the first week of administration. Patients should be warned of the possible hazard when driving or operating machinery.

These effects may be potentiated by alcohol. Other adverse reactions may include a 'hangover' effect, paradoxical excitement, confusion, memory defects and skin rashes in patients who may be sensitive to this type of drug.

Treatment of overdosage: Soneryl overdosage should be treated by gastric lavage, artificial respiration with the administration of oxygen, maintenance of fluid balance and with an antibiotic to prevent pneumonia. Metaraminol may be used to treat hypotension, but if this is unsuccessful, blood volume expanders or intravenous hydrocortisone should be given.

Pharmaceutical precautions Nil.

Legal category CD (Sch 3), POM.

Package quantities Containers of 56 tablets (OP).

Further information Barbiturates have a high addiction potential. Long-term use or use of high dosage for short periods may lead to tolerance and subsequently to physical and psychological dependence. Symptoms of dependence include confusion, defective judgement and loss of emotional control. Withdrawal symptoms occur after long-term normal use (and particularly after abuse) on rapid cessation of barbiturate treatment. Symptoms include nightmares, irritability and insomnia and in severe cases, tremors, delirium, convulsions and death. Withdrawal symptoms have been reported in neonates after barbiturate treatment during pregnancy and labour.

Product licence number 0012/5262.

STEMETIL*

Presentation Stemetil tablets are off-white to cream uncoated tablets containing 5 mg or 25 mg prochlorperazine maleate. The 5 mg tablets are impressed Stemetil 5 on one face, reverse plain.

The 25 mg tablets are impressed Stemetil 25 on one face, with a breakline on the reverse. Both the 5 mg and 25 mg tablets contain lactose.

Stemetil 1.25% Injection – colourless solution containing 12.5 mg prochlorperazine mesylate per ml in ampoules of 1 ml and 2 ml. The injection solution also contains sodium sulphite, sodium metabisulphite, sodium chloride and ethanolamine.

Stemetil Suppositories – cream-coloured suppositories containing base equivalents to 5 mg and 25 mg of maleate.

Stemetil Syrup – a dark straw-coloured syrupy liquid which contains 5 mg prochlorperazine mesylate in each 5 ml. The syrup contains 68% w/v of sugars, sodium sulphite, sodium metabisulphite and sodium benzoate.

Uses Stemetil is a potent phenothiazine neuroleptic. It is used in vertigo due to Meniere's syndrome, labyrinthitis and other causes, and for nausea and vomiting from whatever cause including that associated with migraine. It may also be used for schizophrenia (particularly in the chronic stage), acute mania and as an adjunct to the short term management of anxiety.

There is little information about blood levels, distribution and excretion in humans. The rate of metabolism and excretion of phenothiazines decreases in old age.

Dosage and administration

Oral Administration
Adults

Indication	*Dosage*
Prevention of nausea and vomiting.	5 to 10 mg b.d. or t.d.s.
Treatment of nausea and vomiting.	20 mg stat, followed if necessary by 10 mg two hours later.
Vertigo and Meniere's syndrome.	5 mg t.d.s. increasing if necessary to a total of 30 mg daily. After several weeks dosage may be reduced gradually to 5–10 mg daily.
Adjunct in the short-term management of anxiety.	15–20 mg daily in divided doses initially but this may be increased if necessary to a maximum of 40 mg daily in divided doses.
Schizophrenia and other psychotic disorders.	Usual effective daily oral dosage is in the order of 75–100 mg daily. Patients vary widely in response. The following schedule is suggested: Initially 12.5 mg twice daily for 7 days, the daily amount being subsequently increased by 12.5 mg at four to seven day intervals until a satisfactory response is obtained. After some weeks at the effective dosage, an attempt should be made to reduce this dosage. Total daily amounts as small as 50 mg or even 25 mg have sometimes been found to be effective.

Intramuscular Administration
Adults

Indication	*Dosage*
Treatment of nausea and vomiting.	12.5 mg by deep i.m. injection followed by oral medication six hours later, if necessary.
Schizophrenia and other psychotic disorders.	12.5 mg to 25 mg two or three times a day by deep i.m. injection until oral treatment becomes possible.

Rectal Administration
Adults

Indication	*Dosage*
Treatment of nausea and vomiting.	25 mg followed by oral medication 6 hours later if necessary.
Schizophrenia and psychotic disorders.	25 mg b.d. or t.d.s. until oral treatment possible.
Nausea and vomiting due to migraine	5 mg t.d.s. In acute cases treatment may be initiated by intramuscular injection.
Prevention of post-operative vomiting	10 mg before the operation then 10 mg every two hours for up to 20 hours thereafter.

Children's Dosage. Oral route only	
Indication	*Dosage*
Prevention and treatment of nausea and vomiting	If it is considered unavoidable to use Stemetil for a child, the dosage is 250 micrograms/kg bodyweight two or three times a day. Stemetil has been associated with dystonic reactions particularly after a cumulative dosage of 500 micrograms/kg. It should therefore be used cautiously in children. Stemetil is not recommended for children weighing less than 10 kg.

When treating children, it is recommended that the syrup or 5 mg tablets are used.

Stemetil should not be given to children by the rectal or intramuscular route.

Elderly: A lower initial dosage is recommended. Please see precautions.

Contra-indications, warnings, etc

Pregnancy: Stemetil is contra-indicated in pregnancy. There is inadequate evidence of the safety of Stemetil in human pregnancy but it has been widely used for many years without apparent ill consequence. There is evidence of harmful effects in animals. Like other drugs it should be avoided in pregnancy unless the physician considers it essential. Neuroleptics may occasionally prolong labour and at such a time should be withheld until the cervix is dilated 3–4 cm. Possible adverse effects on the neonate include lethargy or paradoxical hyper-excitability, tremor and low Apgar score. Phenothiazines may be excreted in milk, breastfeeding should be suspended during treatment.

Precautions: Stemetil should be avoided in patients with liver or renal dysfunction, epilepsy, Parkinson's disease, hypothyroidism, phaeochromocytoma, myasthenia gravis, prostate hypertrophy. It should be avoided in patients known to be hypersensitive to phenothiazines or with a history of narrow angle glaucoma. It should be used with caution in the elderly, particularly during very hot or very cold weather (risk of hyper-, hypothermia).

Patients should be warned about drowsiness during the early days of treatment, and advised not to drive or operate machinery.

Postural hypotension with tachycardia as well as local pain or nodule formation may occur after i.m. administration.

The elderly are particularly susceptible to postural hypotension. Stemetil should be used cautiously in the elderly owing to their susceptibility to drugs acting centrally on the nervous system. There is an increased risk of drug-induced Parkinsonism in the elderly particularly after prolonged use. Care should also be taken not to confuse the adverse effects of Stemetil e.g. orthostatic hypotension with effects due to the underlying disorder.

Interactions of phenothiazine neuroleptics: The CNS depressant actions of neuroleptic agents may be intensified (additively) by alcohol, barbiturates and other sedatives. Respiratory depression may occur.

The hypotensive effect of most antihypertensive drugs especially alpha adrenoceptor blocking agents may be exaggerated by neuroleptics.

The mild anticholinergic effect of neuroleptics may be enhanced by other anticholinergic drugs possibly leading to constipation, heat stroke, etc.

The action of some drugs may be opposed by phenothiazine neuroleptics; these include amphetamine, levodopa, clonidine, guanethidine, adrenaline.

Anticholinergic agents may reduce the antipsychotic effect of neuroleptics.

Some drugs interfere with absorption of neuroleptic agents: antacids, anti-parkinson, lithium. Increases or decreases in the plasma concentrations of a number of drugs, e.g. propranolol, phenobarbitone have been observed but were not of clinical significance.

High doses of neuroleptics reduce the response to hypoglycaemic agents the dosage of which might have to be raised.

Adrenaline must *not* be used in patients overdosed with Stemetil. Most of the above interactions are of a theoretical nature and not dangerous.

Simultaneous administration of desferrioxamine and prochlorperazine has been observed to induce a transient metabolic encephalopathy characterised by loss of consciousness for 48–72 hours.

Minor side effects of neuroleptics are nasal stuffiness, dry mouth, insomina, agitation.

Adverse effects of neuroleptics: Liver function: Jaundice, usually transient, occurs in a very small percentage of patients taking neuroleptics. A premonitory sign may be a sudden onset of fever after one to three weeks of treatment followed by the development of jaundice. Neuroleptic jaundice has the biochemical and other characteristics of obstructive jaundice and is associated with obstructions of the canaliculi by bile thrombi; the frequent presence of an accompanying eosinophilia indicates the allergic nature of this phenomenon. Treatment should be withheld on the development of jaundice.

Cardiorespiratory: Hypotension, usually postural, commonly occurs. Elderly or volume depleted subjects are particularly susceptible; it is more likely to occur after intramuscular administration.

Cardiac arrhythmias, including atrial arrhythmia, A-V block, ventricular tachycardia and fibrillation have been reported during neuroleptic therapy, possibly related to dosage. Pre-existing cardiac disease, old age, hypokalemia and concurrent tricyclic antidepressants may predispose. ECG changes, usually benign, include widened QT interval, ST depression, U-waves and T-wave changes.

Respiratory depression is possible in susceptible patients.

Blood picture: A mild leukopenia occurs in up to 30% of patients on prolonged high dosage. Agranulocytosis may occur rarely; it is not dose related. The occurrence of unexplained infections or fever requires immediate haematological investigation.

Extrapyramidal: Acute dystonias or dyskinesias, usually transitory are more common in children and young adults, and usually occur within the first 4 days of treatment or after dosage increases.

Akathisia characteristically occurs after large initial doses.

Parkinsonism is more common in adults and the elderly. It usually develops after weeks or months of treatment. One or more of the following may be seen: tremor, rigidity, akinesia or other features of Parkinsonism. Commonly just tremor.

Tardive dyskinesia: If this occurs it is usually, but not necessarily, after prolonged or high dosage. It can even occur after treatment has been stopped. Dosage should therefore be kept low whenever possible.

Skin and eyes: Contact skin sensitisation is a serious but rare complication in those frequently handling preparations of certain phenothiazines; the greatest care must be taken to avoid contact of the drug with the skin. Skin rashes of various kinds may also be seen in patients treated with the drug. Patients on high dosage should be warned that they may develop photosensitivity in sunny weather and should avoid exposure to direct sunlight.

Ocular changes and the development of a metallic greyish-mauve coloration of exposed skin have been noted in some individuals mainly females, who have received chlorpromazine continuously for long periods (four to eight years). This could possibly happen with Stemetil.

Endocrine: hyperprolactinaemia which may result in galactorrhoea, gynaecomastia, amenorrhoea; impotence.

Neuroleptic malignant syndrome (hyperthermia, rigidity, autonomic dysfunction and altered consciousness) may occur with any neuroleptic.

Toxicity and treatment of overdosage; Symptoms of phenothiazine overdosage include drowsiness or loss of consciousness, hypotension, tachycardia, E.C.G. changes, ventricular arrhythmias and hypothermia. Severe extra-pyramidal dyskinesias may occur.

If the patient is seen sufficiently soon (up to 6 hours) after ingestion of a toxic dose, gastric lavage may be attempted. Pharmacological induction of emesis is unlikely to be of any use. Activated charcoal should be given. There is no specific antidote. Treatment is supportive.

Generalised vasodilatation may result in circulatory collapse; raising the patient's legs may suffice. In severe cases, volume expansion by intravenous fluids may be needed; infusion fluids should be warmed before administration in order not to aggravate hypothermia.

Positive inotropic agents such as dopamine may be tried if fluid replacement is insufficient to correct the circulatory collapse. Peripheral vasoconstrictor agents are not generally recommended; avoid the use of adrenaline.

Ventricular or supraventricular tachy-arrhythmias usually respond to restoration of normal body temperature and correction of circulatory or metabolic disturbances. If persistent or life threatening, appropriate anti-arrhythmic therapy may be considered. Avoid lignocaine and, as far as possible, long acting anti-arrhythmic drugs.

Pronounced central nervous system depression requires airway maintenance or, in extreme circumstances, assisted respiration. Severe dystonic reactions usually respond to procyclidine (5–10 mg) or orphenadrine (20–40 mg) administered intramuscularly or intravenously. Convulsions should be treated with intravenous diazepam.

Neuroleptic malignant syndrome should be treated with cooling. Dantrolene sodium may be tried.

Pharmaceutical precautions Protect from light. Stemetil injection solution rapidly discolours on exposure to light; any such solution should be discarded. Stemetil suppositories, should be stored in a cool, dark place.

Legal category POM.

Package quantities Tablets 5 mg in containers of 84 (OP).

Tablets 25 mg in containers of 56 (OP).

Injection solution of 1.25% in boxes of 10 × 1 ml and 10 × 2 ml.

Syrup presentation of 5 mg per 5 ml in bottles of 100 ml (OP).

Suppositories of 5 mg and 25 mg in boxes of 10.

Further information Nil.

Product licence numbers

Tablets 5 mg	0012/5263
Tablets 25 mg	0012/5316
Injection	0012/5008
Suppositories 5 mg	0012/5117
Suppositories 25 mg	0012/5013
Syrup	0012/5022

STEMETIL Eff*

Presentation Sachets, each containing 5 mg prochlorperazine mesylate incorporated in a white granular powder which dissolves in water to produce a lemon flavoured effervescent solution. The granules are sweetened with aspartame.

Uses Stemetil is a potent phenothiazine neuroleptic. It is used in vertigo due to Meniere's syndrome, labyrinthitis and other causes, and for nausea and vomiting from whatever cause including that associated with migraine. It may also be used as an adjunct to the short term management of anxiety.

Kinetics: There is little information about blood levels, distribution and excretion of humans. The rate of metabolism and excretion of phenothiazines decreases in old age.

Dosage and administration The contents of one or two sachets of Stemetil Eff should be dissolved in about 50 ml cold water and taken once the effervescence has subsided.

Adults

Indication	*Dosage*
Prevention of nausea and vomiting	5 to 10 mg b.d. or t.d.s.
Vertigo and Meniere's syndrome	5 mg t.d.s increasing if necessary to a total of 30 mg daily. After several weeks dosage may be reduced gradually to 5–10 mg daily.
Adjunct in the short-term management of anxiety	15–20 mg daily in divided doses initially but this may be increased if necessary to maximum of 40 mg daily in divided doses.

Children: Not recommended.

Elderly: A lower initial dose is recommended. Please see precautions.

Contra-indications, warnings, etc

Pregnancy and lactation: There is inadequate evidence of the safety of Stemetil in human pregnancy but it has been widely used for many years without apparent ill consequence. There is evidence of harmful effects in animals. Like other drugs it should be avoided in pregnancy unless the physician considers it essential. Neuroleptics may occasionally prolong labour and at such a time should be withheld until the cervix is dilated 3–4 cm. Possible adverse effects on the neonate include lethargy or paradoxical hyperexcitability, tremor and low Apgar score. Phenothiazines may be excreted in milk, breastfeeding should be suspended during treatment.

Precautions: Stemetil should be avoided in patients with liver or renal dysfunction, epilepsy, Parkinson's disease, hypothyroidism, phaeochromocytoma, myasthenia gravis, prostate hypertrophy. It should be avoided in patients known to be hypersensitive to phenothiazines or with a history of narrow angle glaucoma. It should be used with caution in the elderly, particularly during very hot or very cold weather (risk of hyper-, hypothermia).

Patients should be warned about drowsiness during the early days of treatment, and advised not to drive or operate machinery.

Due to its aspartame content, Stemetil Eff should not be given to patients with phenylketonuria.

The elderly are particularly susceptible to postural hypotension. Stemetil should be used cautiously in the elderly owing to their susceptibility to drugs acting centrally on the nervous system and a lower initial dosage is recommended. There is an increased risk of drug-induced Parkinsonism in the elderly particularly after prolonged use. Care should also be taken not to confuse the adverse effects of Stemetil e.g. orthostatic hypotension with effects due to the underlying disorder.

Interactions of phenothiazine neuroleptics: The CNS depressant actions of neuroleptic agents may be intensified (additively) by alcohol, barbiturates and other sedatives. Respiratory depression may occur.

The hypotensive effect of most antihypertensive drugs especially alpha adrenoceptor blocking agents may be exaggerated by neuroleptics.

The mild anticholinergic effect of neuroleptics may be enhanced by other anticholinergic drugs possibly leading to constipation, heat stroke, etc.

The action of some drugs may be opposed by phenothiazine neuroleptics; these include amphetamine, levodopa, clonidine, guanethidine, adrenaline.

Anticholinergic agents may reduce the antipsychotic effect of neuroleptics.

Some drugs interfere with absorption of neuroleptic agents: antacids, anti-Parkinson, lithium. Increases or decreases in the plasma concentrations of a number of drugs, e.g. propranolol, phenobarbitone have been observed but were not of clinical significance.

High doses of neuroleptics reduce the response to hypoglycaemic agents the dosage of which might have to be raised.

Adrenaline must *not* be used in patients overdosed

with Stemetil. Most of the above interactions are of a theoretical nature and not dangerous.

Simultaneous administration of desferrioxamine and prochlorperazine has been observed to induce a transient metabolic encephalopathy characterised by loss of consciousness for 48–72 hours.

Minor side-effects of neuroleptics are nasal stuffiness, dry mouth, insomnia, agitation.

Adverse effects of neuroleptics:

Liver function: Jaundice, usually transient, occurs in a very small percentage of patients taking neuroleptics. A premonitory sign may be a sudden onset of fever after one to three weeks of treatment followed by the development of jaundice. Neuroleptic jaundice has the biochemical and other characteristics of obstructive jaundice and is associated with obstruction of the canaliculi by bile thrombi; the frequent presence of an accompanying eosinophilia indicates the allergic nature of this phenomenon. Treatment should be withheld on the development of jaundice.

Cardiorespiratory: Hypotension, usually postural, commonly occurs. Elderly or volume depleted subjects are particularly susceptible.

Cardiac arrhythmias, including atrial arrhythmia, A-V block, ventricular tachycardia and fibrillation have been reported during neuroleptic therapy, possibly related to dosage. Pre-existing cardiac disease, old age, hypokalaemia and concurrent tricyclic antidepressants may predispose. ECG changes, usually benign, include widened QT interval, ST depression, U-waves and T-wave changes.

Respiratory depression is possible in susceptible patients.

Blood picture: A mild leukopaenia occurs in up to 30% of patients on prolonged high dosage. Agranulocytosis may occur rarely; it is not dose related. The occurrence of unexplained infections or fever requires immediate haematological investigation.

Extrapyramidal: Acute dystonias or dyskinesias, usually transitory, are more common in children and young adults, and usually occur within the first 4 days of treatment or after dosage increases.

Akathisia characteristically occurs after large initial doses.

Parkinsonism is more common in adults and the elderly. It usually develops after weeks or months of treatment. One or more of the following may be seen: tremor, rigidity, akinesia or other features of Parkinsonism. Commonly just tremor.

Tardive dyskinesia: If this occurs it is usually, but not necessarily, after prolonged or high dosage. It can even occur after treatment has been stopped. Dosage should therefore be kept low whenever possible.

Skin and eyes: Contact skin sensitisation is a serious but rare complication in those frequently handling preparations of certain phenothiazines; the greatest care must be taken to avoid contact of the drug with the skin. Skin rashes of various kinds may also be seen in patients treated with the drug. Patients on high dosage should be warned that they may develop photosensitivity in sunny weather and should avoid exposure to direct sunlight.

Ocular changes and the development of a metallic greyish-mauve coloration of exposed skin have been noted in some individuals mainly females, who have received chlorpromazine continuously for long periods (four to eight years). This could possibly happen with Stemetil.

Endocrine: hyperprolactinaemia which may result in galactorrhoea, gynaecomastia, amenorrhoea; impotence.

Neuroleptic malignant syndrome (hyperthermia, rigidity, autonomic dysfunction and altered consciousness) may occur with any neuroleptic.

Toxicity and treatment of overdosage: Symptoms of phenothiazine overdosage include drowsiness or loss of consciousness, hypotension, tachycardia, E.C.G. changes, ventricular arrhythmias and hypothermia. Severe extra-pyramidal dyskinesias may occur.

If the patient is seen sufficiently soon (up to 6 hours) after ingestion of a toxic dose, gastric lavage may be attempted. Pharmacological induction of emesis is unlikely to be of any use. Activated charcoal should be given. There is no specific antidote. Treatment is supportive.

Generalised vasodilatation may result in circulatory collapse; raising the patient's legs may suffice. In severe cases, volume expansion by intravenous fluids may be needed; infusion fluids should be warmed before administration in order not to aggravate hypothermia.

Positive inotropic agents such as dopamine may be tried if fluid replacement is insufficient to correct the circulatory collapse. Peripheral vasoconstrictor agents are not generally recommended; avoid the use of adrenaline.

Ventricular or supraventricular tachy-arrhythmias usually respond to restoration of normal body temperature and correction of circulatory or metabolic disturbances. If persistent or life threatening, appropriate anti-arrhythmic therapy may be considered. Avoid lignocaine and, as far as possible, long acting anti-arrhythmic drugs.

Pronounced central nervous system depression requires airway maintenance or, in extreme circumstances, assisted respiration. Severe dystonic reactions usually respond to procyclidine (5–10 mg) or orphenadrine (20–40 mg) administered intramuscularly or intravenously. Convulsions should be treated with intravenous diazepam.

Neuroleptic malignant syndrome should be treated with cooling. Dantrolene sodium may be tried.

Pharmaceutical precautions Store in a cool place.

Legal category POM.

Package quantities 5 mg sachets in boxes of 21 (OP).

Further information Nil.

Product licence number 0012/0177.

SULPHADIAZINE INJECTION

Presentation A colourless solution containing sulphadiazine sodium 27.2% w/v. Each 4 ml ampoule contains the equivalent of 1 g sulphadiazine. The injection solution also contains sodium thiosulphate.

Uses Sulphadiazine has a bacteriostatic action on a wide range of Gram-negative and Gram-positive micro-organisms including *Neisseria meningitidis*, pneumococcus, B-haemolytic streptococcus, *Haemophilus influenzae*, nocardia and other sulphonamide sensitive organisms.

Sulphadiazine injection is indicated for the treatment of infections due to sulphonamide sensitive organisms.

Dosage and administration Sulphadiazine injection should preferably be administered intravenously. Because of the alkalinity of the solution, it should be diluted to a strength not exceeding 5% sulphadiazine with Water for Injections, or added to an appropriate volume of saline for infusion. The undiluted solution may be administered by deep intramuscular injection if the intravenous route is not available.

Adults: Initially 2–3 g followed by 1 g four times a day for the first two days of the infection. Subsequent treatment should be given by mouth continuing for 2–3 days after clinical recovery.

Elderly: There are no specific dosage recommendations for the elderly but since sulphadiazine is contraindicated in the presence of mild renal failure, caution is advised in this age group.

Children: Over 2 months: 50 mg/kg initially followed by 25 mg/kg four times a day.

Sulphadiazine injection should be administered four times a day during the first two days of the infection after which the drug should be given orally.

Contra-indications, warnings, etc

Contra-indications: In the presence of renal or hepatic disease, in acute porphyria and in patients known to be hypersensitive to sulphonamides. In premature and newborn babies owing to the danger of kernicterus.

Sulphadiazine injection must never be given intrathecally or subcutaneously, as its high alkalinity can cause necrosis.

Precautions: A high fluid intake (5–6 pints in 24 hours) should be maintained and urinary output should be not less than half that amount. In addition the urine should be rendered alkaline.

Use in pregnancy and lactation: There is epidemiological evidence of the safety of sulphadiazine in human pregnancy, but the clinician should assess the risk benefit factors before administering sulphadiazine injection to pregnant women. There is evidence of embryotoxicity and teratogenicity in animals at high dosage, especially during the first trimester. It is generally considered that sulphonamides should not be given in late pregnancy because of the risk of kernicterus in the newborn. However recent work suggests that sulphadiazine may be used in late pregnancy with no ill effect on the newborn. Sulphonamides are excreted in the milk in small amounts and should be used with exteme caution in nursing mothers.

Drug interactions: Sulphonamides potentiate the effects of anticoagulants, thiazide diuretics, methotrexate, phenytoin, chlorpropamide, tolbutamide and some uricosuric agents. Sulphonamides are displaced by indomethacin, salicylates and probenecid. The above interactions are of a theoretical nature and are unlikely to be clinically significant. The antibacterial activity of sulphonamides may be antagonised by local anaesthetics or para-amino benzoic acid. Sulphonamides are physically incompatible with chloramphenicol, aminoglycosides, tetracycline, synthetic penicillins, noradrenaline and insulin.

Side-effects: Those common to all sulphonamides may occur, including nausea, vomiting, diarrhoea, cyanosis, headache, depression and mental confusion. Haemolytic anaemia has been reported, especially in patients with glucose-6-phosphate dehydrogenase deficiency. Other blood dyscrasias include agranulocytosis, aplastic anaemia, leukopenia and thrombocytopenia. Hypersensitivity reactions such as erythema nodosum and drug rashes rarely occur. Other uncommon adverse effects include vasculitis-like polyarteritis nodosa, Stevens-Johnson syndrome and anaphylaxis.

Other side-effects include hepatitis, jaundice, hepatic necrosis, interstitial nephritis, tubular necrosis, necrotizing angiitis with hypersensitivity and crystalluria. If crystalluria followed by haematuria or oliguria occurs, sulphadiazine should be discontinued and large volumes of fluids administered (by intravenous infusion if necessary) followed by effective alkalinisation of the urine with intravenous sodium bicarbonate.

Treatment of overdosage: Continuous forced fluids may be necessary and the urine should be rendered alkaline. Otherwise treatment is symptomatic.

Pharmaceutical precautions Protect from light. Store below 25°C but do not freeze. Sulphadiazine injection is incompatible with acids, laevulose, iron salts and salts of heavy metals.

Legal category POM.

Package quantities Box of 10 × 4 ml ampoules.

Further information Nil.

Product licence number 0012/5057

VALLERGAN*

Presentation *Tablets:* Dark blue, film-coated, one face impressed $^{V}_{10}$, the reverse face plain, each containing 10 mg trimeprazine tartrate. Vallergan tablets contain lactose.

Syrup: A clear bright straw-coloured apricot-flavoured syrupy liquid containing 7.5 mg trimeprazine tartrate in each 5 ml. It contains 68% w/v sugars, ethanol, sodium sulphite, sodium metabisulphite and sodium benzoate.

Forte syrup: A clear colourless/pale yellow apricot-flavoured syrupy liquid containing 30 mg trimeprazine tartrate in each 5 ml. It contains 68% w/v of sugars, ethanol, sodium sulphite, sodium metabisulphite and sodium benzoate.

Uses Trimeprazine has a central sedative effect comparable to that of chlorpromazine, but largely devoid of the latter's anti-adrenaline action. It has powerful antihistamine and anti-emetic actions.

Vallergan is used in:

- Urticaria and pruritus.
- premedication for anaesthesia.

Kinetics: There is little information about blood levels, distribution and excretion in humans. The rate of metabolism and excretion of phenothiazines decreases in old age.

Dosage and administration Not recommended for infants less than 2 years old.

Urticaria and pruritus

Adults: 10 mg two or three times daily; up to 100 mg per day have been used in intractable cases.

Elderly: Dosage should be reduced to 10 mg once or twice daily.

Children: 2.5–5 mg three or four times daily.

Pre-anaesthetic medication (children aged 2–7 years): The maximum dosage of Vallergan or Vallergan Forte syrup recommended for this indication is 2 mg per kg bodyweight.

Contra-indications, warnings, etc *Use in pregnancy and lactation:* There is inadequate evidence of the safety of Vallergan in human pregnancy, but it has been widely used for many years without apparent ill consequence. Some phenothiazines have shown evidence of harmful effects in animals. Vallergan, like other drugs, should be avoided in pregnancy unless the physician considers it essential. Neuroleptics may occasionally prolong labour and at such a time should be withheld until the cervix is dilated 3–4 cm. Possible adverse effects on the neonate include lethargy or paradoxical hyperexcitability, tremor and low Apgar score. Phenothiazines may be excreted in milk; breast feeding should be suspended during treatment.

Contra-indications: Vallergan should be avoided in patients with hepatic or renal dysfunction, epilepsy, Parkinson's disease, hypothyroidism, phaeochromocytoma, myasthenia gravis, prostatic hypertrophy. It should be avoided in patients known to be hypersensitive to phenothiazines or with history of narrow angle glaucoma.

Precautions: It should be used with caution in the elderly, particularly during very hot or very cold weather (risk of hyper-hypothermia). Patients should be warned about drowsiness during the early days of treatment, and advised not to drive or operate machinery. The elderly are particularly susceptible to postural hypotension.

Interactions of phenothiazines: The CNS depressant actions of these agents may be intensified (additively) by alcohol, barbiturates and other sedatives. Respiratory depression may occur.

The hypotensive effect of most antihypertensive drugs especially alpha adrenoreceptor blocking agents may be exaggerated by phenothiazines.

The mild anticholinergic effect of phenothiazines may be enhanced by other anticholinergic drugs possibly leading to constipation, heat stroke, etc.

The action of some drugs may be opposed by phenothiazines; these include amphetamine. laevodopa clonidine, guanethidine, adrenaline.

Anticholinergic agents may reduce the antipsychotic effect of phenothiazines.

Some drugs interfere with absorption of phenothiazines: antacids, anti-Parkinson, lithium. Increases or decreases in the plasma concentrations of a number of drugs, e.g. propranolol, phenobarbitone have been observed but were not of clinical significance.

High doses of phenothiazines reduce the response to hypoglycaemic agents, the dosage of which might have to be raised. Adrenaline must not be used in patients overdosed with phenothiazines. Most of the above interactions are of a theoretical nature and not dangerous.

Adverse effects: Minor side-effects of phenothiazines are nasal stuffiness, dry mouth, insomnia, agitation.

Liver function: Jaundice, usually transient, occurs in a very small percentage of patients taking phenothiazines. A premonitory sign may be a sudden onset of fever after one to three weeks of treatment followed by the development of jaundice. Neuroleptic jaundice has the biochemical and other characteristics of obstructive jaundice and is associated with obstructions of the canaliculi by bile thrombi; the frequent presence of an accompanying eosinophilia indicates the allergic nature of this phenomenon. Treatment should be withheld on the development of jaundice.

Cardiorespiratory: Hypotension, or pallor may occur in children. Elderly or volume depleted subjects are particularly susceptible to postural hypotension.

Cardiac arrhythmias, including atrial arrhythmia, A-V block, ventricular tachycardia and fibrillation have been reported during phenothiazine therapy, possibly related to dosage. Pre-existing cardiac disease, old age, hypokalaemia and concurrent tricyclic antidepressants may predispose. ECG changes, usually benign, include widened QT interval, ST depression, U-waves and T-wave changes.

Respiratory depression is possible in susceptible patients.

Blood picture: A mild leukopaenia occurs in up to 30% of patients on prolonged high dosage of phenothiazines. Agranulocytosis may occur rarely; it is not dose related. The occurrence of unexplained infections or fever requires immediate haematological investigation.

Extrapyramidal: Acute dystonias or dyskinesias, usually transitory are more common in children and young adults, and usually occur within the first 4 days of treatment or after dosage increases.

- Akathisia characteristically occurs after large doses.
- Parkinsonism is more common in adults and the elderly. It usually develops after weeks or months of treatment. One or more of the following may be seen: tremor, rigidity, akinesia or other features of Parkinsonism. Commonly just tremor.
- Tardive dyskinesia: If this occurs it is usually, but not necessarily, after prolonged or high dosage. It can even occur after treatment has been stopped. Dosage should therefore be kept low whenever possible.

Skin and eyes: Contact skin sensitisation is a serious but rare complication in those frequently handling preparations of certain phenothiazines; care must be taken to avoid contact of the drug with the skin. Skin rashes of various kinds may also be seen in patients treated with the drug. Patients on high dosage should be warned that they may develop photosensitivity in sunny weather and should avoid exposure to direct sunlight. Ocular changes and the development of a metallic greyish-mauve coloration of exposed skin have been noted in some individuals mainly females, who have received chlorpromazine continuously for long periods (four to eight years).

Endocrine: Hyperprolactinaemia which may result in galactorrhoea, gynaecomastia, amenorrhoea; impotence.

Neuroleptic malignant syndrome (hyperthermia, rigidity, autonomic dysfunction and altered consciousness) may occur with any phenothiazine.

Toxicity and treatment of overdosage: Symptoms of phenothiazine overdosage include drowsiness or loss of consciousness, hypotension, tachycardia, E.C.G. changes, ventricular arrhythmias and hypothermia. Severe extra-pyramidal dyskinesias may occur.

If the patient is seen sufficiently soon (up to 6 hours) after ingestion of a toxic dose, gastric lavage may be attempted. Pharmacological induction of emesis is unlikely to be of any use. Activated charcoal should be given. There is no specific antidote. Treatment is supportive.

Generalised vasodilation may result in circulatory collapse; raising the patient's legs may suffice, in severe cases, volume expansion by intravenous fluids may be needed; infusion fluids should be warmed before administration in order not to aggravate hypothermia.

Positive inotropic agents such as dopamine may be tried if fluid replacement is insufficient to correct the circulatory collapse. Peripheral vasoconstrictor agents are not generally recommended; avoid the use of adrenaline.

Ventricular or supraventricular tachy-arrhythmias usually respond to restoration of normal body temperature and correction of circulatory or metabolic disturbances. If persistent or life threatening, appropriate anti-arrhythmic therapy may be considered. Avoid lignocaine and, as far as possible, long acting anti-arrhythmic drugs.

Pronounced central nervous system depression requires airway maintenance or, in extreme circumstances, assisted respiration. Severe dystonic reactions usually respond to procyclidine (5–10 mg) or orphenadrine (20–40 mg) administered intramuscularly or intravenously. Convulsions should be treated with intravenous diazepam.

Neuroleptic malignant syndrome should be treated with cooling. Dantrolene sodium may be tried.

Pharmaceutical precautions Protect from light. Store below 25°C. Vallergan Syrup and Vallergan Forte Syrup may be diluted if required, using simple syrup (without preservative).

Legal category POM.

Package quantities Tablets: Containers of 28 (OP).
Syrup: Bottles of 100 ml (OP).
Forte syrup: Bottles of 100 ml (OP).

Further information Nil.

Product licence numbers

Tablets	0012/5303
Syrup	0012/5019
Forte syrup	0012/5018.

ZIMOVANE*▼

Presentation White, or almost white, film-coated, elliptical tablets indented 'ZM' with a break line on one face and with the other face plain. Each tablet contains 7.5 mg zopiclone. The tablets also contain lactose.

Uses

Pharmacology: Zopiclone is a non-benzodiazepine hypnotic agent, a member of the cyclopyrrolone group of compounds which is structurally unrelated to existing hypnotics and tranquillisers. It has a high affinity for CNS binding sites of the GABA macromolecular receptor complex, inducing conformational changes which differ from those of established hypnotics. Thus zopiclone rapidly initiates sleep, without reduction of total REM sleep, and then sustains it with preservation of normal slow wave sleep. Zopiclone has a short elimination half life, typically 3.5 to 6 hours, with no significant accumulation of drug substance or metabolites on repeated dosage.

Indications: Zimovane tablets are indicated for the short term treatment of insomnia, including difficulties in falling asleep, nocturnal awakening and early awakening, transient, situational or chronic insomnia, and insomnia secondary to psychiatric disturbances, in situations where the insomnia is debilitating or is causing severe distress for the patient.

Experience with other hypnotics indicates that the risk of dependence increased with higher doses and longer term use and is further increased in patients with a history of alcoholism or drug abuse and in patients with marked personality disorders. Thus, as with all hypnotics, long term continuous treatment is not recommended and a course of treatment should be no longer than 4 weeks in duration.

Dosage and administration

Adults: The recommended dose is 1 Zimovane tablet (7.5 mg zopiclone) by the oral route shortly before retiring. The dose may be increased to 2 tablets (15 mg zopiclone) for patients who do not respond to the lower dose because of severe or persistent insomnia.

Elderly: A lower dose of 3.75 mg zopiclone should be employed to start treatment in the elderly. Depending on effectiveness and acceptability, the dosage subsequently may be increased if clinically necessary.

Children: An appropriate dosage has not been established.

Patients with hepatic insufficiency: As elimination of zopiclone may be reduced in patients with hepatic dysfunction a lower dose of 3.75 mg zopiclone nightly is recommended. Whilst the standard dose of 7.5 mg zopiclone may be used with caution in some cases, depending on effectiveness and acceptability, higher doses should always be avoided.

Contra-indications, warnings, etc
Use during pregnancy: Experience of use of zopiclone during pregnancy in humans is limited although there have been no adverse findings in animals. Use in pregnancy should be avoided if a safer alternative is known.

Use during lactation: Zopiclone is excreted in breast milk and use in nursing mothers must be avoided.

Use in hepatic insufficiency: A reduced dosage is recommended, see above.

Withdrawal of treatment: When used at the appropriate recommended dose for short term treatment of insomnia the abrupt termination of treatment with zopiclone is unlikely to be associated with withdrawal effects although patients should be closely monitored.

Interactions: As with all hypnotics, caution should be exercised over the concomitant use of alcohol or of other centrally-acting depressant drugs. There is limited evidence that zopiclone may reduce absorption, or increase the rate of elimination, of trimipramine. This effect could decrease the antidepressant activity of trimipramine or related tricyclic drugs although the clinical relevance remains unclear.

Adverse effects: A mild bitter or metallic after-taste is the most frequently reported adverse effect. Less commonly, mild gastrointestinal disturbances, including nausea and vomiting.

Psychological and behavioural disturbances, such as irritability, confusion, depressed mood, anterograde amnesia and hallucinations have been reported.

Allergic and allied manifestations such as urticaria or rashes have been observed very rarely. Drowsiness on waking may occur occasionally and, more rarely, dizziness, light-headedness and incoordination. Although such residual effects are rare and generally of minor significance, patients should be advised not to drive or operate machinery the day after treatment until it is established that their performance is unimpaired.

Overdosage: No serious or lasting effects have been associated with the few recorded cases of accidental overdosage. Drowsiness, lethargy and ataxia were the principal effects reported. Treatment should be supportive and in response to clinical signs and symptoms.

Pharmaceutical precautions Protect from light. Store in a dry place below 30°C.

Legal category POM.

Package quantities Zimovane tablets are available in blister packs of 28 tablets (OP) suitable for original pack dispensing.

Further information Nil.

Product licence number 0012/0162.

**Trade Mark*

A. H. Robins Company Limited
A Division of Wyeth Laboratories
Huntercombe Lane South
Taplow
Maidenhead
Berks SL6 0PH

A·H·ROBINS

ANTEPSIN* TABLETS AND SUSPENSION

Presentation Antepsin Tablets 1 gram are white, oblong, biconvex, uncoated tablets engraved 'Antepsin' on one side and 'WY' breakbar '39' on the other.

Each tablet contains 1 gram sucralfate, a basic aluminium salt of sucrose octa sulphate.

Antepsin Suspension is a white to off-white viscous suspension with an odour of aniseed/caramel. Every 5 ml dose contains 1 gram sucralfate.

Uses

Antepsin Tablets: For the treatment of duodenal ulcer, gastric ulcer, chronic gastritis.

Antepsin Suspension: For the treatment of duodenal ulcer, gastric ulcer, chronic gastritis, and the prophylaxis of gastrointestinal haemorrhage from stress ulceration in seriously ill patients.

Mode of action: The action of Antepsin is non-systemic as the drug is only minimally absorbed from the gastrointestinal tract. The small amounts that are absorbed are excreted primarily in the urine.

Antepsin exerts a generalized cytoprotective effect by preventing gastrointestinal mucosal injury.

Studies in humans and animal models show that Antepsin forms an ulcer adherent complex with the proteinaceous exudate of the ulcer site. This property enables Antepsin to form a protective barrier over the ulcer lesion giving sustained protection against the penetration and action of gastric acid, pepsin and bile.

Studies both in humans and animals demonstrate that Antepsin protects the gastric mucosa against various irritants such as alcohol, acetylsalicylic acid and sodium taurocholate.

Antepsin also directly inhibits pepsin activity and absorbs bile salts. It has only weak antacid activity. It does not alter gastric emptying time, nor normal digestive function.

Antepsin has no demonstrated pharmacological effect on the cardiovascular or central nervous systems.

Dosage and administration For oral administration.

Duodenal ulcer, gastric ulcer and chronic gastritis
Adults: Usual dose 2 grams twice daily to be taken on rising and at bedtime, or 1 gram 4 times a day to be taken 1 hour before meals and at bedtime. Maximum daily dose 8 grams. For ease of administration Antepsin tablets may be dispersed in 10-15 ml of water.

Four to six weeks' treatment is usually needed for ulcer healing, but up to twelve weeks may be necessary in resistant cases.

Prophylaxis of gastrointestinal haemorrhage from stress ulceration:
Adults: The usual dose is 1 gram six times a day. A maximum dose of 8 grams daily should not be exceeded.

Antacids may be used as required for relief of pain, but should not be taken half an hour before or after Antepsin.

Elderly: There are no special dosage requirements for elderly patients but as with all medicines, the lowest effective dose should be used.

Children: Safety and effectiveness in children have not been established.

Contra-indications, warnings, etc

Contra-indications: There are no known contra-indications.

Precautions: 1. The product should only be used with caution in patients with renal dysfunction.

2. *Use in pregnancy:* Teratogenicity studies in mice, rats, and rabbits at doses up to 50 times the human dose have revealed no evidence of harm to the foetus. Safety in pregnant women has not been established and Antepsin should be used during pregnancy only if clearly needed.

3. It is not known whether this drug is excreted in human milk. Caution should be exercised when sucralfate is administered to a nursing woman.

Drug interactions: Concomitant administration of Antepsin may reduce the bioavailability of certain drugs as has been observed in animal studies with tetracycline, phenytoin, and cimetidine, and in human studies with digoxin. The bioavailability of these agents may be restored by separating the administration of these agents from Antepsin by two hours. This interaction appears to be nonsystemic in origin presumably resulting from these agents being bound by Antepsin in the gastrointestinal tract. Because of the potential of Antepsin to alter the absorption of some drugs from the gastrointestinal tract, the separate administration of Antepsin from that of other agents should be considered when alterations in bioavailability are felt to be critical for concomitantly administered drugs.

Side-effects: Adverse reactions to Antepsin in clinical trials were minor and only rarely led to discontinuation of the drug.

Constipation was the most frequent complaint. Other adverse effects reported were diarrhoea, nausea, gastric discomfort, indigestion, dry mouth, rash, pruritus, back pain, dizziness, sleeplessness, vertigo and drowsiness.

Overdosage: There is no experience in humans with overdosage. Acute oral toxicity studies in animals, however, using doses up to 12 g/kg body weight, could not find a lethal dose. Risks associated with overdosage, should, therefore, be minimal.

Pharmaceutical precautions No special requirements for storage are necessary.

Legal category POM.

Package quantities Antepsin Tablets 1 gram: Securitainers of 100. Antepsin Suspension 1 g/5 ml: 560 ml bottles.

Further information Antepsin is a unique agent, chemicaly unrelated to antacids, anticholinergics, or H_2 receptor antagonists.

Product licence numbers

Antepsin Tablets	0011/0176
Antepsin Suspension	0011/0160

DIMOTANE* L.A.
DIMOTANE* TABLETS
DIMOTANE* ELIXIR

Presentation *Dimotane L.A.:* Sugar-coated, peach-coloured tablet monogrammed 'AHR' in black. Each tablet contains Brompheniramine Maleate USP 12.0 mg (one-third of active ingredient in coating for immediate release: two-thirds of active ingredient in delayed-release core).

This product also contains Sucrose PhEur 132 mg per tablet.

Dimotane Tablets: Scored, peach-coloured compressed tablet stamped AHR. Each tablet contains Brompheniramine Maleate USP 4.0 mg.

Dimotane Elixir: Cola-flavoured, pale yellow-green-coloured liquid. Each 5 ml contains Brompheniramine Maleate USP 2.0 mg.

This product also contains Sucrose PhEur 2050 mg per 5 ml, Ethanol (96%) BP 3.2% v/v, Sodium Benzoate PhEur and quinoline yellow (E104).

Uses Antihistaminic in the treatment of allergic conditions and reactions such as hay fever and urticaria.

Dosage and administration Oral.

Dimotane LA:

Adults and older patients: 1 to 2 tablets night and morning.

Children: 6–12 years: 1 tablet at night on retiring, a further tablet may be taken in the morning if necessary.

Dimotane Tablets:

Adults and older patients: 1 to 2 tablets three or four times daily.

Children: 6–12 years: ½ to 1 tablet three or four times daily.

Dimotane Elixir:

Adults and older patients: 10 to 20 ml three or four times daily.

Children: 6–12 years: 5 to 10 ml three or four times daily.

3–6 years: 5 ml three or four times daily.

Under 3 years: 0.4–1 mg/kg per 24 hours in four divided doses or at the discretion of the physician.

Contra-indications, warnings, etc

Contra-indications: Hypersensitivity to the active ingredient. This product should be used with care in epileptiform patients.

Precautions and warnings: Drowsiness may occur. Patients receiving Dimotane should not drive nor operate machinery unless it has been shown that their physical and mental capacity remains unaffected. May potentiate the effects of CNS depressants including alcohol. In common with many other antihistamines, brompheniramine has an atropine-like action and should therefore be used with caution in patients with bronchial asthma, especially children. The effects of anti-cholinergic drugs may be potentiated. May act as a cerebral stimulant in children and occasionally in adults. If this occurs, it is possible that insomnia, nervousness, hyperpyrexia and tremors may occur and, very rarely, epileptiform convulsions. Therefore children taking Dimotane should not be left unattended for long periods. This product should not be used during pregnancy unless considered essential by the physician.

Treatment of overdosage: Gastric lavage together with appropriate supportive therapy dependent upon individual response to the preparation.

Pharmaceutical precautions Discolouration of tablets may occur when exposed to prolonged strong sunlight.

Legal category P.

Package quantities

Dimotane LA:	Bottles of 100 and 500 tablets
Dimotane Tablets:	Bottles of 100 tablets
Dimotane Elixir:	Bottles of 500 ml

Further information Dimotane Tablets, Dimotane LA and Dimotane Elixir are tartrazine free.

Product licence numbers

Dimotane Tablets	0100/5004
Dimotane Elixir	0100/5005
Dimotane LA	0100/5006

DIMOTANE* PLUS LA
DIMOTANE* PLUS
DIMOTANE* PLUS PAEDIATRIC

Presentation

Dimotane Plus LA: Film-coated, white tablet, embossed AHR. Each tablet contains: Brompheniramine Maleate USP 12.0 mg and Pseudoephedrine Hydrochloride BP 120.0 mg in a controlled release formulation.

Dimotane Plus: Clear brown liquid with an odour of grape. Each 5 ml contains: Brompheniramine Maleate USP 4.0 mg and Pseudoephedrine Hydrochloride BP 30.0 mg.

This product also contains Ethanol (96%) BP 2.5% v/v and Sodium Benzoate PhEur.

Dimotane Plus Paediatric: Clear brown liquid with an odour of grape. Each 5 ml contains: Brompheniramine Maleate USP 2.0 mg and Pseudoephedrine Hydrochloride BP 15.0 mg.

This product also contains Ethanol (96%) BP 2.5% v/v and Sodium Benzoate PhEur.

Uses Symptomatic relief of allergic rhinitis.

Dosage and administration Oral.

Dimotane Plus LA

Adults, older patients, and children over 12 years: 1 tablet night and morning.

Children: Under 12 years: Not recommended.

Dimotane Plus and Dimotane Plus Paediatric are suitable for children aged 2 to 12 years.

Dimotane Plus

Adults and older patients: 10 ml three times daily.

Children: 6–12 years: 5 ml three times daily.

2–5 years: 2.5 ml three times daily.

Dimotane Plus Paediatric is recommended.

Under 2 years: Not recommended.

The dosage interval should not be less than 4 hours. Do not exceed three doses per day.

Dimotane Plus Paediatric

Children: 6–12 years: 10 ml three times daily.

2–5 years: 5 ml three times daily.

Under 2 years: Not recommended.

The dosage interval should not be less than 4 hours. Do not exceed three doses per day.

Contra-indications, warnings, etc

Contra-indications: Hypersensitivity to the active ingredients. Coma or pre-coma states. Known brain damage or epilepsy. Use in patients with acute ischaemic heart disease, thyrotoxicosis, glaucoma or urinary retention. Patients currently receiving or who have within two weeks received, monoamine oxidase inhibitors or tricyclic antidepressants. Patients receiving other sympathomimetic drugs. Hypertension or patients receiving antihypertensive therapy.

Precautions and warnings: Drowsiness may occur. Patients receiving these products should not drive nor operate machinery unless it has been shown that their physical and mental capability remain unaffected. May potentiate the effects of CNS depressants including alcohol. In common with many other antihistamines, brompheniramine has an atropine-like action and should therefore be used with caution in patients with bronchial asthma, especially children. The effects of anticholinergic drugs may be potentiated. May act as a cerebral stimulant in children and occasionally in adults. If this occurs, it is possible that insomnia, nervousness, hyperpyrexia or tremor may occur and very rarely epileptiform convulsions. Therefore, children taking this product should not be left unattended for long periods. Should be used with caution in patients receiving digitalis, adrenergic blockers or non-steroidal anti-inflammatory drugs. These products should not be used during pregnancy unless considered essential by the physician.

Treatment of overdosage: Gastric lavage together with appropriate supportive therapy dependent upon individual response to the various constituents of the preparations.

Pharmaceutical precautions Nil.

Legal category

Dimotane Plus LA	POM.
Dimotane Plus	P.
Dimotane Plus Paediatric	P.

Package quantities
Dimotane Plus LA: Bottles of 14 or 56 tablets (OP).
Dimotane Plus: Bottles of 500 ml.
Dimotane Plus Paediatric: Bottles of 500 ml.

Further information The recommended diluent for Dimotane Plus and Dimotane Plus Paediatric is 70% Glycerol.

Dimotane Plus LA, Dimotane Plus and Dimotane Plus Paediatric do not contain sucrose. Dimotane Plus and Dimotane Plus Paediatric contain a sugar substitute (carbohydrate content approx. 1 g per 5 ml) which is unlikely to affect diabetic control. This sweetener will not cause dental caries.

Product licence numbers
Dimotane Plus LA: 0100/0097.
Dimotane Plus: 0100/0085.
Dimotane Plus Paediatric: 0100/0086.

DOPRAM* INFUSION DOPRAM* INJECTION

Presentation
Dopram infusion: Clear colourless solution. Each 500 ml flexible plastic bag contains Doxapram Hydrochloride BP 2 mg per ml in 5% Glucose Intravenous Infusion BP.

Dopram injection: Clear colourless solution. Each 5 ml ampoule contains Doxapram Hydrochloride BP 20 mg per ml in Water for Injections PhEur.

Uses Ventilatory stimulant.

The principal pharmacological action of Dopram is an increase in minute volume produced primarily by an increase in tidal volume and to a lesser extent by changes in respiratory rate. Neuropharmacological studies have shown that the primary sites of action of Dopram are the peripheral chemoreceptors. It is considered that this site of action of Dopram is responsible for its relative specificity of action; it is only following large doses of doxapram hydrochloride that non-specific central nervous system stimulation occurs.

Dopram is specifically indicated in the following situations:

Acute respiratory failure (Dopram Infusion):

1. To stimulate ventilation in patients whose blood gas status or clinical condition suggests that severe carbon dioxide retention would occur during controlled oxygen therapy.
2. To stimulate ventilation in patients showing a progressive increase in PCO_2 with mental status changes during or after controlled oxygen therapy.

Following anaesthesia:

1. To stimulate ventilation in the postoperative period as an aid to the reduction of postoperative pulmonary complications. (Dopram Infusion or Dopram Injection.)
2. To permit the use of effective doses of narcotic analgesics without associated problems of ventilatory depression. (Dopram Infusion or Dopram Injection.)
3. To increase the rate of recovery from inhalational anaesthesia, when this would be beneficial. (Dopram Injection.)

Dosage and administration For intravenous use only.

Adults and older patients:
Acute respiratory failure: Dopram Infusion 1.5 mg per minute to 4.0 mg per minute dependent upon the condition and response of the patient. Administer concurrently with oxygen. Whenever possible the condition of the patient should be monitored by frequent measurement of blood gas tensions.

The following dosage regimen has been shown to result in the rapid production of a steady state plasma concentration of doxapram.

0–15 mins	4.0 mgs/min
15–30 mins	3.0 mgs/min
30–60 mins	2.0 mgs/min
60 mins onwards	1.5 mgs/min

Following anaesthesia: Dopram Injection 1.0 to 1.5 mg/kg body weight administered over a period of 30 seconds or more to reduce possible CNS or cardiovascular stimulation. This may be repeated at one hour intervals if necessary. Alternatively, Dopram Infusion may be given at a rate of 2 to 3 mg per minute. Appropriate adjustments to the administration rate should be made according to the response of the patient.

Children: The use of Dopram in children is not recommended.

Contra-indications, warnings, etc
Contra-indications: Severe hypertension, status asthmaticus, coronary artery disease, thyrotoxicosis, epilepsy, physical obstruction of the respiratory tract.

Precautions and warnings: Dopram should be administered concurrently with oxygen to patients with severe irreversible airways obstruction or severely decreased lung compliance, due to the increased work of breathing in these patients. In patients presenting with bronchoconstriction, Dopram should always be used in conjunction with β-adrenoceptor bronchodilator drugs in order to reduce the amount of respiratory effort. As doxapram is metabolised primarily by the liver, use with care in patients with hepatic dysfunction.

Use in pregnancy: Although there is no recognised hazard, this product is not recommended for use in pregnancy unless there are compelling clinical reasons to do so.

Interactions: Clinical data suggest that there may be interaction between doxapram and aminophylline which is manifested by agitation and increased skeletal muscle activity. Care should thus be taken when these two drugs are used concomitantly. Dopram should also be administered with great care to patients being treated concurrently with monoamineoxidase inhibitors. Animal studies have shown that the action of doxapram, in common with a large number of drugs, is potentiated after pretreatment with a monoamineoxidase inhibitor. Dopram potentiates the effects of sympathomimetic agents.

Side-effects: On recommended dosage a moderate increase in blood pressure and a slight increase in heart rate have been reported. This should be borne in mind when Dopram is considered for use in those patients with hypertension or with impaired cardiac functional reserves. Dizziness and perineal warmth have also been reported. Other side effects have been reported in the post anaesthetic period but these are also commonly observed during recovery from anaesthesia, and include muscle fasciculation, hyperactivity, sweating, confusion, hallucinations, cough, dyspnoea, laryngospasm, bronchospasm, sinus tachycardia, bradycardia, extrasystoles, nausea and/or vomiting and salivation.

Treatment of overdosage: Gross overdosage may result in hypertension, tachycardia, and increased skeletal muscle activity. The hypertension should be treated with appropriate supportive therapy and the increase in skeletal muscle activity controlled with intravenous barbiturates.

Pharmaceutical precautions Dopram is incompatible with alkaline solutions such as aminophylline, frusemide and thiopentone sodium. Store at room temperature. Do not refrigerate Dopram Injection.

Legal category POM.

Package quantities Dopram infusion: Packs of 5 flexible plastic bags each containing 500 ml.
Dopram injection: Packs of 5 ampoules each containing 5 ml.

Further information It has been shown that, when used in the postoperative situation, Dopram does not affect the quality of analgesia produced by narcotics such as morphine or pethidine.

Product licence numbers

Dopram Infusion	0100/5019
Dopram Injection	0100/5018

RHEUMOX* 600
RHEUMOX* CAPSULES

Presentation
Rheumox 600: Pale orange, film coated, capsule shaped tablets. One side scored with a breakline and the other engraved 'AHR', containing Azapropazone Dihydrate 600 mg.

This product also contains sunset yellow (E110) and quinoline yellow (E104).

Rheumox Capsules: Two-tone orange size 1 capsule, monogrammed 'AHR Rheumox' containing Azapropazone Dihydrate 300 mg.

This product also contains sunset yellow (E110) and erythrosine lake (E127).

Uses Rheumox is a non-steroidal anti-inflammatory analgesic agent indicated in the treatment of osteoarthrosis, rheumatoid arthritis and ankylosing spondylitis and acute musculoskeletal conditions. Rheumox is also indicated in attacks of acute gouty arthritis and in the long term prophylaxis of gout and the control of hyperuricaemia.

Dosage and administration
Route of administration: Oral.

Adults under 60 years old: These dosages apply to patients with normal renal function. Azapropazone should be used with caution and at a reduced dosage in patients with reduced renal function. In such cases the lower dosage recommended for adults over 60 years old should be followed.

Acute musculoskeletal conditions:

Rheumox 600 Tablets:	One 600 mg tablet night and morning.
Rheumox Capsules:	Two 300 mg capsules night and morning. Continue therapy until acute symptoms have subsided.

Osteoarthrosis, rheumatoid arthritis and ankylosing spondylitis:

Rheumox 600 Tablets:	One 600 mg tablet night and morning.
Rheumox Capsules:	One 300 mg capsule four times daily or two 300 mg capsules night and morning.

Chronic gout: Azapropazone reduces serum urate levels by enhancing urate excretion. The usual dosage for this purpose is 600 mg night and morning (either Rheumox 600 or Rheumox Capsules may be used).

Older-patients over 60 years:
Acute musculoskeletal conditions, osteoarthrosis, rheumatoid arthritis and ankylosing spondylitis, chronic gout: In patients over 60, a daily dosage of 900 mg azapropazone should not be exceeded. Renal function in patients over 60 may be deteriorating. A clinically significant decrease in the rate of elimination of azapropazone has been observed in elderly patients whose creatinine clearance was less than 60 ml per minute. Consequently, in patients over 60 years of age, dosage of azapropazone should be 300 mg twice daily. If creatinine clearance is more than 60 ml per minute, this may be increased to 900 mg daily in divided doses if necessary, but should not be exceeded.

If any abnormality is suspected, renal function should be fully investigated, before commencing therapy with Rheumox.

Acute gout:
Patients under 60 years: 2,400 mg in divided doses during the first 24 hours followed by 1,800 mg per day until the attack is resolving after which 1,200 mg per day is used until symptoms have disappeared. In treating acute gout it is good practice to ensure that the patient increases his fluid intake.

Patients over 60 years: 2,400 mg in divided doses during the first 24 hours followed by 1,800 mg per day. A maximum maintenance dose of 900 mg per day in divided doses should be achieved as early as possible preferably by the fourth day. Azapropazone should be used with caution and close monitoring in patients with a creatinine clearance of less than 60 ml per minute.

Children: Not recommended.

Contra-indications, warnings, etc
Contra-indications: Use in patients with a history or evidence of peptic ulceration or ulcerative colitis.

Use in patients with a history or evidence of blood dyscrasias.

Use in patients with severe renal insufficiency.

Rheumox should not be given to patients known to be hypersensitive to this drug.

Rheumox increases the plasma concentration of phenytoin and should not be given to patients taking this drug.

Rheumox should not be given to patients taking methotrexate.

Rheumox significantly potentiates the action of warfarin in many patients and must not be used with this or other oral anticoagulants.

Precautions and warnings: Azapropazone is excreted unchanged mainly by the kidney and should therefore be used with caution in older patients and in adults with any reduced renal function. Non-steroidal anti-inflammatory drugs in general inhibit renal prostaglandin synthesis and in patients with reduced renal function this action may result in overt renal decompensation. It is advisable to commence treatment at a reduced dosage in these patients. In such cases, the dosage recommendations for the treatment of older patients over 60 years should be followed. See also Contraindications.

If any abnormality is suspected, renal function should be fully investigated, before commencing therapy with Rheumox.

Patients on long-term treatment should be regularly reviewed.

Inhibition of renal lithium clearance by Rheumox has not been reported but the possibility of this occurring should be borne in mind.

Many non-steroidal anti-inflammatory drugs may precipitate bronchospasm in patients with bronchial asthma or allergic disease, and this has been reported in association with Rheumox.

Use in pregnancy and lactation: Animal reproduction studies did not result in fetal abnormalities but safety in human pregnancy cannot be assumed and its use should be avoided in pregnancy whenever possible. Azapropazone is excreted in small quantities in breast milk and should not therefore be used in breastfeeding women.

Interactions: Consult the section 'Contra-indications' regarding interactions with phenytoin, warfarin and methotrexate.

Since azapropazone is highly protein bound it may displace other protein bound drugs. It may therefore interfere with the blood sugar lowering effect of oral hypoglycaemic agents. Concurrent use of these drugs is not recommended. Data at present available does not indicate that interaction occurs with sulphonamides but adjustments of the dosage of these drugs may be necessary in some instances.

Side-effects: A high proportion of reported skin reactions are light induced. Fluid retention and gastro-intestinal upsets also occur occasionally. Gastro-intestinal bleeding, gastric and duodenal ulceration and perforation have been reported as has angioneurotic oedema.

Rarely, non-steroidal anti-inflammatory drugs may cause toxic nephropathies and such reactions have been reported in association with Rheumox.

Haemolytic anaemia has been reported rarely and some patients may develop a positive direct Coombs test without haemolytic anaemia. If haemolytic anaemia is present, Rheumox should be discontinued and this is also advised in the presence of a positive direct Coombs test.

Fibrosing alveolitis has been reported rarely and if this occurs, Rheumox should be discontinued.

Treatment of overdosage: If overdosage should occur, two specific courses of action are suggested on theoretical grounds. Since Rheumox is poorly soluble in gastric juice, stomach lavage should recover any gastric residue of the drug, provided of course that it is done early enough. Since Rheumox is predominantly excreted by the kidney, forced alkaline diuresis is theoretically indicated.

Pharmaceutical precautions Protect from light.

Legal category POM.

Package quantities
Rheumox 600 Tablets: Amber glass bottles of 100 and 500 tablets.

Rheumox Capsules: Amber glass bottles of 100 and 500 capsules.

Further information Nil.

Product licence numbers

Rheumox 600 Tablets	0100/0059
Rheumox Capsules	0100/0037

ROBAXIN*-750

Presentation Scored white film-coated capsule-shaped tablet engraved 'AHR' containing:
Methocarbamol USP 750 mg.

Uses As a short-term adjunct to the symptomatic treatment of acute musculoskeletal disorders associated with painful muscle spasms.

Dosage and administration *Oral:*
Adults: The usual dosage is 2 tablets four times daily (6.0 g) but therapeutic response has been achieved with doses as low as 1 tablet three times daily.

Older patients: Half the maximum adult daily dose, or less, may be sufficient to produce a therapeutic response in the elderly.

Children: Not recommended.

Contra-indications, warnings, etc
Contra-indications: Hypersensitivity to methocarbamol. Coma or pre-coma states. Known brain damage or epilepsy. Myasthenia gravis.

Use in pregnancy: There is no evidence of safety in human pregnancy, nor is there evidence from animal work that it is free from hazard. Do not use during pregnancy, especially the first trimester, or lactation, unless there are compelling reasons to do so.

Precautions and warnings: Robaxin should be used with caution in patients with renal and hepatic insufficiency.

Interactions: This product may potentiate the effects of other central nervous system depressants and stimulants including alcohol, barbiturates, anaesthetics and appetite suppressants. The effects of anticholinergics, e.g. atropine and some psychotropic drugs may be potentiated by methocarbamol. Little is known about the possibility of interaction with other drugs.

Side-effects: This product may cause drowsiness and patients receiving it should not drive nor operate machinery unless their physical and mental capacities remain unaffected – especially if other medication capable of causing drowsiness is also being taken.

Robaxin may give rise to manifestations of allergy including skin rash, urticaria and angioneurotic oedema. This product may very rarely give rise to restlessness, anxiety, vertigo, tremor, confusion and convulsions. Lightheadedness and dizziness have been reported. Nausea and vomiting have also been reported during use of Robaxin.

Treatment of overdosage: Gastric lavage with appropriate supportive therapy for 24 hours as methocarbamol is excreted within that time.

Pharmaceutical precautions Nil.

Legal category POM.

Package quantities Bottles of 100 tablets.

Further information Nil.

Product licence number 0100/5026.

ROBAXIN* INJECTABLE

Presentation 10 ml sterile ampoules each containing:
Methocarbamol USP 1.0 g
Vehicle 50% aqueous polyethylene glycol 300.
This product also contains Sodium Metabisulphite BP.

Uses In the treatment of acute painful muscle spasm, due to musculoskeletal disorders or trauma.

Dosage and administration For intravenous use only.

Adults: 10–30 ml dependent on the severity of the condition and therapeutic response. Should not exceed 30 ml per day. Not to be administered for more than three consecutive days.

Older patients: Half the maximum adult dose or less may be sufficient for a therapeutic response in the elderly.

Children: Not recommended.

Rate of administration: Administer by slow intravenous injection or infusion directly into the vein at a maximum rate of 3 ml per minute.

Diluent: May be added to an intravenous drip of sterile isotonic saline, or sterile 5% dextrose. 10 ml of Robaxin Injectable should not be diluted to more than 250 ml.

Contra-indications, warnings, etc
Contra-indications: Hypersensitivity to methocarbamol or sulphite. Coma or pre-coma states. Known brain damage or epilepsy. Myasthenia gravis.

Use in pregnancy: There is no evidence of safety in human pregnancy, nor is there any evidence from animal work that it is free from hazard. Do not use during pregnancy, especially the first trimester, or lactation, unless there are compelling reasons to do so.

Precautions and warnings: Robaxin Injectable should be used with extreme caution in patients with impaired renal function, as the solvent used may cause raised urea levels and acidosis. Robaxin should be used with caution in patients with hepatic insufficiency.

Since Robaxin Injectable is hypertonic, vascular extravasation must be avoided. A recumbent position will reduce the likelihood of side-effects. Blood aspirated into the syringe does not mix with the hypertonic solution. The blood may be safely injected with the methocarbamol, or the injection may be stopped when the plunger reaches the blood, whichever the physician prefers.

Interactions: This product may potentiate the effects of other central nervous system depressants and stimulants including alcohol, barbiturates, anaesthetics and appetite suppressants. The effects of anticholinergics, e.g. atropine, and some psychotropic drugs, may be potentiated by methocarbamol. Little is known about the possibility of interaction with other drugs.

Side-effects: This product may cause drowsiness and patients receiving it should not drive or operate machinery unless their physical and mental capabilities remain unaffected – especially if other medication capable of causing drowsiness is also being taken.

Robaxin may give rise to manifestations of allergy

including skin rash, urticaria and angioneurotic oedema. This product may very rarely give rise to restlessness, anxiety, vertigo, tremor, confusion and convulsions. Lightheadedness and dizziness have been reported. Nausea and vomiting have also been reported during use of Robaxin.

Treatment of overdosage: Appropriate supportive therapy for 24 hours as methocarbamol is excreted within that time.

Pharmaceutical precautions Nil.

Legal category POM.

Package quantities Boxes containing 5 ampoules.

Further information Nil.

Product licence number 0100/5027.

ROBAXISAL* FORTE

Presentation A two-layer, pink and white compressed tablet scored and stamped AHR, containing:

Methocarbamol USP 400 mg
Acetylsalicylic Acid PhEur 325 mg

This product also contains erythrosine (E127).

Uses In the short term management of pain and skeletal muscle spasm associated with musculoskeletal disorders such as lumbago, fibrositis, sprains, strains etc.

Dosage and administration *Oral:*
Adults: 2 tablets four times daily.

Older patients: Half the adult dose may be sufficient to produce a therapeutic response.

Children: Not recommended.

Contra-indications, warnings, etc
Contra-indications: Hypersensitivity to methocarbamol or aspirin. Coma or pre-coma states. Known brain damage or epilepsy. Myasthenia gravis. Active peptic ulceration and haemophilia.

Use in pregnancy: There is no evidence of safety in human pregnancy, nor is there evidence from animal work that it is free from hazard. Do not use during pregnancy especially the first trimester, or lactation, unless there are compelling reasons to do so.

Robaxisal Forte contains aspirin and is therefore best avoided at term because of possible effect on platelet function in the newborn. It may enhance the effects of anticoagulants.

Precautions and warnings: Robaxisal Forte should be used with caution in patients with renal and hepatic insufficiency.

Robaxisal Forte contains aspirin and therefore may give rise to gastrointestinal bleeding, and may precipitate bronchospasm especially in asthmatic patients. Patients currently on anti-coagulant therapy should have blood coagulation parameters regularly monitored.

Interactions: This product may potentiate the effects of other central nervous system depressants and stimulants including alcohol, barbiturates, anaesthetics and appetite suppressants. The effects of anti-cholinergics, e.g. atropine, and some psychotropic drugs, may be potentiated by methocarbamol. Little is known about the possibility of interaction with other drugs.

Side-effects: This product may cause drowsiness and patients receiving it should not drive nor operate machinery unless their physical and mental capacities remain unaffected – especially if other medication capable of causing drowsiness is also being taken.

Robaxisal Forte may give rise to manifestations of allergy including skin rash, urticaria and angioneurotic oedema. This product may give rise to restlessness, anxiety, vertigo, tremor, confusion and convulsions. Nausea and vomiting have been reported.

Treatment of overdosage: Supportive therapy for 24 hours, as methocarbamol is excreted within that time. If salicylate intoxication occurs, especially in children, the hyperpnoea may be controlled with sodium bicarbonate. Judicious use of 5% CO_2 with 95% O_2 may be of benefit. Abnormal electrolyte patterns should be corrected with appropriate fluid therapy.

Pharmaceutical precautions Nil.

Legal category POM.

Package quantities Bottles of 100 tablets.

Further information Nil.

Product licence number 0100/5028.

ROBINUL* INJECTION

Presentation 3 ml and 1 ml ampoule (snap-open ampoule) of isotonic aqueous solution containing in each 1 ml:

Glycopyrrolate USP 200 micrograms (0.2 mg)

This product also contains Sodium Chloride PhEur and Water for Injections PhEur.

Uses *Properties:* Robinul (glycopyrrolate) is a quaternary ammonium anticholinergic agent. The quaternary ammonium moiety renders Robinul highly ionised at physiological pH and it thus penetrates the blood brain and placental barriers poorly. The effect of Robinul on secretory organs is particularly marked and prolonged and good control of salivary and pharyngeal secretions can be obtained with doses which do not produce marked changes in heart rate. Gastric secretions are, similarly, reduced by Robinul.

Indications: 1. To protect against the peripheral muscarinic actions of anticholinesterases such as neostigmine and pyridostigmine, used to reverse residual neuromuscular blockade produced by nondepolarising muscle relaxants.

2. As a preoperative antimuscarinic agent to reduce salivary, tracheobronchial and pharyngeal secretions, and to reduce the acidity of the gastric contents.

3. As a preoperative or intra-operative antimuscarinic to attenuate or prevent intraoperative bradycardia associated with the use of suxamethonium or due to cardiac vagal reflexes.

Dosage and administration
Premedication
Adults and older patients: 200 to 400 micrograms (0.2 to 0.4 mg) intravenously or intramuscularly before the induction of anaesthesia. Alternatively, a dose of 4 to 5 micrograms/kg (0.004 to 0.005 mg/kg) up to a maximum of 400 micrograms (0.4 mg) may be used. Larger doses may result in a profound and prolonged antisialogogue effect which may be unpleasant for the patient.

Children: 4 to 8 micrograms/kg (0.004 to 0.008 mg/kg) up to a maximum of 200 micrograms (0.2 mg) intravenously or intramuscularly before the induction of anaesthesia. Larger doses may result in a profound and prolonged antisialogogue effect which may be unpleasant for the patient.

Intraoperative use
Adults and older patients: A single dose of 200 to 400 micrograms (0.2 to 0.4 mg) by intravenous injection should be used. Alternatively, a single dose of 4 to 5 micrograms/kg (0.004 to 0.005 mg/kg) up to a maximum of 400 micrograms (0.4 mg) may be used. This dose may be repeated if necessary.

Children: A single dose of 200 micrograms (0.2 mg) by intravenous injection should be used. Alternatively, a single dose of 4 to 8 micrograms/kg (0.004 to 0.008 mg/kg) up to a maximum of 200 micrograms (0.2 mg) may be used. This dose may be repeated if necessary.

Reversal of residual nondepolarizing neuromuscular block
Adults and older patients: 200 micrograms (0.2 mg) intravenously per 1000 micrograms (1 mg) neostigmine or the equivalent dose of pyridostigmine. Alternatively, a dose of 10 to 15 micrograms/kg (0.01 to 0.015 mg/kg) intravenously with 50 micrograms/kg (0.05 mg/kg) neostigmine or equivalent dose of pyridostigmine. Robinul may be administered simultaneously from the same

syringe with the anticholinesterase; greater cardiovascular stability results from this method of administration (see also 'Further information').

Children: 10 micrograms/kg (0.01 mg/kg) intravenously with 50 micrograms/kg (0.05 mg/kg) neostigmine or the equivalent dose of pyridostigmine. Robinul may be administered simultaneously from the same syringe with the anticholinesterase; greater cardiovascular stability results from this method of administration (see also 'Further information').

Contra-indications, warnings, etc
Contra-indications: Apart from established hypersensitivity to glycopyrrolate, there are no absolute contra-indications to Robinul.

Precautions and warnings: Because of the increase in heart rate produced by the administration of anticholinergics, use with caution in patients with coronary artery disease; congestive heart failure; cardiac arrhythmias; hypertension; thyrotoxicosis. This product should be used very cautiously in pyrexial patients due to inhibition of sweating.

Large doses of quaternary ammonium anticholinergic compounds have been shown to block end plate nicotinic receptors. This should be considered before using glycopyrrolate in patients with myasthenia gravis.

It is known that the administration of anticholinergic agents during inhalation anaesthesia can result in ventricular arrhythmias.

Use in pregnancy: Reproduction studies in rats and rabbits revealed no teratogenic effects from glycopyrrolate. Safety in human pregnancy and lactation has not been established. Diminished rates of conception and of survival at weaning were observed in rats, in a dose-related manner. Studies in dogs suggest that this may be due to diminished seminal secretion which is evident at high doses of glycopyrrolate. The significance of this for man is not clear.

Side-effects: Robinul may produce the following effects which are extensions of its fundamental pharmacological actions; dry mouth, difficulty in micturition, disturbances in visual accommodation, tachycardia, palpitation, inhibition of sweating.

Treatment of overdosage: Since glycopyrrolate is a quarternary ammonium agent symptoms of overdosage are peripheral rather than central in nature. To combat peripheral anticholinergic effects a quaternary ammonium anticholinesterase such as neostigmine methyl sulphate may be given in a dose of 1000 micrograms (1.0 mg) for each 1000 micrograms (1.0 mg) of glycopyrrolate known to have been administered by the parenteral route.

Pharmaceutical precautions Robinul Injection has been shown to be physically compatible with the following agents commonly used in anaesthetic practice: Butorphanol, Lorazepam, Droperidol and Fentanyl Citrate, Levorphanol Tartrate, Pethidine Hydrochloride, Morphine Sulphate, Neostigmine, Promethazine and Pyridostigmine.

Robinul Injection has been shown to be physically incompatible with the following agents commonly used in anaesthetic practice: Diazepam, Dimenhydrinate, Methohexitone Sodium, Pentazocine, Pentobarbitone Sodium, Thiopentone Sodium.

Robinul Injection should be stored at ambient temperature.

Legal category POM.

Package quantities Packs of 10 ampoules each containing 1 ml or 3 ml.

Further information Robinul Injection has been used successfully as an adjunct to reversal by neostigmine when atropine has been used as the preoperative anticholinergic.

The use of Robinul Injection as a preoperative anticholinergic is associated with less effect on the cardiovascular system, compared to atropine.

The use of Robinul Injection as an adjunct to reversal by neostigmine of non depolarising muscle relaxants is associated with less initial tachycardia and better protection against the cholinergic effects of neostigmine compared to reversal with a mixture of neostigmine and atropine.

Greater cardiovascular stability results from simultaneous administration of Robinul (glycopyrrolate) and neostigmine methylsulphate from the same syringe. A ready formulated mixture, Robinul-Neostigmine Injection, is available for this purpose. Each 1 ml ampoule contains Glycopyrrolate USP 500 micrograms and Neostigmine Methylsulphate BP 2500 micrograms.

Product licence number 0100/0054.

ROBINUL*-NEOSTIGMINE INJECTION

Presentation 1 ml glass ampoule containing:
Glycopyrrolate USP 500 micrograms (0.5 mg)
(Glycopyrronium Bromide INN)
Neostigmine Methylsulphate BP 2500 micrograms (2.5 mg)

This product also contains Sodium Phosphate PhEur, Citric Acid PhEur and Water for Injections PhEur.

Uses
Properties: Robinul (glycopyrrolate) is a quaternary ammonium anticholinergic agent. The quaternary ammonium moiety renders Robinul highly ionised at physiological pH and it thus penetrates the blood brain and placental barriers poorly. Robinul has a more gradual onset and longer duration of action than atropine. Neostigmine methylsulphate is a quaternary ammonium anticholinesterase. Robinul-Neostigmine Injection is associated with less initial tachycardia and better protection against the subsequent cholinergic effects of neostigmine methylsulphate than a mixture of atropine and neostigmine methylsulphate. In addition, residual central anticholinergic effects are minimised due to the limited penetration of Robinul into the central nervous system. Administration of glycopyrrolate with neostigmine methylsulphate is associated with greater cardiostability than administration of glycopyrrolate and neostigmine methylsulphate separately.

Indications: Reversal of residual non-depolarising (competitive) neuromuscular block.

Dosage and administration
Adults and older patients: 1–2 ml intravenously over a period of 10–30 seconds [equivalent to neostigmine methylsulphate 2500 micrograms (2.5 mg) with glycopyrrolate 500 micrograms (0.5 mg) to neostigmine methylsulphate 5000 micrograms (5 mg) with glycopyrrolate 1000 micrograms (1 mg)]. Alternatively 0.02 ml/kg intravenously over a period of 10–30 seconds may be used [equivalent to neostigmine methylsulphate 50 micrograms/kg (0.05 mg/kg) with glycopyrrolate 10 micrograms/kg (0.01 mg/kg)].

Children: 0.02 ml/kg intravenously over a period of 10–30 seconds [equivalent to neostigmine methylsulphate 50 micrograms/kg (0.05 mg/kg) with glycopyrrolate 10 micrograms/kg (0.01 mg/kg)]. Alternatively, dilute to 10 ml with Water for Injections BP or Sodium Chloride Injection BP 0.9% w/v and administer 1 ml per 5 kg body weight.

These doses may be repeated if adequate reversal of neuromuscular blockade is not achieved. Total doses in excess of 2 ml are not recommended as this dose of neostigmine may produce depolarising neuromuscular block.

Contra-indications, warnings, etc
Contra-indications: Robinul-Neostigmine Injection should not be given to patients with known hypersensitivity to either of the two active ingredients. Robinul-Neostigmine Injection should not be given to patients with mechanical obstruction of the gastrointestinal or urinary tracts.

Robinul-Neostigmine Injection should not be given in conjunction with suxamethonium as neostigmine potentiates the depolarising myoneural blocking effects of this agent.

Precautions and warnings: Administer with caution to patients with bronchospasm, severe bradycardia or glaucoma. Administration of anticholinesterase agents to patients with intestinal anastomoses may produce rupture of the anastomosis or leakage of intestinal contents. Although Robinul-Neostigmine Injection has been shown to have less impact on the cardiovascular system than atropine with neostigmine methylsulphate, use with caution in patients with coronary artery disease, congestive heart failure, cardiac dysrhythmias, hypertension or thyrotoxicosis.

Use with caution in patients with epilepsy or Parkinsonism. This product should be used cautiously in pyrexial patients due to inhibition of sweating.

Use in pregnancy: Reproduction studies in rats and rabbits revealed no teratogenic effects from glycopyrrolate. Safety in human pregnancy and lactation has not been established. However, diminished rates of conception and of survival at weaning were observed in rats, in a dose-related manner. Studies in dogs suggest that this may be due to diminished seminal secretion which is evident at high doses of glycopyrrolate. The significance of this for man is not clear. The safety of neostigmine methylsulphate in pregnancy and lactation has not been established.

Side-effects: The glycopyrrolate component of Robinul-Neostigmine Injection can give rise to dry mouth, difficulty in micturition, cardiac dysrhythmias, disturbances of visual accommodation and inhibition of sweating.

The neostigmine component of Robinul-Neostigmine Injection can give rise to bradycardia, increased oropharyngeal secretions, cardiac dysrhythmias and increased gastrointestinal activity.

If severe neostigmine-induced muscarinic side effects occur (bradycardia, increased oropharyngeal secretions, decreased cardiac conduction rate, bronchospasm or increased gastrointestinal activity etc), these may be treated by the intravenous administration of Robinul Injection (glycopyrrolate) 200–600 micrograms (0.2–0.6 mg) or atropine 400–1200 micrograms (0.4–1.2 mg).

Treatment of overdosage: The treatment of overdosage depends upon whether signs of anticholinesterase or anticholinergic overdosage are the predominant presenting features. Signs of neostigmine overdosage (bradycardia, increased oropharyngeal secretions, bronchospasm etc) may be treated by the administration of Robinul Injection (glycopyrrolate) 200–600 micrograms (0.2–0.6 mg) or atropine 400–1200 micrograms (0.4–1.2 mg). In severe cases, respiratory depression may occur and artificial ventilation may be necessary in such patients. Signs of glycopyrrolate overdosage (tachycardia, ventricular irritability etc) may be treated by the administration of neostigmine methylsulphate 1000 micrograms (1.0 mg) for each 1000 micrograms (1.0 mg) of glycopyrrolate known to have been administered. As glycopyrrolate is a quaternary ammonium agent, symptoms of overdosage are peripheral rather than central in nature; centrally acting anticholinesterase drugs such as physostigmine are therefore unnecessary to treat glycopyrrolate overdosage.

Pharmaceutical precautions Do not mix Robinul-Neostigmine Injection with any other preparation. Protect from light.

Legal category POM.

Package quantities Packs of 10 ampoules.

Further information Robinul-Neostigmine Injection can be used when atropine has been used as a pre-operative anticholinergic.

Product licence number 0100/0099.

ROBINUL* POWDER

Presentation A white, crystalline powder, Glycopyrrolate USP

Uses Iontophoretic treatment of the plantar and palmar skin for idiopathic hyperhidrosis.

Dosage and administration A 0.05% solution in distilled water of Glycopyrrolate USP is applied to palmar or plantar skin. When treating the foot or hand sufficient solution to cover the palm or sole is placed in a non-metallic container and the anode, of sheet metal larger in area than the part being treated, is placed in the solution. The sole or palm is separated from the anode by 5 mm of plastic foam or a layer of lint or sponge sheet.

In all cases an electrical circuit is completed by placing another limb in lukewarm tap water containing the cathode, similarly shielded from direct contact with the skin.

Recommended average conditions are 90 volts DC at 10–20 mA for adults (including older patients) and 2–10 mA for children, for 12 minutes at each site, depending on the patient's skin tolerance, body weight and size. Only one site should be treated at a time, and only two sites in any one day. Treatments should not be repeated within seven days, but may be repeated later varying the precise conditions according to the recurrence and severity of hyperhidrosis. See also Warnings section below.

Contra-indications, warnings, etc

Contra-indications: Glaucoma. Do not use during pregnancy.

Precautions and warnings: This product should be used with great caution in patients with cardiovascular disease, thyrotoxicosis and obstructive disorders of the lower urinary tract. Patients with mycotic or other skin infection should not be treated.

Exercise care in patients with prostatic hypertrophy. Due to the effect of anticholinergics on mucous secretions, it is advisable not to treat people with chronic bronchitis.

A mild tingling feeling may occur in the immersed areas during treatment and any recent cuts or cracks in the skin may smart when the current is increased at the start of iontophoresis. The latter can be avoided by covering the lesion with a thin smear of petroleum jelly. Avoid over-exertion, especially in hot weather, until any side-effects have disappeared.

The product should only be used by specialist units experienced in iontophoretic technique.

The electrodes and treated skin areas must be placed in non-metallic containers and separated carefully by layers of, for example, sponge or lint. Direct contact between electrodes and skin must be avoided, otherwise burns can result.

The current must be very slowly increased from zero mA and decreased to zero mA at the beginning and end of the treatment period respectively to avoid any Faradic discharge between the electrode and skin on removal of the patient's limb from the container of solution. Instruct patient that contact must not be broken during treatment.

There is only limited experience of the use of this product in children.

Use in pregnancy and lactation: Do not use during pregnancy or lactation as safety in this condition has not been established. Reproduction studies in rats and rabbits revealed no teratogenic effects from glycopyrrolate. However, diminished rates of conception and of survival at weaning were observed in rats, in a dose related manner. Studies in dogs suggest that this may be due to diminished seminal secretion which is evident at high doses of glycopyrrolate. The significance of this for man is not clear.

Side-effects: Glycopyrrolate may cause tachycardia. Since this drug may cause drowsiness, patients receiving glycopyrrolate should not drive nor operate machinery immediately after treatment unless it has been shown not to affect their physical or mental ability.

Dryness of the mouth, blurred vision and mild abdominal discomfort may occur.

Occasionally difficulty in eating may occur and micturition may be temporarily affected for some hours after treatment.

Pharmaceutical precautions Robinul Powder is supplied in amber-glass bottles containing 5 grams. The powder is slightly hygroscopic and the container should not be left open. For use by iontophoresis the powder should be dissolved in freshly distilled or deionised water to the recommended concentration.

Prior to use a stock solution (e.g. 0.1% or 0.5% w/v) may be made up with freshly boiled and cooled distilled or deionised water. This stock solution should be stored in a refrigerator to minimise possible microbial growth and should be kept in thoroughly clean amber-glass, capped containers. Glycopyrrolate does hydrolyse very slowly at pH 7 and room temperature and it is recommended that stock solutions be kept for no more than 14 days. Do not keep solutions once used for iontophoretic treatment. The solution must not be alkaline, otherwise the glycopyrrolate will hydrolyse more rapidly.

Legal category POM.

Package quantities Supplied in amber-glass bottles containing 5 grams Glycopyrrolate USP.

Further information Further recommendations concerning treatment are given in the package insert.

Product licence number 0100/0052.

**Trade Mark*

Roche Products Limited
PO Box 8
Welwyn Garden City
Hertfordshire AL7 3AY

ALCOBON*

Presentation Round, white tablets with 'ROCHE' imprinted on one face and a single break bar on the other, containing 500 mg flucytosine.

Infusion bottles containing 2.5 g flucytosine in 250 ml aqueous saline solution. The solution is colourless to slightly yellow.

Uses *Properties:* Alcobon is a fluorinated pyrimidine effective in the treatment of certain systemic fungal infections. In fungi sensitive to the preparation it acts as a competitive inhibitor of uracil metabolism.

Pharmacokinetics: Alcobon tablets are rapidly and well absorbed from the gastrointestinal tract. Alcobon is widely distributed in body tissues and fluids (including cerebrospinal fluid). Binding to plasma proteins is minimal. Half-life of elimination is 3–6 hours in patients with normal renal function but this value increases in renal failure. The majority of the dose administered is excreted unchanged in the urine. Flucytosine can be removed by haemodialysis.

Indications: Alcobon is indicated for the treatment of systemic yeast and fungal infections due to sensitive organisms: such infections include cryptococcosis, candidiasis, chromomycosis and infections due to Torulopsis glabrata and Hansenula.

In the treatment of cryptococcal meningitis and severe systemic candidiasis it is recommended that Alcobon should be given in combination with amphotericin-B. Amphotericin-B may also be given in combination with Alcobon in severe or long-standing infections due to other organisms.

Alcobon for Infusion is indicated only when the patient is unable to accept oral Alcobon.

Dosage and administration For severe infections the total daily oral dose in adults and children is 200 mg/kg body weight divided into 4 doses. In patients harbouring extremely sensitive organisms a total daily dose of 100–150 mg/kg body weight may be sufficient.

Alcobon for Infusion should be administered using a giving set incorporating a 15 micron filter. It may be administered directly into a vein, through a central venous catheter, or by intraperitoneal infusion. The recommended dosage is the same as for oral Alcobon, the total daily dose being divided over the 24 hours. Adequate effects can, however, often be obtained with a lower dose of Alcobon when the intravenous route is used.

It is suggested that the duration of the infusion should be of the order of 20 to 40 minutes provided this is balanced with the fluid requirements of the patient. As a rule, treatment with Alcobon for Infusion should rarely be required for periods of more than one week. The patient should be started on oral therapy with Alcobon tablets as soon as this becomes practicable.

Since Alcobon is excreted primarily by the kidneys, patients with renal impairment should be given smaller doses. The following is suggested as a guide for dosage in patients with severe infection associated with renal impairment:

In patients with creatinine clearance
<40 to >20 ml/min: 50 mg/kg every 12 hours.
<20 to >10 ml/min: 50 mg/kg every 24 hours.
<10 ml/min: an initial single dose of 50 mg/kg; subsequent doses should be calculated according to the results of regular monitoring of the serum concentration of the drug, which should not be allowed to exceed 80 microgram/ml. Blood levels of 25–50 microgram/ml are normally effective.

The duration of treatment should be determined on an individual basis. The outcome of therapy will be affected by variations in the sensitivity of the infecting organism, its accessibility and its susceptibility to Alcobon, as well as by differences in the response of individual patients. In cases of cryptococcal meningitis, treatment should last for at least four months.

Elderly: Although no specific studies have been performed to establish the use of Alcobon in the elderly, documented use indicates that dosage requirements and side-effects profile are similar to those of younger patients. Particular attention should be paid to renal function in this group.

Alcobon tablets are for oral administration.

Alcobon for Infusion is for intravenous or intraperitoneal administration.

Alcobon for Infusion may be given concurrently with other infusions of normal saline, glucose or glucose/saline. No other agent should be added to or mixed with Alcobon for Infusion.

Contra-indications, warnings, etc
Contra-indications: Alcobon is contra-indicated in patients who have shown hypersensitivity to the drug.

Use in pregnancy: Teratogenic effects have been seen in rats, in which species flucytosine is metabolised to fluorouracil. The metabolism may differ in man; nevertheless, the use of Alcobon in pregnancy and in women of childbearing age requires that the potential benefits of therapy be weighed against its possible hazards.

Precautions: Blood counts and tests of renal and hepatic function should be performed before and during treatment. This should occur at least weekly in patients with renal insufficiency or blood dyscrasias.

If drug serum levels are to be measured it should be noted that levels of the drug in blood samples, taken during or immediately after administration of Alcobon for Infusion, are not a reliable guide to subsequent levels; it is advisable to remove blood for monitoring of blood levels of Alcobon shortly before starting the next infusion.

In calculating the fluid and electrolyte intake of patients with impaired renal function, cardiac failure or electrolyte imbalance, due allowance should be made for the volume and sodium content (138 millimole/litre) of Alcobon for Infusion.

There is contradictory evidence concerning a drug interaction between Alcobon and cytarabine. Strict monitoring of blood levels is required if the two medicines are given concurrently.

Side-effects: Nausea, vomiting, diarrhoea and skin rashes have occurred but are usually of a transient nature.

Less frequently observed side effects include confusion, hallucinations, convulsions, headache, sedation and vertigo. Alterations in tests of liver function are generally dose related and reversible but hepatitis and hepatic necrosis have been reported. Bone marrow depression with leucopenia, thrombocytopenia, agranulocytosis or aplastic anaemia have been reported. This is more common when serum levels of flucytosine are high in patients with renal impairment and when amphotericin B has been co-prescribed. Local irritation or phlebitis does not appear to be a problem with Alcobon for Infusion.

Treatment of overdosage: In the event of overdosage with Alcobon, it is recommended that gastric lavage should be performed and measures taken to encourage diuresis. Haemodialysis produces a rapid fall in the serum concentration of Alcobon.

Pharmaceutical precautions *Storage:* Alcobon tablets should be stored in a well-closed container, protected against moisture and from light.

Alcobon for Infusion should be stored between 18 and 25°C. If stored below 18°C, precipitation of Alcobon substance may occur, which should be redissolved by heating to 80°C for not more than 30 minutes. Prolonged storage above 25°C could lead to the decomposition of Alcobon resulting in the formation of 5-fluorouracil.

Additives: Alcobon for Infusion may be given concurrently with other infusions of Sodium Chloride Intravenous infusion (0.9% w/v) BP, Glucose Intravenous Infusion (5% w/v) BP, or Sodium Chloride (0.18% w/v) and Glucose (4% w/v) Intravenous Infusion BP. No other agent should be added to or mixed with Alcobon for Infusion.

Legal category POM.

Package quantities Alcobon tablets are available in packs of 100.

Alcobon for Infusion 2.5 g in 250 ml in packs of 5.

Further information *Availability:* Alcobon tablets and Alcobon for Infusion are available to hospitals only.

Sensitivity testing: It is recommended that cultures for sensitivity testing be taken before treatment and repeated at regular intervals during therapy. However, it is not necessary to delay treatment until results of these tests are known. To determine sensitivities, the methods of Shadomy (Appl. Microbiol., 1969, *17*, 871) and Scholer (Mykosen, 1970, *13*, 179) are recommended.

For sensitivity testing it is essential that culture media are free of antagonists to flucytosine.

Product licence numbers

Tablets 0031/0069R

Infusion 0031/0094R

ALLOFERIN*

Presentation Ampoules containing 10 mg alcuronium chloride in 2 ml. The ampoule solution is almost colourless to pale yellow.

Uses *Properties:* Alloferin is a medium-acting neuromuscular blocking agent. It is a derivative of toxiferine, an alkaloid of calabash curare producing muscle relaxation of the non-depolarising type.

Indications: Muscle relaxation: Alloferin is used for surgical and anaesthetic procedures in which a muscle relaxant is required.

Dosage and administration Response to Alloferin, as to other non-depolarising relaxants, is subject to individual variation; underlying disease conditions or concurrently administered agents may significantly alter dosage requirements (see Precautions). The following doses are intended only as a guide.

Adults: An initial dose of 200–250 micrograms/kg bodyweight intravenously is usually adequate to achieve 95 per cent neuromuscular block. If endotracheal intubation is to be performed after administration of Alloferin, adequate laryngeal relaxation may be expected after a pause of 90–120 seconds. Profound muscle relaxation will continue for approximately 20–30 minutes when non-potentiating anaesthetic agents are employed. With an initial dose of 300 micrograms/kg body-weight, which may be used when intubating before longer procedures, muscle relaxation is obtained for approximately 40 minutes.

Incremental doses of one-sixth to one-quarter of the initial dose should provide relaxation for additional periods of similar duration to the first.

The following table is given as a more detailed guide to doses for a 70 kg patient:

Anaesthetic	*Intubation with Alloferin (mg)*	*Intubation with suxamethonium*		
		Abdominal (mg)	*Pelvic floor (mg)*	*Upper abdomen and thorax (mg)*
N_2O/O_2	14–17.5	9	7	11
Halothane 1.5 to 2 vol. %	8.5–11	6	4.5	6.5

Elderly: No specific data are available on the use of Alloferin in the elderly. However, there is no indication from the published literature that the problems encountered in the elderly need be any greater than with the younger adult.

Children: There is insufficient information to recommend a dosage for Alloferin in neonates (up to 28 days of age). Older infants and children should be given 125–200 micrograms/kg body-weight.

Alloferin ampoules are for intravenous injection.

Alloferin ampoule solution may be diluted with Water for Injections immediately before use.

Maintenance of stability cannot be guaranteed when Alloferin ampoule solution is diluted.

Contra-indications, warnings, etc

Contra-indications: Alloferin is contra-indicated in patients with a history of hypersensitivity to the agent. Use of muscle relaxants is preferably avoided in patients with myasthenia gravis or myasthenic (Eaton-Lambert) syndrome.

Use in pregnancy: No information is available on the effects of Alloferin on the developing foetus and its use in pregnancy should therefore be avoided. Studies indicate that Alloferin does not cross the placenta in amounts that would affect the foetus at or near term.

Precautions: Like other neuromuscular blocking agents, Alloferin should only be administered in the presence of an experienced anaesthetist. The patient's ventilation should be controlled.

Alloferin is mainly excreted in the urine and may therefore accumulate in patients with renal impairment when repeated doses are given. Dosage should be reduced accordingly.

Alloferin is partly bound to serum albumin. Dosage requirements may therefore be altered in patients with hepatic or other diseases in which serum protein levels are disturbed.

Increased sensitivity to non-depolarising drugs may be seen in most neuromuscular diseases, especially amyotrophic lateral sclerosis, poliomyelitis, Duchenne muscular dystrophy and multiple neurofibromatosis.

Patients with carcinomatosis, especially when this is associated with bronchial carcinoma, may exhibit marked sensitivity; the neuromuscular block may be difficult to reverse with neostigmine.

Sensitivity to non-depolarising relaxants may be increased by the following drugs: Antibiotics of the polymyxin and aminoglycoside groups (including streptomycin, neomycin, kanamycin, gentamicin, amikacin, tobramycin) and lincomycin; volatile anaesthetics (including ether, halothane, methoxyflurane, cyclopropane, isoflurane, enflurane); drugs with local anaesthetic properties (including quinidine, beta-blocking drugs, phenytoin, penicillamine); narcotic analgesics; ganglion-blocking agents (e.g. trimetaphan); diazepam.

In high concentrations, Mg may increase, whilst K, Na and Ca decrease non-depolarising neuromuscular block. The action of Alloferin is reportedly not significantly altered by changes in blood pH within the physiological range. Where marked electrolyte or acid-base disturbances are present these should be corrected, if possible, before Alloferin is administered. Care should be taken with dosage especially in acidosis.

During hypothermia non-depolarising neuromuscular blockade may be decreased. However, care is required during subsequent re-warming to ensure that increased effect does not lead to recurrence of paralysis.

In common with other non-depolarising muscle relaxants, lack of effect has been reported.

Side-effects: At doses producing adequate neuromuscular block, Alloferin does not have marked ganglion-blocking, histamine-releasing or vagolytic actions. Nevertheless, its administration is usually followed by a transient (2–5 minute) lowering of blood pressure due to a fall in peripheral vascular resistance. Less regularly, there may be a moderate increase in heart rate; cardiac output is not significantly altered. Intraocular pressure remains stable.

A few cases of anaphylactoid reaction, with hypotension and/or bronchospasm, have been recorded following administration of Alloferin, in most cases in patients who have had previous anaesthesia or a history of allergy.

Treatment of overdosage: Prolonged respiratory and muscular paralysis are symptoms of overdosage. Artificial ventilation must be continued, and the patient kept under observation until neuromuscular function is restored and there is no risk of recurrence of paralysis.

Prostigmin (neostigmine methylsulphate), given in a dose of 1–5 mg (50–70 micrograms/kg in children) with atropine 400–1250 micrograms (20–30 micrograms/kg in children) by intravenous injection, is routinely used to speed reversal of the neuromuscular block. Patients should not be left unattended until it is ascertained that adequate spontaneous respiration is present.

Pharmaceutical precautions *Storage:* The recommended maximum storage temperature for Alloferin ampoules is 25°C.

Alloferin ampoules should be protected from light.

Alloferin should not be administered in the same syringe as thiopentone.

Legal category POM.

Package quantities Alloferin ampoules in packs of 10.

Further information Nil.

Product licence number 0031/5000R.

ANEXATE*

Presentation Ampoules containing 500 micrograms flumazenil in 5 ml. The ampoule solution is almost colourless.

Uses

Properties: Anexate, an imidazobenzodiazepine, is a specific competitive inhibitor of substances which act via the benzodiazepine receptors, specifically blocking their central effects. The hypnotic-sedative effects of the agonist are rapidly reversed by Anexate and may then reappear gradually within a few hours, depending on the half-life and dose ratio of the agonist and antagonist.

Indications: Anexate is indicated for the complete or partial reversal of the central sedative effects of benzodiazepines. It may therefore be used in anaesthesia and intensive care in the following situations:

Termination of general anaesthesia induced and/or maintained with benzodiazepines.

Reversal of benzodiazepine sedation in short diagnostic and therapeutic procedures.

For the specific reversal of the central effects of benzodiazepines, to allow return to spontaneous respiration and consciousness, in patients in intensive care.

Dosage and administration Anexate is for slow intravenous injection or infusion. It should only be administered under the supervision of an experienced physician.

Anexate ampoule solution may be diluted with Sodium Chloride Intravenous Infusion BP, Sodium Chloride 0.45% and Dextrose 2.5% Intravenous Infusion BP or Dextrose 5% Intravenous Infusion BP. The resultant infusion solution should be used within 24 hours.

No preparations other than those recommended should be added to the Anexate ampoule or mixed with the Anexate infusion solution.

Anexate may be used concurrently with other resuscitative procedures.

Adults: The recommended initial dose is 200 micrograms administered intravenously over 15 seconds. If the desired level of consciousness is not obtained within 60 seconds a further dose of 100 micrograms can be injected and repeated at 60-second intervals where necessary, up to a maximum total dose of 1 mg or in intensive care situations, 2 mg. The usual dose required is 300–600 micrograms.

If drowsiness recurs, an intravenous infusion of 100–400 micrograms per hour may be employed. The rate of infusion should be individually adjusted to achieve the desired level of arousal.

The individually titrated, slow injections or infusions of Anexate should not produce withdrawal symptoms, even in patients exposed to high doses of benzodiazepines for long periods of time. If, however, unexpected signs of overstimulation occur, an individually titrated dose of diazepam (Valium* Roche) or midazolam (Hypnovel*) should be given by slow intravenous injection.

If a significant improvement in consciousness or respiratory function is not obtained after repeated doses of Anexate, a non-benzodiazepine aetiology must be assumed.

Elderly: No specific data are available on the use of Anexate in the elderly, but it should be remembered that this population is more sensitive to the effects of benzodiazepines and should be treated with due caution.

Children: There are insufficient data to make dosage recommendations for Anexate in children. It should, therefore, be administered only if the potential benefits to the patient outweigh the possible risks.

Use in renal and hepatic insufficiency: No dosage adjustments are necessary in patients with renal impairment. However, since flumazenil is primarily metabolised in the liver, careful titration of dosage is recommended in patients with impaired hepatic function.

Contra-indications, warnings, etc

Contra-indications: Anexate is contra-indicated in patients with known hypersensitivity to benzodiazepines.

The use of Anexate is not recommended in epileptic patients who have been receiving benzodiazepine treatment for a prolonged period. Although Anexate exerts a slight intrinsic anticonvulsant effect, its abrupt suppression of the protective effect of a benzodiazepine agonist can give rise to convulsions in epileptic patients.

Use in pregnancy and lactation: Like other benzodiazepine compounds, Anexate is expected to cross the placenta and to enter into breast milk, although the total quantities involved would be small. There has been little human usage but animal studies have shown no teratogenic potential. The established medical principle of only administering drugs in early pregnancy when considered absolutely necessary should be observed.

Emergency use of Anexate during lactation is not contra-indicated.

Precautions: In view of the short duration of action of Anexate and the possible need for repeat doses, the patient should remain under close observation until all possible central benzodiazepine effects have subsided.

Benzodiazepine agonists have a dependence potential when used chronically. Symptoms such as depression, nervousness, rebound insomnia, irritability, sweating and diarrhoea may arise following abrupt cessation of benzodiazepine agonists in patients treated for prolonged periods of time. Rapid injection of Anexate in such patients may trigger these withdrawal symptoms and should therefore be avoided.

Anexate should not be given in anaesthesia reversal until the effects of any neuromuscular blockade have cleared.

In high-risk patients, the advantages of counteracting the central nervous system depression associated with benzodiazepines should be weighed against the drawbacks of rapid awakening.

The dosage of Anexate should be adjusted individually to the needs of patients suffering from pre-operative anxiety or having a history of chronic or episodic anxiety. In anxious patients, particularly those with coronary heart disease, it is preferable to maintain a degree of sedation throughout the early post-operative period rather than bring about complete arousal.

The pain felt by patients in the post-operative period must be taken into account. Following a major intervention, it is preferable to maintain a moderate degree of sedation.

Patients who have received Anexate to reverse the effects of benzodiazepine sedation should be warned not to drive, to operate machinery or to engage in any other physically or mentally demanding activity for at least 24 hours, since the effect of the benzodiazepine may return.

Drug interactions: Anexate blocks the central effects of benzodiazepines by competitive interaction at the receptor level; the effects of non-benzodiazepines acting via the benzodiazepine receptor, such as zopiclone, are also blocked by Anexate. However, Anexate is ineffective when unconsciousness is due to other substances.

Interaction with other central nervous system depressants has not been observed. However, particular caution is necessary when using Anexate in cases of intentional overdosage since the toxic effects of other psychotropic drugs (especially tricyclic antidepressants) taken concurrently may increase with the subsidence of the benzodiazepine effect.

The pharmacokinetics of benzodiazepines are unaltered in the presence of Anexate.

Side-effects and adverse reactions: Anexate is generally well tolerated. In post-operative use, nausea and/or vomiting are occasionally observed, particularly if opiates have also been employed. Flushing has also been noted. If patients are awakened too rapidly, they may become agitated, anxious or fearful. Very rarely, seizures have been reported, particularly in patients known to suffer from epilepsy. Transient increases in blood pressure and heart rate may occur on awakening in intensive care patients.

Any side-effects associated with Anexate usually subside rapidly without the need for special treatment.

Excessive and/or rapidly injected doses of Anexate may induce benzodiazepine withdrawal symptoms such as anxiety attacks, tachycardia, dizziness and sweating in patients on long-term benzodiazepine treatment. Such symptoms may be treated by slow intravenous injection of diazepam or midazolam (see 'Dosage and Administration').

Treatment of overdosage: Even when given intravenously at doses of 100 mg, no symptoms of overdosage attributable to Anexate have been observed.

Pharmaceutical precautions
Storage: The recommended maximum storage temperature for Anexate ampoules is 30°C.

Diluents: Anexate ampoule solution may be diluted with Sodium Chloride Intravenous Infusion BP, Sodium Chloride 0.45% and Dextrose 2.5% Intravenous Infusion BP or Dextrose 5% Intravenous Infusion BP. The resultant infusion solution should be used within 24 hours.

No preparations other than those recommended should be added to the Anexate ampoule or mixed with the Anexate infusion solution.

Legal category POM.

Package quantities Anexate ampoules 500 micrograms per 5 ml in packs of 5.

Further information
Pharmacokinetics: Flumazenil is moderately bound to plasma proteins. The distribution of the drug parallels that of the benzodiazepines. It is extensively metabolised in the liver, primarily to the inactive carboxylic acid form, and has an elimination half-life of approximately 50 minutes.

Availability: Anexate ampoules are available through hospitals, clinics or retail pharmacies.

Product licence number 0031/0228.

ARFONAD*

Presentation Ampoules containing 250 mg trimetaphan camsylate in 5 ml. The ampoule solution is colourless to pale yellow.

Uses *Properties:* Arfonad is a ganglion-blocking agent which also has a direct dilator effect on peripheral vessels. It has a rapid, short and readily reversible action, which permits minute-to-minute control of the blood pressure.

Pharmacokinetics: Trimetaphan crosses the placenta. Further pharmacokinetic data are unavailable as there is no acceptable assay procedure for the determination of trimetaphan in biological specimens, however most of a parenteral dose is excreted unchanged by the kidney.

Indications: Arfonad is used to induce controlled hypotension during certain surgical procedures. These may include: neurosurgery; vascular surgery; prostatectomy; chest surgery; thyroidectomy; bone and joint surgery.

Dosage and administration *Adults and children:*

(a) Dilution to 250 ml with normal saline or dextrose-saline gives a 0.1% solution (1 mg per ml) which is the strength usually used for an intravenous drip. The Arfonad drip is started at an average of 60 drops (approximately 3 to 4 mg) per minute and, having ascertained the patient's response, the rate of administration is then adjusted to maintain the desired level of hypotension. Since there is marked variation in individual response, continuous blood pressure monitoring is essential to maintain proper control.

(b) If a weaker solution is preferred, a 0.05% solution can be prepared by diluting the 5% ampoule solution to 500 ml.

(c) It may be necessary to use a more concentrated solution in operations in which intravenous fluid should be restricted. For such patients a solution containing 0.25% Arfonad should be prepared by diluting the original 5% solution to 100 ml with normal saline or dextrose-saline. The rate at which the drip is given should be correspondingly reduced.

(d) The undiluted solution has also been used by intermittent intravenous injection.

As with other hypotensive drugs, Arfonad should be stopped before wound closure to allow the blood pressure to rise.

Arfonad ampoules are for administration by intravenous drip and intermittent intravenous injection.

Arfonad ampoule solution may be diluted with Water for Injection, normal saline or dextrose-saline immediately before use.

Contra-indications, warnings, etc
Contra-indications: Arfonad should not be used for hypotensive surgery in patients with severe arteriosclerosis, severe cardiac disease, or pyloric stenosis.

Precautions: Arfonad should be used with caution in the elderly, in patients with cerebral or coronary vascular insufficiency, diabetes mellitus, hepatic or renal insufficiency, and in adrenal insufficiency.

Care should also be taken in patients receiving neuromuscular blocking agents (especially suxamethonium), other anti-hypertensive agents, myocardial depressants or systemic corticosteroids.

Since the effect of Arfonad is neutralised by vasopressor drugs such as adrenaline, noradrenaline and ephedrine, local adrenaline infiltration at the site of incision is contra-indicated.

Arfonad may sensitise patients to the cardiovascular effects of sympathomimetic agents.

Use in pregnancy: Use of Arfonad in pregnancy should

be avoided due to the risk of producing paralytic ileus or meconium ileus in the newborn.

Use in elderly: No specific data are available on the use of Arfonad in the elderly. Whilst there is no indication that this is accompanied by particular problems, it is known that the elderly may be more sensitive to hypotensive drugs. Arfonad should be used with particular caution in patients with coronary artery disease, prostatic hypertrophy or glaucoma (cf pupillary dilatation effect).

Use in other special groups: Extreme caution should also be exercised when using Arfonad in patients with degenerative disease of the central nervous system, Addison's disease and diabetes. Owing to its histamine-releasing effects, Arfonad should be used with caution in subjects with a history of allergy.

Side-effects: Ganglionic blockade due to Arfonad may reduce gastro-intestinal motility and bladder function and affect visual accommodation. Constipation, mydriasis, increased intra-ocular pressure, decreased oral and nasal secretion, respiratory arrest (on rapid infusion of greater than 5 mg/minute), hypoglycaemia and hypokalaemia may also rarely occur.

Treatment of overdosage: The major effect will be a marked fall in blood pressure below the desired level of hypotension. Tachycardia and respiratory depression may result, particularly if Arfonad is used concomitantly with a muscle relaxant. Vasopressor agents such as phenylephrine, ephedrine or noradrenaline are antidotes and may be used to effect a rapid return to normotensive level.

Pharmaceutical precautions *Storage:* The recommended maximum storage temperature is 6°C; avoid freezing.

Additives: It is inadvisable to use the Arfonad drip as a vehicle for administering other drugs. Arfonad is known to be incompatible with thiopentone, gallamine triethiodide, strongly alkaline solutions, iodides and bromides.

Legal category POM.

Package quantities Arfonad ampoules in packs of 10.

Further information Nil.

Product licence number 0031/5001R.

BACTRIM* ROCHE

Approved name: Co-trimoxazole

Presentation

Bactrim Drapsules: capsuliform, yellow-orange, film-coated tablets with ROCHE imprinted on one side, containing 80 mg trimethoprim and 400 mg sulphamethoxazole (Co-trimoxazole Tablets BP).

Bactrim Double Strength Tablets: oval, biconvex, white tablets with ROCHE 800+160 imprinted on one face, a single break bar on the other, containing 160 mg trimethoprim and 800 mg sulphamethoxazole.

Bactrim Dispersible Tablets: round, greenish-yellow tablets with ROCHE in a hexagon imprinted on one face, a single break bar on the other, containing 80 mg trimethoprim and 400 mg sulphamethoxazole (Dispersible Co-trimoxazole Tablets BP).

Bactrim Paediatric Tablets: round, white tablets with ROCHE imprinted on one face, containing 20 mg trimethoprim and 100 mg sulphamethoxazole (Paediatric Co-trimoxazole Tablets BP).

Bactim suspension (adult): pale brownish-cream, aniseed-flavoured suspension, containing 80 mg trimethoprim and 400 mg sulphamethoxazole in 5 ml (Co-trimoxazole Mixture BP).

Bactrim Paediatric Syrup: sugar-free, pale creamy-yellow, fruit-flavoured suspension, containing 40 mg trimethoprim and 200 mg sulphamethoxazole in 5 ml (Paediatric Co-trimoxazole Mixture BP).

Uses

Properties: Bactrim is bactericidal *in vitro* to a wide range of Gram-positive and Gram-negative organisms, including *Streptococcus, Staphylococcus, Pneumococcus, Neisseria, B. catarrhalis, Escherichia coli, Klebsiella, Proteus* spp., *Haemophilus, Salmonella, Shigella, Vibrio cholerae, Brucella, Pneumocystis carinii, Nocardia* and *Bordetella.* A particularly high degree of activity is exhibited against *Haemophilus influenzae, E. coli* and *Proteus* spp., making Bactrim particularly suitable for the treatment of chronic bronchitis and urinary tract infections.

Bactrim exerts its bactericidal action by the sequential blockade of two bacterial enzyme systems in the biosynthesis of folinic acid in the micro-organism. The synergy thus produced accounts for the high degree of bactericidal activity.

Pharmacokinetics: Trimethoprim and sulphamethoxazole are pharmacokinetically compatible, i.e. the two components are absorbed and eliminated at similar rates. This enables the two drugs to be given, as Bactrim, in repeated doses without undue changes to their relative concentrations in the body.

Absorption and distribution – Following oral administration, peak blood levels occur at 1 to 4 hours, then both compounds are eliminated with half-lives of approximately 12 hours. Both compounds are only moderately bound to plasma proteins (45% for trimethoprim and 60% for sulphamethoxazole), and the free drugs are considered to be the therapeutically active forms *in vivo.* Distribution studies, in animals and humans, have shown that both components are detectable in interstitial and extravascular fluids such as CSF, milk, synovial fluid, sputum and aqueous humour. High concentrations are achieved in the urine.

Elimination – Sulphamethoxazole and trimethoprim are both excreted unchanged and as metabolites, mainly by the kidneys.

Renal impairment – Because both compounds are cleared largely via the kidneys, their half-lives are significantly increased in patients with creatinine clearance less than 30 ml per min. Thus reduction of dosage is required when patients with renal impairment are treated with Bactrim (see 'Dosage and administration').

Indications

Respiratory tract infections, including acute and chronic bronchitis (treatment and prophylaxis), also bronchiectasis, lung abscess, lobar and bronchopneumonia, *Pneumocystis carinii* pneumonitis, sinusitis and otitis media.

Genito-urinary tract infections, including urethritis, acute and chronic cystitis, pyelitis, pyelonephritis and prostatitis. Male and female gonorrhoea.

Gastro-intestinal tract infections caused by *Salmonella typhi* and *paratyphi,* including the chronic carrier state.

Other infections caused by a wide range of organisms confirmed to be susceptible to Bactrim and where the therapeutic benefits are considered to outweigh the possible occurrence of adverse events. Such infections include acute and chronic osteomyelitis, acute brucellosis, skin infections including pyoderma, abscesses and wound infections, septicaemias, bacillary dysentery and cholera (as an adjuvant to fluid and electrolyte replacement), nocardiosis, actinomycetoma and in South African blastomycosis.

Dosage and administration

Duration of therapy: In acute infections, apart from gonorrhoea, Bactrim should be given for at least five days or until the patient has been symptom-free for two days. Treatment for prostatis and acute brucellosis should be maintained for a period of at least four weeks, whilst nocardiosis, actinomycetoma and South American blastomycosis require long-term therapy.

Adults and children over 12 years

Bactrim Drapsules and Bactrim Double Strength tablets

Usual dosage	Two drapsules or one Double Strength tablet, twice daily.
High dosage for severe infections and septicaemia	Three drapsules or one and a half Double Strength tablets, twice daily.
Uncomplicated gonorrhoea	Four doses of four drapsules or two Double Strength tablets, at 12-hourly intervals over two days or Two doses of five drapsules or two and a half Double Strength tablets, with 8–12 hours between the doses.
Minimum dosage and dosage for long-term treatment (> 14 days)	One drapsule or half a Double Strength tablet, twice daily.

Bactrim dispersible tablets and Bactrim adult suspension: Dispersible tablets or adult suspension may be given instead of the drapsules: 1 drapsule = 1 dispersible tablet = 5 ml of adult suspension

The dosage required for the treatment of *Pneumocystis carinii* pneumonitis is generally higher than that recommended for other conditions. A dosage of 20 mg trimethoprim/kg body-weight/day, plus 100 mg sulphamethoxazole/kg body-weight/day, given in equally divided doses every six hours for 14 days, is suggested. For this reason, treatment should be undertaken only if facilities for regular monitoring of plasma concentrations of the sulphamethoxazole component are available.

Elderly: If there is renal impairment in the elderly patient then the dosage recommendations given for patients with renal impairment apply. Since elderly patients are more susceptible to blood dyscrasias and adverse reactions in general, caution is recommended when treating these patients (see Contra-indications and Warnings – Precautions section).

Children up to 12 years

Bactrim paediatric tablets, Bactrim paediatric syrup and Bactrim dispersible tablets

Recommended dosage	
6 weeks to 5 months	2.5 ml of paediatric syrup, twice daily
6 months to 2 years	5 ml of paediatric syrup, twice daily
2 to 5 years	5 ml of paediatric syrup or two paediatric tablets, twice daily
6 to 12 years	10 ml of paediatric syrup or four paediatric tablets or one dispersible tablet, twice daily

In children this corresponds to an approximate dose of 6 mg trimethoprim/kg body-weight/day plus 30 mg sulphamethoxazole/kg body-weight/day, divided into two equal doses.

Patients with impaired renal function

Creatinine clearance (ml/min)	*Recommended dosage*
>30	Usual dosage
15–30	Half the usual dosage
<15	Use of Bactrim not recommended

Other information: All dosage forms are for oral administration. Bactrim dispersible tablets may be dispersed in water or swallowed whole. Bactrim should be taken with fluid, preferably after a meal.

Dilution of Bactrim adult suspension and Bactrim paediatric syrup is not recommended.

Contra-indications, warnings, etc

Contra-indications: Bactrim is contra-indicated in patients showing marked liver parenchymal damage, blood dyscrasias, severe renal insufficiency and glucose 6-phosphate dehydrogenase deficiency. Bactrim should not be given to patients with a history of sensitivity to sulphonamides or trimethoprim. Treatment must be immediately discontinued on the appearance of a skin rash, or if any element of the blood count is reduced.

Bactrim should not be given to premature babies nor to full term infants during the first six weeks of life.

Use in pregnancy and lactation: The safety of Bactrim in human pregnancy has not been established. There is some evidence of Bactrim, at extremely high doses, having harmful effects in pregnancy in animals. Bactrim should not therefore be given during pregnancy. Sulphonamide-containing products should not be administered in late pregnancy because of the risk of kernicterus. The usual caution in prescribing any drug for women of childbearing age should also be exercised with Bactrim.

Both trimethoprim and sulphamethoxazole are excreted in breast milk. This does not contra-indicate the use of Bactrim in lactating mothers but due account should be taken of the age of the infant being breast-fed.

Precautions: An adequate fluid intake should be ensured to maintain an adequate urinary output in order to prevent crystalluria and stone formation. In cases with renal impairment the dose should be adjusted as indicated in the Dosage and Administration section, to avoid accumulation of the drugs. In such patients, measurement of the plasma concentration of the drugs is advisable. Bactrim should be given with caution to patients with impaired hepatic function and to those patients with severe allergy or bronchial asthma.

There is an increased risk of severe, possibly fatal adverse reactions in elderly patients or when complicating conditions exist. In order to minimise the risk of undesirable reactions, the duration of Bactrim treatment should not be unnecessarily prolonged, particularly in elderly patients.

Regular monthly blood counts are necessary whenever long-term therapy is used. This is particularly advisable if Bactrim is to be given to elderly patients for a prolonged period (i.e. exceeding three months), since it has been suggested that the elderly are more susceptible to blood dyscrasias.

Urine analysis and renal function tests should be performed during long-term therapy.

Special caution should be exercised in treating patients with conditions predisposing to folate deficiency.

Drug interactions: An increased incidence of thrombocytopenia with purpura has been observed in elderly patients concurrently receiving certain diuretics, primarily thiazides.

Care should be taken when giving Bactrim to patients receiving strongly serum protein-bound drugs such as oral hypoglycaemic agents or coumarin anticoagulants as the action of these drugs may be increased. It has been reported that Bactrim may prolong the prothrombin time in patients receiving the anticoagulant warfarin. This interaction should be borne in mind when Bactrim is given to patients already on anticoagulant therapy. In such cases, the coagulation time should be re-determined.

Sulphonamides can displace methotrexate from plasma protein binding sites, thus increasing free methotrexate concentrations.

Bactrim may inhibit the hepatic metabolism of phenytoin. A 39 per cent increase in phenytoin half-life and a 27 per cent decrease in the metabolic clearance rate of phenytoin has been observed following administration of Bactrim at normal clinical dosages. If the two drugs are given concurrently, it is important to remain alert for signs of phenytoin toxicity.

Special caution should be exercised in treating patients who are receiving other preparations containing folate inhibitors (e.g. antimalarial drugs containing pyrimethamine; methotrexate) or anticonvulsant drugs. Occasional reports suggest that patients receiving pyrimethamine as malarial prophlylaxis in doses exceeding 25 mg weekly may develop megaloblastic anaemia if Bactrim is prescribed concurrently.

Reversible deterioration of renal function has been observed in patients treated with co-trimoxazole and cyclosporin following renal transplantation.

Side-effects and adverse reactions: At the recommended dosage Bactrim is usually well tolerated. The most common side-effects are gastro-intestinal disturbances and allergic skin reactions. Hypersensitivity reactions have occasionally been reported.

Gastro-intestinal effects include nausea, vomiting, glossitis, pancreatitis, stomatitis, diarrhoea and rarely, cases of pseudomembranous enterocolitis have been reported.

Other allergic reactions include anaphylactoid reactions, drug fever, photosensitivity, serum sickness, Henoch-Schoenlein purpura, allergic myocarditis and angiooedema. In addition periarteritis nodosa and systemic lupus erythematosus have been reported.

Rarely, cases of hepatitis have been reported.

Skin rashes are generally mild and quickly reversible on withdrawal of the drug; however, in some cases erythema multiforme (Stevens-Johnson syndrome) and toxic epidermal necrolysis (Lyell syndrome) can occur. The latter condition is associated with a high mortality.

As Bactrim contains a sulphonamide, the possibility of blood dyscrasias like those associated with sulphonamides should be borne in mind. The changes reported with Bactrim mainly consist of thrombocytopenia, purpura, leucopenia, neutropenia, haemolytic anaemia, eosinophilia, and methaemoglobinaemia and, very rarely, agranulocytosis, pancytopenia and megaloblastic anaemia. They have usually proved to be reversible on withdrawal of the drug. It has been suggested that elderly patients are more susceptible to these blood dyscrasias. The isolated cases of megaloblastic changes reported in the bone marrow during long-term therapy are reversible by folinic acid therapy.

Neurological effects reported include headache, tinnitus, vertigo, ataxia, convulsions and aseptic meningitis.

Musculoskeletal effects include arthralgia and myalgia.

Genito-urinary tract effects include interstitial nephritis, toxic nephrosis, crystalluria, blood urea nitrogen and serum creatinine elevation.

Raised serum levels of SGOT, SGPT and bilirubin have been reported.

Pulmonary infiltrates such as eosinophilic or allergic alveolitis have been reported in rare instances, which may manifest themselves through symptoms such as cough or shortness of breath. Should such symptoms appear unexpectedly or worsen during Bactrim therapy, the patient should be re-evaluated and discontinuation of the drug should be considered.

Treatment of overdosage: Symptoms and signs of overdosage may include nausea, vomiting, mental and visual disturbances, pyrexia, petechiae, purpura, jaundice, anorexia, colic, bone-marrow depression and abdominal pain. Blood dyscrasias are potential late manifestations. Haematuria, crystalluria and anuria may occur in severe cases.

Treatment is symptomatic and may include gastric lavage and forced diuresis. Alkalinisation of the urine may aid the elimination of the sulphamethoxazole component of Bactrim but may decrease the elimination of the trimethoprim component.

Hypersensitivity reactions may require treatment with steroids. Calcium folinate, 3 to 6 mg intramuscularly for five to seven days, may be given to counteract the effects of trimethoprim on haemopoiesis.

Pharmaceutical precautions
Storage: The recommended maximum storage temperature for Bactrim adult suspension and paediatric syrup is 30°C. No special precautions are required for the other presentations.

Legal category POM.

Package quantities
Bactrim Drapsules in packs of 100 and 500.
Bactrim Double Strength tablets in packs of 100.
Bactrim dispersible tablets in packs of 100.
Bactrim paediatric tablets in packs of 100.
Bactrim adult suspension and paediatric syrup in bottles of 100 ml (OP).

Further information
Laboratory test interactions: Bactrim, specifically the trimethoprim component, can interfere with a serum methotrexate assay using the competitive binding protein technique when a bacterial dihydrofolate reductase is used as the binding protein. No interference occurs, however, if methotrexate is measured by radioimmunoassay.

The presence of trimethoprim and sulphamethoxazole may also interfere with the Jaffe alkaline picrate reaction assay for creatinine, causing values in the normal range to be increased by about 10%.

Parenteral formulations: To hospitals only, Bactrim Roche for Infusion is also available for patients in whom parenteral administration is indicated. See separate prescribing literature.

Product licence numbers

Film-Coated Drapsules	0031/5044
Double Strength Tablets	0031/0110
Dispersible Tablets	0031/0075R
Paediatric Tablets	0031/5045
Adult Suspension	0031/5047
Paediatric Syrup	0031/5046.

BACTRIM* ROCHE FOR INFUSION
Approved name: Co-trimoxazole

Presentation Each 5 ml ampoule contains 80 mg trimethoprim and 400 mg sulphamethoxazole in a vehicle containing 40 per cent propylene glycol.

The solution, which is almost colourless to slightly yellow, has a pH of approximately 9 to 10.

Uses
Properties: Bactrim is bactericidal *in vitro* to a wide range of Gram-positive and Gram-negative organisms, including *Streptococcus, Staphylococcus, Pneumococcus, Neisseria, B. catarrhalis, Escherichia coli, Klebsiella, Proteus* spp., *Haemophilus, Salmonella, Shigella, Vibrio cholerae, Brucella, Pneumocystis carinii, Nocardia* and *Bordetella.* A particularly high degree of activity is exhibited against *Haemophilus influenzae, E. coli* and *Proteus* spp., making Bactrim particularly suitable for the treatment of chronic bronchitis and urinary tract infections.

Bactrim exerts its bactericidal action by the sequential blockade of two bacterial enzyme systems in the biosynthesis of folinic acid in the micro-organism. The synergy thus produced accounts for the high degree of bactericidal activity.

Pharmacokinetics: Trimethoprim and sulphamethoxazole are pharmaco-kinetically compatible. This enables the two drugs to be given, as Bactrim, in repeated doses without undue changes to their relative concentrations in the body.

Distribution – Intravenous infusion of Bactrim enables high blood levels to be achieved very quickly. Both components are only moderately bound to plasma proteins (45% for trimethoprim and 60% for sulphamethoxazole), and the free drugs are considered to be the therapeutically active forms *in vivo.* Distribution studies, in animals and humans, have shown that both components are detectable in interstitial and extravascular fluids such as CSF, milk, synovial fluid, sputum and aqueous humour. High concentrations are achieved in the urine.

Elimination – Sulphamethoxazole and trimethoprim are both excreted unchanged and as metabolites, mainly by the kidneys. Both compounds have elimination half-lives of approximately 12 hours.

Renal impairment – Because both compounds are cleared largely via the kidneys, their half-lives are significantly increased in patients with creatinine clearance less than 30 ml per min. Thus reduction of dosage is required when patients with renal impairment are treated with Bactrim (see 'Dosage and administration').

Indications: Clinical experience with oral Bactrim indicates its therapeutic value in the following conditions: Respiratory tract infections, renal and urinary tract infections, gastro-intestinal tract infections caused by *Salmonella typhi* and *paratyphi*. Osteomyelitis, acute brucellosis, skin and wound infections, septicaemias, bacillary dysentery and cholera (as an adjuvant to fluid and electrolyte replacement), nocardiosis and other infections caused by sensitive organisms.

Parenteral administration of Bactrim for Infusion is indicated where oral dosage is not possible, for example:

Pre- and post-operative infections and severe trauma.

Other clinical situations where the patient is unable to take or tolerate oral therapy.

Dosage and administration Bactrim for Infusion is only to be given when diluted in an intravenous infusion as described below.

Duration of therapy: It is intended that Bactrim for Infusion should be used only during such a period as the patient is unable to accept oral therapy with Bactrim. In general, administration is unlikely to be required for more than a few days. At present, it is recommended that the maximum dosage (as indicated below) should not be administered for more than three successive days.

Adults and children over 12 years: 10 ml twice daily.

Maximum dosage (for severe infections): 15 ml twice daily.

The dosage required for the treatment of *Pneumocystis carinii* pneumonitis is generally higher than that recommended for other conditions. A dosage of 20 mg trimethoprim/kg body-weight/day plus 100 mg sulphamethoxazole/kg body-weight/day, given in equally divided doses every six hours for 14 days, is suggested. For this reason, treatment should be undertaken only if facilities for regular monitoring of plasma concentrations of the sulphamethoxazole component are available.

Elderly: If there is renal impairment in the elderly patient then the dosage recommendations given for patients with renal impairment apply. Since elderly patients are more susceptible to blood dyscrasias and adverse reactions in general, caution is recommended when treating these patients (see 'Contra-indications, warnings, etc'—Precautions section).

Children up to 12 years: The recommended dosage is approximately 6 mg trimethoprim/kg body-weight/day plus 30 mg sulphamethoxazole/kg body-weight/day, divided into two equal doses. As a guide, the following dosage regimens may be used.

Age	*Recommended dosage*
6 weeks to 5 months	1.25 ml twice daily
6 months to 5 years	2.5 ml twice daily
6 to 12 years	5 ml twice daily

Patients with impaired renal function

Creatinine clearance (ml/min)	*Recommended dosage*
>30	Usual dosage
15–30	Half the usual dosage
<15	Use of Bactrim not recommended

Mode of administration of Bactrim for Infusion: Bactrim for Infusion is suitable only for use as described below after addition to intravenous infusions. It is *not* suitable for any other route or method of administration.

Bactrim for Infusion must *only* be given by the intravenous route and *must be diluted* according to the schedule given below.

Bactrim for Infusion should only be mixed with one of the following infusion solutions:

Dextrose Injection BP 5% and 10%

Compound Sodium Chloride Injection BPC 1959 (Ringer's Solution)

Sodium Chloride Injection BP

Sodium Chloride and Dextrose Injection BP (0.45% sodium chloride and 2.5% dextrose)

Dextran 70 Injection BP

No other agent should be added to or mixed with the infusion.

Dilution should be carried out as follows:

One ampoule Bactrim for Infusion (5 ml) to 125 ml infusion solution.

Two ampoules Bactrim for Infusion (10 ml) to 250 ml infusion solution.

Three ampoules Bactrim for Infusion (15 ml) to 500 ml infusion solution.

Dilution should be carried out *immediately* before use. After addition of Bactrim for Infusion to the infusion solution, the mixture should be well shaken in order to ensure thorough mixing. Should visible turbidity or crystallisation appear in the solution at any time before or during the infusion, the mixture should be discarded. Infusion solutions containing Bactrim should be used with six hours of their preparation.

It is suggested that the duration of the infusion should be of the order of 1 hour but this should be balanced against the fluid requirements of the patient.

Bactrim Roche for Infusion should be administered intravenously only in the form of the infusion solutions described above, and may not be injected undiluted either intravenously or direct into the infusion tubing.

Contra-indications, warnings, etc

Contra-indications: Bactrim is contra-indicated in patients showing marked liver parenchymal damage, blood dyscrasias, severe renal insufficiency and glucose 6-phosphate dehydrogenase deficiency. Bactrim should not be given to patients with a history of sensitivity to sulphonamides or trimethoprim. Treatment must be immediately discontinued on the appearance of a skin rash or if any element of the blood count is reduced.

Bactrim should not be given to premature babies nor to full term infants during the first six weeks of life.

Use in pregnancy and lactation: The safety of Bactrim in human pregnancy has not been established. There is some evidence of Bactrim, at extremely high doses, having harmful effects in pregnancy in animals. Bactrim should not therefore be given during pregnancy. Sulphonamide-containing products should not be administered in late pregnancy because of the risk of kernicterus. The usual caution in prescribing any drug for women of childbearing age should also be exercised with Bactrim.

Both trimethoprim and sulphamethoxazole are excreted in breast milk. This does not contra-indicate the use of Bactrim in lactating mothers but due account should be taken of the age of the infant being breast-fed.

Precautions: An adequate fluid intake should be ensured to maintain an adequate urinary output in order to prevent crystalluria and stone formation. In cases with renal impairment the dose should be adjusted as indicated in the Dosage and Administration section, to avoid accumulation of the drugs. In such patients, measurement of the plasma concentration of the drugs is advisable. Bactrim should be given with caution to patients with impaired hepatic function and to those patients with severe allergy or bronchial asthma.

There is an increased risk of severe, possible fatal adverse reactions in elderly patients or when complicating conditions exist. In order to minimise the risk of undesirable reactions, the duration of Bactrim treatment should not be unnecessarily prolonged, particularly in elderly patients.

Regular monthly blood counts are necessary whenever long-term therapy is used. This is particularly advisable if Bactrim is to be given to elderly patients for a prolonged period (i.e. exceeding three months), since it has been suggested that the elderly are more susceptible to blood dyscrasias.

Urine analysis and renal function tests should be performed during long-term therapy.

Special caution should be exercised in treating patients with conditions predisposing to folate deficiency.

Bactrim Roche for Infusion contains propylene glycol

and metabisulphite as preservative which can cause hypersensitivity reactions in susceptible individuals.

Drug interactions: An increased incidence of thrombocytopenia with purpura has been observed in elderly patients concurrently receiving certain diuretics, primarily thiazides.

Care should be taken when giving Bactrim to patients receiving strongly serum protein-bound drugs such as oral hypoglycaemic agents or coumarin anticoagulants as the action of these drugs may be increased. It has been reported that Bactrim may prolong the prothrombin time in patients receiving the anticoagulant warfarin. This interaction should be borne in mind when Bactrim is given to patients already on anticoagulant therapy. In such cases, the coagulation time should be re-determined.

Sulphonamides can displace methotrexate from plasma protein binding sites, thus increasing free methotrexate concentrations.

Bactrim may inhibit the hepatic metabolism of phenytoin. A 39 per cent increase in phenytoin half-life and a 27 per cent decrease in the metabolic clearance rate of phenytoin has been observed following administration of Bactrim at normal clinical dosages. If the two drugs are given concurrently, it is important to remain alert for signs of phenytoin toxicity.

Special caution should be exercised in treating patients who are receiving other preparations containing folate inhibitors (e.g. antimalarial drugs containing pyrimethamine; methotrexate) or anticonvulsant drugs. Occasional reports suggest that patients receiving pyrimethamine as malarial prophylaxis in doses exceeding 25 mg weekly may develop megaloblastic anaemia if Bactrim is prescribed concurrently.

Reversible deterioration of renal function has been observed in patients treated with co-trimoxazole and cyclosporin following renal transplantation.

Side-effects and adverse reactions: At the recommended dosage Bactrim is usually well tolerated. The most common side-effects are gastro-intestinal disturbances and allergic skin reactions. Hypersensitivity reactions have occasionally been reported.

Gastro-intestinal effects include nausea, vomiting, glossitis, pancreatitis, stomatitis, diarrhoea and rarely, cases of pseudomembranous enterocolitis have been reported.

Other allergic reactions include anaphylactoid reactions, drug fever, photosensitivity, serum sickness, Henoch-Schoenlein purpura, allergic myocarditis and angiooedema. In addition periarteritis nodosa and systemic lupus erythematosus have been reported.

Rarely, cases of hepatitis have been reported.

Skin rashes are generally mild and quickly reversible on withdrawal of the drug; however, in some cases erythema multiforme (Stevens-Johnson syndrome) and toxic epidermal necrolysis (Lyell syndrome) can occur. The latter condition is associated with a high mortality.

As Bactrim contains a sulphonamide, the possibility of blood dyscrasias like those associated with sulphonamides should be borne in mind. The changes reported with Bactrim mainly consist of thrombocytopenia, purpura, leucopenia, neutropenia, haemolytic anaemia, eosinophilia, and methaemoglobinaemia, and, very rarely, agranulocytosis, pancytopenia and megaloblastic anaemia. They have usually proved to be reversible on withdrawal of the drug. It has been suggested that elderly patients are more susceptible to these blood dyscrasias. The isolated cases of megaloblastic changes reported in the bone marrow during long-term therapy are reversible by folinic acid therapy.

Neurological effects reported include headache, tinnitus, vertigo, ataxia, convulsions and aseptic meningitis.

Musculoskeletal effects include arthralgia and myalgia.

Genito-urinary tract effects include interstitial nephritis, toxic nephrosis, crystalluria, blood urea nitrogen and serum creatinine elevation.

Raised serum levels of SGOT, SGPT, and bilirubin have been reported.

Pulmonary infiltrates such as eosinophilic or allergic alveolitis have been reported in rare instances, which may manifest themselves through symptoms such as cough or shortness of breath. Should such symptoms appear unexpectedly or worsen during Bactrim therapy, the patient should be re-evaluated and discontinuation of the drug should be considered.

Bactrim for Infusion has occasionally given rise to local side-effects in the form of pain and phlebitis.

Treatment of overdosage: Symptoms and signs of overdosage may include nausea, vomiting, mental and visual disturbances, pyrexia, petechiae, purpura, jaundice, anorexia, colic, bone-marrow depression and abdominal pain. Blood dyscrasias are potential late manifestations. Haematuria, crystalluria and anuria may occur in severe cases.

Treatment is symptomatic and may include gastric lavage and forced diuresis. Alkalinisation of the urine may aid the elimination of the sulphamethoxazole component of Bactrim but may decrease the elimination of the trimethoprim component.

Hypersensitivity reactions may require treatment with steroids. Calcium folinate, 3 to 6 mg intramuscularly for five to seven days, may be given to counteract the effects of trimethoprim on haemopoiesis.

Pharmaceutical precautions
Storage: Bactrim for Infusion should be protected from light.

Legal category POM.

Package quantities Bactrim for Infusion, ampoules containing 80 mg trimethoprim and 400 mg sulphamethoxazole in 5 ml, in packs of 10.

Further information
Laboratory test interactions: Bactrim, specifically the trimethoprim component, can interfere with a serum methotrexate assay using the competitive binding protein technique when a bacterial dihydrofolate reductase is used as the binding protein. No interference occurs, however, if methotrexate is measured by radioimmunoassay.

The presence of trimethoprim and sulphamethoxazole may also interfere with the Jaffe alkaline picrate reaction assay for creatinine, causing values in the normal range to be increased by about 10%.

Availability: Bactrim for Infusion is available to hospitals only.

Bactrim is also available as dispersible tablets, film-coated tablets (Drapsules*), Double Strength tablets, paediatric tablets, adult suspension and paediatric syrup. See separate prescribing literature.

Product licence number 0031/0070.

BECOSYM* SYRUP

Presentation Dark red-orange, fruit-flavoured syrup containing thiamine hydrochloride 5 mg, riboflavine 2 mg, nicotinamide 20 mg and pyridoxine hydrochloride 2 mg.

Uses
Properties: The Vitamin B-complex comprises a group of water-soluble factors more or less closely associated in their natural occurrence. It is known that nearly every vitamin of the B-complex forms part of a co-enzyme essential for the metabolism of protein, carbohydrate or fatty acid.

Indications: Treatment of clinical and sub clinical vitamin deficiency states (manifestations of which include glossitis, stomatitis, cheilosis, the heart manifestations of beriberi, the skin manifestations of pellagra, corneal vascularisation and polyneuritis).

Dosage and administration

Adults and children:	5–15 ml daily
Infants:	5 ml daily

Contra-indications, warnings, etc
Contra-indications: Known hypersensitivity to any of the active constituents.

Use in pregnancy: In high doses, pyridoxine may interfere

with prolactin release and should only be used with caution in nursing mothers.

Precautions: Pyridoxine may increase the peripheral metabolism of levodopa, reducing therapeutic efficacy of the latter drug. Therefore patients with Parkinson's disease who are receiving treatment with plain levodopa should not take vitamin B6 in doses that greatly exceed the daily requirement. This does not apply when levodopa is combined with a peripheral decarboxylase inhibitor.

Pharmaceutical precautions The recommended maximum storage temperature is 25°C. Becosym Syrup should be protected from light.

Legal category GSL.

Package quantities Packings of 100 ml.

Further information Nil.

Product licence number 0031/0147.

DALMANE*

Presentation Capsules with opaque grey cap and opaque yellow body with 'ROCHE 15' printed in red on both cap and body, containing 16.4 mg flurazepam monohydrochloride (equivalent to 15 mg flurazepam). Capsules with black cap and opaque grey body with 'ROCHE 30' printed in red on both cap and body, containing 32.8 mg flurazepam monohydrochloride (equivalent to 30 mg flurazepam).

Uses *Properties:* Dalmane is a benzodiazepine drug with hypnotic properties.

Indications: Short-term treatment of insomnia when it is severe, disabling or subjecting the individual to extreme distress. Dalmane is helpful in overcoming difficulties in getting to sleep and also in the problem of frequent nocturnal awakenings. Its properties make it particularly indicated where the total duration of sleep is less than adequate.

Dosage and administration *Adults:* The dosage of Dalmane should be determined on an individual basis taking into account the severity of the insomnia and the patient's response to treatment. Dosage is important in determining the duration of effect and the occurrence of residual effects. For most patients the optimum dose is 15 mg – this will ensure a full night's sleep with minimal residual effects on wakening. Patients with severe insomnia may require 30 mg but residual effects on awakening, associated with an anxiolytic effect, are more frequent at this dose.

ELDERLY OR DEBILITATED PATIENTS: THE INITIAL DOSE SHOULD NOT EXCEED 15 mg.

Treatment should, if possible, be on an intermittent basis. The lowest dose which can control symptoms should be used. Treatment should not be continued at the full dose beyond four weeks. Long-term chronic use is not recommended. Treatment should always be tapered off gradually. Patients who have taken benzodiazepines for a prolonged time may require a longer period during which doses are reduced. Specialist help may be appropriate.

Dalmane is not for paediatric use.

Dalmane capsules are for oral administration.

Contra-indications, warnings, etc *Contra-indications:* Patients with known sensitivity to benzodiazepines; acute pulmonary insufficiency; respiratory depression; phobic or obsessional states; chronic psychosis.

Use in pregnancy: There is no evidence as to drug safety in human pregnancy, nor is there evidence from animal work that it is free from hazard. Do not use during pregnancy, especially during the first and last trimesters, unless there are compelling reasons.

The administration of high doses or prolonged administration of low doses of benzodiazepines in the last trimester of pregnancy has been reported to produce irregularities in the foetal heart rate, and hypotonia, poor sucking and hypothermia in the neonate.

No data regarding the passage of flurazepam in breast milk are available. However, in common with other benzodiazepines, its passage into breast milk might be expected. If possible, the use of Dalmane during lactation should be avoided.

Precautions: In patients with chronic pulmonary insufficiency, and in patients with chronic renal or hepatic disease, dosage may need to be reduced.

Dalmane should not be used alone to treat depression or anxiety associated with depression, since suicide may be precipitated in such patients.

In cases of loss or bereavement, psychological adjustment may be inhibited by benzodiazepines.

Patients should be advised that, like all medicaments of this type, Dalmane may modify patients' performance at skilled tasks (driving, operating machinery, etc.) to a varying degree depending upon dosage, administration and individual susceptibility. Patients should further be advised that alcohol may intensify any impairment, and should, therefore be avoided during treatment. If the patient is awoken during the period of maximum drug activity recall may be impaired.

The dependence potential of the benzodiazepines is low, particularly when limited to short-term use, but this increases when high doses are used, especially when given over long periods. This is particularly so in patients with a history of alcoholism or drug abuse or in patients with marked personality disorders. Regular monitoring in such patients is essential, routine repeat prescriptions should be avoided and treatment should be withdrawn gradually. Symptoms such as depression, nervousness, rebound insomnia, irritability, sweating, and diarrhoea have been reported following abrupt cessation of treatment in patients receiving even normal therapeutic doses for short periods of time.

In rare instances, withdrawal following excessive dosages may produce confusional states, psychotic manifestations and convulsions.

Abnormal psychological reactions to benzodiazepines have been reported. Rare behavioural effects include paradoxical aggressive outbursts, excitement, confusion and the uncovering of depression with suicidal tendencies. Extreme caution should therefore be used in prescribing benzodiazepines to patients with personality disorders.

If Dalmane is combined with centrally-acting drugs such as neuroleptics, tranquillisers, antidepressants, hypnotics, analgesics and anaesthetics, the sedative effects are likely to be intensified. The elderly require special supervision.

When Dalmane is used in conjunction with antiepileptic drugs, side-effects and toxicity may be more evident, particularly with hydantoins or barbiturates or combinations including them. This requires extra care in adjusting dosage in the initial stages of treatment.

Side-effects and adverse reactions: Common adverse effects include drowsiness, sedation, unsteadiness and ataxia; these are dose-related and may persist into the following day, even after a single dose. The elderly are particularly sensitive to the effects of central depressant drugs and may experience confusion, especially if organic brain changes are present; therefore dosage in these patients should not exceed 15 mg.

Other adverse effects are rare and include headache, vertigo, hypotension, gastro-intestinal upsets, skin rashes, visual disturbances, changes in libido, and urinary retention. Isolated cases of blood dyscrasias and jaundice have also been reported

Occasionally patients treated with Dalmane experience a bitter after-taste.

Treatment of overdosage: When taken alone in overdosage, Dalmane presents few problems in management. Signs may include drowsiness, ataxia and dysarthria, with coma in severe cases. Treatment is symptomatic. Gastric lavage is useful only if performed soon after ingestion. Anexate* is a specific IV antidote for use in emergency situations. Patients requiring such intervention should be monitored closely in hospital (see separate prescribing information).

When taken with centrally-acting drugs, especially

alcohol, the effects of overdosage are likely to be more severe and, in the absence of supportive measures, may prove fatal.

Pharmaceutical precautions *Storage:* Dalmane capsules in blister packings should be stored in a dry place. The recommended maximum storage temperature is 25°C.

Legal category CD (Sch. 4), POM.

Package quantities Dalmane capsules 15 mg and 30 mg in blister packs of 30 (OP).

Further information The pharmacokinetic properties of Dalmane make it particularly indicated for patients whose total duration of sleep is less than adequate. The dosage of the drug is important in balancing the duration of effect with the occurrence of residual effects. On repeated dosing there is accumulation of an active metabolite, desalkylflurazepam, with steady state levels being reached within two to three weeks. Psychomotor studies have demonstrated, however, that a dose of 15 mg given for seven consecutive nights did not significantly affect performance on the morning after final administration. However, impairment of performance was recorded on the morning after final administration of 30 mg for seven consecutive nights. This dose is associated with daytime anxiolytic effects.

The elderly, and patients with impaired renal and/or hepatic function, will be particularly susceptible to the adverse effects listed above. It is advisable to review treatment regularly and to discontinue use as soon as possible.

Treatment should be kept to minimum and given only under close medical supervision. Little is known regarding the efficacy or safety of benzodiazepines in long-term use.

An underlying cause for insomnia should be sought before deciding upon the use of benzodiazepines for symptomatic relief.

Product licence numbers
Capsules 15 mg 0031/0065
Capsules 30 mg 0031/0066

DECLINAX*

Presentation Round, white tablets with 'ROCHE 10' imprinted on one face and a single break bar on the other, containing 12.8 mg debrisoquine sulphate (equivalent to 10 mg base).

Round, pale blue tablets with 'ROCHE 20' imprinted on one face and two break bars on the other, containing 25.6 mg debrisoquine sulphate (equivalent to 20 mg base).

Uses *Properties:* Declinax lowers blood pressure markedly and promptly in the hypertensive patient. It does this by blocking the transmission of sympathetic nerve impulses at the nerve terminals, thereby decreasing peripheral vascular resistance. Reduction in post-ganglionic sympathetic transmission is achieved by interfering with the physiological release of noradrenaline, without depleting major catecholamine stores in cardiovascular tissues and without impairing the cardiac contractile mechanism. The action, as with other adrenergic neurone blocking agents, is most marked in the standing position. Declinax normally acts within 4–10 hours and its effects usually last for 9–24 hours, although an occasional patient may show a longer response. There is no accumulation on maintenance dosage.

Indications: Declinax is indicated for the treatment of all grades of hypertension. It can be given either alone or together with other antihypertensive drugs or diuretics.

Dosage and administration *Adults: Mild to moderate hypertension:* 10 mg once or twice daily. This dose can be increased by 10 mg at three-day intervals. The total dose usually falls within the range 20–60 mg daily.

Adults: Severe hypertension: 20 mg once or twice daily. This dose can be increased, depending on response, by 10–20 mg every three or four days provided a close check is kept on the blood pressure. When initially treating severe hypertension with Declinax, the diastolic pressure should not be reduced below 110 mmHg as impaired autoregulatory mechanisms may lead to impaired perfusion of vital organs. The total dose usually falls within the range 40–120 mg, but in cases of severe hypertension 300 mg or more daily may be given. Although some tolerance to the drug may occur during long-term therapy, requiring increased dosage, this has usually been moderate and not posed special problems.

Should postural hypotension occur with a dosage that controls the blood pressure, the total daily dose should be adjusted to give a small dose in the morning, a relatively large dose at midday and a moderate evening dose. Adequate control of blood pressure is frequently obtained with Declinax alone but, if necessary, its effects can be enhanced by the addition of therapy with a diuretic or another antihypertensive drug (e.g. a beta-adrenergic blocking agent).

Elderly: There is inadequate evidence of the safety of Declinax in the elderly, although it has been in wide use for many years without apparent ill consequence specifically relating to elderly populations. However, as with other potent hypotensive agents, including alpha-adrenergic blockers, the possibility of postural hypotension occurring should be borne in mind.

Children: There is inadequate evidence of the safety of Declinax in children although it has been in wide use for many years without apparent ill consequence specifically relating to childhood.

Declinax tablets are for oral administration.

Contra-indications, warnings, etc
Contra-indications: Declinax should not be given to patients with a phaeochromocytoma or with a recent history of cerebral or myocardial infarction. It is contra-indicated in patients who have shown hypersensitivity to the drug.

Use in pregnancy: There is inadequate evidence of safety of Declinax in human pregnancy but it has been in wide use for many years without apparent ill consequence, animal studies having shown no hazard.

Precautions: Declinax should be used with caution in patients with renal or hepatic insufficiency; smaller or more widely spread doses may be appropriate.

Declinax may give rise to exertional and postural hypotension (see *Side-effects*). Caution should therefore be exercised in patients with coronary or cerebral insufficiency.

The possibility of an enhanced hypotensive effect should be borne in mind when any drug with a tendency to lower blood pressure is given concomitantly with Declinax.

As with other potent hypotensive agents, including alpha-adrenergic blockers, the possibility of postural hypotension occurring in the elderly should be borne in mind.

Patients on antihypertensive drugs often have a lower blood pressure in warm weather, therefore in hot climates their dose of Declinax may need to be reduced. Evidence from both animal experiments and clinical observation suggests that the hypotensive action of adrenergic neurone-blocking drugs such as Declinax may be inhibited by simultaneous treatment with tricyclic antidepressants, monoamine oxidase inhibitors, and fenfuramine. Extra care should be taken when prescribing antihypertensive drugs in patients being treated with levodopa. Patients taking Declinax are sensitive to sympathomimetic drugs.

If anaesthesia for surgery or dentistry is necessary, the anaesthetist should be informed that the patient is being treated with Declinax.

Abrupt cessation of Declinax should be avoided as this may lead to rebound hypertension.

Side-effects: Declinax is well tolerated. Overdosage causes postural hypotension, most noticeable in the early morning or with long standing and associated with weakness, giddiness, fatigue and rarely syncope. The patient should be warned of the possibility of these symptoms occurring. This can be minimised by reducing the dose. Other reported side-effects include malaise, nausea, headache, sweating, oedema, muscle weakness, failure of ejaculation in the male, and sometimes disturbances of micturition and nocturia. Diarrhoea, common with some other antihypertensive agents, is seen only very rarely. Aggravation of angina pectoris has been reported in a few cases.

Effects of overdosage and their treatment: Excessive fall in blood pressure will be shown by orthostatic collapse. This will usually respond rapidly to placing the patient in a recumbent position. Patients receiving Declinax are particularly sensitive to the effects of catecholamines. Sympathomimetic agents should therefore be administered only with great caution.

Pharmaceutical precautions *Storage:* No special storage precautions required.

Legal category POM.

Package quantities Declinax tablets 10 mg in packings of 100.

Declinax tablets 20 mg in packings of 100.

Further information The metabolism of debrisoquine is subject to genetic polymorphism such that non-metabolisers may show a marked response (e.g. orthostatic hypotension) to doses that have little or no effect in metabolisers.

New patients should be carefully monitored during the initial treatment to determine possible non-metabolisers (approximately 8% of Caucasian populations).

Product licence numbers
Tablets 10 mg 0031/5059R
Tablets 20 mg 0031/5060R

EFUDIX*

Presentation White, opaque cream containing 5% w/w fluorouracil.

Uses *Properties:* Efudix is a topical cytostatic preparation which exerts a beneficial therapeutic effect on neoplastic and pre-neoplastic skin lesions without damaging normal skin. The pattern of response follows this sequence: erythema, vesiculation, erosion, ulceration, necrosis and epithelisation.

Indications: Efudix is used for the topical treatment of superficial pre-malignant and malignant skin lesions; keratoses, including senile, actinic and arsenical forms; keratoacanthoma; Bowen's disease; superficial basal-cell carcinoma.

Deep, penetrating or nodular basal cell and squamous cell carcinomas do not usually respond to Efudix therapy. It should be used only as a palliative therapy in such cases where no other form of treatment is possible.

Dosage and administration *Pre-malignant conditions:* The cream should be applied thinly to the affected area once or twice daily; an occlusive dressing is not essential.

Malignant conditions: The cream should be applied once or twice daily under an occlusive dressing where this is practicable.

The cream should not harm healthy skin. Treatment should be continued until there is a marked inflammatory response from the treated area, preferably with some erosion in the case of pre-malignant conditions. Severe discomfort may be alleviated by the use of topical steroid cream. The usual duration of treatment for an initial course of therapy is three to four weeks, but this may be prolonged. Lesions on the face usually respond more quickly than those on the trunk or lower limbs whilst lesions on the hands and forearms respond more slowly. Healing may not be complete until one or two months after therapy is stopped.

Elderly: Many of the conditions for which Efudix is indicated are common in the elderly. No special precautions are necessary.

Children: In view of the lack of clinical data available, Efudix is not recommended for use in children.

Efudix cream is for topical application.

Contra-indications, warnings, etc
Contra-indications: Efudix is contra-indicated in patients with known hypersensitivity to Efudix or parabens.

Use in pregnancy: There is evidence from animal work that fluorouracil is teratogenic and there is no evidence as to drug safety in human pregnancy. Therefore the use of Efudix is contra-indicated during pregnancy. It should also be regarded as contra-indicated in mothers who are breast-feeding.

Precautions: Efudix is for topical use only and care should be taken to avoid contact with mucous membranes or the eyes. The hands should be washed carefully after applying the cream.

The total area of skin being treated with Efudix at any one time should not exceed 500 cm^2 (approx 23 × 23 cm). Larger areas should be treated a section at a time.

Side-effects: Efudix is well tolerated. Transient erythema may occur in healthy skin surrounding the area being treated. Pre-existing subclinical lesions may become apparent. Exposure to sunlight may increase the intensity of the reaction.

Percutaneous absorption of fluorouracil has not led to clinically significant systemic toxicity when Efudix is administered as directed. However, this possibility should be borne in mind if the product is used excessively, especially on ulcerated or broken skin.

Effects of overdosage and their treatment: If Efudix is accidentally ingested, signs of fluorouracil overdosage may include nausea, vomiting and diarrhoea. Stomatitis and blood dyscrasias may occur in severe cases. Appropriate measures should be taken for the prevention of systemic infection and daily white cell counts should be performed.

Pharmaceutical precautions *Storage:* The recommended maximum storage temperature for Efudix cream is 30°C.

Dilution: Efudix cream should not be diluted.

Legal category POM.

Package quantities Efudix cream in tubes of 20 g (OP).

Further information
Availability: Efudix cream is available through hospital pharmacies for use in hospitals and hospital clinics and can be supplied to retail pharmacies for dispensing prescriptions for patients whose treatment has been initiated by a specialist in oncology or dermatology, in the NHS or otherwise, whose bona fide can be identified by the dispensing pharmacist.

Efudix should be used only under specialist medical supervision.

Product licence number 0031/0027

EPHYNAL* SUSPENSION

Presentation A water miscible suspension of tocopheryl acetate, 500 mg/5 ml.

Uses
Properties: Ephynal suspension contains a synthetic vitamin E preparation. The exact role of vitamin E in the animal organism has not yet been established. Vitamin E is known to exert an important physiological function as an antioxidant for fats, with a sparing action on vitamin A, carotenoids and on unsaturated fatty acids. Other work has demonstrated that vitamin E is connected with the maintenance of certain factors essential for the normal metabolic cycle.

Vitamin E is absorbed from the gastro-intestinal tract. Most of the vitamin appears in the lymph and is then widely distributed to all tissues. Most of the dose is slowly excreted in the bile and the remainder is eliminated in the urine as glucuronides of tocopheronic acid or other metabolites.

Indications: Ephynal suspension is indicated for the

correction of vitamin E deficiency occurring in malabsorption disorders, i.e. cystic fibrosis, chronic cholestasis and abetalipoproteinaemia.

Dosage and administration
Adults and the elderly: For the treatment of malabsorption disorders the following doses should be administered:

cystic fibrosis	100–200 mg/day
abetalipoproteinaemia	50–100 mg/kg/day

Children: For the treatment of cystic fibrosis a dose of 50 mg/day should be given to children less than 1 year and 100 mg/day to children 1 year and over.

The adult dosage should be used for the treatment of abetalipoproteinaemia (50–100 mg/kg/day).

Infants with vitamin E deficiency which is secondary to chronic cholestasis may be treated with doses of 150–200 mg/kg/day.

Ephynal suspension may be diluted with Syrup BP but should be used immediately and not stored.

Ephynal suspension is for oral administration.

Contra-indications, warnings, etc
Contra-indications: Known hypersensitivity to vitamin E.

Use in pregnancy and lactation: There is no evidence of the safety of high doses of vitamin E in pregnancy nor is there evidence from animal work that it is free from hazard, therefore do not use in pregnancy especially in the first trimester.

No information is available on excretion into breast milk, therefore it is advisable not to use during lactation.

Precautions: Vitamin E has been reported to increase the risk of thrombosis in patients who are predisposed to this condition, including patients taking oestrogens. This finding has not been confirmed but should be borne in mind when selecting patients for treatment with Ephynal suspension, in particular women taking oral contraceptives containing oestrogens.

A higher incidence of necrotising enterocolitis has been noted in lower weight premature infants (less than 1.5 kg) treated with vitamin E.

Side-effects and adverse reactions: Diarrhoea and abdominal pain may occur with doses greater than 1 g daily.

Treatment of overdosage: Transient gastro-intestinal disturbances have been reported with doses greater than 1 g daily and, where necessary, general supportive measures should be employed.

Pharmaceutical precautions Ephynal suspension may be diluted with Syrup BP but the diluted suspension should be used immediately and not stored.

Storage: Ephynal suspension should be stored at or below 25°C and should be used within 1 month after opening the bottle.

Legal category GSL.

Package quantities Bottles of 100 ml.

Further information Nil.

Product licence number 0031/5076R.

FANSIDAR*

Presentation Round, white tablets with ROCHE and a hexagon imprinted on one face and two break bars on the other, containing 500 mg sulfadoxine and 25 mg pyrimethamine.

Uses *Properties:* The mode of action of Fansidar is based on the reciprocal potentiation of its two components. Fansidar blocks the action of two enzymes which catalyse consecutive stages in the biosynthesis of folinic acid in malaria parasites. Larger doses of the components of Fansidar are necessary if they are given independently and the effect obtained is inferior to that of the combination.

Fansidar is effective against plasmodial strains which are resistant to chloroquine and/or pyrimethamine and other antifolate preparations.

With Fansidar, the danger of emergence of resistance is reduced. However, in certain malarious areas, particularly South-East Asia and South America, strains of *Plasmodium falciparum* may be encountered which have developed resistance to Fansidar. Fansidar affects all developmental stages of the parasites. It has a prolonged action, yet effective plasma concentrations are rapidly attained after a single dose. Trophozoites and schizonts quickly disappear from the blood. Pre-erythrocytic stages are also affected and the gametocytes, although increased in number, are rendered much less infective for the vector. A protective effect persists for up to two to four weeks depending on the dose given and the immune state of the subject.

Indications: Treatment and prophylaxis of *Plasmodium falciparum* malaria.

Treatment of malaria: Fansidar is indicated for the treatment of *Plasmodium falciparum* malaria when the infection is contracted in an area of chloroquine resistance.

Prophylaxis of malaria: Malaria prophylaxis with Fansidar is indicated for travellers to areas where chloroquine-resistant *Plasmodium falciparum* malaria is endemic. Whenever malaria prophylaxis is prescribed, the malaria situation and in particular, resistance trends at the traveller's destination and any stop-over point must be considered. At present, there is no antimalarial agent which provides absolute protection against malaria, but conscientiously performed drug prophylaxis can usually prevent serious progression of the disease.

Dosage and administration
Curative treatment of malaria: The appropriate amount of the drug is given in one single dose. This dose should not be repeated for at least seven days.

Adults (higher dose for persons over 60 kg)			2 to 3 tablets
Children	10–14 years	(31–45 kg)	2 tablets
	7–9 years	(21–30 kg)	1½ tablets
	4–6 years	(11–20 kg)	1 tablet
	under 4 years	(5–10 kg)	½ tablet

In very severe cases, quinine may be added, preferably parenterally. An adequate supply of fluids and electrolytes should be maintained.

Prophylactic management: The following dose of Fansidar should be taken every seven days:

Adults			1 tablet
Children	9–14 years	(30–45 kg)	¾ tablet
	4–8 years	(11–29 kg)	½ tablet
	under 4 years	(5–10 kg)	¼ tablet

Regular dosage is important for continuous protection to be maintained.

Routine measures to protect against mosquito bites should not be omitted.

Fansidar prophylaxis should be started about one week before entering the endemic area in order to assess tolerance; this will enable an alternative drug to be selected in the infrequent case where Fansidar is poorly tolerated.

IMPORTANT: Fansidar prophylaxis should be continued for four to six weeks after returning to a non-malarious area to ensure elimination of possible falciparum infections (malignant malaria). However, as with other prophylactic drugs, infections of benign malaria (vivax and malariae infections) may give rise to clinical attacks up to several months after return, despite regular prophylaxis.

Travellers should be instructed to report to a doctor any fever that occurs during or after their stay in a malarious area.

Use in the elderly: Although no specific studies have been performed to establish the use of Fansidar in the elderly, it has been used extensively and the dosage requirements and side-effects appear to be similar to those of younger adults.

Fansidar tablets are for oral administration.

Contra-indications, warnings, etc
Contra-indications: Patients with known sulphonamide hypersensitivity.

Prophylactic (repeated) use of Fansidar is contra-indicated in patients with severe renal insufficiency, marked liver parenchymal damage or blood dyscrasias.

Treatment must be immediately discontinued upon the appearance of any mucocutaneous signs or symptoms such as pruritus, erythema, rash, orogenital lesions or pharyngitis and a medical practitioner consulted.

The possibility of an adverse drug reaction should be considered in patients developing a rash, jaundice, fever or severe generalized malaise during treatment with Fansidar.

Like all other preparations containing sulphonamides, Fansidar is contra-indicated in premature babies and during the first two months of life.

Use in pregnancy: Foetal damage has been observed in the rat when any drug containing a folate inhibitor, including Fansidar, is administered in early gestation. The damage is caused by the folic acid antagonist, pyrimethamine, a component of Fansidar; the damage can be prevented by the concomitant administration of folinic acid.

However, no such adverse effects attributed to Fansidar have been reported during human clinical use and the preparation is, therefore, not contra-indicated during pregnancy. The usual medical practice of avoiding the use of Fansidar during early pregnancy should be followed unless considered essential by a medical practitioner. Pregnant women should be made aware of the particular risks of contracting malaria during pregnancy, and should be advised not to undertake unnecessary journeys to endemic areas. A folate supplement should be given to pregnant women receiving Fansidar.

Although no cases have been documented to date, there is a possibility that use of Fansidar during pregnancy at term may produce kernicterus in the neonate.

Both pyrimethamine and sulfadoxine are excreted in maternal breast milk. Nursing mothers should not take Fansidar.

Precautions: Excessive exposure to the sun should be avoided.

Regular blood counts are recommended during long-term prophylactic use (over three months) of Fansidar.

Drug interactions: Concurrent administration of other preparations containing folate antagonists (e.g. co-trimoxazole, methotrexate, anticonvulsants) can result in increased impairment of folic acid metabolism which leads to haematological side-effects. Such concomitant therapy should be avoided if possible. There is evidence which may indicate an increase in incidence and severity of adverse reactions when chloroquine is used with Fansidar, as compared to the use of Fansidar alone.

Side-effects and adverse reactions: Fansidar is usually well tolerated at the recommended dosage.

As with other drugs containing sulphonamides and/or pyrimethamine, the following side-effects and hypersensitivity reactions may occur:

Skin reactions: Drug rash, pruritus and slight hair loss have been observed. These reactions are usually mild and disappear spontaneously upon withdrawal of the drug. In very rare instances, particularly in hypersensitive patients, cases of erythema multiforme, Stevens–Johnson syndrome and Lyell's syndrome have occurred, some of which have been fatal.

Gastro-intestinal reactions: Feeling of fullness, nausea, rarely vomiting, stomatitis. There have been isolated reports of hepatitis occurring conjointly with administration of Fansidar.

Haematological changes: In rare cases, leucopenia (usually asymptomatic), thrombocytopenia and megaloblastic anaemia have been observed. In extremely rare cases, they take the form of agranulocytosis or purpura. As a rule, all these changes disappear after withdrawal of the drug.

Other side-effects: Fatigue, headache, fever and polyneuritis may occasionally occur.

Pulmonary infiltrates such as eosinophilic or allergic alveolitis have been reported in rare instances. If symptoms such as cough or shortness of breath should occur during Fansidar therapy, the drug should be discontinued.

Adverse reactions occurring after the administration of the sulfadoxine component of Fansidar are not normally more prolonged than those occurring after shorter-acting sulphonamides despite the continued presence of the drug in the body.

Treatment of overdosage: Possible symptoms of overdosage include anorexia, nausea, vomiting, signs of excitation, and possibly convulsions and haematological changes (megaloblastic anaemia, leucopenia, thrombocytopenia).

Treatment is symptomatic and may include forced diuresis. Vigorous gastric lavage should be carried out as early as possible after ingestion. Alkalinization of the urine may aid elimination of the sulfadoxine component of Fansidar. Possible convulsions due to the pyrimethamine components of Fansidar should be watched for and may require anticonvulsant therapy.

Hypersensitivity reactions may require treatment with steroids. Calcium folinate may be given to counteract the effects of pyrimethamine on haemopoiesis.

Pharmaceutical precautions *Storage:* No special precautions are required.

Legal category POM.

Package quantities Fansidar tablets are available in foil strips in packs of 10.

Further information
Pharmacokinetics

Absorption: After administration of 1 tablet, peak plasma levels for pyrimethamine (0.21 mg per litre) and for sulfadoxine (63.2 mg per litre) are reached after about four hours (means obtained from 14 test subjects).

Elimination: A relatively long elimination half-life is characteristic of both components. The mean values are 96 hours for pyrimethamine and 184 hours for sulfadoxine. Both pyrimethamine and sulfadoxine are eliminated mainly via the kidneys.

Accumulation: Patients taking 1 tablet a week (recommended adult dose for malaria prophylaxis) can be expected to have mean steady state plasma concentrations of 0.15 mg per litre for pyrimethamine (after about four weeks) and 98.4 mg per litre for sulfadoxine (after about seven weeks).

Protein binding: The following values were determined for binding to plasma protein: pyrimethamine 84.9% and sulfadoxine 91.4%.

Product licence number 0031/5097R.

FLUORO-URACIL ROCHE

Presentation Ampoules containing 250 mg fluoro-uracil in the form of the sodium salt in 10 ml Water for Injection BP. The ampoule solution is colourless to slightly yellow.

Capsules with powder blue opaque cap and orange opaque body with ROCHE printed in black along both cap and body, containing 250 mg fluorouracil.

Uses *Properties:* Fluoro-uracil Roche, a cytostatic agent, is a fluorinated pyrimidine belonging to the category of antimetabolites. It inhibits cell division by interfering with the synthesis of deoxyribonucleic acid (DNA) and to a lesser extent of ribonucleic acid (RNA).

Indications: The palliative treatment of carcinoma.

Dosage and administration Various techniques are employed when using Fluoro-uracil Roche in the treatment of carcinoma. The following examples are given for guidance.

Adults: By the intravenous route: Fluoro-uracil Roche may be administered by intravenous infusion or by intravenous injection. Dosages are generally based on the patient's body weight. If the patient is obese or there has been a spurious gain due to oedema, ascites or other forms of fluid retention, the patient's ideal weight should be used in calculating the dosage. The initial doses given below should be reduced by one-third to a half if the following conditions are present: poor nutritional state; after major surgery (within the previous 30 days); poor bone-marrow function (anaemia, leucopenia, thrombocytopenia); impaired hepatic or renal function.

Initial treatment: This may be in the form of an infusion or injection, the former usually being preferred because of lesser toxicity.

Infusion: A daily dose of 15 mg/kg but not more than 1 g per infusion is diluted in 500 ml dextrose 5% solution or 500 ml 0.9% sodium chloride solution and given by intravenous infusion at the rate of 40 drops per minute over four hours. Alternatively, the daily dose may be infused over 30–60 minutes, or given as a continuous infusion over 24 hours. This daily dose is given on successive days until toxicity occurs or until 12–15 g has been given. This sequence of injections constitutes a 'course' of therapy. Some patients have received up to 30 g at a maximum rate of 1 g daily. The daily dose should never exceed 1 g. An interval of four to six weeks should be allowed between any two 'courses' of Fluoro-uracil Roche.

Injection: A dose of 12 mg/kg i.v. daily on three consecutive days. If there are no signs of toxicity the patient receives 6 mg/kg i.v. on the fifth, seventh and ninth days. If toxicity occurs the signs should be allowed to regress before further doses are administered.

Maintenance therapy consists of 5–15 mg/kg i.v. once weekly.

A more recent alternative method is to give 15 mg/kg i.v. once a week throughout the course of treatment.

This obviates the need for an initial period of daily administration.

Regional perfusion intra-arterially: Continuous infusion of Fluoro-uracil Roche into an artery supplying a localised growth has been shown to produce a better result in some tumours than would have been expected from systemic administration by the intravenous route, together with a decrease in toxicity. The usual dose is 5–7.5 mg/kg daily.

In combination with radiotherapy: Irradiation combined with Fluoro-uracil Roche has been found to be useful in the treatment of certain types of metastatic lesions in the lungs and for relief of pain caused by recurrent, inoperable growth. The standard dose of Fluoro-uracil Roche is used.

By the oral route: Fluoro-uracil Roche may be administered orally using either the capsule or the ampoule solution.

Oral administration is not recommended when Fluoro-uracil Roche is being used initially as the sole agent in palliative treatment of carcinoma. Oral administration may be useful in: palliative therapy employing a combination of drugs; long-term maintenance or post-operative prophylactic therapy in weekly doses; and where therapy with Fluoro-uracil Roche is indicated, but it is impracticable to administer the drug parenterally.

The usual dosage for maintenance treatment is 15 mg/kg once weekly. For palliative therapy a more rapid onset of therapeutic effect may be obtained by giving a daily dose of 15 mg/kg on six successive days. This is followed by maintenance therapy of 15 mg/kg once weekly. The daily dose should not exceed 1 g.

The capsules should be taken with water after a meal.

The solution may be mixed with fruit juice or other similar beverages immediately before oral ingestion to mask its rather bitter taste. Multi-dose preparations must not be made up.

Elderly: Fluoro-uracil Roche should be used in the elderly with similar consideration as in younger adults, notwithstanding that incidence of concomitant medical illness is higher in the former group.

Children: No dosage recommendations are made for the administration of Fluoro-uracil Roche to children.

Fluoro-uracil Roche ampoules are for intra-arterial, intravenous or oral administration.

Fluoro-uracil Roche capsules are for oral administration.

Contra-indications, warnings, etc

Contra-indications: Fluoro-uracil Roche should not be used in the management of non-malignant disease.

Use in pregnancy: Fluoro-uracil Roche has been shown to be teratogenic. It therefore should not normally be administered to patients who are pregnant. Fluoro-uracil Roche should also be regarded as contra-indicated in mothers who are breast-feeding.

Precautions: It is recommended that Fluoro-uracil Roche be given only by or under the supervision of a physician who is experienced in cancer chemotherapy and who is well versed in the use of potent antimetabolites. Because of the possibility of severe toxic reactions, all patients should be admitted to hospital for initial treatment. Fluoro-uracil Roche should be used with great care in debilitated patients.

The margin between the effective and toxic doses of Fluoro-uracil Roche is narrow and a therapeutic response is unlikely without some evidence of toxicity. Even with meticulous selection of patients and careful adjustment of dosage, there may be severe haematological toxicity and gastro-intestinal haemorrhage. Severe toxicity is more likely in poor-risk patients.

Treatment should be discontinued promptly whenever one of the following signs of toxicity appears: Leucopenia (WBC under 3,500 per mm^3). Thrombocytopenia (platelets under 100,000 per mm^3). Stomatitis (the first small ulceration at the inner margin of the lips is a signal for stopping treatment). Severe diarrhoea (frequent bowel movements and watery stools). Gastro-intestinal ulceration and bleeding. Haemorrhage at any site.

Isolated cases of angina, ECG abnormalities and rarely myocardial infarction have been reported following Fluoro-uracil Roche administration. Caution should therefore be exercised in treating patients who experience chest pain during courses of therapy, or patients with a history of heart disease.

The carcinogenic potential of Fluoro-uracil Roche has not been evaluated but, as with all cystostatic drugs, this possibility should be borne in mind when designing long-term management of patients.

Side-effects: During treatment, diarrhoea, nausea and vomiting commonly occur, but may be controlled by the use of appropriate drugs.

Leucopenia usually follows an adequate course of treatment with Fluoro-uracil Roche. The lowest white cell count commonly occurs between the seventh and fourteenth days after the first dose, but it may be delayed for as long as the twentieth day. By the thirtieth day, the count has usually returned to the normal range. Because of the importance of leucopenia, the white cell count should be checked frequently throughout the course. If it falls, it is advisable to obtain differential counts. If the total is less than 2,000 per mm^3, and especially if there is granulocytopenia, it is recommended that the patient be placed in protective isolation in the hospital and treated with appropriate measures for the prevention of systemic infection.

Alopecia and dermatitis may occur in a substantial proportion of cases. Female patients particularly should be warned as to the possibility of alopecia. Since the alopecia appears to be reversible, special measures do not seem to be indicated.

Treatment of overdosage: Signs and symptoms are qualitatively similar to the side-effects, and similar measures should be taken to treat them.

Handling precautions: Fluorouracil is irritant, contact with skin and mucous membranes should be avoided.

Handling guidelines: Ampoules: Fluorouracil ampoules should only be opened by trained staff and as with all cytotoxic agents, precautions should be taken to avoid exposing staff during pregnancy.

Preparation of solution for administration should be carried out in a designated handling area and working over a washable tray or disposable plastic-backed absorbent paper.

Suitable eye protection, disposable gloves, face mask and disposable apron should be worn.

Syringes and infusion sets should be assembled carefully to avoid leakage (use of Luer lock fittings is recommended).

On completion, any exposed surface should be thoroughly cleaned and hands and face washed.

Capsules: Undamaged capsules present minimal risk of contamination but in accordance with good hygiene requirements, direct handling should be avoided. As with all cytotoxic agents, precautions should be taken to avoid exposing staff during pregnancy.

Disposal guidelines: All sharps should be placed in an appropriate container and all other disposable items in a sealed plastic bag which should be incinerated with other clinical waste.

Waste material may be disposed of by incineration. Waste ampoule solution may first be absorbed onto cotton wool and double wrapped in sealed polythene bags.

First aid: Eye Contact: Irrigate immediately with water and seek medical advice.

Skin Contact: Wash thoroughly with soap and water and remove contaminated clothing.

Inhalation, Ingestion: Seek immediate medical attention.

Pharmaceutical precautions *Storage:* Fluoro-uracil Roche ampoule solution should be stored between 15°C and 25°C.

Fluorouracil Roche capsules in blister packings should be stored in a dry place; the recommended maximum storage temperature is 25°C.

Additives: Fluoro-uracil Roche ampoule solution may be diluted with Dextrose Injection, Sodium Chloride Injection or Water for Injection BP immediately before parenteral use.

Fluoro-uracil Roche ampoule solution may be diluted with fruit juice or other similar beverages immediately before use to facilitate ingestion by the oral route. Fluoro-uracil Roche ampoule solution must not be made up into multi-dose preparations.

Legal category POM.

Package quantities Fluoro-uracil Roche ampoules in packings of 10.

Fluoro-uracil Roche capsules in blister packings of 30.

Further information *Availability:* Fluoro-uracil Roche ampoules are available through hospital pharmacies for use in hospitals and hospital clinics and can be supplied to retail chemists for dispensing prescriptions for patients whose treatment has been initiated in hospital practice.

Product licence numbers
Ampoules 0031/5079R
Capsules 0031/0139

HYPNOVEL* AMPOULES 10 mg/2 ml

Presentation Colourless glass ampoules containing 10 mg of midazolam base as the hydrochloride in 2 ml aqueous solution. The ampoule solution is colourless.

Uses *Properties:* Midazolam is a potent imidazobenzodiazepine, forming water-soluble salts which are stable and well tolerated by injection. Midazolam possesses the typical pharmacological properties of the benzodiazepines, namely hypnotic, anxiolytic, muscle-relaxant and anticonvulsant activity. In clinical use the induction of sleep is the main action.

At sedative and anaesthetic doses, given intravenously, the action is rapid in onset and of short duration; anterograde amnesia frequently accompanies the period of peak sedation.

When given by intramuscular injection, Hypnovel is very rapidly absorbed and has a bioavailability of greater than 90%. The onset of action is relatively rapid and may be accompanied by anterograde amnesia. On intramuscular injection, Hypnovel is well tolerated locally.

The mean elimination half-life of midazolam is about 2 hours.

Indications: As intravenous sedative cover before and during minor medical, dental and surgical procedures such as gastroscopy, endoscopy, cystoscopy, bronchoscopy and cardiac catheterization.

As an intramuscular premedication for patients with physical status ASA I-IV who are to undergo surgical procedures.

As an alternative intravenous agent for the induction of anaesthesia in high risk and elderly patients, especially where cardiovascular stability is of particular importance. Induction is more reliable when heavy opiate premedication has been administered or when Hypnovel is given with a narcotic analgesic such as fentanyl.

Dosage and administration *Intravenous sedation:* One or more intravenous administrations over a single operating session.

In most circumstances, the 10 mg/5 ml formulation is more convenient for titration purposes.

Adults: An assessment should be made of the degree of sedation necessary for the planned procedure.

The dose should be titrated against the response of the patient. The desired titration end point will depend upon the procedure. Full sedation will be evident by drowsiness, slurred speech but response to commands will be maintained.

As a guide it is recommended that 0.4 ml of Hypnovel 10 mg/2 ml solution (equivalent to 2 mg midazolam) be administered intravenously over 30 seconds. If after 2 minutes, sedation is not adequate, incremental doses of 0.1 ml to 0.2 ml of Hypnovel 10 mg/2 ml solution (0.5 to 1 mg midazolam) should be given.

Usual dosage range 2.5 mg–7.5 mg total dose (equivalent to around 0.07 mg/kg body weight).

Elderly: THE ELDERLY ARE MORE SENSITIVE TO THE EFFECTS OF BENZODIAZEPINES AND IN THESE PATIENTS LOW DOSES AS LITTLE AS 1 mg–2 mg (0.2–0.4 ml) MAY BE ADEQUATE. THE INITIAL DOSE SHOULD NOT EXCEED 1–1.5 mg (0.2–0.3 ml).

Children: Hypnovel has not been evaluated for use as an intravenous sedative in children.

Combination therapy: Where analgesia is provided by a narcotic analgesic the latter should be administered first, the dose of Hypnovel should be carefully titrated and low doses 1 mg–2 mg (0.2–0.4 ml Hypnovel) may be adequate. In the elderly smaller doses as little as 0.5–1 mg (0.1–0.2 ml Hypnovel) may be adequate.

Mode of administration: For the administration of Hypnovel the patient should be placed in a supine position and remain there throughout the procedure. Resuscitation facilities should always be available and a second person fully trained in the use of such equipment should always be present. It is recommended that patients should remain under medical supervision until at least 1 hour has elapsed from the time of injection. They should always be accompanied home by a responsible adult.

Patients who have received Hypnovel alone for IV sedation prior to minor procedures should be warned not to drive or operate machinery for 8 hours. Where Hypnovel is used concurrently with other central nervous system depressants (e.g. potent analgesics) recovery may be prolonged. Patients should therefore be assessed carefully before being allowed to go home or resume normal activities.

Intravenous induction of anaesthesia: One or more bolus intravenous injections over a single anaesthetic session.

Adults: The dose should be titrated against the individual response of the patient. Hypnovel should be given by slow intravenous injection until there is a loss of eyelid reflex, response to commands and voluntary movements.

In anticipating the required dose of Hypnovel, both the premedication already given and the age of the patient are important. Young, fit unpremedicated patients may require at least 0.3 mg/kg body-weight, whereas patients premedicated with an opiate usually require only 0.2 mg/kg body-weight.

Elderly: THE ELDERLY ARE MORE SENSITIVE TO THE EFFECTS OF BENZODIAZEPINES. INDUCTION MAY BE ADEQUATE WITH 0.1 mg/kg BODY-WEIGHT IN PREMEDICATED PATIENTS AND 0.2 mg/kg BODY-WEIGHT IN UNPREMEDICATED PATIENTS.

Children over 7 years: Hypnovel has been shown to be an effective agent for induction of anaesthesia in children over 7 years of age, at a dose of 0.15 mg/kg body-weight.

Intramuscular premedication: Adults: A single intramuscular injection of 0.07–0.1 mg/kg body-weight, administered 30–60 minutes pre-operatively, has been shown to be adequate in most cases. The usual dose is about 5 mg.

Atropine or hyoscine hydrobromide may be given concomitantly, bearing in mind that hyoscine hydrobromide will enhance and prolong the sedative and amnesic effects of Hypnovel.

Hypnovel can be combined with atropine or hyoscine hydrobromide in the same syringe to be given as a single intramuscular injection.

Elderly: THE ELDERLY ARE MORE SENSITIVE TO THE EFFECTS OF BENZODIAZEPINES AND IN THESE PATIENTS THE LOWER DOSE OF 2.5 mg MAY BE ADEQUATE.

Children: Hypnovel has not been evaluated for use as an intramuscular premedicant in children.

Contra-indications, warnings, etc
Contra-indications: Benzodiazepine sensitivity; acute pulmonary insufficiency; respiratory depression.

Use in pregnancy: Animal experiments have not indicated any teratogenic risk with Hypnovel but evaluation in human pregnancy has not been undertaken. Therefore Hypnovel should not be used during pregnancy unless this is considered essential by the physician.

The administration of high single doses of benzodiazepines in the last trimester of pregnancy has been reported to produce irregularities in the foetal heart rate, and hypotonia, poor sucking and hypothermia in the neonate. Hypnovel ampoule solution should not, therefore, be used during the last trimester.

Hypnovel may pass into breast milk and caution should be exercised with its use in lactating mothers.

Precautions: When Hypnovel is given along with central nervous system depressants, such as potent analgesics, the sedative effect may be intensified and the possibility of severe respiratory or cardiovascular depression should be considered.

Patients should be instructed to avoid alcohol before and for at least 8 hours after administration of Hypnovel since the individual response cannot be foreseen.

Hypnovel should be given with caution to patients with pulmonary insufficiency, impairment of renal or hepatic function, to elderly or debilitated patients, and to patients with myasthenia gravis.

Disinhibiting effects have been noted, even after a single dose. This should therefore be borne in mind if treating patients with a history of personality disorders.

Side-effects: Changes in cardiovascular parameters are slight but can include a decrease in mean arterial pressure, cardiac output, stroke volume and systemic vascular resistance. Such changes may be important in patients with impaired myocardial oxygen delivery capacity and hypovolaemia.

Following intravenous application of Hypnovel, respiratory depression and respiratory arrest have occurred. These life-threatening incidents may occur especially in elderly patients or patients with pre-existing respiratory insufficiency, particularly if excessive or too rapidly-injected doses are administered.

Other side effects reported include headache, dizziness and hiccoughs. Local effects on veins are infrequent. However, pain on injection and thrombophlebitis may occur.

Treatment of overdosage: Overdosage may produce airway obstruction, apnoea, hypotension and cardiopulmonary collapse in severe cases. Anexate* is a specific IV antidote for use in emergency situations. Patients requiring such intervention should be monitored closely in hospital (see separate prescribing information).

Pharmaceutical precautions *Additives:* Hypnovel ampoule solution is stable, both physically and chemically, for up to 1 hour at room temperature when mixed in the same syringe with Atropine Sulphate Injection 500 mcg/ml, or Hyoscine Hydrobromide Injection 0.4 mg/ml.

There is no evidence of the adsorption of midazolam into the plastic of infusion apparatus or syringes.

Legal category CD (Sch. 4) POM.

Package quantities Hypnovel ampoules 10 mg/2 ml in packings of 10.

Further information The 'second peak' effect, which is known to occur following intravenous diazepam, has not been observed with Hypnovel.

The metabolites of Hypnovel do not contribute significantly to the clinical effects of the drug.

Although admixture with large-volume parenteral fluids is not recommended for use in the indications described above, Hypnovel ampoule solution is stable, both physically and chemically, for up to 24 hours at room temperature when mixed with 500 ml infusion fluids containing Dextrose 4% with Sodium Chloride 0.18%, Dextrose 5% or Sodium Chloride 0.9%.

Admixture with Hartmann's solution is not recommended, as the potency of midazolam decreases.

Hypnovel ampoules 10 mg/5 ml are also available, and are recommended especially for intravenous administration of the drug where careful dosage titration is required (see separate literature).

Product licence number 0031/0126

HYPNOVEL* AMPOULES 10 mg/ 5 ml

Presentation Colourless glass ampoules containing 10 mg of midazolam base as the hydrochloride in 5 ml aqueous solution. The ampoule solution is colourless.

Uses
Properties: Midazolam is a potent imidazobenzodiazepine, forming water-soluble salts which are stable and well tolerated by injection. Midazolam possesses the typical pharmacological properties of the benzodiazepines, namely hypnotic, anxiolytic, muscle-relaxant and anticonvulsant activity. In clinical use the induction of sleep is the main action.

At sedative and anaesthetic doses, given intravenously, the action is rapid in onset and of short duration; anterograde amnesia frequently accompanies the period of peak sedation.

The mean elimination half-life of midazolam is about 2 hours.

Indications: As intravenous sedative cover before and during minor medical, dental and surgical procedures such as gastroscopy, endoscopy, cystoscopy, bronchoscopy and cardiac catheterisation.

As an alternative intravenous agent for the induction of anaesthesia in high risk and elderly patients, especially where cardiovascular stability is of particular importance. Induction is more reliable when heavy opiate premedication has been administered or when Hypnovel is given with a narcotic analgesic such as fentanyl.

Dosage and administration
Intravenous sedation: One or more intravenous administrations over a single operating session.

Adults: An assessment should be made of the degree of sedation necessary for the planned procedure.

The dose should be titrated against the response of the patient. The desired titration end point will depend upon the procedure. Full sedation will be evident by drowsiness, slurred speech but response to commands will be maintained.

As a guide it is recommended that 1 ml of Hypnovel 10 mg/5 ml solution (equivalent to 2 mg midazolam) be administered intravenously over 30 seconds. If after 2 minutes, sedation is not adequate, incremental doses of 0.25 ml to 0.5 ml of Hypnovel 10 mg/5 ml solution (0.5 to 1 mg midazolam) should be given.

Usual dosage range 2.5 mg–7.5 mg total dose (equivalent to around 0.07 mg/kg body weight).

Elderly: THE ELDERLY ARE MORE SENSITIVE TO THE EFFECTS OF BENZODIAZEPINES AND IN THESE PATIENTS LOW DOSES AS LITTLE AS 1 mg–2 mg (0.5–1.0 ml) MAY BE ADEQUATE. THE INITIAL DOSE SHOULD NOT EXCEED 1–1.5 mg (0.5–0.75 ml).

Children: Hypnovel has not been evaluated for use as an intravenous sedative in children.

Combination therapy: Where analgesia is provided by a narcotic analgesic the latter should be administered first, the dose of Hypnovel should be carefully titrated and low doses 1 mg–2 mg (0.5–1.0 ml Hypnovel) may be adequate. In the elderly smaller doses as little as 0.5–1 mg (0.25–0.5 ml Hypnovel) may be adequate.

Mode of administration: For the administration of Hypnovel the patient should be placed in a supine position and remain there throughout the procedure. Resuscitation facilities should always be available and a second person fully trained in the use of such equipment should always be present. It is recommended that patients should remain under medical supervision until at least 1 hour has elapsed from the time of injection. They should always be accompanied home by a responsible adult.

Patients who have received Hypnovel alone for IV sedation prior to minor procedures should be warned not to drive or operate machinery for 8 hours. Where Hypnovel is used concurrently with other central nervous system depressants (e.g. potent analgesics) recovery may be prolonged. Patients should therefore be assessed carefully before being allowed to go home or resume normal activities.

Intravenous induction of anaesthesia: One or more bolus intravenous injections over a single anaesthetic session.

Adults: The dose should be titrated against the individual response of the patient. Hypnovel should be given by slow intravenous injection until there is a loss of eyelid reflex, response to commands and voluntary movements.

In anticipating the required dose of Hypnovel, both the premedication already given and the age of the patient are important. Young, fit unpremedicated patients may require at least 0.3 mg/kg body-weight, whereas patients premedicated with an opiate usually require only 0.2 mg/kg body-weight.

Elderly: THE ELDERLY ARE MORE SENSITIVE TO THE EFFECTS OF BENZODIAZEPINES. INDUCTION MAY BE ADEQUATE WITH 0.1 mg/kg BODY-WEIGHT IN PREMEDICATED PATIENTS AND 0.2 mg/kg BODY-WEIGHT IN UNPREMEDICATED PATIENTS.

Children over 7 years: Hypnovel has been shown to be an effective agent for induction of anaesthesia in children over 7 years of age, at a dose of 0.15 mg/kg body-weight.

Contra-indications, warnings, etc
Contra-indications: Benzodiazepine sensitivity; acute pulmonary insufficiency; respiratory depression.

Use in pregnancy: Animal experiments have not indicated any teratogenic risk with Hypnovel but evaluation in human pregnancy has not been undertaken. Therefore Hypnovel should not be used during pregnancy unless this is considered essential by the physician.

The administration of high single doses of benzodiazepines in the last trimester of pregnancy has been reported to produce irregularities in the foetal heart rate, and hypotonia, poor sucking and hypothermia in the neonate. Hypnovel ampoule solution should not, therefore, be used during the last trimester.

Hypnovel may pass into breast milk and caution should be exercised with its use in lactating mothers.

Precautions: When Hypnovel is given along with central nervous system depressants, such as potent analgesics, the sedative effect may be intensified and the possibility of severe respiratory or cardiovascular depression should be considered.

Patients should be instructed to avoid alcohol before and for at least 8 hours after administration of Hypnovel since the individual response cannot be foreseen.

Hypnovel should be given with caution to patients with pulmonary insufficiency, impairment of renal or hepatic function, to elderly or debilitated patients, and to patients with myasthenia gravis. Disinhibiting effects have been noted, even after a single dose. This possibility should therefore be borne in mind if treating patients with a history of personality disorders.

Side-effects: Changes in cardiovascular parameters are slight but can include a decrease in mean arterial pressure, cardiac output, stroke volume and systemic vascular resistance. Such changes may be important in patients with impaired myocardial oxygen delivery capacity and hypovolaemia.

Following intravenous application of Hypnovel, respiratory depression and respiratory arrest have occurred. These life-threatening incidents may occur especially in elderly patients or patients with pre-existing respiratory insufficiency, particularly if excessive or too rapidly injected doses are administered.

Other side-effects reported include headache, dizziness and hiccoughs. Local effects on veins are infrequent. However, pain on injection and thrombophlebitis may occur.

Treatment of overdosage: Overdosage may produce airway obstruction, apnoea, hypotension and cardiopulmonary collapse in severe cases. Anexate* is a specific IV antidote for use in emergency situations. Patients requiring such intervention should be monitored closely in hospital (see separate prescribing information).

Pharmaceutical precautions *Additives:* There is no evidence of the adsorption of midazolam onto the plastic of infusion apparatus or syringes.

Legal category CD (Sch. 4) POM.

Package quantities Hypnovel ampoules 10 mg/5 ml in packings of 10.

Further information The second peak effect, which is known to occur following intravenous diazepam, has not been observed with Hypnovel.

The metabolites of Hypnovel do not contribute significantly to the clinical effects of the drug.

Although admixture with large-volume parenteral fluids is not recommended for use in the indications described above, Hypnovel ampoule solution is stable, both physically and chemically, for up to 24 hours at room temperature when mixed with 500 ml infusion fluids containing Dextrose 4% with Sodium Chloride 0.18%, Dextrose 5% or Sodium Chloride 0.9%.

Admixture with Hartmann's solution is not recommended, as the potency of midazolam decreases.

Hypnovel ampoules 10 mg/2 ml are also available, and are recommended especially for use as an intramuscular premedication (see separate literature).

Product licence number 0031/0189.

KONAKION*

Presentation White, sugar-coated tablets printed ROCHE in black across one face, containing 10 mg phytomenadione.

Ampoules containing 1 mg phytomenadione in 0.5 ml.

Ampoules containing 10 mg phytomenadione in 1 ml.

The ampoule solution, which is clear to opalescent greenish-yellow in colour, contains a polyethoxylated castor oil as a non-ionic surfactant.

Uses *Properties:* Konakion is a synthetic preparation of vitamin K_1. The presence of vitamin K (i.e. vitamin K_1 itself or substances with vitamin K activity) is essential for the formation within the body of prothrombin, factor

VII, factor IX and factor X. Lack of vitamin K leads to increased tendency to haemorrhage. When an antidote to an anticoagulant is necessary it is essential to use vitamin K_1 itself, as vitamin K analogues are much less effective.

Indications: Konakion is indicated in the treatment of haemorrhage or threatened haemorrhage associated with a low blood level of prothrombin or factor VII. The main indications are: An antidote to anticoagulant drugs of the coumarin type. Prevention and treatment of neonatal haemorrhage.

Dosage and administration *Adults: As an antidote to anticoagulant drugs*

For potentially fatal and severe haemorrhage: Konakion therapy should be accompanied by a more immediate effective treatment such as transfusions of whole blood or blood clotting factors. The anticoagulant should be withdrawn and an intravenous injection of Konakion given slowly in a dose of 10–20 mg (1 to 2 ampoules). The prothrombin level should be estimated three hours later, and if the response has been inadequate, the dose should be repeated. Not more than 40 mg of Konakion should be given intravenously in 24 hours.

Less severe haemorrhage: Konakion is given orally in doses of 10–20 mg (1 to 2 tablets). The prothrombin level is estimated 8 to 12 hours later, and if the response has been inadequate, the dose should be repeated. Intramuscular injections of Konakion may also be given in doses of 10–20 mg (1 to 2 ampoules), repeated if necessary.

Lowering of prothrombin to dangerous level but no haemorrhage: A dose of 5–10 mg Konakion orally may be given to bring the prothrombin level back to within safe limits. In such instances it is not usually necessary to discontinue the anticoagulant.

Adults: Other indications: Doses of 10–20 mg as required.

Use in the elderly: Elderly patients tend to be more sensitive to reversal of anticoagulation with Konakion; dosage in this group should be at the lower end of the ranges recommended for adults.

Children: If, on the recommendation of a physician, a children's dosage is required, then it is suggested that 5–10 mg be given.

Treatment of newborn infants: Prophylactic: 1 mg by intramuscular injection.

Therapeutic: 1 mg by intramuscular injection, repeated at eight-hourly intervals if necessary.

Konakion tablets are for oral administration and should be chewed or allowed to dissolve slowly in the mouth.

Konakion ampoules are for intramuscular or intravenous injection.

Konakion ampoule solution should not be diluted.

Contra-indications, warnings, etc
Contra-indications: Use in patients with a known hypersensitivity to any of the constituents (see *Precautions*).

Use in pregnancy: There is no specific evidence regarding the safety of Konakion in early pregnancy, but as with most drugs, the administration during pregnancy should only occur if the benefits outweigh the risks.

Precautions: Konakion ampoules contain a polyethoxylated castor oil as a non-ionic surfactant. In animal studies, polyethoxylated castor oil can produce severe anaphylactoid reactions associated with histamine release. There is strong circumstantial evidence that similar reactions occurring in patients may have been caused by polyethoxylated castor oil. Polyethoxylated castor oil, when given to patients over a period of several days, can also produce abnormal lipoprotein electrophoretic patterns, alterations in blood viscosity and erythrocyte aggregation.

In potentially fatal and severe haemorrhages due to overdosage of coumarin anticoagulants, intravenous injections of Konakion must be administered slowly and not more than 40 mg should be given during a period of 24 hours. Konakion therapy should be accompanied by a more immediate effective treatment such as transfusions of whole blood or blood clotting factors. When patients with prosthetic heart valves are given transfusions for the treatment of severe or potentially fatal haemorrhages, fresh frozen plasma should be used.

Side-effects: The too rapid intravenous administration of vitamin K_1 has caused reactions, including flushing of the face, sweating, a sense of chest constriction, cyanosis and peripheral vascular collapse.

Repeated intramuscular injection of vitamin K_1 preparations, usually over prolonged periods in patients with hepatic disease, may give rise to local cutaneous and subcutaneous changes.

Pharmaceutical precautions *Storage:* Konakion ampoule solution should be protected from light; it should not be allowed to freeze. The recommended maximum storage temperature for Konakion ampoules is 30°C.

Konakion tablets should be stored in well-closed containers, and protected from light.

Legal category POM.

Package quantities Konakion tablets in packs of 25.

Konakion ampoules 1 mg in 0.5 ml and 10 mg in 1 ml, in packs of 10.

Further information Large doses of Konakion should be avoided if it is intended to continue with anticoagulant therapy. Vitamin K_1 is not an antidote to heparin.

Product licence numbers

Tablets	0031/5022R
Ampoules 1 mg	0031/5023R
Ampoules 10 mg	0031/5077R

LARIAM* ▼

Presentation Tablets containing 274.09 mg mefloquine hydrochloride, equivalent to 250 mg mefloquine base.

Uses *Pharmacological properties:* The effectiveness of Lariam in the therapy and prophylaxis of malaria is due essentially to destruction of the asexual blood forms of the malarial pathogens that affect humans (*Plasmodium falciparum, P. vivax, P. malariae, P. ovale*).

Lariam is also effective against malarial parasites resistant to other antimalarials such as chloroquine and other 4-aminoquinoline derivatives, proguanil, pyrimethamine and pyrimethamine-sulfonamide combinations.

Pharmocokinetics: Absorption: The maximum plasma concentration is reached within two to twelve hours after a single oral dose of Lariam. The level in nanograms per millilitre is roughly equivalent to the dose in milligrams (for example, approximately 1,000 ng per ml after a dose of 1,000 mg).

Maximum steady-state plasma concentrations of 1,000 ng per ml have been recorded at a weekly dosage of 250 mg (prophylactic maintenance dosage). The RBC concentration is almost twice as high as the plasma level. 98.2% of mefloquine is bound to plasma protein.

Elimination: The average half-life of mefloquine in Europeans is 21 days. Investigations in humans carried out to date have shown that only a minute proportion of the active ingredient is excreted unchanged in the urine. Animal studies (in rats) suggest that excretion is primarily via the bile and faeces.

Indications: Therapy and prophylaxis of malaria.

Therapy: Lariam is especially indicated for therapy of *P. falciparum* malaria in which the pathogen has become resistant to other antimalarial agents.

Following treatment of *P. vivax* malaria with Lariam, relapse prophylaxis with an 8-amino-quinoline derivative, for example primaquine, should be considered in order to eliminate parasites in the hepatic phase.

Prophylaxis: Malaria prophylaxis with Lariam is particularly recommended for travellers to malarious areas in which multiple resistant *P. falciparum* strains occur.

Dosage and administration
Curative treatment: The total dosage of Lariam for adults and for children weighing over 45 kg is 1,250 to 1,500 mg. A lower total dosage of 750–1,000 mg Lariam is sufficient for patients living in malarious areas, because they are already partially immune. Children of less than 45 kg bodyweight (irrespective of immunity status) receive 25 mg per kg. The following dosage schedules are used:

Non-immune patients	*Up to 60 kg*	*Over 60 kg*
Loading dose	3 tablets	3 tablets
After 6–8 hours	2 tablets	2 tablets
After a further 6–8 hours	—	1 tablet
Semi-immune patients		
Loading dose	3 tablets	3 tablets
After 6–8 hours	—	1 tablet
Children, irrespective of immunity status	*Under 45 kg*	
Single dose	25 mg per kg bodyweight = 1 tablet per 10 kg = ¼ tablet per 2.5 kg	

Malaria prophylaxis: Prophylaxis of malaria with Lariam should be initiated one week before arrival in a malarious area. The following dosage schedules are given as a guide:

(a) Dosage for brief stays (one to three weeks in the endemic area):

	Dosage	*Course of prophylaxis*
Adults and children of more than 45 kg bodyweight	1 tablet	Stated dose to be given once weekly, always on the same day, for six weeks. First dose one week before departure. Further doses at weekly intervals during and after visiting the malarious area.
Children (over 15 kg)		
15–19 kg	¼ tablet	
20–30 kg	½ tablet	
31–45 kg	¾ tablet	

(b) Dosage for prolonged stays (more than three weeks in the endemic area)†:

	Dosage	*Course of prophylaxis*
Adults and children of more than 45 kg bodyweight	1 tablet	First to fourth dose once weekly, always on the same day. After the fourth dose, further doses at two-weekly intervals. First dose one week before arriving in malarious area, last two doses at a two-weekly interval after leaving malarious area.
Children (over 15 kg)		
15–19 kg	¼ tablet	
20–30 kg	½ tablet	
31–45 kg	¾ tablet	

† To prevent selection of resistant Plasmodium strains, administration of Lariam should be restricted to three months.

The tablets should be swallowed whole with plenty of liquid (if possible, not on an empty stomach).

Contra-indications, warnings, etc
Contra-indications: Prophylactic use in patients with renal insufficiency or severe impairment of liver function should be regarded for the time being as a contra-indication as no experience has been gained in such patients.

Patients with a history of psychiatric disturbances or convulsions should not be prescribed Lariam prophylactically.

Use in pregnancy and lactation: There is too little clinical experience in humans to assess any possible damaging effects of Lariam during pregnancy. However, mefloquine is teratogenic when administered to rats and mice in early gestation. Therefore, Lariam should be used in pregnancy only if there are compelling medical reasons. In the absence of clinical experience, prophylactic use during pregnancy should be avoided as a matter of principle.

As mefloquine is secreted into the breast milk, nursing mothers should not breast-feed while taking Lariam.

Precautions: Women of childbearing potential travelling to malarious areas in which multiple resistant *P. falciparum* is found and who are receiving Lariam for the treatment and prophylaxis of malaria should take reliable contraceptive precautions for the entire duration of therapy and for three months after the last dose of Lariam.

As yet no experience has been gained with the use of Lariam in young children.

In rare cases if a second dose is considered necessary for treatment this should not be taken before 7 days have elapsed.

Patients should not disregard the possibility that re-infection or recrudescence may occur after effective antimalarial therapy.

Effects on ability to drive and to use machines.
Treatment: Mefloquine can cause dizziness or disturbed sense of balance. It is consequently recommended not to drive or to carry out tasks demanding fine coordination and spatial discrimination during treatment with mefloquine. Patients should avoid such tasks for at least two weeks following therapeutic use.

Prophylactic use: Caution should be exercised with regard to driving, piloting aircraft and operating machines, as dizziness or disturbed sense of balance have been reported during use of Lariam.

Side-effects and adverse reactions: Curative treatment: On administration of Lariam in the higher doses required, the following side-effects have been observed (listed in descending order of frequency): dizziness or disturbed sense of balance (therefore caution should be exercised with regard to driving, piloting aircraft and operating machines), nausea, vomiting, loose stools or diarrhoea, abdominal pain, loss of appetite; other, rare reactions: headache, bradycardia, rash or pruritus, feeling of weakness; extremely rare: transient elevation of transaminases, psychological changes (eg depressive mood, confusion, anxiety, hallucinations, paranoid reactions).

Malaria prophylaxis: In the dosage range recommended for prophylaxis side effects are rare. However, there have been occasional reports of psychological changes similar to those seen with curative therapy. During prophylactic use, therefore, if signs of unexplained anxiety, restlessness or confusion are noticed, these may be considered prodromal to a more serious event. In these cases the drug must be stopped.

Drug interactions: Lariam must not be administered concurrently with quinine since this could increase the risk of convulsions. In severe cases, however, patients may be treated initially for one or more days with quinine given intravenously, and subsequently with Lariam. Aggravation of side-effects can be largely precluded by delaying administration of Lariam until at least twelve hours after the last dose of quinine.

There are no known cases of interactions with antipyretics or analgesics (acetylsalicyclic acid and paracetamol, for example).

Experience is insufficient as yet to rule out the possibility of interactions with cardioactive agents, for example, beta blockers. Since interactions with oral antidiabetics and oral anticoagulants have not so far been excluded, the relevant parameters should be checked before the patient's departure when Lariam is taken for malaria prophylaxis.

Treatment of overdosage: In cases of overdosage with Lariam, the symptoms mentioned under 'Side-effects' may be more pronounced. Countermeasures: gastric lavage, close monitoring of cardiac function (ECG).

Pharmaceutical precautions
Storage: Protect from moisture.

Legal category POM.

Package quantities Tablets (cross-scored) in packs of 6.

Product licence number 0031/0236.

LARODOPA*

Presentation Round, white tablets with 'ROCHE' in a hexagon imprinted on one face and two break bars on the other, containing 500 mg levodopa.

Uses *Properties:* Larodopa is an anti-Parkinsonian agent. Levodopa is the metabolic precursor of dopamine. The latter is severely depleted in the striatum, pallidum and substantia nigra of Parkinsonian patients and it is considered that administration of Larodopa raises the level of available dopamine in these centres.

Treatment with Larodopa gives worthwhile sustained relief in about two-thirds of these patients. Akinesia usually responds first, then rigidity and then tremor. Amelioration may be seen in other symptoms, including oculogyric crises. It may take six months or more before maximal improvement is achieved.

Indications: Parkinsonism – idiopathic, post-encephalitic and arteriosclerotic. Previous neurosurgery is not a contra-indication to Larodopa.

Dosage and administration Dosage and administration are variable and no more than a guide can be given.

Adults: Hospitalised patients: Initially 0.25–1 g daily in up to five divided doses immediately after food. Dosage should be increased by 0.5–1 g every three to four days until adequate improvement results or intolerable side-effects appear. If severe side-effects appear, the dosage should be gradually decreased to the maximum tolerated. The majority of patients will tolerate the rapid dose increase outlined above, but occasionally intolerance may prevent patients from reaching effective dosage levels. When patients discontinue therapy due to intolerance they should be restarted on 0.25 to 0.5 g daily in small divided doses, increasing by 0.125 to 0.5 g at weekly intervals.

Adults: General practice patients and out-patients: Initially 0.125 g twice daily immediately after food. After one week, the dose may be increased to 0.125 g four or five times daily. Thereafter dosage should be increased at weekly intervals by 0.375 g daily, the total daily dose being given in four or five divided doses. The response of individual patients varies and some patients may tolerate a more rapid rate of increase, e.g. by 0.25–0.5 g daily at intervals of three to four days.

Improvement is usually seen in two to three weeks with the normal dosage range being 2.5–8g daily, but further improvement may occur up to six months or even longer.

When the optimum daily dosage for any particular patient has been reached, it may need to be redistributed throughout the day to meet fluctuations in the individual's requirements. Most patients find a four or five times daily dosage scheme satisfactory; some obtain a smoother effect with two-hourly administration; others, who develop akinetic crises at particular times of the day, learn by experience the daily dosage scheme most suited to their needs.

After a period at the maximum tolerated dosage level, side-effects may slowly develop, usually in the form of involuntary movements. These generally regress without loss of therapeutic effect if the dosage is slightly reduced.

Anticholinergic drugs should be continued during Larodopa therapy. As treatment with Larodopa proceeds and the therapeutic effect is found, the dosage of the anticholinergic drugs may need to be changed.

Elderly: Elderly patients with Parkinson's disease have been treated with Larodopa. However, Larodopa tolerance is less in the elderly and produces more severe hypotensive side effects in older patients with Parkinson's disease especially those with a history of myocardial infarction.

Children: No dosage recommendations are made for the administration of Larodopa to children.

Larodopa tablets are for oral administration.

Contra-indications, warnings, etc

Contra-indications: Larodopa is contra-indicated in narrow-angle glaucoma (it may be used in wide-angle glaucoma provided that the intra-ocular pressure remains under control); severe psychoneuroses or psychoses; severe endocrine, renal, hepatic or cardiac disorders.

It should not be given in conjunction with monoamine oxidase inhibitors or within two weeks of their withdrawal.

It should not be given to patients under 25 years of age.

Suspicion has arisen that levodopa may activate a malignant melanoma. Therefore Larodopa should not be used in persons who have a history of, or who may be suffering from, a malignant melanoma.

Use in pregnancy: There is no, or inadequate evidence of safety of the drug in human pregnancy; it has been in wide use for many years without apparent ill-consequence; there is evidence of harmful effects in pregnancy in animals.

Levodopa therapy may interfere with lactation; this should be borne in mind if treatment is required in breast-feeding mothers.

Precautions: Pyridoxine (vitamin B_6) which is often included in multivitamin preparations is known to block the effects of levodopa.

Drugs which interfere with central amine mechanisms, such as rauwolfia alkaloids (reserpine), tetrabenazine (Nitoman), metoclopramide, phenothiazines, thioxanthenes, butyrophenones and amphetamines, and papaverine should be avoided where possible. If, however, their administration is considered essential, extreme care should be exercised and a close watch kept for any signs of potentiation, antagonism or other interactions and for any unusual side-effects.

In the event of general anaesthesia being required, Larodopa therapy may be continued as long as the patient is able to take fluids and medication by mouth. If therapy is temporarily interrupted, the usual daily dosage may be administered as soon as the patient is able to take oral medication. Whenever therapy has been interrupted for longer periods, dosage should again be adjusted gradually; however, in many cases the patient can rapidly be returned to his previous therapeutic dosage.

There have been occasional reports of a neuroleptic malignant-like syndrome, involving hyperthermia, on abrupt withdrawal of levodopa preparations. Sudden discontinuation of Larodopa without close supervision, or 'drug holidays' should therefore be avoided.

Care should be taken when using Larodopa in the following circumstances: in endocrine, renal, pulmonary or cardiovascular disease, particularly where there is a history of myocardial infarction or arrhythmia; psychiatric disturbances; hepatic disorder; peptic ulcer; osteomalacia; where sympathomimetic drugs may be required (e.g. bronchial asthma), due to possible potentiation of the cardiovascular effects of levodopa; where antihypertensive drugs are being used, due to possible increased hypotensive action.

Periodic evaluation of hepatic, haemopoietic, renal and cardiovascular functions is advised.

Patients who improve on Larodopa therapy should be advised to resume normal activities gradually as rapid mobilisation may increase the risk of injury.

Side-effects: Tolerance to Larodopa varies widely between patients and is often related to the rate of dosage increase. Post-encephalitic Parkinsonian patients tolerate the drug less well. Side-effects, usually dose-related, occur at some time in most patients. During the initiation of therapy nausea and vomiting, anorexia, weakness and hypotension, which is usually postural (but a labile hypertension may rarely be seen), are most frequent. Nausea and vomiting may be minimised by administering Larodopa immediately after food; an anti-emetic, e.g. cyclizine hydrochloride 50 mg three times daily, may also be helpful.

Psychiatric disturbances are common in Parkinsonian patients, including those being treated with levodopa. They include mild elation, anxiety, agitation, insomnia, depression, aggression, delusions, hallucinations and 'unmasking' of psychoses. Although there have been rare reports of possible antagonism of levodopa by diazepam, in general diazepam (Valium Roche) and nitrazepam (Mogadon) have been found to be useful in the treatment of anxiety and insomnia, respectively, occurring in Parkinsonism. Depression may be treated with tricyclic antidepressants although isolated cases of hypertensive crisis have been reported with the concomitant use of tricyclic drugs. ECT may be administered if appropriate. MAO inhibitors, except selective MAO-B inhibitors, must not be used.

Involuntary movements, commonly in the form of oral dyskinesia, often accompanied by 'paddling' foot movements, or of the choreo-athetoid type, are common, particularly on long-term administration. These are usually dose-dependent and may disappear or become tolerable after dose adjustment.

With long-term administration, fluctuations in the therapeutic response may be encountered. They include 'freezing' episodes, end-of-dose deterioration and the so-called 'on-off' effect. Patients may be helped by dosage reduction or by giving smaller and more frequent doses.

Other side-effects which have occasionally been reported with levodopa therapy include gastrointestinal bleeding, flushing, sweating and drowsiness.

On some occasions the urine passed during Larodopa treatment may be altered in colour; usually red-tinged, this will turn dark on standing. These changes are due to metabolites and are no cause for concern.

Transient rises in SGOT, SGPT and alkaline phosphatase values have been noted; serum uric acid and blood urea nitrogen levels are occasionally increased.

In rare instances, haemolytic anaemia, mild transient leucopenia and thrombocytopenia have been reported.

Also, in rare instances, headache and peripheral neuropathy have been reported.

Treatment of overdosage: Symptoms of overdosage are qualitatively similar to the side-effects but may be of greater magnitude.

Treatment should include gastric lavage, general supportive measures, intravenous fluids and the maintenance of an adequate airway. Electrocardiographic monitoring should be instituted and the patient carefully observed for the possible development of arrhythmias. If necessary, anti-arrhythmic therapy should be given and other symptoms treated as they arise.

Pharmaceutical precautions *Storage:* Larodopa tablets should be stored in well-closed containers, protected from light.

Legal category POM.

Package quantities Larodopa tablets in packings of 200.

Further information Nil.

Product licence number 0031/5063R.

LEXOTAN*

Presentation Lilac, hexagonal biconvex tablets having L1.5 imprinted on one face and a single break bar on the other, containing 1.5 mg bromazepam.

Pink, hexagonal biconvex tablets having L3 imprinted on one face and a single break bar on the other, containing 3 mg bromazepam.

Uses *Properties:* Lexotan is a pyridylbenzodiazepine compound with anxiolytic properties.

Indications: Lexotan is indicated for the short-term (2–4 weeks) symptomatic treatment of anxiety that is severe, disabling or subjecting the individual to unacceptable distress, occurring alone or in association with insomnia or short-term psychosomatic, organic or psychotic illness.

Dosage and administration *Adults:* The optimum dosage and frequency of administration of Lexotan should be based on the individual patient, the severity of symptoms and previous psychotropic drug history.

The usual dosage in general practice is from 3 mg to 18 mg daily in divided doses.

In exceptional circumstances, in hospitalised patients, up to the maximum daily dosage of 60 mg, in divided doses, may be given.

Elderly: ELDERLY PATIENTS ARE MORE SENSITIVE TO THE ACTIONS OF LEXOTAN; DOSES SHOULD NOT EXCEED HALF THOSE NORMALLY RECOMMENDED.

The lowest dose which can control symptoms should be used. Treatment should not be continued at the full dose beyond four weeks. Long-term chronic use is not recommended. Treatment should always be tapered off gradually. Patients who have taken benzodiazepines for a prolonged time may require a longer period during which doses are reduced. Specialist help may be appropriate.

Children: Lexotan is not for paediatric use.

Lexotan tablets are for oral administration.

Contra-indications, warnings, etc

Contra-indications: Patients with known sensitivity to benzodiazepines; acute pulmonary insufficiency; respiratory depression; phobic or obsessional states; chronic psychosis.

Use in pregnancy: There is no evidence as to drug safety in human pregnancy, nor is there evidence from animal work that it is free from hazard. Do not use during pregnancy, especially during the first and last trimesters unless there are compelling reasons.

The administration of high doses or prolonged administration of low doses of benzodiazepines in the last trimester of pregnancy has been reported to produce irregularities in the foetal heart rate, and hypotonia, poor sucking and hypothermia in the neonate.

Benzodiazepines have been detected in breast milk. If possible, the use of Lexotan should be avoided during lactation.

Precautions: In patients with chronic pulmonary insufficiency, and in patients with chronic renal or hepatic disease, dosage may need to be reduced.

Lexotan should not be used alone to treat depression or anxiety associated with depression, since suicide may be precipitated in such patients.

Amnesia may occur.

In cases of loss or bereavement, psychological adjustment may be inhibited by benzodiazepines.

If Lexotan is combined with centrally-acting drugs such as neuroleptics, tranquillisers, antidepressants, hypnotics, analgesics and anaesthetics, the sedative effects may be intensified. The elderly require special supervision.

Patients should be advised that, like all medicaments of this type, Lexotan may modify patients' performance at skilled tasks (driving, operating machinery, etc.) to a varying degree depending upon dosage and individual susceptibility. Patients should further be advised that alcohol may intensify any impairment and should therefore be avoided during treatment.

The dependence potential of the benzodiazepines is low, particularly when limited to short-term use, but this increases when high doses are used, especially when given over long periods. This is particularly so in patients with a history of alcoholism or drug abuse or in patients with marked personality disorders. Regular monitoring in such patients is essential, routine repeat prescriptions should be avoided and treatment should be withdrawn gradually. Symptoms such as depression, nervousness, rebound insomnia, irritability, sweating and diarrhoea have been reported following abrupt cessation of treatment in patients receiving even normal therapeutic doses for short periods of time. In rare instances, withdrawal following excessive dosages may produce confusional states, psychotic manifestations and convulsions.

Abnormal psychological reactions to benzodiazepines have been reported. Rare behavioural effects include paradoxical aggressive outbursts, excitement, confusion, and the uncovering of depression with suicidal tendencies. Extreme caution should therefore be used in prescribing benzodiazepines to patients with personality disorders.

When Lexotan is used in conjunction with anti-epileptic drugs, side-effects and toxicity may be more evident, particularly with hydantoins or barbiturates or combinations including them. This requires extra care in adjusting dosage in the initial stages of treatment.

Side-effects: Common adverse effects include drowsiness, sedation, unsteadiness and ataxia; these are dose-related and may persist into the following day, even after a single dose. Drowsiness may be a particular problem when Lexotan is used in higher dosage in some patients, especially if they are unused to this form of therapy. The elderly are particularly sensitive to the effects of central depressant drugs and may experience confusion, especially if organic brain changes are present; the dosage of Lexotan should not exceed one-half that recommended for other adults.

Other adverse effects are rare and include headache, vertigo, hypotension, gastro-intestinal upsets, skin rashes, visual disturbances, changes in libido, and urinary retention. Isolated cases of blood dyscrasias and jaundice have also been reported.

Treatment of overdosage: When taken alone in overdosage Lexotan presents few problems in management. Signs may include drowsiness, ataxia and dysarthria, with coma in severe cases. Treatment is symptomatic. Gastric lavage is useful only if performed soon after ingestion. Anexate* is a specific IV antidote for use in emergency situations. Patients requiring such intervention should be monitored closely in hospital (see separate prescribing information).

When taken with centrally acting drugs, especially alcohol, the effects of overdosage are likely to be more severe and, in the absence of supportive measures, may prove fatal.

Pharmaceutical precautions *Storage:* Lexotan tablets should be stored in well-closed containers in a dry place, protected from light.

Legal category CD (Sch. 4), POM.

Package quantities Lexotan tablets 1.5 mg in original blister packings of 60 (OP).
Lexotan tablets 3 mg in blister packings of 60 (OP).

Further information Lexotan is rapidly absorbed from the gastro-intestinal tract. The mean half-life for elimination of Lexotan in man is about 16 hours. Metabolites of Lexotan do not contribute significantly to the effects of the drug.

The elderly, and patients with impaired renal and/or hepatic function, will be particularly susceptible to the adverse effects listed above. It is advisable to review treatment regularly and to discontinue use as soon as possible.

Treatment should be kept to a minimum and given only under close medical supervision. Little is known regarding the efficacy or safety of benzodiazepines in long-term use.

Product licence numbers
Tablets 1.5 mg 0031/0127
Tablets 3 mg 0031/0128.

LIBRIUM*

Presentation Capsules with opaque green cap and opaque yellow body with $^{\text{LIB}}_{5}$ printed in red-brown along both cap and body, containing 5 mg chlordiazepoxide hydrochloride.

Capsules with black cap and opaque green body with $^{\text{LIB}}_{10}$ printed in red-brown along both cap and body, containing 10 mg chlordiazepoxide hydrochloride.

Round, yellowish-green, film-coated tablets with $^{\text{LIB}}_{5}$ imprinted around the periphery, containing 5 mg chlordiazepoxide.

Round, light bluish-green, film-coated tablets with $^{\text{LIB}}_{10}$ imprinted around the periphery, containing 10 mg chlordiazepoxide.

Round, dark bluish-green, film-coated tablets with $^{\text{LIB}}_{25}$ imprinted around the periphery, containing 25 mg chlordiazepoxide.

Uses *Properties:* Librium has anxiolytic and central muscle-relaxant properties. It has little autonomic activity.

Indications: Capsules and tablets: Short-term (2–4 weeks) symptomatic treatment of anxiety that is severe, disabling or subjecting the individual to unacceptable distress, occurring alone or in association with insomnia or short-term psychosomatic, organic or psychotic illness.

Muscle spasm of varied aetiology.

Symptomatic relief of acute alcohol withdrawal.

Dosage and administration
Adults: Capsules and tablets

Anxiety states	
Usual dose	Up to 30 mg daily in divided doses
Maximum dose	Up to 100 mg daily in divided doses Adjusted on an individual basis.
Insomnia associated with anxiety	10–30 mg before retiring
Symptomatic relief of acute alcohol withdrawal	25 to 100 mg repeated if necessary in 2 to 4 hours
Muscle spasm of varied aetiology	10 to 30 mg daily in divided doses

ELDERLY AND DEBILITATED PATIENTS: DOSES SHOULD NOT EXCEED HALF THOSE NORMALLY RECOMMENDED.

The lowest dose which can control symptoms should be used. Treatment should not be continued at the full dose beyond four weeks. Long-term chronic use is not recommended.

Treatment should always be tapered off gradually. Patients who have taken benzodiazepines for a prolonged time may require a longer period during which doses are reduced. Specialist help may be appropriate.

Librium capsules and tablets are for oral administration.

Contra-indications, warnings, etc
Contra-indications: Patients with known sensitivity to benzodiazepines; acute pulmonary insufficiency; respiratory depression; phobic or obsessional states; chronic psychosis.

Use in pregnancy: There is no evidence as to drug safety in human pregnancy, nor is there evidence from animal work that it is free from hazard. Do not use during pregnancy, especially during the first and last trimesters, unless there are compelling reasons.

The administration of high doses or prolonged administration of low doses of benzodiazepines in the last trimester of pregnancy has been reported to produce irregularities in the foetal heart rate, and hypotonia, poor sucking and hypothermia in the neonate.

Chlordiazepoxide may appear in breast milk. If possible, the use of Librium should be avoided during lactation.

Precautions: In patients with chronic pulmonary insufficiency, and in patients with chronic renal or hepatic disease, dosage may need to be reduced.

Librium should not be used alone to treat depression or anxiety associated with depression, since suicide may be precipitated in such patients.

Amnesia may occur.

In cases of loss or bereavement, psychological adjustment may be inhibited by benzodiazepines.

Patients should be advised that, like all medicaments of this type, Librium may modify patients' performance at skilled tasks (driving, operating machinery, etc.) to a varying degree depending upon dosage, administration and individual susceptibility. Patients should further be advised that alcohol may intensify any impairment and should therefore be avoided during treatment.

The dependence potential of the benzodiazepines is low, particularly when limited to short-term use, but this increases when high doses are used, especially when given over long periods. This is particularly so in patients with a history of alcoholism or drug abuse or in patients with marked personality disorders. Regular monitoring in such patients is essential, routine repeat prescriptions should be avoided and treatment should be withdrawn gradually. Symptoms such as depression, nervousness, rebound insomnia, irritability, sweating, and diarrhoea have been reported following abrupt cessation of treatment in patients receiving even normal therapeutic doses for short periods of time.

In rare instances, withdrawal following excessive dosages may produce confusional states, psychotic manifestations and convulsions.

Abnormal psychological reactions to benzodiazepines have been reported. Rare behavioural effects include paradoxical aggressive outbursts, excitement, confusion, and the uncovering of depression with suicidal tendencies. Extreme caution should therefore be used in prescribing benzodiazepines to patients with personality disorders.

If Librium is combined with centrally-acting drugs such as neuroleptics, tranquillizers, antidepressants, hypnotics, analgesics and anaesthetics, the sedative effects are likely to be intensified. The elderly require special supervision.

When Librium is used in conjunction with anti-epileptic drugs, side-effects and toxicity may be more evident, particularly with hydantoins or barbiturates or combinations including them. This requires extra care in adjusting dosage in the initial stages of treatment.

Side-effects and adverse reactions: Common adverse effects include drowsiness, sedation, unsteadiness and ataxia; these are dose-related and may persist into the following day even after a single dose. The elderly are particularly sensitive to the effects of central depressant-drugs and may experience confusion, especially if organic brain changes are present; the dosage of Librium should not exceed one-half that recommended for other adults.

Other adverse effects are rare and include headache, vertigo, hypotension, gastrointestinal upsets, skin rashes, visual disturbances, changes in libido, and urinary retention. Isolated cases of blood dyscrasias and jaundice have also been reported.

Treatment of overdosage: When taken alone in overdosage Librium presents few problems in management. Signs may include drowsiness, ataxia and dysarthria, with coma in severe cases. Treatment is symptomatic. Gastric lavage is useful only if performed soon after ingestion. Anexate* is a specific IV antidote for use in emergency situations. Patients requiring such intervention should be monitored closely in hospital (see separate prescribing information).

When taken with centrally-acting drugs, especially alcohol, the effects of overdosage are likely to be more severe and, in the absence of supportive measures, may prove fatal.

Pharmaceutical precautions *Storage:* The recommended maximum storage temperature of Librium capsules is 30°C and of tablets is 25°C.

Legal category CD (Sch. 4), POM.

Package quantities Librium capsules 5 mg and 10 mg and Librium tablets 5 mg, 10 mg and 25 mg in packings of 100.

Further information Librium is well absorbed, with peak blood levels being achieved one or two hours after administration. The drug has a half-life of 6–30 hours. Steady-state levels are usually reached within three days.

Chlordiazepoxide is metabolised to desmethyl-chlordiazepoxide. Demoxepam and desmethyldiazepam are also found in the plasma of patients on continuous treatment. The active metabolite desmethyl-chlordiazepoxide has an accumulation half-life of 10–18 hours; that of demoxepam has been recorded as 21–78 hours.

Steady-state levels of these active metabolites are reached after 10–15 days, with metabolite concentrations which are similar to those of the parent drug.

No clear correlation has been demonstrated between the blood levels of Librium and its clinical effects.

The elderly and patients with impaired renal and/or hepatic function will be particularly susceptible to the adverse effects listed above. It is advisable to review treatment regularly and to discontinue use as soon as possible.

Treatment should be kept to a minimum and given only under close medical supervision. Little is known regarding the efficacy of benzodiazepines in long-term use.

Product licence numbers

Capsules 5 mg	0031/5025R
Capsules 10 mg	0031/5026R
Tablets 5 mg	0031/5027R
Tablets 10 mg	0031/5028R
Tablets 25 mg	0031/5029R

LIMBITROL*

Presentation Limbitrol 5 capsules with opaque green cap and opaque pink body marked 'LOL 5' printed in red-brown along the cap and body, containing 5 mg chlordiazepoxide and 14.15 mg amitriptyline hydrochloride (equivalent to 12.5 mg amitriptyline base).

Limbitrol 10 capsules with opaque, dark green cap and opaque pink body marked 'LOL 10' printed in red-brown along the cap and body, containing 10 mg chlordiazepoxide and 28.3 mg amitriptyline hydrochloride (equivalent to 25 mg amitriptyline base).

Uses *Properties:* Limbitrol combines the anxiolytic effect of chlordiazepoxide with the antidepressant action of amitriptyline. Chlordiazepoxide is a benzodiazepine which has anxiolytic and central muscle-relaxant properties. It has little autonomic activity. Amitriptyline is a tricyclic antidepressant. Its mode of action in man is believed to result from inhibition of re-uptake of monoamines from the synaptic cleft into the neuron after central transmission.

Indications: The treatment of the symptoms of depressive illness with associated anxiety.

Dosage and administration *Adults:* It is recommended that patients should be started on one capsule Limbitrol 5 three times daily. If the response is inadequate the dose should be increased to one capsule Limbitrol 10 three times daily.

In more severe cases it may be necessary to initiate treatment with one capsule Limbitrol 10 three times daily. If necessary, dosage may be increased to two or three capsules three times daily.

Elderly patients: Limbitrol is not for geriatric use.

Children: Limbitrol is not for paediatric use.

Limbitrol capsules are for oral administration.

Contra-indications, warnings, etc

Contra-indications: Patients with known sensitivity to benzodiazepines; acute pulmonary insufficiency; respiratory depression.

Recent myocardial infarction; heart block of any degree; cardiac arrhythmias. Patients with mania, whose condition may be exacerbated by tricyclic antidepressants.

Because of its anticholinergic effects, Limbitrol should not be given to patients suffering from narrow-angle glaucoma or symptoms suggestive of prostatic hypertrophy. Limbitrol should not be taken with monoamine oxidase inhibitors. A minimum of 14 days should elapse between discontinuation of an MAOI and starting Limbitrol, which should be introduced cautiously and dosage increased gradually.

Use in pregnancy: The use of Limbitrol during pregnancy, especially in the first trimester, should be avoided.

The administration of high doses or prolonged administration of low doses of benzodiazepines in the last trimester of pregnancy and during labour has been reported to produce irregularities in the foetal heart rate, and hypotonia, poor sucking and hypothermia in the neonate.

Tricyclic antidepressants, when administered during the last trimester of pregnancy, have also been associated with adverse effects such as withdrawal symptoms, respiratory depression and agitation in the foetus.

Chlordiazepoxide and amitriptyline may appear in breast milk. Limbitrol should therefore be avoided during lactation.

Precautions: In patients with chronic pulmonary insufficiency, and patients with chronic renal or hepatic disease, dosage may need to be modified.

Limbitrol should be used with caution in patients with a history of urinary retention or blood dyscrasias and in patients with hyperthyroidism or cardiovascular disorders.

Limbitrol should be avoided in patients with a history of epilepsy.

If Limbitrol is combined with centrally-acting drugs such as neuroleptics, tranquillizers, antidepressants, hypnotics, analgesics and anaesthetics, the sedative effects may be intensified.

Patients should be advised that, like all medicaments of this type, Limbitrol may modify patients' performance at skilled tasks (driving, operating machinery, etc.) to a varying degree depending on dosage, administration and individual susceptibility. Patients should further be advised that alcohol may intensify any impairment and should therefore be avoided during treatment.

Anaesthesia given during tricyclic antidepressant therapy may increase the risk of arrhythmias and hypotension. If anaesthesia is necessary, the anaesthetist should be informed that the patient is being treated with Limbitrol.

Amitriptyline may decrease the antihypertensive effect of adrenergic neurone-blocking drugs such as guanethidine, bethanidine or debrisoquine, and possibly also clonidine. It is advisable to review all antihypertensive therapy during treatment with Limbitrol.

Limbitrol should not be given with sympathomimetic agents such as adrenaline, ephedrine, isoprenaline, noradrenaline, phenylephrine and phenylpropanolamine.

Barbiturates may decrease and methylphenidate may increase the antidepressant action of amitriptyline.

The antidepressant effect of amitriptyline may not become apparent for the first 2–4 weeks of therapy, although the anxiolytic effect of chlordiazepoxide should begin within several hours of the first dose of Limbitrol.

The possibility of suicide in depressed patients should be borne in mind, and patients should be carefully supervised, especially during the early stages of treatment.

The dependence potential of the benzodiazepines is low but this increases when high doses are used, especially when given over long periods. This is particularly so in patients with a history of alcoholism or drug abuse or in patients with marked personality disorders. Regular monitoring in such patients is essential, routine repeat prescriptions should be avoided and treatment should be withdrawn gradually. Symptoms such as depression, nervousness, rebound insomnia, irritability, sweating, and diarrhoea have been reported following abrupt cessation of treatment in patients receiving even normal therapeutic doses for short periods of time.

In rare instances, withdrawal following excessive dosages may produce confusional states, psychotic manifestations and convulsions.

Treatment should be kept to a minimum and given only under close medical supervision. Little is known regarding the efficacy of benzodiazepines or tricyclic antidepressants in long-term use.

Abnormal psychological reactions to benzodiazepines have been reported. Rare behavioural effects include paradoxical aggressive outbursts, excitement, confusion, and the uncovering of depression with suicidal tendencies.

The efficacy and safety of Limbitrol in elderly patients has not been demonstrated.

The fixed dosage of chlordiazepoxide and amitriptyline provided in Limbitrol may not be appropriate for some patients, for whom the alternative of prescribing the two active ingredients separately in the necessary amounts should be considered.

Side-effects and adverse reactions: The most common side-effects are drowsiness, dry mouth and dizziness during the first few days of treatment, and anticholinergic effects such as constipation, disturbances of accommodation, tachycardia and hesitancy of micturition, which also usually lessen or disappear with time.

Other adverse effects are rare and include headache, hypotension, gastro-intestinal upsets, skin rashes, tremor, interference with sexual function, and urinary retention. Isolated cases of blood dyscrasias, jaundice, hypomania, convulsions, and peripheral neuropathy have also been reported.

Cardiac arrhythmias and severe hypotension are likely to occur with high dosage and in deliberate overdosage of amitriptyline. They may also occur with normal dosage in patients with pre-existing heart disease.

Psychotic manifestations, including mania and paranoid delusions, may be exacerbated during treatment with tricyclic antidepressants.

Treatment of overdosage: Deaths by deliberate or accidental overdosage of amitriptyline have occurred. Symptoms of amitriptyline overdosage may include drowsiness, stupor and coma; tachycardia and other cardiac arrhythmias including ventricular fibrillation; severe hypotension and congestive cardiac failure; agitation, hyper-reflexia and convulsions; hyperpyrexia, dilated pupils and paralytic ileus.

Symptoms of chlordiazepoxide overdosage may include drowsiness, ataxia and dysarthria, with coma in severe cases.

Treatment is symptomatic and supportive. Gastric lavage should be performed as quickly as possible and followed by the use of activated charcoal. Maintain an open airway and adequate fluid intake. Continuous ECG monitoring is essential; serious cardiac arrhythmias may be treated with neostigmine, pyridostigmine or propranolol. Intravenous fluids may be required to maintain the blood pressure. Body temperature should be regulated. Intravenous diazepam is recommended for the control of convulsions.

There is no specific antidote to amitriptyline and chlordiazepoxide overdosage but the intravenous administration of physostigmine (1 to 3 mg) has been reported to reverse the symptoms. This dose should be repeated as indicated.

When taken with centrally-depressant drugs, especially alcohol, the effects of overdosage are likely to be more severe.

Pharmaceutical precautions *Storage:* Limbitrol capsules should be stored in a dry place. Recommended maximum storage temperature 30°C.

Legal category CD (Sch. 4), POM.

Package quantities Limbitrol 5 and Limbitrol 10 capsules in packs of 100.

Further information Chlordiazepoxide is well absorbed, with peak blood levels being achieved one or two hours after administration. The drug has a half life of 6–30 hours. Steady-state levels are usually reached within three days.

Chlordiazepoxide is metabolised to desmethylchlordiazepoxide. Demoxepam and desmethyldiazepam are also found in the plasma of patients on continuous treatment. The active metabolite desmethylchlordiazide has an accumulation half-life of 10–18 hours; that of demoxepam has been recorded as 21–78 hours.

Steady-state levels of these active metabolites are reached after 10–15 days, with metabolite concentrations which are similar to those of parent drug.

Amitriptyline is rapidly and completely absorbed when

given orally. It is metabolised predominantly in the liver and excreted in the bile and urine and has an elimination half-life of about 40 hours.

Steady-state levels of amitriptyline are usually reached in approximately 10–15 days.

No clear correlation has been demonstrated between the plasma concentrations of chlordiazepoxide and of amitriptyline and their clinical effects.

Product licence numbers

Limbitrol 5 Capsules	0031/5066R
Limbitrol 10 Capsules	0031/5067R

MADOPAR*

Presentation Madopar 62.5 capsules with blue cap and grey body with 'ROCHE' printed in black on both cap and body, containing 50 mg levodopa and 14.25 mg benserazide hydrochloride (equivalent to 12.5 mg of the base).

Madopar 62.5 dispersible tablets: round, white tablets with ROCHE 62.5 imprinted on one face and a single break bar on the other, containing 50 mg levodopa and 14.25 mg benserazide hydrochloride (equivalent to 12.5 mg of the base).

Madopar 125 capsules with blue cap and pink body with 'ROCHE' printed in black on both cap and body, containing 100 mg levodopa and 28.5 mg benserazide hydrochloride (equivalent to 25 mg of the base).

Madopar 125 dispersible tablets: round, white tablets with ROCHE 125 imprinted on one face and a single break bar on the other, containing 100 mg levodopa and 28.25 mg benserazide hydrochloride (equivalent to 25 mg of the base).

Madopar 250 capsules with blue cap and caramel body with 'ROCHE' printed in black on both cap and body, containing 200 mg levodopa and 57 mg benserazide hydrochloride (equivalent to 50 mg of the base).

Uses *Properties:* Madopar is an anti-Parkinsonian agent. Levodopa is the metabolic precursor of dopamine. The latter is severely depleted in the striatum, pallidum and substantia nigra of Parkinsonian patients and it is considered that administration of levodopa raises the level of available dopamine in these centres. However, conversion of levodopa into dopamine by the enzyme dopa decarboxylase also takes place in extracerebral tissues. As a consequence the full therapeutic effect may not be obtained and side-effects occur.

Administration of a peripheral decarboxylase inhibitor, which blocks the extracerebral decarboxylation of levodopa, in conjunction with levodopa has significant advantages; these include reduced gastro-intestinal side-effects, a more rapid response at the initiation of therapy and a simpler dosage regimen.

Madopar is a combination of levodopa and benserazide in the ratio of 4:1 which in clinical trials has been shown to be the most satisfactory. Like every replacement therapy, chronic treatment with Madopar will be necessary.

Indications: Parkinsonism – idiopathic, post-encephalitic. Previous neurosurgery is not a contra-indication to Madopar.

Dosage and administration Dosage and administration are variable and no more than a guide can be given.

Patients not previously treated with levodopa: The recommended initial dose is one capsule or dispersible tablet of Madopar 62.5 three or four times daily. If the disease is at an advanced stage, the starting dose should be one capsule or dispersible tablet of Madopar 125 three times daily. The daily dosage should then be increased by one capsule or dispersible tablet of Madopar 125, or their equivalent, once or twice weekly until a full therapeutic effect is obtained, or side-effects supervene. In some elderly patients, it may suffice to initiate treatment with one capsule or dispersible tablet of Madopar 62.5 once or twice daily, increasing by one capsule or dispersible tablet every third or fourth day.

The effective dose usually lies within the range of 4–8 capsules or dispersible tablets of Madopar 125 (2–4 capsules of Madopar 250) daily in divided doses, most patients requiring no more than 6 capsules or dispersible tablets of Madopar 125 daily.

Optimal improvement is usually seen in one to three weeks, but the full therapeutic effect of Madopar may not be apparent for some time. It is advisable, therefore, to allow several weeks to elapse before contemplating dosage increments above the average dose range. If satisfactory improvement is still not achieved, the dose of Madopar may be increased, but with caution. It is rarely necessary to give more than 10 capsules or dispersible tablets of Madopar 125 (5 capsules of Madopar 250) per day.

Treatment should be continued for at least six months before failure is concluded from the absence of a clinical response.

Madopar 62.5 capsules or dispersible tablets may be used to facilitate adjustment of dosage to the needs of the individual patient. Patients who experience fluctuations in response may be helped by dividing the dosage into smaller, more frequent doses with the aid of Madopar 62.5 capsules or dispersible tablets without, however, altering the total daily dose.

Madopar 250 capsules are only for maintenance therapy once the optimal dosage has been determined using Madopar 125 capsules or dispersible tablets.

Patients previously treated with levodopa: The following procedure is recommended:

Levodopa alone should be discontinued and Madopar started on the following day. The patient should be initiated on a total of one less Madopar 125 capsule or dispersible tablet daily than the total number of 500 mg levodopa tablets or capsules previously taken (for example, if the patient had previously taken 2 g levodopa daily, then he should start on 3 capsules or dispersible tablets Madopar 125 daily on the following day).

Observe the patient for one week and then, if necessary, increase the dosage in the manner described for new patients.

Patients previously treated with other levodopa/decarboxylase inhibitor combinations: Previous therapy should be withdrawn for 12 hours. In order to minimise the potential for any effects of levodopa withdrawal, it may be beneficial to discontinue previous therapy at night and institute Madopar therapy the following morning. The initial Madopar dose should be one capsule or dispersible tablet of Madopar 62.5 three or four times daily. This dose may then be increased in the manner described for patients not previously treated with levodopa.

Other anti-Parkinsonian drugs may be given with Madopar. Existing treatment with other anti-Parkinsonian drugs, e.g. anticholinergics or amantadine, should be continued during initiation of Madopar treatment. However, as treatment with Madopar proceeds and the therapeutic effect becomes apparent, the dosage of the other drugs may need to be reduced or the drugs gradually withdrawn.

Elderly: Although there may be an age-related decrease in tolerance to levodopa in the elderly, Madopar appears to be well-tolerated and side-effects are generally not troublesome.

Children: Not to be given to patients under 25 years of age; therefore, no dosage recommendations are made for the administration of Madopar to children.

Madopar capsules and dispersible tablets are for oral administration. They should be taken with, or immediately after, meals.

Madopar dispersible tablets may be swallowed whole or dispersed in at least 25 ml water per tablet. They may be taken in dilute orange squash (at least 25 ml per tablet) if preferred. However, orange juice should not be used. Madopar dispersible tablets are particularly suitable for patients who dislike taking capsules or have difficulty in swallowing solid dosage forms.

Contra-indications, warnings, etc
Contra-indications: Madopar is contra-indicated in narrow-angle glaucoma (it may be used in wide angle glaucoma provided that the intra-ocular pressure remains under control); severe psychoneuroses or psychoses; severe endocrine, renal, hepatic or cardiac disorders.

It should not be given in conjunction with monoamine oxidase (MAO) inhibitors except selective MAO-B inhibitors, or within two weeks of their withdrawal.

It should not be given to patients under 25 years of age.

Suspicion has arisen that levodopa may activate a malignant melanoma. Therefore Madopar should not be used in persons who have a history of, or who may be suffering from, a malignant melanoma.

Use in pregnancy: Madopar is contra-indicated in pregnancy, since there is evidence of harmful effects in studies in pregnant rabbits and the beserazide component has been found to be associated with skeletal malformations in the rat. In any woman of child-bearing potential the risk of its use, should pregnancy occur, must be weighed against the anticipated benefits of treatment. Patients taking Madopar should not breast-feed their infants.

Precautions: When other drugs must be given in conjunction with Madopar, the patient should be carefully observed for unusual side-effects or potentiating effects.

Drugs which interfere with central amine mechanisms, such as rauwolfia (reserpine), tetrabenazine (Nitoman*), metoclopramide, phenothiazines, thioxanthenes, butyrophenones, amphetamines and papaverine should be avoided where possible. If, however, their administration is considered essential, extreme care should be exercised and a close watch kept for any signs of potentiation, antagonism or other interactions and for any unusual side-effects.

In the event of general anaesthesia being required, Madopar therapy may be continued as long as the patient is able to take fluids and medication by mouth. If therapy is temporarily interrupted, the usual daily dosage may be administered as soon as the patient is able to take oral medication. Whenever therapy has been interrupted for longer periods, dosage should again be adjusted gradually; however, in many cases the patient can rapidly be returned to his previous therapeutic dosage. If a patient has to undergo emergency surgery, when Madopar has not been withdrawn, anaesthesia with cyclopropane or halothane should be avoided.

There have been occasional reports of a neuroleptic malignant-like syndrome, involving hyperthermia, on abrupt withdrawal of levodopa preparations. Sudden discontinuation of Madopar, without close supervision, or 'drug holidays' should therefore be avoided.

Pyridoxine (vitamin B_6) may be given with Madopar, since the presence of a decarboxylase inhibitor protects against the peripheral levodopa transformation facilitated by pyridoxine.

Care should be taken when using Madopar in the following circumstances: in endocrine, renal, pulmonary or cardiovascular disease, particularly where there is a history of myocardial infarction or arrhythmia; psychiatric disturbances; hepatic disorder; peptic ulcer; osteomalacia; where sympathomimetic drugs may be required (e.g. bronchial asthma), due to possible potentiation of the cardiovascular effects of levodopa; where antihypertensive drugs are being used, due to possible increased hypotensive action.

Periodic evaluation of hepatic, haemopoietic, renal and cardiovascular functions is advised.

Patients who improve on Madopar therapy should be advised to resume normal activities gradually as rapid mobilisation may increase the risk of injury.

Side-effects: Tolerance to Madopar varies widely between patients and is often related to the rate of dosage increases. Side-effects such as nausea, vomiting and loss of appetite, which are frequently observed during the initial stages of levodopa therapy, are much less common in patients treated with Madopar. If such side-effects do occur, they can largely be controlled by taking Madopar with, or immediately after, food and by increasing the dosage only slowly. Also, cardiovascular disturbances such as arrhythmias and orthostatic hypotension may occur, but are less frequent than in patients treated with levodopa alone.

Psychiatric disturbances are common in Parkinsonian patients including those being treated with levodopa. They include mild elation, anxiety, agitation, insomnia, depression, aggression, delusions, hallucinations, and 'unmasking' of psychoses.

Although there have been rare reports of possible antagonism of levodopa by diazepam, in general diazepam (Valium Roche*) and nitrazepam (Mogadon*) have been found to be useful in the treatment of anxiety and insomnia, respectively, occurring in Parkinsonism.

Depression may be treated with tricyclic antidepressants although isolated cases of hypertensive crisis have been reported with the concomitant use of tricyclic drugs. ECT may be administered if appropriate. MAO inhibitors, except selective MAO-B inhibitors must not be used.

Involuntary movements, commonly in the form of oral dyskinesias, often accompanied by 'paddling' foot movements, or of the choreoathetoid type, are common, particularly on long-term administration. They are usually dose-dependent and may disappear or become tolerable after dose adjustment.

With long-term administration, fluctuations in the therapeutic response may be encountered. They include 'freezing' episodes, end-of-dose deterioration and the so-called 'on-off' effect. Patients may be helped by dosage reduction or by giving smaller and more frequent doses.

Other side-effects which have occasionally been reported with levodopa therapy include gastro-intestinal bleeding, flushing, sweating, and drowsiness.

On some occasions the urine passed during Madopar treatment may be altered in colour; usually red-tinged, this will turn dark on standing. These changes are due to metabolites and are no cause for concern.

Transient rises in SGOT, SGPT and alkaline phosphatase values have been noted: serum uric acid and blood urea nitrogen levels are occasionally increased. In rare instances, haemolytic anaemia, mild transient leucopenia and thrombocytopenia have been reported.

Levodopa may interfere chemically with several diagnostic laboratory tests including those for glucose, ketone bodies, or catecholamines in urine and for glucose or uric acid in blood. Levodopa therapy has been reported to inhibit the response to protirelin in tests of thyroid function.

Effects of overdosage and their treatment: Symptoms of overdosage are qualitatively similar to the side effects but may be of greater magnitude.

Treatment should include gastric lavage, general supportive measures, intravenous fluids and the maintenance of an adequate airway. Electrocardiographic monitoring should be instituted and the patient carefully observed for the possible development of arrhythmias. If necessary, anti-arrhythmic therapy should be given and other symptoms treated as they arise.

Pharmaceutical precautions *Storage;* Madopar capsules and dispersible tablets should be protected from moisture. The recommended maximum storage temperature is 25°C.

Legal category POM.

Package quantities Madopar 62.5 capsules containing 50 mg levodopa and 12.5 mg benserazide in bottles of 100 (OP).

Madopar 62.5 dispersible tablets containing 50 mg levodopa and 12.5 mg benserazide in bottles of 100 (OP).

Madopar 125 capsules containing 100 mg levodopa and 25 mg benserazide in bottles of 100 (OP).

Madopar 125 dispersible tablets containing 100 mg levodopa and 25 mg benserazide in bottles of 100 (OP).

Madopar 250 capsules containing 200 mg levodopa and 50 mg benserazide in bottles of 100 (OP).

Further information Low levels of endogenous levodopa are detectable in pre-dose blood samples. After oral administration of Madopar, levodopa and benserazide are rapidly absorbed, mainly in the upper regions of the small intestine. Interaction studies indicate that a higher proportion of levodopa is absorbed intact when administered in combination with benserazide, compared with levodopa administered alone.

Maximum plasma concentrations of levodopa are reached approximately 1 hour after ingestion of Madopar.

The elimination half life of levodopa is about 45 minutes.

Product licence numbers

Madopar 62.5 Capsules	0031/0125
Madopar 62.5 dispersible tablets	0031/0220
Madopar 125 Capsules	0031/0073R
Madopar 125 dispersible tablets	0031/0221
Madopar 250 Capsules	0031/0074R

MADOPAR CR*

Presentation Madopar CR 125 capsules with opaque dark green cap and opaque light blue body with 'ROCHE' printed in red on both cap and body, containing 100 mg levodopa and 25 mg benserazide (as 28.5 mg benserazide hydrochloride) in a controlled-release formulation.

Uses

Properties: Madopar consists of levodopa and the peripheral decarboxylase inhibitor benserazide in the ratio 4:1 which in clinical trials has been shown to be the most satisfactory combination. Madopar CR is a controlled-release form which provides more prolonged, but lower, peak plasma concentrations of levodopa than standard Madopar or other conventional formulations of levodopa.

The active ingredients of Madopar CR are released slowly in the stomach and the maximum levodopa plasma concentration is reached approximately 3 hours after ingestion. The plasma concentration-time curve for levodopa shows a longer 'half-duration' (=time-span when plasma concentrations are equal to or higher than half the maximum concentration) than that of standard Madopar, which indicates pronounced controlled-release properties. Madopar CR bioavailability is approximately 60% that of standard Madopar.

Indications: Treatment of Parkinson's disease in patients presenting with fluctuations in response to conventional levodopa preparations. Patients with fluctuations related to levodopa plasma concentrations or timing of dose, e.g. end-of-dose deterioration or wearing-off effects, are more likely to benefit from Madopar CR.

Dosage and administration

Adults, including the elderly

Fluctuations in response to conventional therapy: Dosage and administration are very variable and must be titrated to the needs of the individual patient.

In general, higher doses of Madopar CR will be required than with conventional levodopa-decarboxylase inhibitor combinations as a result of the reduced bioavailability and better tolerance of Madopar CR. Close medical supervision of the patient is advisable during the initial period whilst adjusting the dosage. Patients should be informed that their condition may deteriorate initially until the optimal dosage regimen has been found.

Madopar CR should be substituted for the standard levodopa-decarboxylase inhibitor preparation by one capsule Madopar CR 125 per 100 mg levodopa. For example, where a patient previously received doses of 200 mg levodopa with a decarboxylase inhibitor, then therapy should be initiated with two capsules Madopar CR 125. Therapy should continue with the same frequency of doses as previously.

With Madopar CR, *on average*, a 50% increase in daily levodopa dosage compared with previous therapy has been found to be appropriate. The dosage should be titrated every 2 to 3 days using dosage increments of Madopar CR 125 capsules and a period of up to 4 weeks should be allowed for optimisation of dosage.

Some patients may require a supplementary dose of conventional Madopar together with the first morning dose of Madopar CR to compensate for the more gradual onset of effect of the latter.

In cases of poor response to Madopar CR at total daily doses of Madopar CR plus any supplementary conventional Madopar corresponding to 1,200 mg levodopa, administration of Madopar CR should be discontinued and alternative therapy considered.

Madopar CR capsules must always be swallowed whole, preferably with a little water. They may be taken with or without food but antacid preparations should be avoided.

Children: Not to be given to patients under 25 years of age: therefore, no dosage recommendations are made for the administration of Madopar CR to children.

Contra-indications, warnings, etc

Contra-indications: Madopar is contra-indicated in narrow-angle glaucoma (it may be used in wide-angle glaucoma provided that the intra-ocular pressure remains under control); severe psychoneuroses or psychoses; severe endocrine, renal, hepatic or cardiac disorders.

It should not be given in conjunction with monoamine oxidase (MAO) inhibitors except selective MAO-B inhibitors or within 2 weeks of their withdrawal.

It should not be given to patients under 25 years of age.

Suspicion has arisen that levodopa may activate a malignant melanoma. Therefore, Madopar should not be used in persons who have a history of, or who may be suffering from, a malignant melanoma.

Use in pregnancy: Madopar is contra-indicated in pregnancy, since there is evidence of harmful effects in studies in pregnant rabbits and the benserazide component has been found to be associated with skeletal malformations in the rat. In any woman of childbearing potential the risk of its use, should pregnancy occur, must be weighed against the anticipated benefits of treatment. Patients taking Madopar should not breastfeed their infants.

Precautions: When other drugs must be given in conjunction with Madopar, the patient should be carefully observed for unusual side-effects or potentiating effects.

Drugs which interfere with central amine mechanisms, such as rauwolfia alkaloids (reserpine), tetrabenazine (Nitoman*), metoclopramide, phenothiazines, thioxanthenes, butyrophenones, amphetamines and papaverine, should be avoided where possible. If, however, their administration is considered essential, extreme care should be exercised and a close watch kept for any signs of potentiation, antagonism or other interactions and for unusual side-effects.

In the event of general anaesthesia being required, Madopar therapy may be continued as long as the patient is able to take fluids and medication by mouth. If therapy is temporarily interrupted, the usual daily dosage may be administered as soon as the patient is able to take oral medication. Whenever therapy has been interrupted for longer periods, dosage should again be adjusted gradually; however, in many cases the patient can rapidly be returned to his previous therapeutic dosage.

If a patient has to undergo emergency surgery, when Madopar has not been withdrawn, anaesthesia with cyclopropane or halothane should be avoided.

There have been occasional reports of a neuroleptic malignant-like syndrome, involving hyperthermia, on abrupt withdrawal of levodopa preparations. Sudden discontinuation of Madopar, without close supervision, or 'drug holidays' should therefore be avoided.

Pyridoxine (vitamin B_6) may be given with Madopar since the presence of a decarboxylase inhibitor protects against the peripheral levodopa transformation facilitated by pyridoxine.

Care should be taken when using Madopar in the following circumstances: in endocrine, renal, pulmonary or cardiovascular disease, particularly where there is a history of myocardial infarction or arrhythmia; psychiatric disturbances; hepatic disorder; peptic ulcer; osteomalacia; where sympathomimetic drugs may be required (e.g. bronchial asthma), due to possible potentiation of the cardiovascular effects of levodopa; where antihypertensive drugs are being used, due to possible increased hypotensive action.

Periodic evaluation of hepatic, haemopoietic, renal and cardiovascular functions is advised.

Patients who improve on Madopar therapy should be advised to resume normal activities gradually as rapid mobilisation may increase the risk of injury.

Drug interactions: It should be noted that when Madopar CR is given with antacid preparations, the bioavailability of levodopa is reduced, in comparison with conventional Madopar.

Side-effects and adverse reactions: Tolerance to Madopar varies widely between patients and is often related to the rate of dosage increases. Side-effects such as nausea, vomiting and loss of appetite, which are frequently observed during the initial stages of levodopa therapy, are much less common in patients treated with Madopar. If such side-effects do occur, they can largely be controlled by taking Madopar with, or immediately after, food and by increasing the dosage only slowly. Also, cardiovascular disturbances such as arrhythmias and orthostatic hypotension may occur, but are less frequent than in patients treated with levodopa alone.

Psychiatric disturbances are common in Parkinsonian patients, including those being treated with levodopa. They include mild elation, anxiety, agitation, insomnia, depression, aggression, delusions, hallucinations, and 'unmasking' of psychoses.

Although there have been rare reports of possible antagonism of levodopa by diazepam, in general diazepam (Valium Roche*) and nitrazepam (Mogadon*) have been found to be useful in the treatment of anxiety and insomnia, respectively, occurring in Parkinsonism.

Depression may be treated with tricyclic antidepressants although isolated cases of hypertensive crisis have been reported with the concomitant use of tricyclic drugs. ECT may be administered if appropriate. MAO inhibitors, except selective MAO-B inhibitors must not be used.

Involuntary movements, commonly in the form of oral dyskinesias, often accompanied by 'paddling' foot movements, or of the choreo-athetoid type, are common, particularly on long-term administration. These are usually dose-dependent and may disappear or become tolerable after dose adjustment.

Other side-effects which have occasionally been reported with levodopa therapy include gastro-intestinal bleeding, flushing, sweating, and drowsiness.

On some occasions the urine passed during Madopar treatment may be altered in colour; usually red-tinged, this will turn dark on standing. These changes are due to metabolites and are no cause for concern.

Transient rises in SGOT, SGPT and alkaline phosphatase values have been noted: serum uric acid and blood urea nitrogen levels are occasionally increased. In rare instances, haemolytic anaemia, mild transient leucopenia and thrombocytopenia have been reported.

Levodopa may interfere chemically with several diagnostic laboratory tests including those for glucose, ketone bodies, or catecholamines in urine and for glucose or uric acid in blood. Levodopa therapy has been reported to inhibit the response to protirelin in tests of thyroid function.

Treatment of overdosage: Symptoms of overdosage are qualitatively similar to the side-effects but may be of greater magnitude.

Treatment should include gastric lavage, general supportive measures, intravenous fluids and the maintenance of an adequate airway. Electrocardiographic monitoring should be instituted and the patient carefully observed for the possible development of arrhythmias. If necessary, anti-arrhythmic therapy should be given and other symptoms treated as they arise.

Pharmaceutical precautions
Storage: Madopar CR capsules should be protected from moisture. The recommended maximum storage temperature is 25°C.

Legal category POM.

Package quantities Madopar CR capsules containing 100 mg levodopa and 25 mg benserazide in bottles of 100 (OP).

Further information Madopar is an anti-Parkinsonian agent. Levodopa is the metabolic precursor of dopamine. The latter is severely depleted in the striatum, pallidum and substantia nigra of Parkinsonian patients and it is considered that administration of levodopa raises the level of available dopamine in these centres. However, conversion of levodopa into dopamine by the enzyme dopa decarboxylase also takes place in extracerebral tissues. As a consequence, the full therapeutic effect may not be obtained and side-effects occur.

Administration of a peripheral decarboxylase inhibitor, which blocks the extracerebral decarboxylation of levodopa, in conjunction with levodopa has significant advantages; these include reduced gastro-intestinal side-effects, a more rapid response at the initiation of therapy and a simpler dosage regimen.

Product licence number 0031/0227

MARPLAN*

Presentation Round, pink tablets with ROCHE imprinted across one face and a single break bar on the other, containing 10 mg isocarboxazid.

Uses *Properties:* Marplan is a monoamine oxidase inhibitor, effective in small doses. Its antidepressant action is thought to be related to its effect on physiological amines such as serotonin and noradrenaline, and this effect is cumulative and persistent.

Indications Treatment of the symptoms of depressive illness.

Dosage and administration *Adults:* A daily dose of 30 mg, in single or divided doses, should be given until improvement is obtained. The maximal effect is only observed after a period varying from 1–4 weeks. If no improvement has been seen by 4 weeks, doses up to 60 mg may be tried, according to the patient's tolerance, for no longer than 4–6 weeks, provided the patient is closely monitored because of the increased risk of adverse reactions occurring. Once the optimal effect is achieved, the dose should be reduced to the lowest possible amount sufficient to maintain the improvement. Clinical experience has shown this to be usually 10–20 mg daily but up to 40 mg daily may be required in some cases.

Elderly: The elderly are more likely to experience adverse reactions such as agitation, confusion and postural hypotension. Half the normal maintenance dose may be sufficient to produce a satisfactory clinical response.

Children: Marplan is not indicated for paediatric use.

Marplan tablets are for oral administration.

Contra-indications, warnings, etc
Contra-indications: Marplan is contra-indicated in patients with any impairment of hepatic function, cerebrovascular disorders or severe cardiovascular disease, and in those with actual or suspected phaeochromocytoma.

Use in pregnancy: Do not use in pregnancy, especially during the first and last trimesters, unless there are compelling reasons. There is no evidence as to drug safety in human pregnancy, nor is there evidence from animal work that it is free from hazard. In addition, the effect of psychotropic drugs on the fine brain structure of the foetus is unknown. Since there is no information on the secretion of the drug into breast milk, Marplan is contra-indicated during lactation.

Warnings: Like other monoamine oxidase inhibitors, Marplan potentiates the action of a number of drugs and foods. Patients being treated with a monoamine oxidase inhibitor should not receive indirectly-acting sympathomimetic agents, such as amphetamines, metaraminol, fenfluramine or similar anorectic agents, ephedrine or phenylpropanolamine (contained in many proprietary 'cold-cure' medications), dopamine or levodopa.

Patients should also be warned to avoid foodstuffs and beverages with a high tyramine content: mature cheeses (including processed cheeses), hydrolysed yeast or meat extracts, heavy red wines such as Chianti, and other foods which are not fresh and are fermented, pickled, 'hung', 'matured' or otherwise subject to protein degradation before consumption. Broad bean pods (which contain levodopa) and banana skins may also present a hazard.

In extreme cases interactions may result in severe hypertensive episodes. Marplan should therefore be discontinued immediately upon the occurrence of palpitations or frequent headaches.

Pethidine should not be given to patients receiving monoamine oxidase inhibitors as serious, potentially fatal reactions, including central excitation, muscle rigidity, hyperpyrexia, circulatory collapse, respiratory depression and coma, can result. Such reactions are less likely with morphine, but experience of the interaction of Marplan with narcotic analgesics other than pethidine is limited and extreme caution is therefore necessary when administering morphine to patients undergoing therapy with Marplan.

Marplan should not be administered together with, or immediately following, other monoamine oxidase inhibitors or most tricyclic antidepressants (clomipramine, desipramine, imipramine, butriptyline, nortriptyline or protriptyline). Although there is no proof that combined therapy will be effective, refractory cases of depression may be treated with Marplan in combination with amitriptyline or trimipramine, provided appropriate care is taken. Hypotensive and other adverse reactions are likely to be increased.

An interval of 1–2 weeks should be allowed after treatment with Marplan before the administration of antidepressants with a different mode of action or any other drug which may interact. On the other hand, Marplan may be given immediately following treatment with antidepressants having a different mode of action.

Marplan should be discontinued for at least 2 weeks prior to elective surgery requiring general anaesthesia. The anaesthetist should be warned that a patient is being treated with Marplan, in the event of emergency surgery being necessary.

Precautions: Concurrent administration of Marplan with other central nervous system depressants (especially barbiturates and phenothiazines), stimulants, local anaesthetics, ganglion-blocking agents and other hypotensives (including methyldopa and reserpine), diuretics, vasopressors, anticholinergic drugs and hypoglycaemic agents may lead to potentiation of their effects. This should be borne in mind if dentistry, surgery or a change in treatment of a patient becomes necessary during treatment with Marplan.

All patients taking Marplan should be warned against self-medication with proprietary 'cold-cure' preparations and nasal decongestants and advised of the dietary restrictions listed under '*Warnings*'.

With Marplan, as with other drugs acting on the central nervous system, patients should be instructed to avoid alcohol while under treatment, since the individual response cannot be foreseen. Like all medicaments of this type, Marplan may modify patients' reactions (driving ability, operation of machinery, etc.) to a varying extent, depending on dosage and individual susceptibility.

Some monoamine oxidase inhibitors have occasionally caused hepatic complications and jaundice in patients, therefore regular monitoring of liver function should be carried out during Marplan therapy. If there is any evidence of a hepatotoxic reaction, the drug should be withdrawn immediately.

The drug should be used cautiously in patients with impaired renal function, to prevent accumulation taking place, and also in the elderly or debilitated and those with cardiovascular disease, diabetes or blood dyscrasias.

In restless or agitated patients, Marplan may precipitate states of excessive excitement. Marplan appears to have varying effects in epileptic patients; while some have a decrease in frequency of seizures, others have more seizures.

Side-effects: In general, Marplan is well tolerated by the majority of patients. Side-effects, if they occur, are those common to the group of monoamine oxidase inhibitors. The most frequently reported have been orthostatic hypotension, associated in some patients with disturbances in cardiac rhythm, peripheral oedema, complaints of dizziness, dryness of the mouth, nausea and vomiting, constipation, blurred vision, insomnia, drowsiness, weakness and fatigue. These side-effects can usually be controlled by dosage reduction.

There have been infrequent reports of mild headaches, sweating, paraesthesia, peripheral neuritis, hyperreflexia, agitation, overactivity, muscle tremor, confusion and other behavioural changes, difficulty in micturition, impairment of erection and ejaculation, and skin rashes. Although rare, blood dyscrasias (purpura, granulocytopenia) have been reported. Response to Marplan may be accompanied by increased appetite and weight gain.

Treatment of overdosage: The primary symptoms of overdosage include dizziness, ataxia and irritability. In acute cases, hypotension or hypertension, tachycardia, pyrexia, psychotic manifestations, convulsions, respiratory depression and coma may occur and continue for 8–14 days before recovery.

Gastric lavage should be performed soon after ingestion and intensive supportive therapy carried out.

Sympathomimetic agents should not be given to treat hypotension but plasma expanders may be used in severe cases. Hypertensive crises may be treated by pentolinium or phentolamine, severe shock with hydrocortisone. Diazepam may be used to control convulsions or severe excitement. Dialysis is of value in eliminating the drug in severe cases.

Pharmaceutical precautions *Storage:* Marplan tablets should be stored in well-closed containers. The recommended maximum storage temperature is 25°C.

Legal category POM.

Package quantities Marplan tablets in packings of 50.

Further information Nil.

Product licence number 0031/5080R.

MESTINON*

Presentation Round, white tablets with 'ROCHE' imprinted across one face with two break bars on the other, containing 60 mg pyridostigmine bromide.

Uses *Properties:* Mestinon is an antagonist to cholinesterase, the enzyme which normally destroys acetylcholine. The action of Mestinon can briefly be described, therefore, as the potentiation of naturally occurring acetylcholine. Mestinon has a more prolonged action than Prostigmin* (neostigmine), although it is somewhat slower to take effect (generally taking 30–60 minutes). Because it has a weaker 'muscarinic' action than Prostigmin, it is usually much better tolerated by myasthenic patients in whom the longer action is also an advantage.

Oral pyridostigmine is poorly absorbed. Maximum plasma concentrations occur at 1 to 2 hours and it is eliminated by the kidney largely unchanged with a half-life of 3 to 4 hours.

Indications: Myasthenia gravis; paralytic ileus; post-operative urinary retention.

Dosage and administration
Myasthenia gravis: Adults: Doses of 30 to 120 mg are given at intervals throughout the day when maximum strength is needed (for example, on rising and before mealtimes).

The usual duration of action of a dose is three to four

hours in the daytime but a longer effect (six hours) is often obtained with a dose taken on retiring for bed.

The total daily dose is usually in the range of 5–20 tablets but doses higher than these may be needed by some patients.

Children: Children under 6 years old should receive an initial dose of half a tablet (30 mg) of Mestinon; children 6–12 years old should receive one tablet (60 mg). Dosage should be increased gradually, in increments of 15–30 mg daily, until maximum improvement is obtained. Total daily requirements are usually in the range of 30–360 mg.

The requirement for Mestinon is usually markedly decreased after thymectomy or when additional therapy (steroids, immunosuppressant drugs) is given.

When relatively large doses of Mestinon are taken by myasthenic patients it may be necessary to give atropine or other anticholinergic drugs to counteract the muscarinic effects. It should be noted that the slower gastrointestinal motility caused by these drugs may affect the absorption of oral Mestinon.

In all patients the possibility of 'cholinergic crisis', due to overdosage of Mestinon, and its differentiation from 'myasthenic crisis' due to increased severity of the disease, must be borne in mind. Both types of crisis are manifested by increased muscle weakness, but whereas myasthenic crisis may require more intensive anticholinesterase treatment, cholinergic crisis calls for immediate discontinuation of this treatment and institution of appropriate supportive measures, including respiratory assistance.

Other indications: Adults: The usual dose is 1 to 4 tablets (60–240 mg).

Children: 15–60 mg.

The frequency of these doses may be varied according to the needs of the patient.

Elderly: There are no specific dosage recommendations for Mestinon in elderly patients.

Mestinon tablets are for oral administration.

Contra-indications, warnings, etc

Contra-indications: Mestinon should not be given to patients with mechanical gastro-intestinal or urinary obstruction.

Mestinon is contra-indicated in patients with known hypersensitivity to the drug and to bromides.

Use in pregnancy: The safety of Mestinon during pregnancy or lactation has not been established. Although the possible hazards to mother and child must be weighed against the potential benefits in every case, experience with Mestinon in pregnant patients with myasthenia gravis has revealed no untoward effect of the drug on the course of pregnancy.

As the severity of myasthenia gravis often fluctuates considerably, particular care is required to avoid cholinergic crises, due to overdosage of the drug, but otherwise management is no different from that in non-pregnant patients.

Observations indicate that only negligible amounts of Mestinon are excreted in breast milk; nevertheless, due regard should be paid to possible effects on the breast-feeding infant.

Precautions: Extreme caution is required when administering Mestinon to patients with bronchial asthma.

Care should also be taken in patients with bradycardia, recent coronary occlusion, hypotension, vagotonia, epilepsy or Parkinsonism.

There is no evidence to suggest that Mestinon has any special effects in the elderly. However, elderly patients may be more susceptible to dysrhythmias than the younger adult.

Side-effects: These may include nausea and vomiting, increased salivation, diarrhoea and abdominal cramps.

Treatment of overdosage: Signs of overdosage due to muscarinic effects may include abdominal cramps, increased peristalsis, diarrhoea, nausea and vomiting, increased bronchial secretions, salivation, diaphoresis and miosis. Nicotinic effects consist of muscular cramps, fasciculations and general weakness. Bradycardia and hypotension may also occur.

Artificial ventilation should be instituted if respiratory depression is severe. Atropine sulphate 1 to 2 mg intravenously is an antidote to the muscarinic effects.

Pharmaceutical precautions *Storage:* Recommended maximum storage temperature for Mestinon tablets is 25°C. Mestinon tablets should be protected from light and moisture.

Legal category POM.

Package quantities Mestinon tablets in packs of 200.

Further information Nil.

Product licence number
Tablets 0031/5036R

MOBIFLEX*

Presentation Red-brown, film-coated, pentagonal tablets, imprinted MOBIFLEX on one face, containing 20 mg tenoxicam.

Uses

Pharmacological properties: Mobiflex is a non-steroidal anti-inflammatory drug which has marked anti-inflammatory and analgesic activity and some antipyretic activity. As with other non-steroidal anti-inflammatory drugs, the precise mode of action is unknown, though it is probably multifactorial, involving inhibition of prostaglandin biosynthesis and reduction of leucocyte accumulation at the inflammatory site.

Pharmacokinetics: Mobiflex is long-acting; a single daily dose is effective.

After oral administration, Mobiflex is rapidly and completely absorbed as unchanged drug. Concomitant food reduces the rate, but not the extent, of absorption of Mobiflex. Tenoxicam penetrates well into synovial fluid to give concentrations approximately half those in plasma. The mean plasma elimination half-life is approximately 72 hours.

With the recommended dosage regimen of 20 mg once daily, steady-state plasma concentrations are reached within 10–15 days, with no unexpected accumulation.

Mobiflex is strongly bound to plasma proteins.

Mobiflex is cleared from the body almost exclusively by metabolism. Approximately two-thirds of the administered dose is excreted in the urine, mainly as the pharmacologically inactive 5-hydroxypyridyl metabolite, and the remainder in the bile, much of it as glucuronide conjugates of hydroxymetabolites.

No age-specific changes in the pharmacokinetics of Mobiflex have been found although inter-individual variation tends to be higher in elderly persons.

Indications: Mobiflex is indicated for the relief of pain and inflammation in osteoarthritis and rheumatoid arthritis.

Dosage and administration

Adults (including the elderly): A single daily dose of 20 mg Mobiflex should be taken orally, at the same time each day, with water or other fluid. Higher doses should be avoided as they do not usually achieve significantly greater therapeutic effect but may be associated with a higher risk of adverse events.

Use in the elderly: As with other non-steroidal anti-inflammatory drugs, Mobiflex should be used with special caution in elderly patients since they may be less able to tolerate side-effects than younger patients. They are also more likely to be receiving concomitant medication or to have impaired hepatic, renal or cardiovascular function.

Children: There are insufficient data to make a recommendation for administration of Mobiflex to children.

Use in renal and hepatic insufficiency

Creatinine clearance	*Dosage regimen*
Greater than 25 ml/min.	Usual dosage but monitor patients carefully (see 'Precautions').
Less than 25 ml/min.	Insufficient data to make dosage recommendations.

Because of the high plasma protein-binding of tenoxicam, caution is required when plasma albumin concentrations are markedly reduced (e.g. in nephrotic syndrome) or when biliburin concentrations are high.

There is insufficient information to make dosage recommendations for Mobiflex in patients with pre-existing hepatic impairment.

Contra-indications, warnings, etc

Contra-indications:

1. Active peptic ulceration and a past history of peptic ulceration, gastro-intestinal bleeding (melaena, haematemesis) or severe gastritis.

2. Hypersensitivity to Mobiflex. Mobiflex should also be avoided in cases where the patient has suffered a hypersensitivity reaction (symptoms of asthma, rhinitis, angioedema or urticaria) to other non-steroidal anti-inflammatory drugs, including aspirin, as the potential exists for cross-sensitivity to Mobiflex.

Use in pregnancy: The safety of Mobiflex during pregnancy and lactation has not been established and the drug should therefore not be given in these conditions.

Although no teratogenic effects were seen in animal studies, Mobiflex, like other non-steroidal anti-inflammatory drugs, is associated with prolonged and delayed parturition and an adverse influence on neonatal viability when administered to animals in late pregnancy. Non-steroidal anti-inflammatory agents are also known to induce closure of the ductus arteriosus in infants.

No information is available on penetration of Mobiflex into milk in humans; animal studies indicate that significant levels may be achieved.

Precautions: Any patient being treated with Mobiflex who presents with symptoms of gastro-intestinal disease should be closely monitored. If peptic ulceration or gastro-intestinal bleeding occurs, Mobiflex should be withdrawn immediately.

In rare cases, non-steroidal anti-inflammatory drugs may cause interstitial nephritis, glomerulonephritis, papillary necrosis and the nephrotic syndrome. Such agents inhibit the synthesis of renal prostaglandin which plays a supportive role in the maintenance of renal perfusion in patients whose renal blood flow and volume are decreased. In these patients, administration of a non-steroidal anti-inflammatory drug may precipitate overt renal decompensation, which returns to the pre-treatment state upon withdrawal of the drug. Patients at greatest risk of such a reaction are those with pre-existing renal disease (including diabetics with impaired renal function), nephrotic syndrome, volume depletion, hepatic disease, congestive cardiac failure and those patients receiving concomitant therapy with diuretics or potentially nephrotoxic drugs. Such patients should have their renal, hepatic and cardiac functions carefully monitored.

Occasional elevations of serum transaminases or other indicators of liver function have been reported. In most cases these have been small and transient increases above the normal range. If the abnormality is significant or persistent, Mobiflex should be stopped and follow-up tests carried out. Particular care is required in patients with pre-existing hepatic disease.

Mobiflex reduces platelet aggregation and may prolong bleeding time. This should be borne in mind for patients who undergo major surgery (e.g. joint replacement) and when bleeding time needs to be determined.

Particular care should be taken to regularly monitor elderly patients to detect possible interactions with concomitant therapy and to review renal, hepatic and cardiovascular function which may be potentially influenced by non-steroidal anti-inflammatory drugs.

Adverse eye findings have been reported with non-steroidal anti-inflammatory drugs, therefore it is recommended that patients who develop visual disturbances during treatment with Mobiflex have ophthalmic evaluation.

Drug interactions: Antacids may reduce the rate, but not the extent, of absorption of Mobiflex. The differences are not likely to be of clinical significance. No interaction has been found with concomitantly administered cimetidine.

Tenoxicam is highly bound to serum albumin. Although potentiation of warfarin or sulphonylurea compounds such as glibenclamide has not been observed, close monitoring of the effects of anticoagulants or oral hypoglycaemic agents is advised, especially during the initial stages of treatment with Mobiflex. No interaction with digoxin has been observed.

Salicylates can displace tenoxicam from protein-binding sites and so increase the clearance and volume of distribution of Mobiflex. Concurrent treatment with salicylates or other non-steroidal anti-inflammatory drugs should therefore be avoided because of the increased risk of adverse reactions (particularly gastro-intestinal).

Non-steroidal anti-inflammatory drugs have been reported to produce lithium retention. If tenoxicam is prescribed for a patient receiving lithium therapy, the frequency of lithium monitoring should be increased and the patient warned to maintain fluid intake and to be aware of symptoms of lithium intoxication.

Non-steroidal anti-inflammatory drugs may cause sodium, potassium and fluid retention and may interfere with the natriuretic action of diuretic agents. These properties should be kept in mind when treating patients with compromised cardiac function or hypertension since they may be responsible for a worsening of those conditions.

No clinically relevant interaction was found in small numbers of patients receiving treatment with penicillamine or parenteral gold.

Side-effects and adverse reactions: For most patients, any side-effects are transient and resolve without discontinuation of treatment.

The most common side-effects relate to the gastro-intestinal tract. They include dyspepsia, nausea, abdominal pain and discomfort, constipation, diarrhoea, flatulence, indigestion, epigastric distress, stomatitis and anorexia.

As with other non-steroidal anti-inflammatory drugs, there is a risk of peptic ulceration and gastro-intestinal bleeding, both of which have been reported with Mobiflex. Should this occur, Mobiflex is to be discontinued immediately and appropriate treatment instituted.

As with other non-steroidal anti-inflammatory drugs, peripheral oedema of mild or moderate degree and without clinical sequelae occurred in a small proportion of patients and the possibility of precipitating congestive cardiac failure in elderly patients or those with compromised cardiac function should therefore be borne in mind.

Central nervous system reactions of headache and dizziness have been reported in a small number of patients. Somnolence, insomnia, depression, nervousness, dream abnormalities, mental confusion, paraesthesias and vertigo have been reported rarely.

Skin reactions of rash and pruritus have been reported. Nail disorders, alopecia, erythema, urticaria and photosensitivity reactions have been reported rarely. As with other non-steroidal anti-inflammatory drugs, Lyell's syndrome and Stevens-Johnson syndrome may develop in rare instances. Vesiculobullous reactions have also been reported rarely.

Reversible elevations of blood urea nitrogen and creatinine have been reported (see 'Precautions').

Decrease in haemoglobin, unrelated to gastro-intestinal bleeding, have occurred. Anaemia, thrombocytopenia and non-thrombocytopenic purpura, leucopenia and eosinophilia have been reported. Epistaxis has been reported infrequently. Rare cases of agranulocytosis have been reported.

As with most other non-steroidal anti-inflammatory drugs, changes in various liver function parameters have been observed. Some patients may develop raised serum transaminase levels during treatment. Although such reactions are rare, if abnormal liver function tests persist or worsen, if clinical signs and symptoms consistent with liver disease develop or if systemic manifestations occur (e.g. eosinophilia, rash), Mobiflex should be discontinued.

Palpitations and dyspnoea have also been reported rarely. Metabolic abnormalities such as weight decrease or increase and hyperglycaemia have occurred rarely.

Swollen eyes, blurred vision and eye irritation have been reported. Ophthalmoscopy and slit-lamp examination have revealed no evidence of ocular changes. Malaise and tinnitus may occur.

Treatment of overdosage: There is no reported experience of serious overdosage with Mobiflex. No specific measures are available; administration of H_2-antagonist drugs may be of benefit. Gastric lavage should be carried out as soon as possible after drug ingestion and the patient should be closely observed and general supportive measures taken as necessary.

Pharmaceutical precautions
Storage: No special storage precautions are required.

Legal category POM.

Package quantities Mobiflex tablets 20 mg in packs of 28 (OP) and 500.

Further information Nil.

Product licence number 0031/0200.

MOGADON*

Presentation Round, white tablets with ROCHE and two semi-circles imprinted on one face with a single break bar on the other, containing 5 mg nitrazepam.

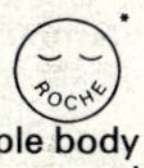

Capsules with black cap and translucent purple body with ROCHE printed in red-brown along both cap and body, containing 5mg nitrazepam.

Uses *Properties:* Mogadon is a benzodiazepine compound with sedative properties.

Indications: Short-term treatment of insomnia when it is severe, disabling or subjecting the individual to unacceptable distress, where daytime sedation is acceptable.

Dosage and administration *Adults:* 5 mg before retiring. This dose may, if necessary, be increased to 10 mg.

Elderly and debilitated patients: DOSES SHOULD NOT EXCEED HALF THOSE NORMALLY RECOMMENDED.

Dosage should be adjusted on an individual basis.

Treatment should, if possible, be on an intermittent basis.

The lowest dose which can control symptoms should be used. Treatment should not be continued at the full dose beyond four weeks. Long-term chronic use is not recommended. Treatment should always be tapered off gradually. Patients who have taken benzodiazepines for a prolonged time may require a longer period during which doses are reduced. Specialist help may be appropriate.

Mogadon 5 mg tablets and 5 mg capsules are not for paediatric use.

Mogadon tablets and capsules are for oral administration.

Contra-indications, warnings, etc
Contra-indications: Patients with known sensitivity to benzodiazepines; acute pulmonary insufficiency; respiratory depression; phobic or obsessional states; chronic psychosis.

Use in pregnancy: There is no evidence as to drug safety in human pregnancy, nor is there evidence from animal work that it is free from hazard. Do not use during pregnancy, especially during the first and last trimesters, unless there are compelling reasons.

The administration of high doses or prolonged administration of low doses of benzodiazepines in the last trimester of pregnancy has been reported to produce irregularities in the foetal heart rate, and hypotonia, poor sucking and hypothermia in the neonate.

Nitrazepam has been detected in breast milk. If possible, the use of Mogadon should be avoided during lactation.

Precautions: In patients with chronic pulmonary insufficiency, and in patients with chronic renal or hepatic disease, dosage may need to be reduced.

Mogadon should not be used alone to treat depression or anxiety associated with depression, since suicide may be precipitated in such patients.

In cases of loss or bereavement, psychological adjustment may be inhibited by benzodiazepines.

Patients should be advised that, like all medicaments of this type, Mogadon may modify patients' performance at skilled tasks (driving, operating machinery, etc.) to a varying degree depending upon dosage and individual susceptibility. Patients should further be advised that alcohol may intensify any impairment, and should, therefore, be avoided during treatment. If the patient is awoken during the period of maximum drug activity recall may be impaired.

The dependence potential of the benzodiazepines is low, particularly when limited to short-term use, but this increases when high doses are used, especially when given over long periods. This is particularly so in patients with a history of alcoholism or drug abuse or in patients with marked personality disorders. Regular monitoring in such patients is essential; routine repeat prescriptions should be avoided and treatment should be withdrawn gradually. Symptoms such as depression, nervousness, rebound insomnia, irritability, sweating, and diarrhoea have been reported following abrupt cessation of treatment in patients receiving even normal therapeutic doses for short periods of time.

In rare instances, withdrawal following excessive dosages may produce confusional states, psychotic manifestations and convulsions.

Abnormal psychological reactions to benzodiazepines have been reported. Rare behavioural effects include paradoxical aggressive outbursts, excitement, confusion and the uncovering of depression with suicidal tendencies. Extreme caution should therefore be used in prescribing benzodiazepines to patients with personality disorders.

If Mogadon is combined with centrally-acting drugs such as neuroleptics, tranquillisers, antidepressants, hypnotics, analgesics and anaesthetics, the sedative effects are likely to be intensified. The elderly require special supervision.

When Mogadon is used in conjunction with anti-epileptic drugs, side-effects and toxicity may be more evident, particularly with hydantoins or barbiturates or combinations including them. This requires extra care in adjusting dosage in the initial stages of treatment.

Side-effects and adverse reactions: Common adverse effects include drowsiness, sedation, unsteadiness and ataxia; these are dose-related and may persist into the following day, even after a single dose. The elderly are particularly sensitive to the effects of central depressant drugs and may experience confusion, especially if organic brain changes are present; the dosage of Mogadon should not exceed one-half that normally recommended for other adults.

Other adverse effects are rare and include headache, vertigo, hypotension, gastro-intestinal upsets, skin rashes, visual disturbances, changes in libido, and urinary retention. Isolated cases of blood dyscrasias and jaundice have also been reported.

Treatment of overdosage: When taken alone in overdosage Mogadon presents few problems in management. Signs may include drowsiness, ataxia and dysarthria, with coma in severe cases. Treatment is symptomatic.

Gastric lavage is useful only if performed soon after ingestion. Anexate* is a specific IV antidote for use in emergency situations. Patients requiring such intervention should be monitored closely in hospital (see separate prescribing information).

When taken with centrally-acting drugs, especially alcohol, the effects of overdosage are likely to be more severe and, in the absence of supportive measures, may prove fatal.

Pharmaceutical precautions *Storage:* Recommended maximum storage temperature for Mogadon tablets and Mogadon capsules is 30°C.

Mogadon tablets and capsules should be protected from light.

Legal category CD (Sch. 4), POM.

Package quantities Mogadon tablets 5 mg and capsules 5 mg in packings of 100.

Further information Mogadon is well absorbed with peak blood levels being achieved within two hours after administration.

The half-life of nitrazepam is on average 24 hours. Steady-state levels are achieved within five days. Nitrazepam undergoes biotransformation to a number of metabolites none of which possesses significant clinical activity.

No clear correlation has been demonstrated between the blood levels of Mogadon and its clinical effects.

The elderly, and patients with impaired renal and/or hepatic function, will be particularly susceptible to the adverse effects listed above. It is advisable to review treatment regularly and to discontinue use as soon as possible.

Treatment should be kept to a minimum and given only under close medical supervision. Little is known regarding the efficacy or safety of benzodiazepines in long-term use.

An underlying cause for insomnia should be sought before deciding upon the use of benzodiazepines for symptomatic relief.

Product licence numbers

Tablets	0031/0062R
Capsules	0031/0083R

NATULAN*

Presentation Capsules with opaque ivory cap and body, containing 58.3 mg procarbazine hydrochloride (equivalent to 50 mg of procarbazine).

Uses *Properties:* Natulan, a methylhydrazine derivative, is a cytostatic agent with weak MAO inhibitor properties. Its exact mode of action on tumour cells is unknown. It may be effective in patients who have become resistant to radiation therapy and other cystostatic agents.

Indications: The main indication is Hodgkin's disease (lymphadenoma).

Natulan may also be useful in other advanced lymphomata and a variety of solid tumours which have proved resistant to other forms of therapy.

Dosage and administration *In combination chemotherapeutic regimens:* Natulan is usually administered concomitantly with other appropriate cytostatic drugs in repeated four- to six-weekly cycles. In most such combination chemotherapy regimens currently in use (e.g. the so-called MOPP schedule with mustine, vincristine and prednisone) Natulan is given daily on the first 10–14 days of each cycle in a dosage of 100 mg per sq. metre of body surface (to nearest 50 mg).

As sole therapeutic agent: Adults: Treatment should begin with small doses which are increased gradually up to a maximum daily dose of 250 or 300 mg divided as evenly as possible throughout the day.

Initial dosage scheme

1st day	50 mg	4th day	200 mg
2nd day	100 mg	5th day	250 mg
3rd day	150 mg	6th day et seq.	250–300 mg

Further procedure: Treatment should be continued with 250 or 300 mg daily until the greatest possible remission has been obtained, after which a maintenance dose is given.

Maintenance dose: 50–150 mg daily. Treatment should be continued until a total dose of at least 6 g has been given; otherwise, a negative result is not significant.

Elderly: Natulan should be used with caution in the elderly. Patients in this group should be observed very closely for signs of early failure or intolerance of treatment.

Children: If, on the recommendation of a physician, a children's dosage is required, 50 mg daily should be given for the first week. Daily dosage should then be maintained at 100 mg per sq metre of body surface (to nearest 50 mg) until leucopenia or thrombocytopenia occurs or maximum response is obtained.

Natulan capsules are for oral administration.

Contra-indications, warnings, etc

Contra-indications: Pre-existing severe leucopenia or thrombocytopenia from any cause; severe hepatic or renal damage.

Natulan should not be used in the management of non-malignant disease.

Use in pregnancy and lactation: Natulan is teratogenic in animals. Isolated human foetal malformations have been reported following MOPP combination therapy. Therefore Natulan should not be administered to patients who are pregnant unless considered absolutely essential by the physician. Natulan should not be given to breast feeding mothers.

Precautions: Natulan should be given only under the supervision of a physician who is experienced in cancer chemotherapy and having facilities for regular monitoring of clinical and haematological effects during and after administration.

Introduction of therapy should only be effected under hospital conditions.

Caution is advisable in patients with hepatic or renal dysfunction, cardiovascular or cerebrovascular disease, phaeochromocytoma, or epilepsy.

Regular blood counts are of great importance. If, during the initial treatment, the total white cell count falls to 3,000 per mm^3 or the platelet count to 80,000 per mm^3, treatment should be suspended temporarily until the leucocyte and/or platelet levels recover, when therapy with the maintenance dose may be resumed.

Treatment should be interrupted on the appearance of allergic skin reactions.

Natulan is a weak MAO inhibitor and therefore interactions with certain foodstuffs and drugs, although very rare, must be borne in mind. Thus, owing to possible potentiation of the effect of barbiturates, narcotic analgesics (especially pethidine), drugs with anticholinergic effects (including phenothiazine derivatives and tricyclic antidepressants), other central nervous system depressants (including anaesthetic agents) and antihypertensive agents, these drugs should be given concurrently with caution and in low doses. Intolerance to alcohol (disulfiram-like reaction) may occur.

Natulan has been shown to be carcinogenic in animals. The increased risk of carcinogenicity in man should be borne in mind when long-term management of patients is proposed.

Side-effects and adverse reactions: Loss of appetite and nausea occur in most cases, sometimes with vomiting. These symptoms are usually confined to the first few days of treatment and then tend to disappear.

Natulan causes leucopenia and thrombocytopenia. These haematological changes are almost always reversible and seldom require complete cessation of therapy.

Treatment of overdosage: Signs of overdosage include severe nausea and vomiting, dizziness, hallucinations, depression and convulsions; hypotension or tachycardia may occur.

Gastric lavage and general supportive treatment should be performed, with prophylactic treatment against possible infection, and frequent blood counts.

Handling guidelines: Undamaged capsules present minimal risk of contamination, but in accordance with good hygiene requirements, direct handling should be avoided. As with all cytotoxics, precautions should be taken to avoid exposing staff during pregnancy. Waste material may be disposed of by incineration.

Pharmaceutical precautions *Storage:* Recommended maximum storage temperature 30°C. Natulan capsules in blister packings should be stored in a dry place.

Legal category POM.

Package quantities Natulan capsules in blister packs of 50.

Further information Nil.

Product licence number 0031/5038R

NEUPOGEN* ▼

Presentation Neupogen contains filgrastim (approved name), chemically known as non-glycosylated recombinant-methionyl human granulocyte-colony stimulating factor (G-CSF).

Filgrastim is produced in a laboratory strain of *Escherichia coli* bacteria which has been genetically altered by the additon of a gene for the granulocyte-colony stimulating factor.

Neupogen is a sterile, clear, colourless liquid. Each single use vial of Neupogen contains 30 million units/ml (300 micrograms/ml) of filgrastim.

Neupogen 30 contains 30 million units (300 micrograms) of filgrastim in 1.0 ml.

Neupogen 48 contains 48 million units (480 micrograms) of filgrastim in 1.6 ml.

Neupogen is formulated in an aqueous sodium acetate buffer at pH 4.0, containing 5% mannitol and 0.004% polysorbate 80.

Uses

Pharmacological properties: Human G-CSF is a glycoprotein which regulates the production and release of functional neutrophils from the bone marrow. Neupogen containing recombinant G-CSF causes marked increases in peripheral blood neutrophil counts within twenty-four hours, with minor increases in monocytes. Elevations of neutrophil counts are dose-dependent at recommended doses. Neutrophils produced in response to Neupogen show normal or enhanced function as demonstrated by tests of chemotactic and phagocytic function. Following termination of Neupogen therapy, circulating neutrophil counts decrease by 50% within 1 to 2 days, and to normal levels within 1 to 7 days.

Use of Neupogen in patients undergong cytotoxic chemotherapy leads to significant reductions in the incidence, severity and duration of neutropenia and febrile neutropenia.

Pharmacokinetics: Clearance of recombinant G-CSF has been shown to follow first-order pharmacokinetics after both subcutaneous and intravenous administration. The serum elimination half-life of recombinant G-CSF is approximately 3.5 hours, with a clearance rate of approximately 0.6 ml/min/kg. Continuous infusion with Neupogen over a period of up to 28 days, in patients recovering from autologous bone-marrow transplantation, resulted in no evidence of drug accumulation and comparable elimination half-lives. There is a positive linear correlation between the dose and the serum concentration of recombinant G-CSF, whether administered intravenously or subcutaneously. Following subcutaneous administration of recommended doses, serum concentrations were maintained above 10 ng/ml for 8 to 16 hours. The volume of distribution in blood is aproximately 150 ml/kg.

Indications: Neupogen is indicated for reduction in the duration of neutropenia and the incidence of febrile neutropenia in patients treated with established cytotoxic chemotherapy for non-myeloid malignancy.

Dosage and administration

Adults: The recommended dose of Neupogen is 0.5 MU (5 micrograms)/kg/day. The first dose of Neupogen should not be administered less than 24 hours following cytotoxic chemotherapy. Neupogen may be given as a daily subcutaneous injection or as a daily intravenous infusion diluted in 5% Glucose Intravenous Solution BP given over 30 minutes (see below section on 'Diluents and additives' for instruction). In randomised clinical trials, a subcutaneous dose of 230 micrograms/m^2/day (4.0–8.4 micrograms/kg/day) was used.

Daily dosing with Neupogen should continue until the expected neutrophil nadir is passed and the neutrophil count has recovered to the normal range. It is expected that the duration of treatment required to fulfil these criteria will be up to 14 days, depending on the type, dose and schedule of cytotoxic chemotherapy used.

In patients receiving cytotoxic chemotherapy, a transient increase in neutrophil counts is typically seen 1 to 2 days after initiation of Neupogen therapy. However, for a sustained therapeutic response, Neupogen therapy should not be discontinued before the expected nadir has passed and the neutrophil count has recovered to the normal range. Premature discontinuation of Neupogen therapy, prior to the time of the expected neutrophil nadir, is not recommended.

Therapy should only be given in collaboration with an oncology centre which has experience in G-CSF treatment and haematology and has the necessary diagnostic facilities.

Use in the elderly: Clinical trials with Neupogen have included a small number of elderly patients but special studies have not been performed in this group and therefore specific dosage recommendations cannot be made.

Children: The safety and efficacy of Neupogen have not been established in children.

Contra-indications, warnings, etc

Contra-indications: Neupogen should not be administered to patients with known hypersensitivity to the product or its constituents. Neupogen should not be used to increase the dose of cytotoxic chemotherapy beyond established dosage regimens.

Use in pregnancy and lactation: The safety of Neupogen has not been established in pregnant women. There is no evidence from studies in rats and rabbits that Neupogen is teratogenic. An increased incidence of embryo-loss has been observed in rabbits, but no malformation has been seen. In pregnancy, the possible risk of Neupogen use to the foetus must be weighed against the expected therapeutic benefit.

It is not known whether Neupogen is excreted in human milk. Neupogen is not recommended for use in nursing women.

Precautions and warnings

Malignant cell growth: Granulocyte-colony stimulating factor can promote growth of myeloid cells *in vitro* and similar effects may be seen on some non-myeloid cells *in vitro*.

The safety and efficacy of Neupogen administration in patients with myelodysplasia, acute myelogenous leukaemia, or chronic myelogenous leukaemia have not been established. Therefore because of the possibility of tumour growth, caution should be exercised in using Neupogen in any malignancy with myeloid characteristics.

Clinical trials have not yet established whether Neupogen influences the progression of myelodysplastic syndromes to acute myeloid leukaemia. Caution should be exercised in using Neupogen in any pre-malignant myeloid condition.

Leucocytosis: White blood cell counts of 100×10^9/l or greater have been observed in less than 5% of patients receiving Neupogen at doses above 0.3 MU/kg/day (3 micrograms/kg/day). No adverse events directly attributable to this degree of leucocytosis have been reported. However, in view of the potential risks associated with severe leucocytosis, a white blood cell count should be performed at regular intervals during Neupogen therapy.

If leucocyte counts exceed 50×10^9/l after the expected nadir, Neupogen should be discontinued immediately.

Risks associated with increased doses of chemotherapy: Special caution should be used when treating patients with high dose chemotherapy, because improved tumour outcome has not been demonstrated and intensified doses of chemotherapeutic agents may lead to increased toxicities including cardiac, pulmonary, neurologic, and dermatologic effects (please refer to the prescribing information of the specific chemotherapy agents used).

Treatment with Neupogen does not preclude thrombocytopenia and anaemia due to myelosuppressive chemotherapy. Because of the potential of receiving higher doses of chemotherapy (e.g. full doses on the prescribed schedule) the patient may be at greater risk of thrombocytopenia and anaemia. Regular monitoring of platelet count and haematocrit is recommended. Special care should be taken when administering single or combination chemotheraputic agents which are known to cause severe thrombocytopenia.

Other special precautions: Monitoring of bone density may be indicated in patients with underlying osteoporotic bone diseases who undergo continuous therapy with Neupogen for more than 6 months.

Studies have not been performed with Neupogen in patients with severe impairment of renal or hepatic function and therefore its use in this patient group cannot be recommended.

The effects of Neupogen in patients with substantially reduced myeloid progenitors have not been studied. Neupogen acts primarily on neutrophil precursors to exert its effect in elevating neutrophil counts. Therefore in patients with reduced precursors (such as those treated with extensive radiotherapy or chemotherapy), neutrophil response may be diminished.

Drug interactions: The safety and efficacy of Neupogen given on the same day as myelosuppressive cytotoxic chemotherapy have not been established. In view of the sensitivity of rapidly dividing myeloid cells to myelosuppressive cytotoxic chemotherapy, the use of Neupogen is not recommended in the period from 24 hours before to 24 hours after chemotherapy. Possible interactions with other haematopoietic growth factors and cytokines have not yet been investigated in clinical trials.

Side-effects and adverse reactions: In clinical trials the most frequent clinical adverse events attributable to Neupogen at the recommended dose were mild to moderate musculoskeletal pain, occurring in 10%, and severe musculoskeletal pain in 3% of patients. Musculoskeletal pain is usually controlled with standard analgesics. Less frequent adverse events include urinary abnormalities (predominantly mild or moderate dysuria).

In randomised, placebo-controlled clinical trials, Neupogen did not increase the incidence of clinical adverse events associated with cytotoxic chemotherapy. Adverse events reported with equal frequency in patients treated with Neupogen/chemotherapy and placebo/chemotherapy included nausea and vomiting, alopecia, diarrhoea, fatigue, anorexia, mucositis, headache, cough, skin rash, chest pain, generalised weakness, sore throat, constipation and unspecified pain.

Reversible, dose-dependent and usually mild or moderate elevations of lactate dehydrogenase, alkaline phosphatase, serum uric acid, and gamma-glutamyl transpeptidase occurred with Neupogen in approximately 50%, 35%, 25%, and 10% of patients, respectively at recommended doses.

Transient decreases in blood pressure, not requiring clinical treatment, have been reported occasionally.

Vascular disorders, including veno-occlusive disease and fluid volume disturbances, have been reported occasionally in patients undergoing high dose chemotherapy followed by autologous bone marrow transplantation. The causal association with Neupogen has not been established.

Treatment of overdosage: The effects of Neupogen overdosage have not been established. Discontinuation of Neupogen therapy usually results in a 50% decrease in circulating neutrophils within 1 to 2 days, with a return to normal levels in 1 to 7 days.

Pharmaceutical precautions
Storage: Neupogen should be stored in a refrigerator at 2–8°C. Do not freeze.

The pack is provided with an indicator to detect possible freezing. Vials which have been frozen (indicator on right-hand side of pack is red) should not be used.

A single brief period (up to 7 days) of exposure to elevated temperatures (up to 37°C) does not affect the stability of Neupogen.

Neupogen should not be used after the given expiry date.

Diluted Neupogen solutions should not be prepared more than 24 hours before administration and should be stored refrigerated at 2–8°C.

Neupogen vials are for single dose use only.

Diluents, additives: If required, Neupogen may be diluted in 5% Glucose Intravenous Solution BP.

Dilute Neupogen may be adsorbed to glass and plastic materials. Dilution to a final concentration less than 0.2 MU (2 micrograms) per ml is not recommended at any time.

For patients treated with Neupogen diluted to concentrations below 1.5 MU (15 micrograms) per ml, human serum albumin (HSA) should be added to a final concentration of 2 mg/ml.

Example: In a final injection volume of 20 ml, total doses of Neupogen less than 30 MU (300 micrograms) should be given with 0.2 ml of 20% HSA added.

When diluted in 5% glucose solution, Neupogen is compatible with a variety of plastics including PVC, polyolefin (a co-polymer of polypropylene and polyethylene) and polypropylene.

Neupogen should not be diluted with saline solutions.

Legal category POM.

Package quantities Neupogen 30: Packages of 5 × 1.0 ml vials. Each 1.0 ml vial contains 30 million units of filgrastim, equivalent to 300 micrograms.

Neupogen 48: Packages of 5 × 1.6 ml vials. Each 1.6 ml vial contains 48 million units of filgrastim, equivalent to 480 micrograms.

Further information In those situations where the physician determines that the patient can safely and effectively self-administer Neupogen, the patient should be instructed as to the proper dosage and method of administration.

Product licence number 0031/0268.

NIPRIDE*

Presentation Ampoules containing the equivalent of 50 mg sodium nitroprusside for reconstitution with 5% Dextrose Injection BP.

Uses *Properties:* Nipride is a potent, rapidly-acting peripheral vasodilator. Vasodilatation is achieved by a balanced action on both arterial and venous blood vessels. The action is directly on vascular musculature and is achieved independently of the autonomic nervous system. The resultant circulatory effects are dose-related and depend on the initial haemodynamic status of the patient. Thus in hypertensive and normotensive patients without heart failure a fall in systemic blood pressure is produced with little or no effect on cardiac output. In patients with heart failure, reduction of resistance to left ventricular ejection ('afterload') and lowering of raised ventricular filling pressure ('preload') regularly lead to increased cardiac output and lowered oxygen requirement of the myocardium, usually without significant hypotension.

Duration of effect is brief due to rapid conversion to cyanide and then thiocyanate. This permits minute-by-minute control of the haemodynamic effects.

Indications: Nipride is indicated for the immediate reduction of blood pressure of patients in hypertensive crises. Oral antihypertensive therapy should be started whilst the blood pressure is being controlled with Nipride.

Nipride may be used for surgical procedures where a hypotensive technique is appropriate.

Nipride may also be used to improve cardiac function in acute myocardial infarction, aortic or mitral valve disease, cardiomyopathy and other associated causes of acute or chronic heart failure. This includes its intra-operative or post-operative administration in patients undergoing surgery. Haemodynamic improvement is generally associated with an improvement in clinical symptoms of cardiac failure.

Dosage and administration Nipride is to be given as an intravenous infusion only. It is not recommended for administration by any other route or method. The infusion rate has to be determined for each individual patient by continuous monitoring of blood pressure. The maximum doses listed below should not be exceeded. Nipride should preferably be administered using a micro-drip regulator, infusion pump or any similar device which allows precise control of the flow rate. To prevent or reduce a marked compensatory reaction – which occurs particularly in younger patients – associated with a sharp rise in plasma catecholamine and renin levels, with tachycardia and corresponding tachyphylaxis of the effect of Nipride, the dose should be *increased slowly* until the desired effect occurs. The infusion *should not be terminated abruptly*, but rather over a period of 10–30 minutes, in order to prevent an excessive rise in blood pressure (rebound effect).

The dose required to achieve a given reduction in blood pressure decreases with increasing age of the patient.

If therapy is required for several days blood and plasma cyanide levels should be monitored regularly to ensure that concentrations of 100 microgram/100 ml (38 micromole/l) and 8 microgram/100 ml (3 micromole/l), respectively, are not exceeded. If an infusion is administered for more than three days, serum thiocyanate concentration should also be monitored and should not exceed 10 mg/100 ml (1.7 millimole/l). It is suggested that the maximum total dose should not exceed 70 mg/kg body-weight for periods of less than 14 days in patients with adequate renal function.

Adults: Hypertensive crises: In patients who are not receiving antihypertensive drugs, treatment with Nipride should be instituted with a dose of 0.3 to 1.0 microgram/kg body-weight/minute.

As soon as a response is obtained the dosage should be adjusted to individual requirements; this will normally be within the range of 0.5 to 6 microgram/kg/minute (average: 3 microgram/kg/minute). Usually, an average of 200 microgram/minute (range of 20 to 400 microgram/minute) is sufficient to maintain the blood pressure at a level 30 to 40 per cent lower than the pre-treatment diastolic blood pressure. The rate of administration should be adjusted to maintain the desired antihypertensive effect, as determined by frequent blood pressure measurements.

In order to avoid excessive levels of cyanide, an end-product of Nipride metabolism, and to lessen the possibility of a precipitous fall in blood pressure, the maximum recommended dose during short-term use (several hours) is 8 microgram/kg/minute. If a marked reduction of blood pressure is not obtained within 10 minutes with the maximum dosage, administration of Nipride should be stopped.

If therapy is required for longer periods, the blood and plasma cyanide and serum thiocyanate levels should be monitored as described above.

Patients who are being treated with antihypertensive drugs are more sensitive to the effects of Nipride and therefore require smaller doses. Nipride is pharmacologically compatible with other drugs commonly used to treat hypertension. The hypotensive effect of Nipride is augmented by ganglion-blocking agents.

Nipride infusion may be continued until the patient can be safely treated with oral antihypertensive agents alone.

Adults: Hypotensive procedures
When Nipride is used for the induction of deliberate hypotension during anaesthesia, lower doses than the above should be employed. The intrinsic hypotensive action of many anaesthetic agents (e.g. halothane) must be borne in mind.

It is suggested that the maximum dose should not exceed 1.5 microgram/kg/minute. The usual practices and precautions for hypotensive techniques should be observed.

Adults: Cardiac failure
Nipride should ideally only be used when facilities for intensive monitoring of the patient are available.

The Nipride infusion should be started at a rate of 10 to 15 microgram/minute and the dosage raised in increments of 10 to 15 microgram/minute every five to ten minutes until an initial response is observed. Thereafter the dosage should be adjusted until the optimal therapeutic effect is achieved. Larger initial increments may be tolerated by hypertensive patients. The therapeutic dosage is usually in the range of 10 to 200 microgram/minute.

It is suggested that dosage should not exceed 280 microgram/minute (4 microgram/kg body-weight/minute); if no significant improvement is achieved with this rate of administration, Nipride infusion should be stopped.

If signs of hypotension or hypoperfusion occur during administration of Nipride, the infusion rate should be reduced or treatment discontinued. Changes in mental status, neurological signs, oliguria, further chest pain or arrhythmias, nausea and vomiting are indications for such dosage adjustment.

Nipride infusion may be given in conjunction with diuretics, inotropic agents or other measures conventionally used in the management of cardiac failure.

Nipride should be continued until the patient can be stabilised on appropriate oral therapy. Normally this should not be for longer than 72 hours.

Elderly: Nipride should be used with caution in the elderly. Treatment should begin with low doses since they may be more sensitive to the hypotensive effects of Nipride.

Children: No dosage recommendations are made for the administration of Nipride to children.

Preparation of Nipride infusion: The infusion solution must be prepared according to the schedule given below.

The contents of a Nipride ampoule should be dissolved in the 2 ml Dextrose Injection BP provided. No other diluent may be used.

The resulting solution should be diluted in 250 ml to 1,000 ml of 5% Dextrose Injection, 0.9% Sodium Chloride Intravenous Infusion, Compound Sodium Lactate Intravenous Infusion, Compound Sodium Chloride Injection or 5% Sorbitol Intravenous Infusion. The infusion bottle should be promptly wrapped in the aluminium foil provided or other opaque materials to protect it from light. A self-adhesive label is provided for attaching to the container of the diluted infusion.

The initial solution should be prepared immediately before use and any unused portion discarded.

The freshly-prepared solution for infusion has a faint orange-brownish tint. If it is highly coloured, it should not be used.

The infusion solution should not be used after a period of twenty-four hours from the time of preparation.

Contra-indications, warnings, etc
Contra-indications: Nipride should not be used in the treatment of compensatory hypertension, e.g. that associated with conditions such as coarctation of the aorta or arteriovenous shunt.

Cyanide and thiocyanate may interfere with the metabolism of cyanocobalamin (vitamin B_{12}). Nipride is therefore contra-indicated in patients who are deficient in this vitamin, have impaired liver function or suffer from Leber's optic atrophy.

Use in pregnancy: The safety of Nipride in pregnant women has not been established.

Precautions: In patients with known disturbance of cerebral blood flow, Nipride should be used to lower blood pressure only with extreme caution.

Caution should be exercised in treating patients with

hypothyroidism because thiocyanate inhibits both the uptake and binding of iodine by the thyroid. Caution is required in treating patients with severe renal impairment as the half life of thiocyanate in plasma may be considerably longer in these patients than in patients with normal renal function.

Blood pressure should be monitored frequently during Nipride administration since the hypotensive effect is rapid. When the rate of infusion is slowed or administration is stopped, the blood pressure usually begins to rise immediately and returns to pre-treatment levels within one to ten minutes.

If higher infusion rates of Nipride are required to control the blood pressure, especially during hypotensive procedures, there is a possibility that a metabolic acidosis may occur.

Side-effects: Nausea, retching, diaphoresis, apprehension, headache, restlessness, muscle-twitching, retrosternal discomfort, palpitations, dizziness and abdominal pain have been noted with a too-rapid reduction in blood pressure. The symptoms rapidly disappear with slowing of the rate of infusion of Nipride or temporary withdrawal of the drug. When administration is continued at a slower rate of infusion symptoms do not usually recur.

Cyanide inhibits cellular oxidative metabolism. Excessive concentrations of cyanide (plasma levels greater than 8 microgram/100 ml), which may occur when levels of available endogenous thiosulphate are depleted, would be manifested by tachycardia, sweating, hyperventilation, cardiac arrhythmias and profound metabolic acidosis. Unexplained cyanosis whilst receiving Nipride may be due to methaemoglobinaemia.

Treatment of overdosage: Overdosage will be manifest by a marked fall in blood pressure below the desired level. The duration of action of Nipride is very short, the hypotensive effects ceasing almost immediately upon discontinuation of the infusion. Pre-treatment blood pressure levels are usually regained within one to ten minutes. Discontinuation of administration or a reduction in the rate of administration are usually sufficient measures for managing overdosage of Nipride.

If cyanide intoxication is diagnosed the following measures should be taken *immediately*:

1. Discontinue the infusion of Nipride.
2. Administer as a cyanide antidote either
   A. Sodium thiosulphate, 12.5 g in 25 ml or 50 ml of 5% Dextrose Injection, infused intravenously over 10 minutes. This dose may be repeated if necessary. (The value of prior administration of sodium nitrite or amyl nitrite has been questioned as this carries the risk that excessive methaemoglobin formation may adversely affect the already critically low oxygen utilisation of a cyanide-poisoned patient.)

   or

   B. Dicobalt edetate, 300 mg in 20 ml, injected intravenously over about one minute, followed by 50 ml of 50% Dextrose Injection. These doses may be repeated immediately if the response is inadequate, and a third dose given after five minutes if necessary.
3. Institute ancillary treatment (oxygen, resuscitation) to support respiration. Haemodialysis enhances removal of thiocyanate and may thereby assist recovery from cyanide poisoning.

Hydroxocobalamin has been suggested as an alternative antidote but is impractical in the acute treatment of cyanide poisoning because of the large dosage requirements. However, hydroxocobalamin 1.5 mg/kg bodyweight or sodium thiosulphate 75 mg/kg body-weight have been used prophylactically to reduce plasma cyanide concentration in patients receiving close to the recommended maximum doses of Nipride.

Pharmaceutical precautions Nipride ampoules and infusion solution should be protected from light. When the infusion solution is prepared, the container should be wrapped in aluminium foil or other opaque material. The infusion solution should not be used after a period of twenty-four hours from the time of preparation.

In aqueous solution Nipride yields the nitroprusside ion which reacts with minute quantities of a wide variety of inorganic or organic substances to form reaction products which are frequently highly coloured. If coloration is observed, the solution should be discarded.

The directions for preparation of Nipride infusion provided under Dosage and Administration should be followed. No preparations other than those recommended should be added to the Nipride ampoule or mixed with the Nipride infusion solution.

Storage: Nipride ampoules and infusion should be protected from light.

Legal category POM.

Package quantities Nipride ampoules 50 mg accompanied by ampoules of 2 ml 5% Dextrose Injection BP in packs of 5 pairs.

Further information At therapeutic doses, nitroprusside is completely metabolised in contact with erythrocytes within a few minutes, with the formation of cyanomethaemoglobin, and cyanide.

Cyanide is mostly retained within the erythrocytes ('bound' cyanide), without significantly affecting the function of the latter, and released only slowly into the plasma ('free' cyanide). In the liver, 'free' cyanide is transformed into relatively non-toxic thiocyanate in the presence of thiosulphate and rhodanase, a high-capacity enzyme. The toxicity of Nipride that has been observed in cases of overdosage and/or absence of endogenous thiosulphate is due almost entirely to the presence of excessive concentrations (>8 micrograms per 100 ml) of 'free' cyanide in the plasma. As a result of its physicochemical similarity to the iodide ion, thiocyanate is subjected to repeated enterohepatic recirculation prior to being eliminated via the kidneys. In patients with normally functioning kidneys, the biological half-life of thiocyanate is several days, but in renal insufficiency the half-life may be considerably longer. When Nipride is administered in high doses for more than three days, potentially toxic levels of thiocyanate (>10 mg per 100 ml) may therefore accumulate.

Availability: Nipride is available to hospitals only.

Product licence number 0031/0102.

NITOMAN*

Presentation Round, yellowish-buff tablets with 'Roche' imprinted across one face and a single break bar on the other, containing 25 mg tetrabenazine.

Uses *Properties:* The central effects of Nitoman closely resemble those of reserpine, but it differs from the latter in having less peripheral activity and being much shorter-acting.

It is known from animal experiments that Nitoman intervenes in the metabolism of biogenic amines, such as serotonin and noradrenaline, and that this activity is mainly limited to the brain. It is thought that the effect of Nitoman on brain amines explains its clinical effects in man.

Indications: Movement disorders associated with organic central nervous system conditions, e.g. Huntington's chorea, hemiballismus and senile chorea.

Dosage and administration *Adults:* Dosage and administration are variable and only a guide is given. An initial starting dose of 25 mg three times a day is recommended. This can be increased by 25 mg a day every three or four days until 200 mg a day is being given or the limit of tolerance, as dictated by unwanted effects, is reached, whichever is the lower dose. If there is no improvement at the maximum dose in seven days, it is unlikely that the compound will be of benefit to the patient, either by increasing the dose or by extending the duration of treatment.

Elderly: No specific studies have been performed in the elderly, but Nitoman has been administered to elderly patients in standard dosage without apparent ill effect.

Children: No specific dosage recommendations are made for the administration of Nitoman to children, although it has been used without ill effect.

Nitoman tablets are for oral administration.

Contra-indications, warnings, etc
Contra-indications: Nitoman blocks the action of reserpine.

Use in pregnancy: There is inadequate evidence of safety of the drug in human pregnancy and no evidence from animal work, but it has been in wide use for many years without apparent ill consequence. Nitoman should be avoided in breast-feeding mothers.

Precautions: Levodopa should be administered with caution in the presence of Nitoman.

Patients should be advised that Nitoman may cause drowsiness and therefore may modify their performance at skilled tasks (driving ability, operation of machinery, etc.) to a varying degree, depending on dose and individual susceptibility.

Side-effects: Side-effects are usually mild with little hypotensive action and few digestive disorders. The main unwanted effect reported to date has been drowsiness, which occurs with higher doses. If depression occurs, it can be controlled by reducing the dose or by giving antidepressant drugs such as the monoamine oxidase inhibitors. However, Nitoman should not be given immediately after a course of any of the monoamine oxidase inhibitors as such treatment may lead to a state of restlessness, disorientation and confusion. In man, a Parkinsonian-like syndrome has been reported on rare occasions, usually in doses above 200 mg per day, but this disappears on reducing the dose.

Effects of overdosage and their treatment: Signs and symptoms of overdosage may include drowsiness, sweating, hypotension and hypothermia. Treatment is symptomatic.

Pharmaceutical precautions *Storage:* Nitoman tablets should be stored in well-closed containers.

Legal category POM.

Package quantities Nitoman tablets in packings of 500.

Further information Nil.

Product licence number 0031/5073R.

NOBRIUM

Presentation Capsules with yellow opaque cap and orange opaque body with 'ROCHE 5' printed in red-brown along both cap and body, containing 5 mg medazepam.

Capsules with black cap and orange opaque body with 'ROCHE 10' printed in red-brown along both cap and body, containing 10 mg medazepam.

Uses *Properties:* Nobrium has anxiolytic properties. It has little autonomic activity.

Indications: Short-term (2–4 weeks) symptomatic treatment of anxiety that is severe, disabling or subjecting the individual to unacceptable distress, occurring alone or in association with insomnia or short-term psychosomatic, organic or psychotic illness.

Dosage and administration
Adults: Up to 40 mg daily in divided doses, adjusted on an individual basis. ELDERLY AND DEBILITATED PATIENTS: DOSES SHOULD NOT EXCEED HALF THOSE NORMALLY RECOMMENDED. The lowest dose which can control symptoms should be used. Treatment should not be continued at the full dose beyond four weeks. Long-term chronic use is not recommended. Treatment should always be tapered off gradually. Patients who have taken benzodiazepines for a prolonged time may require a longer period during which doses are reduced. Specialist help may be appropriate.

Nobrium is not for paediatric use.

Nobrium capsules are for oral administration.

Contra-indications, warnings, etc
Contra-indications: Patients with known sensitivity to benzodiazepines; acute pulmonary insufficiency; respiratory depression; phobic or obsessional states; chronic psychosis.

Use in pregnancy: There is no evidence as to drug safety in human pregnancy, nor is there evidence from animal work that it is free from hazard. Do not use during pregnancy, especially during the first and last trimesters, unless there are compelling reasons.

The administration of high doses or prolonged administration of low doses of benzodiazepines in the last trimester of pregnancy or during labour has been reported to produce irregularities in the foetal heart rate, and hypotonia, poor sucking and hypothermia in the neonate.

Medazepam and its metabolites may appear in breast milk. If possible, the use of Nobrium should be avoided during lactation.

Precautions: In patients with chronic pulmonary insufficiency, and in patients with chronic renal or hepatic disease, dosage may need to be reduced.

Nobrium should not be used alone to treat depression or anxiety associated with depression, since suicide may be precipitated in such patients.

Amnesia may occur.

In cases of loss or bereavement, psychological adjustment may be inhibited by benzodiazepines.

Patients should be advised that, like all medicaments of this type, Nobrium may modify patients' performance at skilled tasks (driving, operating machinery, etc.) to a varying degree depending upon dosage, administration and individual susceptibility. Patients should further be advised that alcohol may intensify any impairment, and should, therefore, be avoided during treatment.

The dependence potential of the benzodiazepines is low, particularly when limited to short-term use, but this increases when high doses are used, especially when given over long periods. This is particularly so in patients with a history of alcoholism or drug abuse or in patients with marked personality disorders. Regular monitoring in such patients is essential, routine repeat prescriptions should be avoided and treatment should be withdrawn gradually. Symptoms such as depression, nervousness, rebound insomnia, irritability, sweating, and diarrhoea have been reported following abrupt cessation of treatment in patients receiving even normal therapeutic doses for short periods of time.

In rare instances, withdrawal following excessive dosages may produce confusional states, psychotic manifestations and convulsions.

Abnormal psychological reactions to benzodiazepines have been reported. Rare behavioural effects include paradoxical aggressive outbursts, excitement, confusion, and the uncovering of depression with suicidal tendencies. Extreme caution should therefore be used in prescribing benzodiazepines to patients with personality disorders.

If Nobrium is combined with centrally-acting drugs such as neuroleptics, tranquillisers, antidepressants, hypnotics, analgesics and anaesthetics, the sedative effects are likely to be intensified. The elderly require special supervision.

When Nobrium is used in conjunction with anti-epileptic drugs, side-effects and toxicity may be more evident, particularly with hydantoins or barbiturates or combinations including them. This requires extra care in adjusting dosage in the initial stages of treatment.

Side-effects and adverse reactions: Common adverse effects include drowsiness, sedation, unsteadiness and ataxia; these are dose-related and may persist into the following day, even after a single dose. The elderly are particularly sensitive to the effects of central depressant drugs and may experience confusion, especially if organic brain changes are present; the dosage of Nobrium should not exceed one-half that recommended for other adults.

Other adverse effects are rare and include headache, vertigo, hypotension, gastro-intestinal upsets, skin rashes, visual disturbances, changes in libido, and urinary retention. Isolated cases of blood dyscrasias and jaundice have also been reported.

Treatment of overdosage: When taken alone in overdosage Nobrium presents few problems in management. Signs may include drowsiness, ataxia and dysarthria, with coma in severe cases. Treatment is symptomatic. Gastric lavage is useful only if performed soon after ingestion. Anexate* is a specific IV antidote for use in emergency situations. Patients requiring such intervention should be monitored closely in hospital (see separate prescribing information).

When taken with centrally-acting drugs, especially alcohol, the effects of overdosage are likely to be more severe and, in the absence of supportive measures, may prove fatal.

Pharmaceutical precautions *Storage:* No special precautions are required.

Legal category CD (Sch. 4), POM.

Package quantities Nobrium capsules 5 mg, 10 mg in packs of 100.

Further information Nobrium is rapidly absorbed, and peak blood levels are reached within two hours of dosing. The drug itself has a short half-life and is metabolised to normedazepam and diazepam, then to N-desmethyldiazepam. These active metabolites have longer half-lives and accumulate during repeated administration.

The active metabolite, N-desmethyldiazepam, accumulates to reach concentrations five to ten times those of the parent compound. Ten to fifteen days continuous administration are thought to produce steady state plasma levels, although a longer period may be required in some individuals, particularly the elderly.

No clear correlation has been demonstrated between the blood levels of Nobrium and its clinical effects.

The elderly, and patients with impaired renal and/or hepatic function, will be particularly susceptible to the adverse effects listed above. It is advisable to review treatment regularly and to discontinue use as soon as possible.

Treatment should be kept to a minimum and given only under close medical supervision. Little is known regarding the efficacy or safety of benzodiazepines in long-term use.

Product licence numbers

Capsules 5 mg	0031/5039R
Capsules 10 mg	0031/5040R

OMNOPON*

Presentation Ampoules containing 20 mg papaveretum in 1 ml. The ampoule solution is colourless to yellowish-brown. Hydroxybenzoates are included in the formulation as preservatives.

Uses *Properties:* Omnopon, a potent analgesic, combines both the phenanthrene and isoquinoline groups of opium alkaloids. The former includes codeine and morphine which exert a marked narcotic action on the central nervous system. The second group is represented by papaverine, which acts mainly at the periphery as an antispasmodic, and noscapine.

Indications: Pre-operative medication; relief of post-operative pain; relief of severe chronic pain, particularly that of inoperable carcinoma, relief of pain in coronary thrombosis.

Dosage and administration Omnopon ampoules are for intramuscular, intravenous or subcutaneous injection. Omnopon ampoule solution contains hydroxybenzoates as preservatives and therefore should not be given by the intrathecal route.

Adults: Single dose of 10 to 20 mg by injection, usually not to be repeated more often than 4 hourly.

Elderly: Elderly patients are more sensitive to the actions of narcotic analgesics: the initial dose of Omnopon should not exceed 10 mg.

Children 1 to 12 years: Usual dosage 0.2–0.3 mg papaveretum/kg body-weight, as a maximum single dose.

Example:

Age	*Weight on 50th centile (approx.)*	*Dose of papaveretum required (0.2–0.3 mg/kg)*	*Quantity of Omnopon 20 mg/ml solution required*
1 year	*10 kg*	*2–3 mg*	*0.10–0.15 ml*
12 years	*40 kg*	*8–12 mg*	*0.4–0.6 ml*

The use of a small graduated syringe is recommended for the accurate administration of dosages given to children. In the absence of graduated syringes, Omnopon ampoule solution should be diluted with Water for Injections before measuring the dose.

Maintenance of stability cannot be guaranteed when Omnopon ampoule solution is diluted.

Omnopon ampoules are not recommended for use in babies under one year of age.

Contra-indications, warnings, etc

Contra-indications: Omnopon should not be given to comatose patients or patients with respiratory depression or obstructive airways disease. It should not be administered to patients who are receiving monoamine oxidase inhibitors or within two weeks of their withdrawal.

Omnopon should not be given to patients with a history of hypersensitivity or idiosyncratic response to opium alkaloids.

Use in pregnancy: There is inadequate evidence of safety of Omnopon in human pregnancy, but the drug has been widely used for many years without apparent ill-consequence, and animal studies have not shown any hazard. Nevertheless, the established medical principle of prescribing medicaments in early pregnancy only when absolutely indicated should be observed.

Omnopon crosses the placenta and is also secreted in breast milk. This should be borne in mind when considering its use in patients during pregnancy or breast feeding. Administration in labour may cause respiratory depression in the newborn infant.

Precautions: Omnopon should only be given with caution, and in reduced dosage, to elderly and debilitated patients, and in patients with head injuries, severe hepatic or renal impairment, biliary tract disorders, hypothyroidism, adrenocortical insufficiency, shock, prostatic hypertrophy, and supraventricular tachycardia.

Caution is also required in patients exhibiting acute alcoholism, raised intracranial pressure or convulsive disorders. Omnopon depresses respiratory function and should be administered with particular care in patients with respiratory insufficiency.

The effects of Omnopon may be potentiated by concurrent administration of other central nervous system depressants, including anaesthetic agents. Concomitant administration of Omnopon with phenothiazines may induce severe hypotension. Patients should be instructed to avoid alcohol while under treatment, since the individual response cannot be foreseen.

Omnopon may modify patients' reactions (driving ability, operation of machinery, etc.) to a varying extent, depending on dosage, administration and individual susceptibility.

Repeated administration of Omnopon may induce tolerance to the drug, with a tendency to increasing dosage requirements to obtain the desired effect, or to physical and psychological dependence of the morphine type, with the development of withdrawal symptoms after abrupt cessation of therapy. Cross-tolerance between narcotic analgesics can occur.

Side-effects: Nausea and vomiting may be troublesome. Constipation and confusion may occur. Late post-operative vomiting may be a problem in paediatrics. Very rarely, neonatal convulsions have been reported.

Treatment of overdosage: Signs of overdosage are similar

to those with morphine; they include pin-point pupils, depressed respiration and coma. In severe poisoning there may be dilatation of the pupils, shock, severe respiratory depression and pulmonary oedema.

Intensive supportive therapy should be carried out. Naloxone is the preferred antidote.

Pharmaceutical precautions *Storage:* Omnopon ampoules should be protected from light. The recommended maximum storage temperature is 25°C.

Legal category CD (Sch. 2), POM.

Package quantities Omnopon ampoules in packings of 10.

Further information Omnopon is also available as Paediatric ampoules (10 mg/ml) to facilitate administration to young children (see separate prescribing information).

Product licence number 0031/5100R

OMNOPON* PAEDIATRIC AMPOULES

Presentation Ampoules containing 10 mg papaveretum in 1 ml. The ampoule solution is colourless to yellowish-brown. Hydroxybenzoates are included in the formulation as preservatives.

Uses *Properties:* Omnopon, a potent analgesic, contains both the phenanthrene and isoquinoline groups of opium alkaloids. The former includes codeine and morphine, which exert a marked narcotic action on the central nervous system. The second group is represented by papaverine, which acts mainly at the periphery as an antispasmodic, and noscapine.

Indications: Pre-operative medication; relief of post-operative pain; relief of severe chronic pain, particularly that of inoperable carcinoma; relief of pain in coronary thrombosis.

Dosage and administration Omnopon paediatric ampoules 10 mg/ml are for intramuscular, intravenous, or subcutaneous injection. Omnopon paediatric ampoule solution 10 mg/ml contains hydroxybenzoates as preservatives and therefore should not be given by the intrathecal route.

Adults: Single dose of 10 to 20 mg by injection, usually not to be repeated more often than four hourly.

Elderly: Elderly patients are more sensitive to the actions of narcotic analgesics: the initial dose should not exceed 10 mg.

Children 1–12 years: Usual dosage: 0.2–0.3 mg/kg body-weight, as a maximum single dose.

Example

Age	*Weight on 50th centile (approx.)*	*Dose of papaveretum required (0.2–0.3 mg/kg)*	*Quantity of Omnopon 10 mg/ml solution required*
1 year	10 kg	2–3 mg	0.2–0.3 ml
12 years	40 kg	8–12 mg	0.8–1.2 ml

Children 1–12 months: Usual dosage: 0.15–0.2 mg/kg body-weight, as a maximum single dose.

Example:

Age	*Weight on 50th centile (approx.)*	*Dose of papaveretum (0.15–0.2 mg/kg) required*	*Quantity of Omnopon 10 mg/ml solution required*
3 months	5 kg	0.75–1 mg	0.075–0.1 ml
12 months	10 kg	1.5–2 mg	0.15–0.2 ml

Neonates aged up to 1 month

Usual dosage: 0.15 mg/kg body-weight, as a maximum single dose.

Example:

Age	*Weight on 50th centile (approx.)*	*Dose of papaveretum (0.15 mg/kg) required*	*Quantity of Omnopon 10 mg/ml solution required*
Newborn	3.5 kg	0.525 mg	0.0525 ml
1 month	4.0 kg	0.6 mg	0.06 ml

The use of a small graduated syringe is recommended for the accurate administration of dosages given to children. In the absence of graduated syringes, Omnopon Paediatric ampoule solution should be diluted with Water for Injections before measuring the dose.

Maintenance of stability cannot be guaranteed when Omnopon Paediatric ampoule solution is diluted.

Omnopon Paediatric ampoules 10 mg/ml are particularly recommended for use in babies under one year of age.

Contra-indications, warnings, etc
Contra-indications: Omnopon should not be given to comatose patients or to patients with respiratory depression or obstructive airways disease. It should not be administered to patients who are receiving monoamine oxidase inhibitors or within two weeks of their withdrawal.

Omnopon should not be given to patients with a history of hypersensitivity or idiosyncratic response to opium alkaloids.

Use in pregnancy: There is inadequate evidence of safety of Omnopon in human pregnancy, but the drug has been widely used for many years without apparent ill-consequence, and animal studies have not shown any hazard. Nevertheless, the established medical principle of prescribing medicaments in early pregnancy only when absolutely indicated should be observed.

Omnopon crosses the placenta and is also excreted in breast milk. This should be borne in mind when considering its use in patients during pregnancy or breast feeding. Administration in labour may cause respiratory depression in the newborn infant.

Precautions: Omnopon should only be given with caution, and in reduced dosage, to neonates and premature infants, elderly and debilitated patients, and in patients with head injuries, severe hepatic or renal impairment, biliary tract disorders, hypothyroidism, adrenocortical insufficiency, shock, prostatic hypertrophy, and supraventricular tachycardia.

Caution is also required in patients exhibiting acute alcoholism, raised intracranial pressure or convulsive disorders. Omnopon depresses respiratory function and should be administered with particular care in patients with respiratory insufficiency.

The effects of Omnopon may be potentiated by concurrent administration of other central nervous system depressants, including anaesthetic agents. Concomitant administration of Omnopon with phenothiazines may induce severe hypotension.

Patients should be instructed to avoid alcohol while under treatment, since the individual response cannot be foreseen.

Omnopon may modify patients' reactions (driving ability, operation of machinery, etc.) to a varying extent, depending on dosage, administration and individual susceptibility.

Repeated administration of Omnopon may induce tolerance to the drug, with a tendency to increasing dosage requirements to obtain the desired effect, or to physical and psychological dependence of the morphine type, with the development of withdrawal symptoms after abrupt cessation of therapy. Cross-tolerance between narcotic analgesics can occur.

Side-effects: Nausea and vomiting may be troublesome. Constipation and confusion may occur. Late post-operative vomiting may be a problem in paediatrics. Very rarely, neonatal convulsions have been reported.

Treatment of overdosage: Signs of overdosage are similar to those with morphine; they include pin-point pupils, depressed respiration and coma. In severe poisoning there may be dilatation of the pupils, shock, severe respiratory depression and pulmonary oedema.

Intensive supportive therapy carried out. Naloxone is the preferred antidote.

Pharmaceutical precautions *Storage:* Omnopon Paediatric ampoules 10 mg/ml should be protected from light; the recommended maximum storage temperature is 25°C.

Legal category CD (Sch. 2), POM.

Package quantities Omnopon Paediatric ampoules 10 mg/ml in packings of 10.

Further information Omnopon is also available as ampoules 20 mg/ml (see separate prescribing information).

Product licence number 0031/0156.

OMNOPON*-SCOPOLAMINE

Presentation Ampoules containing 20 mg of papaveretum and 0.4 mg of hyoscine (scopolamine) hydrobromide in 1 ml. The ampoule solution is almost colourless to pale yellow. Hydroxybenzoates are included in the formulation as preservatives.

Uses *Properties:* Omnopon-scopolamine combines the properties of the opium alkaloids with those of scopolamine. Thus it is an analgesic and sedative and has a marked inhibitory effect on the secretions.

Indication: Pre-anaesthetic medication.

Dosage and administration Omnopon-scopolamine ampoules are for intramuscular or subcutaneous injection. Omnopon-scopolamine ampoule solution contains hydroxybenzoates as preservatives and therefore should not be given by the intrathecal route.

Adults: Usually ½ to one ampoule injected ¾–1 hour before anaesthesia.

Elderly: No specific studies have been performed in the elderly but this group is more sensitive to the actions of narcotic analgesics and hyoscine: the dose of Omnopon-scopolamine should not exceed ½ ampoule.

Children 1–12 years: Usual dosage: 0.2–0.3 mg/kg papaveretum body-weight, as a maximum single dose.

Example:

Age	*Weight on 50th centile (approx.)*	*Dose of papaveretum required (0.2–0.3 mg/kg)*	*Quantity of Omnopon-scopolamine required*
1 year	10 kg	2–3 mg	0.10–0.15 ml
12 years	40 kg	8–12 mg	0.4–0.6 ml

The use of a small graduated syringe is recommended for the accurate administration of dosages given to children. In the absence of graduated syringes, Omnopon-scopolamine ampoule solution should be diluted with Water for Injections before measuring the dose.

Maintenance of stability cannot be guaranteed when Omnopon-scopolamine ampoule solution is diluted.

Omnopon-scopolamine ampoules are not recommended for use in babies under one year.

Contra-indications, warnings, etc

Contra-indications: Omnopon-scopolamine should not be given to comatose patients or to patients with respiratory depression or obstructive airways disease. It should not be administered to patients who are receiving monoamine oxidase inhibitors or within two weeks of their withdrawal.

Omnopon-scopolamine should not be given to patients with a history of hypersensitivity or idiosyncratic response to opium alkaloids.

Use in pregnancy: There is inadequate evidence of safety of Omnopon-scopolamine in human pregnancy, but the drug has been widely used for many years without apparent ill-consequence, and animal studies have not shown any hazard. Nevertheless, the established medical principle of prescribing medicaments in early pregnancy only when absolutely indicated should be observed.

Omnopon-scopolamine crosses the placenta and is also excreted in breast milk. This should be borne in mind when considering its use in patients during pregnancy or breast feeding. Administration in labour may cause respiratory depression in the newborn infant.

Precautions: Omnopon-scopolamine should only be given with caution, and in reduced dosage, to neonates and premature infants, elderly and debilitated patients, and in patients with head injuries, severe hepatic or renal impairment, biliary tract disorders, hypothyroidism, adrenocortical insufficiency, shock, prostatic hypertrophy, and supraventricular tachycardia.

Caution is also required in patients exhibiting acute alcoholism, raised intracranial pressure or convulsive disorders. Omnopon-scopolamine depresses respiratory function and should be administered with particular care in patients with respiratory insufficiency.

The effects of Omnopon-scopolamine may be potentiated by concurrent administration of other central nervous system depressants, including anaesthetic agents. Concomitant administration of Omnopon-scopolamine with phenothiazines may induce severe hypotension. Patients should be instructed to avoid alcohol while under treatment, since the individual response cannot be foreseen.

Omnopon-scopolamine may modify patients' reactions (driving ability, operation of machinery, etc.) to a varying extent, depending on dosage, administration and individual susceptibility.

Repeated administration of Omnopon-scopolamine may induce tolerance to the drug, with a tendency to increasing dosage requirements to obtain the desired effect, or to physical and psychological dependence of the morphine type, with the development of withdrawal symptoms after abrupt cessation of therapy. Cross-tolerance between narcotic analgesics can occur.

Side-effects: Nausea and vomiting may be troublesome. Constipation and confusion may also occur. Late post-operative vomiting may be a problem in paediatrics. Very rarely, neonatal convulsions have been reported. Dryness of the mouth usually occurs.

Treatment of overdosage: Signs of overdosage are similar to those seen with morphine. Pin-point pupils, depressed respiration and impaired level of consciousness or coma may occur. In severe poisoning there may be dilatation of the pupils, shock, severe respiratory depression and pulmonary oedema.

Intensive supportive therapy should be carried out. Naloxone is the preferred antidote. If excitement due to scopolamine occurs, Valium Roche (diazepam) or short-acting barbiturates may be helpful.

Pharmaceutical precautions *Storage:* Omnopon-scopolamine ampoules should be protected from light. The recommended maximum storage temperature is 25°C.

Legal category CD (Sch. 2), POM.

Package quantities Omnopon-scopolamine ampoules in packings of 10.

Further information Nil.

Product licence number 0031/5096R.

PETHIDINE ROCHE

Presentation Round white tablets with 'ROCHE' imprinted on one face, containing 50 mg pethidine hydrochloride.

Ampoules containing 50 mg pethidine hydrochloride in 1 ml. The ampoule solution is colourless to pale yellow.

Ampoules containing 100 mg pethidine hydrochloride in 2 ml. The ampoule solution is colourless to pale yellow.

Uses *Properties:* Pethidine Roche combines analgesic and antispasmodic properties; it is relatively short acting and has little soporific effect. These properties make Pethidine Roche particularly useful for pain relief in labour and as an adjunct to nitrous oxide-oxygen anaesthesia.

Indications: Obstetric analgesia; moderate to severe pain; premedication and analgesia during anaesthesia.

Dosage and administration *Adults:* The normal single dose, usually not to be repeated more often than four-hourly, is as follows:

Oral: 50–150 mg.

Intramuscular or subcutaneous injection: 25–100 mg.

Intravenous injection: 25–50 mg.

Elderly and debilitated patients: Initial doses should not exceed 50 mg orally or 25 mg by injection as elderly and debilitated patients are likely to be particularly sensitive to the central depressant effects of the drug.

Children: Single dose of 0.5–2 mg/kg body weight orally or intramuscularly. This dose may be repeated if clinically necessary but it should not be repeated more often than four-hourly.

The use of a small graduated syringe is recommended for the accurate administration of dosages given to children. In the absence of graduated syringes, Pethidine Roche ampoule solution should be diluted with Water for Injections before measuring the dose.

Pethidine Roche tablets are for oral administration. Pethidine Roche ampoules are for intramuscular, intravenous or subcutaneous injection.

Pethidine Roche ampoule solution may be diluted with Water for Injection.

Maintenance of stability cannot be guaranteed when Pethidine Roche ampoule solution is diluted.

Contra-indications, warnings, etc

Contra-indications: Pethidine Roche should not be given to comatose patients or to patients with respiratory depression or obstructive airways disease. It should not be administered to patients who are receiving monoamine oxidase inhibitors or within two weeks of their withdrawal.

Pethidine Roche should not be given to patients with a history of hypersensitivity or idiosyncratic response to the drug.

Use in pregnancy: There is inadequate evidence of safety of pethidine in human pregnancy, but the drug has been widely used for many years without apparent ill-consequence, and animal studies have not shown any hazard. Nevertheless, the established medical principle of prescribing medicaments in early pregnancy only when absolutely indicated should be observed.

Pethidine Roche crosses the placenta and is also secreted in breast milk. This should be borne in mind when considering its use in patients during pregnancy or breast feeding. Administration in labour may cause respiratory depression in the newborn infant.

Precautions: Pethidine Roche should only be given with caution, and in reduced dosage, to neonates and premature infants, elderly and debilitated patients, and in patients with head injuries, severe hepatic or renal impairment, biliary tract disorders, hypothyroidism, adrenocortical insufficiency, shock, prostatic hypertrophy, and supraventricular tachycardia.

Caution is also required in patients exhibiting acute alcoholism, raised intracranial pressure or convulsive disorders. Pethidine Roche depresses respiratory function and should be administered with particular care in patients with respiratory insufficiency.

The effects of pethidine may be potentiated by concurrent administration of other central nervous system depressants, including anaesthetic agents. Concomitant administration of pethidine with phenothiazines may induce severe hypotension. Pethidine induced neurotoxicity may be seen in patients with renal failure, cancer or sickle cell anaemia, during concomitant administration with anticholinergics or during chronic administration of increasing pethidine doses. Patients should be instructed to avoid alcohol while under treatment, since the individual response cannot be foreseen.

Pethidine may modify patients' reactions (driving ability, operation of machinery, etc.) to a varying extent, depending on dosage, administration and individual susceptibility.

Repeated administration of pethidine may induce tolerance to the drug, with a tendency to increasing dosage requirements to obtain the desired effect, or to physical and psychological dependence of the morphine type, with the development of withdrawal symptoms after abrupt cessation of therapy. Cross-tolerance between narcotic analgesics can occur.

Side-effects: Pethidine Roche may cause mild euphoria, dizziness, nausea and vomiting, hypotension and respiratory depression.

CNS excitation may occur in certain groups.

Treatment of overdosage: In acute overdosage, signs and symptoms may include incoordination, tremors and convulsions followed by respiratory depression and coma.

Gastric lavage should be performed soon after ingestion, and intensive supportive therapy carried out. Naloxone is the preferred antidote. The urinary excretion can be increased by rendering the urine acid by the administration of ammonium chloride.

Patients exhibiting signs of CNS toxicity should be treated by immediate discontinuation of pethidine substituting an alternative narcotic for pain, supporting respiratory function and administering an anticonvulsant if seizures occur. A return to normal neurological function would be expected in three to four days.

Pharmaceutical precautions *Storage:* Pethidine Roche tablets in blister packs should be stored in a dry place. The recommended maximum storage temperature for Pethidine Roche tablets is 35°C.

The recommended maximum storage temperature for Pethidine Roche ampoules is 30°C.

Legal category CD (Sch. 2), POM.

Package quantities Pethidine Roche tablets 50 mg in cartons of 50, containing 5 blister strips of 10 tablets.

Pethidine Roche ampoules containing 50 mg in 1 ml and 100 mg in 2 ml and in packs of 10.

Further information Nil.

Product licence numbers

Tablets 25 mg	0031/5102R
Tablets 50 mg	0031/5103R
Ampoules 50 mg	0031/5105R
Ampoules 100 mg	0031/5106R

PROSTIGMIN*

Presentation Round, white tablets with 'PROSTIGMIN' imprinted on one face with a single break bar on the other, containing 15 mg neostigmine bromide.

Ampoules containing 0.5 mg neostigmine methylsulphate in 1 ml. The ampoule solution is almost colourless to pale yellow.

Ampoules containing 2.5 mg neostigmine methylsulphate in 1 ml. The ampoule solution is almost colourless to pale yellow.

Uses *Properties:* Prostigmin is an antagonist to cholinesterase, the enzyme which normally destroys acetylcholine. The action of Prostigmin can briefly be described, therefore, as the potentiation of naturally occurring acetylcholine.

Indications: Myasthenia gravis; antagonist to non-depolarising neuromuscular blockade; paralytic ileus; post-operative urinary retention.

Dosage and administration Prostigmin has a slower

onset of effect when given orally than when given parenterally, but the duration of action is longer and the intensity of action more uniform.

To facilitate change of treatment from one route of administration to another, the following doses are approximately equivalent in effect:

0.5 mg intravenously = 1–1.5 mg intramuscularly or subcutaneously = 15 mg orally.

Administration of Prostigmin by the intravenous route, if required, should be by very slow injection. When Prostigmin is given by injection a syringe of atropine sulphate should always be available to counteract severe cholinergic reactions, should they occur.

Myasthenia gravis

Adults: Doses of 15 to 30 mg by mouth or 1–2.5 mg by intramuscular or subcutaneous injection are given at intervals throughout the day when maximum strength is needed (for example, on rising and before mealtimes). The usual duration of action of a dose is two to four hours.

The total daily dose is usually in the range of 5–20 tablets (or 5–20 mg by injection) but doses higher than these may be needed by some patients.

Newborn infants: An initial dose of Prostigmin 0.1 mg should be given intramuscularly (or 1–2 mg orally if preferred). Thereafter dosage must be titrated individually but is usually 0.05–0.25 mg by injection or 1–5 mg orally every four hours, given half an hour before feeding.

Treatment is not usually required beyond eight weeks of age except in the rare conditions of congenital and familial infantile myasthenia.

Older children: Children under 6 years old should receive an initial dose of half a tablet (7.5 mg) of Prostigmin; children 6–12 years old should receive one tablet (15 mg). Alternatively, 0.2–0.5 mg may be given by injection as required. Dosage requirements should be adjusted according to the response but are usually in the range of 15–90 mg orally per day.

The requirement for Prostigmin is usually markedly decreased after thymectomy, or when additional therapy (steroids, immunosuppressant drugs) is given.

When relatively large doses of Prostigmin are taken by myasthenic patients, it may be necessary to give atropine or other anticholinergic drugs to counteract the muscarinic effects. It should be noted that the slower gastro-intestinal motility caused by these drugs may affect the absorption of oral Prostigmin.

In all patients the possibility of 'cholinergic crisis', due to overdosage of Prostigmin, and its differentiation from 'myasthenic crisis', due to increased severity of the disease, must be borne in mind. Both types of crisis are manifested by increased muscle weakness, but whereas myasthenic crisis may require more intensive anticholinesterase treatment, cholinergic crisis calls for immediate discontinuation of this treatment and institution of appropriate supportive measures, including respiratory assistance.

Antagonist to non-depolarising neuromuscular blockade

Generally, reversal of neuromuscular block with Prostigmin should not be attempted until there is evidence of spontaneous recovery from paralysis. It is recommended that the patient be well ventilated and a patent airway maintained until complete recovery of normal respiration is assured.

Adults and children: A single dose of Prostigmin 0.05–0.07 mg/kg body-weight and atropine 0.02–0.03 mg/kg body-weight, by slow intravenous injection over one minute, is usually adequate for complete reversal of non-depolarising muscle relaxants within 5–15 minutes. The maximum recommended dose of Prostigmin in adults is 5 mg and in children 2.5 mg. The two drugs are often given simultaneously, but in patients who show bradycardia the pulse rate should be increased to about 80/minute with atropine before administering Prostigmin.

The speed of recovery from neuromuscular blockade is primarily determined by the intensity of the block at the time of antagonism but it is also subject to other factors, including the presence of drugs (e.g. anaesthetic agents, antibiotics, antiarrhythmic drugs) and physiological changes (electrolyte and acid-base imbalance, renal impairment). These factors may prevent successful reversal with Prostigmin or lead to re-curarisation after apparently successful reversal. Therefore it is imperative that patients should not be left unattended until these possibilities have been excluded.

Other indications

Adults: The usual dose is 1 to 2 tablets orally or 0.5 to 2.5 mg by subcutaneous or intramuscular injection.

Children: 2.5–15 mg orally or 0.125–1 mg by injection. The frequency of these doses may be varied according to the needs of the patient.

Elderly: There are no specific dosage recommendations for Prostigmin in elderly patients.

Prostigmin tablets for oral administration, Prostigmin ampoules for intramuscular, intravenous or subcutaneous injection.

Prostigmin ampoule solution may be diluted with Water for Injection. However maintenance of stability cannot be guaranteed when Prostigmin preparations are diluted.

Contra-indications, warnings, etc

Contra-indications: Prostigmin should not be given to patients with mechanical gastro-intestinal or urinary obstruction.

Prostigmin is contra-indicated in patients with known hypersensitivity to the drug and, in the case of Prostigmin tablets, to bromides.

Prostigmin should not be used in conjunction with depolarising muscle relaxants such as suxamethonium as neuromuscular blockade may be potentiated and prolonged apnoea may result.

Use in pregnancy: The safety of Prostigmin during pregnancy or lactation has not been established. Although the possible hazards to mother and child must therefore be weighed against the potential benefits in every case, experience with Prostigmin in pregnant patients with myasthenia gravis has revealed no untoward effect of the drug on the course of pregnancy.

As the severity of myasthenia gravis often fluctuates considerably, particular care is required to avoid cholinergic crisis, due to overdosage of the drug, but otherwise management is no different from that in non-pregnant patients.

Observations indicate that only negligible amounts of Prostigmin are excreted in breast milk; nevertheless due regard should be paid to possible effects on the breast-feeding infant.

Precautions: Extreme caution is required when administering Prostigmin to patients with bronchial asthma.

Care should also be taken in patients with bradycardia, recent coronary occlusion, hypotension, vagotonia, peptic ulcer, epilepsy or Parkinsonism.

Bradycardia may occur, to a possibly dangerous level, on intravenous injection of Prostigmin unless atropine is given simultaneously.

There is no evidence to suggest that Prostigmin has any special effects in the elderly. However, elderly patients may be more susceptible to dysrhythmias than the younger adult.

Prostigmin should not be given during cyclopropane or halothane anaesthesia; however, it may be used after withdrawal of these agents.

Side-effects: These may include nausea and vomiting, increased salivation, diarrhoea and abdominal cramps.

Treatment of overdosage: Signs of overdosage due to muscarinic effects may include abdominal cramps, increased peristalsis, diarrhoea, nausea and vomiting, increased bronchial secretions, salivation, diaphoresis and miosis. Nicotinic effects consist of muscular cramps, fasciculations and general weakness. Bradycardia and hypotension may also occur.

Artificial ventilation should be instituted if respiratory depression is severe. Atropine sulphate 1–2 mg intravenously is an antidote to the muscarinic effects.

Pharmaceutical precautions *Storage:* The recommended maximum storage temperature for Prostigmin ampoules 2.5 mg is 25°C and for Prostigmin tablets is

30°C. Prostigmin preparations should be protected from light.

Legal category
Tablets POM
Ampoules POM

Package quantities Prostigmin tablets in packs of 100.
Prostigmin ampoules 0.5 mg in 1 ml in packs of 10.
Prostigmin ampoules 2.5 mg in 1 ml in packs of 10.

Further information Nil.

Product licence numbers

Ampoules 0.5 mg	0031/5084R
Ampoules 2.5 mg	0031/5085R
Tablets	0031/5086R

REVANIL* ▼

Presentation Round, white, half-scored, convex tablets with CM in a regular hexagon imprinted on one face, containing 200 micrograms lisuride maleate (equivalent to 149 micrograms lisuride).

Uses Revanil is a selective dopamine agonist. Parkinson's disease, which is characterised by a deficiency of dopamine in the nigro-striatal pathway, responds to Revanil, which can be used either alone or in combination with levodopa, for the management of previously untreated patients and those exhibiting 'on-off' phenomena. It is suitable for patients who cannot tolerate levodopa or whose response to levodopa is declining.

Indications: For the treatment of Parkinson's disease.

Dosage and administration The following general rules apply: Revanil should always be taken with food. The initial dose should preferably be taken at bedtime. Dosage should be low initially, increasing gradually to the appropriate final level, as determined by the efficacy and tolerance of the drug.

Initially, one tablet at bedtime. After one week, the dosage may be increased to 200 micrograms at bedtime and 200 micrograms at midday. After a further week, an additional 200 micrograms may be added in the morning. The dosage should continue to be increased by 200 micrograms per week (beginning each sequence of three increases with the bedtime dose) until the optimum dosage is achieved.

The maximum daily dosage should not normally exceed 5 mg (25 tablets).

Contra-indications, warnings, etc
Contra-indications: Severe disturbances of peripheral circulation, coronary insufficiency.

Use in pregnancy: Although many foetuses have been exposed to Revanil, without evidence of teratogenicity, in women of childbearing potential, the potential risks of use must be weighed against the benefits of treatment.

Precautions: Revanil should be given with extreme caution to a patient who has, or has had treated, a pituitary tumour. Enlargement can occur, particularly during pregnancy, which may result in early visual field defects.

Lactation is unlikely to be inhibited if suckling or a breast pump is used.

The possibility of hypotensive reactions demands particular care in activities such as driving or operating machinery.

Psychiatric reactions have been seen with the use of Revanil, and this is more likely with high dosage and in patients who have a history of psychotic disturbance.

The effects of some psychotropic drugs may possibly be impaired by the simultaneous use of Revanil. Dopamine antagonists (e.g. haloperidol, sulpiride and metoclopramide) can weaken the effects and side-effects of Revanil.

Side-effects and adverse reactions: Nausea and vomiting are the most common side-effects experienced in patients with Parkinson's disease. In these patients domperidone can be freely used, since although it is an antidopaminergic drug it does not pass the blood-brain barrier and therefore does not antagonise the anti-Parkinsonian effects of Revanil. A sudden severe fall in blood pressure has been observed in isolated cases. Tolerance is rapidly acquired, and side-effects are most likely during the first few days of treatment. Dizziness, headache, lethargy, malaise and slight drowsiness are possible. There are occasional transient slightly itchy exanthemata. Abdominal pains and constipation occur rarely. Raynaud's phenomenon has been reported in one case so far.

Treatment of overdosage: Expected symptoms of overdosage include severe nausea and vomiting, confusion, hallucinations and postural hypotension. Treatment should include the use of a specific dopamine antagonist as well as general supportive measures and maintenance of the blood pressure. Gastric lavage should be employed if overdosage is discovered soon enough.

Pharmaceutical precautions Recommended maximum storage temperature for Revanil tablets is 25°C. Revanil tablets should be stored in a dry place.

Legal category POM.

Package quantities Bottles of 100 tablets (OP).

Further information Nil.

Product licence number 0053/0164.

RIMIFON*

Presentation Ampoules containing 50 mg isoniazid in 2 ml. The ampoule solution is almost colourless.

Uses *Properties:* Rimifon is a highly active tuberculostatic drug. It is easily absorbed and has a high rate of diffusion so that the tuberculostatic action affects intracellular as well as extracellular bacilli.

Indications: All forms of pulmonary and extra-pulmonary tuberculosis.

Dosage and administration Rimifon ampoules are for intramuscular, intravenous, intrathecal or intrapleural injection.

Adults and children: The usual intramuscular or intravenous dose for adults is 200 to 300 mg as a single daily dose, for children 100 to 300 mg daily (10–20 mg/kg), but doses much larger than these are sometimes given, especially in conditions such as tuberculous meningitis.

Neonates: The recommended intravenous or intramuscular dose for neonates is 3–5 mg/kg with a maximum of 10 mg/kg daily. Isoniazid may be present in the milk of lactating mothers (see Use in Pregnancy).

Elderly: No dosage reduction is necessary in the elderly.

Intrapleural use: 50–250 mg may be instilled intrapleurally after aspiration of pus, the dosage of oral isoniazid on that day being correspondingly reduced. The ampoule solution is also used for the local treatment of tuberculous ulcers, for irrigation of fistulae, etc.

Intrathecal use: It should be noted that CSF concentrations of isoniazid are approximately 90% of plasma concentrations. Where intrathecal use is required 25–50 mg daily has been given to adults and 10–20 mg daily for children, according to age.

It is usual to give Rimifon together with other antituberculous therapy, as determined by current practice and/or sensitivity testing.

It is recommended that pyridoxine 10–50 mg daily be given during Rimifon therapy to minimise adverse reactions, especially in malnourished patients and those predisposed to neuropathy (e.g. diabetics and alcoholics).

Use in renal and hepatic impairment: No dosage reduction of Rimifon is necessary when given to patients with mild renal failure. Patients with severe renal failure (glomerular filtration rate of less than 10 ml/minute) and slow acetylator status might require a dose reduction of about 100 mg to maintain trough plasma levels less than 1 mcg/ml.

The possible risks of administration of Rimifon to patients with pre-existing non-tuberculous hepatic disease should be balanced against the benefits expected from treating tuberculosis.

Contra-indications, warnings, etc
Contra-indications: Rimifon should not be given to patients with a history of sensitivity to isoniazid.

Use in pregnancy: While Rimifon is generally regarded to be safe in pregnancy, there is a possibility of an increased risk of foetal malformations occurring when isoniazid is given in early pregnancy. If pregnancy cannot be excluded possible risks should be balanced against therapeutic benefits.

Isoniazid is excreted in breast milk at concentrations equivalent to those found in maternal plasma, i.e 6–12 mcg/ml. This could result in an infant ingesting up to 2 mg/kg/day.

Precautions: For use in renal and hepatic impairment see *Dosage and administration.*

Care is also required in chronic alcoholism and when prescribing isoniazid for patients with pre-existing hepatitis.

Convulsions and psychotic reactions have occurred, especially in patients with a previous history of these conditions. These manifestations usually subside rapidly when the drug is withdrawn. Isoniazid should therefore be given with caution to patients with convulsive disorders and should be avoided in those with manic or hypomanic psychoses.

Isoniazid may inhibit the metabolism of phenytoin, primidone and carbamazepine. Plasma levels of these drugs should be monitored if concurrent therapy with Rimifon is necessary.

Side-effects: Rimifon is generally well tolerated. Side-effects have been reported mainly in association with high doses or in slow acetylators who develop higher blood levels of the drug. Fever, peripheral neuropathy (preventable with pyridoxine), optic neuritis and atrophy, allergic skin conditions (including erythema multiforme) and, rarely, lupoid syndrome, pellagra, purpura and haematological reactions have occurred during isoniazid therapy.

Hyperglycaemia and gynaecomastia have been reported with isoniazid treatment.

Isoniazid, especially if given with rifampicin, may induce abnormalities in liver function, particularly in patients with pre-existing liver disorders, in the elderly, the very young and the malnourished. Monthly review is suggested to detect and limit the severity of this side-effect by stopping treatment if plasma transaminases exceed three times the upper limit of normal. There is conflicting opinion as to the relationship of this side-effect to acetylator status.

Treatment of overdosage: In severe poisoning the main risk is of epileptiform convulsions. In addition any of the side-effects listed above may occur together with metabolic acidosis and hyperglycaemia. Treatment should be directed to the control of convulsions; large doses of pyridoxine may limit the occurrence of other adverse effects. Metabolic acidosis may require sodium bicarbonate infusion. The drug is removed by dialysis.

Pharmaceutical precautions *Storage:* The recommended maximum storage temperature for Rimifon ampoules is 25°C; the ampoules should be protected from light.

Dilution: Rimifon ampoule solution may be diluted with Water for Injections. Maintenance of stability cannot be guaranteed when Rimifon ampoule solution is diluted.

Legal category POM.

Package quantities Rimifon ampoules in packings of 10.

Further information Isoniazid is metabolised by acetylation, which is subject to genetic variation. The 'slow acetylators' may be more susceptible to drug-induced peripheral neuropathy. However, dose adjustment is not normally required.

Product licence number 0031/5109.

RIVOTRIL*

Presentation Round, dull pinkish-buff tablets with 'RIV 0.5' imprinted on one face and two break bars on the other, containing 0.5 mg clonazepam.

Round, white tablets with 'RIV 2' imprinted on one face and two break bars on the other, containing 2 mg clonazepam.

Ampoules containing 1 mg clonazepam in 1 ml solvent, each accompanied by an ampoule containing 1 ml Water for Injection Ph Eur as a diluent. The ampoule solution is colourless.

Uses *Properties:* Rivotril is a benzodiazepine derivative exhibiting marked anticonvulsant properties. These have been demonstrated in the many tests in animals which are employed to establish the anti-epileptic properties of a drug. Animal experiments and electroencephalographic studies in man have shown that Rivotril prevents generalisation of convulsive activity and raises the seizure threshold. In many cases, abnormal electroencephalograms become normal. Rivotril improves both focal seizures and primarily generalised attacks. Administered intravenously, Rivotril quickly controls status epilepticus.

Rivotril taken orally is well absorbed to give peak levels within four hours. The drug is widely distributed, then eliminated with a half-life generally between one and two days. Clearance is by metabolism in the liver, by nitro-reduction to the corresponding amine, then acetylation. The metabolites are excreted mainly via the urine. Routine monitoring of plasma concentrations of Rivotril is of unproven value since this does not appear to correlate well with either therapeutic response or side-effects.

Indications: Tablets: All clinical forms of epileptic disease and seizures in infants, children and adults, especially absence seizures (petit mal) including atypical absence; primary or secondarily generalised tonic-clonic (grand mal), tonic or clonic seizures; partial (focal) seizures with elementary or complex symptomatology; various forms of myoclonic seizures, myoclonus and associated abnormal movements.

Indications: Ampoules: Status epilepticus in all clinical forms.

Dosage and administration
Tablets: Treatment should be started with low doses. If desired, the total dose may be given at night for the first four days of treatment. The dose may be increased progressively until the maintenance dose suited to the individual patient has been found.

The dosage of Rivotril must be adjusted to the needs of each individual and depends on the individual response to therapy. The maintenance dosage must be determined according to clinical response and tolerance.

Adults: Initial dosage should not exceed 1 mg/day. The maintenance dosage for adults normally falls within the range 4 to 8 mg.

Infants and children: Initial dosage should not exceed 0.25 mg/day for infants and small children (1 to 5 years) and 0.5 mg/day for older children. The maintenance dosage normally falls within the ranges:

School children (5 to 12 years):	3 to 6 mg
Small children (1 to 5 years):	1 to 3 mg
Infants (0 to 1 year):	0.5 to 1 mg

In some forms of childhood epilepsy, certain patients may cease to be adequately controlled by Rivotril. Control may be re-established by increasing the dose, or interrupting treatment with Rivotril for two or three weeks. During the interruption in therapy, careful observation and other drugs may be needed.

Use in elderly: The elderly are particularly sensitive to the effects of central depressant drugs and may experience confusion. It is recommended that the initial dosage of Rivotril should not exceed 0.5 mg/day.

These are total daily dosages which should be divided into three or four doses taken at intervals throughout the day. If necessary, larger doses may be given at the discretion of the physician. The maintenance dose should be attained after two to four weeks of treatment.

Simultaneous administration of more than one anti-epileptic drug is a common practice in the treatment of epilepsy and may be undertaken with Rivotril. The dosage of each drug may be required to be adjusted to obtain the optimum effect. If status epilepticus occurs in a patient receiving oral Rivotril, intravenous Rivotril may still control the status.

Rivotril tablets are for oral administration.

Ampoules: for the treatment of status epilepticus the dose and rate of administration is governed by the response of the patient. As a guide, we suggest:

Adults: 1 mg (1 ampoule of active substance mixed with 1 ampoule of diluent) by slow intravenous injection. Care should be taken with the elderly.

Infants and children: 0.5 mg (equivalent to ½ ampoule of active substance mixed with ½ ampoule of diluent) by slow intravenous injection.

Mode of Administration: Intravenous injection of Rivotril should be into a large vein of the antecubital fossa. The injection should be given slowly – in adults, 1 mg over approximately 30 seconds. This will greatly diminish the rare possibility of hypotension or apnoea occurring. Nevertheless, facilities for resuscitation should always be available.

The contents of the diluent ampoule, which contains 1 ml of Water for Injection PhEur, *must* be added to the contents of the other ampoule, which contains 1 mg clonazepam in 1 ml, *immediately* before injection.

Rivotril ampoule solution may be diluted when given in intravenous infusions of saline or dextrose, such as are customary in the treatment of status epilepticus. Thus, up to 3 mg (3 ampoules) in 250 ml of the following solutions is permissible: Sodium Chloride Injection BP, Dextrose Injection BP 5% and 10%, Sodium Chloride and Dextrose Injection BP (0.45% sodium chloride and 2.5% dextrose). This infusion should be made up freshly and used within 12 hours.

Rivotril ampoules are for intravenous administration.

Maintenance of stability cannot be guaranteed when Rivotril ampoule solution is diluted.

Contra-indications, warnings, etc

Contra-indications: Patients with known sensitivity to benzodiazepines; acute pulmonary insufficiency; respiratory depression.

Use in Pregnancy and lactation: There is little evidence as to the drug safety in human pregnancy nor is there evidence from animal work that it is completely free from hazard. The use of Rivotril during pregnancy or lactation should be avoided unless there are compelling reasons.

The administration of high doses or prolonged administration of low doses of benzodiazepines in the last trimester of pregnancy or during labour has been reported to produce irregularities in the foetal heart rate, and hypotonia, poor sucking and hypothermia in the neonate.

Precautions: Rivotril should be used with caution in patients with chronic pulmonary insufficiency, or with impairment of renal or hepatic function, and the elderly or in the debilitated. In these cases dosage may need to be reduced.

Since alcohol can provoke epileptic seizures, irrespective of therapy, patients should be advised not to drink alcohol while under treatment. In combination with Rivotril, alcohol may modify the effects of the drug, compromise the success of therapy or give rise to unpredictable side-effects.

As a general rule, epileptic patients are not allowed to drive. Even when adequately controlled on Rivotril, it should be remembered that any increase in dosage or alteration in timings of dosage may modify patients' reactions, depending on individual susceptibility. If a patient is allowed to operate machinery, he should also be warned of these possible effects.

When Rivotril is used in conjunction with other anti-epileptic drugs, side-effects and toxicity may be more evident, particularly with hydantoins or phenobarbitone and combinations including them. This requires extra care in adjusting dosage in the initial stages of treatment.

The combination of Rivotril and sodium valproate has, rarely, been associated with the development of absence status epilepticus. Although some patients tolerate and benefit from this combination of drugs, this potential hazard should be borne in mind when its use is considered.

As with all other anti-epileptic drugs, treatment with Rivotril, even if of short duration, must not be abruptly interrupted, but must be withdrawn by gradually reducing the dose in view of the risk of precipitating status epilepticus. This precaution must also be taken when withdrawing another drug while the patient is still receiving Rivotril therapy.

In cases of loss or bereavement, psychological adjustment may be inhibited by benzodiazepines.

Side-effects: The side-effects observed consist of fatigue, somnolence, occasional muscular hypotonia and co-ordination disturbances. Such effects are usually transitory and disappear spontaneously as treatment continues or with dosage reduction. They tend to occur early in treatment and can be greatly reduced, if not avoided, by commencing with low dosages followed by progressive increases.

Rarely respiratory depression may occur with intravenous Rivotril, particularly if other depressant drugs have been administered.

In infants and small children, and particularly those with a degree of mental impairment, Rivotril may give rise to salivary or bronchial hypersecretion with drooling. Supervision of the airway may be required.

As with other benzodiazepines, isolated cases of blood dyscrasias and abnormal liver function tests have been reported.

Rivotril generally has a beneficial effect on behaviour disturbances in epileptic patients. In certain cases, paradoxical effects such as aggressiveness, irritability, agitation, psychotic disorders and activation of new types of seizures may be precipitated. If these occur, the benefit of continuing the drug should be weighed against the adverse effect. The addition to the regimen of another suitable drug may be necessary or, in some cases, it may be advisable to discontinue Rivotril therapy.

Although Rivotril has been given uneventfully to patients with porphyria, rarely it may induce convulsions in these patients.

Treatment of overdosage: As with other benzodiazepine drugs, overdosage should not present undue problems of management or threat to life. Patients have recovered from overdoses in excess of 60 mg without special treatment. Severe somnolence with muscle hypotonia will be present. Treatment is symptomatic and may include the need to maintain an airway. Gastric lavage may be useful if performed soon after ingestion.

Overdosage in non-epileptic patients may be treated with Anexate, a specific IV antidote for use in emergency situations. Patients requiring such intervention should be monitored closely in hospital (see separate prescribing information).

The use of Anexate is not recommended in epileptic patients who have been receiving benzodiazepine treatment for a prolonged period. Although Anexate exerts a slight intrinsic anticonvulsant effect, its abrupt suppression of the protective effect of a benzodiazepine agonist can give rise to convulsions in epileptic patients.

Pharmaceutical precautions *Storage:* Rivotril tablets should be stored in well-closed containers. Rivotril tablets and ampoules should be protected from light.

Legal category CD (Sch. 4), POM.

Package quantities Rivotril tablets 0.5 mg and 2 mg in packings of 100 and 500.

Rivotril ampoules 1 mg in packings of 10, accompanied by 1 ml ampoules Water for Injection PhEur as diluent.

Further information Nil.

Product licence numbers

Tablets 0.5 mg	0031/0076R
Tablets 2 mg	0031/0077R
Ampoules 1 mg	0031/0078

ROACCUTANE*

Presentation Oval, soft-gelatine capsules (spherical diameter approximately 5.8 mm), one-half pale red-violet and the other half white, marked 'R5', containing 5 mg isotretinoin.

Oval, soft-gelatine capsules (spherical diameter approximately 8.2 mm), one-half pale red-violet and the other half white, marked 'R20', containing 20 mg isotretinoin.

Uses *Properties:* Isotretinoin is a stereoisomer of tretinoin (all-*trans*-retinoic acid), an established preparation for topical treatment of acne vulgaris. Taken orally, Roaccutane has marked therapeutic efficacy in severe forms of acne, which are difficult to control with other means. The exact mechanism of action of Roaccutane is not known but clinical improvement is associated with a dose-related suppression of the size and activity of sebaceous glands.

Pharmacokinetics: Following oral administration of Roaccutane, peak blood levels of isotretinoin are achieved within 1–4 hours, and decline with a mean elimination half-life of approximately 10–20 hours.

Terminal elimination of the major metabolite, 4-oxo-isotretinoin, is formation rate limited so that its apparent half-life is similar to that for isotretinoin. The parent compound is highly bound to plasma protein and is excreted via bile and kidney as polar metabolites.

Bioavailability is enhanced by administration with food.

Indications: Roaccutane is indicated for the treatment of cystic and conglobate acne and severe acne which has failed to respond to an adequate course of a systemic antimicrobial agent.

Dosage and administration The therapeutic response to Roaccutane is dose-related and varies between patients. This necessitates individual adjustment of dosage according to the response of the condition and the patient's tolerance of the drug. In most cases complete or near-complete remission of acne is achieved with a 12- to 16-week course of treatment. It is recommended that repeat courses of treatment should not normally be given.

The daily dosage, to the nearest number of whole capsules, should be taken with food either as a single dose or in two divided doses during the day, whichever is more convenient.

Adults: Initial dosage: All patients initially should receive Roaccutane 0.5 mg/kg body-weight daily for a period of 4 weeks, when their responsiveness to the drug will usually be apparent. Acute exacerbation of acne is occasionally seen during the initial period but this subsides, usually within 7–10 days, with continued treatment.

Subsequent dosages: Patients who show early improvement should continue to receive the initial dosage of 0.5 mg/kg body-weight daily for the remainder of the course.

In patients who show little or no initial improvement, and who are tolerating the drug well, dosage should be increased up to 1 mg/kg body-weight daily for the remainder of the course.

In patients who show intolerance to the initial dosage, treatment should be continued with a reduced dosage of 0.1 to 0.2 mg/kg body-weight daily.

Repeated courses of therapy are not normally indicated.

With effective treatment, complete clearing of acne is usually achieved and prolonged remission ensues. However, patients whose acne is not completely cleared at the end of treatment can be expected to show continuing improvement for up to several months thereafter. Only if a definite relapse is seen in the post-treatment period should a repeated course be considered.

Concomitant therapy: As a rule, other treatments conventionally used for the treatment of acne, including antibiotics, keratolytics and exfoliants, are not indicated nor is concurrent radiation therapy with ultraviolet light or prolonged exposure to strong sunlight indicated, but non-irritant topical preparations may be applied if required.

Patients should be instructed to avoid taking preparations containing high doses of vitamin A, i.e. more than the recommended dietary allowance of 4,000–5,000 iu per day.

Elderly: Dosage as for other adults. Older subjects may have a greater risk of drug-induced arthralgia.

Children: Roaccutane is not indicated for the treatment of prepubertal acne.

Roaccutane capsules are for oral administration.

Contra-indications, warnings, etc

Contra-indications: Roaccutane is contra-indicated in hepatic and renal impairment. It should not be given to breast-feeding mothers.

Roaccutane is also contra-indicated in hypervitaminosis A, hyperlipidaemia and hypersensitivity to the drug.

Rare cases of benign intracranial hypertension have been reported after Roaccutane and after tetracyclines. Supplementary treatment with tetracyclines is therefore contra-indicated.

Roaccutane is teratogenic; major foetal abnormalities have been reported in humans. Major foetal abnormalities include: hydrocephalus, microcephalus, abnormalities of the external ear (micropinna, small or absent external auditory canals), microphthalmia, cardiovascular abnormalities, facial dysmorphia, thymus gland abnormalities, parathyroid hormone deficiency and cerebellar malformation. There is also a small risk of spontaneous abortion. Roaccutane is therefore contra-indicated in pregnancy. In any woman of childbearing potential the risk of its use must be weighed against the expected therapeutic benefit under all circumstances, taking into account the precautions specified below.

Precautions: Roaccutane is contra-indicated in a woman of childbearing potential unless she meets the following criteria:

1. Has severe disfiguring cystic acne resistant to standard therapy.

2. Pregnancy should be excluded before instituting therapy with Roaccutane. A negative pregnancy test within two weeks prior to therapy is obtained.

3. Starts Roaccutane therapy only on the second or third day of the next menstrual cycle.

4. Any woman of childbearing potential who is receiving Roaccutane must practise effective contraception for at least four weeks before treatment, during the treatment period and for at least four weeks following its cessation. Even female patients who normally do not practise contraception because of a history of infertility should be advised to do so, while taking Roaccutane.

5. Contraceptive measures must also be taken in the case of repeated courses of treatment.

6. Any pregnancy occurring during treatment with Roaccutane, or immediately following its completion, carries the risk of foetal malformation. This would raise the question of the termination of pregnancy for medical reasons. Therefore, before instituting Roaccutane therapy in a woman of childbearing potential the treating physician must explain clearly and in detail what precautions must be taken. This should include the risks involved and the possible consequences of a pregnancy occurring during Roaccutane treatment or in the first four weeks following its completion.

7. The woman is reliable and capable of understanding the risks and complying with effective contraception and confirms that she has understood the warnings.

In view of the importance of the foregoing precautions,

Roaccutane Patient Information leaflets are available to doctors and it is strongly recommended that these be given to all patients.

Wherever practicable a monthly repetition of the pregnancy test is recommended.

Liver function and blood lipids (fasting value) should be measured in all patients at the start of treatment, after the first month of administration and thereafter at 3-monthly intervals before discontinuation of Roaccutane.

At the completion of a lifespan study in rats there was an increased incidence of phaeochromocytoma in animals given isotretinoin at dosages of 32 and 8 mg/kg/day, but not 2 mg/kg/day. Since rats are particularly prone to develop this tumour type, the significance of this finding for use of Roaccutane in man is uncertain; nevertheless, repeated courses of treatment are not normally recommended.

Patients should not donate blood either during or for at least four weeks following discontinuation of therapy with Roaccutane. Theoretically there would be a small risk to a woman in the first trimester of pregnancy who received blood donated by a patient on Roaccutane therapy.

Side-effects: Most of the clinical side-effects of Roaccutane are dose-related and are usually well-tolerated at the recommended dosages. The side-effects may recede during continued treatment and have generally proved reversible with reduction of dosage or discontinuation of therapy.

The skin and mucous membranes are most commonly affected. Dryness of the skin may be associated with scaling, thinning, erythema (especially of the face) and pruritus. An increase in epidermal fragility has been reported, and frictional trauma may lead to epidermal blistering. Dryness of the nasal mucosa may be associated with mild epistaxis and dryness of the pharyngeal mucosa with hoarseness. Granulomatous lesions have occasionally been reported.

Dryness of the conjunctivae has been reported and may lead to mild to moderate conjunctivitis which may be alleviated by use of topical antibiotics.

Decreased tolerance to contact lenses may occur.

There have been occasional reports of visual disturbances including papilloedema and optic neuritis possibly associated with benign intracranial hypertension; also corneal opacities, cataracts, decreased night vision, photophobia and blurred vision. Patients experiencing visual disturbances should be referred for an expert opthalmological examination and withdrawal of Roaccutane considered.

Isolated cases of hearing deficiency in certain frequencies have been reported.

Hair thinning may occur but is uncommon at dosages below 1 mg/kg/day and is reversible following discontinuation of Roaccutane. Nevertheless, patients should be warned that this is a possibility during treatment.

There have been occasional reports of allergic vasculitis associated with the administration of Roaccutane.

Non-specific symptoms such as nausea, headache, malaise, drowsiness and sweating have been reported infrequently. Benign intracranial hypertension has been reported, particularly in association with concomitant antibiotic therapy.

Some patients have experienced mood changes including both reduction and precipitation of depression. Epileptiform seizures have been reported in patients who are receiving Roaccutane therapy.

Myalgia and arthralgia may occur and may be associated with reduced tolerance to vigorous exercise. Isolated instances of raised serum CPK values have been reported in patients receiving Roaccutane, particularly those undertaking vigorous physical activity. In these cases the clinical significance is unknown.

There have been occasional reports of menstrual irregularities which return to normal after completion of Roaccutane therapy.

A rise in serum levels of liver enzymes may occur. In a few cases significant increases have occurred, necessitating dosage reduction or discontinuation of Roaccutane. Jaundice and hepatitis have occurred rarely.

Elevation of serum triglycerides and cholesterol above the normal range, usually accompanied by decreases in HDL, has been observed, especially where predisposing factors such as a family history of lipid disorders, obesity, alcohol abuse, diabetes mellitus or smoking are present. The changes are dose-related and may be controlled by dietary means (including restriction of alcohol intake) and/or by reduction of dosage of Roaccutane.

Rarely hyperuricemia and inflammatory bowel disease (e.g. colitis, ileitis) have been reported.

Isolated cases of paronychia and local or systemic infections due to Gram positive micro-organisms have been reported.

Rare instances have been reported of elevated blood glucose levels in diabetic patients receiving Roaccutane, therefore, careful monitoring of glucose levels during treatment is advised.

Isolated cases of thrombocytopenia, thrombocytosis, neutropenia and anaemia have been reported.

Isotretinoin has been shown to affect diaphyseal and spongy bone adversely in animals at high doses in excess of those recommended for use in man.

Bone changes, including early epiphyseal closure, have occurred in man after several years' administration of Roaccutane in very high doses for disorders of keratinization. Prospective X-ray examination of some patients treated for severe cystic acne with Roaccutane revealed evidence of skeletal hyperostosis without clinical symptoms.

Treatment of overdosage: Isotretinoin is a derivative of vitamin A and overdosage should be expected to induce symptoms of hypervitaminosis A.

Manifestations of acute vitamin A toxicity include severe headache, nausea or vomiting, drowsiness, irritability, and pruritus. Signs and symptoms of accidental or deliberate overdosage with Roaccutane would probably be similar. They would be expected to be reversible and to subside without need for treatment. Because of the variable absorption of the drug, gastric lavage may be worthwhile in the first few hours after ingestion.

Pharmaceutical precautions *Storage:* Roaccutane capsules should be stored in a well-closed container and protected from light; the recommended maximum storage temperature is 30°C.

Legal category POM.

Package quantities Roaccutane capsules 5 mg in packings of 56 (8 × 7 capsule blister strips) (OP).

Roaccutane capsules 20 mg in packings of 56 (8 × 7 capsule blister strips) (OP).

Further information *Availability:* Roaccutane capsules are available only through hospital pharmacies for use in hospitals and hospital clinics and it is recommended that Roaccutane should be given only by, or under supervision of, a dermatological specialist.

Product licence numbers

Capsules 5 mg	0031/0158
Capsules 20 mg	0031/0160

RO-A-VIT*

Presentation Ampoules containing 100,000 International Units (I.U.) vitamin A as the palmitate (30 mg retinol equivalent) in 2 ml colloidal aqueous solution. The ampoule solution, which is strongly opalescent greenish-yellow in colour, contains a polyethoxylated castor oil as a solubilising agent.

Uses *Properties:* Ro-A-Vit is a synthetic vitamin A preparation. Vitamin A may be considered to act chiefly as a regulator of the growth and activity of epithelial tissues. It plays an essential role in the visual cycle through its participation in the synthesis of rhodopsin by the retina.

The cardinal signs and symptoms of vitamin A deficiency are those affecting the eyes, such as xerosis, swelling and destruction of the cornea and night-blindness. Hyperkeratosis of the skin and keratinising and metaplastic changes in the mucous membranes of the respiratory, digestive and urinary tracts have been reported.

Pharmacokinetics: After a single injection of 100,000 IU of vitamin A palmitate in a water miscible preparation the following results were obtained.

Plasma levels of vitamin A palmitate of up to 6,000 mcg/l were obtained at 10 to 20 hours after administration.

Baseline levels of 10 to 50 mcg/l were reached after approximately 150 hours. Elimination from plasma appears to be governed by non-linear kinetics.

The bioavailability of this water miscible preparation is approximately 50%.

Indications: Prevention and treatment of vitamin A deficiencies.

Ro-A-Vit ampoules are indicated when oral therapy is inappropriate (e.g. in malabsorption syndrome).

Dosage and administration
Adults: A maintenance dose of 100,000 IU by deep intramuscular injection once monthly is usually sufficient.

In acute deficiency states 100,000 IU may be given once weekly. However, if patients are receiving high doses continuously for a prolonged period, it is recommended that Ro-A-Vit be given in courses of no longer than six weeks separated by treatment-free intervals of two weeks in order to minimise the risk of hypervitaminosis A.

In patients with liver disease, a dose of 100,000 IU once every two to four months by deep intramuscular injection is recommended subject to a regular check of vitamin A status.

Children: For children, and infants under one year of age, a dose of 50,000 IU by deep intramuscular injection once monthly is recommended.

Elderly: No specific studies of vitamin A have been performed in elderly patients but Ro-A-Vit has been widely used for many years in the dosages recommended for younger adults without apparent ill consequence.

Due to the greatly enhanced bioavailability of this preparation compared with the previous oil-based formulation, it is possible that some patients previously stabilised on long-term prophylactic treatment with the oil-based presentation might require dosage adjustment of the water-based form.

Ro-A-Vit ampoule solution should not be diluted or mixed with other agents before injection. In particular mixing of the water miscible Ro-A-Vit ampoule solution with oil-based formulations (e.g. Calciferol Injection BP) may be expected to result in emulsification.

Ro-A-Vit ampoule solution is only suitable for deep intramuscular injection.

Contra-indications, warnings, etc
Contra-indication: Use in patients with a known hypersensitivity to any of the constituents (see 'Precautions').

Use in pregnancy: High doses of vitamin A can be teratogenic. Ro-A-Vit is therefore contra-indicated during pregnancy.

Precautions: Small children are sometimes sensitive to single doses of 100,000 iu vitamin A. While children are taking Ro-A-Vit no other vitamin supplement containing vitamin A should be taken, unless under medical supervision.

Massive doses of vitamin A are required to produce toxicity and therefore it is extremely unlikely that even exceptionally large single doses would cause hypervitaminosis A, except possibly in children, and in patients with underlying liver disease where enhanced susceptibility to vitamin A toxicity should be anticipated.

Ro-A-Vit ampoules contain a polyethoxylated castor oil as solubiliser. In animal studies, polyethoxylated castor oil can produce severe anaphylactoid reactions associated with histamine release. There is strong circumstantial evidence that similar reactions occurring in patients may have been caused by polyethoxylated castor oil. If such a reaction should occur the usual measures should be taken (e.g. administration of glucocorticoids and/or antihistamines).

Local injection site reactions have been reported following co-administration of Ro-A-Vit ampoules with oil-based formulations. Ro-A-Vit should not, therefore, be mixed with oil-based formulations.

Side-effects and adverse reactions: Yellowing of skin is one of the signs of toxicity associated with high doses.

Treatment of overdosage: In the event of overdosage the vitamin should be discontinued. Symptoms of acute overdosage subside within 72 hours and of chronic overdosage over a period of several months, without further treatment.

Pharmaceutical precautions *Storage:* Ro-A-Vit ampoules should be protected from light and stored below 15°C. If ampoules show signs of flocculation (as may be in the case of unsuitable storage) they must not be used.

Legal category POM.

Package quantities Ro-A-Vit ampoules in packings of 10.

Further information Nil.

Product licence number 0031/0216

ROCALTROL*

Presentation Soft gelatine capsules, one length red opaque and the other white opaque, containing 0.25 micrograms calcitriol. Soft gelatine capsules, both lengths brown red opaque, containing 0.5 micrograms calcitriol.

Uses *Properties:* Calcitriol has the greatest biological activity of the known vitamin D metabolites and is normally formed in the kidneys from its immediate precursor, 25-hydroxycholecalciferol. In physiological amounts it augments the intestinal absorption of calcium and phosphate and plays a significant part in the regulation of bone mineralisation. The defective production of calcitriol in chronic renal failure contributes to the abnormalities of mineral metabolism found in that disorder.

Rocaltrol is a synthetic preparation of calcitriol. Oral administration of Rocaltrol to patients with chronic renal failure compensates for impaired endogenous production of calcitriol which is decreased when the glomerular filtration rate falls below 30 ml/min. Consequently, intestinal malabsorption of calcium and phosphate and the resulting hypocalcaemia are improved, thereby reversing the signs and symptoms of bone disease.

The onset and reversal of the effects of Rocaltrol are more rapid than those of other compounds with vitamin D activity and adjustment of the dose can be achieved sooner and more precisely. The effects of inadvertent overdosage can also be reversed more readily.

Pharmacokinetics: Rocaltrol is efficiently absorbed following an oral dose, and peak serum levels are reached after 4–6 hours. Calcitriol concentrations return to the basal level with a half-life of 3–6 hours, although the duration of pharmacologic activity is approximately 3–5 days. Following oral administration of 1 mcg radiolabelled calcitriol to normal individuals, approximately 10% of the total radioactivity appears in the urine within 24 hours. Biliary excretion and enterohepatic recirculation also occur.

Indications: Rocaltrol is indicated for the correction of the abnormalities of calcium and phosphate metabolism in patients with renal osteodystrophy.

Dosage and administration The dose of Rocaltrol should be carefully adjusted for each patient according to the biological response so as to avoid hypercalcaemia. The effectiveness of treatment depends in part on an adequate daily intake of calcium, which should be augmented by dietary changes or supplements if necessary. The capsules should be swallowed with a little water.

Adults: It is suggested that treatment should be started with two to four 0.5 microgram capsules of Rocaltrol daily and serum calcium levels monitored at weekly intervals. The daily dose may be increased by increments of 0.25–0.5 micrograms to a total of 2 or 3 micrograms daily according to the biological response. When dose requirements are stable serum calcium levels may be monitored at intervals of two to four weeks.

When there is biochemical or radiographic evidence of bone healing the requirements for Rocaltrol generally decrease. The dose should then be adjusted to avoid hypercalcaemia.

Higher doses of Rocaltrol may be required when barbiturates or anticonvulsants are given concurrently but this should rarely exceed 5 micrograms daily. Reduction of dose is necessary if such drugs are withdrawn.

Elderly: Clinical experience with Rocaltrol in elderly patients indicates that the dosage recommended for use in younger adults may be given without apparent ill consequence.

Children: Dosage in children has not been established.

Rocaltrol capsules are for oral administration only.

Contra-indications, warnings, etc
Contra-indications: Rocaltrol should not be given to patients with hypercalcaemia or evidence of metastatic calcification.

Use in pregnancy: The safety of Rocaltrol during pregnancy has not been established and it should be given only when the potential benefit has been weighed against the possible hazard. The usual caution in prescribing any drug for women of child-bearing age should be observed.

It is not known if calcitriol is excreted in human milk.

Precautions: All other vitamin D compounds and their derivatives, including proprietary compounds or foodstuffs which may be 'fortified' with vitamin D, should be withheld during treatment with Rocaltrol.

Treatment does not obviate the need to control plasma phosphate with phosphate binding agents. Since Rocaltrol affects phosphate transport in the gut and bone, the dose of phosphate binding agent may need to be modified.

Side-effects and adverse reactions: Hypercalcaemia and hypercalciuria are the major side-effects of Rocaltrol and indicate excessive dosage. Patients with tertiary hyperparathyroidism are particularly prone to develop hypercalcaemia. The clinical features of hypercalcaemia include anorexia, nausea, vomiting, headache, weakness, apathy and somnolence. More severe manifestations may include thirst, dehydration, polyuria, nocturia, abdominal pain, paralytic ileus and cardiac arrhythmias. Rarely, overt psychosis and metastatic calcification may occur. The relatively short biological half-life of Rocaltrol permits rapid elimination of the compound when treatment is stopped and hypercalcaemia will recede within two to seven days. The rate of reversal of biological effects is more rapid than when other vitamin D derivatives are used.

Mild, non-progressive and reversible elevations in levels of liver enzymes (SGOT, SGPT) have been noted in a few patients treated with Rocaltrol, but no pathological changes in the liver have been reported.

Effects of overdosage and their treatment: In acute overdose gastric lavage should be considered as soon after ingestion as possible provided that the drug was taken within the previous six to eight hours.

Should hypercalcaemia occur, Rocaltrol should be discontinued until plasma calcium levels have returned to normal. A low-calcium diet will speed this reversal. Rocaltrol can then be restarted at a lower dose or given in the same dose but at less frequent intervals than previously. Severe hypercalcaemia may be treated by ensuring adequate hydration, inducing a diuresis where practicable and by general supportive measures. Calcitonin may increase the rate of fall of serum calcium when bone resorption is increased.

In patients treated by intermittent haemodialysis, a low concentration of calcium in the dialysate may also be used.

Pharmaceutical precautions *Storage:* Rocaltrol capsules should be protected from heat; the recommended maximum storage temperature is 30°C.

Legal category POM.

Package quantities Capsules 0.25 micrograms in packings of 100.

Capsules 0.5 micrograms in packings of 100.

Further information Nil.

Product licence numbers
Capsules 0.25 mcg 0031/0122
Capsules 0.5 mcg 0031/0123

ROFERON-A*

Presentation Roferon-A has the approved name interferon alfa-2a (rbe). It is a highly purified, sterile protein containing 165 amino acids in known sequence. It has an approximate molecular weight of 19,000 daltons. It is produced by recombinant DNA technology using a genetically engineered *E. coli* strain containing DNA that codes for the human protein.

Roferon-A is supplied as a sterile powder for reconstitution in single-dose vials. Each vial contains 3 million, 9 million or 18 million international units (IU) of lyophilised interferon alfa-2a (rbe), 9 mg sodium chloride and 5 mg Human Serum Albumin (PhEur) included as a stabiliser. The solution is reconstituted prior to use by adding the 1 ml of sterile Water for Injections (BP) supplied as solvent.

Uses
Properties: Roferon-A has been shown to possess many of the activities of the so-called "natural" human alpha-interferon preparations.

In particular, Roferon-A has been shown to exert anti-proliferative activity against a variety of human tumours *in vitro* and to inhibit the growth of some human tumour xenografts in nude mice. The degree of anti-proliferative activity is variable, and the essential mechanism responsible for the anti-tumour action is not yet known.

Indications: Roferon-A is indicated for use as a single agent in the treatment of AIDS (Acquired Immune Deficiency Syndrome)-related Kaposi's sarcoma, hairy cell leukaemia and recurrent or metastatic renal cell carcinoma. It is also indicated for the treatment of adult patients (over 18 years) with chronic active hepatitis B who have markers for viral replication, e.g. those who are positive for HBV-DNA, DNA polymerase or HBeAg.

Dosage and administration The following dosage schedules are recommended; these should not be exceeded.

Adults
AIDS-related Kaposi's sarcoma
Induction dose: 36×10^6 IU intramuscularly daily for 4–10 weeks. Maintenance dose: 36×10^6 IU intramuscularly three times per week.

Kaposi's sarcoma patients should be treated for 30 to 90 days before the physician determines the possible benefits of continued therapy.

Hairy cell leukaemia
Induction dose: 3×10^6 IU intramuscularly daily for 16 to 24 weeks. Subcutaneous administration may be utilised in thrombocytopenic patients (platelet count ≤ 50,000) or in patients at risk from bleeding. Maintenance dose: 3×10^6 IU intramuscularly three times per week.

Recurrent or metastatic renal cell carcinoma
Induction dose: escalation from 3 million IU daily to a maximum of 36 million IU daily by intramuscular injection over ten to twelve weeks.

Schedule:
Days 1–3: 3 million IU daily
Days 4–6: 9 million IU daily
Days 7–9: 18 million IU daily, then continue with 18 million IU daily to maximally 36 million IU daily.

Maintenance dose: 18–36 million IU three times per

week. Doses of up to 18 million IU can be given subcutaneously or intramuscularly. Intramuscular injection is recommended for doses of 36 million IU.

The maintenance dose should be given until progressive disease is documented unless it is not in the best interest of the patients.

Chronic active hepatitis B
The optimal schedule of treatment has not yet been established. The dose is usually in the range 2.5 million IU to 5.0 million IU/m^2 body surface area, administered subcutaneously three times per week for 4 to 6 months. If markers of viral replication of HBe antigen do not decrease after 1 month of therapy the dose can be escalated. The dosage may be further adjusted to the patient's tolerance to the medication. If no improvement has been observed after 3 to 4 months of treatment, discontinuation of therapy should be considered.

The appearance of anti-HBe antibody associated with loss of genomic markers for viral replication is indicative of an adequate early response to therapy.

Dosage should be modified to take into account the constitutional symptoms, the myelosuppressive effects, or other clinical or laboratory test abnormalities caused by Roferon-A and other drugs in combination, or the effects of prior X-ray therapy or chemotherapy which may have compromised the bone-marrow reserve.

Elderly: Elderly patients may be more susceptible to the side-effects of Roferon-A and caution is recommended in the treatment of such patients.

Children: Safety and efficacy of Roferon-A in children have not been established. Up to 10 million IU/m^2 has been safely administered to children with chronic hepatitis B. However, efficacy of therapy has not been demonstrated.

Mode of administration: Roferon-A is administered as a deep intramuscular injection or a subcutaneous injection. The injection site should be varied (so that one site is not used for all injections). Subcutaneous administration may be utilised in thrombocytopenic patients (platelet count $\leq$50,000) or in patients at risk from bleeding.

The powder should be reconstituted with the 1 ml of Water for Injections BP supplied as solvent and swirled gently. The reconstituted solution can be stored for 24 hours in a refrigerator (2–8°C) or for 2 hours at room temperature.

Contra-indications, warnings, etc
Contra-indications: Roferon-A is contra-indicated in patients with known histories of hypersensitivity to recombinant interferon alpha-2a, any component of the preparation or mouse immunoglobulin; severe pre-existing cardiac disease; severe renal and/or hepatic impairment; epilepsy and/or compromised central nervous system function.

Additionally, Roferon-A is contra-indicated in chronic active hepatitis patients with advanced, decompensated cirrhosis of the liver and those who are being or have recently been treated with immunosuppressive agents, excluding short term 'steroid withdrawal'.

Use in pregnancy: In pregnancy, Roferon-A should be administered only if the benefit to the woman justifies the potential risk to the foetus. Although animal tests do not indicate that Roferon-A is a teratogen, its effects on the human foetus are unknown. When doses greatly in excess of the recommended clinical dose were administered to pregnant rhesus monkeys in the early to mid-foetal period, an abortifacient effect was observed.

There is no information available on whether interferon is excreted in human milk, nor its effect on lactation.

Precautions: Like other anti-cancer drugs, Roferon-A should not be administered to fertile persons of either sex not practising effective contraception.

Roferon-A should be administered under the supervision of a qualified physician experienced in the management of the respective indication. Appropriate management of the therapy and its complications is possible only when adequate diagnostic and treatment facilities are readily available.

Patients should be informed not only of the possible benefits of therapy but also that they will probably experience adverse reactions.

Efficacy in patients with chronic hepatitis B co-infected with the human immunodeficiency virus (HIV) has not been demonstrated.

When mild to moderate renal or hepatic impairment is present, close monitoring of these functions is required.

Careful periodic neuropsychiatric monitoring of all patients is also recommended.

Extreme caution should be exercised when administering Roferon-A to patients with severe myelosuppression as it has a suppressive effect on the bone marrow, leading to a fall in the white blood count, particularly the granulocytes, the platelet count and less commonly the haemoglobin concentration. This can lead to an increased risk of infection or haemorrhage. It is important to closely monitor these events in patients and periodic complete blood counts should be performed during the course of Roferon-A treatment, both prior to therapy and at appropriate periods during therapy.

Lesions of Kaposi's sarcoma frequently reappear when Roferon-A treatment is discontinued.

Depending on dose and schedule as well as the sensitivity of the individual patient, Roferon-A may have an effect on the speed of reaction which could impair certain operations, e.g. driving, operation of machinery etc.

Drug interactions: Alpha-interferons may affect the oxidative metabolic process; this should be borne in mind when prescribing concomitant therapy with drugs metabolised by this route. However, as yet no specific information is available.

As Roferon-A may affect central nervous function, interactions could occur following concurrent administration of centrally-acting drugs.

Concurrent or previous use of drugs having neurotoxic, haemotoxic, or cardiotoxic effects may increase the toxicity of interferon in these systems.

Side-effects and adverse reactions: Generally, reactions are dose-related and reversible upon dosage reduction, interruption or cessation of therapy. The most frequently reported side-effects consist of influenza-like symptoms; fever, chills (occasionally rigors), headache, malaise, arthralgia and myalgia. These acute side-effects can usually be reduced or eliminated by concurrent administration of paracetamol and tend to diminish with continued therapy or dose moderation although continuing therapy can lead to lethargy, weakness and fatigue. In clinical studies, severe anorexia and weight loss occurred in 17 per cent of patients.

Marked effects on the central nervous system may occur; these include depression, confusion, dizziness, vertigo, drowsiness and nervousness. Convulsions or severe somnolence and coma are rare complications. Paraesthesia, numbness, neuropathy and tremor have occasionally been reported.

The administration of interferon may give rise to transient hypotension or hypertension, oedema, cyanosis, arrhythmias and palpitations in certain individuals. Rarely, severe cardiovascular events have been reported in patients on interferon; these include myocardial infarction, cerebral vascular accidents, congestive cardiac failure, pulmonary oedema and cardiorespiratory arrest.

Many patients experience anorexia and nausea. Other gastrointestinal effects such as diarrhoea and vomiting occur less frequently. In rare instances, reactivation of peptic ulcer and gastrointestinal bleeding have been reported.

The most frequently observed laboratory abnormalities include elevated liver function test parameters and reduction in white blood cells (particularly the myeloid series) and platelet counts; these rarely require dosage reduction. Following severe haematological abnormalities, recovery to pre-treatment values usually occurs within 7–10 days of stopping treatment. Alteration in serum transaminase (ALAT, ASAT) is seen in approximately one half of the patients with chronic hepatitis B and usually signals improvement in the disease.

In rare instances, decreased renal function has occurred.

Electrolyte disturbances have been seen, generally in association with anorexia or dehydration.

Other events occurring infrequently or rarely in patients on interferon include: reactions at injection sites, exacerbation of herpes labialis, rash, pruritis, mild to moderate alopecia, dryness of the skin, rhinorrhoea and epistaxis.

Neutralising antibodies to Roferon-A have been detected in around a quarter of treated patients but as yet no clinical sequelae of their presence have been clearly documented. Antibodies to human leucocyte interferon may occur spontaneously in certain clinical conditions (e.g. malignant disease, systemic lupus erythematosus, herpes zoster) in patients who have never received exogenous interferon.

Transient menstrual cycle irregularities including prolonged menstrual periods have been seen in rhesus monkeys administered doses greatly in excess of the recommended clinical dose. The relevance of these findings to man has not been established.

Inconsequential hypocalcaemia was reported in about one half of the patients. Elevated serum glucose occurred in approximately one third of cancer patients.

Treatment of overdosage: There are no reports of overdosage but repeated large doses of interferon are associated with profound lethargy, fatigue, prostration and coma. Such patients should be hospitalised for observation and appropriate supportive treatment given.

Pharmaceutical precautions The recommended maximum storage temperature for Roferon-A vials is 25°C.

Do not freeze.

Reconstituted vials should not be used after 24 hours storage in a refrigerator (2–8°C) or 2 hours at room temperature.

This product does not contain a preservative and should not normally be used as a multiple-dose vial.

Legal category POM.

Package quantities Vials containing 3, 9 or 18 million international units accompanied by ampoules of 1 ml Water for Injection BP as solvent, in packs of one.

Further information The pharmacokinetics of interferon alfa-2a (rbe) in patients with Kaposi's sarcoma, hairy cell leukaemia or renal cell carcinoma are consistent with those of other patients with metastatic or advanced malignant disease and healthy volunteers.

In healthy man, interferon alfa-2a (rbe) exhibits an elimination half-life of about 5 hours after intravenous administration. The apparent fraction of the dose absorbed after a single intramuscular injection is greater than 80%.

The serum concentrations of interferon alfa-2a (rbe) reflects a large intersubject variation in both healthy volunteers and patients with metastatic or advanced malignant disease. Administration of interferon alfa-2a (rbe) one or more times daily for up to 28 days to some patients resulted in peak plasma concentrations of 2 to 4 times greater than those seen after single doses.

Product licence numbers
Vials 3 million international units: 0031/0201.
Vials 9 million international units: 0031/0215.
Vials 18 million international units: 0031/0202.

ROHYPNOL*

Presentation A purple film-coated, bi-convex diamond-shaped tablet with a single break bar on one side and 'ROHYPNOL' on the other side, containing 1 mg flunitrazepam.

Uses *Properties:* Rohypnol is a benzodiazepine compound with hypnotic properties.

Indications: Short-term treatment of insomnia when it is severe, disabling or subjecting the individual to unacceptable distress, particularly for patients who have difficulty in falling asleep.

May be employed on an intermittent basis for induction of sleep at unusual times on a short-term or irregular basis.

Dosage and administration
Adults: Usual dose 0.5–1 mg. Maximum dose, 2 mg.

Elderly or debilitated patients: It is recommended that the initial dose to be taken before retiring should not exceed 0.5 mg; tolerability at this dosage level is excellent. In exceptional cases, where the hypnotic effect is less than adequate but tolerability is satisfactory, the dose may be increased to 1 mg.

Treatment should, if possible, be on an intermittent basis.

The lowest dose which can control symptoms should be used. Treatment should not be continued at the full dose beyond four weeks. Long-term chronic use is not recommended. Treatment should always be tapered off gradually. Patients who have taken benzodiazepines for a prolonged time may require a longer period during which doses are reduced. Specialist help may be appropriate.

Children: Rohypnol tablets are not for paediatric use.

Rohypnol tablets are for oral administration.

Contra-indications, warnings, etc
Contra-indications: Patients with known sensitivity to benzodiazepines; acute pulmonary insufficiency; respiratory depression; phobic or obsessional states; chronic psychosis.

Use in pregnancy: There is no evidence as to drug safety in human pregnancy, nor is there evidence from animal work that it is free from hazard. Do not use during pregnancy, especially during the first and last trimesters, unless there are compelling reasons.

The administration of high doses or prolonged administration of low doses of benzodiazepines in the last trimester of pregnancy or during labour has been reported to produce irregularities in the foetal heart rate, and hypotonia, poor sucking and hypothermia in the neonate.

Flunitrazepam has been detected in breast milk. If possible, the use of Rohypnol should be avoided during lactation.

Precautions: In patients with chronic pulmonary insufficiency, and in patients with chronic renal or hepatic disease, dosage may need to be reduced.

Rohypnol should not be used alone to treat depression or anxiety associated with depression, since suicide may be precipitated in such patients.

In cases of loss or bereavement, psychological adjustment may be inhibited by benzodiazepines.

Patients should be advised that, like all medicaments of this type, Rohypnol may modify patients' performance at skilled tasks (driving, operating machinery, etc.) to a varying degree depending upon dosage and individual susceptibility. Patients should further be advised that alcohol may intensify any impairment and should, therefore, be avoided during treatment. If the patient is awoken during the period of maximum drug activity, recall may be impaired.

The dependence potential of the benzodiazepines is low, particularly when limited to short-term use, but this increases when high doses are used, especially when given over long periods. This is particularly so in patients with a history of alcoholism or drug abuse or in patients with marked personality disorders. Regular monitoring in such patients is essential; routine repeat prescriptions should be avoided and treatment should be withdrawn gradually. Symptoms such as depression, nervousness, rebound insomnia, irritability, sweating, and diarrhoea have been reported following abrupt cessation of treatment with normal therapeutic doses.

In rare instances, withdrawal following excessive dosages may produce confusional states, psychotic manifestations and convulsions.

Abnormal psychological reactions to benzodiazepines have been reported. Rare behavioural effects include paradoxical aggressive outbursts, excitement, confusion and the uncovering of depression with suicidal tendencies. Extreme caution should therefore be used in prescribing benzodiazepines with personality disorders.

If Rohypnol is combined with centrally-acting drugs such as neuroleptics, tranquillisers, antidepressants, hypnotics, analgesics and anaesthetics, the sedative effects may be intensified. The elderly require special supervision.

When Rohypnol is used in conjunction with anti-epileptic drugs, side-effects and toxicity may be more evident, particularly with hydantoins or barbiturates or combinations including them. This requires extra care in adjusting dosage in the initial stages of treatment.

Side-effects: Adverse effects include drowsiness, unsteadiness and ataxia; these are dose-related and are likely to be uncommon with the recommended dosage. The elderly are particularly sensitive to the effects of central depressant drugs and may experience confusion. If organic brain changes are present, the dosage of Rohypnol should not exceed 0.5 mg in these patients.

Other adverse effects are less common and include headache, vertigo, hypotension, gastro-intestinal upsets, skin rashes, visual disturbances, changes in libido, and urinary retention. Isolated cases of blood dyscrasias and jaundice have also been reported.

Treatment of overdosage: When taken alone in overdosage Rohypnol presents few problems in management. Signs may include drowsiness, ataxia, and dysarthria, with coma in severe cases. Treatment is symptomatic. Gastric lavage is useful only if performed soon after ingestion. Anexate* is a specific IV antidote for use in emergency situations. Patients requiring such intervention should be monitored closely in hospital (see separate prescribing information).

When taken with centrally-acting drugs, especially alcohol, the effects of overdosage are likely to be more severe and, in the absence of supportive measures, may prove fatal.

Pharmaceutical precautions *Storage:* Rohypnol tablets should be stored in a dry place and protected from light.

Legal category CD (Sch. 4), POM.

Package quantities Rohypnol tablets 1 mg are blister-packed in packings of 30 (OP).

Further information The distribution half-life of flunitrazepam is about three hours; the elimination half-life is, on average, 22 hours.

The onset of effect is rapid and the duration of effect is dose-dependent.

Treatment should be kept to a minimum and given only under close medical supervision. Little is known regarding the efficacy or safety of benzodiazepines in long-term use.

An underlying cause for insomnia should be sought before deciding upon the use of benzodiazepines for symptomatic relief.

The elderly and patients with impaired renal and/or hepatic function will be particularly susceptible to the adverse effects listed above. It is advisable to review treatment regularly and to discontinue use as soon as possible.

Product licence number 0031/0104.

RONICOL*

Presentation Round, white tablets with *'RONICOL'* imprinted across one face with a single break bar on the other, containing 60.88 mg nicotinyl alcohol tartrate (equivalent to 25 mg nicotinyl alcohol).

Uses
Properties: Ronicol is the alcohol corresponding to nicotinic acid. Ronicol is rapidly absorbed and metabolised to nicotinic acid. Peak plasma levels of nicotinic acid are reached at about 30 minutes with a subsequent decline to baseline values. Ronicol exerts a direct vasodilator action on the walls of small arteries and arterioles; there is a slight transient tendency towards a fall in blood pressure and slowing of the pulse.

Indications: Treatment of circulatory disorders including peripheral vascular disease without intraluminal obstruction.

Dosage and administration *Adults:* 1–2 tablets four times daily.

Children: No dosage recommendations are made for the administration of Ronicol to children.

Use in elderly: Many studies of Ronicol have included a high proportion of elderly patients. Dosage should be as for younger adults.

Ronicol tablets are for oral administration.

Contra-indications, warnings, etc
Use in pregnancy: There is inadequate evidence of safety of Ronicol in human pregnancy but it has been in wide use for many years without apparent ill consequence, animal studies having showed no hazard. The established medical principle of only administering drugs in early pregnancy when considered absolutely necessary should be observed.

Precautions: Care should be taken in the administration of Ronicol in patients with pre-diabetic or diabetic metabolic disorders as this may lead to an increase in insulin needs of the patient.

Side-effects: At optimal doses it is common for the patient to experience mild, transient flushing of the face and a feeling of warmth in the region of the head. More severe symptoms such as sustained flushing, hypotension, faintness or dizziness due to vasodilation may respond to a reduction in dose. Rashes and symptoms of gastric irritation resolve on discontinuation of treatment. Transient elevations of transaminases and alkaline phosphatase are frequently seen and do not normally require an adjustment of dose. Patients with abnormal values should however be closely monitored since isolated cases of jaundice and hepatic necrosis have been reported.

Treatment of overdosage: Acute overdosage should be treated by gastric lavage and appropriate symptomatic therapy.

Pharmaceutical precautions
Storage: No special storage precautions are required.

Legal category P.

Package quantities Ronicol tablets in packings of 100.

Further information Nil.

Product licence number 0031/5113R.

RONICOL* TIMESPAN*

Presentation Brown-red, sugar-coated tablets containing 357 mg nicotinyl alcohol tartrate (equivalent to 150 mg nicotinyl alcohol).

Uses
Properties: Ronical Timespan tablets are slow-release tablets, the active principle being Ronicol, which is the alcohol corresponding to nicotinic acid. Absorption follows a biphasic pattern with an initial maximum concentration of nicotinic acid in plasma at about 2 hours. Slow release allows plasma levels to be maintained for about 12 hours. The compound exerts a direct vasodilator action on the walls of small arteries and arterioles. There is a slight transient tendency towards a fall in blood pressure and slowing of the pulse.

Indications: Treatment of circulatory disorders including peripheral vascular disease without intraluminal obstruction.

Dosage and administration *Adults:* 1 or 2 tablets night and morning, depending on the severity of the condition. They should be swallowed whole.

Children: No dosage recommendations are made for the administration of Ronicol Timespan to children.

Use in elderly: Many studies of Ronicol have included a high proportion of elderly patients. Dosage should be as for younger adults.

Ronicol Timespan tablets are for oral administration.

Contra-indications, warnings, etc
Use in pregnancy: There is inadequate evidence of safety of Ronicol in human pregnancy but it has been in wide use for many years without apparent ill consequence, animal studies having showed no hazard. The established medical principle of only administering drugs in early pregnancy when considered absolutely necessary should be observed.

Precautions: Care should be taken in the administration of Ronicol in patients with pre-diabetic or diabetic metabolic disorders as this may lead to an increase in the insulin needs of the patient.

Side-effects: At optimal doses it is common for the patient to experience mild, transient flushing of the face and a feeling of warmth in the region of the head. More severe symptoms such as sustained flushing, hypotension, faintness or dizziness due to vasodilation may respond to a reduction in dose. Rashes and symptoms of gastric irritation resolve on discontinuation of treatment. Transient elevations of transaminases and alkaline phosphatase are frequently seen and do not normally require an adjustment of dose. Patients with adnormal values should however be closely monitored since isolated cases of jaundice and hepatic necrosis have been reported.

Treatment of overdosage: Acute overdosage should be treated by gastric lavage and appropriate symptomatic therapy.

Pharmaceutical precautions
Storage: No special storage precautions are required.

Legal category P.

Package quantities Ronicol Timespan tablets in packings of 100.

Further information Nil.

Product licence number 0031/5114R.

SYNKAVIT*

Alternative name: Menadiol sodium diphosphate.

Presentation Round, white tablets with 'SYNKAVIT' imprinted on one face and a single break bar on the other, containing 12.63 mg of the tetra-sodium salt of 2-methyl-1,4-naphthahydroquinone diphosphate (equivalent to 10 mg of the free ester).

Uses *Properties:* Synkavit is a water-soluble vitamin K analogue. The presence of vitamin K is essential for the formation within the body of prothrombin, factor VII, factor IX and factor X. Lack of vitamin K leads to increased tendency to haemorrhage.

Indications: Synkavit is indicated in the treatment of haemorrhage or threatened haemorrhage associated with a low blood level of prothrombin or factor VII.

The main indication is obstructive jaundice (before and after surgery).

Dosage and administration *Adults:* Usual therapeutic dose – 10–40 mg daily.

Children: If, on the recommendation of a physician, a children's dosage is required, it is suggested that 5–20 mg daily be given.

Use in the elderly: Recommendations for use in the elderly do not differ from those for other adults.

Synkavit tablets are for oral administration.

Contra-indications, warnings, etc
Contra-indications: The administration of Synkavit to neonates, infants or to mothers in the pre- and post-natal periods is contra-indicated. Moderate doses of Synkavit have produced haemolytic anaemia, hyperbilirubinaemia and kernicterus, especially in premature infants, even when administered prior to delivery. In the treatment of haemorrhagic disease of the newborn, vitamin K_1 (Konakion) is the preferred drug of choice.

Use in pregnancy: There is no evidence of hazard if Synkavit is used in human pregnancy. It is known to be associated with a small risk of haemolytic anaemia, hyperbilirubinaemia and kernicterus in the infant if administered to the mother in late pregnancy or during labour. Synkavit is therefore contra-indicated during late pregnancy.

Precautions: Large doses of Synkavit may decrease patient sensitivity to anticoagulants.

Side-effects and adverse reactions: Synkavit may induce haemolysis (especially in the newborn infant) in the presence of erythrocyte glucose-6-phosphate dehydrogenase deficiency or low concentrations of alpha-tocopherol in the blood.

Pharmaceutical precautions *Storage:* Recommended maximum storage temperature for Synkavit tablets is 30°C. Synkavit tablets should be protected from light.

Legal category Tablets P

Package quantities Synkavit tablets in packs of 100.

Further information In almost all circumstances Synkavit is as effective as the natural vitamin (vitamin K_1). However, for severe cases of drug-induced hypoprothrombinaemia or bleeding produced in association with coumarin or indanedione anticoagulants or salicylates, Konakion (vitamin K_1) should be used.

Product licence number 0031/5115R.

TENSILON*

Presentation Ampoules containing 10 mg edrophonium chloride in 1 ml. The ampoule solution is almost colourless.

Uses *Properties:* Tensilon is an antagonist to cholinesterase, the enzyme which normally destroys acetylcholine. The action of Tensilon can briefly be described, therefore, as the potentiation of naturally occurring acetylcholine. It differs from Prostigmin* (neostigmine) and Mestinon* (pyridostigmine) in the rapidity and brevity of its action.

Indications: Myasthenia gravis, as a diagnostic test; to distinguish between overdosage and underdosage of cholinergic drugs in myasthenic patients; diagnosis of suspected 'dual block'; antagonist to non-depolarising neuromuscular blockade.

Dosage and administration *Adults – Test for myasthenia gravis:* A syringe is filled with the contents of 1 ampoule Tensilon (10 mg) and 2 mg is given intravenously, the needle and syringe being left *in situ*. If no response occurs within 30 seconds, the remaining 8 mg is injected. In adults with unsuitable veins, 10 mg is given by intramuscular injection.

To differentiate between 'myasthenic' and 'cholinergic' crises: In a myasthenic patient who is suffering from marked muscle weakness, in spite of taking large doses of Mestinon or Prostigmin, a test dose of 2 mg Tensilon is given intravenously one hour after the last dose of the cholinergic compound. If therapy has been inadequate, there is a rapid, transient increase of muscle strength; if the patient has been overtreated, Tensilon causes a transient increase of muscle weakness.

Diagnosis of suspected 'dual block': Tensilon 10 mg intravenously. If the block is due to depolarisation, it is briefly potentiated, whereas in a 'dual block', it is reversed.

Children: Diagnostic tests: A total dose of 100 micrograms/kg body-weight may be given intravenously. One fifth of this dose should be injected initially; if no reaction occurs, the remainder of the dose is administered 30 seconds later.

Antagonist to non-depolarising neuromuscular blockade: Generally, reversal of neuromuscular block with Tensilon should not be attempted until there is evidence of spontaneous recovery from paralysis. It is recommended that the patient be well ventilated and a patent airway maintained until complete recovery of normal respiration is assured.

Adults and children: Tensilon 500–700 micrograms/kg body-weight and atropine 7 micrograms/kg body-weight, by slow intravenous injection over several minutes, is usually adequate for reversal of non-depolarising muscle relaxants within 5–15 minutes. The two drugs are usually given simultaneously, but in patients who show bradycardia the pulse rate should be increased to about 80/minute with atropine before administering Tensilon.

The speed of recovery from neuromuscular blockade is primarily determined by the intensity of the block at the time of antagonism but it is also subject to other factors, including the presence of drugs (e.g. anaesthetic agents, antibiotics, antiarrhythmic drugs) and physiological changes (electrolyte and acid-base imbalance, renal impairment). These factors may prevent successful reversal with Tensilon or lead to recurarisation after apparently successful reversal. Therefore it is imperative that patients should not be left unattended until these possibilities have been excluded.

Elderly: There are no specific dosage recommendations for Tensilon in elderly patients.

Tensilon ampoules are for intramuscular or intravenous injection.

Tensilon ampoules may be diluted with Water for Injections. However, maintenance of stability cannot be guaranteed when Tensilon ampoule solution is diluted.

Contra-indications, warnings, etc

Contra-indications: Tensilon should not be given to patients with mechanical intestinal or urinary obstruction.

Tensilon is contra-indicated in patients with known hypersensitivity to the drug.

With doses above 10 mg, especially the higher dosage employed to antagonise neuromuscular blockade, Tensilon should not be used in conjunction with depolarising muscle relaxants such as suxamethonium as neuromuscular blockade may be potentiated and prolonged apnoea may result.

Use in pregnancy: The safety of Tensilon during pregnancy or lactation has not been established. Although the possible hazards to mother and child must be weighed against the potential benefits in every case, experience with Tensilon in pregnant patients with myasthenia gravis has revealed no untoward effect of the drug on the course of pregnancy.

There is no information on the excretion of Tensilon into breast milk. Although only negligible amounts would be expected to be present, due regard should be paid to possible effects on the breast-feeding infant.

Precautions: Extreme caution is required when administering Tensilon to patients with bronchial asthma.

Care should also be taken in patients with bradycardia, recent coronary occlusion, vagotonia, hypotension, peptic ulcer, epilepsy or Parkinsonism.

In diagnostic uses of Tensilon, a syringe containing 1 mg of atropine should be kept at hand to counteract severe cholinergic reactions, should they occur.

When Tensilon is used as an antagonist to neuromuscular blockade bradycardia may occur, to a possibly dangerous level, unless atropine is given simultaneously. In this indication, Tensilon should not be given during cyclopropane or halothane anaesthesia; however, it may be used after withdrawal of these agents.

There is no evidence to suggest that Tensilon has any special effects in the elderly. However, elderly patients may be more susceptible to dysrhythmias than younger adults.

Side-effects and adverse reactions: These may include nausea and vomiting, increased salivation, diarrhoea and abdominal cramps.

Treatment of overdosage: Tensilon overdosage may give rise to bradycardia, arrhythmias, hypotension and bronchiolar spasm. Perspiration, gastro-intestinal hypermotility and visual disturbances may also occur. Artificial ventilation should be instituted if respiration is severely depressed.

Atropine sulphate 1–2 mg intravenously is an antidote to the muscarinic effects.

Pharmaceutical precautions *Storage:* Tensilon ampoule solution should be protected from light.

Legal category POM.

Package quantities Tensilon ampoules in packings of 10.

Further information Nil.

Product licence number 0031/5095R.

TIGASON*

Presentation Capsules with buff-yellow cap and buff-yellow body with ROCHE printed in black on both cap and body, containing 10 mg etretinate.

Capsules with orange-yellow cap and buff-yellow body with ROCHE printed in black on both cap and body, containing 25 mg etretinate.

Uses *Properties:* Retinol (vitamin A) is known to be essential for normal epithelial growth and differentiation, though the mode of this effect is not yet established.

Both retinol and retinoic acid are capable of reversing hyperkeratotic and metaplastic skin changes. However, these effects are generally only obtained at dosages associated with considerable local or systemic toxicity.

Tigason, a synthetic aromatic derivative of retinoic acid, has a more favourable therapeutic ratio, with a greater and more specific inhibitory effect on psoriasis and disorders of epithelial keratinization. The usual therapeutic response to Tigason consists of desquamation (with or without erythema) followed by more normal re-epithelization.

Tigason is absorbed with a systemic bioavailability of 30–70% and is highly bound to plasma lipoproteins (and to albumin in the case of the major active metabolite, acitretin). It is cleared by metabolism in the gut and liver, and metabolites are eliminated in both urine and faeces. The drug forms depots in adipose tissue and, therefore, has a long elimination half-life (average 120 days).

Indications: Severe extensive psoriasis which is resistant to other forms of therapy.

Palmo-plantar pustular psoriasis.
Severe congenital ichthyosis.
Severe Darier's disease (keratosis follicularis).

Dosage and administration There is a wide variation in the absorption and rate of metabolism of Tigason. This necessitates individual adjustment of dosage. For this reason the following dosage recommendations can serve only as a guide.

Adults: Other dermatological therapy, particularly with keratolytics, should normally be stopped before administration of Tigason, though use of topical corticosteroids or bland emollient ointment may be continued if indicated.

Tigason should be started at a dose of up to 0.75 mg/kg body-weight per day, taken in divided doses, for two to four weeks. By this time involved areas of skin will usually show a marked response and/or side-effects should be apparent. Titration of dose up to 1 mg/kg body-weight may be necessary to achieve adequate clinical results. However, a total daily dose of 75 mg should not be exceeded.

Once a response has been observed, the dosage of Tigason should be reduced to 0.5 mg/kg body-weight per day, taken in divided doses, for a further six to eight weeks, when the maximum therapeutic effect should usually have been obtained.

When maximum clearing of lesions has occurred, especially in patients with psoriasis and Darier's disease, treatment with Tigason should normally be discontinued for an interval in order to assess whether a worthwhile period of remission ensues. Subsequent exacerbations may then be treated intermittently as necessary. However, in some patients, especially those with congenital ichthyosis, the period of remission may be brief and continued maintenance therapy, at the lowest dose which will prevent recurrences (usually 0.25–0.5 mg/kg body-weight per day), may be appropriate. Higher dosages are not normally recommended.

Elderly: Dosage is the same as for younger adults.

Children: Dosage should be administered as outlined above for adults, except that long-term maintenance therapy is not recommended (see Precautions).

Tigason capsules are for oral administration. They should be taken with food.

Contra-indications, warnings, etc

Contra-indications: Tigason is contra-indicated during pregnancy as it is a known human teratogen.

It should not be given to breast-feeding mothers.

Tigason is contra-indicated in patients with hepatic or renal impairment.

Rare cases of benign intracranial hypertension have been reported after Tigason and after tetracyclines. Supplementary treatment with antibiotics such as tetracyclines is therefore contra-indicated.

Use in pregnancy: Tigason is contra-indicated during pregnancy as it is a known human teratogen.

Precautions: Tigason is contra-indicated in a woman of childbearing potential unless she meets the following criteria:

1. Pregnancy has been excluded before instituting therapy with Tigason (negative pregnancy test within two weeks prior to therapy).
2. Starts Tigason therapy only on the second or third day of the next menstrual cycle.
3. Having excluded pregnancy, any woman of childbearing potential who is receiving Tigason must practice effective contraception for at least one month before treatment, during the treatment period and for at least two years following its cessation.

Even female patients who normally do not practice contraception because of a history of infertility should be advised to do so, while taking Tigason.

4. Contraceptive measures must also be taken in the case of repeated courses of treatment.
5. Any pregnancy occurring during treatment with Tigason, or in the two years following its cessation, carries a high risk of foetal malformation. This would raise the question of the termination of pregnancy for medical reasons. Therefore, before instituting Tigason the treating physician must explain clearly and in detail what precautions must be taken. This should include the risks involved and the possible consequences of pregnancy occurring during Tigason treatment or in the two years following its cessation.
6. The woman is reliable and capable of understanding the risk and complying with effective contraception, and confirms that she has understood the warnings.

In view of the importance of the above precautions, Tigason Patient Information leaflets are available to doctors and it is strongly recommended that these be given to all patients.

Patients should not donate blood either during or for at least two years following discontinuation of therapy with Tigason. Theoretically there would be a small risk to a woman in the first trimester of pregnancy who received blood donated by a patient on Tigason therapy.

Etretinate has been shown to affect diaphyseal and spongy bone adversely in animals at high doses in excess of those recommended for use in man. Skeletal hyperostosis and extraosseous calcification have been reported following long-term administration of etretinate to man.

In the treatment of ichthyosis and Darier's disease in adults, when continuous therapy with etretinate may be necessary, consideration should be given to annual lateral thoracic spine and ankle radiographs supplemented by radiographs of symptomatic areas.

There have been occasional reports of bone changes in children, including premature epiphyseal closure, skeletal-hyperostosis and extraosseous calcification, after long-term treatment with Tigason. Long-term therapy in children is not, therefore, recommended. If, in exceptional circumstances, long-term therapy is undertaken the child should be carefully monitored for any abnormalities of musculo-skeletal development.

Any patients complaining of atypical musculo-skeletal symptoms on treatment with Tigason should be promptly and fully investigated to exclude possible etretinate-induced bone changes. If clinically significant bone or joint changes are found, Tigason therapy should be discontinued.

Liver function and blood lipids (fasting value) should be measured at the start of treatment, after the first month of administration and at three-monthly intervals thereafter.

In diabetic patients, retinoids can alter glucose tolerance. Blood sugar levels should therefore be checked frequently at the beginning of the treatment period.

Patients should be warned of the possibility of alopecia occurring (see 'Side-effects').

Patients should also be instructed to avoid taking preparations containing high doses of Vitamin A, i.e. more than the recommended dietary allowance of 4,000–5,000 iu per day.

An increased risk of hepatitis has been reported following the concomitant use of methotrexate and Tigason; this combination should therefore be avoided.

Side-effects: Most of the clinical side-effects of Tigason are dose-related and are usually well-tolerated at the recommended dosages. However, the toxic dose of Tigason is close to the therapeutic dose and most patients experience some side-effects during the initial period whilst dosage is being adjusted. They are reversible with reduction of dosage or discontinuation of therapy.

The skin and mucous membranes are most commonly affected and it is recommended that patients should be so advised before treatment is commenced. Dryness of the mucous membranes, sometimes with erosion, involving the lips, mouth, conjunctivae and nasal mucosa are seen. Dryness of the skin may be associated with scaling, thinning, erythema (especially of the face) and pruritus. Palmar and plantar exfoliation, epistaxis and epidermal fragility have been reported, as well as paronychia. Granulomatous lesions have occasionally been reported. Dryness of the conjunctivae may lead to mild-to-moderate conjunctivitis alleviated by the use of topical antibiotics.

Hair thinning and frank alopecia may occur, usually noted four to eight weeks after starting therapy, and is reversible following discontinuation of Tigason. Full recovery usually occurs within six months of stopping treatment in the majority of patients.

Non-specific symptoms such as nausea, headache, malaise, drowsiness and sweating have been reported infrequently. Myalgia and arthralgia may occur and be associated with reduced tolerance to exercise.

Benign intracranial hypertension has been reported.

There have also been occasional reports of decreased night vision during Tigason therapy.

A rise in serum levels of liver enzymes may occur. When significant, dosage reduction or discontinuation of therapy may be necessary. Jaundice and hepatitis have occurred rarely.

Elevation of serum triglycerides above the normal range has been observed, especially where predisposing factors such as a family history of lipid disorders, obesity, alcohol abuse, use of other drugs which interfere with lipid metabolism, diabetes mellitus or smoking are present.The changes are dose-related and may be controlled by dietary means (including restriction of alcohol intake) and/or by reduction of dosage of Tigason.

Treatment of overdosage: Manifestations of acute vitamin A toxicity include severe headache, nausea or vomiting, drowsiness, irritability and pruritus. Signs and symptoms of accidental or deliberate overdosage with Tigason would probably be similar. They would be expected to be reversible and to subside without need for treatment.

Because of the variable absorption of the drug, gastric lavage may be worthwhile within the first few hours after ingestion.

Pharmaceutical precautions *Storage:* Tigason capsules should be stored in a well-closed container and protected from light. The recommended maximum storage temperature is 30°C.

Legal category POM.

Package quantities Tigason capsules 10 mg in packings of 56 (8 × 7 capsule blister strips) (OP).
Tigason capsules 25 mg in packings of 56 (8 × 7 capsule blister strips) (OP).

Further information *Availability:* Tigason capsules are available only through hospital pharmacies for use in hospitals and hospital clinics.

It is recommended that Tigason be given only by, or under supervision of, a dermatological specialist.

For guidance in advising patients wishing to become pregnant from two years post-treatment, consult the company's Medical Services Department.

Product licence numbers
Capsules 10 mg 0031/0134
Capsules 25 mg 0031/0135

TRH-ROCHE

Approved name: Protirelin.

Presentation Plain glass ampoules containing 200 micrograms TRH-Roche (thyrotrophin-releasing hormone) in 2 ml. The ampoule solution is almost colourless to faintly yellow.

Uses *Properties:* TRH-Roche stimulates the secretion of thyroid stimulating hormone (TSH). Intravenous injection results in a prompt rise in serum TSH levels in normal subjects, peak levels being observed about 20 minutes after administration. There is a concomitant rise in serum levels of prolactin.

TRH rapidly disappears from the plasma after intravenous injection. Over 90% is removed within 20 minutes with a half-life of about 5.3 minutes. About 5.5% of the dose is excreted in the urine, mostly within 30 minutes.

Indications: The administration of TRH-Roche provides a means of assessing thyroid function and the reserve of TSH in the pituitary gland and is recommended as a test procedure where such assessment is indicated.

It is particularly useful as a diagnostic test for:

1. Mild hyperthyroidism.
2. Ophthalmic Graves' disease.
3. Mild or preclinical hypothyroidism.
4. Hypopituitarism.
5. Hypothalamic disease.

It may also be used in place of the T_3 suppression test.

Dosage and administration
Adults: Intravenous injection: Tests employing intravenous TRH-Roche are based on the serum TSH response to a standard dose. They provide a means of both quantitative and qualitative assessment of thyroid function. It is essential for each laboratory to establish its own normal range of values for serum TSH before attempting quantitative assessment of TRH-Roche responses by this means.

Intravenous TRH-Roche test:

1. Blood sample taken for control TSH assay.
2. TRH-Roche 200 micrograms given as a single bolus injection.
3. Blood sample taken 20 minutes after injection for peak TSH assay.
4. If necessary, a further blood sample may be taken 60 minutes after injection to detect a delayed TSH response.

The ampoule solution should not be diluted.

Use in the elderly: The use of TRH-Roche in the elderly has been well documented. Dosage requirements and the side-effects are similar to those of younger adults. The response may be altered in sick elderly subjects.

Children: The procedure for administering TRH-Roche to children are identical with those outlined above. An intravenous dose of 1 microgram/kg body-weight may be used.

Interpretation of results: Interpretation of the responses to TRH-Roche is based on the increase in TSH and/or PBI, T_3 or T_4 levels from the basal values. In normal subjects, there is a prompt rise in serum levels of TSH. The changes observed in various conditions are briefly outlined below:

1. Hyperthyroidism – no rise in serum TSH or thyroid hormone levels.
2. Ophthalmic Graves' disease – often no rise in serum TSH or thyroid hormone levels.
3. Primary hypothyroidism – exaggerated and prolonged rise in serum TSH but no change in thyroid hormone levels.
4. Hypopituitarism – absent or impaired TSH or thyroid hormone response implies diminished TSH reserve.
5. Hypothalamic disease – a rise in serum TSH or thyroid hormone levels can occur in the presence of hypothyroidism; delayed responses are common.

The TRH-Roche test provides, in most instances, information similar to that obtained from a T_3 suppression test in that an absent or impaired response usually correlates with an absent or impaired response to T_3 suppression.

The response to TRH-Roche may be modified in subjects taking T_3, T_4, antithyroid drugs, corticosteroids, oestrogens, theophylline, levodopa, phenothiazines, metoclopramide, bromocriptine, salicylates, benzodiazepines, amiodarone, carbamazepine, lithium or spironolactone.

Contra-indications, warnings, etc
Precautions: There are no absolute contra-indications to TRH-Roche. In view of the postulated effect of bolus injections of TRH-Roche on smooth muscle, patients with bronchial asthma or other types of obstructive airways disease should be closely monitored. Caution should also be observed in patients with myocardial ischaemia and hypopituitarism.

Use in pregnancy: There is some clinical evidence of safety in human pregnancy, animal studies having shown no hazard. Nevertheless, the established medical principle of not administering drugs during early pregnancy should be observed.

Side-effects: TRH-Roche is well tolerated. No impairment of respiratory, hepatic, renal or haematological function has been reported. Following rapid intravenous injection, side-effects of a mild and transient nature may be experienced. They comprise nausea, a desire to micturate, a feeling of flushing, slight dizziness and a peculiar taste, and have been attributed to a local action of the bolus of TRH-Roche on the plain muscle of the gastro-intestinal and genito-urinary tracts. A transient increase in pulse rate and blood pressure may also be noted.

Effects of overdosage: No symptoms of overdosage have been noted in patients receiving up to 1 mg intravenously.

Pharmaceutical precautions *Storage:* The recommended maximum storage temperature for TRH-Roche ampoules is 30°C.

Additives: TRH-Roche ampoule solution should not be diluted.

Legal category POM.

Package quantities TRH-Roche ampoules containing 200 micrograms TRH-Roche in 2 ml in packs of 10.

Further information *Availability:* TRH-Roche is available to hospitals, pharmacies and clinics.

Product licence number
Ampoules 0031/0064

VALIUM* ROCHE TABLETS, SYRUP SUPPOSITORIES

Presentation Round, white tablets with ROCHE 2 imprinted on one face and a single break bar on the other, containing 2 mg diazepam.

Round, pale yellow tablets with ROCHE 5 imprinted on one face and a single break bar on the other, containing 5 mg diazepam.

Round, blue tablets with ROCHE 10 imprinted on one face and a single break bar on the other, containing 10 mg diazepam.

Pink, raspberry-flavoured syrup containing 2 mg diazepam in 5 ml.

Suppositories containing 10 mg diazepam.

Uses *Properties:* Valium Roche has anxiolytic, anticonvulsant and central muscle-relaxant properties. It has little autonomic activity.

Indications: Adults: Short-term (2–4 weeks) symptomatic treatment of anxiety that is severe, disabling or subjecting the individual to unacceptable distress, occurring alone or in association with insomnia or short-term psychosomatic, organic or psychotic illness.

Short-term (2–4 weeks) treatment of conditions where anxiety may be a precipitating or aggravating factor, e.g. tension headaches or migraine attacks.

Muscle spasm. As an adjunct to the control of muscle spasm in tetanus.

May be useful in the management of cerebral spasticity in selected cases.

As an adjunct to the management of some types of epilepsy, e.g. myoclonus.

Premedication.

Symptomatic treatment of acute alcohol withdrawal.

Children: Night terrors and somnambulism.

May be useful in controlling tension and irritability in cerebral spasticity in selected cases.

As an adjunct to the control of muscle spasm in tetanus.

Premedication.

Dosage and administration
Anxiety states: Adults: Usual dose – 2 mg three times daily. Maximum dose, up to 30 mg daily in divided doses, adjusted on an individual basis.

Insomnia associated with anxiety – 5 to 15 mg before retiring.

The lowest dose which can control symptoms should be used. Treatment should not be continued at the full dose beyond four weeks. Long-term chronic use is not recommended. Treatment should always be tapered off gradually. Patients who have taken benzodiazepines for a prolonged time may require a longer period during which doses are reduced. Specialist help may be appropriate.

Symptomatic relief of acute alcohol withdrawal – 5 to 20 mg, repeated if necessary in 2 to 4 hours.

Night terrors and somnambulism: Children: 1 to 5 mg at bedtime.

Conditions associated with muscle spasm: Adults: Muscle spasm – 2 to 15 mg daily in divided doses.

Management of cerebral spasticity in selected cases – 2 to 60 mg daily in divided doses.

Adjunct to control of muscle spasm in tetanus – 3 to 10 mg/kg body-weight daily by nasoduodenal tube. The selected dose should relate to the severity of the case and in extremely severe cases higher doses have been used. Intravenous Valium Roche is recommended initially (see separate data sheet).

Children: Control of tension and irritability in cerebral spasticity in selected cases – 2 to 40 mg daily in divided doses.

As an adjunct to the control of muscle spasm in tetanus – As for adults.

Adjunct to the management of some types of epilepsy: Adults: 2 to 60 mg daily in divided doses.

Premedication:
Adults: 5 to 20 mg.

Children: 2 to 10 mg.

ELDERLY OR DEBILITATED PATIENTS: DOSES SHOULD NOT EXCEED HALF THOSE NORMALLY RECOMMENDED.

Valium Roche tablets and syrup are for oral administration.

Valium Roche suppositories are for rectal administration.

Valium Roche syrup may be diluted with Sorbitol Solution BPC or Syrup BP.

Contra-indications, warnings, etc
Contra-indications: Patients with known sensitivity to benzodiazepines; acute pulmonary insufficiency; respiratory depression; phobic or obsessional states; chronic psychosis.

Use in pregnancy: There is no evidence as to drug safety in human pregnancy, nor is there evidence from animal work that it is free from hazard. Do not use during pregnancy, especially during the first and last trimesters, unless there are compelling reasons.

The administration of high doses or prolonged administration of low doses of benzodiazepines in the last trimester of pregnancy or during labour has been reported to produce irregularities in the foetal heart rate, and hypotonia, poor sucking and hypothermia in the neonate.

Diazepam has been detected in breast milk. If possible, the use of Valium Roche should be avoided during lactation.

Precautions: In patients with chronic pulmonary insufficiency, and in patients with chronic renal or hepatic disease, dosage may need to be reduced.

Valium should not be used alone to treat depression or anxiety associated with depression, since suicide may be precipitated in such patients.

Amnesia may occur.

In cases of loss or bereavement, psychological adjustment may be inhibited by benzodiazepines.

Patients should be advised that, like all medicaments of this type, Valium Roche may modify patients' performance at skilled tasks (driving, operating machinery, etc.) to a varying degree depending on dosage, administration and individual susceptibility. Patients should further be advised that alcohol may intensify any impairment and should, therefore, be avoided during treatment.

The dependence potential of the benzodiazepines is low, particularly when limited to short-term use, but this increases when high doses are used, especially when given over long periods. This is particularly so in patients with a history of alcoholism or drug abuse or in patients with marked personality disorders. Regular monitoring in such patients is essential, routine repeat prescriptions should be avoided and treatment should be withdrawn gradually. Symptoms such as depression, nervousness, rebound insomnia, irritability, sweating, and diarrhoea have been reported following abrupt cessation of treatment in patients receiving even normal therapeutic doses for short periods of time.

In rare instances, withdrawal following excessive dosages may produce confusional states, psychotic manifestations and convulsions.

Abnormal psychological reactions to benzodiazepines have been reported. Rare behavioural effects include paradoxical aggressive outbursts, excitement, confusion, and the uncovering of depression with suicidal tendencies. Extreme caution should therefore be used in prescribing benzodiazepines to patients with personality disorders.

If Valium Roche is given concomitantly with centrally-acting drugs such as neuroleptics, tranquillisers, antidepressants, hypnotics, analgesics and anaesthetics, the sedative effects are likely to be intensified. The elderly require special supervision.

Pharmacokinetic studies on potential interactions between Valium Roche and anti-epileptic drugs have produced conflicting results. Both depression and elevation of drug levels, as well as no change, have been reported. When Valium Roche is used in conjunction with anti-epileptic drugs, side-effects and toxicity may be more evident, particularly with hydantoins or barbiturates or combinations including them. This requires extra care in adjusting dosage in the initial stages of treatment.

Side-effects and adverse reactions: Common adverse effects include drowsiness, sedation, unsteadiness and ataxia, these are dose-related and may persist into the following day, even after a single dose. The elderly are particularly sensitive to the effects of centrally-depressant drugs and may experience confusion, especially if organic brain changes are present; the dosage of Valium Roche should not exceed one-half that recommended for other adults.

Other adverse effects are rare and include headache, vertigo, hypotension, gastrointestinal upsets, skin rashes, visual disturbances, changes in libido, and urinary retention. Isolated cases of blood dyscrasias and jaundice have also been reported.

Treatment of overdosage: When taken alone in overdosage Valium Roche presents few problems in management. Signs may include drowsiness, ataxia and dysarthria, with coma in severe cases. Treatment is symptomatic. Gastric lavage is useful only if performed soon after ingestion. Anexate* is a specific IV antidote for use in emergency situations. Patients requiring such intervention should be monitored closely in hospital (see separate prescribing information).

When taken with centrally-acting drugs, especially alcohol, the effects of overdosage are likely to be more severe and, in the absence of supportive measures, may prove fatal.

Pharmaceutical precautions *Storage:* The recommended maximum storage temperature for Valium Roche syrup and suppositories is 30°C.

All Valium Roche presentations should be protected from light.

Additives and pharmaceutical precautions: Valium Roche syrup may be diluted with Sorbitol Solution BPC or Syrup BP.

Maintenance of stability cannot be guaranteed if this advice is not followed.

Legal category CD (Sch. 4), POM.

Package quantities Valium 2 Roche tablets 2 mg, Valium 5 Roche tablets 5 mg, Valium 10 Roche tablets 10 mg in packs of 100.

Valium Roche syrup in packings of 100 ml.

Valium Roche suppositories 10 mg in packings of 5.

Further information Valium Roche is well absorbed, with peak blood levels being achieved one to two hours after administration, producing a rapid onset of clinical effects.

Diazepam is a long-acting benzodiazepine. It is metabolised to the active metabolites, N-desmethyldiazepam and oxazepam. Excretion is via the kidney in the form of conjugated oxazepam and temazepam. The half-life of diazepam varies from 20 to 50 hours whilst that of desmethyldiazepam ranges up to 100 hours.

Repeated doses will lead to accumulation of whole drug and metabolites. The latter may take two weeks to reach steady state and can reach higher concentrations than the parent compound.

No clear correlation has been demonstrated between the blood levels of Valium Roche and its clinical effects.

The elderly, and patients with impaired renal and/or hepatic function, will be particularly susceptible to the adverse effects listed above. It is advisable to review treatment regularly and to discontinue use as soon as possible.

Treatment should be kept to a minimum and given only under close medical supervision. Little is known regarding the efficacy or safety of benzodiazepines in long-term use.

Availability: Valium Roche is also available as 10 mg ampoules (see separate data sheet).

Product licence numbers

Tablets 2 mg	0031/5121R
Tablets 5 mg	0031/5122R
Tablets 10 mg	0031/5123R
Syrup	0031/5126R
Suppositories 10 mg	0031/0120

VALIUM* ROCHE AMPOULES

Presentation Ampoules containing 10 mg diazepam in 2 ml.

The ampoule solution is greenish-yellow.

Uses *Properties:* Valium Roche has anxiolytic, anticonvulsant and central muscle-relaxant properties. It has little autonomic activity.

Indications: Severe acute anxiety or agitation; delirium tremens.

Acute muscle spasm; tetanus.

Acute convulsions including status epilepticus, those due to poisoning, and febrile convulsions.

Pre-operative medication or premedication for a wide variety of procedures, e.g. in dentistry, surgery, radiology, endoscopy, cardiac catheterisation, cardioversion.

Dosage and administration *Adults:* Severe acute anxiety or agitation – 10 mg by IV or IM injection which may be repeated after an interval of not less than 4 hours.

Delirium tremens – 10 to 20 mg IV or IM. Higher doses may be needed, depending on severity of symptoms.

Acute muscle spasm – 10 mg by IV or IM injection which may be repeated after an interval of not less than 4 hours.

Tetanus – Initially an IV dose of 0.1 to 0.3 mg/kg body-weight, repeated at intervals of 1 to 4 hours. Continuous IV infusion of 3 to 10 mg/kg body-weight per 24 hours can also be used. Alternatively, the same dose of oral Valium Roche may be administered by nasoduodenal tube. The selected dose should relate to the severity of the case and in extremely severe cases higher doses have been used.

Status epilepticus, convulsions due to poisoning – 10 to 20 mg IV or IM, repeated if necessary 30–60 minutes later. If indicated, this may be followed by a slow intravenous infusion (maximum dose: 3 mg/kg body-weight over 24 hours).

Pre-operative medication or premedication – 0.2 mg/kg body-weight. The usual adult dose is 10 to 20 mg but higher doses may be necessary according to the clinical response.

ELDERLY OR DEBILITATED PATIENTS: DOSES SHOULD NOT EXCEED HALF THOSE NORMALLY RECOMMENDED.

Children:

Status epilepticus, convulsions due to poisoning, febrile convulsions – 0.2 to 0.3 mg/kg body-weight IV (or IM) or 1 mg per year of life.

Tetanus – As for adults.

Pre-operative medication or premedication – 0.2 mg/kg body-weight.

In order to reduce the likelihood of untoward effects during intravenous sedation the injection should be given slowly (0.5 ml of the solution per half-minute) until the patient becomes drowsy, the eyelids droop and the speech becomes slurred but the patient is still able to respond to requests.

It is strongly recommended that intravenous injections of Valium Roche should be given into a large vein of the antecubital fossa, the patient having been placed in a supine position and kept there throughout the procedure.

If these conditions are adhered to for administration of Valium Roche intravenously the possibility of hypotension or apnoea occurring will be greatly diminished.

Except in emergencies, a second person should always be present during intravenous use and facilities for resuscitation should always be available. It is recommended that patients should remain under medical supervision until at least one hour has elapsed from the time of injection. They should always be accompanied home by a responsible adult, with a warning not to drive or to operate machinery for 24 hours.

Valium Roche ampoule solution should not normally be diluted. An exception to this is when given slowly in large intravenous infusions of normal saline or dextrose, such as are given in the treatment of tetanus and status epilepticus. Not more than 40 mg (8 ml ampoule solution) should be added to 500 ml of infusion solution. The solution should be freshly made up and used within six hours.

Valium Roche ampoule solution should not be mixed with other drugs in the same infusion solution or in the same syringe.

Maintenance of stability cannot be guaranteed if this advice is not followed.

Valium Roche ampoules are for intravenous or intramuscular administration.

Contra-indications, warnings, etc

Contra-indications: Patients with known sensitivity to benzodiazepines; acute pulmonary insufficiency; respiratory depression; phobic or obsessional states; chronic psychosis.

Use in pregnancy: There is no evidence as to drug safety in human pregnancy, nor is there evidence from animal work that it is free from hazard. Do not use during pregnancy, especially during the first and last trimesters, unless there are compelling reasons.

The administration of high doses or prolonged administration of low doses of benzodiazepines in the last trimester of pregnancy or during labour has been reported to produce irregularities in the foetal heart rate, and hypotonia, poor sucking and hypothermia in the neonate.

Diazepam has been detected in breast milk. If possible the use of Valium Roche should be avoided during lactation.

Precautions: Parenteral Valium Roche should not normally be used in patients with organic brain changes (particularly arteriosclerosis) or with chronic pulmonary insufficiency. However, in emergency or when such patients are treated in hospital, Valium Roche may be given parenterally in reduced dosage. For IV administration, the injection should be given slowly.

In patients with chronic pulmonary insufficiency, and in patients with chronic renal or hepatic disease, dosage may need to be reduced.

Valium Roche should not be used alone to treat depression or anxiety associated with depression, since suicide may be precipitated in such patients.

Amnesia may occur.

In cases of loss or bereavement, psychological adjustments may be inhibited by benzodiazepines.

Patients should be advised that, like all medicaments of this type, Valium Roche may modify patients' performance at skilled tasks (driving, operating machinery, etc.) to a varying degree depending upon dosage, administration and individual susceptibility. Patients should further be advised that alcohol may intensify any impairment and should, therefore, be avoided during treatment.

Abnormal psychological reactions to benzodiazepines have been reported. Rare behavioural effects include paradoxical aggressive outbursts, excitement, confusion, and the uncovering of depression with suicidal tendencies. Extreme caution should therefore be used in prescribing benzodiazepines to patients with personality disorders.

If Valium Roche is combined with centrally-acting drugs such as neuroleptics, tranquillisers, antidepressants, hypnotics, analgesics and anaesthetics, the sedative effects are likely to be intensified. Furthermore, if such centrally-depressant drugs are given parenterally in conjunction with intravenous Valium Roche, severe respiratory and cardiovascular depression may occur. The elderly require special supervision.

When intravenous Valium Roche is to be administered concurrently with a narcotic analgesic agent, e.g. in dentistry, it is recommended that Valium Roche be given after the analgesic and that the dose be carefully titrated to meet the patient's needs.

Pharmacokinetic studies on potential interactions between Valium Roche and anti-epileptic drugs (including valproic acid) have produced conflicting results. Both depression and elevation of drug levels, as well as no change, have been reported. When Valium Roche is used in conjunction with anti-epileptic drugs, side-effects and toxicity may be more evident, particularly with hydantoins or barbiturates or combinations including them. This requires extra care in adjusting dosage in the initial stages of treatment.

Side-effects and adverse reactions: Intravenous injection may be associated with local reactions, and thrombophlebitis and venous thrombosis may occur. In order to minimise the likelihood of these effects, intravenous injections of Valium Roche should be given into a large vein of the antecubital fossa.

Apnoea or hypotension may rarely occur following intravenous injection. The incidence may be minimised by not exceeding the recommended rate of administration. Patients should always be managed in the supine position and kept there throughout the procedure.

Other adverse effects include drowsiness, sedation, unsteadiness and ataxia; these are dose-related and may persist into the following day. The elderly are particularly sensitive to the effects of centrally-depressant drugs and may experience confusion, especially if organic brain symptoms are present. The dosage of Valium Roche in these patients should not exceed one-half that recommended for other adults.

Rare adverse effects include headache, vertigo, hypotension, gastrointestinal upsets, skin rashes, visual disturbances, changes in libido, and urinary retention. Isolated cases of blood dyscrasias and jaundice have also been reported.

Treatment of overdosage: Treatment is symptomatic. Anexate* is a specific IV antidote for use in emergency situations. Patients requiring such intervention should be monitored closely in hospital (see separate prescribing information).

Pharmaceutical precautions *Storage:* The recommended maximum storage temperature for Valium Roche ampoules is 30°C. They should be protected from light.

Dilution, additives and pharmaceutical precautions: Valium Roche ampoule solution should not normally be diluted. An exception to this is when given slowly in large intravenous infusions of normal saline or dextrose such as are given in the treatment of tetanus and status epilepticus. Not more than 40 mg (8 ml ampoule solution) should be added to 500 ml of infusion solution. The solution should be freshly made up and used within six hours.

Over 50% of diazepam in solution may be adsorbed onto the walls of plastic containers of infusion solution; these should not therefore be used for diazepam solutions. Adsorption onto plastic drip tubing causes an initial significant reduction of delivered diazepam concentration which then gradually rises over the next few hours. The drip rate should frequently be titrated against the patient's condition.

Bolus injection allows a more accurate and rapid titration of dosage than slow intravenous infusion. It is therefore to be preferred for the management of acute problems.

Valium Roche ampoule solution should not be mixed with other drugs in the same infusion solution or in the same syringe.

Maintenance of stability cannot be guaranteed if this advice is not followed.

Legal category CD (Sch. 4), POM.

Package quantities Valium Roche ampoules 10 mg in 2 ml in packings of 10.

Further information Diazepam is a long-acting benzodiazepine. It is metabolised to the active metabolites, N-desmethyldiazepam and oxazepam. Excretion is via the kidney in the form of conjugated oxazepam and temazepam. The half-life of diazepam varies from 20 to 50 hours whilst that of desmethyldiazepam ranges up to 100 hours.

Repeated doses will lead to accumulation of whole drug and metabolites. The latter may take two weeks to reach steady state and can reach higher concentrations than the parent compound.

Intramuscular injection of Valium Roche can lead to a rise in serum creatine phosphokinase activity, with a maximum level occurring between 12 and 24 hours after the injection. This fact should be taken into account in the differential diagnosis of myocardial infarction.

The absorption from intramuscular injection of Valium Roche may be variable, particularly from the gluteal muscles. This route of administration should only be used when oral or intravenous dosing is not possible or advisable.

The elderly, and patients with impaired renal and/or hepatic function, will be particularly susceptible to the adverse effects listed above. It is advisable to review treatment regularly and to discontinue use as soon as possible.

Treatment should be kept to a minimum and given only under close medical supervision. Little is known regarding the efficacy or safety of benzodiazepines in long-term use.

Availability: Valium Roche is also available as 2 mg, 5 mg and 10 mg tablets, syrup (2 mg/5 ml) and suppository (10 mg). See separate data sheet.

Product licence number 0031/0068R

VASCACE* ▼

Vascace contains the substance with the approved name cilazapril, as the monohydrate salt. It is chemically described as {9(S)-[1(S)-Ethoxycarbonyl) - 3 - phenyl - propylamino] - octahydro - 10 - oxo -6H-pyridazo [1,2-a] [1,2]diazepine-1(S)-carboxylic acid}.

Presentation White, oval film-coated tablets, scored on one side and marked ROCHE 0.5 on the reverse, containing 0.5 mg anhydrous cilazapril.

Light-yellow, oval film-coated tablets, scored on one side and marked ROCHE 1 on the reverse, containing 1 mg anhydrous cilazapril.

Reddish-pink, oval film-coated tablets scored on one side and marked ROCHE 2.5 on the reverse, containing 2.5 mg anhydrous cilazapril.

Uses

Pharmacological properties: Vascace is a specific, long-acting angiotensin-converting enzyme (ACE) inhibitor which suppresses the renin-angiotensin-aldosterone system and thereby induces a reduction of both supine and standing systolic and diastolic blood pressure, usually with no orthostatic component.

Vascace is effective in all degrees of essential hypertension as well as in renal hypertension. Should the effect of Vascace at the top of the recommended dose be insufficient it can be combined with non-potassium-sparing diuretics.

The antihypertensive effect of Vascace is usually apparent within the first hour after administration, with maximum effect observed between three and seven hours after dosing. In general, the heart rate remains unchanged. Reflex tachycardia is not induced, although small, clinically insignificant alterations of heart rate may occur.

At recommended doses, the antihypertensive effect of Vascace is maintained for up to 24 hours. In some patients blood pressure reduction may diminish toward the end of the dosage interval. The initial dosage seldom achieves the desired therapeutic response. Blood pressure should be assessed and dosage adjusted as required.

The antihypertensive effect of Vascace is maintained during long-term therapy. No rapid increase in blood pressure has been observed after abrupt withdrawal of Vascace.

As with other ACE inhibitors, the blood pressure-lowering effect of Vascace in black patients may be less pronounced than in non-blacks. However, racial differences in response are no longer evident when Vascace is administered in combination with hydrochlorothiazide.

In patients with normal renal function, serum potassium usually remains within the normal range during Vascace treatment. In patients concomitantly taking potassium-sparing diuretics, potassium levels may rise.

In hypertensive patients with moderate to severe renal impairment, the glomerular filtration rate and renal blood flow remained in general unchanged with Vascace despite a clinically significant blood pressure reduction.

Pharmocokinetics: Cilazapril is efficiently absorbed and rapidly converted to the active form, cilazaprilat. Ingestion of food immediately prior to Vascace administration, delays and reduces the absorption to a minor extent which, however, is therapeutically irrelevant. The bioavailability of cilazaprilat from oral cilazapril approximates 60% based on urinary recovery data. Maximum plasma concentrations are reached within two hours after administration and are directly related to dosage.

Cilazaprilat is eliminated unchanged by the kidneys, with an effective half-life of nine hours after once-daily dosing with Vascace. In patients with renal impairment, higher plasma concentrations of cilazaprilat are observed than in patients with normal renal function, since drug clearance is reduced when creatinine clearance is lower. There is no elimination in patients with complete renal failure, but haemodialysis reduces concentrations of both cilazapril and cilazaprilat to a limited extent.

In elderly patients, whose renal function is normal for age, plasma concentrations of cilazaprilat may be up to 40% higher, and the clearance 20% lower than in younger patients. Similar changes in the pharmacokinetics occur in patients with moderate to severe liver cirrhosis.

Indications: All grades of essential hypertension and renovascular hypertension where standard therapy is ineffective or inappropriate because of adverse events.

Dosage and administration

Standard dosage for adults: Vascace should be administered once-daily. As food intake has no clinically significant influence on absorption, Vascace can be administered before or after a meal. The dose should always be taken at about the same time of day.

Essential hypertension: The usual dose range of Vascace is 2.5 to 5 mg once daily. The recommended initial dosage is a 1 mg tablet once a day. This initial dosage seldom achieves the desired therapeutic response. Dosage should be adjusted individually in accordance with the blood pressure response. If the blood pressure is not adequately controlled with 5 mg Vascace once daily, a low dose of non-potassium-sparing diuretic may be administered concomitantly to enhance the antihypertensive effect.

Renovascular hypertension: Treatment with Vascace should be initiated with a dose of 0.5 mg or 0.25 mg since these patients may experience more pronounced decreases in blood pressure in response to ACE inhibitors than patients with essential hypertension. The maintenance dose should be adjusted individually.

Special dosage instructions

Hypertensive patients receiving diuretics: The diuretic should be discontinued two to three days before beginning therapy with Vascace to reduce the likelihood of symptomatic hypotension. It may be resumed later if required. The starting dose in these patients is 0.5 mg.

Cardiac failure: In hypertensive patients who also have congestive heart failure with or without renal insufficiency, severe symptomatic hypotension has been observed after treatment with ACE inhibitors. In these patients Vascace therapy should be started at a dose of 0.5 mg under close medical supervision in hospital. The diuretic should be discontinued two to three days before beginning therapy with Vascace, when possible, to reduce the likelihood of symptomatic hypotension.

Impaired renal function: Reduced dosages may be required for patients with renal impairment, depending on their creatinine clearance.

The following dosage schedules are recommended:

Creatinine clearance	*Initial dose of Cilazapril*	*Maximal dose of Cilazapril*
>40 ml/min	1 mg once daily	5 mg once daily
10–40 ml/min	0.5 mg once daily	2.5 mg once daily
<10 ml/min	0.25–0.5 mg once or twice a week according to blood pressure response	

In patients requiring haemodialysis, Vascace should be administered on days when dialysis is not performed and the dosage should be adjusted according to blood pressure response.

Liver cirrhosis: In the unlikely event that patients with liver cirrhosis should require treatment with cilazapril, it should be initiated with caution at a dose of 0.5 mg or 0.25 mg, because significant hypotension may occur.

Use in the elderly: Treatment with cilazapril should be initiated with a 0.5 mg tablet once daily. Thereafter, the maintenance dose must be adapted to individual response.

Children: Safety and efficacy in children have not been established therefore there is no recommendation for administration of cilazapril to children.

Contra-indications, warnings, etc

Contra-indications: Cilazapril is contra-indicated in patients who are hypersensitive to the drug cilazapril or other ACE inhibitors, in patients with ascites and in pregnancy.

Use in pregnancy and lactation: Vascace is contra-indicated in pregnancy since foetotoxicity has been observed for ACE inhibitors in animals. Although there is no experience with Vascace, other ACE inhibitors in human pregnancy have been associated with oligohydramnios and neonatal hypotension and/or anuria. It is not known whether cilazapril passes into human breast milk, but since animal data show the presence of cilazaprilat in rat milk, Vascace should not be administered to nursing mothers.

Precautions: Occasionally, symptomatic hypotension has been reported with ACE inhibitor therapy, particularly in patients with sodium or volume depletion in connection with conditions such as vomiting, diarrhoea, pretreatment with diuretics, low sodium diet or after dialysis.

Patients with congestive heart failure, especially those taking high doses of loop diuretics, may experience a pronounced blood pressure decrease in response to ACE inhibitors. This should be treated by having the patient rest in the supine position and may require infusion of normal saline or volume expanders. After volume repletion, Vascace therapy may be continued. However, if symptoms persist, the dosage should be reduced or the drug discontinued.

Reduced dosages may be required for patients with renal impairment, depending on their creatinine clearance (see Special Dosage Instructions). As with other ACE inhibitors, increases in blood urea nitrogen and/or serum creatinine may be observed in hypertensive patients with unilateral or bilateral renal artery stenosis. These increases are usually reversible upon discontinuation of cilazapril and/or diuretic therapy.

Since serum potassium may increase in some patients with renal impairment, during ACE inhibitor treatment, potassium levels should be monitored frequently at regular intervals, depending on renal function.

The use of ACE inhibitors in combination with anaesthetic drugs in surgery that also have blood-pressure-lowering effects, can produce arterial hypotension. If this occurs, volume expansion by means of intravenous infusion, or if resistant to these measures – angiotensin II infusion is indicated.

Vascace should not be used in patients with aortic stenosis or outflow obstruction.

Side-effects and adverse reactions: Headache and dizziness were the most frequently reported events in patients taking cilazapril. Undesirable effects occurring in <2% of the patients include fatigue, hypotension, dyspepsia, nausea, rash and coughing. In most cases undesirable effects were transient, mild or moderate in degree, and did not require discontinuation of therapy.

As with other ACE inhibitors, angioneurotic oedema has been reported, although rarely, in patients receiving cilazapril. Since this syndrome can be associated with laryngeal oedema, cilazapril should be discontinued and appropriate therapy instituted without delay when involvement of the face, lips, tongue, glottis and/or larynx occurs.

Clinically relevant changes in laboratory test values possibly or probably related to cilazapril treatment have been observed only rarely. Minor, mostly reversible increases in serum creatinine/urea have been observed in patients treated with cilazapril. Such changes are likely to occur in patients with renal artery stenosis or with renal impairment (see Precautions), but they have also occasionally been observed in patients with normal renal function, particularly in those receiving concomitant diuretics.

In some patients decreases in haemoglobin, haematocrit and/or white blood cell count have been reported, but in no case has a definite causal relationship to cilazapril been established.

Drug interactions: Cilazapril has been administered concomitantly with digoxin, nitrates and H_2-receptor blockers. There was no increase in digoxin plasma concentrations and no other clinically significant drug interactions. An additive effect may be observed when cilazapril is administered in combination with other blood-pressure-lowering agents. Potassium-sparing diuretrics administered together with cilazapril can lead to increases in serum potassium particularly in patients with renal impairment (see Precautions).

As with other ACE inhibitors, use of cilazapril concomitantly with a non-steroidal anti-inflammatory drug (NSAID) may diminish the antihypertensive effect of cilazapril. This does not appear to occur in patients treated with cilazapril prior to the administration of NSAIDs.

Treatment of overdosage: While single doses of up to 160 mg cilazapril have been administered to normal healthy volunteers without untoward effects on blood pressure, only very few data on overdose are available in patients. The most likely event to occur is hypotension, which should be treated by means of volume expansion. If indicated, cilazaprilat, the active form of cilazapril, can be partially removed from the body by haemodialysis.

Pharmaceutical precautions
Storage: Store below 25°C.

Legal category POM.

Package quantities Vascace tablets 0.5 mg, 1 mg and 2.5 mg in packs of 28.

Further information Nil.

Product licence numbers

0.5 mg tablets	0031/0244
1 mg tablets	0031/0245
2.5 mg tablets	0031/0246

**Trade Mark*

Rorer Pharmaceuticals
St Leonards House
St Leonards Road
Eastbourne
East Sussex BN21 3YG

ALGICON* TABLETS AND SUSPENSION

Presentation
Tablets: White tablet marked with the product name on one side and 'RORER' on reverse.

Each tablet contains magnesium alginate 500 mg, aluminium hydroxide/magnesium carbonate co-gel 360 mg, Magnesium Carbonate BP 320 mg, Potassium Bicarbonate USP 100 mg. Other ingredients include sucrose.

Suspension: A yellow suspension with odour and taste of lemon.

Each 5 ml contains: magnesium alginate 250 mg, aluminium hydroxide/magnesium carbonate co-gel 140 mg, Magnesium Carbonate BP 175 mg, Potassium Bicarbonate USP 50 mg. Other ingredients include parabens.

Uses For the relief of heartburn associated with gastric reflux, reflux oesophagitis, hiatis hernia, pregnancy and hyperacidity.

Dosage and administration For oral administration.

Tablets

Adult dose: Chew 1 or 2 tablets four times a day or as directed by a physician. Tablets should be taken after meals and at bedtime, or as needed.

Suspension: 10 to 20 ml four times a day or as directed by a physician. The suspension should be taken after meals and at bedtime, or as needed.

The bottle should be shaken well before use.

Children: Not recommended for children under 12 years.

Elderly: No special precautions required.

Contra-indications, warnings, etc There are no specific contra-indications to Algicon. Products containing antacids should not, however, be administered to patients who are severely debilitated or suffering from kidney disease or to patients who are currently taking an antibiotic drug containing tetracycline.

Due to the high sugar content of the tablets, care should be exercised in the treatment of diabetic patients with this dosage presentation.

Use in pregnancy: It is probably wise to avoid taking preparations containing antacids in the first trimester of pregnancy.

Overdosage: In overdose, abdominal distension is the most likely occurrence and appropriate conservative measures should be taken.

Pharmaceutical precautions
Tablets: Store in a cool, dry place.
Suspension: Mix well before use. Do not freeze.

Legal category P.

Package quantities
Tablets: Cartons containing 60 blister-packed tablets.
Suspension: Bottles containing 500 ml of suspension.

Further information The product contains an alginate combined with an antacid which, on reaction with the gastric contents of the stomach, forms an insoluble gel-like layer above the stomach contents, which impedes reflux and provides a demulcent action.

The product has a low sodium content of less than 10 mg per tablet, and less than 10 mg per 10 ml of suspension.

Product licence numbers

Tablets	5272/0010
Suspension	5272/0009

DIORALYTE* SACHETS PLAIN, BLACKCURRANT AND CITRUS

Presentation Foil-laminate sachets each containing:

Sodium Chloride BP	0.47 g
Potassium Chloride BP	0.30 g
Glucose BP	3.56 g
Disodium Hydrogen Citrate BP	0.53 g

Uses Oral correction of fluid and electrolyte loss in infants, children and adults.

Treatment of watery diarrhoea of various aetiologies, including gastroenteritis, in all age groups.

Dosage and administration
Reconstitution: The contents of each sachet should be dissolved in 200 ml (approximately 7 fluid ounces) of drinking water. Use fresh drinking water for adults and children. For infants, and where drinking water is unavailable, the water should be freshly boiled and cooled. The solution should be made up immediately before use. If refrigerated, the solution may be stored for up to 24 hours, otherwise any solution remaining an hour after reconstitution should be discarded. The solution must not be boiled.

Dosage: The actual volume of reconstituted Dioralyte to be taken should be decided by the clinician, taking into consideration the weight of the patient and the stage and severity of the condition. A basic principle of treatment of diarrhoea is to replace lost fluid and electrolytes and then to maintain sufficient fluid intake to replace fluid loss from stools. Severe dehydration may need to be corrected by parenteral fluids initially followed by oral maintenance with Dioralyte if indicated.

Daily intake may be based on a volume of 150 ml/kg body weight for infants and 20–40 ml/kg body weight for adults and children. A reasonable approximation is:

Infants: One to one and a half times the usual 24 hour feed volume.

Children: One sachet after every loose motion.

Adults (including elderly): One or two sachets after every loose motion.

More may be required initially to ensure early and full volume repletion.

In the initial stages of treatment of diarrhoea all foods, including cow's or artificial milk, should be stopped. However, breast milk need not be witheld. In breast fed infants it is suggested that the infant is given the same volume of Dioralyte as the bottle fed baby and then put to the breast until satisfied. Expression of residual milk from the breasts may be necessary during this period. After 24–48 hours, when symptoms have subsided, the normal diet should be resumed but this should be gradual to avoid exacerbation of the condition.

Where vomiting is present with the diarrhoea, it is advisable that small amounts of Dioralyte be taken frequently. However, it is important that the whole of the required volume of Dioralyte be taken. Where the kidneys are functioning normally, it is difficult to overhydrate by mouth and where there is doubt about the exact dosage, more rather than less should be taken. If no improvement is seen within 36 hours, it is recommended that the patient should be reassessed.

Contra-indications, warnings, etc There are no known contra-indications to Dioralyte. However, there may be a number of conditions where treatment with Dioralyte will be inappropriate, e.g. intestinal obstruction requiring surgical intervention.

Precautions: For oral administration only.

Dioralyte should not be reconstituted in diluents other than water. Each sachet should always be dissolved in 200 ml water. A weaker solution than recommended will not contain the optimal glucose and electrolyte concentration and a stronger solution than recommended may give rise to electrolyte imbalance.

Dioralyte should not be administered to infants under 1 year of age except on medical advice.

Use in the elderly: No specific precautions are necessary. However, care should be taken when administering glucose-electrolyte solutions in cases of severe renal or hepatic impairment or other conditions where the normal electrolyte balance may be disturbed.

Use in pregnancy: Dioralyte therapy is not contra-indicated in pregnancy or lactation.

Overdose: In the event of significant overdose, serum electrolytes should be evaluated as soon as possible, appropriate steps taken to correct any abnormalities and levels monitored until return to normal levels is established. This is particularly important in the very young and in cases of severe hepatic or renal failure.

Pharmaceutical precautions The sachet should be stored in a cool dry place. Shelf life 2 years.

Legal category P.

Package quantities Packs of 20 sachets.

Further information The composition of Dioralyte is based on the observation that a correctly balanced, isotonic solution of glucose and sodium stimulates intestinal water absorption.

A litre of made up solution (5 sachets, 5 × 200 ml quantities) contains 60 mmol sodium (Na^+), 20 mmol potassium (K^+), 60 mmol chloride (Cl^-), 10 mmol citrate and 90 mmol glucose.

The total osmolarity is nominally 240 mmol per litre.

Each sachet of Dioralyte contains 3.56 g of glucose which is equivalent to 13.6 kCal.

Product licence numbers

Dioralyte	5272/0016
Dioralyte Blackcurrant	5272/0022
Dioralyte Citrus	5272/0023

DIORALYTE* EFFERVESCENT TABLETS BLACKCURRANT AND CITRUS

Presentation White/off-white circular tablets each containing:

Anhydrous Glucose BP	1.62 g
Sodium Bicarbonate BP	0.336 g
Potassium Chloride BP	0.186 g
Citric Acid Anhydrous BP	0.384 g
Sodium Chloride BP	0.117 g

Uses Oral correction of fluid and electrolyte loss in infants, children and adults

For the management of watery diarrhoea of various aetiologies, including gastroenteritis in all age groups.

Dosage and administration

Reconstitution: Two tablets should be dissolved in 200 ml (approximately 7 fluid ounces) of drinking water. Use fresh drinking water for adults and children. For infants and where drinking water is unavailable, the water should be freshly boiled and cooled. The solution should be made up immediately before use. If refrigerated, the solution may be stored for up to 24 hours, otherwise any solution remaining an hour after reconstitution should be discarded. The solution must not be boiled.

Dosage: The actual volume of reconstituted Dioralyte effervescent tablets to be taken should be determined by the clinician, depending on the patient's weight and the stage and severity of the condition. A basic principle of treatment of diarrhoea is to replace lost fluid and electrolytes and then to maintain sufficient fluid intake to replace further loss from stools.

Severe dehydration may need to be corrected by parenteral fluids initially followed by oral maintenance with Dioralyte if indicated.

Daily intake may be based on a volume of 150 ml/kg body weight for infants and 20–40 ml/kg body weight for adults and children. A reasonable approximation is:

Infants: One to one and a half times the usual 24 hour feed volume (see 'Precautions').

Children: Two tablets after every loose motion.

Adults (including elderly): Two or four tablets after every loose motion.

More may be required initially to ensure early and full volume repletion.

In the initial stage of treatment of diarrhoea all foods, including's cow's or artificial milk should be stopped. However, breast milk need not be withheld. In breast fed infants it is suggested that the infant is given the same volume of Dioralyte as the bottle fed baby and then put to the breast until satisfied. Expression of residual milk from the breasts may be necessary during this period. After 24 hours, when symptoms are subsiding, the normal diet should be resumed but this should be gradual to avoid worsening or prolonging the diarrhoea.

Where vomiting is present with the diarrhoea it is advisable that small amounts of Dioralyte effervescent be taken frequently. However, it is important that the whole of the required volume of Dioralyte effervescent is taken. With normal renal function it is difficult to overhydrate by mouth and where there is doubt about the exact dosage more rather than less should be taken.

If the diarrhoea does not improve after 36 hours the patient should be reassessed.

Contra-indications, warnings, etc There are no known contra-indications to Dioralyte Effervescent. However, there may be a number of conditions where treatment with Dioralyte Effervescent will be inappropriate, e.g., intestinal obstruction requiring surgical intervention.

Precautions: For oral administration only.

Dioralyte Effervescent tablets should only be taken after dissolution in water (100 ml water per tablet). A weaker solution than recommended will not contain the optimal glucose and electrolyte concentration and a stronger solution than recommended may give rise to electrolyte imbalance.

Because of the tablet effervescence, Dioralyte sachets rather than tablets are recommended for infants under 1 year of age. However, Dioralyte tablets may be used providing the effervescence is allowed to subside before use.

Dioralyte should not be administered to infants under 1 year of age except on medical advice.

Use in the elderly: No specific precautions are necessary. Care should be taken, however, when administering glucose electrolyte solutions in cases of severe renal or hepatic impairment or other conditions where the normal electrolyte balance may be disturbed.

Use in pregnancy: Dioralyte therapy is not contra-indicated in pregnancy or lactation.

Overdosage: In the event of significant overdose serum electrolytes should be evaluated as soon as possible, appropriate steps taken to correct any abnormalities and levels monitored until return to normal levels is established. This is particularly important in the very young and in cases of severe hepatic or renal failure.

Pharmaceutical precautions The tablets should be stored in the original container in a cool, dry place.

The cap should be replaced immediately after removal of tablets from the container.

Legal category P.

Package quantities Pack of 4 tubes of 10 tablets.

Further information The composition of Dioralyte Effervescent tablets is based on the observation that administration of a correctly balanced, isotonic solution of glucose and sodium stimulates intestinal water absorption.

A litre of made-up solution (10 tablets made up to 1 litre) contains 60 mmol sodium (Na^+), 90 mmol glucose, 20 mmol citrate, 25 mmol potassium (K^+) and 45 mmol chloride (Cl^-) (i.e. ionic concentration of solution after dissolution and completion of effervescence).

The total osmolarity is 240 mmol per litre. Each Dioralyte Effervescent tablet contains 1.62 g glucose which is equivalent to 6.2 kcal.

Product licence numbers

Dioralyte Blackcurrant Effervescent Tablets	5272/0025
Dioralyte Citrus Effervescent Tablets	5272/0042

MYOCRISIN*

Presentation Ampoules containing injection solutions of varying strengths of sodium aurothiomalate. The solutions are pale yellow. The injection solution also contains phenylmercuric nitrate.

Uses In the management of active progressive rheumatoid arthritis, and progressive juvenile chronic arthritis especially if polyarticular or seropositive.

Dosage and administration Myocrisin is administered by deep intramuscular injection, followed by gentle massage of the area.

Adults: An initial test dose of 10 mg should be given in the first week followed by weekly doses of 50 mg until signs of remission occur. At this point, 50 mg doses should be given at two week intervals until full remission occurs. With full remission, the interval between injections should be increased progressively to three, four and then (after 18 months to 2 years) to six weeks.

If after reaching a total dose of 1 gram (excluding the test dose) no major improvement has occurred and the patient has not shown any signs of gold toxicity, six 100 mg injections may be administered at weekly intervals. If no signs of remission occur after this time, other forms of treatment ought to be considered.

Elderly: No specific recommendations but elderly patients should be monitored with extra caution.

Children: Progressive juvenile chronic arthritis: Weekly doses of 1 mg/kg should be given but not exceeding a maximum weekly dose of 50 mg. Depending on urgency, this dose may be preceded by a smaller test dose such as $\frac{1}{10}$th or $\frac{1}{5}$th of the full dose for 2–3 weeks. Continue weekly doses until signs of remission appear then increase intervals between injections to two weeks. With full remission increase interval to three then four weeks. In the absence of signs of remission after twenty weeks consider raising the dose slightly or changing to other therapy.

Treatment should be continued for six months. Response can be expected at the 300–500 mg level. If patients respond, maintenance therapy should be continued with the dosage administered over the previous 2–4 weeks for 1–5 years.

Contra-indications, warnings, etc Pregnancy/lactation: The safety of Myocrisin in the foetus and newborn has not been established. Female patients receiving Myocrisin should be instructed to avoid pregnancy. Pregnant patients should not be treated with Myocrisin. Lactating mothers under treatment with Myocrisin excrete significant amounts of gold in their breast milk and should not breast feed their infants.

Myocrisin is contra-indicated in patients with gross renal or hepatic disease, a history of blood dyscrasias, exfoliative dermatitis or systemic lupus erythematosus.

The absolute contra-indications should be positively excluded before considering gold therapy. Myocrisin should be administered with extra caution in the elderly and in patients with a history of urticaria, eczema or colitis. Extra caution should also be exercised if phenylbutazone or oxyphenbutazone are administered concurrently. Gold administration may exacerbate aspirin induced hepatic dysfunction.

Before starting treatment and again before each injection, the urine should be tested for protein, the skin inspected for rash and a full blood count performed, including a numerical platelet count (not an estimate) and the readings plotted. Blood dyscrasias are most likely to occur when between 400 mg and 1 gram of gold have been given, or between the 10th and 20th week of treatment, but can also occur with much lower doses or after only 2–4 weeks of therapy.

The presence of albuminuria, pruritus or rash, or an eosinophilia, are indications of developing toxicity; the Myocrisin should be withheld for one or two weeks until all signs have disappeared when the course may be restarted on a test dose followed by a decreased frequency of gold injections.

A complaint of sore throat, glossitis, buccal ulceration and/or easy bruising or bleeding, demands an immediate blood count, followed, if indicated by appropriate treatment for agranulocytosis, aplastic anaemia and/or thrombocytopenia. Every patient treated with Myocrisin should be warned to report immediately the appearance of pruritus, metallic taste, sore throat or tongue, buccal ulceration or easy bruising, purpura, epistaxis, bleeding gums, menorrhagia or diarrhoea.

Hepatotoxicity with cholestatic jaundice is a rare complication which may occur early in the course of treatment; it subsides on withdrawing Myocrisin. A rare but severe form of enterocolitis has been described.

Diffuse unilateral or bilateral pulmonary fibrosis very rarely occurs. This progressive condition usually responds to drug withdrawal and steroid therapy – annual chest X-ray is recommended and attention should be paid to unexplained breathlessness and dry cough.

Side-effects may be largely avoided by the indicated careful titration of dosage. Minor reactions, usually manifest as skin rashes, are the most frequent and commonly benign, but as such reactions may be the forerunners of severe gold toxicity they must never be treated lightly. Significant skin complications are almost exclusively pruritic. Rare reports of alopoecia exist. Minor side-effects resolve spontaneously on withdrawal of Myocrisin. Symptomatic treatment of pruritus with antihistamines may be helpful. Major skin lesions and serious blood dyscrasias demand hospital admission when dimercaprol or penicillamine may be used to enhance gold excretion. Fresh blood and/or platelet transfusions, corticosteroids and androgenic steroids may be required in the management of severe blood dyscrasias.

Pharmaceutical precautions Protect from light. Discoloured solutions should not be used. Store below 25°C.

Legal category POM.

Package quantities Boxes of 10 × 10 mg, 20 mg and 50 mg ampoules.

Further information Some rheumatologists provide their patients with a 'gold card' on which is recorded the amount of gold salt injected and results of laboratory tests, at the same time issuing a proforma for further treatment to the general practitioner responsible for the management of the patient. These are valuable aids in the early detection, and so reduce the incidence, of toxic reactions.

Product licence numbers

Injection 10 mg	0012/5114
Injection 20 mg	0012/5113
Injection 50 mg	0012/5006

SURMONTIL*

Presentation Surmontil Tablets are compression-coated, white, each containing the equivalent of 10 mg or 25 mg trimipramine (as maleate). The face is indented with the name and strength; the reverse is plain. Surmontil Capsules (body white opaque with green cap, printed 'SU50'), each contain the equivalent of 50 mg trimipramine (as maleate).

Uses Surmontil has a potent antidepressant action similar to that of other tricyclic antidepressants. It also possesses a pronounced sedative action. It is, therefore, indicated in the treatment of depressive illness, especially where sleep disturbance, anxiety or agitation is a presenting symptom. Sleep disturbance is controlled within 24 hours and true antidepressant action follows within 7–10 days.

Dosage and administration *Adults:* Mild/moderate depression in general practice. The recommended dosage is 50–75 mg orally given two hours before bedtime, the larger dose (75 mg) being preferable for those patients with more marked sleep disturbance. Treatment should be continued for at least three weeks.

Moderate/severe depression (patients under psychiatric supervision): Initial dosage – 75 mg orally per day. This is best given as a single dose late in the evening or as 25 mg midday and 50 mg late in the evening. Dosage should then be increased as necessary until the optimal therapeutic level is reached, usually 150–300 mg per day. Treatment at this dosage should be continued for four to six weeks, dosage then being reduced to a maintenance level, usually within the range of 75–150 mg per day, for two to three months.

Giving most of the total daily dosage at night induces a rapid return to normal sleep, reduces the need for night-time sedation and minimises daytime drowsiness.

Elderly: Initially 10–25 mg three times a day. The initial dose should be increased with caution under close supervision. Half the normal maintenance dose may be sufficient to produce a satisfactory clinical response.

Cyclothymic patients with recurrent depression may require maintenance therapy for up to one year or even longer.

Surmontil is not recommended for use in children.

Contra-indications, warnings, etc Recent myocardial infarction. Any degree of heart block or other cardiac arrhythmia. Mania, severe liver disease. During breast feeding.

The elderly are particularly liable to experience adverse reactions, especially agitation, confusion and postural hypotension (see Dosage).

Treatment should be avoided, if possible, in patients with narrow angle glaucoma, symptoms suggestive of prostatic hypertrophy and a history of epilepsy.

Patients posing a high suicidal risk require close initial supervision. The central nervous depressant action of alcohol is potentiated by Surmontil.

Anaesthetics given during tricyclic antidepressant therapy may increase the risk of arrhythmias and hypotension. If surgery is necessary, the anaesthetist should be made aware that a patient is being so treated.

Trimipramine should not be given concurrently with, or within 2 weeks of cessation of therapy with monoamine oxidase inhibitors. The anti-hypertensive effect of guanethidine, debrisoquine, bethanidine and possibly clonidine may be decreased by trimipramine.

It would be advisable to review all anti-hypertensive therapy during treatment with tricyclic anti-depressants. Trimipramine should not be given with sympathomimetic agents such as adrenaline, ephedrine, isoprenaline, noradrenaline, phenylephrine and phenylpropanolamine. Barbiturates may increase the rate of metabolism of Surmontil.

Surmontil should be administered with care in patients receiving therapy for hyperthyroidism.

Patients should be monitored closely during the initial stages of treatment, as improvement may not occur during the first 2–4 weeks. Trimipramine may initially impair alertness. Patients should be warned of the possible hazard when driving or operating machinery. Cardiac arrhythmias and severe hypotension are likely to occur with high dosage or in deliberate overdosage. They may also occur in patients with pre-existing heart disease taking normal dosage. It may be advisable to monitor liver function in patients on long-term treatment with Surmontil.

Side-effects: These are similar to those of other tricyclic anti-depressants; they are usually more evident during the first few days of treatment and are invariably controlled by modification of dosage. Drowsiness may occur, but this is minimised by giving the total daily dosage at night. Atropine-like side effects including dry mouth, disturbances of accommodation, tachycardia, constipation and hesitancy of micturition are common early in treatment, but usually lessen. Other adverse effects include sweating, postural hypotension, tremor and skin rashes.

Interference with sexual function may occur.

Serious adverse effects are rare; the following have been reported: depression of the bone marrow including agranulocytosis, cholestatic jaundice, hypomania, convulsions and peripheral neuropathy. Psychotic manifestations, including mania and paranoid delusions, may be exacerbated during treatment with tricyclic anti-depressants. Withdrawal symptoms may occur on abrupt cessation of therapy and include insomnia, irritability and excessive perspiration. Adverse effects such as withdrawal symptoms, respiratory depression and agitation have been reported in neonates whose mothers had taken trimipramine during the last trimester of pregnancy.

Use in pregnancy and lactation: Do not use during pregnancy, especially during the first and last trimester, unless there are compelling reasons. There is no evidence as to drug safety in human pregnancy nor is there evidence from animal work that it is free from hazard. Trimipramine is contra-indicated during lactation.

Acute overdosage may be accompanied by hypotensive collapse, convulsions and coma. Provided coma is not present, gastric lavage should be carried out without delay even although some time may have passed since the drug was ingested. Patients in coma should have an endotracheal tube passed before gastric lavage is started. Absorption of trimipramine is slow but, as cardiac effects may appear soon after the drug is absorbed, a saline purge should be given. Electrocardiography monitoring is essential.

It is important to treat acidosis as soon as it appears with, for example, 20 ml per kg of M/6 sodium lactate injection by slow intravenous injection. Intubation is necessary and the patient should be ventilated before convulsions develop; convulsions should be treated with diazepam administered intravenously.

Ventricular tachycardia or fibrillation should be treated by electrical defibrillation; if supraventricular tachycardia develops, pyridostigmine bromide 1 mg (adults) intravenously or propranolol 1 mg (adults) intravenously should be administered at intervals as required.

Treatment should be continued for at least three days even if the patient appears to have recovered.

Pharmaceutical precautions Protect from light. Surmontil capsules should be stored in a dry place below 25°C.

Legal category POM.

Package quantities Tablets: Compression-coated – 10 mg in container of 50 (OP), and 25 mg in containers of 50 (OP). Capsules: 50 mg in blister pack of 28 (OP).

Further information Nil.

Product licence numbers

Tablets 10 mg	0012/5296
Tablets 25 mg	0012/5297
Capsules 50 mg	0012/5298

UBRETID*

Presentation *Tablets:* White tablets marked 'UBRETID' with single break line on reverse. Each tablet contains 5 mg distigmine bromide. Other ingredients include lactose.

Ampoules: Clear ampoules each containing 0.5 mg distigmine bromide in 1 ml saline.

Uses Anticholinesterase. Post-operative urinary retention. Post operative ileus and intestinal atony. To assist emptying of the neurogenic bladder. As an adjunct in the treatment of myasthenia gravis.

Distigmine bromide is an anticholinesterase with a much longer duration of action than neostigmine or pyridostigmine. In man, maximum inhibition of plasma cholinesterase occurs nine hours after a single intramuscular dose of 0.5 mg Ubretid, and persists for approximately 24 hours returning to normal after 48 hours.

Dosage and administration *Adults (including the elderly):*

In prevention of urinary retention, ileus or intestinal atony following surgery: 1 Ubretid Ampoule by intramuscular injection given 12 hours after surgery is usually adequate prophylaxis and this may be repeated at 24-hourly intervals until normal function is restored. Caution should be exercised in the timing of this initial dose, where doubt exists as to the integrity of any bowel anastamosis. When injections are not convenient, 1 Ubretid Tablet may be given daily half-an-hour before breakfast.

In neurogenic bladder: 1 Ubretid Tablet daily or on alternate days, half-an-hour before breakfast, on an empty stomach. Intramuscular injections may be given in place of tablets for the first few days of therapy.

In myasthenia gravis – tablets only should be used: Adults: Dosage to be individualised for each patient, dependent upon the severity of the condition, the degree and duration of response and the side-effects encountered. The tablets should always be taken on an empty stomach half an hour before breakfast. Dosage should commence at 1 tablet daily and may be adjusted at intervals of three to four days to a total not exceeding 4 tablets daily.

Children: Up to 2 tablets daily, according to age.

Contra-indications, warnings, etc Ubretid is contra-indicated in cases of severe post-operative shock, serious circulatory insufficiency and serious spastic and mechanical ileus.

Ubretid should be used with caution in conditions where the potentiation of acetylcholine effects is undesirable, e.g. vagotonia, bronchial asthma, cardiac disease, peptic ulcer, epilepsy and Parkinsonism.

In myasthenia gravis, where short-acting cholinergic drugs are taken concurrently, their dosage should be reduced to the minimum required to control symptoms.

The patient should be supervised in the early stages of dosage regulation to guard against the possibility of myasthenic crisis or cholinergic crisis.

Overdosage with Ubretid would be expected to give rise to the signs of anticholinesterase poisoning. Atropine (up to 2 mg i.m.) should be given at once and repeated at intervals indicated by the clinical progress until signs of mild atropinisation appear (dry mouth, mydriasis). The patient is best kept fully atropinised for 24 hours.

Muscarinic side-effects of Ubretid are usually few and mild, and can be controlled with atropine, giving 2 mg intramuscularly and maintaining atropinisation for at least 24 hours.

Use in pregnancy: Ubretid should not be administered to pregnant women.

Treatment of overdosage: Oral absorption is poor unless Ubretid is taken on a completely empty stomach. Observation may be sufficient. Generalised parasympathomimetic symptoms should be antagonised by atropine.

Pharmaceutical precautions No special precautions.

Diluent for ampoules: Water for Injections BP.

Legal category POM.

Package quantities *Tablets:* Containers of 30 and 100 tablets.

Ampoules: Boxes of 10.

Further information Nil.

Product licence numbers

Tablets	5272/0029
Ampoules	5272/0030.

UNIVER*

Presentation Univer capsules are a sustained release formulation of verapamil having clinical efficacy over a full 24 hours with once daily dosing. The product is available in three strengths: 120 mg sustained release Verapamil Hydrochloride BP as a yellow/dark blue capsule, marked V120; 180 mg sustained release Verapamil Hydrochloride BP as a yellow capsule marked V180; and 240 mg sustained release Verapamil Hydrochloride BP as a yellow/dark blue capsule, marked V240.

Uses

Indications: Univer is recommended for the long term treatment of mild to moderate hypertension and angina pectoris.

Mode of action: Calcium antagonists are a group of agents that selectively inhibit calcium influx into cells. In the myocardium two calcium specific channels exist. Fast channels are involved in the initiation of contraction and slow channels in sustaining contraction. Calcium antagonists interfere with calcium movement through slow channels. As a result verapamil tends to increase the refractory period between the contractions of the heart, and reduce excitability.

In smooth vascular muscle this action on calcium channels results in the reduction of muscle tone leading to dilatation of the blood vessels. This effect is most prominent in blood vessels with high tone or in vessels subject to spasm. Verapamil increases arterial blood flow with minimal changes in venous capacitance. This action of verapamil is responsible for the reduction in blood pressure that is observed.

In the coronary artery vasculature verapamil increases blood flow by reducing coronary vessel tone and abolishing vasospasm, increasing oxygen delivery to all areas of the myocardium. This increased level of oxygen delivery results clinically in an effective treatment for angina pectoris.

Dosage and administration

Adults

Hypertension: Initial dose in patients new to verapamil therapy should be 120 mg o.d. This can be increased to 240 mg o.d., which is the normal maintenance dosage. The dose may be further increased to a maximum of 480 mg o.d. if required.

Angina: The usual dose is 360 mg once daily. Dosage may be increased to a maximum of 480 mg daily if required.

Elderly patients: Elderly patients show enhanced bioavailability of verapamil and therapeutic control may be achieved with lower doses in this patient population.

Children: Univer is not recommended in children as no studies have been undertaken.

Contra-indications, warnings, etc

Contra-indications: Significant bradycardia (less than 50 bpm): second or third degree heart block; sick sinus syndrome or uncontrolled heart failure. Verapamil should not be used when atrial flutter/fibrillation complicates Wolff-Parkinson-White syndrome.

Precautions: Verapamil hydrochloride has an action that alters conduction in the heart and should be used with caution in first degree heart block. Patients with atrial flutter/fibrillation in association with Wolff-Parkinson-White Syndrome may develop increased conduction across the anomalous pathway and ventricular tachycardia may be precipitated. It also has an effect that reduces the contractility of the myocardium and this action may aggravate or occasionally precipitate heart failure in borderline cases. In circumstances where there is pre-existing poor ventricular function it is prudent to treat this condition before initiating therapy with Univer.

Special care should be taken in hypotension especially in acute myocardial infarction as this is a condition where atrioventricular conduction defects may develop and contractility may be impaired.

In view of the action of beta-adrenoceptor blocking agents which may tend to interfere with conduction and decrease contractility, verapamil should be used with caution in combination with beta-blocking agents, and a period between stopping beta-blocker therapy and starting Univer Capsules may be advisable.

Verapamil is extensively metabolised in the liver and special care should be taken in cases where liver damage exists, as plasma levels of verapamil may be increased.

Caution is required when verapamil hydrochloride is given with digoxin therapy as the plasma digoxin level may rise.

Use in pregnancy and lactation: The use of all therapeutic agents, including verapamil, requires special care in pregnancy. Although there is no evidence of teratogenicity for verapamil hydrochloride, its use in the first trimester shoud be avoided if at all possible. Verapamil hydrochloride is excreted in breast milk; it is recommended that the product should not be administered to nursing mothers.

Side-effects: Few adverse reactions have been reported in patients taking Univer Capsules. Constipation may occur and flushing has been recorded. Headaches are uncommon. Very infrequently nausea, vomiting and allergic reactions have been observed. On very rare occasions, a reversible impairment of liver function characterised by an increase in transaminases and/or alkaline phosphatase may occur during verapamil treatment and is most probably a hypersensitivity reaction.

Treatment of Overdosage: Normal resuscitation procedures should be initiated in the event of cardiovascular collapse, i.e., if atrioventricular conduction defects such as second or third degree block develop these should be treated in the usual way using atropine, isoprenaline or temporary insertion of a pacemaker, as required. Hypotension may be observed, requiring repositioning of the patient with head tilted down, and if persistent, and in the absence of any conduction defect, treatment with systemic dopaminergic agents, such as dopamine, dobutamine or noradrenaline, should be started.

Pharmaceutical precautions Store in a cool, dry place.

Legal category POM.

Package quantities

For both 120 mg and 240 mg presentations: Blister strips of 14 capsules, two strips per carton of 28 capsules (OP).

For the 180 mg presentation: Blister strips of 14 capsules, four strips per carton of 56 capsules (OP).

Further information In hypertension, patients new to verapamil therapy may be started on 120 mg once daily. Univer Capsules have been found to give good control of blood pressure, with more than 70% of mild to moderate hypertensives showing a good response with up to 240 mg once daily. Two week intervals should be allowed before changing to higher doses, to a maximum of 480 mg once daily. In the few patients who fail to respond to the highest dose, a thiazide may be introduced to produce an additional fall in blood pressure.

Product licence numbers

Univer 120 mg Capsules	5272/0039
Univer 180 mg Capsules	5272/0040
Univer 240 mg Capsules	5272/0041

**Trade Mark*

Roussel Laboratories Limited
Broadwater Park
North Orbital Road
Uxbridge
Middlesex UB9 5HP

ROUSSEL

ACTINAC*

Presentation Actinac is presented as a pale yellow dry powder, together with a solvent for the preparation of a lotion. Each gram of powder contains:

Chloramphenicol BP	40 mg
Hydrocortisone Acetate BP	40 mg
Butoxyethyl nicotinate	24 mg
Allantoin	24 mg
Precipitated Sulphur BP	320 mg

The solvent is Purified Water BP, containing an approved lavender perfume and bacteriostat.

Uses Actinac is for use in the topical treatment of acne vulgaris and other acneiform conditions. It is formulated to control local infection and suppress inflammation with its consequent scarring effects.

Dosage and administration The lotion should be prepared according to the manufacturer's literature and applied with cotton wool or lint night and morning for the first four days and only at night thereafter. In order to prevent recurrence, treatment should be continued for three nights after the lesions have disappeared.

Contra-indications, warnings, etc Actinac is contra-indicated in patients who have a known hypersensitivity to any of the ingredients.

Avoid Actinac coming into contact with the eyes and mouth.

Early in the course of treatment, erythema may occur at the site of application and the patient may experience a sensation of warmth due to the vasodilator action of the nicotinate. In the unlikely event of a severe reaction, the patient is instructed to consult the doctor before further use of Actinac.

In pregnant animals, administration of corticosteroids can cause abnormalities of foetal development. The relevance of this finding to human beings has not been established. However, topical steroids should not be used extensively in pregnancy, i.e. in large amounts or for long periods. It is advisable to remove jewellery before applying the lotion.

Pharmaceutical precautions Store cool. The lotion when constituted will remain active for 21 days. Any lotion remaining after this time must be discarded and a fresh supply of lotion prepared.

Legal category POM.

Package quantities Each pack of Actinac contains two bottles of powder (each 6.25 g), two bottles of solvent (each 20 ml) and an instruction leaflet for the patient.

Further information Actinac powder contains Tragacanth BP, Myrj 53, Syloid 244, Purified talc BP, Titanium dioxide BP. The solvent contains lavender water soluble 0/621970 and Benzoic Acid BP.

Product licence number 0109/0037.

ALTACITE PLUS*
(Approved name: Co-Simalcite)

Presentation *Suspension:* Viscous, slightly off-white aqueous suspension, flavoured with spearmint. Each 5 ml of suspension contains 500 mg of hydrotalcite and 125 mg of activated dimethicone.

Uses Altacite Plus has antacid, mucosal protective and anti-flatulent properties. As an antacid, Altacite Plus buffers in the optimal range of pH 3–5 for over two hours.

It is indicated for symptomatic relief in the following conditions: dyspepsia; flatulence and abdominal distension; hyperacidity; gastritis; peptic ulceration; heartburn, especially when associated with oesophagitis or hiatus hernia; and heartburn in pregnancy.

Dosage and administration *Adults:* 10 ml suspension between meals and at bedtime or as directed by the physician.

Elderly: No specific recommendations in the elderly.

Children (8–12 years): Half the adult dose.

Contra-indications, warnings, etc There are no known contra-indications to Altacite Plus, but it is wise to avoid any drug, including antacids, during the first trimester of pregnancy. As with other compounds containing aluminium or magnesium, Altacite Plus may reduce intestinal absorption of tetracycline. Side-effects are uncommon. Diarrhoea and vomiting have been reported but have ceased on withdrawal of therapy.

Pharmaceutical precautions Store in a cool place.

Legal category P.

Package quantities *Altacite Plus Suspension:* Polyethylene laminate bottle containing 500 ml.

Further information There is no evidence of absorption of hydrotalcite in man. Investigations in healthy human volunteers have shown no elevation of serum aluminium or magnesium levels on administration of hydrotalcite at therapeutic dosage for a continuous period of 28 days.

The sodium content of Altacite Plus suspension is low (0.078 mmol/5 ml).

Product licence number
Altacite Plus Suspension 0109/0062

ASPAV*

Presentation White-coloured, circular, flat bevelled-edge tablets, which disperse in water to give a fine suspension containing the equivalent of Aspirin BP 500 mg and Papaveretum BPC 10 mg.

Uses Analgesic. For the relief of moderate to severe pain in post-operative states and the relief of chronic pain associated with inoperable carcinoma.

Dosage and administration
Adults (not recommended for children under 12 years); One or two tablets dispersed in water every 4–6 hours. (Not more than eight tablets in any 24 hour period).

Contra-indications, warnings, etc
Contra-indications: Not recommended for women of child bearing potential and children under 12 years. Should not be administered to patients with known sensitivity to aspirin or papaveretum. Aspav should not be given to patients with respiratory depression, or obstructive airways disease and should not be given to patients receiving concurrent therapy with monoamaine

oxidase inhibitors, or within two weeks of their withdrawal.

Warnings and adverse effects: Papaveretum is an analgesic with CNS depressant properties; these properties may be enhanced when Aspav is taken in combination with other CNS depressants and/or alcohol. Aspirin may give rise to hypersensitivity reactions, asthma and may induce gastro-intestinal haemorrhage (occasionally major).

Precautions: Aspav should be given with care to patients known to have a lesion of the gastric mucosa. Aspirin may enhance the activity of coumarin anticoagulants and oral hypoglycaemic agents. The activity of methotrexate may be markedly enhanced and its toxicity increased; the toxicity of sulphonamides may also be increased. Aspirin diminishes the effect of uricosuric agents such as probenecid and sulphinpyrazone. Aspirin may precipitate bronchospasm and may induce attacks of asthma in susceptible subjects.

Reduced dosage is advised in elderly and debilitated patients, hypothyroid patients and those with head injuries or chronic hepatic disease. As with all narcotics, patients taking Aspav should avoid alcohol.

Aspav may also modify patients' reactions and they should be advised against driving or performing other complex manual tasks.

Use in pregnancy and lactation: Although Aspav has been used clinically for many years without noticeable ill consequences, noscapine, one of the constituent alkaloids of papaveretum, has been shown to be mutagenic in vitro. Due to the theoretical risk to the developing foetus, the use of Aspav, and all other products containing papaveretum, is contra-indicated in women of child-bearing potential.

Tolerance: Repeated administration of Aspav may give rise to tolerance and dependence of the morphine type.

Side-effects: These include nausea, vomiting, constipation and confusion.

Effects of overdosage: Side-effects of overdosage are similar to those with morphine, but occur to a lesser extent; they may include pin-point pupils, depressed respiration and coma. In severe poisoning there may be dilatation of the pupils, shock, severe respiratory depression and pulmonary oedema.

Gastric lavage should be performed soon after ingestion, and oxygen, intravenous fluids and other intensive supportive therapy carried out, as necessary. Naloxone, is a suitable antidote for papaveretum.

Pharmaceutical precautions Aspav Tablets should be stored in a cool dry place, in a tightly closed container, and protected from light.

Legal category POM.

Package quantities Securitainers of 100 tablets.

Further information Aspav has advantages over morphine combinations, as papaveretum has intrinsic spasmolytic activity in addition to its analgesic properties. Aspav is not subject to the prescribing regulations of the Misuse of Drugs Act. Each tablet contains 1605 mg Lactose BP.

Product licence number 0142/5597.

CIDOMYCIN* EYE/EAR DROPS CIDOMYCIN* EYE OINTMENT

Presentation

Drops: Each millilitre of drops contains Gentamicin Sulphate BP equivalent to 0.3% w/v gentamicin base in sterile buffered isotonic aqueous solution.

Ointment: Each gram of ointment contains Gentamicin Sulphate BP equivalent to 0.3% w/v gentamicin base in Plastibase*.

Uses Cidomycin (gentamicin) is an aminoglycoside antibiotic with broad spectrum bactericidal activity against most Gram positive and Gram negative bacteria.

In the eye: Cidomycin drops and ointment are indicated in the topical treatment of external bacterial infections of the eye, including conjunctivitis, blepharitis, styes, corneal ulcers and for prophylaxis in trauma.

In the ear: Cidomycin drops may also be used effectively in the treatment of external ear infections due to sensitive organisms.

Dosage and administration For adults and children.

In the eye: 1 to 3 drops should be instilled into the affected eye three or four times daily, or as required; alternatively, the ointment may be used applying it to the affected area three or four times daily.

In the ear: Following cleansing of the affected ear, 2 to 4 drops should be instilled three or four times daily and at night.

No specific recommendations for the elderly.

Contra-indications, warnings, etc The product is contra-indicated where there is known hypersensitivity to any of the ingredients. If irritation, sensitisation or superinfection develop, treatment with Cidomycin should be discontinued and appropriate therapy instituted. Use in the ear is contra-indicated if the drum is perforated.

Interactions: Gentamicin is pharmaceutically incompatible with amphotericin, cephalosporins, erythromycin, heparin, penicillins, sodium bicarbonate, and sulphadiazine sodium.

Effects on ability to drive and to use machines: Topical eye preparations may cause transient blurring of vision on instillation. Patients should be warned not to drive or operate hazardous machinery unless vision is clear.

Other undesirable effects: Gentamicin ointment may cause transient eye irritation. Severe dose-related ototoxicity can occur with gentamicin in susceptible patients, particularly those with renal impairment. Vestibular damage is more common than hearing loss.

Use in pregnancy and lactation: There are no proven cases of intrauterine damage caused by gentamicin. However, as with most drugs known to cross the placenta, usage in pregnancy should be considered where benefits outweigh possible risks. In the absence of gastro-intestinal inflammation, the amount of gentamicin ingested from breast milk is unlikely to result in significant blood levels in infants.

Other special warnings and precautions: If irritation, sensitisation, or super-infection develop, treatment with Cidomycin should be discontinued and appropriate therapy instituted.

Overdose: Not applicable.

Pharmaceutical precautions Eye/Ear Drops: Store below 25°C.
Eye Ointment: Store below 30°C.

Legal category POM.

Package quantities Cidomycin Eye/Ear Drops – 8 ml in ophthalmic dispenser.
Cidomycin Eye Ointment – 3 g tube (fitted with ophthalmic nozzle).

Further information Cidomycin eye/ear drops contain disodium edetate BP, benzalkonium chloride solution BP, sodium metabisulphite BP, sodium phosphate EP, sodium acid phosphate BP and purified water EP.

Product licence numbers
Cidomycin Eye/Ear Drops 0109/0114
Cidomycin Eye Ointment 0109/0115

CIDOMYCIN* INJECTIONS Gentamicin Injection BP Gentamicin Intrathecal Injection Gentamicin Sulphate BP

Presentation Cidomycin for parenteral use is available as:

Cidomycin Injection in 2 ml vials or ampoules each containing the equivalent of 80 mg gentamicin base as sulphate.

Cidomycin Injection Paediatric in 2 ml vials each containing the equivalent of 20 mg gentamicin base as sulphate.

Cidomycin Intrathecal Injection in 1 ml ampoules each containing 5 mg gentamicin base as sulphate.

Cidomycin Sterile Powder is whitish in colour and is available in packs of 1 g (base activity).

Uses Gentamicin is an aminoglycoside antibiotic with broad-spectrum bactericidal activity. It is usually active against most strains of the following organisms: *Escherichia coli, Klebsiella spp., Proteus spp.* (indole positive and indole negative), *Pseudomonas aeruginosa,* staphylococci, *Enterobacter spp., Citrobacter spp* and *Providencia spp.*

Gentamicin injection and gentamicin paediatric injection are indicated in urinary-tract infections, chest infections, bacteraemia, septicaemia, severe neonatal infections, infections following burns, infected traumatic or surgical wounds and other systemic infections due to sensitive organisms.

Gentamicin intrathecal injection is indicated as a supplement to systemic therapy in bacterial meningitis, ventriculitis and other bacterial infections of the central nervous system.

Gentamicin sterile powder prepared as a sterile injection may be used for serious intra-ocular infections and prophylactically prior to intra-ocular surgery.

Dosage and administration *Gentamicin injection: Adults: Serious infections:* If renal function is not impaired, 5 mg/kg daily in divided doses at six- or eight-hourly intervals. The total daily dose may be subsequently increased or decreased as clinically indicated.

Systemic infections: If renal function is not impaired, 3–5 mg/kg/day in divided doses according to severity of infection, adjusting according to clinical response and body weight.

Urinary-tract infections: As 'systemic infections'. Or, if renal function is not impaired, 160 mg once daily may be used.

Children: Premature infants or full term neonates up to 2 weeks of age: 3 mg/kg 12-hourly.
2 weeks to 12 years: 2 mg/kg 8-hourly.

The elderly: There is some evidence that elderly patients may be more susceptible to aminoglycoside toxicity whether secondary to previous eighth nerve impairment or borderline renal dysfunction. Accordingly, therapy should be closely monitored by frequent determination of gentamicin serum levels, assessment of renal function and signs of ototoxicity.

Gentamicin intrathecal injection: Bacterial meningitis and ventriculitis: the starting dose of gentamicin intrathecal injection for both children and adults is 1 mg daily, intrathecally or intraventricularly, together with 1 mg/kg every eight hours intramuscularly. The MIC of the infecting organism in the CSF should be assessed and, if necessary, the intrathecal/intraventricular dose increased to 5 mg daily, whilst keeping the intramuscular dose at 1 mg/kg eight-hourly. Treatment should be continued for at least seven days but longer if necessary. Periodic serum and CSF gentamicin assays should be carried out to ensure that adequate antibiotic levels are maintained and that serum and CSF levels do not exceed 10 mg/l.

Renal impairment: Gentamicin is excreted by simple glomerular filtration and therefore reduced dosage is necessary where renal function is impaired. Nomograms are available for the calculation of dose, which depends on the patient's age, weight and renal function. The following table may be useful when treating adults.

The recommended dose and precautions for intramuscular and intravenous administration are identical. Gentamicin when given intravenously should be injected directly into a vein or into the drip set tubing over no less than three minutes. If administered by infusion, this should be over no longer than 20 minutes and in no greater volume of fluid than 100 ml.

Blood urea		*Creatinine clearance (GFR) (ml/min)*	*Dose and frequency of administration*
(mg/100 ml)	*(mmol/l)*		
<40	6–7	>70	80 mg* 8-hourly
40–100	6–17	30–70	80 mg* 12-hourly
100–200	17–34	10–30	80 mg* daily
>200	>34	5–10	80 mg* every 48 hours
Twice-weekly intermittent haemodialysis		<5	80 mg* after dialysis

*60 mg if body weight <60 kg. Frequency of dosage in hours may also be approximated as serum creatinine (mg%) × eight or in SI units, as serum creatinine (μmol/l) divided by 11. If these dosage guides are used peak serum levels must be measured. Peak levels of gentamicin occur approximately one hour after intramuscular injection and intravenous injection. Trough levels are measured just prior to the next injection. Assay of peak serum levels gives confirmation of adequacy of dosage and also serves to detect levels above 10 mg/l, at which the possibility of ototoxicity should be considered. One-hour concentrations of gentamicin should not exceed 10 mg/l (but should reach 4 mg/l), while the pre-dose trough concentration should be less than 2 mg/l.

Gentamicin sterile powder: Serious bacterial intra-ocular infections and prophylaxis prior to surgery: gentamicin sulphate equivalent to 20–40 mg base should be injected subconjunctivally once or twice daily until infection subsides. This may require continuation of therapy for two or more days. In the majority of cases concomitant intramuscular therapy is not required. This dosage regimen is suitable for children and adults.

Contra-indications, warnings, etc
Contra-indications: Hypersensitivity; myasthenia gravis. Pregnancy and lactation: There are no proven cases of intrauterine damage caused by gentamicin. However, in common with most drugs known to cross the placenta, usage in pregnancy should only be considered in life-threatening situations where the expected benefits outweigh possible risks. In the absence of gastro-intestinal inflammation, the amount of gentamicin ingested from the milk is unlikely to result in significant blood levels in breast-fed infants.

Warnings: Ototoxicity has been recorded following the use of gentamicin. Groups at special risk include patients with impaired renal function and possibly the elderly. Consequently, renal, auditory and vestibular functions should be monitored in these patients and serum levels determined so as to avoid peak concentrations above 10 mg/l and troughs above 2 mg/l. As there is some evidence that risk of both ototoxicity and nephrotoxicity is related to the level of total exposure, duration of therapy should be the shortest possible compatible with clinical recovery. In some patients with impaired renal function there has been a transient rise in blood-urea-nitrogen which has usually reverted to normal during or following cessation of therapy. It is important to adjust the frequency of dosage according to the degree of renal function (see table).

Interaction with other substances: Concurrent administration of gentamicin and other potentially ototoxic or nephrotoxic drugs should be avoided. Potent diuretics such as ethacrynic acid and frusemide are believed to enhance the risk of ototoxicity whilst amphotericin B, cis-platinum and cyclosporin are potential enhancers of nephrotoxicity. Any potential nephrotoxicity of cephalosporins, and in particular cephaloridine, may also be increased in the presence of gentamicin. Consequently, if this combination is used monitoring of kidney function is advised.

Neuromuscular blockade and respiratory paralysis have been reported from administration of aminoglycosides to patients who have received curare-type muscle relaxants during anaesthesia.

Overdosage: Haemodialysis and peritoneal dialysis will aid removal from blood but the former is probably more efficient. Calcium salts given intravenously have been used to counter the neuromuscular blockade caused by gentamicin.

Pharmaceutical precautions Gentamicin is a remarkably stable antibiotic and does not require refrigeration. Avoid freezing.

In general gentamicin injection should not be mixed. In particular the following are incompatible in mixed solution with gentamicin injection: penicillins, cephalosporins, erythromycin, Lipiphysan, heparins, sodium bicarbonate.† Dilution in the body will obviate the danger of physical and chemical incompatibility and enable gentamicin to be given concurrently with the drugs listed above either as a bolus injection into the drip tubing, with adequate flushing, or at separate sites. In the case of carbenicillin, administration should only be at a separate site.

Legal category POM.

Package quantities *Cidomycin Injection:* Packs of 25 × 2 ml vials or ampoules.
Cidomycin Injection Paediatric: Packs of 5 × 2 ml vials.
Cidomycin Intrathecal Injection: Packs of 5 × 1 ml ampoules.
Cidomycin Sterile Powder: Bottles containing 1 g.

Further information Cidomycin Adult and Paediatric Injection contains methylhydroxybenzoate, propylhydroxybenzoate and disodium edetate. Cidomycin Intrathecal Injection contains sodium chloride.

Product licence numbers

Cidomycin Injection	0109/5065R
Cidomycin Injection Paediatric	0109/5066R
Cidomycin Intrathecal Injection	0109/0057R
Cidomycin Sterile Powder	0109/5067R

CIDOMYCIN* OINTMENT AND CREAM

Presentation Available as a white cream which contains gentamicin sulphate in a water-miscible base and as a translucent ointment in White Soft Paraffin BP. Each gram of ointment or cream contains gentamicin sulphate equivalent to 3 mg gentamicin base.

Uses Cidomycin is a wide-spectrum antibiotic and the ointment and cream are recommended for the treatment of primary and secondary skin infections due to susceptible bacteria.

Primary infections: Impetigo contagiosa, superficial folliculitis, ecthyma, furunculosis, sycosis barbae and pyoderma gangrenosum.

Secondary infections: Infected, contact, seborrhoeic, and eczematoid dermatitis, pustular acne, infected burns and wounds, ulcers and paronychia.

Dosage and administration For adults, children and the elderly. A small amount of ointment or cream should be applied to the lesions three or four times daily or as prescribed. If necessary this may be covered with a dressing.

Contra-indications, warnings, etc Cidomycin is contra-indicated when there is a known hypersensitivity to any ingredient of the preparation including aminoglycosides.

Precautions: If irritation, sensitisation or super-infection develop, treatment with Cidomycin should be discontinued and appropriate therapy instituted. With application to large wounds, ototoxicity may be a hazard in children and the elderly and those with compromised renal function.

Overdosage: Haemodialysis or peritoneal dialysis will aid the removal of gentamicin from the blood.

† Carbon dioxide may be liberated on addition of the two solutions. Normally this will dissolve in the solution but under some circumstances small bubbles may form.

Pharmaceutical precautions Store cool. In order to preserve their antibacterial activity Cidomycin Cream and Ointment should not be diluted by the addition of excipient.

Legal category POM.

Package quantities *Cidomycin cream:* Tubes of 15 g and 30 g.
Cidomycin ointment: Tubes of 15 g and 30 g.

Further information Cidomycin cream contains Stearic Acid BPC, Propylene Glycol Monostearate, Isopropyl Myristate BP, Tween 40, Butyl Hydroxybenzoate BP, Methyl Hydroxybenzoate PhEur, Sorbitol USP, Propylene Glycol PhEur, Purified Water PhEur.

Product licence numbers

Cidomycin Cream	0109/5063R
Cidomycin Ointment	0109/5064R

CLAFORAN*

Presentation Claforan is available in vials containing 500 mg, 1 g or 2 g of cefotaxime as cefotaxime sodium.

Claforan is a white to slightly creamy powder which, when dissolved in Water for Injections BP forms a straw coloured solution suitable for intravenous or intramuscular administration. Variations in the intensity of colour of the freshly prepared solution do not indicate change in potency or safety.

Uses

Properties: Claforan is a broad spectrum bactericidal cephalosporin antibiotic. Claforan is exceptionally active in vitro against Gram-negative organisms sensitive or resistant to first or second generation cephalosporins. It is similar to other cephalosporins in activity against Gram-positive bacteria.

Indications: Claforan is indicated in the treatment of the following infections either before the infecting organism has been identified or when caused by bacteria of established sensitivity.

Septicaemia

Respiratory tract infections: acute and chronic bronchitis, bacterial pneumonia, infected bronchiectasis, lung abscess and post-operative chest infections.

Urinary tract infections: acute and chronic pyelonephritis, cystitis and asymptomatic bacteriuria.

Soft tissue infections: cellulitis, peritonitis and wound infections.

Bone and joint infections: osteomyelitis, septic arthritis.

Obstetric and gynaecological infections: pelvic inflammatory disease.

Gonorrhoea: particularly where penicillin has failed or is unsuitable.

Other bacterial infections: meningitis and other sensitive infections suitable for parenteral antibiotic therapy.

The administration of Claforan prophylactically may reduce the incidence of certain post-operative infections in patients undergoing surgical procedures that are classified as contaminated or potentially contaminated or in clean operations where infection would have serious effects.

Protection is best ensured by achieving adequate local tissue concentrations at the time contamination is likely to occur. Claforan should therefore be administered immediately prior to surgery and if necessary continued in the immediate post-operative period. Administration should usually be stopped within 24 hours since continuing use of any antibiotic in the majority of surgical procedures does not reduce the incidence of subsequent infections.

Bacteriology: The following organisms have shown in vitro sensitivity to Claforan.

Gram-positive: Staphylococci, including coagulase-positive, coagulase-negative and penicillinase-producing strains. Beta-haemolytic and other streptococci such as *Streptococcus mitis* (*viridans*). Many strains of enterococci, e.g. *Streptococcus faecalis*, are relatively resistant. *Streptococcus* (*Diplococcus*) *pneumoniae*. *Clostridium spp.*

Gram-negative:
Escherichia coli
Haemophilus influenzae including ampicillin-resistant strains
Klebsiella spp.
Proteus spp. both indole-positive and indole-negative
Enterobacter spp.
Neisseria spp. including β-lactamase producing strains of *N. gonorrhoeae*
Salmonella spp. including *Salm. typhi*
Shigella spp.
Providencia spp.
Serratia spp.
Citrobacter spp.

Claforan has frequently exhibited useful in vitro activity against *Pseudomonas* and *Bacteroides* species although some strains of *Bacteroides fragilis* are resistant.

There is in vitro evidence of synergy between Claforan and aminoglycoside antibiotics such as gentamicin against some species of Gram-negative bacteria including some strains of *Pseudomonas*. No in vitro antagonism has been noted. In severe infections caused by *Pseudomonas spp.* the concurrent use of an aminoglycoside antibiotic may be indicated.

Dosage and administration Claforan may be administered intravenously or intramuscularly. Dosage, route and frequency of administration should be determined by severity of infection, sensitivity of causative organisms and condition of the patient. Therapy may be started before the result of sensitivity tests are known.

Adults: The usual dose in adults is 2 to 6 g daily, depending upon the severity of the infection. However, dosage may be varied according to the severity of the infection, sensitivity of causative organisms and condition of the patient. For infections caused by sensitive *Pseudomonas spp.* daily doses of more than 6 g are usually required.

Guidelines for dosage: Moderate to serious infections 1 g every 8 hours. Life threatening infections 2 g every 8 hours.

In exceptional circumstances of life threatening infections caused by an organism less sensitive to cefotaxime, e.g. pseudomonas, up to 12 g per day (in divided dosages) may occasionally be of advantage.

Mild to moderate or uncomplicated infections such as UTI 1 g every 12 hours. Gonorrhoea 1 g single dose.

Children: The usual dosage is 100–150 mg/kg/day in 2 to 4 divided doses. In very severe infections up to 200 mg/kg/day, in divided doses, may be required.

Neonates: The recommended dosage is 50 mg/kg/day in 2 to 4 divided doses. In severe infections, 150–200 mg/kg/day, in divided doses, have been given.

Dosage in renal impairment: Because of extra-renal elimination, it is only necessary to reduce the dosage of Claforan in severe renal failure (GFR <5 ml/min). After an initial loading dose of 1 g, the daily dose should be halved without change in the frequency of dosing, e.g. 1 g 12 hourly becomes 0.5 g 12 hourly, 1 g 8 hourly becomes 0.5 g 8 hourly, 2 g 8 hourly becomes 1 g 8 hourly, etc. As in all other patients, dosage may require further adjustment according to the course of the infection and the general condition of the patient.

Intravenous and intramuscular administration: Dissolve Claforan in Water for Injections BP as shown. Shake well until dissolved and then withdraw the entire contents of the vial into the syringe and use immediately.

Vial size	*Volume of Water for Injections to be added*	*Approx. available volume*
500 mg	*2 ml*	*2.2 ml*
1 g	*4 ml*	*4.5 ml*
2 g	*10 ml*	*11.2 ml*

Intravenous infusion: Claforan may be administerd by intravenous infusion. 1–2 g are dissolved in 40–100 ml of Water for Injections BP or in the infusion fluids listed under 'Pharmaceutical precautions'. The prepared infusion should be administered over 20–60 minutes.

Elderly: No specific recommendations for the elderly.

Contra-indications, warnings, etc
Contra-indications: Known allergy to cephalosporins.

Precautions: Cephalosporin antibiotics may usually be given safely to patients who are hypersensitive to penicillins, although cross reactions have been reported. Special care is indicated in patients who have had an anaphylactic response to penicillin.

Patients with severe renal dysfunction – see 'Dosage and administration'.

As with all cephalosporins, pseudomembranous colitis may rarely occur during treatment. If this occurs, the drug should be stopped and specific treatment instituted.

Interactions: Cephalosporin antibiotics at high dosage should be given with caution to patients receiving aminoglycoside antibiotics or potent diuretics such as frusemide as these combinations are thought to have an adverse effect on renal function. However, at the recommended doses, enhancement of nephrotoxicity is unlikely to be a problem with Claforan.

Interference with laboratory tests: A false-positive reaction to glucose may occur with reducing substances but not with the use of specific glucose oxidase methods.

Pregnancy: Although studies in animals have not shown an adverse effect on the developing foetus, the safety of Claforan in human pregnancy has not been established. Consequently, Claforan should not be administered during pregnancy especially during the first trimester, without carefully weighing the expected benefits against the possible risks.

Lactation: Claforan is excreted in the milk.

Side effects: Adverse reactions to Claforan have occurred relatively infrequently and have generally been mild and transient. Effects reported include diarrhoea, candidiasis, rashes, fever, eosinophilia, leukopenia and transient rises in liver transaminase and/or alkaline phosphatase.

As with other beta-lactam antibiotics, granulocytopenia and more rarely agranulocytosis may develop during treatment with cefotaxime, particularly if given over long periods. A few cases of eosinophilia and neutropenia have been observed, reversible when treatment is ceased. Rare cases of haemolytic anaemia have been reported. For cases of treatment lasting longer than 10 days, blood count should, therefore, be monitored.

Transient pain may be experienced at the site of injection. This is more likely to occur with higher doses. Occasionally, phlebitis has been reported in patients receiving intravenous Claforan. However, this has rarely been a cause for discontinuation of treatment.

Overdosage: Serum levels of Claforan may be reduced by peritoneal dialysis or haemodialysis.

Pharmaceutical precautions The dry powder in vials should be stored away from heat and protected from light. Whilst it is preferable to use only freshly prepared solutions for both intravenous and intramuscular injection, Claforan is compatible with several commonly used intravenous infusion fluids and will retain satisfactory potency for up to 24 hours refrigerated in the following:

Water for Injections BP
Sodium Chloride Injection BP
5% Dextrose Injection BP
Dextrose and Sodium Chloride Injection BP
Compound Sodium Lactate Injection BP (Ringer-Lactate Injection).

After 24 hours any unused solution should be discarded.

Claforan is also compatible with 1% lignocaine. Freshly prepared solutions should be used.

Some increase in colour of prepared solutions may occur on storage. However, provided the recommended storage conditions are observed, this does not indicate change in potency or safety.

Legal category POM.

Package quantities Individually packed vials containing 500 mg or 1 g cefotaxime as cefotaxime sodium (for use by intramuscular or intravenous injection) in packs of 10.

Individually packed vials containing 2 g cefotaxime as cefotaxime sodium (for intravenous use only) in packs of 10.

Further information Each gram of Claforan contains approximately 48 mg (2.09 mmol) of sodium. Claforan has been used with other beta-lactam antibiotics such as carbenicillin in the treatment of neutropenic patients. Claforan may also be administered separately with metronidazole in the treatment of mixed infections caused by anaerobic and aerobic organisms.

Claforan usually passes the blood-brain barrier in levels above the MIC of common sensitive pathogens when the meninges are inflamed.

The laboratory abbreviation for cefotaxime is CTX.

Product licence number 0109/0074

CLORHEXITULLE*

Presentation Clorhexitulle is a sterile, open-mesh gauze dressing impregnated with White Soft Parrafin BP containing 0.5% micronised Chlorhexidine Acetate BP.

Each dressing is enclosed between two pieces of vegetable parchment and presented in individual heat sealed sachets to maintain sterility until opened.

Uses Properties: Chlorhexidine acetate is a potent antiseptic which is bactericidal to a wide range of Gram-positive and Gram-Negative organisms. It also has some activity against yeasts such as Candida and other fungi.

Clorhexitulle is therefore a valuable agent for preventing and for controlling existing infection in a wide range of surgical, traumatic and ulcerative conditions: varicose (gravitational), diabetic and tropical ulcer; lacerations, abrasions, bites, puncture wounds, crush injuries; burns and scalds; pressure sores including bedsores; skin grafts (donor and recipient sites), avulsion of finger and/or toe nails, circumcision, suture lines; secondarily infected skin conditions (e.g. eczema, herpes zoster, colostomies, ileostomies, tracheostomies, incised abscesses, incised paronychia).

Dosage and administration A single layer of Clorhexitulle should be applied to the cleansed lesion, and changed as necessary according to the amount of exudation.

Clorhexitulle is suitable for use on adults, children and infants.

Contra-indications, warnings, etc
Contra-indications: Known allergy to chlorhexidine.
Precautions: Avoid Clorhexitulle coming into contact with the eyes. Clorhexitulle should not be applied to more than 40% of the body surface in adults. In infants, because of the difference in the ratio of surface area to body weight, the maximal area covered should not exceed 20%.

Side-effects: Although no adverse reactions to Clorhexitulle have been recorded, skin sensitivity to chlorhexidine has occasionally been reported.

Use in pregnancy and lactation: The safety of using Chlorhexitulle during pregnancy and lactation has not been established. Consequently, Clorhexitulle should not be used during the first trimester of pregnancy without weighing the expected benefits against the possible risks.

Incompatibilities: Chlorhexidine is incompatible with soaps and other anionic detergents. Chlorhexidine acetate is incompatible with potassium iodide.

Pharmaceutical precautions Clorhexitulle should be stored flat in a cool place.

Legal category P.

Package quantities Cartons of 10 sachets, each sterile sealed sachet containing one dressing (approximately 10 cm × 10 cm).

Further information Nil.

Product licence number 0109/0085.

DIMETRIOSE* ▼

Presentation Size No 4 White, hard gelatin capsules containing 2.5 mg gestrinone.

Uses Gestrinone is indicated for the treatment of endometriosis.

Dosage and administration Gestrinone is for oral administration to adult females only.

The dose is one capsule twice a week.

To ensure that pregnant patients are not treated, it is essential that *the first dose is taken on the first day of the menstrual cycle.*

The second dose should be taken three days later.

Thereafter, gestrinone capsules should be taken on the same two days of the week (preferably at the same time) every week for the duration of the treatment, which will normally be six months.

Should one dose be missed, then a capsule should be taken as soon as possible and the original sequence maintained.

Should two or more doses be missed, treatment should be discontinued and therapy re-started on the first day of the new cycle, following a negative pregnancy test and according to the usual dosage schedule.

Children and elderly adults: Treatment with gestrinone is not appropriate.

Contra-indications, warnings, etc
Contra-indications: Pregnancy. Lactation. Severe cardiac, renal or hepatic insufficiency. Metabolic and/or vascular disorders during previous oestrogen and/or progestogen therapy.

Use in pregnancy and lactation: Gestrinone is specifically contra-indicated in pregnancy and lactation. Administration should be discontinued if a patient is found to be pregnant as animal studies have shown embryotoxicity in some species, albeit at doses well in excess of those used clinically.

Precautions: The possibility of pregnancy must be ruled out before starting treatment, especially in the case of pre-existing amenorrhoea.

Gestrinone, at the recommended dose, may inhibit ovulation in some women but, pregnancies can occur with this treatment and gestrinone must *NOT* be relied on for contraception.

As concurrent administration of oral contraceptives may modify the action of gestrinone, it is, therefore, essential that barrier methods are used throughout treatment as the use of gestrinone is totally contra-indicated in pregnancy.

Because gestrinone may occasionally cause some degree of fluid retention patients with cardiac or renal dysfunction require close monitoring.

Monitor ALAT, ASAT, cholesterol fractions in hyperlipidaemic subjects and blood sugar levels in diabetics.

Gestrinone will cause a decrease in the concentration of thyroid-binding globulin. Hence there will be a decrease in serum total thyroxine levels. This is without clinical significance as free thyroxine levels remain within the reference range as do thyroid-stimulating hormone levels.

Drug interactions: Concomitant administration of anti-epileptic drugs or Rifampicin may result in accelerated metabolism of gestrinone.

Side effects: Spotting has been reported in some patients both during the first few weeks and thoroughout treatment.

Acne, oily skin, fluid retention, weight gain, hirsutism, voice change and other androgen-type effects have been reported by some patients.

Other unwanted reactions recorded during gestrinone therapy include transient increases in liver transaminases, headache, gastro-intestinal disturbances, change in libido, hot flushes, decrease in breast size, nervousness and depression, cramp and change in appetite.

Overdosage: Acute toxicity studies in animals indicate that serious reactions are unlikely as an immediate result of a single excessive dose.

In the case of acute overdosage, the drug should be removed by emesis or gastric lavage if ingestion is recent and the patient kept under observation in case of delayed reaction.

Pharmaceutical precautions Protect from light.

Legal category POM.

Package quantities 8 capsules.

Further information Gestrinone, a synthetic steroid hormone, is an antiprogestin; it is not an oestrogen-progestogen combination.

It is believed to act by reducing gonadotrophin and ovarian steriod production, by increasing free-androgen levels and by a direct antagonistic action on endometrioid tissues.

Product licence number 0109/0207.

EUGLUCON*

Presentation Euglucon is available as:

1. White, circular, biconvex tablets, 6 mm in diameter, marked EU on one side and 2.5 on the reverse. Each tablet contains 2.5 mg Glibenclamide BP.
2. White, oblong 10 mm × 5 mm tablets containing 5 mg Glibenclamide BP. Each side has a breakline and is inscribed BM/EU, such that when a tablet is broken into half, one side is marked BM, and the other EU.

Uses Euglucon is an oral hypoglycaemic agent of the sulphonylurea type.

Euglucon is indicated for the treatment of maturity-onset diabetes which is not adequately controlled by dietary measures alone.

Dosage and administration Euglucon should be taken with or immediately after food. The total daily dosage is preferably given as a single dose at breakfast or with the first main meal, but due consideration should be given to the patient's meal habits and daily activity when apportioning dosage.

1. *New Diabetics*: In maturity-onset diabetes of mild to moderate severity, treatment should be started with 5 mg daily or 2.5 mg in debilitated or elderly patients. If this dosage is not sufficient for proper control it should be increased by 2.5 mg at intervals of one week, or as directed by the clinician. The total daily dose of Euglucon rarely exceeds 15 mg. Increasing dosage beyond this level is unlikely to produce further response.

2. *Transfer from other sulphonylureas:* Transfer to Euglucon can usually be carried out without any break in therapy.

Euglucon treatment should be started with 5 mg daily and, if necessary, adjusted in steps of 2.5 or 5 mg. A dose of 5 mg Euglucon is approximately equivalent to 1000 mg tolbutamide, 250 mg chlorpropamide or 5 mg glipizide.

3. *Changeover from biguanides:* Euglucon treatment should be started with 2.5 mg of Euglucon and the biguanide withdrawn. Dosage should then be adjusted by increments of 2.5 mg to achieve control.

Combination with biguanides: If adequate control is not possible with diet and 15 mg of Euglucon, control can often be re-established by a combination of Euglucon and a biguanide derivative.

4. *Euglucon and insulin:* While it is appreciated that most patients who are on insulin therapy will continue to need it, there may be a few patients, particularly those on low daily dosages, who will remain stabilised if transferred to Euglucon.

No dosage recommendations can be made for the administration of Euglucon to children.

Contra-indications, warnings, etc Euglucon is contra-indicated in:

1. The treatment of juvenile or unstable diabetes.
2. Patients who have had serious metabolic decompensation with ketosis and, in particular, diabetic precoma and coma.
3. Serious impairment of renal, hepatic, thyroid or adrenocortical function.
4. Pregnancy. After delivery, Euglucon therapy can be started or resumed.
5. Hypersensitivity to glibenclamide.

Warnings: The hypoglycaemic action of oral antidiabetic agents including Euglucon may be enhanced by sulphonamides, salicylates, phenylbutazone, coumarin derivatives, beta-blocking agents, monoamine-oxidase inhibitors, cyclophosphamide, bezafibrate, clofibrate, fenfluramine, tetracyclines, sulphinpyrazone and chloramphenicol. Conversely, thiazide diuretics, frusemide, ethacrynic acid, oral contraceptives containing oestrogens/gestagens, phenothiazine derivatives, nicotinic acid (high dosage), sympathomimetics, thyroid hormones and corticosteroids may diminish hypoglycaemic activity. Hypoglycaemic activity may also be affected by tuberculostatics.

Treatment with sulphonylureas has been associated with occasional disturbance of liver function and cholestatic jaundice. If hepatitis or cholestatic clinical jaundice occurs, glibenclamide should be discontinued.

No adverse effect on the ability to drive or use machines is expected in well-controlled patients, but patients should be warned about the possible adverse effects of hypoglycaemia.

In patients suffering from intercurrent infections or trauma, the dosage of Euglucon may need to be increased. If such complications are severe, diabetic control may be lost necessitating withdrawal of Euglucon and maintenance of diabetic control with insulin. Euglucon should be re-introduced when the patient has recovered from the infection or trauma.

Pregnancy: There is no information on the use of Euglucon in human pregnancy but it has been in wide, general use for many years without apparent ill consequence. Animal studies have shown no hazard.

Nursing mothers: It has not been established whether glibencamide is secreted in human milk. Other sulphonylureas have been found in milk. There is no evidence that glibenclamide differs from the group in this respect.

Side-effects: Euglucon is well tolerated and side-effects serious enough to necessitate withdrawal are uncommon. Gastro-intestinal symptoms (nausea, anorexia and diarrhoea) are uncommon and allergic skin reactions are seldom encountered.

Reversible leucopenia and thrombocytopenia have been reported but are rare. Transient changes in liver enzyme concentrations and liver function tests during treatment with glibenclamide have been reported, but these are not known to be directly attributable to the product. As with other agents, hypoglycaemia can occur with Euglucon, but is not usually prolonged and responds to appropriate therapeutic measures.

Effects of overdosage and their treatment: If a hypoglycaemic reaction should occur, the conscious patient may be treated with dextrose or 3–4 lumps of table sugar with water. This may be repeated, if necessary, in 15 minutes.

If the patient is comatose, sucrose or dextrose may be given by stomach tube or dextrose given intravenously. Glucagon may be administered in a dose of 1 mg subcutaneously or intramuscularly to produce consciousness.

Pharmaceutical precautions No special storage requirements.

Legal category POM.

Package quantities 5 mg tablets: OP blister packs of 28. 2.5 mg tablets: OP blister packs of 28.

Further information Absorption studies in healthy

human volunteers using labelled glibenclamide formulated as Euglucon tablets showed a mean absorption of 84±9%.

Excretion was approximately 50% in the urine and 50% in the faeces. Absorbed glibenclamide was completely metabolised and the three isolated metabolites in the concentrations found had no significant hypoglycaemic activity.

Product licence numbers

Euglucon 2.5 mg Tablets	0109/0073
Euglucon 5 mg Tablets	0109/5023R

HYDROTALCITE

Presentation Hydrotalcite (formerly Altacite*) is available as Hydrotalcite Tablets 500 mg: white, buttermint-flavoured tablets marked 'altacite' and 'ROUSSEL', and as Hydrotalcite Suspension 500 mg/5 ml: an aqueous suspension, slightly off-white, viscous and flavoured with peppermint.

Each tablet and each 5 ml of suspension contains 500 mg of hydrotalcite.

Uses Antacid, buffering in the optimum range of pH 3–5 for over two hours.

Hydrotalcite is indicated for symptomatic relief in the following conditions: peptic ulceration; dyspepsia; hyperacidity; gastritis; heartburn, especially when associated with reflux oesophagitis or hiatus hernia, and heartburn in pregnancy.

Dosage and administration *Adults:* 2 tablets or 10 ml of suspension between meals and at bedtime or as directed by a physician.

Elderly: No specific recommendations in the elderly.

Children (6–12 years): Half the adult dose.

The tablets should be chewed or crushed before swallowing.

Contra-indications, warnings, etc There are no contra-indications to hydrotalcite but it is wise to avoid any drug, including antacids, during the first trimester of pregnancy. As with other compounds containing aluminium or magnesium, hydrotalcite may reduce intestinal absorption of tetracycline. Side-effects are uncommon. Diarrhoea and vomiting have been reported but have ceased on withdrawal of therapy.

Pharmaceutical precautions Store in a cool place.

Legal category P.

Package quantities *Hydrotalcite Tablets* are blister packed and presented in OP cartons of 56 tablets.

Hydrotalcite Suspension: Polypropylene bottle containing 500 ml.

Further information There is no evidence of absorption of hydrotalcite in man. Investigations in healthy human volunteers have shown no elevation of serum aluminium or magnesium levels on administering hydrotalcite at therapeutic dosage for a continuous period of 28 days.

The sodium content of hydrotalcite is 0.22 mmol per tablet or 5 ml of suspension.

Product licence numbers

Hydrotalcite Tablets	0109/0040
Hydrotalcite Suspension	0109/0041R

LOPRAZOLAM TABLETS 1 mg

Presentation Loprazolam tablets 1 mg. Yellow, circular tablets, 7 mm in diameter, marked Dormonoct* 1 on one face with breakline on reverse. Each tablet contains loprazolam mesylate equivalent to 1 mg loprazolam.

Uses Loprazolam is indicated for the short-term treatment of insomnia including difficulty in falling asleep and/or frequent nocturnal awakenings. Benzodiazepines should be used to treat insomnia only when it is severe, disabling or subjecting the individual to extreme distress. An underlying cause for insomnia should be sought before deciding upon the use of benzodiazepines for symptomatic relief.

Dosage and administration
Adults: The recommended dose is 1 mg at bedtime. This may be increased to 1.5 mg or 2 mg if necessary.

Elderly: Dosage in the elderly should be limited to 1 mg at bedtime.

Frail, debilitated or aged patients: A starting dose of a half tablet may be appropriate. Dosage should not exceed 1 mg.

Treatment should if possible be intermittent.
The lowest dose to control symptoms should be used.
Treatment should not normally be continued beyond 4 weeks.
Long-term chronic use is not recommended.
Treatment should always be tapered off gradually.
Patients who have taken benzodiazepines for a long time may require a longer period during which doses are reduced.

Children: There is insufficient evidence to recommend the use of Loprazolam in children.

Contra-indications, warnings, etc
Contra-indications: Sensitivity to benzodiazepines, acute pulmonary insufficiency, myasthenia gravis, phobic or obsessional states, monotherapy in depression or anxiety associated with depression and chronic psychosis.

Pregnancy and lactation: The use of loprazolam during pregnancy should be avoided. The possibility of loprazolam being excreted in the milk should also be considered in nursing mothers.

Precautions: As with all CNS-active drugs, patients should be warned of the possible hazard of driving or operating machinery, and that loprazolam may be potentiated by alcohol or other drugs acting on the CNS. Disinhibiting effects may be manifested in various ways. Suicide may be precipitated in patients who are depressed and aggressive behaviour towards self and others may be precipitated. Extreme caution should therefore be used in prescribing benzodiazepines in patients with personality disorders.

In general, the dependence potential of benzodiazepines is low but this increases when high doses are attained, especially when given over long periods, and particularly in patients with a history of alcoholism or drug abuse. However, withdrawal symptoms occur even with normal therapeutic doses given for short periods of time. Withdrawal from benzodiazepines may be associated with physiological and psychological symptoms of withdrawal including depression. Patients receiving benzodiazepines should be regularly monitored.

Loprazolam should be used with caution in chronic pulmonary insufficiency, cerebrovascular disease and chronic renal or hepatic impairment.

Side-effects: In general, loprazolam is very well tolerated. However, the common side effects of benzodiazepines, including headaches, nausea, drowsiness, blurring of vision, dizziness and ataxia may occur on the following day, particularly in unusually sensitive patients or when dosage has been excessive.

Rare behavioural adverse effects of benzodiazepines include paradoxical aggressive outbursts, excitement, confusion, and the uncovering of depression with suicidal tendencies. Even more rare side effects reported with some benzodiazepines have been hypotension, gastrointestinal and visual disturbances, skin rashes, urinary retention, changes in libido, blood dyscrasias and jaundice. Amnesia may occur. In cases of loss or bereavement psychological adjustment may be inhibited by benzodiazepines.

Overdosage: As with other benzodiazepines, overdosage does not usually present a threat to life. Treatment is symptomatic and gastric lavage may be of use if performed shortly after ingestion.

Pharmaceutical precautions Store in a dry place, protected from light.

Legal category CD (Sch 4) POM.

Package quantities Loprazolam Tablets 1 mg are blister packed and presented in OP cartons of 28.

Further information Loprazolam is an intermediate acting benzodiazepine. There are no long-lived sedative metabolites. Therefore there is a reduced likelihood of the occurrence of daytime drowsiness or impairment in the performance of skilled tasks, associated with the long acting products. Equally, there is less likelihood of rebound insomnia, which may occur with the ultra-short acting benzodiazepines.

Loprazolam was previously known as Dormonoct.*

Product licence number 0109/0080.

MOLIPAXIN*

Presentation Molipaxin (trazodone hydrochloride) is available as: Molipaxin 50 mg Size No. 3, opaque violet/green capsules printed R365B and . Each capsule contains 50 mg trazodone hydrochloride.

Molipaxin 100 mg. Size No. 2, opaque violet/fawn capsules printed R365C and . Each capsule contains 100 mg trazodone hydrochloride.

Molipaxin 150 mg, salmon-pink, film coated, round biconvex tablets, approximately 11 mm in diameter with a white core. The tablet is embossed with 'Molipaxin' and '150' on one face and a breakline on the other face.

Molipaxin Liquid for oral use is a clear colourless solution with an orange odour and taste. Each 5 ml contains 50 mg trazodone hydrochloride.

Uses *Properties:* Molipaxin is a potent antidepressant. It also has anxiety reducing activity. Molipaxin is a triazolopyridine derivative chemically unrelated to known tricyclic, tetracyclic and other antidepressant agents. It has negligible effect on noradrenaline re-uptake mechanisms. Whilst the mode of action of Molipaxin is not known precisely, its antidepressant activity may concern noradrenergic potentiation by mechanisms other than uptake blockade. A central anti-serotonin effect may account for the drug's anxiety reducing properties.

Indications: Relief of symptoms in all types of depression including depression accompanied by anxiety. Symptoms of depression likely to respond in the first week of treatment include depressed mood, insomnia, anxiety, somatic symptoms and hypochondriasis.

Dosage and administration The starting dose of Molipaxin is initially 150 mg/day taken in divided doses after food or as a single dose on retiring. This may be increased to 300 mg per day, the major proportion of which is preferably taken on retiring. In hospitalised patients, dosage may be further increased to 600 mg/day in divided doses.

Elderly: Dosage in the elderly or frail should be started at 100 mg/day in divided doses or as a single night time dose. This may be increased, under supervision, according to efficacy and tolerance. Doses above 300 mg/day are unlikely to be required.

In conformity with current psychiatric opinion, it is suggested that Molipaxin be continued for several months after remission. Cessation of Molipaxin treatment should be gradual.

Children: There are insufficient data to recommend the use of Molipaxin in children.

Contra-indications, warnings, etc
Contra-indications: Known sensitivity to trazodone.

Precautions: As with all other drugs acting on the central nervous system, patients should be warned against the risks of handling machinery and driving.

Although no untoward effects have been reported, Molipaxin may enhance the effects of muscle relaxants and volatile anaesthetics. Similar considerations apply to combined administration with sedative and antidepressant drugs, including alcohol. Molipaxin has been well tolerated in depressed schizophrenic patients receiving standard phenothiazine therapy and also in depressed parkinsonian patients receiving therapy with levodopa.

Possible interactions with monoamine oxidase inhibitors have occasionally been reported, therefore, concurrent administration with MAOIs is not recommended. Giving Molipaxin within two weeks of stopping MAOIs or giving MAOIs within one week of stopping Molipaxin are not recommended.

Since Molipaxin is only a very weak inhibitor of noradrenaline re-uptake and does not modify the blood pressure response to tyramine, interference with the hypotensive action of guanethidine-like compounds is unlikely. However, studies in laboratory animals suggest that Molipaxin may inhibit most of the acute actions of clonidine. In the case of other types of antihypertensive drug, although no clinical interactions have been reported, the possibility of potentiation should be considered.

Current clinical experience suggests that Molipaxin does not cause seizures. Nevertheless, care should be exercised when administering Molipaxin to patients suffering from epilepsy, avoiding in particular, abrupt increases or decreases in dosage.

Molipaxin should be administered with care in patients with severe hepatic or renal disease.

Pregnancy and lactation: Although studies in animals have not shown any direct teratogenic effect, the safety of Molipaxin in human pregnancy has not been established. On basic principles, therefore, its use during the first trimester should be avoided. The possibility of Molipaxin being excreted in the milk should also be considered in nursing mothers.

Side-effects: Molipaxin is a sedative antidepressant and drowsiness, sometimes experienced during the first days of treatment, usually disappears on continued therapy.

Anticholinergic-like symptoms do occur but the incidence is similar to placebo.

The following symptoms, most of which are commonly reported in cases of untreated depression, have also been recorded in small numbers of patients receiving Molipaxin therapy: dizziness, headache, nausea and vomiting, weakness, decreased alertness, weight loss, tremor, dry mouth, bradycardia, tachycardia, postural hypotension, oedema, constipation, diarrhoea, blurred vision, restlessness, confusional states, insomnia and skin rash.

As with other drugs with alpha-adrenolytic activity, Molipaxin has been associated with priapism. At the date of issue, there have been a few reports in the UK. However, reports from the United States suggest an association between trazodone and priapism which has on occasion required surgical intervention or led to permanent sexual dysfunction. Priapism should be dealt with as a urological emergency and patients developing this suspected adverse reaction should cease Molipaxin therapy immediately.

Overdosage: There is no specific antidote to Molipaxin. The stomach should be emptied as quickly as possible. Treatment should be symptomatic and supportive in the case of hypotension and excessive sedation.

Pharmaceutical precautions *Molipaxin Capsules:* Store in a dry place.
Molipaxin Tablets: Store in a dry place.
Molipaxin Liquid: Protect from light and store at room temperature. N.B. Molipaxin Liquid is primarily intended for in-patient use. If dispensed for out-patient use a standard childproof cap should be fitted.

Legal category POM.

Package quantities *Molipaxin 50 mg capsules* are blister packed and presented in OP cartons of 84.

Molipaxin 100 mg capsules are blister packed and presented in OP cartons of 56.

Molipaxin 150 mg tablets are blister packed and presented in OP cartons of 28.

Molipaxin Liquid: Bottle of 150 ml oral liquid.

Further information In contrast to the tricyclic antidepressants, Molipaxin is devoid of anticholinergic activity. Consequently, troublesome side effects such as dry mouth, blurred vision and urinary hesitancy have occurred no more frequently than in patients receiving placebo therapy. This may be of importance when treating depressed patients who are at risk from conditions such as glaucoma, urinary retention and prostatic hypertrophy.

Studies in animals have shown that Molipaxin is less cardiotoxic than the tricyclic antidepressants and clinical studies suggest that the drug may be less likely to cause cardiac arrhythmias in man.

Molipaxin has had no effect on arterial blood pCO_2 or pO_2 levels in patients with severe respiratory insufficiency due to chronic bronchial or pulmonary disease.

Product licence numbers

Molipaxin Capsules 50 mg	0109/0045
Molipaxin Capsules 100 mg	0109/0046
Molipaxin Tablets 150 mg	0109/0133
Molipaxin Liquid 50 mg/5 ml	0109/0117

PROCTOSEDYL*

Presentation Proctosedyl is available as smooth, off-white suppositories and as an odourless, yellowish-white, translucent, greasy ointment. Each suppository or gram of ointment contains the following active ingredients:

Cinchocaine Hydrochloride BP	5 mg
Hydrocortisone BP	5 mg

Uses The local anaesthetic cinchocaine relieves pain and relaxes sphincteric spasm. Pruritus and inflammation are relieved by hydrocortisone, which also decreases serous discharge.

Proctosedyl is therefore useful for the short term relief (not more than 7 days) of pain, irritation and pruritus associated with haemorrhoids, pruritus ani.

Dosage and administration A suppository is inserted morning and evening, and after each stool.

Apply the ointment in small quantity with the finger, on the painful or pruritic area, morning and evening and after each stool. For deep application attach cannula to tube, insert to full extent and squeeze tube gently from lower end whilst withdrawing.

The ointment may be used separately or concurrently with the suppositories.

Contra-indications, warnings, etc Known hypersensitivity to any of the ingredients.

In pregnant animals, administration of corticosteroids can cause abnormalities of foetal development. The relevance of this finding to human beings has not been established. However, topical steroids should not be used extensively in pregnancy, i.e. in large amounts or for long periods.

As with all preparations containing topical corticosteroids, the possibility of systemic absorption should be considered. In particular, long-term continuous therapy should be avoided in infants. Adrenal suppression can occur even without occlusion.

Pharmaceutical precautions Ointment: Store cool. Suppositories: Store below 25°C.

Legal category POM.

Package quantities *Proctosedyl Suppositories:* Packs of 12.
Proctosedyl Ointment: Tubes of 30 g (with cannula).

Further information Proctosedyl ointment contains White Soft Paraffin BP, Liquid Paraffin BP and Wool Fat BP. Proctosedyl suppositories contain Suppocire AM.

Product licence numbers

Proctosedyl ointment	0109/5038R
Proctosedyl Suppositories	0109/5039R

RYTHMODAN* CAPSULES
RYTHMODAN* RETARD TABLETS
RYTHMODAN* INJECTION

Presentation
Oral.

Rythmodan Capsules: Capsules with opaque green cap and opaque beige body with 'RY' and 'RL' printed in black, containing 100 mg of disopyramide base.

Capsules with opaque white cap and body with 'RY' and '150' printed in black, containing 150 mg disopyramide base.

Rythmodan Retard Tablets: White, circular biconvex tablets, 12 mm in diameter, film-coated with a break line. Tablets are marked 'RY' and 'R' on one side and on the reverse. Each tablet contains disopyramide phosphate equivalent to 250 mg disopyramide base in a sustained release formulation.

Intravenous Injection.

Rythmodan Injection: Ampoules for intravenous use only. 5 ml ampoules containing disopyramide phosphate equivalent to 50 mg disopyramide base in solution.

Uses *Properties:* Rythmodan is able to prevent and control a wide variety of cardiac arrhythmias, probably by slowing conduction in the His-Purkinje system and by increasing the effective refractory period of the atria and ventricles.

Indications: Oral Rythmodan is indicated in:

1. Maintenance of normal rhythm following conversion by Rythmodan Injection, other parenteral drugs or electroconversion.
2. Prevention of arrhythmias after myocardial infarction.
3. Treatment of persistent ventricular and atrial extrasystoles, paroxysmal supraventricular tachycardia, Wolff-Parkinson-White syndrome.
4. Suppression of arrhythmias during surgical procedures.
5. Control of arrhythmias following the use of digitalis or similar glycosides.

Rythmodan Injection is intended for intravenous use only and is indicated in the following conditions:

1. Conversion of ventricular and supraventricular arrhythmias after myocardial infarction, including those not responding to lignocaine or other i.v. treatment.
2. Control of ventricular and atrial extrasystoles, supraventricular tachycardia, and Wolff-Parkinson-White syndrome.
3. Control of arrhythmias following digitalis or similar glycosides when Rythmodan cannot be administered orally.

Dosage and administration
Oral

Rythmodan Capsules: The recommended daily dosage in adults is 300–800 mg in divided doses adjusted according to the response of the patient.

Rythmodan Retard Tablets: The recommended dose for stabilised patients or those receiving Rythmodan for the first time is 1 to 1½ tablets (250–375 mg) twice daily. Patients being transferred from intravenous therapy with Rythmodan should be stabilised on standard Rythmodan capsules for the first 24 hours (see below). Tablets should be swallowed and not crushed or chewed.

Intravenous Injection

Rythmodan Injection: The recommended dosage can be given by two different regimes.

1. An initial direct intravenous injection of 2 mg/kg (but not exceeding 150 mg (15 ml) irrespective of body weight) should be given SLOWLY OVER NOT LESS THAN FIVE MINUTES, i.e. the rate of injection must not exceed 30 mg (3 ml) per minute in order to reduce or avoid unwanted haemodynamic effects. If conversion occurs during this time the injection should be stopped. If the arrhythmia is to respond to Rythmodan it will usually do so within 10–15 minutes after completion of the injection.

Transfer to oral maintenance therapy is accomplished by giving 200 mg orally, immediately on cessation of intravenous administration, followed by 200 mg every 8 hours for 24 hours. Most patients may be maintained subsequently on a daily dosage of 500–750 mg of Rythmodan, preferably administered as 1 to 1½ Rythmodan Retard tablets (250–375 mg) twice daily. Where the need for lower dosage outweighs the convenience of twice daily administration, appropriate doses of conventional capsules (100 or 150 mg) may be administered.

If conversion is achieved by intravenous Rythmodan but the arrhythmia subsequently recurs, a further slow direct intravenous injection over not less than five minutes may be administered cautiously and preferably under ECG control. The total administration by the intravenous route should not exceed 4 mg/kg (maximum 300 mg) in the first hour, nor should the combined administration by the intravenous and oral routes exceed 800 mg in 24 hours.

2. An initial direct intravenous injection as above, i.e. over not less than five minutes, maintained by intravenous infusion by drip of 20–30 mg/hour (or 0.4 mg/kg/hour) up to a maximum of 800 mg daily. This regime should be employed if the patient is unable to take oral medication or in particularly serious arrhythmias being treated in *coronary care units.*

Heart failure: In determining the intervals between administration of Rythmodan capsules it should be borne in mind that whilst the elimination half-life in normal volunteers is approximately seven hours, in patients with heart failure, half-life values of 12 hours or more have been recorded.

Impaired renal function (Disease state or the elderly): Standard capsules should be used in patients in renal failure. A reduced dosage, preferably accompanied by assay of disopyramide plasma levels in cases of severe renal failure (creatinine clearance <8 ml/min) is recommended. The following table may be helpful as a guide.

Creatinine clearance (ml/min)	*Dosage 100 or 150 mg capsules*
Normal	Normal dosage
20–60	100 mg 8-hourly or 150 mg 12-hourly
8–20	100 mg 12-hourly
<8	150 mg daily

Children: There are insufficient data to recommend the use of Rythmodan in children.

Contra-indications, warnings, etc

Contra-indications: Disopyramide is contra-indicated in second or third degree heart block and sinus node disease if no pacemaker is present, cardiogenic shock and severe uncompensated heart failure and hypersensitivity to disopyramide.

Warnings and precautions: There have been reports of ventricular tachycardia or ventricular fibrillation or Torsade de Pointes in patients receiving disopyramide. These have been usually, but not always, associated with significant widening of the QRS complex or prolonged QT interval. If these ECG changes or arrhythmias develop the drug should be discontinued.

Disopyramide should be used only with caution in patients with atrial flutter or atrial tachycardia with block as conversion of a partial AV block to a 1:1 response may occur. Accordingly, the need for prior digitalisation should be considered.

Owing to its negative inotropic effect, disopyramide should be used with caution in patients suffering from significant cardiac failure. Such patients should be fully digitalised or controlled with other therapy before initiating treatment with disopyramide.

The occurrence of hypotension following disopyramide administration, which has been observed especially in patients with cardiomyopathy or inadequately compensated congestive heart failure, requires prompt discontinuation of the drug. Any resumption of therapy should be at a lower dose with close patient monitoring.

The use of disopyramide in combination with other negative inotropic drugs such as beta adrenoceptor antagonists is not recommended especially in intravenous therapy.

In view of the serious nature of many of the conditions being treated it is suggested that *Rythmodan Injection should only be used when facilities exist for cardiac monitoring or defibrillation, should the need arise.*

Disopyramide should be used with caution in patients receiving concurrent therapy with diuretics likely to give rise to hypokalaemia since this may reduce patient response to disopyramide.

Disopyramide should be used with caution in the treatment of digitalis intoxication.

Care should be taken when prescribing disopyramide for patients with bundle branch block as the effect of disopyramide in this condition is unpredictable. If first degree heart block develops in a patient receiving disopyramide, dosage should be reduced and may require discontinuation if the block persists.

Since disopyramide is eliminated predominantly by glomerular filtration the dose administered to patients with significant renal impairment may require adjustment. Patients with renal impairment should not be treated with sustained release disopyramide.

Hepatic impairment causes an increase in the plasma half-life of Rythmodan and a reduced dosage may be required.

Due to its anticholinergic properties, patients with glaucoma, a tendency to urinary retention, or any patient receiving a drug with anticholinergic activity may be unsuitable for Rythmodan therapy.

Hypoglycaemia has been reported in association with Rythmodan administration. Impaired renal function and cardiac function may be predisposing factors in such patients. Strict adherence to the dosing recommendations is advised and consideration should be given to monitoring blood glucose levels, and if hypoglycaemia occurs treatment with Rythmodan should be stopped.

Pregnancy: Although Rythmodan has undergone animal tests for teratogenicity without evidence of any effect on the developing foetus, the benefits of using Rythmodan in the first trimester of pregnancy should be weighed against possible risks.

Lactation: No data for Rythmodan Injection, but studies have shown that oral disopyramide is secreted in breast milk although no adverse effects to the infant have been noted. However, clinical experience is limited and disopyramide should only be used in lactation if, in the clinicians judgement, it is essential for the welfare of the patient. The infant should be closely supervised, particularly for anti-cholinergic effects and drug levels determined if necessary. Ideally, if the drug is considered essential an alternative method of feeding should be used.

Side effects: Rythmodan is usually well tolerated. Most common side effects (dry mouth, blurred vision, urinary hesitancy) are attributable to the drug's mild anticholinergic action. Exceptionally this may be marked. Gastrointestinal irritation may also occur. Very rarely, disopyramide therapy has been associated with acute psychosis, cholestatic jaundice and hypoglycaemia. Side effects usually disappear rapidly with reduction of dosage or cessation of therapy. Profuse sweating may indicate too rapid intravenous injection.

Overdosage: Animal studies indicate that overdosage may lead to cardiac arrest or atrio-ventricular block or to disorders of ventricular excitability leading to terminal ventricular fibrillation. Intracardiac conduction defects and ventricular hyperexcitability may be controlled by general intensive supportive therapy.

Infusion studies in dogs and man have shown the effectiveness of isoprenaline and dopamine in restoring any marked fall in blood pressure.

Pharmaceutical precautions Store in a cool place. Rythmodan Injection is physically compatible with the following: Sodium Chloride Injection BP, Dextrose

Injection BP, Compound Sodium Chloride Injection BPC, Compound Sodium Lactate Injection BP.

Legal category POM.

Package quantities

Rythmodan Capsules 100 mg	OP packs of 84
Rythmodan Capsules 150 mg	OP packs of 84
Rythmodan Retard 250 mg	OP packs of 56
Rythmodan Injection 50 mg/5 ml	Packs of 5 ampoules

Further information Nil.

Product licence numbers

Rythmodan Capsules 100 mg	0109/0022
Rythmodan Capsules 150 mg	0109/0075
Rythmodan Retard Tablets 250 mg	0109/0094
Rythmodan Injection	0109/0060

SOFRADEX* EAR/EYE DROPS AND OINTMENT

Presentation Sofradex is available as a sterile yellow-white translucent ointment and as sterile, clear colourless drops.

Each gram of ointment contains Framycetin Sulphate BP (Soframycin) 5 mg, gramicidin 0.05 mg and Dexamethasone BP 0.5 mg in Plastibase*.

Each millilitre of drops contains Framycetin Sulphate BP (Soframycin) 5 mg, gramicidin 0.05 mg and dexamethasone 0.5 mg (as sodium metasulphobenzoate salt).

Uses
In the eye: For the short-term treatment of steroid responsive conditions of the eye when prophylactic antibiotic treatment is also required, after excluding the presence of fungal and viral disease.

Application to the eyelid: Blepharitis.

In the ear: Otitis externa.

Dosage and administration
Adults (and the elderly) and children
Sofradex Ear/Eye Drops: In the eye: 1 or 2 drops applied to each affected eye up to six times daily or more frequently if required. In the ear: 2 or 3 drops instilled into the ear three or four times daily.

Sofradex Ear/Eye Ointment: In the eye: Apply sparingly two or three times daily, or at night if drop treatment is given during the day. In the ear: Apply once or twice daily.

Contra-indications, warnings, etc
Contra-indications: Viral, fungal, tuberculous or purulent conditions of the eye. Use is contraindicated if glaucoma is present or herpetic keratitis (e.g. dendritic ulcer) is considered a possibility. Use of topical steroids in the latter conditions can lead to extension of the ulcer and marked visual deterioration.

Otitis externa should not be treated when the ear drum is perforated because of the risk of ototoxicity.

Hypersensitivity to the preparation.

Interactions: Non-relevant to topical use.

Effects on ability to drive and use machines: Use in the eye will cause blurring of vision on application. Warn patients not to drive or operate hazardous machinery unless vision is clear.

Other undesirable effects: Hypersensitivity reactions, usually of the delayed type, may occur leading to irritation, burning, stinging, itching and dermatitis.

Topical steroid use may result in increased intraocular pressure leading to optic nerve damage, reduced visual acuity and visual field defects.

Intensive or prolonged use of topical corticosteroids may lead to formation of posterior subcapsular cataracts.

In those diseases causing thinning of the cornea or sclera, corticosteroid therapy may result in thinning of the globe leading to perforation.

Use in pregnancy and lactation: Safety for use in pregnancy and lactation has not been established. There is inadequate evidence of safety in human pregnancy. Topical administration of corticosteroids to pregnant animals can cause abnormalities of foetal development including cleft palate and intrauterine growth retardation. There may therefore be a very small risk of such effects in the human foetus. There is a risk of foetal ototoxicity if aminoglycoside antibiotic preparations are administered during pregnancy.

Other special warnings and precautions: Topical corticosteroids should never be given for an undiagnosed red eye as inappropriate use is potentially blinding.

Treatment with corticosteroid/antibiotic combinations should not be continued for more than 7 days in the absence of any clinical improvement, since prolonged use may lead to occult extension of infection due to the masking effect of the steroid. Prolonged use may also lead to skin sensitisation and the emergence of resistant organisms.

Prolonged use may lead to the risk of adrenal suppression in infants.

Treatment with corticosteroid preparations should not be repeated or prolonged without regular review to exclude raised intraocular pressure, cataract formation or unsuspected infections.

Aminoglycoside antibiotics may cause irreversible, partial or total deafness when given systemically or when applied topically to open wounds or damaged skin. This effect is dose related and is enhanced by renal or hepatic impairment. Although this effect has not been reported following topical ocular use, the possibility should be considered when high dose topical treatment is given to small children or infants.

Overdosage: Long-term intensive topical use may lead to systemic effects.

Oral ingestion of the contents of one bottle (up to 10 ml) is unlikely to lead to any serious adverse effects.

Incompatibilities: None known.

Pharmaceutical precautions Store cool.

Legal category POM.

Package quantities
Sofradex Ear/Eye Drops: Bottles of 10 ml.
Sofradex Ear/Eye Ointment: Tubes of 5 g (fitted with nozzle).

Further information Sofradex drops also contain 2-Phenyl-ethanol BPC 1963, Tween 80 USP, I.M.S. BP, Citric Acid BP, Sodium Citrate BP, Lithium Chloride BP and Purified Water BP buffered by NaOH and HCl.

Product licence numbers

Sofradex Ear/Eye Drops	0109/0030R
Sofradex Ear/Eye Ointment	0109/0031R

SOFRAMYCIN* STERILE EYE DROPS/OINTMENT

Presentation Soframycin is available as a sterile eye ointment and as colourless, sterile eye drops.

Each gram of ointment contains Framycetin Sulphate BP (Soframycin) 5 mg in Plastibase*.

Each millilitre of drops contains Framycetin Sulphate BP (Soframycin) 5 mg in a sterile, buffered, isotonic, aqueous solution.

Uses Soframycin is used for the treatment of bacterial infections of the eye, such as conjunctivitis and blepharitis, for styes, corneal abrasions and burns, and prophylactically following the removal of foreign bodies. It is also indicated for corneal ulcers.

Dosage and administration *Soframycin Drops:* One or two drops applied to each affected eye up to 6 times daily, or more frequently if required.

Soframycin Ointment: For continued effect, 2 or 3 applications of the ointment daily, or at bedtime if drops have been used during the day.

Contra-indications, warnings, etc
Contra-indications: Known hypersensitivity to Framycetin or to any component of the preparation.

Interactions: None relevant to topical use.

Effects on ability to drive and to use machines: Topical eye drop preparations may cause transient blurring of vision on instillation. Patients should be warned not to drive or operate hazardous machinery unless vision is clear.

Other undesirable effects: Hypersensitivity reactions, usually of the delayed type, may occur with local treatment with Framycetin (cross-sensitivity with other aminoglycoside antibiotics may occur). Irritation, stinging or burning, itching and dermatitis may sometimes occur.

Use in pregnancy and lactation: There is inadequate evidence for the safety of Framycetin in pregnancy and lactation. However, it has been used for may years with no direct evidence for ill consequences. Use should be only when considered essential by the physician.

Other special warnings and precautions:

1. Prolonged use should be avoided as it may lead to skin sensitisation and the emergence of resistant organisms.
2. Contact lenses should be removed during the period of treatment.
3. Aminoglycosides have been reported to cause irreversible partial or total deafness when given systemically, topically to open wounds or broken skin, or intraperitoneally. These effects have not been reported with topical ocular administration of Framycetin. However, the possibility should be considered when using high dose topical treatment in small children, or those patients with renal or hepatic impairment.
4. In cases of severe infections the topical use of Framycetin should be supplemented with appropriate systemic treatment.

Overdosage: Not applicable.

Pharmaceutical precautions Store cool.

Legal category POM.

Package quantities *Soframycin Eye Drops:* 8 ml in ophthalmic dispenser.

Soframycin Eye Ointment: Tubes of 5 g (fitted with ophthalmic nozzle).

Further information Soframycin Eye Drops contain Citric Acid BP, Sodium Chloride PhEur, Sodium Citrate PhEur, Phenylmercuric Nitrate BP, and Purified Water PhEur buffered by Sodium Hydroxide BP and Hydrochloric Acid BP.

Product licence numbers

Soframycin Eye Drops	0109/5040R
Soframycin Eye Ointment	0109/5041R

SOFRA-TULLE*

Presentation Sofra-Tulle is a sterile, lightweight, lanoparaffin gauze dressing impregnated with Framycetin Sulphate BP 1% (Soframycin).

Uses Sofra-Tulle has a wide range of antibacterial activity and is a suitable dressing for immediate use in a variety of infected lesions.

Thermal: Burns, scalds.

Traumatic: Lacerations, abrasions, bites, puncture wounds, crush injuries.

Ulcerative: Varicose, diabetic, decubitus and tropical ulcers.

Elective: Skin grafts (donor and receptor sites), avulsion of finger and/or toe nails, circumcision, suture lines.

Miscellaneous: Secondarily infected skin conditions (e.g. eczema, dermatitis, herpes zoster), colostomies, ileostomies, tracheostomies, incised abscesses, incised paronychia.

Dosage and administration Adults, children and the elderly. If necessary, the lesion should first be cleansed, then a single layer of Sofra-Tulle applied and covered with a suitable dressing. When dressing ulcers, the tulle should be shaped to fit the ulcer crater. If the lesion exudes profusely it is advisable to change the dressings at least once a day.

Contra-indications, warnings, etc Sofra-Tulle is contra-indicated where there is known allergy to lanolin or to framycetin, or where organisms are known to be resistant to the latter.

Precautions: Cross-sensitisation to framycetin may occur in patients known to be allergic to Streptomyces-derived antibiotics (neomycin, paramomycin, kanamycin).

In most cases, absorption of the antibiotic is negligible. However, where large body areas are involved, e.g. 30% or more body burn, the possibility of ototoxicity being produced by prolonged applications should be borne in mind.

Pregnancy and lactation: There is inadequate evidence for the safety of framycetin in pregnancy and lactation. However, it has been used for many years with no direct evidence for ill consequences.

Overdosage: Overdosage is unlikely to occur.

Pharmaceutical precautions Store cool.

Legal category POM.

Package quantities Cartons of 10 and 50 units; each unit pack contains one sterile antibiotic gauze dressing 10 cm × 10 cm placed between two layers of parchment. Also available as a continuous gauze strip 30 cm × 10 cm packed in cartons of 10 units.

Further information Nil.

Product licence number 0109/5047R.

SURGAM*

Presentation Opaque maroon capsules with transparent pink body marked Surgam SA and containing white pellets. Each capsule contains 300 mg tiaprofenic acid in a specially pelleted formulation providing sustained release action.

White, convex tablets, 11 mm in diameter, marked SURGAM 300 on one side and on the reverse. Each tablet contains 300 mg tiaprofenic acid.

White, convex tablets, 10 mm in diameter, marked SURGAM 200 on one side and on the reverse. Each tablet contains 200 mg tiaprofenic acid.

Uses *Properties:* Surgam is a non-steroidal anti-inflammatory agent with marked analgesic properties.

Indications: Rheumatoid arthritis, osteoarthritis; ankylosing spondylitis; low back pain; musculo-skeletal disorders such as fibrositis, capsulitis, epicondylitis and other soft-tissue inflammatory conditions; sprains and strains, post-operative inflammation and pain, and other soft-tissue injuries.

Dosage and administration
Adults: 600 mg daily in divided doses. 300 mg twice daily. Alternatively 200 mg three times daily.

Surgam SA: 2 capsules (600 mg) once daily. Surgam SA capsules should not be crushed or chewed before swallowing.

Elderly: As for adults (see 'precautions'). Non-steroidal anti-inflammatory drugs should be used with particular caution in older patients who generally are more prone to adverse reactions.

Children: There are insufficient data to recommend use of Surgam in children.

Contra-indications, warnings, etc
Contra-indications: Active peptic ulceration, history of peptic ulceration, hypersensitivity to the drug.

Warnings: In patients with renal, cardiac or hepatic impairment caution is required since the use of NSAIDs may result in deterioration of renal function. The dose should be kept as low as possible and renal function should be monitored.

Precautions: Surgam should be used with care in patients with a history of peptic ulceration, severe renal or hepatic insufficiency, asthma or previous sensitivity to aspirin or other non-steroidal anti-inflammatory agents. Non-steroidal anti-inflammatory drugs may cause some sodium and fluid retention and may interfere with the natriuretic action of diuretic agents and reduce the effect of these and other antihypertensive drugs. This should be borne in mind in patients with incipient or actual congestive heart failure and/or hypertension. Since Surgam is highly protein-bound, it may be necessary to modify the dosage of other highly protein-bound drugs, e.g. anticoagulants, sulphonamides, hypoglycaemic agents, phenytoin and certain potent diuretics when these are administered concurrently. As with other non-steroid anti-inflammatory agents, patient monitoring is suggested if Surgam and oral anticoagulants are administered together. Non steroidal and anti-inflammatory drugs have been reported to increase steady state plasma levels of lithium and it is, therefore, recommended that these levels are monitored in patients receiving Surgam therapy.

Pregnancy: Although animal studies have not revealed evidence of teratogenicity, safety in human pregnancy and lactation cannot be assumed and, in common with other non-steroidal anti-inflammatory agents, administration during the first trimester should be avoided.

Lactation: The level of Surgam in mothers milk has been studied and the total daily exposure is very small, approximately 0.2% of the administered dose, and is unlikely to be of pharmacological significance.

Side effects: Reported gastro-intestinal reactions include dyspepsia, nausea, abdominal pain, vomiting, anorexia, indigestion, heartburn, stomatitis, constipation, gastritis, flatulence or diarrhoea. In common with other non-steroidal anti inflammatory agents, peptic ulcers, gastro-intestinal bleeding and perforation have occasionally been reported and in exceptional cases may have been associated with fatalities. Bladder irritation and haematuria have been rarely reported. In such cases it is recommended to discontinue treatment. Headache and drowsiness have occasionally been reported, as have skin reactions which include rash, photosensitivity, urticaria, pruritis, angio-oedema and alopecia.

NSAIDs have been reported to cause nephrotoxicity in various forms and their use can lead to interstitial nephritis, nephrotic syndrome and renal failure.

Treatment of overdosage: In the event of overdosage with Surgam, supportive and symptomatic therapy is indicated.

Pharmaceutical precautions Surgam SA: Store in a dry place below 25°C, protected from light.

Surgam Tablets: Store below 30°C, protected from light.

Legal category POM.

Package quantities Surgam SA 300 mg sustained release action capsules in calender blister packs of 56.

Surgam 300 mg tablets blister packed in OP cartons of 56.

Surgam 200 mg tablets blister packed in OP cartons of 84.

Further information The effects of tiaprofenic acid on articular cartilage have been investigated in in-vivo experiments and in ex-vivo studies using different animal model of arthritis. Ex-vivo experiments on human chondrocyte cultures have also been conducted. In these experiments, tiaprofenic acid, in concentrations equivalent to the therapeutic dose, did not depress the biosynthesis of proteoglycans and did not alter the differentiation of proteoglycans secreted. The degradation of proteoglycan aggregates was inhibited. These results suggest a neutral or possibly beneficial effect of tiaprofenic acid on joint cartilage under experimental conditions. The clinical significance of these findings is not known but is being further investigated.

Product licence numbers

Surgam SA capsules 300 mg	0109/0167
Surgam 300 mg	0109/0109
Surgam 200 mg	0109/0108

TARIVID* ▼

Presentation Tarivid tablets each contain 200 mg ofloxacin. They are yellowish-white oblong tablets, 14 × 7 mm, biconvex with a score mark on one side. Excipients include lactose.

Uses Ofloxacin is a synthetic 4-fluoroquinolone antibacterial agent with bactericidal activity against a wide range of Gram-negative and Gram-positive organisms. It is indicated for the treatment of the following infections when caused by sensitive organisms: Upper and lower urinary tract infections; lower respiratory tract infections; uncomplicated urethral and cervical gonorrhoea; non-gonococcal urethritis and cervicitis.

Microbiological results indicate that the following pathogens may be regarded as sensitive: *Staphylococcus aureus* (including methicillin resistant staph.), *Staphylococcus epidermidis*, Neisseria species, *Escherichia coli*, Citrobacter, Klebsiella, Enterobacter, Hafnia, Proteus (indole-negative and indole-positive strains), *Pseudomonas aeruginosa*, *Haemophilus influenzae*, Chlamydiae, Mycoplasma, Legionella, Gardnerella.

Variable sensitivity is shown by Streptococci, *Serratia marcescens*, Bacteroides species.

Anaerobic bacteria (e.g. Fusobacterium species, Eubacterium species, Peptococci, Peptostreptococci), *Treponema pallidum*, anaerobic bacteria are normally resistant.

Dosage and administration General dosage recommendations: The dose of ofloxacin is determined by the type and severity of the infection. The dosage range for adults is 200 mg to 800 mg daily. Up to 400 mg may be given as a single dose, preferably in the morning, larger doses should be given as two divided doses. Tarivid tablets should be swallowed with liquid; they should not be taken within two hours of magnesium/aluminium containing antacids or iron preparations since reduction of absorption of ofloxacin can occur.

Lower urinary tract infection: 200–400 mg daily.

Upper urinary tract infection: 200–400 mg daily increasing, if necessary, to 400 mg twice a day.

Lower respiratory tract infection: 400 mg daily increasing, if necessary, to 400 mg twice daily.

Uncomplicated urethral and cervical gonorrhoea: A single dose of 400 mg.

Non-gonococcal urethritis and cervicitis: 400 mg daily in single or divided doses.

Impaired renal function: Following a normal initial dose, dosage should be reduced in patients with impairment of renal function. When creatinine clearance is 20–50 ml/minute (serum creatinine 1.5–5.0 mg/dl) the dosage should be reduced by half (100–200 mg daily). If creatinine clearance is less than 20 ml/minute (serum creatinine greater than 5 mg/dl) 100 mg should be given every 48 hours.

In patients undergoing haemodialysis or peritoneal dialysis, 100 mg should be given every 48 hours.

Elderly: No adjustment of dosage is required in the elderly, other than that imposed by consideration of renal function.

Children: Ofloxacin is not indicated for use in children or growing adolescents.

Duration of treatment: Duration of treatment is dependent on the severity of the infection and the response to treatment. The usual treatment period is 5–10 days except in uncomplicated gonorrhoea, where a single dose is recommended.

Treatment should not exceed 2 months duration.

Contra-indications, warnings, etc

Contra-indications: Ofloxacin should not be used in patients with known hypersensitivity to 4-quinolone antibacterials.

Ofloxacin, like other 4-quinolones, is contra-indicated in patients with a history of epilepsy or with a lowered seizure threshold.

Ofloxacin is contra-indicated in children or growing adolescents and in pregnant or breast-feeding women, since animal experiments do not entirely exclude the risk of damage to the cartilage of joints in the growing subject.

Warnings and precautions: Patients being treated with ofloxacin should not expose themselves unnecessarily to strong sunlight and should avoid UV rays (sunlamps, solarium). Caution is recommended if the drug is to be used in psychotic patients or in patients with a history of psychiatric disease.

Use in pregnancy and lactation. Reproduction studies performed in rats and rabbits did not reveal any evidence of teratogenicity, impairment of fertility or impairment of peri-/post-natal development. However, as with other quinolones, ofloxacin has been shown to cause arthropathy in immature animals and therefore its use during pregnancy is not recommended. Studies in rats have indicated that ofloxacin is secreted in milk. It should therefore not be used during lactation.

Interactions: Co-administered magnesium/aluminium antacids or iron can reduce absorption. However, unlike other 4-quinolones, no interactions with theophylline, caffeine or warfarin are known.

Side-effects: Hypersensitivity reactions, immediate or delayed, usually involving the skin, but occasionally with other signs of anaphylaxis, shock, dyspnoea, vasculitic reactions, oedema of the glottis, face or tongue, tachycardia, may occur. Treatment should be stopped immediately, and supportive treatment given. There have been a few cases of skin rections on exposure to strong sunlight and occasionally other severe skin reactions have occurred.

There have been occasional disturbances of the central nervous system, eg. sleep disorders, headaches, dizziness, nightmares, unsteady gait and tremor, neuropathy, numbness and paraesthesia, visual disturbances, disturbances of taste and smell. Restlessness, agitation, anxiety and confusion have been reported, as have hallucinations and psychotic reactions. These reactions have occurred in some patients after the first dose of ofloxacin. In such cases, discontinue treatment immediately.

There have been rare reports of pain in joints and muscles.

There have been rare reports of bone marrow depression, (leukopenia, agranulocytosis, thrombocytopenia and anaemia). Transient increases in liver enzymes and/or bilirubin have been reported, as have disturbances of kidney function including increases in serum creatinine.

As with other antimicrobials, gastrointestinal symptons may occur (gastric symptoms, abdominal pain, loss of appetite, nausea, vomiting, diarrhoea). Pseudomembranous colitis has also been reported.

Ability to drive: Since there have been occasional reports of dizziness and visual disturbances, patients should know how they react to Tarivid before they drive or operate machinery.

Overdosage: Information of overdose is not available. Routine measures such as gastric lavage should be carried out as soon as possible.

Pharmaceutical precautions Keep medicines out of the reach of children. Store in a dry place.

Legal category POM.

Package quantities Blister packs of 10, 20 and 100 tablets.

Further information Crystalluria has not been reported with ofloxacin. Interactions with theophylline metabolism and caffeine are unlikely because of the lack of metabolism of ofloxacin.

Product licence number 0086/0139.

**Trade Mark*

Rybar Laboratories Limited
Amersham
Buckinghamshire HP6 5BX

Rybar

C.A.M.* BRONCHODILATOR SYRUP

Presentation Rybar C.A.M. is a colourless liquid. Each 5 ml contains:

Ephedrine Hydrochloride BP 4 mg
Contains parabens.

Uses C.A.M. is indicated in the symptomatic treatment of bronchospasm in children and adults with asthma or bronchitis. C.A.M.'s antitussive action may also be useful in children with unproductive cough.

Dosage and administration *Age ¼ to 2 years:* half a 5 ml spoonful three times daily.

Age 2–4 years: One 5 ml spoonful three times daily.

Age over 4 years: Two 5 ml spoonsful three times daily.

Adults: Four 5 ml spoonsful, 3–4 times daily.

Contra-indications, warnings, etc C.A.M. is contra-indicated in children and adults with severe heart disease, hypertension, thyrotoxicosis and in patients recently or currently taking monoamine oxidase inhibitors or other sympathomimetics.

Pregnancy: While no evidence of ill consequences have been reported during or following pregnancy, as with most drugs, administration especially during the first and third trimesters, should be avoided if possible.

Overdosage: Patients who have taken an overdosage of C.A.M. should have gastric lavage performed within four hours of the overdosage occurring. If overdosage is extreme, or there is delay in removing the drug from the stomach, symptomatic treatment of cardiac or respiratory embarrassment should be considered.

Pharmaceutical precautions C.A.M. should not be exposed to bright sunlight, as this may cause the chemical degradation of ephedrine hydrochloride.

Legal category P.

Package quantities C.A.M. is available in bottles of 150 ml and 1 litre.

Further information Does not contain colouring agents or sucrose. Contains parabens.

Product licence number 0237/5014R.

FOLEX*-350 TABLETS

Presentation Each pink, sugar-coated Folex-350 Tablet contains:

Ferrous Fumarate BP	308 mg (equivalent to 100 mg ferrous iron)
Folic Acid BP	350 micrograms

Contains lactose.

Each pink tablet is overprinted with the word 'Folex-350'.

Uses The prevention and treatment of iron deficiency anaemia of pregnancy; the prevention of megaloblastic anaemia of pregnancy; nutritional anaemia.

Dosage and administration One tablet a day. In pregnancy it is recommended that Folex-350 should be started at the first ante-natal consultation and continued until 3 months after delivery.

Contra-indications, warnings, etc Folex-350 is contra-indicated in megaloblastic anaemia due to vitamin B_{12} deficiency.

Overdosage: Patients who have taken an overdosage of Folex-350 should have gastric lavage performed, if possible within four hours of the overdosage occurring. In addition, patients should have such symptomatic treatment as appears necessary. In order to eliminate excess free iron, a chelating agent such as desferrioxamine may be administered.

Side-effects: Side-effects of iron and folic acid preparations which have been reported include nausea, vomiting, gastro-intestinal symptoms, constipation and diarrhoea.

Pharmaceutical precautions No special precautions are required.

Legal category P.

Package quantities Folex-350 is supplied in containers of 30 (child-resistant), 100 and 1000 tablets.

Further information The high incidence of iron and folate deficiencies in pregnant women may result in possible obstetrical abnormalities. It is now considered advisable to administer daily iron and folic acid routinely, in one tablet, throughout pregnancy.

Product licence number 0237/5008R.

GUAREM* GRANULES

Presentation Sachets, each containing guar gum granules 5 gramms. The fine pale cream granules, which are tasteless, are readily water-miscible, for the preparation of palatable fluid drinks.

Uses (i) For use in diabetes to help control post-prandial glucose levels, thereby facilitating control, and where appropriate, allowing reduction of insulin or oral hypoglycaemic dosage levels.

(ii) For the relief of the symptoms of the 'dumping syndrome'.

Action: Guar gum which is derived from natural sources is a high molecular weight polysaccharide, galactomannan. In solution it (i) increases gastric transit time, (ii) slows the rate of absorption of other carbohydrates leading to a reduction in post-prandial hyperglycaemia and insulin secretion and (iii) sequesters bile acids. Guar gum is not absorbed and remains chemically unchanged until it reaches the colon where it is broken down before excretion. Reduction in plasma cholesterol (LDL) levels have also been reported.

Dosage and administration
Adults: One 5 g sachet to be taken with each main meal. The contents of a sachet may be simply sprinkled evenly over a meal on the plate or stirred into suitable foods (e.g. tomato juice, yoghurt, muesli, etc), in which case the food must be accompanied by a drink of at least 100 ml (orange juice, etc). Alternatively it may be stirred into a fruit flavoured drink (½ tumbler) and swallowed promptly before each main meal.

Children (12 and over): As for adults.

Children (under 12): Not recommended at present.

Contra-indications, warnings, etc To avoid any risk of oesophageal obstruction or rupture, this product should not be given to patients with a history of oesophageal disease or difficulty in swallowing.

Guarem should not be ingested as dry granules.

In diabetics, during initial therapy, blood glucose levels should be carefully monitored and concurrent treatment adjusted where necessary, to minimise the possibility of hypoglycaemia.

In patients with dumping syndrome, while Guarem may be expected to reduce malabsorption, usual monitoring of nutritional status should be continued.

Side effects: Gastro-intestinal symptoms (flatulence, diarrhoea) are quite common at the commencement of treatment. These can be reduced or avoided by initiating treatment gradually in accordance with pack instructions.

Pregnancy: Guarem has been administered to a very limited number of pregnant diabetic patients without ill consequences.

Elderly: Clinical trials have included patients over 65 years and no adverse reactions specific to this age group have been reported.

Interactions: When given simultaneously with Guarem, the absorption of other drugs may be slowed; total amount absorbed and excreted do not however appear to be significantly affected. With digoxin a study concluded that long term administration of guar gum will not interfere with adequate digitalisation.

When it is important to establish maximum serum levels (e.g. penicillin) administration should precede Guarem by one hour.

Pharmaceutical precautions Guarem should be stored in a dry place.

Legal category P.

Package quantities Cartons of 50 and 100 sachets.

Further information Each sachet is individually printed with simple and clear administration instructions.

Product licence numbers 0237/0023 and 0237/0026.

RBC*CREAM

Presentation Slightly pink cream, in internally lacquered aluminium tubes, containing (W/W):

Antazoline Hydrochloride BP	1.8%
Calamine BP	8.0%
Camphor BP	0.1%
Cetrimide BP	0.5%
Menthol BP	0.1%

Uses For the immediate relief of insect stings and bites, nettle rash, hives and itching due to minor skin irritation.

Dosage and administration Cleanse affected area and apply every 3 hours, as necessary.

Contra-indications, warnings, etc None.

Side effects: In rare cases of sensitivity, application should be discontinued.

Pharmaceutical precautions Store below 25°C.

Legal category P.

Package quantities 25 g.

Further information Nil.

Product licence number 0150/5002R.

**Trade Mark*

Sandoz Pharmaceuticals
A division of Sandoz Products Limited
Frimley Business Park
Frimley
Camberley, Surrey GU16 5SG

SANDOZ

CAFERGOT*

Presentation

Tablets: Whitish, round, coated tablets, 9.5 to 10 mm diameter, 5.4 to 5.6 mm thick, weighing 370 mg. Each tablet contains 1 mg Ergotamine Tartrate PhEur and 100 mg Caffeine PhEur.

Suppositories: Off-white suppositories weighing 1.98 g. Each suppository contains 2 mg Ergotamine Tartrate PhEur and 100 mg Caffeine PhEur.

Uses

Principal actions: Ergotamine aborts attacks of migraine and other vascular headaches by its specific vasoconstrictor effect on distended extracranial arteries. Concomitant administration of caffeine enhances the absorption of ergotamine.

Cafergot suppositories are especially valuable for patients who have nausea and vomiting early in the attack and cannot retain or absorb anything taken by mouth.

To be fully effective the tablets must be taken, or the suppositories used, as early as possible in the attack.

Indications: Acute attacks of migraine and migraine variants unresponsive to simple analgesics.

Dosage and administration There is considerable inter-individual variation in the sensitivity of patients to ergotamine. Care should therefore be exercised in selecting the optimum therapeutic dose for an individual patient which will not give rise to unwanted effects, either acutely or chronically. The maximum recommended dosages should not be exceeded and ergotamine treatment should not be administered at intervals of less than 4 days.

For maximum efficacy, the optimal dose (in the preferred galenical form) should be administered immediately prodromal symptoms are experienced.

Tablets: One or two tablets taken at the first warning of an attack are normally sufficient to obtain migraine relief. Some individuals may require higher dosages which should never exceed 4 tablets (4 mg ergotamine) in 24 hours. It is essential to use the minimum effective dose.

The maximum recommended weekly dose of 10 tablets (10 mg ergotamine) should not be exceeded.

Suppositories: One suppository should be administered at the first warning of an attack. This dose is normally sufficient, although some individuals may require higher dosages which should never exceed 2 suppositories (4 mg ergotamine) in 24 hours. It is essential to use the minimum effective dose.

The maximum recommended weekly dosage of 5 suppositories (10 mg ergotamine) should never be exceeded.

Use in children under 12 years: Not recommended.

Use in the elderly: Whilst there is no evidence to suggest that the elderly require different dosages of Cafergot, nevertheless, the contraindications of this drug are common in the elderly, e.g. coronary heart disease, renal impairment, hepatic impairment and severe hypertension. Caution should therefore be exercised when prescribing for this age group.

Contra-indications, warnings, etc

Contra-indications: Cafergot should not be used for migraine prophylaxis, nor should the recommended dosages be exceeded. Frequent attacks of migraine may be an indication for the use of a suitable prophylatic agent.

Cafergot should not be used in patients with peripheral vascular disease, coronary heart disease, obliterative vascular disease and Raynaud's Syndrome in view of the increased risk of peripheral vasospasm secondary to ergotamine. Impaired hepatic or renal function, sepsis, and severe hypertension are all contraindications for treatment with Cafergot.

Use in pregnancy and lactation: Ergotamine containing products are contraindicated in pregnancy due to oxytocic effects on the pregnant uterus and in breast-feeding mothers due to the risk of the infant developing ergotism. Repeated doses of ergotamine may inhibit lactation.

Precautions: Concomitant use of erythromycin and ergotamine should be avoided, as this can result in an elevated concentration of ergotamine in the plasma.

If symptoms such as tingling in the fingers or toes occur, the drug should be discontinued at once and the physician consulted.

As vasospastic reactions have been reported with beta-blockers alone and in a few patients treated concomitantly with ergotamine and propranolol, caution is advised in the concomitant use of these agents with Cafergot.

The caffeine component of Cafergot may give rise to unwanted stimulant effects.

Side-effects: Side-effects of Cafergot are related in the main to the ergotamine component. Acutely, these may include nausea, vomiting and abdominal pain. Paraesthesia and peripheral vasoconstriction or pain and weakness in the extremities may develop after both acute and chronic dosing. Numbness and tingling of the extremities can be indicative of peripheral vasospasm and treatment must be stopped immediately if signs of circulatory impairment appear. Failure to observe this precaution can lead to the development of ergotism.

Excessive use of ergotamine containing products for prolonged periods may result in fibrotic changes, in particular of the pleura and retroperitoneum.

Overdosage: Symptoms of overdosage are: nausea, vomiting, drowsiness, confusion, tachycardia, dizziness, tingling and numbness in the extremities due to ischaemia, respiratory depression, coma.

Treatment should be directed to the elimination of ingested material by aspiration and gastric lavage.

Rarely, headache may be provoked either by chronic overdosage or by rapid withdrawal of the product. Caffeine is a weak stimulant and excessive use of Cafergot may lead to a state of arousal and anxiety.

If severe arteriospasms occur, vasodilators such as nitroprusside sodium should be administered. General supportive measures should be applied with particular reference to the respiratory and cardiovascular systems.

Pharmaceutical precautions Keep suppositories in a cool place.

Legal category POM.

Package quantities
Tablets: Blister pack of 100 (OP).
Suppositories: Boxes of 30 (OP).

Further information Caffeine is not an active ingredient but enhances the action of ergotamine, probably by facilitating its absorption.

A number of physicians have obtained satisfactory responses in some patients by using only half a suppository.

Product licence numbers
Tablets 0101/5023R
Suppositories 0101/5001R

CALCIUM-SANDOZ AMPOULES 10%

Presentation Clear, colourless solution. Each 10 ml contains 1.375 g calcium glubionate, equivalent to 10% w.v calcium gluconate (93 mg calcium–2.32 mmol: 4.64 mEq Ca^{++}).

Uses
Principal action: Calcium is an essential body electrolyte. It is involved in the maintenance of normal muscle and nerve function, is essential for normal cardiac function and blood coagulation. There is a dynamic equilibrium between the calcium in blood and that in the skeleton. Homeostasis is mainly regulated by parathyroid hormone, by calcitonin and by vitamin D.

Indications: Parenteral therapy should be reserved for occasions where the pharmacological action of a high calcium ion concentration is required, for instance, acute hypocalcaemia, cardiac resuscitation and some cases of neonatal tetany.

Intravenous injections of calcium have been used for the acute colic of lead poisoning.

As an adjunct in treatment of acute fluoride poisoning and prevention of hypocalcaemia in exchange transfusions.

Dosage and administration In health the concentration of calcium in serum is maintained close to 2.5 mmol per litre (normal range 2.25–2.75 mmol or 4.5–5.5 mEq per litre). Treatment should aim to restore or maintain this level.

Serum calcium levels should be closely monitored during administration of parenteral calcium therapy.

Acute hypocalcaemia: 10–20 ml (2.32–4.64 mmol).

Fluoride or lead poisoning: 0.3 ml/kg (0.07 mmol/kg).

Neonatal tetany: 0.3 ml/kg (0.07 mmol/kg).

Cardiac resuscitation: 7–15 ml (1.62–3.45 mmol). It should be noted that the absolute dose of calcium required is difficult to determine for this indication and may vary widely.

Intramuscular injections should be given deep in the gluteus medius muscle using a long needle; this route is not recommended for children. Intravenous injections should be given very slowly (three minutes for 10 ml).

Calcium-Sandoz should not be injected subcutaneously.

Use in the elderly: No evidence exists that tolerance of Calcium-Sandoz is directly affected by advanced age; however, elderly patients should be supervised as factors sometimes associated with ageing, such as poor diet or impaired renal function, may indirectly affect tolerance and may require dosage reduction.

Contra-indications, warnings, etc
Contra-indications: Hypercalcaemia (e.g. in hyperparathyroidism, vitamin D overdosage, decalcifying tumours such as plasmocytoma, bone metastases), severe hypercalciuria, severe renal failure and patients receiving cardiac glycosides.

Precautions: Blood levels and calcium excretion should be monitored when high-dose parenteral calcium therapy is administered, particularly in children, in chronic renal failure or where there is evidence of urinary tract calculi formation. Treatment shoud be discontinued immediately if blood calcium exceeds 2.75 mmol per litre or if the 24-hour urinary calcium excretion exceeds 5 mg/kg. Cardiac dysrhythmias may occur at these calcium levels.

Overdosage: Hypercalcaemia is possible and could be treated with phosphates as necessary. Initial dosage should not exceed 100 mmol or 50 mmol intravenously.

Side-effects: If Calcium-Sandoz injection is administered too rapidly, nausea, vomiting, hot flushes, sweating, hypotension and vasomotor collapse, possibly fatal, may ensue.

Pharmaceutical precautions Protect from light.

Legal category POM.

Package quantities Boxes of 5 × 10 ml.

Further information If oral calcium administration is indicated, Sandocal 400 and 1,000 effervescent tablets and Calcium-Sandoz syrup are available. Details are given on a separate data sheet.

Product licence number 0101/5003R.

CEDILANID*

Presentation White, uncoated tablets weighing 85 mg. Flat and of 6 mm diameter with a bevelled edge, coded GO and scored on one side with SANDOZ engraved on the other. Each tablet contains 250 micrograms lanatoside C.

Uses *Principal action:* In common with all cardio-active glycosides of digitalis, Cedilanid improves cardiac function in the failing heart by increasing the force of myocardial contraction and by correcting disturbances of heart rhythm by a direct effect on the excitatory mechanism and the conduction system probably mediated by ion transport mechanisms.

The onset of action of Cedilanid by the oral route is $1\frac{1}{2}$ to 2 hours.

Indications: Acute heart failure. Atrial fibrilation. Atrial flutter. Paroxysmal tachycardia.

Routine digitalisation and maintenance of the patient in congestive heart failure.

Dosage and administration Dosage should be reduced in the presence of coronary insufficiency, electrolyte disturbances and especially in renal or hepatic insufficiency.

Adults
Digitalisation: 1.5 to 2 mg (6 to 8 tablets) daily over a 3–5 day period.

Maintenance: 250 micrograms to 1.5 mg (1 to 6 tablets) per day as indicated by the patient's requirements.

Children: 10 to 30 micrograms/kg body weight/day in 3 divided doses.

Use in the elderly: Elderly patients may be unusually sensitive to digitalis preparations. Special care is indicated when increasing the dosage and a low initial dose should be used. This sensitivity may be due to a direct effect of ageing but changes in renal function with age may also contribute.

Contra-indications, warnings, etc
Contra-indications: Complete AV block and 2nd degree AV block (especially 2 : 1). Excessive sinus bradycardia (particularly when associated with Stokes-Adams seizures).

Precautions: Recent infarction. During treatment with Cedilanid the patient should be kept under regular supervision; dosage should always be adapted to individual requirements. The dosage of Cedilanid administered should be adjusted to compensate for any other digitalis preparations administered in the recent past. High dose oral calcium supplements, psychotropic drugs (including lithium) and sympathomimetics should be given with caution to digitalised patients. Other drugs which may affect digoxin levels include calcium antagonists, amiodarone, spironolactone, triamterene, antibiotics such as erythromycin and tetracycline, thiazide diuretics, corticosteroids and amphotericin B. Absorption of Cedilanid may be affected by cholestyramine, colestipol, antacids or neomycin. Potassium depletion sensitises the heart to cardiac glycosides. If it is necessary to administer quinidine, the dose of cardiac glycosides should be reduced.

Warnings: Digitalised patients should not be given calcium by parenteral injection. The effects of Cedilanid are enhanced by hypokalaemia, hypomagnesaemia, hypercalcaemia, hypothyroidism, and doses may need to be reduced until these conditions are corrected.

Cedilanid should be given cautiously to patients receiving parathyroid extract or large doses of Vitamin D. In patients with renal insufficiency, it is possible for serum creatinine levels to be normal, due to reduced muscle mass and low creatinine production.

In renal failure, dosage adjustment should be assessed with the aid of digoxin serum levels. If this is not feasible, the following may be of use: the dosage should be decreased by about the same percentage as the reduction in creatinine clearance. If this has not been determined, it may be estimated; in men the formula (140–age) divided by serum creatinine concentration, in women the result should be multiplied by 0.85. In severe renal failure the digoxin serum level should be measured at fortnightly intervals, at least during initial treatment.

Use in pregnancy and lactation: The drug crosses the placenta and may reach therapeutic levels in foetal blood. It is excreted in breast milk but the levels reached are not significant.

Overdosage: Fatalities from ingestion of massive oral doses of Cedilanid are rare because vomiting usually occurs. Common symptoms of overdosage include anorexia, nausea, vomiting, headache, visual disturbances and disorientation. Slow or irregular pulse, fall of blood pressure and a wide range of cardiac arrythmias and conduction defects have been reported as a result of digitalis toxicity. Death is usually due to ventricular fibrillation and is sometimes preceded by delirium and convulsions. Chronic poisoning by cumulation produces gradual onset of these symptoms.

Treatment: Activated charcoal may reduce absorption. Emesis or gastric lavage within eight hours, to empty the stomach. Check and carefully monitor serum potassium. Correct hypo- or hyperkalaemia. Treat arrhythmias.

Atropine, 300 to 600 micrograms, will reverse profound bradycardia. A cardiac pacemaker may be required.

In severe cases treatment with digitalis antibodies may be considered.

Side-effects: Toxic effects occur if the dose of Cedilanid has not been carefully tailored to the specific requirements and tolerance of each individual patient.

The most frequent side-effects noted are:

CNS and gastro-intestinal disturbances: anorexia, nausea, vomiting; in rare instances (especially in elderly arteriosclerotics), confusion, disorientation, aphasia and visual disturbances including chromatopsia.

Cardiac: Disturbances of heart rate, conduction and rhythm (bigeminy), lowering of the S-T segment with preterminal T-wave inversion.

Allergic skin reactions: Pruritus, urticaria, macular rashes occur very occasionally.

Pharmaceutical precautions Protect from light.

Legal category POM.

Package quantities Blister packs of 100 tablets (OP).

Further information Nil.

Product licence number 0101/5025R.

CLOZARIL* ▼

Presentation *25 mg tablets:* Yellow, flat, round tablets of 7 mm diameter with a bevelled edge, scored and coded LO on one side with SANDOZ on the other and weighing approximately 160 mg. Each tablet contains 25 mg clozapine.

100 mg tablets: Yellow, flat, round tablets, of 9 mm diameter with a bevelled edge, scored and coded ZA on one side with SANDOZ on the other and weighing approximately 225 mg. Each tablet contains 100 mg clozapine.

Uses

Principal action: Clozapine is an antipsychotic agent which differs from conventional neuroleptics. In animal experiments, it does not induce catalepsy or inhibit apomorphine- or amphetamine-induced stereotyped behaviour. It has weak dopamine receptor-blocking activity, but potent alpha-adrenoceptor blocking, anticholinergic, antihistaminic and arousal reaction inhibiting effects. It has also been shown to possess antiserotoninergic properties.

Clinically, Clozaril produces rapid and marked sedation, and exerts strong antipsychotic effects. In particular, the antipsychotic effects have been demonstrated in schizophrenic patients resistant to other drug treatment. In such cases, Clozaril has proven effective in relieving both positive and negative schizophrenic symptoms, with about one third of patients showing clinically relevant improvement.

Indications: Clozaril is indicated in treatment-resistant schizophrenic patients, ie patients who are non-responsive to, or intolerant of, conventional neuroleptics.

Non-responsiveness is defined as lack of satisfactory clinical improvement despite the use of adequate doses of at least two marketed neuroleptics prescribed for adequate durations.

Intolerance is defined as the impossibility to achieve adequate benefit with conventional neuroleptic drugs because of severe and untreatable neurological adverse reactions (extrapyramidal symptoms or tardive dyskinesia).

Dosage and administration Initiation of Clozaril treatment must be in hospital in-patients and is restricted to those patients with a normal white blood cell count and differential blood count. *The use of Clozaril is restricted to patients who are registered with the Clozaril Patient Monitoring Service.*

The dosage must be adjusted individually. For each patient the lowest effective dose should be used.

Adults

Initial dose: One or two 25 mg tablets on the first day. The dosage may be increased in daily increments of 25 to 50 mg, achieving a dose level of up to 300 mg/day within 7 to 14 days according to response.

Therapeutic dose range: In most patients, antipsychotic efficacy can be expected with 200 to 450 mg/day in divided doses. The total daily dose may be divided unevenly, with the larger portion at bedtime.

Maximum dose: A few patients may require larger doses to obtain maximum therapeutic benefit. Judicious increments (not exceeding 100 mg per increment) are permissible up to a maximum dose of 900 mg/day. Adverse reactions may increase at doses over 450 mg/day.

Maintenance dose: After achieving maximum therapeutic benefit, many patients can be maintained on lower doses. Careful downward titration to the level of 150 to 300 mg/day given in divided doses is recommended. At daily doses not exceeding 200 mg, a single administration in the evening may be appropriate.

Ending therapy: If termination of Clozaril therapy is planned, a gradual reduction in dose is recommended over a 1 to 2 week period. If abrupt discontinuation is necessary the patient should be carefully observed, particularly in view of the risk of rebound psychosis which may necessitate re-admission.

Re-starting therapy: The original dosage build-up recommendations should be followed.

Children: Not recommended.

Use in the elderly: In elderly patients a lower initial dose of 25 mg and more gradual increments (such as 25 mg/day) are indicated.

Other special patient groups: Patients with a history of epilepsy should be closely monitored during Clozaril therapy since dose-related convulsions have been reported. Therefore in patients with a history of seizures, as well as those suffering from cardiovascular, renal, or hepatic disorders, the initial dose should be low, and any dose increase should be slow.

Contra-indications, warnings, etc

Contra-indications: Patients with a history of drug-induced neutropenia/agranulocytosis, or with myeloproliferative disorders, must not be treated with Clozaril.

Other contra-indications are alcoholic and toxic psychoses, drug intoxication, comatose conditions and other forms of severe central nervous system depression, severe hepatic or renal disease.

Warning: Clozaril can cause agranulocytosis. A fatality rate of up to 1 in 300 has been estimated when Clozaril was used prior to recognition of the risk of agranulocytosis and the need for routine blood monitoring. Since that time careful monitoring of patients has been demonstrated to be effective in markedly reducing the risk of fatality.

Because of the risk associated with Clozaril therapy its use is limited to treatment-resistant schizophrenic patients (see 'indications'):

1. who have normal leucocyte findings (white blood cell count and differential blood count), and
2. in whom regular leucoctye counts can be performed weekly during the first 18 weeks and at least every two weeks thereafter for as long as treatment continues.

Prescribing physicians must register themselves, their patients and a nominated pharmacist with the Clozaril Patient Monitoring Service. This service provides for the required leucocyte counts as well as a drug supply audit so that Clozaril treatment is promptly withdrawn from any patient who develops abnormal leucocyte findings.

Each time Clozaril is prescribed, patients should be reminded to contact the treating physician immediately if any kind of infection begins to develop. Particular attention should be paid to flu-like complaints or other symptoms which might suggest infection, such as fever or sore throat.

Precautions: Clozaril can cause agranulocytosis. The following precautionary measures are mandatory: Clozaril should not be used concurrently with drugs associated with a substantial potential for causing agranulocytosis, such as co-trimoxazole, chloramphenicol, sulphonamides, pyrazolone analgesics, phenylbutazone, penicillamine, carbamazepine or cytotoxic agents. Concomitant use of long-acting depot antipsychotics (which have myelosuppressive potential) is not recommended because these medications cannot rapidly be removed from the body in situations where this may be required eg neutropenia.

Before starting Clozaril treatment, a white blood cell count and a differential count must be performed. Only patients with normal findings may receive the drug.

During Clozaril treatment the white blood cell count and differential count must be monitored weekly for the first 18 weeks and at least at two-week intervals thereafter. Monitoring must continue for as long as the patient is on the drug.

Particular attention should be paid to the white blood cell count and the differential count if any flu-like complaints or other symptoms develop which might suggest infection. Each time Clozaril is prescribed the patient should be reminded to contact the treating physician immediately if any kind of infection begins to develop.

If the white blood cell count falls below 3000/mm^3 and/or the absolute neutrophil count drops below 1500/mm^3, Clozaril must be withdrawn at once and the patient closely monitored.

In the event of an infection or a routine white blood cell count between 3000 and 3500/mm^3 and/or a neutrophil count between 1500 and 2000/mm^3, the patient should be re-evaluated immediately with respect to the white blood cell count and the differential count. Should there be a decline in either, Clozaril must be withdrawn at once. If the blood cell count remains the same or increases, treatment with Clozaril may continue provided that the leucocytes and granulocytes are checked at least twice weekly until it is certain that the patient has a stable leucocyte count within the range 3000 to 3500/mm^3.

If Clozaril has been withdrawn and a further fall of white blood cell count below 1000/mm^3 occurs and/or the neutrophils decrease below 500/mm^3, the patient should be referred immediately for specialised care. Clozaril lowers the seizure threshold – see **'Dosage and administration** – *other special patient groups*'.

Drowsiness may occur, especially at the beginning of therapy. Owing to its sedative action, Clozaril may impair the reactions of the patients e.g. when driving vehicles or operating machinery. Clozaril should be administered with caution to patients who participate in activities requiring complete mental alertness.

Careful supervision is indicated in the presence of prostatic enlargement, narrow-angle glaucoma and paralytic ileus.

In liver diseases, regular monitoring of liver function is necessary.

Concomitant use of Clozaril and lithium may increase the risk of development of neuroleptic malignant syndrome.

Clozaril may enhance the central effects of alcohol, MAO inhibitors, CNS depressants including narcotics, benzodiazepines and antihistamines. Because of the possibility of additive effects, caution should be applied with the concomitant administration of drugs with hypotensive or anticholinergic properties.

Competition for protein binding sites may lead to adverse effects as a result of changes in plasma levels of Clozaril or other highly protein-bound drugs such as warfarin.

Use in pregnancy and lactation: The safe use of Clozaril in pregnancy has not been established and its use is not recommended. Adequate contraceptive measures must therefore be ensured in women of child bearing potential.

Animal studies suggest that Clozaril is excreted in breast milk; therefore, mothers receiving Clozaril must not breast-feed.

Overdosage

Signs and symptoms: drowsiness, lethargy, coma, areflexia, confusion, agitation, delirium, hyperreflexia, convulsions, hypersalivation, mydriasis, blurred vision, thermolability, tachycardia, hypotension, collapse, cardiac arrhythmias, heart block, respiratory depression.

Treatment: gastric lavage followed by the administration of activated charcoal (peritoneal dialysis and haemodialysis are not very effective). Symptomatic treatment under continuous cardiac monitoring, surveillance of respiration, control of electrolytes and acid-base balance. The use of adrenaline and its derivatives should be avoided in the treatment of hypotension because of the possibility of a 'reverse adrenaline' effect. Close medical supervision is necessary for at least four days because of the possibility of delayed reactions.

Side-effects: Neutropenia leading to agranulocytosis is a risk of Clozaril treatment. This reaction can prove fatal. The majority of cases occur in the first 18 weeks of treatment. Because immediate withdrawal of the drug is required to prevent the development of life-threatening agranulocytosis, monitoring of the white blood cell count is mandatory (see 'Warning' and 'Precautions').

Patients on Clozaril may develop unexplained leucocytosis, including eosinophilia, especially in the initial weeks of treatment.

Central nervous system: Drowsiness and fatigue are among the most common side-effects observed. Dizziness or headache may also occur. Clozaril lowers the seizure threshold in a dose-dependent manner and may cause EEG changes, including the occurrence of spike and wave complexes. Convulsions may, therefore, be precipitated in individuals who have epileptogenic potential but no previous history of epilepsy. On rare occasions it may induce episodes of delirium. Extrapyramidal symptoms are limited mainly to tremor, akathisia and rigidity and if such effects occur, they tend to be mild and transient. Neuroleptic malignant syndrome has been reported rarely.

Autonomic nervous system: Dry mouth, disturbances of accommodation and disturbances in sweating and temperature regulation have been reported. Hypersalivation is a common side-effect.

Cardiovascular system: Tachycardia and postural hypotension may occur, especially in the initial weeks of treatment. Less commonly hypertension has been reported. ECG changes may occur and isolated reports of cardiac arrythmias and myocarditis have been received.

Gastro-intestinal system: Nausea, vomiting, constipation and weight gain may occur. Increases in hepatic enzymes and, in rare cases, cholestasis have been reported.

Genito-urinary system: Both urinary incontinence and retention have been reported.

Miscellaneous: Benign hyperthermia may occur, especially in the initial weeks of treatment.

Isolated reports of skin reactions have been received.

Clozaril has not been associated with elevated prolactin levels.

Sudden unexplained deaths are known to occur among psychiatric patients who receive antipsychotic medication as well as those who do not. Isolated cases of such deaths have been reported in patients receiving Clozaril.

Pharmaceutical precautions Nil.

Legal category POM.

Package quantities Containers of 84 tablets.

Further information *Clozaril Patient Monitoring Service: The use of Clozaril is restricted to patients who are registered with the Clozaril Patient Monitoring Service (CPMS).* This service provides for the required leucocyte counts as well as a drug supply audit to ensure that Clozaril is withdrawn from any patient with an abnormal leucocyte count. Full details of the service are available from the Clozaril Patient Monitoring Service Manager at Sandoz Pharmaceuticals, Frimley Business Park, Frimley, Camberley, Surrey GU16 5SG. Tel: 0276 692255.

Supply of Clozaril is restricted to hospital pharmacies registered within the Clozaril Patient Monitoring Service.

Pharmacokinetics: The absorption of orally administered Clozaril is 90 to 95%; the rate or extent of absorption is not influenced by food.

Clozapine is subject to a moderate first-pass metabolism, resulting in an absolute bioavailability of 50 to 60%. In steady-state conditions, when given twice daily, peak blood levels occur on an average at 2.1 hours (range: 0.4 to 4.2 hours). Clozapine is 95% bound to plasma proteins. Its elimination is biphasic with a mean terminal half-life of 12 hours (range: 6 to 26 hours).

Clozapine is almost completely metabolised prior to excretion. Only trace amounts of unchanged drug are detected in the urine and faeces. Approximately 50% of the administered dose is excreted in the urine and 30% in the faeces.

Product licence numbers
25 mg tablets: 0101/0228
100 mg tablets: 0101/0229

DESERIL*

Presentation White, sugar-coated, round, biconvex tablets weighing 100 mg, 6 mm diameter, 3.4 to 3.9 mm thick, branded DSL one side. Each tablet contains 1.33 mg Methysergide Maleate BP (equivalent to 1 mg methysergide base).

Uses *Principal action:* Deseril is a potent serotonin antagonist. In addition to inhibiting the pain-facilitating and permeability-increasing actions of serotonin, Deseril can potentiate the effects of vasoconstrictor stimuli.

Indications: Prophylactic treatment of migraine, cluster headache and other vascular headaches in patients who, despite other attempts at control, experience headaches of such severity or regularity that their social or economic life is seriously disrupted. (Note: Deseril is not recommended for treatment of the acute attack.)

Control of profuse diarrhoea associated with carcinoid disease.

Dosage and administration *Adults: Prophylactic treatment of headache:* 1 or 2 tablets two or three times a day, with meals.

Treatment should start with one tablet at bedtime and dosage should then be increased gradually over about two weeks until effective levels are reached. The minimum effective dose should be used – often that which will prevent 75% of attacks rather than all headaches.

From the outset, patients should understand that regular clinical supervision and periodic withdrawal of treatment are essential so that adverse effects can be recognised and minimised.

Carcinoid syndrome: High doses are usually necessary. In most reported cases dosage ranged between 12 and 20 tablets daily.

Children: Deseril is not recommended for the treatment of children.

Use in the elderly: No evidence exists that elderly patients require different dosages or show different side effects from younger patients.

Contra-indications, warnings, etc
Contra-indications: Pregnancy, lactation, peripheral vascular disorders, progressive arteriosclerosis, severe hypertension, coronary heart disease, valvular heart disease, phlebitis or cellulitis of the lower extremities, pulmonary disease, collagen disease, impaired kidney or liver function, diseases of the urinary tract, cachectic or septic conditions.

Warnings: Continuous Deseril administration should not exceed six months without a drug-free interval of at least one month for reassessment; dosage should be reduced gradually over two or three weeks to avoid rebound headaches. In patients undergoing treatment with Deseril the dose of ergotamine required to control acute attacks may have to be reduced.

Precautions: Regular clinical supervision of patients treated with Deseril is essential. Particular attention should be paid to complaints of urinary dysfunction, pain in the loin, flank or chest, and pain, coldness or numbness in the limbs. Patients should be regularly examined for the presence of cardiac murmurs, vascular bruits, pleural or pericardial friction rubs and abdominal or flank masses or tenderness. Treatment with Deseril should be stopped should any of these symptoms or signs occur.

Caution is also advised during drug administration to patients with a past history of peptic ulceration.

In carcinoid syndrome the risk of adverse reactions due to the higher dosage must be weighed against the therapeutic benefit.

Concomitant use of Deseril and vasoconstrictors or vasopressors may result in enhanced vasoconstriction.

Overdosage: Treatment should be directed to elimination of the ingested material by aspiration and gastric lavage. General supportive measures should be applied. The patient should be carefully observed for peripheral vasospasm which may be treated by warmth, care being taken to protect ischaemic limbs. If there is evidence of impending tissue damage vasodilators may be used.

Side-effects:

General: The most commonly reported side-effects are nausea, heartburn, abdominal discomfort, vomiting, dizziness, lassitude and drowsiness. These side-effects can often be minimised by taking Deseril with food. Tissue oedema, insomnia, leg cramps and weight gain have occurred, and skin eruptions or loss of scalp hair have occasionally been reported. Mental and behavioural disturbances have occurred in isolated instances.

Inflammatory fibrosis: Retroperitoneal fibrosis: Continuous long-term Deseril administration has been associated with the development of retroperitoneal fibrosis. This is very rare when continuous treatment has not exceeded 6 months. Retroperitoneal fibrosis usually presents with symptoms of urinary tract obstruction such as persistent loin or flank pain, oliguria, dysuria, increased blood nitrogen and vascular insufficiency of the lower limbs. Deseril must be withdrawn if retroperitoneal fibrosis develops; drug withdrawal is often associated with clinical improvement over a few days to several weeks.

Fibrosis in other areas: Fibrotic processes involving lungs, pleura, heart valves and major vessels have been reported in a small number of patients. Presenting symptoms include chest pain, dyspnoea or pleural friction rub and pleural effusion. Cardiac murmurs or vascular bruits have also been reported. Appearance of these symptoms demands immediate withdrawal of Deseril. These fibrotic manifestations are often reversible although less readily so than retroperitoneal fibrosis.

Vascular: Vascular reactions, including arterial spasm, have been seen in some patients. The following have all been described: arterial spasm in a limb causing coldness, numbness, pain or intermittent claudication; renal artery spasm giving rise to transitory hypertension; mesenteric artery spasm causing abdominal pain; retinal artery spasm causing reversible loss of vision; coronary artery spasm causing angina and questionably resulting in myocardial infarction. Arterial spasm is rapidly reversible following drug withdrawal.

Pharmaceutical precautions Protect from light.

Legal category POM.

Package quantities Blister pack of 50 tablets (OP).

Further information Deseril tablets no longer contain tartrazine.

Product licence number 0101/5026R.

DIHYDERGOT* INJECTION

Presentation Clear, colourless solution. Each 1 ml ampoule contains 1 mg Dihydroergotamine Mesylate BP.

Uses
Principal action: Dihydroergotamine has a complex pharmacological profile. It possesses affinity for both alpha-adrenergic and serotoninergic receptors with stimulating and blocking properties.

Indication: For the treatment of migraine attack in patients who have failed to respond to analgesics.

Dosage and administration
Adults: 1 ml (1 mg) by intramuscular or subcutaneous injection as early as possible following the first sign of a migraine attack. In refractory cases, a further 1 ml may be administered after 30 to 60 minutes.

Total daily dosage should not exceed 3 ml (3 mg).

Total weekly dosage should not exceed 6 ml (6 mg).

If a patient fails to respond to these maximum daily or weekly dosages, it is recommended that Dihydergot be withdrawn.

Children: Dihydergot injection is not recommended for children.

Use in the elderly: No evidence exists that elderly patients require different dosages or show different side-effects from other adult patients. However, it is probable that many elderly patients will be excluded from treatment by the contra-indications, warnings and precautions.

Contra-indications, warnings, etc
Contra-indications: Known hypersensitivity to ergot alkaloids.

Patients suffering from cardiac failure, coronary artery disease, inadequately controlled hypertension, peripheral vascular disease, septic conditions or shock should not be treated with Dihydergot injections.

Use in pregnancy and lactation: Dihydergot injections are contra-indicated during pregnancy. It is not known whether dihydroergotamine is excreted in the breast milk, and nursing mothers should not, therefore, be treated with Dihydergot.

Precautions: Intra-arterial injection of Dihydergot must be avoided. Should it occur by accident an alpha-blocker should be administered.

Caution is indicated in patients with renal disease and in patients with liver disease. In such cases the dosage may need to be reduced.

Dihydergot is a derivative of ergotamine and may induce vasospastic symptoms including paraesthesia, pain and weakness in the extremities. In rare cases vascular spasms may occur during parenteral Dihydergot therapy, in particular in the lower extremities. Dihydergot should not be used in patients with peripheral vascular disease, obliterating vascular disease or Raynaud's disease, in view of the increased risk of peripheral vasospasm.

Vasospastic reactions have been reported with some beta-blockers alone and in a few patients treated concomitantly with ergotamine and propranolol. Although not reported with dihydroergotamine, caution is advised in the concomitant use of beta-blockers and Dihydergot.

Dihydergot treatment should be withdrawn immediately if symptoms of acute peripheral ischaemia occur. These symptoms may include coldness, numbness and paraesthesia, loss of sensation, paralysis and pallor. If left untreated, these may progress to oedema, ulceration and gangrene. The usual supportive measures must be instituted, including the avoidance of trauma to the ischaemic limb, and the prevention and treatment of infection. In cases unresponsive to these measures, infusion of peripheral vasodilators (such as glyceryl trinitrate or sodium nitroprusside) may be required.

Subcutaneous administration may give rise to local discomfort at the injection site.

There is no evidence that Dihydergot has an adverse effect on driving ability.

Overdosage: Symptoms might include nausea, vomiting, abdominal pain; numbness, tingling, pain and cyanosis of the extremities with absent or diminished peripheral pulses; respiratory depression; hypertension and/or hypotension. Treatment should be directed to general supportive measures with particular reference to the cardiovascular and respiratory systems.

If severe arteriospasms occur vasodilators should be administered.

Side-effects: Nausea and vomiting may occasionally occur. Numbness and tingling of the fingers and toes as well as precordial pain have been reported in a few cases; if these occur, Dihydergot treatment should be withdrawn.

Pharmaceutical precautions Protect from light. Once an ampoule is opened the contents should be used immediately.

Legal category POM.

Package quantities Boxes of 5 × 1 ml ampoules.

Further information Snap ampoules; no file required.

Product licence number 0101/5007R.

HYDERGINE*

Presentation *1·5 mg Tablets:* Hydergine 1.5 mg is available as white, flat, bevel-edged tablets, scored on one side, with HYDERGINE 1.5 engraved on the other, and of 240 mg weight, 9 mm diameter and 2.9 mm thickness. Each tablet contains 1.5 mg Co-dergocrine Mesylate BP.

4·5 mg Tablets: Hydergine 4.5 mg is available as white, round, biconvex tablets coded HYDERGINE on one side with 4.5 engraved on the other, and of 240 mg weight and 9 mm diameter. Each tablet contains 4.5 mg Co-dergocrine Mesylate BP.

Uses *Indications:* As an adjunct in the management of elderly patients with mild to moderate dementia.

Dosage and administration 1.5 mg three times a day or a once daily dosage of 4.5 mg.

Hydergine should be taken before meals.

The effect of Hydergine is not immediate: alleviation of symptoms is usually gradual and may not be apparent for two to three weeks. Continuing improvement may be expected for at least three months.

Hydergine is not intended for use in children.

Contra-indications, warnings, etc
Contra-indications: Known hypersensitivity to the drug.

Precautions: Caution should be exercised in the administration of Hydergine to patients with severe bradycardia.

There are no known drug interactions involving Hydergine.

Overdosage: Symptoms might include nausea, vomiting, nasal stuffiness, flushing of the face, headache, hypotension and collapse. Treatment should be directed to the elimination of the drug from the gastrointestinal tract by gastric lavage, followed by the administration of activated charcoal. General supportive measures should be applied with particular reference to the cardiovascular system.

Side-effects: Side-effects are infrequent following administration of Hydergine and even relatively large doses are well tolerated. Minor side-effects including gastrointestinal disturbances, flushes, rashes, nasal stuffiness, abdominal cramps, headaches, dizziness and postural hypotension in hypertensive patients have on occasion been reported.

Pharmaceutical precautions Protect from light.

Legal category POM.

Package quantities *1.5 mg Tablets:* Blister pack of 100 (OP).
4.5 mg Tablets: Calendar pack of 28 (OP).

Further information Double-blind studies have shown that improvement occurs with all the symptoms listed in the Sandoz Clinical Assessment-Geriatric (SCAG) scale except for hostility; significant improvement can be expected for nine of the symptoms, namely confusion, impairment of recent memory, disorientation, anxiety, depression, emotional lability, irritability, unsociability and the overall impression of the patient.

Product licence numbers

1.5 mg Tablets	0101/0042R
4.5 mg Tablets	0101/0117

LACTULOSE SOLUTION BP

Presentation Lactulose Solution BP is available as a clear, almost colourless to brownish-yellow syrup. Each 5 ml spoonful contains 3.35 g lactulose and 1.34 g of other sugars (lactose, galactose, tagatose and other keto-sugars).

Uses *Principal action:* Lactulose prevents the formation of hard stools and encourages normal bowel movement. Unlike traditional laxative preparations which act either on the innervation or musculature of the intestine or by bulk stimulus, lactulose provides a natural substrate for the saccharolytic bacterial flora in the colon.

Lactulose is a disaccharide which is not hydrolysed in the small intestine. Therefore it cannot be absorbed and is transported to the colon with water to retain the osmotic balance. In the colon, several species of bacteria can hydrolyse lactulose to the monosaccharides galactose and fructose.

By encouraging this normal metabolic activity of the bacteria, the osmotic pressure of the colonic contents is doubled and more water is drawn into the bowel.

Further metabolism of the monosaccharides leads to the production of acetic and lactic acids and the subsequent lowering of colonic pH. This acidification of the colonic contents is considered to be the main reason for the effectiveness of lactulose solution. In chronic portal-systemic encephalopathy it may be associated with the decrease in the relative concentration of free ammonia, the major agent involved in the cerebral disturbance.

Indications: Chronic constipation. Chronic portal-systemic encephalopathy.

Dosage and administration
Chronic constipation: Because lactulose acts naturally to encourage the normal activity of the bowel, it may be two or three days before the full benefit of the treatment is obtained. It is important, therefore, to follow the dosage regimen set out below.

Adults:
Initially: Three to six 5 ml spoonfuls for the first two to three days of treatment. (Nine spoonfuls may be given in obstinate cases).

Maintenance: Two to three 5 ml spoonfuls daily or according to the needs of the patient.

Children:
Initially: Two to five 5 ml spoonfuls for the first two or three days of treatment.

Maintenance: One to three 5 ml spoonfuls daily or according to the needs of the patient.

Chronic portal-systemic encephalopathy: Six to ten 5 ml spoonfuls three times daily according to the requirements of the patient, for adequate acidification of the colonic contents.

Use in the elderly: No evidence exists that elderly patients require different dosages or show different side-effects from younger patients.

Contra-indications, warnings, etc
Contra-indications: In common with other preparations used for the treatment of constipation, lactulose solution should not be used in patients with gastrointestinal obstruction. Lactulose solution should not be given to patients with galactosaemia or lactose intolerance.

Precautions: Lactulose solution should be used with caution during the first trimester of pregnancy.

There are no known drug interactions involving lactulose.

There is no evidence that lactulose affects driving ability.

Overdosage: No cases of intoxication due to deliberate or accidental overdosage with lactulose solution have been reported to the Company.

Side-effects: Side-effects rarely occur after the administration of lactulose solution. Mild transient effects such as abdominal distension or cramps and flatulence, which subside after the initial stages of treatment, have occasionally been reported.

High doses may provoke nausea in some patients. This can be minimised by administration with water, fruit juice, or with meals.

Pharmaceutical precautions Lactulose solution should be stored in a cool place.

Dilution is not recommended.

Legal category P.

Package quantities Bottles of 200 ml, 300 ml, 500 ml and 1 litre.

Further information Lactulose solution has an *absolute* calorific content of approximately 19 kcals/5 ml. However, as lactulose is almost completely unabsorbed from the gastrointestinal tract, the *available* calories will be much lower. Therefore, at the usual maintenance dose for constipation, lactulose solution is unlikely to adversely affect diabetic control.

Product licence number 0101/0076

LAMISIL* TABLETS ▼

Presentation Off-white, bi-convex tablets with a bevelled edge, of 11 mm diameter and weighing 390 mg, scored and coded ST on one side. Each tablet contains 281.25 mg terbinafine hydrochloride, equivalent to 250 mg terbinafine.

Uses
Principal action: Terbinafine is an allylamine which has a broad-spectrum of anti-fungal activity. At low concentrations terbinafine is fungicidal against dermatophytes, moulds and certain dimorphic fungi. The activity against yeasts is fungicidal or fungistatic depending on the species.

Terbinafine interferes specifically with fungal sterol biosynthesis at an early stage. This leads to a deficiency in ergosterol and to an intracellular accumulation of squalene, resulting in fungal cell death. Terbinafine acts by inhibition of squalene epoxidase in the fungal cell membrane.

The enzyme squalene epoxidase is not linked to the cytochrome P-450 system. Terbinafine does not influence the metabolism of hormones or other drugs.

When given orally, the drug concentrates in skin at levels associated with fungicidal activity.

Indications: Fungal infections of the skin caused by *Trichophyton* (eg *T. rubrum, T. mentagrophytes, T. verrucosum, T. violaceum*). *Microsporum canis and Epidermophyton floccosum.*

Oral Lamisil is indicated in the treatment of ringworm (tinea pedis, tinea criris and tinea corporis) where oral therapy is considered appropriate due to the site, severity or extent of the infection.

Dosage and administration
Adults: One 250 mg tablet daily.

The bioavailability of terbinafine is not affected by food.

Duration of treatment: The duration of treatment varies according to the indication and the severity of infection.

Likely durations of treatment are as follows: Tinea pedis (interdigital, plantar/moccasin type): 2 to 6 weeks. Tinea cruris: 2 to 4 weeks. Tinea corporis: 4 weeks.

Complete resolution of the signs and symptoms of infection may not occur until several weeks after mycological cure.

Use in the elderly: There is no evidence to suggest that elderly patients require different dosages or experience side-effects different to those of younger patients. The possibility of impairment of liver or kidney function should be considered in this age group (see 'Precautions').

Children: There is no experience with oral Lamisil in children and its use cannot therefore be recommended.

Contra-indications, warnings, etc
Contra-indications: Hypersensitivity to Lamisil.

Precautions: Patients with severe liver dysfunction or impaired renal function (creatinine clearance less than 50 ml/minute or serum creatinine of more than 300 micromol/l) should receive half the normal dose.

Based on studies undertaken in-vitro and in healthy volunteers, terbinafine shows negligible potential to inhibit or induce the clearance of drugs that are metabolised via the cytochrome P-450 system (e.g. cyclosporin, tolbutamide, oral contraceptives). The plasma clearance of terbinafine may however be accelerated by drugs which induce metabolism (such as rifampicin) and may be inhibited by drugs which inhibit cytochrome P-450 (such as cimetidine). Where coadministration of such agents is necessary the dosage of Lamisil may need to be adjusted accordingly.

Use in pregnancy and lactation: Foetal toxicity and fertility studies in animals suggest no adverse effects.

There is no clinical experience with Lamisil in pregnant women, therefore unless the potential benefits outweigh any potential risks Lamisil should not be administered during pregnancy.

Terbinafine is excreted in breast milk and therefore mothers should not receive Lamisil whilst breast feeding.

Side-effects: Side-effects are mild to moderate, and transient. The most common are gastrointestinal symptoms (fullness, loss of appetite, nausea, mild abdominal pain, diarrhoea) or allergic skin reactions (rash, urticaria). No life-threatening reactions have been reported.

Overdosage: Based on the observed adverse effects in man, the main symptoms of an acute overdosage are likely to be gastrointestinal, eg nausea or vomiting. Gastric lavage and/or symptomatic supportive treatment may be required.

Pharmaceutical precautions Lamisil tablets should be protected from light.

Legal category POM.

Package quantities Calendar packs of 14 and 28.

Further information A single oral dose of 250 mg terbinafine results in mean peak plasma concentrations of 0.97 microgrammes/ml within 2 hours after administration. The absorption half-life is 0.8 hours and the distribution half-life is 4.6 hours.

Terbinafine binds strongly to plasma proteins. It rapidly diffuses through the dermis and concentrates in the lipophilic stratum corneum. Terbinafine is also secreted in sebum thus achieving high concentrations in hair follicles, hair and sebum-rich skins. There is also evidence that terbinafine is distributed into the nail plate within the first few weeks of commencing therapy.

Biotransformation results in metabolites with no antifungal activity, which are excreted predominantly in the urine. The elimination half-life is 17 hours. There is no evidence of accumulation.

No age-dependent changes in pharmacokinetics have been observed but the elimination rate may be reduced in patients with renal or hepatic impairment, resulting in higher blood levels of terbinafine.

Efficacy in tinea capitis has not yet been established.

Oral Lamisil is not effective in Pityriasis versicolor.

Product licence number 0101/0304

MELLERIL*

Presentation
Suspension: An opaque, creamy/white, semi-viscous fluid, available in two strengths: 25 mg in 5 ml (0.5%): Each 5 ml spoonful contains 25 mg thioridazine base equivalent to 27.5 mg of thioridazine hydrochloride.

100 mg in 5 ml (2%): Each 5 ml spoonful contains 100 mg thioridazine base equivalent to 110 mg of thioridazine hydrochloride.

Syrup: A clear, orange liquid. Each 5 ml spoonful contains 27.5 mg of thioridazine hydrochloride equivalent to 25 mg thioridazine base.

Tablets: White, film-coated tablets with a bevel edge, embossed MEL on one side with the strength on the other. They are available in four strengths:

10 mg Thioridazine Tablets BP are 6.3 mm in diameter, 2.9 mm thick and weigh 92 mg.

25 mg Thioridazine Tablets BP are 7.4 mm in diameter, 3.0 mm thick and weigh 143 mg.

50 mg Thioridazine Tablets BP are 9.5 mm in diameter, 4.3 mm thick and weigh 287 mg.

100 mg Thioridazine Tablets BP are 10.5 mm in diameter, 4.5 mm thick and weigh 359 mg.

Uses *Principal action:* Melleril is a phenothiazine antipsychotic.

Although the basic pharmacological actions of Melleril are similar to those of phenothiazines generally, the antipsychotic activity is its principal action, and other effects such as antiemetic and antihistaminic activities are minimal. It has a wide therapeutic margin and is well tolerated in the recommended dosage range.

Indications
Adults: Schizophrenia: treatment of symptoms and prevention of relapse. Mania and hypomania.

As an adjunct to the short-term management of anxiety, moderate to severe psychomotor agitation, excitement, violent or dangerously impulsive behaviour.

Agitation and restlessness in the elderly.

Children: Behaviour disorders and epilepsy – only where there are severe mental or behavioural problems such as senseless hyperactivity, aggressiveness, temper tantrums, self-injury or mutilation, or agitation.

Dosage and administration

Adults	Daily dose range in terms of the hydrochloride (Tablets)†
Schizophrenia, mania, hypomania. For acute schizophrenia, an initial loading dose of 200 mg may be given. In hospitalised, resistant patients under specialist supervision, up to 800 mg daily may be administered *for not more than 4 weeks*.	150–600 mg
Psychomotor agitation, excitement, violent or dangerously impulsive behaviour.	75–200 mg
Anxiety, agitation and restlessness in the elderly.	30–100 mg

There may be great variability in individual response and dosage requirements. In underweight patients, or in those suffering from kidney or liver disease, lower initial doses and more gradual increases are indicated.

Use in the Elderly

In elderly patients lower initial doses and more gradual increases are indicated.

Children	Daily dose range in terms of the hydrochloride (Tablets)†
1 to 5 years of age	1 mg/kg bodyweight
5 years and over	Usually 75–150 mg/day. In severe cases up to 300 mg/day may be used.

† Melleril suspension contains thioridazine base. To convert from hydrochloride to base, multiply by 0.91. As might be expected the in-vitro dissolution profiles of the suspension and tablets differ; bioequivalence of the liquid and solid dose formulations should not, therefore, be assumed.

Contra-indications, warnings, etc

Contra-indications: Comatose states, severe depression of the CNS or a history of blood dyscrasia; severe cardiovascular disease. Phenothiazines can cause sleep apnoea and, because of a possible correlation with sudden infant death syndrome, melleril should not be given to children below one year of age.

Use in pregnancy and lactation: Do not use during pregnancy unless there are compelling reasons. There is inadequate evidence for safety of the drug in human pregnancy, and there is some evidence of harmful effect in a few, but not all, animal studies. The newborn of mothers treated with Melleril in late pregnancy may show signs of intoxication such as excessive sleepiness, tremor and hyperactivity.

Do not use during lactation. If the use of Melleril is considered essential, breast feeding should be discontinued.

Precautions: Melleril should be used with caution in patients with cardiac arrhythmias, cardiac disease, severe respiratory disease, renal failure, Parkinson's disease, a personal or family history of narrow angle glaucoma, in prostatic hypertrophy, myasthenia gravis, epilepsy, phaeochromocytoma and in patients who have shown hypersensitivity to other phenothiazines. In patients with liver disease, regular monitoring of liver function is essential. Phenothiazines should be administered with caution to patients who participate in activities requiring complete mental alertness. They may impair the reactions of the patient e.g. when driving vehicles or operating machinery. Regular blood counts should be carried out during the first three to four months of treatment or if any clinical signs of blood dyscrasias appear. Phenothiazines generally may affect temperature regulation and decrease serum thyroxine concentrations, although this is very unlikely with Melleril.

Acute withdrawal symptoms including nausea, vomiting and insomnia have rarely been described after abrupt cessation of high dose Melleril. Gradual withdrawal is advisable. Drug withdrawal in children may lead to rapid clinical relapse and neurological symptoms, although this is less common with Melleril than with other antipsychotics.

Melleril may enhance the central nervous system depression produced by other CNS depressant drugs including alcohol, hypnotics, sedatives or narcotic analgesics. In common with other phenothiazines, Melleril antagonises the action of adrenaline and other sympathomimetic agents, and may reverse the blood pressure lowering effects of adrenergic-blocking agents such as guanethidine and clonidine. Phenylpropanolamine has been reported to interact with phenothiazines and cause ventricular arrhythmias. Melleril may affect the metabolism of tricyclic antidepressants, phenytoin and other anticonvulsants. It may also impair the antiparkinsonian effects of levodopa; it may possibly affect the control of diabetes or the action of anticoagulants. It may enhance the cardiac depressant effects of quinidine. Antacids should not be used within two hours of taking phenothiazines. Undesirable anticholinergic effects can be enhanced by anticholinergic drugs. Neurotoxicity resulting from combination with lithium has been reported rarely.

Side-effects and warnings: Common side-effects, particularly with higher dosage and at the start of treatment, include drowsiness, sedation, dry mouth and nasal stuffiness. Dose-related postural hypotension may occur, particularly in the elderly. Other dose-related anticholinergic-type side-effects include blurring of vision, tachycardia, constipation and urinary hesitancy or retention.

Even in low dosage, in susceptible (especially non-psychotic) individuals, Melleril may cause feelings of being mentally dulled or slowed down, nausea, dizziness, headache, or paradoxical effects of excitement, agitation or insomnia. Confusional states or epileptic fits can occur.

At higher dose levels, as with other phenothiazines, ECG changes such as prolongation of the Q-T interval, flattening of the T-wave and the appearance of U-waves have been reported. These changes are more likely to occur in the presence of a low potassium blood level. Like all phenothiazines, Melleril may induce arrhythmias.

Pigmentary retinopathy has been observed in a small number of patients receiving long-term therapy with daily doses above the recommended maximum of 600 mg and has been seen rarely in patients taking less. It is characterised by decreased visual acuity, chromatopsia (usually brown-tinted vision) and impairment of dark adaptation; progressive loss of vision may occur. Fundoscopic examination discloses deposits of pigment. The patient should be told of the importance of reporting any change in vision. If prolonged high-dose treatment is envisaged full ophthalmic examinations should be carried out at appropriate intervals.

The possibility of pigmentary retinopathy, together with the possibility of cardiotoxic reactions, emphasises the need not to increase doses beyond the recommended maximum daily dose of 600 mg. Extra-pyramidal reactions may occur but are uncommon within the recommended dosage range; antiparkinsonian agents are therefore rarely required and should be prescribed with caution. Whenever an antipsychotic agent is used, the possible risk of development of tardive dyskinesia should be considered, and the patient monitored for early signs. With Melleril the risk is less than with other phenothiazines, and tardive dyskinesia tends to be seen particularly with prolonged treatment at high doses. The potential seriousness and unpredictability of tardive dyskinesia and the fact that it has occasionally been reported to occur when neuroleptic antipsychotic drugs have been prescribed for relatively short periods in low dosage means that the prescribing of such agents requires especially careful assessment of risks versus benefit. Tardive dyskinesia can be precipitated or aggravated by antiparkinsonian drugs. Short lived dyskinesias may occur after abrupt drug withdrawal.

Antipsychotic drugs such as Melleril may cause hyperprolactinaemia resulting in galactorrhoea and oligo- and amenorrhoea. Sexual function, including erection and ejaculation may be impaired. Weight gain is occasionally seen with Melleril and oedema has been reported. These effects may be prevented by reduction in dosage.

Blood dyscrasias have been reported: transient leucopenia can occur and agranulocytosis has been reported very rarely, most commonly in the first three months of treatment, but occasionally later. Blood counts should be performed if a patient develops signs of persistent infection.

Melleril very rarely may cause a photosensitivity reaction. The critical dose for this to occur is 400 to 600 mg daily. Other rare side-effects include skin rashes, altered seizure control, jaundice, hepatitis and liver dysfunction.

Long-term usage at doses above the recommended maximum can very rarely cause increased melanin pigmentation of the skin, which may be irreversible. Although not reported with Melleril, phenothiazines have been reported to cause raised serum cholesterol, rarely hyperglycaemia, faecal impaction, severe paralytic ileus or megacolon.

Overdosage: Acute overdosage of Melleril usually gives rise to coma with shallow breathing, hypotension and absence of reflexes. Motor restlessness, hyperflexia, cardiac arrhythmias and epileptiform convulsions may occur. Treatment should be directed to the elimination of the ingested material by emesis and gastric lavage. General supportive measures should be applied with particular reference to the cardiovascular and respiratory systems.

Acute hypotension should be treated with plasma expanders. If treatment with a vasopressor (*not* adrenaline) proves necessary (as it might in resistant cases) careful monitoring of the patient, particularly of cardiac function, is indicated. Attention should be paid to symptoms of metabolic acidosis and delayed cardiac effects.

Pharmaceutical precautions Melleril Suspension should not be diluted with any of the usual diluents, but the two strengths may be admixed to give a dosage range of between 25 mg and 100 mg per 5 ml spoonful. If an electric stirrer is used, care should be taken to avoid the incorporation of air.

Melleril Syrup may be diluted with water, sorbitol solution (70%) or preservative free Syrup BP. Diluted Syrup should be used within 14 days of preparation.

Melleril should be protected from light.

Legal category POM.

Package quantities Melleril Suspension 25 mg in 5 ml and 100 mg in 5 ml: Bottles of 1 litre.
Melleril Syrup: Bottles of 100 ml and 500 ml.
Melleril Tablets
10 mg: Blister pack of 100 tablets (OP).
25 mg, 50 mg and 100 mg: Blister pack of 100 (OP) and containers of 1,000 tablets.

Further information Both strengths of Melleril Suspension contain 3.16 g of sucrose per 5 ml spoonful. Approximate calorific value – 13 kcals per 5 ml.

Melleril Syrup contains 2.25 g of sucrose per 5 ml spoonful. Approximate calorific value – 15 kcals per 5 ml.

Melleril Syrup does not contain hydroxybenzoate preservatives.

Product licence numbers

Suspension 25 mg/5 ml	0101/0052R
Suspension 100 mg/5 ml	0101/0053R
Syrup	0101/5034R
Tablets 10 mg	0101/5033R
Tablets 25 mg	0101/5053R
Tablets 50 mg	0101/5054R
Tablets 100 mg	0101/5055R

MIACALCIC*

Presentation clear, colourless parenteral solution of Salcatonin BP (synthetic salmon calcitonin), available as ampoules containing 50 IU in 1 ml or 100 IU in 1 ml and as multidose vials containing 400 IU in 2 ml (ie 200 IU in 1 ml).

Uses
Principal action: Calcitonin is a major regulating factor in mineral and skeletal metabolism; it interferes with the action of parathyroid hormone in the maintenance of skeletal mass, by acting both on the bone and on calcium homeostasis. It markedly reduces the removal of calcium from bone in conditions with a greatly increased rate of resportion and formation, such as Paget's disease and malignant osteolysis. Osteoclast activity is inhibited and osteoblast formation and activity seem to be stimulated. Calcitonin inhibits osteolysis, thus lowering the abnormally increased serum calcium. Additionally, it increases the urinary excretion of calcium, phosphorus and sodium by reducing their tubular re-uptake. Serum calcium is not reduced belore the normal range.

Calcitonin reduces gastric and exocrine pancreatic secretion, without influencing gastrointestinal motility. Clinical experience demonstrates that Miacalcic possesses analgesic activity. Investigations have shown specific salmon calcitonin binding sites in some areas of the central nervous system.

All calcitonin structures show 32 amino-acids in a single chain, the sequence of which differs from species to species. Due to its greater affinity to receptor binding sites than synthetic calcitonins from mammalian species, including the synthetic human calcitonin, Miacalcic is clinically more potent and longer acting.

Indications
Hypercalcaemic crisis:
–due to tumoral osteolysis secondary to breast, lung, kidney and other malignancies
–due to osteolysis induced by myeloma
–due to primary hyperparathyroidism
Short term treatment of chronic hypercalcaemia.

Paget's Disease of bone (osteitis deformans), particularly in cases with:
– bone pain
– neurological complications
–increased bone turnover reflected in elevated alkaline phosphatase and hydroxyproline excretion
–progressive extension of bone lesions
–incomplete or repeated fractures.

Pain associated with advanced metastatic bone cancer.

Dosage and administration Miacalcic may be administered subcutaneously, intramuscularly or by intravenous infusion. The solution provided in multidose vials contains phenol (5 mg/ml) as a preservative, and is not suitable for intravenous bolus injection.

Emergency treatment of hypercalcaemic crisis: Intravenous infusion is the most effective method of administration and should always be used in emergencies or severe cases. However, there is a loss of potency of approximately 20% when Miacalcic is diluted. This should be taken into account when calculating dosage.

5 to 10 IU Miacalcic per kg body weight daily, by slow intravenous infusion in 500 ml physiological saline over at least 6 hours.

Short term treatment of chronic hypercalcaemia: 5 to 10 IU per kg body weight daily by subcutaneous or intramuscular injection as a single dose or in two divided doses. If the volume for injection exceeds 2 ml intramuscular injection is preferable and multiple sites of injection should be used.

Treatment should be adjusted according to the patient's response and should not exceed three months; the definitive treatment should be for the underlying cause.

Paget's Disease: 100 IU daily by subcutaneous or intramuscular injection. In some cases the injections may be given only every second day. In particular after improvement of the objective and subjective symptoms, an injection of 50 IU per day may be sufficient. Clinical improvement is usually seen within three months but may occasionally be delayed for as long as a year.

Treatment should be limited to one course of six

months followed by a treatment free period. A new treatment course of six months can be resumed in the case of biochemical relapse.

Pain associated with advanced metastatic bone cancer: 200 IU, depending on tolerability, up to four times in 24 hours by either the subcutaneous or intramuscular route has been shown to be effective in some patients and to permit reduction in the case of concomitantly administered analgesics. Relief of pain may last for one week or longer. Treatment may be repeated at the discretion of the physician.

Use in children: There is very little experience with use in children. The recommended adult dose should be reduced according to the child's lower body weight.

Miacalcic should not be given to children for periods of more than a few weeks unless the physicians conclude that longer treatment is indicated on compelling grounds. Careful surveillance of bone growth is recommended.

Use in the elderly: There is no evidence to suggests that elderly patients require different dosages or show different side-effects from younger patients. However, elderly patients should be supervised as factors sometimes associated with ageing, such as poor diet or impaired renal function, may affect tolerance and may require dosage reduction.

Contra-indications, warnings, etc
Contra-indications: Hypersensitivity see 'Precautions'.

Use in pregnancy and lactation: Salmon calcitonin has been shown to cause a decrease in foetal birth weight in rabbits when given in doses of 14 to 56 times the dose recommended for human use. Since calcitonin does not cross the placental barrier this finding may be due to metabolic effects of calcitonin on the pregnant animal.

Studies have not been carried out in pregnant women. Whenever possible, treatment should be avoided in women of child-bearing potential. Calcitonin has been shown to inhibit lactation in animals and should not be administered to nursing mothers.

Precautions: Treatment with Miacalcic markedly reduces serum alkaline phosphatase and urinary hydroxyproline excretion, often to normal levels. In rare cases alkaline phosphatase and hydroxyproline excretion levels may rise after an initial fall; the physician must then judge from the clinical picture whether treatment should be continued. Disorders of bone metabolism may recur one or several months after treatment has been discontinued, necessitating a new course of Miacalcic.

Miacalcic is excreted mainly via the kidneys, therefore dosage adjustment may be required in patients with impaired renal function.

Antibodies to salmon calcitonin may develop in a few patients following prolonged therapy. Clinical efficacy, however, is usually not affected. Escape phenomena are sometimes observed following prolonged use but this is not necessarily related to the development of antibodies. Therapeutic response to Miacalcic may be restored after an interruption of treatment.

As Miacalcic is a polypeptide, local or general hypersensitivity reactions are a possibility in rare cases. Symptoms may include local effects at the injection site or generalised skin reactions. Isolated anaphylactic-type reactions resulting in tachycardia, dyspnoea, hypotension and collapse have been reported. If any symptoms observed can definitely be ascribed to the drug, the treatment should be stopped.

In patients with a history of allergic reactions, a skin sensitivity test is advisable before starting treatment. A 1:100 dilution in physiological saline may be used.

Following injections of calcitonin, serum calcium levels may be transiently lowered but usually stay within normal values. This effect is noted most frequently on initiation of therapy where bone turnover is abnormally high, but diminishes as osteoclastic activity is reduced with Miacalcic. This phenomenon does not usually give rise to complications. It is theoretically possible that dosage adjustments may be required in patients receiving concurrent cardiac glycosides as their effect might be modified by changes in cellular electrolyte concentrations.

Side-effects: Nausea and occasional vomiting, slight facial flushing accompanied by a sensation of heat.

Occasional irritation at injection site, skin rash, diarrhoea and dizziness have occurred. Effects are usually dose dependent and occur more frequently after intravenous than after subcutaneous or intramuscular administration. They usually subside spontaneously and a temporary reduction in dosage is only necessary in exceptional cases.

Anti-emetics may be used if necessary during treatment.

Hypersensitivity reactions may occur. (See 'Precautions').

Overdosage: No serious consequences due to overdosage have yet been reported. Treatment would be symptomatic.

Pharmaceutical precautions The ampoules should be stored under refrigeration at a temperature between 2° and 8°C; it should not be allowed to freeze.

Solutions for infusion should be prepared immediately before use and glass or hard plastic containers should not be used.

Allow to reach room temperature before intramuscular or subcutaneous use. Once in use the 400 IU multidose vial may be stored at room temperature for up to one month.

Discard unused portion of contents after one month.

Legal category POM.

Package quantities *50 IU and 100 IU:* Boxes of 5 × 1 ml ampoules
400 IU multidose vials: Boxes of 1 × 2 ml and 5 × 2 ml multidose vials

Further information Pharmacokinetic studies indicate the bioavailability after intramuscular or subcutaneous injection to be about 70%. Maximum plasma concentrations are obtained within one hour. Elimination half-life of 70 to 90 minutes. Miacalcic and its metabolites are excreted up to 95% by the kidney, percentage of parent drug being about 2%. The apparent volume of distribution is 0.15–0.3 litre/kg and the protein binding is 30–40%.

Product licence numbers
50 IU in 1 ml 0101/0202
100 IU in 1 ml 0101/0095R
400 IU in 2 ml 0101/0203

PARLODEL*

Presentation
1 mg tablets: White, round, flat, bevel-edged Bromocriptine Mesylate Tablets BP, impressed PARLODEL 1 on one side and scored on the reverse. The tablets are 8 mm in diameter, with a nominal weight of 180 mg, and provide the equivalent of 1 mg bromocriptine base.

2.5 mg tablets: White, round, flat, bevel-edged Bromocriptine Mesylate Tablets BP, impressed PARLODEL 2.5 on one side and scored on the reverse. The tablets are 7 mm in diameter, with a nominal weight of 140 mg, and provide the equivalent of 2.5 mg bromocriptine base.

5 mg capsules: Opaque, hard gelatin Bromocriptine Mesylate Capsules BP. The capsules are size 3, upper part powder blue, lower part white, printed PARLODEL 5 in red and provide the equivalent of 5 mg bromocriptine base.

10 mg capsules: Opaque, hard gelatin Bromocriptine Mesylate Capsules BP. The capsules are size 1, white, printed PARLODEL 10 in red and provide the equivalent of 10 mg bromocriptine base.

Uses *Principal action:* Parlodel is a dopaminergic-receptor stimulant or dopamine agonist. This pharmacological action is manifest in normal individuals and those with hyperprolactinaemic states by an inhibition of the secretion of prolactin by the pituitary; in many acromegalic patients a lowering of elevated circulating growth hormone levels results.

In patients with prolactin secreting adenomas there is

radiological evidence to indicate tumour regression in some cases. Improvement in visual field defects and in general anterior pituitary function may also occur.

Because of its dopaminergic activity Parlodel is also effective in idiopathic Parkinson's disease, which is characterised by a specific nigro-striatal dopamine deficiency.

Indications: The inhibition or suppression of puerperal lactation for medical reasons.

The treatment of hyperprolactinaemia in men and women with hypogonadism and/or galactorrhoea.

The treatment of hyperprolactinaemic infertility.

Parlodel has been used successfully in the treatment of a number of infertile women who do not have demonstrable hyperprolactinaemia.

In a number of specialized units, patients who have been shown to have prolactin secreting adenomas have been treated successfully with Parlodel.

In particular Parlodel can be considered as a first choice of treatment in patients with macroadenomas and as an alternative to the surgical procedure, transsphenoidal hypophysectomy, in patients with microadenomas.

The treatment of cyclical benign breast disease/cyclical pronounced mastalgia.

Cyclical menstrual disorders have also responded to Parlodel, particularly breast symptomatology, but, in the premenstrual syndrome there is also some evidence that other symptoms, such as headache, mood changes and bloatedness, may be alleviated.

Parlodel has been used in a number of specialized units, as an adjunct to surgery and/or radiotherapy, to reduce circulating growth hormone levels in the management of acromegalic patients.

In the treatment of idiopathic Parkinson's disease, Parlodel has been used both alone and in combination with levodopa in the management of previously untreated patients and those disabled by 'on-off' phenomena. Parlodel has been used with occasional benefit in patients who do not respond to, or are unable to tolerate, levodopa and those whose response to levodopa is declining.

Dosage and administration Parlodel should always be taken during a meal.

A number of disparate conditions are amenable to treatment with Parlodel, and for this reason, the recommended dosage regimens are variable. In most indications, irrespective of the final dosage, the optimum response with the minimum of side-effects is best achieved by gradual introduction of Parlodel. The following scheme is suggested:

Initially 1 mg to 1.25 mg at bedtime, increasing after 2 to 3 days to 2 mg to 2.5 mg at bedtime. Dosage may then be increased by 1 mg to 2.5 mg at 2 to 3 day intervals, until a dosage of 2.5 mg twice daily is achieved. Further dosage increments, if necessary, should be added in a similar manner.

Prevention of lactation: 2.5 mg on the day of delivery, followed by 2.5 mg twice daily for 14 days. Gradual introduction of Parlodel is not necessary in this indication.

Suppression of lactation: 2.5 mg on the first day, increasing after 2 to 3 days to 2.5 mg twice daily for 14 days. Gradual introduction of Parlodel is not necessary in this indication.

Hypogonadism/galactorrhoea syndromes/infertility: Introduce Parlodel gradually according to the suggested scheme.

Most patients with hyperprolactinaemia have responded to 7.5 mg daily, in divided doses, but doses of up to 30 mg daily have been used. In infertile patients without demonstrably elevated serum prolactin levels, the usual dosage is 2.5 mg twice daily.

Prolactinomas: Introduce Parlodel gradually according to the suggested scheme. Dosage may then be increased by 2.5 mg daily at 2 to 3 day intervals as follows: 2.5 mg eight-hourly, 2.5 mg six-hourly, 5 mg six-hourly. Patients have responded to doses of up to 30 mg daily.

Cyclical benign breast disease/cyclical pronounced mastalgia/cyclical menstrual disorders: Introduce Parlodel gradually, according to the suggested scheme, until the recommended dosage of 2.5 mg twice daily is reached.

Acromegaly: Introduce Parlodel gradually, according to the suggested scheme. Dosage may then be increased by 2.5 mg daily at 2 to 3 day intervals as follows: 2.5 mg eight-hourly, 2.5 mg six-hourly, 5 mg six-hourly.

Parkinson's disease: Introduce Parlodel gradually, as follows: Week 1: 1 mg to 1.25 mg at bed time. Week 2: 2 mg to 2.5 mg at bed time. Week 3: 2.5 mg twice daily. Week 4: 2.5 mg three times daily. Thereafter, take three times a day increasing by 2.5 mg every 3 to 14 days depending on the patient's response. Continue until the optimum dose is reached. This will usually be between 10 and 40 mg daily. In patients already receiving levodopa the dosage of this drug may be gradually decreased, while the dosage of Parlodel is increased until the optimum balance is determined.

Use in children: Administration of Parlodel is not appropriate for children less than 15 years old.

Use in the elderly: There is no clinical evidence that Parlodel poses a special risk to the elderly.

Contra-indications, warnings, etc

Contra-indications: Hypersensitivity to bromocriptine or other ergot alkaloids. Toxaemia of pregnancy, hypertension post-partum or in the puerperium. For procedure during pregnancy see 'Use in pregnancy'.

Precautions: Hyperprolactinaemia may be idiopathic, drug-induced, or due to hypothalamic or pituitary disease. The possibility that hyperprolactinaemic patients may have a pituitary tumour should be recognised and complete investigation at specialized units to identify such patients is advisable. Parlodel will effectively lower prolactin levels in patients with pituitary tumours but does not obviate the necessity for radiotherapy or surgical intervention where appropriate in acromegaly.

In women suffering from prolactin-related fertility disorders, treatment with Parlodel results in ovulation. Patients who do not wish to conceive should be advised to practice a reliable method of contraception. Oral contraceptives have, however, been reported to increase serum prolactin levels. When women of child-bearing age are treated with Parlodel for conditions not associated with hyperprolactinaemia the lowest effective dose should be used. This is in order to avoid suppression of prolactin to below normal levels, with consequent impairment of luteal function.

Gynaecological assessment, preferably including cervical and endometrial cytology, is recommended for women receiving Parlodel for extensive periods. Six-monthly assessment is suggested for post-menopausal women and annual assessment for women with regular menstruation.

Hypotensive reactions may be disturbing in some patients during the first few days of treatment and particular care should be exercised when driving vehicles or operating machinery.

Tolerance to Parlodel may be reduced by alcohol.

The concomitant use of erythromycin may increase bromocriptine plasma levels.

In acromegalic patients, whilst Parlodel may effectively lower growth hormone levels, treatment to limit expansion of the tumour is also indicated. Acromegalic patients should be carefully assessed for peptic ulceration prior to treatment with Parlodel and advised to report gastro-intestinal side-effects promptly, as gastro-intestinal bleeding has been reported, though the connection with treatment is not proven.

Caution is required where Parlodel is being given in high doses to patients with a history of psychotic disorders or severe cardiovascular disease.

Among parkinsonian patients on long-term, high-dose Parlodel treatment, pleural effusions have been observed. Patients with unexplained pleuro-pulmonary signs or symptoms should be examined thoroughly and discontinuation of Parlodel therapy should be contemplated.

In a few patients treated for more than a year, with daily doses greater than 30 mg, retroperitoneal fibrosis has been reported. Patients on long-term, high-dose therapy should therefore be observed for manifestations of retroperitoneal fibrosis (e.g. back pain, oedema of the lower limbs or impaired kidney function) so that retroperitoneal fibrosis may be detected at an early stage. Parlodel should be withdrawn if fibrotic changes in the retroperitoneum are diagnosed or suspected.

Use in pregnancy: If pregnancy occurs it is generally advisable to withdraw Parlodel after the first missed menstrual period.

Rapid expansion of pituitary tumours sometimes occurs during pregnancy and this may also occur in patients who have been able to conceive as a result of Parlodel therapy. As a precautionary measure, patients should be monitored to detect signs of pituitary enlargement so that Parlodel may be reintroduced if necessary. Based on the outcome of more than 2,000 pregnancies, the use of Parlodel to restore fertility has not been associated with an increased risk of abortion, premature delivery, multiple pregnancy or malformation in infants. Because this accumulated evidence suggests a lack of teratogenic or embryopathic effect in humans, maintenance of Parlodel treatment during pregnancy may be considered where there is a large tumour or evidence of expansion.

Overdosage: Overdosage with Parlodel is likely to result in vomiting and other symptoms which could be due to over-stimulation of dopaminergic receptors and might include confusion, hallucinations and hypotension. General supportive measures should be undertaken to remove any unabsorbed material and maintain blood pressure if necessary.

Side-effects: Nausea is the most commonly occurring side-effect. Postural hypotension, dizziness, headache, vomiting, and mild constipation have also occasionally been reported. The occurrence of side-effects is minimised by taking Parlodel during a meal and by gradual introduction of the dose. If side-effects do occur, a reduction of dosage, followed in a few days by a more gradual increase, will ameliorate the symptoms.

Episodes of reversible pallor of the fingers and toes induced by cold have occasionally been reported to occur during prolonged treatment, particularly in patients previously exhibiting Raynaud's phenomenon. Drowsiness, and less frequently, confusion, psychomotor excitation, hallucinations, dyskinesia, dry mouth and leg cramps have been reported during high-dose treatment of Parkinson's disease with Parlodel. All these side-effects are dose-dependent and can usually be controlled by a reduction in dosage and a more gradual implementation of dosage increments.

In extremely rare cases (in post partum women treated with Parlodel for the prevention of lactation) serious adverse events including hypertension, myocardial infarction, seizures, stroke, or mental disorders, have been reported although the causal relationship is uncertain. In some patients the occurrence of seizures or stroke was preceded by severe headache and/or visual disturbances.

Pharmaceutical precautions Protect from light.

Legal category POM.

Package quantities 1 mg Tablets: Containers of 100 (OP).
2.5 mg Tablets: Blister pack of 30 (OP) and containers of 100 (OP) and 500.
5 mg Capsules: Containers of 100 (OP).
10 mg Capsules: Containers of 100 (OP).

Further information Nil.

Product licence numbers

1 mg Tablets	0101/0176
2.5 mg Tablets	0101/0061
5 mg Capsules	0101/0131
10 mg Capsules	0101/0108

PHOSPHATE-SANDOZ*

Presentation Flat, round, white, effervescent tablets with a rough surface, weight 3.7 g, 25.4 mm diameter and 4.4 to 4.9 mm thick. Citrus flavoured. Each effervescent tablet contains 1.936 g Anhydrous Sodium Acid Phosphate BP, 350 mg Sodium Bicarbonate PhEur and 315 mg Potassium Bicarbonate BPC. This provides the equivalent of 500 mg elemental phosphorus (16.1 mmol phosphate), 468.8 mg sodium (20.4 mmol: 20.4 mEq Na^+), 123 mg potassium (3.1 mmol: 3.1 mEq K^+), also 800 mg anhydrous citric acid (787.4 mg citrate ion).

Uses *Principal action:* Oral administration of inorganic phosphates produces a fall in serum calcium in patients with hypercalcaemia. The main effect of oral phosphate in hypercalcaemia is to bind calcium in the gut thus reducing absorption.

High-dose phosphate supplement.

Indications: Hypercalcaemia associated with such conditions as hyperparathyroidism, multiple myelomatosis and malignancy. Hypophosphataemia associated with vitamin D resistant rickets and vitamin D resistant hypophosphataemic osteomalacia.

Dosage and administration Phosphate-Sandoz Effervescent Tablets should be dissolved in $\frac{1}{3}$ to $\frac{1}{2}$ a tumblerful of water.

Dosage should be adjusted to suit the requirements of individual patients. Excessive dosage has been reported to produce hypocalcaemia in isolated cases. Particular care should therefore be taken to ensure appropriate dosage in the elderly.

Adults
Hypercalcaemia: Up to 6 tablets daily (adjustment being made according to requirements).
Vitamin D resistant hypophosphataemic osteomalacia: 4 to 6 tablets daily.

Children under 5 years
Hypercalcaemia: Up to 3 tablets daily (adjustment being made according to requirements).
Vitamin D resistant rickets: 2 to 3 tablets daily.

Contra-indications, warnings, etc
Precautions: In cases of impaired renal function associated with hypercalcaemia and in cases where restricted sodium intake is required, e.g. congestive cardiac failure, hypertension or pre-eclamptic toxaemia, the sodium (20.4 mmol per tablet) and potassium (3.1 mmol per tablet) content of Phosphate-Sandoz should be taken into consideration. In cases of hypercalcaemia associated with impaired renal function and hyperphosphataemia, the main effect of oral phosphate is to bind calcium in the gut and thus reduce calcium absorption. The effect of oral phosphate on serum phosphate is likely to be minimal, but close monitoring of serum levels is recommended.

Concurrent administration of antacids, containing agents such as aluminium hydroxide, may result in displacement of calcium from binding to oral phosphate, thus reducing efficacy.

Soft-tissue calcification and nephrocalcinosis have been reported in isolated cases following intravenous therapy with phosphate. This is thought to be a function of dosage and rapidity of phosphate administration. While such effects appear less likely to occur following treatment with oral phosphates, careful surveillance of patients is recommended, especially if on long-term therapy.

Use in pregnancy: The safety of Phosphate-Sandoz in human pregnancy has not been formally studied, but no clinical problems have been encountered during pregnancy or lactation. Nevertheless, the benefit of treatment should be considered in relation to the risks before Phosphate-Sandoz is given to pregnant or nursing women.

Side-effects: Apart from gastro-intestinal upsets, nausea and diarrhoea, very few side-effects have been reported.

Overdosage: Excessive dosage has been reported to produce hypocalcaemia in isolated cases. This has proved reversible when dosage has been adjusted.

Pharmaceutical precautions Protect from heat and moisture. Since Phosphate-Sandoz Tablets are hygroscopic they should be dispensed in their original containers.

Legal category GSL.

Package quantities Boxes of 100 (5 tubes of 20 effervescent tablets).

Further information Phosphate-Sandoz Tablets each contain 136 mg sucrose. Approximate calorific value – 3 kcals per tablet.

Product licence number 0101/5038R

SANDIMMUN*

Presentation
Soft gelatin capsules
25 mg Capsules: Pale-pink, oval capsules, 7.4 mm in diameter and 11.3 mm in length, containing 25 mg cyclosporin.
100 mg Capsules: Dusky-pink, oblong capsules 8.7 mm in diameter and 24.9 mm in length, containing 100 mg cyclosporin.
Oral solution: Clear, yellow, oily solution containing 100 mg cyclosporin per ml.
Concentrate for intravenous infusion: Each ml of concentrate contains 50 mg cyclosporin in a clear, brown-yellow, oily solution containing 650 mg polyethoxylated castor oil and 33% ethanol by volume. Sandimmun concentrate is available in 1 ml (50 mg) and 5 ml (250 mg) ampoules.

Uses *Principal action:* Cyclosporin is a cyclic polypeptide consisting of 11 amino acids. It is a potent immunosuppressive agent which prolongs survival of allogeneic transplants involving skin, heart, kidney, pancreas, bone marrow, cornea, small intestine and lung in animals. Successful solid organ and bone marrow allogeneic transplants have been performed in man using cyclosporin to prevent and treat rejection and graft-versus-host disease.

Studies in animals suggest that cyclosporin inhibits the development of cell-mediated reactions. It appears to block the resting lymphocytes in the G_0 or early G_1 phase of the cell cycle and also inhibits lymphokine production and release, including interleukin 2 (T cell growth factor, TCGF). The available evidence suggests that cyclosporin acts specifically and reversibly on lymphocytes. It does not depress haemopoiesis and has no effect on the function of phagocytic cells.

Indications
Organ transplantation: Prevention of graft rejection following kidney, liver, pancreas, heart or heart-lung transplantation.

Treatment of transplant rejection in patients previously receiving other immunosuppressive agents.

Bone marrow transplantation: Prevention of graft rejection following bone marrow transplantation and prophylaxis of graft-versus-host disease.

Treatment of established graft-versus-host disease.

Dosage and administration
Organ transplantation: Initially, a single oral dose of 14 to 17.5 mg/kg body weight, should be given 4 to 12 hours before transplantation. As a general rule, treatment should continue at a dosage of 14 to 17.5 mg/kg/day for one to two weeks post-operatively. Dosage should then be reduced by about 2 mg/kg/day at monthly intervals until a maintenance dose of 6 to 8 mg/kg/day is reached. Dosage may be adjusted by monitoring cyclosporin blood levels (see 'Further Information'). When Sandimmun is given with corticosteroids, some patients will require doses lower than 5 mg/kg/day as early as one month post-transplant.

The total daily dosage of Sandimmun Capsules or Oral Solution may be given as a single dose or in two divided doses. If the taste of the Oral Solution needs to be masked the solution may be diluted with milk, chocolate drink or fruit juice immediately before being taken.

The Concentrate for intravenous infusion may be used during episodes of gastrointestinal disturbance when absorption of the oral forms might be impaired. It can also be used to initiate Sandimmun therapy but it is recommended that patients be transferred to oral therapy as soon as possible after surgery.

Sandimmun Concentrate should be diluted 1:20 to 1:100 with physiological saline or 5% dextrose before use. The recommended dosage is one third of the previously administered oral dose (3 to 5 mg/kg/day if initiating therapy), given by slow intravenous infusion over 2 to 6 hours.

Bone marrow transplantation/Prevention of graft-versus-host disease (GVHD): Sandimmun Concentrate for intravenous infusion is usually preferred for initiation of therapy, although the oral forms may be used. The recommended dosage by the intravenous route is 3 to 5 mg/kg/day, starting on the day before transplantation and continuing during the immediate post-transplant period of up to two weeks until oral maintenance therapy begins. The Concentrate should be diluted 1:20 to 1:100 with physiological saline or 5% dextrose before use and should be given by slow intravenous infusion over about 2 to 6 hours.

Treatment with Sandimmun should continue using the oral forms at a dosage of 12.5 mg/kg/day for at least three and preferably six months before tailing off to zero, although dosages of up to 25 mg/kg/day have been used. In some cases it may not be possible to withdraw Sandimmun therapy until a year after bone marrow transplantation. If GVHD develops after Sandimmun is withdrawn it should respond to reinstitution of therapy. Low doses should be used for mild, chronic GVHD.

The total daily dosage of Sandimmun Capsules or Oral Solution may be given as a single dose or in two divided doses. If the taste of the Oral Solution needs to be masked the Solution may be diluted with milk, chocolate drink or fruit juice immediately before being taken.

If Sandimmun Capsules or Oral Solution are used to initiate therapy, the recommended dosage is 12.5 to 25 mg/kg/day for about 5 days.

Sandimmun Concentrate for intravenous infusion may be used for maintenance therapy during episodes of gastrointestinal disturbance where absorption of the oral forms might be impaired or where a patient is unable to tolerate the oral preparation. One third of the previously administered oral dose should be given.

Use in the elderly: The indications for Sandimmun make it unlikely that it will be used in elderly patients. Experience in the elderly is, therefore, limited but no particular problems have been reported following the use of the drug at the recommended dose.

Note: Experience with Sandimmun in young children is still limited. Children from three months of age have received the drug at the recommended dosage with no particular problems although at dosages at the upper end of the recommended range, and above, children seem to be more susceptible to fluid retention, convulsions and hypertension. This responds to dosage reduction.

Contra-indications, warnings, etc
Contra-indications: Known hypersensitivity to cyclosporin. Sandimmun concentrate for intravenous infusion should not be used in patients known to be hypersensitive to polyethoxylated castor oils.

Precautions: The concentrate for intravenous infusion contains polyethoxylated castor oil, which has been reported to cause anaphylactoid reactions. Sandimmun should not be administered with other immunosuppressive agents except corticosteroids. Oversuppression can lead to increased susceptibility to infection and the possible development of lymphoma.

Sandimmun may affect liver and kidney function (*see* 'Side-effects'). Close monitoring of serum creatinine, urea, bilirubin and liver enzymes is required and dosage adjustments may be necessary.

A machine perfusion time of more than 24 hours and a reanastomosis time of more than 45 minutes can have a significant effect on renal graft function in Sandimmun treated patients. Both factors appear to enhance the nephrotoxic effect of Sandimmun.

Care should be taken using Sandimmun with systemic

antibiotics or other compounds which are known to have nephrotoxic effects, e.g. aminoglycosides, amphotericin B. The trimethoprim component of co-trimoxazole, given together with Sandimmun may cause a reversible deterioration in renal function.

Ketoconazole, an antifungal agent, has been reported to increase the plasma concentration of cyclosporin. Phenytoin, rifampicin and isoniazid have been reported to decrease serum and blood cyclosporin levels. Intravenous (but not oral) administration of sulphadimidine and trimethoprim has also resulted in a marked reduction of serum cyclosporin levels. Concomitant administration of such drugs with Sandimmun should therefore be avoided. Where combined administration is unavoidable, careful monitoring of cyclosporin blood levels and adjustment of Sandimmun dosage are essential.

Cyclosporin is not teratogenic in animals. As the safety of Sandimmun in human pregnancy has not been fully established it should, therefore, only be used in pregnancy if the benefit outweighs any potential risks.

Cyclosporin passes into the breast milk and mothers receiving treatment with Sandimmun should not, therefore, breast feed their infants.

Side-effects: Side-effects are usually mild to moderate and usually respond to dosage reduction.

The most frequently observed side-effects in organ transplant patients are hypertrichosis, tremor, impaired renal function, hepatic dysfunction, gingival hypertrophy and gastrointestinal disturbances (anorexia, nausea, vomiting). Hyperkalaemia can occur during Sandimmun therapy. It can be treated successfully and has also disappeared spontaneously.

Hypertension has been observed in most heart transplant patients treated with Sandimmun. In renal transplant recipients there is very little difference in the incidence of hypertension between Sandimmun treated and conventionally treated patients.

The most frequently observed side-effects in bone marrow transplant patients are tremor, gastrointestinal disturbances (anorexia, nausea and vomiting), impaired renal function and hypertrichosis. Facial oedema has also been observed. Infrequently, a combination of hypertension, fluid retention and convulsions has occurred, mainly in children.

A dose-dependent and reversible increase in serum creatinine and urea is the most frequent and potentially the most serious complication of Sandimmun therapy. In about one-quarter of patients, reversible impairment of renal function has been observed; this is generally responsive to dosage reduction. Sandimmun may also cause increases in serum bilirubin and liver enzymes and these changes also appear to be dose dependent and reversible.

A subjective burning sensation may occur in the hands and feet usually in the first week of oral administration.

Overdosage: Little experience is available with overdosage. Symptomatic treatment and general supportive measures should be followed in all cases of overdosage. Forced emesis could be of value within the first few hours after intake. Signs of nephrotoxicity might occur which would be expected to resolve following drug withdrawal. Sandimmun is not dialysable to any great extent nor is it well cleared by charcoal haemoperfusion. Hypertension and convulsions have been reported in some patients receiving Sandimmun therapy at dosages above the recommended range and in others with high trough blood levels of cyclosporin. This might, therefore, be expected as a feature of overdosage.

Pharmaceutical precautions Sandimmun Capsules should be left in the blister-pack until required for use. They should not be stored at temperatures above 25°C.

Refrigeration of Sandimmun Oral Solution is not recommended as this may result in precipitation. It should be used within 2 months of opening the bottle.

The polyethoxylated castor oil contained in the Concentrate for intravenous infusion can cause phthalate stripping from PVC. Once an ampoule is opened the contents should be used immediately.

Legal category POM.

Package quantities
Soft Gelatin Capsules (25 mg and 100 mg): Boxes of 30 (OP).
Oral Solution: Bottles of 50 ml (OP).
Concentrate for infusion: Boxes of 10 × 5 ml ampoules. Boxes of 10 × 1 ml ampoules

Further information Sandimmun therapy requires careful monitoring and follow up and the drug should only be used in units with experience of immunosuppressive therapy and organ and bone marrow transplantation where adequate equipment, laboratory and supportive medical resources are available.

A radioimmunoassay kit is available for determining blood cyclosporin levels.

Product licence numbers

25 mg Soft Gelatin Capsules	0101/0207
100 mg Soft Gelatin Capsules	0101/0208
Oral Solution	0101/0124
Concentrate for infusion	0101/0153

SANDOCAL* CALCIUM-SANDOZ*

Presentation
Sandocal 400: White, round, flat-faced, effervescent tablets with a slightly rough surface, weighing 2.92 g, 25 mm diameter and 4.35 mm thick, citrus flavoured. Each effervescent tablet contains 930 mg calcium lactate gluconate and 700 mg calcium carbonate and provides 400 mg calcium (10 mmol: 20 mEq Ca^{++}), and 1.189 g anhydrous citric acid.

Sandocal 1000: White, round, flat-faced effervescent tablets with a slightly rough surface, weighing 7.30 g, 33 mm diameter and 6.4 mm thick, citrus flavoured. Each effervescent tablet contains 2.327 g calcium lactate gluconate, 1.75 g calcium carbonate and provides 1 g calcium (25 mmol: 50 mEq Ca^{++}), 2.973 g anhydrous citric acid.

Calcium-Sandoz Syrup: Colourless to pale straw coloured, fruit flavoured syrup. Each 15 ml contains 3.27 g calcium glubionate and 2.17 g calcium lactobionate. Three 5 ml spoonfuls provide 325 mg calcium (8.1 mmol: 16.2 mEq Ca^{++}).

Uses
Principal action: Calcium is an essential body electrolyte. It is involved in the maintenance of normal muscle and nerve function, is essential for normal cardiac function and is essential to blood coagulation. There is a dynamic equilibrium between the calcium in blood and that in the skeleton. Homeostasis is mainly regulated by parathyroid hormone, by calcitonin and by vitamin D.

Indications

1. As an adjunct to conventional therapy in the arrest or slowing down of bone demineralisation in osteoporosis.
2. In the arrest or slowing down of bone demineralisation in osteoporosis where other effective treatment is contra-indicated.
3. As a supplemental source of calcium in the correction of dietary deficiencies or when normal requirements are high.
4. Calcium-Sandoz syrup is indicated for the treatment of neonatal hypocalcaemia.

Signs of hypocalcaemia may occur when the serum calcium concentration falls below 2.25 mmol per litre (or 4.5 mEq per litre). Symptoms may include paraesthesia, laryngospasm, muscle cramps, increased muscle excitability leading to tetany, prolongation of the Q-T interval on the ECG, convulsions and mental changes (e.g. anxiety, depression, delusions). Also ectodermal changes including loss of hair, grooved and brittle fingernails, defects of dental enamel and fungal infections, typically generalised candidiasis.

Dosage and administration In health the concentration of calcium in serum is maintained close to 2.5 mmol per litre (normal range 2.25–2.75 mmol or 4.5–5.5 mEq per litre). Treatment or therapeutic supplementation should aim to restore or maintain this level.

Effervescent tablets must be dissolved in ⅓ to ½ tumbler full of water.

Indication	*Daily Dose Tablets Sandocal 400*	*Sandocal 1000*	*Syrup (5 ml spoonfuls)*
Adults			
Osteoporosis	3–4	1–2	11–15
Therapeutic supplement (dose dependent upon severity)	1–4	1–2	3–15
Children			
Calcium deficiency	1–2	1	6–9
Dietary supplementation	1	—	2–6
Neonatal hypocalcaemia	108 mg (5 ml of syrup) four hourly mixed with milk feed.		

For the acute state of neonatal hypocalcaemia parenteral calcium may be used (see further information).

Use in the elderly: No evidence exists that tolerance of Sandocal 400, Sandocal 1000 or Calcium-Sandoz is directly affected by advanced age; however, elderly patients should be supervised as factors sometimes associated with ageing, such as poor diet or impaired renal function, may indirectly affect tolerance and may require dosage reduction.

Contra-indications, warnings, etc
Contra-indications: Hypercalcaemia (e.g. in hyperparathyroidism, vitamin D overdosage, decalcifying tumours such as plasmocytoma, severe renal failure, bone metastases), severe hypercalciuria, and renal calculi.

Due to its galactose component Calcium-Sandoz syrup should not be given to patients with galactosaemia.

Precautions: In mild hypercalciuria (exceeding 300 mg (7.5 mmol)/24 hours) or renal failure, or where there is evidence of stone formation in the urinary tract, adequate checks must be kept on urinary calcium excretion; if necessary the dosage should be reduced or calcium therapy discontinued. High vitamin D intake should be avoided during calcium therapy, unless especially indicated.

Thiazide diuretics reduce urinary calcium excretion so the risk of hypercalcaemia should be considered.

Oral calcium supplementation is aimed at restoring normal serum calcium levels. Although it is extremely unlikely that high enough levels will be achieved to adversely affect digitalised patients, this theoretical possibility should be considered.

The sugar content of Calcium-Sandoz syrup should be taken into account in diabetic patients.

Oral calcium administration may reduce the absorption of oral tetracycline or fluoride preparations. An interval of 3 hours should be observed if the two are to be given.

Use in pregnancy and lactation: The likelihood of hypercalcaemia is increased in pregnant women in whom calcium and vitamin D are co-administered. Epidemiological studies with calcium have shown no increase in the teratogenic hazard to the foetus if used in the doses recommended. Although supplemental calcium may be excreted in breast milk, the concentration is unlikely to be sufficient to produce any adverse effect on the neonate.

Side-effects: Mild gastrointestinal disturbances have occurred rarely (e.g. constipation, diarrhoea). Although hypercalcaemia would not be expected in patients unless their renal function were impaired, the following symptoms could indicate the possibility of hypercalcaemia: nausea, vomiting, anorexia, constipation, abdominal pain, bone pain, thirst, polyuria, muscle weakness, drowsiness or confusion.

Overdosage: The amount of calcium absorbed following overdosage with Sandocal 400, Sandocal 1000 or Calcium-Sandoz Syrup will depend on the individual's calcium status. Deliberate overdosage is unlikely with effervescent preparations and acute overdosage has not been reported. It might cause gastrointestinal disturbances but would not be expected to cause hypercalcaemia except in patients treated with excessive doses of vitamin D. Treatment should be aimed at lowering serum calcium levels, e.g. administration of oral phosphates.

Pharmaceutical precautions Sandocal 400 and Sandocal 1000 tablets must be stored in a cool, dry place.

Calcium-Sandoz Syrup may be diluted with Syrup BP; the diluted syrup should be used within 14 days.

Legal category P.

Package quantities
Sandocal 400 Effervescent Tablets: Boxes of 100 (5 tubes of 20).
Sandocal 1000 Effervescent Tablets: Boxes of 30 (3 tubes of 10).
Calcium-Sandoz Syrup: Bottles of 500 ml.

Further information Sandocal 400 and Sandocal 1000 contain aspartame as an artificial sweetener, so that the preparations are free from sucrose. There is no added sodium or potassium in the tablets.

Calcium-Sandoz Syrup contains 1.512 g sucrose per 5 ml (4.536 g sucrose per 15 ml dose). Approximate calorific value of 13 kcals per 5 ml (39 kcals per 15 ml dose).

If parenteral calcium administration is indicated Calcium-Sandoz Ampoules 10% may be used. Details are given on a separate data sheet.

Product licence numbers

Calcium-Sandoz Syrup	0101/5024R
Sandocal 400	0101/5043R
Sandocal 1000	0101/0205

SANDOGLOBULIN*

Presentation Freeze-dried substance for preparation of an intravenous solution of human normal immunoglobulin. Sodium chloride 0.9% w/v (physiological saline) for reconstitution.

Sandoglobulin is a polyvalent antibody preparation containing, in concentrated form, all the antibodies normally occurring in the donor pool. The distribution of IgG subclasses in the preparation corresponds closely to that found in normal plasma.

Sandoglobulin is available in three pack sizes: one containing 1 g protein, 1.67 g sucrose as stabiliser and a 33 ml bottle of saline; one containing 3 g protein, 5 g sucrose and a 100 ml bottle of saline; and one containing 6 g protein, 10 g sucrose and a 200 ml bottle of saline. It does not contain any preservative.

Uses *Principal actions:* Sandoglobulin contains intact immunoglobulin which possesses unchanged Fab and Fc functional activity. The anticomplementary activity of the preparation is only detectable at very low levels, but in the presence of an appropriate antigen it activates complement by the classical pathway.

The exact mechanism of action in idiopathic thrombocytopenic purpura remains to be elucidated. Changes have been shown to occur in the function of Fc receptors in mononuclear phagocytes, leading to a decreased binding affinity and prolonged clearance rates within the reticulo-endothelial system. It would appear that Sandoglobulin may block platelet removal by temporary competitive inhibition.

Indications: Replacement therapy for congenital agammaglobulinaemia and hypogammaglobulinaemia.

Treatment of idiopathic thrombocytopenic purpura.

Dosage and administration
Dosage: Replacement therapy for congenital agammaglobulinaemia and hypogammaglobulinaemia: 0.1 to 0.3 g/kg body weight every 2 to 4 weeks according to severity of clinical signs and symptoms.

Idiopathic thrombocytopenic purpura: 0.4 g/kg body

weight/day on 5 successive days. Maintenance doses of 0.4 g/kg body weight may be given as required in order to maintain platelet count.

Reconstitution: Prepare the solution immediately before use. Dissolve the contents of the bottle in sodium chloride 0.9% w/v (physiological saline) as follows:
1 g in 33 ml to produce a 3% solution.
3 g in 100 ml to produce a 3% solution.
6 g in 200 ml to produce a 3% solution.
1 g in 16.5 ml to produce a 6% solution.
3 g in 50 ml to produce a 6% solution.
6 g in 100 ml to produce a 6% solution.

After disinfecting the stoppers, use the transfer needle provided to connect the bottles of saline and Sandoglobulin. Invert the connected bottles to allow the saline to flow into the Sandoglobulin bottle. Discard the empty saline bottle and transfer needle. Turn the Sandoglobulin bottle to wet any undissolved substance. Avoid frothing and *do not shake the solution.* Sandoglobulin usually dissolves in a few minutes, but in exceptional cases may take up to 20 minutes. When reconstituted Sandoglobulin should appear as an opalescent solution devoid of any particulate matter.

Administration: Sandoglobulin is for intravenous use. Use only solutions at close to body temperature which contain no undissolved Sandoglobulin. The first infusion of Sandoglobulin should be of a 3% solution, infused at a rate not exceeding 10 to 20 drops per minute. This is because the first infusion of immunoglobulin, particularly in previously untreated agammaglobulinaemic patients, may lead to inflammatory side-effects as a result of the reaction between the antibodies administered and the free antigen in the blood and tissues of the recipient. After 15 minutes the rate of infusion may be increased to 20 to 30 drops per minute and, after 30 minutes, it may be further increased to 40 to 50 drops per minute. Subsequent infusions may be administered at a rate of 40 to 50 drops per minute. For repeated administration of high doses a 6% solution may be used. In this case the initial rate of infusion should again be 20 to 30 drops per minute, increasing after 15 minutes to a maximum of 50 drops per minute. Antihistamines may be administered to prevent inflammatory reactions in agammaglobulinaemic patients being treated for the first time.

Note: 20 drops = approximately 1 ml.

Use in the elderly: Since there is an increased susceptibility to left ventricular overload in the elderly, particular caution is required with infusion volumes and infusion rates.

Contra-indications, warnings, etc
Contra-indications: Like all blood products containing IgA, Sandoglobulin is contra-indicated in IgA deficient patients who have circulating antibodies to IgA as anaphylactoid reactions may occur.

Precautions: Live virus vaccines should not normally be given until three months after a dose of normal immunoglobulin injection. If a live virus vaccine has been given, Sandoglobulin should not be given for at least two weeks, except in special circumstances. The risk of transmission of infection, in particular non-A non-B hepatitis, by intravenous immunoglobulin preparations cannot be entirely excluded.

Side-effects: If the correct dosage and administration routine is followed (Dosage and Administration) severe adverse reactions rarely occur. Nevertheless, the patient should be closely monitored for signs of anaphylactoid reactions such as a sensation of pressure in the chest, hypotension and cyanosis. In such cases the infusion should be stopped until the symptoms have passed.

Delayed inflammatory reactions including headache, nausea, mild pyrexia, shivering and tachycardia are more likely to occur in agammaglobulinaemic and hypogammaglobulinaemic patients who have never received immunoglobulin substitution therapy before or who have not received therapy within the previous 8 weeks. These reactions usually occur 30 to 60 minutes after the start of the infusion and disappear after it has been completed.

Overdosage: An overdosage of Sandoglobulin has never been reported, but is unlikely to leave harmful effects either on blood circulation or on other body functions. The only consequence of an abnormally increased level of IgG is the accelerated catabolic rate of this protein.

High infusion rates may produce symptoms resembling shock.

Pharmaceutical precautions Sandoglobulin should be protected from light and stored at a temperature not exceeding 25°C.

Once the freeze-dried substance has been reconstituted it should be used without delay.

Do not shake the Sandoglobulin solution.

Any solution remaining after infusion must be discarded. Open bottles must not be used again because of the danger of bacterial contamination.

Infuse only solutions devoid of any undissolved particulate matter at close to body temperature.

Sodium chloride 0.9% w/v (physiological saline) should be used to reconstitute Sandoglobulin. No other compatibilities have yet been evaluated so due consideration should be given to the advisability of adding other intravenous fluids or medications to Sandoglobulin.

Legal category POM.

Package quantities 1 g pack including 33 ml saline and transfer needle. 3 g pack including 100 ml saline transfer needle and 6 g pack including 200 ml saline and transfer needle.

Further information Sandoglobulin is prepared by cold alcohol fractionation of pooled plasma from blood donors and contains at least 96% IgG.

Individual donor units of plasma are screened for hepatitis B surface antigen and for the presence of antibodies to human immunodeficiency virus (HIV) which, combined with careful donor selection, minimises the risk of viral transmission. To date, no new antigenic properties have been shown to be acquired during fractionation and sensitisation has not been recognised as a clinical problem even after repeated administration. At least 90% of the immunoglobulin is intact monomeric and dimeric (7S) IgG; the remainder consists of a small amount of polymeric IgG and traces of IgA, IgM and immunoglobulin fragments.

Product licence numbers

1 g pack	0101/0181
3 g pack	0101/0182
6 g pack	0101/0186

SANDO-K*

Presentation Flat, round, white, effervescent tablets with a slightly rough surface, weighing 2.4 g and of 22 mm diameter and 4.25 mm thickness. Salty taste. Each tablet contains 600 mg Potassium Chloride PhEur, 400 mg Potassium Bicarbonate BPC and 800 mg of anhydrous citric acid. This provides the equivalent of 470 mg potassium (12 mmol: 12 mEq K^+) and 285 mg chloride (8 mmol: 8 mEq Cl^-). Sodium content 2.6 mg (0.1 mmol: 0.1 mEq Na+).

Uses *Principal action:* Potassium is the major cation in intracellular fluid and is essential for carbohydrate metabolism, glycogen storage and protein synthesis. It is also involved in transmembrane potentials thereby having important effects on muscle.

The concentration of potassium in the plasma is usually maintained between 3.5–5 mmol/l. Signs of hypokalaemia may occur when the plasma concentration falls below 3.5 mmol/l. Signs of deficiency include vomiting, abdominal distention, paralytic ileus, muscular weakness, confusion, reduced reflexes, respiratory failure and cardiac arrythmias.

Administration of potassium salts may cause gastric irritancy, intestinal ulceration has been seen with enteric-coated and matrix-type solid dose form potassium supplements. Sando-K effervescent tablets when dissolved in water prevent such local concentration, thereby minimising irritation.

Indications: Prevention and treatment of hypokalaemic states such as those associated with:
(i) use of drugs which can induce potassium depletion, eg, frusemide, thiazide diuretics, corticosteroids, carbenoxolone and cardiac glycosides, especially in combination with diuretics;
(ii) potassium loss resulting from severe diarrhoea, vomiting or fistulas;
(iii) acid-base disturbances eg alkalosis, renal tubular acidosis, states in which there is aldosterone excess, Cushing's syndrome;
(iv) decreased intake of potassium eg malnutrition, alcoholism, some elderly patients with deficient diets;
(v) since Sando-K effervescent tablets contain Cl- they may be used in the treatment of hypokalaemia associated with hypochloraemic alkalosis.

Dosage and administration Sando-K Effervescent Tablets must be dissolved in $\frac{1}{3}$ to $\frac{1}{2}$ a tumblerful of water and may be taken with food if preferred.

Use in adults and children: Dosage is dependent upon the clinical conditions and diet of the patient, however the administration of 2 to 4 tablets daily (24 to 48 mmol K+) is likely to provide an adequate prophylactic or therapeutic dose in most patients. Large doses may be indicated in more severe hypokalaemic conditions when the dose should be regulated by the patient's response as determined by serum electrolyte levels and acid-base studies.

Dosage guidelines: A drop in serum potassium level of 1 mmol/l represents a loss of about 100–200 mmol of potassium from body stores. While serum potassium levels below 2 mmol/l may warrant intravenous replacement therapy, the following are approximate guidelines in less severe potassium depletion: For serum levels between 2–3 mmol/l, a maximum daily dose of 100–200 mmol K+ (8–16 tablets) and for serum levels between 3–4 mmol/l, a maximum daily dose of 50–100 mmol K+ (4–8 tablets) should be considered.

Use in the elderly: No evidence exists that elderly patients require different dosages or show different side-effects than younger patients. However, such patients should be carefully supervised as factors sometimes associated with ageing, such as poor diet or impaired renal function, may indirectly affect the dosage or tolerability.

Contra-indications, warnings, etc
Contra-indications and precautions: The use of Sando-K is contra-indicated in patients with severe renal impairment with oliguria, inadequately treated Addison's disease, hyperkalaemia from any cause, crush injuries and acute dehydration.

If co-administered with potassium-sparing diuretics and ACE-inhibitors, the risk of hyperkalaemia must be considered.

Use in pregnancy and lactation: No clinical problems have been encountered during pregnancy or lactation. Nevertheless, the benefit of treatment should be considered in relation to the risks before Sando-K is given to pregnant or nursing women.

Warning: Periodic evaluation of the patient's clinical status, serum electrolytes and the ECG should be carried out when replacement therapy is undertaken. This is particularly important in patients with cardiac disease and in those receiving digitalis. Care should be taken to avoid dosage in excess of requirements for patients with impaired renal function. Caution is also necessary in patients receiving potassium-sparing diuretics and ACE-inhibitors and in patients with myotonia congenita or severe haemolysis. In patients with acidosis, the acid-base balance should be monitored. In patients with hypertension, it should be remembered that correction of hypokalaemia may lower blood pressure.

Side-effects: Abdominal discomfort, diarrhoea, nausea and vomiting may occur. If there are any signs of gastric irritancy, Sando-K, in common with all other potassium salts, should be given with or after food. Gastric irritancy has occurred but this is rare since the tablets dissolve in water and are taken in solution thus preventing high local concentrations. Moderate hyperkalaemia may be asymptomatic. If suspected, reference to the section on overdosage is recommended.

Overdosage: Hyperkalaemia. Poisoning is usually minimal below 6.5 mmol/l but may be severe above 8 mmol/l. However, comparatively low doses may cause adverse effects when excretion is delayed as in renal insufficiency. The absolute toxicity is dependent on other electrolytes and acid-base levels.

Hyperkalaemic symptoms include paraesthesia of the extremities, listlessness, mental confusion, weakness, paralysis, hypotension, cardiac arrhythmias, heart block and cardiac arrest.

Hyperkalaemia is often asymptomatic. However, increasing serum potassium levels can be detected by changes in the ECG; initially the appearance of tall, peaked T waves, followed by a widening of the QRS complex blending into the abnormal T waves. P-wave voltage decreases and the PR interval is prolonged.

Severe cardiac toxicity may be treated with calcium gluconate (10–20 ml of a 10% injection given over 1–5 minutes with ECG monitoring). The effect may be transient and the injection may need to be repeated.

Raised serum potassium levels respond to administration of dextrose (300–500 ml/hr of 10 or 25% solution), dextrose and insulin (as for dextrose with 10 units of insulin per 20 g dextrose), or sodium bicarbonate solution.

Cation exchange resins may be used, or in severe cases peritoneal dialysis or haemodialysis may be necessary.

Caution should be exercised in patients who are digitalised and who may experience acute digitalis intoxication in the course of potassium removal.

Pharmaceutical precautions Store in a cool dry place. Sando-K Effervescent Tablets are hygroscopic and should be dispensed in their original containers.

Legal category P.

Package quantities Boxes of 100 (5 × 20 effervescent tablets).

Further information Sando-K Tablets each contain 521.5 mg sucrose. Approximate calorific value – 4 kcals per tablet.

Product licence number 0101/5044R.

SANDOSTATIN* ▼

Presentation
Clear, colourless solution of octreotide acetate, available as ampoules and multidose vials. Ampoules provide 50 micrograms octreotide per ml, 100 micrograms octreotide per ml and 500 micrograms octreotide per ml. Multidose vials provide 1 mg octreotide in 5 ml, phenol 0.5% w/v as preservative.

Uses
Principal actions: Sandostatin is a synthetic octapeptide analogue of naturally occurring somatostatin with similar pharmacological effects, but with a longer duration of action. It inhibits the secretion of peptides of the gastroenteropancreatic endocrine system and of growth hormone.

In animals, Sandostatin is a more potent inhibitor of growth hormone, glucagon and insulin release than somatostatin with greater selectivity for growth hormone and glucagon suppression.

In normal healthy subjects Sandostatin inhibits the release of growth hormone stimulated by arginine, exercise and insulin-induced hypoglycaemia; postprandial release of insulin, glucagon, gastrin, other peptides of the gastroenteropancreatic system; arginine-stimulated release of insulin and glucagon and thyrotropin releasing hormone-stimulated release of thyroid stimulating hormone.

Because of its diverse endocrine effects, Sandostatin modifies different clinical features in patients with tumours of the gastroenteropancreatic endocrine system. Its effects in the different tumour types are as follows:

Carcinoid tumours: Sandostatin may improve symptoms, particularly flush and diarrhoea. In some cases there is a fall in plasma serotonin and reduced urinary excretion of 5-hydroxyindole acetic acid.

VIPomas: In most cases, Sandostatin alleviates the severe secretory diarrhoea typical of the condition, with consequent improvement in quality of life. This is accompanied by an improvement in associated electrolyte abnormalities, e.g. hypokalaemia, enabling enteral and parenteral fluid and electrolyte supplementation to be withdrawn. A reduction in plasma VIP levels, often into the normal reference range, usually accompanies clinical improvement.

Glucagonomas: Sandostatin produces an improvement of the characteristic necrolytic migratory rash in most patients. Its effect on the mild diabetes mellitus which frequently occurs is variable. Sandostatin produces improvement of diarrhoea, in those patients affected, and weight gain. Its administration often leads to an immediate reduction in plasma glucagon levels which is generally not maintained long-term, despite continued symptomatic improvement.

Indications: For the relief of symptoms associated with the gastroenteropancreatic endocrine tumours, carcinoid tumours with features of the carcinoid syndrome, VIPomas, and glucagonomas.

Sandostatin is not an antitumour therapy and is not curative in these patients.

Dosage and administration

Adults: The initial dose is 50 micrograms once or twice daily by subcutaneous injection. Depending on response, dosage can be gradually increased to 200 micrograms three times daily. Under exceptional circumstances higher doses may be required. Maintenance doses are variable.

The recommended route of administration is subcutaneous. However, in instances where a rapid response is required eg carcinoid crises, the initial recommended dose of Sandostatin may be administered by the intravenous route diluted and given as a bolus, whilst monitoring the cardiac rhythm.

For intravenous use Sandostatin should be diluted with sodium chloride 0.9% w/v solution to a ratio of not less than 1:1 and not more than 1:9. Dilution of Sandostatin with glucose solution is not recommended.

In carcinoid tumours, if there is no beneficial effect within a week, continued therapy is not recommended.

Children: Experience with Sandostatin in children is very limited.

Use in the elderly: In elderly patients treated with Sandostatin there is no evidence of reduced tolerability or altered dosage requirements.

Note: To reduce local discomfort, let the solution reach room temperature before injection. Avoid multiple injections at short intervals at the same site.

Contra-indications, warnings, etc

Contra-indications: Hypersensitivity to the drug.

Precautions: Sudden escape of gastroenteropancreatic endocrine tumours from symptomatic control by Sandostatin may occur infrequently, with rapid recurrence of severe symptoms.

Sandostatin may increase the depth and duration of hypoglycaemia in patients with insulinoma. This is because it is relatively more potent in inhibiting growth hormone and glucagon secretion than in inhibiting insulin and because its duration of insulin inhibition is shorter. If Sandostatin is given to a patient with insulinoma, close observation is necessary on introduction of therapy and at each change of dosage. Marked fluctuations of blood glucose concentrations may be reduced by more frequent administration of Sandostatin.

Sandostatin may reduce insulin or oral hypoglycaemic requirements in patients with diabetes mellitus.

Thyroid function should be monitored in patients receiving long-term Sandostatin therapy.

Ultrasonic examination of the gallbladder is recommended before, and at 6 to 12 months intervals during, Sandostatin therapy as gallstones have been reported on long-term Sandostatin treatment.

Sandostatin has been reported to reduce the intestinal absorption of cyclosporin and to delay that of cimetidine.

Use in pregnancy and lactation: Experience with Sandostatin in pregnant or nursing women is not available. Studies in animals showed transient growth retardation of offspring, possibly consequent upon the specific endocrine profiles of the species tested, but there was no evidence of foetotoxic, teratogenic or other reproduction effects. Nevertheless, Sandostatin should not be given during pregnancy except in compelling circumstances.

Women receiving treatment with Sandostatin should not breast feed their infants.

Side-effects: The main side-effects are local and gastrointestinal.

Local reactions include pain, a sensation of stinging, tingling or burning at the site of injection, with redness and swelling. They rarely last more than fifteen minutes. Local discomfort may be reduced by allowing the solution to reach room temperature before injection.

Gastrointestinal side-effects include anorexia, nausea, vomiting, abdominal pain, abdominal bloating, flatulence, loose stools, diarrhoea and steatorrhoea. Although measured faecal fat excretion may increase, there is no evidence to date that long-term treatment with Sandostatin has led to nutritional deficiency due to malabsorption. In rare instances, gastrointestinal side-effects may resemble acute intestinal obstruction with progressive abdominal distention, severe epigastric pain, abdominal tenderness and guarding. Occurrence of gastrointestinal side-effects may be reduced by avoiding meals around the time of Sandostatin administration, that is, by injecting between meals or on retiring to bed.

Formation of gallstones has been reported in patients on long-term Sandostatin treatment.

Because of its inhibitory action on insulin release, Sandostatin may impair postprandial glucose tolerance. In rare instances, with chronic administration, a state of persistent hyperglycaemia may be induced.

There have been isolated reports of hepatic dysfunctions associated with Sandostatin administration. These consist of acute hepatitis, without cholestasis, where transaminase values have normalised on withdrawal of Sandostatin, or slow development of hyperbilirubinaemia in association with elevation of alkaline phosphatase, gamma-glutamyl transferase and, to a lesser extent, transaminases.

Overdosage: No life-threatening reactions have been reported after acute overdosage. The maximum single dose so far given to an adult has been 1 mg by intravenous bolus injection. The observed signs and symptoms were a brief drop in heart rate, facial flushing, abdominal cramps, diarrhoea, an empty feeling in the stomach and nausea, which resolved within twenty-four hours of drug administration.

One patient has been reported to have received an accidental overdosage of Sandostatin by continuous infusion (250 micrograms per hour for forty-eight hours instead of 25 micrograms per hour). He experienced no side-effects.

The management of overdosage is symptomatic.

Pharmaceutical precautions For prolonged storage Sandostatin ampoules and multidose vials should be stored between 2° and 8°C. For day-to-day use they may be stored at room temperature for up to 2 weeks. Unused portion of contents of multidose vials should be discarded after 2 weeks.

When Sandostatin Injection needs to be given by the intravenous route, it should be diluted immediately prior to use.

Legal category POM.

Package quantities

50 micrograms per ml:	boxes of 5 ampoules.
100 micrograms per ml:	boxes of 5 ampoules.

500 micrograms per ml: boxes of 5 ampoules.
1 mg per 5 ml: boxes of 1 × 5 ml multidose vial.

Further information After subcutaneous injection Sandostatin is rapidly and completely absorbed. Peak plasma concentrations are reached within 30 minutes. The elimination after subcutaneous administration takes place with a half-life of 100 minutes. After intravenous injection the elimination is biphasic with half-lives of 10 and 90 minutes respectively. The volume of distribution is 0.27 l/kg and the total body clearance 160 ml/min. Plasma protein binding amounts to 65%. The amount of Sandostatin bound to blood cells is negligible.

Product licence numbers
50 micrograms per ml: 0101/0212.
100 micrograms per ml: 0101/0213.
500 micrograms per ml: 0101/0214.
1 mg per 5 ml: 0101/0300.

SANOMIGRAN*

Presentation
0.5 mg Tablets: Ivory/yellow, coated, bi-convex tablets of 5.5 to 5.6 mm diameter, weighing 90 mg. Printed SMG on one face. Each tablet contains 725 micrograms pizotifen hydrogen malate (equivalent to 500 micrograms pizotifen base).

1.5 mg Tablets: Ivory/yellow, coated, bi-convex tablets of 9.0 mm diameter, weighing 280 mg. Printed SMG 1.5 on one face. Each tablet contains 2.175 mg pizotifen hydrogen malate (equivalent to 1.5 mg pizotifen base).

Elixir 0.25 mg in 5 ml: Clear, colourless, fruit flavoured elixir. Each 5 ml spoonful contains 365 micrograms pizotifen hydrogen malate (equivalent to 250 micrograms pizotifen base).

Uses *Principal action:* Pharmacodynamic studies demonstrate pizotifen to have powerful antiserotonin and antitryptaminic properties, marked antihistaminic effects and some antagonistic activity against kinins. Pizotifen also has weak anticholinergic effects and sedative properties.

Sanomigran also possesses appetite-stimulating properties.

The prophylactic effect of Sanomigran in migraine is associated with its ability to modify the humoral mechanisms of headache. It inhibits the permeability-increasing effect of serotonin and histamine on the affected cranial vessels, thereby checking the transudation of plasmakinin so that the pain threshold of the receptors is maintained at 'normal' levels. In the sequence of events leading to the migraine attack, depletion of plasma serotonin contributes to loss of tone in the extracranial vessels. Pizotifen inhibits serotonin re-uptake by the platelets, thus maintaining plasma serotonin and preventing the loss of tone and passive distension of the extracranial arteries.

Indications: Prophylactic treatment of recurrent vascular headaches, including classical migraine, common migraine and cluster headache (periodic migrainous neuralgia).

Dosage and administration
Adults: Usually 1.5 mg daily. This may be taken as a single dose at night or in three divided doses, using 1.5 mg tablets, 0.5 mg tablets or elixir as appropriate. Dosage should be adjusted to individual patients' requirements up to a maximum of 6 mg daily. Up to 3 mg may be given as a single daily dose.

Children: Up to 1.5 mg daily, usually as a divided dose. Use of the 1.5 mg tablets is not recommended but up to 1 mg has been given as a single daily dose at night. 0.5 mg tablets or elixir may be used.

Use in the elderly: Clinical work with Sanomigran has not shown that elderly patients require different dosages from younger patients. However, dosage adjustment may be required in patients with renal insufficiency.

Contra-indications, warnings, etc
Contra-indications: Hypersensitivity to the drug.

Precautions: Patients should be cautioned about the possibility of drowsiness and informed of its significance in the driving of vehicles and the operation of machinery. The central effects of sedatives, hypnotics, antihistamines (including certain common cold preparations) and alcohol may be enhanced by Sanomigran.

Although the anticholinergic activity of Sanomigran is relatively weak, caution is required in the presence of closed angle glaucoma and in patients with a predisposition to urinary retention. Dosage adjustment may be necessary in patients with kidney insufficiency.

As clinical data with Sanomigran in pregnancy are very limited it should only be administered during pregnancy under compelling circumstances.

Although the concentrations of Sanomigran measured in the milk of treated mothers are not likely to affect the infant, its use in nursing mothers is not recommended.

Side-effects: The most commonly occurring side-effects are drowsiness, a gain in weight and/or an increased appetite. Other side-effects such as dizziness and nausea have been reported infrequently. In children CNS stimulation may occur.

Overdosage: Symptoms of overdosage may include drowsiness, dizziness, hypotension, dryness of the mouth, confusion, excitatory states (in children), ataxia, nausea, vomiting, dyspnoea, cyanosis, tachycardia, convulsions (particularly in children), coma and respiratory paralysis. Treatment should be directed to the elimination of the drug by gastric lavage and diuresis. Severe hypotension must be corrected (*cave:* adrenaline may produce paradoxical effects). Convulsions may be treated with short-acting barbiturates or benzodiazepines. General surveillance measures are indicated.

Pharmaceutical precautions Protect tablets from direct light.

Legal category POM.

Package quantities 0.5 mg tablets: Blister pack of 100 (OP).
1.5 mg tablets: Calendar packs of 28 (OP).
Elixir: Bottles of 300 ml (OP).

Further information Sanomigran elixir does not contain sucrose and neither Sanomigran tablets nor elixir contain tartrazine.

Product licence numbers
0.5 mg tablets 0101/0036
1.5 mg tablets 0101/0129
Elixir 0101/0163

SYNTOCINON* PARENTERAL SOLUTION

Presentation Syntocinon is available as Oxytocin Injection BP containing 2 units in 2 ml, 5 units in 1 ml, 10 units in 1 ml or 50 units in 5 ml.

Uses *Principal action:* Syntocinon is synthetic oxytocin which is identical to the polypeptide hormone released by the posterior lobe of the pituitary gland. Unlike oxytocin from natural sources, Syntocinon is completely free from vasopressin and extraneous animal protein.

At normal therapeutic doses, Syntocinon selectively stimulates the contraction of uterine smooth muscle.

Indications: Syntocinon Parenteral Solution may be used for: Induction of labour; stimulation of labour in hypotonic uterine inertia; management of missed and incomplete abortion; postpartum haemorrhage in the occasional patient who does not respond to ergometrine.

Dosage and administration By intravenous drip infusion: 1 Unit of oxytocin in 1 litre 5% dextrose solution delivers approximately 1 mUnit/min when infused at a rate of 15 drops per minute.

For induction or stimulation of labour:

1. Physiological oxytocin infusion. The range of dosage is between 2 mUnits and 5 mUnit/min.

2. Pharmacological oxytocin infusion. Initially 1½–3 mUnit/min adjusted gradually until contractions occur

every two to five minutes; rate of infusion not exceeding 12 mUnit/min.

3. Oxytocin titration: Initially 1 mUnit/min, then double the rate of flow every 10 minutes until contractions commence. Thereafter double the rate of flow every 20 minutes until contractions lasting 40–50 seconds occur at intervals of two to three minutes. Doses of oxytocin up to 128 mUnit/min have been used.

Missed abortion: 10 to 20 Units per 500 ml of 5% dextrose solution increasing by 10 to 20 Units per 500 ml every hour to a maximum of 100 Units per 500 ml if necessary. The rate of infusion recommended is 10 to 30 drops per minute.

Contra-indications, warnings, etc
Contra-indications: The use of Syntocinon is contra-indicated in hypertonic uterine inertia, mechanical obstruction to delivery, failed trial labour, severe toxaemia, predisposition to amniotic fluid embolism, foetal distress and placenta praevia. Also hypersensitivity.

Precautions: Considerable caution should be exercised in abnormal presentation, multiple pregnancy, excessive parity and previous caesarian section. High doses of oxytocin should only be used in fully equipped centres where patients can be kept under constant observation. In patients with cardiovascular disorders the infusion volume should be low.

Prostaglandins may potentiate the effect of oxytocin.

Overdosage: The fatal dose of Syntocinon has not been established. Syntocinon is subject to inactivation by proteolytic enzymes of the alimentary tract. Hence it is not absorbed from the intestine and is not likely to have toxic effects when ingested.

Where high doses of Syntocinon are given with large volumes of electrolyte-free fluid, the following symptoms of water intoxication may occur:

1. Headache, anorexia, nausea, vomiting and abdominal pain.
2. Lethargy, drowsiness, unconsciousness and grand-mal type seizures.
3. Low blood electrolyte concentration.

Treatment: All fluid intake should be restricted. Diuresis should be promoted as soon as possible and the electrolyte imbalance should be corrected. Convulsions may be controlled by judicious use of diazepam. In the case of coma, a free airway should be maintained with other routine measures normally employed in the nursing of the unconscious patient.

Side-effects: As there is a wide variation in uterine sensitivity, uterine spasm may be caused in some instances by what are normally considered to be low doses.

Very high doses may cause violent uterine contractions leading to uterine rupture, tissue damage and asphyxia of the foetus.

Pharmaceutical precautions Protect from light. Store between 4° and 22°C.

Syntocinon should not be infused via the same apparatus as blood or plasma, because the peptide linkages are rapidly inactivated by oxytocinase. Syntocinon is incompatible with solutions containing sodium metabisulphite as a stabiliser.

Syntocinon is compatible with the following infusion fluids, but due attention should be paid to the advisability of using electrolyte fluids in individual patients: Dextrose 5%, Sodium/potassium chloride (103 mmol Na^+ and 51 mmol K^+), Laevulose 20%, Macrodex 6%, Sodium bicarbonate 1.39%, Sodium chloride 0.9%, Sodium lactate 1.72%, Rheomacrodex 10%, Ringer's solution.

Legal category POM.

Package quantities

2 Units/2 ml:	Boxes of 10.
5 Units/1 ml:	Boxes of 10.
10 Units/1 ml:	Boxes of 10.
50 Units/5 ml:	Boxes of 5.

Further information Nil.

Product licence numbers

2 Units/2 ml	0101/0068
5 Units/1 ml	0101/0069
10 Units/1 ml	0101/0070
50 Units/5 ml	0101/0071

SYNTOMETRINE*

Presentation Syntometrine is available as a parenteral solution containing Ergometrine Maleate PhEur 500 micrograms and 5 Units of oxytocin in 1 ml.

Uses *Principal action:* Designed for intramuscular injection, Syntometrine combines the known sustained oxytocic action of ergometrine with the more rapid action of oxytocin on the uterus. The latent period following an intramuscular injection of Syntometrine is considerably shorter than with any other ergot preparation.

Indications: Syntometrine is indicated in the active management of the third stage of labour or, routinely following the birth of the placenta, to prevent or treat postpartum haemorrhage.

Dosage and administration Intramuscular injection of 1 ml. May also be administered by intravenous injection in a dose of $\frac{1}{2}$ to 1 ml.

Contra-indications, warnings, etc
Contra-indications: Severe disorders of liver or kidney function.

Precautions: When the intravenous route is employed, care should be exercised in patients of doubtful cardiac status.

Caution should be exercised in the presence of hypertension, sepsis, obliterative vascular disorders and liver or kidney failure.

Syntometrine may enhance the effects of vasoconstrictors and of prostaglandins.

Side-effects: Occasional reports of nausea, vomiting and abdominal pain.

Overdosage: No case of maternal intoxication with Syntometrine has been reported to the Company. Inadvertent administration to the newborn infant has proved fatal. In reported accidental neonatal overdosage cases, respiratory and cardiovascular support have been required.

Pharmaceutical precautions For prolonged periods Syntometrine should be stored between 2° and 8°C and protected from light. Syntometrine may be stored at temperatures up to 25°C for two months when protected from light.

Legal category POM.

Package quantities Boxes of 10 × 1 ml.

Further information Snap ampoules: no file required.

Product licence number 0101/5046.

SYNTOPRESSIN* NASAL SPRAY

Presentation Syntopressin is available as a solution containing lypressin 50 Units per ml for use as a nasal spray.

Uses *Principal action:* Syntopressin is synthetic 8-lysine-vasopressin (lypressin). It is completely free of oxytocin and extraneous animal protein. Syntopressin has a direct antidiuretic action. It is used for the control of polyuria in diabetes insipidus.

Indications: Diabetes insipidus, spontaneous or induced.

Dosage and administration One or two applications of the spray (2.5 to 5.0 Units) to one or both nostrils, repeated three to seven times a day according to the response of the patient.

The patient should be advised to hold the bottle upright and to spray the inside of one or both nostrils by squeezing the bottle firmly then removing from the nostril to release the pressure. This should be repeated one or more times at intervals as required to produce the desired dose.

Use in the elderly: No evidence exists that elderly patients require different dosages, or show different side-effects from younger people.

Contra-indications, warnings, etc
Contra-indications: Coronary heart disease, anaesthesia with halothane or cyclopropane.

Precautions: As with other forms of vasopressin, caution is advised in the administration of this drug to patients suffering from advanced arteriosclerosis, peripheral vascular disease, hypertension, epilepsy and during pregnancy, particularly toxaemic.

The antidiuretic effect of Syntopressin may be enhanced by carbamazepine, chlorpropamide or clofibrate and decreased by lithium.

Overdosage: No cases of overdosage have been reported to the Company.

Side-effects: Nausea, abdominal pain or urge to defaecate may follow injudicious use. On rare occasions nasal congestion with ulceration of the nasal mucosa has been reported.

Pharmaceutical precautions Store in a cool place, but do NOT freeze. Use within one month of opening.

Legal category POM.

Package quantities Spray bottles of 5 ml.

Further information Nil.

Product licence number 0101/5047.

TAVEGIL*

Presentation

Tablets: White, uncoated, round tablets, 7 mm in diameter, with bevelled edges, branded TAVEGIL on one side with a single break line on the other. Each tablet contains 1.34 mg clemastine hydrogen fumarate (equivalent to 1 mg clemastine base).

Elixir: A clear, colourless liquid with an odour of peaches. Each 5 ml spoonful contains 670 micrograms (0.67 mg) clemastine hydrogen fumarate (equivalent to 500 micrograms (0.5 mg) clemastine base).

Uses *Principal action:* Tavegil is a potent, specific antihistamine which is innately long-acting.

Indications: Allergic rhinitis, including hay fever and perennial rhinitis, vasomotor rhinitis. Allergic dermatoses, including pruritus, atopic eczema and contact dermatitis. Urticaria. Angioneurotic oedema. Drug allergy.

Dosage and administration
Adults: 1 mg clemastine base (one tablet or two 5 ml spoonfuls of elixir) night and morning.

In individual cases the dose may be increased to 6 mg clemastine base daily if necessary (six tablets or twelve 5 ml spoonfuls of elixir).

Children:

1 to 3 years:	250 micrograms to 500 micrograms clemastine base night and morning.
3 to 6 years:	500 micrograms clemastine base night and morning.
6 to 12 years:	500 micrograms to 1000 micrograms (1 mg) clemastine base night and morning.

For doses less than 500 micrograms Tavegil elixir should be diluted to a dose volume of 5 ml or a multiple thereof. For dilution details see 'Pharmaceutical precautions'.

Use in the elderly: No evidence exists that elderly patients require different dosages or show different side-effects from younger patients.

Contra-indications, warnings, etc
Contra-indications: Tavegil is contra-indicated in patients with a known hypersensitivity to clemastine or other arylalkylamine antihistamines.

Tavegil should not be given to children below one year of age.

Precautions: Patients should be warned not to take charge of vehicles or machinery until the effect of Tavegil treatment on the individual is known. Tavegil may potentiate the effects of sedatives, hypnotics, mono-amine-oxidase inhibitors and alcohol and patients should be advised to avoid alcoholic drinks.

Antihistamines should be used with caution in patients with narrow-angle glaucoma, stenosing peptic ulcer, pyloroduodenal obstruction, prostatic hypertrophy with urinary retention and bladder neck obstruction.

Use in pregnancy and lactation: Tavegil should not be given during pregnancy and breast feeding unless it is strictly indicated.

Overdosage: May give rise to confusion, nausea and vomiting. Treatment should be directed to the removal of ingested material by induced emesis or gastric lavage as appropriate. Routine supportive measures are indicated to combat respiratory depression and hypotension.

Side-effects: Drowsiness, fatigue, occasionally CNS stimulation has been reported, particularly in children. Very occasional miscellaneous side-effects such as weakness, dizziness, dry mouth, headache, palpitations, gastro-intestinal disturbance, heartburn and skin rash have occurred. In general, these adverse effects can be controlled by a diminution of dosage.

Pharmaceutical precautions Protect tablets from light. Tavegil Elixir may be diluted with Syrup BP or Sorbitol Syrup (70%). The diluted elixir should be used within 14 days.

Legal category P.

Package quantities *Tavegil Tablets:* Blister pack of 50 (OP).

Tavegil Elixir: Bottles of 150 ml.

Further information Tavegil Elixir is sucrose free and is suitable for diabetic patients. It has an approximate calorific value of 11 kcals per 5 ml spoonful.

Product licence numbers

Tavegil Tablets	0101/0033
Tavegil Elixir	0101/0058

TERONAC*

Presentation Whitish, flat, bevel-edged tablets of 7 mm diameter, each weighing 125 mg. Scored on one side with TERONAC imprinted on the other side. Each tablet contains 2 mg mazindol base.

Uses *Principal action:* Teronac is an appetite suppressant with potent anorexic activity.

It is unrelated to amphetamine and is not metabolised to an amphetamine derivative.

Indications: An aid to the establishment of a diet in the treatment of obesity, accompanied by close support and supervision.

Teronac may be used in patients with stable heart disease, and in diabetic patients (see Precautions).

Dosage and administration *Adults:* 1 tablet after breakfast or as directed by the physician.

Use in the elderly: Not recommended.

Children: Not recommended.

A continuous treatment period of not more than three months is recommended as an aid to the establishment of a controlled diet. The recommended dosage should not be exceeded in an attempt to increase the effect. Administration should not continue if weight loss does not occur within one month of starting treatment, or if weight loss ceases.

Contra-indications, warnings, etc
Contra-indications: Teronac should not be used in

patients with peptic ulcer or glaucoma, severe renal, hepatic or cardiac insufficiency, cardiac arrhythmias and severe hypertension or in patients who are breast feeding. Teronac is contra-indicated in patients with a history of psychiatric illness, emotional instability, or those who are liable to drug or alcohol abuse.

Teronac does not inhibit monoamine oxidase (MAO) but potentiates the pressor effects of catecholamines. It can therefore be anticipated that Teronac will interact with the following: MAO inhibitors and antihypertensive agents of the adrenergic neurone blocking type, e.g. guanethidine and debrisoquine. These medicinal agents should not be taken until one month has elapsed from the cessation of treatment with Teronac.

Use in Pregnancy: Teronac should not be used during pregnancy. There is no evidence as to the safety of the drug in human pregnancy, nor is there evidence from animal work that it is free from hazard.

Precautions: Teronac should be used with caution in patients with prostatic hypertrophy, coronary heart disease, severely agitated states, and in patients taking thyroid medication, psychostimulants or antihypertensive agents. Patients should be cautioned against taking cough and cold remedies containing sympathomimetic decongestants during treatment with Teronac and for one month after ceasing treatment, without first seeking the doctor's advice. This caution is also applicable to patients undergoing local anaesthesia for dental procedures with products containing adrenaline or other sympathomimetic haemostatics.

Diabetic patients' response to insulin and oral antidiabetic agents may be affected by Teronac and dietary control, and the metabolic status of such patients should therefore be monitored and the dosage of insulin or oral antidiabetic agents adjusted if necessary.

Patients driving vehicles or operating machinery should be alerted to the possibility of impaired reactions and be advised to avoid alcohol.

Overdosage: Treatment should be directed to the removal of ingested material by induced emesis and gastric lavage as appropriate. Hyperactivity and anxiety are major factors of overdosage; excess CNS stimulation should be controlled if necessary with chlorpromazine. There is no reported use of forced acid diuresis, but it may be of theoretical value.

Side-effects: The most commonly occurring side-effects include constipation, sweating, dry-mouth and insomnia. Less frequently nervousness, headache, syncope, dizziness, chills, skin rashes and reversible disturbances of micturition and sexual function may also occur. Mild tachycardia has occasionally been reported at higher dosage levels. On rare occasions, euphoria and hallucinations have been reported in the first few days of therapy.

Pharmaceutical precautions Store in a dry place at a temperature not exceeding 30°C.

Legal category CD (Sch 3), POM.

Package quantities Blister pack of 30 tablets (OP).

Further information Dependence and abuse for stimulant effect have rarely been reported. Weight loss is steady and consistent during treatment with Teronac.

Product licence number 0101/0079R.

TORECAN*

Presentation

Tablets: White, bi-convex, sugar-coated tablets of 7 mm diameter, weighing 180 mg and printed 'SANDOZ' on one face. Each tablet contains thiethylperazine maleate equivalent to 6.33 mg base (10 mg maleate salt).

Ampoules: Clear, colourless to yellow-tinged parenteral solution. Each 1 ml ampoule contains thiethylperazine malate equivalent to 6.5 mg base (10.86 mg malate salt).

Suppositories: White to pale-yellow suppositories weighing 1.93 g. Each suppository contains thiethylperazine maleate equivalent to 6.5 mg base (10.28 mg maleate salt).

Uses *Principal action:* Torecan is an anti-emetic and anti-nauseant. It controls vomiting, nausea and vertigo. Torecan is a phenothiazine derivative which, unlike many other compounds in this group, exhibits specific anti-emetic and anti-vertiginous properties with little or no tranquillising, sedative or other effects.

The present concept of the vomiting mechanism is that emesis may be induced by direct action on the vomiting centre in the medulla or by lowering its threshold to stimulation. Excitation of the vomiting centre may result from direct visceral impulses or be secondary to stimulation of the chemoreceptor trigger zone. Pharmacological studies have shown that Torecan in similar doses will control vomiting induced by stimulation of both the chemoreceptor trigger zone and the vomiting centre.

Indications: Torecan is indicated for the relief of vertigo and the control of nausea and vomiting associated with various causes, notably:

1. Labyrinthine disturbances – Menière's disease, labyrinthitis, surgery, motion sickness, cerebral irritation and damage or disease of the inner ear.
2. Gastro-intestinal disturbances – gastroenteritis.
3. Radiotherapy and treatment with cytostatic agents.
4. Post-operative nausea, vomiting and vertigo.
5. Drug-induced vomiting.

Dosage and administration
Adults:
Tablets: 1 tablet two or three times daily.
Ampoules: 1 ml by intramuscular injection. Effective in 30 to 60 minutes.
Suppositories: 1 suppository night and morning.

Children: Not recommended for children under 15 years.

Use in the elderly: See 'Side-effects'.

Contra-indications, warnings, etc
Contra-indications: Severely depressed or comatose states. Hypersensitivity to phenothiazines. Torecan should not be given to children under 15 years, since this age group is particularly susceptible to extrapyramidal side effects.

Precautions: Phenothiazines undergo extensive and complex metabolic biotransformation in the liver, occasionally to other active metabolites, prior to biliary or urinary excretion. Consequently, caution should be exercised during their use in hepatic and/or renal dysfunction – a dose reduction may be necessary.

On a very few occasions, jaundice has occurred following administration of Torecan but a drug-effect relationship has not been established.

Torecan may cause drowsiness and impair the patient's reactions (e.g. while driving or operating machinery). Torecan can potentiate the effects of CNS depressants including benzodiazepines, opiates and alcohol.

Among elderly patients on long-term treatment with Torecan tardive dyskinesia has been observed on rare occasions. Therefore patients of this age group should in general not be treated for longer than about 2 months and should be carefully monitored for the occurrence of untoward neurological signs.

Phenothiazines are known to cause neuroleptic malignant syndrome, a condition requiring immediate discontinuation of the drug. Torecan, given in the immediate post-operative period, may lead to restlessness and/or CNS depression.

Hypotensive episodes are rare (for treatment see 'Overdosage').

Use in pregnancy and lactation: Torecan has been available for many years and there is no evidence to suggest any associated hazard to the foetus. Nevertheless, as for most drugs, Torecan should be given in pregnancy only if strictly indicated.

Small amounts of phenothiazines may be excreted in breast milk. Although the quantity is probably too small to have any significant effect, breast feeding should be suspended during treatment.

Warning: Intra-arterial injection of Torecan must be strictly avoided.

Side-effects: Thiethylperazine is a phenothiazine and Torecan may to some extent exhibit similar side-effects to the other phenothiazines.

Drowsiness, somnolence, dryness of the mouth, tachycardia and occasional postural hypotension may occur, particularly if the maximum recommended dosage of 30 mg thiethylperazine maleate daily is exceeded.

In isolated cases, liver function abnormalities have been reported. Tardive dyskinesia may rarely occur in elderly patients (see Precautions).

Like other phenothiazine derivatives, Torecan may – although rarely and then usually in younger patients – cause extrapyramidal symptoms (oculogyric crises, difficulties in swallowing and speaking, muscle spasms). However, these symptoms respond promptly to parenteral treatment with an anti-parkinsonian agent. In many cases the extrapyramidal symptoms disappear rapidly following withdrawal of the drug.

The occurrence of neuroleptic malignant syndrome following Torecan administration has to date been reported in one patient.

Overdosage: The symptoms of Torecan overdosage are similar to those of other phenothiazines with the exception that there is less CNS depression with Torecan. Drowsiness, confusion, followed in more severe cases by coma and areflexia, tachycardia, postural hypotension and collapse may result. Respiratory depression is possible as a late manifestation of severe intoxication. Agitation, acute dystonic reactions and convulsions may also occur.

There is no specific antidote for acute phenothiazine poisoning, therefore treatment is directed at minimising the amount of the drug absorbed, eliminating the absorbed drug from the body and combating the toxic effects of the overdose by gastric lavage, maintenance of adequate pulmonary ventilation and general supportive measures. Emetics are obviously of less value. If emetics are given and do not work, then do not exceed the normal dose.

Peritoneal dialysis and haemodialysis are ineffective in the treatment of phenothiazine poisoning.

Symptoms of hypotension should be corrected. If treatment with a vasopressor (adrenaline should be avoided) proves necessary, careful monitoring of cardiovascular function is indicated. Severe extrapyramidal reactions usually respond to intravenous administration of anti-parkinsonian agents, e.g. Benztropine 2 mg i.v. or i.m. If convulsions occur they may be treated with benzodiazepines.

Prophylactic antibiotic therapy is generally favoured. Hypothermia: body temperature should be allowed to recover naturally unless it falls below 30°C.

Pharmaceutical precautions Suppositories should be stored below 30°C. Ampoules should be protected from light.

Legal category POM.

Package quantities Tablets: Blister packs of 50. Ampoules: Boxes of 5 × 1 ml. Suppositories: Boxes of 5.

Further information Nil.

Product licence numbers

Tablets	0101/5048R
Ampoules	0101/5012R
Suppositories	0101/5013R

TREMONIL*

Presentation White, uncoated, bi-convex tablets of 8 mm diameter, each weighing 155 mg. Scored on one side, with TREMONIL imprinted on the other side. Each tablet contains 5 mg methixene hydrochloride.

Uses *Principal actions:* Tremonil is a parasympatholytic agent and has spasmolytic and antihistaminic properties.

Indications: Tremonil is indicated in the treatment of parkinsonism and of drug-induced extra-pyramidal symptoms except tardive dyskinesia. It is more effective in controlling the tremors than in reducing the rigidity of this syndrome.

Tremonil is also indicated in the treatment of senile tremor.

Dosage and administration *Adults:* Treatment should be started with single doses of 2.5 mg (½ tablet) three times daily. The dose may then be slowly and gradually raised by small increments until the most effective dose is reached. The optimum effective dosage lies between 15 mg and 60 mg daily in divided dosage, depending upon the severity of symptoms initially and their response to treatment.

Use in the elderly: In elderly patients, the optimum maintenance dosage is often lower than that required by younger subjects with comparable disease, e.g. 15 to 30 mg daily.

Children: There are no dosage recommendations for children.

Contra-indications, warnings, etc

Contra-indications: Prostatic hypertrophy and other conditions causing urinary retention, narrow angle glaucoma, cardiac arrhythmias, pyloric stenosis, paralytic ileus, intestinal hypotonia, myasthenia gravis, acute intoxication with alcohol, hypnotics, analgesics or psychotropics.

Use in pregnancy and lactation: Tremonil should be given in the early stages of pregnancy and during breast feeding only if strictly indicated.

Precautions: Autonomic disturbances occasionally occur during the initial stages of treatment and due caution should be observed in patients who have to drive or perform tasks requiring precision. If these do not disappear spontaneously as treatment proceeds, the dose should be lowered until the highest well-tolerated dose is reached. Treatment should be continued at this level for several days and then gradually increased.

Special care is needed in the adjustment of the daily dosage in patients with marked autonomic lability.

When changing treatment from another anti-parkinson drug, the small starting dose of Tremonil should be substituted for a part of the dosage of the drug already in use. As the dose of Tremonil is increased, that of the drug for which it is being substituted should be reduced accordingly.

When adding Tremonil to drugs with anticholinergic properties, it is advisable to reduce slightly the dose of the latter for a few days. In this way the occurrence of undesirable side-effects due to the sudden increase in the total dosage of parasympatholytic agents may be avoided. When Tremonil is administered concurrently with phenothiazine tranquillisers to control extra-pyramidal side-effects, the average total daily dose of Tremonil is around 15 mg.

Side-effects: Tremonil is generally well tolerated but signs of autonomic imbalance, e.g. dryness of mucous membranes, transient visual disturbances, tachycardia, flushing and dizziness, may occur in some patients during the early stages of treatment. These symptoms tend to disappear spontaneously during treatment, but a temporary reduction in dosage may be required. (See recommendations under 'Dosage').

Nausea, sensations of abdominal pressure, weakness and fatigue may occur half to one hour after a single dose of 10 to 15 mg.

Constipation and urinary retention have been noted.

Mental confusion may result from the use of synthetic anti-parkinsonian drugs, especially when given in high dosage, or to elderly patients, and the possibility of this side-effect should be borne in mind, especially when several drugs are given concurrently. If signs of mental confusion are observed the drug should be discontinued immediately.

Overdosage: Toxic effects are anticholinergic in nature.

Treatment should consist of gastric lavage, routine supportive measures and giving fluids freely. Atropine antagonists such as neostigmine methylsulphate may relieve the peripheral symptoms.

Although physostigmine (1 to 4 mg i.v.) will antagonise the central effects, it is rarely indicated.

Pharmaceutical precautions Protect from light and heat.

Legal category POM.

Package quantities Blister pack of 50 tablets (OP).

Further information Nil.

Product licence number 0101/5904R.

VISKALDIX*

Presentation White, uncoated, round, flat, bevel-edged tablets of 7 mm diameter and weighing 130 mg. The tablets are marked VISKALDIX on one side with a single break line on the other. Each tablet contains 10 mg Pindolol PhEur and 5 mg clopamide.

Uses *Principal action:* Viskaldix is a combination of the beta-adrenoceptor blocking agent pindolol and the diuretic clopamide; each component lowers blood pressure through a different mechanism of action. Clinical studies have shown that the combination is an effective and well-tolerated antihypertensive agent, that both components contribute to this effect, and that the combination is more effective than pindolol alone.

Pindolol is a specific beta-adrenoceptor blocking agent with some intrinsic sympathomimetic activity which minimises myocardial depression and other undesirable effects of beta-blockade, including bradycardia and bronchoconstriction. Clopamide, in the dosage present in Viskaldix, contributes to a lowering of blood pressure without marked diuresis. The hypotensive effect of the combination is often seen after five to seven days but the maximum effect may not be achieved for two to three weeks.

Indication: Mild to moderate hypertension.

Dosage and administration
Adults: 1 tablet daily in the morning. If blood pressure is not satisfactorily lowered after two to three weeks, two tablets may be taken as a single dose in the morning. A maximum dose of three tablets daily may be taken if necessary.

Children: There is no experience with Viskaldix in children.

Use in the elderly: No evidence exists that the dosage or tolerability of Viskaldix is directly affected by advanced age. However, because of the diuretic component, elderly patients should be carefully supervised as factors sometimes associated with ageing, such as poor diet or impaired renal function, may indirectly affect the dosage or tolerability.

Contra-indications, warnings, etc
Contra-indications: Cardiac failure unless satisfactorily controlled by digitalis (see also 'Precautions'). Atrioventricular block, pronounced bradycardia, obstructive pulmonary disease, cor pulmonale, severe renal or hepatic failure, metabolic acidosis, prolonged fasting, hypokalaemia.

Viskaldix should not be taken in conjunction with agents which inhibit calcium transport, e.g. verapamil, during concomitant administration of lithium, or by patients with known hypersensitivity to sulphonamides.

Use in pregnancy and lactation: Viskaldix is contra-indicated in pregnancy. It should not be used in breast-feeding mothers because of the possibility of sulphonamide sensitivity (due to clopamide) in the infant.

Precautions: Patients with a poor cardiac reserve should be stabilised with digitalis before treatment with Viskaldix to prevent impairment of myocardial contractility. Viskaldix should be used with caution in patients with a history of bronchial asthma or recent myocardial infarction. Caution must be exercised when beta-blocking agents are administered to patients with spontaneous hypoglycaemia and diabetics under treatment with insulin or oral hypoglycaemic agents, since hypoglycaemia may occur during prolonged fasting and some of its symptoms (tachycardia, tremor) are masked.

During treatment with Viskaldix, patients should not undergo anaesthesia with agents causing myocardial depression (e.g. halothane, cyclopropane, trichlorethylene, ether, chloroform). Viskaldix should be gradually withdrawn before elective surgery. In emergency surgery or cases where withdrawal of Viskaldix would cause deterioration in cardiac condition, atropine sulphate 1 to 2 mg intravenously should be given to prevent severe bradycardia.

If a beta-blocker is indicated in a patient with a phaeochromocytoma it must always be given in conjunction with an alpha-blocker. Pre-existing peripheral vascular disorders may be aggravated by beta-blockers.

In severe renal failure a further impairment of renal function following beta-blockade has been reported in a few cases. Potassium levels should be checked in patients with kidney or liver failure, and urate levels in patients suffering from gout.

There have been reports of skin rashes and/or dry eyes associated with the use of beta-adrenoreceptor blocking drugs. The reported incidence is small and in most cases the symptoms have cleared when treatment was withdrawn. Discontinuance of the drug should be considered if any such reaction is not otherwise explicable. Cessation of therapy with a beta-blocker should be gradual.

Because dizziness or fatigue may occur during the initial phase of treatment with antihypertensive drugs, patients driving vehicles or operating machinery should exercise caution until their individual reaction to treatment has been determined.

Side-effects: Few serious side-effects have been reported. Depression, diarrhoea, insomnia, headaches, sleep disturbance, epigastric pain, fatigue, dizziness and hypotension have occurred but are usually transient and disappear if dosage is reduced.

Overdosage: Overdosage may cause alterations in heart rate, nausea, vomiting, orthostatic disturbances, collapse, hypokalaemia and its accompanying disorders.

Treat by elimination of any unabsorbed drug and general supportive measures. Plasma electrolytes should be closely monitored. Marked bradycardia, as a result of overdosage or idiosyncrasy, should be treated with atropine sulphate 1 to 2 mg intravenously. If necessary isoprenaline hydrochloride can be administered by slow intravenous injection, under constant supervision, beginning with 25 micrograms (5 micrograms/min) until the desired effect is achieved. A cardiac pacemaker may be required. Intravenous glucagon (5 to 10 mg) has been reported to overcome some of the features of serious overdosage with beta–blockers and may be useful.

Pharmaceutical precautions Nil.

Legal category POM.

Package quantities Calendar pack of 28 (OP).

Product licence number 0101/0113.

VISKEN*

Presentation *5 mg Tablets:* Visken 5 mg is available as white, round, flat, bevel-edged tablets of 7 mm diameter, and weighing 120 mg. The tablets are marked VISKEN 5 on one side with a single break line on the reverse. Each tablet contains 5 mg Pindolol PhEur.

15 mg Tablets: Visken 15 mg is available as white, round, flat, bevel-edged tablets of 9 mm diameter and weighing 200 mg. The tablets are marked VISKEN 15 on one side, and scored on the reverse. Each tablet contains 15 mg Pindolol PhEur.

Uses *Principal action:* Visken is a specific beta-adrenoceptor blocking agent with low cardiodepressant activity at therapeutic dose. Its beta-blocking activity prevents excessive sympathetic drive to the heart, resulting in a fall in heart rate, and a decrease in cardiac work and myocardial oxygen consumption. Visken possesses some intrinsic sympathomimetic activity even at low dosage which may prevent reduction of resting sympathetic tone to an undesirably low level and minimise myocardial depression.

Indications: Hypertension: For reduction of blood pressure in essential hypertension. Onset of action of Visken is usually rapid, most patients showing a response within the first one to two weeks of treatment. However, maximum response may take several weeks to develop.

Angina pectoris: Prophylactic treatment with Visken reduces the frequency and severity of anginal attacks and increases work capacity.

Dosage and administration *Hypertension:* Initially one 15 mg tablet daily, with breakfast or 5 mg two or three times daily. Most patients respond to a once-daily dose of from 15 mg to 30 mg.

If necessary, dosage may be increased at weekly intervals up to a maximum of 45 mg daily in single or divided doses. Patients not responding after three to four weeks at this dosage level rarely benefit from further elevations in dosage. Addition of Visken to existing diuretic therapy increases the hypotensive effect and combination with other antihypertensives enables reduction in dosage of these agents.

Angina pectoris: Usually half to one 5 mg tablet up to three times a day according to response.

Use in the elderly: No evidence exists that elderly patients require different dosages or show different side-effects from younger patients.

Contra-indications, warnings, etc
Contra-indications: Cardiac failure unless satisfactorily controlled by digitalis (see also 'Precautions'). Atrioventricular block, pronounced bradycardia, obstructive pulmonary disease, cor pulmonale, metabolic acidosis, prolonged fasting, severe renal failure.

Visken should not be taken in conjunction with agents which inhibit calcium transport, e.g. verapamil.

Use in pregnancy and lactation: Visken is contra-indicated in pregnancy and passes in small quantities into breast milk.

Precautions: Patients with a poor cardiac reserve should be stabilised with digitalis before treatment with Visken to prevent impairment of myocardial contractility.

As with all beta-blockers, Visken should be used with caution in patients with a history of bronchial asthma or recent myocardial infarction. Caution must be exercised when beta-blocking agents are administered to patients with spontaneous hypoglycaemia or diabetics under treatment with insulin or oral hypoglycaemic agents, since hypoglycaemia may occur during prolonged fasting and some of its symptoms (tachycardia, tremor) may be masked.

During treatment with Visken, patients should not undergo anaesthesia with agents causing myocardial depression (e.g. halothane, cyclopropane, trichlorethylene, ether, chloroform). Visken should be gradually withdrawn before elective surgery. In emergency surgery or cases where withdrawal of Visken would cause deterioration in cardiac condition, atropine sulphate 1 to 2 mg intravenously should be given to prevent severe bradycardia.

If a beta-blocker is indicated in a patient with a phaeochromocytoma it must always be given in conjunction with an alpha-blocker. Pre-existing peripheral vascular disorders may be aggravated by beta-blockers.

In severe renal failure a further impairment of renal function following beta blockade has been reported in a few cases.

There have been reports of skin rashes and/or dry eyes associated with the use of beta-adrenoceptor blocking drugs. The reported incidence is small and in most cases the symptoms have cleared when treatment was withdrawn. Discontinuance of the drug should be considered if any such reaction is not otherwise explicable. Cessation of therapy with a beta-blocker should be gradual.

Because dizziness or fatigue may occur during the initial phase of treatment with antihypertensive drugs, patients driving vehicles or operating machinery should exercise caution until their individual response to treatment has been determined.

Side-effects: Few serious side-effects have been reported. Depression, diarrhoea, insomnia, headaches, sleep disturbance, epigastric pain, fatigue, dizziness, hypotension have occurred but are usually transient and disappear if dosage is reduced. Allergic skin reactions have occasionally been reported.

Overdosage: Treat by elimination of any unabsorbed drug and general supportive measures. Marked bradycardia as a result of overdosage or idiosyncrasy should be treated with atropine sulphate 1 to 2 mg intravenously. If necessary, isoprenaline hydrochloride can be administered by a slow intravenous injection, under constant supervision, beginning with 25 micrograms (5 micrograms/min) until the desired effect is achieved. A cardiac pacemaker may be required; i.v. glucagon (5 to 10 mg) has been reported to overcome some of the features of serious overdosage and may be useful.

Pharmaceutical precautions Nil.

Legal category POM.

Package quantities *5 mg tablets:* Blister pack of 100 (OP).
15 mg tablets: Blister pack of 30 (OP).

Further information Nil.

Product licence numbers

Tablets 5 mg	0101/0065
Tablets 15 mg	0101/0110

ZADITEN*

Presentation *1 mg capsules:* White, opaque, oblong, gelatin capsules, size 4, weighing 182 mg. Each capsule contains 1.38 mg ketotifen hydrogen fumarate (equivalent to 1 mg ketotifen base). Coded CS in red.

1 mg tablets: Off-white, uncoated, round, flat, bevel-edged tablets weighing 190 mg, 7 mm diameter. The tablets are marked ZADITEN 1 on one side and scored on the other. Each tablet contains 1.38 mg ketotifen hydrogen fumarate (equivalent to 1 mg ketotifen base).

Elixir: Clear, colourless, strawberry flavoured elixir. Each 5 ml spoonful contains 1.38 mg ketotifen hydrogen fumarate (equivalent to 1 mg ketotifen base).

Uses *Principal action:* Zaditen possesses marked anti-anaphylactic properties and is effective in preventing asthmatic attacks.

Laboratory experiments indicate that this anti-anaphylactic activity may be due in the main to the inhibition of release of myotonic mediators from tissue mast cells and basophils, in particular SRS (slow reacting substance) and histamine, to the inhibition of SRS-induced bronchospasms *in vivo* and to calcium antagonistic properties. In addition, Zaditen exerts a sustained inhibitory effect on histamine reactions which can be clearly dissociated from its anti-anaphylactic properties.

Experimental investigations in asthmatic subjects have shown that Zaditen is as effective orally as a selective mast cell stabiliser administered by inhalation: anti-histamines are ineffective in these tests.

The effectiveness of Zaditen in the prevention of bronchial asthma has been studied in long term clinical trials. Asthma attacks were reduced in number, severity and duration and in some cases the patients were completely freed from attacks. Progressive reduction of corticosteroids and/or bronchodilators was also possible.

The prophylactic activity of Zaditen may take several weeks to become fully established.

Zaditen will not abort established attacks of asthma.

Indications: Prophylactic treatment of bronchial asthma. Symptomatic treatment of allergic conditions including rhinitis and conjunctivitis.

Dosage and administration *Adults:* 1 mg twice daily with food. If necessary the dose may be increased to 2 mg twice daily.

Children from two years: 1 mg twice daily with food.

Use in the elderly: No evidence exists that elderly patients require different dosages or show different side effects from younger patients.

Patients known to be easily sedated should begin treatment with 0.5 to 1 mg at night for the first few days.

Contra-indications, warnings, etc
Contra-indications: A reversible fall in the thrombocyte count in patients receiving Zaditen concomitantly with oral antidiabetic agents has been observed in a few cases. This combination of drugs should therefore be avoided until this phenomenon has been satisfactorily explained.

Use in pregnancy and lactation: Although there is no evidence of any teratogenic effect, recommendations for Zaditen in pregnancy or when breast feeding cannot be given.

Precautions: Post-marketing surveillance has shown exacerbation of asthma in approximately 2 per 1000 patients. Since some of these asthmatic attacks might have been related to stopping existing treatment, it is important to continue such treatment for a minimum of two weeks after starting Zaditen. This applies especially to systemic corticosteroids and ACTH because of the possible existence of adrenocortical insufficiency in steroid-dependent patients; in such cases recovery of a normal pituitary-adrenal response to stress may take up to one year.

If intercurrent infection occurs Zaditen treatment must be supplemented by specific antimicrobial therapy.

During the first days of treatment with Zaditen reactions may be impaired. Patients should be warned not to take charge of vehicles or machinery until the effect of Zaditen treatment on the individual is known. Patients should be advised to avoid alcoholic drinks.

Zaditen may potentiate the effects of sedatives, hypnotics, antihistamines and alcohol.

Side-effects: Drowsiness and, in isolated cases, dry mouth and slight dizziness may occur at the beginning of treatment, but usually disappear spontaneously after a few days. Occasionally symptoms of CNS stimulation have been observed. Weight gain has also been reported.

Overdosage: The reported features of overdosage include confusion, drowsiness, nystagmus, headache, disorientation, tachycardia, hypotension, reversible coma, especially in children, hyperexcitability or convulsions. Bradycardia and respiratory depression should be watched for. Elimination of the drug with gastric lavage or emesis is recommended. Otherwise general supportive treatment is all that is required.

Pharmaceutical precautions Protect tablets and capsules from heat and moisture.

Legal category POM.

Package quantities *1 mg capsules:* Blister pack of 60 capsules (OP).
1 mg tablets: Blister pack of 60 tablets (OP).
Elixir 1 mg/5 ml: Bottles of 150 ml.

Further information Zaditen Elixir is sugar free.

Product licence numbers

1 mg capsules	0101/0105
1 mg tablets	0101/0125
Elixir 1 mg/5 ml	0101/0137

**Trade Mark*

Sanofi Pharma
Floats Road
Wythenshawe
Manchester, M23 9NF

Associated companies: Labaz Ltd.
The Dermalex Co. Ltd.

CALCIPARINE*

Presentation Sterile, clear, pyrogen-free solution for subcutaneous injection containing Heparin Calcium BP 2,500 iu per 0.1 ml dissolved in Water for Injections BP.

Contains no preservatives.

Calciparine is presented as a solution of 2,500 iu in each 0.1 ml:

(a) in disposable syringes of
0.2 ml 5,000 iu
0.5 ml 12,500 iu
0.8 ml 20,000 iu

(b) in glass ampoules containing
0.8 ml 20,000 iu

Uses As an anticoagulant for the prophylaxis and treatment of thromboembolic phenomena, especially myocardial infarction, acute arterial embolism or thrombosis, deep vein thrombosis, thrombophlebitis or pulmonary embolism.

Dosage and administration
Administration: Calciparine should be given by subcutaneous injection, using a 26-gauge needle. The best site is the subcutaneous tissue of the lateral abdominal wall. The needle should be inserted perpendicularly into a pinched-up fold of skin and held gently but firmly within the skinfold until injection has been completed.

Standard prophylactic dosage: In patients over 40 years of age undergoing major elective surgery 5,000 iu 2 hours before operation, followed by 5,000 iu every 8 hours for 7 days. In patients still confined to bed at the end of this period, the dosage should be continued until they are ambulant.

Following myocardial infarction 5,000 iu twice daily for 10 days or until the patient is mobile. In other medical conditions in which there is an associated increased risk of thromboembolic phenomena, the same dosage is recommended. These standard prophylactic regimens do not require routine control but see below.

Treatment dosage: For existing thrombosis the standard dose is 0.1 ml Calciparine (2,500 iu) per 10 kg body weight 12 hourly. To enable dosage to be individually adjusted to maintain a coagulation time twice that of control it is recommended that the thrombin clotting time, whole blood clotting time or the activated partial thromboplastin time be measured on blood withdrawn 4 hours after the first injection and then at intervals until the patient is stabilised. During long-term therapy, the test should be repeated at least once each week.

Considerations for dosage: For both prophylaxis and treatment, higher doses are likely to be required in patients of abnormally high body weight and in those suffering from cancer, diabetes mellitus or other diseases associated with marked hypercoagulability. Lower doses are usually indicated in the elderly and in those with low serum albumin or impaired renal or hepatic function. In such patients, coagulation times should be checked frequently and dosage adjusted accordingly.

Children: treatment dosage: Dosage should be individually adjusted according to changes in whole blood clotting time and/or thrombin clotting time and/or APTT. The initial dose should be 0.1 ml Calciparine (2,500 iu) per 10 kg of body weight. The usual interval between doses is 12 hours, but this also may require individual adjustment.

Prophylactic dosage in pregnancy: There is clinical evidence that heparin does not cause foetal damage and may be the anticoagulant of choice when anticoagulation is indicated during pregnancy. However, the risk of maternal bleeding may be increased. Individual control is essential and the aim should be to maintain plasma heparin levels between 0.1 and 0.4 units/ml, as assessed by the Anti-Xa assay, and a whole blood clotting time of 15 to 20 minutes.

A prophylactic dosage of 5,000 iu every 8 hours is a suitable starting dose in the first 3 or 4 months of pregnancy but higher doses are needed as pregnancy progresses, 10,000 iu two or three times daily being usual in the last trimester. Dosage must be reduced during labour and standard prophylactic dosage is suitable post-partum.

Contra-indications, warnings, etc Calciparine is contra-indicated in patients hypersensitive to heparin. Calciparine is contra-indicated in patients with a condition in which there is an increased danger of haemorrhage. Such conditions include haemophilia, thrombocytopenia and other haemorrhagic diatheses; gastric and duodenal ulcer; sub-acute bacterial endocarditis; threatened abortion and major surgery involving the brain, spinal cord and eye.

Calciparine should not be used in patients with advanced renal or hepatic dysfunction, in severe hypertension or patients in shock.

Care should be used in patients receiving salicylates or any drug likely to prolong coagulation.

Special care should be taken when elderly patients and pregnant women are involved.

Side-effects: Hypersensitivity reactions may occur, but are rare. Acute reversible thrombocytopenia has been reported but is rare. Osteoporosis and alopecia have occurred in patients treated over many months.

Treatment of overdosage: If bleeding should occur, the effect of heparin can be reversed immediately by intravenous administration of a 1% protamine sulphate solution. The dose of protamine sulphate required for neutralisation should be determined accurately by titrating the patient's plasma.

It is important to avoid overdosage of protamine sulphate because protamine itself has anticoagulant properties. A single dose of protamine sulphate should never exceed 50 mg. Intravenous injection of protamine may cause a sudden fall in blood pressure, bradycardia, dyspnoea and transitory flushing, but these may be avoided or diminished by slow and careful administration.

Pharmaceutical precautions Store below 25°C but do not freeze. Other preparations should not be mixed with Calciparine.

Legal category POM.

Package quantities Calciparine disposable syringes sterilised ready for use (5,000 iu; 12,500 iu; 20,000 iu) are supplied in cartons of 10. Calciparine ampoules (20,000 iu) are supplied in cartons of 10 individual packs each containing an ampoule and sterile disposable syringe and needle.

Further information Nil.

Product licence number 0623/0010.

CARTROL* TABLETS ▼

Presentation White, round, biconvex tablets marked C10, each containing 10 mg carteolol hydrochloride.

Uses In the management of angina pectoris.

Cartrol is a non-selective beta-adrenoceptor blocking agent with partial agonist activity, otherwise known as intrinsic sympathomimetic activity, but with no significant membrane stabilising activity.

Blockade of beta-adrenoceptors by Cartrol prevents excessive sympathetic drive to the heart, resulting in a fall in heart rate and a decrease in myocardial work and oxygen consumption.

The partial agonist activity of Cartrol maintains a significant degree of stimulation of beta-adrenoceptors, which can prevent reduction of resting sympathetic drive to the heart to an undesirably low level and so minimise the risk of excessive bradycardia and myocardial depression. The significant partial agonist activity of Cartrol results in stimulation of the heart at low levels of sympathetic nervous tone, whilst maintaining an inhibitory effect at high levels of sympathetic drive. Thus inappropriate sympathetic activity is inhibited without serious myocardial depression at rest.

Indication: Angina pectoris: Cartrol is indicated in the prophylactic management of patients with angina pectoris. Exercise tolerance and work capacity increase, in association with a reduction in exercise tachycardia and the frequency and severity of anginal attacks. Due to Cartrol's partial agonist activity however, resting heart rate is not significantly reduced.

Dosage and administration The initial dose of Cartrol for angina pectoris is 10 mg daily. If necessary the dose should be increased gradually. Some patients may require 30 mg daily.

Cartrol is compatible with the concomitant administration of nitrates. However, it is sometimes possible to reduce or even discontinue the use of nitrates when the patient is estabished on Cartrol.

Cartrol is eliminated mainly by renal excretion with only a small amount metabolised in the liver. Lower doses may therefore be necessary in patients with significant renal insufficiency.

Use in the elderly: There is no evidence that elderly patients show different side-effects from younger patients but in elderly patients control of anginal symptoms may be achieved at lower doses.

Contra-indications, warnings, etc

Contra-indications: Second or third degree atrioventricular block, severe bradycardia, cardiogenic shock, uncontrolled heart failure, metabolic acidosis (e.g. diabetic acidotic states; prolonged fasting), severe renal failure.

Precautions: Care should be taken when administering beta-adrenoceptor blocking agents to patients whose cardiac reserve is poor, who have a history of cardiac failure, or who are in cardiac failure following a myocardial infarction. Myocardial contractility should be maintained and signs of cardiac failure controlled before commencing therapy with Cartrol.

As with other beta-adrenoceptor blocking agents Cartrol should not be used in patients with asthma or a history of obstructive airways disease, unless no alternative treatment is available. In such cases the risk of inducing bronchospasm should be appreciated and appropriate precautions taken.

Treatment with beta-adrenoceptor blocking agents is liable to mask symptoms of hypoglycaemia and also to affect carbohydrate metabolism. They should be used with caution in patients with labile or insulin-dependent diabetes under treatment with insulin or oral hypoglycaemic agents, where it may be necessary to readjust the dosage of anti-diabetic medication.

Secondary sympathetic hyperactivity has sometimes been reported following discontinuation of treatment with beta-adrenoceptor blocking agents. Even though the therapeutic effects of Cartrol decrease slowly, withdrawal of the product should be gradual.

Effects on ability to drive and to use machines: As with some other beta-blockers dizziness or fatigue may occur during the initial phase of treatment and patients should exercise caution until their individual response to treatment has been determined.

If clonidine is being administered concurrently it should not be discontinued until several days after withdrawal of the beta-blocker.

Beta-adrenoceptor blocking agents should be used with caution in combination with calcium antagonists of the verapamil type in patients with impaired ventricular function, and such combinations are contra-indicated in patients with conduction disorders.

In the event of surgical intervention, the anaesthetist should be advised in advance that the patient is receiving a beta-blocker. If it is decided to withdraw Cartrol before surgery, 48 hours should be allowed to elapse between the last dose and anaesthesia. If treatment with a beta-blocker is continued care should be taken when using anaesthetic agents which may cause myocardial depression. Vagal dominance, if it occurs, may be corrected with atropine 1–2 mg i.v.

If a beta-adrenoceptor blocking agent is indicated in a patient with phaeochromocytoma it must always be given in conjunction with an alpha-adrenoceptor blocking agent.

Side-effects: Cartrol is well tolerated. In clinical studies with Cartrol the side effects reported are usually attributable to the pharmacological actions and include nausea, lassitude, dizziness, pain in extremities, headache and diarrhoea. These effects are usually mild and transient and do not necessitate withdrawal of therapy.

There have been occasional reports of skin rashes and/or dry eyes associated with the use of beta-adrenoceptor blocking agents. The reported incidence is small and in most cases the symptoms have cleared when treatment was withdrawn. Discontinuation of therapy should be considered if any such reaction is not otherwise explicable.

Pregnancy and lactation: Cartrol should be administered during pregnancy and breast feeding only if there are compelling reasons to do so. Animal studies with Cartrol have shown no evidence of teratogenicity or other harmful effects on the foetus or offspring.

If Cartrol is used during pregnancy and lactation, slowing of the heart rate in the foetus, neonate and breast fed infant should call for vigilance because of the drug's beta-blocking action. Cartrol has been shown in animal studies to pass through the placenta in small amounts, but there is no data regarding foetal bradycardia.

Cartrol has been found in breast milk in rats but there is no data on the detection of Cartrol in human breast milk.

Overdosage: Treat by elimination of any unabsorbed medicine and general supportive measures.

Excessive bradycardia may be countered with atropine 1–2 mg intravenously, followed if necessary by a beta-adrenoceptor stimulant such as isoprenaline, administered with caution by slow intravenous injection.

In cardiogenic shock glucagon administered intravenously (5 to 10 mg) may be useful because of its inotropic and chronotropic properties.

Pharmaceutical precautions Store in a dry place below 25°C.

Legal category POM

Package quantities Blister packs of 28 (OP).

Further information Nil.

Product licence number 0623/0051.

CORDARONE* X

Presentation

1. Cordarone X 200 Tablets: White to off-white scored round biconvex tablets marked with the action potential symbol and 200, approximately 10.5 mm in diameter, each containing 200 mg amiodarone hydrochloride.

2. *Cordarone X 100 Tablets:* White to off-white scored round biconvex tablets marked with the action potential symbol and 100, approximately 9.0 mm in diameter, each containing 100 mg amiodarone hydrochloride.

3. *Cordarone X Intravenous:* Ampoules for intravenous injection: clear, pale yellow solution containing 150 mg amiodarone hydrochloride in 3 ml.

Uses Treatment should be initiated only under hospital or specialist supervision.

Tablets: Tachyarrhythmias associated with Wolff-Parkinson-White syndrome.

Atrial flutter and fibrillation when other drugs cannot be used.

All types of tachyarrhythmias of paroxysmal nature including: supraventricular, nodal and ventricular tachycardias, ventricular fibrillation; when other drugs cannot be used.

Tablets are used for stabilisation and long-term treatment.

Injection for intravenous use: Tachyarrhythmias associated with Wolff-Parkinson-White syndrome. All types of tachyarrhythmias including: supraventricular, nodal and ventricular tachycardias; atrial flutter and fibrillation; ventricular fibrillation; when other drugs cannot be used.

The injection is to be used where a rapid response is required.

Dosage and administration

Tablets: It is particularly important that the minimum effective dose be used. In all cases the patient's management must be judged on the individual response and well being. The following dosage regimen is generally effective.

Initial stabilisation: Treatment should be started with 200 mg, 3 times a day and may be continued for 1 week. The dosage should then be reduced to 200 mg, twice daily for a further week.

Maintenance: After the initial period the dosage should be reduced to 200 mg daily, or less if appropriate. Rarely, the patient may require a higher maintenance dose. The scored 100 mg tablet should be used to titrate the minimum dosage required to maintain control of the arrhythmia. The maintenance dose should be regularly reviewed, especially where this exceeds 200 mg daily.

General considerations: The high initial dose is necessary because of the slow onset of action whilst the necessary tissue levels of amiodarone are achieved. Cordarone X has a low acute toxicity and in this initial treatment period serious problems have not been reported. However, excessive dosage during maintenance therapy can cause side effects which are believed to be related to excessive tissue retention of amiodarone and/or its metabolites. Side effects slowly disappear as the tissue levels fall after the dosage is reduced or the drug withdrawn.

If the drug is withdrawn, residual tissue-bound amiodarone may protect the patient for up to a month, but the likelihood of recurrence of cardiac arrhythmias during this period should be a consideration. The important factor is that the patient requires monitoring regularly to ensure that clinical features of excessive dosage are detected and the dosage adjusted accordingly.

It is particularly important that the minimum effective dose be used.

Intravenous injection: Cordarone X Intravenous should only be used when facilities exist for cardiac monitoring and defibrillation, should the need arise.

The standard recommended dose is 5 mg/kg bodyweight given by intravenous infusion over a period of 20 minutes to 2 hours. Where possible this should be administered as a dilute solution in 250 ml 5% dextrose. This may be followed by repeat infusions up to 1200 mg, i.e. (approximately 15 mg/kg bodyweight) in up to 500 ml 5% dextrose per 24 hours, the rate of infusion being adjusted on the basis of clinical response. In extreme clinical emergency the drug may, at the discretion of the clinician, be given as a slow injection of 150–300 mg in 10–20 ml 5% dextrose over a minimum of 3 minutes. This should not be repeated for at least 15 minutes. Patients treated in this way must be closely monitored, e.g. in an intensive care unit.

When given by infusion Cordarone X may reduce drop size and, if appropriate, adjustments should be made to the rate of infusion.

Repeated or continuous infusion via the peripheral veins may lead to local discomfort and inflammation. When repeated or continuous infusion is anticipated, administration by a central venous catheter is recommended.

Changeover from intravenous to oral therapy: Oral therapy should be initiated concomitantly at the usual loading dose ie 200 mg three times a day, as soon as possible after an adequate response has been obtained using Cordarone X Intravenous which should then be phased out gradually.

Use in the elderly: As with all patients it is important that the minimum effective dose is used. Whilst there is no evidence that dosage requirements are different for this group of patients they may be more susceptible to bradycardia and conduction defects if too high a dose is employed. Particular attention should be paid to monitoring of thyroid function. See Contra-indications, warnings, etc.

Contra-indications, warnings, etc Cordarone X is contra-indicated in patients with evidence or history of thyroid dysfunction. In doubtful cases thyroid function tests should be performed prior to therapy with Cordarone X.

Cordarone X is contra-indicated in patients with sinus bradycardia and sino-atrial heart block. In patients with severe conduction disturbances (high grade AV block, bifascicular or trifascicular block), or sinus node disease Cordarone X should only be used in conjunction with a pacemaker.

One tablet of Cordarone X 200 contains approximately 75 mg iodine and one ampoule of Cordarone X Intravenous contains approximately 56 mg Iodine. Caution is therefore advised when considering administration to patients with known hypersensitivity to iodine.

Too high a dosage may lead to severe bradycardia and to conduction disturbances with the appearance of an idioventricular rhythm, particularly in elderly patients or during digitalis therapy. In these circumstances, Cordarone X treatment should be withdrawn. If necessary beta-adrenostimulants or glucagon may be given.

Oral Cordarone X is not contra-indicated in patients with latent or manifest heart failure, but caution should be exercised as, occasionally, existing heart failure may be worsened. In this case, Cordarone X should be associated with the usual cardiotonic and diuretic treatment.

Cordarone X Intravenous is contra-indicated in severe respiratory failure, circulatory collapse or severe arterial hypotension and may cause moderate and transient reduction in blood pressure. Circulatory collapse may be precipitated by too rapid an administration or overdosage (atropine has been used successfully in such patients presenting with bradycardia).

Congestive heart failure is also a contra-indication when using Cordarone X Intravenous as a bolus injection.

Side effects: Rapid administration of Cordarone X Intravenous has been associated with anaphylactic shock, hot flushes, sweating and nausea. In cases of respiratory failure, notably in asthmatics, bronchospasm and/or apnoea may also occur.

Because some side effects may arise only after long-term treatment patients should be regularly monitored.

Ophthalmological: Patients on continuous therapy may develop microdeposits in the cornea. The deposits are usually discernible only by slit-lamp examination and very rarely give rise to symptoms such as visual haloes.

They regress with termination of treatment and are considered essentially benign in nature. Rare cases of impaired visual acuity due to optic neuritis have been reported. During long-term administration regular ophthalmological examination is recommended.

Cardiac: Bradycardia which is generally moderate and dose dependent has been reported. In some cases (sinus node disease, elderly patients) marked bradycardia or more exceptionally sinus arrest has occurred. There have been rare instances of conduction disturbances (sino-atrial block, various degrees of AV block).

Cordarone X has a low pro-arrhythmic effect. This has usually occurred in combination with other precipitating factors particularly other antiarrhythmic agents, hypokalaemia and digoxin.

Dermatological: Cordarone X may induce photosensitisation in some patients; this can usually be alleviated by the use of total sun block barrier creams and other protective measures. Rarely a slate grey or bluish discolouration of the skin has been reported; resolution may be very slow on discontinuation of the drug. Skin rashes including isolated cases of exfoliative dermatitis have also been reported. Cases of erythema have been reported during the course of radiotherapy.

Thyroid: Both hyper and hypothyroidism have occurred during, or soon after, treatment with Cordarone X. Simple monitoring of the usual biochemical tests is confusing because some (PBI and ^{131}I uptake) are invalidated and others (T_4, T_3 and FTI) may be altered where the patient is clearly euthyroid. Clinical monitoring is therefore recommended and should be continued for some months after discontinuation of Cordarone X treatment. This is particularly important in the elderly. In patients whose history indicates an increased risk of thyroid dysfunction, regular testing is recommended.

Clinical features of hyperthyroidism such as weight loss, asthenia, restlessness, increase in heart rate, recurrence of the cardiac dysrhythmia, angina or congestive heart failure, should alert the clinician. The diagnosis may be supported by the finding of an elevated serum tri-iodothyronine (T_3), a low level of thyroid stimulating hormone (TSH as measured by high sensitivity methods) and a reduced TSH response to thyrotrophin releasing hormone (TRH). Elevation of reverse T_3 (r.T_3) may also be found.

The clinical features of hypothyroidism such as weight gain and reduced activity or excessive bradycardia should alert the clinician. The onset may be abrupt. The diagnosis may be supported by the presence of an elevated serum TSH level and an exaggerated TSH response to TRH. The thyroxine (T_4), T_3 and free thyroxine index (FTI) may be low.

In the case of hyperthyroidism Cordarone X should be withdrawn. Clinical recovery usually occurs within a few weeks.

Courses of anti-thyroid drugs have been used for the treatment of severe thyroid hyperactivity; large doses may be required initially. These may not always be effective and concomitant high dose corticosteroid therapy (eg 1 mg/kg prednisolone) may be required for several weeks.

Thyroid hypofunction, usually resolves within 3 months of cessation of Cordarone X; it may be treated cautiously with L-thyroxine. Concomitant use of Cordarone X should be only in life threatening situations, when TSH levels may provide a guide to L-thyroxine dosage.

Pulmonary: Diffuse pulmonary alveolitis and fibrosis have been reported, sometimes presenting as unexplained or disproportionate dyspnoea whether in isolation or associated with deterioration of general health (fatigue, weight loss, fever). Patients developing dyspnoea without signs of cardiac failure or loss of control of arrhythmias should be carefully evaluated clinically including chest X-ray and lung function testing. Pulmonary alveolitis has usually been reversible with and without corticosteroid therapy following early withdrawal of Cordarone X therapy. Clinical symptoms often resolve within a few weeks followed by slower radiological and lung function improvement.

Hepatic: It is advisable to monitor liver function particularly transaminases before treatment and periodically thereafter.

At the beginning of therapy: elevation of serum transaminases which can be in isolation (1.5 to 3 times normal) may occur. These may return to normal with dose reduction, or sometimes spontaneously. Occasional cases of acute liver disorders with elevated serum transaminases and/or jaundice may occur. These normally regress when treatment is withdrawn.

During long term therapy: There have been reports of chronic liver disease. Alteration of laboratory tests which may be minimal (transaminases elevated 1.5 to 5 times normal) or clinical signs (possible hepatomegaly) during treatment for longer than 6 months should suggest this diagnosis. Routine monitoring of liver function tests is therefore advised. Abnormal clinical and laboratory test results usually regress upon cessation of treatment. A few cases of irreversible progression have been reported. Histological findings may resemble pseudo-alcoholic hepatitis, but they can be variable and include cirrhosis.

Neurological: Peripheral neuropathy and/or myopathy have been reported. These conditions may be serious and ultimately are usually reversible on withdrawal of the drug. Nightmares, vertigo, headaches and sleeplessness may also occur. Tremor and ataxia have also infrequently been reported usually with complete regression after reduction of dose or withdrawal of the drug. Benign raised intracranial pressure has been reported.

Other: Other unwanted effects occasionally reported include nausea, vomiting, metallic taste (which usually occur with loading dosage and which regress on dose reduction), fatigue and epididymo-orchitis. Isolated cases suggesting a hypersensitivity reaction involving vasculitis, renal involvement with moderate elevation of creatinine levels or thrombocytopenia have been observed.

Drug interactions: Administration of Cordarone X to a patient already receiving digoxin may bring about an increase in the plasma digoxin concentration and thus precipitate symptoms and signs associated with high digoxin levels. Monitoring is recommended and digoxin dosage should be adjusted accordingly. A synergistic effect on heart rate and atrioventricular conduction is also possible.

It may potentiate oral anticoagulant therapy by increasing plasma levels of oral anticoagulants. More frequent monitoring of prothrombin time during treatment with and after discontinuation of Cordarone X therapy is indicated. Consideration should be given to the possibility that Cordarone X may alter the plasma concentrations of other drugs particularly those which are highly protein-bound e.g. phenytoin.

Potentiation of the negative chronotropic and dromotropic properties of beta blockers and certain calcium channel inhibitors (verapamil, diltiazem) may occur. Combination therapy should therefore be strictly monitored.

The risk of Torsade de Pointes may be increased when Cordarone X is used in combination with other drugs which directly or indirectly prolong the QT interval eg certain antiarrhythmics (quinidine, disopyramide) or agents which may induce hypokalaemia eg diuretics.

The combination of Cordarone X with other antiarrhythmics (especially Class I) needs particularly careful consideration.

Cordarone X should not be used with sotalol because of the effects on repolarization.

Potentially severe complications have been reported in patients taking amiodarone undergoing general anaesthesia: bradycardia unresponsive to atropine, hypotension, disturbances of conduction, decreased cardiac output. A few cases of acute respiratory distress have been observed in the period immediately after cardiovascular surgery. Possible potentiation of the toxic effect of oxygen has been implicated. The anaesthetist should be informed that the patient is taking Cordarone X.

Women of child-bearing age: Although no teratogenic effects have been observed in animals, there are insufficient data on the use of Cordarone X during pregnancy in humans to judge any possible toxicity. However, in view of the pharmacological properties of the drug on the foetus and its effect on the foetal thyroid gland, its administration in pregnancy should be avoided.

Breast-feeding: Cordarone X is present in the breast milk in significant quantities and breast-feeding is contraindicated.

Treatment of overdosage: Animal studies indicate that Cordarone X has a high LD_{50}, hence it is most unlikely that a patient will ingest an acute toxic dose. In such an event gastric lavage may be employed to reduce absorption in addition to general supportive measures. The patient should be monitored and if bradycardia ensues beta-adrenostimulants or glucagon may be given. Spontaneously resolving attacks of ventricular tachycardia may also occur. Due to the pharmacokinetics of Cordarone X, adequate and prolonged surveillance of the patient, particularly cardiac status is recommended.

Pharmaceutical precautions Tablets and ampoules should be protected from light. Cordarone X Intravenous is incompatible with saline and should be administered solely in 5% Dextrose solution. Solutions containing less than 2 ampoules Cordarone X Intravenous in 500 ml Dextrose 5% are unstable and should not be used.

Legal category POM.

Package quantities *Tablets:* carton of 28 tablets (in blister pack of 14 tablets) (OP).
Intravenous injection: carton of 10 ampoules.

Further information Cordarone X Intravenous may be used prior to DC cardioversion. It has been used to treat successfully atrial, junctional and ventricular tachyarrhythmias. It may be used where a rapid response is required, such as following a myocardial infarction.

Cordarone X induces ECG changes; QT interval lengthening corresponding to prolonged repolarisation; U and deformed T waves may occur because of the fixing of amiodarone in myocardial tissues.

Cordarone X is strongly protein-bound and the plasma half-life is usually of the order of 50 days. However there may be considerable inter-patient variation; in individual patients a half-life of less than 20 days and a half-life of more than 100 days has been reported. High doses of Cordarone X, for example 600 mg/day, should be given initially to achieve effective tissue levels as rapidly as possible. Owing to the long half-life of the drug, a maintenance dose of only 200 mg/day, or less is usually necessary. Sufficient time must be allowed for a new distribution equilibrium to be achieved between adjustments of dose.

The long half-life is a valuable safeguard for patients with potentially lethal arrhythmias as omission of occasional doses does not significantly influence the protection afforded by Cordarone X.

Inactive ingredients include: Cordarone X 200 and Cordarone X 100 Tablets – lactose; Cordarone X Intravenous – Benzyl alcohol and polysorbate 80.

Product licence numbers

Cordarone X 100	0623/0017
Cordarone X 200	0623/0007
Cordarone X Intravenous	0623/0012

DERMALEX* SKIN LOTION

Presentation A white oil-in-water emulsion containing Cosbiol (Squalane) 3.0%, hexachlorophane 0.5%, allantoin 0.2%.

Uses Prevention of pressure sores. Prevention and treatment of incontinence rash and non-specific rashes. Skin antiseptic for preparation of split-skin donor areas. As a hand cream for medical and surgical staff to reduce the risk of cross infection.

Dosage and administration Apply sparingly as a routine procedure every 4 to 6 hours and after washing.

Only a thin film is needed on the skin for good results. Over generous application can occasionally cause redness.

It is important to ensure that no barrier creams are used on a patient using Dermalex skin lotion.

Contra-indications, warnings, etc Dermalex skin lotion should not be applied to broken skin, open pressure sores, seriously burnt skin or mucous membranes. During regular use in the treatment of pressure areas it is inadvisable to apply to areas of the skin in excess of half of the total body surface area.

Dermalex should not be administered except on medical advice to children under two years of age.

Pharmaceutical precautions No special storage requirements.

Legal category P.

Package quantities 100 mls (OP).
250 mls (Pump action dispenser with this size).

Further information Dermalex is a deep penetrating lotion effective against a wide range of organisms and with a long allergy free history. It maintains its deep antiseptic activity in the skin for at least six hours, and in addition Cosbiol provides a beneficial effect for patients with dry skin.

Product licence number 1983/5000.

EPILIM*

Presentation

1. *Epilim 200 Enteric-Coated:* A lilac-coloured enteric-coated tablet containing 200 mg Sodium Valproate BP.
2. *Epilim 500 Enteric-Coated:* A lilac-coloured enteric-coated tablet containing 500 mg Sodium Valproate BP.
3. *Epilim 100 mg Crushable Tablets:* A white scored tablet containing 100 mg Sodium Valproate BP.
4. *Epilim Syrup:* A red, cherry-flavoured syrup containing 200 mg Sodium Valproate BP per 5 ml.
5. *Epilim Liquid:* A red, cherry-flavoured, sugar-free liquid containing 200 mg Sodium Valproate BP per 5 ml.

Uses In the treatment of generalised, partial or other epilepsy. In women of childbearing age Epilim should be used only in severe cases or in those resistant to other treatment.

Dosage and administration Daily dosage requirements vary according to age and body weight.
Monotherapy: Usual requirements are as follows:
Adults: Dosage should start at 600 mg daily increasing by 200 mg at three day intervals until control is achieved. This is generally within the dosage range 1000 mg to 2000 mg per day, i.e. 20–30 mg/kg body weight. Where adequate control is not achieved within this range the dose may be further increased to 2500 mg per day.
Children over 20 kg: Initial dosage should be 400 mg/day (irrespective of weight) with spaced increases until control is achieved; this is usually within the range 20–30 mg/kg body weight per day. Where adequate control is not achieved within this range the dose may be increased to 35 mg/kg body weight per day.
Children under 20 kg: 20 mg/kg of body weight per day; in severe cases this may be increased but only in patients in whom plasma valproic acid levels can be monitored. Above 40 mg/kg/day, clinical chemistry and haematological parameters should be monitored.
Use in the elderly: Although the pharmacokinetics of Epilim are modified in the elderly, they have limited clinical significance and dosage should be determined by seizure control. The volume of distribution is increased in the elderly and, because of decreased binding to serum albumin, the proportion of free drug is increased. This will affect the clinical interpretation of plasma valproic acid levels.
Administration: Epilim tablets, syrup and liquid may be given twice daily. Uncoated tablets may be crushed if necessary.
Combined therapy: In certain cases it may be necessary to raise the dose by 5 to 10 mg/kg/day when used in

combination with anticonvulsants which induce liver enzyme activity, e.g. phenytoin, phenobarbitone, and carbamazepine. Once known enzyme inducers have been withdrawn it may be possible to maintain seizure control on a reduced dose of Epilim. When barbiturates are being administered concomitantly the dosage of barbiturate should be reduced should sedation be observed.

General considerations: Optimum dosage is mainly determined by seizure control and routine measurement of plasma levels is unnecessary. However, a method for measurement of plasma levels is available and may be helpful where there is poor control or side-effects are suspected, see Further Information.

Contra-indications, warnings, etc
Contra-indication: Active liver disease.

Side-effects
Hepatic: Liver dysfunction, including hepatic failure resulting in fatalities, has occurred in patients whose treatment included valproic acid or sodium valproate. Patients most at risk are children under the age of three and those with congenital metabolic disorders, organic brain disease or severe seizure disorders associated with mental retardation. The incidents mainly occurred during the first six months of therapy, the period of maximum risk being 2–12 weeks, and usually involved multiple anticonvulsant therapy. Monotherapy is to be preferred in this group of patients.

Clinical symptoms are more helpful than laboratory investigations in the early stages of hepatic failure. The onset of an acute illness, especially within the first six months, which may include symptoms of vomiting, lethargy or weakness, drowsiness, anorexia, jaundice or loss of seizure control, is an indication for immediate withdrawal of the drug. Patients should be instructed to report any such signs to the clinician should they occur. Available evidence to date does not establish which, if any, investigation could predict this possible adverse effect. However, routine measurement of liver function should be undertaken in the first six months of therapy in those who seem most at risk, and those with a prior history of liver disease; such patients should have close clinical supervision. Raised liver enzymes are not uncommon during treatment with Epilim and are usually transient or respond to reduction in dosage of Epilim. Patients with such biochemical abnormalities should be reassessed clinically and tests of liver function should be monitored until they return to normal.

Metabolic: Hyperammonaemia without hepatic damage can occur in patients during treatment with valproic acid or sodium valproate. This is usually transient, but may occasionally present clinically as vomiting, ataxia and increasing clouding of consciousness. Should these symptoms occur Epilim should be discontinued. Oedema has been reported rarely.

Pancreatic: There have been reports of pancreatitis occurring in patients receiving valproic acid or sodium valproate, usually within the first six months of therapy. Patients experiencing acute abdominal pain should have their serum amylase estimated; if these levels are elevated treatment should be discontinued.

Haematological: Valproic acid inhibits the second stage of platelet aggregation. Reversible prolongation of bleeding time and thrombocytopenia have been reported, but are usually associated with doses above those recommended. Spontaneous bruising or bleeding is an indication for withdrawal of medication pending investigations; it is recommended that patients receiving Epilim be monitored for platelet function before major surgery. Red cell hypoplasia and leucopenia have been reported rarely; the blood picture returned to normal when the drug was discontinued.

Neurological: Ataxia and tremor have been occasionally reported and appear to be dose related effects.

Sedation has been reported occasionally, usually when used in combination with other anticonvulsants. In Epilim monotherapy it occurred early in treatment on rare occasions and is usually transient. Rare cases of lethargy and confusion occasionally progressing to stupor, sometimes with associated hallucinations have been reported. Coma has very rarely been observed. These cases have usually been in association with other anticonvulsants, notably phenobarbitone, and have been reversible on withdrawal of treatment.

An increase in alertness may occur; this is generally beneficial but occasionally aggression, hyperactivity and behavioural deterioration have been reported.

Gastro-intestinal: Increase in appetite may occur and an increase in weight is not uncommon. Minor gastric irritation and, less frequently, nausea have been observed in some patients at the start of treatment, but these problems can usually be overcome by administering Enteric Coated Epilim or administering Epilim with or after food.

Dermatological: Transient hair loss has been noted in some patients. This effect does not appear to be dose-related and regrowth normally begins within six months, although the hair may become more curly than previously. Rashes have been reported rarely.

Endocrine: There have been isolated reports of amenorrhoea.

Drug interactions: Like many other drugs, Epilim may potentiate the effect of monoamine oxidase inhibitors and other antidepressants. The enzyme inducing effect of valproate is appreciably less than that of certain other anticonvulsants and loss of efficacy of oral contraceptive agents does not appear to be a problem.

Caution is recommended when administering anticoagulants and other products which have anticoagulant properties (e.g. warfarin and aspirin). Epilim decreases protein binding of warfarin but this may not lead to clinically significant effects.

Dosage of Epilim may require adjustment when used in combination with other anticonvulsants. See Dosage, Combined Therapy Section.

Diabetic patients: Epilim is eliminated mainly through the kidneys, partly in the form of ketone bodies; this may give false positives in the urine testing of possible diabetics. In addition, care should be taken when treating diabetic patients with Epilim Syrup, as this contains 3.6 g sucrose per 5 ml; Epilim Liquid is, however, sugar-free.

Women of childbearing age: An increased incidence of congenital abnormalities in offspring born to mothers with epilepsy both untreated and treated has been demonstrated.

There have been reports of foetal anomalies including neural tube defects in women receiving valproate during the first trimester. This incidence has been estimated to be in the region of 1%. Such pregnancies should be carefully screened by alpha-foetoprotein measurement and ultrasound and if indicated amniocentesis.

In all pregnancies monotherapy is to be recommended and the benefits of antiepileptic therapy must be evaluated against the possible risks and patients should be informed of these and the need for screening.

Breast feeding: The concentration of valproic acid found in the breast milk is very low, between 1% and 10% of total maternal plasma levels. There appears to be no contra-indication to breast feeding by patients on Epilim. The decision to allow the patients to breast feed should be taken with regard to all the known facts.

Overdosage: Cases of accidental and suicidal overdosage have been reported. At plasma concentrations of up to 5 to 6 times the maximum therapeutic levels, there are unlikely to be any symptoms other than nausea, vomiting and dizziness.

In massive overdose, i.e. with plasma concentrations 10 to 20 times maximum therapeutic levels there may be serious CNS depression and respiration may be impaired. Full recovery is usual following treatment including induced vomiting, gastric lavage, assisted ventilation, and other supportive measures.

Pharmaceutical precautions Epilim tablets are hygroscopic and must be kept in their protective foil until taken; they should be stored in a dry place below 30°C.

Epilim Syrup and Epilim Liquid should be kept below 30°C and away from direct sunlight.

Dilutions: If it is necessary to dilute Epilim Syrup, the recommended diluent is Syrup BP, but syrup containing SO_2 as a preservative should not be used. The diluted product will have a 14 day shelf life. Epilim Liquid should not be diluted.

Legal category POM.

Package quantities Epilim 200 Enteric-Coated, Epilim 500 Enteric-Coated tablets and Epilim 100 mg Crushable tablets are packed in foil, in cartons of 100 tablets. Epilim Syrup and Epilim Liquid are packed in 300 ml bottles.

Further information The beneficial effects of Epilim may not be clearly correlated with the total plasma valproic acid levels. The reported effective range is usually between 40–100 mg/litre (278–694 micro mol/litre) depending on time of sampling and presence of co-medication.

The percentage of free drug then is usually between 6% and 15% of the total levels. Above this range an increased incidence of adverse effects may occur.

The half-life of sodium valproate is usually reported to be within the range of 8–20 hours.

Product licence numbers

Epilim Syrup	0623/0004
Epilim 500 Enteric-Coated	0623/0005
Epilim 200 Enteric-Coated	0623/0006
Epilim 100 mg Crushable tablets	0623/0015
Epilim Liquid	0623/0016

EPILIM* INTRAVENOUS

Presentation Epilim Intravenous. Off-white sterile, freeze dried Sodium Valproate BP 400 mg in a clear glass vial supplied with an ampoule of 4 ml of solvent (Water for Injections).

Uses Epilim Intravenous may be used for epileptic patients who would normally be maintained on oral sodium valproate, and for whom oral therapy is temporarily not possible.

Dosage and administration Daily dosage requirements vary according to age and body weight.

To reconstitute, inject the solvent provided (4 ml) into the vial, allow to dissolve and extract the appropriate dose. Due to displacement of solvent by sodium valproate the concentration of reconstituted sodium valproate is 95 mg/ml.

Each vial of Epilim Intravenous is for single dose injection only. It should be reconstituted immediately prior to use and infusion solutions containing it used within 24 hours. Any unused portion should be discarded.

Epilim Intravenous may be given by direct slow intravenous injection or by infusion using a separate intravenous line in normal saline, dextrose 5%, or dextrose saline.

Patients already satisfactorily treated with Epilim may be continued at their current dosage using continuous or repeated infusion. Other patients may be given a slow intravenous injection over 3–5 minutes, usually 400–800 mg depending on body weight (up to 10 mg/kg) followed by continuous or repeated infusion up to a maximum of 2500 mg/day.

Epilim Intravenous should be replaced by oral Epilim therapy as soon as practicable.

Daily requirement for children is usually in the range 20–30 mg/kg/day and method of administration is as above. Where adequate control is not achieved within this range the dose may be increased up to 40 mg/kg/day but only in patients in whom plasma valproic acid levels can be monitored. Above 40 mg/kg/day clinical chemistry and haematological parameters should be monitored.

Use in the elderly: Although the pharmacokinetics of Epilim are modified in the elderly, they have limited clinical significance and dosage should be determined by seizure control. The volume of distribution is increased in the elderly and because of decreased binding to serum albumin, the proportion of free drug is increased. This will affect the clinical interpretation of plasma valproic acid levels.

Combined therapy: In certain cases it may be necessary to raise the dose by 5 to 10 mg/kg/day when used in combination with anticonvulsants which induce liver enzyme activity, e.g. phenytoin, phenobarbitone, and carbamazepine. Once known enzyme inducers have been withdrawn it may be possible to maintain seizure control on a reduced dose of Epilim. When barbiturates are being administered concomitantly the dosage of barbiturate should be reduced if sedation is observed.

General considerations: Optimum dosage is mainly determined by seizure control and routine measurement of plasma levels is unnecessary. However, a method for measurement of plasma levels is available and may be helpful where there is poor control or side effects are suspected, see further information.

Contra-indications, warnings, etc

Contra-indications: Active liver disease.

Side-effects

Hepatic: Liver dysfunction, including hepatic failure resulting in fatalities has occurred in patients whose treatment included valproic acid or sodium valproate. Patients most at risk are children under the age of three and those with congenital metabolic disorders, organic brain disease or severe seizure disorders associated with mental retardation. The incidents mainly occurred during the first six months of therapy, the period of maximum risk being 2–12 weeks, and usually involved multiple anticonvulsant therapy. Monotherapy is to be preferred in this group of patients.

Clinical symptoms are more helpful than laboratory investigations in the early stages of hepatic failure. The onset of an acute illness, especially within the first six months, which may include symptoms of vomiting, lethargy or weakness, drowsiness, anorexia, jaundice or loss of seizure control, is an indication for immediate withdrawal of the drug. Patients should be instructed to report any such signs to the clinician should they occur. Available evidence to date does not establish which, if any, investigation could predict this possible adverse effect. However, routine measurement of liver function should be undertaken in the first six months of therapy in those who seem most at risk and those with a prior history of liver disease; such patients should have close clinical supervision. Raised liver enzymes are not uncommon during treatment with Epilim and are usually transient or respond to reduction in dosage of Epilim. Patients with such biochemical abnormalities should be reassessed clinically and tests of liver function should be monitored until they return to normal.

Metabolic: Hyperammonaemia without hepatic damage can occur in patients during treatment with valproic acid or sodium valproate. This is usually transient, but may occasionally present clinically as vomiting, ataxia and increasing clouding of consciousness. Should these symptoms occur Epilim should be discontinued. Oedema has been reported rarely.

Pancreatic: There have been reports of pancreatitis occurring in patients receiving valproic acid or sodium valproate, usually within the first six months of therapy. Patients experiencing acute abdominal pain should have the serum amylase estimated; if these levels are elevated treatment should be discontinued.

Haematological: Valproic acid inhibits the second stage of platelet aggregation. Reversible prolongation of bleeding time and thrombocytopenia have been reported, but are usually associated with doses above those recommended. Spontaneous bruising or bleeding is an indication for withdrawal of medication pending investigations; it is recommended that patients receiving Epilim be monitored for platelet function before major surgery. Red cell hypoplasia and leucopenia have been reported rarely; the blood picture returned to normal when the drug was discontinued.

Neurological: Ataxia and tremor have been reported occasionally and appear to be dose-related effects.

Sedation has been occasionally reported, usually in combination with other anticonvulsants. In Epilim monotherapy it occurs on rare occasions early in treatment and is usually transient. It is possible that rare cases of lethargy and confusion occasionally progressing to stupor, sometimes with associated hallucinations may occur.

An increase in alertness may occur; this is generally beneficial but occasionally aggression, hyperactivity and behavioural deterioration have been reported.

Drug interactions: Like many other drugs, Epilim may potentiate the effect of monoamine oxidase inhibitors and other anti-depressants. The enzyme inducing effect of valproate is appreciably less than that of certain other anti-convulsants and loss of efficacy of oral contraceptive agents does not appear to be a problem.

Caution is recommended when administering anticoagulants and other products which have anticoagulant properties (e.g. warfarin and aspirin). Epilim decreases protein binding of warfarin but this may not lead to clinically significant effects.

Dosage of Epilim may require adjustment when used in combination with other anti-convulsants. See 'Dosage, Combined Therapy Section'.

Diabetic patients: Epilim is eliminated mainly through the kidneys, partly in the form of ketone bodies; this may give false positives in the urine testing of possible diabetics.

Pregnancy: An increased incidence of congenital abnormalities in offspring born to mothers with epilepsy both untreated and treated has been demonstrated.

There have been reports of foetal anomalies including neural tube defects in women receiving valproate during the first trimester. This incidence has been estimated to be in the region of 1%. Such pregnancies should be carefully screened by alpha-foetoprotein measurement and ultrasound and if indicated amniocentesis.

In all pregnancies monotherapy is to be recommended and the benefits of antiepileptic therapy must be evaluated against the possible risks and patients should be informed of these and the need for screening.

Breast feeding: The concentration of valproic acid found in the breast milk is very low, between 1% and 10% of total maternal plasma levels. Thus there appears to be no contra-indication to breast feeding by patients on Epilim. The decision to allow the patient to breast feed should be taken with regard to all the known facts.

Overdosage: At plasma concentrations of up to 5 to 6 times the maximum therapeutic levels, there are unlikely to be any symptoms other than nausea, vomiting and dizziness.

In massive overdose, i.e. with plasma concentrations 10 to 20 times maximum therapeutic levels there may be serious CNS depression and respiration may be impaired. Full recovery is usual following treatment including induced vomiting, gastric lavage, assisted ventilation, and other supportive measures.

Pharmaceutical precautions Epilim Intravenous freeze dried powder should be stored below 25°C; infusion solutions at 2–8°C if stored before use, discarding any remaining after 24 hours. Epilim Intravenous should not be administered via the same IV line as other IV additives. The intravenous solution is suitable for infusion in PVC, polythene, or glass containers.

Legal category POM.

Package quantities Epilim Intravenous is supplied as a pack of one vial of 400 mg Sodium Valproate BP and one ampoule containing 4 ml of solvent.

Further information The beneficial effects of Epilim may not be clearly correlated with the total plasma valproic acid levels. The reported effective range is usually between 40–100 mg/litre (278–694 micro mol/litre) depending on time of sampling and presence of comedication.

The percentage of free drug then is usually between 6% and 15% of the total levels. Above this range an increased incidence of adverse effects may occur.

The half life of sodium valproate is usually reported to be within the range 8 –20 hours.

Product licence numbers

Vial of freeze dried powder	0623/0038
Ampoule of solvent	0623/0040

OSSOPAN*

Presentation The active ingredient of Ossopan preparations is microcrystalline hydroxyapatite compound (MCHC), which is a source of calcium and phosphorus in a protein base containing trace elements.

Ossopan 800 tablets: Pale buff, film-coated. Each tablet contains 830 mg MCHC, providing 178 mg calcium and 83 mg phosphorus.

Ossopan granules: Coarse, brown granules, with a taste and odour of malt and cocoa. Each sachet contains 3320 mg MCHC, providing 712 mg calcium and 332 mg phosphorus. Each sachet contains approximately 4 grams, equivalent to 4 Ossopan 800 tablets.

Uses Provision of calcium and phosphorus in osteoporosis, rickets, osteomalacia and during lactation.

Dosage and administration
Ossopan 800: 4–8 tablets to be taken daily in divided doses, before meals.

Ossopan granules: One to two sachets daily with or before food.

Use in the elderly: There are no special dosage recommendations.

Contra-indications, warnings, etc
Contra-indications: Hypercalcaemia, hypercalciuria.

Precautions: Care should be exercised in patients with severe immobilisation, e.g. paraplegia, and in patients with a history of renal calcium stone formation.

Treatment of overdosage: No cases of intoxication with Ossopan due to deliberate or accidental overdosage have been reported to the Company. It is considered that overdosage is unlikely to be a problem.

Pharmaceutical precautions Store in a dry place.

Legal category P.

Package quantities
Ossopan 800: packs of 50 tablets.
Ossopan granules: packs containing 28 sachets (OP).

Further information Hydroxyapatite is the complex biological calcium salt which forms the basis of skeletal structure; its overall formula is $Ca_{10}\ (PO_4)_6(OH)_2$. MCHC contains about 50 per cent hydroxyapatite and X-ray diffraction studies have confirmed the presence and microcrystalline nature of the salt. It also contains many essential trace elements together with natural skeletal protein (collagen), substituent amino acids and glycosaminoglycans. Clinical studies suggest that MCHC may be more readily assimilable than synthetic calcium supplements.

Product licence numbers

Ossopan 800 tablets	0376/0001
Ossopan granules	0623/0045

TRIFYBA*

Presentation Trifyba is a light brown particulate powder containing 80% of fibre, dervied from the husk of wheat (Testa Triticum Tricum). It is presented as single dose sachets each containing 3.5 g.

Uses Colonic and gastro-intestinal disorders where a high-fibre regimen is indicated including simple constipation, uncomplicated diverticular disease, irritable colon, haemorrhoidal disorders and fissures and other conditions where straining at stool should be avoided.

Dosage and administration
Adults: One sachet two to three times daily.

Children: Half to one sachet once or twice daily depending on age and size.

Trifyba should be taken mixed with food or liquids. For maximum effect adequate fluids should be taken.

Contra-indications, warnings, etc Trifyba is contra-indicated in cases of intestinal obstruction. Some patients may experience transient abdominal distention and flatulence, but this rapidly diminishes and usually disappears within two weeks.

Overdosage: Due to the nature of the preparation, overdosage is unlikely. If it does occur, it should be treated conservatively and the patient given copious fluids by mouth.

Pharmaceutical precautions Nil.

Legal category GSL.

Package quantities Cartons containing 56 sachets.

Further information Trifyba is 80% fibre, and therefore represents a highly concentrated source of fibre. It is classified as an insoluble bulk forming laxative acting by retaining water in a cellular network with consequent improvement in colonic function. Trifyba contains clinically insignificant levels of phytic acid and does not interfere with mineral absorption from the gastrointestinal tract. Trifyba is free from sugar and other additives, contains no starch and can be used for diabetics and others on a calorie restricted diet. Trifyba contains negligible amounts of sodium, a factor of importance in the treatment of patients with cardiac or renal disease.

Product licence number 5287/0001.

**Trade Mark*

Schering Health Care Limited
The Brow, Burgess Hill
West Sussex RH15 9NE

ANDROCUR*

Presentation Each round, white, 9 mm tablet is impressed on one side with 'BV' in a regular hexagon, and is scored on the other. It contains 50 mg cyproterone acetate.

Excipients: maize starch, povidone 25000, aerosil, magnesium stearate, lactose.

Uses Control of libido in severe hypersexuality and/or sexual deviation in the adult male.

Dosage and administration The daily dose should be divided and taken after the morning and evening meals. The usual dose is 1 tablet twice daily.

Contra-indications, warnings, etc *Contra-indications:* Liver diseases. Malignant tumours (other than prostatic cancer, for which cyproterone acetate is indicated. See data sheet for Cyprostat*) and wasting diseases (because of transient catabolic action). A history of or existing thrombosis or embolism. Severe diabetes with vascular changes. Sicklecell anaemia. Severe chronic depression. Androcur should not be given to youths under 18 or those whose bone maturation and testicular maturation are incomplete.

Warnings/side-effects: Liver. Cyproterone acetate has been found to cause liver abnormalities in animals, including the development of tumours. Disturbances of liver function, some of them severe, have been reported with high-dosed Androcur treatment. Liver-function tests should be performed regularly during treatment.

In rare cases benign and in even rarer cases malignant liver tumours, leading in isolated cases to life-threatening intra-abdominal haemorrhage, have been observed after the use of sex steroids, to which class cyproterone acetate belongs. If severe upper abdominal complaints, liver enlargement or signs of intra-abdominal haemorrhage occur, a liver tumour should be considered in the differential diagnosis and, if necessary, Androcur should be withdrawn.

Inhibition of spermatogenesis. The sperm count and the volume of ejaculate are reduced. Infertility is usual, and there may be azoospermia after eight weeks. There is usually slight atrophy of the seminiferous tubules. Follow-up examinations have shown these changes to be reversible, spermatogenesis usually reverting to its previous state about three to five months after stopping Androcur, or, in some users, up to 20 months. That spermatogenesis can recover even after very long treatment is not certain. There is evidence that abnormal sperms which might give rise to malformed embryos are produced during treatment with Androcur.

Tiredness. Fatigue and lassitude are common in the first few weeks but become much less from the third month.

Breathlessness: A sensation of shortness of breath may occur under high-dosed treatment with Androcur, owing to the known stimulatory effect of progesterone and synthetic progestogens on breathing, which is accompanied by hypocapnia and compensatory alkalosis, and is not considered to require treatment.

Gynaecomastia. Some patients develop transient or perhaps in some cases permanent enlargement of the mammary glands. In rare cases galactorrhoea and tender benign nodules have been reported. Symptoms mostly subside after discontinuation of treatment or reduction of dosage.

Bodyweight. During long-term treatment, changes in body weight have been reported, chiefly weight gains.

Other changes that have been reported include reduction of sebum production and consequently improvement of existing acne vulgaris, transient patchy loss and reduced growth of body hair, increased growth of scalp hair, lightening of hair colour and female type of pubic hair growth.

Rarely cases of osteoporosis have been reported.

Precautions and special information: Adrenocortical function: During treatment, adrenocortical function should be supervised, since suppression has been observed.

Diabetes: Androcur can influence carbohydrate metabolism. Parameters of carbohydrate metabolism should be examined carefully in all diabetics before and regularly during treatment.

Chronic alcoholism: Alcohol appears to reduce the effect of Androcur, which is of no value in chronic alcoholics.

Haemoglobin: Hypochromic anaemia has been found rarely during long-term treatment, and blood counts before and at regular intervals during treatment are advisable.

Nitrogen balance: A negative nitrogen balance is usual at the start of treatment, but usually does not persist.

Spermatogenesis: A spermatogram should be recorded before starting treatment in patients of procreative age, as a guard against attribution of pre-existing infertility to Androcur at a later stage.

It should be noted that the decline in spermatogenesis is slow, and Androcur should, therefore, not be regarded as a male contraceptive.

Medico-legal considerations: Doctors are advised to ensure that the fully informed consent of the patient to Androcur treatment is obtained and can be verified.

Road safety: The marked lassitude and asthenia that may be experienced, particularly during the first few weeks of treatment, necessitate especial care while driving.

Overdosage: There have been no reports of ill-effects from overdosage, which it is, therefore, generally unnecessary to treat. There are no specific antidotes, and treatment should be symptomatic.

Pharmaceutical precautions Store in cool, dry conditions away from strong sunlight: shelf-life five years.

Legal category POM.

Package quantities Original packs containing 56 tablets (4 blister strips of 14 tablets).

Further information Cyproterone acetate acts as an antiandrogen by blocking androgen receptors. It also has progestogenic activity which exerts a negative feedback effect on the hypothalamic receptors, so leading to a reduction in gonadotrophin release, and hence to diminished production of testicular androgens.

Product licence number 0053/0023.

BILISCOPIN*

Presentation Ampoules or bottles containing sterile solutions of meglumine iotroxate.

Excipients: calcium disodium edetate, sodium bicarbonate, water for injection. Sodium chloride is present in the infusion presentation only.

	Volume ml	Iodine mg/ml	Iodine Total, g	Osmoles/l at 37°C
Biliscopin:	30	180	5.4	0.46
Biliscopin for infusion:	100	50	5.0	0.28

Uses Cholegraphy, infusion cholegraphy.

Intravenous cholegraphy should be performed as the first examination only when there is strong evidence of disease involving the biliary tract. In all other cases for diagnosis – especially in obscure upper abdominal complaints – oral cholegraphy (Biloptin, Solu-Biloptin) is to be preferred.

Dosage and administration
1. Adults: Injection: 30 ml Biliscopin provides good contrast in most normal or overweight adults. In underweight patients, 20 ml is generally sufficient.

Injection time: not less than 5 minutes.

Infusion: one 100 ml bottle of Biliscopin for infusion in not less than 15 minutes.

The infusion should always be started at a low rate and then increased to the final higher rate after three to five minutes. This technique reduces heterotopic excretion and improves tolerance.

2. Children: Because of insufficient experience in the use of Biliscopin in children, optimal paediatric dosages have not been established.

Contra-indications, warnings, etc
Contra-indications: Severe cardiovascular insufficiency, particularly right ventricular failure. Proven or suspected hypersensitivity to iodine-containing contrast media. Manifest thyrotoxicosis. Severe functional disturbance of the liver or kidneys. Monoclonal IgM gammopathy e.g. macroglobulinaemia (Waldenström's disease).

Warnings/side-effects: In patients with multiple myeloma, other severe diseases, poor general health or thyroid hyperfunction, the need for examination merits particularly careful consideration. This applies to patients with a history of allergy (e.g. bronchial asthma, endogenous eczema), since experience has shown that they may exhibit hypersensitivity to drugs. Pre-testing does not give a reliable warning of allergic reactions to iodine-containing contrast media. Some radiologists give an antihistamine or a corticoid prophylactically to patients with a history of allergy. Because of the possibility of precipitation, contrast medium and prophylactic agents must not be administered mixed together. Since radiation should, if possible, be avoided during pregnancy, and moreover it has not yet been demonstrated whether it is safe to use Biliscopin in pregnant patients, Biliscopin should be administered during pregnancy only if the doctor regards the examination as essential.

Thyroid hyperfunction can increase for some time after the administration of biliary contrast media.

If iodine isotopes are to be administered for the diagnosis of thyroid disease, it should be borne in mind that the capacity of the thyroid tissue to take up iodine will be reduced for eight to ten weeks or more by iodinated biliary contrast media.

Some investigators have reported temporary and reversible changes in liver-function tests after Biliscopin. These changes are not thought to reflect liver damage.

The opinion has been expressed that intravenous cholegraphy should not be performed immediately after negative oral cholegraphy. A large number of radiologists do not share this view – provided that the patient is adequately hydrated and renal function is not impaired.

The patient should be recumbent during the administration of Biliscopin. Thereafter, he must be kept under close observation for at least 30 minutes, since about 90% of all severe incidents occur within that time, and must not be left unsupervised until the end of the examination. If the administration does not take place on the X-ray table, any patient with a labile circulation should be brought to the X-ray machine sitting or lying down. Inadvertent paravenous administration of Biliscopin can cause pain, but experience has shown that it is very rarely followed by serious tissue reactions. A local anaesthetic helps to relieve the pain. With more extensive paravenous infiltration, it is recommended that a hyaluronidase preparation be injected into the affected area to hasten absorption.

The greater the rate of administration of Biliscopin, the higher the incidence of common side-effects, such as an unpleasant taste, nausea, vomiting and a sensation of heat. These side-effects are rare if the recommended rate of administration is adhered to. Too rapid an administration may put the patient's life at risk – particularly if he has cardiovascular damage, whether manifest or not, or if his general condition is poor. Each bottle of Biliscopin for infusion should be used for one investigation only, and any remaining medium should be discarded.

Particular caution should be exercised in allergic patients who have previously tolerated injectable iodine-containing contrast media without any complication, since they may have become sensitised to these substances. As with any contrast medium, the possibility of hypersensitivity must always be considered. If marked side-effects or suspected allergic reactions occur during infusion or injection and persist or even worsen when the administration is interrupted, it is probable that the patient has such a hypersensitivity. Therefore, the investigation must be abandoned. The needle or cannula should be left in the vein for some time in order to maintain access for intravenous therapy. Even relatively minor symptoms, such as itching of the skin, sneezing, violent yawns, tickling in the throat, hoarseness or attacks of coughing may be early signs of a severe reaction and, therefore, merit careful attention.

Very rarely, severe or even life-threatening incidents, such as severe hypotension and collapse, circulatory failure, ventricular fibrillation, cardiac arrest, pulmonary oedema, anaphylactic shock or other allergic manifestations, convulsions or other cerebral symptoms may occur.

At present there is no clinical test that is suitable for predicting an incident. It must be emphasised that every use of a contrast medium therefore entails a certain risk and requires appropriate precautions. Ready availability of all drugs and equipment for emergency treatment and familiarity with the various procedures are prerequisites for the effective management of contrast-medium incidents.

Some guidance in the treatment of such incidents is contained in the leaflet supplied with the pack.

Pharmaceutical precautions
Storage: Protect from light and heat.
Shelf-life: Five years.

Legal category POM.

Package quantities *Biliscopin:* Packs of 10 × 30 ml ampoules. *Biliscopin for infusion:* Packs of 10 × 100 ml infusion bottles.

Further information Nil.

Product licence numbers

Biliscopin	0053/0109
Biliscopin for infusion	0053/0110

BILOPTIN* AND SOLU-BILOPTIN*

Presentation *Biloptin:* Capsules of sodium iopodate. 6 Biloptin capsules, containing a total 1.84 g iodine in 3 g of sodium iopodate.

Excipients: soy lecithin, disodium edetate dihydrate, butylated hydroxytoluene, peanut oil, gelatine, glycerin karion 83, purified water, titanium dioxide, ferric oxide pigment, methylparaben, propylparaben.

Solu-Biloptin: Sachets, each containing 1.85 g iodine in 3 g of calcium iopodate.

Excipients: sucrose, myrj 53, carboxymethylcellulose sodium, sodium lauryl sulphate, monastery aroma, curaçao aroma, blackcurrant aroma.

Uses Oral contrast media for cholecystography and cholangiography.

Dosage and administration See table below.

Routine cholecystography

Solu-Biloptin	*Biloptin*
Both media should be taken after the last meal on the evening before the examination.	
Adults	
The contents of 1 sachet.	6 capsules
Children:	
Under 4 yrs or under 20 kg body weight 0.3 g of powder/kg body weight.	Solu-Biloptin is recommended.
Over 4 yrs or over 20 kg body weight 0.15 g of powder/kg body weight.	
Neonates and infants: 0.45 g of Solu-Biloptin powder/kg body weight.	
The results are improved if an enema is given on the preceding evening and another immediately before the examination.	

Other examination techniques in adults only

Biloptin	*Solu-Biloptin*
Rapid cholecystography	
6 capsules or double dose of 12 capsules.	The contents of 1 sachet or double dose of 2 sachets.
Cholangiography	
12 capsules	The contents of 2 sachets.
Fractionated oral cholecystography	
6 capsules 10–12 hrs before the examination and another 6 capsules 3 hrs before the examination.	The contents of 1 sachet 10–12 hrs before the examination and another 1 sachet 3 hrs before the examination.

Contra-indications, warnings, etc
Contra-indications: Proven or suspected hypersensitivity to iodine-containing contrast media. Thyrotoxicosis. Severe impairment of hepatic or renal function.

Warnings/side-effects: Biloptin and Solu-Biloptin are well tolerated, and side-effects, even of a trivial nature, are extraordinarily rare. Sensitive patients may occasionally complain of mild sensations of pressure in the stomach or nausea. Attacks of diarrhoea and vomiting are exceptional. Very few cases of urticaria have been observed.

If iodine isotopes are to be administered for the diagnosis of thyroid disease, it should be borne in mind that the capacity of the thyroid tissue to take up iodine will be reduced for 8–10 weeks or more by iodinated biliary X-ray contrast media.

Since radiation should, if possible, be avoided during pregnancy, and it has not yet been proved that Biloptin and Solu-Biloptin may be safely used in pregnant patients, these media should be administered during pregnancy only if the doctor regards the examination as essential.

Pharmaceutical precautions Store in cool, dry conditions. Shelf-life five years.

Legal category P.

Package quantities
Biloptin capsules. 0.5 g 20 × 6
Solu-Biloptin sachets. 3 g × 20

Further information Nil.

Product licence numbers
Biloptin 0053/5048R
Solu-Biloptin 0053/5049R

CYCLO-PROGYNOVA* 1 mg
CYCLO-PROGYNOVA* 2 mg

Presentation *Cyclo-Progynova 1 mg:* The circular memo-pack holds 11 beige tablets, each containing 1 mg oestradiol valerate, and 10 light-brown tablets, each containing 1 mg oestradiol valerate and 250 micrograms levonorgestrel. All tablets have a lustrous sugar coating, and bear a black B in a black regular hexagon printed on both sides.

Cyclo-Progynova 2 mg: The circular memo-pack holds 11 white tablets, each containing 2 mg oestradiol valerate, and 10 pale brown tablets, each containing 2 mg oestradiol valerate and 500 micrograms norgestrel. All tablets have a lustrous sugar coating and bear a red B in a red regular hexagon printed on both sides.

Excipients: Lactose, maize starch, povidone 25 000, talc, magnesium stearate, sucrose, povidone 700 000, polyethylene glycol 6000, calcium carbonate, titanium dioxide, glycerin, wax E, ferric oxide pigments.

Uses The treatment of the climacteric syndrome. The prophylaxis and treatment of the postmenopausal sequelae of oestrogen withdrawal, e.g. osteoporosis and senile vaginitis.

Cyclo-Progynova 1 mg and Cyclo-Progynova 2 mg are designed to provide hormone replacement therapy during and after the climacteric. The addition of a progestogen in the second half of each course helps to provide good control of the irregular cycles that are characteristic of the premenopausal phase and opposes the production of endometrial hyperplasia. Whilst natural hormone production is little affected, Cyclo-Progynova 1 mg and Cyclo-Progynova 2 mg abolish or improve the characteristic symptoms of the climacteric such as hot flushes, sweating attacks and sleep disorders.

Cyclo-Progynova 1 mg and Cyclo-Progynova 2 mg do not consistently inhibit ovulation and are therefore unsuitable for contraception.

Dosage and administration If the patient is still menstruating, treatment should begin on the 5th day of menstruation. Patients whose periods are very infrequent or who are postmenopausal may start at any time, provided pregnancy has been excluded (see Precautions and special information).

Initial treatment should be with Cyclo-Progynova 1 mg. One beige tablet is taken daily for 11 days, followed by one light-brown tablet daily for 10 days. An interval of seven days follows, during which bleeding will normally occur. Cyclo-Progynova 2 mg should be substituted if the control of climacteric symptoms or dysfunctional bleeding is not fully achieved at the lower dosage. One white tablet is taken daily for 11 days, followed by one pale brown tablet for 10 days. An interval of seven days again follows, during which bleeding is to be expected.

When symptoms have been controlled, Cyclo-Progynova 1 mg will usually suffice for maintenance, but it should be borne in mind that the appropriate dosage will be determined by the rate of metabolism of Cyclo-Progynova, rather than by the initial severity of the symptoms.

Contra-indications, warnings, etc
Contra-indications: Pregnancy, severe disturbances of liver function, previous or existing liver tumours, jaundice or general pruritus during a previous pregnancy, Dubin-Johnson syndrome, Rotor syndrome, existing or previous thromboembolic processes, sickle-cell anaemia, suspected or existing hormone-dependent disorders or tumours of the uterus and breast, congenital disturbances of lipid metabolism, a history of herpes gestationis endometriosis, severe diabetes with vascular changes, otosclerosis with deterioration in previous pregnancies.

Warnings/side-effects: Hormonal contraception should be stopped when Cyclo-Progynova is started and the patient should be advised to take non-hormonal contraceptive precautions. The following symptoms have been reported during treatment: anxiety, increased appetite, bloating, breast symptoms, cardiac symptoms, depressive symptoms, dizziness, dyspepsia, leg pains and swelling, altered libido, nausea, rashes, vomiting and altered weight.

Some women are predisposed to cholestasis during steroid therapy.

Diseases that are known to be subject to deterioration during pregnancy (e.g. multiple sclerosis, epilepsy, diabetes, hypertension, porphyria, tetany and otosclerosis) should be carefully observed during treatment.

Precautions and special information: Before starting treatment, pregnancy must be excluded. If withdrawal bleeding fails to occur at about 28-day intervals, treatment should be stopped until pregnancy has been ruled out.

Treatment should be stopped at once if migrainous or frequent and unusually severe headaches occur for the first time, or if there are other symptoms that are possible prodromata of vascular occlusion.

Treatment should also be stopped if trauma, illness or impending surgery is considered to entail a risk of thrombosis.

Treatment should be stopped at once if jaundice or pregnancy occurs, or if there is a significant rise in blood-pressure or exacerbations of epilepsy.

In patients with mild chronic liver disease, liver function should be checked every 8–12 weeks.

Examination of the pelvic organs, endometrium, breasts and blood-pressure is advised before and periodically during treatment with Cyclo-Progynova.

Irregular bleeding during tablet-taking should be investigated.

Prolonged exposure to unopposed oestrogens may increase the risk of development of endometrial carcinoma. The general consensus of opinion is that the addition of 10–12 days progestogen towards the end of the cycle, as in Cyclo-Progynova, diminishes the possibility of such a risk, and some investigators consider that it might be protective.

In rare cases benign and in even rarer cases malignant liver tumours leading in isolated cases to life-threatening intra-abdominal haemorrhage have been observed after the use of hormonal substances such as those contained in Cyclo-Progynova. If severe upper abdominal complaints, liver enlargement or signs of intra-abdominal haemorrhage occur, a liver tumour should be included in the differential-diagnostic considerations and, if necessary, the preparation withdrawn.

Overdosage: There have been no reports of ill-effects from overdosage which it is, therefore, generally unnecessary to treat. There are no specific antidotes, and treatment should be symptomatic.

Pharmaceutical precautions Store in cool, dry conditions. Shelf-life five years.

Legal category POM.

Package quantities Each outer carton contains a memo-pack containing 21 tablets (OP).

Further information Nil.

Product licence numbers
Cyclo-Progynova 1 mg 0053/0108
Cyclo-Progynova 2 mg 0053/0053

CYPROSTAT*

Presentation Each round white, 9 mm tablet is impressed on one side with 'BV' in a regular hexagon, and is scored on the other. It contains 50 mg cyproterone acetate.

Excipients: maize starch, povidone 25000, aerosil, magnesium stearate, lactose.

Uses Palliative treatment of prostatic carcinoma.

Cyprostat may be used alone or in conjunction with surgery. (See Further Information.)

Dosage and administration The usual daily dose is 300 mg (6 tablets) orally, divided into 2–3 doses and taken after meals. Cyprostat therapy should not be discontinued when remission or improvement occurs. The dose may be reduced if side-effects are troublesome, but should be kept within the range of 200–300 mg daily.

Contra-indications, warnings, etc
Contra-indications: None.

Warnings, Side-effects: Liver: Cyproterone acetate has been found to cause liver abnormalities in animals, including the development of tumours.

In individual cases, disturbances of liver function, some of them severe, have been reported with high-dosed Cyprostat treatment. Liver-function tests should be performed regularly during treatment.

In rare cases benign and in even rarer cases malignant liver tumours, leading in isolated cases to life-threatening intra-abdominal haemorrhage, have been observed after the use of sex steroids, to which class cyproterone acetate belongs. If severe upper abdominal complaints, liver enlargement or signs of intra-abdominal haemorrhage occur, a liver tumour should be considered in the differential diagnosis, and, if necessary, Cyprostat should be withdrawn.

Inhibition of spermatogenesis: The sperm count and the volume of ejaculate are reduced. Infertility is usual, and there may be azoospermia after 8 weeks. There is usually slight atrophy of seminiferous tubules. Follow-up examinations have shown these changes to be reversible, spermatogenesis usually reverting to its previous state about 3–5 months after stopping Cyprostat, or in some users, up to 20 months. That spermatogenesis can recover even after very long treatment is not yet known. There is evidence that abnormal sperms which might give rise to malformed embryos are produced during treatment with Cyprostat.

Thromboembolism: Patients with a history of thrombosis may be at risk of recurrence of the disease during Cyprostat therapy. In patients with a history of thromboembolic processes or suffering from sickle-cell anaemia or severe diabetes with vascular changes, the risk: benefit ratio must be considered carefully in each individual case before Cyprostat is prescribed.

Chronic depression: It has been found that some patients with severe chronic depression deteriorate whilst taking Cyprostat therapy.

Tiredness: Fatigue and lassitude are common in the first few weeks of therapy but usually become much less from the third month. The marked lassitude and asthenia necessitate especial care when driving or operating machinery.

Breathlessness: A sensation of shortness of breath may occur under treatment with Cyprostat, owing to the known stimulatory effect of progesterone and synthetic progestogens on breathing, which is accompanied by hypocapnia and compensatory alkalosis, and is not considered to require treatment.

Gynaecomastia: Transient, and perhaps in some cases permanent, enlargement of the mammary glands has been reported. In rare cases, galactorrhoea and tender benign nodules have been reported. Symptoms generally subside after discontinuation of treatment or on reduction of dosage, but this should be weighed against the risk to the tumour of using inadequate doses.

Body weight: During long-term treatment, changes in body weight have been reported. Both increases and decreases have been seen.

Other changes that have been reported include reduction of sebum production leading to dryness of the skin, and transient patchy loss of body hair.

Adrenocortical function: During treatment adrenocortical function should be supervised, since suppression has been observed.

Diabetes: Cyprostat can influence carbohydrate metabolism. Parameters of carbohydrate metabolism should be examined carefully in all diabetics before and regularly during treatment.

Chronic alcoholism: The chronic abuse of alcohol appears to reduce the effect of cyproterone acetate in male hypersexuality, but the relevance of this to the treatment of prostatic carcinoma is not known.

Haemoglobin: Hypochromic anaemia has been found rarely during long-term treatment, and blood-counts before and at regular intervals during treatment are advisable.

Nitrogen balance: A negative balance is usual at the start of treatment, but usually does not persist.

Overdosage: There have been no reports of ill-effects of overdosage, which it is, therefore, generally unnecessary to treat. There are no specific antidotes, and treatment should be symptomatic.

Pharmaceutical precautions Store in cool, dry conditions away from strong sunlight. *Shelf-life:* five years.

Package quantities: Original packs containing 168 tablets (14 blister strips of 12 tablets). Starter packs containing 84 tablets (7 blister strips of 12 tablets).

Legal category: POM.

Further information: Prostatic carcinoma and its metastases are in general androgen-dependent. Cyprostat exerts a direct antiandrogenic action on the tumour and its metastases, and in addition it exerts a negative feedback effect on the hypothalamic receptors, so leading to a reduction in gonadotrophin release, and hence to diminished production of testicular androgens.

Product licence number 0053/0133.

DEPOSTAT*

Presentation Gestronol hexanoate in oily solution for intramuscular administration. Ampoules containing 200 mg in 2 ml.

Excipients: benzyl benzoate, castor oil.

Uses Advanced endometrial carcinoma. Benign prostatic hyperplasia. Depostat is a depot progestogen, in a concentrated injectable non-aqueous solution, and is 25 times more potent than its parent substance progesterone. In the female, the action of Depostat is concentrated on the endometrium. This action is direct and does not involve suppression via the pituitary. Except in some highly anaplastic tumours, Depostat has a strong antimitotic effect, with regression or arrest of primary endometrial carcinoma and of soft-tissue metastases.

In the male, Depostat has been shown to reduce prostatic weight significantly. It may effect an objective improvement in peak urine flow rates and residual urine and in subjective symptoms such as nocturia.

Dosage and administration Endometrial carcinoma, before hysterectomy and for advanced disease. A well-tolerated adjunct to other therapy. To inhibit metastatic spread before and after operation, 200–400 mg intramuscularly every 5–7 days, starting immediately following diagnosis and continuing for a minimum of 12 weeks.

For treating existing metastases: 200–400 mg intramuscularly every 5–7 days. If the metastases are hormone-responsive, improvement will be observed within 8-12 weeks of therapy. Treatment should then be continued as long as it appears beneficial.

Benign prostatic hyperplasia where a) the patient is an operation risk; b) symptoms are mild; c) there is a waiting list for operation: standard dosage is 200 mg weekly by intramuscular injection, but in view of Depostat's good tolerance, this dosage can confidently be increased. In trials, 300 mg and 400 mg weekly have been used. The full benefit of treatment is unlikely to be established in a shorter period than three months, and trial results suggest that improvement can continue during substantially longer periods.

Contra-indications, warnings, etc
Contra-indications: Pregnancy. History of herpes gestationis (also known as pemphigoid gestationis). Previous or existing liver tumour (in advanced endometrial carcinoma, only if these are not due to metastases).

Warning/side-effects: Rarely, local reactions may occur at the site of injection. Exacerbation of bronchial asthma, epilepsy and migraine may sometimes occur.

Side-effects are infrequent. In males, a reversible depression of libido and mammary discomfort have been reported by a few patients. Spermatogenesis is temporarily inhibited. In rare cases coughing, dyspnoea and circulatory irregularities may develop during or immediately after the injection.

Tolerance: In patients with chronic liver damage it is advisable to check liver function at intervals during long-term treatment or repeated courses of Depostat. Transient moderate rises in bromsulphthalein retention and serum transaminases have occasionally been observed but have always proved harmless.

Pharmaceutical precautions Store in cool dry conditions away from strong sunlight: shelf-life five years.

Legal category POM.

Package quantities 5 ampoules of 2 ml.

Further information Nil.

Product licence number 0053/0018.

DIANETTE*

Presentation Each beige, sugar-coated tablet, bearing a black printed 'c' in a regular hexagon on both sides, contains 2 mg of the anti-androgen cyproterone acetate and 35 micrograms of the oestrogen ethinyloestradiol.

Excipients: lactose, maize starch, povidone 25000, talc, magnesium stearate, sucrose, povidone 700000, polyethylene glycol 6000, calcium carbonate, titanium dioxide, glycerin 85%, wax E, ferric oxide pigment.

Uses *In women only:* (a) Severe acne, refractory to prolonged oral antibiotic therapy and (b) idiopathic hirsutism of mild to moderate degree. Dianette blocks androgen-receptors. It also reduces androgen synthesis by a negative feedback effect on the hypothalamo-pituitary-ovarian systems. Sex-hormone-binding globulin (SHBG) levels are increased by the oestrogen component of Dianette, thus reducing the free, circulating plasma levels of androgens. Unlike some other progestogens, cyproterone acetate has no tendency to reduce SHBG levels.

Although Dianette also acts as an oral contraceptive, it is not recommended in women solely for contraception, but should be reserved for those women requiring treatment for the androgen-dependent skin conditions described.

Complete remission of acne is to be expected in nearly all cases, often within a few months, but in particularly severe cases treatment for longer may be necessary before the full benefit is seen. It is recommended that treatment be withdrawn when the acne or hirsutism has completely resolved. Repeat courses of Dianette may be given if the condition recurs.

Dosage and administration
First treatment course: One tablet daily for 21 days, starting on the 5th day of the menstrual cycle (the first day of menstruation counting as Day 1).

When the contraceptive action of Dianette is also to be employed, it is essential that the above instructions be rigidly adhered to. Other contraceptive precautions (excluding oral contraceptives and other hormonal methods and the rhythm, temperature or cervical-mucus methods) should be taken during the first 14 days of tablet-taking. Should bleeding fail to occur at the usual time, the possibility of pregnancy must be excluded before the next pack is started.

Subsequent courses: Each subsequent course is started after 7 tablet-free days have followed the preceding course.
The following circumstances in which the contraceptive action of Dianette may be diminished should be noted:

Special circumstances requiring additional contraception – incorrect administration: If a tablet is delayed, it should be taken as soon as possible, and if it is taken within 12 hours of the correct time additional contraception is not needed. Further tablets should then be taken at the usual time. However, if the delay exceeds 12 hours, ovulation may occur. In those circumstances, any tablet or tablets delayed more than 12 hours should be omitted, the remaining tablets should be taken on the correct days at the usual time, and extra precautions (except the rhythm, temperature or cervical-mucus methods) should be used until the next withdrawal bleed.

Gastro-intestinal upset: Vomiting or diarrhoea may reduce the contraceptive effectiveness of the tablets by preventing them from being fully absorbed. Therefore, it is advisable that an additional method of contraception be used until the next withdrawal bleed. Mild laxatives do not impair contraceptive action.

Interaction with other drugs: Some drugs taken concurrently accelerate the metabolism of Dianette. Drugs suspected of having the capacity to reduce the contraceptive efficacy of Dianette include barbiturates, phenytoin, phenylbutazone, rifampicin, ampicillin, griseofulvin and other antibiotics. The possibility cannot be ruled out that oral tetracyclines, if used in conjunction with Dianette may have such an effect, although it has not been shown. When drugs of these classes are being taken, it is, therefore, advisable to use additional methods of contraception (excluding oral contraceptives and other hormonal methods) since an extremely high degree of protection must be provided when Dianette is being taken.

Contra-indications, warnings, etc

Contra-indications: Pregnancy (see second paragraph of 'Warnings'). Lactation. Thrombotic disorders and a history of these conditions, sickle-cell anaemia, disorders of lipid metabolism and other conditions in which, in individual cases, there is known or suspected to be a much increased risk of thrombosis. Acute or severe chronic liver diseases. Dubin-Johnson syndrome. Rotor syndrome. History, during pregnancy, of idiopathic jaundice or severe pruritus. History of herpes gestationis (also know as pemphigoid gestationis). Mammary or endometrial carcinoma, or a history of these conditions. Abnormal vaginal bleeding of unknown cause. History of deterioration of otosclerosis during pregnancy.

Warnings: Like many other steroids, cyproterone acetate, when given in very high doses and for the majority of the animal's life-span, has been found to cause an increase in the incidence of tumours, including carcinoma, in the liver of rats. The relevance of this finding to humans is unknown. Dianette has been shown to have good liver tolerance in women given prolonged treatment.

Animal studies have revealed that feminisation of male foetuses may occur if cyproterone acetate is administered during the phase of embryogenesis at which differentiation of the external genitalia occurs. Although the results of these tests are not necessarily relevant to man, the possibility must be considered that administration of Dianette to women after the 45th day of pregnancy could cause feminisation of male foetuses. It follows from this that pregnancy is an absolute contra-indication for treatment with Dianette, and must be excluded before such treatment is begun.

Although its strong anti-androgenic effect is distinctive, Dianette has many properties in common with combined oral contraceptives, which must not be taken during treatment with Dianette. There is a general opinion, based on statistical evidence, that users of combined oral contraceptives experience, more often than non-users, venous thromboembolism, arterial thrombosis, including cerebral and myocardial infarction, and subarachnoid haemorrhage. Full recovery from such disorders does not always occur, and it should be realised that in a few cases they are fatal.

Certain factors may entail some risk of thrombosis, e.g. smoking, obesity, varicose veins, cardiovascular diseases, diabetes and migraine. The risk of arterial thrombosis associated with combined oral contraceptives increases with age, and this risk is aggravated by cigarette-smoking. The suitability of Dianette should be judged according to the severity of such conditions in the individual case, and should be discussed with the patient before she decides to take it.

Numerous epidemiological studies have been reported on the risks of ovarian, endometrial, cervical and breast cancer in women using combined oral contraceptives. The evidence is clear that combined oral contraceptives offer substantial protection against both ovarian and endometrial cancer.

An increased risk of cervical cancer in long-term users of combined oral contraceptives has been reported in some studies, but there continues to be controversy about the extent to which this is attributable to the confounding effects of sexual behaviour and other factors.

The evidence linking combined oral contraceptive use and breast cancer remains inconclusive. The results of some studies suggest an increased risk of breast cancer presenting below the age of about 35, the risk rising with duration of use. Any possible increased risk of breast cancer with combined oral contraceptives is however likely to be small, and may be expected to be less with low-dosage pills. This possible risk should be weighed against the many benefits of combined oral contraceptives, including their protective effects against ovarian and endometrial cancers.

The possibility cannot be ruled out that certain chronic diseases may occasionally deteriorate during the use of Dianette (see '*Precautions*').

Reasons for stopping medication immediately: Occurrence of migraine in patients who have never previously suffered from it. Exacerbation of pre-existing migraine. Any unusually frequent or unusually severe headaches. Any kind of acute disturbances of vision. Suspicion of thrombosis or infarction. Jaundice. Six weeks before elective operations and during immobilisation, e.g. after accidents, etc. Significant rise in blood pressure. Clear exacerbation of conditions known to be capable of deteriorating during oral contraception or pregnancy. Pregnancy is a reason for stopping immediately, not only because of the possible specific risk to a male foetus referred to above, but also because it has been suggested by some investigations that oral contraceptives taken in early pregnancy may slightly increase the risk of foetal malformations in general. Other investigations have failed to support these findings. The possibility therefore cannot be excluded, but it is certain that, if a risk of general malformations exists at all, it is very small.

Precautions: Examinations of the pelvic organs, breasts and blood-pressure should precede the prescribing of Dianette, and should be repeated regularly. The following conditions require careful observation during medication: a history of severe depressive states, varicose veins, diabetes, hypertension, epilepsy, otosclerosis, multiple sclerosis, porphyria, tetany, disturbed liver function, gall-stones, cardiovascular diseases, renal diseases, chloasma, uterine fibroids, asthma, the wearing of contact lenses or any disease that is prone to worsen during pregnancy. The deterioration or first appearance of any of these conditions may indicate that Dianette should be stopped.

It should be borne in mind that the use of ultraviolet lamps for the treatment of acne, or prolonged exposure to sunlight, increases the risk of the deterioration of chloasma.

Side-effects: Occasional side-effects may include: nausea, vomiting, headaches, breast tension, changed body weight or libido, depressive moods, chloasma.

Menstrual changes: 1. Reduction of flow. This is not abnormal and it is to be expected in some patients.
2. Missed menstruation. If withdrawal bleeding does not occur, pregnancy must be excluded by a pregnancy test after a suitable interval before a new course of tablets is started.

Intermenstrual bleeding: Very light 'spotting' or heavier 'breakthrough bleeding' may occur during tablet-taking, especially in the first few cycles. It appears to be generally of no significance, except where it indicates errors of tablet-taking, or where the possibility of interaction with other drugs exists (*q.v.*). However, if irregular bleeding is persistent, an organic cause should be considered.

Effect on thyroid glands: The radio-iodine uptake shows that thyroid function is unchanged. There is a rise in serum protein-bound iodine, similar to that in pregnancy and during the administration of oestrogens. This is due to the increased capacity of the plasma proteins for binding thyroid hormones, rather than to any change in glandular function. In women taking Dianette, the content of protein-bound iodine in blood serum should, therefore, not be used for the evaluation of thyroid function.

Effect on blood chemistry: Dianette may accelerate erythrocyte sedimentation in the absence of any disease. This effect is due to change in the proportion of the plasma protein fractions. Increases in plasma copper, iron and alkaline phosphatase have also been recorded.

Overdosage: There have been no reports concerning overdosage, but, on general principles from a knowledge of the pharmacological actions of the constituents of Dianette, it would seem unnecessary to treat. There are no specific antidotes and treatment should be symptomatic.

Pharmaceutical precautions Storage: cool, dry conditions. Shelf-life: five years.

Legal category POM.

Package quantities Outer carton contains three memo-packs; each containing 21 tablets (OP).

Further information Nil.

Product licence number 0053/0190.

EUGYNON* 30
MICROGYNON* 30

Presentation *Eugynon 30:* Each white sugar-coated tablet bears a printed black C in a regular hexagon on both sides and contains 250 micrograms levonorgestrel and 30 micrograms ethinyloestradiol.

Excipients: lactose, maize starch, povidone 25 000, talc, magnesium stearate, sucrose, povidone 700 000, polyethylene glycol 6000, calcium carbonate, wax E.

Microgynon 30: Each beige sugar-coated tablet bears a black A in a black hexagon printed on both sides and contains 150 micrograms levonorgestrel and 30 micrograms ethinyloestradiol.

Excipients: lactose, maize starch, povidone 25 000, talc, magnesium stearate, sucrose, povidone 700 000, polyethylene glycol 6000, calcium carbonate, talc, titanium dioxide, glycerin, wax E, iron oxide pigment.

Uses Oral contraception and the recognised gynaecological indications for such oestrogen-progestogen combinations. The mode of action includes the inhibition of ovulation by suppression of the mid-cycle surge of luteinising hormone, the inspissation of cervical mucus so as to constitute a barrier to sperm, and the rendering of the endometrium unreceptive to implantation.

Dosage and administration *First treatment cycle:* 1 tablet daily for 21 days, starting on the first day of the menstrual cycle (the first day of menstruation counting as day 1). Contraceptive protection begins immediately.

Subsequent cycles: Each subsequent course is started after seven tablet-free days have followed the preceding course.

Changing from other oral contraceptives: The first tablet of Eugynon 30/Microgynon 30 should be taken on the first day immediately after the end of the previous oral contraceptive course. Additional precautions are not required.

Post-partum and post-abortum use: After pregnancy oral contraception can be started 21 days after a vaginal delivery, provided that the patient is fully ambulant and there are no puerperal complications. After a first-trimester abortion, oral contraception may be started immediately. Since the first post-partum ovulation may precede the first bleeding, another method of contraception should be used in the interval between childbirth and the first course of the pills.

Special circumstances requiring additional contraception: Incorrect administration: A single delayed tablet should be taken as soon as possible, and if this can be done within 12 hours of the correct time, contraceptive protection is maintained.

With larger errors, additional contraception is needed. Only the most recently delayed tablet should be taken, earlier missed tablets being omitted, and additional contraception (barriers and spermicides) should be used for the next 7 days, *while the next 7 tablets are being taken. Additionally,* therefore, if pills have been missed *during the last 7 days* of a pack, there should be no break before the next pack is started (Dept. of Health Handbook of Contraceptive Practice).

Gastro-intestinal upset: Vomiting or diarrhoea may reduce efficacy by preventing full absorption. Barriers and spermicides should be used until 7 days after the upset, and, if those 7 days overrun the end of a pack, the next pack should be started without a break. Mild laxatives do not impair contraceptive action.

Interaction with other drugs: Some drugs accelerate the metabolism of oral contraceptives taken concurrently. Drugs suspected of having the capacity to reduce the efficacy of oral contraceptives include barbiturates, phenytoin, phenylbutazone, rifampicin, ampicillin, griseofulvin and other antibiotics. It is, therefore, advisable to use non-hormonal methods of contraception (except the rhythm, temperature or cervical-mucus methods) in addition to the oral contraceptive as long as an extremely high degree of protection must be provided during treatment with such drugs.

Contra-indications, warnings, etc

Contra-indications: Pregnancy. Thrombotic disorders and a history of these conditions, sickle-cell anaemia, disorders of lipid metabolism and other conditions in which, in individual cases, there is known or suspected to be a much increased risk of thrombosis. Acute or severe chronic liver diseases. Dubin-Johnson syndrome. Rotor syndrome. History, during pregnancy, of idiopathic jaundice or severe pruritus. History of herpes gestationis (also known as pemphigoid gestationis). Mammary or endometrial carcinoma, or a history of these conditions. Abnormal vaginal bleeding of unknown cause. Deterioration of otosclerosis during pregnancy.

Warnings: There is a general opinion, based on statistical evidence, that users of combined oral contraceptives experience, more often than non-users, venous thromboembolism, arterial thrombosis, including cerebral and myocardial infarction, and subarachnoid haemorrhage. Full recovery from such disorders does not always occur, and it should be realised that in a few cases they are fatal. How often these disorders occur in users of the modern low-dose pills is not known, but there are reasons for suggesting that they may occur less often than with older pills.

Certain factors may entail some risk of thrombosis, e.g. smoking, obesity, varicose veins, cardiovascular diseases, diabetes and migraine. The suitability of a combined oral contraceptive should be judged according to the severity of such conditions in the individual case, and should be discussed with the patient before she decides to take it. The risk of arterial thrombosis associated with oral contraceptives increases with age, and this risk is aggravated by cigarette-smoking. The use of combined oral contraceptives by women in the older age-group, especially those who are cigarette-smokers should therefore be discouraged, and alternative methods advised.

Numerous epidemiological studies have been reported on the risks of ovarian, endometrial, cervical and breast cancer in women using combined oral contraceptives. The evidence is clear that combined oral contraceptives offer substantial protection against both ovarian and endometrial cancer.

An increased risk of cervical cancer in long-term users of combined oral contraceptives has been reported in some studies, but there continues to be controversy about the extent to which this is attributable to the confounding effects of sexual behaviour and other factors.

The evidence linking the use of combined oral contraceptives and breast cancer remains inconclusive. The results of some studies suggest an increased risk of breast cancer presenting below the age of about 35, the risk rising with duration of use. Any possible increased risk of breast cancer with combined oral contraceptives is however likely to be small, and may be expected to be less with low-dosage pills. This possible risk should be weighed against the many benefits of combined oral contraceptives, including their protective effects against ovarian and endometrial cancers.

The possibility cannot be ruled out that certain chronic diseases may occasionally deteriorate during the use of combined oral contraceptives (see 'Precautions'). Benign hepatic tumours have been associated with oral contraceptive usage. Malignant hepatic tumours have also been reported on rare occasions in long-term oral contraceptive users. A hepatic tumour should be considered in the differential diagnosis when upper abdominal pain, enlarged liver or signs of intra-abdominal haemorrhage occur.

Reasons for stopping oral contraception immediately: Occurrence of migraine in patients who have never previously suffered from it. Exacerbation of pre-existing migraine. Any unusually frequent or unusually severe headaches. Any kind of acute disturbance of vision. Suspicion of thrombosis or infarction. Six weeks before elective operations and during immobilisation, e.g. after accidents, etc. Significant rise in blood-pressure. Jaundice. Clear exacerbation of conditions known to be capable of deteriorating during oral contraception or pregnancy. Pregnancy is a reason for stopping immediately because it has been suggested by some investigations that oral contraceptives taken in early pregnancy may slightly increase the risk of foetal malformations. Other investigations have failed to support these findings. The possibility therefore cannot be excluded, but it is certain that if a risk exists at all, it is very small.

Precautions: Examination of the pelvic organs, breasts and blood-pressure should precede the prescribing of any combined oral contraceptive, and should be repeated regularly. Before starting treatment, pregnancy must be excluded.

The following conditions require careful consideration: a history of severe depressive states, varicose veins, diabetes, hypertension, epilepsy, otosclerosis, multiple sclerosis, porphyria, tetany, disturbed liver function, gallstones, cardiovascular diseases, renal diseases, chloasma, uterine fibroids, asthma, the wearing of contact lenses, or any disease that is prone to worsen during pregnancy. The first appearance or deterioration of any of these conditions may indicate that the oral contraceptive should be stopped.

The risk of the deterioration of chloasma, which is often not fully reversible, is reduced by the avoidance of excessive exposure to sunlight.

Side-effects: Occasional side-effects may include nausea, vomiting, headaches, breast tension, changed body weight or libido, depressive moods and chloasma.

Menstrual changes:

1. *Reduction of menstrual flow:* This is not abnormal and it is to be expected in some patients. Indeed, it may be beneficial where heavy periods were previously experienced.

2. *Missed menstruation:* Occasionally, withdrawal bleeding may not occur at all. If the tablets have been taken correctly, pregnancy is very unlikely, but should be ruled out before a new course of tablets is started.

Intermenstrual bleeding: Very light 'spotting' or heavier 'breakthrough bleeding' may occur during tablet-taking, especially in the first few cycles. It appears to be generally of no significance, except where it indicates errors of tablet-taking, or where the possibility of interaction with other drugs exists (q.v.). However, if irregular bleeding is persistent, an organic cause should be considered.

Effect on adrenal and thyroid glands: Oral contraceptives have no significant influence on adrenocortical function. The ACTH function test for the adrenal cortex remains unchanged. The reduction in corticosteroid excretion and the elevation of plasma corticosteroids are due to an increased cortisol-binding capacity of the plasma proteins.

The response to metyrapone is less pronounced than in untreated women and is thus similar to that during pregnancy.

The radio-iodine uptake shows that thyroid function is unchanged. There is a rise in serum protein-bound iodine, similar to that in pregnancy and during the administration of oestrogens. This is due to the increased capacity of the plasma proteins for binding thyroid hormones, rather than to any change in glandular function. In women taking oral contraceptives, the content of protein-bound iodine in blood serum should, therefore, not be used for evaluation of thyroid function.

Effect on blood chemistry: Oral contraceptives may accelerate erythrocyte sedimentation in the absence of any disease. This effect is due to a change in the proportion of the plasma protein fractions. Increases in plasma copper, iron and alkaline phosphatase have also been recorded.

Overdosage: There have been no reports of serious ill-effects from overdosage, even when a considerable number of pills have been taken by a small child. In general, it is, therefore, unnecessary to treat overdosage.

There are no specific antidotes and treatment should be symptomatic.

Pharmaceutical precautions Store in cool, dry conditions.

Shelf-life:
Eugynon 30 and Microgynon 30 – 5 years.

Legal category POM.

Package quantities Available in packs containing one month's supply (OP).

Further information Nil.

Product licence numbers

Eugynon 30	0053/0049
Microgynon 30	0053/0064

FEMODENE*

Presentation Each white sugar-coated tablet bears a printed red N in a red regular hexagon on both sides and contains 75 micrograms gestodene and 30 micrograms ethinyloestradiol.

Excipients: lactose, maize starch, povidone 25 000, calcium disodium edetate, magnesium stearate, sucrose, povidone 700 000, polyethylene glycol 6000, calcium carbonate, talc, wax E.

Uses Oral contraception and the recognised gynaecological indications for such oestrogen-progestogen combinations. The mode of action includes the inhibition of ovulation by suppression of the mid-cycle surge of luteinising hormone, the inspissation of cervical mucus so as to constitute a barrier to sperm, and the rendering of the endometrium unreceptive to implantation.

Dosage and administration

First treatment cycle: 1 tablet daily for 21 days, starting on the first day of the menstrual cycle.

Subsequent cycles: Each subsequent course is started when seven tablet-free days have followed the previous course.

Changing from other oral contraceptives: The first tablet of Femodene should be taken on the first day immediately after the end of the previous oral contraceptive course. Additional precautions are not required.

Post-partum use: After pregnancy, oral contraception can be started 21 days after a vaginal delivery, provided that the patient is fully ambulant and there are no puerperal complications. After a first-trimester abortion, oral contraception may be started immediately. Since the first post-partum ovulation may precede the first bleeding, another method of contraception should be used in the interval between childbirth and the first course of pills.

Special circumstances requiring additional contraception: Incorrect administration: A single delayed tablet should be taken as soon as possible, and if this can be done within 12 hours of the correct time, contraceptive protection is maintained. With larger errors, additional contraception is needed. Only the most recently delayed tablet should be taken, earlier missed tablets being omitted, and additional contraception (barriers and spermicides) should be used for the next 7 days, while the next 7 tablets are being taken. Additionally, therefore, if tablets have been missed during the last 7 days of a pack, there should be no break before the next pack is started (Dept of Health Handbook of Contraceptive Practice).

Gastro-intestinal upset: Vomiting or diarrhoea may reduce efficacy by preventing full absorption. Barriers and spermicides should be used until 7 days after the upset, and, if those 7 days overrun the end of a pack, the next pack should be started without a break. Mild laxatives do not impair contraceptive action.

Interaction with other drugs: Some drugs accelerate the metabolism of oral contraceptives taken concurrently. Drugs suspected of having the capacity to reduce the efficacy of oral contraceptives include barbiturates, phenylbutazone, phenytoin, rifampicin, ampicillin, griseofulvin and other antibiotics. It is, therefore, advisable to use non-hormonal methods of contraception (except the rhythm, temperature or cervical-mucus methods) in addition to the oral contraceptive as long as an extremely high degree of protection must be provided during treatment with such drugs.

Contra-indications, warnings, etc

Contra-indications: Pregnancy. Thrombotic disorders and a history of these conditions, sickle-cell anaemia, disorders of lipid metabolism and other conditions in which, in individual cases, there is known or suspected to be a much increased risk of thrombosis. Acute or severe chronic liver diseases, Dubin-Johnson syndrome, Rotor syndrome, History, during pregnancy, of idiopathic jaundice or severe pruritus. History of herpes gestationis. Mammary or endometrial carcinoma, or a history of these conditions. Abnormal vaginal bleeding of unknown cause. History of deterioration of otosclerosis during pregnancy.

Warnings: There is a general opinion, based on statistical evidence, that users of combined oral contraceptives experience, more often than non-users, venous thromboembolism, arterial thrombosis, including cerebral and myocardial infarction, and subarachnoid haemorrhage. Full recovery from such disorders does not always occur, and it should be realised that in a few cases they are fatal. How often these disorders occur in users of the modern low-dose pills is not known, but there are reasons for suggesting that they may occur less often than with older pills.

Certain factors may entail some risk of thrombosis, e.g. smoking, obesity, varicose veins, cardiovascular diseases, diabetes, and migraine. The suitability of a combined oral contraceptive should be judged according to the severity of such conditions in the individual case, and should be discussed with the patient before she decides to take it. The risk of arterial thrombosis associated with combined oral contraceptives increases with age, and this risk is aggravated by cigarette-smoking. The use of combined oral conraceptives by women in the older age-group, especially those who are cigarette smokers, should therefore be discouraged and alternative methods used.

Numerous epidemiological studies have been reported on the risks of ovarian, endometrial, cervical and breast cancer in women using combined oral contraceptives. The evidence is clear that combined oral contraceptives offer substantial protection against both ovarian and endometrial cancer.

An increased risk of cervical cancer in long-term users of combined oral contraceptives has been reported in some studies, but there continues to be controversy about the extent to which this is attributable to the confounding effects of sexual behaviour and other factors.

The evidence linking the use of combined oral contraceptives and breast cancer remains inconclusive. The results of some studies suggest an increased risk of breast cancer presenting below the age of about 35, the risk rising with duration of use. Any possible increased risk of breast cancer with combined oral contraceptives is however likely to be small, and may be expected to be less with low-dosage pills. This possible risk should be weighed against the many benefits of combined oral contraceptives, including their protective effects against ovarian and endometrial cancers.

The possibility cannot be ruled out that certain chronic diseases may occasionally deteriorate during the use of combined oral contraceptives (see 'Precautions'). The combination of ethinyloestradiol and gestodene, like other contraceptive steroids, is associated with an increased incidence of neoplastic nodules in the rat liver, the relevance of which to man is unknown. Malignant liver tumours have been reported on rare occasions in long-term users of oral contraceptives. Benign hepatic tumours have also been associated with oral contraceptive usage. A hepatic tumour should be considered in the differential diagnosis when upper abdominal pain, enlarged liver or signs of intra-abdominal haemorrhage occur.

Reasons for stopping oral contraception immediately: Occurrence of migraine in patients who have never previously suffered from it. Exacerbation of pre-existing migraine. Any unusually frequent or unusually severe headaches. Any kind of acute disturbance of vision. Suspicion of thrombosis or infarction. Six weeks before elective operations and during immobilisation, e.g. after accidents, etc. Significant rise in blood pressure. Jaundice. Clear exacerbation of conditions known to be capable of deteriorating during oral contraception or pregnancy. Pregnancy is a reason for stopping immediately because it has been suggested by some investigations that oral contraceptives taken in early pregnancy may slightly increase the risk of foetal malformations. Other investigations have failed to support these findings. The possibility therefore cannot be excluded, but it is certain that if a risk exists at all, it is very small.

Precautions: Examination of the pelvic organs, breasts and blood-pressure should precede the prescribing of any combined oral contraceptive, and should be repeated regularly. Before starting treatment, pregnancy must be excluded. The following conditions require careful observation during medication: a history of severe depressive states, varicose veins, diabetes, hypertension, epilepsy, otosclerosis, multiple sclerosis, porphyria, tetany, disturbed liver function, gall-stones, cardiovascular diseases, renal diseases, chloasma, uterine fibroids, asthma, the wearing of contact lenses, or any disease that it prone to worsen during pregnancy. The deterioration or first appearance of any of these conditions may indicate that the oral contraceptive should be stopped. The risk of the deterioration of chloasma, which is often not fully reversible, is reduced by the avoidance of excessive exposure to sunlight.

Side-effects: Occasional side-effects may include: nausea, vomiting, headaches, breast tension, changed bodyweight or libido, depressive moods and chloasma.

Menstrual changes:

1. *Reduction of menstrual flow:* This is not abnormal and it is to be expected in some patients. Indeed, it may be beneficial where heavy periods were previously experienced.

2. *Missed menstruation:* Occasionally, withdrawal bleeding may not occur at all. If the tablets have been taken correctly, pregnancy is very unlikely, but should be ruled out before a new course of tablets is started.

Intermenstrual bleeding: 'Spotting' or heavier 'breakthrough bleeding' may occur during tablet-taking, especially in the first few cycles. It appears to be generally of no significance, except where it indicates errors of tablet-taking, or where the possibility of interaction with other drugs exists (q.v.). However, if irregular bleeding is persistent, an organic cause should be considered.

Effect on adrenal and thyroid glands: Oral contraceptives have no significant influence on adrenocortical function. The ACTH function tests for the adrenal cortex remains unchanged. The reduction in corticosteroid excretion and the elevation of plasma corticosteroids are due to an increased cortisol-binding capacity of the plasma proteins.

The response to metyrapone is less pronounced than in untreated women and is thus similar to that during pregnancy.

The radio-iodine uptake shows that thyroid function is unchanged. There is a rise in serum protein-bound iodine, similar to that in pregnancy and during the administration of oestrogens. This is due to the increased capacity of the plasma proteins for binding thyroid hormones, rather than to any change in glandular function. In women taking oral contraceptives, the content of protein-bound iodine in blood serum should, therefore, not be used for the evaluation of thyroid function.

Effect on blood chemistry: Oral contraceptives may accelerate erythrocyte sedimentation in the absence of any disease. This effect is due to a change in the proportion of the plasma protein fractions. Increases in plasma copper, iron and alkaline phosphatase have also been recorded.

Overdose: There have been no reports of serious ill-effects from overdosage, even when a considerable number of tablets have been taken by a small child. In general, it is, therefore, unnecessary to treat overdosage. There are no specific antidotes and treatment should be symptomatic.

Pharmaceutical precautions *Storage* – cool, dry conditions. *Shelf-life* – five years.

Legal category POM.

Package quantities Individual packs containing three months' supply (OP).

Further information Nil.

Product licence number 0053/0179.

FEMODENE* ED

Presentation Each white sugar-coated tablet bears a printed red N in a red regular hexagon on both sides and contains 75 micrograms gestodene and 30 micrograms ethinyloestradiol.

In addition, there are 7 white placebo tablets which are larger and bear a black 0 in a regular hexagon.

Excipients: lactose; maize starch; povidone 25,000; calcium disodium edetate; magnesium stearate; purified water; saccharose; povidone 700,000; polyethylene glycol 6,000; calcium carbonate; talc; wax E.

Uses Oral contraception and the recognised gynaecological indications for such oestrogen-progestogen combinations. The mode of action includes the inhibition of ovulation by suppression of the mid-cycle surge of luteinising hormone, the inspissation of cervical mucus so as to constitute a barrier to sperm, and the rendering of the endometrium unreceptive to implantation.

Dosage and administration

First treatment cycle: 1 tablet daily for 28 days, starting in the red section on the first day of bleeding, the initial tablet being the one marked with the appropriate day of the week. In the first cycle only, an additional method of contraception (except the rhythm, temperature or cervical-mucus methods) must be used for the first 14 days of tablet-taking. A withdrawal bleed should occur when the placebo tablets are being taken.

Subsequent cycles: Each subsequent course is started in the red section on the day after the previous one has been finished. Pack, therefore, follows pack without interval.

Changing from other oral contraceptives: The first tablet of Femodene ED should be taken on the first day immediately after the end of the previous oral contraceptive course. Additional (non-hormonal) precautions other than the rhythm, temperature or cervical mucus methods, should also be used for the first 14 days when changing products.

Post-partum use: Femodene ED can be started 21 days after a vaginal delivery, provided that the patient is fully ambulant and there are no puerperal complications. After a first-trimester abortion, oral contraception may be started immediately. Since the first post-partum ovulation may precede the first bleeding, another method of contraception should therefore be used in the interval between childbirth and the first course of pills.

Special circumstances requiring additional contraception

Incorrect administration: Errors in taking the 7 inactive (large) tablets (i.e. the first 5 tablets in the red section and the 2 immediately before the red section) can, of course, be ignored. A single delayed active (small) tablet should be taken as soon as possible, and if this can be done within 12 hours of the correct time, contraceptive protection is maintained.

With larger errors in taking active tablets, additional contraception is needed. Only the most recently delayed tablet should be taken, earlier missed tablets being omitted, and additional contraception (barriers and spermicides) should be used for the next 7 days, *while the next 7 (active) tablets are being taken*. Therefore, if the 7 days' additional contraception will extend beyond the Friday just before the red section, (i.e. the last active tablet) the user should take the tablets up to and including that Friday, and start a new pack next day with the Saturday tablet in the red section i.e. the first active tablet (Dept. of Health Handbook of Contraceptive Practice).

Gastro-intestinal upset: Vomiting or diarrhoea may reduce efficacy by preventing full absorption. Barriers and spermicides should be used until 7 days after the upset, and, if those 7 days overrun the Friday just before the red section, the user should omit the 7 inactive tablets (as above). Mild laxatives do not impair contraceptive action.

Interaction with other drugs: Some drugs accelerate the metabolism of oral contraceptives taken concurrently. Drugs suspected of having the capacity to reduce the efficacy of oral contraceptives include barbiturates, phenylbutazone, phenytoin, rifampicin, ampicillin and other antibiotics. It is, therefore, advisable to use non-hormonal methods of contraception (except the rhythm, temperature or cervical-mucus methods) in addition to the oral contraceptive as long as an extremely high degree of protection must be provided during treatment with such drugs.

Contra-indications, warnings, etc

Contra-indications: Pregnancy. Thrombotic disorders and a history of these conditions, sickle-cell anaemia, disorders of lipid metabolism and other conditions in which, in individual cases, there is known or suspected to be a much increased risk of thrombosis. Acute or severe chronic liver diseases, Dubin-Johnson syndrome, Rotor syndrome, History, during pregnancy, of idiopathic jaundice or severe pruritus. History of herpes gestationis (also know as pemphigoid gestationis). Mammary or endometrial carcinoma, or a history of these conditions. Abnormal vaginal bleeding of unknown cause. History of deterioration of otosclerosis during pregnancy.

Warnings: There is a general opinion, based on statistical evidence, that users of combined oral contraceptives experience, more often than non-users, venous thromboembolism, arterial thrombosis, including cerebral and myocardial infarction, and subarachnoid haemorrhage. Full recovery from such disorders does not always occur, and it should be realised that in a few cases they are fatal. How often these disorders occur in users of the modern low-dose pills is not known, but there are reasons for suggesting that they may occur less often than with older pills. Certain factors may entail some risk of thrombosis, e.g. smoking, obesity, varicose veins, cardiovascular diseases, diabetes, and migraine. The suitability of a combined oral contraceptive should be judged according to the severity of such conditions in the individual case, and should be discussed with the patient before she decides to take it. The risk of arterial thrombosis associated with combined oral contraceptives increases with age, and this risk is aggravated by cigarette-smoking. The use of combined oral contraceptives by women in the older age-group, especially those who are cigarette smokers, should therefore be discouraged and alternative methods used.

Numerous epidemiological studies have been reported on the risks of ovarian, endometrial, cervical and breast cancer in women using combined oral contraceptives. The evidence is clear that combined oral contraceptives offer substantial protection against both ovarian and endometrial cancer.

An increased risk of cervical cancer in long-term users of combined oral contraceptives has been reported in some studies, but there continues to be controversy about the extent to which this is attributable to the confounding effects of sexual behaviour and other factors.

The evidence linking the use of combined oral contraceptives and breast cancer remains inconclusive. The results of some studies suggest an increased risk of breast cancer presenting below the age of about 35, the risk rising with duration of use. Any possible increased risk of breast cancer with combined oral contraceptives is however likely to be small, and may be expected to be less with low-dosage pills. This possible risk should be weighed against the many benefits of combined oral contraceptives, including their protective effects against ovarian and endometrial cancers.

The possibility cannot be ruled out that certain chronic diseases may occasionally deteriorate during the use of combined oral contraceptives (see 'Precautions').

The combination of ethinyloestradiol and gestodene, like other contraceptive steroids, is associated with an increased incidence of neoplastic nodules in the rat liver, the relevance of which to man is unknown.

Benign hepatic tumours have been associated with oral contraceptive use. Malignant hepatic tumours have also been reported on rare occasions in long-term users of oral contraceptives. A hepatic tumour should be considered in the differential diagnosis when upper abdominal pain, enlarged liver or signs of intra-abdominal haemorrhage occur.

Reasons for stopping oral contraception immediately: Occurrence of migraine in patients who have never previously suffered from it. Exacerbation of pre-existing migraine. Any unusually frequent or unusually severe headaches. Any kind of acute disturbance of vision. Suspicion of thrombosis or infarction. Six weeks before elective operations and during immobilisation, e.g. after accidents, etc. Significant rise in blood pressure. Jaundice. Clear exacerbation of conditions known to be capable of deteriorating during oral contraception or pregnancy. Pregnancy is a reason for stopping immediately because it has been suggested by some investigations that oral contraceptives taken in early pregnancy may slightly increase the risk of foetal malformations. Other investigations have failed to support these findings. The possibility therefore cannot be excluded, but it is certain that if a risk exists at all, it is very small.

Precautions: Examination of the pelvic organs, breasts and blood-pressure should precede the prescribing of any combined oral contraceptive, and should be repeated regularly. Before starting treatment, pregnancy must be excluded. The following conditions require careful observation during medication: a history of severe depressive states, varicose veins, diabetes, hypertension, epilepsy, otosclerosis, multiple sclerosis, porphyria, tetany, disturbed liver function, gall-stones, cardiovascular diseases, renal diseases, chloasma, uterine fibroids, asthma, the wearing of contact lenses, or any disease that it prone to worsen during pregnancy. The deterioration or first appearance of any of these conditions may indicate that the oral contraceptive should be stopped. The risk of the deterioration of chloasma, which is often not fully reversible, is reduced by the avoidance of excessive exposure to sunlight.

Side-effects: Occasional side-effects may include: nausea, vomiting, headaches, breast tension, changed bodyweight or libido, depressive moods and chloasma.

Menstrual changes:

1. *Reduction of menstrual flow:* This is not abnormal and it is to be expected in some patients. Indeed, it may be beneficial where heavy periods were previously experienced.

2. *Missed menstruation:* Occasionally, withdrawal bleeding may not occur at all. If the tablets have been taken correctly, pregnancy is very unlikely, but should be ruled out before a new course of tablets is started.

Intermenstrual bleeding: 'Spotting' or heavier 'breakthrough bleeding' may occur during tablet-taking, especially in the first few cycles. It appears to be generally of no significance, except where it indicates errors of tablet-taking, or where the possibility of interaction with other drugs exists (q.v.). However, if irregular bleeding is persistent, an organic cause should be considered.

Effect on adrenal and thyroid glands: Oral contraceptives have no significant influence on adrenocortical function. The ACTH stimulation test remains unchanged. The reduction in corticosteroid excretion and the elevation of plasma corticosteroids are due to an increased cortisol-binding capacity of the plasma proteins.

The response to metyrapone is less pronounced than in untreated women and is thus similar to that during pregnancy.

The radio-iodine uptake shows that thyroid function is unchanged. There is a rise in serum protein-bound iodine, similar to that in pregnancy and during the administration of oestrogens. This is due to the increased capacity of the plasma proteins for binding thyroid hormones, rather than to any change in glandular function. In women taking oral contraceptives, the content of protein-bound iodine in blood serum should, therefore, not be used for the evaluation of thyroid function.

Effect on blood chemistry: Oral contraceptives may accelerate erythrocyte sedimentation in the absence of any disease. This effect is due to a change in the proportion of the plasma protein fractions. Increases in plasma copper, iron and alkaline phosphatase have also been recorded.

Overdose: There have been no reports of serious ill-effects from overdosage, even when a considerable number of tablets have been taken by a small child. In general, it is, therefore, unnecessary to treat overdosage. There are no specific antidotes and treatment should be symptomatic.

Pharmaceutical precautions *Storage* – cool, dry conditions. *Shelf-life* – five years.

Legal category POM.

Package quantities Individual packs containing three months' supply (OP).

Further information Nil.

Product licence number 0053/0180.

GASTROGRAFIN*

Presentation Gastrografin contains 10% sodium diatrizoate and 66% meglumine diatrizoate in aqueous solution, with added flavouring and wetting agents. The iodine content is 370 mg/ml.

Excipients: disodium edetate, saccharin sodium, aniseed oil, polysorbate 80, water for injection.

Uses Gastrografin is designed for investigation of the gastro-intestinal tract. It can be used either orally or as an enema. Follow-through examinations with barium can often be improved by combining it with Gastrografin. Gastrografin is of considerable value in the following instances.

1. Suspected partial or complete stenosis.

2. Acute haemorrhage.
3. Threatening perforation (peptic ulcer, diverticulum).
4. Megacolon.
5. Foreign bodies or tumours.
6. Gastrocolic fistula.
7. Before endoscopy.

Gastrografin is also recommended for the treatment of uncomplicated meconium ileus.

Dosage and administration *Oral – Adults and children of 10 years of age or over:* 60 ml Gastrografin are sufficient for the visualisation of the stomach. Up to 100 ml may be needed for a follow-through examination of the gastrointestinal tract.

For computed tomography, 1 to 1.5 litres of a 3% solution of Gastrografin in water (30 ml/litre).

For elderly or cachetic patients: Dilution with an equal volume of water is recommended.

Children up to 10 years of age: 15–30 ml are usually sufficient. This dose may be diluted with twice its volume of water.

For infants and young children: It is recommended that the contrast medium be diluted with three times its volume of water.

Rectal – Adults: The contrast medium should be diluted with three to four times its volume of water. Not more than 500 ml of Gastrografin solution should normally be required.

Children: The contrast medium should be diluted with four to five times its volume of water; up to five years of age the weaker dilution should be used.

Gastrografin and Barium Sulphate: Oral and rectal administration.

Adults: 30 ml Gastrografin plus the usual dose of barium should be adequate.

Children: 10 ml Gastrografin may be added to the barium.

For children up to five years of age: from 2–5 ml Gastrografin to 100 ml barium may be preferable. Further dilution which does not affect the contrast may be used if necessary in cases of pylorospasm or pyloric stenosis.

For the early diagnosis of a perforation or anastomosis in the oesophagus or gastrointestinal tract, the patient should drink 100 ml Gastrografin. After 30–60 minutes (later, if the defect is suspected of being in the distal gut), a urine specimen should be taken and 5 ml mixed with 5 drops of concentrated hydrochloric acid. The contrast medium which has undergone renal excretion will appear within two hours as a typical crystal formation in the precipitate.

Technique for the treatment of uncomplicated meconium ileus: Gastrografin can be given by enema to infants for non-operative treatment of uncomplicated meconium ileus, i.e. in the absence of volvulus, gangrene, perforation, peritonitis or atresia, all of which require immediate operation.

A large syringe and soft rubber catheter, No. 8 French, are recommended. The buttocks can be taped tightly together to minimise leakage but a balloon catheter should not be used. The procedure must be carried out slowly and only under fluoroscopic control. Injection should stop as soon as Gastrografin is seen to enter the ileum. Owing to its high osmolarity, Gastrografin may cause the loss of a large amount of fluid into the intestines. An intravenous drip must therefore be set up before the enema is given and plasma should be infused as required. If the Gastrografin is not expelled during the first hour after removal of the rectal catheter, an X-ray should be taken to ensure that overdistension of the bowel as a result of the high osmolarity of Gastrografin has not occurred.

Contra-indications, warnings, etc
Contra-indications: Hypersensitivity to iodine-containing contrast media. Manifest hyperthyroidism.

Warnings/side-effects: The need for examination merits particularly careful consideration in the case of latent hyperthyroidism, benign nodular goitre, in dehydrated patients and in babies and young children. Disturbances in water or electrolyte balance must first be corrected.

Because of its high osmotic pressure and minimal absorption, Gastrografin should not be administered to infants in higher doses than those recommended above.

Caution should be observed in patients with thyroid disease. Aspiration of Gastrografin into the lungs may cause pulmonary oedema. Caution is needed with oesophagotracheal fistulae to avoid passage of the medium into the lungs. Systemic effects are rare, since Gastrografin is only minimally absorbed from the alimentary tract.

Nausea and vomiting occur in exceptional cases. Urticarial skin reactions have occasionally been observed, while anaphylactoid reactions and shock are possible.

Owing to its hypertonicity, Gastrografin may occasionally cause diarrhoea, but this ceases as soon as the intestine has been emptied.

Existing enteritis or colitis may be temporarily exacerbated.

Because of the additives (flavourings and a wetting agent), Gastrografin must not be used intravascularly.

Following the administration of iodinated renal contrast media, the capacity of the thyroid tissue to take up radioisotopes for diagnosing disorders of the thyroid is reduced for up to 2 weeks, and even longer in individual cases.

Overdose: There are no specific antidotes to Gastrografin. Treatment should be symptomatic.

Pharmaceutical precautions *Storage:* Protect from light and heat. Shelf-life five years. At temperatures below 7°C Gastrografin tends to crystallize, but this can be reversed by gently warming and shaking the bottle. This phenomenon has no effect on the effectiveness or stability of the preparation.

Legal category P.

Package quantities Bottles 5 × 100 ml.

Further information Nil.

Product licence number 0053/5023R.

ISOVIST* ▼

Presentation Bottles containing colourless sterile aqueous solutions of various strengths of the non-ionic dimeric contrast medium, iotrolan. Isovist 240 contains 240 mg iodine per ml; Isovist 300 contains 300 mg iodine per ml.

Inactive ingredients: Isovist 240: calcium disodium edetate, sodium bicarbonate, sodium chloride, water for injection.

Isovist 300: calcium disodium edetate, sodium bicarbonate, water for injection.

Uses Isovist is intended for intrathecal use, i.e. radiculography and myelography of all regions, for ventriculography, evaluation of the circulation of cerebrospinal fluid and cisternography by computed tomography, and for use in other body cavities.

Dosage and administration
General information: The patient should attend for myelographic examination fasting but adequately hydrated. Disorders of water and electrolyte balance must be corrected, particularly in patients prone to this type of disorder.

Nervous patients may be given a suitable sedative (e.g. diazepam) prophylactically. No anaesthesia is required if thin puncture needles are used. If antiemetics are administered, they should not possess neuroleptic properties.

After myelographic investigations – particularly of higher regions – the patient should be confined to bed with head raised for at least 6 hours, and remain passive for 24 hours.

Patients with a known or suspected low seizure

threshold must be kept under careful observation for eight hours.

Isovist should not be drawn up into the syringe until immediately before use. Contrast medium not used in one examination must be discarded.

Dosage: The concentration and volume of Isovist chosen depend on the radiological equipment available. If equipment is available that allows films to be taken in all necessary projections without the patient's having to move, and with which the injection can be performed under fluoroscopic control, iodine concentrations and volumes of medium at the lower end of the specified range can be used.

Higher concentrations are indicated if it will be necessary to reposition the patient during a myelographic examination, since the medium becomes diluted more quickly as a result of turbulence, and the clarity of detail deteriorates.

Lumbar myelography (with thoracic transition) – 7–12 ml Isovist 240.

Thoracic myelography – 10–15 ml Isovist 240. 8–12 ml Isovist 300.

Panmyelography (injection in the lumbar region) – 10–15 ml Isovist 300.

Cervical myelography – Direct (lateral access between C_1/C_2). 8–12 ml Isovist 240. 7–10 ml Isovist 300.

Indirect (injection in the lumbar region). 15 ml Isovist 240. 8–15 ml Isovist 300.

Ventriculography – 3–5 ml Isovist 240. 3–5 ml Isovist 300.

CT-cisternography (injection in the lumbar region) – 4–12 ml Isovist 240.

Administration of the contrast medium in myelography: After withdrawal of the volume of cerebrospinal fluid (CSF) needed for examination, the appropriate dose of Isovist is injected. N.B. The more the patient moves after the administration of Isovist, the quicker will the medium mix with the CSF and the density of contrast decrease.

Other body cavities

Indirect lymphography (e.g. lymphoedema) – 2–20 ml Isovist 300.

Arthrography – 2–15 ml Isovist 240/300.

Hysterosalpingography – 7–25 ml Isovist 240/300.

Mammary ducts – 1–3 ml Isovist 240/300.

Endoscopic retrograde cholangiopancreatography – 10–30 ml Isovist 240/300.

Oesophagus - stomach - bowel – 8–100 ml Isovist 300.

In the administration of contrast medium for indirect lymphography, multiple simultaneous interstitial (e.g. intracutaneous) injections are to be preferred.

Contra-indications, warnings, etc

Contra-indications: Manifest thyrotoxicosis, proven or suspected hypersensitivity to iodine-containing contrast media.

Hysterosalpingography must not be carried out during pregnancy or in the presence of acute inflammatory conditions in the pelvic cavity.

Use in pregnancy: X-ray examinations should, if possible, be avoided during pregnancy. It has not yet been proved beyond question that Isovist may be used without hesitation in pregnant patients. Therefore, examination with Isovist during pregnancy should be carried out only if considered essential.

Warnings/side-effects: Epilepsy is a relative contra-indication for myelography. If, after careful consideration, myelography is considered necessary, equipment and drugs necessary to treat any convulsion that may occur must be readily available. Neuroleptics or antidepressants should be discontinued 48 hours before the examination, because they lower the seizure threshold. Alcoholics and drug addicts may have a lowered seizure threshold. Anticonvulsants (e.g. phenobarbitone 200 mg i.m.) may be given prophylactically.

Hyperthyroidism may be exacerbated. Iodinated contrast media reduce the capacity of the thyroid gland to take up radio-isotopes of iodine for up to 2 weeks, and sometimes longer. Patients with a history of allergy may be particularly susceptible to hypersensitivy reactions. Such reactions are possible in any patient, but are rare in the recommended indications.

The most frequently reported symptoms are headache, nausea and vomiting. However, experience shows that their incidence is no higher than after the loss of pressure in the subarachnoid space that results from a diagnostic tap of CSF from the spinal canal. In view of this, an effort should be made to remove only as much CSF as is being replaced by the Isovist solution. On the other hand, administration of an amount of Isovist greater than the amount of CSF removed does not lead to an increase in CSF pressure.

Severe side-effects are extremely rare when Isovist is administered in the recommended dosages. Minor side-effects include pain or an increase in existing pain in the back, nape or extremities, and, rarely, very brief non-specific EEG changes. Slight muscular tension or paraesthesia has been reported in rare cases 2–6 hours after administration of the medium.

Severe headaches lasting several days occur rarely. If convulsions occur, give 10 mg diazepam immediately by slow i.v. injection, followed, 20–30 minutes after the subsidence of the convulsions, by 200 mg phenobarbitone i.m. to prevent recurrence, unless this has been given prophylactically. Diazepam should be injected i.v. as a precaution at the first signs of hyperactivity or muscular twitching.

As with other myelographic agents, the CSF cell-count increases somewhat after intrathecal injection of Isovist. Very rarely, headaches, nausea, vomiting, stiffness of the neck and an increased cell-count in the CSF may mimic aseptic meningitis. All symptoms have usually disappeared after 2–3 days. Arachnoiditis has not been reported.

Isovist is excreted renally. Therefore, for patients with severe impairment of renal function, the need for examination with Isovist merits careful consideration.

Ready availability of all drugs and equipment for emergency treatment and familiarity with the relevant procedures are prerequisites for the effective management of contrast-medium incidents.

Overdosage: Acute symptoms of poisoning are unlikely with intrathecal administration. Treatment is symptomatic.

Pharmaceutical precautions Protect from light and secondary X-rays. Store below 30°C. Shelf-life 3 years.

Legal category POM.

Package quantities Isovist 240: Box containing 10 vials of 10 ml. Box containing 10 vials of 20 ml.

Isovist 300: Box containing 10 vials of 10 ml.

Further information Isovist is a series of non-ionic, dimeric, water-soluble contrast media with osmolalities close to those of normal body fluids. Isovist 240 – 270 mosm/kg H_2O at 37°C. Isovist 300 – 320 mosm/kg H_2O at 37°C.

Product licence numbers

Isovist 240 0053/0201.
Isovist 300 0053/0202.

LOGYNON* (21-day)

Presentation The memo-pack holds six light-brown tablets containing 30 micrograms ethinyloestradiol and 50 micrograms levonorgestrel, five white tablets containing 40 micrograms ethinyloestradiol and 75 micrograms levonorgestrel and ten ochre tablets containing 30 micrograms ethinyloestradiol and 125 micrograms levonorgestrel.

All tablets have a lustrous, sugar coating. The light-brown tablets bear a black C in a regular hexagon on both sides. The white and the ochre tablets bear a black B in a regular hexagon on both sides.

Excipients: lactose, maize starch, povidone 25 000, talc, magnesium stearate, sucrose, povidone 700 000, polyethylene glycol 6000, calcium carbonate, wax E, titanium dioxide, glycerin, ferric oxide pigment yellow.

Uses Oral contraception and the recognised gynaecological indications for such oestrogen-progestogen combinations. The mode of action includes the inhibition of ovulation by suppression of the mid-cycle surge of luteinising hormone, the inspissation of cervical mucus so as to constitute a barrier to sperm, and the rendering of the endometrium unreceptive to implantation.

Dosage and administration *First treatment cycle:* 1 tablet daily for 21 days, starting with the tablet marked number 1, on the first day of the menstrual cycle.

Subsequent cycles: Each subsequent course is started when seven tablet-free days have followed the preceding course.

Changing from other oral contraceptives: The first tablet of Logynon should be taken on the first day immediately after the end of the previous oral contraceptive course. Additional contraceptive precautions are not required.

Post-partum and post-abortum use: After pregnancy oral contraception can be started 21 days after a vaginal delivery, provided that the patient is fully ambulant and there are no puerperal complications. After a first-trimester abortion, oral contraception may be started immediately. Since the first post-partum ovulation may precede the first bleeding, another method of contraception should be used in the interval between childbirth and the first course of pills.

Special circumstances requiring additional contraception: Incorrect administration: A single delayed tablet should be taken as soon as possible, and if this can be done within 12 hours of the correct time contraceptive protection is maintained.

With larger errors, additional contraception is needed. Only the most recently delayed tablets should be taken, earlier missed pills being omitted, and additional contraception (barriers and spermicides) should be used for the next 7 days, *while the next 7 tablets are being taken. Additionally,* therefore, if pills have been missed *during the last 7 days* of a pack, there should be no break before the next pack is started (Dept. of Health Handbook of Contraceptive Practice).

Gastro-intestinal upset: Vomiting or diarrhoea may reduce efficacy by preventing full absorption. Barriers and spermicides should be used until 7 days after the upset, and, if those 7 days overrun the end of a pack, the next pack should be started without a break. Mild laxatives do not impair contraceptive action.

Interaction with other drugs: Some drugs accelerate the metabolism of oral contraceptives taken concurrently. Drugs suspected of having the capacity to reduce the efficacy of oral contraceptives include barbiturates, phenytoin, phenylbutazone, rifampicin, ampicillin, griseofulvin and other antibiotics. It is, therefore, advisable to use non-hormonal methods of contraception (except the rhythm, temperature or cervical-mucus methods) in addition to the oral contraceptive as long as an extremely high degree of protection must be provided during treatment with such drugs.

Contra-indications, warnings, etc
Contra-indications: Pregnancy. Thrombotic disorders and a history of these conditions, sickle-cell anaemia, disorders of lipid metabolism and other conditions in which, in individual cases, there is known or suspected to be a much increased risk of thrombosis. Acute or severe chronic liver diseases. Dubin-Johnson syndrome. Rotor syndrome. History, during pregnancy, of idiopathic jaundice or severe pruritus. History of herpes gestationis (also known as pemphigoid gestationis). Mammary or endometrial carcinoma, or a history of these conditions. Abnormal vaginal bleeding of unknown cause. Deterioration of otosclerosis during pregnancy.

Warnings: There is a general opinion, based on statistical evidence, that users of combined oral contraceptives experience, more often than non-users, venous thromboembolism, arterial thrombosis, including cerebral and myocardial infarction, and subarachnoid haemorrhage. Full recovery from such disorders does not always occur, and it should be realised that in a few cases they are fatal. How often these disorders occur in users of the modern low-dose pills is not known, but there are reasons for suggesting that they may occur less often than with older pills.

Certain factors may entail some risk of thrombosis, e.g. smoking, obesity, varicose veins, cardiovascular diseases, diabetes and migraine. The suitability of a combined oral contraceptive should be judged according to the severity of such conditions in the individual case, and should be discussed with the patient before she decides to take it. The risk of arterial thrombosis associated with oral contraceptives increases with age, and this risk is aggravated by cigarette-smoking. The use of combined oral contraceptives by women in the older age-group, especially those who are cigarette-smokers, should therefore be discouraged, and alternative methods advised.

Numerous epidemiological studies have been reported on the risks of ovarian, endometrial, cervical and breast cancer in women using combined oral contraceptives. The evidence is clear that combined oral contraceptives offer substantial protection against both ovarian and endometrial cancer.

An increased risk of cervical cancer in long-term users of combined oral contraceptives has been reported in some studies, but there continues to be controversy about the extent to which this is attributable to the confounding effects of sexual behaviour and other factors.

The evidence linking the use of combined oral contraceptives and breast cancer remains inconclusive. The results of some studies suggest an increased risk of breast cancer presenting below the age of about 35, the risk rising with duration of use. Any possible increased risk of breast cancer with combined oral contraceptives is however likely to be small, and may be expected to be less with low-dosage pills. This possible risk should be weighed against the many benefits of combined oral contraceptives, including their protective effects against ovarian and endometrial cancers.

The possibility cannot be ruled out that certain chronic diseases may occasionally deteriorate during the use of combined oral contraceptives (see 'Precautions'). Benign hepatic tumours have been associated with oral contraceptive usage. Malignant hepatic tumours have also been reported on rare occasions in long-term users of oral contraceptives. A hepatic tumour should be considered in the differential diagnosis when upper abdominal pain, enlarged liver or signs of intra-abdominal haemorrhage occur.

Reasons for stopping oral contraception immediately: Occurrence of migraine in patients who have never previously suffered from it. Exacerbation of pre-existing migraine. Any unusually frequent or unusually severe headaches. Any kind of acute disturbance of vision. Suspicion of thrombosis or infarction. Six weeks before elective operations and during immobilisation, e.g. after accidents, etc. Significant rise in blood-pressure. Jaundice. Clear exacerbation of conditions known to be capable of deteriorating during oral contraception or pregnancy. Pregnancy is a reason for stopping immediately because it has been suggested by some investigations that oral contraceptives taken in early pregnancy may slightly increase the risk of foetal malformations. Other investigations have failed to support these findings. The possibility therefore cannot be excluded, but it is certain that if a risk exists at all, it is very small.

Precautions: Examination of the pelvic organs, breasts and blood-pressure should precede the prescribing of any combined oral contraceptive, and should be repeated regularly. Before starting treatment, pregnancy must be excluded.

The following conditions require careful consideration: a history of severe depressive states, varicose veins, diabetes, hypertension, epilepsy, otosclerosis, multiple sclerosis, porphyria, tetany, disturbed liver function, gallstones, cardiovascular diseases, renal diseases, chloasma, uterine fibroids, asthma, the wearing of contact lenses, or any disease that is prone to worsen during pregnancy. The first appearance or deterioration of any of these conditions may indicate that the oral contraceptive should be stopped.

The risk of the deterioration of chloasma, which is often not fully reversible, is reduced by the avoidance of excessive exposure to sunlight.

Side-effects: Occasional side-effects may include nausea, vomiting, headaches, breast tension, changed body weight or libido, depressive moods and chloasma.

Menstrual changes:

1. *Reduction of menstrual flow:* This is not abnormal and it is to be expected in some patients. Indeed, it may be beneficial where heavy periods were previously experienced.

2. *Missed menstruation:* Occasionally, withdrawal bleeding may not occur at all. If the tablets have been taken correctly, pregnancy is very unlikely, but should be ruled out before a new course of tablets is started.

Intermenstrual bleeding: Very light 'spotting' or heavier 'breakthrough bleeding' may occur during tablet-taking, especially in the first few cycles. It appears to be generally of no significance, except where it indicates errors of tablet-taking, or where the possibility of interaction with other drugs exists (q.v.). However, if irregular bleeding is persistent, an organic cause should be considered.

Effect on adrenal and thyroid glands: Oral contraceptives have no significant influence on adrenocortical function. The ACTH function test for the adrenal cortex remains unchanged. The reduction in corticosteroid excretion and the elevation of plasma corticosteroids are due to an increased cortisol-binding capacity of the plasma proteins.

The response to metyrapone is less pronounced than in untreated women and is thus similar to that during pregnancy.

The radio-iodine uptake shows that thyroid function is unchanged. There is a rise in serum protein-bound iodine, similar to that in pregnancy and during the administration of oestrogens. This is due to the increased capacity of the plasma proteins for binding thyroid hormones, rather than to any change in glandular function. In women taking oral contraceptives, the content of protein-bound iodine in blood serum should, therefore, not be used for evaluation of thyroid function.

Effect on blood chemistry: Oral contraceptives may accelerate erythrocyte sedimentation in the absence of any disease. This effect is due to a change in the proportion of the plasma protein fractions. Increases in plasma copper, iron and alkaline phosphatase have also been recorded.

Overdosage: There have been no reports of serious ill-effects from overdosage, even when a considerable number of tablets have been taken by a small child. In general, it is, therefore, unnecessary to treat overdosage.

There are no specific antidotes and treatment should be symptomatic.

Pharmaceutical precautions Store in cool, dry conditions: shelf-life five years.

Legal category POM.

Package quantities Available in packs containing one month's supply (OP).

Further information Nil.

Product licence number 0053/0085.

LOGYNON* ED

Presentation The memo-pack holds six light-brown tablets containing 30 micrograms ethinyloestradiol and 50 micrograms levonorgestrel, five white tablets containing 40 micrograms ethinyloestradiol and 75 micrograms levonorgestrel, ten ochre tablets containing 30 micrograms ethinyloestradiol and 125 micrograms levonorgestrel and seven white placebo tablets.

All tablets have a lustrous, sugar coating. The light-brown tablets bear a black C in a regular hexagon printed on both sides. The white active tablets and the ochre tablets bear a black B in a regular hexagon on both sides. The white placebo tablets are larger and bear a black O in a regular hexagon.

Excipients: lactose, maize starch, povidone 25 000, talc, magnesium stearate, sucrose, povidone 700 000, polyethylene glycol 6000, calcium carbonate, wax E, titanium dioxide, glycerin, ferric oxide pigment yellow.

Uses Oral contraception and the recognised gynaecological indications for such oestrogen-progestogen combinations. The mode of action includes the inhibition of ovulation by suppression of the mid-cycle surge of luteinising hormone, the inspissation of cervical mucus so as to constitute a barrier to sperm, and the rendering of the endometrium unreceptive to implantation.

Dosage and administration *First treatment cycle:* 1 tablet daily for 28 days, starting in the red section on the first day of bleeding, the initial tablet being the one marked with the appropriate day of the week. In the first cycle only, an additional form of contraception (except the rhythm, temperature or cervical-mucus methods) must be used for the first 14 days of tablet-taking.

Subsequent cycles: Each subsequent course is started in the red section on the day after the previous one has been finished. Pack, therefore, follows pack without interval.

Changing from other oral contraceptives: The first tablet of Logynon ED should be taken on the first day immediately after the end of the previous oral contraceptive course. Additional (non-hormonal) precautions, other than the rhythm, temperature or cervical-mucus methods, should also be used for the first 14 days when changing products.

Post-partum and post-abortum use: After pregnancy oral contraception can be started 21 days after a vaginal delivery, provided that the patient is fully ambulant and there are no puerperal complications. After a first-trimester abortion, oral contraception may be started immediately. Since the first post-partum ovulation may precede the first bleeding, another method of contraception should be used in the interval between childbirth and the first course of pills.

Special circumstances requiring additional contraception

Incorrect administration: Errors in taking the 7 inactive (large) tablets (i.e. the first 5 tablets in the red section and the 2 immediately before the red section) can, of course, be ignored. A single delayed active (small) tablet should be taken as soon as possible, and if this can be done within 12 hours of the correct time, contraceptive protection is maintained.

With larger errors in taking active tablets, additional contraception is needed. Only the most recently delayed tablet should be taken, earlier missed tablets being omitted, and additional contraception (barriers and spermicides) should be used for the next 7 days, *while the next 7 (active) tablets are being taken.* Therefore, if the 7 days' additional contraception will extend beyond the Friday just before the red section, (i.e. the last active tablet) the user should take the tablets up to and including that Friday, and start a new pack next day with the Saturday tablet in the red section i.e. the first active tablet (Dept. of Health Handbook of Contractive Practice).

Gastro-intestinal upset: Vomiting or diarrhoea may reduce efficacy by preventing full absorption. Barriers and spermicides should be used until 7 days after the upset, and, if those 7 days overrun the Friday just before the red section, the user should omit the 7 inactive tablets (as above). Mild laxatives do not impair contraceptive action.

Interaction with other drugs: Some drugs accelerate the metabolism of oral contraceptives taken concurrently. Drugs suspected of having the capacity to reduce the efficacy of oral contraceptives include barbiturates, phenytoin, phenylbutazone, rifampicin, ampicillin, griseofulvin and other antibiotics. It is, therefore, advisable to use non-hormonal methods of contraception (except the rhythm, temperature or cervical-mucus methods) in addition to the oral contraceptive as long as an extremely high degree of protection must be provided during treatment with such drugs.

Contra-indications, warnings, etc

Contra-indications: Pregnancy. Thrombotic disorders and a history of these conditions, sickle-cell anaemia, disorders of lipid metabolism and other conditions in which, in individual cases, there is known or suspected to be a much increased risk of thrombosis. Acute or severe chronic liver diseases. Dubin-Johnson syndrome. Rotor syndrome. History, during pregnancy, of idiopathic jaundice or severe pruritus. History of herpes gestationis (also known as pemphigoid gestationis). Mammary or endometrial carcinoma, or a history of these conditions. Abnormal vaginal bleeding of unknown cause. Deterioration of otosclerosis during pregnancy.

Warnings: There is a general opinion, based on statistical evidence, that users of combined oral contraceptives experience, more often than non-users, venous thromboembolism, arterial thrombosis, including cerebral and myocardial infarction, and subarachnoid haemorrhage. Full recovery from such disorders does not always occur, and it should be realised that in a few cases they are fatal. How often these disorders occur in users of the modern low-dose pills is not known, but there are reasons for suggesting that they may occur less often than with older pills.

Certain factors may entail some risk of thrombosis, e.g. smoking, obesity, varicose veins, cardiovascular diseases, diabetes and migraine. The suitability of a combined oral contraceptive should be judged according to the severity of such conditions in the individual case, and should be discussed with the patient before she decides to take it. The risk of arterial thrombosis associated with oral contraceptives increases with age, and this risk is aggravated by cigarette-smoking. The use of combined oral contraceptives by women in the older age-group, especially those who are cigarette-smokers should therefore be discouraged, and alternative methods advised.

Numerous epidemiological studies have been reported on the risks of ovarian, endometrial, cervical and breast cancer in women using combined oral contraceptives. The evidence is clear that combined oral contraceptives offer substantial protection against both ovarian and endometrial cancer.

An increased risk of cervical cancer in long-term users of combined oral contraceptives has been reported in some studies, but there continues to be controversy about the extent to which this is attributable to the confounding effects of sexual behaviour and other factors.

The evidence linking the use of combined oral contraceptives and breast cancer remains inconclusive. The results of some studies suggest an increased risk of breast cancer presenting below the age of about 35, the risk rising with duration of use. Any possible increased risk of breast cancer with combined oral contraceptives is however likely to be small, and may be expected to be less with low-dosage pills. This possible risk should be weighed against the many benefits of combined oral contraceptives, including their protective effects against ovarian and endometrial cancers.

The possibility cannot be ruled out that certain chronic diseases may occasionally deteriorate during the use of combined oral contraceptives (see 'Precautions'). Benign hepatic tumours have been associated with oral contraceptive usage. Malignant hepatic tumours have also been reported in long-term oral contraceptive users. A hepatic tumour should be considered in the differential diagnosis when upper abdominal pain, enlarged liver or signs of intra-abdominal haemorrhage occur.

Reasons for stopping oral contraception immediately: Occurrence of migraine in patients who have never previously suffered from it. Exacerbation of pre-existing migraine. Any unusually frequent or unusually severe headaches. Any kind of acute disturbance of vision. Suspicion of thrombosis or infarction. Six weeks before elective operations and during immobilisation, e.g. after accidents, etc. Significant rise in blood-pressure. Jaundice. Clear exacerbation of conditions known to be capable of deteriorating during oral contraception or pregnancy. Pregnancy is a reason for stopping immediately because it has been suggested by some investigations that oral contraceptives taken in early pregnancy may slightly increase the risk of foetal malformations. Other investigations have failed to support these findings. The possibility therefore cannot be excluded, but it is certain that if a risk exists at all, it is very small.

Precautions: Examination of the pelvic organs, breasts and blood-pressure should precede the prescribing of any combined oral contraceptive, and should be repeated regularly. Before starting treatment, pregnancy must be excluded.

The following conditions require careful consideration: a history of severe depressive states, varicose veins, diabetes, hypertension, epilepsy, otosclerosis, multiple sclerosis, porphyria, tetany, disturbed liver function, gallstones, cardiovascular diseases, renal diseases, chloasma, uterine fibroids, asthma, the wearing of contact lenses, or any disease that is prone to worsen during pregnancy. The first appearance or deterioration of any of these conditions may indicate that the oral contraceptive should be stopped.

The risk of the deterioration of chloasma, which is often not fully reversible, is reduced by the avoidance of excessive exposure to sunlight.

Side-effects: Occasional side-effects may include nausea, vomiting, headaches, breast tension, changed body weight or libido, depressive moods and chloasma.

Menstrual changes:

1. *Reduction of menstrual flow:* This is not abnormal and it is to be expected in some patients. Indeed, it may be beneficial where heavy periods were previously experienced.

2. *Missed menstruation:* Occasionally, withdrawal bleeding may not occur at all. If the tablets have been taken correctly, pregnancy is very unlikely, but should be ruled out before a new course of tablets is started.

Intermenstrual bleeding: Very light 'spotting' or heavier 'breakthrough bleeding' may occur during tablet-taking, especially in the first few cycles. It appears to be generally of no significance, except where it indicates errors of tablet-taking, or where the possibility of interaction with other drugs exists (q.v.). However, if irregular bleeding is persistent, an organic cause should be considered.

Effect on adrenal and thyroid glands: Oral contraceptives have no significant influence on adrenocortical function. The ACTH function test for the adrenal cortex remains unchanged. The reduction in corticosteroid excretion and the elevation of plasma corticosteroids are due to an increased cortisol-binding capacity of the plasma proteins.

The response to metyrapone is less pronounced than in untreated women and is thus similar to that during pregnancy.

The radio-iodine uptake shows that thyroid function is unchanged. There is a rise in serum protein-bound iodine, similar to that in pregnancy and during the administration of oestrogens. This is due to the increased capacity of the plasma proteins for binding thyroid hormones, rather than to any change in glandular function. In women taking oral contraceptives, the content of protein-bound iodine in blood serum should, therefore, not be used for evaluation of thyroid function.

Effect on blood chemistry: Oral contraceptives may accelerate erythrocyte sedimentation in the absence of any disease. This effect is due to a change in the proportion of the plasma protein fractions. Increases in plasma copper, iron and alkaline phosphatase have also been recorded.

Overdosage: There have been no reports of serious ill-effects from overdosage, even when a considerable number of tablets have been taken by a small child. In general, it is, therefore, unnecessary to treat overdosage.

There are no specific antidotes and treatment should be symptomatic.

Pharmaceutical precautions Store in cool, dry conditions: shelf-life five years.

Legal category POM.

Package quantities Available in packs containing one month's supply (OP).

Further information Nil.

Product licence number 0053/0115.

MAGNEVIST*

Presentation Each vial contains 20 ml or 15 ml of a colourless sterile aqueous solution of the paramagnetic contrast medium for magnetic resonance imaging, dimeglumine gadopentetate, which is the dimeglumine salt of gadolinium-diethylenetriaminepenta-acetic acid (gadolinium DTPA). A small amount of free DTPA is present to ensure the complete chelation of the gadolinium. 1 ml of Magnevist contains 469.01 mg dimeglumine gadopentetate.

Inactive excipient: water for injection.

Uses Cranial and spinal magnetic resonance imaging (MRI). After the administration of Magnevist, the resulting opacification of areas with dysfunction of the blood-brain barrier (e.g. glioblastoma) and other intracranial and intraspinal lesions of non-cerebral origin provides a greater diagnostic yield than is achieved with a plain scan.

Dosage and administration No special preparation of the patient is required. The usual precautions for MRI (e.g. exclusion of ferromagnetic objects, including vascular clips, etc) must be observed.

Magnevist should not be drawn up into the syringe until immediately before use. Contrast medium not used in one examination must be discarded.

Magnevist is not recommended for children below 18 years of age, owing to the small amount of clinical experience with this age group as yet.

Dosage: 0.1 mmol Magnevist/kg body weight (equivalent to 0.2 ml/kg body weight) is usually sufficient to provide diagnostically-adequate contrast. The required dose should be administered as a single intravenous injection. If required, intravenous bolus administration can be used.

Contrast-enhanced MRI can start immediately after administration of the medium. Optimal opacification is generally observed within 45 minutes of injection of Magnevist. T_1-weighted scanning sequences are particularly suitable for contrast-enhanced examinations with Magnevist. In the investigated range of field-strengths, from 0.14 Tesla up to 1.5 Tesla (resistive or superconductive magnets), the image contrast was found to be independent of the applied field strength.

Contra-indications, warnings, etc
Contra-indications: None known.

Use in pregnancy: There is as yet no evidence of the safety of Magnevist during human pregnancy. With daily dosages in the rat for 10 days of 12.5 times, and in the rabbit for 13 days of at least 7.5 times, the human dose per unit weight, there was slight retardation of foetal growth and ossification. It is advisable to avoid using Magnevist during pregnancy, unless an enhanced MR investigation is essential, and no suitable alternative is available.

Warnings: Magnevist is excreted renally. Therefore the need for Magnevist-enhanced MRI requires careful consideration in patients with severely impaired renal function in view of the potential retention of Magnevist that may occur in these cases.

It is known from animal experiments that minimal amounts of Magnevist (less than 0.2% of the administered dose) enter the breast milk. The clinical relevance of this is not known.

Slightly elevated levels of iron and bilirubin (within the normal range in the majority of cases) have been observed in the serum in some patients after administration of Magnevist. However, the elevations were seldom sustained for more than 24 hours and there was always a return to the initial values. The clinical significance of this, if any, is not known, and all patients in whom this effect was observed remained asymptomatic.

The results of serum iron determinations using complexımetric methods (e.g. bathophenanthroline) may be reduced for up to 24 hours after the administration of Magnevist because of the free DTPA contained in the contrast-medium solution.

Side-effects: Transient sensations of slight warmth at the injection-site or of pain have been reported very rarely. Dermal and mucosal reactions of allergic type have been observed after the administration of Magnevist.

In very rare cases anaphylactoid reactions or shock may occur. Familiarity with the practice of emergency measures is essential for prompt efficient action in the event of contrast-medium incidents. Appropriate drugs and instruments (e.g. endotracheal tube and ventilator) must be readily available. Transient sensations of a sweetish taste may occur after rapid bolus injections.

Inadvertent paravenous injection of Magnevist may cause pain lasting up to 20 minutes.

Overdosage: Acute symptoms of toxicity are unlikely with intravenous administration. Treatment is symptomatic.

Pharmaceutical precautions Do not store above 25°C. Protect from light. Shelf-life 3 years.

Legal category POM.

Package quantities Vials of 20 ml and 15 ml.

Further information Magnevist is excreted by the kidneys.

Osmolality at 37°C 1960.0 (mosm/kg H_2O)
Viscosity at 37°C 2.9 (mPa.s)
20°C 4.9
pH 6.5–8.0

Product licence number 0053/0206.

NEOGEST*

Presentation Each round, dark brown, sugar-coated tablet bears a printed white D in a white regular hexagon on both sides and contains 37.5 micrograms levonorgestrel contained in 75 micrograms norgestrel.

Excipients: lactose, maize starch, povidone 25 000, talc, magnesium stearate, sucrose, povidone 700 000, polyethylene glycol 6000, calcium carbonate, titanium dioxide, ferric oxide, glycerin, wax E.

Uses Oral contraception.

Mode of action: The contraceptive action of Neogest may be explained as follows.

It changes the cervical mucus so that a barrier is formed against the migration of sperm into the uterine cavity. Nidation is impeded because of changes in the structure of the endometrium. As a rule there is no inhibition of ovulation. Evidence suggests that a reduction in corpus-luteum function may also contribute to the contraceptive action.

Dosage and administration The first tablet is taken on the first day of menstrual bleeding or on the day after the end of a course of a different oral contraceptive, at a time chosen by the patient. All subsequent tablets must then be taken at this time. The contraceptive effect is likely to be reduced if a tablet is delayed more than three hours. The tablets are taken daily and pack follows pack without interruption for as long as protection against conception is required. The contraceptive action begins after 14 tablets have been taken.

When starting oral contraception anew with Neogest, additional precautions other than the rhythm or temperature or combined-pill methods must be used for the first 14 days of tablet-taking. In patients switching from other oral contraceptives, additional precautions are not required.

Use after delivery or abortion: Neogest may be started as early as the 7th day post partum.

Use during breast feeding: There is no evidence that Neogest diminishes the yield of breast milk. Radioactivity can be found in the milk after the administration of labelled levonorgestrel. However, it is not known whether the metabolites which appear in minute amounts in the milk and do not accumulate in the infant's tissues are biologically active.

Contra-indications, warnings, etc
Contra-indications: History during pregnancy of idiopathic jaundice or severe pruritus. Dubin-Johnson and Rotor syndromes, acute and severe chronic liver diseases. Pregnancy. History of herpes gestationis (also known as pemphigoid gestationis). Although no association between progestogen-only oral contraceptives and thromboembolic disorders has been shown, it is at present required that a history of such disorders be described as a contra-indication to Neogest, as it is to oestrogen-containing oral contraceptives.

Warnings/side-effects: Clinical investigations indicate that, in general, Neogest is very well tolerated. Symptoms reported in isolated cases include nausea, vomiting, dizziness, headaches, migraine, depressive moods, disturbances of appetite, allergic reactions. Amenorrhoea and changes in the pattern of the menstrual cycle have also been observed (For details see 'Menstrual pattern'.)

Circumstances requiring additional contraceptive precautions, other than the temperature, rhythm and cervical-mucus methods.

1. If a tablet is taken more than three hours late (i.e. if it is more than 27 hours since the last tablet was taken), protection against conception may be impaired. From the time of such an error, extra nonhormonal methods must be employed until 14 consecutive tablets have been taken in the correct manner.

2. Vomiting or diarrhoea may reduce the effectiveness of the tablets by preventing them from being fully absorbed. If vomiting occurs shortly after a tablet has been taken, the contraceptive protection may be maintained if a second tablet is taken within three hours of the normal time, provided that vomiting does not recur. It is advisable to take the last tablet of the pack for this purpose, so as to avoid confusion.

In the case of repeated vomiting, or continued diarrhoea, additional contraceptive measures should be employed until 14 days after the symptoms have subsided.

3. Interaction with other drugs. Some drugs accelerate the metabolism of oral contraceptives taken concurrently. Drugs suspected of having the capacity to reduce the efficacy of oral contraceptives include barbiturates, phenylbutazone, phenytoin, rifampicin, ampicillin, griseofulvin and other antibiotics. It is, therefore, advisable to use non-hormonal methods of contraception (except the rhythm, temperature or cervical-mucus methods) during treatment with such drugs.

Menstrual pattern: A usual feature of all progestogen-only oral contraceptives is that they produce an initial irregularity of the bleeding pattern, but such irregularity tends to decrease with time.

The patient should be informed before starting Neogest that her menstrual pattern is likely to alter.

Procedure in the case of cycle disturbances: Irregular bleeding is from a medical point of view no reason for discontinuing therapy, as long as organic causes and pregnancy can be ruled out.

If amenorrhoea lasts longer than three months, or occurs repeatedly, administration of Neogest should be suspended until regular cyclical bleeding has been re-established.

No attempt must be made to control irregular cycles by the additional administration of oestrogens, since they would reverse the effect of Neogest on the cervical mucus, thus seriously reducing the contraceptive efficacy.

Reasons for stopping oral contraception immediately: First signs of thrombophlebitis or thromboembolism. Jaundice. Pregnancy.

Overdosage: There have been no reports of serious ill-effects from overdosage even when a considerable number of tablets have been taken by a small child. In general, it is, therefore, unnecessary to treat overdosage. There are no specific antidotes and treatment should be symptomatic.

Pharmaceutical precautions Store in cool, dry conditions.

Shelf-life: Seven years.

Legal category POM.

Package quantities Memo-pack containing 35 tablets (OP).

Further information Nil.

Product licence number 0053/0062.

NERICUR* GEL 5
NERICUR* GEL 10

Presentation Nericur Gel is an aqueous gel containing either 5% or 10% benzoyl peroxide.

Excipients: Carbopol 940, polyoxyethylene 23 lauryl ether, propylene glycol, sodium hydroxide, purified water.

Uses All stages of acne vulgaris. Benzoyl peroxide has a strong antibacterial action against Propionibacterium acnes. It also has keratolytic and sebostatic actions, which cause some dryness and desquamation.

Dosage and administration Treatment should be initiated with Nericur Gel 5%. Once daily, the affected areas should be washed with soap and water and then dried, before Nericur Gel is applied. For stubborn cases treatment may be continued with Nericur Gel 10%, provided that Nericur Gel 5% has been well tolerated. For particularly sensitive skin, Nericur Gel 5% should be applied on alternate days.

For optimal effect, Nericur Gel should be applied in the evening, sufficient time being allowed for it to dry before the patient goes to bed, in order to avoid any bleaching of bed-linen.

Contra-indications, warnings, etc
Contra-indications: Known hypersensitivity to benzoyl peroxide.

Precautions: For external use only. Avoid contact with eyes and mucosae. If the skin is exposed to strong or prolonged sunlight, Nericur Gel should be applied at longer intervals, and a highly protective sun-screening agent should be used. Nericur Gel should only be applied to dry skin, to avoid unnecessary irritation.

Side-effects: As with all keratolytic substances, itching, reddening, burning and a feeling of skin tension may occur. This may be relieved by the use of a moisturising cream or by temporary interruption of use.

In rare cases, a contact dermatitis may occur, in which event treatment should be stopped immediately.

Pharmaceutical precautions Store in a cool place. Shelf-life 2 years from date of manufacture.

Legal category P.

Package quantities Tubes containing 30 g (OP).

Further information Nil.

Product licence numbers
Nericur 5 0053/0168
Nericur 10 0053/0169.

NERISONE* CREAM, OILY CREAM AND OINTMENT

Presentation *Cream* (oil-in-water emulsion), *oily cream* (water-in-oil emulsion) and *ointment* (anhydrous base): 1 g of each Nerisone presentation contains 1 mg (0.1%) diflucortolone valerate.

Excipients: Cream: polyoxyl 40 stearate, stearyl alcohol, heavy liquid paraffin, white soft paraffin, disodium edetate dihydrate, carbopol 934, sodium hydroxide, methylparaben, propylparaben, purified water.

Oily cream: bleached wax, heavy liquid paraffin, white soft paraffin, Dehymuls E, purified water.

Ointment: heavy liquid paraffin, white soft paraffin, wax, castor oil.

Uses Corticoid-responsive dermatoses in the absence of infection.

Dosage and administration Initially 2–3 applications daily, according to the severity of the condition. For maintenance, one application daily.

Nerisone is available in three bases. The base chosen for an individual case should depend on the physical characteristics of the lesion. For example, in very dry and chronic skin conditions, the occlusive effect of the Nerisone ointment base aids the healing process.

Contra-indications, warnings, etc

Contra-indications: Rosacea and peri-oral dermatitis. Viral infections. Bacterial or fungal infections of the skin in the absence of appropriate anti-infective therapy. Nerisone is not suitable for the treatment of ophthalmic conditions.

Warnings/side-effects: In infants, long-term continuous therapy with topical corticosteroids should be avoided. Adrenal suppression can occur, even without occlusion.

In common with all other topical corticoids, side-effects may occur when Nerisone is applied to large areas of the body (10% or more) and for long periods of time (more than four weeks), especially if the ointment or an occlusive dressing is being used. These may be local signs such as atrophy of the skin, telangiectasia, striae and acneform changes, or systemic corticoid effects caused by absorption. Therefore, caution should be exercised when using occlusive dressings, as there is a possibility that natural steroid production may be depressed.

Babies and children up to the age of 4 years should not be treated with Nerisone for longer than three weeks – particularly on skin areas covered by napkins.

Nerisone may be applied under an occlusive dressing. However, each dressing should not be left on for more than 24 hours. Although occlusive dressings may be used repeatedly, it should be noted that systemic corticoid absorption is likely to be increased, with a consequent increased risk of adrenal suppression. If secondary infection occurs during treatment, the use of occlusive dressings should be postponed until the infection has been controlled.

Pregnancy warning: There is inadequate evidence of safety in human pregnancy. Topical administration of corticosteroids to pregnant animals can cause abnormalities of foetal development, including cleft palate and intra-uterine growth retardation. There may therefore be a very small risk of such effects on the human foetus.

Pharmaceutical precautions Store in cool, dry conditions.

Shelf-life: Five years.

Legal category POM.

Package quantities 30 g tubes (OP).

Further information Nil.

Product licence numbers

Nerisone Cream	0053/0075
Nerisone Oily Cream	0053/0073
Nerisone Ointment	0053/0074

NERISONE* FORTE OILY CREAM AND OINTMENT

Presentation *Oily cream* (water-in-oil emulsion) and *ointment* (anhydrous base). 1 gram of each Nerisone Forte presentation contains 3 mg (0.3%) diflucortolone valerate.

Excipients: Oily cream: bleached wax, heavy liquid paraffin, white soft paraffin, Dehymuls E, purified water.

Ointment: heavy liquid paraffin, white soft paraffin, wax, castor oil.

Uses Initial and intermittent treatment of severe and recalcitrant corticoid-responsive dermatoses in the absence of infection. These include psoriasis, neurodermatitis (endogenous eczema, atopic dermatitis), lichen planus, discoid lupus erythematosus and severe chronic eczema.

Dosage and administration Initially, two or three thin applications daily, according to the severity of the condition. Once the clinical picture has improved, the patient should be changed from Nerisone Forte to Nerisone, for maintenance therapy.

In view of the high efficacy and potency of Nerisone Forte, no more than 60 g a week should be applied, and it is suggested that treatment for one or two weeks should generally be sufficient to obtain control of even the most refractory lesion, after which a change to Nerisone can usually be made if maintenance therapy is necessary.

Nerisone Forte is available in two bases.

Nerisone Forte Oily Cream: This is an emulsion of water in oil. Because it is an emulsion, it allows heat and exudate to pass freely through, while the oil component protects the skin against undesirable drying out.

Nerisone Forte Ointment: This has an anhydrous fatty base, which is particularly indicated in chronic and dry skin conditions. The softening and occlusive properties of this base often aid the healing process.

Contra-indications, warnings, etc

Contra-indications: Rosacea, acne, peri-oral dermatitis and all other facial diseases. Viral infections. Bacterial or fungal infections of the skin in the absence of appropriate anti-infective therapy. Nerisone Forte is not suitable for the treatment of ophthalmic conditions or of infants and children up to the age of four years.

Warnings/side-effects: In infants, long-term continuous therapy with topical corticosteroids should be avoided. Adrenal suppression can occur, even without occlusion.

Since prolonged therapy with potent topical corticosteroids may cause local atrophic changes such as striae, thinning and telangiectasia, particularly in skin folds and where occlusive dressings are used, it is recommended that the progress of patients under treatment for more than one week with Nerisone Forte be reviewed weekly, and that repeat prescriptions be written only when the prescribing physician has again seen the patient.

Since absorption is increased with the use of occlusive dressings, these should not be left on for more than 24 hours. If secondary infection occurs during treatment, the use of occlusive dressings should be stopped until the infection has been eliminated, and appropriate treatment of the infection should be instituted if it persists.

Pregnancy warning: There is inadequate evidence of safety in human pregnancy. Topical administration of corticosteroids to pregnant animals can cause abnormalities of foetal development, including cleft palate and intra-uterine growth retardation. There may therefore be a very small risk of such effects on the human foetus.

Pharmaceutical precautions Store in cool, dry conditions.

Shelf-life: Five years.

Legal category POM.

Package quantities 15 g tubes (OP).

Further information Nerisone Forte preparations contain neither parabens nor lanolin.

Product licence numbers

Nerisone Forte Oily Cream	0053/0099
Nerisone Forte Ointment	0053/0100

NORGESTON*

Presentation Each round, white, sugar-coated tablet bears a printed black E in a black regular hexagon on both sides and contains 30 micrograms levonorgestrel.

Excipients: lactose, maize starch, povidone 25 000, talc, magnesium stearate, sucrose, povidone 700 000, polyethylene glycol 6000, calcium carbonate, wax E.

Uses Oral contraception.

Mode of action: The contraceptive action of Norgeston may be explained as follows:

It changes the cervical mucus so that a barrier is formed against the migration of sperm into the uterine cavity. Nidation is impeded because of changes in the structure of the endometrium. As a rule there is no inhibition of ovulation. Evidence suggests that a reduction in corpus-luteum function may also contribute to the contraceptive action.

Dosage and administration The first tablet is taken on the first day of menstrual bleeding or on the day after a course of a different oral contraceptive, at a time chosen by the patient. All subsequent tablets must then be taken at this time. The contraceptive effect is likely to be reduced if a tablet is delayed more than three hours. The tablets are taken daily and pack follows pack without interruption for as long as protection against conception is required. The contraceptive action begins after 14 tablets have been taken.

When starting oral contraception anew with Norgeston, additional precautions other than the rhythm or temperature methods must be used for the first 14 days of tablet-taking. In patients switching from other oral contraceptives additional precautions are not required.

Use after delivery or abortion: Norgeston may be started as early as the seventh day post-partum.

Use during breast feeding: There is no evidence that Norgeston diminishes the yield of breast milk. Radioactivity can be found in the milk after the administration of labelled levonorgestrel. However, it is not known whether the metabolites which appear in minute amounts in the milk, and do not accumulate in the infant's tissues, are biologically active.

Contra-indications, warnings, etc

Contra-indications: History, during pregnancy, of idiopathic jaundice or severe pruritus; Dubin-Johnson and Rotor syndromes; acute and severe chronic liver diseases; pregnancy. History of herpes gestationis (also known as pemphigoid gestationis). Although no association between progestogen-only oral contraceptives and thromboembolic disorders has been shown, it is at present required that a history of such disorders be described as a contra-indication to Norgeston, as it is to oestrogen-containing oral contraceptives.

Warnings/side-effects: Clinical investigations indicate that, in general, Norgeston is very well tolerated. Symptoms reported in isolated cases include nausea, vomiting, dizziness, headaches, migraine, depressive moods, disturbances of appetite, allergic reactions. Amenorrhoea and changes in the pattern of the menstrual cycle have been observed. (For details, see 'Menstrual pattern'.)

Circumstances requiring additional contraceptive precautions, other than the temperature, rhythm and cervical-mucus methods.

1. If a tablet is taken more than three hours late (i.e. if it is more than 27 hours since the last tablet was taken), protection against conception may be impaired. From the time of such as error, extra non-hormonal methods must be employed until 14 consecutive tablets have been taken in the correct manner.

2. Vomiting or diarrhoea may reduce the effectiveness of the tablets by preventing them from being fully absorbed. If vomiting occurs shortly after a tablet has been taken, the contraceptive protection may be maintained if a second tablet is taken within three hours of the normal time, provided that vomiting does not recur. It is advisable to take the last tablet of the pack for this purpose, so as to avoid confusion.

In the case of repeated vomiting, or continued diarrhoea, additional contraceptive measures should be employed for a further 14 days after the symptoms have subsided.

3. Interaction with other drugs. Some drugs accelerate the metabolism of oral contraceptives taken concurrently. Drugs suspected of having the capacity to reduce the efficacy of oral contraceptives include barbiturates, phenylbutazone, phenytoin, rifampicin, ampicillin, griseofulvin and other antibiotics. It is, therefore, advisable to use non-hormonal methods of contraception (except the rhythm, temperature or cervical-mucus methods) during treatment with such drugs.

Menstrual pattern: A usual feature of all progestogen-only oral contraceptives is that they produce an initial irregularity of the bleeding pattern, but such irregularity tends to decrease with time.

The patient should be informed before starting Norgeston that her menstrual pattern is likely to alter.

Procedure in the case of cycle disturbances: Irregular bleeding is, from a medical point of view, no reason for discontinuing therapy, as long as organic causes and pregnancy can be ruled out.

If amenorrhoea lasts longer than three months, or occurs repeatedly, administration of Norgeston should be suspended until regular cyclical bleeding has been re-established.

No attempt must be made to control irregular cycles by the additional administration of oestrogens, since they would reverse the effect of Norgeston on the cervical mucus, thus seriously reducing the contraceptive efficacy.

Reasons for stopping oral contraception immediately: First signs of thrombophlebitis or thromboembolism. Jaundice. Pregnancy.

Overdosage: There have been no reports of serious ill-effects from overdosage, even when a considerable number of tablets have been taken by a small child. In general, it is, therefore, unnecessary to treat overdosage. There are no specific antidotes and treatment should be symptomatic.

Pharmaceutical precautions Store in cool, dry conditions.

Shelf-life: Five years.

Legal category POM.

Package quantities Memo-pack containing 35 tablets (OP).

Further information Nil.

Product licence number 0053/0068.

NORISTERAT*

Presentation Norethisterone oenanthate in oily solution for intramuscular administration. Ampoules contain 200 mg in 1 ml.

Excipients: benzyl benzoate, castor oil.

Uses Noristerat is a depot contraceptive. It is intended for short-term use when a high level of efficacy independent of possible errors by the patient is required. It has been licensed for short-term use for wives of men undergoing vasectomy, until the vasectomy is effective, and women immunised against rubella, to prevent pregnancy during the period of activity of the virus.

Use after delivery or abortion: Noristerat can generally be used immediately after delivery or abortion (but see following 'Use during lactation').

Use during lactation: Noristerat has not been reported to inhibit milk production, which is an advantage when the mother wishes to breast-feed. However, traces of the hormone appear in the milk, and although considered harmless to a healthy neonate might theoretically, like other steroids, impair the degradation of bilirubin, especially during the first week of life. If the mother has received Noristerat, breast-feeding should therefore be withheld from neonates with severe or persistent jaundice requiring medical treatment.

Dosage and administration 200 mg Noristerat intramuscularly provides contraception for eight weeks. The first injection should be given within the first five days of a menstrual cycle (the first day of menstruation counting as day 1), unless it is given so soon after delivery or abortion that no possibility of pregnancy exists. The injection may be repeated once, after eight weeks. Noristerat must always be injected deep into the gluteal muscles, care being taken that no liquid runs back from the injection site, which could result in loss of efficacy. The viscosity of the liquid at low temperatures is high, necessitating considerable pressure of injection. Therefore it is suggested that the ampoule be immersed in warm water before injection. A needle of at least medium bore should be used, and care taken to ensure that the needle is securely attached to the syringe.

Contra-indications, warnings, etc
Interaction with other drugs: Some drugs may accelerate the metabolism of Noristerat. Drugs suspected of having this capacity, which may reduce the efficacy of the preparation, include barbiturates, phenytoin and rifampicin.

Contra-indications: Pregnancy. Current thromboembolic disease. Pathologically increased blood pressure. Sickle-cell anaemia. Severe diabetes with vascular changes. Previous or existing liver tumours. Acute and severe chronic liver disease. History, during pregnancy, of idiopathic jaundice or general pruritus, or of herpes gestationis (also known as pemphigoid gestationis). Dubin-Johnson and Rotor syndromes.

Eight weeks before planned operations and during immobilisation (e.g. after accidents).

Warnings: Although there have so far been no observations of thromboembolic disease during the use of Noristerat, as a precaution it is recommended that this preparation should not be used where there is a history of thromboembolic processes. Porphyria and existing impairment of liver function might theoretically be exacerbated by Noristerat.

No further injection should be given if, during treatment, migrainous headaches occur for the first time or recurrent unusually severe headaches develop, if sudden perceptual disorders (e.g. disturbances of vision or hearing) occur, if first signs of thrombophlebitis or thromboembolic disease are noted, or if a feeling of pain and tightness in the chest, a significant rise in blood pressure, recurrence of earlier depression or pathological changes of liver function and hormone levels are experienced.

A reduction of glucose tolerance has been observed in some women using progestogens. Consequently, diabetics and women with a tendency to diabetes should be carefully supervised during the use of Noristerat. In the case of diabetes, it may be necessary to reassess the required doses of antidiabetics or insulin.

Like all nortestosterone derivatives used for contraception, Noristerat has slight androgenic activity, and a virilising effect on the external genitalia of a female foetus exposed to Noristerat after the first month of pregnancy cannot be totally ruled out on theoretical grounds. However, no such virilisation has been observed after the few pregnancies that have occurred during the use of Noristerat.

There is a general opinion, based on statistical evidence, that users of hormonal contraceptives experience, more often than non-users, venous thromboembolism, arterial thrombosis, including cerebral and myocardial infarction, and subarachnoid haemorrhage. Full recovery from such disorders does not always occur, and it should be realised that in a few cases they are fatal.

The relative risk of arterial thromboses (e.g. stroke and myocardial infarction) appears to increase further when heavy smoking, increasing age and the use of hormonal contraceptives coincide.

In rare cases benign and in even rarer cases malignant liver tumours, leading in isolated cases to life-threatening intra-abdominal haemorrhage, have been observed after the use of hormonal substances such as the one contained in Noristerat. If severe upper abdominal complaints, liver enlargement or signs of intra-abdominal haemorrhage occur, a liver tumour should be considered in the differential diagnosis and, if necessary, the preparation should be withdrawn.

In rare cases coughing, dyspnoea and circulatory irregularities may occur during or immediately after the injection. Experience has shown that these reactions can be avoided by injecting Noristerat very slowly.

Side-effects: Subjective symptoms reported consist mainly of bloating, breast discomfort, headaches, dizziness and transient nausea. Marked increases of weight are rare.

Menstrual pattern: The patient should be informed before starting Noristerat that her menstrual pattern is likely to alter.

Menstrual changes: These, in the form of spotting, breakthrough bleeding and delayed menstruation are relatively frequent, and generally do not require treatment. With persistent bleeding, however, it may be expedient to administer progestogen/oestrogen tablets, e.g. combined oral contraceptives, for 10 days to create a withdrawal bleed 1–4 days later.

Amenorrhoea: If, when the second injection is due, bleeding has not occurred in the preceding eight weeks, the second injection should not be given until pregnancy has been ruled out.

Precautions: Women with a history of severe depressive states, disturbed liver function or any disease that is prone to worsen during pregnancy should be carefully observed during medication.

Effect on blood chemistry: No influence of Noristerat on basal plasma cortisol, the ACTH test or the metyrapone test has been observed. In the acute dexamethasone suppression test, however, a higher plasma cortisol value than expected was found in four out of 10 women, although there were no clinical indications of disturbed adrenocortical function. A shortening of the recalcification time and of the thromboplastin time (Quick's test) were observed in studies of the blood coagulation system.

Pharmaceutical precautions Store away from strong sunlight. Shelf-life 5 years.

Legal category POM.

Package quantities Single packs of 1 ampoule.

Further information Nil.

Product licence number 0053/0095.

NOVA-T*

Presentation Nova-T is an intra-uterine contraceptive device (IUCD) in the form of a T, made of polyethylene impregnated with barium sulphate to make the device radio-opaque. Around the stem is wound a wire of surface area about 200 square mm, the outer layer consisting of 107–141 mg of copper, and the core of 11–29 mg of silver. The silver core, which is resistant to corrosion, is designed to prevent fracture of the wire when the copper is substantially corroded, and to enable the device to be retained for up to five years.

Uses Intra-uterine contraception.

Administration After a pelvic examination to exclude contra-indications, and to determine the size and position of the uterus, the presterilised device is inserted into the uterus by means of the inserter, and according to the instructions provided, using non-touch technique.

After delivery or abortion, an IUCD is best inserted when the uterus has reverted to its normal size, i.e. after 4–6 weeks.

Contra-indications, warnings, etc

Contra-indications: Pregnancy. Known or suspected malignant tumours in the genital tract. Large or multiple fibroids. Uterine polyps. Hypoplasia (external os to fundus, less than 6.5 cm), malformation, or extreme malposition of the uterus. Severe dysmenorrhoea. Genital infections. Postpartum endometritis or infected abortion in the last three months. Endometriosis. Active pelvic inflammatory disease. History of repeated pelvic inflammatory disease. Genital bleeding of unknown origin. Menorrhagia and/or intermenstrual bleeding. Coagulation deficiencies. Wilson's disease. Allergy to copper.

Conditions that can lead to or promote bacteraemia (e.g. cardiac valve defects, congenital heart disease). Immunodeficiency. A history of ectopic pregnancy.

Warnings: Medical diathermy must not be applied to the user's abdomen or sacral region, since heating of the copper may cause injury.

Perforation of the uterus may occur during insertion or subsequently, and demands early removal of the device, the copper of which may cause peritoneal adhesions.

Caution is advised in patients with a history of uterine perforation or surgery, especially tubal, or any abdominal or pelvic surgery, since the risks of ectopic pregnancy and uterine perforation may be increased. Insertion of an IUCD before the uterus has reverted to its normal size (i.e. after 4–6 weeks) after delivery or abortion increases the risks of expulsion or uterine perforation.

IUCD's may, in general, predispose to uterine infections. The use of IUCD's may rarely jeopardise subsequent fertility. IUCD's should be used with caution in patients with anaemia and those receiving anticoagulants, in whom additional menstrual bleeding may be of clinical consequence. Caution is necessary in patients receiving steroid therapy, which may mask pelvic inflammatory disease.

In very young women and nulliparae, the benefit/risk ratio must be weighed particularly carefully, since reports exist of higher failure-rates and complications. Epidemiological studies suggest that nulliparous IUCD-users and users with a multiplicity of sexual partners may be at a greater risk of pelvic infection and subsequently becoming infertile.

Pregnancy: The user must be instructed to inform her doctor at once if she suspects herself to be pregnant.

If a pregnancy should occur, the possibility that it is ectopic should be carefully considered, since intra-uterine contraceptive devices provide less protection against ectopic than against intra-uterine pregnancies, and a pregnancy occurring with an IUCD in situ is therefore more likely to be ectopic than a pregnancy occurring without an IUCD in situ.

The device should be removed by traction on the threads, since, although this procedure may itself entail some risk of increasing abortion, retention of the device in the uterus may increase the risk of sepsis and spontaneous abortion at a later stage. Moreover, the long-term effects of the intra-uterine copper on the foetus are not fully known. If the device cannot be removed, termination of the pregnancy should be considered.

If, after the discussion of the above recommendation, the patient insists on continuing a pregnancy with the device still present, she should be closely observed and told to report all abnormal symptoms such as flu-like symptoms, fever, cramping pain, vaginal bleeding or discharge, since the onset of septicaemia associated with septic abortion may be insidious, with initial general symptoms rather than localising symptoms and signs of spontaneous abortion.

Precautions: Appropriate precautions, including administration of antibiotics, should be considered when inserting an IUCD in patients with known or suspected rheumatic or congenital heart disease. The possibility of a seizure's being precipitated in an epileptic patient at or shortly after the insertion of an IUCD should be borne in mind. The efficacy of IUCDs may be reduced by long-term treatment with nonsteroidal anti-inflammatory drugs (especially aspirin), antibiotics (especially tetracyclines) and systemic corticosteroids, but is not apparently reduced by short-term treatment of dysmenorrhoea with nonsteroidal anti-inflammatory drugs.

Follow-up examinations are recommended after 6 weeks and thereafter about once a year. The user should feel for the presence of the threads at least after each period. Symptoms suggestive of inflammation (e.g. discharge) require bacteriological investigation and possibly treatment of infection. If actinomyces is found in cytological smears, even in asymptomatic users, removal of the IUCD and treatment should be considered, especially if the IUCD has been in the uterus for some time.

Side-effects: Insertion and removal may be associated with some pain and bleeding, and rarely a vasovagal attack. Otherwise pain, especially cramps, in the lower abdomen or sacral area, is most common in the first few days after insertion. Menses are often somewhat heavier than before, especially in patients who are taking anticoagulants. Iron-deficiency anaemia occasionally results. Intermenstrual bleeding or spotting is usually transient. Dysmenorrhoea may occur. Rashes, disappearing on removal of the device, and probably due to allergy to copper, have been reported.

Medical indications for removal of the device: Persistent pain or heavy bleeding. Differential diagnosis of persistent irregular uterine bleeding. Signs and symptoms of uterine infections or other pelvic inflammatory disease. Pregnancy. Displacement of the device. Development of allergy to copper.

Pharmaceutical precautions Nova-T is supplied in a sterile pack, which should not be opened until just before insertion of the device, which must be handled with aseptic precautions. If the seal of the sterile envelope is broken, the device inside should not be used.

Shelf-life 5 years.

Legal category POM.

Package quantities 1 IUCD per envelope.

Further information Nil.

Product licence number 0053/0128.

PRIMOLUT N*

Presentation Each white, uncoated tablet is impressed with 'AN' in a regular hexagon on one side and contains 5 mg norethisterone BP.

Excipients: lactose, maize starch, magnesium stearate.

Uses Metropathia haemorrhagica. Premenstrual syndrome. Postponement of menstruation. Endometriosis. Menorrhagia.

A total dose of about 100–150 mg Primolut N (10–15 mg on each of 10 consecutive days) will produce complete secretory transformation of an endometrium that has been subjected to the proliferative effect of oestrogens.

A particular advantage is that menstruation-like withdrawal bleeding occurs consistently two to three days after Primolut N is stopped.

During treatment with Primolut N the basal body temperature rises, as it does under the influence of endogenous progesterone in the second half of the menstrual cycle.

Dosage and administration The use of Primolut N is restricted to patients in whom there is no possibility of early pregnancy in the cycle concerned.

Metropathia haemorrhagica (dysfunctional uterine bleeding): 1 tablet 3 times daily for 10 days. Bleeding is arrested usually within 1–3 days. A withdrawal bleeding resembling normal menstruation occurs within 2–4 days after discontinuing treatment.

Prophylaxis against recurrence of dysfunctional bleeding: If there are no signs of resumption of normal ovarian function (no rise in the second half of the cycle of the morning temperature, which should be measured daily) recurrence must be anticipated. Cyclical bleeding can be established with 1 tablet twice daily from the 19th to the 26th day of the cycle.

Premenstrual syndrome (including premenstrual mastalgia): Premenstrual symptoms such as headache, migraine, breast discomfort, water retention, tachycardia and psychological disturbances may be relieved by the administration of 2–3 tablets daily from the 19th to the 26th day of the cycle. Treatment should be repeated for several cycles. When treatment is stopped, the patient may remain symptom-free for a number of months.

Postponement of menstruation: In cases of too frequent menstrual bleeding, and in special circumstances (e.g. operations, travel, sports) the postponement of menstruation is possible. 1 tablet Primolut N three times daily, starting 3 days before the expected onset of menstruation. A normal period should occur 2–3 days after the patient has stopped taking tablets.

Endometriosis (pseudo-pregnancy therapy): Longterm treatment is commenced on the 5th day of the cycle with 2 tablets Primolut N daily for the first few weeks. In the event of spotting, the dosage is increased to 4 and, if necessary, 5 tablets daily.

After bleeding has ceased, the initial dose is usually sufficient. Duration of treatment: 4–6 months continuously, or longer if necessary.

Menorrhagia (hypermenorrhoea): 1 tablet 2–3 times a day from the 19th to the 26th day of the cycle (counting the first day of menstruation as day 1).

Note: If menstrual bleeding should fail to follow a course of Primolut N, the possibility of pregnancy must be ruled out before a further course is given.

Contra-indications, warnings, etc
Contra-indications
Pregnancy: Severe disturbances of liver function. Dubin-Johnson and Rotor syndromes. Previous or existing liver tumours. History during pregnancy of idiopathic jaundice, severe pruritus or herpes gestationis (also known as pemphigoid gestationis). Current thromboembolic processes.

Reasons for immediate discontinuation of the tablets: Occurrence for the first time of migrainous headaches or more frequent occurrence of unusually severe headaches, sudden perceptual disorders (e.g. disturbances of vision or hearing), first signs of thrombophlebitis or thromboembolic symptoms, a feeling of pain and tightness in the chest, pending operations (six weeks beforehand), immobilisation (for instance, following accidents), onset of jaundice, hepatitis, general pruritus, significant rise in blood pressure, pregnancy.

Warnings: There is a general opinion, based on statistical evidence that users of combined oral contraceptives experience, more often than non-users, venous thromboembolism, arterial thrombosis, including cerebral and myocardial infarction, and subarachnoid haemorrhage. Full recovery from such disorders does not always occur, and it should be realised that in a few cases they are fatal. Although Primolut N does not contain oestrogen, one should keep the possibility of an increased thromboembolic risk in mind, particularly where there is a history of thromboembolic disease or in the presence of severe diabetes with vascular changes or sickle-cell anaemia.

Primolut N can influence carbohydrate metabolism. Parameters of carbohydrate metabolism should be examined carefully in all diabetics before and regularly during treatment.

In rare cases benign and in even rarer cases malignant liver tumours, leading in isolatad cases to life-threatening intra-abdominal haemorrhage, have been observed after the use of hormonal substances such as the one contained in Primolut N. If severe upper abdominal complaints, liver enlargement or signs of intra-abdominal haemorrhage occur, a liver tumour should be considered in the differential diagnosis and, if necessary, the preparation should be withdrawn.

Side-effects: Rarely occur in doses of 15 mg daily. Amongst those recorded are slight nausea, exacerbation of epilepsy and migraine. With extremely high dosage there may be cholestatic liver changes.

Overdosage: There have been no reports of ill-effects from overdosage and treatment is generally unnecessary.

There are no special antidotes, and treatment should be symptomatic.

Pharmaceutical precautions Store in cool dry conditions: shelf-life five years.

Legal category POM.

Package quantities Bottles of 100 tablets and 500 tablets with tamper-evident tops.

Further information Nil.

Product licence number 0053/5033R.

PRIMOTESTON* DEPOT 250 mg

Presentation Primoteston Depot 250 mg contains testosterone oenanthate 250 mg per ml in clear non-aqueous solution for intramuscular injection.

Excipients: Benzyl benzoate, castor oil.

Uses Advanced mammary carcinoma in the female. Androgen deficiency in the male.

Primoteston Depot is a depot androgen for use when male sex hormones are indicated. Testosterone oenanthate has not only a sustained androgenic effect but also a very powerful one, since testosterone in this depot form is particularly well utilised by the body.

Dosage and administration *In the female. Advanced mammary carcinoma:* 250 mg Primoteston depot by slow intra-muscular injection every two to three weeks. In advanced mammary carcinoma with metastases or recurrences, high-dosage therapy causes objective remission in some cases and frequently subjective improvement. In responsive cases, pain is diminished and the general condition considerably improved. Bone metastases are often affected favourably. In order to sustain a remission for as long as possible, it is sometimes necessary after a time to shorten the interval between injections. If hypercalcaemia occurs, treatment must be discontinued. In women over 60 years of age, treatment with oestrogens is often more effective.

In the male: Hypogonadism: To stimulate development of underdeveloped androgen-dependent organs and for initial treatment of deficiency symptoms, 250 mg Primoteston Depot intramuscularly every two to three weeks.

For maintenance treatment: 250 mg Primoteston Depot intramuscularly every three to six weeks, according to individual requirement.

Contra-indications, warnings, etc
Contra-indications: Prostatic carcinoma and pregnancy.

Previous or existing liver tumours (in advanced mammary carcinoma in the female only if these are not due to metastases).

Warnings/side-effects: Androgens should not be used for enhancing muscular development in healthy individuals or for increasing physical ability.

High-dosed or long-term administration of testosterone occasionally increases the tendency to water retention and oedema. Caution should therefore be exercised in patients predisposed to oedema.

In rare cases benign and in even rarer cases malignant liver tumours, leading in isolated cases to life-threatening intra-abdominal haemorrhage, have been observed after the use of hormonal substances such as the one contained in Primoteston Depot. If severe upper abdominal complaints, liver enlargement or signs of intra-abdominal haemorrhage occur, a liver tumour should be considered in the differential diagnosis and, if necessary, the preparation should be withdrawn.

Women treated with Primosteston Depot may develop signs of virilisation (e.g. acne, hirsutism, voice changes). Particular care is therefore necessary in women whose occupations involve singing or speaking.

Spermatogenesis is inhibited by long-term and high-dosed treatment with Primoteston Depot.

Regular examination of the prostate is advisable for men receiving androgen therapy.

If, in individual cases, frequent or persistent erections occur, the dose should be reduced or the treatment discontinued in order to avoid injury to the penis.

In women: If hypercalcaemia develops, therapy must be discontinued.

In rare cases coughing, dyspnoea and circulatory irregularities may occur during or immediately after the injection. Experience has shown that these reactions can be avoided by injecting very slowly.

Pharmaceutical precautions Store in cool, dry conditions away from strong sunlight: shelf-life five years.

Legal category POM.

Package quantities Ampoules of 250 mg, 3 × 1 ml.

Further information Nil.

Product licence number 0053/5037R.

PROGYNOVA* 1 mg
PROGYNOVA* 2 mg

Presentation *Progynova 1 mg:* Each beige, sugar-coated tablet bears a printed black B in a black regular hexagon and contains 1 mg of oestradiol valerate.

Progynova 2 mg: Each pale blue, sugar-coated tablet bears a printed red B in a red regular hexagon and contains 2 mg of oestradiol valerate.

Excipients: lactose, maize starch, povidone 25 000, talc, magnesium stearate, sucrose, povidone 700 000, polyethylene glycol 6000, calcium carbonate, titanium dioxide, glycerin, wax E, ferric oxide pigment, indigo carmine.

Uses The treatment of climacteric symptoms in the short term in postmenopausal women (i.e. who have had no uterine bleeding for at least 12 months).

Dosage and administration One tablet of Progynova 1 mg daily for 21 days, followed by an interval of at least seven days before the next course. If the response is inadequate, Progynova 2 mg may be substituted, but the lowest dose compatible with the control of symptoms should always be used, and an attempt should be made to revert to Progynova 1 mg after symptoms have been satisfactorily controlled. However, it should be realised that the appropriate dosage will be determined by the individual patient's rate of metabolism of Progynova, rather than by the initial severity of the symptoms.

Alternatively, if the response to Progynova 1 mg is inadequate, Cyclo-Progynova 2 mg can be substituted, and in general when high-dose oestrogen therapy is required, oestrogen-progestogen combinations are recommended.

Bleeding: If possible, a dosage should be found that will abolish climacteric symptoms without inducing endometrial bleeding. Non-recurrent bleeding of short duration in the tablet-free intervals is usually due to oestrogen withdrawal. Any recurrent bleeding occurring during tablet-taking should be investigated to exclude endometrial hyperplasia or carcinoma. If recurrent bleeding is found to be non-pathological, then Cyclo-Progynova, which produces controlled shedding of the endometrium, should be substituted. (For further information, see the data sheet for Cyclo-Progynova.)

The treatment of recurrences: If, after completion of short-term treatment and the withdrawal of Progynova, climacteric symptoms should recur, further treatment should be with Cyclo-Progynova (except in hysterectomised patients).

Contra-indications, warnings, etc

Contra-indications: Pregnancy. Severe disturbances of liver function, previous or existing liver tumours, jaundice or general pruritus during a previous pregnancy, Dubin-Johnson syndrome, Rotor syndrome, existing or previous thromboembolic processes, sickle-cell anaemia, suspected or existing hormone-dependent disorders or tumours of the uterus or breast, congenital disturbances of lipid metabolism, endometriosis, severe diabetes with vascular changes, otosclerosis with deterioration in previous pregnancies.

Warnings/side-effects: Prolonged exposure to unopposed oestrogens may increase the risk of the development of endometrial carcinoma. The following have been reported during treatment: dyspepsia, flatulence, nausea, vomiting, abdominal pain and bloating, weight-gain, breast tension and pain, palpitations, cardiac symptoms, increased libido, headaches, dizziness, vertigo, epistaxis, biliary stasis, hypertension, urticaria and other rashes, thrombophlebitis, uterine bleeding, mucous vaginal discharge, general pruritus.

Diseases that are known to be subject to deterioration during pregnancy (e.g. multiple sclerosis, epilepsy, diabetes, hypertension, porphyria, tetany and otosclerosis) should be carefully observed during treatment.

Precautions and special information: Treatment should be stopped at once if migrainous or frequent and unusually severe headaches occur for the first time, or if there are any other symptoms that are possible prodromata of vascular occlusion.

Treatment should also be stopped if trauma, illness or impending surgery is considered to entail a risk of thrombosis.

Treatment should be stopped at once if jaundice occurs, or if there is a significant rise in blood-pressure.

In patients with mild chronic liver disease, liver function should be checked every 8–12 weeks.

Women with a family history of endometrial carcinoma should be carefully observed.

Examination of the pelvic organs, endometrium, breasts and blood-pressure is advised before and periodically during treatment with Progynova.

Overdosage: There have been no reports of ill-effects from overdosage, which it is, therefore, generally unnecessary to treat. There are no specific antidotes, and treatment should be symptomatic.

Pharmaceutical precautions Store in cool, dry conditions:

Shelf-life:
Progynova 1 mg 5 years.
Progynova 2 mg 7 years.

Legal category POM.

Package quantities Memo-packs of 21 tablets (OP).

Further information Nil.

Product licence numbers
Progynova 1 mg 0053/0057
Progynova 2 mg 0053/0058

PROLUTON* DEPOT
(*formerly* PRIMOLUT DEPOT)

Presentation Hydroxyprogesterone hexanoate BP 250 mg and 500 mg in ampoules for intramuscular injection.

Excipients: Benzyl benzoate, castor oil.

Uses Habitual abortion, when associated with proven progesterone-deficiency.

Dosage and administration 250–500 mg Proluton Depot at weekly intervals during the first half of pregnancy.

Contra-indications, warnings, etc

Contra-indications: A history of herpes gestationis (also known as pemphigoid gestationis). Previous or existing liver tumours.

Warnings: Many medicinal products, including female sex hormones, have been suspected of being capable of affecting the normal development of a child in the early stages of pregnancy. Many researchers consider that in relation to sex hormones such a suspicion is ill founded but one has to accept that for no medicinal product can teratogenic activity be excluded with absolute certainty. Therefore, the general principle is now widely accepted that inessential use of drugs during pregnancy should be avoided. Following this general principle, Proluton Depot should be used to maintain pregnancy only if it is strictly indicated, i.e. if there is an urgent desire to have a child, and luteal insufficiency is present.

Since Proluton Depot may prevent spontaneous evacuation of a dead foetus (missed abortion) the progress of the pregnancy should be regularly monitored by appropriate means, including immunological tests.

Proluton Depot can influence carbohydrate metabolism. Parameters of carbohydrate metabolism should be examined carefully in all diabetics before and regularly during treatment.

In rare cases benign and in even rarer cases malignant liver tumours, leading in isolated cases to life-threatening intra-abdominal haemorrhage, have been observed after the use of hormonal substances such as the one contained in Proluton Depot. If severe upper abdominal complaints, liver enlargement or signs of intra-abdominal haemorrhage occur, a liver tumour should be considered in the differential diagnosis and, if necessary, the preparation should be withdrawn.

In rare cases coughing, dyspnoea and circulatory irregularities may occur during or immediately after the injection. Experience has shown that these reactions can be avoided by injecting very slowly.

Side-effects: Very rarely, local reactions may occur at the site of injection.

Pharmaceutical precautions Store in cool, dry conditions away from strong sunlight. Shelf-life five years.

Legal category POM.

Package quantities *250 mg:* Packs of 3 ampoules 1 ml.

500 mg: Packs of 3 ampoules 2 ml.

Further information Nil.

Product licence numbers
Proluton Depot 250 mg 0053/5031R
Proluton Depot 500 mg 0053/5032R

PRO-VIRON*

Presentation Each white tablet has AX in a regular hexagon impressed on one side and is scored on the reverse. It contains 25 mg mesterolone.

Excipients: lactose, starch, povidone 25 000, methylparaben, propylparaben, magnesium stearate.

Uses Androgen deficiency. Male infertility.

Pro-viron is an orally active androgen with properties quite distinct from those of older products. It offers unusual therapeutic possibilities because it can be given in high dosage over long periods. The presence of a methyl group at C-1 confers special properties on this steroid which, unlike testosterone and all its derivatives that are used for androgen therapy, is not metabolised to oestrogen.

This difference almost certainly accounts for the observation that, in its usual therapeutic dosage in normal men, Pro-viron does not significantly depress the release of gonadotrophins from the pituitary. Hence (1) spermatogenesis is unimpaired (2) unlike other androgens, which suppress and therefore replace endogenous androgens, Pro-viron supplements endogenous androgens.

Furthermore, in contrast to other orally active androgens, liver tolerance is excellent (a fact probably related to the absence of 17-alkyl substitution of the steroid nucleus).

Dosage and administration *Androgen deficiency:* Initially: 1 tablet three to four times daily, i.e. 75–100 mg daily for several months, followed by maintenance therapy of 2–3 tablets (50–75 mg) daily.

Male infertility: 100 mg daily for several months.

Contra-indications, warnings, etc
Contra-indications: Previous or existing liver tumours. In common with other androgens, Pro-viron is contraindicated in the presence of prostatic carcinoma, since androgens can stimulate the growth of an existing carcinoma.

Warnings/side-effects: Androgens should not be used for enhancing muscular development in healthy individuals or for increasing physical ability. Reported side-effects have been rare, transient and minor. Regular examination of the prostate during treatment is advised, in order to exclude prostatic carcinoma. In rare cases benign and in even rarer cases malignant liver tumours, leading in isolated cases to life-threatening intra-abdominal haemorrhage, have been observed after the use of hormonal substances such as the one contained in Pro-viron. If severe upper abdominal complaints, liver enlargement or signs of intra-abdominal haemorrhage occur, a liver tumour should be considered in the differential diagnosis and, if necessary, the preparation should be withdrawn.

If, in individual cases, frequent or persistent erections occur, the dose should be reduced or the treatment discontinued in order to avoid injury to penis.

Overdosage: There have been no reports of ill-effects from overdosage and treatment is generally unnecessary. There are no special antidotes and treatment should be symptomatic.

Pharmaceutical precautions Store in cool, dry conditions, away from strong sunlight. Shelf-life five years.

Legal category POM.

Package quantities Bottles of 50 tablets.

Further information Nil.

Product licence number 0053/0030.

SCHERING PC4*

Presentation Four white sugar-coated tablets, each containing 250 micrograms levonorgestrel (in 500 micrograms dl-norgestrel) and 50 micrograms ethinyloestradiol.

Excipients: lactose, maize starch, povidone 25 000, talc, magnesium stearate, sucrose, povidone 700 000, polyethylene glycol 6000, calcium carbonate, wax E.

Uses Post-coital contraception within 72 hours of unprotected coitus as an occasional emergency measure. Schering PC4 is primarily aimed to prevent implantation of the fertilised ovum in the endometrium.

Dosage and administration The first two tablets should be taken as soon as possible after coitus (up to a maximum of 72 hours afterwards) and the remaining two tablets twelve hours after the first two.

Contra-indications, warnings, etc
Contra-indications: Therapy should not be administered to a patient whose menstrual bleeding is overdue. Treatment is inappropriate also for a patient who has had unprotected intercourse more than 72 hours previously in the current menstrual cycle.

Other contra-indications: Thrombotic disorders and a history of these conditions, sickle-cell anaemia, disorders of lipid metabolism and other conditions in which, in individual cases, there is known or suspected to be a much increased risk of thrombosis. Acute or severe chronic liver diseases. Dubin-Johnson syndrome. Rotor syndrome. History, during pregnancy, of idiopathic jaundice or severe pruritus. History of herpes gestationis. Mammary or endometrial carcinoma, or a history of these conditions. Abnormal vaginal bleeding of unknown cause. Deterioration of otosclerosis during pregnancy.

Warnings: Schering PC4 does not appear to be as effective as some regularly-used methods of contraception and is suitable only as an occasional emergency measure. Schering PC4 is not effective if started later than 72 hours after coitus and should not be so used.

Patients who become pregnant despite post-coital contraception should be carefully evaluated for possible ectopic pregnancy. Since Schering PC4 appears to affect only endometrial implantation, tubal pregnancy may occur at the expected rate, and it is thus possible that there will be a relative increase in ectopic pregnancy in patients who become pregnant despite the use of Schering PC4.

The safety of use during lactation has not been established.

The effect of Schering PC4 on the conceptus in the event of failure to prevent conception is not definitely known. Some investigators have suggested that sex hormones taken in the first trimester of pregnancy may slightly increase the risk of foetal malformations, but numerous other investigators have failed to support these findings. The consensus of opinion amongst teratologists is that even known teratogens will not produce malformations before organogenesis starts, which is much later than the 72 hours after fertilisation to which the use of Schering PC4 is restricted.

Malabsorption: Vomiting, severe diarrhoea or other causes of malabsorption might impair the efficacy of Schering PC4.

Drug interactions: The efficacy of Schering PC4 might be impaired by interaction with concurrently-used drugs including barbiturates, phenylbutazone, phenytoin, rifampicin, ampicillin, griseofulvin and other antibiotics.

Precautions: Examination of the pelvic organs, breasts and blood pressure should normally precede the prescribing of any combined oral contraceptive. The following conditions require careful consideration: a history of severe depressive states, diabetes, hypertension, epilepsy, porphyria, tetany, disturbed liver function, gallstones, cardiovascular diseases, renal diseases.

The importance of follow-up and the possibility of an early or late onset of the next period should be explained to the patient. The practice of abstinence or careful use of a barrier method until the onset of the next period should also be advised. Follow-up should be carried out 3 weeks after administration of therapy to assess the effectiveness of the method, to discuss future management if a period has not occurred, and to counsel the patient about future contraception.

Side-effects: Nausea and vomiting are common side-effects, and the latter may reduce the efficacy of therapy if it occurs within about 2 hours after the ingestion of either dose of tablets, in which event consideration should be given to the taking of more pills.

The concomitant administration of an anti-emetic has been favoured by some practitioners.

The pattern of menstrual bleeding is often temporarily disturbed. Breast discomfort and headaches also may occur.

Overdosage: There have been no reports of serious ill-effects from overdosage. Treatment is symptomatic.

Pharmaceutical precautions Store in cool, dry conditions: shelf-life five years.

Legal category POM.

Package quantities Single pack of four tablets (OP).

Further information Nil.

Product licence number 0053/0162.

SCHERIPROCT* OINTMENT AND SUPPOSITORIES

Presentation Each white suppository contains:

Prednisolone hexanoate	1.3 mg
Dibucaine hydrochloride	1.0 mg

Excipient: solid fat.

A white ointment containing in 1 g:

Prednisolone hexanoate	1.9 mg
Dibucaine hydrochloride	5.0 mg

Excipients: polyethylene glycol 400, monoricinoleate, castor oil, eutanol G, perfume.

Uses For the symptomatic relief of haemorrhoids and pruritus ani and vulvae in the short term (5–7 days).

Dosage and administration *Suppositories:* 1 Scheriproct Suppository to be inserted daily. In severe cases 1 suppository two to three times daily at the beginning of treatment. The suppositories should be inserted after defaecation.

Ointment: Apply in a thin layer twice daily. In order to obtain a rapid improvement, Scheriproct Ointment may be applied three to four times on the first day. To avoid relapses, Scheriproct Ointment should be applied once a day for a few days after complete disappearance of the symptoms. The nozzle provided facilitates intra-rectal application.

Contra-indications, warnings, etc
Contra-indications: Viral infections. Primary bacterial or fungal infections. Secondary infections of the skin in the absence of appropriate anti-infective therapy. Known sensitivity to local anaesthetics.

Warnings/side-effects: In infants, long-term continuous therapy with topical corticosteroids should be avoided. Occlusion is not appropriate on the perineum. Adrenal suppression can occur, even without occlusion. As with all topical steroids, there is a risk of developing skin atrophy following extensive therapy. The application of unusually large quantities of topical corticoids may result in the absorption of systemically active amounts of corticoid. Infections or secondarily infected dermatoses definitely require additional therapy with antibiotics or chemotherapeutic agents. This treatment can often be topical, but for heavy infections systemic antibacterial therapy may be necessary. If fungal infections are present, a topically active antimycotic should be applied.

Pregnancy warning: There is inadequate evidence of safety in human pregnancy. Topical administration of corticosteroids to pregnant animals can cause abnormalities of foetal development, including cleft palate and intra-uterine growth retardation. There may therefore be a very small risk of such effects on the human foetus.

Pharmaceutical precautions In order to restore the consistency of suppositories which have become soft owing to warm temperature, they should be put into cold water before the covering is removed.

Store in cool, dry conditions: shelf-life five years.

Legal category POM.

Package quantities *Suppositories:* Packs of 12 (OP). *Ointment:* Tubes of 30 g (OP).

Further information Nil.

Product licence numbers

Scheriproct Suppositories	0053/5001R
Scheriproct Ointment	0053/5002R

SH420*

Presentation Each uncoated, white tablet has AR in a regular hexagon impressed on one side, with quarter-scoring on the reverse. It contains 10 mg norethisterone acetate.

Excipients: lactose, maize starch, povidone 25 000, talc, magnesium stearate.

Uses Inoperable mammary carcinoma. As an adjunct to surgery and/or radiotherapy.

Note: Hormone therapy can never replace surgery or radiotherapy.

SH420 is a potent progestogen with a clinical efficacy which appears to be at least comparable to that of androgens and oestrogens in the treatment of inoperable mammary carcinoma. It does not, however, have the disadvantage of virilisation as with androgens and is unlikely to cause uterine bleeding as is the case with oestrogens. It may be used in the treatment of both pre- and post-menopausal women.

Although the mode of action of the various classes of hormone in inhibiting the growth of mammary carcinoma is not well understood, the very important role of the pituitary seems to be generally agreed on, as is shown by the response to pituitary ablation and hence to pituitary suppression by hormonal means.

SH420 is a powerful inhibitor of the pituitary. The effect of the progestogen may not depend wholly, however, on pituitary inhibition and it may be that an anti-oestrogenic effect as well as a direct effect on the tumour plays a part. Clinically SH420 has yielded subjective improvement (relief of pain and improvement in the general condition) and objective improvement (regression of tumour and/or bone and soft-tissue metastases).

Dosage and administration The recommended initial dosage of SH420 is 1 tablet three times a day (30 mg norethisterone acetate daily). If, after 6 weeks, no response is apparent, this can be increased to 2 tablets three times daily (60 mg daily).

Any remission obtainable should be apparent by the end of two months. If regression or arrest of tumour growth is obtained, treatment should be maintained as long as it continues to appear beneficial. If after about 9 weeks no response is apparent, none is to be expected and some other form of therapy should be tried.

Contra-indications, warnings, etc

Contra-indications:
Pregnancy. History of herpes gestationis (also known as pemphigoid gestationis).

Warnings/side-effects: The great advantage of SH420 over oestrogens and androgens is the almost complete freedom from side-effects.

Side-effects such as nausea, uterine bleeding and reversible cholestatic liver changes have occasionally been observed.

Overdosage: There have been no reports of ill-effects from overdosage and treatment is generally unnecessary.

There are no special antidotes and treatment should be symptomatic.

Pharmaceutical precautions Store in cool, dry conditions, away from strong sunlight. Shelf-life: five years.

Legal category POM.

Package quantities Bottles of 100 tablets.

Further information Nil.

Product licence number 0053/5012R.

TRAVOGYN

Presentation (a) *Vaginal tablets:* White, almond-shaped vaginal tablets, impressed with CT in a regular hexagon on one side, and containing 300 mg isoconazole nitrate.

Excipients: lactose, cellulose, magnesium stearate.

(b) *Cream:* A white cream containing 1% isoconazole nitrate.

Excipients: polyethylene glycol, sorbitan stearate, cetostearyl alcohol, white soft paraffin, purified water.

Uses Travogyn exhibits a broad spectrum of activity against fungal pathogens, including yeasts and yeast-like fungi (particularly those belonging to Candida spp. and Torulopsis glabrata), and against dermatophytes and hyphomycetes. Travogyn also has bactericidal activity against some gram-positive bacteria, including staphylococci, streptococci and micrococci, which may cause secondary infection of inflammatory skin lesions.

(a) *Vaginal tablets:* Travogyn vaginal tablets may be used for vaginal mycoses, particularly those due to Candida, or for mixed infections with fungi and gram-positive bacteria.

(b) *Cream:* Travogyn cream should be used, in conjunction with Travogyn vaginal tablets, to treat vulval or perianal spread of susceptible vaginal infections. It may be used to treat balanitis of possible candidal origin and its prophylactic use in the partners of infected women is advisable.

Travogyn cream may be used alone for perineal or intertriginous infections of probable fungal origin that do not appear to be secondary to vaginal mycoses.

N.B. Travogyn formulations should not be the treatment of first choice for pure trichomonal infections.

Dosage and administration (a) *Vaginal tablets:* Two 300 mg vaginal tablets should be inserted together deep into the vagina. Only one application is required and may be done by the doctor at the time of consultation, or by the patient, preferably at night.

(b) *Cream:* Where treatment of the external genital or peri-anal regions, or simultaneous treatment of the partner, is required, Travogyn cream should be applied twice daily until symptoms have disappeared.

Contra-indications, warnings, etc There are no known contra-indications.

Occasionally during the first 12 to 24 hours, symptoms of intolerance, such as burning or itching of the vagina and vulva, may occur. Although, in order to avoid any possibility of adverse effects on the foetus, the general principle is now widely accepted that the administration of drugs to women during pregnancy should, as far as possible, be avoided, nothing that is known about the effect of isoconazole nitrate, either from animal experiments, or from clinical experience, suggests that Travogyn therapy should not be used during pregnancy.

Pharmaceutical precautions Store in a cool place. Shelf-life: five years.

The cream should be used within 28 days of opening.

Legal category POM.

Package quantities Two vaginal tablets in foil-backed blister packs (OP).

Tubes of 20 g cream (OP).

Further information Nil.

Product licence numbers
Vaginal tablets: 0053/0124
Cream: 0053/0122

ULTRABASE*

Presentation Ultrabase is a white oil-in-water cream for topical application.

Components: Polyoxyl 40 stearate, white soft paraffin, liquid paraffin, stearyl alcohol, carbopol 934, sodium hydroxide, methylhydroxybenzoate (methyl-paraben), propylhydroxybenzoate (propyl-paraben), disodium-edetate, demineralised water, crematest perfume oil.

Uses Ultrabase is intended for general use as an emollient and as a diluent for dermatological preparations and a vehicle for other medicaments. Additionally, it may be alternated with topical corticosteroids when the latter are being gradually withdrawn, and may be continued alone after complete withdrawal of the topical corticosteroid.

Dosage and administration The cream should be smoothed into the skin as often as required.

Contra-indications, warnings, etc There are no specific contra-indications to the use of Ultrabase, other than known allergy to any of the components.

Side-effects: No side-effects have been reported.

Pharmaceutical precautions Store in cool, dry conditions, away from strong sunlight: shelf-life five years.

Legal category GSL.

Package quantities Tubes containing 50 g. Jars containing 500 g.

Further information Ultrabase is suitable as a diluent

for Schering's corticoid cream preparations and as a vehicle for coal tar solutions, urea, resorcinol, zinc oxide and precipitated sulphur.

Product licence number 0053/0063.

ULTRADIL* OINTMENT PLAIN AND CREAM PLAIN
ULTRALANUM* OINTMENT PLAIN AND CREAM PLAIN

Presentation White creams (oil-in-water emulsions) and ointments (water-in-oil emulsions) with the following ingredients.

Ultradil Ointment plain and Cream plain: 0.1% fluocortolone pivalate BP and 0.1% fluocortolone hexanoate BP.

Ultralanum Ointment plain: 0.25% fluocortolone and 0.25% fluocortolone hexanoate BP.

Ultralanum Cream plain: 0.25% fluocortolone pivalate BP and 0.25% fluocortolone hexanoate BP.

Ultradil plain and Ultralanum plain are dilute and full-strength preparations respectively of the corticoid, fluocortolone, and its esters.

Excipients: ointments; white wax, lanolin, heavy liquid paraffin, white soft paraffin, Amphocerin KS, Dehymuls E perfume, purified water.

Creams; polyoxyl 40 stearate, stearyl alcohol, heavy liquid paraffin, white soft petroleum jelly, disodium edetate dihydrate, carbopol 934, sodium hydroxide, methylparaben, propylparaben, water perfume.

Uses *Ultradil Cream and Ointment plain:* Eczema and dermatitis of all types including atopic eczema, photodermatitis and primary irritant and allergic dermatitis, prurigo nodularis and insect bite reactions. Lichen planus, lichen simplex, discoid lupus erythematosus, necrobiosis lipoidica, pretibial myxoedema, erythroderma, psoriasis of the scalp, chronic plaque psoriasis of hands and feet.

Ultralanum Cream and Ointment plain: More severe corticoid-responsive skin conditions in the absence of infection.

Dosage and administration *Ultradil plain: (ointment and cream):* The usual initial dosage is 1 application three times a day, reducing to 1 application twice daily.

For maintenance one application daily.

Ultralanum plain: (ointment and cream): Initially 2–3 applications daily, according to severity of condition. For maintenance one application daily.

Contra-indications, warnings, etc
Contra-indications: Rosacea and peri-oral dermatitis, acne vulgaris, perianal and genital pruritus, napkin rashes. Viral infections. Primary bacterial or fungal infections of the skin. Secondary infections in the absence of appropriate anti-infective therapy. Not suitable for the treatment of ophthalmic conditions.

Warnings/side-effects: In all patients long-term continuous therapy with topical corticosteroids should be avoided. Adrenal suppression can occur even without occlusion. As with all topical steroids, there is a risk of skin atrophy following extensive therapy. The application of unusually large quantities of topical corticoids may result in the absorption of systemically active amounts of corticoid. If used in childhood or on the face, courses should be limited to 5 days, and occlusion should not be used. Long-term continuous therapy should be avoided irrespective of age. Occlusion should be restricted to dermatoses involving limited areas. Topical corticosteroids may be hazardous in psoriasis for a number of reasons, including rebound relapses following development of tolerance, risk of generalised pustular psoriasis, and local and systemic toxicity due to impaired barrier function of the skin. Steroids may have a place in psoriasis of the scalp and chronic plaque psoriasis of the hands and feet. Careful supervision of patients is important in psoriasis. Infections or secondarily infected dermatoses definitely require additional therapy with antibiotics or chemotherapeutic agents. This treatment can often be topical, but for heavy infections systemic antibacterial therapy may be necessary. If fungal infections are present, a topically active antimycotic should be applied.

Pregnancy warning: There is inadequate evidence of safety in human pregnancy. Topical administration of corticosteroids to pregnant animals can cause abnormalities of foetal development, including cleft palate and intra-uterine growth retardation. There may therefore be a very small risk of such effects on the human foetus.

Pharmaceutical precautions Store in cool, dry conditions: shelf-life five years.

Legal category POM.

Package quantities *Ultradil Ointment plain:* Tubes of 50 g (OP).

Ultradil Cream plain: Tubes of 50 g (OP).

Ultralanum Ointment plain: Tubes of 50 g (OP).

Ultralanum Cream plain: Tubes of 50 g (OP).

Further information Nil.

Product licence numbers

Ultradil Ointment plain	0053/5015
Ultradil Cream plain	0053/5017R
Ultralanum Cream plain	0053/5011
Ultralanum Ointment plain	0053/5005

ULTRAPROCT* OINTMENT
ULTRAPROCT* SUPPOSITORIES

Presentation Each white suppository contains:

Fluocortolone pivalate BP	0.61 mg
Fluocortolone hexanoate BP	0.63 mg
Dibucaine hydrochloride	1.00 mg

Excipient: solid fat.

A white ointment containing in 1 g:

Fluocortolone pivalate BP	0.92 mg
Fluocortolone hexanoate BP	0.95 mg
Dibucaine hydrochloride	5.00 mg

Excipients: polyethylene glycol 400 monoricinoleate, castor oil, eutanol G, perfume.

Uses For the symptomatic relief of haemorrhoids and of pruritus ani and vulvae in the short term (5–7 days).

Dosage and administration *Suppositories:* 1 Ultraproct Suppository to be inserted daily. In severe cases 1 suppository two to three times daily at the beginning of treatment. The suppositories should be inserted after defaecation.

Ointment: Apply in a thin layer twice daily. In order to obtain a rapid improvement, Ultraproct Ointment may be applied three or four times on the first day. The nozzle provided facilitates intra-rectal application.

Contra-indications, warnings, etc
Contra-indications: Viral infections. Primary bacterial or fungal infections. Secondary infections of the skin in the absence of appropriate anti-infective therapy. Known sensitivity to local anaesthetics.

Warnings/side-effects: In infants, long-term continuous therapy with topical corticosteroids should be avoided. Occlusion is not appropriate on the perineum. Adrenal suppression can occur even without occlusion. As with all topical steroids, there is a risk of skin atrophy following extensive therapy. The application of unusually large quantities of topical corticoids may result in the absorption of systemically active amounts of corticoid. Infections or secondarily-infected dermatoses definitely require additional therapy with antibiotics or chemotherapeutic agents. This treatment can often be topical but for heavy infections systemic antibacterial therapy may be necessary. If fungal infections are present, a topically active antimycotic should be applied.

Pregnancy warning: There is inadequate evidence of safety in human pregnancy. Topical administration of corticosteroids to pregnant animals can cause abnormalities of foetal development, including cleft palate and intra-uterine growth retardation. There may therefore be a very small risk of such effects on the human foetus.

Pharmaceutical precautions In order to restore the consistency of suppositories which have become soft owing to warm temperature, they should be put into cold water before the covering is removed.

Store in cool dry conditions: shelf-life five years.

Legal category POM.

Package quantities *Suppositories:* Packs of 12 (OP). *Ointment:* Tubes of 30 g (OP).

Further information Nil.

Product licence numbers

Ultraproct Suppositories	0053/5009R
Ultraproct Ointment	0053/5008R

ULTRAVIST*

Presentation Ampoules or bottles containing colourless, sterile solutions of various strengths of iopromide. Ultravist 150 contains 150 mg iodine per ml. Ultravist 240 contains 240 mg iodine per ml, Ultravist 300 contains 300 mg iodine per ml, Ultravist 370 contains 370 mg iodine per ml.

Excipients: calcium disodium edetate, tromethamine, hydrochloric acid, water for injection.

Uses Non-ionic X-ray contrast media for computed tomography, digital subtraction angiography, intravenous urography, venography, arteriography, visualization of body cavities (e.g. arthrography, hysterosalpingography and fistulography), checking the function of dialysis shunts. Ultravist should not be used for myelography (see 'Further information').

Dosage and administration

Intravenous urography

Dosage

Adults: The minimum dose is 0.8 ml/kg body weight Ultravist 370, (1 ml/kg Ultravist 300 or 1.3 ml/kg Ultravist 240). These doses should provide adequate filling of the ureters. It may be necessary to increase the dose in individual cases e.g. obesity or impaired renal function.

Children: The poor concentrating ability of the immature nephron of infantile kidneys necessitates the use of relatively high doses of contrast medium, i.e. Ultravist 300:

Neonates:	4.0 ml/kg body weight
Babies:	3.0 ml/kg body weight
Small children:	1.5 ml/kg body weight

Computed tomography

Cranial CT: The following dosages are recommended for cranial CT:

Ultravist 240: 1.5–2.5 ml/kg body weight
Ultravist 300: 1–2 ml/kg body weight
Ultravist 370: 1–1.5 ml/kg body weight

Whole-body CT: For whole-body computed tomography, the doses of the contrast medium and the rates of administration depend on the organs under investigation, the diagnostic problem and, in particular, the different scan and image-reconstruction times of the scanners in use. Infusion is preferable for slow scanners and injection for fast scanners.

Angiography: The dosage depends on the age, weight, cardiac output and general condition of the patient, the clinical problem, examination technique and the nature and volume of the vascular region to be investigated.

The following dosages may serve as a guide:

Cerebral angiography	
Aortic arch angiography	50–80 ml Ultravist 300/inj.
Selective angiography	6–15 ml Ultravist 300/inj.
Thoracic aortography:	50–80 ml Ultravist 300/inj.
Abdominal aortography:	40–60 ml Ultravist 300/inj.
Bifemoral arteriography:	40–60 ml Ultravist 300/inj.
Peripheral angiography:	
Upper extremities:	
Arteriography	8–12 ml Ultravist 300/inj.
Venography	50–60 ml Ultravist 240/inj.
	15–30 ml Ultravist 300/inj.
Lower extremities:	
Arteriography	20–30 ml Ultravist 300/inj.
Venography	50–80 ml Ultravist 240/inj.
	30–60 ml Ultravist 300/inj.
Angiocardiography: Cardiac-ventriculography	
	40–60 ml Ultravist 370/inj.
Coronary angiography:	5– 8 ml Ultravist 370/inj.

Digital subtraction angiography (DSA): I.V. injection of 30–60 ml Ultravist 300 or 370 as a bolus (flow-rate: 8–12 ml/second into the cubital vein; 10–20 ml/second into the vena cava) is recommended for high-contrast demonstrations of the great vessels, of the pulmonary arteries and of the arteries of the neck, head, kidneys and extremities.

Intra-arterial digital subtraction angiography requires smaller volumes and lower iodine concentrations than the intravenous technique.

The more selective the angiography, the lower the dose of contrast medium can be. This method is therefore recommended for patients with impaired renal function. For high-contrast demonstration of the arteries of the head, neck and limbs, several injections of 10–40 ml Ultravist 150, depending on the size of the vessels, are usually given directly or via a catheter. Larger volumes of contrast medium (about 200 ml) may be necessary in some cases to demonstrate the vessels of the lower limbs, particularly if both legs are to be examined.

Dialysis shunt: Ultravist 150 is also suitable for checking the function of a dialysis shunt. About 10 ml of contrast medium is required for this.

Contra-indications, warnings, etc

Contra-indications: Proven or suspected hypersensitivity to iodine-containing contrast media, manifest thyrotoxicosis and decompensated cardiac insufficiency.

Hysterosalpingography must not be carried out during pregnancy or in patients with acute inflammatory conditions in the pelvic cavity.

Use in pregnancy: X-ray examinations should, if possible, be avoided during pregnancy. It has not yet been proved beyond question that Ultravist may be used without hesitation in pregnant patients. Therefore, an examination with Ultravist during pregnancy should be carried out only if considered absolutely necessary by the physician.

Warning/side-effects: For patients with severe impairment of hepatic or renal function, cardiac or circulatory insufficiency, cerebral arteriosclerosis, cerebral spasmodic conditions, epilepsy, juvenile-onset diabetes, long-standing diabetes, pulmonary emphysema, poor general health, hyperthyroidism or multiple myeloma, the need for examination with X-ray contrast media merits careful consideration.

This also applies to patients with a history of allergy, e.g. bronchial asthma, since experience shows that they may exhibit hypersensitivity to drugs. Because of possible precipitation, X-ray contrast media and prophylactic agents must not be injected as mixed solutions.

Particular caution should be exercised in allergic patients who have previously tolerated an injectable iodine-containing contrast medium without any complications, because they may have become sensitised to these substances in the meantime.

Nonionic contrast media have less anticoagulant activity in vitro than ionic media. Meticulous attention should therefore be paid to angiographic technique. Nonionic media should not be allowed to remain in contact with blood in a syringe, and intravascular catheters should be flushed frequently, to minimise the risk of clotting, which rarely has led to serious thromboembolic complications of the procedures.

The patient should be recumbent during the administration of Ultravist, and thereafter, must be kept under close observation for at least 30 minutes, since the majority of severe incidents occur within that time. If the administration does not take place on the X-ray table, any patient with a labile circulation should be brought to the X-ray machine sitting or lying down.

The fluid supply should not be restricted, and existing disturbances of the balance of water and electrolytes must be corrected before the administration of Ultravist.

Premedication with an alpha-blocker is recommended in patients with phaeochromocytoma, because of the risk of hypertensive crisis.

If iodine isotopes are to be administered for the diagnosis of thyroid disease, it should be borne in mind that after the administration of iodised contrast media which are excreted via the kidneys, the capacity of the thyroid tissue to take up iodine will be reduced for a few days, and sometimes up to six weeks.

Symptoms, such as feelings of heat and nausea may occur, but disappear rapidly when the injection is slowed down or briefly interrupted. Transient pain may occur, in particular during the examination of peripheral vascular regions. Extravasations give rise to serious tissue reactions only in very rare cases.

If marked side-effects or suspected allergic reactions occur during injection and do not disappear, or even get worse, when the injection is briefly interrupted, it is probable that the patient is hypersensitive and the investigation must be abandoned. Even relatively minor symptoms such as itching of the skin, sneezing, violent yawns, tickling in the throat, hoarseness or attacks of coughing may be early signs of a severe reaction and, therefore, merit careful attention.

Very rarely, severe or even life-threatening side-effects such as severe hypotension and collapse, circulatory failure, ventricular fibrillation, cardiac arrest, pulmonary oedema, anaphylactic shock or other allergic manifestations, convulsions, or other cerebral symptoms may occur.

Ready availability of all drugs and equipment for emergency treatment and familiarity with the respective procedures are prerequisites for the effective management of contrast-medium incidents. Some guidance in the treatment of such incidents is contained in the leaflet supplied with the pack.

Overdosage: Acute symptoms of poisoning are unlikely with intravascular administration. In special cases, e.g. if renal function is impaired, the contrast medium may be removed by dialysis, and, in cases of intravascular administration of 300 ml or more, the balance of water and electrolytes should be corrected.

Pharmaceutical precautions Protect from light and secondary X-rays. Store below 30°C. Shelf-life: two years. Because of possible precipitation, X-ray contrast media and prophylactic agents must not be injected as mixed solutions.

Legal category POM.

Package quantities
Ultravist 150: Bottles of 50 ml.
Ultravist 240: Bottles of 50 ml
Ultravist 300: Ampoules of 20 ml. Bottles of 50 ml, 75 ml and 100 ml
Ultravist 370: Ampoules of 30 ml. Bottles of 50 ml, 75 ml, 100 ml and 200 ml

Further information The Ultravist range consists of non-ionic contrast media with osmotic pressures that are relatively low for contrast media.
Ultravist 150: 0.34 osm/kg H_2O at 37°C
Ultravist 240: 0.48 osm/kg H_2O at 37°C
Ultravist 300: 0.62 osm/kg H_2O at 37°C
Ultravist 370: 0.78 osm/kg H_2O at 37°C

Although it showed excellent neural tolerance in animal studies, the intrathecal administration of iopromide has not been investigated in clinical studies. Ultravist should not therefore be used for myelographic examinations.

Product licence numbers
Ultravist 150 0053/0209
Ultravist 240 0053/0173
Ultravist 300 0053/0174
Ultravist 370 0053/0175

UROGRAFIN*

Presentation Ampoules, vials or bottles containing colourless sterile solutions of varying strengths of meglumine diatrizoate and meglumine/sodium diatrizoates.

Urografin 150: An intravenous injection of meglumine diatrizoate 26.1% w/v and sodium diatrizoate 3.9% w/v, containing 146 mg iodine per ml.

Urografin 290: An intravascular injection of meglumine diatrizoate 52.1% w/v and sodium diatrizoate 7.9% w/v, containing 292 mg iodine per ml.

Urografin 325: An intravenous injection of meglumine diatrizoate 18% w/v and sodium diatrizoate 40% w/v, containing 325 mg iodine per ml.

Urografin 370: An intravascular injection of meglumine diatrizoate 66% w/v and sodium diatrizoate 10% w/v, containing 370 mg iodine per ml.
Excipients: calcium disodium edetate, water for injection.

Uses X-ray contrast media for the delineation of the vascular and renal systems.

Dosage and administration See table on following pages.

Contra-indications, warnings, etc
Contra-indications: Proven or suspected hypersensitivity to iodine-containing contrast media, manifest thyrotoxicosis and decompensated cardiac insufficiency.

Hysterosalpingography must not be carried out during pregnancy or in patients with acute inflammatory conditions in the pelvic cavity.

Warnings/side-effects: For patients with severe impairment of hepatic or renal function, cardiac or circulatory insufficiency, cerebral arteriosclerosis, cerebral spasmodic conditions, epilepsy, juvenile-onset diabetes, long-standing diabetes, pulmonary emphysema, poor general health, hyperthyroidism or multiple myeloma the need for examination with X-ray contrast media merits careful consideration.

This also applies to patients with a history of allergy, e.g. bronchial asthma, since experience shows that they may exhibit hypersensitivity to drugs. Because of possible precipitation, X-ray contrast media and prophylactic agents must not be injected as mixed solutions.

Particular caution should be exercised in allergic persons who have previously tolerated an injectable iodine-containing contrast medium without any complication because they may have become sensitized to these substances in the meantime.

The patient should be recumbent during the administration of Urografin. Thereafter, the patient must be kept under close observation for at least 30 minutes, since about 90% of all severe incidents occur within that time. If the administration does not take place on the X-ray table, any patient with a labile circulation should be brought to the X-ray machine sitting or lying down.

In patients with multiple myeloma, juvenile-onset diabetes, long-standing diabetes, polyuria, oliguria or gout, and in infants, young children and marasmic patients the fluid supply should not be restricted. Existing disturbances of the balance of water and electrolytes must be corrected before the administration of a hypertonic contrast-medium solution.

Premedication with an alpha-blocker is recommended in patients with phaeochromocytoma, because of the risk of hypertensive crisis.

X-ray examinations should if possible be avoided during pregnancy. It has not yet been proved beyond question that Urografin may be used without hesitation in pregnant patients. Therefore an examination with a contrast medium during pregnancy should be carried out only if considered absolutely necessary by the physician.

If iodine isotopes are to be administered for the diagnosis of thyroid disease, it should be borne in mind that after the administration of iodised contrast media which are excreted via the kidneys, the capacity of the thyroid tissue to take up iodine will be reduced for a few days, and sometimes up to 6 weeks.

Mild subjective symptoms, such as a feeling of heat and nausea, occur very seldom and disappear rapidly when the injection is slowed down or briefly interrupted. Transient pain may occur, in particular during the examination of peripheral vascular regions. Extravasations give rise to serious tissue reactions only in very rare cases.

If marked side-effects or suspected allergic reactions occur during injection and do not disappear, or even get worse, when the injection is briefly interrupted, it is probable that the patient has such a hypersensitivity and the investigation must be abandoned. Even relatively minor symptoms such as itching of the skin, sneezing, violent yawns, tickling in the throat, hoarseness or attacks of coughing may be early signs of a severe reaction and, therefore, merit careful attention.

Very rarely, severe or even life-threatening side-effects such as severe hypotension and collapse, circulatory failure, ventricular fibrillation, cardiac arrest, pulmonary oedema, anaphylactic shock or other allergic manifestations, convulsions, or other cerebral symptoms may occur.

Ionic iodinated contrast media inhibit blood coagulation in vitro more than non-ionic contrast media. Nevertheless medical personnel performing vascular catheterisation procedures should pay meticulous attention to the angiographic technique and catheter flushing so as to minimise the risk of procedure-related thrombosis and embolisation.

Ready availability of all drugs and equipment for emergency treatment and familiarity with the respective procedures are prerequisites for the effective management of contrast-medium incidents. Some guidance in the treatment of such incidents is contained in the leaflet supplied with the pack.

Overdosage: Acute symptoms of poisoning are unlikely with intravascular administration. In special cases, e.g. if renal function is impaired, the contrast medium may be removed by dialysis, and the balance of water and electrolytes should be corrected.

UROGRAFIN MEDIA – DOSAGE AND ADMINISTRATION

1. Adults only

The table on this page shows the medium/media Schering suggest for each investigation. Alternative medium/media (shown by asterisk) may be used in the same dose. Schering media may be used at the discretion of the radiologist for other established permutations of medium and examination which, for the sake of simplicity, have been omitted from the table.

Examination	*150*	*290*	*325*	*370*
Intravenous urography		Up to 70 ml	Up to 70 ml	Up to 70 ml
High-dose urography		100 ml	100 ml	
Drip-infusion urography	2–4 ml/kg body wt up to 250 ml			
Retrograde urography	5–10 ml			
Cystography	Up to 500 ml			
Angiocardiography				30–50 ml
Right-heart catheterisation				40–80 ml
Left-heart catheterisation				40–60 ml
Pulmonary angiography				30–40 ml
Coronary arteriography				4–8 ml per artery[a]
Renal arteriography		*		5–8 ml
Coeliac-axis arteriography		*		35–80 ml
Thoracic aortography				30–60 ml
Pelvic aortography				20–25 ml
Translumbar abdominal aortography				20–30 ml
Placentography				25 ml
Pelvic venography		*	25–30 ml	
Venacavography				
Inferior			30–50 ml	
Superior			25–35 ml	
Splenoportography				40–50 ml
Hysterosalpingography				4–7 ml
Arthrography		*	1–10 ml	
Percutaneous cholangiography		20–30 ml		

[a] 100 ml and 200 ml vials are available for coronary arteriography

(Other indications include selective visceral angiography, limb venography, jugular venography, vesiculography, sialography, sinusography, amniography, lymphangiography, intramuscular urography, operative cholangiography, fistulography, oesophageal and anal atresia.)

Urografin media are not suitable for myelography

2. Children and neonates

Intravenous urography: The fact that urograms of infants and young children generally show a lower contrast density than those of adults is explained by the physiologically less effective function of the immature nephron. Relatively high doses of media are therefore indicated.

	Urografin 290		*Urografin 325/370*
Up to 1 year	8–12 ml	Up to 1 year	7–10 ml
1–2 years	12–15 ml	1–2 years	10–12 ml
2–6 years	15–20 ml	2–6 years	12–15 ml
6–10 years	20–25 ml	6–12 years	15–20 ml
10–15 years	25–30 ml	over 12 years	adult dose

Drip-infusion urography: Dosage of Urografin 150 should not exceed 4 ml/kg body weight.

Angiocardiography: In neonates up to 5 kg body weight, 8 ml of Urografin 370. Infants over 5 kg body weight, 1 ml/kg body weight up to 25 ml per injection.

Right- and left-heart catheterisation: 1–1.2 ml/kg body weight of Urografin 370, with a maximum of 15 ml per injection for the right heart and 25 ml per injection for the left heart.

Pulmonary angiography: 0.5–0.6 ml/kg body weight up to 8 ml Urografin 370 per injection.

Pharmaceutical precautions *Storage:* Protect from light and heat. Shelf-life five years.

Legal category POM.

Package quantities
Urografin 150: Packs of 10 × 10 ml ampoules and 10 × 20 ml ampoules.

Urografin 150 for Infusion: Packs of 1 × 250 ml bottles and 1 × 500 ml bottles.

Urografin 290: Packs of 10 × 20 ml ampoules.

Urografin 325: Packs of 10 × 20 ml ampoules and 10 × 50 ml vials.

Urografin 370: Packs of 10 × 20 ml ampoules and 10 × 50 ml vials. In addition packs of 1 × 100 ml vials and 1 × 200 ml vials.

Further information Nil.

Product licence numbers

Urografin 150	0053/5041R
Urografin 150 for infusion	0053/5007R
Urografin 290	0053/5043R
Urografin 325	0053/5006R
Urografin 370	0053/5044R

**Trade Mark*

Schering-Plough Ltd
Mildenhall
Bury St Edmunds
Suffolk IP28 7AX

Schering-Plough

CLARITYN*

Presentation Clarityn tablets each containing 10 mg micronised loratadine. The tablets are white, oval plain on one side, and deep score, flask and dish logo with number 10 below on the other.

Uses

Mode of action: Clarityn is a long acting tricyclic antihistamine with selective peripheral H_1-receptor antagonistic activity and no central sedative or anticholinergic effects.

Indications: Clarityn tablets are indicated for the relief of symptoms associated with seasonal and perennial allergic rhinitis, such as sneezing, nasal discharge and itching and ocular itching and burning. Nasal and ocular signs and symptoms are relieved rapidly after oral administration. Clarityn tablets are also indicated for the relief of the symptoms associated with idiopathic chronic urticaria.

Dosage and administration

Adults and children 12 years of age and over: One Clarityn 10 mg tablet once daily. Safety and efficacy of Clarityn tablets in children under 12 years of age has not yet been established.

Contra-indications, warnings, etc

Contra-indications: Clarityn tablets are contra-indicated in patients who have shown hypersensitivity or idiosyncrasy to their components.

Use in the elderly: Clarityn is not recommended as studies to establish safety and efficacy in the elderly are not yet completed.

Preganancy and lactation: Clarityn tablets should not be administered during pregnancy. There is no experience of the use of Clarityn in human pregnancy. In animal studies loratadine was not teratogenic, at high doses some embryotoxic effects were observed. Since loratadine is excreted in breast milk it should not be administered to lactating women.

Side effects: During controlled clinical studies the incidence of adverse events, including sedation and anticholinergic effects observed with 10 mg Clarityn was comparable to that observed with placebo. Fatigue, nausea and headache were reported rarely.

Interactions: When administered concurrently with alcohol, Clarityn tablets have no potentiating effects as measured by psychomotor performance studies. Interactions with other drugs have not been reported.

Drug/laboratory test interactions: Antihistamines should be discontinued about four days prior to skin testing procedures, since these drugs may prevent or diminish otherwise positive reactions to dermal reactivity indicators.

Overdosage: In the event of overdosage, treatment which should be started immediately is symptomatic and supportive. The patient should be induced to vomit, even if emesis has occurred spontaneously (ipecacuanha is a preferred method), but not in patients with impaired consciousness. Administration of activated charcoal as a slurry with water may be attempted following emesis. If vomiting is unsuccessful or contra-indicated, gastric lavage should be performed. Loratadine is not dialysable to any appreciable extent. After emergency treatment, the patient should continue to be under medical supervision.

Pharmaceutical precautions None.

Legal category POM.

Package quantities Blister strips of 10 in OP cartons of 30 tablets.

Further information Nil.

Product licence number 0201/0095

CONGESTEZE*

Presentation
White sugar-coated tablets. Each contains 1 mg Azatadine Maleate USP and 60 mg Pseudoephedrine Sulphate USP in the coating and 60 mg Pseudoephedrine Sulphate USP in the barrier-coated core. The two active ingredients in the coating are quickly liberated, release of the decongestant in the core is delayed for several hours after ingestion.

Uses Antihistamine and decongestant.

Azatadine maleate is a long-acting antihistamine with anti-serotonin and anticholinergic properties. Pseudoephedrine, an orally administered vasoconstrictor, produces a gradual but sustained decongestant effect causing little, if any, 'rebound congestion' and facilitates shrinkage of congested mucosa in upper respiratory areas.

Congesteze is indicated for the relief of symptoms of upper respiratory mucosal congestion in allergic rhinitis.

Dosage and administration
Adults, the elderly and children over 12 years of age: The usual dose is one tablet taken twice a day ie one tablet morning and evening.

Contra-indications, warnings, etc Congesteze is contra-indicated in patients receiving MAO inhibitor therapy, cardiac asthma or with a known hypersensitivity to any of the constituents.

Although pseudoephedrine causes virtually no pressor effect in patients with normal blood pressure, Congesteze should be used with caution in patients with cardiovascular disorders and those being treated with beta-blocking agents.

Use with caution in patients with prostatic hypertrophy, urinary retention, glaucoma, stenosing peptic ulcer or pyloroduodenal obstructions.

Although drowsiness is infrequent and impairment of psychomotor function is not manifested at the recommended dosage of azatadine maleate, patients should be warned about engaging in mechanical operations requiring mental alertness, such as driving a car or operating machinery etc., until individual response has been determined.

Congesteze should not be given to pregnant women or nursing mothers.

Side-effects: Congesteze has caused no serious or unusual adverse effects either reported or determined by laboratory tests. The tablets are well tolerated and side effects are generally dose-related and transient. Side-effects most frequently reported are those commonly associated with antihistamine/decongestant preparations such as drowsiness, epigastric distress, weakness and nervousness, etc.

Overdosage: In the event of overdosage, emergency treatment should be started immediately. Treatment of signs and symptoms of overdosage is symptomatic and supportive.

Pharmaceutical precautions No special precautions.

Legal category POM.

Package quantities Tablets in OP Cartons of 28 containing 2 blister strips of 14 tablets.

Further information Nil.

Product licence number 0201/0134

DIPROBASE*

Presentation Diprobase Cream is a smooth, uniform white cream containing chlorocresol (0.1% w/w) as preservative. Diprobase Ointment is a smooth white preservative-free ointment, containing 5% w/w Liquid Paraffin BP and 95% White Soft Paraffin BP.

Diprobase presentations, because of their emollient and soothing properties, are particularly suitable for the care of the skin. They are also exceptionally well tolerated.

Uses Diprobase Cream and Ointment are emollients, with moisturizing and protective properties, indicated for follow-up treatment with topical steroids or in spacing such treatment. They may also be used as diluents for topical steroids. Diprobase products are recommended for the symptomatic relief of red inflamed, damaged, dry or chapped skin, the protection of raw skin areas and as a pre-bathing emollient for dry/eczematous skin to alleviate drying effects.

Dosage and administration The Cream or Ointment should be thinly applied to cover the affected area completely, massaging gently and thoroughly into the skin. Frequency of application should be established by the physician. Generally, Diprobase Cream and Ointment can be used as often as required.

Contra-indications, warnings, etc Hypersensitivity to any of the components of the Cream or Ointment is a contra-indication to their use.

Side-effects: No side-effects have been reported.

Pharmaceutical precautions Store in a cool place.

Legal category GSL.

Package quantities Diprobase Cream is supplied in 50 g tubes and 500 g dispensers. Diprobase Ointment is supplied in 50 g tubes.

Further information Nil.

Product licence numbers
Cream 0201/0076
Ointment 0201/0075

DIPROSALIC*

Presentation Diprosalic Ointment contains 0.05% betamethasone as the dipropionate ester and 3% salicylic acid. It is a smooth white, preservative-free ointment.

Diprosalic Scalp Application contains 0.05% betamethasone as the dipropionate ester and 2% salicylic acid in a preservative-free isopropyl alcohol base. It is formulated to spread easily without adherence to the hair.

Uses Betamethasone dipropionate is a synthetic fluorinated corticosteroid. In combination with salicylic acid it is indicated for the treatment of chronic lichenified eczema, lichen planus, lichen simplex, non bullous ichthyosiform erythroderma. It is also effective in the less responsive conditions such as psoriasis of the scalp and chronic plaque psoriasis of the hands and feet but excluding widespread plaque psoriasis.

Topical salicylic acid softens keratin, loosens cornified epithelium and desquamates the epidermis.

Diprosalic presentations are therefore indicated for the treatment of hyperkeratotic and dry corticosteroid-responsive dermatoses where the cornified epithelium may resist penetration of the steroid. The salicylic acid constituent of Diprosalic preparations, as a result of its descaling action, allows access of the corticosteroid to the underlying diseased areas of the dermis more rapidly than by applying steroid alone.

Dosage and administration Once to twice daily.

Diprosalic Ointment: In most cases a thin film should be applied to cover the affected area once or twice daily.

Diprosalic Scalp Application: In most cases a few drops should be applied to the affected areas once or twice daily and massaged gently and thoroughly into the skin.

For some patients adequate maintenance therapy may be achieved with less frequent application.

It is recommended that Diprosalic preparations are prescribed for 2 weeks, and that treatment is reviewed at that time. The maximum weekly dose should not exceed 60 g.

Contra-indications, warnings, etc Rosacea, acne, peri-anal and genital pruritus and peri-oral dermatitis. Hypersensitivity to any of the ingredients of the Diprosalic presentations contra-indicates their use as do tuberculous and most viral lesions of the skin, particularly herpes simplex, vaccinia, varicella. Diprosalic Ointment and Scalp Application should not be used in napkin eruptions, fungal or bacterial skin infections without suitable concomitant anti-infective therapy.

Occlusion must not be used, since under these circumstances the keratolytic action of salicylic acid may lead to enhanced absorption of the steroid.

Warnings: Local and systemic toxicity is common, especially following long continued use on large areas of damaged skin, in flexures or with polythene occlusion. If used in children or on the face, courses should be limited to five days. Long term, continuous therapy should be avoided in all patients irrespective of age.

Topical corticosteroids may be hazardous in psoriasis for a number of reasons, including rebound relapses following development of tolerance, risk of generalised, pustular psoriasis and local systemic toxicity due to impaired barrier function of the skin. Careful patient supervision is important.

It is dangerous if Diprosalic presentations come into contact with the eyes. Avoid contact with eyes and mucous membranes.

There is inadequate evidence of safety in human pregnancy. Topical administration of corticosteroids to pregnant animals can cause abnormalities of foetal development including cleft palate and intra-uterine growth retardation. There may therefore, be a very small risk of such effects in the human foetus.

The systemic absorption of betamethasone dipropionate and salicylic acid may be increased if extensive body surface areas or skin folds are treated for prolonged periods or with excessive amounts of steroids. Suitable precautions should be taken in these circumstances, particularly with infants and children.

Side-effects: Diprosalic skin preparations are generally well tolerated and side-effects are rare. Continuous application without interruption may result in local atrophy of the skin, striae and superficial vascular dilatation, particularly on the face. In addition prolonged use of salicylic acid preparations may cause dermatitis.

Overdosage: Excessive prolonged use of topical corticosteroids can suppress pituitary-adrenal functions resulting in secondary adrenal insufficiency which is usually reversible. In such cases appropriate symptomatic treatment is indicated.

With topical preparations containing salicylic acid excessive prolonged use may result in symptoms of salicylism. Treatment is symptomatic.

The steroid and salicylic acid content of each tube is so low as to have little or no toxic effect in the unlikely event of accidental oral ingestion.

Pharmaceutical precautions Nil.

Legal category POM.

Package quantities Diprosalic Ointment is supplied

in 30 g and 100 g tubes. Diprosalic Scalp Application is supplied in 30 ml and 100 ml bottles.

Further information Diprosalic Ointment and Scalp Application are formulated to avoid the problems of incompatibility normally experienced between steroids and salicylic acid.

Product licence numbers

Diprosalic Ointment	0201/0070
Diprosalic Scalp Application	0201/0069

DIPROSONE*

Presentation The Diprosone skin preparations contain 0.05% betamethasone as the dipropionate ester.

Diprosone Cream is a smooth white cream. It contains chlorocresol as the preservative.

Diprosone Ointment is a smooth white preservative free ointment.

Diprosone Lotion is a slightly gelled solution containing isopropyl alcohol, which has antibacterial activity. It is formulated to spread without adherence to hair.

Uses Betamethasone dipropionate is a synthetic fluorinated corticosteroid. It is active topically and produces a rapid and sustained response in eczema and dermatitis of all types, including atopic eczema, photo-dermatitis, primary irritant and allergic dermatitis, lichen planus, lichen simplex, prurigo nodularis, discoid lupus erythematosus, necrobiosis lipoidica, pretibial myxoedema and erythroderma. It is also effective in the less responsive conditions such as psoriasis of the scalp and chronic plaque psoriasis of the hands and feet, but excluding widespread plaque psoriasis.

Diprosone Lotion is indicated for serious steroid responsive dermatoses of the scalp.

Dosage and administration Once to twice daily. In most cases a thin film of Diprosone Cream or Ointment should be applied to cover the affected area once or twice daily. For some patients adequate maintenance therapy may be achieved with less frequent application.

Diprosone Cream is especially appropriate for moist or weeping surfaces and the ointment for dry, lichenified or scaly lesions but this is not invariably so.

Control over the dosage regimen may be achieved during intermittent and maintenance therapy by using Diprobase Cream or Ointment (PL 0201/0076 and 0201/0075) the base vehicles of Diprosone Cream and Ointment. Such control may be necessary in mild and improving dry skin conditions requiring low dose steroid treatment.

A few drops of Diprosone Lotion should be applied to the affected areas twice daily and massaged gently and thoroughly into the scalp. For some patients adequate maintenance therapy may be achieved with less frequent application.

Contra-indications, warnings, etc

Contra-indications: Rosacea, acne, perioral dermatitis, perianal and genital pruritus. Hypersensitivity to any of the ingredients of the Diprosone presentations contra-indicates their use as does tuberculous and most viral lesions of the skin, particularly herpes simplex, vaccinia, varicella. Diprosone should not be used in napkin eruptions, fungal or bacterial skin infections without suitable concomitant anti-infective therapy.

Warnings: Local and systemic toxicity is common, especially following long continued use on large areas of damaged skin, in flexures or with polythene occlusion. If used in children or on the face courses should be limited to five days. Long term continuous therapy should be avoided in all patients irrespective of age. Occlusion must not be used.

Topical corticosteroids may be hazardous in psoriasis for a number of reasons, including rebound relapses following development of tolerance, risk of generalised pustular psoriasis and local systemic toxicity due to impaired barrier function of the skin. Careful patient supervision is important.

There is inadequate evidence of safety in human pregnancy. Topical administration of corticosteroids to pregnant animals can cause abnormalities of foetal development including cleft palate and intra-uterine growth retardation. There may, therefore, be a very small risk of such effects in the human foetus.

Side effects: Diprosone skin preparations are generally well tolerated and side effects are rare. The systemic absorption of betamethasone dipropionate may be increased if extensive body surface areas of skin folds are treated for prolonged periods or with excessive amounts of steroids. Suitable precautions should be taken in these circumstances, particularly with infants and children.

Continuous application without interruption may result in local atrophy of the skin, striae and superficial vascular dilatation, particularly on the face.

Overdosage: Excessive prolonged use of topical corticosteroids can result in suppression of pituitary-adrenal function resulting in secondary adrenal insufficiency which is usually reversible. In such cases appropriate symptomatic treatment is indicated.

The steroid content of each tube is so low as to have little or no toxic effect in the unlikely event of accidental oral ingestion.

Pharmaceutical precautions Store in a cool place.

Legal category POM.

Package quantities Diprosone Cream and Ointment are supplied in 30 g and 100 g tubes.

Diprosone Lotion is supplied in 30 ml and 100 ml plastic bottles.

Further information These preparations do not contain lanolin or parabens.

Product licence numbers

Cream	0201/0072
Ointment	0201/0074
Lotion	0201/0073

DROGENIL*▼

Presentation Each round, yellow, scored tablet contains 250 mg flutamide.

Uses

Properties; In animal studies, flutamide demonstrates potent antiandrogenic effects. It exerts its antiandrogenic action by inhibiting androgen uptake and/or by inhibiting nuclear binding of androgens in target tissues. When Drogenil is given in combination with surgical or medical castration, suppression of both testicular and adrenal androgen activity is achieved. Because flutamide is non-steroidal, Drogenil tablets demonstrate a low potential for cardiovascular side-effects.

Indications: Treatment of advanced prostatic carcinoma in which suppression of testosterone effects is indicated: as initial treatment in combination with an LHRH agonist; as adjunctive therapy in patients already receiving LHRH agonist therapy; in surgically castrated patients; in the treatment of patients who have not responded to other forms of hormonal manipulation or in patients who cannot tolerate such treatment.

Dosage and administration One tablet three times daily.

When used as initial treatment with an LHRH agonist, a greater reduction in the incidence and severity of the LHRH agonist flare reaction may be achieved if Drogenil is introduced before rather than concomitantly with the agonist. It is, therefore, recommended that Drogenil one tablet three times daily should be started at least three days before an LHRH agonist and continued thereafter at the same dose.

Contra-indications, warnings, etc

Contra-indications: Patients exhibiting sensitivity reactions to flutamide.

Drug interactions: Increases in prothrombin time have been reported in patients receiving long-term warfarin therapy after flutamide monotherapy was initiated.

Adjustment of the anticoagulant dose may be necessary when Drogenil is administered concomitantly with warfarin.

Precautions: Hepatic injury: Transaminase abnormalities, cholestatic jaundice, hepatic necrosis, and hepatic encephalopathy have been reported with the use of flutamide. The hepatic conditions were usually reversible after discontinuing therapy, although there have been occasional reports of a fatal outcome following severe hepatic injury in patients receiving flutamide. Periodic liver function tests should be considered in all patients and performed in patients on long-term treatment.

In addition in patients who have not received medical or surgical castration, periodic sperm count determinations may be considered during long-term treatment. In such patients flutamide administration tends to elevate plasma testosterone and oestradiol levels, fluid retention may occur, thus the drug should be used with caution in cardiac disease.

Adverse effects: The most frequently reported adverse reactions to Drogenil tablets are gynaecomastia and/or breast tenderness, sometimes accompanied by galactorrhoea. These reactions disappear upon discontinuation of treatment or reduction in dosage.

Less frequent adverse reactions include nausea, vomiting, diarrhoea, increased appetite, insomnia and tiredness.

Rare reactions include hepatic injury (see Precautions Section). In addition skin reactions including photosensitivity, erythema, ulcerations, bullous eruptions, epidermal necrolysis, ecchymoses, herpes zoster, pruritus and lupus-like syndrome; gastro-intestinal symptoms including anorexia, constipation, dyspepsia and heartburn; reports of a more general nature include decreased libido, headache, hypertension, dizziness, weakness, malaise, blurred vision, thirst, chest pain, anxiety, lymphoedema, depression and thrombocytopenia. These reports have been observed in clinical studies and are not necessarily drug related, but may be due to the underlying clinical condition.

Usually these reactions have not been of sufficient severity to require dosage reduction or discontinuation of therapy.

Laboratory abnormalities reported include changes in liver function tests (see Precautions Section) haemolytic anaemia, macrocytic anaemia and methaemoglobinaemia. No abnormalities in renal function have been detected although elevated serum creatinine levels have been reported. Reduced sperm counts have been observed during long term treatment.

In combination therapy additional adverse events may be observed which are related to concomitant treatment. However, during clinical investigation of flutamide/LHRH agonist combination therapy, the incidence of gynaecomastia was one third of that generally observed with flutamide monotherapy.

Overdosage: The Drogenil dose associated with symptoms of overdosage, or considered to be life-threatening has not been established. One patient survived after taking more than 5 g as a single dose – no adverse effects were observed.

If vomiting does not occur spontaneously, it should be induced if the patient is alert. General supportive care including frequent monitoring of the vital signs and close observation of the patient, is indicated.

Pharmaceutical precautions None.

Legal category POM.

Package quantities Boxes of 100 tablets in blister packs.

Further information Patients may rarely experience an asymptomatic change in the colour of urine to an amber or yellow-green appearance, which can be attributed to flutamide and/or its metabolites.

Product licence number 0201/0062.

INTRON A* INJECTION

Presentation Intron A is a highly purified sterile, stable lyophilised formulation of interferon alfa-2b(rbe). It is a white to cream coloured powder.

Intron A is a water soluble human protein produced by recombinant DNA techniques. Its activity is expressed in International Units (IU) with 10 million IU corresponding to 0.05 mg of interferon alfa-2b(rbe) protein.

Each vial of Intron A contains either 3 million, 5 million, 10 million or 30 million IU of interferon alfa-2b(rbe), together with aminoacetic acid, sodium phosphate dibasic and sodium phosphate monobasic as buffering agents and human albumin as a stabiliser.

Uses Treatment of hairy cell leukaemia, chronic myelogenous leukaemia, condyloma acuminatum and in patients with Kaposi's sarcoma developing as a consequence of acquired immune deficiency syndrome (AIDS).

Dosage and administration

1. Subcutaneous administration

Hairy cell leukaemia: The recommended dose is 2 million IU/m^2 Intron A administered subcutaneously three times per week (i.e. every other day). The dosage may be adjusted according to the patient's tolerance to the medication. The normalisation of one or more haematologic variables begins within one month of therapy. Improvement in all three haematologic variables (granulocyte count, platelet count and haemoglobin level) may require six months or more. The regimen should be maintained unless the disease progresses rapidly or severe intolerance is manifested.

Chronic myelogenous leukaemia: The recommended dose is 4 to 5 million IU/m^2 Intron A, administered subcutaneously daily. When the white blood cell count is controlled, the dosage may be administered every other day.

The dosage may be adjusted according to the patient's tolerance to the medication. The regimen should be maintained unless the disease progresses rapidly or severe intolerance is manifested.

AIDS-related Kaposi's sarcoma: The recommended dose of Intron A is 30 million IU/m^2 administered subcutaneously three times per week (i.e. every other day). The regimen should be maintained indefinitely unless the disease progresses rapidly or severe intolerance develops.

If adverse reactions develop, the dosage should be modified, or therapy temporarily discontinued until the adverse reactions abate. If persistent or recurrent intolerance develops following adequate dosage adjustment, or disease progresses, treatment with Intron A should be discontinued.

Reconstitution of lyophilised Intron A: Hairy cell leukaemia, chronic myelogenous leukaemia, AIDS-related Kaposi's sarcoma: The powder is reconstituted with Water for Injections BP. The volume of Water for Injections added should be 1 ml. The appropriate dose is then withdrawn and injected subcutaneously. The colourless to light yellow reconstituted solution is stable for 24 hours at 2°C to 8°C.

Laboratory Tests: The laboratory tests listed below should be carried out during treatment:

- Standard haematologic tests (including complete blood counts and differential as well as platelet counts)
- Blood chemistries (including calcium and liver function)
- Serum electrophoresis
- Urinalysis
- Renal function tests

Patients with pre-existing cardiac abnormalities and/or in advanced stages of cancer should have an ECG taken frequently during treatment.

2. Intralesional administration

Condyloma acuminatum: The lesion or lesions to be injected should be cleaned first with a sterile alcohol pad. The intralesional injection should be made at the base of the lesion using a fine needle (30 gauge). Inject

0.1 ml of sterile solution containing 1.0 million IU Intron A injection into the lesion three times per week on alternate days, for three weeks. As many as five lesions can be treated at one time. The maximum total dose administered weekly should not exceed 15 million IU.

Large lesions may be treated by multiple injections (up to a total of 5.0 million IU of Intron A per day) or by sequentially injecting different areas of the lesions.

Re-treatment: Improvement usually occurs four to eight weeks after initiation of the first treatment course. If results at this time are not satisfactory, a second course of treatment at the same dosage schedule may be instituted providing that clinical signs and symptoms or changes in laboratory parameters do not preclude re-treatment.

Reconstitution of lyophilised Intron A: Condyloma acuminatum: Using a sterile syringe and needle, inject sufficient Water for Injections BP into the vial to provide a solution containing 1.0 million IU per 0.1 ml solution e.g. 0.5 ml Water for Injections BP into the 5 million IU vial. The appropriate dose should then be withdrawn with a sterile syringe and injected intralesionally.

Laboratory tests: The laboratory tests listed below should be carried out during treatment.

- Standard haematologic tests (including complete blood counts and differential as well as platelet counts).
- Liver function tests.

Contra-indications, warnings, etc
Contra-indications: In patients with a history of hypersensitivity to Interferon Alfa-2b(rbe) or any of the components of Intron A.

Warnings and precautions: Serious, acute hypersensitivity reactions to Intron A have not been observed, but if such a reaction develops the drug should be discontinued immediately. Moderate to severe adverse experiences may require modification of the dosage regimen, or, in some cases, termination of Intron A therapy.

Adverse cardiovascular effects have been observed in some patients and appeared to be correlated with pre-existing condition, age, prior cardiotoxic therapy, as well as Intron A dosage. These effects were controlled by modification of the dosage or discontinuation of treatment. Hypotension may occur during, or up to two days post treatment and may require supportive treatment. Cardiac arrhythmias usually respond to conventional therapy, but may require discontinuation of Intron A. Patients with a recent history of myocardial infarction and/or previous or current arrhythmic disorder should be closely monitored.

Adequate hydration of patients should be maintained during treatment.

In a few cases CNS effects commonly manifested by confusion have been seen, usually at higher dose levels. These are reversible but full resolution may take up to three weeks. Discontinuation of Intron A therapy may be required. Very rarely, seizures have occurred at high doses Narcotics, hypnotics or sedatives should be administered with caution concomitantly with Intron A.

Concurrent or previous use of neurotoxic, haemotoxic or cardiotoxic drugs may increase the toxicity of interferon and significant renal dysfunction may require dosage adjustment. There is evidence to suggest that interferons may affect the oxidative metabolic process and this should be taken into consideration in concomitant therapy with drugs metabolised by this route.

If interferon is administered to patients who are taking xanthine derivatives such as theophylline or aminophylline, the xanthine derivative levels should be monitored and dosage adjusted as necessary.

Although not clearly related to Intron A therapy, bleeding, sometimes severe, has been observed.

Safety in patients below the age of 18 has not been established.

It is not known whether Intron A can cause foetal harm when administered to pregnant women or whether its components are excreted in human milk and therefore it should only be given to pregnant women or nursing mothers if the potential benefit to the mother clearly outweighs the potential hazard to the foetus or nursing infant.

Side-effects: The most frequently observed laboratory abnormalities, especially at doses above 10 million IU daily, include elevated liver function tests, reduction in white blood cell, granulocyte and platelet counts. These were reversible on cessation of therapy. Other reported laboratory findings include increases in serum creatinine, LDH and alkaline phosphatase.

Studies in patients and healthy volunteers showed the most common adverse effects were "flu-like" symptoms, leukopaenia or thrombocytopaenia and CNS effects. These should be ameliorated by adjusting the dosage level or schedule and all were reversible on interruption or cessation of treatment. The reactions were generally dose-related.

Paracetamol can be used successfully to alleviate the flu-like symptoms of fever and headache which can occur with Intron A therapy.

Intralesional administration is generally well tolerated. Injection-site reactions appear to be due to manipulation of the lesion rather than to Intron A therapy. Most reported adverse reactions were mild to moderate, transient and rapidly reversible and appear to increase in proportion to the number of lesions treated.

Pharmaceutical precautions Store in a refrigerator at 2–8°C. Reconstituted solutions should be used immediately and examined by visual inspection for particulate matter; solutions not for immediate use should be prepared under aseptic conditions, kept refrigerated at 2–8°C and any portion remaining after 24 hours discarded.

Package quantities. Intron A is supplied in vials containing 3 million, 5 million, 10 million or 30 million international units of interferon alfa-2b(rbe) per vial.

Further information For treatment of Condyloma acuminatum, lignocaine gel may be used if the patient is especially sensitive.

Product licence numbers

3 million IU	0201/0064
5 million IU	0201/0065
10 million IU	0201/0066
30 million IU	0201/0067

LOTRIDERM CREAM*

Presentation Smooth uniform white to off-white cream free of foreign matter, containing 0.05% betamethasone as the dipropionate ester and 1% clotrimazole.

Uses Lotriderm cream combines the broad spectrum antifungal activity of clotrimazole with the sustained anti-inflammatory, antipruritic and vasoconstrictive actions of betamethasone dipropionate and is indicated for short-term topical treatment of the following dermal infections: *Trichophyton rubrum, T. mentagrophytes, Epidermophyton floccosum* and *Microsporum canis*; candidiasis due to *Candida albicans.*

Dosage and administration Gently massage sufficient Lotriderm cream into the affected and surrounding skin areas twice daily, in the morning and evening for two weeks in tinea cruris, tinea corporis and candidiasis and four weeks in tinea pedis.

Clinical improvement, with relief of erythema and pruritis, usually occurs within the first 3 to 5 days of treatment. If a patient with tinea cruris, tinea corporis or candidiasis shows no clinical improvement after one week of treatment with Lotriderm, the diagnosis should be reviewed. Similarly in tinea pedis diagnosis should be reviewed if no improvement is shown after two weeks of treatment.

Contra-indications, warnings, etc Lotriderm is contra-indicated in those patients with history of sensitivity to any of its components or to other corticosteroids or imidazoles.

If irritation or sensitisation develops with the use of

Lotriderm cream, treatment should be discontinued and appropriate therapy instituted.

Lotriderm is contra-indicated in facial rosacea, acne vulgaris, perioral dermatitis, perianal and genital pruritus, napkin eruptions and bacterial or viral infections.

In the presence of bacterial or viral infections, appropriate concomitant therapy should be administered. If a favourable response does not occur promptly, treatment with Lotriderm should be discontinued until the infection has been controlled adequately.

Any of the side-effects that are reported following systemic use of corticosteroids, including adrenal suppression, may also occur with topical steroids, especially in infants and children.

Local and systemic toxicity is common especially following long continued use on large areas of damaged skin, and in flexures. If used in children or on the face courses should be limited to 5 days. Long term continuous therapy should be avoided in all patients irrespective of age.

Lotriderm Cream should not be used with occlusive dressing.

The safety and effectiveness of Lotriderm cream has not been established in children below the age of 12.

Lotriderm cream is not intended for ophthalmic use.

Topical corticosteroids may be hazardous in psoriasis for a number of reasons including rebound relapses following the development of tolerance, risk of generalised pustular psoriasis and local and systemic toxicity due to impaired barrier function of the skin.

There is inadequate evidence of safety in pregnancy. Clotrimazole has shown no teratogenic effect in animals but is foetotoxic at high oral doses. Topical administration of corticosteroids to pregnant animals can cause abnormalities of foetal development including cleft palate and intra uterine growth retardation. There may therefore be a very small risk of such effects in the human foetus. Hence Lotriderm cream should only be used in pregnancy if the benefit justifies the potential risk to the foetus and such use should not be extensive, i.e. in large amounts or for long periods.

It is not known whether the components of Lotriderm are excreted in human milk and therefore caution should be exercised when treating nursing mothers.

Adverse reactions reported for Lotriderm include, burning and stinging, maculopapular rash, oedema and secondary infection.

Reported reactions to clotrimazole include erythema, stinging, blistering, peeling, oedema, pruritis, urticaria and general irritation of the skin.

Reactions to betamethasone dipropionate include: burning, itching, irritation, dryness, folliculitis, hypertrichosis, acneiform eruptions, hyperpigmentation, perioral dermatitis, allergic contact dermatitis, maceration of the skin, secondary infection, skin atrophy, striae and miliaria.

Pharmaceutical precautions Store in a cool place.

Legal category POM.

Package quantities Tubes of 15 g.

Further information Nil.

Product licence number 0201/0081.

MODRASONE* CREAM AND OINTMENT

Presentation Modrasone Cream contains 0.05% alclometasone dipropionate in a smooth white emollient cream base. It contains chlorocresol as the preservative.

Modrasone Ointment contains 0.05% alclometasone dipropionate in a preservative-free ointment base.

Uses Alclometasone dipropionate is a non-fluorinated, topically active synthetic corticosteroid.

Modrasone cream or ointment is indicated for the treatment of inflammatory and pruritic manifestations of corticosteroid responsive dermatoses.

Dosage and administration For adults and children, a thin film of Modrasone Cream or Ointment should be applied to the affected skin area two or three times daily or as directed by the physician. Massage gently into the skin until the medication disappears.

Contra-indications, warnings, etc

Contra-indications: Hypersensitivity to any of the ingredients. Rosacea, acne and peri-oral dermatitis. Tuberculous and viral lesions of the skin, particularly herpes simplex, vaccina, varicella. Modrasone should not be used in fungal or bacterial skin infections.

Warnings: As with all topical steroids, long term continuous therapy should be avoided where possible, particularly in infants and children as adrenal suppression may occur even without occlusion. In infants the napkin may act as an occlusive dressing and thus increase absorption.

Topical administration of corticosteroids to pregnant animals can cause abnormalities to foetal development. The relevance of this finding to human beings has not been established; however, topical steroids should not be used extensively in pregnancy, i.e. in large amounts or for long periods.

Side-effects: Excessive prolonged use may result in local atrophy of the skin, striae and superficial vascular dilatation, particularly on the face.

Overdosage: Excessive prolonged use of topical corticosteroids may result in suppression of pituitary-adrenal function resulting in secondary adrenal insufficiency which is usually reversible. In such cases appropriate symptomatic treatment is indicated.

The total steroid content of each tube is low and is unlikely to have any toxic effect in the unlikely event of accidental oral ingestion.

Pharmaceutical precautions Store in a cool place.

The dilution of Modrasone Cream and Ointment is not recommended.

Legal category POM.

Package quantities Modrasone Cream or Ointment are supplied in 15 g and 50 g tubes.

Further information Nil.

Product licence numbers
Cream 0201/0060
Ointment 0201/0061

NETILLIN* Injection

Presentation Netillin Injection for parenteral use is an aqueous solution of netilmicin sulphate. Each millilitre contains netilmicin sulphate equivalent to 100 mg, 50 mg or 10 mg of netilmicin base, and is available in ampoules.

Uses Netilmicin sulphate is a semi-synthetic, water-soluble antibiotic of the aminoglycoside group. It is a rapidly acting bactericidal antibiotic which probably acts by inhibiting normal protein synthesis in susceptible organisms. It is active at low concentrations against many strains of a wide variety of pathogenic bacteria including *Escherichia coli, Klebsiella-Enterobacter-Serratia* species, *Citrobacter* species, *Proteus* species (indole-positive and indole-negative), including *Proteus mirabilis, Proteus morganii, Proteus rettgeri, Proteus vulgaris; Pseudomonas aeruginosa*, and *Staphylococcus* species (coagulase-positive and coagulase-negative, including penicillin and methicillin-resistant strains).

Netillin Injection is indicated in: bacteraemia, septicaemia (including neonatal sepsis), serious infections of the respiratory tract, kidney and genitourinary tract infections, skin and soft tissue infections, bone and joint infections, burns, wounds and peri-operative infections, intra-abdominal infections (including peritonitis) and infections of the gastro-intestinal tract.

A single Netillin Injection has been shown to be effective in the treatment of gonorrhoea.

Netillin Injection has also been effective in the treatment of infections caused by organisms resistant to other aminoglycosides, such as kanamycin, gentamicin, tobramycin and amikacin.

Netillin Injection is recommended for prophylactic use.

Dosage and administration The recommended dosage for intramuscular and intravenous administration is identical and should be calculated on mg/kg lean body weight. Netillin Injection should usually be administered intramuscularly. For i.v. administration see below.

The usual duration of treatment is seven to fourteen days. Longer courses have been well tolerated but it is important that patients treated beyond the usual period be carefully monitored for changes in renal, auditory and vestibular function. Dosage should be reduced if clinically indicated.

Serum levels: The measurement of peak and trough serum levels is of value to assure adequate levels and to avoid potentially toxic levels. Once daily administration of Netillin may lead to transient peak concentrations of 20–30 mcg/ml. Other dosage regimens will result in peak levels generally not exceeding 12 mcg/ml. Prolonged levels above 16 mcg/ml should be avoided. If trough levels are monitored (just prior to next dose) they will usually be 3 mcg/ml or less with the recommended dosage. Trough concentrations above 4 mcg/ml should be avoided.

The regular monitoring of serum levels is particularly important for patients with impaired renal function or where a longer duration of treatment is necessary.

I.V. administration: If i.v. administration is required, the dose may be injected directly into a vein or i.v. tubing over a period of 3 to 5 minutes or administered as an infusion. For infusion in adults, a single dose of Netillin injection may be diluted in 50 to 200 ml of sterile normal saline or in a sterile solution of dextrose 5% in water; in infants and children the volume of diluent should be dependant on the patients fluid requirements. The solution may be infused over a period of one half to two hours.

Netillin injection should not be physically pre-mixed with other drugs, but should be administered separately in accordance with the recommended route of administration and dosage schedule. Netillin injection is physically compatible with the following parental solutions: Sterile Water for Injections, Normal Saline, 5% and 10% Dextrose in Water.

Patients with normal renal function:
Adults: Urinary tract or non-life threatening systemic infections: The recommended dose is 4.0–6 mg/kg/day given once daily. The dose may also be given in equal sub doses 12 hourly or eight hourly. In general within this dose range, lower dosage will be used for urinary tract infections and higher dosage for systemic infections. Dosage should be adjusted for both uses depending on severity of infection and patient condition.

Patients with urinary tract infections may be treated with a single daily dose of 150 mg administered for five days.

Netillin in a single dose of 300 mg may be used in the treatment of gonorrhoea.

Life threatening infections: Dosages up to 7.5 mg/kg/day may be administered in three equal doses every eight hours. This dosage should be reduced to 6 mg/kg/day or less as soon as clinically indicated, usually within 48 hours.

Children: 6.0–7.5 mg/kg/day (2.0 to 2.5 mg/kg administered every eight hours).

Infants and neonates: over one week of age: 7.5 to 9.0 mg/kg/day (2.5 to 3.0 mg/kg administered every eight hours).

Premature or full term neonates: One Week of Age or Less: 6 mg/kg/day (3.0 mg/kg administered every 12 hours).

Patients with impaired renal function: The usual daily dose should be given on the first day as a loading dose (divided into three equal doses every 8 hrs). Dosage must then be adjusted. Whenever possible netilmicin serum concentrations should be monitored and used as the basis for dosage adjustment (see serum levels). If serum levels cannot be measured directly, serum creatinine or creatinine clearance rate may be used as a guide to dosage adjustment, as shown in the Table below.

Haemodialysis: For patients on haemodialysis the recommended dose is 2 mg/kg at the end of each dialysis period. In children a dose of 2–2.5 mg/kg may be administered depending on the severity of infection.

Peritoneal dialysis: Netillin has been used sucessfully in doses of 7.5–10 mg/l at each change of dialysing fluid without elevation of serum levels.

Concomitant therapy: Dosages recommended above for patients with normal or impaired renal function should not be reduced when netilmicin is administered concomitantly with other antibiotics (but see Warnings).

Contra-indications, warnings, etc
Contra-indications: Hypersensitivity to netilmicin contra-indicates its use. A history of hypersensitivity or serious toxic reactions to other aminoglycosides may also be a contra-indication.

Dosage Adjustment Guide for Patients with Renal Function Impairment
(Daily dose to be divided into three equal doses every 8 hours)

Administer the usual dose on the first day as follows:

1. Adults, urinary tract and systemic infections 4–6 mg/kg/day.
2. Adults, life-threatening infections 7.5 mg/kg/day.
3. Children, 6–7.5 mg/kg/day.
4. Infants and neonates over 1 week of age, 7.5–9 mg/kg/day.
5. Premature or full term neonates one week of age or less, 6 mg/kg/day.

On subsequent days, administer a percent of the usual dose, based on serum creatinine or creatinine clearance rate as follows:

Approx. creatinine clearance rate (ml/min/1.73 sq m)	*Serum creatinine level*		*Percent of usual dose*
	mg/100 ml	*S.I. Units μmol/l*	
100	≤1.0	80	100
71–100	1.1–1.3	100–120	80
56–70	1.4–1.6	130–150	65
46–55	1.7–1.9	160–175	55
41–45	2.0–2.2	180–190	50
36–40	2.3–2.5	210–220	40
31–35	2.6–3.0	230–260	35
26–30	3.1–3.5	270–310	30
21–25	3.6–4.0	320–360	25
16–20	4.1–5.1	365–450	20
10–15	5.2–6.6	460–580	15
<10	6.7–8.0	600–700	10

Warnings: Patients treated with aminoglycosides should be under close clinical observation because of the potential toxicity associated with their use. Monitoring of renal and eighth cranial nerve functions is desirable during therapy, particularly for patients with known or suspected reduced renal function.

Evidence of ototoxicity requires dosage adjustment or discontinuance of the drug.

Serum concentration assays of aminoglycosides are of value to assure adequate levels and to avoid potentially toxic levels. Once daily administration of Netillin may lead to transient peak concentrations of 20–30 mcg/ml. Other dosages regimens will result in peak levels not exceeding 12 mcg/ml. Prolonged levels above 16 mcg/ml should be avoided. If trough levels are monitored (just prior to next dose) they will usually be 3 mcg/ml or less with the recommended dosage. Increasing trough concentrations above 4 mcg/ml should be avoided.

In patients with extensive body surface burns, altered pharmocokinetics may result in reduced serum concentrations of aminoglycosides. Measurement of netilmicin serum concentrations is particularly important in these patients as a basis for dosage adjustment.

Concurrent and/or sequential systemic or topical use of other potentially neurotoxic and/or nephrotoxic drugs, such as polymyxin B, colistin, cephaloridine, kanamycin, gentamicin, amikacin, tobramycin, neomycin, streptomycin and vancomycin should be avoided. Advanced age and dehydration may also increase the risk of toxicity.

Increased nephrotoxicity has been reported following concomitant administration of aminoglycoside antibiotics and cephalothin.

Neurotoxic or nephrotoxic antibiotics may be absorbed from body surfaces after local irrigation or application. The potential toxic effect of such antibiotics administered in this fashion should be considered.

The concurrent use of netilmicin with potent diuretics, such as ethacrynic acid or frusemide, should be avoided since these diuretics by themselves may cause ototoxicity. In addition, when administered intravenously, diuretics may enhance aminoglycoside toxicity by altering the antibiotic concentrations in serum and tissue.

Patients should be well hydrated during treatment.

Neuromuscular blockade has been reported in animals receiving netilmicin at doses considerably above those clinically recommended. The possibility of this phenomenon occurring in man should be considered, particularly if aminoglycosides are administered to patients receiving anaesthetics, neuromuscular blocking agents (such as succinylcholine or tubocurarine), or massive transfusions of citrate-anticoagulated blood. If blockade occurs, calcium salts may reverse it.

Aminoglycosides should be used with caution in patients with neuromuscular disorders, such as myasthenia gravis or parkinsonism, since these drugs theoretically may aggravate muscle weakness because of their potential curare-like effects on the neuromuscular junction.

Elderly patients may have reduced renal function which might not be evident by routine screening tests, such as BUN or serum creatinine. A creatinine clearance determination may be more useful. Monitoring of renal function during netilmicin treatment, as with other aminoglycosides, is particularly important in these patients.

Cross-allergenicity among aminoglycosides has been demonstrated.

Although the *in vitro* mixing of netilmicin and carbenicillin results in a rapid and significant inactivation of netilmicin, this interaction has not been demonstrated in patients with normal renal function who received both drugs by different routes of administration. In patients with severe renal impairment receiving carbenicillin concomitantly with an aminoglycoside, a reduction in aminoglycoside serum half-life has been reported.

Treatment with netilmicin may result in overgrowth of non-susceptible organisms. If this occurs, appropriate therapy is indicated.

Safety for use in pregnancy has not been established.

Netilmicin is not intended for intrathecal use.

Side-effects: Adverse renal effects, generally mild in nature, have been reported infrequently after netilmicin administration. They occur more frequently in patients with a history of renal impairment, in patients treated with larger than the recommended dosage, and are most often reversible. While eighth cranial nerve toxicity has been reported with netilmicin, the incidence is lower and the severity appears milder than with other aminoglycosides. Some clinical studies indicate that at therapeutic dosage, netilmicin may have less effect than other aminoglycosides on eighth cranial nerve function. Adverse effects on both the vestibular and auditory branches of the eighth cranial nerve occur primarily in patients with renal impairment and in patients on high doses and/or prolonged therapy. Symptoms which are often transient may include dizziness, vertigo, tinnitus, roaring in the ears and hearing loss. The latter is usually manifested by diminution of high-tone acuity. Total deafness has not been reported.

Some patients who have had previous ototoxic reactions to other aminoglycosides have been treated safely with Netillin Injection.

Other rarely reported adverse reactions possibly related to netilmicin include: headache, malaise, visual disturbances, disorientation, tachycardia, paraesthesia, rash, chills, fever, fluid retention, vomiting and diarrhoea.

Laboratory abnormalities possibly related to netilmicin include: increased blood sugar, increased alkaline phosphatase, increased SGOT or SGPT; other abnormal liver function studies; decreased haemoglobin, WBCs, and platelets; eosinophilia and increase in prothrombin time.

While local tolerance of Netillin Injection is generally excellent, there has been an occasional report of pain at the injection site or local reaction.

Overdosage: In the event of overdose or toxic reaction, haemodialysis or peritoneal dialysis will aid the removal of netilmicin from the blood.

Pharmaceutical precautions Netillin Injection should be stored at 2°C to 30°C (35.6°F to 86°F). Protect from freezing.

Netillin Injections should not be physically premixed with other drugs, but should be administered separately in accordance with the recommended route of administration and dosage schedule.

Legal category POM.

Package quantities All the presentations of Netillin are colour coded on both cartons and the containers. The 100 mg/ml strength is available in 2 ml (colour coded red), 1.5 ml (orange) and 1 ml (yellow) ampoules. The 50 mg/ml and 10 mg/ml strengths are available in 1 ml (green) and 1.5 ml (blue) ampoules respectively. All ampoules are supplied in packs of ten.

Further information Nil.

Product licence numbers

Netillin Injection 100 mg/ml	3478/0041
Netillin Injection 50 mg/ml	3478/0040
Netillin Injection 10 mg/ml	3478/0039

OPTIMINE*

Presentation *Optimine Tablets:* Each white tablet, with score mark on one side and Schering Corporation USA Trademark on the other, contains 1.0 mg Azatadine Maleate USP.

Optimine Syrup: Each 5 ml of clear, colourless syrup which has the characteristic odour and flavour of blackcurrant, contains 0.5 mg of Azatadine maleate USP.

Indications Optimine Tablets and Syrup are indicated for the symptomatic relief of allergic conditions such as hayfever, vasomotor rhinitis, urticaria, pruritus of allergic origin and allergic reactions associated with insect bites and stings.

Dosage and administration *Adults, the elderly and children over 12 years of age:* In most conditions, 1 mg of azatadine maleate (1 tablet or 10 ml of syrup) in the morning and evening is recommended in the majority of patients. In refractory or more severe cases, 2 mg twice daily may be used.

Children 6–12 years of age: 0.5 to 1.0 mg of azatadine maleate ($\frac{1}{2}$ to 1 tablet or 5 to 10 ml of syrup) twice daily.

Children 1–6 years of age: 0.25 mg azatadine maleate (2.5 ml of syrup) twice daily.

Optimine Syrup may be diluted with Syrup BP.

Contra-indications, warnings, etc Until the safety of azatadine maleate concerning adverse effects on human foetal development has been established, the drug is not recommended for use in pregnant or lactating women.

Patients taking azatadine maleate should be cautioned against ingestion of alcohol. The drug may potentiate central nervous system depressants.

Although drowsiness is infrequent and impairment of psychomotor function is not manifested at the recommended dosage, patients should be cautioned against engaging in mechanical operations requiring mental alertness until individual response to azatadine maleate has been determined.

Due to the anticholinergic effect of azatadine maleate, the drug should be used with caution in patients with prostatic hypertrophy, urinary retention, glaucoma, stenosing peptic ulcer or pyloroduodenal obstructions.

Mono-amine oxidase inhibitors, which are known to intensify or prolong the anticholinergic and sedative action of drugs, should not be used concomitantly with azatadine maleate.

Side Effects: Azatadine maleate is well tolerated and side-effects are generally dose-related and transient. Among these are: weakness, nervousness, dry mouth, increased appetite, anorexia, nausea, headache, drowsiness, dysuria and blurring of vision.

Overdosage: Symptoms may vary from central nervous system depression to stimulation, the latter is particularly likely in children. Atropine-like symptoms may also occur. If vomiting has not occurred spontaneously the patient should be induced to vomit. If unsuccessful the stomach should be emptied by aspiration and lavage. Stimulants should not be used and vasopressors may be used to treat hypotension.

Pharmaceutical precautions None.

Legal category P.

Package quantities Optimine Tablets are supplied in OP cartons of 56 tablets containing 4 blister strips of 14 tablets. Optimine syrup is supplied in a 120 ml bottle.

Further information Azatadine maleate possesses potent antihistamine and antiserotonin activity. It has an inherently long action which enables effective and sustained control of symptoms from twice a day administration.

Product licence numbers

Optimine Tablets	0201/0128
Optimine Syrup	0201/0129

PALACOS LV-40 with GENTAMICIN* PALACOS LV-30 with GENTAMICIN*

Presentation Palacos LV with Gentamicin low viscosity cement is a radiopaque bone cement formed from the mixture of two separate pre-measured sterilised components. Each pack contains two sachets of powder and 2 ampoules. One component is supplied in a polyethylene coated paper packet and consists of a powder (polymer) with the following composition:

	Palacos LV-40	*Palacos LV-30*
Gentamicin sulphate	1.67 g	1.25 g
Methyl methacrylate/ methylacrylate copolymer	33.12 g	24.78 g
Benzoyl peroxide	0.62 g	0.47 g
Zirconium dioxide	6.26 g	4.68 g
Chlorophyll	1.0 mg	0.8 mg

The other component is supplied in an amber glass ampoule and consists of a liquid (monomer) with the following composition:

	Palacos LV-40	*Palacos LV-30*
Methylmethacrylate (stabilised with hydroquinone)	18.424 g	13.818 g
N,N-Dimethyl-p-toluidine	0.376 g	0.282 g
Chlorophyll	0.4 mg	0.3 mg

Palacos LV with Gentamicin is pigmented light green to make it clearly visible in the operative field.

The liquid monomer is sterile filtered and the powder is sterilised by ethylene oxide gas. The polyethylene coated paper packet containing the powder as well as the exterior of the ampoule containing the liquid are also sterilised with ethylene oxide.

Note: Palacos LV powder is double packaged. The outer aluminium protective foil which is NON-STERILE contains a polyethylene peel-pack, enclosing a STERILE polyethylene paper coated packet of Palacos LV Powder.

The STERILE ampoule containing the liquid monomer is packaged in a protective plastic blister pack.

When the powder (polymer) and the liquid (monomer) are mixed, the dimethyl-p-toluidine in the liquid activates the benzoyl peroxide catalyst in the powder, initiating polymerisation of the monomer which then binds together granules of polymer. As polymerisation proceeds, a dough-like mass is formed which hardens over eight to ten minutes into a mechanically uniform solid. Polymerisation is an exothermic reaction with temperatures rising as high as 80°C. Although the generation of heat accelerates the reaction, polymerisation of this self-curing resin occurs even if the temperature is reduced by irrigation with cool physiological saline solution.

Uses Palacos LV with Gentamicin bone cement is indicated for fixation of prostheses to bone in partial or total arthroplastic procedures of the hip, knee or other joints.

Dosage and administration A dose is prepared by mixing the entire contents of one packet of powder with one ampoule of liquid. One or two doses will usually suffice, although this will depend upon the specific surgical procedure and the techniques employed. (At least one extra unit of Palacos LV should be available before starting a surgical procedure.) The amount of material required and the timing of insertion are determined by the clinical judgement of the surgeon in each individual case.

The following are required for preparation of the bone cement: Sterile working area; sterile porcelain or stainless steel bowls; sterile porcelain or stainless steel mixing spoons or spatulas.

The polyethylene peel package and the blister pack are opened by a circulating nurse or assistant and the sterile paper packet and ampoule are aseptically placed on a sterile table. The paper packet and the ampoule are opened under sterile conditions.

The liquid is poured into a bowl and the powder is added.

Application: Low viscosity cements tend to be too fluid for convenient handling, and generally a higher viscosity form of the cement is recommended for manual insertion into the femoral canal and into the prepared acetabulum.

Application by hand: The mixture is stirred carefully for 20–30 seconds and left to stand until a dough-like mass is formed which does not adhere to rubber gloves. At this stage, the mass is kneadable and will remain so for about 2–3 minutes. The ideal working consistency of the Palacos LV for application to bone is best determined by the surgeon's experience. When the desired consistency is obtained, the preparation may be applied to bone and prosthesis as required. To ensure adequate fixation, the prosthesis should be inserted by five minutes and held securely in place without movement until the bone cement has fully hardened, generally eight to ten minutes after the start of mixing.

Injection from a cement gun: Mixing in the barrel of the cement gun may be difficult because Palacos LV with Gentamicin is rather liquid in the early stage of mixing and the bottom of the barrel is often not a tight enough fit to prevent leakage.

Hence, when using a cement gun, the same initial

procedure for mixing as described above is adopted. A double dose will generally be required. After 1 minute, the cement can be poured into the syringe. Cement can be injected from the gun from about 1.5 minutes onwards, but has to be controlled carefully by the surgeon, or it may flow out of the bony cavity as it is still runny at this stage. The use of a bone cement restrictor or a bone plug in the femoral canal is recommended. If the femoral canal is filled from the distal end, an air vent is not necessary. The implant should be in place by approximately 5½ minutes. The cement heats up at about 7½ minutes and polymerises generally by 9½ minutes.

Pressure should be applied to the cement, whether applied by hand or cement gun, until the prosthesis is inserted. Excess cement must be removed while it is still soft.

The longer time intervals when using a cement gun are due to reduced handling of the cement. Handling the cement warms it slightly during the early stages of polymerisation and accelerates the process.

The times given above for doughing, working and setting apply at approximately 23°C (73°F). Higher temperatures will shorten these times and lowering temperatures will prolong the times. If, during the surgical procedure, additional cement is required, another packet of powder and ampoule of liquid may be mixed as described above. The kneadable mass must be applied to the hardened cement without delay to form a continuous mass; delay will increase the risk of laminations forming in the relatively unsupported proximal end of the femur, with the possibility of resultant weakness in the cement core.

Since each pack contains premeasured quantities of components, care should be taken to mix the entire contents of one packet with the entire contents of one ampoule.

Kneading of the cement will produce evaporation of the volatile monomer, thereby reducing the amount to which the patient is exposed; however, if the kneading process is too long, the polymerisation may proceed to a point where the mass is no longer soft and pliable, making manipulation and application to bone difficult.

Contra-indications, warnings, etc
Contra-indications: Palacos LV with Gentamicin is contra-indicated in patients allergic to any of the components including gentamicin sulphate. If gentamicin or other aminoglycosides are needed prior to surgery, monitoring of trough serum concentrations should be performed on the day before operation. If serum concentrations are above 1 mcg/ml gentamicin, Palacos LV with gentamicin should not be used in surgery.

Warnings: Before using Palacos LV with Gentamicin, surgeons should be thoroughly familiar with its properties, handling characteristics and application to arthroplasty. (See Presentation, Precautions, and Dosage and Administration.) It is advisable for the surgeon to go through the entire mixing, handling and setting process before using the material in an actual surgical procedure.

The liquid monomer is highly volatile and flammable and appropriate caution should be taken with its use. It is also a potent lipid solvent, may irritate the respiratory tract and eyes and may possibly be harmful to the liver. Direct contact of the monomer with any part of the body or with rubber, including surgical rubber gloves, should be avoided. Care should be taken during the mixing to prevent excessive exposure to concentrated monomer vapours; mixing should take place in a well ventilated part of the operating theatre, or a vacuum device or protective mask should be used.

The completion of polymerisation occurs in the patient and is associated with the liberation of heat. The long-term effects of this heat on the tissues surrounding the bone cement are not known.

Long-term durability, wearability and stability of the polymerised bone cement *in situ* are unknown. The long-term effects of this preparation are unknown. Safety of use in children has not been established. This should be considered in light of the expected longevity of the patients for whom the substance will be used. Thus the physician should decide whether the benefits expected from its use outweigh any possible long-term adverse effects.

There is no evidence of the safety of use of bone cement, gentamicin or associated surgical procedures in pregnancy or lactation.

If use of systemic aminoglycosides is necessary post operatively, these should only be given with simultaneous monitoring and not within 24 h following the operation.

The low viscosity characteristics of Palacos LV result in greater penetration of the cement with resulting increase in surface area. This results in increased release of gentamicin. Thus there may be a potential transient risk affecting renal function; in this event serum monitoring is recommended.

Neuromuscular blockade and respiratory paralysis has been reported with systemic gentamicin, especially in patients receiving concomitant neuromuscular blocking agents. This effect may be reversed by calcium salts.

Precautions: Blood pressure, pulse and respiration should be carefully monitored during and immediately after the operation. Any significant alteration in these vital signs should be corrected with appropriate measures. Thus it is advisable that the surgeon informs the anaesthetist at the time of insertion.

Palacos LV with Gentamicin should be applied to clean dry bone.

Adverse reactions: Transient fall in blood pressure immediately after implantation of the bone cement and endo-prosthesis is frequently observed. Rare cases have been reported in which the hypotension was associated with cardiac arrest and sudden death.

The following additional adverse reactions have been reported with joint replacement surgery involving acrylic bone cements. The contribution of the cementing procedure to these is not established: Thrombophlebitis; pulmonary embolism; superficial wound infection; haemorrhage and haematoma; loosening or displacement of the prosthesis; heterotopic new bone; short-term irregularities in cardiac conduction; deep wound infection; trochanteric bursitis; trochanteric separation; myocardial infarction; cerebrovascular accident.

Pharmaceutical precautions Do not store the liquid component above 30°C (86°F) or in direct sunlight to prevent premature polymerisation. Sterility is only guaranteed if the containers are undamaged. Resterilisation of any of the components should not be attempted.

Legal category POM.

Package quantities
Palacos LV-40 with Gentamicin: Carton consisting of 2 packets, each containing 41.7 g sterilised powder (polymer); 2 ampoules, each containing 20 ml of sterilised liquid monomer.
Palacos LV-30 with Gentamicin: Carton consisting of: 2 packets, each containing 31.3 g sterilised powder (polymer); 2 ampoules, each containing 15 ml of sterilised liquid monomer.

Further information Nil.

Product licence number 0201/0085.

PALACOS* R

Presentation Palacos R is a radio-opaque, rapidly setting bone cement. It is water soluble and heat stable.

Two separate, premeasured, sterilised components are mixed to form the cement, which is pigmented light green in order to make it more clearly visible in the operative field.

Component 1 is a powder (polymer) with the following composition:

Methylmethacrylate-methylacrylate co-polymer	33.80 g
Benzoyl peroxide	0.20 g
Zirconium dioxide	6.00 g
Chlorophyll	0.001 g

Component 2, supplied in an amber ampoule, is a liquid (monomer) with the following composition:

Methylmethacrylate monomer (stabilised with hydroquinone)	18.40 g
N,N-dimethyl-p-toluidine	0.40 g
Chlorophyll	0.0004 g

The liquid monomer is sterile filtered. The powder polymer is sterilised by ethylene oxide.

Note: Component 1 – Palacos R powder polymer is double packaged. Each polyethylene peel pack is contained in an outer aluminium/paper protective foil which is NON-STERILE. Each peel-pack contains a STERILE polyethylene paper coated packet of powder polymer.

Component 2 – Palacos R liquid monomer is contained in an ampoule enclosed in a protective plastic blister pack, the inside of which is STERILE.

When the powder (polymer) and liquid (monomer) are mixed, the polymerisation catalyst (benzoyl peroxide) is activated initiating polymerisation of the monomer and binding together of polymer granules. As polymerisation continues to take place a dough-like mass is formed which, after 5 to 6 minutes hardens into a solid, mechanically uniform complex. The temperature of the reaction rises as high as 80°C accelerating polymerisation. However, self-curing of the resin takes place even if the temperature is reduced by irrigation with a cool physiological saline solution.

Uses Palacos R is indicated for fixation of prostheses to bone in partial or total arthroplastic procedures of the hip, knee or other joints.

Dosage and administration One dose is prepared by mixing the entire contents of one packet of powder polymer (Component 1) with the entire contents of one ampoule of liquid monomer (Component 2) i.e. 40 g powder plus 20 ml liquid. Each dose must be prepared separately. The number of doses prepared will depend on the surgical procedure and technique to be used.

The following items will be required for preparation of the bone cement: Sterile working area; sterile porcelain or stainless steel bowls; sterile porcelain or stainless steel mixing spoons or spatulas.

The following steps should be followed:

1. The polyethylene peel package and the blister pack are opened by a circulating nurse or assistant, placing the sterile paper inner packet and ampoule on to a sterile table.
2. Paper packet and ampoule are opened under sterile conditions.
3. The liquid is poured into a bowl.
4. The powder is added to the liquid.

(*NB* The liquid *must not* be added to the powder).

5. Stir the mixture vigorously, but carefully, for 30–40 seconds until a dough-like mass, which does not adhere to rubber gloves, is formed.

At this stage the mass is kneadable and will only remain so for 4–5 minutes. The ideal working consistency of the bone cement for application is best determined by the surgeon's experience with the preparation.

6. When the desired consistency is obtained the preparation can be applied to bone and prosthesis as required. It is important to apply adequate pressure.
7. The prosthesis should be held securely in place without movement until the bone cement has fully hardened (7–8 minutes after mixing the powder and liquid).
8. Excessive cement is removed whilst it is still soft.

The above doughing, working and setting times apply at approximately 23°C (73°F). An increase in temperature will shorten and a decrease will lengthen these times.

Kneading of the material will assist in the evaporation of excess monomer, and hence decrease the amount to which the patient will be exposed. However, excessive kneading will produce a non-pliable mass, which is very difficult to manipulate and to apply to bone successfully.

Heat continues to be released when the material has been applied, as polymerisation proceeds and the cement hardens. The long term effects of this heat on surrounding tissues is not known, but irrigation of the site with cool physiological saline solution will help to dissipate the heat more rapidly.

To prepare additional amounts of cement use another whole packet of powder polymer and a whole ampoule of liquid monomer using the procedure described above. The entire contents of each must be used. The kneadable mass should then be applied immediately to previously hardened bone cement to ensure reliable fixation.

Contra-indications, warnings, etc
Contra-indications: Palacos R is contra-indicated in patients allergic to any of its components.

Warnings: Prior to using Palacos R surgeons should be thoroughly familiar with its properties, handling characteristics and application to arthroplasty (see Presentation; Precautions; Dosage and Preparation).

Surgeons are advised to perform the entire mixing, handling and setting procedure prior to using the materials in an actual surgical procedure. The liquid monomer is highly volatile and flammable. Care must be exercised during the mixing of the two components, which should take place in a well ventilated area. This will help to prevent excessive exposure to the concentrated vapours of the monomer, which can irritate the respiratory tract, the eyes and may be harmful to the liver. If possible a proprietary vacuum extractor or appropriate masks can be used.

The monomer is also a potent lipid solvent and should not be allowed to come into direct contact with the body. Skin reactions have been reported after contact with the monomer. Contact of the liquid monomer with rubber, including surgical gloves, should also be avoided.

The long-term effects of this preparation are unknown. Thus the physician should decide whether the benefits of its use outweigh any possible adverse effects. The long term durability, stability and wearability of the bone cement *in situ* have not been examined. This should be considered in light of the expected longevity of the prospective patient.

Precautions: Any significant alteration in blood pressures, pulse and respiration should be corrected immediately with appropriate measures. Monitoring of these vital signs should take place during and immediately after implantation of bone cement.

Adverse reactions: Transient fall in blood pressure immediately after implantation of bone cement and endo-prosthesis is frequently observed. Rare cases have been reported in which the hypotension was associated with cardiac arrest and sudden death.

The following adverse reactions have been associated with joint replacement surgery:

Thrombophlebitis	Superficial wound infection
Pulmonary embolism	Deep wound infection
Haemorrhage and haematoma	Trochanteric bursitis
Loosening or displacement of the prosthesis	Trochanteric separation

Others which have been observed:

Heterotopic new bone	Myocardial infarction
Short term irregularities in cardiac conduction	Cerebrovascular accident

Pharmaceutical precautions To prevent premature polymerisation, do not store components above 30°C (86°F) or in direct sunlight. Resterilisation of any of the components must not be attempted under any circumstances.

Legal category POM.

Package quantities Palacos R – Two 40 g packets of radio-opaque sterile powder polymer. Two 20 ml ampoules of sterile liquid monomer.

Further information Nil.

Product licence number 3478/0008.

PALACOS* R WITH GENTAMICIN PALACOS* R-20 WITH GENTAMICIN

Presentation Palacos R with Gentamicin and Palacos R-20 with Gentamicin is a radio-opaque, rapidly setting bone cement, which contains the antibiotic gentamicin. Gentamicin is a broad spectrum bactericidal aminoglycoside antibiotic having activity against Gram-negative and some Gram-positive bacteria. It is water soluble and heat stable.

Two separate, premeasured, sterilised components are mixed to form the cement, which is pigmented light green in order to make it more clearly visible in the operative field.

Component 1 is a powder (polymer) with the following composition:

	Palacos R with Gentamicin	Palacos R-20 with Gentamicin
Methylmethacrylate–methylacrylate co-polymer	33.80 g	16.9 g
Benzoyl peroxide	0.20 g	0.10 g
Zirconium dioxide	6.00 g	3.00 g
Chlorophyll	0.001 g	0.0005 g
Gentamicin (as the sulphate)	0.50 g	0.25 g

Component 2, supplied in an amber ampoule, is a liquid (monomer) with the following composition:

	Palacos R with Gentamicin	Palacos R-20 with Gentamicin
methylmethacrylate monomer (stabilised with hydroquinone)	18.40 g	9.20 g
N,N-dimethyl-p-toluidine	0.40 g	0.20 g
Chlorophyll	0.0004 g	0.0002 g

The liquid monomer is sterile filtered. The powder polymer and Gentamicin mixture is sterilised by ethylene oxide.

Note: Component 1 – powder polymer plus Gentamicin is double packaged. Each polyethylene peel pack is contained in an outer aluminium/paper protective foil which is NON-STERILE. Each peel-pack contains a STERILE polyethylene paper coated packet of powder polymer plus Gentamicin.

Component 2 – liquid monomer is contained in an ampoule enclosed in a protective plastic blister pack, the inside of which is STERILE.

When the powder (polymer) and liquid (monomer) are mixed, the polymerisation catalyst (benzoyl peroxide) is activated, initiating polymerisation of the monomer and binding together of polymer granules. As polymerisation continues to take place a dough-like mass is formed which, after 5 to 6 minutes hardens into a solid, mechanically uniform complex. The temperature of the reaction rises as high as 80°C accelerating polymerisation. However, self-curing of the resin takes place even if the temperature is reduced by irrigation with a cool physiological saline solution.

In man, following total hip replacement where Palacos R with Gentamicin was used, the antibiotic has been found in joint fluid, blood and urine. Concentrations in the urine have been detected for up to 3 weeks after surgery, suggesting good release of antibiotic. In vitro, Gentamicin has been shown to be released in active form from the bone cement complex for periods of greater than one year.

Uses Palacos R with Gentamicin and Palacos R-20 with Gentamicin bone cement is indicated for fixation of prostheses to bone in partial or total arthroplastic procedures of the hip, knee or other joints when infection by Gentamicin-sensitive organisms is a potential risk.

Dosage and administration One dose is prepared by mixing the entire contents of one packet of powder polymer (Component 1) with the entire contents of one ampoule of liquid monomer (Component 2) i.e. 40 g powder plus 20 ml liquid OR 20 g powder plus 10 ml liquid. Each dose must be prepared separately. The number of doses prepared will depend on the surgical procedure and technique to be used.

The following items will be required for preparation of the bone cement: Sterile working area; sterile porcelain or stainless steel bowls; sterile porcelain or stainless steel mixing spoons or spatulas.

The following steps should be followed:

1. The polyethylene peel package and the blister pack are opened by a circulating nurse or assistant, placing the sterile paper inner packet and ampoule on to a sterile table.
2. Paper packet and ampoule are opened under sterile conditions.
3. The liquid is poured into a bowl.
4. The powder is added to the liquid.

(*NB.* The liquid *must not* be added to the powder).

5. Stir the mixture vigorously, but carefully, for 30–40 seconds until a dough-like mass, which does not adhere to rubber gloves, is formed.

At this stage the mass is kneadable and will only remain so for 4–5 minutes. The ideal working consistency of the bone cement for application is best determined by the surgeon's experience with the preparation.

6. When the desired consistency is obtained the preparation can be applied to bone and prosthesis as required. It is important to apply adequate pressure.
7. The prosthesis should be held securely in place without movement until the bone cement has fully hardened (7–8 minutes after mixing the powder and liquid).
8. Excessive cement is removed whilst it is still soft.

The above doughing, working and setting times apply at approximately 23°C (73°F). An increase in temperature will shorten and a decrease will lengthen these times.

Kneading of the material will assist in the evaporation of excess monomer, and hence decrease the amount to which the patient will be exposed. However, excessive kneading will produce a non-pliable mass, which is very difficult to manipulate and to apply to bone successfully.

Heat continues to be released when the material has been applied, as polymerisation proceeds and the cement hardens. The long term effects of this heat on surrounding tissues is not known, but irrigation of the site with cool physiological saline solution will help to dissipate the heat even more rapidly.

To prepare additional amounts of cement use another whole packet of powder polymer and a whole ampoule of liquid monomer using the procedure described above. The entire contents of each must be used. The kneadable mass should then be applied immediately to previously hardened bone cement to ensure reliable fixation.

Contra-indications, warnings, etc
Contra-indications: Palacos R with Gentamicin and Palacos R-20 with Gentamicin is contra-indicated in patients allergic to any of its components.

Warnings: Prior to using Palacos R with Gentamicin or Palacos R-20 with Gentamicin surgeons should be thoroughly familiar with its properties, handling characteristics and application to arthroplasty (see Presentation; Precautions; Dosage and Preparation).

Surgeons are advised to perform the entire mixing, handling and setting procedure prior to using the materials in an actual surgical procedure. The liquid monomer is highly volatile and flammable. Care must be exercised during the mixing of the two components, which should take place in a well ventilated area. This will help to prevent excessive exposure to the concentrated vapours of the monomer, which can irritate the respiratory tract, the eyes and may be harmful to the liver. If possible a proprietary vacuum extractor or appropriate masks can be used.

The monomer is also a potent lipid solvent and should not be allowed to come into direct contact with the body. Skin reactions have been reported after contact with the monomer. Contact of the liquid monomer with rubber, including surgical gloves, should also be avoided.

The long term effects of this preparation are unknown. Thus the physician should decide whether the benefits of its use outweigh any possible adverse effects. The long term durability, stability and wearability of the bone cement *in situ* have not been examined. This should be considered in light of the expected longevity of the prospective patient.

Precautions: Any significant alteration in blood pressure, pulse and respiration should be corrected immediately with appropriate measures. Monitoring of these vital signs should take place during and immediately after implantation of the bone cement.

Adverse reactions: Transient fall in blood pressure immediately after implantation of bone cement and endo-prosthesis is frequently observed. Rare cases have been reported in which the hypotension was associated with cardiac arrest and sudden death.

The following adverse reactions have been associated with joint replacement surgery:

Thrombophlebitis	Superficial wound infection
Pulmonary embolism	Deep wound infection
Haemorrhage and haematoma	Trochanteric bursitis
Loosening or displacement of the prosthesis	Trochanteric separation

Others which have been observed:

Heterotopic new bone	Myocardial infarction
Short-term irregularities in cardiac conduction	Cerebrovascular accident

Since the concentration of gentamicin reaching the VIII nerve and the kidney will be quite low, ototoxic and nephrotoxic reactions are very unlikely to result from the use of Palacos R with Gentamicin and Palacos R-20 with Gentamicin. No such events have been reported for these products. Hypersensitivity to gentamicin has been reported only rarely.

Pharmaceutical precautions To prevent premature polymerisation, do not store components above 30°C (86°F) or in direct sunlight. Resterilisation of any of the components must not be attempted under any circumstances.

Legal category POM.

Package quantities Palacos R with Gentamicin – Two 40 g packets of radio-opaque sterile powder polymer containing 0.5 g Gentamicin base per packet. Two 20 ml ampoules of sterile liquid monomer.

Palacos R-20 with Gentamicin – Two 20 g packets of radio-opaque sterile powder polymer containing 0.25 g Gentamicin base per packet. Two 10 ml ampoules of sterile liquid monomer.

Further information Nil.

Product licence number 3478/0009.

TINADERM*-M CREAM

Presentation Each gram of Tinaderm-M Cream contains 10 mg of tolnaftate and 100,000 units of Nystatin in a white, water-washable, vanishing cream base.

Uses Tinaderm-M Cream is recommended for the topical treatment of cutaneous mycotic infections such as Tinea pedis, Tinea cruris, Tinea corporis, Tinea barbae and Tinea manuum due to Trichophyton rubrum, T. mentagrophytes, T. tonsurans, Microsporum canis, M. audouinii, Epidermophyton floccosum, Candida (monilia) albicans and Tinea versicolor (Malassezia furfur).

If Candida albicans is the primary cause of infections, such conditions as 'Athlete's foot' (dermatophytosis), perleche, paronychia, intertrigo, 'nappy rash' and other cutaneous lesions can be successfully treated with Tinaderm-M.

Tinaderm-M is particularly recommended for the treatment of fungal infections localised in intertriginous and other moist areas of the skin where Candida infections are present or likely to develop.

Dosage and administration A sufficient quantity of Tinaderm-M should be applied to completely cover the affected area two or three times daily until healing is complete. Lesions generally begin to clear during the first treatment week and disappear completely after two to three weeks of treatment. If thickening of skin has occurred, treatment for as long as 4–6 weeks may be required. The concomitant use of a mild keratolytic agent may be indicated in areas where the skin has become hyperkeratotic. Use of wet compresses prior to application of Tinaderm-M aids in the healing of exudative lesions and does not interfere with the fungicidal action of the medication. Surgical debridement of dead skin and treatment of calluses is advised when necessary.

If after four weeks of therapy there has not been a progressive improvement, diagnosis should be reconfirmed. Mycosis complicated by bacterial infections may require additional antibiotic treatment.

Contra-indications, warnings, etc Tinaderm-M should not be administered to patients with known hypersensitivity to any ingredients. Should sensitivity occur, discontinue use.

Keep away from eyes and mucous membranes. In mixed infections caused by non-susceptible bacteria or fungi, supplementary topical or systemic anti-infective therapy is indicated.

Tinaderm-M is for dermatological use only.

Side-effects: A few cases of mild irritation and sensitisation have been reported.

Pharmaceutical precautions There are no pharmaceutical precautions for Tinaderm-M.

Legal category POM.

Package quantities Tinaderm-M is available in 20 g tubes.

Further information Tolnaftate is a highly active, nonsensitising, fungicidal agent that is very effective in the treatment of superficial fungal infections of the skin. Nystatin, an antibiotic with antifungal activity, provides specific therapy for all localised forms of moniliasis.

Tinaderm-M Cream does not ordinarily sting or irritate intact or broken skin and is inactive systemically. Tinaderm-M Cream will not stain or discolour skin, hair, nails or clothing.

Product licence number 0201/0071.

**Trade Mark*

Schwarz Pharma Limited
Schwarz House
East Street
Chesham
Bucks HP5 1DG

SCHWARZ PHARMA

DEPONIT* 5
DEPONIT* 10

Presentation Deponit is a transdermal drug delivery system in the form of a self-adhesive, clear patch. Deponit contains 1 mg of glyceryl trinitrate per cm^2 of surface area. Deponit 5 has a surface area of 16 cm^2 (containing 16 mg glyceryl trinitrate), and Deponit 10 has a surface area of 32 cm^2 (containing 32 mg glyceryl trinitrate). Each patch is designed to release glyceryl trinitrate at the average fixed rates of 5 mg and 10 mg respectively per 24 hours.

Uses Deponit is indicated for the prophylaxis of angina pectoris either alone, or in combination with other anti-anginal therapy. The glyceryl trinitrate is formulated in the adhesive layer in the form of dissolved and adsorbed molecules. By simple diffusion across the skin, the active constituent is thus released at a fixed rate per 24 hours.

Glyceryl trinitrate reduces the tone of vascular smooth muscle. This action is more marked on the venous capacitance vessels than the arterial vessels. There is a reduction in venous return to the heart and a lowering of elevated filling pressure. This lowering of filling pressure reduces the left ventricular end diastolic volume and preload. The net effect is a reduction in myocardial oxygen consumption.

Systemic vascular resistance, pulmonary vascular resistance and arterial pressure are also reduced and there is a net reduction in afterload.

Glyceryl trinitrate improves the myocardial oxygen supply by redistributing the blood flow along collateral channels and from the epicardial to the endocardial regions.

Dosage and administration
Adults: One patch to be applied to the lateral chest wall daily. The treatment should be started with Deponit 5. If the patient response is considered inadequate, the larger Deponit 10 patch should be substituted.

Children: The safety and efficacy of Deponit in children has yet to be established.

Each patch is packaged in individually sealed sachets and should only be removed prior to administration. There is a convenient break in the covering foil which can be easily peeled off by the patient. The exposed patch may then be applied to the lateral chest wall and should be removed after no longer than 24 hours.

Subsequent applications should always be made to a new area of skin and several days should be allowed to elapse before applying a fresh patch to the same area.

There is evidence to suggest that tolerance or an attenuation of effect with all nitrates can occur during long-term therapy unless blood levels of the drug are sufficiently low during several hours of each day. Whilst Deponit is designed to avoid levels normally associated with this phenomenon there may be some patients who would benefit from a dosage regimen in which the daily patch is applied 1–2 hours after removal of the previous one.

Use in the elderly: No specific information on use in the elderly is available, but there is no evidence to suggest that an alteration in dose is required.

Contra-indications, warnings, etc
Contra-indications: Deponit should not be given to patients who are sensitive to nitrates or with increased intracranial pressure. Marked anaemia, acute circulatory failure (shock) or severe hypotension are other contra-indications to Deponit.

Side-effects: Headaches may develop initially, but these will usually disappear after a few days. There is also the possibility of reflex tachycardia. Postural hypotension, syncope and dizziness occur rarely, and these effects may be potentiated by alcohol. Nausea may also occur infrequently.

Allergic reactions may occur in sensitive patients.

When the patch is removed, there may be a slight reddening of the skin which will usually subside in a few hours.

Precautions: Deponit should not be used during pregnancy or lactation unless considered absolutely essential by the physician.

Deponit is not suitable for acute anginal attacks. If these occur during therapy then additional medication should be considered. Deponit dilates peripheral blood vessels and may increase the antihypertensive properties of vasodilators, calcium antagonists, tricyclic antidepressants and alcohol.

In patients with a recent history of myocardial infarction or acute heart failure, Deponit should be used with caution. As with all anti-anginal nitrate preparations, withdrawal of treatment should be gradual (over 4–6 weeks) by replacement with decreasing doses of long-acting oral nitrates. This product should be used with extreme caution in patients pre-disposed to closed angle glaucoma.

Pharmaceutical precautions Store below 25°C.

Legal category P.

Package quantities Deponit 5 and 10 are packaged in cartons of 30 patches.

Further information Deponit consists of an adhesive layer containing glyceryl trinitrate which is approximately 300 μm thick.

When applied to the skin, Deponit adheres to the whole area of application without risk of becoming detached even during activities like swimming and bathing.

Glyceryl trinitrate is also known as nitroglycerin, trinitrin or trinitroglycerin.

Product licence numbers
Deponit 5 4438/0014
Deponit 10 4438/0016

ELANTAN* 10
ELANTAN* 20
ELANTAN* 40

Presentation White tablets with break-score containing isosorbide mononitrate. The tablets are available in three strengths: Elantan 10 (marked E10), Elantan 20 (marked E20) and Elantan 40 (marked E40) containing isosorbide mononitrate 10 mg, 20 mg and 40 mg respectively.

Uses
Prophylaxis of angina pectoris: Elantan 10, 20 and 40 are indicated for the prophylaxis of angina pectoris.

Congestive heart failure: Elantan 20 and 40 are indicated as adjunctive therapy in chronic congestive heart failure not responding to cardiac glycosides or diuretics.

Dosage and administration The tablets should be taken unchewed with a little water after meals.

Adults:
Angina prophylaxis: Elantan 20, one tablet two or three times a day. Elantan 40, one tablet to be taken twice a day. For patients not already receiving prophylactic nitrate therapy it is recommended that the initial dose be one tablet of Elantan 10 twice a day.

Congestive heart failure: Elantan 20, one tablet to be taken two or three times a day. Elantan 40, one tablet to be taken twice a day. The dosage may be increased up to 120 mg per day.

Elderly: There is no evidence to suggest that an adjustment of the dosage is necessary.

Children: The safety and efficacy of Elantan has yet to be established in children.

Contra-indications, warnings, etc
Contra-indications: Elantan should not be used in cases of acute myocardial infarction with low filling pressures, acute circulatory failure (shock, vascular collapse) or very low blood pressure.

This product should not be given to patients with a known sensitivity to nitrates.

Elantan should not be used in patients with marked anaemia, head trauma, cerebral haemorrhage, severe hypotension or hypovolaemia.

Precautions and warnings: This preparation may give rise to postural hypotension and syncope. In order to avoid precipitating symptoms in patients at risk, treatment should be started with one tablet of Elantan 10 morning and evening.

Some of the effects of alcohol may be potentiated by this agent.

Elantan should be used with caution in patients who are pre-disposed to closed angle glaucoma.

Headache may occur as a side-effect, it is also a sign of overdose. Usually the headache subsides after a few days.

Elantan should be used with caution in patients suffering from hypothyroidism, hypothermia, malnutrition, severe liver or renal disease.

Symptoms of circulatory collapse may arise after the first dose in patients with labile circulation and patients already taking ACE inhibitors.

Use in pregnancy and lactation: There is inadequate evidence of safety of the drug in human pregnancy but nitrates have been used widely in the treatment of angina for many years without apparent ill consequence, animal studies having shown no hazard. Nevertheless it is not advisable to use this drug during pregnancy and lactation.

Overdose: Overdosage may lead to vascular collapse and gastric lavage is indicated in severe cases. Further measures to support the circulation are recommended, e.g. elevating the legs and/or treatment with hypertensive agents.

Pharmaceutical precautions None.

Legal category
Elantan 10 P.
Elantan 20 and 40 POM.

Package quantities Elantan 10 is blister packed in cartons of 50 tablets. Elantan 20 and 40 are blister packed in cartons of 50 and 100 tablets.

Further information Isosorbide mononitrate is the British approved name for Isosorbide 5-mononitrate.

Elantan lacks any significant first pass metabolism providing consistently uniform plasma levels of Isosorbide mononitrate thereby laying the foundation for improved clinical response.

Product licence numbers
Elantan 10 4438/0018
Elantan 20 4438/0005
Elantan 40 4438/0008

ELANTAN* LA50

Presentation Pink/dark pink, opaque gelatin capsules containing 50 mg Isosorbide mononitrate, in a slow release formulation.

Use For the prophylaxis of angina pectoris.

Dosage and administration The capsules are for oral administration and should be swallowed whole.

Adults: One capsule to be taken in the morning.

Children: The safety and efficacy of Elantan LA 50 has yet to be established in children.

Elderly: There is no evidence to suggest an adjustment of the dosage is necessary.

Contra-indications, warnings, etc
Contra-indications: Elantan LA 50 should not be used in cases of acute myocardial infarction with low filling pressures, acute circulatory failure (shock, vascular collapse), severe hypotension or hypovolemia.

Elantan LA 50 should not be given to patients with a known sensitivity to nitrates, marked anaemia, head trauma, cerebral haemorrhage, or cardiovascular insufficiency.

Warnings: A headache may occur at the start of treatment but this usually disappears after a few days.

Precautions: Elantan LA 50 should be used with caution in patients who are pre-disposed to closed angle glaucoma or are suffering from hypothyroidism, hypothermia, malnutrition, severe liver or severe renal disease.

Symptoms of circulatory collapse may arise after the first dose, particularly in patients with labile circulation.

Symptoms of postural hypotension and synope may result in some patients.

Interactions: Some of the effects of alcohol, and the action of hypotensive drugs may be potentiated by this product.

Use in pregnancy and lactation: There is inadequate evidence of safety and efficacy of isosorbide mononitrate in human pregnancy. The use of this product should therefore be avoided during pregnancy, and by breast-feeding mothers.

Overdosage: Overdosage may lead to vascular collapse and gastric lavage is indicated in severe cases. Further measures to support the circulation are recommended, such as elevating the legs and/or treatment with hypertensive agents.

Pharmaceutical precautions None.

Legal category P.

Package quantities Elantan LA 50 are available in 'original packs' of 28 capsules.

Further information Isosorbide mononitrate lacks any significant first pass metabolism providing consistently uniform plasma levels.

Elantan LA 50 capsules are designed to release 30% of the dose initially, to ensure rapid attainment of therapeutic nitrate plasma levels. The remaining 70% is released over a prolonged period to provide long lasting effect, thus giving the convenience of once-daily dosing. Nitrate plasma levels, 17 hours after an oral dose, fall below 100 nanograms/millilitre, thus reducing the risk of tolerance development during chronic therapy.

Isosorbide mononitrate is the British Approved Name for isosorbide 5-mononitrate.

Product licence number 4438/0015.

HYPERTANE* 50

Presentation White, round, flat, bevel-edged tablets marked HYPERTANE 50 with break-line on the reverse, each containing 5 mg amiloride hydrochloride and 50 mg Hydrochlorothiazide BP.

Uses Hypertane 50 is an antihypertensive and potassium-conserving diuretic.

Hypertane 50 is indicated in patients with congestive heart failure, hypertension, or hepatic cirrhosis with ascites, particularly where potassium balance is important.

Dosage and administration The dosage should be determined by rate of weight loss (ideal target being 0.5 to 1.0 kg per day) and serum electrolyte level.

Adults: Usually 1 or 2 tablets once a day, or in divided doses. The dosage should not exceed 4 tablets a day.

After initial diuresis has been achieved, a reduction in dosage should be attempted for maintenance therapy.

Children: Hypertane 50 is not recommended for use in children.

Elderly: Hypertane 50 should be used with particular care in the elderly since they are more susceptible to electrolyte imbalances. The dosage should be carefully adjusted to renal function and clinical response.

Contra-indications, warnings, etc

Contra-indications: Hyperkalaemia (serum potassium over 5.5 mmol/l): hypercalcaemia: other potassium-conserving diuretics and potassium supplements; severe progressive renal disease and acute renal failure; severe hepatic failure; Addison's disease; diabetic nephropathy; anuria; patients with blood urea over 10 mmol/l or serum creatinine over 130 micromol/l in whom serum electrolyte and blood urea levels cannot be monitored frequently or carefully; concurrent administration with lithium; known sensitivity to amiloride or hydrochlorothiazide.

Precautions

Diabetes mellitus: Hyperkalaemia can occur in diabetics on amiloride hydrochloride, especially those with chronic renal disease. Renal function status should be determined before Hypertane 50 is given to known or suspected diabetics. Hypertane 50 should be discontinued before giving a glucose-tolerance test. Adjustments to the insulin requirements of diabetic patients may be necessary. Latent diabetes mellitus may become manifest during thiazide therapy.

Hyperkalaemia: (serum potassium level over 5.5 mmol/l). Hyperkalaemia has been observed in patients receiving amiloride hydrochloride (either alone or in combination with other diuretics), particularly in the aged; diabetics; and seriously ill patients who were undergoing vigorous diuretic therapy. Careful observation of such patients for manifestation of hyperkalaemia using clinical, laboratory and ECG evidence should be undertaken.

In the event hyperkalaemia develops, Hypertane 50 should be discontinued immediately and, if necessary, active measures should be taken to reduce the serum potassium levels to normal.

Metabolic or respiratory acidosis: Potassium-conserving therapy should be initiated with caution in severely ill patients likely to experience respiratory or metabolic acidosis, e.g. with decompensated diabetes or cardiopulmonary disease. The development of acidosis may be associated with rapid increases in serum potassium.

Effects in cirrhotic patients: Patients with hepatic cirrhosis are intolerant of acute shifts in electrolyte balance and often have pre-existing hypokalaemia, as a result of associated aldosteronism. These patients are more likely to experience adverse reactions with diuretic therapy. Hepatic encephalopathy manifested by confusion, tremors and coma have been reported in patients on amiloride hydrochloride. Patients with liver disease should be observed for this complication when Hypertane 50 is given. A deepening of jaundice has occurred in cirrhotic patients receiving amiloride hydrochloride alone, but the relationship to treatment is uncertain.

Other precautions: In post-sympathectomy patients, the antihypertensive action of thiazides may be enhanced.

Orthostatic hypotension may occur. Serum uric acid levels may rise during treatment with Hypertane 50 and may precipitate acute attacks of gout.

Serum PBI levels may be decreased without signs of thyroid disturbance.

Thiazides should be discontinued before carrying out tests for parathyroid function.

Use in pregnancy and lactation: Thiazides appear in breast milk and cross the placental barrier, appearing in cord blood.

Pregnancy: Hypertane 50 is not recommended for use during pregnancy. Benefits of treatment must be weighed against possible hazards to the foetus which include thrombocytopaenia, foetal or neonatal jaundice, bone marrow depression.

Lactation: Mothers should stop nursing during treatment.

Drug interactions: The hypotensive effects of other antihypertensive agents, alcohol, barbiturates and narcotics may be potentiated. The dosage of concurrently administered cardiac glycosides or antihypertensive agents may require adjustment.

Risk of lithium toxicity is increased with Hypertane 50 (see 'Contra-indications').

Arterial responsiveness to noradrenaline may be slightly decreased by Hypertane 50.

Side-effects: Sensitivity reactions to thiazides may occur.

Gastrointestinal upsets (e.g. nausea, vomiting, diarrhoea, constipation, anorexia), minor psychiatric disturbances (e.g. restlessness, insomnia) and disturbances in liver function tests have been reported.

Effects related to dehydration through diuresis (e.g. muscle cramps, dry mouth, etc) may also occur.

Skin rashes, photosensitivity reactions and blood dyscrasias including thrombocytopenia have infrequently been reported, in which cases treatment should be withdrawn.

Overdosage: No specific antidote is available. Treatment of overdosage should be aimed at reversing dehydration and correcting electrolyte imbalance. Supportive measures include emesis or gastric lavage. In particular, if hyperkalaemia occurs, measures should be taken to reduce serum potassium levels.

Pharmaceutical precautions Store below 25°C in a dry place, protected from light.

Legal category POM.

Package quantities Containers of 500 tablets (for hospital use only).

Further information Nil.

Product licence number 0225/0064

Product licence holder: DDSA Pharmaceuticals Limited, 10 Old Brompton Road, London SW5 9JO.

ISOKET* 0.1%
ISOKET* 0.05%

Presentation

Isoket 0.1% (Isosorbide dinitrate 1 mg/ml) in 10 ml ampoules, 50 ml, 100 ml bottles.

Isoket 0.05% (Isosorbide dinitrate 0.5 mg/ml) in 50 ml bottles.

Both Isoket 0.1% and 0.05% contain Isosorbide dinitrate in sterile isotonic saline, no other additives (e.g. potassium, alcohol, propylene glycol) are present.

Uses

1. Isoket (0.1% and 0.05%) is indicated in the treatment of unresponsive left ventricular failure, secondary to acute myocardial infarction, or of various aetiology.
2. Osoket (0.1% and 0.05%) is indicated in the treatment of severe or unstable angina pectoris.
3. Isoket (0.1% and 0.05%) is indicated for intracoronary use during Percutaneous Transluminal Coronary Angioplasty, to facilitate prolongation of balloon inflation and to prevent or relieve coronary spasm.

Dosage and administration

Dosage

1. Intravenous

Adults and Elderly: The dose employed must be adjusted

according to patient response. Generally a dose of between 2 mg and 12 mg per hour is suitable, although doses as high as 20 mg per hour may be required.

Children: The safety and efficacy of Isoket has not yet been established in children.

2. Intra-coronary
The usual dose is 1 mg given as a bolus, prior to balloon inflation. Further doses may be given not exceeding 5 mg, within a 30 minute period.

Administration *1. Isoket 0.1%*—This is a concentrated solution, it should never be injected directly and *must be diluted.* Suitable vehicles to form an admixture are Sodium Chloride injection BP or Dextrose injection BP.

For example, if a dose of 6 mg per hour is required, 50 ml of Isoket 0.1% should be added to 450 ml of a suitable vehicle under aseptic conditions. The resultant admixture (500 ml), contains 100 micrograms/ml (1 mg/10 ml) Isosorbide dinitrate. To achieve the required dosage of 6 mg per hour, an infusion rate of 60 ml per hour (equivalent to 60 paediatric microdrops *or* 20 standard drops per minute) is required. At such an infusion rate, this admixture would provide an infusion time of 8 hours 20 minutes.

Should it be necessary to reduce fluid intake, 100 ml of Isoket 0.1% may be diluted to 500 ml using a suitable vehicle. The resultant solution now contains 200 micrograms/ml, (2 mg/10 ml) Isosorbide dinitrate. The required dose (6 mg/hour) can be achieved with an infusion rate of 30 ml/hour (equivalent to 30 paediatric microdrops or 10 standard drops per minute).

In cases where fluid intake is strictly limited, or for intra-coronary administration, a dilution of 50% is advocated to produce a solution containing 0.5 mg/ml.

2. Isoket 0.05%—Can be administered undiluted using a syringe pump. It is compatible with infusion vehicles such as Sodium Chloride injection BP or Dextrose injection BP, and can be administered as an admixture if required.

3. Bottles of Isoket are for single use only and should not be regarded as multi-dose containers.

4. For details on compatibility of Isoket see 'Pharmaceutical precautions'.

Contra-indications, warnings, etc
Contra-indications:
1. Isoket should not be used in the treatment of cardiogenic shock, unless some means of maintaining an adequate diastolic aortic pressure are undertaken.
2. Use in circulatory collapse, severe hypotension or low filling pressure, is contra-indicated.
3. Isoket should not be used in patients with known hypersensitivity to nitrates.
4. Isoket should not be used in patients with marked anaemia, trauma, cerebral haemorrhage, sever hypotension or hypovolaemia.

Precautions:
1. Close attention to pulse and blood pressure is necessary during administration of Isoket, and the dose should be adjusted according to patient response.
2. Isoket should be used with caution in patients suffering from hypothyroidism, malnutrition, severe liver or renal disease or hypothermia, or those who are pre-disposed to closed angle glaucoma.
3. The effects of anti-hypertensive drugs may be enhanced.
4. Some of the effects of alcohol may be potentiated by this agent.

Pregnancy and lactation: No data have been reported which would indicate the possibility of adverse effects resulting from the use of Isosorbide dinitrate in pregnancy. Safety in pregnancy however has not been established.

Isosorbide dinitrate should only be used in pregnancy and during lactation if, in the opinion of the physician, the possible benefits of treatment outweigh the possible hazards.

Adverse effects: Whilst sharp falls in systemic arterial pressure can give rise to symptoms of cerebral flow deficiency and decreased coronary perfusion, clinical experience with Isoket has shown that this is not normally a problem. The effect is consistent with the known vasodilatory effects of Isosorbide dinitrate which occur predominantly on the venous rather than the arterial side of the circulation.

In common with other nitrates, heachache and nausea may occur during administration.

Treatment of overdosage:
If arterial systolic blood pressure drops below 90 mmHg and if heart rate increases above 10% of its initial value, the infusion should be discontinued to allow a return to pretreatment levels. If hypotension persists or in more severe cases, measures should be taken to increase blood pressure, e.g. raising the foot of the bed and/or treatment with hypertensive agents, e.g. methoxamine and phenylephrine.

Pharmaceutical precautions
Compatibility: Isoket contains Isosorbide dinitrate in isotonic saline and is compatible with commonly employed infusion fluids, no incompatibilities have so far been demonstrated.

Compatibility with giving sets: Isoket is compatible with glass infusion bottles and infusion packs made from polyethylene, e.g. Polyfusor (Kendall).

Isoket may be infused slowly using a syringe pump with a glass or plastic syringe (Gillette Sabre Syringe, BP Plastipak Syringe or Monoject disposable syringe, Sherwood Medical Limited).

Isoket is incompatible with infusion bags and administration sets made from PVC, a loss of activity up to 40% is possible on prolonged contact (e.g. 8 hours). Loss after 1 hour may be up to 30%. The use of PVC containers should therefore be avoided, e.g. Viaflex (Travenol) or Steriflex (Kendall). A high pressure tubing known to be compatible with Isoket is available from Vygon UK under the name Lectrocath. Alternatively Avon Sureset administration sets may be used.

Legal category POM

Package quantities *Isoket 0.1%:* Packs of ten 10 ml ampoules (Isosorbide dinitrate 10 mg/10 ml); 50 ml bottle (Isosorbide dinitrate 50 mg/50 ml); 100 ml bottle (Isosorbide dinitrate 100 mg/100 ml).
Isoket 0.05%: 50 ml bottle (Isosorbide dinitrate 25 mg/50 ml)

Further information Isoket 0.1% and 0.05% contain no potassium, alcohol, propylene glycol, these substances have been shown to have deleterious effects in patients with coronary heart disease.

Product licence numbers
Isoket 0.1% 4438/0001
Isoket 0.05% 4438/0017

ISOKET* RETARD 20
ISOKET* RETARD 40

Presentation Tablets containing isosorbide dinitrate in a sustained release formulation.

Isoket Retard 20: Yellow tablets, scored on one side, and containing 20 mg isosorbide dinitrate.

Isoket Retard 40: Orange tablets, scored on one side, and containing 40 mg isosorbide dinitrate.

Uses For the prophylaxis of angina pectoris.

Dosage and administration The tablets are for oral administration.

Adults: The usual dose for long term treatment is one tablet (20–40 mg) every 12 hours; the tablets should be swallowed without chewing. No more than 4 tablets should be taken daily.

Children: The safety and efficacy of Isoket Retard Tablets has yet to be established.

Elderly: There is no evidence to suggest an adjustment of the dosage is necessary.

Contra-indications, warnings, etc
Contra-indications: A history of sensitivity to the drug. Very low blood pressure and acute circulatory failure. Isoket Retard Tablets should not be used in patients with acute myocardial infarction with low filling pressure, marked anaemia, head trauma, cerebral haemorrhage, severe hypotension or hypovolaemia.

Warnings: Headaches may develop in sensitive persons and these may be minimised by commencing with low, gradually increasing doses. Cutaneous vasodilatation, postural hypotension and dry rashes may occasionally occur. Tolerance may occasionally occur.

Isoket Retard Tablets should be used with caution in patients who are predisposed to closed angle glaucoma.

Precautions: Alcohol intake may enhance the effect of the drug and induce hypotension. Isoket Retard Tablets should be used with caution in patients suffering from hypothyroidism, hypothermia, malnutrition, severe liver or renal disease.

Use in pregnancy and lactation: This product should not be used during pregnancy or lactation unless considered essential by the physician.

Management of overdosage: Overdosage may lead to vascular collapse and gastric lavage is indicated in severe cases. Further measures to support the circulation are recommended e.g. elevating the legs and/or treatment with hypertensive agents.

Pharmaceutical precautions None.

Legal category P.

Package quantities The tablets are supplied in blister-packs of 50 tablets.

Further information Nil.

Product licence numbers
Isoket Retard 20 Tablets 4438/0004
Isoket Retard 40 Tablets 4438/0002

MENZOL*

Presentation Each white, uncoated tablet is impressed with NE5 on one side, has a breakline on the other side, and contains 5 mg norethisterone BP.

Menzol 8-day: 8-day treatment with 3 tablets daily (in divided doses) (24 tablets in total) in a Planapak wallet.

Menzol 20-day: 20-day treatment with 3 tablets daily (in divided doses) (60 tablets in total) in a Planapak wallet.

Uses Menorrhagia. Premenstrual syndrome. Dysmenorrhoea.

Menzol will produce secretory transformation of an endometrium which has been previously exposed to the proliferative effect of oestrogens. During treatment with Menzol the basal body temperature rises, as it does under the influence of endogenous progesterone in the second half of the menstrual cycle.

Menstruation-like withdrawal bleeding occurs consistently two to three days after stopping Menzol.

Dosage and administration The use of Menzol must be restricted to patients in whom there is no possibility of early pregnancy in the cycle concerned.

The following dosages should be used for the following indications.

Menorrhagia (hypermenorrhoea): 1 tablet 2-3 times daily from the 19th to the 26th day of the cycle (counting the first day of menstruation as Day 1).

Premenstrual syndrome (including premenstrual mastalgia): Premenstrual symptoms such as headache, migraine, breast discomfort, water retention, tachycardia, and psychic disturbances may be relieved by the administration of 1 tablet 2-3 times daily from the 19th to the 26th day of the cycle. Treatment should be repeated for several cycles. When treatment is stopped, the patient may remain symptom-free for a number of months.

Dysmenorrhoea: Functional or primary dysmenorrhoea is almost invariably relieved by the suppression of ovulation. 1 tablet three times daily for 20 days, starting on the fifth day of the cycle (the first day of menstruation counting as Day 1). Treatment should be maintained for three to four cycles followed by treatment-free cycles. A further course of therapy may be employed if symptoms return.

Note: If menstrual bleeding should fail to follow a course of menzol, the possibility of pregnancy must be ruled out before a further course is given.

Contra-indications, warnings, etc
Contra-indications: Pregnancy. History during pregnancy of idiopathic jaundice, severe pruitus or herpes gestationis. Severe disturbances of liver function. Dubin-Johnson and Rotor syndromes.

Interactions: The effects of Menzol may be altered if other sex hormones are prescribed simultaneously.

Adsverse effects: Side effects rarely occur in doses of 10 mg or 15 mg daily. The commonest side effect is breakthrough bleeding, particularly when treatment is continuous over a long period. Other reported side effects are nausea, vomiting, acne, oedema, weight gain, headache and depression. Androgenic effects with deepening of the voice and hirsutism, and oestrogenic effects, have been reported after prolonged therapy.

Warning and precautions: Alterations in liver function have been reported. In common with other steroids, Menzol should be given with care to patients with liver disturbances.

Overdosage: there have been no reports of ill-effects from overdosage and treatment is generally unnecessary. There are no special antidotes, and further treatment should be symptomatic.

Pharmaceutical precautions Protect from heat, light and moisture. Keep out of the reach of children.

Legal category POM.

Package quantities *Menzol 8-day:* Planapak wallet of 24 tablets (3 daily × 8). Three packs per carton.

Menzol 20-day: Planapak wallet of 60 tablets (3 daily × 20). Three packs per carton.

Further information The Planapak wallet is designed to enhance compliance by enabling the patient to calculate easily the first day of treatment and complete the course of medication.

Product licence number 4438/0025

NITROCINE*

Presentation Nitrocine is presented as ampoules containing 10 mg nitroglycerin in 10 ml isotonic sterile solution or as glass bottles containing 50 mg nitroglycerin in 50 ml isotonic sterile solution. Nitrocine contains no alcohol or potassium.

Uses
Actions: Nitroglycerin reduces the tone of vascular smooth muscle. This action is more marked on the venous capacitance vessels than the arterial vessels. There is a reduction in venous return to the heart and a lowering of elevated filling pressure. This lowering of filling pressure reduces the left ventricular end diastolic volume and preload. The net effect is a lowering of myocardial oxygen consumption.

Systemic vascular resistance, pulmonary vascular resistance and arterial pressure are also reduced by nitroglycerin and there is a net reduction in afterload.

Nitroglycerin reduces the work load on the heart by reducing the preload and the afterload.

Nitroglycerin improves the myocardial oxygen supply by redistributing blood flow along collateral channels and from epicardial to endocardial regions.

Surgery: Nitrocine may be used for the rapid control of hypertension during cardiac surgery.

Nitrocine may be used to reduce blood pressure and

maintain controlled hypotension during surgical procedures.

Nitrocine may also be used to control myocardial ischaemia during and after cardiovascular surgery.

Unresponsive congestive heart failure: Nitrocine may be used to treat unresponsive congestive heart failure secondary to acute myocardial infarction.

Unstable angina: Nitrocine may be used to treat unstable angina which is refractory to treatment with beta blockers and sublingual nitrates.

Dosage and administration Nitrocine can be administered undiluted by slow intravenous infusion using a syringe pump. Alternatively, Nitrocine may be administered intravenously as an admixture using a suitable vehicle such as Sodium Chloride Injection BP or Dextrose Injection BP.

Admixtures are prepared by exchanging the required volume of Nitrocine with an equal volume of infusion vehicle. For example to obtain an admixture of nitroglycerin at a concentration of 100 micrograms/ml 50 ml, Nitrocine solution (containing 50 mg nitroglycerin) is added to 450 ml of the infusion vehicle to give a final volume of 500 ml. If a dosage of 100 micrograms/min is required, this can be obtained by giving 60 ml of the admixture per hour. This is equivalent to a drip rate of 60 paediatric microdrops per minute or 20 standard drops per minute. At this drip rate, the admixture provides enough solution for an infusion time of 8 hours 20 minutes. For full details it is advisable to consult the dosage chart on the package insert.

Prepared admixtures should be given by intravenous infusion or with the aid of a syringe pump to ensure a constant rate of infusion. During Nitrocine administration there should be close haemodynamic monitoring of the patient.

Compatibility: Nitrocine is compatible with glass infusion bottles and with rigid infusion packs made of polyethylene, e.g. Polyfusor (Boots). Nitrocine may also be infused slowly using a syringe pump with a glass or plastic syringe (Gillette Sabre syringe, B.D. Plastipak syringe or Monoject disposable syringe, Sherwood Medical Ltd.)

Nitrocine is incompatible with PVC and severe losses of nitroglycerin (over 40%) may occur if this material is used. Contact with PVC bags such as Viaflex (Travenol) or Steriflex (Boots) should be avoided. A high pressure tubing known to be compatible with nitroglycerin is Lectrocath tubing from Vygon U.K. Limited.

Dosage: The dose of Nitrocine should be adjusted to meet the individual needs of the patient and the responses of the monitored haemodynamic parameters.

The recommended dosage range is 10–200 micrograms/min but up to 400 micrograms/min may be necessary during some surgical procedures.

Surgery: A starting dose of 25 micrograms/min is recommended for the control of hypertension, or to produce hypotension during surgery. This may be increased by increments of 25 micrograms/min at 5 minute intervals until the blood pressure is stabilized. Doses between 10–200 micrograms are usually sufficient during surgery although doses of up to 400 micrograms/min have been required in some cases.

The treatment of perioperative myocardial ischaemia may be started with a dose of 15–20 micrograms/min, with subsequent increments of 10–15 micrograms/min until the required effect is obtained.

Unresponsive congestive heart failure: The recommended starting dose is 20–25 micrograms/min. This may be decreased to 10 micrograms/min or increased in steps of 20–25 micrograms/min every 15–30 minutes until the desired effect is obtained.

Unstable angina: An initial dose of 10 micrograms/min is recommended with increments of 10 micrograms/min being made at approximately 30 minute intervals according to the needs of the patient.

Children: The safety and efficacy of Nitrocine has not yet been established in children.

Contra-indications, warnings, etc
Contra-indications: Nitrocine should not be used in the following cases:

Known hypersensitivity to nitrates.

Marked anaemia, severe cerebral haemorrhage, uncorrected hypovolaemia or severe hypotension.

Patients predisposed to closed angle glaucoma.

The safety of Nitrocine during pregnancy and lactation has not yet been established, therefore it should not be used unless considered absolutely essential.

Precautions: Close attention to pulse and blood pressure is necessary during the administration of Nitrocine infusions.

Nitrocine should be used with caution in patients suffering from hypothyroidism, severe liver or renal disease, hypothermia and malnutrition.

Adverse effects: In common with other nitrates, headaches and nausea may occur during administration. Other possible adverse reactions include hypotension, tachycardia, retching, diaphoresis, apprehension, restlessness, muscle twitching, retrosternal discomfort, palpitations, dizziness and abdominal pain. Paradoxical bradycardia has also been observed. Mild overdose usually results in hypotension and tachycardia. This may be reversed by elevating the legs and decreasing or terminating the infusion. In the event of severe overdose, intravenous administration of methoxamine or phenylephrine is recommended.

Pharmaceutical precautions Admixtures are stable for approximately 24 hours at room temperature in the recommended containers. Open ampoules or bottles should be used immediately and any unused drug discarded. Nitrocine contains nitroglycerin and no drug incompatibilities have been reported so far.

Legal category POM.

Package quantities
Ampoules: Each pack contains 10 × 10 ml ampoules of Nitrocine.
Bottles: Each pack contains 1 × 50 ml bottle of Nitrocine.

Further information Nitrocine contains no alcohol since small amounts of this substance are known to be deleterious to patients with coronary heart disease. The effects reported include diminished left ventricular function, shown by a decrease in stroke volume and a rise in end diastolic pressure, with associated deterioration in the electrocardiograph.

The effects of alcohol are known to persist beyond 5 hours.

Nitroglycerin is also known as glyceryl trinitrate, trinitroglycerin or trinitrin.

Product licence number 4438/0006.

**Trade Mark*

Scotia Pharmaceuticals Ltd

Woodbridge Meadows
Guildford
Surrey GU1 1BA

EPOGAM* CAPSULES
EPOGAM* PAEDIATRIC CAPSULES

Presentation Epogam is available in capsule form containing a clear yellow to yellow-green oil.

Each capsule is printed with EPOGAM. Two sizes are available containing either 40 mg or 80 mg gamolenic acid (gamma-linolenic acid, GLA) provided by evening primrose oil.

Epogam: The oblong soft gelatin capsule contains 40 mg gamolenic acid provided by evening primrose oil.

Epogam Paediatric: The oblong soft gelatin capsule with a snip-off neck contains 80 mg gamolenic acid provided by evening primrose oil.

Uses Epogam is indicated for the symptomatic relief of atopic eczema. All features of the disease may improve but Epogam is particularly effective in relieving the generalised itch of atopic eczema.

Dosage and administration Oral.
Epogam
Children aged 1–12 years: 2–4 capsules twice daily, providing a total daily dose of 4–8 capsules.

Adults: 4–6 capsules twice daily, providing a total daily dose of 8–12 capsules.

Elderly: The usual adult dose.

These capsules may be snipped open and the oil swallowed directly, or mixed with milk or another drink, or put onto bread or other food.

Epogam Paediatric
These capsules have been specifically designed for children (and also incidentally for older people) who have difficulty in swallowing the 40 mg Epogam capsules. The snip-off neck should be cut off and the capsule squeezed to express the contents which may be swallowed directly or mixed with milk or another drink or put onto bread or other food.

Children aged 1–12 years: 1–2 capsules twice daily, providing a total daily dose of 2–4 capsules.

Adults: 2–3 capsules twice daily, providing a total daily dose of 4–6 capsules.

Elderly: The usual adult dose.

No formal studies have been carried out in children under the age of 1 year.

It is suggested that patients start treatment at the highest recommended dose.

Some patients may not begin to show a clinical response to treatment for 8–12 weeks due to the gradual onset of action of Epogam. Once a clinical response has been achieved the treatment may be stopped or continued at a lower maintenance dose.

Contra-indications, warnings, etc
Contra-indications: None known.

Interactions: Epogam may have the potential to make manifest undiagnosed temporal lobe epilepsy, especially in schizophrenic patients and/or those who are receiving known epileptogenic drugs such as the phenothiazines. Physicians are advised to monitor carefully the effects of Epogam in patients on epileptogenic drugs, or in any individuals with a history of epilepsy. No epileptic events have been reported in patients not being treated with phenothiazines.

Pregnancy: No teratogenic effects have been observed in animal studies. However, as with all medicines, caution is advised concerning administration in the first trimester of pregnancy.

Lactation: Epogam may be taken while breast feeding.

Adverse effects: No major adverse effects have been reported. Nausea, indigestion and headaches have occurred occasionally.

Overdosage: The only symptom noted in a few cases has been loose stools sometimes accompanied by abdominal pains. No special treatment is required.

There is a high degree of tolerance to evening primrose oil. Up to 25 ml of oil (equivalent to 50 capsules) has been administered daily for one year to children aged 5–12 years, without adverse effects other than occasional loose stools.

Pharmaceutical precautions Store in a dry place, protected from heat.

Legal category POM.

Package quantities
Epogam: Containers of 240 capsules.
Epogam Paediatric: Containers of 60 capsules.

Further information Gamolenic acid (gamma-linolenic acid, GLA) is normally formed within the body from the dietary polyunsaturated fatty acid, linoleic acid.

Patients with atopic eczema have been reported to have lower than normal levels of GLA and its metabolites. Since GLA and its metabolites are required for normal skin health, this biochemical abnormality may contribute to the skin problems in atopic eczema. Administration of Epogam raises the blood levels of GLA and substances derived from it.

Epogam also contains 10 mg Vitamin E (d-alpha tocopheryl acetate) as an *in vivo* antioxidant.

Epogam Paediatric also contains 20 mg Vitamin E (d-alpha tocopheryl acetate) as an *in vivo* antioxidant.

Product licence numbers

Epogam	4382/0005.
Epogam Paediatric	4382/0013

EFALITH* OINTMENT

Presentation Efalith Ointment is a white to off-white water in oil emulsion containing lithium succinate 8% w/w and zinc sulphate 0.05% w/w.

Uses Efalith is indicated for the topical treatment and symptomatic relief of seborrhoeic dermatitis.

Dosage and administration Efalith may be administered to adults, the elderly and children of 12 years of age and over.

The ointment should be applied thinly and evenly to affected areas and rubbed in gently, twice daily in the morning and evening. This dosage regime should be continued until improvement occurs, usually within four weeks. It may then be possible to maintain this improvement in the long-term by applying the ointment less frequently or on an intermittent basis.

Contra-indications, warnings, etc
Contra-indications: Administration to children under 12 years of age. Known sensitivity to wool alcohols or paraffins.

Precautions: Caution should be used when applying Efalith to or near eyelids and mucous membranes. Psoriasis may be exacerbated by oral lithium therapy. No formal studies have been conducted in patients with psoriasis and, therefore, Efalith should be used with caution in such patients.

Pregnancy: As with all medicines, Efalith should not be used during the first trimester of pregnancy if this can be avoided. Teratogenic effects in animals are known to occur following oral administration of lithium salts. However, animal and clinical studies have shown that Efalith, applied topically, is not systemically absorbed or accumulated.

Lactation: Efalith may be administered to breast-feeding mothers if care is taken not to apply it to the breasts so as to avoid possible oral ingestion by infants.

Adverse effects: Mild and transient irritation to skin and eyelids at sites of application have been reported occasionally.

Pharmaceutical precautions Store in a cool place.

Legal category POM.

Package quantities Each tube contains 20 g.

Further information Efalith also contains wool alcohols and hard, soft and liquid paraffins as excipients.

Product licence number 4382/0009.

EFAMAST* CAPSULES

Presentation Oblong soft gelatin capsules containing a clear yellow to yellow-green oil, printed with EFAMAST. Each capsule contains 40 mg gamolenic acid (gamma-linolenic acid, GLA), provided by evening primrose oil.

Uses Efamast is indicated for the symptomatic relief of premenstrual breast pain (cyclical mastalgia) and non-cyclical mastalgia.

Dosage and administration Oral. 3–4 capsules twice daily.

It is suggested that patients start treatment at the highest recommended dose.

Some patients may not begin to show a clinical response to treatment for 8–12 weeks due to the gradual onset of action of Efamast. Once a clinical response has been achieved the treatment may be stopped or continued at a lower maintenance dose.

Contra-indications, warnings, etc

Contra-indications: None known.

Warnings: Breast pain may occasionally be a symptom of breast cancer. The doctor should be satisfied that the patient does not have breast cancer.

Interactions: Efamast may have the potential to make manifest undiagnosed temporal lobe epilepsy, especially in schizophrenic patients and/or those who are receiving known epileptogenic drugs such as the phenothiazines. Physicians are advised to monitor carefully the effects of Efamast in patients on epileptogenic drugs, or in any individuals with a history of epilepsy. No epileptic events have been reported in patients not being treated with phenothiazines.

Pregnancy: No teratogenic effects have been observed in animal studies. However, as with all medicines, caution is advised concerning administration in the first trimester of pregnancy.

Lactation: Efamast may be taken while breast feeding.

Adverse effects: No major adverse effects have been reported. Nausea, indigestion and headaches have occurred occasionally.

Overdosage: The only symptom noted in a few cases has been loose stools sometimes accompanied by abdominal pains. No special treatment is required.

Pharmaceutical precautions Store in a dry place, protected from heat.

Legal category POM.

Package quantities 224 capsules as an original dispensing pack (14 strips of 16 capsules).

Further information Gamolenic acid (gamma-linolenic acid, GLA) is normally formed within the body from the dietary polyunsaturated fatty acid, linoleic acid. Patients with mastalgia have been reported to have lower than normal levels of GLA and its metabolites. Polyunsaturated fatty acids can modulate the binding of steroid hormones to their receptors. Therefore low levels of GLA and its metabolites may lead to exaggerated peripheral effects of normal concentrations of ovarian hormones. Administration of Efamast raises the blood levels of GLA and substances derived from it.

Efamast also contains 10 mg Vitamin E (d-alpha tocopheryl acetate) as an *in vivo* antioxidant.

Product licence number 4382/0010.

**Trade Mark*

Searle Pharmaceuticals
Division of G. D. Searle & Company Limited
PO Box 53
Lane End Road
High Wycombe
Bucks HP12 4HL

SEARLE

ALDACTONE* 100 mg
ALDACTONE* 50 mg
ALDACTONE* 25 mg

Presentation *Aldactone 100 mg:* Buff, film-coated tablets engraved SEARLE 134 on one side. Each tablet contains Spironolactone BP 100 mg.

Aldactone 50 mg: Off-white, film-coated tablets engraved SEARLE 916 on one side. Each tablet contains Spironolactone BP 50 mg.

Aldactone 25 mg: Buff, film-coated tablets engraved SEARLE 39 on one side. Each tablet contains Spironolactone BP 25 mg.

Uses Congestive cardiac failure; hepatic cirrhosis with ascites and oedema; malignant ascites; nephrotic syndrome; diagnosis and treatment of primary aldosteronism.

Dosage and administration Administration of Aldactone once daily with a meal is recommended.

Adults: Congestive cardiac failure: Usual dose – 100 mg/day. In difficult or severe cases the dosage may be gradually increased up to 400mg/day. When oedema is controlled, the usual maintenance level is 75–200 mg/day.

Hepatic cirrhosis with ascites and oedema: If urinary Na^+ /K^+ ratio is greater than 1.0, 100 mg/day. If the ratio is less than 1.0, 200–400 mg/day. Maintenance dosage should be individually determined.

Malignant ascites: Initial dose usually 100–200 mg/day. In severe cases the dosage may be gradually increased up to 400 mg/day. When oedema is controlled, maintenance dosage should be individually determined.

Nephrotic syndrome: Usual dose – 100–200 mg/day. Spironolactone has not been shown to be anti-inflammatory, nor to affect the basic pathological process. Its use is only advised if glucocorticoids by themselves are insufficiently effective.

Diagnosis and treatment of primary aldosteronism: Aldactone may be employed as an initial diagnostic measure to provide presumptive evidence of primary hyperaldosteronism while patients are on normal diets.

Long test: Aldactone is administered at a daily dosage of 400 mg for three to four weeks. Correction of hypokalaemia and of hypertension provides presumptive evidence for the diagnosis of primary hyperaldosteronism.

Short test: Aldactone is administered at a daily dosage of 400 mg for four days. If serum potassium increases during Aldactone administration but drops when Aldactone is discontinued, a presumptive diagnosis of primary hyperaldosteronism should be considered.

After the diagnosis of hyperaldosteronism has been established by more definitive testing procedures, Aldactone may be administered in doses of 100 mg to 400 mg daily in preparation for surgery. For patients who are considered unsuitable for surgery, Aldactone may be employed for long-term maintenance therapy at the lowest effective dosage determined for the individual patient.

Elderly: It is recommended that treatment is started with the lowest dose and titrated upwards as required to achieve maximum benefit. Care should be taken in severe hepatic and renal impairment which may alter drug metabolism and excretion.

Children: Initial daily dosage should provide 3 mg of spironolactone per kilogram body weight, given in divided doses. Dosage should be adjusted on the basis of response and tolerance. If necessary a suspension may be prepared by crushing Aldactone tablets. A suitable suspending vehicle is methylcellulose mixture '450' (900 mg/10 ml) [Cologel*] 20% v/v, purified water to 100%. Such a suspension is chemically stable for one month when refrigerated.

Contra-indications, warnings, etc
Contra-indications: Aldactone is contra-indicated in patients with anuria, acute renal insufficiency, rapidly deteriorating or severe impairment of renal function, hyperkalaemia, Addison's disease and in patients who are hypersensitive to spironolactone.

Aldactone should not be administered concurrently with other potassium-conserving diuretics and potassium supplements should not be given routinely with Aldactone as hyperkalaemia may be induced.

Warnings: Carcinogenicity: Spironolactone has been shown to produce tumours in rats when administered at high doses over a long period of time. The significance of these findings with respect to clinical use is not certain. However, the long-term use of spironolactone in young patients requires careful consideration of the benefits and the potential hazard involved.

Precautions: Fluid and electrolyte balance: Fluid and electrolyte status should be regularly monitored, particularly in the elderly and in those with significant renal and hepatic impairment.

Hyperkalaemia may occur in patients with impaired renal function or excessive potassium intake and can cause cardiac irregularities which may be fatal. Should hyperkalaemia develop Aldactone should be discontinued, and if necessary, active measures taken to reduce the serum potassium to normal.

Hyponatraemia may be induced, especially when Aldactone is administered in combination with other diuretics.

Reversible hyperchloraemic metabolic acidosis usually in association with hyperkalaemia has been reported to occur in some patients with decompensated hepatic cirrhosis, even in the presence of normal renal function.

Urea: Reversible increases in blood urea have been reported in association with Aldactone therapy, particularly in the presence of impaired renal function.

Drug interactions: Spironolactone has been reported to increase serum digoxin concentration and to interfere with certain serum digoxin assays. In patients receiving digoxin and spironolactone the digoxin response should be monitored by means other than serum digoxin concentrations, unless the digoxin assay used has been proven not to be affected by spironolactone therapy. If it proves necessary to adjust the dose of digoxin patients should be carefully monitored for evidence of enhanced or reduced digoxin effect.

Potentiation of the effect of antihypertensive drugs

occurs and their dosage may need to be reduced when Aldactone is added to the treatment regime, and then adjusted as necessary.

Since ACE inhibitors decrease aldosterone production they should not routinely be used with Aldactone, particularly in patients with marked renal impairment.

As carbenoxolone may cause sodium retention and thus decrease the effectiveness of Aldactone, concurrent use should be avoided.

Nonsteroidal anti-inflammatory drugs may attenuate the natriuretic efficacy of diuretics due to inhibition of intrarenal synthesis of prostaglandins.

Spironolactone reduces vascular responsiveness to noradrenaline. Caution should be exercised in the management of patients subjected to regional or general anaesthesia while they are being treated with Aldactone.

In fluorimetric assays spironolactone may interfere with the estimation of compounds with similar fluorescence characteristics.

Pregnancy: Spironolactone or its metabolites may cross the placental barrier. With spironolactone feminisation has been observed in male rat foetuses. The use of Aldactone in pregnant women requires that the anticipated benefit be weighed against the possible hazards to the mother and foetus.

Nursing mothers: Metabolites of spironolactone have been detected in breast milk. If use of Aldactone is considered essential, an alternative method of infant feeding should be instituted.

Adverse effects: Gynaecomastia may develop in association with the use of spironolactone. Development appears to be related to both dosage level and duration of therapy and is normally reversible when spironolactone is discontinued. In rare instances some breast enlargement may persist. Other adverse reactions reported in association with spironolactone include: gastrointestinal intolerance, drowsiness, lethargy, headache, mental confusion, ataxia, drug fever, skin rashes, breast-soreness, menstrual irregularities, impotence and mild androgenic effects.

Overdosage: Acute overdosage may be manifested by drowsiness, mental confusion, nausea, vomiting, dizziness or diarrhoea. Hyponatraemia or hyperkalaemia may be induced but these effects are unlikely to be associated with acute overdosage. Symptoms of hyperkalaemia may manifest as paraesthesia, weakness, flaccid paralysis or muscle spasm and may be difficult to distinguish clinically from hypokalaemia. Electrocardiographic changes are the earliest specific signs of potassium disturbances. No specific antidote has been identified. Improvement may be expected after withdrawal of the drug. General supportive measures including replacement of fluids and electrolytes may be indicated. For hyperkalaemia, reduce potassium intake, administer potassium-excreting diuretics, intravenous glucose with regular insulin, or oral ion-exchange resins.

Pharmaceutical precautions Store in a dry place below 30°C (86°F).

Legal category POM.

Package quantities *Aldactone 100 mg:* Calendar blister pack of 28 tablets (OP); blister pack of 100 tablets; bottle of 500 tablets.

Aldactone 50 mg: Blister pack of 100 tablets.

Aldactone 25 mg: Blister pack of 100 tablets; bottle of 500 tablets.

Further information Aldactone, as a competitive aldosterone antagonist increases sodium excretion whilst reducing potassium loss at the distal renal tubule. It has a gradual and prolonged action, maximum response being usually attained after 2–3 days' treatment.

Combination of Aldactone with a conventional, more proximally acting diuretic usually enhances diuresis without excessive potassium loss.

Product licence numbers
Aldactone 100 mg 0020/0048
Aldactone 50 mg 0020/0088
Aldactone 25 mg 0020/5000

CYTOTEC*

Presentation White/off-white, hexagonal tablet, scored on both sides, engraved 'SEARLE 1461' on one side. Each tablet contains misoprostol 200 micrograms.

Uses
Indications: Cytotec is indicated for the healing of duodenal ulcer and gastric ulcer including those induced by nonsteroidal anti-inflammatory drugs (NSAID) in arthritic patients at risk, whilst continuing their NSAID therapy. In addition Cytotec can be used for the prophylaxis of NSAID-induced ulcers.

Actions: Cytotec is an analogue of naturally occurring prostaglandin E_1 which promotes peptic ulcer healing and symptomatic relief.

Cytotec protects the gastroduodenal mucosa by inhibiting basal, stimulated and nocturnal acid secretion and by reducing the volume of gastric secretions, the proteolytic activity of the gastric fluid, and increasing bicarbonate and mucus secretion.

Dosage and administration
Adults:
Healing of duodenal ulcer, gastric ulcer and NSAID-induced peptic ulcer: 800 micrograms daily in two or four divided doses taken with breakfast and/or each main meal and at bedtime.

Treatment should be given initially for at least 4 weeks even if symptomatic relief has been achieved sooner. In most patients ulcers will be healed in 4 weeks but treatment may be continued for up to 8 weeks if required. If the ulcer relapses further treatment courses may be given.

Prophylaxis of NSAID-induced peptic ulcer: 200 micrograms twice daily, three times daily or four times daily. Treatment can be continued as required. Dosage should be individualised according to the clinical condition of each patient.

Elderly: The usual dosage may be used.

Renal impairment: Available evidence indicates that no adjustment of dosage is necessary in patients with renal impairment.

Hepatic impairment: Cytotec is metabolised by fatty acid oxidising systems present in organs throughout the body. Its metabolism and plasma levels are therefore unlikely to be affected markedly in patients with hepatic impairment.

Children: Use of Cytotec in children has not yet been evaluated in the treatment of peptic ulceration or NSAID-induced peptic ulcer disease.

Contra-indications, warnings, etc
Contra-indications: Cytotec is contra-indicated in pregnant women and in women planning a pregnancy as it increases uterine tone and contractions in pregnancy which may cause partial or complete expulsion of the products of conception. It is also contra-indicated in patients with a known allergy to prostaglandins.

Warnings
Use in pre-menopausal women (see also Contra-indications): Cytotec should not be used in pre-menopausal women unless the patient requires nonsteroidal anti-inflammatory (NSAID) therapy and is at high risk of complications from NSAID-induced ulceration.

In such patients it is advised that Cytotec should only be used if the patient:
—takes effective contraceptive measures
—has been advised of the risks of taking Cytotec if pregnant (see Contra-indications).

Precautions: The results of clinical studies indicate that Cytotec does not produce hypotension at dosages effective in promoting the healing of gastric and duodenal ulcers. Nevertheless, Cytotec should be used with caution in the presence of disease states where hypotension might precipitate severe complications, eg, cerebrovascular disease, coronary artery disease or severe peripheral vascular disease including hypertension.

There is no evidence that Cytotec has adverse effects on glucose metabolism in human volunteers or patients with diabetes mellitus.

Drug interactions: Cytotec is predominantly metabolised via fatty acid oxidising systems and has shown no adverse effect on the hepatic microsomal mixed function oxidase (P450) enzyme system. In specific studies no clinically significant pharmacokinetic interaction has been demonstrated with antipyrine, diazepam and propranolol. In extensive clinical studies no drug interactions have been attributed to Cytotec. Additional evidence shows no clinically important pharmacokinetic or pharmacodynamic interaction with nonsteroidal anti-inflammatory drugs including aspirin, diclofenac and ibuprofen.

Pregnancy: See Contra-indications.

Lactation: It is not known if the active metabolite of Cytotec is excreted in breast milk, therefore Cytotec should not be administered during breast feeding.

Adverse effects:

Gastrointestinal system: Diarrhoea has been reported and is occasionally severe and prolonged and may require withdrawal of the drug. It can be minimised by using single doses not exceeding 200 micrograms with food and by avoiding the use of predominantly magnesium containing antacids when an antacid is required.

Abdominal pain with or without associated dyspepsia or diarrhoea can follow misoprostol therapy.

Other gastrointestinal adverse effects reported include dyspepsia, flatulence, nausea and vomiting.

Female reproductive system: Menorrhagia, vaginal bleeding and intermenstrual bleeding have been reported in pre- and post-menopausal women.

Other adverse events: Skin rashes have been reported. Dizziness has been infrequently reported.

The pattern of adverse events associated with Cytotec is similar when an NSAID is given concomitantly.

Overdosage: Intensification of pharmacological effects may occur with overdose. In the event of overdosage symptomatic and supportive therapy should be given as appropriate. In clinical trials patients have tolerated 1200 micrograms daily for three months without significant adverse effects.

Pharmaceutical precautions Store in a dry place below 30°C (86°F).

Legal category POM.

Package quantities Foil/foil blister pack of 56 (OP) or 112 tablets.

Further information Cytotec in multiples of the recommended therapeutic dose in animals has produced gastric mucosal hyperplasia. This characteristic response of E prostaglandins reverts to normal on discontinuation of the compound. In patients, histological examination of gastric biopsies taken before and after treatment with misoprostol after up to one year's duration have shown no adverse tissue response attributable to misoprostol.

Inhibition of gastric secretion by Cytotec is achieved by a combination of local and systemic effects. Cytotec is rapidly absorbed following oral administration, with peak plasma levels of the active metabolite (misoprostol acid) occurring after about 30 minutes. The plasma elimination half-life of misoprostol acid is 20–40 minutes. No accumulation of misoprostol acid in plasma occurs after repeated dosing of 400 micrograms twice daily.

Product licence number 0020/0115.

REHIDRAT*

Presentation Foil/laminate sachet containing 14 g of lemon and lime flavoured greyish-white granular powder with green particles. Each sachet contains:

Sodium Chloride PhEur	0.44 g
Potassium Chloride PhEur	0.38 g
Sodium Bicarbonate PhEur	0.42 g
Citric Acid PhEur	0.44 g
Glucose	4.09 g
Sucrose PhEur	8.07 g
Fructose	0.07 g
Plus flavourings	

Uses Oral electrolyte mixture for prevention and correction of mild and moderate dehydration. In the management of diarrhoea in infants, children and adults.

Maintenance and replacement of fluid and electrolytes following corrective parenteral therapy for dehydration. As a supplement to corrective parenteral therapy for dehydration.

Dosage and administration

General advice: The contents of one 14 g sachet should be dissolved in 250 ml of drinking water. For infants the water should be freshly boiled and cooled. The solution should be freshly made immediately prior to use. Any unused solution remaining an hour after reconstitution should be discarded unless stored in a refrigerator where it may be kept and used for up to 24 hours. Advise patients that the solution should not be boiled after reconstitution, and that it should be used at the recommended dilution.

The degree of dehydration should be assessed. Patients with mild or moderate dehydration may appear almost normal, they may be thirsty and may have normal or slightly diminished skin elasticity or, in children, slightly sunken fontanelle. Urine flow may be reduced. Patients with signs of severe dehydration who are usually too weak to drink will initially require parenteral therapy. Oral therapy should only be instituted when shock is corrected.

The volume of reconstituted Rehidrat required will depend on the weight of the patient.

General guidelines for oral therapy

1. Rehydration: Replacement of fluid and electrolyte losses. Mild or moderate dehydration – 50–120 ml per kilogram body weight orally, usually given in divided doses over 4 to 6 hours. Adults may need up to 1000 ml per hour. A continuous nasogastric infusion may be used if necessary.

2. Maintenance: Mild to moderate diarrhoea – 100–200 ml per kilogram body weight orally over a period of 24 hours in divided doses. Continuing diarrhoea – 15 ml per kilogram body weight orally every hour. Observe carefully to confirm adequate maintenance of hydration.

Where nausea or vomiting is present Rehidrat should be administered in small frequent doses, in sips. If vomiting persists appropriate intravenous therapy should be instituted. The patient instruction leaflet included in each carton advises patients to consult their doctor if there is no improvement in 24–48 hours.

Elderly: Administer Rehidrat in amounts appropriate to correct dehydration. Also see Precautions.

Infants and children: For bottle fed infants advise mothers to make the feed up for a 24 hour period and to store the reconstituted solution in the refrigerator.

Diarrhoea can have serious consequences in children under 3 years old. For this age group, the patient instruction leaflet included in each carton, advises that management should be on medical advice. Breast feeding should continue and Rehidrat should be given after feeds. In other infants and children administration of Rehidrat should begin with discontinuation of cow's milk and solids for 24 hours. Regrading of feeds is advisable and should be adjusted to meet individual needs. Cow's milk should gradually be introduced over a period of about five days as treatment with Rehidrat continues.

A suggested regimen for regrading of feeds in infants is given below. Regrading may be carried out more quickly for older children.

Day	Volume of Rehidrat solution (ml)	Volume of milk (ml)	Total volume in 24 hours (ml)
1	150 × wt†	0	150 × wt
2	120 × wt	30 × wt	150 × wt
3	90 × wt	60 × wt	150 × wt
4	60 × wt	90 × wt	150 × wt
5	30 × wt	120 × wt	150 × wt
6	0	150 × wt	150 × wt

† Weight in kilograms

Solids are usually reintroduced when the infant is receiving full strength milk but introduction may be sooner to suit individual needs.

Simplified oral dosage guidelines: For mild diarrhoea a simplified dosage scheme may be suggested. Young children may be given Rehidrat solution in quantities usual for their normal feeds, in conjunction with an appropriate graduated feeding regimen.

Older children and adults may be allowed to drink Rehidrat solution to satisfy their thirst.

Contra-indications, warnings, etc Rehidrat is contra-indicated in patients with renal impairment manifesting as oliguria or anuria, intestinal obstruction, paralytic ileus, intractable vomiting and in patients with severe dehydration which requires parenteral fluid therapy. Rehidrat should not be mixed or given with electrolyte-containing solutions. Salt or sugar should not be added to Rehidrat.

Precautions: When Rehidrat is used as a supplement to parenteral fluid therapy, care must be taken not to exceed the total water and electrolyte requirements.

The sugar content of Rehidrat should be considered when treating diabetics.

Administration of oral sugar-electrolyte solutions to patients with sugar malabsorption may worsen diarrhoea.

Adverse effects: Incorrect dilution could result in abnormalities of carbohydrate and electrolyte balance.

Overdosage: Toxicity resulting from overdosage of oral electrolyte solutions is rare. In the event of overdosage hypernatraemia or hyperkalaemia could occur.

Pharmaceutical precautions Store in a dry place below 30°C (86°F).

Legal category P.

Package quantities Boxes of 24 sachets with instructions for use (OP).

Further information The reconstituted Rehidrat and water solution has the following composition:

	mmol/l
Sodium	50
Potassium	20
Chloride	50
Bicarbonate	20
Citrate	9
Glucose	91
Sucrose	94
Fructose	2
Total osmolarity	336

Product licence number 0020/0093.

REHIDRAT* ORANGE

Presentation Foil/laminate sachet containing 14 g of orange flavoured white granular powder with yellow particles. Each sachet contains:

Sodium Chloride PhEur	0.44 g
Potassium Chloride PhEur	0.38 g
Sodium Bicarbonate PhEur	0.42 g
Citric Acid PhEur	0.44 g
Glucose	4.09 g
Sucrose PhEur	8.07 g
Fructose	0.07 g
Plus flavourings	

Uses Oral electrolyte mixture for prevention and correction of mild and moderate dehydration. In the management of diarrhoea in infants, children and adults.

Maintenance and replacement of fluid and electrolytes following corrective parenteral therapy for dehydration. As a supplement to corrective parenteral therapy for dehydration.

Dosage and administration
General advice: The contents of one 14 g sachet should be dissolved in 250 ml of drinking water. For infants the water should be freshly boiled and cooled. The solution should be freshly made immediately prior to use. Any unused solution remaining an hour after reconstitution should be discarded unless stored in a refrigerator where it may be kept and used for up to 24 hours. Advise patients that the solution should not be boiled after reconstitution, and that it should be used at the recommended dilution. The degree of dehydration should be assessed. Patients with mild or moderate dehydration may appear almost normal, they may be thirsty and may have normal or slightly diminished skin elasticity or, in children, slightly sunken fontanelle. Urine flow may be reduced. Patients with signs of severe dehydration who are usually too weak to drink will initially require parenteral therapy. Oral therapy should only be instituted when shock is corrected. The volume of reconstituted Rehidrat required will depend on the weight of the patient.

General guidelines for oral therapy
1. Rehydration – Replacement of fluid and electrolyte losses. Mild or moderate dehydration – 50–120 ml per kilogram body weight orally, usually given in divided doses over 4 to 6 hours. Adults may need up to 1000 ml per hour. A continuous nasogastric infusion may be used if necessary.

2. Maintenance: Mild to moderate diarrhoea – 100–200 ml per kilogram body weight orally over a period of 24 hours in divided doses. Continuing diarrhoea – 15 ml per kilogram body weight orally every hour. Observe carefully to confirm adequate maintenance of hydration.

Where nausea or vomiting is present Rehidrat Orange should be administered in small frequent doses, in sips. If vomiting persists appropriate intravenous therapy should be instituted. The patient instruction leaflet included in each carton advises patients to consult their doctor if there is no improvement in 24–48 hours.

Elderly: Administer Rehidrat Orange in amounts appropriate to correct dehydration. Also see Precautions.

Infants and children: For bottle fed infants advise mothers to make the feed up for a 24 hour period and to store the reconstituted solution in the refrigerator.

Diarrhoea can have serious consequences in children under 3 years old. For this age group, the patient instruction leaflet included in each carton, advises that management should be on medical advice. Breast feeding should continue and Rehidrat Orange should be given after feeds. In other infants and children administration of Rehidrat Orange should begin with discontinuation of cow's milk and solids for 24 hours. Regrading of feeds is advisable and should be adjusted to meet individual needs. Cow's milk should gradually be introduced over a period of about five days as treatment with Rehidrat Orange continues.

A suggested regimen for regrading of feeds in infants is given below. Regrading may be carried out more quickly for older children.

Day	Volume of Rehidrat Orange solution (ml)	Volume of milk (ml)	Total volume in 24 hours (ml)
1	150 × wt†	0	150 × wt
2	120 × wt	30 × wt	150 × wt
3	90 × wt	60 × wt	150 × wt
4	60 × wt	90 × wt	150 × wt
5	30 × wt	120 × wt	150 × wt
6	0	150 × wt	150 × wt

† Weight in kilograms.

Solids are usually reintroduced when the infant is receiving full strength milk but introduction may be sooner to suit individual needs.

Simplified oral dosage guidelines: For mild diarrhoea a simplified dosage scheme may be suggested. Young children may be given Rehidrat Orange solution in quantities usual for their normal feeds, in conjunction with an appropriate graduated feeding regimen.

Older children and adults may be allowed to drink Rehidrat Orange solution to satisfy their thirst.

Contra-indications, warnings, etc Rehidrat Orange is contra-indicated in patients with renal impairment manifesting as oliguria or anuria, intestinal obstruction, paralytic ileus, intractable vomiting and in patients with severe dehydration which requires parenteral fluid therapy. Rehidrat Orange should not be mixed or given with electrolyte-containing solutions. Salt or sugar should not be added to Rehidrat Orange.

Precautions: When Rehidrat Orange is used as a supplement to parenteral fluid therapy, care must be taken not to exceed the total water and electrolyte requirements.

The sugar content of Rehidrat Orange should be considered when treating diabetics.

Administration of oral sugar-electrolyte solutions to patients with sugar malabsorption may worsen diarrhoea.

Adverse effects: Incorrect dilution could result in abnormalities of carbohydrate and electrolyte balance.

Overdosage: Toxicity resulting from overdosage of oral electrolyte solutions is rare. In the event of overdosage hypernatraemia or hyperkalaemia could occur.

Pharmaceutical precautions Store in a dry place below 30°C (86°F).

Legal category P.

Package quantities Boxes of 24 sachets with instructions for use (OP).

Further information The reconstituted Rehidrat Orange and water solution has the following composition:

	mmol/l
Sodium	50
Potassium	20
Chloride	50
Bicarbonate	20
Citrate	9
Glucose	91
Sucrose	94
Fructose	2
Total osmolarity	336

Product licence number 0020/0120.

REHIDRAT* BLACKCURRANT

Presentation Foil laminate sachets containing 14 g of blackcurrant flavoured white powder. Each sachet contains:

Sodium Chloride PhEur	0.44 g
Potassium Chloride PhEur	0.38 g
Sodium Bicarbonate PhEur	0.42 g
Citric Acid PhEur	0.44 g
Glucose	4.13 g
Sucrose PhEur	8.17 g
Fructose	0.01 g
Plus flavourings	

Uses Oral electrolyte mixture for the prevention and correction of mild and moderate dehydration in the management of diarrhoea in infants, children and adults.

Maintenance and replacement of fluid and electrolytes following corrective parenteral therapy for dehydration. As a supplement to corrective parenteral therapy for dehydration.

Dosage and administration

General advice: The contents of one 14 g sachet should be dissolved in 250 ml of drinking water. For infants the water should be freshly boiled and cooled. The solution should be freshly made immediately prior to use. Any unused solution remaining an hour after reconstitution should be discarded unless stored in a refrigerator where it may be kept and used for up to 24 hours. Advise patients that the solution should not be boiled after reconstitution, and that it should be used at the recommended dilution. The degree of dehydration should be assessed. Patients with mild or moderate dehydration may appear almost normal; they may be thirsty and may have normal or slightly diminished skin elasticity or, in children, slightly sunken fontanelle. Urine flow may be reduced. Patients with signs of severe dehydration who are usually too weak to drink will initially require parenteral therapy. Oral therapy should only be instituted when shock is corrected. The volume of reconstituted Rehidrat Blackcurrant required will depend on the weight of the patient.

General guidelines for oral therapy

1. Rehydration – Replacement of fluid and electrolyte losses. Mild or moderate dehydration: 50–120 ml per kilogram body weight orally, usually given in divided doses over 4 to 6 hours. Adults may need up to 1000 ml per hour. A continuous nasogastric infusion may be used if necessary.

2. Maintenance – Mild to moderate diarrhoea: 100–200 ml per kilogram body weight orally over a period of 24 hours in divided doses. Continuing diarrhoea: 15 ml per kilogram body weight orally every hour. Observe carefully to confirm adequate maintenance of hydration.

Where nausea or vomiting is present Rehidrat Blackcurrant should be administered in small frequent doses, in sips. If vomiting persists appropriate intravenous therapy should be instituted. The patient instruction leaflet included in each carton advises patients to consult their doctor if there is no improvement in 24–48 hours.

Elderly: Administer Rehidrat Blackcurrant in amounts appropriate to correct dehydration. Also see Precautions.

Infants and children: For bottle fed infants advise mothers to make the feed up for a 24 hour period and to store the reconstituted solution in the refrigerator.

Diarrhoea can have serious consequences in children under 3 years old. For this age group, the patient instruction leaflet included in each carton, advises that management should be on medical advice. Breast feeding should continue and Rehidrat Blackcurrant should be given after feeds. In other infants and children administration of Rehidrat Blackcurrant should begin with discontinuation of cow's milk and solids for 24 hours. Regrading of feeds is advisable and should be adjusted to meet individual needs. Cow's milk should gradually be introduced over a period of about five days as treatment with Rehidrat Blackcurrant continues.

A suggested regimen for regrading of feeds in infants is given below. Regrading may be carried out more quickly for older children.

Day	*Volume of Rehidrat Blackcurrant solution (ml)*	*Volume of milk (ml)*	*Total volume in 24 hours (ml)*
1	150 × wt†	0	150 × wt
2	120 × wt	30 × wt	150 × wt
3	90 × wt	60 × wt	150 × wt
4	60 × wt	90 × wt	150 × wt
5	30 × wt	120 × wt	150 × wt
6	0	150 × wt	150 × wt

† Weight in kilograms.

Solids are usually reintroduced when the infant is receiving full strength milk but introduction may be sooner to suit individual needs.

Simplified oral dosage guidelines: For mild diarrhoea a simplified dosage scheme may be suggested. Young children may be given Rehidrat Blackcurrant solution in quantities usual for their normal feeds, in conjunction with an appropriate graduated feeding regimen.

Older children and adults may be allowed to drink Rehidrat Blackcurrant solution to satisfy their thirst.

Contra-indications, warnings, etc
Contra-indications: Rehidrat Blackcurrant is contra-indicated in patients with renal impairment manifesting as oliguria or anuria, intestinal obstruction, paralytic ileus, intractable vomiting and in patients with severe dehydration which requires parenteral fluid therapy.

Precautions: When Rehidrat Blackcurrant is used as a supplement to parenteral fluid therapy, care must be taken not to exceed the total water and electrolyte requirements.

The sugar content of Rehidrat Blackcurrant should be considered when treating diabetics.

Administration of oral sugar-electrolyte solutions to patients with sugar malabsorption may worsen diarrhoea.

Drug interactions: Rehidrat Blackcurrant should not be mixed or given with electrolyte-containing solutions. Salt or sugar should not be added to Rehidrat Blackcurrant.

Adverse effects: Incorrect dilution could result in abnormalities of carbohydrate and electrolyte balance.

Overdosage: Toxicity resulting from overdosage of oral electrolyte solutions is rare. In the event of overdosage hypernatraemia or hyperkalaemia could occur.

Pharmaceutical precautions Store in a dry place below 30°C (86°F).

Legal category P.

Package quantities Boxes of 24 sachets with instructions for use.

Further information When reconstituted Rehidrat Blackcurrant and water solution has the following composition:

	mmol/l
Sodium	50
Potassium	20
Chloride	50
Bicarbonate	20
Citrate	9
Glucose	92
Sucrose	96
Fructose	<1
Total osmolarity	337

Product licence number 0020/0127.

REHIDRAT* MULTIPACK

Presentation Foil/laminate sachets containing 14 g of fruit flavoured powder. Each sachet contains:

Sodium Chloride PhEur	0.44 g
Potassium Chloride PhEur	0.38 g
Sodium Bicarbonate PhEur	0.42 g
Citric Acid PhEur	0.44 g
Glucose	4.09–4.13 g
Sucrose PhEur	8.07–8.17 g
Fructose	0.01–0.07 g
Plus flavourings	

Uses Oral electrolyte mixture for the prevention and correction of mild and moderate dehydration in the management of diarrhoea in infants, children and adults.

Maintenance and replacement of fluid and electrolytes following corrective parenteral therapy for dehydration. As a supplement to corrective parenteral therapy for dehydration.

Dosage and administration
General advice: The contents of one 14 g sachet should be dissolved in 250 ml of drinking water. For infants the water should be freshly boiled and cooled. The solution should be freshly made immediately prior to use. Any unused solution remaining an hour after reconstitution should be discarded unless stored in a refrigerator where it may be kept and used for up to 24 hours. Advise patients that the solution should not be boiled after reconstitution, and that it should be used at the recommended dilution. The degree of dehydration should be assessed. Patients with mild or moderate dehydration may appear almost normal; they may be thirsty and may have normal or slightly diminished skin elasticity or, in children, slightly sunken fontanelle. Urine flow may be reduced. Patients with signs of severe dehydration who are usually too weak to drink will initially require parenteral therapy. Oral therapy should only be instituted when shock is corrected. The volume of reconstituted Rehidrat required will depend on the weight of the patient.

General guidelines for oral therapy

1. Rehydration – Replacement of fluid and electrolyte losses. Mild or moderate dehydration: 50–120 ml per kilogram body weight orally, usually given in divided doses over 4 to 6 hours. Adults may need up to 1000 ml per hour. A continuous nasogastric infusion may be used if necessary.
2. Maintenance – Mild to moderate diarrhoea: 100–200 ml per kilogram body weight orally over a period of 24 hours in divided doses. Continuing diarrhoea: 15 ml per kilogram body weight orally every hour. Observe carefully to confirm adequate maintenance of hydration.

Where nausea or vomiting is present Rehidrat should be administered in small frequent doses, in sips. If vomiting persists appropriate intravenous therapy should be instituted. The patient instruction leaflet included in each carton advises patients to consult their doctor if there is no improvement in 24–48 hours.

Elderly: Administer Rehidrat in amounts appropriate to correct dehydration. Also see Precautions.

Infants and children: For bottle fed infants advise mothers to make the feed up for a 24 hour period and to store the reconstituted solution in the refrigerator.

Diarrhoea can have serious consequences in children under 3 years old. For this age group, the patient instruction leaflet included in each carton, advises that management should be on medical advice. Breast feeding should continue and Rehidrat should be given after feeds. In other infants and children administration of Rehidrat should begin with discontinuation of cow's milk and solids for 24 hours. Regrading of feeds is advisable and should be adjusted to meet individual needs. Cow's milk should gradually be introduced over a period of about five days as treatment with Rehidrat continues.

A suggested regimen for regrading of feeds in infants is given below. Regrading may be carried out more quickly for older children.

Day	*Volume of Rehidrat solution (ml)*	*Volume of milk (ml)*	*Total volume in 24 hours (ml)*
1	150 × wt†	0	150 × wt
2	120 × wt	30 × wt	150 × wt
3	90 × wt	60 × wt	150 × wt
4	60 × wt	90 × wt	150 × wt
5	30 × wt	120 × wt	150 × wt
6	0	150 × wt	150 × wt

† Weight in kilograms.

Solids are usually reintroduced when the infant is receiving full strength milk but introduction may be sooner to suit individual needs.

Simplified oral dosage guidelines: For mild diarrhoea a simplified dosage scheme may be suggested. Young children may be given Rehidrat solution in quantities usual for their normal feeds, in conjunction with an appropriate graduated feeding regimen.

Older children and adults may be allowed to drink Rehidrat solution to satisfy their thirst.

Contra-indications, warnings, etc
Contra-indications: Rehidrat is contra-indicated in patients with renal impairment manifesting as oliguria or anuria, intestinal obstruction, paralytic ileus, intractable vomiting and in patients with severe dehydration which requires parenteral fluid therapy.

Precautions: When Rehidrat is used as a supplement to parenteral fluid therapy, care must be taken not to exceed the total water and electrolyte requirements.

The sugar content of Rehidrat should be considered when treating diabetics.

Administration of oral sugar-electrolyte solutions to patients with sugar malabsorption may worsen diarrhoea.

Drug interactions: Rehidrat should not be mixed or given with electrolyte-containing solutions. Salt or sugar should not be added to Rehidrat.

Adverse effects: Incorrect dilution could result in abnormalities of carbohydrate and electrolyte balance.

Overdosage: Toxicity resulting from overdosage of oral electrolyte solutions is rare. In the event of overdosage hypernatraemia or hyperkalaemia could occur.

Pharmaceutical precautions Store in a dry place below 30°C (86°F).

Legal category P.

Package quantities Cartons of 16 sachets with instructions for use. Each carton contains 6 sachets each of Rehidrat Orange and Rehidrat Blackcurrant and 4 sachets of Rehidrat Lemon & Lime.

Further information When reconstituted with 250 ml water the solution has the following composition:

	mmol/l
Sodium	50
Potassium	20
Chloride	50
Bicarbonate	20
Citrate	9
Glucose	91–2
Sucrose	94–6
Fructose	< 1–2
Total osmolarity	336–337

Product licence number 0020/0134.

SERENACE* AMPOULES
SERENACE* TABLETS
SERENACE* LIQUID
SERENACE* CAPSULES

Presentation *Serenace 5 mg and 20 mg Ampoules:* Clear glass ampoules containing Haloperidol BP 5 mg in 1 ml aqueous solution.

Clear glass ampoules containing Haloperidol BP 20 mg in 2 ml aqueous solution.

Serenace 1.5 mg; 5 mg; 10 mg and 20 mg Tablets:

White, biconvex, scored tablets engraved 'SEARLE 41' on one side, containing Haloperidol BP 1.5 mg.

Bright pink, biconvex, scored tablets engraved 'SEARLE 12' on one side, containing Haloperidol BP 5 mg.

Pale pink, biconvex, scored tablets engraved 'SEARLE 919' on one side, containing Haloperidol BP 10 mg.

Dark pink, biconvex, scored tablets engraved 'SEARLE 920' on one side, containing Haloperidol BP 20 mg.

Serenace Liquid: Clear, odourless, colourless liquid containing Haloperidol BP 2 mg per ml.

Serenace Capsules: Two-tone green capsules printed 'SEARLE' on both halves, containing Haloperidol BP 500 micrograms.

Uses Psychotic disorders – schizophrenia, mania and hypomania, especially paranoid psychoses. Mental or behavioural problems such as aggression, hyperactivity and self-mutilation in the mentally retarded. Moderate to severe psychomotor agitation, excitement, violent or dangerously impulsive behaviour. Gilles de la Tourette syndrome and severe tics. Childhood behaviour disorders, especially when associated with hyperactivity and aggression. Restlessness and agitation in the elderly. Adjunct to short-term management of anxiety.

Dosage and administration There is considerable variation from patient to patient in the response to treatment and the dosage required. As with all antipsychotics, dosage should be individualised according to the needs and response of each patient.

To determine the initial dosage, consideration should be given to the patient's age, severity of symptoms and previous response to other antipsychotic therapy. Oral dosage may be given in single or divided doses. Administration twice daily is sufficient in most cases.

Adults: Psychotic disorders; mental or behavioural problems; moderate to severe psychomotor agitation or impulsive behaviour.

Initial treatment: Parenteral administration; For rapid emergency treatment 5 or 10 mg or, infrequently, up to 30 mg by intramuscular injection may be required. Depending on the response of the patient, subsequent doses may be given as frequently as every 30 to 60 minutes, although 6–12 hourly intervals may be satisfactory. There is a wide variation among individual patients, so that cumulative dosage is not predictable in advance. Some patients may have an optimal early response after as little as 10 mg, whereas others may require up to 40 or 50 mg. Higher doses are not usually necessary.

Serenace injection may also be administered intravenously.

Oral administration: Initial dosage may range from as little as 1.5 mg daily to 20 mg daily, dependent on the characteristics, severity of symptoms and response of each individual patient. It may be necessary to increase the dosage gradually to obtain maximum control of symptoms. Severely disturbed or resistant patients may require up to 100 mg daily or, infrequently, up to 200 mg daily.

Maintenance treatment: Once a satisfactory therapeutic response has been achieved, dosage should be reduced gradually to the lowest effective maintenance level which is often as low as 3 to 10 mg daily, dependent on the characteristics and response of each individual patient.

Gilles de la Tourette Syndrome: Initial dosage is usually 2 mg daily. During the acute phase of treatment, dosage can be increased gradually to obtain maximum control of symptoms and may range between 6 and 50 mg or, exceptionally, up to 180 mg daily.

Once a satisfactory therapeutic response has been achieved dosage should be reduced gradually to the lowest effective maintenance level which for most patients is 4 mg daily.

Elderly: Half the recommended adult starting dose may be sufficient for a therapeutic response in the elderly. The maximum and maintenance dose will generally be lower for debilitated or geriatric patients who may be more sensitive to Serenace.

Anxiety: 500 micrograms (one capsule) twice daily.

Children: Oral administration: 25 to 50 micrograms per kg body weight per day to a maximum of 10 mg, although adolescents may require up to 30 mg or, exceptionally, up to 60 mg daily.

Parenteral administration: Not recommended.

Contra-indications, warnings, etc
Contra-indications: Comatose states, patients with Parkinson's disease or a sensitivity to haloperidol and use during breast feeding.

Precautions: Liver disease, renal failure, phaeochromocytoma, conditions predisposing to epilepsy (e.g. alcohol withdrawal or brain damage). May be given to epileptics, but usual anticonvulsant therapy should be continued.

Use cautiously in thyrotoxic patients and those with arteriosclerosis who may have occult or manifest lesions of the basal ganglia. Such patients may be more prone to develop extrapyramidal symptoms.

Administer with care to patients with severe cardiovascular disorders, because of the possibility of transient hypotension. Should hypotension occur and a vasopressor be required, adrenaline should not be used since haloperidol may block its vasopressor activity and paradoxical further lowering of the blood pressure may occur.

Drug interactions: Serenace may potentiate the central nervous system depression produced by other CNS-depressant drugs including alcohol, hypnotics, sedatives or strong analgesics.

Enhanced CNS effects (sedation, mental disturbances) have been reported with the combined use of methyldopa and haloperidol.

Severe neuromuscular symptoms with impairment of consciousness and fever have been reported with combined use of lithium and haloperidol. A causal relationship has not been established, however, patients receiving such combined therapy should be carefully observed for early evidence of neurological toxicity and treatment should be discontinued if such signs appear.

Serenace may antagonise the action of adrenaline and other sympathomimetic agents.

Pregnancy: The safety of Serenace in pregnancy has not been established.

Reproduction studies in rodents have shown an increased incidence of resorption, reduced fertility and pup mortality. No specific teratogenic effect has been reported in rats, rabbits or dogs but cleft palate and open eye syndrome have been observed in mice.

No well controlled studies of haloperidol use in pregnant women have been conducted. Two cases of foetal limb malformation have been reported following maternal use of haloperidol combined with other drugs during the first trimester. No causal relationship has been established. Use of haloperidol during pregnancy requires that the anticipated benefit be weighed against the possible hazards to mother and foetus.

Lactation: Haloperidol has been detected in breast milk. If use of haloperidol is considered essential, breast feeding should be discontinued.

Warnings and adverse effects: Haloperidol may impair alertness, especially at the start of treatment. These effects may be potentiated by alcohol. Patients should be warned of the risks of sedation and advised not to drive or operate machinery during treatment, until their susceptibility is known.

Extrapyramidal symptoms such as Parkinson-like symptoms, akinesia, akathisia, dyskinesia, dystonia may develop during haloperidol treatment. Very rarely dystonia has been reported to produce laryngeal/pharyngeal spasm associated with gagging, cyanosis, respiratory distress and asphyxia. Such symptoms may be promptly controlled by parenteral administration of a short-acting barbiturate, an antihistamine or an antiparkinsonian drug. The occurrence and severity of most extrapyramidal symptoms are generally, but not always, dose related. Extrapyramidal reactions have on occasions been reported during treatment at relatively low dose levels in both children and adults. Administration of anti-Parkinsonian drugs may be required for control of such reactions.

In common with other antipsychotics haloperidol has been associated with persistent dyskinesia. Tardive dyskinesia may develop in some patients on long term therapy, possibly in relation to total cumulative dose, or may develop after drug therapy has been discontinued. The risk is reported to be greater in elderly patients on high dose therapy. Characteristic symptoms are rhythmical involuntary movements of the tongue, face, mouth or jaw sometimes accompanied by involuntary movements of the extremities. They may persist for many months or even years and, while they gradually disappear in some patients, they appear to be permanent in others. At the first signs of tardive dyskinesia which may be orofacial dyskinesia the benefit of continued treatment should be carefully assessed against the risk of the development of persistent dyskinesia. Withdrawal of treatment with careful observation of the dyskinesia and psychotic condition has been suggested in order to assess the need for continued neuroleptic therapy and to reveal persisting dyskinesia. Should it be necessary to reinstate treatment, the antipsychotic agent may mask the syndrome. Anti-Parkinsonian agents have proved of little value in this syndrome.

In schizophrenia, the response to antipsychotic drug treatment may be delayed. If drugs are withdrawn, recurrence of symptoms may not become apparent for several weeks or months.

Some degree of sedation may occur, particularly with higher doses and at the start of treatment. The elderly appear more susceptible. At low doses in susceptible (especially non-psychotic) individuals, haloperidol may cause unpleasant subjective feelings of being mentally dulled or slowed down, dizziness, headaches or paradoxical effects of excitement, agitation or insomnia.

Other adverse effects reported include gastrointestinal symptoms, nausea, loss of appetite, dyspepsia, autonomic effects such as blurring of vision and, infrequently, tachycardia. Dose-related hypotension is uncommon, but can occur, particularly in the elderly or after parenteral administration.

Impairment of sexual function, including erection and ejaculation; oedema; blood dyscrasias, including agranulocytosis and transient leucopenia; skin reactions including exfoliative dermatitis, erythema multiforme and photosensitisation and jaundice, are rarely reported. Transient abnormalities of liver function tests may occur in the absence of jaundice.

Impairment of body temperature could occur at high doses. In common with other antipsychotics, hormonal effects include hyperprolactinaemia which could cause galactorrhoea, gynaecomastia and oligo- or amenorrhoea. Abrupt discontinuation of high doses of antipsychotics has very rarely resulted in acute withdrawal symptoms, including nausea, vomiting and insomnia. Gradual withdrawal is advisable.

Rare cases of sudden and unexplained death have been reported in psychiatric patients receiving treatment with antipsychotics including haloperidol. The nature of the evidence makes it impossible to determine the contributory role, if any, of the drug.

In common with other antipsychotics, haloperidol has been associated with rare cases of neuroleptic malignant syndrome, an idiosyncratic response characterised by hyperthermia, muscle rigidity, autonomic instability, altered consciousness and coma. Signs of autonomic dysfunction such as tachycardia, labile arterial pressure, and sweating may precede the onset of hyperthermia, acting as early warning signs. Recovery usually occurs within five to seven days of antipsychotic withdrawal. Affected patients should be carefully monitored.

Overdosage: Intensification of the known pharmacological and adverse effects may occur. The most prominent would be severe extrapyramidal symptoms, hypotension or sedation. The patient may appear comatose with respiratory depression and hypotension which could be severe enough to produce a shock-like state. Extrapyramidal reactions may include muscular weakness or rigidity and a generalised or localised tremor. With accidental overdosage hypothermia, bradycardia, sinus arrhythmia and hypertension have been reported in young children.

No specific antidote has been identified.

In the event of overdosage the stomach should be emptied by aspiration and lavage. Emetics should not be used. Establishment of a patent airway and artificial ventilation may be needed. Hypotension may be counteracted by placing the patient in the head-down position and by use of a plasma expander and careful use of a vasopressor agent such as noradrenaline. Adrenaline should not be used. Severe extrapyramidal reactions should be treated with parenteral antihistamines or antiparkinsonian drugs. The relatively long plasma elimination half-life of haloperidol should be considered. (See Further Information).

Pharmaceutical precautions Store in a dry place below 30°C (86°F). Serenace Ampoules and Liquid should be protected from light.

Serenace Liquid can be diluted to meet individual patient requirements. The diluted solution should be stored in amber glass, screw-cap bottles at 4°C. If a concentration of 100 micrograms haloperidol per 5 ml diluted solution or less is required, Syrup B.P. is the recommended diluent. If a concentration greater than 100 micrograms haloperidol per 5 ml diluted solution is required, Syrup B.P. or distilled water are the recommended diluents. When following these recommendations the diluted solution has been found to be chemically stable for at least 8 weeks. However, it is advised that it be used as soon as possible. It may be considered advisable to restore the concentration of preservatives to original levels of 500 micrograms/ml and 50 micrograms/ml methyl- and propylhydroxybenzoate respectively.

Legal category POM.

Package quantities
5 mg Ampoules: Boxes of 6.
20 mg Ampoules: Boxes of 10.
1.5 mg Tablets: Blister strips of 100, bottles of 1000.
5 mg Tablets: Blister strips of 100, bottles of 1000.
10 mg Tablets: Blister strips of 100, bottles of 1000.
20 mg Tablets: Blister strips of 100.
2mg/ml Liquid: Bottles of 100 ml and 500 ml.
500 microgram Capsules: Blister strips of 100, bottles of 1000.

Further information Haloperidol is a butyrophenone. Its pharmacological profile of activity includes a pronounced capacity to induce extrapyramidal reactions and a low incidence of autonomic side-effects, such as hypotension.

The pharmacokinetics of haloperidol have been studied in healthy volunteers and patients. In volunteers, following a single intravenous or oral dose, serum elimination half-life ranged from 10 to 19 hours and 12 to 38 hours respectively. Similar elimination half-lives were observed in patients after administration of a single oral or intramuscular dose of the drug or after withdrawal of the drug from patients who were in a steady-state. Steady-state serum levels were usually achieved within 6 days on a fixed oral dosage.

Product licence numbers

5 mg Ampoules	0020/5036
20 mg Ampoules	0020/0078
1.5 mg Tablets	0020/5033
5 mg Tablets	0020/5034
10 mg Tablets	0020/0076
20 mg Tablets	0020/0079
2 mg/ml Liquid	0020/5035
500 microgram Capsules	0020/5038

**Trade Mark*

Serono Laboratories (UK) Ltd
99 Bridge Road East
Welwyn Garden City
Hertfordshire AL7 1BG

Serono

ARES-SERONO GROUP

METRODIN*

Presentation Metrodin ampoules contain urofollitrophin in a freeze-dried, sterile powder form. Urofollitrophin is the Approved Name given to a gonadotrophin preparation, extracted from urine of menopausal women, which possesses follicle-stimulating hormone (FSH) although virtually no luteinising hormone (LH) activity.

Each ampoule of Metrodin contains:

Human follicle-stimulating hormone (FSH)	75 IU
Lactose	10 mg

Each Metrodin ampoule is accompanied by a solvent ampoule containing:

Sodium Chloride Injection BP	1 ml

Uses

(i) Women with hypothalamic-pituitary dysfunction who present with either oligomenorrhoea or amenorrhoea: Metrodin, followed by chorionic gonadotrophin (hCG, Profasi*), is recommended for the induction of follicular development and ovulation in women with hypothalamic-pituitary dysfunction who present with either oligomenorrhoea or amenorrhoea. These women are normally classified as WHO Group II patients. They have evidence of endogenous oestrogen production and thus will either spontaneously menstruate or experience withdrawal bleeding after progestagen administration. In the majority of these patients there is evidence of polycystic ovarian syndrome (PCOS).

(ii) Women undergoing superovulation for in vitro fertilisation (IVF) and other assisted conception techniques: Metrodin and Profasi are indicated, either alone or combined with Serophene therapy, for the induction of multiple follicular development in patients undergoing an assisted conception technique, such as IVF. The induction of multiple follicular growth is also known as 'superovulation'. Tubal occlusion, unexplained infertility and male factor infertility are common indications for IVF.

Children: Metrodin is not recommended for use in children.

Elderly: Metrodin is not recommended for use in the elderly.

Dosage and administration The injection should be reconstituted immediately prior to use with the solvent provided. In order to avoid the intramuscular injection of large volumes, up to 5 ampoules of Metrodin may be dissolved in 1 ml of solvent.

(i) Women with hypotyhalamic-pituitary dysfunction who present with either oligomenorrhoea or amenorrhoea: The object of Metrodin therapy is to develop a single mature Graafian follicle from which the ovum will be liberated after the administration of Profasi.

Metrodin may be given as a course of daily or alternate day injections. In menstruating patients treatment should commence within the first 7 days of the menstrual cycle.

Daily therapy: Treatment should be commenced at 1 to 2 ampoules (75–150 IU FSH) daily and increased or decreased by 1 ampoule (75 IU)/day at approximately weekly intervals if necessary, to obtain an adequate, but not excessive, response. If a patient fails to respond adequately after 3 weeks' treatment that cycle should be abandoned.

Alternate day therapy: Treatment should be commenced at 3 to 5 ampoules (225–375 IU FSH) per dose and increased or decreased by 1 to 2 ampoules (75–150 IU) per injection at approximately weekly intervals until an adequate, but not excessive response is obtained. If a patient fails to respond adequately after 3 weeks of treatment that cycle should be abandoned.

When an optimal response is obtained, following daily or alternate-day therapy, a single intramuscular injection of up to 10,000 IU Profasi should be administered 24–48 hours after the last Metrodin injection. The patient is recommended to have coitus on the day of and that following Profasi administration.

If an excessive response is obtained, treatment should be stopped and Profasi withheld. Treatment should recommence in the next cycle at a dosage of 1–2 ampoules (75–150 IU) lower than that of the previous cycle.

Monitoring of Metrodin therapy: The dose of Metrodin required to evoke the desired response is critical and varies both from patient to patient and in the same patient from cycle to cycle. Monitoring of Metrodin therapy is, therefore, essential.

Several methods are available for monitoring gonadotrophin therapy. Follicular development may be judged by the concentration of oestrogen measured in blood or urine and/or by ultrasonic visualisation of follicle-size—ideally both methods should be used concurrently. Although seldom adequate alone, clinical assessment of response to Metrodin, including pelvic examination and cervical mucus studies are a useful adjunct to monitoring and may be performed.

The amount of oestrogen excreted in a 24-hour collection of urine should be estimated at regular intervals throughout treatment. Urinary oestrogen levels between 180 nmol/24 hr (50 micrograms/24 hr) and 514 nmol/24 hr (140 micrograms/24 hr) generally indicate an optimum response. Values below this therapeutic range may indicate inadequate follicular development. In cases where the levels are in excess of 514 nmol/24 hr there is an increased risk of ovarian hyperstimulation. A very steep rise in oestrogen levels generally indicates an increased risk of hyperstimulation. In cycles in which an excessive oestrogen response has occurred, Profasi should not be given (see 'Warnings') and the patient should refrain from having coitus for at least the next 4 days.

Plasma oestradiol-17β: The level of plasma oestradiol-17β should be estimated at regular intervals throughout treatment with Metrodin. Levels between 1100 pmol/l (300 pg/ml) and 3000 pmol/l (800 pg/ml) generally indicate an optimum response. Values below this therapeutic range may indicate inadequate follicular development. In cases where the oestradiol-17β level exceeds 3000 pmol/l there is an increased risk of hyperstimulation and Profasi should be withheld (see Warnings) and the patient should refrain from having coitus for at least the next 4 days. A very steep rise in oestradiol levels generally indicates an increased risk of hyperstimulation.

Ultrasound: When monitoring Metrodin therapy by serial ultrasonic visualisation of follicle size, a follicular diameter of 16–25 mm should indicate the presence of a mature follicle and therefore the optimum time for the administration of Profasi. If the follicular diameter of the dominant follicle is less than 16 mm further Metrodin may be required.

Profasi should not be given if several mature follicles are visualised as there is a risk of multiple ovulation and the occurrence of hyperstimulation syndrome.

(ii) Women undergoing superovulation for in-vitro ferilisation (IVF) and other assisted conception techniques: The objective of superovulation is to stimulate multiple follicular growth, thereby increasing the number of eggs available for fertilisation.

The most frequently used regimen for superovulation involves pretreatment with Serophene followed by Metrodin and Profasi. A commonly used combined dosage regimen involves the administration of 100 mg Serophene daily on cycle days 2–6, followed by 2–3 ampoules (150–225 IU FSH) per day commencing on day 5 of the cycle and continuing at a dose dependent upon the patient's response, until adequate follicular development has been achieved.

An alternative regimen using Metrodin and Profasi involves the administration of 2–3 ampoules (150–225 IU FSH) daily commencing on days 2 or 3 of the cycle. Treatment is continued, with the dose adjusted according to the patient's response, until adequate follicular development has been achieved.

For both Metrodin+Profasi and Serophene+Metrodin+Profasi regimens, a single injection of up to 10,000 IU Profasi is administered 24–48 hours after the last Metrodin injection to coincide with the expected onset of the (endogenous) LH surge.

Monitoring of superovulation: The administration of Metrodin for superovulation is usually monitored by plasma oestradiol-17β and ultrasound. One recommendation is that the diameter of at least 3 follicles should be equal to or greater than 16 mm, with the diameter of the leading follicle being 18 mm, and the plasma oestradiol-17β level at least 3500 pmol/l (920 pg/ml).

Profasi should not be administered unless there is evidence of adequate follicular development as evidenced by progressively rising oestrogen levels and concomitant follicular growth on ultrasound.

Egg retrieval: Egg retrieval is carried out, either by laparoscopy or ultrasound guided aspiration, about 34–36 hours following the Profasi injection. Ideally, all follicles should be aspirated at egg retrieval (see 'Warnings').

Further details concerning Metrodin dosage and monitoring are available on request.

Contra-indications, warnings, etc

Contra-indications: Metrodin therapy is precluded in women in whom a satisfactory outcome cannot be expected e.g. women with ovarian dysgenesis, absent uterus, premature menopause and also in women with tubal occlusion unless they are undergoing superovulation for an assisted conception technique.

Appropriate treatment should first be given for other endocrine disorders, e.g hypothyroidism, adrenocortical deficiency, hyperprolactinaemia or pituitary tumour and other possible causes of infertility in either partner. An acceptable semen analysis should be available.

Warnings: Metrodin may cause local reaction at the injection site.

Allergic-type reactions have occasionally been reported, in which lactose intolerance has been suspected, although not proven. It is therefore important to consider the effect of the lactose component of Metrodin, if administered to lactose-sensitive patients.

Although adherence to recommended Metrodin dosages will minimise the incidence of ovarian hyperstimulation in patients undergoing ovulation induction, the possibility of hyperstimulation and multiple ovulation should be considered and careful monitoring performed during treatment in order to minimise their occurrence. Excessive oestrogenic responses seldom give rise to significant hyperstimulation unless Profasi is administered to induce ovulation. It is therefore prudent to withhold Profasi in such cases and advise the patient to refrain from coitus for at least 4 days (also see 'Overdosages').

One might expect patients undergoing superovulation to be at an increased risk of developing hyperstimulation in view of the excessive oestrogen response and multiple follicular development. Aspiration of all follicles, prior to ovulation, may reduce the incidence of hyperstimulation.

The risk of multiple pregnancy following assisted conception techniques is related to the number of oocytes/embryos replaced. In other patients the incidence of multiple pregnancies and births is increased by Metrodin therapy; however, the majority of multiple conceptions are twins.

Pregnancy loss is higher than that in the normal population, but comparable with the rates found in women with other fertility problems.

Precautions: In those patients not undergoing superovulation the occurrence of smaller, secondary follicles in the presence of more than one dominant follicle, as visualised by ultrasonography, is reported to be associated with an increased incidence of hyperstimulation.

Side-effects: Local reaction at injection site; allergic-type reaction possibly due to lactose component; hyperstimulation; multiple pregnancy. There have been no reports of congenital abnormalities associated with Metrodin therapy.

Overdosage (and treatment): There are no reports of toxic effects occurring as a result of overdosage.

Hyperstimulation may result from overdosage with Metrodin. Hyperstimulation is generally categorised as mild, moderate or severe and symptoms usually appear 3–6 days after hCG administration.

Mild hyperstimulation—symptoms may include some abdominal swelling and pain, ovaries enlarged up to 5 cm diameter. Therapy—rest; careful observation and symptomatic relief. Ovarian enlargement declines rapidly.

Moderate hyperstimulation—symptoms include more pronounced abdominal distension and pain; nausea; vomiting; occasional diarrhoea; ovaries enlarged up to 12 cm diameter. Therapy—bed rest; close observation, in the case of conception occurring, to detect any progression to severe hyperstimulation. Pelvic examination of enlarged ovaries should be gentle in order to avoid rupture of the cysts. Symptoms subside spontaneously over 2–3 weeks.

Severe hyperstimulation—this is a very rare but serious complication—symptoms include pronounced abdominal distension and pain; ascites; pleural effusion; decreased blood volume; reduced urine output; electrolyte imbalance and sometimes shock; ovaries enlarged to in excess of 12 cm diameter. Therapy—hospitalisation, treatment should be conservative and concentrate on restoring the blood volume and preventing shock. Acute symptoms subside over several days and ovaries return to normal over 20–40 days if conception does not occur—symptoms may be prolonged if conception occurs.

Pharmaceutical precautions Metrodin should be stored below 25°C and protected from light.

Legal category POM.

Package quantities Boxes containing:
(i) 1 ampoule Metrodin plus 1 ampoule solvent
(ii) 3 ampoules Metrodin plus 3 ampoules solvent
(iii) 50 ampoules Metrodin plus 50 ampoules solvent

Further information One IU of human urinary FSH is defined as the activity contained in 0.11388 mg of the 1st International Standard.

Product licence numbers
Metrodin 3400/0012
Profasi 3400/0003–6
Serophene 3400/0009
Sodium Chloride Injection BP 3400/0024

PERGONAL*

Presentation Pergonal ampoules contain human menopausal gonadotrophin (HMG) in a freeze-dried, sterile powder form (Approved Name: Menotrophin).

Each Pergonal ampoule contains:

Human follicle-stimulating hormone (FSH)	75 IU
Human luteinising hormone (LH)	75 IU
Lactose	10 mg

Each Pergonal ampoule is accompanied by a solvent ampoule containing:

Sodium Chloride Injection BP	1 ml

Uses Pergonal is used for the treatment of infertile patients under the guidance of clinicians familiar with infertility problems.

(i) Amenorrhoeic anovulatory women: Pergonal followed by chorionic gonadotrophin (hCG, Profasi*) are indicated for the induction of ovulation in the amenorrhoeic patient or anovulatory woman with regular or irregular cycles.

(ii) Women undergoing superovulation for in vitro fertilisation (IVF) and other assisted conception techniques: Pergonal and Profasi are also indicated, either alone or combined with Serophene therapy, for the induction of multiple follicular development in patients undergoing an assisted conception technique, such as IVF. The induction of multiple follicular growth is also known as 'superovulation'. Tubal occlusion, unexplained infertility and male subfertility are common indications for IVF.

(iii) Hypogonadotrophic hypogonadism in men: Pergonal with concomitant Profasi therapy is indicated for the stimulation of spermatogenesis in men who have primary or secondary hypogonadotrophic hypogonadism.

Elevated endogenous FSH levels are indicative of primary testicular failure. Such patients are usually unresponsive to Pergonal/Profasi therapy.

Dosage and administration Pergonal is given by intramuscular injection only. In order to avoid the intramuscular injection of large volumes, up to 5 ampoules of Pergonal may be dissolved in 1 ml of solvent.

(i) Amenorrhoeic/anovulatory women: The object is to develop a single mature Graafian follicle with individually tailored doses of Pergonal over several days. Stimulated follicles will not always liberate ova spontaneously, therefore follicular rupture has to be achieved by injecting Profasi, which simulates the normal mid-cycle surge of LH.

Pergonal may be given as a course of daily or alternate day injections. In menstruating patients treatment should commence within the first 7 days of the menstrual cycle.

Two Pergonal dosage schedules are commonly employed:

Alternate day therapy: Three equal doses of Pergonal are given on alternate days followed by up to 10,000 IU Profasi one week after the first injection of Pergonal, provided an adequate but not excessive response has been obtained (see 'Monitoring'). Coitus is recommended on the day of and that following Profasi injection.

The recommended dosage for the initial course of treatment is:

WHO Group I patients (women with little or no evidence of endogenous oestrogen activity)—5 ampoules per injection.

WHO Group II patients (women with evidence of some oestrogen activity)—3 ampoules per injection.

In both groups of patients, the dosage in subsequent courses should be adjusted if necessary, depending upon the patient's response to the previous course.

Daily therapy: Pergonal is given as a course of daily injections. Treatment should be commenced at 2 ampoules per day (Group I patients) or 1 ampoule per day (Group II patients) and increased or decreased at approximately weekly intervals if necessary, to obtain an adequate, but not excessive, response (see Monitoring). Up to 10,000 IU Profasi should be given 24–48 hours after the last Pergonal injection. Coitus is recommended on the day of and that following Profasi injection. If a patient fails to respond adequately after 3 weeks' treatment that cycle should be abandoned.

The dosage in subsequent cycles should be adjusted if necessary depending upon the patient's response to the previous treatment course.

Monitoring of Pergonal therapy: The dose of Pergonal required to evoke the desired response is critical and varies both from patient to patient and in the same patient from cycle to cycle. Monitoring of Pergonal therapy is, therefore, essential.

Several methods are available for monitoring of gonadotrophin therapy. Follicular development may be judged by the concentration of oestrogen measured in blood or urine and/or by ultrasonic visualisation of follicle size—ideally both methods should be used concurrently. Although seldom adequate alone, clinical assessment of response to Pergonal, including pelvic examination and cervical mucus studies are a useful adjunct to monitoring and may be performed.

Urinary oestrogens: The amount of oestrogen excreted in a 24 hour collection of urine shoud be estimated at regular intervals throughout treatment. Urinary oestrogen levels between 180 nmol/24 hr and 514 nmol/24 hr generally indicate an optimum response. Values below this therapeutic range may indicate inadequate follicular development. In cases where the levels are in excess of 514 nmol/24 hr or where a very steep rise in oestrogen levels occur there is an increased risk of hyperstimulation. In cycles in which an excessive oestrogen response has occurred, Profasi should be withheld (see 'Warnings') and the patient should refrain from having coitus for at least the next 4 days.

Plasma oestradiol-17β. The level of plasma oestradiol-17β should be estimated at regular intervals throughout treatment with Pergonal. Levels between 1100 pmol/l and 3000 pmol/l generally indicate an optimum response. Values below this therapeutic range may indicate inadequate follicular development. In cases where the oestradiol-17β level exceeds 3000 pmol/l or where a very steep rise occurs, there is an increased risk of hyperstimulation. Profasi should be withheld (see 'Warnings') and the patient should refrain from having coitus for at least the next 4 days.

Ultrasound: When monitoring Pergonal therapy by serial ultrasonic visualisation of the follicle size, a follicular diameter of 16–25 mm should indicate the presence of a mature follicle and therefore the optimum time for the administration of Profasi. If the follicular diameter of the dominant follicle is less than 16 mm, further Pergonal may be required.

Profasi should not be given if several mature follicles are visualised as there is a risk of multiple ovulation and the occurrence of hyperstimulation syndrome.

(ii) Women undergoing superovulation for in-vitro fertilisation (IVF) and other assisted conception techniques: The objective of superovulation is to stimulate multiple follicular growth, thereby increasing the number of eggs available for fertilisation.

Serophene pretreatment combined with Pergonal and Profasi can be used for superovulation. A commonly used combined dosage regimen involves the administration of 100 mg Serophene daily on cycle days 2–6, followed by 2–3 ampoules Pergonal (150–225 IU FSH+LH) per day commencing on day 5 of the cycle and continuing, at a dose dependent upon the patient's response, until adequate follicular development has been achieved.

One regimen using Pergonal and Profasi alone involves the administration of 2–3 ampoules Pergonal (150–225 IU FSH+LH) daily commencing on day 2 or 3 of the cycle. Treatment is continued, with the dose adjusted according to the patient's response, until adequate follicular development has been achieved.

For both Pergonal+Profasi and Serophene+Pergonal+Profasi regimens, a single injection of up to 10,000 IU Profasi is administered 24–48 hours after the last Pergonal injection to coincide with the expected onset of the (endogenous) LH surge.

Monitoring of superovulation: The administration of Pergonal for superovulation is usually monitored by plasma oestradiol-17β and ultrasound. One recommendation is that the diameter of at least 3 follicles should be equal to or greater than 15 mm, with the diameter of the leading follicle being 18 mm and the plasma oestradiol-17β level at least 3500 pmol/l (920 pg/ml).

Profasi should not be administered unless there is evidence of adequate follicular development as evidenced by progressively rising oestrogen levels and concomitant follicular growth on ultrasound.

Egg retrieval: Egg retrieval is carried out, either by laparoscopy or ultrasound guided aspiration, about 34–36 hours following Profasi injection. All follicles should be aspirated at egg retrieval (see 'Warnings').

Further details concerning Pergonal dosage and monitoring for both amenorrhoeic/anovulatory women and superovulation are available on request.

(iii) Hypogonadotrophic hypogonadism in men: Treatment should begin with Profasi 2000 IU 2–3 times a week to produce evidence of adequate masculinisation.

If the only response to Profasi is androgenic in nature, Pergonal (1 ampoule 3 times a week) and Profasi 2000 IU (twice a week) should be given for a minimum period of four months.

If the patient has not responded with evidence of increased spermatogenesis at the end of four months, therapy may be continued with Pergonal (1 or 2 ampoules 3 times a week) and Profasi 2000 IU (twice a week).

Children: Not recommended for use in children.

Elderly: Not recommended for use in the elderly.

Contra-indications, warnings, etc

Contra-indications: Pergonal therapy is precluded in women in whom a satisfactory outcome cannot be expected, e.g. women with ovarian dysgenesis, absent uterus, premature menopause and also in women with tubal occlusion unless they are undergoing superovulation for assisted conception.

Appropriate treatment should first be given for other endocrine disorders, e.g. hypothyroidism, adrenocortical deficiency, hyperprolactinaemia or pituitary tumour and other possible causes of infertility in either partner. An acceptable semen analysis should be available for those couples undergoing ovulation induction or in vitro fertilisation. However, certain types of male infertility can be successfully treated by assisted conception techniques.

Warnings: Pergonal may occasionally cause local reactions at the injection site. Fever and joint pains have been reported rarely.

Allergic-type reactions have occasionally been reported, in which lactose intolerance has been suspected, although not proven.

Hyperstimulation: Adherence to recommended Pergonal dosages and monitoring schedules will minimise the possibility of ovarian hyperstimulation in amenorrhoeic and anovulatory women. Excessive oestrogenic responses to Pergonal do not generally give rise to significant side effects unless Profasi is given to induce ovulation. Hormone assays will detect an excessive oestrogen response to Pergonal and ultrasound will reveal any excessive follicular development; Profasi administration should be withheld in this event. (Also see 'Overdosage').

One might expect patients undergoing superovulation to be at an increased risk of developing hyperstimulation in view of the excessive oestrogen response and multiple follicular development. Aspiration of all follicles, prior to ovulation, may reduce the incidence of hyperstimulation syndrome.

Multiple pregnancy: The incidence of multiple births following Pergonal/Profasi therapy in anovulatory and amenorrhoeic women has been variously reported between 10% and 40%. However, the majority of multiple conceptions are twins: high order multiple births are extremely rare when accurate monitoring is employed.

The incidence of multiple pregnancies following assisted conception techniques, is related to the number of oocytes/embryos replaced.

Pregnancy loss, in both amenorrhoeic/anovulatory patients and women undergoing assisted conception techniques, is higher than that in the normal population, but comparable with the rates found in women with other fertility problems.

The risks of congenital abnormalities are not increased by Pergonal.

Precautions: In amenorrhoeic/anovulatory patients the occurrence of smaller, secondary follicles in the presence of more than one dominant follicle, as visualised by ultrasonography, is reported to be associated with an increased incidence of hyperstimulation syndrome.

Side-effects: Local reaction at injection site, allergic-type reaction possibly due to lactose component, fever and joint pains, hyperstimulation, multiple pregnancy.

Overdosage and treatment: There are no reports of toxic effects occurring as a result of overdosage. However, hyperstimulation syndrome may result from overdosage with Pergonal. Hyperstimulation is generally categorised as mild, moderate or severe and symptoms usually appear 3–6 days after hCG administration.

Mild hyperstimulation—Symptoms may include some abdominal swelling and pain; ovaries enlarged to about 5 cm diameter. Therapy—rest; careful observation and symptomatic relief. Ovarian enlargement declines rapidly.

Moderate hyperstimulation—Symptoms include more pronounced abdominal distension and pain; nausea; vomiting; occasional diarrhoea; ovaries enlarged up to 12 cm diameter. Therapy—bed rest; close observation, in the case of conception occurring, to detect any progression to severe hyperstimulation. Pelvic examination of enlarged ovaries should be gentle in order to avoid rupture of the cysts. Symptoms subside spontaneously over 2–3 weeks.

Severe hyperstimulation—This is a rare but serious complication—symptoms include pronounced abdominal distension and pain; ascites; pleural effusion; decreased blood volume; reduced urine output; electrolyte imbalance and sometimes shock; ovaries enlarge to in excess of 12 cm diameter. Therapy—hospitalisation; treatment should be conservative and concentrate on restoring blood volume and preventing shock. Acute symptoms subside over several days and ovaries return to normal over 20–40 days if conception does not occur—symptoms may be prolonged if conception occurs.

Pharmaceutical precautions Pergonal should be stored below 25°C. The injection should be reconstituted immediately prior to use with the solvent provided.

Legal category POM.

Package quantities Boxes containing:
(i) 1 ampoule Pergonal plus 1 ampoule solvent.
(ii) 10 ampoules Pergonal plus 10 ampoules solvent.

Further information One IU of human urinary FSH and one IU of human urinary LH are defined as the activities contained in 0.11388 mg and 0.13369 mg of the 1st International Standard, respectively.

Product licence numbers
Pergonal 3400/0007
Profasi 3400/0003–6
Serophene 3400/0009
Sodium Chloride Injection BP 3400/0024.

PROFASI*

Presentation Profasi ampoules contain human chorionic gonadotrophin (hCG) in a sterile, freeze-dried, powder form. The Chorionic Gonadotrophin Injection BP monograph applies to a hormonal preparation extracted from the urine of pregnant women, which possesses predominantly luteinising properties.

Profasi is available in four strengths (500, 1000, 2000 and 5000 IU). Ampoules of Profasi contain either:

500 IU chorionic gonadotrophin + 20 mg mannitol
1000 IU chorionic gonadotrophin + 20 mg mannitol
2000 IU chorionic gonadotrophin + 20 mg mannitol
5000 IU chorionic gonadotrophin + 20 mg mannitol

Each Profasi ampoule is accompanied by a solvent ampoule containing:

Sodium Chloride Injection BP 1 ml

Uses The action of human chorionic gonadotrophin is predominantly luteinising. Profasi is used in the treatment of infertility where its administration forms part of a recognised treatment regimen.

(i) Anovulatory women: Briefly, follicular development and endometrial proliferation are first stimulated with a suitable agent, e.g. Serophene, Pergonal* (Menotrophin Injection BP, HMG) or Metrodin* (Urofollitrophin, FSH), Profasi is then given to simulate the LH surge and induce ovulation.

(ii) Women undergoing superovulation for an assisted conception technique: Profasi is used as part of a superovulation programme in women undergoing an assisted conception technique. Multiple follicular development is stimulated with Pergonal or Metrodin, either alone or in combination with Serophene, Profasi is then administered to bring about final maturation of the follicles. Follicles are aspirated prior to spontaneous ovulation.

(iii) Hypogonadotrophic hypogonadism in men: Profasi stimulates the interstitial (Leydig) cells of the testes and consequently the secretion of androgens and the development of secondary sexual characteristics. With concomitant Pergonal therapy, Profasi stimulates the induction and maintenance of spermatogenesis.

(iv) Cryptorchidism: Profasi stimulates the Leydig cells of the testes and effects the secretion of androgens. The combined action of hCG and intratesticular testosterone leads to the descent of cryptorchid testes.

Dosage and administration Profasi is given by intramuscular injection only.

(i) Anovulatory women: Up to 10,000 IU Profasi in midcycle or as indicated following Serophene, Pergonal or Metrodin, according to a recognised scheme, provided an adequate but not excessive response has been obtained. (See appropriate Data Sheet for details of dosage and monitoring).

(ii) Women undergoing superovulation for an assisted conception technique: Up to 10,000 IU Profasi is given following the induction of multiple follicular development with Pergonal or Metrodin, either alone or in combination with Serophene, according to a recognised treatment scheme. (See appropriate Data Sheet for details of dosage and monitoring). Egg retrieval is carried out 34–36 hours following Profasi administration.

(iii) Hypogonadotrophic Hypogonadism in men: 2,000 IU Profasi twice weekly to bring about the development of secondary sexual characteristics and a testosterone level within the normal range.

Elevated endogenous FSH levels are indicative of primary testicular failure. Such patients are usually unresponsive to Pergonal/Profasi therapy.

If the induction of spermatogenesis is required, but the only response to Profasi has been androgenic, therapy should be continued with Profasi 2,000 IU twice weekly, and one ampoule of Pergonal three times a week. This regimen should be continued for a minimum of four months.

If, after the four months, the patient has not responded with evidence of increased spermatogenesis, therapy may be continued with Profasi 2,000 IU twice weekly and 1 or 2 ampoules Pergonal three times a week.

Although no specific monitoring is required in the male patient, semen analysis is useful in assessing the response to treatment.

(iv) Cryptorchidism: 500–1,000 IU Profasi, dependent upon age, on alternate days for several weeks.

Children—girls: Profasi is not recommended for use in girls.

Contra-indications, warnings, etc

Contra-indications: Profasi is precluded in women in whom stimulation of follicular maturation is not indicated because of the expectations of an unsatisfactory outcome. For example, women with ovarian dysgenesis, absent uterus, premature menopause and also in women with tubal occlusion unless they are undergoing superovulation for IVF.

Appropriate treatment should first be given for other endocrine disorders, e.g. hypothyroidism, adrenocortical deficiency, hyperprolactinaemia or pituitary tumour and other possible causes of infertility in either partner. An acceptable semen analysis should be available, however certain types of male infertility can be successfully treated by assisted conception techniques.

Hyperstimulation: In women undergoing ovulation induction, an excessive response to follicular stimulating agents (e.g. Serophene, Metrodin or Pergonal) may lead to the development of hyperstimulation syndrome, particularly if Profasi is given to induce ovulation; Profasi should be withheld in such cycles. (See 'Overdosage').

Warnings: Profasi may occasionally cause local reactions at the injection site.

In men, high doses of Profasi may lead to oedema and in such cases the dosage should be considerably reduced.

The risk of hyperstimulation developing in women undergoing superovulation for an assisted conception technique may be reduced by aspiration of all the follicles prior to ovulation.

The risk of multiple pregnancy following assisted conception techniques, is related to the number of oocytes/embryos replaced. In other patients the incidence of multiple pregnancies and births is increased by gonadotrophin therapy; however, the majority of multiple pregnancies are twins.

Sexual precocity: Profasi may cause sexual precocity. If signs are observed, treatment should be stopped. If continued therapy is considered necessary, a reduced dosage regimen should be instituted.

Pregnancy loss, in both anovulatory patients and women undergoing assisted conception techniques, is higher than that found in the normal population, but comparable with the rates observed in women with other fertility problems.

The risk of congenital abnormalities is not increased by Profasi.

Precautions: In those patients not undergoing superovulation the occurrence of smaller, secondary follicles in the presence of more than one dominant follicle, as visualised by ultrasonography, is reported to be associated with an increased incidence of hyperstimulation.

Side-effects: Hyperstimulation (see 'Overdosage'); multiple pregnancy; oedema; sexual precocity; local reaction at injection site.

Overdosage: There are no reports of toxic effects occurring as a result of overdosage. However, hyperstimulation syndrome may result from overdosage with follicle stimulating/ovulation inducing agents. Hyperstimulation is generally categorised as mild, moderate or severe and symptoms usually appear 3–6 days after hCG administration.

Mild hyperstimulation—Symptoms may include some abdominal swelling and pain; ovaries enlarged to about 5 cm diameter. Therapy—rest; careful observation and symptomatic relief. Ovarian enlargement declines rapidly.

Moderate hyperstimulation—Symptoms include more pronounced abdominal distension and pain; nausea; vomiting; occasional diarrhoea; ovaries enlarged up to 12 cm diameter. Therapy—bed rest; close observation, in the case of conception occurring, to detect any progression to severe hyperstimulation. Pelvic examination of enlarged ovaries should be gentle, in order to avoid rupture of the cysts. Symptoms subside spontaneously over 2–3 weeks.

Severe hyperstimulation—This is a rare but serious complication. Symptoms include pronounced abdominal distension and pain; ascites; pleural effusion; decreased blood volume; reduced urine output; electrolyte imbalance and sometimes shock; ovaries enlarge to in excess of 12 cm diameter. Therapy—hospitalisation, treatment should be conservative and concentrate on restoring blood volume and preventing shock. Acute symptoms subside over several days and ovaries return to normal over 20–40 days, if conception has not occurred. Symptoms may be prolonged if conception has occurred.

Pharmaceutical precautions Profasi should be stored below 25°C and protected from light. Solutions of Profasi should be used immediately after preparation.

Legal category POM.

Package quantities Boxes containing:
3 ampoules of Profasi 500 IU, 1000 IU or 2000 IU plus 3 ampoules solvent.
1 ampoule Profasi 5000 IU plus 1 ampoule solvent.
10 ampoules Profasi 5000 IU plus 10 ampoules solvent.

Further information One IU of chorionic gonadotrophin is defined as the activity contained in 0.001279 mg of the 2nd International Standard Preparation.

Product licence numbers
Profasi 500 3400/0003
Profasi 1000 3400/0004
Profasi 2000 3400/0005
Profasi 5000 3400/0006
Pergonal 3400/0007
Metrodin 3400/0012
Sodium Chloride Injection BP 3400/0024
Serophene 3400/0009

REHIBIN*

Presentation White, uncoated, scored, flat tablets with bevelled edges. Each tablet contains cyclofenil 100 mg.

Uses Rehibin is indicated for the treatment of anovulatory infertility attributed to dysfunction of the hypothalamo-pituitary ovarian axis.

Best response is generally obtained in patients with anovulatory cycles or oligomenorrhoea.

Rehibin is prescribable under the supervision of clinicians involved in the treatment of infertility.

Dosage and administration Rehibin 200 mg (2 tablets) twice daily (morning and evening) for 10 days. Treatment should be commenced 3 days after the onset of spontaneous or induced menstruation.

Treatment should be continued for at least 3 cycles. Coitus is recommended around the expected time of ovulation. (see Monitoring.)

If the patient remains anovulatory after 3 cycles of treatment, further assessment should be carried out and gonadotrophin therapy considered.

If ovulation is induced, but pregnancy has not occurred within 6 treatment cycles, the patient should be reassessed and considered for gonadotrophin therapy.

Rehibin is not recommended for use in children.

Monitoring of rehibin therapy: Monitoring may be used to determine the efficacy of treatment and to aid the timing of coitus.

The daily recording of basal body temperature (BBT) by the patient is a useful monitoring method. A BBT chart showing a mid-cycle dip followed by a rise in temperature is suggestive of ovulation. Coitus is recommended around the time of the 'dip' as this represents the time of ovulation.

The measurement of mid-luteal plasma progesterone may be used to assess the ovulatory response to treatment. Progesterone levels (7 days after ovulation approx. cycle day 21) in excess of 30 nmol/l are suggestive of ovulation.

If a patient shows presumptive evidence of ovulation and menstruation does not follow, pregnancy should be excluded before treatment is recommenced.

Contra-indications, warnings, etc
Contra-indications: Liver disease; a history of liver dysfunction; pregnancy (see Warnings); pituitary tumours and/or endocrine disorders (see Warnings).

Rehibin therapy is precluded in women in whom a satisfactory outcome cannot be expected e.g., women with ovarian dysgenesis, absent uterus, premature menopause and also women with tubal occlusion.

Warnings: Appropriate treatment should first be given for other endocrine disorders e.g. hypothyroidism, adrenocortical deficiency, hyperprolactinaemia or pituitary tumour and other possible causes of infertility in either partner. An acceptable semen analysis should be available prior to commencing treatment.

Administration of Rehibin during pregnancy should be avoided, although no adverse effects on the foetus have been reported.

Administration of Rehibin may inhibit lactation.

Side-effects: Infrequent reversible jaundice has only been reported with continuous administration of cyclofenil, at higher than recommended doses.

Minor complaints such as nausea, hot flushes and slight abdominal pain have been reported occasionally.

Overdosage: There have been no reports of serious ill effects from overdosage. Necessary treatment would be symptomatic and supportive.

Pharmaceutical precautions Store below 25°C.

Legal category POM.

Package quantities Rehibin is packed in amber glass bottles each containing 100 × 100 mg tablets.

Further information Rehibin has been shown to increase gonadotrophin secretion in patients with anovulation. There is also evidence that Rehibin acts directly on the ovary by enhancing the response to pituitary gonadotrophins.

Cervical mucus becomes copious and thin during Rehibin treatment, which favours conception.

Hyperstimulation syndrome has not been reported.

Pregnancy loss is higher than that in the normal population, but comparable with the rates found in women with fertility problems.

Product licence number 5305/0001.

Product licence holder: Pharmacia AB, Box 839, 20180 Malmo, Sweden.

SAIZEN* ▼

Presentation Saizen vials contain somatropin (rmc) in a freeze-dried, sterile powder form.

Each single-use vial of Saizen contains rhGH, 4IU along with sodium phosphate; disodium hydrogen phosphate; sodium chloride and mannitol. Each vial is accompanied by an ampoule of diluent containing 1 ml of 0.9% w/v sodium chloride solution.

Uses The treatment of short stature resulting from growth failure caused by decreased or absent secretion of endogenous growth hormone. The diagnosis should be confirmed by appropriate investigations of pituitary function. It is recommended that Saizen treatment should be initiated/given under the guidance of a physician experienced in the diagnosis and management of GH deficiency.

Dosage and administration The dosage must be individualised for each patient.

The recommended dose is 0.6 IU/kg body weight (or 12 IU/m^2 body surface area) per week. The dosage can be increased to 0.8 IU/kg (or 20 IU/m^2) if the response is poor.

The lyophilised material should be reconstituted with 0.5–1 ml of the solvent ampoule and dissolved using a gentle, swirling motion. Vigorous shaking should be avoided as this can lead to a cloudiness of the solution.

Route of administration: Subcutaneous or intramuscular injection.

(a) Subcutaneous injection: The weekly dose can be divided into 3 single doses (corresponding to 0.2 IU/kg/injection) or into 6 or 7 single daily doses (corresponding to 0.08 to 0.07 IU/kg/injection or 2 to 1.7 IU/m^2/

injection). The injection site should be alternated to prevent lipoatrophy.

(b) Intramuscular injection: The weekly dose should be divided into 3 single injections (corresponding to 0.2 IU/kg or 4 IU/m² per injection).

Treatment should be continued until the patient has reached a satisfactory adult height or the epiphyses are closed.

Contra-indications, warnings, etc

Contra-indications: Patients in whom epiphyseal fusion has occurred should not be treated with Saizen.

Saizen is also contra-indicated in patients who show recurrence or progression of an underlying intracranial lesion.

Saizen is not recommended for use during pregnancy and lactation.

Precautions: Saizen treatment should be carried out under regular medical supervision.

In patients with diabetes mellitus the treatment should be carried out under strict medical control with laboratory monitoring of their diabetic status as hypoglycaemia has been associated with the growth response. Adjustment of anti-diabetic therapy may be required.

Patients with growth hormone deficiency secondary to a treated intracranial lesion should be examined frequently for recurrence of the underlying disease process.

The possible appearance of hypothyroidism in the course of the therapy with growth hormone should be corrected with thyroid hormone in order to obtain a sufficient growth promoting effect.

When growth hormone is administered subcutaneously at the same site over a longer period, local tissue atrophy may result. This can be avoided by rotating the injection site daily.

Pregnancy and lactation: There are no data from either human or animal studies relating to the use of Saizen during pregnancy. In the event of pregnancy occurring, treatment must be discontinued. There is no knowledge regarding the secretion of growth hormone into human breast milk.

Overdose: Acute overdosage can produce transient hypoglycaemia followed by hyperglycaemia. Long term overdosage may result in the clinical features of acromegaly.

Side-effects: Some patients may experience redness and itching at the site of injection, particularly when the subcutaneous route is used.

Antibodies to somatropin can form in some patients; the clinical significance of these antibodies is unknown. In very rare instances, where short stature is due to deletion of the growth hormone gene complex, treatment with growth hormone may induce growth attenuating antibodies.

Interaction with other medicines: Concomitant corticosteroid therapy may inhibit the growth promoting effects of growth hormone. Interactions with other medicines are, at present, unknown.

Also see 'Precautions' re: insulin-dependent diabetes mellitus.

Pharmaceutical precautions Saizen has a shelf life of two years when stored at 2–8°C. Reconstituted solution should be used immediately or within 24 hours when stored in a refrigerator.

Legal category POM.

Package quantities Each box contains: 1 vial of Saizen and 1 ml solvent ampoule.

Further information Saizen is produced by recombinant DNA technology, using a mammalian cell line. The physical, chemical and biological profiles of Saizen are identical to those of pituitary growth hormone.

Actions: The administration of Saizen stimulates an increase in growth velocity.

Product licence numbers
Saizen 3400/0023
Sodium Chloride Injection BP 3400/0024

SEROPHENE*

Presentation White, round, flat, bevelled tablet, single score on one side and the letter 'S' imprinted on the other, each containing 50 mg Clomiphene Citrate B.P.

Uses Serophene is indicated for the induction of ovulation in women with:

(i) hypothalamic-pituitary dysfunction (including polycystic ovaries (PCO))

(ii) the induction of multiple follicular development in women undergoing superovulation for an assisted conception technique.

Serophene is prescribable under the supervision of clinicians involved in the treatment of infertility.

Dosage and administration

(i) Hypothalamic pituitary dysfunction (including PCO): Serophene is given as a 5 day course of tablets, commencing within the first 5 days of spontaneous or progesterone-induced menstrual bleeding. In patients who have not experienced recent uterine bleeding the commencement date is arbitrary.

A suggested dosage schedule is presented in the following table:

	dose mg/day	*Result after 1 cycle*			*Result after 6 cycles—no pregnancy*
		ovulation pregnancy	*ovulation no pregnancy*	*no ovulation*	
Cycle 1	50	cease therapy	continue 6 cycles (max)	increase dose (cycle 2)	
Cycle 2	100	cease therapy	continue 6 cycles (max)	same dose with hCG may be considered (cycle 3) *or*	reassess patient and consider gonadotrophin therapy
Cycle 3	100† +hCG	cease therapy	continue for 6 cycles (max)	reassess patient and consider gonadotrophin therapy	

†This dose of Serophene should not be exceeded.

If ovulation does not occur naturally, a single intramuscular injection of up to 10,000 IU Profasi (chorionic gonadotrophin, hCG) may be given 7 to 10 days after the last Serophene tablet.

Coitus is recommended around the expected time of ovulation (approximately 8–12 days after the last dose of Serophene).

Monitoring of treatment: The daily recording of basal body temperature (BBT) by the patient is a useful monitoring method. A BBT chart showing a mid-cycle dip followed by a rise in temperature sustained throughout the luteal phase is suggestive of ovulation. Coitus is recommended around the time of the 'dip' as this represents the time of ovulation.

The measurement of mid-luteal plasma progesterone is the best way to assess the ovulatory response to treatment. On cycle day 21, serum progesterone levels in excess of 30 nmol/l are suggestive of ovulation.

If a patient shows presumptive evidence of ovulation and menstruation does not follow, pregnancy should be excluded before treatment is recommenced.

(ii) Superovulation for an assisted conception technique: The objective of superovulation is to stimulate multiple follicular growth, thereby increasing the number of eggs available for fertilisation.

Serophene is usually administered in combination with gonadotrophins to induce multiple follicular maturation. A commonly used dosage regimen involves the administration of 100 mg (two tablets) Serophene daily on cycle days 2–6, followed by daily injections of Pergonal or Metrodin (150–225 IU FSH) commencing on day 5 of the cycle and continuing, at a dose dependent upon the response of the patient, until adequate follicular development has been achieved. (See Pergonal, Metrodin and Profasi Data Sheets for further details).

A single injection of up to 10,000 IU Profasi is administered 24–48 hours after the last gonadotrophin injection to coincide with the expected onset of the (endogenous) LH surge.

Monitoring of superovulation: Superovulation is monitored by plasma oestradiol-17β estimations and by ultrasonography.

One recommendation is that the diameter of at least 3 follicles should be equal to or greater than 15 mm, with the diameter of the leading follicle 18 mm or more and a plasma oestradiol-17β level greater than 3500 pmol/l.

hCG should not be administered unless there is evidence of adequate follicular development as evidenced by progressively rising oestrogen levels and concomitant follicular growth on ultrasound.

Egg retrieval: Egg retrieval is carried out, either by laparoscopy or ultrasound guided aspiration, about 24–36 hours following Profasi injection. All follicles should be aspirated at egg retrieval (see 'Warnings').

Further details concerning Serophene dosage and monitoring, are available on request.

Contra-indications, warnings, etc

Contra-indications: Liver disease and liver dysfunction; hereditary defect in bilirubin metabolism; pregnancy; abnormal uterine bleeding; ovarian cysts (except polycystic ovaries); ovarian endometriosis.

Serophene therapy is precluded in women in whom a satisfactory outcome cannot be expected, e.g., women with ovarian dysgenesis, absent uterus, premature menopause, hypothalamic pituitary failure and also in women with tubal occlusion unless thay are undergoing superovulation for IVF.

Although Serophene has been shown to be embryotoxic in animals at high doses, there is no evidence to suggest that it increases the incidence of congenital malformations in humans at therapeutic levels. Treatment with Serophene has not been shown to alter the incidence of congenital malformations observed in the offspring of women with fertility problems.

Warnings

Hyperstimulation:

(i) Hypothalamic pituitary dysfunction (including PCO): Patients receiving Serophene should be instructed to report any abdominal discomfort immediately and a pelvic examination should be performed to determine whether or not ovarian enlargement has occurred. Whilst the incidence of clinically significant hyperstimulation is low with the recommended Serophene dosage scheme, the presence of excessive ovarian enlargement may require the dosage scheme to be modified (see Overdosage). Rare occurrences of lutein cyst rupture with intraperitoneal haemorrhage have been reported.

(ii) Superovulation for an assisted conception technique: The incidence of hyperstimulation is minimised in patients undergoing superovulation by the aspiration of all follicles prior to ovulation.

Visual symptoms: Clomiphene citrate should be withdrawn if visual disturbances occur, e.g., blurring, spots or flashes (in rare cases scotomata). Patients should not drive or operate machinery if their vision is adversely affected.

Multiple pregnancy: The multiple pregnancy rate in patients with hypothalamic pituitary dysfunction or PCO is approximately 8%, twins representing 90% of this figure.

The multiple pregnancy rate following assisted conception techniques is related to the number of oocytes/embryos replaced.

Although a higher spontaneous abortion rate than that found in the normal population has been reported, this is comparable to the abortion rate in women with other fertility problems. A causal relationship with clomiphene has not been established.

Precautions; Appropriate treatment should first be given for other endocrine disorders, e.g., hypothyroidism, adrenocortical deficiency, hyperprolactinaemia or pituitary tumours and other possible causes of infertility in either partner. An acceptable semen analysis should be available for those couples undergoing ovulation induction.

Side-effects: Side-effects are usually dose-related and generally reversible on drug withdrawal. The following side-effects have been reported:

Ovarian enlargement and abdominal/pelvic discomfort, vasomotor symptoms (hot flushes).

Nausea, vomiting, breast discomfort and visual symptoms have been reported occasionally.

Nervousness, insomnia, headache, dizziness, increased urination, heavier menses, depression, fatigue, skin reactions (dermatitis and urticaria), weight gain and temporary hair loss have been reported rarely.

Overdosage (and treatment): There is no experience of acute poisoning with Serophene.

Hyperstimulation may occasionally result from an excessive response to clomiphene citrate therapy. Hyperstimulation is categorised as mild, moderate or severe. Generally hyperstimulation will be mild or, very rarely, moderate after clomiphene citrate treatment. Symptoms usually appear 3–6 days after ovulation or hCG administration.

Mild hyperstimulation—Symptoms may include some abdominal swelling and pain; ovaries enlarged to 5 cm diameter. Therapy—rest; careful observation and symptomatic relief. Ovarian enlargement declines rapidly.

Moderate hyperstimulation—Symptoms include more pronounced abdominal distension and pain; nausea; vomiting; occasional diarrhoea; ovaries enlarged up to 12 cm diameter. Therapy—bed rest; close observation, in the case of conception occurring, to detect any progression to severe hyperstimulation. Pelvic examination should be gentle in order to avoid rupture of the cysts. Symptoms subside spontaneously over 2–3 weeks.

Severe hyperstimulation—A rare but serious complication—symptoms include pronounced abdominal distention and pain; ascites; pleural effusion; decreased blood volume; reduced urine output; electrolyte imbalance and sometimes shock; ovaries enlarged to in excess of 12 cm diameter and may contain cysts. Therapy—hospitalisation, treatment should be conservative concentrating on restoring the blood volume and preventing shock. Acute symptoms subside over several days and ovaries return to normal after 20–40 days if conception does not occur—symptoms may be prolonged if conception has occurred.

Pharmaceutical precautions Serophene should be stored below 25°C and protected from light and moisture.

Legal category POM.

Package quantities Serophene is blister packed in boxes of 10, 30 and 100 tablets.

Further information The mode of action of Serophene at the recommended dose appears to be through competition for available oestrogen receptor sites in the hypothalamus. Oestrogen is displaced from these sites and the hypothalamus perceives an apparent lack of circulating oestrogen. This results in gonadotrophin releasing hormone stimulated secretion of FSH and LH, which initiates the normal menstrual cycle.

Patients with very low baseline levels of endogenous gonadotrophins and oestrogens are usually less responsive to Serophene treatment, and consideration should be given to gonadotrophin therapy.

Clomiphene citrate is readily absorbed from the gastrointestinal tract and slowly excreted through the liver into the bile. The biological half-life is reported to be five days. Enterohepatic recirculation takes place.

There is evidence that some women ovulate spontaneously for some cycles after cessation of Serophene treatment.

Product licence numbers
Serophene 3400/0009
Pergonal 3400/0007
Profasi 3400/0003–6
Metrodin 3400/0012

UKIDAN*

Presentation Ukidan 5 000, 25 000 and 100 000 are available in single vials containing 5 000, 25 000 or 100 000 International Units (IU) of urokinase in a sterile, white, freeze-dried powder form.

Uses Ukidan is a preparation of urokinase, which is an enzyme extracted from human adult male urine. As Ukidan is of human origin, it is not antigenic in man.

Mode of action: Ukidan brings about the dissolution of blood clots by promoting the activation of plasminogen; the latter is the inactive precursor of plasmin, the proteolytic enzyme responsible for the breakdown of fibrin into small soluble peptides which are dispersible through the blood stream.

Ukidan is indicated for the lysis of clots in the following conditions:

(i) Thromboembolic occlusive vascular disease such as deep vein thrombosis (DVT), pulmonary embolism (PE) and peripheral vascular occlusion.

(ii) Hyphaema (haemorrhage into the anterior chamber of the eye).

(iii) Arterio-venous haemodialysis shunts and intravenous cannulae which are blocked by fibrin clots.

Urokinase has been used experimentally in the treatment of coronary thrombosis.

Dosage and administration Ukidan should be reconstituted with a small amount of sterile water for injection or saline and then further diluted with normal saline to the desired volume for administration.

Adults

(i) Thromboembolic occlusive vascular disease

Deep vein thrombosis: A recommended dosage regimen consists of an initial loading dose of 4400 IU/kg body weight in 15 ml solution, given over 10 minutes followed by an intravenous infusion of 4400 IU/kg/hour for 12–24 hours.

Pulmonary embolism: A recommended dosage regimen consists of an initial loading dose of 4400 IU/kg body weight in 15 ml solution, given over 10 minutes followed by an intravenous infusion of 4400 IU/kg/hour for 12 hours.

Alternatively, a 50 ml bolus injection of Ukidan into the pulmonary artery, repeated for up to 3 doses, at 24 hour intervals, has been employed. The initial dosage of 15,000 IU/kg body weight may be adjusted if necessary for subsequent injections, dependent upon the plasma fibrinogen concentration produced by the previous injection.

Peripheral vascular occlusion: A recommended dosage regimen involves the infusion of a 2500 IU/ml solution of Ukidan (500,000 IU in 200 ml) into the clot, using angiography to monitor the progress of treatment. Ukidan should be infused into the clot at a dose rate of 4000 IU/minute (96 ml/hr) for 2 hours followed by repeat angiography. The catheter is then advanced into the remaining occluded segment and Ukidan infused at 4000 IU/min for a further 2 hours; this may be repeated up to 4 times if antegrade flow has not occurred. After lysing a channel through the occlusion the catheter is withdrawn until it is proximal to the remaining clot lining the vessel wall. Ukidan is given at a dose rate of 1000 IU/min (0.4 ml) until the clot has completely lysed. A dose of 500,000 IU given over approximately 8 hours should be sufficient to achieve this.

If the clot is not reduced in length by more than 25% after the initial infusion of 500,000 IU and by an incremental 10% by subsequent infusions of 500,000 IU, consideration should be given to discontinuation of treatment.

After fibrinolytic therapy has been completed, treatment may be continued with suitable anticoagulant therapy.

(ii) Hyphaema: When saline irrigation is unsuccessful in removing the blood clot, Ukidan may be considered for the management of hyphaema, particularly when the clot completely fills the anterior chamber and there is an accompanying rise in intra-ocular pressure. The following general technique is used: an incision of about 3 mm is made inside the temporal limbus of the cornea. 5000 IU Ukidan is dissolved in Sodium Chloride Injection (2 ml) and drawn up into a syringe fitted with a suitable irrigator. The tip of the irrigator is introduced through the incision so as to be over the iris rather than the pupillary space (thus avoiding risk of damage to the lens), with the aperture directed towards the corneal endothelium or parallel to the plane of the iris. The solution is injected and withdrawn repeatedly with minimal pressure. Clot disintegration commonly begins within five minutes, facilitating injection of the solution and aspiration of the clot. The chamber is then washed out with saline. If residual clot remains, a small quantity of the solution (e.g. 0.3 ml) may be left in the anterior chamber to facilitate further dissolution of the clot over the next 24–48 hours.

(iii) Clotted arterio—venous shunts: Generally, 5 000–25 000 IU Ukidan in 2–3 ml Sodium Chloride Injection is instilled into the affected limb of the shunt which is then clamped off for 2–4 hours. The lysate is then aspirated. This may be repeated if necessary. For the venous side an infusion of 5000 IU in 200 ml, run in over 30 minutes, has been used but this may be less satisfactory than the use of more concentrated solutions.

Dosage in the elderly: Initially no dosage alterations are recommended, however, thereafter, the dosage should be adjusted as necessary, according to response.

Dosage in children: Initially no dosage alterations are recommended, however, thereafter, the dosage should be adjusted as necessary, according to response.

Use in pregnancy: The use of Ukidan is contra-indicated in pregnancy and the immediate post-partum period.

Monitoring of treatment: The need for haematological monitoring arises only when Ukidan is used systemically to induce a state of whole-body fibrinolysis (e.g. in the treatment of thromboembolic occlusion). Several tests may be needed to give an overall picture of the biochemical state, because there is no simple way of measuring an induced thrombolytic state.

Suitable tests include: measurement of euglobin lysis time, assay of thrombolytic state using ^{131}I-fibrinogen; assay for plasminogen and fibrinogen; measurements of thrombin clotting time; prothrombin time; platelet counts and detection of fibrin degradation products.

Local use of Ukidan in 'closed situations' does not require haematological monitoring.

Contra-indications, warnings, etc

Contra-indications: Ukidan is contra-indicated in any situation where bleeding has occurred, or is likely to occur.

Recent surgery (including biopsy): administration of Ukidan for thromboembolic occlusive vascular disease is not recommended for 72 hours following surgery because of the risk of bleeding from the operation site.

Severe hypertension (with systolic bp > 200 mmHg and/or diastolic bp > 120 mmHg): in patients with severe hypertension, administration of Ukidan carries the risk of cerebral haemorrhage.

Pregnancy: Ukidan is contra-indicated in pregnancy and the immediate post-partum period.

Severe hepatic or renal insufficiency.

When used in 'local' situations, the above contra-indications may not be relevant.

Warnings: If bleeding occurs following systemic use, the infusion should be stopped immediately. However, this contra-indication is relative. The benefits of the continued use of Ukidan must be weighed against the risks of stopping therapy, for example, in the situation where vascular occlusion can be life-threatening. For treatment of bleeding see 'Overdosage'.

When used in the eye, a normal gonioscopy result should be evident.

Precautions: Systemic Ukidan should be used with caution in patients with gastrointestinal lesions such as peptic ulceration, which may be prone to haemorrhage, and in patients who have had multiple intracardiac and intravascular punctures as a consequence of cardiopulmonary resuscitation.

Interactions: In glucose solution there is a measurable (< 10%) reduction in the activity of Ukidan after 8 hours. Concomitant administration of dextran sulphate may prolong the activity of Ukidan.

Side-effects: The following side-effects have been associated with Ukidan use in the listed indications.

Hyphaema—none reported.

Arteriovenous shunts—warmth, initial severe pain and dull ache in shunt limb have been reported occasionally.

Thromboembolic occlusive vascular disease—overt bleeding, haemorrhagic complications may occur. Temporary increase in temperature (when a high yield of lysis degradation products are produced) and haematuria have been reported occasionally.

Overdosage: If severe haemorrhage occurs, treatment with Ukidan must be stopped. Aprotinin and synthetic inhibitors such as epsilon-aminocaproic acid, tranexamic acid or p-aminomethylbenzoic acid can be used to inhibit the fibrinolytic action of Ukidan. In serious cases, human fibrinogen, Factor XIII, Cohn-Fraction I, packed red cells or whole blood can be given, as appropriate.

Pharmaceutical precautions Ukidan, in the lyophilised form, has a shelf-life of two years when stored at 0–6°C. When reconstituted, Ukidan is stable for 12 hours at room temperature.

Legal category POM.

Package quantities Ukidan injections (all strengths) are packed as single vials.

Further information The activity of Ukidan is expressed in International Units (IU). One IU is approximately equivalent to one CTA unit, and to about 0.7 Ploug units.

Product licence numbers
Ukidan 5 000 IU 3400/0001
Ukidan 25 000 IU 3400/0026
Ukidan 100 000 IU 3400/0027

**Trade Mark*

Servier Laboratories Limited
Fulmer Hall
Windmill Road
Fulmer, Slough SL3 6HH

ADIFAX* ▼

Presentation No. 3 size opaque white capsules marked S 5614, each containing 15 mg of dexfenfluramine hydrochloride, which is the dextrorotatory isomer of fenfluramine (+)-2-ethylamino-1-(3-trifluoromethylphenyl) propane hydrochloride.

Uses As an adjunct to continued dietary treatment of severe obesity in patients who have not responded to an appropriate weight reducing diet alone (see 'Further information'). Patients should be given close support and supervision.

Dosage and administration
Adults: 2 capsules of 15 mg daily taken orally, one capsule in the morning and one capsule in the evening, preferably at meal time.

Elderly: Not recommended in absence of clinical studies in elderly.

Children: Not recommended.

Duration of treatment: Weight reduction starts after two weeks' treatment and continues at three months. Treatment duration should not exceed three months.

Contra-indications, warnings, etc
Contra-indications: Dexfenfluramine hydrochloride produces mild mydriasis in some patients and Adifax should not be used in obese patients with glaucoma.

Adifax should not be used in obese patients with a history of anorexia nervosa, psychiatric illness, depressive illness or with known history of drug or alcohol abuse.

No specific studies have been carried out in patients with renal or hepatic impairment and in such cases administration of Adifax should be avoided.

Precautions and warnings: Dexfenfluramine has a specific serotoninergic action and Adifax should not be used concomitantly with monoamine oxidase inhibitors (MAOIs). There should be at least a 2 week interval after stopping MAOIs before commencing treatment with Adifax.

Adifax should not be used concomitantly with any centrally acting appetite suppressant.

Adifax may potentiate the action of anti-hypertensive, anti-diabetic or sedative drugs and the hypotensive effect of tricyclic anti-depressive drugs.

Depression has occurred in some patients after abrupt cessation of fenfluramine-containing preparations most commonly about 4 days after cessation of treatment. Therefore steady reduction of dosage of Adifax over one or more weeks is recommended.

Depression has also been reported in patients taking fenfluramine-containing preparations although clinical studies show that incidence of depression was not significantly different in patients taking Adifax compared with placebo.

Pregnancy and lactation: Use in pregnancy: Animal studies with dexfenfluramine hydrochloride have shown no evidence of teratogenicity; there is, however, no clinical evidence of safety in human pregnancy and Adifax is not therefore recommended in human pregnancy unless the benefits outweigh any possible risk. Also it would not be good clinical practice to treat pregnant women with an anorectic agent.

Use in lactation: Dexfenfluramine hydrochloride may be excreted in breast milk and administration of Adifax during lactation is not therefore recommended.

Side-effects: Most commonly reported are dry mouth, nausea, constipation and diarrhoea, disappearing on continuing treatment. Drowsiness, dizziness, urinary frequency, headache, asthenia, mood disturbance, symptoms of depression, insomnia, nervousness and conjunctivitis are also reported but more rarely.

Rarely, schizophrenia-like reactions have been reported with the racemate fenfluramine (Ponderax). So far there have been no reports with the d-isomer Adifax.

Overdosage: No case of overdosage has been reported during clinical trials.

Actions to be taken in the event of overdosage: (i) gastric lavage; (ii) provoked diuresis with acidification of urine, to accelerate elimination of the drug; (iii) intensive care, with cardiac monitoring.

(Unlike overdosage with sympathomimetic anorectic drugs, overdosage with Adifax does not necessitate routine administration of a barbiturate.)

Pharmaceutical precautions Nil.

Legal category POM.

Package quantities Carton of 60 capsules (containing two push-through blister strips of 30 capsules).

Further information Adifax has been found to be effective adjunctive treatment in severe obesity associated with disorders of eating behaviour (carbohydrate craving).

Dexfenfluramine hydrochloride is extensively metabolised with formation of an active metabolite, d-norfenfluramine. No major metabolite has an amphetamine-like structure. Experimental studies have shown that the mode of action of dexfenfluramine hydrochloride is specifically serotoninergic and that it has no psychostimulating action, no hypertensive effect and no addiction potential (its racemic, fenfluramine hydrochloride, is not subject to control under the Misuse of Drugs Act 1971 nor under the Misuse of Drugs Regulations 1985).

Product licence number 5815/0003.

Product licence holder: Les Laboratoires Servier, Gidy, 45400 Fleury-les-Aubrais, France.

COVERSYL* ▼

Presentation
Coversyl Tablets 2 mg: round, white, biconvex tablets containing 2 mg of perindopril tert-butylamine salt.

Coversyl Tablets 4 mg: white, oblong tablets, half-scored on one side, containing 4 mg of perindopril tert-butylamine salt.

Uses
Actions: Perindopril tert-butylamine salt, 1-((2S) 2-((1S) 1-carbotoxybutyl amino) 1-oxopropyl) (2S, 3aS, 7aS) perhydroindole 2-carboxylic acid, tert-butylamine salt, is an inhibitor of angiotensin I-converting enzyme, the enzyme which converts angiotensin I into vasoconstrictive angiotensin II and degrades vasodilatory bradykinin into an inactive heptapeptide.

Perindopril acts through its active metabolite, perindoprilat, the other metabolites being inactive.

Indications: Essential and renovascular hypertension where standard therapy is ineffective or inappropriate because of adverse effects.

Dosage and administration

Dosage: 2 mg once a day is the normal starting dose. Optimum control of blood pressure is achieved by increasing the dose, titrating it against the blood pressure. The usual maintenance dose of 4–8 mg given once daily may be combined with diuretic therapy.

The maximum daily dose is 8 mg.

Coversyl should be taken before a meal as ingestion of food decreases conversion to perindoprilat.

Combinations with diuretic: There may be excessive fall in blood pressure when Coversyl treatment is initiated in patients receiving diuretic treatment, in particular if treatment was begun only a short time before.

It is therefore recommended to discontinue the diuretic 3 days before beginning treatment with Coversyl at the starting dose of 2 mg.

Addition of a diuretic potentiates the anti-hypertensive effects of Coversyl.

If co-treatment with a diuretic is thought necessary in patients on Coversyl therapy, the diuretic should be initiated at the lowest dose.

Potassium sparing diuretics should be avoided or used with extreme caution (see 'Warnings').

Elderly: Since elderly patients may have renal impairment and/or other organ dysfunction, Coversyl treatment should be initiated at 2 mg daily under close supervision.

Patients with impaired renal function (see 'Precautions'): Perindoprilat is excreted by the kidney. Coversyl should therefore be used with caution in patients with renal impairment and the dose adjusted to the degree of renal failure. Normal medical follow-up will include periodic control of potassium and creatinine. The following dosages are recommended:

Creatinine clearance	*Recommended dosage*
Between 30 and 60 ml/min	2 mg per day
Between 15 and 30 ml/min	2 mg every other day
< 15 ml/min	2 mg on the day of dialysis On days when the patients are not on dialysis the dose should be tailored to the blood pressure response.

Children: Coversyl is not recommended in children as paediatric use has not been studied.

Contra-indications, warnings, etc

Contra-indications: Patients with a history of hypersensitivity to Coversyl.

Pregnancy: Coversyl is contra-indicated in pregnancy and should not be used in women of child-bearing potential, unless protected by effective contraception. Maternal and foetal toxicity has been shown at high doses in rodents and rabbits although not in monkeys.

Neither embryotoxicity not teratogenicity was observed.

Oligohydramnios, neonatal hypotension and anuria have been reported following use of ACE inhibitors in the 2nd and 3rd trimester of pregnancy.

Lactation: In animals, very little perindopril crosses into maternal milk. No data are available in humans. Coversyl should not be used in nursing mothers.

Precautions:

Pre-treatment assessment of renal function: Evaluation of patients should include assessment of renal function both prior to initiation of Coversyl therapy, and during treatment where appropriate.

Warnings:

Hypotension: Symptomatic hypotension was seen rarely in uncomplicated hypertensive patients. Symptomatic hypotension with ACE inhibitors is more likely to occur in patients who have been volume depleted by diuretics, salt restriction, dialysis, diarrhoea or vomiting.

Some patients may experience symptomatic hypotension with the first one or two doses. The occurrence of first dose hypotension does not preclude restarting Coversyl cautiously and subsequent dose titration against the blood pressure after correction of hypovolaemia and hypotension.

Exaggerated hypotensive responses may occur after the initial dose of Coversyl in patients receiving diuretic treatment. The possibility of such an occurrence is reduced by discontinuing diuretic therapy 3 days prior to initiating Coversyl.

In most instances, symptoms are relieved simply by the patient lying down, but volume repletion with oral fluids or intravenous infusion with normal saline may be required.

Renal: Renal function of patients with renal failure or insufficiency should be closely monitored.

Marked water and sodium depletion (salt-free diet and/or diuretic treatment) or stenosis of the renal arteries stimulate the renin-angiotensin system; blockage of this system by an ACE inhibitor, especially upon initial dosing and during the first 2 weeks of treatment, may lead to an abrupt fall in blood pressure and/or to functional and possibly acute renal failure, although the latter is uncommon and the time interval variable. Discontinuation of Coversyl or discontinuation or reduction of the diuretic may be required.

Renovascular hypertension: Coversyl can be used when surgery is not indicated or prior to surgery. Renal function of patients with renovascular hypertension should be closely monitored.

Surgery/anaesthesia: In patients undergoing major surgery or during anaesthesia with agents that produce hypotension, Coversyl blocks angiotensin II formation secondary to compensatory renin release. This may lead to hypotension which can be corrected by volume expansion.

Plasma potassium: Combination of potassium supplements or potassium-sparing diuretics with Coversyl is not recommended, particularly in patients with renal impairment, since this may lead to significant increase in plasma potassium.

However, if combination with these agents is necessary, caution should be exercised and plasma potassium frequently monitored.

Side-effects:

Haematological: Decreases in haemoglobin, red cells and platelets have been reported in a few patients with Coversyl, as with other inhibitors, but a causal relationship has not been established.

Renal: Increased blood urea and creatinine may be observed but are reversible on discontinuation of treatment. Proteinuria has been observed in some patients.

Skin: Localised skin rashes, pruritus or flushing may occur. Angioneurotic oedema has been reported with Coversyl as with other ACE inhibitors.

Where swelling is confined to the face, lips and mouth, the condition will usually resolve on withdrawal without further treatment, although antihistamines may be useful in relieving symptoms.

Where there is involvement of the tongue, glottis or larynx, likely to cause airways obstruction, subcutaneous adrenaline (0.5 ml 1:1,000) should be administered promptly. The patient should be closely monitored until swelling has resolved.

Cardiovascular: Some patients may experience hypotension, usually with the first one or two doses of Coversyl, when the dose is increased, or when a diuretic is also given (see 'Dosage and administration' and 'Warnings').

Gastro-intestinal: Taste impairment, epigastric discomfort, nausea and abdominal pain have been reported.

Other: Fatigue, asthenia, malaise, headache, disturbances of mood and/or sleep have been reported. Most of these effects occurred on initiating treatment and were transient. Cough (described as dry and irritating) may sometimes be observed but is usually mild.

Drug interactions: Combination with other antihypertensive agents such as betablockers, methyldopa, calcium antagonists or diuretics may increase the antihypertensive efficacy;

Combination with potassium supplements and potassium-sparing diuretics can lead to elevated plasma potassium (see Warnings);

As with all antihypertensive agents, combination with

a neuroleptic or an imipramine-type antidepressant may increase the risk of postural hypotension;

Concomitant therapy with lithium may increase serum lithium concentration.

Overdosage: To date, no case of overdosage has been reported. Signs and symptoms expected in cases of overdosage would be related to hypotension and should be relieved by intravenous infusion of isotonic saline solution.

Gastric lavage should be considered.

Perindopril is dialysable (70 ml/min).

Pharmaceutical precautions Store below 25°C.

Legal category POM.

Package quantities Tablets 4 mg: PVC aluminium blister strip of 30 tablets packaged in a carton box. Tablets 2 mg: PVC aluminium blister strip of 30 tablets packaged in a carton box.

Further information Nil.

Product licence numbers
2 mg 5815/0001
4 mg 5815/0002.

DIAMICRON*

Presentation *Diamicron tablets:* White, circular, flat compressed tablets with flat bevelled edges and a cross on one face, each containing 80 mg gliclazide. Gliclazide is 1-(3-azabicyclo (3,3,0) oct-3-yl)-3-(p-tolylsulphonyl) urea.

Uses
Indication: For the treatment of maturity onset diabetes mellitus.

Mode of action: Gliclazide is a hypoglycaemic sulphonylurea differing from other related compounds by the addition of an azabicyclo octane ring. The drug is well absorbed and its half-life in man is approximately 10–12 hours. Gliclazide is metabolised in the liver; less than 5% of the dose is excreted unchanged in the urine.

In man, apart from having similar hypoglycaemic effect to the other sulphonylureas, gliclazide has been shown to reduce platelet adhesiveness and aggregation and increase fibrinolytic activity. These factors are thought to be implicated in the pathogenesis of long term complications of diabetes mellitus.

Gliclazide primarily enhances the first phase of insulin secretion, but also to a lesser degree its second phase. Both phases are diminished in non-insulin dependent diabetes mellitus.

Dosage and administration *Adults:* The total daily dose may vary from 40 to 320 mg taken orally. The dose should be adjusted according to the individual patient's response, commencing with 40–80 mg daily ($\frac{1}{2}$–1 tablet) and increasing until adequate control is achieved. A single dose should not exceed 160 mg (2 tablets). When higher doses are required, Diamicron should be taken twice daily and according to the main meals of the day.

In obese patients or those not showing adequate response to Diamicron alone, additional therapy may be required.

Elderly: Plasma clearance of gliclazide is not altered in the elderly and steady state plasma levels can therefore be expected to be similar to those in adults under 65 years. Clinical experience in the elderly to date shows that Diamicron is effective and well tolerated. Care should be exercised, however, when prescribing sulphonylureas in the elderly due to a possible age-related increased risk of hypoglycaemia.

Children: Diamicron, as with other sulphonylureas, is not indicated for the treatment of juvenile onset diabetes mellitus.

Route of administration: Oral.

Contra-indications, warnings, etc
Contra-Indications: Diamicron should not be used in:

Juvenile onset diabetes.

Diabetes complicated by ketosis and acidosis.

Pregnancy.

Diabetics undergoing surgery, after severe trauma or during infections.

Patients known to have hypersensitivity to other sulphonylureas and related drugs.

Diabetic pre-coma and coma.

Severe renal or hepatic insufficiency.

Precautions and warnings: Care should be exercised in patients with hepatic and/or renal impairment and a small starting dose should be used with careful patient monitoring. As with other sulphonylureas, hypoglycaemia will occur if the patients' dietary intake is reduced or if they are receiving a larger dose of Diamicron than required.

Interactions with other medicaments: Care should be taken when giving Diamicron with drugs which are known to alter the diabetic state or potentiate the drug's action. The hypoglycaemic effect of Diamicron may be potentiated by phenylbutazone, salicylates, sulphonamides, coumarin derivatives, MAOIs, beta adrenergic blocking agents, tetracycline compounds, chloramphenicol, clofibrate, disopyramide, miconazole (oral forms) and cimetidine.

It may be diminished by corticosteroids, oral contraceptives, thiazide diuretics, phenothiazine derivatives, thyroid hormones and abuse of laxatives.

Use in pregnancy and lactation:

Pregnancy: See 'Contra-indications'.

Nursing mothers: It has not yet been established whether gliclazide is transferred to human milk. However, other sulphonylureas have been found in milk and there is no evidence to suggest that gliclazide differs from the group in this respect.

Effects on ability to drive and use machines: Patients should be informed that their concentration may be affected if their diabetes is not satisfactorily controlled, especially at the beginning of treatment (see other special warnings and precautions).

Other special warnings and precautions: Hypoglycaemia: all sulphonylureas drugs are capable of producing moderate or severe hypoglycaemia, particularly in the following conditions:
- in patients controlled by diet alone;
- in cases of accidental overdose;
- when calorie or glucose intake is deficient;
- in patients with hepatic and/or renal impairment, however, in long-term clinical trials, patients with renal insufficiency have been treated satisfactorily, using Diamicron at reduced doses.

In order to reduce the risk of hypoglycaemia it is therefore recommended:
- to initiate treatment for non-insulin dependent diabetics by diet alone, if this is possible;
- to take into account the age of the patient: blood sugar levels not strictly controlled by diet alone might be acceptable in the elderly;
- to adjust the dose of Diamicron according to the blood glucose response and to the 24 hour urinary glucose during the first days of treatment.

Dosage adjustments may be necessary:
- on the occurence of mild symptoms of hypoglycaemia (sweating, pallor, hunger pangs, tachycardia, sensation of malaise. Such findings should be treated with oral glucose and adjustments made in drug dosage and/or meal patterns;
- on the occurrence of severe hypoglycaemic reactions (coma or neurological impairment, see overdose);
- loss of control of blood glucose (hyperglycaemia). When a patient stabilised on any diabetic regimen is exposed to stress such as fever, trauma, infection or surgery, a loss of control may occur. At such times, it may be necessary to progressively increase the dosage of Diamicron and if this is insufficient, to discontinue the treatment with Diamicron and to administer insulin.

Incompatibilities (major): Non stated.

Side effects: Hypoglycaemia (see other special warnings and precautions).

Abnormalities of hepatic function are not uncommon

during glicazide therapy. There are rare reports of hepatic failure, hepatitis, and jaundice following treatment with gliclazide.

Mild gastro-intestinal disturbances including nausea, dyspepsia, diarrhoea and constipation have been reported, but this type of adverse reaction can be avoided if Diamicron is taken during a meal.

Skin reactions including rash, pruritus, erythema, bullous eruption; blood dyscrasia including anaemia, leucopaenia, thrombocytopaenia and granulocytopaenia have been observed during treatment with Diamicron but are not known to be directly attributable to the drug.

Overdosage: The symptom to be expected with an overdose would be hypoglycaemia. The treatment is gastric lavage and correction of the hypoglycaemia by appropriate means with continued monitoring of the patient's blood sugar until the effect of the drug has ceased.

Pharmaceutical precautions Nil.

Legal category POM.

Package quantities Cartons of 60 tablets (containing three push-through blister strips of 20 tablets).

Further information Nil.

Product licence number 0093/0024.

FLUZONE*

Presentation Single dose disposable syringe with a 25 ga. needle containing 0.5 ml of Fluzone, Inactivated Influenza Vaccine, (Split Virion) BP, which is a sterile aqueous suspension of highly purified influenza virus subvirions and contains the haemagglutinin and neuraminidase antigens of the A and B strains currently recommended by the WHO.

Fluzone is colourless, but slightly opalescent. Triton* X-100 detergent is used in the course of the purification process. It is stabilised with gelatin 0.05% and preserved with thiomersal 0.01%. No antibiotics are used during manufacture.

Uses Active immunisation for the prevention of influenza, for use in adults and children over 6 months of age.

The recommendation to doctors on the use of influenza vaccine are issued by the Department of Health in an annual letter from the Chief Medical Officer (see Further Information).

Dosage and administration
Adults (including elderly): One 0.5 ml dose

Children:
13 years and older: One 0.5 ml dose
3–12 years of age: Two 0.5 ml doses
6–35 months of age: Two 0.25 ml doses

Where more than one dose is to be given, they should be administered 4 or more weeks apart. Both doses are recommended for maximum protection; however, if in previous years the person received any influenza vaccine one dose is sufficient.

Administer by intramuscular injection only.

Contra-indications, warnings, etc
Contra-indications: Do not administer to persons with known allergy to eggs, egg products or thiomersal.

Do not administer in patients with acute respiratory or other active infections or illnesses.

Defer immunisation in a patient with an active neurological disorder.

Use in pregnancy: Animal reproduction studies have not been conducted, hence it is not known if influenza virus vaccine can cause fetal harm or affect reproduction capacity. The vaccine should be given to pregnant women only if clearly needed.

Interactions: Do not administer within 3 days of immunisation with DTP. Possible interactions with coumarins, theophylline and phenytoin have been reported.

Other undesirable effects (frequency and seriousness): Soreness around the injection site lasting 1–2 days has been seen in less than $\frac{1}{3}$ of vaccinees. Fever, malaise, myalgia and other systemic symptoms of toxicity may occur infrequently, generally 6–12 hours after vaccination and lasting 1–2 days.

Other special warnings and precautions: Adrenaline injection (1:1000) should be immediately available for the control of anaphylactic reactions which may occur.

The vaccine may not result in sero-conversion of all patients and protection is only against the strains of virus contained in the vaccine or those closely related.

Overdose: Is unlikely to have any specific adverse effect.

Incompatibilities (major): None.

Effect on ability to drive and use machines: None.

Pharmaceutical precautions Store between 2°–8°C. Do not freeze. Shake well before administration.

Legal category POM.

Package quantities Syringes of 0.5 ml, packed singly, or in tens.

Further information The Chief Medical Officer has advised that vaccination should be *considered for persons at special risk,* including those, especially the elderly, suffering from: Chronic pulmonary disease; chronic heart disease; chronic renal failure; diabetes mellitus and other endocrine disorders associated with adrenal suppression; other conditions which may themselves, or as a result of treatment, give rise to immunosuppression; elderly persons living in residential homes and long stay accommodation where rapid spread of infection is likely; children age 4 years or over who live in hospital or residential establishments; children with conditions which render them at special risk; at the direction of the doctor concerned.

Product licence number 4788/0008.

Product licence holder: Connaught Laboratories Inc, Swiftwater, PA18370, USA.

LOCABIOTAL*

Presentation 10 ml of 0.25% solution of fusafungine in a pressurised aerosol container designed to give approximately 200 metered doses. Each metered dose contains approximately 125 micrograms fusafungine. Two attachments, one for nasal use, one for oral use, are supplied.

Fusafungine is an antibiotic produced by *Fusarium lateritium* strain 437.

Other constituents: Saccharin, eucalyptol, pure alcohol, isopropyl myristate, dichlorodifluoromethane.

Uses
Indications: The treatment of infections and inflammatory conditions of the upper respiratory tract.

Mode of action: A topical antibiotic with anti-inflammatory properties. It is bacteriostatic.

Dosage and administration *Administration:* By inhalation (via mouth or nose) using the appropriate attachment.

Duration of treatment: Depending on severity, one week to ten days, under medical supervision. Should there be no relief of symptoms and signs in one week, alternative treatment should be considered.

Adults and the elderly: Nasal: 3 metered doses in each nostril 5 times a day.

Oral: 5 metered doses 5 times a day.

Children

	Number of metered doses		
	3–5 years	*6–12 years*	*12 years*
Nasal (in each nostril 5 times daily	1	2	3
Oral (3 times a day)	2	3	4

Route of administration: Oral or nasal.

Contra-indications, warnings, etc
Contra-indications: Hypersensitivity to fusafungine or excipients.

Precautions and warnings: Use with caution in patients with allergic tendencies. Prolonged use may encourage superinfection.

Avoid directing the spray towards the eyes as the aerosol can cause irritation. If symptoms and signs do not improve in one week, alternative therapy should be considered.

Interactions with other medicaments: There have been no documented reports of any interactions with fusafungine used topically. In particular, no interactions have been reported with systemic antibiotics.

Use in pregnancy and lactation: There are no reports of safety of fusafungine in pregnancy or lactation. In general, fusafungine should be used in these conditions only when benefits clearly exceed potential unknown risks.

Effects on ability to drive and use machines: No evidence of any adverse effect on mental alertness.

Incompatibilities (major): None known.

Side-effects: Side-effects observed are mainly local reactions including coughing, sneezing, dryness of nose or throat, unpleasant taste in mouth and congestion of eyes. Very rarely, general reactions have been observed, particularly in patients with allergic tendencies. These include cutaneous allergy, attacks of asthma, urticaria and nausea.

Overdosage: There are no reports of any overdosage and the management should be symptomatic and supportive.

Pharmaceutical precautions *Storage:* Store at room temperature.

Note. Do not throw full or empty aerosol containers into a fire or subject them to excessive heat.

Legal category POM.

Package quantities Unit pack of one 10 ml aerosol container with one oral and one nasal attachment.

Further information An insert leaflet for patients is included in each pack.

Product licence number 0093/5003R.

NATRILIX*

Presentation Pink biconvex sugar-coated tablets each containing 2.5 mg indapamide hemihydrate.

Uses *Indication:* For the treatment of essential hypertension. Natrilix may be used as sole therapy or combined with other antihypertensive agents.

Mode of Action: Natrilix is a non-thiazide indole derivative of chlorosulphonamide. The mechanism of action of Natrilix in hypertensive patients includes reduction in peripheral arterial resistance and normalisation of vascular hyper-reactivity.

Dosage and administration *Adults:* The dosage is one tablet, containing 2.5 mg indapamide hemihydrate, daily to be taken in the morning. The action of Natrilix is progressive and the reduction in blood pressure may continue and not reach a maximum until several months after the start of therapy. A larger dose than 2.5 mg Natrilix daily is not recommended as there is no appreciable additional antihypertensive effect but a diuretic effect may become apparent. If a single daily tablet of Natrilix does not achieve a sufficient reduction in blood pressure, another antihypertensive agent may be added; those which have been used in combination with Natrilix include beta-blockers, ACE inhibitors, methyldopa, clonidine and other adrenergic blocking agents. The co-administration of Natrilix with diuretics may cause hypokalaemia and, therefore, is not recommended.

There is no evidence of rebound hypertension on withdrawal of Natrilix.

Elderly: There are no significant changes in the pharmacokinetics of Natrilix in the elderly. Numerous clinical studies have shown that it can be used without problems and indeed has a particular benefit on systolic blood pressure in the elderly.

Children: There is no experience of the use of this drug in children.

Route of administration: Oral.

Contra-indications, warnings, etc
Contra-indications: Natrilix is not recommended in patients with recent cerebrovascular accident, severe hepatic failure or a known history of allergy to sulphonamide derivatives.

Precautions and warnings: Studies in functionally anephric patients for one month undergoing chronic haemodialysis, have not shown evidence of drug accumulation despite the fact that Natrilix is not dialysable.

Although Natrilix 2.5 mg daily (one tablet) can be safely administered to hypertensive patients with impaired renal function, the treatment should be discontinued if there are signs of increasing renal insufficiency.

Interactions with other medicaments: The concomitant administration of the following medicaments with Natrilix is not recommended:

Diuretics (risk of electrolyte imbalance);

Antiarrhythmics such as quinidine derivatives, cardiac glycosides, corticoids or laxatives, in case of hypokalaemia;

Lithium (increase in blood levels due to a diminished urinary excretion of lithium).

Use in pregnancy and lactation: Pregnancy: no teratological effects have been seen in animals but because animal reproduction studies are not always predictive of human response, Natrilix should be used during pregnancy only if clearly needed.

Nursing mothers: It is not known if Natrilix is excreted in human milk, therefore, if use of Natrilix is deemed essential, the patient should stop nursing.

Effects on ability to drive and use machines: No evidence of any adverse effect on mental alertness.

Other special warnings and precautions: Blood potassium and urate levels should be closely monitored:
- in patients predisposed or sensitive to hypokalaemia (cardiac patients treated with glycosides, elderly, or patients suffering from hyperaldosteronism);
- in patients suffering from gout.

If pre-existing renal insufficiency is aggravated, treatment with Natrilix should be stopped.

If hypercalcaemia occurs in patients with hyperparathyroidism, treatment with Natrilix should be stopped.

Incompatibilities (major): None stated.

Side-effects: Hypokalaemia, headache, dizziness, fatigue, muscular cramps, nausea, anorexia, diarrhoea, constipation, dyspepsia and cutaneous rash may occur as a result of treatment with Natrilix. There have been some rare reports of orthostatic hypotension, metabolic alkalosis, hyperglycaemia, increase in blood urate levels, paraesthesia, erythema multiforme, epidermal necrolysis, photosensitivity, impotence, renal insufficiency and reversible acute myopia. At the dosage recommended for hypotension, Natrilix does not usually adversely influence plasma triglycerides, LDL cholesterol or the LDL-HDL cholesterol ratio. Natrilix does not appear to adversely affect glucose tolerance when used in patients, with or without diabetes.

Overdosage: Symptoms of overdosage would be those associated with a diuretic effect: electrolyte disturbances, hypotension and muscular weakness. Treatment would be symptomatic, directed at correcting the electrolyte abnormalities and gastric lavage or emesis should be considered.

Pharmaceutical precautions Nil.

Legal category POM.

Package quantities Cartons of 30 and 60 tablets (containing respectively blister strips of 2 × 15 and 3 × 20 tablets).

Further information Nil.

Product licence number 0093/0022.

PONDERAX PACAPS*

Presentation Prolonged action formulation in hard gelatine capsule with clear body and opaque blue cap, printed in black with PxPA 60 containing small white pellets. Each prolonged action capsule contains 60 mg Fenfluramine Hydrochloride BP.

Uses As an adjunct to continued dietary treatment of severe obesity, including severe obesity associated with maturity onset diabetes, in patients who have not responded to an appropriate weight reducing diet alone (see 'Further information').

Patients should be given close support and supervision.

Dosage and administration
Adults: One 60 mg capsule daily.

Treatment with Ponderax Pacaps should not be stopped suddenly. Steady reduction of dosage over one or more weeks, e.g. one capsule every other day, is recommended to avoid the possibility of precipitating depression which occasionally has been severe.

If possible, the capsules should be taken half an hour before food.

Elderly: Care should be taken when prescribing for patients over 65 years of age because drowsiness is more likely to occur.

Children: Not recommended.

Duration of treatment: Weight reduction starts after two weeks treatment and still continues at three months. Treatment duration should not exceed three months.

Contra-indications, warnings, etc
Contra-indications: History of depressive illness and concurrent treatment with antidepressants.

History of drug or alcohol abuse.

Ponderax should not be used in epilepsy, although exacerbation of this condition has only been reported very infrequently.

Precautions and warnings: Ponderax should not be used concomitantly with neuroleptic or antidepressant therapy especially MAOI's. There should be an interval of three weeks between stopping MAOI's and starting Ponderax.

Ponderax should not be used concomitantly with other appetite suppressants. There should be an interval of two weeks between stopping any other appetite suppressant and starting Ponderax to allow for any possible withdrawal symptoms to subside.

Ponderax may potentiate the action of anti-hypertensive, anti-diabetic and sedative drugs. The dosage of these drugs should be re-assessed when Ponderax is prescribed.

Ponderax may cause drowsiness. It may affect the ability to drive or operate machinery and increase the effects of alcohol.

Dependence has been rarely reported and has occurred very seldom in subjects without a history of drug abuse. Although fenfluramine is chemically related to amphetamine, the introduction of a CF_3 groups into the molecule alters the pharmacological characteristics of the compound which is evident from its lack of central nervous system stimulation and its low risk of abuse or dependence.

Care should be exercised in patients with a history of psychiatric illness and those in whom there is underlying emotional instability.

Following sudden withdrawal of Ponderax, severe depression has occasionally been reported. This risk may be avoided by a gradual reduction of dosage.

Pregnancy and lactation: Medicines should not be used in pregnancy, especially the first trimester, unless the benefits outweigh any possible risk. Although no harmful effects on the foetus have been demonstrated, it is not recommended that Ponderax be administered during pregnancy. Fenfluramine may be excreted in breast milk and administration during lactation is not recommended.

Side-effects: The most common side-effects are diarrhoea, drowsiness, dizziness and lethargy. Dry mouth, urinary frequency, nausea, vomiting, nervousness, irritability and headache have also been reported. Depression may occur after abrupt withdrawal and most commonly about 4 days after cessation of treatment although it has also been reported during therapy. Infrequent occurrences of insomnia, bad dreams, visual disorder, hypotension, impotence and loss of libido have been reported. Rashes, reversible pulmonary hypertension, purpura and blood dyscrasias have been rarely reported. Rarely, schizophrenic-like reactions have been reported with Ponderax.

Overdosage: The following symptoms have been reported: Dilated pupils, tachycardia, facial flushing, hypertension, agitation, fine tremor; these can progress to vomiting, convulsions, unconsciousness, hyperpyrexia, depression of respiration, cardiac arrhythmias, ventricular fibrillation and death may occur.

Action to be taken in the event of overdosage:

(i) continuously monitor ECG
(ii) use diazepam to control convulsions
(iii) reduce hyperthermia
(iv) use anti-arrhythmic drugs (e.g. beta-blockers) to control cardiac tachyarrhythmias.

Pharmaceutical precautions Ponderax Pacaps should be stored in a cool, dry place.

Legal category POM.

Package quantities Push-through blister strips of fifteen capsules. Carton of 60 capsules (four strips).

Further information Ponderax is not a controlled drug under the Misuse of Drugs Act 1971 and the Misuse of Drugs Regulations 1985.

The 29th session of the U.N. Commission on Narcotic Drugs endorsed the WHO recommendation that 'fenfluramine does not have amphetamine-like abuse potential nor is there evidence of significant public health or social problems arising from its use'.

Product licence number
Pacaps 0093/0013R.

SERVIER TETANUS VACCINE*

Presentation Adsorbed Tetanus Vaccine BP is a suspension of purified formol toxoid, prepared by formalin detoxification of Clostridium tetani exotoxin, adsorbed on aluminium hydroxide. Each 0.5 ml dose has an immunising potency of not less than 40 International Units.

Uses Active immunisation against tetanus. Reinforcement of immunity to tetanus.

Dosage and administration The vaccine should be administered by deep subcutaneous or intramuscular injection. The container should be shaken before withdrawing the prescribed dose.

Primary immunisation: A course consists of 3 doses each of 0.5 ml and in line with the current DoH recommendation, the interval between each dose is one month. This will increase the degree of patient compliance compared to the previous regime. If the course is interrupted it should be resumed where it left off, without starting at the beginning again.

Reinforcing doses: A reinforcing dose of 0.5 ml should be given 10 years after the basic course. A further dose 10 years later provides a satisfactory degree of protection which will probably be life-long.

After a basic course has been given, a single reinforcing dose will provide protection in the event of an injury which is considered might give rise to tetanus. Reinforcing doses should not be given at too frequent intervals as they may provoke hypersensitivity reactions.

Tetanus vaccine should not routinely be given to any patient who has received a reinforcing dose in the preceding 10 years, unless the wound is regarded as carrying an unusually high risk of tetanus, and even then vaccine is not necessary if a reinforcing dose has been given during the preceding year.

Patients presenting with a tetanus prone wound who have not received a primary course or whose immunisation status is not known, should receive one injection of antitetanus immunoglobulin at one site, and the first dose of a primary course of adsorbed tetanus vaccine at another site.

Patients who have completed a primary course or received a reinforcing dose more than 10 years previously should receive one injection each of antitetanus immunoglobulin and absorbed tetanus vaccine.

Contra-indications, warnings, etc
Contra-indications: Acute infection is a contra-indication to routine tetanus immunisation, except in the presence of a tetanus-prone wound.

Warnings: A sterile syringe and adrenaline injection should be ready for use, in case the need arises for emergency treatment of an allergic reaction. Not for intradermal use.

Side-effects: Local reactions including pain, redness and swelling may occur at the injection site and last for several days. Systemic reactions may include headache, malaise, lethargy, myalgia and pyrexia. A small painless nodule may form at the injection site. Severe anaphylactoid reactions are rare. Neurological symptoms have been reported occasionally.

Pharmaceutical precautions Protect from light. Store in a refrigerator between 2°C and 8°C (36°F and 46°F).

Do not freeze.

Legal category POM.

Package quantities Cartons of 5 × 0.5 ml single dose ampoules.

Further information Nil.

Product licence number 0039/0115.

Manufacturer and product licence holder: Evans Medical Ltd, Langhurst, Horsham, West Sussex RH12 4QD.

**Trade Mark*

Shire Pharmaceuticals Ltd
1 Viscount Court
Andover
Hampshire SP10 5NW

CALCICHEW* TABLETS

Presentation Round, white, slightly speckled, biconvex, chewable tablet, containing 1260 mg Calcium Carbonate PhEur equivalent to 500 mg calcium.

Uses To be chewed, as a supplemental source of calcium in the correction of dietary deficiencies or when normal requirements are high. As an adjunct to conventional therapy in osteoporosis. Phosphate binding agent in the management of renal failure in patients on renal dialysis.

Dosage and administration
Adults and elderly:
Adjunct to osteoporosis therapy: 2 to 3 tablets daily.
Dietary deficiency: 2 to 3 tablets daily.
Osteomalacia: 2 to 6 tablets daily.
Phosphate binder: Dose as required by the individual patient depending on serum calcium and phosphate levels.

Children:
Dietary deficiency: As for adults.
Phosphate binder: As for adults.

Contra-indications, warnings, etc
Contra-indications: Severe hypercalcaemia and hypercalciuria for example in hyperparathyroidism, vitamin D overdose, decalcifying tumours such as plasmacytoma and skeletal metastases, in severe renal failure untreated by renal dialysis, and in osteoporosis due to immobilisation.

Precautions: May impair absorption of other drugs e.g. tetracyclines, fluoride preparations.

Thiazide diuretics reduce urinary calcium excretion so the risk of hypercalcaemia should be considered.

Oral calcium supplementation is aimed at restoring normal serum calcium levels. Although it is extremely unlikely that high enough levels will be achieved to adversely affect digitalised patients, this theoretical possibility should be considered. Vitamin D causes an increase in calcium absorption and plasma calcium levels may continue to rise after stopping Vitamin D therapy. Patients treated with high doses of Vitamin D or who are receiving prolonged calcium treatment, should undergo regulatory measurements of plasma calcium levels which should be interpreted in conjunction with measurements of plasma protein levels.

When used as a phosphate binder in patients on renal dialysis serum phosphate and calcium levels should be monitored regularly.

Side-effects: Constipation and wind. Rebound acid production. Hypercalcaemia – although hypercalcaemia would not be expected in patients unless their renal function were impaired, the following symptoms could indicate the possibility of hypercalcaemia: nausea, vomiting, anorexia, constipation, abdominal pain, bone pain, thirst, polyuria, muscle weakness, drowsiness or confusion. Alkalosis with high doses and in patients on renal dialysis. On long term phosphate binding therapy there are rare reports of tissue calcification.

Use in pregnancy and lactation: There is epidemiological and clinical evidence of safety of calcium carbonate in human pregnancy.

Overdosage: There are no reports of overdose. Alkalosis is a theoretical risk.

Pharmaceutical precautions No special storage is required.

Legal category P.

Package quantities Containers of 100 tablets.

Further information Calcichew contains no lactose, no sodium or potassium and no artificial colours.

Product licence number 8557/0003.

CALCIDRINK* SACHETS

Presentation Calcidrink sachets contain granules to prepare a fresh orange flavoured drink containing 2.52 g Calcium Carbonate PhEur equivalent to 1 g calcium.

Uses Orally for the treatment of calcium deficiency.

Dosage and administration
Adults, elderly and children: One sachet to be taken daily, dispersed in water.

Contra-indications, warnings, etc
Contra-indications: Severe hypercalcaemia and hypercalciuria, for example in hyperparathyroidism, vitamin D overdose, decalcifying tumours such as plasmacytoma and skeletal metastases, in severe renal failure, renal calculi and in osteoporosis due to immobilisation.

Precautions: May impair absorption of other drugs eg tetracyclines, fluoride preparations.

Thiazide diuretics reduce urinary calcium excretion so the risk of hypercalcaemia should be considered.

Oral calcium supplementation is aimed at restoring normal serum calcium levels. Although it is extremely unlikely that high enough levels will be achieved to adversely affect digitalised patients, this theoretical possibility should be considered. Vitamin D causes an increase in calcium absorption and plasma calcium levels may continue to rise after stopping Vitamin D therapy. Patients treated with high doses of Vitamin D or who are receiving prolonged calcium treatment, should undergo regulatory measurements of plasma calcium levels which should be interpreted in conjunction with measurements of plasma protein levels.

Side-effects: Constipation and wind. Rebound acid production. Hypercalcaemia – although hypercalcaemia would not be expected in patients unless their renal function were impaired, the following symptoms could indicate the possibility of hypercalcaemia: nausea, vomiting, anorexia, constipation, abdominal pain, bone pain, thirst, polyuria, muscle weakness, drowsiness or confusion. Alkalosis with high doses.

Use in pregnancy and lactation: There is epidemiological and clinical evidence of safety of calcium carbonate in human pregnancy.

Overdosage: There are no reports of overdose. Acute hypercalcaemia and alkalosis are a theoretical risk.

Pharmaceutical precautions There are no special requirements.

Legal category P.

Package quantities Boxes of 30 sachets.

Further information When dispersed in water the calcium carbonate reacts with the citric acid to produce effervesence and calcium citrate. Calcidrink contains no potassium and clinically insignificant amounts of sodium (0.11 mg).

Product licence number 8557/0018.

CITRICAL* SACHETS

Presentation Citrical sachets contain granules to prepare a pleasantly flavoured drink containing 1260 mg Calcium Carbonate PhEur equivalent to 500 mg calcium.

Uses Orally for the treatment of calcium deficiency.

Dosage and administration
Adults and elderly: One sachet to be taken three times a day, dispersed in water.

Children: Not indicated.

Contra-indications, warnings, etc
Contra-indications: Severe hypercalcaemia and hypercalciuria, for example in hyperparathyroidism, vitamin D overdose, decalcifying tumours such as plasmacytoma and skeletal metastases, in severe renal failure and in osteoporosis due to immobilisation.

Precautions: May impair absorption of other drugs eg tetracyclines, fluoride preparations.

Thiazide diuretics reduce urinary calcium excretion so the risk of hypercalcaemia should be considered.

Oral calcium supplementation is aimed at restoring normal serum calcium levels. Although it is extremely unlikely that high enough levels will be achieved to adversely affect digitalised patients, this theoretical possibility should be considered. Vitamin D causes an increase in calcium absorption and plasma calcium levels may continue to rise after stopping Vitamin D therapy. Patients treated with high doses of Vitamin D or who are receiving prolonged calcium treatment, should undergo regulatory measurements of plasma calcium levels which should be interpreted in conjunction with measurements of plasma protein levels.

Side-effects: Constipation and wind. Rebound acid production. Hypercalcaemia – although hypercalcaemia would not be expected in patients unless their renal function were impaired, the following symptoms could indicate the possibility of hypercalcaemia: nausea, vomiting, anorexia, constipation, abdominal pain, bone pain, thirst, polyuria, muscle weakness, drowsiness or confusion. Alkalosis with high doses.

Use in pregnancy and lactation: There is epidemiological and clinical evidence of safety of calcium carbonate in human pregnancy.

Overdosage: There are no reports of overdose. Acute hypercalcaemia and alkalosis are a theoretical risk.

Pharmaceutical precautions There are no special requirements.

Legal category P.

Package quantities Boxes of 90 sachets.

Further information When dispersed in water the calcium carbonate reacts with the citric acid to produce effervesence and calcium citrate. Citrical contains no potassium and clinically insignificant amounts of sodium (0.055 mg).

Product licence number 8557/0004.

HORMONIN*

Presentation Each pink, round, scored tablet contains:
Oestriol PhEur 0.27 mg.
Oestradiol USP 0.6 mg.
Oestrone USP 1.40 mg.

Uses Hormonin has been designed for replacement therapy in oestrogen-deficiency states, particularly those associated with the menopause such as nocturnal sweating, vasomotor disturbances, atrophic vaginitis and pruritus vulvae.

Prevention of postmenopausal osteoporosis.

Dosage and administration Hormonin is given by mouth. The dosage for the relief of menopausal symptoms range from 2 tablets per day to half tablet per day. In general, the maximum dosage is required for not more than three weeks to initiate therapy.

For maintenance the lowest effective dose should be used. If the patient has not menstruated within the last two months or more, cyclic administration is started arbitrarily. If the patient is menstruating cyclic administration is started on day five of bleeding.

For prophylactic use in post-menopausal women, a dosage of 1 tablet is recommended daily or on alternate days, according to the needs of the individual patient. Cyclic therapy is recommended (3 weeks treatment followed by 1 weeks treatment free). In women with an intact uterus the addition of an adequate dose and duration a progestogen (for 12 to 13 days) is recommended.

Before therapy commences, the patient should have a complete physical and gynaecological examination with special emphasis on blood pressure, breasts, abdomen and pelvic organs. In women with an intact uterus, endometrial assessments should be carried out whenever possible. Any breakthrough bleeding is an indication for endometrial evaluation.

Regular follow up examinations are recommended every 6 to 12 months.

Contra-indications, warnings, etc Pregnancy. Cardiovascular or cerebrovascular disorders e.g. thrombophlebitis, thrombosis or thromboembolic disorders, moderate to severe hypertension, hyperlipoproteinaemia, or a history of these conditions.

Known or suspected oestrogen-dependent tumours. Endometrial hyperplasia, uterine fibromyomata, undiagnosed vaginal bleeding.

Severe liver disease. Porphyria.

Precautions: In patients with mild hypertension or a history of it, blood pressure should be monitored at regular intervals.

If hypertension develops in patients receiving oestrogens, treatment should be stopped.

Risk of deep vein thrombosis is temporarily increased when undergoing major surgery or prolonged immobilisation, therefore treatment should be stopped before surgery.

If any signs of thrombosis develop in patients receiving oestrogens, discontinue treatment. Caution should be exercised in prescribing to women with a strong familial history of breast carcinoma, breast nodules or abnormal breast mammograms.

Glucose tolerance may be lowered and may, therefore, increase the need for insulin or other anti-diabetic drugs in diabetics.

Thyrotoxicosis. Thyroid hormone binding globulin may be increased leading to increased circulating total thyroid hormone, therefore care must be taken in interpreting thyroid function tests.

History of gall stones, cholestatic jaundice in pregnancy or jaundice due to oral contraceptives.

If liver function tests become abnormal during oestrogen therapy discontinue treatment.

Endometriosis. Renal dysfunction. Major depression. Contact lens wearers.

Warnings: Unopposed oestrogens predispose to endometrial neoplasia.

Severe varicose veins—the benefits of oestrogen-containing preparations must be weighed against the possible risks.

Cardiac failure, latent or overt.

Epilepsy or migraine or otosclerosis or a history of these conditions.

Sickle cell haemoglobinopathy, since under certain circumstances e.g. infections or anoxia, oestrogen-containing preparations may induce thromboembolic processes in patients with this condition.

Untreated polycythaemia or pulmonary hypertension.

Side-effects: Genito-urinary tract: Endometrial neoplasia, intermenstrual bleeding, increase in the size of uterine fibromyomata, endometrial proliferation or aggravation of endometriosis, excessive production of cervical mucus.

Breast: Tenderness, pain enlargement, secretion.

Gastro-intestinal tract: Nausea, vomiting, cholelithiasis, cholestatic jaundice.

Cardiovascular system: Hypertension, thrombosis, thrombophlebitis, thromboembolism.

Skin: Erythema nodosum, rash, chloasma, hirsutism loss of scalp hair.

Eyes: Corneal discomfort if contact lenses are used.

CNS: Headache, migraine, mood changes (elation or depression).

Metabolic: Sodium and water retention, reduced glucose tolerance, and change in body weight.

Pharmaceutical precautions Store in a closed container in a cool, dry place.

Legal category POM.

Package quantities Securitainers of 100 tablets.

Further information Nil.

Product licence number 0271/5000R.

Product licence holder: G. W. Carnrick Co Ltd, 431 Victoria House, Bloomsbury Square, London WC1B 4EB.

MIDRID*

Presentation Scarlet capsules containing 65 mg isometheptene mucate and 325 mg paracetamol PhEur.

Uses In the treatment of migraine and other vascular headaches. Midrid contains isometheptene mucate, a cerebral vasoconstrictor, which provides prompt relief of vascular head pain by reducing the underlying cerebrovascular disturbances.

The inclusion of paracetamol as the analgesic in Midrid is designed to bring relief to the throbbing head pain of migraine that is the first consideration of the patient.

Dosage and administration
Adults: 2 capsules at once, followed by 1 capsule every hour until relief is obtained. Up to 5 capsules within a 12-hour period.

Children: Not recommended.

Contra-indications, warnings, etc
Contra-indications: Midrid is contraindicated in severe renal, hepatic or organic heart disease, severe hypertension, glaucoma, and in those patients who are on monoamine-oxidase inhibitor therapy.

Precautions: Diabetes mellitus, hyperthyroidism.

Interactions: On theoretical grounds care should be taken with patients receiving cardiac glycosides, quinidine, and tricyclic antidepressants.

Side-effects: Transient dizziness may appear in hypersensitive patients. This can usually be eliminated by reducing the dose. Use in pregnancy: There is no evidence on the drug safety in human pregnancy nor is there evidence from animal work that it is free from hazard. Avoid in pregnancy.

Overdosage: Gastric lavage plus appropriate supportive treatment. Assessment of severity of paracetamol poisoning by measurement of plasma paracetamol levels. Administration of cysteamine, methionine or N-acetylcl-steine within 10–12 hours to protect the liver from damage due to paracetamol poisoning.

Pharmaceutical precautions Store in a closed container in a cool, dry place.

Legal category P.

Package quantities Securitainers of 100 capsules.

Further information Nil.

Product licence number 0271/5001R.

Product licence holder: G. W. Carnrick Co Ltd, 431 Victoria House, Bloomsbury Square, London WC1B 4EB.

**Trade Mark*

Smith & Nephew Pharmaceuticals Ltd
Bampton Road,
Harold Hill,
Romford,
Essex RM3 8SL

Smith+Nephew

BALMANDOL* BATH OIL

Presentation A clear straw coloured solution containing Almond Oil BP 30% w/w and Light Liquid Paraffin BP 69.6% w/w with butylated hydroxyanisole 0.1% as a preservative.

Uses Balmandol bath oil has emollient properties and is indicated for the treatment of dermatoses characterised by dry, scaly or fissured skin including atopic eczema, contact dermatitis, psoriasis, ichthyosis, senile pruritus, eczema craquelé, and neurodermatitis.

Dosage and administration Suitable for all ages. Baths: Using the enclosed measure, add 15–30 mls of Balmandol to a bath of warm water and mix well. Soak for 10–15 minutes. Do not use soap. Pat dry.

Showers: Apply to wet skin after showering.

May also be used as an emollient – apply to affected areas and rub in.

Contra-indications, warnings, etc Discontinue use if irritation occurs. Keep away from the eyes. Guard against slipping. Not for use in patients sensitive to any of the ingredients.

Pharmaceutical precautions Store at room temperature.

Legal category GSL.

Package quantities 225 ml and 500 ml bottles.

Further information Also contains poloxamer, cyclomethicone, citric acid monohydrate and perfume. Contains no detergents, emulsifiers or lanolin. Clean the bath or shower with detergent after use.

Product licence number 0033/0138

CLINITAR* CREAM

Presentation Greenish-brown oil in water cream containing 1% w/w Stantar*.

Uses Stantar is an antipruritic and keratoplastic agent and is used for the treatment of sub-acute and chronic psoriasis and eczema.

Dosage and administration *All age groups:* Apply to the affected areas once or twice daily.

Contra-indications, warnings, etc The use of Clinitar Cream is not recommended in generalised pustular psoriasis, infections of the skin, or for patients allergic to coal tar.

Coal tar can sensitise the skin to UV light, leading to sunburn. Clinitar Cream should therefore be used cautiously in the sun. Before any irradiation treatment, Clinitar Cream should be removed completely.

Clinitar Cream has been in wide use for a number of years without apparent ill consequence in pregnancy and lactation.

Pharmaceutical precautions Store at room temperature.

Legal category P.

Package quantities 60 g tube.

Further information Stantar 1% is an extract of coal tar with a photosensitising activity equivalent to 1% crude coal tar in a formulation designed to improve patient compliance. Also contains propylene glycol, cetostearyl alcohol, glyceryl monostearate and isopropyl palmitate. Fragrance free.

Product licence number 0033/0110.

CLINITAR* SHAMPOO

Presentation A clear, brown shampoo with a slight greenish fluorescence, containing 2% w/w Stantar*.

Uses Stantar is an antipruritic and keratoplastic agent and is used for the treatment of psoriasis of the scalp, seborrhoeic dermatitis of the scalp and dandruff.

Dosage and administration Wet the hair and apply the shampoo. Massage until a lather is produced. Rinse. Reapply the shampoo and leave for 5 minutes. Rinse carefully. Use up to 3 times a week.

Contra-indications, warnings, etc Not to be used on coal tar sensitive skin. Avoid getting shampoo into the eyes. Clinitar shampoo has been in wide use for a number of years without apparent ill-consequence in pregnancy and lactation.

Pharmaceutical precautions Store at room temperature.

Legal category P.

Package quantities 60 g tube.

Further information Stantar 2% is an extract of coal tar with a photosensitising activity equivalent to 2% crude coal tar in a perfumed formulation designed to improve patient compliance. Also contains sodium laurylethersulphate, triethanolamine laurylsulphate, polyoxyethylene glycerol monostearate, polysorbate, fatty acid surfactants and perfume.

Product licence number 0033/0109.

CUPLEX*

Presentation A clear, brownish-yellow viscous gel containing Salicylic Acid PhEur 11% w/w, Lactic Acid PhEur 4% w/w and copper acetate (equivalent to 1.1 mg of copper per 100 g), collodion, colophony and venice turpentine.

Uses Topical treatment of common, juvenile, plantar and mosaic warts; corns and calluses.

Dosage and administration Soak the wart nightly for 5 minutes in hot water. Dry thoroughly. Apply sufficient Cuplex gel to cover the wart. Each morning, remove elastic film and re-apply. Gently rub the wart surface 2–3 times weekly with an emery board or pumice. Excessive rubbing can cause stinging. Suitable for all ages, except infants.

Contra-indications, warnings, etc Do not apply to

facial or anogenital warts. Not for use in patients sensitive to colophony. Avoid contact with the eyes. Only apply to the affected area. Keep away from naked flames.

Pharmaceutical precautions Store in a cool place. Highly inflammable.

Legal category P.

Package quantities 5 g tubes.

Further information Warts are contagious and any person suffering from warts should always use their own towel.

Most warts will disappear after 6 to 12 weeks of treatment with Cuplex Gel, providing instructions are carefully and consistently followed. Where, however, the wart continues to increase in size after 6 weeks treatment and the patient has not consulted a doctor, the patient should be advised to do so.

Product licence number 0033/0100.

DITROPAN*▼

Presentation *Ditropan tablets 5 mg:* Pale blue bi-convex circular tablets, 8 mm in diameter, marked Ditropan on one side, scored on reverse and marked S&N 5. Each tablet containing 5 mg oxybutynin hydrochloride.

Ditropan tablets 2.5 mg: Pale blue bi-convex oval tablets 8.5 mm by 5.8 mm marked Ditropan on one side, scored on reverse and marked S&N 2.5. Each tablet containing 2.5 mg oxybutynin hydrochloride.

Uses Urinary incontinence, urgency and frequency in the unstable bladder, whether due to neurogenic bladder disorders (detrusor hyperreflexia) in conditions such as multiple sclerosis and spina bifida, or to idiopathic detrusor instability (motor urge incontinence).

Children over 5 years of age: In addition to neurogenic bladder disorders, Ditropan may also be used in nocturnal enuresis in conjunction with non-drug therapy where this alone, or in conjunction with other drug treatment, has failed.

Dosage and administration *Adult:* The usual dose is 5 mg two or three times a day. This may be increased to a maximum of 5 mg four times a day to obtain a clinical response provided that the side effects are tolerated.

Elderly: The elimination half-life is increased in the elderly therefore a dose of 5 mg twice a day, particularly if the patient is frail, is likely to be adequate.

Children (under 5 years of age): Not recommended.

Children (over 5 years of age): Neurogenic bladder instability: The usual dose is 5 mg twice a day. This may be increased to 5 mg three times a day to obtain a clinical response provided that the side effects are tolerated. Nocturnal enuresis: The usual dose is 5 mg two or three times a day. The last dose should be given before bedtime.

Contra-indications, warnings, etc

Contra-indications: Ditropan is contra-indicated in patients with obstruction of the bowel and in patients with a significant degree of bladder outflow obstruction where urinary retention may be precipitated.

It is also contra-indicated in patients with intestinal atony, severe ulcerative colitis or toxic megacolon, myasthenia gravis or glaucoma.

Precautions: Ditropan should be used with caution in the frail elderly and in patients with autonomic neuropathy, hepatic or renal disease.

The symptoms of hyperthyroidism, coronary artery disease, congestive cardiac failure, cardiac arrhythmias, tachycardias and prostatic hypertrophy may be aggravated following administration of Ditropan.

Special care should be taken in patients with hiatus hernia associated with reflux oesophagitis, as anticholinergic drugs may aggravate this condition.

As Ditropan may produce drowsiness or blurred vision, the patient should be cautioned regarding activities requiring mental alertness such as driving, operating machinery or performing hazardous work while taking this drug

Pregnancy: There is no evidence as to the safety of Ditropan in human pregnancy nor is there evidence from animal work that it is totally free from hazard. Avoid in pregnancy unless there is no safer alternative.

Lactation: Ditropan has been detected in breast milk and should therefore not be taken by breast-feeding mothers.

Side-effects: The most frequently reported side effects (>1%) to oxybutynin are: dry mouth (about 22%), constipation, blurred vision, nausea, abdominal discomfort, facial flushing and difficulty in micturition. The incidence of facial flushing is more marked in children than adults. The occurrence of these effects may be reduced by lowering the dose. Those side effects reported less frequently include: headache, urinary retention, dizziness, drowsiness, dry skin, diarrhoea and cardiac arrhythmias.

Drug interactions: Care should be taken if other anticholinergic agents are administered together with Ditropan, as potentiation of anticholinergic effects could occur.

Occasional cases of interaction between anticholinergics and phenothiazines, amantidine, butyrophenones, L.dopa, digitalis and tricyclic antidepressants have been reported and care should be taken if Ditropan is administered concurrently with such drugs.

Overdosage: The symptoms of overdosage with Ditropan progress from an intensification of the usual side-effects of CNS disturbances (from restlessness and excitement to psychotic behaviour), circulatory changes (flushing, fall in blood-pressure, circulatory failure etc), respiratory failure, paralysis and coma.

Measures to be taken are: (1) Immediate gastric lavage, and (2) Slow intravenous injection of 1.0 to 2.0 mg of physostigmine, repeated as necessary up to a total of 5 mg.

Fever should be treated symptomatically with tepid sponging or ice packs.

In pronounced restlessness or excitation, diazepam 10 mg may be given in intravenous injection, tachycardia may be treated with intravenous injection of propranolol, and urinary retention can be managed by catheterisation.

In the event of progression of the curare-like effect to the paralysis of the respiratory muscles, mechanical ventilation will be required.

Pharmaceutical precautions Store under dry ambient conditions.

Legal category POM.

Package quantities Original packs containing 4 opaque blister strips of 21 tablets each.

Further information Oxybutynin has both direct antispasmodic action on the smooth muscle of the bladder detrusor as well as anticholinergic action in blocking the muscarinic effects of acetylcholine on smooth muscle.

These properties cause relaxation of the detrusor muscle of the bladder and in patients with an unstable bladder, Ditropan increases bladder capacity and reduces the incidence of spontaneous contractions of the detrusor muscle.

Product licence numbers 2.5 mg tablets 0033/0124
5.0 mg tablets 0033/0125

EPPY*

Presentation L-adrenaline base 1% in an isotonic buffered ophthalmic solution, containing phenylmercuric acetate 0.002% w/v as the preservative.

Uses Indicated for the treatment of elevated intraocular pressure in open-angle (chronic simple) glaucoma.

It may be used in combination with miotics, beta-adrenergic blocking agents or carbonic anhydrase inhibitors where indicated.

Dosage and administration
Adults (including the elderly): One or two drops to each eye, usually once or twice daily. (May be given as infrequently as every three days). Determine the frequency of instillation by tonometry.

When used in conjunction with miotics, instil this drug five or ten minutes after the miotic drops.

Children: As directed by a physician. Safety and efficacy of use in children has not been established.

Contra-indications, warnings, etc
Contra-indications: Narrow-angle glaucoma (unless previously treated with iridectomy).

Patients with a narrow-angle prone to angle block precipitated by mydriatics.

Hypersensitivity to adrenaline or any other component of the preparation.

Interactions

Monoamine oxidase inhibitors: There is an increased risk of adrenergic reactions when used simultaneously with, or up to three weeks after, the administration of MAOIs.

Tricyclic anti-depressants: The pressor response to adrenergic agents and the risk of cardiac arrhythmia may be potentiated in patients receiving tricyclic anti-depressants, (or within several days of their discontinuation).

Cyclopropane or halothane: Because of the increased risk of ventricular fibrillation, adrenaline should not be given during general anaesthesia with anaesthetic agents which sensitise the myocardium to sympathomimetics.

Effect on the ability to drive and use machines: May cause temporarily blurred vision. Warn patients not to drive or operate hazardous machinery unless vision is clear.

Other undesirable effects

Local: Severe smarting on instillation, blurred vision, photophobia, eye pain, conjunctival hyperaemia (resulting in a red eye as a frequent response). Conjunctival sensitisation and allergy and local skin reactions occur occasionally. Pigmentary deposits in the conjunctiva, cornea or eyelids may occur after prolonged use.

CNS: Headache or browache are also common but usually diminish as treatment is continued.

Systemic: Systemic adverse reactions are rare following topical use at normal dosage. However, palpitations, tachycardia, raised blood pressure, extrasystoles, cardiac arrhythmias, faintness, sweating, pallor, trembling and perspiration may occur.

Use in pregnancy and lactation: Safety for use in pregnancy and lactation has not been established. This product should not be used during pregnancy unless it is considered essential by a physician.

Other special warnings and precautions: Do not use until the diagnosis of glaucoma has been verified and the nature of the glaucoma has been confirmed. (As contra-indicated in narrow-angle glaucoma).

To reduce the risk of precipitating an attack of narrow-angle glaucoma, evaluate the anterior chamber angle by gonioscopy before initiating therapy.

Adrenaline eyedrops should be used with caution by patients with hypertension, cardiac disease, aneurysms, arrhythmia or tachycardia, hyperthyroidism, cerebral arteriosclerosis and diabetes mellitus.

Long-term use with soft contact lenses is not recommended.

Maculopathy with a central scotoma may occur following use in aphakic patients. Discontinue use in such patients if visual acuity deteriorates.

Systemic absorption of adrenaline from eye drops may be minimised by compressing the lacrimal sac at the medial canthus for a minute during and following the instillation of the drops. (This blocks the passage of the drops via the naso-lacrimal duct to the wide absorptive area of the nasal and pharyngeal mucosa. It is especially advisable in children).

Overdose: Systemic reactions to topical adrenaline are unlikely at normal doses. Greater caution is necessary in children and the elderly and those patients predisposed to such reactions, eg hypertensive cardiac disease or thyrotoxicosis.

A severe reaction to adrenaline is of rapid onset and short duration.

The treatment of a severe toxic reaction is an immediate intravenous injection of a quick acting alpha-adrenoceptor blocking agent (such as 5 mg to 10 mg of phentolamine) followed by a beta-adrenoceptor blocking agent (such as 2.5 mg to 5 mg of propranolol).

Adrenaline is almost totally inactive when given by mouth as a result of enzymic degradation in the gut and first pass metabolism in the liver.

Incompatibilities: None known.

Pharmaceutical precautions Eppy should not be diluted or dispensed from any container other than the original bottle. It should be stored, in its carton, in a cool place away from strong light. Eppy should not be used if the solution has become dark amber. Eppy should be discarded one month after opening.

Legal category P.

Package quantities Eppy is supplied as a sterile ophthalmic solution in a 7.5 ml bottle, with a separate sterile dropper.

Further information In common with other sympathomimetic agents Eppy does not affect accommodation.

Product licence number 0033/5022.

FLAMAZINE*

Presentation A white hydrophilic cream containing micronised silver sulphadiazine 1% w/w in a semi-solid oil in water emulsion.

Uses Flamazine cream is indicated for the prophylaxis and treatment of infection in burn wounds. Flamazine cream may also be used as an aid to the short-term treatment of infections in leg ulcers and pressure sores, and as an aid to the prophylaxis of infection in skin graft donor sites and extensive abrasions.

Dosage and administration *Burns:* The burn wound should be cleaned and Flamazine cream applied over all the affected areas to a depth of 3–5 mm.

This application is best achieved with a sterile gloved hand and/or sterile spatula. Where necessary, the cream should be re-applied to any area from which it has been removed by patient activity.

In burns, Flamazine cream should be re-applied at least every 24 hours, or more frequently if the volume of exudate is large.

Hand burns: Flamazine cream can be applied to the burn and the whole hand enclosed in a clear plastic bag or glove which is closed at the wrist.

The patient should be encouraged to move the hand and fingers. The dressing should be changed when an excessive amount of exudate has accumulated in the bag.

Leg ulcers/pressure sores: The cavity of the ulcer should be filled with Flamazine cream to a depth of at least 3-5 mm. As Flamazine cream can cause maceration of normal skin on prolonged contact, care should be taken to prevent spread onto non-ulcerated areas.

Application of Flamazine cream should be followed by an absorbent pad or gauze dressing, with further application of pressure bandaging as appropriate for the ulcer.

The dressings should normally be changed daily but for wounds which are less exudative, less frequent changes (every 48 hours) may be acceptable. Cleansing and debriding should be performed before application of Flamazine cream.

Flamazine cream is not recommended for use in leg or pressure ulcers that are very exudative.

The contents of one container are for the treatment of one person on one occasion and any remaining cream should be discarded.

Contra-indications, warnings, etc As sulphonamides are known to cause kernicterus, Flamazine cream should not be used at, or near term pregnancy, on premature infants or on newborn infants during the first months of life. Flamazine cream is also contra-indicated in patients known to be hypersensitive to silver sulphadiazine or to other components of the preparation such as cetyl alcohol or propylene glycol.

As silver may inactivate enzymatic debriding agents, their concomitant use may be inappropriate.

In large-area burns where serum sulphadiazine levels may approach therapeutic levels, it should be noted that the effects of systemically administered drugs may be altered. This can especially apply to oral hypoglycaemic agents, and to phenytoin. In the case of these drugs, it is recommended that blood levels should be monitored as their effects can be potentiated.

Local reactions such as burning, itching and skin rash may occur in about 2% of patients.

Leucopenia has been reported in 3–5% of burns patients treated with Flamazine cream. This may be a drug-related effect, and often manifests itself 2–3 days after treatment has commenced. It is usually self-limiting and therapy with Flamazine cream does not usually need to be discontinued, although the blood count must be carefully monitored to ensure that it returns to normal within a few days.

Systemic absorption of silver sulphadiazine may very rarely result in any of the adverse reactions attributable to systemic sulphonamide therapy.

Safety of use in pregnancy and lactation has not been established. Although animal studies have not shown any hazard, adequate studies in pregnant women have not been performed. Use in pregnancy only if benefit is likely to be greater than possible risk to the foetus. Since all sulphonamides increase the possibility of kernicterus, caution is required in nursing mothers.

Flamazine cream should be used with caution in the presence of significant hepatic or renal impairment. Caution of use is required in patients known to be sensitive to systemic sulphonamides and in individuals known to have glucose-6-phosphate dehydrogenase deficiency.

Use of Flamazine cream may delay separation of burn eschar and may alter the appearance of the burn wounds.

Pharmaceutical precautions The container should be stored in a cool place away from light.

Legal category POM.

Package quantities Flamazine cream is available in plastic tubes containing 50 g, and in jars of 250 g and 500 g.

Further information Silver sulphadiazine is an effective topical antimicrobial agent, active against most strains of gram positive and gram negative bacteria found as wound pathogens, as well as some types of yeasts and fungi.

Flamazine cream is a sterile product and contains no preservatives.

Other ingredients of Flamazine are glycerol monoester, polysorbates, cetyl alcohol, liquid paraffin, propylene glycol and purified water.

Product licence number 0033/0056R.

FLUORETS*

Presentation Sterile, individually wrapped paper strips each impregnated with approximately 1 mg Fluorescein Sodium BP.

Uses Fluorescein is a corneal stain and can be used in diagnostic examinations including Goldmann tonometry and the fitting of hard contact lenses.

Dosage and administration
Adults and children: One Fluoret moistened with tear fluid; sterile water or sterile ophthalmic solution should be sufficient to provide adequate corneal staining. Pull tabs apart at right-hand end of envelope and withdraw Fluoret. Moisten tip as above, then gently stroke the Fluoret across the conjunctiva. For the best result the patient should blink several times.

Contra-indications, warnings, etc Not to be used with soft contact lenses. The applicator should be used once and then discarded. Care should be taken to handle the strip by the non-impregnated end only.

Pharmaceutical precautions No special precautions.

Legal category P.

Package quantities Gravity-delivered cartons of 100 individually wrapped Fluorets.

Further information Fluorescein does not stain a normal cornea but conjunctival abrasions are stained yellow or orange, corneal abrasions or ulcers are stained a bright green and foreign bodies are surrounded by a green ring.

Product licence number 0033/5095R.

GANDA*

Presentation Ganda is a clear, viscous, colourless to almost colourless liquid, available in two strengths.

Ganda 1+0.2 (Guanethidine Monosulphate PhEur 1% w/v+Adrenaline BP 0.2% w/v)

Ganda 3+0.5 (Guanethidine Monosulphate PhEur 3% w/v+Adrenaline BP 0.5% w/v)

in a buffered solution containing benzalkonium chloride 0.01% w/v as the preservative. It is supplied in a plastic dropper bottle packed in a nitrogen-filled pouch.

Uses For the treatment of primary open angle or secondary glaucoma. It may be used in conjunction with miotics or carbonic anhydrase inhibitor therapy.

Dosage and administration *Adults (including the elderly):* One drop to be instilled into the eye once or twice daily or at the discretion of the physician.

Children: At the discretion of the physician. Light pressure may be applied for a few minutes to the inner canthus to reduce systemic absorption via the nasolacrimal duct.

When used in conjunction with miotics, Ganda should follow the miotic after an interval of 5–10 minutes.

Contra-indications, warnings, etc Ganda should not be used in the case of a narrow angle between the iris and cornea as pupillary dilation may precipitate angle closure.

Miotics and other forms of glaucoma treatment produce an enhancement of the therapeutic effect of Ganda. Monoamine oxidase inhibitors increase the effect of adrenaline.

After prolonged treatment with Ganda (more than 9–12 months) cicatrising changes of the conjunctiva and cornea leading to corneal ulceration and scarring have been reported in some patients. If the initial changes are detected on slit lamp examination, treatment with Ganda should be stopped. These cicatrising changes develop slowly and six-monthly examination of the conjunctiva and cornea will enable Ganda to be withdrawn in any patients who are starting to show conjunctival damage.

Occasionally a patient may complain of orbital discomfort or red eye. Rarely, headache, irritation and local skin reactions may occur. As with other adrenaline preparations, melanosis may occasionally occur, but this has no pathological significance. Topical adrenaline has been shown to occasionally cause macular oedema in aphakic eyes and thus the use of adrenaline-containing eye drops in aphakic patients is not recommended. Systemic effects are rare but can include tachycardia, extrasystoles, and elevation of blood pressure. Although no reports of such reactions to Ganda have been received, caution is recommended in patients with thyrotoxicosis, hypertension or cardiovascular problems including tachycardia.

One clinical investigator has reported that in two cases out of 21, a paradoxical increase of intra-ocular pressure occurred for which no explanation was offered.

Some degree of ptosis may represent an adverse effect

in glaucoma, but will usually respond to a reduction in dosage or in the frequency of administration.

At prolonged high dosage a tendency to superficial punctate keratitis has been reported, responding either to a reduction in dosage or termination of treatment.

No data are available on the use of Ganda in pregnancy and lactation, therefore Ganda cannot be recommended in pregnancy or during lactation unless the therapeutic benefit exceeds the potential risk and there is no safer alternative.

Pharmaceutical precautions Ganda is supplied in a plastic dropper bottle in a nitrogen-filled pouch, inside a carton. It should be stored in its carton in a cool place away from strong light. The carton only should be removed before supplying to the patient. Ganda should not be diluted, nor should it be dispensed from any container other than the original bottle. Ganda should not be used if the solution has become dark amber. The contents of the bottle should be discarded one month after removal from the pouch.

Legal category POM.

Package quantities Ganda is supplied as a sterile ophthalmic solution in a 7.5 ml plastic dropper bottle. Each bottle is enclosed in a nitrogen-filled, nylon/aluminium foil pouch inside a carton.

Further information The use of the nitrogen-filled overwrap ensures the long shelf-life of Ganda.

Ganda is a unique combination of Adrenaline BP and Guanethidine Monosulphate PhEur in a plastic dropper bottle which has been specially designed for patient convenience. Its special formulation gives improved stability, and includes a viscoliser to enhance comfort and effectiveness.

In common with other sympathomimetic agents Ganda does not affect accommodation.

Product licence numbers

Ganda 1+0.2	0033/0075
Ganda 3+0.5	0033/0071

GLAULINE*

Presentation A clear, colourless solution in a plastic dropper bottle. Glauline is available in two strengths containing 0.1% or 0.3% w/v metipranolol together with benzalkonium chloride 0.01% w/v as a preservative.

Uses Glauline is a beta adrenoceptor blocking agent used in the topical treatment of chronic open-angle glaucoma and other conditions in which intra-ocular pressure is elevated above normal levels.

Dosage and administration *Adults and the elderly:* The recommended dosage is one drop instilled into the affected eye(s) twice daily.

Children: Not recommended.

Newly diagnosed patients with ocular hypertension or chronic open-angle glaucoma should be treated with Glauline 0.1%, changing to the higher strength if adequate control is not achieved or maintained.

Patients on existing therapy, whether or not this is to be continued, should receive Glauline 0.3%.

Contra-indications, warnings, etc

Contra-indications: Bronchial asthma, history of bronchial asthma, chronic obstructive airways disease, sinus bradycardia, second or third degree atrio-ventricular block, cardiac failure, cardiogenic shock, hypersensitivity to any of the components of the preparation.

Precautions and warnings: As with other topically applied beta-blockers, systemic absorption may occur giving adverse reactions similar to those of orally administered beta-blockers.

Cardiac and respiratory reactions have been reported with topically applied beta-blockers including, rarely, death due to bronchospasm or cardiac failure.

Congestive cardiac failure should be adequately controlled before starting therapy with Glauline. If the patient has a history of cardiac disease, pulse rate should be monitored.

Diabetic control should be monitored during Glauline therapy in patients with labile diabetes.

There have been reports of granulomatous anterior uveitis occuring in patients using Glauline. In any case, where a patient shows symptoms or signs suggestive of anterior uveitis, Glauline should be withdrawn and an alternative ocular hypotensive agent substituted.

Glauline contains benzalkonium chloride as a preservative and should therefore not be used in patients continuing to wear soft (hydrophilic) contact lenses.

Use in pregnancy: Although there is no evidence to suggest that metipranolol has teratogenic properties, its use during pregnancy should be avoided, unless the potential benefits are considered to outweigh the possible hazards.

Use in lactation: As beta-blockers can pass into breast milk, consideration should be given to stopping breast-feeding if therapy with Glauline is considered necessary.

Side-effects:

Ocular: Transient burning or stinging on instillation, blurred vision, superficial punctate keratitis, blepharo-conjunctivitis and anterior uveitis have been reported.

Cardiovascular: Bradycardia and hypotension can occasionally occur following the systemic absorption of topically applied beta-blockers.

Respiratory: Bronchospasm can occur, predominantly in patients with a history of reversible obstructive airways disease. Dyspnoea and respiratory failure have also been reported with topically applied beta-blockers.

CNS: Headache, ataxia, weakness and lethargy can occur.

Dermatological: Local manifestations of contact sensitivity reactions around the eyes can involve skin rashes on the lower lids and cheeks, and peri-orbital oedema.

Drug interactions: Caution should be exercised if used in conjunction with oral beta-blockers as additive effects on systemic beta blockade may occur.

Overdosage: Overdosage is unlikely by the ocular route. If excess drug is accidentally administered to the eye, the affected eye(s) should be immediately flushed with water or saline.

If accidental or deliberate systemic ingestion has taken place, bronchospasm, bradycardia, hypotension and cardiac failure may result, and treatment for overdosage of a beta-receptor blocking agent should be initiated.

Pharmaceutical precautions Glauline should not be diluted or dispensed from any container other than the original bottle. As with other eye drops the contents of each bottle should be discarded one month after opening.

Legal category POM.

Package quantities Glauline is supplied as a sterile ophthalmic solution in a 5 ml plastic dropper bottle.

Further information Glauline reduces intra-ocular pressure with little or no effect on pupil size or accommodation.

For newly diagnosed glaucoma patients, clinical trial experience suggests that approximately 85% will achieve adequate control of their intra-ocular pressure with Glauline 0.1%.

Product licence numbers

Glauline 0.1%	0033/0104
Glauline 0.3%	0033/0105

MINIMS* AMETHOCAINE HYDROCHLORIDE

Presentation Single-use, clear, colourless, sterile eye drops. Two strengths are available: Amethocaine (Tetracaine) Hydrochloride PhEur 0.5% and 1% w/v solutions.

Uses As a topical anaesthetic.

Dosage and administration One drop as required.

Each Minims unit should be discarded after a single use.

Contra-indications, warnings, etc Amethocaine may give rise to dermatitis in hypersensitive patients. Amethocaine is hydrolysed in the body to p-aminobenzoic acid and should not therefore be used in patients being treated with sulphonamides. On instillation an initial burning sensation may be complained of but this passes off in less than half a minute. The anaesthetised eye should be protected from dust and bacterial contamination. The cornea may be damaged by prolonged application of anaesthetic eye drops.

Pharmaceutical precautions Minims should be stored in a cool place (8–15°C), and should not be exposed to strong light.

Legal category POM.

Package quantities Cartons of 20 units, each containing approximately 0.5 ml.

Further information Nil.

Product licence numbers

Amethocaine Hydrochloride 0.5%	0033/5000R
Amethocaine Hydrochloride 1%	0033/5001R

MINIMS* ARTIFICIAL TEARS

Presentation Single-use, clear, colourless, sterile eye drops containing hydroxyethylcellulose 0.44% w/w and Sodium Chloride PhEur 0.35% w/w. No preservatives are included in the formulation.

Uses For the relief of dry eye syndromes associated with deficient tear secretion.

Dosage and administration One or two drops instilled into the affected eye three or four times daily, or as required. Each Minims unit should be discarded after a single dose.

Contra-indications, warnings, etc May cause transient blurring on instillation, do not drive or operate hazardous machinery unless vision is clear. May cause transient mild stinging. There is no, or inadequate evidence of safety of the drug in human pregnancy but it has been in wide use for many years without apparent ill consequence. If therapy is needed in pregnancy, this preparation can be used if recommended by a physician.

If irritation persists or worsens or continued redness occurs, discontinue use and consult a physician.

Pharmaceutical precautions Minims Artificial Tears should be stored in a cool place (8–15°C), and should not be exposed to strong light.

Legal category P.

Package quantities Cartons of 20 units, each containing approximately 0.5 ml.

Further information Nil.

Product licence number 0033/0137.

MINIMS* ATROPINE SULPHATE

Presentation Single-use, clear, colourless, sterile eye drops, available as a 1% w/v solution of Atropine Sulphate PhEur.

Uses As a mydriatic and cycloplegic.

Dosage and administration One drop as required.

Each Minims unit should be discarded after a single use.

Contra-indications, warnings, etc The protracted mydriasis which is difficult to reverse, may be a disadvantage. All mydriatics and cycloplegics are contra-indicated in eyes where the filtration angle is narrow, as an acute attack of angle closure glaucoma may be precipitated. If in doubt it is recommended that homatropine is used, since its action can be reversed by eserine (physostigmine).

Pharmaceutical precautions Minims should be stored in a cool place (8–15°C), and should not be exposed to strong light.

Legal category POM.

Package quantities Cartons of 20 units, each unit containing approximately 0.5 ml.

Further information Dilation of the pupil occurs within half an hour after application.

Product licence number 0033/5002R.

MINIMS* BENOXINATE (OXYBUPROCAINE) HYDROCHLORIDE

Presentation Single-use, clear, colourless, sterile eye drops, available as a 0.4% w/v solution of Benoxinate (Oxybuprocaine) Hydrochloride USP.

Uses As a topical anaesthetic.

Dosage and administration One drop of benoxinate 0.4% is sufficient when dropped into the conjunctival sac to anaesthetise the surface of the eye to allow tonometry after one minute. A further drop after 90 seconds provides adequate anaesthesia for the fitting of contact lenses.

Three drops at 90 second intervals provides sufficient anaesthesia after five minutes for a foreign body to be removed from the corneal epithelium, or for incision of a Meibomian cyst through the conjunctiva.

Corneal sensitivity is normal again after about one hour.

Each Minims unit should be discarded after a single use.

Contra-indications, warnings, etc The anaesthetised eye should be protected from dust and bacterial contamination. The cornea may be damaged by prolonged application of anaesthetic eye drops.

Pharmaceutical precautions Minims should be stored in a cool place (8–15°C), and should not be exposed to strong light.

Legal category POM.

Package quantities Cartons of 20 units, each unit containing approximately 0.5 ml.

Further information When applied to the conjunctiva benoxinate is less irritant than amethocaine in normal concentrations.

Product licence number 0033/5004R.

MINIMS* CASTOR OIL

Presentation Single-use, clear, almost colourless or slightly yellow, viscous sterile eye drops.

Uses In first-aid treatment to aid the removal of non-penetrating ocular foreign bodies.

Dosage and administration One or more drops as required.

Each Minims unit should be discarded after a single use.

Contra-indications, warnings, etc Minims Castor Oil should not be used in injuries where there is evidence of actual damage to the conjunctiva or cornea, in penetrating injuries, injuries caused by high velocity metal or stone particles, or in the presence of thermal or caustic burns. As castor oil can damage the conjunctival epithelium, prolonged use is not recommended.

Pharmaceutical precautions Minims should be stored in a cool place (8–15°C) and should not be exposed to strong light.

Legal category P.

Package quantities Cartons of 20 units, each unit containing approximately 0.5 ml.

Further information Nil.

Product licence number 0033/5018.

MINIMS* CHLORAMPHENICOL

Presentation Single-use, clear, colourless, sterile eye drops, available as a 0.5% w/v solution of Chloramphenicol PhEur containing buffering agents.

Uses Chloramphenicol is a broad spectrum bacteriostatic antibiotic. It is active against a wide variety of Gram-negative and Gram-positive organisms as well as rickettsiae and spirochaetes. It is indicated for use as a topical antibacterial in the treatment of superficial ocular infections.

Dosage and administration
Adults (including the elderly) and children: One to two drops applied to each affected eye up to six times daily or more frequently if required. (Severe infections may require one to two drops every fifteen to twenty minutes initially, reducing the frequency of instillation gradually as the infection is controlled).

Each Minims unit should be discarded after a single use.

Contra-indications, warnings, etc
Contra-indications: Hypersensitivity to chloramphenicol or to any component of the preparation.

Interactions: Chymotrypsin will be inhibited if given simultaneously with chloramphenicol.

Effects on ability to drive and use machines: May cause transient blurring of vision on instillation. Warn patients not to drive or operate hazardous machinery unless vision is clear.

Other undesirable effects
Local: Sensitivity reactions such as transient irritation, burning, stinging, itching and dermatitis.

Systemic: Several cases of major adverse haematological events (bone marrow depression, aplastic anaemia and death) have been reported following ocular use of chloramphenicol.

Use in pregnancy and lactation: Safety for use in pregnancy and lactation has not been established. Therefore, use only when considered essential by the physician.

Other special warnings and precautions: In severe infections topical use of chloramphenicol should be supplemented with appropriate systemic treatment.

Aplastic anaemia has followed topical use of chloramphenicol eye drops and, whilst this hazard is a rare one, it should be considered when the benefits of the use of chloramphenicol are assessed.

Prolonged use should be avoided as it may increase the likelihood of sensitisation and the emergence of resistant organisms.

Contact lenses should be removed during the period of treatment.

Overdose: Not applicable.

Incompatibilities: None known.

Pharmaceutical precautions Minims Chloramphenicol should be stored between 2°C and 8°C. Do not freeze.

Legal category POM.

Package quantities Cartons of 20 units, each unit containing approximately 0.5 ml.

Further information Nil.

Product licence number 0033/0055.

MINIMS* CYCLOPENTOLATE HYDROCHLORIDE

Presentation Single-use, clear, colourless, sterile eye drops. Two strengths are available: Cyclopentolate Hydrochloride BP 0.5% and 1% w/v solutions.

Uses As a mydriatic and cycloplegic.

Dosage and administration *Adults (including the elderly):* One or two drops as required. Maximum effect is induced 30–60 minutes after instillation. In iritis or iridocyclitis 1 or 2 drops of a 0.5% w/v solution are instilled every six to eight hours. One or two drops of a 0.5% w/v solution are also used for breaking down adhesions of the iris to the lens. For refraction the instillation of 1 drop of a 0.5% w/v solution repeated after five minutes is usually sufficient. Deeply pigmented eyes may require a 1% w/v solution.

Children: At the discretion of the physician.

Each Minims unit should be discarded after a single use.

Contra-indications, warnings, etc Recovery of accommodation occurs within 24 hours.

All mydriatics and cycloplegics are contra-indicated in eyes where the filtration angle is narrow, as an acute attack of angle closure glaucoma may be precipitated.

Minims Cyclopentolate should not be used in neonates except where, on expert evaluation, the need is considered to be compelling.

Pharmaceutical precautions Minims should be stored in a cool place (8–15°C), and should not be exposed to strong light.

Legal category POM.

Package quantities Cartons of 20 units, each unit containing approximately 0.5 ml.

Further information Nil.

Product licence numbers

Cyclopentolate Hydrochloride 0.5%	0033/5005R
Cyclopentolate Hydrochloride 1%	0033/5006R

MINIMS* FLUORESCEIN SODIUM

Presentation Single-use, clear, orange-red, sterile eye drops. Two strengths are available: Fluorescein Sodium BP 1% and 2% w/v solutions.

Uses Fluorescein is a corneal stain and can be used in diagnostic examinations including Goldmann tonometry and the fitting of hard contact lenses.

Dosage and administration Sufficient solution should be applied to stain the damaged areas. Excess may be washed away with sterile saline solution.

Each Minims unit should be discarded after a single use.

Contra-indications, warnings, etc Not to be used with soft contact lenses.

Pharmaceutical precautions Minims should be stored in a cool place(8–15°C), and should not be exposed to strong light.

Legal category P.

Package quantities Cartons of 20 units, each unit containing approximately 0.5 ml.

Further information Fluorescein does not stain a normal cornea but conjunctival abrasions are stained yellow or orange, corneal abrasions or ulcers are stained a bright green and foreign bodies are surrounded by a green ring.

Product licence numbers

Fluorescein Sodium 1%	0033/0079
Fluorescein Sodium 2%	0033/5008R

MINIMS* GENTAMICIN SULPHATE

Presentation Single-use, clear, colourless sterile eye drops containing Gentamicin Sulphate BP equivalent to 0.3% w/v gentamicin base, and additional ingredients.

Uses As a broad-spectrum bactericidal antibiotic, for the treatment of ocular infections caused by both Gram-positive and Gram-negative organisms.

Dosage and administration *Adults (including the elderly):* One drop as required.

Children: At the discretion of the physician.

Each Minims unit should be discarded after a single use.

Contra-indications, warnings, etc Gentamicin should not be used in patients with hypersensitivity to gentamicin and/or other aminoglycosides.

Gentamicin has been used topically without any evidence of significant absorption of the drug to cause systemic reactions. Gentamicin is well tolerated when applied topically to the eye.

The use of sulphacetamide with gentamicin in the treatment of eye infections is not recommended. Concomitant administration of frusemide and gentamicin may reduce the renal clearance of gentamicin but this is unlikely to be of significance with topical use.

Gentamicin is incompatible with amphotericin, cephalosporins, erythromycin, heparin, penicillins, sodium bicarbonate and sulphadiazine sodium. This is unlikely to be relevant regarding topical use.

The use of gentamicin during pregnancy is not recommended.

Gentamicin should not be the first choice antibiotic for minor infections in order to minimise the possibility of bacterial resistance.

Pharmaceutical precautions Minims Gentamicin Sulphate should be stored in a cool place (8–15°C), but not frozen, and should not be exposed to strong light.

Legal category POM.

Package quantities Cartons of 20 units, each unit containing approximately 0.5 ml.

Further information Nil.

Product licence number 0033/0094.

MINIMS* HOMATROPINE HYDROBROMIDE

Presentation Single-use, clear, colourless, sterile eye drops, available as a 2% w/v solution of Homatropine Hydrobromide PhEur.

Uses As a mydriatic and cycloplegic.

Dosage and administration One drop as required.

Each Minims unit should be discarded after a single use.

Contra-indications, warnings, etc All mydriatics and cycloplegics are contra-indicated in eyes where the filtration angle is narrow, as an acute attack of angle closure glaucoma may be precipitated.

Minims Homatropine should not be used in patients allergic to atropine.

Pharmaceutical precautions Minims should be stored in a cool place(8–15°C), and should not be exposed to strong light.

Legal category POM.

Package quantities Cartons of 20 units, each unit containing approximately 0.5 ml.

Further information Homatropine hydrobromide has properties similar to those of atropine and is often used in preference to the latter because its action is more rapid in onset and it has a less prolonged mydriatic action.

Product licence number 0033/5010R.

MINIMS* LIGNOCAINE AND FLUORESCEIN

Presentation Single-use, clear, yellow, sterile eye drops containing Lignocaine (Lidocaine) Hydrochloride PhEur 4.0% w/v, Fluorescein Sodium BP 0.25% w/v and stabilising agents.

Uses As a diagnostic stain and topical anaesthetic combined. Minims Lignocaine and Fluorescein units are used in the measurement of intra-ocular pressure by Goldman tonometry.

Dosage and administration *Adult:* One or more drops as required.

Children: At the discretion of the physician.

Each Minims unit should be discarded after a single use.

Contra-indications, warnings, etc Known hypersensitivity to lignocaine and other local anaesthetics.

Special care should be taken to protect the anaesthetised eye from foreign body contamination, particularly in elderly patients in whom the duration of anaesthesia may exceed 30 minutes. This combination has been in use during pregnancy and lactation for a number of years without apparent ill consequence.

Overdose is not expected to cause adverse effects. However, over-use of local anaesthetics can cause keratitis, with loss of corneal epithelium and stromal opacity.

Pharmaceutical precautions Store in a cool place (8–15°C). Protect from light.

Legal category POM.

Package quantities Cartons of 20 units, each unit containing approximately 0.5 ml.

Further information Nil.

Product licence number 0033/0073.

MINIMS* METIPRANOLOL

Presentation Single-use, clear, colourless, sterile eye drops. Three strengths are available: 0.1% w/v, 0.3% w/v and 0.6% w/v as metipranolol.

No preservatives are included in the formulation.

Uses Metipranolol is a non-selective beta adrenoreceptor blocking agent.

Minims Metipranolol is indicated for the treatment of raised intra-ocular pressure. It is particularly suitable for the treatment of patients who are allergic to preservatives, for control of post-operative increases in intra-ocular pressure and as an initial test for responsiveness to metipranolol therapy.

Dosage and administration The recommended dose is one drop instilled into the affected eye twice daily. Newly diagnosed patients should be treated in the first instance with the 0.1% w/v strength changing to a higher strength if adequate control is not achieved or maintained.

If used as a diagnostic agent before planning a treatment programme then only one drop need be instilled.

In the treatment of post-operative rises in intra-ocular pressure the dosage and frequency should be at the discretion of the physician.

Each Minims unit should be discarded after a single use.

Contra-indications, warnings, etc The use of Minims Metipranolol is not recommended in patients with obstructive airways disease, cardiac failure or hypersensitivity to metipranolol. Beta blockers should not be given with verapamil and neither drug should be administered within several days of discontinuing the other. As absorption into the circulation is possible, Minims Metipranolol should only be used with caution in patients already receiving similar drugs by mouth. In particular, care should be taken in patients with sinus bradycardia and greater than first degree heart block.

Although there is no evidence to suggest that metipranolol has teratogenic properties, its use during pregnancy should be avoided, unless the potential benefits are considered to outweigh the possible hazards. No clinical trials in children have been carried out.

Intra-ocular pressure should be determined at frequent and regular intervals.

Ophthalmic solutions should only be used in patients fitted with contact lenses at the discretion of the physician.

Pharmaceutical precautions Minims should be stored in a cool place (8°–15°C) and should not be exposed to strong light.

Legal category POM.

Package quantities Cartons of 20 units, each unit containing approximately 0.5 g of solution.

Further information Metipranolol has little or no effect on pupil size or accommodation. Metipranolol is generally well tolerated but some patients may experience slight, transient stinging. Transient headaches have been reported.

Product licence numbers
0.1% w/v 0033/0121
0.3% w/v 0033/0122
0.6% w/v 0033/0123

MINIMS* NEOMYCIN SULPHATE

Presentation Single-use, clear, colourless, sterile eye drops, available as a 0.5% w/v solution of Neomycin Sulphate PhEur. Contains stabilising agents.

Uses For the topical treatment of superficial ocular infections caused by sensitive pathogens.

Dosage and administration *Adults (including the elderly) and children:* One or two drops applied to each affected eye up to six times daily or more frequently if required. (Severe infections may require one or two drops every fifteen to twenty minutes initially, reducing the frequency of instillation gradually as the infection is controlled).

Each Minims unit should be discarded after a single use.

Contra-indications, warnings, etc Should not be used in patients with a known hypersensitivity to the constituents or to other aminoglycosides.

Effects on ability to drive: May cause transient blurring of vision on instillation. Patients should be advised not to drive or operate hazardous machinery until vision is clear.

Other undesirable effects: Hypersensitivity reactions, usually of the delayed type, occur frequently with local treatment with neomycin. Irritation, burning, stinging, itching and dermatitis may occur.

Use in pregnancy and lactation: Safety for use in pregnancy and lactation has not been established. Use only when it is considered essential by the physician.

Other special warnings and precautions: In severe infections, topical use of neomycin should be supplemented with appropriate systemic treatment. Prolonged use should be avoided as it may lead to skin sensitisation and the emergence of resistant organisms.

Neomycin may cause irreversible partial or total deafness when given systemically or applied topically to open wounds or damaged skin. This effect is dose-related and is enhanced by renal or hepatic impairment. Although this effect has not been reported following topical ocular use, the possibility should be considered when high-dose topical treatment is given to small children or infants.

Contact lenses should be removed during the period of treatment.

Pharmaceutical precautions Minims should be stored in a cool place (8–15°C), and should not be exposed to strong light.

Legal category POM.

Package quantities Cartons of 20 units, each unit containing approximately 0.5 ml.

Further information Neomycin sulphate has a broad spectrum of antibiotic activity, being effective against most strains of staphylococci and some strains of *Proteus vulgaris* and *Pseudomonas aeruginosa*. It has no action against fungi and viruses.

Product licence number 0033/5012R.

MINIMS* PHENYLEPHRINE HYDROCHLORIDE

Presentation Single-use, clear, colourless, sterile eye drops. Two strengths are available: Phenylephrine Hydrochloride BP 2.5% and 10% w/v solutions, containing stabilising agents.

Uses Phenylephrine is a directly acting sympathomimetic agent used topically in the eye as a mydriatic. It may be indicated to dilate the pupil in diagnostic or therapeutic procedures.

Dosage and administration
Adults: Apply one drop to each eye. If necessary this dose may be repeated once only, at least one hour after the first drop.

NB The use of a drop of topical anaesthetic a few minutes before instillation of phenylephrine is recommended to prevent stinging.

Children and the elderly: The use of phenylephrine 10% solution is contra-indicated in these groups because of the increased risks of systemic toxicity. One drop of the 2.5% w/v solution may be used. It is not usually necessary to exceed this dosage.

Each Minims unit should be discarded after a single use.

Contra-indications, warnings, etc
Contra-indications: Patients with cardiac disease, hypertension, aneurysms, thyrotoxicosis, long-standing insulin-dependant diabetes and tachycardia.

Patients on monoamine oxidase inhibitors, tricyclic anti-depressants and anti-hypertensive agents (including beta-blockers).

Patients with closed angle glaucoma (unless previously treated with iridectomy) and patients with a narrow angle prone to glaucoma precipitated by mydriatics.

Hypersensitivity to phenylephrine or any component of the preparation.

Interactions

Anti-hypertensive agents: Topical phenylephrine should not be used as it may reverse the action of many anti-hypertensive agents with possibly fatal reactions.

Monoamine oxidase inhibitors: There is an increased risk of adrenergic reactions when used simultaneously with, or up to three weeks after, the administration of MAOIs.

Tricyclic anti-depressants: The pressor response to adrenergic agents and the risk of cardiac arrhythmia may be potentiated in patients receiving tricyclic anti-depressants, (or within several days of their discontinuation).

Cyclopropane or halothane: Because of the increased risk of ventricular fibrillation, phenylephrine should be used with caution during general anaesthesia with anaesthetic agents which sensitise the myocardium to sympathomimetics.

Cardiac glycosides or quinidine: There is an increased risk of arrhythmias.

Effects on the ability to drive and use machines: May cause stinging and temporarily blurred vision. Warn patients not to drive or operate hazardous machinery until vision is clear.

Other undesirable effects

Local: Eye pain and stinging on instillation (use of a drop of topical anaesthetic a few minutes before the instillation of phenylephrine is recommended), temporarily blurred vision and photophobia, conjunctival sensitisation and allergy may occur.

Systemic: Palpitations, tachycardia, extrasystoles, cardiac arrhythmias and hypertension.

Serious cardiovascular reactions including coronary artery spasm, ventricular arrhythmias and myocardial infarctions have occurred following topical use of 10% phenylephrine. These sometimes fatal reactions have usually occurred in elderly patients with pre-existing cardiovascular disease.

Use in pregnancy and lactation: Safety for use in pregnancy and lactation has not been established. This product should only be used during pregnancy if it is considered by the physician to be essential.

Other special warnings and precautions: Use with caution in the presence of diabetes, cerebral arteriosclerosis or long standing bronchial asthma.

To reduce the risk of precipitating an attack of narrow angle glaucoma evaluate the anterior chamber angle before use.

Corneal clouding may occur if phenylephrine 10% is instilled when the corneal epithelium has been denuded or damaged.

Systemic absorption may be minimised by compressing the lacrimal sac at the medial canthus for one minute during and after the instillation of the drops.

Overdose: Because a severe toxic reaction to phenylephrine is of rapid onset and short duration, treatment is primarily supportive. Prompt injection of a rapidly acting alpha-adrenergic blocking agent such as phentolamine (dose 5 to 10 mg iv) has been recommended.

Incompatibilities: None relevant.

Pharmaceutical precautions Minims should be stored in a cool place (8–15°C) and should not be exposed to strong light.

Legal category P.

Package quantities Cartons of 20 units, each unit containing approximately 0.5 ml of solution.

Further information Nil.

Product licence numbers

Phenylephrine hydrochloride 2.5% w/v 0033/0117
Phenylephrine hydrochloride 10% w/v 0033/5021R

MINIMS* PILOCARPINE NITRATE

Presentation Single-use, clear, colourless, sterile eye drops. Three strengths are available: Pilocarpine Nitrate PhEur 1%, 2%, and 4% w/v solutions.

Uses As a miotic for reversing the action of the weaker mydriatics and in emergency treatment of glaucoma.

Dosage and administration To induce miosis one or two drops should be used. In cases of emergency treatment of acute narrow angle glaucoma, one drop should be used every five minutes until miosis is achieved.

Each Minims unit should be discarded after a single use.

Contra-indications, warnings, etc Pilocarpine induces spasm of the ciliary muscle which may last up to two hours.

Pharmaceutical precautions Minims should be stored in a cool place (8–15°C), and should not be exposed to strong light.

Legal category POM.

Package quantities Cartons of 20 units, each unit containing approximately 0.5 ml.

Further information Nil.

Product licence numbers

Pilocarpine Nitrate 1% 0033/5013R
Pilocarpine Nitrate 2% 0033/5014R
Pilocarpine Nitrate 4% 0033/5016R

MINIMS* PREDNISOLONE SODIUM PHOSPHATE

Presentation Single-use, clear, colourless, sterile eye drops, available as a 0.5% w/v solution of Prednisolone Sodium Phosphate BP containing additional ingredients.

Uses Non-infected inflammatory conditions of the eye.

Dosage and administration

Adults (including the elderly): One or two drops as required.

Children: At the discretion of the physician.

Each Minims unit should be discarded after a single use.

Contra-indications, warnings, etc Use is contra-indicated in viral, fungal, tuberculous and other bacterial infections. Care should be taken to ensure that the eye is not infected before Minims Prednisolone is used. Prolonged application to the eye of preparations containing corticosteroids has caused increased intra-ocular pressure and therefore the drops should not be used in patients with glaucoma. Topical administration of corticosteroids to pregnant animals can cause abnormalities of foetal development and although the relevance of this finding to human beings has not been established, the use of Minims Prednisolone during pregnancy should be avoided. Prolonged treatment with corticosteroids in high dosage is occasionally associated with subcapsular cataract. The systemic effects of steroids are possible following the use of Minims Prednisolone, but are however unlikely due to the reduced absorption of topical eye drops.

In children, long-term continuous topical corticosteroid therapy should be avoided due to possible adrenal suppression.

Pharmaceutical precautions Minims should be stored in a cool place (8–15°C), and should not be exposed to strong light.

Legal category POM.

Package quantities Cartons of 20 units, each unit containing approximately 0.5 ml.

Further information Corticosteroids are known to increase the effects of barbiturates, sedatives, hypnotics and tricyclic antidepressants. They will, however, decrease the effects of anticholinesterases, antiviral eye preparations and salicylates.

Product licence number 0033/0091.

MINIMS* ROSE BENGAL

Presentation Single-use, clear, dark-red, sterile eye drops, available as a 1% w/v solution of rose bengal.

Uses As a diagnostic stain. Rose bengal solution stains degenerated conjunctival and corneal epithelial cells. It is particularly useful in demonstrating these changes in Sjogren's syndrome, where lack of tears has caused damage. Pressure marks from contact lenses are shown by rose bengal indicating that alteration of the lens may be necessary.

Dosage and administration One or two drops as required.

Each Minims unit should be discarded after a single use.

Contra-indications, warnings, etc Rose bengal can produce severe stinging in dry eyes where it should be used with care.

Rose bengal may discolour the eye lids and/or conjunctiva. The use of rose bengal in pregnancy and lactation over many years has not shown any adverse effects.

In the absence of any teratology studies, however, rose bengal is not recommended in pregnancy unless the therapeutic benefit exceeds the potential risk.

Rose bengal solution should not be instilled into the eye when the patient is wearing contact lenses.

Pharmaceutical precautions Minims should be stored in a cool place (8–15°C), and should not be exposed to strong light.

Legal category P.

Package quantities Cartons of 20 units, each unit containing approximately 0.5 ml.

Further information Nil.

Product licence number 0033/0048R.

MINIMS* SODIUM CHLORIDE

Presentation Single-use, clear, colourless, sterile eye drops, available as a 0.9% w/v solution of Sodium Chloride PhEur.

Uses As an irrigating solution.

Dosage and administration Adequate solution should be used to irrigate the eye.

Each Minims unit should be discarded after a single use.

Contra-indications, warnings, etc Nil.

Pharmaceutical precautions Minims should be stored in a cool place (8–15°C), and should not be exposed to strong light.

Legal category P.

Package quantities Cartons of 20 units, each unit containing approximately 0.5 ml.

Further information Nil.

Product licence number 0033/5017R.

MINIMS* SULPHACETAMIDE SODIUM

Presentation Single-use, clear, colourless or slightly yellow, sterile eye drops, available as a 10% w/v solution of Sulphacetamide Sodium PhEur containing stabilising agents.

Uses For the treatment of bacterial conjunctivitis caused by organisms sensitive to sodium sulphacetamide.

Dosage and administration *Adult:* One or two drops every one to two hours.

Children: At the discretion of the physician.

Each Minims unit should be discarded after a single use.

Contra-indications, warnings, etc Local application to the eye may cause burning or stinging, but this is rarely severe enough to necessitate discontinuation of treatment. Sulphacetamide sodium should not be used in persons who have shown hypersensitivity to sulphonamides.

Pharmaceutical precautions Minims should be stored in a cool place (8–15°C), and should not be exposed to strong light.

Legal category POM.

Package quantities Cartons of 20 units, each unit containing approximately 0.5 ml.

Further information Nil.

Product licence number 0033/5019.

MINIMS* THYMOXAMINE HYDROCHLORIDE

Presentation Single-use, clear, colourless, sterile eye drops, available as a 0.5% w/v solution of Thymoxamine Hydrochloride BP.

Uses As a miotic for the acute reversal of the mydriasis caused by phenylephrine and other sympathomimetics.

Dosage and administration One or more drops as required. Each Minims unit should be discarded after a single use.

Contra-indications, warnings, etc Any known hypersensitivity to thymoxamine. Upon instillation an initial transient burning sensation may be experienced. Minimal conjunctival hyperaemia generally occurs but this passes after a few hours. A transient ptosis may occasionally occur.

Although there is no evidence to suggest that thymoxamine has teratogenic properties, its use in pregnancy should be avoided unless the potential benefits are considered to outweigh possible hazards.

Pharmaceutical precautions Thymoxamine Minims should be stored between 2°C and 8°C. Do not freeze. Do not expose to strong light.

Legal category POM.

Package quantities Cartons of 20 units, each unit containing approximately 0.5 ml.

Further information Clinical studies with thymoxamine have shown that it produces miosis without causing a significant change in the depth of the anterior chamber or altering facility of outflow. Alpha-blocking agents reduce the effect of sympathomimetics. Unlike parasympathomimetic miotics thymoxamine does not cause spasm of the ciliary muscle.

Product licence number 0033/0101.

MINIMS* TROPICAMIDE

Presentation Single-use, clear, colourless, sterile eye drops. Two strengths are available: Tropicamide BP 0.5% and 1% w/v solutions.

Uses As a mydriatic and cycloplegic.

Dosage and administration *Adult:* 2 drops at five minute intervals, with a further 1 or 2 drops after 30 minutes if required.

Children: At the discretion of the physician.

Each Minims unit should be discarded after a single use.

Contra-indications, warnings, etc All mydriatics and cycloplegics are contra-indicated in eyes where the filtration angle is narrow, as an acute attack of angle closure glaucoma may be precipitated.

Patients who receive a mydriatic may suffer from photophobia and this may impair their ability to drive under certain circumstances.

There is no evidence as to the drug safety in human pregnancy nor is there evidence from animal work that it is free from hazard. This product should only be used during pregnancy if considered essential by the physician.

Systemic effects from Minims Tropicamide are not expected. Should an overdosage occur causing local effects eg sustained mydriasis, physostigmine 0.25% w/v should be applied.

Pharmaceutical precautions Minims units should be stored in a cool place (8–15°C) and should not be exposed to strong light.

Legal category POM.

Package quantities Cartons of 20 units, each unit containing approximately 0.5 ml.

Further information The 0.5% solution in particular may be expected to cause little or no cycloplegia.

Product licence numbers
Tropicamide 0.5% 0033/0077
Tropicamide 1.0% 0033/0078

NARPHEN*

Presentation Narphen is available as white, biconvex compressed tablets embossed SNP/2 on one side and scored on the reverse. Each tablet contains 5 mg Phenazocine Hydrobromide BP (1973).

Uses Narphen is a powerful analgesic for the relief of severe pain. Pain relief usually occurs within 20 minutes and lasts for five to six hours. Narphen is indicated for acute and chronic pain, including pre- and postoperative pain and for obstetric analgesia. Narphen is particularly suitable for the treatment of intractable pain such as that of carcinoma as it produces minimal sedation.

In treating biliary or pancreatic pain constriction of the Sphincter of Oddi is undesirable and the low spasmogenic activity of Narphen may be advantageous.

Dosage and administration *Adults (including the elderly):* One tablet every four to six hours sublingually or orally; up to 20 mg may be administered in a single dose if necessary.

Children: Paediatric dosage not established.

Contra-indications, warnings, etc Narphen is contra-indicated in coma, convulsive disorders, delirium tremens, myxoedema, alcoholism, respiratory depression and obstructive airways disease. Narphen should not be given concurrently with monoamine oxidase inhibitors, nor within two weeks of discontinuation of treatment with them.

It is wise to reduce dosage in the elderly, and in hypothyroidism or chronic hepatic disease. Administration in labour may cause respiratory depression in the new-born infant.

Care is required in the presence of renal insufficiency or concurrent administration of other narcotic analgesics, sedatives/hypnotics or anaesthetics.

At the commencement of dosage some patients may experience a feeling of light-headedness or dizziness which soon passes but if affected the patient should not attempt to drive or operate machinery.

Nausea and vomiting may be troublesome although emetic symptoms and constipation are less than with other narcotic analgesics. If nausea and vomiting occur anti-emetics such as those of the phenothiazine type may be effective.

Pruritus and occasionally dryness of the mouth and sweating have occurred. Hypotension is rare. As with other narcotics respiratory depression, tolerance and dependence may occur.

Although there is insufficient evidence of the safety of this drug in human pregnancy, animal studies have not shown any hazard. Nevertheless the use of phenazocine during pregnancy is not recommended.

Treatment of overdosage: Naloxone may be used as an antidote to overdosage or to antagonise any respiratory depression that may occur.

Incompatibilities: Should not be used concomitantly with MAOIs.

Pharmaceutical precautions Protect from light.

Legal category CD (Sch 2) POM.

Package quantities Tablets of 5 mg in securitainers of 100.

Further information Nil.

Product licence number 0033/5047R.

SIMPLENE*

Presentation Simplene is a clear, viscous, colourless to almost colourless liquid, containing Adrenaline BP in a buffered solution preserved with benzalkonium chloride 0.01% w/v. It is supplied in a plastic dropper bottle packed in a nitrogen-filled pouch and is available in two strengths:

Simplene 0.5% (Adrenaline BP 0.5% w/v)
Simplene 1.0% (Adrenaline BP 1.0% w/v)

Uses Indicated for the treatment of elevated intraocular pressure in open-angle (chronic simple) glaucoma.

It may be used in combination with miotics, beta-adrenergic blocking agents or carbonic anhydrase inhibitors where indicated.

Dosage and administration
Adults (including the elderly): One or two drops to each eye, usually once or twice daily (may be given as infrequently as every three days). Determine the frequency of instillation by tonometry.

When used in conjunction with miotics, instil this drug five or ten minutes after the miotic drops.

Children: As directed by a physician. Safety and efficacy of use in children has not been established.

Contra-indications, warnings, etc
Contra-indications: Closed-angle glaucoma (unless previously treated with iridectomy).

Patients with a narrow-angle prone to angle block precipitated by mydriatics.

Hypersensitivity to adrenaline or any other component of the preparation.

This product contains benzalkonium chloride and should not be used when soft contact lenses are worn.

Interactions

Monoamine oxidase inhibitors: There is an increased risk of adrenergic reactions when used simultaneously with, or up to three weeks after, the administration of MAOIs.

Tricyclic anti-depressants: The pressor response to adrenergic agents and the risk of cardiac arrhythmia may be potentiated in patients receiving tricyclic anti-depressants, (or within several days of their discontinuation).

Cyclopropane or halothane: Because of the increased risk of ventricular fibrillation, adrenaline should not be given during general anaesthesia with anaesthetic agents which sensitise the myocardium to sympathomimetics.

Effects on the ability to drive and use machines: May cause temporarily blurred vision. Warn patients not to drive or operate hazardous machinery unless vision is clear.

Other undesirable effects

Local: Severe smarting on instillation, blurred vision, photophobia, eye pain, conjunctival hyperaemia (resulting in a red eye as a frequent response). Conjunctival sensitisation and allergy and local skin reactions occur occasionally. Pigmentary deposits in the conjunctiva, cornea or eyelids may occur after prolonged use.

CNS: Headache or browache are also common but usually diminish as treatment is continued.

Systemic: Systemic adverse reactions are rare following topical use at normal dosage. However, palpitations, tachycardia, raised blood pressure, extrasystoles, cardiac arrhythmias, faintness, sweating, pallor, trembling and perspiration may occur.

Use in pregnancy and lactation: Safety for use in pregnancy and lactation has not been established. This product should not be used during pregnancy unless it is considered essential by a physician.

Other special warnings and precautions: Do not use until the diagnosis of glaucoma has been verified and the nature of the glaucoma has been confirmed (as contra-indicated in narrow-angle glaucoma).

To reduce the risk of precipitating an attack of narrow-angle glaucoma, evaluate the anterior chamber angle by gonioscopy before initiating therapy.

Adrenaline eye drops should be used with caution by patients with hypertension, cardiac disease, aneurysms, arrhythmia or tachycardia, hyperthyroidism, cerebral arteriosclerosis and diabetes mellitus.

Maculopathy with a central scotoma may occur following use in aphakic patients. Discontinue use in such patients if visual acuity deteriorates.

Systemic absorption of adrenaline from eye drops may be minimised by compressing the lacrimal sac at the medial canthus for a minute during and following the instillation of the drops (this blocks the passage of the drops via the naso-lacrimal duct to the wide absorptive area of the nasal and pharyngeal mucosa. It is especially advisable in children).

Overdose: Systemic reactions to topical adrenaline are unlikely at normal doses. Greater caution is necessary in children and the elderly and those patients predisposed to such reactions, e.g. hypertensive cardiac disease or thyrotoxicosis.

A severe reaction to adrenaline is of rapid onset and short duration.

The treatment of a severe toxic reaction is an immediate intravenous injection of a quick acting alpha-adrenoceptor blocking agent (such as 5 mg to 10 mg of phentolamine) followed by a beta-adrenoceptor blocking agent (such as 2.5 mg to 5 mg of propranolol).

Adrenaline is almost totally inactive when given by mouth as a result of enzymic degradation in the gut and first pass metabolism in the liver.

Incompatibilities: None known.

Pharmaceutical precautions Simplene is supplied in a plastic dropper bottle in a nitrogen-filled pouch, inside a carton. It should be stored in its carton in a cool place away from strong light. The carton only should be removed before supplying to the patient. Simplene should not be diluted, nor should it be dispensed from any container other than the original bottle. Simplene should not be used if the solution has become dark amber. The contents of the bottle should be discarded one month after removal from the pouch.

Legal category POM.

Package quantities Simplene is supplied as a sterile ophthalmic solution in a 7.5 ml plastic dropper bottle. Each bottle is enclosed in a nitrogen-filled, nylon/aluminium foil pouch, inside a carton.

Further information The use of the nitrogen-filled overwrap ensures the long shelf-life of Simplene.

Simplene is a unique presentation of adrenaline in a plastic dropper bottle, which has been specially designed for patient convenience. Its special formulation gives improved stability, and includes a viscoliser to enhance comfort and effectiveness.

In common with other sympathomimetic agents Simplene does not affect accommodation.

Product licence numbers
Simplene 1.0% 0033/0057R
Simplene 0.5% 0033/0072

SNO* PHENICOL

Presentation Multi-dose, colourless to pale straw coloured eye drops containing Chloramphenicol PhEur 0.5% w/v supplied in a plastic dropper bottle. This solution contains chlorhexidine acetate 0.01% w/v as the preservative.

Uses Chloramphenicol is a broad spectrum antibiotic. It is active against a wide variety of gram-negative and gram-positive organisms as well as rickettsiae and spirochaetes. It is indicated for use as a topical antibacterial in the treatment of superficial ocular infections.

Dosage and administration
Adults (including the elderly): One or two drops applied to each affected eye up to six times daily or more frequently if required. (Severe infections may require one to two drops every fifteen to twenty minutes initially, reducing the frequency of instillation gradually as the infection is controlled).

Children: One drop as required.

Contra-indications, warnings, etc
Contra-indications: This product is not intended as a long term treatment for dry eye syndromes.

Hypersensitivity to chloramphenicol or to any component of the preparation.

Interactions: Chymotrypsin will be inhibited if given simultaneously with chloramphenicol.

Effects on ability to drive and use machines: May cause transient blurring of vision on instillation. Warn patients not to drive or operate hazardous machinery unless vision is clear.

Other undesirable effects

Local: Sensitivity reactions such as transient irritation, burning, stinging, itching and dermatitis.

Systemic: Several cases of major adverse haematological events (bone marrow depression, aplastic anaemia and death) have been reported following ocular use of chloramphenicol.

Use in pregnancy and lactation: Safety for use in pregnancy and lactation has not been established. Therefore, use only when considered essential by the physician.

Other special warnings and precautions: In severe infections topical use of chloramphenicol should be supplemented with appropriate systemic treatment.

Aplastic anaemia has followed topical use of chloramphenicol eye drops and, whilst this hazard is a rare one, it should be considered when the benefits of the use of chloramphenicol are assessed.

Prolonged use should be avoided as it may increase the likelihood of sensitisation and the emergence of resistant organisms.

Contact lenses should be removed during the period of treatment.

Incompatibilities: None known.

Pharmaceutical precautions Sno phenicol should not be diluted or dispensed from any container other than the original bottle and should be stored at 2°C–8°C. Do not freeze.

Sno phenicol, like other eye drops, should be discarded one month after opening.

Legal category POM.

Package quantities Sno phenicol is supplied as a sterile ophthalmic solution in a 10 ml plastic dropper bottle.

Further information The solution is formulated with a viscoliser for patient comfort.

Product licence number 0033/0076.

SNO* PILO

Presentation Multi-dose, clear, colourless to pale yellow, eye drops supplied in a plastic dropper bottle. Three strengths are available: 1.0%, 2.0% and 4.0% w/v Pilocarpine Hydrochloride BP preserved with 0.01% benzalkonium chloride.

Uses Sno pilo is a directly-acting miotic used for the treatment of glaucoma. For topical instillation into the eye, indicated for:

Chronic simple glaucoma

Acute (closed-angle) glaucoma: Pilocarpine may be used alone or in conjunction with other agents to decrease intraocular pressure prior to surgical treatment.

Miosis: To counter the effects of cycloplegic and mydriatic eye drops.

Dosage and administration
Adults (including the elderly): One or two drops up to four times daily or as prescribed.

The frequency of instillation and concentration of drops used are determined by the severity of the glaucoma and the response to treatment.

Children: At the discretion of the physician. Safety and efficacy of use in children has not been established.

Contra-indications, warnings, etc
Contra-indications: Conditions where pupillary constriction is undesirable e.g. acute iritis, anterior uveitis and some forms of secondary glaucoma.

Hypersensitivity to any component of the preparation.

Patients with soft contact lenses should not use this preparation.

Interactions: Although clinically not proven, the miotic effects of pilocarpine may be antagonised by long-term topical or systemic corticosteroid therapy, systemic anticholinergics, antihistamines, pethidine, sympathomimetics or tricyclic antidepressants. Concomitant administration of two miotics is not recommended because of interdrug antagonism, and unresponsiveness may develop to both drugs.

Effects on ability to drive and use machines: Causes difficulty with dark adaptation, therefore, caution is necessary with night driving and when hazardous tasks are undertaken in poor illumination. May cause accommodation spasm. Patients should be advised not to drive or use machinery if vision is not clear.

Other undesirable effects

Local: Burning, itching, smarting, blurring of vision, ciliary spasm, conjunctival vascular congestion, induced myopia, sensitisation of the lids and conjunctiva, reduced visual acuity in poor illumination, lens changes with chronic use, increased pupillary block, retinal detachments and vitreous haemorrhages.

CNS: Browache and headache (especially in younger patients who have recently started therapy).

Systemic: Systemic reactions rarely occur in the treatment of chronic simple glaucoma but they may include hypertension, tachycardia, bronchial spasm, pulmonary oedema, salivation, sweating, nausea, vomiting, diarrhoea and lacrimation.

Use in pregnancy and lactation: Safety for use in pregnancy and lactation has not been established, therefore, use only when clearly indicated.

Other special warnings and precautions: Although systemic reactions rarely occur in the treatment of chronic simple glaucoma with the usual doses used, in the treatment of acute closed-angle glaucoma the possibility of systemic reactions must be considered because of the higher doses given. Caution is particularly advised with patients with acute heart failure, bronchial asthma, peptic ulceration, hypertension, urinary tract obstruction and Parkinson's disease.

Retinal detachments have been caused in susceptible individuals and those with pre-existing retinal disease, therefore, fundus examination is advised in all patients prior to the initiation of therapy.

Patients with chronic simple glaucoma on long-term pilocarpine therapy should have regular monitoring of intraocular pressure and visual fields.

Overdose: If accidentally ingested, induce emesis or perform gastric lavage. Observe for signs of toxicity (salivation, lacrimation, sweating, nausea, vomiting and diarrhoea).

Incompatibilities: None known.

Pharmaceutical precautions Sno pilo should not be diluted or dispensed from any container other than the original bottle and should be stored in a cool place. Sno pilo, like other eye drops, should be discarded one month after opening.

Legal category POM.

Package quantities Sno pilo is supplied as a sterile ophthalmic solution in a 10 ml plastic dropper bottle.

Further information The solution is formulated with a viscoliser for patient comfort.

Product licence numbers

Sno pilo 1.0% w/v 0033/0065
Sno pilo 2.0% w/v 0033/0066
Sno pilo 4.0% w/v 0033/0068

SNO* TEARS

Presentation Sno tears is a clear, colourless slightly viscous solution in a plastic dropper bottle. It contains polyvinyl alcohol 1.4% w/v together with benzalkonium chloride 0.004% w/v and disodium edetate 0.02% w/v as an antibacterial system.

Uses Sno tears is used topically to provide tear-like lubrication for the symptomatic relief of dry eyes and eye irritation associated with deficient tear production (usually in cases of keratoconjunctivitis sicca and xerophthalmia).

Also used as an ocular lubricant for artificial eyes.

Dosage and administration

Adults, children and the elderly: The dose depends on the need for lubrication. Usually one or more drops as required or as prescribed.

Contra-indications, warnings, etc

Contra-indications: Hypersensitivity to any component of the preparation.

Contains benzalkonium chloride and should not be used when soft contact lenses are worn.

Interactions: None known.

Effects on the ability to drive and use machines: May cause transient blurring of vision on instillation. Do not drive or operate hazardous machinery unless vision is clear.

Other undesirable effects: May cause transient mild stinging or temporarily blurred vision.

Use in pregnancy and lactation: There is no, or inadequate, evidence of safety of the drug in human pregnancy but it has been in wide use for many years without apparent ill consequence. If drug therapy is needed in pregnancy this preparation can be used if recommended by a physician.

Other special warnings and precautions: If irritation persists or worsens, or headache, eye pain, vision changes or continued redness occur, discontinue use and consult a physician.

To preserve sterility do not allow the dropper to touch the eye or any other surface.

Incompatibilities: None known.

Pharmaceutical precautions Sno tears should not be diluted or dispensed from any container other than the original bottle and should be stored in a cool place.

Sno tears, as with other eye drops, should be discarded one month after opening.

Legal category P.

Package quantities Sno tears is supplied as a sterile ophthalmic solution in a 10 ml plastic dropper bottle.

Further information Nil.

Product licence number 0033/0097.

WELLDORM*

Presentation An elongated, oval, bluish-purple, film-coated tablet. Each tablet contains 707 mg chloral betaine, equivalent to 414 mg of chloral hydrate. The tablets are packed in opaque blister strips.

Uses Welldorm Tablets are used for the short-term treatment of insomnia.

Dosage and administration

Adults: The hypnotic dose is one to two tablets taken 15–30 minutes before bedtime with water or milk. Dose should not exceed 2 g of chloral hydrate per day.

Elderly: Dosage as for adults except in the frail elderly or those with hepatic impairment, where a reduction in dose may be appropriate.

Children: Welldorm tablets are not suitable for use in children under the age of 12, for such patients Welldorm Elixir is recommended (please refer to separate data sheet for dosage recommendations).

Contra-indications, warnings, etc Should not be used in patients with marked hepatic or renal impairment, or in patients who have severe cardiac disease. Best avoided in the presence of gastritis and in patients who have previously exhibited an idiosyncracy or hypersensitivity to chloral hydrate. Should not be used in patients susceptible to acute attacks of porphyria. Should not be used in pregnancy and lactation.

Interactions may occur in patients taking anticoagulants. When chloral hydrate is added to or withdrawn from the drug regimen, or its dosage changed, careful monitoring of the prothrombin time is required.

Patients should be warned that their ability to drive or use machinery may be impaired by drowsiness.

Side-effects: Gastric irritation, abdominal distension and flatulence may occur. Excitement, tolerance, allergic skin reactions, headache and ketonuria have occasionally been reported.

Alcohol potentiates the sedative effect. Chloral hydrate followed by intravenous frusemide may result in sweating, hot flushes and variable blood pressure including hypertension due to a hypermetabolic state caused by displacement of thyroid hormone from its bound state.

Delirium may occur, especially in the elderly, particularly when used in conjunction with psychotropics or anticholinergics.

Abuse and chronic intoxication: There is a danger of abuse or chronic intoxication and the possibility that habituation may develop. In such patients gastritis and parenchymatous renal injury may develop. After long term use sudden withdrawal may result in delirium.

Overdosage: The signs and symptoms of overdosage involve the CNS, cardiovascular and respiratory systems. These may include: respiratory depression, arrhythmias, hypothermia, pin-point pupils, hypotension or coma. Gastric irritation may result in vomiting and even gastric necrosis. If the patient survives, icterus due to hepatic damage and albuminuria from renal damage may appear. Serious problems have arisen with doses as little as 4 g and 10 g can be fatal. Overdosage should be treated with gastric lavage or inducing vomiting to empty the stomach. Supportive measures must be used. Haemodialysis, and in some cases haemoperfusion, have been reported to be effective in promoting the clearance of trichloroethanol.

Pharmaceutical precautions The tablets should be stored in a dry place at 15–25°C.

Legal category POM.

Package quantities The tablets are packed in blister strips of 15, two strips (30 tablets) per carton.

Further information Chloral hydrate and its metabolite trichloroethanol act as central nervous system depressants.

Welldorm is a chloral hydrate derivative, which leads to a decrease in sleep latency and in the number of awakenings. A near natural sleep is induced and the REM/NON-REM ratio is not altered.

Chloral hydrate is rapidly absorbed from the stomach, and starts to act within 30 minutes. It is widely distributed throughout the body, and is metabolised to trichloroethanol, also an active hypnotic, and trichloroacetic acid in the erythrocytes, liver and other tissues. It is excreted partly in the urine as trichloroethanol and its glucuronide, urochloric acid, and as trichloroacetic acid. Significant amounts are also excreted in bile. Trichloroethanol has a plasma half-life of the order of 8 hours. Trichloroacetic acid has a half-life of several days.

Product licence number 0033/0032R.

WELLDORM* ELIXIR

Presentation Welldorm Elixir is a clear red syrup, with a pleasant passion-fruit flavour. Welldorm Elixir contains Chloral Hydrate BP 143 mg/5 ml.

Uses Welldorm Elixir is for the short-term treatment of insomnia.

Dosage and administration
Adults: 15–45 ml taken 15–30 minutes before bedtime with water or milk. Dose should not exceed 2 g chloral hydrate per day.

Elderly: Dosage as for adults except in the frail elderly or those with hepatic impairment, where a reduction in dose may be appropriate.

Children: 30–50 mg/kg (1.0–1.7 ml/kg). Dose should not exceed 1 g chloral hydrate per day (35 ml).

Contra-indications, warnings, etc Should not be used in patients with marked hepatic or renal impairment, or in patients with severe cardiac disease. Best avoided in the presence of gastritis and in patients who have previously exhibited an idiosyncrasy or hypersensitivity to chloral hydrate. Should not be used in patients susceptible to acute attacks of porphyria.

Interactions may occur in patients taking anticoagulants. When chloral hydrate is added to or withdrawn from the regimen, or its dosage changed, careful monitoring of the prothrombin time is required.

Patients should be warned that their ability to drive or use machinery may be impaired by drowsiness.

It is contra-indicated in pregnancy and lactation.

Side-effects: Gastric irritation, abdominal distension and flatulence may occur. Excitement, tolerance, allergic skin reactions, headache and ketonuria have occasionally been reported.

Alcohol potentiates the sedative effect. Chloral hydrate followed by intravenous frusemide may result in sweating, hot flushes and variable blood pressure including hypertension due to a hypermetabolic state caused by displacement of thyroid hormone from its bound state. Delirium may occur, especially in the elderly, particularly when used in conjunction with psychotropics or anticholinergics.

Abuse and chronic intoxication: There is a danger of abuse or chronic intoxication and the possibility that habituation may develop. In such patients gastritis and parenchymatous renal injury may develop. After long term use sudden withdrawal may result in delirium.

Overdosage: The signs and symptoms of overdosage involve the CNS, cardiovascular and respiratory systems. These may include: respiratory depression, arrhythmias, hypothermia, pin-point pupils, hypotension or coma. Gastric irritation may result in vomiting and even gastric necrosis. If the patient survives, icterus due to hepatic damage and albuminuria from renal damage may appear. Serious problems have arisen with doses as little as 4 g and 10 g can be fatal. Overdosage should be treated with gastric lavage or inducing vomiting to empty the stomach. Supportive measures must be used. Haemodialysis, and in some cases haemoperfusion, have been reported to be effective in promoting the clearance of trichloroethanol.

Pharmaceutical precautions Syrup BP can be used as a diluent. Welldorm elixir should be stored in a well-stoppered bottle away from direct sunlight.

Legal category POM.

Package quantities Welldorm elixir is supplied in bottles containing 150 ml.

Further information Chloral hydrate and its metabolite trichloroethanol act as a central nervous system depressant.

Chloral hydrate leads to a decrease in sleep latency and in the number of awakenings. A near natural sleep is induced and the REM/NON-REM ratio is not altered.

Chloral hydrate is rapidly absorbed from the stomach, and starts to act within 30 minutes. It is widely distributed throughout the body, and is metabolised to trichloroethanol, also an active hypnotic, and trichloroacetic acid in the erythrocytes, liver and other tissues. It is excreted partly in the urine as trichloroethanol and its glucuronide, urochloralic acid, and as trichloroacetic acid. Significant amounts are also excreted in bile. Trichloroethanol has a plasma half-life of the order of 8 hours. Trichloroacetic acid has a half-life of several days.

Product licence number 0033/5025R.

**Trade Mark*

Smith Kline & French Laboratories
Welwyn Garden City
Hertfordshire AL7 1EY

SK&F

AC VAX*
Meningococcal vaccine BP (groups A and C polysaccharides)

Presentation AC Vax meningococcal meningitis vaccine is a lyophylised preparation of purified polysaccharides from *Neisseria meningitidis* (meningococcus) of groups A and C. It is presented as a white pellet in a glass vial together with a separate ampoule or vial of clear, colourless, sterile diluent. Each 0.5 ml dose of reconstituted vaccine contains 50 micrograms of group A polysaccharide and 50 micrograms of group C polysaccharide dissolved in isotonic sodium chloride (0.9 per cent). The diluent for the 10-dose preparation contains 0.25 per cent phenol.

Uses Active immunisation against meningococcal meningitis caused by group A and group C meningococci.

AC Vax is particularly recommended for subjects at risk, for example those living in areas or travelling to countries where the disease is epidemic or highly endemic. It is also recommended in epidemic situations and for close contacts of patients with this disease.

Dosage and administration
Adults and children aged two months and over: 0.5 ml of the reconstituted vaccine administered by deep subcutaneous injection only. The vaccine must not be given intravenously under any circumstances.

The vaccine should be reconstituted with the diluent supplied by adding the entire contents of the diluent vial to the vaccine vial.

Contra-indications, warnings, etc
Contra-indications: Do not use in subjects hypersensitive to any component of the vaccine or in those with febrile conditions.

Precautions: AC Vax gives no protection against meningococcal meningitis caused by meningococci belonging to groups other than A and C.

If administered to subjects with impaired immune responses, the vaccine may not induce an effective response.

As with all vaccinations, a solution of 1:1000 adrenaline should be available for injection should an anaphylactic reaction occur.

Use in pregnancy: No studies in animals have been performed . Since the effect of the vaccine on the foetus is not known, it should not be given during pregnancy unless there is a definite risk from groups A and C meningococcal disease.

Adverse reactions: These are mild and short-lasting. Local reactions may consist of erythema, slight induration and tenderness or pain at the site of injection. Febrile reactions and chills have been observed rarely in the first 24 hours after vaccination.

Pharmaceutical precautions AC Vax should be stored between 2°C and 8°C, its shelf life then being 4 years. The reconstituted vaccine should be used immediately, and certainly within one hour. The reconstituted 10-dose presentation may be kept between 2°C and 8°C, but it must be used within 4 hours or otherwise discarded.

Legal category POM.

Package quantities Monodose vials (OP) and 10-dose vials, each with a separate ampoule/vial of diluent.

Further information One dose of AC Vax will elicit a protective response in over 90 per cent of older children and adults within 2 to 3 weeks.

In adults and children over 5 years of age, immunity will persist for up to 5 years. In younger children, particularly those below the age of 2 years, immunity against group C meningococci is unlikely to persist for more than 1 to 2 years.

Inactive ingredients in the reconstituted vaccine are lactose and sodium chloride, together with phenol in the 10-dose presentation.

Product licence numbers

AC Vax vaccine	0002/0192.
Saline diluent (0.9 per cent) for monodose presentation	0002/0194.
Saline diluent (0.9 per cent with 0.25 per cent phenol) for 10-dose presentation	0002/0193.

ALGITEC* SUSPENSION
ALGITEC* CHEWTAB* TABLETS

Presentation A white suspension with an odour of fruit and mint, each 10 ml of which contains 500 mg Sodium Alginate BPC and 200 mg cimetidine.

Circular, off-white, flat-faced chewable tablets with an odour of butterscotch and with a characteristic pattern and 'Algitec' on both sides. Each tablet contains 500 mg Alginic Acid BPC and 200 mg cimetidine.

Uses Algitec combines sodium alginate or alginic acid, which forms a barrier to the reflux of gastric contents, with cimetidine, an H_2-receptor antagonist, which reduces the volume and acidity of gastric juice.

Algitec is indicated in the treatment of gastro-oesophageal reflux disease.

Dosage and administration
Adults only: Oral: 10 ml suspension or one tablet four times a day, after meals and at bedtime, for four to eight weeks. If the response is inadequate, the dosage may be increased to 20 ml suspension or two tablets four times a day. The tablets should be thoroughly chewed and may be followed by a drink of water.

Elderly: The normal adult dosage may be used unless renal function is markedly impaired (see *Precautions* and *Adverse reactions*).

Children: Algitec is not recommended for children.

Contra-indications, warnings, etc
Contra-indication: Hypersensitivity to cimetidine.

Precautions: Because of the need to reduce the dose of cimetidine in patients with marked renal impairment, Algitec is not recommended for such patients.

Cimetidine can prolong the elimination of drugs metabolised by oxidation in the liver. Although pharmacological interactions with a number of drugs, e.g. diazepam, propranolol, have been demonstrated, only those with oral anticoagulants, phenytoin, theophylline and intravenous lignocaine appear, to date, to be of clinical significance. Close monitoring of patients on 'Algitec' receiving oral anticoagulants or phenytoin is recommended and a reduction in the dosage of these drugs may be necessary.

Clinical trials with cimetidine of over six years' continuous treatment and more than thirteen years' widespread use have not revealed unexpected adverse reactions related to long-term therapy. The safety of prolonged use is not, however, fully established and care should be taken to observe periodically patients given prolonged treatment.

Cimetidine treatment can mask the symptoms and allow transient healing of gastric cancer. The potential delay in diagnosis should particularly be borne in mind in patients of middle age and over with new or recently changed dyspeptic symptoms.

In patients on drug treatment or with illnesses that could cause falls in blood cell count, the possibility that H_2-receptor antagonism could potentiate this effect should be borne in mind.

Use in pregnancy and lactation: Although tests in animals and clinical evidence have not revealed any hazards from the administration of cimetidine during pregnancy and lactation, both animal and human studies have shown that it does cross the placental barrier and is excreted in milk. As with most drugs, the use of Algitec should be avoided during pregnancy and lactation unless essential.

Adverse reactions: More than 35 million patients have been treated with cimetidine worldwide and adverse reactions have been infrequent. Diarrhoea, dizziness or rash, usually mild and transient, and tiredness have been reported. Gynaecomastia has been reported and is almost always reversible on discontinuing treatment. Biochemical or biopsy evidence of reversible liver damage has been reported occasionally. Reversible confusional states have occurred, usually in elderly or already very ill patients, e.g. those with renal failure. There have been very rare reports of interstitial nephritis, acute pancreatitis, thrombocytopenia, agranulocytosis (see *Precautions*), headache, myalgia, arthralgia, sinus bradycardia, tachycardia and heart block, all reversible on withdrawal of treatment, and aplastic anaemia. Alopecia has been reported but no causal relationship has been established. Reversible impotence has also been very rarely reported but no causal relationship has been established at usual therapeutic doses. Isolated increases of plasma creatinine have been of no clinical significance.

Overdosage: Acute overdosage of up to 20 grams of cimetidine has been reported several times with no significant ill effects. Overdosage with sodium alginate or alginic acid presents virtually no hazard, though abdominal bloating may be present. Induction of vomiting and/or gastric lavage may be employed together with symptomatic and supportive therapy.

Pharmaceutical precautions Store the suspension below 25°C but do not refrigerate. Shake the bottle before use. Dilution is not recommended. Store the tablets below 30°C.

Legal category POM.

Package quantities White plastic bottles (OP) containing 600 ml suspension. Cartons (OP) containing 120 Chewtab Tablets in 6 tubes of 20.

Further information Algitec allows the simultaneous use of two distinct and complementary methods, both of proven utility, of treating gastro-oesophageal reflux disease. Alginate and sodium or potassium bicarbonate are converted in the stomach to a viscous frothy gel of alginic acid which floats on the gastric contents to prevent reflux. Should reflux still occur, the gel itself may be refluxed to protect the oesophageal mucosa and allow any inflammation to heal. Cimetidine inhibits gastric secretion of acid and pepsin, reducing both the damaging gastric acidity and the volume available for reflux.

The absorption of cimetidine is not significantly affected by the sodium alginate or alginic acid in Algitec.

Each 10 ml suspension contains 65.8 mg (2.86 mmol) sodium and 1200 mg sorbitol.

Each tablet contains 47 mg (2.05 mmol) sodium, 330 mg lactose and 680 mg sorbitol.

Inactive ingredients include aspartame in the Chewtab Tablets and disodium edetate and parabens in the Suspension.

Product licence numbers

Algitec Suspension	0002/0176.
Algitec Chewtab Tablets	0002/0149.

ASACOL* TABLETS
ASACOL* SUPPOSITORIES

Presentation Red, oblong tablets containing 400 mg mesalazine (5-aminosalicylic acid) coated with an acrylic based resin (Eudragit S) formulated to release the active ingredient in the terminal ileum and colon.

Opaque, beige suppositories, containing 250 mg or 500 mg mesalazine.

Uses For the treatment of mild to moderate acute exacerbations of ulcerative colitis.

For the maintenance of remission of ulcerative colitis.

The suppositories are particularly appropriate in patients with distal disease.

Dosage and administration
Tablets:
Adults: Acute disease: Six tablets a day in divided doses, with concomitant corticosteroid therapy where clinically indicated.

Maintenance therapy: Three to six tablets a day in divided doses.

Children: There is no dosage recommendation.

Suppositories:
Adults: 250 mg Suppositories: Three to six suppositories a day in divided doses, with the last dose at bedtime.

500 mg Suppositories: A maximum of three suppositories a day in divided doses, with the last dose at bedtime.

Children: There is no dosage recommendation.

Contra-indications, warnings, etc
Contra-indications: A history of sensitivity to salicylates. Severe renal impairment (GFR less than 20 ml/min). Children under 2 years of age.

Precautions: Renal disorder: mesalazine is excreted rapidly by the kidney, mainly as its metabolite, N-acetyl-5-aminosalicylic acid. In rats, large doses of mesalazine injected intravenously produce tubular and glomerular toxicity. Asacol is best avoided in patients with established renal impairment, but if necessary, it should be used with caution.

Asacol Tablets should not be given with lactulose or similar preparations which lower stool pH and may prevent release of mesalazine.

Use during pregnancy and lactation: No information is available with regard to teratogenicity; however, negligible quantities of mesalazine are transferred across the placenta and are excreted in breast milk following sulphasalazine therapy. Use of Asacol during pregnancy should be with caution, and only if, in the opinion of the physician, the potential benefits of treatment are greater than the possible hazards. Asacol should, unless essential, be avoided by nursing mothers.

Elderly: Use in the elderly should be cautious and subject to patients having a normal renal function (see *Precautions*).

Adverse reactions: The side-effects are predominantly gastrointestinal. Nausea, diarrhoea, abdominal pain and headache have been reported.

Asacol may be associated with the exacerbation of the symptoms of colitis in those patients who have previously had such problems with sulphasalazine. There have been reports of leucopenia, neutropenia, thrombocytopenia, pancreatitis, hepatitis, interstitial nephritis, nephrotic syndrome and renal failure with oral treatment, usually reversible on withdrawal. Mesalazine-induced nephrotoxicity should be suspected in patients developing renal failure during treatment.

Other side effects observed with sulphasalazine such as depression of sperm count and function, have not been reported with Asacol.

Treatment of overdosage: Following tablet ingestion, gastric lavage and intravenous transfusion of electrolytes to promote diuresis. There is no specific antidote.

Pharmaceutical precautions Store tablets in a dry place below 25°C and protect from direct sunlight. Store suppositories below 25°C and protect from light.

Legal category POM.

Package quantities Tablets in cartons (OP) of 120, each containing 12 opaque blister packs of 10 tablets. Suppositories in cartoned plastic moulds (OP), each containing 20 suppositories (250 mg) or 10 suppositories (500 mg).

Further information Mesalazine is one of the two components of sulphasalazine, the other being sulphapyridine. It is the latter which is responsible for the majority of side-effects associated with sulphasalazine therapy whilst mesalazine is known to be the active moiety in the treatment of ulcerative colitis. Asacol consists only of this active component which is released topically in the colon from the tablets or delivered directly by the suppositories.

Asacol Tablets contain 400 mg of available mesalazine. This is released in the terminal ileum and large bowel by the effect of pH. Above pH 7 the Eudragit coat disintegrates and releases the active constituent.

Asacol Tablets contain, in a single tablet, an equivalent quantity of mesalazine to that theoretically available from the complete azoreduction of 1 g of sulphasalazine.

Inactive ingredients in the tablets include lactose.

The inactive ingredient in the suppositories is Witepsol W45 (Hard Fat).

Product licence numbers

Asacol Tablets	0002/0173
Asacol Suppositories 250 mg	0002/0158
Asacol Suppositories 500 mg	0002/0195

DEXEDRINE* TABLETS

Presentation Half-scored, white tablets, marked SK&F, each containing 5 mg dexamphetamine sulphate.

Uses Dexedrine is a sympathomimetic amine with central stimulant and anorectic activity.

It is indicated in narcolepsy. It is also indicated for children with refractory hyperkinetic states under the supervision of a physician specialising in child psychiatry.

Dosage and administration *Adults:* In narcolepsy, the usual starting dosage is 10 mg Dexedrine a day, given in divided doses. Dosage may be increased if necessary by 10 mg a day at weekly intervals to a suggested maximum of 60 mg a day.

Elderly: Start with 5 mg a day, and increase by increments of 5 mg at weekly intervals.

Children: In hyperkinetic states, the usual starting dosage for children aged 3–5 years is 2.5 mg a day, increased if necessary by 2.5 mg at weekly intervals; for children aged 6 years and over, the usual starting dosage is 5–10 mg a day, increasing if necessary by 5 mg at weekly intervals. The usual upper limit is 20 mg a day, though some older children have needed 40 mg or more for optimal response.

Contra-indications, warnings, etc

Contra-indications: Do not use in patients known to be intolerant of sympathomimetic amines, during, or for 14 days after, treatment with an MAO inhibitor, in those with a history of drug abuse, with symptomatic cardiovascular disease and/or moderate or severe hypertensive disease, in those suffering from hyperthyroidism or hyperexcitability or in those with glaucoma.

Precautions: Use with caution in patients on guanethidine, since the action of this drug may be antagonised by Dexedrine; and in patients with mild hypertension.

Height and weight should be carefully monitored in children as growth retardation may occur.

In common with other drugs acting on the CNS, Dexedrine may affect ability to drive or operate machinery.

Use in pregnancy and lactation: Dexamphetamine has been thought to produce embryotoxic effects in rodents, and retrospective evidence of uncertain significance in man has suggested a similar possibility. Dexedrine should therefore be avoided in pregnancy, especially during the first trimester. Dexedrine passes into breast milk.

Adverse reactions: Insomnia (especially with dosage later in the day), restlessness, irritability, euphoria, tremor, dizziness, headache and other symptoms of overstimulation have been reported. Also dry mouth, anorexia and other gastro-intestinal symptoms, sweating, and cardiovascular effects such as tachycardia, palpitation and minor increases in blood pressure. There have been isolated reports of cardiomyopathy associated with chronic amphetamine use.

Drug dependence, with consumption of increasing doses to levels many times those recommended, may occur as tolerance develops. At such levels, a psychosis, which may be clinically indistinguishable from schizophrenia, can occur. Treatment should be stopped gradually since abrupt cessation may produce extreme fatigue and mental depression.

Overdosage: Symptoms of overdosage include excitement, hallucinations, convulsions leading to coma; tachycardia and cardiac arrhythmias; and respiratory depression. Treatment consists of the induction of vomiting and/or gastric lavage, together with supportive and symptomatic measures. Excessive stimulation or convulsions may be treated with diazepam. Excretion of dexamphetamine may be increased by forced acid diuresis.

Pharmaceutical precautions No special storage precautions are required.

Legal category CD (Sch 2), POM.

Package quantities Containers of 100 tablets.

Further information Inactive ingredients include lactose and sucrose.

Product licence number 0002/5008R.

DIBENYLINE* CAPSULES

Presentation Opaque white capsules with clear ruby-red caps, double-marked SKF, each containing 10 mg phenoxybenzamine hydrochloride as a white powder.

Uses Dibenyline is a non-competitive long-acting α-adrenergic receptor antagonist.

It is indicated in the short-term management of severe hypertensive episodes associated with phaeochromocytoma. Dibenyline should only be used after careful consideration of the likely benefit of treatment compared with the mutagenic and carcinogenic risk (see *Precautions* below).

Dosage and administration *Adults:* The usual starting dose is 10 mg daily. This may be increased by 10 mg daily until control of hypertensive episodes is achieved, or postural hypotension occurs. Usually the dosage required is 1 to 2 mg/kg body weight daily in two doses. Concomitant β-adrenergic blockade may be necessary to control tachycardia and arrhythmias notably when tumours are secreting an appreciable amount of adrenaline as well as noradrenaline.

Elderly: Use with caution (see *Contra-indications* and *Precautions* below).

Children: There is little experience in children, but doses of 1 to 2 mg/kg daily have been used successfully.

Contra-indications, warnings, etc

Contra-indications: Do not use in patients who have had a cerebrovascular accident; or in the recovery period (usually 3 to 4 weeks) after acute myocardial infarction.

Precautions: Use with great caution in patients in whom a fall in blood pressure and/or tachycardia may be undesirable, such as the elderly or those with severe heart disease, congestive heart failure, cerebrovascular disease or renal damage. The mode of action should be borne in mind if used concurrently with α-sympathomimetics or myocardial depressants.

Phenoxybenzamine is carcinogenic in the rat and has shown mutagenic activity in the bacterial Ames test and the mouse lymphoma assay. It should, therefore, be used only after very careful consideration of the risks, in patients in whom alternative treatment is inappropriate.

Use in pregnancy: There is little evidence as to the safety of Dibenyline in pregnancy and it should not be used in pregnancy unless essential.

Adverse reactions: Side-effects are generally mild and transient, but may include postural hypotension with dizziness and compensatory tachycardia, nasal congestion, inhibition of ejaculation, miosis and lassitude. Gastro-intestinal upset has also been reported.

Overdosage: The main effect of overdosage is profound hypotension, which may last several hours, tachycardia and collapse. Treatment consists of the induction of vomiting and/or gastric lavage together with appropriate symptomatic and supportive measures. Treat hypotension with plasma expanders and the 'head down' position. Noradrenaline is of little value when α-adrenergic receptors are blocked. Adrenaline should not be used since stimulation of β-adrenergic receptors will further decrease blood pressure.

Pharmaceutical precautions Store in a dry place and protect from light.

Legal category POM.

Package quantities Opaque blister packs (OP) of 30 (2 × 15) capsules.

Further information Treatment should be started as soon as possible after diagnosis, and time allowed for stabilisation of the condition before invasive investigations or operations are carried out. Operative cover with intravenous phenoxybenzamine may be given. In a few inoperable cases long-term treatment with Dibenyline has been used.

Inactive ingredients include lactose.

Product licence number 0002/5009R.

DYAZIDE* TABLETS

Presentation Peach-coloured, half-scored, circular tablets bearing the mark SKF E93, each containing 50 mg triamterene and 25 mg hydrochlorothiazide.

Uses Dyazide is a potassium-conserving diuretic preparation with antihypertensive activity.

It is recommended for the treatment of mild to moderate hypertension, alone or in combination with other antihypertensive drugs. It is also indicated in the control of oedema in cardiac failure, cirrhosis of the liver or the nephrotic syndrome and in that associated with corticosteroid treatment.

Dosage and administration

Adults only: In hypertension: Initially 1 tablet a day after the morning meal, thereafter adjusted to the patient's needs. If Dyazide is added to already established therapy with another antihypertensive drug, the dosage of the latter should be reduced, and later adjusted if necessary. If another antihypertensive drug is added to Dyazide therapy, the dosage of the latter will not normally be reduced.

In oedema: The usual starting dosage is 1 Dyazide tablet twice a day after meals. The optimal dosage may be 3 tablets a day, 2 after breakfast and 1 after lunch. Maintenance dosage: Once a diuresis has been established, dosage should be reduced. Usually 1 tablet a day, or 2 tablets on alternate days, will suffice.

A dosage of 4 tablets a day should not be exceeded; at this level adverse reactions such as raised blood urea are more likely.

Elderly: Dosage as above. Dyazide has been widely used and is usually well tolerated in patients over the age of 60 years. The normally occurring reduction in glomerular filtration with age should be borne in mind.

Contra-indications, warnings, etc

Contra-indications: Do not give Dyazide to patients with hyperkalaemia, progressive renal failure, increasing hepatic dysfunction, hypercalcaemia, diabetic ketoacidosis, Addison's disease or known hypersensitivity to either constituent of the product. Potassium supplements, or other potassium-conserving drugs, including ACE inhibitors, should not be given routinely with Dyazide.

Precautions: Use Dyazide with caution in patients with hepatic or renal insufficiency, and in those predisposed to gout since both components can elevate uric acid levels. Folate antagonists combined with triamterene are inadvisable in patients with hepatic cirrhosis because of the increased theoretical risk of folate deficiency. Since thiazide diuretics can provoke hyperglycaemia and glycosuria, diabetic patients should be treated with care, as should patients with diabetic nephropathy due to an increased risk of hyperkalaemia; the dosage of any concomitant sulphonylurea may need increasing. Pancreatitis may be aggravated.

It is advisable to monitor blood urea, serum potassium levels and electrolytes periodically. This is important in the elderly, those with renal impairment and those receiving concomitant treatment with NSAIDs (see 'Adverse reactions').

Triamterene and thiazides reduce excretion of lithium and may thus precipitate intoxication. There may be increased responsiveness to tubocurarine. Cholestyramine may delay or reduce the absorption of many drugs including diuretics.

Caution should be exercised if 'Dyazide' is used in conjunction with hypotensive agents. Also use with caution in conjunction with corticosteroids since an additive effect may result in excess potassium loss: with cardiac glycosides and antiarrhythmic drugs whose toxicity potential is enhanced by hypokalaemia which may result from diuretic treatment; and with carbenoxolone which may antagonise the diuretic action of 'Dyazide'.

Use in pregnancy and lactation: Animal studies have not suggested foetal abnormalities. Nevertheless, both triamterene and thiazides have been shown to pass through the placenta in humans and also to pass into breast milk. In rare instances, thrombocytopenia, pancreatitis or hypoglycaemia have been reported in newborn infants of mothers treated with thiazides. Dyazide is best avoided in pregnancy unless used for a pre-existing illness and then only after assessing risk versus benefit. It should also not be used in breast-feeding mothers. Folate antagonists combined with triamterene are inadvisable during pregnancy because of the increased theoretical risk of folate deficiency.

Adverse reactions: Nausea, vomiting, diarrhoea, muscle cramps, weakness, dizziness, headache, dry mouth, thirst, undesirable decreases in blood pressure and rash have been reported. Photosensitivity is rare. Anaphylaxis is a remote possibility.

Minor serum electrolyte changes have been observed infrequently, and marked fluctuations in serum potassium levels are uncommon. Long-term use has confirmed that little change occurs in serum potassium and sodium levels in most patients. Metabolic acidosis occasionally occurs. Electrolyte imbalance may also indicate excessive dosage or be secondary to the condition under treatment. Hyperglycaemia, increased uric acid levels which sometimes lead to gout, and hypercalcaemia that does not lead to tertiary hyperparathyroidism may also occur.

In common with most diuretics, 'Dyazide' may reduce glomerular filtration rate and cause a temporary increase in blood urea and creatinine levels; again this may also indicate excessive dosage or be secondary to the condition under treatment. It can also cause increases in plasma lipid levels.

Triamterene has been found in renal stones both alone and in association with other usual calculus components. There is no evidence that stone formation is increased in patients taking triamterene-containing drugs.

Renal failure, reversible on stopping treatment, has been reported very rarely and has been due to acute interstitial nephritis or an interaction between triamterene and some NSAIDs.

Rare cases of thrombocytopenic purpura and megaloblastic anaemia have been reported with triamterene; thiazides alone have caused jaundice, acute pancreatitis and, rarely, blood dyscrasias including agranulocytosis, thrombocytopenia and leucopenia. Very rare cases of SLE have been reported associated with Dyazide.

Overdosage: Symptoms of electrolyte imbalance, especially hyperkalaemia, are likely. Symptoms include nausea, vomiting, weakness, lassitude, muscular weakness, hypotension and cardiac arrhythmias. Treatment consists of gastric lavage with careful monitoring of electrolytes and fluid balance. Cardiac rhythm should be monitored and appropriate measures taken to correct hyperkalaemia as necessary. There is no specific antidote. Renal dialysis may be of some benefit in cases of severe overdosage.

Pharmaceutical precautions No special storage precautions are required.

Legal category POM.

Package quantities Calendar packs (OP) of 30 (2 × 15) and containers of 500 tablets.

Further information Triamterene may cause a blue fluorescence of the urine under certain light conditions.

Dyazide interferes with some laboratory tests of thyroid and parathyroid functions and bioassay of folic acid.

Inactive ingredients include aluminium lake of E110.

Product licence number 0002/0050R.

ENGERIX* B
Hepatitis B Vaccine (rby)

Presentation Engerix B is a suspension of hepatitis B surface antigen produced by yeast cells using a recombinant DNA technique. It is available in vials containing a fine white suspension. Each 1 ml contains 20 micrograms of protein, comprising at least 95 per cent hepatitis B surface antigen, adsorbed on aluminium hydroxide adjuvant, together with thiomersal 1:20,000 as preservative.

Uses Active immunisation against infections caused by hepatitis B virus.

Preference should be given to those at increased risk of infection, primarily those likely to be exposed to blood, blood products or other body fluids (see Further information). In addition, those who live in or travel to high endemic hepatitis B areas such as Africa or the Far East and their close contacts are at a generally increased risk of infection, and should be considered for vaccination.

Engerix B may be used as a booster in patients previously immunised with other hepatitis B vaccines.

Dosage and administration Engerix B is for intramuscular use only, and must not be given intravenously or intradermally. The vial should be shaken well before use.

The immunisation regimen consists of three doses of vaccine, the second dose at one month and the third at six months after the initial dose. Where more rapid immunisation is required, for example with travellers, the third dose may be given at two months after the initial dose, with a booster dose at twelve months. Specific humoral antibodies against the surface antigen of hepatitis B appear in almost 100 per cent of those who have received 3 doses.

Adults and children over 12 years: 20 micrograms (1 ml) given intramuscularly.

Neonates and children 12 years and under: 10 micrograms (0.5 ml) given intramuscularly.

The vaccine should be administered in the deltoid region or the antero-lateral aspect of the thigh but not the gluteal region. In patients with severe bleeding tendencies such as haemophiliacs, subcutaneous injection may be considered.

In neonates born to HBsAg positive mothers, hepatitis B immunoglobulin should be given simultaneously with the vaccine at different sites within a few hours of birth. For other subjects at particular risk, similar simultaneous administration may be considered.

Contra-indications, warnings, etc

Contra-indications: Hypersensitivity to any component of the vaccine. Severe febrile infections.

Precautions: In patients having renal dialysis, or those who are immunocompromised, response may be impaired and further vaccinations may be necessary.

Because of the prolonged incubation period of hepatitis B, infection may be present at the time of vaccination. If so, Engerix B may be ineffective.

As with all vaccinations, a solution of 1:1000 adrenaline should be available for injection should an anaphylactic reaction occur.

Use in pregnancy: No studies in pregnant animals have been done. Engerix B is not recommended in pregnancy unless there is a definite risk of hepatitis B.

Adverse reactions: These are usually mild. The most common reactions, occurring in up to half of vaccinees, are mild transient local soreness, erythema and induration at the injection site.

Less common systemic complaints, not necessarily related to vaccine, include low-grade fever, malaise, fatigue, arthralgia, myalgia, headache, dizziness, nausea, vomiting, abdominal pain and rashes, rarely including urticaria. These have been mild and usually confined to the first few days after injection. Very rarely, transient arthralgia and urticaria have been reported, appearing one week or more after injection. A causal relationship has not been established.

Pharmaceutical precautions Engerix B should be stored between 2°C and 8°C, its shelf life then being 3 years, and must not be frozen. It should not be diluted. Protect from light.

Legal category POM.

Package quantities Monodose vials containing 1 ml suspension in packs of 1, 3 (OP) and 10; paediatric monodose vials containing 0.5 ml suspension in packs of 3 (OP).

Further information In areas of low prevalence of hepatitis B, the following examples of subjects at increased risk of infection should be considered for vaccination: health care personnel; patients and patient contacts; persons at particular risk by nature of their work; persons at increased risk due to their sexual practices; drug abusers; neonates born to carrier mothers; consorts or spouses of carrier individuals; patients on entry to institutions where there is a high prevalence of hepatitis B.

It is expected that immunity will persist for at least 5 years following the last dose of vaccine.

Engerix B must *not* be mixed in the same syringe or injected at the same site as other vaccines.

Inactive ingredients are dried aluminium hydroxide, sodium chloride, sodium monohydrogen phosphate dihydrate, sodium dihydrogen phosphate dihydrate, hydrochloric acid, water for injection, and also thiomersal (see **Presentation**).

Product licence number 0002/0160.

ERVEVAX*
Rubella vaccine, live BP (RA27/3 strain)

Presentation Ervevax rubella vaccine is a live attenuated vaccine prepared in human diploid cells. It is presented as a pink pellet in a glass vial; clear, colourless sterile diluent is provided in a separate container. Each 0.5 ml dose of the reconstituted vaccine contains not less than 1,000 $TCID_{50}$ of the RA27/3 live attenuated strain of rubella virus with not more than 25 micrograms (17 i.u.) neomycin sulphate.

Uses Routine immunisation of pre-pubertal girls against rubella. Also indicated in seronegative women of child-bearing age *who are not pregnant* and in whom the possibility of pregnancy can be excluded for at least one month following vaccination, including post-partum mothers, and for immunisation of children and adults to prevent transmission of rubella to the at-risk pregnant woman.

Dosage and administration
Adults and children: 0.5 ml of the reconstituted vaccine administered subcutaneously or intramuscularly.

The vaccine should be reconstituted using only the sterile diluent supplied. The whole of the sterile diluent should be transferred into the vial containing the vaccine, keeping the latter upright. The vaccine pellet should be completely dissolved by shaking. The syringe should be dry sterilised; the vaccine is readily inactivated by alcohol and other chemical disinfectants and antiseptics, and care is needed to avoid contact with these substances when sterilising skin before vaccination.

Contra-indications, warnings, etc
Contra-indications: **Never give to pregnant women, or to women of child-bearing age not fully aware of the need to avoid pregnancy for one month after vaccination,** since theoretically the vaccine virus could have an effect on the foetus.

Do not use in the presence of acute febrile illness, in states of altered immunity including those which may accompany conditions such as leukaemia, lymphoma or generalised malignancy or treatment with corticosteroids, cytotoxic drugs or irradiation. Do not give to those with known systemic hypersensitivity to this vaccine or to neomycin. Although anaphylactic reactions are rare, facilities for management should always be available.

Precautions: Transmission of vaccine virus to susceptible contacts, while accepted as a theoretical possibility, has not been regarded as a significant risk.

The possibility of interference from passive antibodies following administration of gamma globulin or anti-D immunoglobulin or blood transfusion should be borne in mind. Serum antibodies may be checked three months after injection.

At least 3 weeks should normally intervene between the administration of any two live vaccines. Ervevax can, however, be given simultaneously with poliomyelitis, measles and mumps vaccines. In this case the injectable vaccines should be given at different sites.

Adverse reactions: Mild rash, temperature elevation and slight enlargement of the posterior cervical glands, transient arthralgia and arthritis with or without joint effusion, and extremely rarely transient polyneuropathy or thrombocytopenic purpura could occur. Such effects are more common and tend to be more marked in adults than in children. Symptoms, when they do occur, usually begin 1 to 3 weeks following vaccination and are normally transient.

Overdosage: Not a problem.

Pharmaceutical precautions Protect from light. The vaccine should be stored between 2°C and 8°C, its shelf life then being 2 years (lower temperatures will not harm the vaccine, but may damage the diluent container). At room temperature (20–25°C) the unreconstituted vaccine is stable for up to 10 weeks.

Reconstitute only with the diluent supplied. The reconstituted vaccine should be used immediately, and certainly within one hour. The reconstituted vaccine may vary in colour from light orange to light red.

Legal category POM.

Package quantities Monodose vials (OP), each with a separate ampoule of sterile diluent, or 10-dose vials, each with a separate vial of sterile diluent. The diluent is Water for Injections PhEur.

Further information Latest data indicate that satisfactory antibody titres have persisted for up to 18 years so far.

Because of possible interference from persisting maternal antibodies, there is little value in giving the vaccine to infants under one year of age.

Inactive ingredients are human albumin, lactose, sorbitol, dextran 10, casein hydrolysate, and also neomycin sulphate (see **Presentation**).

Product licence number 0002/0125.

ESKAMEL* CREAM

Presentation A smooth, brown, non-greasy cream, which dries rapidly to a flesh colour when applied to the skin. It contains 2% w/w resorcinol and 8% w/w precipitated sulphur.

Uses Eskamel has mild antiseptic, keratolytic and exfoliative properties, and is indicated in the treatment of acne.

Dosage and administration *Adults and children:* Wash the affected areas with soap and water, and dry carefully. Apply Eskamel thinly to the skin with the fingers but do not rub in. Once a day is usually enough, but if the patient has a very oily skin, the cream may be applied more often. Eskamel may be used under make-up to mask the spots and lesions of acne.

Contra-indications, warnings, etc
Contra-indications: Do not use in patients who are sensitive to sulphur or resorcinol, or in the presence of acute local infection.

Precautions: Use with care on acutely inflamed areas or near the eyes and mouth.

Adverse reactions: Moderate erythema and scaling are the expected effects of Eskamel. If these are excessive, stop treatment until the reaction has subsided, and then apply Eskamel less often. If inflammation occurs, treatment should also be stopped since this may indicate hypersensitivity. The prolonged use of high doses of resorcinol may produce hypothyroidism.

Overdosage: If ingestion occurs, mild gastro-intestinal disturbance might occur. Treatment consists of rinsing out the mouth together with symptomatic measures if required.

Pharmaceutical precautions Store at a temperature not exceeding 30°C. Keep in the original specially lined tubes to prevent evaporation.

Legal category P.

Package quantities Tubes (OP) containing 25 g.

Further information Inactive ingredients are propylene glycol, ethyl alcohol (90%), bentonite, purified water, potassium hydroxide pellets, 17841 brown iron oxide (Anstead; E172), perfume bouquet 3522 and titanium dioxide.

Product licence number 0002/5000R.

ESKORNADE* SPANSULE* CAPSULES
ESKORNADE* SYRUP

Presentation Clear, colourless capsules, grey-capped and filled with a mixture of red, grey and white pellets. Each Spansule sustained-release capsule contains 50 mg phenylpropanolamine hydrochloride and 5 mg diphenylpyraline hydrochloride. Two-thirds of the phenylpropanolamine and diphenylpyraline is formulated for sustained release over a period of six to eight hours.

A pale green syrup, greengage-flavoured, each 5 ml dose containing 12.5 mg phenylpropanolamine hydrochloride and 1.5 mg diphenylpyraline hydrochloride.

Uses Eskornade is a combination of an oral nasal decongestant and an antihistamine (H_1-receptor antagonist).

It is indicated in the relief of congestion and hypersecretion in the nasal cavity and paranasal sinuses, associated with the common cold, allergic rhinitis, acute and chronic rhinitis, sinusitis and influenza.

Dosage and administration The stated dose should not be exceeded. *Adults:* One Eskornade Spansule capsule every 12 hours or two 5 ml doses of Eskornade syrup up to four times a day.

Elderly: Use with great caution (see *Contra-indications* and *Precautions* below).

Eskornade Spansule capsules are not recommended in children under 12 years, and Eskornade syrup is not recommended in children under 2 years.

Children aged 2 to 5 years: One 2.5 ml dose of Eskornade syrup up to four times a day.

Children aged 6 to 12 years: One 5 ml dose up to four times a day.

Contra-indications, warnings, etc
Contra-indications: Do not use in patients with hypertensive disease, including those treated with antihypertensive drugs, whose action may be impaired by phenylpropanolamine, severe heart disease, or hyperthyroidism; or hypersensitivity to either of the ingredients; or during, or for 14 days after, treatment with an MAO inhibitor.

Precautions: Patients who drive or operate machinery should be warned of the possibility of drowsiness. Alcoholic drinks should be avoided. Administer with caution to patients with organic heart disease or angina of effort or with prostatic hypertrophy or glaucoma. Potentiation may occur if this product is used with other CNS depressants.

Use in pregnancy: Eskornade has been available since 1960. Based on animal studies and clinical experience, there is no evidence to suggest any associated hazard to the foetus. Nevertheless, drugs should be avoided in pregnancy unless essential, especially during the first trimester.

Adverse reactions: Blurred vision, dry mouth, urinary hesitancy or retention, palpitations, drowsiness or insomnia, and dizziness may occur.

Overdosage: Signs and symptoms may be related to either of the product's constituents and may include nausea and vomiting, irritability, convulsions, fever, tachycardia, arrhythmias or increased blood pressure. Absorption of phenylpropanolamine and diphenylpyraline from the sustained-release Spansule capsule is likely to be prolonged, and this should be borne in mind. Treatment consists of gastric lavage, together with appropriate supportive and symptomatic measures. Central excitation or convulsions may require treatment with diazepam. Excretion of phenylpropanolamine may be increased by forced acid diuresis.

Pharmaceutical precautions Store Spansule capsules and syrup below 25°C and Spansule Capsules in a dry place. The syrup should not be refrigerated; if stored below about 15°C, cloudiness may occur, which readily disappears if the product is stored at normal room temperature. Dilute only with Sorbitol Solution BP; a 50/50 dilution is stable for one month at temperatures of up to 30°C.

Legal category P.

Package quantities Opaque blister packs (OP) of 30 (2 × 15) Spansule capsules. Bottles (OP) containing 150 ml syrup.

Further information Inactive ingredients in the Spansule capsules include sucrose and E110 and in the syrup sucrose, ethyl alcohol, methyl paraben and propyl paraben.

Product licence numbers

Eskornade Spansule capsules	0002/5019R
Eskornade syrup	0002/5020R

FEFOL* SPANSULE* CAPSULES

Presentation Clear, colourless capsules, transparent green-capped and filled with a mixture of red, pale yellow and white pellets. Each Spansule sustained-release capsule contains 150 mg dried ferrous sulphate (47 mg elemental iron) and 500 micrograms folic acid. The iron is specially formulated for sustained release over a period of several hours.

Uses Fefol is a haematinic preparation for prophylaxis of iron and folic-acid deficiency during pregnancy.

Dosage and administration *Adults only:* 1 Fefol Spansule capsule a day during pregnancy. Some pregnant patients may need a higher prophylactic dose of iron because of dietary or other factors.

Contra-indications, warnings, etc
Contra-indications: Do not use in patients hypersensitive to the product or those with iron overload.

Precautions: Care should be taken in patients who may develop iron overload, such as those with haemochromatosis, haemolytic anaemia or red cell aplasia.

Failure to respond to treatment may indicate other causes of anaemia and should be further investigated.

The folic acid content of one capsule a day is unlikely to mask pernicious anaemia should this condition be present; pregnancy during pernicious anaemia is very rare.

Iron chelates with tetracyclines, and absorption of both agents may be impaired. Absorption of iron may be impaired by penicillamine and by antacids. Such potential interactions can be reduced by separating administration of each product by several hours.

Use in pregnancy: Fefol should not be used during the first trimester of pregnancy. Prophylaxis of iron and folate deficiency during the remainder of pregnancy is justified.

Adverse reactions: Dark stools are usual during iron therapy, and nausea and other symptoms of gastrointestinal irritation, such as anorexia, vomiting, discomfort, constipation and diarrhoea are sometimes encountered. Fefol Spansule capsules are designed to reduce the possibility of gastrointestinal irritation. There have been rare reports of allergic reactions.

Overdosage: Iron overdosage is dangerous, particularly in children, and requires immediate attention. Treatment is necessary if more than 30 mg elemental iron per kilogram body weight has been ingested. In the first phase, 30 minutes to 6 hours after ingestion, symptoms may include abdominal pain, vomiting, diarrhoea and haematemesis, with in more severe cases, coma, convulsions and shock. Symptoms then abate, with either recovery, or within 12 hours after ingestion, deterioration. Symptoms can then include severe lethargy or coma, gastrointestinal haemorrhage, severe shock, metabolic acidosis, convulsions, jaundice, coagulation disorders, hypoglycaemia, renal failure and pulmonary oedema. These may last up to 48 hours after ingestion. In the last phase, 2 to 5 weeks after ingestion, effects such as encephalopathy, hepatic necrosis and pyloric stenosis may occur. The sustained-release Spansule capsule presentation of ferrous sulphate may delay excessive absorption of iron and allow more time for initiation of appropriate countermeasures. Gastric lavage should be carried out in the early stages, or if this is not possible, vomiting should be induced. Give oral desferrioxamine (2 g for a child or 5 g for an adult) and demulcents. If serum iron levels at 4 hours or more post-ingestion are over 5 mg/l in a child or 8 mg/l in an adult, or if the patient is in shock or coma, intramuscular or intravenous desferrioxamine should be used according to instructions for this product. Symptomatic and supportive measures should be given as required.

Pharmaceutical precautions Store in a dry place below 25°C and protect from light.

Legal category P.

Package quantities Opaque calendar packs (OP) of 30 (2 × 15) Spansule capsules.

Further information Fefol Spansule capsules are formulated to release the iron in the small intestine where absorption is greatest rather than in the stomach where gastric irritation may be caused.

Inactive ingredients include sucrose and alumiunium lake of E110.

Product licence number 0002/5022R.

FEFOL Z* SPANSULE* CAPSULES

Presentation Clear, colourless capsules, transparent dark blue-capped and filled with a mixture of red, pale yellow and white pellets. Each Spansule sustained-release capsule contains 150 mg dried ferrous sulphate (47 mg elemental iron), 61.8 mg zinc sulphate monohydrate (22.5 mg elemental zinc) and 500 micrograms folic acid. The iron is specially formulated for sustained release over several hours. The zinc sulphate is formulated for release over one to two hours.

Uses Fefol Z is an oral iron, zinc and folic acid preparation for the prophylaxis of iron and folic acid deficiency during pregnancy for use when inadequate diet calls for supplementary zinc and when the need for such therapy has been determined by a physician.

Dosage and administration
Adults only: 1 Fefol Z Spansule Capsule a day during pregnancy. Some pregnant patients may need a higher prophylactic dose of iron because of dietary or other factors.

Contra-indications, warnings, etc
Contra-indications: Do not use in patients hypersensitive to the product or those with iron overload.

Precautions: Care should be taken in patients who may develop iron overload, such as those with haemochromatosis, haemolytic anaemia or red cell aplasia.

Failure to respond to treatment may indicate other causes of anaemia and should be further investigated.

The folic acid content of one capsule a day is unlikely to mask pernicious anaemia should this condition be present; pregnancy during pernicious anaemia is very rare.

Iron and zinc chelate with tetracyclines and absorption of all three agents may be impaired. The absorption of zinc may be reduced in the presence of iron. Absorption of iron may be impaired by penicillamine and by antacids. Such potential interactions can be reduced by separating administration of each product by several hours.

In patients with renal failure, a risk of zinc accumulation could exist.

Use in pregnancy: Fefol Z should not be used during the first trimester of pregnancy. Prophylaxis of iron and folate deficiency where inadequate diet calls for supplementary zinc is justified during the remainder of pregnancy.

Adverse reactions: Dark stools are usual during iron therapy, and nausea and other symptoms of gastrointestinal irritation, such as anorexia, vomiting, discomfort, constipation and diarrhoea are sometimes encountered. Zinc may also produce gastrointestinal upset. Fefol Z Spansule capsules are designed to reduce the possibility of gastrointestinal irritation. There have been rare reports of allergic reactions.

Overdosage: Iron overdosage is dangerous, particularly in children, and requires immediate attention. Treatment is necessary if more than 30 mg elemental iron per kilogram body weight has been ingested. In the first phase, 30 minutes to 6 hours after ingestion, symptoms may include abdominal pain, vomiting, diarrhoea and haematemesis, with in more severe cases, coma, convulsions and shock. Symptoms then abate, with either recovery, or within 12 hours after ingestion, deterioration. Symptoms can then include severe lethargy or coma, gastrointestinal haemorrhage, severe shock, metabolic acidosis, convulsions, jaundice, coagulation disorders, hypoglycaemia, renal failure and pulmonary oedema. These may last up to 48 hours after ingestion. In the last phase, 2 to 5 weeks after ingestion, effects such as encephalopathy, hepatic necrosis and pyloric stenosis may occur. Gastric lavage should be carried out in the early stages, or if this is not possible, vomiting should be induced. These procedures should not be undertaken where signs of the corrosive effect of zinc are present (see below). Give oral desferrioxamine (2 g for a child or 5 g for an adult) and demulcents. If serum iron levels at 4 hours or more post-ingestion are over 5 mg/l in a child or 8 mg/l in an adult, or if the patient is in shock or coma, intramuscular or intravenous desferrioxamine should be used according to instructions for this product.

Zinc sulphate in gross overdosage is corrosive. Symptoms are those of gastro-intestinal irritation, leading in severe cases to haemorrhage, corrosion of the mucosa and possible later stricture formation. Gastric lavage or emesis should be avoided. Demulcents such as milk should be given. Chelating agents such as dimercaprol, penicillamine or edetic acid have been recommended.

Symptomatic and supportive measures should be given as required. The sustained-release Spansule capsule presentation may delay excessive absorption of iron and zinc and allow more time for initiation of appropriate countermeasures.

Pharmaceutical precautions Store in a dry place below 25°C and protect from light.

Legal category P.

Package quantities Containers (OP) of 30 Spansule capsules.

Further information Inactive ingredients include sucrose and aluminium lake of E110.

Product licence number 0002/0100.

FEFOL-VIT* SPANSULE* CAPSULES

Presentation Clear, colourless capsules, opaque white-capped and filled with a mixture of red, orange-yellow, pale yellow and white pellets. Each Spansule sustained-release capsule contains 150 mg dried ferrous sulphate (47 mg elemental iron), 500 micrograms folic acid, 2 mg thiamine mononitrate, 2 mg riboflavine, 1 mg pyridoxine hydrochloride, 10 mg nicotinamide and 50 mg ascorbic acid. The iron is specially formulated for sustained release over a period of several hours.

Uses Fefol-Vit is a haematinic with added vitamins, for prophylaxis of iron and folic-acid deficiency during pregnancy, particularly when inadequate diet calls for supplementary vitamins B and C.

Dosage and administration *Adults only:* 1 Fefol-Vit Spansule capsule a day during pregnancy. Some pregnant patients may need a higher prophylactic dose of iron because of dietary or other factors.

Contra-indications, warnings, etc
Contra-indications: Do not use in patients hypersensitive to the product or those with iron overload.

Precautions: Care should be taken in patients who may develop iron overload, such as those with haemochromatosis, haemolytic anaemia or red cell aplasia.

Failure to respond to treatment may indicate other causes of anaemia and should be further investigated.

The folic acid content of one capsule a day is unlikely to mask pernicious anaemia should this condition be present; pregnancy during pernicious anaemia is very rare.

Iron chelates with tetracyclines, and absorption of both agents may be impaired. Absorption of iron may be impaired by penicillamine and by antacids. Such potential interactions can be reduced by separating administration of each product by several hours.

Use in pregnancy: Fefol-Vit should not be used during the first trimester of pregnancy. Prophylaxis of iron and folate deficiency where inadequate diet calls for supplementary vitamins B and C is justified during the remainder of pregnancy.

Adverse reactions: Dark stools are usual during iron therapy, and nausea and other symptoms of gastrointestinal irritation, such as anorexia, vomiting, discomfort, constipation and diarrhoea are sometimes encountered. Fefol-Vit Spansule capsules are designed to reduce the possibility of gastrointestinal irritation. There have been rare reports of allergic reactions.

Overdosage: Iron overdosage is dangerous, particularly in children, and requires immediate attention. Treatment is necessary if more than 30 mg elemental iron per kilogram body weight has been ingested. In the first phase, 30 minutes to 6 hours after ingestion, symptoms may include abdominal pain, vomiting, diarrhoea and haematemesis, with in more severe cases, coma, convulsions and shock. Symptoms then abate, with either recovery, or within 12 hours after ingestion, deterioration. Symptoms can then include severe lethargy or coma, gastrointestinal haemorrhage, severe shock, metabolic acidosis, convulsions, jaundice, coagulation disorders, hypoglycaemia, renal failure and pulmonary oedema. These may last up to 48 hours after ingestion. In the last phase, 2 to 5 weeks after ingestion, effects such as encephalopathy, hepatic necrosis and pyloric stenosis may occur. The sustained-release Spansule capsule presentation of ferrous sulphate may delay excessive absorption of iron and allow more time for initiation of appropriate countermeasures. Gastric lavage should be carried out in the early stages, or if this is not possible, vomiting should be induced. Give oral desferrioxamine (2 g for a child or 5 g for an adult) and demulcents. If serum iron levels at 4 hours or more post-ingestion are over 5 mg/l in a child or 8 mg/l in an adult, or if the patient is in shock or coma, intramuscular or intravenous desferrioxamine should be used according to instructions for this product. Symptomatic and supportive measures should be given as required.

Pharmaceutical precautions Store in a dry place below 25°C and protect from light.

Legal category P.

Package quantities Containers (OP) of 30 Spansule capsules.

Further information Fefol-Vit Spansule capsules are formulated to release the iron in the small intestine where absorption is greatest rather than in the stomach where gastric irritation may be caused.

Inactive ingredients include sucrose and aluminium lake of E110.

Product licence number 0002/0049R.

FENBID* SPANSULE* CAPSULES

Presentation Opaque maroon capsules, opaque pink-capped, containing off-white pellets. Each capsule contains 300 mg ibuprofen in a sustained release formulation which provides a prolonged therapeutic effect.

Uses Ibuprofen is a non-steroidal anti-inflammatory agent with analgesic and antipyretic properties. Fenbid is indicated for the treatment of rheumatoid arthritis, osteoarthritis, ankylosing spondylitis and other sero-negative (non-rheumatoid) arthropathies. It is also indicated in acute periarticular disorders such as bursitis, capsulitis of the shoulder, tendinitis, tenosynovitis and for the relief of mild to moderate pain in sprains, strains, low back pain, dysmenorrhoea and dental and post-operative pain.

Dosage and administration
Adults and children over 12 years: Usual starting dose is two capsules (600 mg) twice daily, taken night and morning. This may be increased to three capsules (900 mg) twice daily until the acute phase is controlled. Maintenance dose: One or two capsules twice daily.

Elderly: Dosage as above.

Patients should be instructed not to chew or suck the capsules as this destroys the sustained release properties. Providing this is ensured, the contents of a capsule may be sprinkled onto a spoonful of soft food, yoghurt, or similar substance, for patients who experience difficulty in swallowing the capsules.

The evening dose of Fenbid Spansule capsules will maintain a prolonged therapeutic effect throughout the night and help to prevent morning stiffness.

Contra-indications, warnings, etc
Contra-indication: Active peptic ulceration. Bronchospasm may be precipitated in patients suffering from, or with a previous history of, bronchial asthma or allergic disease. Fenbid should not be given to patients in whom aspirin and other non-steroidal anti-inflammatory drugs induce the symptoms of asthma, rhinitis or urticaria.

Precautions: Fenbid may be used, with caution, in patients with gastrointestinal disease, but may be tolerated by patients with intolerance to other anti-rheumatic drugs. The possibility of cross-sensitivity with aspirin and other non-steroidal anti-inflammatory agents should be borne in mind.

In patients with renal, cardiac, or hepatic impairment caution is required since the use of NSAIDS may result in deterioration of renal function. The dose should be kept as low as possible and renal function should be monitored.

If given to patients receiving anticoagulant therapy, prothrombin time should be monitored daily for the first few days of combined treatment. Ibuprofen may interfere with the efficacy of antihypertensive drugs. In therapeutic doses, no evidence of significant interactions with other commonly used drugs has been observed. However, as with other non-steroidal anti-inflammatory drugs, caution should be exercised in patients receiving thiazide diuretics.

Use in pregnancy and lactation: Based on animal studies and clinical experience, there is no evidence to suggest associated foetal abnormalities. However, as with other non-steroidal anti-inflammatory agents, Fenbid Spansule capsules should be avoided during pregnancy and lactation unless essential. Traces of ibuprofen have been detected in breast milk, but no adverse effects have been reported.

Adverse reactions: Generally well-tolerated with a low incidence of side-effects. Adverse effects may include gastrointestinal upsets, rashes, headache, nervousness, tinnitus and oedema. Gastrointestinal haemorrhage may rarely occur. Blurred vision, toxic amblyopia and thrombocytopenia have been reported during ibuprofen treatment, but were resolved on cessation of treatment. NSAIDS have been reported to cause nephrotoxicity in various forms and their use can lead to interstitial nephritis, nephrotic syndrome and renal failure.

Overdosage: The following signs and symptoms have been reported: headache, vomiting, drowsiness, loss of consciousness and hypotension. Symptomatic treatment is recommended, directed at maintaining normal blood pressure and correcting any electrolyte imbalance, particularly potassium. In children, emesis, and in adults, gastric lavage, may need to be considered, but only after careful assessment of the patient's condition, in particular the level of consciousness.

Pharmaceutical precautions Store in a dry place at a temperature not exceeding 30°C and protect from light.

Legal category POM.

Package quantities Containers (OP) of 120 Spansule capsules.

Further information Inactive ingredients include sucrose.

Product licence number 0002/0111.

FEOSPAN* SPANSULE* CAPSULES

Presentation Clear, colourless capsules, ruby-red-capped and filled with a mixture of green and red pellets. Each Spansule sustained-release capsule contains 150 mg dried ferrous sulphate (47 mg elemental iron). The iron is specially formulated for sustained release over a period of several hours.

Uses Feospan is a haematinic for the prevention and treatment of iron deficiency.

Dosage and administration *Adults:* 1 Feospan Spansule capsule a day. In more severe cases, 2 capsules a day may be required.

Elderly: Dosage as above.

Children aged over 1 year: 1 capsule a day. The capsule may be opened and the pellets mixed with soft, cool food, but they must not be chewed.

Treatment should continue for at least 3 months after correction of anaemia and then be reviewed.

Contra-indications, warnings, etc
Contra-indications: Do not use in patients hypersensitive to the product or those with iron overload.

Precautions: Care should be taken in patients who may develop iron overload, such as those with haemochromatosis, haemolytic anaemia or red cell aplasia.

Failure to respond to treatment may indicate other causes of anaemia and should be further investigated.

Iron chelates with tetracyclines, and absorption of both agents may be impaired.

Absorption of iron may be impaired by penicillamine and by antacids. Such potential interactions can be reduced by separating administration of each product by several hours.

Use in pregnancy: Use of any drug during the first trimester of pregnancy should be avoided if possible. Thus administration of iron during the first trimester requires definite evidence of iron deficiency. Prophylaxis of iron deficiency during the remainder of pregnancy is justified.

Adverse reactions: Dark stools are usual during iron therapy, and nausea and other symptoms of gastrointestinal irritation, such as anorexia, vomiting, discomfort, constipation and diarrhoea are sometimes encountered. Feospan Spansule capsules are designed to reduce the possibility of gastrointestinal irritation. There have been rare reports of allergic reactions.

Overdosage: Iron overdosage is dangerous, particularly in children, and requires immediate attention. Treatment is necessary if more than 30 mg elemental iron per kilogram body weight has been ingested. In the first phase, 30 minutes to 6 hours after ingestion, symptoms may include abdominal pain, vomiting, diarrhoea and haematemesis, with in more severe cases, coma, convulsions and shock. Symptoms then abate, with either recovery, or within 12 hours after ingestion, deterioration. Symptoms can then include severe lethargy or coma, gastrointestinal haemorrhage, severe shock, metabolic acidosis, convulsions, jaundice, coagulation disorders, hypoglycaemia, renal failure and pulmonary oedema. These may last up to 48 hours after ingestion. In the last phase, 2 to 5 weeks after ingestion, effects such as encephalopathy, hepatic necrosis and pyloric stenosis may occur. The sustained-release Spansule capsule presentation of ferrous sulphate may delay excessive absorption of iron and allow more time for initiation of appropriate countermeasures. Gastric lavage should be carried out in the early stages, or if this is not possible, vomiting should be induced. Give oral desferrioxamine (2 g for a child or 5 g for an adult) and demulcents. If serum iron levels at 4 hours or more post-ingestion are over 5 mg/l in a child or 8 mg/l in an adult, or if the patient is in shock or coma, intramuscular or intravenous desferrioxamine should be used according to instructions for this product. Symptomatic and supportive measures should be given as required.

Pharmaceutical precautions Store in a dry place below 25°C.

Legal category P.

Package quantities Opaque blister packs (OP) of 30 (2 × 15) Spansule capsules.

Further information Feospan Spansule capsules are formulated to release the iron in the small intestine where absorption is greatest rather than in the stomach where gastric irritation may be caused.

Inactive ingredients include sucrose and aluminium lake of E110.

Product licence number 0002/5023R.

FESOVIT Z* SPANSULE* CAPSULES

Presentation Clear, colourless capsules, transparent orange-capped and filled with a mixture of red, orange-yellow and white pellets. Each Spansule sustained-release capsule contains 150 mg dried ferrous sulphate (47 mg elemental iron), 61.8 mg zinc sulphate monohydrate (22.5 mg elemental zinc), 2 mg thiamine mononitrate, 2 mg riboflavine, 1 mg pyridoxine hydrochloride, 10 mg nicotinamide, and 50 mg ascorbic acid. The iron is specially formulated for sustained release over several hours. The zinc sulphate is formulated for release over one to two hours.

Uses Fesovit Z is an oral iron and zinc preparation, with added vitamins, for the prevention of iron deficiency for use when inadequate diet calls for supplementary zinc and vitamins B and C and when the need for such therapy has been determined by a physician.

Dosage and administration
Adults: 1 Fesovit Z Spansule capsule a day. In more severe cases, 2 capsules a day may be required.

Elderly: Dosage as above.

Children aged over 1 year: 1 capsule a day. The capsule may be opened and the pellets mixed with soft, cool food, but they must not be chewed.

Contra-indications, warnings, etc
Contra-indications: Do not use in patients hypersensitive to the product or those with iron overload

Precautions: Care should be taken in patients who may develop iron overload, such as those with haemochromatosis, haemolytic anaemia or red cell aplasia.

Failure to respond to treatment may indicate other causes of anaemia and should be further investigated.

Iron and zinc chelate with tetracyclines and absorption of all three agents may be impaired. The absorption of zinc may be reduced in the presence of iron. Absorption of iron may be impaired by penicillamine and by antacids. Such potential interactions can be reduced by separating administration of each product by several hours.

In patients with renal failure, a risk of zinc accumulation could exist.

Use in pregnancy: Use of any drug during the first trimester of pregnancy should be avoided if possible. Thus administration of iron during the first trimester requires definite evidence of iron deficiency. Prophylaxis of iron deficiency where inadequate diet calls for supplementary zinc and vitamins B and C is justified during the remainder of pregnancy.

Adverse reactions: Dark stools are usual during iron therapy, and nausea and other symptoms of gastrointestinal irritation, such as anorexia, vomiting, discomfort, constipation and diarrhoea are sometimes encountered. Zinc may also produce gastrointestinal upset. Fesovit Z Spansule capsules are designed to reduce the possibility of gastrointestinal irritation. There have been rare reports of allergic reactions.

Overdosage: Iron overdosage is dangerous, particularly in children, and requires immediate attention. Treatment is necessary if more than 30 mg elemental iron per kilogram body weight has been ingested. In the first phase, 30 minutes to 6 hours after ingestion, symptoms may include abdominal pain, vomiting, diarrhoea and haematemesis, with in more severe cases, coma, convulsions and shock. Symptoms then abate, with either recovery, or within 12 hours after ingestion, deterioration. Symptoms can then include severe lethargy or coma, gastrointestinal haemorrhage, severe shock, metabolic acidosis, convulsions, jaundice, coagulation disorders, hypoglycaemia, renal failure and pulmonary oedema. These may last up to 48 hours after ingestion. In the last phase, 2 to 5 weeks after ingestion, effects such as encephalopathy, hepatic necrosis and pyloric stenosis may occur. Gastric lavage should be carried out in the early stages, or if this is not possible, vomiting should be induced. These procedures should not be undertaken where signs of the corrosive effect of zinc are present (see below). Give oral desferrioxamine (2 g for a child or 5 g for an adult) and demulcents. If serum iron levels at 4 hours or more post-ingestion are over 5 mg/l in a child or 8 mg/l in an adult, or if the patient is in shock or coma, intramuscular or intravenous desferrioxamine should be used according to instructions for this product.

Zinc sulphate in gross overdosage is corrosive. Symptoms are those of gastro-intestinal irritation, leading in severe cases to haemorrhage, corrosion of the mucosa and possible later stricture formation. Gastric lavage or emesis should be avoided. Demulcents such as milk should be given. Chelating agents such as dimercaprol, penicillamine or edetic acid have been recommended.

Symptomatic and supportive measures should be given as required. The sustained-release Spansule capsule presentation may delay excessive absorption of iron and zinc and allow more time for initiation of appropriate countermeasures.

Pharmaceutical precautions Store in a dry place below 25°C and protect from light.

Legal category P.

Package quantities Containers (OP) of 30 Spansule capsules.

Further information Inactive ingredients include sucrose and aluminium lake of E110.

Product licence number 0002/0101.

LISKONUM* TABLETS

Presentation White, oblong, film-coated tablets, with convex faces and a breakline on both sides, each containing 450 mg lithium carbonate (12.2 mmol Li^+) in controlled-release form.

Uses Liskonum is a controlled-release tablet, designed to reduce fluctuations in serum lithium levels and the likelihood of adverse reactions.

It is indicated for the treatment of acute episodes of mania or hypomania and for the prophylaxis of recurrent manic-depressive illness.

Dosage and administration *Adults only:* Liskonum should be given twice a day.

Treatment of acute mania or hypomania: Patients should be started on one or one and a half tablets twice a day. Dosage should then be adjusted to achieve a serum lithium level of 0.8 to a maximum of 1.5 mmol/l. Serum concentration of lithium should be measured after four to seven days' treatment and then at least once a week until dosage has remained constant for 4 weeks. When the acute symptoms have been controlled, recommendations for prophylaxis should be followed.

Prophylaxis: The usual starting dosage is one tablet twice a day. Dosage should then be adjusted until a serum level of 0.5 to 1.0 mmol/l is maintained. Serum concentration of lithium should be measured after four to seven days' treatment and then every week until dosage has remained constant for four weeks. Frequency of monitoring may then be gradually decreased to a minimum of once every two months but should be increased following any situation where changes in lithium levels are possible (see *Precautions*).

Blood samples for measurement of serum lithium concentration should be taken just before a dose is due and not less than 12 hours after the previous dose.

Levels of more than 2 mmol/l *must* be avoided.

Tablets may be halved but should not be chewed or broken up.

Elderly: Use with caution. Start with half a tablet twice a day and adjust serum levels to the lower end of the above ranges (see also *Precautions*).

The full prophylactic effect of lithium may not be evident for 6 to 12 months, and treatment should be continued through any recurrence of the illness.

Contra-indications, warnings, etc

Contra-indications: Do not use in patients with impaired renal function, cardiac disease, or untreated hypothyroidism. Lithium should not be given to patients with low body sodium levels, including, for example, dehydrated patients, those on low sodium diets, or those with Addison's disease.

Precautions: Vomiting, diarrhoea, intercurrent infection, fluid deprivation and drugs likely to upset electrolyte balance, such as diuretics, may all reduce lithium excretion and thereby precipitate intoxication; reduction of dosage may be required. In elderly patients, lithium excretion may also be reduced. Diuretics should only be used with caution during treatment; thiazides show a paradoxical antidiuretic effect resulting in possible water retention and lithium intoxication. Lithium retention may also follow combined use with indomethacin and other prostaglandin-synthetase-inhibiting drugs. The possibility of hypothyroidism and of renal dysfunction arising during prolonged treatment should be borne in mind and periodic assessments made.

There have been reports of interaction between lithium and some neuroleptics, particularly haloperidol at higher dosages, also between lithium and methyldopa or phenytoin. Fluvoxamine and fluoxetine should be combined with lithium with care.

Patients should be warned of the symptoms of impending intoxication (see below), of the urgency of immediate action should these symptoms appear, and also of the need to maintain a constant and adequate salt and water intake.

Use in pregnancy and lactation: Lithium crosses the placental barrier. In animal studies, lithium has been reported to interfere with fertility, gestation and foetal development. There is epidemiological evidence that the drug may be harmful in human pregnancy. Lithium therapy should not be used during pregnancy, especially during the first trimester, unless considered essential. In certain cases where a severe risk to the patient could exist if treatment were to be stopped, lithium has been continued during pregnancy. If given, however, serum levels should be measured frequently because of the changes in renal function associated with pregnancy and parturition.

Since lithium is secreted in breast milk, bottle feeding is advisable.

Adverse reactions: At therapeutic serum levels, mild nausea and diarrhoea, fine tremor of the hands, muscle weakness, vertigo, giddiness, weight gain, oedema, and a dazed feeling may occur. Hypothyroidism has been reported. Rarely hyperthyroidism may occur and mild hyperparathyroidism has been reported. Mild polyuria and polydipsia are not infrequent and, occasionally, nephrogenic diabetes insipidus may be present. Histological renal changes, with interstitial fibrosis, have been observed in some patients on long-term treatment; while there may be an association with impaired reabsorption, a relationship between these changes and a reduction in glomerular filtration rate or development of renal insufficiency has not been established.

Skin reactions including acne or acneiform eruptions, papular skin disorders, rashes, and exacerbation of psoriasis have been reported.

Intoxication: Vomiting, diarrhoea, drowsiness, lack of co-ordination and/or a coarse tremor of the extremities and lower jaw may occur, especially with serum levels above the therapeutic range. Ataxia, giddiness, blurred vision, dysarthria, tinnitus, muscle hyperirritability, choreoathetoid movements and toxic psychosis have also been described.

If any of the above symptoms appear, treatment should be stopped immediately and arrangements made for serum lithium measurement.

Overdosage: Symptoms are similar to those listed above under *Intoxication* but more marked, particularly those of central nervous system origin. In severe cases, seizures, coma and death may ensue.

Treatment consists of the induction of vomiting and/or gastric lavage together with supportive and symptomatic measures. Particular attention should be paid to maintenance of fluid and electrolyte balance and of adequate renal function. Where convulsions are present, diazepam may be used. Forced alkaline diuresis, peritoneal dialysis or haemodialysis may help eliminate the lithium ion. The latter method is preferable, particularly where serum lithium exceeds 4 mmol/l.

Pharmaceutical precautions Store in a dry place.

Legal category POM.

Package quantities Opaque blister packs (OP) of 60 (6 × 10) and containers of 1,000 tablets.

Further information Inactive ingredients include lactose.

Product licence number 0002/0083.

OCTOVIT* TABLETS

Presentation Maroon, oblong, film-coated tablets, engraved SK&F on one side, each containing: 2500 i.u. vitamin A present as the acetate, 1 mg thiamine present as the mononitrate, 1.5 mg riboflavine, 20 mg nicotinamide, 2 mg pyridoxine present as the hydrochloride, 2 micrograms cyanocobalamin, 30 mg ascorbic acid, 100 i.u. cholecalciferol, 10 mg tocopherol present as the acetate, 100 mg calcium present as the hydrogenphosphate dihydrate, 10 mg iron present as dried ferrous sulphate, 10 mg magnesium present as the hydroxide, and 5 mg zinc present as the sulphate monohydrate.

Uses Octovit is a multivitamin/mineral product indicated where supplementation with the vitamins and minerals specified above may be of benefit and for those at risk of developing a deficiency state.

Dosage and administration *Adults and children over 12 years:* One tablet a day or as prescribed by the physician.

Contra-indications, warnings, etc
Precaution: Iron and zinc chelate with tetracyclines and absorption of all three agents may be impaired.

Use in pregnancy: Excessive vitamin A taken in pregnancy has been reported to be potentially dangerous. The recommended daily dose of Octovit has a vitamin content within the advised maximum daily intake in pregnancy and does not present a hazard. This should however be considered in the context of total dietary vitamin A.

Overdosage: Overdosage is unlikely to occur. However, prolonged administration of extremely large doses of vitamin A and cholecalciferol may result in hypervitaminosis. Early symptoms include irritability, nausea and vomiting, loss of appetite, headache, and dry and pruritic skin.

Pharmaceutical precautions Store in a dry place at a temperature not exceeding 25°C and protect from light.

Legal category P.

Package quantities Opaque blister packs of 14 (1 × 14) (OP) and 70 (5 × 14) tablets.

Further information Inactive ingredients include sugar stearate.

Product licence number 0002/0113.

PARNATE* TABLETS

Presentation Geranium-red, sugar-coated tablets, marked SKF, each containing 10 mg tranylcypromine present as the sulphate.

Uses Parnate is a non-hydrazine monoamine oxidase inhibitor for the treatment of symptoms of depressive illness especially where phobic symptoms are present or where treatment with other types of antidepressant has failed. It is not recommended for mild depressive states resulting from temporary situational difficulties.

Dosage and administration *Adults only:* Initially, one tablet morning and afternoon. If the response is not adequate after the first week, add a further tablet at midday, and continue for at least a week. A dosage of 3 tablets a day should only be exceeded with caution. When a satisfactory response has been obtained, dosage may be reduced to a maintenance level, often of 1 tablet a day.

When given with a tranquilliser, the dosage of Parnate is not affected. When given concurrently with electroconvulsive therapy, the usual dosage is 1 tablet twice a day during the series and 1 tablet a day afterwards as maintenance therapy.

Elderly: Use with great caution (see *Contra-indications* and *Precautions* below).

Contra-indications, warnings, etc
Contra-indications: Do not give Parnate less than a week after stopping treatment with any other antidepressant drug including other MAO inhibitors, because of persisting effects, then give half the usual dosage for the first week. Similarly, after stopping Parnate, allow at least two weeks to elapse before starting treatment with any drug or ingesting any food that may interact.

Do not give Parnate with indirectly-acting sympathomimetic amines such as amphetamine, fenfluramine or similar anti-obesity agents, ephedrine or phenylpropanolamine (certain 'cold-cures' may contain such agents), or with levodopa or dopamine, as severe hypertensive reactions may result; with pethidine and closely related narcotic analgesics as potentiation may occur; with dextromethorphan as a similar reaction has been reported; with other MAO inhibitors, as symptoms of overdosage are possible; or with buspirone, since increased blood pressure may occur.

Reports of hyperactivity, hypertonicity, hyperpyrexia, coma and death have been associated with the use of Parnate in combination with tricyclic antidepressants; tetracyclic antidepressants should also be avoided. The use of clomipramine in patients already on Parnate may be particularly hazardous. Use of MAO inhibitors with or after fluvoxamine or fluoxetine has been reported to produce a serotonin syndrome, sometimes fatal.

Do not use Parnate in patients with actual or suspected cerebrovascular disease or severe cardiovascular disease; in those with actual or suspected phaeochromocytoma, or with hyperthyroidism; or in those with known liver damage or blood dyscrasias.

Dietary precautions: High levels of tyramine in certain foods have been the cause of severe hypertensive reactions in patients on MAO inhibitor therapy (see *Adverse reactions*). Accordingly, patients must be warned to avoid the following: matured cheeses, hydrolysed protein extracts such as Marmite or Bovril, alcoholic drinks, particularly red wines such as Chianti, non-alcoholic beer and lager, and protein foods that are not fresh or whose preparation involved hydrolysis, fermentation, pickling, or 'hanging'; also broad-bean pods, which contain levodopa, and banana skins.

Precautions: Caution should be exercised when giving Parnate with the following: guanethidine, as its action may be antagonised; reserpine, as hyperactivity may occur; methyldopa, as central excitation may result; other hypotensive agents because of possible additive effects; oral hypoglycaemic agents or insulin, as their action may be potentiated; anticholinergic antiparkinsonism drugs, as potentiation has been reported; narcotic analgesics, except pethidine which is contra-indicated (see above), because of possible potentiation; and carbamazepine, which has similarities with tricyclic antidepressants. Although the effects of barbiturates may be enhanced, and this possibility should be borne in mind, they have frequently been given with Parnate, particularly at night. Metrizamide should be avoided in patients on MAO inhibitors since they may lower the seizure threshold. Although MAO inhibitors have been used therapeutically with L-tryptophan, a neuromotor syndrome has been reported with this combination.

Patients should be specifically asked if they are taking any other medication because of the possibility of drug interactions.

Use Parnate with great caution in elderly patients; in those with cardiovascular disease in whom physical activity should be regulated, as the drug may suppress anginal pain; and in epileptic patients, as tranylcypromine has a variable effect on the convulsive threshold in animals. Parnate may aggravate some co-existing symptoms in depression such as anxiety and agitation. Parnate should preferably be withdrawn at least two weeks before elective surgery because of possible drug interaction.

Caution should be exercised in prescribing Parnate for patients with a previous history of dependence on drugs or alcohol.

In common with other drugs acting on the CNS, Parnate may affect ability to drive or operate machinery.

Use in pregnancy and lactation: Do not use in pregnancy, especially during the first and last trimesters, unless there are compelling reasons. There is no evidence as to drug safety in human pregnancy nor is there evidence from animal work that it is free from hazard. Tranylcypromine passes into the milk of lactating dogs.

Adverse reactions: Severe hypertensive reactions may occur, notably in association with foods containing tyramine (see *Dietary precautions*). Such reactions may be presaged by palpitations and unusually frequent headaches; patients should be warned to discontinue the drug if such symptoms occur. As well as a rapid rise in blood pressure, severe occipital headache, which may radiate frontally, is virtually always present, and pain and stiffness in the neck are usual; other features include multiple extrasystoles, often with bradycardia though sometimes with tachycardia, other arrhythmias, substernal pain, nausea and vomiting, sweating, pallor, sometimes followed by flushing, mydriasis and photophobia. Rarely, hypotension may dominate the clinical picture. ECG changes may be seen. The symptoms can mimic subarachnoid haemorrhage or may actually be associated with intracranial bleeding. Exceptionally, hemiparesis, hemiplegia or death has resulted.

Severe hypertensive reactions should be treated at once by reducing the blood pressure; slow intravenous injection of 5 mg phentolamine mesylate should be effective. Injectable or oral chlorpromazine is suitable for milder reactions. Acute symptoms generally subside within 24 hours.

Insomnia is the most frequent side-effect; it may usually be overcome by giving the last dose of the day not later than 3 pm, by reducing dosage, or by prescribing a mild hypnotic.

Mild headache, drowsiness, weakness, dizziness, palpitation, transient restlessness, dry mouth, blurred vision, nausea, oedema, weight gain, increased appetite and rash have been reported. Overstimulation, including anxiety and agitation, developing rarely into hypomania, has also been observed; the dosage should be reduced. Hypotension, which may be postural, may occur; it is usually temporary, but if it persists the drug should be stopped. Peripheral neuritis and difficulty in micturition have occurred rarely.

Dependence on Parnate, with tolerance to high doses, has been reported rarely, and can occur in patients without a past history of drug dependence. This should be distinguished from the return of features of the original illness on cessation of treatment.

Liver dysfunction has occurred very rarely, and isolated instances of purpura and blood dyscrasias have been reported.

Overdosage: Signs and symptoms are usually of the type already described as adverse reactions, but may be more intense, may include hyperpyrexia, tremor and convulsions, and may follow a latent period. Treatment consists of the induction of vomiting and/or gastric lavage together with supportive and symptomatic measures. External cooling is recommended for hyperpyrexia. Treat hypotension with fluid replacement; if severe or persistent, noradrenaline may be considered. Hypertension, if it occurs, may be relieved by slow intravenous injection of phentolamine mesylate. Pancuronium with mechanical ventilation may help reverse muscle spasm and pyrexia. Beta-adrenergic receptor blockade has been used successfully.

Pharmaceutical precautions Store in a dry place at a temperature not exceeding 25°C and protect from light.

Legal category POM.

Package quantities Containers of 100 tablets.

Further information It is generally considered that no particular hazard is attached to the use of local anaesthetics containing small amounts of adrenaline in patients receiving Parnate unless cardiovascular disease is present.

Inactive ingredients include sucrose and aluminium lakes of E122 and E124.

Product licence number 0002/5040R.

PARSTELIN* TABLETS

Presentation Leaf-green, sugar-coated tablets, marked SKF, each containing 10 mg tranylcypromine present as the sulphate and 1 mg trifluoperazine present as the hydrochloride.

Uses Parstelin is a combination of a non-hydrazine monoamine oxidase inhibitor and a phenothiazine tranquilliser, for the treatment of symptoms of depressive illness complicated by anxiety, especially where phobic symptoms are present or where treatment with other types of antidepressant has failed. It is not recommended for mild depressive states resulting from temporary situational difficulties.

Dosage and administration *Adults only:* Initially, 1 tablet morning and afternoon. If the response is not adequate after the first week, add a further tablet at midday, and continue for at least a week. A dosage of 3 tablets a day should only be exceeded with caution. When a satisfactory response has been obtained, dosage may be reduced to a maintenance level, often of 1 tablet a day.

Elderly: Use with great caution (see *Contra-indications* and *Precautions* below).

Contra-indications, warnings, etc

Contra-indications: Do not give Parstelin less than a week after stopping treatment with any other antidepressant drug including other MAO inhibitors, because of persisting effects, then give half the usual dosage for the first week. Similarly, after stopping Parstelin, allow at least two weeks to elapse before starting treatment with any drug or ingesting any food that may interact.

Do not give Parstelin with indirectly-acting sympathomimetic amines such as amphetamine, fenfluramine, or similar anti-obesity agents, ephedrine or phenylpropanolamine (certain 'cold-cures' may contain such agents), or with levodopa or dopamine, as severe hypertensive reactions may result; with pethidine and closely related narcotic analgesics, as potentiation may occur; with dextromethorphan as a similar reaction has been reported; with other MAO inhibitors, as symptoms of overdosage are possible; or with buspirone, since increased blood pressure may occur.

Reports of hyperactivity, hypertonicity, hyperpyrexia, coma and death have been associated with the use of tranylcypromine in combination with tricyclic antidepressants; tetracyclic antidepressants should also be avoided. The use of clomipramine in patients already on Parstelin may be particularly hazardous. Use of MAO inhibitors with or after fluvoxamine or fluoxetine has been reported to produce a serotonin syndrome, sometimes fatal.

Do not use Parstelin in patients with actual or suspected cerebrovascular disease or severe cardiovascular disease; in those with actual or suspected phaeochromocytoma, or with hyperthyroidism; in those with existing blood dyscrasias or known liver damage; or in those hypersensitive to the ingredients.

Dietary precautions: High levels of tyramine in certain foods have been the cause of severe hypertensive reactions in patients on MAO inhibitor therapy (see *Adverse reactions*). Accordingly, patients must be warned to avoid the following: matured cheese, hydrolysed protein extracts such as Marmite or Bovril, alcoholic drinks, particularly red wines such as Chianti, non-alcoholic beer and lager, and protein foods that are not fresh or whose preparation involved hydrolysis, fermentation, pickling, or 'hanging'; also broad-bean pods, which contain levodopa, and banana skins.

Precautions: Caution should be exercised when giving Parstelin with the following: guanethidine, as its action may be antagonised; reserpine, as hyperactivity may occur; methyldopa, as central excitation may result; other hypotensive agents because of possible additive effects; oral hypoglycaemic agents or insulin, as their action may be potentiated; anticholinergic antiparkinsonism drugs, as potentiation has been reported; narcotic analgesics, except pethidine which is contra-indicated (see above), because of possible potentiation; and carbamazepine, which has similarities with tricyclic antidepressants. Although the effects of barbiturates may be enhanced, and this possibility should be borne in mind, they have frequently been given with Parstelin, particularly at night. Metrizamide should be avoided in patients on MAO inhibitors since they may lower the seizure threshold. Although MAO inhibitors have been used therapeutically with L-tryptophan, a neuromotor syndrome has been reported with this combination. Potentiation may occur if trifluoperazine is used with other CNS depressants.

Patients should be specifically asked if they are taking any other medication because of the possibility of drug interactions.

Use Parstelin with great caution in elderly patients; in those with cardiovascular disease in whom physical activity should be regulated, as tranylcypromine may suppress anginal pain; and in epileptic patients as tranylcypromine has a variable effect on the convulsive threshold in animals. Tranylcypromine may aggravate some co-existing symptoms in depression such as anxiety and agitation. Parstelin should preferably be withdrawn at least two weeks before elective surgery because of possible drug interaction.

Nausea and vomiting as a sign of organic disease may be masked by the anti-emetic action of trifluoperazine.

Caution should be exercised in prescribing Parstelin for patients with a previous history of dependence on drugs or alcohol.

In common with other drugs acting on the CNS, Parstelin may affect ability to drive or operate machinery.

Use in pregnancy and lactation: Do not use in pregnancy, especially during the first and last trimesters, unless there are compelling reasons. There is no evidence as to drug safety in human pregnancy nor is there evidence from animal work that it is free from hazard. Both tranylcypromine and trifluoperazine pass into the milk of lactating dogs.

Adverse reactions: Severe hypertensive reactions may occur, notably in association with foods containing tyramine (see *Dietary precautions*). Such reactions may be presaged by palpitations and unusually frequent headaches; patients should be warned to discontinue the drug if such symptoms occur. As well as a rapid rise in blood pressure, severe occipital headache, which may radiate frontally, is virtually always present, and pain and stiffness in the neck are usual; other features include multiple extrasystoles, often with bradycardia though sometimes with tachycardia, other arrhythmias, substernal pain, nausea and vomiting, sweating, pallor, sometimes followed by flushing, mydriasis and photophobia. Rarely, hypotension may dominate the clinical picture. ECG changes may be seen. The symptoms can mimic subarachnoid haemorrhage or may actually be associated with intracranial bleeding. Exceptionally, hemiparesis, hemiplegia or death has resulted.

Severe hypertensive reactions should be treated at once by reducing the blood pressure; slow intravenous injection of 5 mg phentolamine mesylate should be effective. Injectable or oral chlorpromazine is suitable for milder reactions. Acute symptoms generally subside within 24 hours.

Insomnia is the most frequent side-effect; it may usually be overcome by giving the last dose of the day not later than 3 pm, by reducing dosage, or by prescribing a mild hypnotic.

Mild headache, drowsiness, weakness, dizziness, palpitation, transient restlessness, dry mouth, blurred vision, nausea, oedema, weight gain, increased appetite and rash have been reported. Overstimulation, including anxiety and agitation, developing rarely into hypomania, has also been observed; the dosage should be reduced. Hypotension, which may be postural, may occur; it is usually temporary, but if it persists the drug should be stopped. Peripheral neuritis and difficulty in micturition have occurred rarely.

Dependence on tranylcypromine, with tolerance to high doses, has been reported rarely, and can occur in patients without a past history of drug dependence. This should be distinguished from the return of features of the original illness on cessation of treatment.

Extrapyramidal symptoms due to the trifluoperazine component are very unlikely at the recommended dosage. Extremely rarely, long-term therapy with trifluoperazine in low dosage has been associated with tardive dyskinesia, which can be long-lasting or even irreversible.

Liver dysfunction has occurred very rarely, and isolated instances of purpura and blood dyscrasias have been reported.

Overdosage: Signs and symptoms are usually of the type already described as adverse reactions to tranylcypromine, but may be more intense, may include hyperpyrexia, tremor and convulsions, and may follow a latent period. In the unlikely event of symptoms from the trifluoperazine component, these are extrapyramidal in type. Treatment consists of gastric lavage together with supportive and symptomatic measures. Do not induce vomiting. External cooling is recommended for hyperpyrexia. Treat hypotension with fluid replacement; if severe or persistent, noradrenaline may be considered; adrenaline is contra-indicated. Hypertension, if it occurs, may be relieved by slow intravenous injection of phentolamine mesylate. Pancuronium with mechanical ventilation may help reverse muscle spasm and pyrexia. Beta-adrenergic receptor blockade has been used successfully.

Pharmaceutical precautions Store in a dry place at a temperature not exceeding 25°C and protect from light.

Legal category POM.

Package quantities Containers of 100 tablets.

Further information It is generally considered that no particular hazard is attached to the use of local anaesthetics containing small amounts of adrenaline in patients receiving tranylcypromine unless cardiovascular disease is present.

Inactive ingredients include sucrose and aluminium lake of E110.

Parstelin should normally only be used on the recommendation of a specialist in psychiatry.

Product licence number 0002/5041R.

PLUSERIX* MMR

Presentation Pluserix MMR is a mixed preparation of the highly attenuated live measles virus (Schwarz strain) and mumps virus (Urabe Am 9 strain), both prepared in chick embryo tissue, and rubella virus (RA 27/3 strain), prepared in human diploid cell culture, presented as a pink pellet in a glass vial with a separate ampoule or vial of clear, colourless, sterile diluent. Each 0.5 ml dose of the reconstituted vaccine contains not less than 1,000 $TCID_{50}$ of the Schwarz, 20,000 $TCID_{50}$ of the Urabe Am 9 and 1,000 $TCID_{50}$ of the RA 27/3 virus strains and not more than 25 micrograms (17 i.u.) of neomycin sulphate.

Uses Pluserix MMR is indicated for active immunisation of children and susceptible adults against measles, mumps and rubella.

Dosage and administration
Adults and children: 0.5 ml of the reconstituted vaccine, given subcutaneously or intramuscularly. *Do not give intravenously.* The vaccine should be reconstituted using the sterile diluent provided.

In children of under 12 months, persisting maternal measles antibodies may interfere with immune response. However, in situations where severe measles is common in children under this age, the benefit of vaccination at, for example, nine months may outweigh the risk of vaccine failure.

Vaccination up to 72 hours after exposure to natural measles may offer some protection, though this may not be provided after exposure to rubella or mumps.

The vaccine is quickly inactivated by ether, alcohol and detergents and care should be taken to avoid contact with these substances when cleaning skin prior to vaccination. Syringes need to be dry sterilised.

Contra-indications, warnings, etc
Contra-indications: Never give to pregnant women, or women of child-bearing age not fully aware of the need to avoid pregnancy for one month after vaccination, since theoretically the vaccine virus could have an effect on the foetus.

Do not use Pluserix MMR in the presence of acute febrile illness, whether active or expected, following exposure to infection other than measles, mumps or rubella. This applies particularly to active tuberculosis and respiratory tract infection. It is also contra-indicated in states of altered immunity including those which may accompany conditions such as leukaemia, lymphoma, generalised malignancy or treatment with corticosteroids, cytotoxic drugs or irradiation.

Pluserix MMR may contain traces of chick embryo protein, but this does not normally contra-indicate its use except in cases of severe hypersensitivity to eggs (past anaphylactoid reactions to egg ingestion). Pluserix MMR should not be given to those known to be hypersensitive to neomycin. A solution of 1:1000 adrenaline should be available for injection in rare cases of anaphylactic reaction. Pluserix MMR should not be given to those who have previously had severe reactions to measles, mumps or rubella vaccines.

Precautions: Since pyrexia may occur 5 to 10 days after vaccination, parents, especially of children with a personal or close family history of febrile convulsions, should be given advice about reducing fever. For example should the child appear unwell and develop a temperature, measures such as removal of clothing, tepid sponging and administration of paracetamol may be indicated.

Because of the possibility of interference from passive antibodies, the vaccine should not normally be given to subjects who have received blood or human plasma transfusions or human immunoglobulin within the previous three months. If the vaccine is given in these circumstances, serum antibodies should be checked at a later date.

Tuberculin testing may be carried out before or at the same time as vaccination with Pluserix MMR. It should otherwise be delayed for about eight weeks after vaccination since false-negative results may be obtained during this period.

At least three weeks should normally intervene between the administration of any two live vaccine preparations. Pluserix MMR can however be given simultaneously with live oral poliomyelitis vaccine and with DTP vaccine, but at a different site.

Adverse reactions: These are usually mild and similar in incidence to those seen after separate administration of the respective monovalent vaccines. They are usually delayed for several days and may include rash, mild irritability, malaise, cough, pharyngitis, coryza, pyrexia, headache and slight enlargement of the posterior cervical glands. In a very few subjects, convulsions may accompany the fever. Rarely parotid swelling, pruritus, purpura or transient arthralgia and arthritis with or without effusion may occur. Immediate allergic-type reactions have been reported rarely. Very rarely meningitis or meningoencephalitis has been reported in temporal association with the vaccine and, in these rare cases, complete recovery was observed. Extremely rarely transient polyneuropathy, unilateral nerve deafness or thrombocytopenic purpura could occur. Reactions at the site of injection are rare and usually mild.

Pharmaceutical precautions Protect from light. Pluserix MMR vaccine should be stored between 2°C and 8°C, its shelf life then being 2 years, and should not be frozen (lower temperatures will not harm the vaccine but may damage the diluent container). At 37°C Pluserix MMR is stable for at least 7 days.

The vaccine should be reconstituted using the sterile diluent provided and the pellet should be completely dissolved. The colour of reconstituted vaccine may vary from yellow to light red. Once reconstituted Pluserix MMR should be used immediately, and certainly within one hour.

Legal category POM.

Package quantities Monodose vials (OP), each with a separate ampoule containing sterile diluent. The diluent is Water for Injections PhEur.

Further information A single dose of Pluserix MMR has been shown in clinical studies to induce seroconversion rates of over 95 per cent against measles, mumps and rubella when given to triple seronegative subjects, similar to the seroconversion rates induced by the monovalent vaccines in seronegative subjects.

Current policy recommends that measles/mumps/rubella vaccine should be given to all children aged 1 to 2 years for whom there is no valid contra-indication. Children of 4 to 5 years who have not previously had the vaccine and for whom there is no valid contra-indication should also be vaccinated.

Inactive ingredients are human albumin, lactose, sorbitol, dextran 10, casein hydrolysate, and also neomycin sulphate (see **Presentation**).

Product licence number 0002/0166.

POLIOMYELITIS VACCINE, LIVE (ORAL) BP (Sabin strains)

Presentation Poliomyelitis Vaccine, Live (Oral) BP, as supplied by Smith Kline & French, is a light orange to pink liquid stabilised with molar magnesium chloride. Each dose (the entire contents of a monodose tube or 3 drops from a 10-dose tube) provides at least 10^6TCID$_{50}$ type 1 (LS-c,2ab), 10^5TCID$_{50}$ type 2 (P712, Ch, 2ab) and $10^{5.5}$TCID$_{50}$ type 3 (Leon 12a$_1$b) live attenuated strains of poliomyelitis virus grown in monkey kidney cell cultures, and contains not more than 7 micrograms (5 i.u.) neomycin sulphate.

Uses Active immunisation against poliomyelitis.

Dosage and administration *Adults and children: For oral use only:* NOT FOR INJECTION. The contents of a monodose tube or 3 drops of vaccine from a 10-dose tube constitute one dose which may be given with syrup or on a lump of sugar to mask the bitter salty taste of the magnesium chloride.

For a complete schedule, three doses of the vaccine should be given at intervals of at least four weeks (see also **Further information**).

Other unvaccinated members of the same household (including adults) should be advised vaccination at the same time as the vaccinee.

Contra-indications, warnings, etc
Contra-indications: The vaccine should not be used in the presence of acute febrile illness or intercurrent infection, diarrhoea, vomiting or other gastro-intestinal disturbance, neither should it be given in the presence of impaired immune response including leukaemia, lymphoma, generalised malignancy or treatment with corticosteroids, cytotoxic drugs or irradiation. Do not give to those known to be hypersensitive to neomycin (see also *Precautions*).

Precautions: The vaccine may contain trace amounts of penicillin and streptomycin which should not contra-indicate its use except in those with a history of severe anaphylaxis due to either antibiotic.

At least 3 weeks should normally intervene between the administration of any two live vaccines. Poliomyelitis vaccine can, however, be given simultaneously with measles, mumps and rubella vaccines and with DTP vaccine. In this case the injectable vaccines should be given at different sites.

Use in pregnancy: Pregnant women should not be given oral poliomyelitis vaccine unless they are at definite risk from poliomyelitis.

Adverse reactions: Paralysis temporally associated with vaccination has been reported very rarely in recipients or contacts.

Overdosage: Not applicable.

Pharmaceutical precautions Protect from light and store between 2°C and 6°C. Under these conditions there is no significant loss of virus titre for 12 months.

When tubes of vaccine have been opened there is a risk of contamination with bacteria and moulds which may result in a reduction of vaccine potency. It is good practice, therefore, to discard vaccine remaining in opened 10-dose tubes at the end of the vaccinating session. Any unopened vaccine should be returned to storage between 2°C and 6°C as soon as possible. Potency is maintained for two weeks at room temperature (20°C to 25°C).

Legal category POM.

Package quantities Plastic monodose dropper tubes in packs of 10; individual plastic 10-dose dropper tubes.

Further information Current policy recommends that the first dose of oral poliomyelitis vaccine should be given from two months of age. The primary course consists of three separate doses with intervals of one month between each dose, given at the same time as DTP vaccine.

It is currently recommended that a reinforcing dose of poliomyelitis vaccine should be given at school entry and at 15 to 19 years of age. Adults need not be offered a reinforcing dose unless they are at special risk.

Inactive ingredients are magnesium chloride, polysorbate 80, purified water, and also neomycin sulphate (see **Presentation**).

Product licence numbers

Monodose tubes	0002/0075
10-dose tubes	0002/0076

REDEPTIN* INJECTION

Presentation Each ampoule or vial of Redeptin contains an opalescent white aqueous suspension containing 2 mg fluspirilene in each 1 ml.

Uses Fluspirilene is a major tranquilliser of the diphenylbutylpiperidine group. It is slowly absorbed after intramuscular injection. Detectable blood levels are reached within four hours of injection, and the antipsychotic action usually lasts for about a week, with a range of 5 to 15 days.

Redeptin is recommended for the symptomatic treatment of schizophrenia, and has proved especially useful for maintenance therapy. It is of particular value in patients who are unreliable in taking oral medication.

Dosage and administration *Adults only:* The recommended starting dose is 2 mg a week by deep intramuscular injection; this may be increased by 2 mg a week according to response. Do not massage the injection site. The maintenance dosage for most patients is from 2 to 8 mg a week, but some may require up to 12 mg a week. Dosage should not exceed 20 mg a week. Gradual withdrawal from high dosage treatment is advisable.

Elderly: A quarter to half the usual starting dosage may be sufficient. See also *Precautions.*

Because individual response and dosage requirements can vary considerably, treatment should be started and dosage increased under close supervision.

As with all major tranquillisers clinical improvement may not be evident for several weeks after starting treatment, and there may also be delay before recurrence of symptoms after stopping treatment.

Administration: Before administration the container should be shaken well. The 6 ml vial should be used on one occasion only.

Contra-indications, warnings, etc

Contra-indications: Do not use in patients who have suffered uncontrollable adverse effects during previous treatment with diphenylbutylpiperidine derivatives or in those hypersensitive to such compounds.

Do not use in pregnancy, especially during the first and last trimesters, unless there are compelling reasons. There is no evidence of safety in human pregnancy, and there is some evidence of harmful effects in animal studies. Fluspirilene may be excreted into breast milk. Since the effect of even small quantities of fluspirilene on the infant brain is not established, nursing mothers should be advised to stop breast feeding.

Precautions: Patients who drive or operate machinery should be warned of the possibility of drowsiness.

Potentiation may occur if antipsychotic drugs are combined with CNS depressants such as alcohol, hypnotics and strong analgesics.

Elderly patients may be particularly sensitive, especially as regards extrapyramidal effects.

Care should be exercised in patients with known liver damage, and, because Redeptin contains povidone, in those with kidney damage.

In patients with Parkinson's disease, symptoms may be worsened, and the effects of levodopa reversed. Since fluspirilene may lower the convulsive threshold, patients with epilepsy or conditons pre-disposing to epilepsy, such as alcohol or brain damage, should be treated with caution, and metrizamide avoided; the effect of anticonvulsants may be impaired.

Although no neurotoxic interactions with lithium have been reported, this possibility should be borne in mind.

Nausea and vomiting as a sign of organic disease may be masked by the anti-emetic action of fluspirilene.

The possibilities of interaction with anticoagulants and of effects on control of diabetes have been raised with antipsychotic drugs but there have been no reports to date of such effects with fluspirilene.

Adverse reactions: The majority of side-effects occur during the first two days after injection. Extrapyramidal reactions are common in moderate to high dosage, and include especially dyskinesia and akathisia but also tremor, salivation, acute dystonias and oculogyric crises. They may occur within 6 to 12 hours after injection and usually disappear within 48 hours; they can normally be controlled by reduction of dosage or, when necessary, by the use of anticholinergic antiparkinsonism drugs.

Tardive dyskinesia may occur during or after long-term treatment with antipsychotic drugs. Symptoms (persistent dyskinesia of facial muscles, sometimes with involuntary movements of the extremities) may persist for prolonged periods, in some cases being irreversible. Elderly patients and those with organic brain damage are at particular risk. Periodic gradual reduction of dosage to reveal persisting dyskinesia has been suggested so that treatment may be stopped if necessary. Anticholinergic antiparkinsonism drugs may aggravate the condition. Since the occurrence of tardive dyskinesia may be related to length of treatment and dosage, Redeptin should be given for as short a time and at as low a dose as possible.

Subcutaneous nodules at the site of injection have been reported, usually in patients on high doses for long periods. These nodules tend to disappear when treatment is stopped. They may be minimised by using as many different injection sites as possible. Other reactions reported include fatigue and drowsiness, which may be dose-related and be particularly marked at the start of treatment, upper gastro-intestinal symptoms such as nausea and vomiting, insomnia, restlessness, excitement, anxiety, headache and sweating. There have also been occasional reports of autonomic symptoms such as blurred vision, hypotension and dizziness, rash, weight gain, and EEG and ECG changes. Increased prolactin levels, with galactorrhoea, gynaecomastia or amenorrhoea have been reported; certain hormone-dependent breast neoplasms may be affected. In some patients side-effects may become progressively more marked over a period of weeks or months; these signs of accumulation can be eliminated by omitting one injection every four or five weeks.

The neuroleptic malignant syndrome is a rare but occasionally fatal complication of treatment with various neuroleptic drugs, and is characterised by hyperpyrexia, muscle rigidity, altered consciousness and autonomic instability. Intensive symptomatic treatment should include cooling. Intravenous dantrolene has been suggested for muscle rigidity.

Jaundice has been rarely reported during treatment with Redeptin; transient abnormalities of liver function tests have also occurred.

Overdosage: In the unlikely event of accidental overdosage, signs and symptoms are likely to be predominantly extrapyramidal, possibly with some excitation. Treatment would consist of supportive and symptomatic measures. Extrapyramidal symptoms should be treated with an anticholinergic antiparkinsonism drug. The long-acting properties of the presentation should be borne in mind.

Pharmaceutical precautions Redeptin ampoules and vials should be stored upright at room temperature and protected from light.

Legal category POM.

Package quantities Redeptin ampoules, each containing either 2 mg fluspirilene in 1 ml or 6 mg fluspirilene in 3 ml, are available in boxes of 10. Redeptin vials, each containing 12 mg fluspirilene in 6 ml, are available in packs of 5.

Further information Maximal plasma levels of fluspirilene are found 4 to 8 hours after administration; it has a very prolonged excretion half-life of approximately 3 weeks.

Inactive ingredients are benzyl alcohol, polysorbate 80, sodium monohydrogen phosphate anhydrous, sodium dihydrogen phosphate monohydrate, povidone K17 and water for injection.

Product licence number 0002/0056R.

STELAZINE* TABLETS
STELAZINE* SPANSULE* CAPSULES
STELAZINE* SYRUP
STELAZINE* CONCENTRATE
STELAZINE* INJECTION

Presentation Blue, sugar-coated tablets, marked SKF, containing either 1 mg or 5 mg trifluoperazine present as the hydrochloride.

Clear, colourless capsules, opaque yellow-capped and filled with a mixture of dark and light blue and white pellets. Each Spansule capsule contains 2 mg, 10 mg or 15 mg trifluoperazine present as the hydrochloride; the capsules are double-marked 2, 10 and 15 respectively. Two-thirds of the dose of trifluoperazine is formulated for release over a period of six to eight hours.

A clear, pale yellow, peach-flavoured syrup, each 5 ml dose containing 1 mg trifluoperazine present as the hydrochloride.

A clear, pale yellow, peach-flavoured concentrate with a bitter numbing after-taste. Before dilution, each 1 ml of concentrate contains 10 mg trifluoperazine present as the hydrochloride.

Ampoules containing 1 mg trifluoperazine present as the hydrochloride in 1 ml.

Uses Stelazine is a piperazine phenothiazine tranquilliser with potent antipsychotic, anxiolytic, and anti-emetic activity, and a pharmacological profile of moderate sedative and hypotensive properties, and fairly pronounced tendency to cause extrapyramidal reactions.

Low dosage: Stelazine is indicated as an adjunct in the short term management of anxiety states, depressive symptoms secondary to anxiety, and agitation. It is also indicated in the symptomatic treatment of nausea and vomiting.

High dosage: Stelazine is indicated for the treatment of symptoms and prevention of relapse in schizophrenia and in other psychoses, especially of the paranoid type, but not in depressive psychoses. It may also be used as an adjunct in the short term management of severe psychomotor agitation and of dangerously impulsive behaviour in, for example, mental subnormality.

Dosage and administration *Adults: Low dosage:* 2–4 mg a day as tablets or syrup, given in divided doses, or one or two 2 mg Spansule capsules a day, according to the severity of the patient's condition. If necessary, dosage may be increased to 6 mg a day, but above this level extrapyramidal symptoms are more likely to occur in some patients.

High dosage: The recommended starting dose for physically fit adults is 5 mg twice a day (or one 10 mg Spansule capsule a day); after a week this may be increased to 15 mg a day (which may be given as one 15 mg Spansule capsule). If necessary, further increases of 5 mg may be made at three-day intervals, but not more often. When satisfactory control has been achieved, dosage should be reduced gradually until an effective maintenance level has been established. Stelazine Spansule capsules are particularly useful for such maintenance therapy.

As with all major tranquillisers clinical improvement may not be evident for several weeks after starting treatment, and there may also be delay before recurrence of symptoms after stopping treatment. Gradual withdrawal from high dosage treatment is advisable.

Intramuscular use: For a more rapid and intense effect or when oral administration presents difficulties, Stelazine may be given by deep intramuscular injection; the recommended dosage is 1–3 mg a day, given in divided doses. Higher dosages may sometimes be necessary up to a suggested maximum of 6 mg a day. Oral therapy should be substituted as soon as possible.

Elderly: Reduce starting dose in elderly or frail patients by at least half.

Children: Low dosage: For children aged 3–5 years, up to 1 mg a day as the syrup, given in divided doses. For children aged 6–12 years, the dosage may be increased to a maximum of 4 mg a day.

High dosage: For children aged under 12 years, the initial oral dosage should not exceed 5 mg a day, given in divided doses. Any subsequent increase should be made with caution, at intervals of not less than three days, and taking into account age, body weight and severity of symptoms.

Intramuscular use: There has been little experience in the use of intramuscular Stelazine in children. If required, a starting dose of 1 mg per 20 kg (44 lb) body weight a day, given in divided doses, is suggested.

Use of liquid presentations: Dilute Stelazine Concentrate before use with either purified water containing 0.1% benzoic acid or Sorbitol Solution BP. Dilution at the rate of 1 in 10 volumes gives a concentration of 5 mg trifluoperazine in each 5 ml dose. Stelazine Syrup may be diluted with Sorbitol Solution BP.

Both Stelazine Syrup and Concentrate may be administered with a drink of demineralised water or orange juice.

Contra-indications, warnings, etc

Contra-indications: Do not use Stelazine in comatose patients, or in those with existing blood dyscrasias or known liver damage, or in those hypersensitive to the active ingredient or related compounds.

Precautions: Care should be taken when treating elderly patients, and initial dosage should be reduced. Such patients can be especially sensitive, particularly to extrapyramidal and hypotensive effects. Patients with cardiovascular disease including arrhythmias should also be treated with caution. Because Stelazine may increase activity, care should be taken in patients with angina pectoris.

In patients with Parkinson's disease, symptoms may be worsened, and the effects of levodopa reversed. Since phenothiazines may lower the convulsive threshold, patients with epilepsy should be treated with caution, and metrizamide avoided. Although Stelazine has minimal anticholinergic activity, this should be borne in mind when treating patients with narrow angle glaucoma, myasthenia gravis or prostatic hypertrophy.

Nausea and vomiting as a sign of organic disease may be masked by the anti-emetic action of Stelazine.

Potentiation may occur if antipsychotic drugs are combined with CNS depressants such as alcohol, hypnotics and strong analgesics. Phenothiazines may antagonise the action of guanethidine.

Desferrioxamine should not be used in combination with Stelazine, since prolonged unconsciousness has occurred after combination with the related prochlorperazine.

Patients who drive or operate machinery should be warned of the possibility of drowsiness.

Use in pregnancy and lactation: Stelazine has been available since 1958. There are some animal studies that indicate a teratogenic effect, but results are conflicting. There is no clinical evidence (including follow-up surveys in over 800 women who had taken low-dosage Stelazine during pregnancy) to indicate that trifluoperazine has a teratogenic effect in man. Nevertheless, drug treatment should be avoided in pregnancy unless essential, especially during the first trimester. Trifluoperazine passes into the milk of lactating dogs.

Adverse reactions: Lassitude, drowsiness, dizziness, transient restlessness, insomnia, dry mouth, blurred vision, muscular weakness, anorexia, mild postural hypotension, skin reactions including photosensitivity reactions, weight gain, oedema and confusion may occasionally occur. Tachycardia, constipation, urinary hesitancy and retention, and hyperpyrexia have been reported very rarely. Adverse reactions tend to be dose related and to disappear. Hyperprolactinaemia may occur at higher dosages with associated effects such as galactorrhoea or amenorrhoea; certain hormone-dependent breast neoplasms may be affected. Phenothiazines can produce ECG changes with prolongation of the QT interval and T-wave changes; serious arrhythmias have been reported. Such effects are rare with Stelazine. In some patients, especially non-psychotic patients, Stelazine even at low dosage may cause unpleasant symptoms of being dulled or paradoxically of being agitated.

Extrapyramidal symptoms are rare at daily dosages of 6 mg or less; they are considerably more common at higher dosage levels. These symptoms include parkinsonism; akathisia, with motor restlessness and difficulty in sitting still; and acute dystonia or dyskinesia, which may occur early in treatment and may present with torticollis, facial grimacing, trismus, tongue protrusion and abnormal eye movements including oculogyric crises. Such reactions may often be controlled by reducing the dosage or by stopping medication. In more severe dystonic reactions, an anticholinergic antiparkinsonism drug should be given.

Tardive dyskinesia of the facial muscles, sometimes with involuntary movements of the extremities, has occurred in some patients on long-term high dosage and, more rarely, low-dosage phenothiazine therapy, including Stelazine. Symptoms may appear for the first time either during or after a course of treatment; they may become worse when treatment is stopped. The symptoms may persist for many months or even years, and while they gradually disappear in some patients, they appear to be permanent in others. Patients have most commonly been elderly, with organic brain damage. Particular caution should be observed in treating such patients. Periodic gradual reduction of dosage to reveal persisting dyskinesia has been suggested, so that treatment may be stopped if necessary. Anticholinergic antiparkinsonism agents may aggravate the condition. Since the occurrence of tardive dyskinesia may be related to length of treatment and dosage, Stelazine should be given for as short a time and at as low a dosage as possible.

The neuroleptic malignant syndrome is a rare but occasionally fatal complication of treatment with various neuroleptic drugs, and is characterised by hyperpyrexia, muscle rigidity, altered consciousness and autonomic instability. Intensive symptomatic treatment should include cooling. Intravenous dantrolene has been suggested for muscle rigidity.

Mild cholestatic jaundice, and blood dyscrasias such as agranulocytosis, pancytopenia, leucopenia and thrombocytopenia have been reported very rarely. Signs of persistent infection should be investigated.

Very rare cases of skin pigmentation and lenticular opacities have been reported with Stelazine.

Overdosage: Signs and symptoms will be predominantly extrapyramidal; hypotension may occur. Absorption of trifluoperazine from the Spansule capsule is likely to be prolonged, and this should be borne in mind. Treatment consists of gastric lavage together with supportive and symptomatic measures. Do not induce vomiting. Extrapyramidal symptoms may be treated with an anticholinergic antiparkinsonism drug. Treat hypotension with fluid replacement; if severe or persistent, noradrenaline may be considered. Adrenaline is contra-indicated.

Pharmaceutical precautions Store tablets in a dry place and protect from light. Store Spansule capsules in a dry place below 25°C and protect from light. Store syrup in carton and protect from light. If it is necessary to dilute the syrup use Sorbitol Solution BP; the diluted syrup is stable for 4 weeks. Store diluted syrup in the dark. Store concentrate at a temperature not exceeding 30°C and protect from light by storage in carton. The concentrate must be diluted before use, if possible with Sorbitol Solution BP; alternatively it may be diluted with purified water containing 0.1% w/v benzoic acid. If the concentrate is diluted with Sorbitol Solution BP and refrigerated or stored below 15°C, crystallisation of the diluent may occur. However this readily disappears if the product is stored at room temperature. The diluted concentrate when stored in the dark at a temperature not exceeding 30°C is stable for up to 3 months. Cloudiness may result if diluents containing sodium salts of parahydroxybenzoic acid esters are used. Protect ampoules from light.

Legal category POM.

Package quantities Tablets, 1 mg, in opaque blister packs of 100 (4 × 25). Tablets, 5 mg, in opaque blister packs of 100 (4 × 25) and containers of 5000.

Spansule Capsules, 2 mg, in opaque blister packs (OP) of 60 (4 × 15) and containers of 5000. Spansule Capsules, 10 mg, in opaque blister packs (OP) of 30 (2 × 15). Spansule Capsules, 15 mg, in opaque blister packs (OP) of 30 (2 × 15).

Syrup, in bottles (OP) containing 200 ml.

Concentrate, in bottles containing 100 ml and one litre.

Ampoules, each containing 1 ml, in boxes of 10.

Further information Inactive ingredients in the tablets include sucrose, in the Spansule capsules sugar and in the concentrate and syrup sodium benzoate. Inactive ingredients in the injection are sodium D tartrate, sodium dihydrogen phosphate, saccharin sodium, sodium chloride and water for injection.

Product licence numbers

Stelazine tablets, 1 mg	0002/5081R
Stelazine tablets, 5 mg	0002/5082R
Stelazine Spansule capsules, 2 mg	0002/5077R
Stelazine Spansule capsules, 10 mg	0002/5078R
Stelazine Spansule capsules, 15 mg	0002/5079R
Stelazine syrup	0002/5080R
Stelazine concentrate	0002/5076R
Stelazine injection	0002/5075R

TAGAMET* TABLETS
TAGAMET* EFFERVESCENT TABLETS
TAGAMET* SYRUP
TAGAMET* INJECTION
TAGAMET* INFUSION

Presentation Pale green, oval, film-coated Tiltab* tablets, engraved SK&F T800 on one side, containing 800 mg cimetidine.

Pale green, oblong, film-coated tablets, engraved TAGAMET on one side and SK&F 400 on reverse, containing 400 mg cimetidine.

Pale green, circular, film-coated Tiltab tablets, engraved TAGAMET on one side and SK&F 200 on reverse, containing 200 mg cimetidine.

White, circular, effervescent tablets with a raspberry odour, containing 400 mg cimetidine.

A clear, orange-coloured, peach-flavoured syrup, each 5 ml dose containing 200 mg cimetidine.

Ampoules containing 200 mg cimetidine in 2 ml solution.

Infusion bags (flexible plastic containers) containing 400 mg cimetidine in 100 ml 0.9% w/v sodium chloride.

Uses Tagamet is a histamine H_2-receptor antagonist which rapidly inhibits both basal and stimulated gastric secretion of acid and reduces pepsin output.

Tagamet is indicated in the treatment of duodenal and benign gastric ulceration, including that associated with non-steroidal anti-inflammatory agents, recurrent and stomal ulceration, oesophageal reflux disease and other conditions where reduction of gastric acid by Tagamet has been shown to be beneficial: persistent dyspeptic symptoms with or without ulceration, particularly meal-related upper abdominal pain, including such symptoms associated with non-steroidal anti-inflammatory agents; the prophylaxis of gastro-intestinal haemorrhage from stress ulceration in seriously ill patients; before general anaesthesia in patients thought to be at risk of acid aspiration (Mendelson's) syndrome, particularly obstetric patients during labour; to reduce malabsorption and fluid loss in the short bowel syndrome; and in pancreatic insufficiency to reduce degradation of enzyme supplements. Tagamet is also recommended in the management of the Zollinger-Ellison syndrome.

Dosage and administration Tagamet is usually given orally, but parenteral or nasogastric dosing may be substituted for all or part of the recommended oral dose in cases where oral dosing is impracticable or considered inappropriate.

The total daily dose by any route should not normally exceed 2.4 g. Dosage should be reduced in patients with impaired renal function (see *Precautions*).

Adults: Oral: For patients with duodenal or benign gastric ulceration, a single daily dose of 800 mg at bedtime is recommended. Otherwise the usual dosage is 400 mg twice a day with breakfast and at bedtime. Other effective regimens are 200 mg three times a day with meals and 400 mg at bedtime (1.0 g/day) and, if inadequate, 400 mg four times a day (1.6 g/day) also with meals and at bedtime.

Symptomatic relief is usually rapid. Treatment should be given initially for at least four weeks (six weeks in benign gastric ulcer, eight weeks in ulcer associated with continued non-steroidal anti-inflammatory agents). Most ulcers will have healed by that stage, but those which have not will usually do so after a further course of treatment.

Treatment may be continued for longer periods in those patients who may benefit from reduction of gastric secretion and the dosage may be reduced as appropriate to 400 mg at bedtime or 400 mg in the morning and at bedtime.

In patients with benign peptic ulcer disease, relapse may be prevented by continued treatment, usually with 400 mg at bedtime; 400 mg in the morning and at bedtime has also been used.

In oesophageal reflux disease, 400 mg four times a day, with meals and at bedtime, for four to eight weeks is recommended to heal oesophagitis and relieve associated symptoms.

In patients with very high gastric acid secretion (e.g. Zollinger-Ellison syndrome) it may be necessary to increase the dose to 400 mg four times a day, or in occasional cases further.

Antacids can be made available to all patients until symptoms disappear.

In the prophylaxis of haemorrhage from stress ulceration in seriously ill patients, doses of 200–400 mg can be given every four to six hours by oral, nasogastric or parenteral routes. By direct intravenous injection a dose of 200 mg should not be exceeded: see below.

In patients thought to be at risk of acid aspiration syndrome an oral dose of 400 mg can be given 90–120 minutes before induction of general anaesthesia or, in obstetric practice, at the start of labour. While such a risk persists, a dose of up to 400 mg may be repeated (parenterally if appropriate) at four-hourly intervals as required up to the usual daily maximum of 2.4 g. Tagamet syrup should not be used. The usual precautions to avoid acid aspiration should be taken.

In the short bowel syndrome, e.g. following substantial resection for Crohn's disease, the usual dosage range (see above) can be used according to individual response.

To reduce degradation of pancreatic enzyme supplements, 800–1600 mg a day may be given according to response in four divided doses, one to one and a half hours before meals.

Administration of effervescent tablets: The tablets should be dissolved in a glass of water.

Parenteral: Tagamet may be given intramuscularly or intravenously.

The dose by intramuscular injection is normally 200 mg which may be repeated at four- to six-hourly intervals.

The usual dosage for intravenous administration is 200–400 mg which may be repeated four- to six-hourly.

If direct intravenous injection cannot be avoided, 200 mg should be given **slowly** over at least 2 minutes, and may be repeated four- to six-hourly. Rapid intravenous injection has been associated with cardiac arrhythmias. If there is cardiovascular impairment, or if a larger dose is needed, the dose should be diluted and given over at least 10 minutes. In such cases infusion is preferable.

For intermittent intravenous infusion, the contents of one Tagamet Infusion bag (containing cimetidine 400 mg in 100 ml 0.9% w/v sodium chloride) should be infused over 30 minutes to 1 hour, and may be repeated every four to six hours.

If continuous intravenous infusion is required, Tagamet may be given at an average rate of 50 to 100 mg/hour over 24 hours.

Elderly: The normal adult dosage may be used unless renal function is markedly impaired (see *Precautions* and *Adverse reactions*).

Children: Experience in children is less than that in adults. In children more than one year old, Tagamet 25–30 mg/kg body weight per day in divided doses may be administered by either the oral or parenteral route.

The use of Tagamet in infants under one year old is not fully evaluated; 20 mg/kg body weight per day in divided doses has been used.

Contra-indications, warnings, etc

Contra-indication: Hypersensitivity to cimetidine.

Precautions: Dosage should be reduced in patients with impaired renal function according to creatinine clearance. The following dosages are suggested: creatinine clearance of 0 to 15 ml per minute, 200 mg twice a day; 15 to 30 ml per minute, 200 mg three times a day; 30 to 50 ml per minute, 200 mg four times a day; over 50 ml per minute, normal dosage. Cimetidine is removed by haemodialysis, but not to any significant extent by peritoneal dialysis.

Tagamet can prolong the elimination of drugs metabolised by oxidation in the liver. Although pharmacological interactions with a number of drugs, e.g. diazepam, propranolol, have been demonstrated, only those with oral anticoagulants, phenytoin, theophylline and intravenous lignocaine appear, to date, to be of clinical significance. Close monitoring of patients on Tagamet receiving oral anticoagulants or phenytoin is recommended and a reduction in the dosage of these drugs may be necessary.

Clinical trials of over six years' continuous treatment and more than thirteen years' widespread use have not revealed unexpected adverse reactions related to long-term therapy. The safety of prolonged use is not, however, fully established and care should be taken to observe periodically patients given prolonged treatment.

Tagamet treatment can mask the symptoms and allow transient healing of gastric cancer. The potential delay in diagnosis should particularly be borne in mind in patients of middle age and over with new or recently changed dyspeptic symptoms.

Care should be taken that patients with a history of peptic ulcer, particularly the elderly, being treated with Tagamet and a non-steroidal anti-inflammatory agent are observed regularly.

In patients on drug treatment or with illnesses that could cause falls in blood cell count, the possibility that H_2-receptor antagonism could potentiate this effect should be borne in mind.

Use in pregnancy and lactation: Although tests in animals and clinical evidence have not revealed any hazards from the administration of Tagamet during pregnancy or lactation, both animal and human studies have shown that it does cross the placental barrier and is excreted in milk. As with most drugs, the use of Tagamet should be avoided during pregnancy and lactation unless essential.

Adverse reactions: More than 35 million patients have been treated with Tagamet worldwide and adverse reactions have been infrequent. Diarrhoea, dizziness or rash, usually mild and transient, and tiredness have been reported. Gynaecomastia has been reported and is almost always reversible on discontinuing treatment. Biochemical or biopsy evidence of reversible liver damage has been reported occasionally. Reversible confusional states have occurred, usually in elderly or already very ill patients, e.g. those with renal failure. There have been very rare reports of interstitial nephritis, acute pancreatitis, thrombocytopenia, agranulocytosis (see *Precautions*), headache, myalgia, arthralgia, sinus bradycardia, tachycardia and heart block, all reversible on withdrawal of treatment, and aplastic anaemia. Alopecia has been reported but no causal relationship has been established. Reversible impotence has also been very rarely reported but no causal relationship has been established at usual therapeutic doses. Isolated increases of plasma creatinine have been of no clinical significance.

Overdosage: Acute overdosage of up to 20 grams has been reported several times with no significant ill effects. Induction of vomiting and/or gastric lavage may be employed together with symptomatic and supportive therapy.

Pharmaceutical precautions Store effervescent tablets in a dry place, and replace cap after use. Store syrup below 25°C, and ampoules below 30° C, protected from light. Store infusion bags below 25°C, and protect from light except during use.

Legal category POM.

Package quantities Tiltab Tablets, 800 mg, in opaque calendar packs (OP) of 30 (2 × 15) and 150 (10 × 15). Tablets, 400 mg, in opaque calendar packs (OP) of 60 (4 × 15), ward packs of 1000 (20 × 50) and containers of 2500. Tiltab Tablets, 200 mg, in opaque blister packs (OP) of 120 (4 × 30) and containers of 5000. Effervescent Tablets, 400 mg, in containers (OP) of 60 (3 tubes each containing 20 tablets). Syrup in bottles (OP) containing 600 ml. Ampoules in boxes of 20. Infusion bags in boxes of 20.

Further information Tagamet has been shown to be compatible with electrolyte and dextrose solutions commonly used for intravenous infusion.

Inactive ingredients in the effervescent tablets include aspartame and sodium benzoate. These tablets also contain sodium bicarbonate and sodium dihydrogen citrate, and the total sodium content per tablet is 178 mg. Inactive ingredients in the syrup include ethanol, methyl paraben, propyl paraben, sucrose and E110. Inactive ingredients in the injection are hydrochloric acid and water for injection and in the infusion are sodium chloride, hydrochloric acid, sodium hydroxide and water for injection.

Tagamet Effervescent Tablets may be particularly suitable for patients with difficulty in swallowing.

Product licence numbers

Tagamet Tiltab tablets 800 mg	0002/0128
Tagamet tablets 400 mg	0002/0092
Tagamet Tiltab tablets 200 mg	0002/0063R
Tagamet Effervescent Tablets 400 mg	0002/0206
Tagamet syrup	0002/0073R
Tagamet injection	0002/0059R
Tagamet infusion	0002/0112

VERTIGON* SPANSULE* CAPSULES

Presentation Clear, colourless capsules, opaque purple-capped and filled with a mixture of yellow-green and white pellets, in two strengths. Each Spansule sustained-release capsule, size No. 4, contains 10 mg, and each capsule, size No. 3, 15 mg prochlorperazine present as the maleate. Two-thirds of the dose is specially formulated for sustained release over a period of six to eight hours.

Uses Vertigon is a potent phenothiazine tranquilliser, anti-emetic, and vestibular sedative.

Vertigon Spansule capsules are indicated in the short term symptomatic treatment of vertigo due to Menière's disease, labyrinthitis or other causes; nausea and vomiting associated with vertigo or other causes; and as an adjunct in the short term management of anxiety states.

Dosage and administration *Adults and children aged 12 years and over:* Usually one 15 mg Vertigon Spansule capsule once or twice a day. In less severe cases one 10 mg capsule once or twice a day may be adequate. When satisfactory control has been achieved, a daily maintenance dosage of one 10 mg or 15 mg capsule may be given.

Elderly: Start with 10 mg once a day (see *Precautions*).

Contra-indications, warnings, etc

Contra-indications: Do not use Vertigon in patients with existing blood dyscrasias, known liver damage, phaeochromocytoma or in those hypersensitive to the active ingredient or related compounds.

Precautions: Care should be taken when treating elderly patients, and initial dosage should be reduced. Such patients can be especially sensitive, particularly to extrapyramidal and hypotensive effects. Patients with cardiovascular disease including arrythmias should also be treated with caution.

In patients with Parkinson's disease, symptoms may be worsened, and the effects of levodopa reversed. Since phenothiazines may lower the convulsive threshold, patients with epilepsy should be treated with caution, and metrizamide avoided. Although Vertigon has only slight anticholinergic activity, this should be borne in mind when treating patients with narrow angle glaucoma, myasthenia gravis or prostatic hypertrophy.

Nausea and vomiting as a sign of organic disease may be masked by the anti-emetic action of Vertigon.

Potentiation may occur if neuroleptic drugs are combined with CNS depressants such as alcohol, hypnotics and strong analgesics. Phenothiazines may antagonise the action of guanethidine and of clonidine. Avoid drugs that depress leucopoeisis.

Simultaneous administration of desferrioxamine and prochlorperazine has been observed to induce a transient metabolic encephalopathy characterised by loss of consciousness for 48 to 72 hours.

Patients who drive or operate machinery should be warned of the possibility of drowsiness.

Use in pregnancy and lactation: Prochlorperazine has been widely used for many years without apparent deleterious effects in pregnancy. There is however evidence of harmful effects in animals. Vertigon should be avoided in pregnancy especially during the first trimester except in cases of nausea and vomiting so intractable that the physician considers the benefit to outweigh the risk. Prochlorperazine passes into the milk of lactating dogs.

Adverse reactions: At dosages of 30 mg a day or less, side-effects may include drowsiness, dizziness, skin reactions, dry mouth and, rarely, hypotension. Hyperprolactinaemia may occur at higher dosages with associated effects such as galactorrhoea or amenorrhoea, but is extremely unusual at this dosage level.

Phenothiazines can produce ECG changes with prolongation of the QT interval and T-wave changes; serious arrhythmias have been reported. Such effects are rare with prochlorperazine at lower dosages. In some patients, especially non-psychotic patients, neuroleptics even at low dosage may cause unpleasant symptoms of being dulled or paradoxically of being agitated.

Extrapyramidal symptoms are rare at daily dosages of 30 mg or less. These symptoms include Parkinsonism; akathisia, with motor restlessness and difficulty in sitting still; and acute dystonia or dyskinesia, which may occur early in treatment and may present with torticollis, facial grimacing, trismus, tongue protrusion and abnormal eye movement including oculogyric crises. Such reactions may often be controlled by reducing the dosage or by stoppping medication. In more severe dystonic reactions, an anticholinergic antiparkinsonism drug should be given.

Tardive dyskinesia of the facial muscles, sometimes with involuntary movements of the extremities, has occurred in some patients on long-term high-dosage and, more rarely, low-dosage phenothiazine therapy, including prochlorperazine. Symptoms may appear for the first time either during or after a course of treatment; they may become worse when treatment is stopped. The symptoms may persist for many months or even years, and while they gradually disappear in some patients, they appear to be permanent in others. Patients have more commonly been elderly, with organic brain damage. Particular caution should be observed in treating such patients. Periodic gradual reduction of dosage to reveal persisting dyskinesia has been suggested, so that treatment may be stopped if necessary. Anticholinergic antiparkinsonism agents may aggravate the condition. Since the occurrence of tardive dyskinesia may be related to length of treatment and dosage, Vertigon should be given for as short a time and at as low a dosage as possible.

The neuroleptic malignant syndrome is a rare but occasionally fatal complication of treatment with various neuroleptic drugs, and is characterised by hyperpyrexia, muscle rigidity, altered consciousness and autonomic instability. Intensive symptomatic treatment should include cooling. Intravenous dantrolene has been suggested for muscle rigidity.

Rare cases of toxic hepatitis of a cholestatic type, and leucopenia and agranulocytosis have been reported with prochlorperazine. Signs of persistent infection should be investigated.

Skin pigmentation and lenticular opacities have been reported with long-term treatment with higher dosages of phenothiazines.

Overdosage: Signs and symptoms will be predominantly extrapyramidal; hypotension may occur. Absorption of prochlorperazine from the sustained-release Spansule capsule is likely to be prolonged, and this should be borne in mind. Treatment consists of gastric lavage together with appropriate supportive and symptomatic measures. Do not induce vomiting. Extrapyramidal symptoms may be treated with an anticholinergic antiparkinsonism drug. Treat hypotension with fluid replacement; if severe or persistent, noradrenaline may be considered. Adrenaline is contra-indicated.

Pharmaceutical precautions Store in a dry place below 25°C and protect from light.

Legal category POM.

Package quantities Both strengths in opaque blister packs (OP) of 60 (4 × 15) Spansule capsules.

Further information Inactive ingredients include sucrose and aluminium lake of E110.

Product licence numbers
Vertigon Spansule capsules, 10 mg 0002/0036R
Vertigon Spansule capsules, 15 mg 0002/0037R

Z SPAN* SPANSULE* CAPSULES

Presentation Clear, colourless capsules, opaque light blue-capped and filled with a mixture of white and grey pellets. Each Spansule sustained-release capsule contains 61.8 mg zinc sulphate monohydrate (22.5 mg elemental zinc) formulated for release over one to two hours.

Uses Z Span is an oral zinc preparation for use when inadequate diet calls for supplementary zinc and when the need for such therapy has been determined by a physician, and for the treatment of zinc deficiency which has been demonstrated.

Dosage and administration *Adults and children over 1 year:* As a dietary supplement, 1 Z Span Spansule capsule a day. For the treatment of frank zinc deficiency, 1 capsule three times a day, to be adjusted thereafter according to response. The capsule may be opened and the pellets mixed with soft, cool food, but they must not be chewed.

Elderly: Dosage as above.

Contra-indications, warnings, etc
Precautions: Zinc chelates with tetracyclines and absorption of both agents may be impaired.

Excessive zinc intake over long periods may affect absorption of other metals such as iron or copper, but no clinically significant effect is expected at the dose of one capsule a day.

In patients with renal failure, a risk of accumulation could exist.

Adverse reactions: Mild gastro-intestinal upset is occasionally produced by zinc sulphate but the sustained-release presentation is designed to minimise this effect.

Overdosage: A single dose in excess of 10 capsules may be emetic. A fatal dose of zinc sulphate is unlikely to be less than 10 g (equivalent to more than 150 capsules). Zinc sulphate in gross overdosage is corrosive. Symptoms are those of gastro-intestinal irritation, leading in severe cases to haemorrhage, corrosion of the mucosa and possible later stricture formation. Gastric lavage or emesis should be avoided. Demulcents such as milk should be given. Chelating agents such as dimercaprol, penicillamine or edetic acid have been recommended.

Symptomatic and supportive therapy should be given. Absorption of zinc may be slowed by the sustained-release presentation.

Pharmaceutical precautions Store in a dry place at a temperature not exceeding 30°C.

Legal category P.

Package quantities Opaque blister packs (OP) of 30 (2 × 15) Spansule capsules.

Further information Inactive ingredients include sucrose.

Product licence number 0002/0098.

**Trade Mark*

SmithKline Beecham Pharmaceuticals
Welwyn Garden City
Hertfordshire AL7 1EY

SmithKline Beecham Pharmaceuticals

SEROXAT* ▼ TABLETS

Presentation
20 mg tablets: White, film-coated, modified oval, biconvex tablets engraved 'Seroxat 20' on one side and having a breakline on the reverse. Each tablet contains paroxetine hydrochloride equivalent to 20 mg paroxetine free base.
30 mg tablets: Blue, film-coated, modified oval, biconvex tablets engraved 'Seroxat 30' on one side and having a breakline on the reverse. Each tablet contains paroxetine hydrochloride equivalent to 30 mg paroxetine free base.

Uses Treatment of symptoms of depressive illness of all types including depression accompanied by anxiety.

Dosage and administration For oral administration the recommended dose is 20 mg daily. In some patients it may be necessary to increase the dose. This should be done gradually by 10 mg increments to a maximum of 50 mg according to the patient's response.

It is recommended that Seroxat be administered once daily in the morning with food.

The tablet should be swallowed rather than chewed. As with all antidepressant drugs, dosage should be reviewed and adjusted if necessary within two to three weeks of initiation of therapy and thereafter as judged clinically appropriate. It is recommended that a course of antidepressant treatment should continue for a sufficient period, which may be several months. As with any psychoactive medicine, it is advisable to discontinue therapy gradually as abrupt or sudden discontinuation may lead to symptoms such as disturbed sleep, irritability or dizziness.

Elderly: Increased plasma concentrations of Seroxat occur in elderly subjects.

The recommended dose is 20 mg daily. In some patients it may be necessary to increase the dose. This should be done gradually by 10 mg increments to a maximum of 40 mg according to the patient's response.

Children: The use of Seroxat in children is not recommended as safety and efficacy have not been established in this population.

Renal/hepatic impairment: Increased plasma concentrations of Seroxat occur in patients with severe renal impairment (creatinine clearance <30 ml/min) or severe hepatic impairment. Therefore dosage should be restricted to the lower end of the dosage range.

Contra-indications, warnings, etc
Contra-indication: Known hypersensitivity to paroxetine.

Use during pregnancy and lactation: Although animal studies have not shown any teratogenic or selective embryotoxic effects, the safety of Seroxat in human pregnancy has not been established and it should not be used during pregnancy or by nursing mothers unless the potential benefit outweighs the possible risk.

Warnings: MAO inhibitors: As with most antidepressants, Seroxat should not be used in combination with MAO inhibitors or within two weeks of terminating treatment with MAO inhibitors. Thereafter treatment should be initiated cautiously and dosage increased gradually until optimal response is reached.

MAO inhibitors should not be introduced within two weeks of cessation of therapy with Seroxat.

History of mania: As with all antidepressants, Seroxat should be used with caution in patients with a history of mania.

Patients receiving oral anticoagulants: Seroxat should be administered with great caution to patients receiving oral anticoagulants. (See 'Interactions').

Precautions: Cardiac conditions: Seroxat does not produce clinically significant changes in blood pressure, heart rate and ECG. Nevertheless, as with all psychoactive drugs, caution is advised when treating patients with cardiac conditions.

Epilepsy: As with other antidepressants, Seroxat should be used with caution in patients with epilepsy.

Seizures: Overall, the incidence of seizures is <0.1% in patients treated with Seroxat. Seroxat should be discontinued in any patient who develops seizures.

ECT: There is little clinical experience of concurrent administration of Seroxat with ECT.

Ability to drive/use machines: Clinical experience has shown that therapy with Seroxat is not associated with impairment of cognitive or psychomotor function. However, as with all psychoactive drugs, patients should be cautioned about their ability to drive a car and operate machinery.

Interactions: Food/antacids: The absorption and pharmacokinetics of Seroxat are not affected by food or antacids.

Tryptophan: As with other 5-HT re-uptake inhibitors, animal studies indicate that an interaction between Seroxat and tryptophan may occur, resulting in a 'serotonin syndrome' suggested by a combination of agitation, restlessness and gastrointestinal symptoms including diarrhoea.

Drug metabolising enzyme inducers/inhibitors: The metabolism and pharmacokinetics of Seroxat may be affected by drugs which induce or inhibit hepatic drug metabolising enzymes.

When Seroxat is to be co-administered with a known drug metabolising inhibitor, consideration should be given to using doses at the lower end of the range. No initial dosage adjustment of Seroxat is considered necessary when it is to be co-administered with known drug metabolising enzyme inducers. Any subsequent dosage adjustment should be guided by clinical effect (tolerability and efficacy).

Alcohol: Although Seroxat does not increase the impairment of mental and motor skill caused by alcohol, the concomitant use of Seroxat and alcohol in depressed patients is not advised.

Haloperidol/amylobarbitone/oxazepam: Experience in a limited number of healthy subjects has shown that Seroxat did not increase the sedation and drowsiness associated with haloperidol, amylobarbitone or oxazepam when given in combination.

MAOIs: As with other 5-HT re-uptake inhibitors, animal studies indicate that an interaction between Seroxat and monoamine oxidase (MAO) inhibitors may occur (see 'Warnings' section).

Lithium: Since there is little clinical experience, and there have been reports of interaction of lithium with other 5-HT re-uptake inhibitors, the concurrent administration of Seroxat and lithium should be undertaken with caution. Lithium levels should be monitored.

Phenytoin/anticonvulsants: Co-administration with Seroxat and phenytoin is associated with decreased plasma concentrations of Seroxat and increased adverse experiences.

Co-administration of Seroxat with other anticonvulsants may also be associated with an increased incidence of adverse experiences.

Warfarin: Preliminary data suggest that there may be a pharmacodynamic interaction between Seroxat and warfarin which may result in increased bleeding in the presence of unaltered prothrombin times. Seroxat should therefore be administered with great caution to patients receiving oral anticoagulants.

Side effects: The most commonly observed adverse events associated with the use of Seroxat and not seen at an equivalent incidence among placebo-treated patients were: nausea, somnolence, sweating, tremor, asthenia, dry mouth, insomnia and sexual dysfunction. Adverse experiences may decrease in intensity and frequency with continued treatment and do not generally lead to cessation of therapy.

Clinical experience has shown that Seroxat is not associated with tachycardia or postural hypotension. Seroxat is less likely than tricyclic antidepressants to be associated with dry mouth, constipation and somnolence.

Overdose: Data on Seroxat overdose are limited.

Symptoms of overdose with Seroxat include nausea, vomiting, tremor, dilated pupils, dry mouth and irritability.

Overdose attempts have been reported with Seroxat in 16 patients who took up to 850 mg alone or in combination with other agents.

In these patients, there are no reports of ECG abnormalities, coma or convulsions and recovery was medically uneventful.

No specific antidote is known.

Treatment should consist of those general measures employed in the management of overdose with any antidepressant. Early administration of activated charcoal may delay the absorption of Seroxat.

Pharmaceutical precautions Store at room temperature.

Legal category POM.

Package quantities 20 mg and 30 mg tablets. Available in Original Packs of 30 (two calendar strips of 15 tablets).

Further information Seroxat is a potent and selective inhibitor of 5-hydroxytryptamine re-uptake (5-HT, serotonin) and its antidepressant action is thought to be related to its specific inhibition of 5-HT re-uptake in brain neurones.

Seroxat is chemically unrelated to the tricyclic, tetracyclic and other available antidepressants.

The principal metabolites of Seroxat are polar and conjugated products of oxidation and methylation which are readily cleared. In view of their relative lack of pharmacological activity, it is most unlikely that they contribute to the therapeutic effects of Seroxat.

Seroxat is well absorbed after oral dosing and undergoes first-pass metabolism.

The elimination half-life is variable but is generally about one day. Steady state systemic levels are attained by 7–14 days after starting treatment and pharmacokinetics do not appear to change during long-term therapy.

Seroxat inhibits the hepatic cytochrome P450 isozyme responsible for the metabolism of debrisoquine and sparteine. This may lead to enhanced plasma levels of those co-administered drugs which are metabolised by this isozyme. Such drugs may include certain tricyclic antidepressants, phenothiazine neuroleptics and type Ic anti-arrhythmics.

Long-term treatment with Seroxat has shown that efficacy is maintained for periods of at least one year.

Product licence numbers

Seroxat 20 mg Tablets	10592/0001
Seroxat 30 mg Tablets	10592/0002

**Trade Mark*

Solco Basle (UK) Ltd
3 Cliveden Office Village
Lancaster Road
High Wycombe
Bucks HP12 3YZ

GYNATREN*

Presentation A white sterile suspension for intramuscular injection. Each 0.5 ml ampoule of the vaccine contains 7×10^9 inactivated *Lactobacillus acidophilus* organisms in isotonic saline with 0.25% w/v of phenol as preservative.

Uses Gynatren is a vaccine that stimulates antibody production against aberrant coccoid forms of lactobacilli associated with trichomoniasis and also, by cross-reaction, against the trichomonads themselves. The normal vaginal flora and acidity is restored.

Indication: Prophylaxis of recurrent trichomoniasis in women.

Dosage and administration Three intramuscular injections of 0.5 ml at an interval of two weeks between each dose. Shake the ampoule before opening.

Contra-indications, warnings, etc
Contra-indications: Gynatren should not be administered during acute febrile infections nor in the presence of significant haematopoietic, renal nor heart disease with decompensation.

Precautions: Although anaphylaxis following Gynatren injections has never been reported, facilities for its management should always be available during vaccination.

Side- and adverse-effects: Local inflammation at the injection site has been reported and fever may occur concurrently.

Use in pregnancy: There is no recorded experience of use during pregnancy or lactation.

Pharmaceutical precautions Gynatren should be stored refrigerated at 4–8°C. Do not freeze.

Legal category POM.

Package quantities In packs of 3 × 0.5 ml ampoules.

Further information A trichomonacide preparation may be given at the time of first injection.

Product licence number 1317/0001.

SOLCO* ALBU-RES

Presentation A kit contains 5 vials. Each vial contains 2.5 mg Human Albumin BP as a microcolloid and 0.4 mg stannous chloride dihydrate. The sterile, pyrogen-free formulation is freeze-dried and sealed under nitrogen.

Uses Addition of sodium pertechnetate (^{99m}Tc) injection to a maximum of 5.55 GBq (150 mCi) labels the microcolloid for liver and spleen scintigraphy.

Dosage and administration
Scintigraphy of liver and spleen
Adults: Dose range 40–80 MBq (1–2.2 mCi) by intravenous injection. Imaging is started 10–60 minutes after injection.

Elderly patients: As adult dose.

Children: Solco Albu-Res is not recommended for use in children.

Preparation of the ^{99m}Tc Solco Albu-Res injection should use aseptic technique as follows:
1. Wipe the closure of a vial with a sterilising swab, place the vial in a lead shield.
2. Using a 10 ml sterile syringe inject 1–5 ml of sterile, pyrogen-free ^{99m}Tc eluate into the vial. Remove an equal volume of the inert gas from the vial with the syringe to normalize the pressure.

Note: To minimise the level of ionic aluminium from undiluted ^{99m}Tc eluates, use a minimum volume and adjust the final volume with oxidant-free normal saline for injection.

3. Resuspend the contents of the vial by gently swirling the milky-white colloid suspension and allow it to incubate at room temperature for at least 5 minutes.

Contra-indications, warnings, etc Use is contra-indicated in persons with a history of hyper-sensitivity to products containing human albumin.

Side-effects: No adverse effects occurred during clinical trials of Solco Albu-Res.

Use in pregnancy and lactation: There is no evidence on the drug's safety in human pregnancy nor is there evidence from animal work that it is free from hazard. Avoid in pregnant or nursing women unless there is no safer alternative.

In any woman of child-bearing age the potential risk of its use, should pregnancy occur, must be weighed against the anticipated benefits.

It is not recommended that Solco Albu-Res should be administered to breast-feeding mothers.

Precautions: Solco Albu-Res should be used only by persons experienced in the use of radio-pharmaceutical products and in units with adequate equipment and facilities.

Overdosage: The administration of a complete vial i.e. 2.5 mg human albumin, would not be likely to cause any adverse pharmacological effect.

Pharmaceutical precautions Store the Solco Albu-Res kit at 2–8°C.

Store the prepared injection at room temperature and use within 6 hours. Contains no preservatives.

Legal category POM.

Package quantities Each pack contains 5 vials.

Further information Nil.

Product licence number 1317/0003.

Product licence holder: Solco Basle Ltd, CH-4127 Birsfelden, Switzerland.

SOLCO* NANOCOLL

Presentation A kit contains 5 vials. Each vial contains 0.5 mg Human Albumin BP as a nanocolloid and 0.2 mg stannous chloride dihydrate. The sterile, pyrogen-free formulation is freeze-dried and sealed under nitrogen.

Uses Addition of sodium pertechnetate ^{99m}Tc injection to a maximum of 5.55 GBq (150 mCi) labels the nanocolloid for bone marrow imaging and lymphoscintigraphy.

Dosage and administration
Bone marrow scintigraphy

Adults: Dose range 185–400 MBq (5–11 mCi) by intravenous injection. Imaging is started 45–60 minutes post injection.

Elderly patients: As adult dose.

Children: Solco Nanocoll is not recommended for children.

Lymphoscintigraphy
Adults: Dose range by single or multiple subcutaneous injection 18–40 MBq (0.5–1 mCi) per investigation. The dose is dependent on the anatomical areas to be investigated and upon the time interval between injection and imaging. A maximum volume of 0.5 ml per injection site should not be exceeded. Recommended volumes are 0.2–0.3 ml. When performing lymphoscintigraphy of the lower limbs, dynamic imaging can start immediately after the injections, static imaging 30–60 minutes later. Additional images can be taken up to several hours later, i.e. using repeated injections separated by several hours.

Elderly patients: As adult dose.

Children: Solco Nanocoll is not recommended for use in children.

Preparation of the Tc-99m Solco Nanocoll injection should use aseptic technique as follows:

1. Wipe the closure of a vial with a sterilising swab, place the vial in a lead shield.
2. Using a 10 ml sterile syringe inject 1–5 ml of sterile, pyrogen-free Tc-99m eluate into the vial. Remove an equal volume of the inert gas from the vial with the syringe to normalise the pressure.

Note: To minimise the level of ionic aluminium from undiluted Tc-99m eluates, use a minimum volume and adjust the final volume with oxidant-free normal saline for injection.

3. Resuspend the contents of the vial by gently swirling the colloid suspension and allow it to incubate at room temperature for 5–10 minutes.

Contra-indications, warnings, etc Use is contra-indicated in persons with a history of hyper-sensitivity to products containing human albumin.

Lymphoscintigraphy can be considered as contra-indicated in patients with complete blockage of the lymphatic system, particularly in the lower extremities because of the potential radiation hazard at the injection sites e.g. after contrast angiography.

Side-effects: No adverse effects have been reported following the use of Solco Nanocoll.

Use in pregnancy and lactation: There is no evidence on the drug's safety in human pregnancy nor is there evidence from animal work that it is free from hazard. Avoid in pregnant or nursing women unless there is no safer alternative.

In any woman of child-bearing age the potential risk of its use, should pregnancy occur, must be weighed against the anticipated benefits.

It is not recommended that Solco Nanocoll be administered to breast-feeding mothers.

Precautions: Solco Nanocoll should be used only by persons experienced in the use of radio-pharmaceutical products and in units with adequate equipment and facilities.

Overdosage: The administration of a complete vial i.e. 0.5 mg human albumin, would not be likely to cause any adverse pharmacological effects.

Pharmaceutical precautions Store the Solco Nanocoll Kit at 2–8°C.

Store the prepared injection at room temperature and use within 6 hours. Contains no preservatives.

Legal category POM.

Package quantities Each pack contains 5 vials.

Further information Nil.

Product licence number 1317/0002.

Product licence holder: Solco Basle Ltd, CH-4127 Birsfelden, Switzerland.

SOLCO* VENTICOLL

Presentation A kit contains 5 vials. Each vial contains 0.5 mg Human Albumin BP as a colloid and 0.2 mg stannous chloride dihydrate. The freeze-dried formulation is conditioned to be low in bacterial contents and free of pathogenic microorganisms and is sealed under nitrogen.

Uses Addition of sodium pertechnetate (^{99m}Tc) injection to a maximum of 5.55 GBq (150 mCi) labels the colloid for use in lung ventilation scintigraphy by aerosol inhalation.

Dosage and administration
Route of administration: Solco Venticoll is conditioned for inhalaltion scintigraphy only. The contents of the kit are tested to ensure that they are low in bacterial contents and free of pathogenic microorganisms to meet the specific requirements for substances intended for inhalation. Hence the contents of the Solco Venticoll kit are not sterile nor pyrogen-free and may *not be used for injection.*

Ventilation scintigraphy
Adults: The adult dose is 11 MBq (300 μCi) to be deposited in the lungs. The dose to be introduced into the nebuliser to yield this deposit depends on the characteristics of the aerosol generator used and, to a certain extent, on the condition of the patient to be investigated.

Imaging is started immediately after inhalation of the aerosol.

Elderly patients: As adult dose.

Children: Solco Venticoll is not recommended for use in children.

Preparation of the ^{99m}Tc Solco Venticoll suspension should use aseptic technique as follows:

1. Wipe the closure of a vial with a sterilising swab, place the vial in a lead shield.
2. Using a 10 ml sterile syringe inject 3–6 ml of sterile, pyrogen-free Tc-99m eluate into the vial. Remove an equal volume of the inert gas from the vial with the syringe to normalise the pressure.

Note: To minimise the level of ionic aluminium from undiluted Tc-99m eluates, use a minimum volume and adjust the final volume with oxidant-free normal saline for injection.

3. Resuspend the contents of the vial by gently swirling the colloid suspension and allow it to incubate at room temperature for 5–10 minutes.

Contra-indications, warnings, etc Use is contra-indicated in persons with a history of hypersensitivity to products containing human albumin.

Side-effects: No adverse effects have been reported.

Use in pregnancy and lactation: There is no evidence on the drug's safety in human pregnancy nor is there evidence from animal work that it is free from hazard. Avoid in pregnant or nursing women unless there is no safer alternative.

In any woman of child-bearing age the potential risks of its use, should pregnancy occur, must be weighed against the anticipated benefits.

It is not recommended that Solco Venticoll should be administered to breast-feeding mothers.

Precautions: Solco Venticoll should be used only by persons experienced in the use of radio-pharmaceutical products and in units with adequate equipment and facilities.

Overdosage: Overdosage of human albumin by this route of administration would not be likely to cause any adverse pharmacological effect.

Pharmaceutical precautions Store the Solco Venticoll kit at 2–8°C.

Store the prepared suspension at room temperature and use within 6 hours. Contains no preservatives.

Legal category POM.

Package quantities Each pack contains 5 vials.

Further information Nil.

Product licence number 1317/0004

Product licence holder: Solco Basle Ltd, CH-4127 Birsfelden, Switzerland.

**Trade Mark*

E. R. Squibb & Sons Limited
Bristol-Myers Squibb House
Staines Rd
Hounslow TW3 3JA

SQUIBB

ACEPRIL*

Presentation

Acepril tablets 12.5 mg: Slightly mottled, white, flat faced, capsule shaped tablets, each containing captopril 12.5 mg. Engraved with "A" on one side with a bisecting bar on the other.

Acepril tablets 25 mg: Slightly mottled, white, round, biconvex tablets each containing captopril 25 mg. Engraved with "ACE 25" on one side and with quadrisect bars (for identification only) on the other.

Acepril tablets 50 mg: Slightly mottled, white, round, biconvex tablets each containing captopril 50 mg. Engraved with "ACE 50" on one side with a bisecting bar on the other.

Other ingredients: Lactose, maize starch, microcrystalline cellulose, stearic acid.

Uses

Actions: Captopril, 1–[(2S)-3-mercapto-2-methyl-propionyl]-L-proline, is a highly specific competitive inhibitor of angiotensin I-converting enzyme, the enzyme responsible for the conversion of angiotensin I to angiotensen II.

Indications

Hypertension: Acepril is indicated for the first line treatment of mild to moderate hypertension.

In severe hypertension it should be used where standard therapy is ineffective or inappropriate.

Congestive heart failure: Acepril is indicated for the treatment of congestive heart failure. The drug should be used together with diuretics and, where appropriate digitalis.

Dosage and administration

Hypertension: Treatment with Acepril should be at the lowest effective dose which should be titrated according to the needs of the patient.

Mild to moderate hypertension: The starting dose is 12.5 mg twice daily. The usual maintenance dose is 25 mg twice daily which can be increased incrementally, at 2-4 week intervals, until a satisfactory response is achieved, to a maximum of 50 mg twice daily.

A thiazide diuretic may be added to Acepril if satisfactory response has not been achieved. The dose of diuretic may be increased at 1-2 week intervals to the level of optimum response or until the maximum dose is reached.

Severe hypertension: In severe hypertension where standard therapy is ineffective or inappropriate because of adverse affects, the starting dose is 12.5 mg b.d. The dosage may be increased incrementally to a maximum of 50 mg t.i.d. Acepril should be used together with other anti-hypertensive agents but the dose of these should be individually titrated. A daily dose of 150 mg of Acepril should not normally be exceeded.

Heart failure: Acepril therapy must be started under close medical supervision. Acepril should be introduced when diuretic therapy (such as frusemide 40-80 mg or equivalent) is insufficient to control symptoms. A starting dose of 6.25 mg or 12.5 mg may minimise a transient hypotensive effect. The possibility of this occuring can be reduced by discontinuing or reducing diuretic therapy if possible, prior to initiating Acepril. the usual maintenance dose is 25 mg two or three times a day which can be increased incrementally, with intervals of at least two weeks, until a satisfactory response is achieved. The usual maximum dose is 150 mg daily.

Elderly: The dose should be titrated against the blood pressure response and kept as low as possible to achieve adequate control. Since elderly patients may have reduced renal function and other organ dysfunctions, it is suggested that a low dose of Acepril be used initially.

Children: Acepril is not recommended for the treatment of mild to moderate hypertension in children.

Experience in neonates, particularly premature infants, is limited. Because renal function in infants is not equivalent to that of older children and adults, lower doses of Acepril should be used with the patients under close medical supervision.

The starting dose should be 0.3 mg per Kg bodyweight up to a maximum of 6 mg per Kg bodyweight daily in divided doses. The dose should be individualised according to the response and may be given two or three times daily.

Patients with renal impairment: Acepril is not recommended in patients with renal impairment. Where it is clinically indicated in severly hypertensive patients with impaired renal function, the dose should be kept as low as possible to maintain adequate blood pressure control. The dose can be titrated against the response but adequate time should be allowed between dosage adjustments. In these patients a loop-diuretic rather than a thiazide should be the diuretic of choice.

Acepril is readily eliminated by haemodialysis.

Contra-indications, warnings, etc

Contra-indications: A history of previous hypersensitivity to the product.

Pregnancy: Acepril has been shown to be lethal to rabbit and sheep foetuses. There were no foetotoxic effects to hamster or rat foetuses.

Acepril is contra-indicated in pregnancy and should not be used in women of child bearing potential unless protected by effective contraception.

Exposure of the mother in the second and third trimesters of pregnancy has been associated with oligohydramnois and neonatal hypotension and/or anuria.

Precautions: Evaluation of the patient should include assessment of renal function prior to initiation of therapy and at appropriate intervals thereafter. Patients with renal impairment should not normally be treated with captopril.

Acepril should not be used in patients with aortic stenosis or outflow tract obstruction.

As limited experience has been obtained in the treatment of acute hypertensive crises, the use of Acepril should be avoided in these patients.

Warnings: The incidence of adverse reactions to captopril is principally associated with renal function since the drug is excreted primarily by the kidney. The dose should not exceed that necessary for adequate control and should be reduced in patients with impaired renal function.

Hypotension: With the first one or two doses some patients may experience symptomatic hypotension. In most instances, symptoms are relieved simply by the patient lying down.

In patients with severe and renin dependent hypertension (e.g. renovascular hypertension) or severe congestive heart failure who are receiving large doses of diuretic, exaggerated hypotensive responses have occured usually within one hour of the initial dose of Acepril. In these patients, by discontinuing diuretic therapy or significantly reducing the diuretic dose for four to seven days prior to initiating Acepril the possibility of this occurence is reduced. By commencing Acepril therapy with small doses (6.25 mg or 12.5 mg) the duration of any hypotensive effect is lessened. Some patients may benefit from an infusion of saline.

The occurence of first dose hypotension does not preclude subsequent dose titration with Acepril.

Hypotension has been occasionally reported in patients on Acepril due to causes of acute volume depletion such as vomiting and diarrhoea.

Serum potassium: Since Acepril decreases aldosterone production, serum potassium is usually maintained in patients on diuretics. Potassium sparing diuretics or potassium supplements should not therefore be used routinely. In patients with marked renal impairment a significant elevation of serum potassium may occur.

Renal: Proteinuria in patients with prior normal renal function is rare.

Where proteinuria has occured it has usually been in patients with severe hypertension and evidence of prior renal disease. Nephrotic syndrome occured in some of these patients.

In patients with evidence of prior renal disease, monthly urinary protein estimations (dip stick) are recommended for the first 9 months of therapy. If repeated determinations show increasing amounts of urinary protein, a 24-hour quantitative determination should be obtained, and if this exceeds 1 g/day, the benefits and risks of continuing Acepril should be evaluated.

Although membranous glomerulopathy was found in biopsies taken from some proteinuric patients, a causal relationship to Acepril has not been established.

Some patients with renal disease, particularly those with bilateral renal artery stenosis or unilateral renal artery stenosis in a single functioning kidney, have developed increased concentrations of blood urea and serum creatinine. Acepril dosage reduction and/or discontinuation of diuretic may be required. For some of these patients it may not be possible to normalise blood pressure and maintain adequate renal perfusion.

Haematological: Neutropenia/agranulocytosis, thromboyctopenia and anaemia have been reported in patients receiving Acepril.

In patients with normal renal function and no other complicating factors, neutropenia occurs rarely.

Acepril should not be used routinely in patients with pre-existing impaired renal function, collagen vascular disease, immunosuppressant therapy, treatment with allopurinol or procainamide, or a combination of these complicating factors. Some of these patients developed serious infections which in a few instances did not respond to intensive antibiotic therapy.

If Acepril is used in such patients, it is advised that white blood cell count and differential counts should be performed prior to therapy, every 2 weeks during the first 3 months of Acepril therapy, and periodically thereafter.

During treatment all patients should be instructed to report any sign of infection (e.g. sore throat, fever), when a differential white blood cell count should be performed. Acepril and other concomitant medication should be withdrawn if neutropenia (neutrophils less than 1000/mm^3) is detected or suspected.

In most patients neutrophil counts rapidly returned to normal upon discontinuing Acepril.

Nursing mothers: Because captopril is excreted in breast milk, Acepril should not be used in nursing mothers.

Surgery anaesthesia: In patients undergoing major surgery, or during anaesthesia with agents which produced hypotension, captopril will block angiotensin II formation secondary to compensatory renin release. This may lead to hypotension which can be corrected by volume expansion.

Clinical chemistry: Acepril may cause a false-positive urine test for acetone.

Side-effects

Idiosyncratic: angioedema involving the extremities, face lips, mucous membranes, tongue, glottis or larynx has been seen in patients treated with ACE inhibitors, including captoporil. In this situation, the ACE inhibitors, should be discontinued. Where swelling is confined to the face, lips and mouth the condition will usually resolve without further treatment, although antihistamines may be useful in relieving symptoms. These patients should be followed carefully until the swelling has resolved. However, where there is involvement of the tongue, glottis or larynx, likely to cause airway obstruction, subcutaneous adrenaline (0.5 ml, 1:1,000) should be administered promptly where indicated.

Haematological: Neutropenia, anaemia and thrombocytopenia (see Warnings). Rarely a positive ANA has been reported.

Renal: Proteinuria, elevated blood urea and creatinine, elevated serum potassium and acidosis (see Warnings).

Cardiovascular: Hypotension (see Warnings), tachycardia.

Skin: Rashes, usually pruritic, may occur. They are usually mild, maculopapular, rarely urticarial and disappear within a few days of dosage reduction, short-term treatment with an antihistamine and/or discontinuing therapy. In a few cases the rash has been associated with fever. Pruritus, flushing, vesicular or bullous rash, and photosensitivity have been reported.

Gastrointestinal: Reversible and usually self-limiting taste impairment has been reported. Weight loss may be associated with the loss of taste. Stomatitis, resembling aphthous ulcers, has been reported. Elevation of liver enzymes has been noted in a few patients. Rare cases of hepatocellular injury and cholestatic jaundice have been reported. Gastric irritation and abdominal pain may occur.

Other: Paraesthesias of the hands, serum sickness, cough, bronchospasm and lymphadenopathy have been reported.

Overdosage: In the event of overdosage, blood pressure should be monitored and if hypotension develops volume expansion is the treatment of choice. Captopril is removed by dialysis.

Drug interactions

Diuretics: Diuretics potentiate the anti-hypertensive effectiveness of Acepril.

Potassium-sparing diuretics (triamterene, amiloride and spironolactone), or potassium supplements may cause significant increase in serum potassium.

Indomethacin: A reduction of anti-hypertensive effectiveness may occur. This is probably also the case with other non-steroidal anti-inflammatory drugs.

Vasodilators: Acepril has been reported to act synergistically with peripheral vasodilators such as minoxidil. Awareness of this interaction may avert an initial hypotensive response.

Clondine: It has been suggested that the anti-hypertensive effect of Acepril can be delayed when patients treated with clonidine are changed to Acepril.

Allopurinol & procainamide: There have been reports of neutropenia and/or Stevens-Johnson syndrome in patients on Acepril plus either allopurinol or procainamide. Although a causal relationship has not been established, these combinations should only be used with caution, especially in patients with impaired renal function.

Immunosuppressants: Azathioprine and cyclophosphamide have been associated with blood dyscrasias in patients with renal failure who were also taking Acepril.

Probenecid: The renal clearance of Acepril is reduced in the presence of probenecid.

Pharmaceutical precautions Store at room temperature.

Legal category POM.

Package quantities

Tablets 12.5 mg: Bottles of 100 tablets.

Tablets 25 and 50 mg: Blister packs of 56 and 90 and bottles of 100 tablets.

Further information Nil.

Product licence numbers

Acepril Tablets 12.5 mg	0034/0298
Acepril Tablets 25 mg	0034/0299
Acepril Tablets 50 mg	0034/0300

ACEZIDE*

Presentation
Acezide 50 mg/25 mg, white biconvex, round tablets with possible slight mottling, each containing captopril 50 mg and hydrochlorothiazde 25 mg. Engraved with "AZE 50/25" on one side with a bisect bar on the other.

Other ingredients: Lactose, magnesium stearate, maize starch, microcrystalline cellulose, stearic acid.

Uses
Actions: Captopril, designated chemically as 1–[(2S)-3-mercapto-2-methyl-propionyl]-L-proline, is a specific competitive inhibitor of angiotensin I-converting enzyme, and hydrochlorothiazide is a diuretic-antihypertensive agent.

Captopril and hydrochlorothiazide lower blood pressure by different, though complementary, mechanisms. With diuretic treatment, blood pressure and blood volume fall resulting in a rise in angiotensin II levels which tend to blunt the hypotensive effect. Captopril blocks this rise in angiotensin II. The anti-hypertensive effects of captopril and hydrochlorothiazide are additive.

Indications: For the treatment of mild to moderate hypertension in patients who have been stabilised on the individual components given in the same proportions.

Dosage and administration
Adults: The usual dose of Acezide is one tablet daily. A daily dose of two tablets should not be exceeded.

Elderly: The dose should be kept as low as possible to achieve adequate blood pressure control. In some patients half a tablet daily may be sufficient.

Children: Safety and effectiveness of Acezide has not been established.

Patients with renal failure: Acezide is not recommended for use in patients with significant renal impairment.

Contra-indications, warnings, etc
Contra-indications: Acezide is contra-indicated in patients with anuria or hypersensitivity to captopril, thiazdes, or any sulphonamide-derived drug.

Pregnancy: Captopril has been shown to be lethal to rabbit and sheep foetuses. There were no foetotoxic effects to hamster or rat foetuses.

Acezide is contra-indicated in pregnancy and should not be used in women of childbearing potential unless protected by effective contraception.

Exposure of the mother in the second and third trimesters of pregnancy has been associated with oligohydramnois and neonatal hypotension and/or anuria.

Precautions: Acezide should not be used in patients with aortic stenosis or outflow tract obstruction.

Warnings
Haematological: Neutropenia agranulocytosis, thrombocytopenia and anaemia have been reported in patients receiving captopril.

In patients with normal renal function and no other complicating factors, neutropenia occurs rarely.

Captopril should not be used routinely in patients with pre-existing impaired renal function, collagen vascular disease, immunosuppressant therapy, treatment with allopurinol or procainamide, or a combination of these complicating factors, because neutropenia has been limited almost exclusively to this group. Some of these patients developed serious infections which in a few instances did not respond to intensive antibiotic therapy.

During treatment, all patients should be instructed to report any sign of infection (e.g. persistent sore throat, fever), when a differential white blood cell count should be performed. Acezide and other concomitant medication should be withdrawn if neutropenia (neutrophils less than 1000/mm^3) is detected or suspected.

In most patients neutrophil counts rapidly returned to normal upon discontinuing captopril.

Renal: Proteinura is a rare complication of captopril therapy.

Some patients with renal disease, particularly those with bilaterial renal artery stenoses or unilateral renal artery stenoses in a single functioning kidney, have developed increased concentrations of blood urea and serum creatine. Discontinuation of Acezide may be required.

Hepatic: Acezide should be used with caution in patients with impaired hepatic function or progressive liver disease because of the known risks associated with alterations in fluid and electrolyte balance resulting from thiazide treatment in such patients.

Electrolyte imbalance: Patients receiving Acezide should be observed for clinical signs of thiazide-induced fluid or electrolyte imbalance. In such patients periodic determinations of serum electrolytes should be performed. Because captopril reduces the production of aldosterone, its combination with hydrochlorothiazide may minimise diuretic-induced hypokalaemia. However, some patients may still require potassium supplements. Potassium-sparing diuretics should not be used in conjunction with Acezide.

Nursing mothers: Acezide shold not be used in nursing mothers.

Surgery anaesthesia: In patients undergoing major surgery, or during anaesthesia with agents which produce hypotension, captopril will block angiotensin II formation secondary to compensastory renin release. this may lead to hypotension which can be corrected by volume expansion.

Thiazides may decrease the arterial response to noradrenaline. In emergency surgery, pre-anaesthetic agents should be administered in reduced doses. Thiazides may increase the response to tubocurarine.

Metabolic disorders: Hyperuricaemia may occur, or frank gout be precipitated by thiazides in certain patients. Insulin requirements in diabetic patients may be altered by thiazides and latent diabetes mellitus may emerge. The captopril component of Acezide has been shown to ameliorate these effects of thiazides.

Clinical chemistry: Acezide may cause a false-positive urine test for acetone.

Side-effects
Haematological: With captopril, anaemia and thrombocytopenia have been reported (see Warnings).

With thiazides, leucopenia, agranulocytosis, thrombocytopoenia an aplastic anaemia have occured.

Renal: Proteinuria, elevated blood urea and creatinine, elevated serum potassium and acidosis (see Warnings).

Cardiovascular: Hypotension has been reported in volume depleted patients. Tachycardia.

Skin: With captopril, rashes, usually pruritic may occur. They are usually mild, transient and maculopapular, rarely urticarial. In a few cases the rash has been associated with fever and some patients have developed angioneurotic oedema. Pruritis, flushing vesicular rash, and photosensitivity have been reported.

With thiazides, purpura, photosensitivity, rash, urticaria, necrotising angiitis, Stevens-Johnson syndrome and other hypersensitivity reactions have been observed.

Gastrointestinal: Reversible and usually self-limiting taste impairment has been reported. Weight loss may be associated with the loss of taste. Stomatitis, resembling aphthous ulcers, has been reported. Elevation of liver enzymes has been noted in a few patients receiving captopril. Rare cases of hepatocellular injury and cholestatic jaundice have been reported. Gastric irritation and abdominal pain may occur.

Other: Paraesthesias of the hands, serum sickness, cough, bronchospasm and lymphadenopathy have been reported.

With thiazides, dizziness, vertigo, headache, xanthopsia, hyperglycaemia, hypokalaemia, glycosuria, hyperuricaemia, hypercalcaemia, muscle spasm, weakness and restlessness have been reported.

Overdosage: In the event of overdosage, blood pressure should be monitored and if hypotension develops volume expansion is the treatment of choice.

Captopril is removed by dialysis.

Drug interactions:

Diuretics: Potassium-sparing diuretics (triamterene, amiloride and spironolactone), or potassium supplements may cause significant increase in serum potassium.

Indomethacin: A reduction of anti-hypertensive effectiveness may occur. This is probably also the case with other non-steroidal anti-inflammatory drugs.

Vasodilators: Acezide has been reported to act synergistically with peripheral vasodilators such as minoxidil. This may improve blood pressure control, and awareness of this interaction may avert an initial hypotensive response.

Clonidine: It has been suggested that the anti-hypertensive effect of captopril can be delayed when patients treated with clonidine are changed to Acezide.

Allopurinol & procainamide: There have been reports of neutropenia and/or Stevens–Johnson syndrome in patients on captopril plus either allopurinol or procainamide. Although a causal relationship has not been established, these combinations should only be used with caution, especially in patients with impaired renal function.

Immunosuppressants: Azathioprine and cyclophosphamide have been associated with blood dyscrasias in patients with renal failure who were also taking captopril.

Probenecid: the renal clearance of captopril is reduced in the presence of probenecid.

Pharmaceutical precautions Do not store above 30°C (86°F).

Legal category POM.

Package quantities Calendar packs of 28.

Further information Acezide is designed to aid drug compliance by providing a convenient once daily preparation of captopril combined with hydrochlorothiazide for the treatment of mild to moderate hypertension. Significant antihypertensive activity is detectable throughout a 24 hour period following oral therapy.

By combining lower doses than might be required if each component were used alone, side effects, especially the hypokalaemia associated with diuretics, can be minimised.

Product licence number 0034/0301.

ADCORTYL* CREAM, AND OINTMENT

Presentation

Cream: White cream containing triamcinolone acetonide 0.1% in an aqueous vanishing cream base.

Other ingredients: Benzyl alcohol, cetyl alcohol, glyceryl monostearate, isopropyl palmitate, polysorbate 60, propylene glycol, water.

Ointment: Almost translucent ointment, containing triamcinolone acetonide 0.1% in Plastibase* (liquid paraffin and polyethylene resin)

Uses

Actions: Triamcinolone acetonide is a potent fluorinated corticosteroid with rapid anti-inflammatory, antipruritic and anti-allergic actions.

Indications: Adcortyl Cream and Ointment are recommended in steroid-responsive conditions which include: atopic eczema, contact eczema, follicular eczema, infantile eczema, otitis externa without frank infection, anogenital eczema, nummular eczema, seborrhoeic or flexural eczema, neurodermatitis, psoriasis of the scalp, chronic plaque psoriasis of the palms and soles and in other selected forms of psoriasis (excluding widespread plaque psoriasis) – 'Precautions'.

Dosage and administration *Adults and children:*

Cream: To be applied to moist, weeping lesions two to four times daily.

Ointment: To be applied to dry, scaly lesions two to four times daily.

Elderly: Corticosteroids should be used sparingly and for short periods of time, as natural thinning of the skin occurs in the elderly.

Contra-indications, warnings, etc

Contra-indications: In tuberculous and most viral lesions of the skin, particularly herpes simplex and varicella. The products should not be used in fungal or bacterial skin infections without suitable concomitant anti-infective therapy.

Should not be used for facial rosacea, acne vulgaris, perioral dermatitis or napkin eruptions.

Precautions: Adrenal suppression can occur, even without occlusion. If used in childhood, or on the face, courses should be limited to 5 days and occlusion should not be used.

Topical corticosteroids may be hazardous in psoriasis for a number of reasons including rebound relapses following development of tolerance, risk of generalised pustular psoriasis and local and systemic toxicity due to impaired barrier function of the skin. Steroids may have a place in psoriasis of the scalp and chronic plaque psoriasis of the hands and feet. Careful patient supervision is important.

Children: In infants, long-term, continuous topical steroid therapy should be avoided. Courses should be limited to 5 days and occlusion should not be used.

Pregnancy: There is inadequate evidence of safety in human pregnancy. Topical administration of corticosteroids to pregnant animals can cause abnormalities of foetal development including cleft palate and intrauterine growth retardation. There may, therefore, be a very small risk of such effects in the human foetus.

Side-effects: Triamcinolone acetonide is well tolerated. Where adverse reactions occur they are usually reversible on cessation of therapy. However the following side-effects have been reported usually with prolonged usage:

Dermatological: impaired wound healing, thinning of the skin, petechiae and ecchymoses, facial erythema and telangiectasia, increased sweating, purpura, striae, hirsutism, acneiform eruptions, lupus erythematosus-like lesions and suppressed reactions to skin tests.

These effects may be enhanced with occlusive dressings.

Signs of systemic toxicity such as oedema and electrolyte imbalance have not been observed even when high topical dosage has been used. The possibility of the systemic effects which are associated with all steroid therapy should be considered.

Overdosage: Topically applied corticosteroids can be absorbed in sufficient amounts to produce systemic effects (see Side-effects).
In the event of accidental ingestion, the patient should be observed and treated symptomatically.

Pharmaceutical precautions

Storage:
Cream: At room temperature; avoid freezing.
Ointment: At room temperature.
Dilution:
Cream: Cetomacrogol Cream (formula B) BPC or Aqueous Cream BP. Preservative cover may be reduced depending on the diluent. Diluted creams should be stored below 25°C and should be discarded two weeks after dilution.
Ointment: White soft paraffin.

Legal category POM.

Package quantities *Cream:* Tubes of 30 g. *Ointment:* Tubes of 30 g.

Further information Nil.

Product licence numbers
Adcortyl Cream 0034/5000R
Adcortyl Ointment 0034/5004R

ADCORTYL* IN ORABASE*

Presentation White to light tan crystalline paste containing triamcinolone acetonide 0.1% in Orabase formulated for adhesion to mucous membrane.

Other ingredients: Gelatin, liquid paraffin, pectin, polyethylene resin, sodium carboxymethylcellulose.

Uses
Actions: Triamcinolone acetonide is a potent fluorinated corticosteroid with rapid anti-inflammatory, antipruritic and anti-allergic actions.

Indications: Adcortyl in Orabase is indicated for aphthous ulcers, ulcerative stomatitis, denture stomatitis, desquamative gingivitis, erosive lichen planus and lesions of the oral mucosa of traumatic origin.

Dosage and administration Adults and children. To be applied to the oral lesion two to four times daily. Apply to the affected area; do not rub in.

Elderly: Corticosteroids should be used sparingly and for short periods of time.

Contra-indications, warnings, etc
Contra-indications: In tuberculous and most viral lesions, particularly herpes simplex and varicella. The products should not be used in fungal or bacterial infections without suitable concomitant anti-infective therapy.

Precautions: Adrenal suppression can occur, and dentures may act in the same way as an occlusive dressing. If used in childhood, courses should be limited to 5 days.

Children: In infants, long-term, continuous topical steroid therapy should be avoided. Courses should be limited to 5 days.

Pregnancy: There is inadequate evidence of safety in human pregnancy. Topical administration of corticosteroids to pregnant animals can cause abnormalities of foetal development including cleft palate and intra-uterine growth retardation. There may, therefore, be a very small risk of such effects in the human foetus.

Side-effects: Triamcinolone acetonide is well tolerated. Where adverse reactions occur they are usually reversible on cessation of therapy.

Signs of systemic toxicity such as oedema and electrolyte imbalance have not been observed even when high topical dosage has been used. The possibility of the systemic effects which are associated with all steroid therapy should be considered.

Overdosage: Topically applied corticosteroids can be absorbed in sufficient amounts to produce systemic effects (see side-effects).

In the event of accidental ingestion, the patient should be observed and treated symptomatically.

Pharmaceutical precautions
Storage: At room temperature.

Dilution: Should not be diluted.

Legal category POM.

Package quantities Tubes of 10 g.

Further information Nil.

Product licence number 0034/5006R.

ADCORTYL* INTRA-ARTICULAR/INTRADERMAL

Presentation Sterile aqueous suspension containing triamcinolone acetonide 10 mg per ml.

Other ingredients: Benzyl alcohol, polysorbate 80, sodium carboxymethylcellulose, sodium chloride, water.

Uses *Actions:* Triamcinolone acetonide is a synthetic glucocorticoid with marked anti-inflammatory and anti-allergic actions. Following local injection of Adcortyl, relief of pain and swelling and greater freedom of movement are usually obtained within a few hours; such administration avoids the more severe systemic side-effects which may accompany parenteral or oral corticosteroid administration.

Indications: Intra-articular use: for alleviating the joint pain, swelling and stiffness associated with rheumatoid arthritis and osteoarthrosis with an inflammatory component; also for bursitis, epicondylitis, and tenosynovitis.

Intradermal use: for lichen simplex chronicus (neurodermatitis), granuloma annulare, lichen planus, keloids, alopecia areata and hypertrophic scars.

Dosage and administration Adcortyl injection is not for intravenous use. Strict aseptic precautions should be observed. Since the duration of effect is variable, subsequent doses should be given when symptoms recur and not at set intervals.

Adults: The dose of Adcortyl injection for intra-articular administration, and injection into tendon sheaths and bursae, is dependent on the size of the joint to be treated and on the severity of the condition. Doses of 2.5-5 mg (0.25-0.5 ml) for smaller joints and 5-15 mg (0.5-1.5 ml) for larger joints usually alleviate the symptoms. Triamcinolone acetonide 40 mg/ml (Kenalog) is available to facilitate administration of larger doses. (See Precautions re Achilles tendon).

Intradermal dosage is usually 2-3 mg (0.2-0.3 ml), depending on the size of the lesion. No more than 5 mg (0.5 ml) should be injected at any one site. If several sites are injected the total dosage administered should not exceed 30 mg (3 ml). The injection may be repeated, if necessary, at one or two week intervals.

Children: Adcortyl is not recommended in children under 6 years. Adcortyl intra-articular/intradermal may be used in older children in suitably adjusted dosages. Growth and development of children on prolonged corticosteroid therapy should be carefully observed.

Elderly: Treatment of elderly patients, particularly if long term, should be planned bearing in mind the more serious consequences of the common side effects of corticosteroids in old age, especially osteoporosis, diabetes, hypertension, susceptibility to infection and thinning of the skin.

Contra-indications, warnings, etc
Contra-indications: None.

Precautions: In common with other steroids Adcortyl injection should be used with caution in patients with recent intestinal anastomoses, thrombophlebitis, psychotic tendencies, exanthematous disease, chronic nephritis, metastatic carcinoma, osteoporosis, in patients with an active peptic ulcer (or a history of peptic ulcer). Latent or healed tuberculosis; in the presence of local or systemic viral infection, systemic fungal infections or in active infections not controlled by antibiotics. In acute psychoses; in acute glomerulonephritis. Hypertension; glaucoma (or a family history of glaucoma), previous steroid myopathy or epilepsy.

Intra-articular injection should not be carried out in the presence of active infection in or near joints. The preparation should not be used to alleviate joint pain arising from infectious states such as gonococcal or tubercular arthritis.

Diabetes may be aggravated, necessitating a higher insulin dosage. Latent diabetes mellitus may be precipitated.

Menstrual irregularities may occur, and this possibility should be mentioned to female patients.

Patients on long-term systemic therapy with Adcortyl may require supportive corticosteroid therapy in times of stress, both during the treatment period and for a year afterwards.

During corticosteroid therapy antibody response will be reduced and therefore affect the patient's response to vaccines.

Rare instances of anaphylactoid reactions have occurred in patients receiving parenteral corticosteroids, especially when a patient has a history of drug allergies.

All corticosteroids increase calcium excretion.

Avoid abrupt cessation of corticosteroids.

Aspirin should be used cautiously in conjunction with corticosteroids in patients with hypoprothrombinaemia.

Corticosteroid effects may be enhanced in patients with hypothyrodism or cirrhosis.

Pregnancy: Corticosteroids are not recommended for pregnant patients, particularly in the first trimester, or for nursing mothers, except when the disease for which they are indicated warrants their use. There is inadequate evidence of safety in human pregnancy and there may be a very small risk of cleft palate and intra-uterine growth retardation in the foetus; there is evidence of harmful effects on pregnancy in animals.

Intra-articular injection: Patients should be specifically warned to avoid over-use of joints in which symptomatic benefit has been obtained. Severe joint destruction with necrosis of bone may occur if repeated intra-articular injections are given over a long period of time. Care should be taken if injections are given into tendon sheaths to avoid injection into the tendon itself.

Due to the absence of a true tendon sheath, the Achilles tendon should not be injected with depot corticosteroids.

Side-effects: Where adverse reactions occur they are usually reversible on cessation of therapy. Absorption of triamcinolone following Adcortyl injection, especially when given by the intra-articular route, is rare. However, the possibility of the systemic effects which are associated with all steroid therapy should be considered. These may include:

Dyspepsia, peptic ulceration with perforation and haemorrhage, abdominal distension, oesophageal ulceration, oesophageal candidiasis, acute pancreatitis.

Proximal myopathy, osteoporosis, vertebral and long bone fractures, avascular osteonecrosis, tendon rupture.

Sodium and water retention, hypertension, hypokalaemic alkalosis.

Impaired healing, skin atrophy, bruising, striae, telangiectasia, acne.

Suppression of the hypothalamo-pituitary adrenal axis, growth suppression in childhood and adolescence, menstrual irregularity and amenorrhoea. Cushingoid facies, hirsutism, weight gain, impaired carbohydrate tolerance with increased requirement for antidiabetic therapy, negative nitrogen balance.

Euphoria, psychological dependence, depression, insomnia. Intracranial hypertension has been reported in children on cessation of long term steroid therapy. Aggravation of schizophrenia.

Increased intra-ocular pressure, glaucoma, papilloedema, cataracts, corneal or scleral thinning, exacerbation of ophthalmic viral disease.

Opportunistic infection, recurrence of dormant tuberculosis, leucocytosis, hypersensitivity, thromboembolism, increased appetite, nausea, malaise.

On withdrawal fever, myalgia, arthralgia or adrenal insufficiency may occur.

Intra-articular injection: Reactions following intra-articular administration have been rare. In a few instances transient flushing and dizziness have occurred. Pain and other local symptoms may continue for a short time before effective relief is obtained, but an increase in joint discomfort has seldom occurred. Local fat atrophy may occur if the injection is not given into the joint space, but is temporary and disappears within a few weeks to months.

Intradermal injection: Sterile abscesses, hyper- and hypo-pigmentation and subcutaneous and cutaneous atrophy (which usually disappears unless the basic disease process is itself atrophic) have occurred.

Pharmaceutical precautions *Storage:* In an upright position at room temperature: avoid freezing.

Legal category POM.

Package quantities Multidose vials of 5 ml. Ampoules 5 × 1 ml.

Further information Nil.

Product licence number 0034/5002R.

ADCORTYL* WITH GRANEODIN* CREAM AND OINTMENT

Presentation
Cream: White vanishing cream.

Other ingredients: Benzyl alcohol, cetyl alcohol, ethanol, glyceryl monostearate, isopropyl palmitate, polysorbate 60, propylene glycol.

Ointment: Smooth, soft, translucent ointment in Plastibase* (liquid paraffin and polyethylene resin).

Each gram of the cream and ointment contains:

Triamcinolone acetonide	0.1%
Neomycin (as sulphate)	0.25%
Gramicidin	0.025%

Uses *Actions:* Triamcinolone acetonide is a potent fluorinated corticosteroid with rapid anti-inflammatory, antipruritic and anti-allergic actions.

The combined action of the antibiotics neomycin and gramicidin provides comprehensive antibacterial therapy against a wide range of Gram-positive and Gram-negative bacteria, including those micro-organisms responsible for most bacterial skin infections.

Indications: For the treatment of inflammatory dermatoses, which are complicated or threatened by secondary infection such as: atopic eczema, contact eczema, follicular eczema, infantile eczema, otitis externa, anogenital pruritus (pruritus ani et vulvae), psoriasis, nummular eczema, post-traumatic infective eczema, seborrhoeic or flexural eczema, neurodermatitis.

Dosage and administration *Adults and children:* Apply to the affected areas two to four times daily.

Elderly: Natural thinning of the skin occurs in the elderly; hence corticosteroids should be used sparingly and for short periods of time.

Contra-indications, warnings, etc
Contra-indications: In tuberculous and most viral lesions of the skin, particularly herpes simplex, vaccinia, varicella. The products should not be used in fungal or bacterial skin infections without suitable concomitant anti-infective therapy.

In patients with hypersensitivity to any of the components.

Should not be applied to the external auditory canal in patients with perforated eardrums.

Precautions: Adrenal suppression can occur, even without occlusion. The use of occlusive dressings should be avoided because of the increased risk of sensitivity reactions and increased percutaneous absorption. The possibility of sensitivity to neomycin should be taken into consideration especially in the treatment of patients suffering from leg ulcers.

Children: In infants, long-term, continuous topical steroid therapy should be avoided.

Pregnancy: Topical administration of corticosteroids to pregnant animals can cause abnormalities of foetal development. The relevance of this finding to humans has not been established. However, topical steroids should not be used extensively in pregnancy, i.e. in large amounts or for long periods. Topical corticosteroids should be used during pregnancy only if the potential benefit justifies the potential risk to the foetus.

Side-effects: Triamcinolone acetonide: Is well tolerated. Where adverse reactions occur they are usually reversible on cessation of therapy. However the following side-effects have been reported, usually with prolonged usage:

Dermatologic – impaired wound healing, thinning of the skin, petechiae and ecchymoses, facial erythema and telangiectasia, increased sweating, purpura, striae, hirsutism, acneiform eruptions, lupus erythematosus-like lesions and suppressed reactions to skin tests.

These effects may be enhanced with occlusive dressings.

Signs of systemic toxicity such as oedema and electrolyte imbalance have not been observed even when high topical dosage has been used. The possibility of the systemic effects which are associated with all steroid therapy should be considered.

Neomycin: Sensitivity reactions may occur especially with prolonged use. Ototoxicity and nephrotoxicity have been reported. Large amounts of this product should be avoided in the treatment of skin infections following extensive burns, trophic ulceration and other conditions where absorption of neomycin is possible.

Gramicidin: Sensitivity has occasionally been reported.

Overdosage: Topically applied corticosteroids can be absorbed in sufficient amounts to produce systemic effects (see Side-effects).

Pharmaceutical precautions *Storage: Cream:* At room temperature; avoid freezing.

Ointment: At room temperature.

Dilution: Not recommended, as this would reduce the concentration of the antibiotics to below therapeutic levels.

Legal category POM.

Package quantities
Cream: 25 g tube (OP)
Ointment: 15 g tube (OP).

Further information Nil.

Product licence numbers

Adcortyl with Graneodin Cream	0034/5015
Adcortyl with Graneodin Ointment	0034/5017

AZACTAM* FOR INJECTION

Presentation Azactam for Injection is a sterile white to off-white, sodium-free, powder blend of aztreonam and L-arginine (780 mg per g of aztreonam). After reconstitution, Azactam for Injection provides 500 mg, 1.0 g and 2.0 g of aztreonam activity in 15 ml vials, and 2.0 g of aztreonam activity in 100 ml infusion bottles.

Uses
Microbiology: Aztreonam is a monocyclic beta-lactam antibiotic with potent bactericidal activity against a wide spectrum of Gram-negative aerobic pathogens.

Unlike the majority of beta-lactam antibiotics, it is not an inducer *in vitro* of beta-lactamase activity. Aztreonam is usually active *in vitro* against those resistant aerobic organisms whose beta-lactamases hydrolyse other antibiotics.

Aztreonam is active *in vitro* against most strains of the following Gram-negative micro-organisms:

Escherichia coli, Enterobacter species, Klebsiella species (including *K. pneumoniae* and *K. oxytoca*), *Proteus mirabilis*, *Proteus vulgaris*, *Morganella morganii*, Providencia species (including *P. stuartii* and *P. rettgeri*), Pseudomonas species (including *Ps. aeruginosa*), *Serratia marcescens*, *Neisseria gonorrhoeae* (including penicillinase-producing strains), *Haemophilus influenzae* (including ampicillin-resistant and other penicillinase-producing strains), *Neisseria meningitidis*, Citrobacter species.

The majority of these organisms are susceptible to an aztreonam concentration of less than 1 mg/L. Most Pseudomonas and Enterobacter species are also susceptible but at higher concentrations *in vitro*.

Aztreonam and aminoglycosides are synergistic *in vitro* for many strains of Enterobacteriaceae and for most strains of *Ps. aeruginosa*.

Indications: The treatment of the following infections caused by susceptible aerobic Gram-negative microorganisms:

Urinary tract infections: including pyelonephritis and cystitis (initial and recurrent) and asymptomatic bacteriuria, including those due to pathogens resistant to the aminoglycosides, cephalosporins or penicillins.

Gonorrhoea: acute uncomplicated urogenital or anorectal infections due to beta-lactamase producing or non-producing strains of *N. gonorrhoeae*.

Lower respiratory tract infections: including pneumonia, bronchitis and lung infections in patients with cystic fibrosis.

Bacteraemia/septicaemia.

Meningitis caused by *Haemophilus influenza* or *Neisseria meningitis*. Since Azactam provides only Gram-negative cover, it should not be given alone as initial blind therapy, but may be used with an antibiotic active against Gram-positive organisms until the results of sensitivity tests are known.

Bone and joint infections.

Skin and soft tissue infections: including those associated with postoperative wounds, ulcers and burns.

Intra-abdominal infections: peritonitis.

Gynaecological infections: pelvic inflammatory disease, endometritis, and pelvic cellulitis.

Azactam is indicated for adjunctive therapy to surgery in the management of infections caused by susceptible organisms, including abscesses, infections complicating hollow viscus perforations, cutaneous infections and infections of serous surfaces.

Bacteriological studies to determine the causative organism(s) and their sensitivity to aztreonam should be performed. Therapy may be instituted prior to receiving the results of the sensitivity test.

In patients at risk of infections due to non-susceptible pathogens, additional antibiotic therapy should be initiated concurrently with Azactam to provide broad-spectrum coverage before identification and susceptibility testing results of the causative organism(s) are known. Based on these results, appropriate antibiotic therapy should be continued.

Patients with serious Pseudomonas infections may benefit from concurrent use of Azactam and an aminoglycoside because of their synergistic action. If such concurrent therapy is considered in these patients, susceptibility tests should be performed *in vitro* to determine the activity in combination. The usual monitoring of serum levels and renal function during aminoglycoside therapy applies.

Dosage and administration Intramuscular or intravenous injection, or intravenous infusion.

Adults: The dose range of Azactam is 1 to 8 g daily in equally divided doses. The usual dose is 3 to 4 g daily. The maximum recommended dose is 8 g daily. The dosage and route of administration should be determined by the susceptibility of the causative organisms, severity of infection, and the condition of the patient.

Dosage Guide: Adults

Type of infection[1]	*Dosage (g)*	*Frequency (hr)*	*Route*
Urinary tract	0.5–1	8–12	IM or IV
Gonorrhoea/cystitis	1	single dose	IM
Cystic Fibrosis	2	6–8	IV
Severe or life-threatening infections	2	6–8	IV
Other infections either	1	8	IM or IV
or	2	12	IV

[1] Because of the serious nature of infections due to *Pseudomonas aeruginosa*, a dose of 2 g every 6 or 8 hours is recommended, at least for initial therapy in systemic infections caused by this organism.

The intravenous route is recommended for patients requiring single doses greater than 1 g, or those with bacterial septicaemia, localised parenchymal abscess (e.g. intra-abdominal abscess), peritonitis, meningitis or other severe systemic or life-threatening infections.

Children: The usual dosage for patients older than one week is 30 mg/kg/dose every 6 or 8 hours. For severe infections in patients 2 years of age or older, 50 mg/kg/dose every 6 or 8 hours is recommended. The total daily dose should not exceed 8 g. Dosage information is not yet available for new-borns less than 1 week old.

Elderly: In the elderly, renal status is the major determinant of dosage. Estimated creatinine clearance should be used to determine appropriate dosage, since serum creatinine is not an accurate measurement of renal function in these patients.

Elderly patients normally have a creatinine clearance in excess of 30 ml/min and therefore would receive the normal recommended dose. If renal function is below this level, the dosage schedule should be adjusted (see Renal impairment).

Renal impairment: In patients with impaired renal function, the normal recommended initial dose should be given. This should be followed by maintenance doses as shown in the following table.

Estimated creatinine clearance (ml/min)	*Maintenance dose*
10–30	Half the initial dose
Less than 10	One quarter of the initial dose

The normal dose interval should not be altered.

In patients on haemodialysis a supplementary one eighth of the initial dose should be given after each dialysis.

Reconstitution: Azactam for Injection is supplied in 15 ml vials or in an infusion bottle of 100 ml. Upon the addition of the diluent the contents should be shaken immediately and vigorously. Vials of reconstituted Azactam are not intended for multi-dose use, and any unused solution from a single dose must be discarded. Depending on the type and amount of diluent, the pH ranges from 4.5 to 7.5, and the colour may vary from colourless to light straw-yellow, which may develop a slight pink tint on standing; however this does not affect the potency.

For intramuscular injection: For each gram of aztreonam add at least 3 ml Water for Injections PhEur or 0.9% Sodium Chloride Injection BP and shake well.

Single-dose vial size	*Volume of diluent to be added*
0.5 g	1.5 ml
1.0 g	3.0 ml

Azactam is given by deep injection into a large muscle mass, such as the upper outer quadrant of the gluteus maximus or the lateral part of the thigh.

For intravenous injection: To the contents of the vial add 6 to 10 ml Water for Injections PhEur, and shake well. Slowly inject directly into the vein over a period of 3 to 5 minutes.

For intravenous infusion

Vials: For each gram of aztreonam add at least 3 ml of Water for Injections PhEur and shake well.

Infusion bottle: To the contents of the infusion bottle, add 6 ml of Water for Injections PhEur and shake well.

Dilute this initial solution with an appropriate infusion solution to a final concentration less than 2% w/v (at least 50 ml solution per gram of aztreonam). The infusion should be administered over 20–60 minutes.

Appropriate infusion solutions include:
0.9% Sodium Chloride Injection BP
5% Glucose Intravenous Infusion BP
5% or 10% Mannitol Intravenous Infusion BP
Sodium Lactate Intravenous Infusion BP
0.9%, 0.45% or 0.2% Sodium Chloride and 5% Glucose Intravenous Infusion BP
Compound Sodium Chloride Injection BPC 1959 (Ringer's Solution for Injection).
Compound Sodium Lactate Intravenous Infusion BP (Hartmanns Solution for Injection).

A volume control administration set may be used to deliver the initial solution of Azactam into a compatible infusion solution being administered. With use of a Y-tube administration set, careful attention should be given to the calculated volume of Azactam solution required so that the entire dose will be infused.

With intermittent infusion of Azactam and another drug via a common delivery tube, the tube should be flushed before and after delivery of Azactam with any appropriate infusion solution compatible with both drug solutions. Except for the antibiotics described below, the drugs should not be delivered simultaneously.

Intravenous infusion solutions of Azactam for Injection prepared with 0.9% Sodium Chloride Injection BP or 5% Glucose Intravenous Infusion BP, in PVC or glass containers, to which clindamycin phosphate, gentamicin sulphate, tobramycin sulphate, or cephazolin sodium have been added at concentrations usually used clinically, are stable for up to 24 hours in a refrigerator (4–7°C). Ampicillin sodium admixtures with aztreonam in 0.9% Sodium Chloride Injection BP are stable for 24 hours in a refrigerator (4–7°C); stability in 5% Glucose Intravenous Infusion BP is eight hours under refrigeration.

If aztreonam and metronidazole are to be used together, they should be administered separately as a cherry red colour has been observed after storage of solutions containing combinations of the two products.

Contra-indications, warnings, etc

Contra-indications: Patients with a known hypersensitivity to aztreonam.

Aztreonam is contra-indicated in pregnancy. Aztreonam crosses the placenta and enters the foetal circulation.

Precautions: Specific studies have not shown significant cross-reactivity between Azactam and antibodies to penicillins or cephalosporins. The incidence of hypersensitivity to Azactam in clinical trials has been low but caution should be exercised in patients with a history of hypersensitivity to beta-lactam antibiotics until further experience is gained.

Experience in patients with impaired hepatic function is limited. Appropriate liver function monitoring in these patients is recommended.

Concurrent therapy with other antimicrobial agents and Azactam is recommended as initial therapy in patients who are at risk of having an infection due to pathogens that are not susceptible to aztreonam.

Therapy with Azactam may result in overgrowth of nonsusceptible organisms which may require additional antimicrobial therapy. In comparative studies, the number of patients treated for super-infections was similar to that of the control drugs used.

It is recommended that prothrombin times should be monitored if the patient is on concomitant anticoagulant therapy.

Aztreonam is excreted in breast milk in concentrations that are less than 1% of those in simultaneously obtained maternal serum. Lactating mothers should refrain from breast feeding during the course of therapy.

Side-effects: Azactam is generally well tolerated. The following side-effects have been reported from Azactam therapy:

Dermatological: Rash; pruritus, urticaria, erythema, petechiae and exfoliative dermatitis.

Haematological: Eosinophilia. Increases in prothrombin and partial thromboplastin time have occurred. There have been isolated reports of thrombocytopenia, neutropenia, anaemia and bleeding.

Hepatobiliary: Jaundice and hepatitis; transient elevations of hepatic transaminases and alkaline phosphatase (without overt signs or symptoms of hepatobiliary dysfunction).

Gastro-intestinal: Diarrhoea, nausea and/or vomiting, abdominal cramps, mouth ulcer and altered taste.

Local reations: Phlebitis and discomfort at the i.v. injection site; discomfort at the i.m. injection site.

Rare instances of the following events have been reported: vaginitis, candidosis, anaphylaxis, hypotension, weakness, confusion, dizziness, vertigo, sweating, headache, breast tenderness, halitosis, muscle aches, fever, malaise, sneezing and nasal congestion, transient increases in serum creatinine.

Treatment of overdosage: There have been no reported cases of overdosage.

Pharmaceutical precautions

Storage before reconstitution: At room temperature (15–25°C).

Stability after reconstitution: It is good practice to reconstitute immediately before use. If this is not possible,

Azactam is stable for 24 hours if stored in a refrigerator (4–7°C).

Azactam should not be physically mixed with any other drug, antibiotic or diluent except those listed in the 'Dosage and administration' section under reconstitution for intravenous infusion.

Legal category POM.

Package quantities

500 mg vial:	pack of 5
1 g vial:	single-dose pack
2 g vial:	single-dose pack
2 g infusion bottle:	single-dose pack

Further information Aztreonam is the first member of a new class of antibiotics, the monobactams. It has been synthesised as a monocylic beta-lactam antibiotic in which the sulphonic acid substituent in the 1-position of the nuclear ring activates the beta-lactam moiety.

Single 30-minute i.v. infusions of 0.5 g, 1.0 g and 2.0 g in healthy volunteers produced peak serum levels of 54, 90 and 204 mg/L, and single 3-minute i.v. injections of the same doses produced peak levels of 58, 125 and 242 mg/L. Peak levels of aztreonam are achieved at about one hour after i.m. administration. After identical single i.m. or i.v. doses, the serum concentrations are comparable at 1 hour (1.5 hours from the start of i.v. infusion), with similar slopes of serum concentrations thereafter.

The serum half-life of aztreonam averaged 1.7 hours in subjects with normal renal function, independent of the dose and route. In healthy subjects 60–70% of a single i.m. or i.v. dose was recovered in the urine by 8 hours, and urinary excretion was essentially complete by 12 hours.

Single-dose pharmacokinetic studies have not shown any significant interaction between aztreonam and gentamicin, cephradine, clindamycin or metronidazole.

As with other antibiotics, in the treatment of acute pulmonary exacerbations in patients with cystic fibrosis, while clinical improvement is usually noted, lasting bacterial eradications may not be achieved.

Unlike broad spectrum antibiotics, aztreonam produces no effects on the normal anaerobic intestinal flora. No disulfiram-like reactions with alcohol ingestion have been reported.

Product licence numbers

500 mg vial	0034/0250
1 g vial	0034/0251
2 g vial	0034/0252
2 g bottle	0034/0255

CAPOTEN* TABLETS

Presentation

Capoten Tablets 12.5 mg: Slightly mottled, white, flat-faced, bevel edged, capsule shaped, tablets, each containing captopril 12.5 mg. Engraved with "Squibb" and "450" on one side with a bisecting bar on the other.

Capoten Tablets 25 mg: Slightly mottled, white, square biconvex tablets each containing captopril 25 mg. Engraved with "Squibb" and "452" on one side and with quadrisect bars (for identification only) on the other.

Capoten Tablets 50 mg: Slightly mottled, white, oval, biconvex tablets each containing captopril 50 mg. Engraved with "Squibb" and "482" on one side with a bisecting bar on the other.

Other ingredients: Lactose, maize starch, microcrystalline cellulose, stearic acid.

Uses

Actions: Captopril, 1-[(2S)-3-mercapto-2-methyl-propionyl]-L-proline, is a highly specific competitive inhibitor of angiotensin I-converting enzyme, the enzyme responsible for the conversion of angiotensin I to angiotensin II.

Indications

Hypertension: Capoten is indicated for the first line treatment of mild to moderate hypertension.

In severe hypertension it should be used where standard therapy is ineffective or inappropriate.

Congestive heart failure: Capoten is indicated for the treatment of congestive heart failure. The drug should be used together with diuretics and, where appropriate, digitalis.

Dosage and administration

Recommended dose and dosage schedule

Hypertension: Treatment with Capoten should be at the lowest effective dose which should be titrated according to the needs of the patient.

Mild to moderate hypertension: The starting dose is 12.5 mg twice daily. The usual maintenance dose is 25 mg twice daily which can be increased incrementally, at 2–4 week intervals, until a satisfactory response is achieved, to a maximum of 50 mg twice daily.

A thiazide diuretic may be added to Capoten if satisfactory response has not been achieved. The dose of diuretic may be increased at 1-2 week intervals to the level of optimum response or until the maximum dose is reached.

Severe hypertension: In severe hypertension where standard therapy is ineffective or inappropriate because of adverse effects, the starting dose is is 12.5 mg b.d. The dosage may be increased incrementally to a maximum of 50 mg t.i.d. Capoten should be used together with other anti-hypertensive agents but the dose of these should be individually titrated. A daily dose of 150 mg of Capoten should not normally be exceeded.

Heart failure: Capoten therapy must be started under close medical supervision. Capoten should be introduced when diuretic therapy (such as frusemide 40–80 mg or equivalent) is insufficient to control symptoms. A starting dose of 6.25 mg or 12.5 mg may minimise a transient hypotensive effect. The possibility of this occurring can be reduced by discontinuing or reducing diuretic therapy if possible, prior to initiating Capoten. The usual maintenance dose is 25 mg two or three times a day, which can be increased incrementally, with intervals of at least two weeks, until a satisfactory response is achieved. The usual maximum dose is 150 mg daily.

Elderly: The dose should be titrated against the blood pressure response and kept as low as possible to achieve adequate control. Since elderly patients may have reduced renal function and other organ dysfunctions, it is suggested that a low dose of Capoten be used initially.

Children: Capoten is not recommended for the treatment of mild to moderate hypertension in children.

Experience in neonates, particularly premature infants, is limited. Because renal function in infants is not equivalent to that of older children and adults, lower doses of Capoten should be used with the patients under close medical supervision.

The starting dose should be 0.3 mg per Kg bodyweight up to a maximum of 6 mg per Kg bodyweight daily, in divided doses. The dose should be individualised according to the response and may be given two or three times daily.

Patients with renal impairment: Capoten is not recommended in patients with renal impairment.

Where it is clinically indicated in severely hypertensive patients with impaired renal function, the dose should be kept as low as possible to maintain adequate blood pressure control. The dose can be titrated against the response but adequate time should be allowed between dosage adjustments. In these patients a loop-diuretic rather than a thiazide should be the diuretic of choice.

Capoten is readily eliminated by haemodialysis.

Contra-indications, warnings, etc

Contra-indications: A history of previous hypersensitivity to the product.

Pregnancy: Capoten has been shown to be lethal to rabbit and sheep foetuses. There were no foetotoxic effects to hamster or rat foetuses.

Capoten is contraindicated in pregnancy and should not be used in women of child bearing potential unless protected by effective contraception.

Exposure of the mother in the second and third trimesters of pregnancy has been associated with oligohydramnios and neonatal hypotension and/or anuria.

Precautions: Evaluation of the patient should include assessment of renal function prior to initiation of therapy and at appropriate intervals thereafter. Patients with renal impairment should not normally be treated with captopril.

Capoten should not be used in patients with aortic stenosis or outflow tract obstruction.

As limited experience has been obtained in the treatment of acute hypertensive crises, the use of Capoten should be avoided in these patients.

Warnings: The incidence of adverse reactions to Capoten is principally associated with renal function since the drug is excreted primarily by the kidney. The dose should not exceed that necessary for adequate control and should be reduced in patients with impaired renal function.

Hypotension: With the first one or two doses some patients may experience symptomatic hypotension. In most instances, symptoms are relieved simply by the patient lying down.

In patients with severe and renin dependent hypertension (e.g. renovascular hypertension) or severe congestive heart failure, who are receiving large doses of diuretic, exaggerated hypotensive responses have occurred, usually within one hour of the initial dose of Capoten. In these patients, by discontinuing diuretic therapy or significantly reducing the diuretic dose for four to seven days prior to initiating Capoten the possibility of this occurrence is reduced. By commencing Capoten therapy with small doses (6.25 mg or 12.5 mg) the duration of any hypotensive effect is lessened. Some patients may benefit from an infusion of saline.

The occurrence of first dose hypotension does not preclude subsequent dose titration with Capoten.

Hypotension has been occasionally reported in patients on Capoten due to causes of acute volume depletion such as vomiting and diarrhoea.

Serum potassium: Since Capoten decreases aldosterone production, serum potassium is usually maintained in patients on diuretics. Potassium sparing diuretics or potassium supplements should not therefore be used routinely. In patients with marked renal impairment a significant elevation of serum potassium may occur.

Renal: Proteinuria in patients with prior normal renal function is rare.

Where proteinuria has occurred it has usually been in patients with severe hypertension and evidence of prior renal disease. Nephrotic syndrome occurred in some of these patients.

In patients with evidence of prior renal disease, monthly urinary protein estimations (dip stick) are recommended for the first 9 months of therapy. If repeated determinations show increasing amounts of urinary protein, a 24-hour quantitative determination should be obtained, and if this exceeds 1 g/day, the benefits and risks of continuing Capoten should be evaluated.

Although membranous glomerulopathy was found in biopsies taken from some proteinuric patients, a causal relationship to Capoten has not been established.

Some patients with renal disease, particularly those with bilateral renal artery stenosis or unilateral renal artery stenosis in a single functioning kidney, have developed increased concentrations of blood urea and serum creatinine. Capoten dosage reduction and/or discontinuation of diuretic may be required. For some of these patients it may not be possible to normalise blood pressure and maintain adequate renal perfusion.

Haematological: Neutropenia/agranulocytosis, thrombocytopenia and anaemia have been reported in patients receiving Capoten.

In patients with normal renal function and no other complicating factors, neutropenia occurs rarely.

Capoten should not be used routinely in patients with pre-existing impaired renal function, collagen vascular disease, immunosuppressant therapy, treatment with allopurinol or procainamide, or a combination of these complicating factors. Some of these patients developed serious infections which in a few instances did not respond to intensive antibiotic therapy.

If Capoten is used in such patients, it is advised that white blood cell count and differential counts should be performed prior to therapy, every 2 weeks during the first 3 months of Capoten therapy, and periodically thereafter.

During treatment, all patients should be instructed to report any sign of infection (e.g. sore throat, fever), when a differential white blood cell count should be performed. Capoten and other concomitant medication should be withdrawn if neutropenia (neutrophils less than 1000/mm^3) is detected or suspected.

In most patients neutrophil counts rapidly returned to normal upon discontinuing Capoten.

Nursing mothers: Because captopril is excreted in breast milk, Capoten should not be used in nursing mothers.

Surgery/anaesthesia: In patients undergoing major surgery, or during anaesthesia with agents which produce hypotension, captopril will block angiotensin II formation secondary to compensatory renin release. This may lead to hypotension which can be corrected by volume expansion.

Clinical chemistry: Capoten may cause a false-positive urine test for acetone.

Side-effects

Idiosyncratic: Angioedema involving the extremities, face, lips, mucous membranes, tongue, glottis, or larynx has been seen in patients treated with ACE inhibitors, including captopril. In this situation, the ACE inhibitors should be discontinued. Where swelling is confined to the face, lips and mouth the condition will usually resolve without further treatment, although antihistimines may be useful in relieving symptoms. These patients should be followed carefully until the swelling has resolved. However, where there is involvement of the tongue, glottis or larynx, likely to cause airway obstruction, subcutaneous adrenaline (0.5 ml, 1:1,000) should be administered promptly where indicated.

Haematological: Neutropenia, anaemia and thrombocytopenia (see Warnings). Rarely a positive ANA has been reported.

Renal: Proteinuria, elevated blood urea and creatinine, elevated serum potassium and acidosis (see Warnings).

Cardiovascular: Hypotension (see Warnings), tachycardia.

Skin: Rashes, usually pruritic, may occur. They are usually mild, transient and maculopapular, rarely urticarial and disappear within a few days of dosage reduction, short-term treatment with an antihistamine and/or discontinuing therapy. In a few cases the rash has been associated with fever. Pruritus, flushing, vesicular or bullous rash, and photosensitivity have been reported.

Gastro-intestinal: Reversible and usually self-limiting taste impairment has been reported. Weight loss may be associated with the loss of taste. Stomatitis, resembling aphthous ulcers, has been reported. Elevation of liver enzymes has been noted in a few patients. Rare cases of hepatocellular injury and cholestatic jaundice have been reported. Gastric irritation and abdominal pain may occur.

Other: Paraesthesias of the hands, serum sickness, cough, bronchospasm and lymphadenopathy have been reported.

Overdosage: In the event of overdosage, blood pressure should be monitored and if hypotension develops volume expansion is the treatment of choice. Captopril is removed by dialysis.

Drug interactions

Diuretics: Diuretics potentiate the anti-hypertensive effectiveness of Capoten.

Potassium-sparing diuretics (triamterene, amiloride and spironolactone), or potassium supplements may cause significant increase in serum potassium.

Indomethacin: A reduction of anti-hypertensive effectiveness may occur. This is probably also the case with other non-steroidal anti-inflammatory drugs.

Vasodilators: Capoten has been reported to act synergistically with peripheral vasodilators such as minoxidil. Awareness of this interaction may avert an initial hypotensive response.

Clonidine: It has been suggested that the anti-hypertensive effect of Capoten can be delayed when patients treated with clonidine are changed to Capoten.

Allopurinol and procainamide: There have been reports of neutropenia and/or Stevens-Johnson syndrome in patients on Capoten plus either allopurinol or procainamide. Although a causal relationship has not been established, these combinations should only be used with caution, especially in patients with impaired renal function.

Immunosuppressants: Azathioprine and cyclophosphamide have been associated with blood dyscrasias in patients with renal failure who were also taking Capoten.

Probenecid: The renal clearance of Capoten is reduced in the presence of probenecid.

Pharmaceutical precautions Store at room temperature.

Legal category POM.

Package quantities
Tablets 12.5 mg: Bottles of 100 tablets.
Tablets 25 and 50 mg: Blister packs of 56 and 90 and bottles of 100 tablets.

Further information Nil.

Product licence numbers

Capoten Tablets 12.5 mg	0034/0221
Capoten Tablets 25 mg	0034/0193
Capoten Tablets 50 mg	0034/0194

CAPOZIDE* TABLETS

Presentation Capozide 50 mg/25 mg: White, biconvex, round tablets with possible slight mottling, each containing captopril 50 mg and hydrochlorothiazide 25 mg. Engraved with 'Squibb' and 390 on one side with a bisect bar on the other.

Other ingredients: Lactose, magnesium stearate, maize starch, microcrystalline cellulose, stearic acid.

Uses
Actions: Captopril, designated chemically as l-[(2S)-3-mercapto-2-methyl-propionyl]-L-proline, is a specific competitive inhibitor of angiotensin I-converting enzyme, and hydrochlorothiazide is a diuretic-antihypertensive agent.

Captopril and hydrochlorothiazide lower blood pressure by different, though complementary, mechanisms. With diuretic treatment, blood pressure and blood volume fall resulting in a rise in angiotensin II levels which tend to blunt the hypotensive effect. Captopril blocks this rise in angiotensin II. The anti-hypertensive effects of captopril and hydrochlorothiazide are additive.

Indications: For the treatment of mild to moderate hypertension in patients who have been stabilised on the individual components given in the same proportions.

Dosage and administration
Adults: The usual dose of Capozide is one tablet daily. A daily dose of two tablets should not be exceeded.

Elderly: The dose should be kept as low as possible to achieve adequate blood pressure control. In some patients half a tablet daily may be sufficient.

Children: Safety and effectiveness of Capozide has not been established.

Patients with renal failure: Capozide is not recommended for use in patients with significant renal impairment.

Contra-indications, warnings, etc
Contra-indications: Capozide is contra-indicated in patients with anuria or hypersensitivity to captopril, thiazides, or any sulphonamide-derived drug.

Pregnancy: Captopril has been shown to be lethal to rabbit and sheep foetuses. There were no foetotoxic effects to hamster or rat foetuses.

Capozide is contra-indicated in pregnancy and should not be used in women of child bearing potential unless protected by effective contraception.

Exposure of the mother in the second and third trimesters of pregnancy has been associated with oligohydramnios and neonatal hypotension and/or anuria.

Precautions: Capozide should not be used in patients with aortic stenosis or outflow tract obstruction.

Warnings
Haematological: Neutropenia/agranulocytosis, thrombocytopenia and anaemia have been reported in patients receiving captopril.

In patients with normal renal function and no other complicating factors, neutropenia occurs rarely.

Captopril should not be used routinely in patients with pre-existing impaired renal function, collagen vascular disease, immunosuppressant therapy, treatment with allopurinol or procainamide, or a combination of these complicating factors, because neutropenia has been limited almost exclusively to this group. Some of these patients developed serious infections which in a few instances did not respond to intensive antibiotic therapy.

During treatment, all patients should be instructed to report any sign of infection (e.g. persistent sore throat, fever), when a differential white blood cell count should be performed. Capozide and other concomitant medication should be withdrawn if neutropenia (neutrophils less than 1000/mm^3) is detected or suspected.

In most patients neutrophil counts rapidly returned to normal upon discontinuing captopril.

Renal: Proteinuria is a rare complication of captopril therapy.

Some patients with renal disease, particularly those with bilateral renal artery stenoses or unilateral artery stenoses in a single functioning kidney, have developed increased concentrations of blood urea and serum creatinine. Discontinuation of Capozide may be required.

Hepatic: Capozide should be used with caution in patients with impaired hepatic function or progressive liver disease because of the known risks associated with alterations in fluid and electrolyte balance resulting from thiazide treatment in such patients.

Electrolyte imbalance: Patients receiving Capozide should be observed for clinical signs of thiazide-induced fluid or electrolyte imbalance. In such patients periodic determinations of serum electrolytes should be performed. Because captopril reduces the production of aldosterone, its combination with hydrochlorothiazide may minimise diuretic-induced hypokalaemia. However, some patients may still require potassium supplements. Potassium-sparing diuretics should not be used in conjunction with Capozide.

Nursing mothers: Capozide should not be used in nursing mothers.

Surgery/anaesthesia: In patients undergoing major surgery, or during anaesthesia with agents which produce hypotension, captopril will block angiotensin II formation secondary to compensatory renin release. This may lead to hypotension which can be corrected by volume expansion.

Thiazides may decrease the arterial response to noradrenaline. In emergency surgery, pre-anaesthetic and anaesthetic agents should be administered in reduced doses. Thiazides may increase the response to tubocurarine.

Metabolic disorders: Hyperuricaemia may occur, or frank gout be precipitated by thiazides in certain patients. Insulin requirements in diabetic patients may be altered by thiazides and latent diabetes mellitus may emerge. The captopril component of Capozide has been shown to ameliorate these effects of thiazides.

Clinical chemistry: Capozide may cause a false-positive urine test for acetone.

Side-effects:
Haematological: With captopril, neutropenia, anaemia and thrombocytopenia have been reported (see Warnings).

With thiazides, leucopenia, agranulocytosis, thrombocytopenia and aplastic anaemia have occurred.

Renal: Proteinuria, elevated blood urea and creatinine, elevated serum potassium and acidosis (see Warnings).

Cardiovascular: Hypotension has been reported in volume depleted patients. Tachycardia.

Skin: With captopril, rashes, usually pruritic, may occur. They are usually mild, transient and maculopapular, rarely urticarial. In a few cases the rash has been associated with fever and some patients have developed angio-neurotic oedema. Pruritus, flushing, vesicular rash, and photosensitivity have been reported.

With thiazides, purpura, photosensitivity, rash, urticaria, necrotising angiitis, Stevens-Johnson syndrome and other hypersensitivity reactions have been observed.

Gastro-intestinal: Reversible and usually self-limiting taste impairment has been reported. Weight loss may be associated with the loss of taste. Stomatitis, resembling aphthous ulcers, has been reported. Elevation of liver enzymes has been noted in a few patients receiving captopril. Rare cases of hepatocellular injury and cholestatic jaundice have been reported. Gastric irritation and abdominal pain may occur.

Other: Paraesthesias of the hands, serum sickness, cough, bronchospasm and lymphadenopathy have been reported.

With thiazides, dizziness, vertigo, headache, xanthopsia, hyperglycaemia, hypokalaemia, glycosuria, hyperuricaemia, hypercalcaemia, muscle spasm, weakness and restlessness have been reported.

Overdosage: In the event of overdosage, blood pressure should be monitored and if hypotension develops volume expansion is the treatment of choice.

Captopril is removed by dialysis.

Drug interactions

Diuretics: Potassium-sparing diuretics (triamterene, amiloride and spironolactone), or potasssium supplements may cause significant increase in serum potassium.

Indomethacin: A reduction of anti-hypertensive effectiveness may occur. This is probably also the case with other non-steroidal anti-inflammatory drugs.

Vasodilators: Capozide has been reported to act synergistically with peripheral vasodilators such as minoxidil. This may improve blood pressure control and awareness of this interaction may avert an initial hypotensive response.

Clonidine: It has been suggested that the anti-hypertensive effect of captopril can be delayed when patients treated with clonidine are changed to Capozide.

Allopurinol and procainamide: There have been reports of neutropenia and/or Stevens-Johnson syndrome in patients on captopril plus either allopurinol or procainamide. Although a causal relationship has not been established, these combinations should only be used with caution, especially in patients with impaired renal function.

Immunosuppressants: Azathioprine and cyclophosphamide have been associated with blood dyscrasias in patients with renal failure who were also taking captopril.

Probenecid: The renal clearance of captopril is reduced in the presence of probenecid.

Pharmaceutical precautions Do not store above 30°C (86°F).

Legal category POM.

Package quantities Calendar packs of 28 tablets (OP).

Further information Capozide is designed to aid drug compliance by providing a convenient once daily preparation of captopril combined with hydrochlorothiazide for the treatment of mild to moderate hypertension. Significant antihypertensive activity is detectable throughout a 24 hour period following oral therapy.

By combining lower doses than might be required if each component were used alone, side-effects, especially the hypokalaemia associated with diuretics, can be minimised.

Product licence number 0034/0263.

CORGARD* TABLETS

Presentation Pale blue, round, biconvex tablets. The 80 mg nadolol tablet is scored on one side and engraved 'Squibb' and '241' while the 40 mg nadolol tablet is unscored with 'Squibb' and '207' engraved on one side.

Other ingredients: Citric acid anhydrous, indigo carmine, magnesium stearate, maize starch, microcrystalline cellulose, polyvinylpyrrolidone.

Uses *Actions:* Nadolol is a beta-adrenergic receptor blocking agent with a prolonged activity, permitting once-daily dosage in angina, hypertension, cardiac arrhythmias, the prophylaxis of migraine, and the relief of hyperthyroid symptoms.

Nadolol is not metabolised. It has no membrane stabilising or intrinsic sympathomimetic activity, and its only effect on the autonomic nervous system is one of beta-adrenergic blockade. Nadolol is nonselective.

Receptor blockade by nadolol results in protection from excessive inappropriate sympathetic activity. Nadolol reduces the number and severity of attacks of angina pectoris by blocking response to catecholamine stimulation and thus lowers the oxygen requirement of the heart at any given level of effort.

Nadolol reduces both supine and erect blood pressure. Like other beta-blockers nadolol exerts an antiarrhythmic action. Nadolol has been shown to reduce the rapid ventricular response which accompanies atrial fibrillation/flutter by slowing conduction through the A-V node. Beta-blockade is of particular value in arrhythmias caused by increased levels of, or sensitivity of the heart to, circulating catecholamines, e.g. arrhythmias associated with phaeochromocytoma, thyrotoxicosis, or exercise. Nadolol is effective in reducing ventricular premature beats in selected patients.

Nadolol exerts an effect in the prophylaxis of migraine by a mechanism which may involve prevention of vasoconstriction in the area served by the internal carotid artery and prevention of excessive adrenergic vasodilation in the external carotid artery.

Nadolol alleviates the symptoms of thyrotoxicosis and provides symptomatic control before and during thyroid surgery.

Beta-blocking agents have been shown in large scale studies to reduce mortality by preventing reinfarction and sudden death in patients surviving their first myocardial infarction.

Indications: Corgard is indicated in the management of:

Angina pectoris: For the long-term management of patients with angina pectoris by continuous medication.

Hypertension: For the long-term management of essential hypertension, either alone or in combination with other antihypertensive agents, especially thiazide-type diuretics.

Arrhythmias: For the treatment of cardiac tachyarrhythmias.

Migraine: For the prophylactic management of migraine headache. The efficacy of Corgard in the treatment of a migraine attack that has already started has not been established, and nadolol is not indicated for such use.

Thyrotoxicosis: For the relief of the symptoms of hyperthyroidism and the pre-operative preparation of patients for surgery. Nadolol may be used in conjunction with conventional antithyroid therapy.

Dosage and administration Dosage should be titrated gradually with at least a week between increments to assess response; individuals show considerable variation in their response to beta-adrenergic blockade.

Corgard may be given in a once daily dosage without regard to meals. The dosage interval should be increased when creatinine clearance is below 50 ml/min/1.73m^2.

If Corgard is to be discontinued, reduce dosage over a period of at least two weeks (see Warnings).

Angina pectoris: Initially 40 mg once daily. This may be increased at weekly intervals until an adequate response is obtained or excessive bradycardia occurs. Most patients respond to 160 mg or less daily. The value and safety of daily doses exceeding 240 mg have not been established.

Hypertension: Initially 80 mg once daily. This may be increased by a weekly increment of 80 mg or less until an optimum response is obtained. Many patients respond to 80 mg daily and most patients respond to 240 mg or less, daily, but higher doses have been required for a few patients. In some patients it is necessary to administer a diuretic, peripheral vasodilator and/or other antihypertensive agents in conjunction with nadolol in order to achieve satisfactory response.

Treatment of hypertension associated with phaeochromocytoma may require the addition of an alpha-blocking agent.

Cardiac tachyarrhythmias: Initially 40 mg once daily. This may be increased if necessary to 160 mg once daily. If bradycardia occurs dosage should be reduced to 40 mg once daily.

Migraine: The initial dose of nadolol is 40 mg once daily. Dosage may be gradually increased in 40 mg increments until optimum migraine prophylaxis is achieved. The usual maintenance dose is 80 to 160 mg administered once daily. After 4 to 6 weeks at the maximum dose if a satisfactory response is not obtained, therapy with nadolol should be withdrawn gradually.

Thyrotoxicosis: The dosage range is 80–160 mg once daily. It has been found that most patients require a dose of 160 mg once daily. Nadolol may be used together with conventional anti-thyroid treatment. For the preparation of patients for partial thyroidectomy, nadolol should be administered in conjunction with potassium iodide for a period of 10 days prior to operation. Nadolol should be administered on the morning of operation. Post operatively nadolol dosage should be slowly reduced and then withdrawn following clinical stability.

Elderly patients: In elderly patients a low initial dose should be used so that sensitivity to side-effects may be assessed. As with all drugs, patients with impaired renal or hepatic function should be monitored.

Children: Safety and effectiveness in children have not been established.

Administration in renal failure: In patients with decreased renal function, dosage adjustment is necessary. The recommended dosage intervals are:

Creatinine Clearance ($ml/min/1.73\ m^2$)	*Dosage Interval (Hours)*
<10	40–60
10–30	24–48
31–50	24–36
>50	24

Contra-indications, warnings, etc

Contra-indications: Like other drugs in this class, nadolol is contra-indicated in bronchial asthma or a history of asthma; sinus bradycardia and second and third degree heart block; cardiogenic shock; right ventricular failure secondary to pulmonary hypertension; congestive heart failure.

Warnings: Exacerbation of angina and myocardial infarction have occurred after abrupt discontinuation of therapy with beta-adrenergic blocking agents in patients with angina pectoris or other evidence of coronary artery insufficiency. When discontinuing long-term treatment with nadolol, the dosage should be reduced gradually over a period of at least two weeks and the patient carefully monitored.

Beta-adrenergic blockade carries the potential hazard of precipitating cardiac failure. Should this occur and it is not controlled by digitalisation, nadolol should be withdrawn, consideration being given to the foregoing warning.

Beta-blockade impairs the ability of the heart to respond to stress. It has been the usual practice to recommend withdrawal of beta-blockers several days prior to surgery.

However, this may render the patient's blood pressure unstable and difficult to control during anaesthesia and the anaesthetist may wish to advise on discontinuation of therapy. In no circumstances should beta-blockers be discontinued prior to surgery in patients with phaeochromocytoma or thyrotoxicosis. In the event of emergency surgery, the effects of nadolol may be reversed by isoprenaline or noradrenaline. However, such patients may be subject to protracted severe hypotension. General anaesthetics which can cause myocardial depression, such as cyclopropane, trichloroethylene, chloroform and ether, should be avoided if nadolol is continued during surgery.

Nadolol should be administered with caution to patients with chronic obstructive airways disease. Discontinue therapy if condition relapses.

Care should be exercised in the administration of nadolol to diabetic patients since early signs of acute hypoglycaemia may be masked. It may also be necessary to adjust the dosage of hypoglycaemic drugs or insulin doses.

There have been reports of skin rashes (including a psoriasiform type) and/or ocular changes (conjunctivitis and 'dry eye') associated with the use of beta-adrenergic blocking drugs. The reported incidence is small and in most cases the symptoms have cleared when the treatment was withdrawn. Discontinuance of the drug should be considered if any such reaction is not otherwise explicable. Cessation of therapy with a beta-adrenergic blocker should be gradual.

Beta-blockade may mask certain clinical signs (e.g. tachycardia) of hyperthyroidism. Patients suspected of developing thyrotoxicosis should be managed carefully to avoid abrupt withdrawal of beta-blockade which might precipitate a thyroid storm.

Precautions: Occasionally, beta-blockade with drugs such as nadolol may produce hypotension and/or marked bradycardia, resulting in vertigo, syncope or orthostatic hypotension.

Nadolol should be used with caution in patients with impaired renal or hepatic function.

Administration in renal failure: In patients with decreased renal function, dosage adjustment is necessary (see Dosage).

Use in pregnancy and nursing mothers: The safety of nadolol in pregnancy has not been established and animal studies have shown some foetotoxicity. Use of any drug in pregnancy or women of childbearing potential requires that the possible risk to the mother and/or foetus be weighed against the expected therapeutic benefit.

Nadolol is excreted in human milk; therefore nursing mothers should only receive nadolol if deemed essential.

Side-effects: Most patients tolerate nadolol well. Side-effects resemble those reported with other beta-blocking drugs and rarely require withdrawal of treatment. Those reported infrequently include gastrointestinal effects, bradycardia, fatigue, light-headedness, cold extremities, depression, insomnia, paraesthesia, dryness of the mouth and alopecia. Cardiac insufficiency, hypotension and AV block have occurred on rare occasions.

Overdosage or exaggerated response: Excessive bradycardia should be treated initially with atropine. If there is no response, isoprenaline may be administered with caution.

Cardiac failure should be managed by digitalisation and diuretics. Glucagon has also been reported to be useful.

Hypotension may be managed with vasopressors such as adrenaline.

Bronchospasm may be counteracted by isoprenaline and aminophylline.

Drug interactions:

General anaesthetics: Those which cause myocardial depression such as chloroform, cyclopropane, trichloroethylene and ether should be avoided as the patient may be subject to protracted severe hypotension.

Myocardial depressants: Myocardial depressants such as lignocaine and procainamide may potentiate the hypotensive action of nadolol and lead to severe hypotension.

Adrenoceptor stimulants: Beta-adrenoceptor stimulants such as isoprenaline and verapamil, or alpha-adrenoceptor stimulants such as noradrenaline, adrenaline, will reverse the hypotensive effects and increase vasoconstrictor activity.

Calcium antagonists: e.g. verapamil, should not be given concurrently with Corgard. Several days should be allowed after their discontinuation before administering nadolol.

Catecholamine depleting drugs: eg: reserpine. Excessive reduction in sympathetic drive to the heart might occur. Close observation is advised.

Antihypertensives (eg, neurone-blocking drugs, vasodilators, diuretics): Additive hypotensive effect.

Clonidine: If Corgard and clonidine are given concurrently, clonidine should not be discontinued until several days after Corgard withdrawal.

Hypoglycaemics, insulin: Possible dosage adjustment, see warnings.

Monoamine oxidase inhibitors: Administration of nadolol during and within 2 weeks of administration of adrenergic augmenting psychotropic drugs such as monoamine oxidase inhibitors, should be avoided, although the clinical significance is undetermined.

Pharmaceutical precautions Store at room temperature, protected from excessive heat and moisture in a tightly closed container.

Legal category POM.

Package quantities Calendar packs of 28 (OP).

Further information The lipid solubility of beta-blocking agents has been correlated with the extent to which these agents cross the blood-brain barrier and cause central nervous system-related side-effects. Corgard has a low lipid solubility.

Corgard has been demonstrated in both animal and clinical studies to preserve, and in some cases, increase renal blood flow upon acute and long-term administration in spite of a concurrent decrease in arterial pressure and cardiac output. Glomerular filtration rate remains unchanged, and renal vascular resistance is reduced, even in the presence of diuretic pretreatment. The exact mechanism of this effect of Corgard on the renal circulation has not been elucidated.

About 30 per cent of an oral dose of Corgard is absorbed. Peak serum concentrations usually occur in 3 to 4 hours after drug administration. The presence of food in the gastrointestinal tract does not affect the rate or extent of Corgard absorption. Approximately 30 per cent of the Corgard present in serum is reversibly bound to plasma protein. Unlike most available beta-blocking agents, Corgard is not metabolised, and is excreted unchanged principally by the kidneys. The serum half-life of therapeutic doses of Corgard is relatively long, ranging from 20 to 24 hours (permitting once daily dosage). A significant correlation between minimum steady-state serum concentrations of Corgard and total oral daily dose has been demonstrated in hypertensive patients; however, the observed dose-response range is wide and proper dosage requires individual titration.

Corgard can be efficiently removed from the general circulation by haemodialysis.

Product licence numbers
80 mg 0034/0186
40 mg 0034/0185.

CORGARETIC* TABLETS

Presentation White, blue-speckled, round, biconvex tablets, in two strengths.

Corgaretic 40: nadolol 40 mg with bendrofluazide 5 mg is engraved 'Squibb' and '283' on one side with a bisect bar on the other.

Corgaretic 80: nadolol 80 mg with bendrofluazide 5 mg is engraved 'Squibb' and '284' on one side with a bisect bar on the other.

Other ingredients: Indigo carmine, lactose, magnesium stearate, maize starch, microcrystalline cellulose, polyvinylpyrrolidone, sodium starch glycollate, sucrose.

Uses *Actions:* Nadolol is a beta-adrenergic receptor blocking agent with a prolonged activity, permitting once-daily dosage.

Nadolol is not metabolised. It has no membrane stabilising or intrinsic sympathomimetic activity, and its only effect on the autonomic nervous system is one of beta-adrenergic blockade. Nadolol is nonselective.

Receptor blockade by nadolol results in protection from excessive or inappropriate sympathetic activity.

Nadolol reduces both supine and erect blood pressure.

Bendrofluazide is a thiazide diuretic which interferes with renal tubular electrolyte reabsorption, thereby increasing sodium and water excretion.

Indications: For the treatment of hypertension. The combination of a diuretic and a beta-blocker may be of particular value in patients whose blood pressure has not been adequately controlled with either component given alone.

Dosage and administration One or two tablets once daily to a maximum of 160 mg nadolol and 10 mg bendrofluazide. For doses of nadolol in excess of 160 mg, the combination product may not be appropriate because an excessive dose of the thiazide component may be administered.

The dosage should be titrated gradually with at least a week between increments to assess response; individuals show considerable variation in their response to beta-adrenergic blockade.

Corgaretic may be given in a once-daily dosage without regard to meals.

If Corgaretic is to be discontinued, reduce dosage over a period of at least two weeks (see Warnings).

Elderly patients: In elderly patients a low initial dose should be used so that sensitivity to side-effects may be assessed. As with all drugs, patients with impaired renal or hepatic function should be monitored.

Children: Safety and effectiveness in children have not been established.

Contra-indications, warnings, etc
Contra-indications: In bronchial asthma or a history of asthma; sinus bradycardia and second and third degree heart block; cardiogenic shock; right ventricular failure secondary to pulmonary hypertension; congestive heart failure, anuria, past sensitivity to thiazide diuretics or any sulphonamide-derived drugs.

Warnings: Exacerbation of angina and myocardial infarction have occurred after abrupt discontinuation of therapy with beta-adrenergic blocking agents in patients with angina pectoris or other evidence of coronary artery insufficiency. When discontinuing long-term treatment with nadolol, the dosage should be reduced gradually over a period of at least two weeks and the patient carefully monitored. If acute coronary insufficiency develops, temporarily reinstitute therapy with Corgard (nadolol) promptly.

Beta-adrenergic blockade carries the potential hazard of precipitating cardiac failure. Should this occur and it is not controlled by digitalisation, Corgaretic should be withdrawn, consideration being given to the foregoing warning.

Beta-blockade impairs the ability of the heart to respond to stress. It has been the usual practice to recommend withdrawal of beta-blockers several days prior to surgery. However, this may render the patient's blood pressure unstable and difficult to control during anaesthesia and the anaesthetist may wish to advise on discontinuation of therapy. In no circumstances should beta-blockers be discontinued prior to surgery in patients with phaeochromocytoma or thyrotoxicosis. In the event of emergency surgery, the effects of nadolol may be reversed by isoprenaline or noradrenaline. However, such patients may be subject to protracted severe hypotension. General anaesthetics which can cause myocardial depression, such as cyclopropane, trichloroethylene, chloroform and ether, should be avoided if Corgaretic is continued during surgery.

Corgaretic should be administered with caution to

patients with chronic obstructive airways disease. Discontinue therapy if condition relapses.

Diabetic patients should be monitored closely as nadolol may mask the early signs of acute hypoglycaemia, and thiazide diuretics can lower insulin tolerance. Therefore, dosages of hypoglycaemic drugs or insulin doses may need adjustment.

There have been reports of skin rashes (including a psoriasiform type) and/or ocular changes (conjunctivitis and 'dry eye') associated with the use of beta-adrenergic blocking drugs. The reported incidence is small and in most cases the symptoms have cleared when the treatment was withdrawn. Discontinuance of the drug should be considered if any such reaction is not otherwise explicable. Cessation of the therapy with a beta-adrenergic blocker should be gradual.

Beta-blockade may mask certain clinical signs (e.g., tachycardia) of hyperthyroidism. Patients suspected of developing thyrotoxicosis should be managed carefully to avoid abrupt withdrawal of beta-blockade which might precipitate a thyroid storm.

Precautions: Occasionally, beta-blockade with drugs such as nadolol may produce hypotension and/or marked bradycardia, resulting in vertigo, syncope or orthostatic hypotension.

Nadolol should be used with caution in patients with impaired renal or hepatic function.

Periodic determination of serum electrolytes to detect possible imbalance, e.g. hyponatraemia, hypochloric alkalosis and hypokalaemia, should be performed at regular intervals.

Potassium depletion is a danger to digitalised patients or those with hepatic cirrhosis with ascites. In patients with renal disease, thiazides may precipitate azotaemia and cumulative effects of the drug may develop. In patients with impaired hepatic function, minor alterations of fluid and electrolyte balance may precipitate hepatic coma.

Thiazide diuretics may raise serum uric acid levels, thus exacerbating gout in susceptible patients.

Pathologic changes in the parathyroid gland with hypercalcaemia and hypophosphataemia have been observed in a few patients during prolonged thiazide therapy.

The possibility that thiazides may exacerbate or activate systemic lupus erythematosus has been reported.

Administration in renal failure: Increased blood levels of nadolol occur in the presence of renal failure. Although non-renal elimination does occur, dosage adjustments are necessary in this patient group. The total daily dose of Corgaretic should be reduced or the dose interval increased. Corgaretic, however, would not be appropriate for patients with severe renal impairment since loop diuretics (e.g. frusemide) rather than a thiazide are preferred for such patients.

Use in pregnancy and nursing mothers: The safety of nadolol in pregnancy has not been established and animal studies have shown some foetotoxicity. The use of diuretics in otherwise healthy pregnant women with or without mild oedema is contra-indicated. The hazards of using thiazides include foetal or neonatal jaundice, thrombocytopenia and possibly other adverse reactions which have occurred in the adult. Nadolol and bendrofluazide are excreted in human milk.

Corgaretic is therefore not considered suitable for pregnant patients or nursing mothers.

Side-effects: Most patients tolerate Corgaretic well.

Nadolol: Side-effects resemble those reported with other beta-blocking drugs and rarely require withdrawal of treatment. Those reported infrequently include gastro-intestinal effects, bradycardia, fatigue, light-headedness, cold extremities, depression, insomnia, paraesthesia, dryness of the mouth and alopecia. Cardiac insufficiency, hypotension and AV block have occurred on rare occasions.

Thiazides: Those reported with the use of thiazides include hypokalaemia, anorexia, gastric irritation, nausea, vomiting, cramping, diarrhoea, intrahepatic cholestatic jaundice, pancreatitis, dizziness, vertigo, headache, xanthopsia, leucopenia, agranulocytosis, thrombocytopenia, aplastic anaemia, purpura, photosensitivity, rash, urticaria, necrotising angiitis, hyperglycaemia, glycosuria, hyperuricaemia, muscle spasm, weakness and restlessness.

Overdosage or exaggerated response: Excessive bradycardia should be treated initially with atropine. If there is no response, isoprenaline may be administered with caution.

Cardiac failure should be managed by digitalisation and diuretics. Glucagon has also been reported to be useful.

Hypotension may be managed with vasopressors such as adrenaline.

Bronchospasm may be counteracted by isoprenaline and aminophylline.

Drug interactions:

General anaesthetics: Those which cause myocardial depression such as chloroform, cyclopropane, trichloroethylene and ether should be avoided as the patient may be subject to protracted severe hypotension.

Myocardial depressants: Myocardial depressants such as lignocaine and procainamide may potentiate the hypotensive action of nadolol and lead to severe hypotension.

Adrenoceptor stimulants: Beta-adrenoceptor stimulants such as isoprenaline and verapamil, or alpha-adrenoceptor stimulants such as noradrenaline, adrenaline, will reverse the hypotensive effects and increase vasoconstrictor activity. Thiazides may decrease the arterial responsiveness to noradrenaline.

Calcium antagonists: e.g. verapamil, should not be given concurrently with Corgard. Several days should be allowed after their discontinuation before administering nadolol.

Catecholamine depleting drugs (eg, reserpine): Excessive reduction in sympathetic drive to the heart might occur. Close observation is advised.

Antihypertensives (eg, neurone-blocking drugs, vasodilators, diuretics): Additive hypotensive effect.

Clonidine: If Corgard and clonidine are given concurrently, clonidine should not be discontinued until several days after Corgard withdrawal.

Hypoglycaemics, insulin: Possible dosage adjustment, see warnings.

Monoamine oxidase inhibitors: Administration of nadolol during and within 2 weeks of administration of adrenergic augmenting psychotropic drugs such as monoamine oxidase inhibitors, should be avoided, although the clinical significance is undetermined.

Tubocurarine: Thiazides may increase the responsiveness to tubocurarine.

Pharmaceutical precautions Store at room temperature, protected from excessive heat and moisture in a tightly closed container.

Legal category POM.

Package quantities Calendar packs of 28 (OP).

Further information Corgaretic tablets simplify the treatment of hypertension by increasing patient acceptability and dosage flexibility. The two available strengths allow increasing the dose of the beta-blocker nadolol, without necessarily increasing the bendrofluazide dosage.

The lipid solubility of beta-blocking agents has been correlated with the extent to which these agents cross the blood-brain barrier and cause central nervous system-related side-effects. Nadolol has a low lipid solubility.

Nadolol has been demonstrated in both animal and clinical studies to preserve, and in some cases, increase renal blood flow upon acute and long-term administration in spite of a concurrent decrease in arterial pressure and cardiac output. Glomerular filtration rate remains unchanged, and renal vascular resistance is reduced, even in the presence of diuretic pretreatment.

The exact mechanism of this effect of nadolol on the renal circulation has not been elucidated. The net effect on glomerular filtration rate of the simultaneous administration of nadolol/bendrofluazide as initial therapy has not been investigated.

About 30 per cent of an oral dose of nadolol is absorbed. Peak serum concentrations usually occur in 3 to 4 hours after drug administration. The presence of food in the gastrointestinal tract does not affect the rate or extent of nadolol absorption. Approximately 30 per cent of the nadolol present in serum is reversibly bound to plasma protein. Unlike most available beta-blocking agents, nadolol is not metabolised, and is excreted unchanged. The serum half-life of therapeutic doses of nadolol is relatively long, ranging from 20 to 24 hours (permitting once daily dosage). A significant correlation between minimum steady-state serum concentrations of nadolol and total oral daily dose has been demonstrated in hypertensive patients; however, the observed dose-response range is wide and proper dosage requires individualised titration.

Bendrofluazide is almost completely absorbed from the gastro-intestinal tract. It is extensively metabolised, 30 per cent being excreted unchanged in the urine. Its plasma half-life is 3 to 4 hours, its biological half-life being much longer.

Product licence numbers

Corgaretic 40	0034/0212
Corgaretic 80	0034/0213

DOLMATIL† TABLETS

Presentation Plain white round tablets with a transverse breaking line on one side and the mark D200 on the other. Each tablet contains 200 mg sulpiride.

Other ingredients: Hydrated silica, lactose, magnesium stearate, methyl cellulose, potato starch, talc.

Uses *Acute and chronic schizophrenia:* One of the characteristics of Dolmatil is its bimodal activity, as it has both antidepressant and neuroleptic properties. Schizophrenia characterised by a lack of social contact can benefit strikingly. Mood elevation is observed after a few days treatment, followed by disappearance of the florid schizophrenic symptoms. The sedation and lack of affect characteristically associated with classical neuroleptics of the phenothiazine or butyrophenone type are not features of Dolmatil therapy.

Dosage and administration *Adults:* A starting dose of 400 mg to 800 mg daily, given as one or two tablets twice daily (morning and early evening) is recommended.

Predominantly positive symptoms (formal thought disorder, hallucinations, delusions, incongruity of affect) respond to higher doses, and a starting dose of at least 400 mg twice daily is recommended, increasing if necessary up to a suggested maximum of 1200 mg twice daily. Increasing the dose beyond this level has not been shown to produce further improvement.

Predominantly negative symptoms (flattening of affect, poverty of speech, anergia, apathy), as well as depression, respond to doses below 800 mg daily; therefore, a starting dose of 400 mg twice daily is recommended. *Reducing* this dose towards 200 mg twice daily will normally *increase* the alerting affect of Dolmatil.

Patients with mixed positive and negative symptoms, with neither predominating, will normally respond to dosage of 400–600 mg twice daily.

Elderly: The same dose ranges may be required in the elderly, but should be reduced if there is evidence of renal impairment.

Children: Clinical experience in children under 14 years of age is insufficient to permit specific recommendations.

Contra-indications, warnings, etc
Contra-indications: The only absolute contra-indication is phaeochromocytoma. There are no cardiovascular contra-indications.

Warnings: Increased motor agitation has been reported at high dosage in a small number of patients: in aggressive, agitated or excited phases of the disease process, Dolmatil may aggravate symptoms. Care should be exercised where hypomania is present.

Extrapyramidal reactions, principally akathisia have been reported in a small number of cases. If warranted, reduction in dosage or anti-parkinsonian medication may be necessary.

After over a decade of widespread use in many countries, tardive dyskinesia has occurred rarely.

Insomnia has been reported.

As with all neuroleptic drugs, the presence of unexplained hyperthermia could indicate the neuroleptic malignant syndrome (NMS). In this event Dolmatil and any associated neuroleptic treatment should be discontinued until the origin of the fever has been determined.

Many medicines, including neuroleptics, raise serum prolactin levels, which may be associated with galactorrhoea and amenorrhoea, and less frequently with gynaecomastia. In long-term animal studies with neuroleptic drugs, including sulpiride, an increased incidence of various endocrine tumours (some of which have occasionally been malignant) has been seen in some but not all strains of rats and mice studied. The significance of these findings to man is not known; there is no evidence of an association between Dolmatil use and tumour risk in man. However, when prescribing neuroleptics to patients with existing mammary neoplasia or a history of this disease, possible risks should be weighed against benefits of therapy.

Precautions: While no drug interactions are known, unnecessary polypharmacy should be avoided. Although Dolmatil only induces slight EEG modifications, caution is advised in prescribing it for patients with unstable epilepsy. Patients requiring Dolmatil who are receiving anti-convulsant therapy should continue unchanged on the latter medication. Dolmatil has no significant anticholinergic or cardiovascular activity. As with all drugs for which the kidney is the major elimination pathway, the usual precautions should be taken in cases of renal failure.

Use in pregnancy: Despite the negative results of teratogenicity studies in animals and the lack of teratogenic effects during widespread clinical use in other countries, Dolmatil should not be considered an exception to the general principle of avoiding drug treatment during pregnancy, particularly during the first 16 weeks, with potential benefits being weighed against possible hazards.

Toxicity and treatment of overdose: Dolmatil is very well tolerated and only minor side-effects occur, if at all, at the recommended doses. The range of single toxic doses is 1 to 16 g but no death has occurrred even at the 16 g dose.

The clinical manifestations of poisoning vary depending upon the size of the dose taken. After single doses of 1 to 3 g restlessness and clouding of consciousness have been reported and (rarely) extrapyramidal symptoms. Doses of 3 to 7 g may produce a degree of agitation, confusion and extrapyramidal symptoms; more than 7 g can cause, in addition, coma and low blood pressure.

The duration of intoxication is generally short, the symptoms disappearing within a few hours. Comas which have occurred after large doses have lasted up to four days.

There are no specific complications from overdose. In particular no haematological or hepatic toxicity has been reported.

Overdose may be treated with alkaline osmotic diuresis and, if necessary, anti-parkinsonian drugs. Coma needs appropriate nursing. Emetic drugs are unlikely to be effective in Dolmatil overdosage.

Pharmaceutical precautions Store at room temperature.

Legal category POM.

Package quantities Cardboard cartons containing 10 bubble blister strips, each of which contains 10 tablets.

Further information Dolmatil is a member of the group of substituted benzamides, which are structurally distinct from the phenothiazines, butyrophenones and thioxanthenes. Current evidence suggests that the actions of Dolmatil hint at an important distinction between different types of dopamine receptors or receptor mechanisms in the brain. Behaviourally and biochemically, Dolmatil shares with these classical neuroleptics a number of properties indicative of cerebral dopamine receptor antagonism. Essential and intriguing differences include lack of catalepsy at doses active in other behavioural tests, lack of effect in the dopamine sensitive adenylate cyclase systems, lack of effect upon noradrenaline or 5HT turnover, negligible anticholinesterase activity, no effect on muscarinic or GABA receptor binding, and a radical difference in the binding of tritiated sulpiride to striatal preparations in-vitro, compared to ^{3}H-spiperone or ^{3}H-haloperidol. These findings indicate a major differentiation between Dolmatil and classical neuroleptics which lack such specificity.

The plasma half-life in man is approximately 8 hours.

Product licence number 5299/0006.

†DOLMATIL-SESIF Trade Mark: Authorised User Delagrange Limited.

ECONACORT* CREAM

Presentation White cream containing 1% w/w econazole nitrate and 1% w/w hydrocortisone.

Other ingredients: Benzoic acid, butylated hydroxyanisole, hard fat, liquid paraffin; esters of stearic acid, ethylene glycol and polyethylene glycol; glycerol and polyoxyethylene glycol esters.

Uses *Actions:* Econazole nitrate is a broad spectrum antifungal and antibiotic agent, active against dermatophytes (*Trichophyton rubrum, Trichophyton mentagrophytes, Epidermophyton floccosum* and *Malassezia furfur*); pathogenic yeasts; *Candida albicans* and other *Candida* species. It is also active against Gram-positive bacteria.

Hydrocortisone is a widely used topical anti-inflammatory agent of value in the treatment of inflammatory skin conditions including atopic and infantile eczema, contact sensitivity reactions and intertrigo.

Indications: Econacort is indicated for the topical treatment of inflammatory dermatoses where infection by susceptible organisms co-exists e.g. inflammatory fungal infections including ringworm and Candida and infected eczema where Gram-positive organisms are commonly associated with exacerbations and chronicity.

Dosage and administration
Adults and children: To be massaged gently into the affected and surrounding skin area morning and evening. The cream is particularly suitable for moist and weeping lesions.

Elderly: Natural thinning of the skin occurs in the elderly, hence corticosteroids should be used sparingly and for short periods of time.

Contra-indications, warnings, etc
Contra-indications: Hypersensitivity to either of the active ingredients.

In tuberculous and most viral lesions of the skin, particularly herpes simplex, vaccinia and varicella.

Precautions: Econacort cream should not be used in or near the eyes.

Children: As with any topical corticosteroid, care is advised with infants and children where the preparation is to be applied to extensive areas or under occlusive dressing. However, continuous prolonged treatment should not be necessary.

Pregnancy: Topical administration of corticosteroids to pregnant animals can cause foetal abnormalities. The relevance of this finding to humans has not been established. However, topical corticosteroids should not be used extensively in pregnancy, i.e. in large amounts or for long periods. Topical corticosteroids should be used during pregnancy only if the potential benefit justifies the potential risk to the foetus.

Side-effects: Econazole nitrate and hydrocortisone are well tolerated. Where adverse reactions occur they are usually reversible on cessation of therapy.

Side-effects of econazole nitrate are limited to occasional local irritation manifested by erythema, burning or stinging sensation, and pruritis, but these may be minimised by the hydrocortisone component.

The possibility of the systemic effects which are associated with all steroid therapy should be considered. These effects may be enhanced with occlusive dressings.

Overdosage: Topically applied corticosteroids can be absorbed in sufficient amounts to produce systemic effects.

Pharmaceutical precautions Store in a cool place. Dilution is not recommended, as this would reduce the concentration of the antibiotic to below therapeutic levels.

Legal category POM.

Package quantities Tubes of 30 g (OP).

Further information Nil.

Product licence number 0034/0249.

ECOSTATIN* CREAM, LOTION, POWDER, SPRAY POWDER, AND SPRAY SOLUTION

Presentation
Cream: White cream containing 1% w/w econazole nitrate.

Other ingredients: Benzoic acid, butylated hydroxyanisole, liquid paraffin, perfume; esters of stearic acid, ethylene glycol and polyethylene glycol; glycerol and polyoxyethylene glycol esters.

Lotion: Milky white homogeneous lotion containing 1% w/w econazole nitrate.

Other ingredients: Benzoic acid, butylated hydroxyanisole, colloidal silicon dioxide, liquid paraffin, perfume; esters of stearic acid, ethylene glycol and polyethylene glycol; glycerol and polyoxyethylene glycol esters.

Powder: White powder containing 1% w/w econazole nitrate in talc base.

Other ingredients: Colloidal silicon dioxide, zinc oxide, talc, perfume.

Spray powder: White powder containing 1% w/w econazole nitrate in talc base.

Other ingredients: Colloidal silicon dioxide, zinc oxide, talc, perfume, with dichlorodifluoromethane, trichloromonofluoromethane.

Spray Solution: Alcoholic solution containing 1% w/w econazole nitrate.

Other ingredients: Ethanol, perfume, propylene glycol, with dichlorodifluoromethane, trichloromonofluoromethane, tris hydroxymethyl aminomethane.

Uses *Actions:* Econazole nitrate is a broad spectrum antifungal agent, active against dermatophytes (*Trichophyton rubrum, Trichophyton mentagrophytes, Epidermophyton floccosum* and *Malassezia furfur*); pathogenic yeasts; *Candida albicans* and other *Candida* species. Also active against some Gram-positive bacteria, e.g. staphylococci and streptococci.

Indications All fungal skin infections due to dermatophytes (e.g. *Trichophyton* species), yeasts (e.g. *Candida* species), moulds and other fungi. These include ringworm (tinea) infections, athlete's foot, paronychia, pityriasis versicolor, erythrasma, intertrigo, fungal nappy rash, candidal vulvitis and candidal balanitis. Bacterial skin infections due to Gram-positive organisms.

Dosage and administration *Adults and Children: Cream:* To be massaged gently into the affected and surrounding skin area morning and evening. The cream is particularly suitable for moist or weeping lesions.

Lotion: To be applied twice daily to the affected and surrounding skin area. In the treatment of fungal infections of the nail, apply once daily with an occlusive dressing.

Powder and spray powder: To be applied to the affected area twice daily. The powder is particularly suitable for use in skin folds, e.g. inguinal and interdigital.

Spray solution: To be applied twice daily. See precautions.

Clinical improvement usually occurs promptly; however, complete disappearance of the symptoms of the disease may require prolonged treatment. Therapy should continue for several days following both clinical and mycological cure in order to prevent relapse.

Elderly: No specific dosage recommendations.

Contra-indications, warnings, etc
Contra-indications: Patients with a history of sensitivity to any of the components of the preparations.

Precautions: Ecostatin cream, lotion, powder, spray powder or spray solution should not be used in or near the eyes. Ecostatin spray solution should not be used on mucous membranes.

Pregnancy: No specific precautions apply; systemic absorption is likely to be negligible.

Side-effects: Ecostatin is well tolerated. Side-effects are limited to occasional local irritation manifested by erythema, burning or stinging sensations and pruritus.

Pharmaceutical precautions *Storage: Cream, lotion, powder:* Store at room temperature.

Spray powder, spray solution: Store in a cool place.

Legal category P.

Package quantities *Ecostatin cream:* Tubes of 30 g and 15 g (OP).
Ecostatin lotion: 30 ml (OP).
Ecostatin powder: 30 g (OP).
Ecostatin spray powder: 200 g (OP).
Ecostatin spray solution: 150 g (OP).

Further information Nil.

Product licence numbers

Ecostatin Cream	0034/0231
Ecostatin Lotion	0034/0232
Ecostatin Powder	0034/0234
Ecostatin Spray Powder	0034/0235
Ecostatin Spray Solution	0034/0236

ECOSTATIN* PESSARIES AND TWIN PACK

Presentation
Pessaries: White, opaque, oval pessaries each containing 150 mg econazole nitrate in an hydrogenated vegetable oil base. 3 pessary treatment pack.

Other ingredients: Hard fat.

Twin pack: Three Ecostatin pessaries with applicator plus 15 g Ecostatin cream (containing 1% w/w econazole nitrate).

The Cream also contains: Benzoic acid, butylated hydroxyanisole, liquid paraffin, perfume; esters of stearic acid, ethylene glycol and polyethylene glycol; glycerol and polyoxyethylene glycol esters.

Uses *Actions:* Econazole nitrate has a broad spectrum of antifungal activity. It is highly active against *Candida albicans* and other *Candida* species and is effective in controlling infections of the vagina and vulva caused by such organisms (thrush).

Indications: Vulvovaginal candidosis. In addition to vaginal treatment the Twin Pack contains cream for topical application to the anogenital area.

Dosage and administration *Adults: Pessaries:* One pessary to be inserted at bedtime for three consecutive nights. Administration should be continued even if menstruation occurs, and despite the disappearance of signs and symptoms of the infection.

The pessary should be inserted high into the vagina while the patient is supine.

Cream: The cream is applied twice daily, in the morning and evening, to the anogenital area.

Note: To prevent re-infection with *Candida*, the male consort should be treated concurrently with Ecostatin cream, applied twice daily to the external genital area during the treatment period.

Although a three day course of therapy usually suffices, it may be necessary to institute a second course of therapy.

Children: Vulvovaginal candidosis is not normally a problem in children, therefore there are no specific dosage recommendations.

Elderly: No specific dosage recommendations or precautions apply.

Contra-indications, warnings, etc
Contra-indications: Patients with a history of sensitivity to any of the components of the preparation.

Precautions: Avoid contact between this product and contraceptive diaphragms and condoms since the rubber may be damaged by the preparation.

Pregnancy: Ecostatin pessaries are effective in the candidal vaginitis associated with pregnancy. Safety of systemic econazole has not been established but percutaneous absorption following topical application is likely to be low. However, as with other agents, Ecostatin should not be used during the first trimester of pregnancy unless the physician deems its use essential for the welfare of the patient. In pregnancy, extra care should be taken in using an applicator to prevent the possibility of mechanical trauma.

Side-effects: Patients may rarely complain of discomfort; this is usually transitory and disappears with continued treatment. Seldom is it necessary to discontinue econazole pessary treatment.

Ecostatin cream is well tolerated. Side-effects are limited to occasional local irritation manifested by erythema, burning or stinging sensation, and pruritus.

Pharmaceutical precautions *Storage:* Store at room temperature.

Legal category Cream P.
Pessaries POM.

Package quantities *Pessaries:* Pack of three pessaries with applicator (OP).
Twin pack: Three pessaries with applicator plus 15 g cream (OP).

Further information Nil.

Product licence numbers

Ecostatin Pessaries	0034/0233
Ecostatin Cream	0034/0231

ECOSTATIN*-1 PESSARY

Presentation A white, opaque, oval pessary containing 150 mg econazole nitrate in a long-acting formulation and melting at 37°C. Single dose treatment pack.

Other ingredients: Colloidal silicon dioxide, hard fat, natural polysaccharides, stearyl heptanoate.

Uses
Actions: Econazole nitrate has a broad spectrum of antifungal activity. It is highly active against *Candida albicans* and other Candida species and is effective in controlling infections of the vagina and vulva caused by such organisms (thrush).

Indications: The treatment of vaginitis due to *Candida albicans* and other yeasts.

Dosage and administration
Adults: The recommended dose is one pessary inserted at bedtime. The pessary should be inserted as high as possible into the vagina, using the applicator, with the patient in the supine position.

Note: To prevent re-infection with Candida, the male consort should be treated concurrently with Ecostatin cream.

Although one course of therapy usually suffices, it may be necessary to institute a second course of therapy.

Children: Vulvovaginal candidosis is not normally a problem in children, therefore there are no specific dosage recommendations.

Elderly: No specific dosage recommendations or precautions apply.

Contra-indications, warnings, etc
Contra-indications: Patients with a known history of sensitivity to any of the components of the preparation.

Precautions: Avoid contact between this product and contraceptive diaphragms and condoms since the rubber may be damaged by the preparation.

Pregnancy: Ecostatin-1 Pessaries are effective in the candidal vaginitis associated with pregnancy. Safety of systemic econazole has not been established but percutaneous absorption following topical application is likely to be low. However, as with other agents, Ecostatin should not be used during the first trimester of pregnancy unless the physician deems its use essential for the welfare of the patient. In pregnancy, extra care should be taken in using an applicator to prevent the possibility of mechanical trauma.

Side-effects: Patients may rarely complain of transitory discomfort.

Overdosage: There have been no recorded cases of overdose.

Pharmaceutical precautions Store in a cool place.

Legal category POM.

Package quantities Each pack contains one pessary with an applicator (OP).

Further information Patients should be advised of the importance of anogenital hygiene to help prevent reinfection.

Product licence number 0034/0266.

FLORINEF* TABLETS

Presentation Round, pale pink tablets, scored on one side and engraved Squibb and 429 on reverse, containing 0.1 mg fludrocortisone acetate.

Other ingredients: Dicalcium phosphate, erythrosin, lactose, magnesium stearate, maize starch, sodium benzoate, talc.

Uses *Actions:* Qualitatively, the physiological action of fludrocortisone acetate is similar to hydrocortisone. In very small doses, fludrocortisone maintains life in adrenalectomised animals, enhances the deposition of liver glycogen and produces thymic involution, eosinopenia, retention of sodium and increased urinary excretion of potassium.

Indications: For partial replacement therapy for primary and secondary adrenocortical insufficiency in Addison's disease and for the treatment of salt-losing adrenogenital syndrome.

Dosage and administration
Adult dosage: A daily dosage range of 0.05–0.3 mg Florinef tablets orally. Supplementary parenteral administration of sodium-retaining hormones is not necessary. When an enhanced glucocorticoid effect is desirable, cortisone or hydrocortisone by mouth should be given concomitantly with Florinef tablets.

Children: May be used adjusted to the age and weight of the child according to the severity of the condition (see 'Precautions').

Elderly: No specific dosage recommendations or precautions.

Contra-indications, warnings, etc
Contra-indications: Because of its marked effect on sodium retention, the use of Florinef in the treatment of conditions other than those indicated, is not advised.

Since Florinef is a potent mineralocorticoid both the dosage and salt intake should be carefully monitored to avoid the development of hypertension, oedema or weight gain. Periodic checking of serum electrolyte levels is advisable during prolonged therapy.

Precautions: Florinef is a potent mineralocorticoid and is used predominantly for replacement therapy. Although glucocorticoid side effects may occur, these can be reduced by reducing the dosage.

In common with other steroids Florinef should be used with caution in patients with diverticulitis, recent intestinal anastomoses, thrombophlebitis, psychotic tendencies, exanthematous disease, chronic nephritis, metastatic carcinoma, osteoporosis, in patients with an active peptic ulcer (or a history of peptic ulcer), and myasthenia gravis. Latent or healed tuberculosis; in the presence of local or systemic viral infection, systemic fungal infections or in active infections not controlled by antibiotics. In acute psychoses; in acute glomerulonephritis. Hypertension; glaucoma (or a family history of glaucoma), previous steroid myopathy or epilepsy. Diabetes may be aggravated, necessitating a higher insulin dosage. Latent diabetes mellitus may be precipitated.

Menstrual irregularities may occur, and this possibility should be mentioned to female patients.

Patients on long-term systemic therapy with Florinef may require supportive corticosteroid therapy in times of stress (such as trauma, surgery or severe illness), both during the treatment period and for a year afterwards.

During corticosteroid therapy antibody response will be reduced and therefore affect the patient's response to vaccines.

Rare instances of anaphylactoid reactions have occurred in patients receiving corticosteroids, especially when a patient has a history of drug allergies.

All corticosteroids increase calcium excretion.

Avoid abrupt cessation of corticosteroids.

Aspirin should be used cautiously in conjunction with corticosteroids in patients with hypoprothrombinaemia.

Corticosteroid effects may be enhanced in patients with hypothyroidism or cirrhosis.

Children: Growth and development of children on prolonged corticosteroid therapy should be carefully observed.

Pregnancy and nursing mothers: It may be decided to continue a pregnancy in a woman requiring replacement mineralocorticoid therapy, despite the risk to the foetus.

There is evidence of harmful effects in pregnancy in animals. There is inadequate evidence of safety of the foetus in human pregnancy and there may be a very small risk of cleft palate and intra-uterine growth retardation.

Infants born of mothers who have received substantial doses of fludrocortisone acetate during pregnancy should be carefully observed for signs of hypoadrenalism. Maternal treatment should be carefully documented in the infant's medical records to assist in follow up.

Corticosteroids are found in breast milk.

Side-effects: Where adverse reactions occur they are usually reversible on cessation of therapy.

Patients should be watched closely for the following adverse reactions which may be associated with any corticosteroid therapy:

Fluid and electrolyte disturbances: Sodium retention, fluid retention, congestive heart failure in susceptible patients, potassium loss, cardiac arrhythmias or ECG changes due to potassium deficiency, hypokalaemic alkalosis, increased calcium excretion and hypertension.

Musculoskeletal: Muscle weakness, fatigue, steroid myopathy, loss of muscle mass, osteoporosis, vertebral compression fractures, delayed healing of fractures, aseptic necrosis of femoral and humeral heads, pathological fractures of long bones and spontaneous fractures.

Gastro-intestinal: Peptic ulcer with possible subsequent perforation and haemorrhage, pancreatitis, abdominal distension and ulcerative oesophagitis.

Dermatologic: Impaired wound healing, thin fragile skin, petechiae and ecchymoses, facial erythema, increased sweating, purpura, striae, hirsutism, acneiform eruptions, lupus erythematosus-like lesions and suppressed reactions to skin tests.

Neurological: Convulsions, increased intracranial pressure with papilloedema (pseudo-tumour cerebri) usually after treatment, vertigo, headache, neuritis or paraesthesias and aggravation of pre-existing psychiatric conditions.

Endocrine: Menstrual irregularities; development of the Cushingoid state; suppression of growth in children; secondary adrenocortical and pituitary unresponsiveness, particularly in times of stress (e.g. trauma, surgery or illness); decreased carbohydrate tolerance; manifestations of latent diabetes mellitus and increased requirements for insulin or oral hypoglycaemic agents in diabetes.

Ophthalmic: Posterior subcapsular cataracts, increased intraocular pressure, glaucoma and exopthalmos.

Metabolic: Hyperglycaemia, glycosuria and negative nitrogen balance due to protein catabolism.

Others: Necrotising angiitis, thrombophlebitis, thromboembolism, aggravation or masking of infections, insomnia, syncopal episodes and anaphylactoid reactions, particularly where there is a history of drug allergies.

Overdosage: A single large dose should be treated with plenty of water by mouth. Careful monitoring of serum electrolytes is essential, with particular consideration being given to the need for administration of potassium chloride and restriction of dietary sodium intake.

Pharmaceutical precautions *Storage:* At room temperature.

Legal category POM.

Package quantities Bottles of 100.

Further information Nil.

Product licence numbers
Florinef Tablets 0.1 mg 0034/5027R

FUNGILIN* LOZENGES, SUSPENSION AND TABLETS

Presentation
Lozenges: Round, pale yellow, engraved '929' and 'Squibb', containing 10,000 units (10 mg) amphotericin.

Other ingredients: Acacia powder, d-mannitol, flavours, magnesium stearate, polyvinyl alcohol, talc.

Suspension: Orange-flavoured, viscous suspension containing 100,000 units (100 mg) amphotericin per ml.

Other ingredients: Citric acid, ethanol, glycerin, flavours, methyl hydroxybenzoate, propyl hydroxybenzoate, sodium benzoate, sodium carboxymethylcellulose, sodium phosphate, potassium chloride, water.

Tablets: Yellow to tan, scored one side and engraved Squibb and 430 on reverse, containing 100,000 units (100 mg) amphotericin.

Other ingredients: Ethyl cellulose, lactose, maize starch, magnesium stearate, talc.

Uses *Actions:* Amphotericin is an antifungal antibiotic active against a wide range of yeasts and yeast-like fungi including *Candida albicans.* Absorption from the gastrointestinal tract is negligible even with very large doses. Extensive clinical experience has not shown problems of toxicity or sensitisation.

Indications: Lozenges/Suspension: For the treatment of candidal lesions (thrush) of the oral and perioral areas. The suspension may be used in the treatment of denture stomatitis.

Suspension/Tablets: For the treatment of intestinal candidosis and the suppression of the intestinal reservoir of *C. albicans* which may precipitate cutaneous or vaginal candidosis.

Dosage and administration *Adult dosage: Lozenges:* Dissolve 1 slowly in the mouth four times a day. Depending on the severity of infection, the dose may be increased to 8 lozenges daily.

To clear the condition fully may require 10-15 days' treatment.

Suspension: For denture stomatitis and oral infections caused by *C. albicans,* 1 ml should be placed in the mouth four times daily; it should be kept in contact with lesions for as long as possible.

For the treatment or suppression of intestinal candidosis, 2 ml four times daily.

Tablets: 1 or 2 tablets four times daily.

Administration of Fungilin for oral and intestinal candidosis should be continued for 48 hours after clinical cure to prevent relapse.

Infants and children: Suspension: For intestinal and oral candidosis, 1 ml should be dropped into the mouth four times daily. The suspension should be held in contact with oral lesions for as long as possible before swallowing.

For prophylaxis in the newborn, the suggested dose is 1 ml daily.

Elderly: No specific dosage recommendations or precautions.

Contra-indications, warnings, etc
Contra-indications: There are no known contra-indications to the use of these products.

Precautions: No specific precautions apply.

Pregnancy/Children: Absorption of amphotericin from the gastrointestinal tract is negligible, therefore no special precautions apply.

Side-effects: Gastro-intestinal side-effects have occasionally been reported following continuous administration of amphotericin for several months in daily doses in excess of 3 g. These have been mild in nature and have readily cleared on cessation of treatment. No systemic toxic effects or allergic reactions have been associated with its oral use.

Overdosage: Since absorption of amphotericin from the gastro-intestinal tract is negligible, overdosage causes no systemic toxicity.

Pharmaceutical precautions *Storage: Lozenges/Tablets:* At room temperature.

Suspension: Cool place; protect from direct sunlight. Discard any unused suspension 4 days after opening.

Dilution: Fungilin Suspension should not be diluted prior to use; it is formulated to coat and adhere to the oral lesions being treated.

Legal category POM.

Package quantities *Lozenges:* Blister packs of 60 (OP).
Tablets: Bottles of 56 (OP).
Suspension: 12 ml bottles with graduated dropper (OP).

Further information Nil.

Product licence numbers

Fungilin Lozenges	0034/5034R
Fungilin Suspension	0034/5038R
Fungilin Tablets	0034/5039R

FUNGIZONE* INTRAVENOUS

Presentation Each vial contains a yellow, fluffy powder: amphotericin 50,000 units (50 mg).

Other ingredients: Desoxycholic acid, sodium phosphates, sodium hydroxide, phosphoric acid.

Uses *Actions:* Amphotericin is a polyene antifungal antibiotic active against a wide range of yeasts and yeast-like fungi including Candida albicans. Crystalline amphotericin is insoluble in water; therefore, the antibiotic is solubilised by the addition of sodium desoxycholate to form a mixture which provides a colloidal dispersion for parenteral administration. Amphotericin is fungistatic rather than fungicidal in concentrations obtainable in body fluids. It probably acts by binding to sterols in the fungal cell membrane with a resultant change in membrane permeability which allows leakage of intracellular components. Mammalian cell membranes also contain sterols and it has been suggested that the damage to human and fungal cells may share common mechanisms. No strains of Candida resistant to amphotericin have been reported in clinical use, and although in vitro testing does produce a small number of resistant isolates this occurs only following repeated subcultures.

Clinical pharmacology: An initial intravenous infusion of 1 to 5 mg of amphotericin per day, gradually increased to 0.65 mg/kg daily, produces peak plasma concentrations of approximately 2 to 4 mg/l which can persist between doses since the plasma half-life of amphotericin is about 24 hours. It has been reported that amphotericin is highly bound (more than 90%) to plasma proteins and is poorly dialysable.

Amphotericin is excreted very slowly by the kidneys with 2 to 5% of a given dose being excreted in biologically active form. After treatment is discontinued the drug can be detected in the urine for at least seven weeks. The cumulative urinary output over a seven day period amounts to approximately 40% of the amount of drug infused.

Details of tissue distribution and possible metabolic pathways are not known.

Indications: Fungizone Intravenous should be administered primarily to patients with progressive, potentially fatal infections. This potent drug should not be used to treat the common forms of fungal disease which show only positive skin or serological tests.

Fungizone Intravenous is specifically intended to treat cryptococcosis (torulosis); North American blastomycosis; the disseminated forms of candidosis, coccidioidomycosis and histoplasmosis; mucormycosis (phycomycosis) caused by species of the genera *Mucor, Rhizopus, Absidia, Entomophthora*, and *Basidiobolus sporotrichosis (Sporotrichum schenckii)*, aspergillosis *(Aspergillus fumigatus)*.

Amphotericin may be helpful in the treatment of American mucocutaneous leishmaniasis but is not the drug of choice in primary therapy.

Dosage and administration *Adults and children:* Fungizone should be administered by slow intravenous infusion over a period of six hours. Initial daily dose should be 0.25 mg/kg of body weight gradually increasing to a level of 1.0 mg/kg of body weight depending on individual response and tolerance. Within the range of 0.25-1.0 mg/kg the daily dose should be maintained at the highest level which is not accompanied by unacceptable toxicity.

In seriously ill patients the daily dose may be gradually increased up to a total of 1.5 mg/kg. Since amphotericin is excreted slowly, therapy may be given on alternate days in patients on the higher dosage schedule. Several months of therapy are usually necessary; a shorter period of therapy may produce an inadequate response and lead to relapse.

Whenever medication is interrupted for a period longer than seven days, therapy should be resumed by starting with the lowest dosage level, i.e. 0.25 mg/kg of body weight, and increased gradually.

Caution: Under no circumstances should a total daily dose of 1.5 mg/kg be exceeded. The recommended concentration for intravenous infusion is 10 mg/100 ml (100 units per ml).

Elderly: No specific dosage recommendations or precautions.

Preparation of solutions: Reconstitute as follows: An initial concentrate of 5 mg amphotericin per ml is first prepared by rapidly expressing 10 ml sterile water for injection, without a bacteriostatic agent, directly into the lyophilised cake, using a sterile needle (minimum diameter: 20 gauge) and syringe. Shake the vial immediately until the colloidal solution is clear. The infusion solution, providing 10 mg/100 ml is obtained by further dilution (1:50) with 5% Glucose Injection of pH above 4.2. The pH of each container of Glucose Injection should be ascertained before use. Commercial Glucose Injection usually has a pH above 4.2; however, if it is below 4.2 then 1 or 2 ml of buffer should be added to the Glucose Injection before it is used to dilute a concentrated solution of amphotericin. The recommended buffer has the following composition:

Dibasic sodium phosphate (anhydrous)	1.59 g
Monobasic sodium phosphate (anhydrous)	0.96 g
Water for Injection BP	qs 100 ml

The buffer should be sterilised before it is added to the Glucose Injection, either by filtration through a bacterial filter, or by autoclaving for 30 mins at 15 lb pressure (121° C).

Caution: Aseptic technique must be strictly observed in all handling, since no preservative or bacteriostatic agent is present. Do not reconstitute with saline solutions. The use of any diluent other than the ones recommended or the presence of a bacteriostatic agent in the diluent may cause precipitation of the amphotericin. Do not use the initial concentrate or the infusion solution if there is any evidence of precipitation of foreign matter.

An in-line membrane filter may be used for intravenous infusion of amphotericin; however the mean pore diameter of the filter should not be less than 1.0 micron in order to assure passage of the amphotericin dispersion.

Other preparations for injection should not be added to the infusion solution or administered via the cannula being used to administer Fungizone Intravenous.

Contra-indications, warnings, etc
Contra-indications: Those patients who are hypersensitive to amphotericin, unless, in the opinion of the physician, the condition requiring treatment is life-threatening and amenable only to such therapy.

Precautions: Prolonged therapy with amphotericin is usually necessary. Unpleasant reactions are quite common when the drug is given parenterally at therapeutic dosage levels. Some of these reactions are potentially dangerous. Hence amphotericin should be used parenterally only in hospitalised patients, or those under close clinical observation. If the BUN exceeds 6.5 mmol/l, or the serum creatinine exceeds 260 micromol/l, the drug should be discontinued or the dosage markedly reduced until renal function is improved. Weekly blood counts and serum potassium determinations are also advisable. Low serum magnesium levels have also been noted during treatment with amphotericin. Therapy should be discontinued if liver function test results (elevated bromsulphalein, alkaline phosphatase and bilirubin) are abnormal.

Corticosteroids should not be administered concomitantly unless they are necessary to control drug reactions. Other nephrotoxic antibiotics and antineoplastic agents should not be given concomitantly except with great caution.

Pregnancy: Safety for use in pregnancy has not been established; therefore it should be used during pregnancy only if the possible benefits to be derived outweigh the potential risks involved.

Side-effects: While some patients may tolerate full intravenous doses of amphotericin without difficulty, most will exhibit some intolerance, often at less than the full therapeutic dosage. They may be made less severe by giving aspirin, antihistamines or antiemetics. Administration of the drug on alternate days may decrease anorexia and phlebitis. Intravenous administration of small doses of adrenal corticosteroids just prior to or during the amphotericin infusion may decrease febrile reactions. The dosage and duration of such corticosteroid therapy should be kept to a minimum. Adding a small amount of heparin to the infusion may lessen the incidence of thrombophlebitis and coagulation problems. Extravasation may cause chemical irritation. The adverse reactions that are most commonly observed are: fever (sometimes with shaking chills), headache, anorexia, weight loss, nausea and vomiting, malaise, muscle and joint pains, dyspepsia, cramping epigastric pain, diarrhoea, local venous pain at the injection site with phlebitis and thrombophlebitis, normochromic normocytic anaemia and hypokalaemia. Abnormal renal function, including hypokalaemia, azotaemia, hyposthenuria, renal tubular acidosis or nephrocalcinosis, is also commonly observed and usually improves upon interruption of therapy; however, some permanent impairment often occurs, especially in those patients receiving large amounts (over 5 g) of amphotericin. The following adverse reactions occur less frequently or rarely: anuria (oliguria); cardiovascular toxicity including arrhythmias, ventricular fibrillation, cardiac arrest, hypotension, hypertension; coagulation defects; thrombocytopenia; leucopenia; agranulocytosis; eosinophilia; leucocytosis; melaena or haemorrhagic gastroenteritis; maculopapular rash and pruritus; hearing loss, tinnitus; transient vertigo; blurred vision, or diplopia; peripheral neuropathy, convulsions and other neurologic symptoms; anaphylactoid reactions, acute liver failure and flushing.

Drug interactions: Concomitant administration of nephrotoxic drugs or anti-neoplastics should be avoided if at all possible.

The hypokalaemia following amphotericin therapy may potentiate the toxicity of digitalis glycosides or enhance the curariform actions of skeletal muscle relaxants.

Corticosteroids may increase the potassium loss due to amphotericin.

Pharmaceutical precautions *Storage:* Vials of powder for reconstitution should be stored in a refrigerator. The concentrate (5 mg per ml after reconstitution with 10 ml sterile Water for Injection) should be stored protected from light. The absence of microbial preservative and the risk of contamination during reconstitution mean that the product should be stored for no more than 8 hours at room temperature or 24 hours in a refrigerator. Should the need arise and a validated aseptic reconstitution technique is applied, the product is chemically stable when stored for 24 hours at room temperature or one week in a refrigerator. It is not intended as a multidose vial. Any unused material should be discarded. Solutions prepared for intravenous infusion (i.e. 10 mg or less amphotericin per 100 ml) should be used promptly after preparation and should be protected from light during administration.

Legal category POM.

Package quantities Vials of 50 mg.

Further information The use of Fungizone intravenous by other routes has been documented in the published literature:

Bladder irrigation/installation (e.g. candiduria). Continuous irrigation with 50 mg Fungizone in 1 litre sterile water each day until urinary cultures are negative. Intermittent use of volumes of 100–400 ml (concentrations of 37.5–200 microgram/ml) has also been reported. The urine should be alkalinised (with potassium citrate) and antifungal ointment applied to the perineal area.

Lung inhalation (e.g. pulmonary aspergillosis). 8–40 mg amphotericin (nebulised in sterile water or 5% dextrose) has been given daily in divided doses. Concurrent eradication of oral and intestinal yeasts reservoirs is recommended.

Intrathecal (e.g. coccidiodal meningitis). Current published dosage recommendations are for maintenance 0.25–1.0 mg amphotericin 2–4 times weekly following initiation with a low dose (0.025 mg) and cautious increases. Amphotericin is irritating when injected into the CSF.

Other: Other uses of solutions prepared using Fungizone intravenous include local instillations for the treatment of fungal infections of the ear, eye, peritoneum, lung cavities and joint spaces.

Product licence number 0034/5041R.

GRANEODIN* OINTMENT

Presentation Graneodin Ointment is soft, slightly opaque, colourless, containing neomycin (as sulphate) 0.25% and gramicidin 0.025% in Plastibase* (liquid paraffin, and polyethylene resin).

Uses *Actions:* Neomycin is active against a wide range of Gram-positive and Gram-negative bacteria, including many of the organisms responsible for bacterial skin infections.

Gramicidin is active against Gram-positive bacteria and supplements the action of neomycin against the many common skin pathogens found in this group.

Indications–Topical: Superficial bacterial infections such as impetigo; impetiginised eczema; infected eczema; furuncles; sycosis barbae; folliculitis; ecthyma; chronic ulcers of the skin; scratches or abrasions; bacterial infections of the ear. (See Contra-indications.)

For prophylaxis against infections following minor surgery.

Dosage and administration *Adults and children–Topical:* To be applied two to four times a day. Any crusts should be removed and the ointment rubbed well in.

Elderly: No specific dosage recommendations or precautions.

Contra-indications, warnings, etc
Contra-indications: Fungal or viral infections of the skin or for the treatment of deep-seated infections. This preparation is contra-indicated in persons with known sensitivity to neomycin. Should not be applied to the external auditory canal in patients with perforated eardrums.

Precautions: The possibility of sensitivity to neomycin should be taken into consideration especially in the treatment of patients suffering from leg ulcers. Since the use of occlusive dressings may increase the risk of sensitivity reactions such dressings should be avoided.

Pregnancy/Children: No specific precautions apply.

Side-effects: Neomycin: Sensitivity reactions may occur especially with prolonged use. Ototoxicity and nephrotoxicity have been reported. Large amounts of this product should be avoided in the treatment of skin infections following extensive burns, trophic ulceration, and other conditions where absorption of neomycin is possible.

Gramicidin: Sensitivity has occasionally been reported.

Pharmaceutical precautions *Storage:* At room temperature.

Dilution: Not recommended.

Legal category POM.

Package quantities *Ointment:* Tubes of 25 g (OP).

Further information Nil.

Product licence number 0034/5042

HALCIDERM* TOPICAL

Presentation A white topical preparation containing halcinonide 0.1% in a water-miscible base.

Other ingredients: Benzyl alcohol, castor oil, colloidal silicon dioxide, macrogol ether, propylene glycol, stearates, white soft paraffin.

Uses *Actions:* Halcinonide is a potent corticosteroid with rapid anti-inflammatory, antipruritic and anti-allergic actions.

Halciderm is suitable for both wet and dry lesions.

Indications: Halciderm is indicated in acute and chronic corticosteroid-responsive conditions which may include: psoriasis, atopic eczema, contact eczema, follicular eczema, infantile eczema, neurodermatitis, anogenital eczema (pruritus ani et vulvae), nummular eczema, seborrhoeic or flexural eczema, otitis externa.

Dosage and administration *Adults:* Halciderm should be applied to the affected area two, or occasionally three, times daily. In long-term therapy, or where lower strength preparations are required, do not dilute but use intermittently.

Children: In infants, long-term continuous topical steroid therapy should be avoided.

Elderly: Natural thinning of the skin occurs in the elderly; hence corticosteroids should be used sparingly and for short periods of time.

Contra-indications, warnings, etc
Contra-indications: Halciderm is not intended for ophthalmic use, nor should it be applied in the external auditory canal of patients with perforated eardrums.

In tuberculous and most viral lesions of the skin, particularly herpes simplex, vaccinia, varicella. The product should not be used in fungal or bacterial skin infections without suitable concomitant anti-infective therapy.

Precautions: Adrenal suppression can occur, even without occlusion.

Pregnancy: Topical administration of corticosteroids to pregnant animals can cause abnormalities of foetal development. The relevance of this finding to humans has not been established. However, topical steroids should not be used extensively in pregnancy, i.e. in large amounts or for long periods. Topical corticosteroids should be used during pregnancy only if the potential benefit justifies the potential risk to the foetus.

Side-effects: Halcinonide is well tolerated. Where adverse reactions occur they are usually reversible on cessation of therapy. However the following side-effects have been reported usually with prolonged usage:

Dermatologic – impaired wound healing, thinning of the skin, petechiae and ecchymoses, facial erythema and telangiectasia, increased sweating, purpura, striae, hirsutism, acneiform eruptions, lupus erythematosus-like lesions and suppressed reaction to skin tests. These effects may be enhanced with occlusive dressings.

Signs of systemic toxicity such as oedema and electrolyte imbalance have not been observed even when high topical dosage has been used. The possibility of the systemic effects which are associated with all steroid therapy should be considered.

Overdosage: Topically applied corticosteroids can be absorbed in sufficient amounts to produce systemic effects (see Side-effects).

Pharmaceutical precautions *Storage:* Halciderm should be stored in a cool place.

Dilution: Due to special formulation of topical Halciderm, normal dermatological diluents should not be used. For further information consult the manufacturer.

Legal category POM.

Package quantities Tubes containing 30 g (OP).

Further information Halciderm contains halcinonide 0.1%, dissolved in the non-aqueous phase of the formulation.

Product licence number 0034/0160.

HYDREA* CAPSULES

Presentation Pink, opaque capsule body with green, opaque cap, both parts printed Squibb and 830 in black, containing hydroxyurea 500 mg.

Other ingredients: Citric acid, lactose, magnesium stearate, sodium phosphate; gelatin/glycerin capsules contain erythrosine, iron oxide, Patent Blue V, quinoline yellow, titanium dioxide.

Uses *Actions:* Hydroxyurea is an orally active antineoplastic agent. Although the mechanism of action has not yet been clearly defined, hydroxyurea appears to act by interfering with synthesis of DNA.

Indications: The treatment of chronic myeloid leukaemia.

The treatment of cancer of the cervix in conjunction with radiotherapy.

Dosage and administration Treatment regimens can be continuous or intermittent. The continuous regimen is particularly suitable for chronic myeloid leukaemia, while the intermittent regimen, with its diminished effect on the bone marrow, is more satisfactory for the management of cancer of the cervix.

Hydrea should be started 7 days before concurrent irradiation therapy.

An adequate trial period for determining the antineoplastic effect of Hydrea is six weeks.

Continuous therapy: Hydrea 20-30 mg/kg should be given daily in single doses. Dosage should be based on the patient's actual or ideal weight, whichever is the less. Therapy should be monitored by repeat blood counts.

Intermittent therapy: Hydrea 80 mg/kg in single doses should be given every third day. Using the intermittent regimes the likelihood of WBC depression is diminished, but if low counts are produced, 1 or more doses of Hydrea should be omitted.

Children: Because of the rarity of these conditions in children, dosage regimens have not been established.

Elderly: Elderly patients may be more sensitive to the effects of hydroxyurea, and may require a lower dosage regimen.

N.B. If the patient prefers, or is unable to swallow capsules, the contents of the capsules may be emptied into a glass of water and taken immediately.

Contra-indications, warnings, etc
Contra-indications: Marked leucopenia, thrombcytopenia, severe anaemia and those who have previously shown hypersensitivity to Hydrea.

Precautions: The myelosuppressive activity may be potentiated by previous or concomitant radiotherapy or cytotoxic therapy.

The complete status of the blood, including bone marrow examination, if indicated, as well as kidney function and liver function should be determined prior to, and repeatedly during, treatment. The determination of haemoglobin level, total leucocyte counts, and platelet counts should be performed at least once a week throughout the course of hydroxyurea therapy.

Severe anaemia must be corrected with whole blood replacement before initiating therapy with hydroxyurea. Erythrocytic abnormalities; megaloblastic erythropoeisis, which is self-limiting, is often seen early in the course of hydroxyurea therapy. The morphologic change resembles pernicious anaemia, but is not related to Vitamin B_{12} or folic acid deficiency. Hydroxyurea may also delay plasma iron clearance and reduce the rate of iron utilisation by erythrocytes but it does not appear to alter the red blood cell survival time.

Hydroxyurea should be used with caution in patients with marked renal dysfunction.

The possibility of an increase in serum uric acid, resulting in the development of gout or, at worst, uric acid nephropathy, should be borne in mind in patients treated with hydroxyurea, especially when used with other cytotoxic agents. It is therefore important to monitor uric acid levels regularly and maintain a high fluid intake during treatment.

Pregnancy: Drugs which affect DNA synthesis, such as hydroxyurea, may be potent mutagenic agents. The physician should carefully consider this possibility before administering this drug to male or female patients who may contemplate conception. Since Hydrea is a cytotoxic agent it has produced a teratogenic effect in some animal species. This product should not normally be administered to patients who are pregnant, or to mothers who are breast feeding, unless the potential benefits outweigh the possible hazards.

Side-effects: Bone-marrow suppression is the major toxic effect of Hydrea, while leucopenia, thrombocytopenia and anaemia may occur in that order. Other side-effects are generally rare, but the following have been reported; anorexia, nausea, vomiting, diarrhoea, constipation, headache, drowsiness, dizziness, stomatitis, alopecia, skin rash, melaena, abdominal pain, disorientations, pulmonary oedema, hallucinations, convulsions, potentiation of the erythema caused by irradiation, dysuria and impairment of renal tubular function accompanied by elevation in serum uric acid, BUN, and creatinine levels. Abnormal BSP retention and fever, chills, malaise and elevation of hepatic enzymes have been reported.

Overdosage: Immediate treatment consists of gastric lavage, followed by supportive therapy for the cardio-respiratory systems if required. In the long term, careful monitoring of the haemopoietic system is essential and, if necessary, blood should be transfused.

Pharmaceutical precautions *Storage:* At room temperature. Bottles should be kept tightly closed since hydroxyurea is hygroscopic.

Legal category POM.

Package quantities Bottles of 100.

Further information Nil.

Product licence number 0034/5044R.

IPRAL* TABLETS

Presentation
Tablets: Round, white tablets engraved Squibb and 513, containing 100 mg trimethoprim.

Round, white tablets engraved Squibb and 514, containing 200 mg trimethoprim.

Other ingredients: Gelatin, lactose, magnesium stearate, maize starch, talc.

Uses *Actions:* Trimethoprim is bactericidal in-vitro against most pathogenic Gram-positive and Gram-negative bacteria. Exceptions are *Nocardia* species, *Treponema pallidum, Pseudomonas aeruginosa*, anaerobic bacteria and possibly *Mycobacterium* and *Neisseria* species and *Brucella abortus.*

Indications: Urinary tract: In the treatment of acute and chronic urinary tract infections and for prophylactic treatment of patients with a tendency to recurrent urinary infections.

Respiratory tract: In the treatment of acute and chronic bronchitis, bronchopneumonia and lobar pneumonia.

Ipral is particularly useful for patients sensitive to sulphonamides.

Dosage and administration
Ipral Tablets: Adults and Children over 12 years: For acute urinary tract and respiratory tract infections, 200 mg twice daily. For long-term and prophylactic therapy of urinary tract infections, 100 mg at night.

6 to 12 years: 100 mg twice daily

Elderly: There are no specific dosage recommendations or precautions for use in the elderly except, as with other drugs, to monitor those patients with impaired renal or hepatic function.

Contra-indications, warnings, etc
Contra-indications: Ipral should not be given to patients with severe renal insufficiency where blood levels cannot be monitored regularly. Trimethoprim should not be given to patients with a history of sensitivity to the drug. It should not be administered to pregnant women, premature infants nor during the first two months of life. Blood dyscrasias.

Precautions: Care is necessary in administration to patients with impaired renal function. Regular haematological examinations should be performed during long-term therapy. Special precautions should be exercised in patients with a predisposition to folate deficiency.

Pregnancy and nursing mothers: Contra-indicated during pregnancy and in nursing mothers. Ipral is excreted in breast milk.

Side-effects: Ipral is well tolerated at therapeutic doses with few side-effects. Nausea, vomiting, gastro-intestinal upset and dermatological reactions such as pruritus and rash have been reported. Given over a prolonged period, Ipral may depress haemopoiesis due to an effect on folic acid metabolism. This effect may be reversed by calcium folinate.

Treatment of overdosage: Symptoms of overdosage include diarrhoea and vomiting. Treatment is symptomatic and gastric lavage and forced diuresis may be used. Calcium folinate may be used to counteract any effect of Ipral on bone-marrow.

Pharmaceutical precautions *Storage:* Ipral tablets should be stored in closed containers at room temperature.

Legal category POM.

Package quantities
100 mg Tablets: Packs of 100 and 500 tablets.
200 mg Tablets: Packs of 100 tablets.

Further information Absorption from the oral route is rapid, and peak plasma levels are obtained between one and four hours. Ipral is well distributed throughout the tissues and is excreted, predominantly unchanged, in the urine.

Nearly all of an oral dose of trimethoprim is excreted within 48 hours both unchanged and as metabolites.

Product licence numbers

Ipral Tablets 100 mg	0034/0190.
Ipral Tablets 200 mg	0034/0204.

KENALOG* INTRA-ARTICULAR/ INTRA-MUSCULAR

Presentation Sterile, aqueous suspension of triamcinolone acetonide 40 mg per ml.

Other ingredients: Benzyl alcohol, sodium carboxymethylcellulose, polysorbate 80, sodium chloride, water.

Uses Triamcinolone acetonide is a synthetic glucocorticoid with marked anti-inflammatory and anti-allergic actions.

Intra-articular injection: Following the local injection of Kenalog, relief of pain and swelling, with greater freedom of movement, is usually obtained within a few hours.

Intramuscular injection: Provides an extended duration of therapeutic effect and fewer side-effects of the kind associated with oral corticosteroid therapy, particularly gastro-intestinal reactions such as peptic ulceration. Studies indicate that, following a single intramuscular dose of 80 mg triamcinolone acetonide, adrenal suppression occurs within 24-48 hours and then gradually returns to normal, usually in approximately three weeks. This finding correlates closely with the extended duration of therapeutic action of triamcinolone acetonide.

Indications
Intra-articular use: For alleviating the joint pain, swelling and stiffness associated with rheumatoid arthritis and osteoarthrosis with an inflammatory component; also for bursitis, epicondylitis, and tenosynovitis.

Intramuscular use: Where sustained systemic corticosteroid treatment is required: *Allergic states*, eg bronchial asthma, seasonal or perennial allergic rhinitis. In seasonal allergies, patients who do not respond to conventional therapy may achieve a remission of symptoms over the entire period with a single intramuscular injection (see Dosage); *Endocrine disorders*, eg primary or secondary adrenocortical insufficiency. *Collagen disorders*, eg during an exacerbation of maintenance therapy of selected cases of SLE or acute rheumatic carditis; *Dermatologic diseases*, eg pemphigus, severe dermatitis and Stevens Johnson Syndrome; *Rheumatic, gastrointestinal or respiratory disorders* – as an adjunctive, short-term therapy; *Haematological disorders*, eg acquired (autoimmune) haemolytic anaemia; *Neoplastic diseases*, eg palliative management of leukaemia and lymphomas; *Renal disease*, such as acute interstitial nephritis, minimal change nephrotic syndrome or lupus nephritis.

Dosage and administration
Kenalog intra-articular/intramuscular injection is not for intravenous use.

Strict aseptic precautions should be observed. Since the duration of effect is variable, subsequent doses should be given when symptoms recur and not at set intervals.

Intra-articular injection: For intra-articular administration or injection into tendon sheaths and bursae, the dose of Kenalog injection may vary from 5 mg to 10 mg (0.125-0.25 ml) for smaller joints and up to 40 mg (1 ml) for larger joints, depending on the specific disease entity being treated. Single injections into several sites for multiple joint involvement, up to a total of 80 mg, have been given without undue reactions.

It is recommended that, when injections are given into the sheaths of short tendons, Adcortyl injection (triamcinolone acetonide 10 mg/ml) should be used. (See under Precautions re Achilles tendon.)

Intramuscular injection: Adults and children over 12 years: The suggested initial dose is 40 mg (1 ml) injected deeply into the upper, outer quadrant of the gluteal muscle. Subsequent dosage depends on the patient's response and period of relief. Patients with hay fever or pollen asthma who do not respond to conventional therapy may obtain a remission of symptoms lasting throughout the pollen season after a dose of 40-100 mg given when allergic symptoms appear.

For children from 6-12 years of age: The suggested initial dose of 40 mg (1 ml) injected deeply into the gluteal muscle should be scaled according to the severity of symptoms and the age and weight of the child. Kenalog is not recommended for children under six years (see Precautions).

Elderly: Treatment of elderly patients, particularly if long term, should be planned bearing in mind the more serious consequences of the common side effects of corticosteroids in old age, especially osteoporosis, diabetes, hypertension, susceptibility to infection and thinning of the skin.

Contra-indications, warnings, etc
Contra-indications: None.

Precautions: In common with other steroids Kenalog injection should be used with caution in patients with recent intestinal anastomoses, thrombophlebitis, psychotic tendencies, exanthematous disease, chronic nephritis, metastatic carcinoma, osteoporosis, in patients with an active peptic ulcer (or a history of peptic ulcer). Latent or healed tuberculosis; in the presence of local or systemic viral infection, systemic fungal infections or in active infections not controlled by antibiotics. In acute psychoses; in acute glomerulonephritis. Hypertension; glaucoma (or a family history of glaucoma), previous steroid myopathy or epilepsy.

Intra-articular injection should not be carried out in the presence of active infection in or near joints. The preparation should not be used to alleviate joint pain arising from infectious states such as gonococcal or tubercular arthritis.

Diabetes may be aggravated, necessitating a higher insulin dosage. Latent diabetes mellitus may be precipitated.

Menstrual irregularities may occur, and this possibility should be mentioned to female patients.

Patients on long-term systemic therapy with Kenalog may require supportive corticosteroid therapy in times of stress, both during the treatment period and for a year afterwards.

During corticosteroid therapy antibody response will be reduced and therefore affect the patient's response to vaccines.

Rare instances of anaphylactoid reactions have occurred in patients receiving parenteral corticosteroids, especially when a patient has a history of drug allergies.

All corticosteroids increase calcium excretion.

Avoid abrupt cessation of corticosteroids.

Aspirin should be used cautiously in conjunction with corticosteroids in patients with hypoprothrombinaemia.

Corticosteroid effects may be enhanced in patients with hypothyroidism or cirrhosis.

Pregnancy: Corticosteroids are not recommended for pregnant patients, particularly in the first trimester, or for nursing mothers, except when the disease for which they are indicated warrants their use. There is inadequate evidence of safety in human pregnancy and there may be a very small risk of cleft palate and intra-uterine growth retardation in the foetus; there is evidence of harmful effects on pregnancy in animals.

Children: Kenalog is not recommended for children under six years. Growth and development of children on prolonged corticosteroid therapy should be carefully observed.

Intra-articular injection: Patients should be specifically warned to avoid over-use of joints in which symptomatic benefit has been obtained. Severe joint destruction with necrosis of bone may occur if repeated intra-articular injections are given over a long period of time. Care should be taken if injections are given into tendon sheaths to avoid injection into the tendon itself.

Due to the absence of a true tendon sheath, the Achilles tendon should not be injected with depot corticosteroids.

Intra-muscular injection: During prolonged therapy a liberal protein intake is essential to counteract the tendency to gradual weight loss sometimes associated with negative nitrogen balance and wasting of skeletal muscle.

N.B. To avoid the danger of subcutaneous fat atrophy, it is important to ensure that deep intramuscular injection is given into the gluteal site. The deltoid should not be used. Alternate sides should be used for subsequent injections.

Side-effects: Where adverse reactions occur they are usually reversible on cessation of therapy. Absorption of triamcinolone following injection by the intra-articular route is rare. However, the possibility of the systemic effects which are associated with all steroid therapy should be considered with both routes of administration. These may include:

Dyspepsia, peptic ulceration with perforation and haemorrhage, abdominal distension, oesophageal ulceration, oesophageal candidiasis, acute pancreatitis.

Proximal myopathy, osteoporosis, vertebral and long bone fractures, avascular osteonecrosis, tendon rupture.

Sodium and water retention, hypertension, hypokalaemic alkalosis.

Impaired healing, skin atrophy, bruising, striae, telangiectasia, acne.

Suppression of the hypothalamo-pituitary adrenal axis, growth suppression in childhood and adolescence, menstrual irregularity and amenorrhoea. Cushingoid facies, hirsutism, weight gain, impaired carbohydrate tolerance with increased requirement for antidiabetic therapy, negative nitrogen balance.

Euphoria, psychological dependence, depression, insomnia. Intracranial hypertension has been reported in children on cessation of long term steroid therapy. Aggravation of schizophrenia.

Increased intra-ocular pressure, glaucoma, papilloedema, cataracts, corneal or scleral thinning, exacerbation of ophthalmic viral disease.

Opportunistic infection, recurrence of dormant tuberculosis, leucocytosis, hypersensitivity, thromboembolism, increased appetite, nausea, malaise.

On withdrawal fever, myalgia, arthralgia or adrenal insufficiency may occur.

Intra-articular injection: Reactions following intra-articular administration have been rare. In a few instances transient flushing and dizziness have occurred. Pain and other local symptoms may continue for a short time before effective relief is obtained, but an increase in joint discomfort has seldom occurred. Local fat atrophy may occur if the injection is not given into the joint space, but is temporary and disappears within a few weeks to months.

Pharmaceutical precautions *Storage:* At room temperature; avoid freezing.

Legal category POM.

Package quantities 1 ml and 2 ml ready filled syringes (Intramuscular use only). 1 ml vials: pack of 5 (Intra-articular and Intramuscular use).

Further information Nil.

Product licence number 0034/5045R.

LIPOSTAT* TABLETS ▼

Presentation

Lipostat tablets 10 mg: Pink, oblong, biconvex tablets each containing pravastatin sodium 10 mg. Engraved with "SQUIBB" and 154 on one side.

Lipostat tablets 20 mg: Pink, oblong, biconvex tablets each containing pravastatin sodium 20 mg. Engraved with "SQUIBB" and 178 on one side.

Other ingredients: croscarmellose sodium, erythrosine E127, lactose, magnesium stearate, microcrystalline cellulose, povidone.

Uses

Indications: For use in patients with primary hypercholesterolaemia, intolerant or not responsive to other forms of therapy, with a cholesterol level in excess of 7.8 mmol/L.

Mode of action: Lipostat (pravastatin sodium) is an HMG-CoA reductase inhibitor that reduces cholesterol biosynthesis and has been shown to be tissue selective such that inhibitory activity is highest in those tissues (e.g. liver, ileum) with the highest rates of cholesterol synthesis. Unlike other HMG-CoA reductase inhibitors, Lipostat has little effect on cholesterol synthesis in other tissues (e.g. lens, adrenal glands).

Pravastatin sodium is a competitive inhibitor of 3-hydroxy-3-methylglutaryl-coenzyme A (HMG-CoA) reductase, the enzyme catalysing the early rate-limiting step in cholesterol biosynthesis, and produces its lipid-lowering effect in two ways. First, it effects modest reductions in intracellular pools of cholesterol which results in an increased number of LDL-receptors on cell surfaces, enhanced receptor-mediated catabolism and clearance of circulating LDL-C. Second, pravastatin inhibits LDL-C production by inhibiting hepatic synthesis of very low density lipoprotein cholesterol (VLDL-C), the LDL-C precursor. These effects result in a reduction of total cholesterol (Total-C), low density lipoprotein cholesterol (LDL-C), very low density lipoprotein cholesterol (VLDL-C), apolipoprotein B and triglycerides, whilst increasing high density lipoprotein cholesterol (HDL-C) and apolipoprotein A.

Pharmacokinetics: Pravastatin is administered orally in the active form. Pravastatin undergoes extensive first-pass extraction in the liver which is its primary site of action, and the primary site of cholesterol synthesis and of LDL-C clearance. Since it is excreted in the bile, plasma levels are of limited value in prediciting therapeutic efficacy. Approximately 50% of the circulating drug is bound to plasma proteins. There are dual routes of elimination and the potential exists for compensatory excretion by the alternate route in patients with renal or hepatic insufficiency. The plasma elimination half life of pravastatin is between $1\frac{1}{2}$ and 2 hours.

Dosage and administration

Adults: The usual dosage range is 10 to 40 mg administered once a day at bedtime.

Prior to initiating Lipostat, secondary causes of hypercholesterolaemia should be excluded and the patient should be placed on a standard cholesterol-lowering diet which should be continued during treatment.

A dose response effect is apparent within one or two weeks with maximal effects of a given dose usually seen within four weeks, and maintained during extended periods of therapy. Periodic lipid determinations should be performed and dosage adjusted according to the patient's response.

Elderly patients and patients with hepatic or renal impairment: There is no clinical evidence to suggest the dose range needs to be different in these patients. In common with other treatments, treatment should be initiated at the lower end of the dosage range.

Children: There are insufficient clinical data to recommend use in individuals less than 18 years old.

Concomitant therapy: Some patients may require combination therapy with one or more lipid-lowering agents. The effect of Lipostat on lowering total and LDL cholesterol are enhanced when combined with a bile acid-binding resin. When administering a bile acid-binding resin (e.g. cholestyramine, colestipol) Lipostat should be given either one hour or more before or at least four hours after the resin. The bioavailability of pravastatin is not altered by concurrent administration with nicotinic acid, probucol and gemfibrozil (see Precautions, Skeletal Muscle).

Contra-indications, warnings, etc

Contra-indications: Hypersensitivity to any component of this medication.

Active liver disease or unexplained persistent elevations in liver function tests.

Pregnancy: There have been no teratogenic effects in animal studies. There are no data available on the use of Lipostat in pregnant women. As cholesterol and other products of cholesterol biosynthesis are essential components for foetal development Lipostat is contra-indicated in pregnancy and women of childbearing potential unless protected by appropriate contraception. An interval of one month should elapse between the end of therapy with Lipostat and planned conception.

Nursing mothers: A negligible amount of pravastatin is excreted in human breast milk hence Lipostat should not be used in nursing mothers.

Precautions

General: As with other lipid-lowering therapy, Lipostat is not indicated when hypercholesterolaemia is due to elevated high density lipoprotein cholesterol (HDL-C).

Lipostat has not been evaluated in patients with the rare homozygous familial hypercholesterolaemia. In this group of patients, it has been reported that that HMG-CoA reductase inhibitors are less effective because the patients lack functional LDL receptors.

Liver function: As with other lipid-lowering agents, including HMG-CoA reductase inhibitors and nonabsorbable bile acid-binding resins, increases in liver enzymes have occured during therapy with pravastatin. The significance of these changes, which usually appear during the first few months of treatment, is not known. In the majority of patients treated with pravastatin in clinical trials, these increased values declined to pretreatment levels despite continuation of therapy at the same dose.

In clinical trials 0.5% of patients treated with pravastatin had marked persistent increases (greater than 3 times the upper limit of normal) in the serum transaminases. These elevations were not associated with clinical signs and symptoms of liver disease and usually declined to pretreatment levels upon discontinuation of therapy.

As with other lipid-lowering agents, liver function tests should be performed periodically. Special attention should be given to patients who develop increased transaminase levels and therapy should be discontinued if increases in alanine aminotransferase (ALT) and aspartate aminotransferase (AST) exceed three times the upper limit of normal and persist.

Caution should be exercised when pravastatin is administered to patients with a history of liver disease or heavy alcohol ingestion.

Skeletal muscle: As with other HMG-CoA reductase inhibitors, sporadic elevations of creatine phosphokinase levels (CPK [MM fraction]) have been observed. If a markedly elevated (greater than 10 times upper limit of normal) serum CPK develops, discontinuation of pravastatin therapy is recommended. An increase in the incidence of myositis and myopathy has been seen in patients receiving other HMG-CoA reductase inhibitors, especially those being treated concomitantly with cyclosporin, fibric acid derivatives and nicotinic acid. Until further experience has been gained, pravastatin should be used with caution in these patients.

Ophthalmological: Pravastatin was not associated with cataract formation in patients treated for up to a year or more in clinical studies nor in long-term animal studies.

Drug interactions: No clinically significant effects were seen in a range of interaction studies.

Cholestyramine/colestipol: There was no clinically significant decrease in bioavailability or therapeutic effect when pravastatin was administered one hour before or four hours after cholestyramine or one hour before colestipol and a standard meal. Concomitant administration resulted in approximately 40 to 50% decrease in the bioavailability of pravastatin.

Antipyrine: Clearance by the cytochrome P450 system was unaltered by concomitant administration of pravastatin. Since pravastatin does not appear to induce hepatic drug-metabolising enzymes, it is not expected that any significant interaction of pravastatin with other drugs (e.g. phenytoin, quinidine) metabolised by the cytochrome P450 system will occur.

Warfarin: Bioavailability parameters at steady state for pravastatin were not altered following administration with warfarin. Chronic dosing of the two drugs did not produce any changes in the anticoagulant action of warfarin.

In interaction studies with aspirin, antacids (one hour prior to Lipostat) cimetidine, gemfibrozil, nicotinic acid or probucol, no statistically significant differences in bioavailability were seen. Although blood levels were altered after administration of antacids and cimetidine, this did not affect the clinical efficacy of Lipostat.

Other drugs: During clinical trials, no noticeable drug interactions were reported when Lipostat was added to: diuretics, antihypertensives, digitalis, converting-enzyme inhibitors, calcium channel blockers, beta-blockers, or nitroglycerins.

Side-effects: Lipostat is generally well tolerated. Adverse events, both clinical and laboratory are usually mild and transient.

In placebo controlled studies, the following events showed a small increase in incidence over placebo: rash, myalgia, headache, non-cardiac chest pain, nausea/vomiting, diarrhoea, fatigue.

Pravastatin has been administered concurrently with cholestyramine, colestipol, nicotinic acid and probucol. No adverse reactions unique to the combination or in addition to those previously reported for each drug alone have been reported.

Overdosage: There have been no reports of overdoses with pravastatin.

Should an accidental overdose occur, treat symptomatically and institute supportive measures as required.

Pharmaceutical precautions Store below 30°C. Protect from light and moisture.

Legal category POM.

Package quantities Blister packs of 28 tablets.

Product licence numbers

10 mg	0034/0286
20 mg	0034/0287

MODECATE* INJECTION MODECATE* CONCENTRATE INJECTION

Presentation *Modecate injection:* Straw-coloured viscous liquid containing fluphenazine decanoate 25 mg per ml.

Other ingredients: Benzyl alcohol, sesame oil.

Modecate Concentrate injection: Straw-coloured, viscous liquid containing fluphenazine decanoate 100 mg per ml. Other ingredients: Benzyl alcohol, sesame oil. Ampoules are marked with a distinctive blue band.

Uses

Indications: For the treatment and maintenance of schizophrenic patients and those with paranoid psychoses. While Modecate injection has been shown to be effective in acute states, it is particularly useful in the maintenance treatment of chronic patients who are unreliable at taking their oral medication, and also of those who do not absorb their oral phenothiazines in adequate amounts.

Modecate Concentrate injection provides a high concentration of fluphenazine decanoate in a small volume which may be injected without discomfort to the patient and it is therefore particularly suitable for those patients who require higher doses for effective antipsychotic control.

Dosage and administration It is preferable that patients be stabilised on the injection in hospital.

Recommended dosage regimes for all indications:

1. *Modecate injection 25 mg/ml*

a) *Patients without previous exposure to a depot fluphenazine formulation:* Initially 0.5 ml (0.25 ml for patients over 60) by deep intramuscular injection into the gluteal region.

The onset of action generally appears between 24 and 72 hours after injection and the effects of the drug on psychotic symptoms become significant within 48 to 96 hours. Subsequent injections and the dosage interval are determined in accordance with the patient's response. When administered as maintenance therapy, a single injection may be effective in controlling schizophrenic symptoms up to four weeks or longer.

It is desirable to maintain as much flexibility in the dose as possible to achieve the best therapeutic response with the least side-effects; most patients are successfully maintained within the dose range 0.5 ml to 4 ml given at a dose interval of 2 to 5 weeks.

Patients previously maintained on oral fluphenazine: It is not possible to predict the equivalent dose of depot formulation in view of the wide variability of individual response.

b) *Patients previously maintained on depot fluphenazines:* Patients who have suffered a relapse following cessation of depot fluphenazine therapy may be restarted on the same dose as they were receiving formerly, although the frequency of injections may need to be increased in the early weeks of treatment until satisfactory control is obtained.

2. *Modecate Concentrate injection 100 mg/ml:* Where a smaller volume of injection is desirable, patients may be transferred directly to the equivalent dose of Modecate Concentrate on the basis that 1 ml Modecate Concentrate Injection is equivalent to 4 ml Modecate injection.

Elderly: Elderly patients may be particularly susceptible to extrapyramidal reactions. Therefore, reduced maintenance dosage may be required and a smaller initial dose (see above).

Children: Not recommended for children.

Note: The dosage should not be increased without close supervision and it should be noted that there is a variability in individual response.

The response to antipsychotic drug treatment may be delayed. If drugs are withdrawn, recurrence of symptoms may not become apparent for several weeks or months.

Contra-indications, warnings, etc

Contra-indications: Comatose states; marked cerebral atherosclerosis; phaeochromocytoma; renal failure; liver failure; severe cardiac insufficiency; and severely depressed states.

Precautions: Liver disease; cardiac arrhythmias, cardiac disease; thyrotoxicosis; severe respiratory disease; epilepsy, conditions predisposing to epilepsy (e.g. alcohol withdrawal or brain damage); Parkinson's disease; patients who have shown hypersensitivity to other phenothiazines; personal or family history of narrow angle glaucoma; in very hot weather; the elderly, particularly if frail or at risk of hypothermia; hypothyroidism; myasthenia gravis; prostatic hypertrophy.

Use in pregnancy: The safety for the use of this drug during pregnancy has not been established; therefore, the possible hazards should be weighed against the potential benefits when administering this drug to pregnant patients.

Nursing mothers: Breast feeding is not recommended during treatment with depot fluphenazines, owing to the possibility that fluphenazine is excreted in the milk of nursing mothers.

Drug interactions: The possibility should be borne in mind that phenothiazines may:

(1) Increase the central nervous system depression produced by drugs such as alcohol, hypnotics, sedatives or strong analgesics.

(2) Antagonise the action of adrenaline and other sympathomimetic agents and reverse the blood-pressure-lowering effects of adrenergic-blocking agents such as guanethidine and clonidine.

(3) Impair
  (a) the anti-Parkinsonian effect of L-Dopa
  (b) the effect of anti-convulsants
  (c) metabolism of tricyclic antidepressants
  (d) the control of diabetes

(4) Increase the effect of anticoagulants.

(5) Interact with lithium.

Anticholinergic effects may be enhanced by anti-Parkinsonian or other anticholinergic drugs.

Phenothiazines may enhance: The cardiac-depressant effects of quinidine; the absorption of corticosteroids, and digoxin, and neuromuscular blocking agents.

Side-effects: Acute dystonic reactions occur infrequently, as a rule within the first 24–48 hours, although delayed reactions may occur. In susceptible individuals they may occur after only small doses. These may include such dramatic manifestations as oculogyric crises and opisthotonos. They are rapidly relieved by intravenous administration of an anti-Parkinsonian agent such as procyclidine.

Parkinsonian-like states may occur particularly between the second and fifth days after each injection, but often decrease with subsequent injections. These reactions may be reduced by using smaller doses more frequently, or by the concomitant use of anti-Parkinsonian drugs such as benzhexol, benztropine or procyclidine. Anti-Parkinsonian drugs should not be prescribed routinely, because of the possible risks of aggravating anti-cholinergic side-effects or precipitating toxic confusional states, or of impairing therapeutic efficacy.

With careful monitoring of the dose the number of patients requiring anti-Parkinsonian drugs can be minimised.

Tardive dyskinesia: As with all antipsychotic agents, tardive dyskinesia may appear in some patients on long term therapy or may occur after drug therapy has been discontinued. The risk seems to be greater in elderly patients on high dose therapy, especially females. The symptoms are persistent and in some patients appear to be irreversible.

The syndrome is characterised by rhythmical involuntary movements of the tongue, face, mouth or jaw (e.g. protrusion of tongue, puffing of cheeks, puckering of mouth, chewing movements). Sometimes these may be accompanied by involuntary movements of the extremities. There is no known effective treatment for tardive dyskinesia; anti-Parkinsonian agents usually do not alleviate the symptoms of this syndrome. It is suggested that all antipsychotic agents be discontinued if these symptoms appear. Should it be necessary to reinstitute treatment, or increase the dosage of the agent, or switch to a different antipsychotic agent, the syndrome may be masked. It has been reported that fine vermicular movements of the tongue may be an early sign of the syndrome and if the medication is stopped at that time, the syndrome may not develop.

As with other phenothiazines, drowsiness, lethargy, blurred vision, dryness of the mouth, constipation, urinary hesitancy or incontinence, mild hypotension, impairment of judgement and mental skills, and epileptiform attacks are occasionally seen.

The use of this drug may impair the mental and physical abilities required for driving a car or operating heavy machinery.

Blood dyscrasias have rarely been reported with phenothiazine derivatives. Blood counts should be performed if the patient develops signs of persistent infection. Transient leucopenia and thrombocytopenia have been reported. Antinuclear antibodies and SLE have been reported very rarely.

Jaundice has rarely been reported. Transient abnormalities of liver function tests may occur in the absence of jaundice.

A transient rise in serum cholesterol has been reported very occasionally in patients on oral fluphenazine.

Abnormal skin pigmentation and lens opacities have sometimes been seen following long-term administration of high doses of phenothiazines.

Phenothiazines are known to cause photosensitivity reactions but this has not been reported for fluphenazine. Skin rashes have occasionally been reported.

Elderly patients may be more susceptible to the sedative and hypotensive effects.

The effects of phenothiazines on the heart are dose-related. ECG changes, with prolongation of the QT interval and T-wave changes have been reported commonly in patients treated with moderate to high dosage; they are reversible on reducing the dose. In a very small number of cases, they have been reported to precede serious arrhythmias, including ventricular tachycardia and fibrillation, which have also occurred after overdosage. Sudden, unexpected and unexplained deaths have been reported in hospitalised psychotic patients receiving phenothiazines.

Phenothiazines may impair body temperature regulation. Cases of severe hypothermia or hyperpyrexia have been reported in association with moderate or high dosage of phenothiazines.

Elderly or hypothyroid patients may be particularly susceptible to hypothermia. The hazard of hyperpyrexia may be increased by especially hot or humid weather, or by drugs such as anti-Parkinsonian agents, which impair sweating.

Rare occurrences of neuroleptic malignant syndrome (NMS) have been reported in patients on neuroleptic therapy. The syndrome is characterised by hyperthermia, together with some or all of the following: muscular rigidity, autonomic instability (labile blood pressure, tachycardia, diaphoresis), akinesia, and altered consciousness, sometimes progressing to stupor or coma. Leucocytosis, elevated CPK, liver function abnormalities, and acute renal failure may also occur. Neuroleptic therapy should be discontinued immediately and vigorous symptomatic treatment implemented since the syndrome is potentially fatal.

Hormonal effects of phenothiazines include hyperprolactinaemia, which may cause galactorrhoea, gynaecomastia and oligo- or amenorrhoea. Sexual function may be impaired.

Oedema has been reported with phenothiazine medication.

Overdosage: It should be treated symptomatically and supportively. Extrapyramidal reactions will respond to oral or parenteral anti-Parkinsonian drugs such as procyclidine or benztropine. In cases of severe hypotension, all procedures for the management of circulatory shock should be instituted, e.g. vasconstrictors and/or intravenous fluids. However, only the vasoconstrictors metaraminol or noradrenaline should be used, as adrenaline may further lower the blood pressure through interaction with the phenothiazine.

Pharmaceutical precautions *Storage:* At room temperature. Do not store in a refrigerator, since this will cause precipitation of triglycerides from the sesame oil. If precipitation does occur, warming the product to 37° C will dissolve the precipitate without harming the active ingredient. The 10 ml multidose vial should be discarded 28 days after it is first used. Protect from direct sunlight.

Mixing: Modecate and Modecate Concentration should not be mixed in the same syringe.

Legal category POM.

Package quantities *Modecate Injection 25 mg/ml:*
Ampoules 0.5 ml, pack of 5
Ampoules 1 ml, pack of 10
Ampoules 2 ml, pack of 5
Ready filled syringes 1 ml, pack of 5

Ready filled syringes 2 ml, pack of 5
Multidose vial 10 ml, pack of 1
Modecate Concentrate Injection 100 mg/ml:
Ampoules 0.5 ml, pack of 10
Ampoules 1 ml, pack of 5

Further information Fluphenazine decanoate is an ester of the potent neuroleptic fluphenazine, a phenothiazine derivative of the piperazine type. The ester is slowly absorbed from the intramuscular site of injection and is then hydrolysed in the plasma to the active therapeutic agent, fluphenazine.

Extrapyramidal reactions are not uncommon, but fluphenazine does not have marked sedative or hypotensive properties.

Pharmacokinetics: Plasma level profiles of fluphenazine following Modecate injection have shown half-lives of plasma clearance ranging from 2½–16 weeks, emphasising the importance of adjusting dose and interval to the individual requirements of each patient. The slow decline of plasma levels in most patients means that a reasonably stable plasma level can usually be achieved with injections spaced at 2–4 week intervals.

Product licence numbers

Modecate Injection 25 mg/ml	0034/5046R
Modecate Concentrate Injection 100 mg/ml	0034/0189

MODITEN* ENANTHATE INJECTION

Presentation Straw-coloured viscous liquid containing fluphenazine enanthate 25 mg per ml in sesame oil.

Other ingredients: Benzyl alcohol, sesame oil.

Uses *Indications:* For the treatment and maintenance of schizophrenic patients and those with paranoid psychoses.

While Moditen Enanthate Injection has been shown to be effective in acute states, it is particularly useful in the maintenance treatment of chronic patients who are unreliable at taking their oral medication, and also of those who do not absorb their oral phenothiazines in adequate amounts.

Dosage and administration It is preferable that patients be stabilised on the injection in hospital.

Recommended dosage regimes for all indications:

(a) *Patients without previous exposure to a depot fluphenazine formulation:* Initially 0.5 ml (0.25 ml for patients over 60) by deep intramuscular injection into the gluteal region.

The onset of action generally appears between 24 and 72 hours after injection and the effects of the drug on psychotic symptoms become significant within 48 to 96 hours. Subsequent injections and the dosage interval are determined in accordance with the patient's response. When administered as maintenance therapy, a single injection may be effective in controlling schizophrenic symptoms up to three weeks or longer.

It is desirable to maintain as much flexibility in the dose as possible to achieve the best therapeutic response with the least side-effects; most patients are successfully maintained within the dose range 0.5 ml to 4.0 ml given at a dose interval of 10 days to 3 weeks.

Patients previously maintained on oral fluphenazine: It is not possible to predict the equivalent dose of depot formulation in view of the wide variability of individual response.

(b) *Patients previously maintained on depot fluphenazine:* Patients who have suffered a relapse following cessation of depot fluphenazine therapy may be restarted on the same dose as they were receiving formerly, although the frequency of injections may need to be increased in the early weeks of treatment until satisfactory control is obtained.

Elderly: Elderly patients may be particularly susceptible to extrapyramidal reactions. Therefore reduced maintenance may be required and a smaller initial dose. (See above).

Children: Not recommended for children.

Note: The dosage should not be increased without close supervision and it should be noted that there is a variability in individual response.

The response to antipsychotic drug treatment may be delayed. If drugs are withdrawn, recurrence of symptoms may not become apparent for several weeks or months.

Contra-indications, warnings, etc

Contra-indications: Comatose states; marked cerebral atherosclerosis; phaeochromocytoma; renal failure; liver failure; severe cardiac insufficiency; severely depressed states.

Precautions: Liver disease; cardiac arrhythmias, cardiac disease; thyrotoxicosis; severe respiratory disease; epilepsy, conditions predisposing to epilepsy (e.g. alcohol withdrawal or brain damage); Parkinson's disease; patients who have shown hypersensitivity to other phenothiazines; personal or family history of narrow angle glaucoma; in very hot weather; the elderly, particularly if frail or at risk of hypothermia; hypothyroidism; myasthenia gravis; prostatic hypertrophy.

Use in pregnancy: The safety for the use of this drug during pregnancy has not been established; therefore, the possible hazards should be weighed against the potential benefits when administering this drug to pregnant patients.

Nursing mothers: Breast feeding is not recommended during treatment with depot fluphenazines, owing to the possibility that fluphenazine is excreted in the milk of nursing mothers.

Drug interactions: The possibility should be borne in mind that phenothiazines may:

(1) Increase the central nervous system depression produced by drugs such as alcohol, hypnotics, sedatives or strong analgesics.

(2) Antagonise the action of adrenaline and other sympathomimetic agents and reverse the blood-pressure-lowering effects of adrenergic-blocking agents such as guanethidine and clonidine.

(3) Impair (a) the anti-Parkinsonian effect of L-Dopa; (b) the effect of anti-convulsants; (c) metabolism of tricyclic antidepressants; (d) the control of diabetes.

(4) Increase the effect of anticoagulants.

(5) Interact with lithium.

Anticholinergic effects may be enhanced by anti-Parkinsonian or other anticholinergic drugs.

Phenothiazines may enhance: The cardiac-depressant effects of quinidine; the absorption of corticosteroids, and digoxin, and neuromuscular blocking agents.

Side-effects: Acute dystonic reactions occur infrequently but nearly always within the first 24–48 hours, and may include such dramatic manifestations as oculogyric crises and opisthotonos. They are rapidly relieved by intravenous administration of an anti-Parkinsonian agent such as procyclidine.

Parkinsonian-like states may occur particularly between the second and fifth days after each injection, but often decrease with subsequent injections. These reactions may be reduced by using smaller doses more frequently, or by the concomitant use of anti-Parkinsonian drugs such as benzhexol, benztropine or procyclidine. Anti-Parkinsonian drugs should not be prescribed routinely, because of the possible risks of aggravating anti-cholinergic side-effects or precipitating toxic confusional states, or of impairing therapeutic efficacy.

With careful monitoring of the dose the number of patients requiring anti-Parkinsonian drugs can be minimised.

Tardive dyskinesia: As with all antipsychotic agents, tardive dyskinesia may appear in some patients on long term therapy or may occur after drug therapy has been discontinued. The risk seems to be greater in elderly patients on high dose therapy, especially females. The symptoms are persistent and in some patients appear to be irreversible. The syndrome is characterised by rhythmical involuntary movements of the tongue, face, mouth or jaw (e.g. protrusion of tongue, puffing of cheeks, puckering of mouth, chewing movements). Sometimes these may be accompanied by involuntary movements of the extremities. There is no known effective treatment for tardive dyskinesia; anti-Parkinsonian agents usually do not alleviate the symptoms of this syndrome. It is suggested that all antipsychotic agents be discontinued if these symptoms appear. Should it be necessary to reinstitute treatment, or increase the dosage of the agent, or switch to a different antipsychotic agent, the syndrome may be masked. It has been reported that fine vermicular movements of the tongue may be an early sign of the syndrome and if the medication is stopped at that time, the syndrome may not develop.

As with other phenothiazines, drowsiness, lethargy, blurred vision, dryness of the mouth, constipation, urinary hesitancy or incontinence, mild hypotension, impairment of judgement and mental skills, and epileptiform attacks are occasionally seen.

The use of this drug may impair the mental and physical abilities required for driving a car or operating heavy machinery.

Blood dyscrasias have rarely been reported with phenothiazine derivatives. Blood counts should be performed if the patient develops signs of persistent infection. Transient leucopenia and thrombocytopenia have been reported. Antinuclear antibodies and SLE have been reported very rarely.

Jaundice has rarely been reported. Transient abnormalities of liver function tests may occur in the absence of jaundice.

A transient rise in serum cholesterol has been reported very occasionally in patients on oral fluphenazine.

Abnormal skin pigmentation and lens opacities have sometimes been seen following long-term administration of high doses of phenothiazines.

Phenothiazines are known to cause photosensitivity reactions but this has not been reported for fluphenazine. Skin rashes have occasionally been reported.

Elderly patients may be more susceptible to the sedative and hypotensive effects.

The effects of phenothiazines on the heart are dose-related. ECG changes, with prolongation of the QT interval and T-wave changes have been reported commonly in patients treated with moderate to high dosage; they are reversible on reducing the dose. In a very small number of cases, they have been reported to precede serious arrhythmias, including ventricular tachycardia and fibrillation, which have also occurred after overdosage. Sudden, unexpected and unexplained deaths have been reported in hospitalised psychotic patients receiving phenothiazines.

Phenothiazines may impair body temperature regulation. Cases of severe hypothermia or hyperpyrexia have been reported in association with moderate or high dosage of phenothiazines.

Elderly or hypothyroid patients may be particularly susceptible to hypothermia. The hazard of hyperpyrexia may be increased by especially hot or humid weather, or by drugs such as anti-Parkinsonian agents, which impair sweating.

Rare occurrences of neuroleptic malignant syndrome (NMS) have been reported in patients on neuroleptic therapy. The syndrome is characterised by hyperthermia, together with some or all of the following: muscular rigidity, autonomic instability (labile blood pressure, tachycardia, diaphoresis), akinesia, and altered consciousness, sometimes progressing to stupor or coma. Leucocytosis, elevated CPK, liver function abnormalities, and acute renal failure may also occur. Neuroleptic therapy should be discontinued immediately and vigorous symptomatic treatment implemented since the syndrome is potentially fatal.

Hormonal effects of phenothiazines include hyperprolactinaemia, which may cause galactorrhoea, gynaecomastia and oligo- or amenorrhoea. Sexual function may be impaired.

Oedema has been reported with phenothiazine medication.

Overdosage: It should be treated symptomatically and supportively. Extrapyramidal reactions will respond to oral or parenteral anti-Parkinsonian drugs such as procyclidine or benztropine. In cases of severe hypotension, all procedures for the management of circulatory shock should be instituted, e.g. vasoconstrictors and/or intravenous fluids. However, only the vasoconstrictors metaraminol or noradrenaline should be used, as adrenaline may further lower the blood pressure through interaction with the phenothiazine.

Pharmaceutical precautions *Storage:* At room temperature. Do not store in a refrigerator, since this will cause precipitation of triglycerides from the sesame oil. If precipitation does occur, warming the product to 37°C will dissolve the precipitate without harming the active ingredient. Protect from direct sunlight.

Legal category POM.

Package quantities Ampoules of 1 ml.

Further information Fluphenazine enanthate is an ester of the potent neuroleptic fluphenazine, a phenothiazine derivative of the piperazine type. The ester is slowly absorbed from the intramuscular site of injection and is then hydrolysed in the plasma to the active therapeutic agent, fluphenazine.

Extrapyramidal reactions are not uncommon, but fluphenazine does not have marked sedative or hypotensive properties.

Product licence number 0034/5048R.

MODITEN* TABLETS

Presentation

Tablets 1.0 mg: Round, pink, sugar-coated tablets containing 1 mg fluphenazine hydrochloride.

Tablets 2.5 mg: Round, yellow, sugar-coated tablets containing 2.5 mg fluphenazine hydrochloride.

Tablets 5 mg: Round, white, sugar-coated tablets containing 5 mg fluphenazine hydrochloride.

Other ingredients: Acacia powder, castor oil, carnauba wax, chalk, curcumin (in 2.5 mg tablet), erythrosine (in 1 mg tablet), lactose, magnesium stearate, maize starch, polyvinylpyrrolidone, shellac, sodium benzoate, sucrose, talc, titanium dioxide.

Uses *Adults:* Moditen Tablets are indicated: As an adjunct to the short-term management of anxiety, severe psychomotor agitation, excitement, violent or dangerously impulsive behaviour; in schizophrenia – treatment of symptoms and prevention of relapse; in other psychoses, especially paranoid; in mania and hypomania.

Dosage and administration

1. Adults: Anxiety and other non-psychotic behavioural disturbances: Initially 1 mg twice daily rising to 2 mg twice daily, if necessary, according to response.

Schizophrenia, mania, hypomania, and other psychoses: Initially 2.5–10 mg daily divided into 2 or 3 doses, depending on the severity and duration of symptoms, rising to 20 mg daily, as necessary. Doses exceeding 20 mg daily (10 mg in the elderly) should be used with caution.

2. Elderly: Elderly patients may be particularly susceptible to extrapyramidal reactions. Dosage at the lower end of the range is likely to be sufficient for elderly patients.

3. Children: Not recommended for children.

Note: The dosage should not be increased without close supervision and it should be noted that there is a variability in individual response.

The response to antipsychotic drug treatment may be delayed. If drugs are withdrawn, recurrence of symptoms may not become apparent for several weeks or months.

Contra-indications, warnings, etc

Contra-indications: Comatose states; marked cerebral atherosclerosis; phaeochromocytoma; renal failure; liver failure; severe cardiac insufficiency; severely depressed states.

Precautions: Liver disease; cardiac arrhythmias, cardiac

disease; thyrotoxicosis; severe respiratory disease; epilepsy, conditions predisposing to epilepsy (e.g. alcohol withdrawal or brain damage); Parkinson's disease; patients who have shown hypersensitivity to other phenothiazines; personal or family history of narrow angle glaucoma; in very hot weather; the elderly, particularly if frail or at risk of hypothermia; hypothyroidism; myasthenia gravis; prostatic hypertrophy.

Use in pregnancy: The safety for the use of this drug during pregnancy has not been established; therefore, the possible hazards should be weighed against the potential benefits when administering this drug to pregnant patients.

Nursing mothers: Breast feeding is not recommended during treatment with fluphenazines, owing to the possibility that fluphenazine is excreted in the milk of nursing mothers.

Drug interactions: The possibility should be borne in mind that phenothiazines may:

(1) Increase the central nervous system depression produced by drugs such as alcohol, hypnotics, sedatives or strong analgesics.

(2) Antagonise the action of adrenaline and other sympathomimetic agents and reverse the blood-pressure-lowering effects of adrenergic-blocking agents such as guanethidine and clonidine.

(3) Impair: (a) the anti-Parkinsonian effect of L-Dopa; (b) the effect of anti-convulsants; (c) metabolism of tricyclic antidepressants; (d) the control of diabetes.

(4) Increase the effect of anticoagulants.

(5) Interact with lithium.

Tea and coffee form insoluble precipitates with fluphenazine in vitro, but there is conflicting evidence as to whether this reduces absorption in man.

Antacids may impair absorption.

Anticholinergic effects may be enhanced by anti-Parkinsonian or other anticholinergic drugs.

Phenothiazines may enhance: The cardiac-depressant effects of quinidine; the absorption of corticosteroids, digoxin and neuromuscular blocking agents.

Side-effects: Extrapyramidal reactions are common at higher doses and occasionally occur at low dosage. Acute dystonias may occur early in treatment, and oculogyric crises have been reported. Both usually respond rapidly to an i.v. or i.m. administration of an anti-Parkinsonian agent. Parkinsonian rigidity, tremor, akathisia, tend to appear less rapidly, and may be reduced by using a smaller dose or by the concomitant use of an oral anti-Parkinsonian drug such as benzhexol, benztropine or procyclidine. However, anti-Parkinsonian agents should not be prescribed routinely, because of the possible risks of aggravating anticholinergic side-effects of fluphenazine, of precipitating toxic-confusional states or of impairing its therapeutic efficacy.

Numerous surveys of schizophrenic patients receiving phenothiazine medication have reported varying prevalences of irregularly repetitive involuntary movements, which collectively have been termed 'tardive dyskinesia'. The movements most commonly involve the tongue and facial muscles, but sometimes affect the limbs and trunk. Although the only two surveys which assessed the prevalence of involuntary movements among schizophrenic patients never treated with neuroleptics found similar prevalence to that among the neuroleptic-treated patients, phenothiazines as well as other antipsychotics have been implicated in the emergence of these syndromes.

Tardive dyskinesia: As with all antipsychotic agents, tardive dyskinesia may appear in some patients on long term therapy or may occur after drug therapy has been discontinued. The risk seems to be greater in elderly patients on high dose therapy, especially females. The symptoms are persistent and in some patients appear to be irreversible. The syndrome is characterised by rhythmical involuntary movements of the tongue, face, mouth or jaw (e.g. protrusion of tongue, puffing of cheeks, puckering of mouth, chewing movements). Sometimes these may be accompanied by involuntary movements of the extremities. There is no known effective treatment for tardive dyskinesia; anti-Parkinsonian agents usually do not alleviate the symptoms of this syndrome. It is suggested that all antipsychotic agents be discontinued if these symptoms appear. Should it be necessary to reinstitute treatment, or increase the dosage of the agent, or switch to a different antispsychotic agent, the syndrome may be masked. It has been reported that fine vermicular movements of the tongue may be an early sign of the syndrome and if the medication is stopped at that time, the syndrome may not develop.

As with other phenothiazines, drowsiness, lethargy, blurred vision, dryness of the mouth, constipation, urinary hesitancy and incontinence, mild hypotension, impairment of judgement and mental skills, and epileptiform attacks are occasionally seen, but extremely rarely in doses used for non-psychotic conditions.

The use of this drug may impair the mental and physical abilities required for driving a car or operating heavy machinery.

Blood dyscrasias have rarely been reported with phenothiazine derivatives. Blood counts should be performed if the patient develops signs of persistent infection. Transient leucopenia and thrombocytopenia have been reported. Antinuclear antibodies and SLE have been reported very rarely.

Jaundice has rarely been reported. Transient abnormalities of liver function tests may occur in the absence of jaundice.

A transient rise in serum cholesterol has been reported very occasionally in patients on oral fluphenazine.

Abnormal skin pigmentation and lens opacities have sometimes been seen following long-term administration of high doses of phenothiazines.

Phenothiazines are known to cause photosensitivity reactions but this has not been reported for fluphenazine. Skin rashes have occasionally been reported.

Elderly patients may be more susceptible to the sedative and hypotensive effects.

The effects of phenothiazines on the heart are dose-related. ECG changes, with prolongation of the QT interval and T-wave changes have been reported commonly in patients treated with moderate to high dosage; they are reversible on reducing the dose. In a very small number of cases, they have been reported to precede serious arrhythmias, including ventricular tachycardia and fibrillation, which have also occurred after overdosage. Sudden, unexpected and unexplained deaths have been reported in hospitalised psychotic patients receiving phenothiazines.

Phenothiazines may impair body temperature regulation. Cases of severe hypothermia or hyperpyrexia have been reported in association with moderate or high dosage of phenothiazines.

Elderly or hypothyroid patients may be particularly susceptible to hypothermia. The hazard of hyperpyrexia may be increased by especially hot or humid weather, or by drugs such as anti-Parkinsonian agents, which impair sweating.

Rare occurrences of neuroleptic malignant syndrome (NMS) have been reported in patients on neuroleptic therapy. The syndrome is characterised by hyperthermia, together with some or all of the following: muscular rigidity, autonomic instability (labile blood pressure, tachycardia, diaphoresis), akinesia, and altered consciousness, sometimes progressing to stupor or coma. Leucocytosis, elevated CPK, liver function abnormalities, and acute renal failure may also occur. Neuroleptic therapy should be discontinued immediately and vigorous symptomatic treatment implemented since the syndrome is potentially fatal.

Hormonal effects of phenothiazines include hyperprolactinaemia, which may cause galactorrhoea, gynaecomastia and oligo- or amenorrhoea. Sexual function may be impaired.

Oedema has been reported with phenothiazine medication.

Acute withdrawal symptoms including nausea, vomiting and insomnia, have very rarely been described after abrupt cessation of high doses of phenothiazines. Gradual withdrawal is advisable.

Overdosage: It should be treated symptomatically and supportively. Extrapyramidal reactions will respond to oral or parenteral anti-Parkinsonian drugs such as procyclidine or benztropine. In cases of severe hypotension, all procedures for the management of circulatory shock should be instituted, e.g. vasoconstrictors and/or intravenous fluids. However, only the vasoconstrictors metaraminol or noradrenaline should be used, as adrenaline may further lower the blood pressure through interaction with the phenothiazine.

Pharmaceutical precautions *Storage:* At room temperature.

Legal category POM.

Package quantities Bottles of 100.

Further information Fluphenazine hydrochloride is a salt of the potent neuroleptic fluphenazine, a phenothiazine derivative of the piperazine type. Extrapyramidal reactions, are not uncommon, but fluphenazine does not have marked sedative or hypotensive properties.

Product licence numbers

Moditen Tablets 1 mg	0034/5049R
Moditen Tablets 2.5 mg	0034/5050R
Moditen Tablets 5 mg	0034/5051R

MOTIPRESS* TABLETS MOTIVAL* TABLETS

Presentation
Motival: Each pink, triangular-shaped, sugar-coated tablet contains nortriptyline hydrochloride equivalent to 10 mg nortriptyline base and fluphenazine hydrochloride 0.5 mg.

Other ingredients: Acacia, caster oil, chalk, curcumin, dicalcium phosphate, erythrosine, gelatin, lactose, magnesium stearate, maize, starch, shellac, sucrose, talc, titanium dioxide.

Motipress: Each yellow, triangular-shaped, sugar-coated tablet contains nortriptyline hydrochloride equivalent to 30 mg nortriptyline base and fluphenazine hydrochloride 1.5 mg.

Other ingredients: Acacia, caster oil, chalk, curcumin, dicalcium phosphate, gelatin, lactose, magnesium stearate, maize starch, shellac, sucrose, talc, titanium dioxide.

Uses *Actions:* Nortriptyline hydrochloride is a tricyclic antidepressant with more rapid activity and less sedation than the majority of the drugs of its class. It possesses some atropine-like properties. It is not a monoamine oxidase inhibitor.

Fluphenazine hydrochloride is a phenothiazine derivative of the piperazine type, its principal actions being those of tranquillization and anti-emesis.

Indications: Motival and Motipress are indicated for the treatment of patients suffering from mild to moderate mixed anxiety depressive states.

Dosage and administration *Adults:* Motival: The dose is 1 tablet three times daily.

Motipress: The dose is 1 tablet daily, preferably before retiring.

A course of treatment with either Motival or Motipress should be limited to three months. If the patient does not respond after four weeks an alternative treatment should be given.

Elderly: Elderly patients should be started on Motival one tablet twice daily. If Motival one tablet, three times daily, is required, subsequently Motipress may be substituted.

Children: These formulations are not indicated for the treatment of children.

Contra-indications, warnings, etc
Contra-indications: Phenothiazines and tricyclic antidepressants have been shown to lower the threshold for electrically induced convulsions in animals, hence Motival and Motipress are not recommended for patients with a history of epilepsy or brain damage. It is further contra-indicated in patients with blood dyscrasias, severe cardiac insufficiency, renal or liver damage.

It is inadvisable to give monoamine oxidase inhibitors (MAOIs) with Motival or Motipress, nor should they be given within two weeks after cessation of treatment with MAOIs.

Precautions: Motival and Motipress should be given with caution to patients with glaucoma and to those who have a propensity for urinary retention. Interaction with barbiturates, alcohol and narcotic drugs may occur, so central nervous depressants should be administered with caution. Motival and Motipress may diminish the antihypertensive effect of adrenergic blocking agents and could potentiate the pressor response to locally injected sympathomimetic agents.

Tardive dyskinesias have been reported in association with phenothiazine therapy, usually after prolonged courses given at doses adequate to treat psychotic illness. Consequently Motival and Motipress treatment should be limited to three months (see Dosage and Administration).

The use of Motival or Motipress may impair alertness and abilities required for driving a car or operating machinery.

Motival or Motipress should be used with caution in patients with cardiac failure, especially when there is evidence of rhythm disturbance, and in patients with recent myocardial infarction.

Pregnancy: Do not use during pregnancy, especially the first and last trimesters, unless there are compelling reasons. There is no evidence as to drug safety in human pregnancy nor are the results of animal studies conclusive.

Nursing mothers: Breast feeding is not recommended in women receiving Motival and Motipress.

Side-effects: Dryness of mouth, drowsiness, faintness and constipation. Occasionally tachycardia, nasal congestion, blurred vision and excitement are seen.

Extrapyramidal reactions are unlikely to occur with this dose of fluphenazine alone, and it is probable that the anticholinergic activity of nortriptyline affords protection against such effects.

Motival and Motipress contain the phenothiazine, fluphenazine. As with all neuroleptic drugs, the presence of unexplained hyperthermia could indicate neuroleptic malignant syndrome (NMS). In this event, Motival/Motipress and any associated neuroleptic treatment should be discontinued until the origin of the fever has been determined.

Overdosage: Overdosage should be treated symptomatically and supportively. If the patient is conscious, prompt gastric lavage, dilution of the stomach contents to delay absorption, or stimulation of vomiting should be attempted. An open airway should be maintained. Extrapyramidal symptoms are amenable to antiparkinsonian drugs. In severe hypotension, all the standard procedures for the management of circulatory shock should be instituted, e.g. vasoconstrictors and/or intravenous fluids. If vasoconstrictors are required, metaraminol, mephentermine or noradrenaline should be administered, but not adrenaline, as this will further lower the blood pressure through interaction with the phenothiazine.

Pharmaceutical precautions *Storage:* At room temperature.

Legal category POM.

Package quantities Motival: Bottles of 100 and 500 tablets.
Motipress: 28 day calendar pack (OP).

Further information Nil.

Product licence numbers

Motival Tablets	0034/0219
Motipress Tablets	0034/0220.

MYSTECLIN* TABLETS

Presentation Orange, sugar-coated tablet containing tetracycline hydrochloride 250 mg and nystatin 250,000 units.

Other ingredients: Ac-di-sol (cellulose gum), castor oil, chalk, erythrosine, indigo carmine, magnesium stearate, microcrystalline cellulose, polyvinylpyrrolidone, quinoline yellow, shellac, sucrose, talc, titanium dioxide.

Uses *Actions:* Tetracycline has a broad antimicrobial activity against pathogenic organisms including many Gram-positive and Gram-negative bacteria, spirochaetes, certain rickettsiae, large viruses, *Mycoplasma pneumoniae* and *Entamoeba histolytica.* After oral administration therapeutically effective blood and urinary levels are obtained in a short period of time. It diffuses readily into most body tissues.

Nystatin is an antifungal antibiotic active against a wide range of yeasts and yeast-like fungi, including *Candida albicans.* Following wide use over many years, no clinical isolates resistant to this compound have emerged. Repeated subculture, *in vitro,* produces a small number of resistant isolates, but with reduced growth rate and pathogenicity. The possibility of these organisms causing disease in man is remote.

Indications: For infections caused by organisms sensitive to tetracycline, particularly in patients who may be susceptible to candidal overgrowth. These may include elderly or debilitated patients, diabetics, women taking hormonal contraceptive agents, patients with malignant disease especially if receiving cytotoxic drugs and those patients receiving high doses or prolonged courses of antibiotics or corticosteroids. Representative infections due to susceptible organisms, including chronic bronchitis and other respiratory tract infections, urinary tract infections, brucellosis, acne and many mixed infections.

Dosage and administration *Adult dosage:* One Mysteclin tablet four times daily. This dose may be doubled in severe infections.

Children over 12 years: A divided daily dose equivalent to 22–44 mg tetracycline per kg should be given according to the type and severity of the infection (see 'Precautions').

Elderly: No specific dosage recommendations, but see 'Precautions' re renal and hepatic failure.

All patients: Absorption of tetracycline from the gut is diminished by milk, salts of calcium, magnesium, aluminium and iron. Lowered absorption also results from alkalis, and concomitant administration of antacids should therefore be avoided.

Mysteclin should preferably be taken one hour before, or two hours after meals.

Contra-indications, warnings, etc

Contra-indications: The tetracycline group of antibiotics is normally contra-indicated during pregnancy and childhood except in certain severe infections where tetracycline may be the drug of choice, and the risk involved is justified (see 'Precautions'). Mysteclin should not be used in patients with a history of hypersensitivity to the tetracycline group of antibiotics.

There are no known contra-indications to the use of nystatin.

Precautions: There are no special precautions for the oral use of nystatin.

If renal impairment exists, even usual oral or parenteral doses of tetracycline may lead to excessive systemic accumulation of the drug and possible liver toxicity.

During long-term therapy periodic assessment of organ system function, including renal, hepatic and haemopoeitic systems, should be made.

The effects of anticoagulants are not usually altered by concurrent treatment with tetracycline, although a few isolated cases of enhancement have been described. Therefore, occasionally, reduction in doses of concurrent anticoagulants may be required.

Pregnancy and breast feeding: Tetracycline crosses the placental barrier and, in the last half of pregnancy may cause permanent discoloration of the teeth and depression of bone growth in the foetus. Similarly, tetracycline is excreted in breast milk which may also affect the infant. Therefore tetracyclines, as a class, are contra-indicated during pregnancy and breast feeding.

Infants and children: Tetracyclines may be deposited in areas of calcification in bones and teeth. The use of drugs of the tetracycline class during tooth development (last half of pregnancy, infancy and childhood to the age of twelve years) may cause permanent discoloration of the teeth (yellow-grey-brown). This reaction is more common during long-term use of the drugs but has been observed following repeated short-term courses. Enamel hypoplasia has also been reported. Tetracycline drugs, therefore, should not be used in this age group unless other drugs are not likely to be effective or are contra-indicated.

Bulging fontanelles in infants and benign intracranial hypertension in adults have been reported with therapeutic doses of tetracycline. These occurrences are rare and signs and symptoms have disappeared on cessation of treatment. Hence treatment should cease if evidence of raised intracranial pressure develops.

Side-effects: Mysteclin is generally well tolerated, but a few patients may experience skin rashes or gastro-intestinal side-effects such as nausea, vomiting and diarrhoea. A phototoxic reaction may be produced in some patients, although such reactions are less common with tetracycline than with other members of the group. Rise in BUN has been reported and is apparently dose-related.

No systemic effects or allergic reactions have been associated with the oral use of nystatin.

Overdosage: The most common symptoms are nausea, vomiting and diarrhoea. The possibility of liver and renal failure should be borne in mind.

Pharmaceutical precautions *Storage:* At room temperature.

Legal category POM.

Package quantities Bottles of 100.

Further information By the inclusion of nystatin with tetracycline, the fungal overgrowth frequently associated with broad-spectrum antibiotic therapy is avoided.

Product licence number 0034/5056R.

NOCTEC* CAPSULES

Presentation Clear, orange-red gelatin capsules, each containing 500 mg chloral hydrate in solution.

Other ingredients: Erythrosine, quinoline yellow, methyl hydroxybenzoate, polyethylene glycol, propyl hydroxybenzoate, gelatin/glycerin capsule.

Uses *Actions:* The hypnotic, chloral hydrate, in doses of 0.5-1 g, produces sedation in approximately 15 minutes followed by sleep in about half an hour. The drug has virtually no effect on REM sleep. It is generally believed that the central depressant effects are due to the principal pharmacologically active metabolite, trichloroethanol, which has a plasma half-life of 7–10 hours.

Blood pressure and respiration are depressed only slightly more than in normal sleep, and reflexes are not significantly depressed.

Indications: Insomnia.

Dosage and administration

Adults: 500 mg to 1 g taken 15 to 30 minutes before bedtime. Daily dose should not exceed 2 g. The capsules should be taken with water, to avoid gastro-intestinal upset.

Children: Not recommended.

Elderly: No specific dosage recommendations (see 'Precautions').

Contra-indications, warnings, etc

Contra-indications: In patients with marked hepatic or renal impairment, or in patients with severe cardiac disease. Noctec is best avoided in the presence of marked gastritis and in patients who have previously exhibited an idiosyncrasy or hypersensitivity to chloral hydrate.

Chloral hydrate should not be used in patients susceptible to acute attacks of porphyria.

Chloral hydrate is contra-indicated in pregnancy and breastfeeding.

Precautions: Alcohol potentiates the sedative effect.

In patients taking anticoagulants, when Noctec is added or withdrawn from the drug regimen, or its dosage changed, careful monitoring of the prothrombin time is required.

Chloral hydrate followed by intravenous frusemide may result in sweating, hot flushes and variable blood pressure including hypertension due to a hypermetabolic state caused by displacement of thyroid hormone from its bound state.

Delirium may occur, especially in the elderly, particularly when used in conjunction with psychotropics or anticholinergics.

Abuse and chronic intoxication: There is a danger of misuse and the possibility that habituation may develop. In such patients gastritis and parenchymatous renal injury may develop. After long term use sudden withdrawal may result in delirium.

Side-effects: Gastric irritation, abdominal distension and flatulence may occur. Excitement, tolerance, allergic skin reactions, headache and ketonuria have occasionally been reported.

Overdosage: The signs and symptoms of chloral hydrate overdosage affect the CNS, cardiovascular and respiratory systems. These may include: respiratory depression, arrhythmias, hypothermia, pin-point pupils, hypotension or coma. Gastric irritation may result in vomiting and even gastric necrosis. If the patient survives, icterus due to hepatic damage and albuminuria from renal damage may appear.

Serious problems have arisen with doses as little as 4 g and 10 g can be fatal.

Overdosage should be treated with gastric lavage or inducing vomiting to empty the stomach. Supportive measures must be used. Haemodialysis, and in some cases haemoperfusion, have been reported to be effective in promoting the clearance of trichloroethanol.

Pharmaceutical precautions *Storage:* In a cool place; avoid freezing.

Legal category POM.

Package quantities Bottles of 50 capsules.

Further information Nil.

Product licence number 0034/5057R.

NYSTADERMAL* CREAM

Presentation A yellow to light buff cream containing in each gram nystatin 100,000 units and triamcinolone acetonide 0.1%.

Other ingredients: Aluminium hydroxide, antifoam emulsion, benzyl alcohol, macrogol ether, perfume, propylene glycol, sorbitol, titanium dioxide, white soft paraffin.

Uses *Actions:* Triamcinolone acetonide is a potent fluorinated corticosteroid with rapid anti-inflammatory, antipruritic and anti-allergic actions. Nystatin is an antifungal antibiotic active against a wide range of yeasts and yeast-like fungi, including Candida albicans. The cream is formulated for use on moist weeping lesions.

Indications: Nystadermal Cream is indicated for those cases of cutaneous candidosis where the addition of a corticosteroid to the antifungal antibiotic may be beneficial in controlling the commonly associated inflammation and pruritus. Nystadermal Cream will also be of benefit in those cases of eczema where Candida is either the precipitating cause, or present as a secondary invader.

Dosage and administration *Adults and children:* To be applied to moist weeping lesions two to four times daily.

Elderly: Corticosteroids should be used sparingly and for short periods of time, as natural thinning of the skin occurs in the elderly: hence, if, after about 7 days application, little or no improvement has occurred, cultural isolation of the offending organism should be followed by appropriate local or systemic antimicrobial therapy.

Contra-indications, warnings, etc

Contra-indications: There are no known contra-indications or special precautions for topical application of nystatin. Corticosteroids are contra-indicated in tuberculous and most viral lesions of the skin, particularly herpes simplex and varicella. The products should not be used in fungal lesions not susceptible to nystatin or bacterial skin infections without suitable concomitant anti-infective therapy.

In patients with hypersensitivity to any of the components.

Should not be used for facial rosacea, acne vulgaris or perioral dermatitis.

Precautions: Adrenal suppression can occur, even without occlusion. The use of occlusive dressings should be avoided because of the increased risk of sensitivity reactions and increased percutaneous absorption.

If used in childhood, or on the face, courses should be limited to 5 days and occlusion should not be used.

Children: In infants, long-term continuous topical steroid therapy should be avoided. Courses should be limited to 5 days and occlusion should not be used.

Pregnancy: There is inadequate evidence of safety in human pregnancy. Topical administration of corticosteroids to pregnant animals can cause abnormalities of foetal development including cleft palate and intra-uterine growth retardation There may, therefore, be a very small risk of such effects in the human foetus.

Side-effects: There have been no substantiated reports of sensitivity associated with topical nystatin.

Triamcinolone acetonide is well tolerated. Where adverse reactions occur they are usually reversible on cessation of therapy. However the following side-effects have been reported usually with prolonged usage:

Dermatologic – impaired wound healing, thinning of the skin, petechiae and ecchymoses, facial erythema and telangiectasia, increased sweating, purpura, striae, hirsutism, acneiform eruptions, lupus erythematosus-like lesions and suppressed reactions to skin tests.

These effects may be enhanced with occlusive dressings.

Signs of systemic toxicity such as oedema and electrolyte imbalance have not been observed even when high topical dosage has been used. The possibility of the systemic effects which are associated with all steroid therapy should be considered.

Overdosage: Topically applied corticosteroids can be absorbed in sufficient amounts to produce systemic effects (see 'Side-effects').

In the event of accidental ingestion, the patient should be observed and treated symptomatically.

Pharmaceutical precautions *Storage:* At room temperature; avoid freezing.

Dilution: Not recommended, as this may reduce therapeutic efficacy of nystatin. If necessary, refer to the manufacturer.

Legal category POM.

Package quantities 15 g tubes.

Further information Nil.

Product licence number 0034/0131R

NYSTAN* CREAM, OINTMENT, AND GEL

Presentation

Gel: Yellow to amber, opaque, containing 100,000 units nystatin per gram. Other ingredients: Carbopol, chlorocresol, perfume, potassium phosphates, sodium hydroxide.

Cream: Pale buff, containing 100,000 units per gram nystatin in a vanishing-cream base. Other ingredients: Aluminium hydroxide, antifoam emulsion, benzyl alcohol, macrogol ether, perfume, propylene glycol, sorbitol, titanium dioxide, white soft paraffin.

Ointment: Yellow to amber containing 100,000 units nystatin per gram in Plastibase* (liquid paraffin and polyethylene resin).

Uses *Actions:* Nystatin is an antifungal antibiotic active against a wide range of yeasts and yeast-like fungi, including *Candida albicans.*

Indications: For the treatment of cutaneous and mucocutaneous mycoses, particularly those caused by *C. albicans.*

Dosage and administration *Adults and children:* To be applied two to four times daily.

Elderly: No specific dosage recommendations or precautions.

Contra-indications, warnings, etc
Contra-indications: There are no known contra-indications or special precautions for topical application of nystatin.

Pregnancy/children: No specific precautions apply; systemic absorption is negligible.

Side-effects: There have been no substantiated reports of sensitivity associated with topical nystatin.

Overdosage: Since absorption of nystatin from the gastro-intestinal tract is negligible, accidental ingestion causes no systemic toxicity.

Pharmaceutical precautions *Storage:*
Gel: In a cool place; avoid freezing.

Cream: At room temperature; avoid freezing.

Ointment: At room temperature.

Dilution: Nystan topicals should not be diluted as this may reduce therapeutic efficacy.

Legal category POM.

Package quantities *Cream/Ointment:* Tubes of 30 g (OP).
Gel: Tubes of 30 g (OP).

Further information Nil.

Product licence numbers

Nystan Cream	0034/5058R
Nystan Ointment	0034/0161R
Nystan Gel	0034/0142R

NYSTAN* ORAL SUSPENSION, NYSTAN* FOR SUSPENSION AND TABLETS

Presentation
Nystan Oral Suspension: Yellow, cherry-mint flavoured suspension providing 100,000 units nystatin per ml. N.B. Suspension contains sugar.

Other ingredients: Ethyl alcohol, flavours, glycerin, hydrochloric acid, methyl parahydroxybenzoate, propyl parahydroxybenzoate, sodium carboxymethylcellulose, sodium phosphate, sodium hydroxide, sucrose.

Nystan For Suspension: A powder for reconstitution to provide oral suspension containing 100,000 units nystatin per ml. N.B. Reconstituted suspension is sugar-free.

Other ingredients: Methyl hydroxybenzoate, propyl hydroxybenzoate, saccharin, saccharin sodium, sodium benzoate, sodium carboxymethylcellulose, wood cellulose.

Nystan Tablets: Sugar-coated, chocolate-brown tablets containing 500,000 units nystatin.

Other ingredients: Carnauba wax, castor oil, chalk, iron oxide, lactose, magnesium stearate, maize starch, polyvinylpyrrolidone, shellac, sucrose, talc, white beeswax.

Uses *Actions:* Nystatin is an antifungal antibiotic active against a wide range of yeasts and yeast-like fungi, including Candida albicans.

Indications: Suspension for the prevention and treatment of candidal infections of the oral cavity, oesophagus and intestinal tract. It provides effective prophylaxis against oral candidosis in those born of mothers with vaginal candidosis.

Tablets for intestinal candidosis. Also for use in patients who may be susceptible to candidal overgrowth, e.g. patients with malignant disease especially if receiving cytotoxic drugs, and those patients receiving high doses or prolonged courses of antibiotics or corticosteroids.

Dosage and administration Reconstitution of Granules For Suspension: Add 23 ml water to the bottle and shake vigorously.

Adults: Suspension (Nystan Oral and Nystan For Suspensions): For the treatment of denture sores, and oral infections in adults caused by *C. albicans,* 1 ml of the suspension should be dropped into the mouth four times daily; it should be kept in contact with the affected areas as long as possible.

Tablets: For the treatment of intestinal candidosis 1 tablet four times daily, but this dose may be doubled. For prophylaxis a total daily dosage of 1 million units has been found to suppress the overgrowth of *C. albicans* in patients receiving broad-spectrum antibiotic therapy.

Older people with intestinal candidosis who are unable to swallow tablets should be given 5 ml of the suspension four times a day.

Administration should be continued for 48 hours after clinical cure to prevent relapse.

Children: Suspension: In intestinal and oral candidosis (thrush) in infants and children, 1 ml should be dropped into the mouth four times a day. The longer the suspension is kept in contact with the affected area in the mouth, before swallowing, the greater will be its effect.

For prophylaxis in the newborn the suggested dose is 1 ml once daily.

Elderly: No specific dosage recommendations or precautions.

Contra-indications, warnings, etc
Contra-indications: There are no known contra-indications to the use of nystatin.

Precautions: Nystan Oral Suspension contains sugar. For children with disaccharide intolerance the sugar-free formulation, Nystan For Suspension, is recommended.

Pregnancy: Absorption of nystatin from the gastro-intestinal tract is negligible, therefore no special precautions apply in pregnancy.

Side-effects: Nausea, vomiting and diarrhoea have occasionally been reported with doses of nystatin exceeding 4 to 5 million units daily. No systemic effects or allergic reactions have been associated with its oral use.

Overdosage: Since the absorption of nystatin from the gastro-intestinal tract is negligible, overdosage causes no systemic toxicity.

Pharmaceutical precautions *Storage: Nystan Suspension:* At room temperature; avoid freezing. *Nystan For Suspension:* The reconstituted suspension will remain suitable for use for 7 days at room temperature or 10 days under refrigeration. Store the dry powder at room temperature. *Nystan Tablets:* At room temperature.

Dilution: Not recommended as this may reduce therapeutic efficacy.

If necessary, refer to the manufacturer.

Legal category POM.

Package quantities
Nystan Oral Suspension: Bottles of 30 ml with graduated dropper (OP).
Nystan For Suspension: Bottles of 24 ml when reconstituted, with graduated dropper (OP).
Nystan Tablets: Bottles of 56 (OP) and 100.

Further information Nil.

Product licence numbers

Nystan Oral Suspension	0034/0130R
Nystan For Suspension	0034/5061R
Nystan Tablets	0034/5063R

NYSTAN* PASTILLES

Presentation Yellow-brown, aniseed flavoured soft pastille providing 100,000 units nystatin per pastille; containing sugar and cinnamon.

Other ingredients: Aniseed oil, antifoam emulsion, cinnamon oil, dextrose monohydrate, gelatin, hydrochloric acid, liquid glucose, potassium hydroxide, silicone, sucrose.

Uses *Actions:* Nystatin is an antifungal antibiotic active against a wide range of yeasts and yeast-like fungi, including Candida albicans.

Indications: For the treatment of oral candidosis.

Dosage and administration No food or drink should be taken for five minutes before or one hour after consumption of the pastille. The pastilles should be sucked slowly and retained in the mouth for as long as possible in accordance with the doctors instructions.

Adults and children: One pastille to be sucked slowly, four times a day for 7–14 days.

Elderly: No specific dosage recommendations or precautions.

Contra-indications, warnings, etc
Contra-indications: There are no known contra-indications to the use of nystatin.

Precautions: Pregnancy: Absorption of nystatin from the gastro-intestinal tract is negligible, therefore no special precautions apply in pregnancy.

Side-effects: Nausea, vomiting and diarrhoea have occasionally been reported with doses of nystatin exceeding 4 to 5 million units daily. No systemic effects or allergic reactions have been associated with its oral use.

Overdosage: Since the absorption of nystatin from the gastro-intestinal tract is negligible, overdosage causes no systemic toxicity.

Pharmaceutical precautions *Storage:* At room temperature.

Legal category POM.

Package quantities Packs of 28 pastilles (OP).

Further information The pastille allows longer contact of the active ingredient nystatin with the mucous membrane than liquid formulations.

Successful treatment of oral candidosis also includes good oral hygiene. Patients with dentures are advised to remove them whilst sucking the pastilles.

Product licence number 0034/0248.

NYSTAN* PESSARIES AND VAGINAL CREAM

Presentation *Pessaries:* Pale yellow to tan, diamond-shaped, with Squibb logo and 457 engraved on one side, containing 100,000 units nystatin.

Other ingredients: Lactose, magnesium stearate, maize starch, modified cellulose gum, stearic acid.

Vaginal Cream: Pale buff containing in each 4 g application 100,000 units nystatin.

Other ingredients: Aluminium hydroxide, antifoam emulsion, benzyl alcohol, hydrochloric acid, macrogol ether, propylene glycol, sodium hydroxide, sorbitol, water, white soft paraffin.

Uses *Actions:* Nystatin is an antifungal antibiotic active against a wide range of yeasts and yeast-like fungi, including *Candida albicans*.

Indications: For the treatment of candidal vaginitis.

Dosage and administration
Pessaries: Adults: 1 or 2 pessaries should be inserted high into the vagina for 14 consecutive nights or longer, regardless of any intervening menstrual period.

Vaginal Cream: Adults: Insert 1 or 2 applications (of 4 g each) high into the vagina for 14 consecutive nights, or longer, regardless of any intervening menstrual period. Reinfection from the candidal content of the intestinal tract may be prevented by concomitant therapy with oral nystatin.

Nystatin Cream, Gel or Ointment should be applied to the perineal region 2–4 times daily, if necessary.

Note: To prevent reinfection with *Candida*, the male consort should be treated concurrently with Nystan Gel or Cream applied to the external genital area 2–4 times daily during the treatment period.

Children: Vulvovaginal candidosis is rarely a problem in children. It is suggested that the vaginal cream is the most acceptable formulation for children, together with concomitant oral medication where necessary.

Elderly: No specific dosage recommendations or precautions.

Contra-indications, warnings, etc
Contra-indications: There are no known contra-indications to the use of these products.

Precautions: Avoid contract between the cream and contraceptive diaphragms and condoms, since the rubber may be damaged by the preparation.

Pregnancy: There is no evidence that nystatin is absorbed systemically from the vagina. However, as with all drugs, caution should be exercised in pregnancy. Care should be taken while using an applicator to prevent the possibility of mechanical trauma.

Side-effects: Nystan is well tolerated and no substantiated sensitivity reactions have been associated with its use. Some transient local discomfort may be experienced.

Overdosage: Since the absorption of nystatin from the gastro-intestinal tract is negligible, overdosage or accidental ingestion causes no systemic toxicity.

Pharmaceutical precautions *Storage: Pessaries:* At room temperature.

Vaginal Cream: At room temperature: avoid freezing.

Dilution: Not recommended for Vaginal Cream as this may reduce therapeutic efficacy.

Legal category POM.

Package quantities *Pessaries:* Foiled, in packs of 28 and 100 with applicators.
Vaginal Cream: Tubes of 60 g with applicator (OP).

Further information Nil.

Product licence numbers

Nystan Pessaries	0034/5062R
Nystan Vaginal Cream	0034/0137R

OPHTHAINE* SOLUTION

Presentation Sterile, aqueous ophthalmic solution containing:

Proxymetacaine hydrochloride	0.5%
Chlorbutol	0.2%
Benzalkonium chloride	0.01%

Other ingredients: Glycerin, hydrochloric acid, sodium hydroxide, water.

Uses *Actions:* Proxymetacaine hydrochloride is a rapidly acting local anaesthetic. With a single drop the onset of anaesthesia occurs in an average of 13 seconds and will persist for an average of 15 minutes.

Indications: Topical anaesthesia in ophthalmic practice.

Dosage and administration *Adults and children:* Administered by topical instillation into the eye. The recommended doses are as follows:

Deep anaesthesia: Instil 1 drop every five to ten minutes for 5–7 doses.

Removal of sutures: Instil 1 or 2 drops two or three minutes before removal of stitches.

Removal of foreign bodies: Instil 1 or 2 drops prior to operating.

Tonometry: Instil 1 or 2 drops immediately before measurement.

Elderly: No specific dosage recommendations or precautions.

Contra-indications, warnings, etc
Contra-indications: Patients with known hypersensitivity to proxymetacaine or constituents.

Precautions: Ophthaine solution is not intended for long-term use.

Ophthaine Solution is not miscible with fluorescein. However, the eye can be anaesthetised with Ophthaine Solution before fluorescein is administered.

Use cautiously and sparingly in patients with known allergies, cardiac disease, or hyperthyroidism.

Regular and prolonged use of a topical ocular anaesthetic, e.g. in conjunction with contact lens insertion, may cause softening and erosion of the corneal epithelium, which could produce corneal opacification with accompanying loss of vision.

Protection of the eye from irritating chemicals, foreign bodies and rubbing during the period of anaesthesia is very important. Tonometers soaked in sterilising or detergent solutions should be thoroughly rinsed with sterile distilled water prior to use. Patients should be advised to avoid touching the eye until the anaesthesia has worn off.

Side-effects: Pupillary dilatation or cycloplegic effects have rarely been observed with Ophthaine Solution. Irritation of the conjunctiva or other toxic reactions attributable to the preparation have occurred only rarely. A severe, immediate-type apparently hyperallergic corneal reaction may rarely occur which includes acute, intense and diffuse epithelial keratitis; a grey ground-glass appearance; sloughing of large areas of necrotic epithelium; corneal filaments and sometimes, iritis with descemetitis.

Pharmaceutical precautions *Storage:* In a refrigerator. Do not freeze. Protect from light. If solution shows more than a very pale yellow colour, it should be discarded. The product should not be used one month after first opening the container.

Legal category POM.

Package quantities Bottles of 15 ml.

Further information Nil.

Product licence number 0034/5064R.

PRONESTYL* TABLETS

Presentation
Tablets: White, engraved Squibb and 754 on one side and scored on reverse, containing 250 mg procainamide hydrochloride.

Other ingredients: Ethylcellulose, lactose, magnesium stearate, maize starch, stearic acid, sucrose.

Uses
Actions: Procainamide is a class I anti-arrhythmic agent (Vaughan Williams classification). Abnormal automaticity and excitability are reduced: the former by a slowing of the rate of diastolic phase 4 depolarisation; the latter by a reduction of the rate of rise of phase 0 depolarisation.

Action potention duration is prolonged but the effect on refractory period is greater.

These actions are apparent throughout the myocardium, and are most pronounced within the atria. Abnormal ectopic foci may be suppressed by the slowing of phase 4 depolarisation, while re-entrant tachyarrhythmias may be inhibited both by the reduced excitability of the myocardium and by the prolongation of the refractory period. In those arrhythmias not fully suppressed, procainamide is likely to slow the tachycardia.

Following oral administration therapeutic levels (3 to 10 mcg/ml, with those for a majority of patients in the range of 4 to 8 mcg/ml) are usually obtained by 30 minutes, with maximal levels occuring after 60 minutes.

Indications: The treatment of atrial tachycardia.

The treatment of symptomatic or potentially malignant ventricular arrhythmias (i.e. extrasystoles or tachycardia).

The treatment or prophylaxis of symptomatic or potentially malignant ventricular arrhythmias following acute myocardial infarction.

Dosage and administration
Children: Pronestyl is not recommended.

Adults: Oral Pronestyl can be used for maintenance therapy once control of arrhythmias is achieved. Intravenous therapy is available for more serious tachyarrhythmias.

Plasma concentrations correlate well with therapeutic and toxic effects; consequently plasma level assays should be carried out if facilities are available. The usual effective antiarrhythmic serum concentration is 4 to 8 mcg/ml. Toxic manifestations are rare in concentrations less than 12 mcg/ml.

Oral therapy is preferred for treatment of arrhythmias which do not require immediate suppression, and for prevention of recurrence of serious arrhythmias after initial control by cardioversion, by intravenous Pronestyl Injection or by other antiarrhythmic therapy.

Ideally, the oral dose and interval of administration should be adjusted for the individual patient, based on clinical assessment of the degree of underlying myocardial disease, the patient's age, and renal function.

As a general guide, for younger patients with normal renal function, an initial total daily oral dose of up to 50 mg/kg of body weight of Pronestyl Tablets may be used, given in divided doses, every three hours, to maintain therapeutic blood levels. For older patients, especially those over 50 years of age, or for patients with renal, hepatic, or cardiac insufficiency, lesser amounts or longer intervals may produce adequate blood levels. The initial total daily dose should be divided for administration at three, four, or six hour intervals as estimated for the patient's needs; then, the dose and interval should be adjusted for the individual.

To provide up to 50 mg per kg of body weight per day:

Patients weighing	
40–50 kg	250 mg 3 hrly to 500 mg 6 hrly
60–70 kg	375 mg 3 hrly to 750 mg 6 hrly
80–90 kg	500 mg 3 hrly to 1 g 6 hrly
More than 100 kg	625 mg 3 hrly to 1.25 g 6 hrly

Atrial arrhythmias: Higher dosages, than for ventricular arrhythmias, may be required (see 'Warnings and precautions').

Elderly: Reduction in dose or increase in dosage interval may be necessary to maintain constant blood levels without accumulation (see above).

Contra-indications, warnings, etc
Contra-indications: Hypersensitivity to the drug is an absolute contra-indication. In this connection, cross sensitivity to procaine and related drugs must be borne in mind.

Procainamide should not be administered to patients with complete atrioventricular heart block or a high degree of A-V block or bifasicular block unless an electrical pacemaker is operative.

Systemic lupus erythematosus:

'Torsade de Pointes', a variant form of ventricular tachycardia associated with a prolonged QT interval, should not be treated with Pronestyl which may aggravate rather than suppress this arrhythmia.

Warnings and precautions: Myasthenia gravis: Patients with myasthenia gravis may show worsening of symptoms from procainamide due to its procaine-like effect on diminishing acetylcholine release at skeletal muscle motor nerve endings, so that procainamide administration may be hazardous without optimal adjustment of anticholinesterase medications and other precautions.

Digitalis intoxication: Procainamide may further depress conduction and ventricular asystole or fibrillation may result.

If the patient develops first degree heart block, dosage reduction and/or discontinuation of procainamide should be considered.

Caution in patients with congestive heart failure, acute ischaemic heart disease, cardiogenic shock or cardiomyopathy as even slight depression in myocardial contractility may reduce the cardiac output of the damaged heart.

Cardiotoxicity may be reflected by hypotension, excessive widening of the QRS complex or prolongation of the PR interval or the appearance of proarrhythmic effects.

In patients with significant impairment of renal or hepatic function, accumulation of Pronestyl may occur, leading to drug toxicity.

The electrophysiological action of procainamide may be affected by electrolyte imbalance.

Pregnancy and nursing mothers: Safety has not been established; therefore, Pronestyl should be used during pregnancy only if the possible benefits outweigh the potential risks involved. Procainamide crosses the placenta but the extent is unknown. Procainamide is excreted in breast milk; therefore, it should not be given to nursing mothers because of the potential risk of adverse reactions in the infant.

Side-effects: A Lupus-like syndrome has been reported after prolonged courses of Pronestyl. The Lupus-like syndrome seldom appears in less than two months, but is very common after six months. It is virtually completely reversible and tests for antinuclear factors are usually positive before clinical signs appear. It is perhaps more often observed in patients who are slow acetylators. If long-term treatment is considered desirable, it is advisable to undertake serological tests at no less than monthly intervals and to continue treatment for no longer than absolutely necessary.

Agranulocytosis is a rare side effect of prolonged procainamide therapy. Susceptibility to this is greater in the period following coronary bypass surgery. The patient should be instructed to report any soreness of the mouth, throat, or gums, unexplained fever or any symptoms of upper respiratory tract infection. If any of these should occur, and leucocyte counts indicate cellular depression, Pronestyl therapy should be discontinued, and appropriate treatment should be instituted immediately.

Nausea, vomiting, diarrhoea, anorexia, bitter taste, mental depression, psychoses with hallucinations, dizziness, headache, pruritus, chills, fever, hepatitis and allergic reactions (such as vasculitis, eosinophilia, skin reactions or angioneurotic oedema) may occur infrequently. They are usually not sufficiently severe to discontinue treatment.

Neutropenia, thrombocytopenia or haemolytic anaemia may rarely be encountered.

As with all other class 1 agents, pro-arrhythmic effects may occur.

Drug interactions:

Other antiarrhythmic drugs: Additive effects can occur and dosage reduction may be necessary.

Antihypertensive agents: Procainamide may produce an additive effect and dosage adjustment may be necessary.

Anticholinergic drugs: Additive antivagal effects on A-V nodal conduction may occur.

Neuromuscular blocking agents: Possibly reduce dosage of Neuromuscular blocking drugs as procainamide may reduce acetylcholine release.

Captopril: There have been reports of neutropenia and/or Stevens Johnson syndrome in patients on procainamide plus captopril. Although a causal relationship has not been established, this combination should only be used with caution, especially in patients with impaired renal function.

Sulphonamides: p-amino benzoic acid is a metabolite of procainamide and can inhibit the action of sulphonamides.

Pharmacokinetic interactions: The elimination of procainamide may be decreased by cimetidine or propranolol, and increased by alcohol.

Overdosage: After intravenous administration, but seldom after oral, hypotension may occur. Progressive widening of the QRS or AV conduction block may be seen as may increased ventricular extrasystoles or even ventricular tachycardia or fibrillation. Procainamide and n-acetyl procainamide are removed by haemodialysis but not by peritoneal dialysis. No specific antidote is known.

Overdosage should be managed by general supportive measures and close observation. Fluid expansion and the infusion of noradrenaline (8 micrograms/ml in Sodium Chloride Injection BP) may be useful for hypotension; insertion of a temporary ventricular pacing system may be beneficial.

Pharmaceutical precautions
Storage: At room temperature.

Legal category POM.

Package quantities Bottles of 100.

Further information Procainamide is less readily hydrolysed than procaine and plasma levels decline slowly – about 10–20% per hour. The drug is excreted primarily in the urine, about 10% as free and conjugated p-aminobenzoic acid and about 60% in the unchanged form. The remainder is mainly excreted as n-acetyl procainamide.

The formation of n-acetyl procainamide will depend upon the acetylator status of the patient. As this metabolite also has significant anti-arrhythmic activity and a somewhat slower renal clearance than procainamide, both acetylation rate capability and renal function will affect the duration of action.

Product licence number 0034/5066R

PRONESTYL* SOLUTION FOR INJECTION

Presentation
Solution for Injection: A sterile, aqueous solution containing 100 mg/ml procainamide hydrochloride. Other ingredients: Benzyl alcohol, sodium hydroxide, sodium metabisulphite, water.

Uses
Actions: Procainamide is a class I anti-arrhythmic agent (Vaughan Williams classification). Abnormal automaticity and excitability are reduced: the former by a slowing of the rate of diastolic phase 4 depolarisation; the latter by a reduction of the rate of rise of phase 0 depolarisation.

Action potention duration is prolonged but the effect on refractory period is greater.

These actions are apparent throughout the myocardium, and are most pronounced within the atria. Abnormal ectopic foci may be suppressed by the slowing of phase 4 depolarisation, while re-entrant tachyarrhythmias may be inhibited both by the reduced excitability of the myocardium and by the prolongation of the refractory period. In those arrhythmias not fully suppressed, procainamide is likely to slow the tachycardia.

The action of procainamide begins almost immediately after intravenous administration with maximal effects being observed at 30 minutes.

Indications: The treatment of symptomatic or potentially malignant ventricular arrhythmias (i.e. extrasystoles or tachycardia).

The treatment or prophylaxis of symptomatic or potentially malignant ventricular arrhythmias following acute myocardial infarction.

Dosage and administration
Children: Pronestyl is not recommended.

Adults: Intravenous therapy should be reserved for more serious tachyarrhythmias, in which case administration should be under continuous ECG monitoring. Once control is achieved oral Pronestyl can be substituted (see data sheet for Pronestyl Tablets).

Plasma concentrations correlate well with therapeutic and toxic effects; consequently plasma level assays should be carried out if facilities are available. The usual effective antiarrhythmic serum concentration is 4 to 8 mcg/ml. Toxic manifestations are rare in concentrations less than 12 mcg/ml.

Administration: To initiate therapy, the dose should be diluted in 5% Dextrose Injection BP immediately prior to administration to facilitate control of dosage rate; the dose should be given at a rate no greater than 50 mg per minute under ECG control, and blood pressure must be taken before each dose (see Precautions). Slow administration allows for some initial tissue distribution.

Acute control of tachyarrhythmia: 100 mg may be given every 5 minutes by slow injection, at a rate not exceeding 50 mg in any one minute, until the arrhythmia is suppressed or a maximum dosage of 1 gram has been administered.

Some effects may be seen after the first 100 or 200 mg and it is unusual to require more than 500 to 600 mg to achieve satisfactory antiarrhythmic effects.

Chronic suppression of arrhythmias: An alternative approach to achieving and then maintaining a therapeutic plasma concentration is to infuse 500 to 600 mg of procainamide at a constant rate over a period of 25 to 30 minutes and then change to another infusion for maintenance at a rate of 2 to 6 mg/min (see Table below).

Intravenous therapy should be terminated as soon as the patient's basic cardiac rhythm appears to be stabilized and, if indicated, the patient should be placed on oral antiarrhythmic maintenance therapy. A period of 3 to 4 hours (one half-life) should elapse after the last intravenous dose of procainamide before administering the first oral dose of procainamide.

Dilutions and rates for intravenous infusions†

Approximate final concentration	*Infusion bottle size (ml)*	*ml of Pronestyl (100 mg/ml) to be added*	*Infusion rate*
0.2% (2 mg/ml)	500	10	1–3
	250	5	ml/min
0.4% (4 mg/ml)	500	20	0.5–1.5
	250	10	ml/min

†*Caution:* The flow rate of all intravenous infusion solutions must be closely monitored. These dilutions are calculated to deliver 2–6 mg per minute at the infusion rates listed.

Elderly: Reduction in dose or increase in dosage interval may be necessary to maintain constant blood levels without accumulation (see above).

Contra-indications, warnings, etc

Contra-indications: Hypersensitivity to the drug is an absolute contra-indication. In this connection, cross sensitivity to procaine and related drugs must be borne in mind.

Procainamide should not be administered to patients with complete atrioventricular heart block or a high degree of A-V block or bifasicular block unless an electrical pacemaker is operative.

'Torsade de Pointes', a variant form of ventricular tachycardia associated with a prolonged QT interval, should not be treated with Pronestyl which may aggravate rather than suppress this arrhythmia.

Warnings and precautions: Myasthenia gravis: Patients with myasthenia gravis may show worsening of symptoms from procainamide due to its procaine-like effect on diminishing acetylcholine release at skeletal muscle motor nerve endings, so that procainamide administration may be hazardous without optimal adjustment of anticholinesterase medications and other precautions.

Digitalis intoxication: Procainamide may further depress conduction and ventricular asystole or fibrillation may result.

If the patient develops first degree heart block, dosage reduction and/or discontinuation of procainamide should be considered.

Caution in patients with congestive heart failure, acute ischaemic heart disease, cardiogenic shock or cardiomyopathy as even slight depression in myocardial contractility may reduce the cardiac output of the damaged heart.

Hypotension may occur when Pronestyl is administered intravenously. Patients should be kept in a supine position and blood pressure readings made frequently. If hypotension occurs the rate of injection should be reduced or temporarily discontinued and, if necessary, a vasopressor agent administered cautiously.

Intravenous administration should be monitored by ECG. Excessive widening of the QRS complex or prolongation of the P-R interval suggests the occurrence of myocardial toxicity and Pronestyl administration should be stopped. Cardiotoxicity may also be reflected by the appearance of proarrhythmic effects.

In patients with significant impairment of renal or hepatic function, accumulation of Pronestyl may occur, leading to drug toxicity.

The electrophysiological action of procainamide may be affected by electrolyte imbalance.

Pregnancy and nursing mothers: Safety has not been established: therefore, Pronestyl should be used during pregnancy only if the possible benefits outweigh the potential risks involved. Procainamide crosses the placenta but the extent is unknown. Procainamide is excreted in breast milk; therefore, it should not be given to nursing mothers because of the potential risk of adverse reactions in the infant.

Side-effects: A Lupus-like syndrome has been reported after prolonged courses of Pronestyl. The Lupus-like syndrome seldom appears in less than two months, but is very common after six months. It is virtually completely reversible and tests for antinuclear factors are usually positive before clinical signs appear. It is perhaps more often observed in patients who are slow acetylators. If long-term treatment is considered desirable, it is advisable to undertake serological tests at no less than monthly intervals and to continue treatment for no longer than absolutely necessary.

Agranulocytosis is a rare side effect of prolonged procainamide therapy. Susceptibility to this is greater in the period following coronary bypass surgery. The patient should be instructed to report any soreness of the mouth, throat, or gums, unexplained fever or any symptoms of upper respiratory tract infection. If any of these should occur, and leucocyte counts indicate cellular depression, Pronestyl therapy should be discontinued, and appropriate treatment should be instituted immediately.

Nausea, vomiting, diarrhoea, anorexia, bitter taste, mental depression, psychoses with hallucinations, dizziness, headache, pruritus, chills, fever, hepatitis and allergic reactions (such as vasculitis, eosinophilia, skin reactions or angioneurotic oedema) may occur infrequently. They are usually not sufficiently severe to discontinue treatment.

Neutropenia, thrombocytopenia or haemolytic anaemia may rarely be encountered.

As with all other class 1 agents, pro-arrhythmic effects may occur.

Pronestyl injection contains sodium metabisulphite. This ingredient has been associated with allergic reacations in sensitive individuals.

Drug interactions:

Other antiarrhythmic drugs: Additive effects can occur and dosage reduction may be necessary.

Antihypertensive agents: Procainamide may produce an additive effect and dosage adjustment may be necessary.

Anticholinergic drugs: Additive antivagal effects on A-V nodal conduction may occur.

Neuromuscular blocking agents: Possibly reduce dosage of Neuromuscular blocking drugs as procainamide may reduce acetylcholine release.

Captopril: There have been reports of neutropenia and/or Stevens Johnson syndrome in patients on procainamide plus captopril. Although a causal relationship has not been established, this combination should only be used with caution, especially in patients with impaired renal function.

Sulphonamides: p-amino benzoic acid is a metabolite of procainamide and can inhibit the action of sulphonamides.

Pharmacokinetic interactions: The elimination of procainamide may be decreased by cimetidine or propranolol, and increased by alcohol.

Overdosage: After intravenous administration, but seldom after oral, hypotension may occur. Progressive widening of the QRS or AV conduction block may be seen as may increased ventricular extrasystoles or even ventricular tachycardia or fibrillation. Procainamide and n-acetyl procainamide are removed by haemodialysis but not by peritoneal dialysis. No specific antidote is known.

Overdosage should be managed by general supportive measures and close observation. Fluid expansion and the infusion of noradrenaline (8 micrograms/ml in Sodium Chloride Injection BP) may be useful for hypotension; insertion of a temporary ventricular pacing system may be beneficial.

Pharmaceutical precautions
Storage: At room temperature.

Legal category POM.

Package quantities Solution 100 mg/ml: 10 ml multidose vials.

Further information Procainamide is less readily hydrolysed than procaine and plasma levels decline slowly – about 10–20% per hour. The drug is excreted primarily in the urine, about 10% as free and conjugated p-aminobenzoic acid and about 60% in the unchanged form. The remainder is mainly excreted as n-acetyl procainamide.

The formation of n-acetyl procainamide will depend upon the acetylator status of the patient. As this metabolite also has significant anti-arrhythmic activity and a somewhat slower renal clearance than procainamide, both acetylation rate capability and renal function will affect the duration of action.

Product licence number 0034/5065R

STARIL* TABLETS ▼

Presentation
Staril tablets 10 mg: White, flat end, diamond tablets each containing fosinopril sodium 10 mg. Engraved with Squibb and unilog number 158 on one face and a star design on the other.

Staril tablets 20 mg: White round biconvex tablets each containing fosinopril sodium 20 mg. Engraved with Squibb and unilog number 609 on one face and a star design on the other.

Other ingredients: Crospovidone, lactose, magnesium stearate, microcrystalline cellulose, povidone.

Uses
Indications: Staril is indicated in the treatment of hypertension where standard therapy is ineffective or inappropriate because of adverse effects. Staril may be used alone as initial therapy or in combination with other antihypertensive agents. The antihypertensive effects of Staril and diuretics used concomitantly are approximately additive.

Mode of action: Fosinopril, [(4*S*)-4-Cyclohexyl-1-[*RS*)-2-methyl-1-(propionyloxy) propoxy] (4-phenylbutyl) = phosphinoylacetyl]-L-proline; sodium salt, is the ester prodrug of an angiotensin converting enzyme (ACE) inhibitor, fosinoprilat, which maintains blood pressure control.

Pharmacokinetics: The absolute absorption of fosinopril averaged 36% of an oral dose, and was not affected by the presence of food. Rapid and complete hydrolysis to active fosinoprilat occurs in the gastrointestinal mucosa and liver.

The time to reach C max is independent of dose, achieved in approximately three hours and consistent with peak inhibition of the angiotensin I pressor response 3 to 6 hours following administration.

The effective $T\frac{1}{2}$ for accumulation of fosinoprilat averaged 11.5 hours. Fosinoprilat is highly protein bound (> 95%), has a relatively small volume of distribution and negligible binding to cellular components in blood. Unlike other ACE inhibitors, elimination of fosinopril is by both hepatic and renal routes allowing compensatory excretion by the alternative route in patients with renal or hepatic insufficiency.

Dosage and administration
Recommended dose and dosage schedule
Hypertensive patients not being treated with diuretics: The normal starting dose for patients is 10 mg once a day. The dose range is 10 to 40 mg per day administered in a single dose and without regard to meals. The usual maintenance dose is 20 mg once a day. No additional blood pressure lowering is achieved with doses greater than 40 mg daily. Dosage may need to be adjusted after approximately 4 weeks according to blood pressure response. If blood pressure is not adequately controlled with Staril alone, a diuretic can be added.

Use with concomitant diuretic therapy: The diuretic should preferably be discontinued for several days prior to beginning therapy with Staril to reduce the risk of an excessive hypertensive response. If blood pressure is inadequately controlled after an observation period of approximately 4 weeks, diuretic therapy may be resumed. Alternatively, if diuretic therapy cannot be discontinued, an initial dose of 10 mg of Staril should be used with careful medical supervision for several hours, until blood pressure has stabilised. In diuretic treated hypersensitive patients, mean cerebral blood flow is maintained between 4 and 24 hours after Staril, despite significant reduction in blood pressure.

Use in the elderly (over 65 years): No dosage reduction is necessary in patients with clinically normal renal and hepatic function as no significant differences in the phamacokinetic parameters or antihypertensive effect of fosinoprilat have been found compared with younger subjects.

Use in impaired renal function: It is advisable to initiate treatment at a dose of 10 mg. Depending on the response, the dose should then be titrated to achieve the desired therapeutic effect.

Absorption, bioavailability, protein binding, biotransformation and metabolism are not appreciably altered by reduced renal function. In patients with impaired renal function, the total body clearance of fosinoprilat is approximately 50% slower than that in patients with normal renal function. However, since hepatobiliary elimination compensates at least partially for diminished renal elimination, the body clearance of fosinoprilat is not appreciably different over a wide range of renal insufficiency (creatinine clearances ranging from < 10 to 80 ml/min, i.e. including end-stage renal failure).

Clearance of fosinoprilat by haemodialysis and peritoneal dialysis averages 2% and 7%, respectively, of urea clearances.

Uae in hepatic insufficiency (alcoholic or biliary cirrhosis): It is advisable to initiate treatment at a dose of 10 mg. Although the rate of hydrolysis may be slowed, the extent of hydrolysis is not appreciably reduced in patients with hepatic impairment. In this group of patients, there is evidence of reduced hepatic clearance of fosinoprilat with compensatory increase in renal excretion.

Use in children: The paediatric use of Staril has not been established.

Contra-indications, warnings, etc
Contra-indications: A history of hypersensitivity to Staril.

Pregnancy: Staril is contra-indicated in pregnancy. It has been shown to be lethal to rabbit foetuses at doses that were maternally toxic. Oligohydramnios and neonal hypotension and/or anuria have been reported following use of ACE inhibitors in the second and third trimester of pregnancy.

Nursing mothers: Staril should not be given to nursing mothers as fosinoprilat has been detected in human breast milk.

Precautions
Pretreatment assessment of renal function: Evaluation of the hypertensive patient should include assessement of renal function prior to initiation of therapy and during treatment where appropriate.

Warnings
Hypotension: Rarely, as with all ACE inhibitors, a hypotensive response may be observed. If this occurs it is usually associated with the first dose and in most instances, symptoms are relieved simply by the patient lying down. A transient hypotensive episode is not a contraindication to continuing therapy once the patient's blood pressure has been stabilised.

As with other ACE inhibitors, patients at risk of an excessive hypotensive response, sometimes associated with renal dysfunction, include those with: congestive heart failure, renovascular hypertension, renal dialysis, or volume and/or salt depletion of any aetiology. In patients with any one of these risk factors, it may be prudent to discontinue or reduce the dose of diuretic therapy or take other measures to ensure adequate hydration prior to initiating fosinopril treatment. Treatment of these high risk patients should be initiated under careful medical supervision and they should be followed closely, particularly if it becomes necessary to resume or increase the the dose of diuretic or Staril.

Impaired renal function: When treated with ACE inhibitors, patients with pre-existing congestive heart failure, renovascular hypertension (especially renal artery stenosis), and salt or volume depletion of any aetiolgy are at increased risk of developing findings indicative of renal dysfunction, including: increases in BUN and serum creatinine and potassium; proteinuria; changes in urine volume (including oliguria/anuria); and an abnormal urinalysis. Dosage reduction and/or discontinuation of diuretic and/or fosinopril may be required.

Hyperkalaemia: When treated with ACE inhibitors, patients at risk of developing hyperkalaemia include those with renal insufficiency, diabetes mellitus, and those using concomitant potassium-sparing diuretics, potassium supplements and/or potassium-containing salt substitutes.

Surgery/anaesthesia: ACE inhibitors may augment the hypotensive effects of anaesthetics and analgesics. If hypotension occurs in patients undergoing surgery/anaesthesia and concomitantly receiving ACE inhibitors, it can usually be corrected by intravenous administration of fluid.

Idiosyncratic: Angioedema involving the extremities, face, lips, mucous membranes, tongue, glottis or larynx has been seen in patients treated with other ACE inhibitors. If such symptoms occur during treatment with Staril, therapy should be discontinued.

Side-effects: In placebo controlled studies, there were no significant differences in clinical adverse experiences.

The most commonly reported side effects with Staril were dizziness, cough, upper respiratory symptoms, gastrointestinal disturbances, palpatations/chest pain, rash/pruritus, musculoskeletal pain/paraesthesia, fatigue and taste disturbance, Rarely, pancreatitis has been reported, but its relationship to the drug is uncertain.

The incidence and type of side effects did not differ between elderly and younger patients.

Laboratory test findings showed some modest, usually transient, decreases in haemoglobin and haematocrit values.

Overdosage: Blood pressure should be monitored and if hypotension develops, volume expansion is the treatment of choice. Fosinoprilat cannot be removed from the body by dialysis.

Drug interactions
Diuretics: As with all ACE inhibitors, an exaggerated hypotensive response may be expected when Staril is administered concomitantly with diuretics.

Since increases in serum potassium have been observed with ACE inhibitors, including fosinopril, the potassium wasting effect of most diuretics may be blunted by concomitant ACE inhibitor therapy.

Decreases in serum sodium and increases in serum creatinine occurred more frequently in patients receiving concomitant diuretics than in those treated with fosinopril alone. Concomitant administration with potassium sparing diuretics may lead to hyperkalaemia.

Antacids: Coadministration of antacids with Staril has been shown to reduce serum levels and urinary excretion of fosinoprilat as compared with Staril administered alone, suggesting that antacids may impair absorption of fosinopril.

NSAIs: NSAI drugs may interefere with the anti-hypertensive effect. However, concomitant administration of a single dose of 325 mg aspirin did not result in a clinically significant reduction in anti-hypertensive effect.

Lithium: Concomitant therapy with lithium may increase the serum lithium concentration.

Other anti-hypersensitive agents: Combination with other anti-hypertensive agents such as beta blockers, methyldopa, calcium antagonists, and diuretics may increase the anti-hypertensive efficacy.

Other drugs: In pharmacokinetic studies with nifedipine, propranolol, cimetidine, metoclopramide and propantheline the bioavailability of fosinoprilat was not altered by coadministration of Staril with any one of these drugs.

Pharmaceutical precautions Store below 30°C in a dry place.

Legal category POM.

Package quantities Bottles of 28.

Product licence numbers

10 mg	0034/0293
20 mg	0034/0294

TRI-ADCORTYL* CREAM, OINTMENT AND OTIC OINTMENT

Presentation Cream, Ointment and Otic Ointment. Containing in each gram the following:

Triamcinolone acetonide	0.1%
Neomycin (as sulphate)	0.25%
Gramicidin	0.025%
Nystatin	100,000 units

Cream: Pale buff. Other ingredients: Aluminium hydroxide, antifoam emulsion, benzyl alcohol, ethyl alcohol, ethylene diamine, hydrochloric acid, macrogol ether, perfume, polysorbate 60, propylene glycol, sorbitol, titanium dioxide, white soft paraffin.

Ointment: Yellow to amber in Plastibase* (liquid paraffin, polyethylene resin).

Otic Ointment: Presentation for aural use in Plastibase* (liquid paraffin, polyethylene resin).

Uses *Actions:* Triamcinolone acetonide is a potent fluorinated corticosteroid with rapid anti-inflammatory, antipruritic and anti-allergic actions.

The combined action of the antibiotics neomycin and gramicidin provides comprehensive antibacterial therapy against a wide range of Gram-positive and Gram-negative bacteria, including those micro-organisms responsible for most bacterial skin infections.

Nystatin is an antifungal antibiotic, active against a wide range of yeasts and yeast-like fungi, including *Candida albicans.*

Indications: The topical treatment of superficial bacterial infections, cutaneous candidosis and dermatological conditions known to respond to topical steroid therapy when threatened or complicated by bacterial or candidal superinfections. These include: atopic eczema, contact eczema, follicular eczema, infantile eczema, otitis externa, anogenital pruritus (pruritus ani et vulvae), nummular eczema, post-traumatic infective eczema, seborrhoeic or flexural eczema, neurodermatitis, psoriasis.

Dosage and administration *Adults and children: Cream, ointment:* Apply to the affected areas two to four times daily.

Otic Ointment: After cleaning, apply the nozzle to the aural canal and squeeze a small amount into the canal two to four times daily.

Elderly: Natural thinning of the skin occurs in the elderly; hence corticosteroids should be used sparingly and for short periods of time.

Contra-indications, warnings, etc
Contra-indications: In tuberculous and most viral lesions of the skin, particularly herpes simplex, vaccinia and varicella. Also in fungal lesions not susceptible to nystatin.

In patients with hypersensitivity to any of the components.

Should not be applied to the external auditory canal in patients with perforated eardrums.

Precautions: Adrenal suppression can occur, even without occlusion. The use of occlusive dressings should be avoided because of the increased risk of sensitivity reactions and increased percutaneous absorption. The possibility of sensitivity to neomycin should be taken into consideration especially in the treatment of patients suffering from leg ulcers.

Pregnancy: Topical administration of corticosteroids to pregnant animals can cause abnormalities of foetal development. The relevance of this finding to humans has not been established. However, topical steroids should not be used extensively in pregnancy, i.e. in large amounts or for long periods. Topical corticosteroids should be used during pregnancy only if the potential benefit justifies the potential risk to the foetus.

Children: In infants, long-term continuous topical steroid therapy should be avoided.

Otic ointment: Care is necessary in applying this preparation if perforation of the eardrum is suspected.

Not for ophthalmic use.

Side-effects: Triamcinolone acetonide is well tolerated. Where adverse reactions occur they are usually reversible on cessation of therapy. However the following side-effects have been reported usually with prolonged usage:

Dermatologic – impaired wound healing, thinning of the skin, petechiae and ecchymoses, facial erythema and telangiectasia, increased sweating, purpura, striae, hirsutism, acneiform eruptions, lupus erythematosus-like lesions and suppressed reactions to skin tests.

These effects may be enhanced with occlusive dressings.

Signs of systemic toxicity such as oedema and electrolyte imbalance have not been observed even when high topical dosage has been used. The possibility of the systemic effects which are associated with all steroid therapy should be considered.

Neomycin: Sensitivity reactions may occur especially with prolonged use. Ototoxicity and nephrotoxicity have been reported. Large amounts of this product should be avoided in the treatment of skin infections following extensive burns, trophic ulceration and other conditions where absorption of neomycin is possible.

Gramicidin: Sensitivity has occasionally been reported.

Nystatin: There have been no substantiated reports of sensitivity associated with topical nystatin.

Overdosage: Topically applied corticosteroids can be absorbed in sufficient amounts to produce systemic effects (see Side-effects).

Pharmaceutical precautions *Storage: Cream:* At room temperature; avoid freezing.

Ointment: At room temperature.

Dilution: Not recommended, as this would reduce the concentration of the antibiotics to below therapeutic levels.

Legal category POM.

Package quantities Tubes of and 30 g (OP).
Otic Ointment: Tubes of 10 g (OP).

Further information Tri-Adcortyl Ointment is preservative-free, and avoids the risk of allergic reactions to preservatives.

Product licence numbers

Tri-Adcortyl Cream	0034/5093R
Tri-Adcortyl Ointment	0034/5094R
Tri-Adcortyl Otic Ointment	0034/5095R

VELOSEF* CAPSULES
VELOSEF* SYRUP

Presentation
Capsules 250 mg: Opaque, orange body with opaque blue cap printed Squibb and 113 in white on each half. Each capsule contains 250 mg cephradine. Other ingredients: Erythrosine, gelatin capsules, indigo carmine, iron oxide, lactose, magnesium stearate, titanium dioxide.

Capsules 500 mg: Opaque blue printed in white with Squibb and 114 on each half. Each capsule contains 500 mg cephradine. Other ingredients: Gelatin capsules, indigo carmine, lactose, magnesium stearate, titanium dioxide.

Syrup 250 mg: When reconstituted contains 250 mg cephradine per 5 ml. Other ingredients: Citric acid, flavours, guar gum, methylcellulose, sodium citrate, sucrose.

Uses *Actions:* Cephradine is a broad-spectrum, bactericidal antibiotic active against both Gram-positive and Gram-negative bacteria. It is also highly active against most strains of penicillinase-producing *Staphylococci.*

Microbiology: The following organisms have shown *in vitro* sensitivity to cephradine:

Gram-positive – *Staphylococci* (both penicillin sensitive and resistant strains), *Streptococci*, both *Streptococcus pyogenes* (beta haemolytic) and Group D *Streptococci* (enterococci) and *Streptococcus pneumoniae.*

Gram-negative – *E. coli, Klebsiella, P. mirabilis, Haemophilus influenzae, Shigella* spp., *Salmonella* spp. (including *Salmonella typhi*) and *Neisseria* spp.

Enterococci (S. faecalis) may be susceptible to the high levels of cephradine achieved in the urine.

Because cephradine is unaffected by penicillinase, many strains of *E. coli* and *Staphylococcus aureus* which produce this enzyme are susceptible to cephradine but resistant to ampicillin.

Indications: In the treatment of infections of the urinary, respiratory and gastro-intestinal tracts and of the skin and soft tissues. These include:

Upper respiratory infections – pharyngitis, sinusitis, otitis media, tonsilitis, laryngo-tracheo bronchitis.

Lower respiratory infections – acute and chronic bronchitis, lobar and bronchopneumonia.

Urinary tract infections – cystitis, urethritis, pyelonephritis.

Skin and soft tissue infections – abscess, cellulitis, furunculosis, impetigo.

Gastro-intestinal tract – bacillary dysentery, enteritis, peritonitis.

Velosef has been shown to be effective in reducing the incidence of postoperative infections in patients undergoing surgical procedures associated with a high risk of infection. It is also of value where postoperative infections would be disastrous and where patients have a reduced host resistance to bacterial infection. Protection is best ensured by achieving adequate local tissue concentrations at the time contamination is likely to occur. Thus, Velosef should be administered immediately prior to surgery and continued during the postoperative period.

Bacteriology studies to determine the causative organisms and their sensitivity to cephradine should be performed. Therapy may be instituted prior to receiving the results of the sensitivity test.

Dosage and administration Velosef may be given without regard to meals.

Adults: For urinary tract infections the usual dose is 500 mg four times daily or 1 g twice daily; severe or chronic infections may require larger doses. Prolonged intensive therapy is needed for complications such as prostatitis and epididymitis. For respiratory tract infections and skin and soft tissue infections the usual dose is 250 mg or 500 mg four times daily or 500 mg or 1 g twice daily depending on the severity and site of infections. For gastro-intestinal tract infections, 500 mg three or four times daily may be employed.

Children: The usual dose is from 25 to 50 mg/kg/day total, given in two or four equally divided doses.

For otitis media daily doses from 75 to 100 mg/kg in divided doses every 6 to 12 hours are recommended. Maximum dose 4 g per day.

Elderly: There are no specific dosage recommendations or precautions for use in the elderly except, as with other drugs, to monitor those patients with impaired renal or hepatic function.

All patients, irrespective of age and weight: Larger doses (up to 1 g four times daily) may be given for severe or chronic infections. Therapy should be continued for a minimum of 48-72 hours after the patient becomes asymptomatic or evidence of bacterial eradication has been obtained. In infections caused by haemolytic strains of streptococci, a minimum of 10 days treatment is recommended to guard against the risk of rheumatic fever or glomerulonephritis. In the treatment of chronic urinary tract infections, frequent bacteriological and clinical appraisal is necessary during therapy and may be necessary for several months afterwards. Persistent infections may require treatment for several weeks. Smaller doses than those indicated above should not be used. Doses for children should not exceed doses recommended for adults. As Velosef is available in both injectable and oral form, patients may be changed from the Velosef injectable to the Velosef oral at the same dosage level.

Renal impairment dosage: A modified dosage schedule in patients with decreased renal function is necessary. Each patient should be considered individually; the following reduced dosage schedule is recommended as a guideline, based on the creatinine clearance (ml/min/1.73 m^2). In adults, the initial loading dose is 750 mg of Velosef and the maintenance dose is 500 mg at the time intervals listed below:

Creatinine clearance	*Time interval*
more than 20 ml/min	6–12 hours
15–19 ml/min	12–24 hours
10–14 ml/min	24–40 hours
5–9 ml/min	40–50 hours
less than 5 ml/min	50–70 hours

Further modification of the dosage schedule may be necessary in children.

Contra-indications, warnings, etc

Contra-indications: Patients with known hypersensitivity to the cephalosporin antibiotics.

Precautions: There is evidence of partial cross-allergenicity between the penicillins and the cephalosporins. Therefore cephradine should be used with caution in those patients with known hypersensitivity to penicillins.

After treatment with Velosef, a false positive reaction for glucose in the urine may occur with Benedict's or Fehling's solution or with reagent tablets such as Clinitest*, but not with enzyme-based tests such as Clinistix* or Diastix*.

As with all antibiotics, prolonged use may result in overgrowth of non-susceptible organisms.

Administration in renal failure: A modified dosage schedule in patients with decreased renal function is necessary (see Dosage).

Pregnancy and breast feeding: Although animal studies have not demonstrated any teratogenicity, safety in pregnancy has not been established. Cephradine is excreted in breast milk and should be used with caution in lactating mothers.

Side-effects: Limited essentially to gastro-intestinal disturbances and on occasion to hypersensitivity phenomena. The latter are more likely to occur in individuals who have previously demonstrated hypersensitivity and those with a history of allergy, asthma, hay fever or urticaria. The majority of reported side-effects have been mild. Skin reactions have occasionally been reported.

Adverse reaction reports are rare, but include glossitis, heartburn, dizziness, tightness in the chest, nausea, vomiting, diarrhoea, abdominal pain, vaginitis, candidal overgrowth. Skin and hypersensitivity reactions include urticaria, skin rashes, joint pains, oedema.

As with other cephalosporins, mild transient eosinophilia, leucopenia and neutropenia, positive direct Coombs tests and pseudomembraneous colitis have been reported.

Clinical chemistry: Isolated instances of elevated SGOT, SGPT, total bilirubin and alkaline phosphatase have been observed; in most patients, the values were only mildly elevated and tended to return to normal at the end of therapy. No consistent pattern was observed that would suggest hepatocellular damage.

Mild elevations of BUN have been reported. In most cases, however, the values tended to return to normal. In adults for whom serum creatinine determinations were performed, the rise in BUN was not accompanied by a rise in serum creatinine, which would suggest an extrarenal mechanism for the elevation of BUN.

Pharmaceutical precautions *Storage: Capsules:* In a cool place.

Powder for syrup: A cool place. After reconstitution; discard unused syrup after 14 days if stored in refrigerator, or seven days at room temperature.

Dilution: Velosef Syrup may be diluted with Syrup BP. The diluted syrup should be used within seven days.

Legal category POM.

Package quantities *Capsules:* Boxes of 20 in blisters (OP) and bottles of 100.
Syrup: Bottles of 100 ml.

Further information Cephradine has a high degree of stability to many beta-lactamases. It has a low degree of protein-binding and a large volume of distribution. Therefore, tissue levels are generally found to be high. Oral cephradine can be given twice or four times daily, and is well absorbed.

Human pharmacology: Cephradine is acid stable and is rapidly absorbed following oral administration in the fasting state. Following doses of 250 mg, 500 mg and 1000 mg average peak serum levels of approximately 9, 16.5, and 24.2 micrograms/ml, respectively, were obtained at one hour. The presence of food in the gastrointestinal tract delays the absorption but does not affect the total amount of cephradine absorbed. Measurable serum levels are present six hours after administration. Over 90% of the drug is excreted unchanged in the urine within 6 hours. Peak urine concentrations are approximately 1600 micrograms/ml following a 250 mg dose, 3200 micrograms/ml following a 500 mg dose, and 4000 micrograms/ml following a 1000 mg dose. After 48 hours' administration of 100 mg/kg/day of cephradine for the treatment of otitis media, cephradine has been measured in the middle ear exudate at an average level of 3.6 microgram/ml.

Product licence numbers

Velosef Capsules 250 mg	0034/0133R
Velosef Capsules 500 mg	0034/0134R
Velosef Syrup 250 mg/5 ml	0034/0136R

VELOSEF* FOR INJECTION

Presentation Velosef for Injection is a sterile powder blend of cephradine and L-arginine. After reconstitution, Velosef for Injection 500 mg and 1.0 g vials provide 500 mg and 1.0 g of cephradine activity, respectively.

Uses *Actions:* Cephradine is a broad-spectrum bactericidal antibiotic active against both Gram-positive and Gram-negative bacteria. It is also highly active against most strains of penicillinase-producing staphylococci.

Microbiology: The following organisms have shown *in vitro* sensitivity to cephradine:

Gram-positive – *Staphylococci* (both penicillin sensitive and resistant strains), *Streptococci*, both *Streptococcus pyogenes* (beta haemolytic) and Group D *Streptococci* (enterococci) and *Streptococcus pneumoniae.*

Gram-negative – *E. coli, Klebsiella, P. mirabilis, Haemophilus influenzae, Shigella* spp., *Salmonella* spp. (including *Salmonella typhi*) and *Neisseria* spp.

Enterococci (*S. faecalis*) may be susceptible to the high levels of cephradine achieved in the urine.

Because cephradine is unaffected by penicillinase, many strains of *E. coli* and *Staphylococcus aureus* which produce this enzyme are susceptible to cephradine but resistant to ampicillin.

Indications: The treatment of infections of the urinary, respiratory and gastro-intestinal tracts and of the skin and soft tissues, bones and joints; also septicaemia and endocarditis. These include:

Upper respiratory infections – pharyngitis, sinusitis, otitis media, tonsillitis, laryngo-tracheo-bronchitis.

Lower respiratory infections – acute and chronic bronchitis, lobar and bronchopneumonia.

Urinary tract infections – cystitis, urethritis, pyelonephritis.

Skin and soft tissue infections – abscess, cellulitis, furunculosis, impetigo.

Gastro-intestinal tract – bacillary dysentery, enteritis, peritonitis.

Velosef has been shown to be effective in reducing the incidence of postoperative infections in patients undergoing surgical procedures associated with a high risk of infection. It is also of value where post-operative infection would be disastrous and where patients have a reduced host resistance to bacterial infection. Protection is best ensured by achieving adequate local tissue concentrations at the time contamination is likely to occur. Thus, Velosef should be administered immediately prior to surgery and continued during the postoperative period.

Bacteriological studies to determine the causative organisms and their sensitivity to cephradine should be performed. Therapy may be instituted prior to receiving the results of the sensitivity test.

Sterile Velosef for injection is indicated primarily for those patients unable to tolerate oral medication. It is also indicated for intravenous use either by direct injection or by intravenous infusion for the treatment of serious and life-threatening infections.

Dosage and administration Intramuscular or intravenous injection and intravenous infusion.

Adults: Treatment: The usual dose range of Velosef for injection is 2-4 g daily in four equally divided doses. This may be increased up to 8 g a day for severe infections, e.g. septicaemia and endocarditis. For the majority of infections, the usual dose is 500 mg q.i.d. in equally spaced doses; severe or chronic infections may require larger doses. Prolonged intensive therapy is needed for complications such as prostatitis and epididymitis. Patients who are severely ill and who require high serum levels of cephradine for treating their infections should be started on intravenous therapy.

Limited experience indicates that intraperitoneal administration of Velosef may be effective after surgery in cases of peritonitis where a surgical drainage system has been established.

Prophylaxis: The recommended dose for surgical prophylaxis is a single, pre-operative 1–2 g IM or IV dose. Subsequent parenteral or oral doses can be administered as appropriate.

Children: The usual dose is 50-100 mg/kg/day total given in four equally divided doses. More serious illnesses (e.g. typhoid fever) may require 200-300 mg/kg/day.

Elderly: There are no specific dosage recommendations or precautions for use in the elderly except, as with other drugs, to monitor those patients with impaired renal or hepatic function.

All patients, regardless of age and weight: Therapy should be continued for a minimum of 48-72 hours after the patient becomes asymptomatic or evidence of bacterial eradication has been obtained. In infections caused by haemolytic strains of streptococci, a minimum of 10 days of treatment is recommended to guard against the risk of rheumatic fever or glomerulonephritis. In the treatment of chronic urinary tract infections, frequent bacteriological and clinical appraisal is necessary during therapy and may be necessary for several months afterwards. Persistent infections may require treatment for several weeks. Smaller doses than those indicated above should not be used. Doses for children should not exceed doses recommended for adults. As Velosef is available in both injectable and oral form, patients may be changed from Velosef injectable to Velosef oral at the same dosage level.

Renal impairment dosage: A modified dosage schedule in patients with decreased renal function is necessary. Each patient should be considered individually; the following reduced dosage schedule is recommended as a guideline, based on the creatinine clearance (ml/min/1.73 m^2). In adults, the initial loading dose is 750 mg of Velosef and the maintenance dose is 500 mg at the time intervals listed below:

Creatinine clearance	*Time interval*
more than 20 ml/min	6–12 hours
15–19 ml/min	12–24 hours
10–14 ml/min	24–40 hours
5–9 ml/min	40–50 hours
less than 5 ml/min	50–70 hours

Further modification of the dosage schedule may be necessary in children.

Reconstitution: For intramuscular use: Aseptically add sterile water for injection or 0.9% sodium chloride injection according to the following table:

Single dose vial size*	*Volume of diluent to be added*
500 mg	2.0 ml
1 g	4.0 ml

* Preparation contains no bactericide and is not intended for multiple dose use.

Shake to effect solution and withdraw the entire contents. Intramuscular solutions should be used within 2 hours at room temperature; when stored in a refrigerator at 5°C, solutions retain full potency for 12 hours. Reconstituted solutions may vary in colour from light to straw yellow; however, this does not affect the potency.

For intravenous use: Velosef for injection may be administered by direct intravenous injection or by infusion. A 3 microgram/ml serum concentration can be maintained for each milligram of cephradine per kg body weight per hour of infusion.

For direct intravenous administration: Suitable intravenous injection solutions are Sterile Water for Injection, 5% Glucose Injection or 0.9% Sodium Chloride Injection.

Aseptically add 5 ml of diluent to the 500 mg vial or 10 ml to the 1 g vial. Shake to effect solution and withdraw the entire contents. The solution may be slowly injected directly into a vein over a 3 to 5 minute period. The solution should be used within 2 hours when kept at room temperature; if stored at 5°C, solutions retain full potency for 12 hours.

For continuous or intermittent intravenous infusion: Suitable intravenous infusion solutions are Sterile Water for Injection (50 mg/ml cephradine solutions are approximately isotonic); 5% or 10% Glucose Injection; 0.9% Sodium Chloride Injection; Sodium Lactate Injection (M/6 sodium lactate); Glucose and Sodium Chloride Injection; Lactated Ringer's Injection; Ringer's Injection; 5% Glucose in Lactated Ringer's Injection; 5% Glucose in Ringer's Injection.

Aseptically add 10 ml of the diluent to the 1 g vial and shake to effect solution. Aseptically transfer the entire contents to the IV infusion diluent. Intravenous infusions prepared remain potent for 24 hours at room temperature or 1 week at 5°C at concentrations up to 10 mg/ml (1%), and for 10 hours at room temperature or 48 hours at 5°C at concentrations up to 50 mg/ml (5%). For prolonged infusion, replace 5% infusions every 10 hours and 1% infusions every 24 hours with freshly-prepared solutions.

N.B. Only cephradine solubilised with arginine may be reconstituted with solutions containing calcium salts, such as Ringer's Solutions.

For further information on compatibilities consult the manufacturer.

Protect solutions of cephradine from concentrated light or direct sunlight.

Contra-indications, warnings, etc
Contra-indications: Patients with known hypersensitivity to the cephalosporin antibiotics.

Precautions: There is evidence of partial cross-allergenicity between the penicillins and the cephalosporins. Therefore Velosef should be used with caution in those patients with known hypersensitivity to penicillins.

After treatment with Velosef a false positive reaction for glucose in the urine may occur with Benedict's solution or Fehling's solution or with reagent tablets such as Clinitest*, but not with enzyme-based tests such as Clinistix* or Diastix*.

As with all antibiotics, prolonged use may result in overgrowth of non-susceptible organisms.

Administration in renal impairment: A modified dosage schedule in patients with decreased renal function is necessary (see Dosage).

Pregnancy and breast feeding: Although animal studies have not demonstrated any teratogenicity, safety in pregnancy has not been established. Cephradine is excreted in breast milk and should be used with caution in lactating mothers.

Side-effects: Limited essentially to gastro-intestinal disturbances and on occasion to hypersensitivity phenomena. The latter are more likely to occur in individual's who have previously demonstrated hypersensitivity and those with a history of allergy, asthma, hay fever or urticaria. The majority of reported side-effects have been mild. Skin reactions have occasionally been reported.

Adverse reaction reports are rare, but include glossitis, heartburn, headache, dizziness, dyspnoea, paraesthesia, nausea, vomiting, diarrhoea, abdominal pain, candidal overgrowth, vaginitis. Skin and hypersensitivity reactions include urticaria, skin rashes, joint pains, oedema.

As with other cephalosporins, mild transient eosinophilia, leucopenia and neutropenia, rarely positive direct Coombs tests and pseudomembranous colitis have been reported.

Clinical chemistry: Isolated instances of elevated SGOT, SGPT, total bilirubin and alkaline phosphatase have been observed; in most patients, the values were only mildly elevated and tended to return to normal at the end of therapy. No consistent pattern was observed that would suggest hepatocellular damage.

Mild elevations of BUN have been reported. In most cases, however, the values tended to return to normal. In adults for whom serum creatinine determinations were performed, the rise in BUN was not accompanied by a rise in serum creatinine, which would suggest an extrarenal mechanism for the elevation of BUN.

Injection: As with other parenterally administered antibiotics, transient pain may be experienced at the injection site, but is seldom the cause for discontinuing treatment. Thrombophlebitis has been reported following intravenous injection.

Since sterile abscesses have been reported following accidental subcutaneous injection, the preparation should be administered by deep intramuscular injection.

Pharmaceutical precautions *Storage (before reconstitution):* At room temperature. Not for multidose use.

Legal category POM.

Package quantities *500 mg single-dose vials:* Pack of 5.

1 g single-dose vials: Single-vial pack.

Further information Cephradine has a high degree of stability to beta-lactamases. It has a low degree of protein binding and a large volume of distribution. Therefore, tissue levels are generally found to be high.

Human pharmacology: Following intramuscular administration of a single 0.5 g dose of cephradine to normal volunteers, the average peak serum concentration was 8.41 microgram/ml with the time to peak concentration being 0.93 hours. The serum half-life averaged 1.25 hours. A single 1 g intravenous dose resulted in serum concentrations of 86 microgram/ml at 5 minutes and 12 microgram/ml at 1 hour; these concentrations declined to 1 microgram/ml at 4 hours. Continuous infusion of 500 mg per hour into a 70 kg man maintained a concentration of about 21.4 microgram/ml cephradine activity; this study showed that a serum concentration of approximately 3 microgram/ml can be obtained for each milligram of cephradine administered per kg of body weight per hour of infusion.

Cephradine is excreted unchanged in the urine. The kidneys excrete 57% to 80% of an intramuscular dose in the first six hours; this results in a high urine concentration, e.g. 880 microgram/ml of urine after a 500 mg intramuscular dose. Probenecid slows tubular secretion and almost doubles peak serum concentration.

Assays of bone obtained at surgery have shown that cephradine penetrates bone tissue.

Product licence numbers

Velosef Injection 500 mg	0034/0198R
Velosef Injection 1 g	0034/0199R

**Trade Mark*

Stafford-Miller Limited
45 Broadwater Road
Welwyn Garden City
Herts AL7 3SP

ALPHOSYL* LOTION AND CREAM

Presentation The lotion is a light free-flowing emulsion and the cream is smooth and homogeneous. Both are light tan in colour and contain:

Alcoholic extract of coal tar	5%
Allantoin	2%

Uses The treatment of psoriasis and psoriasis of the scalp.

Alphosyl Lotion is the basic treatment for widespread psoriasis of the body and scalp.

Alphosyl Cream is for the treatment of psoriasis and its moisturising capability makes it particularly useful on flexures.

Dosage and administration
Lotion and Cream: Apply liberally two to four times daily. Rub vigorously into the affected areas. Alphosyls do not stain, and can be applied freely, even to the scalp. Where hard scales exist, apply after a hot bath. Optimum results may take several weeks of daily application. After the lesions have been brought under control continue use to prevent recurrence.

Contra-indications, warnings, etc Alphosyl Lotion and Cream are contra-indicated in patients with acute psoriasis, and those with a known sensitivity to coal tar. Skin irritation, acne-like eruptions or photosensitivity may occur in patients who are sensitive to coal tar. These undesirable effects resolve when treatment is stopped.

Use in pregnancy and lactation: Safety in pregnancy and lactation has not been established, and hence, use in the first trimester of pregnancy is best avoided.

Warnings: For external use only. Discontinue if irritation occurs or in cases of sensitivity to coal tar.

Pharmaceutical precautions Store at room temperature. Do not refrigerate.

Legal category P.

Package quantities
Alphosyl Lotion: Bottles of 250 ml.
Alphosyl Cream: Tube of 100 g.

Further information Nil.

Product licence numbers

Alphosyl Lotion	0036/5008R
Alphosyl Cream	0036/5006R

ALPHOSYL* HC CREAM

Presentation A cream containing refined alcoholic extract of coal tar 5%, allantoin 2% and hydrocortisone PhEur 0.5% in a greaseless aqueous cream base. The cream is smooth, homogeneous, and light tan in colour.

Uses The treatment of psoriasis. The anti-inflammatory action of the hydrocortisone in Alphosyl HC Cream enhances the basic Alphosyl action.

Dosage and administration
Adults, including elderly: Apply cream sparingly twice daily to psoriatic plaques. Rub in well. Not recommended for children under 5 years.

Contra-indications, warnings, etc
Contra-indications: Tuberculosis or fungal lesions of the skin, herpes simplex, vaccinia or varicella, and a history of hypersensitivity to any of the ingredients.

Other undesirable effects: Hypersensitivity reactions may occasionally occur. See special warnings below.

Use in pregnancy and lactation: Topical administration of corticosteroids to pregnant animals can cause abnormality of foetal development. Topical steroids should not be used extensively in pregnancy, i.e., in large amounts or for long periods because of the risk of teratogenic effects or significant absorption causing suppression of the HPA axis.

Other special warnings and precautions: For external use only. Avoid contact with the eyes. Use sparingly. Discontinue use if sensitivity occurs.

The following results of steroid use are uncommon at this dosage, however:

— When used over large areas or for prolonged periods systemic side effects can result.
— Under occlusive dressings or in intertriginous areas, topical steroids may cause skin atrophy manifesting as striae, thinning and telangiectasia.
— Viral, bacterial or fungal infection of the skin may be substantially exacerbated by topical steroid treatment unless accompanied by appropriate therapy.
— Wound healing can be significantly retarded.

Pharmaceutical precautions Store at room temperature. Do not refrigerate.

Legal category POM.

Package quantities Tubes of 30 g and 100 g.

Further information Nil.

Product licence number 0036/0026R.

ALPHOSYL* SHAMPOO

Presentation Alphosyl Shampoo is a pale green lotion shampoo with a herbal fragrance containing:

Alcoholic extract of coal tar	5%
Allantoin	0.2%

Uses Alphosyl Shampoo is indicated for the treatment of scalp disorders such as, psoriasis, seborrheic dermatitis and scaling and itching (often associated with eczema).

Dosage and administration Wet hair thoroughly then briskly rub a liberal amount of shampoo into the hair and scalp. Rinse thoroughly and repeat the procedure massaging the scalp for several minutes and working the shampoo into a rich lather. Rinse thoroughly.

Dandruff: Once or twice weekly as necessary, or as directed by the physician.

Psoriasis, seborrheic dermatitis, scaling and itching: Use every two or three days, or as directed by the physician.

Contra-indications, warnings, etc Discontinue if irritation develops. Avoid contact with eyes. If necessary rinse with warm water.

Legal category GSL.

Package quantities Bottles of 125 ml and 250 ml.

Further information Alphosyl Shampoo is also of value in the removal of ointments and pastes used in the treatment of psoriasis of the scalp. It is prescribable on

FP10 for psoriasis, seborrheic dermatitis and scaling and itching of the scalp.

Product licence number 0036/0019.

COLIFOAM*

Presentation An aerosol can releasing a white odourless foam containing hydrocortisone acetate PhEur 10%.

Uses Anti-inflammatory corticosteroid therapy for the topical treatment of ulcerative colitis, proctosigmoiditis and granular proctitis.

Dosage and administration One applicatorful inserted into the rectum once or twice daily for two or three weeks and every second day thereafter. Shake can vigorously before use (illustrated instructions are enclosed in each pack).

Contra-indications, warnings, etc
Contra-indications: Local contra-indications to the use of intrarectal steroids include obstruction, abscess, perforation, peritonitis, fresh intestinal anastomoses and extensive fistulae and tuberculous, fungal or viral infections.

Pregnancy: Systemic and topical administration of corticosteroids to pregnant animals can cause abnormalities of foetal development. The relevance of this finding to human beings has not been established, but at present steroids should not be used extensively in pregnancy, that is in large amounts or for prolonged periods.

Warnings: General precautions common to all corticosteroid therapy should be observed during treatment with Colifoam especially in the case of young children. Treatment should be administered with caution in patients with severe ulcerative disease because of their predisposition to perforation of the bowel wall.

For external use only.

Pharmaceutical precautions Pressurized container. Protect from sunlight and do not expose to temperatures above 50°C. Do not pierce or burn even after use.

Do not refrigerate. Shake vigorously before use.

Legal category POM.

Package quantities Aerosol canister containing 25 g (approx. 14 applications) plus a plastic applicator and illustrated leaflet.

Further information One applicatorful of Colifoam provides a dose of approximately 125 mg of hydrocortisone acetate.

Product licence number 0036/0021.

EPIFOAM*

Presentation An aerosol can releasing a muco-adherent, white, odourless aerosol foam containing:

Hydrocortisone acetate PhEur	1%
Pramoxine hydrochloride USP	1%

Uses For the topical treatment of perineal trauma including post-episiotomy pain and discomfort.

Dosage and administration A suitable quantity of foam should be dispensed onto a pad, preferably sterile, and applied to the site or affected areas 3–4 times daily.

If an absorbent pad is used, a piece of porous but non-absorbent material should be placed between the foam and the pad in order to maximise contact of the foam with the wound.

Contra-indications, warnings, etc
Contra-indications: Do not use on infected lesions unless accompanied by appropriate anti-infective agents.

Pregnancy: Systemic and topical administration of corticosteroids to pregnant animals can cause abnormalities of foetal development. The relevance of this finding to human beings has not been established, but at present steroids should not be used extensively in pregnancy, that is in large amounts or for prolonged periods.

No consequences are expected to result from the use of Epifoam in lactation.

Pharmaceutical precautions Pressurised container. Protect from sunlight and do not expose to temperatures above 50°C. Do not pierce or burn even after use.

Do not refrigerate. Shake vigorously before use. Use at room temperature.

Legal category POM.

Package quantities Aerosol canister containing 12 g of foam.

Further information An illustrated instruction leaflet is enclosed with each pack.

Product licence number 0036/0043.

OTOMIZE* EAR SPRAY

Presentation A non-pressurised pump action aerosol spray containing Dexamethasone PhEur 0.1%, and Neomycin Sulphate PhEur 3250 IU/ml as a mobile milky aqueous suspension.

Uses Otomize is indicated for the treatment of otitis externa.

The product provides a rapid and convenient means of treatment. It is also easy to administer because of its unique spray form.

Dosage and administration
Adults, children and the elderly: One metered dose (60 mg) to be administered directly into each affected ear three times daily.

Treatment should be continued until two days after symptoms have disappeared.

Discontinue treatment if there is no clinical improvement after 7 days.

Contra-indications, warnings, etc
Contra-indications: The product should not be used in patients with a known sensitivity to neomycin. Treatment should be discontinued if sensitivity develops during use. Neomycin is ototoxic and should not be used where perforated ear drum has been diagnosed or is suspected.

Interactions: None known.

Effect on ability to drive or to use machines: None known.

Other undesirable effects: Some patients may experience a transient stinging or burning sensation for the first few days of treatment.

Use in pregnancy and lactation: There is inadequate evidence of safety in human pregnancy. Topical administration of corticosteroids to pregnant animals can cause abnormalities of foetal development including cleft palate and intra-uterine growth retardation. There may therefore be a very small risk of such effects in the human foetus.

Other special warnings and precautions: See pharmaceutical precautions.

Overdose: Not applicable.

Incompatibilities: None known.

Pharmaceutical precautions Store upright in the carton below 25°C. Do not freeze. Before using the product for the first time, prime the pump by depressing actuator 6–10 times until a fine spray is obtained. Use within 1 month of first actuation. If more than one week has elapsed since the last use, dispose of the contents of the pump chamber by 1 or 2 depressions of the actuator. An expiry date is given on the package.

Legal category POM.

Package quantities 5 ml bottles.

Product licence number 0036/0042.

PROCTOFOAM HC*

Presentation An aerosol can releasing a muco-adherent, white, odourless aerosol foam containing:

Hydrocortisone acetate PhEur	1%
Pramoxine hydrochloride USP	1%

Uses Anti-inflammatory, antipruritic, anaesthetic. For the relief of inflammation, pruritus, pain and swelling associated with haemorrhoids, proctitis, cryptitis, fissures, post-operative pain and pruritus ani.

Dosage and administration One applicatorful per rectum two or three times daily and after each bowel evacuation. Not indicated in infants and young children.

Contra-indications, warnings, etc
Contra-indications: Do not use on infected lesions unless accompanied by appropriate anti-infective treatment.

Pregnancy: Systemic and topical administration of corticosteroids to pregnant animals can cause abnormalities of foetal development. The relevance of this finding to human beings has not been established, but at present steroids should not be used extensively in pregnancy, that is in large amounts or for prolonged periods.

Warnings: A complete rectal examination to rule out serious pathology should be completed before instituting therapy. Discontinue use if sensitivity develops.

For external use only.

Pharmaceutical precautions Pressurized container. Protect from sunlight and do not expose to temperatures above 50°C. Do not pierce or burn even after use.

Do not refrigerate. Shake vigorously before use. Use at room temperature.

Legal category POM.

Package quantities Aerosol canister containing 24 g of foam (approximately 40 doses), plus a plastic applicator.

Further information One applicatorful of Proctofoam HC provides a dose of approximately 4–6 mg of both hydrocortisone acetate and pramoxine hydrochloride.

An illustrated instruction leaflet is enclosed with each pack.

Product licence number 0036/5002.

QUELLADA* APPLICATION PC

Presentation A clear yellow foaming shampoo base containing Gamma Benzene Hexachloride BP 1%.

Uses Gamma benzene hexachloride (Lindane) is an insecticide, larvicide, acaricide and an ovacide. Quellada Application PC is indicated for the treatment of head and pubic lice infestation (Pediculus capitis and Phthirus pubis).

Dosage and administration Adults and children should apply Quellada Application PC to dry hair, in quantities sufficient to thoroughly wet the hair and skin of the infested and adjacent hairy areas. Work thoroughly into the hair and allow to remain in place for 4 minutes. Add small quantities of water until a good lather forms. Rinse thoroughly. Towel dry and then, if required, remove any remaining nits or nit shells from hair by fine tooth combing, or from pubic hair with tweezers.

Contra-indications, warnings, etc For external use only. Contact with eyes can cause stinging, flush immediately with water. Do not use as a routine shampoo, or on broken or infected skin. Quellada Application PC should be used with caution especially on infants and children. Lindane penetrates human skin and has potential for CNS irritation. Studies indicate that the potential for toxic effects after the topical application of lindane is greater in the young. However, for a shampoo, this difference is likely to be insignificant. The reported incidence of toxic effects is every low and has, in most cases, been related to misuse. Seizures have been reported after the use of lindane but a cause and effect relationship has not been established. Simultaneous application of cream, ointments or oils may enhance the percutaneous absorption of lindane.

Pregnancy: At very high doses foetal toxicity has been demonstrated in animals (rats and dogs). Quellada Application PC has been in wide use for many years without apparent ill consequence. However, the safety of Quellada Application PC during pregnancy and lactation has not been established, and use is not recommended unless there is no safer alternative.

Overdosage: Acute poisoning (ingestion). Emesis should be induced with syrup of ipecac unless the patient is comatose or has lost the gag reflex when gastric lavage should be performed, followed by activated charcoal and then sodium or magnesium sulphate cathartics. Do not administer sympathomimetics, atropine or oils. Artificial respiration may be indicated to counteract pulmonary failure. Convulsions may be treated with i.v. diazepam.

Chronic poisoning (topical) may occur when patients use the product regularly (misuse), or apply the shampoo regularly to others without gloves. The patient should be withdrawn from the product.

Side effects: Very rarely – skin irritation.

Pharmaceutical precautions Do not refrigerate, store at room temperature.

Legal category P.

Package quantities Bottles of 100 ml or 500 ml.

Further information Nursing or medical staff who apply Quellada Application PC to patients regularly should wear surgical gloves during the application.

Product licence number 0036/5001R.

QUELLADA* LOTION

Presentation A pleasantly perfumed pearly white lotion base containing Gamma Benzene Hexachloride BP 1%.

Uses Gamma benzene hexachloride (Lindane) is an insecticide, larvicide, acaricide and an ovacide. Quellada Lotion is indicated for the treatment of scabies and body lice infestation (Sarcoptes scabiei and Pediculus corporis).

Dosage and administration
Adults: A thin layer of Quellada Lotion should be applied to the whole body surface excluding face and scalp. It is important that areas such as soles of the feet, toe webs and finger webs should not be missed. Quellada Lotion should be left on the body for 24 hours, and then washed off thoroughly. If evidence of viable mites or lice is present 7 days after treatment, the dosage schedule should be repeated. Do not use more than twice in any one infestation or in any one week.

Children: Under 1 month Quellada Lotion is not recommended. Children 1–6 months treated (under appropriate supervision) as adults but the lotion should be washed off after 8–12 hours. Children over 6 months should be treated as adults.

All children should be under supervision, constant or as required, to ensure that they do not lick the lotion off and ingest it.

Contra-indications, warnings, etc For external use only. Avoid contact with eyes and other mucous membranes. Do not use on broken or infected skin. Quellada Lotion should be used with caution especially on infants and children. Lindane penetrates human skin and has potential for CNS irritation. Studies indicate that the potential for toxic effects after the topical application of lindane is greater in the young. The reported incidence of toxic effects is very low and has, in most cases, been related to misuse. Seizures have been reported after the use of lindane but a cause and effect relationship has not been established. Simultaneous application of cream, ointments or oils may enhance the percutaneous absorption of lindane.

Pregnancy: At very high doses foetal toxicity has been demonstrated in animals (rats and dogs). Quellada Lotion has been in wide use for many years without apparent ill consequence. However, the safety of Quellada Lotion during pregnancy and lactation has not been established, and use is not recommended unless there is no safer alternative.

Overdosage: Acute poisoning (ingestion). Emesis should be induced with syrup of ipecac unless the patient is comatose or has lost the gag reflex when gastric lavage should be performed, followed by activated charcoal and then sodium or magnesium supphate cathartics. Do not administer sympathomimetics, atropine or oils. Artificial respiration may be indicated to counteract pulmonary failure. Convulsions may be treated with i.v. diazepam.

Chronic poisoning (topical) may occur when patients use the product regularly (misuse), or apply the shampoo regularly to others without gloves. The patient should be withdrawn from the product.

Side effects: Very rarely – skin irritation.

Pharmaceutical precautions Do not refrigerate, store at room temperature.

Legal category P.

Package quantities Bottles of 100 ml or 500 ml.

Further information Nursing or medical staff who apply Quellada Lotion to patients regularly should wear surgical gloves during the application.

Product licence number 0036/5000R.

TARCORTIN*

Presentation Hydrocortisone PhEur 0.5% and refined alcoholic extract of coal tar 5% in a vanishing cream base. It is a light tan, homogeneous cream.

Uses Tarcortin Cream is a stimulating antipruritic. It is indicated for sub-acute and chronic eczema, localised neurodermatitis, seborrhoea, dermatitis venenata and psoriasis, excluding widespread plaque psoriasis.

Dosage and administration Apply twice daily or more frequently to the affected area by gentle massage until the cream has vanished into the skin. No dressing is needed.

Contra-indications, warnings, etc

Contra-indications: The use of Tarcortin is contra-indicated in the presence of viral or fungal infections, tubercular or syphilitic lesions, and in bacterial infections, unless used in conjunction with appropriate chemotherapy.

Interactions: No interactions are known or suspected.

Adverse effects: The use of coal tar can cause skin irritation, acne-like eruptions and photosensitivity.

Use in pregnancy and lactation: There is inadequate evidence of safety of topical steroids in human pregnancy. Topical administration of corticosteroids to pregnant animals can cause abnormalities of foetal development, including cleft palate and intra-uterine growth retardation. There may, therefore, be a very small risk of such effects in the human foetus.

Other special warnings and precautions: The cream should be massaged well into the affected area to prevent a temporary discolouration of skin, hair or fabric. Although generally regarded as safe, even for long term administration in adults, there is a potential for overdose in infancy. Extreme caution is required in dermatoses of infancy including napkin eruption. In such patients, courses of treatment should not normally exceed 7 days. Topical corticosteroids may be hazardous in psoriasis for a number of reasons, including rebound relapses following development of tolerance, risk of generalised pustular psoriasis and local systemic toxicity due to impaired barrier function of the skin. Careful patient supervision is important.

Pharmaceutical precautions Do not refrigerate. Store at room temperature.

Legal category POM.

Product licence number 0036/5007.

**Trade Mark*

STD Pharmaceutical Products Ltd
Fields Yard, Plough Lane
Hereford HR4 0EL

STD* INJECTION 3%, 1% and ½% Sodium Tetradecyl Sulphate Injection

Presentation STD Injection is a sterile aqueous solution of Sodium Tetradecyl Sulphate available in three strengths 3%, 1% and ½% and each containing 2% Benzyl Alcohol and buffered to pH 7.6.

Uses The solution is designed for intravenous use and is used as a sclerosant in the treatment of varicose veins of the leg by compression sclerotherapy.

The action of sodium tetradecyl sulphate in this technique is considered to be that of irritation to the intima of the vein wall, so that on compression of the vein fibrosis takes place and the vein is permanently occluded by the development of fibrosis in the wall, and across the lumen of the compressed vein.

Dosage and administration
Dosage
STD Injection 3%
Adults and the elderly (not recommended for use in chldren): 0.25 to 1.0 ml of 3% STD Injection injected intravenously into the lumen of an isolated segment of emptied superficial vein, followed by immediate continuous compression. A maximum of four sites (4 ml total) may be injected during one treatment session.

STD Injection 1%
Adults and the elderly (not recommended for use in children): 0.25–1 ml at each of 10 sites (maximum 10 ml).

The uses and principles behind the treatment using STD Injection 1% is the same as described for STD Injection 3%. However, the 1% Injection is designed for the treatment of small varicose veins and the larger venules by empty vein techniques.

STD Injection ½%
Adults and the elderly (not recommended for use in children); 0.1–1.0 ml at each of 10 sites (maximum 10 ml).

STD Injection ½% is produced specifically for the treatment of sclerotherapy of minor venules and spider veins (Venous Flares).

Administration: The technique of injection followed by immediate uninterrupted compression is of supreme importance. The following procedure is recommended for the treatment of medium to large veins using 1% and 3% STD Injection:

Diagnosis and determination of proposed injection sites. Prepare to inject most distal site first. Needle recommended 25G × ⅝" (27G × ½" for 1%) with transparent hub. Venepuncture whilst leg is horizontal. Elevation of leg prior to injection. Isolation of empty segment of vein using ring and index fingers. Slow injection of 0.25–1.0 ml into empty isolated segment. Maintain isolation of segment for 30 seconds. Immediate compression. Compression uninterrupted until next visit. Re-examination at 7–14 days – further injections if necessary. Reapply compression. Daily walking (2–3 miles). Avoid standing still during treatment period (6–8 weeks).

Compression is enhanced by the application of foam rubber pads over the sites of injection, held in place by firmly applied Cotton Crepe bandages and secured by the application of a Class 1 Elastic Stocking over the bandages. This compression regime should be maintained until intramural fibrosis is complete.

Minor venules and spider veins are treated using STD Injection ½% by the following technique: Needle recommended – 30G × ½" with transparent hub. Use illuminated magnifying lens. Sterile needle can be 'cranked' about 30° to allow easier venepuncture. Venepuncture and injection with leg horizontal. Slow injection, observe blanching. Immediate compression – uninterrupted until next visit. Re-examine and further injections at 7 days. Maintain compression for at least 2 weeks. Encourage walking and avoid standing still.

Compression of injected minor venules may be achieved using a small foam rubber pad secured over the site of injection and a Class 2 Elastic Stocking applied immediately and worn during the daytime.

Contra-indications, warnings, etc
Contra-indications:
1. Allergy to Sodium Tetradecyl Sulphate or to any component of the preparation.
2. Patients unable to walk due to any cause.
3. Patients currently taking oral contraceptives.
4. Significant obesity.
5. Acute superficial thrombophlebitis.
6. Local or systematic infection.
7. Varicosities caused by pelvic or abdominal tumours.
8. Uncontrolled systematic disease e.g. diabetes mellitus.
9. Significant valvular incompetence requiring surgical treatment.

Side-effects:
1. (a) Allergy and anaphylaxis – rarely (see 'Precautions' below). (b) Allergy – Urticaria (see 'Precautions' below).
2. Extravascular injection will give rise to pain, and may produce necrosis and ulceration (if close to surface).
3. Other undesirable effects: (a) Local – Pain or burning. Skin pigmentation. Tissue necrosis and ulceration may occur with extravasation. Parasthesiae and anaesthesia may occur if an injection effects a cutaneous nerve.
(b) Vascular – Superficial Thrombophlebitis. Deep vein Thrombosis and Pulmonary Embolism are very rare. Inadvertent Intra-arterial injection is very rare, but may lead to gangrene. Most cases have involved the posterior tibial artery above the medial maleolus.

Use in pregnancy and lactation: Safety for use in pregnancy has not been established. Use only when clearly needed for symptomatic relief and when the potential benefits outweigh the potential hazards to the foetus.

It is not known whether Sodium Tetradecyl Sulphate is excreted in human milk. Caution should be exercised when used in nursing mothers.

Special warnings and precautions
1. STD Injection should only be administered by practitioners familiar with an acceptable injection technique. Thorough pre-injection assessment for valvular competence and deep vein patency must be carried out. Extreme care in needle placement and slow injection of the minimal effective volume at each injection site are essential for safe and efficient use.
2. Allergy and anaphylaxis – (a) History of allergy should be taken from all patients prior to treatment. In particular allergic reactions to previous injection of Sodium Tetradecyl Sulphate should be noted (see 'Contra-indications' above).
(b) A higher incidence of allergic reaction is thought

to result from repeated treatment involving Sodium Tetradecyl Sulphate injection and may involve intervals of several years between courses of injection.

(c) Where special caution is indicated a test dose of 0.25 to 0.5 ml STD Injection should be given up to 24 hours before any further therapy.

3. Equipment of clinic – The treatment of Anaphylaxis may require, depending on severity of attack, some or all of the following: Injection of adrenaline (epinephrine), injection of hydrocortisone, antihistamine injection, endotracheal tube, laryngoscope mucus extraction pump. The treatment of varicose veins by STD Injection should not be undertaken in clinics where these items are not readily available.

4. Special care should be exercised when injecting above and posterior to the median malleous where extra vascular injection is in danger of being close to the posterior and tibial artery.

5. Pigmentation can result if blood is extravasated at the injection site, particularly when treating the smaller surface veins, and compression is not used.

6. Extreme caution in use is required in patients with arterial disease such as severe peripheral atherosclerosis of thromboangiitis obliterans (Buerger's disease).

Incompatibilities (Major): Do not use with Heparin in the same syringe.

Pharmaceutical precautions Store in a cool place, away from direct sunlight.

The in-use period of each multidose vial is a single session of therapy and for use in the treatment of a single patient. Unused vial contents should be discarded immediately after use.

Legal category POM.

Package quantities
3% 5 ml multidose (pack of 10).
3% 5 × 2 ml single dose ampoules.
1% 5 × 2 ml single dose ampoules.
½% 5 × 2 ml single dose ampoules.

Further information The use of a small dose, the isolation of the injection within the vein segment and the application of immediate, adequate and lasting compression are of supreme importance in obtaining a good result.

Product licence numbers
3% 0398/5000R
1% 0398/0003
½% 0398/0002

**Trade Mark*

Sterling-Winthrop Group Limited
Sterling-Winthrop House
Onslow Street
Guildford
Surrey GU1 4YS

Sterling Winthrop

AT10*

Presentation A clear, deep straw-coloured, oily solution with a faint nut-like odour containing 250 micrograms/ml Dihydrotachysterol BP.

Uses AT10 is recommended for use in the acute, chronic and latent forms of hypocalcaemic tetany due to hypoparathyroidism where its action is to increase the rate of absorption and utilisation of calcium.

Dosage and administration AT10 is for oral administration only.

Adults including the elderly: In acute cases 3–5 ml may be given on each of the first three days of treatment, followed two or three days later by blood and urinary calcium estimations. The maintenance dose of AT10 is usually in the range of 1–7 ml each week, but the precise amount depends on the results of serum and urinary calcium determinations.

In chronic cases an initial dose of 2 ml of AT10 daily, or on alternate days, may be sufficient to maintain normocalcaemia in moderate cases. The dose of AT10 usually has to be increased during menstruation and periods of unusual activity.

Children: No specific dosage recommendations.

Contra-indications, warnings, etc As with calciferol, uncontrolled, prolonged administration of AT10 can result in hypercalcaemia which may lead to nephrocalcinosis. Therefore accurate blood calcium determinations must be made at the beginning of treatment and then periodically until the required maintenance dose has been established. The serum calcium level should subsequently be kept between 2.25–2.5 mmol/litre. Serum phosphate, magnesium and alkaline phosphatase should also be measured periodically to monitor progress. If nausea and vomiting are present, serum calcium levels should be checked.

The Sulkowitch test (for urinary calcium) is a convenient supplement to blood calcium determinations, but it should not be regarded as a substitute, because in hypoparathyroid patients treated with AT10, hypercalcuria can occur in the presence of hypocalcaemia.

Certain individuals, particularly those suffering from sarcoidosis, are very sensitive to the effect of Vitamin D and it is advisable to consult a physician in cases of doubt.

Use in pregnancy and lactation: The safety of AT10 in pregnancy is not established. There is some evidence that its injudicious and unsupervised use during pregnancy could lead to foetal damage and hypercalcaemia in the newborn.

Dihydrotachysterol is excreted in breast milk and may cause hypercalcaemia in the suckling infant.

Interactions: Several classes of medicine interact with vitamin D analogues calling for adjustment in the dosage of AT10. Thyroid replacement therapy may increase clearance of dihydrotachysterol; cholestyramine may impair its absorption; thiazide diuretics may enhance the calcaemic response leading to hypercalcaemia; barbiturates, anticonvulsants, rifampicin and isoniazid may reduce the effectiveness of AT10. Hypercalcaemia induced by excessive dosaging of AT10 may enhance the toxic effects of cardiac glycosides.

Side-effects: Side-effects are most likely to be due to overdosage leading to hypercalcaemia, the first signs of which are loss of appetite, listlessness and nausea. More severe manifestations include vomiting, urgency of micturition, polyuria, dehydration, thirst, vertigo, stupor, headache, abdominal cramps and paralysis. The calcium and phosphorus concentrations of serum and urine are increased. With chronic overdosage, calcium may be deposited in many tissues including arteries and the kidneys, leading to hypertension and renal failure. Plasma cholesterol may also be increased.

Overdosage: The symptoms of hypercalcaemia in chronic overdosage will usually respond to withdrawal of medication, bed rest, liberal fluid intake, and the use of laxatives.

In acute overdosage, consideration should be given to recovery of AT10 by emesis or gastric lavage if ingestion is recent. Serum calcium estimations should be helpful in determining management.

In massive overdosage of vitamin D, corticosteroids have been found useful and also neutral phosphate in resistant cases. Several months management may be needed in such cases.

Pharmaceutical precautions Store in well-closed containers protected from heat and light.

Legal category P.

Package quantities AT10 is supplied in bottles containing 15 ml with a 1 ml dropper.

Further information The hypercalcaemic action of AT10 is slower in onset and more prolonged than that of parathyroid hormone, but faster in onset and less persistent in action than calciferol. In patients who have become resistant to large doses of calciferol it may be possible to control blood calcium levels with AT10.

Product licence number 0071/5020.

BENORAL*

Presentation 1. Benoral Suspension is a white suspension, 10 ml of which contains 4 g Benorylate BP. Benoral Suspension contains sorbitol.

2. Benoral Granules: sachets filled with a white, free-flowing powder which disperses readily in water. The contents of each sachet are equivalent to 2 g Benorylate BP. Benoral Granules contain 550 mg sucrose in each sachet.

3. Benoral Tablets are white, capsule-shaped tablets marked 'Benoral' on one side only, each containing 750 mg Benorylate BP.

Uses Benoral is an anti-inflammatory analgesic and antipyretic. It is recommended for the treatment of rheumatoid arthritis, osteoarthritis and painful musculoskeletal conditions. It may also be used to treat mild to moderate pain due to many other causes and as an antipyretic in febrile conditions.

Dosage and administration Benoral is for oral administration only.

Benoral Suspension may be administered undiluted or taken in hot or cold beverages. Benoral Granules should be stirred into half a glass of water or milk, if preferred.

Adults (except elderly) The maximum daily dosage of benorylate is 8 g. The maximum individual dose is 4 g.
Suspension: To treat active rheumatoid arthritis 10 ml of suspension (4 g benorylate) twice daily is normally required.

For osteoarthritis, quiescent rheumatoid arthritis or soft tissue (non-articular) rheumatism 5 ml (2 g benorylate) twice daily may suffice.

For mild to moderate pain and as an antipyretic the normal dosage is 5 ml suspension (2 g benorylate) twice daily.

Tablets: In osteoarthritis, quiescent rheumatoid arthritis and soft tissue rheumatism six to eight 750 mg tablets (4.5 to 6 g benorylate) per day, in divided doses, are recommended.

Sachets: For acute rheumatic conditions up to four sachets (8 g benorylate) daily in divided doses may be required but three sachets (6 g benorylate) daily are often adequate. For milder rheumatic conditions and for the relief of non-rheumatic pain one sachet (2 g benorylate) twice daily is recommended.

Elderly: In elderly patients, especially those with impaired renal function, symptoms of salicylism may arise at dosages not normally associated with this effect. In elderly patients it is recommended that the adult dose of Benoral be reduced and that total daily dosage does not exceed 6 g benorylate. For example, dose reduction of Benoral Suspension to a 5 ml (2 g benorylate) morning dose with 10 ml (4 g benorylate) at bedtime may be instituted. Further reduction to 5 ml (2 g benorylate) twice daily may be necessary in some cases.

Dose reduction of Benoral Sachets to three (6 g benorylate) daily in divided doses may be instituted. Further reduction to one sachet (2 g benorylate) twice daily may be necessary in some cases.

Children: Benoral is not recommended for children.

Contra-indications, warnings, etc
Contra-indications: Benoral should not be given to patients with active peptic ulcer, nor to patients known to be sensitive to aspirin including those with asthma, or haemophilia and similar coagulation disorders.

The safety of benorylate has not been established in human pregnancy. Whilst there is clinical and epidemiological evidence that its metabolic products, salicylate and paracetamol, are safe in pregnancy, it is also known that benorylate, in high doses, may have an aspirin-like effect on platelet function. As with aspirin therefore, benorylate should be avoided in the last trimester and at term because of a potential risk of contributing to maternal and neonatal bleeding.

Because salicylate is excreted in breast milk, benorylate should also be avoided by breast feeding mothers.

Because of the possible association between Reye's syndrome and aspirin use, Benoral labelling contains the statement 'Do not give to children under 12 unless your doctor tells you to'.

Patients taking Benoral should be advised against taking analgesics containing aspirin or paracetamol.

Precautions: Care is needed in prescribing Benoral for patients with impaired renal or hepatic function and for those with a history of peptic ulcer.

Patients who are taking anticoagulants should have their prothrombin time checked.

Concomitant administration of carbonic anhydrase inhibitors may increase salicylate level and dispose to toxicity, whilst corticosteroids may reduce salicylate level. Salicylate may diminish the diuretic efficiency of frusemide. These possible interactions should be borne in mind in determining respective dosages when initiating or discontinuing concomitant therapy.

Side-effects: Overall tolerability is excellent. Minor disturbances including nausea, constipation or diarrhoea, indigestion or heartburn have occurred from time to time and drowsiness and skin rashes have also been reported. The possibility that gastro-intestinal haemorrhage may be induced by Benoral cannot be excluded. The high salicylate levels obtained with Benoral may give rise to dizziness, tinnitus and deafness. If this happens, the dose should be reduced.

Overdosage: Symptoms are likely to resemble those caused by salicylate overdosage. Treatment should be based on the levels of salicylate and paracetamol found in the blood. The possibility that overdosage may cause hepatic necrosis due to accumulation of a highly reactive intermediate metabolite of paracetamol, must be considered. Management may therefore need to include gastric lavage, forced alkaline diuresis, correction of acid-base balance and the use of N-acetyl cysteine intravenously or methionine orally, which, with paracetamol, have been shown to protect the liver if given within 10–12 hours of an overdose.

Pharmaceutical precautions Nil.

Legal category P.

Package quantities Benoral Suspension – bottles of 300 ml. Benoral Granules – cartons of 60 sachets (OP). Benoral Tablets – bottles of 100.

Further information Benorylate is a prodrug which is metabolised to salicylate and paracetamol by esterases after absorption. It does not give rise to detectable levels of acetylsalicylic acid in the plasma. In chemical terms, 2 g benorylate is equivalent to 1.15 g aspirin and 0.97 g paracetamol.

Product licence numbers

Benoral Suspension	0071/5022
Benoral Granules	0071/0149
Benoral Tablets	0071/5901

BIOGASTRONE*

Presentation White, flat, round, bevelled-edged tablets 9.5 mm in diameter, marked BG and scored on one side and unmarked on the other with a slight odour of peppermint. Each tablet contains Carbenoxolone Sodium BP 50 mg. Biogastrone Tablets contain lactose.

Uses For the treatment of benign gastric ulcers in young and middle-aged patients, ie those within the age range of 16 to 65 years.

Dosage and administration For oral administration only.

Adults: Two tablets three times daily after meals for the first week. Thereafter, one tablet should be taken three times a day until the ulcer has healed.

Patients taking antacids should continue to do so until symptoms disappear but anticholinergic drugs should be discontinued. Despite early relief of symptoms, treatment should continue for at least six weeks and should usually be extended to 12 weeks to ensure maximum healing effect.

Elderly: Not recommended for adults over 65 years.

Children: Not recommended for children under 16 years.

Contra-indications, warnings, etc
Contra-indications: Biogastrone is contra-indicated in the elderly and in children.

Biogastrone should not be administered to patients suffering from cardiac, renal or hepatic failure nor to patients on digitalis glycosides unless serum electrolyte levels are monitored at weekly intervals and measures taken to avoid the development of hypokalaemia. Biogastrone is contra-indicated in established hypokalaemia.

Although animal studies have shown no hazard, there is inadequate evidence of the safety of carbenoxolone in human pregnancy. Biogastrone should be avoided in patients who are pregnant.

Precautions: Special care should be exercised with patients predisposed to sodium and water retention, potassium loss and hypertension (e.g. those with cardiac, renal or hepatic disease) since carbenoxolone can induce similar changes. Potassium supplements should be considered for those at risk from developing hypokalaemia.

Regular monitoring of weight, blood pressure and clinical condition is advisable for all patients. Biogastrone should be withdrawn if hypokalaemia or oedema develop or a clinically significant rise in blood pressure occurs. Potassium loss should be corrected by the administration of supplements.

Interactions: Biogastrone may provoke digitalis glycoside toxicity by inducing hypokalaemia.

Most classes of diuretics will induce hypokalaemia which may be exacerbated by concomitant administration of carbenoxolone as may the mineralocorticoid effects of steroids.

Although spironolactone and amiloride will antagonise the hypokalaemia induced by carbenoxolone, they also inhibit its healing actions and, therefore, should not be prescribed with Biogastrone.

There is a theoretical possibility of a pharmacodynamic interaction with anti-hypertensive drugs, carbenoxolone possibly making hypertension more difficult to control.

Side-effects: Biogastrone may induce sodium and water retention and potassium loss, provoking hypertension and cardiac failure in those so predisposed. If profound hypokalaemia is permitted to develop, it may lead to widespread impairment of neuromuscular function and to muscle damage. Prolonged hypokalaemia may cause renal damage.

Overdosage: If the tablets have been recently ingested, the stomach should be emptied by gastric lavage. Serum electrolytes should be monitored and any deficiency in potassium should be corrected, using the intravenous route if necessary, or slow-release or effervescent potassium chloride tablets. Should water and sodium retention require correction with a diuretic, careful monitoring of potassium levels is mandatory.

Pharmaceutical precautions Nil.

Legal category POM.

Package quantities Bottles of 100 tablets.

Further information Carbenoxolone has been shown to exert a healing effect on gastric ulcers, possibly by improving mucus synthesis and by prolonging the life-span of gastric epithelium through local rather than systemic action. Systemic absorption of carbenoxolone is extensive. There is more than 99.95% binding to plasma proteins. There appears to be entero-hepatic circulation which delays clearance. Excretion is mainly via the faeces. Plasma elimination half life increases with age.

Product licence number 0071/5902.

BRONCHILATOR*

Presentation Bronchilator is an aerosol inhalant in the form of an oral nebuliser, delivering 250 metered doses by finger depression of an actuator. Each metered dose (0.05 ml) contains 350 micrograms isoetharine mesylate and 70 micrograms Phenylephrine Hydrochloride BP. Bronchilator aerosol contains ethyl alcohol, ascorbic acid, saccharin, menthol, dichlorodifluoromethane and dichlorotetrafluoroethane.

Uses Bronchilator is indicated for effective and relatively long-lasting relief of bronchospasm in bronchial asthma and chronic bronchitis.

Dosage and administration Bronchilator is for oral inhalation only.

Adults including the elderly: The usual dose is 1 or 2 inhalations and it is not normally necessary to repeat this dose at less than half-hourly intervals. In bronchial asthma 1 or 2 inhalations more may be required, but it is important to wait one full minute after the initial 1 or 2 inhalations, to be certain that relief has not been obtained. Not more than eight inhalations should be taken in 24 hours.

Children: Bronchilator should only be administered to children under the supervision of a responsible adult and strictly as recommended by the doctor. The usual dose is one inhalation. This may be increased to two inhalations if necessary. As with adults, adequate time should be allowed to assess the response before further dosing and no more than eight inhalations should be taken in 24 hours.

Contra-indications, warnings, etc

Contra-indications: Bronchilator should not be given to patients taking MAO inhibitors.

Precautions: As with all medicines, Bronchilator should not be used in pregnancy unless the expected benefit is thought to outweigh any possible risk to the foetus.

Potentially serious hypokalaemia may result from beta 2 agonist therapy. Particular caution is advised in severe asthma as this effect may be potentiated by concomitant treatment with xanthine derivatives, corticosteroids, diuretics and by hypoxia. It is recommended that serum potassium levels are monitored in such situations.

As with other sympathomimetic amines, too frequent use of Bronchilator may cause tachycardia, palpitations, nausea, headache, changes in blood pressure, anxiety, tension, restlessness, insomnia, tremor, weakness, dizziness and excitement. Patients should therefore be advised not to exceed the recommended dose.

As with other inhalational adrenergic therapy, the potential for paradoxical bronchospasm should be borne in mind. If it occurs, Bronchilator therapy should be discontinued immediately and alternative therapy instituted.

Caution should be exercised and dosage carefully adjusted, in patients with hyperthyroidism, hypertension, coronary artery disease, cardiac asthma, limited cardiac reserve and in individuals sensitive to sympathomimetic amines.

Side-effects: Potentially serious hypokalaemia may result from beta 2 agonist therapy. When used as recommended, sympathomimetic side-effects are unlikely to occur. A small drop in pulse rate and blood pressure may rarely follow from inhalation of Bronchilator.

Overdosage: Serious symptoms are unlikely except after massive overdosage. They may be treated in the same way as those due to adrenaline overdosage (i.e. injection of piperoxan or phentolamine). Slow intravenous procaine or procainamide should be used for fibrillation, and artificial respiration and oxygen for cyanosis and respiratory embarrassment. Particular attention should be paid to the detection and correction of hypokalaemia.

Pharmaceutical precautions Keep away from extreme heat.

Legal category POM.

Package quantities Complete nebuliser containing 12.5 ml of solution (equivalent to 250 doses).

Further information Nil.

Product licence number 0071/0196.

CALCIUM RESONIUM*

Presentation Calcium Resonium contains 99.93% calcium polystyrene sulphonate ground and flavoured to a buff-coloured fine powder with a pleasant vanilla odour and sweet taste.

Uses Calcium Resonium is an ion-exchange resin. It is recommended for the treatment of hyperkalaemia associated with anuria or severe oliguria. It is also used to treat hyperkalaemia in patients requiring dialysis and in patients on regular haemodialysis or on prolonged peritoneal dialysis.

Dosage and administration Calcium Resonium is for oral or rectal administration only. The dosage recommendations detailed below are a guide only; the precise requirements should be decided on the basis of regular serum electrolyte determinations.

Adults, including the elderly:

1. *Oral:* Usual dose 15 g three or four times a day. The resin is given by mouth in a little water, or it may be made into a paste with some sweetened vehicle.

2. *Rectal:* In cases where vomiting may make oral administration difficult, the resin may be given rectally as a suspension of 30 g resin in 100 ml 2% Methylcellulose 450 BP (medium viscosity) and 100 ml water, as a daily retention enema. In the initial stages administration by this route as well as orally may help to achieve a more rapid lowering of the serum potassium level.

The enema should if possible be retained for at least nine hours following which the colon should be irrigated to remove the resin. If both routes are used initially it is probably unnecessary to continue rectal administration once the oral resin has reached the rectum.

Children: 1 g/kg body weight daily in divided doses in acute hyperkalaemia. For maintenance therapy dosage may be reduced to 0.5 g/kg body weight daily in divided doses.

The resin is given orally, preferably with a drink (not a fruit squash because of the high potassium content) or a little jam or honey. When refused by mouth it should be given rectally using a dose at least as great as that which would have been given orally, diluted in the same ratio as described for adults. Following retention of the enema, the colon should be irrigated to ensure adequate removal of the resin.

Neonates: Calcium Resonium should not be given by the oral route. With rectal administration, the minimum effective dosage within the range 0.5 g/kg to 1 g/kg should be employed, diluted as for adults and with adequate irrigation to ensure recovery of the resin.

Contra-indications, warnings, etc

Contra-indications: Calcium Resonium should not be administered orally to neonates and is contraindicated in neonates with reduced gut motility (e.g. post-operatively or drug induced). Calcium Resonium is also contraindicated in patients with hyperparathyroidism, multiple myeloma, sarcoidosis or metastatic carcinoma who may present with renal failure and hypercalcaemia and in the presence of obstructive bowel disease.

Precautions: The possibility of severe potassium depletion should be considered and adequate clinical and biochemical control is essential during treatment especially in patients on digitalis.

Administration of the resin should be stopped when the serum potassium falls to 5 mmol/litre. Serum calcium levels should be estimated at weekly intervals to detect the early development of hypercalcaemia, and the dose of resin adjusted to levels at which hypercalcaemia and hypokalaemia are prevented. In the event of clinically significant constipation, treatment should be discontinued until normal bowel movement is resumed. In children and neonates, particular care is needed with rectal administration as excessive dosage or inadequate dilution could result in impaction of the resin. Cation donating agents may reduce the potassium binding effectiveness of Calcium Resonium.

Side-effects: Nausea, vomiting and constipation occasionally occur. Faecal impaction following rectal administration has been reported in children, and gastrointestinal concretions following oral administration to neonates. Intestinal obstruction has also been reported although this has been extremely rare and, possibly, a reflection of co-existing pathology, excessive dosage or inadequate dilution of the resin. Hypokalaemia may occur.

Hypercalcaemia has been reported in well-dialysed patients receiving calcium resin, and in the occasional patient with chronic renal failure. Many patients in chronic renal failure have low serum calcium and high serum phosphate, but some, who cannot be screened out beforehand, show a sudden rise in serum calcium to high levels after therapy. The risk emphasises the need for adequate biochemical control.

Overdosage: Hypokalaemia may be manifest clinically by signs of irritable confusion, delayed thought processes, severe muscle weakness or paralysis. ECG abnormalities may be evident and cardiac arrhythmias may occur. In the event of overdosage the resin should be removed from the alimentary tract by the use of laxatives or enemas, and appropriate measures should be taken to restore serum potassium levels to normal, and to reduce blood calcium levels if these are raised.

Pharmaceutical precautions Store in a dry place. Suspensions of the resin should be freshly prepared and not stored beyond 24 hours.

Legal category P.

Package quantities HDPE containers of 300 g each containing a plastic scoop which, when filled level, contains approximately 15 g.

Further information Theoretically, each gram of Calcium Resonium should take up 1.3 to 2 mmol of potassium. However, in vivo, the actual amount of potassium bound will be less than this. The sodium content of Calcium Resonium is less than 1 mg/g. Calcium content is about 8% w/w (1.6–2.4 mmol/g).

Product licence number 0071/5025.

DANOL*

Presentation

Danol 200 mg capsules: Pink/white No. 1 hard gelatin capsules printed in black ink with Danol 200 and filled with a white or almost white powder containing 200 mg danazol and lactose.

Danol 100 mg capsules: Grey/white No. 3 hard gelatin capsules printed in black ink with Danol 100 and filled with a white or almost white powder containing 100 mg danazol and lactose.

Pharmacology: Danazol, 17 alpha-pregna-2,4-dien-20-yno[2,3-d]-isoxazol-17-ol, is a synthetic steroid derived from ethisterone. Its pharmacological properties include:
1. Relatively marked affinity for androgen receptors, less marked affinity for progesterone receptors and least affinity for oestrogen receptors. Danazol is a weak androgen but in addition antiandrogenic, progestogenic, antiprogestogenic, oestrogenic and antioestrogenic actions have been observed.
2. Interference with the synthesis of gonadal steroids, possibly by inhibition of the enzymes of steroidogenesis, including 3 beta hydroxysteroid dehydrogenase, 17 beta hydroxysteroid dehydrogenase, 20 hydroxysteroid dehydrogenase, 17 hydroxylase, 17, 20 lyase, 11 beta hydroxylase, 21 hydroxylase and cholesterol side chain cleavage enzymes or alternatively by inhibition of the cyclic AMP accumulation usually induced by gonadotrophic hormones in granulosa and luteal cells.
3. Inhibition of the mid-cycle surge of FSH and LH as well as alterations in the pulsatility of LH. Danazol can also reduce the mean plasma levels of these gonadotrophins after the menopause.
4. A wide range of actions on plasma proteins, including increasing prothrombin, plasminogen, antithrombin III, alpha-2 macroglobulin, C1 esterase inhibitor, erythropoietin and reducing fibrinogen, thyroid binding and sex hormone binding globulin. Danazol increases the proportion and concentration of testosterone carried unbound in the plasma.

Uses Danol is recommended in the treatment of:
1. Endometriosis, to control pain, pelvic tenderness and other associated symptoms and to resolve or reduce the extent of endometriotic foci. Danol may be used as sole therapy or in preparation for, or following, surgery.
2. For the treatment of severe cyclical mastalgia with or without nodularity (fibrocystic disease), unresponsive to counselling or simple analgesics, to reduce pain, tenderness and nodularity.
3. For the control of benign, multiple or recurrent breast cysts in conjunction with aspiration.
4. Dysfunctional uterine bleeding presenting as menorrhagia, to control excessive blood loss and to control associated dysmenorrhoea.
5. Severe symptomatic gynaecomastia, both idiopathic as well as drug induced, to reduce the size of the breast and to control associated pain and tenderness.

Dosage and administration For oral administration only.

Adults: The usual dosage range is 200–800 mg daily in up to four divided doses.

Specific recommendations for each indication are set out below. Danol should be given as a continuous course, dosage being adjusted according to the patient's response. A reduction in dosage once a satisfactory response has been achieved may prove possible. In fertile females, Danol should be started during menstruation, preferably on the first day, to avoid exposing a pregnancy to its possible effects. Where doubt exists, appropriate checks should be made to exclude pregnancy before starting medication. Females of child bearing age should employ non-hormonal contraception throughout the course of treatment.

In endometriosis, the recommended dosage is initially 400 mg daily in a course of treatment lasting normally six months, although up to nine months may be necessary in some cases. Dosage should be increased, if normal cyclical bleeding still persists after two months therapy; a higher dosage may also be needed for severe disease.

In severe cyclical mastalgia, treatment should commence at a dose of 200–300 mg daily, according to the severity of the symptoms, a course of treatment normally lasting 3–6 months.

In benign breast cysts, treatment should commence at a dose of 300 mg daily, a course of treatment normally lasting 3 to 6 months.

For dysfunctional uterine bleeding presenting as menorrhagia the dosage should be 200 mg daily, normally for 3 months.

In gynaecomastia a six month course of therapy is recommended at a dose of 200 mg daily in adolescents which may be increased to 400 mg daily if no response is obtained after two months. Adults may be given 400 mg daily.

Elderly: Danol is not recommended.

Children: Danol is not recommended.

Renal and hepatic dysfunction: No special dose requirements have been defined, however see Warnings.

Contra-indications, warnings, etc

Contra-indications: Pregnancy.

Breast feeding: Danol may be excreted in breast milk.
Markedly impaired hepatic, renal or cardiac function.
Porphyria: Danol can induce ALA synthetase activity and hence porphyrin metabolism.
Thromboembolic disease.
Androgen dependent tumour.
Abnormal vaginal bleeding that has not been fully investigated.

Warnings:

Use in pregnancy: There is epidemiological and toxicological evidence of hazard in human pregnancy. Danazol is known to be associated with the risk of virilisation to the female foetus if administered during human pregnancy. Danazol should not be used during pregnancy. Women of child bearing age should be advised to use an effective, non-hormonal method of contraception.

Use during lactation: Danazol has the theoretical potential for androgenic effects in breast-fed infants and therefore either danazol therapy or breast feeding should be discontinued.

Particular care should be observed when using Danol in patients with hepatic or renal disease, hypertension or other cardiovascular disease and in any state which may be exacerbated by fluid retention as well as in diabetes mellitus, polycythaemia, epilepsy, lipoprotein disorder, in those with a history of thrombosis and in those who have shown marked or persistent androgenic reaction to previous gonadal steroid therapy. Adjustment in concomitant therapy may be called for particularly in patients with hypertension, diabetes mellitus or epilepsy, when introducing or discontinuing Danol as well as during Danol treatment.

Caution is advised in patients with migraine. Until more is known, caution is also advised in the use of Danol in the presence of known or suspected malignant disease (see also contra-indications). The presence of carcinoma should be excluded before continuing Danol therapy if breast nodules persist or enlarge during treatment.

In the event of virilisation, Danol should be withdrawn. Whilst androgenic reactions will generally prove reversible, continued use of Danol in the face of evident virilisation is likely to cause irreversible change.

In addition to clinical monitoring in all patients, appropriate laboratory monitoring should be considered which may include periodic measurement of hepatic function and haematological state.

Experience of long term therapy with Danol is limited. Whilst a course of therapy may need to be repeated, care should be observed. The long term risk of 17-alkylated steroids (including benign hepatic adenomata and peliosis hepatis), should be considered when danazol, which is chemically related to these compounds is used for periods longer than those normally recommended.

Interactions: Anti-convulsant therapy: Danol may affect the plasma level of carbamazepine and, possibly, the patient's response to this agent and to phenytoin. With phenobarbitone it is likely that similar interaction would occur.

Anti-diabetic therapy: Danol can cause insulin resistance.

Anti-coagulant therapy: Danol can potentiate the action of warfarin.

Anti-hypertensive therapy: possibly through promotion of fluid retention, Danol can oppose the action of anti-hypertensive agents.

Cyclosporin: Danol can increase the plasma level of cyclosporin.

Concomitant steroids: although specific instances have not been described, it is likely that interactions will occur between Danol and gonadal steroid therapy.

Migraine therapy: Danol may itself provoke migraine and possibly reduce the effectiveness of medication to prevent that condition.

Ethyl alcohol: subjective intolerance in the form of nausea and shortness of breath has been reported.

Alpha calcidol: Danol may increase the calcaemic response in primary hypoparathyroidism necessitating a reduction in dosage of this agent.

Side-effects: The possible causal relationship between Danol and many of the following events reportedly associated with its use remains to be defined.

Androgenic effects include weight gain, acne and seborrhoea. Hirsutism, hair loss, voice change, which may take the form of hoarseness, sore throat or of instability or deepening of pitch, may occur. Hypertrophy of the clitoris is rare.

Other possible endocrine effects include menstrual disturbances in the form of spotting, alteration of the timing of the cycle and amenorrhoea. Although cyclical bleeding and ovulation usually return within 60–90 days after Danol, persistent amenorrhoea has occasionally been reported. Flushing, vaginal dryness and irritation and reduction in breast size, may reflect lowering of oestrogen. In the male a modest reduction in spermatogenesis may be evident during treatment.

Insulin resistance may be increased in diabetes mellitus, but symptomatic hypoglycaemia in non-diabetic patients has also been reported as has an increase in plasma glucagon level.

Danol may aggravate epilepsy and expose the condition in those so predisposed.

Cutaneous reactions include rashes, which may be maculopapular, petechial, or purpuric or may take an urticarial form and may be accompanied by facial oedema. Associated fever has also been reported. Rarely, sun-sensitive rash has been noted. Inflammatory erythematous nodules, changes in skin pigmentation and exfoliative dermatitis have also been reported.

Musculo-skeletal reactions include backache and muscle cramps which can be severe. Creatine phosphokinase levels may also rise. Muscle tremors, fasciculation, limb pain, joint pain and joint swelling have also been reported.

Cardiovascular reactions may include exacerbation of hypertension, palpitation and tachycardia.

Benign intracranial hypertension, visual disturbances

which may take the form of blurring or difficulty in focusing and in wearing contact lenses or need for temporary alteration in refractive correction, have been noted.

Haematological responses include an increase in red cell and platelet count. Reversible erythrocytosis or polycythaemia may be provoked. Eosinophilia, leucopenia and thrombocytopenia have also been noted.

Arterial or venous thrombosis is unlikely because danazol activates both the fibrinolytic system and inhibitors in the clotting cascade. Clinical and epidemiological evidence supports this conclusion. Rare occurrences of sagittal sinus and cerebrovascular thrombosis have been observed but their association with danazol is unclear.

Hepatic reactions include modest increases in serum transaminase levels, and, rarely, cholestatic jaundice. Benign hepatic adenomata and peliosis hepatis have been observed with long term use.

Fluid retention may explain the occasional reports of carpal tunnel syndrome. Danol may also provoke migraine.

Possible psychical reactions include increased appetite, emotional lability, anxiety, depressed mood, nervousness and changes in libido. Dizziness, vertigo, nausea, headache, fatigue and epigastric and pleuritic pain have also been noted.

A temporary alteration of lipoproteins in the form of an increase in LDL cholesterol, a decrease in HDL, affecting all subfractions, and a decrease in apolipoproteins AI and AII, is likely with Danol in the female. The clinical significance of these changes is not established.

Reduction in thyroid binding globulin, T4, with increased uptake of T3 but without disturbance of thyroid stimulating hormone or free thyroxin index, is also likely during therapy.

Haematuria has rarely been reported with prolonged use in patients with hereditary angioedema.

Overdosage: In animal tests, doses of 16,000 mg/kg body weight produced no fatalities and it is unlikely that any immediate serious reactions would be seen from a single excessive dose in man.

In the case of acute overdosage, the drug should be removed by emesis or stomach pump (if ingestion is recent) and the patient should be kept under observation in case of any delayed reactions.

Pharmaceutical precautions Nil.

Legal category POM.

Package quantities Danol 200 mg capsules are supplied in cartons of 50 and 100 in blisters and as Danol 200 C-Pak in calendar packs of 56 (OP).
Danol 100 mg capsules are supplied in cartons of 50 and 100 in blisters.

Further information Nil.

Product licence numbers

Danol 200 mg	0071/0095
Danol 100 mg	0071/0094

ERADACIN*

Presentation Eradacin capsules are No. 1 opaque, red/yellow capsules filled with a white powder. Each capsule contains 150 mg acrosoxacin (rosoxacin I.N.N.) Eradacin capsules contain lactose.

Uses Eradacin is for the treatment of acute gonorrhoea infection in both male and female patients.

Dosage and administration Eradacin is for oral administration only.

Adults including the elderly: A single dose of two capsules (300 mg) preferably on an empty stomach.

Children: Not recommended.

Contra-indications, warnings, etc Safe use during human pregnancy has not yet been established and Eradacin should be used only when necessitated by the anticipated bacteriological and clinical benefits.

It should be used with caution in patients with impaired renal or hepatic function.

Because Eradacin may cause dizziness and drowsiness, patients should be warned not to drive or operate machinery if affected.

Eradacin has been shown to induce lesions in weight-bearing joints of young animals receiving high, single or repeated doses. The relevance of this to man is unknown but it is recommended that frequent, repeated doses should not be given to those under 18 years of age.

Side-effects: Occasionally headaches, gastro-intestinal upsets, dizziness and drowsiness may occur.

Overdosage: Animal toxicity studies suggest that CNS depression is a likely symptom of overdosage. If vomiting does not occur, the drug should be removed by emesis or gastric lavage, if ingestion is recent, and symptomatic treatment applied.

Pharmaceutical precautions None.

Legal category POM.

Package quantities Eradacin is supplied in blister packs of 20 capsules.

Further information A single dose of 300 mg Eradacin has been shown to produce a cure rate of over 90% in cases of uncomplicated gonococcal urethritis. Treatment with Eradacin may be successful in patients infected with *N. gonorrhoeae* strains resistant to penicillin and other antibiotics.

Product licence number 0071/0168.

FERGON*

Presentation Fergon Tablets are smoothly polished, red, sugar-coated tablets with no markings, each containing 300 mg Ferrous Gluconate PhEur, which provides 35 mg elemental iron. Fergon Tablets contain dextrose, sucrose, Carmoisine (E122) and Ponceau 4R(E124).

Uses Fergon Tablets are recommended for the treatment and prophylaxis of uncomplicated iron deficiency anaemia.

Dosage and administration Fergon is for oral administration. It is best administered about one hour before meals.

Adults (including the elderly and pregnant women from the second trimester):
Prophylactic: 2 tablets (600 mg) daily.

Therapeutic: 4–6 tablets (1.2–1.8 g) daily in divided doses.

Children: Children aged 6–12 years may be given 1–3 tablets daily for therapeutic purposes. A smaller dose may be sufficient for prophylaxis. Not recommended for children under 6 years.

Contra-indications, warnings, etc
Contra-indications: Fergon tablets should not be given to patients receiving repeated blood transfusions or those with haemosiderosis, haemochromatosis, haemolytic anaemia, active peptic ulcer, regional enteritis, ulcerative colitis or hypersensitivity to ferrous gluconate.

Precautions: Fergon should be used with caution in patients with iron-absorption diseases, for example post-gastrectomy, or those with haemoglobinopathies, existing gastrointestinal disease or history of peptic ulcer.

Iron preparations may have a constipating effect in the elderly.

Duration of treatment should generally not exceed 3 months after correction of anaemia. Co-existing deficiency of vitamin B12 or folic acid should be excluded. Iron deficiency in males should be carefully investigated to determine primary treatment.

Administration of drugs during the first trimester of pregnancy requires careful assessment of potential risks versus benefits to be gained and should not be undertaken unless clearly indicated. For the remainder of pregnancy, iron therapy may be indicated but only on the advice of a physician.

Interactions: The absorption of iron is decreased when iron salts are given concomitantly with antacids, zinc salts, tetracyclines, penicillamine, cholestyramine, tea, eggs or milk. Conversely, iron salts decrease the absorption of zinc salts, ciprofloxacin, tetracycline, penicillamine and methyldopa. Chloramphenicol delays plasma clearance of iron and incorporation of iron into red cells by interfering with erythropoiesis.

Side-effects: Side-effects to iron salts are mainly gastrointestinal and include anorexia, nausea, vomiting, heartburn, epigastric pain, diarrhoea, constipation, dark stools and allergic reactions. They occur in 15–20% of patients and are usually mild or moderate. Neutropenia has also been reported.

Overdosage: Iron overdosage is an acute emergency requiring urgent medical attention. An acute intake of 75 mg/kg elemental iron is considered extremely dangerous in young children.

Initial symptoms include nausea, vomiting, diarrhoea, abdominal pain, haematemesis, rectal bleeding, lethargy and circulatory collapse. Hyperglycaemia and metabolic acidosis may also occur. In severe cases, after a latent phase, relapse may occur after 24–48 hours, manifest by hypotension, coma, hypothermia, hepatocellular necrosis, renal failure, pulmonary oedema, diffuse vascular congestion, coagulopathy and/or convulsions. Full recovery may be complicated by long term effects such as hepatic necrosis, toxic encephalitis, CNS damage and pyloric stenosis.

If overdose is suspected, treatment should be implemented immediately as follows and serum iron levels monitored throughout:

Children:

1. Administer an emetic such as syrup of ipecac.
2. Gastric lavage should be undertaken with desferrioxamine solution (2 g/l) followed by the introduction and retention in the stomach of desferrioxamine 5 g in 50–100 ml water. Inducing diarrhoea in young children may be dangerous and should therefore not be undertaken. Keep the patient under constant surveillance (to detect possible aspiration of vomitus) with suction apparatus and emergency oxygen to hand.
3. Severe poisoning: in the presence of shock and/or coma with high serum iron levels (>90 micromol/l) institute immediate supportive measures and administer desferrioxamine 15 mg/kg/hour by slow iv infusion to a maximum 80 mg/kg/24 hours. Hypotension may occur if the infusion rate is too rapid.
4. Less severe poisoning: administer desferrioxamine intramuscularly 1 g 4–6 hourly.

Adults:

1. Initial management is similar to that for children (see 1 and 2 above), but small bowel emptying may also be induced by giving mannitol or sorbitol.
2. Severe poisoning; in the presence of shock and/or coma with high serum levels (>142 micromol/l), institute immediate supportive measures and administer desferrioxamine 5 mg/kg/hour by slow iv infusion to a maximum of 80 mg/kg/24 hours. Hypotension may occur if the infusion rate is too rapid.
3. Less severe poisoning: administer desferrioxamine intramuscularly 50 mg/kg to a maximum dose of 4 g.

Pharmaceutical precautions Protect from light.

Legal category P.

Package quantities Fergon is supplied in bottles of 100 tablets.

Further information Following administration as ferrous salt, iron is absorbed throughout the gastrointestinal tract but mainly in the duodenum and proximal jejunum. It is transported in the blood, bound to a plasma protein transferrin. Peak plasma-iron concentrations in healthy subjects occur about 2 hours after the administration of ferrous sulphate.

Approximately 5–10% dietary iron is absorbed during prophylaxis and 10–30% in iron deficient subjects. Transfer of iron across the placenta is an active process. Excess iron ingested is stored as ferritin and haemosiderin.

Product licence number 0071/5032.

FORTAGESIC*

Presentation White tablets with bevelled edges 12.7 mm diameter, marked with an ankh on one side and FORTAGESIC on the other. Each tablet provides Pentazocine BP 15 mg (as the hydrochloride) and Paracetamol PhEur 500 mg. Fortagesic tablets contain sodium metabisulphite.

Uses Fortagesic is a compound analgesic for the relief of moderate pain associated with musculoskeletal disorders or injuries, such as bursitis, sprains, strains, fibrositis, sciatica and osteoarthritis, and for rheumatoid arthritis in patients sensitive to aspirin.

Dosage and administration Fortagesic is for oral administration only.

Adults including the elderly: 2 tablets up to four times daily.

Children: 7–12 years: 1 tablet every three to four hours. Not more than 4 doses to be taken in any 24 hour period. Not recommended for children under 7 years of age.

Contra-indications, warnings, etc

Contra-indications: Fortagesic should not be administered to patients with established respiratory depression, especially in the presence of cyanosis and excessive bronchial secretion and is also contraindicated in the presence of acute alcoholism, head injuries, conditions in which intracranial pressure is raised, acute bronchial asthma, in heart failure, secondary to chronic lung disease and in patients known to be hypersensitive to pentazocine or paracetamol.

Warnings:

Use in pregnancy and lactation: There is epidemiological evidence for the safety of paracetamol in human pregnancy. No such evidence exists for pentazocine but it has been widely used for many years without apparent ill consequences. In rodents, harmful effects in the foetus have been observed but only at doses high enough to cause maternal toxicity. Pentazocine can enter the foetal circulation and has the potential to cause opioid effects including central depression and abstinence syndrome in the foetus (see below). It does not appear to have significant adverse effects on uterine function at parturition. Nonetheless, careful consideration should be given to the use of Fortagesic during pregnancy, particularly during the first trimester, or at term.

There are insufficient data on the secretion of pentazocine in breast milk so it is recommended that infants of nursing mothers who are receiving high doses of Fortagesic be appropriately monitored.

Precautions:

Particular caution should be observed in administering Fortagesic to patients with porphyria, since it may provoke an acute attack in susceptible individuals, as well as in its use in patients who are receiving monoamine oxidase inhibitors or who have received them within the preceding 14 days.

Pentazocine can both depress as well as elevate blood pressure possibly through the release of endogenous catecholamines. Particular caution should be observed therefore in using Fortagesic in the presence of phaeochromocytoma, in the acute phase following myocardial infarction when it may increase pulmonary and systemic blood pressure and vascular resistance and in other clinical situations where alteration of vascular resistance or blood pressure might be particularly undesirable.

Caution should be observed in patients with renal or hepatic impairment and in elderly patients, who may additionally be especially sensitive to the effects of opioids, as both conditions may lead to an increase in bioavailability of pentazocine and call for a reduction in dosage.

Caution should also be observed in patients who are

prone to seizures and in the presence of other opioids or opioid-dependence since the weak opioid antagonistic effects of pentazocine may provoke withdrawal symptoms.

Caution should also be observed in patients with hypothyroidism, adrenocortical insufficiency, prostatic hypertrophy and in patients with inflammatory or obstructive bowel disorders.

Pentazocine may produce sedation, so ambulant patients should be warned not to operate machinery or drive if affected.

In chronic usage, care should be exercised to avoid any unnecessary increase in dosage since prolonged use of high doses of pentazocine may produce dependence.

Interactions: Monoamine oxidase inhibitors may enhance the opioid effects of pentazocine and the agents may interact through their respective effects on catecholamine breakdown and release. Agents with sedative action including phenothiazines and ethyl alcohol can enhance the central depressant effects of pentazocine which are opposed by respiratory stimulants such as doxapram. Tobacco smoking appears to enhance the metabolic clearance rate of pentazocine reducing the clinical effectiveness of a standard dose of pentazocine.

Pentazocine can antagonise the effects of stronger opioid agonists such as diamorphine, morphine and heroin and is itself antagonised by naloxone.

Side-effects: At normal therapeutic doses side-effects are generally of a minor nature. Paracetamol is extremely well tolerated. Any side-effects to Fortagesic are likely to be due to pentazocine which may cause lightheadedness, dizziness, nausea and vomiting, sedation and sweating. Pentazocine may also cause headache, dry mouth, constipation, flushing of the skin, tachycardia, mood changes, nightmares, paraesthesia, pruritus, biliary tract spasm and urinary retention. Respiratory depression, raised intracranial pressure, hypotension, transient hypertension can also occur. Altered uterine contractions, muscle tremor, insomnia, disorientation, hallucinations, disturbances of vision, transient depression of white blood cells, chills and allergic reactions have also been reported. After large intravenous doses, grand mal convulsions have been noted.

Abrupt discontinuation of pentazocine in patients receiving large parenteral doses over a prolonged period of time may result in withdrawal symptoms, which can also occur in the newborn following prolonged in utero exposure. The abstinence syndrome of pentazocine is not typical of opiate dependence. Symptoms include mild abdominal cramps, nausea, vomiting, nervousness or restlessness, dizziness, fever and chills, but are mild compared with symptoms of opiate withdrawal. Managing the abstinence syndrome of pentazocine has raised few problems. Supportive therapy with tranquillisers may sometimes be required. It should be emphasised that the majority of patients reported to have become dependent on pentazocine had previously been dependent on opiates or had misused other drugs.

Overdose: The symptoms and clinical signs of Fortagesic overdose are likely to resemble those of the individual ingredients. Thus with pentazocine, as with morphine and other opioids, there may be somnolence, respiratory depression and hypotension. Circulatory failure and deepening coma may occur in more severe cases, as may convulsions. Adequate measures to maintain ventilation and general circulatory support should be employed. Anti-convulsant therapy may be necessary and the specific antagonist naloxone should be employed appropriately to reverse any CNS depression.

With paracetamol overdose, patients may appear well for the first three days, then succumb with liver damage. The hepatic changes produced by overdosage of paracetamol result from the accumulation of a highly active intermediate metabolite in the hepatocytes.

N-acetylcysteine intravenously or methionine orally protects the liver if administered within 10–12 hours of ingesting an overdose.

In managing Fortagesic overdose, consideration should be given to gastric lavage and aspiration.

Pharmaceutical precautions Nil.

Legal category CD (Sch 3) POM.

Package quantities Fortagesic is supplied in bottles of 100 tablets.

Further information Paracetamol is rapidly and completely absorbed from the gastro-intestinal tract, it is relatively uniformly distributed throughout most body fluids and exhibits variable protein binding. Excretion is almost exclusively renal, in the form of conjugated metabolites.

Pentazocine is a strong opioid analgesic with weak opioid antagonist properties. By mouth, pentazocine has a bioavailability of about 47%. In the plasma it is 50–75% bound to protein and has an elimination half-life of about 4.6 hours. Peak plasma concentrations are obtained in 1 to 3 hours. Pentazocine diffuses across the placenta and appears in cerebro-spinal fluid in concentrations reaching 30–50% of those in plasma. It is metabolised by the liver, only a small proportion of a dose being excreted unchanged in the urine.

Product licence number 0071/0022.

FORTRAL* (pentazocine)

Presentation 1. A sterile, isotonic aqueous solution for intramuscular, intravenous or subcutaneous injection containing Pentazocine BP 30 mg/ml as the lactate in 1 ml or 2 ml ampoules. Fortral injection contains sodium chloride and lactic acid.

2. No. 4 hard gelatine, grey/yellow capsules marked FORTRAL 50. Each capsule contains Pentazocine Hydrochloride BP 50 mg (equivalent to 44.3 mg base). Fortral capsules contain lactose.

3. White, torpedo-shaped suppositories, average weight 1.9 g, for rectal administration. Each suppository contains Pentazocine BP 50 mg as the lactate.

4. White, bi-convex film-coated tablets, 9.5 mm diameter, marked fortral on one face and with an ankh on the other. Each tablet contains Pentazocine Hydrochloride BP 25 mg (equivalent to 22.17 mg base). Fortral tablets contain sodium metabisulphite and lactose.

Uses Fortral is a strong analgesic for the relief of moderate to severe pain.

Dosage and administration 1. *Fortral Ampoules: Adults:* Fortral injections may be administered subcutaneously, intramuscularly or intravenously. The usual starting dose is 30 mg to 60 mg according to pain severity. The dose should be adjusted according to response and repeated as necessary every three to four hours.

A dose should not normally exceed 1 mg/kg body weight subcutaneously or intramuscularly or 500 microgrammes/kg intravenously.

Children: In the case of patients between the ages of 1 year and 12 years, the maximum single dose of parenteral Fortral should be calculated on the basis of 1 mg/kg body weight by subcutaneous or intramuscular injection or 500 microgrammes/kg body weight intravenously. There are no dosage recommendations for children less than one year old.

Elderly: Since impaired renal or hepatic function is often associated with ageing, elderly patients may require smaller doses of Fortral.

As with most parenteral drugs, when frequent daily injections are needed over long periods, intramuscular administration is preferable to subcutaneous. To reduce the risk of local tissue damage it is recommended that intramuscular sites of injection be rotated, e.g. deltoid areas, upper outer quadrants of the buttocks and midlateral aspects of the thighs.

2. Fortral Capsules: Adults: The usual recommended dosage is one to two 50 mg capsules every three to four hours after meals according to the response of the patient. Dosage is best tailored to the individual patient and to the response.

Children: For children under 12 years of age, it is

recommended that other dosage forms of Fortral, tablets or injection, be used as appropriate.

Elderly: Since impaired renal or hepatic function is often associated with ageing, elderly patients may require smaller doses of Fortral.

3. *Fortral Suppositories: Adults:* 1 suppository at any one time. It will not normally be necessary to exceed 4 suppositories daily.

Children: Fortral Suppositories are not suitable for administration to children under 12 years of age.

Elderly: Since impaired renal or hepatic function is often associated with ageing, elderly patients may require smaller doses of Fortral.

4. *Fortral Tablets: Adults:* The usual starting dose is two 25 mg tablets every four hours after meals, but dosage is best tailored to the individual patient and to the degree of pain within the range of 25–100 mg every three to four hours.

Children: 6–12 years: One 25 mg tablet every three to four hours as required.

1–6 years: The recommended dosage is such that Fortral injection is considered to be a more convenient dosage form.

Under 1 year: Fortral tablets are not recommended for children less than 1 year old.

Elderly: Since impaired renal or hepatic function is often associated with ageing, elderly patients may require smaller doses of Fortral.

Contra-indications, warnings, etc

Contra-indications: Fortral should not be administered to patients with established respiratory depression, especially in the presence of cyanosis and excessive bronchial secretion and is also contraindicated in the presence of acute alcoholism, head injuries, conditions in which intracranial pressure is raised, acute bronchial asthma, in heart failure, secondary to chronic lung disease and in patients known to be hypersensitive to pentazocine.

Warnings

Use in pregnancy and lactation: There is no epidemiological evidence for the safety of pentazocine in human pregnancy but it has been widely used for many years without apparent ill consequences. In rodents, harmful effects in the foetus have been observed but only at doses high enough to cause maternal toxicity. Pentazocine can enter the foetal circulation and has the potential to cause opioid effects including central depression and abstinence syndrome in the foetus (see below). It does not appear to have significant adverse effects on uterine function at parturition. Nonetheless, careful consideration should be given to the use of Fortral during pregnancy, particularly during the first trimester, or at term.

There are insufficient data on the secretion of pentazocine in breast milk so it is recommended that infants of nursing mothers who are receiving high doses of Fortral be appropriately monitored.

Precautions: Particular caution should be observed in administering Fortral to patients with porphyria since it may provoke an acute attack in susceptible individuals as well as in its use in patients who are receiving monoamine oxidase inhibitors or who have received them within the preceding 14 days.

Pentazocine can both depress as well as elevate blood pressure possibly through the release of endogenous catecholamines. Particular caution should be observed therefore in using it in the presence of phaeochromocytoma, in the acute phase following myocardial infarction when it may increase pulmonary and systemic arterial pressure and vascular resistance, and in other clinical situations where alteration of vascular resistance and blood pressure might be particularly undesirable.

Caution should be observed in patients with renal or hepatic impairment and in elderly patients, who may additionally be especially sensitive to the effects of opioids, as both conditions may lead to an increase in bioavailability of pentazocine and call for a reduction in dosage.

Caution should also be observed in patients who are prone to seizures and in the presence of other opioids or opioid-dependence since the weak opioid antagonistic effects of pentazocine may provoke withdrawal symptoms.

Caution should also be observed in patients with hypothyroidism, adrenocortical insufficiency, prostatic hypertrophy and in patients with inflammatory or obstructive bowel disorders.

Pentazocine may produce sedation, so ambulant patients should be warned not to operate machinery or drive if affected.

In chronic usage, care should be exercised to avoid any unnecessary increase in dosage since prolonged use of high doses of pentazocine may produce dependence.

Interactions: Monoamine oxidase inhibitors may enhance the opioid effects of pentazocine and the agents may interact through their respective effects on catecholamine breakdown and release. Agents with sedative action including phenothiazines and ethyl alcohol can enhance the central depressant effects of pentazocine which are opposed by respiratory stimulants such as doxapram. Tobacco smoking appears to enhance the metabolic clearance rate of pentazocine reducing the clinical effectiveness of a standard dose of Fortral.

Pentazocine can antagonise the effects of stronger opioid agonists such as diamorphine, morphine and heroin and is itself antagonised by naloxone.

Side-effects: At normal therapeutic doses side effects are generally of a minor nature. The most frequent side effects of Fortral are lightheadedness, dizziness, nausea and vomiting, sedation and sweating. It may also cause headache, dry mouth, constipation, flushing of the skin, tachycardia, mood changes, nightmares, paraesthesia, pruritus, biliary tract spasm and urinary retention. Respiratory depression, raised intracranial pressure, hypotension, transient hypertension can also occur. Altered uterine contractions, muscle tremor, insomnia, disorientation, hallucinations, disturbances of vision, transient eosinophilia, depression of white cells, chills and allergic reactions have also been reported. After large intravenous doses, grand mal convulsions have been noted. Local tissue damage at injection sites has been reported, particularly after subcutaneous injection or multiple doses.

Abrupt discontinuation in patients receiving large parenteral doses over a prolonged period of time may result in withdrawal symptoms, which can also occur in the newborn following prolonged in utero exposure to pentazocine. The abstinence syndrome of pentazocine is not typical of opiate dependence. Symptoms include mild abdominal cramps, nausea, vomiting, nervousness or restlessness, dizziness, fever and chills, but are mild compared with symptoms of opiate withdrawal. Managing the abstinence syndrome of pentazocine has raised few problems. Supportive therapy with tranquillisers may sometimes be required. It should be emphasised that the majority of patients reported to have become dependent on Fortral had previously been dependent on opiates or had misused other drugs.

Overdosage: The symptoms and clinical signs of Fortral overdose will resemble those of morphine and other opioids. They may therefore include somnolence, respiratory depression and hypotension. Circulatory failure and deepening coma may occur in more severe cases as may convulsions. Adequate measures to maintain ventilation and general circulatory support should be employed and consideration given to gastric lavage and gastric aspiration.

Anti-convulsant therapy may be necessary and the specific antagonist naloxone should be employed appropriately.

Pharmaceutical precautions Fortral injection appears to be compatible for up to seven days with most commonly used infusion solutions. The exceptions are those which contain sodium bicarbonate, where the high pH causes immediate precipitation of pentazocine base.

Fortral is chemically compatible with atropine sulphate, hyoscine hydrobromide and promethazine hydrochloride. Precipitation will occur if Fortral injection is mixed in the same syringe with soluble barbiturates, diazepam or with chlordiazepoxide.

Fortral Suppositories should be stored in a cool place and the ampoules should be protected from light.

Legal category CD (Sch 3), POM.

Package quantities
1. Ampoules in boxes of ten 1 ml or 2 ml.
2. Capsules in bottles of 100.
3. Suppositories in PVC/PE laminate strips. Boxes of 20.
4. Tablets in bottles of 100.

Further information Pentazocine is a strong opioid analgesic with weak opioid antagonist properties. By mouth, pentazocine has a bioavailability of about 47%. In the plasma it is 50–75% bound to protein and has an elimination half-life of about 4.6 hours. With rectal administration, peak plasma concentrations of 50–100 nanograms/ml are obtained in about 2.5 hours and with oral administration in 1–3 hours. Pentazocine diffuses across the placenta and appears in cerebrospinal fluid in concentrations reaching 30–50% of those in plasma. It is metabolised by the liver, only a small proportion of a dose being excreted unchanged in the urine.

Product licence numbers

Fortral Ampoules	0071/5033
Fortral Capsules	0071/5034
Fortral Suppositories	0071/0064
Fortral Tablets	0071/5035

FRANOL*

Presentation Franol Tablets are flat, white tablets with bevelled edges, 8.7 mm in diameter, marked F on one side and with an ankh symbol on the other side. Each tablet contains 120 mg Theophylline PhEur and 11 mg Ephedrine Hydrochloride PhEur.

Uses Franol Tablets are recommended for the management of bronchospasm in reversible airway-obstruction associated with stable asthma or chronic bronchitis.

Dosage and administration Oral administration only. *Adults:* Dosage varies with individual requirements and should be adjusted accordingly. The usual dosage is 3 tablets daily (morning, midday and evening). For the patient who suffers nocturnal attacks, an extra tablet taken at bedtime is recommended.

Elderly: As for adults but see 'Use in special groups'.

Children: Not recommended for children under 12 years of age.

If more than four tablets a day are required, it is advisable to monitor plasma theophylline levels during dose titration to ensure that levels are kept below 20 micrograms/ml.

Contra-indications, warnings, etc
Contra-indications: Franol should not be given to patients who are sensitive to either of its ingredients or to patients with unstable angina, cardiac arrhythmias, severe hypertension, severe coronary artery disease, porphyria or to those receiving other xanthines. Franol should not be used during pregnancy.

Precautions: Avoid or use only with special caution in patients with cardiovascular disease, hypertension, agitation, phaeochromocytoma, hyperthyroidism, closed-angle glaucoma, prostatic hypertrophy, peptic ulceration, underlying seizure disorders, patients receiving anti-depressant drugs, or patients on MAO inhibitors within the previous 14 days. Special caution is also needed in the elderly, those with hepatic, renal, or cardiac dysfunction and during lactation. Ephedrine has a potential for tachyphylaxis, and abuse with dependence has been reported.

Potentially serious hypokalaemia can result from the use of $beta_2$ agonists and xanthines in combination particularly when hypoxia is present. The effect may be enhanced by concomitant diuretics or corticosteroids. Care should be observed and serum potassium levels monitored in patients receiving Franol who develop severe asthma, particularly if concomitant diuretic, corticosteroid or $beta_2$ agonist therapy is being employed.

Use in special groups:

Pregnancy: Although caffeine has been implicated as a teratogen, adequate animal teratogenic studies have not been conducted with theophylline nor with ephedrine. The safety of ephedrine and of theophylline, which crosses the placental barrier, have not been established in human pregnancy. Franol should not therefore be prescribed for patients who are pregnant.

Lactation: Theophylline distributes readily into breast milk therefore Franol should be used with caution in nursing women.

Hepatic dysfunction: Theophylline is eliminated primarily by metabolism in the liver. Thus in patients with severe liver disease, theophylline clearance may be decreased. If Franol is used in such patients, dosage may need to be reduced.

Renal dysfunction: Ephedrine is excreted largely unchanged in the urine, therefore Franol should be used with caution in patients with severe renal impairment.

Cardiac dysfunction: Theophylline clearance may be decreased in patients with congestive cardiac failure, acute pulmonary oedema or cor pulmonale, and theophylline may cause arrhythmias or worsen existing arrhythmias, thus caution should be exercised if Franol is used in such patients.

Elderly (over 65 years): Theophylline clearance decreases slightly with age. Elderly patients will tend therefore to have higher serum theophylline levels than younger adults at a given dose. They should be monitored closely for signs of toxicity during dose adjustment.

Others: Theophylline clearance may be increased in heavy smokers, decreased in patients with respiratory infection or those on a high carbohydrate – low protein diet, therefore the dose of Franol may need to be adjusted appropriately in these groups.

Drug interactions: Theophylline clearance may be decreased by concurrent administration of cimetidine, macrolide antibiotics, oral contraceptives, interferons, diltiazem, verapamil and viloxazine. Ciprofloxacin also increases plasma theophylline concentrations and if concomitant use is essential, the dose of theophylline should be reduced and plasma concentrations closely monitored to avoid toxicity. Theophylline clearance may be increased by concurrent administration of barbiturates, carbamazepine, phenytoin, rifampicin, sulphinpyrazone, aminoglutethimide, phenobarbitone and primidone.

Lithium excretion is accelerated by theophylline.

The effects of ephedrine are diminished by guanethidine, reserpine, and probably methyldopa, and may be diminished or enhanced by tricyclic anti-depressants. Ephedrine may also diminish the effects of guanethidine and may increase the possibility of arrhythmias in digitalised patients.

Side-effects: Potentially serious hypokalaemia may result from $beta_2$ agonists and xanthines in combination.

Large doses of Franol may give rise to the following side effects: arrhythmias, tachycardia, palpitation, flushing, giddiness, headache, tremor, anxiety, restlessness, insomnia, muscular weakness, nausea, vomiting, dyspepsia, thirst, sweating, difficulty in micturition.

Some patients may exhibit one or more such symptoms with therapeutic doses.

Overdosage: The symptoms and signs of overdosage with Franol are likely to include excessive irritability, sweating, nausea and vomiting, tachycardia, arrhythmias, hypertension, profuse diuresis with fever, flushing and hyperglycaemia, opisthotonus, hallucinations, convulsions and respiratory difficulty. In general the management of overdosage with Franol involves supportive and symptomatic therapy with particular attention being paid to the detection and correction of hypokalaemia, and should include serial assay of plasma potassium and theophylline levels, cardiac monitoring with electrocardiogram, and maintenance of fluid and electrolyte balance.

Gastric aspiration and lavage may be employed. Convulsions and other CNS stimulation can usually be controlled by intravenous diazepam, or if that fails other anti-convulsants may be used. Marked excitement or hallucinations may be managed with chlorpromazine. Severe hypertension may necessitate the use of an alpha-adrenoreceptor blocking agent and a beta-adrenoreceptor blocking agent may be required to control arrhythmias. Beta 1-receptor agonists such as dopamine should be avoided. Charcoal haemoperfusion may be indicated to remove theophylline, but forced diuresis or peritoneal dialysis are inadequate for this purpose.

Pharmaceutical precautions Nil.

Legal category POM.

Package quantities Franol Tablets are supplied in bottles of 100 and 500.

Further information The bronchodilator action of ephedrine is through direct agonism at beta adrenoceptors and, indirectly, through sympathetic amine release. Bronchodilatation with theophylline is attributable to adenosine antagonism or phosphodiesterase inhibition which would be pharmacologically complementary to the action of ephedrine. Theophylline is variably absorbed from the gastrointestinal tract. It is excreted via the urine mainly as 1,3-dimethyluric acid. About 10% is unchanged. Ephedrine is readily absorbed. Its action is evident within one hour. With a plasma elimination half life of about 4 hours, 60–75% is excreted unchanged in the urine.

Product licence number 0071/5036R.

FRANOL* PLUS

Presentation Franol Plus Tablets are flat, white tablets with bevelled edges, 8.7 mm in diameter, marked F+ on one side and with an ankh symbol on the other. Each tablet contains 120 mg Theophylline PhEur and 15 mg Ephedrine Sulphate USP.

Uses Franol Plus Tablets are recommended for the management of bronchospasm in reversible airway-obstruction associated with stable asthma or chronic bronchitis.

Dosage and administration Oral administration only. *Adults:* Dosage varies with individual requirements and should be adjusted accordingly. The usual dosage is 3 tablets daily (morning, midday and evening). For the patient who suffers from nocturnal attacks, an extra tablet at bedtime is recommended.

Elderly: As for adults but see 'Use in special groups'.

Children: Not recommended for children under 12 years of age.

If more than four tablets a day are required, it is advisable to monitor plasma theophylline levels during dose titration to ensure that levels are kept below 20 micrograms/ml.

Contra-indications, warnings, etc
Contra-indications: Franol Plus should not be given to patients who are sensitive to either of its ingredients or to patients with unstable angina, cardiac arrhythmias, severe hypertension, severe coronary artery disease, porphyria or to those receiving other xanthines. Franol Plus should not be used during pregnancy.

Precautions: Avoid or use only with special caution in patients with cardiovascular disease, hypertension, agitation, phaeochromocytoma, hyperthyroidism, closed-angle glaucoma, prostatic hypertrophy, peptic ulceration, underlying seizure disorders, patients receiving anti-depressant drugs, or patients on MAO inhibitors within the previous 14 days. Special caution is also needed in the elderly, those with hepatic, renal, or cardiac dysfunction and during lactation. Ephedrine has a potential for tachyphylaxis, and abuse with dependence has been reported.

Potentially serious hypokalaemia can result from the use of beta$_2$ agonists and xanthines in combination particularly when hypoxia is present. The effect may be enhanced by concomitant diuretics or corticosteroids. Care should be observed and serum potassium levels monitored in patients receiving Franol who develop severe asthma, particularly if concomitant diuretic, corticosteroid or beta$_2$ agonist therapy is being employed.

Use in special groups:
Pregnancy: Although caffeine has been implicated as a teratogen, adequate animal teratogenic studies have not been conducted with theophylline nor with ephedrine. The safety of ephedrine and of theophylline, which crosses the placental barrier, have not been established in human pregnancy. Franol Plus should not therefore be prescribed for patients who are pregnant.

Lactation: Theophylline distributes readily into breast milk therefore Franol Plus should be used with caution in nursing women.

Hepatic dysfunction: Theophylline is eliminated primarily by metabolism in the liver. Thus in patients with severe liver disease, theophylline clearance may be decreased. If Franol Plus is used in such patients, dosage may need to be reduced.

Renal dysfunction: Ephedrine is excreted largely unchanged in the urine, therefore Franol Plus should be used with caution in patients with severe renal impairment.

Cardiac dysfunction: Theophylline clearance may be decreased in patients with congestive cardiac failure, acute pulmonary oedema or cor pulmonale, and theophylline may cause arrhythmias or worsen existing arrhythmias, thus caution should be exercised if Franol Plus is used in such patients.

Elderly (over 65 years): Theophylline clearance decreases slightly with age. Elderly patients will tend therefore to have higher serum theophylline levels than younger adults at a given dose. They should be monitored closely for signs of toxicity during dose adjustment.

Others: Theophylline clearance may be increased in heavy smokers, decreased in patients with respiratory infection or those on a high carbohydrate – low protein diet, therefore the dose of Franol Plus may need to be adjusted appropriately in these groups.

Drug interactions: Theophylline clearance may be decreased by concurrent administration of cimetidine, macrolide antibiotics, oral contraceptives, interferons, diltiazem, verapamil and viloxazine. Ciprofloxacin also increases plasma theophylline concentrations and if concomitant use is essential, the dose of theophylline should be reduced and plasma concentrations closely monitored to avoid toxicity. Theophylline clearance may be increased by concurrent administration of barbiturates, carbamazepine, phenytoin, rifampicin, sulphinpyrazone, aminoglutethimide, phenobarbitone and primidone.

Lithium excretion is accelerated by theophylline.

The effects of ephedrine are diminished by guanethidine, reserpine, and probably methyldopa, and may be diminished or enhanced by tricyclic anti-depressants. Ephedrine may also diminish the effects of guanethidine and may increase the possibility of arrhythmias in digitalised patients.

Side-effects: Potentially serious hypokalaemia can result from beta$_2$ agonists and xanthines in combination. Large doses of Franol Plus may give rise to the following side effects: arrhythmias, tachycardia, palpitation, flushing, giddiness, headache, tremor, anxiety, restlessness, insomnia, muscular weakness, nausea, vomiting, dyspepsia, thirst, sweating, difficulty in micturition.

Some patients may exhibit one or more such symptoms with therapeutic doses.

Overdosage: The symptoms and signs of overdosage with Franol Plus are likely to include excessive irritability, sweating, nausea and vomiting, tachycardia, arrhythmias, hypertension, profuse diuresis with fever, flushing and hyperglycaemia, opisthotonus, hallucinations, convulsions and respiratory difficulty. In general the management of overdosage with Franol Plus involves supportive and symptomatic therapy with particular attention being paid to the detection and correction of hypokalaemia, and should include serial assay of plasma potassium and theophylline levels, cardiac monitoring with electro-cardiogram, and maintenance of fluid and electrolyte balance.

Gastric aspiration and lavage may be employed. Convulsions and other CNS stimulation can usually be controlled by intravenous diazepam, or if that fails other anti-convulsants may be used. Marked excitement or hallucinations may be managed with chlorpromazine. Severe hypertension may necessitate the use of an alpha-adrenoreceptor blocking agent and a beta-adrenoreceptor blocking agent may be required to control arrhythmias. Beta 1-receptor agonist agents such as dopamine should be avoided. Charcoal haemoperfusion may be indicated to remove theophylline, but forced diuresis or peritoneal dialysis are inadequate for this purpose.

Pharmaceutical precautions Nil.

Legal category POM.

Package quantities Franol Plus Tablets are supplied in bottles of 250.

Further information The bronchodilator action of ephedrine is through direct agonism at beta adrenoceptors and, indirectly, through sympathetic amine release. Bronchodilatation with theophylline is attributable to adenosine antagonism or phosphodiesterase inhibition which would be pharmacologically complementary to the action of ephedrine. Theophylline is variably absorbed from the gastrointestinal tract. It is excreted via the urine mainly as 1,3-dimethyluric acid. About 10% is unchanged. Ephedrine is readily absorbed. Its action is evident within one hour. With a plasma elimination half life of about 4 hours, 60–75% is excreted unchanged in the urine.

Product licence number 0071/5037.

GASTRON*

Presentation Off-white, round, strawberry-flavoured, chewable tablets 22.2 mm in diameter, marked GASTRON on one side and with an ankh symbol on the other. Each tablet contains:

Alginic Acid BPC	600 mg
Dried Aluminium Hydroxide PhEur	240 mg
Sodium Bicarbonate PhEur	210 mg
Magnesium Trisilicate BP	60 mg

Uses To alleviate heartburn and other epigastric and retrosternal symptoms arising from gastro-oesophageal reflux.

Dosage and administration
Adults: One or two tablets to be chewed three times a day immediately after meals and two at bedtime. The tablets may be followed by a drink of water.

Elderly: As for adults.

Children: Not recommended.

Contra-indications, warnings, etc There are no specific contra-indications to the use of Gastron.

There is no evidence of the safety of Gastron in human pregnancy. The active ingredients have been in wide use for many years without apparent ill consequence. However, careful consideration should be given before prescribing Gastron to women who are pregnant, particularly during the first trimester.

The sodium content of each tablet (70 mg) should be taken into account when prescribing for patients in whom sodium restriction is needed.

Interactions: Antacids can interact with a wide variety of medications generally through effects on their absorption or excretion. These include:

Antiarrhythmics – the urinary excretion of flecainide, mexiletine and quinidine may be reduced.

Analgesics – the absorption of diflunisal is reduced and urinary excretion of aspirin may be increased.

Antibacterials – the absorption of ciprofloxacin, ofloxacin, pivampicillin, rifampicin and most tetracyclines may be reduced as may the absorption of itraconazole and ketoconazole.

Other agents – the absorption of chloroquine, hydroxychloroquine, phenothiazines, oral iron, dipyridamole and penicillamine may all be reduced whilst excretion of lithium may be increased.

Overdosage: Because of the nature of the product, overdosage should not be a problem. Ingestion of a larger number of tablets than recommended may result in abdominal distension.

Pharmaceutical precautions Store in a dry place.

Legal category GSL.

Package quantities Packs of 100 tablets in foil strips.

Further information The alginate-antacid in Gastron tablets forms a viscous foam which has buffering capacity. This is designed to relieve symptoms on contact with the oesophageal wall, and to impede oesophageal reflux. The tablets are sweetened with mannitol and saccharin.

Product licence number 0071/0257.

GLURENORM*

Presentation Flat, white, bevelled-edged tablets, 9 mm in diameter, scored on one side and with G on the other, each containing 30 mg gliquidone. Glurenorm tablets contain lactose.

Uses For the treatment of non-insulin dependent diabetes mellitus which does not respond adequately to dietary measures.

Dosage and administration For oral administration only. Glurenorm should be taken up to half an hour before a meal. The dose and frequency of administration should be adjusted, together with the diet, to obtain the best possible control throughout the day.

Adults including the elderly: Most patients respond to a total daily dose of 45–60 mg given in two or three divided doses, of which the largest dose is usually taken in the morning with breakfast. The recommended maximum single dose is 60 mg (2 tablets). The maximum daily dose 180 mg (6 tablets).

During stabilisation, dosage adjustment should be based on frequent blood (random and postprandial) and urinary glucose determinations.

Stabilisation of previously untreated cases: Normally, treatment should begin with 15 mg (half a tablet) before breakfast and this should be gradually increased by 15 mg increments prior to mealtimes.

Change-over in patients previously treated with other oral anti-diabetic agents: Patients can be changed over from other sulphonylureas to Glurenorm without interruption. It is usual to start with 30 mg Glurenorm before breakfast, increasing as necessary by increments of 15 mg at mealtimes.

In terms of comparative potency of single doses, 30 mg Glurenorm corresponds approximately to 1,000 mg tolbutamide, 5 mg glibenclamide, 250 mg chlorpropamide or 500 mg acetohexamide. However, in estimating equivalent total daily doses, the half-lives and duration of action of the respective sulphonylureas must be taken into consideration. Thus it will usually be necessary to administer Glurenorm more frequently than a long-acting sulphonylurea.

Change-over in non-insulin dependent diabetics previously treated with insulin: In patients treated with up to 30 i.u. of insulin daily, change-over to Glurenorm may be attempted with an initial dose of 30 mg accompanied by a simultaneous gradual reduction of the amount of insulin, provided the pancreas still contains some functioning β cells. Patients who change from insulin to Glurenorm should be strictly supervised and response assessed by frequent and regular blood-glucose determinations.

It may be possible to reduce the insulin requirements of patients who require more than 30 i.u. daily by the concurrent administration of Glurenorm. Blood-glucose should be monitored frequently during the change-over period.

Combined treatment: The administration of metformin with Glurenorm to patients who cannot be adequately controlled by Glurenorm alone may achieve satisfactory stabilisation of blood-glucose levels.

Children: Not recommended.

Contra-indications, warnings, etc
Contra-indications: Do not use for diabetes complicated by acidosis or ketosis nor in patients subject to the stress of surgery or acute infections. Glurenorm should not be used in pregnancy or breast feeding nor in patients with severe hepatic or renal failure, or porphyria.

Precautions: Patients who miss a meal (particularly the elderly or debilitated) should be warned not to take their dose of Glurenorm, in order to reduce the risk of a hypoglycaemic reaction.

Special care should be observed in the concomitant use of Glurenorm with many other medications because interactions with sulphonylureas are common.

The effect of Glurenorm may be increased by physical exertion.

Interactions: The effect of Glurenorm may be increased by alcohol, salicylates, sulphonamides, phenylbutazone, ethionamide, coumarin anticoagulants, chloramphenicol, tetracyclines, cyclophosphamide, MAO inhibitors, tuberculostatics, β-adrenergic blocking agents, azapropazone, co-trimoxazole, miconazole and sulphinpyrazone.

It may be necessary to increase the dose of Glurenorm when any of the following are administered concurrently: oral contraceptives, chlorpromazine, sympathomimetic agents, corticosteroids, thyroid hormones, nicotinic acid preparations, rifampicin, diazoxide and loop or thiazide diuretics.

The effects of barbiturates, vasopressin and oral anticoagulants are potentiated by the administration of Glurenorm.

Side-effects: Glurenorm is generally well tolerated, but minor skin allergies, gastric upsets and other non-specific symptoms have been noted.

Reversible leucopenia has been reported and also reversible thrombocytopenia, but in neither has a causal connection with Glurenorm been established.

Hypoglycaemic reactions are infrequent, but may be accompanied by malaise, impaired concentration and altered consciousness. They may be treated with oral carbohydrate or with intravenous dextrose if the oral route is impractical. Glucagon (1 mg subcutaneously) could also be given.

Overdosage: In the conscious patient, hypoglycaemia may be managed by the oral administration of glucose. In the comatose patient, parenteral administration of glucose by intravenous infusion should be instituted. The patient should be kept under observation for further signs of hypoglycaemia. Consideration may be given to the recovery of ingested tablets by gastric lavage.

Pharmaceutical precautions Nil.

Legal category POM.

Package quantities Bottles of 100 tablets.

Further information Gliquidone is a sulphonylurea hypoglycaemic agent. Following oral administration it is rapidly absorbed. Its action normally starts within one hour and its optimal effect lasts two to three hours. The plasma elimination half-life is about 1.4 hours. It is almost completely metabolised in the liver by hydroxylation and demethylation, and excreted principally via the bile. Since only approximately 5% of the administered dose appears in the urine, mainly as inactive metabolites, there is little risk of hypoglycaemia due to drug accumulation in patients with impaired renal function.

Sold under licence from Boehringer Ingelheim International GmbH.

Product licence number 0071/0155.

HEXOPAL* TABLETS AND SUSPENSION HEXOPAL FORTE

Presentation 1. Hexopal Tablets are white or almost white, flat tablets with bevelled edges, 12.7 mm in diameter and marked with a stylised Hv on one side and scored on the other. Each tablet contains 500 mg Inositol Nicotinate BP.

2. Hexopal Suspension is a smooth white fluid with a sweet odour and taste which contains 1000 mg Inositol Nicotinate BP in each 5 ml.

3. Hexopal Forte. White or almost white, oval, biconvex tablets marked HEX750 on one side and scored on the other. Each tablet contains 750 mg Inositol Nicotinate BP.

Uses Hexopal is indicated for the symptomatic relief of severe intermittent claudication and Raynaud's phenomenon.

Dosage and administration Hexopal is for oral administration only.

Adults including the elderly: The usual dose is 3 g daily (5 ml Hexopal Suspension or two Hexopal tablets three times a day or two Hexopal Forte tablets twice daily). The dose may be increased to 4 g daily if necessary.

Children: Not recommended.

Contra-indications, warnings, etc There are no known contra-indications or precautions associated with the use of Hexopal, and side-effects are uncommon.

There is no evidence of the safety of Hexopal in human pregnancy, nor is there adequate evidence from animal work that it is free from hazard. The use of Hexopal in pregnancy should therefore be avoided unless there is no safer alternative. Hexopal appears to be virtually non-toxic to animals even in doses up to 100 times the normal therapeutic level.

Despite extensive clinical experience in Britain since 1959, no case of poisoning or overdosage with Hexopal has been reported. In an emergency, it is suggested that the stomach should be emptied by gastric lavage and the patient be treated symptomatically.

Pharmaceutical precautions Nil.

Legal category P.

Package quantities Hexopal Tablets: Blister packs of 100 and bottles of 500. Hexopal Suspension: Bottles of 300 ml. Hexopal Forte: Bottles of 250 and as Hexopal Forte C-Pak in calendar packs of 112 (OP).

Further information Patients with peripheral vascular disease are likely to benefit from stopping or reducing smoking and from control of their weight. It is recommended that patients be so advised.

Product licence numbers

Hexopal Tablets	0071/5043
Hexopal Suspension	0071/0090
Hexopal Forte	0071/0164

HYPAQUE* 25% AND 45%

Presentation Hypaque is a sterile, almost colourless aqueous solution in clear glass ampoules or infusion bottles containing either 25% w/v or 45% w/v Sodium Diatrizoate BP. Hypaque 25% and 45% contain sodium calcium edetate.

Uses A radiographic contrast medium suitable for intravenous and retrograde urography, angiography, venography and many other specialised procedures including examination of the gastro-intestinal tract.

Dosage and administration The route of administration of Hypaque, which may be parenteral, oral or rectal, and the volume and concentration employed depend on the procedure being undertaken.

Parenteral administration: suggested strength and quantity according to procedure.

Procedure	*Strength (%)*	*Amount of medium used (ml)*	
		Adults and elderly	*Children*
Urography:			
i.v.	45	0.5–2.0/kg	as adult
infusion	25	4.0/kg	as adult
retrograde	25–45	5–20	as adult
Cystography	10–45	500–1500	100–300
Peripheral arteriography	45	20–40	10–20
Haemorrhoidal portal venography	45	30–40	15–20
Renal cyst puncture	25–45	5–60	5–20
Orbital phlebography	45	2–4	1–2
Intraosseous venography	45	20–45	—
Choledochography:			
percutaneous transhepatic	25–45	15	5
operative	25–45	5–20	5
post-op. 'T' tube	25–45	5–20	5
Hysterosalpingography	45	10	—
Arthrography	25–45	5–20	3–10
Sinography	45	20–40	—
Tube screening (gastric)	25	5–20	—
Abdominal stab wounds	25	q.s.	q.s.
Dacryocystography	45	1–3	—
Vesiculography	45	1.5–2.0 to a total of 10–12 each side	—
Myography	45	3	—
Duct mammography	25	1–2	—
Discography	45	0.5 max. 2.0	—

Oral and rectal administration in examination of the gastro-intestinal tract: For adults including the elderly an average dose of 100 ml to 150 ml of a 25–45% solution is suggested when given by mouth or tube. From 500 ml to 1,000 ml of 20–35% solution is suggested as an enema.

For infants or children the dose by mouth or tube may vary from 50 ml to 120 ml of a 10–25% solution, and by enema from 100 ml to 500 ml of a 10–15% solution may be used.

Contra-indications, warnings, etc Serious, rarely fatal, thromboembolic events causing myocardial infarction and stroke have been reported during angiographic procedures with both ionic and nonionic contrast media. Therefore, meticulous intravascular administration technique is necessary, particularly during angiographic procedures, to minimise thromboembolic events. Numerous factors, including length of procedure, catheter and syringe material, underlying disease state and concomitant medications may contribute to the development of thromboembolic events. For these reasons, meticulous angiographic techniques are recommended including close attention to guidewire and catheter manipulation, use of manifold systems and/or three-way stopcocks, frequent catheter flushing with heparinised saline solutions and minimising the length of the procedure. The use of plastic syringes in place of glass syringes has been reported to decrease but not eliminate the likelihood of in vitro clotting.

Hypaque should not be used for myelography. Injection of even a small amount into the subarachnoid space may produce convulsions and result in fatality.

Patients with a history of allergy, especially to iodine, require careful consideration. There is no satisfactory way of pre-testing which will allow the prediction of a severe reaction, but the following precautions may help to minimise reactions, according to some workers:

(a) Obtain a history of personal or familial allergies, of previous iodine studies, and of sensitivity to iodine and other drugs.
(b) Make a preliminary sensitivity test by injecting intravenously a small dose (0.5 to 1 ml) followed by a period of observation long enough to detect delayed reactions. (Although allergic reactions generally occur quickly, on very rare occasions they may not appear for 10 or even 15 minutes).
(c) Give preliminary antihistamine or corticosteroid medication.
(d) Have drugs on hand for emergency use.

It was formerly believed that the use of contrast media was contra-indicated in patients with advanced renal destruction associated with severe uraemia, and in those with severe hepatic and cardiac disorders. However, one review concludes that although there appear to be no definite contra-indications, potentially hazardous situations requiring particular care are oliguric renal failure, myeloma and combined renal and hepatic failure. No attempt should be made to dehydrate the uraemic patient, nor should dehydration be carried out in a patient with myeloma. Evidence suggests that, in the latter case, it is dehydration rather than the presence of myeloma protein which has been the cause of adverse effects. Prior purgation should be avoided.

Contrast media may promote sickling in individuals who are homozygous for sickle cell disease when the material is injected intravenously or intra-arterially.

Administration of radiopaque materials to patients known or suspected of having phaeochromocytoma should be performed with extreme caution. If, in the opinion of the physician, the possible benefits of such procedures outweigh the considered risks, the procedures may be performed; however, the amount of radiopaque medium injected should be kept to an absolute minimum. The blood pressure should be assessed throughout the procedure and measures for treatment of a hypertensive crisis should be available.

Recent reports of thyroid storm occurring following the intravascular use of iodinated radiopaque diagnostic agents in patients with hyperthyroidism or with an autonomously functioning thyroid nodule suggest that this additional risk be evaluated in such patients before use of Hypaque.

In patients with subarachnoid haemorrhage, a rare association between contrast administration and clinical deterioration, including convulsions and death, has been reported. Therefore, administration of intravascular iodated ionic contrast media to these patients should be undertaken with caution.

In examinations of the gastro-intestinal tract, Hypaque should be used with caution in infants and debilitated elderly patients because hypovolaemia may develop due to the osmotic activity of the contrast material in the intestines.

Caution should be observed in patients with tuberculosis since it has been suggested that iodine could exacerbate active tuberculosis, although this has not been reported with Hypaque.

Because of the possibility of inducing a temporary suppression of urine, it is wise to allow an interval of at least 24 hours before repeating excretory or retrograde pyelography in patients with unilateral reduction of normal renal function.

Use in pregnancy and lactation: X-ray examinations should be avoided during pregnancy. Animal reproduction studies have not been carried out with Hypaque, and it is not known whether it can cause foetal harm when administered to a pregnant woman. Hypaque can be transferred across the placenta to the foetus, and may also appear in breast milk. Hypaque therefore should only be administered to pregnant women when absolutely necessary. Caution should be observed in its administration to nursing mothers.

Interactions: Organic iodine contrast media are known to remain in the blood serum of patients for periods varying from two days to several years in concentrations sufficient to interfere with tests of thyroid function such as protein-bound iodine determinations. It has been reported that sodium diatrizoate remains in the serum for four days. It is therefore advisable to perform such thyroid function tests before any examination involving the use of Hypaque.

Other tests which may be affected by sodium diatrizoate, and for which an interval of 2 or 3 days should be allowed between administration and testing include:

Blood tests: Diatrizoate salts significantly inhibit all stages of coagulation. The fibrinogen concentration, and factors V, VII and VIII are decreased. Prothrombin time and thromboplastin time are increased.

Platelet aggregation: High levels of plasma diatrizoates inhibit platelet aggregation.

Serum calcium: Diatrizoate salts may decrease serum calcium levels. However, this depletion of serum calcium may also be the result of the addition of chelating agents (edetate disodium) in the preparation of certain contrast media.

Red cell counts: Transitory decreases in red cell counts. Technetium-99m-RBC labelling interference.

Leukocyte counts: Decrease following injection.

Urea nitrogen (BUN): Transitory increase.

Serum creatinine: Transitory increase.

Urine tests: Urine osmolality and specific gravity may be decreased due to induced diuresis. Diatrizoate in urine cultures may inhibit bacterial growth.

Albumin: crystals of diatrizoic acid may separate out on acidification with mineral acid but these crystals are easily distinguished from the amorphous albumin precipitate. Hypaque does not affect the acetic acid or heat coagulation tests.

Side-effects: Approximately 95 per cent of adverse reactions accompanying the intravascular use of diatrizoate salts are of mild to moderate severity. However, life-threatening reactions and fatalities, mostly of cardiovascular origin, have occurred.

Adverse reactions to injectable contrast media fall into two categories: chemotoxic reactions and idiosyncratic reactions.

Chemotoxic reactions result from the physicochemical properties of the contrast media, the dose, and the speed of injection. All haemodynamic disturbances and injuries to organs or vessels perfused by the contrast medium are included in this category.

Idiosyncratic reactions include all other reactions. They occur more frequently in patients 20 to 40 years old. Idiosyncratic reactions may or may not be dependent on the amount of dose injected, the speed of injection, the mode of injection, and the radiographic procedure. Idiosyncratic reactions are subdivided into minor, intermediate, and severe. The minor reactions are self-limited and of short duration; the severe reactions are life-threatening and treatment is urgent and mandatory.

The reported incidence of adverse reactions to contrast media in patients with a history of allergy are twice that of the general population. Patients with a history of previous reactions to a contrast medium are three times more susceptible than other patients. However, sensitivity to contrast media dose not appear to increase with repeated examinations.

Most adverse reactions to injectable contrast media appear within one to three minutes after the start of injection, but delayed reactions may occur.

Adverse reactions are grouped by organ system and listed below by decreasing order of occurrence and with an approximate incidence of occurrence. Significantly more severe reactions are listed before the other reactions regardless of frequency.

Greater than 1 in 100 patients

Body as a whole: Reported incidences of death range from 6.6 per 1 million (0.00066 percent) to 1 in 10,000 patients (0.01 percent). Most deaths occur during injection or 5 to 10 minutes later, the main feature being cardiac arrest with cardiovascular disease as the main aggravating factor.

Isolated reports of hypotensive collapse and shock following urography are found in the literature. The incidence of shock is estimated to occur in 1 out of 20,000 (0.005 percent) patients.

Cardiovascular system: The most frequent adverse reaction to diatrizoate salts is vasodilation (feeling of warmth). The estimated incidence is 49 percent.

Digestive system: Nausea 6 percent, vomiting 3 percent.

Nervous system: Paraesthesia 6 percent, dizziness 5 percent.

Respiratory system: Rhinitis 1 percent, increased cough 2 percent.

Skin and appendages: Urticaria 1 percent. Pain at the injection site is estimated to occur in about 12 percent of the patients undergoing urography. Pain is usually due to extravasation.

Painful hot erythematous swelling above the venipuncture site was estimated to occur in more than one percent of the patients undergoing phlebography.

Special senses: Perversion of taste 11 percent, and numbness.

Urogenital system: Osmotic nephrosis of the proximal tubular cells is estimated to occur in 23 percent of patients following excretory urography.

Less than 1 in 100 patients

Other infrequently reported reactions without accompanying incidence rates are listed below, grouped by organ system.

Body as a whole: Malaria relapse, uraemia, high creatinine and BUN, thrombocytopenia, leukopenia and anaemia.

Cardiovascular system: Cerebral haematomas, haemodynamic disturbances, sinus brachycardia, transient electrocardiographic abnormalities, ventricular fibrillation, and petechiae.

Digestive system: Severe unilateral or bilateral swelling of the parotid and submaxillary glands.

Nervous system: Convulsions, paralysis, coma and agitation.

Respiratory system: Asthma, dyspnoea, laryngeal oedema, pulmonary oedema, bronchospasm and respiratory arrest.

Skin and appendages: Extravasation necrosis, urticaria with or without pruritus, mucocutaneous oedema, and angioneurotic oedema.

Special senses: Bilateral ocular irritation, lacrimation, itching, conjunctival chemosis, infection, and conjunctivitis.

Urogenital: Renal failure, pain.

Pharmaceutical precautions The sterile aqueous solutions are clear and almost colourless. Hypaque is relatively thermostable and may be autoclaved if 0.0125% w/v sodium calcium edetate is added to the solution, but sterile Hypaque solution should not be re-autoclaved because of the possibility of free amine production. Solutions should be protected from light.

Legal category POM.

Package quantities *Hypaque 25%:* 20 ml ampoules in boxes of 5. Infusion bottles of 250 ml or 350 ml.
Hypaque 45%: 20 ml ampoules in boxes of 20.

Further information The radio-opacity of sodium diatrizoate is due to the presence of iodine which absorbs x-rays.

Product licence numbers

Hypaque 25%	0071/5044
Hypaque 45%	0071/5045

HYPAQUE* SODIUM

Presentation Hypaque Sodium is a white, odourless powder with a saline taste, consisting of Sodium Diatrizoate BP. The anhydrous material contains 59.8% of iodine. Hypaque Sodium powder contains sodium calcium edetate.

Uses Hypaque Sodium Powder is used in the preparation of radiographic contrast media for examination of the gastro-intestinal tract and for use in retrograde cystography and micturating urethrography.

Dosage and administration Hypaque Sodium Powder is only used for the preparation of solutions for oral and rectal administration and for introduction into the bladder via a urinary catheter. Hypaque Sodium Powder is not suitable for the preparation of injectable solutions for intravascular or other applications.

(a) Examination of the gastro-intestinal tract:
Adults: For adults an average dose of from 100 to 150 ml of a 25–50% solution is suggested when given by mouth or by tube. From 500 ml to 1,000 ml of a 20–35% solution is suggested as an enema.

Elderly: As for adults, but see 'Precautions'.

Children: The dose by mouth or tube may vary from 50 ml to 120 ml of a 10–25% solution, and by enema from 100 ml to 500 ml of a 10–15% solution.

The solvent may be water, saline or Ringer's solution. For oral use, suitable flavouring such as vanilla or chocolate syrup may be helpful in masking the taste of Hypaque.

(b) Retrograde cystography and micturating urethrography: There is some variation in the strength and quantity of medium employed. However, for urethrography 5 ml to 20 ml of a 25–45% solution is recommended for both adults and children. For cystography the recommendation for adults is 500 ml to 1500 ml of a 10–45% solution, and the recommendation for children is 100 ml–300 ml of a 10–45% solution.

To sterilise, 0.012% w/v sodium calcium edetate should be added to the solution which is then autoclaved at 10 lb per sq in (115–116°C) for 30 minutes.

Contra-indications, warnings, etc
There are no specific contra-indications to the use of Hypaque Sodium.

Precautions: Patients with a history of allergy, especially to iodine, require careful consideration since Hypaque may be absorbed, though in very small amounts, through the intestinal wall. A solution of Hypaque Sodium in water greater than 10% is hypertonic. Therefore, care should be taken when such solutions are used to examine the gastro-intestinal tracts of infants and debilitated elderly patients, since hypovolaemia may develop due to the osmotic activity of the contrast material in the intestines. It is advisable to correct any electrolyte disturbances before using solutions that are extremely hypertonic.

Caution is advised in patients with tuberculosis since it has been suggested that iodine could exacerbate active tuberculosis although this has not been reported with Hypaque.

Use in pregnancy and lactation: X-ray examinations should be avoided during pregnancy. Animal reproduction studies have not been carried out with Hypaque, and it is not known whether Hypaque can cause foetal harm when administered to a pregnant woman. Hypaque can be transferred across the placenta to the foetus, and may also appear in breast milk. Hypaque therefore should only be administered to pregnant women when absolutely necessary. Caution should be observed in its administration to nursing mothers.

Interactions: The presence of sodium diatrizoate in the serum may interfere with tests of thyroid function such as protein bound iodine determinations. It is therefore advisable to perform such thyroid function tests before any examination involving the use of Hypaque.

Side-effects: Nausea and diarrhoea have been occasionally reported with Hypaque Sodium Powder and dehydration from fluid loss in such cases must be borne in mind. Rarely, the following have been reported: pulmonary oedema following accidental aspiration, colonic overdistension and perforation, mucosal damage due to prolonged contact, and precipitation of the medium as a solid mass in the stomach. Irritation of the urethral and vesicular mucosa has occasionally followed administration into the bladder.

Minor allergic disturbances such as sneezing, rhinorrhoea, lacrimation and pruritus or urticarial rashes may occasionally occur, and should respond to antihistamine treatment.

Pharmaceutical precautions Hypaque is relatively thermostable and may be autoclaved if 0.012% w/v sodium calcium edetate is added to the solution.

Legal category P.

Package quantities Bottles of 500 g.

Further information The radio-opacity of sodium diatrizoate is due to the presence of iodine which absorbs X-rays.

Following oral administration to adults, Hypaque passes unchanged through the gastro-intestinal tract. A very small amount is absorbed through the intestinal wall, since traces of iodine are excreted by the kidney. Absorption from the gastro-intestinal tract occurs to a greater extent in infants.

Product licence number 0071/5048.

INTEGRIN* CAPSULES

Presentation Integrin Capsules are No. 4 white, opaque, hard gelatine capsules marked Integrin 10 on both cap and body and filled with a fine, off-white powder. Each capsule contains 10 mg oxypertine. Integrin Capsules contain lactose.

Uses Integrin Capsules are recommended for the short-term treatment of acute and chronic anxiety states and psychosomatic conditions whether or not accompanied by depressive overlay, tension, apprehension or sleep disturbance.

Dosage and administration For oral administration only.

Adults: 10 mg three or four times daily, usually after meals. In certain cases up to 60 mg daily in divided doses may be needed.

Children: Not recommended.

Elderly: Doses lower than those for other adults are recommended.

Contra-indications, warnings, etc
Contra-indications: Bone marrow depression, closed-angle glaucoma and hypersensitivity to phenothiazines. Because oxypertine can bring about the release of small amounts of catecholamines in experimental animals, it would be wise not to give Integrin with or within three weeks of the use of monoamine oxidase inhibitors.

Precautions: Integrin should be used with caution in patients with: cardiovascular disease, respiratory disease, phaeochromocytoma, Parkinsonism, epilepsy, acute infections, renal and hepatic impairment, history of jaundice, hypothyroidism, myasthenia gravis and prostatic hypertrophy. Observe caution also in very hot or very cold weather because oxypertine, like phenothiazines may affect temperature regulation. Elderly patients are more susceptible to side-effects and lower doses are recommended.

Patients should be warned to observe caution in car driving and similar activities. If affected by sedation or drowsiness, patients should not drive or operate machinery.

Use in pregnancy and lactation: There is no information on the use of oxypertine in human pregnancy and lactation. Although tests on pregnant rabbits (Somers' test) have revealed no teratogenic effects of oxypertine, the benefits of using Integrin in pregnancy, particularly in the first trimester, should be weighed against the possible risks.

Clinical experience with other phenothiazine derivatives has shown that their use in pregnancy is occasionally associated with extrapyramidal effects in the neonate, and their use during lactation with drowsiness in the suckling infant.

Interactions: Oxypertine can interact with monoamine oxidase inhibitors, leading to CNS excitation and hypertension. Oxypertine may potentiate the central depressant effect of antihypertensives, alcohol and other CNS depressants. There are conflicting reports on the effect of oxypertine on urinary excretion of vanilmandelic acid.

Side-effects: Oxypertine would be expected to share the side-effect profiles of phenothiazines. Compared to phenothiazines, however, oxypertine has fewer sedative, anticholinergic and possibly extrapyramidal effects. Low doses may produce agitation and hyperactivity, while higher doses are sedative.

Other side-effects reported with either oxypertine or with phenothiazines include gastro-intestinal disturbances, nasal congestion, dry mouth, hypotension, hypothermia, photophobia and photosensitivity, rashes, eosinophilia and other blood dyscrasias, positive LE cell phenomenon, insomnia, dizziness, abnormal liver function tests and jaundice, myalgia, extrapyramidal signs and disturbances of endocrine function, e.g. hyperglycaemia, hyperprolactinaemia, menstrual disorders and disturbed sexual function. Malignant neuroleptic syndrome, although not reported to date with oxypertine, is a rare but potentially fatal side-effect of some antipsychotic drugs.

Overdosage: Symptoms and signs include CNS depression, respiratory depression, hypotension, arrhythmias, hypothermia, convulsions and severe Parkinsonism. Treatment is gastric lavage but use of emetics should be avoided. Hypotension is treated by plasma expanders. Adrenaline should be avoided. Treatment of other features is symptomatic and supportive. Dialysis is probably not effective at removing the drug.

Pharmaceutical precautions Protect from moisture and heat.

Legal category POM.

Package quantities Integrin 10 mg Capsules are available in bottles of 100.

Further information Integrin is a potent neuroleptic, similar in many respects to the piperazine phenothiazines. It causes depletion of monoamines (especially noradrenaline) in the brain, but there is some evidence of dopamine-receptor blockade.

Product licence number 0071/5049.

INTEGRIN* TABLETS

Presentation Integrin 40 mg Tablets are white, slightly speckled, flat tablets with bevelled edges, 8.7 mm in diameter, marked 'int' on one side and scored on the other. Each tablet contains 40 mg oxypertine. Integrin Tablets contain lactose.

Uses Integrin 40 mg Tablets are recommended for the treatment of psychotic patients and are particularly useful in withdrawn schizophrenic patients. Integrin 40 mg Tablets may also be used in acute incidents of mental disturbances such as acute agitation, behavioural disturbances, delirium, and acute or subacute psychoses, including the manic phase of manic-depressive psychoses.

Dosage and administration For oral administration only.

Adults: The usual dose is 2–3 tablets (80–120 mg) daily in divided doses. This may be varied according to the mental state and clinical response of the patient, but the total daily dosage should not exceed 300 mg.

Children: Not recommended.

Elderly: Doses lower than those for other adults are recommended.

Contra-indications, warnings, etc

Contra-indications: Bone marrow depression, closed-angle glaucoma and hypersensitivity to phenothiazines. Because oxypertine can bring about the release of small amounts of catecholamines in experimental animals, it would be wise not to give Integrin with or within three weeks of the use of monoamine oxidase inhibitors.

Precautions: Integrin should be used with caution in patients with: cardiovascular disease, respiratory disease, phaeochromocytoma, Parkinsonism, epilepsy, acute infections, renal and hepatic impairment, history of jaundice, hypothyroidism, myasthenia gravis and prostatic hypertrophy. Observe caution also in very hot or very cold weather because oxypertine, like phenothiazines, may affect temperature regulation. Elderly patients are more susceptible to side-effects and lower doses are recommended.

Patients should be warned to observe caution in car driving and similar activities. If affected by sedation or drowsiness, patients should not drive or operate machinery.

Use in pregnancy and lactation: There is no information on the use of oxypertine in human pregnancy and lactation. Although tests on pregnant rabbits (Somers' test) have revealed no teratogenic effects of oxypertine, the benefits of using Integrin in pregnancy, particularly in the first trimester, should be weighed against the possible risks.

Clinical experience with other phenothiazine derivatives has shown that their use in pregnancy is occasionally associated with extrapyramidal effects in the neonate, and their use during lactation with drowsiness in the suckling infant.

Interactions: Oxypertine may interact with monoamine oxidase inhibitors, leading to CNS excitation and hypertension. Oxypertine may potentiate the central depressant effect of antihypertensives, alcohol and other CNS depressants. There are conflicting reports on the effect of oxypertine on urinary excretion of vanilmandelic acid.

Side-effects: Oxypertine would be expected to share the side-effect profile of phenothiazines. Compared to phenothiazines however, oxypertine has fewer sedative, anticholinergic and possibly extrapyramidal effects. Low doses may produce agitation and hyperactivity, while higher doses are sedative.

Other side-effects reported with either oxypertine or with phenothiazines include gastro-intestinal disturbances, nasal congestion, dry mouth, hypotension, hypothermia, photophobia and photosensitivity, rashes, eosinophilia and other blood dyscrasias, positive LE cell phenomenon, insomnia, dizziness, abnormal liver function tests and jaundice, myalgia, extrapyramidal signs and disturbances of endocrine function, e.g. hyperglycaemia, hyperprolactinaemia, menstrual disorders and disturbed sexual function. Malignant neuroleptic syndrome, although not reported to date with oxypertine, is a rare but potentially fatal side-effect of some antipsychotic drugs.

Overdosage: Symptoms and signs include CNS depression, respiratory depression, hypotension, arrhythmias, hypothermia, convulsions and severe Parkinsonism. Treatment is gastric lavage but use of emetics should be avoided. Hypotension is treated by plasma expanders. Adrenaline should be avoided. Treatment of other features is symptomatic and supportive. Dialysis is probably not effective at removing the drug.

Pharmaceutical precautions Nil.

Legal category POM.

Package quantities Integrin Tablets are available in bottles of 250.

Further information Integrin is a potent neuroleptic, similar in many respects to the piperazine phenothiazines. It causes depletion of monoamines (especially noradrenaline) in the brain, but there is some evidence of dopamine-receptor blockade.

Product licence number 0071/5050.

KANNASYN*

Presentation Kannasyn Powder is a sterile, white, or almost white, crystalline powder. The powder is filled into vials to contain Kanamycin Acid Sulphate PhEur equivalent to 1 g kanamycin base. Kannasyn Powder contains no excipients.

Uses Kannasyn is recommended for the treatment of serious infections due to susceptible Gram-negative organisms which have proved resistant to other antibiotics.

It may also be used in the treatment of certain staphylococcal infections due to multiple-resistant strains and in gonorrhoea.

Dosage and administration Kannasyn Powder is used for the preparation of solutions for intravenous or intramuscular administration.

1. *Intramuscular injection:* Kannasyn should be given as a solution containing 250 mg/ml. This can be prepared by dissolving the contents of a 1 g vial in 4 ml Water for Injections B.P.

Adults: In acute infections: 1 g daily in two to four equally divided doses. Therapy should normally be limited to six days' treatment and should not exceed a total dose of 10 g.

In chronic infections: 3 g weekly (1 g every three or four days) or 1 g twice a day, twice weekly (4 g weekly). The total amount administered should not exceed 50 g.

Elderly: A reduced dosage may be required. See under warnings.

Children: In acute infections: 15mg/kg body weight daily in 2–4 equally divided doses for no more than six days.

In chronic infections: there are no specific dosage recommendations.

2. *Intravenous use:* This route is recommended only for gravely ill patients with overwhelming infections or with impending cardiovascular collapse. Kannasyn may be given as a solution containing 2.5 mg/ml by slow intravenous infusion at the rate of 3–4 ml per minute. This solution may be prepared by dissolving the contents of a 1 g vial in 400 ml Sodium Chloride Intravenous Infusion B.P. or Glucose Intravenous Infusion B.P. The dosage for both adults and children is 15–30 mg/kg body weight daily in 2 or 3 divided doses.

Contra-indications, warnings, etc

Contra-indications: Kannasyn should not be used during pregnancy or lactation. It is also contra-indicated in patients with a history of hypersensitivity or toxic reaction to kanamycin or other aminoglycosides.

Precautions: Kannasyn should always be administered with caution and preferably only in severe or resistant infections caused by organisms known to be sensitive to the compound. Plasma levels should not be allowed to rise above 30 microgrammes/ml.

In cases of impaired renal function, the kidney may be unable to eliminate kanamycin effectively and as a result the serum level will rise quickly. In these conditions reduced doses are necessary to avoid toxic effects. It has been reported that kanamycin is retained in the serum of patients with renal disease for a considerable time. If it is necessary to give the antibiotic to anuric patients, they should not receive increments more frequently than every three to four days and these increments should be one-half the loading dose used. The safest procedure, however, is to control the dosage by monitoring plasma level to prevent it rising above 30 microgrammes per ml.

Particular caution should be observed in those with hearing loss. In common with certain other antibiotics, kanamycin can damage the eighth cranial nerve when used in large doses or for long periods. The resultant hearing loss, which may be permanent, is usually but not always preceded by tinnitus. Vestibular damage is less common. Should tinnitus or other sign of auditory toxicity appear, the dose of kanamycin should be reduced or it should be discontinued.

Caution should be observed also in myasthenia gravis because kanamycin has a weak curare-like action.

Interactions: The use of potent diuretics such as ethacrynic acid or frusemide with kanamycin should be avoided because they are known to potentiate the toxic action of aminoglycoside antibiotics.

As with other aminoglycoside antibiotics, apnoea and respiratory depression have been reported following the intraperitoneal use of kanamycin because of its curare-like effect. In addition, motor and sensory neuropathy has occurred following local application of kanamycin during spinal surgery. It has also produced slight weakening in muscle strength in a patient with myasthenia gravis. Because of these effects, it has been suggested that kanamycin should not be given intraperitoneally during surgery to patients who have received neuromuscular blocking agents. Calcium gluconate has been suggested to counteract this curare-like action of kanamycin, but neostigmine appears to be more effective.

It has been shown that calcium can inhibit the antibacterial activity of kanamycin against certain organisms and for this reason the routine prophylactic use of calcium solutions with intraperitoneal kanamycin should be discouraged.

Concurrent aminoglycosides may increase the risk of ototoxicity as may anti-emetics by masking its development. The dose of concurrent oral anticoagulant may require alteration because kanamycin may affect endogenous vitamin K. It should be noted that prior treatment with streptomycin or viomycin may increase the likelihood of a nephrotoxic reaction with kanamycin.

Side-effects: Apart from the possibility of eighth cranial nerve damage and a curare-like action (see above), hyaline and granular casts are sometimes observed in urine samples collected in the first 16 hours after administration in patients who have been given high doses of kanamycin. In these cases no permanent impairment of renal function occurs and the casts disappear within a few days of stopping treatment. Although nephrotoxic effects have been reported in some studies, serious renal toxicity is not a frequent problem with the doses now used.

Local intolerance to intramuscular injection has sometimes been reported, but it is transient and does not require interruption of therapy. Ecchymoses have also been observed at the site of injection in a few patients. It has been suggested that in concentrations above those achieved in the blood at therapeutic dosage, kanamycin has anticoagulant action which may explain haematomas at the site of injection. Sensitivity rashes appear to be uncommon.

Intravenous injections are well tolerated and pain is not a problem. Thrombophlebitis has only been reported once in a patient who was receiving 50 million units of penicillin with the kanamycin.

Overdosage: In cases of overdosage or toxic reaction, haemodialysis or peritoneal dialysis will aid the removal of kanamycin from the blood.

Pharmaceutical precautions Kannasyn should be protected from light. The powder may be stored at room temperature but should be used within three years of assay. Solutions of Kannasyn should be used immediately or stored at 2–8°C for not more than 24 hours.

Infusion solutions containing kanamycin have been reported to be incompatible with the following substances: amphotericin, barbiturates, cephalothin sodium, chlorpromazine, electrolytes (Ca^{++}, Mg^{++}, citrate or phosphate ions), heparin, hydrocortisone, methicillin sodium, methohexitone, nitrofurantoin, phenytoin, prochlorperazine, sulphafurazole.

Legal category POM.

Package quantities Boxes of 5 vials.

Further information Nil.

Product licence number 0071/5052.

LEVOPHED*

Presentation Levophed is a clear, colourless or almost-colourless solution containing 2 mg/ml Noradrenaline Acid Tartrate PhEur which is equivalent to 1 mg/ml noradrenaline base. Levophed Solution also contains sodium metabisulphite and sodium chloride.

Uses Levophed is for intravenous use only. It is recommended for use as an emergency measure in the restoration of blood pressure in cases of acute hypotension.

Dosage and administration Levophed should be diluted and administered as an intravenous infusion, preferably through a fine polythene catheter inserted into a large vein in the arm or leg in which blood flow is rapid. It is recommended that Levophed be administered in 5% dextrose or dextrose-saline solution.

Adults: A suitable initial concentration is obtained by adding 4 ml Levophed to a litre of infusion fluid to give a concentration of 8 microgram/ml of noradrenaline acid tartrate which is equivalent to 4 microgram/ml of noradrenaline base. There is a direct relationship between the drip rate and the blood pressure. After observing the response to an initial dose of 2 ml or 3 ml per minute, the rate of flow should be adjusted to establish and maintain a low normal blood pressure (100–120 mm Hg systolic), or somewhat higher in previously hypertensive patients. In patients with severe haemorrhagic or hypovolaemic shock, when blood or fluid replacement has not been completed, it is preferable to maintain the pressure at a lower level sufficient to maintain the circulation to vital organs. The average maintenance dose ranges from 0.5 ml to 1 ml per minute, but there is great individual variation in the dose required to attain and maintain normotension. Infusion should be continued until adequate blood pressure is maintained without the help of Levophed. The infusion should be reduced gradually avoiding abrupt withdrawal.

The dilution of Levophed should be decided in the light of the patient's intravenous fluid requirement. Concentrations greater than 4 ml Levophed per litre of infusion fluid may need to be employed in, for example, congestive heart failure if fluid intake is to be restricted. Conversely, where a large volume of infusate is required, dilutions greater than 4 ml Levophed per litre of fluid may be needed to avoid excessive dosaging of the pressor agent. With prolonged therapy, Levophed may deplete plasma volume. Appropriate monitoring and correction is therefore needed.

Elderly: As for adults but see Precautions.

Children: Not recommended.

Contra-indications, warnings, etc Levophed should be used only in conjunction with appropriate blood volume replacement.

The use of pressor amines during cyclopropane or halothane anaesthesia may cause serious cardiac arrhythmias. Because of the possibility of increasing the risk of ventricular fibrillation, Levophed should be used with caution in patients receiving these or any other cardiac sensitising agent or who exhibit profound hypoxia or hypercarbia.

Levophed should be used with extreme caution in patients receiving monoamine oxidase inhibitors or tricyclic antidepressants because severe, prolonged hypertension may result. The elderly may be especially sensitive to the effects of noradrenaline. Particular caution should be observed in patients with coronary, mesenteric or peripheral vascular thrombosis because noradrenaline may increase the ischaemia and extend the area of infarction. Similar caution should be observed in patients with hypotension following myocardial infarction and in patients with Prinzmetal's variant angina.

When infusing Levophed, the blood pressure and rate of flow should be checked frequently to avoid hypertension.

Extravasation of the solution may cause local tissue necrosis. This may be preceded by blanching along the course of the infused vein, suggesting a need to change the infusion site, which should be checked frequently. If extravasation occurs, the area should be infiltrated with phentolamine without delay. It has been suggested that phentolamine may be added directly to the infusion flask to act as an antidote against sloughing without affecting the vasopressor activity of the Levophed.

Pregnancy: Noradrenaline may impair placental perfusion and induce foetal bradycardia. It may also exert a contractile effect on the pregnant uterus and lead to foetal asphyxia in late pregnancy. These possible risks to the foetus should therefore be weighed against the potential benefit to the mother.

Side-effects: Hypertension may occur, which may be associated with bradycardia as well as headache and peripheral ischaemia, including gangrene of the extremities. Cardiac arrhythmias may arise when Levophed is used in conjunction with cardiac sensitising agents, and may be more likely in patients with hypoxia or hypercarbia. Prolonged administration may result in plasma volume depletion.

Overdosage: Overdosage may result in severe hypertension, reflex bradycardia, marked increase in peripheral resistance and decreased cardiac output. These may be accompanied by violent headache, photophobia, retrosternal pain, pallor, intense sweating and vomiting.

In the event of overdosage, treatment should be withdrawn. The judicious use of phentolamine may be considered.

Pharmaceutical precautions Protect from light. Store below 25°C. The solution should not be used if it is brown in colour. Levophed is best administered in 5% dextrose or dextrose saline solution because the dextrose protects against significant loss of potency due to oxidation. Deterioration occurs more rapidly in normal saline than in dextrose solution.

Infusion solutions containing noradrenaline acid tartrate have been reported to be incompatible with the following substances: alkalis and oxidising agents, barbiturates, chlorpheniramine, chlorothiazide, nitrofurantoin, novobiocin, phenytoin, sodium bicarbonate, sodium iodide, streptomycin.

Legal category POM.

Package quantities Boxes of six 2 ml or 4 ml ampoules.

Further information Nil.

Product licence number
0071/5056

LEVOPHED* SPECIAL

Presentation Levophed Special is a clear, colourless or almost colourless, sterile solution providing 200 micrograms/ml Noradrenaline Acid Tartrate PhEur which is equivalent to 100 micrograms/ml of noradrenaline base. Levophed Special also contains sodium metabisulphite and sodium chloride.

Uses Levophed Special is for parenteral use only. It is recommended as an emergency measure in the management of cardiac arrest to help restore and maintain blood pressure.

Dosage and administration
Adults: In cases of cardiac standstill the rapid intravenous or intracardiac injection of 0.50–0.75 ml of Levophed Special may restore a recordable blood pressure for one to four minutes. After intravenous injection the solution should be massaged towards the heart.

A similar dose may be repeated when the blood pressure starts to fall again, or blood pressure can be maintained with a normal Levophed drip (see Levophed data sheet). If there is no response to Levophed Special administered intravenously, cardiac massage should be started with the injection of 0.50–0.75 ml Levophed Special into the ascending aorta or into the left atrium. Injection into the ventricle should be avoided because of the possible risk of inducing fibrillation. If the myocardium is fibrillating, a dose of Levophed Special may be injected after normal rhythm has been restored by massage or by electrical defibrillation.

Elderly: As for adults but see Precautions.

Children: Not recommended.

Contra-indications, warnings, etc Levophed Special should be used only in conjunction with appropriate blood volume replacement.

The use of pressor amines during cyclopropane or halothane anaesthesia may cause serious cardiac arrhythmias. Because of the possibility of increasing the risk of ventricular fibrillation, Levophed Special should be used with caution in patients receiving these or any other cardiac sensitising agent or who exhibit profound hypoxia or hypercarbia.

Levophed Special should be used with caution in patients receiving monoamine oxidase inhibitors or tricyclic antidepressants because severe, prolonged hypertension may result. The elderly may be especially sensitive to the effects of noradrenaline. Caution should be observed in patients with coronary, mesenteric, or peripheral vascular thrombosis because noradrenaline may increase the ischaemia and extend the area of infarction.

Pregnancy: Noradrenaline may impair placental perfusion and induce foetal bradycardia. It may also exert a contractile effect on the pregnant uterus and lead to foetal asphyxia in late pregnancy. These possible risks to the foetus should therefore be weighed against the potential benefit to the mother.

Side-effects: Hypertension may occur, which may be associated with bradycardia as well as headache and peripheral ischaemia, including gangrene of the extremities. Cardiac arrhythmias may arise when Levophed Special is used in conjunction with cardiac sensitising agents, and may be more likely in patients with hypoxia or hypercarbia. Extravasation may cause local tissue necrosis.

Overdosage: Overdosage may result in severe hypertension, reflex bradycardia, marked increase in peripheral resistance and decreased cardiac output. These may be accompanied by violent headache, photophobia, retrosternal pain, pallor, intense sweating and vomiting.

In the event of overdosage, treatment should be withdrawn. The judicious use of phentolamine may be considered.

Pharmaceutical precautions Protect from light. Store below 25°C. The solution should not be used if it is brown in colour.

Legal category POM.

Package quantities Box of five 2 ml ampoules.

Further information Nil.

Product licence number 0071/5057.

LINGRAINE*

Presentation Lingraine Tablets are light green, biconvex tablets, 6.4 mm in diameter, with no markings. Each tablet contains 2.0 mg Ergotamine Tartrate PhEur. Lingraine Tablets also contain lactose.

Uses Lingraine Tablets are recommended for the relief of migraine and other vascular headaches.

Dosage and administration Lingraine Tablets are for sublingual administration only.

Adults: One tablet to be taken at the first sign of an attack of migraine. If necessary another tablet may be taken half an hour to an hour later. No more than three tablets should be taken in 24 hours and not more than six tablets in any one week.

Elderly: As for adults but see warnings.

Children: Not recommended.

Contra-indications, warnings, etc Since (like other ergot alkaloids) ergotamine tartrate causes contraction of uterine muscle it should not be used during pregnancy. Avoid during breast feeding.

Because ergotamine brings about constriction of peripheral blood vessels Lingraine should not be used in the presence of severe arteriosclerosis, coronary artery disease, thrombophlebitis, Raynaud's syndrome or Buerger's disease. Furthermore, Lingraine should not be used where there is liver or kidney dysfunction, nor in the presence of severe hypertension, hyperthyroidism or porphyria. Concomitant use with beta blockers may increase the risk of peripheral vasoconstriction, whilst with erthromycin, the risk of ergotism.

Side-effects: These are a relatively minor problem if the dose is carefully regulated. Nausea and vomiting are most frequently reported; other side-effects encountered include abdominal pain, leg cramps, vertigo, diarrhoea and, occasionally, increased headache. If such symptoms are profound or accompanied by cardiovascular or neurological disturbances, they are indicative of chronic overdosage (see below).

Overdosage: Like all the natural amino-acid alkaloids of ergot, ergotamine is a highly toxic substance which may cause chronic or acute poisoning, although the latter is less frequent.

The oral administration of 26 mg over several days has proved fatal, and there have also been deaths from as little as 0.5 mg to 1.5 mg in a single injection.

The principal signs of chronic overdosage are circulatory disturbances, due to vasoconstriction and thrombiformation, including coldness of the skin, severe muscle pains, and vascular stasis resulting in dry peripheral gangrene. Anginal pain, tachycardia or bradycardia and hypertension or hypotension may occur. Other symptoms include headache, nausea, vomiting, diarrhoea and weakness of the legs. Confusion, drowsiness, hemiplegia and convulsions may also occur.

The main symptoms of acute poisoning consist of nausea, vomiting, diarrhoea, unquenchable thirst, tingling, itching and coldness of the skin, a rapid and weak pulse, confusion and unconsciousness. Treatment: Amyl nitrate inhalations (0.2–0.3 ml) are suggested to counteract arterial spasm.

Pharmaceutical precautions Nil.

Legal category POM.

Package quantities Lingraine Tablets are available in P.F.P. laminate strips in boxes of 12 tablets (OP).

Further information Ergotamine is an ergot alkaloid, and acts by antagonism of alpha adrenoceptors.

Product licence number 0071/5058.

LOBAK*

Presentation Lobak Tablets are white, flat tablets with bevelled edges, 12.7 mm in diameter marked LOBAK on one side and scored on the other. Each tablet contains 450 mg Paracetamol PhEur and 100 mg chlormezanone.

Uses For the treatment of painful conditions where the combination of an analgesic and a mild tranquilliser/muscle relaxant would be of value. Such conditions include the short-term symptomatic treatment of acute musculoskeletal disorders associated with painful muscle spasm.

Dosage and administration For oral administration only.

Adults: The usual dose is 1 or 2 tablets three times daily. The dosage should be adjusted to the patient's response, but should not exceed 8 tablets daily.

Elderly: Half the normal adult dose or less may be sufficient for a therapeutic response in the elderly.

Children: Not recommended.

Contra-indications, warnings, etc
Contra-indications: Lobak tablets are contra-indicated in patients sensitive to chlormezanone or paracetamol and in individuals taking monoamine oxidase inhibitors.

Precautions: Lobak should be used with caution in patients with hepatic or renal insufficiency or with porphyria.

Day-time sedation is a relatively uncommon effect of Lobak but may lead to modification of patient's reactions (performance at skilled tasks, alertness etc.) to a varying extent depending on individual susceptibility. Therefore patients should be advised not to drive or operate machinery during treatment.

The dependence potential of chlormezanone is not known. As with sedative drugs, dependence may possibly occur when chlormezanone is given in high dosage or for prolonged periods, especially in patients with a history of alcoholism or drug dependence, or in patients with marked personality disorders. The possibility of withdrawal reactions to abrupt termination of chlormezanone after long term treatment has not been studied. Gradual withdrawal may be more appropriate.

Chormezanone has a prolonged half-life in man and hence prolonged duration of action. The possibility of cumulative effects has not been studied. Safety and efficacy have not been established beyond short-term use.

Use in pregnancy: There is insufficient evidence of the safety of Lobak in human pregnancy nor is there evidence from animal work that it is free from hazard. Do not use during pregnancy, especially in the first trimester, nor during breast feeding, unless there are compelling reasons.

Interactions: Patients should be warned that the sedative effect of Lobak tablets is potentiated by alcohol. The concurrent use of other CNS depressant drugs should be avoided because their sedative effect may be intensified.

Side-effects: Drowsiness and dizziness have been the commonest side-effects, particularly at higher doses.

Other reported side-effects include nausea, lightheadedness, headache, lethargy, and dryness of the mouth. Cholestatic jaundice has occurred. Less common adverse effects include ataxia, depression, flushing, 'hangover' and blurring of vision or diplopia. Slight skin reactions of the urticaria or erythematous type can occur. Cases of fixed drug rash and various forms of exudative erythema multiforme have been reported; these are very uncommon but in certain cases can be serious.

Overdosage: The signs and symptoms of overdose with the chlormezanone component of Lobak will probably resemble those of other central depressant drugs, for example somnolence, prostration, muscular inco-ordination and memory disturbances. In severe cases, hypotension, respiratory depression and loss of consciousness may occur. Symptomatic treatment is suggested with gastric lavage if ingestion was recent.

Patients who have taken an overdose of paracetamol may appear well for the first three days then succumb with liver damage. The hepatic changes produced by overdose of paracetamol result from the accumulation of a highly reactive intermediate metabolite in the hepatocytes. N-acetyl-cysteine intravenously or l-methionine orally protect the liver if administered within 10–12 hours of ingesting an overdose.

Pharmaceutical precautions The product should be stored at room temperature.

Legal category POM.

Package quantities Lobak is supplied in bottles of 50.

Further information Chlormezanone appears to act by central depression of polysynaptic reflexes and to possess some peripheral inhibiting effects at neuromuscular junctions. Paracetamol is a well established analgesic which appears to act peripherally.

In healthy adults, peak plasma levels of 5–6 microgram/ml are seen within 1–2 hours of a 400 mg oral dose of chlormezanone. Mean plasma elimination half life is 24 hours (range 19–30 hours). About 1% of the dose is excreted unchanged in the urine within 24 hours. The majority appears to undergo hydrolysis followed by oxidation and conjugation to 4-chlorohippuric acid which appears in the urine.

Paracetamol is rapidly and almost completely absorbed, peak plasma concentrations being reached in 30 to 60 minutes. Plasma half life is 1 to 4 hours. Excretion is almost exclusively renal in the form of conjugated metabolites.

Product licence number 0071/5059.

MICTRAL*

Presentation A mixture of granules containing particles varying in colour from white to yellow. When added to water, they disperse with slight effervescence, yielding a citrus-flavour suspension. Each 7 g of granules contains Nalidixic Acid BP 660.0 mg and Sodium Citrate PhEur, Citric Acid PhEur and Sodium Bicarbonate PhEur with a combined citrate content equivalent to 4.1 g Sodium Citrate PhEur. Mictral granules contain sucrose, invert sugar and dextrose.

Uses For the treatment of cystitis and lower urinary tract infections caused by pathogens sensitive to nalidixic acid.

Dosage and administration For oral administration only.

Adults including the elderly: The contents of one sachet should be dissolved in a tumblerful of water and taken three times a day. A 3-day course is normally sufficient.

Children: Not recommended.

Contra-indications, warnings, etc
Contra-indications: Mictral is contra-indicated for patients with a history of convulsive disorders, renal impairment, porphyria or hypersensitivity to nalidixic acid or related compounds.

Precautions: Use with caution in patients with liver disease since nalidixic acid is mainly metabolised by the liver. Observe caution also in those with allergic disposition. Patients should avoid excessive exposure to sunlight (including sunbathing).

Mictral may precipitate a haemolytic reaction in G-6-PD deficient individuals.

Each sachet contains 950 mg (41.3 mEq) of sodium. This should be taken into account when prescribing for patients for whom sodium restriction is indicated, especially the elderly.

Use in pregnancy and lactation: Animal studies have not shown any hazard in pregnancy, although in some species nalidixic acid has been seen to be taken up by growing cartilage. Particular consideration should be given before prescribing Mictral for pregnant women, especially during the first trimester and also during lactation since traces of nalidixic acid may be excreted in human milk.

Interactions: Serious gastro-intestinal toxicity may be provoked if Mictral is given concomitantly with melphalan.

If Mictral is given to patients on anticoagulant therapy, it may be necessary to reduce the anticoagulant dosage because nalidixic acid may interact with anticoagulants by competing for protein binding sites. Monitoring of prothrombin time and appropriate adjustment of anticoagulant dosage following introduction and also withdrawal of Mictral is recommended.

Active proliferation of the organisms is a necessary condition for the antibacterial action of nalidixic acid; the action of Mictral may therefore be inhibited by the presence of other antibacterial substances especially bacteriostatic agents such as tetracycline, chloramphenicol and nitrofurantoin which is antagonistic to nalidixic acid in vitro.

Probenecid may reduce the efficacy of Mictral by inhibiting tubular secretion of nalidixic acid.

It is possible that there will be an increased risk of nephrotoxicity with cyclosporin.

When testing for glycosuria in patients receiving Mictral, glucose specific methods based on glucose oxidase should be used since copper reduction methods may give false-positive results.

Mictral may interfere with the estimation of urinary 17-ketosteroids causing high results in the assay of urinary vanilmandelic acid (Pisano method).

Side-effects: In keeping with the reduced systemic exposure to nalidixic acid which Mictral therapy entails, it is unlikely that Mictral will give rise to the full spectrum of adverse events reported with conventional oral nalidixic acid therapy, which include:

CNS: drowsiness, weakness, headache, dizziness and vertigo; subjective visual disturbances such as over-brightness of lights, changed colour perception, difficulty in focusing, decreased visual acuity and double vision, which are infrequent and usually disappear promptly on reducing dosage or stopping therapy.

Toxic psychosis or brief convulsions, which are rare, have usually followed excessive dosage in patients predisposed by epilepsy or cerebral arteriosclerosis. Very rarely, 6th cranial nerve palsy, has been observed. The mechanism for these reactions is unknown but following withdrawal of treatment, rapid resolution without sequelae has usually occurred.

Gastro-intestinal: abdominal pain, nausea, vomiting and diarrhoea.

Allergic: rash, pruritus, urticaria, angio-oedema, eosinophilia, arthralgia with joint stiffness and swelling and, rarely, anaphylactoid reactions; photosensitivity reactions which include erythema and bullae on exposed surfaces are likely to resolve within 2–8 weeks of stopping therapy but bullae may continue to appear for up to 12 weeks after therapy, with mild skin trauma or exposure to sunlight (see Warnings).

Other: rarely, cholestasis, paraesthesia, metabolic acidosis, thrombocytopenia, leucopenia or haemolytic anaemia, sometimes associated with glucose-6-phosphate dehydrogenase deficiency.

Overdosage: Because of the nature of the product, serious overdosage is unlikely. An excessive amount of granules is likely to cause vomiting.

Pharmaceutical precautions Store in a dry place.

Legal category POM.

Package quantities Cartons containing nine 7 g sachets (OP).

Further information Sodium citrate raises the urinary pH thereby increasing the amount of free nalidixic acid and of its active metabolite hydroxynalidixic acid which appear in the urine.

Nalidixic acid acts by selectively inhibiting bacterial DNA synthesis.

Product licence number 0071/0126.

MOTILIUM*

Presentation Motilium tablets are white film-coated tablets with 63 and L embossed on one face and the ankh symbol on the reverse, containing domperidone maleate, equivalent to 10 mg domperidone base. Motilium tablets contain lactose.

Motilium suppositories are white and each contains domperidone 30 mg.

Motilium suspension is a sweet tasting, sugar free white suspension containing domperidone 1 mg/ml. The suspension also contains methyl and propyl parabens and sorbitol.

Uses

Adults: 1. Motilium is indicated for the acute treatment of nausea and vomiting of any aetiology, in adults. Motilium is not recommended for chronic administration.

2. Motilium is indicated for the treatment of nausea and vomiting caused by L-dopa and bromocriptine.

Children: Motilium is not recommended for use in children unless indicated for the management of nausea and vomiting following cancer chemotherapy or irradiation.

Dosage and administration Dose, route and frequency of administration should be adjusted according to severity and duration of symptoms.

The maximum duration of treatment with Motilium for nausea and vomiting due to L-dopa and bromocriptine use is 12 weeks.

Tablets and Suspension

Adults (including the elderly): 10–20 mg orally at 4–8 hourly intervals depending on clinical response.

Children: 0.2–0.4 mg/kg suspension by mouth at 4–8 hourly intervals.

Suppositories:

Adults (including the elderly): 1 or 2 suppositories at 4–8 hourly intervals.

Children aged 2–12 yrs:

Weight (kg)	*Maximum daily dose suppositories/day (mg/day)*
10 –15	1 (30 mg)
15.5–25	2 (60 mg)
25.5–35	3 (90 mg)
35.5–45	4 (120 mg)

Contra-indications, warnings, etc No specific contra-indications.

Precautions: Use in pregnancy: Safe use in pregnant women has not been established, although studies in animals have not demonstrated teratogenic effects. It is therefore not advisable to administer Motilium in pregnancy.

Interactions: Whilst adverse interactions have not been reported in general clinical use it is clear that there is a theoretical potential for domperidone to interact with several classes of agent. Domperidone may, therefore, alter the peripheral actions of dopamine agonists such as bromocriptine, including its hypoprolactinaemic action. The actions of domperidone on gastro-intestinal function may be antagonised by antimuscarinics and opioid analgesics. Domperidone may enhance the absorption of concomitantly administered drugs particularly in patients with delayed gastric emptying.

Side-effects: In common with other dopamine antagonists Motilium produces a rise in serum prolactin which may be associated with galactorrhoea and less frequently with gynaecomastia.

Motilium does not readily cross the normally functioning blood brain barrier and therefore is unlikely to interfere with central dopaminergic function. However, acute extrapyramidal dystonic reactions have been reported.

Overdosage: No case of overdosage with oral domperidone has been reported. There is no specific antidote to Motilium but in the event of overdosage gastric lavage may be useful.

Pharmaceutical precautions Motilium suppositories should be stored in a cool place.

Legal category POM.

Package quantities *Motilium tablets:* Cartons of 30 and 100 tablets in blister strips of 10 tablets.

Motilium Suppositories: Unit Carton: 10 suppositories.

Motilium Suspension: Bottles of 200 ml (1 mg/ml).

Further information Nil.

Product licence numbers

Motilium tablets	0071/0287
Motilium suppositories	0071/0290
Motilium suspension	0071/0292

MYCARDOL*

Presentation Mycardol Tablets are white, flat tablets with bevelled edges, 7.9 mm in diameter, marked M on one side and scored on the other. Each tablet contains 30 mg pentaerythritol tetranitrate. Mycardol Tablets also contain lactose and dextrose.

Uses Mycardol Tablets are recommended for the symptomatic treatment of angina pectoris. They are not recommended as a single measure for the treatment of anginal attacks, but rather as an adjunct to glyceryl trinitrate.

Dosage and administration For oral administration only.

Adults including the elderly: The usual dosage is 2 tablets three times a day, though some may need 2 tablets four times daily. If there is nocturnal pain, the last dose should be taken before retiring. The tablets should be taken before meals.

Children: Not recommended.

Contra-indications, warnings, etc Mycardol should not be used immediately following a coronary thrombosis or in patients with marked anaemia, cerebral haemorrhage or head trauma.

Mycardol should be used with caution in cases of closed angle glaucoma, and in patients liable to hypotension.

There is no evidence of the safety of Mycardol in human pregnancy, nor is there evidence from animal work that it is free from hazard. It should be avoided in pregnancy unless there is no safer alternative.

Mycardol may potentiate the effect of anti-hypertensive drugs. Tolerance to nitrates may occur and tolerance to glyceryl trinitrate may occur during treatment with Mycardol. Alcohol may enhance some of the effects of Mycardol.

Side-effects: Side-effects most commonly reported are headaches (8.3% in one study), nausea (4.6%), rash (3.7%), lethargy and drowsiness. They are usually mild and often resolve on reducing the dose.

Overdosage: Symptoms of overdose are likely to be similar to those of glyceryl trinitrate: flushing, dizziness, tachycardia, headache, vomiting, restlessness, hypotension, syncope, cyanosis and methaemoglobinaemia, followed by coldness of skin, impairment of respiration and bradycardia. Treatment involves: gastric lavage, oxygen and assisted ventilation if necessary. Intravenous methylene blue, 1-4 mg/kg, is given if methaemoglobinaemia is present.

Pharmaceutical precautions Store in a cool place and protect from light.

Legal category P.

Package quantities Mycardol Tablets are supplied in bottles of 100.

Further information The clinical effects of pentaerythritol tetranitrate may be explained by improved oxygenation of ischaemic areas of the myocardium, and reduction in its oxygen demand, through a vasodilatory action on coronary and systemic vessels. It can be detected in the blood within 15 minutes of dosing, and peak levels occur within 4 to 8 hours. It is estimated in the faeces and urine. Its trinitrate metabolite is very active and may contribute substantially to its activity.

Product licence number 0071/5065.

NEGRAM*

Presentation Negram Suspension is a deep pink, viscous suspension with a raspberry odour and taste. It contains 300 mg Nalidixic Acid BP per 5 ml dose. Negram Suspension contains methyl, propyl and butyl p-hydroxybenzoate and amaranth (E123).

Negram Tablets are beige, bi-convex tablets, 12.7 mm in diameter, marked 'NEGRAM' on one side and with an ankh symbol on the other. Each tablet contains 500 mg Nalidixic Acid BP.

Uses Negram is recommended for the treatment of acute or chronic infections, especially those of the urinary tract caused by Gram-negative organisms, other than *Pseudomonas* species, sensitive to nalidixic acid. It may also be used for the treatment of selected cases of gastrointestinal Gram-negative infections sensitive to nalidixic acid.

Dosage and administration For oral administration only.

Adults including the elderly: For acute infections, 1 g four times daily for at least seven days, reducing to 0.5 g four times a day for chronic infections.

Children: For those over the age of three months, the maximum recommended dose is 50 mg/kg body weight per day in divided doses. When prolonged treatment is necessary it may be possible to reduce the dose to 30 mg/kg body weight without loss of therapeutic benefit.

Not recommended for infants less than three months of age.

Contra-indications, warnings, etc

Contra-indications: Negram is contra-indicated for patients with a history of convulsive disorders, porphyria or hypersensitivity to nalidixic acid or related compounds.

Precautions: Particular caution is advised in patients with a known allergic disposition.

Patients taking Negram should avoid excessive exposure to sunlight (including sunbathing).

Negram is mainly metabolised by the liver and should therefore be used with caution in patients with liver disease. Although care should be exercised in treating patients with renal failure, the full dosage of Negram may be administered in patients with creatinine clearance of more than 20 ml/min and half the normal dosage in patients with creatinine clearance less than this.

When Negram is given to patients on anticoagulant therapy, it may be necessary to reduce the anticoagulant dosage.

Nalidixic acid has been shown to induce lesions in weight-bearing joints of young animals. The relevance of this to man is unknown. The possible risk of late degenerative joint changes in young patients receiving nalidixic acid preparations should therefore be considered. If symptoms of arthralgia occur, treatment with nalidixic acid should be stopped.

Blood count, renal and liver function should be monitored periodically if treatment is continued for more than two weeks.

Use in pregnancy and lactation: Animal studies have not shown any hazard in pregnancy, although in some species nalidixic acid has been seen to be taken up by growing cartilage. Particular consideration should be given before prescribing Negram for pregnant women, especially during the first trimester. When treating women who are breast feeding, consideration should be given to the fact that traces of nalidixic acid are excreted in the milk.

Interactions: Negram may interact with anticoagulants due to competition for protein binding sites and it may therefore be necessary to reduce the anticoagulant dosage and monitor the prothrombin time during co-administration, until a satisfactory prothrombin ratio is achieved.

There have been reports of serious gastro-intestinal toxicity following the concomitant use of Negram and melphalan.

Nalidixic acid in therapeutic doses can interfere with the estimation of urinary 17-ketosteroids and may cause high results in the assay of urinary vanilmandelic-acid (Pisano method).

When testing for glycosuria in patients receiving Negram, glucose-specific methods based on glucose oxidase should be used because copper reduction methods may give false-positive results.

Active proliferation of the organisms is a necessary condition for the antibacterial activity of nalidixic acid: the action of Negram may therefore be inhibited by the presence of other antibacterial substances especially bacteriostatic agents such as tetracycline, chloramphenicol, and nitrofurantoin which is antagonistic to nalidixic acid in vitro.

Negram also interacts with probenecid, which inhibits the tubular secretion of nalidixic acid. This may reduce the efficacy of the product in the treatment of urinary tract infections and increase the risk of systemic side-effects. It is possible that there will be an increased risk of nephrotoxicity with cyclosporin.

Side-effects: Reactions reported after oral administration of Negram include:

CNS: drowsiness, weakness, headache, and dizziness and vertigo. Reversible subjective visual disturbances without objective findings have occurred infrequently (generally with each dose during the first few days of treatment). These reactions include overbrightness of lights, change in colour perception, difficulty in focusing, decrease in visual acuity, and double vision. They usually disappear promptly when dosage is reduced or therapy is discontinued. Toxic psychosis or brief convulsions have been reported rarely, usually following excessive doses. In general, the convulsions have occurred in patients with predisposing factors such as epilepsy or cerebral arteriosclerosis. In infants and children receiving therapeutic doses of Negram, increased intracranial pressure with bulging anterior fontanelle, papilloedema, and headache has occasionally been observed. A few cases of 6th cranial nerve palsy have been reported. Although the mechanisms of these reactions are unknown, the signs and symptoms usually disappear rapidly with no sequelae when treatment is discontinued.

Gastro-intestinal: abdominal pain, nausea, vomiting and diarrhoea.

Allergic: rash, pruritus, urticaria, angio-oedema, eosinophilia, arthralgia with joint stiffness and swelling, and rarely, anaphylactoid reaction. Photosensitivity reactions consisting of erythema and bullae on exposed skin surfaces usually resolve completely in 2 weeks to 2 months after Negram is discontinued; however, bullae may continue to appear with successive exposures to sunlight or with mild skin trauma for up to 3 months after discontinuation of the drug. (See Warnings).

Other: rarely cholestasis, paraesthesia, metabolic acidosis, thrombocytopenia, leucopenia, or haemolytic anaemia, sometimes associated with glucose-6-phosphate dehydrogenase deficiency.

Overdosage: In adults, symptoms of overdosage have been noted following single doses of 20 and 25 g. These have included toxic psychosis and convulsions.

Occasional reports of metabolic acidosis have occurred in association with overdosage, use in infants under the age of three months, or overdose with concurrent use of probenecid.

In an emergency, it is suggested that the stomach should be emptied, and symptomatic treatment applied as necessary, a particular watch being kept for central or respiratory depression.

Pharmaceutical precautions Where doses of less than 5 ml of Negram suspension are required, the suspension may be diluted with Syrup BP so that the standard 5 ml spoonful can be given. Such dilutions will remain stable for two or three weeks.

Legal category POM.

Package quantities *Negram Suspension:* Bottles of 150 ml.
Negram Tablets: Boxes of 56 tablets (7 strips of 8 tablets) (OP).

Further information Nalidixic acid acts by selectively inhibiting bacterial DNA synthesis. It is well absorbed following oral administration, and almost all is excreted by the kidneys, about 80% being recovered in the urine. Effective antibacterial concentrations are readily obtainable in the urine: in human volunteers, single 0.5 and 1 g oral doses produce peak urine levels varying from 25 to 250 microgram/ml.

Product licence numbers
Negram Suspenion 0071/5067
Negram Tablets 0071/5068.

PAMETON*

Presentation White, unmarked, capsule-shaped tablets 19 mm long and 8 mm wide, with a characteristic odour of methionine. Each tablet contains Paracetamol PhEur 500 mg and D.L-methionine 250 mg.

Uses A mild analgesic and antipyretic suitable for use in most painful and febrile conditions: for example headache, toothache, colds, influenza, rheumatic pain and dysmenorrhoea. This formulation should prove particularly useful where the possibility of misuse or overdosage exists.

Dosage and administration Pameton is for oral administration only.

Adults including the elderly: Two tablets up to four times a day as required.

Children: 6–12 years: Half to one tablet. Allow at least 4 hours between doses. Do not give more than four doses in any 24-hour period.

Not suitable for children under 6 years of age.

Contra-indications, warnings, etc Pameton should be avoided in those hypersensitive to paracetamol. Because of the methionine content, Pameton should be used with care in patients with severe liver damage. Although there is epidemiological evidence of the safety of paracetamol in human pregnancy and methionine is an essential amino acid, Pameton should be used with caution in pregnancy.

Concurrent administration of methionine and levodopa may inhibit the effect of the latter drug.

Overdosage: Death from paracetamol overdosage invariably results from hepatic necrosis caused by a reactive metabolite of paracetamol which only becomes toxic when liver glutathione stores are exhausted. Concurrent ingestion of methionine (a precursor of glutathione) in these tablets is designed to help protect the liver against the hepatotoxic effect of excessive amounts of paracetamol. If a patient is seen within 4 hours of ingestion of an overdose of Pameton, the stomach should be emptied by gastric lavage or emesis and, if indicated by blood levels of paracetamol, treatment should be continued with either oral methionine or N-acetyl-cysteine intravenously taking into account the amount of methionine already ingested by the patient.

Pharmaceutical precautions Protect from light.

Legal category P.

Package quantities Cartons of 60 tablets in blisters (OP).

Further information Nil.

Product licence number 0071/0216.

PARACETAMOL SOLUBLE (PANADOL* SOLUBLE)

Presentation Paracetamol Soluble consists of white, bevelled-edged, unmarked, scored tablets which effervesce vigorously when placed in water. Each is 25.4 mm in diameter and contains 500 mg Paracetamol PhEur.

Uses Paracetamol is a mild analgesic and antipyretic. The tablets are recommended for the treatment of most painful and febrile conditions, for example, headache including migraine headache, toothache, sore throat, colds, influenza, rheumatic pain and dysmenorrhoea.

Dosage and administration Paracetamol Soluble is for oral administration only and should be dissolved in a tumblerful of water before taking.

Adults: One to two tablets.

Elderly: As for adults but see warnings.

Children: 6–12 years: Half to one tablet.
Under 6 years: Not recommended.

These dosages may be repeated as required, but should be given no more frequently than every 4 hours. Not more than 4 doses should be taken in any 24 hours.

Contra-indications, warnings, etc Apart from hypersensitivity to paracetamol, which is rare, there are no known contra-indications associated with the use of paracetamol and side-effects are unusual.

There is epidemiological evidence of the safety of paracetamol in human pregnancy. Each Paracetamol Soluble tablet contains 425 mg (18.5 mmol) of sodium. This sodium content should be taken into account when prescribing for patients for whom sodium restriction is indicated.

Overdosage: It should be noted that patients who have taken an overdose of paracetamol may appear well for the first three days then succumb with liver damage. The hepatic changes produced by overdosage of paracetamol result from the accumulation of a highly reactive intermediate metabolite in the hepatocytes.

N-acetyl-cysteine intravenously, or methionine orally protects the liver if administered within 10–12 hours of ingesting the overdose.

Patients in whom oxidative liver enzymes have been induced, including alcoholics, those receiving barbiturates and patients who are chronically malnourished, may be more sensitive to the toxic effects of paracetamol.

Pharmaceutical precautions Nil.

Legal category P.

Package quantities Paracetamol Soluble tablets are packed in PFP laminate strips in cartons of 60 tablets (OP).

Further information Nil.

Product licence number 0071/0072

pHiso-MED*

Presentation A white solution which forms suds when added to water. It contains 21.2% w/w Chlorhexidine Gluconate Solution BP (equivalent to 4% w/w chlorhexidine gluconate) and 2% Benzyl Alcohol BP as preservative. In addition, pHiso-MED contains a blend of compatible mild surfactants consisting of ethoxylated glycerides and bis 2 hydroxyethylcocamine oxide. It also contains a triglyceride ester of fatty wax acids, polyethylene glycol ethoxy distearate and a selected fraction of lanolin alcohol.

Uses

1. Pre-operative preparation of surgeons' and nurses' hands and the skin of patients.
2. As an antiseptic skin cleanser for routine hand washing and for spots and acne on the face, shoulders and chest.
3. For use in maternity units by nurses and mothers, and for bathing babies, as a measure to prevent cross-infection.

Dosage and administration pHiso-Med is for topical use only.

Adults including the elderly:

1. *Pre-operative hand preparation:* Wet the hands and forearms, apply about 5 ml of solution and wash for one minute. Thoroughly clean finger-nails with a brush or scraper. Rinse, and repeat the wash for two minutes. Rinse thoroughly and dry.
2. *Preparation of patients for elective surgery:* Using a sterile swab, the solution is rubbed over the site and surrounding skin for two minutes, adding a little sterile water to work up a lather. Wipe off and dry thoroughly with fresh sterile swabs. Subsequently, at the time of operation, a 0.5% solution of chlorhexidine in alcohol should be applied to the site with sterile gauze swabs. The site and the surrounding skin should be rubbed vigorously for two minutes and until dry.
3. *As an antiseptic skin cleanser:* Wet the area to be cleaned, apply 5 ml of solution and wash for one minute. Rinse thoroughly and dry.

Children: For bathing infants in maternity units: A 1 in 10 dilution of the solution is applied over the baby's body with a swab or with the palm of the hand. Rinse thoroughly with warm water and dry in the usual way.

Contra-indications, warnings, etc Chlorhexidine should not be allowed to come into contact with the brain, meninges or middle ear. During use, ensure that the solution is kept away from the eyes and ears. Material which has been in contact with the solution may be stained brown by hypochlorite bleaches.

Overdosage: If the solution is swallowed, it should be removed from the stomach by gastric lavage and symptomatic treatment applied as necessary.

Pharmaceutical precautions Protect from heat and light.

Legal category GSL.

Package quantities Containers of 150 ml.

Further information Chlorhexidine is a disinfectant effective against a wide range of vegetative bacteria. It is more effective against Gram positive than Gram negative bacteria, some species of *Pseudomonas* and *Proteus* being relatively less susceptible. Chlorhexidine is most active at a neutral or slightly alkaline pH. Its activity is reduced by blood and other organic matter.

Product licence number 0071/0178.

PLAQUENIL*

Presentation Plaquenil Tablets are smoothly polished, orange-coloured, biconvex, sugar-coated tablets with no markings. Each tablet contains 200 mg Hydroxychloroquine Sulphate BP.

Uses Plaquenil Tablets are recommended for the treatment of rheumatoid arthritis, juvenile chronic arthritis, discoid and systemic lupus erythematosus and dermatological conditions caused or aggravated by sunlight.

Dosage and administration Plaquenil tablets are for oral administration only.

In rheumatoid arthritis, juvenile chronic arthritis, discoid and systemic lupus erythematosus, treatment should be discontinued if there is no improvement by 6 months. In light-sensitive diseases, treatment should only be given during periods of maximum exposure to light.

Adults including the elderly: Initially 400 mg daily in divided doses. The dose can be reduced to 200 mg when no further improvement is evident. The maintenance dose should be increased to 400 mg daily if the response lessens. The minimum effective dose should be employed and should not exceed 6.5 mg/kg/day (calculated from ideal body weight and not actual body weight).

Children: The minimum effective doses should be employed and should not exceed 6.5 mg/kg/day. The Plaquenil 200 mg tablet is therefore not suitable for use in children with a body weight of less than 33 kg.

Contra-indications, warnings, etc

Contra-indications: Plaquenil should not be used in patients with pre-existing maculopathy nor should it be used in those sensitive to 4-aminoquinoline compounds. A chemically related compound, chloroquine phosphate, has been found to cause foetal cochlear damage when taken in high doses during pregnancy; therefore Plaquenil should not be used in pregnancy.

Precautions: All patients should have an ophthalmological examination before treatment with Plaquenil is initiated. Thereafter, ophthalmological examinations must be repeated at least every 6 months. The examination should include testing visual acuity, careful ophthalmoscopy and central visual field testing with a red target. Plaquenil should be discontinued immediately in any patient who develops a pigmentary abnormality or visual field defect or any other abnormality not explainable by difficulty in accommodation or presence of corneal opacities. Patients should continue to be observed for possible progression of the changes.

The occurrence of retinopathy is very uncommon if the recommended daily doses are not exceeded. The administration of doses in excess of the recommended maximum is likely to increase the risk of retinopathy and accelerate its onset.

Impaired visual accommodation soon after the start of treatment has been reported and patients should be warned regarding driving or operating machinery. If the condition is not self-limiting it will resolve on reducing the dose or stopping treatment.

Plaquenil should be used with caution in patients taking medicines which may cause adverse ocular or skin reactions. Caution should also be applied when it is used in patients with hepatic or renal disease, in those taking medicines known to affect those organs and in patients with severe gastro-intestinal, neurological or blood disorders. Estimation of plasma hydroxychloroquine levels should be undertaken in patients with severely compromised renal or hepatic function and dosage adjusted accordingly.

Caution is also advised in patients with a sensitivity to quinine, those with glucose-6-phosphate dehydrogenase deficiency, those with porphyria cutanea tarda which can be exacerbated by hydroxychloroquine and in patients with psoriasis since it appears to increase the risk of skin reactions.

Although the risk of bone-marrow depression is low, periodic blood counts are advisable and Plaquenil should be discontinued if abnormalities develop.

Small children are particularly sensitive to the toxic effects of 4-aminoquinolines; therefore, patients should be warned to keep Plaquenil out of the reach of children.

Interactions: Plaquenil has been reported to increase plasma digoxin levels.

Plaquenil may also be subject to several of the known interactions of chloroquine even though specific reports have not appeared. These include: potentiation of its direct blocking action at the neuromuscular junction by aminoglycoside antibiotics; inhibition of its metabolism by cimetidine which may increase plasma concentration of the antimalarial; antagonism of effect of neostigmine and pyridostigmine; reduction of the antibody response to primary immunisation with intradermal human diploid-cell rabies vaccine.

As with chloroquine, antacids may reduce absorption of hydroxychloroquine so it is advised that a 4 hour interval be observed between Plaquenil and antacid dosaging.

Side-effects: Retinopathy with changes in pigmentation and visual field defects can occur, but appears to be uncommon if the recommended daily dose is not exceeded. In its early form, it appears reversible on discontinuation of Plaquenil. If allowed to develop, there may be a risk of progression even after treatment withdrawal.

Corneal opacities have been reported. They are either symptomless or may cause disturbances such as haloes, blurring of vision or photophobia. They are reversible on stopping treatment.

Skin rashes sometimes occur; pigmentary changes in skin and mucous membranes, bleaching of hair, and hair loss have also been reported. These usually resolve readily on stopping treatment.

Other adverse effects include gastrointestinal disturbances such as nausea, diarrhoea, anorexia, abdominal cramps and, rarely, vomiting. These symptoms usually resolve immediately on reducing the dose or on stopping the treatment. Less frequently, muscle weakness, vertigo, tinnitus, nerve deafness, headache, nervousness and emotional upsets have been reported. Rarely, there have been reports of bone marrow depression, neuromyotoxicity, and toxic psychosis.

Plaquenil can also precipitate porphyria.

Overdosage: Recovery under treatment has followed the ingestion of 36 Plaquenil tablets, while an estimated dose of 54 tablets has proved rapidly fatal. Overdosage with the 4-aminoquinolines is particularly dangerous in infants, as little as 1–2 g having proved fatal.

The symptoms of overdosage may include headache, visual disturbance, cardiovascular collapse, and convulsions, followed by sudden and early respiratory and cardiac arrest. Since these effects may appear soon after taking a massive dose, treatment should be prompt and symptomatic. The stomach should be immediately evacuated, either by emesis or by gastric lavage. Finely powdered charcoal in a dose at least five times that of the overdose may inhibit further absorption if introduced into the stomach by tube, following lavage and within 30 minutes of ingestion of the overdose.

Parenteral diazepam should be administered in all cases of overdosage; it has been shown to reverse chloroquine cardiotoxicity.

Respiratory support may be needed and need for intubation or tracheostomy considered. Shock should be treated by the administration of fluid (with plasma expanders if necessary) with central venous pressure monitoring. In severe cases, the administration of dopamine should be considered.

A patient who survives the acute phase and is asymptomatic should be closely observed for at least six hours.

Pharmaceutical precautions Nil.

Legal category POM.

Package quantities Plaquenil is supplied in bottles of 56 tablets (OP).

Further information Hydroxychloroquine has several pharmacological actions which may be involved in its therapeutic effect. These include interaction with sulphydryl groups, interference with enzyme activity (including phospholipase, NADH – cytochrome C reductase, cholinesterase, proteases and hydrolases), DNA binding, stabilisation of lysosomal membranes, inhibition of prostaglandin formation, polymorphonuclear cell chemotaxis and phagocytosis, possible interference with interleukin 1 production from monocytes and inhibition of neutrophil superoxide release.

Following oral administration, hydroxychloroquine is almost completely absorbed. In one study, mean peak plasma hydroxychloroquine concentrations following a single dose of 400 mg in healthy subjects ranged from 53–208 ng/ml with a mean of 105 ng/ml. The mean time to peak plasma concentration was 1.83 hours.

The mean plasma elimination half-life varied: 5.9 hours (at C_{max}–10 hours), 26.1 hours (at 10–48 hours) and 299 hours (at 48–504 hours). The parent compound and metabolites are widely distributed in the body and elimination is mainly via the urine.

Product licence number 0071/5083.

PRIMACOR* INJECTION ▼

Presentation Primacor Injection is a sterile, clear, colourless to pale yellow solution, each 10 ml ampoule containing 10 mg milrinone as the lactate. Primacor also contains dextrose and lactic acid.

Uses Primacor Injection is indicated for the short-term treatment of severe congestive heart failure unresponsive to conventional maintenance therapy.

Milrinone is a positive inotrope and vasodilator, with little chronotropic activity. It also improves left ventricular diastolic relaxation. It differs in structure and mode of action from the digitalis glycosides, catecholamines or angiotensin-converting enzyme inhibitors.

It is a selective inhibitor of peak III phosphodiesterase isoenzyme in cardiac and vascular muscle. It produces slight enhancement of A–V node conduction, but no other significant electrophysiological effects.

In clinical studies Primacor Injection has been shown to produce improvements in the haemodynamic indices of congestive heart failure, including cardiac output, pulmonary capillary wedge pressure and vascular resistance, without clinically significant effect on heart rate or myocardial oxygen consumption. These improvements are related to both dose and plasma concentration. Haemodynamic improvement during intravenous Primacor therapy is accompanied by clinical symptomatic improvement, as measured by changes in New York Heart Association classification.

Dosage and administration For intravenous administration.

Adults: Primacor Injection should be given as a loading dose of 50 micrograms/kg administered over a period of 10 minutes followed usually by continuous maintenance infusion of 0.5 micrograms/kg/min.

Maintenance infusion dosage may be titrated between 0.375 micrograms/kg/min and 0.75 micrograms/kg/min to a maximum haemodynamic effect but should not exceed 1.13 mg/kg/day total dose.

Note: In impaired renal function, lower rates of

maintenance infusion are advised: See 'Use in impaired renal function.'

The following provides a guide to maintenance infusion delivery rate based upon a solution containing milrinone 200 micrograms/ml.†

Primacor Injection Dose (micrograms/kg/min)	*Infusion delivery rate (ml/kg/hr)*
0.375	0.11
0.400	0.12
0.500	0.15
0.600	0.18
0.700	0.21
0.750	0.22

† A 200 micrograms/ml solution is prepared by adding 40 ml diluent per 10 ml ampoule Primacor Injection.

0.45% saline, 0.9% saline or 5% dextrose may be used as diluents.

Solutions of different concentrations may be used according to patient fluid requirements.

The duration of therapy should depend upon the patient's response. The usual period is 48 to 72 hours, although some patients have been maintained on the infusion for up to 5 days.

Use in impaired renal function: Data obtained from patients with severe renal impairment but without congestive heart failure have demonstrated that the presence of renal impairment significantly increases the terminal elimination half-life of milrinone. For patients with clinical evidence of renal impairment, the following infusion rates are recommended:

Creatinine Clearance (ml/min/ 1.73m²)	*Primacor Injection Dose (micrograms/ kg/min)*	*Infusion delivery rate (for solution of milrinone 200 micrograms/ml) ml/kg/hr*
5	0.20	0.06
10	0.23	0.07
20	0.28	0.08
30	0.33	0.10
40	0.38	0.11
50	0.43	0.13

Adjustment of the infusion rate should be made according to haemodynamic response.

Use in elderly patients: Experience so far suggests that no special dosage recommendations for the elderly patient are necessary.

Use in children: Safety and effectiveness in children have not been established.

Contra-indications, warnings, etc
Contra-indications: Hypersensitivity to Primacor Injection is a contra-indication to its use.

Precautions: The use of Primacor Injection is not recommended immediately following acute myocardial infarction until safety and efficacy have been established in this situation.

In patients with severe obstructive aortic or pulmonary valvular disease or hypertrophic subaortic stenosis, Primacor Injection should not be used in place of surgical relief of the obstruction. In these conditions it is possible that a drug with inotropic/vasodilator properties might aggravate outflow obstruction.

Supraventricular and ventricular arrhythmias have been observed in the high risk population treated with Primacor Injection. In some patients an increase in non-sustained ventricular tachycardia has been observed which did not affect patient safety or outcome. Patients receiving Primacor Injection should therefore be closely monitored during infusion.

As Primacor Injection produces a slight enhancement in A–V node conduction, there is a possibility of an increased ventricular response rate in patients with uncontrolled atrial flutter/fibrillation. In these patients, digitalisation or treatment with other agents to prolong A–V node conduction time should be considered prior to the institution of Primacor Injection therapy.

Milrinone may induce hypotension as a consequence of its vasodilatory activity. Therefore during therapy with Primacor Injection, blood pressure and heart rate should be monitored and the rate of infusion slowed or stopped in patients showing excessive decreases in blood pressure.

If prior vigorous diuretic therapy is suspected to have caused significant decreases in cardiac filling pressure, Primacor Injection should be cautiously administered with monitoring of blood pressure, heart rate and clinical state.

Fluid balance, electrolytes and renal function should be carefully monitored during Primacor Injection therapy. Improvement in cardiac output with resultant diuresis may necessitate a reduction in the dose of diuretic. Potassium loss due to excessive diuresis may predispose digitalised patients to arrhythmias. Therefore, hypokalaemia should be corrected by potassium supplementation in advance of, or during, the use of Primacor Injection.

Use in pregnancy and lactation: Although animal studies have not revealed evidence of drug-induced foetal damage or other deleterious effects on reproductive function, the safety of milrinone in human pregnancy has not yet been established. It should be used during pregnancy only if the potential benefit justifies the potential risk to the foetus.

Caution should be exercised when Primacor Injection is administered to nursing women, since it is not known whether milrinone is excreted in human milk.

Side-effects: Supraventricular and ventricular arrhythmias have been reported during treatment with Primacor Injection. The incidence has not been related to dose or plasma levels of milrinone. Other reported side-effects include hypotension, angina/chest pain and headaches. Hypokalaemia, tremor, and thrombocytopenia have been reported with an incidence similar to placebo and have not been definitely related to the administration of Primacor injection.

Drug interactions: No untoward clinical manifestations of drug interaction have been observed during Primacor Injection therapy.

Whilst there is a theoretical potential interaction with calcium channel blockers, there has been no evidence of a clinically significant interaction to date.

Milrinone has a favourable inotropic effect in fully digitalised patients without causing signs of glycoside toxicity.

Chemical compatibility: Precipitation occurs immediately when frusemide or bumetanide is mixed with milrinone solution. Therefore, frusemide or bumetanide should not be administered in intravenous lines containing Primacor Injection. Sodium Bicarbonate Intravenous Infusion should not be used for dilution.

Other drugs should not be mixed with Primacor Injection until further compatibility data are available.

Overdosage: Overdoses of intravenous Primacor Injection may produce hypotension because of its vasodilatory effect. If this occurs, Primacor Injection administration should be reduced or temporarily discontinued until the patient's condition stabilises. No specific antidote is known, but general measures for circulatory support should be taken.

Pharmaceutical precautions Store at room temperature; avoid freezing. Infusion solutions diluted as recommended with 0.45% saline, 0.9% saline or 5% dextrose should be freshly prepared before use.

Parenteral drug products should be examined visually and should not be used if particulate matter or discolouration are present.

Legal category POM.

Package quantities Boxes of 10 ampoules.

Further information In congestive heart failure, milrinone, on intravenous administration, has a volume of distribution of about 0.4 l/kg, a terminal elimination half-life of about 2.3 hours and a clearance of about

0.13 l/kg/h. These pharmacokinetic parameters are not dose-dependent. Milrinone is approximately 70% bound to plasma protein and the primary route of excretion is via the urine.

Product licence number 0071/0323.

PROMINAL*

Presentation Prominal Tablets 30 mg are white, biconvex tablets, 6.4 mm in diameter, marked P30 on one side and plain on the other. Each tablet contains 30 mg Methylphenobarbitone PhEur.

Prominal Tablets 60 mg are white, biconvex tablets, 7.9 mm in diameter, marked P60 on one side and plain on the other. Each tablet contains 60 mg Methylphenobarbitone PhEur.

Prominal Tablets 200 mg are white, biconvex tablets, 10.3 mm in diameter, marked P200 on one side and plain on the other. Each tablet contains 200 mg Methylphenobarbitone PhEur.

Prominal Tablets 30 mg, 60 mg and 200 mg contain lactose.

Uses

Indications: Prominal Tablets are recommended for the treatment of epilepsy except absence seizures.

Pharmacology: Barbiturates reversibly depress the activity of all excitable tissues, the central nervous system being exquisitely sensitive to their effects.

Methylphenobarbitone undergoes N-demethylation by hepatic microsomal enzymes, forming phenobarbitone, to which most of its activity in chronic medication can be attributed.

Dosage and administration Prominal is for oral administration only.

Adults: The daily dosage must be determined individually. The average range is 200–400 mg. The maximum daily dose is 600 mg.

Elderly: As for adults but see 'Precautions'.

Children: 5–15 mg/kg/day but see 'Precautions'.

Dosing: Dosage should be adjusted carefully with gradual increments at intervals of two to three weeks until fits are controlled or toxicity supervenes. Plateau-state at a given dosage is only achieved after some weeks of medication. Unless serious toxicity dictates otherwise, any reduction in dosage should proceed very gradually to avoid provoking status epilepticus. Monitoring plasma phenobarbitone levels may be helpful when therapy is switched from phenobarbitone to Prominal or vice versa.

Contra-indications, warnings, etc

Contra-indications: Acute intermittent and variegate porphyria; hypersensitivity or idiosyncrasy to barbiturates, states of debilitation, senility, alcohol or other drug abuse or history of abuse; hyperkinetic children; severe renal or hepatic disease.

Precautions: Prominal should be avoided or used only with particular caution and appropriate supervision in children and the elderly who are likely to be specially sensitive to its effects and may react paradoxically.

Prominal should also be avoided or used with special care in patients with hepatic or renal disease whose ability to excrete phenobarbitone may be impaired. Similar caution should be observed in patients with respiratory insufficiency who may prove specially sensitive to the depressant effects of barbiturate on respiration.

Patients who drive or operate machinery should be warned that Prominal can reduce alertness and impair performance. If affected, patients should not undertake these tasks.

Alcohol should be avoided when taking Prominal since as with other CNS depressants, its depressant effect is likely to be additive to that of the barbiturate. In view of the extensive range of inter-reactions between barbiturates and other drugs (see below) caution is advised whenever Prominal is to be co-administered with another medication.

Vitamin D supplement may be needed during long-term Prominal therapy, since Vitamin D catabolism may be increased. Vitamin K supplement may be needed for neonates exposed to barbiturate (see below).

Abuse and dependence: Prominal, like other barbiturates, may lead to psychical and physical dependence in which tolerance and dose increment may be marked features. Symptoms of chronic intoxication include confusion, poor judgement, irritability, insomnia and somatic complaints. Prominal intake should be reduced with great care and under appropriate supervision. Abrupt cessation may precipitate convulsions and can be fatal. Neonates may also suffer from withdrawal symptoms (see below) even in the face of therapeutic dosaging.

Use in pregnancy: Anticonvulsant drugs are as useful to an epileptic during pregnancy as they are at other times and for the individual epileptic mother the chance of an abnormal baby due to drug treatment is small. However, several reports have appeared in the literature suggesting the possible implication of the epileptic state, anticonvulsants and folic acid deficiency as causative agents in certain congenital abnormalities. Scientific knowledge does not yet permit an adequate definition to be made of the respective roles of these three factors. It is recommended therefore, that if anticonvulsant therapy with Prominal is judged necessary during pregnancy, adequate folic acid supplements should be given and the epilepsy controlled as completely as possible with the lowest effective dose.

Neonates: Barbiturates may be transferred to the foetus in utero, as well as to the suckling neonate. Therefore the possibility of barbiturate effects in the neonate, including respiratory depression, sedation and withdrawal reaction, and of the need to give Vitamin K to counteract possible hypoprothrombinaemia, should be borne in mind.

Interactions with other drugs: Barbiturates can affect the actions of a wide range of other drugs principally through an increase in their disposal by stimulation of hepatic microsomal enzymes with usually a resultant decrease but in some instances, an increase, in their therapeutic effect or toxicity. The interactions may be mutual, the plasma levels and activities of barbiturates being also subject to influence by other drugs. Apart from kinetic and metabolic interactions, there may be an addition of effect, for example, the severe depression that may occur when barbiturates are combined with ethanol or other CNS depressants. For these reasons particular care should be observed when administering Prominal in combination with CNS depressants such as sedatives and antihistamines, coumarin-type anticoagulants, antidepressants, including mono-amine oxidase inhibitors, systemic steroids (including oral contraceptives), anticonvulsants such as phenytoin and valproate, antibiotics such as chloramphenicol, rifampicin, metronidazole, doxycycline and also griseofulvin, antihypertensive agents including beta-blockers such as metoprolol and propranolol, but also frusemide and digoxin, opioids such as pethidine and dextropropoxyphene, and many other agents including theophylline, cimetidine, and some oral hypoglycaemic drugs.

Side-effects: Drowsiness and other evidence of sedation is likely to be the most common side effect, but unsteadiness, vertigo and inco-ordination may occur. Paradoxical excitement, restlessness and confusion may occur in the elderly or in the presence of pain; irritability and hyperexcitability may occur in children. Respiratory depression may also occur even at therapeutic dosage and with chronic medication there may be disorientation, mental confusion, ataxia, depression and dependence.

Allergic reactions particularly affecting the skin are not uncommon, including maculopapular rash, fixed drug eruptions and photosensitivity. Occasionally exfoliative dermatitis, erythema multiforme and toxic epidermal necrolysis have been reported. Megaloblastic anaemia associated with folate deficiency has developed during chronic administration and hypoprothrombinaemia may occur in neonates exposed to the barbiturate. Other reported side effects associated with barbiturate include stomatitis, arthritis, acute interstitial nephritis and hepatitis in patients who may be sensitive to this type of drug.

Overdosage: The signs and symptoms of acute overdosage include varying degrees of cardiorespiratory depression, hypotension, absent bowel sounds, renal failure, hypothermia, CNS depression including coma and areflexia. In this setting, a flat EEG may not indicate irreversible brain damage. The aims in treating poisoning by Prominal are to maintain respiration, treat any shock and prevent further absorption of the drug. Where patients are seen within four hours of taking an overdose, gastric aspiration or lavage may be beneficial in adults, while children who are conscious may be given an emetic (e.g. Ipecacuanha Emetic Mixture Paediatric BP). Severely poisoned patients who continue to deteriorate despite supportive treatment may require additional active measures including forced alkaline diuresis, peritoneal dialysis, haemodialysis and haemoperfusion.

Pharmaceutical precautions Nil.

Legal category CD (Sch 3) POM.

Package quantities Prominal Tablets (30 mg, 60 mg and 200 mg) are supplied in bottles of 100.

Further information Nil.

Product licence numbers

Prominal Tablets 30 mg	0071/5084
Prominal Tablets 60 mg	0071/5085
Prominal Tablets 200 mg	0071/5086

PYROGASTRONE* TABLETS PYROGASTRONE* LIQUID

Presentation *Pyrogastrone tablets* are white, round, strawberry-flavoured chewable tablets, 22.2 mm in diameter, marked with an ankh symbol on one side and PG on the other. Each tablet contains:

Carbenoxolone Sodium BP	20 mg
Dried Aluminium Hydroxide PhEur	240 mg
Magnesium Trisilicate BP	60 mg

in a base containing 210 mg Sodium Bicarbonate PhEur and 600 mg Alginic Acid BPC.

Pyrogastrone Liquid is presented in bottles containing a white powder for the preparation of 533 ml of suspension. The suspension is prepared by reconstitution with 450 ml distilled water. When prepared as instructed, each 10 ml contains Carbenoxolone Sodium BP 20 mg and Dried Aluminium Hydroxide PhEur 300 mg in a vehicle with Sodium Alginate BPC and Potassium Bicarbonate BPC. Pyrogastrone Liquid contains sodium methylhydroxybenzoate, sodium propylhydroxybenzoate and sucrose.

Each Pyrogastrone tablet contains 59.2 mg (2.6 mmol) sodium, and Pyrogastrone Liquid provides 117 mg (3.0 mmol) potassium and 38.8 mg (1.7 mmol) sodium per 10 ml dose.

Uses For the treatment of oesophageal inflammation, erosions and ulcers due to hiatus hernia or other conditions causing gastro-oesophageal reflux and for the relief of heartburn, flatulence and other symptoms associated with reflux oesophagitis.

Dosage and administration For oral administration only.

Adults: Pyrogastrone Tablets: 1 tablet to be chewed three times daily immediately after meals and 2 tablets to be chewed at bedtime. The tablets may be followed by a drink of water. *Pyrogastrone Liquid:* 10 ml to be taken three times daily immediately after meals and 20 ml at bedtime.

Treatment should be continued for at least six weeks, but up to 12 weeks' treatment may be necessary to ensure maximum healing effect.

Elderly: Not recommended for patients over 75 years. Otherwise, as for adults.

Children: Not recommended.

Contra-indications, warnings, etc

Contra-indications: Pyrogastrone is contra-indicated in patients over 75 years, in children and in pregnancy. Pyrogastrone should not be administered to patients suffering from cardiac, renal or hepatic failure nor to patients on digitalis glycosides unless serum electrolyte levels are monitored at weekly intervals and measures taken to avoid the development of hypokalaemia. It is contra-indicated in established hypokalaemia.

Precautions: Special care should be exercised with patients pre-disposed to sodium and water retention, potassium loss and hypertension (e.g. the elderly and those with cardiac, renal or hepatic disease) since carbenoxolone can induce similar changes. Potassium supplements should be considered for those at risk from developing hypokalaemia.

Regular monitoring of weight, blood pressure and clinical condition is advisable for all patients. Pyrogastrone should be withdrawn if hypokalaemia or oedema develops or a clinically significant rise in blood pressure occurs. Potassium loss should be corrected by the administration of supplements.

Pregnancy: Although animal studies have shown no hazard, there is inadequate evidence of the safety of carbenoxolone in human pregnancy. Pyrogastrone should be avoided in patients who are pregnant.

Interactions: Pyrogastrone may provoke digitalis glycoside toxicity by inducing hypokalaemia.

There is a theoretical possibility of a pharmacodynamic interaction with anti-hypertensive drugs, carbenoxolone possibly making hypertension more difficult to control.

Most classes of diuretics will induce hypokalaemia which may be exacerbated by concomitant administration of carbenoxolone as may the mineralocorticoid effects of steroids.

Although spironolactone and amiloride will antagonise the hypokalaemia induced by carbenoxolone they also inhibit its healing action and, therefore, should not be prescribed with Pyrogastrone.

Antacids can interact with a wide variety of medications generally through effects on their absorption or excretion. These include:

Analgesics – the absorption of diflunisal is reduced and urinary excretion of aspirin may be increased.

Antiarrhythmics – the urinary excretion of flecainide, mexiletine and quinidine may be reduced.

Antibacterials – the absorption of ciprofloxacin, ofloxacin, pivampicillin, rifampicin and most tetracyclines may be reduced as may the absorption of itraconazole and ketoconazole.

Other agents – the absorption of chloroquine, hydroxychloroquine, phenothiazines, oral iron, dipyridamole and penicillamine may all be reduced whilst excretion of lithium may be increased.

Side-effects: Pyrogastrone may induce sodium and water retention and potassium loss, provoking hypertension and cardiac failure in those so predisposed. If profound hypokalaemia is permitted to develop it may lead to widespread impairment of neuromuscular function and to muscle damage. Prolonged hypokalaemia may cause renal damage.

Overdosage: If recently ingested the stomach should be emptied by gastric lavage. Serum electrolytes should be monitored and any deficiency in potassium should be corrected, using the intravenous route if necessary, or slow-release or effervescent tablets of potassium chloride. Should water and sodium retention require correction with a diuretic, careful monitoring of potassium levels is mandatory.

Pharmaceutical precautions Store tablets in a dry place.

Legal category POM.

Package quantities *Pyrogastrone Tablets:* Boxes containing 25 foil strips of 4 tablets.

Pyrogastrone Liquid: Bottles containing sufficient powder to prepare 533 ml Pyrogastrone Liquid.

Further information The alginate antacid base of Pyrogastrone forms a clinging viscous foam which has buffering capacity. This relieves symptoms, either by coating the oesophageal wall, by impeding gastro-oesophageal reflux, or the foam may reflux instead of the acid gastric contents. The incorporation of carbenoxolone into the formulation has been shown to exert an additional healing effect on oesophageal ulcers possibly by improving mucus synthesis and/or by increasing the life-span of oesophageal epithelium.

Systemic absorption of carbenoxolone is extensive. There is more than 99.95% binding to plasma proteins. There appears to be enterohepatic circulation which delays clearance. Excretion is mainly via the faeces. Plasma elimination half life increases with age. Aluminium hydroxide is not generally absorbed from the gastrointestinal tract, while alginic acid is not digested and passes unchanged into the faeces.

Product licence numbers
Pyrogastrone Tablets: 0071/0138
Pyrogastrone Liquid: 0071/0236

RESONIUM* A

Presentation Resonium A contains 99.93% sodium polystyrene sulphonate ground and flavoured to a buff-coloured powder with a pleasant vanilla odour and sweet taste.

Uses Resonium A is an ion-exchange resin which is recommended for the treatment of hyperkalaemia associated with anuria or severe oliguria. It is also used to treat hyperkalaemia in patients requiring dialysis and in patients on regular haemodialysis or on prolonged peritoneal dialysis.

Dosage and administration Resonium A is for oral or rectal administration only. The dosage recommendations detailed in this section are a guide only, the precise requirements should be decided on the basis of regular serum electrolyte determinations.

Adults including the elderly:
1. *Oral:* Usual dose 15 g three or four times a day. The resin is given by mouth in a little water, or it may be made into a paste with some sweetened vehicle.
2. *Rectal:* In cases where vomiting may make oral administration difficult, the resin may be given rectally as a suspension of 30 g resin in 100 ml 2% Methylcellulose 450 BP (medium viscosity) and 100 ml water, as a daily retention enema. In the initial stages administration by this route as well as orally may help to achieve a more rapid lowering of the serum potassium level.

The enema should if possible be retained for at least nine hours following which the colon should be irrigated to remove the resin. If both routes are used initially it is probably unnecessary to continue rectal administration once the oral resin has reached the rectum.

Children: 1 g/kg body weight daily in divided doses in acute hyperkalaemia. Dosage may be reduced to 0.5 g/kg body weight in divided doses for maintenance therapy. The resin is given orally, preferably with a drink (not a fruit squash because of the high potassium content) or a little jam or honey. When refused by mouth it should be given rectally, using a dose at least as great as that which would have been given orally, diluted in the same ratio as described for adults. Following retention of the enema, the colon should be irrigated to ensure adequate removal of the resin.

Neonates: Resonium A should not be given by the oral route. With rectal administration, the minimum effective dosage within the range 0.5 g/kg to 1 g/kg should be employed diluted as for adults and with adequate irrigation to ensure recovery of the resin.

Contra-indications, warnings, etc
Contra-indications: Resonium A should not be administered orally to neonates and is contra-indicated in neonates with reduced gut motility (e.g. post-operatively or drug induced). Resonium A is also contra-indicated in the presence of obstructive bowel disease.

Precautions: The possibility of potassium depletion should be considered and adequate clinical and biochemical control is essential during treatment, especially in patients on digitalis. Administration of the resin should be stopped when the serum potassium level falls to 5 mmol/litre.

In the event of clinically significant constipation treatment should be discontinued until normal bowel movement has resumed.

In children and neonates particular care is needed with rectal administration as excessive dosage or inadequate dilution could result in impaction of the resin. Care should be taken when administering to patients in whom an increase in sodium load may be detrimental (i.e. congestive heart failure, hypertension, renal damage or oedema). In such cases, Calcium Resonium (calcium polystyrene sulphonate) may be used in place of Resonium A.

Interactions: There have been reports of metabolic alkalosis following concurrent administration of aluminium and magnesium containing antacids. Cation donating agents may reduce the potassium binding effectiveness of Resonium A.

Side-effects: Nausea, vomiting and constipation occasionally occur. Faecal impaction following rectal administration has been reported in children, and gastrointestinal concretions following oral administration to neonates.

Intestinal obstruction has been reported with calcium polystyrene sulphonate. Although extremely rare and possibly a reflection of co-existing pathology, excessive dosage or inadequate dilution of the resin, a similar risk may exist with Resonium A.

Hypokalaemia may occur. In some patients with renal failure, serum sodium levels have increased and led to oedema, hypertension and congestive heart failure. A small reduction in serum calcium levels has also been reported.

Overdosage: Hypokalaemia may be manifest clinically by signs of irritable confusion, delayed thought processes, severe muscle weakness or paralysis. ECG abnormalities may be evident and cardiac arrhythmias may occur. In the event of overdosage the resin should be removed from the alimentary tract by the use of laxatives or enemas and appropriate measures should be taken to restore serum levels of potassium and other electrolytes to normal.

Pharmaceutical precautions Store in a dry place. Suspensions of the resin should be freshly prepared and not stored beyond 24 hours.

Legal category P.

Package quantities Supplied in HDPE containers containing 454 g Resonium A together with a plastic scoop which, when filled level, contains approximately 15 g.

Further information Theoretically, each gram of Resonium A should take up 2.8 to 3.4 mmol of potassium. However, in vivo, the actual amount of potassium bound will be less than this. The sodium content of Resonium A is 4.1 to 4.8 mmol/g.

Product licence number 0071/5087.

SOLPADOL*

Presentation White bevelled-edged soluble tablets, plain on the reverse and scored on the obverse, which effervesce vigorously when placed in water. Each tablet is 25.4 mm in diameter and contains Paracetamol PhEur 500 mg and Codeine Phosphate PhEur 30 mg.

Uses Solpadol is an analgesic, the effect being produced by a combination of the peripheral action of paracetamol and the central action of codeine at opioid binding sites. It is recommended for the relief of severe pain.

Dosage and administration Solpadol is for oral administration only and should be dissolved in at least half a tumblerful of water before taking.

Adults: Two tablets not more frequently than every 4 hours, up to a maximum of 8 tablets in any 24 hour period.

Elderly: A reduced dose may be required – see warnings.

Children: Not recommended for children under 12 years of age.

Contra-indications, warnings, etc
Contra-indications: Hypersensitivity to paracetamol or codeine, which is rare. Conditions where morphine and opioids are contra-indicated e.g. acute asthma, respiratory depression, acute alcoholism, head injuries, raised intra-cranial pressure and following biliary tract surgery; monoamine oxidase inhibitor therapy, concurrent or within 14 days.

Warnings: Patients should be advised not to drive or operate machinery if affected by dizziness or sedation.

Care should be taken in administering the product to any patient whose condition may be exacerbated by opioids, particularly the elderly, who are specially sensitive to their central and gastro-intestinal effects, those on concurrent CNS depressant drugs, those with prostatic hypertrophy and those with inflammatory or obstructive bowel disorders.

Care should also be taken if prolonged therapy is contemplated.

There is inadequate evidence of the safety of codeine in human pregnancy, but there is epidemiological evidence of the safety of paracetamol. Both substances have been used for many years without apparent adverse effect and animal studies have not shown any hazard. Nonetheless, careful consideration should be given before prescribing Solpadol for pregnant patients. Opioid analgesics may depress neonatal respiration and cause withdrawal effects in neonates of dependent mothers.

Each tablet contains 426.8 mg sodium (18.56 mEq). This sodium content should be taken into account when prescribing for patients for whom sodium restriction is indicated.

Interactions: Paracetamol may increase the elimination half-life of chloramphenicol. The absorption of paracetamol may be increased by metoclopramide and decreased by cholestyramine. Oral contraceptives may increase its rate of clearance. The effects of CNS depressants (including alcohol) may be potentiated by codeine.

Side-effects: Adverse effects to paracetamol are rare, but hypersensitivity has been reported. Codeine can produce typical opioid effects, including constipation, nausea, vomiting, dizziness, light headedness, confusion, drowsiness and urinary retention. The frequency and severity are determined by dosage, duration of treatment and individual sensitivity.

Tolerance and dependence can occur, especially with prolonged high dosage of codeine.

Overdosage: Nausea and vomiting are prominent symptoms of codeine toxicity and there is evidence of circulatory and respiratory depression. Suggested treatment is gastric lavage and catharsis. If CNS depression is severe, assisted ventilation, oxygen and parenteral naloxone may be needed.

Patients who have taken an overdose of paracetamol may appear well for the first three days, then succumb to liver damage. The hepatic changes produced by overdosage of paracetamol result from the accumulation of a highly reactive intermediate metabolite in the hepatocytes. N-acetylcysteine intravenously or methionine orally protects the liver if administered within 12 hours of ingesting an overdose.

Patients in whom oxidative liver enzymes have been induced, including alcoholics and those receiving barbiturates and patients who are chronically malnourished, may be particularly sensitive to the toxic effects of paracetamol in overdosage.

Pharmaceutical precautions Store in a cool dry place.

Legal category POM.

Package quantities Cartons of 60 tablets (15 laminate strips of 4 tablets). (OP)

Further information Nil.

Product licence number 0071/0332.

STROMBA*

Presentation Stromba Tablets are flat, white tablets 9.5 mm in diameter, marked STROMBA on one side and scored in quarters on the other side. Each tablet contains 5 mg Stanozolol BP. Stromba tablets also contain lactose.

Uses
1. For the vascular manifestations of Behcet's disease.
2. For the prevention of spontaneous attacks of proven hereditary angio-oedema.

Dosage and administration Stromba is for oral administration only.
1. Behcet's disease
Adults: 10 mg daily.

2. Hereditary angio-oedema: The initial dosage should be adjusted to control the occurrence of attacks. Thereafter, the dosage may be reduced for maintenance therapy according to patient response.

Adults: Initially 2.5–10 mg daily. Dosage as low as 2.5 mg three times a week has been effective maintenance therapy.

Children: Not suitable for children less than one year old. 1–6 years, initially 2.5 mg daily. 6–12 years, initially 2.5–5 mg daily.

Contra-indications, warnings, etc
Contra-indications: Stromba is not intended for the treatment of loss of appetite, unexplained weight loss or failure to thrive in children. Such cases should be referred to the appropriate centre for investigation.

Because of possible virilising effects on a female foetus, Stromba should not be administered to pregnant women. There are no available data on the excretion of stanozolol in breast milk. Lactating mothers should not breast feed if Stromba treatment is necessary.

Stromba should not be administered to patients with established liver disease. Patients with a history of jaundice should have liver function tests checked prior to commencing treatment.

Stromba should not be used in cases of cancer of the prostate because the condition is androgen-dependent.

Stromba increases ALA synthetase activity and hence porphyrin metabolism. It is therefore not recommended in patients with a history of porphyria as its use may precipitate an acute attack.

Stromba has been used in patients with non-insulin dependent diabetes without adverse consequences. However, it may be advisable to avoid its use in insulin dependent diabetics.

Precautions: Prolonged use in children may lead to premature closure of the epiphyses.

In hereditary angio-oedema:

(a) long-term use of Stromba should be restricted to well established cases who had experienced serious attacks.
(b) Stromba should not be used in pre-menopausal women except in life-threatening situations.

Stromba should be used with caution in the presence of impaired renal or cardiac function as it may encourage sodium and water retention that could result in cardiac failure.

Peliosis hepatis and tumours of the liver have been reported occasionally in patients subject to prolonged treatment with androgenic anabolic steroids. The tumours are not typical of primary hepatocellular carcinoma and in some cases discontinuation of steroids has resulted in tumour regression without other therapy. The possibility that Stromba may induce or enhance the development of peliosis hepatis and hepatic tumours cannot be excluded and this should be considered when long-term treatment is carried out.

Caution should also be observed in treating patients with breast cancer since anabolic steroids may induce hypercalcaemia in this condition. Periodic assessment of liver function, haematocrit and haemoglobin is advised during treatment.

Interactions: Anabolic steroids increase sensitivity to warfarin type anti-coagulants; therefore, the dose of the latter should be decreased by approximately a half in order to maintain the prothrombin time at the desired therapeutic level.

Dosage of oral hypoglycaemic agents may require adjustment when initiating or discontinuing Stromba therapy.

Side-effects: Because of the structural relationship to the male hormones, some androgenic side-effects e.g. acne, hirsutism, amenorrhoea, are to be expected. Because the ratio of anabolic to androgenic properties is high, these effects should be minimal at the recommended dosage and those reported have been generally mild and reversible on stopping treatment. On rare occasions, usually with higher dosage, voice change has been reported; if observed, treatment should be discontinued. Other effects, such as menstrual irregularity, headache, muscle cramp, dyspepsia, skin rash and occasionally hair loss, euphoria and depression have occurred. An increase in haematocrit and haemoglobin level may also occur. There have been occasional reports of cholestatic jaundice, and very rarely, peliosis hepatis and hepatic tumours.

In children, prolonged use may lead to premature closure of the epiphyses.

Stromba may raise levels of aspartate transaminase (AST) and alanine transaminase (ALT) and in some patients these may rise above laboratory normal ranges. These levels return to normal on withdrawing Stromba.

Elevations of creatine phospho-kinase and of alkaline phosphatase have also occasionally been reported.

The use of this preparation may temporarily result in an alteration in the ratio of high and low density lipoproteins. The significance of this is not understood.

Some patients taking Stromba may show increased T3 uptake, decreased T4 levels and a decrease in throxine binding globulin although they are clinically euthyroid.

Overdosage: There are no reports of chronic or acute overdosage with Stromba. By analogy with other substances of this type, one would expect chronic overdosage to be associated with the signs and symptoms caused by excessive circulating androgens. It is unlikely that any immediate serious reactions would be seen in a single excessive dose (in animals acute toxicity cannot be measured). In such an event, however, the patient should be kept under observation and liver function monitored, in case of delayed reactions.

Pharmaceutical precautions Nil.

Legal category POM.

Package quantities Calendar packs of 56 tablets (OP).

Further information Stanozolol is an anabolic agent with fibrinolytic properties which are of therapeutic value in modifying the vascular manifestations of Behcet's disease. In patients with hereditary angio-oedema, stanozolol alters the functional level of plasma C1 esterase inhibitor which is depressed in this condition.

Stanozolol given by mouth is readily absorbed into the bloodstream. Within the serum it is highly protein bound. Metabolism is carried out to a large extent in the liver and the conjugated metabolites are excreted in both the faeces and urine.

Product licence number 0071/5092

TELEPAQUE*

Presentation Telepaque Tablets are off-white to buff, bi-convex tablets, 10.3 mm in diameter and plain on both sides. Each tablet contains 500 mg Iopanoic Acid BP.

Uses Telepaque Tablets are recommended for oral cholecystography and cholangiography.

Dosage and administration Telepaque Tablets are for oral administration only. Telepaque Tablets are usually given 10–14 hours before cholecystography.

Adults:

1. The usual dose is 6 Telepaque Tablets swallowed whole with at least one full glass of water on the evening before the examination with a low-fat supper. Eight tablets may be given to very obese patients. For repeat examinations on the same day as the original procedure, an additional 6 tablets may be administered. However, if the repeat examination is to be performed with a double dose of Telepaque tablets, a period of five to seven days should be allowed between the two examinations. No more than 12 tablets should be taken during a 24-hour period.

2. In order to obtain better visualisation of the extra-hepatic ducts, three to six Telepaque tablets are given four hours after a fatty meal on the day preceding the examination, then a full dose of 6 tablets after a fat-free meal that evening.

Another technique is to administer a double dose (12 tablets) of Telepaque after a 12-hour fast, followed by 8 ml Camphorated Opium Tincture BP to close the sphincter of Oddi. Films may be taken 5–14 hours later, and any sphincter pain caused by the tincture may be eased with an anticholinergic. As noted above, 12 tablets is the maximum dose which should be administered in 24 hours.

3. Certain biliary calculi only become radiographically opaque after prolonged exposure to the contrast medium. Such prolonged exposure to Telepaque can be obtained by the following regimen. Patients are instructed to take two Telepaque Tablets after each of the three main meals of the day for four days. During this time the meals should be relatively fat-free. The X-ray examination is made on the morning of the fifth day, the patient fasting.

Elderly: As for adults except that the use of repeat dosage should be avoided.

Children: A dosage of 0.15 g/kg body weight has been suggested for children.

Contra-indications, warnings, etc

Contra-indications: Telepaque is contra-indicated in patients with advanced hepatorenal disease or severe impairment of renal function. It should not be given to patients with gastro-intestinal disorders which interfere with absorption and result in inadequate visualisation. Telepaque may also be contra-indicated in patients who are sensitive to iodine compounds.

Precautions: Caution is necessary in patients suffering from cholangitis or marked hyperthyroidism. In patients with severe advanced liver disease, renal function should be assessed before cholecystography, and renal output and hepatic function should be observed for a few days after the procedure. Observation of renal function after multiple doses of the contrast medium has also been recommended. Iopanoic acid has a uricosuric effect approximately equivalent to that of probenecid. Although this action cannot be definitely linked with nephrotoxicity, it has been strongly recommended that adequate hydration should be encouraged as a possible means of decreasing the risk of renal complications.

Elderly patients and those patients with pre-existing renal disease should not receive double doses of cholecystographic media. It is possible that renal irritation in susceptible individuals could result in reflex vascular spasm with partial or complete renal shutdown. It is therefore suggested that kidney function in patients with renal disease should be assessed before administration of cholecystographic media, and for several days afterwards.

Fatal coronary occlusion in four patients with arteriosclerotic heart disease who had taken a cholecystographic agent has been reported and premedication with atropine is a reasonable prophylactic measure against vagal stimulation if cholecystography is necessary in patients with recent symptoms of coronary artery disease. However, the connection between these fatalities and the administration of the contrast media (iopanoic acid in two cases and iodoalphionic acid in the other two) may have been wholly fortuitous.

Use in pregnancy and lactation: Elective contrast radiography of the abdomen should be avoided during pregnancy.

Animal reproduction studies have not been carried out with Telepaque. It is not known whether Telepaque can cause foetal harm when administered to a pregnant woman. It can be transferred across the placenta, and may also appear in breast milk. Telepaque therefore should only be administered to pregnant patients when absolutely necessary, and caution should be observed in its administration to nursing mothers.

Interactions: Concomitant treatment with cholestyramine may interfere with the action of iopanoic acid. At least one week should be allowed between discontinuing cholestyramine and radiographic examination with Telepaque.

It has also been suggested that the administration of large doses of other aromatic iodine compounds like urographic and angiographic agents with or shortly following cholecystographic agents may increase the likelihood of toxic reactions.

The results of PBI and RAI uptake studies, which depend on iodine estimations, will not reflect thyroid function for several months following administration of cholecystographic media. However, function tests not depending on iodine estimations, e.g. T_3 resin uptake or free thyroxine assays, are not affected.

Bilirubin, thymol turbidity, cephalin flocculation, and serum enzyme values are unaffected but Telepaque may delay BSP clearance values for up to two days.

Pseudoalbuminuria may be present for three days in response to certain chemical protein precipitation tests. Positive reactions should be verified by the heat-and-acetic acid or colourimetric dip-strip methods.

Side-effects: The most frequently reported adverse reactions have been mild and transient nausea, vomiting, diarrhoea and cramps. A stinging sensation during micturition occurs occasionally and has been attributed to urethral irritation. It does not indicate any renal or upper urinary tract toxicity. Skin reactions such as urticaria, pruritus and flushing rarely occur.

A few cases of transitory thrombocytopenia with petechiae have been reported. Very rarely, hepatorenal, cardiovascular and thyroid function may be disturbed, but usually only in patients with pre-existing renal disease (see Precautions).

Overdosage: Acute renal failure with complete recovery has been reported in four patients, three of whom were given doses of Telepaque which were higher than those recommended.

Patients should be treated conservatively or using standard procedures. High fluid intake and alkalinisation may help urinary clearance of the drug and avoidance of its precipitation in the renal tract. Cholestyramine may help reduce absorption.

Pharmaceutical precautions Nil.

Legal category P.

Package quantities Cartons of 36 tablets packed in aluminium foil strips of 6.

Further information Iopanoic acid is absorbed from the gastrointestinal tract and is strongly bound to plasma protein. It is conjugated in the liver to the glucuronide, 65% being excreted in the bile, the remainder in the urine. It appears in the gall-bladder within about 4 hours of dosaging, achieving maximum concentration within 10–14 hours. Excretion of 50% of the dose is obtained within about 24 hours, the remainder within 5 days.

Product licence number 0071/5095.

TRANCOPAL*

Presentation Trancopal tablets are flat, yellow tablets with bevelled edges 9.5 mm in diameter, marked with a stylised TR on one side and plain on the reverse. Each tablet contains 200 mg chlormezanone.

Uses Trancopal tablets are recommended for the short-term symptomatic treatment of anxiety states where muscle tension is prominent and as an adjunct to the treatment of acute musculo-skeletal disorders associated with painful muscle spasm. Trancopal tablets are also recommended for the short-term treatment of insomnia, whether or not due to these conditions.

Dosage and administration For oral administration only.

Adults: States of anxiety and skeletal muscle tension: usually 200 mg repeated up to 3 or 4 times daily or a single dose of 400 mg at night. *Sleep disturbances:* usually 400 mg at night.

Elderly: Half the normal adult dose or less may be sufficient for a therapeutic response in the elderly.

Children: Not recommended.

Contra-indications, warnings, etc *Contra-indications:* Trancopal tablets are contra-indicated in patients sensitive to chlormezanone, and in those taking monoamine oxidase inhibitors.

Precautions

Use in pregnancy and lactation: There is insufficient evidence of safety of chlormezanone in human pregnancy nor is there evidence from animal work that it is free from hazard. Do not use during pregnancy, especially the first trimester, nor during breast-feeding, unless there are compelling reasons.

Use in renal and hepatic disease: Trancopal should be given with caution to patients with hepatic or renal insufficiency.

Effect on ability to drive and use machines: Day-time sedation is a relatively uncommon effect of Trancopal, but may lead to modification of patients' reactions (performance at skilled tasks, alertness, etc.) to a varying extent depending on individual susceptibility. Therefore patients should be advised not to drive or operate machinery during treatment if affected.

Interactions: The concurrent use of other CNS depressant drugs should be avoided because their sedative effect may be intensified, and the sedative effect of Trancopal tablets is potentiated by alcohol.

Other warnings: Observe caution in patients with porphyria. The dependence potential of chlormezanone is not known. As with sedative drugs, dependence may possibly occur when chlormezanone is given in high dosage or for prolonged periods, especially in patients with a history of alcoholism or drug dependence, or in patients with marked personality disorders. The possibility of withdrawal reactions to abrupt termination of chlormezanone after long term treatment has not been studied. Gradual withdrawal may be more appropriate.

Chlormezanone has a prolonged half-life in man and hence prolonged duration of action. The possibility of cumulative effects has not been studied. Safety and efficacy have not been established beyond short-term use.

Side effects: Drowsiness and dizziness have been the commonest side-effects, particularly at higher doses. Other reported side-effects include nausea, lightheadedness, headache, lethargy and dryness of the mouth. Less common adverse effects include ataxia, depression, flushing, 'hangover' and blurring of vision or diplopia. Slight skin reactions of the urticaria or erythematous type can occur. Cases of fixed drug rash and various forms of exudative erythema multiforme have been reported; these are very uncommon but in certain cases can be serious.

Cholestatic jaundice has also occurred.

Overdosage: The signs and symptoms of overdosage with chlormezanone resemble those seen with other central depressant drugs, for example, somnolence, prostration, muscular incoordination and memory disturbances. In severe cases, there may be hypotension, respiratory depression and loss of consciousness, but recovery is to be expected. Treatment should be symptomatic but gastric lavage may be useful if performed soon after ingestion.

Pharmaceutical precautions Nil.

Legal category POM.

Package quantities Trancopal tablets are available in bottles of 60.

Further information Evidence suggests that chlormezanone acts by central depression of polysynaptic reflexes, and that it possesses some peripheral inhibiting effect at the neuromuscular junction

In healthy adults, peak plasma levels of 5–6 microgram/ml chlormezanone are seen within 1–2 hours of a 400 mg oral dose. Mean plasma elimination half life is 24 hours (range 19–30 hours). About 1% of the dose is excreted unchanged in the urine within 24 hours. The majority appears to undergo hydrolysis followed by oxidation and conjugation to 4-chlorohippuric acid which appears in the urine.

Product licence number 0071/5098.

URISAL*

Presentation A mixture of white and yellow granules which dissolve in water with slight effervescence to give a solution with an orange flavour.

Each 7 g sachet of granules contains the equivalent of 4.4 g Sodium Citrate PhEur. Urisal granules contain sucrose, invert sugar and dextrose.

Uses For the relief of cystitis in adult women.

Dosage and administration For oral administration only.

Adult women: One sachet three times a day for three days. Urisal should not be taken for more than 72 hours.

The contents of one sachet should be added to a glass of water and stirred vigorously until dispersed.

Elderly: Not recommended.

Children: Not recommended.

Contra-indications, warnings, etc Each sachet of Urisal contains approximately 41 mmol (950 mg) sodium and 2.3 g sucrose. Urisal should not be used in pregnancy or lactation, nor in patients with heart disease, hypertension or a history of renal disease.

Non-specific side effects, e.g. nausea, have been reported but are rare. Because of the nature of the product, overdosage is unlikely. In case of overdosage, patients should be treated symptomatically.

Pharmaceutical precautions Store in a dry place.

Legal category GSL.

Package quantities Cartons of nine sachets (OP).

Further information Sodium citrate renders the urine less acidic.

Supplied through doctors and registered pharmacies on prescription.

Product licence number 0071/0248.

VERIPAQUE*

Presentation Veripaque Powder is a fine, white powder containing 50 mg oxyphenisatin in 3 g. Veripaque Powder contains lactose.

Uses Veripaque is recommended: a) for adding to barium enemas in radiological examination of the large intestine; b) as a cleansing enema to remove colonic gas and faeces before proctosigmoidoscopy and various radiological examinations of the abdomen including barium enema, cholecystography, excretory urography and double-air contrast examination of the colon; c) for pre-operative cleansing of the large intestine.

Dosage and administration

Veripaque is for rectal administration.

Adults: Veripaque enemas should be administered slowly over a period of five to eight minutes with the fluid level 18–24 inches above the hips.

As a cleansing enema prior to diagnostic or surgical procedures, 3 g of Veripaque Powder is dissolved in 2 litres of water.

When used as an adjuvant to a barium enema, 3 g Veripaque Powder is mixed thoroughly with 2 litres of barium enema suspension.

Elderly: As for adults but see 'precautions'.

Children: Not recommended.

Contra-indications, warnings, etc

Contra-indications: As with all enemas Veripaque is not recommended in cases of appendicitis, gross bleeding from the bowel, intestinal obstruction, severe spasm or severe diarrhoea, or when there is danger of intestinal perforation.

Precautions: Care is needed in patients with an irritable colon or inflammatory diseases of the large intestine; in such cases Veripaque should be used in smaller than usual doses. Caution is also advised in elderly or debilitated patients because of the possibility of dehydration. There is no evidence of harmful effects resulting from use during pregnancy. However, as with all medicines, Veripaque should not be used in pregnancy unless the expected benefit is thought to outweigh any possible risk to the foetus. Although when used in small and infrequent doses and in preparations for radiography it may well be harmless, regular, prolonged use should be discouraged because of the possibility of liver toxicity.

Side-effects: Minor side-effects such as cramps, diarrhoea, nausea and vomiting, sweating and tachycardia may occur infrequently and can usually be obviated by decreasing the dosage. The cramps, which occur in about 8% of cases, usually produce only mild discomfort and do not interfere with the completion of the procedure.

As with tannic acid, more serious side-effects such as syncope may occur occasionally; they are usually caused by administration of too large a dose.

Overdosage: Because of the nature of the product, overdosage is unlikely.

Pharmaceutical precautions Nil.

Legal category P.

Package quantities Boxes of 6 vials each containing 3 g Veripaque Powder.

Further information Oxyphenisatin is a purgative.

Product licence number 0071/5099.

**Trade Mark*

Stiefel Laboratories (UK) Limited
Holtspur Lane
Wooburn Green
High Wycombe
Buckinghamshire HP10 0AU

ACETOXYL* 2.5
ACETOXYL* 5

Presentation White, viscous gels containing benzoyl peroxide 2.5 and 5% w/w in an aqueous acetone base.

Excipients: carbomer, triethanolamine, propylene glycol, sodium lauryl sulphate, acetone, purified water.

Uses Acetoxyl 2.5 and 5 are each indicated for use in the treatment of acne vulgaris.

Dosage and administration Treatment should normally commence with Acetoxyl 2.5. Apply the gel to the affected areas once daily. Washing with soap and water prior to application greatly enhances the efficacy of the preparation.

The reaction of the skin to benzoyl peroxide differs in individual patients. The higher concentration in Acetoxyl 5 may be required to ensure a satisfactory response.

Contra-indications, warnings, etc Acetoxyl should not be prescribed for patients with known hypersensitivity to benzoyl peroxide.

Avoid contact with the eyes, mouth and other mucous membranes. Care should be taken when applying the product to the neck and other sensitive areas. In normal use, a mild burning sensation will probably be felt on first application and a moderate reddening and peeling of the skin will occur within a few days. During the first weeks of treatment a sudden increase in peeling will occur in most patients, this is not harmful and will normally subside within a day or two if treatment is temporarily discontinued.

There are no restrictions on the use of Acetoxyl during pregnancy and lactation.

Acetoxyl may bleach dyed fabrics.

Pharmaceutical precautions Store in a cool place.

Legal category P.

Package quantities Tubes of 40 g.

Further information Benzoyl peroxide has sebostatic and keratolytic activity coupled with antibacterial activity against Propionibacterium acnes, the organism implicated in acne vulgaris. Its use in the treatment of acne is well established.

Product licence numbers
Acetoxyl 2.5 0174/0041
Acetoxyl 5 0174/0039

ACNEGEL*
ACNEGEL* FORTE

Presentation Acnegel and Acnegel Forte contain respectively 5% and 10% w/w benzoyl peroxide in an ethanolic base.

Excipients: magnesium aluminium silicate, hypromellose, macrogol lauryl ether, ethanol, citric acid, fragrance 6565A and purified water.

Uses Acnegel and Acnegel Forte are indicated for the treatment of acne.

Dosage and administration
Adults, the elderly and children over 12 years: Treatment should normally commence with Acnegel. Apply the gel to the affected areas once daily. Washing with soap and water prior to application greatly enhances the efficacy of the preparation.

The reaction of the skin to benzoyl peroxide differs in individual patients and for this reason the higher percentage of benzoyl peroxide in Acnegel Forte may be required in order to provide a satisfactory drying and desquamative action.

Children under 12 years: Not recommended.

Contra-indications, warnings, etc Avoid contact with eyes, mouth and mucous membranes. Take care when applying to the neck and other sensitive areas. Do not use in patients with known hypersensitivity to benzoyl peroxide.

In normal use a mild burning sensation will probably be felt on first application and a moderate reddening and peeling of the skin will occur within a few days. During the first few weeks of treatment a sudden increase in peeling will occur in most patients.

There are no restrictions on the use of Acnegel and Acnegel Forte during pregnancy and lactation.

Acnegel and Acnegel Forte may bleach dyed clothing and fabrics.

Pharmaceutical precautions Store in a cool place.

Legal category P.

Package quantities Acnegel and Acnegel Forte are supplied in tubes each containing 50 g.

Further information Benzoyl peroxide has sebostatic and keratolytic activity coupled with antibacterial activity against Propionibacterium acnes, the organism implicated in acne vulgaris. Its use in the treatment of acne is well established.

Product licence numbers
Acnegel 0174/0019R
Acnegel Forte 0174/0020R

ANTHRANOL* 0.4
ANTHRANOL* 1.0
ANTHRANOL* 2.0

Presentation Smooth soft yellow ointments containing Dithranol BP 0.4% w/w, 1.0% w/w and 2.0% w/w respectively.

Excipients: white soft paraffin, light liquid paraffin, cetyl alcohol, sodium lauryl sulphate, salicylic acid.

Uses For the topical treatment of sub-acute and chronic psoriasis, including psoriasis of the scalp, by the *short contact therapy* method.

Dosage and administration Treatment should begin with Anthranol 0.4. Clinical response and tolerance will determine the necessity for progression to Anthranol 1.0 and subsequently Anthranol 2.0.

Apply the ointment once daily, sparingly, to the psoriatic plaques. Surrounding normal skin should be protected with white soft paraffin. Leave the ointment on for the required time then remove excess ointment with a paper tissue and wash off the remainder thoroughly.

If Anthranol has been applied to the scalp, the ointment should be removed by shampooing.

The initial daily treatment time with each strength should not exceed 10 minutes. The time may be increased gradually over a period of 7 days to a maximum of 30 minutes. The daily treatment time should not normally exceed 30 minutes.

In the event of undue irritation, stop treatment for 2 days and resume on alternate days.

Treatment should be continued at the optimum tolerated strength and leave-on time, depending on patient response.

Anthranol is not suitable for the treatment of infants and young children.

Contra-indications, warnings, etc Anthranol ointments are contra-indicated for pustular psoriasis and are not suitable for acute psoriasis or use on inflamed skin. The products should not be used in patients with renal disease.

Anthranol ointments should not be applied to the face, the inside of the thighs, the genital region or skinfold areas. Should contact with the eyes occur, bathe immediately with water and seek medical advice.

Dithranol is a strong irritant; always wash the hands after using Anthranol ointment. The ointment will cause staining and discolouration to the skin, clothing and bathroom ware. Use gloves to avoid staining fingernails. Stains on clothing should be assumed to be permanent. Stains on bathroom ware may be removed by bleach.

Although there is no experimental evidence to support the safety of Anthranol in pregnancy and lactation, no adverse effects have been reported.

Pharmaceutical precautions Store in a cool place.

Legal category
Anthranol 0.4 P.
Anthranol 1.0 P.
Anthranol 2.0 POM.

Package quantity Anthranol ointments are supplied in tubes of 50 g.

Further information Anthranol 0.4 can also be used for treatment of psoriasis by the overnight method. Use a plastic cap at night to prevent staining of the pillow.

Product licence numbers

Anthranol 0.4 ointment	0174/0018R
Anthranol 1.0 ointment	0174/0057
Anthranol 2.0 ointment	0174/0058

BENOXYL* 5
BENOXYL* 10

Presentation Benoxyl 5 is available as a white lotion or cream containing benzoyl peroxide 5% w/w.

Benoxyl 10 is a white lotion containing benzoyl peroxide 10% w/w.

Excipients: macrogol 1000 monostearate, stearic acid, glyceryl monostearate, isopropyl palmitate, propylene glycol, zinc caproate, zinc laurate, zinc myristate, purified water.

Uses Benoxyl 5 and 10 are each indicated for use in the treatment of acne vulgaris.

Dosage and administration Treatment should normally commence with Benoxyl 5. Apply the lotion or cream to the affected areas once daily. Washing with soap and water prior to application greatly enhances the efficacy of the preparation.

The reaction of the skin to benzoyl peroxide differs in individual patients. The higher concentration in Benoxyl 10 may be required to ensure a satisfactory response.

Contra-indications, warnings, etc Benoxyl should not be prescribed for patients with a known hypersensitivity to benzoyl peroxide.

Avoid contact with the eyes, mouth and other mucous membranes. Care should be taken when applying the product to the neck and other sensitive areas. In normal use, a mild burning sensation will probably be felt on first application and a moderate reddening and peeling of the skin will occur within a few days. During the first weeks of treatment a sudden increase in peeling will occur in most patients, this is not harmful and will normally subside within a day or two if treatment is temporarily discontinued.

There are no restrictions on the use of the product during pregnancy and lactation.

Benoxyl may bleach dyed fabrics.

Pharmaceutical precautions Store in a cool place.

Legal category P.

Package quantities Lotion: Bottles of 30 ml.
Cream: Tubes of 40 g.

Further information Benzoyl peroxide has sebostatic and keratolytic activity coupled with antibacterial activity against Propionibacterium acnes, the organism implicated in acne vulgaris. Its use in the treatment of acne is well established.

Product licence numbers

Benoxyl 5 lotion	0174/5003R
Benoxyl 5 cream	0174/5007R
Benoxyl 10 lotion	0174/0034

BRĀSIVOL*

Presentation Brāsivol is an abrasive cleansing paste in two grades, each containing graded particles of fused synthetic aluminium oxide in a non-irritant soap-detergent base.

Brāsivol No. 1 Fine is an off-white paste containing 38% aluminium oxide.

Brāsivol No. 2 Medium is a light-blue paste containing 52% aluminium oxide.

Excipients: glycerol, polyethylene glycol, stearic acid, lauric acid, myristic acid, quaternium 15, bentonite, sodium lauryl sulphate, colour: fine E172, medium E131, fragrance BV-2, purified water.

Uses Brāsivol is a cleansing and abrading agent which effectively removes debris from blocked pores. It is used in the management of acne vulgaris, either as a sole agent or as an adjunct to other treatment.

Dosage and administration The product is intended for use in adults and children over 12 years of age. The patient should commence treatment with Brāsivol No. 1 Fine. The product should be applied top wetted skin and rubbed gently but firmly over the affected area with a circular motion for 15–20 seconds, then rinsed off thoroughly with water. This routine may be repeated 2 or 3 times daily, replacing ordinary soap and water.

If the condition does not improve after 2 to 3 weeks, the treatment should be repeated using Brāsivol No. 2 Medium in place of Brāsivol No. 1.

Once you have established the most suitable grade for your condition and skin type, continue treatment for 2 to 3 months.

Contra-indications, warnings, etc Brāsivol is contra-indicated in the presence of superficial venules, telangiectasia, cystic acne and rosacea.

Care should be taken to avoid using Brāsivol close to the eyes or mouth and male patients using an electric razor should shave before applying Brāsivol.

A degree of dryness and redness will be seen during the first few days of treatment. Over-enthusiastic use, however, can cause irritation and, if this occurs, treatment should be interrupted for a day or two and then resumed.

There is no experimental evidence of the safety of the drug in human pregnancy but it has been in wide use for many years without ill consequence.

Pharmaceutical precautions Nil.

Legal category GSL.

Package quantities
Brāsivol No. 1 Fine. 75 g.

Brāsivol No. 2 Medium. 75 g.

Further information Brāsivol assists in the treatment of acne by exerting a debrading effect on the skin surface, unblocking the follicles, thus allowing the removal of retained sebum and permitting the sebaceous glands to return to normal size and activity.

Product licence numbers

Brāsivol No. 1 Fine	0174/5000R
Brāsivol No. 2 Medium	0174/5001R

DRICLOR*

Presentation Driclor is a clear colourless alcoholic solution containing Aluminium Chloride Hexahydrate USP 20% w/w.

Excipients: ethanol, purified water.

Uses Driclor is indicated for the treatment of hyperhidrosis.

Dosage and administration Apply Driclor last thing at night after drying the affected areas carefully. Wash off in the morning. Do not re-apply the product during the day.

Initially the product may be applied each night until sweating stops during the day. The frequency of application may then be reduced to twice a week or less.

Contra-indications, warnings, etc Ensure that the affected areas to be treated are completely dry before application.

Do not apply Driclor to broken, irritated, or recently shaven skin. Do not apply within one hour of bathing.

Driclor may cause irritation which may be alleviated by the use of a weak, corticosteroid cream.

Avoid contact with the eyes.

There are no restrictions on the use of Driclor during pregnancy and lactation.

Avoid direct contact with clothing and polished metal surfaces.

Pharmaceutical precautions Store upright in a cool place.

Replace cap tightly after use.

Inflammable – keep away from naked flame.

Legal category POM.

Package quantities 60ml in roll-on applicator plastic bottle.

Further information Aluminium chloride hexahydrate acts locally, in the stratum corneum and in the terminal duct, to relieve hyperhidrosis.

Product licence number 0174/0044.

DUOFILM*

Presentation Duofilm is a clear mobile liquid containing:

Salicylic Acid BP	16.7% w/w
Lactic Acid BP	16.7% w/w

in Flexible Collodion BP.

Uses Duofilm is for topical application only and is indicated in the treatment of warts.

Dosage and administration For application to the affected areas on the surface of the skin.

Adults (including the elderly): Apply daily to the affected areas only.

Children under 12: Children over two years are to be treated under supervision, but treatment of infants is not recommended.

Contra-indications, warnings, etc Avoid applying to normal skin.

Duofilm should not be used on the face or anogenital regions.

There are no restrictions on the use of Duofilm during pregnancy and lactation.

Pharmaceutical precautions Store upright in a cool place.

Replace cap tightly after use.

Highly inflammable – keep away from naked flame.

Legal category P.

Package quantities Duofilm is available in an amber screw-capped applicator bottle containing 15 ml.

Further information Lactic acid affects the keratinisation process, reducing the hyperkeratosis which is characteristic of warts. It is caustic, leading to the destruction of the keratotic tissue of the wart and of the causative virus. Salicylic acid is keratolytic, producing desquamation by solubilising the intercellular cement in the stratum corneum.

Product licence number 0174/0025R.

LACTICARE*

Presentation Lacticare contains lactic acid 5% w/w and sodium pyrrolidone carboxylate 2.5% w/w in an oil-in-water viscous lotion base.

Excipients: imidurea, dehydroacetic acid, carbomer, macrogol ether complex, glyceryl monostearate, cetyl alcohol, isopropyl palmitate, light liquid paraffin, myristyl lactate, fragrance antaria 78/82, purified water.

Uses Lacticare is indicated for the symptomatic relief of hyperkeratotic and other chronic dry skin conditions and for dry skin conditions caused by low humidity or the use of detergents.

Dosage and administration Use as required on affected areas. Shake well before use.

Contra-indications, warnings, etc Occasionally a transient mild stinging sensation may occur. Should prolonged irritation develop when used on abraded or inflamed skin, discontinue use.

Keep away from the eyes and mucous membranes. Should contact with the eyes occur, remove with water.

Although there is no experimental evidence to support the safety of the drug during pregnancy and lactation, no adverse effects have been reported.

Pharmaceutical precautions Nil.

Legal category P.

Package quantities Bottles containing 150 ml.

Further information Both lactic acid and sodium pyrrolidone carboxylate are hygroscopic. They enhance the ability of the stratum corneum to retain water and counteract the tendency of the skin to dry out. Lactic acid also modulates epidermal keratinisation and increases skin extensibility.

Product licence number 0174/0038.

OILATUM* CREAM

Presentation Oilatum Cream is a white, oil-in-water cream containing Arachis Oil BP, 21% w/w.

Excipients: potassium sorbate, magnesium aluminium silicate, citric acid, sodium phosphate, glyceryl monostearate, quaternium 15, fragrance 2174-H, purified water.

Uses Oilatum Cream is indicated in cases of dry, sensitive skin, lanolin sensitivity, alkali intolerance, ichthyosis and similar conditions.

The use of Oilatum Cream in such conditions reduces moisture loss from the stratum corneum and thus restores skin flexibility.

The use of an inert plastic in the oil phase ensures a continuous residual film which tends to be more occlusive and longer-lasting than ordinary vegetable oil films.

Dosage and administration Oilatum Cream may be used as often as required. Apply to the affected area and rub in well. It is especially effective immediately after washing, when the normal acid condition of the skin may be disturbed and when the sebum content of the stratum corneum may be depleted.

The product is suitable for use in adults, children and the elderly.

Contra-indications, warnings, etc There is no evidence of the safety of Oilatum Cream in human pregnancy or lactation, but it has been in wide use for many years without apparent ill consequence.

Pharmaceutical precautions Nil.

Legal category P.

Package quantities Oilatum Cream is available in tubes containing 40 g and 80 g.

Further information Arachis oil exerts an emollient effect by forming an occlusive film which reduces transepidermal water loss thus restoring normal skin humidity levels.

Product licence number 0174/5014R.

OILATUM* EMOLLIENT

Presentation Oilatum Emollient is a liquid bath additive. Active ingredient: Liquid paraffin 63.4% w/w.

Excipients: acetylated wool alcohols, isopropyl palmitate, macrogol 400 dilaurate, macrogol ester, fragrance floral spice.

Uses Oilatum Emollient is indicated in the treatment of contact dermatitis, atopic dermatitis, senile pruritus, ichthyosis and related dry skin conditions. Oilatum Emollient replaces oil and water and hydrates the keratin. Oilatum Emollient is particularly suitable for infant bathing. The preparation also overcomes the problem of cleansing the skin in conditions where the use of soaps, soap substitutes and colloid or oat-meal baths proves irritating.

Dosage and administration Oilatum Emollient should always be used with water, either added to water or applied to wet skin.

Adult bath: Add 10–20 mls (1–3 capfuls) to an 8 inch bath of water. Soak for 10–20 minutes. Pat dry.

Infant bath: Add 5–10 mls ($\frac{1}{2}$–2 capfuls) to a basin of water. Apply gently over entire body with a sponge. Pat dry.

Skin cleansing: Rub a small amount of oil into wet skin. Rinse and pat dry.

Where conditions permit, and particularly in cases of extensive areas of dry skin, Oilatum Emollient should be used as a bath oil, ensuring complete coverage by immersion. In addition to the therapeutic benefits, this method of use provides a means of sedating tense patients, particularly relevant in cases of acute pruritic dermatoses where relaxation of tension appears to relieve symptoms.

The product is suitable for use in adults, children and the elderly.

Contra-indications, warnings, etc The patient should be advised to use care to avoid slipping in the bath. If a rash or skin irritation occurs, stop using the product and consult your doctor.

Contains acetylated lanolin alcohols; avoid use in individuals with known lanolin hypersensitivity.

There is no evidence of the safety of Oilatum Emollient in human pregnancy or lactation, but it has been in wide use for many years without ill consequence.

Pharmaceutical precautions Nil.

Legal category GSL.

Package quantities Oilatum Emollient is available in bottles containing 150 ml, 350 ml and 1 litre.

Further information Light liquid paraffin exerts an emollient effect by forming an occlusive film in the stratum corneum. This prevents excessive evaporation of water from the skin surface and aids in the prevention of dryness.

Product licence number 0174/5010R.

PANOXYL* 5
PANOXYL* 10

Presentation White viscous gels containing benzoyl peroxide 5 and 10% w/w in an ethanolic base.

Excipients: magnesium aluminium silicate, hypromellose, macrogol lauryl ether, ethanol, citric acid, fragrance 6565A, purified water.

Uses PanOxyl 5 and 10 are each indicated for use in the treatment of acne vulgaris.

Dosage and administration
Adults, the elderly and children over 12 years: Treatment should normally commence with PanOxyl 5. Apply the gel to the affected areas once daily. Washing prior to application greatly enhances the efficacy of the preparation. The reaction of the skin to benzoyl peroxide differs in individual patients, and for this reason the higher percentage of benzoyl peroxide in PanOxyl 10 may be required in order to provide a satisfactory drying and desquamative action.

Children under 12 years: Not recommended.

Contra-indications, warnings, etc Avoid contact with eyes, mouth and mucous membranes. Take care when applying to the neck and other sensitive areas. Do not use in patients with known hypersensitivity to benzoyl peroxide.

In normal use, a mild burning sensation will probably be felt on first application and a moderate reddening and peeling of the skin will occur within a few days. During the first few weeks of treatment a sudden increase in peeling will occur in most patients.

There are no restrictions on the use of PanOxyl 5 and PanOxyl 10 during pregnancy and lactation.

PanOxyl 5 and PanOxyl 10 may bleach dyed fabrics.

Pharmaceutical precautions Store in a cool place.

Legal category P.

Package quantities PanOxyl 5 and PanOxyl 10 are supplied in tubes each containing 40 g.

Further information Benzoyl peroxide has sebostatic and keratolytic activity coupled with antibacterial activity against Propionibacterium acnes, the organism implicated in acne vulgaris. Its use in the treatment of acne is well established.

Product licence numbers
PanOxyl 5 0174/0019R
PanOxyl 10 0174/0020R

PANOXYL AQUAGEL* 2.5
PANOXYL AQUAGEL* 5
PANOXYL AQUAGEL* 10

Presentation White viscous gels containing benzoyl peroxide 2.5, 5 and 10% w/w in an aqueous, non alcoholic base.

Excipients: carbomer, diisopropanolamine, propylene glycol, macrogol lauryl ether, sodium lauryl sulphate, purified water.

Uses PanOxyl Aquagel 2.5, 5 and 10 are each indicated for use in the topical treatment of acne vulgaris.

Dosage and administration Treatment should normally begin with PanOxyl Aquagel 2.5. Apply to the affected areas once daily. Washing prior to application enhances the efficacy of the preparation.

The reaction of the skin to benzoyl peroxide differs in individual patients. The higher concentration in PanOxyl Aquagel 5 or 10 may be required to produce a satisfactory response.

Contra-indications, warnings, etc PanOxyl Aquagel should not be prescribed for patients with a known hypersensitivity to benzoyl peroxide.

Avoid contact with the eyes, mouth and mucous membranes. Care should be taken when applying the product to the neck and other sensitive areas. In normal use, a mild burning sensation will probably be felt on first application and a moderate reddening and peeling of the skin will occur within a few days. During the first weeks of treatment a sudden increase in peeling will occur in most patients, this is not harmful and will normally subside within a day or two if treatment is temporarily discontinued. If excessive irritation, redness or peeling occurs discontinue use.

There are no restrictions on the use of PanOxyl Aquagel during pregnancy and lactation.

These products may bleach dyed fabrics.

Pharmaceutical precautions Store in a cool place.

Legal category P.

Package quantities Tubes of 40 g.

Further information Benzoyl peroxide has sebostatic and keratolytic activity coupled with antibacterial activity against Propionibacterium acnes, the organism implicated in acne vulgaris. Its use in the treatment of acne is well established.

Product licence numbers

PanOxyl Aquagel 2.5	0174/0049
PanOxyl Aquagel 5	0174/0050
PanOxyl Aquagel 10	0174/0051

PANOXYL* WASH

Presentation A white viscous lotion containing benzoyl peroxide 10% w/w.

Excipients: magnesium aluminium silicate, macrogol lauryl ether, hypromellose, citric acid, sodium alkyl aryl polyether sulphonate, sodium lauryl sulphoacetate, purified water.

Uses PanOxyl Wash is a skin cleanser for use in the topical treatment of acne vulgaris.

Dosage and administration Wet the affected area with water and wash thoroughly with PanOxyl Wash. Rinse well with warm water, then rinse with cold water. Pat dry with a clean towel. Use once a day, preferably in the morning.

Contra-indications, warnings, etc PanOxyl Wash should not be prescribed for patients with a known hypersensitivity to benzoyl peroxide.

Avoid contact with the eyes, mouth and mucous membranes. Care should be taken when using the product on the neck and other sensitive areas. After a few days, the area being treated may show mild to moderate redness or peeling.

There are no restrictions on the use of PanOxyl Wash during pregnancy.

PanOxyl Wash can cause bleaching of dyed fabrics, such as towels. It is important to emphasise thorough rinsing with water after use.

Pharmaceutical precautions Store in a cool place.

Legal category P.

Package quantity 150 ml.

Further information Benzoyl peroxide has sebostatic and keratolytic activity coupled with antibacterial activity against Propionibacterium acnes, the organism implicated in acne vulgaris. Its use in the treatment of acne is well established.

Product licence number 0174/0048.

POLYTAR* EMOLLIENT

Presentation Polytar Emollient is a liquid bath additive. The active ingredients are as follows:

Polytar†	25% w/w
Light Liquid Paraffin	35% w/w

(†Polytar consists of: Pine Tar BP, 30% w/w; Cade Oil BPC, 30%w/w; Coal Tar Solution BP, 10% w/w; Arachis Oil Extract of Coal Tar BP, 30% w/w.)

Excipients: octoxinol, sorbitan mono-oleate, polysorbate 80, isopropyl palmitate, macrogol 400 dilaurate, purified water.

Uses Polytar Emollient is indicated in the treatment of psoriasis, eczema, atopic and pruritic dermatoses. The use of Polytar Emollient may be combined with ultraviolet radiation and other adjunctive therapy.

Polytar Emollient is also of value in removing loose psoriatic scales and paste following dithranol treatment.

Dosage and administration 15–30 mls (2–4 capfuls) of Polytar Emollient should be added to an 8 inch bath and the patient instructed to soak for 20 minutes.

Contra-indications, warnings, etc Patients should be instructed to guard against slipping when entering or leaving the bath.

Tar products may cause skin irritation, rashes and rarely, photosensitivity. In the event of such a reaction, discontinue use and consult your doctor. Tar products may stain baths and fabrics.

There is no evidence of the safety of Polytar Emollient in human pregnancy but it has been in wide use for many years without apparent ill consequence.

Pharmaceutical precautions Nil.

Legal category GSL.

Package quantities Polytar Emollient is available in bottles of 350 ml and 1 litre.

Further information Tar preparations have keratoplastic and antipruritic activity and are widely used as topical therapy for a range of dermatoses. The use of emollient bath oils in the management of dry and itching skin is well established. Mineral oil exerts its emollient effect by skin absorption.

Polytar Emollient is prescribable on FP10 for the treatment of psoriasis, eczema, atopic and pruritic dermatoses.

Product licence number 0174/5011R.

POLYTAR* LIQUID

Presentation Polytar Liquid is a medicated shampoo containing the following active ingredients:

Polytar†	1% w/w
Oleyl Alcohol	1% w/w

(†Polytar consists of: Pine Tar BP, 30% w/w; Cade Oil BPC, 30%/w/w; Coal Tar Solution BP, 10%/w/w; Arachis Oil Extract of Coal Tar BP, 30% w/w.)

Excipients: coconut diethanolamide, hexylene glycol, polysorbate 80, triethanolamine lauryl sulphate, sodium chloride, citric acid, octoxinol, fragrance 5412, purified water.

Uses Polytar Liquid is indicated in the treatment of scalp disorders such as psoriasis, dandruff, seborrhoea, eczema and pruritus. Polytar Liquid is also of value in the removal of ointments and pastes used in the treatment of psoriasis.

Dosage and administration

Adults, children and the elderly: The hair should be wetted and sufficient Polytar Liquid applied to produce an abundant lather. The scalp and adjacent areas should be vigorously massaged with the fingertips. The hair should then be thoroughly rinsed and the procedure repeated.

Polytar Liquid should be used once or twice weekly.

Contra-indications, warnings, etc Tar products may cause skin irritation, rashes and rarely, photosensitivity. In the event of such a reaction, discontinue use and consult your doctor.

There is no evidence of the safety of Polytar Liquid in human pregnancy but it has been in wide use for many years without apparent ill consequence.

Pharmaceutical precautions Nil.

Legal category GSL.

Package quantities Polytar Liquid is available in bottles of 65 ml, 150 ml, 350 ml and 1 litre.

Further information Tars suppress DNA synthesis in hyperplastic skin, this inhibits mitotic activity and protein synthesis. By decreasing epidermal proliferation and dermal infiltration, they promote a return to normal keratinisation. Tars also have vasoconstricting, astringent and antipruritic properties.

Polytar Liquid is prescribable on FP10 for psoriasis, eczema and seborrhoea of the scalp and dandruff.

Product licence number 0174/5016R.

POLYTAR PLUS*

Presentation Polytar Plus is a concentrated antiseptic, tar medicated scalp cleanser adjusted to pH 5.5, containing the following active ingredient: Polytar† 1% w/w.

(†Polytar consists of: Pine Tar BP, 30% w/w; Cade Oil BPC, 30% w/w; Coal Tar Solution BP, 10% w/w; Arachis Oil Extract of Coal Tar BP, 30% w/w.)

Excipients: coconut diethanolamide, hexylene glycol, macrogol oleyl ether, polysorbate 80, polypeptide SF, oleyl alcohol, triethanolamine lauryl sulphate, citric acid, hypromellose, imidurea, fragrance 5412, purified water.

Uses Polytar Plus is indicated in the treatment of scalp disorders such as dandruff, psoriasis, seborrhoea, eczema and pruritus. Polytar Plus is also of value in the removal of ointments and pastes used in the treatment of psoriasis.

Dosage and administration
Aduts, children and the elderly: The hair should be wetted and sufficient Polytar Plus applied to produce an abundant lather. The scalp and adjacent areas should be vigorously massaged with the fingertips. The hair should then be thoroughly rinsed and the procedure repeated.

Polytar Plus should be used once or twice weekly.

Contra-indications, warnings, etc Tar products may cause skin irritation, rashes and rarely, photosensitivity. In the event of such a reaction, discontinue use and consult your doctor.

There are no restrictions on the use of Polytar Plus during pregnancy or lactation.

Pharmaceutical precautions Nil.

Legal category P.

Package quantities Polytar Plus is available in bottles of 350 ml.

Further information While the mode of action of tars is not fully established, their therapeutic effect has been observed over many years. It has been postulated that tars work by exerting a cytostatic action following an initial cytoproliferative effect. This slowing of the keratinisation process in the epidermal layer and reduction in the rate of epidermal turnover promoting a return to normal keratinisation.

Polytar Plus is prescribable on FP10 for psoriasis, eczema and seborrhoea of the scalp and for dandruff.

Product licence number 0174/0037.

SPECTRABAN* 4

Presentation SpectraBAN 4 contains Padimate O 3.2% w/w in an ethanolic base. The product, which is non-greasy and invisible on the skin, is blue in colour.

Excipients: ethanol, carbomer, polyoxyethylene cocoamine, colour: E131, oleyl alcohol, fragrance A-3012, purified water.

Uses SpectraBAN 4 is a protective sunscreen lotion indicated in patients at risk from exposure to ultraviolet light within the UVB wavelength range (280–315 nanometres). It is this narrow waveband of ultraviolet light which is responsible for burning and tanning of the skin in man. Use of the product should allow 4 times normal exposure to sunlight before burning.

SpectraBAN 4 is indicated in sun-sensitive conditions such as polymorphic light eruptions and solar urticaria and any condition made worse by UVB light such as lupus erythematosus.

Dosage and administration Apply carefully and evenly to areas to be exposed or protected only by light clothing. Allow to dry before dressing. Allow 45 minutes before swimming or sweat producing exercise. A single application may give day long protection but the product should be re-applied during prolonged sunning or after swimming or excessive sweating.

The product is intended for use in adults, children and the elderly.

Contra-indications, warnings, etc Sunscreen agents occasionally produce a sensitivity reaction and can cause contact dermatitis. Treatment should be discontinued if a skin rash or irritation develops. Do not apply to broken skin. Avoid contact with the eyes, mouth and other mucous membranes.

Although there is no experimental evidence to support the safety of the drug in pregnancy and lactation, no adverse effects have been reported.

Pharmaceutical precautions Avoid flame.

Legal category P.

Package quantities SpectraBAN 4 is available in bottles containing 150 ml.

Further information Nil.

Product licence number 0174/5013R.

SPECTRABAN* 15

Presentation SpectraBAN 15 contains Padimate O 3.2% w/w and Para Aminobenzoic Acid USP 5% w/w in an ethanolic base. The product, which is non-greasy and invisible on the skin, is pink in colour.

Excipients: ethanol, carbomer, polyoxyethylene cocoamine, colour E122, oleyl alcohol, fragrance A3012, purified water.

Uses SpectraBAN 15 is a protective sunscreen lotion indicated in patients at risk from exposure to ultraviolet light within the UVB wavelength range (280–315 nanometres). It is this narrow waveband of ultraviolet light which is responsible for burning and tanning of the skin in man. Use of the product should allow 15 times normal exposure to sunlight before burning.

SpectraBAN 15 is indicated in sun-sensitive conditions such as polymorphic light eruptions and solar urticaria and any condition made worse by UVB light such as lupus erythematosus.

Dosage and administration Apply carefully and evenly to areas to be exposed or protected only by light clothing. Allow to dry before dressing. Allow 45 minutes before swimming or sweat producing exercise. A single application may give day long protection but the product should be re-applied during prolonged sunning or after swimming or excessive sweating.

Contra-indications, warnings, etc Sunscreen preparations occasionally produce a sensitivity reaction. Treatment should be discontinued if a skin rash or irritation develops. Do not apply to broken skin. Avoid contact with the eyes, mouth and other mucous membranes.

The product can stain clothing and other items permanently.

There is no evidence of the safety of the drug in human pregnancy but it has been in wide use for many years without apparent ill consequence.

Pharmaceutical precautions Avoid flame.

Legal category P.

Package quantities SpectraBAN 15 is available in bottles containing 150 ml.

Further information SpectraBAN 15 is prescribable on FP10 for patients who require protection from ultraviolet radiation in photodermatoses.

Product licence number 0174/0035.

STIEDEX*

Presentation Stiedex contains 0.25% w/w desoxymethasone in an oily cream base.

Excipients: isopropyl myristate, wool alcohols ointment, edetic acid, purified water.

Uses Stiedex contains a potent corticosteroid, desoxymethasone.

Stiedex is indicated for the treatment of severe acute inflammatory and allergic conditions and for chronic skin disorders such as psoriasis which have proved intractable to other treatment.

Stiedex is indicated for short courses of treatment only, in view of the risks of adverse steroid effects which frequently occur with the continuous administration of potent steroids.

Dosage and administration Stiedex should be applied sparingly to the affected area and rubbed gently into the skin. Initially, application should be 2–3 times daily; as the condition of the skin improves it may be possible to reduce the frequency of administration.

Contra-indications, warnings, etc

Contra-indications: Stiedex is not suitable for infants or young children. Stiedex is contra-indicated in facial rosacea, acne vulgaris, perioral dermatitis, perianal and genital pruritus, napkin eruptions, bacterial (e.g. impetigo), viral (e.g. *Herpes simplex*) and fungal (e.g. *Candida* and dermatophyte) infections.

Stiedex is not suitable for use in the treatment of inflammatory disorders of the eye.

Stiedex is contra-indicated in patients with hypersensitivity to the preparation.

There is inadequate evidence of safety in human pregnancy. Topical administration of corticosteroids to pregnant animals can cause abnormalities of foetal development including cleft palate and intrauterine growth retardation. There may therefore be a very small risk of such effects in the human foetus.

Precautions: The continuous administration of topical steroids over prolonged periods may result in adrenal suppression. The use of occlusive dressings is not recommended in view of the risks of significant steroid absorption.

The prolonged administration of potent corticosteroids may diminish skin collagen and cause subcutaneous atrophy; thinning of the epidermal layer and dilation of superficial blood vessels may occur, especially when corticosteroids are used on the face.

Warning: The product is a potent corticosteroid formulation with a greater likelihood of causing the adverse effects commonly associated with these preparations.

Pharmaceutical precautions Stiedex should be stored in a cool, dry place in containers similar to those of the manufacturer.

Legal category POM.

Package quantities Stiedex is available in tubes of 30 g.

Further information Stiedex contains no preservative. Stiedex may be diluted by admixture with Oily Cream BP.

Product licence number 0174/0052.

STIEDEX* LOTION

Presentation Stiedex Lotion contains desoxymethasone USP 0.25% w/w, Salicylic Acid PhEur 1.0% w/w.

Excipients: Polyol fatty acid ester, 1,2-propylene glycol, ethanol, sodium hydroxide, disodium edetate, purified water.

Uses Stiedex Lotion contains a potent corticosteroid and is indicated for the treatment of psoriasis, particularly of the scalp (but excluding widespread plaque psoriasis),seborrhoeic eczema, chronic lichenified eczema, lichen planus, lichen simplex, non-bullous ichthyosiform erythroderma.

Stiedex Lotion is especially suitable for use in hairy regions such as scalp, cheeks, neck and chest and for skin areas difficult to reach such as the auditory meatus.

Dosage and administration Stiedex Lotion should be applied to the affected areas once or twice daily, preferably morning and/or night. When the skin condition improves, application may be reduced to once daily. In order to prevent recurrence, treatment with Stiedex Lotion should be continued for some days after complete control of the condition. If the lotion is being used on the face or in children, courses should be limited to five days duration.

Contra-indications, warnings, etc *Contra-indications:* Stidex Lotion is contra-indicated in infants and young children, in facial rosacea, acne vulgaris, perioral dermatitis, perianal and genital pruritis, napkin eruptions, bacterial (e.g. impetigo), viral (e.g. Herpes simplex), and fungal (e.g. Candida or dermatophyte) infections.

Stiedex Lotion contains propylene glycol and should not be used in patients with a known hypersensitivity to this, or any of the other ingredients.

Precautions: The continuous administration of topical steriods over prolonged periods may result in adrenal suppression; in infants and children, this may cause growth retardation. The use of occlusive dressings enhances the absorption of the steroid, and in consequence, systemic effects are more likely to occur. Salicyclic acid may enhance absorption of the steroid or itself be absorbed. Adrenal suppression is unlikely in short courses of treatment or with doses not exceeding 10 g daily.

Long term continuous therapy should be avoided in all patients irrespective of age. The lotion should not be applied to extensive skin surfaces and application under occlusion should be restricted to dermatoses involving limited areas.

The use of topical corticosteroids may be hazardous in psoriasis for a number of reasons including rebound relapses following development of tolerance, risk of generalised pustular psoriasis and local and systemic toxicity due to impaired barrier function of the skin. Careful patient supervision is important if Stiedex Lotion is used in psoriasis.

Prolonged administration of potent corticosteroids has been shown also to cause a thinning in skin collagen and subcutaneous atrophy, resulting in striae, thinning and dilation of superficial blood vessels. These changes are particularly liable to occur on the face.

Percutaneous absorption of salicylic acid due to extensive use could lead to salicylism.

Salicylic acid may alter the permeability of the skin to other substances applied simultaneously. The use of other preparations, cosmetics etc., on skin treated with Stiedex Lotion should be avoided.

Stiedex Lotion should not be applied to or near the eye.

Use in pregnancy: There is inadequate evidence of safety in human pregnancy. Topical administration of corticosteroids to pregnant animals can cause abnormalities of foetal development including cleft palate and intrauterine growth retardation. There may therefore be a very small risk of such effects in the human foetus.

Pharmaceutical precautions Stiedex Lotion should be protected from heat and stored below 25°C.

Legal category POM.

Package quantities 50 ml.

Further information Nil.

Product licence number 0174/0062.

STIEDEX* LP

Presentation Stiedex LP contains 0.05% w/w desoxymethasone in an oily cream base.

Excipients: isopropyl myristate, wool alcohols ointment, edetic acid, purified water.

Uses Stiedex LP contains a potent corticosteroid and is indicated for the treatment of a wide range of acute inflammatory and allergic conditions, and chronic skin disorders.

Stiedex LP is specifically indicated for the treatment of eczema (including atopic, seborrhoeic and nummular eczema), intertrigo, psoriasis, pompholyx, lichen planus and discoid lupus erythematosus; acute and chronic allergic dermatoses, neurodermatitis; erythroderma, and may also be used in the non-specific treatment of sunburn, insect bites and anogenital pruritus.

Dosage and administration Stiedex LP should be applied sparingly to the affected area and rubbed gently into the skin. Initially, application should be made 2–3 times daily and the frequency of administration reduced as the conditions subsides.

Stiedex LP may be applied under an occlusive dressing. The affected area should be thoroughly cleansed prior to administration of cream and dressing to prevent infection.

Contra-indications, warnings, etc
Contra-indications: Stiedex LP is not suitable for infants and young children. Stiedex LP is contra-indicated in facial rosacea, acne vulgaris, perioral dermatitis, perianal and genital pruritus, napkin eruptions, bacterial (e.g. impetigo), viral (e.g. *Herpes simplex*) and fungal (e.g. *Candida* and dermatophyte) infections.

Stiedex LP is contra-indicated in patients with hypersensitivity to the preparation.

Stiedex LP is not suitable for use in the treatment of inflammatory disorders of the eye.

There is inadequate evidence of safety in human pregnancy. Topical administration of corticosteroids to pregnant animals can cause abnormalities of foetal development including cleft palate and intrauterine growth retardation. There may therefore be a very small risk of such effects in the human foetus.

Precautions: The continuous administration of topical steroids over prolonged periods may result in adrenal suppression; in infants and children, this may cause growth retardation. The use of occlusive dressings enhances the absorption of the active substance, desoxymethasone, and in consequence systemic effects are more likely to occur. Adrenal suppression is unlikely in short courses of treatment or with doses not exceeding 10 g daily.

Prolonged administration of potent corticosteroids has been shown also to cause a reduction in skin collagen and subcutaneous atrophy, resulting in striae, thinning and dilation of superficial blood vessels. These changes are particularly liable to occur on the face.

Pharmaceutical precautions Stiedex LP should be stored in a cool, dry place.

Legal category POM.

Package quantities Stiedex LP is available in tubes of 30 g and 100 g.

Further information Stiedex LP contains no preservative. Stiedex LP may be diluted by admixture with Oily Cream BP.

Product licence number 0174/0053.

STIEDEX* LPN

Presentation Stiedex LPN contains 0.05% w/w desoxymethasone and 0.5% w/w neomycin (as the sulphate) in an oily cream base.

Excipients: isopropyl myristate, wool alcohols ointment, edetic acid, purified water.

Uses Stiedex LPN contains a potent corticosteroid and is indicated for the treatment of a wide range of acute inflammatory and allergic conditions, and chronic skin disorders. Neomycin sulphate is a broad spectrum antibiotic effective against the majority of bacteria commonly associated with skin infections.

Stiedex LPN is specifically indicated for the treatment of steroid-responsive dermatoses complicated by bacterial infection. Such conditions would include eczema (atopic, seborrhoeic and nummular), intertrigo, psoriasis, pompholyx, lichen planus and discoid lupus erythematosus; acute and chronic allergic dermatoses, neurodermatitis; and erythroderma, and may also be used in the non-specific treatment of insect bites, sunburn, and anogenital pruritus.

Dosage and administration Stiedex LPN should be applied sparingly to the affected area and rubbed gently into the skin. Initially, application should be made 2–3 times daily and the frequency of administration reduced as the conditions subside.

In the treatment of more resistant lesions, the effect of Stiedex LPN may be enhanced by application of occlusive dressings. The affected area should be thoroughly cleansed prior to administration of cream and dressing.

Contra-indications, warnings, etc
Contra-indications: Stiedex LPN is not suitable for infants and young children. Stiedex LPN is contra-indicated in facial rosacea, acne vulgaris, perioral dermatitis, perianal and genital pruritus, napkin eruptions, viral (e.g. *Herpes simplex*) and fungal (e.g. *Candida* and dermatophyte) infections.

Stiedex LPN is contra-indicated in patients with hypersensitivity to the preparation.

Stiedex LPN is not suitable for use in the treatment of inflammatory disorders of the eye and should not be applied in the region of the external auditory meatus when the eardrum is perforated, because of the risk of ototoxicity.

Stiedex LPN should not be used in the treatment of tuberculous, fungal or viral infections of the skin, in which conditions topical corticosteroids are contra-indicated.

There is inadequate evidence of safety in human pregnancy. Topical administration of corticosteroids to pregnant animals can cause abnormalities of foetal development including cleft palate and intrauterine growth retardation. There may therefore be a very small risk of such effects in the human foetus.

Precautions: The continuous administration of topical steroids over prolonged periods may result in adrenal suppression; in infants and children, this may cause growth retardation. The use of occlusive dressings enhances the absorption of the active substance, desoxymethasone, and in consequence systemic effects are more likely to occur. Adrenal suppression is unlikely in short courses of treatment or with doses not exceeding 10 g daily.

Prolonged administration of potent corticosteroids has been shown also to cause a reduction in skin collagen and subcutaneous atrophy, resulting in striae, thinning and dilation of superficial blood vessels. These changes are particularly liable to occur on the face.

Pharmaceutical precautions Stiedex LPN should be stored in a cool, dry place.

Legal category POM.

Package quantities Stiedex LPN is available in tubes of 15 g.

Further information Stiedex LPN contains no preservative.

Product licence number 0174/0054.

STIEMYCIN*

Presentation A clear colourless solution in an amber glass screw capped applicator bottle. The applicator allows the product to be applied directly to the involved skin.

Each ml contains 20 mg erythromycin base PhEur in an amount equivalent to 20 mg of erythromycin base 1st International Standard, in an ethanol base also containing propylene glycol and Laureth 4.

Uses Stiemycin is indicated for use in the topical treatment of acne vulgaris.

Dosage and administration To be applied to the affected area twice daily after washing.

Contra-indications, warnings, etc Stiemycin is contra-indicated in patients with known sensitivity to any of the ingredients.

Concomitant topical acne therapy should be used with caution because a cumulative irritant effect may occur.

Avoid contact with eyes and other mucous membranes.

This product is for external use only.

There is no evidence of hazard from erythromycin in human pregnancy. It has been in wide use for many years without apparent ill consequence.

Pharmaceutical precautions Store in a cool place.

Legal category POM.

Package quantity 50 ml (2 × 25 ml).

Further information Nil.

Product licence number 0174/0047.

ZEASORB* POWDER

Presentation ZeaSORB is an off-white, highly absorbent, soft, antiseptic dusting powder containing the following:

Chloroxylenol BPC	0.5% w/w
Aluminium dihydroxyallantoinate	0.2% w/w

Excipients: talc, fragrance 6A, microcrystalline cellulose.

Uses Intertrigo, hyperhidrosis, bromidrosis, prevention of tinea pedis and related conditions.

Dosage and administration The affected areas should be dried as thoroughly as possible before applying ZeaSORB Powder. The powder should be smoothed over the surface of the skin, between joints and in folds.

ZeaSORB is intended for use in adults, the elderly and, with supervision, in children. Special care should be taken when using the product in children to avoid inhalation.

Contra-indications, warnings, etc Can be irritant to the eyes. Problems of granuloma have been associated with contact of talc with broken skin. As with all powders, take care to avoid inhalation.

There are no restrictions on the use of ZeaSORB in pregnancy and lactation.

Pharmaceutical precautions Store in a cool dry place.

Legal category P.

Package quantities ZeaSORB Powder is available in sifter-top plastic containers of 50 g.

Further information ZeaSORB Powder is non-caking and remains soft on saturation, preventing irritation.

Product licence number 0174/5015R.

**Trade Mark*

Stuart Pharmaceuticals
King's Court
Water Lane
Wilmslow
Cheshire SK9 5AZ

STUART

CORWIN* ▼

Presentation Corwin tablets containing xamoterol fumarate equivalent to 200 mg xamoterol are round, biconvex, dark yellow, film coated tablets impressed with 'CORWIN' on one face and the Stuart logo on the reverse. The impressions are highlighted in white. The inactive ingredients are calcium phosphate, gelatin, iron oxide, lactose, macrogol, magnesium carbonate, magnesium stearate, methylhydroxypropylcellulose, sodium starch glycollate and titanium dioxide.

Uses Chronic mild heart failure: Corwin is recommended for the treatment of patients who are not breathless at rest but who are limited by symptoms on exertion (eg breathlessness and fatigue). Treatment with Corwin should be initiated under hospital supervision only after the patient has been fully assessed [see 'Initiation of treatment' below]. After initiation of treatment the appropriate follow-up should be provided by hospital or general practitioners.

Corwin is contra-indicated in patients with moderate to severe heart failure. Some patients with moderate to severe heart failure have shown deterioration on Corwin. See 'Contra-indications' below.

Mode of action: Corwin is a $beta_1$-selective partial agonist. At rest and under conditions of low sympathetic drive Corwin acts predominantly as a beta adrenoceptor agonist. On exercise and under conditions of increased sympathetic drive, eg severe heart failure, Corwin acts as a beta adrenoceptor antagonist. In mild heart failure, Corwin improves cardiac efficiency by modestly increasing myocardial contractility, improving diastolic relaxation and lowering left ventricular filling pressure. The improved ventricular function results in increased cardiac output with no attendant increase in myocardial oxygen demand. This improvement in myocardial performance is maintained on exercise.

Many heart failure patients suffer from concomitant ischaemic heart disease. In patients with angina pectoris, a reduction in myocardial ischaemia on exercise has been demonstrated with Corwin at the dose levels recommended for heart failure.

Dosage and administration
Adults: Treatment should be started with 200 mg once a day for a week; dosage should then be increased to 200 mg twice daily provided that there are no adverse effects. The usual effective dose is 200 mg twice daily (but see renal impairment warning below). Improvement in symptoms of heart failure (eg dyspnoea, fatigue) may be progressive over a period of several weeks.

Elderly patients: No specific dosage reduction is necessary except in those with suspected or established renal impairment (see below).

Initiation of treatment: Treatment should be initiated under hospital supervision after full assessment of the patient who has completed an exercise test which excludes diagnosis of moderate or severe heart failure. In addition to other exclusion criteria under 'Contra-indications' and depending on the method used, the patient should be able to complete one of the following exercise tests (equivalent to 3.6 kilojoules).

- For a bicycle ergometer; two minutes of exercise starting with a load of 20 W for the first minute and at a load of 40 W for the second minute.
- For an exercise treadmill; two minutes of exercise at a treadmill speed of 4 km/h with the treadmill level (ie 0% incline).
- For a corridor walk test; 150 yards on the level in two minutes.
- Alternatively, any other standardised exercise test in which the patient achieves a basal workload equivalent to one of the tests defined above (equivalent to 3.6 kilojoules).

Patients who are unable to complete the minimum of two minutes exercise on the bicycle ergometer or equivalent should not be given Corwin. Assessment of the patient's heart failure status should also include such tests as an ECG and a chest X-ray. Additional investigations such as an echocardiogram may be necessary.

Children: There is no paediatric experience with Corwin and for this reason it is not recommended for use in children.

Contra-indications, warnings, etc
Contra-indications: Corwin is contra-indicated in patients with moderate to severe heart failure because some patients with moderate to severe heart failure have shown deterioration on Corwin.

Corwin should, therefore, not be used in patients with the following features:

- Those who are short of breath or fatigued at rest or limited on minimal exercise.
- Those who have a resting tachycardia (>90 beats per minute) or hypotension (systolic BP <100 mmHg).
- Those who present with acute pulmonary oedema or who have a history of repeated episodes of acute pulmonary oedema.
- Those with peripheral oedema, a raised jugular venous pressure, an enlarged liver or a third heart sound.
- Those who require treatment with doses of diuretics in excess of frusemide 40 mg per day or equivalent.
- Those who require treatment with an ACE inhibitor.

Precautions: Deterioration of disease: Corwin should be withdrawn from patients whose mild heart failure deteriorates whilst on the drug, for example, if the patient develops worsening symptoms (shortness of breath and/ or fatigue), diminishing effort tolerance, or the appearance of signs such as peripheral oedema, a raised jugular venous pressure, an enlarged liver or a third heart sound. If Corwin is withdrawn, the patient should be carefully observed.

Renal impairment: Since Corwin is excreted by the kidneys, dosage should be adjusted in cases of severe impairment of renal function. No significant accumulation of Corwin occurs at a GFR greater than 35 ml/min/ 1.73 m^2. Significant accumulation of Corwin occurs only when GFR decreases to 15–35 ml/min/1.73 m^2. This level of renal impairment is usually clinically evident and approximates to a doubling of the serum creatinine (eg greater than 250 micromol/l or 3 mg/dl). The dose of Corwin is 200 mg daily when clinical evidence indicates suspected or established renal impairment (approximate doubling of serum creatinine value or a GFR of 15–35 ml/min/1.73 m^2).

Obstructive airways disease: Due to the beta adrenoceptor antagonist effects of Corwin, an increase in airways resistance may be provoked in patients with asthma or chronic obstructive airways disease. In such an event, Corwin should be withdrawn and increased airways resistance may be reversed by the use of inhaled bronchodilator preparations such as salbutamol. Corwin should be used with caution in patients with co-existing obstructive airways disease.

Liver function: Elevations of liver enzymes have been reported rarely in patients receiving Corwin but in such cases no relationship to the drug has been established.

Aortic stenosis/hypertrophic obstructive cardiomyopathy: As with other drugs which increase the force of myocardial contraction, Corwin should be used with caution in patients with outflow obstruction.

Cardiac arrhythmias: Cardiac arrhythmias are common in patients with heart failure. Occasional cases of ventricular arrhythmias have been reported during Corwin therapy and, in some patients, Corwin cannot be excluded as a contributory factor. Ambulatory (Holter) ECG monitorinig studies have not shown any evidence that Corwin therapy promotes arrhythmias. In patients with atrial fibrillation, concurrent therapy with a cardiac glycoside must be maintained.

Pregnancy and lactation: There is no evidence for the safety of the drug in human pregnancy. When high doses of Corwin were given to rats and rabbits during the second half of pregnancy, the cardiovascular effects of the drug led to deformations. It is recommended, therefore, that administration of the drug is avoided in pregnancy unless the condition itself carries sufficient risks to the mother and foetus to warrant use.

Studies in rats show that Corwin is excreted in the breast milk of lactating females. Its use in lactating women who are breast feeding should be avoided.

Side-effects: Rarely bronchospasm, worsening of obstructive airways diseases and hypotension have been observed after introduction of Corwin.

Adverse experiences in controlled studies showed a small excess in incidence over placebo of gastrointestinal complaints, headache and dizziness.

Although there was also an apparent excess of angina/chest pain such events are not uncommon and are to be expected in heart failure patients. Other controlled studies with Corwin in patients with angina pectoris showed reduced incidence of myocardial ischaemia during exercise.

Rash, palpitations and muscle cramp were also reported.

Overdosage: There is no experience of overdosage with Corwin. Effects are unlikely to be life threatening; symptomatic conservative management is recommended.

Pharmaceutical precautions Corwin tablets should be stored at room temperature.

Legal category POM.

Package quantities Corwin tablets (200 mg) in calendar packs of 56 tablets (OP).

Further information Corwin should not be co-administered with other beta$_1$ adrenoceptor agonists or antagonists because of competition between these drugs and Corwin for the beta$_1$ adrenoceptor.

Corwin has been co-administered without evidence of incompatibility with a range of other therapies including thiazide and potassium-sparing diuretics, cardiac glycosides, warfarin, antiplatelet drugs and non-steroidal anti-inflammatory drugs.

Product licence number 0029/0207.

DISADINE* DP

Presentation Disadine DP is presented as a dry powder aerosol spray containing 0.5% Povidone Iodine USP in BP propellants. The inactive ingredients are dichlorodifluoromethane, povidone, and trichlorofluoromethane.

Uses Disadine DP is a broad spectrum antiseptic for topical application in the treatment and prevention of infection in wounds, including burns, varicose ulcers and bed sores.

Dosage and administration Shake the can before use and spray the treatment area from a distance of 6–10 inches (15–25 cm) until a light dusting of powder is deposited. Disadine DP should be used directly from the aerosol container.

Adults: The recommended usual maximum daily adult application for regular use on broken skin is 150 mg available iodine. This is equivalent to the use of two cans of Disadine DP (each containing a total of 750 mg of povidone iodine yielding 75 mg of available iodine) per day.

Children and elderly patients: There are no special dosage recommendations for either elderly patients or children. However, povidone iodine is not recommended for regular use in neonates and is contra-indicated in very low-birth-weight infants (below 1500 grams).

Contra-indications, warnings, etc Disadine DP is contra-indicated for patients with non-toxic nodular colloid goitre.

Disadine DP must not be used in deep wounds or in clean surgical wounds.

Disadine DP should be used with caution in neonates.

For topical application only, keep out of the eyes and nose.

Care must be taken when Disadine DP is used on known iodine-sensitive subjects although these do not normally react to povidone-iodine.

Iodine can be absorbed systemically especially when large areas of broken skin are treated and caution is necessary if the product is used for prolonged periods.

Since iodine can cross the placenta and can be secreted into breast milk, prolonged use should be avoided in pregnant or lactating women.

Treatment of patients with severe and extensive burns may cause metabolic acidosis, hypernatraemia and renal impairment.

Absorption of povidone iodine may interfere with thyroid function tests by causing an increase in protein bound iodine levels.

Side-effects: Local irritation and sensitivity can occasionally occur.

Overdosage: High serum levels resulting from excessive use can be reduced by haemodialysis.

Accidental ingestion: The amount of povidone iodine contained in an aerosol can of Disadine DP is unlikely to have any toxic effects if ingested.

Pharmaceutical precautions Store at room temperature and away from direct heat and sunlight. Do not autoclave. The container must not be punctured or destroyed by burning, even when empty.

Legal category P.

Package quantities Disadine DP is supplied in a 150 g aerosol can (OP).

Further information Nil.

Product licence number 0029/5903.

KALTEN*

Presentation Hard gelatin capsules with opaque red caps and opaque cream bodies.

Each capsule is imprinted KALTEN and with the Stuart logo in black. Each capsule contains Atenolol BP 50 mg, Hydrochlorothiazide PhEur 25 mg and Amiloride Hydrochloride BP (dihydrate) 2.84 mg (equivalent to amiloride hydrochloride 2.5 mg). The inactive ingredients are gelatin, ink, iron oxide, lactose, magnesium stearate, maize starch, sodium lauryl sulphate, sodium starch glycollate and titanium dioxide.

Uses Management of hypertension.

Mode of action: Atenolol preferentially blocks the cardiac beta$_1$-adrenergic receptors. This beta$_1$-selectivity permits treatment of patients with simultaneous respiratory function problems. Atenolol is devoid of intrinsic sympathomimetic activity and membrane stabilising effect. It does not cross the blood-brain barrier. Treatment is characterised by a simple dosage regimen with rapid effect.

Hydrochlorothiazide is a thiazide diuretic acting on the distal tubule. It exerts its effect on sodium and water excretion by inhibiting sodium absorption thereby impeding the capacity of the kidneys to concentrate the urine. It has a relatively flat dose-response curve.

Amiloride is a potassium sparing diuretic which although having a mild antihypertensive effect is used primarily for its potassium conserving effects. It acts on the early distal tubule. Studies show that the combination of hydrochlorothiazide and amiloride in the ratio of 10 to 1 is optimal to achieve these effects.

Atenolol, hydrochlorothiazide and amiloride have compatible pharmacokinetics. All three drugs are rapidly but incompletely absorbed following oral administration. However, because none of them is significantly metabolised by the liver, the blood levels of the drugs are consistent and subject to little variability. They are eliminated unmetabolised by the kidney with elimination half-lives between 6 and 10 hours. When given together no clinically significant pharmacokinetic interactions occur.

Dosage and administration

Adults including the elderly: One capsule daily. Kalten is recommended for use in hypertensive patients where monotherapy with a beta-adrenoceptor blocker or diuretic proves inadequate. Where necessary another antihypertensive drug, such as a vasodilator, can be added. Patients can be transferred to preparations containing beta-adrenoceptor blocking drugs from other antihypertensive treatments with the exception of clonidine (see 'Warnings' below).

Kalten contains low effective doses of both a beta-adrenoceptor blocking agent and a combination of diuretics with a potassium-sparing action, and may be suited to older patients where higher doses of these drugs may be considered inappropriate.

Children: There is no paediatric experience with Kalten; therefore this is not recommended for use in children.

Contra-indications, warnings, etc

Kalten should not be given to patients with second or third degree heart block, with hyperkalaemia (serum potassium over 5.5 mmol/L) or where potassium-sparing diuretics or potassium supplements are already being given. Kalten is contra-indicated in anuria, acute renal failure, severe progressive renal disease, diabetic nephropathy; patients with blood urea over 10 mmol/L or serum creatinine over 130 micro mol/L in whom serum electrolyte and blood urea levels cannot be monitored carefully and frequently. Kalten should not be used in patients with cardiogenic shock.

In renal impairment, use of a potassium-conserving agent may result in rapid development of hyperkalaemia.

Kalten should not be given to those with prior sensitivity to hydrochlorothiazide or amiloride hydrochloride.

Special care should be taken with patients whose cardiac reserve is poor. Beta-adrenoceptor blockers should be avoided in overt heart failure. However, they may be used in patients whose signs of failure have been controlled.

One of the pharmacological actions of beta-adrenoceptor blocking drugs is to reduce heart rate. In the rare instance that symptoms may be attributable to the slow heart rate, the dose of the beta-adrenoceptor blocker may be reduced.

Kalten contains the cardioselective beta-adrenoceptor blocking drug atenolol. Although cardioselective ($beta_1$) beta-blockers may have less effect on lung function than non-selective beta-blockers, as with all beta-blockers, these should be avoided in patients with reversible obstructive airways disease, unless there are compelling clinical reasons for their use. Where such reasons exist, Kalten may be used with caution. Occasionally, some increase in airways resistance may occur in asthmatic patients, however, and this may usually be reversed by commonly used dosage of bronchodilators such as salbutamol or isoprenaline.

Cessation of therapy with preparations containing a beta-adrenoceptor blocking drug in patients with ischaemic heart disease should be gradual.

Caution should be exercised when transferring patients from clonidine to beta-adrenoceptor blocking drugs. If beta-adrenoceptor blocking drugs and clonidine are given concurrently, clonidine should not be discontinued until several days after withdrawal of the beta-adrenoceptor blocking drug (also see prescribing information for clonidine).

Care should be taken in prescribing a beta-adrenoceptor blocking drug with Class 1 antidysrhythmic agents such as disopyramide.

Beta-adrenoceptor blocking drugs should be used with caution in combination with verapamil in patients with impaired ventricular function. The combination should not be given to patients with conduction abnormalities. Neither drug should be administered intravenously within 48 hours of discontinuing the other.

Preparations containing lithium generally should not be given with diuretics because they may reduce its renal clearance.

Kalten, as with other preparations containing a potassium conserving diuretic, must be used with great caution in severely ill patients in whom metabolic or respiratory acidosis may occur (e.g. decompensated diabetes or cardiopulmonary disease). Acidosis may be associated with rapid increases in serum potassium. Kalten may be associated with minor increases in uric acid.

Measurement of potassium levels is appropriate, especially in the older patient, those receiving digitalis preparations for cardiac failure, taking abnormal (low in potassium) diet, or suffering from gastrointestinal complaints.

Kalten should be used with caution in diabetic patients, or those with a known pre-disposition to diabetes, particularly those with abnormal renal function. Hyperkalaemia has commonly occurred in diabetic patients on amiloride, especially those with chronic renal disease or pre-renal azotaemia. The status of renal function should therefore be determined before Kalten is given to known or suspected diabetics. Lowering of glucose tolerance may occur and the insulin dosage of the diabetic patient may require adjustment.

Kalten should be discontinued at least 3 days before glucose tolerance testing. Kalten modifies the tachycardia of hypoglycaemia.

Hyponatraemia and hypochloraemia may occur, although the likelihood of hypochloraemic alkalosis is reduced. Any chloride deficiency may be corrected by ammonium chloride (except in hepatic disease) and largely prevented by a near normal salt intake.

Kalten should be used with caution in patients with renal or hepatic impairment and in those patients in whom fluid and electrolyte balance is critical. Hyperkalaemia or hypokalaemia has been observed in patients receiving amiloride hydrochloride, particularly in the aged, in diabetics, and in hospital patients with hepatic cirrhosis or congestive heart failure, who had known renal impairment, were seriously ill, or were undergoing vigorous diuretic therapy. Such patients should be carefully observed for clinical, laboratory, and ECG evidence of hyperkalaemia (not always associated with an abnormal ECG). Should hyperkalaemia develop, discontinue treatment immediately, and if necessary, take active measures to reduce the serum potassium to normal.

Kalten should be used with caution in those with impaired renal function. Special care should be taken to avoid cumulative or toxic effects due to a reduced excretion of the components of Kalten. In addition, azotaemia may be precipitated or increased by hydrochlorothiazide. If increasing azotaemia and oliguria occur, treatment should be discontinued.

In liver disease amiloride has been reported to precipitate hepatic encephalopathy, and deepening jaundice has also occurred in cirrhotic patients receiving amiloride.

Pregnancy and lactation: As clinical experience is limited,

Kalten is not recommended for use during pregnancy. Tenormin and thiazides appear in breast milk and also cross the placental barrier and appear in cord blood. In patients treated with Tenormin there were no apparent detrimental effects in the baby at birth or during breast feeding. However the use of Kalten where pregnancy is present or suspected requires that the benefits of the drug be weighed against possible hazards to the foetus. The hazards of thiazides include foetal or neonatal jaundice, thrombocytopenia, and possibly other side-effects that have occurred in the adult. If the use of the drug is deemed essential, the patient should stop nursing.

Anaesthesia: Care should be taken when using anaesthetic agents with Kalten. The anaesthetist should be informed and the choice of anaesthetic should be the agent with as little negative inotropic activity as possible.

Side-effects: With atenolol cold extremities, muscular fatigue and, in isolated cases, bradycardia may occur. Sleep disturbances of the type noted with other beta-adrenoceptor blocking drugs have rarely been reported.

There have been reports of skin rashes and/or dry eyes associated with the use of beta-adrenergic blocking drugs. The reported incidence is small and in most cases the symptoms have cleared when treatment was withdrawn. Discontinuance of the drug should be considered if any such reaction is not otherwise explicable and cessation of therapy should be gradual.

With amiloride hydrochloride and hydrochlorothiazide gastrointestinal effects including anorexia, nausea, vomiting, gastric irritation, cramps, pain, constipation and diarrhoea may occur. Dry mouth, thirst and paraesthesia, transient blurred vision, salivary gland inflammation, vertigo, fatigue, muscle cramps and orthostatic hypotension may also occur secondary to diuresis. Dizziness and headache may occur. Skin rashes with associated photosensitivity, necrotising vasculitis, acute pancreatitis and blood dyscrasias have been reported.

Rarely, hypersensitivity reactions, including pulmonary oedema with symptoms of shock, have been reported with hydrochlorothiazide.

Overdosage: Dehydration, electrolyte imbalance and hepatic coma are treated by the established procedures. There is no specific antidote. If ingestion is recent, emesis should be induced or gastric lavage performed. If hyperkalaemia occurs, active measures should be taken to reduce the serum potassium levels. For respiratory impairment, oxygen or artificial respiration should be administered.

Excessive bradycardia may be countered by atropine 1–2 mg intravenously, followed, if necessary, by a bolus dose of glucagon 10 mg intravenously. If required, this may be repeated or followed by an intravenous infusion of glucagon 1–10 mg/hour depending on response. If no response to glucagon occurs or if glucagon is unavailable, a beta-adrenoceptor stimulant such as prenalterol 5 mg intravenously, followed if necessary by an intravenous infusion of 5 mg/hour or dobutamine 2.5 to 10 microgram/kg/minute by intravenous infusion may be given.

Any risk of hypotension occurring following the use of beta-adrenoceptor agonists will be reduced by the use of the more selective agents, e.g. prenalterol and dobutamine. Excessive diuresis should be countered by maintaining normal fluid and electrolyte balance.

Pharmaceutical precautions Kalten capsules should be stored at room temperature, protected from light and moisture.

Legal category POM.

Package quantities Calendar packs of 28 (OP).

Further information *Effect on ability to drive or operate machinery:* Since there are only rare reports of beta-blockers causing symptomatic hypotension and bradycardia, the use of Kalten is unlikely to result in any impairment of the ability of patients to drive or operate machinery.

When the combined antihypertensive effect of a beta-blocker and a potassium-conserving diuretic is required, Kalten is a simple, convenient and acceptable therapy which may be expected to improve patient compliance. The effect of Kalten following a one capsule oral dose is sustained for at least 24 hours.

Product licence number 0029/0186.

METOSYN* FAPG CREAM
METOSYN* OINTMENT

Presentation Metosyn consists of the corticosteroid fluocinonide presented as FAPG Cream and as Ointment. In Metosyn FAPG Cream, fluocinonide 0.05% w/w is dissolved completely in propylene glycol with fatty alcohols added to produce a white, homogeneous, semi-solid preparation. Inactive ingredients in Metosyn FAPG Cream are citric acid, hexanetriol, polyethylene glycol, propylene glycol, and stearyl alcohol. Metosyn Ointment contains fluocinonide 0.05% w/w completely dissolved in a petroleum base. Inactive ingredients contained in Metosyn ointment are amerchol CAB, propylene carbonate, propylene glycol and white soft paraffin.

Uses Metosyn contains an effective topical corticosteroid, and is suitable for treating a wide variety of local inflammatory, pruritic and allergic disorders of the skin. It is indicated for topical application in the following conditions:

Eczema and dermatitis, atopic eczema, seborrhoeic dermatitis, discoid eczema, contact dermatitis, neurodermatitis, prurigo. Psoriasis (excluding widespread plaque psoriasis). Lichen planus. Discoid lupus erythematosus.

Metosyn FAPG Cream may be used for wet or dry lesions. Metosyn Ointment, with its emollient effects, is particularly suitable for dry scaly lesions.

Dosage and administration *All age groups:* A small quantity of Metosyn FAPG Cream or Metosyn Ointment should be applied three to four times daily to the affected area and massaged well in.

Once improvement is apparent, usage may be reduced to twice or even once daily.

It is recommended that Metosyn is used undiluted (see Pharmaceutical precautions).

Contra-indications, warnings, etc
Contra-indications: Metosyn is contra-indicated in rosacea, acne and peri-oral dermatitis, all of which can be treated with oral tetracyclines and hydrocortisone if a topical steroid is required. As with all topical steroids, Metosyn is contra-indicated in tuberculous, syphilitic, fungal and viral infections of the skin. The product should not be used for napkin eruptions or anogenital pruritus.

Precautions: Where there is bacterial infection associated with an inflammatory skin condition, Metosyn should only be administered if adequate antibacterial cover is also given.

Pregnancy: There is inadequate evidence of safety in human pregnancy. Topical administration of corticosteroids to pregnant animals can cause abnormalities of foetal development, including cleft palate and intra-uterine growth retardation. There may therefore be a very small risk of such effects on the human foetus.

Lactation: When topical steroid treatment is considered necessary during breast feeding, both the amount applied and the length of treatment should be minimised.

Long-term continuous topical steroid therapy should be avoided since adrenal suppression can occur, particularly when infants are being treated. It is recommended that treatment on the face and for children should not normally be extended beyond five days, and occlusion in such cases should not be used. Very occasionally hypersensitivity reactions may occur.

When using topical corticosteroids to treat psoriasis there are risks of rebound relapse following the development of tolerance, and of generalised pustular psoriasis. Impairment of the barrier function of the skin may lead to local and systemic toxicity. Careful patient supervision is important.

Side-effects: As with all topical steroids, striae may occur after extensive use of Metosyn. Irritation at the site of application may occur infrequently.

Overdosage: A 25 g tube of Metosyn FAPG Cream or Ointment contains 12.5 mg of fluocinonide. Toxic effects are not likely to occur following accidental ingestion. Similarly, the components of the vehicles, singly or collectively, have not been shown to produce toxic effects in these quantities.

Pharmaceutical precautions Metosyn should be stored in the original tube at room temperature. It is recommended that the product be used undiluted. However, if dilution of Metosyn Ointment is required, white soft paraffin should be used and special FAPG diluent should be used to dilute Metosyn FAPG Cream.

Legal category POM.

Package quantities Tubes of 25 g (OP) and 100 g FAPG Cream.
Tubes of 25 g (OP) and 100 g Ointment.

Further information Metosyn FAPG Cream and Metosyn Ointment do not contain lanolin or parabens.

Product licence numbers

Metosyn FAPG Cream	0029/5071
Metosyn Ointment	0029/0133

METOSYN* SCALP LOTION

Presentation Metosyn Scalp Lotion is a clear, colourless, slightly viscous solution containing 0.05% w/v fluocinonide in a vehicle containing citric acid, ethanol, di-isopropyl adipate and propylene glycol.

Uses Steroid-responsive dermatoses of the scalp such as psoriasis (excluding widespread plaque psoriasis), seborrhoeic dermatitis and severe dandruff.

Dosage and administration *All age groups:* A small quantity of Metosyn Scalp Lotion should be applied to the scalp morning and night until improvement is noticeable. Improvement may then be maintained with application once a day or less frequently. However, Metosyn Scalp Lotion should be prescribed for short courses of therapy and not used by patients on a continuous basis. In childhood, courses should be limited to five days.

Contra-indications, warnings, etc
Contra-indications: Infections of the scalp. Hypersensitivity to the preparation.

Precautions: Care must be taken to keep Metosyn Scalp Lotion away from the eyes and it must not be used near a naked flame.

If hypersensitivity develops treatment should be discontinued.

Long-term continuous therapy should be avoided particularly in infants and children, as adrenal suppression can occur even without occlusion.

Development of secondary infection requires withdrawal of therapy and commencement of appropriate antimicrobial therapy.

When using topical corticosteroids to treat psoriasis there are risks both of rebound relapse following the development of tolerance, and of generalised pustular psoriasis. Impairment of the barrier function of the skin may lead to local and systemic toxicity. Careful patient supervision is important.

Pregnancy: There is inadequate evidence of safety in human pregnancy. Topical administration of corticosteroids to pregnant animals can cause abnormalities of foetal development, including cleft palate and intrauterine growth retardation. There may therefore be a very small risk of such effects on the human foetus.

Lactation: When topical steroid treatment is considered necessary during breast feeding, both the amount applied and the length of treatment should be minimised.

Side-effects: As with all topical steroids, treatment of large areas such as the scalp can allow sufficient absorption to give systemic steroidal effects. This is more likely with children or infants, where occlusive dressing is used or treatment is prolonged. Atrophic skin changes can take place on continued application.

Irritation at the site of application may occur infrequently.

A burning feeling may be noticed on application and this may, on occasion, warrant discontinuation of therapy.

Overdosage: A 30 ml bottle of Metosyn Scalp Lotion contains 15 mg of fluocinonide and 30% w/v ethanol. Toxic effects unlikely to occur following accidental oral ingestion.

Pharmaceutical precautions Metosyn Scalp Lotion should be stored in its original bottle at room temperature. The bottle should not be stored or opened near a naked flame. Use undiluted.

Legal category POM.

Package quantities Glass bottles containing 30 ml with plastic applicator (OP).

Further information Nil.

Product licence number 0029/0163.

MONIT* TABLETS
MONIT* LS TABLETS

Presentation Monit tablets are white, round tablets imprinted 'Stuart 20' on one face and bisected on the reverse. Each tablet contains 20 mg isosorbide mononitrate.

Monit LS tablets are white, round tablets with '10' on one face and 'STUART' on the reverse. Each tablet contains 10 mg isosorbide mononitrate.

Inactive ingredients in Monit and Monit LS tablets are lactose, magnesium stearate, microcrystalline cellulose, povidone, sodium starch glycollate, and silicon dioxide.

Uses *Angina prophylaxis:* Monit and Monit LS tablets are indicated for the prophylaxis of angina.

Congestive heart failure: Monit tablets are indicated as adjunctive therapy in congestive heart failure which does not respond adequately to cardiac glycosides and/or diuretics.

Mode of action: Isosorbide 5-mononitrate is an active metabolite of isosorbide dinitrate. The predominant action is that of a vasodilator with effects on both arteries and veins.

Isosorbide 5-mononitrate is completely absorbed after oral administration. The elimination half-life is approximately 5 hours. The volume of distribution is about 0.62 l/kg. The time to maximum plasma level is approximately 1 hour and peak plasma concentrations are approximately 250 and 500 ng/ml for Monit LS and Monit respectively. In patients with renal failure, the half-life is unchanged, remaining at approximately 5 hours.

Dosage and administration
Adults
Angina pectoris: Usually one tablet twice or three times daily. Patients already accustomed to prophylactic nitrate therapy (for example with isosorbide dinitrate) may normally be transferred directly to a therapeutic dose of Monit. For patients not receiving prophylactic nitrate therapy, it is recommended that the initial dose should be one Monit LS tablet twice daily. Maintenance dose in individual patients will be between 20 and 120 mg daily.

Congestive cardiac failure: In severe congestive cardiac failure Monit tablets may be taken in doses of 20 mg two to three times daily depending on patient requirements. In this situation optimal individual dose is best determined by continuous haemodynamic monitoring. The use of Monit in severe congestive cardiac failure should be considered adjunctive therapy to more conventional treatment (e.g. cardiac glycosides, diuretics etc).

Elderly patients: Dosage requirements may be reduced, especially when hepatic or renal function is impaired.

The tablets should be swallowed whole with a little fluid.

Contra-indications, warnings, etc
Contra-indications: Monit and Monit LS are contra-indicated in patients with a known sensitivity to the drug or to isosorbide dinitrate.

Pregnancy and lactation: Since its safety and efficacy during pregnancy and lactation have not been established, Monit like other drugs should not be administered to pregnant women and nursing mothers unless considered essential. No data are available on the presence of isosorbide mononitrate in breast milk.

Nitrate preparations can act as physiological antagonists to noradrenaline, acetylcholine, histamine and other agents.

Side-effects: The following adverse effects may be seen with nitrate therapy:

Cutaneous vasodilatation, headache, dizziness and weakness may occur, and are usually controlled by lowering the dose. The incidence of these effects is highest at commencement of treatment and tends to decline with time. If headache is a problem a temporary lowering of the Monit dose and the use of analgesics may be necessary.

Postural hypotension may occur, especially with high doses.

Dry rash and/or exfoliative dermatitis have been described rarely with isosorbide dinitrate and similar reactions might be expected occasionally.

Overdosage: Overdosage should be treated symptomatically. The main symptom is likely to be hypotension and this may be treated by elevation of the legs to promote venous return.

Pharmaceutical precautions Store at room temperature. Protect from moisture.

Legal category

Monit	P.
Monit LS	P.

Package quantities Monit tablets are supplied in calendar packs of 56 tablets (OP) and bottles of 100. Monit LS tablets are supplied in calendar packs of 14 and 56 tablets (OP).

Further information *Effect on ability to drive or operate machinery:* The effect of isosorbide mononitrate upon an individual's performance of skilled and potentially dangerous tasks, such as car driving and the operation of machinery, has not been evaluated. However, there have been no published reports of impaired performance of such tasks.

Isosorbide mononitrate is the British Approved name for isosorbide-5-mononitrate.

Beta-blocking drugs have a different pharmacological action in angina and may have a complementary effect when co-administered with Monit.

Product licence numbers

Monit	0029/0174
Monit LS	0029/0194

MONIT* SR TABLETS

Presentation Monit SR tablets are white, round, sugar coated tablets each containing 40 mg isosorbide mononitrate in a sustained release form. Inactive ingredients are Eudragit E, glucose, kaolin, lactose, macrogol, magnesium stearate, montanic acid/ethylene glycol ester, povidone, silicon dioxide, sucrose, talc and titanium dioxide.

Uses Monit SR is indicated for the prophylaxis of angina pectoris.

Mode of action: Monit SR has been developed to provide a convenient, once daily dosage form of isosorbide mononitrate. It is designed to achieve therapeutic blood concentrations within 30 minutes which persist up to 17 hours. A nitrate free interval of up to 7 hours makes the development of anti-anginal tolerance during chronic therapy unlikely.

Dosage and administration The tablets should be swallowed whole without chewing.

Adults: One tablet daily, to be taken in the morning.

Elderly patients: There is no evidence to suggest an adjustment of dose is necessary. However, caution may be required in elderly patients who are known to be susceptible to the effects of hypotensive medication.

Children: The safety and efficacy of Monit SR in children has not been established.

Contra-indications, warnings, etc
Contra-indications: Monit SR is contra-indicated in patients with a known hypersensitivity to isosorbide mononitrate or isosorbide dinitrate.

Precautions: Monit SR is not indicated for relief of acute anginal attacks. In the event of an acute attack, sublingual or buccal glyceryl trinitrate tablets or spray should be used.

Patients who have not previously received nitrates may be started with a low dose which should be increased gradually before introducing Monit SR.

Caution is required in patients with increased susceptibility to hypotension and in patients with marked hepatic or renal insufficiency, closed angle glaucoma, marked anaemia and hypothyroidism.

Some of the effects of alcohol and the action of hypotensive agents may be potentiated by isosorbide mononitrate.

Pregnancy and lactation: There is inadequate evidence of safety of the drug in human pregnancy although nitrates have been in wide use for many years without ill consequence, animal studies having shown no adverse effects on the foetus. Nevertheless, it is not advisable to use this drug during pregnancy and lactation.

Side-effects: A number of nitrate-related adverse effects may occur during treatment, including headache and feelings of dizziness. Other reactions, such as those associated with isosorbide dinitrate (eg flushing, postural hypotension, skin reactions) may occur occasionally.

Overdosage: In the event of overdosage with Monit SR the main sign is likely to be hypotension. The stomach should be aspirated to remove any remaining tablets. The patient should be placed in a supine position with the legs elevated to promote venous return. Any other treatment should be symptomatic.

Pharmaceutical precautions Store at room temperature. Protect from light and moisture.

Legal category P.

Package quantities Monit SR tablets are supplied in calendar packs of 28 tablets (OP).

Further information Nil.

Product licence number 0029/0225.

SORBICHEW*

Presentation Sorbichew tablets contain isosorbide dinitrate.

The chewable tablets are round, green, scored tablets marked 'S' on one face and marked 810 on the reverse, each containing 5 mg isosorbide dinitrate. The inactive ingredients are D & C yellow No. 10, F D & C Blue No. 1, hydrogenated vegetable oil, lime flavour, magnesium stearate, mannitol, povidone, starch, sugar and water.

Uses Sorbichew is indicated in the management of angina pectoris to prevent or abort the acute attack.

Mode of action: The predominant mode of action of isosorbide dinitrate is that of a vasodilator with effects on both arteries and veins.

Following systemic absorption isosorbide dinitrate is metabolised by the liver to isosorbide 2-mononitrate and isosorbide 5-mononitrate. The elimination half-life of isosorbide dinitrate is approximately 0.8 hours. The bioavailability is $22 \pm 14\%$ after oral administration because of significant first-pass metabolism. The volume of distribution is 1.5 ± 0.8 l/kg with around 30% binding to plasma proteins. Clearance has been shown to be 45 ± 20 ml/min/kg. Isosorbide 2-mononitrate has a half-life of approximately 2 hours with that of isosorbide 5-mononitrate being 5 hours.

Dosage and administration *Adults including the elderly:*

Treatment of the acute attack: Either one or two Sorbichew tablets should be chewed until dissolved completely and swallowed.

Prevention of an expected attack: Immediately prior to the stressful event either one or two Sorbichew tablets should be chewed until dissolved completely and swallowed.

Sorbichew tablets are scored for easier dose adjustment.

Contra-indications, warnings, etc
Sorbichew is contra-indicated in patients with a known sensitivity to the drug.

Pregnancy and lactation: As with other drugs, nitrates should not be administered to pregnant women and nursing mothers unless essential. No data are available on the presence of isosorbide dinitrate in breast milk.

Nitrate preparations can act as physiological antagonists to noradrenaline, acetylcholine, histamine and other agents.

Side-effects: The following adverse effects may be seen with isosorbide dinitrate.

Cutaneous vasodilatation, headache, dizziness and weakness may occur. If headache is a problem, a temporary lowering of the dose, and the use of analgesics, may be necessary. In the majority of patients, headache diminishes or disappears after 1–3 weeks and optimum dosage may be achieved.

Postural hypotension.

Dry rash and/or exfoliative dermatitis may occasionally occur.

Overdosage: Overdosage should be treated symptomatically. The main symptom is likely to be hypotension and this may be treated by elevation of the legs to promote venous return.

Pharmaceutical precautions Although Sorbichew tablets are stable and no special storage precautions are required, it is advised that in accordance with good pharmaceutical practice the tablets should be stored at room temperature protected from moisture.

Legal category P.

Package quantities Sorbichew: 5 mg chewable tablets are supplied in containers of 100 (OP).

Further information *Effect on ability to drive or operate machinery:* The effect of isosorbide dinitrate upon an individual's performance of skilled and potentially dangerous tasks, such as car driving and the operation of machinery, has not been evaluated. However, there have been no published reports of impaired performance of such tasks.

Unlike glyceryl trinitrate, Sorbichew tablets are stable and therefore loss of potency when carried by the patient does not normally occur.

Sorbichew has an approximate onset of action of two minutes and duration of action up to two hours.

Product licence number
Sorbichew 5 mg 0029/0109

SORBID*-20 SA and SORBID*-40 SA CAPSULES

Presentation Sorbid-20 SA capsules and Sorbid-40 SA capsules contain isosorbide dinitrate.

Sorbid-20 SA is presented as transparent red/yellow capsules containing 20 mg isosorbide dinitrate in a sustained release spheroid formulation. Sorbid-40 SA is presented as transparent red/colourless capsules containing 40 mg isosorbide dinitrate in a sustained release spheroid formulation. Sorbid-40 SA capsules contain the following inactive ingredients: erythrosine, ethanol, gelatin, iron oxide, maize starch, shellac, sucrose and talc. Sorbid-20 SA capsules also contain Quinoline Yellow.

Uses Prophylaxis of angina pectoris.

Mode of action: The predominant mode of action of isosorbide dinitrate is that of a vasodilator with effects on both arteries and veins.

Following oral dosing with Sorbid-20 SA and Sorbid-40 SA, the peak blood levels of isosorbide dinitrate are approximately 8 and 15 ng/ml respectively. Isosorbide dinitrate is metabolised by the liver to isosorbide 2-mononitrate and isosorbide 5-mononitrate. The corresponding values for the peak blood levels of the 2-mononitrate are approximately 25 and 45 ng/ml and for the 5-mononitrate 135 and 286 ng/ml respectively. The elimination half-life of isosorbide dinitrate is 2–3 hours, the half-life of isosorbide 2-mononitrate is 4–5 hours and the half-life of isosorbide 5-mononitrate is 5–6 hours.

Dosage and administration
Adults: 1–2 Sorbid-20 SA capsules twice daily, or when higher doses are required, 1–2 Sorbid-40 SA capsules, should be swallowed twice daily.

Elderly patients: Dosage requirements may be reduced, especially when hepatic or renal function is impaired.

Contra-indications, warnings, etc
Sorbid SA is contraindicated in patients with a known sensitivity to the drug.

Pregnancy and lactation: As with other drugs, nitrates should not be administered to pregnant women and nursing mothers unless essential. No data are available on the presence of isosorbide dinitrate in breast milk.

Nitrate preparations can act as physiological antagonists to noradrenaline, acetylcholine, histamine and other agents.

Side-effects: The following adverse effects may be seen with isosorbide dinitrate:

Cutaneous vasodilatation, headache, dizziness and weakness may occur. If headache is a problem, a temporary lowering of the dose and the use of analgesics may be necessary. In the majority of patients, headache diminishes or disappears after 1–3 weeks and optimum dosage may be achieved.

Postural hypotension.

Dry rash and/or exfoliative dermatitis may occasionally occur.

Overdosage: Overdosage should be treated symptomatically. The main symptom is likely to be hypotension and this may be treated by elevation of the legs to promote venous return.

Pharmaceutical precautions Store at room temperature, protected from light and moisture.

Legal category P.

Package quantities Sorbid-20 SA and Sorbid-40 SA capsules are supplied in calendar packs of 56 capsules (OP).

Further information *Effect on ability to drive or operate machinery:* The effect of isosorbide dinitrate upon an individual's performance of skilled and potentially dangerous tasks, such as car driving and the operation of machinery, has not been evaluated. However, there have been no published reports of impaired performance of such tasks.

Unlike glyceryl trinitrate, Sorbid-20 SA and Sorbid-40 SA capsules are very stable and therefore loss of potency when carried by patients does not normally occur.

The duration of action of the capsules is estimated to be up to 12 hours.

Product licence numbers
Sorbid-20 SA capsules 0029/0161
Sorbid-40 SA capsules 0029/0162

SORBITRATE*

Presentation Sorbitrate tablets contain isosorbide dinitrate. Sorbitrate tablets are available containing 10 mg and 20 mg isosorbide dinitrate. The 10 mg tablets are oval, yellow, scored tablets marked 'S' on one face and marked '780' on the reverse. Inactive ingredients in Sorbitrate Tablets 10 mg are D & C Yellow No. 10, lactose, magnesium stearate and starch. The 20 mg tablets are oval, blue, scored tablets marked 'S' on one face and marked '820' on the reverse. Inactive ingredients in Sorbitrate Tablets 20 mg are FD & C Blue No. 1, lactose, magnesium stearate and starch.

Uses Sorbitrate is indicated for:

(a) prophylaxis of angina pectoris
(b) congestive cardiac failure – as adjunctive therapy in the management of severe acute or chronic congestive cardiac failure.

Mode of action: The predominant mode of action of isosorbide dinitrate is that of a vasodilator with effects on both arteries and veins.

Following systemic absorption isosorbide dinitrate is metabolised by the liver to isosorbide 2-mononitrate and isosorbide 5-mononitrate. The elimination half-life of isosorbide dinitrate is approximately 0.8 hours. The bioavailability is $22 \pm 14\%$ after oral administration because of significant first-pass metabolism. The volume of distribution is 1.5 ± 0.8 l/kg with around 30% binding to plasma proteins. Clearance has been shown to be 45 ± 20 ml/min/kg. Isosorbide 2-mononitrate has a half-life of approximately 2 hours with that of isosorbide 5-mononitrate being 5 hours.

Dosage and administration *Adults:*

Angina Prophylaxis: 10–40 mg, three to four times daily depending on individual requirement.

Congestive Cardiac Failure: In severe congestive cardiac failure Sorbitrate tablets may be taken in doses of 10–40 mg three to four times daily depending on patient requirements. In this situation optimal individual dose is best determined by continuous haemodynamic monitoring. The use of Sorbitrate in severe congestive cardiac failure should be considered adjunctive therapy to more conventional treatment (e.g. digitalis, diuretics, etc.).

Elderly patients: Dosage requirements may be reduced, especially when hepatic or renal function is impaired. The tablets are scored for easier dose adjustment.

Contra-indications, warnings, etc
Sorbitrate is contra-indicated in patients with a known sensitivity to the drug.

Pregnancy and lactation: As with other drugs, nitrates should not be administered to pregnant women and nursing mothers unless essential. No data are available on the presence of isosorbide dinitrate in breast milk.

Nitrate preparations can act as physiological antagonists to noradrenaline, acetylcholine, histamine and other agents.

Side-effects: The following adverse effects may be seen with isosorbide dinitrate.

Cutaneous vasodilatation, headache, dizziness and weakness may occur. If headache is a problem, a temporary lowering of the dose, and the use of analgesics, may be necessary. In the majority of patients, headache diminishes or disappears after 1–3 weeks and optimum dosage of Sorbitrate may be achieved.

Postural hypotension.

Dry rash and/or exfoliative dermatitis may occasionally occur.

Overdosage: Overdosage should be treated symptomatically. The main symptom is likely to be hypotension and this may be treated by elevation of the patient's legs to promote venous return.

Pharmaceutical precautions Store at room temperature protected from moisture.

Legal category P.

Package quantities Sorbitrate tablets: 20 mg tablets are supplied in containers of 100 (OP).

10 mg tablets are supplied in containers of 100 (OP) and 500.

Further information *Effect on ability to drive or operate machinery:* The effect of isosorbide dinitrate upon an individual's performance of skilled and potentially dangerous tasks, such as car driving and the operation of machinery, has not been evaluated. However, there have been no published reports of impaired performance of such tasks.

Unlike glyceryl trinitrate, Sorbitrate tablets are stable and therefore loss of potency when carried by the patient does not normally occur. The duration of action of the tablets is estimated to be four to six hours.

Product licence numbers

Sorbitrate Tablets 20 mg	0029/0145
Sorbitrate Tablets 10 mg	0029/0111

TENIF*

Presentation Tenif is presented as reddish brown capsules bearing the name Tenif with the Stuart logo. Each capsule contains Atenolol BP 50 mg and a slow release formulation of nifedipine 20 mg. The inactive ingredients are gelatin, iron oxide, lactose, macrogol, magnesium carbonate, magnesium stearate, maize starch, methylhydroxypropyl cellulose, microcrystalline cellulose, polysorbate, sodium lauryl sulphate and titanium dioxide.

Uses Management of hypertension where therapy with either a calcium channel blocker or a beta-blocker proves inadequate.

Management of angina pectoris where therapy with either a calcium channel blocker or a beta-blocker proves inadequate.

Mode of action: Atenolol effects a marked negative inotropic and chronotropic effect thereby reducing cardiac output, myocardial oxygen demand and blood pressure, particularly during exercise. Nifedipine is a powerful coronary and peripheral vasodilator which increases myocardial oxygen supply and reduces blood pressure (afterload) and peripheral resistance. Concomitant use of $beta_1$-blockade, therefore, ameliorates the reflex sympathetic response to nifedipine monotherapy by blocking the rise in heart rate, while atenolol's tendency to increase peripheral resistance is balanced by the vasodilatation and increased sympathetic tone induced by the calcium antagonist. Consequently, greater antihypertensive or antianginal efficacy is achieved by the concomitant use of nifedipine and atenolol than either drug alone.

Dosage and administration
Adults: Hypertension: One capsule daily. If necessary, the dosage may be increased to one capsule dosed twice daily. Patients can be transferred to the combination from other antihypertensive treatments with the exception of clonidine (see 'Precautions' below).

Angina: One capsule dosed twice daily. Where additional efficacy is necessary, prophylactic nitrate therapy or additional nifedipine may be of benefit.

Children: There is no paediatric experience with Tenif and therefore Tenif should not be used in children.

Elderly: Dosage should not exceed one capsule daily in hypertension or one capsule twice daily in angina.

Contra-indications, warnings, etc
Contra-indications: Tenif must not be administered to women capable of childbearing or to nursing mothers.

Tenif must not be used in the presence of second or third degree heart block.

Tenif must not be used in patients with cardiogenic shock or evidence of overt heart failure.

Tenif must not be used in conjunction with other drugs with a cardio-depressant action eg verapamil, as conduction disturbances may ensue.

Precautions:
Cardiac: Particular care should be taken with patients with conduction defects or whose cardiac reserve is

poor. However, in patients already treated with a beta-adrenoceptor antagonist, and/or where signs of cardiac failure have been controlled, Tenif may be substituted with care if necessary.

Care should be taken in prescribing a beta-adrenoceptor blocking drug with Class I antidysrhythmic agents such as disopyramide.

One of the pharmacological actions of beta-adrenoceptor blocking drugs is to reduce heart rate. In the rare instance when symptoms may be attributable to the slow heart rate at a dose of one capsule daily, the drug should be discontinued.

Cessation of therapy with a beta-adrenoceptor blocking drug in patients with ischaemic heart disease should be gradual.

Caution should be exercised when transferring patients from clonidine to beta-adrenoceptor blocking drugs. If beta-adrenoceptor blocking drugs are given concurrently, clonidine should not be discontinued until several days after withdrawal of the beta-adrenoceptor blocking drug.

Obstructive airways disease: Tenif contains the cardioselective beta-adrenoceptor blocking drug atenolol. Although cardioselective ($beta_1$) beta-blockers may have less effect on lung function than non-selective beta-blockers, as with all beta-blockers, these should be avoided in patients with reversible obstructive airways disease, unless there are compelling clinical reasons for their use. Where such reasons exist, Tenif may be used with caution. Occasionally, some increase in airways resistance may occur in asthmatic patients, however, and this may usually be reversed by commonly used dosage of bronchodilators such as salbutamol or isoprenaline.

Renal impairment: In patients with marked renal impairment (ie creatinine clearance below 15 ml/min/1.73 m^2, serum creatinine greater than 600 mcmol/litre) the use of the combination is considered inappropriate.

Hepatic impairment: Care should be taken in patients with marked hepatic impairment. Although no dosage adjustment is suggested from the systemic availability of the monocomponents in patients with cirrhosis, hypertensive patients with clinically significant liver disease have not been studied.

Anaesthesia: It is not advisable to withdraw beta-adrenoceptor blocking drugs prior to surgery in the majority of patients. However, care should be taken when using anaesthetic agents such as ether, cyclopropane and trichloroethylene. Vagal dominance, if it occurs, may be corrected with atropine (1–2 mg i.v.).

Diabetes: The use of nifedipine in diabetic patients may require adjustment of their control.

Tenif modifies the tachycardia of hypoglycaemia.

Interactions: The antihypertensive effect of nifedipine can be potentiated by simultaneous administration of cimetidine.

When used in combination with nifedipine serum quinidine levels may be suppressed regardless of dosage of quinidine.

Side-effects: Side-effects which have been reported during treatment with the combination include headache, flushing, fatigue, dizziness and oedema. Side effects of nifedipine such as flushing and headache may occur at the beginning of the treatment. They are however, mostly slight and diminish with continuous use. Rare cases of hypersensitivity type jaundice have been reported with nifedipine. There are reports of gingival hyperplasia with nifedipine which may regress on withdrawal of therapy.

There have been reports of skin rashes and/or dry eyes associated with the use of beta-adrenoceptor blocking drugs. The reported incidence is small. Discontinuance of the drug should be considered if any such reaction is not otherwise explicable.

Overdosage: Excessive bradycardia can be countered with atropine 1–2 mg intravenously. If necessary, this may be followed by a bolus dose of glucagon 10 mg intravenously. If required, this may be repeated or followed by an intravenous infusion of glucagon 1–10 mg/hour depending on response. If no response to glucagon occurs or if glucagon is unavailable, a beta-adrenoceptor stimulant such as prenalterol 5 mg intravenously, followed if necessary by an intravenous infusion of 5 mg/hour or dobutamine 2.5 to 10 microgram/kg/minute by intravenous infusion may be given.

There is a possibility of hypotension occurring following the use of beta-adrenoceptor agonists but this will be reduced by the more selective agents, prenalterol and dobutamine. In severe cases, cardiac pacing with appropriate cardiorespiratory support may be necessary.

Intravenous calcium gluconate combined with metaraminol may be beneficial for hypotension induced by nifedipine.

Pharmaceutical precautions Tenif capsules should be stored at room temperature, protected from light and moisture.

Legal category POM.

Package quantities Calendar packs of 28 capsules (OP).

Further information When the combined antihypertensive effect or antianginal effect of a beta-adrenoceptor antagonist and calcium antagonist is required, Tenif is a convenient and acceptable therapy. The combination of atenolol and the slow release formulation of nifedipine, given once daily, provides control of raised blood pressure over a 24 hour period and may be expected to improve patient compliance. Given twice daily the combination provides control of angina.

The use of Tenif is unlikely to result in any impairment of the ability of patients to drive or operate machinery.

Product licence number 0029/0202.

TENORETIC*

Presentation Tenoretic tablets are round, bi-convex, brown, film-coated tablets impressed TENORETIC on one face and with the Stuart logo on the reverse. The impressions are highlighted in white. Each tablet contains 100 mg Atenolol BP and 25 mg Chlorthalidone PhEur. The inactive ingredients are gelatin, iron oxide, macrogol, magnesium carbonate, magnesium stearate, methyl hydroxypropyl cellulose, sodium lauryl sulphate and starch.

Uses Management of hypertension.

Mode of action: Tenoretic combines the antihypertensive activity of two agents, a beta-adrenergic receptor blocking agent (atenolol) and a diuretic (chlorthalidone). Atenolol predominantly blocks $beta_1$ receptors and does not possess membrane stabilising or intrinsic sympathomimetic (partial agonist) activities. The mechanism of the antihypertensive effect of atenolol has not been established.

Chlorthalidone, a monosulfonamyl diuretic, increases excretion of sodium and chloride. Natriuresis is accompanied by some loss of potassium. The mechanism by which chlorthalidone reduces blood pressure is not fully known but may be related to the excretion and redistribution of body sodium. Chlorthalidone usually does not decrease normal blood pressure.

The combination of atenolol with thiazide-like diuretics has been shown to be compatible and generally more effective than either drug used alone as an antihypertensive agent.

Co-administration of chlorthalidone and atenolol has little effect on the pharmacokinetics of either. Approximately 50% of an oral dose of atenolol and 60% of an oral dose of chlorthalidone is absorbed from the gastro-intestinal tract. Atenolol is only poorly bound to plasma proteins. Chlorthalidone is 75% plasma protein bound. The t_{max} for atenolol is 3 hours and the t_{max} for chlorthalidone is 12 hours. Metabolism of atenolol occurs to only a very minor extent and both atenolol and chlorthalidone are excreted predominantly via the kidney. A pharmacologically active metabolite of atenolol is present in urine of man but represents only 2% of the dose. This metabolite is not detected in plasma. Information is not available on chlorthalidone. The elimination half-life of atenolol is 6–9 hours and that for chlorthalidone is approximately 50 hours.

Dosage and administration *Adults:* One tablet daily. Most patients with hypertension will give a satisfactory response to a single tablet daily of Tenoretic. There is little or no further fall in blood pressure with increased dosage, and where necessary another antihypertensive drug, such as a vasodilator, can be added.

Elderly patients: Dosage requirements are often lower in this age group (see data sheet for Tenoret 50).

Children: There is no paediatric experience with Tenoretic, therefore this preparation is not recommended for children.

Renal failure: In patients with severe renal impairment a reduction in daily dose or in frequency of administration may be necessary.

Contra-indications, warnings, etc
Tenoretic should not be given to patients with second or third degree heart block. Tenoretic should not be used in patients with cardiogenic shock.

Special care should be taken with patients whose cardiac reserve is poor. Beta-adrenoceptor blockers should be avoided in overt heart failure. However, they may be used in patients whose signs of failure have been controlled.

One of the pharmacological actions of beta-adrenoceptor blocking drugs is to reduce heart rate. In the rare instance when symptoms may be attributable to the slow heart rate the dose may be reduced.

Tenoretic modifies the tachycardia of hypoglycaemia.

Tenoretic contains the cardioselective beta-adrenoceptor blocking drug atenolol. Although cardioselective ($beta_1$) beta-blockers may have less effect on lung function than non-selective beta-blockers, as with all beta-blockers, these should be avoided in patients with reversible obstructive airways disease, unless there are compelling clinical reasons for their use. Where such reasons exist, Tenoretic may be used with caution. Occasionally, some increase in airways resistance may occur in asthmatic patients, however, and this may usually be reversed by commonly used dosage of bronchodilators such as salbutamol or isoprenaline.

In patients suffering from ischaemic heart disease, as with other beta-blocking agents, treatment should not be discontinued abruptly.

Caution should be exercised when transferring patients from clonidine to beta-adrenoceptor blocking drugs. If beta-adrenoceptor blocking drugs and clonidine are given concurrently, clonidine should not be discontinued until several days after withdrawal of the beta-adrenoceptor blocking drug. (See also prescribing information on clonidine.)

Care should be taken in prescribing a beta-adrenoceptor blocking drug with Class I antidysrhythmic agents such as disopyramide.

Beta-adrenoceptor blocking drugs should be used with caution in combination with verapamil in patients with impaired ventricular function. The combination should not be given to patients with conduction abnormalities. Neither drug should be administered intravenously within 48 hours of discontinuing the other.

Preparations containing lithium generally should not be given with diuretics because they may reduce its renal clearance.

The metabolic effects of chlorthalidone are dose-related and, at the low dose contained in the Tenoretic tablet, are unlikely to be troublesome.

As with other combinations of beta-adrenoceptor blocking drugs and diuretics, hypokalaemia may occur with Tenoretic. In most patients this appears to be of little clinical significance. Measurement of potassium levels is appropriate, especially in the older patient, those receiving digitalis preparations for cardiac failure, taking abnormal (low in potassium) diets, or suffering from gastro-intestinal complaints.

Tenoretic is generally associated with only a minor increase in serum uric acid. In cases of prolonged elevation the concurrent use of a uricosuric agent will reverse the hyperuricaemia.

Tenoretic contains chlorthalidone which may decrease glucose tolerance. During prolonged therapy regular tests for glycosuria should be carried out.

Because Tenoretic contains chlorthalidone, care should be taken in patients with severe renal failure or with a history of sensitivity to chlorthalidone.

Pregnancy: Like other drugs Tenoretic should not be given during pregnancy unless its use is essential.

Lactation: Tenoretic should not be given during lactation unless its use is essential.

Anaesthesia: Care should be taken when using anaesthetic agents with Tenoretic. The anaesthetist should be informed and the choice of anaesthetic should be the agent with as little negative inotropic activity as possible.

Side-effects: Tenoretic is well tolerated. Side effects associated with it are infrequent and generally mild.

Minor side effects include cold extremities, muscular fatigue and, in isolated cases, bradycardia. Sleep disturbances of the type noted with other beta-adrenoceptor blocking drugs have rarely been reported.

There have been reports of skin rashes and/or dry eyes associated with the use of beta-adrenergic blocking drugs. The reported incidence is small and in most cases the symptoms have cleared when treatment was withdrawn. Discontinuance of the drug should be considered if any such reaction is not otherwise explicable. Cessation of therapy with a beta-blocker should be gradual.

Nausea and dizziness have been reported occasionally with chlorthalidone and idiosyncratic drug reactions such as thrombocytopenia and leucopenia have occurred rarely.

Overdosage: Excessive bradycardia may be countered with atropine 1–2 mg intravenously, followed, if necessary, by a bolus dose of glucagon 10 mg intravenously. If required, this may be repeated or followed by an intravenous infusion of glucagon 1–10 mg/hour depending on response. If no response to glucagon occurs or if glucagon is unavailable, a beta-adrenoceptor stimulant such as prenalterol 5 mg intravenously, followed if necessary by an intravenous infusion of 5 mg/hour or dobutamine 2.5 to 10 microgram/kg/minute by intravenous infusion may be given.

Any risk of hypotension occurring following the use of beta-adrenoceptor agonists will be reduced by the use of the more selective agents, e.g. prenalterol and dobutamine.

Excessive diuresis should be countered by maintaining normal fluid and electrolyte balance.

Pharmaceutical precautions Tenoretic should be stored at room temperature, protected from light and moisture.

Legal category POM.

Package quantities Calendar packs of 28 tablets (OP) and blister packs of 30 tablets.

Further information *Effect on ability to drive or operate machinery:* Since there are only rare reports of beta-blockers causing symptomatic hypotension and bradycardia, the use of Tenoretic is unlikely to result in any impairment of the ability of patients to drive or operate machinery.

When the combined antihypertensive effect of a beta-blocker and a diuretic is required, Tenoretic is a simple, convenient and acceptable therapy which may be expected to improve patient compliance. The effect of Tenoretic following a single oral dose is sustained for at least twenty-four hours.

Product licence number 0029/0139.

TENORET* 50

Presentation Tenoret 50 tablets are round, bi-convex, brown, film-coated tablets impressed TENORET 50 on one face and with the Stuart logo on the reverse. The impressions are highlighted in white. Each tablet contains

50 mg Atenolol BP and 12.5 mg Chlorthalidone PhEur. The inactive ingredients are gelatin, iron oxide, macrogol, magnesium carbonate, magnesium stearate, methyl hydroxypropyl cellulose, sodium lauryl sulphate and starch.

Uses *Hypertension:* Particularly suited to the older patient. The combination of low effective doses of a beta-blocking drug and diuretic may be suited to older patients where full doses of both may be considered inappropriate.

Mode of action: Tenoret 50 combines the antihypertensive activity of two agents, a beta-adrenergic receptor blocking agent (atenolol) and a diuretic (chlorthalidone). Atenolol predominantly blocks $beta_1$ receptors and does not possess membrane stabilising or intrinsic sympathomimetic (partial agonist) activities. The mechanism of the antihypertensive effect of atenolol has not been established.

Chlorthalidone, a monosulfonamyl diuretic, increases excretion of sodium and chloride. Natriuresis is accompanied by some loss of potassium. The mechanism by which chlorthalidone reduces blood pressure is not fully known but may be related to the excretion and redistribution of body sodium. Chlorthalidone usually does not decrease normal blood pressure.

The combination of atenolol with thiazide-like diuretics has been shown to be compatible and generally more effective than either drug used alone as an antihypertensive agent.

Co-administration of chlorthalidone and atenolol has little effect on the pharmacokinetics of either. Approximately 50% of an oral dose of atenolol and 60% of an oral dose of chlorthalidone is absorbed from the gastro-intestinal tract. Atenolol is only poorly bound to plasma proteins. Chlorthalidone is 75% plasma protein bound. The t_{max} for atenolol is 3 hours and the t_{max} for chlorthalidone is 12 hours. Metabolism of atenolol occurs to only a very minor extent and both atenolol and chlorthalidone are excreted predominantly via the kidney. A pharmacologically active metabolite of atenolol is present in urine of man but represents only 2% of the dose. This metabolite is not detected in plasma. Information is not available on chlorthalidone. The elimination half-life of atenolol is 6–9 hours and that for chlorthalidone is approximately 50 hours.

Dosage and administration *Adults including the elderly:* One tablet daily. Older patients with hypertension who do not respond to low dose therapy with a single agent should have a satisfactory response to a single tablet daily of Tenoret 50. Where hypertensive control is not achieved addition of a small dose of a third agent, e.g. a vasodilator, may be appropriate.

Children: There is no paediatric experience with Tenoret 50, therefore this preparation is not recommended for children.

Renal failure: In patients with severe renal impairment a reduction in daily dose or in frequency of administration may be necessary.

Contra-indications, warnings, etc Tenoret 50 should not be given to patients with second or third degree heart block.

Tenoret 50 should not be used in patients with cardiogenic shock.

Special care should be taken with patients whose cardiac reserve is poor. Beta-adrenoceptor blockers should be avoided in overt heart failure. However, they may be used in patients whose signs of failure have been controlled.

One of the pharmacological actions of beta-adrenoceptor blocking drugs is to reduce heart rate. In the rare instance when symptoms may be attributable to the slow heart rate the dose may be reduced.

Tenoret 50 modifies the tachycardia of hypoglycaemia.

Tenoret 50 contains the cardioselective beta-adrenoceptor blocking drug atenolol. Although cardioselective ($beta_1$) beta-blockers may have less effect on lung function than non-selective beta-blockers, as with all beta-blockers, these should be avoided in patients with reversible obstructive airways disease, unless there are compelling clinical reasons for their use. Where such reasons exist, 'Tenoret' 50 may be used with caution. Occasionally, some increase in airways resistance may occur in asthmatic patients, however, and this may usually be reversed by commonly used dosage of bronchodilators such as salbutamol or isoprenaline.

In patients suffering from ischaemic heart disease, as with other beta-blocking agents, treatment should not be discontinued abruptly.

Caution should be exercised when transferring patients from clonidine to beta-adrenoceptor blocking drugs. If beta-adrenoceptor blocking drugs and clonidine are given concurrently, clonidine should not be discontinued until several days after withdrawal of the beta-adrenoceptor blocking drug (see also prescribing information on clonidine).

Care should be taken in prescribing a beta-adrenoceptor blocking drug with Class I antidysrhythmic agents such as disopyramide.

Beta-adrenoceptor blocking drugs should be used with caution in combination with verapamil in patients with impaired ventricular function. The combination should not be given to patients with conduction abnormalities. Neither drug should be administered intravenously within 48 hours of discontinuing the other.

Preparations containing lithium generally should not be given with diuretics because they may reduce its renal clearance.

The metabolic effects of chlorthalidone are dose-related and, at the low dose contained in a Tenoret 50 tablet, are most unlikely to be troublesome.

As with other combinations of beta-adrenoceptor blocking drugs and diuretics hypokalaemia may occur with Tenoret 50. In most patients this appears to be of little clinical significance. Measurement of potassium levels is appropriate, especially in the older patient, those receiving digitalis preparations for cardiac failure, taking abnormal (low in potassium) diets, or suffering from gastro-intestinal complaints.

Experience with Tenoretic has generally been associated with only a minor increase in serum uric acid. In cases of prolonged elevation the concurrent use of a uricosuric agent will reverse the hyperuricaemia.

Tenoret 50 contains chlorthalidone which may decrease glucose tolerance. During prolonged therapy regular tests for glycosuria should be carried out.

Because Tenoret 50 contains chlorthalidone, care should be taken in patients with severe renal failure or with a history of sensitivity to chlorthalidone.

Pregnancy: Like other drugs Tenoret 50 should not be given during pregnancy unless its use is essential.

Lactation: Tenoret 50 should not be given during lactation unless its use is essential.

Anaesthesia: Care should be taken when using anaesthetic agents with Tenoret 50. The anaesthetist should be informed and the choice of anaesthetic should be the agent with as little negative inotropic activity as possible.

Side-effects: Tenoret 50 is well tolerated. Side effects associated with it are infrequent and generally mild.

Minor side effects include cold extremities, muscular fatigue and, in isolated cases, bradycardia. Sleep disturbances of the type noted with other beta-adrenoceptor blocking drugs have rarely been reported.

There have been reports of skin rashes and/or dry eyes associated with the use of beta-adrenergic blocking drugs. The reported incidence is small and in most cases the symptoms have cleared when treatment was withdrawn. Discontinuance of the drug should be considered if any such reaction is not otherwise explicable. Cessation of therapy with beta-adrenoceptor blocking drugs should be gradual.

Nausea and dizziness have been reported occasionally with chlorthalidone and idiosyncratic drug reactions such as thrombocytopenia and leucopenia have occurred rarely.

Overdosage: Excessive bradycardia can be countered with atropine 1–2 mg intravenously, followed, if necessary, by a bolus dose of glucagon 10 mg intravenously. If required, this may be repeated or followed by an intravenous infusion of glucagon 1–10 mg/hour depending on response. If no response to glucagon occurs or if glucagon is unavailable, a beta-adrenoceptor stimulant such as prenalterol 5 mg intravenously, followed if necessary by an intravenous infusion of 5 mg/hour or dobutamine 2.5 to 10 microgram/kg/minute by intravenous infusion may be given.

Any risk of hypotension occurring following the use of beta-adrenoceptor agonists will be reduced by the use of the more selective agents, e.g. prenalterol and dobutamine.

Excessive diuresis should be countered by maintaining normal fluid and electrolyte balance.

Pharmaceutical precautions Tenoret 50 should be stored at room temperature, protected from light and moisture.

Legal category POM.

Package quantities Calendar packs of 28 tablets (OP) and blister packs of 30 tablets.

Further information *Effect on ability to drive or operate machinery:* Since there are only rare reports of beta-blockers causing symptomatic hypotension and bradycardia, the use of Tenoret 50 is unlikely to result in any impairment of the ability of patients to drive or operate machinery.

When the combined antihypertensive effect of a beta-blocker and a diuretic is required, Tenoret 50 one tablet daily is a simple, convenient and acceptable therapy which may be expected to improve patient compliance.

Product licence number 0029/0156.

TENORMIN* TABLETS
TENORMIN* LS TABLETS
TENORMIN* 25 TABLETS

Presentation Tenormin tablets, containing Atenolol BP 100 mg are round, bi-convex, orange, film-coated tablets impressed with TENORMIN on one face and the Stuart logo on the reverse. The impressions are highlighted in white.

Tenormin LS tablets, containing Atenolol BP 50 mg are round, bi-convex, orange, film-coated tablets impressed with TENORMIN LS on one face and bisected on the reverse. The impressions are highlighted in white.

Tenormin 25 tablets, containing Atenolol BP 25 mg, are round, biconvex, white, film-coated tablets impressed with TENORMIN 25 on one face and the Stuart logo on the reverse.

The inactive ingredients are gelatin, glycerol, magnesium carbonate, magnesium stearate, methylhydroxypropylcellulose, sodium lauryl sulphate, starch and titanium dioxide. In addition, Tenormin and Tenormin LS tablets also contain ethylcellulose, macrogol, stearic acid, sunset yellow lake and talc.

Uses

i) Management of hypertension
ii) Management of angina pectoris
iii) Management of cardiac dysrhythmias
iv) Myocardial infarction: early intervention in the acute phase.

Mode of action: Tenormin (atenolol) is a beta-adrenoceptor blocking drug which is $beta_1$ selective (i.e. acts preferentially on $beta_1$-adrenergic receptors in the heart). It is without intrinsic sympathomimetic and membrane stabilising activities. Human studies indicate that it crosses the blood brain barrier only to a negligible extent.

As with other beta-adrenoceptor blocking drugs, its mode of action in the treatment of hypertension is unclear. It is probably the action of Tenormin in reducing cardiac rate and contractility which makes it effective in eliminating or reducing the symptoms of patients with angina.

Early intervention with Tenormin in acute myocardial infarction reduces infarct size and decreases morbidity and mortality. Fewer patients with a threatened infarction progress to frank infarction; the incidence of ventricular arrhythmias is decreased and marked pain relief may result in reduced need of opiate analgesics. Early mortality is decreased. Tenormin is an additional treatment to standard coronary care.

Absorption of atenolol following oral dosing is consistent but incomplete (approximately 40–50%) with peak plasma concentrations occurring 2–4 hours after dosing. There is no significant hepatic metabolism of atenolol and more than 90% of that absorbed reaches the systemic circulation unaltered. The plasma half-life is about 6 hours but this may rise in severe renal impairment since the kidney is the major route of elimination. Atenolol penetrates tissues poorly due to its low lipid solubility and its concentration in brain tissue is low. Plasma protein binding is low (approximately 3%).

Dosage and administration *Adults: Hypertension:* One tablet daily. Most patients respond to 100 mg daily given orally as a single dose. Some patients, however, will respond to 50 mg given as a single daily dose. The effect will be fully established after one to two weeks. A further reduction in blood pressure may be achieved by combining Tenormin with other antihypertensive agents. For example, co-administration of Tenormin with a diuretic, as in Tenoretic, provides a highly effective and convenient antihypertensive therapy.

Angina: Most patients with angina pectoris will respond to 100 mg given orally once daily or 50 mg given twice daily. It is unlikely that additional benefit will be gained by increasing the dose.

Dysrhythmias: A suitable initial dose of Tenormin is 2.5 mg (5 ml) injected intravenously over a 2.5 minute period (i.e. 1 mg/minute). (See also prescribing information for Tenormin Injection.) This may be repeated at 5 minute intervals until a response is observed up to a maximum dosage of 10 mg. If Tenormin is given by infusion, 0.15 mg/kg bodyweight may be administered over a 20 minute period. If required, the injection or infusion may be repeated every 12 hours. Having controlled the dysrhythmias with intravenous 'Tenormin', a suitable oral maintenance dosage is 50–100 mg daily, given as a single dose.

Myocardial infarction: For patients suitable for treatment with intravenous beta-blockade and presenting within 12 hours of the onset of the chest pain, Tenormin 5–10 mg should be given by slow intravenous injection (1 mg/minute) followed by Tenormin 50 mg orally about 15 minutes later provided no untoward effects occur from the intravenous dose. This should be followed by a further 50 mg orally 12 hours after the intravenous dose and then 12 hours later by 100 mg orally to be given once daily. If bradycardia and/or hypotension requiring treatment, or any other untoward effects occur, Tenormin should be discontinued.

Elderly patients: Dosage requirements may be reduced, especially in patients with impaired renal function.

Children: There is no paediatric experience with Tenormin and for this reason it is not recommended for use in children.

Renal failure: Since Tenormin is excreted via the kidneys dosage should be adjusted in cases of severe impairment of renal function. No significant accumulation of Tenormin occurs in patients who have a creatinine clearance greater than 35 ml/min/1.73 m^2 (normal range is 100–150 ml/min/1.73 m^2). For patients with a creatinine clearance of 15–35 ml/min/1.73 m^2 (equivalent to serum creatinine of 300–600 mcmol/litre) the oral dose should be 50 mg daily and the intravenous dose should be 10 mg once every two days. For patients with a creatinine clearance of <15 ml/min/1.73 m^2 (equivalent to serum creatinine of >600 mcmol/litre) the oral dose should be 25 mg daily or 50 mg on alternate days and the intravenous dose should be 10 mg once every four days. Patients on haemodialysis should be given 50 mg orally after each dialysis; this should be done under hospital supervision as marked falls in blood pressure can occur.

Contra-indications, warnings, etc
Tenormin is contra-indicated in patients with second

degree or third-degree heart block. Tenormin should not be used in patients with cardiogenic shock.

Special care should be taken with patients whose cardiac reserve is poor. Beta-adrenoceptor blockers should be avoided in overt heart failure. However, they may be used in patients whose signs of failure have been controlled.

One of the pharmacological actions of Tenormin is to reduce heart rate. In the rare instance when symptoms may be attributable to the slow heart rate, the dose may be reduced.

Tenormin modifies the tachycardia of hypoglycaemia.

Although cardioselective ($beta_1$) beta-blockers may have less effect on lung function than non-selective beta-blockers, as with all beta-blockers, these should be avoided in patients with reversible obstructive airways disease, unless there are compelling clinical reasons for their use. Where such reasons exist, 'Tenormin' may be used with caution. Occasionally, some increase in airways resistance may occur in asthmatic patients, however, and this may usually be reversed by commonly used dosage of bronchodilators such as salbutamol or isoprenaline.

In patients suffering from ischaemic heart disease, as with other beta-blocking agents, treatment should not be discontinued abruptly.

Caution should be exercised when transferring patients from clonidine to beta-adrenoceptor blocking drugs. If beta-adrenoceptor blocking drugs and clonidine are given concurrently, clonidine should not be discontinued until several days after the withdrawal of the beta-adrenoceptor blocking drug (see also prescribing information on clonidine).

Care should be taken in prescribing a beta-adrenoceptor blocking drug with Class I antidysrhythmic agents such as disopyramide.

Beta-adrenoceptor blocking drugs should be used with caution in combination with verapamil in patients with impaired ventricular function. The combination should not be given to patients with conduction abnormalities. Neither drug should be administered intravenously within 48 hours of discontinuing the other.

Anaesthesia: Care should be taken when using anaesthetic agents with Tenormin. The anaesthetist should be informed and the choice of anaesthetic should be the agent with as little negative inotropic activity as possible.

Pregnancy and lactation: Tenormin has been used effectively under close supervision for the treatment of pregnancy-associated hypertension. There was no evidence of any foetal abnormalities although Tenormin was generally given after 20 weeks gestation.

Tenormin crosses the placental barrier and appears in cord blood. There is an approximate three-fold accumulation of Tenormin in the breast milk. However, there were no apparent detrimental effects in the baby at birth or during breast feeding.

The possibility of foetal injury cannot be excluded and the use of the drug in women who are, or may become pregnant or who are nursing the newborn infant, requires that anticipated benefits be weighed against possible risks.

Side-effects: In clinical studies, the side effects reported are usually attributable to its pharmacological actions and include coldness of the extremities, muscular fatigue and, in isolated cases, bradycardia. Sleep disturbances of the type noted with other beta-blockers have rarely been reported.

There have been reports of skin rashes and/or dry eyes associated with the use of beta-adrenergic blocking drugs. The reported incidence is small and in most cases the symptoms have cleared when treatment was withdrawn. Discontinuance of the drug should be considered if any such reaction is not otherwise explicable. Cessation of therapy with a beta-blocker should be gradual.

Overdosage: From first principles, excessive bradycardia may be countered by atropine 1–2 mg intravenously, followed, if necessary, by a bolus dose of glucagon 10 mg intravenously. If required, this may be repeated or followed by an intravenous infusion of glucagon 1–10 mg/hour depending on response. If no response to glucagon occurs or if glucagon is unavailable, a beta-adrenoceptor stimulant such as prenalterol 5 mg intravenously, followed if necessary by an intravenous infusion of 5 mg/hour or dobutamine 2.5 to 10 microgram/kg/minute by intravenous infusion may be given.

Any risk of hypotension occurring following the use of beta-adrenoceptor agonists will be reduced by the use of the more selective agents, e.g. prenalterol and dobutamine.

Pharmaceutical precautions Tenormin, Tenormin LS and Tenormin 25 Tablets should be stored at room temperature, protected from light and moisture.

Legal category POM.

Package quantities Tenormin Tablets: 100 mg in Calendar packs of 28 (OP) and blister packs of 30. Tenormin LS Tablets: 50 mg in Calendar packs of 28 (OP) and blister packs of 30. Tenormin 25 Tablets: 25 mg in calendar packs of 28 (OP).

Further information *Effect on ability to drive or operate machinery:* Since there are only rare reports of beta-blockers causing symptomatic hypotension and bradycardia, the use of Tenormin is unlikely to result in any impairment of the ability of patients to drive or operate machinery.

Tenormin is effective for at least 24 hours after a single oral dose. The drug facilitates compliance by its acceptability to patients and simplicity of dosing. The narrow dose range and early patient response ensure that the effect of the drug in individual patients is quickly demonstrated. Tenormin is compatible with diuretics, other hypotensive agents and antianginals (but see Warnings). Since it acts preferentially on beta-receptors in the heart, Tenormin may, with care, be used successfully in the treatment of patients with respiratory disease who cannot tolerate non-selective beta-blockers.

Product licence numbers

Tenormin Tablets	0029/0122
Tenormin LS Tablets	0029/0086
Tenormin 25 Tablets	0029/0218

TENORMIN* INJECTION

Presentation Tenormin Injection contains 5 mg Atenolol BP in 10 ml isotonic, citrate buffered aqueous solution. The inactive ingredients are citric acid/sodium citrate, sodium chloride and water.

Uses Management of dysrhythmias and for the early intervention treatment of acute myocardial infarction.

Tenormin (atenolol) is a beta-adrenoceptor blocking drug which is $beta_1$ selective (i.e. acts preferentially on $beta_1$-adrenergic receptors in the heart). It is without intrinsic sympathomimetic and membrane stabilising activities. Human studies indicate that it crosses the blood-brain barrier only to a negligible extent.

Early intervention with Tenormin in acute myocardial infarction reduces infarct size and decreases morbidity and mortality. Fewer patients with a threatened infarction progress to frank infarction; the incidence of ventricular arrhythmias is decreased and marked pain relief may result in reduced need for opiate analgesics. Early mortality is decreased. Tenormin is an additional treatment in standard coronary care.

Absorption of atenolol following oral dosing is consistent but incomplete (approximately 40–50%) with peak plasma concentrations occurring 2–4 hours after dosing. There is no significant hepatic metabolism of atenolol and more than 90% of that absorbed reaches the systemic circulation unaltered. The plasma half-life is about 6 hours but this may rise in severe renal impairment since the kidney is the major route of elimination. Atenolol penetrates tissues poorly due to its low lipid solubility and its concentration in brain tissue is low. Plasma protein binding is low (approximately 3%).

Dosage and administration *Adults: Dysrhythmias:* A suitable initial dose of Tenormin is 2.5 mg (5 ml) injected intravenously over a 2.5 minute period (i.e. 1 mg/minute). This may be repeated at 5 minute intervals until a response is observed up to a maximum dosage of 10 mg. If Tenormin is given by infusion, 0.15 mg/kg body weight may be administered over a 20 minute period. If required, the injection or infusion may be repeated every 12 hours. Having controlled the dysrhythmias with intravenous Tenormin a suitable oral maintenance dosage is 50–100 mg daily (see prescribing information for Tenormin and Tenormin LS Tablets).

Myocardial infarction: For patients suitable for treatment with intravenous beta-blockade and presenting within 12 hours of the onset of the chest pain, Tenormin 5–10 mg should be given by slow intravenous injection (1 mg per minute) followed by Tenormin 50 mg orally after about 15 minutes provided no untoward effects occur from the intravenous dose. This should be followed by a further 50 mg orally 12 hours after the intravenous Tenormin and then 12 hours later by 100 mg orally to be given once daily. If bradycardia and/or hypotension requiring treatment or any other untoward effects occur, Tenormin should be discontinued.

Elderly patients: Dosage requirements may be reduced, especially in patients with impaired renal function.

Children: There is no paediatric experience with Tenormin and for this reason it is not recommended for children.

Renal failure: Since Tenormin is excreted via the kidneys dosage should be adjusted in cases of severe impairment of renal function. No significant accumulation of Tenormin occurs in patients who have a creatinine clearance greater than 35 ml/min/1.73 m^2 (normal range is 100–150 ml/min/1.73 m^2). For patients with a creatinine clearance of 15–35 ml/min/1.73 m^2 (equivalent to serum creatinine of 300–600 mcmol/litre) the oral dose should be 50 mg daily and the intravenous dose should be 10 mg once every two days. For patients with a creatinine clearance of <15 ml/min/1.73 m^2 (equivalent to serum creatinine of >600 mcmol/litre) the oral dose should be 25 mg daily or 50 mg on alternate days; and the intravenous dose should be 10 mg once every four days.

Patients on haemodialysis should be given 50 mg orally after each dialysis; this should be done under hospital supervision as marked falls in blood pressure can occur.

Contra-indications, warnings, etc Tenormin is contra-indicated in patients with second-degree or third-degree heart block.

Tenormin Injection should not be used in patients with cardiogenic shock.

Special care should be taken with patients whose cardiac reserve is poor. Beta-adrenoceptor blockers should be avoided in overt heart failure. However, they may be used in patients whose signs of failure have been controlled.

One of the pharmacological actions of Tenormin is to reduce heart rate. In the rare instances when symptoms may be attributable to the slow heart rate, the dose may be reduced.

Tenormin modifies the tachycardia of hypoglycaemia.

Although cardioselective (beta$_1$) beta-blockers may have less effect on lung function than non-selective beta-blockers, as with all beta-blockers, these should be avoided in patients with reversible obstructive airways disease, unless there are compelling clinical reasons for their use. Where such reasons exist, Tenormin may be used with caution. Occasionally, some increase in airways resistance may occur in asthmatic patients, however, and this may usually be reversed by commonly used dosage of bronchodilators such as salbutamol or isoprenaline.

In patients suffering from ischaemic heart disease, as with other beta-blocking agents, treatment should not be discontinued abruptly.

Caution should be exercised when transferring patients from clonidine to beta-adrenoceptor blocking drugs. If beta-adrenoceptor blocking drugs and clonidine are given concurrently, clonidine should not be discontinued until several days after the withdrawal of the beta-adrenoceptor blocking drug (see also prescribing information on clonidine).

Care should be taken in prescribing a beta-adrenoceptor blocking drug with Class I antidysrhythmic agents such as disopyramide.

Beta-adrenoceptor blocking drugs should be used with caution in combination with verapamil in patients with impaired ventricular function. The combination should not be given to patients with conduction abnormalities. Neither drug should be administered intravenously within 48 hours of discontinuing the other.

Anaesthesia: Care should be taken when using anaesthetic agents with Tenormin. The anaesthetist should be informed and the choice of anaesthetic should be the agent with as little negative inotropic activity as possible.

Pregnancy and lactation: Tenormin has been used effectively under close supervision for the treatment of pregnancy-associated hypertension. There was no evidence of any foetal abnormalities although Tenormin was generally given after 20 weeks gestation.

Tenormin crosses the placental barrier and appears in cord blood. There is an approximate three-fold accumulation of Tenormin in the breast milk. However, there were no apparent detrimental effects in the baby at birth or during breast feeding.

The possibility of foetal injury cannot be excluded and the use of the drug in women who are, or may become pregnant or who are nursing the newborn infant, requires that anticipated benefits be weighed against possible risks.

Side-effects: In clinical studies, the side effects reported are usually attributable to its pharmacological actions and include coldness of the extremities, muscular fatigue and, in isolated cases, bradycardia. Sleep disturbances of the type noted with other beta-blockers have rarely been reported.

There have been reports of skin rashes and/or dry eyes associated with the use of beta-adrenergic blocking drugs. The reported incidence is small and in most cases the symptoms have cleared when treatment was withdrawn. Discontinuance of the drug should be considered if any such reaction is not otherwise explicable. Cessation of therapy with a beta-blocker should be gradual.

Overdosage: From first principles, excessive bradycardia may be countered by atropine 1–2 mg intravenously, followed, if necessary, by a bolus dose of glucagon 10 mg intravenously. If required, this may be repeated or followed by an intravenous infusion of glucagon 1–10 mg/hour depending on response. If no response to glucagon occurs or if glucagon is unavailable, a beta-adrenoceptor stimulant such as prenalterol 5 mg intravenously, followed if necessary by an intravenous infusion of 5 mg/hour or dobutamine 2.5 to 10 microgram/kg/minute by intravenous infusion may be given.

Any risk of hypotension occurring following the use of beta-adrenoceptor agonists will be reduced by the use of the more selective agents, e.g. prenalterol and dobutamine.

Pharmaceutical precautions Tenormin Injection should be protected from light.

Dilutions of Tenormin Injection in Dextrose Injection BP, Sodium Chloride Injection BP, or Sodium Chloride and Dextrose Injection BP may be used.

Legal category POM.

Package quantities *Injection:* 10 ml ampoules in boxes of 10.

Further information *Effect on ability to drive or operate machinery:* Since there are only rare reports of beta-blockers causing symptomatic hypotension and bradycardia, the use of Tenormin is unlikely to result in any impairment of the ability of patients to drive or operate machinery.

The narrow dose range and early patient response to Tenormin ensure that the effect of the drug in individual patients is quickly demonstrated. Tenormin is fully compatible with diuretics, other hypotensive agents and antianginals (but see Warnings). Since it acts preferentially on beta-receptors in the heart, Tenormin may, with care, be used successfully in the treatment of patients with respiratory disease who cannot tolerate non selective beta blockers.

Product licence number 0029/0087.

TENORMIN* SYRUP

Presentation Tenormin Syrup is a clear, colourless, lemon and lime flavoured syrup containing 0.5% w/v Atenolol BP (equivalent to 25 mg/5 ml). The inactive ingredients are citric acid, flavour, methyl hydroxybenzoate, propyl hydroxybenzoate, saccharin sodium, sodium citrate, sorbitol and water.

Uses
(i) Management of hypertension.
(ii) Management of angina.
(iii) Management of cardiac dysrhythmias.
(iv) Myocardial infarction: early intervention in the acute phase.

Mode of action: Tenormin (atenolol) is a beta-adrenoceptor blocking drug which is $beta_1$ selective (i.e. acts preferentially on $beta_1$-adrenergic receptors in the heart). It is without intrinsic sympathomimetic and membrane stabilising activities. Human studies indicate that it crosses the blood brain barrier only to a negligible extent.

As with other beta-adrenoceptor blocking drugs, its mode of action in the treatment of hypertension is unclear. It is probably the action of Tenormin in reducing cardiac rate and contractility which makes it effective in eliminating or reducing the symptoms of patients with angina.

Early intervention with Tenormin in acute myocardial infarction reduces infarct size and decreases morbidity and mortality. Fewer patients with a threatened infarction progress to frank infarction; the incidence of ventricular arrhythmias is decreased and marked pain relief may result in reduced need of opiate analgesics. Early mortality is decreased. Tenormin is an additional treatment to standard coronary care.

Absorption of atenolol following oral dosing is consistent but incomplete (approximately 40–50%) with peak plasma concentrations occurring 2–4 hours after dosing. There is no significant hepatic metabolism of atenolol and more than 90% of that absorbed reached the systemic circulation unaltered. The plasma half-life is about 6 hours but this may rise in severe renal impairment since the kidney is the major route of elimination. Atenolol penetrates tissues poorly due to its low lipid solubility and its concentration in brain tissue is low. Plasma protein binding is low (approximately 3%).

Dosage and administration

Adults: Hypertension: Two or four 5 ml spoonfuls daily i.e. 50 mg or 100 mg in patients unable to take 50 mg or 100 mg tablets.

Most patients respond to 100 mg once daily. Some patients, however, will respond to 50 mg given as a single daily dose. The effect will be fully established after one to two weeks. A further reduction in blood pressure may be achieved by combining Tenormin with other antihypertensive agents.

Angina: Most patients with angina pectoris will respond to 100 mg (four 5 ml spoonfuls) given orally once a day or 50 mg (two 5 ml spoonfuls) given twice daily. It is unlikely that additional benefit will be gained by increasing the dose.

Dysrhythmias: A suitable initial dose of Tenormin is 2.5 mg (5 ml) injected intravenously over a 2.5 minute period (i.e. 1 mg/minute). (See also prescribing information for Tenormin Injection). This may be repeated at 5 minute intervals until a response is observed up to a maximum dosage of 10 mg. If Tenormin is given by infusion, 0.15 mg/kg bodyweight may be administered over a 20 minute period. If required, the injection or infusion may be repeated every 12 hours. Having controlled the dysrhythmias with intravenous Tenormin a suitable oral maintenance dosage is 50–100 mg (two to four 5 ml spoonfuls) daily given as a single dose.

Myocardial infarction: For patients suitable for treatment with intravenous beta-blockade and presenting within 12 hours of the onset of the chest pain, Tenormin 5–10 mg should be given by slow intravenous injection (1 mg/minute) followed by Tenormin 50 mg (two 5 ml spoonfuls) orally about 15 minutes later provided no untoward effects occur from the intravenous dose. This should be followed by a further 50 mg orally 12 hours after the intravenous dose and then 12 hours later by 100 mg (four 5 ml spoonfuls) orally to be given once daily. If bradycardia and/or hypotension requiring treatment, or any other untoward effects occur, Tenormin should be discontinued.

Elderly patients: Dosage requirements may be reduced, especially in patients with impaired renal function.

Children: There is no paediatric experience with Tenormin and for this reason it is not recommended for use in children.

Renal failure: Since Tenormin is excreted via the kidneys dosage should be adjusted in cases of severe impairment of renal function. No significant accumulation of Tenormin occurs in patients who have a creatinine clearance greater than 35 ml/min/1.73 m^2 (normal range is 100–150 ml/min/1.73 m^2). For patients with a creatinine clearance of 15–35 ml/min/1.73 m^2 (equivalent to serum creatinine of 300–600 mcmol/litre) the oral dose should be 50 mg daily and the intravenous dose should be 10 mg once every two days. For patients with a creatinine clearance of <15 ml/min/1.73 m^2 (equivalent to serum creatinine of >600 mcmol/litre) the oral dose should be 25 mg daily or 50 mg on alternate days and the intravenous dose should be 10 mg once every four days.

Patients on haemodialysis should be given 50 mg orally after each dialysis: this should be done under hospital supervision as marked falls in blood pressure can occur.

Contra-indications, warnings, etc Tenormin is contra-indicated in patients with second degree or third degree heart block. Tenormin should not be used in patients with cardiogenic shock.

Special care should be taken with patients whose cardiac reserve is poor. Beta-adrenoceptor blockers should be avoided in overt heart failure. However, they may be used in patients whose signs of failure have been controlled.

One of the pharmacological actions of Tenormin is to reduce heart rate. In the rare instances when symptoms may be attributable to the slow heart rate, the dose may be reduced.

Tenormin modifies the tachycardia of hypoglycaemia.

Although cardioselective ($beta_1$) beta-blockers may have less effect on lung function than non-selective beta-blockers, as with all beta-blockers, these should be avoided in patients with reversible obstructive airways disease, unless there are compelling clinical reasons for their use. Where such reasons exist, 'Tenormin' may be used with caution. Occasionally, some increase in airways resistance may occur in asthmatic patients, however, and this may usually be reversed by commonly used dosage of bronchodilators such as salbutamol or isoprenaline.

In patients suffering from ischaemic heart disease, as with other beta-blocking agents, treatment should not be discontinued abruptly.

Caution should be exercised when transferring patients from clonidine to beta-adrenoceptor blocking drugs. If beta-adrenoceptor blocking drugs and clonidine are given concurrently, clonidine should not be discontinued until several days after the withdrawal of the beta-adrenoceptor blocking drug (see also prescribing information on clonidine).

Care should be taken in prescribing a beta-adrenoceptor blocking drug with Class 1 antidysrhythmic agents such as disopyramide.

Beta-adrenoceptor blocking drugs should be used with caution in combination with verapamil in patients with impaired ventricular function. The combination should not be given to patients with conduction abnormalities. Neither drug should be administered intravenously within 48 hours of discontinuing the other.

Anaesthesia: Care should be taken when using anaesthetic agents with Tenormin. The anaesthetist should be informed and the choice of anaesthetic should be the agent with as little negative inotropic activity as possible.

Pregnancy and lactation: Tenormin has been used effectively under close supervision for the treatment of pregnancy-associated hypertension. There was no evidence of any foetal abnormalities although Tenormin was generally given after 20 weeks gestation.

Tenormin crosses the placental barrier and appears in cord blood. There is an approximate three-fold accumulation of Tenormin in the breast milk. However, there were no apparent detrimental effects upon the baby at birth or during breast feeding.

The possibility of foetal injury cannot be excluded and the use of the drug in women who are, or may become pregnant or who are nursing the newborn infant, requires that anticipated benefits be weighed against possible risks.

Side-effects: In clinical studies, the side effects reported are usually attributable to its pharmacological actions and include coldness of the extremities, muscular fatigue and, in isolated cases, bradycardia. Sleep disturbances of the type noted with other beta-blockers have rarely been reported.

There have been reports of skin rashes and/or dry eyes associated with the use of beta-adrenergic blocking drugs. The reported incidence is small and in most cases the symptoms have cleared when treatment was withdrawn. Discontinuance of the drug should be considered if any such reaction is not otherwise explicable. Cessation of therapy with a beta-blocker should be gradual.

Overdosage: From first principles, excessive bradycardia may be countered by atropine 1–2 mg intravenously, followed, if necessary, by a bolus dose of glucagon 10 mg intravenously. If required, this may be repeated or followed by an intravenous infusion of glucagon 1–10 mg/hour depending on response. If no response to glucagon occurs or if glucagon is unavailable, a beta-adrenoceptor stimulant such as prenalterol 5 mg intravenously, followed if necessary by an intravenous infusion of 5 mg/hour or dobutamine 2.5 to 10 microgram/kg/minute by intravenous infusion may be given.

Any risk of hypotension occurring following the use of beta-adrenoceptor agonists will be reduced by the use of the more selective agents, e.g. prenalterol and dobutamine.

Pharmaceutical precautions Tenormin Syrup should be stored at room temperature, protected from light.

Legal category POM.

Package quantities 300 ml bottle (OP).

Further information *Effect on ability to drive or operate machinery:* Since there are only rare reports of beta-blockers causing symptomatic hypotension and bradycardia, the use of Tenormin is unlikely to result in any impairment of the ability of patients to drive or operate machinery.

Tenormin Syrup is intended for patients unable to swallow Tenormin tablets. Tenormin is effective for at least 24 hours after once daily dosing with 10 ml or 20 ml Tenormin Syrup. Tenormin Syrup facilitates compliance by its acceptability to patients and the once-daily dosing regimen. The narrow dose range and early patient response ensure that the effect of the drug in individual patients is quickly demonstrated. Tenormin is compatible with diuretics, other hypotensive agents and antianginals (but see Warnings). Since it acts preferentially on beta-receptors in the heart, Tenormin may, with care, be used successfully in the treatment of patients with respiratory disease who cannot tolerate non-selective beta-blockers.

Product licence number 0029/0195.

**Trade Mark*

Syntex Pharmaceuticals Limited
St Ives Road
Maidenhead
Berkshire SL6 1RD

SYNTEX

ANAPOLON* 50

Presentation Each Anapolon 50 Tablet contains Oxymetholone BP 50 mg. The white tablets are scored and stamped with '50' and a breakline on one side and SYNTEX on the other.

Uses Anapolon 50 is recommended for the treatment of aplastic and refractory anaemias (including acquired, idiopathic and congenital aplasias).

Anapolon 50 should not replace other supportive measures such as transfusion, correction of iron, folic acid, vitamin B12 or pyridoxine deficiency, antibacterial therapy and the appropriate use of corticosteroids.

Oxymetholone has a potent haemopoietic activity. Oxymetholone stimulates the production of erythropoietin, which in turn acts on the primitive stem cells increasing the rate of differentiation into red cell precursors. It has also been demonstrated that oxymetholone increases the mitotic rate of the stem cells, stimulating the extension of healthy tissue into hypoplastic areas of the bone marrow. Oxymetholone has a beneficial effect on haemoglobin synthesis as shown by an increased plasma iron clearance.

Dosage and administration The recommended dosage when treating aplasias is from 2 mg to 5 mg per kg body weight daily for adults, and from 2 mg to 4 mg per kg body weight daily for children in divided doses. The selected dose will depend on the severity of the condition.

1. Initial therapy should be continued for a period of six months or until a response is seen (whichever is the shorter time). Therapy must be maintained for at least three months before a response can be expected.
2. From the time of response the same dose should be continued for a further three months.
3. At this time the dose should be halved and, if the remission is maintained, continued for three months.
4. During the next three months gradual withdrawal should be attempted.
5. Should a relapse occur at any time whilst the dose is being reduced the initial dosage regime should be reinstituted.

Use in the elderly: The usual adult regimen is recommended.

Contra-indications, warnings, etc

Contra-indications: Carcinoma of the prostate or breast in male patients; carcinoma of the breast in women with hypercalcaemia (androgenic anabolic steroids may stimulate osteolytic resorption of bones); pregnancy or lactation; infancy; nephrosis or the nephrotic phase of nephritis; severe hepatic dysfunction; hypersensitivity to oxymetholone.

Warnings and precautions: Because of serious side-effects, anabolic steroids should not be used to enhance athletic ability.

Tumours of the liver have been reported occasionally in patients subjected to prolonged treatment with androgenic-anabolic steroids. The possibility that these compounds may induce or enhance the development of hepatic tumours cannot at present be excluded and this should be considered when the use of this product is proposed, especially in young people who are not suffering from life-threatening disorders.

Hepatotoxic effects, including jaundice, are common with the prescribed dosage. Clinical jaundice may be painless, with or without pruritus. It may also be associated with acute hepatic enlargement and right-upper quadrant pain, which has been mistaken for acute (surgical) obstruction of the bile duct. Drug-induced jaundice is usually reversible when the medication is discontinued. Continued therapy has been associated with hepatic coma and death. Because of the hepatotoxicity associated with oxymetholone administration, periodic liver function tests are recommended. Disturbance of liver function tests, elevation of serum bilirubin and jaundice may occur, together with other signs of liver disturbance. Should this happen, the dosage should be halved. If liver function tests do not improve within one week then oxymetholone therapy should be withdrawn.

Caution is required in administering these agents to patients with cardiac, renal or hepatic disease. Oedema, with or without congestive heart failure, may occur occasionally. Concomitant administration with adrenal steroids or ACTH may add to the oedema. This is generally controllable with appropriate diuretic and/or digitalis therapy. Anabolic steroids should be used with caution in patients with benign prostatic hypertrophy. Geriatric male patients treated with androgenic anabolic steroids maybe at an increased risk for the development of prostrate hypertrophy and prostatic carcinoma.

When anticoagulant therapy is used concomitantly, dosage of the anticoagulant may have to be decreased in order to maintain the prothrombin time at the desired therapeutic level. This is because Anapolon 50, like other anabolic steroids, may enhance blood fibrinolytic activity.

Oxymetholone exhibits only slight androgenic activity in low doses, but in the high dosage levels employed in the treatment of aplastic anaemias, it may lead to virilisation in women and prepubertal children.

Amenorrhoea usually occurs in the adult female, even in the presence of thrombocytopenia. Concomitant administration of large doses of progestational agents to control menorrhagia is not recommended. Hypercalcaemia may develop both spontaneously and as a result of hormonal therapy in women with disseminated breast carcinoma. If it develops while on this agent, the drug should be stopped.

The development of iron deficiency anaemia manifested by a low serum iron and decreased percent saturation of transferrin, has been observed in some patients treated with oxymetholone. Periodic determination of the serum iron and iron binding capacity is recommended. If iron deficiency is detected, it should be appropriately treated with supplementary iron.

Leukaemia has been observed in patients with aplastic anaemia treated with oxymetholone. The role, if any, of oxymetholone is unclear since malignant transformation has been seen in blood dyscrasias and leukaemia has been reported in patients with aplastic anaemia who have not been treated with oxymetholone.

Anabolic steroids have been shown to alter glucose tolerance tests. Diabetics should be followed carefully and the insulin or oral hypoglycaemic dosage adjusted accordingly.

Serum cholesterol may increase or decrease during therapy. Therefore, caution is required in administering these agents to patients with a history of myocardial infarction or coronary artery disease. Serial determinations of serum cholesterol should be made and therapy adjusted accordingly.

Alterations in these clinical laboratory tests may occur:

(a) The metyrapone test.

(b) The fasting blood sugar and glucose tolerance test.
(c) The thyroid function tests: a decrease in the PBI, in thyroxine-binding capacity and radioactive iodine uptake and an increase in T3 uptake by the rbc's or resin may occur. Free thyroxine (T4) is normal. Altered tests usually persist for 2–3 weeks after stopping anabolic therapy.
(d) The electrolytes; retention of sodium, chlorides, water, potassium, phosphates and calcium.
(e) Increased or decreased serum cholesterol.
(f) Suppression of clotting factors II, V, VII, and X.
(g) Increased creatinine excretion lasting up to two weeks after discontinuing therapy.
(h) Decreased 17-ketosteroid excretion.

The following adverse reactions may occur:

1. Hepatotoxicity is the most serious adverse reaction associated with anabolic steroid therapy. Reversible increase in BSP retention occurs early and appears to be directly related to the dose. Increase in serum bilirubin, with or without an increase in the serum alkaline phosphatase and transaminases (SGOT and SGPT) indicate a higher degree of excretory dysfunction. Clinical jaundice, which is reversible when the drug is discontinued, may occur. The histologic picture is one of intrahepatic cholestasis with little or no cellular damage. Continued therapy may be associated with hepatic coma and death.

2. Virilisation is the most common undesirable effect associated with anabolic steroid therapy. Acne occurs frequently in all age groups.

Prepubertal male: The first signs of virilisation in the prepubertal male are phallic enlargement and an increase in frequency of erection. Hirsutism and increased skin pigmentation may also occur.

Postpubertal male: Inhibition of testicular function with oligospermia; decrease in seminal volume, alteration in libido, and impotence may occur with prolonged or intensive anabolic therapy. Gynaecomastia, and testicular atrophy may occur. Chronic priapism, hair loss, epididymitis and bladder irritability have been reported.

In females, hirsutism, hoarseness or deepening of the voice, clitoral enlargement, alteration of libido, and menstrual irregularities and male-pattern baldness may occur. The voice change and clitoral enlargement are usually irreversible even after prompt discontinuation of therapy. The use of oestrogens in combination with androgens will not prevent virilisation in females.

3. *Other adverse reactions associated with anabolic/androgenic therapy include:*
(a) Muscle cramps.
(b) Nausea.
(c) Excitation and sleeplessness.
(d) Chills.
(e) Bleeding in patients on concomitant anticoagulant therapy.
(f) Premature closure of epiphyses in children.
(g) Vomiting.
(h) Diarrhoea.

Hepatocellular carcinoma and peliosis hepatis have been observed in patients with congenital and acquired aplastic anaemia treated with oxymetholone and other oral androgens for prolonged periods. In some cases withdrawal of the drug has been associated with regressions of the hepatic lesions.

Use in pregnancy and lactation: Anapolon 50 is contra-indicated in pregnancy (primarily because of masculinisation of the fetus). It is not known whether anabolic steroids are excreted in human milk. Because of the potential for serious adverse reactions from anabolics in breast-fed infants, women who take Anapolon 50 should not breast feed.

Treatment of overdosage: There are no reports of chronic or acute overdosage with Anapolon 50. Gastric lavage may be helpful if performed soon after ingestion.

Pharmaceutical precautions Anapolon 50 should be kept under normal storage conditions.

Legal category POM.

Package quantities Anapolon 50 is available in containers of 100 tablets.

Further information Nil.

Product licence number 0286/5009.

BREVINOR*

Presentation White, flat, circular, bevel-edged tablets inscribed 'B' on one face and SYNTEX on the reverse. Each tablet contains Norethisterone BP 500 micrograms and Ethinyloestradiol BP 35 micrograms.

Uses Brevinor is indicated for oral contraception.

The mode of action of Brevinor is similar to that of other progestogen/oestrogen oral contraceptives; its activity is exerted through a combined effect on one or more of the following: hypothalamus, anterior pituitary, ovary, endometrium and cervical mucus.

Dosage and administration The dosage of Brevinor for the initial cycle of therapy is 1 tablet taken daily from the 5th to the 25th day of the menstrual cycle, counting the first day of menstrual flow as 'Day 1'. For subsequent cycles, no tablets are taken for seven days, then a new course is started of 1 tablet daily for 21 days. This sequence of 21 days on treatment, seven days off treatment is repeated for as long as contraception is required.

When starting oral contraception with Brevinor, additional precautions must be used for the first 14 days of tablet-taking.

Tablet omissions: Tablets must be taken daily in order to maintain adequate hormone levels. If a tablet is missed, it should be taken as soon as possible, within 24 hours of the correct time even if this means that 2 tablets are taken together. If 2 tablets are missed, a tablet should be taken as soon as possible so medication is re-established. An additional method of contraception should be used for the remainder of that tablet cycle. If more than 2 tablets have been missed, oral contraceptive therapy should be discontinued immediately and a method of non-hormonal contraception should be used until menses has appeared or pregnancy has been excluded.

Changing from another oral contraceptive: Brevinor should be started seven days after completing the last course of the other product. An additional mechanical or chemical contraceptive should be used for the first 14 days of tablet-taking.

Use after childbirth, miscarriage or abortion: After childbirth, oral contraception is usually started when spontaneous menstruation has resumed. Another method of contraception should be used in the meantime, unless the first course of tablets is started within seven days of delivery. After a miscarriage or abortion, oral contraception can normally be started on the fifth day.

Contra-indications, warnings, etc
Contra-indications: As with all combined progestogen/oestrogen oral contraceptives, the following conditions should be regarded as contra-indications:
(a) Thrombophlebitis, thromboembolic disorders, cerebrovascular disorders, coronary artery disease, or a history of these conditions.
(b) Acute or severe chronic liver disease, Dubin-Johnson or Rotor syndrome, history during pregnancy of idiopathic jaundice or severe pruritus.
(c) Known or suspected breast or genital cancer.
(d) Known or suspected oestrogen-dependent neoplasia.
(e) Undiagnosed abnormal vaginal bleeding.
(f) Pregnancy.

Side-effects and precautions: As with all oral contraceptives, there may be slight nausea at first, weight gain or breast discomfort, which soon disappear.

Other side-effects known or suspected to occur with oral contraceptives include gastrointestinal symptoms, changes in libido and appetite, headache, exacerbation of existing uterine fibroid disease, depression, and changes in carbohydrate, lipid and vitamin metabolism.

Spotting or bleeding may occur during the first few cycles. Usually menstrual bleeding becomes light and occasionally there may be no bleeding during the tablet-free days.

Hypertension, which is usually reversible on discontinuing treatment, has occurred in a small percentage of women taking oral contraceptives. Oestrogen-progestogen preparations should be used with caution in patients with a history of hepatic dysfunction or hypertension.

A statistical association between the use of oral contraceptives and the occurrence of thrombosis, embolism or haemorrhage has been reported. Patients on such treatments should be kept under regular surveillance, in view of the possibility of development of such conditions as thromboembolism.

Risk of coronary artery disease in women taking oral contraceptives is increased by the presence of other predisposing factors such as cigarette smoking, hypercholesterolaemia, obesity, diabetes, history of pre-eclamptic toxaemia and increasing age. After the age of thirty-five years, the patient and physician should carefully re-assess the risk/benefit ratio of using combined oral contraceptives as opposed to alternative methods of contraception.

Benign and malignant liver tumours have been associated with oral contraceptive use. The relationship between occurrence of liver tumours and use of female sex hormones is not known at present. These tumours are very rare but they may rupture causing intra-abdominal bleeding. If the patient presents with a mass or tenderness in the right upper quadrant or an acute abdomen, the possible presence of a tumour should be considered.

The use of this product in patients suffering from epilepsy, migraine, asthma or cardiac dysfunction may result in exacerbation of these disorders, because of fluid retention. Caution should also be observed in patients who wear contact lenses.

Decreased glucose tolerance may occur in diabetic patients on this treatment, and their control must be carefully supervised.

The use of oral contraceptives has also been associated with a possible increased incidence of gallbladder disease.

An increased risk of congenital anomalies, including heart defects and limb defects, has been reported following the use of sex hormones, including oral contraceptives, in pregnancy. If the patient does not adhere to the prescribed schedule, the possibility of pregnancy should be considered at the time of the first missed period and further use of oral contraceptives should be withheld until pregnancy has been ruled out. It is recommended that for any patient who has missed two consecutive periods, pregnancy should be ruled out before continuing the contraceptive regimen. If pregnancy is confirmed the patient should be apprised of the potential risks to the foetus and the advisability of continuing the pregnancy should be discussed in the light of these risks. It is advisable to discontinue Brevinor three months before a planned pregnancy.

Gastro-intestinal upsets may interfere with the absorption of the tablets. Some drugs may modify the metabolism of Brevinor reducing its effectiveness; these include certain sedatives, antibiotics, anti-epileptic and anti-arthritic drugs. During the time such agents are used concurrently, it is advisable that mechanical contraceptives also be used.

Women taking oral contraceptives require careful observation if they have or have had any of the following conditions: breast nodules; fibrocystic disease of the breast or an abnormal mammogram; uterine fibroids; a history of severe depressive states; varicose veins; sickle-cell anaemia; diabetes; hypertension; high blood cholesterol levels; epilepsy; asthma; otosclerosis; multiple sclerosis; porphyria; tetany; disturbed liver functions; gallstones; cardiovascular disease; kidney disease; chloasma; herpes of pregnancy or any disease that is prone to worsen during pregnancy. The worsening or first appearance of any of these conditions may indicate that the oral contraceptive should be stopped. Discontinue treatment if there is a gradual or sudden, partial or complete loss of vision or any evidence of ocular changes, onset or aggravation of migraine or development of headache of a new kind which is recurrent, persistent or severe.

Brevinor should be discontinued at least six weeks before elective operations and during immobilisation.

Women with a history of oligomenorrhoea or secondary amenorrhoea or young women without regular cycles may have a tendency to remain anovulatory or to become amenorrhoeic after discontinuation of oral contraceptives. Women with these pre-existing problems should be advised of this possibility and encouraged to use other contraceptive methods.

The risk of arterial thrombosis associated with combined oral contraceptives increases with age, and this risk is aggravated by cigarette smoking. The use of combined oral contraceptives by women in the older age group, especially those who are cigarette smokers, should therefore be discouraged and alternative methods advised.

Numerous epidemiological studies have been reported on the risks of ovarian, endometrial, cervical and breast cancer in women using combined oral contraceptives. The evidence is clear that combined oral contraceptives offer substantial protection against both ovarian and endometrial cancer.

An increased risk of cervical cancer in long-term users of combined oral contraceptives has been reported in some studies, but there continues to be controversy about the extent to which this is attributable to the confounding effects of sexual behaviour and other factors.

The evidence linking combined oral contraceptive use and breast cancer remains inconclusive. The results of some studies suggest an increased risk of breast cancer presenting below the age of about 35, the risk rising with duration of use. Any possible increased risk of breast cancer with combined oral contraceptives is however likely to be small, and may be expected to be less with low dosage pills. This possible risk should be weighed against the many benefits of combined oral contraceptives, including their protective effects against ovarian and endometrial cancers.

Use during breast-feeding: Active ingredients or their metabolites have been detected in the milk of mothers taking oral contraceptives. The effect of Brevinor on breast-fed infants has not been determined.

Treatment of overdose: Overdosage may be manifested by nausea, vomiting, breast enlargement and vaginal bleeding. There is no specific antidote and treatment should be symptomatic. Gastric lavage may be employed if the overdose is large and the patient is seen sufficiently early (within four hours).

Pharmaceutical precautions Brevinor should be stored in a cool, dry place away from direct sunlight.

Legal category POM.

Package quantities Brevinor is available in calendar packs of 3 × 21 tablets.

Further information Nil.

Product licence number 0286/0054.

CARDENE*

Presentation Capsules with opaque blue cap and opaque white body, marked CARDENE 20, each capsule containing 20 mg nicardipine hydrochloride.

Capsules with opaque blue cap and opaque pale blue body, marked CARDENE 30, each capsule containing 30 mg nicardipine hydrochloride.

Uses

Mode of action: Cardene is a calcium ion influx inhibitor (slow channel blocker or calcium ion antagonist). Studies suggest that its main mode of action is to cause smooth muscle relaxation of both peripheral and coronary arterioles. Clinical studies have shown that cardiac performance is improved after the administration of Cardene, presumably in part due to the effect of afterload reduction and increased myocardial blood flow.

In man Cardene produces a significant decrease in systemic vascular resistance, the degree of vasodilatation being more predominant in hypertensive patients than in normotensive subjects. Haemodynamic studies in patients with coronary artery disease and normal left ventricular function have shown significant increases in cardiac index and coronary blood flow, with little if any increase in left ventricular end-diastolic pressure.

Pharmacokinetics and metabolism: Nicardipine is rapidly and completely absorbed following oral doses in capsules. Plasma levels are detectable as early as 20 minutes following an oral dose and maximal plasma levels are observed within 30 minutes to two hours (mean $T_{max} = 1$ hour). When given with high fat meal, the area under the concentration-time curve and peak plasma levels were reduced by 20 and 30%, respectively. The clinical trials with nicardipine were done in non-fasting subjects. While nicardipine is completely absorbed, it is subject to saturable first pass metabolism and the bioavailability is about 35% following a 30 mg oral dose at steady state.

The pharmacokinetics of nicardipine are nonlinear due to saturable hepatic first pass metabolism. Steady state plasma levels are achieved after about 3 days of dosing (at 20 and 30 mg tid) and are two- to three-fold higher at steady state than after a single dose. Once steady state was achieved, plasma levels remained relatively constant over 28 days of dosing at 30 mg tid. Increasing doses result in a disproportionate increase in plasma levels. Steady state peak plasma levels following 20, 30, and 40 mg (tid) averaged 36, 88, and 113 ng/ml, respectively. Hence, increasing the dose from 20 to 30 mg (tid) more than doubled plasma levels and increasing the dose from 20 to 40 mg (tid) increased plasma levels more than three-fold. Considerable intersubject variability in plasma levels was also observed. Following dosing to steady state using doses of 30 mg and 40 mg tid, the terminal plasma half-life of nicardipine averaged 8.6 hours. Nicardipine is highly protein bound (>99%) in human plasma over a wide concentration range.

Nicardipine is metabolized extensively by the liver, little or no (<1%) intact drug is detected in the urine, and none of the metabolites possesses significant biological activity. Following a radioactive oral solution dose, 60% of the radioactivity was recovered in the urine and 35% in faeces. Most of the dose (>90%) was recovered within 48 hours of dosing. Nicardipine does not induce its own metabolism and does not induce hepatic microsomal enzymes.

Electrophysiologic effects: Nicardipine prolongs the corrected QT interval to a minor degree. The sinus node recovery times and SA conduction times are not affected by the drug. Most importantly, the PA, AH, and HV intervals† and the functional and effective refractory periods of the His-Purkinje system are not prolonged by nicardipine.

Indications: Cardene is indicated for the management of patients with chronic stable angina and for the treatment of mild to moderate hypertension.

Dosage and administration

Adults

Angina: The dose for each patient should be individually adjusted by titration. The usual effective dose is 30 mg three times a day, with a range between 60 mg to 120 mg per day. A starting dose of 20 mg three times a day is recommended, titrating rapidly upwards as necessary. At least three days should be allowed before increasing the Cardene dose to ensure achievement of steady state plasma drug concentration.

Many studies have shown that Cardene and beta-blockers show additive efficacy when used concomitantly.

†PA = conduction time from high to low right atrium, AH = conduction time from low right atrium to His bundle deflection, or AV nodal conduction time, HV = conduction time through the His bundle and bundle branch-Purkinje system.

Hypertension: Therapy should be adjusted individually for each patient. The usual effective dose is 30 mg three times a day, with a range between 60 mg to 120 mg per day. A starting dose of 20 mg three times a day is recommended titrating rapidly upwards as necessary to achieve or maintain adequate control of blood pressure. In patients whose hypertension is successfully controlled at a dose of 20 to 30 mg three times a day a maintenance dose of 30 mg or 40 mg twice a day may be effective.

Cardene has been shown to be effective as sole therapy in patients with mild to moderate hypertension. Where appropriate, it may also be used concomitantly with diuretics or beta-blockers. In order to avoid excessive blood pressure reductions, careful titration of Cardene is advised when it is to be added to existing therapies.

For either indication, treatment may be required indefinitely.

Caution is advised when titrating Cardene dosage in patients with congestive heart failure, hepatic insufficiency or renal insufficiency.

Use in the elderly: Clinical and pharmacokinetic studies in the elderly generally showed no significant differences from the younger adult population. However nicardipine may lower systolic blood pressure more than diastolic blood pressure in these patients and therefore careful titration of the dose in elderly patients, starting with 20 mg three times a day, is advised.

Children: Safety and efficacy in patients under the age of 18 have not been established.

Contra-indications, warnings, etc

Contra-indications:

(i) Pregnancy and lactation.
(ii) Hypersensitivity to nicardipine hydrochloride.
(iii) Because part of the effect of nicardipine is secondary to reduced afterload, the drug should not be given to patients with advanced aortic stenosis. Reduction of diastolic pressure in these patients may worsen rather than improve myocardial oxygen supply.

Warnings and precautions: Where it is intended to substitute nicardipine for beta-blocker therapy, it should be noted that nicardipine gives no protection against the dangers of abrupt beta-blocker withdrawal; any such withdrawal should be by gradual reduction of the dose of beta-blocker, preferably over 8–10 days.

Ocasionally, patients have developed increased frequency, duration or severity of angina on starting nicardipine, at the time of dosage increases, or during the course of treatment. Patients experiencing this effect should discontinue Cardene.

Use in patients with congestive heart failure or poor cardiac reserve: Haemodynamic studies in patients with heart failure have shown that nicardipine reduces afterload and improves overall haemodynamics. In one study, intravenous nicardipine reduced myocardial contractility in patients with severe heart failure despite increases in cardiac index and ejection fraction noted in the same patients.

Use in patients with impaired hepatic function: Since the liver is the major site of biotransformation and since Cardene is subject to first pass metabolism the drug should be used with caution in patients having impaired liver function or reduced hepatic blood flow.

Patients with severe liver disease showed elevated blood levels and the half-life of nicardipine was prolonged. The drug should be administered cautiously in these patients, with a suggested starting dose of 20 mg twice a day, and individually titrated based on clinical findings maintaining the twice a day schedule.

Nicardipine administered intravenously has been reported to increase hepatic venous pressure gradient by 4 mmHg in cirrhotic patients at high doses (5 mg/20 min). Cardene should therefore be used with caution in patients with portal hypertension.

Use in patients with impaired renal function: Limited information suggests that Cardene blood levels may be elevated in some renally-impaired patients. Careful dose titration beginning with 20 mg three times a day is advised when treating such patients.

Laboratory tests: Transient elevations of alkaline phosphatase, serum bilirubin, SGPT, SGOT and glucose, have been observed. BUN and creatinine may also become elevated. While out-of-range values were seen in T_3, T_4, and TSH, the lack of consistent alterations suggest that any changes were not drug-related.

Hypotension: Cardene, like other calcium channel blockers, may occasionally produce hypotension. As with other antihypertensive agents, caution is advised to avoid systemic hypotension when administering the drug to patients who have sustained an acute cerebral infarction or haemorrhage.

Drug interactions: Some calcium blockers may increase the concentration of digitalis preparations in the blood. Nicardipine does not usually alter the plasma levels of digoxin, however, serum digoxin levels should be re-evaluated when concomitant therapy with nicardipine is initiated.

The binding of nicardipine to plasma proteins *in vitro* is not changed by the therapeutic concentrations of frusemide or propranolol.

Clinical studies have shown that Cardene may be used concomitantly with nitrates, beta-blockers or diuretics where appropriate.

Cimetidine increases nicardipine plasma levels. Patients receiving the two drugs concomitantly should be carefully monitored.

Severe hypotension has been reported during fentanyl anaesthesia with concomitant use of a beta-blocker and calcium blockade. Even though such interactions have not been seen in clinical trials, such hypotensive episodes should be vigorously treated with conventional therapy such as intravenous fluids.

Concomitant administration of nicardipine and cyclosporine results in elevated plasma cyclosporine levels. Plasma concentration of cyclosporine should therefore be closely monitored, and its dosage reduced accordingly, in patients treated with nicardipine.

Side-effects: Side-effects reported are generally not serious but occasionally require dosage adjustment or less frequently, discontinuation of therapy. Most are expected consequences of the vasodilator effects of Cardene.

The most frequent occurrences are dizziness, headache, oedema of the lower limbs, heat sensation and flushing, palpitations, nausea and less commonly hypotension.

In addition, adverse events were observed with either oral or intravenous nicardipine which are not readily distinguishable from the natural history of the disease in these patients. It remains possible, however, that some of these events were drug-related: Increased angina; sustained tachycardia; syncope; ventricular tachycardia; supraventicular tachycardia; myocardial infarction; intracranial haemorrhage; atrioventricular block; sinus node dysfunction.

The following have been reported: abdominal pain, diarrhoea, constipation, vomiting, anorexia, heartburn, tinnitus, drowsiness, heavy head, insomnia, lassitude, depression, nervousness, sweating, supraventricular arrhythmias, dyspnoea, skin itching, rash, salivation, dry mouth, backache, myalgia, paraesthesia, frequent micturition, renal and hepatic impairment.

Carcinogenesis: Rats treated with high doses of nicardipine for two years showed a dose-dependent increase in thyroid hyperplasia and neoplasia. Studies in the rat have indicated these results are linked to a combination of pharmacologic effects on the thyroid and liver leading to a reduction in plasma T_4. This results in a chronic elevation of TSH causing hyperstimulation of the thyroid. In animal safety studies these effects occurred only in the rat. In man nicardipine does not have an analogous combination of effects on the liver and thyroid and in clinical studies no effects on thyroid function tests have been reported even after long-term treatment. Carcinogenicity studies in mice and long-term studies in dogs have shown no evidence of neoplasia of any tissue, and no evidence of thyroid changes.

Overdosage: Several overdosages with nicardipine have been reported. One adult patient allegedly ingested 600 mg of nicardipine (standard capsules), and another patient, 2,160 mg of the sustained release formulation of nicardipine. Symptoms included marked hypotension, bradycardia, palpitations, flushing, drowsiness, confusion and slurred speech. All symptoms resolved without sequelae. An overdosage occurred in a one year old child who ingested half of the powder in a 30 mg nicardipine standard capsule. The child remained asymptomatic. Based on results obtained in laboratory animals, lethal overdosage may cause systemic hypotension, bradycardia (following initial tachycardia) and progressive atrioventricular conduction block. Reversible hepatic function abnormalities and sporadic focal hepatic necrosis were noted in some animal species receiving very large doses of nicardipine.

For treatment of overdose, standard measures including monitoring of cardiac and respiratory functions should be implemented. The patient should be positioned so as to avoid cerebral anoxia. Frequent blood pressure determinations are essential. Intravenous calcium gluconate may help reverse the effects of calcium entry blockade. Vasopressors are clinically indicated for patients exhibiting profound hypotension.

Pharmaceutical precautions No special precautions are required.

Legal category POM.

Package quantities Cardene 20 mg and 30 mg capsules are supplied in packs of 100 capsules.

Further information Nil.

Product licence numbers
Cardene 20 mg capsules: 0286/0089.
Cardene 30 mg capsules: 0286/0090.

CYMEVENE*

Presentation Each vial of Cymevene sterile powder contains 546 mg of sterile, freeze-dried ganciclovir sodium equivalent to 500 mg ganciclovir. It is a white to off-white powder. When reconstituted as directed, Cymevene has a pH of about 11.

Uses

Pharmacology: Cymevene (9-(1, 3-Dihydroxy-2-propoxymethyl guanine) is a synthetic nucleoside analogue of guanine which inhibits replication of herpes viruses both *in vitro* and *in vivo*. Sensitive human viruses include cytomegalovirus (CMV), herpes simplex virus-1 and -2 (HSV-1 and HSV-2), Epstein-Barr virus (EBV) and varicella zoster virus (VZV). Clinical studies have been limited to assessment of efficacy in patients with CMV infection.

Intracellular ganciclovir is phosphorylated to ganciclovir monophosphate by a cellular deoxyguanosine kinase. Further phosphorylation occurs by several cellular kinases resulting in ganciclovir triphosphate. In CMV-infected cells there is approximately a 10-fold increased concentration of both cellular kinases and ganciclovir triphosphate. Thus, there is a preferential phosphorylation of ganciclovir in virus-infected cells. In such cells ganciclovir triphosphate is metabolised slowly, with 60 to 70% remaining 18 hours after removal of ganciclovir from the extracellular fluid. The antiviral activity of ganciclovir is the result of inhibition of viral DNA synthesis by: (1) competitive inhibition of incorporation of deoxyguanosine triphosphate into DNA polymerase. (2) This means that incorporation of ganciclovir triphosphate into viral DNA causes subsequent termination or very limited viral DNA elongation.

Pharmacokinetics: In patients with normal renal function

the plasma half-life of ganciclovir following an i.v. infusion of 5 mg/kg averaged 2.9 hours with a mean systemic clearance of 3.64 ml/min/kg. Twice-daily administration of 5 mg/kg for 14 days did not cause accumulation in plasma. Renal impairment leads to altered kinetics of ganciclovir as indicated below.

Serum creatinine (micromol/l)		*Ganciclovir*	
		Systemic plasma clearance (ml/min/kg)	*Plasma half life (hours)*
<124	(n=22)	3.64	2.9
125–225	(n=9)	2.0	5.3
226–398	(n=3)	1.11	9.7
>398	(n=5)	0.33	28.5

Indications: Cymevene is indicated for the treatment of life-threatening or sight-threatening cytomegalovirus (CMV) infections in immunocompromised individuals. These states might include acquired immunodeficiency syndrome (AIDS), iatrogenic immunosuppression associated with organ transplantation, or chemotherapy for neoplasia. Life- or sight-threatening CMV infections might include retinitis, colitis, oesophagitis, pneumonia, other visceral involvement or severe systemic infection without documented visceral involvement.

Special considerations for use: Safety and efficacy of ganciclovir have not been evaluated in the treatment of less than severe CMV infections; nor for congenital or neonatal CMV disease; nor for the treatment of CMV infections in non-immunocompromised individuals.

The adverse effects of Cymevene include leucopenia and thrombocytopenia. In animals and in *in vitro* studies Cymevene caused aspermatogenesis, mutagenicity and teratogenicity and should be considered a potential carcinogen. Cymevene is indicated for use *only* in immunocompromised patients with life-threatening or sight-threatening CMV infections where the potential benefit outweighs these risks.

Dosage and administration THE RECOMMENDED DOSAGE, FREQUENCY OR INFUSION RATES SHOULD NOT BE EXCEEDED.

Because of individual patient variations in the clinical response of CMV infections and the sensitivity to the myelosuppressive effects of Cymevene, the treatment of each patient with Cymevene should be considered individually. Changes in dose should be based on regular clinical evaluations as well as regular haematological monitoring.

Initial (induction) treatment: 5 mg/kg infused at a constant rate over 1 hour every 12 hours (10 mg/kg/day) for 14 to 21 days for patients with normal renal function.

Long-term (maintenance) treatment: For immunocompromised patients at risk of relapse of CMV retinitis a course of maintenance therapy may be given. The recommended dose is 6 mg/kg daily given 5 days per week, or 5 mg/kg daily 7 days per week.

Treatment of disease progression: Indefinite treatment may be required in patients with AIDS, but even with continued maintenance treatment, patients may have progression of retinitis. Any patient in whom the retinitis progresses, either while on maintenance treatment or because treatment with Cymevene has been withdrawn, may be re-treated using the induction treatment regimen.

For patients with renal insufficiency the dose should be modified as follows:

Serum creatinine (micromol/l)	*Dose (mg/kg)*	*Dosing interval (hours)*
<124	5.0	12
125–225	2.5	12
226–398	2.5	24
>398	1.25	24

Use in the elderly. No studies on the efficacy or safety of Cymevene specifically in elderly patients have been conducted. Since elderly individuals often have reduced renal function, Cymevene should be administered to elderly patients with special consideration for their renal status (see above).

Use in children: There has been limited clinical experience in treating cytomegalovirus infections with Cymevene in patients under the age of 12 years. Reported adverse events were not markedly different in this group compared to treated adult patients. However, the use of Cymevene in children warrants extremely careful consideration, due to the probability of long-term carcinogenicity and reproductive toxicity.

Administration to children should be undertaken only after careful evaluation and only if, in the opinion of the physician, the potential benefits of treatment outweigh these considerable risks. Cymevene is not indicated for the treatment of congenital or neonatal CMV infections.

Method of administration: Caution – Intramuscular or subcutaneous injection may result in severe tissue irritation due to the high pH of ganciclovir solution.

Caution – Rapid or bolus intravenous injection must be avoided, as the toxicity of ganciclovir may be increased as a result of excessive plasma levels.

Reconstitution of the vial: The contents of the vial should be reconstituted when required for preparation of the infusion solution. Each vial (containing the equivalent of 500 mg ganciclovir) should be reconstituted by the addition of 10 ml Water for Injections BP. Do not use bacteriostatic water for injection containing para-hydroxybenzoates, since these are incompatible with ganciclovir sterile powder and may cause recipitation.

When reconstituting the contents of the vial, caution in handling and preparation of the solution should be exercised. The use of polythene gloves and safety glasses is recommended to avoid exposure in case of breakage of the vial. If the solution contacts skin or mucosa, immediately wash thoroughly with soap and water. Rinse eyes for at least 15 minutes with plain water.

The vial should be shaken to dissolve the drug. Reconstituted solution should be inspected for particulate matter.

Infusion solution preparation and administration: Based on patient weight and therapeutic indication, the appropriate calculated dose volume should be removed from the vial (ganciclovir concentration 50 mg/ml) and added to an acceptable infusion fluid (typically 100 ml) for delivery over the course of one hour. Infusion concentrations greater than 10 mg/ml are not recommended. The following infusion fluids are compatible with ganciclovir: normal saline; dextrose 5% in water; Ringer's solution (sodium chloride, potassium chloride and calcium chloride in water for injections); Ringer-Lactate solution for Injection (calcium chloride, potassium chloride, sodium chloride and sodium lactate in water for injections).

Because non-bacteriostatic infusion solution must be used, each infusion solution containing ganciclovir must be used within 24 hours of dilution to reduce the risk of bacterial contamination. The infusion solution should be stored in a refrigerator, but for no longer than 24 hours. Freezing is not recommended.

Diagnosis: The diagnosis of CMV retinitis should be made by an ophthalmologist using indirect ophthalmoscopy. In the differential diagnosis of CMV retinitis there are other conditions, e.g. cotton wool spots, candidiasis, or toxoplasmosis, which may produce a retinal appearance similar to CMV. For this reason it is essential that the diagnosis of CMV be confirmed by an ophthalmologist familiar with the retinal presentation of these diseases. The diagnosis of CMV retinitis may be aided by culture of CMV from urine, blood, throat, or other tissues or fluids. A CMV culture that is subsequently found to be negative does not exclude CMV retinitis.

Laboratory tests should be performed to confirm the diagnosis of CMV disease. Such diagnosis should not be based solely on the presence of antibodies to CMV, since many individuals have antibodies without active CMV infection. Confirmation of CMV should be by viral culture, identification of CMV antigen using CMV-specific immunochemical reagents (e.g. specific antibodies to CMV), or CMV-specific DNA hybridization probe reagents. In the absence of any confirmatory tests for active CMV infection, caution should be exercised in basing a diagnosis of CMV disease solely on histologic features, such as viral inclusions in biopsy specimens.

Contra-indications, warnings, etc

Contra-indications: (i) Pregnancy. (ii) Patients with known hypersensitivity to Cymevene or to acyclovir.

Warnings and precautions: Approximately 40% of patients receiving intravenous Cymevene develop neutropenia (neutrophil count less than 1000/microlitre). Cymevene should, therefore, be used with caution in those patients with pre-existing cytopenias, with a history of cytopenic reactions to other drugs or with a history of exposure to irradiation or known myelosuppressive drugs or chemicals. Cymevene should not be administered if the absolute neutrophil count falls below 500 cells/microlitre. However, in a clinical study of 314 patients (5 of whom died while neutropenic), no relationship between baseline neutrophil counts and frequency of neutropenia was observed; therefore the risk of neutropenia may not necessarily be predicted from pretreatment cell counts. Neutropenia typically occurs during the first or second week of induction therapy and prior to administration of a total cumulative dose of 200 mg/kg. Cell counts usually normalise within 2 to 5 days after either discontinuing the drug or decreasing the dose.

Thrombocytopenia (platelet count less than 50,000/microlitre) was observed in 20% of patients treated with Cymevene. Patients with iatrogenic immunosuppression following treatment with immunosuppressive drugs were more likely to develop lowered platelet counts than patients with AIDS. Patients with platelet counts less than 100,000/microlitre are also at increased risk of this toxicity of ganciclovir.

Animal data indicate that an additional likely side-effect is inhibition of spermatogenesis, which is reversible at lower doses and irreversible at higher doses. Clinical data have not yet been obtained regarding this side-effect. It is considered likely that intravenous Cymevene in the recommended doses will result in temporary or permanent inhibition of spermatogenesis. Animal data have also indicated that permanent suppression of fertility in women may occur.

Men and women of childbearing potential should be advised to use effective contraception during treatment. Men should be advised to practice barrier contraception for 90 days following treatment.

Use in patients with renal impairment: Cymevene should be used with caution in patients with impaired renal function. Both the plasma half-life of ganciclovir as well as peak plasma levels may be increased in patients with decreased creatinine clearance. In a small number of patients who were undergoing dialysis, ganciclovir plasma levels were reduced by approximately 50% following dialysis.

Administration of Cymevene by intravenous infusion should be accompanied by adequate hydration, since ganciclovir is excreted by the kidneys and normal clearance depends upon adequate renal function. If renal function is impaired, dosage adjustments are required. Such adjustments should be based on serum creatinine (see 'Dosage and administration').

In clinical studies with Cymevene, the maximum dose administered was 6 mg/kg given by intravenous infusion over a duration of one hour. It is likely that larger doses, or more rapid infusions, could result in increased toxicity, and therefore the data sheet recommendations should be followed.

Cymevene solutions have a high pH (range 9 to 11) and may cause phlebitis and/or pain at the site of intravenous infusion. Care must be taken to infuse ganciclovir solutions only into veins with adequate blood flow to allow rapid dilution and distribution.

Side-effects: Both neutropenia and thrombocytopenia have been observed frequently in patients treated with Cymevene. The frequency and severity of these events is summarised in the table below.

Absolute neutrophil count (cells/microlitre)	*Percentage of patients*
<500	16
500 to 1000	22
Platelet count (cells/microlitre)	
<20,000	9
20,000 to 50,000	10

Anaemia occurred in 3% of patients and eosinophilia in 2%.

Safety data involving body systems other than the haematopoietic system have been derived from adverse events reported during treatment with ganciclovir. These data include events reported as 'probably related', 'probably not related' and of 'unknown' relationship to treatment. Evaluation and attribution of cause and effect has been particularly difficult because of patients' underlying disease and multiple treatments.

The most frequent events, reported by 3% of patients, were fever, rash and abnormal liver function tests, followed by raised BUN or serum creatinine which were reported for 2% of patients.

Adverse events which occurred in 1% or less of the patients (but in more than one patient) are listed by body systems below:

General: Malaise, sepsis, facial oedema, sore throat, epistaxis.

Cardiovascular: Syncope, hypotension, tachycardia, hypertension, haemorrhage, generalised oedema, arrhythmias, chest pain, cardiac arrest, myocardial infarction, phlebitis.

Central nervous system: A wide variety of CNS events has been recorded. They may include: headache and dizziness; increases in excitability (anxiety states); decreases in excitability (drowsiness and coma); thought disorders (confusion, hallucinations) and neurological phenomena including ataxia, paraesthesiae and fits. Overall, CNS events occurred in 9% of patients.

Special senses: Deafness, retinal detachment.

Digestive system: Abdominal pain, feelings of fullness, anorexia, constipation, diarrhoea, haemorrhage, melaena.

Metabolic/nutritional disorders: Acidosis. Increases in plasma levels of alkaline phosphatase, bilirubin, LDH, SGOT, SGPT, potassium, glucose, or uric acid. Decreases in plasma levels of glucose, potassium, or sodium.

Musculoskeletal: Arthralgia, myalgia, muscular twitching.

Respiratory system: Asthma, cough, dyspnoea.

Skin and hair: Pruritus, urticaria, alopecia.

Urogenital system: Anuria, haematuria, urinary incontinence.

Infusion site reactions: Hypersensitivity, inflammation and pain.

Drug interactions: Binding of ganciclovir to plasma proteins is only about 1–2% and drug interactions involving binding site displacement are not anticipated. It is possible that probenecid, as well as other drugs which inhibit renal tubular secretion or resorption, may reduce renal clearance of ganciclovir and could increase the plasma half-life of ganciclovir. It is also possible that drugs which inhibit replication of rapidly dividing cell populations such as bone marrow, spermatogonia, and germinal layers of skin and gastrointestinal mucosa might have combined additive toxic effects when used concomitantly with, before, or after Cymevene. Because of the possibility of additive toxicity with co-administration of drugs such as dapsone, pentamidine, fluocytosine, vincristine, vinblastine, adriamycin, amphotericin B, trimethoprim/sulpha combinations or other nucleoside analogues combination with Cymevene therapy should be used only if the potential benefits outweigh the risks.

Patients with AIDS may be receiving, or have received, treatment with zidovudine. Since both zidovudine and Cymevene can result in neutropenia, it is recommended that these two drugs not be given concomitantly during induction treatment with ganciclovir. If maintenance treatment with Cymevene is undertaken, zidovudine therapy may be reinstituted at the discretion of the treating physician. Data from a small number of patients studied to date indicate that maintenance ganciclovir treatment plus zidovudine at the recommended dose resulted in severe neutropenia in most individuals.

Generalised seizures have been reported in patients taking Cymevene and imipenem-cilastatin concomitantly. These drugs should only be used concomitantly with Cymevene after careful consideration of the risks involved.

Laboratory testing: Due to the frequency of neutropenia or leucopenia observed in patients receiving Cymevene (see 'side-effects'), it is recommended that white blood cell counts be performed every two days for the first 14 days of ganciclovir administration. In patients in whom ganciclovir has previously resulted in leucopenia, or in whom white blood cell counts are less than 2000 cells/ microlitre at the beginning of treatment, white blood cell counts should be performed daily.

Mutagenesis/carcinogenesis: Ganciclovir caused point mutations and chromosomal damage in mammalian cells *in vitro* and *in vivo*, but did not cause point mutations in bacterial or yeast cells or dominant lethality in mice. Although morphologically transformed cells were not elicited *in vitro*, ganciclovir should be considered a potential carcinogen. The carcinogenic potential of ganciclovir is being evaluated in a lifetime bioassay in mice.

Impairment of fertility: Female mice exhibited decreased fertility, decreased mating behaviour, and increased embryo death after daily intravenous doses of 90 mg/kg. Daily intravenous doses of up to 20 mg/kg and daily oral doses of up to 1000 mg/kg did not impair female fertility.

In male mice, fertility was decreased after daily intravenous doses of 2–10 mg/kg, and daily oral doses of 10–1000 mg/kg. These effects were reversible. They became irreversible or partly reversible after daily intravenous doses of 10 mg/kg and daily oral doses of 100 or 1000 mg/kg.

Ganciclovir has also caused hypospermatogenesis in rats after daily oral doses of 100 mg/kg and over, and in dogs after daily intravenous doses of 0.4 mg/kg and over, and a daily oral dose of 0.2 mg/kg.

Use in pregnancy and lactation

Pregnancy: teratogenic effects – There have been no studies of ganciclovir in pregnant women. Cymevene should not be given to pregnant women as there is a high likelihood of damage to the developing fetus.

Ganciclovir had no effects on developing mouse fetuses at daily intravenous doses of 36 mg/kg, but caused maternal/fetal toxicity and embryo death at daily doses of 108 mg/kg (see also 'Nursing mothers').

Ganciclovir had no effects on developing rabbit fetuses at daily intravenous doses of 6 mg/kg, but caused fetal growth retardation, embryo death, teratogenicity, and/ or maternal toxicity at daily doses of 20 or 60 mg/kg. Teratogenic changes seen included cleft palate, anophthalmia, microphthalmia, aplastic organs (kidney and pancreas), hydrocephaly, and brachygnathia.

Nursing mothers: It is not known if ganciclovir is excreted in human milk. Since many drugs are, Cymevene should not be given to lactating mothers. Nursing should not be resumed until 72 hours after the last dose of Cymevene.

Daily intravenous doses of 90 mg/kg ganciclovir administered to female mice prior to mating, and during gestation and lactation, caused hypoplasia of the testes and seminal vesicles in the month-old offspring, as well as pathological changes in the non-glandular region of the stomach. It is not known whether these effects are attributable to maternal treatment during gestation or during nursing. The histological changes in the non-glandular stomach cannot be extrapolated to man as human beings do not have an analogous region.

Toxicity and treatment of overdosage: Overdosage with Cymevene has been reported in five instances. These patients include: A 34-year-old man with AIDS who received 7 doses at 22 mg/kg; a 34-year-old man with AIDS who received 18 mg/kg for 3 days and a 21-month-old girl who received 2 doses of 500 mg. In these three patients, no adverse events were observed after the overdosage. However, a 42-year-old man with AIDS who received an initial dose of 5 mg/kg followed by a dose of 8 mg/kg given once daily and a 34-year-old woman who received a single dose of approximately 24 mg/kg both developed reversible neutropenia.

In studies on anephric patients ganciclovir has been found to be dialysable by peritoneal as well as haemodialysis. In the event of overdose, dialysis and hydration may be of benefit in more quickly reducing plasma levels of ganciclovir.

Toxic manifestations seen in animals given very high single doses of ganciclovir (500 mg/kg) included emesis, hypersalivation, anorexia, bloody diarrhoea, inactivity, cytopenia, abnormal liver function tests and blood urea nitrogen, testicular atrophy, and death.

Pharmaceutical precautions Store the vials at room temperature, avoid excessive heat. Infusion solutions containing ganciclovir may be stored for up to 24 hours, provided they are refrigerated. Freezing is not recommended.

Legal category POM.

Package quantities Pack of 25 vials.

Further information Nil.

Product licence number 0286/0100.

NAPROSYN* TABLETS
NAPROSYN* 375 TABLETS
NAPROSYN* 500 TABLETS
NAPROSYN* SUPPOSITORIES
NAPROSYN* SUSPENSION
NAPROSYN* GRANULES

Presentation Naprosyn (naproxen) is d-2(6′-methoxy-2-naphthyl) propionic acid, a non-steroidal anti-inflammatory agent, developed by Syntex Research. It is presented as:

(i) A round, scored, buff, low excipient tablet containing 250 mg Naproxen BP inscribed NAPROSYN 250 on one side and SYNTEX with a breakline on the other.
(ii) An oval, scored, pink, low excipient tablet containing 375 mg of Naproxen BP inscribed 'NAPROSYN 375' on one side and 'SYNTEX' on the other.
(iii) An oblong, buff tablet containing 500 mg Naproxen BP in a low excipient formulation, inscribed NAPROSYN 500 on one side and SYNTEX with a breakline on the other.
(iv) Suppositories each containing 500 mg Naproxen BP.
(v) A flavoured orange suspension containing 25 mg/ ml Naproxen BP.
(vi) A dry powder formulation containing 500 mg Naproxen BP which is to be dispersed in water to form a white, flavoured suspension.

Uses Naprosyn is indicated for the treatment of rheumatoid arthritis, osteoarthrosis (degenerative arthritis), ankylosing spondylitis, juvenile rheumatoid arthritis, acute gout, and acute musculoskeletal disorders (such as sprains and strains, direct trauma, lumbosacral pain, cervical spondylitis, tenosynovitis and fibrositis).

Naprosyn has been shown to have striking anti-inflammatory, analgesic and antipyretic properties when tested in classical animal test systems. It exhibits its anti-inflammatory effect even in adrenalectomised animals, indicating that its action is not mediated through the pituitary-adrenal axis. It inhibits prostaglandin synthetase, as do other non-steroidal anti-inflammatory agents. As with other agents, however, the exact mechanism of its anti-inflammatory action is not known.

Dosage and administration *Adults:* Rheumatoid arthritis, osteoarthrosis and ankylosing spondylitis: the usual dose is 500 mg to 1 g daily taken in two doses at 12-hour intervals or alternatively as a single administration of two tablets, morning or evening. Alternatively some patients may find it more convenient to use Naprosyn Granules twice daily. Patients should be advised to add the contents of the sachet to half a tumblerful of water, stir vigorously and drink the whole contents of the glass immediately.

In the following cases a loading dose of 750 mg or 1 g per day for the acute phase is recommended:

(a) In patients reporting severe night-time pain and/or morning stiffness.
(b) In patients being switched to Naprosyn from a high dose of another anti-rheumatic compound.
(c) In osteoarthritis where pain is the predominant symptom.

For the patient who requires 750 mg per day, the size of the morning and evening doses can be adjusted on the basis of the predominant symptoms, i.e. night-time pain or morning stiffness.

Naprosyn suppositories are recommended for patients in whom rectal administration may be preferable. One suppository is to be inserted at night. If necessary another suppository or up to 500 mg oral Naprosyn therapy, can be used in the morning.

Acute gout: the recommended dosage is 750 mg initially, then 250 mg every eight hours until the attack has passed.

Acute musculoskeletal disorders: the recommended dose is 500 mg initially followed by 250 mg at 6–8 hour intervals as needed, with a maximum daily dose after the first day of 1250 mg.

Use in the elderly: Studies indicate that although total plasma concentration of naproxen is unchanged, the unbound plasma fraction of naproxen is increased in the elderly. The implication of this finding for Naprosyn dosing is unknown. As with other drugs used in the elderly it is prudent to use the lowest effective dose. For the effect of reduced elimination in the elderly refer to the section 'Use in patients with impaired renal function'.

Children: Naprosyn is effective in the treatment of juvenile rheumatoid arthritis in children over five years of age at a dose of 10 mg/kg/day taken in two doses at 12-hour intervals. Naprosyn is not recommended for use in any other indication in children under 16 years of age.

Contra-indications, warnings, etc

Contra-indications: Active peptic ulceration. Hypersensitivity to naproxen or naproxen sodium formulations. Since the potential exists for cross-sensitivity reactions, Naprosyn should not be given to patients in whom aspirin or other non-steroidal anti-inflammatory/analgesic drugs induce asthma, rhinitis or urticaria.

Special precautions and warnings: Episodes of gastro-intestinal bleeding have been reported in patients with Naprosyn therapy. Naprosyn should be given under close supervision to patients with a history of gastro-intestinal disease.

Bronchospasm may be precipitated in patients suffering from, or with a history of, bronchial asthma or allergic disease.

Sporadic abnormalities in laboratory tests (e.g. liver function tests) have occurred in patients on Naprosyn therapy, but no definite trend was seen in any test indicating toxicity.

Naprosyn decreases platelet aggregation and prolongs bleeding time. This effect should be kept in mind when bleeding times are determined.

Mild peripheral oedema has been observed in a few patients receiving Naprosyn. Although sodium retention has not been reported in metabolic studies, it is possible that patients with questionable or compromised cardiac function may be at a greater risk when taking Naprosyn.

Naprosyn suspension contains sodium chloride (20 mg/ml). This should be considered in patients whose overall intake of sodium must be restricted.

Use in patients with impaired renal function: As naproxen is eliminated to a large extent (95%) by urinary excretion via glomerular filtration it should be used with great caution in patients with impaired renal function and the monitoring of serum creatinine and/or creatinine clearance is advised in these patients. Naprosyn is not recommended in patients having baseline creatinine clearance less than 20 ml/minute.

Certain patients, specifically those whose renal blood flow is compromised because of extracellular volume depletion, cirrhosis of the liver, sodium restriction, congestive heart failure, and pre-existing renal disease, should have renal function assessed before and during Naprosyn therapy. Some elderly patients in whom impaired renal function may be expected could also fall within this category. A reduction in daily dosage should be considered to avoid the possibility of excessive accumulation of naproxen metabolites in these patients.

Use in patients with impaired liver function: Chronic alcoholic liver disease and probably also other forms of cirrhosis reduce the total plasma concentration of naproxen but the plasma concentration of unbound naproxen is increased. The implication of this finding for Naprosyn dosing is unknown, but it is prudent to use the lowest effective dose.

Interactions with other drugs: Due to the high plasma protein binding of Naprosyn, patients simultaneously receiving hydantoins, anticoagulants or a highly protein-bound sulphonamide should be observed for signs of overdosage of these drugs. No interactions have been observed in clinical studies with Naprosyn and anti-coagulants or sulphonylureas, but caution is nevertheless advised since interaction has been seen with other non-steroidal agents of this class.

The natriuretic effect of frusemide has been reported to be inhibited by some drugs of this class.

Inhibition of renal lithium clearance leading to increases in plasma lithium concentrations has also been reported.

Naprosyn and other non-steroidal anti-inflammatory drugs can reduce the anti-hypertensive effect of propranolol and other beta-blockers.

Probenecid given concurrently increases Naprosyn plasma levels and extends its half-life considerably.

Caution is advised where methotrexate is administered concurrently because of possible enhancement of its toxicity, since Naprosyn, among other non-steroidal anti-inflammatory drugs, has been reported to reduce the tubular secretion of methotrexate in an animal model.

It is suggested that Naprosyn therapy be temporarily discontinued 48 hours before adrenal function tests are performed because Naprosyn may artifactually interfere with some tests for 17-ketogenic steroids. Similarly, Naprosyn may interfere with some assays of urinary 5-hydroxyindoleacetic acid.

Side-effects:

Gastro-intestinal: The more frequent reactions are nausea, vomiting, abdominal discomfort and epigastric distress. More serious reactions which may occur occasionally are gastro-intestinal bleeding, peptic ulceration (sometimes with haemorrhage and perforation) and colitis.

Dermatological/hypersensitivity: Skin rashes, urticaria, angio-oedema. Anaphylactic reactions to naproxen and naproxen sodium formulations, eosinophilic pneumonitis, alopecia, erythema multiforme, Stevens Johnson syndrome, epidermal necrolysis and photosensitivity reactions, including rare cases in which the skin resembles porphyria cutanea tarda ('pseudoporphyria') or epidermolysis bullosa, may occur rarely.

CNS: Headache, insomnia, inability to concentrate and cognitive dysfunction have been reported.

Haematological: Thrombocytopenia, granulocytopenia, aplastic anaemia and haemolytic anaemia may occur rarely.

Other: Tinnitus, hearing impairment, vertigo, mild peripheral oedema. Jaundice, fatal hepatitis, nephropathy, haematuria, visual disturbances, vasculitis, aseptic meningitis and ulcerative stomatitis have been reported rarely.

Naprosyn Suppositories: The following minor side-effects have been reported with the use of Naprosyn suppositories: rectal discomfort, soreness, burning and itching. Also isolated cases of rectal bleeding, tenesmus and proctitis have been reported. However, the incidence of local side-effects in clinical trials was low.

Use in pregnancy and in breast feeding: Teratology studies in rats and rabbits, at dose levels equivalent on a human multiple basis to those which have produced fetal abnormality with certain other non-steroidal anti-inflammatory agents, e.g. aspirin, have not produced evidence of fetal damage with Naprosyn. As with other drugs of this type Naprosyn delays parturition in animals (the relevance of this finding to human patients is unknown) and also affects the human fetal cardiovascular system (closure of the ductus arteriosus). Good medical practice indicates minimal drug usage in pregnancy, and use of this class of therapeutic agent requires cautious balancing of possible benefit against potential risk to the mother and fetus especially in the first and third trimesters.

Naprosyn has been found in the milk of lactating mothers. The use of Naprosyn should therefore be avoided in patients who are breast feeding.

Overdosage: Significant overdosage of the drug may be characterised by drowsiness, heartburn, indigestion, nausea or vomiting. A few patients have experienced seizures, but it is not clear whether these were naproxen related or not. It is not known what dose of the drug would be life-threatening.

Should a patient ingest a large amount of Naprosyn accidentally or purposefully, the stomach may be emptied and usual supportive measures employed. Animal studies indicate that the prompt administration of activated charcoal in adequate amounts would tend to reduce markedly the absorption of the drug.

Haemodialysis does not decrease the plasma concentration of naproxen because of the high degree of protein binding. However, haemodialysis may still be appropriate in a patient with renal failure who has taken naproxen.

Pharmaceutical precautions Protect from light and store below 30°C. Naprosyn suppositories should be stored at not more than 15°C in a dry place.

Legal category POM.

Package quantities Naprosyn Low Excipient Tablets are supplied in packs of 250 tablets. Naprosyn 375 Low Excipient tablets are supplied in packs of 60 tablets. Naprosyn 500 Low Excipient Tablets are supplied in packs of 60 tablets (OP) and 100 tablets. Naprosyn Suppositories are supplied in packs containing 10 suppositories. Naprosyn Suspension is supplied in 500 ml bottles. Naprosyn Granules are supplied in packs containing 60 sachets.

Further information Nil.

Product licence numbers

Naprosyn Low Excipient Tablets	0286/0103
Naprosyn 375 Low Excipient Tablets	0286/0104
Naprosyn 500 Low Excipient Tablets	0286/0105
Naprosyn Suppositories	0286/0053
Naprosyn Suspension	0286/0047
Naprosyn Granules	0286/0098

NORIDAY*

Presentation White, flat, circular, bevel-edged tablets inscribed NORIDAY on one side and SYNTEX on the other. Each tablet contains Norethisterone BP 350 micrograms.

Uses Noriday is a progestogen-only oral contraceptive. It is particularly useful for women for whom oestrogens may not be appropriate. Although the mode of action of Noriday tablets has not yet been fully defined it is thought that alterations occur in the cervical mucus which inhibit the penetration of sperm, there is substantial inhibition of ovulation, and changes occur in the endometrium which inhibit implantation of the fertilised egg.

Dosage and administration The first Noriday tablet is taken on the FIRST DAY of menstrual bleeding. Thereafter, 1 tablet is taken continuously at the same time every day even during menstrual bleeding.

When starting oral contraception with Noriday, additional precautions must be used for the first 14 days of tablet-taking. Suitable methods are sheaths, caps plus spermicides, and intra-uterine devices. The rhythm, temperature and cervical-mucus methods cannot be used.

Tablet omissions: Tablets must be taken daily in order to maintain adequate hormone levels. If a tablet is missed, it should be taken as soon as possible, with the next tablet being taken at the usual time so that two tablets are taken on that date. An additional method of contraception should be used for the next 14 days. If two or more tablets are missed, Noriday should be discontinued immediately and a method of non-hormonal contraception should be used until menses has appeared or pregnancy has been excluded.

Contra-indications, warnings, etc

Contra-indications: A history during pregnancy of idiopathic jaundice or severe pruritus; Dubin-Johnson or Rotor syndrome; acute or severe chronic liver diseases; undiagnosed irregular vaginal bleeding; a history of thromboembolic disorders; pregnancy. Special caution should be observed in the presence of pre-existing breast or genital-tract cancer.

Warnings, side-effects: Hypertension, which is usually reversible on discontinuing treatment, has occurred in a small percentage of women taking oral contraceptives. Noriday should be used with caution in patients with a history of hepatic dysfunction or hypertension.

A statistical association between the use of oral contraceptives and the occurrence of thrombosis, embolism or haemorrhage has been reported. Patients on such treatments should be kept under regular surveillance, in view of the possibility of development of such conditions as thromboembolism. Risk of coronary artery disease in women taking oral contraceptives is increased by the presence of other predisposing factors such as cigarette smoking, hypercholesterolaemia, obesity, diabetes, history of pre-eclamptic toxaemia and increasing age. After the age of thirty-five years, the patient and physician should carefully re-assess the risk/benefit ratio of using oral contraceptives as opposed to alternative methods of contraception.

It is advisable to discontinue Noriday at least six weeks before elective operations and during immobilisation.

Benign and malignant liver tumours have been associated with oral contraceptive use. The relationship between occurrence of liver tumours and use of female sex hormones is not known at present. These tumours may rupture causing intra-abdominal bleeding. If the patient presents with a mass or tenderness in the right upper quadrant or an acute abdomen, the possible presence of a tumour should be considered.

An increased risk of congenital anomalies, including heart defects and limb defects, has been reported following the use of sex hormones, including oral contraceptives, in pregnancy. If the patient does not adhere to the prescribed schedule, the possibility of pregnancy should be considered at the time of the first missed period and further use of oral contraceptives should be withheld until pregnancy has been ruled out. It is recommended that for any patient who has missed two consecutive periods, pregnancy should be ruled out before continuing the contraceptive regimen. If pregnancy is confirmed the patient should be apprised of the potential risks to the fetus and the advisability of continuing the pregnancy should be discussed in the light of these risks. It is advisable to discontinue the use of oral contraceptives three months before a planned pregnancy.

Progestogen-only oral contraceptives such as Noriday may offer less protection against ectopic pregnancy than against intra-uterine pregnancy.

The incidence of side-effects in clinical trials was lower than that experienced with oestrogen-containing oral contraceptives. Side-effects which did occur included some cycle irregularity during the first few months of therapy, spotting or breakthrough bleeding, amenorrhoea, breast discomfort, gastro-intestinal symptoms, headaches, migraine, depression, fatigue, nervousness, disturbance of appetite, changes in weight and libido, rash.

Circumstances requiring additional contraceptive precautions other than the temperature, rhythm and cervical-mucus methods:

1. When changing to Noriday tablets from other hormonal contraceptives, additional contraceptive measures should be employed until 14 consecutive tablets have been taken regularly.
2. Vomiting or diarrhoea may reduce the effectiveness of the tablets by preventing them from being fully absorbed. In the case of repeated vomiting or continued diarrhoea, additional contraceptive measures should be employed for 14 days after the symptoms have subsided.
3. Interaction with other drugs. Some drugs accelerate the metabolism of oral contraceptives taken concurrently. Drugs suspected of having the capacity to reduce the efficacy of oral contraceptives include certain sedatives, antibiotics, anti-epileptic and anti-arthritic drugs.

It is therefore advisable to use non-hormonal methods of contraception during treatment with such drugs.

Menstrual pattern: A usual feature of all progestogen-only oral contraceptives is that they produce an initial irregularity of the bleeding pattern, but such irregularity tends to decrease with time. The patient should be informed before starting Noriday tablets that her menstrual pattern is likely to alter.

Irregular bleeding is, from a medical point of view, no reason for discontinuation of therapy, as long as organic causes and pregnancy can be ruled out. The patient should be instructed that if two or more consecutive periods are missed, she should consult her physician in order to rule out pregnancy.

Use after delivery or abortion: Although after delivery or abortion it is customary to start oral contraception at the end of the first biphasic menstrual cycle, Noriday tablets may be started as early as the seventh day post-partum. Additional contraceptive measures should be employed for the first 14 days of tablet-taking.

Use during breast feeding: There is no evidence that Noriday tablets diminish the yield of breast milk. Small amounts of steroid materials appear in the milk; their effect on the breast-fed child has not been determined.

Reasons for stopping oral contraception immediately: First signs of thrombophlebitis or thromboembolism, jaundice or pregnancy.

Overdosage: Overdosage may be manifested by nausea, vomiting, breast enlargement and vaginal bleeding. There is no specific antidote and treatment should be symptomatic. Gastric lavage may be employed if the overdosage is large and the patient is seen sufficiently early (within four hours).

Pharmaceutical precautions Noriday tablets should be stored in a cool, dry place away from direct sunlight.

Legal category POM.

Package quantities Noriday tablets are available in calendar packs of 3 × 28 tablets.

Further information Nil.

Product licence number 0286/0024.

NORIMIN*

Presentation Yellow, flat, circular bevel-edged tablets inscribed SYNTEX on one face. Each tablet contains Norethisterone BP 1.0 mg and Ethinyloestradiol BP 35 micrograms.

Uses Norimin is indicated for oral contraception.
The mode of action of Norimin is similar to that of other progestogen/oestrogen oral contraceptives; its activity is exerted through a combined effect on one or more of the following: hypothalamus, anterior pituitary, ovary, endometrium and cervical mucus.

Dosage and administration The dosage of Norimin for the initial cycle of therapy is 1 tablet taken daily from the 5th to the 25th day of the menstrual cycle, counting the first day of menstrual flow as 'Day I'. For subsequent cycles, no tablets are taken for seven days, then a new course is started of 1 tablet daily for 21 days. This sequence of 21 days on treatment, seven days off treatment is repeated for as long as contraception is required.

When starting oral contraception with Norimin, additional precautions must be used for the first 14 days of tablet-taking.

Tablet omissions: Tablets must be taken daily in order to maintain adequate hormone levels. If a tablet is missed, it should be taken as soon as possible within 24 hours of the correct time even if this means that 2 tablets are taken together. If 2 tablets are missed, a tablet should be taken as soon as possible so medication is re-established. An additional method of contraception should be used for the remainder of that tablet cycle. If more than 2 tablets have been missed, oral contraceptive therapy should be discontinued immediately and a method of non-hormonal contraception should be used until menses has appeared or pregnancy has been excluded.

Changing from another oral contraceptive: Norimin should be started seven days after completing the last course of the other product. An additional mechanical or chemical contraceptive should be used for the first 14 days of tablet-taking.

Use after childbirth, miscarriage or abortion: After childbirth, oral contraception is usually started when spontaneous menstruation has resumed. Another method of contraception should be used in the meantime, unless the first course of tablets is started within seven days of delivery. After a miscarriage or abortion, oral contraception can normally be started on the fifth day.

Contra-indications, warnings, etc
Contra-indications: As with all combined progestogen/oestrogen oral contraceptives, the following conditions should be regarded as contra-indications:

(a) Thrombophlebitis, thromboembolic disorders, cerebrovascular disorders, coronary artery disease, or a history of these conditions.
(b) Acute or severe chronic liver disease, Dubin-Johnson or Rotor syndrome, history during pregnancy of idiopathic jaundice or severe pruritus.
(c) Known or suspected breast or genital cancer.
(d) Known or suspected oestrogen-dependent neoplasia.
(e) Undiagnosed abnormal vaginal bleeding.
(f) Pregnancy.

Side-effects and precautions: As with all oral contraceptives, there may be slight nausea at first, weight gain or breast discomfort, which soon disappear.

Other side-effects known or suspected to occur with oral contraceptives include gastro-intestinal symptoms, changes in libido and appetite, headache, exacerbation of existing uterine fibroid disease, depression, and changes in carbohydrate, lipid and vitamin metabolism.

Spotting or bleeding may occur during the first few cycles. Usually menstrual bleeding becomes light and occasionally there may be no bleeding during the tablet-free days.

Hypertension, which is usually reversible on discontinuing treatment, has occurred in a small percentage of women taking oral contraceptives. Progestogen/oestrogen preparations should be used with caution in patients with a history of hepatic dysfunction or hypertension.

A statistical association between the use of oral contraceptives and the occurrence of thrombosis, embolism or haemorrhage has been reported. Patients on such treatments should be kept under regular surveillance in view of the possibility of development of such conditions as thromboembolism.

Risk of coronary artery disease in women taking oral

contraceptives is increased by the presence of other predisposing factors such as cigarette smoking, hypercholesterolaemia, obesity, diabetes, history of pre-eclamptic toxaemia and increasing age. After the age of thirty-five years, the patient and physician should carefully re-assess the risk/benefit ratio of using combined oral contraceptives as opposed to alternative methods of contraception.

Benign and malignant liver tumours have been associated with oral contraceptive use. The relationship between occurrence of liver tumours and use of female sex hormones is not known at present. These tumours are very rare but they may rupture causing intra-abdominal bleeding. If the patient presents with a mass or tenderness in the right upper quadrant or an acute abdomen, the possible presence of a tumour should be considered.

The use of this product in patients suffering from epilepsy, migraine , asthma or cardiac dysfunction may result in exacerbation of these disorders, because of fluid retention. Caution should also be observed in patients who wear contact lenses.

Decreased glucose tolerance may occur in diabetic patients on this treatment, and their control must be carefully supervised.

The use of oral contraceptives has also been associated with a possible increased incidence of gallbladder disease.

An increased risk of congenital anomalies, including heart defects and limb defects, has been reported following the use of sex hormones, including oral contraceptives, in pregnancy. If the patient does not adhere to the prescribed schedule, the possibility of pregnancy should be considered at the time of the first missed period and further use of oral contraceptives should be withheld until pregnancy has been ruled out. It is recommended that for any patient who has missed two consecutive periods, pregnancy should be ruled out before continuing the contraceptive regimen. If pregnancy is confirmed the patient should be apprised of the potential risks to the fetus and the advisability of continuing the pregnancy should be discussed in the light of these risks. It is advisable to discontinue Norimin three months before a planned pregnancy.

Gastro-intestinal upsets may interfere with the absorption of the tablets. Some drugs may modify the metabolism of Norimin reducing its effectiveness; these include certain sedatives, antibiotics, anti-epileptic and anti-arthritic drugs. During the time such agents are used concurrently, it is advisable that mechanical contraceptives also be used.

Women taking oral contraceptives require careful observation if they have or have had any of the following conditions: breast nodules; fibrocystic disease of the breast or an abnormal mammogram; uterine fibroids; a history of severe depressive states; varicose veins; sickle-cell anaemia; diabetes; hypertension; high blood cholesterol levels; epilepsy; asthma; otosclerosis; multiple sclerosis; porphyria; tetany; disturbed liver functions; gallstones; cardiovascular disease; kidney disease; chloasma; herpes of pregnancy or any disease that is prone to worsen during pregnancy. The worsening or first appearance of any of these conditions may indicate that the oral contraceptive should be stopped. Discontinue treatment if there is a gradual or sudden, partial or complete loss of vision or any evidence of ocular changes, onset or aggravation of migraine or development of headache of a new kind which is recurrent, persistent or severe.

Norimin should be discontinued at least six weeks before elective operations and during immobilisation.

Women with a history of oligomenorrhoea or secondary amenorrhoea or young women without regular cycles may have a tendency to remain anovulatory or to become amenorrhoeic after discontinuation of oral contraceptives. Women with these pre-existing problems should be advised of this possibility and encouraged to use other contraceptive methods.

The risk of arterial thrombosis associated with combined oral contraceptives increases with age, and this risk is aggravated by cigarette smoking. The use of combined oral contraceptives by women in the older age group, especially those who are cigarette smokers, should therefore be discouraged and alternative methods advised.

Numerous epidemiological studies have been reported on the risks of ovarian, endometrial, cervical and breast cancer in women using combined oral contraceptives. The evidence is clear that combined oral contraceptives offer substantial protection against both ovarian and endometrial cancer.

An increased risk of cervical cancer in long-term users of combined oral contraceptives has been reported in some studies, but there continues to be controversy about the extent to which this is attributable to the confounding effects of sexual behaviour and other factors.

The evidence linking combined oral contraceptive use and breast cancer remains inconclusive. The results of some studies suggest an increased risk of breast cancer presenting below the age of about 35, the risk rising with duration of use. Any possible increased risk of breast cancer with combined oral contraceptives is however likely to be small, and may be expected to be less with low dosage pills. This possible risk should be weighed against the many benefits of combined oral contraceptives, including their protective effects against ovarian and endometrial cancers.

Use during breast feeding: Active ingredients or their metabolites have been detected in the milk of mothers taking oral contraceptives. The effect of Norimin on breast-fed infants has not been determined.

Treatment of overdosage: Overdosage may be manifested by nausea, vomiting, breast enlargement and vaginal bleeding. There is no specific antidote and treatment should be symptomatic. Gastric lavage may be employed if the overdose is large and the patient is seen sufficiently early (within four hours).

Pharmaceutical precautions Norimin should be stored in a cool, dry place away from direct sunlight.

Legal category POM.

Package quantities Norimin is available in calendar packs of 3 × 21 tablets.

Further information Nil.

Product licence number 0286/0059.

NORINYL*-1

Presentation White, flat, circular, bevel-edged tablets inscribed NORINYL on one side and SYNTEX on the other. Each tablet contains Norethisterone BP 1 mg and Mestranol BP 50 micrograms.

Uses Norinyl-1 is indicated for oral contraception and is also useful in the treatment of certain menstrual disorders, e.g. heavy, irregular or painful periods. Activity is exerted through a combined effect on one or more of the following: hypothalamus, anterior pituitary, ovary, endometrium and cervical mucus.

Dosage and administration The first tablet is taken on the *fifth* day of a menstrual period. One tablet is then taken at the same time of day, every day, until all 21 tablets are used. The next pack is started after *seven tablet-free* days: this sequence is repeated for as long as contraception is required.

When starting oral contraception with Norinyl-1, additional precautions must be used for the first 14 days of tablet-taking.

Tablet omissions: Tablets must be taken daily in order to maintain adequate hormone levels. If a tablet is missed, it should be taken as soon as possible within 24 hours of the correct time even if this means that 2 tablets are taken together. If 2 tablets are missed, a tablet should be taken as soon as possible so medication is re-established. An additional method of contraception should be used for the remainder of that tablet cycle. If more than 2 tablets have been missed, oral contraceptive therapy should be discontinued immediately and a method of non-hormonal contraception should be used until menses has appeared or pregnancy has been excluded.

Changing from another oral contraceptive: Norinyl-1 should be started seven days after completing the last course of the other product. An additional mechanical or chemical contraceptive should be used for the first 14 days of tablet-taking.

Use after childbirth, miscarriage or abortion: After childbirth, oral contraception is usually started when spontaneous menstruation has resumed. Another method of contraception should be used in the meantime, unless the first course of tablets is started within seven days of delivery. After a miscarriage or abortion, oral contraception can normally be started on the fifth day.

Contra-indications, warnings, etc

Contra-indications: As with all combined progestogen/oestrogen oral contraceptives, the following conditions should be regarded as contra-indications:

(a) Thrombophlebitis, thromboembolic disorders, cerebrovascular disorders, coronary artery disease, or a history of these conditions.
(b) Acute or severe chronic liver disease, Dubin-Johnson or Rotor syndrome, history during pregnancy of idiopathic jaundice or severe pruritus.
(c) Known or suspected breast or genital cancer.
(d) Known or suspected oestrogen-dependent neoplasia.
(e) Undiagnosed abnormal vaginal bleeding.
(f) Pregnancy.

Side-effects and precautions: As with all oral contraceptives, there may be slight nausea at first, weight gain or breast discomfort, which soon disappear.

Other side-effects known or suspected to occur with oral contraceptives include gastro-intestinal symptoms, changes in libido and appetite, headache, exacerbation of existing uterine fibroid disease, depression, and changes in carbohydrate, lipid and vitamin metabolism.

Spotting or bleeding may occur during the first few cycles. Usually menstrual bleeding becomes light and occasionally there may be no bleeding during the tablet-free days.

Hypertension, which is usually reversible on discontinuing treatment, has occurred in a small percentage of women taking oral contraceptives. Oestrogen-progestogen preparations should be used with caution in patients with a history of hepatic dysfunction or hypertension.

A statistical association between the use of oral contraceptives and the occurrence of thrombosis, embolism or haemorrhage has been reported. Patients on such treatments should be kept under regular surveillance, in view of the possibility of development of such conditions as thromboembolism.

Risk of coronary artery disease in women taking oral contraceptives is increased by the presence of other predisposing factors such as cigarette smoking, hypercholesterolaemia, obesity, diabetes, history of pre-eclamptic toxaemia and increasing age. After the age of thirty-five years, the patient and physician should carefully re-assess the risk/benefit ratio of using combined oral contraceptives as opposed to alternative methods of contraception.

Benign and malignant liver tumours have been associated with oral contraceptive use. The relationship between occurrence of liver tumours and use of female sex hormones is not known at present. These tumours are very rare but they may rupture causing intra-abdominal bleeding. If the patient presents with a mass or tenderness in the right upper quadrant or an acute abdomen, the possible presence of a tumour should be considered.

The use of this product in patients suffering from epilepsy, migraine, asthma or cardiac dysfunction may result in exacerbation of these disorders, because of fluid retention. Caution should also be observed in patients who wear contact lenses.

A decreased glucose tolerance may occur in diabetic patients on this treatment, and their control must be carefully supervised.

The use of oral contraceptives has also been associated with a possible increased incidence of gall bladder disease.

An increased risk of congenital anomalies, including heart defects and limb defects, has been reported following the use of sex hormones, including oral contraceptives, in pregnancy. If the patient does not adhere to the prescribed schedule, the possibility of pregnancy should be considered at the time of the first missed period and further use of oral contraceptives should be withheld until pregnancy has been ruled out. It is recommended that for any patient who has missed two consecutive periods, pregnancy should be ruled out before continuing the contraceptive regimen. If pregnancy is confirmed the patient should be apprised of the potential risks to the foetus and the advisability of continuing the pregnancy should be discussed in the light of these risks. It is advisable to discontinue Norinyl-1 three months before a planned pregnancy.

Gastro-intestinal upsets may interfere with the absorption of the tablets. Some drugs may modify the metabolism of Norinyl-1 reducing its effectiveness; these include certain sedatives, antibiotics, anti-epileptic and anti-arthritic drugs. During the time such agents are used concurrently, it is advisable that mechanical contraceptives also be used.

Women taking oral contraceptives require careful observation if they have or have had any of the following conditions: breast nodules; fibrocystic disease of the breast or an abnormal mammogram; uterine fibroids; a history of severe depressive states; varicose veins; sickle-cell anaemia; diabetes; hypertension; high blood cholesterol levels; epilepsy; asthma; otosclerosis; multiple sclerosis; porphyria; tetany; disturbed liver functions; gallstones; cardiovascular disease; kidney disease; chloasma; herpes of pregnancy or any disease that is prone to worsen during pregnancy. The worsening or first appearance of any of these conditions may indicate that the oral contraceptive should be stopped. Discontinue treatment if there is a gradual or sudden, partial or complete loss of vision or any evidence of ocular changes, onset or aggravation of migraine or development of headache of a new kind which is recurrent, persistent or severe.

Norinyl-1 should be discontinued at least 6 weeks before elective operations and during immobilisation.

Women with a history of oligomenorrhoea or secondary amenorrhoea or young women without regular cycles may have a tendency to remain anovulatory or to become amenorrhoeic after discontinuation of oral contraceptives. Women with these pre-existing problems should be advised of this possibility and encouraged to use other contraceptive methods.

The risk of arterial thrombosis associated with combined oral contraceptives increases with age, and this risk is aggravated by cigarette smoking. The use of combined oral contraceptives by women in the older age group, especially those who are cigarette smokers, should therefore be discouraged and alternative methods advised.

Numerous epidemiological studies have been reported on the risks of ovarian, endometrial, cervical and breast cancer in women using combined oral contraceptives. The evidence is clear that combined oral contraceptives offer substantial protection against both ovarian and endometrial cancer.

An increased risk of cervical cancer in long term users of combined oral contraceptives has been reported in some studies, but there continues to be controversy about the extent to which this is attributable to the confounding effects of sexual behaviour and other factors.

The evidence linking combined oral contraceptive use and breast cancer remains inconclusive. The results of some studies suggest an increased risk of breast cancer presenting below the age of about 35, the risk rising with duration of use. Any possible increased risk of breast cancer with combined oral contraceptives is however likely to be small, and may be expected to be less with low dosage pills. This possible risk should be weighed against the many benefits of combined oral contraceptives, including their protective effects against ovarian and endometrial cancers.

Use during breast feeding: Active ingredients or their metabolites have been detected in the milk of mothers taking oral contraceptives. The effect of Norinyl-1 on breast-fed infants has not been determined.

Treatment of overdose: Overdosage may be manifested by nausea, vomiting, breast enlargement and vaginal bleeding. There is no specific antidote and treatment should be symptomatic. Gastric lavage may be employed if the overdose is large and the patient is seen sufficiently early (within four hours).

Pharmaceutical precautions Norinyl-1 should be stored in a cool, dry place away from direct sunlight.

Legal category POM.

Package quantities Norinyl-1 is available in packs of 3 × 21 tablets.

Further information Nil.

Product licence number 0286/5000.

STAYCEPT* PESSARIES

Presentation Smooth, torpedo-shaped, solid white, translucent, waxy pessaries containing nonoxynol-9 6% w/w (equivalent to 96 mg nonoxynol-9 per pessary).

Uses Spermicidal contraceptive agent. As with other spermicidal preparations, additional methods of contraception, for example, diaphragm, cap, sheath or intra-uterine device, must be used with Staycept pessaries.

When pregnancy is medically contra-indicated, the choice of contraceptive should be made in consultation with a doctor.

Dosage and administration Adult Females: one to be inserted into the vagina 10 minutes before intercourse. When used with a diaphragm or cap, one pessary should be placed inside the diaphragm or cap before it is put into position; a second pessary is then inserted into the vagina as far as possible.

If coitus is delayed for longer than 1 hour, another pessary should be inserted. Another pessary should be used each time intercourse takes place.

Contra-indications, warnings, etc
Contra-indication: Known hypersensitivity to nonoxynol-9 and polyethylene glycol.

Precautions and warnings: If irritation of the vagina or penis occurs, the use of the product should be discontinued.

Side effects: Local irritation. No reports have been received on Staycept Pessaries but nonoxynol-9 products have a potential to cause dysuria and excessive vaginal discharge.

Use in pregnancy and breastfeeding: Staycept Pessaries should not be used during pregnancy.

No data on the safety or on the use of Staycept Pessaries in lactating women are available.

Overdosage: Staycept Pessaries are intended for intravaginal use only. If taken orally this may cause gastric irritation as the product contains a surfactant. General supportive measures, together with monitoring of renal and hepatic function should be implemented as medically indicated.

Pharmaceutical precautions Store in a cool place.

Legal category GSL.

Package quantities Pack of 10 pessaries.

Further information Nil.

Product licence number 0286/5012.

STAYCEPT* JELLY

Presentation A smooth, clear jelly containing octoxynol 1% w/w.

Uses Spermicidal contraceptive agent. As with other spermicidal preparations, additional methods of contraception, for example, diaphragm, cap, sheath or intra-uterine device, must be used with Staycept Jelly.

Staycept Jelly can be used as a lubricant by women who experience difficulty with intercourse because of a dry vagina.

When pregnancy is medically contra-indicated, the choice of contraceptive should be made in consultation with a doctor.

Dosage and administration Adult Females:

(a) Used with diaphragm. Two 1-inch strips of jelly to be applied to either side of diaphragm and spread in a thin layer over cap and rim.
(b) Used with intra-uterine device or sheath. Two to three inches applied into the vagina, from an applicator 10 minutes before intercourse.

If coitus is delayed for longer than 1 hour, more jelly should be used. More jelly should be used each time intercourse takes place.

Contra-indications, warnings, etc
Contra-indication: Known hypersensitivity to octoxynol.

Precautions and warnings: If irritation of the vagina or penis occurs, the use of the product should be discontinued.

Use in pregnancy and in breastfeeding: Staycept Jelly should not be used during pregnancy. No data on the safety or on the use of Staycept Pessaries in lactating women are available.

Overdosage: Staycept Jelly is intended for intravaginal use only. If taken orally this may cause gastric irritation as the product contains a surfactant. General supportive measures, together with monitoring of renal and hepatic function should be implemented as medically indicated.

Pharmaceutical precautions Store in a cool place.

Legal category GSL.

Package quantities 80 g tube.

Further information Nil.

Product licence number 0286/5011.

SYNFLEX*

Presentation Opaque, orange, film-coated oval tablet marked SYNTEX on one face, containing naproxen sodium 275 mg (equivalent to naproxen 250 mg).

Uses Synflex is an anti-inflammatory analgesic for the treatment of musculoskeletal disorders (including sprains and strains, direct trauma and lumbo-sacral pain, cervical spondylitis, fibrositis, bursitis and tendinitis); post-operative pain; post-partum pain; uterine pain following IUCD insertion; dysmenorrhoea. Synflex is also indicated for the relief of migraine.

Dosage and administration
Adults: For musculoskeletal disorders, postoperative pain and pain following IUCD insertion the recommended dose is 550 mg (2 tablets) twice daily. Not more than 1100 mg should be taken per day.

For post-partum pain a single dose of 550 mg is recommended.

For dysmenorrhoea the recommended dose is 550 mg initially followed by 275 mg at 6–8 hour intervals as needed. This represents a maximum dose on the first day of 1375 mg (5 tablets) and 1100 mg (4 tablets) per day thereafter.

For the relief of migraine, the recommended dose is 825 mg at the first symptom of an impending attack. 275–550 mg can be taken in addition throughout the day, if necessary, but not before half an hour after the initial dose. A total dose of 1375 mg per day should not be exceeded.

Use in the elderly: Studies indicate that although total plasma concentration of naproxen is unchanged, the unbound plasma fraction of naproxen is increased in the elderly. The implication of this finding for Synflex dosing is unknown. As with other drugs used in the elderly it is prudent to use the lowest effective dose. For the effect of reduced elimination in the elderly refer to the section 'Use in patients with impaired renal function'.

Children: Synflex is not recommended for use in children under 16 years of age.

Contra-indications, warnings, etc

Contra-indications: Active peptic ulceration. Hypersensitivity to naproxen or naproxen sodium formulations. Since the potential exists for cross-sensitivity reactions, Synflex should not be given to patients in whom aspirin or other non-steroidal anti-inflammatory/analgesic drugs induce asthma, rhinitis or urticaria.

Special precautions and warnings: Synflex should be given under close supervision to patients with a history of gastro-intestinal disease.

Serious gastrointestinal adverse reactions can occur at any time in patients on therapy with non-steroidal anti-inflammatory drugs. The risk of their occurrence does not seem to change with duration of therapy. Studies to date have not identified any subset of patients not at risk of developing peptic ulcer and bleeding, however elderly and debilitated patients tolerate gastrointestinal ulceration or bleeding less well than others. Most of the fatal gastrointestinal events associated with non-steroidal anti-inflammatory drugs occurred in this patient population.

Bronchospasm may be precipitated in patients suffering from, or with a history of, bronchial asthma or allergic disease.

Sporadic abnormalities in laboratory tests (e.g. liver function tests) have occurred in patients on Synflex therapy, but no definite trend was seen in any test indicating toxicity.

Synflex decreases platelet aggregation and prolongs bleeding time. This effect should be kept in mind when bleeding times are determined.

Mild peripheral oedema has been observed in a few patients receiving Synflex. Although sodium retention has not been reported in metabolic studies, it is possible that patients with questionable or compromised cardiac function may be at a greater risk when taking Synflex.

Each Synflex tablet contains approximately 25 mg (about 1 m Eq) sodium. This should be considered in patients whose overall intake of sodium must be markedly restricted.

Use in patients with impaired renal function: As Synflex is eliminated to a large extent (95%) by urinary excretion via glomerular filtration it should be used with great caution in patients with impaired renal function and the monitoring of serum creatinine and/or creatinine clearance is advised in these patients. Synflex is not recommended in patients having baseline creatinine clearance less than 20 ml/minute.

Certain patients, specifically those whose renal blood flow is compromised, such as in extracellular volume depletion, cirrhosis of the liver, sodium restriction, congestive heart failure, and pre-existing renal disease, should have renal function assessed before and during Synflex therapy. Some elderly patients in whom impaired renal function may be expected as well as patients using diuretics could also fall within this category. A reduction in daily dosage should be considered to avoid the possibility of excessive accumulation of naproxen metabolites in these patients.

Use in patients with impaired liver function: Chronic alcoholic liver disease and probably also other forms of cirrhosis reduce the total plasma concentration of naproxen but the plasma concentration of unbound naproxen is increased. The implication of this finding for Synflex dosing is unknown, but it is prudent to use the lowest effective dose.

Interactions with other drugs: Due to the high plasma protein binding of Synflex, patients simultaneously receiving hydantoins, anticoagulants or a highly protein-bound sulphonamide should be observed for signs of overdosage of these drugs. No interactions have been observed in clinical studies with naproxen sodium or naproxen and anticoagulants or sulphonylureas, but caution is nevertheless advised since interaction has been seen with other non-steroidal agents of this class.

The natriuretic effect of frusemide has been reported to be inhibited by some drugs of this class.

Inhibition of renal lithium clearance leading to increases in plasma lithium concentrations has also been reported.

Synflex and other non-steroidal anti-inflammatory drugs can reduce the anti-hypertensive effect of propranolol and other beta-blockers.

Probenecid given concurrently increases Synflex plasma levels and extends its half-life considerably.

Caution is advised when methotrexate is given concurrently because of possible enhancement of its toxicity, since Synflex, among other non-steroidal anti-inflammatory drugs, has been reported to reduce the tubular secretion of methotrexate in an animal model.

It is suggested that Synflex therapy be temporarily discontinued 48 hours before adrenal function tests are performed because Synflex may artifactually interfere with some tests for 17-ketogenic steroids. Similarly, Synflex may interfere with some assays of urinary 5-hydroxyindoleacetic acid.

Side-effects:

Gastro-intestinal: The more frequent reactions are nausea, vomiting, abdominal discomfort and epigastric distress. More serious reactions which may occur occasionally are gastro-intestinal bleeding, non-peptic gastro-intestinal ulceration, peptic ulceration (sometimes with haemorrhage and perforation) and colitis.

Dermatological/hypersensitivity: Skin rash, urticaria, angio-oedema. Anaphylactic reactions to naproxen and naproxen sodium formulations, eosinophilic pneumonitis, alopecia, erythema multiforme, Stevens Johnson syndrome, epidermal necrolysis and photosensitivity reactions, including rare cases in which the skin resembles porphyria cutanea tarda ('pseudo-porphyria') or epidermolysis bullosa, may occur rarely.

Renal: Glomerular nephritis, interstitial nephritis, nephrotic syndrome, haematuria, renal papillary necrosis, renal failure.

CNS: Headache, insomnia, inability to concentrate and cognitive dysfunction have been reported.

Haematological: Thrombocytopenia, granulocytopenia, aplastic anaemia and haemolytic anaemia may occur rarely.

Other: Tinnitus, hearing impairment, vertigo, mild peripheral oedema. Jaundice, fatal hepatitis, visual disturbances, vasculitis, aseptic meningitis, hyperkalemia and ulcerative stomatitis have been reported rarely.

Use in pregnancy and in breast feeding: Teratology studies in rats and rabbits, at dose levels equivalent on a human multiple basis to those which have produced fetal abnormality with certain other non-steroidal anti-inflammatory agents, e.g. aspirin, have not produced evidence of fetal damage with Synflex. As with other drugs of this type Synflex delays parturition in animals (the relevance of this finding to human patients is unknown) and also affects the human fetal cardiovascular system (closure of the ductus arteriosus). Good medical practice indicates minimal drug usage in pregnancy, and use of this class of therapeutic agent requires cautious balancing of possible benefit against potential risk to the mother and fetus especially in the first and third trimesters.

The use of Synflex should be avoided in patients who are breast feeding.

Overdosage: Significant overdosage of the drug may be characterised by drowsiness, heartburn, indigestion, nausea or vomiting. A few patients have experienced seizures, but it is not clear whether these were naproxen related or not. It is not known what dose of the drug would be life-threatening.

Should a patient ingest a large amount of Synflex accidentally or purposefully, the stomach may be emptied and usual supportive measures employed. Animal studies indicate that the prompt administration of activated charcoal in adequate amounts would tend to reduce markedly the absorption of the drug.

Haemodialysis does not decrease the plasma concentration of naproxen because of the high degree of its protein binding.

Pharmaceutical precautions Protect from light and moisture.

Legal category POM.

Package quantities Synflex Tablets are supplied in packs of 100 tablets.

Further information Nil.

Product licence number 0286/0063.

SYNPHASE*

Presentation A 21-tablet memo pack consisting of 7 white tablets containing Norethisterone BP 500 micrograms and Ethinyloestradiol BP 35 micrograms, marked 'B' on one side and SYNTEX on the other; then 9 yellow tablets containing Norethisterone BP 1 mg and Ethinyloestradiol BP 35 micrograms, inscribed SYNTEX on one face; then 5 white tablets containing Norethisterone BP 500 micrograms and Ethinyloestradiol BP 35 micrograms, marked 'B' on one side and SYNTEX on the other.

Uses Synphase is indicated for oral contraception.

The mode of action of Synphase is similar to that of other progestogen/oestrogen oral contraceptives; its activity is exerted through a combined effect on one or more of the following: hypothalamus, anterior pituitary, ovary, endometrium and cervical mucus.

Dosage and administration For the initial cycle of therapy one tablet is taken daily from 5th–25th day of the menstrual cycle, counting the first day of menstrual flow as 'Day 1'. No tablets are taken for 7 days, then a new course of one tablet daily for 21 days is started. Tablets must be taken in numerical order as indicated on the pack. This sequence of 21 days on treatment, 7 days off treatment is repeated for as long as contraception is required.

When starting oral contraception with Synphase, additional precautions must be used for the first 14 days of tablet-taking.

Tablet omissions: Tablets must be taken daily in order to maintain adequate hormone levels. If a tablet is missed, it should be taken as soon as possible, within 24 hours of the correct time even if this means that 2 tablets are taken together. If 2 tablets are missed, a tablet should be taken as soon as possible so medication is re-established. An additional method of contraception should be used for the remainder of that tablet cycle. If more than 2 tablets have been missed, oral contraceptive therapy should be discontinued immediately and a method of non-hormonal contraception should be used until menses has appeared or pregnancy has been excluded.

Changing from another oral contraceptive: Synphase should be started 7 days after completion of the previous course of tablets. An additional mechanical or chemical contraceptive should be used for the first 14 days of tablet-taking.

Use after childbirth, miscarriage or abortion: After childbirth, oral contraception is usually started when spontaneous menstruation has resumed. Another method of contraception should be used in the meantime, unless the first course of tablets is started within 7 days of delivery. After a miscarriage or abortion, oral contraception can normally be started as early as the fifth day.

Contra-indications, warnings, etc

Contra-indications: As with all combined progestogen/oestrogen contraceptives, the following conditions should be regarded as contra-indications:

(i) Thrombophlebitis, thromboembolic disorders, cerebrovascular disorders, coronary artery disease, or a history of these conditions.

(ii) Acute or severe chronic liver disease, Dubin-Johnson or Rotor syndrome, history during pregnancy of idiopathic jaundice or severe pruritus.

(iii) Known or suspected breast or genital cancer.

(iv) Known or suspected oestrogen-dependent neoplasia.

(v) Undiagnosed abnormal vaginal bleeding.

(vi) Pregnancy.

Side-effects, precautions and warnings: As with all oral contraceptives, there may be slight nausea at first, weight gain or breast discomfort, which soon disappear.

Other side-effects known or suspected to occur with oral contraceptives include gastro-intestinal symptoms, changes in libido and appetite, headache, exacerbation of existing uterine fibroid disease, depression, and changes in carbohydrate, lipid and vitamin metabolism.

Spotting or bleeding may occur during the first few cycles. Usually menstrual bleeding becomes light and occasionally there may be no bleeding during the tablet-free days.

Hypertension, which is usually reversible on discontinuing treatment, has occurred in a small percentage of women taking oral contraceptives. Oestrogen-progestogen preparations should be used with caution in patients with a history of hepatic dysfunction or hypertension.

A statistical association between the use of oral contraceptives and the occurrence of thrombosis, embolism or haemorrhage has been reported. Patients on such treatments should be kept under regular surveillance, in view of the possibility of development of such conditions as thromboembolism.

Risk of coronary artery disease in women taking oral contraceptives is increased by the presence of other predisposing factors such as cigarette smoking, hypercholesterolaemia, obesity, diabetes, history of pre-eclamptic toxaemia and increasing age. After the age of thirty-five years, the patient and physician should carefully re-assess the risk/benefit ratio of using combined oral contraceptives as opposed to alternative methods of contraception.

Benign and malignant liver tumours have been associated with oral contraceptive use. The relationship between occurrence of liver tumours and use of female sex hormones is not known at present. These tumours are very rare but they may rupture causing intra-abdominal bleeding. If the patient presents with a mass or tenderness in the right upper quadrant or an acute abdomen, the possible presence of a tumour should be considered.

The use of this product in patients suffering from epilepsy, migraine, asthma or cardiac dysfunction may result in exacerbation of these disorders, because of fluid retention. Caution should also be observed in patients who wear contact lenses.

Decreased glucose tolerance may occur in diabetic patients on this treatment, and their control must be carefully supervised.

The use of oral contraceptives has also been associated with a possible increased incidence of gall bladder disease.

An increased risk of congenital anomalies, including heart defects and limb defects, has been reported following the use of sex hormones, including oral contraceptives, in pregnancy. If the patient does not adhere to the prescribed schedule, the possibility of pregnancy should be considered at the time of the first missed period and further use of oral contraceptives should be withheld until pregnancy has been ruled out. It is recommended that for any patient who has missed two consecutive periods, pregnancy should be ruled out before continuing the contraceptive regimen. If pregnancy is confirmed the patient should be apprised of the potential risks to the foetus and the advisability of continuing the pregnancy should be discussed in the light of these risks. It is advisable to discontinue Synphase three months before a planned pregnancy.

Gastro-intestinal upsets may interfere with the absorption of the tablets. Some drugs may modify the metabolism of Synphase reducing its effectiveness; these include certain sedatives, antibiotics, anti-epileptic and anti-arthritic drugs. During the time such agents are used concurrently, it is advisable that mechanical contraceptives also be used.

Women taking oral contraceptives require careful observation if they have or have had any of the following conditions: breast nodules; fibrocystic disease of the breast or an abnormal mammogram; uterine fibroids; a history of severe depressive states; varicose veins; sickle-cell anaemia; diabetes; hypertension; high blood cholesterol levels; epilepsy; asthma; otosclerosis; multiple sclerosis; porphyria; tetany; disturbed liver functions; gallstones; cardiovascular disease; kidney disease; chloasma; herpes of pregnancy or any disease that is prone to worsen during pregnancy. The worsening or first appearance of any of these conditions may indicate that the oral contraceptive should be stopped. Discontinue treatment if there is a gradual or sudden, partial or complete loss of vision or any evidence of ocular changes, onset or aggravation of migraine or development of headache of a new kind which is recurrent, persistent or severe.

Synphase should be discontinued at least six weeks before elective operations and during immobilisation.

Women with a history of oligomenorrhoea or secondary amenorrhoea or young women without regular cycles may have a tendency to remain anovulatory or to become amenorrhoeic after discontinuation of oral contraceptives. Women with these pre-existing problems should be advised of this possibility and encouraged to use other contraceptive methods.

The risk of arterial thrombosis associated with combined oral contraceptives increases with age, and this risk is aggravated by cigarette smoking. The use of combined oral contraceptives by women in the older age group, especially those who are cigarette smokers, should therefore be discouraged and alternative methods advised.

Numerous epidemiological studies have been reported on the risks of ovarian, endometrial, cervical and breast cancer in women using combined oral contraceptives. The evidence is clear that combined oral contraceptives offer substantial protection against both ovarian and endometrial cancer.

An increased risk of cervical cancer in long-term users of combined oral contraceptives has been reported in some studies, but there continues to be controversy about the extent to which this is attributable to the confounding effects of sexual behaviour and other factors.

The evidence linking combined oral contraceptive use and breast cancer remains inconclusive. The results of some studies suggest an increased risk of breast cancer presenting below the age of about 35, the risk rising with duration of use. Any possible increased risk of breast cancer with combined oral contraceptives is however likely to be small, and may be expected to be less with low dosage pills. This possible risk should be weighed against the many benefits of combined oral contraceptives, including their protective effects against ovarian and endometrial cancers.

Use during breast feeding: Active ingredients or their metabolites have been detected in the milk of mothers taking oral contraceptives. The effect of Synphase on breast-fed infants has not been determined.

Treatment of overdosage: Overdosage may be manifested by nausea, vomiting, breast enlargement and vaginal bleeding. There is no specific antidote and treatment should be symptomatic. Gastric lavage may be employed if the overdose is large and the patient is seen sufficiently early (within four hours).

Pharmaceutical precautions Synphase should be stored in a cool dry place, away from direct sunlight.

Legal category POM.

Package quantities Synphase is available in packs of 21 tablets.

Further information Nil.

Product licence number 0286/0085.

SYNTARIS* NASAL SPRAY

Presentation A buffered, clear, colourless, slightly viscous aqueous solution in a bottle fitted with a metered pump device which delivers 25 micrograms of flunisolide (6 α-fluoro-11 β, 16α, 17, 21-tetrahydroxypregna-1, 4-dien-3, 20-dione, 16, 17-acetonide) per actuation via a nozzle which is inserted into the nostril.

Uses Syntaris Nasal Spray is indicated for the prophylaxis and treatment of perennial and seasonal allergic rhinitis including hay fever.

Flunisolide has marked anti-inflammatory and anti-allergic activity, as shown in classical animal test systems. It is a corticosteroid which is several hundred times more potent in animal anti-inflammatory assays than the cortisol standard.

At the low doses used, clinical studies with flunisolide have shown a topical activity on the nasal mucous membrane with minimal associated systemic activity.

Dosage and administration Syntaris Nasal Spray is for administration by the intranasal route only.

Usual starting dose: Adults (including the elderly): 2 sprays into each nostril twice daily. If symptoms are severe, or if an exacerbation occurs, the physician may recommend 2 sprays into each nostril three times daily. *Children:* For children five years of age and over, 1 spray (approximately 25 micrograms) into each nostril three times daily.

Maintenance dose: After the desired clinical effect is obtained, the maintenance dose should be the smallest amount necessary to control the symptoms. Some patients may be maintained on as little as 1 spray (approximately 25 micrograms) to each nostril per day.

The maximum daily dose should not exceed 6 sprays in each nostril for adults, and 3 sprays in each nostril for children five years of age and over.

Syntaris Nasal Spray is not recommended for use in children under five years of age.

The effect of Syntaris Nasal Spray, unlike that of vasoconstrictor preparations, is not immediate. Full therapeutic benefit requires regular usage. The absence of an immediate effect should be explained to the patient in order to ensure co-operation and continuation of treatment with the regular dosage schedule.

There is no evidence that exceeding the maximum recommended dosage is more effective; higher dosage should therefore be avoided.

For full information on using the device, see patient instruction insert.

Contra-indications, warnings, etc
Contra-indications:

1. Untreated fungal, bacterial or viral infections of the nose or eyes.
2. Hypersensitivity to the formulation.

Warnings, precautions, side-effects etc: Glucocorticoids may mask some signs of infection and new infections may appear during their use.

Since systemic activity has not been seen with therapeutic doses of Syntaris Nasal Spray, care must be taken when transferring patients from systemic steroid therapy to Syntaris Nasal Spray if there is reason to suspect that their adrenal function is impaired.

Although adrenal suppression or atrophy of the nasal mucosa have not been observed in clinical trials, the potential for these effects should be considered with prolonged excessive usage.

Because of the inhibitory effect of corticosteroids in wound healing in patients who have experienced recent nasal septal ulcers, recurrent epistaxis, nasal surgery or trauma, a nasal corticosteroid should be used with caution until healing has occurred.

Side-effects: Adverse reactions noted in clinical trials with Syntaris Nasal Spray have been consistent with what one would expect when applying topical medication to an already inflamed membrane. The most frequently observed side-effect was aftertaste and a mild transient nasal burning and stinging which was occasionally severe enough to warrant discontinuation of treatment. Other side-effects noted, in order of decreasing prevalence were: nasal irritation, epistaxis, runny and stuffy nose, sore throat, hoarseness, throat irritation and rarely, alteration of smell and/or taste, nasal septal perforation. If severe these may require discontinuation of therapy.

Use in pregnancy and lactation: Syntaris Nasal Spray is not recommended in the first three months of pregnancy. If used in the second or third trimester, the expected benefits should be weighed against the potential hazards to the fetus.

Carcinogenesis: A 22-month study in mice and a 24-month study in rats showed some evidence of tumour formation that was not consistent between the two species and is not believed to be biologically meaningful to man.

Treatment of overdosage: Administration of large amounts of flunisolide over a short period may produce suppression of hypothalamic-pituitary-adrenal function. In such event, Syntaris Nasal Spray should be reduced immediately to the recommended dosage.

Pharmaceutical precautions Store at room temperature below 30°C.

Legal category POM.

Package quantities Each pack of Syntaris Nasal Spray contains one 24 ml bottle and the metered pump device.

Further information Nil.

Product licence number 0286/0057.

SYNTEX MENOPHASE*

Presentation Syntex Menophase consists of 28 tablets in a bubble pack. This is a sequential oestrogen-progestogen product comprising six different formulations arranged so that 1 tablet is taken daily starting with 5 pink, and continuing with 8 orange, 2 yellow, 3 green, 6 blue and 4 lavender tablets. Each tablet is inscribed SYNTEX on one face.

Composition: Syntex Menophase comprises six formulations:

	(*mg*)	(*microgram*)	*Tablets*
1. Mestranol BP	0.0125	(12.5)	5 pink
2. Mestranol BP	0.025	(25.0)	8 orange
3. Mestranol BP	0.050	(50.0)	2 yellow
4. Norethisterone BP	1.00		
Mestranol BP	0.025	(25.0)	3 green
5. Norethisterone BP	1.50		
Mestranol BP	0.030	(30.0)	6 blue
6. Norethisterone BP	0.75		
Mestranol BP	0.020	(20.0)	4 lavender

Uses Syntex Menophase is indicated for the treatment of menopausal symptoms and allied disorders. These include hot flushes and sweats, depression, lack of concentration, emotional lability, nervousness, lethargy, insomnia, loss of libido, senile vaginitis, pruritus and dry skin. Syntex Menophase may also be of use in the prophylaxis of post-menopausal osteoporosis in females who are at risk from developing fractures.

Dosage and administration The patient is advised to take her first tablet on a Sunday and thereafter to take one tablet at the same time each day in sequential order round the pack. She starts a new pack the day after she has taken her last lavender tablet from the previous pack.

Though menopausal symptoms are likely to improve during the first month of treatment, it will be necessary to maintain therapy for 6–12 months. If symptoms recur after discontinuation, further courses can be prescribed.

Contra-indications, warnings, etc

Contra-indications: Pregnancy (see also 'Precautions'); benign and malignant liver tumours; severe disturbances of liver function; jaundice or general pruritus during a previous pregnancy; Dubin-Johnson syndrome; Rotor syndrome; cardiovascular or cerebrovascular disorders eg. thrombophlebitis, thromboembolic processes or a history of these conditions; sickle-cell anaemia; porphyria; existing or previous moderate to severe hypertension; existing or previous breast or uterine cancer or oestrogen-dependent neoplasia; undiagnosed irregular vaginal bleeding; congenital disturbances of lipid metabolism; existing or previous hyperlipoproteinaemia; a history of herpes or otosclerosis made worse by pregnancy.

Warnings: Syntex Menophase is not an oral contraceptive. Syntex Menophase provides sequential graded doses of hormones; the post-menopausal patient with an intact uterus may therefore experience a small, regular monthly bleed but if forewarned of this possibility it usually causes no distress. Hormonal contraception should be stopped when Syntex Menophase is started and the patient should be advised to take non-hormonal contraceptive precautions during the prescribing period.

Treatment should be stopped at once if jaundice or pregnancy occurs. If pregnancy is confirmed the patient should be told of the potential risk to the fetus and the advisability of continuing the pregnancy should be discussed.

The use of this product in patients suffering from epilepsy, migraine, asthma or cardiac dysfunction may result in exacerbation of these disorders because of fluid retention; these patients should be carefully observed during treatment. Because of the possibility of corneal oedema caution should also be observed in patients who wear contact lenses.

Discontinue treatment if there is gradual or sudden, partial or complete loss of vision or any evidence of ocular changes, onset or aggravation of migraine or development of headache of a new kind which is recurrent, persistent or severe.

Diseases known to deteriorate during pregnancy (eg. multiple sclerosis, epilepsy, diabetes, hypertension, porphyria, tetany and otosclerosis) should be carefully observed during treatment.

Caution should be observed in patients with severe varicose veins, sickle cell haemoglobinopathy, untreated polycythaemia or pulmonary hypertension.

Forgotten tablets: Since Syntex Menophase is not an oral contraceptive, in the event of a missed tablet the patient should be advised to discard the tablet(s) missed and take only the tablet appropriate to the day of the week.

Side-effects and precautions: Pregnancy must be excluded before starting treatment with Syntex Menophase.

Measurement of blood pressure, along with examination of breasts and pelvic organs is advised before and periodically during treatment. Examination of the endometrium may also be considered. Treatment should be discontinued if there is a consistent rise in blood pressure.

Treatment should be stopped if trauma, illness or impending surgery is considered to entail a risk of thrombosis. Syntex Menophase should be discontinued at least six weeks before elective operations and during immobilisation.

A statistical association between the use of long-term oestrogen therapy (e.g. oral contraceptives) and the occurrence of thrombosis, embolism or haemorrhage (including myocardial infarct and stroke) has been reported. Patients on such treatments should be kept under regular surveillance in view of the possibility of development of such conditions as thromboembolism. This risk is aggravated by cigarette smoking and therefore use of Syntex Menophase in this group of women requires careful consideration.

Benign and malignant liver tumours have also been associated with long-term oestrogen therapy. The relationship between occurrence of liver tumours and the use of female sex hormones is not known at present. These tumours are very rare but they may rupture, causing intra-abdominal bleeding. If the patient presents with a mass or tenderness in the right upper quadrant or an acute abdomen, the presence of a tumour should be considered.

Decreased glucose tolerance may occur in diabetic patients on this treatment and their control must be carefully supervised. Changes in lipid metabolism may also be observed.

Thyroid hormone binding globulin may be increased, leading to increased circulating total thyroid hormone. Hence, care must be taken in interpreting thyroid function tests.

Caution should be observed in patients with a history of gall stones. Some women are predisposed to cholestasis during steroid therapy. Caution should also be observed in patients with renal dysfunction.

The following symptoms have been reported during treatment: anxiety, increased appetite, bloating, breast symptoms, cardiac symptoms, depression, dizziness, headaches, dyspepsia, leg pains and swelling, altered libido, excessive production of cervical mucus, intermenstrual bleeding, nausea, rashes, vomiting and altered weight.

The following have also been observed: endometrial neoplasia, increase in the size of uterine fibromyomata, endometrial proliferation and aggravation of endometriosis.

Drug interactions: Syntex Menophase may alter the effectiveness of anti-convulsants, antihypertensive agents, beta-blockers, hypnotics, hypoglycaemic agents, oral anticoagulants, theophylline, tranquillisers, tricyclic antidepressants and vitamins.

Overdosage: This may be manifested by nausea, vomiting, breast enlargement and vaginal bleeding. There is no specific antidote and treatment should be symptomatic. Gastric lavage may be employed if the overdose is large and the patient is seen sufficiently early (within four hours).

Pharmaceutical precautions Syntex Menophase should be stored in a cool place.

Legal category POM.

Package quantities Push-through bubble pack containing 28 tablets.

Further information Nil.

Product licence number 0286/0027.

TOPILAR*
TOPILAR* OINTMENT

Presentation Topilar and Topilar Ointment contain fluclorolone acetonide, a topical anti-inflammatory corticosteroid.

Topilar contains Fluclorolone Acetonide BP 0.025% w/w completely dissolved in the specially formulated FAPG cream base (a combination of fatty alcohols and propylene glycol). The FAPG cream base is a white, soft, non-aqueous hydrophilic, semi-solid vehicle with a slight pearly sheen.

Topilar Ointment contains Fluclorolone Acetonide BP 0.025% w/w dissolved in an emollient ointment base.

Uses Topilar and Topilar Ointment are indicated for the treatment of eczema and dermatitis of all types (atopic eczema, photodermatitis, primary irritant and allergic dermatitis), lichen planus, lichen simplex, prurigo nodularis, discoid lupus erythematosus, necrobiosis lipoidica, pretibial myxoedema and erythroderma. They may be useful in the treatment of chronic plaque psoriasis of the palms and soles. However, topical corticosteroids are not generally indicated in psoriasis; see 'Precautions' below.

Dosage and administration *Adults (including the elderly):* A thin smear is applied to the affected areas twice daily. This regimen should be followed until the acute phase has passed. Treatment should be continued for at least one week thereafter with one application daily. The course is completed by a further short period, e.g. two weeks, during which one application is made on alternate days.

Polythene occlusion may be required for difficult cases.

Children: The use of potent topical steroids on children should be avoided if at all possible, but if mild or moderately potent steroids have failed, use of this product should be limited to 5 days and occlusion (including nappies) should not be used.

Contra-indications, warnings, etc
Contra-indications:

(i) Viral, bacterial and fungal infections of the skin.
(ii) Facial rosacea, acne vulgaris, perioral dermatitis, perianal and genital pruritus and napkin eruptions.
(iii) Hypersensitivity to the formulation.

Precautions and warnings: Long-term, continuous, topical steroid therapy can produce atrophic skin changes. Prolonged use of topical steroids on large areas of damaged skin, in flexures and under occlusion, can result in sufficient absorption of the steroid to produce the features of adrenal suppression. If used on children or on the face treatment should be limited to 5 days and occlusion should not be used.

Long-term continuous therapy should be avoided in all patients irrespective of age. Application under occlusion should be restricted to dermatoses involving limited areas.

Topical steroids may be hazardous in psoriasis. When using topical corticosteroids to treat psoriasis there are risks of both rebound relapse following the development of tolerance and of generalised pustular psoriasis. Impairment of the barrier function of the skin may lead to local and systemic toxicity. Careful patient supervision is important.

In the presence of an infection, the use of an appropriate antibacterial, antiviral or antifungal agent should be instituted. If a favourable response does not occur promptly, Topilar or Topilar Ointment should be discontinued until the infection has been adequately controlled.

These preparations are not for ophthalmic use.

Use in pregnancy: There is insufficient evidence of safety in human pregnancy. Topical administration of corticosteroids to pregnant animals can cause abnormalities of fetal development, including cleft palate and intrauterine growth retardation. There may therefore be a very small risk of such effects on the human fetus.

Side-effects: The following local adverse reactions have been reported with topical corticosteroids: burning, itching, irritation, dryness, folliculitis, hypertrichosis, acneiform eruptions, hypopigmentation, perioral dermatitis, allergic contact dermatitis, maceration of the skin, secondary infection, skin atrophy, striae, miliaria.

Pharmaceutical precautions Topilar and Topilar Ointment should be stored in a cool place. The propylene glycol in the FAPG base may separate at temperatures above 35°C. Topilar Ointment may be diluted in white soft paraffin when a weaker preparation is required.

Legal category POM.

Package quantities Topilar and Topilar Ointment are available in tubes of 30 g and 100 g.

Further information Nil.

Product licence numbers

Topilar	0286/0026
Topilar Ointment	0286/5002

URISPAS*

Presentation Each Urispas Tablet contains flavoxate hydrochloride 100 mg. The white, sugar-coated tablets are overprinted with the name URISPAS.

Uses Urispas is indicated for the symptomatic relief of dysuria, urgency, nocturia, vesical suprapubic pain, frequency and incontinence as may occur in cystitis, prostatitis, urethritis, urethrocystitis and urethro-trigonitis.

In addition the preparation is indicated for the relief of vesico-urethral spasms due to catheterisation, cystoscopy or indwelling catheters; prior to cystoscopy or catheterisation; sequelae of surgical intervention of the lower urinary tract.

Urispas is an antispasmodic, selective to the urinary tract. In animal and human studies, Urispas has been shown to have a direct antispasmodic action on smooth muscle fibres. In addition, animal studies have shown Urispas to have analgesic and local anaesthetic properties.

Where evidence of urinary infection is present, appropriate anti-infective therapy should be instituted concomitantly.

Dosage and administration *Adults (including the elderly):* The recommended adult dosage is 2 tablets three times a day for as long as required.

Children: Not recommended for children under 12 years of age.

Contra-indications, warnings, etc
Contra-indications: The following obstructive conditions: pyloric or duodenal obstruction, obstructive intestinal lesions, or ileus, achalasia, gastro-intestinal haemorrhage and obstructive uropathies of the lower urinary tract.

Special precautions: Urispas should be used with caution in patients with suspected glaucoma.

In the event of drowsiness and blurred vision, the patient should not operate a motor vehicle or machinery.

Side-effects: In clinical trials comparing Urispas with other antispasmodic agents, the incidence of side-effects was low. The following adverse reactions have been observed:

Gastro-intestinal: Nausea, vomiting, dry mouth, diarrhoea.

CNS: Vertigo, headache, mental confusion, especially in the elderly, drowsiness, fatigue and nervousness.

Haematologic: Leucopenia (one case which was reversible upon discontinuation of the drug).

Cardiovascular: Tachycardia and palpitation.

Allergic: Urticaria and other dermatoses, eosinophilia and hyperpyrexia.

Ophthalmic: Increased ocular tension, blurred vision, disturbance in eye accommodation.

Renal: Dysuria.

Use in pregnancy and breast feeding: Since there is no evidence as to the drug's safety in human pregnancy, nor is there any evidence from animal work that it is free from hazard, Urispas should be avoided in pregnancy unless there is no safer alternative. It is not known whether flavoxate is excreted in human milk. Because many drugs are excreted in human milk, caution should be exercised when Urispas is administered during breast feeding.

Overdosage: Patients who have taken an overdosage of Urispas should have gastric lavage performed within four hours of the overdosage occurring. If overdosage is extreme, or there is delay in removing the drug from the stomach, administration of a para-sympathomimetic drug should be considered.

Pharmaceutical precautions No special precautions are required.

Legal category POM.

Package quantities Containers of 100.

Further information Nil.

Product licence number 0286/5005.

UTOVLAN*

Presentation Each Utovlan Tablet contains Norethisterone BP 5 mg. The white tablets are marked SYNTEX on one side with a breakline on the other.

Uses At low dosage Utovlan is indicated for dysfunctional uterine bleeding, endometriosis, polymenorrhoea, menorrhagia, metropathia haemorrhagica, postponement of menstruation, and premenstrual syndrome. At high dosage Utovlan is recommended for disseminated carcinoma of the breast.

Dosage and administration
Low dosage
Dysfunctional Uterine Bleeding, Polymenorrhoea, Menorrhagia, Dysmenorrhoea and Metropathia Haemorrhagica: 1 tablet three times daily for 10 days; bleeding usually stops within 48 hours. Withdrawal bleeding resembling true menstruation occurs a few days after the end of treatment. One tablet twice daily, from days 19 to 26 of the two subsequent cycles, should be given to prevent recurrence of the condition.

Endometriosis: 1 tablet three times daily for a minimum treatment period of six months. The dosage should be increased to 4 or 5 tablets a day if spotting occurs. The initial dosage should be resumed when bleeding or spotting stops.

Postponement of menstruation: 1 tablet three times daily, starting three days before the expected onset of menstruation. Menstruation usually follows within three days of finishing the treatment.

Premenstrual syndrome: 1 tablet daily from days 16 to 25 of the menstrual cycle.

High dosage
For disseminated breast carcinoma the starting dose is 8 tablets (40 mg) per day increasing to 12 tablets (60 mg) if no regression is noted.

Contra-indications, warnings, etc
Contra-indications: Pregnancy, disturbance of liver function, history during pregnancy of idiopathic jaundice, severe pruritus, herpes, undiagnosed irregular vaginal bleeding.

Side-effects: These rarely occur at the usual dosage levels of 15 mg per day. Mild nausea has been reported. High dosage treatment, even over long periods, is well tolerated; transitory digestive upsets and jaundice have rarely been reported.

If menstrual bleeding should fail to follow a course of Utovlan, the possibility of pregnancy must be ruled out before a further course is given.

Overdosage: Overdosage may be manifested by nausea, vomiting, breast enlargement and later vaginal bleeding. There is no specific antidote and treatment should be symptomatic.

Gastric lavage may be employed if the overdosage is large and the patient is seen sufficiently early (within four hours).

Pharmaceutical precautions No special precautions.

Legal category POM.

Package quantities Containers of 100 and 1,000 tablets.

Further information Nil.

Product licence number 0286/5007.

**Trade Mark*

Thames Laboratories Ltd

Abbey Road
Wrexham Industrial Estate
Wrexham
Clwyd LL 13 9PW

THAMES LABORATORIES

BIOPLEX*

Presentation White or off-white granules flavoured with peppermint, containing 1% w/w Carbenoxolone Sodium BP. Other ingredients include lactose.

Uses The treatment of mouth ulcers.

Dosage and administration
Adults and children: 2 g of Mouthwash Granules (one sachet) dissolved in 30–50 ml warm water and used as a mouthwash 3 times daily and at night until the ulcers have healed.

Contra-indications, warnings, etc The mouthwash must not be swallowed and, when used as directed, no side-effects have been reported and no contra-indications are anticipated. However, the daily dosage of carbenoxolone (80 mg) in the mouthwash if ingested may, in elderly patients and those suffering from cardiovascular, renal or hepatic disease, cause sodium and water retention, increased blood pressure and hypokalaemia. It is therefore important, particularly in long-term treatment of recurrent ulceration, to warn patients not to swallow the mouthwash.

Overdosage: Problems are not anticipated from the accidental ingestion of a single dose of the mouthwash.

If large quantities of the granules or the mouthwash have been recently ingested the stomach may be emptied by gastric lavage. Serum electrolytes should be monitored and any potassium deficiency remedied by the intravenous route if necessary or by slow-release or effervescent tablets of potassium chloride. Water retention and sodium balance should be corrected by means of a diuretic.

Pharmaceutical precautions Store in a cool dry place.

Legal category POM.

Package quantities Boxes containing of 24 2 g sachets.

Further information Nil.

Product licence number 0181/0029

BRITIAZIM*

Presentation White flat, bevelled edge tablets embossed T on one side and 60 on the other. Each tablet contains 60 mg diltiazem hydrochloride in a modified release formulation. Other ingredients include lactose.

Uses
Actions: Britiazim is a calcium antagonist. It inhibits the slow channel entry of extracellular calcium during membrane depolarisation of cardiac and vascular smooth muscle. The resulting reduction in intracellular calcium modifies myocardial contractility, thus reducing myocardial oxygen demand. This increases exercise capacity. The inhibition of calcium entry into the smooth muscle of vascular tissue causes vasodilatation, particularly of the coronary blood vessels. This increases blood supply to the myocardium and relieves coronary artery spasm.

Indications: For the prophylaxis and treatment of angina pectoris.

Dosage and administration
Adults: The usual dose is one tablet (60 mg) three times daily. However, patient responses may vary and dosage requirements can differ significantly between individual patients. If necessary the dose can be increased to 360 mg daily in divided doses. Higher doses up to 480 mg/day have been used with benefit in some patients especially in unstable angina. There is no evidence of any decrease in efficacy at these high doses. Diltiazem has not been reported to precipitate angina.

Elderly patients with impaired hepatic or renal function: Treatment should be started with one tablet (60 mg) twice daily. Heart rate should be monitored regularly. The dose should not be increased if the heart rate falls below 50 beats per minute.

Children: Not recommended.

Contra-indications, warnings, etc
Contra-indications: Britiazim is contra-indicated in patients with bradycardia, second or third degree heart block or sick sinus syndrome. Britiazim should not be used in pregnant women or women of children-bearing potential.

Drug interactions: When Britiazim is used with a beta-blocker, the dosage of both should be reduced. Britiazim may increase blood levels of beta-blockers which have a low bioavailability.

Britiazim may cause small increases in plasma levels of digitalis.

Side-effects: Possible side effects include bradycardia, ankle oedema and more rarely headache, nausea and skin rash.

Overdosage: If overdosage should occur the patient should be observed in a coronary care unit. It is reported that spontaneous recovery usually occurs.

Pharmaceutical precautions Store in a cool, dry place. Protect from heat, light and moisture.

Legal category POM.

Package quantities Containers of 100 tablets.

Further information There is little information on the pharmacokinetics of diltiazem but it is understood that this substance has a short half-life. Diltiazem is metabolised primarily in the liver. The mean half-life of Britiazim and its metabolites are reported to be 4–6 hours in healthy volunteers.

Product licence number 4408/0023

CHENOFALK*

Presentation White opaque hard gelatin capsules containing 250 mg chenodeoxycholic acid (CDCA). Other ingredients include gluten.

Uses Dissolution of radiolucent gallstones measuring up to 15 mm diameter, as assessed on X-ray films, in patients whose gall bladder opacifies on oral cholecystrography. Chenofalk lowers biliary cholesterol secretion, reduces cholesterol saturation in bile, and facilitates transfer of cholesterol from gallstones to bile.

Dosage and administration The following dose

regime is recommended to provide a daily dosage of 13–17.5 mg CDCA/kg.

Body weight (kg)	*Dose of Chenofalk*	
	Capsules daily (2 doses)	*mg/kg/day*
45–57	3	13.2–16.6
58–75	4	13.3–17.2
76–95	5	13.2–16.5

If doses are unequal the larger dose should be taken in late evening to counteract the rise in biliary cholesterol saturation which occurs in the early hours of the morning.

The late evening dose may usefully be taken with food to help maintain bile flow overnight.

The time required for dissolution of gallstones is likely to range from 6 to 24 months depending on stone size and composition. Follow-up cholecystograms or ultrasound investigation may be useful at six month intervals until the gallstones have disappeared.

Treatment should be continued until two successive cholecystograms and/or ultrasound investigation 4–12 weeks apart have failed to demonstrate gallstones. This is because these techniques do not permit reliable visualisation of stones less than 2 mm diameter.

The likelihood of recurrence of gallstones after dissolution by bile acid treatment has been estimated as up to 50% as 5 years.

The efficacy of Chenofalk in treating radio-opaque or partially radio-opaque gallstones has not yet been tested but these are generally thought to be less soluble than radiolucent stones. Non-cholesterol stones may not be dissolved by bile acids. These account for 10–15% of radiolucent stones.

Obese patients may require a higher dose of Chenofalk for gallstone dissolution, for example up to 20 mg/kg daily.

Contra-indications, warnings, etc Radio-opaque stones; non-functioning gall-bladder; biliary colic; complete or incomplete biliary obstruction; chronic liver disease; liver cirrhosis; gastric or duodenal ulcer; or inflammatory bowel disease.

Warnings: Chenodeoxycholic acid given in long-term studies at doses of 600 mg/kg/day to rats and 1,000 mg/kg/day for mice, induced malignant liver cell tumours in female rats and benign liver cell tumours in female rats and male mice. The clinical significance of these findings is not known.

Drug interactions: The following drugs bind bile acids in vitro and may therefore interfere with the absorption of Chenofalk: cholestyramine, charcoal, colestipol and certain antacids, e.g. aluminium hydroxide.

Hormonal contraceptives may increase the lithogenicity of bile and therefore should not be prescribed concomitantly except at the discretion of the physician who should monitor hepatic function. There is no clinical evidence of any adverse reaction between chenodeoxycholic acid and hormonal contraceptives.

Use in pregnancy: Chenodeoxycholic acid has been shown to cause liver damage in the fetuses of certain species of experimental animals when given in doses equivalent to 5–10 times that normally recommended for use in humans. A toxic metabolite of chenodeoxycholic acid has been found in these species which does not arise in humans. However, if chenodeoxycholic is given to women of childbearing age, measures should be taken to prevent pregnancy. A non-hormonal contraceptive method is indicated. Should pregnancy occur treatment should be immediately discontinued.

Side-effects: Chenodeoxycholic acid is generally well tolerated. In some patients diarrhoea may occur at the start of treatment, but this can usually be controlled by a slight dosage reduction and the dose can subsequently be gradually increased again to an optimum level. Some instances of pruritus and transient rises in liver transaminases have been reported.

Pharmaceutical precautions Store in a cool dry place.

Legal category POM.

Package quantities Chenofalk 250 mg capsules in packs of 60.

Further information Many patients report a reduction in severity and frequency of biliary colic during bile acid treatment.

The following methods of post-dissolution treatment have been used: (a) continued treatment with a reduced dose or (b) intermittent treatment with the standard recommended dose. Another approach is to give no continuing therapy, but to maintain regular monitoring of the patient for the recurrence of gallstones by means of cholecystograms.

Product licence number 4408/0002.

COLGEN* COMPRESS

Presentation A rectangular compress of non-denatured collagen 7 cm × 5 cm, creamy white in colour, presented individually in a double wrapped sachet, sterilised by gamma-irradiation.

Uses As a contact anti-haemorrhagic and haemostat. Intended for use in surgical procedures as a local haemostat, where other haemostat may be ineffective.

Dosage and administration Apply one or more compresses to the site of the haemorrhage.

Contra-indications, warnings, etc The product should not be used in patients sensitive to collagen; no other contra-indications are known.

The product should be used dry; moistening or wetting with saline or thrombin impairs the haemostatic activity of the product. Handle with dry instruments.

Side-effects: No side-effects have been reported in clinical practice.

Pharmaceutical precautions Check the integrity of the sachet before use, do not re-sterilise. Discard any unused portion.

Legal category P.

Package quantities Cartons, each containing 10 individually wrapped compresses.

Further information Nil.

Product licence number 5842/0002.

COLGEN* POWDER

Presentation A plastic screw capped vial, fitted with a sprinkler top, containing approximately 0.4 g non-denatured collagen, creamy white in colour, presented individually in a double wrapped sachet, sterilised by gamma-irradiation.

Uses As a contact anti-haemorrhagic and haemostat. Primarily intended for topical application as a contact anti-haemorrhagic and haemostat.

Dosage and administration Apply the contents of one or more vials to the site of the haemorrhage.

Contra-indications, warnings, etc The product should not be used in patients sensitive to collagen; no other contra-indications are known.

The product should be used dry; moistening or wetting with saline or thrombin impairs the haemostatic activity of the product. Handle with dry instruments.

Side-effects: No side-effects have been reported in clinical practice.

Pharmaceutical precautions Check the integrity of the sachet before use, do not re-sterilise. Discard any unused portion.

Legal category P.

Package quantities Cartons, each containing 10 individually wrapped vials.

Further information Nil.

Product licence number 5842/0001.

PSORIN* OINTMENT

Presentation A sand-coloured ointment containing Dithranol BP (0.11% w/w), Coal Tar BP (1% w/w) and Salicylic Acid BP (1.6% w/w) in a high density emollient vanishing base. Other ingredients are yellow beeswax, white soft paraffin, cod liver oil, lanolin, zinc oxide and corn starch.

Uses The topical treatment of sub-acute and chronic (stable) psoriasis. Dithranol and coal tar both suppress the proliferation of psoriatic tissue. Salicylic acid acts as a keratolytic. The emollient base helps to promote healing of psoriatic areas.

Dosage and administration
Adults children and elderly: Following a 24 hour skin test, a small quantity of Psorin should be applied to the affected areas morning and evening for seven days. If no redness occurs, it may then be applied more liberally twice daily. The ointment should be rubbed well into the skin.

Contra-indications, warnings, etc Psorin should not be used to treat patients with unstable psoriasis which tends to deteriorate in the sunlight and where the skin is hot to the touch and itchy.

Patients sensitive to dithranol, coal tar or salicylic acid should not be treated with Psorin; a 24-hour skin test is recommended prior to treatment.

Contact with the eyes should be avoided.

It is not recommended that users of Psorin should spend long periods in direct sunlight.

Use should be discontinued if irritation of the skin occurs.

There is no evidence to support the safe use of Psorin in pregnant or lactating women.

Pharmaceutical precautions Store in a cool place away from light.

Legal category P.

Package quantities Tubes of 25 g, 50 g and 100 g.

Further information The concentration of both dithranol and coal tar is low in Psorin which helps to minimise problems of staining commonly caused by these substances.

Product licence number 4408/0008

SOLVAZINC*

Presentation White to faintly yellow, flat, effervescent tablet containing zinc sulphate 200 mg, corresponding to 45 mg Zn^{2+}. Other ingredients are sorbitol, carbowax 6000, sodium bicarbonate, citric acid and saccharin sodium.

Uses Zinc deficiency. Severe zinc deficiency has been observed in acrodermatitis enteropathica. Marginal zinc deficiency has been observed in connection with many conditions such as poor wound healing, major surgical procedures, or may be due to inadequate intake of zinc in the diet. Zinc deficiency should be demonstrated before treatment is given.

Dosage and administration
Adults: One tablet dissolved in water once to three times daily after meals.

Children: More than 30 kg: One tablet dissolved in water once to three times daily after meals.

10–30 kg: Half a tablet dissolved in water once to three times daily after meals.

Less than 10 kg: Half a tablet in water once daily after a meal.

Contra-indications, warnings, etc Zinc may inhibit the absorption of concurrently administered tetracyclines; when both are given an interval of at least 3 hours should be allowed.

Accumulation of zinc could occur in cases of renal failure.

Pharmaceutical precautions The effervescent tablets must be protected from moisture. A dessicant capsule is included in the tube cap. The tablets must be dissolved in water before intake.

Legal category P.

Package quantities 30 tablets per metal tube. Packed in cartons of three tubes.

Further information When Solvazinc tablets are dissolved in water, a zinc citrate complex is formed which is well tolerated and causes little of the gastrointestinal irritation usually associated with zinc sulphate preparations.

Product licence number 4408/0004

URSOFALK*

Presentation White opaque hard gelatin capsules containing 250 mg ursodeoxycholic acid (UDCA). Other ingredients include gluten.

Uses Dissolution of radiolucent gallstones measuring up to 15 mm diameter, as assessed on X-ray films in patients whose gall bladder opacifies on oral cholecystrography. Ursofalk lowers biliary cholesterol secretion, reduces cholesterol saturation in bile, and facilitates transfer of cholesterol from gallstones to bile.

Dosage and administration The following dose regime is recommended to provide a daily dosage of 8–12 mg UDCA/kg.

Body weight (kg)	*Dose of Ursofalk*	
	Capsules daily (in 2 doses)	*mg/kg/day*
50–62	2	8.1–10
63–85	3	8.8–11.9
86–120	4	8.3–11.6

If doses are unequal the larger dose should be taken in late evening to counteract the rise in biliary cholesterol saturation which occurs in the early hours of the morning.

The late evening dose may usefully be taken with food to help maintain bile flow overnight.

The time required for dissolution of gallstones is likely to range from 6 to 24 months depending on stone size and composition. Follow-up cholecystograms or ultrasound investigation may be useful at six month intervals until the gallstones have disappeared.

Treatment should be continued until two successive cholecystograms and/or ultrasound investigations 4–12 weeks apart have failed to demonstrate gallstones. This is because these techniques do not permit reliable visualisation of stones less than 2 mm diameter.

The likelihood of reccurrence of gallstones after dissolution by bile acid treatment has been estimated as up to 50% at 5 years.

The efficacy of Ursofalk in treating radio-opaque or partially radio-opaque gallstones has not yet been tested but these are generally thought to be less soluble than radiolucent stones.

Non-cholesterol stones may not be dissolved by bile acids. These account for 10–15% of radiolucent stones.

Obese patients may require a higher dose of Ursofalk for gallstone dissolution, for example up to 15 mg/kg daily.

Contra-indications, warnings, etc Like other bile acids, Ursofalk is absorbed from the intestine, passed to the liver, conjugated and excreted into the bile. Little information is available on the effects and tolerance of

Ursofalk in the presence of hepatic damage or inflammatory bowel disease.

The following drugs bind bile acids in vitro and may therefore interfere with the absorption of Ursofalk: cholestyramine, charcoal, colestipol and certain antacids, e.g. aluminium hydroxide.

The use of Ursofalk in early pregnancy is contra-indicated. (In the rabbit, but not in the rat embryotoxicity has been observed.) A product of this class has been found to be carcinogenic in animals. The relevance of these findings to the clinical use of UDCA has not been established. When treating women of child-bearing potential, non-hormonal or low oestrogen oral contraceptive measures are recommended.

Overdosage: Doses of up to 4 g UDCA/day have been used therapeutically.

The compound is almost entirely excreted in the stool as UDCA or bacterial metabolites. Serious toxicity from a gross overdose is not to be expected although some looseness of the bowels may occur.

Pharmaceutical precautions Store in a cool dry place.

Legal category POM.

Package quantities Ursofalk 250 mg capsules in packs of 60.

Further information Many patients report a reduction in severity and frequency of biliary colic during bile acid treatment.

Product licence number 4408/0001

**Trade Mark*

Tillotts Laboratories
23 Grosvenor Road
St Albans
Hertfordshire AL 1 3AW

CAVED-S* TABLETS

Presentation Brown mottled tablets embossed Caved-S. Each tablet contains:

Deglycyrrhizinated liquorice	380 mg
Aluminium hydroxide gel	100 mg
Magnesium carbonate	200 mg
Sodium bicarbonate	100 mg
Bismuth subnitrate	100 mg

Uses *Action and indications:* For treatment of peptic ulcer.

The main active ingredient of Caved-S is deglycyrrhizinated liquorice, which has peptic ulcer healing and spasmolytic activity and is free from deoxycortone like actions (i.e. does not alter serum levels of sodium, potassium or chloride). Deglycyrrhizinated liquorice primarily enhances the defence mechanism of the mucosa by increasing the number of mucus secreting cells. The cell proliferation rate is also increased. The spasmolytic activity and the action of the added antacids, alleviates gastric distress.

The special deglycyrrhizination process of Caved-liquorice, ensures that side effects, such as oedema, hypertension and hypokalaemia, normally associated with crude liquorice or liquorice derivatives, have been eliminated.

Dosage and administration Oral administration. The tablets should be taken between meals.

Adult dose for gastric ulcer: 2 tablets three times a day.

Adult dose for duodenal ulcer: Increase to 2 tablets six times a day when necessary.

Prophylactic dose: 1 tablet three times a day for gastric ulcer, 2 tablets three times a day for duodenal ulcer.

No dose recommended for children.

Dosage for the elderly: Clinical and metabolic studies have demonstrated that the recommended adult dose for Caved-S is suitable for use in elderly patients.

The tablets should be lightly chewed and swallowed but in exceptional cases of objection to taste the tablets should be broken into a few pieces and then swallowed with a drink of water. No additional antacids need be taken.

Contra-indications, warnings, etc
Precautions; The tablets should be lightly chewed before swallowing.

Prolonged use of Caved-S, in doses higher than recommended for prophylaxis, should be avoided in patients with colostomies.

Caved-S is not recommended for patients with poor renal function or those on dialysis—hyperaluminaemia and/or hypermagnesaemia may result.

Drug interactions: The absorption of a number of drugs is impaired or delayed by antacids. These drugs include digoxin, tetracyclines, ciprofloxacin, rifampicin, chlorpromazine, diflunisal, penicillamine, warfarin, quinidine and anticholingergic drugs.

Concomitant use of alcohol should be avoided.

In the event of combination therapy of Caved-S with sucralfate, it should be noted that sucralfate works most efficiently in acid medium and its efficacy is likely to be impaired by concurrent administration of antacids.

Administration of high doses of aluminium hydroxide antacids to patients on low phosphate diet may lead to phosphate depletion and hypercalcaemia.

Adverse effects: Rare cases of mild diarrhoea have been reported.

The gastro-intestinal absorption of insoluble bismuth compounds such as bismuth subnitrate, taken orally is limited and acute toxic effects are unlikely. However, the effects of acute bismuth intoxication, as observed after intramuscular injection of bismuth salts, include gastrointestinal disturbances, anorexia, headache, malaise, skin reactions, discolourations of mucus membranes and occasionally mild jaundice. If albuminuria or stomatitis occurs, therapy should be immediately withdrawn as serious ulceration stomatitis or renal failure may result.

A reversible neurological syndrome characterised by deterioration of mental ability, confusion, tremor and impaired co-ordination has occurred in colostomy and ileostomy patients after long term oral intake of more than 5 grammes per day of bismuth salts. Intestinal bacteria may reduce bismuth subnitrate to nitrite, causing nitrite poisoning with sufficiently large doses.

Uses in pregnancy and lactation: The safety of Caved-S in pregnancy has not been established. Its use during pregnancy is not recommended unless a physician considers that the benefits outweigh potential risks and no other alternatives are available.

No data on levels of deglycyrrhizinated liquorice (DGL) or bismuth subnitrate in breast milk are available, but in view of the extremely low toxicity of Caved-S, use in lactating mothers would not seem to be a contra-indication.

Treatment of overdosage: No cases of overdosage have been reported. If excessive amounts are ingested, gastric lavage and supportive symptomatic treatment are recommended. In the event of acute bismuth intoxication (see section on Adverse effects for symptoms), hepatic and renal function should be monitored. Severe bismuth intoxication may be treated with dimercaprol. Induction of acidosis by ammonium chloride may promote mobilisation of bismuth from tissue depots.

Pharmaceutical precautions *Storage:* Protect from excessive heat and moisture.

Legal category GSL.

Package quantities Blister packs of 180 tablets (OP).

Further information Nil.

Product licence number 0424/5000R.

CEDOCARD*-5

Presentation Round white tablets, embossed 'CC' reverse side scored, containing 5 mg isosorbide dinitrate.

Uses For the treatment and prophylaxis of angina pectoris and for the long term management of coronary insufficiency.

Cedocard-5 is a coronary vasodilator having a marked anti-anginal effect when administered sublingually as well as orally.

The mode of action depends on the reduced work load following vasodilation and reduced venous return.

Dosage and administration *Sublingual administration:* Adult dose: For treatment of acute attack of angina pectoris – 1 tablet as required.

Oral administration: Adult dose: For prophylaxis of

angina pectoris 1–2 tablets three or four times a day as required.

To prevent nocturnal attacks of angina pectoris – 1–2 tablets before retiring to sleep.

Onset of action sublingually – one to two minutes and duration of up to two hours.

Onset of action orally – 20/30 minutes and duration of four to six hours.

Dosage for the elderly: The dosage of nitrates in cardiovascular disease is usually determined by patient response and stabilisation. Clinical experience has not necessitated alternative advice for use in elderly patients. The pharmacokinetics of isosorbide dinitrate in patients with severe renal failure and liver cirrhosis are similar to those in normal subjects.

No recommended dose for children.

Contra-indications, warnings, etc
Contra-indications: A history of sensitivity to nitrates; severe anaemia; head trauma; cerebral haemorrhage.

Adverse reactions: Cutaneous vasodilation with flushing, transient episodes of dizziness and weakness and other signs of cerebral ischaemia, may occur with postural hypotension.

Interactions: Cedocard-5 may potentiate the effects of antihypertensive agents. The effect of sublingual Cedocard-5 may be diminished when used concurrently with anticholinergic drugs or tricyclic antidepressants due to failure to dissolve sublingual preparations.

Warnings: Side effects include throbbing head and dizziness. Patients are advised not to drive or operate machinery if so affected.

Precautions: Use with caution in patients with hypotension or closed-angle glaucoma. Tolerance to this drug and cross tolerance to other nitrates and nitrites may develop.

Use in pregnancy: No data have been reported which would indicate the possibility of adverse effects resulting from the use of isosorbide dinitrate in pregnancy. Safety in pregnancy, however, has not been established. Isosorbide dinitrate should only be used in pregnancy if, in the opinion of the physician, the possible benefits of treatment outweigh the possible hazards.

Treatment of overdosage: Symptoms and signs of overdosage include vomiting, hypotension, restlessness, syncope, cyanosis, headache, flushing, dizziness, collapse, convulsions and methaemoglobinaemia. Treatment should include emesis or gastric lavage if appropriate. Symptomatic and supportive measures should be provided. Syncope should be treated by keeping the patient in recumbent position. Fluid replacement with or without vasopressors may be indicated. Methaemoglobinaemia should be treated with intravenous injection of 1–4 mg/kg of methylene blue.

Pharmaceutical precautions *Storage:* Protect from heat and moisture.

Legal category P.

Package quantities Containers of 60 and 180.

Further information Cedocard-5 rapidly dissolves after sublingual administration to bring quick relief from acute anginal attack.

If the tablet is swallowed a more prolonged action is achieved for prophylaxis.

Cedocard-5 is more stable than glyceryl trinitrate and has a shelf life of 5 years.

Product licence number 0424/5001R.

CEDOCARD-10*

Presentation Round, rose coloured tablets, scored on one side and imprinted with CC on the other side. Each tablet contains 10 mg isosorbide dinitrate.

Uses For the prophylaxis of angina pectoris.

Cedocard-10 relaxes vascular smooth muscle, dilates coronary vessels, reduces peripheral resistance and venous return, resulting in alteration of myocardial metabolism and reduction of myocardial oxygen demand.

Dosage and administration For oral administration.

Adult dose: 1–3 tablets four times daily. Onset of action 20–30 minutes and duration of four to six hours.

Dosage for the elderly: The dosage of nitrates in cardiovascular disease is usually determined by patient response and stabilisation. Clinical experience has not necessitated alternative advice for use in elderly patients. The pharmacokinetics of isosorbide dinitrate in patients with severe renal failure and liver cirrhosis are similar to those in normal subjects.

There is no recommended dose for children.

Contra-indications, warnings, etc
Contra-indications: A history of sensitivity to the drug.

Precautions: Tolerance and cross-tolerance to other nitrates may occur.

Adverse reactions: Transient headaches, these can usually be controlled by temporary dosage reduction.

Cutaneous vasodilation with flushing, transient episodes of dizziness and weakness and other signs of cerebral ischaemia, may occur with postural hypotension.

Use in pregnancy: No data have been reported which would indicate the possibility of adverse effects resulting from the use of isosorbide dinitrate in pregnancy. Safety in pregnancy, however, has not been established. Isosorbide dinitrate should only be used in pregnancy if, in the opinion of the physician, the possible benefits of treatment outweigh the possible hazards.

Treatment of overdosage: In rare cases of overdosage, gastric lavage is indicated. Passive exercise of the extremities of the recumbent patient will promote venous return.

Pharmaceutical precautions *Storage:* Protect from heat and moisture.

Legal category P.

Package quantity Containers of 100 and 1000 tablets.

Further information Nil.

Product licence number 0424/0015.

CEDOCARD-20*

Presentation Round, flat, bevel-edged blue tablets, scored on one side and imprinted CC on the other side, containing 20 mg isosorbide dinitrate per tablet.

Uses For the treatment of severe congestive heart failure. Cedocard-20 reduces elevated left ventricular filling pressure in patients with congestive heart failure and lowers peripheral resistance, which leads to a reduced after load; therefore, the heart has to perform less work to overcome the peripheral resistance.

For the prophylaxis of angina pectoris.

Dosage and administration Oral administration.

Severe congestive heart failure: After determination of peripheral resistance, arterial and pulmonary pressure, and stroke volume, half a tablet of Cedocard-20 is administered. On the basis of its effect on these parameters, an effective dose of Cedocard-20 is established. This dose can vary between ½ and 2 tablets, and is then administered every 4 hours. Haemodynamic monitoring of the treatment should be carried out.

Angina prophylaxis: One half to 2 tablets three or four times daily.

Dosage for the elderly: The dosage of nitrates in cardiovascular disease is usually determined by patient response and stabilisation. Clinical experience has not necessitated alternative advice for use in elderly patients. The pharmacokinetics of isosorbide dinitrate in patients with severe renal failure and liver cirrhosis are similar to those in normal subjects.
No recommended dose for children.

Contra-indications, warnings, etc
Contra-indications: Hypotension, cardiac shock. A known sensitivity to the drug.

Precautions: Treatment of severe congestive heart failure with Cedocard-20 should be checked haemodynamically, by measuring the intra-arterial pressure, pulmonary artery pressure, stroke volume and peripheral resistance.

Tolerance to this drug and cross tolerance to other nitrates and nitrites may develop. To be used with caution in patients with hypotension or closed-angle glaucoma.

Interactions: Isosorbide Dinitrate may potentiate the effects of antihypertensive agents.

Warnings: Side-effects include throbbing head and dizziness. Patients are advised not to drive or operate machinery if so affected.

Adverse reactions: Transient headaches at the start of therapy; these can usually be controlled by temporary dosage reduction. Less frequently cutaneous vasodilation with flushing, transient episodes of dizziness and weakness and other signs of cerebral ischaemia can occur with postural hypotension.

Use in pregnancy: No data have been reported which would indicate the possibility of adverse effects resulting from the use of isosorbide dinitrate in pregnancy. Safety in pregnancy, however, has not been established. Isosorbide dinitrate should only be used in pregnancy if, in the opinion of the physician, the possible benefits of treatment outweigh the possible hazards.

Treatment of overdosage: Symptoms and signs of overdosage include vomiting, hypotension, restlessness, syncope, cyanosis, headache, flushing, dizziness, collapse, convulsions and methaemoglobinaemia. Treatment should include emesis or gastric lavage if appropriate. Symptomatic and supportive measures should be provided. Syncope should be treated by keeping the patient in recumbent position. Fluid replacement with or without vasopressors may be indicated. Methaemoglobinaemia should be treated with Intravenous injection of 1–4 mg/kg of Methylene Blue.

Pharmaceutical precautions *Storage:* Protect from heat and moisture.

Legal category P.

Package quantities Containers of 100 and 1000 tablets.

Further information Nil.

Product licence number 0424/0008.

CEDOCARD*-40

Presentation Round, green, bevel-edged tablets, scored on one side and imprinted 'CC' on the other side. Each tablet contains 40 mg isosorbide dinitrate.

Uses For the prophylaxis of angina pectoris. Cedocard-40 relaxes vascular smooth muscle, dilates coronary vessels, reduces peripheral resistance and venous return, resulting in alteration of myocardial metabolism and reduction of myocardial oxygen demand.

For the treatment of severe congestive heart failure. Cedocard-40 reduces elevated left ventricular filling pressure in congestive heart failure patients, lowers peripheral resistance, leading to a reduced after-load.

Dosage and administration Oral administration.

For prophylaxis of angina: Adult dose: One tablet three to four times daily.

For congestive heart failure: Doses of 10–40 mg isosorbide dinitrate three or four times daily may be given depending on patient requirement. The optimal individual dose is determined by haemodynamic monitoring. A low dose should be administered at the initiation of treatment in order to assess the required dosage.

Dosage for the elderly: The dosage of nitrates in cardiovascular disease is usually determined by patient response and stabilisation. Clinical experience has not necessitated alternative advice for use in elderly patients. The pharmacokinetics of isosorbide dinitrate in patients with severe renal failure and liver cirrhosis are similar to those in normal subjects.

There is no recommended dose for children.

Contra-indications, warnings, etc
Contra-indications: A history of sensitivity to the drug.

Precautions: Tolerance and cross-tolerance to other nitrates may occur.

Adverse reactions: Transient headaches; these can usually be controlled by temporary dosage reduction.

Cutaneous vasodilation with flushing, transient episodes of dizziness and weakness and other signs of cerebral ischaemia, may occur with postural hypotension.

Use in pregnancy: No data have been reported which would indicate the possibility of adverse effects resulting from the use of isosorbide dinitrate in pregnancy. Safety in pregnancy, however, has not been established. Isosorbide dinitrate should only be used in pregnancy if, in the opinion of the physician, the possible benefits of treatment outweigh the possible hazards.

Treatment of overdosage: In rare cases of overdosage, gastric lavage is indicated. Passive exercise of the extremities of the recumbent patient will promote venous return.

Pharmaceutical precautions *Storage:* Protect from heat and moisture.

Legal category P.

Package quantities Containers of 120 tablets.

Further information Nil.

Product licence number 0424/0067.

CEDOCARD RETARD*-20

Presentation Round yellow sustained-release tablets, embossed CC, SR and scored on reverse side, each containing 20 mg isosorbide dinitrate.

Uses For the prophylaxis of angina pectoris.

The active principle of Cedocard Retard-20 is isosorbide dinitrate which relaxes vascular smooth muscle and produces coronary vasodilation, reduction in peripheral resistance and venous return, alteration of myocardial metabolism, and reduction of the myocardial oxygen demand.

Dosage and administration For oral administration.

Adult dose: One tablet in the morning and 1 tablet before retiring to sleep. Onset of action 20–30 minutes and the duration of action is 10–12 hours.

Dosage for the elderly: The dosage of nitrates in cardiovascular disease is usually determined by patient response and stabilisation. Clinical experience has not necessitated alternative advice for use in elderly patients. The pharmacokinetics of isosorbide dinitrate in patients with severe renal failure and liver cirrhosis are similar to those in normal subjects.

There is no recommended dose for children.

Contra-indications, warnings, etc
Contra-indication: A history of sensitivity to the drug.

Precautions: Tolerance and cross-tolerance to other nitrates may occur.

Adverse reactions: Cutaneous vasodilation with flushing, transient episodes of dizziness and weakness, and other signs of cerebral ischaemia, may occur with postural hypotension.

Use in pregnancy: No data have been reported which would indicate the possibility of adverse effects resulting from the use of isosorbide dinitrate in pregnancy. Safety in pregnancy, however, has not been established. Isosorbide dinitrate should only be used in pregnancy if, in the opinion of the physician, the possible benefits of treatment outweigh the possible hazards.

Treatment of overdosage: In rare cases of overdosage,

gastric lavage is indicated. Passive exercise of the extremities of the recumbent patient will promote venous return.

Pharmaceutical precautions *Storage:* Protect from heat and moisture.

Legal category P.

Package quantities Containers of 60 and 1000 tablets.

Further information Nil.

Product licence number 0424/0007.

CEDOCARD* RETARD-40

Presentation Round, orange/red, sustained-release tablets, embossed CCSR and scored on reverse side, each containing 40 mg isosorbide dinitrate.

Uses For the prophylaxis of angina pectoris. The active principle of Cedocard Retard-40 is isosorbide dinitrate which relaxes vascular smooth muscle and produces coronary vasodilation, reduction in peripheral resistance and venous return, alteration of myocardial metabolism, and reduction of the myocardial oxygen demand.

Dosage and administration For oral administration.

Adult dose: 1–2 tablets in the morning and 1–2 tablets before retiring to sleep. Onset of action is 20–30 minutes and the duration of action is 10–12 hours.

There is no dose recommendation for children.

Contra-indications, warnings, etc
Contra-indications: A history of sensitivity to the drug.

Precautions: Tolerance and cross-tolerance to other nitrates may occur.

Adverse reactions: Headache; cutaneous vasodilation with flushing; transient episodes of dizziness, weakness and other signs of cerebral ischaemia associated with hypotension may occur.

Treatment of overdosage: In rare cases of overdosage, gastric lavage is indicated. Passive exercise of the extremities of the recumbent patient will promote venous return.

Pharmaceutical precautions *Storage:* Protect from heat and moisture.

Legal category P.

Package quantities Containers of 60 tablets (OP).

Further information Nil.

Product licence number 0424/0050.

CEDOCARD* IV

Presentation Clear glass 10 ml ampoules, 50 ml bottles and 100 ml bottles each containing 1 mg/ml isosorbide dinitrate in colourless isotonic saline solution.

Uses For the treatment of unresponsive congestive heart failure, particularly after myocardial infarction.

Cedocard infusion reduces elevated left ventricular filling pressure in patients with congestive heart failure.

For the control of refractory angina pectoris.

Dosage and administration Administration by intravenous infusion only, or as a diluted solution via a syringe pump.

Adult dose: The dosage must be determined individually. Doses of 2–10 mg per hour (33–167 microgram per min) are recommended.

Dosage for the elderly: The dosage of nitrates in cardiovascular disease is usually determined by patient response and stabilisation. Clinical experience has not necessitated alternative advice for use in elderly patients. The pharmacokinetics of isosorbide dinitrate in patients with severe renal failure and liver cirrhosis are similar to those in normal subjects.

There is no recommended dose for children.

Start the infusion with 2 mg/hour and increase progressively according to the evolution of haemodynamic parameters and the clinical condition of the patient. Gradually decrease the concentration of infusion and switch to oral or sublingual isosorbide dinitrate. There should be no abrupt interruption of the infusion except for severe hypotension. Continuous haemodynamic supervision during the infusion is required.

Preparation of solution for infusion: The contents of Cedocard IV must be administered by intravenous infusion only, or as a diluted solution via a syringe pump.

Cedocard IV can be diluted with sodium chloride 0.9% or dextrose injection 5–30%. The diluted solution should be well mixed before administration.

Contra-indications, warnings, etc
Contra-indications: Hypotension, cardiogenic shock.

Precautions: Close supervision of the patient is necessary for safe and optimum treatment. Cedocard IV must be administered by intravenous infusion only, or as a diluted solution via a syringe pump.

If PVC infusion bags (e.g. Travenol Viaflex, Boots Steriflex) and administration sets are used for Cedocard infusion, 15–30% of the drug can be lost by adsorption. There is no loss of active constituent from solution in glass, polyethylene or polybutadiene apparatus.

It is recommended that Cedocard IV is administered using a syringe pump (glass or rigid plastic) with short sections of polyethylene tubing. Alternatively, a polyethylene infusion bag (e.g. Boots Polyfusor) may be used. Polybutadiene administration sets (Avon A2001) are recommended.

Should only PVC infusion bags be available, then it is important to carry out close haemodynamic monitoring of the patient; infusion rate should be modified according to required haemodynamic response. PVC bags of 500 ml volume should be used to minimise adsorption of isosorbide dinitrate.

Adverse reactions: Headache. In the case of an excessive reduction in blood pressure, symptoms of cerebral ischaemia may appear.

Use in pregnancy: No data have been reported which would indicate the possibiity of adverse effects resulting from the use of isosorbide dinitrate in pregnancy. Safety in pregnancy, however, has not been established. Isosorbide dinitrate should only be used in pregnancy if, in the opinion of the physician, the possible benefits of treatment outweigh the possible hazards.

Treatment of overdosage: If arterial systolic blood pressure drops below 90 mm. Hg and if heart rate increases above 10% of its initial value, the infusion should be discontinued to allow a return to pretreatment levels. Passive exercise of the extremities of the recumbent patient will promote venous return.

Pharmaceutical precautions Protect from exposure to excessive heat. The Cedocard dilution for infusion is stable up to 24 hours.

The diluted solution should be well mixed before intravenous administration. Bottles of Cedocard IV should be used once only and discarded. (Do not multidose.)

Legal category POM.

Package quantities Packs of 10 ampoules, 1 × 50 ml bottle and 4 × 100 ml bottles.

Further information Nil.

Product licence number 0424/0012.

COLPERMIN*

Presentation A light blue/dark blue enteric-coated hard gelatin capsule size 1, with a green band between cap and body. Each capsule contains 0.2 ml standardised peppermint oil BP in a sustained-release gel matrix.

Uses For the treatment of symptoms of discomfort and

of abdominal colic and distension experienced by patients with irritable bowel syndrome.

Dosage and administration For oral administration.

Adult dose: One capsule three times a day, taken 30–60 minutes before food with a small quantity of water. The capsules should *not* be taken immediately after food.

The dose may be increased to two capsules, three times a day when discomfort is more severe.

The capsules should be taken until symptoms resolve, usually within one or two weeks. At times when symptoms are more persistent, the capsules can be continued for longer periods of between 2 to 3 months.

Dosage for the elderly: The mode of action of peppermint oil is local rather than systemic. Clinical experience and known pharmacology do not necessitate alternative advice for elderly patients.

Children: There is no experience in the use of these capsules in children under the age of 15 years.

Contra-indications, warnings, etc
Precautions: Patients should be instructed not to break or chew the capsules because this would release the peppermint oil prematurely, possibly causing local irritation of the mouth and oesophagus.

Patients who already suffer from heartburn, sometimes experience an exacerbation of these symptoms when taking the capsule. Treatment should be discontinued in these patients.

Antacids should not be administered at the same time of day as Colpermin.

There are no data available to establish the safety of Colpermin in pregnancy, therefore, it should be used only if, in the opinion of the physician, the possible benefits of treatment outweigh the possible hazards.

Adverse effects: Occasional heartburn, perianal irritation; allergic reactions to menthol, which are rare, and include erythematous skin rash, headache, bradycardia, muscle tremor and ataxia.

Treatment of overdosage: If capsules have been recently ingested, the stomach should be emptied by gastric lavage. Patients should be observed and symptomatic treatment carried out if necessary.

Pharmaceutical precautions Store in a cool place. Avoid direct sunlight.

Legal category P.

Package quantities Containers of 100 capsules.

Further information The enteric-coating of the capsule delays release of the peppermint oil until it reaches the distal small bowel. The oil exerts local effects of colonic relaxation and a fall of intracolonic pressure. The gel matrix ensures both the sustained release of the peppermint oil and its slow transit through the lower bowel.

Product licence number 0424/0009.

MONO-CEDOCARD*-10

Presentation Round orange tablets, embossed 'C MONO C', reverse side scored, containing 10 mg isosorbide-5-mononitrate.

Uses For the prophylaxis of angina pectoris.

Isosorbide Mononitrate, the active constituent of Mono-Cedocard-10, is the major active metabolite of isosorbide dinitrate. It has significant vasodilator activity, the strongest effect being exerted on the venous system and a lesser effect on the arterial circulation. As a consequence, the heart has less work to perform against diminished resistance and therefore oxygen requirement is reduced.

Dosage and administration For oral administration.

Adult dose: One tablet two to three times a day. The tablet should be swallowed (without chewing) with a little water. The daily dosage may be increased to 120 mg if necessary, taken in divided doses. Mono-Cedocard-10 is suitable when lower dosage is used at the start of treatment.

Dosage for the elderly: The dosage of nitrates in cardiovascular disease is usually determined by patient response and stabilisation. Clinical experience has not necessitated alternative advice for use in elderly patients.

There is no dose recommendation for children.

Contra-indications, warnings, etc
Contra-indications: Acute myocardial infarction with low filling pressures. Acute circulatory failure (shock, vascular collapse). When blood pressure is very low. During the first three months of pregnancy.

Warnings/precautions: Some of the effects of alcohol and the action of hypotensive agents may be potentiated by isosorbide dinitrate.

Adverse effects: Generally, no serious adverse effects are to be expected. Headache, dizziness, fatigue, palpitations, orthostatic hypotension and flushing may occur, especially at the beginning of treatment. These reactions can usually be controlled by a temporary dosage reduction.

Patients who experience throbbing headache and dizziness, should be advised not to drive or operate machinery, if so affected.

Use in pregnancy: Mono-Cedocard-10 should not be used in the first trimester of pregnancy. Although no data have been reported which would indicate the possibility of adverse effects resulting from the use of isosorbide mononitrate during pregnancy, safety has not been established. Use of the drug in the second and third trimesters of pregnancy, should only occur if considered essential by the physician.

Treatment of overdosage: Gastric lavage: passive exercise of the extremities of the recumbent patient will promote venous return.

Pharmaceutical precautions
Storage: Protect from heat and moisture.

Legal category P.

Package quantities Packs of 60 tablets (OP).

Further information The plasma half-life of isosorbide mononitrate is 4.2 hours. After oral administration, isosorbide mononitrate is well absorbed, a haemodynamic effect being measurable within 15–20 minutes. In contrast to isosorbide dinitrate, the mononitrate is not subject to first-pass metabolism.

Product licence number 0424/0072.

MONO-CEDOCARD*-20

Presentation Round white tablets, embossed 'MONO CC', reverse side scored, containing 20 mg isosorbide 5-mononitrate.

Uses For the prophylaxis of angina pectoris.

Isosorbide mononitrate, the active constituent of Mono-Cedocard-20, is the major active metabolite of isosorbide dinitrate. It has significant vasodilator activity, the strongest effect being exerted on the venous system and a lesser effect on the arterial circulation. As a consequence, the heart has less work to perform against diminished resistance and therefore oxygen requirement is reduced.

Dosage and administration For oral administration.

Adult dose: One tablet two or three times a day taken after meals. The tablet should be swallowed (without chewing) with a little water. The dosage may be increased to two tablets three times a day.

Dosage for the elderly: The dosage of nitrates in cardiovascular disease is usually determined by patient response and stabilisation. Clinical experience has not necessitated alternative advice for use in elderly patients.

There is no dose recommendation for children.

Contra-indications, warnings, etc
Contra-indications: In acute myocardial infarction with low filling pressures. Acute circulatory failure (shock, vascular collapse). When blood pressure is very low. During the first three months of pregnancy.

Warnings/precautions: Consumption of alcohol should be avoided during treatment, as reaction capacity may be reduced, and the vasodilator activity of isosorbide mononitrate may be enhanced. Symptoms of circulatory collapse can arise in patients already taking ACE inhibitors.

Adverse effects: Generally, no serious adverse effects are to be expected. Headache, dizziness, fatigue, palpitations, orthostatic hypotension and flushing may occur, especially at the beginning of treatment. These reactions can usually be controlled by a temporary dosage reduction.

Treatment of overdosage: Gastric lavage; passive exercise of the extremities of the recumbent patient will promote venous return.

Pharmaceutical precautions
Storage; Protect from heat and moisture.

Legal category P.

Package quantities Packs of 100 tablets (OP).

Further information The plasma half-life of isosorbide mononitrate is 4.2 hours.

After oral administration, isosorbide mononitrate is well absorbed, a haemodynamic effect being measurable within 15–20 minutes. In contrast to isosorbide dinitrate, the mononitrate is not subject to first-pass metabolism.

Product licence number 0424/0040.

MONO-CEDOCARD*-40

Presentation Round white tablets, embossed '40 MONO 40', reverse side scored, containing 40 mg isosorbide 5-mononitrate.

Uses For the prophylaxis of angina pectoris. Isosorbide mononitrate, the active constituent of Mono-Cedocard-40, is the major active metabolite of isosorbide dinitrate. It has significant vasodilator activity, the strongest effect being exerted on the venous system, and a lesser effect on the arterial circulation. As a consequence, the heart has less work to perform against diminished resistance and therefore oxygen requirement is reduced.

Dosage and administration For oral administration.

Adult dose: One tablet twice a day taken after meals. The tablets should be swallowed (without chewing) with a little water.

Dosage for the elderly: The dosage of nitrates in cardiovascular disease is usually determined by patient response and stabilisation. Clinical experience has not necessitated alternative advice for use in elderly patients.

There is no dose recommendation for children.

Contra-indications, warnings, etc
Contra-indications: In acute myocardial infarction with low filling pressures. In acute circulatory failure (shock, vascular collapse). When blood pressure is very low. During the first three months of pregnancy.

Warnings/precautions: Consumption of alcohol should be avoided during treatment, as reaction capacity may be reduced and the vasodilator activity of isosorbide mononitrate may be enhanced.

Adverse effects: Generally, no serious adverse effects are to be expected. Headache, dizziness, fatigue, palpitations, orthostatic hypotension and flushing may occur, especially at the beginning of treatment. These reactions can usually be controlled by a temporary dosage reduction.

Treatment of overdosage: Gastric lavage; passive exercise of the extremities of the recumbent patient will promote venous return.

Pharmaceutical precautions Storage: Protect from heat and moisture.

Legal category P.

Package quantities Packs of 60 tablets (OP).

Further information The plasma half-life of isosorbide mononitrate is 4.2 hours.

After oral administration, isosorbide mononitrate is well absorbed, a haemodynamic effect being measurable within 15–20 minutes. In contrast to isosorbide dinitrate, the mononitrate is not subject to first-pass metabolism.

Product licence number 0424/0054.

MCR-50* (MONO CEDOCARD RETARD-50)

Presentation Hard gelatin slow release capsules containing 50mg isosorbide mononitrate. Each capsule contains white micro pellets which are specially formulated to release 30% of the dose initially and the remaining 70% as a maintenance dose.

Uses For the prophylaxis of angina pectoris.

Dosage and administration The capsules are for oral administration and should be swallowed whole.

Adults: One capsule to be taken in the morning. For patients with higher nitrate requirements the dose may be increased to two capsules daily.

Elderly patients: The dosage of nitrates in cardiovascular disease is usually determined by patient response and stabilisation. Clinical experience has not necessitated alternative advice for use in elderly patients.

Children: The safety and efficacy of MCR-50 in children has yet to be established.

Contra-indications, warnings, etc
Contra-indications: MCR-50 should not be used in cases of acute myocardial infarction with low filling pressures, acute circulatory failure (shock, vascular collapse) or very low pressure.

This product should not be given to patients with a known sensitivity to nitrates.

MCR-50 should not be used in patients with marked anaemia, head trauma, cerebral haemorrhage, severe hypotension or hypovolaemia.

Precautions and warnings: This preparation may give rise to postural hypotension and syncope at higher doses. This may be avoided if treatment is started with the lowest dose possible.

Some of the effects of alcohol and the action of hypotensive agents may be potentiated by this product. MCR-50 should be used with caution in patients who are pre-disposed to closed angle glaucoma.

A headache may occur at the start of the treatment but this usually disappears after a few days.

This product should not be used during pregnancy or lactation unless considered essential by the physician. MCR-50 should be used with caution in patients suffering from hypothyroidism, hypothermia, malnutrition, severe liver or renal disease.

Symptoms of circulatory collapse may arise after the first dose, particularly in patients with labile circulation.

Pharmaceutical precautions None.

Legal category P.

Package quantities MCR-50 is calendar packed in cartons of 28 capsules (OP).

Further information MCR-50 is a long-acting nitrate which is effective for twenty four hours. The total amount of drug is divided into micro pellets which distribute themselves throughout the gastro-intestinal tract, thus giving a controlled and predictable release of isosorbide 5-mononitrate.

Each micro pellet releases 30% of the dose initially and the remaining 70% as a maintenance dose.

Isosorbide mononitrate is the British Approved Name for isosorbide 5-mononitrate.

MCR-50 lacks any significant first pass metabolism providing consistently uniform plasma levels of isosorbide mononitrate thereby laying the foundation for improved clinical response.

Product licence number 0424/0081.

NIFEREX* ELIXIR

Presentation Niferex is a non-ionic polysaccharide-iron complex. The elixir is brown, flavoured, containing the equivalent to 100 mg elemental iron per 5 ml teaspoonful.

Uses Haemopoietic. For the prophylaxis and treatment of uncomplicated iron-deficiency anaemia.

Dosage and administration
Prophylactic dose: 2.5 ml (50 mg elemental iron) elixir daily.

Therapeutic dose: 5 ml (100 mg elemental iron) elixir once or twice daily.

Children 6–12 years: 5 ml (100 mg elemental iron) elixir daily.

Children 2–6 years: 2.5 ml (50 mg elemental iron) elixir daily.

Infants (including premature babies): 1 drop elixir (from paediatric dropper) per 0.45 kg body weight three times a day (5.33 mg elemental iron per kg body weight daily). One drop, from paediatric dropper contains approximately 500 micrograms elemental iron.

Elderly patients: The adult dose is appropriate for elderly patients.

Pregnant patients (during second and third trimester only): 5 ml daily (100 mg elemental iron daily).

Contra-indications, warnings, etc
Contra-indications: Hypersensitivity to the product or ingredients. Haemosiderosis and haemochromatosis. Active peptic ulcer. Repeated blood transfusion. Regional enteritis and ulcerative colitis. Haemolytic anaemias. Known iron overload.

Drug interactions: Iron and tetracyclines interfere with absorption of each other.

Absorption of iron is impaired by penicillamine, antacids, neomycin cholestyramine, tea, eggs or milk.

Chloramphenicol delays plasma clearance of iron and incorporation of iron into red blood cells by interfering with erythropoiesis.

Side-effects: Anorexia, nausea, vomiting, gastro-intestinal discomfort, constipation, diarrhoea, dark stools and allergic reactions. These side-effects may be minimised by taking the elixir after food.

Use in pregnancy and lactation: Administration of drugs during the first trimester of pregnancy requires careful assessment of potential risks versus benefits to be gained and should not be administered unless clearly indicated. For the remainder of the pregnancy, iron therapy may be indicated but only on advice of a physician.

Iron is excreted in breast milk, but not in clinically significant concentrations (about 500 micrograms per day).

Precautions and warnings: Patients post-gastrectomy have poor absorption of iron.

Caution is advised when prescribing iron preparations to individuals with history of peptic ulcer.

Duration of treatment should generally not exceed 3 months *after* correction of anaemia.

Co-existing deficiency of vitamin B_{12} or folic acid should not be ruled out since combined deficiencies produce microcytic blood film.

Iron deficiency in a male patient warrants careful investigation to determine its cause which forms the basis of primary treatment.

Treatment of overdosage: Iron overdosage is an acute emergency requiring urgent medical attention. An acute intake of 75 mg/kg of elemental iron is considered extremely dangerous in young children.

Symptoms: initial symptoms of iron overdosage include, nausea, vomiting, diarrhoea, abdominal pain, haematemesis, rectal bleeding, lethargy and circulatory collapse. Hyperglycaemia and metabolic acidosis may also occur. However, if overdosage is suspected, treatment should be implemented immediately. In severe cases, after a latent phase, relapse may occur after 24–48 hours, manifested by hypotension, coma, hypothermia, hepatocellular necrosis, renal failure, pulmonary oedema, diffuse vascular congestion, coagulopathy and/or convulsions. In many cases, full recovery may be complicated by long-term effects such as hepatic necrosis, toxic encephalitis, CNS damage and pyloric stenosis.

Treatment: The following steps are recommended to minimise or prevent further absorption of the medication.

CHILDREN
1. Administer an emetic such as syrup of ipecac.
2. Emesis should be followed by gastric lavage with desferrioxamine solution (2 g/l). This should then be followed by the installation of desferrioxamine 5 g in 50–100 ml water, to be retained in the stomach. Inducing diarrhoea in children may be dangerous and should not be undertaken in young children. Keep the patient under constant surveillance to detect possible aspiration of vomitus – maintain suction apparatus and standby emergency oxygen in case of need.
3. Severe poisoning: in the presence of shock and/or coma with high serum iron levels (serum iron>90 micromol/l) immediate supportive measures plus i.v. infusion of desferrioxamine should be instituted. Desferrioxamine 15 mg/kg body weight should be administered every hour by slow i.v. infusion to a maximum 80 mg/kg/24 hours.
Warning: hypotension may occur if the infusion rate is too rapid.
4. Less severe poisoning: i.m. desferrioxamine 1 g 4–6 hourly is recommended.
5. Serum iron levels should be monitored throughout.

ADULTS
1. Administer an emetic.
2. Gastric lavage may be necessary to remove drug already released into the stomach. This should be undertaken using a desferrioxamine solution (2 g/l).
Desferrioxamine 5 g in 50–100 ml water should be introduced into the stomach following gastric emptying. Keep the patient under constant surveillance to detect possible aspiration of vomitus; maintain suction apparatus and standby emergency oxygen in case of need.
3. A drink of mannitol or sorbitol should be given to induce small bowel emptying.
4. Severe poisoning: in the presence of shock and/or coma with high serum iron levels (>142 micromol/l) immediate supportive measures plus i.v. infusion of desferrioxamine should be instituted. The recommended dose of desferrioxamine is 5 mg/kg/hour by slow i.v. infusion up to a maximum of 80 mg/kg/24 hours.
Warning: hypotension may occur if the infusion rate is too rapid.
5. Less severe poisoning: i.m. desferrioxamine 50 mg/kg up to a maximum dose of 4 g should be given.
6. Serum iron levels should be monitored throughout.

Pharmaceutical precautions Store in a cool place.

Legal category P.

Package quantities Bottle of 240 ml and paediatric dropper bottle of 30 ml.

Further information Niferex is a highly water-soluble polysaccharide-iron complex which is stable in the range pH 4.5–11.0 and disassociates only after leaving the stomach. The iron is released over a period of one hour, circumventing the nausea associated with sudden doses of free iron. In elixir form, the complex remains in solution and does not precipitate in gastric or duodenal fluid.

Product licence number 0546/5001.

NIFEREX-150*

Presentation Size 1, hard gelatin capsule, brown opaque body and orange opaque cap, imprinted "Central" in white ink on both cap and body, containing 150 mg elemental iron (as polysaccharide-iron complex) per capsule.

Uses Haemopoietic. For the treatment of uncomplicated iron-deficiency anaemia.

Dosage and administration Oral administration.

Adults: One or two capsules daily.

Children: Niferex elixir is recommended for children.

Contra-indications, warnings, etc Niferex-150 capsules should not be given to patients with haemochromatosis and haemosiderosis, and to those with a known hypersensitivity to any of the ingredients.

Use in pregnancy: As with other oral iron preparations, Niferex-150 may be used for prophylaxis against anaemia during pregnancy.

Pharmaceutical precautions Niferex-150 capsules should be protected from heat and moisture.

Legal category P.

Package quantities Packs of 100 capsules in plastic containers.

Further information Polysaccharide-iron complex has relatively low toxicity, and few, if any, of the gastrointestinal side-effects associated with iron therapy, thus permitting full therapeutic dosage (150 to 300 mg elemental iron daily) in a single dose if desirable. There is no staining of teeth and no metallic after taste.

Product licence number 6171/0001.

SALBUVENT* INHALER

Presentation Salbuvent Inhaler: Pressurised aerosol delivering 100 micrograms Salbutamol base BP per metered dose.

Uses Prophylaxis and treatment of bronchospasm associated with asthma, bronchitis and emphysema.

Dosage and administration
Adults: For treatment of acute attack of bronchospasm and for managing intermittent episodes of asthma, one or two inhalations as a single dose. As a prophylactic maintenance therapy, one or two inhalations three or four times a day. For prevention of exercise-induced bronchospasm, two inhalations before exertion.

Children: For treatment of the acute attack of bronchospasm, one inhalation. In the management of episodic asthma or before exercise, one inhalation. As a prophylactic maintenance therapy, one inhalation three or four times a day. This may be increased to two inhalations if necessary.

The Salbuvent Rondo spacer device is recommended to enable patients with difficulty co-ordinating conventional aerosols to derive greater therapeutic benefit.

Patients whose asthma fails to respond to the recommended dosage should be warned not to exceed this dosage, but to consult their doctor.

Dosage for the elderly: As for other adults.

Contra-indications, warnings, etc
Contra-indications: None

Warnings: Patients whose asthma fails to respond to the recommended dosage should be warned not to exceed this dosage but to consult their doctor.

Precautions: Care should be taken if Salbuvent is prescribed for patients with thyrotoxicosis or hypersensitivity to the drug. Potentially serious hypokalaemia may result from $beta_2$ agonist therapy. Particular caution is advised in severe asthma as this effect may be potentiated by concomitant treatment with xanthine derivatives, steroids, diuretics and by hypoxia. It is recommended that serum potassium levels are monitored in such situations.

Adverse effects: Although salbutamol has been shown to increase tremor due to its direct action upon skeletal muscle, it is unlikely that the quantities delivered by Salbuvent Inhaler will produce any adverse effect. Potentially serious hypokalaemia may result from $beta_2$ agonist therapy.

Use in pregnancy: The use of inhaled salbutamol during the first trimester of pregnancy is not recommended unless the clinical need outweighs the risk. Salbuvent Inhaler should not be used for threatened abortion during the first or second trimesters of pregnancy. Salbutamol has been shown to reduce uterine contraction and is used to prevent premature delivery.

Overdosage: Overdosage is characterised by tremor and tachycardia. Administer an alpha adrenergic blocker by intravenous injection, and an oral beta blocking agent. Non-selective beta blocking agents must not be given to asthmatics because of the risk of bronchoconstriction.

Pharmaceutical precautions Salbuvent Inhaler should be stored below 20°C out of direct sunlight, and protected from frost. The canister should not be burnt, broken or punctured, even if thought to be empty.

Legal category POM.

Package quantities Salbuvent Inhaler is supplied as a 200 dose metered aerosol in a single unit pack (OP).

Further information The Salbuvent Rondo spacer device is recommended for patients who have difficulty co-ordinating inhalation with actuation so that they may obtain a more certain delivery of the drug.

Product licence number 4984/0004.

SALBUVENT* INJECTION AND INFUSION

Presentation Salbuvent injection 50 micrograms/ml is a clear, colourless solution containing 50 micrograms Salbutamol BP (as sulphate) per millilitre.

Salbuvent injection 500 micrograms/ml is a clear, colourless solution containing 500 micrograms of Salbutamol BP (as sulphate) per millilitre.

Salbuvent infusion 1000 micrograms/ml is a clear, colourless solution containing 1000 micrograms Salbutamol BP (as sulphate) per millilitre.

Uses Treatment of bronchospasm associated with asthma, emphysema and chronic bronchitis.

For the reduction of uterine contractions in third trimester premature labour.

Dosage and administration
Bronchospasm.
Adults: Salbuvent 0.5 mg/ml and 0.05 mg/ml injection solutions: 8 micrograms per kg to be given intramuscularly or subcutaneously every four hours as necessary.

It may also be given by slow intravenous injection in a dosage of 4 micrograms per kg body weight. Repeat if necessary. It may be given by intravenous infusion at an initial rate of 5 micrograms per minute (as Salbuvent infusion 1 mg/ml). The dosage may then be altered according to the patient's response. Dosages of greater than 20 micrograms per minute should only be employed in exceptional cases.

Children: There are insufficient data to recommend a suitable dosage for children.

Elderly patients: As adult dosage.

Premature labour
Reduce uterine contraction rates by initial infusion rate of 10 micrograms per minute increasing by 5 micrograms per minute every ten minutes until the contraction rate slows. The dosage should then be gradually increased until contractions are stopped. Dosage should not exceed 45 micrograms per minute. The maternal pulse rate must not exceed 140 beats per minute.

After halting uterine contractions maintain dosage for one hour, then administer at half this concentration for a further six hours. Thereafter reduce the level of dosage by 50% decrements at six-hourly intervals. Treatment may be continued orally with Salbuvent tablets.

Contra-indications, warnings, etc Premature labour associated with toxaemia or haemorrhage.

Precautions: Care should be taken if Salbuvent is prescribed for patients with thyrotoxicosis. Potentially serious hypokalaemia may result from $beta_2$ agonist therapy. Particular caution is advised in severe asthma as this effect may be potentiated by concomitant treatment with xanthine derivatives, steroids, diuretics and by hypoxia. It is recommended that serum potassium levels are monitored in such situations.

Use in pregnancy: Caution should be exercised as uterine contractility will be modified under the normal conditions of use. Salbuvent should not be used for threatened abortion during first or second trimester of pregnancy.

Side-effects: Increased physiological tremor and increased heart rate may occur. Potentially serious hypokalaemia may result from $beta_2$ agonist therapy.

Overdosage: Overdosage is characterised by tremor and tachycardia. Administer an alpha-adrenergic blocker by intravenous injection and a beta-blocker per os. Non-selective beta-blockers must not be given to asthmatics because of the risk of bronchoconstriction.

Pharmaceutical precautions Store all three injectable products at or below 25°C. Protect from light.

Salbuvent Infusion 1000 micrograms/ml must be diluted before use. The maximum concentration of Salbuvent Injection for parenteral use is 500 micrograms/ml. Recommended diluents for Salbuvent parenteral preparations are as follows:

Sodium Chloride Injection 0.9% BP
Dextrose Injection 5.0% BP
Sodium Chloride 0.45% and Dextrose 2.5% Injection BP.

Salbuvent parenteral preparations should not be administered in the same syringe or infusion as any other medication.

Legal category POM.

Package quantities Salbuvent Injection 50 micrograms/ml 10 × 5 ml ampoules
Salbuvent Injection 500 micrograms/ml 5 × 1 ml ampoules
Salbuvent Infusion 1000 micrograms/ml 10 × 5 ml ampoules

Product licence numbers
Salbuvent Injection 50 micrograms/ml 4984/0006
Salbuvent Injection 500 micrograms/ml 4984/0007
Salbuvent Infusion 1000 micrograms/ml 4984/0008.

SALBUVENT* RESPIRATOR SOLUTION

Presentation Clear, colourless solution containing 5 mg/ml Salbutamol BP as sulphate, adjusted to pH 3.5. Contains 0.1 mg/ml of benzalkonium chloride as preservative.

Uses For the treatment of bronchospasm associated with asthma (administration by nebulisers or intermittent positive-pressure ventilators).

Dosage and administration
Adults: Salbuvent Respirator Solution may be continually administered as a 1:99 or 1:49 dilution of Salbuvent Respirator Solution to isotonic saline for injection (50–100 micrograms of salbutamol per ml; 1–2 ml solution made up to 100 ml of diluent). Administer as an aerosol, (via a nebuliser) at a rate of one or two milligrams per hour.

For intermittent administration Salbuvent Respirator Solution is administered via a nebuliser or ventilator in 10 mg aliquots three or four times a day.

Children: Children of two to six years should receive a maximum of 0.5 mg per hour or 2.5 mg by intermittent ventilation three or four times a day. Children aged six to twelve should be given 0.5 mg to 1.0 mg per hour or 2.5 mg to 5 mg three or four times a day.

Elderly: The same dosage as in other adults.

Contra-indications, warnings, etc
Pregnancy: The use of inhaled salbutamol during the first trimester of pregnancy is not recommended unless the clinical needs outweigh the risk. Salbuvent should not be used for threatened abortion during the first or second trimester of pregnancy.

Salbutamol has been shown to reduce uterine contractions and is used to prevent premature delivery.

Warning: This product contains benzalkonium chloride which is associated with paradoxical broncho-constriction as an infrequent reaction. Hypotonicity and/or low pH (3.5) may also infrequently be associated with paradoxical bronchospasm.

Precautions: Care should be taken if Salbuvent is prescribed for patients with thyrotoxicosis, hypersensitivity to the drug or in patients known to have received large doses of sympathomimetic drugs. Potentially serious hypokalaemia may result from $beta_2$ agonist therapy. Particular caution is advised in severe asthma as this effect may be potentiated by concomitant treatment with xanthine derivatives, steroids, diuretics and by hypoxia. It is recommended that serum potassium levels are monitored in such situations.

Salbuvent Respirator Solution is to be used with a respirator or nebuliser, only under the direction of a physician. It is not to be injected or administered orally. If patients are using Salbuvent Respirator Solution at home, they should be warned that if the effect of their usual dose is diminished, they should not exceed the recommended dosage, but consult their doctor.

Side-effects: Tremor and slight increase in heart rate may occur. Potentially serious hypokalaemia may result from $beta_2$ agonist therapy.

Overdosage: Overdosage is characterised by tremor and tachycardia. Administer an alpha-adrenergic blocker by intravenous injection and a beta-blocking agent per os. Non-selective beta-blocking agents must not be given to asthmatics because of the risk of bronchospasm.

Pharmaceutical precautions Salbuvent Respirator Solution should be stored below 25°C. Do not expose to strong sunlight. Once the bottle has been opened the contents should be discarded after one month.

Diluted solutions should be discarded after twenty four hours.

Legal category POM.

Package quantities Bottles of 20 ml.

Product licence number 4984/0005.

SALBUVENT* TABLETS AND SYRUP

Presentation
Salbuvent Tablets 2 mg: White, scored tablets containing 2 mg Salbutamol BP as sulphate. Each tablet is marked L42 on one side.

Salbuvent Tablets 4 mg: White, scored tablets containing 4 mg Salbutamol BP as sulphate. Each tablet is marked L47 on one side.

Salbuvent Syrup: Colourless, strawberry flavoured syrup containing 2 mg Salbutamol BP as sulphate in each 5 ml of syrup.

Uses Prophylaxis and treatment of bronchospasm associated with asthma, bronchitis and emphysema.

Dosage and administration Salbuvent Tablets 2 mg, 4 mg and syrup:

Adults: The normal dose for adults is 2–4 mg three or four times a day. The optimal single dose for many patients is 4 mg. If sufficient bronchodilation is not obtained the dose may be raised to a maximum of 32 mg per day, taken as four divided doses.

Elderly patients: In elderly patients and those with known sensitivity to the drug, treatment should be commenced with the lower recommended dosage.

Children:
2 to 6 years: 1–2 mg (2.5–5 ml of syrup or 0.5–1 tablet 2 mg) three to four times a day.
6 to 12 years: 2 mg (5 ml of syrup or 1 tablet 2 mg) three to four times a day.

Contra-indications, warnings, etc
Contra-indications; Premature labour associated with toxaemia or haemorrhage.

Use in pregnancy: Although intravenous salbutamol and occasionally salbutamol tablets are used in the management of uncomplicated labour, Salbuvent presentations should not be used for threatened abortion during the first or second trimesters of pregnancy.

Precautions: Care should be taken if Salbuvent is prescribed for patients with thyrotoxicosis or hypersensitivity to the drug. Potentially serious hypokalaemia may result from $beta_2$ agonist therapy. Particular caution is advised in severe asthma as this effect may be potentiated by concomitant treatment with xanthine derivatives, steroids, diuretics and by hypoxia. It is recommended that serum potassium levels are monitored in such situations.

Side-effects: Increased tremor may occur owing to the direct action of salbutamol upon skeletal muscle. In doses higher than recommended and in hypersensitive patients, peripheral vasodilation and a slight tachycardia have been observed. Headaches (occasional), tenderness and muscle cramps have been reported. Potentially serious hypokalaemia may result from $beta_2$ agonist therapy.

Overdosage: Overdosage is characterised by tremor and tachycardia. Administer an alpha-adrenergic blocker by intravenous injection and a beta-blocking agent per os. Non-selective beta-blocking agents must not be given to asthmatics because of the risk of broncho-constriction.

Pharmaceutical precautions Salbuvent Tablets should be stored below 25°C in a dry place.
Salbuvent Syrup should be stored below 20°C.

Legal category POM.

Package quantities Salbuvent Tablets are available in pack sizes of 90 and 500.
Salbuvent Syrup is available in 150 ml bottles.

Further information Nil.

Product licence numbers
Salbuvent Tablets 2 mg 4984/0001
Salbuvent Tablets 4 mg 4984/0002
Salbuvent Syrup 4984/0003

SULPITIL*

Presentation Round, white tablets with bevelled edge, marked 'L113' on one side and scored on reverse. Each tablet contains 200 mg sulpiride.

Uses For the treatment of acute and chronic schizophrenia. Sulpiride belongs to a new class of neuroleptics, the benzamides. Its pharmacodynamic properties differ from those of the known neuroleptic and antidepressive agents. Sulpiride does not influence the absolute concentrations of serotonin, noradrenaline and dopamine receptors as do the classic neuroleptics, but stimulates dopamine turnover without producing catalepsy or other extrapyramidal symptoms markedly.

Clinical studies have indicated a broad therapeutic usefulness of sulpiride in different areas of mental pathology. The neuroleptic effects of the drug appear, in general, at doses above 400 mg daily. At these dose levels, sulpiride is suitable for the treatment of schizophrenia and similar psychoses.

The sedative effect normally associated with neuroleptics rarely occurs with sulpiride therapy.

Dosage and administration For oral administration.
Adult dose: In mild cases, 400 mg to 800 mg daily given as one or two tablets twice daily. In severe cases, a maximum dosage of 1200 mg to 1800 mg per day may be given. A maintenance dose of 400 mg to 800 mg is recommended.

Children: 3 mg to 5 mg/kg body weight daily is recommended. Clinical experience in children under the age of 14 years is insufficient to permit specific recommendations.

Dosage in the elderly: Elderly patients are usually more sensitive to all centrally-acting drugs, therefore an initial dose of 50 mg to 100 mg is recommended, increasing gradually to the normal adult dose. Reduced dosage should be used in patients with renal impairment.

Contra-indications, warnings, etc
Contra-indications: Phaeochromocytoma. Severe hepatic, renal or blood disease. Alcoholic intoxication and other disorders which depress CNS function.

Warnings and precautions: Sulpiride should be given with caution to patients suffering from extrapyramidal disturbances, hypertension, and to patients with tumours.

Patients should be warned against taking alcohol with sulpiride as reaction capacity may be impaired.

Patients should be advised not to drive or operate machinery if they experience symptoms of slowing of reaction time or loss of concentration.

Increased motor agitation has been reported at high doses in a small number of patients, i.e. in excessively agitated or excited phases of the disease process, this drug may aggravate symptoms. Care should be exercised when hypomania is present. If warranted, reduction in dosage or anti-parkinsonian medication is sufficient.

In long term animal studies with neuroleptic drugs, including sulpiride, an increased incidence of various endocrine tumours, some of which have occasionally been malignant, has been seen in some, but not all, strains of rats and mice studied. The significance of these findings to man is not known. There is no current evidence of an association between neuroleptic use and tumour risk in man.

Although no drug interactions are known, unnecessary polypharmacy should be avoided.

Sulpiride has no epileptogenic, anticholinergic or significant cardiovascular activity.

As with all drugs of which the kidney is the major elimination pathway, the usual precautions should be taken in cases of renal failure.

Adverse effects: Extrapyramidal symptoms can occur: tremor, tardive dyskinesia (rare), and akathisia. Insomnia and other sleep disturbances have been reported.

As is usual with neuroleptic and psychotropic drugs, sulpiride increases serum prolactin levels, sometimes causing gynaecomastia and galactorrhoea.

Sulpiride has a low toxicity and, unlike other neuroleptics, does not produce serious adverse effects on the autonomic nervous system.

Use in pregnancy: Despite the negative results of teratogenicity studies in animals sensitive to the effects of thalidomide, and the lack of teratogenic effects during widespread clinical use in other countries, this drug should not be considered an exception to the general principle of avoiding drug treatment during pregnancy, particularly during the first sixteen weeks, with potential benefits being weighed against possible hazards.

Treatment of overdosage: Overdosage may be treated with alkaline osmotic diuresis and anti-parkinsonian drugs to treat any extrapyramidal symptoms. An overdose of more than 7 g may cause coma which has been observed to last for up to four days and which should receive suitable treatment.

Pharmaceutical precautions Store in a dry place below 25°C.

Legal category POM.

Package quantities Containers of 28 and 112.

Further information Sulpiride can be given to patients with glaucoma. The plasma half-life of sulpiride is 8–9 hours.

Product licence number 0424/0066.

TAMOFEN*

Presentation Round, convex, off-white tablets, scored on one side and marked T10 on the reverse. Each tablet contains 15.2 mg Tamoxifen Citrate BP equivalent to 10 mg tamoxifen.

Uses For the treatment of: (i) Breast cancer; (ii) Anovulatory infertility.

Tamoxifen is an anti-oestrogenic drug which binds to oestrogen receptors preventing the stimulating effects of oestrogen on nucleic acid synthesis. The metabolites of tamoxifen are also anti-oestrogens.

Dosage and administration For oral administration.

(1) *Breast cancer:* One tablet twice a day. This may be increased to two tablets twice a day in unresponsive cases.

(2) *Anovulatory infertility:* In women with regular menstruation but anovular cycles, treatment should start with one tablet twice a day given on the second, third, fourth and fifth days of the menstrual cycle. If treatment is unsuccessful, further courses may be given during subsequent menstrual periods, increasing the dosage to two, and then four tablets, twice daily.

In women with irregular menstruation, treatment can be initiated on any day. If there are no signs of ovulation, a subsequent course of treatment, may be started 45 days later, at the higher dosage level increased as necessary (two or four tablets twice a day). If a patient responds with menstruation then the next course of treatment is started on the second day of the cycle.

Contra-indications, warnings, etc
Contra-indications: Pregnancy.

Precautions: Tamoxifen may be given to pre-menopausal women only after thorough examination has excluded the possibility of pregnancy.

Adverse effects: Side effects are generally mild. The following effects have been reported – hot flushes, mild nausea, mild thrombocytopenia and leucopenia.

Occasionally occurring side effects are vaginal bleeding, pruritus vulvae, skin rash, fluid retention, gastrointestinal pain, pain from metastases and tumour pain.

A number of cases of visual disturbance including corneal changes, cataracts and retinopathy have been described in patients receiving tamoxifen therapy.

In breast cancer patients, temporary reductions in platelet count (usually to 80,000–90,000 but sometimes lower) have been observed during treatment with tamoxifen. The platelet counts have recovered during treatment and no haemorrhagic tendency has been reported.

Hypercalcaemia has been reported in patients with bone metastases.

The adverse reactions can sometimes be controlled by a reduction of dosage.

In a proportion of pre-menopausal women treated for breast cancer, there is a suppression of menstruation; reversible cystic ovarian swelling has occasionally been observed in this group of patients receiving 40 mg of tamoxifen twice a day for short periods.

A small number of endometrial hyperplasia, endometrial polyps and endometrial carcinomas have been reported in association with tamoxifen treatment. A definitive relationship to tamoxifen therapy has not been established.

Treatment of overdosage: Overdosage causes anti-oestrogenic effects. In animals, extremely high doses (over 100 times the recommended daily dose) have caused oestrogenic effects. There is no specific antidote to overdosage, and treatment should therefore be symptomatic.

Pharmaceutical precautions *Storage:* Protect from moisture and heat (store below 25°C).

Legal category POM.

Package quantities Containers of 30 (OP) and 250 tablets.

Further information Maximum plasma levels of tamoxifen occur at 4–7 hours after administration. The elimination half-life is about 7 days. Considerable enterohepatic circulation is a probable reason for the slow elimination.

Product licence number 0424/0031.

TAMOFEN-20*

Presentation Round, convex, off-white tablets marked T20 on one side. Each tablet contains 30.4 mg Tamoxifen Citrate BP equivalent to 20 mg tamoxifen.

Uses For the treatment of: (i) Breast cancer; (ii) anovulatory infertility.

Tamoxifen is an anti-oestrogenic drug which binds to oestrogen receptors preventing the stimulating effects of oestrogen on nucleic acid synthesis. The metabolites of tamoxifen are also anti-oestrogens.

Dosage and administration For oral administration.

(1) *Breast cancer:* One tablet (20 mg) once daily. This may be increased to two tablets (40 mg) once daily in unresponsive cases.

(2) *Anovulatory infertility:* In women with regular menstruation but anovular cycles, treatment should start with one tablet (20 mg) once daily given on the second, third, fourth and fifth days of the menstrual cycle. If treatment is unsuccessful, further courses may be given during subsequent menstrual periods, increasing the dosage to two (40 mg), and then four (80 mg) tablets daily.

In women with irregular menstruation, treatment can be initiated on any day. If there are no signs of ovulation, a subsequent course of treatment, may be started 45 days later, at the higher dosage level increased as necessary (two or four tablets daily). If a patient responds with menstruation then the next course of treatment is started on the second day of the cycle.

Contra-indications, warnings, etc *Contra-indications:* Pregnancy.

Precautions: Tamoxifen may be given to pre-menopausal women only after thorough examination has excluded the possibility of pregnancy.

Adverse effects: Side-effects are generally mild. The following effects have been reported – hot flushes, mild nausea, mild thrombocytopenia and leucopenia.

Occasionally occurring side-effects are vaginal bleeding, pruritus vulvae, skin rash, fluid retention, gastro-intestinal pain, pain from metastases and tumour pain.

A number of cases of visual disturbance including corneal changes, cataracts and retinopathy have been described in patients receiving tamoxifen therapy.

In breast cancer patients, temporary reductions in platelet count (usually to 80,000–90,000 but sometimes lower) have been observed during treatment with tamoxifen. The platelet counts have recovered during treatment and no haemorrhagic tendency has been reported.

Hypercalcaemia has been reported in patients with bone metastases.

The adverse reactions can sometimes be controlled by a reduction of dosage.

In a proportion of pre-menopausal women treated for breast cancer, there is a suppression of menstruation; reversible cystic ovarian swelling has occasionally been observed in this group of patients receiving 40 mg of tamoxifen twice a day for short periods.

A small number of endometrial hyperplasia, endometrial polyps and endometrial carcinomas have been reported in association with tamoxifen treatment. A definitive relationship to tamoxifen therapy has not been established.

Treatment of overdosage: Overdosage causes anti-oestrogenic effects. In animals, extremely high doses (over 100 times the recommended daily dose) have caused oestrogenic effects. There is no specific antidote to overdosage, and treatment should therefore be symptomatic.

Pharmaceutical precautions *Storage:* protect from moisture and heat.

Legal category POM.

Package quantities Containers of 30 (OP)and 250 tablets.

Further information Maximum plasma levels of tamoxifen occur at 4–7 hours after administration. The elimination half-life is about 7 days. Considerable enterohepatic circulation is a probable reason for the slow elimination.

Product licence number 0424/0043.

TAMOFEN-40*

Presentation Round, convex, off white tablets marked T40 on one side. Each tablet contains 60.8 mg Tamoxifen Citrate BP equivalent to 40 mg tamoxifen.

Uses For the treatment of: (1) Breast cancer; (2) anovulatory infertility.

Tamoxifen is an anti-oestrogenic drug which binds to oestrogen receptors preventing the stimulating effects of oestrogen on nucleic acid synthesis. The metabolities of tamoxifen are also anti-oestrogens.

Dosage and administration For oral administration

(1) *Breast cancer:* The daily dose is 20 to 40 mg as a single dose.

(2) *Anovulatory infertility:* In women with regular menstruation but anovular cycles, treatment should start with 20 mg once daily given on the second, third, fourth and fifth days of the menstrual cycle. If treatment is unsuccessful, further courses may be given during subsequent menstruation periods, increasing the dosage to 40 mg, and then to 80 mg daily.

In women with irregular menstruation, treatment can be initiated on any day. If there are no signs of ovulation, a subsequent course of treatment may be started 45 days later, at the higher dosage level increased as necessary (40 mg or 80 mg daily). If a patient responds with menstruation then the next course of treatment is started on the second day of the cycle.

Contra-indications, warnings, etc

Contra-indications: Pregnancy.

Precautions: Tamoxifen may be given to pre-menopausal women only after thorough examination has excluded the possibility of pregnancy.

Adverse effects: Side effects are generally mild. The following effects have been reported – hot flushes, mild nausea, mild thrombocytopenia and leucopenia.

Occasionally occurring side effects are vaginal bleeding, pruritus vulvae, skin rash, fluid retention, gastrointestinal pain, pain from metastases and tumour pain.

A number of cases of visual disturbance including corneal changes, cataracts and retinopathy have been described in patients receiving tamoxifen therapy.

In breast cancer patients, temporary reductions in platelet count (usually to 80,000–90,000 but sometimes lower) have been observed during treatment with tamoxifen. The platelet counts have recovered during treatment and no haemorrhagic tendency has been reported.

Hypercalcaemia has been reported in patients with bone metastases.

The adverse reactions can sometimes be controlled by a reduction of dosage.

In a proportion of pre-menopausal women treated for breast cancer, there is a suppression of menstruation; reversible cystic ovarian swelling has occasionally been observed in this group of patients receiving 40 mg of tamoxifen twice a day for short periods.

A small number of endometrial hyperplasia, endometrial polyps and endometrial carcinomas have been reported in association with tamoxifen treatment. A definitive relationship to tamoxifen therapy has not been established.

Treatment of overdosage: Overdosage causes anti-oestrogenic effects. In animals, extremely high doses (over 100 times the recommended daily dose) have caused oestrogenic effects. There is no specific antidote to overdosage, and treatment should therefore be symptomatic.

Pharmaceutical precautions Protect from moisture and heat. Store below 25°C.

Legal category POM.

Package quantities Containers of 30 tablets (OP).

Further information Maximum plasma levels of tamoxifen occur at 4–7 hours after administration. The elimination half-life is about 7 days. Considerable enterohepatic circulation is a probable reason for the slow elimination.

Product licence number 0424/0055.

**Trade Mark*

Typharm Limited
14 Parkstone Road
Poole
Dorset

CAFADOL*

Presentation Yellow tablet, bisected, reverse side embossed with name 'Cafadol'. Each tablet contains paracetamol 500 mg and caffeine citrate 30 mg.

Uses For analgesia without sedation, mild to moderate pain associated with muscular disorders, tension, headaches, dysmenorrhoea, colds, arthritis and rheumatism.

Dosage and administration
Adult dose: Two tablets every 3–4 hours. As necessary.
Children 5–12 years: One tablet.

Contra-indications, warnings, etc None.

Pharmaceutical precautions Store in cool dry place.

Legal category P.

Package quantities 100.

Further information Nil.

Product licence number 0551/5001.

EFFERCITRATE* TABLETS

Presentation White, circular, flat, effervescent tablets with a slightly rough surface, weighing about 2.7 g, 19 mm in diameter and having the odour of lemon and lime.

Each tablet contains the equivalent of 1.5 g of Potassium Citrate BP and 250 mg Citric Acid BP in a pleasantly flavoured effervescent base.

Uses Effective relief from the symptoms of cystitis.

Dosage and administration *Adults and children over 6 years of age:* Two tablets in a tumblerful of water up to three times daily.

Children Age 1–6 years: One tablet in a tumblerful of water up to three times daily.

Not recommended for children under 1 year.

Sufficient should be given in all cases to render and maintain the urine alkaline.

Contra-indications, warnings, etc A mild diuresis usually follows treatment with Potassium Citrate.

Each tablet contains 13.9 mmol potassium. Care should be taken to prevent hyperkalaemia particularly in patients with impaired renal function.

Side-effects: In common with other potassium salts Effercitrate may give rise to gastric irritation and the tablets must always be taken well diluted with water. Gastric effects may be minimized by giving doses with or after meals.

Overdosage: Hyperkalaemia. Below 6.5 mmol per litre poisoning is minimal, moderate up to 8 mmol per litre and severe above 8 mmol per litre. Absolute toxicity is governed by pH and sodium levels. Hyperkalaemia symptoms, may be transiently controlled with calcium gluconate, glucose or glucose and insulin, sodium bicarbonate or hypertonic sodium infusions, cationic exchange resins, or haemo and peritoneal dialysis. Patients who are digitalized may experience acute digitalis intoxication during potassium removal.

Pharmaceutical precautions Store in a cool dry place below 20°C. Effercitrate tablets are hygroscopic and should be dispensed in the original containers which include a desiccant, and should be kept closed.

Legal category P.

Package quantities Tubes contain 12 tablets.

Further information Each Effercitrate tablet contains the equivalent of the Potassium Citrate and Citric acid content of 5 ml Potassium Citrate Mixture BPC 1973.

Product licence number 0551/0002.

VERACUR* GEL

Presentation Clear, water-miscible gel in a tube. Veracur Gel contains 0.75% w/w formaldehyde.

Uses Treatment of warts, particularly plantar warts (verrucae).

Dosage and administration To be applied directly on to the wart (verruca) and covered with a plaster, twice a day. Remove the outer dead layers with an emery board or pumice stone as the treatment progresses.

Contra-indications, warnings, etc If required protect surrounding skin with a thin film of Vaseline petroleum jelly before application.

For external use only.

Not to be applied to broken skin.

Pharmaceutical precautions Store in cool dry place.

Legal category GSL.

Package quantities 15 g.

Further information Nil.

Product licence number 0551/5000.

**Trade Mark*

Upjohn Limited
Fleming Way
Crawley
West Sussex RH10 2NJ

AMBAXIN*

Presentation White to off-white, rod-shaped, scored tablets with parallel sides and rounded ends, containing 400 mg bacampicillin hydrochloride, one side marked Upjohn, the other side 130 on each side of the score.

Uses Antibacterial. Ambaxin is indicated in the treatment of infections due to susceptible strains of the following: Gram-positive organisms – streptococci (including *Streptococcus faecalis*), pneumococci, non-penicillinase-producing staphylococci, *Clostridia* spp. and *Listeria monocytogenes*. Gram-negative organisms – *Haemophilus influenzae*, meningococci, *Neisseria gonorrhoeae*, *Escherichia coli*, *Proteus mirabilis*, *Shigella* spp. and *Salmonella* spp.

The indications for Ambaxin include the following: sinusitis, tonsillitis, peritonsillitis, acute and chronic bronchitis, pneumonia, skin and soft tissue infections, urinary infections, gonorrhoea, otitis media, pleurisy, acute endometritis, post-operative infections and paratyphoid fever. *In vitro* studies should be performed to determine causative organisms and their susceptibility to Ambaxin. Therapy may be initiated prior to obtaining results of susceptibility testing.

Penetration into the cerebrospinal fluid and brain occurs only when the meninges are inflamed.

Ampicillin, 10 microgram discs, should be used to determine the *in vitro* susceptibility of organisms to Ambaxin.

Ambaxin has no appreciable antibacterial activity itself but is rapidly hydrolysed to ampicillin *in vivo*, thus its antibacterial spectrum is the same as that of ampicillin.

Cross-resistance with cephalosporins and penicillins may occur.

Dosage and administration Ambaxin tablets should be taken with a drink of water. The usual dosage for adults is one 400 mg tablet two or three times a day. Dosage may be doubled in severe infections or where infection is caused by less sensitive pathogens.

The dose for uncomplicated gonorrhoea is 1600 mg plus 1 gram probenecid in a single dose.

Elderly patients: There is no information to suggest that a change in dosage is warranted in the elderly. Side effects do not appear to be more common or severe in elderly patients.

Children: The dosage for children over 5 years is one half a 400 mg tablet (200 mg) three times daily.

Contra-indications, warnings, etc

Contra-indications: A history of previous hypersensitivity to any of the penicillins is a contra-indication.

Warnings and precautions: Bacampacillin is hydrolysed to ampicillin *in vivo* and the possibility of encountering those adverse reactions seen either with ampicillin e.g. antibiotic-associated diarrhoea or, rarely, pseudomembranous colitis or with the penicillins in general, particularly serious hypersensitivity reactions such as anaphylaxis, should be borne in mind. Particular care should be taken in the treatment of atopic individuals.

The possibility of superinfection with mycotic organisms or bacterial pathogens should be kept in mind during therapy. The risk of skin reaction is particularly high in patients with infectious mononucleosis or lymphatic leukaemia. As with other potent antibiotics, periodic assessment of organ system function, including renal, hepatic and haemopoietic, should be made during prolonged therapy.

Side-effects: Ambaxin is well tolerated, side-effects being generally mild and of the usual penicillin type. Interruption of treatment is not usually necessary. The incidence of diarrhoea as a side-effect is lower than that seen with oral ampicillin.

Interactions: Probenecid decreases the renal tubular secretion of ampicillin. Concurrent use with bacampicillin may result in increased and prolonged blood levels of ampicillin.

Ambaxin may be given without regard to time of food intake.

Use in pregnancy and lactation: Safety for use in pregnancy has not been established. Bacampacillin has been reported to appear in breast milk following oral administration.

Overdosage: Since Ambaxin is a penicillin, problems of overdosage are unlikely to be encountered.

Pharmaceutical precautions Store at room temperature (15–25°C).

Legal category POM.

Package quantities Packs of 100 tablets.

Further information Ambaxin is more rapidly absorbed than equimolar amounts of ampicillin, and achieves three times the serum levels of ampicillin in ½ to 1 hour, thereby increasing its penetration into tissues and body fluids such as sinus mucosa and sputum, achieving concentrations greatly exceeding MIC's of susceptible pathogens. Ambaxin may be taken without regard to time of food intake.

Product licence number 0032/0070.

COLESTID*

Presentation Light yellow, tasteless and odourless granules consisting of colestipol hydrochloride with 0.2% colloidal silicon dioxide. Each sachet contains 5 g colestipol hydrochloride.

Uses Ion-exchange resin which lowers plasma cholesterol levels through binding with bile acids in the intestinal lumen.

Colestid is indicated as adjunctive therapy to diet in the management of patients with elevated cholesterol levels who have not responded adequately to diet. It may be used alone or in combination with additional lipid lowering agents. Colestid may elevate serum triglyceride levels when used as sole therapy. This elevation is generally transient but may persist in some individuals.

Although Colestid is effective in all types of hypercholesterolaemia, it is medically most appropriate in patients with Fredrickson's type II hyperlipoproteinaemia.

Dietary therapy specific for the type of hypercholesterolaemia should be the initial treatment of choice. Excess body weight may be an important factor and weight reduction should be attempted prior to drug therapy in the over-weight. The use of drugs should be considered only when reasonable attempts have been made to obtain satisfactory results with non-drug methods. When drug therapy is begun, the patient should be instructed of the importance of adhering to the correct diet.

Dosage and administration
Preparation: Colestid granules should always be taken mixed in a liquid such as orange or tomato juice, water, skimmed milk or non-carbonated beverage. The contents of the sachet should be added to 100 ml or more of the preferred aqueous vehicle and mixed thoroughly until dispersed. Colestid may also be taken in soups or with cereals, pulpy fruits with a high water content or yoghurt.

The recommended initial daily adult dosage of Colestid is 5 grams either once or twice daily.

For adults, Colestid is recommended in doses of 5–30 grams taken as one dose or two divided doses. Initiation of therapy is recommended at 5 grams either once or twice daily with 5 gram increments at one to two month intervals. Appropriate use of lipid profiles including LDL-cholesterol and triglycerides is advised so that optimal, but not excessive doses are used to obtain the desired therapeutic effect on LDL-cholesterol level. If the desired therapeutic effect is not obtained at a dose of 5–30 grams/day with good compliance and acceptable side effects, combined therapy or alternate treatment should be considered. Patients should take other drugs at least one hour before or four hours after Colestid to minimise possible interference with their absorption (see Precautions).

Elderly patients: At present there are no extensive clinical studies with colestipol in patients over the age of 65. Review of available data does not suggest that the elderly are more predisposed to side-effects attributable to colestipol than the general population; however, therapy should be individualised and based on each patient's clinical characteristics and tolerance to the medication.

Contra-indications, warnings, etc
Contra-indications: Colestipol is contra-indicated in individuals who have previously demonstrated hypersensitivity to its use.

Warnings: Before instituting therapy with Colestid, diseases contributing to increased blood cholesterol such as hypothyroidism, diabetes mellitus, nephrotic syndrome, dysproteinaemias and obstructive liver diseases should be looked for and specifically treated.

To avoid accidental inhalation or oesophageal distress, Colestid should not be taken in its dry form.

Safety for use in pregnant women has not been established. The use of Colestid in pregnancy or lactation or by women of childbearing age requires that the potential benefits of treatment be weighed against the possible hazards to the mother and child.

The use of colestipol in children has been limited; however, it does appear to be effective in lowering serum cholesterol in older children and young adults. Dosage and long term safety in children have not been established.

Precautions: In man, Colestid may delay or reduce the absorption of certain concomitant oral drugs (digitalis and its alkaloids, propranolol, chlorothiazide and hydrochlorothiazide, tetracycline hydrochloride, penicillin G). Particular caution should be taken with digitalis preparations since conflicting results have been obtained for the effect of Colestid on the availability of digoxin and digitoxin. Colestid has been shown not to interfere with the absorption of clindamycin, clofibrate, aspirin, tolbutamide, warfarin, methyldopa and phenytoin. The clinical response to concomitant medication should be closely monitored and appropriate adjustments made.

Because it sequesters bile acids, Colestid may interfere with normal fat absorption and thus may alter absorption of fat soluble vitamins such as A, D, E and K. A study in humans found only one patient in whom a prolonged prothombin time was noted. Most studies did not show a decrease in vitamin A, D, or E levels during the administration of Colestid; however, if Colestid is to be given for a long period these vitamin levels should be monitored and supplements given if necessary.

Both clinical usage and animal studies with Colestid have provided no evidence of drug related intestinal neoplasms. Colestid is not mutagenic in the Ames test.

Side-effects: The most common adverse reactions reported with Colestid have been of a functional gastrointestinal nature. The most frequent is constipation, which is usually mild, transient and responsive to the usual adjunctive measures. At times, constipation can be severe and may be accompanied by impaction. As such, haemorrhoids can be aggravated. Less frequent gastrointestinal complaints are abdominal discomfort, belching, flatulence, nausea, vomiting and diarrhoea. Rarely, peptic ulceration and bleeding, cholelithiasis and cholecystitis have been reported, although these are not necessarily drug related.

Transient and modest elevation of SGOT and alkaline phosphatase have been observed. No medical significance is attached to these observed changes. Urticaria and dermatitis have been noted rarely.

Overdosage: No toxic effects due to overdosage have been reported. Should overdosage occur, obstruction of the gastrointestinal tract would be expected to occur. Treatment would be determined by the location and degree of obstruction.

Pharmaceutical precautions None.

Legal category POM.

Package quantities Box containing 30 × 5 gram foil sachets.

Further information Colestid is not absorbed; its action is limited to the lumen of the gastrointestinal tract, and it is passed in the faeces. It binds bile acids in the intestinal lumen and causes them to be excreted in the faeces together with the polymer. When the enterohepatic circulation of bile acids is interrupted, cholesterol conversion to bile acids is enhanced and plasma cholesterol levels are thereby lowered.

Product licence number Foil sachet 0032/0055.

CYTOSAR*

Presentation Off-white, sterile, freeze-dried cake of 100 mg or 500 mg cytarabine (cytosine arabinoside) in a vial.

Uses Cytotoxic. For induction of remission in acute myeloid leukaemia in adults and for other acute leukaemias of adults and children.

Dosage and administration By intravenous infusion or injection, or subcutaneous injection. Water for Injections, 0.9% saline or 5% dextrose should be used for preparing a solution of cytarabine in the vial. When the accompanying diluent (Water for Injections) is used, such solution contains 20 mg/ml (100 mg vial) or 50 mg/ml (500 mg vial) cytarabine.

The physician is reminded that in practice Cytosar has been administered in combination with a variety of other cytotoxic agents using a number of different dosage schedules, and reference to the current literature before commencing treatment is recommended.

Dosage recommendations may be converted from those in terms of bodyweight to those related to surface area by means of nomograms such as are presented in Documenta Geigy.

1. Remission induction:

(a) Continuous treatment:

(i) Rapid injection – 2 mg/kg/day is a judicious starting dose. Administer for 10 days. Obtain daily blood counts. If no antileukaemic effect is noted and there is no apparent toxicity, increase to 4 mg/kg/day and maintain until therapeutic response or toxicity is evident. Almost all patients can be carried to toxicity with these doses.

(ii) 0.5–1.0 mg/kg/day may be given in an infusion of up to 24 hours duration. Results from one-hour infusions have been satisfactory in the majority of patients. After 10 days this initial daily dose may be increased to 2 mg/kg/day subject to toxicity. Continue to toxicity or until remission occurs.

(b) Intermittent treatment:

3–5 mg/kg/day is administered intravenously on each of five consecutive days. After a two to nine-day rest period, a further course is given. Continue until response or toxicity occurs.

The first evidence of marrow improvement has been reported to occur 7–64 days (mean 28 days) after the beginning of therapy.

In general, if a patient shows neither toxicity nor remission after a fair trial, the cautious administration of higher doses is warranted. As a rule patients have been seen to tolerate higher doses when given by rapid intravenous injection as compared with slow infusion. This difference is due to the rapid metabolism of Cytosar and the consequent short duration of action of the high dose.

2. Maintenance therapy: Remissions which have been induced by cytarabine, or by other drugs, may be maintained by intravenous or subcutaneous injection of 1 mg/kg once or twice weekly.

Children: Children appear to tolerate higher doses than adults and, where dose ranges are quoted, the children should receive the higher dose and the adults the lower.

Elderly patients: There is no information to suggest that a change in dosage is warranted in the elderly. Nevertheless, the elderly patient does not tolerate drug toxicity as well as the younger patient, and particular attention should thus be given to drug induced leucopenia, thrombocytopenia and anaemia with appropriate initiation of supportive therapy when indicated.

Contra-indications, warnings, etc

Contra-indications: Therapy with Cytosar should not be considered in patients with pre-existing drug-induced bone marrow suppression, unless the clinician feels that such management offers the most hopeful alternative for the patient. Cytosar should not be used in the management of non-malignant disease, except for immunosuppression.

Warning: Cytosar is a potent bone marrow suppressant. Therapy should be started cautiously in patients with pre-existing drug-induced bone marrow suppression. Patients receiving this drug must be under close medical supervision and, during induction therapy, should have leucocyte and platelet counts performed daily. Bone marrow examinations should be performed frequently after blasts have disappeared from the peripheral blood. Facilities should be available for management of complications, possibly fatal, of bone marrow suppression (infection resulting from granulocytopenia and other impaired body defences, and haemorrhage secondary to thrombocytopenia). One case of anaphylaxis that resulted in acute cardiopulmonary arrest and required resuscitation has been reported. This occurred immediately after the intravenous administration of Cytosar.

Severe and at times fatal CNS, GI and pulmonary toxicity (different from that seen with conventional therapy regimens of Cytosar) has been reported following some experimental Cytosar dose schedules. These reactions include reversible corneal toxicity; cerebral and cerebellar dysfunction, usually reversible; severe gastrointestinal ulceration, including pneumatosis cystoides intestinalis, leading to peritonitis; sepsis and liver abscess; and pulmonary oedema.

Cytosar is known to be teratogenic in some animal species. The use of Cytosar in women who are, or who may become, pregnant should be undertaken only after due consideration of the potential benefits and hazards.

This product should not normally be administered to patients who are pregnant or to mothers who are breast-feeding.

Cytosar has been shown to be carcinogenic in animals. The possibility of a similar effect should be borne in mind when designing the long-term management of the patient.

Precautions: Patients receiving Cytosar must be monitored closely. Frequent platelet and leucocyte counts are mandatory. Suspend or modify therapy when drug-induced marrow depression has resulted in a platelet count under 50,000 or a polymorphonuclear count under 1,000 per cubic mm. Counts of formed elements in the peripheral blood may continue to fall after the drug is stopped and reach lowest values after drug-free intervals of five to seven days. If indicated, restart therapy when definite signs of marrow recovery appear (on successive bone marrow studies). Patients whose drug is withheld until 'normal' peripheral blood values are attained may escape from control.

When intravenous doses are given quickly, patients are frequently nauseated and may vomit for several hours afterwards. This problem tends to be less severe when the drug is infused.

The human liver apparently detoxifies a substantial fraction of an administered dose. Use the drug with caution and at reduced dose in patients whose liver function is poor.

Periodical checks of bone marrow, liver and kidney functions should be performed in patients receiving Cytosar.

The safety of this drug for use in infants is not established.

Like other cytotoxic drugs, Cytosar may induce hyperuricaemia secondary to rapid lysis of neoplastic cells. The clinician should monitor the patient's blood uric acid level and be prepared to use such supportive and pharmacological measures as may be necessary to control this problem.

Side-effects: Adverse reactions seen with cytarabine treatment have included those seen with cytotoxic agents having an effect on bone marrow, such as: leucopenia, thrombocytopenia, anaemia, bone marrow suppression and megaloblastosis. Other side-effects have included: nausea, vomiting, diarrhoea, oral ulceration, hepatic dysfunction. Occasional adverse experiences have been reported as follows: renal dysfunction, anorexia, sepsis, gastro-intestinal haemorrhage, irritation or sepsis at site of injection, neuritis or neurotoxicity, rash, freckling, oesophagitis, skin and mucosal bleeding, chest pain, joint pain and reduction in reticulocytes.

A Cytosar syndrome has been described. It is characterised by fever, myalgia, bone pain, occasionally chest pain, maculopapular rash, conjunctivitis and malaise. It usually occurs 6–12 hours following drug administration. Corticosteroids have been shown to be beneficial in treating or preventing this syndrome. If the symptoms of the syndrome are serious enough to warrant treatment, corticosteroids should be contemplated as well as continuation of therapy with Cytosar.

Overdosage: Cessation of therapy, followed by management of ensuing bone marrow depression including whole blood or platelet transfusion and antibiotics as required.

Pharmaceutical precautions Solutions reconstituted with Water for Injections, 0.9% saline, or 5% dextrose must be used immediately and not stored. Discard any solution in which a slight haze develops.

Legal category POM.

Package quantities Cytosar is supplied as a single vial containing 100 mg or 500 mg cytarabine sterile powder together with an ampoule of diluent (Water for Injections).

Cytosar is also available as 10 × 100 mg vials or 10 × 500 mg vials without diluent.

Further information Published work indicates that Cytosar is effective in the indications for which it is recommended. However, a greater treatment success has been achieved in certain studies by the combination of Cytosar with other agents. The literature should be referred to in determining whether this latter course of action should be considered.

Product licence numbers 0032/5037 (100 mg)
0032/0109 (500 mg)

DALACIN* C

Presentation Hard-filled gelatine capsules (lavender/lavender) containing 75 mg clindamycin (as clindamycin hydrochloride).

Hard-filled gelatine capsules (maroon/lavender) containing 150 mg clindamycin (as clindamycin hydrochloride).

Pink, sucrose-based granules for paediatric suspension, with pineapple flavour. Each 5 ml reconstituted suspension contains 75 mg clindamycin (as clindamycin palmitate hydrochloride).

Uses Antibacterial. Serious infections caused by susceptible Gram-positive organisms, staphylococci (both penicillinase and non-penicillinase producing), streptococci (except *Streptococcus faecalis),* and pneumococci. It is also indicated in serious infections caused by susceptible anaerobic pathogens.

Clindamycin does not penetrate the blood/brain barrier in therapeutically effective quantities.

Dosage and administration Oral. Absorption of Dalacin C is not appreciably modified by the presence of food.

Capsules: *Adults:* Moderately severe infection, 150–300 mg every six hours. Severe infection, 300–450 mg every six hours. Dalacin C Capsules should always be taken with a glass of water.

Paediatric: To each 100 ml bottle of granules add 74 ml purified water and shake.

Children: 3–6 mg/kg every six hours depending on the severity of the infection.

In children under one year or weighing 10 kg or less the minimum recommended dose is 2.5 ml (37.5 mg) every eight hours.

The following paediatric dose regime is recommended as a guide:

Moderately severe infection: 0–11 months: 3.5–9.0 kg: 2.5 ml every eight hours.

1–3 years: 10–15 kg: 2.5 ml every six hours.

4–7 years: 16–25 kg: 5 ml every six hours.

8–12 years: 26–38 kg: 7.5 ml every six hours.

Severe infection: 0–11 months: 3.5–9.0 kg: 2.5 ml every six hours.

1–3 years: 10–15 kg: 5 ml every six hours.

4–7 years: 16–25 kg: 7.5 ml every six hours.

8–12 years: 26–38 kg: 10 ml every six hours.

Adults: Moderately severe infection: 10 ml every six hours. Severe infection: 20 ml every six hours.

Note: In cases of β-haemolytic streptococcal infection, treatment with Dalacin C should continue for at least 10 days to diminish the likelihood of subsequent rheumatic fever or glomerulonephritis.

Elderly patients: The half-life, volume of distribution and clearance, and extent of absorption after administration of clindamycin hydrochloride is not altered by increased age. Analysis of data from clinical studies has not revealed any age-related increase in toxicity. Therefore, dosage requirements in elderly patients should not be influenced by age alone. See *Precautions* for other factors which should be taken into consideration.

Contra-indications, warnings, etc

Contra-indications: Dalacin C is contra-indicated in patients previously found to be hypersensitive to this antibiotic. Although cross-sensitisation to lincomycin has not been demonstrated, it is recommended that Dalacin C is not used in patients who have demonstrated lincomycin sensitivity.

Warnings: Dalacin C should only be used in the treatment of serious infections. In considering the use of the product the practitioner should bear in mind the type of infection and the potential hazard of the diarrhoea which may develop since cases of colitis have been reported. The appearance of marked diarrhoea should be regarded as an indication that the product should be discontinued immediately.

Studies indicate a toxin(s) produced by clostridia (especially *Clostridium difficile)* is the principal direct cause of antibiotic-associated colitis. These studies also indicate that this toxigenic clostridium is usually sensitive *in vitro* to vancomycin. When 125 mg to 500 mg of vancomycin is administered orally four times a day, there is a rapid observed disappearance of the toxin from faecal samples and a coincident clinical recovery from the diarrhoea.

Precautions: Care should be observed in the use of Dalacin C in atopic individuals, e.g. asthma and allergy.

Clindamycin has been shown to have neuromuscular blocking properties that may enhance the action of other neuromuscular blocking agents. Therefore it should be used with caution in patients receiving such agents.

Periodic liver function tests and blood counts should be carried out during prolonged therapy. Such monitoring is also recommended in neonates and infants. Safety and appropriate dosage in infants less than one month old have not been established.

The dosage of Dalacin C may require reduction in patients with renal or hepatic impairment due to prolongation of the serum half-life of the antibiotic.

Safety for use in pregnancy has not yet been established.

Side-effects: In general Dalacin C is well tolerated. Side-effects referable to the gastro-intestinal tract include abdominal discomfort, loose stools or diarrhoea or colitis (see 'Warnings'), nausea or occasional vomiting. Hypersensitivity reactions are rare, even in patients sensitive to penicillins. A low incidence of skin rash has been observed. Dalacin C has been shown to be free from major toxicity; no direct relationship to ototoxicity, nephrotoxicity, neurotoxicity, liver disease or haematopoietic damage has been established.

Overdosage: In cases of overdosage no specific treatment is indicated.

The serum biological half-life of clindamycin is 2.4 hours. Clindamycin cannot be readily removed from the blood by dialysis or peritoneal dialysis.

If an allergic adverse reaction occurs, therapy should be with the usual emergency treatments, including corticosteroids, adrenaline and antihistamines.

Pharmaceutical precautions Dalacin C Paediatric Granules are stable at room temperature (18–25°C) for at least 24 months.

Following reconstitution the paediatric suspension is stable for up to two weeks at room temperature.

Where further dilution is required use purified water.

Legal category POM.

Package quantities 75 mg capsules in packs of 16 and 100.

150 mg capsules in packs of 16, 100 and 500.

Paediatric granules to make 100 ml suspension.

Further information Rapid absorption gives peak serum levels within 45 minutes and such levels exceed the *in vitro* minimum inhibitory concentrations for most sensitive bacteria.

Clindamycin demonstrates cross-resistance with lincomycin. When tested by *in vitro* methods, some staphylococcal strains originally resistant to erythromycin rapidly developed resistance to clindamycin.

Product licence numbers

Dalacin C Capsules 75 mg	0032/5006
Dalacin C Capsules 150 mg	0032/5007
Dalacin C Paediatric	0032/0023

DALACIN* C PHOSPHATE STERILE SOLUTION

Presentation Clear, colourless, sterile solution of clindamycin phosphate containing the equivalent of 150 mg clindamycin base per ml.

Uses Antibacterial. Dalacin C Phosphate is indicated in serious infections caused by susceptible Gram-positive organisms, staphylococci (both penicillinase and non-penicillinase-producing), streptococci (except *Streptococcus faecalis)*, and pneumococci. It is also indicated in serious infections caused by susceptible anaerobic pathogens, such as *Bacteroides* spp., *Fusobacterium* spp., *Propionibacterium* spp., *Peptostreptococcus* spp. and microaerophilic streptococci.

Clindamycin does not penetrate the blood/brain barrier in therapeutically effective quantities.

Dosage and administration Dalacin C Phosphate *must* be diluted prior to IV administration (see Package Insert) and should be infused over at least 10–60 minutes.

Adults: Parenteral (IM or IV administration).

Serious infections: 600 mg–1.2 g/day in two, three or four equal doses.

More severe infections: 1.2–2.7 g/day in two, three or four equal doses.

Single IM injections of greater than 600 mg are not recommended nor administration of more than 1.2 g in a single one-hour infusion.

For more serious infections, these doses may have to be increased. In life-threatening situations doses as high as 4.8 g daily have been given intravenously to adults.

Alternatively, the drug may be administered in the form of a single rapid infusion of the first dose followed by continuous IV infusion.

For details of dilution and infusion rates see package insert.

Children (over 1 month of age): Parenteral (IM or IV administration).

Serious infections: 15–25 mg/kg/day in three or four equal doses.

More severe infections: 25–40 mg/kg/day in three or four equal doses.

In severe infections it is recommended that children be given no less than 300 mg/day regardless of body weight.

Note: In cases of β-haemolytic streptococcal infections, treatment should continue for at least 10 days.

Elderly patients: The half-life, volume of distribution and clearance, and extent of absorption after administration of clindamycin phosphate is not altered by increased age. Analysis of data from clinical studies has not revealed any age related increase in toxicity. Therefore, dosage requirements in elderly patients should not be influenced by age alone. See *Precautions* for other factors which should be taken into consideration.

Contra-indications, warnings, etc

Contra-indications: Dalacin C Phosphate is contra-indicated in patients previously found to be hypersensitive to preparations containing clindamycin. Although cross-sensitisation to lincomycin has not been demonstrated, it is recommended that Dalacin C Phosphate should not be used in patients who have demonstrated lincomycin sensitivity.

Warnings: Dalacin C Phosphate should only be used in the treatment of serious infections. In considering the use of this product the practitioner should bear in mind the type of infection and the potential hazard of the diarrhoea that may develop since cases of colitis have been reported. The appearance of marked diarrhoea should be regarded as an indication that the drug should be discontinued immediately.

Studies indicate a toxin(s) produced by clostridia (especially *Clostridium difficile*) is the principal direct cause of antibiotic-associated colitis. These studies also indicate that this toxigenic clostridium is usually sensitive *in vitro* to vancomycin. When 125 mg to 500 mg of vancomycin is administered orally four times a day, there is a rapid observed disappearance of the toxin from faecal samples and a coincident clinical recovery from the diarrhoea.

Precautions: Care should be observed in the use of Dalacin C Phosphate in atopic individuals, e.g. asthma and allergy.

Periodic liver function tests and blood counts should be carried out during prolonged therapy. Such monitoring is also recommended in neonates and infants. Safety and appropriate dosage in infants less than one month old have not been established.

The dosage of Dalacin C Phosphate may require reduction in patients with renal or hepatic impairment due to prolongation of the serum half-life of the drug.

Safety for use in pregnancy has not yet been established.

Clindamycin has been shown to have neuromuscular blocking properties that may enhance the action of other neuromuscular blocking agents. Therefore, it should be used with caution in patients receiving such agents.

Side-effects: In general Dalacin C Phosphate is well tolerated. Side-effects referable to the gastro-intestinal tract include abdominal discomfort, loose stools, diarrhoea or colitis (see Warnings), nausea or occasional vomiting. Hypersensitivity reactions are rare, even in patients sensitive to penicillins though a few cases of anaphylactoid reactions have been reported. A low incidence of skin rash has been observed.

Jaundice and abnormalities in liver function tests have been observed during clindamycin therapy. Transient neutropenia (leukopenia) and eosinophilia have been reported, and occasional reports of agranulocytosis and thrombocytopenia have been made.

Pain, induration and sterile abscess have been reported after intramuscular injection and thrombophlebitis after intravenous infusion. Reactions can be minimised or avoided by giving deep IM injections and avoiding prolonged use of indwelling intravenous catheters.

Overdosage: In cases of overdosage that may have led to adverse reactions, therapy should be discontinued and the usual emergency treatment, including corticosteroids, adrenaline and antihistamines, instituted. The serum biological half-life of clindamycin is 2.4 hours. Clindamycin cannot be readily removed from the blood by dialysis or peritoneal dialysis.

Pharmaceutical precautions *In vitro* compatibility studies monitored for 24 hours at room temperature using a concentration no greater than 6 mg/ml have demonstrated no inactivation or physical incompatibility with the use of Dalacin C Phosphate in IV solutions containing sodium chloride, glucose or potassium usually used clinically.

The following drugs are physically incompatible with Dalacin C Phosphate: ampicillin, diphenylhydantoin, barbiturates, aminophylline, calcium gluconate and magnesium sulphate.

Compatibility or incompatibility with other drugs besides the ones already mentioned has not been determined.

Store at room temperature. Avoid refrigeration.

Legal category POM.

Package quantities 5 × 2 ml and 5 × 4 ml ampoules.

Further information Biologically inactive clindamycin phosphate is rapidly converted to active clindamycin following injection.

Clindamycin demonstrates cross-resistance with lincomycin. When tested by *in vitro* methods some staphylococcal strains originally resistant to erythromycin rapidly developed resistance to clindamycin.

Product licence number 0032/0042

DALACIN* T TOPICAL SOLUTION

Presentation Clear, colourless solution containing 10 mg/ml clindamycin as clindamycin phosphate. The solution contains isopropyl alcohol, propylene glycol, and water.

Uses Treatment of moderate to severe acne vulgaris.

Dosage and administration Apply a thin film of Dalacin T Topical Solution twice daily to the affected area.

Contra-indications, warnings, etc

Contra-indications: Dalacin T is contra-indicated in

patients previously found to be hypersensitive to this antibiotic. Although cross-sensitisation to lincomycin has not been demonstrated, it is recommended that Dalacin T is not used in patients who have demonstrated lincomycin sensitivity.

Warnings and precautions: Oral and parenteral clindamycin, as well as most other antibiotics, have been associated with severe pseudomembranous colitis. However, post-marketing studies have indicated a very low incidence of colitis with Dalacin T Topical Solution. The physician should, nonetheless, be alert to the development of antibiotic-associated diarrhoea or colitis. If diarrhoea occurs, the product should be discontinued immediately.

Studies indicate a toxin(s) produced by *Clostridium difficile* is the major cause of antibiotic-associated colitis. Colitis is usually characterised by persistent, severe diarrhoea and abdominal cramps. Endoscopic examination may reveal pseudomembranous colitis. Stool culture for *C. difficile* and/or assay for *C. difficile* toxin may be helpful to diagnosis.

Vancomycin is effective in the treatment of antibiotic-associated colitis produced by *C. difficile*. The usual dose is 125–500 mg orally every 6 hours for 7–10 days. Additional supportive medical care may be necessary.

Mild cases of colitis may respond to discontinuance of clindamycin alone. Cholestyramine and colestipol resins have been shown to bind *C. difficile* toxin *in vitro*, and cholestyramine has been effective in the treatment of some mild cases of antibiotic-associated colitis. Cholestyramine resins have been shown to bind vancomycin; therefore, when both cholestyramine and vancomycin are used concurrently, their administration should be separated by at least two hours.

Dalacin T Topical Solution contains an alcohol base which can cause burning and irritation of the eye. In the event of accidental contact with sensitive surfaces (eye, abraded skin, mucous membranes), bathe with copious amounts of cool tap water. The solution has an unpleasant taste and caution should be exercised when applying medication around the mouth.

Safety for use in pregnancy has not been established.

Reproduction studies have been performed in rats and mice using subcutaneous and oral doses of clindamycin ranging from 100 to 600 mg/kg/day and have revealed no evidence of impaired fertility or harm to the foetus due to clindamycin. There are, however, no adequate and well-controlled studies in pregnant women. Because animal reproduction studies are not always predictive of human response, this drug should be used during pregnancy only if clearly needed.

It is not known whether clindamycin is excreted in human milk following use of Dalacin T Topical Solution. However, orally and parenterally administered clindamycin has been reported to appear in breast milk. As a general rule, nursing should not be undertaken while a patient is on a drug since many drugs are excreted in breast milk.

Products containing benzoyl peroxide should not be used concurrently with Dalacin T Topical Solution.

Side-effects: Skin dryness is the most common side effect reported. Other side effects include skin irritation, contact dermititis, oily skin, stinging of the eye, gram-negative folliculitis, gastro-intestinal disturbances, and abdominal pain.

Pharmaceutical precautions Store at room temperature. This product is flammable.

Legal category POM.

Package quantities 30 ml bottle with integral applicator.

Further information Clindamycin *in vitro* inhibited all *Propionibacterium acnes* cultures tested (MIC 0.4 microgram/ml). The mean concentration of clindamycin in comedone samples from patients treated for 4 weeks with Dalacin T was 597 microgram/g.

Product licence number 0032/0135.

DALACIN* T TOPICAL LOTION

Presentation White to off white emulsion containing 10 mg/ml clindamycin as clindamycin phosphate in an aqueous base.

Uses Treatment of acne vulgaris.

Dosage and administration Apply a thin film of Dalacin T Topical Lotion twice daily to the affected area.

Contra-indications, warnings, etc
Contra-indications: Dalacin T is contra-indicated in patients previously found to be hypersensitive to this antibiotic. Although cross-sensitisation to lincomycin has not been demonstrated, it is recommended that Dalacin T is not used in patients who have demonstrated lincomycin sensitivity.

Warnings and precautions: Oral and parenteral clindamycin, as well as most other antibiotics, have been associated with severe pseudomembranous colitis. However, post-marketing studies have indicated a very low incidence of colitis with Dalacin T Solution. The physician should, nonetheless, be alert to the development of antibiotic-associated diarrhoea or colitis. If diarrhoea occurs, the product should be discontinued immediately.

Studies indicate a toxin(s) produced by *Clostridium difficile* is the major cause of antibiotic-associated colitis. Colitis is usually characterised by persistent, severe diarrhoea and abdominal cramps. Endoscopic examination may reveal pseudomembranous colitis. Stool culture for *C. difficile* and/or assay for *C. difficile* toxin may be helpful to diagnosis.

Vancomycin is effective in the treatment of antibiotic-associated colitis produced by *C. difficile*. The usual dose is 125–500 mg orally every 6 hours for 7–10 days. Additional supportive medical care may be necessary.

Mild cases of colitis may respond to discontinuance of clindamycin alone. Cholestyramine and colestipol resins have been shown to bind *C. difficile* toxin *in vitro*, and cholestyramine has been effective in the treatment of some mild cases of antibiotic-associated colitis. Cholestyramine resins have been shown to bind vancomycin; therefore, when both cholestyramine and vancomycin are used concurrently, their administration should be separated by at least two hours.

The lotion has an unpleasant taste and caution should be exercised when applying medication around the mouth.

Safety for use in pregnancy has not been established.

Reproduction studies have been performed in rats and mice using subcutaneous and oral doses of clindamycin ranging from 100 to 600 mg/kg/day and have revealed no evidence of impaired fertility or harm to the foetus due to clindamycin. There are, however, no adequate and well-controlled studies in pregnant women. Because animal reproduction studies are not always predictive of human response, this drug should be used during pregnancy only if clearly needed.

It is not known whether clindamycin is excreted in human milk following use of Dalacin T Topical Lotion. However, orally and parenterally administered clindamycin has been reported to appear in breast milk. As a general rule, nursing should not be undertaken while a patient is on a drug since many drugs are excreted in human milk.

Side-effects: Adverse reactions reported in clinical trials have been minor and of a similar incidence to placebo.

Pharmaceutical precautions Store at room temperature.

Legal category POM.

Package quantities 30 ml bottles with dispensing top.

Further information Dalacin T Topical Lotion does not contain alcohol. It is non-drying and particularly useful for those with dry skins or who live in cold climates.

Product licence number 0032/0156.

DEPO-MEDRONE*

Presentation White, sterile aqueous suspension for injection containing 40 mg per ml methylprednisolone acetate.

Uses Depo-Medrone may be used locally or systemically, particularly where oral therapy is not feasible.

Depo-Medrone may be used by any of the following routes: intramuscular, intra-articular, periarticular, intrabursal, intralesional or into the tendon sheath. It *must not* be used by the intrathecal or intravenous routes (see Contra-indications).

Intramuscular administration

1. *Rheumatic disorders:* Rheumatoid arthritis.
2. *Collagen diseases/arteritis:* Systemic lupus erythematosus.
3. *Dermatological diseases:* Severe erythema multiforme (Stevens–Johnson syndrome).
4. *Allergic states:* Bronchial asthma; severe seasonal and perennial allergic rhinitis; drug hypersentivity reactions; angioneurotic oedema.
5. *Gastro-intestinal diseases:* Ulcerative colitis; Crohn's disease.
6. *Respiratory diseases:* Fulminating or disseminated tuberculosis (with appropriate anti-tuberculous chemotherapy); aspiration of gastric contents.
7. *Miscellaneous:* TB meningitis (with appropriate antituberculous chemotherapy).

Intra-articular administration: Rheumatoid arthritis; osteoarthritis with an inflammatory component.

Soft tissue administration (intrabursal, periarticular, into tendon sheath): Synovitis not associated with infection; epicondylitis; tenosynovitis; plantar fasciitis; bursitis.

Intralesional: Keloids; localised lichen planus; localised lichen simplex; granuloma annulare; discoid lupus erythematosus; alopecia areata.

Dosage and administration Depo-Medrone should not be mixed with any other suspending agent or solution. Parenteral drug products should be inspected visually for particulate matter and discoloration prior to administration, whenever suspension and container permit. Depo-Medrone may be used by any of the following routes: intramuscular, intra-articular, periarticular, intrabursal, intralesional and into the tendon sheath. It must not be used by the intrathecal or intravenous routes.

Depo-Medrone vials are intended for single dose use only.

Intramuscular – for sustained systemic effect:

Allergic conditions (severe seasonal and perennial allergic rhinitis, asthma, drug reactions), 80–120 mg (2–3 ml).

Dermatological conditions, 40–120 mg (1–3 ml).

Rheumatic disorders and Collagen diseases (rheumatoid arthritis, SLE), 40–120 mg (1–3 ml) per week.

Dosage must be individualised and depends on the condition being treated and its severity.

Note: Depo-Medrone is not intended for the prophylaxis of severe seasonal and perennial allergic rhinitis or other seasonal allergies and should be administered only when symptoms are present.

The frequency of intramuscular injections should be determined by the duration of clinical response.

In the case of seasonal allergic rhinitis a single injection is frequently sufficient. If necessary, however, a second injection may be given after two to three weeks.

On average the effect of a single 2 ml (80 mg) injection may be expected to last approximately two weeks.

Intra-articular: Rheumatoid arthritis, osteo-arthritis. The dose of Depo-Medrone depends upon the size of the joint and the severity of the condition. Repeated injections, if needed, may be given at intervals of one to five or more weeks depending upon the degree of relief obtained from the initial injection. A suggested dosage guide is: large joint (knee, ankle, shoulder), 20–80 mg (0.5–2 ml); medium joint (elbow, wrist), 10–40 mg (0.25–1 ml); small joint (metacarpophalangeal, interphalangeal, sternoclavicular, acromioclavicular), 4–10 mg (0.1–0.25 ml).

Intrabursal: Subdeltoid bursitis, prepatellar bursitis, olecranon bursitis. For administration directly into bursae, 4–30 mg (0.1–0.75 ml). In most cases, repeat injections are not needed.

Intralesional: Keloids, localised lichen planus, localised lichen simplex, granuloma annulare, alopecia areata, and discoid lupus erythematosus. For administration directly into the lesion for local effect in dermatological conditions, 20–60 mg (0.5–1.5 ml). For large lesions, the dose may be distributed by repeated local injections of 20–40 mg (0.5–1 ml). One to four injections are usually employed. Care should be taken to avoid injection of sufficient material to cause blanching, since this may be followed by a small slough.

Periarticular: Epicondylitis. Infiltrate 4–30 mg (0.1–0.75 ml) into the affected area.

Into the tendon sheath: Tenosynovitis, epicondylitis. For administration directly into the tendon sheath, 4–30 mg (0.1–0.75 ml). In recurrent or chronic conditions, repeat injections may be necessary.

Special precautions should be observed when administering Depo-Medrone. Intramuscular injections should be made deeply into the gluteal muscles. The usual technique of aspirating prior to injection should be employed to avoid intravascular administration. Doses recommended for intramuscular injection must not be administered superficially or subcutaneously.

Intra-articular injections should be made using precise, anatomical localisation into the synovial space of the joint involved. The injection site for each joint is determined by that location where the synovial cavity is most superficial and most free of large vessels and nerves. Suitable sites for intra-articular injection are the knee, ankle, wrist, elbow, shoulder, phalangeal and hip joints. The spinal joints, unstable joints and those devoid of synovial space are not suitable. Treatment failures are most frequently the result of failure to enter the joint space. Intra-articular injections should be made with care as follows; ensuring correct positioning of the needle into the synovial space and aspirating a few drops of joint fluid. The aspirating syringe should then be replaced by another containing Depo-Medrone. To ensure position of the needle synovial fluid should be aspirated and the injection made. After injection the joint is moved slightly to aid mixing of the synovial fluid and the suspension. Subsequent to therapy care should be taken for the patient not to overuse the joint in which benefit has been obtained. Negligence in this matter may permit an increase in joint deterioration that will more than offset the beneficial effects of the steroid.

Intrabursal injections should be made as follows: the area around the injection site is prepared in a sterile way and a wheal at the site made with 1 per cent procaine hydrochloride solution. A 20 to 24 gauge needle attached to a dry syringe is inserted into the bursa and the fluid aspirated. The needle is left in place and the aspirating syringe changed for a small syringe containing the desired dose. After injection, the needle is withdrawn and a small dressing applied. In the treatment of tenosynovitis care should be taken to inject Depo-Medrone into the tendon sheath rather than into the substance of the tendon. Due to the absence of a true tendon sheath, the Achilles tendon should not be injected with Depo-Medrone.

Children: Dosage may be reduced for infants and children but should be governed more by the severity of the condition and response of the patient, than by age or size.

Elderly patients: When used according to instructions, there is no information to suggest that a change in dosage is warranted in the elderly. However for prolonged treatment the serious consequences of corticosteroid side-effects should be taken into consideration for elderly patients.

Contra-indications, warnings, etc

Contra-indications: The usual contra-indications to the

systemic or local use of corticosteroids should be observed. These include; known hypersensitivity to components and in systemic fungal infections. Immunisation procedures should not be undertaken in patients who are on corticosteroids, especially on high doses, due to the possibility of neurological complications and lack of antibody response.

Due to its potential for neurotoxicity, Depo-Medrone *must not* be given by the intrathecal route. In addition, as the product is a suspension it must not be given by the intravenous route.

Warnings: Corticosteroids may mask some signs of infection, and new infections may appear during their use. There may be decreased resistance and inability to localise infection when corticosteroids are used.

Depo-Medrone vials are intended for single dose use only. Any multidose use of the product may lead to contamination.

While crystals of adrenal steroids in the dermis suppress inflammatory reactions, their presence may cause disintegration of the cellular elements and physiochemical changes in the ground substance of the connective tissue. The resultant infrequently occurring dermal and/or subdermal changes may form depressions in the skin at the injection site. The degree to which this reaction occurs will vary with the amount of adrenal steroid injected. Regeneration is usually complete within a few months or after all crystals of the adrenal steroid have been absorbed. In order to minimise the incidence of dermal and subdermal atrophy, care must be exercised not to exceed recommended doses in injections. Multiple small injections into the area of the lesion should be made whenever possible. The technique of intra-articular and intramuscular injection should include precautions against injection or leakage into the dermis. Injection into the deltoid muscle should be avoided because of a high incidence of subcutaneous atrophy.

Depo-Medrone is not recommended for epidural, intranasal, intraocular, or any other unapproved route of administration. See Side-effects section for details of side-effects reported from some non-recommended routes of administration.

Due to the absence of a true tendon sheath, the Achilles tendon should not be injected with Depo-Medrone.

Intra-articular corticosteroids are associated with a substantially increased risk of inflammatory response in the joint, particularly bacterial infection introduced with the injection. Charcot like arthropathies have been reported particularly after repeated injections. Appropriate examination of any joint fluid present is necessary to exclude any bacterial infection, prior to injection.

In patients on corticosteroid therapy subjected to unusual stress, increased dosage of rapidly acting corticosteroids before, during and after the stressful situation is indicated.

Prolonged use of corticosteroids may produce posterior subcapsular cateracts, glaucoma with possible damage to the optic nerves, and may enhance the establishment of secondary ocular infections due to fungi or viruses.

The use of Depo-Medrone in active tuberculosis should be restricted to those cases of fulminating or disseminated tuberculosis in which the corticosteroid is used for the management of the disease in conjunction with appropriate antituberculous regimen. If corticosteroids are indicated in patients with latent tuberculosis or tuberculin reactivity, close observation is necessary as reactivation of the disease may occur. During prolonged corticosteroid therapy, these patients should receive chemoprophylaxis.

Because rare instances of anaphylactic reactions have occurred in patients receiving parenteral corticosteroid therapy, appropriate precautionary measures should be taken prior to administration, especially when the patient has a history of allergy to any drug.

Allergic skin reactions have been reported apparently related to the excipients in the formulation. Rarely has skin testing demonstrated a reaction to methylprednisolone acetate, per se.

Following a single dose of Depo-Medrone, plasma cortisol levels are reduced and there is evidence of hypothalamic–pituitary–adrenal (HPA) axis suppression as judged by Synacthen test or insulin induced hypoglycaemic response. This suppression lasts for a variable period of up to 4 weeks. The amount and duration of HPA axis suppression is generally proportional to the dose of methylprednisolone administered and the length of therapy, although there is wide individual variation. Multiple doses would therefore be expected to produce greater and more prolonged suppression. The usual dynamic tests of HPA axis function can be used to diagnose evidence of impaired activity (e.g. Synacthen test).

Systemic absorption of methylprednisolone occurs following intra-articular injection of Depo-Medrone. Systemic as well as local effects can therefore be expected.

Precautions: Depo-Medrone should be used with caution in the presence of diabetes, osteoporosis, chronic psychotic reactions, glaucoma, previous steroid myopathy, peptic ulceration, epilepsy, predisposition to thrombophlebitis, hypertension, congestive heart failure, renal insufficiency, infection, non-specific ulcerative colitis if there is a probability of impending perforation, abscess or other pyogenic infection, and in patients with ocular herpes simplex for fear of corneal perforation.

Psychic derangements may appear when corticosteroids are used, ranging from euphoria, insomnia, mood swings, personality changes, and severe depression to frank psychotic manifestations. Also, existing emotional instability or psychotic tendencies may be aggravated by corticosteroids.

Intralesional doses should not be placed too superficially, particularly in easily visible sites in patients with deeply pigmented skins, since there have been rare reports of subcutaneous atrophy and depigmentation.

No evidence exists showing that corticosteroids are carcinogenic or mutagenic.

The following additional precautions apply for parenteral corticosteroids: Following intra-articular injection, the occurrence of a marked increase in pain accompanied by local swelling, further restriction of joint motion, fever, and malaise are suggestive of septic arthritis. If this complication occurs and the diagnosis of sepsis is confirmed, appropriate antimicrobial therapy should be instituted.

Local injection of a steroid into a previously infected joint is to be avoided.

Corticosteroids should not be injected into unstable joints.

Sterile technique is necessary to prevent infections or contamination.

The slower rate of absorption by intramuscular administration should be recognised.

Use in pregnancy and lactation: The use of corticosteroids, in general, during pregnancy involves balancing the clinical benefit against the possible risks. There is inadequate evidence of safety in human pregnancy and there may be a very small risk of cleft palate and intrauterine growth retardation in the foetus: there is evidence of harmful effects on pregnancy in animals. Also neonates of mothers who received such therapy during pregnancy should be observed for signs of hypoadrenalism and appropriate measures instituted if such signs exist.

Because prednisolone is excreted in breast milk, it is reasonable to assume that all corticosteroids are. No specific data are known for methylprednisolone acetate. Therefore, the use of corticosteroids in pregnancy, nursing mothers and women of childbearing potential requires that the possible benefits of the drug be weighed against the potential hazards to the mother, embryo or foetus.

Use in children: Corticosteroids cause growth retardation in infancy, childhood and adolescence. Treatment should be limited to the minimum dosage for the shortest possible time.

Side-effects: Side-effects associated with the use of corticosteroids may be observed, including:

Gastro-intestinal: Dyspepsia, peptic ulceration with perforation and haemorrhage, abdominal distension, oesophageal ulceration, oesophageal candidiasis, acute pancreatitis, perforation of bowel.

Musculoskeletal: Proximal myopathy, osteoporosis, vertebral and long bone fractures, avascular osteonecrosis, tendon rupture.

Fluid and electrolyte disturbance: Sodium and water retention, hypertension, hypokalaemic alkalosis, congestive heart failure in susceptible patients, potassium loss.

Dermatological: Impaired healing, skin atrophy, bruising, striae, telangiectasia, acne, may suppress reactions to skin tests.

Endocrine/metabolic: Suppression of the hypothalamo-pituitary-adrenal axis, growth suppression in childhood and adolescence, menstrual irregularity and amenorrhoea. Cushingoid facies, hirsutism, weight gain, impaired carbohydrate tolerance with increased requirement for antidiabetic therapy, negative nitrogen balance.

Neuropsychiatric: Euphoria, psychological dependence, depression, convulsions, insomnia. Intracranial hypertension in children. Aggravation of schizophrenia.

Ophthalmic: Increased intra-ocular pressure, glaucoma, papilloedema, cataracts, corneal or scleral thinning, exacerbation of ophthalmic viral disease, exophthalmos.

General: Opportunistic infection, recurrence of dormant tuberculosis, leucocytosis, hypersensitivity, thrombo-embolism, increased appetite, nausea, vertigo, malaise.

Withdrawal symptoms: Fever, myalgia, arthralgia, adrenal insufficiency.

Parenteral corticosteroid therapy: Anaphylactic reaction or allergic reactions, hypopigmentation or hyperpigmentation, subcutaneous and cutaneous atrophy, sterile abscess, post injection flare (following intra-articular use), Charcot like arthropathy, rare instances of blindness associated with intralesional therapy around the face and head.

Certain side-effects reported with some non *recommended routes of administration*

Intrathecal: Usual systemic corticoid adverse reactions, headache, meningismus, meningitis, paraplegia, spinal fluid abnormalities, nausea, vomiting, sweating, arachnoiditis, convulsions.

Extradural: Wound dehiscence, loss of sphincter control.

Intranasal: Permanent/temporary blindness, rhinitis.

Ophthalmic (Subconjunctival): Redness and itching, abscess, slough at injection site, residue at injection site, increased intra-ocular pressure, decreased vision – blindness, infection.

Miscellaneous injection sites: Scalp, tonsillar fauces, sphenopalantine ganglion: blindness.

Overdosage: No known antidote. Following overdosage the possibility of adrenal suppression should be guarded against by gradual diminution of dose levels over a period of time. In such event the patient may require to be supported during any further traumatic episode.

Pharmaceutical precautions Depo-Medrone should be protected from freezing. Depo-Medrone should not be mixed with any other fluid. Discard any remaining solution after use.

Legal category POM.

Package quantities 1 ml, 2 ml and 3 ml vials packed singly and as 6-vial clinic packs.

Further information Methylprednisolone has achieved a clinically acceptable split between glucocorticoid effect and undesired mineralocorticoid effect. Methylprednisolone has five times the anti-inflammatory activity of hydrocortisone but has little tendency to cause salt and water retention. Depo-Medrone affords advantages in treatment which include high concentration in low fluid volume, greater gastric tolerance in avoidance of the GI tract and complete physician control of dosage.

Product licence number 0032/5038

DEPO-MEDRONE* WITH LIDOCAINE

Presentation White, sterile aqueous suspension for injection containing 40 mg per ml methylprednisolone acetate and 10 mg per ml lidocaine hydrochloride.

Uses Corticosteroid (glucocorticoid). Depo-Medrone with Lidocaine is indicated in conditions requiring a glucocorticoid effect: e.g. anti-inflammatory or anti-rheumatic. It is recommended for local use where the added anaesthetic effect would be considered advantageous.

Therapy with Depo-Medrone with Lidocaine does not obviate the need for the conventional measures usually employed. Although this method of treatment will ameliorate symptoms, it is in no sense a cure and the hormone has no effect on the cause of the inflammation.

Depo-Medrone with Lidocaine may be used as follows:

Intra-articular administration: Rheumatoid arthritis; osteoarthritis with an anti-inflammatory component.

Peri-articular administration: Epicondylitis.

Intrabursal administration: Subacromial bursitis; prepatellar bursitis; olecranon bursitis.

Tendon sheath administration: Tendinitis; tenosynovitis; epicondylitis.

Dosage and administration Depo-Medrone with Lidocaine should not be mixed with any other preparations as flocculation of the product may occur. Parenteral drug products should be inspected visually for particulate matter and discoloration prior to administration whenever suspension and container permit. Depo-Medrone with Lidocaine may be used by any of the following routes: intra-articular, peri-articular, intrabursal, and into the tendon sheath.

Depo-Medrone with Lidocaine vials are intended for single dose use only.

Intra-articular: Rheumatoid arthritis, osteo-arthritis. The dose of Depo-Medrone with Lidocaine depends on the size of the joint and the severity of the condition. Repeated injections, if needed, may be given at intervals of one to five or more weeks depending upon the degree of relief obtained from the initial injection. A suggested dosage guide is: large joint (knee, ankle, shoulder), 0.5–2 ml (20–80 mg of steroid); medium joint (elbow, wrist), 0.25–1 ml (10–40 mg of steroid); small joint (metacarpophalangeal, interphalangeal, sternoclavicular, acromioclavicular), 0.1–0.25 ml (4–10 mg of steroid).

Peri-articular: Epicondylitis. Infiltrate 0.1–0.75 ml (4–30 mg of steroid) into the affected area.

Intrabursal: Subdeltoid bursitis, prepatellar bursitis, olecranon bursitis. For administration directly into bursae, 0.1–0.75 ml (4–30 mg of steroid). In most acute cases, repeat injections are not needed.

Into the tendon sheath: Tendinitis, tenosynovitis, epicondylitis. For administration directly into the tendon sheath, 0.1–0.75 ml (4–30 mg of steroid). In recurrent or chronic conditions, repeat injections may be necessary.

Special precautions should be observed when administering Depo-Medrone with Lidocaine:

Intra-articular injections should be made using precise, anatomical localisation into the synovial space of the joint involved. The injection site for each joint is determined by that location where the synovial cavity is most superficial and most free of large vessels and nerves. Suitable sites for intra-articular injection are the knee, ankle, wrist, elbow, shoulder, phalangeal and hip joints. The spinal joints, unstable joints and those devoid of synovial space are not suitable. Treatment failures are most frequently the result of failure to enter the joint space. Intra-articular injections should be made with care as follows; ensuring correct positioning of the needle into the synovial space and aspirating a few drops of joint fluid. The aspirating syringe should then be replaced by another containing Depo-Medrone with Lidocaine. To ensure position of the needle synovial fluid should be aspirated and the injection made.

After injection the joint is moved slightly to aid mixing

of the synovial fluid and the suspension. Subsequent to therapy care should be taken for the patient not to overuse the joint in which benefit has been obtained. Negligence in this matter may permit an increase in joint deterioration that will more than offset the beneficial effects of the steroid. Intrabursal injections should be made as follows: the area around the injection site is prepared in a sterile way and a wheal at the site made with 1 percent procaine hydrochloride solution. A 20 to 24 gauge needle attached to a dry syringe is inserted into the bursa and the fluid aspirated. The needle is left in place and the aspirating syringe changed for a small syringe containing the desired dose. After injection, the needle is withdrawn and a small dressing applied. In the treatment of tenosynovitis and tendinitis, care should be taken to inject Depo-Medrone with Lidocaine into the tendon sheath rather than into the substance of the tendon. Due to the absence of a true tendon sheath, the Achilles tendon should not be injected with Depo-Medrone with Lidocaine.

Children: For infants and children, the recommended dosage should be reduced, but dosage should be governed by the severity of the condition rather than by strict adherence to the ratio indicated by age or body weight.

Elderly patients: When used according to instructions, there is no information to suggest that a change in dosage is warranted in the elderly.

Contra-indications, warnings, etc

Contra-indications: The usual contra-indications to systemic or local use of corticosteroids should be observed.

Depo-Medrone with Lidocaine is contra-indicated in patients who exhibit heart block, in the presence of systemic fungal infections, or cases of known hypersensitivity to methylprednisolone acetate, Lidocaine or other local anaesthetics of the amide type.

Immunisation procedures should not be undertaken in patients who are on corticosteroids, especially on high doses, due to the possibility of neurological complications and lack of antibody response.

Due to its potential for neuro-toxicity, Depo-Medrone with Lidocaine *must not* be given by the intrathecal route. In addition, as the product is a suspension it must not be given by the intravenous route.

Warnings: Corticosteroids may mask some signs of infection, and new infections may appear during their use. There may be decreased resistance and inability to localise infection when corticosteroids are used. Hence all patients receiving methylprednisolone should be watched for evidence of intra-current infection. Should infection occur, it must be brought under control by the use of appropriate antibacterial therapy or administration of corticosteroids should be discontinued. Do not use intrasynovial, intrabursal or intratendinous administration for local effect in the presence of acute infection.

Depo-Medrone with Lidocaine vials are intended for single dose use only. Any multidose use of the product may lead to contamination.

Due to the absence of a true tendon sheath, the Achilles tendon should not be injected with Depo-Medrone with Lidocaine.

Depo-Medrone with Lidocaine is not recommended for epidural, intranasal, intra-ocular, or any other unapproved route of administration. See Side-effects section for details of side-effects reported from some non-recommended routes of administration.

While crystals of adrenal steroids in the dermis suppress inflammatory reactions, their presence may cause disintegration of the cellular elements and physiochemical changes in the ground substance of the connective tissue. The resultant infrequently occurring dermal and/or subdermal changes may form depressions in the skin at the injection site and the possibility of depigmentation. The degree to which this reaction occurs will vary with the amount of adrenal steroid injected. Regeneration is usually complete within a few months or after all crystals of the adrenal steroid have been absorbed.

In order to minimise the incidence of dermal and subdermal atrophy, care must be exercised not to exceed recommended doses in injections. Multiple small injections into the area of the lesion should be made whenever possible. The technique of intra-articular injection should include precautions against injection or leakage into the dermis.

Intra-articular corticosteroids are associated with a substantially increased risk of inflammatory response in the joint, particularly bacterial infection introduced with the injection. Charcot-like arthropathies have been reported particularly after repeated injections. Appropriate examination of any joint fluid present is necessary to exclude any bacterial infection, prior to injection.

In patients on corticosteroid therapy subjected to unusual stress, increased dosage of rapidly acting corticosteroids before, during and after the stressful situation is indicated.

Prolonged use of corticosteroids may produce posterior subcapsular cataracts, glaucoma with possible damage to the optic nerves, and may enhance the establishment of secondary ocular infections due to fungi or viruses.

If corticosteroids are indicated in patients with latent tuberculosis or tuberculin reactivity, close observation is necessary as reactivation of the disease may occur. During prolonged corticosteroid therapy, these patients should receive chemoprophylaxis.

Because rare instances of anaphylactic reactions have occurred in patients receiving parenteral corticosteroid therapy, appropriate precautionary measures should be taken prior to administration, especially when the patient has a history of allergy to any drug.

Allergic skin reactions have been reported apparently related to the excipients in the formulation. Rarely has skin testing demonstrated a reaction to methylprednisolone acetate, per se.

Following a single dose of Depo-Medrone with Lidocaine, plasma cortisol levels are reduced and there is evidence of hypothalamic–pituitary–adrenal (HPA) axis suppression as judged by Synacthen test or insulin induced hypoglycaemic response. This suppression lasts for a variable period of up to 4 weeks. The amount and duration of such suppression is generally proportional to the dose of methylprednisolone administered and the length of therapy, although there is a wide individual variation. Repeated dosing would therefore be expected to produce greater and more prolonged suppression. The usual dynamic tests of HPA axis function can be used to diagnose evidence of impaired activity e.g.: – Synacthen test.

Systemic absorption of methylprednisolone occurs following intra-articular injection of Depo-Medrone with Lidocaine. Systemic as well as local effects can therefore be expected.

Precautions: Depo-Medrone with Lidocaine should be used with caution in the presence of diabetes, osteoporosis, chronic psychotic reactions, glaucoma, previous steroid myopathy, peptic ulceration, epilepsy, predisposition to thrombophlebitis, congestive heart failure, renal insufficiency, infection, non-specific ulcerative colitis if there is a probability of impending perforation, abscess or other pyogenic infection, diverticulitis, fresh intestinal anastomoses, myasthenia gravis, Cushing's syndrome, hypertension, and in patients with ocular herpes simplex for fear of corneal perforation.

Psychic derangements may appear when corticosteroids are used, ranging from euphoria, insomnia, mood swings, personality changes, and severe depression to frank psychotic manifestations. Also, existing emotional instability or psychotic tendencies may be aggravated by corticosteroids.

No evidence exists showing that corticosteroids are carcinogenic or mutagenic.

Since complications of treatment with glucocorticoids are dependent on the size of the dose and the duration of treatment, a risk/benefit decision must be made in each individual case as to dose and duration of treatment.

This product contains benzyl alcohol. Benzyl alcohol has been reported to be associated with a fatal 'Gasping Syndrome' in premature infants.

The following additional precautions apply for parenteral corticosteroids: Following intra-articular injection, a marked increase in pain accompanied by local swelling, further restriction of joint motion, fever, and malaise are suggestive of septic arthritis. If this complication occurs and the diagnosis of sepsis is confirmed, appropriate antimicrobial therapy should be instituted.

No additional benefit derives from the intramuscular administration of Depo-Medrone with Lidocaine. Where parenteral corticosteroid therapy for sustained systemic effect is desired, plain Depo-Medrone should be used.

Local injection of a steroid into a previously infected joint is to be avoided.

Corticosteroids should not be injected into unstable joints.

Sterile technique is necessary to prevent infections or contamination.

Use in pregnancy and lactation: The use of corticosteroids, in general, during pregnancy involves balancing the clinical benefit against the possible risks. There is inadequate evidence of safety in human pregnancy and there may be a very small risk of foetal malformations; there is evidence of harmful effects on pregnancy in animals. Also neonates of mothers who received such therapy during pregnancy should be observed for signs of hypoadrenalism and appropriate measures instituted if such signs exist.

Because prednisolone is excreted in breast milk, it is reasonable to assume that all corticosteroids are. No specific data are known for methylprednisolone acetate. Therefore, the use of corticosteroids in pregnancy, nursing mothers and women of childbearing potential requires that the possible benefits of the drug be weighed against the potential hazards to the mother, embryo or foetus.

The use of local anaesthetics such as lidocaine during labour and delivery may be associated with adverse effects on mother and foetus. Lidocaine readily crosses the placenta.

It is not known whether lidocaine is excreted in human breast milk.

Use in children: Corticosteroids cause growth retardation in infancy, childhood and adolescence. Treatment should be limited to the minimum dosage for the shortest possible time.

Side-effects: Side-effects associated with the use of corticosteroids may be observed, including for the Depo-Medrone component:

Gastro-intestinal: Dyspepsia, peptic ulceration with perforation and haemorrhage, abdominal distension, oesophageal ulceration, oesophageal candidiasis, acute pancreatitis, perforation of bowel.

Musculoskeletal: Proximal myopathy, osteoporosis, vertebral and long bone fractures, avascular osteonecrosis, tendon rupture, aseptic necrosis.

Fluid and electrolyte disturbance: Sodium and water retention, hypertension, hypokalaemic alkalosis, congestive heart failure in susceptible patients, potassium loss.

Dermatologic: Impaired healing, petechiae and ecchymosis, thin fragile skin, skin atrophy, bruising, striae, telangiectasia, acne, may suppress reactions to skin tests, sterile abscess.

Endocrine/metabolic: Suppression of the hypothalamo–pituitary–adrenal axis, growth suppression in childhood and adolescence, menstrual irregularity and amenorrhoea. Cushingoid syndrome, moon facies, hirsutism, weight gain, impaired carbohydrate tolerance with increased requirement for antidiabetic therapy, negative nitrogen balance.

Neuropsychiatric: Euphoria, pseudotumor cerebri, psychological dependence, depression, convulsions, insomnia. Intracranial hypertension in children. Aggravation of schizophrenia.

Ophthalmic: Increased intra-ocular pressure, glaucoma, papilloedema, cataracts, corneal or scleral thinning, exacerbation of ophthalmic viral disease, exophthalmos.

General: Opportunistic infection, recurrence of dormant tuberculosis, leucocytosis, hypersensitivity, thrombo-embolism, increased appetite, nausea, vertigo, malaise, supraclavicular pads of fat, weakness, headache.

Withdrawal symptoms: Fever, myalgia, arthralgia, adrenal insufficiency.

Parenteral corticosteroid therapy: Anaphylactic reaction or allergic reactions, hypopigmentation or hyperpigmentation, subcutaneous and cutaneous atrophy, sterile abscess, post injection flare (following intra-articular use), Charcot-like arthropathy.

Side effects for the Lidocaine component include:

Central nervous system: Lightheadedness, nervousness, apprehension, euphoria, confusion, dizziness, drowsiness, tinnitus, blurred or double vision, vomiting, sensation of heat, cold, numbness, twitching, tremors, convulsions, loss of consciousness, respiratory depression, respiratory arrest.

Cardiovascular system: Bradycardia, hypotension, cardiovascular collapse, cardiac arrest.

Allergic reactions: Cutaneous lesions, urticaria, oedema, anaphylactic reactions.

Certain side-effects reported with some non *recommended routes of administration*

Intrathecal: Usual systemic corticoid adverse reactions, headache, meningismus, meningitis, paraplegia, spinal fluid abnormalities, nausea, vomiting, sweating, arachnoiditis, convulsions.

Extradural: Wound dehiscence, loss of sphincter control.

Intranasal: Temporary/permanent impairment including visual blindness, allergic reactions, rhinitis.

Ophthalmic (Subconjunctival): Redness and itching, abscess, slough at injection site, residue at injection site, increased intra-ocular pressure, decreased vision – blindness, infection.

Miscellaneous: Scalp, tonsillar fauces, sphenopalantine ganglion: blindness.

Overdosage: There is no clinical syndrome of acute overdosage with Depo-Medrone with Lidocaine.

Repeated frequent doses (daily or several times per week) over a protracted period may result in a Cushingoid state and other complications of chronic steroid therapy.

Following overdosage the possibility of adrenal suppression should be guarded against by gradual diminution of dose levels over a period of time. In such event the patient may require to be supported during any further traumatic episode.

Pharmaceutical precautions Depo-Medrone with Lidocaine should be protected from freezing. Depo-Medrone with Lidocaine should not be mixed with any other fluid. Discard any remaining solution after use.

Legal category POM.

Package quantities 2 ml vials and 6 × 1 ml vial clinic pack.

Further information Methylprednisolone has achieved a clinically acceptable split between glucocorticoid effect and undesired mineralocorticoid effect. Methylprednisolone has five times the anti-inflammatory activity of hydrocortisone but has little tendency to cause salt and water retention. Depo-Medrone affords advantages in treatment which include high concentration in low fluid volume and a predictable pharmacokinetic profile.

Product licence number 0032/0076.

DEPO-PROVERA* 50 mg/ml

Presentation White, sterile aqueous suspension containing 50 mg/ml medroxyprogesterone acetate.

Uses Progestogen: for the treatment of endometriosis.

Dosage and administration The sterile aqueous suspension of Depo-Provera should be vigorously shaken just before use to ensure that the dose being given represents a uniform suspension of Depo-Provera.

Doses should be given by deep intramuscular injection.

A dose of 50 mg i.m. once a week or 100 mg i.m. every two weeks should be given for six months or longer.

Contra-indications, warnings, etc

Contra-indications: Depo-Provera is contra-indicated in patients with a known sensitivity to medroxyprogesterone acetate.

Depo-Provera should not be used in pregnancy, either for diagnosis or therapy.

Warnings, precautions, side-effects: Whether administered alone or in combination with oestrogen, Depo-Provera should not be employed in patients with abnormal uterine bleeding until a definite diagnosis has been established and the possibility of genital tract malignancy eliminated.

Doctors should therefore check that patients are not pregnant before initial injection, and also if administration of any subsequent injection is overdue. Congenital anomalies, including female foetal masculinisation and clitoral hypertrophy, have been observed following larger doses of progestogens.

Medroxyprogesterone and/or its metabolites are secreted in breast milk but there is no evidence to suggest that this presents any hazard to the child.

A few cases of breast cancer have been reported in women taking Depo-Provera, but no causal relationship has been established.

Endometrial tumours have developed in monkeys given fifty times the human contraceptive dose but the relevance of this to man has not been established.

A very low incidence of anaphylactoid reactions has been reported.

For patients with a history of endogenous depression, the physician should bear in mind the prolonged action of the product when considering the use of Depo-Provera.

A decrease in glucose tolerance has been observed in some patients treated with progestogens. The mechanism for this decrease is obscure. For this reason, diabetic patients should be carefully observed while receiving progestogen therapy.

Rare cases of thromboembolism have been reported with the use of Depo-Provera, but causality has not been established.

Interaction with other medicinal treatment has not been reported, but the possibility should be borne in mind in patients receiving concurrent treatment with other drugs.

Patients receiving Depo-Provera may be subject to the side-effects normally associated with the use of progestogens. In addition, it is likely that some or all of the following effects may occur:

1. Delay in return to normal menstrual cycling and transient infertility lasting up to two years or longer may occur following continuous treatment with Depo-Provera.
2. Depo-Provera may be expected to cause disruption of the normal menstrual cycle. Irregular, prolonged or heavy vaginal bleeding or spotting may be experienced during the first two or three cycles of treatment. The frequency of occurrence of bleeding usually decreases with subsequent injections. After one year of treatment some women are amenorrhoeic.
3. Back pain.
4. Weight gain.
5. Fluid retention.

Overdosage: No positive action is required.

Pharmaceutical precautions Store at room temperature and protect from freezing. Do not mix with other agents. Discard any remaining contents after use.

Legal category POM.

Package quantities 1 ml, 3 ml and 5 ml vials.

Further information Provera is a potent progestational agent with very low toxicity. Depo-Provera is ideally suited to the patient with endometriosis in whom oestrogen and androgen treatment may be considered to offer too many drawbacks on grounds of intolerance or masculinisation.

A 150 mg/ml strength of Depo-Provera is also available in a 3.3 ml vial and a 1 ml vial for alternative indications.

Product licence number 0032/0056

DEPO-PROVERA* 150 mg/ml

Presentation White, sterile aqueous suspension containing 150 mg/ml medroxyprogesterone acetate.

Uses Progestogen: for short-term and long-term contraception.

a. Short-term contraception:

Depo-Provera may be used for short-term contraception when an oral contraceptive is contra-indicated or considered inappropriate in the following circumstances:

(i) For wives of men undergoing vasectomy, for protection until the vasectomy becomes effective.

(ii) In women who are being immunised against rubella, to prevent pregnancy during the period of activity of the virus.

b. Long-term contraception:

Depo-Provera is intended for long-term use only in women in whom other contraceptives are contra-indicated or have caused unacceptable side-effects or are otherwise unsatisfactory.

It is of the greatest importance that adequate explanations of the long-term nature of the product, of its possible side-effects and of the impossibility of reversing the effects of each injection are given to potential users and that every effort is made to ensure that each patient receives such counselling as to enable her to fully understand these explanations.

Consistent with good clinical contraceptive practice a general medical as well as gynaecological examination should be undertaken before administration of Depo-Provera and at yearly intervals thereafter.

As with other long-term hormonal contraceptives, regular consideration should be given to whether the previous treatment has resulted in:

1. First time migraine or unusually severe headaches, acute visual disturbances of any kind.
2. Re-appearance of depression.
3. Pathological changes in liver function and hormone levels.

Dosage and administration The sterile aqueous suspension of Depo-Provera should be vigorously shaken just before use to ensure that the dose being given represents a uniform suspension of Depo-Provera.

Doses should be given by deep intramuscular injection.

To provide contraceptive cover in the first cycle of use, an injection of 150 mg i.m. should be given during the first five days of a normal menstrual cycle. If the injection is carried out according to these instructions, no additional contraceptive cover is required. A similar injection should be given before the sixth week postpartum for immediate contraceptive cover. Further doses should be given at 3-month intervals. (N.B. For wives of men undergoing vasectomy a second injection of 150 mg i.m. three months after the first may be necessary in a small proportion of patients where the husband's sperm count has not fallen to zero).

Because of the risk of heavy or prolonged bleeding in some women, the drug should be used with caution in the puerperium.

If the puerperal woman will be breast-feeding, the initial injection should be delayed until six weeks postpartum, when the infant's enzyme system is more fully developed. Further injections should be given at 3-month intervals.

Contra-indications, warnings, etc

Contra-indications: Depo-Provera is contra-indicated as a contraceptive at the above dosage in known or suspected hormone-dependent malignancy of breast or genital organs, and in patients with a known sensitivity to medroxyprogesterone acetate.

Depo-Provera should not be used in pregnancy, either for diagnosis or therapy.

Warnings, precautions, and side-effects: Whether administered alone or in combination with oestrogen, Depo-Provera should not be employed in patients with abnormal uterine bleeding until a definite diagnosis has been established and the possibility of genital tract malignancy eliminated.

Doctors should therefore check that patients are not pregnant before initial injection, and also if administration of any subsequent injection is overdue. Congenital anomalies, including female foetal masculinisation and clitoral hypertrophy, have been observed following larger doses of progestogens.

Medroxyprogesterone and/or its metabolites are secreted in breast milk but there is no evidence to suggest that this presents any hazard to the child.

A few cases of breast cancer have been reported in women taking Depo-Provera, but no causal relationship has been established.

Endometrial tumours have developed in monkeys given fifty times the human contraceptive dose but the relevance of this to man has not been established.

For patients with a history of endogenous depression, the physician should bear in mind the prolonged action of the product when considering the use of Depo-Provera.

A decrease in glucose tolerance has been observed in some patients treated with progestogens. The mechanism for this decrease is obscure. For this reason, diabetic patients should be carefully observed while receiving progestogen therapy.

Rare cases of thromboembolism have been reported with use of Depo-Provera, but causality has not been established.

Interaction with other medicinal treatment has not been reported, but the possibility should be borne in mind in patients receiving concurrent treatment with other drugs.

Patients receiving Depo-Provera may be subject to the side-effects normally associated with the use of progestogens. In addition, it is likely that some or all of the following effects may occur:

1. Delay in return to normal menstrual cycling and transient infertility lasting up to two years or longer may occur following continuous treatment with Depo-Provera.
2. Depo-Provera may be expected to cause disruption of the normal menstrual cycle. Irregular, prolonged or heavy vaginal bleeding or spotting may be experienced during the first two or three cycles of treatment. The frequency of occurrence of bleeding usually decreases with subsequent injections. After one year of treatment some women are amenorrhoeic.
3. Back pain.
4. Weight gain.
5. Fluid retention.

Overdosage: No positive action is required.

Pharmaceutical precautions Store at room temperature and protect from freezing. Do not mix with other agents. Discard any remaining contents after use.

Legal category POM.

Package quantities 1 ml vial.

Further information The contraceptive effect of 150 mg i.m. Depo-Provera lasts approximately 90 days.

The 150 mg/ml strength of Depo-Provera is also available in a 3.3 ml vial for alternative indications.

A 50 mg/ml strength of Depo-Provera is available in 1 ml, 3 ml and 5 ml vials for the treatment of endometriosis.

Product licence number 0032/0082.

DEPO-PROVERA* 150 mg/ml

Presentation White sterile aqueous suspension. Each 1 ml contains 150 mg medroxyprogesterone acetate.

Uses Progestogen.

A proportion of certain classes of malignant tumours have been shown to respond to hormone administration or ablative hormonal surgery. These classes include carcinoma of endometrium, carcinoma of kidney and carcinoma of breast. Depo-Provera has been shown to be effective as adjunctive therapy in carcinoma of endometrium, carcinoma of kidney and carcinoma of breast in post-menopausal women.

Dosage and administration The sterile aqueous suspension of Depo-Provera should be vigorously shaken just before each use to ensure that the dose being given represents a uniform suspension of Depo-Provera. Doses should be given intramuscularly, deep into the gluteal muscle.

Endometrial or renal carcinoma: The normal initial dose lies in the range 400–1000 mg per week, but doses in excess of 1000 mg per day have been used without serious adverse effects. If improvement is noted within a few weeks or months and the disease appears stabilised, it may be possible to maintain the improvement with as little as 400 mg per month. Depo-Provera is not recommended as primary therapy but as adjunctive and palliative treatment in advanced inoperable cases including those with recurrent or metastatic disease.

Breast carcinoma: The recommended schedule is 500 mg/day for 28 days. The patient should then be placed on a maintenance schedule of 500 mg twice weekly as long as the patient is responding to treatment.

Progression of disease at any time during therapy indicates treatment with Depo-Provera should be terminated, although response to hormonal therapy may not be evident until after at least 8–10 weeks of therapy.

Where large doses are being administered consideration should be given to dividing the dose between two separate sites.

Elderly patients: Depo-Provera has been extensively used in both the young (20–35) and older age groups (50–75). Its use in the young has been primarily for contraception while its use in the older age group has been for the treatment of malignancies. There appears to be no evidence to suggest that the older aged patient is less well prepared to handle the drug metabolically than is the younger aged patient. Therefore the same dosage, contra-indications, and precautions would apply to either age group.

Contra-indications, warnings, etc

Contra-indications: Depo-Provera is contra-indicated in patients with a known sensitivity to medroxyprogesterone acetate and in patients with liver dysfunction or disease. It should not be used during pregnancy, either for diagnosis or therapy.

Warnings and precautions: Doctors should check that patients are not pregnant before initial injection, and also if administration of any subsequent injection is overdue. Congenital anomalies, including female foetal masculinisation and clitoral hypertrophy, have been observed following larger doses of progestogens.

In the treatment of carcinoma of breast occasional cases of hypercalcaemia have been reported.

Any patient who develops an acute impairment of vision, proptosis, diplopia or migraine headache should be carefully evaluated ophthalmologically to exclude the presence of papilloedema or retinal vascular lesions before continuing medication.

Animal studies show that Depo-Provera possesses adrenocorticoid activity. This has also been reported in man, therefore patients receiving large doses continuously and for long periods should be observed closely.

Medroxyprogesterone acetate and/or its metabolites are secreted in breast milk but there is no evidence to suggest that this presents a hazard to the child.

Because progestogens may cause some degree of fluid retention, conditions which might be influenced by this factor, such as epilepsy, migraine, asthma, cardiac or renal dysfunction, require careful observation.

A very low incidence of anaphylactoid reactions has been reported.

For patients with a history of endogenous depression, the physician should bear in mind the prolonged action of the product when considering the use of Depo-Provera.

A decrease in glucose tolerance has been observed in some patients on progestogens. The mechanism for this decrease is obscure. For this reason diabetic patients should be carefully observed while receiving progestogen therapy.

Rare cases of thromboembolism have been reported with use of Depo-Provera, but causality has not been established.

Gynaecomastia, hirsutism and other evidence of virilisation may develop after prolonged courses.

This form of therapy should only be administered under the direction of specialist units having facilities for appropriate surveillance of the patient.

Interactions with other medicinal treatments have not been reported, but the possibility should be borne in mind in patients receiving concurrent treatment with other drugs.

Side-effects: Depending on the volume injected, some patients may be expected to show undesirable sequelae at the site of injection such as residual lump, change in colour of skin or sterile abscess. Other adverse reactions noted, particularly with large doses, have been:

Breast: In a few instances breast tenderness or galactorrhoea has occurred.

Psychic: An occasional patient has experienced nervousness, insomnia, somnolence, fatigue or dizziness.

Skin and Mucous Membranes: Sensitivity reactions ranging from pruritus, urticaria, angioneurotic oedema, to generalised rash and anaphylaxis have occasionally been reported. Acne, alopecia or hirsutism have been reported in a few cases.

Gastro-intestinal: Rarely nausea has been reported. Jaundice has been noted in a few instances.

Miscellaneous: Hyperpyrexia, weight gain and moon facies.

Overdosage: No action required other than cessation of therapy.

Pharmaceutical precautions Store at room temperature and protect from freezing. Do not mix with other agents. Discard any remaining contents after use.

Legal category POM.

Package quantities 3.3 ml vial.

Further information The results of certain laboratory tests may be affected by the use of Depo-Provera; these include gonadotrophin levels, plasma progesterone levels, urinary pregnanediol levels, plasma testosterone levels (in the male), plasma oestrogen levels (in the female), plasma cortisol levels, glucose tolerance and metyrapone tests.

The 150 mg/ml strength of Depo-Provera is also available in a 1 ml vial for contraceptive use.

A 50 mg/ml strength of Depo-Provera is available in 1 ml, 3 ml and 5 ml vials for the treatment of endometriosis.

Product licence number 0032/0082

HALCION*

Presentation Blue flat oval tablets scored on one side and imprinted Upjohn 17 on the other side, each containing 250 micrograms (0.25 mg) triazolam.

Pale lavender flat oval tablets imprinted Upjohn 10 on one side, otherwise plain, each containing 125 micrograms (0.125 mg) triazolam.

Uses Halcion is indicated for the short-term (up to 4 weeks) treatment of insomnia when it is severe, disabling, or subjecting the individual to extreme distress, particularly for patients with transient sleep disorders. As with all hypnotics, long term chronic use is not recommended.

Dosage and administration The lowest dose which can control symptoms should be used. It should not be continued beyond 4 weeks. Treatment should be intermittent, if possible. The usual dose for adults is 125–250 micrograms (0.125–0.25 mg) before retiring. A dose of 250 micrograms should not be exceeded.

Treatment in all patients should be withdrawn gradually.

Elderly patients: The initial dose for geriatric patients is 125 micrograms (0.125 mg) and this may be increased to 250 micrograms (0.25 mg) if necessary.

Contra-indications, warnings, etc

Contra-indications: Halcion is contra-indicated in patients with known hypersensitivity to benzodiazepines, acute pulmonary insufficiency, phobic or obsessional states or chronic psychosis.

Warnings: As with all medicaments of this type, avoidance of alcohol in patients receiving Halcion is recommended since the individual response cannot be foreseen. Similarly, during its period of activity, Halcion may modify patients' reactions (driving, operating machinery) to a varying extent depending on dosages and individual susceptibility.

When used at the appropriate recommended dose for short-term treatment, the dependence potential is low. However, as with all benzodiazepines, the risk of dependence increases with higher doses and longer-term use and is further increased in patients with a history of alcoholism, drug abuse, or in patients with marked personality disorders.

Precautions: Abnormal psychological reactions to most benzodiazepines have been reported. Rare behavioural adverse effects include: paradoxical aggressive outbursts; excitement; inappropriate behaviour, sometimes with amnesia; and the uncovering of depression with suicidal tendencies. Extreme caution, therefore, should be used in prescribing benzodiazepines in patients with personality disorders.

In elderly and/or debilitated patients, it is recommended that treatment with Halcion be initiated at 125 micrograms (0.125 mg) to decrease the possibility of development of over-sedation, dizziness, or impaired co-ordination. If Halcion is to be combined with other drugs having known hypnotic properties or CNS depressant effects, consideration should be given to potential additive effects.

An underlying cause for insomnia should be sought before deciding upon the use of benzodiazepines for symptomatic relief.

As with other benzodiazepines, Halcion should not be used alone to treat depression or anxiety associated with depression. Suicide may be precipitated in such patients. Under these circumstances, limiting the prescription size is recommended.

The usual precautions should be observed in patients with impaired renal or hepatic function or chronic pulmonary insufficiency.

Safety for use during pregnancy has not yet been established.

Use in nursing mothers: Human studies have not been performed; however, studies in rats have indicated that Halcion and its metabolites are secreted in milk. Therefore administration to nursing mothers is not recommended.

Safety and effectiveness in patients under the age of 18 have not been established.

Benzodiazepines should be used with extreme caution in patients who are prone to substance abuse.

In cases of loss or bereavement, psychological adjustment may be inhibited by benzodiazepines.

Triazolam plasma concentrations may double when cimetidine is co-administered. The co-administration of triazolam and cimetidine results in a reduction of triazolam clearance without a change in elimination half-life in most subjects. The elimination half-life may be prolonged in some subjects but does not result in drug accumulation on once daily dosing.

Triazolam plasma concentrations may double when erythromycin is co-administered. The co-administration of triazolam and erythromycin results in a reduction of triazolam clearance and an increase in the elimination half-life.

Increased clinical observation and consideration of dose reduction may be appropriate in patients concomitantly taking triazolam with cimetidine, or erythromycin or other macrolide antibiotics.

Side-effects: Drowsiness, dizziness, light-headedness, confusion and impaired co-ordination have occurred. The incidence and severity of these pharmacological events are generally dose-related. Cases of amnesia (sometimes with inappropriate behaviour) have been reported in association with Halcion use. Headache has occurred in some patients. Less frequently taste alterations, CNS depression, falling, transient insomnia after drug treatment is discontinued, hallucinations and somnambulism have been reported. Adverse reactions which have been reported rarely are pruritus, skin rash, blurred vision, hiccups, palpitations, epigastric discomfort, diarrhoea and burning eyes. Severe sedation and impaired co-ordination are indicative of drug intolerance or overdose.

Overdosage: Manifestations of Halcion overdosage include extensions of its pharmacological activity, namely somnolence and hypnosis. As in all cases of drug overdosage, respiration, pulse and blood pressure should be monitored and supported by general measures when necessary. Immediate gastric lavage should be performed. Intravenous fluids should be administered and an adequate airway maintained.

Experiments in animals have indicated that cardiopulmonary collapse can occur with massive intravenous doses of Halcion (over 100 mg/kg, greater than 20,000 times the maximum daily human dose). This could be reversed with positive mechanical respiration and the intravenous infusion of noradrenaline or metaraminol. Other animal experiments have suggested that haemodialysis and forced diuresis are probably of little value.

Pharmaceutical precautions Keep container tightly closed and protect from light.

Legal category CD (Sch 4) POM.

Package quantities Packs of 30 (OP), 250 and 1,000 tablets.

Further information Nil.

Product licence numbers

250 micrograms (0.25 mg) Tablet	0032/0058
125 micrograms (0.125 mg) Tablet	0032/0063

HEMABATE* STERILE SOLUTION ▼

Presentation Colourless, sterile, aqueous solution containing 250 micrograms/ml carboprost as the tromethamine salt.

The product also contains sodium chloride and benzyl alcohol.

Uses Treatment of post-partum haemorrhage due to uterine atony and refractory to conventional methods of treatment with oxytocic agents and ergometrine used either alone or in combination.

Conventional therapy should usually consist of 0.5–1 mg ergometrine with up to 50 units of oxytocin infused intravenously over periods of time from 20 minutes to 12 hours. The dosage and duration of administration should reflect the seriousness of the clinical situation.

Dosage and administration Parenteral drug products should be inspected visually for particulate matter and discolouration prior to administration whenever solution and container permit.

An initial dose of 250 micrograms (1.0 ml) of Hemabate should be administered as a deep intramuscular injection by means of a tuberculin syringe.

If necessary further doses of 250 micrograms may be administered at intervals of approximately 1.5 hours. In severe cases the interval between doses may be reduced at the discretion of the attending physician, but it should not be less than 15 minutes. The total dose of Hemabate should not exceed 12 mg (48 doses).

Contra-indications, warnings, etc

Contra-indications: There are no absolute contra-indications to the use of Hemabate. However, its use is not recommended in the following circumstances:

(1) Hypersensitivity to any of the components of the preparation.

(2) Acute pelvic inflammatory disease.

(3) Patients with known cardiac, pulmonary, renal, or hepatic disease.

Warnings: This preparation should not be used for induction of labour.

Hemabate, as with other potent oxytocic agents, should be used only with strict adherence to recommended dosages. Hemabate should be used by medically trained personnel, and is available only to hospitals and clinics with specialised obstetric units where 24 hour resident medical cover is provided.

Hemabate must not be given intravenously.

Since prostaglandins may potentiate the effect of oxytocin, it is recommended that the use of these drugs simultaneously or in sequence should be carefully monitored.

Very rare cases of cardiovascular collapse have been reported following the use of prostaglandins. This should always be considered when using Hemabate.

Precautions:

(1) Hemabate should be used with caution in patients with a history of glaucoma or raised intra-ocular pressure, asthma, hypertension or hypotension, cardiovascular disease, renal disease, hepatic disease, anaemia, jaundice, diabetes or past history of epilepsy.

(2) As with other oxytocic agents, Hemabate should be used with care in patients with compromised (scarred) uteri. The possibility of uterine rupture should be borne in mind where high tone myometrial contractions are sustained.

(3) Animal studies lasting several weeks at high doses have shown that prostaglandins of the E and F series can induce proliferation of bone. Such effects have also been noted in newborn infants who have received prostaglandin E1 during prolonged treatment. There is no evidence that short-term administration of Hemabate can cause similar bone effects.

(4) Decreases in maternal arterial oxygen content have been observed in patients treated with carboprost tromethamine. A causal relationship to carboprost tromethamine has not been established, however, it is recommended that patients with pre-existing cardiopulmonary problems receiving Hemabate are monitored during treatment and given additional oxygen if necessary.

Side-effects: The adverse effects of Hemabate are generally transient and reversible when therapy ends.

The most frequent side-effects observed with the use of Hemabate are related to its contractile effect on smooth muscle. Thus nausea, vomiting and diarrhoea have been reported as commmonly encountered. The incidence of vomiting and diarrhoea may be decreased by pretreatment and concomitant use during treatment of antiemetic and antidiarrhoeal agents.

Hyperthermia and flushing have been observed after intramuscular Hemabate, but if not complicated by endometritis, the temperature elevation will usually return to normal within several hours of the last injection.

Asthma and wheezing have been noted with Hemabate treatment.

Less frequent but potentially more serious adverse effects are elevated blood pressure, dyspnoea and pulmonary oedema. Other less serious adverse effects noted include chills, headache, diaphoresis, dizziness and injection site erythema and pain.

Overdosage: Treatment of overdose must be, at this time, symptomatic, as clinical studies with prostaglandin antagonists have not progressed to the point where recommendations may be made.

If evidence of excessive uterine activity or side-effects appear, the frequency of administration should be decreased or discontinued.

In cases of massive overdosage resulting in extreme uterine hypertonus, appropriate obstetric procedures are indicated.

Pharmaceutical precautions Hemabate must be stored in a refrigerator between 0 and 6°C. At 4°C it has a shelf life of 24 months.

Legal category POM.

Package quantities Pack containing 2 × 1 ml ampoules of Hemabate Sterile Solution 250 micrograms/ml.

Further information Carboprost tromethamine stimulates the myometrium of the gravid uterus to contract in a manner that is similar to that observed in the term uterus during labour. Whether or not this action results from a direct effect of carboprost tromethamine on the myometrium has not been determined with certainty at this time.

When Hemabate is given post-partum, the resulting myometrial contractions provide haemostasis at the site of placentation and hence prevent further blood loss.

Product licence number 0032/0152.

KAOPECTATE*

Presentation Off-white suspension. Each 5 ml contains 1.03 g Kaolin BP in an aromatic and carminative vehicle.

Uses Antidiarrhoeal.
Diarrhoea of non-specific origin.

Dosage and administration Oral.
Adult: 10–30 ml every 4 hours.

Children: Up to 1 year – 5 ml every 4 hours.
1–5 years – 10 ml every 4 hours.

Elderly patients: There is no information to suggest that a change in dosage is warranted in the elderly. Side-effects do not appear to be more common or severe in elderly patients.

Contra-indications, warnings, etc
Contra-indications: Intestinal obstruction.

Warnings: None.

Precautions: None.

Interactions: The absorption of other drugs from the gastro-intestinal tract may be reduced if given concomitantly.

Use in pregnancy and lactation: No restrictions.

Side-effects: None.

Overdosage: The possibility of intestinal obstruction should be investigated.

Pharmaceutical precautions None.

Legal category GSL.

Package quantities Bottles of 180 ml and 500 ml.

Further information Nil.

Product licence number 0032/5040R

LONITEN*

Presentation Round white biconvex tablets with the dosage strength imprinted on one side and scored on the other with a U on either side of the score. Each tablet contains 2.5 mg, 5 mg or 10 mg minoxidil.

Uses Loniten is indicated for the treatment of severe hypertension.

It should not be used as the sole agent to initiate therapy. It is a peripheral vasodilator and should be given in conjunction with a diuretic, to control salt and water retention, and a beta-adrenergic blocking agent, or appropriate substitute to control reflex tachycardia.

Dosage and administration *Adults and patients over 12 years of age:* An initial daily dose of 5 mg, which may be given as a single or divided dosage is recommended. This dose may first be increased to 10 mg daily and subsequent increases should be by increments of 10 mg in the daily dose. Dosage adjustments should be made at intervals of not less than three days, until optimum control of blood pressure is achieved. It is seldom necessary to exceed 50 mg per day although, in exceptional circumstances, doses up to 100 mg per day have been used. Twice-daily dosage is satisfactory. Where diastolic pressure reduction of less than 30 mm Hg is required, once daily dosing has been reported as effective.

Dosage requirements may be lower in dialysis patients. Minoxidil is removed from the blood by dialysis, but its pharmacological action, once established is not reversed. Therefore haemodialysis patients should take Loniten either after or at least two hours before dialysis.

Children: For patients of 12 years of age or under, the initial dose should be 200 micrograms per kilogram (0.2 mg/kg) given as a single or divided daily dosage. Incremental increases of 100–200 micrograms per kilogram (0.1–0.2 mg/kg) in the daily dose are recommended at intervals of not less than three days until optimum blood pressure control has been achieved or the maximum daily dose of 1.0 mg/kg has been reached.

Rapid reduction of blood pressure: Rapid reduction of blood pressure can be achieved using continuous blood pressure monitoring and incremental doses of 5 mg every six hours.

Concomitant antihypertensive therapy: It is recommended that, where possible, antihypertensive therapy, other than a beta-adrenergic blocking agent and a diuretic be discontinued before Loniten treatment is started. It is recognised that some antihypertensive agents should not be abruptly discontinued. These drugs should be gradually discontinued during the first week of Loniten treatment.

Loniten causes sodium retention and if used alone can result in several hundred milli-equivalents of salt being retained together with a corresponding volume of water.

Therefore, in all patients who are not on dialysis, Loniten must be given in conjunction with a diuretic in sufficient dosage to maintain salt and water balance. Examples of the daily dosages of diuretics commonly used when starting therapy with Loniten include:

1. Hydrochlorothiazide (100 mg) – or other thiazides at equi-effective dosage.
2. Chlorthalidone (100 mg).
3. Frusemide (80 mg).

If excessive water retention results in a weight gain of more than 3 pounds when a thiazide or chlorthalidone is being used, diuretic therapy should be changed to frusemide, the dose of which may be increased in accordance with the patients' requirements. Diuretic dosage in children should be proportionally less in relation to weight.

Patients will require a sympathetic nervous system suppressant to limit a Loniten-induced rise in heart rate. The preferred agent is a beta-blocker equivalent to an adult propranolol dosage of 80–160 mg/day. Higher doses may be required when pre-treated patients have an increase in heart rate exceeding 20 beats per minute or when simultaneous introduction causes an increase exceeding 10 beats per minute. When beta-blockers are contra-indicated, alternatives such as methyldopa may be used instead and should be started 24 hours prior to Loniten.

Elderly patients: At present there are no extensive clinical studies with minoxidil in patients over age 65. There is data indicating that elevated systolic and diastolic pressures are important risk factors for cardiovascular disease in individuals over age 65. However, elderly patients may be sensitive to the blood pressure lowering effect of minoxidil and thus caution is urged in initiating therapy as orthostatic hypotension may occur. It is suggested that 2.5 mg per day be used as the initial starting dose in patients over 65 years of age.

Contra-indications, warnings, etc
Contra-indications: Loniten is contra-indicated in patients with a phaeochromocytoma.

Warnings: If used alone, Loniten can cause a significant retention of salt and water leading to positive physical signs such as oedema, and to clinical deterioration of some patients with heart failure. Diuretic treatment alone, or in combination with restricted salt intake is, therefore, necessary for all patients taking Loniten.

Patients who have had myocardial infarction should only be treated with Loniten after a stable post-infarction state has been established.

The physician should bear in mind that if not controlled by sympathetic suppressants, the rise in cardiac rate and output that follows the use of potent vasodilators may induce anginal symptoms in patients with undiagnosed coronary artery disease, or may aggravate pre-existing angina pectoris.

The effect of Loniten may be additive to concurrent antihypertensive agents. The interaction of Loniten with sympathetic-blocking agents such as guanethidine or bethanidine may produce excessive blood pressure reduction and/or orthostasis.

Precautions: The safety of Loniten in pregnancy remains to be established.

Hypertrichosis occurs in most patients treated with Loniten and all patients should be warned of this possibility before starting therapy. Spontaneous reversal to the pre-treatment state can be expected one to three months after cessation of therapy.

Soon after starting Loniten therapy approximately 60% of patients exhibit ECG alterations in the direction and magnitude of their T waves. Large changes may encroach on the ST segment, unaccompanied by evidence of ischaemia. These asymptomatic changes usually disappear with continuing Loniten treatment. The ECG reverts to the pre-treatment state if Loniten is discontinued.

Pericardial effusion has been detected in patients treated with a Loniten-containing regime. A cause and effect relationship has not been established. Most effusions have either been present before Loniten was given, or occurred among uraemic patients. However, it is suggested that Loniten-treated patients should be periodically monitored for signs or symptoms of pericardial effusion and appropriate therapy instituted if necessary.

Salt and water retention in excess of 2 to 3 pounds may diminish the effectiveness of Loniten. Patients should, therefore, be carefully instructed about compliance with diuretic therapy and a detailed record of body weight should be maintained.

Side-effects: Most patients receiving Loniten experience a diminution of pre-existing side-effects attributable to their disease or previous therapy. New events or side-effects likely to increase include peripheral oedema, associated with or independent of weight gain; increases in heart rate; hypertrichosis; and a temporary rise in creatinine and blood urea nitrogen. Gastro-intestinal intolerance, rash, and breast tenderness are infrequently reported side-effects of Loniten therapy.

Overdosage: If exaggerated hypotension is encountered, it is most likely to occur in association with residual sympathetic nervous system blockade (guanethidine-like effects or alpha-adrenergic blockade). Recommended treatment is intravenous administration of 0.9% saline. Sympathomimetic drugs, such as noradrenaline or adrenaline, should be avoided because of their excessive cardiac-stimulating action. Phenylephrine, angiotensin II and vasopressin, which reverse the effect of Loniten, should be used only if inadequate perfusion of a vital organ is evident.

Pharmaceutical precautions None.

Legal category POM.

Package quantities 2.5 mg, 5 mg and 10 mg Loniten tablets supplied as packs of 100.

Further information Loniten is a potent vasodilator which probably exerts its action after binding to the smooth muscle of the blood vessel wall. At least 90% of an oral dose is rapidly absorbed and the average plasma half-life in man is 4.2 hours. The clinical duration of action is up to 72 hours. Approximately 90% of administered drug is metabolised and excreted in the urine within 24 hours. Drug-related materials can be removed by dialysis.

Product licence numbers

2.5 mg	0032/0064
5 mg	0032/0065
10 mg	0032/0066

MEDRONE* TABLETS 2 MG AND 4 MG

Presentation Oval double-scored white tablet containing 4 mg methylprednisolone: oval double-scored pink tablet containing 2 mg methylprednisolone.

Uses Medrone is a potent corticosteroid with an anti-inflammatory activity at least five times that of hydrocortisone. An enhanced separation of glucocorticoid and mineralocorticoid effect results in a reduced incidence of sodium and water retention.

Medrone is indicated for conditions requiring glucocorticoid activity such as:

Endocrine disorders: Primary and secondary adrenal insufficiency; congenital adrenal hyperplasia.

Rheumatic disorders: Rheumatoid arthritis; juvenile chronic arthritis; ankylosing spondylitis.

Collagen diseases/arteritis: Systemic lupus erythematosus; systemic dermatomyositis (polymyositis); rheumatic fever with severe carditis; giant cell arteritis/polymyalgia rheumatica.

Dermatological diseases: Pemphigus vulgaris.

Allergic states: Severe seasonal and perennial allergic rhinitis; drug hypersensitivity reactions; serum sickness; allergic contact dermatitis; bronchial asthma.

Ophthalmic diseases: Anterior uveitis (iritis, iridocyclitis); posterior uveitis; optic neuritis.

Respiratory diseases: Pulmonary sarcoid; fulminating or disseminated tuberculosis (with appropriate anti-tuberculous chemotherapy); aspiration of gastric contents.

Haematological disorders: Idiopathic thrombocytopenia purpura; haemolytic anaemia (autoimmune).

Neoplastic diseases: Leukaemia (acute and lymphatic); malignant lymphoma.

Gastro-intestinal diseases: Ulcerative colitis; Crohn's disease.

Miscellaneous: Tuberculous meningitis (with appropriate anti-tuberculous chemotherapy); transplantation.

Dosage and administration The dosage recommendations shown in the table below are suggested initial daily doses and are intended as guides. The average total daily dose recommended should be given in 3 or 4 equally divided doses (excepting in alternate day therapy when the minimum effective daily dose is double and given every other day at 8.00 a.m.)

The initial suppressive dose level may vary depending on the condition being treated. This is continued until a satisfactory clinical response is obtained, a period usually of three to seven days in the case of rheumatic diseases (except for acute rheumatic carditis), allergic conditions affecting the skin or respiratory tract and ophthalmic diseases. If a satisfactory response is not obtained in seven days, re-evaluation of the case to confirm the original diagnosis should be made. As soon as a satisfactory clinical response is obtained, the daily dose should be reduced gradually, either to termination of treatment in the case of acute conditions (e.g. seasonal asthma, exfoliative dermatitis, acute ocular inflammations) or to the minimal effective maintenance dose level in the case of chronic conditions (e.g. rheumatoid arthritis, systemic lupus erythematosus, bronchial asthma, atopic dermatitis). In chronic conditions, and in rheumatoid arthritis especially, it is important that the reduction in dosage from initial to maintenance dose levels be accomplished slowly. Decrements of not more than 2 mg at intervals of 7–10 days are suggested. In rheumatoid arthritis, maintenance steroid therapy should be at the lowest possible level.

In alternate-day therapy, the minimum daily corticoid requirement is doubled and administered as a single dose every other day at 8.00 a.m. Dosage requirements depend on the condition being treated and response of the patient.

Elderly patients: Treatment of elderly patients, particularly if long-term, should be planned bearing in mind the more serious consequences of the common side-effects of corticosteroids in old age, particularly osteoporosis, diabetes, hypertension, susceptibility to infection and thinning of skin.

Children: Treatment should be limited to the minimum dosage for the shortest period of time. If possible treatment should be administered as a single dose on alternate days. In general, dosage for children should be based upon clinical response and is at the discretion of the clinician.

Dosage recommendations

Indications	*Recommended initial daily dosage*
Rheumatoid arthritis	
severe	12–16 mg
moderately severe	8–12 mg
moderate	4–8 mg
children	4–8 mg
Systemic dermatomyositis	48 mg
Systemic lupus erythematosus	20–96 mg
Acute rheumatic fever	48 mg until ESR normal for one week
Allergic diseases	12–40 mg
Bronchial asthma	up to 64 mg single dose/ alternate day up to 80 mg maximum
Ophthalmic diseases	12–40 mg
Haematological disorders and leukaemias	16–96 mg
Ulcerative colitis	16–60 mg
Crohn's disease	up to 48 mg per day in acute episodes
Organ transplantation	up to 3.6 mg/kg/day
Pulmonary sarcoid	32–48 mg on alternate days
Giant cell arteritis/ polymyalgia rheumatica	64 mg
Pemphigus vulgaris	80–360 mg

Contra-indications, warnings, etc

Contra-indications: Medrone is contra-indicated in known hypersensitivity to components and in systemic fungal infections. Immunisation procedures should not be undertaken in patients who are on corticosteroids, especially on high doses, due to the possibility of neurological complications and lack of antibody response.

Warnings: Drug induced adrenocortical insufficiency may be minimised by gradual reduction of dosage. This type of relative insufficiency may persist for months after discontinuation of therapy; therefore, in any situation of stress occurring during that period, hormone therapy should be reinstituted. Since mineralocorticoid secretion may be impaired, salt and/or a mineralocorticoid should be administered concurrently.

Corticosteroids may mask some signs of infection, and new infections may appear during their use. There may be a decreased resistance and inability to localise infection when corticosteroids are used.

In patients on corticosteroid therapy subjected to unusual stress increased dosage of rapidly acting corticosteroids before, during and after the stressful situation is indicated.

The use of Medrone in active tuberculosis should be restricted to those cases of fulminating or disseminated tuberculosis in which the corticosteroid is used for the management of the disease in conjunction with an appropriate antituberculous regimen. If corticosteroids are indicated in patients with latent tuberculosis or tuberculin reactivity, close observation is necessary as reactivation of the disease may occur. During prolonged corticosteroid therapy, these patients should receive chemoprophylaxis.

Corticosteroids should be used with caution in nonspecific ulcerative colitis if there is a probability of impending perforation, abscess or other pyogenic infection.

There is no evidence that corticosteroids are carcinogenic or mutagenic.

Prolonged use of corticosteroids may produce posterior subcapsular cataracts, glaucoma with possible damage to the optic nerves, and may enhance the establishment of secondary ocular infections due to fungi or viruses. Allergic reactions may occur.

Average and large doses of hydrocortisone or cortisone can cause elevation of blood pressure, salt and water retention, and increased excretion of potassium. These effects are less likely to occur with the synthetic derivatives except when used in large doses. Dietary salt restriction and potassium supplementation may be necessary. All corticosteroids increase calcium excretion.

Osteoporosis is a common but infrequently recognised adverse effect associated with long-term use of large doses of glucocorticoids.

Host defences are impaired in patients receiving large doses of glucocorticoids and this effect increases susceptibility to fungal infections as well as bacterial and viral infections.

Precautions: The presence of diabetes, ocular herpes simplex, osteoporosis, diverticulitis, fresh intestinal anastomoses, active or latent peptic ulcer, myasthenia gravis, chronic psychotic reactions, glaucoma, previous steroid myopathy, epilepsy, predisposition to thrombophlebitis, hypertension, congestive heart failure and renal insufficiency necessitate the carefully controlled use of methylprednisolone. There is an enhanced effect of corticosteroids on patients with hypothyroidism and in those with cirrhosis.

Psychic derangements may appear when corticosteroids are used ranging from euphoria, insomnia, mood swings, personality changes, and severe depression to frank psychotic manifestations. Also, existing emotional instability or psychotic tendencies may be aggravated by corticosteroids.

Aspirin and non-steroidal anti-inflammatory agents should be used cautiously in conjunction with corticosteroids in patients with hypoprothrombinaemia.

Because complications of treatment with glucocorticoids are dependent on the size of the dose and the duration of treatment, a risk/benefit decision must be made in each individual case as to dose and duration of treatment and as to whether daily or intermittent therapy should be used.

Use in pregnancy: The use of corticosteroids, in general, in pregnancy involves balancing the clinical benefit against the possible risks. There is inadequate evidence of safety in human pregnancy and there may be a very small risk of cleft palate and intra-uterine growth retardation in the foetus; there is evidence of harmful effects on pregnancy in animals. Neonates of mothers who have received such therapy during pregnancy should be observed for signs of hypoadrenalism and appropriate measures instituted if such signs exist.

Because prednisolone is excreted in breast milk, it is reasonable to assume that all corticosteroids are.

Use in children: Corticosteroids cause growth retardation in infancy, childhood and adolescence. Treatment should be limited to the minimum dosage for the shortest possible time. In order to minimise suppression of the hypothalamo-pituitary-adrenal axis and growth retardation, treatment should be administered where possible as a single dose on alternate days.

Side-effects: Side-effects associated with the use of corticosteroids may be observed, including:

Gastro-intestinal: Dyspepsia, peptic ulceration with perforation and haemorrhage, abdominal distension, oesophageal ulceration, oesophageal candidiasis, acute pancreatitis, perforation of bowel.

Musculoskeletal: Proximal myopathy, osteoporosis, vertebral and long bone fractures, avascular osteonecrosis, tendon rupture, muscle weakness.

Fluid and electrolyte disturbance: Sodium and water retention, hypertension, hypokalaemic alkalosis, potassium loss, congestive heart failure in susceptible patients.

Dermatological: Impaired healing, skin atrophy, bruising, striae, telangiectasia, acne, petechiae and ecchymosis.

Endocrine/metabolic: Suppression of the hypothalamo-pituitary-adrenal axis, growth suppression in childhood and adolescence, menstrual irregularity and amenorrhoea. Cushingoid facies, hirsutism, weight gain, impaired carbohydrate tolerance with increased requirement for antidiabetic therapy, negative nitrogen balance.

Neuropsychiatric: Euphoria, psychological dependence, depression, insomnia. Intracranial hypertension in children. Aggravation of schizophrenia. Pseudotumour cerebri, seizures.

Ophthalmic: Increased intra-ocular pressure, glaucoma, papilloedema, cataracts, corneal or scleral thinning, exacerbation of ophthalmic viral or fungal disease, exophthalmos.

Immune system: Masking of infections, hypersensitivity reactions including anaphylaxis, may suppress reactions to skin tests.

General: Opportunistic infection, recurrence of dormant tuberculosis, leucocytosis, hypersensitivity, thrombo-embolism, increased appetite, nausea, malaise.

Withdrawal symptoms: Fever, myalgia, arthralgia, adrenal insufficiency.

Overdosage: Administration of Medrone should not be discontinued abruptly but tailed off over a period of time. Appropriate action should be taken to alleviate the symptoms produced by any side-effect that may become apparent. It may be necessary to support the patient with corticosteroids during any further period of trauma occurring within two years of overdosage.

There is no clinical syndrome of acute overdosage with Medrone. Methylprednisolone is dialysable.

Pharmaceutical precautions No special precautions are required.

Legal category POM.

Package quantities 2 and 4 mg tablets in packs of 30 and 100.

Further information Medrone has achieved a clinically acceptable split between glucocorticoid effect and undesired mineralocorticoid effect. Weight for weight, methylprednisolone has five times the anti-inflammatory activity of hydrocortisone but has little tendency to cause salt and water retention.

A separate data sheet is available for Medrone Tablets 16 mg, which details those indications for which high dose oral steroid therapy is appropriate.

Product licence numbers
Medrone Tablets 2 mg 0032/5017
Medrone Tablets 4 mg 0032/5018

MEDRONE* TABLETS 16 MG

Presentation Oval single-scored white tablet marked 'Upjohn 73' containing 16 mg methylprednisolone.

Uses Medrone is a potent corticosteroid with an anti-inflammatory activity at least five times that of hydrocortisone. An enhanced separation of glucocorticoid and mineralocorticoid effect results in a reduced incidence of sodium and water retention.

Medrone 16 mg is indicated for conditions requiring glucocorticoid activity such as:

Collagen diseases/arteritis: Systemic lupus erythematosus; systemic dermatomyositis (polymyositis); rheumatic fever with severe carditis; giant cell arteritis/polymyalgia rheumatica.

Dermatological diseases: Pemphigus vulgaris.

Allergic states: Bronchial asthma.

Respiratory diseases: Pulmonary sarcoid.

Haematological disorders: Idiopathic thrombocytopenia purpura; haemolytic anaemia (autoimmune).

Neoplastic diseases: Leukaemia (acute and lymphatic); malignant lymphoma.

Gastro-intestinal diseases: Crohn's disease.

Miscellaneous: Tuberculous meningitis (with appropriate anti-tuberculous chemotherapy); transplantation.

Dosage and administration The dosage recommendations shown in the table below are suggested initial daily doses and are intended as guides. The average total daily dose recommended should be given in 3 or 4 equally divided doses (excepting in alternate day therapy when the minimum effective daily dose is doubled and given every other day at 8.00 a.m.).

The initial suppressive dose level may vary depending on the condition being treated. As soon as a satisfactory clinical response is obtained, the daily dose should be reduced gradually, either to termination of treatment in the case of acute conditions or to the minimal effective maintenance dose level in the case of chronic conditions. In chronic conditions it is important that the reduction in dosage from initial to maintenance dose levels be accomplished slowly.

In alternate-day therapy, the minimum daily corticoid requirement is doubled and administered as a single dose every other day at 8.00 a.m. Dosage requirements depend on the condition being treated and response of the patient.

Elderly patients: Treatment of elderly patients, particularly if long-term, should be planned bearing in mind the more serious consequences of the common side-effects of corticosteroids in old age, particularly osteoporosis, diabetes, hypertension, susceptibility to infection and thinning of skin.

Children: In general, dosage for children should be based upon clinical response and is at the discretion of the clinician. Treatment should be limited to the minimum dosage for the shortest period of time. If possible, treatment should be administered as a single dose on alternate days.

Dosage recommendations

Indications	*Recommended initial daily dosage*
Systemic lupus erythematosus	20–96 mg
Systemic dermatomyositis	48 mg
Acute rheumatic fever	48 mg until ESR normal for one week.
Giant cell arteritis/ polymyalgia rheumatica	64 mg
Pemphigus vulgaris	80–360 mg
Bronchial asthma	up to 64 mg single dose/ alternate day up to 80 mg maximum.
Pulmonary sarcoid	32–48 mg on alternate days.
Haematological disorders and leukaemias	16–96 mg
Malignant lymphoma	16–96 mg
Crohn's disease	up to 48 mg per day in acute episodes
Organ transplantation	up to 3.6 mg/kg/day

Contra-indications, warnings, etc

Contra-indications: Medrone is contra-indicated in known hypersensitivity to components and in systemic fungal infections. Immunisation procedures should not be undertaken in patients who are on corticosteroids, especially on high doses, due to the possibility of neurological complications and lack of antibody response.

Warnings: Drug induced adrenocortical insufficiency may be minimised by gradual reduction of dosage. This type of relative insufficiency may persist for months after discontinuation of therapy; therefore, in any situation of stress occurring during that period, hormone therapy should be reinstituted. Since mineralocorticoid secretion may be impaired, salt and/or a mineralocorticoid should be administered concurrently.

Corticosteroids may mask some signs of infection, and new infections may appear during their use. There may be a decreased resistance and inability to localise infection when corticosteroids are used.

In patients on corticosteroid therapy subjected to unusual stress increased dosage of rapidly acting corticosteroids before, during and after the stressful situation is indicated.

The use of Medrone in active tuberculosis should be restricted to those cases of fulminating or disseminated tuberculosis in which the corticosteroid is used for the management of the disease in conjunction with an appropriate antituberculous regimen. If corticosteroids are indicated in patients with latent tuberculosis or tuberculin reactivity, close observation is necessary as reactivation of the disease may occur. During prolonged corticosteroid therapy, these patients should receive chemoprophylaxis.

Corticosteroids should be used with caution in non-specific ulcerative colitis if there is a probability of impending perforation, abscess or other pyogenic infection.

There is no evidence that corticosteroids are carcinogenic or mutagenic.

Prolonged use of corticosteroids may produce posterior subcapsular cataracts, glaucoma with possible damage to the optic nerves, and may enhance the establishment of secondary ocular infections due to fungi or viruses. Allergic reactions may occur.

Average and large doses of hydrocortisone or cortisone can cause elevation of blood pressure, salt and water retention, and increased excretion of potassium. These effects are less likely to occur with the synthetic derivatives except when used in large doses. Dietary salt restriction and potassium supplementation may be necessary. All corticosteroids increase calcium excretion.

Osteoporosis is a common but infrequently recognised adverse effect associated with long-term use of large doses of glucocorticoids.

Host defences are impaired in patients receiving large doses of glucocorticoids and this effect increases susceptibility to fungal infections as well as bacterial and viral infections.

Precautions: The presence of diabetes, ocular herpes simplex, osteoporosis, diverticulitis, fresh intestinal anastomoses, active or latent peptic ulcer, myasthenia gravis, chronic psychotic reactions, glaucoma, previous steroid myopathy, epilepsy, predisposition to thrombophlebitis, hypertension, congestive heart failure and renal insufficiency necessitate the carefully controlled use of methylprednisolone. There is an enhanced effect of corticosteroids on patients with hypothyroidism and in those with cirrhosis.

Psychic derangements may appear when corticosteroids are used ranging from euphoria, insomnia, mood swings, personality changes, and severe depression to frank psychotic manifestations. Also, existing emotional instability or psychotic tendencies may be aggravated by corticosteroids.

Aspirin and non-steroidal anti-inflammatory agents should be used cautiously in conjunction with corticosteroids in patients with hypoprothrombinaemia.

Because complications of treatment with glucocorticoids are dependent on the size of the dose and the duration of treatment, a risk/benefit decision must be made in each individual case as to dose and duration of treatment and as to whether daily or intermittent therapy should be used.

Use in pregnancy: The use of corticosteroids, in general, in pregnancy involves balancing the clinical benefit against the possible risks. There is inadequate evidence of safety in human pregnancy and there may be a very small risk of cleft palate and intra-uterine growth retardation in the foetus; there is evidence of harmful effects on pregnancy in animals. Neonates of mothers who have received such therapy during pregnancy should be observed for signs of hypoadrenalism and appropriate measures instituted if such signs exist.

Because prednisolone is excreted in breast milk, it is reasonable to assume that all corticosteroids are.

Use in children: Corticosteroids cause growth retardation in infancy, childhood and adolescence. Treatment should be limited to the minimum dosage for the shortest possible time. In order to minimise suppression of the hypothalamo-pituitary-adrenal axis and growth retardation, treatment should be administered where possible as a single dose on alternate days.

Side-effects: Side-effects associated with the use of corticosteroids may be observed, including:

Gastro-intestinal: Dyspepsia, peptic ulceration with perforation and haemorrhage, abdominal distension, oesophageal ulceration, oesophageal candidiasis, acute pancreatitis, perforation of bowel.

Musculoskeletal: Proximal myopathy, osteoporosis, vertebral and long bone fractures, avascular osteonecrosis, tendon rupture, muscle weakness.

Fluid and electrolyte disturbance: Sodium and water retention, hypertension, hypokalaemic alkalosis, potassium loss, congestive heart failure in susceptible patients.

Dermatological: Impaired healing, skin atrophy, bruising, striae, telangiectasia, acne, petechiae and ecchymosis.

Endocrine/metabolic: Suppression of the hypothalamo-pituitary-adrenal axis, growth suppression in childhood and adolescence, menstrual irregularity and amenorrhoea. Cushingoid facies, hirsutism, weight gain, impaired carbohydrate tolerance with increased requirement for antidiabetic therapy, negative nitrogen balance.

Neuropsychiatric: Euphoria, psychological dependence, depression, insomnia. Intracranial hypertension in children. Aggravation of schizophrenia. Pseudotumour cerebri, seizures.

Ophthalmic: Increased intra-ocular pressure, glaucoma, papilloedema, cataracts, corneal or scleral thinning, exacerbation of ophthalmic viral or fungal disease, exophthalmos.

Immune system: Masking of infections, hypersensitivity reactions including anaphylaxis, may suppress reactions to skin tests.

General: Opportunistic infection, recurrence of dormant tuberculosis, leucocytosis, hypersensitivity, thrombo-embolism, increased appetite, nausea, malaise.

Withdrawal symptoms: Fever, myalgia, arthralgia, adrenal insufficiency.

Overdosage: Administration of Medrone should not be discontinued abruptly but tailed off over a period of time. Appropriate action should be taken to alleviate the symptoms produced by any side-effect that may become apparent. It may be necessary to support the patient with corticosteroids during any further period of trauma occurring within two years of overdosage.

There is no clinical syndrome of acute overdosage with Medrone. Methylprednisolone is dialysable.

Pharmaceutical precautions No special precautions are required.

Legal category POM.

Package quantities 16 mg tablets in bottles of 14 (OP).

Further information Medrone has achieved a clinically acceptable split between glucocorticoid effect and undesired mineralocorticoid effect. Weight for weight, methylprednisolone has five times the anti-inflammatory activity of hydrocortisone but has little tendency to cause salt and water retention. The 16 mg tablet gives opportunity for use of alternate day therapy in long term use in chronic conditions.

A separate data sheet is available for Medrone Tablets

2 mg and 4 mg and includes additional indications in which low dose therapy is appropriate.

Product licence number 0032/0024.

MOTRIN*

Presentation Film-coated tablets containing Ibuprofen BP:
200 mg – round, biconvex, red tablet marked U on one side;
400 mg – round, biconvex, orange tablet marked U on one side;
600 mg – elliptical, peach tablet marked U on one side;
800 mg – elliptical, capsule shaped, bright orange tablet marked MOTRIN and 800 mg on one side.

Uses Non-steroidal, anti-inflammatory agent with analgesic and antipyretic properties. Motrin is indicated for the relief of the signs and symptoms of rheumatoid arthritis (including Still's Disease), osteo-arthritis, ankylosing spondylitis and seronegative (non-rheumatoid) arthropathies. It may also be used in non-articular rheumatic conditions and soft tissue injuries; these include low back pain, capsulitis, bursitis, tenosynovitis, sprains and strains.

Dosage and administration
Adults: 1200–1800 mg daily in three divided doses; up to 2400 mg daily may be given in severe conditions.

Children: 20 mg/kg daily in divided doses. In juvenile rheumatoid arthritis, up to 40 mg/kg daily in divided doses may be taken. In those children weighing less than 30 kg, the total dose in 24 hours should not exceed 500 mg.

Elderly patients: It appears that advanced age has a minimal influence on the pharmacokinetics of ibuprofen. However, the following should be considered:

Ibuprofen may increase levels of digoxin concentration, presumably from reduced renal excretion of digoxin.

Ibuprofen has been reported to have an antagonistic effect on frusemide-induced diuresis in cardiac failure.

Ibuprofen has been reported to be associated with cognitive dysfunction in the elderly.

Although ibuprofen is probably one of the safer non-steroidal anti-inflammatory drugs to use in association with anticoagulants (warfarin), it should be used with caution.

Contra-indications, warnings, etc
Contra-indications: Active peptic ulceration. Motrin Tablets should not be given to patients who have previously shown hypersensitivity to the drug, or to those patients in whom aspirin, Motrin or other non-steroidal anti-inflammatory drugs induce the syndrome of nasal polyps, bronchospastic reactivity or angioedema. Anaphylactoid reactions have occurred in such patients.

Precautions: Reproductive studies conducted in rats and rabbits at doses somewhat less than the clinical maximum dose did not demonstrate any evidence of developmental abnormalities. As there are no adequate and well-controlled studies in pregnant women, this drug should be used during pregnancy only if clearly needed. Because of the known effects of non-steroidal anti-inflammatory drugs on the foetal cardiovascular system (closure of ductus arteriosus), use during late pregnancy should be avoided. As with other drugs known to inhibit prostaglandin synthesis, an increased incidence of dystocia and delayed parturition occurred in rats. Administration of Motrin is not recommended during pregnancy.

In limited studies, an assay capable of detecting 1 microgram/ml did not demonstrate ibuprofen in the milk of lactating women. However, due to the limited nature of the studies and the possible adverse effects of prostaglandin-inhibiting drugs on neonates, Motrin is not recommended for use in nursing mothers.

Fluid retention and oedema have been reported in association with Motrin; therefore, the drug should be used with caution in patients with a history of cardiac decompensation or hypertension.

As with other non-steroidal anti-inflammatory drugs, long-term administration of ibuprofen to animals has resulted in renal papillary necrosis and other abnormal renal pathology. In humans, there have been reports of acute interstitial nephritis with haematuria, proteinuria and occasionally nephrotic syndrome.

A second form of renal toxicity has been seen in patients with prerenal conditions leading to a reduction in renal blood flow or blood volume, where the renal prostaglandins have a supportive role in the maintenance of renal perfusion. In these patients, administration of a non-steroidal anti-inflammatory drug may cause a dose dependent reduction in prostaglandin formation and may precipitate overt renal decompensation. Patients at greatest risk of this reaction are those with impaired renal function, heart failure, liver dysfunction, those taking diuretics and the elderly. Discontinuation of non-steroidal anti-inflammatory drug therapy is typically followed by recovery to the pre-treatment state.

Since ibuprofen is eliminated primarily by the kidneys, patients with significantly impaired renal function should be closely monitored and a reduction in dosage should be anticipated to avoid drug accumulation.

Those patients at high risk of developing renal dysfunction during long-term treatment should have renal function monitored periodically.

Ibuprofen, like other non-steroidal anti-inflammatory drugs, can inhibit platelet aggregation, but the effect is quantitatively less and of shorter duration than that seen with aspirin. Motrin has been shown to prolong bleeding time (but within the normal range) in normal subjects. Because this prolonged bleeding effect may be exaggerated in patients with underlying haemostatic defects, Motrin should be used with caution in persons with intrinsic coagulation defects and those on anticoagulant therapy.

Patients on Motrin should report to their physicians signs or symptoms of gastro-intestinal ulceration or bleeding, blurred vision or other eye symptoms, skin rash, weight gain or oedema.

The antipyretic and anti-inflammatory activity of ibuprofen may reduce fever and inflammation, thus diminishing their utility as diagnostic signs in detecting complications of presumed non-infectious, non-inflammatory painful conditions.

Warnings: Use with extreme caution in those patients with asthma.

Peptic ulceration and gastro-intestinal bleeding, sometimes severe, have been reported in patients receiving ibuprofen.

Motrin should be given under close supervision to patients with a history of upper gastro-intestinal tract disease.

Treatment should be discontinued in patients reporting blurred or diminished vision, scotomata and/or changes in colour vision.

Adverse reactions: A decrease in haemoglobin content of 1 gram or more has been observed in 20% of patients.

Gastro-intestinal effects are a frequent adverse reaction to Motrin Tablets.

The following adverse reactions may occur in 3–9% of patients taking Motrin Tablets: nausea, epigastric pain, dizziness, non-specific rash, elevated serum creatinine levels and anaemia.

The following rarely occurring adverse reactions have been reported in patients taking Motrin Tablets: renal failure, lupus erythematosus syndrome with aseptic meningitis, jaundice, abnormal liver function tests, blood dyscrasias including thrombocytopenia. Aseptic meningitis is probably more common in patients with systemic lupus erythematosus and related connective tissue diseases.

Drugs interactions:
Coumarin-type anticoagulants: Several short-term controlled studies failed to show that Motrin significantly affected prothrombin times, or a variety of other clotting factors, when administered to individuals on coumarin-type anticoagulants.

Aspirin: Animal studies show that aspirin given with non-steroidal anti-inflammatory drugs, including Motrin, causes a net decrease in anti-inflammatory activity with lowered blood levels of the non-aspirin drug.

Methotrexate: Motrin and other non-steroidal anti-inflammatory drugs have been reported to reduce renal tubular secretion of methotrexate *in vitro*. This may lead to enhanced toxicity of methotrexate. Caution should be used if Motrin is administered concomitantly with methotrexate.

Frusemide: Motrin has been shown to reduce the natriuretic effect of frusemide and thiazide diuretics in some patients, probably due to inhibition of renal prostaglandin synthesis by Motrin and other non-steroidal anti-inflammatory drugs. Patients being treated concomitantly with Motrin and frusemide or thiazides should therefore be observed closely.

Lithium: Motrin has been shown to produce a clinically relevant elevation of plasma lithium levels and a reduction in renal lithium clearance in a volunteer study. This effect has been attributed to inhibition of renal prostaglandin synthesis. Thus, when Motrin and lithium are administered concurrently, subjects should be carefully observed for signs of lithium toxicity.

Treatment of overdosage: Gastric lavage. No specific antidote. It is theoretically advantageous to administer alkali and induce diuresis as the drug is acidic and excreted in the urine.

Pharmaceutical precautions Motrin tablets should be stored at room temperature (15–30°C) in a well-closed container.

Legal category POM.

Package quantities Packs of 100 tablets.

Further information The absorption profile shows Motrin to be of particular value in relieving morning stiffness.

Product licence numbers

200 mg	0032/0104
400 mg	0032/0105
600 mg	0032/0106
800 mg	0032/0134

NEO-CORTEF* EYE/EAR DROPS NEO-CORTEF* EYE/EAR OINTMENT

Presentation White, sterile aqueous suspension containing hydrocortisone acetate 15 mg and neomycin sulphate 5 mg (0.5%) per ml. Yellow soft ointment containing hydrocortisone acetate 15 mg and neomycin sulphate 5 mg (0.5%) per gram.

Uses

Eye: Short term treatment of steroid responsive conditions of the eye when prophylactic antibiotic treatment is also required, after excluding the presence of fungal and viral disease.

Eyelid: Blepharitis.

Ear: Otitis externa.

Dosage and administration

Adults and children:

Eye: One or two drops to be applied to each eye up to six times daily or more frequently if required.

Apply ointment sparingly two or three times daily, or at night if drops are used during the day.

Ear: Two or three drops to be instilled into the ear three to four times daily.

Apply ointment once or twice daily.

Elderly patients: There is no information to suggest that a change in dosage is warranted in the elderly.

Contra-indications, warnings, etc

Contra-indications: Viral, fungal, tuberculous or purulent conditions of the eye. Use is contra-indicated if glaucoma is present or herpetic keratitis (eg dendritic ulcer) is considered a possibility.

Use of topical steroids in the latter condition can lead to extension of the ulcer and marked visual deterioration.

Otitis externa should not be treated when the eardrum is perforated because of the risk of ototoxicity.

Hypersensitivity to the preparation.

Warnings:

Effects on ability to drive and use machines: Transient blurring of vision on instillation or application. Warn patients not to drive or operate hazardous machinery unless vision is clear.

Use in pregnancy and lactation: Safety for use in pregnancy and lactation has not been established. There is inadequate evidence of safety in human pregnancy. Topical administration of corticosteroids to pregnant animals can cause abnormalities of foetal development including cleft palate and intrauterine growth retardation. There may therefore be a very small risk of such effects in the human foetus. There is a risk of foetal ototoxicity if aminoglycoside antibiotic preparations are administered during pregnancy.

Other special warnings and precautions: Topical corticosteroids should never be given for an undiagnosed red eye as inappropriate use is potentially blinding.

Treatment with corticosteroid/antibiotic combinations should not be continued for more than 7 days in the absence of any clinical improvement, since prolonged use may lead to occult extension of infection due to the masking effect of the steroid. Prolonged use may also lead to skin sensitisation and the emergence of resistant organisms.

Prolonged use may lead to the risk of adrenal suppression in infants.

Treatment with corticosteroid preparations should not be repeated or prolonged without regular review to exclude raised intraocular pressure, cataract formation or unsuspected infections.

Aminoglycoside antibiotics may cause irreversible, partial or total deafness when given systemically or when applied topically to open wounds or damaged skin. This effect is dose related and is enhanced by renal or hepatic impairment. Although this effect has not been reported following topical ocular use, the possibility should be considered when high dose topical treatment is given to small children or infants.

Side-effects: Hypersensitivity reactions, usually of the delayed type, may occur leading to irritation, burning, stinging, itching and dermatitis.

Topical steroid use may result in increased intraocular pressure leading to optic nerve damage, reduced visual acuity and visual field defects.

In those diseases causing thinning of the cornea or sclera, corticosteroid therapy may result in thinning of the globe leading to perforation.

Overdosage: Long-term intensive topical use may lead to systemic effects.

Oral ingestion of the contents of one bottle or tube is unlikely to lead to any serious adverse effects.

Pharmaceutical precautions None.

Legal category POM.

Package quantities Neo-Cortef Eye/Ear Drops supplied as 5 ml plastic squeeze bottles with applicator tip.

Neo-Cortef Eye/Ear Ointment is supplied in tubes of 3.9 g with applicator tip.

Further information Nil.

Product licence numbers

Neo-Cortef Eye/Ear Drops	0032/5026
Neo-Cortef Eye/Ear Ointment	0032/5027

PREPIDIL* GEL 500 MICROGRAMS

Presentation Translucent, thixotropic, sterile gel containing 500 micrograms dinoprostone per 3 g (2.5 ml).

Uses Pre-induction cervical softening and dilation in pregnant women with at term, or near term, gestation and unfavourable induction features, when there are no foetal or maternal contra-indications.

Dosage and administration The entire contents of

the syringe are administered into the cervical canal just below the level of the internal cervical os using the accompanying catheter. The patient should be instructed to remain recumbent for 10–15 minutes.

Contra-indications, warnings, etc
Contra-indications: There are no absolute contra-indications to the use of Prepidil Gel but its use is not recommended for the following:

1. Patients in whom oxytocic drugs are generally contra-indicated or where prolonged contractions of the uterus are considered inappropriate such as:

Cases with a history of caesarean section or major uterine surgery;

Cases in which major degrees of cephalopelvic disproportion may be present;

Cases in which there is clinical suspicion or definite evidence of pre-existing foetal distress;

Cases in which there is a history of difficult labour and/or traumatic delivery;

Grand multiparae with six or more previous term pregnancies.

2. Patients with ruptured membranes.
3. Patients with a known sensitivity to prostaglandins.
4. Patients with unexplained vaginal bleeding during this pregnancy.
5. Patients with non-vertex presentations.

Warnings: Since it has been found that prostaglandins may potentiate the effect of oxytocin, it is recommended that if these drugs are used in sequence the patient's uterine activity should be carefully monitored.

The product is available only to hospitals and clinics with specialised obstetric units.

Precautions: Care should be taken not to administer Prepidil Gel above the level of the internal os as placement of the gel into the extra-amniotic space has been associated with uterine hyperstimulation.

Caution should be exercised in the administration of Prepidil Gel to patients with:
(i) glaucoma or raised intraocular pressure.
(ii) asthma or a history of asthma.

Foeto-pelvic relationships should be carefully evaluated before use of the gel. During use uterine activity, foetal status and cervical dilation and effacement should be carefully monitored to detect possible evidence of undesired responses e.g. hypertonus, sustained uterine contractions or foetal distress. In cases where there is a known history of hypertonic uterine contractility or tetanic uterine contractions it is recommended that uterine activity and the state of the foetus should be continuously monitored. The possibility of uterine rupture should be borne in mind where high-tone myometrial contractions are sustained. Animal studies lasting several weeks at high doses have shown that prostaglandins of the E and F series can induce proliferation of bone. Such effects have also been noted in newborn infants who have received prostaglandin E_1 during prolonged treatment. There is no evidence to suggest that short term administration of Prepidil Gel can cause similar bone effects.

Side-effects: Occasional gastro-intestinal upsets with vomiting and/or diarrhoea have occurred. Intrapartum foetal heart rate changes and unclassified foetal distress have been reported. Uterine contractile abnormalities either with or without foetal heart rate changes have also occurred. Apgar scores below 7 at birth have been reported.

Overdosage: Treatment of overdosage must, at this time, be symptomatic since clinical studies with prostaglandin antagonists have not progressed to the point where recommendations may be made.

Pharmaceutical precautions Store in a refrigerator at 2–8°C. Use the total contents of the syringe for one patient only. Discard after use.

Legal category POM.

Package quantities Prepidil Gel is supplied as a 2.5 ml pre-filled disposable syringe containing 500 micrograms dinoprostone.

Further information Prepidil Gel exhibits the capacity of other prostaglandins to influence uterine activity at any stage of gestation. Other forms of dinoprostone (Prostin E2) are available for induction of labour (oral, vaginal and i.v. routes), foetal death in utero (i.v. route), therapeutic termination of pregnancy (i.v. and extra amniotic routes), missed abortion and hydatidiform mole (i.v. route).

Product licence number 0032/0138.

PROSTIN E2* STERILE SOLUTIONS 1 MG/ML, 10 MG/ML

Presentation Colourless sterile solutions in ampoules containing 1 mg/ml or 10 mg/ml dinoprostone, prostaglandin E2, in ethanol.

Uses Oxytocic agent.

Indications for Prostin E2 are: induction of labour, foetal death in utero, therapeutic termination of pregnancy, missed abortion and hydatidiform mole.

1. 0.75 ml ampoule of a 1 mg/ml solution of dinoprostone in ethanol – for induction of labour and foetal death in utero (intravenous).
2. 0.5 ml ampoule of a 10 mg/ml solution of dinoprostone in ethanol – for therapeutic termination of pregnancy, missed abortion and hydatidiform mole (intravenous).
3. 0.5 ml ampoule of a 10 mg/ml solution of dinoprostone in ethanol (plus a 50 ml vial of saline diluent) – for therapeutic termination of pregnancy (extra-amniotic).

Dosage and administration Prostin E2 Sterile Solution may be administered by two routes, intravenous or extra-amniotic, depending on dose form and indication as shown above. *In each case the ampoule contents must be diluted before use and full instructions on method of dilution and dosage are given on the package insert which should be consulted prior to initiation of therapy.* Continuous administration of the drug for more than two days is not recommended (See Precautions). The following is a guide to dosage:

1. *Prostin E2 1 mg/ml solution (in ethanol). Intravenous for induction of labour:* Dilute with normal saline or 5% dextrose according to the package insert to produce a 1.5 micrograms/ml solution. The 1.5 micrograms/ml solution is infused at 0.25 micrograms/minute for 30 minutes and then maintained or increased. Cases of foetal death in utero may require higher doses. An initial rate of 0.5 micrograms/minute may be used with stepwise increases, at intervals of not less than one hour.

2. *Prostin E2 10 mg/ml solution (in ethanol). Intravenous for therapeutic termination of pregnancy, missed abortion and hydatidiform mole:* Dilute with normal saline or 5% dextrose according to package insert to produce a 5 micrograms/ml solution. The 5 micrograms/ml solution is infused at 2.5 micrograms/minute for 30 minutes and then maintained or increased to 5 micrograms/minute. The rate should be maintained for at least four hours before increasing further.

3. *Prostin E2 10 mg/ml solution (in ethanol). Extra-amniotic for therapeutic termination of pregnancy:* Dilute with the 50 ml of diluent provided according to the package insert to produce a 100 micrograms/ml solution. The 100 micrograms/ml solution is instilled via a 12–14 French-gauge Foley catheter. Initial instillation is 1 ml, then, dependent on uterine response, 1 or 2 ml usually at two-hour intervals.

Contra-indications, warnings, etc
Contra-indications: There are no absolute contra-indications to the use of Prostin E2 Sterile Solution. However, its use is not recommended in the following circumstances:

1. Where the patient is sensitive to prostaglandins.
2. For patients in whom oxytocic drugs are generally contra-indicated or where prolonged contractions of the uterus are considered inappropriate, such as: cases with a history of Caesarean section or major uterine surgery;

cases in which major degrees of cephalopelvic disproportion may be present; cases in which foetal malpresentation is present; cases in which there is clinical suspicion or definite evidence of pre-existing foetal distress; cases in which there is a history of difficult labour and/or traumatic delivery; grand multiparae with six or more previous term pregnancies; cases with a history of pelvic inflammatory disease.

3. In therapeutic termination of pregnancy where known pelvic infection exists, unless adequate prior treatment has been instituted.

4. The extra-amniotic route should not be employed in the presence of cervicitis or vaginal infections.

Warnings: There is some evidence in animals of a low order of teratogenicity, therefore, if abortion does not occur or is suspected to be incomplete as a result of prostaglandin therapy, the appropriate treatment for complete evacuation of the uterus should be instituted in all instances.

Since prostaglandins may potentiate the effect of oxytocin it is recommended that the use of these drugs simultaneously or in sequence be carefully monitored.

It is advised that Prostin E2 Sterile Solution should not be administered by the intramyometrial route since there have been reports of a possible association between this route of administration and cardiac arrest in severely ill patients.

The products are available only to hospitals and clinics with specialised obstetric units and should only be used where 24-hour resident medical cover is provided.

Precautions: Caution should be exercised in the administration of Prostin E2 in patients with: (i) glaucoma or raised intra-ocular pressure; (ii) asthma or a history of asthma.

In addition, in labour induction, cephalopelvic relationships should be carefully evaluated before use of Prostin E2. During use, uterine activity, foetal status and the progression of cervical dilatation should be carefully monitored to detect possible evidence of undesired responses, e.g. hypertonus, sustained uterine contractions or foetal distress. In cases where there is a known history of hypertonic uterine contractility or tetanic uterine contractions, it is recommended that uterine activity and the state of the foetus should be continuously monitored throughout labour. The possibility of uterine rupture should be borne in mind where high-tone myometrial contractions are sustained.

Animal studies lasting several weeks at high doses have shown that prostaglandins of the E and F series can induce proliferation of bone. Such effects have also been noted in newborn infants who received prostaglandin E1 during prolonged treatment. There is no evidence that short term administration of Prostin E2 can cause similar bone effects.

Side-effects: Clinical studies have not revealed any life-threatening adverse reactions. The incidence of side-effects is directly dose-related.

Nausea, vomiting and diarrhoea have been reported as commonly encountered at dose levels required to induce therapeutic termination of pregnancy by the intravenous route; however, these side-effects are markedly less frequent with doses used by either the extra-amniotic route for therapeutic termination of pregnancy, or intravenously for induction of labour. Transient vasovagal symptoms, including flushing, shivering, headache and dizziness, have been recorded. On intravenous use of Prostin E2 local tissue irritation and erythema have occurred.

No evidence of thrombophlebitis has been recorded and local tissue erythema at the infusion site has disappeared within two to five hours after infusion. A temporary pyrexia and elevated WBC are not unusual, but both have reverted after termination of infusion. In extra-amniotic therapy the possibility of local infection must be considered and appropriate therapy initiated if necessary.

Overdosage: Treatment of overdosage must be, at this time, symptomatic, as clinical studies with prostaglandin antagonists have not progressed to the point where recommendations may be made. However, the following guidelines are recommended:

If evidence of excessive uterine activity or side-effects appear, the rate of infusion should be decreased or discontinued.

In cases of massive overdosage resulting in extreme uterine hypertonus appropriate obstetric procedures are indicated.

Pharmaceutical precautions Prostin E2 Sterile Solutions (in ethanol) must be refrigerated at 4°C. They should be diluted before use only with the diluents stated. Diluted solutions should be used within 24 hours (48 hours for extra-amniotic).

Legal category POM.

Package quantities

1. Pack containing 1 × 0.75 ml ampoule of Prostin E2 Sterile Solution 1 mg/ml (IV induction).
2. Pack containing 1 × 0.5 ml ampoule of Prostin E2 Sterile Solution 10 mg/ml (IV termination).
3. Pack containing 1 × 0.5 ml ampoule of Prostin E2 Sterile Solution 10 mg/ml plus 50 ml diluent (EA termination).

Further information Oral Prostin E2 Tablets, Prostin E2 Vaginal Tablets and Prostin E2 Vaginal Gel are also available for the induction of labour.

Product licence numbers

0.75 ml ampoule (1 mg/ml i.v.)	0032/0020R
0.5 ml ampoule (10 mg/ml i.v.)	0032/0021R
0.5 ml ampoule (10 mg/ml e.a.)	0032/0026R

PROSTIN E2* ORAL TABLETS

Presentation Prostin E2 Oral Tablets are presented as white, roughly rectangular tablets embossed on one side to resemble the letter 'U' and marked '76' on the other side. Each tablet contains 500 micrograms (0.5 mg) dinoprostone.

Uses Oxytocic agent. Prostin E2 Oral Tablets are indicated for the induction of labour when there are no foetal or maternal contra-indications.

Dosage and administration The dosage of Prostin E2 must be adapted to the patient's response and should always be maintained at the lowest level which will produce satisfactory uterine response. All doses should be taken with a small glass of water.

An initial dose of 500 micrograms (1 tablet) should be given. Thereafter, doses should be given hourly. The usual dose will be 500 micrograms (1 tablet), but if uterine activity is inadequate, 1 mg (2 tablets) may be given hourly until such time as adequate uterine activity is established.

Thereafter it may be possible to reduce the dosage to 500 micrograms (1 tablet) hourly. It is recommended that a total single dose of 1.5 mg (3 tablets) not be exceeded.

Continuous administration of the drug for more than two days is not recommended. (See Precautions.)

Contra-indications, warnings, etc

Contra-indications: There are no absolute contra-indications to the use of Prostin E2. However, its use is not recommended in the following circumstances:

1. Where the patient is sensitive to prostaglandins.
2. For patients in whom oxytocic drugs are generally contra-indicated or where prolonged contractions of the uterus are considered inappropriate, such as:

Cases with a history of Caesarean section or major uterine surgery.

Cases in which major degrees of cephalopelvic disproportion may be present.

Cases in which there is clinical suspicion or definite evidence of pre-existing foetal distress.

Cases in which there is a history of difficult labour and/or traumatic delivery.

Grand multiparae with six or more previous term pregnancies.

3. Cases with a history of pelvic inflammatory disease.

Warnings: Since it has been found that prostaglandins may potentiate the effect of oxytocin, it is recommended that these drugs should not be used together, and, if used in sequence, that the patient's uterine activity should be carefully monitored.

The product is available only to hospitals and clinics with specialised obstetric units and should only be used where 24-hour resident medical cover is provided.

Precautions: Caution should be exercised in the administration of Prostin E2 Oral Tablets for the induction of labour in patients with: (i) glaucoma or raised intraocular pressure; (ii) asthma or a history of asthma. In addition, in labour induction, cephalopelvic relationships should be carefully evaluated before use of Prostin E2. During use, uterine activity, foetal status, and the progression of cervical dilatation should be carefully monitored to detect possible evidence of undesired responses, e.g. hypertonus, sustained uterine contractions, or foetal distress. In cases where there is a known history of hypertonic uterine contractility or tetanic uterine contractions, it is recommended that uterine activity and the state of the foetus should be continuously monitored throughout labour. The possibility of uterine rupture should be borne in mind where high-tone myometrial contractions are sustained.

Animal studies lasting several weeks at high doses have shown that prostaglandins of the E and F series can induce proliferation of bone. Such effects have also been noted in newborn infants who received prostaglandin E1 during prolonged treatment. There is no evidence that short term administration of Prostin E2 can cause similar bone effects.

Side-effects: Clinical studies have not revealed any life-threatening adverse reactions. The incidence of side-effects is directly dose-related. Nausea, vomiting and diarrhoea have been noted following oral administration of Prostin E2, but have seldom been severe enough to necessitate discontinuation of medication.

Overdosage: Uterine hypertonus or unduly severe uterine contractions have rarely been encountered, but might be anticipated to result from overdosage. In the rare instance where temporary discontinuation of therapy is not effective in reversing foetal distress or uterine hypertonus then prompt delivery is indicated. Treatment of overdosage must be, at this time, symptomatic, since clinical studies with prostaglandin antagonists have not progressed to the point where recommendations may be made. It is currently believed that vomiting produced by overdosage may act as a self-limiting factor in protecting the patient.

Pharmaceutical precautions Store in a refrigerator. The tablets should be used within three months of opening the bottle.

Legal category POM.

Package quantities Packs of 10 tablets.

Further information Unlike other oxytocics, Prostin E2 exhibits the capacity of the prostaglandins to influence uterine activity at any stage of gestation. Other Prostin E2 dose forms are available for a number of indications, including induction of labour.

Product licence number 0032/0040

PROSTIN E2* VAGINAL GEL 1 MG AND 2 MG

Presentation Translucent thixotropic gel containing 1 or 2 mg dinoprostone per 3 g (2.5 ml).

Uses Oxytocic. Prostin E2 Vaginal Gel is indicated for the induction of labour, when there are no foetal or maternal contra-indications.

Dosage and administration In primigravida patients with unfavourable induction features (Bishop score of 4 or less), an initial dose of 2 mg should be administered vaginally. In other patients an initial dose of 1 mg should be administered vaginally.

In both groups of patients, a second dose of 1 mg or 2 mg may be administered after 6 hours as follows:

1 mg should be used where uterine activity is insufficient for satisfactory progress of labour.

2 mg may be used where response to the initial dose has been minimal.

Maximum dose 4 mg in unfavourable primigravida patients or 3 mg in other patients (see Precautions).

The gel should be inserted high into the posterior fornix avoiding administration into the cervical canal. The patient should be instructed to remain recumbent for at least 30 minutes.

Contra-indications, warnings, etc

Contra-indications: There are no absolute contra-indications to the use of Prostin E2. However, its use is not recommended in the following circumstances:

1. For patients in whom oxytocic drugs are generally contra-indicated or where prolonged contractions of the uterus are considered inappropriate such as:
   - Cases with a history of Caesarean section or major uterine surgery;
   - Cases in which major degrees of cephalopelvic disproportion may be present;
   - Cases in which there is clinical suspicion or definite evidence of pre-existing foetal distress;
   - Cases in which there is a history of difficult labour and/or traumatic delivery;
   - Grand multiparae with six or more previous term pregnancies.
2. Patients with ruptured membranes.
3. Patients with a known sensitivity to prostaglandins.

Warnings: Since it has been found that prostaglandins may potentiate the effect of oxytocin, it is recommended that, if these drugs are used together or in sequence the patient's uterine activity should be carefully monitored. The product is available only to hospitals and clinics with specialised obstetric units.

Precautions: Prostin E2 Vaginal Gel and Prostin E2 Vaginal Tablets are not bioequivalent. Caution should be exercised in the administration of Prostin E2 Vaginal Gel for the induction of labour in patients with:

(i) glaucoma or raised intra-ocular pressure;
(ii) asthma or history of asthma.

In addition, in labour induction, cephalopelvic relationships should be carefully evaluated before use of Prostin E2. During use, uterine activity, foetal status and the progression of cervical dilatation should be carefully monitored to detect possible evidence of undesired responses, e.g. hypertonus, sustained uterine contractions, or foetal distress. In cases where there is a known history of hypertonic uterine contractility or tetanic uterine contractions, it is recommended that uterine activity and the state of the foetus should be continuously monitored throughout labour. The possibility of uterine rupture should be borne in mind where high-tone myometrial contractions are sustained. Animal studies lasting several weeks at high doses have shown that prostaglandins of the E and F series can induce proliferation of bone. Such effects have also been noted in newborn infants who have received prostaglandin E1 during prolonged treatment. There is no evidence that short term administration of Prostin E2 Vaginal Gel can cause similar bone effects.

Side-effects: Very occasional gastro-intestinal disturbance. Uterine hypertonus or unduly severe uterine contractions have rarely been encountered.

Overdosage: Treatment of overdosage must be, at this time, symptomatic since clinical studies with prostaglandin antagonists have not progressed to the point where recommendations may be made.

Pharmaceutical precautions Store in a refrigerator at 2–8°C. The contents of one syringe to be used for one patient. Discard after use.

Legal category POM.

Package quantities Prostin E2 Vaginal Gel is available in single packs of 1 mg or 2 mg.

Further information Unlike other oxytocics, Prostin E2 exhibits the capacity of the prostaglandins to influence uterine activity at any stage of gestation. Other Prostin E2 dosage forms are available for induction of labour (oral, vaginal and i.v. routes), foetal death in utero (i.v. route), therapeutic termination of pregnancy (i.v. and extra-amniotic routes), missed abortion and hydatidiform mole (i.v. route).

Product licence numbers

Prostin E2 Vaginal Gel 1 mg	0032/0123
Prostin E2 Vaginal Gel 2 mg	0032/0124

PROSTIN E2* VAGINAL TABLETS

Presentation Prostin E2 Vaginal Tablets are presented as white biconvex oblong tablets with radiused corners debossed with 'UPJOHN' and '715' on one side. Each tablet contains 3 mg dinoprostone.

Uses Oxytocic. Prostin E2 Vaginal Tablets are indicated for the induction of labour, especially in patients with favourable induction features, when there are no foetal or maternal contra-indications.

Dosage and administration One tablet (3 mg) to be inserted high into the posterior fornix. A second tablet may be inserted after six to eight hours if labour is not established. Maximum dose 6 mg.

Contra-indications, warnings, etc
Contra-indications: There are no absolute contra-indications to the use of Prostin E2. However, its use is not recommended in the following circumstances:

1. For patients in whom oxytocic drugs are generally contra-indicated or where prolonged contractions of the uterus are considered inappropriate, such as:

Cases with a history of Caesarean section or major uterine surgery.

Cases in which major degrees of cephalopelvic disproportion may be present.

Cases in which there is clinical suspicion or definite evidence of pre-existing foetal distress.

Cases in which there is a history of difficult labour and/or traumatic delivery.

Grand multiparae with six or more previous term pregnancies.

2. Patients with ruptured membranes.
3. Patients with known hypersensitivity to prostaglandins.

Warnings: Since it has been found that prostaglandins may potentiate the effect of oxytocin, it is recommended that, if these drugs are used together or in sequence, the patient's uterine activity should be carefully monitored.

The product is available only to hospitals and clinics with specialised obstetric units.

Precautions: Caution should be exercised in the administration of Prostin E2 Vaginal Tablets for the induction of labour in patients with:

(i) glaucoma or raised intra-ocular pressure;
(ii) asthma or a history of asthma.

In addition, in labour induction, cephalopelvic relationships should be carefully evaluated before use of Prostin E2. During use, uterine activity, foetal status, and the progression of cervical dilatation should be carefully monitored to detect possible evidence of undesired responses, e.g. hypertonus, sustained uterine contractions, or foetal distress. In cases where there is a known history of hypertonic uterine contractility or tetanic uterine contractions, it is recommended that uterine activity and the state of the foetus should be continuously monitored throughout labour. The possibility of uterine rupture should be borne in mind where high-tone myometrial contractions are sustained.

Animal studies lasting several weeks at high doses have shown that prostaglandins of the E and F series can induce proliferation of bone. Such effects have also been noted in newborn infants who have received prostaglandin E1 during prolonged treatment. There is no evidence that short-term administration of Prostin E2 Vaginal Tablets can cause similar bone effects.

Side Effects: Very occasional nausea and vomiting. Uterine hypertonus or unduly severe uterine contractions have rarely been encountered.

Overdosage: Treatment of overdosage must be, at this time, symptomatic, since clinical studies with prostaglandin antagonists have not progressed to the point where recommendations may be made.

Pharmaceutical precautions Prostin E2 Vaginal Tablets have a shelf-life of 24 months when stored at 4°C. Store in a refrigerator.

Legal category POM.

Package quantities Prostin E2 Vaginal Tablets are supplied in packs of 8 tablets.

Further information Tablet disintegration and release of prostaglandin is moisture dependent. In a small proportion of women tablet remains may be seen in the vagina a few hours after insertion and may contain some prostaglandin. However, this is rarely of clinical significance.

Unlike other oxytocics, Prostin E2 exhibits the capacity of the prostaglandins to influence uterine activity at any stage of gestation.

Other Prostin E2 dose forms are available for a number of indications, including induction of labour.

Product licence number 0032/0074

PROSTIN VR* STERILE SOLUTION

Presentation Ampoule containing 500 micrograms (0.5 mg) alprostadil in 1 ml dehydrated ethanol.

Uses Prostin VR is indicated to temporarily maintain the patency of the ductus arteriosus until corrective or palliative surgery can be performed in infants who have congenital defects and who depend upon the patent ductus for survival. Such congenital heart defects include pulmonary atresia, pulmonary stenosis, tricuspid atresia, tetralogy of Fallot, interruption of the aortic arch, coarctation of the aorta, aortic stenosis, aortic atresia, mitral atresia, or transposition of the great vessels with or without other defects.

Dosage and administration For administration by intravenous drip or constant-rate infusion pump.

In infants with lesions restricting pulmonary blood flow (blood is flowing through the ductus arteriosus from the aorta to the pulmonary artery), Prostin VR may be administered by continuous infusion through an umbilical artery catheter placed at or just above the junction of the descending aorta and the ductus arteriosus, or intravenously. Adverse effects have occurred with both routes of administration, but the types of reactions are different. A higher incidence of flushing has been associated with intra-arterial than with intravenous administration.

The infusion is generally initiated at a rate of 0.05 to 0.1 micrograms alprostadil per kilogram of body weight per minute. The most experience has been with 0.1 micrograms/kg/min. After a therapeutic response (an increase in pO_2 in neonates with restricted pulmonary blood flow or an increase in systemic blood pressure and blood pH in neonates with restricted systemic blood flow) has been obtained, the infusion rate should be reduced to the lowest possible dosage that will maintain the desired response.

Dilution Instructions: To prepare infusion solutions, dilute 1 ml of Prostin VR Sterile Solution with sterile 0.9% Sodium Chloride Intravenous Infusion or sterile 5% Dextrose Intravenous Infusion. Dilute to volumes appropriate for the delivery system available. Prepare fresh infusion solutions every 24 hours. Discard any solution more than 24 hours old.

Sample dilutions and infusion rates to provide a dosage of 0.1 micrograms/kg body weight/minute

Add 1 ml ampoule (500 micrograms alprostadil) to:	Concentration of resulting solution (micrograms/ml)	Infusion rate (ml/min/kg)
250 ml	2	0.05
100 ml	5	0.02
50 ml	10	0.01
25 ml	20	0.005

Example: To provide 0.1 micrograms/kg/min to a 2.8 kg neonate, using a concentration of 5 micrograms/ml;
Infusion rate = 0.02 ml/min/kg × 2.8 kg = 0.056 ml/min or 3.36 ml/hr.

Change the dosage from 0.1 micrograms per kilogram of body weight per minute to 0.05 micrograms per kilogram of body weight per minute by reducing the pump rate to one-half the original rate.

PARTICULAR CARE SHOULD BE TAKEN IN CALCULATING AND PREPARING DILUTIONS OF PROSTIN VR

Contra-indications, warnings, etc
Contra-indications: None.

Warnings: Only the recommended Prostin VR dosages should be administered and only by medically trained personnel in hospitals or other facilities with immediately available intensive care.

Approximately 10–12% of neonates with congenital heart defects treated with Prostin VR Sterile Solution experienced apnoea. Apnoea is most often seen in neonates weighing less than 2 kg at birth and usually appears during the first hour of drug infusion. Therefore, Prostin VR Sterile Solution should be used where ventilatory assistance is immediately available.

Precautions: Prostin VR Sterile Solution (alprostadil) should be infused for the shortest time and at the lowest dose which will produce the desired effects. The risk of long-term infusion of Prostin VR should be weighed against the possible benefits that critically ill infants may derive from its administration.

Cortical proliferation of the long bones has followed long-term infusions of alprostadil in infants and dogs. The proliferation in infants regressed after withdrawal of the drug.

Use Prostin VR Sterile Solution cautiously in neonates with histories of bleeding tendencies.

Care should be taken to avoid the use of Prostin VR Sterile Solution in neonates with respiratory distress syndrome (hyaline membrane disease), which sometimes can be confused with cyanotic heart disease. If full diagnostic facilities are not immediately available, cyanosis (pO_2 less than 40 mmHg) and restricted pulmonary blood flow apparent on an X-ray are good indicators of congenital heart defects.

In all infants, commencing when infusion starts, intermittently monitor arterial pressure by umbilical artery catheter, auscultation, or with a Doppler transducer. Should arterial pressure fall significantly, decrease the rate of infusion immediately.

A weakening of the wall of the ductus arteriosus and pulmonary artery has been reported, particularly during prolonged administration.

Long-term carcinogenicity and fertility studies have not been done. The Ames and Alkaline Elution assays reveal no potential for mutagenesis.

No drug interactions have been reported to occur between Prostin VR and the standard therapy employed in neonates with congenital heart defects. Standard therapy includes antibiotics, such as penicillin or gentamicin; vasopressors, such as dopamine or isoproterenol; cardiac glycosides; and diuretics, such as frusemide.

Side-effects and adverse reactions: The most frequent adverse reactions observed with Prostin VR infusion in neonates with ductal-dependent congenital heart defects are related to the drug's known pharmacological effects. These include, in decreasing frequency, transient pyrexia, apnoea, bradycardia, seizures, hypotension, tachycardia, and diarrhoea. The relationship of the following adverse events, in decreasing frequency, to the drug is unknown: sepsis, cardiac arrest, disseminated intravascular coagulation, hypokalaemia and oedema. Cutaneous vasodilation (flushing) is the only event related to the route of administration, occurring more frequently during intra-arterial administration.

Overdosage: Apnoea, bradycardia, pyrexia, hypotension and flushing may be signs of drug overdose. If apnoea or bradycardia occur, the infusion should be discontinued and the appropriate medical treatment initiated. Caution should be used if the infusion is restarted. If pyrexia or hypotension occur, the infusion rate should be reduced until these symptoms subside. Flushing is usually attributed to incorrect intra-arterial catheter placement and is usually alleviated by repositioning the tip of the catheter.

Pharmaceutical precautions Prostin VR must be stored in a refrigerator. See dilution instructions for shelf-life of diluted solutions.

Diluted solutions of Prostin VR should be infused from glass or hard plastic containers; use with soft plastic such as PVC has not been established.

Legal category POM.

Package quantities Pack containing 5 × 1 ml ampoules Prostin VR Sterile Solution.

Further information Starting dosages lower than those recommended in the section 'Dosage and administration' have been used with apparent good response, and this experience has been published. Alprostadil (formerly known as prostaglandin E1) dilates the ductus arteriosus in neonates, probably by relaxing smooth muscle, thereby helping to maintain patency. It also relaxes smooth muscle in other parts of the vascular system, and can thus lower blood pressure.

Product licence number 0032/0083

PROVERA*TABLETS 5 MG and 10 MG

Presentation 5 mg: White compressed tablets scored on one face, embossed 286 on either side of score, and marked 'U' on other face, containing 5 mg medroxyprogesterone acetate.

10 mg: White, round, half-oval tablets marked Upjohn 50 on one side and singly scored on the other, containing 10 mg medroxyprogesterone acetate.

Uses Progestogen.

Indicated for dysfunctional (anovulatory) uterine bleeding, secondary amenorrhoea, and for mild to moderate endometriosis.

Dosage and administration Oral.

Dysfunctional (anovulatory) uterine bleeding: 2.5–10 mg daily for 5–10 days commencing on the assumed or calculated sixteenth to twenty-first day of the cycle. Treatment should be given for two consecutive cycles. When bleeding occurs from a poorly developed proliferative endometrium, conventional oestrogen therapy may be employed in conjunction with medroxyprogesterone acetate in doses of 5–10 mg for 10 days.

Secondary Amenorrhoea: 2.5–10 mg daily for 5–10 days beginning on the assumed or calculated sixteenth to twenty-first day of the cycle. Repeat treatment for three consecutive cycles. In amenorrhoea associated with a poorly developed proliferative endometrium, conventional oestrogen therapy may be employed in conjunction with medroxyprogesterone acetate in doses of 5–10 mg for 10 days.

Mild to moderate endometriosis: Beginning on the first day of the menstrual cycle, 10 mg three times a day for 90 consecutive days.

Contra-indications, warnings, etc
Contra-indications: Use in patients with a history of, or existing thrombo-embolic disorders.

Use in patients with a known sensitivity to medroxyprogesterone acetate.

Use in patients with impaired liver function, or with active liver disease.

Before using Provera, the general medical condition of the patient should be carefully evaluated. This evaluation should exclude the presence of genital or breast neoplasia before considering the use of Provera.

Precautions: A negative pregnancy test should be demonstrated before starting therapy with Provera.

Whether administered alone or in conjunction with oestrogens, Provera should not be employed in patients with abnormal uterine bleeding until a definite diagnosis has been established and the possibility of genital malignancy eliminated.

Provera, especially in the high doses used for cancer therapy, may cause weight gain and fluid retention and there have been some reports of thrombo-embolic events. With this in mind, caution should be exercised in treating any patient with a pre-existing medical condition, such as epilepsy, migraine, asthma, cardiac or renal dysfunction, that might be adversely affected by weight gain or fluid retention.

Some patients receiving Provera may exhibit a decreased glucose tolerance. The mechanism for this is not known. This fact should be borne in mind when treating all patients and especially known diabetics.

Patients with a history of treatment for mental depression should be carefully monitored while receiving Provera therapy. Some patients may complain of premenstrual like depression while on Provera therapy.

Medroxyprogesterone acetate and its metabolites are secreted in breast milk but there is no evidence to suggest that this presents any hazard to the child.

Side-effects: The following medical events, listed in order of seriousness rather than frequency of occurrence, have been occasionally to rarely associated with the use of progestogens:

Rare anaphylactoid-like reactions.
There have been some reports of thrombo-embolic disorders, especially with higher doses.
Psychic – nervousness, insomnia, somnolence, fatigue, depression, dizziness and headache.
Skin and mucous membranes – urticaria, pruritus, rash, acne, hirsutism and alopecia.
Gastro-intestinal – nausea.
Breast tenderness and galactorrhoea.
Miscellaneous – change in weight.

Overdosage: In animals Provera has been shown to be capable of exerting an adreno-corticoid effect but this has not been reported in the human, following usual dosages. The oral administration of Provera at a rate of 100 mg per day has been shown to have no effect on adrenal function.

Pharmaceutical precautions None.

Legal category POM.

Package quantities 5 mg: Packs of 100, also dosepak of 20 tablets.
10 mg: Packs of 50.

Further information Pathologists should be informed of the patients ingestion of Provera if endometrial or endocervical tissue is submitted for examination.

The results of certain laboratory tests may be affected by the use of Provera, these include gonadotrophin levels, plasma progesterone levels, urinary pregnanediol levels, plasma testosterone levels (in the male), plasma oestrogen levels (in the female), plasma cortisol levels, glucose tolerance test, and metyrapone tests.

Product licence numbers
5 mg: 0032/5035R
10 mg: 0032/0151

PROVERA* TABLETS 100 MG, 200 MG and 400 MG PROVERA* ORAL SUSPENSION 80 MG/ML

Presentation *Tablets: 100 mg:* White, circular, flat bevelled tablets marked 'U 467' on one side and scored on the reverse, containing 100 mg medroxyprogesterone acetate.

200 mg: White, circular, biconvex tablets marked 'U 320' on one side and scored on the reverse, containing 200 mg medroxyprogesterone acetate.

400 mg: White, capsule shaped, compressed tablets marked 'Upjohn 421' on one side only, containing 400 mg medroxyprogesterone acetate.

Suspension: 80 mg/ml: White to off-white homogeneous suspension with an odour and flavour of peppermint.

Uses Progestogen.

Indicated for the treatment of certain hormone dependent neoplasms, such as endometrial carcinoma, renal cell carcinoma and carcinoma of breast in post-menopausal women.

Dosage and administration Oral.

For endometrial and renal cell carcinoma: 200–400 mg daily.

For breast carcinoma: 400–800 mg per day. Doses of 1000 mg daily have been given although the incidence of minor side effects, such as indigestion and weight gain, increase with the increase in dose. Response to hormonal therapy may not be evident until after at least 8–10 weeks of therapy.

Provera Oral Suspension may be diluted with Purified Water BP but should be used within 28 days.

Elderly patients: These products have been used primarily in the older age group for the treatment of malignancies. There is no evidence to suggest that the older aged group is any less prepared to handle the drug metabolically than is the younger aged patient. Therefore, the same dosage, contra-indications and precautions would apply to either age group.

Contra-indications, warnings, etc

Contra-indications: Use in patients with a history of, or existing thromboembolic disorders.

Use in patients with a known sensitivity to medroxyprogesterone acetate.

Use in patients with impaired liver function or active liver disease.

Warnings: In the treatment of carcinoma of the breast occasional cases of hypercalcaemia have been reported.

Any patient who develops an acute impairment of vision, proptosis, diplopia or migraine headache should be carefully evaluated ophthalmologically to exclude the presence of papilloedema or retinal vascular lesions before continuing medication.

Medroxyprogesterone acetate and/or its metabolites are secreted in breast milk but there is no evidence to suggest that this presents any hazard to the child.

Precautions: Animal studies show that Provera possesses adrenocorticoid activity. This has also been reported in man, therefore patients receiving large doses continuously and for long periods should be observed closely. The administration of large doses to pregnant women has resulted in the observation of some instances of female foetal masculinisation. Doctors should therefore check that patients are not pregnant before commencing treatment. Because progestogens may cause some degree of fluid retention, conditions which might be influenced by this factor, such as epilepsy, migraine, asthma, cardiac or renal dysfunction, require careful observation.

Patients who have a history of mental depression should be carefully observed and the drug discontinued if the depression recurs to a serious degree. A decrease in glucose tolerance has been observed in some patients on progestogens. The mechanism of this decrease is obscure. For this reason diabetic patients should be carefully observed while receiving progestogen therapy. Before using Provera the general medical condition of the patient should be carefully evaluated.

This product should be used under the supervision of a specialist and the patients kept under regular surveillance.

Side-effects: Reactions occasionally associated with the use of progestogens, particularly in high doses, are:

Breast: tenderness or galactorrhoea.

Psychic: nervousness, insomnia, somnolence, fatigue, dizziness, depression and headache.

Skin and Mucous Membranes: sensitivity reactions ranging from pruritus, urticaria, angioneurotic oedema, to generalised rash and anaphylaxis have occasionally been reported. Acne, alopecia or hirsutism have been reported in a few cases.

Thromboembolic disorders.

Gastro-intestinal: nausea and indigestion have been noted particularly with the higher doses.

Miscellaneous: hyperpyrexia, weight gain, moon facies, increased blood pressure.

Overdosage: No action required other than cessation of therapy.

Pharmaceutical precautions Keep containers tightly closed.

Provera Tablets and Provera Oral Suspension should be stored at controlled room temperature (15–30°C).

Legal category POM.

Package quantities Bottles of 100 ml suspension together with a 5 ml spoon.

Tablets:	*Pack available:*
100 mg	100, 30*
200 mg	100, 60, 30*
400 mg	60, 30*

* depicts original packs.

Further information The results of certain laboratory tests may be affected by the use of Provera; these include gonadotrophin levels, plasma progesterone levels, urinary pregnanediol levels, plasma testosterone levels (in the male), plasma oestrogen levels (in the female), plasma cortisol levels, glucose tolerance and metyrapone tests.

Pathologists should be informed of the patient's ingestion of Provera if endometrial or endocervical tissue is submitted for examination.

Product licence numbers

100 mg Tablet	0032/0111
200 mg Tablet	0032/0112
400 mg Tablet	0032/0131
80 mg/ml suspension	0032/0141

REGAINE* TOPICAL SOLUTION 2%

Presentation Clear, colourless to light yellow liquid containing minoxidil 20 mg per ml in a solution of ethanol, propylene glycol and water.

Uses Regaine Topical Solution is indicated for the treatment of alopecia androgenetica. There is also evidence that Regaine slows hair loss in patients with diagnosed male pattern baldness.

After only four months of treatment, little regrowth of terminal hair should be expected (the average length of the scalp hair cycle is three years). Physicians observed 8% of subjects to have moderate or dense terminal hair regrowth after four months, increasing to 39% of the subjects after treatment for 12 months. Twenty-six per cent of patients assessed themselves as having moderate to dense hair regrowth after four months, increasing to 48% of subjects treated for 12 months. At 12 months, 36% of patients had minimal regrowth as assessed by both the patients themselves as well as the treating physicians. In these patients loss of hair from affected areas was considered to be reduced. Onset and degree of hair regrowth may be variable amongst patients and it may take at least four months of continuous twice daily use before evidence of hair regrowth can be expected. Although trends in the data suggest that those patients who are younger, who have been balding for a shorter period of time or who have a smaller area of baldness on the vertex are more likely to respond to Regaine, individual response cannot be predicted. If hair regrowth occurs, twice daily applications of Regaine are necessary for continued hair growth. Anecdotal reports indicate that regrown hair may disappear three to four months after stopping Regaine application and the balding process will continue. Patients should discontinue treatment if there is no improvement after one year.

Dosage and administration Hair and scalp should be thoroughly dry prior to topical application of Regaine. A dose of 1 ml Regaine Topical Solution should be applied to the total affected areas of the scalp twice daily. The total dosage should not exceed 2 ml. If fingertips are used to facilitate drug application, hands should be washed afterwards.

The method of application varies according to the disposable applicator used:

Pump spray applicator: This is useful for large areas. Aim the pump at the centre of the bald area, press once and spread with fingertips over the entire bald area. Repeat for a total of 6 times to apply a dose of 1 ml. Avoid breathing spray mist.

Extended spray tip applicator: This is useful for small areas, or under hair. The pump spray applicator must be in place in order to use this additional applicator. Use in the same way as the pump spray.

Rub-on applicator: Squeeze the upright bottle once to fill the 1 ml chamber to the black line. Invert bottle, dab on scalp, and spread Regaine over the entire bald area until chamber is empty.

Contra-indications, warnings, etc
Contra-indications: Regaine is contra-indicated in patients with a history of sensitivity to minoxidil, ethanol or propylene glycol.

Warnings: Use of Regaine Topical Solution results in slight absorption (an average of 1.4% of the applied topical dose) of minoxidil from the skin surface. Although not causally related to the use of Regaine in clinical trials, the following potential systemic effects should be considered: sodium and water retention, tachycardia, aggravation of pre-existing angina pectoris or the induction of anginal symptoms in patients with undiagnosed coronary artery disease. Patients should be instructed to discontinue use of Regaine and contact their physician if any of the above systemic effects occurs.

Precautions: Patients with hypertension, including those under treatment with antihypertensive agents, should be monitored closely when treated with Regaine Topical Solution.

Regaine contains an alcohol base which will cause burning and irritation of the eye. In the event of accidental contact with sensitive surfaces (eye, abraded skin and mucous membranes) the area should be bathed with large amounts of cool tap water.

Inhalation of the spray mist should be avoided. Regaine should not be used in conjunction with the other topical agents including corticosteroids, retinoids and petrolatum or agents that are known to enhance cutaneous drug absorption.

As is the case with other topically applied drugs, decreased integrity of the epidermal barrier caused by inflammation or disease processes in the skin (e.g. excoriations of the scalp, scalp psoriasis, or severe sunburn) may increase percutaneous absorption of minoxidil.

Regaine is for external use only. Do not apply to areas of the body other than the scalp.

The safety and effectiveness of Regaine in patients under 18 or over 65 years of age has not been established.

There is no evidence as to drug safety in human pregnancy nor is there evidence from animal work that it is free from hazard. Regaine should not be used during pregnancy or lactation.

Side-effects: When incidences of medical events in placebo-controlled trials of topical minoxidil were compared, they revealed that only reports involving the dermatological system were present at a significantly greater level in the minoxidil group than in the placebo group. In both groups in all body systems, the overall incidence of medical events reported by females was approximately five times that of males.

Details of percentage occurrences after 4–8 months treatment with minoxidil (n=3857) or placebo (n=2717) were as follows:

Body system	*Minoxidil % occurrence*	*Placebo % occurrence*
Respiratory (bronchitis, URTI, sinusitis)	7.16	8.58
Dermatological (irritant dermatitis, allergic contact dermatitis)	7.36	5.41
Gastrointestinal (diarrhoea, nausea, vomiting)	4.33	6.55
Neurology (headache, dizziness, faintness, lightheadedness)	3.42	3.46
Musculoskeletal (fractures, back pain, tendinitis, aches and pains)	2.59	2.21
Cardiovascular (oedema, chest pain, blood pressure increases/ decreases, palpitations, pulse rate increases/decreases)	1.53	1.55

In other systems monitored (allergy, special senses, metabolic-nutritional, urinary tract, genital tract, psychiatric, haematology, endocrine) occurrences were all below 1.5% (range 0.31–1.29).

Interactions: There are currently no known drug interactions associated with the use of Regaine Topical Solution. Although it has not been clinically demonstrated, there exists the theoretical possibility of absorbed minoxidil potentiating orthostatic hypotension caused by guanethidine.

Overdosage: Increased systemic absorption of minoxidil may potentially occur if higher-than-recommended doses of Regaine are applied to larger surface areas of the body or areas other than the scalp. There are no known cases of minoxidil overdosage resulting from topical administration of Regaine.

Because of the concentration of minoxidil in Regaine, accidental ingestion has the potential of producing systemic effects related to the pharmacological action of the drug (5 ml of Regaine contains 100 mg minoxidil, the maximum recommended adult dose for oral minoxidil administration in the treatment of hypertension). Signs and symptoms of minoxidil overdosage would most likely be cardiovascular effects associated with sodium and water retention and tachycardia. Fluid retention can be managed with appropriate diuretic therapy. Clinically significant tachycardia can be controlled by administration of a beta adrenergic blocking agent.

If encountered, hypotension should be treated by intravenous administration of 0.9% saline. Sympathomimetic drugs, such as noradrenaline and adrenaline should be avoided because of their excessive cardiac stimulating activity.

Pharmaceutical precautions Regaine Topical Solution should be stored at room temperature. The solution is flammable.

Legal category POM.

Package quantities Regaine Topical Solution is supplied in bottles of 60 ml with one or more of the following disposable applicators: pump spray, extended tip, or rub-on assemblies.

Further information The mechanism of action of minoxidil in the treatment of male pattern baldness is currently not known.

Following application of Regaine, minoxidil is poorly absorbed from normal intact skin with an average of 1.4% (range 0.3–4.5%) of the total applied dose reaching the systemic circulation. Therefore, a 1 ml dose of Regaine Topical Solution, delivering 20 mg of minoxidil solution to the skin, would result in absorption of approximately 0.28 mg minoxidil. This compares with greater than 95% absorption from the gastrointestinal tract of orally administered minoxidil as tablets. Serum levels resulting from administration of Regaine are governed by the drug's percutaneous absorption rate. Following cessation of topical dosing of Regaine approximately 95% of systemically absorbed minoxidil is eliminated within four days.

Product licence numbers
0032/0136
0032/0157

SOLU-CORTEF*

Presentation White, freeze dried powder of hydrocortisone sodium succinate, equivalent to 100 mg hydrocortisone, supplied in vials.

Uses Anti-inflammatory agent.

Solu-Cortef is indicated for any condition in which rapid and intense corticosteroid effect is required such as:

1. *Endocrine disorders:* Primary or secondary adrenocortical insufficiency.
2. *Collagen diseases:* Systemic lupus erythematosus.
3. *Dermatological diseases:* Severe erythema multiforme (Stevens-Johnson syndrome).
4. *Allergic states:* Bronchial asthma; anaphylactic reactions.
5. *Gastrointestinal diseases:* Ulcerative colitis; Crohn's disease.
6. *Respiratory diseases:* Aspiration of gastric contents.
7. *Medical emergencies:* Solu-Cortef is indicated in the treatment of shock secondary to adrenocortical insufficiency or shock unresponsive to conventional therapy when adrenocortical insufficiency may be present.

Dosage and administration Solu-Cortef may be administered by intravenous injection, by intravenous infusion, or by intramuscular injection, the preferred method for initial emergency use being intravenous injection. Following the initial emergency period, consideration should be given to employing a longer-acting injectable preparation or an oral preparation.

Dosage usually ranges from 100 mg to 500 mg depending on the severity of the condition, administered by intravenous injection over a period of one to ten minutes. This dose may be repeated at intervals of 2, 4 or 6 hours as indicated by the patient's response and clinical condition.

In general high-dose corticosteroid therapy should be continued only until the patient's condition has stabilised—usually not beyond 48 to 72 hours. If hydrocortisone therapy must be continued beyond 48 to 72 hours hypernatraemia may occur, therefore it may be preferable to replace Solu-Cortef with a corticosteroid such as methylprednisolone sodium succinate as little or no sodium retention occurs. Although adverse effects associated with high dose, short-term corticoid therapy are uncommon, peptic ulceration may occur. Prophylactic antacid therapy may be indicated.

Patients subjected to severe stress following corticoid therapy should be observed closely for signs and symptoms of adrenocortical insufficiency.

While the dose may be reduced for infants and children, it is governed more by the severity of the condition and response of the patient than by age or body weight but should not be less than 25 mg daily.

Corticosteroid therapy is an adjunct to, and not a replacement for, conventional therapy.

Elderly patients: Solu-Cortef is primarily used in acute

short-term conditions. There is no information to suggest that a change in dosage is warranted in the elderly. See Contra-indications, Warnings and Precautions for other factors which should be taken into account.

Preparation of solutions: For intravenous or intramuscular injection prepare the solution aseptically by adding not more than 2 ml of Sterile Water for Injection to the contents of one vial of Solu-Cortef 100 mg, shake and withdraw for use.

For intravenous infusion, first prepare the solution by adding not more than 2 ml of Sterile Water for Injection to the vial; this solution may then be added to 100 ml – 1000 ml (but not less than 100 ml) of 5% dextrose in water (or isotonic saline solution or 5% dextrose in isotonic saline solution if patient is not on sodium restriction).

When reconstituted as directed the pH of solution will range from 7.0 to 8.0.

Contra-indications, warnings, etc

Contra-indications: Solu-Cortef is contra-indicated where there is known hypersensitivity to components and in systemic fungal infections. Immunization procedures should not be undertaken in patients who are on corticosteroids, especially on high doses, due to the possibility of neurological complications and lack of antibody response.

Warnings:

1. Corticosteroids may mask some signs of infection, and new infections may appear during their use. There may be decreased resistance and inability to localize infection when corticosteroids are used.
2. In patients on corticosteroid therapy subjected to unusual stress, increased dosage of rapidly acting corticosteroids before, during and after the stressful situation is indicated.
3. Rarely anaphylactoid reactions have been reported following parenteral Solu-Cortef therapy. Physicians using the drug should be prepared to deal with such a possibility.
4. There is no evidence that corticosteroids are carcinogenic or mutagenic.
5. Average and large doses of hydrocortisone can cause elevation of blood pressure, salt and water retention, and increased excretion of potassium. These effects are less likely to occur with the synthetic derivatives except when used in large doses. Dietary salt restriction and potassium supplementation may be necessary. All corticosteroids increase calcium excretion.

Use in pregnancy and lactation: The use of corticosteroids in general during pregnancy involves balancing the clinical benefit against the possible risks. There is inadequate evidence of safety in human pregnancy and there may be a very small risk of cleft palate and intrauterine growth retardation in the foetus; there is evidence of harmful effects on pregnancy in animals. Also neonates of mothers who received such therapy during pregnancy should be observed for signs of hypoadrenalism, and appropriate measures instituted if such signs exist.

Because prednisolone is excreted in breast milk, it is reasonable to assume that all corticosteroids are. No specific data are known for hydrocortisone sodium succinate. Therefore the use of corticosteroids in pregnancy, nursing mothers and women of childbearing potential requires that the possible benefits of the drug be weighed against the potential hazards to the mother, embryo or foetus.

Use in children: Corticosteroids cause growth retardation in infancy, childhood and adolescence. Treatment should be limited to the minimum dosage for the shortest possible time. Therefore the use of steroids should be restricted to the most serious indications.

Precautions:

1. The existence of congestive heart failure, hypertension, peptic ulceration, glaucoma, previous steroid myopathy, epilepsy, diabetes mellitus, osteoporosis, chronic psychotic reactions or previous history of tuberculosis necessitate caution in the administration of Solu-Cortef.
2. The lowest possible dose of corticosteroid should be used to control the condition under treatment, and when reduction of dosage is possible, the reduction must be gradual in order to minimize drug induced secondary adrenocortical insufficiency.
3. Steroids should be used with caution in non-specific ulcerative colitis, if there is a probability of impending perforation, abscess or other pyogenic infections, also in diverticulitis, fresh intestinal anastomoses, active or latent peptic ulcer, renal insufficiency, hypertension, osteoporosis, and myasthenia gravis.
4. There is an enhanced effect of corticosteroids in patients with hypothyroidism and cirrhosis.
5. Aspirin should be used cautiously in conjunction with corticosteroids in hypoprothrombinaemia.
6. Corticosteroids should be used cautiously in patients with ocular herpes simplex for fear of corneal perforation.

Side-effects: Since Solu-Cortef is normally employed on a short-term basis it is unlikely that side-effects will occur; however, the possibility of side-effects attributable to corticosteroid therapy should be recognised. Such side-effects include:

Gastrointestinal—Dyspepsia, peptic ulceration with perforation and haemorrhage, abdominal distension, oesophageal ulceration, oesophageal candidiasis, acute pancreatitis.

Musculoskeletal—Proximal myopathy, osteoporosis, vertebral and long bone fractures, avascular osteonecrosis, tendon rupture.

Fluid and electrolyte disturbance—Sodium and water retention, potassium loss, hypertension, hypokalaemic alkalosis, congestive heart failure in susceptible patients.

Dermatological—Impaired healing, skin atrophy, bruising, striae, increased sweating, telangiectasia, acne.

Endocrine/metabolic—Suppression of the hypothalamo-pituitary-adrenal axis, growth suppression in childhood and adolescence, menstrual irregularity and amenorrhoea, Cushingoid facies, hirsutism, weight gain, impaired carbohydrate tolerance with increased requirement for antidiabetic therapy, negative nitrogen balance.

Neuropsychiatric—Euphoria, psychological dependence, mood swings, depression, insomnia, convulsions. Intracranial hypertension in children. Aggravation of schizophrenia.

Ophthalmic—Increased intra-ocular pressure, glaucoma, exophthalmos, papilloedema, cataracts, corneal or scleral thinning, exacerbation of ophthalmic viral or fungal diseases.

General—Opportunistic infection, recurrence of dormant tuberculosis, leucocytosis, hypersensitivity, thrombo-embolism, increased appetite, nausea, malaise.

Withdrawal symptoms—Fever, myalgia, arthralgia, adrenal insufficiency.

Parenteral corticosteroid therapy—Anaphylactoid reaction e.g. bronchospasm, hyperpigmentation or hypopigmentation, subcutaneous and cutaneous atrophy, sterile abscess, laryngeal oedema and urticaria.

Overdosage: There is no clinical syndrome of acute overdosage with Solu-Cortef. Hydrocortisone is dialysable.

Pharmaceutical precautions Store at controlled room temperature (15–30°C). Reconstituted solutions should be used immediately. No diluents other than those referred to are recommended. Parenteral drug products should be inspected visually for particulate matter and discoloration prior to administration.

Legal category POM.

Package quantities Solu-Cortef is supplied as a 100 mg vial with accompanying Sterile Water for Injection diluent.

Also packs of 10 × 100 mg vials without diluent.

Further information Solu-Cortef has the same metabolic and anti-inflammatory actions as hydrocortisone. When given parenterally and in equimolar quantities, the two compounds are equivalent in biological activity. Following the intravenous injection of hydrocortisone sodium succinate, demonstrable effects are evident within one hour and persist for a variable period. Excretion of the administered dose is nearly complete within 12 hours. Thus, if constantly high blood levels are required, injections should be made every 4 to 6 hours. This preparation is also rapidly absorbed when administered intramuscularly and is excreted in a pattern similar to that observed after intravenous injection.

Product licence number 100 mg vial 0032/5019.

SOLU-MEDRONE*

Presentation 40 mg, 125 mg, 500 mg, 1 g and 2 g vials of methylprednisolone (as the sodium succinate).

Uses Medrone is a potent corticosteroid with an anti-inflammatory activity at least five times that of hydrocortisone. An enhanced separation of glucocorticoid and mineralocorticoid effect results in a reduced incidence of sodium and water retention.

Solu-Medrone is indicated for any condition in which rapid and intense corticosteroid effect is required such as:

1. Dermatological disease: Severe erythema multiforme (Stevens-Johnson syndrome).

2. Allergic states: Bronchial asthma; severe seasonal and perennial allergic rhinitis; angioneurotic oedema; anaphylaxis.

3. Gastro-intestinal diseases: Ulcerative colitis; Crohn's disease.

4. Respiratory diseases: Aspiration of gastric contents; fulminating or disseminated tuberculosis (with appropriate anti-tuberculous chemotherapy).

5. Neurological disorders: Cerebral oedema secondary to cerebral tumour.

6. Miscellaneous: T.B. meningitis (with appropriate anti-tuberculous chemotherapy); transplantation.

Dosage and administration Solu-Medrone may be administered intravenously or intramuscularly, the preferred method for emergency use being intravenous injection given over a suitable time interval. When administering Solu-Medrone in high doses intravenously it should be given over a period of at least 30 minutes. Doses up to 250 mg should be given intravenously over a period of at least five minutes.

For intravenous infusion the initially prepared solution may be diluted with 5% dextrose in water, isotonic saline solution, or 5% dextrose in isotonic saline solution.

Parenteral drug products should wherever possible be visually inspected for particulate matter and discoloration prior to administration.

Adults: Dosage should be varied according to the severity of the condition, initial dosage will vary from 10–500 mg. In the treatment of graft rejection reactions following transplantation, a dose of up to 1 g/day may be required. Although doses and protocols have varied in studies using methylprednisolone sodium succinate in the treatment of graft rejection reactions, the published literature supports the use of doses of this level, with 500 mg–1 g most commmonly used for acute rejection. Treatment at these doses should be limited to a 48–72 hour period until the patient's condition has stabilised, as prolonged high dose corticosteroid therapy can cause serious corticosteroid induced side-effects.

Children: In the treatment of high dose indications, such as haematological, rheumatic, renal and dermatological conditions, a dosage of 30 mg/kg/day to a maximum of 1 g/day is recommended. This dosage may be repeated for three pulses either daily or on alternate days. In the treatment of graft rejection reactions following transplantation, a dosage of 10–20 mg/kg/day for up to 3 days, to a maximum of 1 g/day, is recommended. In the treatment of status asthmaticus, a dosage of 1–4 mg/kg/day for 1–3 days is recommended.

Elderly patients: Solu-Medrone is primarily used in acute short-term conditions. There is no information to suggest that a change in dosage is warranted in the elderly. See Contra-indications, Warnings and Precautions for other factors which should be taken into account.

Detailed recommendations for adult dosage are as follows:

In *anaphylactic reactions* adrenaline or noradrenaline should be administered first for an immediate haemodynamic effect, followed by intravenous injection of Solu-Medrone (methylprednisolone sodium succinate) with other accepted procedures. There is evidence that corticosteroids through their prolonged haemodynamic effect are of value in preventing recurrent attacks of acute anaphylactic reactions.

In *sensitivity reactions* Solu-Medrone is capable of providing relief within one half to two hours. In patients with status asthmaticus Solu-Medrone may be given at a dose of 40 mg intravenously, repeated as dictated by patient response. In some asthmatic patients it may be advantageous to administer by slow intravenous drip over a period of hours.

In *graft rejection reactions following transplantation* doses of up to 1 g per day have been used to suppress rejection crises, with doses of 500 mg–1 g most commonly used for acute rejection. Treatment should be continued only until the patient's condition has stabilised; usually not beyond 48–72 hours.

In *cerebral oedema* corticosteroids are used to reduce or prevent the cerebral oedema associated with brain tumours (primary or metastatic).

In patients with oedema due to tumour, tapering the dose of corticosteroid appears to be important in order to avoid a rebound increase in intracranial pressure. If brain swelling does occur as the dose is reduced (intracranial bleeding having been ruled out), restart larger and more frequent doses parenterally. Patients with certain malignancies may need to remain on oral corticosteroid therapy for months or even life. Similar or higher doses may be helpful to control oedema during radiation therapy.

The following are suggested dosage schedules for oedemas due to brain tumour:

Schedule A (1)	*Dose (mg)*	*Route*	*Interval in hours*	*Duration*
Pre-operative:	20	IM	3–6	
During surgery:	20–40	IV	hourly	
Post-operative:	20	IM	3	24 hours
	16	IM	3	24 hours
	12	IM	3	24 hours
	8	IM	3	24 hours
	4	IM	3	24 hours
	4	IM	6	24 hours
	4	IM	12	24 hours

Schedule B (2)	*Dose (mg)*	*Route*	*Interval in hours*	*Days Duration*
Pre-operative:	40	IM	6	2–3
Post-operative:	40	IM	6	3–5
	20	oral	6	1
	12	oral	6	1
	8	oral	8	1
	4	oral	12	1
	4	oral		1

Aim to discontinue therapy after a total of 10 days.

REFERENCES

1. Fox, J L, M.D. 'Use of Methylprednisolone in Intracranial Surgery' Medical Annals of the District of Columbia, 34: 261–265, 1965.

2. Cantu, R C, M.D. Harvard Neurological Service, Boston, Massachusetts. Letter on file, The Upjohn Company (February 1970).

In other indications, initial dosage will vary from 10 to

500 mg depending on the clinical problem being treated. Larger doses may be required for short-term management of severe, acute conditions. The initial dose, up to 250 mg, should be given intravenously over a period of at least 5 minutes, doses exceeding 250 mg should be given intravenously over a period of at least 30 minutes. Subsequent doses may be given intravenously or intramuscularly at intervals dictated by the patient's response and clinical condition. Corticosteroid therapy is an adjunct to, and not replacement for, conventional therapy.

Contra-indications, warnings, etc
Contra-indications: Solu-Medrone is contra-indicated where there is known hypersensitivity to components, in systemic fungal infections and in cerebral oedema in malaria. Immunization procedures should not be undertaken in patients who are on corticosteroids, especially on high doses, due to the possibility of neurological complications and lack of antibody response.

Warnings:
1. Although Solu-Medrone is not approved in the U.K. for use in any shock indication, the following warning statement should be adhered to. Data from a clinical study conducted to establish the efficacy of Solu-Medrone in septic shock, suggest that a higher mortality occurred in subsets of patients who entered the study with elevated serum creatinine levels or who developed a secondary infection after therapy began. Therefore this product should not be used in the treatment of septic syndrome or septic shock.
2. There have been a few reports of cardiac arrhythmias and/or circulatory collapse and/or cardiac arrest associated with the rapid intravenous administration of large doses of Solu-Medrone (greater than 500 mg administered over a period of less than 10 minutes). Bradycardia has been reported during or after the administration of large doses of methylprednisolone sodium succinate, and may be unrelated to the speed and duration of infusion.
3. In patients on corticosteroid therapy subjected to unusual stress, increased dosage of rapidly acting corticosteroids before, during and after the stressful indication is indicated.
4. Rarely anaphylactoid reactions have been reported following parenteral Solu-Medrone therapy. Physicians using the drug should be prepared to deal with such a possibility.
5. Corticosteroids may mask some signs of infection and new infections may appear during their use. There may be decreased resistance and inability to localize infection when corticosteroids are used.
6. The use of Solu-Medrone in active tuberculosis should be restricted to those cases of fulminating or disseminated tuberculosis in which the corticosteroid is used for the management of the disease in conjunction with appropriate anti-tuberculous regimen. If corticosteroids are indicated in patients with latent tuberculosis or tuberculin reactivity, close observation is necessary as reactivation of the disease may occur. During prolonged corticosteroid therapy, these patients should receive chemoprophylaxis.
7. Solu-Medrone does not appear to be carcinogenic or mutagenic.

Use in pregnancy and lactation: The use of corticosteroids, in general, during pregnancy involves balancing the clinical benefit against the possible risks. There is inadequate evidence of safety in human pregnancy and there may be a very small risk of cleft palate and intra-uterine growth retardation in the foetus: there is evidence of harmful effects on pregnancy in animals. Also neonates of mothers who received such therapy during pregnancy should be observed for signs of hypoadrenalism and appropriate measures instituted if such signs exist.

Because prednisolone is excreted in breast milk, it is reasonable to assume that all corticosteroids are. No specific data are known for methylprednisolone sodium succinate. Therefore, the use of corticosteroids in pregnancy, nursing mothers or women of childbearing potential requires that the possible benefits of the drug be weighed against the potential hazards to the mother, embryo or foetus.

Use in children: Corticosteroids cause growth retardation in infancy, childhood and adolescence. Treatment should be limited to the minimum dosage for the shortest possible time. In order to minimise suppression of the hypothalamo-pituitary-adrenal axis and growth retardation, treatment should be administered where possible as a single dose on alternate days.

Precautions:
1. Corticosteroids should be used with caution in nonspecific ulcerative colitis if there is a probability of impending perforation, abscess or other pyogenic infection, diverticulitis, fresh intestinal anastomoses, active or latent peptic ulcer, renal insufficiency, hypertension, osteoporosis, myasthenia gravis, diabetes, glaucoma, previous steroid myopathy or epilepsy.
2. Corticosteroids should be used cautiously in patients with ocular herpes simplex because of possible corneal perforation.
3. Psychic derangements may appear when corticosteroids are used, ranging from euphoria, insomnia, mood swings, personality changes, and severe depression to frank psychotic manifestations. Also, existing emotional instability or psychotic tendencies may be aggravated by corticosteroids.
4. Since complications of treatment with glucocorticoids are dependent on the size of the dose and the duration of treatment, a risk/benefit decision must be made in each individual case as to dose and duration of treatment and as to whether daily or intermittent therapy should be used.

Adverse reactions and side-effects: Under normal circumstances Solu-Medrone therapy would be considered as short-term. However, the possibility of side-effects and adverse reactions common to corticosteroids must be considered, particularly when high-dose therapy is being used. Such reactions include:

Gastrointestinal – Dyspepsia, peptic ulceration with perforation and haemorrhage, abdominal distension, oesophageal ulceration, oesophageal candidiasis, acute pancreatitis. Nausea, vomiting and bad taste in mouth may occur especially with rapid administration.

Musculoskeletal – Proximal myopathy, osteoporosis, vertebral and long bone fractures, avascular osteonecrosis, tendon rupture.

Fluid and electrolyte disturbance – Sodium and water retention, hypertension, hypokalaemic alkalosis.

Dermatological – Impaired healing, skin atrophy, bruising, striae, telangiectasia, acne.

Endocrine/metabolic – Suppression of the hypothalamo-pituitary-adrenal axis, growth suppression in childhood and adolescence, menstrual irregularity and amenorrhoea. Cushingoid facies, hirsutism, weight gain, impaired carbohydrate tolerance with increased requirement for antidiabetic therapy, negative nitrogen balance.

Neuropsychiatric – Euphoria, psychological dependence, depression, insomnia. Intracranial hypertension in children. Aggravation of schizophrenia.

Ophthalmic – Increased intra-ocular pressure, glaucoma, papilloedema, cataracts, corneal or scleral thinning, exacerbation of ophthalmic viral disease.

General – Opportunistic infection, recurrence of dormant tuberculosis, leucocytosis, hypersensitivity, thrombo-embolism, increased appetite, nausea, malaise.

Withdrawal symptoms – Fever, myalgia, arthralgia, adrenal insufficiency.

Parenteral corticosteroid therapy – Anaphylactic reaction with or without circulatory collapse, cardiac arrest, bronchospasm, cardiac arrhythmias, hypotension or hypertension.

Overdosage: There is no clinical syndrome of acute overdosage with Solu-Medrone. Methylprednisolone is dialysable. Following chronic overdosage the possibility of adrenal suppression should be guarded against by gradual diminution of dose levels over a period of time. In such event the patient may require to be supported during any further stressful episode.

Pharmaceutical precautions Solu-Medrone should

be stored at controlled room temperature (15–30°C). Solutions prepared using Sterile Water for Injection should be used immediately.

Dilute concentrations of Solu-Medrone in 5% dextrose solution, isotonic saline solution or 5% dextrose in saline (250 micrograms per ml or less) are physically and chemically stable for 24 hours. In high concentrations in the above infusion fluids Solu-Medrone is physically and chemically stable for at least six hours.

Legal category POM.

Package quantities Packs of 40 mg, 125 mg, 500 mg, 1 g and 2 g supplied with Sterile Water for Injection diluent.

Further information To prepare solutions for intravenous infusion, first prepare the solution for injection. This solution may then be added to indicated amounts of 5% dextrose in water, isotonic saline solution or 5% dextrose in isotonic saline solution. To avoid compatibility problems with other drugs Solu-Medrone should be administered separately, only in the solutions mentioned.

Product licence numbers

40 mg/1 ml	0032/0033
125 mg/2 ml	0032/0034
500 mg/8 ml	0032/0035
1 g/16 ml	0032/0039
2 g/32 ml	0032/0073

TOLANASE*

Presentation White, scored, convex tablets marked 'UPJOHN 70' on the opposite side, containing 100 mg tolazamide.

White, scored, convex tablet marked 'UPJOHN 114' on the opposite side, containing 250 mg tolazamide.

Uses Sulphonylurea.

Indicated in maturity-onset diabetes of mild to moderate severity.

Dosage and administration Oral.

100–250 mg daily, or up to 1 g daily in divided doses if necessary. It is doubtful whether doses greater than 1 g daily will result in improved control. (For dose conversion from other oral hypoglycaemic agents see literature.)

Depending on the results of urinary glucose tests and blood sugar determinations the daily dose should be either raised or lowered by amounts of one tablet (100 mg or 250 mg) at weekly intervals.

Elderly patients: These agents have had their primary use in the older aged group. The contra-indications and precautions that appear in the data sheet should be carefully observed for all aged patients and any patient with significantly compromised liver or renal function should be very carefully followed if it is the election of the physician to use oral agents.

Contra-indications, warnings, etc

Contra-indications: Tolanase is not indicated in juvenile or labile (brittle) diabetes, or in patients with infections or those undergoing surgery or trauma. It is contra-indicated in patients with ketosis, acidosis or in coma, or who have a history of such.

Since Tolanase has not been studied extensively in diabetes complicated by pregnancy or in diabetics with liver, kidney or endocrine disease, it is not recommended in these instances.

Warnings: The appearance of significant acetonuria in a patient transferred from insulin to tolazamide makes return to insulin therapy mandatory.

Interactions: The hypoglycaemic action of sulphonylureas may be potentiated by certain drugs including phenylbutazone, oxyphenbutazone, salicylates, sulphonamides, chloramphenicol, probenecid, coumarins, monoamine oxidase inhibitors, and beta adrenergic blocking agents. When such drugs are administered to a patient receiving Tolanase, the patient should be closely observed for hypoglycaemia. When such drugs are withdrawn from a patient receiving Tolanase, the patient should be observed closely for loss of control.

Certain drugs tend to produce hyperglycaemia and may lead to loss of control. These drugs include the thiazides and other diuretics, corticosteroids, phenothiazines, thyroid products, oestrogens, oral contraceptives, phenytoin, nicotinic acid, sympathomimetics and isoniazid. When such drugs are administered to a patient receiving Tolanase, the patient should be observed for loss of control. When such drugs are withdrawn from a patient receiving Tolanase, the patients should be observed closely for hypoglycaemia.

Side-effects: The most commonly encountered symptoms are gastro-intestinal (1.8%), including nausea, anorexia, diarrhoea. Other minor occurrences, such as dizziness, weakness, insomnia, lethargy, have been reported. A disulfiram-like action after taking alcohol has been reported.

Overdosage: Action should be taken to counteract the ensuing hypoglycaemic period. No known antidote.

Pharmaceutical precautions Store at room temperature.

Legal category POM.

Package quantities Containers of 100 tablets.

Further information The half-life of seven hours makes Tolanase an ideal agent for a single or twice-daily dose regime.

Product licence numbers

Tablets 100 mg	0032/5043R
Tablets 250 mg	0032/5044R

TROBICIN*

Presentation Vial containing Spectinomycin Hydrochloride BP, equivalent to spectinomycin 2 g, as a sterile powder. Also ampoule containing Water for Injections BP, for use as a diluent.

Uses Antibiotic for intramuscular injection in the treatment of ano-genital gonorrhoea.

Dosage and administration Add 3.2 ml water for injections to the vial containing Trobicin as the sterile powder. Shake the vial vigorously immediately after adding diluent and before withdrawing dose. When reconstituted according to direction, each vial yields 5 ml of a suspension containing 400 mg spectinomycin per millilitre.

Adults: A single dose of 2 grams (5 ml) by deep intramuscular injection. Up to 4 grams (10 ml) have been administered in difficult-to-treat cases and in areas where antibiotic resistance is known to occur. Intramuscular injections should be made deep into the upper outer quadrant of the gluteal muscle. The dose may be divided between two injection sites.

Elderly: There is no evidence to suggest that Trobicin is less well tolerated by patients of advanced age. The normal adult dose should be given.

Children: There are insufficient data to recommend the use of Trobicin in children. Doses of 40 mg/kg are reported to be effective in children of over 2 years of age and may be used where no alternative therapy exists. There are no data to support the use of Trobicin in infants.

Contra-indications, warnings, etc

Contra-indications: Trobicin is contra-indicated for patients previously found to be hypersensitive to it. Trobicin is not indicated for the treatment of syphilis.

Interactions with other medicaments: Spectinomycin increases lithium effect and toxicity due to decreased lithium clearance. This interaction is clinically significant.

Side-effects: The following reactions have been observed during single dose clinical trials: soreness at the injection site; urticaria; dizziness; nausea; chills; fever; and a reduction in urine output (without renal function changes indicative of renal toxicity).

The following reactions have been observed during multiple-dose tolerance studies in healthy volunteers: a decrease in haemoglobin, haematocrit and creatinine clearance; and an elevation of alkaline phosphatase, blood urea nitrogen and serum glutamic pyruvic transaminase.

Anaphylaxis or anaphylactoid reactions have been reported on rare occasions.

Use in pregnancy and lactation: There are no adequate or well-controlled studies in pregnant women. Trobicin has been used successfully, at the standard adult dose level, to treat gonorrhoea in pregnant women where either the strain of *Neisseria gonorrhoeae* was resistant to penicillin or in whom penicillin had produced an allergic reaction. Reproductive studies conducted in rats, mice and rabbits, at doses above the clinical dose level, did not demonstrate any evidence of developmental abnormalities. Nevertheless, Trobicin should only be used during pregnancy if clearly needed.

Animal studies have demonstrated that only minute quantities of Trobicin are excreted in breast milk. There are, however, insufficient data to support the use of Trobicin in nursing mothers.

Other special warnings and precautions: Spectinomycin is excreted renally and where renal impairment exists there has been shown to be a significant prolonging of the excretion time. As Trobicin is given as single-dose therapy the increased excretion time is not considered to be a contra-indication to its use in renally impaired patients, nevertheless Trobicin should be used only where alternative therapies are inappropriate. The standard adult dosage should be used. The safety of use in patients with hepatic dysfunction has not been established.

Antibiotics used in high doses for short periods of time to treat gonorrhoea may mask or delay the symptoms of incubating syphilis. Since the treatment of acute syphilis demands prolonged therapy with an effective antibiotic, patients being treated for gonorrhoea should be closely observed clinically for a period of four to six weeks. Appropriate serological follow-up for at least four months should be instituted if a diagnosis of syphilis is suspected.

Development of resistance to antibiotics has been observed with *N. gonorrhoeae*. This appears, so far, to occur only rarely with Trobicin, however, the clinical effectiveness of Trobicin should be monitored to detect evidence of resistance development.

Overdosage: Overdosage is unlikely to be a problem in practice.

Pharmaceutical precautions Shake vial vigorously immediately after adding diluent and before withdrawing dose. Dilution of the reconstituted suspension should not be necessary. Prepare suspension immediately before use. Discard any unused suspension.

Legal category POM.

Package quantities 1 × 2 g vial plus diluent.

Further information Trobicin bears no structural or antigenic relationship to the penicillins. It is an inhibitor of protein synthesis in the bacterial cell, the site of action being the 30 S ribosomal subunit. Trobicin is rapidly absorbed after intramuscular injection, a single 2 g dose producing peak serum concentrations averaging 103 microgram/ml at one hour. Serum concentrations inhibitory to most gonococcal strains persist for up to eight hours. Up to 100% of the administered dose is excreted in the urine within 48 hours in a biologically active form.

Product licence number 0032/0032.

XANAX*

Presentation White, oval, biconvex tablets containing 250 micrograms (0.25 mg) alprazolam, scored on one side and marked 'Upjohn 29' on the other. Pink, oval, biconvex tablets containing 500 micrograms (0.5 mg) alprazolam, scored on one side and marked 'Upjohn 55' on the other.

Uses Xanax is indicated for the short-term treatment of moderate or severe anxiety states and anxiety associated with depression. Xanax should not be used to treat short term mild anxiety, such as anxiety or tension associated with the stress of everyday life. As the efficacy of Xanax in depression, and in phobic or obsessional states has yet to be established, specific treatment may have to be considered.

Xanax tablets are recommended for short-term use. It is recommended that the patient be reassessed at the end of no longer than 4 weeks' treatment and the need for continued treatment be established. As with all benzodiazepines, physicians should be aware that long-term use may lead to dependence in certain patients.

Dosage and administration The optimum dosage of Xanax should be based upon the severity of the symptoms and individual patient response. The lowest dose which can control symptoms should be used. Dosage should be reassessed at intervals of no more than 4 weeks. Xanax should not be used for long-term chronic treatment. The usual dosage is stated below; in the few patients who require higher doses, the dosage should be increased cautiously to avoid adverse effects. When higher dosage is required, the evening dose should be increased before the daytime doses. In general, patients who have not previously received psychotropic medications will require lower doses than those so treated, or those with a history of chronic alcoholism. Treatment should always be tapered off gradually. Patients who have taken benzodiazepines for a long time may require a longer period during which doses are reduced.

There is a reduced clearance of the drug and, as with other benzodiazepines, an increased sensitivity to the drug in elderly patients.

Anxiety: 250 micrograms (0.25 mg) to 500 micrograms (0.5 mg) three times daily increasing if required to a total of 3 mg daily.

Geriatric patients or in the presence of debilitating disease: 250 micrograms (0.25 mg) two to three times daily to be gradually increased if needed and tolerated.

If side-effects occur, the dose should be lowered. It is advisable to review treatment regularly and to discontinue use as soon as possible. Should longer term treatment be necessary then intermittent treatment may be considered to minimise the risk of dependence.

Contra-indications, warnings, etc
Contra-indications: Xanax should not be used in patients with a known sensitivity to benzodiazepines or patients with acute pulmonary insufficiency.

Warnings and precautions:

1. Xanax is not recommended as the primary treatment for psychotic patients and should not be used in lieu of appropriate treatment for psychosis.
2. There is no evidence as to drug safety in human pregnancy nor is there evidence from animal work that it is free from hazard. Do not use during pregnancy, especially during the first and last trimesters, unless there are compelling reasons.
3. Products should be used with caution in chronic pulmonary insufficiency and chronic renal or hepatic disease.
4. In labour. High single doses or repeated low doses have been reported to produce hypotonia, poor sucking and hypothermia in the neonate and irregularities in the foetal heart.
5. Avoid if possible in lactation.
6. The concurrent use of other CNS depressant drugs should be avoided.
7. The safety and efficacy of Xanax in patients less than 18 years old has not been established.
8. As with other benzodiazepines disinhibiting effects and aggressive behaviour towards self and others may be manifested in various ways. Extreme caution should therefore be used in prescribing benzodiazepines in patients with personality disorders.

9. Administration to severely depressed or suicidal patients should be done with appropriate precautions and appropriate size of prescriptions.
10. In cases of loss or bereavement, psychological adjustment may be inhibited by benzodiazepines.

Adverse effects: Common adverse effects include drowsiness, sedation, blurring of vision, unsteadiness and ataxia. These effects occur following single as well as repeated dosage and may persist well into the following day. Performance at skilled tasks and alertness may be impaired. Patients should be warned of this hazard and advised not to drive or operate machinery during treatment. These effects are potentiated by alcohol. The elderly are particularly liable to experience these symptoms together with confusion especially if organic brain symptoms are present. Amnesia may occur. See also *Dependence potential and withdrawal symptoms* below.

Abnormal psychological reactions to benzodiazepines have been reported. Rare behavioural adverse effects include paradoxical aggressive outbursts, excitement, and confusion.

Other rare adverse effects including hypotension, gastro-intestinal and visual disturbances, skin rashes, urinary retention, headache, vertigo, changes in libido, blood dyscrasias and jaundice have also been reported.

Dependence potential and withdrawal symptoms: In general the dependence potential of benzodiazepines is low, but this increases when high dosage is attained, especially when given over long periods. This is particularly so in patients with a history of alcoholism, drug abuse or in patients with marked personality disorders. Regular monitoring of treatment in such patients is essential and routine repeat prescriptions should be avoided.

Treatment in all patients should be withdrawn gradually as symptoms such as depression, nervousness, rebound insomnia, irritability, sweating and diarrhoea have been reported following abrupt cessation of treatment, even in patients receiving normal therapeutic doses for short periods of time.

Abrupt withdrawal following excessive dosage may produce confusion, toxic psychosis, convulsions or a condition resembling delirium tremens.

Overdosage: Manifestations of Xanax overdosage include extensions of its pharmacological activity, namely ataxia and somnolence. Induced vomiting and/or gastric lavage are indicated. As in all cases of drug overdosage, respiration, pulse, and blood pressure should be monitored and supported by general measures when necessary. Intravenous fluids may be administered and an adequate airway maintained.

Animal experiments have suggested that forced diuresis or haemodialysis are probably of little value in treating overdosage.

As with the management of any overdosage, the physician should bear in mind that multiple agents may have been ingested.

Pharmaceutical precautions Protect from light.

Legal category CD (Sch 4) POM.

Package quantities Packs of 60 (OP).

Further information Alprazolam is readily absorbed. Following oral administration, peak concentrations in the plasma occur after 1–2 hours. The mean half-life is 12–15 hours. Repeated dosage may lead to accumulation and this should be borne in mind in elderly patients and those with impaired renal or hepatic function. Alprazolam and its metabolites are excreted primarily in the urine. Xanax did not affect the prothrombin times or plasma warfarin levels in male volunteers administered sodium warfarin orally.

Product licence numbers

250 micrograms (0.25 mg) Tablets	0032/0092
500 micrograms (0.5 mg) Tablets	0032/0093

**Trade Mark*

Vifor (UK) Ltd
Bridgegate Pavilion
Chester Business Park
Chester CH4 9QH

Vifor

GELOFUSINE*

Presentation Sterile 4% w/v succinylated Gelatin (Modified Fluid Gelatin) in Saline.

Gelatin (MFG)	40.0 gm/litre
Sodium	154 mmol/litre
Chloride	125 mmol/litre
Av Mw	30,000
Av Mn	22,600
pH	7.4±0.3
Relative viscosity at 37°C	1.9
Iso-electric point	pH 4.5±0.3
Colloid osmotic pressure	465 mmH_2O
Gel point	0°C
Osmolalrity	279 mOsm/litre

Description: Gelofusine is prepared by hydrolysis and succinylation of bovine collagen.

Uses
Actions: Gelofusine is a colloidal plasma volume substitute. When used in the treatment of hypovolaemia it produces significant increases in blood volume, cardiac output, stroke volume, blood pressure, urinary output and oxygen delivery. The half-life of Gelofusine is about 4 hours, with the majority of the dose administered being eliminated by renal excretion within 24 hours.

Indications: As a plasma volume substitute in the initial management of hypovolaemic shock due to, for example, haemorrhage, acute trauma or surgery, burns, sepsis, peritonitis, pancreatitis or crush injury.

Dosage and administration Gelofusine is given intravenously. The volume and the rate of administration will depend upon the condition of the patient. The rate of administration can be increased by the application of pressure to the container or by use of a giving set pump. When given rapidly it should be warmed to no more than 37°C if possible. In severe acute blood loss 500 ml may be given in 5–10 minutes until signs of hypovolaemia are relieved. When large volumes are infused, suitable monitoring should be employed to ensure that an adequate haematocrit is maintained, (the haematocrit should not be allowed to fall below 25%), and that dilutional effects upon coagulation are avoided (expert haematological advice should be sought especially in cases of massive blood loss).

For massive fluid loss, Gelofusine may be used concomitantly with blood, the rate and amount of which would depend upon the clinical condition of the patient. The haemodynamic status of the patient should be monitored.

If blood is to be given at the same time as Gelofusine it can be given through the same giving set since Gelofusine has a negligible calcium content and therefore does not clot blood. Gelofusine can also be used to reconstitute packed red cells.

Contra-indications, warnings, etc Known hypersensitivity to Gelofusine.

In common with other colloidal plasma volume expanders, mild urticarial reactions have been reported.

Severe anaphylactic reactions following use of Gelofusine occur with a reported incidence of between 1 in 6,000 and 1 in 13,000 units administered. Such reactions are related to the release of vasoactive substances and can be assumed to be more frequent and particularly hazardous in patients with known allergic conditions such as asthma. *Treatment:* The infusion of Gelofusine should be stopped. Further treatment will depend upon the severity of the anaphylactic reaction. Administration of supplemental oxygen; an alternative intravenous fluid; and the parenteral administration of adrenaline (e.g. 0.5 to 1 ml of a 1:1,000 solution intramuscularly, repeated every 15 minutes as necessary, or 5 to 10 ml of a 1:100,000 solution slowly intravenously), and an antihistamine (e.g. chloropheniramine 10–20 mg slowly intravenously) should be considered.

Gelofusine should be given with care to patients who are susceptible to circulatory overloading (e.g. severe congestive cardiac failure or renal failure with oliguria or anuria) since excessive volumes may give rise to circulatory overload and electrolyte imbalance. *Treatment:* The infusion should be stopped and the patient treated symptomatically. Electrolytes should be monitored. If necessary a diuretic may be given to promote fluid loss. Decreased urinary output secondary to shock is not a contra-indication unless there is no improvement in urine output after the initial dose of Gelofusine.

Pregnancy and lactation: There is very little information available on the use of plasma substitutes in pregnant or lactating women. As with all drugs, the benefits and risks of use should be assessed in the light of the patients condition: Gelofusine may be used in the initial treatment of blood loss during pregnancy where plasma volume replacement is needed.

Pharmaceutical precautions The bottle overwrap is not sterile. If it is damaged, or fluid is present in the space between the wrap and the plastic bottle, the bottle should be assumed to be damaged and should therefore be discarded. The cap covering the giving set entry port should not be replaced after it has been removed, and the entry port area should be disinfected prior to insertion of the giving set.

Gelofusine is stable for five years and can be stored at room temperature. Only clear solution should be used; it contains no preservative and any unused Gelofusine should be discarded once the seal has been opened.

Although water soluble drugs can be given in Gelofusine, experience is limited. If essential, they may be given through the giving set, close to the intravenous cannula. The small calcium content of Gelofusine does not give rise to clotting in the giving set when citrated blood precedes or follows its administration.

Legal category POM.

Package quantities Plastic infusion containers of 500 ml. Packs of 10.

Further information Gelofusine promotes an osmotic diuresis, thereby helping protect the kidneys from the adverse effects of hypovolaemia. It does not interfere with blood grouping or cross-matching.

Product licence number 0183/5025R.

Product licence holder: Conslidated Chemicals Ltd., The Industrial Estate, Wrexham, Clwyd, LL13 9PS.

NUTRIFLEX* 32

Presentation A clear colourless solution of amino acids and electrolytes for intravenous infusion presented in a Twinflex PVC container. Sterile and pyrogen free.

Nutriflex 32 has the following composition per litre:

32 g of amino acids (4.5 g nitrogen)
180 g of glucose = 2800 non-protein kJ (670 kcal)

8 mmol phosphate which can be used directly
1400 mosm/litre

Full details of the composition are given in the following table.

Uses Parenteral nutrition with Nutriflex 32 is indicated when nutritional supplementation is required and enteral nutrition is inadequate or impossible. Such situations may occur following surgery, trauma or burns, or when gastro-intestinal absorption of nutrients is impaired.

Nutriflex 32 contains a balanced mixture of essential and non-essential amino acids, together with electrolytes and glucose. The glucose provides 150 kcal/g nitrogen.

Dosage and administration Shock, and major acid-base of electrolyte imbalance, should be corrected before parenteral nutrition is commenced. Monitoring of nutritional and electrolyte status should be performed, and trace element and vitamin levels should be assessed, particularly in the critically ill, or those patients receiving prolonged parenteral nutrition.

The dose should be adapted to individual patient requirements:

Volume of Nutriflex 32/day (ml)	*Non-protein kcal*	*Nitrogen g*
500	335	2.3
1000	670	4.5
1500	1005	6.8
2000	1340	9.0
3000	2010	13.5

In order to provide an appropriate input of calories, additional glucose or a lipid emulsion may be administered. Supplementation with further electrolytes, and trace elements and vitamins may be required.

Nutriflex 32 has an osmolarity of about 1400 mosm/l. It should therefore be administered by continuous infusion over 24 hours through a central vein. The rate of infusion should be controlled so as to avoid rapid administration of large volumes: 1000 ml of Nutriflex 32 should not be administered in less than 6 to 8 hours.

Contra-indications, warnings, etc

Contra-indications: Parenteral nutrition is contra-indicated in the case of irreversible hepatic failure; renal failure where facilities for dialysis do not exist.

As with all large volume infusion fluids, Nutriflex 32 should be administered with caution to patients with cardiac or renal dysfunction.

Care should be exercised in the administration of parenteral nutrition solutions containing amino acids to patients with altered amino acid metabolism, or with hepatic dysfunction.

Precautions, warnings, side-effects: As with other solutions containing glucose, administration of Nutriflex 32 may lead to hyperglycaemia. Blood glucose levels should be monitored, and the rate of infusion adjusted, or insulin administered, if hyperglycaemia occurs.

Fluid, electrolyte and acid-base balance should be monitored. Administration of amino-acid solutions may cause acute folate deficiency, and supplementary folic acid shoud be administered. Vitamin B_{12} status should be monitored, and supplementation given if necessary.

Nausea may occasionally occur. If the recommended infusion rate is exceeded, vomiting, sweating and flushing may occur. Abnormal results of liver function tests and cholestasis have been reported in some patients receiving parenteral nutrition.

As with all parenteral solutions administered through a central venous catheter, strict aseptic precautions should be taken when Nutriflex 32 is infused. Care should be taken to avoid complications of catheterisation including air embolism and central venous thrombosis.

Overdosage: Gross overdosage of patients during total parenteral nutrition may lead to complications such as acidosis, hyperosmolar coma, hyperammonaemia. If Nutriflex is administered at the recommended rates no such problems are to be anticipated.

Pharmaceutical precautions Store between 4°C and 25°C. Use only clear solution from an undamaged container. Never use a previously opened and partly

Composition (g/litre)

	Before mixing		*After mixing*	*Before mixing*		*After mixing*
	Upper compartment 600 ml	*Lower compartment 400 ml*	*1000 ml*	*Upper compartment 300 ml*	*Lower compartment 200 ml*	*500 ml*
L-Isoleucine		1.88 g	1.88 g		0.94 g	0.94 g
L-Leucine		2.50 g	2.50 g		1.25 g	1.25 g
L-Lysine		1.82 g	1.82 g		0.91 g	0.91 g
L-Methionine		1.56 g	1.56 g		0.78 g	0.78 g
L-Phenylalanine		2.81 g	2.81 g		1.41 g	1.41 g
L-Threonine		1.45 g	1.45 g		0.73 g	0.73 g
L-Tryptophane		0.46 g	0.46 g		0.23 g	0.23 g
L-Valine		2.08 g	2.08 g		1.04 g	1.04 g
L-Arginine		2.16 g	2.16 g		1.08 g	1.08 g
L-Histidine		1.00 g	1.00 g		0.50 g	0.50 g
L-Alanine		3.88 g	3.88 g		1.94 g	1.94 g
L-Aspartic Acid		1.20 g	1.20 g		0.60 g	0.60 g
L-Glutamic Acid		2.80 g	2.80 g		1.40 g	1.40 g
Glycine		1.32 g	1.32 g		0.66 g	0.66 g
L-Proline		2.72 g	2.72 g		1.36 g	1.36 g
L-Serine		2.40 g	2.40 g		1.20 g	1.20 g
Total amino acids		32.0 g	32.0 g		16.0 g	16.0 g
Glucose anhydrous	180.0 g		180.0 g	90.0 g		90.0 g
Na^+	21.0 mmol	13.9 mmol	35.0 mmol	10.5 mmol	7 mmol	17.5 mmol
K^+		25.2 mmol	25.2 mmol		12.6 mmol	12.6 mmol
Ca^{++}	3.6 mmol		3.6 mmol	1.8 mmol		1.8 mmol
Mg^{++}		5.7 mmol	5.7 mmol		2.9 mmol	2.9 mmol
Cl^-	28.2 mmol	18.9 mmol	47.1 mmol	14.1 mmol	9.5 mmol	23.6 mmol
$H_2PO_4^-$		8.0 mmol	8.0 mmol		4.0 mmol	4.0 mmol
Acetate		22.9 mmol	22.9 mmol		11.5 mmol	11.5 mmol
Nitrogen (N)			4.5 g			2.25 g
kJ (kcal)			2800 (670)			1400 (335)

used Nutriflex 32 Solution. Always throw away any remaining solution.

Only mixtures of known compatibility should be prepared. Information on the compatibiity of Nutriflex 32 with vitamins, trace elements and insulin is available from the manufacturer, and if necessary these may be added aseptically just prior to use. Following their addition the bag should be thoroughly agitated to ensure complete mixing. The solution should be used within 24 hours. The compatibility with other additives has not been verified and none should be added to the solution.

Legal category POM.

Package quantities 10 units of 500 ml and 1000 ml of Nutriflex 32. Twinflex: flexible, single PVC container with two compartments separated by an internal obturator.

Further information Nutriflex 32 is a nutritional solution containing amino acids and electrolytes for parenteral administration to patients who are unable to tolerate oral or nasogastric feeding.

The large number of substances which must be supplied and the incompatibilities existing between certain of these substances present a number of difficulties in the preparation of such a solution. These have been overcome with the aid of the Twinflex system. This comprises a twin compartment container in which the upper compartment contains the electrolytes in glucose solution and the lower compartment the amino acids.

Product licence number 5249/0008.

NUTRIFLEX* 48

Presentation A clear colourless solution of amino acids and electrolytes for intravenous infusion presented in a Twinflex PVC container. Sterile and pyrogen free.

Nutriflex 48 has the following composition per litre:

48.1 g of amino acids (6.8 g nitrogen)
300 g of glucose = 4680 non-protein kJ (1120 kcal)
20 mmol phosphate which can be used directly
2300 mosm/litre

Full details of the composition are given in the following table.

Uses Parenteral nutrition with Nutriflex 48 is indicated when nutritional supplementation is required and enteral nutrition is inadequate or impossible. Such situations may occur following surgery, trauma or burns, or when gastro-intestinal absorption of nutrients is impaired.

Nutriflex 48 contains a balanced mixture of essential and non-essential amino acids, together with electrolytes and glucose. The glucose provides 165 kcal/g nitrogen.

Dosage and administration Shock, and major acid-base of electrolyte imbalance, should be corrected before parenteral nutrition is commenced. Monitoring of nutritional and electrolyte status should be performed, and trace element and vitamin levels should be assessed, particularly in the critically ill, or those patients receiving prolonged parenteral nutrition.

The dose should be adapted to individual patient requirements:

Volume of Nutriflex 48/day (ml)	*Non-protein kcal*	*Nitrogen g*
500	560	3.4
1000	1120	6.8
1500	1680	10.2
2000	2240	13.6

In order to provide an appropriate input of calories, additional glucose or a lipid emulsion may be administered. Supplementation with further electrolytes, and trace elements and vitamins may be required.

Nutriflex 48 has an osmolarity of about 2300 mosm/l. It should therefore be administered by continuous infusion over 24 hours through a central vein. The rate of infusion should be controlled so as to avoid rapid administration of large volumes: 1000 ml of Nutriflex 48 should not be administered in less than 6 to 8 hours.

Composition (g/litre)

	Before mixing		*After mixing*	*Before mixing*		*After mixing*
	Upper compartment 600 ml	*Lower compartment 400 ml*	*1000 ml*	*Upper compartment 300 ml*	*Lower compartment 200 ml*	*500 ml*
L-Isoleucine		2.82 g	2.82 g		1.41 g	1.41 g
L-Leucine		3.76 g	3.76 g		1.88 g	1.88 g
L-Lysine		2.73 g	2.73 g		1.37 g	1.37 g
L-Methionine		2.35 g	2.35 g		1.18 g	1.18 g
L-Phenylalanine		4.21 g	4.21 g		2.11 g	2.11 g
L-Threonine		2.18 g	2.18 g		1.09 g	1.09 g
L-Tryptophane		0.68 g	0.68 g		0.34 g	0.34 g
L-Valine		3.12 g	3.12 g		1.56 g	1.56 g
L-Arginine		3.24 g	3.24 g		1.62 g	1.62 g
L-Histidine		1.50 g	1.50 g		0.75 g	0.75 g
L-Alanine		5.82 g	5.82 g		2.91 g	2.91 g
L-Aspartic Acid		1.80 g	1.80 g		0.90 g	0.90 g
L-Glutamic Acid		4.21 g	4.21 g		2.11 g	2.11 g
Glycine		1.98 g	1.98 g		0.99 g	0.99 g
L-Proline		4.08 g	4.08 g		2.04 g	2.04 g
L-Serine		3.60 g	3.60 g		1.80 g	1.80 g
Total amino acids		48.1 g	48.1 g		24.1 g	24.1 g
Glucose anhydrous	300.0 g		300.0 g	150.0 g		150.0 g
Na^+		37.2 mmol	37.2 mmol		18.6 mmol	18.6 mmol
K^+		25.0 mmol	25.0 mmol		12.5 mmol	12.5 mmol
Ca^{++}	3.6 mmol		3.6 mmol	1.8 mmol		1.8 mmol
Mg^{++}		5.7 mmol	5.7 mmol		2.9 mmol	2.9 mmol
Cl^-	7.2 mmol	28.3 mmol	35.5 mmol	3.6 mmol	14.2 mmol	17.8 mmol
$H_2PO_4^-$		20.0 mmol	20.0 mmol		10.0 mmol	10.0 mmol
Acetate		22.9 mmol	22.9 mmol		11.5 mmol	11.5 mmol
Nitrogen (N)			6.8 g			3.4 g
kJ (kcal)			4680 (1120)			2340 (560)

Contra-indications, warnings, etc
Contra-indications: Parenteral nutrition is contra-indicated in the case of irreversible hepatic failure; renal failure where facilities for dialysis do not exist.

As with all large volume infusion fluids, Nutriflex 48 should be administered with caution to patients with cardiac or renal dysfunction.

Care should be exercised in the administration of parenteral nutrition solutions containing amino acids to patients with altered amino acid metabolism, or with hepatic dysfunction.

Precautions, warnings, side-effects: As with other solutions containing glucose, administration of Nutriflex 48 may lead to hyperglycaemia. Blood glucose levels should be monitored, and the rate of infusion adjusted, or insulin administered, if hyperglycaemia occurs.

Fluid, electrolyte and acid-base balance should be monitored. Administration of amino-acid solutions may cause acute folate deficiency, and supplementary folic acid shoud be administered. Vitamin B_{12} status should be monitored, and supplementation given if necessary.

Nausea may occasionally occur. If the recommended infusion rate is exceeded, vomiting, sweating and flushing may occur. Abnormal results of liver function tests and cholestasis have been reported in some patients receiving parenteral nutrition.

As with all parenteral solutions administered through a central venous catheter, strict aseptic precautions should be taken when Nutriflex 48 is infused. Care should be taken to avoid complications of catheterisation including air embolism and central venous thrombosis.

Overdosage: Gross overdosage of patients during total parenteral nutrition may lead to complications such as acidosis, hyperosmolar coma, hyperammonaemia. If Nutriflex is administered at the recommended rates no such problems are to be anticipated.

Pharmaceutical precautions Store between 4°C and 25°C. Use only clear solution from an undamaged container. Never use a previously opened and partly used Nutriflex 48 Solution. Always throw away any remaining solution.

Only mixtures of known compatibility should be prepared. Information on the compatibiity of Nutriflex 48 with vitamins, trace elements and insulin is available from the manufacturer, and if necessary these may be added aseptically just prior to use. Following their addition the bag should be thoroughly agitated to ensure complete mixing. The solution should be used within 24 hours. The compatibility with other additives has not been verified and none should be added to the solution.

Legal category POM.

Package quantities 10 units of 500 ml and 1000 ml of Nutriflex 48. Twinflex: flexible, single PVC container with two compartments separated by an internal obturator.

Further information Nutriflex 48 is a nutritional solution containing amino acids and electrolytes for parenteral administration to patients who are unable to tolerate oral or nasogastric feeding.

The large number of substances which must be supplied and the incompatibilities existing between certain of these substances present a number of difficulties in the preparation of such a solution. These have been overcome with the aid of the Twinflex system. This comprises a twin compartment container in which the upper compartment contains the electrolytes in glucose solution and the lower compartment the amino acids.

Product licence number 5249/0009.

NUTRIFLEX* 70

Presentation A clear colourless solution of amino acids and electrolytes for intravenous infusion presented in a Twinflex PVC container. Sterile and pyrogen free.

Nutriflex 70 has the following composition per litre:

70.1 g of amino acids (10 g nitrogen)
240 g of glucose = 3750 non-protein kJ (900 kcal)
15 mmol phosphate which can be used directly
2100 mosm/litre

Full details of the composition are given in the following table.

Uses Parenteral nutrition with Nutriflex 70 is indicated when nutritional supplementation is required and enteral nutrition is inadequate or impossible. Such situations may occur following surgery, trauma or burns, or when gastro-intestinal absorption of nutrients is impaired.

Nutriflex 70 contains a balanced mixture of essential and non-essential amino acids, together with electrolytes and glucose. The glucose provides 90 kcal/g nitrogen.

Dosage and administration Shock, and major acid-base of electrolyte imbalance, should be corrected before parenteral nutrition is commenced. Monitoring of nutritional and electrolyte status should be performed, and trace element and vitamin levels should be assessed, particularly in the critically ill, or those patients receiving prolonged parenteral nutrition.

The dose should be adapted to individual patient requirements:

Volume of Nutriflex 70/day (ml)	*Non-protein kcal*	*Nitrogen g*
500	450	5
1000	900	10
1500	1350	15
2000	1800	20

In order to provide an appropriate input of calories, additional glucose or a lipid emulsion may be administered. Supplementation with further electrolytes, and trace elements and vitamins may be required.

Nutriflex 70 has an osmolarity of about 2100 mosm/l. It should therefore be administered by continuous infusion over 24 hours through a central vein. The rate of infusion should be controlled so as to avoid rapid administration of large volumes: 1000 ml of Nutriflex 70 should not be administered in less than 6 to 8 hours.

Contra-indications, warnings, etc
Contra-indications: Parenteral nutrition is contra-indicated in the case of irreversible hepatic failure; renal failure where facilities for dialysis do not exist.

As with all large volume infusion fluids, Nutriflex 70 should be administered with caution to patients with cardiac or renal dysfunction.

Care should be exercised in the administration of parenteral nutrition solutions containing amino acids to patients with altered amino acid metabolism, or with hepatic dysfunction.

Precautions, warnings, side-effects: As with other solutions containing glucose, administration of Nutriflex 70 may lead to hyperglycaemia. Blood glucose levels should be monitored, and the rate of infusion adjusted, or insulin administered, if hyperglycaemia occurs.

Fluid, electrolyte and acid-base balance should be monitored. Administration of amino-acid solutions may cause acute folate deficiency, and supplementary folic acid shoud be administered. Vitamin B_{12} status should be monitored, and supplementation given if necessary.

Nausea may occasionally occur. If the recommended infusion rate is exceeded, vomiting, sweating and flushing may occur. Abnormal results of liver function tests and cholestasis have been reported in some patients receiving parenteral nutrition.

As with all parenteral solutions administered through a central venous catheter, strict aseptic precautions should be taken when Nutriflex 70 is infused. Care should be taken to avoid complications of catheterisation including air embolism and central venous thrombosis.

Overdosage: Gross overdosage of patients during total parenteral nutrition may lead to complications such as acidosis, hyperosmolar coma, hyperammonaemia. If Nutriflex is administered at the recommended rates no such problems are to be anticipated.

Composition (g/litre)

	Before mixing		*After mixing*	*Before mixing*		*After mixing*
	Upper compartment 600 ml	*Lower compartment 400 ml*	*1000 ml*	*Upper compartment 300 ml*	*Lower compartment 200 ml*	*500 ml*
L-Isoleucine		4.11 g	4.11 g		2.06 g	2.06 g
L-Leucine		5.48 g	5.48 g		2.74 g	2.74 g
L-Lysine		3.98 g	3.98 g		1.99 g	1.99 g
L-Methionine		3.42 g	3.42 g		1.71 g	1.71 g
L-Phenylalanine		6.15 g	6.15 g		3.08 g	3.08 g
L-Threonine		3.18 g	3.18 g		1.59 g	1.59 g
L-Tryptophane		1.00 g	1.00 g		0.50 g	0.50 g
L-Valine		4.54 g	4.54 g		2.27 g	2.27 g
L-Arginine		4.73 g	4.73 g		2.37 g	2.37 g
L-Histidine		2.19 g	2.19 g		1.10 g	1.10 g
L-Alanine		8.49 g	8.49 g		4.25 g	4.25 g
L-Aspartic Acid		2.63 g	2.63 g		1.32 g	1.32 g
L-Glutamic Acid		6.14 g	6.14 g		3.07 g	3.07 g
Glycine		2.89 g	2.89 g		1.45 g	1.45 g
L-Proline		5.95 g	5.95 g		2.98 g	2.98 g
L-Serine		5.25 g	5.25 g		2.63 g	2.63 g
Total amino acids		70.1 g	70.1 g		35.1 g	35.1 g
Glucose anhydrous	240.0 g		240.0 g	120.0 g		120.0 g
Na^+		40.5 mmol	40.5 mmol		20.3 mmol	20.3 mmol
K^+		25.7 mmol	25.7 mmol		12.9 mmol	12.9 mmol
Ca^{++}	4.1 mmol		4.1 mmol	2.1 mmol		2.1 mmol
Mg^{++}		5.0 mmol	5.0 mmol		2.5 mmol	2.5 mmol
Cl^-	8.2 mmol	41.3 mmol	49.5 mmol	4.1 mmol	20.7 mmol	24.8 mmol
$H_2PO_4^-$		14.7 mmol	14.7 mmol		7.4 mmol	7.4 mmol
Acetate		22.0 mmol	22.0 mmol		11.0 mmol	11.0 mmol
Nitrogen (N)			10.0 g			5.0 g
kJ (kcal)			3750 (900)			1875 (450)

Pharmaceutical precautions Store between 4°C and 25°C. Use only clear solution from an undamaged container. Never use a previously opened and partly used Nutriflex 70 Solution. Always throw away any remaining solution.

Only mixtures of known compatibility should be prepared. Information on the compatibiity of Nutriflex 70 with vitamins, trace elements and insulin is available from the manufacturer, and if necessary these may be added aseptically just prior to use. Following their addition the bag should be thoroughly agitated to ensure complete mixing. The solution should be used within 24 hours. The compatibility with other additives has not been verified and none should be added to the solution.

Legal category POM.

Package quantities 10 units of 500 ml and 1000 ml of Nutriflex 70. Twinflex: flexible, single PVC container with two compartments separated by an internal obturator.

Further information Nutriflex 70 is a nutritional solution containing amino acids and electrolytes for parenteral administration to patients who are unable to tolerate oral or nasogastric feeding.

The large number of substances which must be supplied and the incompatibilities existing between certain of these substances present a number of difficulties in the preparation of such a solution. These have been overcome with the aid of the Twinflex system. This comprises a twin compartment container in which the upper compartment contains the electrolytes in glucose solution and the lower compartment the amino acids.

Product licence number 5249/0010.

**Trade Mark*

Wellcome Medical Division
The Wellcome Foundation Limited
Crewe Hall
Crewe,
Cheshire
CW1 1UB

Wellcome

1989
THE QUEEN'S AWARD FOR EXPORT ACHIEVEMENT

1990
THE QUEEN'S AWARD FOR TECHNOLOGICAL ACHIEVEMENT TO THE WELLCOME RESEARCH LABORATORIES OF THE WELLCOME FOUNDATION LTD

1991
THE QUEEN'S AWARD FOR EXPORT ACHIEVEMENT

ACTIDIL* TABLETS AND ELIXIR

Presentation Each tablet contains 2.5 mg Triprolidine Hydrochloride BP. Scored and coded 'WELLCOME L2A'. White in colour.

Each 5 ml of orange-coloured elixir contains 2 mg Triprolidine Hydrochloride BP and has a flavour of mandarin orange.

Uses Antihistamine.

Actidil is indicated for the symptomatic relief of allergic conditions normally responsive to antihistamines, e.g. hay fever, and allergic skin conditions, e.g. urticaria and pruritus.

Actidil Elixir is particularly suitable for use in children.

Dosage and administration *Adults:* 1–2 tablets or 5–10 ml elixir three times a day.

Children: Over 12 years: As for adults.

6–12 years: 5–7.5 ml three times a day.

1–6 years: 5 ml three times a day.

Under 1 year: 2.5 ml three times a day.

Actidil Elixir may be diluted 1:1 (1 in 2) or 1:3 (1 in 4) with Syrup BP, and these dilutions have a shelf life of 4 weeks if stored at 25°C.

Use in the elderly: No specific studies have been carried out in the elderly, but Actidil has been widely used in older people. However, it may be advisable to monitor renal or hepatic function and if there is serious impairment then caution should be exercised.

Contra-indications, warnings, etc
Contra-indications: Contra-indicated in patients with known hypersensitivity to triprolidine.

Precautions: May cause drowsiness. Patients should not drive a vehicle or operate machinery until they have determined their own response. In some patients the drowsiness induced by antihistamines may be potentiated by alcohol or other central sedatives.

There have been no specific studies of Actidil in patients with hepatic and/or renal dysfunction. The major metabolite identified in human volunteers is the carboxylated derivative of triprolidine. This accounts for approximately 50% of the dose excreted in the urine.

Since antihistamines have some anticholinergic properties, Actidil should be used with care in patients with elevated intraocular pressure and in patients with prostatic hypertrophy.

Side- and adverse effects: Triprolidine may cause drowsiness. Lichenoid skin eruptions due to triprolidine have rarely been reported

Use in pregnancy and lactation: Although triprolidine has been in widespread use for many years without apparent ill consequence, there are no specific data on its use during pregnancy. Caution should therefore be exercised by balancing the potential benefit of treatment against any possible hazards. Systemic administration of triprolidine in rats and rabbits up to 75 times the human dose did not produce teratogenic effects.

It has been estimated that approximately 0.06–0.2% of a single dose of triprolidine ingested by a mother will be excreted in the breast milk over 24 hours, but the effect of this on breast-fed infants is not known.

Toxicity and treatment of overdosage: Drowsiness, lethargy, dizziness, ataxia, weakness, hypotonicity and respiratory depression may occur. Atropine-like symptoms such as dryness of the skin and mucous membranes, tachycardia, hyperpyrexia, hyperactivity and convulsions may also occur.

Necessary measures should be taken to maintain and support respiration. Gastric lavage should be performed if indicated and convulsions controlled with diazepam.

Pharmaceutical precautions *Tablets:* Store below 25°C. Protect from light.

Elixir: Store below 25°C. Protect from light.

Legal category P.

Package quantities Bottle of 100 tablets. Bottle of 500 ml elixir.

Further information Nil.

Product licence numbers
Tablets 0003/5001R
Elixir 0003/5002R

ACTIFED* COMPOUND LINCTUS

Presentation Each 5 ml of bright-red-coloured linctus contains 10 mg Dextromethorphan Hydrobromide BP, 30 mg Pseudoephedrine Hydrochloride BP, and 1.25 mg Triprolidine Hydrochloride BP and has a fruity flavour.

Uses Relief of unproductive cough accompanied by congestion of the upper respiratory tract, including congestion with an allergic component.

Dosage and administration
Adults and children over 12 years: 10 ml three times a day.

Children 6–12 years: 5 ml three times a day.
2–5 years: 2.5 ml three times a day.

Actifed Compound Linctus may be diluted 1:1 (1 in 2) or 1:3 (1 in 4) with Syrup BP, and these dilutions have a shelf life of 4 weeks if stored at 25°C.

Use in the elderly: No specific studies have been carried out in the elderly, but Actifed Compound Linctus has been widely used in older people. However, it may be advisable to monitor renal or hepatic function and if there is serious impairment then caution should be exercised.

Pharmacology: Pseudoephedrine has direct and indirect sympathomimetic activity and is an orally effective upper respiratory tract decongestant. Pseudoephedrine is substantially less potent than ephedrine in producing both tachycardia and elevation in systolic blood pressure, and is considerably less potent in causing stimulation of the central nervous system. Triprolidine provides antihistamine activity by antagonising H_1 receptors. Dextromethorphan provides antitussive activity by acting on the medullary cough centre.

Contra-indications, warnings, etc
Contra-indications: Contra-indicated in patients with a known hypersensitivity to pseudoephedrine, triprolidine, or dextromethorphan. Contra-indicated in persons under

treatment with monoamine oxidase inhibitors or within 2 weeks of stopping such treatment.

Actifed Compound Linctus is contra-indicated in patients with severe hypertension or severe coronary artery disease.

Actifed Compound Linctus should not be administered to patients where cough is associated with asthma or where cough is accompanied by excessive secretions.

Dextromethorphan, in common with other centrally acting antitussive agents, should not be given to patients in or at risk of developing respiratory failure.

Precautions: Although pseudoephedrine has virtually no pressor effect in patients with normal blood pressure Actifed Compound Linctus should be used with caution in patients taking antihypertensive agents, tricyclic antidepressants, other sympathomimetic agents, such as decongestants, appetite suppressants and amphetamine-like psychostimulants. The effects of a single dose of Actifed Compound Linctus on the blood pressure of these patients should be observed before recommending repeated or unsupervised treatment.

As with other sympathomimetic agents, caution should be exercised in patients with uncontrolled diabetes, hyperthyroidism, elevated intraocular pressure and prostatic enlargement.

Drug interactions: Concomitant use of Actifed Compound Linctus with sympathomimetic agents, such as decongestants, tricyclic antidepressants, appetite suppressants and amphetamine-like psychostimulants or with monoamine oxidase inhibitors which interfere with the catabolism of sympathomimetic amines, may occasionally cause a rise in blood pressure.

Because of its pseudoephedrine content, the effect of antihypertensive agents which modify sympathetic activity may be partially reversed by Actifed Compound Linctus.

It has been reported that a fatality was probably due to a toxic reaction resulting from the combination of dextromethorphan with a monoamine oxidase inhibitor.

The antibacterial agent furazolidone is known to cause a dose-related inhibition of monoamine oxidase and although there are no reports of a hypertensive crisis having occurred, it should not be administered concurrently with Actifed Compound Linctus.

Side- and adverse effects: In some patients, pseudoephedrine may occasionally cause insomnia. Rarely, sleep disturbance and hallucinations have been reported. Triprolidine may cause drowsiness and patients should not drive a vehicle or operate machinery until they have determined their own response. In some patients, the drowsiness induced by antihistamines may be potentiated by alcohol or other central sedatives. Fixed drug eruption due to pseudoephedrine, taking the form of erythematous nummular patches, and lichenoid skin eruption due to triprolidine, have been reported but both these reactions should be regarded as rare events.

Urinary retention may occasionally occur in male patients in whom prostatic enlargement could be an important predisposing factor.

Side-effects attributed to dextromethorphan are uncommon; occasionally nausea, vomiting or gastrointestinal disturbance may occur.

Use in pregnancy and lactation: Although pseudoephedrine, triprolidine and dextromethorphan have been in widespread use for many years without apparent ill consequence, there are no specific data on their use during pregnancy. Caution should therefore be exercised by balancing the potential benefit of treatment against any possible hazards. Systemic administration of triprolidine in rats and rabbits up to 75 times the human dose did not produce teratogenic effects.

Systemic administration of pseudoephedrine, up to 50 times the human dose in rats and up to 35 times the human dose in rabbits, did not produce teratogenic effects.

It has been estimated that approximately 0.5–0.7% of a single dose of pseudoephedrine and approximately 0.06–0.2% of a single dose of triprolidine ingested by a mother will be excreted in the breast milk over 24 hours, but the effect of this on breast-fed infants is not known.

It is not known whether dextromethorphan or its metabolites are excreted in human milk.

Toxicity and treatment of overdosage: The effects of acute toxicity from Actifed Compound Linctus may include drowsiness, lethargy, dizziness, ataxia, nystagmus, weakness, hypotonicity, respiratory depression, dryness of the skin and mucous membranes, tachycardia, hypertension, hyperpyrexia, hyperactivity, irritability, visual and auditory hallucinations, convulsions, difficulty with micturition, nausea and vomiting.

Necessary measures should be taken to maintain and support respiration and control convulsions. Gastric lavage should be performed if indicated. Catheterisation of the bladder may be necessary. If desired, the elimination of pseudoephedrine can be accelerated by acid diuresis or by dialysis.

Naloxone has been used successfully as a specific antagonist to dextromethorphan toxicity in a child.

Pharmaceutical precautions Store below 25°C. Protect from light.

Legal category P.

Package quantities Bottles of 100 ml and 200 ml.

Further information Nil.

Product licence number 0003/0160.

ACTIFED* EXPECTORANT

Presentation Each 5 ml of clear orange syrup contains 1.25 mg Triprolidine Hydrochloride BP, 30 mg Pseudoephedrine Hydrochloride BP and 100 mg Guaiphenesin BP.

Uses Actifed Expectorant is indicated for the symptomatic relief of upper respiratory tract disorders accompanied by productive cough, which benefit from the administration of a nasal decongestant, a histamine H_1-receptor antagonist and an expectorant combination.

Dosage and administration

Adults and children over 12 years: 10 ml three times a day.

Children 6–12 years: 5 ml three times a day.

Children 2–5 years: 2.5 ml three times a day.

Actifed Expectorant may be diluted 1:1 (1 in 2) or 1:3 (1 in 4) with unpreserved Syrup BP, and these dilutions have a shelf life of 4 weeks if stored at 25°C.

Use in the elderly: No specific studies have been carried out in the elderly. Experience has indicated that normal adult dosage is appropriate, although it may be advisable to monitor renal and/or hepatic function. If there is serious impairment then caution should be exercised.

Mode of action: Triprolidine provides symptomatic relief in conditions believed to depend wholly or partly upon the triggered release of histamine. It is a potent competitive histamine H_1-receptor antagonist of the pyrrolidine class with mild central nervous system depressant properties which may cause drowsiness. Pseudoephedrine has direct and indirect sympathomimetic activity and is an effective upper respiratory decongestant. Pseudoephedrine is substantially less potent than ephedrine in producing both tachycardia and elevation of systolic blood pressure and considerably less potent in causing stimulation of the central nervous system. Guaiphenesin has an expectorant action. It is thought to reduce sputum viscosity by increasing the volume and water content of the bronchial secretion, thereby facilitating the expectoration of sputum.

Contra-indications, warnings, etc

Contra-indications: Actifed Expectorant is contra-indicated in individuals who have previously exhibited intolerance to it or to any of its constituents.

Actifed Expectorant is contra-indicated in patients who are taking or have taken monoamine oxidase inhibitors within the preceding two weeks. The concomitant use of pseudoephedrine and this type of product may occasionally cause a rise in blood pressure.

Actifed Expectorant is contra-indicated in patients

with severe hypertension or severe coronary artery disease.

The antibacterial agent furazolidone is known to cause a dose-related inhibition of monoamine oxidase. Although there are no reports of hypertensive crises caused by the concurrent administration of Actifed Expectorant and furazolidone, they should not be taken together.

Precautions: Actifed Expectorant may cause drowsiness and impair performance in tests of auditory vigilance. Patients should not drive or operate machinery until they have determined their own response.

Although there are no objective data, users of Actifed Expectorant should avoid the concomitant use of alcohol or other centrally acting sedatives.

Although pseudoephedrine has virtually no pressor effect in patients with normal blood pressure, Actifed Expectorant should be used with caution in patients taking antihypertensive agents, tricyclic antidepressants, or other sympathomimetic agents, such as decongestants, appetite suppressants and amphetamine-like psychostimulants. The effects of a single dose of Actifed Expectorant on the blood pressure of these patients should be observed before recommending repeated or unsupervised treatment.

As with other sympathomimetic agents caution should be exercised in patients with hypertension, heart disease, diabetes, hyperthyroidism, elevated intraocular pressure and prostatic enlargement.

There have been no specific studies of Actifed Expectorant in patients with hepatic and/or renal dysfunction. Caution should be exercised in the presence of severe renal or hepatic impairment.

Actifed Expectorant should not be used for persistent or chronic cough such as occurs with smoking, asthma or emphysema or where cough is accompanied by excessive secretions unless directed by a physician.

There is insufficient information available to determine whether triprolidine, pseudoephedrine or guaiphenesin have mutagenic or carcinogenic potential.

Drug interactions: Concomitant use of Actifed Expectorant with sympathomimetic agents, such as decongestants, tricyclic antidepressants, appetite suppressants and amphetamine-like psychostimulants or with monoamine oxidase inhibitors which interfere with the catabolism of sympathomimetic amines, may occasionally cause a rise in blood pressure.

Because of its pseudoephedrine content, Actifed Expectorant may partially reverse the hypotensive action of drugs which interfere with sympathetic activity including bretylium, bethanidine, guanethidine, debrisoquine, methyldopa, alpha- and beta-adrenergic blocking agents.

Side- and adverse effects: Central nervous system (CNS) depression or excitation may occur, drowsiness being reported most frequently. Sleep disturbance and, rarely, hallucinations have been reported.

Skin rashes with or without irritation, tachycardia, dryness of mouth, nose and throat have occasionally been reported. Urinary retention has been reported occasionally in men receiving pseudoephedrine; prostatic enlargement could have been an important predisposing factor.

Use in pregnancy and lactation: Although pseudoephedrine, triprolidine and guaiphenesin have been in widespread use for many years without apparent ill consequence, there are no specific data on their use during pregnancy. Caution should therefore be exercised by balancing the potential benefit of treatment to the mother against any possible hazards to the developing foetus.

In rats and rabbits systemic administration of triprolidine up to 75 times the human daily dosage did not produce teratogenic effects.

Systemic administration of pseudoephedrine, up to 50 times the human daily dosage in rats and up to 35 times the human daily dosage in rabbits, did not produce teratogenic effects.

There is no information available on whether or not guaiphenesin has teratogenic potential.

No studies have been conducted in animals to determine whether triprolidine, pseudoephedrine or guaiphenesin have potential to impair fertility. There is no information on the effect of Actifed Expectorant on human fertility.

Pseudoephedrine and triprolidine are excreted in breast milk in small amounts but the effect of this on breast-fed infants is not known. It has been estimated that 0.5 to 0.7% of a single dose of pseudoephedrine ingested by a mother will be excreted in the breast milk over 24 hours.

Guaiphenesin is excreted in breast milk in small amounts with no expected effect on the infant.

Toxicity and treatment of overdosage: The effects of acute toxicity from Actifed Expectorant may include gastro-intestinal discomfort, nausea, vomiting, drowsiness, lethargy, dizziness, ataxia, weakness, hypotonicity, respiratory depression, dryness of the skin and mucous membranes, tachycardia, hypertension, hyperpyrexia, hyperactivity, irritability, convulsions and difficulty with micturition.

Necessary measures should be taken to maintain and support respiration and control convulsions. Gastric lavage should be performed up to 3 hours after ingestion if indicated. Catheterisation of the bladder may be necessary. If desired, the elimination of pseudoephedrine can be accelerated by acid diuresis or by dialysis.

Pharmaceutical precautions Store below 25°C. Do not refrigerate. Protect from light.

Legal category P.

Package quantities Bottles of 100 ml and 200 ml.

Further information Nil.

Product licence number 0003/0152.

ACTIFED* TABLETS AND SYRUP

Presentation Each tablet contains 2.5 mg Triprolidine Hydrochloride BP and 60 mg Pseudoephedrine Hydrochloride BP. Scored and coded 'WELLCOME M2A'. White in colour.

Each 5 ml of clear, golden-yellow syrup contains 1.25 mg Triprolidine Hydrochloride BP and 30 mg Pseudoephedrine Hydrochloride BP, and has a pleasant flavour.

Uses Decongestant and antihistamine.

For decongestion of the upper respiratory tract including the sinuses, antra and Eustachian tubes in the common cold, hay fever, allergic rhinitis and vasomotor rhinitis.

Dosage and administration *Adults, and children over 12 years:* 1 tablet or 10 ml three times a day.

6–12 years: 5 ml three times a day.

2–5 years: 2.5 ml three times a day.

Actifed Syrup may be diluted 1:1 (1 in 2) or 1:3 (1 in 4) with Syrup BP, and these dilutions have a shelf life of 4 weeks if stored at 25°C.

Use in the elderly: No specific studies have been carried out in the elderly, but Actifed has been widely used in older people. However, it may be advisable to monitor renal or hepatic function and if there is serious impairment then caution should be exercised.

Pharmacology: Pseudoephedrine has direct and indirect sympathomimetic activity and is an orally effective upper respiratory tract decongestant. Pseudoephedrine is substantially less potent than ephedrine in producing both tachycardia and elevation in systolic blood pressure and considerably less potent in causing stimulation of the central nervous system. Triprolidine provides antihistamine activity by antagonising H_1 receptors.

Contra-indications, warnings, etc
Contra-indications: Contra-indicated in patients with known hypersensitivity to pseudoephedrine or triprolidine.

Contra-indicated in persons under treatment with

monoamine oxidase inhibitors, and within two weeks of stopping such treatment.

It is also contra-indicated in patients with severe hypertension or severe coronary heart disease.

Precautions: Although pseudoephedrine has virtually no pressor effect in patients with normal blood pressure, Actifed should be used with caution in patients taking anti-hypertensive agents, tricyclic antidepressants, other sympathomimetic agents, such as decongestants, appetite suppressants and amphetamine-like psychostimulants. The effects of a single dose on the blood pressure of these patients should be observed before recommending repeated or unsupervised treatment.

As with other sympathomimetic agents, caution should be exercised in patients with uncontrolled diabetes, hyperthyroidism, elevated intraocular pressure and prostatic enlargement.

Drug interactions: Concomitant use of Actifed with sympathomimetic agents, such as decongestants, tricyclic antidepressants, appetite suppressants and amphetamine-like psychostimulants or with monoamine oxidase inhibitors which interfere with the catabolism of sympathomimetic amines, may occasionally cause a rise in blood pressure.

Because of its pseudoephedrine content, the effect of antihypertensive agents which modify sympathetic activity may be partially reversed by Actifed.

The antibacterial agent furazolidone is known to cause a dose-related inhibition of monoamine oxidase and although there are no reports of hypertensive crises having occurred, it should not be administered concurrently with Actifed.

Side- and adverse effects: In some patients, pseudoephedrine may occasionally cause insomnia. Rarely, sleep disturbance and hallucinations have been reported. Triprolidine may cause drowsiness. Patients should not drive a vehicle or operate machinery until they have determined their own response. In some patients the drowsiness induced by antihistamines may be potentiated by alcohol or other central sedatives. Fixed drug eruption due to pseudoephedrine taking the form of erythematous nummular patches and lichenoid skin eruption due to triprolidine have been reported but these are rare events.

Urinary retention may occasionally occur in male patients in whom prostatic enlargement could be an important predisposing factor.

Use in pregnancy and lactation: Although pseudoephedrine and triprolidine have been in widespread use for many years without apparent ill consequence, there are no specific data on their use during pregnancy. Caution should therefore be exercised by balancing the potential benefit of treatment against any possible hazards.

Systemic administration of triprolidine in rats and rabbits up to 75 times the human dose did not produce teratogenic effects.

Systemic administration of pseudoephedrine, up to 50 times the human dose in rats and up to 35 times the human dose in rabbits, did not produce teratogenic effects.

It has been estimated that approximately 0.5–0.7% of a single dose of pseudoephedrine and approximately 0.06–0.2% of a single dose of triprolidine ingested by a mother will be excreted in the breast milk over 24 hours, but the effect of this on breast-fed infants is not known.

Toxicity and treatment of overdosage: The effects of acute toxicity from Actifed may include drowsiness, lethargy, dizziness, ataxia, weakness, hypotonicity, respiratory depression, dryness of the skin and mucous membranes, tachycardia, hypertension, hyperpyrexia, hyperactivity, irritability, convulsions and difficulty with micturition. Gastric lavage and supportive measures for respiration and circulation should be performed if indicated. Convulsions should be controlled with an anticonvulsant. Catheterisation of the bladder may be necessary.

If desired, the elimination of pseudoephedrine can be accelerated by acid diuresis or by dialysis.

Pharmaceutical precautions *Tablets:* Store below 25°C in a dry place. Protect from light.

Syrup: Store below 25°C. Protect from light.

Legal category P.

Package quantities Pack of 12 tablets in a blister strip. Bottles of 100 ml.

Further information Nil.

Product licence numbers

Tablets	0003/5003R
Syrup	0003/5004R

AEROSPORIN*

Presentation Each rubber-capped vial contains 500,000 i.u. of sterile freeze-dried Polymyxin B Sulphate BP.

Uses Bactericidal antibiotic.

As an alternative therapy in severe systemic infections caused by a wide range of susceptible Gram-negative organisms, particularly *Pseudomonas aeruginosa*, pulmonary infections due to *Ps. aeruginosa, E. coli*, and *H. influenzae*.

Dosage and administration

Intravenous administration – Adults and children: 15,000–25,000 units per kg. bodyweight per day. Total daily dosage must not exceed 2,000,000 units.

No dosage information is available for intravenous administration in neonates.

The total daily dose may be given as a continuous infusion or as 2 infusions per day each for 1–2 hours and given 12 hours apart. 5% Dextrose in water is recommended as the diluent.

Intramuscular administration – Adults and children: 15,000 to 25,000 units per kg bodyweight per day. Total daily dosage must not exceed 2,000,000 units.

Neonates: 15,000–45,000 units per kg bodyweight per day.

The total daily dose should be given in 4 equally divided doses at 6-hourly intervals. 1–2 mls of water for injection, 0.9% sterile sodium chloride or 1% sterile procaine hydrochloride solution should be used as diluent.

The monitoring of serum polymyxin levels is a sensible precaution in this age group.

Dosage in renal failure:

Creatinine clearance	*Dosage (units/kg/day)*
Normal or 80% of normal	25,000
80% to 30% of normal	1st day: 25,000 Daily thereafter 10,000–15,000
25% of normal	1st day: 25,000 Every 2–3 days thereafter 10,000–15,000
Anuria	1st day: 25,000 Every 5–7 days thereafter 10,000

Patients with impaired renal function excrete the drug more slowly and an appropriate adjustment in the intravenous or intramuscular dosage should be made. The table above gives guidelines based on creatinine clearance. Additional guidance should be obtained by regular monitoring of serum levels of polymyxin B and renal function. The serum level of polymyxin B should be kept below 10 μg/ml.

Subconjunctival injection: Up to 100,000 units per day is recommended, administered in water for injection or sterile 0.9% sodium chloride solution. A concentration of 500,000 units per ml is suggested and not more than 1 ml of diluent should be administered per injection.

Use of a local anaesthetic should be considered when Aerosporin is administered by this route.

Use in the elderly: No specific studies have been carried out in the elderly, but the drug has been widely used in older people. However, it may be advisable to monitor renal function in these patients and if there is any impairment then serum levels should be monitored.

Contra-indications, warnings, etc
Contra-indications: Hypersensitivity to polymyxins.

Precautions: Nephropathy and neuropathy may result from the use of this drug. It may therefore be advisable to monitor renal function before and during parenteral therapy.

The concomitant use of other potentially nephrotoxic drugs should be avoided if possible.

Due to the possibility of neuromuscular blockade leading to respiratory paralysis and apnoea, caution is advised in the administration of other agents with a similar action (eg muscle relaxants, general anaesthetics, antibiotics with muscle relaxant properties).

Side- and adverse effects: Occasionally mild drug fever and a variety of skin eruptions, including urticaria, have been reported after parenteral therapy.

Local pain at the injection site may occur when the drug is given intramuscularly. Subconjunctival injection may also be painful.

Polymyxin B may cause nephrotoxicity. This effect is dose-related and rarely a serious clinical problem in patients with adequate renal function receiving recommended doses; it is usually reversible on discontinuation. As with all antibacterial preparations prolonged use may result in the overgrowth of non-susceptible organisms including fungi.

Neurological symptoms of varying intensity may occur. There may be circumoral and peripheral paraesthesia, some dizziness and a feeling of weakness without, however, any objective signs. These effects are transient and disappear within 48 hours of stopping treatment.

At parenteral dose levels of 25,000 units per kg/day (2.5 mg/kg per day) or more, proteinuria, casts and microscopic haematuria are frequently found. This does not constitute a reason for cessation of therapy.

At dose levels above 30,000 units/kg/day (3 mg/kg per day) nitrogen retention often develops and the glomerular filtration rate may be reduced leading to oliguria. Increasing nitrogen retention is an indication to reduce dosage and oliguria is an indication to stop therapy. Nephrotoxicity is usually reversible on discontinuation of the drug.

Polymyxin B sulphate can cause neuromuscular blockade leading to respiratory paralysis and apnoea. This latter problem is often preceded by dyspnoea and restlessness. It is *not* antagonised by neostigmine or reliably reversed by calcium salts. The only reliable treatment for respiratory paralysis is the institution of artificial respiration and the discontinuation of the drug.

Apnoea due to neuromuscular blockade by polymyxin B sulphate is a rare sequel of therapy and is only likely to occur in the circumstances of overdosing, renal insufficiency, concomitant administration of other neuromuscular blocking drugs or the presence of disease with neuromuscular effects, such as myasthenia gravis.

Electrolyte imbalance, including hyponatraemia, hypochloraemia, hypokalaemia and hypocalcaemia, has been reported during parenteral polymyxin B sulphate therapy in patients with serious underlying malignant disease.

Eosinophilia, occurring during the course of polymyxin B sulphate therapy has been reported. The significance of this finding is not clearly established.

Drug interactions: Due to the possibility of neuromuscular blockade leading to respiratory paralysis and apnoea, great care must be exercised if Aerosporin has to be given at the same time as muscle relaxants, general anaesthetics or other antibiotics which have muscle relaxant properties.

Use in pregnancy and lactation: The active ingredient of Aerosporin, polymyxin B sulphate, has been used for several years without any evidence of untoward effect in pregnancy. The clinical benefit of the treatment to the mother must be balanced against any possible, but unknown hazards to the developing foetus.

No information is available regarding the excretion of the active ingredient or its metabolites in human breast milk and its use in lactating mothers is not recommended.

Toxicity and treatment of overdosage: Antihistamines may relieve some of the subjective symptoms. If respiratory paralysis occurs, artificial respiration should be instituted. There is some evidence that haemodialysis lowers serum levels of the drug. However, the value of this procedure is open to doubt due to tissue localisation of the antibiotic.

Pharmaceutical precautions Store in a dry place, below 25°C. Protect from light. Use immediately after reconstitution. Aerosporin should not be mixed with solutions containing heparin, prednisolone, protein hydrolysate, or other antibiotics.

Legal category POM.

Package quantities Rubber-capped vial of 500,000 i.u.

Further information It is desirable to continue therapy until the lesions are healed; otherwise infecting organisms may reappear if the antibiotic is withdrawn too soon.

Product licence number 0003/5006R.

ALCOPAR* DISPERSIBLE GRANULES

Presentation Each 5 g of the dispersible yellow-green granules contains the equivalent of 2.5 g bephenium ion as Bephenium Hydroxynaphthoate BP.

Uses For the treatment of hookworm infestation by *Ancylostoma duodenale.* Also concurrent ascariasis (roundworm infection), and trichostrongyliasis.

Dosage and administration The required dose of Alcopar should be mixed in water or in a flavoured drink and swallowed immediately.

Adults: The contents of 1 sachet.

Children: Over 2 years: The contents of 1 sachet.

In the presence of heavy infections it is recommended that treatment be repeated after three days.

No purgation or dietary restriction is necessary.

Oral iron may be given concurrently with Alcopar to patients with iron deficiency anaemia.

Use in the elderly: Alcopar is poorly absorbed from the intestinal tract, it is, therefore, unlikely to affect elderly patients in apparently good health.

Contra-indications, warnings, etc
Contra-indications: Alcopar should not be given to patients with persistent vomiting.

Side- and adverse effects: Nausea, vomiting, headache, vertigo, abdominal discomfort and diarrhoea have occasionally been observed.

Use in pregnancy and lactation: There is inadequate evidence of safety of Alcopar in human pregnancy although animal studies have shown no hazard except at doses that cause maternal toxicity. Alcopar has been in wide use for many years without apparent untoward effect. However, caution should be exercised by balancing the potential benefit of treatment against any possible hazards.

As only minimal amounts of bephenium are absorbed from the gut, Alcopar would not be expected to present a hazard to the suckling infant.

Toxicity and treatment of overdosage: No data available. When administered orally, only a small fraction is absorbed from the gastro-intestinal tract. Thus symptoms are likely to be similar to those listed under side- and adverse effects. Gastric lavage followed by symptomatic and general supportive therapy is recommended.

Pharmaceutical precautions Store below 35°C.

Legal category P.

Package quantities Box of 25 × 5 g sachets.

Further information Nil.

Product licence number 0003/5007R.

ALKERAN* TABLETS AND INJECTION

Presentation *Alkeran Tablets:* 2 mg Melphalan BP coloured white with a pink core and coded 'WELLCOME A2A'.

5 mg Melphalan BP coloured white with a pink core and coded 'WELLCOME B2A'.

Alkeran Injection: Each vial contains the equivalent of 100 mg sterile anhydrous Melphalan BP. 1.8 ml ampoule of Wellcome Acid-Alcohol Solvent and 9 ml ampoule of Wellcome Diluent are included in the unit pack.

Uses Cytotoxic agent. Alkylating agent.

Alkeran tablets are indicated in the treatment of multiple myeloma and advanced ovarian adenocarcinoma. Alkeran has a significant therapeutic effect in a proportion of patients suffering from advanced breast cancer or polycythaemia vera. Alkeran has been used as an adjuvant to surgery in the management of breast carcinoma.

Alkeran injection is indicated in the treatment of localised malignant melanoma of the extremities and localised soft tissue sarcoma of the extremities, when treated by regional perfusion.

Dosage and administration

Adults: The absorption of Alkeran after oral administration is variable and in some patients it is poorly absorbed. Dosage may need to be cautiously increased until myelosuppression is seen, in order to ensure that potentially therapeutic levels have been reached.

Use in the elderly: There is no specific information on the use of Alkeran in the elderly. However, caution should be taken where there is renal impairment.

Multiple myeloma: The administration of Alkeran and prednisone is more effective than Alkeran alone. The combination is usually given on an intermittent basis, although the superiority of this technique over continuous therapy is not established. A typical dosage schedule is 0.15 mg/kg bodyweight/day in divided doses for 4 days together with 40 mg prednisone daily for 4 days, repeated at intervals of six weeks. Numerous regimes have been used and the literature should be consulted for details. Prolonging treatment beyond one year in responders does not appear to improve results.

Ovarian adenocarcinoma: The usual regime is 0.2 mg/kg bodyweight/day, given orally in divided doses, three times daily, for 5 days. This is repeated every 4–8 weeks, provided the bone marrow has recovered. Similar results have been reported following a single intravenous infusion of 1 mg/kg bodyweight over 8 hours every 4 weeks.

Advanced carcinoma of the breast: Alkeran may be given orally at a dose of 200–300 micrograms/kg bodyweight daily or 6 mg/m^2 body surface area daily for 4–6 days and repeated every 3–6 weeks.

Malignant melanoma: Regional perfusion with Alkeran has been used as an adjuvant to surgery for early malignant melanoma and as palliative treatment for advanced but localised disease. The literature should be consulted for details of perfusion technique and dosage.

Soft tissue sarcoma: Regional perfusion with Alkeran has been used in the management of all stages of localised soft tissue sarcoma, usually in combination with surgery. Alkeran has frequently been given with actinomycin D and the literature should be consulted for details of dose regimes.

Polycythaemia vera: For remission induction the usual dose is 6–10 mg daily for 7–10 days, the maintenance dose is 2–4 mg daily. During maintenance careful haematological control is essential with dosage adjustment according to the results of frequent blood counts.

Children: Alkeran is very rarely indicated in children and dosage guidelines cannot be stated.

Administration of injection: Alkeran is unstable in infusion fluids. It should not be given in dextrose solutions. Infusions may be given with saline but, at room temperature, administration of the infusion should be completed within 2 hours of reconstitution of Alkeran. Alternatively, Alkeran may be injected into the tubing of a fast running infusion. Do not administer by syringe pump.

When using Alkeran injection precautions should be taken to avoid contact with it. It is recommended that the handling of Alkeran injection follows the 'Guidelines for the Handling of Cytotoxic Drugs', issued by the RPSGB.

Preparation of Alkeran Melphalan Injection: 1.8 ml Wellcome Acid-Alcohol Solvent should be added to the vial containing 100 mg anhydrous melphalan. The vial should be shaken at once and the melphalan will dissolve in up to 2 minutes. When it has dissolved, 9 ml Wellcome Diluent should be added to give a resulting solution with a pH of about seven which will remain clear for some time. The solution has limited stability and should be prepared as required and used within 30 minutes.

Contra-indications, warnings, etc

Contra-indications: In view of the seriousness of the indications there are no absolute contra-indications.

Precautions: Alkeran is an active cytotoxic agent for use only under the direction of physicians experienced in the administration of such agents.

Careful attention should be paid to the monitoring of blood counts to avoid the possibility of excessive myelosuppression and the risk of irreversible bone marrow aplasia.

The main side-effect of Alkeran treatment is bone marrow depression, leading to leucopenia and thrombocytopenia. Blood counts may continue to fall after treatment is stopped, so at the first sign of an abnormally large fall in leucocyte or platelet counts treatment should be temporarily interrupted.

Alkeran should not be given to patients who have recently received radiotherapy or other cytotoxic agents.

In patients with moderate to severe renal impairment, the initial dose of the intravenous preparation should be reduced by 50%. Subsequent dosage should be determined according to haematological response. Currently available pharmacokinetic data does not justify an absolute recommendation on dosage reduction when administering the oral preparation to these patients, but it may be prudent to use a reduced dose initially.

Patients with renal impairment should be closely observed as they may have uraemic marrow suppression. Temporary significant elevation of the blood urea has been seen in the early stages of Alkeran therapy in myeloma patients with renal damage.

Alkeran is mutagenic in animals and chromosome aberrations have been observed in patients being treated with the drug.

The evidence is growing that Alkeran in common with other alkylating agents may be leukaemogenic in man. There have been reports of acute leukaemia occurring after prolonged Alkeran treatment for diseases such as amyloid, malignant melanoma, macroglobulinaemia, cold agglutinin syndrome and ovarian cancer.

A comparison of patients with ovarian cancer who received alkylating agents with those who did not showed that the use of alkylating agents, including Alkeran, significantly increased the incidence of acute leukaemia. The leukaemogenic risk must be balanced against the potential therapeutic benefit when considering the use of Alkeran.

Alkeran causes suppression of ovarian function in premenopausal women resulting in amenorrhoea in a significant number of patients.

Simultaneous administration of nalidixic acid with Alkeran should be avoided. The combination of high dose Alkeran and cyclosporin is known to cause a deterioration in renal function and can be potentially dangerous.

Side- and adverse effects: The most common side-effect is bone marrow depression.

Gastro-intestinal effects such as nausea and vomiting occur in up to 30 per cent of patients receiving Alkeran. Diarrhoea and stomatitis may occasionally occur. Gastro-intestinal disturbance is usually mild and occurs less frequently than with combination cytotoxic therapy.

Alopecia has been reported but is uncommon. Maculopapular rashes and pruritus have occasionally been noted. There have also been case reports of pulmonary fibrosis and haemolytic anaemia occurring after melphalan treatment.

A life-threatening immediate allergic reaction has been reported after intravenous administration.

Use in pregnancy and lactation: Although there are no data available the possibility that melphalan may be teratogenic should be borne in mind because of its similarity to other alkylating agents which are potentially teratogenic.

The use of Alkeran should be avoided whenever possible during pregnancy, particularly during the first trimester. In any individual case the potential hazard to the foetus must be balanced against the expected benefit to the mother.

Mothers receiving Alkeran should not breastfeed.

Toxicity and treatment of overdosage: The principal toxic effect is on the bone marrow and as there is no known antidote the blood picture should be closely monitored for two weeks.

General supportive measures, together with appropriate blood transfusion, should be instituted if necessary.

Pharmaceutical precautions *Alkeran Tablets:* Store below 25°C in a dry place.

Alkeran Injection: Store below 25°C. Protect from light. Do not refrigerate.

Legal category POM.

Package quantities *Tablets 2 mg:* Bottle of 25.

Tablets 5 mg: Bottle of 25.

Unit Pack: 1 vial containing the equivalent of Melphalan BP 100 mg; 1 ampoule of 1.8 ml Wellcome Acid-Alcohol Solvent for Alkeran; 1 ampoule of 9 ml Wellcome Diluent for Alkeran.

Further information Alkeran has the general pharmacological properties of nitrogen mustard compounds. It is well absorbed by the oral route, both in animals and in man.

Product licence numbers

Tablets 2 mg	0003/5008R
Tablets 5 mg	0003/5009R
Injection	0003/5010R

ALMEVAX* RUBELLA VACCINE, LIVE BP

Presentation A live attenuated Wistar RA 27/3 rubella virus strain, propagated in human diploid cells, and freeze-dried. The vaccine is manufactured and tested in accordance with the requirements of the United Kingdom control authorities and the World Health Organization. It also complies with the European Pharmacopoeia (1982).

0.5 ml of the reconstituted vaccine contains not less than 1,000 $TCID_{50}$ (tissue culture infective dose, 50).

This vaccine contains not more than 2 i.u. neomycin sulphate and 5 i.u. polymyxin B sulphate per 0.5 ml reconstituted vaccine.

Uses For active immunisation against rubella. Vaccination may be carried out at any age; preferably, however, it should be postponed beyond the first year of life since, below one year, the presence of maternal antibodies may impair the immune response. It should be noted that a past history of clinical rubella is an unreliable guide to immune status.

As with any other live attenuated virus vaccine, vaccination does not always result in seroconversion of 100% of susceptible subjects.

Dosage and administration *Adults:* 0.5 ml of the reconstituted vaccine.

Children: As for adults.

A single dose constitutes a full immunising course.

0.5 ml of the reconstituted vaccine is injected subcutaneously. If the injection site is swabbed, only acetone, ether or isopropyl alcohol should be used and allowed to dry before the injection is made.

Use in the elderly: No special comment.

Method of use: For reconstitution, use only the special sterile diluent. Almevax diluent has been tested to ensure that it does not inhibit the live attenuated virus.

Use only sterile disposable syringes and needles which are free from traces of disinfectants or spirits. Use a fresh syringe and needle for each injection.

To ensure satisfactory reconstitution add the diluent slowly. The reconstituted vaccine should be colourless to light pink. See *Pharmaceutical Precautions* for handling of reconstituted vaccine.

Do not attempt to obtain more than the stated number of doses from the vial. It is good practice to record the title, dose and lot numbers of all vaccines and dates of administration. Any untoward reactions should be reported to the regulatory authorities and to the manufacturer.

Reconstitution: Pack size – volume of special sterile diluent required for reconstitution of vaccine.
One-dose: The contents of the diluent container.
Ten-dose: The contents of the diluent container.

Contra-indications, warnings, etc
Contra-indications: Pregnant women must not be vaccinated. Vaccination should not be carried out within three weeks of other live vaccines or within 3 months following administration of human immune serum globulin, whole blood or plasma.

In the rare cases where anti-D immunoglobulin and rubella vaccine are required in the immediate postpartum period, it is advisable to test for rubella antibodies at 6–8 weeks after vaccination to ensure that the anti-D immunoglobulin has not interfered with the response to the vaccine. Data on the persistence of antibody following concurrent administration of rubella vaccine and anti-D immunoglobulin are not available.

The vaccine should not be given to persons suffering from febrile conditions, any active or suspected infection, malignant disease, severe chronic disease, gammaglobulin deficiency or to those with impaired immune responsiveness, whether idiopathic or as a result of treatment with steroids, radiotherapy, cytotoxic drugs or other agents. Vaccination of subjects with thrombocytopenia should be avoided. The vaccine should not be administered to a subject who has experienced a serious reaction (e.g. anaphylaxis) to a previous dose of this vaccine or who is known to be hypersensitive to any component thereof. The vaccine contains a small amount of neomycin and polymyxin and should not be given to individuals known to be hypersensitive to either of them.

Precautions: Attenuated rubella virus vaccine may temporarily depress tests for cell-mediated immunity.

Caution should be exercised should it become necessary to administer a second dose of rubella vaccine, if there has been a severe local or general reaction to a previous injection of the vaccine.

Rubella virus has been implicated as a possible aetiological factor in juvenile rheumatoid arthritis. The rubella immune status of any child with a history of juvenile arthritis should be determined by serological testing before vaccination. Vaccine should be withheld from seropositive children. Vaccination of seronegative children should be deferred until the disease is in remission since, as with other chronic illness, juvenile rheumatoid arthritis may be exacerbated by intercurrent infection.

Although anaphylaxis is rare, facilities for its management should always be available during vaccination.

Side- and adverse effects: Side-effects are uncommon, but mild symptoms may occur about the ninth day after vaccination. Symptoms relate to those seen following natural infection, but in the majority of cases are slight and transient. They include lymphadenopathy, rash, malaise, sore throat, mild fever, headache and occasionally temporary arthràlgia, infrequently associated with signs of inflammation. Marked joint symptoms are more often seen in adult females than in children or adolescents. Nevertheless, even in adults, joint symptoms do not usually interfere with normal activities. Local pain and, rarely, erythema at the site of injection may occur.

Falls in platelet counts, unassociated with symptoms, have been described after vaccination. Serious neurological symptoms have been reported rarely following vaccination. However, a cause and effect relationship has not been established.

Use in pregnancy and lactation: There is a possibility that live attenuated virus administered during pregnancy could infect and damage the foetus, producing congenital abnormalities. Therefore, *pregnant women must not be vaccinated* and pregnancy should be excluded before vaccination is undertaken. This danger to the developing foetus equally applies in the case of a pregnancy conceived within three months following vaccination. Women of childbearing age must be warned that, for at least three months after vaccination, they must take strict contraceptive precautions. If there is any possibility that they may become pregnant within this period, they should not be vaccinated.

Toxicity and treatment of overdosage: Not applicable.

Pharmaceutical precautions Store at 2–8°C. Use special Almevax diluent for reconstitution. After reconstitution the vaccine should be kept cool (2–20°C), protected from light, and used within one hour.

Legal category POM.

Package quantities Ampoule of 1 dose, with container of special diluent.

Rubber-capped vial of 10 doses, with container of special diluent.

Further information Rubella vaccination policy differs from country to country. In the UK the vaccine is offered routinely to all girls between their 11th and 14th birthdays and to susceptible adult females of childbearing age, including post-partum women.

Product licence number 0003/5123.

ANECTINE* INJECTION

Presentation Each ampoule of Anectine contains 100 mg Suxamethonium Chloride Injection BP (succinylcholine chloride) in 2 ml sterile aqueous solution. The pH is 3.0 to 5.0.

Uses Anectine is a short-acting depolarising neuromuscular blocking agent. It is used in anaesthesia as a muscle relaxant to facilitate endotracheal intubation, mechanical ventilation and a wide range of surgical and obstetric procedures.

It is also used to reduce the intensity of muscular contractions associated with pharmacologically or electrically-induced convulsions.

Dosage and administration The usual method of Anectine Injection administration is by bolus intravenous injection.

Adults: The dose of Anectine is dependent on body weight, the degree of muscular relaxation required, the route of administration, and the response of individual patients.

To achieve endotracheal intubation Anectine is usually administered intravenously in a dose of 1 mg/kg. This dose will usually produce muscular relaxation in about 30–60 seconds and has a duration of action of about 2–6 minutes. Larger doses will produce more prolonged muscular relaxation, but doubling the dose does not necessarily double the duration of relaxation. Supplementary doses of Anectine of 50%–100% of the initial dose administered at 5–10 minutes intervals will maintain muscle relaxation during short surgical procedures performed under general anaesthesia.

For prolonged surgical procedures Anectine may be given by intravenous infusion as a 0.1% to 0.2% solution, diluted in 5% glucose solution or sterile isotonic saline solution, at a rate of 2.5 to 4 mg per minute. The infusion rate should be adjusted according to the response of individual patients.

The total dose of Anectine given by repeated intravenous injection or continuous infusion should *not* exceed 500 mg per hour.

Children: Infants and young children are more resistant to Anectine compared with adults.

The recommended intravenous dose of Anectine for neonates and infants is 2 mg/kg. A dose of 1 mg/kg in older children is recommended.

When Anectine is given as intravenous infusion in children, the dosage is as for adults with a proportionately lower initial infusion rate based on body weight.

Anectine may be given intramuscularly to infants at doses up to 4–5 mg/kg and in older children up to 4 mg/kg. These doses produce muscular relaxation within about 3 minutes. A total dose of 150 mg should *not* be exceeded.

Use in the elderly: Dosage requirements of Anectine in the elderly are comparable to those for younger adults.

The elderly may be more susceptible to cardiac arrythmias, especially if digitalis-like drugs are also being taken. See also *'Precautions'*.

Contra-indications, warnings, etc

Contra-indications: Anectine has no effect on the level of consciousness and should not be administered to a patient who is not fully anaesthetised.

Hypersensitivity to suxamethonium may exist in rare instances, and Anectine should not be administered to patients known to be hypersensitive to the drug.

As suxamethonium can act as a trigger of sustained myofibrillar contraction in susceptible individuals, Anectine is contra-indicated in patients with a personal or family history of malignant hyperthermia. If this condition occurs unexpectedly, all anaesthetic agents known to be associated with its development (including Anectine) must be immediately discontinued, and full supportive measures must be immediately instituted. Intravenous dantrolene sodium is the primary specific therapeutic drug and is recommended as soon as possible after the diagnosis is made.

Anectine is contra-indicated in patients known to have an inherited atypical plasma cholinesterase activity.

An acute transient rise in serum potassium often occurs following the administration of Anectine in normal individuals; the magnitude of this rise is of the order of 0.5 mmol/litre. In certain pathological states or conditions this increase in serum potassium following Anectine administration may be excessive and cause serious cardiac arrhythmias and cardiac arrest. For this reason the use of Anectine is contra-indicated in:

- Patients recovering from major trauma; the potential for potassium release is not seen immediately but begins 5–15 days after injury. It persists for 2–3 months or longer if there is associated sepsis.
- Patients recovering from severe burns; the potential for potassium release is not seen immediately but during the period from about the 10th to 66th day post-burn or longer if there is associated sepsis.
- Patients with neurological deficits involving acute major muscle wasting (upper and/or lower motor neurone lesions); the potential for potassium release occurs within the first 6 months after the acute onset of the neurological deficit and correlates with the degree and extent of muscle paralysis. Patients who have been immobilised for prolonged periods of time may be at similar risk.
- Patients with pre-existing hyperkalaemia. In the absence of hyperkalaemia and neuropathy, renal failure is not a contra-indication to the administration of a normal single dose of Anectine Injection, but multiple or large doses may cause clinically significant rises in serum potassium and should not be used.

Suxamethonium causes a slight transient rise in intraocular pressure, and should therefore not be used in the presence of open eye injuries or where an increase in intra-ocular pressure is undesirable unless the potential benefit of its use outweighs the potential risk to the eye.

Anectine should be avoided in patients with congenital myotonic diseases such as myotonia congenita and dystrophia myotonica since its administration may on occasion be associated with severe myotonic spasms and rigidity.

Anectine should be avoided in patients with Duchenne muscular dystrophy since its administration may be associated with rigidity, hyperthermia, hyperkalaemia, myoglobinaemia, cardiac arrest, and post-operative respiratory depression.

Precautions: Anectine should be administered only by or under close supervision of an anaesthetist familiar with its action, characteristics and hazards, who is skilled in the management of artificial respiration and only where there are adequate facilities for immediate endotracheal intubation with administration of oxygen by intermittent positive pressure ventilation.

During prolonged administration of Anectine, it is recommended that the patient is fully monitored with a peripheral nerve stimulator in order to avoid overdosage.

Anectine is rapidly hydrolysed by plasma cholinesterases which thereby limits the intensity and duration of the neuromuscular blockade.

Prolonged and intensified neuromuscular blockade following Anectine Injection may occur secondary to reduced plasma cholinesterase activity in the following states or pathological conditions: Physiological variation as in pregnancy and the puerperium; Genetically determined abnormal plasma cholinesterase; Severe generalised tetanus, tuberculosis, other severe or chronic infections; Following severe burns; Chronic debilitating disease, malignancy, chronic anaemia and malnutrition; End-stage hepatic failure, acute or chronic renal failure; Autoimmune diseases: myxoedema, collagen diseases; Iatrogenic: following plasma exchange, plasmapheresis, cardiopulmonary bypass, and as a result of concommitant drug therapy (see *Drug Interactions*).

If Anectine is given over a prolonged period, the characteristic depolarising neuromuscular (or Phase I) block may change to one with characteristics of a non-depolarising (or Phase II) block.

Although the characteristics of a developing Phase II block resemble those of a true non-depolarising block, the former cannot always be fully or permanently reversed by anticholinesterase agents.

When a Phase II block is fully established, its effects will then usually be fully reversible with standard doses of neostigmine accompanied by an anticholinergic agent.

Tachyphylaxis occurs after repeated administration of Anectine.

It is inadvisable to administer Anectine to patients with advanced myasthenia gravis. Although these patients are resistant to suxamethonium they develop a state of Phase II block which can result in delayed recovery. Patients with myasthenic Eaton–Lambert syndrome are more sensitive than normal to Anectine, necessitating dosage reduction.

In healthy adults, Anectine occasionally causes a mild transient slowing of the heart rate on initial administration. Bradycardias are more commonly observed in children and on repeated administration of suxamethonium in both children and adults. Pre-treatment with intravenous atropine or glycopyrrolate significantly reduces the incidence and severity of suxamethonium-related bradycardia.

Anectine may induce cardiac arrhythmias. The effects of digitalis may be enhanced with increased ventricular irritability.

Drug interactions: Certain drugs or chemicals are known to reduce normal plasma cholinesterase activity and may therefore prolong the neuromuscular blocking effects of Anectine. These include: organophosphorous insecticides and metriphonate; ecothiopate eye drops; trimetaphan; specific anticholinesterase agents: neostigmine, pyridostigmine, physostigimine, edrophonium; cytotoxic compounds: cyclophosphamide, mechlorethamine, triethylene-melamine, and thiotepa; psychiatric drugs: phenelzine, promazine and chlorpromazine; anaesthetic agents and drugs: ketamine, morphine and morphine antagonists, pethidine, pancuronium, propanidid.

Other drugs with potentially deleterious effects on plasma cholinesterase activity include aprotinin, diphenhydramine, promethazine, oestrogens, oxytocin, high-dose steroids, and oral contraceptives.

Certain drugs or substances may enhance or prolong the neuromuscular effects of Anectine by mechanisms unrelated to plasma cholinesterase activity. These include: magnesium salts; lithium carbonate; azathioprine; quinine and chloroquinine; antibiotics such as the aminoglycosides, clindamycin and polymyxins; Antiarrhythmic drugs: quinidine, procainamide, verapamil, beta-blockers, lignocaine and procaine; volatile inhalational anaesthetic agents: halothane, enflurane, isoflurane, diethylether and methoxyflurane have little effect on the Phase I block of Anectine injection but will accelerate the onset and enhance the intensity of a Phase II suxamethonium-induced block.

Side- and adverse effects: Muscle pains are frequently experienced 1–2 days after administration of suxamethonium and most commonly occur in ambulatory patients undergoing short surgical procedures under general anaesthesia. There appears to be no direct connection between the degree of visible muscle fasciculation after Anectine administration and the incidence of severity of pain. The use of small doses of non-depolarising muscle relaxants given minutes before suxamethonium administration has been advocated for the reduction of incidence and severity of suxamethonium-associated muscle pains. This technique may require the use of doses of suxamethonium in excess of 1 mg/kg to achieve satisfactory conditions for endotracheal intubation.

The following adverse reactions have been reported after administration of Anectine:

- Cardiovascular: bradycardia, tachycardia, hypertension, hypotension, arrhythmias;
- Respiratory: bronchospasm, prolonged respiratory depression and apnoea;
- Musculoskeletal: muscle fasciculation, post-operative muscle pains, myoglobinaemia, myoglobinuria;
- Other: hyperthermia, increased intraocular pressure, increased intragastric pressure, rash, excessive salivation.

There are case reports of hyperkalaemia-related cardiac arrests following the administration of suxamethonium to patients with congenital cerebral palsy, tetanus, Duchenne muscular dystrophy, and closed head injury.

Use in pregnancy and lactation: Although Anectine does not readily cross the placental barrier it should not be administered to pregnant women unless the potential benefit outweighs possible hazards.

Plasma cholinesterase levels fall during the first trimester of pregnancy to about 70–80% of their pre-pregnancy values; a further fall to about 60–70% of the pre-pregnancy levels occurs within 2–4 days after delivery. Plasma cholinesterase levels then increase to reach normal over the next 6 weeks. Consequently, a high proportion of pregnant and puerperal patients may exhibit mildly prolonged neuromuscular blockade following Anectine injection.

Toxicity and treatment of overdosage: Apnoea and prolonged muscle paralysis are the main and serious effects of overdosage. It is essential, therefore, to maintain the airway and adequate ventilation until spontaneous respiration occurs.

The dicision to use neostigmine to reverse a Phase II suxamethonium-induced block depends on the judgement of the clinician in the individual case. Valuable information in regard to this dicision will be gained by monitoring neuromuscular function. If neostigmine is used its administration should be accompanied by appropriate doses of an anticholinergic agent such as atropine.

Pharmaceutical precautions Anectine should not be mixed in the same syringe with any other agent, especially thiopentone. Store below 4°C and protect from light. Do not freeze. Do not resterilise.

Legal category POM.

Package quantities Box of 5 × 2 ml ampoules.

Further information Nil.

Product licence number 0003/5203R.

ANTEPAR* TABLETS AND ELIXIR

Presentation Each tablet contains Piperazine Phosphate BP equivalent to 500 mg Piperazine Hydrate BP, coloured yellow and scored, with the word 'ANTEPAR' embossed on the reverse side.

The elixir is a pineapple-flavoured, clear, orange-coloured syrup containing a stable combination of Piperazine Hydrate BP and Piperazine Citrate BP equivalent to 750 mg Piperazine Hydrate BP in each 5 ml.

Uses For the treatment of enterobiasis (pinworm, threadworm infection) and ascariasis (roundworm infection).

Antepar Elixir is especially suitable for administration to infants and children.

Dosage and administration The tablets should be chewed.

Antepar Elixir may be diluted with Syrup BP. The shelf-life of the diluted product is four weeks when stored at 25°C and protected from light.

Enterobiasis: The dose should be calculated according to age or weight and given once daily for seven days.

Age (years)	*Approx. weight*	*Elixir*	*Tablets*
Adults	Over 55 kg	15 ml	4
Children:			
Over 12	Over 40 kg	15 ml	4
5–12	17–40 kg	10 ml	3
2–4	13–16 kg	5 ml	1½
Under 2	Under 13 kg	50–75 mg piperazine hydrate/kg bodyweight	

It may be necessary to repeat the course after a week's interval.

No special dietary regimen is needed.

Attention to general cleanliness is essential in order to prevent reinfection.

Owing to the facility with which pinworm infection is transmitted, it is advisable to examine all other members of a household once one is known to be infected. Treatment of all positive cases should be carried out simultaneously.

Ascariasis: A single dose taken preferably in the morning will usually produce complete clearance of worms from the gut.

Age (years)	*Approx. weight*	*Elixir*	*Tablets*
Adults	Over 55 kg	30 ml	8
Children:			
Over 10	Over 34 kg	30 ml	8
6–10	21–33 kg	20 ml	6
5–6	17–20 kg	15 ml	4½
2–4	13–16 kg	10 ml	3
Under 2	Under 13 kg	120 mg piperazine hydrate/kg bodyweight	

Use in the elderly: No specific studies have been carried out in the elderly, although Antepar has been widely used in older people. However, it may be advisable to monitor renal or hepatic function and if there is serious impairment then caution should be exercised. Antepar should not be given to elderly patients with symptomatic abnormalities of the kidney or CNS.

Contra-indications, warnings, etc

Contra-indications: Patients with a history of piperazine hypersensitivity or patients with renal failure.

Precautions: Caution should be exercised in treating patients with renal or significant hepatic impairment, or chronic disorders of the central nervous system.

Precipitation of grand mal attacks in patients with a known history of epilepsy has been reported.

Care should be taken in administration of piperazine to patients receiving phenothiazines as it has been suggested that piperazine potentiates the extrapyramidal effects of chlorpromazine in man and animals.

Side- and adverse effects: These are uncommon when Antepar is given at the recommended dosage but the following reactions have been reported:

Gastro-intestinal: nausea, vomiting, colic and diarrhoea.

Central nervous system: transient headache and dizziness. More severe reactions, including ataxia, muscle hypotonia, clonic contractions, drowsiness and impaired consciousness, seldom occur at the recommended dosage in individuals without a previous history of neurological abnormalities or renal disease.

Hypersensitivity reactions: urticaria, bullous eruptions, oedema, arthralgia, fever and tachycardia.

Case reports of purpura, a viral hepatitis-like disorder and acute haemolysis in a glucose-6-phosphate dehydrogenase deficient individual after piperazine administration, appear in the medical literature.

Use in pregnancy and lactation: The safety of Antepar for use during pregnancy has not been determined. Studies in animals demonstrated teratogenesis in rabbits given high doses of piperazine but not in rats. Although no causal relationship has been established, isolated instances of foetal malformation following the administration of piperazine have been reported. Accordingly, piperazine should not be used during pregnancy unless, in the judgement of the physician, immediate treatment is warranted and alternative therapy inappropriate. No information is available on the excretion of piperazine or its metabolites in breast milk.

Toxicity and treatment of overdosage: Symptoms of overdosage are likely to be similar in character to the side-effects listed above. These may be expected to resolve spontaneously. Gastric lavage should be carried out only if Antepar has been recently ingested. Adequate fluids and routine supportive measures should be given, including the administration of anti-convulsants when necessary.

Pharmaceutical precautions *Tablets:* Store below 25°C. Keep dry. Protect from light.

Elixir: Store below 25°C. Protect from light.

Legal category P.

Package quantities 28 tablets as 7 foil strips of 4 tablets. Bottles of 100 ml and 500 ml elixir.

Further information Nil.

Product licence numbers
Tablets 0003/5016R
Elixir 0003/5015R

ARILVAX* YELLOW FEVER VACCINE, LIVE BP (17D strain live freeze-dried) (Yel/Vac)

Presentation A specially stabilised freeze-dried preparation of the living attenuated 17D strain of yellow fever virus. The strain of virus used in this preparation is free of avian leucosis viruses and is propagated in leucosis-free chick embryos. The vaccine fulfils the requirements of the World Health Organisation.

Each 0.5 ml dose of reconstituted vaccine contains the equivalent of not less than 1,000 mouse LD_{50} units as defined by the World Health Organisation requirements, and not more than 2 i.u. of neomycin sulphate and 5 i.u. of polymyxin B sulphate.

The diluent consists of sterile water which has been specially tested to ensure that it does not inhibit the vaccine virus.

Uses For active immunisation of residents in yellow

fever endemic areas and travellers to and from such areas, for the issue of an International Certificate of Vaccination, as required by the national health authorities of certain countries which consider these zones as infected areas (although the 'yellow-fever endemic zones' are in fact no longer included in the International Health Regulations). Yellow fever endemic areas are limited to the African and South American continents and Central America. The International Health Regulations define the form of certificate of vaccination to be used which, in the case of primary vaccination, is valid for a period of 10 years from the 10th day after vaccination. In the case of revaccination within 10 years, the certificate is valid at once.

Dosage and administration *Adults and children over age of 9 months:* The dose shall be the same for persons of all ages, 0.5 ml of reconstituted vaccine, given subcutaneously.

Use in the elderly: No special comment.

For reconstitution use only the special sterile diluent supplied.

Arilvax diluent has been tested to ensure that it does not inhibit the vaccine virus. Using a sterile syringe and needle inject the contents of the appropriate Arilvax diluent container into the vaccine vial and gently agitate to ensure reconstitution. The vaccine vial is sealed under vacuum to enhance stability and some users may prefer to break this vacuum to facilitate withdrawal of the vaccine solution. Any frothing will then subside.

See *Pharmaceutical precautions* for handling of reconstituted vaccine.

Use a fresh sterile disposable syringe and needle free from traces of spirit and disinfectants for each injection.

Do not attempt to obtain more than the stated number of doses from the vial. It is good practice to record the title, dose and lot numbers of all vaccines and dates of administration. Any untoward reactions should be reported to the regulatory authorities and to the manufacturer.

Contra-indications, warnings, etc
Contra-indications: The vaccine should not be administered to a subject who has experienced a serious reaction (e.g. anaphylaxis) to a previous dose of this vaccine or who is known to be hypersensitive to any component thereof. It is advisable to avoid vaccination during an acute infection. Since the vaccine is prepared in chick embryos and contains small quantities of neomycin and polymyxin, it should not be administered to individuals who are hypersensitive to egg or chick protein or to these antibiotics.

The vaccine should not be given to those with impaired immune responsiveness, whether idiopathic or as a result of treatment with steroids, radiotherapy, cytotoxic drugs or other agents.

Precautions: The vaccine is not recommended for use in children under the age of 9 months. The decision to vaccinate infants under this age must depend on the anticipated risk of exposure to the disease, since the small number of cases of encephalitis that have been reported have nearly all occurred in infants under this age.

It is advisable to avoid administration of the vaccine within 6 weeks following the administration of immune globulin on general principles. Similarly, on theoretical grounds it is advisable to avoid the administration of immune globulin within 2 weeks following vaccination. Although anaphylaxis is rare, facilities for its management should always be available during vaccination.

An interval of not less than 3 weeks should normally be allowed to lapse between the administration of any two live vaccines. If time does not permit then they might be given simultaneously at separate sites.

Side- and adverse effects: Reactions to the vaccine are extremely rare. Occasionally some redness and swelling may occur at the site of injection, and headache has been reported.

One or two cases of urticaria, bursitis, jaundice and neuritis have been reported in a temporal relationship to vaccination.

Use in pregnancy and lactation: On theoretical grounds the vaccine should not be administered during pregnancy.

Toxicity and treatment of overdosage: Not applicable.

Pharmaceutical precautions The freeze-dried vaccine should be stored between 2–8°C and protected from light. Diluent should not be frozen but should be stored upright below 25°C.

After reconstitution the vaccine should be kept cool, protected from light and used within one hour.

Any remaining vaccine should be disposed of by incineration or by treatment with disinfectant such as strong hypochlorite solution.

Legal category POM.

Package quantities Freeze-dried vaccine in packs of 10 × 1-dose vials with separate diluent; 10 × 5-dose vials with separate diluent.

Further information Nil.

Product licence number 0003/0100.

BANOCIDE* TABLETS

Presentation Each round, white, biconvex tablet contains 50 mg Diethylcarbamazine Citrate BP, is scored and impressed 'WELLCOME S2A'.

Uses For the treatment of filarial infections due to: *Wuchereria bancrofti, Brugia malayi, Brugia timori* and *Loa loa.*

For the prophylaxis of bancroftian and malayan filariasis and loiasis.

Dosage and administration *Adults: Treatment of the indicated filariases:* 6 mg/kg body weight daily in 3 divided doses for three weeks. In order to reduce the incidence and severity of allergic manifestations (see below), an initial dose of 1 mg/kg body weight, gradually increased over three days, is recommended. Full dosage should be maintained for 21 days.

Prophylaxis: Bancroftian and malayan filariasis – 50 mg monthly.

Loiasis – 5 mg/kg for three successive days each month.

Children: As for adults.

Use in the elderly: There is no information on the effect of Banocide on elderly individuals. The same pattern of adverse reactions associated with the use of Banocide in the treatment of filarial infections should be expected. Therefore, older patients should be treated with careful attention to the normal precautions.

Dosage in renal impairment: Diethylcarbamazine citrate and its metabolites are excreted in the urine. The plasma half life of diethylcarbamazine is increased in patients with impaired renal function. Allowance should therefore be made for a more gradual increase in dosage.

Contra-indications, warnings, etc
Contra-indications: None known.

Precautions: During the first few days of treatment of filarial infections with Banocide, patients should be monitored carefully for the reactions described below. The dosage should be increased, as outlined under dosage and administration, in individuals showing no or mild reactions. The dosage increase should be slower in individuals showing more severe reactions. In the large majority of cases, reactions resolve during treatment.

In the event of a severe hypersensitivity reaction, administration of a corticosteroid, such as betamethasone, is recommended.

Fatalities have been reported, rarely, after treatment of encephalitis due to loiasis.

Side- and adverse effects: In the absence of a filarial infection the only side-effects of Banocide, when given at the recommended dosage, are nausea and vomiting.

Reactions associated with the microfilaricidal action of Banocide resolve during treatment.

B. malayi and B. timori infection: Fever associated with chills, rigor, dizziness and/or anorexia occurs with varying severity in the majority of individuals treated for *B. malayi* and *B. timori* infections with Banocide.

Less common reactions include lymphadenitis, lymphangitis, myalgia, arthralgia, headache, nausea and vomiting.

Loa loa infection: More than half of the individuals treated for loiasis with Banocide develop allergic manifestations in the skin. The most common complaint is pruritus, although rashes of different types have been reported.

Fever, oedema, arthralgia, headache, nausea and vomiting are also commonly associated with treatment of loiasis.

Very rarely, exacerbation of encephalitis due to loiasis following treatment with diethylcarbamazine citrate may prove fatal.

W. bancrofti infection: Treatment of bancroftian filariasis with Banocide results in the development of fewer and milder reactions than those seen following therapy of malayan filariasis and loiasis. Fever is the most frequent reaction.

Less common reactions include headache, nausea, vomiting and chills.

Use in pregnancy and lactation: In view of the severe reactions that may follow diethylcarbamazine administration, it is advisable to postpone treatment of pregnant women until after parturition. No information is available on the excretion of diethylcarbamazine in breast milk.

Toxicity and treatment of overdosage

Symptoms: There are no reports of overdosage with Banocide following treatment of the indicated filariases in the literature. However, symptoms are likely to consist of nausea, vomiting, headache, dizziness and drowsiness.

Treatment: In view of the rapid absorption of diethylcarbamazine, gastric lavage should be considered only if the patient is seen within 2 hours of excessive ingestion of Banocide.

Adequate fluids should be given to ensure optimal diuresis.

Acidification of urine should enhance the excretion of diethylcarbamazine.

Routine supportive measures should be given when necessary.

Pharmaceutical precautions Store below 35°C. Keep dry.

Legal category P.

Package quantities Bottle of 100 tablets.

Further information Nil.

Product licence number 0003/5018R.

BRETYLATE* INJECTION

Presentation A colourless, sterile, aqueous solution containing 50 mg/ml bretylium tosylate in a 10 ml ampoule.

Uses Bretylate Injection is indicated primarily for the treatment of ventricular fibrillation and has often proved effective in ventricular fibrillation resistant to direct current countershock, with or without additional use of other anti-arrhythmic drugs such as lignocaine. Consideration should be given at an early stage to the use of Bretylate Injection in resuscitation from ventricular fibrillation.

Bretylate Injection is also indicated for ventricular tachycardia and has proved successful in restoring sinus rhythm where other anti-arrhythmics have failed.

Anti-arrhythmic effectiveness of Bretylate Injection has been demonstrated in:

– acute myocardial infarction or chronic ischaemic heart disease;

– ventricular fibrillation complicating severe hypothermia;

– and, ventricular arrhythmias following cardiac surgery.

Dosage and administration

Adults: For ventricular fibrillation or ventricular tachycardia with associated haemodynamic disturbance, the minimal suggested initial dose is 5 mg/kg bodyweight administered undiluted by rapid intravenous injection. Resuscitation should be continued with further attempts at electrical cardioversion. The anti-fibrillatory effect in responding patients will usually be apparent within 5 to 15 minutes.

If no response is evident after 5 minutes, the dose of bretylium may be repeated or increased to 10 mg/kg by bolus injection. There is little experience with total dosages greater than 40 mg/kg, although with such dosage, adverse effects have not been apparent. In some patients the full anti-arrhythmic effect of Bretylate Injection may require several hours to develop.

If Bretylate Injection is to be used for less serious ventricular rhythm disturbances, it should be given more slowly and in diluted form to reduce the risk of vomiting.

Dilution: Bretylate Injection should be diluted with one of the recommended infusion fluids (see below) in the ratio of 1 part Bretylate Injection added to not less than 4 parts of infusion fluid, i.e. to give a final concentration of not more than 10 mg/ml.

When diluted with either Glucose Intravenous Infusion BP (5% w/v) or Sodium Chloride Intravenous Infusion BP (0·9% w/v) in the ratios recommended, Bretylate Injection is stable for up to 24 hours.

Administration by infusion: The diluted solution (prepared as recommended above) should be infused initially over a period of at least 8 minutes, preferably over 15 to 30 minutes, so as to provide a total dose of 5 to 10 mg/kg bodyweight. If the arrhythmia persists, this initial dose may be repeated at one to two hour intervals.

Once control of the arrhythmia has been established, maintenance therapy using the diluted solution can be given either as a continuous infusion at the rate of 1 to 2 mg per minute, or with a dosage of 5 to 10 mg/kg bodyweight infused over a period of 15 to 30 minutes every 6 hours.

Intramuscular administration: Bretylate Injection has been administered by intramuscular injection. A dose of 5 to 10 mg/kg bodyweight is recommended and this is administered undiluted at intervals of 6 to 8 hours. The site of injection should be varied on repeated injection and not more than 5 ml given into any one site.

Dosage in renal impairment: With repeated bolus doses or continuous intravenous infusions of Bretylate Injection in patients with impaired renal function, it is necessary to reduce the dosage in proportion to the reduction in creatinine clearance. The use of a nomogram is recommended for administration of Bretylate Injection as an infusion to patients with renal impairment, and the literature should be consulted for details.

The following table is intended to be used as a guide for administering Bretylate Injection by continuous infusion.

Creatinine clearance (ml/minute)	*Rate of infusion (mg/hour)*
40 – <90	10 – 40
10 – <40	2 – 10
1 – <10	0·6 – 2

Children: Information on the use of Bretylate Injection as an anti-arrhythmic agent in children is sparse and there are no data on its use in doses in excess of 5 mg/kg bodyweight.

Use in the elderly: The decision to treat with Bretylate rests on the balance between the expected anti-arrhythmic effect and the disadvantages of inappropriate dosing, taking into account the degree of reduction in cardiac and renal function.

Pharmacokinetics: The anti-arrhythmic effects of a single dose of bretylium last for up to 12 hours. After a single intravenous dose bretylium appears to be eliminated from serum with an elimination half life of about 13·5 hours. Apart from the particular effect of the drug on ventricular fibrillation, which seems to be exerted within 5 to 15 minutes of initial intravenous bolus administration, the anti-arrhythmic effects of bretylium seem to be related to tissue concentrations rather than serum or plasma concentrations of the drug and the latter are therefore probably not useful indicators during acute treatment.

Pharmacology: Bretylium is a Class III anti-arrhythmic agent. It may produce pharmacological defibrillation, but more usually it facilitates electrical conversion to sinus rhythm in patients with ventricular fibrillation.

Acute administration of bretylium in both animals and man leads to a biphasic cardiovascular response. Monitoring of heart rate and blood pressure is therefore recommended. An initial release or noradrenaline from adrenergic nerve endings is accompanied by an acute rise in systemic arterial pressure and heart rate, followed within 20 to 30 minutes by reductions in vascular resistance, systemic arterial pressure and heart rate. The hypotension caused by Bretylate is orthostatic and was found to occur rarely in recumbent patients with acute myocardial infarction receiving the drug in a coronary care unit.

Contra-indications, warnings, etc
Contra-indications: Bretylate Injection is likely to cause a severe hypertensive response in patients with phaeochromocytoma and is therefore contra-indicated in this condition.

Precautions: Bretylate Injection is not recommended as a prophylactic agent to prevent serious ventricular arrhythmias, but data are conflicting.

Orthostatic hypotension may occur 20 to 30 minutes after acute administration of Bretylate Injection, and in patients with poor cardiac function clinically significant hypotension may occur even in the supine position. An asymptomatic fall in blood pressure usually need not be treated unless the systolic pressure falls below 75 to 80 mm Hg. Hypotension may also be troublesome after cardiac surgery.

Hypovolaemia will augment the hypotensive response to Bretylate Injection. If the blood pressure does not respond to simple postural manoeuvres intravenous fluid should be given. Hypotension requiring such treatment may also respond to vasopressors. Hypersensitivity to infused catecholamines must, however, be anticipated and caution exercised.

Intramuscular administration of bretylium may cause tissue necrosis at the site of injection; this is rare if the site of injection is varied and the injected volume limited to 5 ml.

Side- and adverse effects: The most common side effect following the administration of bretylium is hypotension, especially in patients whose initial haemodynamic state and/or cardiac function are poor. Hypotension with increased pulmonary vascular resistance has also been reported.

Immediately after commencement of bretylium administration, more ectopic beats may arise, but this effect does not usually lead to serious problems.

Nausea and vomiting may occur following rapid intravenous administration of bretylium.

Moderate increases in blood pressure, heart rate and a positive inotropic effect may occur on commencement of bretylium administration.

Drug interactions: Parenteral administration of bretylium may exacerbate ventricular tachyarrhythmias caused by digitalis toxicity.

Hypersensitivity to infused catecholamines would be expected after Bretylate administration because it blocks their normal mechanism of metabolism, namely neuronal uptake and subsequent degradation by monoamine oxidase. For this reason, when it is necessary to increase perfusion pressure to vital organs after bretylium-induced hypotension, noradrenaline or other sympathomimetics should only be given under expert supervision.

The hypotension resulting from adrenergic neurone blockade has been prevented by inhibition of the noradrenaline uptake mechanism, principally by tricyclic antidepressants.

Use in pregnancy and lactation: There is no reference to the use of bretylium as an anti-arrhythmic in pregnancy in the published literature.

No information is available on the excretion of bretylium into breast milk or, therefore, on its effects on the breastfed infant.

Toxicity and treatment of overdosage: Bretylium overdose has been reported in a patient with recurrent ventricular fibrillation and tachycardia who was inadvertently given an intravenous bolus of 2 g (approximately 30 mg/kg bodyweight). The authors reported ultimately successful control of the ventricular tachyarrhythmias but the patient exhibited marked hypertension with peak blood pressure of 310/90 mm Hg, followed within an hour or so by marked hypotension refractory to intravenous dobutamine and volume-expansion therapy.

Bretylate can be eliminated by haemodialysis.

Pharmaceutical precautions Store below 25°C. Do not freeze. Protect from light.

Legal category POM.

Package quantities 1 × 10 ml ampoule.

Further information Patients generally receive Bretylate Injection after many other anti-arrhythmic agents have failed. Nevertheless, clinical observations suggest that Bretylate is a more effective anti-arrhythmic and anti-fibrillatory agent when given alone rather than in combination with other anti-arrhythmics.

Despite concern on theoretical grounds and data from animal experiments suggesting that Bretylate may be inapproprate in cardiac arrhythmias associated with digitalis toxicity, there is a report of effective control of ventricular arrhythmias refractory to lignocaine when Bretylate was given to 2 patients in this situation and no adverse effects were observed.

Bretylate Injection has been successful in treatment of the unusual ventricular arrhythmia *torsade de pointes*, ventricular flutter associated with prolongation of the electrocardiographic QT interval after quinidine therapy and in ventricular fibrillation unresponsive to electrical cardioversion in a child with the long QT syndrome.

Product licence number 0003/0038R.

CALPOL* INFANT SUSPENSION
SUGAR-FREE CALPOL* INFANT SUSPENSION
CALPOL* SIX PLUS SUSPENSION

Presentation *Calpol Infant Suspension and Sugar-Free Calpol Infant Suspension:* Each 5 ml dose of viscous, pink, strawberry flavoured suspension contains 120 mg Paracetamol BP.

Calpol Six Plus Suspension: Each 5 ml dose of viscous, orange coloured and orange flavoured suspension contains 250 mg Paracetamol BP.

Uses Calpol products are indicated for the treatment of mild to moderate pain (including teething pain), and as antipyretics.

Dosage and administration *Adults:* The optimal dosage range is 500 mg to 1 g paracetamol, i.e. 10–20 ml Calpol Six Plus Suspension (maximum 1 g), which may be repeated every 4 hours to a maximum of 4 g paracetamol (80 ml Calpol Six Plus Suspension), per day.

	Calpol Infant Suspension and Sugar-Free Calpol Infant Suspension	*Calpol Six Plus Suspension*
Children 6 to 12 years	Use Calpol Six Plus	5 to 10 ml (250 mg–500 mg paracetamol)
1 to under 6 years	5 to 10 ml (120 mg–240 mg paracetamol)	2.5 to 5 ml (125 mg–250 mg paracetamol)
3 months to under 1 year	2.5 to 5 ml (60 mg–120 mg paracetamol)	Use Calpol Infant Suspension
Infants under 3 months	A 2.5 ml dose is suitable for babies who develop a fever following vaccination at 2 months. In other cases, use only under medical supervision.	Not recommended

Repeat every four hours, if necessary, up to a maximum of 4 doses per 24 hours.

Use in the elderly: In the elderly the rate and extent of paracetamol absorption is normal but plasma half-life is longer and paracetamol clearance is lower than in young adults.

Dilution: Calpol Infant Suspension may be diluted 1:1 with Syrup BP. Sugar-Free Calpol Infant Suspension may be diluted 1:1 with either Sorbitol Solution BPC (non-crystallising) or Glycerol BP. In all cases dilutions should be freshly-prepared, stored below 25°C and used within 28 days.

Where a dilution of Calpol Six Plus Suspension is prescribed, one of the Calpol Infant Suspensions should be dispensed.

Contra-indications, warnings, etc

Contra-indications: Calpol is contra-indicated in patients with known hypersensitivity to paracetamol.

Precautions: Calpol should be used with caution in the presence of severe hepatic or renal dysfunction.

Side- and adverse effects: Paracetamol has been widely used and, when taken at the usual recommended dosage, side-effects are mild and infrequent and reports of adverse reactions are rare. Skin rashes and other allergic reactions occur rarely.

Most reports of adverse reactions to paracetamol relate to overdosage with the drug.

Isolated cases of thrombocytopenic purpura, haemolytic anaemia and agranulocytosis have been recorded.

Chronic hepatic necrosis has been reported in a patient who took daily therapeutic doses of paracetamol for about a year and liver damage has been reported after daily ingestion of excessive amounts for shorter periods. A review of a group of patients with chronic active hepatitis failed to reveal differences in the abnormalities of liver function in those who were long-term users of paracetamol nor was the control of their disease improved after paracetamol withdrawal.

Nephrotoxicity following therapeutic doses of paracetamol is uncommon, but papillary necrosis has been reported after prolonged administration.

Drug interactions: Patients who have taken barbiturates, tricyclic antidepressants and alcohol may show diminished ability to metabolise large doses of paracetamol, the plasma half-life of which can be prolonged.

Alcohol can increase the hepatotoxicity of paracetamol overdosage and may have contributed to the acute pancreatitis reported in one patient who had taken an overdose of paracetamol.

Chronic ingestion of anticonvulsants or oral steroid contraceptives induces liver enzymes and may prevent attainment of therapeutic paracetamol levels by increasing first pass metabolism or clearance.

Use in pregnancy and lactation: Data are not available on the use of Calpol during pregnancy. There is epidemiological evidence of safety of paracetamol in human pregnancy.

A pharmacokinetic study in 12 nursing mothers revealed that less than 1% of the dose ingested by a nursing mother appears in human milk, therefore maternal ingestion of therapeutic doses does not present a risk to the infant.

Toxicity and treatment of overdosage; Pallor, anorexia, nausea and vomiting are frequent early symptoms of paracetamol overdosage. Hepatic necrosis is a dose-related complication of paracetamol overdosage. Hepatic enzymes may become elevated and prothrombin time prolonged within 12–48 hours but clinical symptoms may not be apparent until 1 to 6 days after ingestion. Toxicity is likely in adults who have taken more than 10 g.

To protect the patient against delayed hepatotoxicity, paracetamol overdosage should be treated promptly by gastric lavage followed by intravenous N-acetylcysteine or oral methionine. Additional therapy (further methionine or intravenous cysteamine or intravenous N-acetylcysteine) is normally considered in the light of blood paracetamol content and the time elapsed since ingestion. Fulminant hepatic failure which may follow paracetamol overdosage requires specialised management.

In paracetamol overdosage with liver cell damage paracetamol half life is often prolonged from around 2 hours in normal adults to 4 hours or longer. However liver cell damage has been found in patients with a paracetamol half life less than 4 hours. Diminution in $^{14}CO_2$ excretion after oral ^{14}C-aminopyrine has been reported to correlate better with liver cell damage in paracetamol overdosage than do either plasma paracetamol concentration or half life or conventional liver function test measurements. Concomitant renal failure due to acute tubular necrosis may accompany paracetamol-induced fulminate hepatic failure. The incidence is, however, no more frequent in these patients than in others with fulminant hepatic failure from other causes.

Pharmaceutical precautions Store below 25°C. Protect from light.

Legal category P.

Package quantities *Calpol Infant Suspension:* bottles of 70 ml, 140 ml, and 1 litre.

Sugar-Free Calpol Infant Suspension: bottles of 140 ml and 1 litre.

Calpol Six Plus Suspension: bottles of 100 ml (OP).

Further information The viscous consistency of Calpol suspensions helps keep the medicine on the spoon and so makes it easier to administer.

Paracetamol does not cause the gastro-intestinal side-effects often seen after standard doses of aspirin.

Product licence numbers

Calpol Infant Suspension:	0003/5067R
Sugar-Free Calpol Infant Suspension:	0003/0244
Calpol Six Plus Suspension:	0003/0182R

CEFIZOX* INJECTION

Presentation Vials containing 500 mg, 1 g and 2 g of ceftizoxime as its sterile sodium salt. Ceftizoxime sodium is a white to pale yellow crystalline powder. For each gram of ceftizoxime there is approximately 60 mg (2.6 mmol) of sodium.

Uses Broad-spectrum, bactericidal, cephalosporin antibiotic indicated for the treatment of infections either before the infecting organism has been identified, or when caused by bacteria of known sensitivity. Indications include lower respiratory tract infections, genito-urinary tract infections including gonorrhoea, intra-abdominal infections, septicaemia, skin and soft tissue infections.

Many infections caused by aerobic and anaerobic, Gram-negative and Gram-positive organisms resistant to other cephalosporins, aminoglycosides, or penicillins, have responded to treatment with Cefizox. Cefizox has been effective in the treatment of seriously ill, immunocompromised patients e.g. those with neutropenia and granulocytopenia.

Bacteriology: Cefizox is active *in vitro* against a wide range of Gram-positive and Gram-negative organisms. These include the following:

Gram-positive aerobes – staphylococci including *Staph. pyogenes* and *Staph. epidermidis,* streptococci including *Strep. pneumoniae* and *Strep. pyogenes, Corynebacterium diphtheriae.* Most strains of enterococci are resistant.

Gram-negative aerobes – Esch. coli, Klebsiella spp., Proteus spp. both indole positive and negative, Serratia spp., Enterobacter spp., Providencia spp., many strains of Pseudomonas spp., Citrobacter spp., *Haemophilus influenzae* including ampicillin-resistant strains, Neisseria spp. including β-lactamase-producing strains, Salmonella spp., Shigella spp., *Aeromonas hydrophila, Yersinia enterocolitica.*

Anaerobes – Bacteroides spp. including many, but not all strains of *B.fragilis.,* Peptococcus spp., Eubacterium spp., Clostridium spp.

Cefizox is stable to a broad spectrum of beta-lactamases produced by both aerobic and anaerobic organisms.

Dosage and administration Cefizox may be given by slow intravenous injection, by continuous or intermittent intravenous infusion or by deep intramuscular injection. Dosage and route of administration should be determined by the condition of the patient, severity of the infection and susceptibility of the causative organisms.

General guidelines: Adults:

Type of infection	*Dosage*	*Route*
Urinary tract	0.5–1 g 12-hourly	IM or IV
Gonorrhoea	1 g single dose	IM
Other infections	1–2 g 8–12 hourly	IM* or IV
Severe or life-threatening infections	2–3 g 8-hourly	IM* or IV

* When administering 2 g intramuscularly, the dose should be divided and given in different large muscle masses.

Dosages in excess of 4 g daily are rarely necessary but, exceptionally, dosages up to 8 g per day have been given and were well tolerated.

Children over the age of 3 months: 30–60 mg/kg bodyweight/day in 2–4 divided doses, increased in severe or life-threatening infections to 100–150 mg/kg bodyweight/day. The total dose should not exceed the adult dose.

Children under the age of 3 months: There are insufficient data to recommend the use of Cefizox.

Dosage in renal impairment: Modification of dosage is necessary in patients with impaired renal function. For an adult, following an initial loading dose of 500 mg–1.0 g, IM or IV, the maintenance dosing schedule shown below should be followed (no data are available for children):

Creatinine clearance ml/min.	*Less severe infections*	*Severe or life-threatening infections*
50–79	500 mg 8-hourly	0.75–1.5 g 8-hourly
5–49	250–500 mg 12-hourly	0.5–1.0 g 12-hourly
0–4 (dialysis patients)	500 mg 48-hourly or 250 mg 24-hourly	0.5–1.0 g 48-hourly or 0.5 g 24-hourly

In patients undergoing haemodialysis, no additional supplemental dosing is required following haemodialysis; however, dosing should be timed so that the patient receives the dose (according to the table above), at the end of the dialysis.

Preparation of parenteral solutions: Reconstitute with Water for Injections BP in the minimum volumes shown below. Shake well. Further dilutions may be used. See 'Administration'.

Vial size	*Vol. diluent*
500 mg	2.0 ml
1 g	3.0 ml
2 g	6.0 ml

These solutions are stable for 8 hours at 25°C and for 24 hours at 5°C. When freshly reconstituted, Cefizox is a colourless to pale yellow solution with a pH of 6.0 to 8.0. Reconstituted solutions may discolour. Yellow discolouration will not alter potency or therapeutic efficacy. Discard solution if markedly discoloured.

Administration: IM injection: Inject deep within the body of a relatively large muscle. When administering 2 g, the dose should be divided and given in different large muscle masses. For intramuscular injection, Cefizox may be diluted with 0.5% lignocaine.

IV injection: Inject slowly over 3 to 5 mins. either directly or via the tubing of an established intravenous infusion (see list below).

IV infusion: For intermittent or continuous infusion, dilute Cefizox reconstituted with Water for Injections BP, or Sodium Chloride Injection BP in 50 to 100 ml of one of the following solutions:

Glucose Intravenous Infusion BP (5% and 10% w/v)
Sodium Chloride Intravenous Infusion BP
Sodium Chloride and Glucose Intravenous Infusion BP (0.18% and 4% w/v, 0.45% or 0.9% and 5% w/v)
Compound Sodium Chloride Injection BPC 1959 (Ringer's Solution for Injection)
Compound Sodium Lactate Intravenous Infusion BP

Cefizox in these fluids is stable for 8 hours at 25°C and for 24 hours at 5°C.

Use in the elderly: It is recommended that the dose is reduced even though the serum creatinine level shows a normal value. In the presence of renal impairment doses should be reduced according to the table above, on the basis of creatinine clearance values.

Contra-indications, warnings, etc

Contra-indications: Hypersensitivity to cephalosporin antibiotics.

Precautions: Cefizox should be given cautiously to penicillin-sensitive patients. Although cephalosporin antibiotics may usually be given safely to such patients, cross reactions have been reported. Special care is required in patients who have had an anaphylactic reaction to penicillin.

Patients with impaired renal function – see 'Dosage and Administration'.

Cefizox has not been shown to alter renal function, but renal status should be monitored, especially in seriously ill patients receiving maximum dose therapy and co-administration of aminoglycoside antibiotics. Although the occurrence has not been reported with Cefizox, nephrotoxicity has been reported following concomitant administration of other cephalosporins and aminoglycosides.

As with any antibiotic, prolonged use may result in overgrowth of non-susceptible organisms.

Side- and adverse effects: Cefizox is generally well tolerated. The most common adverse reactions have been local, following IM or IV injection. These include burning, cellulitis, pain, induration, tenderness, paraesthesia and phlebitis. Other adverse reactions include hypersensitivity reactions (rash, pruritus, fever), gastro-intestinal disturbance (diarrhoea, nausea and vomiting), vaginitis, transient eosinophilia, and thrombocytosis. Neutropenia, leucopenia and thrombocytopenia have been reported rarely. Some individuals have developed a positive Coombs' test. Transient elevation in SGOT, SGPT, alkaline phosphatase, BUN and serum creatinine have occasionally been observed.

Use in pregnancy and lactation: Animal studies have not revealed evidence of an adverse effect on the developing foetus but there are no data in pregnant women. Thus the benefit of using Cefizox in pregnancy should be weighed against the possible hazard. Ceftizoxime is excreted in human milk in low concentrations. Caution should therefore be exercised if Cefizox is administered to a nursing mother.

Toxicity: None has been reported.

Treatment of overdosage: Not applicable.

Pharmaceutical precautions Store below 25°C. Protect from light.

Legal category POM.

Package quantities Individual vials containing 500 mg, 1 gram or 2 gram packed singly.

Further information Ceftizoxime is not metabolised and is excreted virtually unchanged by the kidneys within 24 hours, thus providing high urinary concentrations. It passes readily into various body fluids and tissues including those of the full-term foetus.

Interference with laboratory tests: a false-positive reaction to glucose may occur with reducing substances but not with the use of specific glucose oxidase methods.

Product licence numbers

500 mg	0003/0174
1 g, 2 g	0003/0175

CHOLERA VACCINE BP WELLCOME* (Cho/Vac)

Presentation Cholera vaccine contains heat-killed phenol-preserved *Vibrio cholerae,* serotypes Inaba and Ogawa, at a concentration of not less than 8,000 million per ml. The phenol concentration is 0.5% w/v.

Uses Immunisation against cholera including cholera El Tor. Although this vaccine does not contain the El Tor biotypes of the classical Inaba and Ogawa serotypes, carefully controlled field studies have shown that the classical biotype equally protects against both classical and El Tor.

Dosage and administration Primary vaccination consists of two doses of vaccine given subcutaneously or intramuscularly, preferably separated by a period of over a month. This interval may be reduced even to seven days, though the response may be poorer, when rapid immunisation is necessary.

Age	*First dose*	*All subsequent doses*
1–5 years	0.1 ml	0.3 ml
5–10 years	0.3 ml	0.5 ml
Over 10 years	0.5 ml	1.0 ml

The container should on all occasions be well shaken before withdrawing material for injection.

Immunity is short-lived so that booster doses are required every six months under conditions of continued exposure. A single booster dose will suffice even if considerably longer than six months has elapsed since the last dose was administered.

For second and subsequent doses, particularly if there has been some reaction to a previous dose, it may be preferable to give the vaccine intradermally, in a volume of 0.1 ml where the subcutaneous dose is 0.5 ml or less, and 0.2 ml in other cases. However, it is possible that some countries may be unwilling to accept travellers who have not received the larger subcutaneous doses.

Travellers to or from certain countries which have reported cholera infection may be required to produce written evidence of cholera vaccination during the previous six months. A single dose normally meets these requirements and the International Certificate becomes valid six days after the first dose of vaccine was administered, but some countries may demand two doses. The certificate becomes valid immediately after a booster dose within six months of primary immunisation.

It is good practice to record the title, dose and lot numbers of all vaccines and dates of administration. Any untoward reactions should be reported to the regulatory authorities and to the manfacturer.

Use in the elderly: No special comment.

Contra-indications, warnings, etc
Contra-indications: The vaccine should not be administered to a subject who has experienced a serious reaction (e.g. anaphylaxis) to a previous dose of this vaccine or who is known to be hypersensitive to any component thereof. It is advisable to avoid vaccination during acute infection or chronic illness.

Precautions: Repeated vaccination may result in the development of hypersensitivity to protein constituents of the vaccine. Although anaphylaxis is rare, facilities for its management should always be available during vaccination.

Cholera vaccine is not recommended for administration to infants under the age of one year as reactions are more frequent in this age group.

Intradermal administration of the first dose of a primary course is not recommended.

Side- and adverse effects: Local reactions consisting of pain, redness and swelling may develop within hours of vaccination resulting in discomfort at the site of injection for one or two days. They may be accompanied by fever, malaise and headache. Persons who have received numerous doses of cholera vaccine are particularly susceptible to such reactions even if many years have elapsed since the last vaccination was carried out. Occasionally delayed reactions occur. Serious reactions are uncommon but may include collapse, and rarely neurological symptoms such as neuritis, polyneuritis and various other manifestations of cerebral and meningeal involvement.

Use in pregnancy and lactation: This vaccine has been in wide use for many years without apparent ill consequence. However, as with any agent which may produce a systemic reaction, such as pyrexia, vaccination is, if possible, to be avoided in pregnancy.

Toxicity and treatment of overdosage: Not applicable.

Pharmaceutical precautions Store at 2 8°C. Protect from light. *Do not freeze.* When multidose containers are employed it is good practice to discard any partly used vaccine vials at the end of the vaccinating session.

This preparation on standing has a tendency to settle out in a gelatinous form. This is the nature of the organism in the vaccine and vigorous shaking as a rule will yield a homogenous suspension for injection. The container should on all occasions be well shaken before withdrawing material for injection.

Legal category POM.

Package quantities Vials of 1.5 ml and 10 ml.

Further information Nil.

Product licence number 0003/5126.

CICATRIN* AEROSOL

Presentation Each gram contains:

Neomycin Sulphate BP	16,500 units
Zinc Bacitracin BP	1,250 units
l-Cysteine	12 mg
Glycine	60 mg

Uses Topical broad-spectrum antibacterial. Superficial bacterial infections of skin.

Dosage and administration *Adults:* A thin, uniform spray should be applied to affected areas, as required. This can be obtained from a spray of about one second's duration to the wound surface at a distance of not less than 20 cm. The application of one can of spray daily for a maximum period of 10–12 weeks should not be exceeded in adults. After such a course, treatment should not be repeated for at least three months.

Children: The maximum dosage should be reduced in proportion to body weight.

Use in the elderly: No specific studies have been carried out in the elderly, however, it may be advisable to monitor renal function in these patients and if there is any impairment then caution should be exercised.

Contra-indications, warnings, etc
Contra-indications: Hypersensitivity to bacitracin or the neomycin group of antibiotics or to l-cysteine or glycine.

The presence of pre-existing nerve deafness is a contra-indication to the use of Cicatrin Aerosol in circumstances where significant systemic absorption could occur.

Cicatrin Aerosol should not be used on pre-term infants.

Precautions: Absorption of the active ingredients can occur following the application of Cicatrin Aerosol to raw or broken skin.

Neomycin sulphate is the dose-limiting ingredient of Cicatrin Aerosol because it can cause irreversible nerve deafness following significant systemic absorption.

Following significant systemic absorption neomycin sulphate and bacitracin zinc have nephrotoxic potential.

In cases where there is established partial nerve deafness and where a significant degree of neomycin absorption could occur it might be inappropriate to use any neomycin-containing product and treatment with an antibacterial without an aminoglycoside constituent should be used if possible. In renal impairment the plasma clearance of neomycin is reduced, therefore a reduction in dose should be made that relates to the degree of renal impairment.

The inappropriate use of topical antibiotics has been associated with the emergence of resistant strains of bacteria.

The spray should not be used on large denuded areas (e.g. burns or ulcers) because of the risk of systemic absorption. Patients with hypostatic leg ulcers or hypostatic leg eczemas may have an increased sensitivity to a large number of topically applied drugs, including neomycin.

Concurrent administration of other aminoglycoside antibiotics is not recommended.

As neomycin has a neuromuscular blocking effect, patients concurrently receiving other agents with a similar action should be observed for signs of possible respiratory insufficiency.

As with all aerosol products not specifically intended for respiratory tract therapy, care should be taken to avoid inhalation of spray mist.

Avoid spraying Cicatrin Aerosol into the eyes.

Side- and adverse effects: Allergic hypersensitivity to neomycin is generally uncommon following topical use but may manifest itself as a reddening and scaling of the affected skin, as an eczematous exacerbation of the lesion, or as a failure of the lesion to heal.

Allergic hypersensitivity, including anaphylaxis, following topical administration of bacitracin has been reported rarely.

A transient, mild, burning sensation on the skin has occasionally been reported following the administration of Cicatrin Aerosol. As with all antibacterial preparations prolonged use may result in the overgrowth of non-susceptible organisms including fungi.

Use in pregnancy and lactation: Due to a lack of detailed information, the use of Cicatrin during pregnancy and lactation cannot be recommended in circumstances where significant systemic absorption of the active ingredients may occur.

No information is available regarding the excretion of the active ingredients or their metabolites in human milk.

Toxicity and treatment of overdosage: In the event of signs of toxicity developing following significant systemic absorption of the active ingredients of Cicatrin aerosol the patient's general status, hearing acuity, renal function and neuromuscular function should be monitored and blood levels of neomycin and zinc bacitracin determined. Serum levels of neomycin may be reduced by haemodialysis.

Pharmaceutical precautions Store below 25°C. Keep away from heat. Do not puncture or incinerate can.

Legal category POM.

Package quantities Pressurised aerosol powder spray. Net content of powder 3 g approx (OP).

Further information Nil.

Product licence number 0003/5083

CICATRIN* POWDER
CICATRIN* CREAM

Presentation Each gram of powder/cream contains:

Neomycin Sulphate BP	3,300 units
Zinc Bacitracin BP	250 units
l-Cysteine	2 mg
Glycine	10 mg
dl-Threonine	1 mg

Uses Topical broad-spectrum antibacterial.

Superficial bacterial infection of skin, such as in impetigo, varicose ulcers, pressure sores, trophic ulcers and burns.

Dosage and administration *Adults:* A light dusting of the powder or thin layer of the cream should be applied to the affected skin area up to three times daily. See Contra-indications, warnings, etc.

Children: As for adults. The maximum dosage should be reduced in proportion to body weight.

Use in the elderly: No specific studies have been carried out in the elderly, however, it may be advisable to monitor renal function in these patients and if there is any impairment then caution should be exercised.

Contra-indications, warnings, etc
Contra-indications: Hypersensitivity to bacitracin or the neomycin group of antibiotics or to l-cysteine, glycine or threonine.

The presence of pre-existing nerve deafness is a contra-indication to the use of Cicatrin Powder and Cicatrin Cream in circumstances in which significant systemic absorption could occur.

Precautions: Following the application of Cicatrin Powder or Cicatrin Cream to substantial areas of burned, raw or broken skin, significant systemic absorption of active ingredients may occur. Neomycin sulphate is the dose-limiting ingredient of Cicatrin Powder and Cicatrin Cream because it can cause irreversible nerve deafness following significant systemic absorption. The maximum recommended application of two 30 g tubes of the cream daily for three weeks, or one 50 g puffer pack of the powder daily for four weeks should *not* be exceeded in adults. After such a course, treatment should not be repeated for at least three months.

In renal impairment the plasma clearance of neomycin is reduced, therefore a reduction in dose should be made that relates to the degree of renal impairment.

In cases where there is established partial nerve deafness and where a significant degree of neomycin absorption could occur it might be inappropriate to use any neomycin-containing product and treatment with an antibacterial without an aminoglycoside constituent should be used if possible.

Concurrent administration of other aminoglycoside antibiotics is not recommended.

As neomycin has a neuromuscular blocking effect, patients concurrently receiving other agents with a similar action should be observed for signs of possible respiratory insufficiency.

Patients with hypostatic leg ulcers or hypostatic leg eczemas may have an increased sensitivity to a large number of topically applied drugs, including neomycin.

Side- and adverse effects: Allergic hypersensitivity to neomycin is generally uncommon following topical use but may manifest itself as a reddening and scaling of the affected skin, as an eczematous exacerbation of the lesion, or as a failure of the lesion to heal.

Allergic hypersensitivity, including anaphylaxis, following topical administration of bacitracin has been reported rarely.

A transient, mild, burning sensation on the skin has occasionally been reported following the administration of Cicatrin. As with all antibacterial preparations prolonged use may result in the overgrowth of non-susceptible organisms including fungi.

Use in pregnancy and lactation: Due to a lack of detailed information, the use of Cicatrin during pregnancy and lactation cannot be recommended in circumstances where significant systemic absorption of the active ingredients may occur.

No information is available regarding the excretion of the active ingredients or their metabolites in human milk.

Toxicity and treatment of overdosage: In the event of signs of toxicity developing following significant systemic absorption of the active ingredients of Cicatrin Powder/Cream the patient's general status, hearing acuity, renal function and neuromuscular function should be monitored and blood levels of neomycin and zinc bacitracin determined. Serum levels of neomycin may be reduced by haemodialysis.

Pharmaceutical precautions Store below 25°C. Keep dry.

Legal category POM.

Package quantities *Cicatrin Powder:* Puffer packs of 15 g (OP) and 50 g (OP).
Cicatrin Cream: Tubes of 15 g (OP) and 30 g (OP).

Further information Nil.

Product licence numbers
Powder 0003/5081.
Cream 0003/5082.

COPARVAX*

Presentation Each vial contains 7 mg (dry weight of the *Corynebacterium parvum* organisms (inactivated) WFL strain CN 6134) in a freeze-dried form. Thiomersal and glycine are added to concentrations of 0.01% and 2.3% prior to freeze-drying.

Uses Coparvax is indicated for the alleviation of malignant pleural effusions and malignant ascites.

Dosage and administration The recommended dose is 7–14 mg, although some patients have responded to lower doses.

Freeze-dried Coparvax should be reconstituted with 1 ml of physiological saline for injection and diluted in a further volume of 10–20 ml prior to injection into the pleural or peritoneal cavity.

Coparvax is injected into the pleural or peritoneal cavity via the paracentesis needle immediately after the effusion has been aspirated. Instillation of Coparvax may be repeated, if necessary, at intervals of one to four weeks.

The suspension should be administered within 24 hours of reconstitution.

Use in the elderly: No special comment.

Contra-indications, warnings, etc
Contra-indications: There are no specific contra-indications.

Precautions: The incidence and severity of side-effects attributable to Coparvax administered intrapleurally appears to be intensified if given within 10 days of thoracotomy and lung resection probably due to enhanced systemic absorption of Coparvax. It should not be given during the immediate post-operative period.

Following intrapleural or intra-abdominal administration, leakage of Coparvax into subcutaneous tissues may result in local tenderness. Intense fibrinous reaction in the pleural and peritoneal cavities has been observed following local administration of Coparvax. Intestinal obstruction due to the formation of adhesions is a theoretical possibility, although it has not been reported as a complication of Coparvax administration.

Side- and adverse effects: Fever occurs in 10 to 60% of patients following intracavitary injection of Coparvax.

Abdominal pain or mild abdominal discomfort has been reported in some 20% of patients following intraperitoneal injection of Coparvax. Nausea and vomiting may occur in a minority of patients following intracavitary administration of Coparvax.

Use in pregnancy and lactation: Since there are no laboratory or clinical data on mutagenicity or teratogenicity, Coparvax should not be administered during pregnancy or lactation.

Pharmaceutical precautions Store between 2 and 8°C. Do not freeze. Protect from light.

Legal category POM.

Package quantities Vial of 7 mg.

Further information Nil.

Product licence number 0003/0097.

CYCLIMORPH* 10 INJECTION
CYCLIMORPH* 15 INJECTION

Presentation Cyclimorph 10 Injection contains morphine tartrate 10 mg, cyclizine tartrate 50 mg, in 1 ml.

Cyclimorph 15 Injection contains morphine tartrate 15 mg, cyclizine tartrate 50 mg, in 1 ml.

Uses Cyclimorph Injection is indicated in all medical and surgical conditions where cyclizine is needed in addition to morphine. Cyclimorph contains cyclizine, a non-phenothiazine anti-emetic, which minimises the nausea and vomiting which may be caused by the narcotic. It is particularly useful in the management of myocardial infarction where control of nausea and vomiting is also clearly desirable. Cyclimorph can also be used for the relief of severe pain; left ventricular failure, pulmonary oedema, shock, and post-operative sedation.

Dosage and administration *Adults and children over 12 years:* Usual adult dose – 10–20 mg morphine tartrate subcutaneously, intramuscularly or intravenously.

Children 6–12 years: 5–10 mg morphine tartrate as a maximum single dose.

1–5 years: 2.5–5 mg morphine tartrate as a maximum single dose.

Use in the elderly: Use reduced dosage.

If required, repeat not more often than 4-hourly with not more than 3 doses (representing 150 mg cyclizine tartrate) in any 24-hour period.

Contra-indications, warnings, etc
Contra-indications: Respiratory depression; obstructive airways disease. Concurrent administration with monoamine oxidase inhibitors or within 2 weeks of their discontinuation.

Precautions: Use reduced dosage in the elderly, in hypothyroidism and chronic hepatic disease. Administration during labour may cause respiratory depression in the new-born infant.

Side- and adverse effects: Tolerance and dependence may occur. Drowsiness, dry mouth and blurred vision may occur in a small number of patients, due to the cyclizine component.

Use in pregnancy and lactation:
Morphine: There is inadequate evidence of safety in human pregnancy but the drug has been widely used for many years without apparent ill consequence and animal studies have not shown any hazard. No data available on its excretion in breast milk.

Cyclizine: There is some clinical evidence of safety in human pregnancy. No data available on its excretion in breast milk.

Toxicity and treatment of overdosage: Symptoms are likely to consist of respiratory depression, hypotension, with circulatory failure and deepening coma.

Naloxone, given intravenously, intramuscularly or

subcutaneously, effectively antagonises the toxic effects of morphine. The circulation should be maintained with infusions of dextrose and suitable electrolyte solutions. Assisted respiration may be required.

Note: The use of the specific antidote in addicts tolerant to morphine may produce withdrawal symptoms.

Pharmaceutical precautions Store below 30°C. Protect from light. Do not freeze.

Legal category CD (Sch 2), POM.

Package quantities *Cyclimorph 10 Injection;* 1 ml ampoules: Box of 5.
Cyclimorph 15 Injection; 1 ml ampoules: Box of 5.

Further information Nil.

Product licence numbers
Cyclimorph 10 0003/5022R
Cyclimorph 15 0003/5023R

DARAPRIM* TABLETS

Presentation Each tablet contains 25 mg of Pyrimethamine BP, Scored and coded 'WELLCOME A3A' and white in colour.

Uses Daraprim acts as a causal prophylactic and suppressive agent against malaria caused by Plasmodium falciparum. It also acts as a suppressant against Plasmodium vivax infections. In areas of known or suspected resistance to pyrimethamine or related compounds, another prophylactic should be used.

Dosage and administration *Adults:* 1 tablet regularly each week.

Children: Over 10 years: 1 tablet regularly each week.

5–10 years: ½ tablet regularly each week.

Under 5 years: Formulation not applicable.

Daraprim is rapidly absorbed and therefore prophylactic cover can be expected shortly after the first dose. Prophylaxis should commence before arrival in an endemic area and be continued once weekly. On returning to a non-malarious area dosage should be maintained for a further four weeks.

Use in the elderly: No specific studies have been carried out in the elderly, however, it may be advisable to monitor renal or hepatic function and if there is serious impairment then caution should be exercised.

Daraprim, at the doses recommended for the prevention of Malaria is unlikely to have any adverse effect on older people normally of good health.

Contra-indications, warnings, etc
Contra-indications: Daraprim should not be given to patients with a history of pyrimethamine sensitivity.

Precautions: The recommended dosage should not be exceeded.

Daraprim should be used with caution in patients with hepatic or renal disorders.

During pregnancy and in other conditions predisposing to folate deficiency, a folate supplement should be given.

Daraprim, by its mode of action, may further depress folate metabolism in patients receiving treatment with other folate inhibitors. Occasional reports suggest that individuals taking pyrimethamine as malarial prophylaxis at doses in excess of 25 mg weekly may develop megaloblastic anaemia if co-trimoxazole is prescribed concurrently.

The concurrent administration of lorazepam and Daraprim may induce hepatotoxicity.

Daraprim may exacerbate folate deficiency due to innate disease or malnutrition.

Side- and adverse effects: At the recommended dose, side-effects are rare. Occasionally, rashes have been observed which disappeared when the administration of Daraprim was stopped. Excessive doses may produce a macrocytic anaemia resembling that of folic acid deficiency. Insomnia has been reported when pyrimethamine has been given at weekly doses above those recommended.

Use in pregnancy and lactation: While there is a theoretical risk of foetal abnormality with all folate inhibitors given during pregnancy, no such adverse effects have been reported with Daraprim in humans. A folate supplement should be given to pregnant women receiving Daraprim. The amount of pyrimethamine excreted in breast milk is insufficient to contra-indicate its use in lactating mothers, but breast-fed infants should not receive other anti-folate agents.

Toxicity and treatment of overdosage: Symptoms reported have included vomiting, cyanosis, respiratory distress, convulsions and tachycardia. Routine supportive treatment, including maintenance of a clear airway and control of convulsions, should be given. Adequate fluids should be given to ensure optimal diuresis. Gastric lavage may be of value only if instituted within two hours of ingestion, in view of the rapid absorption of Daraprim. Fresh blood transfusions to counteract blood dyscrasias should be available.

To counteract possible folate deficiency, calcium folinate 9 to 15 mg daily should be given until the signs of toxicity have subsided. There may be a delay of 7 to 10 days before the full leucopenic side-effects become evident, therefore calcium folinate therapy should be continued for the period at risk.

Pharmaceutical precautions Store below 35°C. Protect from light.

Legal category P.

Package quantities 30 tablets as 5 foil strips of 6 tablets.

Further information When taken as directed Daraprim is an effective antimalarial, but it may be rendered ineffective by the development of drug resistance from time to time in certain regions. Local medical advice about the suitability of the product should, therefore, be obtained immediately on arrival in a malarious region.

Product licence number 0003/5026R.

DICONAL* TABLETS

Presentation Each tablet contains 10 mg of Dipipanone Hydrochloride BP and 30 mg of Cyclizine Hydrochloride BP, coloured deep pink, scored and coded 'WELLCOME F3A'.

Uses Analgesic with anti-emetic action.

Indicated in those medical and surgical conditions where morphine would normally be used. It also contains cyclizine, an anti-emetic which effectively overcomes the nausea and vomiting which may be caused by the narcotic. Often effective in patients who have ceased to respond to morphine or pethidine.

Dosage and administration *Adults:* In all cases an initial dose of 1 tablet should not be exceeded. The onset of action is within an hour and adequate relief from a single dose will last about six hours. The dose can be repeated every six hours if necessary. Should the initial dose prove inadequate, as in cases of severe intractable pain or where other potent analgesics have been used previously, the dose may be increased subsequently by ½ tablet increments. It will seldom be necessary to exceed a dose of 3 tablets.

Children: Not applicable.

Use in the elderly: Although there is no absolute contra-indication to the use of Diconal in the elderly, opioid drugs may cause confusion in this age group and careful monitoring should be ensured.

Contra-indications, warnings, etc
Contra-indications: Respiratory depression, obstructive airways disease. Concurrent administration with mono-amine oxidase inhibitors or within 2 weeks of their discontinuation.

Precautions: Use with caution in patients with severe liver or kidney diseases.

As with all potent analgesics the possibility of addiction cannot be excluded and the usual precautions should be observed.

Misuse of Diconal has been reported, particularly by young addicts who have previously been dependent on, or have misused other agents, both opiate and non-opiate. Extreme caution is warranted when prescribing Diconal to this group of patients.

As with morphine-type drugs respiratory depression is a hazard. Particular care should therefore be taken when increasing the dosage and when treating patients with impaired respiration. Concurrent administration with other CNS depressants including alcohol may enhance the central effects of Diconal.

Side- and adverse effects: Cyclizine may cause drowsiness, dryness of the mouth and blurred vision in a small number of patients. Diconal may cause confusion in the elderly.

Use in pregnancy and lactation: No data are available on the use of Diconal in human pregnancy nor of the excretion of it or its metabolites in human milk. Its administration to pregnant or lactating mothers is best avoided unless there are compelling reasons for its use.

Administration during labour may cause respiratory distress in the newborn.

Toxicity and treatment of overdosage: The main problem with overdosage is likely to be respiratory depression. Depressed respiration can be counteracted by the administration of naloxone. Gastric lavage. Oxygen and respiratory support if necessary.

Pharmaceutical precautions Store below 25°C. Protect from light. Keep dry.

Legal category CD (Sch 2), POM.

Package quantities Blister pack of 50 tablets as 5 blister strips of 10 tablets.

Further information Nil.

Product licence number 0003/5027R.

DIGIBIND*
Digoxin-specific antibody fragments (Fab)

Presentation Each vial of Digibind contains a sterile, lyophilised, crystalline, off-white powder, comprising 40 mg of antigen-binding fragments (Fab) derived from specific antidigoxin antibodies raised from sheep, approximately 75 mg Sorbitol BP and approximately 28 mg Sodium Chloride BP.

Uses Digoxin-specific antibody fragments are indicated for the treatment of known or strongly suspected digoxin or digitoxin toxicity, where measures beyond the withdrawal of the digitalis glycoside and correction of any serum electrolyte abnormality are felt to be necessary.

Dosage and administration Fab dosage is governed by the body load of digoxin (or digitoxin) to be counteracted. The load can be estimated in two ways:

either (i) from information on the acutely ingested dose, the amount of which, in mg, should be multiplied by 0.80 to take account of incomplete absorption;

or (ii) from the plasma or serum concentration in the quasi-steady state, which can be assumed for any interval longer than 6 hours after ingesting a dose.

Using the latter method, the following formulae are employed:

digoxin

plasma (serum) concentration (ng/ml) × *0.0056* × bodyweight (kg) = estimated total body load (mg)

Thus, for a plasma (serum) concentration of 20 ng/ml in a patient weighing 70 kg:

body load = 20 × (0.0056 × 70) = 7.84 mg

digitoxin

plasma (serum) concentration (ng/ml) × *0.00056* × bodyweight (kg) = estimated total body load (mg)

Thus, for a plasma (serum) concentration of 250 ng/ml in a patient weighing 65 kg:

body load = 250 × (0.00056 × 65) = 9.1 mg

The plasma concentration factor is derived from the volume of distribution (L/kg body weight) divided by 1000 to reduce the body load estimate to mg.

The approximate molecular weight ratio of Fab and digoxin (or digitoxin) is 60. Hence the approximate dose of Fab required is 60 times the load, rounded up to the nearest 40 mg, since this is the amount of Fab contained in a single vial. Hence, in the examples above, 480 mg (12 vials) and 560 mg (14 vials) would be required respectively.

The content of each vial to be used should be dissolved in 4 ml of Water for Injections BP, thus producing an approximately isosmotic solution with a protein concentration of between 9 and 11 mg/ml. This may then be diluted further to any convenient volume with Sodium Chloride Intravenous Infusion BP. The final solution of Fab should be administered intravenously over a 20-minute period through a 0.22 micron Millipore filter, which is recommended to remove any incompletely dissolved aggregates.

If there is incomplete reversion, or a recurrence of toxicity, further Fab can be given after a few hours at a dose suggested from the earlier clinical experience.

Use in children and the elderly: There is no information to suggest that the treatment of children or the elderly presents any special risk in an already grave situation – thus they should be dosed in the same way.

Pharmacology: The affinity constant (K_D) of Fab for digoxin is high (10^{-10}M) and greater than that of digoxin for its receptor (Na-K ATPase), which is implicated in the digoxin toxic effects. The affinity constant of Fab for digitoxin is also high (10^{-9}M). Digoxin (and digitoxin) are therefore attracted away from the receptor on heart tissue (and presumably other tissues as well, though this has not been studied) and their rate of elimination is changed from that governed by the kinetics of receptor binding to that governed by the kinetics of access and elimination of Fab.

In animals Fab reverses digoxin effects much more quickly than does IgG. There is a suggestion that reversal of inotropy with Fab lags behind reversal of electrical dysrhythmic effects. This could possibly be due to cellular differences between contractile and conducting tissue, or to differences in accessibility.

The plasma disappearance half-life of Fab in the baboon is 9–13 h and that of the parent IgG antibody is 61 h. The total volume of distribution of Fab in the baboon is 8.7 times greater than that of IgG and the readier diffusion of the smaller moiety sufficiently accounts for this.

About 93% of radioactively labelled Fab, injected into baboons, appeared in the urine within 24 h and the corresponding amount of digoxin-specific IgG was less than 1%. However, much of the urinary Fab was not intact. Small molecular weight proteins are catabolised by the kidney, as after filtration they are taken up into proximal tubular cells. Fab elimination is greatly prolonged in nephrectomised rats, but is actually enhanced in rats whose renal tubules have been damaged by the specific toxin maleate.

Corresponding information on human patients is sparse, but the close relationship of the therapeutic performance to predictions suggests that the animal data will be helpful. The human plasma disappearance half-life after intravenous administration of Fab is about 16 h with good renal function.

Several patients with renal dysfunction have received digoxin-specific Fab. The time course of therapeutic effect was not distinguishable from that in patients with good function. In the patient with virtually no renal excretory function, the reticuloendothelial system might be expected to eliminate the complex. Whether elimination would be accomplished with the digoxin still bound, rendered inactive, is not known.

Ordinarily, following administration of Fab, improvements in signs and symptoms begin within 30 minutes. At the same time, the plasma digoxin concentration rises sharply. The digoxin is protein-bound and pharmacologically inactive. The free digoxin remains less than 0.2 ng/ml in intoxicated dogs treated with IgG.

Contra-indications, warnings, etc
Contra-indications: None known.

Precautions: Patients with mild to moderate renal dysfunction have been successfully treated with digoxin-specific antibody fragments. The elimination half-life in the presence of renal failure has not been clearly defined but is expected to be substantially prolonged. The time course of therapeutic effect has not been different in these patients, but excretion of the antibody fragment-digoxin complex from the body should be delayed.

Patients previously dependent on the inotropism of digoxin could develop signs of heart failure when treated with Digibind. After successful management of poisoning, digoxin has had to be reinstituted in some cases. During management, additional inotropic support can be obtained from intravenous dopamine or dobutamine, but caution is required as catecholamines can aggravate arrhythmias caused by cardiac glycosides.

Laboratory tests: Patients should be closely monitored, including blood pressure and electrocardiogram, at all times during and after administration of Digibind. Presence of the exogenous antibody fragments will interfere with radioimmunoassay measurements of digoxin.

Potassium concentrations should be followed carefully, since severe digitalis intoxication can cause life-threatening elevation in serum potassium concentration by shifting it from within the cells. Such patients often have a total body deficit of potassium, and when the effect of digitalis is reversed by Digibind, potassium reuptake by the cells causes a reduction in the serum potassium levels. Hypokalaemia can develop rapidly in this situation unless corrective action is taken.

Side- and adverse effects: Although allergic responses have been reported rarely, the possibility of anaphylactic, hypersensitivity or febrile reactions should be borne in mind. Patients allergic to ovine proteins would be particularly at risk, as might individuals who have previously received digoxin-specific antibody fragments raised in sheep. Since the Fab fragment of the antibody lacks the antigenic determinants of the Fc fragment, it should pose less of an immunogenic threat to patients than does an intact immunoglobulin molecule.

Use in pregnancy and lactation: Animal reproduction studies have not been conducted with Digibind. Whether Digibind can cause foetal damage when administered to a pregnant woman or can affect reproductive capacity is not known. Hence digoxin-specific antibody fragments should be given to a pregnant woman only if clearly needed.

Carcinogenesis, mutagenesis, impairment of fertility: There have been no long-term studies performed in animals to evaluate carcinogenic or mutagenic potential or effects on fertility.

Toxicity and treatment of overdosage: Not relevant.

Pharmaceutical precautions Store at 2–8°C. Protect from light.

Legal category POM.

Package quantities Single vial of lyophilised powder containing 40 mg of antigen-binding fragments (Fab).

Further information Digoxin-specific antibody fragments (Fab) have been used successfully to treat a case of lanatoside C intoxication.

Product licence number 0003/0207.

ADSORBED DIPHTHERIA VACCINE BP, WELLCOME* (Dip/Vac/Ads)

Presentation Adsorbed Diphtheria Vaccine is a suspension of highly purified toxoid prepared from the exotoxin of *Corynebacterium diphtheriae* adsorbed onto hydrated aluminium phosphate. The aluminium content does not exceed 1.25 mg/dose. Thiomersal BP is added as a preservative to a concentration of 0.01%.

Each 0.5 ml dose has an immunising potency of not less than 30 International Units (IU).

The immunising potency of this vaccine is now expressed in International Units in accordance with the requirements of the European and British Pharmacopoeias. These units measure the immunising activity of the vaccine whereas the previously used Lf units expressed the quantity of toxoid present. There is no simple numerical relationship between IU and Lf. No change has been made to the potency although it is now expressed in IU.

Uses For active immunisation against diphtheria.

Primary immunisation against diphtheria in infancy is usually carried out by the administration of combined adsorbed diphtheria and tetanus (DT/Vac/Ads) or Trivax* (DTPer/Vac) or Trivax-Ad* (DTPer/Vac/Ads). Primary immunisation against diphtheria alone for children under the age of 10 years may be carried out with adsorbed diphtheria vaccine. It may also be used in Schick-positive adults and children over the age of 10 years who are at particular risk.

Dosage and administration The primary course of immunisation is two doses given by intramuscular or deep subcutaneous injection separated by an interval of at least four weeks.

In the UK and many other countries a third dose is advised in order to ensure long-lasting immunity.

Adults and children over 10 years of age: Two doses of 0.2 ml.

Children under 10 years of age: Two doses of 0.5 ml.

A reinforcing dose of 0.5 ml should be administered at about five years of age to children immunised in infancy.

Oral Poliomyelitis Vaccine BP may be given at the same time as Diphtheria Vaccine.

Shake well before each dose is withdrawn. It is good practice to record the title, dose and lot numbers of all vaccines and the dates of administration. Any untoward reactions should be reported to the regulatory authorities and to the manufacturer.

Use in the elderly: No special comment.

Contra-indications, warnings, etc
Contra-indications: Adsorbed diphtheria vaccine should not be administered intradermally. The vaccine should not be administered to a subject who has experienced a serious reaction (e.g. anaphylaxis) to a previous dose of this vaccine or who is known to be hypersensitive to any component thereof. It is advisable to avoid vaccination during an acute infection.

Precautions: Adsorbed Diphtheria Vaccine should not be administered to children over the age of 10 years or to adults without a preliminary Schick test, to avoid giving vaccine to persons who are already immune or to those who are hypersensitive, i.e. those who show a negative-or-pseudo-Schick reaction.

Although anaphylaxis is rare, facilities for its management should always be available during vaccination.

Side- and adverse effects: Local reactions consisting of swelling, redness and tenderness at the injection site may occur and occasionally may be severe. They may be more frequent and severe after the second than the first injection. Local reactions are uncommon in children under two years of age.

General reactions consisting of transient fever, malaise and headache may occur.

Allergic reactions, urticaria, pallor and dyspnoea have been reported following injection of adsorbed diphtheria vaccine.

A small painless nodule may form at the injection site but usually disappears without sequelae. However, persistent nodules at the injection site may occasionally follow the administration of this vaccine especially if the inoculation is introduced into the superficial layers of subcutaneous tissue.

Use in pregnancy and lactation: Accurate information is not available on the safety of the vaccine in pregnancy.

Toxicity and treatment of overdosage: Not applicable.

Pharmaceutical precautions Store at 2–8°C. Protect from light.
Do not freeze.

Legal category POM.

Package quantities Box of 5 × 0.5 ml ampoules.

Further information Nil.

Product licence number 0003/5128R.

DIPHTHERIA AND TETANUS VACCINE BP, WELLCOME* (DT/Vac/FT)

Presentation Diphtheria and tetanus vaccine is a mixture of purified diphtheria and tetanus toxoids which are prepared by formalin detoxification of *Corynebacterium diphtheriae* and *Clostridium tetani* exotoxins. Thiomersal BP is added as a preservative to a concentration of 0.01%. Each 0.5 ml dose contains not less than 25 Lf diphtheria toxoid and not less than 3.5 Lf tetanus toxoid.

The antigenic content and formulation of this vaccine has not been changed, although the labelled content of the tetanus component has been altered to conform with the flocculation equivalence of the new British reference antitoxin preparation.

Uses For reinforcement of immunity at five years or over in children who were immunised in infancy with either adsorbed diphtheria-tetanus vaccine (DT/Vac/Ads) or with Trivax* (DTPer/Vac) or Trivax-Ad* (DTPer/Vac/Ads) and who do not require continued immunisation against whooping cough.

The more potent antigen, Adsorbed Diphtheria and Tetanus Vaccine is preferred for primary immunisation against diphtheria and tetanus, but either preparation of combined diphtheria-tetanus vaccine may be used for reinforcement of immunity.

Simultaneous reinforcement of immunity to diphtheria and tetanus in adults and children over 10 years of age is rarely needed. Diphtheria-containing vaccines should not be given to these subjects unless a Schick test has been carried out to avoid giving the vaccine to persons who are already immune or to those who are hypersensitive, i.e. those who show a negative-or-pseudo-Schick reaction.

Dosage and administration The vaccine is given by intramuscular or deep subcutaneous injection.

Children under 10 years: 0.5 ml.

Adults and children over 10 years: 0.2 ml.

Use in the elderly: No special comment.

In subjects who suffered a reaction to a previous dose of adsorbed vaccine it may be preferable to administer 0.1 ml of Diphtheria and Tetanus vaccine in Simple Solution intradermally. Oral Poliomyelitis Vaccine BP may be given at the same time as Diphtheria and Tetanus Vaccine.

Shake well before withdrawing a dose. It is good practice to record the title, dose and lot numbers of all vaccines and the dates of administration. Any untoward reactions should be reported to the regulatory authorities and to the manufacturer.

Contra-indications, warnings, etc
Contra-indications: The vaccine should not be administered to a subject who has experienced a serious reaction (e.g. anaphylaxis) to a previous dose of this vaccine or who is known to be hypersensitive to any component thereof. It is advisable to avoid vaccination during an acute infection.

Precautions: Although anaphylaxis is rare, facilities for its management should always be available during vaccination.

Side- and adverse effects: Local reactions, swelling, redness and tenderness at the injection site, and general reactions, transient fever, malaise and headache may be caused by either or both component toxoids. Acute allergic reactions – anaphylaxis, urticaria, angioneurotic oedema, pallor and dyspnoea have been reported. Serum sickness, polyradicular neuritis, and peripheral neuropathy have also occurred following administration of diphtheria or tetanus vaccines.

Transverse myelitis has been reported after simultaneous administration of diphtheria and tetanus vaccine and oral polio vaccine, but a cause and effect relationship has not been established.

Use in pregnancy and lactation: Since simultaneous vaccination against diphtheria and tetanus in adults is uncommon, there is no accurate information on the safety of this vaccine in pregnancy.

Toxicity and treatment of overdosage: Not applicable.

Pharmaceutical precautions Store at 2–8°C. Protect from light.
Do not freeze.
When multi-dose containers are employed it is good practice to discard any partly used vaccine vials at the end of the vaccinating session.

Legal category POM.

Package quantities Vial of 5 ml.

Further information Nil.

Product licence number 0003/5130.

ADSORBED DIPHTHERIA AND TETANUS VACCINE BP, WELLCOME* (DT/Vac/Ads)

Presentation Adsorbed diphtheria and tetanus vaccine is a mixture of highly purified diphtheria and tetanus toxoids which are prepared by formalin detoxification of *Corynebacterium diphtheriae* and *Clostridium tetani* exotoxins. The toxoids are adsorbed onto aluminium hydroxide. The aluminium content does not exceed 1.25 mg/dose. Thiomersal BP is added as a preservative to a concentration of 0.01%. Each 0.5 ml dose contains not less than 30 i.u. diphtheria toxoid and not less than 40 i.u. tetanus toxoid.

The immunising potency of this vaccine is now expressed in International Units in accordance with the requirements of the European and British Pharmacopoeias. These units measure the immunising activity of the vaccine whereas the previously used Lf units expressed the quantity of toxoid present. There is no simple numerical relationship between IU and Lf. No change has been made to the potency although it is now expressed in IU.

Uses For active immunisation against diphtheria and tetanus.

Adsorbed diphtheria and tetanus vaccine is used principally for the primary immunisation of infants and children under ten years of age against tetanus and diphtheria where the use of pertussis-containing vaccines (DTPer/Vac, DTPer/Vac/Ads) is contra-indicated or not required. It is also given to reinforce immunity in children under 10 years of age immunised in infancy with diphtheria and tetanus vaccine. Trivax* or Trivax-Ad* (DT/Vac/Ads, DTPer/Vac, DTPer/Vac/Ads).

Simultaneous primary immunisation or reinforcement of immunity to diphtheria and tetanus in adults and children over 10 years of age is rarely needed. Diphtheria-containing vaccines should not be given to these subjects unless a Schick test has been carried out to avoid immunising persons who are already immune and/or hypersensitive, i.e., those who show a negative-and/or-pseudo-Schick reaction.

Dosage and administration For primary immunisation two intramuscular or deep subcutaneous injections separated by an interval of at least four weeks are recommended.

In the UK and many other countries a third dose is advised in order to ensure long-lasting immunity.

Children under 10 years: Two doses of 0.5 ml.

Adults and children over 10 years: Two doses of 0.2 ml.

A single dose of adsorbed tetanus vaccine should be administered 6 to 12 months after the second dose of the combined diphtheria and tetanus vaccine to complete the primary course of immunisation against tetanus.

A reinforcing dose of 0.5 ml of adsorbed or simple diphtheria and tetanus vaccines should be administered at about five years of age to children immunised in infancy with diphtheria and tetanus vaccine or combined diphtheria, tetanus and pertussis vaccine.

It may be preferable to administer 0.1 ml of Diphtheria and Tetanus vaccine in simple solution intradermally to adults and children who have suffered a reaction to a previous dose of adsorbed vaccine.

Poliomyelitis vaccine (oral) may be given at the same time as diphtheria and tetanus vaccine.

Shake thoroughly before withdrawing each dose. It is good practice to record the title, dose and lot numbers of all vaccines and the dates of administration. Any untoward reactions should be reported to the regulatory authorities and to the manufacturer.

Use in the elderly: No special comment.

Contra-indications, warnings, etc
Contra-indications: Adsorbed Diphtheria and Tetanus vaccine should not be administered intradermally.

The vaccine should not be administered to a subject who has experienced a serious reaction (e.g. anaphylaxis) to a previous dose of this vaccine or who is known to be hypersensitive to any component thereof. It is advisable to avoid vaccination during an acute infection.

Precautions: Although anaphylaxis is rare, facilities for its management should always be available during vaccination.

Side- and adverse effects: Local reactions, swelling, redness and tenderness at the injection site, and general reactions, transient fever, malaise and headache may be caused by either or both component toxoids. Acute allergic reactions – anaphylaxis, urticaria, angioneurotic oedema, pallor and dyspnoea have been reported. Serum sickness, polyradicular neuritis, and peripheral neuropathy have also occurred following administration of diphtheria or tetanus vaccines.

Persistent nodules at the injection site may occasionally follow administration of adsorbed vaccine, especially if the inoculation is into the superficial layers of subcutaneous tissue.

Transverse myelitis has been reported after simultaneous administration of diphtheria and tetanus vaccine and oral polio vaccine, but a cause and effect relationship has not been established.

Use in pregnancy and lactation: Since simultaneous vaccination against diphtheria and tetanus in adults is uncommon there is no accurate information on the safety of this vaccine in pregnancy.

Toxicity and treatment of overdosage: Not applicable.

Pharmaceutical precautions Store at 2–8°C. Protect from light.

Do not freeze.

It is good practice to discard any partly used vaccine vials at the end of the vaccinating session.

Legal category POM.

Package quantities Box of 5 × 0.5 ml ampoules. Vial of 5 ml.

Further information Nil.

Product licence number 0003/5131.

ESBATAL* TABLETS

Presentation Esbatal Tablets containing 10 mg Bethanidine Sulphate BP in each tablet. Peach coloured, scored and coded 'WELLCOME P3A'.

Esbatal Tablets containing 50 mg Bethanidine Sulphate BP in each tablet. Peach coloured, scored and coded 'WELLCOME T3A'.

Uses Antihypertensive agent.

Esbatal is an adrenergic neurone blocking agent which acts selectively on peripheral sympathetic nerves.

It is indicated for all grades of hypertension. Because of its speed of action, it is of special value in malignant hypertension, hypertensive crises and hypertensive heart disease.

Adrenergic neurone blockade is apparent within two hours, with peak effect two to four hours later, and usually disappears within 10–12 hours. There may be some cumulative effect where renal function is impaired.

Esbatal has been used successfully in combination with other established antihypertensive agents.

Dosage and administration *Adults:* Blood pressure should be recorded when the patient is standing.

Starting dose – one 10 mg tablet three times daily, after meals. Where necessary the dosage should be increased by half a tablet three times daily, at intervals, until effective control is obtained. Doses should not exceed 200 mg daily. Diuretics may be given concurrently. For the elderly and patients with a history of a cerebrovascular accident, half the starting dose is recommended.

Where rapid lowering of blood pressure is urgently needed, an initial dose of 20 mg should be increased by 10–20 mg every four to six hours until control is achieved.

Children: Not applicable.

Use in the elderly: Use half the usual starting dose in the elderly. Use with caution in those with renal, coronary, or cerebral impairment.

Contra-indications, warnings, etc
Contra-indications: Patients become very sensitive to any circulating sympathomimetic agent after adrenergic neurone blockade. Hence Esbatal is contra-indicated for patients with phaeochromocytoma. Adrenaline, amphetamine or any other sympathomimetic such as, for example, appetite suppressants, should not be used in patients on Esbatal except on the very rare occasion that its action requires antagonising.

Precautions: Special care should be taken when treating hypertension in patients with disease of cerebral or coronary vasculature or with severe renal damage. As Esbatal is excreted mainly by the kidneys, reduced doses may suffice in renal impairment.

Tricyclic antidepressants antagonise the activity of Esbatal thus necessitating larger doses. If simultaneously prescribed tricyclic antidepressants are discontinued, a substantial reduction in Esbatal requirements must be anticipated.

Side- and adverse effects: The beneficial effects of Esbatal derive from reduced peripheral vascular resistance and are most marked in the erect posture. Transient symptoms of a further reduction in resistance such as faintness, sweating, muscle fatigue and headache may occur with sudden changes in posture, excessive exercise and extremes of temperature, all of which should be avoided. Regularly repeated symptoms can be managed by reducing the size of the dose preceding their onset or by taking the dose after a meal. Sometimes Esbatal disturbs the normal ejaculation of semen. After omission of one or two doses normal sexual function returns. Nasal stuffiness and disturbed micturition may occur. It rarely causes diarrhoea.

Use in pregnancy and lactation: Esbatal may exacerbate placental insufficiency, and its benefits must be balanced against the risks of its use. There are no data on its use in lactating mothers.

Toxicity and treatment of overdosage: The main problem with overdosage would be severe hypotension. Treatment of overdosage is by means of general supportive measures with intravenous injection of plasma. *Slow* intravenous injection of noradrenaline or phenylephrine may be given under expert supervision.

Pharmaceutical precautions Store below 25°C in a dry place.

Legal category POM.

Package quantities *Tablets 10 mg:* Bottle of 100 tablets.
Tablets 50 mg: Bottle of 100 tablets.

Further information Nil.

Product licence numbers
Tablets 10 mg 0003/5037R
Tablets 50 mg 0003/5038R

EXOSURF* NEONATAL ▼

Presentation Exosurf Neonatal is supplied as a vial of white, sterile, freeze-dried powder stored under vacuum together with a vial containing 8 ml preservative-free, sterile Water for Injections BP.

Each vial of powder contains 108 mg colfosceril palmitate. The sodium content per vial is 18.4 mg.

The reconstituted product is an opaque, white suspension.

Uses Exosurf Neonatal is indicated for the treatment of newborn babies with birthweight of 700 g or greater undergoing mechanical ventilation for respiratory distress syndrome, whose heart rate and arterial oxygenation are continuously monitored.

Dosage and administration
Dosage: A dose of 5 ml/kg birthweight of reconstituted Exosurf Neonatal should be given via the endotracheal tube. If the baby is still intubated, a second equal dose should be given 12 hours later by the same route. Each dose corresponds to 67.5 mg of colfosceril palmitate per kg birthweight.

Reconstitution: Exosurf Neonatal should be reconstituted immediately before use as it contains no antibacterial preservatives. Once reconstituted, it should be used within 8 hours.

ONLY preservative-free, sterile Water for Injections should be used for reconstitution, which should be performed as follows:

1. Fill a sterile syringe with 8 ml preservative-free, sterile Water for Injections.
2. Allow the vacuum in the vial of Exosurf Neonatal to draw the preservative-free, sterile Water for Injections through a sterile needle into the vial.
3. Aspirate the resulting suspension back into the syringe and then release the syringe plunger to allow the suspension to return into the Exosurf Neonatal vial.
4. Repeat aspiration and return three or four times to ensure adequate mixing of the vial contents. If the suspension appears to separate, gently shake or swirl the vial to resuspend.
5. Withdraw the required volume of Exosurf Neonatal suspension from the vial with the tip of the withdrawing needle well below the froth on the surface of the suspension.

Administration: Exosurf Neonatal should be administered only by those trained and experienced in the care and resuscitation of preterm infants.

Exosurf Neonatal can only be administered endotracheally to intubated infants undergoing mechanical ventilation. Infants should NOT be intubated solely for the administration of Exosurf Neonatal.

The infant's airway should be cleared by suction prior to the administration of Exosurf Neonatal.

Exosurf Neonatal is administered from a syringe into the endotracheal tube via the side-port on a special endotracheal adaptor, without interrupting mechanical ventilation. The part of the endotracheal tube outside the infant should be aligned vertically during administration (see diagram below).

The total dose should be administered at a rate slow enough to allow the reconstituted Exosurf Neonatal suspension to pass into the lungs through the endotracheal tube without accumulation. The minimum recommended time for administration of the full dose is 4 minutes.

Dosing should be slowed or interrupted if the infant's skin colour deteriorates, the heart rate slows, arterial oxygen monitors indicate more than transitory depression of arterial oxygen concentration or if Exosurf Neonatal accumulates in the endotracheal tube.

Contra-indications, warnings, etc
Contra-indications: There are no known contra-indications to treatment with Exosurf Neonatal.

Precautions: Exosurf Neonatal should only be administered with adequate facilities for ventilation and monitoring of babies with respiratory distress syndrome (RDS).

Preterm birth is hazardous. Surfactant administration can be expected to diminish the severity of RDS and hence to diminish complications of the intensive care, especially of the ventilatory support required for the treatment of RDS, but cannot be expected to eliminate entirely the mortality and morbidity associated with preterm delivery. Infants who but for the administration of surfactant might have died from RDS may be exposed to other complications of their immaturity.

As a consequence of the surfactant properties of

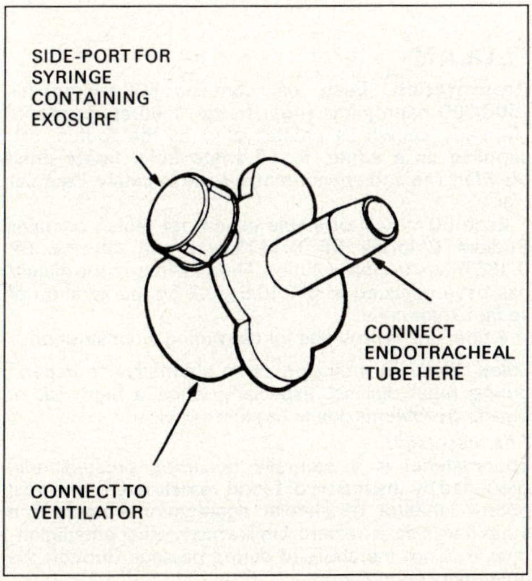

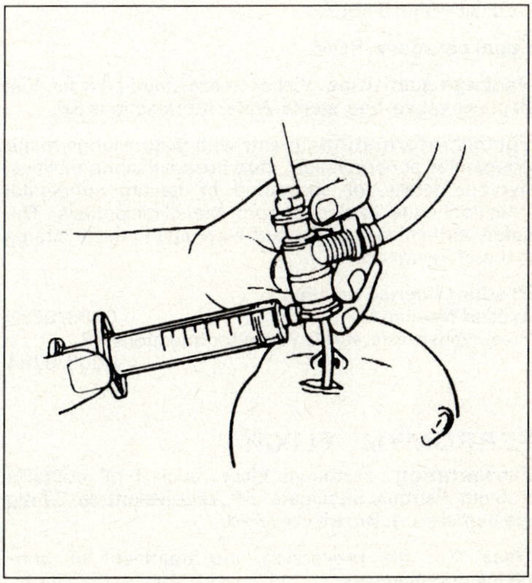

Exosurf Neonatal, chest expansion may improve rapidly after dosing, necessitating rapid reduction in peak ventilator inspiratory pressure.

The improvement in lung mechanics resulting from Exosurf Neonatal administration may result in rapid improvement in arterial oxygen concentration. After any appropriate reduction in ventilator pressure, rapid reduction in inspired oxygen concentration may be needed to avoid hyperoxaemia.

Infants no longer requiring positive pressure ventilation may require treatment for apnoea of prematurity. In clinical trials infants treated with Exosurf Neonatal had a higher incidence of apnoea, probably as a consequence of earlier ending of positive pressure ventilation. There were no adverse consequences in terms of increased mortality or long-term morbidity as a consequence of this increased incidence.

Exosurf Neonatal was non-mutagenic in the Ames Salmonella assay.

No long-term studies have been performed in animals to determine whether Exosurf Neonatal has carcinogenic potential.

The effects of Exosurf Neonatal on fertility have not been studied.

Side- and adverse effects: Pulmonary haemorrhage, the incidence of which increases the more immature the infant, is a rare and sometimes fatal complication of preterm delivery. Although no single trial of Exosurf Neonatal has demonstrated a significant increase in pulmonary haemorrhage, summation of all available results from controlled trials suggests that Exosurf Neonatal administration may be associated with an increase from 1 to 2% in the incidence of pulmonary haemorrhage. As might be expected, this association appears to be more marked the more immature the infant.

In occasional infants (approximately 3 per thousand) Exosurf Neonatal administration has been associated with obstruction of the endotracheal tube by mucous secretions. In infants in whom endotracheal tube obstruction is suspected this should be treated, according to normal practice, by suction of the tube, followed by replacement of the tube if this is unsuccessful.

Pregnancy and lactation: Not relevant with this product.

Drug interactions: No specific drug interactions have been identified.

Toxicity and treatment of overdosage: There have been no reports of overdosage with Exosurf Neonatal.

In case of accidental overdose, as much as possible of the suspension should be aspirated and the baby should then be managed with supportive treatment, with particular attention to fluid and electrolyte balance.

Pharmaceutical precautions Store below 30°C. Do not freeze. Once reconstituted, Exosurf Neonatal should be used within 8 hours.

Legal category POM.

Package quantities Vial of freeze-dried powder. Vial of preservative-free, sterile Water for Injections BP.

Further information Infants with mature lungs, major congenital abnormalities, chromosomal abnormalities, hydrops fetalis, or suspected of having congenital infection were excluded from the clinical trials. The safety and efficacy of Exosurf Neonatal in these infants is therefore unknown.

Product licence numbers
Exosurf Neonatal 0003/0283
Preservative-free, sterile Water for Injections BP 0003/0284

FERROMYN* ELIXIR

Presentation Ferromyn Elixir: each 5 ml contains 106 mg Ferrous Succinate BP (equivalent to 37 mg elemental iron). Brown coloured.

Uses For the prevention and treatment of iron-deficiency anaemias.

Dosage and administration *Adults:* 5 ml elixir three times a day.

Children up to 2 years: Up to 1 ml twice daily.

2–5 years: 2.5 ml three times daily.

5–10 years: 5 ml twice daily.

Over 10 years: As for adults.

Use in the elderly: No special comment.

Contra-indications, warnings, etc
Contra-indications: No special comments.

Precautions: May be less well absorbed if taken with food. Iron absorption may be impaired by magnesium trisilicate and carbonates.

If Ferromyn and oral tetracycline are given concomitantly, absorption and therefore serum levels of the antibiotic will be reduced. As with other conventional iron preparations, Ferromyn should not be given within 2 to 3 hours of an oral dose of tetracycline.

Side- and adverse effects: Side-effects are generally uncommon at the recommended dose. Occasionally abdominal discomfort, nausea and diarrhoea may occur. Chronic usage may lead to constipation, particularly in the elderly.

Use in pregnancy and lactation: As pregnancy is frequently an indication for iron therapy there is no reason to expect problems with Ferromyn therapy. Iron is excreted in breast milk but not in clinically significant amounts (about 0.5 mg/day).

Toxicity and treatment of overdosage: The initial symptoms of acute overdosage with iron are acute gastric disturbance with epigastric pain, nausea, vomiting and diarrhoea. Haematemesis may occur. These features may be followed by profound cardiovascular collapse and acute encephalopathy.

If serum iron levels exceed 5 mg/l within six hours of dosing, then treatment is a matter of urgency.

Lavage should be carried out using a solution of desferrioxamine (2 g/l of warm water) and 5 g of desferrioxamine (in 50 to 100 ml water) should be left in the stomach. In addition, 1 g should be given twice daily by intramuscular injection. The antidote may be administered by continuous infusion (15 mg/kg/hr) but blood pressure should be monitored to avoid desferrioxamine hypotension.

It is important to maintain an adequate urine flow.

Pharmaceutical precautions Store below 25°C. Protect from light.

Legal category P.

Package quantities Bottle of 100 ml.

Further information Nil.

Product licence number 0003/5088R.

FLOLAN*

Presentation Each vial contains 500 micrograms (500,000 nanograms (ng)) freeze-dried epoprostenol (formerly known as prostacyclin) as the sodium salt supplied as a white, to off-white fluffy freeze-dried powder. The sodium content is approximately 1 mg per vial.

Each 50 ml vial of sterile diluent for Flolan contains Sodium Chloride BP 0.147% w/v and Glycine BP 0.188% w/v in clear solution. The alkalinity of the diluent has been adjusted to pH 10.5 ± 0.3 by the addition of sodium hydroxide.

A filter unit is provided for use during reconstitution.

Uses Flolan is indicated as an alternative to heparin during renal dialysis, especially when a high risk of bleeding problems due to heparin exists.

Pharmacology:
Epoprostenol is a naturally occurring prostaglandin produced by the intima of blood vessels and is the most potent inhibitor of platelet aggregation known. The inhibition is dose-related. Unlike many other prostaglandins, it is not metabolised during passage through the pulmonary circulation.

Epoprostenol sodium is a potent vasodilator. The cardiovascular effects disappear within 30 minutes of the end of infusion.

It inhibits platelet aggregation by elevating platelet cyclic adenosine monophosphate. The action is dose-related above 2 nanograms/kg/min, following intravenous administration. Significant inhibition of aggregation induced by adenosine diphosphate is observed after intravenous administration of 4 or more nanograms/kg/min. Effects on platelets usually disappear within 30 minutes of discontinuing infusion of epoprostenol sodium.

Higher doses of epoprostenol sodium (20 nanograms/kg/min) disperse circulating platelet aggregates and increase by up to twofold the cutaneous bleeding time.

Epoprostenol sodium reduces platelet procoagulant activity and the release of heparin neutralising factor.

The fate of epoprostenol sodium in man is not fully established. At normal physiological pH and temperature, epoprostenol sodium is hydrolysed with a half-life of 2–3 minutes to 6-keto prostaglandin $F_{1\alpha}$.

Dosage and administration Flolan is suitable for continuous infusion only, either intravascularly or into the blood supplying dialyser.

The following schedules of infusion have been found effective in adults:

Prior to dialysis: 5 nanograms/kg/min intravenously.

During dialysis: 5 nanograms/kg/min into the arterial inlet of the dialyser.

The infusion should be stopped at the end of dialysis.

The recommended doses should be exceeded only with appropriate patient monitoring.

Use in children:
There is no specific information on the use of Flolan in children.

Use in the elderly: There is no specific information available on the use of Flolan in elderly patients.

Reconstitution:
Only the diluent provided for the purpose should be used. The enclosed filter unit must be used once only and then discarded after use.

To reconstitute Flolan, a strict aseptic technique must be used. *Particular care should be taken in calculating dilutions*, and in diluting Flolan the following procedure is recommended:

1. Withdraw approximately 10 ml of the sterile diluent into a sterile syringe.
2. Inject the contents of the syringe into the vial containing Flolan and dissolve the contents completely.
3. Draw up all the Flolan solution into the syringe.
4. Re-inject the entire contents into the residue of the original 50 ml of sterile diluent.
5. Mix well. This solution is now referred to as the *concentrated solution* and contains Flolan 10,000 nanograms per millilitre. The *concentrated solution* is normally further diluted before use. It may be diluted with physiological saline (0.9%), provided a ratio of 6 volumes of saline to 1 volume of *concentrated solution* is not exceeded; e.g. 50 ml of *concentrated solution* further diluted with a maximum of 300 ml saline.

Other common intravenous fluids are unsatisfactory for the dilution of the *concentrated solution* as the required pH is not attained. Flolan solutions are less stable at low pH. For administration using a pump capable of delivering small volume constant infusions, suitable aliquots of concentrated solution may be diluted with sterile physiological saline.

6. Before further dilution, draw up the *concentrated solution* into a larger syringe.
7. The filter provided should then be attached to the syringe and the *concentrated solution* is dispensed by filtration using firm but not excessive pressure. The typical time taken for filtration of 50 ml of solution is 70 seconds.

Infusion Rate Guidance:
In general, the infusion rate may be calculated by the following formula:

Infusion rate (ml/min)

$$= \frac{\text{Dosage (ng/kg/min)} \times \text{body weight (kg)}}{\text{Concentration of infusion (ng/ml)}}$$

(See Table below for examples).

Contra-indications, warnings, etc

Contra-indications:
There are no recognised contra-indications to the administration of Flolan in renal dialysis.

Precautions:
Because of the high pH of the final infusion solutions, care should be taken to avoid extravasation during their administration and consequent risk of tissue damage.

Epoprostenol sodium is a potent vasodilator. The cardiovascular effects disappear within 30 minutes of the end of the infusion.

Flolan sodium is not a conventional anticoagulant.

INFUSION RATE FORMULAE—EXAMPLES

Flolan may be administered in diluted form (1) or as the *concentrated solution* (2)

1. *Diluted:* A commonly used dilution is:
10 ml *concentrated solution* + 40 ml physiological saline (0.9%).
Resultant concentration = 2000 ng/ml epoprostenol.

		Body weight (kilograms)							
		30	40	50	60	70	80	90	100
Dosage (ng/kg/min)	1	0.90	1.20	1.50	1.80	2.10	2.40	2.70	3.00
	2	1.80	2.40	3.00	3.60	4.20	4.80	5.40	6.00
	3	2.70	3.60	4.50	5.40	6.30	7.20	8.10	9.00
	4	3.60	4.80	6.00	7.20	8.40	9.60	10.80	12.00
	5	4.50	6.00	7.50	9.00	10.50	12.00	13.50	15.00

Flow rates in mls/hr

2. Using *concentrated solution*, i.e. 10 000 ng/ml epoprostenol:

		Body weight (kilograms)							
		30	*40*	*50*	*60*	*70*	*80*	*90*	*100*
Dosage (ng/kg/min)	1	0.18	0.24	0.30	0.36	0.42	0.48	0.54	0.60
	2	0.36	0.48	0.60	0.72	0.84	0.96	1.08	1.20
	3	0.54	0.72	0.90	1.08	1.26	1.44	1.62	1.80
	4	0.72	0.96	1.20	1.44	1.68	1.92	2.16	2.40
	5	0.90	1.20	1.50	1.80	2.10	2.40	2.70	3.00

Flow rates in mls/hr

Flolan has been successfully used instead of heparin in renal dialysis, but in a small proportion of dialyses clotting has developed in the dialysis circuit, requiring termination of dialysis.

Haemorrhagic complications have not been encountered with Flolan but the possibility should be considered when the drug is administered to patients with spontaneous or drug-induced haemorrhagic diatheses.

Blood pressure and heart rate should be monitored during administration of Flolan. Tachycardia, bradycardia and hypotension may occur during infusions of Flolan.

The effects of Flolan on heart-rate may be masked by concomitant use of drugs which affect cardiovascular reflexes.

If excessive hypotension occurs during administration of Flolan, the dose should be reduced or the infusion discontinued. The hypotensive effect of Flolan may be enhanced by the use of acetate buffer in the dialysis bath during renal dialysis.

Elevated serum glucose levels have been reported during infusion of Flolan in man but these are not inevitable.

Drug interactions: Flolan may potentiate the action of heparin, and standard anticoagulant monitoring is advisable when Flolan is admininistered to patients receiving concomitant anticoagulants.

The vasodilator effect of Flolan may augment or be augmented by concomitant use of other vasodilators.

Use in pregnancy and lactation:
In the absence of adequate experience of administration of Flolan to pregnant women, the potential benefit to the mother must be weighed against the unknown risks to the foetus.

There is no information on the use of Flolan during lactation.

Side- and adverse effects:
Facial flushing is commonly seen, even in the anaesthetised patient.

Headache and gastro-intestinal symptoms including nausea, vomiting and abdominal colic have occurred in some conscious individuals.

Jaw pain, dry mouth, lassitude, reddening over the infusion site, chest pain and tightness have been reported with varying frequency.

Bradycardia, accompanied by pallor, nausea, sweating and sometimes abdominal discomfort and orthostatic hypotension, has occurred in healthy volunteers at doses of epoprostenol sodium greater than 5 nanograms/kg/min. Bradycardia associated with a considerable fall in systolic and diastolic blood pressure has followed intravenous administration of a dose of epoprostenol sodium equivalent to 30 nanograms/kg/min in healthy conscious volunteers.

Toxicity and treatment of overdosage:
The main feature of overdosage is likely to be hypotension.

Reduce the dose or discontinue the infusion and initiate appropriate supportive measures as necessary; for example, plasma volume expansion and/or adjustment to pump flow.

Pharmaceutical precautions Store Flolan vials at a temperature between 2°C and 8°C. Protect from light. Keep dry.

Under these conditions, freeze-dried Flolan in an unopened vial should not be affected by moisture present in the atmosphere.

Store the sterile glycine buffet diluent at a temperature between 2°C and 8°C. Do not freeze.

The stability of solutions of Flolan is pH dependent. Only the diluent supplied should be used for reconstitution of freeze-dried Flolan and only the recommended infusion solutions, in the stated ratio, should be used for further dilution, otherwise the required pH may not be maintained.

The reconstituted *concentrated solution* when prepared as directed using the sterile glycine buffer provided, contains 10,000 nanograms epoprostenol per ml and is suitable for further dilution as recommended.

Reconstitution and dilution should be carried out immediately prior to use. (See *'Reconstitution and dilution'*).

Glycine buffer diluent contains no preservative, consequently a vial should be used only once and then discarded.

Legal category POM.

Package quantities 1 vial of 500 micrograms epoprostenol with 1 × 50 ml vial of sterile diluent.

Further information The stability of the concentrated solution is not enhanced by refrigeration.

Product licence number 0003/0151.

HUMOTET* ANTITETANUS IMMUNOGLOBULIN INJECTION BP

Presentation Purified immunoglobulin obtained from the sera of healthy human donors known to have high levels of tetanus antitoxin following active immunisation with tetanus vaccine.

Humotet is a clear, colourless, semi-viscous liquid containing thiomersal 0.01% as a preservative, and glycine 2.25%. Each vial contains 250 i.u. of tetanus antitoxin in 1.0 ml solution.

Uses For passive immunisation against tetanus, in conjunction with adsorbed tetanus vaccine as soon as practicable after a tetanus-susceptible person has sustained a wound. Also for the treatment of tetanus.

Dosage and administration *Prevention of tetanus following injury: Adults and children:* Humotet should be administered by intramuscular injection usually in a dose of 250 i.u. – see table on next page.

Persons not immunised, or inadequately immunised, with tetanus vaccine are susceptible to tetanus and all wounds are prone to tetanus infection. In cases of doubt a person should be regarded as inadequately immunised.

Administration of immunoglobulin does not obviate the need for debridement and wound cleansing, nor does it contra-indicate the use of antibiotics.

The prophylactic immunisation schedule against tetanus (see table) should be carried out as soon as possible after a person has sustained a wound. Passive immunisation with immunoglobulin should be accompanied by simultaneous active immunisation with adsorbed tetanus vaccine.

If more than 24 hours have elapsed since the wound was sustained or if there is a risk of heavy contamination with *Clostridium tetani* 2 ml (500 i.u.). Humotet should be given, irrespective of immunisation history.

Humotet and adsorbed tetanus vaccine should be administered with separate syringes and into separate sites. Tetanus vaccine in simple solution is unsuitable for administration concurrently with Humotet.

A single dose of Humotet usually provides a protective level of tetanus antitoxin, over 0.01 i.u. per ml serum, for a period of four weeks. Long-term immunity against tetanus is conferred by giving further doses of vaccine; see table below.

Treatment of tetanus: Adults and children: 30–300 i.u. per kilogram body weight given intramuscularly.

Use in the elderly: No special comment.

Contra-indications, warnings, etc
Contra-indications: Humotet should not be given intravenously. The administration of immunoglobulin may be contra-indicated by a history of anaphylaxis resulting from administration of a previous dose of human gammaglobulin.

Precautions: Humotet should not be given concurrently with tetanus vaccine in simple solution.

Although anaphylaxis is rare, facilities for its management should always be available during vaccination.

Side- and adverse effects: A local reaction, consisting of a small area of inflammation and tenderness, may occur

Patient's history		*Immediate action*	*Follow-up action*
Previous record of receiving tetanus vaccine	*Administer Humotet*	*Administer adsorbed tetanus vaccine*	*Administer tetanus vaccine (adsorbed or in simple solution)*
None or Not known	1.0 ml (250 i.u.)	0.5 ml	0.5 ml after 6–12 weeks and 6–12 months
One dose (during last 6 weeks)	1.0 ml (250 i.u.)	0.5 ml to be given 4–6 weeks after first dose of vaccine	0.5 ml 6–12 months after second dose
One dose (more than 6 weeks ago)	1.0 ml (250 i.u.)	0.5 ml	0.5 ml 6–12 months after second dose
Two doses	Nil	0.5 ml to be given if more than 6 weeks after second dose of vaccine	Nil
Three doses	Nil	0.5 ml if more than 1 year since third dose of vaccine	Nil

after administration of the immunoglobulin, but this rarely constitutes more than a temporary inconvenience. Constitutional upsets, and particularly anaphylactic reactions, are uncommon. Patients with antibody deficiency syndromes may be liable to have local reactions after administration of the immunoglobulin.

Use in pregnancy and lactation: Accurate information is not available on the safety of Humotet in pregnancy.

Toxicity and treatment of overdosage: Not applicable.

Pharmaceutical precautions Store at 2–8°C. *Do not freeze.* Protect from light.

Legal category POM.

Package quantities 1 dose vial.

Further information Nil.

Product licence number 0003/0087.

HYPON* TABLETS

Presentation Each tablet contains:

Acetylsalicylic Acid BP	325 mg
Caffeine BP	10 mg
Codeine Phosphate BP	5 mg

The tablets are yellow and impressed with the word 'HYPON' on one side.

Uses Analgesic and antipyretic.

For symptomatic relief of pain and fever associated with acute and chronic rheumatism, dysmenorrhoea, neuralgia, tonsillitis, influenza, coryza, headaches, and all conditions where an analgesic is indicated.

Dosage and administration *Adults and children over 12 years:* 2 tablets every four hours.

Children under 12 years: Not recommended.

A maximum of 12 tablets to be taken in 24 hours.

Use in the elderly: Use with caution in those with renal impairment.

Contra-indications, warnings, etc

Contra-indications: Hypersensitivity to any of the constituents. Contra-indicated in haemophiliacs and in those with active peptic ulcers.

Precautions: Aspirin may prolong labour and contribute to maternal and neonatal bleeding, and is best avoided at term. Aspirin may enhance the effects of oral hypoglycaemics and anticoagulants and inhibit the action of uricosurics. It may precipitate bronchospasm or asthma in susceptible patients. Caution is necessary in renal impairment.

Side- and adverse effects: Occasionally, aspirin may induce hypersensitivity or asthmatic reactions. Gastrointestinal haemorrhages, (occasionally major) have been reported with aspirin. Codeine may sometimes cause constipation.

Use in pregnancy and lactation: No data are available on the use of Hypon in human pregnancy or on the excretion of it or its metabolites in human milk.

Toxicity and treatment of overdosage: Acute aspirin toxicity would be characterised mainly by vomiting, abdominal pain, tinnitus and hyperventilation. In severe cases, there may be pyrexia and convulsions. Hypoglycaemia and convulsions occur most commonly in children. Respiratory depression from the codeine content may occur.

Treatment comprises gastric aspiration with thorough lavage. Replace fluids and electrolytes as necessary. Forced alkaline diuresis is the treatment of choice for accelerating elimination of absorbed salicylate.

Pharmaceutical precautions Store below 25°C in a dry place.

Legal category CD (Sch 5), P.

Package quantities 12 tablets as 2 foil strips of 6 tablets. Drum of 300.

Further information Nil.

Product licence number 0003/0119.

IMURAN* TABLETS AND INJECTION

Presentation Each yellow film-coated tablet containing 50 mg Azathioprine BP is imprinted 'Imuran' on one face and '50' inside a shield on the obverse. Each orange film-coated tablet containing 25 mg Azathioprine BP is imprinted 'Imuran' on one face and '25' inside a shield on the obverse.

Each vial of injection contains the equivalent of 50 mg Azathioprine BP as its sodium salt, a yellow to amber freeze-dried powder. The sodium ion content is approximately 4.5 mg.

Uses Imuran Tablets are used as an immunosuppressant antimetabolite either alone, or more commonly, in combination with other agents (usually corticosteroids) and procedures which influence the immune response. Therapeutic effect may be evident only after weeks or months and can include a steroid-sparing effect, thereby reducing the toxicity associated with high dosage and prolonged usage of corticosteroids.

Imuran Injection and Tablets, in combination with corticosteroids and/or other immunosuppressive agents and procedures, are indicated in the management of patients receiving organ transplants.

Imuran Tablets, either alone or more usually in combination with corticosteroids and/or other procedures, have been used with clinical benefit which may include reduction of dosage or discontinuation of corticosteroids, in a proportion of patients suffering from the following: severe rheumatoid arthritis; systemic lupus erythematosus; dermatomyositis/polymyositis; autoimmune chronic active hepatitis; pemphigus vulgaris; polyarteritis nodosa; autoimmune haemolytic anaemia and chronic refractory idiopathic thrombocytopenic purpura.

Dosage and administration Imuran Injection should be used ONLY when the oral route is impractical and should be discontinued as soon as oral therapy is tolerated.

Specialist medical literature should be consulted for guidance as to clinical experience in particular conditions.

Transplantation: Adults and children: Depending on the immunosuppressive regimen adopted, a loading dose of up to 5 mg/kg bodyweight/day either orally or intravenously is usually given.

Maintenance dosage may range from 1 to 4 mg/kg bodyweight/day orally (or intravenously ONLY if oral therapy is not tolerated) and must be adjusted according to clinical requirements and haematological tolerance.

Evidence indicates that Imuran therapy should be maintained indefinitely, even if only low doses are necessary, because of the risk of graft rejection.

Other conditions: Adults and children: In general, starting dosage rarely exceeds 3 mg/kg bodyweight/day, and should be reduced depending on the clinical response (which may not be evident for weeks or months) and haematological tolerance.

When therapeutic response is evident, consideration should be given to reducing the maintenance dosage to the lowest level compatible with maintenance of that response. If no improvement occurs in the patient's condition within three months, consideration should be given to withdrawing Imuran.

The maintenance dosage required may range from less than 1 mg/kg bodyweight/day to 3 mg/kg bodyweight/day, depending on the clinical condition being treated and the individual patient response, including haematological tolerance.

Use in the elderly: The rapid *in vivo* cleavage of the azathioprine molecule followed by tissue fixation makes it impossible to relate plasma drug levels to toxicity. There are no specific data as to the tolerance of Imuran in elderly patients. It is recommended that the dosages used are at the lower end of the range given for adults and children.

Particular care should be taken to monitor haematological response and to reduce the maintenance dosage to the minimum required for clinical response.

Renal and/or hepatic insufficiency: It is impossible to relate plasma levels of azathioprine or 6-mercaptopurine to therapeutic efficacy or toxicity. Conversion of 6-thioinosinic acid to 6-thiouric acid by xanthine oxidase is not dependent on intact hepatic and/or renal function. Nevertheless, it is recommended that the dosages used are at the lower end of the normal range and that haematological response is carefully monitored.

The maintenance dosage used for the treatment of liver disorders is at the low end of the recommended range.

Reconstitution and dilution of Imuran Injection: The contents of each vial should be reconstituted by the addition of 5 ml to 15 ml Water for Injections BP. The reconstituted solution is stable for up to 5 days when stored between 5°C and 25°C.

When diluted on the basis of 5 ml of reconstituted solution added to a volume of between 20 ml and 200 ml of one of the following infusion solutions, Imuran is stable for up to 24 hours at room temperature (15°C to 25°C): Sodium Chloride Intravenous Infusion BP (0.45% w/v and 0.9% w/v); Sodium Chloride (0.18% w/v) and Glucose (4.0% w/v) Intravenous Infusion BP.

No antimicrobial preservative is included, therefore reconstitution and dilution must be carried out under full aseptic conditions, preferably immediately before use, and any unused solution discarded.

Should any visible turbidity or crystallisation appear in the reconstituted or diluted solution the preparation must be discarded.

Addition of reconstituted Imuran Injection to any other infusion solution or an intravenous admixture is not recommended.

Administration: Imuran Injection, when reconstituted as directed, results in a very irritant solution with a pH of 10 to 12.

When the reconstituted solution is diluted as directed above, the pH of the resulting solution may be expected to be within the range pH 8.0 to 9.5 (the greater the dilution, the lower the pH).

Where dilution is not practicable, the reconstituted solution should be injected slowly over a period of not less than one minute and followed immediately by not less than 50 ml of one of the recommended infusion solutions.

Care must be taken to avoid perivenous injection which may produce tissue damage. Should this occur accidentally, the injection/infusion should be stopped immediately and appropriate local therapy instituted.

It is recommended that the handling of Imuran Injection follows the 'Guidelines for the Handling of Cytotoxic Drugs' issued by the Royal Pharmaceutical Society of Great Britain Working Party on the Handling of Cytotoxic Drugs.

Imuran Tablets should not be divided.

Provided that the film coating is intact, there is no risk in handling film-coated Imuran Tablets.

Contra-indications, warnings, etc

Contra-indications: Imuran is contra-indicated in patients known to be hypersensitive to azathioprine. Hypersensitivity to 6-mercaptopurine (6-MP) should alert the prescriber to probable hypersensitivity to Imuran.

Imuran therapy should not be initiated in patients known to be pregnant.

Precautions: There are potential hazards in the use of this preparation. Therefore, it should not be prescribed unless the patient can be adequately monitored for toxic effects throughout the duration of the therapy.

During the first eight weeks of therapy with Imuran complete blood counts, including platelet counts, must be performed at least weekly (and more frequently when higher dosages are used or in the presence of disturbed renal or hepatic function). The blood count frequency may be reduced later in therapy, but it is recommended that complete blood counts are repeated at intervals of not longer than three months.

Patients receiving Imuran should be instructed to report immediately any evidence of infections, unexpected bruising or bleeding or other manifestations of bone marrow depression.

Chromosomal abnormalities, which can occur independently of the influence of Imuran, have been demonstrated in both male and female transplant recipients.

Chromosomal abnormalities which disappear in time have been demonstrated in offspring of transplant recipients. Except in extremely rare cases, no overt physical evidence of abnormality has been observed in these offspring.

There is no clear evidence that, in therapeutic dosages, azathioprine *per se* is oncogenic in man, but the issue remains unresolved.

Immunosuppressed patients are at greater risk of developing atypical lymphomata than the general population. Renal transplant recipients in some geographical areas are at greater risk of skin cancers than those in other areas.

Drug interactions: Allopurinol/oxipurinol/thiopurinol: Xanthine oxidase activity is inhibited by allopurinol, oxipurinol and thiopurinol which results in reduced conversion of biologically active 6-thioinosinic acid to biologically inactive 6-thiouric acid. When allopurinol, oxipurinol and/or thiopurinol are given concomitantly with 6-mercaptopurine (6-MP) or azathioprine, the dose of 6-MP and azathioprine should be reduced to one-quarter of the original dose.

Neuromuscular blocking agents: Imuran can potentiate the neuromuscular blockade produced by depolarising agents such as succinylcholine and reduce the blockade produced by non-depolarising agents such as tubocurarine.

Cytostatic agents: Imuran should be used with caution in patients receiving, or who have recently received, other bone marrow suppressive agents.

Others: Interactions between Imuran and cimetidine, penicillamine and frusemide have been alleged, but the nature and clinical significance has yet to be defined.

Side- and adverse effects: Several different clinical syndromes, which appear to be of an idiosyncratic hypersensitivity nature, have been described occasionally. They include general malaise, dizziness, vomiting, fever, rigors, muscular pains, arthralgia, disturbed liver function, cholestatic jaundice, cardiac dysrhythmia and hypotension. In many cases, re-challenge has confirmed an association with Imuran.

It has been suggested that the imidazole side-chain gives rise to hypersensitivity, whereas the 6-mercaptopurine (6-MP) molecule gives rise to cholestasis.

Immediate withdrawal of azathioprine and supportive circulatory measures have led to recovery in the majority of cases. Other marked underlying pathology has contributed to the very rare deaths reported.

Imuran should be PERMANENTLY withdrawn after any such clinical syndrome.

Therapeutic use of Imuran is associated with reversible, dose-related increases in mean corpuscular volume and red cell haemoglobin content. Megaloblastic bone marrow changes have been observed, but severe megaloblastic anaemia and erythroid hypoplasia are rare.

Therapeutic use of Imuran is associated with a reversible, dose-related reduction in numbers of circulating total white cells, granulocytes and lymphocytes, an effect which has been used to monitor patient response.

Therapeutic use of Imuran is associated with a dose-related, generally reversible, depression of bone marrow function, most frequently expressed as leucopenia, but also sometimes as anaemia and thrombocytopenia.

Failure to reduce the dosage of Imuran in the presence of allopurinol can result in severe bone marrow suppression and pancytopenia.

Hair loss has been described in 50% of renal transplant recipients receiving Imuran and corticosteroids, but does not appear to be a major problem when Imuran is used for other indications. It is reversible in over 80% of cases despite continuing immunosuppression.

Transplant recipients receiving Imuran and corticosteroids have shown increased susceptibility to viral, fungal and bacterial infections evident both in skin and other body systems. The use of Imuran in other conditions does not appear to give rise to increased susceptibility to such infections.

A minority of patients experience nausea when first given Imuran. This appears to be relieved by administering the tablets after meals.

Serious complications, including bowel perforation, have been described in transplant recipients and appear to relate to high dosage of corticosteroids rather than to Imuran *per se*.

Pancreatitis has been reported in a small percentage of patients on Imuran therapy, particularly in renal transplant patients and those diagnosed as having inflammatory bowel disease. There are difficulties in relating the pancreatitis to the administration of one particular drug, although re-challenge has confirmed an association with Imuran on occasions.

Reversible pneumonitis has been described very rarely.

Use in pregnancy and lactation: The decision to maintain or discontinue Imuran during pregnancy, or to terminate the pregnancy, depends on the condition under treatment in which the maternal wellbeing has to be weighed against possible risks to the foetus. As a general rule, Imuran therapy should not be initiated in patients known to be pregnant.

Azathioprine and/or its metabolites have been found in low concentrations in foetal blood and amniotic fluid.

The rare possibility of neonatal leucopenia and/or thrombocytopenia which may not be clinically evident appears to be preventable by reducing maternal dosage of Imuran if, at 32 weeks' gestation, the maternal leucocyte count is at or below 8.6×10^9 per litre.

Studies in pregnant rats, mice and rabbits using azathioprine in dosages from 5–15 mg/kg bodyweight/day over the period of organogenesis have shown varying degrees of foetal abnormalities. Teratogenicity was evident in rabbits at 10 mg/kg bodyweight/day.

Epidemiological evidence in man indicates that the frequency of occurrence of congenital abnormalities in the offspring of maternal transplant recipients is similar to that in the general population.

Azathioprine and/or its metabolites have not been demonstrated in the breast milk of patients receiving Imuran.

Relief of chronic progressive renal failure by renal transplantation involving the use of Imuran has been accompanied by increased fertility in both male and female transplant recipients.

Toxicity and treatment of overdosage: Unexplained infection, ulceration of the throat, bruising and bleeding are the main signs of overdosage with Imuran and result from bone marrow depression which may be maximal after 9–14 days. These signs are more likely to be manifest following chronic overdosage, rather than after a single acute overdose. Occasional reports describe ingestion of from 0.5–7.5 g Imuran on a single occasion with apparently uneventful recovery.

Treatment is symptomatic and has included gastric lavage. Azathioprine is dialysable but the procedure is of doubtful value since azathioprine is rapidly metabolised with entry of metabolites into tissue cells.

Pharmaceutical precautions

Tablets: Store below 25°C. Protect from light.
Injection: Store below 25°C. Protect from light. Keep dry.

Legal category POM.

Package quantities

Imuran Tablets 25 mg: Blister packs of 100 as 10 blister strips of 10 tablets.
Imuran Tablets 50 mg: Blister packs of 100 as 10 blister strips of 10 tablets and 1000 tablets.
Imuran Injection: Single vials.

Further information Nil.

Product licence numbers

Tablets 25 mg	0003/0225
Tablets 50 mg	0003/0226
Injection	0003/5043R

NOVO NORDISK WELLCOME INSULINS

HUMAN VELOSULIN* HUMAN INSULATARD* HUMAN MIXTARD* 30/70 HUMAN INITARD* 50/50

Presentation

Human Velosulin (Neutral Insulin Injection) is a clear neutral solution of highly purified human insulin (emp).

Human Insulatard (Isophane Insulin Injection, NPH) is a cloudy neutral suspension of highly purified microcrystalline human insulin (emp).

Human Mixtard 30/70 is a cloudy neutral suspension of highly purified human insulin (emp) comprising 30% Neutral Insulin in solution and 70% Isophane Insulin in microcrystalline form.

Human Initard 50/50 is a cloudy neutral suspension of highly purified human insulin (emp) comprising 50% Neutral Insulin in solution and 50% Isophane Insulin in microcrystalline form.

All the above insulins are available in 10 ml vials containing 100 IU/ml and are buffered with Sodium Phosphate PhEur 2.4 mg/ml. Human Velosulin is preserved with m-Cresol BP 3.0 mg/ml; and Human Insulatard, Human Mixtard 30/70 and Human Initard 50/50 are preserved with m-Cresol BP 1.5 mg/ml and Phenol BP 0.6 mg/ml.

The vials are fitted with tamper evident orange-coloured disposable plastic caps as a security safeguard. No attempt should be made to refit the caps after removal. Additionally, to aid identification, by those with visual impairment, Human Velosulin has one, Human Insulatard two, Human Mixtard 30/70 three and Human Initard 50/50 four raised tactile marks on the aluminium closure ring.

Uses For the treatment of insulin-requiring diabetic patients.

Human Velosulin has a rapid onset and a short duration of action, making it particularly suitable for the treatment of diabetic coma and pre-coma.

Human Mixtard 30/70 contains 30% soluble insulin and 70% isophane insulin designed to avoid the necessity for self titration in the majority of patients requiring a combination of quick and intermediate acting insulin.

Human Initard 50/50 contains a higher ratio of neutral insulin in solution and should be used when a more intense initial effect is required.

Dosage and administration The dosage of insulin is determined by the physician according to the needs of the patient.

Human Velosulin may be given by subcutaneous, intramuscular or intravenous injection, or infusion.

Human Insulatard, Human Mixtard 30/70 and Human Initard 50/50 may be given by subcutaneous or intramuscular injection. The suspension should be well mixed by gently inverting the vial several times prior to drawing up the insulin. The patient should then check that the insulin suspension appears a uniform cloudy grey/white which indicates that the isophone crystals have been completely resuspended. Care should be taken to avoid accidental intravascular injection.

Human Velosulin and Human Insulatard may be mixed together, or with Human Mixtard 30/70 and Human Initard 50/50 in all proportions without changing the characteristic effect of any of the types of insulin.

The injection site should be changed regularly according to a set routine.

Subcutaneous injection: Human Velosulin has an onset of action of approximately half an hour after subcutaneous injection with a duration of about 8 hours, the maximum effect being exerted between 1 and 3 hours after injection.

Human Insulatard has an onset of action of approximately $1\frac{1}{2}$ hours with a duration of action of up to 24 hours, the maximum effect being exerted 4 to 12 hours after injection.

Human Mixtard 30/70 and Human Initard 50/50 have an onset of action of about half an hour with a duration of action of up to 24 hours. A maximum effect is exerted 4–8 hours after injection, Human Initard 50/50 having a stronger initial effect than Human Mixtard 30/70.

Intramuscular injection: Following intramuscular injection, the onset of action is more rapid, while the overall duration of action is shorter, provided the injection site is well perfused muscle.

Use in pregnancy and lactation: It is important to maintain continuous good glycaemic control during conception and throughout pregnancy. In insulin-requiring pregnant diabetic patients, insulin requirements generally fall during the first trimester and increase during the second and third trimesters.

Use in the elderly: Clearance rates may be reduced in the elderly due to declining renal function. Insulin may therefore have a more prolonged action. Dose requirements should be regularly reviewed.

Contra-indications, warnings, etc

Contra-indications: Insulin is contra-indicated in hypoglycaemia.

Precautions: Variations in lifestyle and other factors, e.g. infection and pregnancy, can affect insulin requirements.

Patients whose blood glucose control is greatly improved, e.g. by intensified insulin therapy, may lose some or all of the warning symptoms of hypoglycaemia, and should be advised accordingly.

Some patients previously treated with insulin of beef or pork origin may require a dosage adjustment on transfer to highly purified human insulin (emp). This is more likely in patients previously treated with beef or mixed beef/port insulin.

Hypoglycaemia may be precipitated by some drugs including the following: – aspirin; sulphonylureas and agents affecting them; and certain steroids. Hypoglycaemia may also occur following excessive physical activity, alcohol intake or reduced food intake.

Hyperglycaemia can be enhanced by drugs including the following: triiodothyronine; thyroxine; various natural and synthetic steroids, including some oral contraceptives; diuretics including thiazides; and cyclophosphamide.

Certain beta-blockers, especially propranolol, may affect insulin requirements and mask the signs of hypoglycaemia mediated by the sympathetic nervous system. Monoamine oxidase inhibitors (MAOI) may potentiate the action of insulin.

A few patients have reported that after being transferred to human insulin, their early warning symptoms for hypoglycaemia were less pronounced than they had been with beef or porcine insulin. Patients should be alerted to this possibility on being transferred to human insulin.

Side-and adverse effects: The most important side-effect is hypoglycaemia. Reduction of hyperglycaemia in newly diagnosed diabetic patients may alter visual refraction.

Insulin, and protamine, like any other injected proteins are potentially immunogenic. This may or may not have clinical implications. Local reactions at the injection site may include transient erythema, induration, urticaria and oedema. The incidence is minimal with highly purified human insulin (emp) and these usually resolve with continuing insulin usage. True generalised hypersensitivity reactions approaching anaphylaxis are very rare.

Clinical evidence suggests that highly purified human insulins (emp) is unlikely to cause localised lipodystrophy. However, at present, this possibility cannot be totally excluded.

Toxicity and treatment of overdosage: The symptoms and signs of hypoglycaemia depend on the patient's clinical state and on the rate and extent of the fall in blood glucose levels.

If possible, glucose, sucrose, or rapidly absorbable carbohydrate should be taken by mouth. Failing this, hypoglycaemia should be reversed as rapidly as possible by intravenous injection of glucose 50% solution. Alternative emergency treatments include the subcutaneous injection of up to 1 ml of adrenaline solution 1:1000 or the subcutaneous, intramuscular or intravenous injection of lyophilised glucagon 0.5–1.0 mg (1 unit = 1.0 mg). Both adrenaline and glucagon injections mobilise hepatic glycogen, but this effect is short lived and must be supplemented by freely available carbohydrate as soon as possible.

Pharmaceutical precautions Store at a temperature between 2 and 8°C, protected from sunlight. The shelf life is 3 years from the date of manufacture. Insulin which has been frozen should not be used.

Legal category P.

Package quantities 10 ml glass vials in individual cartons.

Further information Nil.

Product licence numbers

Human Velosulin	3132/0031
Human Insulatard	3132/0034
Human Mixtard 30/70	3132/0037
Human Initard 50/50	3132/0040

Product licence holder: Novo Nordisk Pharmaceuticals Ltd, Crawley.

VELOSULIN* INSULATARD* MIXTARD* 30/70 INITARD* 50/50

Presentation Velosulin (Neutral Insulin Injection BP) is a clear neutral solution of highly purified pork insulin.

Insulatard (Isophane Insulin Injection BP [NPH]) is a cloudy neutral suspension of highly purified microcrystalline pork insulin.

Mixtard 30/70 is a cloudy neutral suspension of highly purified pork insulin comprising 30% Neutral Insulin in solution and 70% Isophane Insulin in microcrystalline form.

Initard 50/50 is a cloudy neutral suspension of highly purified pork insulin comprising 50% Neutral Insulin in solution and 50% Isophane Insulin in microcrystalline form.

All the above insulins are available in 100 units/ml strength and are buffered with Sodium Phosphate PhEur 2.4 mg/ml. Velosulin is preserved with m-Cresol BP 3 mg/ml and Insulatard, Mixtard 30/70 and Initard 50/50 are preserved with m-Cresol BP 1.5 mg/ml and Phenol BP 0.6 mg/ml. The vials are fitted with orange coloured disposable plastic caps as a security safeguard. No attempt should be made to refit the caps after removal. Additionally, to aid identification, Velosulin has one, Insulatard two, Mixtard 30/70 three and Initard 50/50 four raised tactile marks on the aluminium closure ring.

Uses The treatment of insulin-requiring diabetic patients. Velosulin has a rapid onset and a short duration of action making it particularly suitable for the treatment of diabetic coma and pre-coma.

Dosage and administration The dosage of insulin is determined by the physician according to the needs of the patient. Velosulin, Insulatard, Mixtard 30/70 and Initard 50/50 may be mixed in all proportions without changing the characteristic effect of any of the types of insulin.

Velosulin may be given by subcutaneous, intramuscular or intravenous injection or infusion. It has an onset of action of approximately 30 minutes after subcutaneous injection with duration of about 8 hours, the maximum effect being 1 to 3 hours after injection.

Insulatard, Mixtard 30/70 and Initard 50/50 should be well mixed by gently inverting the vial several times before being given by subcutaneous or intramuscular injection. Insulatard, Mixtard 30/70 and Initard 50/50 should not be given intravenously.

Insulatard has an onset of action of approximately $1\frac{1}{2}$ hours after subcutaneous injection with an overall duration of action which may extend to 24 hours, the maximum effect occurring 4 to 12 hours after injection.

Mixtard 30/70 and Initard 50/50 each have a duration of action of some $\frac{1}{2}$ to 24 hours after subcutaneous injection, the maximum effect occurring 4 to 8 hours after injection. Initard 50/50 has a stronger initial effect than Mixtard 30/70.

Onset of action is more rapid and overall duration of action shorter following intramuscular injection than with the subcutaneous route assuming adequate vascular perfusion.

Use in pregnancy and lactation: It is essential to maintain continuous good glycaemic control throughout pregnancy. In the insulin-treated (gestational or insulin-dependent) pregnant diabetic patient, the insulin requirements fall during the first trimester and increase during the second and third trimesters.

Use in the elderly: Clearance rates may be reduced in the elderly due to falling renal function. Insulin may therefore have a more prolonged action. Dose requirements should be regularly reviewed.

Contra-indications, warnings, etc
Contra-indications: Insulin is contra-indicated in hypoglycaemia.

Precautions: Variations in lifestyle and other factors, eg. infection and pregnancy, can affect insulin requirements.

Patients whose blood glucose control is greatly improved, e.g. by intensified insulin therapy, may lose some or all of the warning symptoms of hypoglycaemia, and should be advised accordingly.

Some patients previously treated with insulin of beef or mixed beef/pork origin may require a dosage adjustment on transfer to highly purified pork insulin.

Hypoglycaemia can be enhanced by drugs including the following: aspirin; sulphonylureas and agents affecting them; certain steroids.

Hyperglycaemia can be enhanced by drugs including the following: triiodothyronine; thyroxine; various natural and synthetic steroids, including some oral contraceptives; diuretics, including thiazides; cyclophosphamide.

Certain beta-blockers, especially propranolol, may affect insulin requirements and mask the signs of hypoglycaemia mediated by the sympathetic nervous system.

Monoamine oxidase inhibitors (MAOI) may potentiate the action of insulin.

Side-and adverse effects: The most important side-effect is hypoglycaemia. Reduction of hyperglycaemia in newly diagnosed diabetics may alter visual refraction.

Insulin, and protamine, like any other injected proteins, are potentially immunogenic. This may or may not have clinical implications. Local reactions at the injection site may include transient erythema, induration, urticaria and oedema. The incidence is minimal with highly purified pork insulin. These usually resolve with continuing usage of insulin. True generalised hypersensitivity reactions approaching anaphylaxis are very rare.

Clinical evidence suggests that highly purified pork insulins are unlikely to cause localised lipodystrophies. However, at present, this possibility cannot be totally excluded.

Toxicity and treatment of overdosage: The symptoms and signs of hypoglycaemia depend on the patient's clinical state and on the rate and extent of the fall in blood glucose levels.

If possible, glucose, sucrose, or rapidly absorbable carbohydrate should be taken by mouth. Failing this, hypoglycaemia should be reversed as rapidly as possible by intravenous injection of glucose 50% solution. Alternative emergency treatments include the subcutaneous injection of up to 1 ml of adrenaline solution 1:1000 or the subcutaneous, intramuscular or intravenous injection of lyophilised glucagon 0.5–1.0 mg (1 unit = 1.0 mg). Both adrenaline and glucagon injections mobilise hepatic glycogen, but the effect is short lived and must be supplemented by freely available carbohydrate as soon as possible.

Pharmaceutical precautions Nordisk Wellcome highly purified pork insulins should be stored between 2 and 8°C, protected from sunlight. Under these storage conditions Nordisk Wellcome highly purified pork insulins have a shelf life of 3 years from date of manufacture. Insulin which has been frozen should not be used.

Legal category P.

Package quantities 10 ml glass vials.

Further information Mixing of these highly purified pork insulins with preparations of other species is not recommended.

Product licence numbers

Velosulin	3132/0019
Insulatard	3132/0018
Mixtard 30/70	3132/0021
Initard 50/50	3132/0020

Product licence holder: Novo Nordisk Pharmaceuticals Ltd, Crawley.

VELOSULIN* CARTRIDGE
Neutral Insulin Injection BP, highly purified pork

Presentation Velosulin Cartridge is a clear neutral solution of highly purified pork insulin available in 5.7 ml glass cartridge vials containing 100 iu/ml for use only in the Nordisk Infuser*. Other ingredients include buffer (Sodium Phosphate PhEur 2.4 mg/ml) and preservative (Phenol BP 0.6 mg/ml).

Uses The treatment of insulin-requiring diabetic patients. To be used only with the Nordisk Infuser.

Dosage and administration Velosulin Cartridge is intended to be administered as subcutaneous infusion using the Nordisk Wellcome Infuser System.

Basal rate and prandial doses are to be determined by the physician according to the needs of the patient.

Velosulin Cartridge should only be used with the infusion set supplied with the Nordisk Infuser. No attempt should be made to refill the cartridges. When empty, they should be discarded and a fresh cartridge inserted. In order to minimise the risk of infusion site irritation or infection, it is recommended that the infusion set is changed every 2–3 days. The infusion site should be cleansed thoroughly and the needle taped securely in place. The infusion site should be changed according to a suitable routine and should be cleansed regularly. The procedure (given in the User's Manual) should be followed when the cartridge or infusion set is changed. The maximum in-use life of Velosulin Cartridge used in the Nordisk Infuser is 14 days.

Velosulin Cartridge is stable at normal Infuser operating temperatures (30–37°C if worn under outdoor clothing), although care must be taken to avoid extremes of temperature, eg. when sunbathing, winter sports, etc.

Use in pregnancy and lactation: It is essential to maintain continuous good glycaemic control throughout pregnancy. In the insulin-treated (gestational or insulin-dependent) pregnant diabetic patient, the insulin requirements fall in the first trimester and increase during the second and third trimesters.

Use in the elderly: No specific studies regarding continuous subcutaneous insulin infusion (CSII) in the elderly have yet been conducted. Clearance rates may be reduced in the elderly due to falling renal function. Insulin may therefore have a more prolonged action. Dose requirements should be regularly reviewed.

Contra-indications, warnings, etc

Contra-indications: Insulin is contra-indicated in hypoglycaemia.

Precautions: Variations in lifestyle and other factors, eg. infection and pregnancy, can affect insulin requirements.

Patients whose blood glucose control is greatly improved, e.g. by intensified insulin therapy, may lose some or all of the warning symptoms of hypoglycaemia, and should be advised accordingly.

Patients previously treated by subcutaneous insulin injection may require a dosage adjustment when transferred to subcutaneous infusion.

Hypoglycaemia can be enhanced by drugs including the following: aspirin; sulphonylureas, and agents affecting them; certain steroids.

Hyperglycaemia can be enhanced by drugs including the following: triiodothyronine; thyroxine; various natural and synthetic steroids, including some oral contraceptives; diuretics, including thiazides; cyclophosphamide.

Certain beta-blockers, especially propranolol, may affect insulin requirements and mask the signs of hypoglycaemia mediated by the sympathetic nervous system.

Monoamine oxidase inhibitors (MAOI) may potentiate the action of insulin.

Side-and adverse effects: The most important side-effect is hypoglycaemia. Reduction of hyperglycaemia in newly diagnosed diabetics may alter visual refraction.

Insulin, like many other injected substances, is potentially immunogenic. This may or may not have clinical implications. Local reactions at the infusion site may include transient erythema, induration, urticaria and oedema. The incidence is minimal with highly purified pork insulin. These usually resolve with continuing usage of insulin. True generalised hypersensitivity reactions approaching anaphylaxis are very rare.

Clinical evidence suggests that highly purified pork insulins are unlikely to cause localised lipodystrophies. However, at present, this possibility cannot be totally excluded.

Toxicity and treatment of overdosage: The symptoms and signs of hypoglycaemia depend on the patient's clinical state and on the rate and extent of the fall in blood glucose levels.

Infusion with Velosulin Cartridge should be reduced or suspended until normal blood glucose levels are restored.

If possible, glucose, sucrose, or rapidly absorbable carbohydrate should be taken by mouth. Failing this, hypoglycaemia should be reversed as rapidly as possible by intravenous injection of glucose 50% solution. Alternative emergency treatments include the subcutaneous injection of up to 1 ml of adrenaline solution 1:1000 or the subcutaneous, intramuscular or intravenous injection of lyophilised glucagon 0.5–1.0 mg (1 unit = 1.0 mg). Both adrenaline and glucagon injections mobilise hepatic glycogen, but the effect is short lived and must be supplemented by freely available carbohydrate as soon as possible.

Pharmaceutical precautions Velosulin Cartridge should be stored between 2 and 8°C, protected from sunlight. Insulin which has been frozen should not be used. Velosulin Cartridge insulin which appears turbid (cloudy) should not be used.

Legal category P.

Package quantities 1 × 5.7 ml glass cartridge vials.

Further information Nil.

Product licence number 3132/0043

Product licence holder: Novo Nordisk Pharmaceuticals Ltd, Crawley.

KEMADRIN* TABLETS AND INJECTION

Presentation *Tablets:* Each white tablet containing 5 mg Procyclidine Hydrochloride BP is scored and coded 'WELLCOME S3A'.

Injection: Each 2 ml ampoule contains 10 mg Procyclidine Hydrochloride BP.

Uses Kemadrin is indicated in all forms of Parkinson's disease: idiopathic (paralysis agitans), postencephalitic and arteriosclerotic.

Symptoms often responding well to Kemadrin include: rigidity, akinesia, tremor, speech and writing difficulties, gait, sialorrhoea and drooling, sweating, oculogyric crises and depressed mood.

Kemadrin is also used to control troublesome extrapyramidal symptoms induced by neuroleptic drugs including pseudo-parkinsonism, acute dystonic reactions and akathisia.

Dosage and administration The variation in optimum dosage from one patient to another should be taken into consideration by the physician. Treatment is usually started at 2.5 mg three times a day, increasing by 2.5–5 mg daily at intervals of two or three days until the optimum clinical response is achieved. The usual maximum total daily dose is 30 mg. However, at the discretion of the attending physician where appropriate this total may be as high as 60 mg.

The daily dosage used in the control of neuroleptic-induced extrapyramidal symptoms is usually not more than 20 mg daily. After a period of 3–4 months, Kemadrin should be stopped and the patient observed to see if the neuroleptic-induced extrapyramidal symptoms recur. Cessation of treatment periodically is to be recommended even in patients who appear to require the drug for longer periods.

Avoid abrupt discontinuation of treatment.

Kemadrin may be combined with levodopa or amantadine in patients who are inadequately controlled on a single agent.

In acute dystonia 5 mg Kemadrin intravenously is frequently effective within 5 minutes. An occasional patient may need 10 mg or more and may require up to half an hour to obtain relief.

Kemadrin Injection may be given intramuscularly in doses of 5–10 mg repeated after 20 minutes if necessary, up to a daily maximum of 20 mg.

Children: Not applicable.

Use in the elderly: Elderly patients are more sensitive to anticholinergics, and a reduced dose may be required.

Pharmacology: Procyclidine is a synthetic anticholinergic agent which blocks the excitatory effects of acetylcholine at the muscarinic receptor.

Idiopathic Parkinson's disease is now thought to result from degeneration of neurones in the substantia nigra whose axons project and inhibit cells in the corpus striatum. Blockade by neuroleptic drugs of the dopamine released by these terminals produces a similar clinical picture. The cell bodies in the corpus striatum also receive cholinergic innervation which is excitatory. Relief of the parkinsonian syndrome can be achieved either by potentiation of the dopaminergic system or blockade of the cholinergic input by anticholinergics. It is by a central action of this latter type that procyclidine exerts its effect.

Procyclidine is adequately absorbed from the gastro-intestinal tract and disappears rapidly from the tissues. After intravenous administration it acts within 5 to 20 minutes with a duration of up to 4 hours. After both oral and IV dosing the mean values for volume of distribution, total body clearance and plasma elimination half-life of procyclidine were of the order of 1 litre/kg, 68 ml/min and 12 hours respectively.

Contra-indications, warnings, etc
Contra-indications: Tardive dyskinesias.

Precautions: As with all anticholinergics such as Kemadrin, cautious prescribing is indicated in patients predisposed to glaucoma, obstructive disease of the gastro-intestinal tract, those with urinary symptoms associated with prostatic hypertrophy and in hepatic and renal impairment.

In a proportion of patients undergoing neuroleptic treatment, tardive dyskinesias will occur. While anticholinergic agents do not cause this syndrome, when given in combination with neuroleptics they may reduce the threshold at which dyskinesias appear in patients predisposed to this abnormality. In such individuals subsequent adjustment of neuroleptic therapy is indicated.
Drug interactions: The anticholinergic activity of Kemadrin may be increased by agents having anticholinergic activity, e.g. antidepressants (e.g. amitriptyline), phenothiazines, (e.g. thioridazine), amantadine and disopyramide. The absorption of ketoconazole may be reduced by concomitant administration of Kemadrin.

Use in pregnancy and lactation: The safety of using Kemadrin during pregnancy has not been established. However, extensive clinical use has not given any evidence that it in any way compromises the normal course of pregnancy. No data are available on the excretion of this drug in breast milk.

Side- and adverse effects: The main side-effects are those to be expected from any anticholinergic agent. Dry mouth, blurring of vision and constipation are most commonly recorded. At higher doses dizziness, mental confusion and hallucinations may occur. The unwanted anticholinergic effects are easily reversed by reducing the dosage.

In rare instances, Kemadrin administered for the treatment of neuroleptic-induced symptoms was associated with an apparent worsening of the patient's state.

Toxicity and treatment of overdosage: Reports of overdosage are relatively rare. Symptoms of overdosage are agitation, restlessness and confusion with severe sleeplessness lasting up to 24 hours or more. Visual and occasionally auditory hallucinations are likely. Most subjects are euphoric but the occasional patient may be anxious and aggressive. The pupils are widely dilated and unreactive to light. In recorded cases, the disorientation has lasted 1 to 4 days and ended in recuperative sleep.

If procyclidine has been ingested within the previous hour or two (or possibly longer in view of its likely effects on gastric motility) then gastric lavage is probably indicated. Other active measures such as the use of cholinergic agents or haemodialysis are extremely unlikely to be of clinical value, although if convulsions occur they should be controlled by injections of diazepam.

Pharmaceutical precautions *Tablets and injection:* Store below 25°C.

Legal category POM.

Package quantities Bottles of 100 and 500 tablets. Ampoules of 10 mg in 2 ml. Box of 5 ampoules.

Further information Nil.

Product licence numbers
Tablets 0003/5255R
Injection 0003/5256R

LANOXIN* TABLETS
LANOXIN-125* TABLETS
LANOXIN-PG* TABLETS
LANOXIN* INJECTION
LANOXIN-PG* ELIXIR

Presentation Lanoxin tablets each contain 250 micrograms (0.25 mg) of Digoxin BP, scored and coded 'WELLCOME X3A', white in colour.

Lanoxin-125 Tablets each contain 125 micrograms (0.125 mg) of Digoxin BP coded 'WELLCOME Y3B', white in colour.

Lanoxin-PG (Paediatric/Geriatric) Tablets each contain 62.5 micrograms (0.0625 mg) of Digoxin BP, coded 'WELLCOME U3A' and coloured blue.

Lanoxin Injection contains 250 micrograms (0.25 mg) of Digoxin BP per ml in each 2 ml ampoule.

Lanoxin-PG (Paediatric/Geriatric) Elixir contains 50 micrograms (0.050 mg) of Digoxin BP in each ml. Clear bright yellow in colour and lime flavoured.

Uses Lanoxin is indicated in the management of heart failure.

Lanoxin is indicated in the management of certain supraventricular arrhythmias, particularly atrial flutter and fibrillation, where its major beneficial effect is the reduction of the ventricular rate.

Dosage and administration The dose of Lanoxin for each patient has to be tailored individually according to age, lean body weight and renal function. Suggested doses are intended only as an initial guide.

Lanoxin PG Elixir, 50 micrograms in 1 ml, is supplied with a graduated pipette and this should be used for measurement of all doses.

Adults and children over 10 years
Rapid oral loading: 750 to 1500 micrograms (0.75 to 1.5 mg) as a single dose.

Where there is less urgency, or a greater risk of toxicity e.g. in the elderly, the oral loading dose should be given in divided doses 6 hours apart, assessing clinical response before giving each additional dose (see *Precautions*).

Slow oral loading: 250 to 750 micrograms (0.25 to 0.75 mg) should be given daily for 1 week followed by an appropriate maintenance dose. A clinical response should be seen within one week.

NOTE: The choice between slow and rapid oral loading depends on the clinical state of the patient and the urgency of the condition.

Maintenance: The maintenance dosage should be based upon the percentage of the peak body stores lost each day through elimination. The following formula has had wide clinical use:

$$\text{Maintenance dose} = \text{Peak body stores} \times \frac{\%\ \text{daily loss}}{100}$$

Where: Peak body stores = loading dose
% daily loss = 14 + creatinine clearance (C_{cr})/5

C_{cr} is creatinine clearance corrected to 70 kg bodyweight or 1.73 m^2 body surface area. If only serum creatinine (S_{cr}) concentrations are available, a C_{cr} (corrected to 70 kg bodyweight) may be estimated in men as

$$C_{cr} = \frac{(140 - \text{age})}{S_{cr}}$$

For women, this result should be multiplied by 0.85.

NOTE: This formula cannot be used for creatinine clearance in children.

In practice, this will mean that most patients will be maintained on 0.125 to 0.75 mg digoxin daily; however in those who show increased sensitivity to the adverse effects of digoxin, a dosage of 0.0625 mg (62.5 microgram) daily or less may suffice.

Emergency parenteral loading (In patients who have not been given cardiac glycosides within the preceding two weeks).

The loading of parenteral Lanoxin is 500 to 1000 micrograms (0.5 to 1.0 mg) depending on age, lean body weight and renal function.

The loading dose should be administered in several portions with roughly half of the total dose given as the first dose and further fractions of the total dose given at intervals of 4 to 8 hours, assessing clinical response before giving each additional dose. Each dose should be given by intravenous infusion (see *Dilution*) over 10 to 20 minutes as more rapid administration may cause generalised vasoconstriction.

Neonates, infants and children up to 10 years of age (if cardiac glycosides have not been given in the preceding two weeks): The *intravenous loading dose* in the above groups should be administered in accordance with the following schedule:

	microgram/kg over 24 hours
Preterm neonates 1.5 kg	20
Preterm neonates 1.5 kg–2.5 kg	30
Term neonates to 2 years	35
2 to 5 years	35
5 to 10 years	25

The loading dose should be administered in several portions with roughly half the total dose given as the first dose and further fractions of the total dose given at intervals of 4 to 8 hours, assessing clinical response before giving each additional dose. Each dose should be given by intravenous infusion (see *Dilution*) over 10 to 20 minutes as more rapid administration may cause generalised vasoconstriction.

Oral loading dose: This should be administered in accordance with the following schedule:

	microgram/kg over 24 hours
Preterm neonates 1.5 kg	25
Preterm neonates 1.5 kg–2.5 kg	30
Term neonates to 2 years	45
2 to 5 years	35
5 to 10 years	25

The loading dose should be administered in several portions with roughly half the total dose given as the first dose and further fractions of the total dose given at intervals of 4 to 8 hours, assessing clinical response before giving each additional dose.

Maintenance: The maintenance dose should be administered in accordance with the following schedule:

Preterm neonates: daily dose = 20% of 24-hour loading dose (intravenous or oral)

Term neonates and children up to 10 years: daily dose = 25% of 24-hour loading dose (intravenous or oral)

These dosage schedules are meant as guidelines and careful clinical observations and monitoring of plasma digoxin levels (see *Monitoring*) should be used as a basis for adjustment of dosage in these paediatric patient groups.

If cardiac glycosides have been given in the two weeks preceding commencement of Lanoxin therapy, it should be anticipated that optimum loading doses of Lanoxin will be less than those recommended above.

Dose Recommendations in Renal Disorder or with Diuretic Therapy: The dosing recommendations should be reconsidered if patients are elderly or there are other reasons for the renal clearance of digoxin being reduced, such as renal disease or renal function impairment secondary to cardiovascular disease. The prolongation of excretion in these cases requires a reduction in both initial and maintenance doses and also a greater awareness of the possibility of intoxication.

Dilution: Lanoxin Injection, 250 micrograms per ml when diluted in the ratio of 1 with 250 (i.e. one 2 ml ampoule containing 500 micrograms added to 400 ml of infusion solution) is known to be compatible with the following infusion solutions and stable for up to 48 hours at room temperature (20 to 25°C):

Sodium Chloride Intravenous Infusion BP 0.9% w/v
Sodium Chloride (0.18% w/v) and Glucose (4% w/v) Intravenous Infusion BP
Glucose Intravenous Infusion BP 5% w/v

Dilution should be carried out either under full aseptic conditions or immediately before use. Any unused solution should be discarded.

Monitoring: The plasma concentration of digoxin can be determined by radioimmunassay. Blood should be taken 6 hours or more after the last dose of Lanoxin. There are no rigid guidelines as to the range of plasma concentrations that are most efficacious but most patients will benefit, with little risk of toxic symptoms developing, with digoxin concentrations from 0.8 nanogram/ml (ng/ml) (1.00 nanoMol/litre, nM/L) to 2.0 ng/ml (2.56 nM/L). Above this range toxic symptoms and signs become more frequent and levels above 3.0 ng/ml (3.74 nM/L) are quite likely to be toxic. However, in deciding whether a patient's symptoms are due to digoxin, the patient's clinical state together with the potassium level and thyroid function are important factors.

Other glycosides including metabolites of digoxin can interfere with the assays that are available and one should always be wary of values which do not seem commensurate with the clinical state of the patient.

Use in the elderly: The dosing recommendations should be reconsidered if patients are elderly or there are other reasons for the renal clearance of digoxin being reduced, such as renal disease or renal function impairment secondary to cardiovascular disease. The prolongation of excretion in these cases requires a reduction in both initial and maintenance doses and also a greater awareness of the possibility of intoxication.

Contra-indications, warnings, etc

Contra-indications: Lanoxin is contra-indicated in intermittent complete heart block or second degree atrioventricular block, especially if there is a history of Stokes Adams attacks.

Lanoxin is contra-indicated in arrhythmias caused by cardiac glycoside intoxication.

Lanoxin is contra-indicated in supraventricular arrhythmias associated with Wolff-Parkinson-White syndrome unless the precise electrophysical characteristics of the accessory tract are known.

Lanoxin is contra-indicated in hypertrophic obstructive cardiomyopathy, unless there is concomitant atrial fibrillation and heart failure, but even then caution should be exercised if digoxin is to be used.

Precautions: Arrhythmias may be precipitated by digoxin toxicity, some of which can resemble arrhythmias for which the drug could be advised. For example, atrial tachycardia with varying atrioventricular block requires particular care as clinically the rhythm resembles atrial fibrillation.

Determination of the plasma digoxin concentration may be very helpful in making a decision to treat with further digoxin, but toxic doses of other glycosides may cross-react in the assay and wrongly suggest apparently satisfactory measurements. Observations during the temporary withholding of digoxin might be more appropriate.

In cases where cardiac glycosides have been taken in the preceding two weeks the recommendations for initial dosing of a patient should be reconsidered and a reduced dose is advised.

Hypokalaemia sensitises the myocardium to the cardiac glycosides. Hypokalaemia may arise from treatment with diuretics, corticosteroids, peritoneal or haemodialysis, suction of gastro-intestinal secretions, ion-exchange resins and carbenoxolone treatment. Hypokalaemia may accompany malnutrition, diarrhoea, vomiting, long standing wasting diseases and cardiac failure.

Hypercalcaemia and hypomagnesaemia may increase myocardial sensitivity but are probably of less clinical importance.

Rapid intravenous injection can cause vasoconstriction producing hypertension and/or reduced coronary flow. A slow injection rate is therefore important in hypertensive heart failure and acute myocardial infarction.

Administering Lanoxin to a patient with thyroid disease requires care. Initial and maintenance doses of Lanoxin should be reduced when thyroid function is subnormal. In hyperthyroidism there is relative digoxin resistance and the dose may have to be increased. If Lanoxin is prescribed during the course of treatment of thyrotoxicosis, the dosage should be reduced as the thyrotoxicosis comes under control.

Patients with malabsorption syndrome or gastro-intestinal reconstructions may require larger doses of digoxin.

The risk of provoking dangerous arrhythmias with direct current cardioversion is greatly increased in the presence of digitalis toxicity and is in proportion to the cardioversion energy used.

For elective direct current cardioversion of a patient who is taking digoxin, the drug should be withheld for 24 hours before cardioversion is performed. In emergencies, such as cardiac arrest, when attempting cardioversion the lowest effective energy should be applied.

Direct current cardioversion is inappropriate in the treatment of arrhythmias thought to be caused by cardiac glycosides.

Many beneficial effects of digoxin on arrhythmias result from a degree of atrioventricular conduction blockade. However, when incomplete atrioventricular block already exists the effects of a rapid progression in the block should be anticipated. In complete heart block the idioventricular escape rhythm may be suppressed.

The administration of digoxin in the period immediately following myocardial infarction is not contra-indicated. However, the possibility of arrhythmias arising in patients who may be hypokalaemic after myocardial infarction and are likely to be cardiologically unstable must be borne in mind. The limitations imposed thereafter on direct current cardioversion must also be remembered.

Although many patients with chronic congestive cardiac failure benefit from acute administration of digoxin, there are some in whom it does not lead to constant, marked or lasting haemodynamic improvement. It is therefore important to evaluate the response of each patient individually when Lanoxin is continued long-term.

The intramuscular route is painful and is associated with muscle necrosis. This route cannot be recommended.

No data are available on whether or not digoxin has mutagenic, carcinogenic or teratogenic effects; however, maternally-administered digoxin has been used to treat foetal tachycardia and congestive heart failure.

There is no information available on the effect of digoxin on human fertility.

Use in pregnancy and lactation: The use of digoxin in pregnancy is not contra-indicated, although the dosage and control may be less predictable in pregnant than in non-pregnant women and some women may require an increased dosage of digoxin during pregnancy. As with all drugs, use should be considered only when the expected clinical benefit of treatment to the mother outweighs any possible risk to the developing foetus.

Although digoxin is excreted in breast milk, the quantities are minute and breast feeding is not contra-indicated.

Drug interactions: These may arise from effects on the renal excretion, tissue binding, plasma protein binding, distribution within the body, gut absorption capacity and sensitivity to Lanoxin. Consideration of the possibility of an interaction whenever concomitant therapy is contemplated is the best precaution and a check on plasma digoxin concentration is recommended when any doubt exists.

Agents causing hypokalaemia or intracellular potassium deficiency may cause increased sensitivity to Lanoxin; they include diuretics, lithium salts, corticosteroids and carbenoxolone.

Spironolactone has been reported to increase serum digoxin levels by up to 100%. Serum digoxin levels should be monitored and dose reduction anticipated when spironolactone is given with digoxin.

Quinidine reduces renal clearance of digoxin and also displaces digoxin from tissues so decreasing its volume of distribution. Concomitant administration of quinidine with Lanoxin thus raises steady-state digoxin concentration in proportion to the quinidine concentration achieved. At usual quinidine dosing the digoxin concentration thereby rises by roughly 50%. Halving the Lanoxin dosage on commencing quinidine and adjusting it later according to need is prudent because the raised digoxin concentrations can be toxic. Extra inotropy is not always observed because quinidine is a cardiac depressant.

Prazosin increases serum levels of digoxin by 50% by reducing its volume of distribution and renal clearance. Serum digoxin levels should be monitored when prazosin is co-administered.

Antacids, kaolin-pectin, some bulk laxatives and cholestyramine decrease absorption of digoxin by interaction in the gut lumen. This can be avoided by temporal separation in the dosage of the drugs. Some compounds decrease or retard absorption by decreasing motility, e.g. propantheline, diphenoxylate, or by impairing absorptive capacity, e.g. sulphasalazine, neomycin, cytostatics and phenytoin. Metoclopramide can reduce digoxin absorption by increasing its speed of transit through the intestine.

Digoxin plasma levels can be lowered by neomycin and rifampicin but other antibiotics, in individuals whose gut flora normally metabolise digoxin, may cause an increase in plasma levels and possible toxicity. Tetracycline and erythromycin have been shown to affect digoxin absorption in this way and it is possible that several other antibiotics have this effect.

Co-administration of the calcium channel blockers verapamil or nifedipine with digoxin results in elevated plasma digoxin levels. Similar effects have been reported with diltiazem, although data are conflicting.

Concurrent administration of amiodarone results in elevated plasma digoxin levels, especially in children.

It has been reported that concomitant administration of captopril may reduce digoxin clearance and cause a rise in plasma digoxin levels. Measurement of plasma digoxin levels in these circumstances would seem prudent.

Serum digoxin levels may be decreased by penicillamine, although the clinical significance of this interaction is unclear.

Side- and adverse effects: Non-cardiac: These are principally associated with overdosage but may occur from a temporarily high serum concentration due to rapid absorption. They include anorexia, nausea and vomiting and usually disappear within a few hours of taking the drug. Diarrhoea can also occur. It is inadvisable to rely on nausea as an early warning of excessive digoxin dosage as arrhythmias may occur first.

Weakness, apathy, fatigue, malaise, headache, visual disturbances, depression and even psychosis have been reported as adverse central nervous system effects. Some of these symptoms could arise in prolonged illness in which digoxin was coincidentally required. However, the possibility of too high a maintenance dose should be considered.

Oral digoxin has also been associated with intestinal ischaemia and, rarely, with intestinal necrosis.

Gynaecomastia can occur with long-term administration.

Skin rashes of urticarial or scarlatiniform character are rare reactions to digoxin, and may be accompanied by pronounced eosinophilia.

Very rarely, digoxin can cause thrombocytopenia.

Cardiac: A characteristic feature of digoxin intoxication is a combination of arrhythmias. Usually an early sign is the occurrence of ventricular premature contractions. They can proceed to bigeminy or even trigeminy. Atrial tachycardias, frequently an indication for digoxin, may nevertheless occur with excessive dosage of the drug. Atrial tachycardia with some degree of atrioventricular block is particularly characteristic, and the pulse rate may not necessarily be fast. Persistent bigeminy at rest but not on exercise when the sinus rate increases has traditionally been acceptable in the management of some arrhythmias, but it suggests approaching toxicity and a lower dose of digoxin plus a small dose of beta blocker may give better control. There are comprehensive reviews of the cardiac manifestations of digoxin toxicity in the medical literature. (See also *Precautions.*)

Toxicity and treatment of overdosage: For symptoms and signs see Side- and Adverse Effects.

Treatment: After recent ingestion, such as accidental or deliberate self-poisoning, the load awaiting absorption may be reduced by gastric lavage.

An overdosage of more than 10 mg of Lanoxin in previously healthy adults or 4 mg in previously healthy children, or overdosage resulting in steady-state concentrations greater than 10 ng/ml (7.8 microMol/L), often gives rise to life-threatening arrhythmias.

If hypokalaemia is present, it should be corrected with supplements either orally or intravenously depending on the urgency of the situation. In cases where a large amount of digoxin has been ingested, hyperkalaemia may be present due to release of potassium from skeletal muscle. Before administering potassium in digoxin overdose the plasma potassium level must be known.

Bradyarrhythmias may be treated with atropine but temporary cardiac pacing may be required in cases of severe overdosage. Atrial tachyarrhythmias may be associated with a degree of atrioventricular block and may not require treatment. Ventricular arrhythmias may respond to lignocaine or phenytoin.

Dialysis is not particularly effective in removing digoxin from the body in potentially life-threatening poisoning.

Rapid reversal of the complications that are associated with serious poisoning by digoxin, digitoxin and related glycosides has followed intravenous administration of digoxin-specific (ovine) antibody fragments (Fab) when other therapies have failed. Digibind* is the only specific treatment for digoxin toxicity and is very effective. For details consult the literature supplied with Digibind.

Pharmaceutical precautions
Tablets: Store below 25°C.
Elixir: Store below 25°C. Protect from light. Do not dilute.
Injection: Store below 25°C. Protect from light. Dilution should be carried out either under full aseptic conditions or immediately before use. Any unused solution should be discarded.

Legal category POM.

Package quantities
Lanoxin Tablets: Bottles of 500 and 1,000; container of 5,000.
Lanoxin-125 Tablets: Bottle of 500.
Lanoxin-PG Tablets: Bottles of 100 and 500.
Lanoxin Injection: Ampoule of 2 ml; box of 5 ampoules.
Lanoxin-PG Elixir: Bottle of 60 ml (OP).

Further information Intravenous administration of a loading dose produces an appreciable pharmacological effect within 5 to 30 minutes; this reaches a maximum in 1 to 5 hours.

Using the oral route, the onset of effect occurs in 0.5 to 2 hours and reaches its maximum at 2 to 6 hours.

The terminal elimination half life of digoxin in patients with normal renal function is 30 to 40 hours. It will be prolonged in patients with impaired renal function and in anuric patients will be of the order of 100 hours.

Product licence numbers

Tablets	0003/0090R
125 Tablets	0003/0102R
PG Tablets	0003/0091R
Injection	0003/5259R
PG Elixir	0003/5260R

LANVIS* TABLETS

Presentation Each pale greenish yellow biconvex tablet, scored and coded 'WELLCOME U3B', contains 40 mg Thioguanine BP.

Uses Cytotoxic agent.

The main indication is acute myeloblastic leukaemia, but it has also been used in acute lymphoblastic and chronic granulocytic (myelocytic, myeloid, myelogenous) leukaemia.

Cross-resistance exists between Lanvis and Puri-Nethol* (6-mercaptopurine) and it is not to be expected that patients who no longer respond to Puri-Nethol will respond to Lanvis or vice versa.

Dosage and administration The dosage and duration of its administration must be carefully adjusted to obtain optimum benefit without undue toxic effects.

Adults: The usual dosage of Lanvis is between 2.0 and 2.5 mg/kg body weight/day, the total daily doses being calculated to the nearest multiple of 20 mg and given at one time. The duration of drug administration will depend on the nature and dosage of other antineoplastic drugs administered with thioguanine, the patient's condition and whether early signs of toxicity occur. For induction therapy thioguanine is usually administered as one of a number of drugs for periods of 5–20 days according to the regimen adopted and the patient's tolerance.

For maintenance therapy, the usual dosage of thioguanine is 2.0 mg/kg body weight/day, but the patient must be monitored for bone-marrow toxicity, particularly if other cytotoxic drugs are given conjointly.

Children: As for adults.

Use in the elderly: No specific studies have been carried out in the elderly, however, it may be advisable to monitor renal or hepatic function and if there is serious impairment then caution should be exercised.

Consult the literature for details of various combination chemotherapy.

Contra-indications, warnings, etc
Contra-indications: In view of the seriousness of the indications there are no absolute contra-indications.

Precautions: Lanvis is an active cytotoxic agent for use only under the direction of physicians experienced in the administration of such agents.

Since Lanvis is strongly myelosuppressive, full blood counts must be taken daily during remission induction. Patients must be carefully monitored during therapy.

The main side-effect of treatment with Lanvis is bone marrow suppression leading to leucopenia and thrombocytopenia. The leucocyte and platelet counts continue to fall after treatment is stopped, so at the first sign of an abnormally large fall in the counts, treatment should be temporarily interrupted. Bone marrow suppression is readily reversible if the drug is withdrawn early enough. During remission induction in acute myelogenous leukaemia the patient may frequently have to survive a period of relative bone marrow aplasia and it is important that adequate supportive facilities are available.

Patients on myelosuppressive chemotherapy are particularly susceptible to a variety of infections.

During remission induction, particularly when rapid cell lysis is occurring, adequate precautions should be taken to avoid hyperuricaemia and/or hyperuricosuria and the risk of uric acid nephropathy.

In view of its action on cellular DNA, Lanvis is potentially mutagenic and carcinogenic, and consideration should be given to the theoretical risk of carcinogenesis when Lanvis therapy is given. It is advised that care be taken when handling or halving these tablets not to contaminate hands or to inspire drug.

Side- and adverse effects: Gastro-intestinal intolerance has been reported. Similar intolerance has been noted with Puri-Nethol but individual patients may tolerate either Lanvis or Puri-Nethol better than the other. At high doses gastro-intestinal symptoms may be more apparent and stomatitis has also been reported. Intestinal necrosis and perforation has been reported in patients who received combination chemotherapy including Lanvis.

Liver function abnormalities and jaundice have been reported during treatment with Lanvis and may be reversible if therapy is withdrawn. There has been a report of veno-occlusive disease of the liver occurring in patients who received combination chemotherapy including Lanvis.

Use in pregnancy and lactation: Lanvis like other cytotoxic agents is potentially teratogenic. Its use should be avoided whenever possible during pregnancy, particularly during the first trimester. In any individual case the potential hazard to the foetus must be balanced against the expected benefit to the mother. There have been isolated cases where men who have received combinations of cytotoxic agents including Lanvis have fathered children with congenital abnormalities and consideration should be given to this potential risk when treating male patients.

Mothers receiving Lanvis should not breast feed.

Toxicity and treatment of overdosage: The principal toxic effect is on the bone marrow and haematological toxicity is likely to be more profound with chronic overdosage than with a single ingestion of Lanvis. As there is no known antidote the blood picture should be closely monitored and general supportive measures instituted together with appropriate blood transfusion if necessary.

Pharmaceutical precautions Store below 25°C. Protect from light. Keep dry.

Legal category POM.

Package quantities Bottle of 25 tablets.

Further information The concomitant use of Zyloric* (allopurinol) to inhibit uric acid formation does not necessitate reduction of the dosage of Lanvis as is necessary with Puri-Nethol* (6-mercaptopurine) and Imuran* (azathioprine).

Product licence number 0003/0083.

LEUKERAN* TABLETS

Presentation *Leukeran Tablets:* 2 mg Chlorambucil BP, coded 'WELLCOME C2A'. Coloured yellow with white core.

5 mg Chlorambucil BP, coded 'WELLCOME H2A'. Coloured yellow with white core.

Uses Cytotoxic agent.

Leukeran is indicated in the treatment of Hodgkin's disease, certain forms of non-Hodgkin's lymphoma, chronic lymphocytic leukaemia, Waldenstrom's macroglobulinaemia and advanced ovarian adenocarcinoma. Leukeran has a significant therapeutic effect in a proportion of patients with breast cancer.

Dosage and administration *Adults: Hodgkin's disease:* Used as a single agent a typical dosage is 0.2 mg/kg/day for 4–8 weeks. Leukeran is usually included in combination therapy and a number of regimes have been used. Leukeran has been used as an alternative to nitrogen mustard with a reduction in toxicity but similar therapeutic results.

Non-Hodgkin's lymphoma: Used as a single agent the usual dosage is 0.1–0.2 mg/kg/day for 4–8 weeks initially; maintenance therapy is then given either by a reduced daily dosage or intermittent courses of treatment. Leukeran is useful in the management of patients with advanced diffuse lymphocytic lymphoma and those who have relapsed after radiotherapy. There is no significant difference in the overall response rate obtained with chlorambucil as a single agent and combination chemotherapy in patients with advanced non-Hodgkin's lymphocytic lymphoma.

Chronic lymphocytic leukaemia: Treatment with Leukeran is usually started after the patient has developed symptoms or when there is evidence of impaired bone marrow function (but not marrow failure) as indicated by the peripheral blood count. Initially Leukeran is given at a dosage of 0.15 mg/kg/day until the total leucocyte count has fallen to 10,000 per µl. Treatment may be resumed 4 weeks after the end of the first course and continued at a dosage of 0.1 mg/kg/day. In a proportion of patients, usually after about 2 years of treatment, the blood leucocyte count is reduced to the normal range, enlarged spleen and lymph nodes become impalpable and the proportion of lymphocytes in the bone marrow is reduced to less than 20 per cent. Patients with evidence of bone marrow failure should first be treated with prednisolone and evidence of marrow regeneration should be obtained before commencing treatment with Leukeran. Intermittent high dose therapy has been compared with daily Leukeran but no significant difference in therapeutic response or frequency of side effects was observed between the two treatment groups.

Waldenstrom's macroglobulinaemia: Leukeran is the treatment of choice in this indication. Starting doses of 6–12 mg daily until leucopenia occurs are recommended followed by 2–8 mg daily indefinitely.

Ovarian carcinoma: Used as a single agent a typical dosage is 0.2 mg/kg/day for 4–6 weeks. A dosage of 0.3 mg/kg/day has been given until leucopenia had been induced. Maintenance dosage of 0.2 mg/kg/day has been given aiming to keep the total leucocyte count below 4,000/mm^3. In practice, maintenance courses tend to last 2–4 weeks with intervals of 2–6 weeks between each course.

Advanced breast cancer: Used as a single agent a typical dosage is 0.2 mg/kg bodyweight per day for 6 weeks. Leukeran may be given in combination with prednisolone at a dose range of 14–20 mg daily, regardless of bodyweight, over 4–6 weeks provided there is no serious haemopoietic depression. Leukeran may be given in combination with methotrexate, 5-fluorouracil, and prednisolone at a dosage of 5 to 7.5 mg/m^2/day.

Children: Leukeran may be used in the management of Hodgkin's disease and non-Hodgkin's lymphomas in children. The dosage regimens are similar to those used in adults.

Use in the elderly: No specific studies have been carried out in the elderly, however, it may be advisable to monitor renal or hepatic function and if there is serious impairment then caution should be exercised.

Contra-indications, warnings, etc
Contra-indications: In view of the seriousness of the indications there are no absolute contra-indications.

Precautions: Leukeran is an active cytotoxic agent for use only under the direction of physicians experienced in the administration of such agents.

Since Leukeran is capable of producing irreversible bone marrow suppression, blood counts should be closely monitored in patients under treatment.

At therapeutic dosage Leukeran depresses lymphocytes and has less effect on neutrophil and platelet counts and on haemoglobin levels. Discontinuation of Leukeran is not necessary at the first sign of a fall in neutrophils but it must be remembered that the fall may continue for 10 days or more after the last dose.

Leukeran should not be given to patients who have recently undergone radiotherapy or received other cytotoxic agents.

When lymphocytic infiltration of the bone marrow is present or the bone marrow is hypoplastic, the daily dose should not exceed 0.1 mg/kg body weight.

Patients with evidence of impaired renal function should be carefully monitored as they are prone to additional myelosuppression associated with azotaemia.

The metabolism of Leukeran is still under investigation

and consideration should be given to dose reduction in patients with gross hepatic dysfunction.

Leukeran has been shown to cause chromatid or chromosome damage in man. Development of acute leukaemia after Leukeran therapy for chronic lymphocytic leukaemia has been reported. However, it was not clear whether the acute leukaemia was part of the natural history of the disease or if the chemotherapy was the cause.

A comparison of patients with ovarian cancer who received alkylating agents with those who did not, showed that the use of alkylating agents, including Leukeran, significantly increased the incidence of acute leukaemia.

Acute myelogenous leukaemia has been reported in a small proportion of patients receiving Leukeran as long-term adjuvant therapy for breast cancer.

The leukaemogenic risk must be balanced against the potential therapeutic benefit when considering the use of Leukeran.

Chlorambucil may cause suppression of ovarian function and amenorrhoea has been reported following chlorambucil therapy.

Azoospermia has been observed as a result of therapy with Leukeran although it is estimated that a total dose of at least 400 mg is necessary.

Varying degrees of recovery of spermatogenesis have been reported in patients with lymphoma following treatment with Leukeran in total doses of 410–2,600 mg. Patients receiving phenylbutazone may require a reduced dose of Leukeran.

Side- and adverse effects: The most common side-effect is bone marrow suppression. Although this frequently occurs, it is usually reversible if Leukeran is withdrawn early enough. However, irreversible bone marrow failure has been reported.

Gastro-intestinal disturbances such as nausea and vomiting, diarrhoea and oral ulceration occur infrequently. Other side-effects may be encountered but usually only when the therapeutic dosage has been exceeded.

Severe interstitial pulmonary fibrosis has occasionally been reported in patients with chronic lymphocytic leukaemia on long-term Leukeran therapy. However, this may be reversible on withdrawal of Leukeran.

Hepatotoxicity and jaundice have been reported after Leukeran treatment.

Other reported adverse reactions include fever, skin hypersensitivity, peripheral neuropathy, interstitial pneumonia and sterile cystitis.

Seizures have occurred in children with nephrotic syndrome treated with Leukeran and dose-related focal fits in adults have been reported.

Use in pregnancy and lactation: As with other cytotoxic agents Leukeran is potentially teratogenic. The use of Leukeran should be avoided whenever possible during pregnancy, particularly during the first trimester. In any individual case, the potential hazard to the foetus must be balanced against the expected benefit to the mother.

Mothers receiving Leukeran should not breast feed.

Toxicity and treatment of overdosage: Reversible pancytopenia was the main finding of inadvertent overdoses of Leukeran. Neurological toxicity ranging from agitated behaviour and ataxia to multiple grand mal seizures has also occurred. As there is no known antidote the blood picture should be closely monitored and general supportive measures should be instituted, together with appropriate blood transfusion if necessary.

Pharmaceutical precautions Store at 2–8°C in a dry place.

Legal category POM.

Package quantities *2 mg:* Bottle of 25 tablets. *5 mg:* Bottle of 25 tablets.

Further information Leukeran has the pharmacological properties of the nitrogen mustard compounds. The drug is only partly radiomimetic, affecting chiefly the lymphoid tissues. Experimental studies have shown that chlorambucil is well absorbed and well tolerated by the oral route.

Product licence numbers
Tablets 2 mg 0003/5264R
Tablets 5 mg 0003/5265R

LYCLEAR* CREME RINSE

Presentation Lyclear Creme Rinse contains 1% w/w permethrin plus 20% w/w isopropanol in a creme rinse base. It is orange in colour.

Uses Lyclear is indicated for the treatment of infections with the head louse *Pediculus humanus capitis*.

Dosage and administration
Adults and children over 2 years of age: Treatment: Shampoo the hair with a proprietary shampoo according to the manufacturer's instructions. After the final rinse, towel dry the hair so that it remains damp.

Shake Lyclear Creme Rinse thoroughly before using.

Apply enough Lyclear to all the scalp and hair so that they are both well coated. A single bottle of Lyclear is sufficient to treat shoulder-length hair of normal thickness.

Leave the Lyclear on the hair for 10 minutes, then rinse the hair thoroughly with water and dry in the usual way.

Eggs (nits) remain cemented to the hair even when dead and are, therefore, not a sign of treatment failure. Combing of the hair to remove nits is not required for therapeutic efficacy, but may be done for cosmetic or other reasons.

Use in the elderly: No special comment.

Pharmacology: Permethrin is rapidly absorbed across the insect cuticle. The principal physiological lesion is the induction of electrochemical abnormalities across the membranes of excitable cells, leading to sensory hyperexcitability, incoordination and prostration. When presented in an aqueous base the ovicidal activity of permethrin is increased by the addition of an alcohol.

Contra-indications, warnings, etc
Contra-indications: The use of Lyclear is contra-indicated in individuals with a known hypersensitivity to permethrin, other synthetic pyrethroids, the pyrethrins or chrysanthemums.

Precautions: For external use only.

It is good practice for nursing staff involved in multiple applications of Lyclear to wear gloves.

Lyclear should only be applied to children of less than 2 years of age under medical supervision.

There are no data on the use of Lyclear by patients with co-existing skin disease.

Lyclear is not an eye irritant. However patients should avoid contact with eyes during application. In the event of accidental contamination, the eyes should be rinsed immediately with plenty of water.

Side- and adverse effects: Adverse reactions are infrequent, mild and transitory. The most commonly reported symptom after treatment with Lyclear is pruritus. In the majority of cases this was also reported prior to treatment as a feature of the infection. A few individuals may experience mild erythema and/or stinging of the scalp. Rarely, a very mild self-limiting rash or oedema of the scalp has been reported.

Use in pregnancy and lactation: Although animal reproductive studies have not revealed any evidence of impaired fertility or harm to the foetus from the administration of permethrin during pregnancy, they have shown that this compound crosses the placental barrier and is excreted in milk. Animal reproductive studies are not always predictive of the human response. As with most drugs, the use of Lyclear should be avoided during pregnancy and lactation.

Drug interactions: There are no known interactions with permethrin.

Toxicity and treatment of overdose: No instance of accidental ingestion of Lyclear has been reported. The results of animal studies suggest that the permethrin content of Lyclear would be insufficient to cause serious toxicity in a child who consumed the contents of a bottle. However, it is possible that the isopropanol content may lead to alcoholic intoxication on ingestion by small children.

In view of the rapid absorption of isopropanol, gastric lavage should be considered within 2 hours of ingestion but would probably not be of value thereafter. Management should relate to alcoholic intoxication and include maintenance of the fluid balance using suitable electrolyte solutions, monitoring of blood glucose levels and keeping the patient warm. In extreme cases haemodialysis or peritoneal dialysis to remove isopropanol from the blood may be of value.

Pharmaceutical precautions Shake well before use. Store below 25°C. Protect from light.

Legal category P.

Package quantities Plastic bottle of 59 ml.

Further information Clinical work has shown that residual activity may persist for up to 6 weeks, following a single application. Permethrin is not affected by the chlorine in swimming baths, so normal swimming activities may continue after use. Similarly, there should be no reason to change normal shampooing routines.

Product licence number 0003/0252.

MALOPRIM* TABLETS

Presentation *Tablets:* Each white tablet is scored and contains 12.5 mg Pyrimethamine BP and 100 mg Dapsone BP, coded 'WELLCOME H9A'.

Uses Maloprim is effective as a causal prophylactic and suppressive agent against malaria caused by *Plasmodium falciparum* and probably other malaria parasites, notably *P. vivax.* Since potentiation takes place between its two active constituents Maloprim is recommended particularly when resistance to pyrimethamine or other antifolate preparations is known or suspected. It is also effective in chloroquine-resistant areas.

Note: Maloprim should not be used for treatment of the acute attack.

Dosage and administration *Adults:* 1 tablet each week.

Children: Over 10 years: 1 tablet each week.

5–10 years: ½ tablet each week.

Under 5 years: Formulation not applicable.

THE RECOMMENDED DOSE MUST NOT BE EXCEEDED.

The constituents are rapidly absorbed and prophylactic cover can be expected shortly after taking the first dose. Prophylaxis should commence before arrival in an endemic area and be continued once weekly. On returning to a non-malarious area dosage should be maintained for a further four weeks.

Use in the elderly: No specific studies have been carried out in the elderly, however, it may be advisable to monitor renal or hepatic function and if there is serious impairment then caution shold be exercised.

Maloprim, at the doses recommended for the prevention of Malaria is unlikely to have any adverse effect on older people normally of good health.

Contra-indications, warnings, etc

Contra-indications: Maloprim should not be given to individuals with a known history of sensitivity to sulphonamides or sulphones or pyrimethamine.

Precautions: Short-term usage of Maloprim is unlikely to carry excess risk in patients with renal or hepatic impairment. However, patients with significant kidney or liver disease taking Maloprim for prolonged periods should be monitored regularly for signs of bone marrow depression.

During pregnancy and in the presence of other conditions predisposing to folate deficiency a folic acid supplement should be given.

Maloprim, through its mode of action, may further depress folate metabolism in patients already receiving treatment with other folate inhibitors, including combinations of trimethoprim and sulphonamides.

Similarly, Maloprim may exacerbate folate deficiency in individuals predisposed to this condition through disease or malnutrition.

Side- and adverse effects: Side-effects caused by Maloprim at the recommended doses are rare. Agranulocytosis has been reported, particularly in association with doses of one tablet twice weekly.

Cyanosis, attributable to methaemoglobinaemia, has occurred.

Inadvertent administration of excessive doses over a prolonged period may produce megaloblastic or haemolytic anaemia.

The haemolytic effect of dapsone is dose related and greater in glucose-6-phosphate dehydrogenase deficiency. Consequently, the dosage of dapsone as used in Maloprim is insufficient to cause clinically apparent disease in the majority of individuals. However, rare cases of haemoglobinuria have been reported in glucose-6-phosphate dehydrogenase deficient individuals, following Maloprim administration.

Skin sensitivity reactions have occurred.

Insomnia has been reported when pyrimethamine has been given at weekly doses above those recommended.

Use in pregnancy and lactation: While there is a theoretical risk of foetal malformation with all folate inhibitors given during pregnancy, no such adverse effects have been reported with Maloprim in humans. A folate supplement should be given to pregnant women receiving Maloprim. The amount of the components of Maloprim excreted in breast milk is insufficient to contraindicate its use in lactating mothers, but breast-fed infants should not receive other anti-folate agents.

Toxicity and treatment of overdosage: Symptoms are likely to be nausea, vomiting, hyperexcitability, methaemoglobinaemia and haemolytic anaemia. Convulsions may be apparent and megaloblastic anaemia may ensue. Routine supportive treatment, including maintenance of a clear airway and control of convulsions should be given. Adequate fluids should be given to enhance optimal diuresis. Gastric lavage may be of value only if instituted within two hours in view of the rapid absorption of Maloprim. Provision should be made for fresh blood transfusions. To counteract possible folate deficiency calcium folinate 9–15 mg daily should be administered. There may be a delay of 7 to 10 days before the full leucopenic side effects become evident, therefore calcium folinate should be continued for the period at risk. Methaemoglobinaemia should be treated with ascorbic acid, 200 mg three times daily, or, except in patients with G-6-PD deficiency, by intravenous administration of methylene blue, 2 mg/kg body weight.

Pharmaceutical precautions Store below 25°C. Protect from light.

Legal category POM.

Package quantities Strip pack of 30 tablets as 5 foil strips of 6 tablets.

Further information Nil.

Product licence number 0003/5117.

MIGRIL* TABLETS

Presentation White, round, biconvex compression-coated tablets with a pink core, scored and impressed 'WELLCOME A4A', with each tablet containing 2 mg Ergotamine Tartrate BP, 50 mg Cyclizine Hydrochloride BP and Caffeine BP equivalent to 100 mg Caffeine Hydrate BP.

Uses MIGRIL is indicated for the relief of the acute migraine attack.

Dosage and administration

Adults: Migril should be taken as soon as possible after

the first warning of an attack of migraine and repeated if necessary at the prescribed intervals.

The usual initial dose is one tablet.

Additional doses of a half to one tablet may then be required at half-hourly intervals.

No more than 4 tablets (8 mg ergotamine) should be taken in any one attack.

No more than 6 tablets (12 mg ergotamine) should be given in any one week.

Children: There are no absolute contra-indications to the use of Migril in children but its use is not recommended.

Use in the elderly: There are no absolute contra-indications to the use of Migril in the elderly, but see 'Contra-indications' and 'Precautions'.

Contra-indications, warnings, etc

Contra-indications: Migril is contra-indicated during pregnancy because of a direct effect of ergotamine on the uterus. In animals, ergotamine has been reported to inhibit implantation, cause peri-natal mortality and foetal retardation.

Migril is contra-indicated during lactation and breast-feeding; it may suppress milk production and may also be excreted in milk at levels high enough to cause pharmacological effects in breast-fed infants.

Migril is contra-indicated in pre-existing vascular disease including angina, claudication, peripheral ischaemia, Raynaud's syndrome and hypertension.

Migril should not be taken if there is a hypersensitivity to any of its constituents.

Precautions: Migril should not be used for migraine prophylaxis because of the risk of inducing ergotism.

The use of ergotamine-containing compounds carries the risk of precipitating arterial constriction and other manifestations of ergotism.

Use the *minimum* effective dosage of Migril necessary since individual sensitivity to the arterial effects of ergotamine varies considerably.

Discontinue the use of Migril if symptoms of arterial insufficiency develop.

Doses of ergotamine as small as 2 mg have caused signs of arterial insufficiency but this is a very rare occurrence.

Migril should be used with caution in patients with infective hepatitis because of an increased risk of precipitating peripheral ischaemia.

Repeated doses of egotamine have occasionally been associated with renal artery spasm and loss of renal function.

Alcohol and Migril should not be taken concurrently.

Ergotamine should be used with care when hyperthyroidism, sepsis or anaemia are present.

Cyclizine, in common with other antihistamines, may cause sedation; patients should be cautioned about driving or operating machinery.

Drug interactions: The concomitant use of ergot alkaloids and beta-blocking agents increases the risks of peripheral vasoconstriction.

Vomiting and peripheral ischaemia have been reported after concomitant use of ergot alkaloids and the antibiotics erythromycin and oleandomycin.

Side- and adverse effects: Habitual use of ergotamine-containing preparations can produce a syndrome of non-migrainous rebound headaches in which case Migril should be discontinued.

Side-effects seen with Migril are usually due to the ergotamine components of the preparation and are more common if the dosage recommendations are exceeded. They include intermittent claudication, coldness and whiteness of the extremities, dysaesthesia, paraesthesia, formication and precordial pain.

Other side-effects seen with ergotamine include muscle cramps, joint pains, raised blood pressure, pulselessness, cyanosis, thrombophlebitis, peripheral arterial thrombosis, gangrene, abdominal pain, coronary infarction, cerebral thrombosis, nausea, dyspnoea, decreased visual acuity, vertigo and diarrhoea. These effects have mostly occurred following habitual chronic use exceeding the recommended dose; they may occasionally occur however at the therapeutic dose.

Arterial vasospasm severe enough to threaten the viability of the limbs has been reported after routine therapy but it is more normally to be expected after prolonged overdosage.

Use in pregnancy and lactation: See '*Contra-indications*'.

Toxicity and treatment of overdosage
Acute overdosage:
Symptoms; Acute overdosage with an ergotamine-containing preparation is characterised by nausea, vomiting, tachycardia, hypotonia and peripheral ischaemia. Blood pressure may be difficult to measure.

Treatment: If vomiting has not occurred, efforts should be made to clear the stomach contents. General supportive measures should be applied and intravenous vasodilators may be necessary to relieve vasospasm.

Peritoneal dialysis and forced diuresis may help to eliminate ergotamine from the body.

Chronic overdosage:
Symptoms:
Chronic overdosage with ergotamine-containing preparations usually presents as peripheral ischaemia threatening the viability of the affected limb.

Treatment: Withdraw Migril immediately.

Intravenous vasodilators such as nitroprusside and nitroglycerin may be used to re-establish normal blood flow. Captopril has also been used to reverse the effects of chronic overdosage with ergotamine.

Re-establishment of blood flow may be associated with intense burning sensations in the affected areas but these usually resolve after several weeks.

Pharmaceutical precautions Store below 25°C. Keep dry. Protect from light.

Legal category POM.

Package quantities Bottle of 100 tablets.

Further information Nil.

Product licence number 0003/5114R

M-M-R$_{II}$*
Measles, Mumps and Rubella Vaccine, Live, Attenuated

Presentation A lyophilised powder for subcutaneous or intramuscular injection after reconstitution that offers protection against measles, mumps, and rubella. M-M-R$_{II}$ is prepared from (1) a more attenuated line of measles virus derived from Enders' attenuated Edmonston Strain and (2) the Jeryl Lynn (B level) mumps strain and (3) The Wistar RA27/3 strain of live, attenuated rubella vaccine. When reconstituted, each 0.5 ml dose contains not less than the equivalent of 1,000 TCID$_{50}$ (tissue culture infectious dose) of the US Reference Measles Virus; 5,000 TCID$_{50}$ of the US Reference Mumps Virus; and 1,000 TCID$_{50}$ of the US Reference Rubella Virus. Each 0.5 ml dose contains approximately 25 micrograms neomycin. The product contains no preservative. Sorbitol, hydrolysed gelatin and human albumin are added as stabilisers.

Uses For simultaneous immunisation against measles, mumps, and rubella.

Children: In the United Kingdom, M-M-R$_{II}$ is recommended for the immunisation of both boys and girls over 12 months of age. No booster is needed. Infants who are less than 15 months of age may fail to respond to the measles component of the vaccine due to presence in the circulation of residual measles antibody of maternal origin – the younger the infant, the lower the likelihood of seroconversion. In geographically isolated or other relatively inaccessible populations for whom immunisation programs are logistically difficult, and in population groups in which natural measles infection may occur in a significant proportion of infants before 15 months of age, it may be desirable to give the vaccine to infants at an earlier age. Infants vaccinated under these conditions at less than 12 months of age should be revaccinated after reaching 15 months of age. There is some evidence to suggest that infants immunised at less than one year of age may not develop sustained antibody levels when later reimmunised. The advantage of early protection must be weighed against the chance for failure to respond adequately on reimmunisation.

Pregnant females: Pregnant females must NOT be given M-M-R_{II}. Furthermore, pregnancy should be avoided for three months following vaccination (see 'Use in pregnancy and lactation').

Animal reproduction studies have not been conducted with M-M-R_{II}. It is also not known whether M-M-R_{II} can cause foetal harm when given to a pregnant woman or affect reproductive capacity.

If a pregnant woman is inadvertently vaccinated or if she becomes pregnant within three months of vaccination, she should be counselled by her physician. It has been established that: (1) in a ten-year study involving 700 pregnant women who received rubella vaccination within three months of conception, none of their newborn infants had abnormalities compatible with a congenital rubella syndrome; (2) although mumps virus is capable of infecting the placenta and foetus, there is no good evidence that it causes congenital malformations in humans.

Mumps vaccine virus has also been shown to affect the placenta, but the virus has not been isolated from foetal tissues taken from susceptible women who were vaccinated and underwent elective abortions; and (3) reports indicate that contracting natural measles during pregnancy increases the rates of spontaneous abortion, stillbirth, congenital defects, and prematurity. Although there are no adequate studies on the attenuated (vaccine) strain in pregnancy, it would be prudent to assume that the strain of virus in the vaccine is also capable of inducing adverse foetal effects.

Non-pregnant adolescent and adult females: Immunisation of susceptible non-pregnant adolescent and adult females of child-bearing age with live attenuated rubella vaccine is indicated when the potential vaccinee:

(a) agrees not to become pregnant for the next three months after vaccination and is informed of the reason for this precaution (this precaution also applies to women in the immediate post-partum period when it may be found most convenient to vaccinate – but see 'Nursing mothers');
(b) is told of the frequent occurrence of generally self-limiting arthralgia and/or arthritis beginning two to four weeks after vaccination.

It is also prudent, where practicable, to carry out blood tests on subjects of child-bearing age, in order to determine their immune status.

Vaccinating susceptible post-pubertal females confers individual protection against acquired rubella infection during pregnancy. This in turn prevents infection of the foetus and consequent congenital rubella injury.

Use in the elderly: No special comment.

Revaccination: Based on available evidence, there is no reason to revaccinate children who were vaccinated originally when 12 months of age or older; however, children vaccinated when younger than 12 months of age should be revaccinated. (M-M-R_{II} is not recommended for infants under 12 months of age.)

Vaccinees should be revaccinated if there is evidence to suggest that initial immunisation was ineffective.

Use with other vaccines: Vaccines containing diphtheria, tetanus, and pertussis antigens and/or oral poliomyelitis vaccine can be administered at the same time as M-M-R_{II}. For concurrent parenteral vaccination, separate syringes and separate sites for injection should be used. M-M-R_{II} should not be given less than one month before or after immunisation with other live virus vaccines.

Dosage and administration

Adults and children: After suitably cleansing the injection site, 0.5 ml of reconstituted vaccine should be injected subcutaneously or intramuscularly, preferably into the outer aspect of the arm. M-M-R_{II} must not be given intravenously. If the injection site is swabbed, it should be allowed to dry before the injection is given.

Do not give immunoglobulin with M-M-R_{II}.

Warning: A sterile syringe and Adrenaline Injection BP (1:1,000) should be available for immediate use should an anaphylactoid reaction occur.

Reconstitution: To reconstitute the vaccine, all the diluent provided should be injected into a vial of lyophilised vaccine, and this agitated to ensure thorough mixing. 0.5 ml of the reconstituted vaccine is then injected subcutaneously or intramuscularly.

Only the diluent supplied should be used for reconstitution, since it is free of preservatives and other antiviral substances that may inactivate the vaccine.

When reconstituted, the vaccine is yellow. It is acceptable for use only when clear and free from particulate matter.

The vaccine should be used as soon as possible and not later than one hour after reconstitution.

A separate sterile disposable needle and syringe should be used for each vaccine.

It is good practice to record the title, dose and lot number of all vaccines and dates of administration.

Contra-indications, warnings, etc

Contra-indications: Do not give M-M-R_{II} to pregnant females; the possible effects of the vaccine on foetal development are unknown at this time. Pregnancy must be avoided for three months following vaccination of post-pubertal females.

Anaphylactoid reaction to neomycin or other vaccine constituent. (Each dose of reconstituted vaccine contains approximately 25 micrograms neomycin.)

History of anaphylactoid reaction to eggs (see 'Hypersensitivity to eggs, chicken, or chicken feathers').

Any febrile respiratory illness, or other active or suspected infection.

Those with impaired immune responsiveness, whether occurring naturally or as a result of therapy with steroids, radiotherapy, cytotoxic or other agents. This contraindication does not apply to patients receiving corticosteroids as replacement therapy, e.g. for Addison's disease.

Patients with active untreated tuberculosis, blood dyscrasias such as thrombocytopenia, leukaemia, malignant disease including lymphomas or any type or other malignant neoplasms affecting the bone marrow or lymphatic systems.

Primary immunodeficiency states, including cellular immune deficiencies, hypogammaglobulinaemic and dysgammaglobulinaemic states.

Those patients with a family history of congenital or hereditary immunodeficiency until their immune competence has been demonstrated.

Hypersensitivity to eggs, chicken, or chicken feathers: Live measles and live mumps vaccine are produced in cell cultures of chick embryo.

Patients with a history of anaphylactoid or other immediate reactions to eating eggs (e.g. hives, swelling of the mouth and throat, difficult breathing, hypotension and shock) should not be vaccinated. Evidence indicates, however, that patients with egg allergies that are not anaphylactoid may be vaccinated in the usual way. There is also no evidence to suggest that allergy to chicken or feathers increases the risk of reaction.

Children below 12 months of age: Children below the age of 12 months should not normally be given M-M-R_{II} unless they are at special risk, since the presence of maternal antibody may interfere with their ability to respond. Where immunisation below the age of 12 months is deemed necessary, a second dose should be given after the child has reached 15 months of age.

Precautions: Adrenaline should be available for immediate use should an anaphylactic reaction occur.

M-M-R_{II} should be given with caution to those with a history of febrile convulsions, cerebral injury or any other condition in which stress due to fever should be avoided. The physician should be alert to the rise in temperature that may follow vaccination.

Vaccination should be deferred for at least three

months following blood or plasma transfusions, or administration of human immune serum globulin. If any of these substances has been used near to the time of vaccination with M-M-R_{II}, a test should subsequently be made to confirm successful seroconversions.

Where anti-Rh_0 (D) globulin (human) and rubella vaccine are required in the immediate post-partum period, rubella vaccine alone and not M-M-R_{II} should be used.

Excretion of small amounts of live attenuated rubella virus from the nose and throat has occurred in the majority of susceptible individuals 7–28 days after vaccination. There is no definite evidence to indicate that such virus is transmitted to susceptible persons who are in contact with vaccinated individuals. Consequently, transmission, while accepted as a theoretical possibility, has not been regarded as a significant risk. However, transmission of the vaccine virus via breast milk has been documented.

There are no reports of transmission of live attenuated measles or mumps viruses from vaccinees to susceptible contacts.

It has been reported that live attenuated measles, mumps, and rubella vaccine may temporarily depress tuberculin skin sensitivity. If a tuberculin test is to be done, therefore, it should be administered before or simultaneously with M-M-R_{II}.

Nursing mothers: Caution should be exercised when M-M-R_{II} is given to a nursing mother. Although it is not known whether measles or mumps vaccine virus is secreted in human milk, studies have shown that nursing mothers immunised with live attenuated RA 27/3 strain rubella vaccine may transmit the virus via breast milk. In those babies with serological evidence of rubella, none showed clinical disease.

Parents of children with a personal or family history of convulsions or idiopathic epilepsy should be advised that such children have a small increased risk of seizures following vaccination and informed in advance of procedures for their management.

Adverse reactions: Because the vaccine is slightly acidic (pH 6.2–6.6), patients may complain or burning and/or stinging at the injection site for a short time.

Adverse reactions associated with M-M-R_{II} are similar to those to be expected from administration of monovalent vaccines given separately. These may include malaise, sore throat, headache, fever and rash, nausea and vomiting; mild local reactions such as erythema, induration, tenderness and regional lymphadenopathy; parotitis, orchitis, nerve deafness, thrombocytopenia and purpura; allergic reactions such as wheal and flare at the injection site or urticaria; polyneuritis; and arthralgia and/or arthritis (usually transient and rarely chronic). Cough, coryza and pharyngitis have also occurred.

Moderate fever (38.3°C/101°F) or high fever (above 39.4°C/103°F) may occur following vaccination, predominantly between days 5 and 10. On rare occasions, children developing fever may exhibit febrile convulsions. Rash occurs infrequently and is usually minimal, but rarely may be generalised.

Forms of optic neuritis, inlcuding retrobulbar neuritis, papillitis and retinitis have infrequently been reported one to three weeks after inoculation with some live virus vaccines.

Very rarely, encephalitis and other CNS reactions have been associated with measles, mumps, and rubella vaccines when given individually. These reactions might be reported with M-M-R_{II}.

Experience from more than 80 million doses of all live measles vaccines given in the USA up to 1975 indicates that significant central nervous system reactions such as encephalitis and encephalopathy, occurring within 30 days after vaccination, have been temporally associated with measles vaccine approximately once for every million doses. In no cases has it been shown that reactions were actually caused by vaccine. The risk of such serious neurological disorders following live measles virus vaccine administration remains far less than that for encephalitis and encephalopathy caused by natural measles (one per two thousand reported cases).

There have been isolated reports of both the Guillain-Barre syndrome being seen after vaccination and ocular palsies occurring 3–24 days after vaccination with a live attenuated measles virus vaccine, but no definite causal relationship between the vaccine and the disease syndromes has been established. Isolated cases of polyneuropathy, including Guillain-Barre syndrome, have also been reported after immunisation with rubella-containing vaccines.

There have been reports of subacute sclerosing panencephalitis (SSPE) in children who did not have a history of natural measles but did receive measles vaccine. Some of these cases may have resulted from unrecognised measles in the first year of life or possibly from the measles vaccination. Based on estimated nationwide measles vaccine distribution in the USA, the association of SSPE cases to measles vaccination is about one case per million vaccine doses distributed. This is far less than the association with natural measles: 6–22 cases of SSPE per million cases of measles.

A study suggests that the overall effect of measles vaccine has been to protect against SSPE by preventing measles with its inherent higher risk of SSPE.

Local reactions characterised by marked swelling, redness and vesiculation at the injection site of attenuated live virus measles vaccines, and systemic reactions including atypical measles have occurred in vaccinees who had previously received killed measles vaccine. Rarely, there have been reports of more severe reactions, including prolonged high fevers and extensive local reactions requiring hospitalisation. Panniculitis has also been reported rarely following vaccination with measles vaccines.

Arthralgia or arthritis, or both, are usually transient and rarely chronic features of natural rubella. Like the polyneuritis that is also a feature of natural infection, their frequency and severity vary with age and sex, being greatest in adult females and least in prepubertal children. This type of involvement as well as myalgia and paraesthesiae have also been reported with the separate use of the rubella vaccine.

The chronic arthritis associated with natural rubella has been related to virus and/or viral antigen found in body tissues. Only rarely have vaccinees developed chronic joint symptoms.

Following vaccination in children, reactions in joints are uncommon and generally of brief duration. In women, incidence rates for arthritis and arthralgia are generally higher than those seen in children (children: 0–3%; women: 12–20%) and the reactions tend to be more marked and of longer duration. Symptoms may persist for a matter of months or, on rare occasions, for years. In adolescent girls, the reactions appear to be intermediate in incidence between those seen in children and in adult women. Even in older women (35–45 years) these reactions are generally well tolerated and rarely interfere with normal activities.

Overdosage: Poisoning is unlikely. Swallowing M-M-R_{II} would render the live attenuated vaccine benign, and the content of neomycin (25 micrograms/ml) is not likely to cause toxicity. No case of overdose has been reported.

Pharmaceutical precautions During shipment, the vaccine must be maintained at a temperature of 10°C (50°F) or less to ensure no loss of potency.

Before reconstitution, M-M-R_{II} should be stored between 2° to 8°C (35.6° to 46.4°F) and protected from light. Do not freeze.

A separate sterile disposable needle and syringe should be used for each vaccinee.

Only the diluent supplied should be used for reconstitution since it is free of preservatives and other antiviral substances that may inactivate the vaccine.

When reconstituted, the vaccine is yellow. It is acceptable for use only when clear and free from particulate matter.

The vaccine should be used as soon as possible and not later than one hour after reconstitution.

Legal category POM.

Package quantities 10 Single-dose vials of freeze-dried vaccine powder with vials of sterile diluent.

Further information M-M-R_{II} is highly immunogenic and generally well tolerated. Clinical studies suggest that a single injection of the vaccine will induce measles HI antibodies in 95%, mumps neutralising antibodies in 96%, and rubella HI antibodies in 99% of susceptible vaccinees.

Product licence number 0025/0078.

*Trademark of Merck & Co Inc, Rahway, N.J., USA (subject to application). Used under licence from Merck & Co Inc.

MYLERAN* TABLETS

Presentation *Myleran Tablets:* 0.5 mg Busulphan BP, coded 'WELLCOME F2A'. Coloured white with yellow core.

2.0 mg Busulphan BP, coded 'WELLCOME K2A'. Coloured white with yellow core.

Uses Myleran is indicated for the palliative treatment of the chronic phase of chronic granulocytic leukaemia. Although not curative, Myleran is very effective in reducing the total granulocyte mass, relieving the symptoms of disease and improving the clinical state of the patient.

Myleran has been shown to be superior to splenic irradiation when judged by survival times and maintenance of haemoglobin levels and is as effective in controlling spleen size.

Myleran is ineffective once blast transformation has occurred.

Myleranis is effective in producing prolonged remission in polycythaemia vera, particularly in cases with marked thrombocytosis.

Myleran may be useful in selected cases of essential thrombocythaemia and myelofibrosis.

Mode of action: Busulphan (1,4-butanediol dimethanesulfonate) is a bifunctional alkylating agent. Binding to DNA is believed to play a role in its mode of action, and di-guanyl derivatives have been isolated, but interstrand crosslinking has not been conclusively demonstrated.

The basis for the uniquely selective effect of busulphan on granulocytopoiesis is not fully understood.

Pharmacology: Early studies were carried out with radioactively labelled busulphan. More recently, gas liquid chromatography with selected ion monitoring has been used to quantitate busuphan in biological fluids. Busulphan doses of 2 to 6 mg were well absorbed and the kinetic data could be fitted to a zero-order absorption, one compartment open model. The mean half life for drug elimination was 2.57 hours.

The pharmacokinetics of busulphan have also been studied in patients following high-dose administration (1 mg/kg every 6 hours for 4 days). Drug was assayed either using gas liquid chromatography with electron capture detection or by high-performance liquid chromatography (HPLC). Using the former technique, the mean elimination half life was found to be 2.3 hours after the final busulphan dose, but 3.4 hours after the first dose. This suggests that busulphan may increase its own metabolic rate on repeated treatment. The mean steady-state plasma concentration was 1.1 microgram/ml after dosing. Due to the variable absorption kinetics observed, it was not possible to evaluate the order of kinetics.

Using HPLC, steady-state plasma levels of busulphan were found to range from 2 to 8 microM (approximately 0.5 to 2 microgram/ml respectively). Peak plasma levels ranged from 3.1 to 5.9 microgram/ml in a patient treated with a total dose of 16 mg/kg, or from 3.8 to 9.7 microgram/ml in two patients treated with a total of 20 mg/kg.

The urinary metabolites of busulphan have been identified as 3-hydroxysulpholane, tetrahydrothiophene 1-oxide and sulpholane, in patients treated with high-dose busulphan. Very little (1–2%) busulphan is excreted unchanged in the urine.

Busulphan given in high doses has recently been shown to enter the cerebrospinal fluid (CSF) in concentrations comparable to those found in plasma, with a mean CSF:plasma ratio of 1.3:1. The saliva:plasma distribution of busulphan was found to be 1.1:1.

The level of busulphan bound reversibly to plasma proteins has been variably reported to be insignificant or approximately 55%. Irreversible binding of drug to blood cells and plasma proteins has been reported to be 47% and 32% respectively.

Dosage and administration
Chronic granulocytic leukaemia:
Induction in adults: Treatment is usually initiated as soon as the condition is diagnosed. The dose is 0.06 mg/kg/day with an initial daily maximum of 4 mg, which may be given as a single dose.

There is individual variation in the response to Myleran and in a small proportion of patients the bone marrow may be extremely sensitive. (See *Precautions*).

The blood count must be monitored at least weekly during the induction phase and it may be helpful to plot counts on semilog graph paper.

The dose should be increased only if the response is inadequate after three weeks.

Treatment should be continued until the total leucocyte count has fallen to between 15 and 25 × 10^9 per litre (typically 12 to 20 weeks). Treatment may then be interrupted, following which a further fall in the leucocyte count may occur over the next two weeks. Continued treatment at the induction dose after this point or following depression of the platelet count to below 100 × 10^9 per litre is associated with a significant risk of prolonged and possibly irreversible bone marrow aplasia.

Maintenance in adults: Control of the leukaemia may be achieved for long periods without further Myleran treatment; further courses are usually given when the leucocyte count rises to 50 × 10^9 per litre, or symptoms return.

Some clinicians prefer to give continuous maintenance therapy. Continuous treatment is more practical when the duration of unmaintained remissions is short. The usual maintenance dosage is 0.5–2 mg/day, but individual requirements may be much less. The aim is to maintain a leucocyte count of 10–15 × 10^9 per litre and blood counts must be performed at least every 4 weeks. The maintenance dose may also be adjusted by reducing the number of treatment days per week.

NOTE: Lower doses of Myleran should be used if it is administered in conjunction with other cytotoxic agents. (See also '*Side-effects*' and '*Drug interactions*'.)

Children: Chronic granulocytic leukaemia is rare in the paediatric age group. Myleran may be used to treat Philadelphia chromosome positive (Ph' positive) disease, but the Ph' negative juvenile variant responds poorly.

Polycythaemia vera: The usual dose is 4 to 6 mg daily, continued for 4 to 6 weeks, with careful monitoring of the blood count, particularly the platelet count.

Further courses are given when relapse occurs; alternatively maintenance therapy may be given using approximately half the induction dose.

If the polycythaemia is controlled primarily by venesection, short courses of Myleran may be given solely to control the platelet count.

Myelofibrosis: The usual initial dose is 2 to 4 mg daily.

Very careful haematological control is required because of the extreme sensitivity of the bone marrow in this condition.

Essential thrombocythaemia: The usual dose is 2 to 4 mg per day.

Treatment should be interrupted if the total leucocyte count falls below 5 × 10^9 per litre or the platelet count below 500 × 10^9 per litre.

Use in the elderly: No special comment.

Contra-indications, warnings, etc

Contra-indications: Myleran should not be used in patients whose disease has demonstrated resistance to busulphan.

Myleran should not be given to patients who have previously suffered a hypersensitivity reaction to the drug.

Precautions: MYLERAN IS AN ACTIVE CYTOTOXIC AGENT FOR USE *ONLY* UNDER THE DIRECTION OF PHYSICIANS EXPERIENCED IN THE ADMINISTRATION OF SUCH AGENTS.

Myleran should be discontinued if lung toxicity develops (See *Side-effects*).

Myleran should not generally be given in conjunction with or soon after radiotherapy.

If anaesthesia is required in patients with possible pulmonary toxicity, the concentration of inspired oxygen should be kept as low as safely possible and careful attention given to post-operative respiratory care.

Hyperuricaemia and/or hyperuricosuria are not uncommon in patients with chronic granulocytic leukaemia and should be corrected before starting treatment with Myleran. During treatment, hyperuricaemia and the risk of uric acid nephropathy should be prevented by adequate prophylaxis, including adequate hydration and the use of allopurinol.

Very careful consideration should be given to the use of Myleran for the treatment of polycythaemia vera and essential thrombocythaemia in view of the drug's carcinogenic potential. The use of Myleran for these indications should be avoided in younger or asymptomatic patients. If the drug is considered necessary treatment courses should be kept as short as possible.

Careful attention must be paid to monitoring the blood counts throughout treatment to avoid the possibility of excessive myelosuppression and the risk of irreversible bone marrow aplasia.

It is recommended that the handling of Myleran Tablets follows the 'Guidelines for the Handling of Cytotoxic Drugs' issued by the Royal Pharmaceutical Society of Great Britain Working Party on the Handling of Cytotoxic Drugs.

If halving of a tablet is required, care should be taken not to contaminate the hands or inhale the drug.

Busulphan has been shown to be mutagenic in various experimental systems, including bacteria, fungi, *Drosophila* and cultured mouse lymphoma cells.

In vivo cytogenetic studies in rodents have shown an increased incidence of chromosome aberrations in both germ cells and somatic cells after busulphan treatment.

Various chromosome aberrations have been noted in cells from patients receiving Myleran.

On the basis of short-term tests, Myleran has been classified as potentially carcinogenic by the IARC. The World Health Association has concluded that there is a causal relationship between busulphan exposure and cancer.

Widespread epithelial dysplasia has been observed in patients treated with long-term Myleran, with some of the changes resembling precancerous lesions.

A number of malignant tumours have been reported in patients who have received Myleran treatment.

The evidence is growing that Myleran, in common with other alkylating agents, is leukaemogenic. In a controlled prospective study in which 2 years' Myleran treatment was given as an adjuvant to surgery for lung cancer, long-term follow-up showed an increased incidence of acute leukaemia compared with the placebo-treated group. The incidence of solid tumours was not increased.

Although acute leukaemia is probably part of the natural history of polycythaemia vera, prolonged alkylating agent therapy may increase the incidence.

Ovarian suppression and amenorrhoea with menopausal symptoms commonly occur in pre-menopausal patients. In one case, recovery of ovarian function has been reported with continuing treatment.

Myleran treatment in a pre-adolescent girl prevented the onset of puberty due to ovarian failure.

Busulphan interferes with spermatogenesis in experimental animals, and there have been clinical reports of sterility, azoospermia and testicular atrophy in male patients.

Side- and adverse effects: The main adverse reaction of Myleran treatment is bone marrow depression, particularly thrombocytopenia.

Gastro-intestinal effects such as nausea, vomiting and diarrhoea have been reported rarely at normal therapeutic doses and may possibly be ameliorated by using divided doses.

Diffuse interstitial pulmonary fibrosis, with progressive dyspnoea and a persistent, non-productive cough has occurred rarely, usually after prolonged treatment over a number of years. Histological features include atypical changes of the alveolar and bronchiolar epithelium and the presence of giant cells with large hyperchromatic nuclei. Once pulmonary toxicity is established the prognosis is poor despite Myleran withdrawal and there is little evidence that corticosteroids are helpful. The onset is usually insidious but may also be acute. The lung pathology may be complicated by superimposed infections. Pulmonary ossification and dystrophic calcification have also been reported. It is possible that subsequent radiotherapy can augment subclinical lung injury caused by Myleran. Other cytotoxic agents may cause additive lung toxicity.

Hyperpigmentation is the most common skin reaction and occurs in 5–10% of patients, particularly those with a dark complexion. It is often most marked on the neck, upper trunk, nipples, abdomen and palmar creases. In a few cases following prolonged Myleran therapy, hyperpigmentation occurs as part of a clinical syndrome resembling adrenal insufficiency (Addison's disease). It is characterised by weakness, severe fatigue, anorexia, weight loss, nausea and vomiting and hyperpigmentation of the skin, but without biochemical evidence of adrenal impairment or mucous membrane hyperpigmentation or hair loss. The syndrome has sometimes resolved when Myleran has been withdrawn.

Other rare skin reactions include urticaria, erythema multiforme, erythema nodosum, alopecia, porphyria cutanea tarda, an 'allopurinol-type' rash and excessive dryness and fragility of the skin with complete anhydrosis, dryness of the oral mucous membranes and cheilosis. Sjogren's syndrome has also been reported.

An increased cutaneous radiation effect has been observed in patients receiving radiotherapy soon after high-dose Myleran.

There have been occasional reports of cholestatic jaundice and liver function abnormalities, but Myleran is not generally considered to be significantly hepatotoxic at normal therapeutic doses. However, retrospective review of postmortem reports of patients who had been treated with low-dose Myleran for at least two years for chronic granulocytic leukaemia showed evidence of centrilobular sinusoidal fibrosis. The combination of Myleran and thioguanine is associated with significant hepatotoxicity (see *Drug interactions*). Hyperbilirubinaemia, jaundice, hepatic veno-occlusive disease and centrilobular sinusoidal fibrosis and hepatocellular atrophy and necrosis have been observed after high-dose Myleran treatment.

Lens changes and cataracts, which may be bilateral, have been reported during Myleran therapy. Corneal thinning has been reported after bone marrow transplantation preceded by high-dose Myleran treatment.

Convulsions have been observed in adults who have received high-dose Myleran.

Gynaecomastia has been reported as a side effect of Myleran, as have myasthenia gravis and haemorrhagic cystitis.

Many histological and cytological changes have been observerd in patients treated with Myleran, including widespread dysplasia, affecting uterine cervical, bronchial and other epithelia. Most reports relate to long-term treatment but transient epithelial abnormalities have been observed following short-term, high-dose treatment.

Use in pregnancy and lactation: As with all cytotoxic

chemotherapy, adequate contraceptive precautions should be advised when either partner is receiving Myleran.

Busulphan is teratogenic in animal studies and potentially teratogenic in humans. A few cases of congenital abnormalities, not necessarily attributable to busulphan, have been reported and third trimester exposure may be associated with impaired intra-uterine growth. However, there have also been many reported cases of apparently normal children born after exposure to Myleran *in utero*, even during the first trimester.

The use of Myleran should be avoided whenever possible during pregnancy, particularly during the first trimester. In every individual case the expected benefit of treatment to the mother must be weighed against the possible risks to the foetus.

It is not known whether Myleran or its metabolites are excreted in human breast milk. Mothers receiving Myleran should not breast feed their infants.

Drug interactions: The combination of Myleran and thioguanine has resulted in the development of nodular regenerative hyperplasia, portal hypertension and oesophageal varices.

The effects of other cytotoxics producing pulmonary toxicity may be additive.

Toxicity and treatment of overdosage: The acute dose-limiting toxicity of Myleran in man is myelosuppression. If high-dose Myleran is used in association with bone marrow transplantation, gastro-intestinal toxicity becomes dose-limiting, with mucositis, nausea, vomiting, diarrhoea and anorexia. The main effect of chronic overdosage is bone marrow depression and pancytopenia.

There is no known antidote to Myleran. There are no data about the possible value of dialysis. Appropriate supportive treatment should be given during the period of haematological toxicity.

Pharmaceutical precautions 0.5 mg: Store at 2–8°C. Keep dry. 2.0 mg: Store below 25°C. Keep dry.

Legal category POM.

Package quantities 0.5 mg: Bottle of 25 tablets. 2.0 mg: Bottle of 25 tablets.

Further information Nil.

Product licence numbers
Tablets 0.5 mg 0003/5113R
Tablets 2.0 mg 0003/5112R

NEOSPORIN* EYE DROPS

Presentation A colourless to very pale yellow, slightly hazy solution. Each ml contains:

Polymyxin B Sulphate BP	5,000 units
Neomycin Sulphate BP	1,700 units
Gramicidin USP	25 units

Also contains Thiomersal BP (0.001%) as preservative.

Uses Topical antibacterial agent.

For the prophylaxis and treatment of external bacterial infections of the eye. Prophylactically, it is useful following removal of foreign bodies, and before and after ophthalmic surgery, to help provide and maintain a sterile field.

Dosage and administration *Adults:* 1 or 2 drops in the affected eye, two to four times daily or more frequently as required. In severe infections, therapy should be started with 1 or 2 drops every 15 to 30 minutes, reducing the frequency of instillation gradually as the infection is controlled.

Children: As for adults.

Use in the elderly: No special comment.

Contra-indications, warnings, etc
Contra-indications: Hypersensitivity to polymyxins, gramicidin or the neomycin group of antibiotics.

Precautions: Neomycin is ototoxic and nephrotoxic if absorbed from open surfaces. Polymyxin B and gramicidin are also nephrotoxic. However, these effects are unlikely with ocular administration.

Neosporin Eye Drops should not be used during surgical procedures nor before surgery in circumstances where access of the product to intra-ocular fluids could occur.

Side- and adverse effects: Allergic reactions following the topical application of neomycin have been reported in the literature, but such reactions following the application of polymyxin B and gramicidin are rare events.

As with all antibacterial preparations prolonged use may result in the overgrowth of non-susceptible organisms including fungi.

Use in pregnancy and lactation: Neosporin Eye Drops have been in use for many years. There has been no evidence of untoward effects in pregnancy. However, caution should be exercised by balancing the potential benefits of treatment against any possible hazard.

No information is available regarding the excretion of the active ingredients or their metabolites in human breast milk.

Toxicity and treatment of overdosage: Not applicable.

Pharmaceutical precautions Store below 15°C. Keep dry. Protect from light.

Not suitable for injection. Discard four weeks after opening.

Legal category POM.

Package quantities Special dropper bottle of 5 ml (OP).

Further information Neosporin is a non-irritating isotonic solution and is well tolerated by the sensitive structures of the eye.

Product licence number 0003/5108R.

OTOSPORIN* EAR DROPS

Presentation Each ml of milky-white liquid contains 10,000 IU Polymyxin B Sulphate BP, 3,400 IU Neomycin Sulphate BP, and 1% w/v Hydrocortisone BP, in an aqueous base.

Uses Topical antibacterial and anti-inflammatory for use in the treatment of bacterial infection and inflammation of the external auditory meatus.

Dosage and administration *Adults:* 3 drops should be instilled into the affected ear three or four times daily. Alternatively, a gauze wick may be introduced into the external auditory canal and kept saturated with the solution; the wick may be left in place for 24 to 48 hours. The external auditory meatus and canal should be thoroughly cleansed and carefully dried before each application, but soap should not be used as the antibiotics may be inactivated by it.

Children: As for adults.

Use in the elderly: No special comment.

Contra-indications, warnings, etc
Contra-indications: Hypersensitivity to polymyxins the neomycin group of antibiotics or corticosteroids.

Otosporin should not be used in patients with perforation of the ear drum. It is also contra-indicated in untreated viral, fungal and tubercular conditions.

Precautions: Occasionally, delayed hypersensitivity to corticosteroids may occur. Treatment with topical steroid antibiotic combinations should not be continued for more than seven days in the absence of any clinical improvement, since prolonged use may lead to occult extension of infection due to the masking effect of the steroid.

Prolonged use may also lead to skin sensitisation and the emergence of resistant organisms.

In infants long-term continuous topical steroid therapy should be avoided. Adrenal suppression can occur, even without occlusion.

Prolonged, unsupervised, use should be avoided as it may lead to irreversible partial or total deafness, especially in the elderly and in patients with impaired renal function.

Use in the immediate pre- and post-operative period is not advised as neomycin may rarely cause neuromuscular block; because it potentiates skeletal muscle relaxant drugs, it may cause respiratory depression and arrest.

Side- and adverse effects: Allergic reactions e.g. rash following the topical application of neomycin have been reported in the literature, but such reactions following the application of polymyxin B are rare events.

Use in pregnancy and lactation: Safety for use in pregnancy and lactation has not been established. There is inadequate evidence of safety in human pregnancy. Topical administration of corticosteroids to pregnant animals can cause abnormalities of foetal development, including cleft palate and intra-uterine growth retardation. There may be a very small risk of such effects in the human foetus.

As well as suppression of the neonatal HPA axis, there is a risk of foetal toxicity if aminoglycoside antibiotic preparations are administered during pregnancy.

No information is available regarding the excretion of polymyxin B sulphate or neomycin sulphate or their metabolites in human breast milk, following the use of Otosporin Ear Drops.

Toxicity and treatment of overdosage: There is no experience of overdosage with Otosporin.

Pharmaceutical precautions Store below 15°C. Protect from light.

Legal category POM.

Package quantities Plastic drop-dose bottles of 5 ml (OP) and 10 ml (OP).

Further information Nil.

Product licence number 0003/5106R.

PARAHYPON* TABLETS

Presentation Each tablet contains:

Paracetamol BP	500 mg
Codeine Phosphate BP	5 mg
Caffeine BP	10 mg

The tablets are pink, scored on one side and impressed with the word 'PARA-HYPON' on the other.

Uses Analgesic.

For the relief of pain associated with arthritis, rheumatism and other diseases of the skeletal system, headache, toothache, colds and influenza and other conditions where simple analgesia is required.

Dosage and administration *Adults and children over 12 years:* 2 tablets up to four times daily.

Children 6–12 years: 1 tablet up to four times daily.

Not more than 4 doses should be administered in any 24-hour period; do not repeat dose more frequently than 4-hourly.

Use in the elderly: Use with caution in those with renal or hepatic impairment.

Contra-indications, warnings, etc

Contra-indications: Hypersensitivity to any of the constituents.

Precautions: Use with caution in the presence of renal or hepatic dysfunction.

Drug interactions: In cases of paracetamol overdosage, liver microsomal inducing agents such as barbiturates, tricyclic antidepressants, and alcohol may increase the hepatotoxicity of paracetamol.

Side- and adverse effects: Side-effects with Parahypon are rare in therapeutic doses. Paracetamol has been widely used and reports of adverse reactions are rare, and are generally associated with overdosage. Isolated cases of thrombocytopenic purpura, methaemoglobinaemia, and agranulocytosis have been recorded. Isolated cases of chronic hepatic necrosis, acute pancreatitis and nephrotoxicity have been reported after overdosage or prolonged administration.

Codeine may sometimes cause constipation.

Use in pregnancy and lactation: No data are available on the use of Parahypon in human pregnancy or on the excretion of it or its metabolites in human milk.

Toxicity and treatment of overdosage: Even in severe cases, initial symptoms are likely to be mild and may comprise pallor, nausea and vomiting. Liver damage may not become apparent for 24 hours to 6 days after ingestion.

Overdosage should therefore be treated promptly by gastric lavage followed by i.v. N-acetylcysteine or oral methionine. Additional therapy (further methionine, i.v. N-Acetylcysteine or i.v. cysteamine) is normally considered in the light of blood paracetamol content and the time elapsed since ingestion. Such therapy is probably best undertaken in a specialised unit.

Pharmaceutical precautions Store below 25°C. Keep dry. Protect from light.

Legal category CD (Sch 5), P.

Package quantities Strip-pack of 12 as 2 foil strips of 6 tablets. Container of 100 tablets.

Further information Nil.

Product licence number 0003/0118.

PENTOSTAM* INJECTION

Presentation Pentostam is a faintly yellow, sterile, aqueous solution containing Sodium Stibogluconate BP equivalent to 100 mg pentavalent antimony in each ml.

Uses Pentostam is indicated for the following diseases: Visceral leishmaniasis (kala azar); cutaneous leishmaniasis; South American mucocutaneous leishmaniasis.

Note: Cutaneous and diffuse cutaneous leishmaniasis caused by *Leishmania aethiopica* infections are unresponsive to treatment with pentavalent antimony compounds, including Pentostam, at conventional dosage, but may respond slowly at higher dosage.

Mode of action: The mode of action of Pentostam is unknown. *In vitro* exposure of amastigotes to 500 mg Sb^{5+}/ml results in a greater than 50% decrease in parasite DNA, RNA protein and purine nucleoside triphosphate levels. It has been postulated that the reduction in ATP (adenosine triphosphate) and GTP (guanosine triphosphate) synthesis contributes to decreased macromolecular synthesis.

Pharmacokinetics: Following intravenous or intramuscular administration of sodium stibogluconate, antimony is excreted rapidly via the kidneys, the majority of the dose being detected in the first 12-hour urine collection. This rapid excretion is reflected by a marked fall in serum or whole blood antimony levels to approximately 1–4% of the peak level by 8 hours after an intravenous dose. During daily administration, there is a slow accumulation of sodium stibogluconate into the central compartment so that tissue concentrations reach a theoretical maximum level after at least 7 days.

Dosage and administration Except where otherwise stated, all doses should be given by the intravenous or intramuscular route. (See *Precautions*).

All dosage recommendations are based on the findings of the WHO Expert Committee on leishmaniasis which met in 1984. There are no special recommendations for different age groups.

Visceral leishmaniasis: 10–20 mg Sb^{5+} (0.1–0.2 ml Pentostam)/Kg bodyweight to a maximum of 850 mg (8.5 ml Pentostam) daily for a minimum period of 20 days.

Patients should be examined for evidence of relapse after 2 and 6 months, and in Africa after 12 months.

Cutaneous leishmaniasis NOT caused by L. aethiopica: The dosage regimen outlined for visceral leishmaniasis is recommended. Alternatively, single, non-inflamed nodular lesions known not to be due to *L. braziliensis* may be treated with intralesional injections of 100–300 mg Sb^{5+} (1–3 ml Pentostam) repeated once or twice if necessary at intervals of 1–2 days. Infiltration must be thorough and produce complete blanching of the base of the lesion.

Individuals with cutaneous leishmaniasis due to *L. braziliensis* should be treated systemically for several days after the lesion is healed.

Note: After successful treatment of *L. braziliensis*, anti-leishmania antibody titres decline steadily over 4–24 months.

Muco-cutaneous leishmaniasis: Patients with parasitologically confirmed leishmaniasis should be treated with 20 mg Sb^{5+} (0.2 ml Pentostam)/kg bodyweight to a maximum of 850 mg (8.5 ml Pentostam) daily, continuing this dosage for several days longer than it takes to achieve parasitological and clinical cure.

In the event of relapse, a further course should be given for at least twice the previous duration.

Diffuse cutaneous leishmaniasis in the New World and leishmaniasis recidivans: Owing to the rarity of these conditions, precise data on dosage are not available. A dose of 10–20 mg Sb^{5+} (0.1–0.2 mg Pentostam)/kg bodyweight to a maximum of 850 mg (8.5 ml Pentostam) may be given daily for 2–3 weeks. If there is a response, then treatment should be maintained until several days after clinical cure of leishmaniasis recidivans and for several months after clinical and parasitological cure of diffuse cutaneous leishmaniasis.

Use in the elderly: There is little information on the effects of Pentostam on elderly individuals. If treatment of cutaneous leishmaniasis is necessary then local infiltration is preferred. The normal precautions should be strictly adhered to when treating older patients for visceral leishmaniasis.

Contra-indications, warnings, etc

Contra-indications: Pentostam should not be given to any patient with significantly impaired renal function.

Pentostam should not be given to any patient who has experienced a serious adverse reaction to a previous dose.

Precautions: Intravenous injection should be administered very slowly over 5 minutes to reduce the risk of local thrombosis. In the unlikely event of coughing, vomiting or substernal pain occurring, administration should be discontinued immediately. In such cases, extreme care should be taken if Pentostam is re-administered by this route.

Successful treatment of mucocutaneous leishmaniasis may induce severe inflammation around the lesion. In cases of pharyngeal or tracheal involvement, this may be life-threatening. Under such circumstances, corticosteroids may be used.

Very rarely, anaphylactic shock may develop during treatment for which adrenaline injection and appropriate supportive measures should be given immediately.

Pentostam should be used cautiously in patients with heart disease.

Electrocardiographic changes, notably alterations in T wave amplitude, may be expected in the majority of patients given Pentostam and are not of serious significance. Where electrocardiograms have been done in patients receiving doses in excess of 20 mg/kg bodyweight/day, modest increases in the rate-corrected QT interval have been observed. There is no firm evidence of drug-induced arrhythmias in patients receiving Pentostam, but it is recommended that treatment is withdrawn if conduction disturbances occur.

Patients who have recently received other antimonial drugs should be monitored closely for signs of antimony intoxication such as bradycardia and cardiac arrhythmias during administration of Pentostam.

Intercurrent infections, such as pneumonia, should be sought and treated concomitantly.

High concentrations of antimony are found in the livers of animals after repeated dosage with pentavalent antimony. Pentostam should therefore be used with caution in patients with hepatic disease. However, some abnormalities of liver function may be expected in cases of visceral leishmaniasis. In such patients the benefit of pentavalent antimony treatment outweighs the risk. Pentostam may induce mild elevation of hepatic enzymes in serum which later return to normal; in these cases, treatment should not be stopped.

Drug interactions: No interactions with Pentostam have been reported.

Side- and adverse effects: The majority of side-effects are transitory in nature.

Approximately 1–2% of patients complain of nausea, vomiting and/or diarrhoea and a slightly higher number of abdominal pain.

Other common side-effects include anorexia, malaise, myalgia, headache and lethargy.

Transient coughing immediately following injection was reported with varying frequency during several trials.

Intravenous injection of Pentostam may cause transient pain along the course of the vein and eventually thrombosis of that vein.

During some early trials of sodium stibogluconate, pneumonia occurred in a small number of patients treated for visceral leishmaniasis and this occasionally proved fatal. Pneumonia is a feature of the visceral leishmaniasis disease process; however, it has been associated with the toxicity profile of trivalent antimony. It is, therefore, not possible to determine whether these cases were due to the disease or to Pentostam.

Other (rarely reported) side-effects include fever, rigor, sweating, vertigo, facial flushing, worsening of lesions on the cheek, bleeding from the nose or gum, substernal pain, jaundice and rash.

Use in pregnancy and lactation: Although no effects on the foetus have been reported, Pentostam should be withheld during pregnancy unless the potential benefits to the patient outweigh the possible risk to the foetus.

Children should not be breast-fed by mothers receiving Pentostam.

Toxicity and treatment of overdosage: Main symptoms of antimony overdosage are gastro-intestinal disturbances (nausea, vomiting and severe diarrhoea). Haemorrhagic nephritis and hepatitis may also occur.

There is only limited information on the use of chelating agents in the treatment of intoxication with antimony compounds. Dimercaprol has been reported to be effective: a dose of 200 mg by intramuscular injection, every six hours until recovery is complete, is suggested. 2,3-dimercaptosuccinic acid (DMSA) may also be effective treatment.

Pharmaceutical precautions Store below 25°C and protect from light.

Legal category POM.

Package quantities Rubber-capped bottle of 100 ml.

Further information There is no information on whether Pentostam interferes with the accuracy of routine biochemical tests.

Product licence number 0003/5105R.

PHYSEPTONE* INJECTION
PHYSEPTONE* TABLETS

Presentation Physeptone Injection contains 10 mg Methadone Hydrochloride BP in each ml.

Physeptone Tablets each contain 5 mg Methadone Hydrochloride BP, scored, coded 'WELLCOME L4A' and white in colour.

Uses *Analgesic:* In conditions where morphine would make a reasonable alternative, particularly for the relief of pain of visceral origin. It is not recommended for use in ambulant patients.

Dosage and administration *Analgesic use: Adults:* Usual single dose 5–10 mg by mouth, subcutaneous or intramuscular injection.

Owing to its long plasma half-life caution with repeated dosage should be observed in the very ill or elderly. The usual initial dose should be 5–10 mg, 6–8 hourly, later adjusted to the degree of pain relief obtained.

Children: Not suitable.

Where the drug is given by mouth for the control of pain associated with a chronic condition it is wise to restrict the dose to the smallest amount which adequately controls the symptoms.

Physeptone has less hypnotic effect than morphine.

If it is necessary to give a patient a potent analgesic for a prolonged period, some increase in dose may be found necessary; in such circumstances it is probably sound practice to change to another drug (codeine, morphine, pethidine) for a time. Physeptone may then be resumed in diminished doses.

Use in the elderly: Use caution with repeated dosage in elderly and ill patients.

Contra-indications, warnings, etc
Contra-indications: Respiratory depression, obstructive airways disease. Concurrent administration with monoamine oxidase inhibitors, or within 2 weeks of discontinuation of treatment with them. Obstetric use is not recommended.

Precautions: The possibility of addiction cannot be excluded and patients should be reminded of the necessity of adhering to the prescribed dosage.

Side- and adverse effects: Euphoria, dizziness, drowsiness, vomiting or nausea, and respiratory depression may occur in some patients. In rare cases a hypersensitive subject may react with a sudden transient fall in blood pressure; this is short-lived and self-terminating. Side-effects are more common and more severe in ambulant patients. Nausea and vomiting appear to be more frequent after oral administration than after injection.

In known drug addicts, Physeptone has produced withdrawal symptoms but these are mild. Tolerance and dependence of the morphine type may occur.

Use in pregnancy and lactation: There is no, or inadequate, evidence of safety in human pregnancy but the drug has been widely used for many years without apparent ill-consequence and animal studies have not shown any hazard. From theoretical considerations methadone is likely to be excreted in breast milk.

Toxicity and treatment of overdosage: Toxic doses of methadone cause unconsciousness, pin-point pupils, slow, shallow respiration, cyanosis and weak pulse. Often there is a 2–3 hour delay between ingestion and the appearance of symptoms. Lavage, dialysis and CNS stimulation are contra-indicated. Intravenous naloxone should be given and repeated at 5–10 minute intervals to attain full benefit.

Acidification of the urine will increase the rate of elimination of the drug via the kidney.

Pharmaceutical precautions *Tablets:* Store below 25°C.

Injection: Store below 25°C, protect from light.

Legal category CD (Sch 2), POM.

Package quantities *Physeptone Injection:* 10 mg in 1 ml ampoules. Boxes of 5 and 100 ampoules.

Physeptone Tablets: Blister pack of 50 tablets as 5 blister strips of 10 tablets.

Further information Nil.

Product licence numbers
Injection 0003/5100R
Tablets 0003/5099R

POLIOMYELITIS VACCINE, LIVE (ORAL) BP WELLCOME* 10 DOSE OPV TRIVALENT SABIN TYPE (Pol/Vac (Oral))

Presentation This vaccine is a stabilised sterile aqueous suspension of suitable live attenuated strains of poliomyelitis virus, types 1, 2 and 3, grown in cultures of human diploid cells.

The attenuated vaccine strain of each type of poliovirus has antibody-inducing characteristics similar to its virulent counterpart. Extensive studies have shown that there is little risk of Sabin attenuated virus reverting to a virulent condition.

The vaccine may vary in colour from clear to light pink.

Each dose of Poliomyelitis Vaccine, Live (Oral) contains up to 6 i.u. polymyxin and up to 3 i.u. neomycin. In common with all vaccine derived from Sabin seed, it may also contain traces of penicillin and streptomycin.

Use For active immunisation against poliomyelitis.

Dosage and administration *Dosage: Adults and children:* Three drops constitute one dose. The primary course consists of three doses of poliomyelitis vaccine at intervals of not less than four weeks.

Use in the elderly: No special comment.

Administration: For oral use only. The container should be shaken. To ensure the correct drop size is obtained, the container should be held vertically with the nozzle pointing downwards. Although between batches of containers the drop size, and hence the fill volume, may vary, the virus dose provided remains constant.

In the United Kingdom, oral polio vaccine is usually given in infancy at the same time as routine immunisation against diphtheria, tetanus and pertussis. Thereafter it is recommended that all immunised children be given a single reinforcing dose of oral poliomyelitis vaccine at school entry at the time they receive their reinforcing dose of diphtheria/tetanus vaccine, and again at 15 to 19 years of age or on leaving school. Further reinforcing doses are given to adults if they are likely to be exposed to special risk of contracting the disease.

Administration of oral poliomyelitis vaccine induces circulating antibodies and local antibody responses in the intestine. However, one type of poliovirus in the vaccine may inhibit another from establishing immunity. Thus, when only a single dose of trivalent oral polio vaccine is given successful immunisation against all three types of poliovirus may not occur. Therefore in the primary course the vaccine is administered on at least three occasions to ensure that each type of vaccine poliovirus is given an opportunity of establishing immunity.

If parents or siblings of an infant due for immunisation have never been immunised then, provided there is no contra-indication, it is preferable to vaccinate them with Poliomyelitis Vaccine, Live (Oral) at the same time in order to reduce the remote risk of contact paralysis.

Alternatively, two doses of inactivated poliomyelitis vaccine, one month apart, may be given to the adults *before* administration of Poliomyelitis Vaccine, Live (Oral) to the infant.

It is good practice to record the title, dose and lot numbers of all vaccines and dates of administration. Any untoward reactions should be reported to the regulatory authorities and to the manufacturer.

Contra-indications, warnings, etc
Contra-indications: The antibiotic content of the vaccine does not normally contra-indicate use except in cases of extreme hypersensitivity, e.g. anaphylaxis following its administration.

The efficacy of the vaccine may be impaired if given while the subject has diarrhoea or vomiting. In common with other live vaccines, it should not be administered to subjects with an acute febrile illness or severe chronic illness or widespread malignancy or impaired immune responsiveness whether idiopathic, or as a result of treatment with steroids, radiotherapy, cytotoxic drugs or other agents.

Vaccinees, parents and other household contacts should be made aware of the possible risk of recipient and contact paralysis prior to vaccination.

Any patient who has previously experienced a serious reaction to the vaccine or any component thereof should not be re-vaccinated.

Precautions: Although anaphylaxis is rare, facilities for its management should always be available during vaccination.

Side- and adverse effects: Vaccine-related paralysis in recipients or contacts may occur on very rare occasions.

Use in pregnancy and lactation: Routine oral poliomyelitis vaccination in pregnancy should be avoided, particularly in the first 4 months. If rapid protection must be achieved during pregnancy because of exposure to poliomyelitis, then oral poliomyelitis vaccine may be given. There is some evidence that polio virus is not teratogenic and does not cross the placental barrier.

Poliomyelitis Vaccine Live (Oral) may be administered as early as six weeks of age and the response has been shown to be unaffected by breast feeding from this age onwards.

Toxicity and treatment of overdosage: Not applicable.

Pharmaceutical precautions If stored between 0° and 4°C oral poliomyelitis vaccine can be expected to retain its potency for six months. If stored at or just below 25°C, oral poliomyelitis vaccine can be expected to retain its potency for one week. When tubes of vaccine have been opened there is a risk of contamination with bacteria and moulds which may result in a reduction of vaccine potency. It is good practice, therefore, to discard vaccine remaining in opened tubes at the end of the vaccinating session.

Legal category POM.

Package quantities Polythene dropper tube of 10 doses.

Product licence number 0003/0116

POLIOMYELITIS VACCINE, LIVE (ORAL) BP, WELLCOME* SINGLE DOSE OPV TRIVALENT SABIN TYPE (Pol/Vac (Oral))

Presentation This vaccine is a stabilised sterile aqueous suspension of suitable live attenuated strains of poliomyelitis virus, types 1, 2 and 3, grown in cultures of human diploid cells.

The attenuated vaccine strain of each type of poliovirus has antibody-inducing characteristics similar to its virulent counterpart. Extensive studies have shown that there is little risk of Sabin attenuated virus reverting to a virulent condition.

The vaccine may vary in colour from clear to light pink.

Each dose of Poliomyelitis Vaccine, Live (Oral) contains up to 6 i.u. polymyxin and up to 3 i.u. neomycin. In common with all vaccine derived from Sabin seed, it also may contain traces of penicillin and streptomycin.

Uses For active immunization against poliomyelitis.

Dosage and administration
Dosage: Adults and children: The contents of one single dose polythene tube constitute one dose. The primary course consists of three doses of poliomyelitis vaccine at intervals of not less than four weeks.

Use in the elderly: No special comment.

Administration: For oral use only. Separate a single-dose tube from the strip. The tube should be held by the large tab and shaken down, as with a thermometer, to propel the entire contents to the corrugated end. The tube should be held upright without applying pressure to the tube, and the narrow end removed by twisting the top. Incline tube and shake gently to move the vaccine to the open end. The contents are then expelled by exerting gentle pressure to the tube just above the surface of the liquid (a small residue of vaccine may remain). Since the vaccine contains live attenuated poliomyelitis virus, care should be taken to avoid transfer of virus to immunodeficient subjects. Caution should be exercised to avoid spillage. Both parts of the container should be subject to disposal, e.g. by incineration, while the spoon may be either incinerated or sterilised in a 0.1% aqueous hypochlorite solution yielding 1000 ppm available chlorine (e.g. 1:10 Milton* 1%) and then rinsed thoroughly in water.

In the United Kingdom, oral polio vaccine is usually given in infancy at the same time as routine immunization against diphtheria, tetanus and pertussis. Thereafter it is recommended that all immunized children be given a single reinforcing dose of oral poliomyelitis vaccine at school entry at the time they receive their reinforcing dose of diphtheria/tetanus vaccine, and again at 15 to 19 years of age or on leaving school. Further reinforcing doses are given to adults if they are likely to be exposed to special risk of contracting the disease.

Administration of oral poliomyelitis vaccine induces circulating antibodies and local antibody responses in the intestine. However, one type of poliovirus in the vaccine may inhibit another from establishing immunity. Thus, when only a single dose of trivalent oral polio vaccine is given, successful immunization against all three types of poliovirus may not occur. Therefore in the primary course the vaccine is administered on at least three occasions to ensure that each type of vaccine poliovirus is given an opportunity of establishing immunity.

If parents or siblings of an infant due for immunization have never been immunized then, provided there is no contra-indication, it is preferable to vaccinate them with Poliomyelitis Vaccine, Live (Oral) BP at the same time in order to reduce the remote risk of contact paralysis.

Alternatively, two doses of inactivated poliomyelitis vaccine, one month apart, may be given to the adults *before* administration of Poliomyelitis Vaccine, Live (Oral) BP to the infant.

It is good practice to record the title, dose and lot numbers of all vaccines and dates of administration. Any untoward reactions should be reported to the regulatory authorities and to the manufacturer.

Contra-indications, warnings, etc
Contra-indications: The antibiotic content of the vaccine does not normally contra-indicate use except in cases of extreme hypersensitivity, e.g. anaphylaxis following its administration.

The efficacy of the vaccine may be impaired if given while the subject has diarrhoea or vomiting. In common with other live vaccines, it should not be administered to subjects with an acute febrile illness or severe chronic illness or widespread malignancy or impaired immune responsiveness whether idiopathic, or as a result of treatment with steroids, radiotherapy, cytotoxic drugs or other agents.

Vaccinees, parents and other household contacts should be made aware of the possible risk of recipient and contact paralysis prior to vaccination.

Any patient who has previously experienced a serious reaction to the vaccine or any component thereof should not be re-vaccinated.

Precautions: Although anaphylaxis is rare, facilities for its management should always be available during vaccination.

Side- and adverse effects: Vaccine-related paralysis in recipients or contacts may occur on very rare occasions.

Use in pregnancy and lactation: Routine oral poliomyelitis vaccination in pregnancy should be avoided particularly in the first 4 months, but it may be given if rapid protection during pregnancy is indicated because of exposure to poliomyelitis. There is some evidence that polio virus is not teratogenic and does not cross the placental barrier.

Poliomyelitis Vaccine Live (Oral) BP may be administered as early as six weeks of age and the response has been shown to be unaffected by breast feeding from this age onwards.

Toxicity and treatment of overdosage: Not applicable.

Pharmaceutical precautions If stored between 0° and 4°C, oral poliomyelitis vaccine can be expected to retain its potency for six months. If stored at or just below 25°C, oral poliomyelitis vaccine can be expected to retain its potency for one week.

Legal category POM.

Package quantities Strip of 10 polythene dropper tubes each containing one dose.

Product licence number 0003/0116.

POLYBACTRIN* SOLUBLE GU

Presentation One vial contains, in sterile dry powder:

Polymyxin B Sulphate BP	75,000 units
Neomycin Sulphate BP	20,000 units
Bacitracin BP 1968	1,000 units

Uses Antibacterial for bladder irrigation only.

To treat and prevent bacteriuria and prevent Gram-negative rod bacteraemia associated with the use of indwelling catheters. For temporary retention in the bladder following intermittent catheterisation and following cystoscopy.

Dosage and administration Reconstitute in 10 ml of isotonic saline then transfer to the appropriate volume of isotonic saline and mix. *Adults:* For continuous irrigation of the bladder for periods up to 10 days, a three-way catheter should be used. Two vials of powder dissolved in 500 ml of isotonic saline provide for a slow drip to be delivered over 24 hours. For patients with a urine output exceeding 2 litres per day, it is recommended that the drip rate be doubled.

Following intermittent catheterisation or cystoscopy, 1 vial of powder dissolved in 10–40 ml of isotonic saline may be introduced into the bladder and retained for an hour. This treatment may be used twice daily. See Contra-indications, warnings, etc.

Children: Proportionate reduction in dose according to weight.

Use in the elderly: No specific studies have been carried out in the elderly, however, it may be advisable to monitor renal function in these patients and if there is any impairment then caution should be exercised.

Contra-indications, warnings, etc

Contra-indications: Hypersensitivity to polymyxins, bacitracin or the neomycin group of antibiotics.

The presence of pre-existing nerve deafness is a contra-indication to the use of Polybactrin Soluble GU or any aminoglycoside in circumstances in which significant systemic absorption could occur.

Precautions: Polybactrin Soluble GU may be absorbed after administration to the bladder, particularly if it is denuded, and therefore excessive use should be avoided in order to prevent complications from systemic absorption of excess amounts of the antibiotic constituents.

Neomycin sulphate is the dose-limiting ingredient of Polybactrin Soluble GU because it can cause irreversible nerve deafness following significant systemic absorption; the recommended dosages should *not* be exceeded.

In adult patients with normal renal function, the maximum recommended *parenteral* dosage of neomycin sulphate is 1 g/day for not more than 7 days. This amount would be provided by 4 vials of Polybactrin Soluble GU administered daily for 21 days. After such a maximum course, further treatment with Polybactrin Soluble GU, must *not* be administered for at least three months.

In renal impairment the plasma clearance of neomycin is reduced, therefore a reduction in dose should be made that relates to the degree of renal impairment.

In cases where there is established partial nerve deafness and where a significant degree of neomycin absorption could occur it might be inappropriate to use any neomycin-containing product and treatment with an antibacterial without an aminoglycoside constituent should be used if possible.

Concurrent administration of other aminoglycoside antibiotics is not recommended.

As neomycin and polymyxin have a neuromuscular blocking effect, patients concurrently receiving other agents with a similar action should be observed for signs of possible respiratory insufficiency.

Side- and adverse effects: Allergic reactions following the topical application of neomycin have been reported in the literature, but such reactions following the application of polymyxin B and bacitracin are rare events.

Anaphylactic reactions following the topical administration of bacitracin zinc have been reported, however this is a rare occurrence.

Following significant systemic absorption, neomycin sulphate, polymyxin B sulphate and bacitracin zinc have nephrotoxic potential and polymyxin B sulphate has neurotoxic potential.

Use in pregnancy and lactation: Due to a lack of detailed information the use of Polybactrin Soluble GU during pregnancy and lactation cannot be recommended in circumstances where significant systemic absorption of the active ingredients may occur.

No information is available regarding the excretion of the active ingredients or their metabolites in human milk.

Toxicity and treatment of overdosage: In the event of signs of toxicity developing following significant systemic absorption of the active ingredients of Polybactrin Soluble GU, the patient's general status, hearing acuity, renal function and neuromuscular function should be monitored and blood levels of polymyxin B, neomycin, and bacitracin determined. Serum levels of neomycin may be reduced by haemodialysis.

Pharmaceutical precautions Store below 25°C. Keep dry.

Solutions should be used within 24 hours of their preparation.

Legal category POM.

Package quantities Pack of 5 sterile vials.

Further information Nil.

Product licence number 0003/5055.

POLYBACTRIN* SPRAY

Presentation A sterile powder. Each 115 ml pressurised canister contains:

Polymyxin B Sulphate BP	150,000 units
Neomycin Sulphate BP	495,000 units
Zinc Bacitracin BP	37,500 units

in aerosol propellant.

Uses Topical antibacterial powder.

Prevention of wound infection in surgery. Treatment of infected skin.

Dosage and administration *Adults:* A thin, uniform spray should be applied to affected areas, as required. This can be obtained from a spray of about one second's duration to the wound surface at a distance of not less than 20 cm. The application of one can of spray daily for seven days should not be exceeded. After such a course, treatment should not be repeated for at least three months.

Children: The maximum dosage should be reduced in proportion to body weight.

Use in the elderly: No specific studies have been carried out in the elderly, however, it may be advisable to monitor renal function in these patients and if there is any impairment then caution should be exercised.

Contra-indications, warnings, etc

Contra-indications: Hypersensitivity to polymyxins, bacitracin or the neomycin group of antibiotics.

Polybactrin Spray should not be used on pre-term infants.

Precautions: Absorption of the active ingredients can occur following the application of Polybactrin Spray to serous membranes or raw broken skin.

Neomycin sulphate is the dose-limiting ingredient of Polybactrin Spray because it can cause irreversible nerve deafness following significant systemic absorption.

In cases where there is established partial nerve deafness and where a significant degree of neomycin absorption could occur it might be inappropriate to use any neomycin-containing product and treatment with an antibacterial without an aminoglycoside constituent should be used if possible.

In renal impairment the plasma clearance of neomycin is reduced, therefore a reduction in dose should be made that relates to the degree of renal impairment.

The inappropriate use of topical antibiotics has been associated with the emergence of resistant strains of bacteria.

The spray should not be used on large denuded areas (e.g. burns or ulcers) because of the risk of systemic absorption. Patients with hypostatic leg ulcers may have an increased sensitivity to a large number of topically applied drugs, including Neomycin.

Concurrent administration of other aminoglycoside antibiotics is not recommended.

As neomycin and polymyxin have a neuromuscular blocking effect, patients concurrently receiving other agents with a similar action should be observed for signs of possible respiratory insufficiency.

As with all aerosol products not specifically intended for respiratory tract therapy, care should be taken to avoid inhalation of spray mist.

Avoid spraying Polybactrin Spray into the eyes.

Side- and adverse effects: Allergic reactions following the topical application of neomycin have been reported in the literature, but such reactions following the application of polymyxin B and bacitracin are rare events.

Allergic hypersensitivity to neomycin is generally uncommon following topical use but may manifest itself as a reddening and scaling of the affected skin, as an eczematous exacerbation of the lesion, or as a failure of the lesion to heal.

Allergic hypersensitivity, including anaphylaxis, following topical administration of bacitracin has been reported rarely.

Following significant systemic absorption, neomycin sulphate, polymyxin B sulphate and bacitracin zinc have nephrotoxic potential and polymyxin B sulphate has neurotoxic potential.

A transient, mild burning sensation on the skin has occasionally been reported following the administration of Polybactrin Spray.

Use in pregnancy and lactation: Due to a lack of detailed information the use of Polybactrin Spray during pregnancy and lactation cannot be recommended in circumstances where significant systemic absorption of the active ingredients may occur.

No information is available regarding the excretion of the active ingredients or their metabolites in human milk.

Toxicity and treatment of overdosage: In the event of signs of toxicity developing following significant systemic absorption of the active ingredients of Polybactrin Spray, the patient's general status, hearing acuity, renal function and neuromuscular function should be monitored and blood levels of polymyxin B, neomycin, and bacitracin determined. Serum levels of neomycin may be reduced by haemodialysis.

Pharmaceutical precautions Do not expose to temperatures over 25°C. Do not puncture or incinerate even after use. Do not autoclave.

Legal category POM.

Package quantities Pressurised aerosol powder spray (OP).

Further information Nil.

Product licence number 0003/5056.

POLYFAX* OINTMENT

Presentation Polyfax Ointment contains 10,000 units of Polymyxin B Sulphate BP and 500 units of Zinc Bacitracin BP per gram, in a stable petrolatum base. The translucent ointment is off-white in colour.

Uses Topical antibacterial agent.

Polyfax Ointment is indicated for the treatment of infected wounds, burns, skin grafts, ulcers, pyoderma, sycosis barbae, impetigo, and in secondarily infected skin lesions of scabies, pediculosis, tinea pedis and contact and allergic dermatitis.

Dosage and administration *Adults:* Polyfax Ointment should be applied thinly over the affected area, which is best left exposed. Two or more applications a day may be necessary, depending on the severity of the condition.

Children: As for adults.

Use in the elderly: No specific studies have been carried out in the elderly, however, it may be advisable to monitor renal function in these patients and if there is any impairment then caution should be exercised.

Contra-indications, warnings, etc
Contra-indications: Hypersensitivity to bacitracin, polymyxins or cross-sensitising substances.

Precautions: The following statements take into account the possibility that the constituent drugs of Polyfax Ointment may be absorbed to a significant degree after topical application. However, the normal use of Polyfax is unlikely to present any risk of systemic toxicity unless the application were excessive, e.g. more than 200 g per day in adults or proportionately less in children and in patients with compromised renal function.

Nephrotoxicity may result from the absorption of bacitracin, and nephrotoxicity and neurotoxicity from polymyxin B.

As with all antibacterial preparations prolonged use may result in the overgrowth of non-susceptible organisms including fungi.

Side- and adverse effects: Allergic reactions following topical application of polymyxin B and zinc bacitracin have rarely been reported.

Anaphylactic reactions have been reported, as rare events, following topical application of zinc bacitracin.

Following significant systemic absorption, polymyxin B can intensify and prolong the respiratory depressant effects of neuromuscular blocking agents.

Use in pregnancy and lactation: Due to a lack of detailed information, the use of Polyfax Ointment during pregnancy and lactation cannot be recommended in circumstances where significant systemic absorption of the active ingredients may occur.

No information is available regarding the excretion of the active ingredients or their metabolites in human milk.

Toxicity and treatment of overdosage: In the unlikely event of significant systemic absorption of the active ingredients of Polyfax Ointment occurring, signs of neurotoxicity and nephrotoxicity may be noted. In such an event, the patient's general status and renal function should be monitored and blood levels of polymyxin B and zinc bacitracin determined.

Pharmaceutical precautions Store below 25°C.

Legal category POM.

Package quantities Tube of 20 g (OP).

Further information Nil.

Product licence number 0003/5230.

POLYFAX* OPHTHALMIC OINTMENT

Presentation An off-white, translucent ointment. Each gram of ointment contains:

Polymyxin B Sulphate BP	10,000 IU
Bacitracin Zinc BP	500 IU

in a sterile, anhydrous, stable paraffin base.

Uses Polyfax Ophthalmic Ointment is indicated for the treatment of bacterial infections of the eye and its adnexa, including, conjunctivitis, keratitis, corneal ulceration and ulcerative blepharitis.

Polyfax Ophthalmic Ointment may be applied both pre- and post-operatively to prevent ocular infection following surgical procedures, including the removal of foreign bodies from the eye.

The use of Polyfax does not exclude concomitant systemic therapy or other forms of local therapy where appropriate.

In vitro activity: Polyfax Ophthalmic Ointment is a bactericidal preparation active against the majority of bacterial eye pathogens including:

GRAM-POSITIVE
Staphylococcus spp
Streptococcus spp including *S. pyogenes* (B haemolytic streptococcus)
S. pneumoniae (pneumococcus)
Corynebacterium spp

GRAM-NEGATIVE
Pseudomonas spp (including *P. aeruginosa*)
Haemophilus spp
Klebsiella spp
Enterobacter spp
Escherichia spp
Neisseria spp

Dosage and administration
Adults: A thin film of ointment should be applied to the affected part or inside the lower eyelid two or more times a day depending on the severity of the condition.

Treatment should be continued until at least two days after the eye has apparently recovered.

Children: As for adults.

Use in the elderly: No special comment.

Contra-indications, warnings, etc
Contra-indications: Hypersensitivity to bacitracin zinc, polymyxin B sulphate or to cross-sensitising substances.

Precautions: Ocular administration of Polyfax Ophthalmic Ointment is extremely unlikely to lead to significant absorption of the constituents and therefore presents no risk of systemic toxicity.

Side- and adverse effects: Allergic reactions following topical (dermatological) application of polymyxin B and bacitracin zinc is rare but has been reported.

As with other antibacterial preparations, prolonged use may result in the overgrowth of non-susceptible organisms, including fungi.

Use in pregnancy and lactation: Polyfax has been used for several years without any untoward effect in pregnancy. The clinical benefit of the treatment to the patient must be balanced against any possible but unknown hazards to the developing foetus.

No information is available regarding the excretion of the active ingredients or their metabolites in human milk.

Toxicity and treatment of overdosage: Not applicable.

Pharmaceutical precautions Store below 25°C. Discard the tube within one month of first opening.

Legal category POM.

Package quantities Tube of 4 g (OP).

Further information In widespread and long established clinical use, Polyfax Ophthalmic Ointment has an excellent record in terms of non-irritancy and non-allergenicity.

Product licence number 0003/5229R.

POLYTRIM* EYE DROPS

Presentation A clear, colourless, sterile, aqueous solution containing in each ml: Trimethoprim BP 1 mg; Polymyxin B Sulphate BP 10,000 units. Thiomersal BP (0.05 mg per ml) is included as a preservative.

Uses Antibacterial agent. For the treatment and prophylaxis of external bacterial infections of the eye including conjunctivitis, keratitis, corneal ulceration, ulcerative blepharitis with associated conjunctivitis, and chronic dacryocystitis. Prophylactically, it is useful following removal of foreign bodies, and before and after ophthalmic surgery to help provide and maintain a sterile field. Use of Polytrim does not exclude concomitant systemic therapy or other forms of local therapy, where appropriate.

Dosage and administration *Adults:* 1 drop in the affected eye four times daily. *Children:* As for adults.

More frequent administration may be required, depending on the severity of the condition. Treatment should normally be continued for at least forty-eight hours after the eye has apparently returned to normal.

Use in the elderly: No special precautions.

Contra-indications, warnings, etc
Contra-indications: Contra-indicated in individuals who have a history of hypersensitivity to trimethoprim, polymyxins, or cross-sensitising substances.

Precautions: As with all antibacterial preparations, prolonged use may result in the overgrowth of non-susceptible organisms including fungi.

Side- and adverse effects: Polytrim is isotonic with tear fluid and is well tolerated in the eye. No local adverse effects are to be expected, except rarely, a hypersensitivity reaction. If one is suspected during treatment, administration should be discontinued.

Use in pregnancy and lactation: The active ingredients of Polytrim Eye Drops have been used for several years without any evidence of untoward effect in pregnancy, however the clinical benefit of treatment to the patient must be balanced against any possible hazard to the developing foetus.

No information is available regarding the excretion of polymyxin B sulphate or its metabolites in human breast milk.

Trimethoprim is excreted in breast milk following *systemic* administration but this presents a negligible risk to the suckling infant. No information, however, is available on the excretion of trimethoprim or its metabolites in human breast milk following topical application.

Toxicity and treatment of overdosage: Not applicable.

Pharmaceutical precautions Do not use if the container seal has been broken. Use within one month of opening container: Store below 25°C, and protect from light. Not suitable for injection.

Legal category POM.

Package quantities Screw-capped plastic dropper bottle containing 5 ml (OP).

Further information The combination is effective against a wide variety of Gram-positive and Gram-negative bacterial ocular pathogens, including *Pseudomonas aeruginosa.*

Product licence number 0003/0153.

POLYTRIM* OPHTHALMIC OINTMENT

Presentation A white to off-white sterile ointment containing Trimethoprim BP 0.5% w/w and Polymyxin B Sulphate BP 10,000 units per gram in a sterile, anhydrous, soft paraffin base.

Uses An antibacterial agent for the treatment and prophylaxis of external bacterial infections of the eye and surrounding tissues including conjunctivitis, keratitis, corneal ulceration, ulcerative blepharitis and chronic dacryocystitis. Prophylactically, it can be used following removal of foreign bodies, and before and after ophthalmic surgery to help provide and maintain a sterile field.

Dosage and administration
Dosage in adults: Apply a thin film of ointment either directly to the affected part or inside the lower conjunctival sac 3 to 4 times a day depending on the severity of the condition.

Dosage in children: As for adults. Suitable for use in subjects of all ages including infants.

Treatment should normally be continued until at least forty-eight hours after the eye has apparently returned to normal. Debris such as crusts or pus should be removed prior to application of the ointment.

Use in the elderly: No specific studies have been carried out in the elderly, although no special precautions are expected to be applied to this group.

Contra-indications, warnings, etc
Contra-indications: Contra-indicated in individuals who have a history of hypersensitivity to trimethoprim or to polymyxins.

Precautions: As with all antibacterial preparations prolonged use may result in the overgrowth of non-susceptible organisms including fungi.

Side- and adverse effects: Rarely, hypersensitivity reactions may occur. If one is suspected during treatment, administration should be discontinued.

Use in pregnancy and lactation: There is no evidence of safety of Polytrim Ophthalmic Ointment in human pregnancy, however the active ingredients have been in use for many years without apparent ill consequence. In high systemic dosage (40 times the human systemic dose), trimethoprim has been shown to be teratogenic in rats. Although the topical application is unlikely to be associated with risk, the clinical benefit of treatment to the patient must be balanced against any possible but unknown hazards to the developing foetus.

No information is available on the excretion of polymyxin in breast milk.

Excretion of trimethoprim into breast milk has been noted after oral administration to lactating women, but this represents negligible risk to the suckling infant.

Toxicity and treatment of overdosage: Not applicable.

Pharmaceutical precautions Do not use if container seal has been broken. Use within one month of opening container. Store below 25°C.

Legal category POM.

Package quantities Tubes of 4 g (OP).

Further information The combination is effective against a wide variety of Gram-positive and Gram-negative bacterial ocular pathogens, including *Pseudomonas aeruginosa*, but not *Neisseria gonorrhoeae*.

Product licence number 0003/0223.

PRO-ACTIDIL* TABLETS

Presentation Each tablet contains 10 mg of Triprolidine Hydrochloride BP divided between three layers to give a rapid onset of action, followed by a sustained release of the drug to give a therapeutic effect lasting up to 24 hours in most patients. Each tablet is coded 'WELLCOME M4A' and is white with blue core and pink middle layer.

Uses Prolonged action antihistamine.

Pro-Actidil is indicated for the symptomatic relief of allergic conditions normally responsive to antihistamines, e.g. hay fever and allergic skin conditions, e.g. urticaria and pruritus.

Dosage and administration *Adults and children over 12 years:* 1 tablet swallowed whole with a little water in the early evening, or five to six hours before retiring. A few patients with very severe symptoms may need two tablets during 24 hours.

Under 12 years: Pro-Actidil is not recommended for children under 12 years.

Use in the elderly: No specific studies have been carried out in the elderly, however, it may be advisable to monitor renal or hepatic function and if there is serious impairment then caution should be exercised.

Contra-indications, warnings, etc
Contra-indications: Contra-indicated in patients with known hypersensitivity to triprolidine.

Pro-Actidil is contra-indicated in individuals with severe hepatic or renal dysfunction because of its long duration of action, but consideration may be given to the cautious use of Actidil.

Precautions: May cause drowsiness. Patients should not drive a vehicle or operate machinery until they have determined their own response. In some patients the drowsiness induced by antihistamines may be potentiated by alcohol or other central sedatives.

Since antihistamines have some anticholinergic properties, Pro-Actidil should be used with care in patients with elevated intraocular pressure and in patients with prostatic hypertrophy.

Side- and adverse effects: Triprolidine may cause drowsiness. Lichenoid skin eruptions due to triprolidine have rarely been reported.

Use in pregnancy and lactation: Although triprolidine has been in widespread use for many years without apparent ill consequence, there are no specific data on its use during pregnancy. Caution should therefore be exercised by balancing the potential benefit of treatment against any possible hazards. Systemic administration of triprolidine in rats and rabbits up to 75 times the human dose did not produce teratogenic effects.

It has been estimated that approximately 0.06–0.2% of a single dose of triprolidine ingested by a mother will be excreted in the breast milk over 24 hours.

Toxicity and treatment of overdosage: Symptoms of acute toxicity from Pro-Actidil arise from its effects on the central nervous system and may include drowsiness, lethargy, dizziness, ataxia, weakness, hypotonicity and respiratory depression. Atropine-like symptoms such as dryness of the skin and mucous membranes, tachycardia, hyperpyrexia, hyperactivity and convulsions may also occur.

Necessary measures should be taken to maintain and support respiration. Gastric lavage should be performed if indicated and convulsions controlled with diazepam.

Pharmaceutical precautions Store below 15°C. Protect from light.

Legal category P.

Package quantities Bottle of 100 tablets.

Further information Nil.

Product licence number 0003/5228R.

PRO-VENT*

Presentation Each Pro-Vent capsule contains 300 mg of Theophylline BP in specially formulated pellets to provide continuous therapeutic effect for 12 hours. Each capsule has a white opaque cap and a clear colourless body and is marked in blue with 'Wellcome' and the code 'B7C'.

Uses Pro-Vent capsules are indicated for the prevention and treatment of bronchial smooth-muscle constriction in patients with asthma and chronic bronchitis.

Dosage and administration The dose should be adjusted according to the need and response of the patient. Since theophylline pharmacokinetics are very variable between individuals, serum levels should be monitored wherever possible particularly in smokers and other fast clearers of theophylline. The conventional therapeutic range is 10–20 mg/l although bronchodilation has been demonstrated with serum levels below this range.

Adults and children over 12 years: A typical starting dose is one 300 mg capsule 12 hourly.

Pharmacokinetic studies with Pro-Vent do not indicate

that any special consideration needs to be given to the timing of doses in relation to meals, although morning and evening mealtimes may be convenient markers to remind patients to take a dose.

Children under 12 years: Formulations not applicable.

Use in the elderly: There are no specific studies with Pro-Vent although, for theophylline generally, there is evidence that a decrease in total body clearance together with an increase in elimination half-life parallels increase in age of patient. Serum levels should therefore be monitored, as a lower dose may be necessary.

Pharmacology: Theophylline inhibits phosphodiesterase, leading to an increase in intracellular cyclic AMP which results in smooth-muscle relaxation.

Pharmacokinetics: Pro-vent capsules provide a completely available controlled oral dose of theophylline. In fasted young (mean age 25 y) male and female healthy non-smokers, the bioavailability of a single 300 mg capsule relative to theophylline solution was 105%. The peak concentration (Cmax) of the mean theophylline profile was reduced and delayed, relative to solution, from 7.4 mg/l at 3 h, to 4.6 mg/l at 8 h. Multiple dosing for 5 days with Pro-Vent 300 mg b.d. compared with theophylline solution 200 mg t.i.d. in these subjects indicated bioavailability of 102%, a mean Cmax of 11.1 mg/l at 3.6 h post dose and 12 h trough (Cmin) of 5.7 mg/l, with an average theophylline concentration of 7.6 mg/l.

Multiple dosing of Pro-Vent for 5 days (escalating from 1 × 300 mg b.d. to 2 × 300 mg b.d. in increments) in selected fast-clearing young healthy smokers and non-smokers (mean age 24 y, male and females) showed dose proportionality with each increase, with smokers producing lower theophylline levels than non-smokers. At 300 mg b.d. steady state average plasma theophylline levels were 3.3 mg/l, with Cmax 5.1 mg/l and Cmin 1.9 mg/l, rising to an average of 8.3 mg/l, Cmax of 11.4 mg/l and Cmin of 5.4 mg/l at 600 mg b.d.

Contra-indications, warnings, etc

Contra-indications: Pro-Vent is contra-indicated in patients who are hypersensitive to theophylline or to other xanthines.

Pro-Vent should not be used in conjunction with other xanthine-containing preparations.

Precautions: Duration of action of theophylline is reduced by smoking, which increases clearance of the drug. A higher dosage may therefore be required.

Caution should be exercised when prescribing theophylline for patients with heart failure or liver failure or chronic alcoholism. These diseases may reduce the clearance of theophylline and lead to higher than normal serum levels and a greater risk of toxicity.

Viral infections, influenza vaccination and BCG inoculation can impair metabolism of theophylline, leading to increased serum concentrations.

Renal failure does not affect theophylline dosing requirements, although plasma concentrations may be reduced by haemodialysis or peritoneal dialysis.

Where patients receiving oral theophylline require parenteral theophylline therapy, this should ideally be deferred until a serum theophylline measurement is obtained.

Serum theophylline levels should also be used to guide conversion from intravenous theophylline therapy to sustained release preparations.

Caution should be exercised in patients with peptic ulcer, cardiac arrhythmias, hyperthyroidism, hypertension or epilepsy.

The total dose of theophylline may need to be reduced when converting from an immediate release to a sustained-release preparation.

Dosage adjustment may be necessary when switching between brands of sustained release theophylline, since bioavailability may not be constant.

Xanthines can potentiate hypokalaemia resulting from $beta_2$ agonist therapy, steroids, diuretics and hypoxia. Particular caution is advised in severe asthma. It is recommended that serum potassium levels are monitored in such situations.

Side- and adverse effects: Nausea, dyspepsia, vomiting, haematemesis and anorexia may occur in some patients. Central nervous stimulation, dizziness, light-headedness, nervousness, headache and insomnia are rarely seen unless plasma levels rise above 20 mg/l. Convulsions may occur when blood levels exceed 25 mg/l.

Palpitations, tachycardia and urinary retention have also been reported. Peptic ulcer disease may be exacerbated through theophylline stimulation of gastric acid secretion.

The correct use of a sustained-release preparation means that potentially toxic peaks in theophylline serum levels are avoided.

Drug interactions: Theophylline may interact with other xanthine derivatives or sympathomimetics to produce exaggerated effects. The excretion of lithium carbonate may be increased by theophylline. Increased theophylline plasma levels have been described when erythromycin, clindamycin, lincomycin, cimetidine, allopurinol, influenza vaccine, propanolol, thiabendazole, troleandomycin, hydrocortisone, methylprednisolone, interferon or ciprofloxacin are administered concurrently.

Decreased plasma levels of theophylline have been attributed to concurrent use of sulphinpyrazone, rifampicin, phenytoin, carbamazepine, isoprenaline, phenobarbitone and quinalbarbitone.

Theophylline has been reported to decrease steady-state levels of phenytoin by decreasing absorption of phenytoin when the two are co-administered orally.

Use in pregnancy and lactation: There is inadequate evidence of safety of theophylline in human pregnancy but it has been in wide use for many years without apparent ill consequence. If drug therapy is needed in pregnancy this drug can be used if there is no safer alternative.

Although no long term adverse effects have been reported in infants of mothers receiving theophylline throughout pregnancy, a single case of transplacental aminophylline toxicity in a neonate (irritability, vomiting and jitteriness) has been reported.

Theophylline is excreted in human milk. Tachycardia and transient jitteriness have been reported in three newborn infants whose mothers had blood concentrations of theophylline within the therapeutic range. Care should thus be exercised with theophylline therapy for nursing mothers.

Toxicity and treatment of overdosage: The clinical presentations of chronic and acute toxicity differ although in both cases seizures may be the major symptom. Chronic toxicity can reveal itself through tachycardia, tachypnoea, nausea, irritability, anorexia and seizures. Acute toxicity can present with the above symptoms but also metabolic disturbance, cardiac arrhythmias and circulatory failure.

Gastric lavage and supportive measures for respiration and circulation should be performed if necessary. Convulsions should be controlled with an anticonvulsant. Charcoal haemoperfusion has been used to facilitate rapid removal of theophylline from serum in cases of gross overdosage.

Pharmaceutical precautions Store below 25°C. Keep dry.

Legal category P.

Package quantities Container of 100 capsules.

Further information The specially formulated pellets in Pro-Vent capsules give both rapid and predictable absorption along with prolonged therapeutic blood levels of theophylline for up to 12 hours.

Product licence number 0003/0167.

PURI-NETHOL* TABLETS

Presentation Each tablet contains 50 mg Mercaptopurine BP, fawn coloured, scored and coded 'WELLCOME 04A'.

Uses Cytotoxic agent.

Puri-Nethol is indicated for the treatment of acute

leukaemia. It is of value in remission induction and is particularly indicated for maintenance therapy in acute lymphoblastic leukaemia and acute myelogenous leukaemia. Puri-Nethol is used in the treatment of chronic granulocytic leukaemia.

Dosage and administration For adults and children the usual dose is 2.5 mg/kg bodyweight per day, but the dose and duration of administration depend on the nature and dosage of other cytotoxic agents given in conjunction with Puri-Nethol. The dosage should be carefully adjusted to suit the individual patient. Puri-Nethol has been used in various combination therapy schedules for acute leukaemia and the literature should be consulted for details. Consideration should be given to reducing the dosage in patients with impaired hepatic or renal function. When Zyloric (allopurinol) and mercaptopurine are administered concomitantly it is essential that only a quarter of the usual dose of mercaptopurine is given since Zyloric (allopurinol) decreases the rate of catabolism of mercaptopurine.

Use in the elderly: No specific studies have been carried out in the elderly, however, it is advisable to monitor renal and hepatic function in these patients, and if there is any impairment consideration should be given to reducing the Puri-Nethol dosage.

Contra-indications, warnings, etc
Contra-indications: In view of the seriousness of the indications there are no absolute contra-indications.

Precautions: Puri-Nethol is an active cytotoxic agent for use only under the direction of physicians experienced in the administration of such agents.

Since Puri-Nethol is strongly myelosuppressive full blood counts must be taken daily during remission induction. Patients must be carefully monitored during therapy.

Treatment with Puri-Nethol causes bone marrow suppression leading to leucopenia and thrombocytopenia.

The leucocyte and platelet counts continue to fall after treatment is stopped, so at the first sign of an abnormally large fall in the counts, treatment should be interrupted immediately.

Bone marrow suppression is reversible if Puri-Nethol is withdrawn early enough.

During remission induction in acute myelogenous leukaemia the patient may frequently have to survive a period of relative bone marrow aplasia and it is important that adequate supportive facilities are available.

Puri-Nethol is hepatotoxic and liver function tests should be monitored weekly during treatment. More frequent monitoring may be advisable in those with pre-existing liver disease or receiving other potentially hepatotoxic therapy. The patient should be instructed to discontinue Puri-Nethol immediately if jaundice becomes apparent.

During remission induction when rapid cell lysis is occurring, uric acid levels in blood and urine should be monitored as hyperuricaemia and/or hyperuricosuria may develop, with the risk of uric acid nephropathy.

Puri-Nethol in common with other antimetabolites is potentially mutagenic and chromosome damage has been reported in rats and man.

In view of its action on cellular deoxyribonucleic acid (DNA) mercaptopurine is potentially carcinogenic and consideration should be given to the theoretical risk of carcinogenesis with this treatment.

It is advised that care be taken when handling or halving these tablets not to contaminate hands or to inspire drug.

Side- and adverse effects: The main side-effect of treatment with Puri-Nethol is bone marrow suppression leading to leucopenia and thrombocytopenia. Puri-Nethol is hepatotoxic in animals and man. The histological findings in man have shown hepatic necrosis and biliary stasis. The incidence of hepatotoxicity varies considerably and can occur with any dose but more frequently when the recommended dose of 2.5 mg/kg bodyweight daily is exceeded. Monitoring of liver function tests may allow early detection of liver toxicity. This is usually reversible if Puri-Nethol therapy is stopped soon enough. However, irreversible liver damage leading to a fatal outcome has occurred.

Anorexia, nausea and vomiting have occasionally been noted.

Oral ulceration has been reported during Puri-Nethol therapy and rarely intestinal ulceration has occurred.

Rare complications are drug fever and skin rash.

Drug interactions: When Zyloric [allopurinol] and Puri-Nethol are administered concomitantly it is essential that only a quarter of the usual dose of Puri-Nethol is given since Zyloric decreases the rate of catabolism of Puri-Nethol.

Inhibition of the anticoagulant effect of warfarin, when given with Puri-Nethol, has been reported.

Use in pregnancy and lactation: Puri-Nethol is embryotoxic in rats. This effect is dose dependent.

Normal offspring have been born after Puri-Nethol therapy during human pregnancy, but abortion, prematurity and malformation have been reported. The small numbers involved do not allow an evaluation of the degree of risk of Puri-Nethol therapy during pregnancy and the possible hazard to the foetus must be balanced against the expected benefit in individual cases.

Mothers receiving Puri-Nethol should not breast feed.

Toxicity and treatment of overdosage: The principal toxic effect is on the bone marrow and haematological toxicity is likely to be more profound with chronic overdosage than with a single ingestion of Puri-Nethol. The risk of overdosage is also increased when Zyloric is being given concomitantly with Puri-Nethol. As there is no known antidote the blood picture should be closely monitored and general supportive measures, together with appropriate blood transfusion, instituted if necessary.

Pharmaceutical precautions Store below 25°C. Keep dry, protect from light.

Legal category POM.

Package quantities Bottle of 25 tablets.

Further information Puri-Nethol is an analogue of adenine and hypoxanthine, and microbiological studies have shown it to be an antagonist of these; its mode of action differs thus from that of the folic acid antagonists.

Product licence number 0003/5227R.

RETROVIR* CAPSULES

Presentation Each opaque capsule containing 250 mg zidovudine has a blue cap and a white body; the cap is marked with 'Wellcome' and a unicorn, the body is marked '250' and the code 'H2F'. The waist of the capsule is sealed with a dark blue band.

Each opaque capsule containing 100 mg zidovudine has a white cap and body; the cap is marked with 'Wellcome' and a unicorn, the body is marked '100' and the code 'Y9C'. The waist of the capsule is sealed with a dark blue band.

Uses Retrovir Capsules are indicated for the management of patients with advanced HIV disease, such as those with the acquired immune deficiency syndrome (AIDS) or AIDS-related complex (ARC).

In patients with HIV infection, Retrovir Capsules are also indicated in early symptomatic patients with CD4 counts of less than 500/mm^3, or in asymptomatic patients with markers indicating risk of progressive disease including repeated CD4 counts of less than 200/mm^3, or with CD4 counts between 500/mm^3 and 200/mm^3 which are rapidly falling.

Mode of action: Zidovudine is an antiviral agent which is highly active *in vitro* against retroviruses including the Human Immunodeficiency Virus (HIV).

Zidovudine is phosphorylated in both infected and uninfected cells to the monophosphate (MP) derivative by cellular thymidine kinase. Subsequent phosphorylation of zidovudine-MP to the diphosphate, and then the triphosphate (TP) derivative is catalysed by cellular thymidylate kinase and non-specific kinases, respectively. Zidovudine-TP acts as an inhibitor of, and substrate for, the viral reverse transcriptase. The formation of further proviral DNA is blocked by incorporation of zidovudine-TP into the chain and subsequent chain termination.

Competition by zidovudine-TP for HIV reverse transcriptase is approximately 100-fold greater than for cellular DNA polymerase alpha.

Pharmacokinetics: Zidovudine is well absorbed from the gut and at all dose levels studied the bioavailability was 60–70%. Mean steady state peak (C^{ss} max) and trough (C^{ss} min) plasma concentrations following oral doses of 5 mg zidovudine in solution per kg body weight every four hours were 7.1 and 0.4 microMolar (or 1.9 and 0.1 micrograms/ml) respectively. Limited data with Retrovir Capsules suggest C^{ss} max and C^{ss} min levels following a dosage of 200 mg every four hours are about 3.5 and less than 0.5 microMolar (or about 1.0 and less than 0.1 micrograms/ml), respectively; the corresponding levels following a dosage of 250 mg every four hours are about 4.4 and 0.4 microMolar (or 1.2 and 0.1 micrograms/ml).

From studies with intravenous zidovudine the terminal plasma half-life was approximately 1.1 hours. Renal clearance of zidovudine greatly exceeds creatinine clearance, indicating that significant tubular secretion takes place.

The 5'-glucuronide of zidovudine is the major metabolite in both plasma and urine and accounts for about 50–80% of the dose eliminated by renal excretion. No other metabolites have been observed.

There are limited data concerning the pharmacokinetics of zidovudine in children and in patients with renal or hepatic impairment (see *Dosage and administration*). No data are available on the pharmacokinetics of zidovudine in the elderly.

Cerebrospinal fluid levels of zidovudine averaged approximately 50% of corresponding plasma levels following chronic dosing. Plasma protein binding is relatively low (34 to 38%) and so drug interactions involving binding site displacement are not anticipated.

Dosage and administration

Dosage in adults: The optimal dosage remains unknown and may vary from patient to patient and may depend on the stage of infection.

For asymptomatic patients a dosage of 500 mg to 1500 mg daily has been used. Treatment can be initiated with 500 mg daily, however, if the disease progresses, it is recommended to increase the dose, if tolerated (see below).

For symptomatic patients a dose of 200 mg every 4 hours (1200 mg/day) is generally recommended for a 70 kg patient. For patients with advanced HIV disease who are likely to tolerate the drug less well a maintenance dosage of 100 mg every 4 hours (600 mg/day) may be preferred. For patients with early symptomatic disease the effectiveness of reduced dosages is unknown. The effectiveness of lower dosages in the treatment or prevention of HIV-associated neurological dysfunction and malignancies is unknown.

In practice, daily dosages can be administered in 4 or 5 divided doses.

Dosage adjustments may be necessary in patients with possible haematological toxicity. This is more likely in patients with poor bone marrow reserve prior to treatment, particularly in patients with advanced HIV disease. If the haemoglobin level falls to between 7.5 g/decilitre and 9 g/decilitre or the neutrophil count falls to between 0.75×10^9/litre and 1.0×10^9/litre, the daily dosage should be halved (e.g. the recommended dose should be taken every 8 hours). Recovery may be enhanced by a brief interruption of zidovudine therapy. Provided there is recovery, the dosage may subsequently be increased up to the original daily dosage.

Therapy with Retrovir Capsules should be discontinued if the haemoglobin level falls below 7.5 g/decilitre or the neutrophil count falls to less than 0.75×10^9/litre. Recovery is usually observed within two weeks, after which time zidovudine therapy at a reduced dosage (i.e. recommended dose every 8 hours) may be reinstituted. After a further 2 to 4 weeks the dosage may be gradually increased, depending on patient tolerance, until the original dosage is reached.

Dosage in children: Limited data are available on the use of zidovudine by mouth in children. Although still experimental, starting dosages of 150 to 180 mg/m^2 every 6 hours (four times daily) have been most widely employed.

Dosage in the elderly: No data are available but special care is advised because of the increased likelihood of renal impairment in the elderly.

Dosage in renal impairment: Limited data in patients with renal impairment do not suggest a particular need for initial dosage adjustment since zidovudine levels are not notably increased. However, accumulation of the glucuronide metabolite can be expected in the presence of renal impairment and may increase the risk of toxicity. Monitoring of plasma zidovudine (and its glucuronide) levels is advisable and, in conjunction with haematological parameters, may indicate the need for subsequent dosage adjustment. Haemodialysis appears to have a limited effect on elimination of zidovudine but enhances the elimination of the glucuronide metabolite.

Dosage in hepatic impairment: Limited data in patients with cirrhosis suggest that accumulation of zidovudine may occur in patients with hepatic impairment because of decreased glucuronidation. Dosage adjustments may be necessary but precise recommendations cannot be made at present. If monitoring of plasma zidovudine levels is not feasible, physicians will need to pay particular attention to signs of intolerance and increase the interval between doses as appropriate.

Contra-indications, warnings, etc

Contra-indications: Retrovir Capsules are contra-indicated in patients known to be hypersensitive to zidovudine.

Retrovir Capsules should not be given to patients with abnormally low neutrophil counts (less than 0.75×10^9/litre) or abnormally low haemoglobin levels (less than 7.5 g/decilitre).

Precautions: Patients should be cautioned about the concomitant use of self-administered medications (see *Drug interactions*).

Patients should be advised that zidovudine therapy has not been shown to reduce the risk of transmission of HIV to others through sexual contact or blood contamination.

No evidence of mutagenicity was observed in the Ames test. However, zidovudine was weakly mutagenic in a mouse lymphoma cell assay and was positive in an *in vitro* cell transformation assay. Clastogenic effects (chromosome damage) were observed in an *in vitro* study in *human* lymphocytes and in *in vivo* oral repeat dose micronucleus studies in rats and mice. An *in vivo* cytogenetic study in rats did not show chromosomal damage. The clinical significance of these findings is unclear.

Haematological toxicity: Anaemia (usually occurring after six weeks of zidovudine therapy but occasionally earlier), neutropenia (usually occurring at any time after 4 weeks' therapy but sometimes earlier) and leucopenia (usually secondary to neutropenia) can be expected to occur frequently in patients with advanced HIV disease receiving Retrovir Capsules. Therefore haematological parameters should be carefully monitored. It is recommended that blood tests are performed at least every two weeks for the first three months of therapy and at least monthly thereafter.

If severe anaemia or myelosuppression occurs dose adjustments are suggested (see *Dosage and administration*). Such abnormalities are usually rapidly reversible on stopping therapy.

Particular care should be taken in patients with pre-existing bone marrow compromise (e.g. haemoglobin less than 9 g/decilitre or neutrophil count less than 1.0×10^9/litre). Lower daily dosages from the start of treatment may be appropriate for some such patients.

In patients with early HIV disease (where bone marrow

reserve is generally good), haematological toxicity is less frequent. Depending on the overall condition of the patient, blood tests may be performed less often, for example every one to three months.

Carcinogenicity: Zidovudine was administered orally at three dosage levels to separate groups of mice and rats (60 females and 60 males in each group). Initial single daily doses were 30, 60 and 120 mg/kg/day and 80, 220 and 600 mg/kg/day in mice and rats, respectively. The doses in mice were reduced to 20, 30 and 40 mg/kg/day after day 90 because of treatment-related anaemia, whereas in rats, only the high dose was reduced (to 450 and then 300 mg/kg/day on days 91 and 279, respectively).

In mice, seven late-appearing (after 19 months) vaginal neoplasms (5 squamous cell carcinomas, one squamous cell papilloma and one squamous polyp) occurred at the highest dose. One late-appearing squamous cell papilloma occurred in the vagina of a middle-dose animal. No vaginal tumours were found at the lowest dose.

In rats, two late-appearing (after 20 months) vaginal squamous cell carcinomas occurred in animals given the highest dose. No vaginal tumours occurred at the middle or low doses in rats.

There were no other drug-related tumours observed in either sex of either species.

The predictive value of rodent carcinogenicity studies for humans in uncertain and thus the clinical significance of these findings is unclear.

Side- and adverse effects: The most serious adverse reactions include anaemia (often requiring transfusions), neutropenia and leucopenia. These occur more frequently at higher dosages (1200 to 1500 mg/day) and in patients with advanced HIV disease (especially when there is poor bone marrow reserve prior to treatment), and particularly in patients with low T_4 (T-helper) cell counts less than 100/mm^3. Dosage reduction or cessation of therapy may become necessary (see *Dosage and administration*). The incidence of neutropenia was also increased in patients with pre-existing neutropenia or anaemia, those with low vitamin B_{12} levels and those taking paracetamol concomitantly (see *Drug interactions*).

Other frequent adverse events reported in large placebo-controlled clinical trials included nausea, vomiting, anorexia, abdominal pain, headache, rash, fever, myalgia, paraesthesia, insomnia, malaise, asthenia and dyspepsia. Apart from nausea, which was significantly more common in all studies in patients receiving Retrovir Capsules, the other adverse events were not consistently reported to be more common than in the placebo recipients. Severe headaches, myalgia and insomnia were more common in patients with advanced HIV disease, whilst vomiting, anorexia, malaise and asthenia were more common in patients with early HIV disease.

Other adverse events have included somnolence, diarrhoea, dizziness, sweating, dyspnoea, flatulence, taste perversion, chest pain, loss of mental acuity, anxiety, urinary frequency, depression, generalised pain, chills, cough, urticaria, pruritus and influenza-like syndrome. The incidence of these, and other less frequent adverse events, was similar in both Retrovir- and placebo-treated patients.

The following events have been reported in patients treated with Retrovir. They may also occur as part of the underlying disease process. The relationship between these events and the use of Retrovir is therefore difficult to evaluate, particularly in the medically complicated situations which characterise advanced HIV infection: convulsions and other cerebral events; myopathy; nail pigmentation; pancytopenia with marrow hypoplasia and isolated thrombocytopenia; and liver disorders such as hepatomegaly, fatty change and raised blood levels of liver enzymes and bilirubin.

Use in pregnancy and lactation: Studies in pregnant rats and rabbits given zidovudine orally at dosage levels up to 450 and 500 mg/kg/day respectively during the major period of organogenesis have revealed no evidence of teratogenicity. There was, however, a statistically significant increase in foetal resorptions in rats given 150 to 450 mg/kg/day and in rabbits given 500 mg/kg/day.

Zidovudine did not impair male or female fertility in rats given oral dosages of up to 450 mg/kg/day. It is not known whether zidovudine can affect human fertility, or whether it can cause foetal harm when administered to a pregnant woman. The use of zidovudine during pregnancy should be considered only if clearly indicated.

Limited data indicate that zidovudine is excreted in animal milk. It is not known if zidovudine is excreted in human milk. Since the drug may pass into breast milk and could cause serious toxicity in nursing infants, it is recommended that mothers taking Retrovir Capsules do not breast feed their infants.

Drug interactions: As experience of drug interactions with zidovudine is still limited, care should be taken in combining other drug regimens with Retrovir Capsules. The interactions listed below should not be considered exhaustive but are representative of the classes of drug where caution should be exercised.

Phenytoin blood levels have been reported to be low in some patients receiving zidovudine, while in one patient a high level was noted. These observations suggest that phenytoin levels should be carefully monitored in patients receiving both drugs.

Paracetamol use during treatment with Retrovir Capsules increased the incidence of neutropenia especially following chronic therapy, presumably by reducing metabolism of zidovudine.

Other drugs (such as aspirin, codeine, morphine, indomethacin, ketoprofen, naproxen, oxazepam, lorazepam, cimetidine, clofibrate, dapsone and isoprinosine) may also alter the metabolism of zidovudine by competitively inhibiting glucuronidation or directly inhibiting hepatic microsomal metabolism. Careful thought should be given to the possibilities of drug interactions before using such drugs, particularly for chronic therapy, in combination with Retrovir Capsules.

Concomitant therapy with potentially nephrotoxic or myelosuppressive drugs (e.g. dapsone, pentamidine, amphotericin, flucytosine, ganciclovir, interferon, vincristine, vinblastine and doxorubicin) may also increase the risk of toxicity with Retrovir Capsules.

Some nucleoside analogues (e.g. ribavirin) antagonise the *in vitro* antiviral activity of zidovudine and so concomitant use of such drugs should be avoided.

Since some patients receiving zidovudine may continue to experience opportunistic infections, concomitant use of prophylactic antimicrobial therapy may have to be considered. Such drugs might include co-trimoxazole, pyrimethamine and acyclovir. Limited data do not indicate an increased risk of toxicity with these drugs.

Limited data suggest that probenecid increases the mean half-life and area under the plasma concentration curve of zidovudine, by decreasing renal excretion. Glucuronidation of the drug may also be reduced in the presence of probenecid.

Toxicity and treatment of overdosage: Limited data are available on the consequences of ingestion of acute overdoses. No specific symptoms have been identified following such overdosage.

Dosages as high as 1250 mg Retrovir taken orally every four hours for four weeks have been administered to two patients. One experienced anaemia and neutropenia while the other had no untoward effects.

Patients should be observed closely for evidence of toxicity (see *Side- and adverse effects*) and given the necessary supportive therapy.

Haemodialysis appears to have a limited effect on elimination of zidovudine but enhances the elimination of the glucuronide metabolite.

Pharmaceutical precautions Store below 30°C. Protect from light. Keep dry.

Legal category POM.

Package quantities
Retrovir Capsules 100 mg: pack of 100 capsules.
Retrovir Capsules 250 mg: pack of 40 capsules as 5 blister strips of 8 capsules.

Further information Nil.

Product licence numbers
Retrovir Capsules 100 mg 0003/0239
Retrovir Capsules 250 mg 0003/0240

SCHICK TEST TOXIN BP AND SCHICK CONTROL BP WELLCOME*

Presentation Schick Test Toxin is the sterile diluted filtrate from a culture of *Corynebacterium diphtheriae*. The Control Fluid is the same material heated sufficiently to inactivate the toxin but not sufficiently to destroy the more heat-stable bacterial proteins and broth constituents.

Schick Test Toxin contains thiomersal 0.004% as preservative.

Uses The Schick test is used to demonstrate whether or not a certain degree of immunity to diphtheria is present, either initially or after immunisation. The toxin produces a local skin reaction in those who are susceptible to the disease, while in those who are satisfactorily immune it is neutralised by the subject's antitoxin and no reaction results. The concurrent injection of Control Fluid at another, comparable site provides a means of distinguishing between true, positive reactions due to toxin and other reactions of an allergic nature due to non-specific constituents. During the first few months of life babies usually have maternally derived immunity. Those between 6 months and 8 years old rarely suffer from untoward reactions after primary immunisation. Therefore, the Schick test is not usually given to infants or children up to 8 or even 10 years of age. In children over 10 years and adults, the state of immunity varies, so a preliminary Schick test should always be performed before injection of a vaccine, the main purpose being to detect those giving a negative-and-pseudo reaction, for they may experience a reaction after a dose of vaccine.

Dosage and administration *Technique:* A dose of 0.2 ml of the Toxin is injected *intradermally* into the anterior surface of the left forearm, and 0.2 ml of the Control Fluid into the corresponding position on the right forearm.

Separate syringes and needles should be used for the Toxin and Control Fluid. It is a practical advantage, when dealing with groups of subjects, to identify each syringe; a rubber band around the barrels of, say, those for the Control Fluid is suggested. Any unused portion of a container should be discarded.

Readings: Results may be read at 24–48 (possibly up to 72) hours, and again at five to seven days to detect late reactors and to reconsider earlier, doubtful readings. By comparing the appearance of the two arms it is possible to judge how far any reaction is due to the toxin and how far to the other constituents. Four types of result may be seen:

Negative (= immune). No reaction visible on either arm.

Negative-and-pseudo (= immune). Both arms show somewhat similar flushes which usually fade more rapidly than that of a true positive reaction. They are due to non-specific constituents and not to toxin.

Positive (= susceptible). The left arm shows a flush from 10–50 mm in diameter; this fades and becomes brown and fine desquamation may occur. The staining may persist for several weeks.

Positive-and-pseudo (= susceptible) (also called 'combined'). Both arms show a flush but the left is larger, deeper and more persistent than the right. The pseudo effect develops more rapidly than any positive response and may be at its maximum at 24–72 hours. By the fifth to sixth day, the pseudo effect has faded considerably or disappeared, whereas the positive reaction has increased in size and intensity.

Distinction must be made between those with a well-marked pseudo reaction, which may be slightly greater on the left arm, and those with a positive-and-pseudo result, which will be markedly greater on the left arm. The true positive-and-pseudo reaction is extremely rare and most subjects showing a large flush on both arms are immune, even if there is some difference between the two arms. Persons showing a well-marked pseudo reaction are almost invariably immune to diphtheria and should not be immunised further because they may react severely to the vaccine.

The Schick test may be vitiated by the following: the reading of Schick tests performed from 12 hours before to four weeks after the administration of diphtheria, tetanus or of any other equine antitoxin or of convalescent human serum or gammaglobulin may be erroneous and should, if negative, be disregarded.

Use in the elderly: No special comment.

Contra-indications, warnings, etc
Contra-indications: Subjects with a history of hypersensitivity to previous doses of Schick Test materials or with a known hypersensitivity to diphtheria vaccine should not be tested.

Precautions: Although anaphylaxis associated with the Schick Test is extremely rare, facilities for the management of anaphylaxis should be available during its administration.

The validity of the Schick Test may be impaired if the test is performed within 12 hours to 4 weeks following the administration of any equine antitoxin or of human sera or gamma globulin. Negative results obtained during this period are not indicative of immunity to diphtheria and should be disregarded.

Use in pregnancy and lactation: The Schick Test has been in wide use for many years without apparent ill consequence.

Toxicity and treatment of overdosage: Not applicable.

Pharmaceutical precautions Store at 2–8°C. *Do not freeze.*

Legal category POM.

Package quantities Set of 2 ml.

Further information Nil.

Product licence number 0003/5139.

SEMPREX* CAPSULES

Presentation Each opaque white capsule contains 8 mg acrivastine. Markings include 'Wellcome' and a unicorn printed in black, and 'SEMPREX' printed in reddish-brown.

Uses Antihistamine. Semprex is indicated for the symptomatic relief of allergic rhinitis, including hay fever. Semprex is also indicated for chronic idiopathic urticaria, symptomatic dermographism, cholinergic urticaria and idiopathic acquired cold urticaria.

Dosage and administration
Adults, and children over 12 years: One 8 mg capsule three times a day.

Use in the elderly: As yet, no specific studies have been carried out in the elderly. Until further information is available, Semprex should not be given to elderly patients.

Pharmacology: Acrivastine provides symptomatic relief in conditions believed to depend wholly or partly upon the triggered release of histamine.

It is a potent competitive histamine H_1 antagonist which lacks significant anticholinergic effects, and has a low potential to penetrate the central nervous system.

After oral administration of a single dose of 8 mg acrivastine to adults, the onset of action, as determined by the ability to antagonise histamine-induced weals and flares in the skin, is within 1 hour. Peak effects occur at 2 hours, and although activity declines slowly thereafter, significant inhibition of histamine-induced weals and flares still occurs 8 hours after dose.

In patients, relief from the symptoms of allergic rhinitis is apparent within 1 hour after the systemic administration of the drug.

Pharmacokinetics: Acrivastine is well absorbed from the gut. In healthy adult volunteers, the peak plasma concentration (Cmax) is approximately 150 ng/ml, occurring at about 1.5 hours (Tmax) after the administration of 8 mg acrivastine. The plasma half-life is approximately 1.5 hours. In multiple dose studies over 6 days, no accumulation of acrivastine was observed.

Contra-indications, warnings, etc Semprex is contra-indicated in individuals with known hypersensitivity to acrivastine or triprolidine. Renal excretion is the principal route of elimination of acrivastine. Until specific studies have been carried out Semprex should not be given to patients with significant renal impairment (creatinine clearance less than 50 ml per minute or serum creatinine greater than 150 micromoles per litre).

Precautions: Most patients do not experience drowsiness with Semprex. Nevertheless, as there is individual variation in response to all medication, it is sensible to caution all patients about engaging in activities requiring mental alertness, such as driving a car or operating machinery, until patients are familiar with their own response to the drug.

It is usual to advise patients not to undertake tasks requiring mental alertness whilst under the influence of alcohol and other C.N.S. depressants. Concomitant administration of acrivastine may, in some individuals, produce additional impairment.

Side- and adverse effects: Reports of drowsiness directly attributable to Semprex are extremely rare. Indeed for the great majority of patients, treatment with Semprex is not associated with clinically significant anticholinergic or sedative side-effects.

Use in pregnancy and lactation: No data are available on the use of Semprex during pregnancy, therefore caution should be exercised by balancing the potential benefits of treatment against any possible hazard. Systemic administration of acrivastine in animal reproductive studies did not produce embryotoxic or teratogenic effects and did not impair fertility.

There is no information on the levels of acrivastine which may appear in human breast milk after administration of Semprex.

Toxicity and treatment of overdosage: There is no experience of overdosage with Semprex. Appropriate supportive therapy, including gastric lavage, should be initiated if indicated.

Pharmaceutical precautions Protect from light. Keep dry. Store below 25°C.

Legal category POM.

Package quantities 84 capsules as 4 blister strips of 21 tablets.

Further information Nil.

Product licence number 0003/0254.

SEPTRIN* TABLETS
SEPTRIN* DISPERSIBLE TABLETS
SEPTRIN* FORTE TABLETS
SEPTRIN* ADULT SUSPENSION
SEPTRIN* PAEDIATRIC SUSPENSION
SEPTRIN* PAEDIATRIC DISPERSIBLE TABLETS

Presentation Septrin Tablets (Co-trimoxazole Tablets BP) each contain 80 mg Trimethoprim BP and 400 mg Sulphamethoxazole BP. Coded 'SEPTRIN Y2B WELLCOME'. White in colour.

Septrin Dispersible Tablets (Dispersible Co-trimoxazole Tablets BP) each contain 80 mg Trimethoprim BP and 400 mg Sulphamethoxazole BP. Coded 'SEPTRIN Y2B WELLCOME'. Orange in colour.

Septrin Forte Tablets (Co-trimoxazole Tablets BP) each contain 160 mg Trimethoprim BP and 800 mg Sulphamethoxazole BP. Scored and coded 'SEPTRIN FORTE O2C'. White in colour.

Septrin Adult Suspension (Co-trimoxazole Mixture BP) contains 80 mg Trimethoprim BP and 400 mg Sulphamethoxazole BP in each 5 ml. Off-white in colour.

Septrin Paediatric Suspension (Paediatric Co-trimoxazole Mixture BP) contains 40 mg Trimethoprim BP and 200 mg Sulphamethoxazole BP in each 5 ml. Off-white in colour. Sugar-free.

Septrin Paediatric Dispersible Tablets (Dispersible Co-trimoxazole Tablets BP Paediatric) each contain 20 mg Trimethoprim BP and 100 mg Sulphamethoxazole BP. Scored and coded 'WELLCOME H4B'. Orange in colour.

Uses Septrin is an antibacterial agent. Septrin is effective *in vitro* against a wide range of Gram-positive and Gram-negative organisms. It is not active against *Mycobacterium tuberculosis, Mycoplasma* or *Treponema pallidum, Pseudomonas aeruginosa* is usually insensitive.

Septrin is of value in the treatment of the following:

Respiratory tract: Acute and chronic bronchitis, bronchiectasis, lobar and broncho-pneumonia, *Pneumocystis carinii* pneumonitis, otitis media and sinusitis.

Genito-urinary tract: Acute upper and lower urinary tract infections, bacterial prostatitis and male and female gonorrhoea.

Gastro-intestinal tract: Typhoid and paratyphoid fevers, chronic carriage of *Salmonella typhi* and *paratyphi*, cholera and shigellosis.

Skin infections: Pyoderma, abscesses and wound infections.

Other bacterial infections: Acute and chronic osteomyelitis, acute brucellosis, septicaemias and other infections caused by sensitive organisms.

Dosage and administration *Septrin Tablets* and *Septrin Dispersible Tablets – Adults:* Standard dosage: 2 twice daily.

For severe infections: 3 twice daily.

Children over 12 years: As for adults.

6–12 years: 1 twice daily.

Septrin Forte Tablets – Adults: Standard dosage: 1 twice daily.

For severe infections: 1½ twice daily.

Children over 12 years: As for adults.

Children under 12 years: Not applicable.

Septrin Adult Suspension – Adults: Standard dosage: 10 ml twice daily.

For severe infections: 15 ml twice daily. For long-term treatment (more than 14 days): 5 ml twice daily.

Children over 12 years: As for adults.

Septrin Paediatric Suspension

Children 6–12 years: 10 ml twice daily.

6 months to 6 years: 5 ml twice daily.

6 weeks to 6 months: 2.5 ml twice daily.

Septrin Adult and Paediatric Suspensions may be diluted 1:1 with Syrup BP. In addition, Septrin Paediatric Suspension may be diluted 1:1 with Sorbitol Solution BPC, non-crystallising grade – particularly where it is desirable to retain its sugar-free property. In all cases dilutions should be freshly prepared, stored below 25°C, and used within 14 days.

Septrin Paediatric Dispersible Tablets

Children 6–12 years: 4 twice daily.

2–6 years: 2 twice daily.

Paediatric dosage may be increased by 50% for severe infections.

Septrin Dispersible Tablets should be taken in a little water or swallowed whole.

Septrin may be taken with some food to minimise the possibility of GI disturbances.

Special Dosage Recommendations: Unless stated, standard dosage applies.

In acute infections, Septrin should be given for at least five days or until the patient has been symptom-free for two days. If clinical improvement is not evident after seven days' therapy, the patient should be reassessed. As an alternative to standard therapy for acute uncomplicated lower urinary tract infections, short-term therapy of one to three days' duration has been shown to be effective.

Impaired renal function: If Septrin is given to patients with renal impairment then the following dosage scheme is suggested (no information is available for children with renal failure).

Creatinine clearance (ml/min)	*Serum creatinine (µmol/l)*	*Dosage*
Above 25	men <265 women <175	Standard dosage.
15–25	men 265–620 women 175–400	Standard dosage for a maximum of three days followed by half the standard dosage.
Below 15	men >620 women >400	Not to be administered unless haemodialysis facilities are available. Under this condition half the standard dosage may be given.

Measurements of plasma concentrations of sulphamethoxazole at intervals of two to three days are recommended in samples obtained 12 hours after administration of Septrin. If the concentration of total sulphamethoxazole exceeds 150 micrograms/ml, then treatment should be interrupted until the value falls below 120 micrograms/ml.

Long-term prophylaxis of recurrent or suppression of chronic infection following sterilisation of the urine:

Adults and children over 12 years: 1 tablet nightly.

Children under 12 years: A single nightly dose of 2 mg trimethoprim and 10 mg sulphamethoxazole per kg body weight.

Treatment may be continued for 3 to 12 months or more as appropriate.

Chronic prostatitis: It may be advisable to use a *higher* than standard dose initially. The course of treatment should last for three months to reduce the risk of relapse.

Pneumocystis carinii *pneumonitis:*

Treatment: 20 mg trimethoprim and 100 mg sulphamethoxazole per kg body weight per day in two or more divided doses for two weeks. The steady state or serum level of trimethoprim should be maintained at 5 mcg/ml or higher for maximum efficacy.

Prevention: Standard dosage for the duration of the period at risk.

Gonorrhoea: In uncomplicated cases 4 tablets every 12 hours for two days *or* 5 tablets followed by a further dose of 5 tablets eight hours later.

Acute brucellosis: It may be advisable to use a *higher* than standard dose initially. Treatment should continue for a period of at least four weeks and repeated courses may be beneficial.

Typhoid and paratyphoid carriage: Treatment should be continued for at least 1–3 months.

Use in the elderly: No specific studies have been carried out in the elderly, although Septrin has been widely used in older people. See 'Precautions' for further information.

Contra-indications, warnings, etc

Contra-indications: Septrin should not be given to patients with a history of sulphonamide, trimethoprim or co-trimoxazole hypersensitivity.

Contra-indicated in patients showing marked liver parenchymal damage.

Except in certain circumstances it should not be given to patients with serious haematological disorders. The combination has been administered to patients receiving cytotoxic agents without evidence of an adverse effect on the bone marrow or peripheral blood.

Contra-indicated in severe renal insufficiency where repeated measurements of the plasma concentration cannot be performed.

Septrin should not be given to premature babies nor to full-term infants during the first six weeks of life.

Precautions: Septrin should be discontinued if a skin rash appears.

In cases with renal impairment a modified dosage schedule as described above is indicated. In such patients, measurements of the plasma concentration of the drug is advisable. An adequate urinary output should be maintained.

Use in the elderly: Particular care is always advisable when treating elderly patients because, as a group, they are more susceptible to adverse reactions and more likely to suffer serious effects as a result.

A folate supplement should be considered when treating potentially folate deficient patients such as the elderly. A folate supplement should also be considered with prolonged high dosage of Septrin.

If Septrin treatment is prolonged, especially in patients with suspected impairment of folate metabolism, it is suggested that complete blood counts including thrombocytes be performed at monthly intervals.

Drug interactions: Co-trimoxazole has been shown to potentiate the anticoagulant activity of warfarin via stereo-selective inhibition of its metabolism. Sulphamethoxazole may displace warfarin from plasma-albumin protein-binding sites in vitro. Careful control of the anticoagulant therapy during treatment with Septrin is advisable.

Co-trimoxazole prolongs the half life of phenytoin and if co-administered the prescriber should be alert for excessive phenytoin effect. Close monitoring of the patient's condition and serum phenytoin levels are advisable.

Interaction with sulphonylurea hypoglycaemic agents is uncommon but potentiation has been reported.

Concurrent use of rifampicin and Septrin results in a shortening of the plasma half life of trimethoprim after a period of about one week. This is not thought to be of clinical significance.

Reversible deterioration in renal function has been observed in patients treated with co-trimoxazole and cyclosporin following renal transplantation.

Occasional reports suggest that patients receiving pyrimethamine as malarial prophylaxis at doses in excess of 25 mg weekly may develop megaloblastic anaemia should co-trimoxazole be prescribed concurrently.

In elderly patients concurrently receiving diuretics, mainly thiazides, there appears to be an increased risk of thrombocytopenia with or without purpura.

Side- and adverse effects: As Septrin contains trimethoprim and a sulphonamide, the type and frequency of adverse effects associated with such compounds may be expected.

Nausea, vomiting, diarrhoea, glossitis and skin rashes can occur. Pseudomembranous colitis has been reported rarely. Severe skin sensitivity reactions such as erythema multiforme bullosa (Stevens-Johnson syndrome) and toxic epidermal necrolysis (Lyell syndrome) have occurred rarely; the latter condition carries a high mortality.

As Septrin contains a sulphonamide, the possibility of blood dyscrasias like those associated with sulphonamides should be borne in mind. The changes reported with Septrin mainly consist of thrombocytopenia, purpura, leucopenia, neutropenia and very rarely agranulocytosis. They have usually proved to be reversible on withdrawal of the drug. Elderly patients are more susceptible to these blood changes. Septrin may induce haemolysis in certain susceptible glucose-6-phosphate dehydrogenase deficient patients. Jaundice and, very rarely, hepatic necrosis have been reported.

There have been a few reports of subjective experiences such as headache, depression, dizziness and hallucinations but their relationship to therapy remains unproven.

During long-term therapy, isolated cases of megaloblastic changes in the bone marrow have been reported; these are reversible by folinic acid therapy.

At the high dosages used for the therapy of *Pneumocystis carinii pneumonitis* in patients with Acquired Immune Deficiency Syndrome, rash, fever, neutropenia, thrombocytopenia and raised liver enzymes have been reported, necessitating cessation of therapy.

Use in pregnancy and lactation: The safety of Septrin in human pregnancy has not been established. The drug should not be given during pregnancy. Animal studies have shown teratogenic effects typical of a folate antagonist in rats but not rabbits at high doses; these were prevented by administration of dietary folates. Sulphonamide-containing products should not be administered in late pregnancy because of the risk of kernicterus.

The usual caution in prescribing any drug for women of child-bearing age should be exercised with Septrin.

Both sulphamethoxazole and trimethoprim may be found in breast milk but the administration of Septrin to lactating women represents a negligible risk to the suckling infant.

Toxicity and treatment of overdosage: The maximum tolerated dose in humans is unknown. Symptoms of acute overdosage are likely to be nausea, vomiting, abdominal pain, dizziness and confusion. In cases of known, suspected or accidental overdosage, stop therapy. Treatment should consist of gastric lavage if within an hour of ingestion. Absorption of trimethoprim from the gastro-intestinal tract is normally complete in approximately 2 hours, but this may not be the case in gross overdosage. Increased fluid intake will increase the elimination of sulphamethoxazole. Alkalinisation of the urine will also increase the elimination of sulphamethoxazole but decrease that of the trimethoprim. Calcium folinate (3–6 mg/day) given orally or intramuscularly for five to seven days should reverse any folate deficiency effect of trimethoprim. General supportive measures are recommended.

Both trimethoprim and sulphamethoxazole are dialysable by renal dialysis.

Pharmaceutical precautions *Tablets:* Store below 25°C. Protect from light.

Dispersible Tablets: Store below 25°C. Keep dry, protect from light.

Adult and Paediatric Suspension: Store below 25°C. Protect from light.

Legal category POM.

Package quantities *Septrin Tablets:* packs of 100 and 500 tablets.
Septrin Dispersible Tablets: packs of 100 and 500 tablets.
Septrin Forte Tablets: pack of 100 tablets.
Septrin Adult Suspension: bottle of 100 ml.
Septrin Paediatric Suspension: bottle of 100 ml.
Septrin Paediatric Dispersible Tablets: pack of 100 tablets.

Further information Absorption by the oral route is rapid: significant plasma levels are obtained within an hour. Peak levels are reached between two and four hours and are maintained over a period of 12 hours.

In the treatment of tonsillo-pharyngitis due to Group A beta-haemolytic streptococci, eradication of these organisms from the oro-pharynx is less rapid than with some other antibiotics.

Trimethoprim may cause an apparent rise in serum creatinine levels due to (a) competition for the tubular secretory mechanisms; (b) chemical interference with the visual auto-analyser method of estimating creatinine.

Trimethoprim does not induce its own metabolism and therefore no dose modification is required on this account during long-term treatment.

Co-trimoxazole may cause a fall in circulating thyroid hormone levels but the clinical significance requires confirmation.

Trimethoprim has been noted to impair phenylalanine metabolism but this is of no significance in phenylketonuric patients on appropriate dietary restriction.

Plasma or serum levels of sulphamethoxazole and trimethoprim may be determined by high performance liquid chromatography.

Septrin for Infusion and Septrin Intra-muscular Injection are also available.

Product licence numbers

Tablets	0003/0109R
Dispersible Tablets	0003/0099R
Forte Tablets	0003/0121
Adult Suspension	0003/5223R
Paediatric Suspension	0003/5222R
Paediatric Dispersible Tablets	0003/0238

SEPTRIN* FOR INFUSION

Strong Sterile Co-trimoxazole Solution To make Co-trimoxazole Intravenous Infusion BP.

Presentation Septrin for Infusion contains 80 mg Trimethoprim BP and 400 mg Sulphamethoxazole BP in each 5 ml ampoule. The infusion is faintly yellow and contains 40 per cent w/v propylene glycol together with ethyl alcohol and a small amount of benzyl alcohol. It has a pH of approximately 10.

Uses Septrin is an antibacterial agent. Septrin is effective *in vitro* against a wide range of Gram-positive and Gram-negative organisms. It is not active against *Mycobacterium tuberculosis, Mycoplasma* or *Treponema pallidum. Pseudomonas aeruginosa* is usually insensitive.

In general, the indications for the use of Septrin for Infusion are the same as those for oral presentations. Septrin for Infusion is for use when oral dosage is not possible.

Clinical experience with oral Septrin indicates its value in the following:

Respiratory tract: Acute and chronic bronchitis, bronchiectasis, lobar and broncho-pneumonia, *Pneumocystis carinii* pneumonitis, otitis media and sinusitis.

Genito-urinary tract: Acute upper and lower urinary tract infections, bacterial prostatitis and male and female gonorrhoea.

Gastro-intestinal tract: Typhoid and paratyphoid fevers, chronic carriage of *Salmonella typhi* and *paratyphi*, cholera, and shigellosis.

Skin infections: Pyoderma, abscesses and wound infections.

Other bacterial infections: Acute and chronic osteomyelitis, acute brucellosis, septicaemias and other infections caused by sensitive organisms.

Dosage and administration
Adults and children over 12 years: Standard dosage: 10 ml twice daily, morning and evening.

For severe infections: 15 ml twice daily, morning and evening.

Children up to 12 years: The recommended dosage is approximately 6 mg trimethoprim and 30 mg sulphamethoxazole per kg body weight per 24 hours, divided into two equal doses. As a guide the following doses of Septrin for Infusion may be used:

6 weeks to 6 months: 1.25 ml twice daily.
6 months to 6 years: 2.5 ml twice daily.
6–12 years: 5.0 ml twice daily.

Paediatric dosage may be increased by 50% for severe infections.

It is intended that Septrin for Infusion should be used only during such a period as the patient is unable to accept oral therapy.

Dosage in Pneumocystis carinii *pneumonitis:* The dosage is 20 mg trimethoprim, 100 mg sulphamethoxazole/kg/day in two or more divided doses. The course is two weeks, but oral therapy should be substituted as soon as it is appropriate. The steady state or serum level of trimethoprim should be maintained at 5 mcg/ml or higher for maximum efficacy.

Dosage recommendations in renal impairment: If Septrin

is given to patients with renal impairment then the following dosage scheme is suggested (no information is available for children with renal failure); see table below.

Creatinine clearance (ml/min)	*Serum creatinine (μmol/l)*	*Dosage*
Above 25	men < 265 women < 175	Standard dosage.
15–25	men 265–620 women 175–400	Standard dosage for a maximum of three days followed by half the standard dosage.
Below 15	men > 620 women > 400	Not to be administered unless haemodialysis facilities are available. Under this condition half the standard dosage may be given.

Measurements of plasma concentrations of sulphamethoxazole at intervals of two to three days after recommended in samples obtained 12 hours after administration of Septrin. If the concentration of total sulphamethoxazole exceeds 150 micrograms/ml then treatment should be interrupted until the value falls below 120 micrograms/ml.

Use in the elderly: No specific studies have been carried out in the elderly, although Septrin has been widely used in older people. See 'Precautions' for further information.

Administration: Septrin for Infusion must be given by the intravenous route ONLY and MUST BE DILUTED before administration, according to the following schedules:

One ampoule Septrin for Infusion (5 ml) to 125 ml infusion solution.

Two ampoules Septrin for Infusion (10 ml) to 250 ml infusion solution.

Three ampoules Septrin for Infusion (15 ml) to 500 ml infusion solution.

DILUTION SHOULD BE CARRIED OUT DIRECTLY BEFORE USE. After the addition of Septrin for Infusion to the infusion solution the mixture should be shaken to ensure thorough mixing. Should visible turbidity or crystallisation appear in the solution at any time before or during an infusion the mixture should be discarded.

Septrin for Infusion is known to be compatible, when diluted in accordance with the schedules above, with the following fluids:

Glucose Intravenous Infusion BP 5% and 10%.

Fructose Intravenous Infusion BP 5%.

Sodium Chloride Intravenous Infusion BP (0.9%).

Sodium Chloride (0.18%) and Glucose (4%) Intravenous Infusion BP.

Dextran 70 Injection BP 6% in glucose 5% or normal saline.

Dextran 40 Injection BP 10% in glucose 5% or normal saline.

Ringer's Solution for Injection BPC 1959.

No other substance should be mixed with the infusion.

It is suggested that the duration of the infusion should be approximately one and a half hours, but this should be balanced against the fluid requirements of the patient.

When fluid restriction is necessary, Septrin for Infusion may be given in a higher concentration such as one 5 ml ampoule in 50 ml or 75 ml of 5% w/v glucose in water.

Discard any unused diluted solution.

Contra-indications, warnings, etc

Contra-indications: Septrin should not be given to patients with a history of sulphonamide, trimethoprim or co-trimoxazole hypersensitivity.

Contra-indicated in patients showing marked liver parenchymal damage.

Except in certain circumstances it should not be given to patients with serious haematological disorders. The combination has been administered to patients receiving cytotoxic agents without evidence of an adverse effect on the bone marrow or peripheral blood.

Contra-indicated in severe renal insufficiency where repeated measurements of the plasma concentration cannot be performed.

Septrin should not be given to premature babies nor to full-term infants during the first six weeks of life.

Precautions: Septrin for Infusion should be discontinued if a skin rash appears.

Fluid overload is possible, especially when very high doses are being administered to patients with underlying cardiopulmonary disease. In cases with renal impairment a modified dosage schedule as described above is indicated. In such patients, measurement of the plasma concentration of the drug is advisable. An adequate urinary output should be maintained.

Use in the elderly: Particular care is always advisable when treating elderly patients because, as a group, they are more susceptible to adverse reactions and more likely to suffer serious effects as a result.

A folate supplement should be considered when treating potentially folate deficient patients such as the elderly. A folate supplement should also be considered with prolonged high dosage of Septrin.

If Septrin treatment is prolonged, especially in patients with suspected impairment of folate metabolism, it is suggested that complete blood counts including thrombocytes be performed at monthly intervals.

Drug interactions: Co-trimoxazole has been shown to potentiate the anticoagulant activity of warfarin via stereo-selective inhibition of its metabolism. Sulphamethoxazole may displace warfarin from plasma-albumin protein-binding sites in vitro. Careful control of the anticoagulant therapy during treatment with Septrin is advisable.

Co-trimoxazole prolongs the half life of phenytoin and if co-administered the prescriber should be alert for excessive phenytoin effect. Close monitoring of the patient's condition and serum phenytoin levels is advisable.

Interaction with sulphonylurea hypoglycaemic agents is uncommon but potentiation has been reported.

Concurrent use of rifampicin and Septrin results in a shortening of the plasma half life of trimethoprim after a period of about one week. This is not thought to be of clinical significance.

Reversible deterioration in renal function has been observed in patients treated with co-trimoxazole and cyclosporin following renal transplantation.

Occasional reports suggest that patients receiving pyrimethamine as malarial prophylaxis at doses in excess of 25 mg weekly may develop megaloblastic anaemia should co-trimoxazole be prescribed concurrently.

In elderly patients concurrently receiving diuretics, mainly thiazides, there appears to be an increased risk of thrombocytopenia with or without purpura.

Side- and adverse effects: As Septrin contains trimethoprim and a sulphonamide, the type and frequency of adverse effects associated with such compounds may be expected.

Nausea, vomiting, diarrhoea, glossitis and skin rashes can occur. Pseudomembranous colitis has been reported rarely. Severe skin sensitivity reactions such as erythema multiforme bullosa (Stevens-Johnson syndrome) and toxic epidermal necrolysis (Lyell syndrome) have occurred rarely; the latter condition carries a high mortality.

As Septrin contains a sulphonamide, the possibility of blood dyscrasias like those associated with sulphonamides should be borne in mind. The changes reported with Septrin mainly consist of thrombocytopenia, purpura, leucopenia, neutropenia and very rarely agranulocytosis. They have usually proved to be reversible on withdrawal of the drug. Elderly patients are more susceptible to these blood changes. Septrin may induce haemolysis in certain susceptible glucose-6-phosphate dehydrogenase deficient patients.

Jaundice and, very rarely hepatic necrosis have been reported.

There have been a few reports of subjective experiences such as headache, depression, dizziness and hallucinations but their relationship to therapy remains unproven.

During long-term therapy, isolated cases of megaloblastic changes in the bone marrow have been reported; these are reversible by folinic acid therapy.

At the high dosages used for the therapy of *Pneumocystis carinii* pneumonitis in patients with Acquired Immune Deficiency Syndrome, rash, fever, neutropenia, thrombocytopenia and raised liver enzymes have been reported, necessitating cessation of therapy. Concomitant administration of intravenous diphenhydramine may permit continued infusion.

Use in pregnancy and lactation: The safety of Septrin in human pregnancy has not been established. The drug should not be given during pregnancy. Animal studies have shown teratogenic effects typical of a folate antagonist in rats but not rabbits at high doses; these were prevented by administration of dietary folates. Sulphonamide-containing products should not be administered in late pregnancy because of the risk of kernicterus.

The usual caution in prescribing any drug for women of child-bearing age should be exercised with Septrin.

Both sulphamethoxazole and trimethoprim may be found in breast milk, but the administration of Septrin to lactating women represents a negligible risk to the suckling infant.

Toxicity and treatment of overdosage: The maximum tolerated dose in humans is unknown.

Nausea, vomiting, dizziness and confusion are likely symptoms of overdosage.

In cases of known, suspected, or accidental overdosage stop therapy.

Acidification of the urine will increase the elimination of trimethoprim. Inducing diuresis plus alkalinisation of urine will enhance the elimination of sulphamethoxazole. Alkalinisation will reduce the rate of elimination of trimethoprim. Calcium folinate (3–6 mg/day) given orally or intramuscularly for five to seven days should reverse any folate deficiency effect of trimethoprim. General supportive measures are recommended.

Both trimethoprim and sulphamethoxazole are dialysable by renal dialysis.

Pharmaceutical precautions Store below 25°C. Protect from light.

Legal category POM.

Package quantities Box of 10 × 5 ml ampoules.

Further information In the treatment of tonsillopharyngitis due to Group A beta-haemolytic streptococci, eradication of these organisms from the oropharynx is less rapid than with some other antibiotics.

Trimethoprim may cause an apparent rise in serum creatinine levels due to (a) competition for the tubular secretory mechanisms; (b) chemical interference with the visual auto-analyser method of estimating creatinine.

Trimethoprim does not induce its own metabolism and therefore no dose modification is required on this account during long-term treatment.

Co-trimoxazole may cause a fall in circulating thyroid hormone levels but the clinical significance requires confirmation.

Trimethoprim has been noted to impair phenylalanine metabolism but this is of no significance in phenylketonuric patients on appropriate dietary restriction.

Plasma or serum levels of sulphamethoxazole and trimethoprim may be determined by high performance liquid chromatography.

Septrin is available also as: Tablets, Dispersible Tablets, Forte Tablets, Adult Suspension, Paediatric Suspension, Paediatric Dispersible Tablets, and Intramuscular Injection.

Product licence number 0003/0095.

SEPTRIN* INTRAMUSCULAR INJECTION

Presentation Septrin IM Injection contains 160 mg Trimethoprim BP and 800 mg Sulphamethoxazole BP in each 3 ml ampoule.

The sterile solution is faintly yellow and contains the active substances in a 52 per cent v/v solution of glycofurol.

The pH of the solution is approximately 9.0–10.5.

Uses Septrin is an antibacterial agent. Septrin is effective *in vitro* against a wide range of Gram-positive and Gram-negative organisms. It is not active against *Mycobacterium tuberculosis, Mycoplasma* or *Treponema pallidum. Pseudomonas aeruginosa* is usually insensitive.

In general, the indications for the use of Septrin Intramuscular are the same as for oral presentations. Septrin Intramuscular should be used when the intramuscular route is considered preferable.

Clinical experience with oral Septrin indicates its value in the following:

Respiratory tract: Acute and chronic bronchitis, bronchiectasis, lobar and broncho-pneumonia, *Pneumocystis carinii* pneumonitis, otitis media and sinusitis.

Genito-urinary tract: Acute upper and lower urinary tract infections, bacterial prostatitis, male and female gonorrhoea.

Gastro-intestinal tract: Typhoid and paratyphoid fevers, chronic carriage of *Salmonella typhi* and *paratyphi,* cholera and shigellosis.

Skin infections: Pyoderma, abscesses and wound infections.

Other bacterial infections: Acute and chronic osteomyelitis, acute brucellosis, septicaemias and other infections caused by sensitive organisms.

Dosage and administration *Adults and children over 12 years:* Standard dosage: One 3 ml ampoule 12-hourly, morning and evening.

Maximum dosage (for severe infections): One and a half ampoules (4.5 ml) 12-hourly, morning and evening, or one 3 ml ampoule three times daily.

Children aged 6–12 years: The usual recommended dose is half an ampoule (1.5 ml) 12-hourly, morning and evening (this dose is based on an average of 6 mg trimethoprim plus 30 mg sulphamethoxazole per kg body weight daily). Paediatric dosage may be increased by 50% for severe infections.

Slight adjustment of this dose may be necessary for children whose body weights approach the extremes of the range for their height and age.

It is NOT recommended that Septrin Intramuscular Injection be given to children under the age of six years because of their small muscle mass.

It is intended that Septrin IM Injection should be used only during such a period as the patient is unable to accept oral therapy. It is recommended that the standard dosage (above) should not normally be administered for more than five successive days nor the maximum dosage (above) for more than three successive days.

Dosage in *Pneumocystis carinii* pneumonitis: Since the volume containing the suggested dose exceeds the maximum recommended, the use of Septrin Intramuscular is inappropriate. Septrin for Infusion should be administered if parenteral therapy is required.

Dosage recommendations in renal impairment: If Septrin is given to patients with renal impairment then the dosage scheme below is suggested (no information is available for children with renal failure).

Creatinine clearance (ml/min)	*Serum creatinine (μmol/l)*	*Dosage*
Above 25	men < 265 women < 175	Standard dosage.
15–25	men 265–620 women 175–400	Standard dosage for a maximum of three days followed by half the standard dosage.
Below 15	men > 620 women > 400	Not to be administered unless haemodialysis facilities are available. Under this condition half the standard dosage may be given.

Measurements of plasma concentration of sulphamethoxazole at intervals of two to three days are recommended in samples obtained 12 hours after administration of Septrin. If the concentration of total sulphamethoxazole exceeds 150 mcg/ml, then treatment should be interrupted until the value falls below 120 mcg/ml.

Use in the elderly: No specific studies have been carried out in the elderly, although Septrin has been widely used in older people. See 'Precautions' for further information.

Administration: Septrin IM Injection must be given by this route ONLY and ONLY when an intramuscular formulation is indicated by the clinical condition.

The injection should be made deep into the upper and outer quadrant of the buttock, and injections should be given into each buttock alternately.

If the total contents of an ampoule are not used after opening then the remainder should be destroyed.

Contra-indications, warnings, etc

Contra-indications: Septrin should not be given to patients with a history of sulphonamide, trimethoprim or co-trimoxazole hypersensitivity.

Contra-indicated in patients showing marked liver parenchymal damage.

Except in certain circumstances it should not be given to patients with serious haematological disorders. The combination has been administered to patients receiving cytotoxic agents without evidence of an adverse effect on the bone marrow or peripheral blood.

Contra-indicated in severe renal insufficiency where repeated measurements of the plasma concentration cannot be performed.

Septrin should not be given to premature babies nor to full-term infants during the first six weeks of life.

Precautions: Septrin Intramuscular Injection should be discontinued if a skin rash appears.

In cases with renal impairment a modified dosage schedule as described above is indicated. In such patients, measurements of the plasma concentration of the drug is advisable. An adequate urinary output should be maintained.

Use in the elderly: Particular care is always advisable when treating elderly patients because, as a group, they are more susceptible to adverse reactions and more likely to suffer serious effects as a result.

A folate supplement should be considered when treating potentially folate deficient patients or with prolonged high dosage of Septrin.

If Septrin treatment is prolonged, especially in patients with suspected impairment of folate metabolism, it is suggested that complete blood counts including thrombocytes be performed at monthly intervals.

Drug interactions: Co-trimoxazole has been shown to potentiate the anticoagulant activity of warfarin via stereo-selective inhibition of its metabolism. Sulphamethoxazole may displace warfarin from plasma-albumin protein-binding sites in vitro. Careful control of the anticoagulant therapy during treatment with Septrin is advisable.

Co-trimoxazole prolongs the half life of phenytoin and if co-administered the prescriber should be alert for excessive phenytoin effect. Close monitoring of the patient's condition and serum phenytoin levels is advisable.

Interaction with sulphonylurea hypoglycaemic agents is uncommon but potentiation has been reported.

Concurrent use of rifampicin and Septrin results in a shortening of the plasma half life of trimethoprim after a period of about one week. This is not thought to be of clinical significance.

Reversible deterioration in renal function has been observed in patients treated with co-trimoxazole and cyclosporin following renal transplantation.

Occasional reports suggest that patients receiving pyrimethamine as malarial prophylaxis at doses in excess of 25 mg weekly may develop megaloblastic anaemia should co-trimoxazole be prescribed concurrently.

In elderly patients concurrently receiving diuretics, mainly thiazides, there appears to be an increased risk of thrombocytopenia with or without purpura.

Side- and adverse effects: Local reactions mainly vary from mild to moderate pain at the injection site; induration is uncommon. As Septrin contains trimethoprim and a sulphonamide, the type and frequency of adverse effects associated with such compounds may be expected.

Nausea, vomiting, diarrhoea, glossitis and skin rashes can occur. Pseudomembranous colitis has been reported rarely. Severe skin sensitivity reactions such as erythema multiforme bullosa (Stevens-Johnson syndrome) and toxic epidermal necrolysis (Lyell syndrome) have occurred rarely; the latter condition carries a high mortality.

As Septrin contains a sulphonamide, the possibility of blood dyscrasias like those associated with sulphonamides should be borne in mind. The changes reported with Septrin mainly consist of thrombocytopenia, purpura, leucopenia, neutropenia and very rarely agranulocytosis. They have usually proved to be reversible on withdrawal of the drug. Elderly patients are more susceptible to these blood changes. Septrin may induce haemolysis in certain susceptible glucose-6-phosphate dehydrogenase deficient patients.

Jaundice and, very rarely, hepatic necrosis have been reported.

There have been a few reports of subjective experiences such as headache, depression, dizziness and hallucinations but their relationship to therapy remains unproven.

During long-term therapy, isolated cases of megaloblastic changes in the bone marrow have been reported: these are reversible by folinic acid therapy.

Use in pregnancy and lactation: The safety of Septrin in human pregnancy has not been established. The drug should not be given during pregnancy. Animal studies have shown teratogenic effects typical of a folate antagonist in rats but not rabbits at high doses; these were prevented by administration of dietary folates. Sulphonamide-containing products should not be administered in late pregnancy because of the risk of kernicterus.

The usual caution in prescribing any drug for women of child-bearing age should be exercised with Septrin.

Both sulphamethoxazole and trimethoprim may be found in breast milk, but the administration of Septrin to lactating women represents a negligible risk to the suckling infant.

Toxicity and treatment of overdosage: Nausea, vomiting, dizziness and confusion are likely symptoms of overdosage.

In cases of known, suspected or accidental overdosage, stop therapy.

Acidification of the urine will increase the elimination of trimethoprim. Inducing diuresis plus alkalinisation of urine will enhance the elimination of sulphamethoxazole. Alkalinisation will reduce the rate of elimination of trimethoprim. Calcium folinate (3–6 mg/day) given orally or intramuscularly for five to seven days should reverse any folate deficiency effect of trimethoprim. General supportive measures are recommended.

Both trimethoprim and sulphamethoxazole are dialysable by renal dialysis.

Pharmaceutical precautions Do not use if the injection solution is cloudy or if precipitation has occurred. Store below 25°C. Do not freeze. Protect from light.

Legal category POM.

Package quantities Box of 10 × 3 ml ampoules.

Further information In the treatment of tonsillopharyngitis due to Group A beta-haemolytic streptococci, eradication of these organisms from the oropharynx is less rapid than with some other antibiotics.

Trimethoprim may cause an apparent rise in serum creatinine levels due to (a) competition for the tubular secretory mechanisms; (b) chemical interference with the visual auto-analyser method of estimating creatinine.

Trimethoprim does not induce its own metabolism and therefore no dose modification is required on this account during long-term treatment.

Co-trimoxazole may cause a fall in circulating thyroid hormone levels but the clinical significance requires confirmation.

Trimethoprim has been noted to impair phenylalanine metabolism but this is of no significance in phenylketonuric patients on appropriate dietary restriction.

Plasma or serum levels of sulphamethoxazole and trimethoprim may be determined by high performance liquid chromatography.

Septrin is available also as: Tablets, Dispersible Tablets, Forte Tablets, Adult Suspension, Paediatric Suspension, Paediatric Dispersible Tablets and Septrin for Infusion.

Product licence number 0003/0124.

SUDAFED* TABLETS
SUDAFED* ELIXIR

Presentation Each orange to red, biconvex, film-coated tablet contains 60 mg Pseudoephedrine Hydrochloride BP and is imprinted 'WELLCOME SUDAFED' on one side.

Each 5 ml of red elixir contains 30 mg Pseudoephedrine Hydrochloride BP and has a raspberry flavour.

Uses Sudafed is a decongestant of the mucous membranes of the upper respiratory tract, especially the nasal mucosa and sinuses, and is indicated for the symptomatic relief of conditions such as allergic rhinitis, vasomotor rhinitis, the common cold and influenza.

Dosage and administration *Adults and children over 12 years:* 1 tablet or 10 ml elixir three times a day.

Children: 6–12 years: 5 ml elixir three times a day.

2–5 years: 2.5 ml elixir three times a day.

Sudafed Elixir may be diluted 1:1 (1 in 2) or 1:3 (1 in 4) with Syrup BP. These dilutions are stable for 4 weeks if stored at 25°C.

Use in the elderly: No specific studies have been carried out in the elderly, but Sudafed has been widely used in older people. However, it may be advisable to monitor renal and hepatic function, and if there is serious impairment then caution should be exercised.

Pharmacology: Pseudoephedrine has direct and indirect sympathomimetic activity and is an orally effective upper respiratory tract decongestant. Pseudoephedrine is substantially less potent than ephedrine in producing both tachycardia and elevation in systolic blood pressure and considerably less potent in causing stimulation of the central nervous system.

Contra-indications, warnings, etc
Contra-indications: Contra-indicated in patients who have previously shown intolerance to pseudoephedrine. It is contra-indicated in persons under treatment with monoamine oxidase inhibitors and within two weeks of stopping such treatment.

It is also contra-indicated in patients with severe hypertension or severe coronary artery disease.

Precautions: Although pseudoephedrine has virtually no pressor effects in patients with normal blood pressure, Sudafed should be used with caution in patients taking antihypertensive agents, tricyclic anti-depressants, other sympathomimetic agents, such as decongestants, appetite suppressants and amphetamine-like psycho-stimulants. The effects of a single dose on the blood pressure of these patients should be observed before recommending repeated or unsupervised treatment.

As with other sympathomimetic agents, caution should be exercised in patients with uncontrolled diabetes, hyperthyroidism, elevated intraocular pressure and prostatic enlargement.

Drug interactions: The effect of antihypertensive agents which modify sympathetic activity may be partially reversed by Sudafed.

Concomitant use of Sudafed with other sympathomimetic agents such as decongestants, tricyclic antidepressants, appetite suppressants and amphetamine-like psychostimulants or with monoamine oxidase inhibitors, which interfere with the catabolism of sympathomimetic amines, may occasionally cause a rise in blood pressure.

The antibacterial agent furazolidone is known to cause a dose-related inhibition of monoamine oxidase and although there are no reports of hypertensive crises having occurred, it should not be administered concurrently with Sudafed.

Side- and adverse effects: Side-effects are uncommon. In some patients pseudoephedrine may occasionally cause insomnia. Rarely, sleep disturbances and hallucinations have been reported.

A fixed drug eruption to pseudoephedrine, taking the form of erythematous nummular patches has been reported, but is a rare occurrence.

Urinary retention has been reported in male patients in whom prostatic enlargement could have been an important predisposing factor.

Use in pregnancy and lactation: Although pseudoephedrine has been in widespread use for many years without apparent ill consequence, there are no specific data on its use during pregnancy. Caution should, therefore be exercised by balancing the potential benefit of treatment against any possible hazards. Systemic administration of pseudoephedrine, up to 50 times the human dose in rats and up to 35 times the human dose in rabbits, did not produce teratogenic effects.

It has been estimated that approximately 0.5%–0.7% of a single dose of pseudoephedrine ingested by a mother will be excreted in the breast milk over 24 hr, but the effect of this on breast-fed infants is not known.

Toxicity and treatment of overdosage: As with other sympathomimetic agents, symptoms of overdosage include irritability, restlessness, tremor, convulsions, palpitations, hypertension and difficulty in micturition. Gastric lavage and supportive measures for respiration and circulation should be performed if indicated. Convulsions should be controlled with an anticonvulsant. Catheterisation of the bladder may be necessary.

If desired, the elimination of pseudoephedrine can be accelerated by acid diuresis or by dialysis.

Pharmaceutical precautions
Tablets: Store below 25°C. Keep dry.
Elixir: Store below 25°C. Protect from light.

Legal category P.

Package quantities *Sudafed Tablets:* Container of 100 tablets. 12 tablets in a blister strip.
Sudafed Elixir: Bottles of 100 ml and 1 litre.

Further information Nil.

Product licence numbers
Tablets 0003/5061R
Elixir 0003/5062R

SUDAFED* SA

Presentation Each Sudafed SA capsule has a red cap and a clear colourless body, is marked 'SUDAFED SA' 'Wellcome' and with a unicorn, and contains 120 mg

Pseudoephedrine Hydrochloride USP in specially formulated pellets designed to provide continuous therapeutic effect for 12 hours.

Uses For the symptomatic relief of allergic rhinitis, vasomotor rhinitis, and congestion associated with the common cold.

Dosage and administration
Adults and children over 12 years: One capsule every 12 hours.

Children 6–12 years: It is recommended that Sudafed Elixir be used.

Use in the elderly: No specific studies have been carried out in the elderly, however, it may be advisable to monitor renal function in these patients and if there is serious impairment then caution should be exercised.

Pharmacology: Pseudoephedrine has direct and indirect sympathomimetic activity and is an orally effective upper respiratory tract decongestant.

Pseudoephedrine is substantially less potent than ephedrine in producing both tachycardia and elevation in systolic blood pressure and considerably less potent in causing central nervous system stimulation.

Contra-indications, warnings, etc
Contra-indications: Contra-indicated in patients who have previously shown intolerance to pseudoephedrine and in persons under treatment with monoamine oxidase inhibitors or within two weeks of stopping such treatment. It is also contra-indicated in patients with severe hypertension or severe coronary artery disease.

Precautions: Although pseudoephedrine has virtually no pressor effect in patients with normal blood pressure, Sudafed SA should be used with caution in patients taking antihypertensive agents, tricyclic anti-depressants, other sympathomimetic agents, such as decongestants, appetite suppressants and amphetamine-like psychostimulants. The effects of a single dose on the blood pressure of these patients should be observed before recommending repeated or unsupervised treatment.

As with other sympathomimetic agents, caution should be exercised in patients with uncontrolled diabetes, hyperthyroidism, elevated intraocular pressure and prostatic enlargement.

Drug interactions: The effect of antihypertensive agents which modify sympathetic activity may be partially reversed by Sudafed.

Concomitant use of Sudafed with other sympathomimetic agents such as decongestants, tricyclic antidepressants, appetite suppressants and amphetamine-like psychostimulants or with monoamine oxidase inhibitors, which interfere with the catabolism of sympathomimetic amines, may occasionally cause a rise in blood pressure.

The antibacterial agent furazolidone is known to cause a dose-related inhibition of monoamine oxidase and, although there are no reports of a hypertensive crisis having occurred, it should not be administered concurrently with Sudafed SA.

Side- and adverse effects: Side-effects are uncommon. In some patients pseudoephedrine may occasionally cause insomnia. Rarely, sleep disturbances and hallucinations have been reported. A fixed drug eruption to pseudoephedrine, taking the form of erythematous nummular patches, has been reported, but should be regarded as a rare occurrence.

Urinary retention has been reported in male patients in whom prostatic enlargement could have been an important predisposing factor.

Use in pregnancy and lactation: Although pseudoephedrine has been in widespread use for many years without apparent ill consequence, there are no specific data on its use during pregnancy. Caution should, therefore be exercised by balancing the potential benefit of treatment against any possible hazards. Systemic administration of pseudoephedrine, up to 50 times the human dose in rats and up to 35 times the human dose in rabbits, did not produce teratogenic effects.

It has been estimated that approximately 0.5%–0.7% of a single dose of pseudoephedrine ingested by a mother will be excreted in the breast milk over 24 hr, but the effect of this on breast-fed infants is not known.

Toxicity and treatment of overdosage: As with other sympathomimetic agents, symptoms of overdosage include irritability, restlessness, tremor, convulsions, palpitations, hypertension and difficulty in micturition. Gastric lavage and supportive measures for respiration and circulation should be performed if indicated. Convulsions should be controlled with an anti-convulsant. Catheterization of the bladder may be necessary.

If desired, the elimination of pseudoephedrine can be accelerated by acid diuresis or by dialysis.

Pharmaceutical precautions Store below 25°C in a dry place. Protect from light.

Legal category POM.

Package quantities Container of 100 capsules.

Further information Nil.

Product licence number 0003/0158.

SUDAFED*-CO TABLETS

Presentation White scored tablets coded 'WELLCOME A7C' containing 500 mg Paracetamol BP and 60 mg Pseudoephedrine Hydrochloride BP.

Uses For the relief of conditions where upper respiratory congestion is associated with pyrexia or pain. These conditions include the common cold, influenza, sinusitis and nasopharyngitis.

Dosage and administration *Adults and children over 12 years:* One tablet three times a day.

Children 6–12 years: Half a tablet three times a day.

Children under 6 years: Not recommended.

Use in the elderly: No specific studies have been carried out in the elderly, but Sudafed-Co has been widely used in older people. However, it may be advisable to monitor renal and hepatic function, and if there is serious impairment then caution should be exercised.

Pharmacology: Pseudoephedrine has direct and indirect sympathomimetic activity and is an orally effective upper respiratory tract decongestant. Pseudoephedrine is substantially less potent than ephedrine in producing both tachycardia and elevation in systolic blood pressure and considerably less potent in causing stimulation of the central nervous system. Paracetamol provides analgesic and antipyretic activity, probably by antagonising cerebral prostaglandin synthetase.

Contra-indications, warnings, etc
Contra-indications: Contra-indicated in patients with a known hypersensitivity to paracetamol or pseudoephedrine. It is contra-indicated in persons under treatment with monoamine oxidase inhibitors and within two weeks of stopping such treatment. It is also contra-indicated in patients with severe hypertension or severe coronary artery disease.

Precautions: Although pseudoephedrine has virtually no pressor effects in patients with normal blood pressure, Sudafed-Co should be used with caution in patients taking antihypertensive agents, tricyclic anti-depressants, other sympathomimetic agents, such as decongestants, appetite suppressants and amphetamine-like psychostimulants. The effects of a single dose on the blood pressure of these patients should be observed before recommending repeated or unsupervised treatment.

As with other sympathomimetic agents, caution should be exercised in patients with uncontrolled diabetes, hyperthyroidism, elevated intraocular pressure and prostatic enlargement.

Drug interactions: The effect of antihypertensive agents which modify sympathetic activity may be partially reversed by Sudafed-Co.

Concomitant use of Sudafed-Co with other sympathomimetic agents such as decongestants, tricyclic antidepressants, appetite suppressants and amphetamine-like psychostimulants or with monoamine oxidase inhibitors, which interfere with the catabolism of sympathomimetic amines, may occasionally cause a rise in blood pressure.

The antibacterial agent furazolidone is known to cause a dose-related inhibition of monoamine oxidase and, although there are no reports of a hypertensive crisis having occurred, it should not be administered concurrently with Sudafed-Co.

In cases of paracetamol overdosage, liver microsomal inducing agents such as barbiturates, tricyclic antidepressants, and alcohol may increase the hepatotoxicity of paracetamol.

Side- and adverse effects: Side-effects are uncommon. In some patients pseudoephedrine may occasionally cause insomnia. Rarely, sleep disturbances and hallucinations have been reported. A fixed drug eruption to pseudoephedrine taking the form of erythematous nummular patches has been reported but is a rare occurrence. Paracetamol has been widely used and reports of adverse reactions are rare, and are generally associated with overdosage.

Isolated cases of chronic hepatic necrosis, acute pancreatitis or nephrotoxicity have been reported, after overdosage or prolonged administration of paracetamol. Isolated cases of thrombocytopenic purpura, methaemoglobinaemia, haemolytic anaemia, and agranulocytosis have been recorded. Nephrotoxic effects are uncommon and have not been reported in association with therapeutic doses, except after prolonged administration.

Urinary retention has been reported in male patients in whom prostatic enlargement could have been an important predisposing factor.

Use in pregnancy and lactation: Although pseudoephedrine and paracetamol have been in widespread use for many years without apparent ill consequence, there are no specific data on their use during pregnancy. Caution should, therefore, be exercised by balancing the potential benefit of treatment against any possible hazards. Systemic administration of pseudoephedrine, up to 50 times the human dose in rats and up to 35 times the human dose in rabbits, did not produce teratogenic effects.

It has been estimated that approximately 0.5%–0.7% of a single dose of pseudoephedrine ingested by a mother will be excreted in the breast milk over 24 hr, but the effect of this on breast-fed infants is not known.

Toxicity and treatment of overdosage: Pallor, nausea and vomiting may occur due to the paracetamol component. With pseudoephedrine, symptoms of overdosage may include irritability, convulsions, palpitations, hypertension, and difficulty in micturition. Hepatoxicity may be a complication from the paracetamol content but may not be apparent from 24 hours–6 days after ingestion.

Overdosage should, therefore, be treated promptly by gastric lavage followed by i.v. N-acetylcysteine, or oral methionine. Additional therapy (further methionine or i.v. cysteamine or i.v. N-acetylcysteine) is normally considered in the light of blood paracetamol content and the time elapsed since ingestion. Such therapy is probably best undertaken in a specialised unit. Supportive measures for respiration and circulation should be performed if indicated. Convulsions should be controlled with an anticonvulsant. Catheterisation of the bladder may be necessary. If desired, the elimination of pseudoephedrine can be accelerated by acid diuresis or by dialysis.

Pharmaceutical precautions Store below 25°C in a dry place. Protect from light.

Legal category P.

Package quantities 12 tablets in a blister strip.

Further information Nil.

Product licence number 0003/0157.

SUDAFED* EXPECTORANT

Presentation Each 5 ml of orange red syrup contains 100 mg Guaiphenesin BP and 30 mg Pseudoephedrine Hydrochloride BP.

Uses Conditions where an expectorant and upper respiratory tract decongestant are required.

Dosage and administration *Adults and children over 12 years:* 10 ml three times a day.

6–12 years: 5 ml three times a day.

2–5 years: 2.5 ml three times a day.

Sudafed Expectorant may be diluted 1:1 (1 in 2) or 1:3 (1 in 4) with Syrup BP. These dilutions are stable for 4 weeks if stored at 25°C.

Use in the elderly: No specific studies have been carried out in the elderly, but Sudafed Expectorant has been widely used in older people. However, it may be advisable to monitor renal and hepatic function, and if there is serious impairment then caution should be exercised.

Pharmacology: Pseudoephedrine has direct and indirect sympathomimetic activity and is an orally effective upper respiratory tract decongestant. Pseudoephedrine is substantially less potent than ephedrine in producing both tachycardia and elevation in systolic blood pressure and considerably less potent in causing stimulation of the central nervous system. On the basis of widespread and long established clinical use, guaiphenesin is recognised as an expectorant in bronchitis.

Contra-indications, warnings, etc

Contra-indications: Contra-indicated in patients who have previously shown intolerance to pseudoephedrine or guaiphenesin. Sudafed Expectorant is contra-indicated in persons under treatment with monoamine oxidase inhibitors and within two weeks of stopping such treatment.

It is also contra-indicated in patients with severe hypertension or severe coronary artery disease.

Precautions: Although pseudoephedrine has virtually no pressor effect in patients with normal blood pressure, Sudafed Expectorant should be used with caution in patients taking antihypertensive agents, tricyclic antidepressants, other sympathomimetic agents, such as decongestants, appetite suppressants and amphetamine-like psychostimulants. The effects of a single dose of Sudafed Expectorant on the blood pressure of these patients should be observed before recommending repeated or unsupervised treatment.

As with other sympathomimetic agents, caution should be exercised in patients with uncontrolled diabetes, hyperthyroidism, elevated intraocular pressure and prostatic enlargement.

Drug interactions: The effect of antihypertensive agents which modify sympathetic activity may be partially reversed by Sudafed Expectorant.

Concomitant use of Sudafed Expectorant with other sympathomimetic agents such as decongestants, tricyclic antidepressants, appetite suppressants and amphetamine-like psychostimulants or with monoamine oxidase inhibitors, which interfere with the catabolism of sympathomimetic amines, may occasionally cause a rise in blood pressure.

The antibacterial agent furazolidone is known to cause a dose-related inhibition of monoamine oxidase and, although there are no reports of hypertensive crises having occurred, it should not be administered concurrently with Sudafed Expectorant.

Side- and adverse effects: Side-effects are uncommon. In some patients pseudoephedrine may occasionally cause insomnia. Rarely, sleep disturbances and hallucinations have been reported.

A fixed drug eruption to pseudoephedrine, taking the form of erythematous nummular patches has been reported, but is a rare occurrence.

Urinary retention has been reported in male patients in whom prostatic enlargement could have been an important predisposing factor.

Use in pregnancy and lactation: Although pseudoephedrine and guaiphenesin have been in widespread use for many years without apparent ill consequence, there are no specific data on their use during pregnancy. Caution should, therefore, be exercised by balancing the potential benefit of treatment against any possible hazards. Systemic administration of pseudoephedrine, up to 50 times the human dose in rats and up to 35 times the human dose in rabbits, did not produce teratogenic effects.

It has been estimated that approximately 0.5%–0.7% of a single dose of pseudoephedrine ingested by a mother will be excreted in the breast milk over 24 hr, but the effect of this on breast-fed infants is not known.

Toxicity and treatment of overdosage: As with other sympathomimetic agents, symptoms of overdosage include irritability, restlessness, tremor, convulsions, palpitations, hypertension and difficulty in micturition. Gastric lavage and supportive measures for respiration and circulation should be performed if indicated. Convulsions should be controlled with an anticonvulsant. Catheterisation of the bladder may be necessary.

If desired, the elimination of pseudoephedrine can be accelerated by acid diuresis or by dialysis.

Pharmaceutical precautions Store below 25°C. Protect from light. Do not refrigerate.

Legal category P.

Package quantities Bottle of 100 ml.

Further information Nil.

Product licence number 0003/0145.

SUDAFED LINCTUS*

Presentation Each 5 ml of clear red linctus contains 10 mg Dextromethorphan Hydrobromide BP and 30 mg Pseudoephedrine Hydrochloride BP.

Uses Relief of unproductive cough accompanied by congestion of the upper respiratory tract.

Dosage and administration

Adults and children over 12 years: 10 ml three times a day.

Children 6–12 years: 5 ml three times a day.

2–5 years: 2.5 ml three times a day.

Sudafed Linctus may be diluted 1:1 (1 in 2) or 1:3 (1 in 4) with Syrup BP, these dilutions have a shelf life of 4 weeks if stored at 25°C.

Use in the elderly: No specific studies have been carried out in the elderly, but pseudoephedrine and dextromethorphan has been widely used in older people. However, it may be advisable to monitor renal or hepatic function and if there is serious impairment then caution should be exercised.

Pharmacology: Pseudoephedrine has direct and indirect sympathomimetic activity and is an orally effective upper respiratory tract decongestant. Pseudoephedrine is substantially less potent than ephedrine in producing both tachycardia and elevation in systolic blood pressure, and is considerably less potent in causing stimulation of the central nervous system. Dextromethorphan provides antitussive activity by acting on the medullary cough centre.

Contra-indications, warnings, etc

Contra-indications: Contra-indicated in patients with a known hypersensitivity to pseudoephedrine or dextromethorphan. Contra-indicated in persons under treatment with monoamine oxidase inhibitors or within 2 weeks of stopping such treatment.

Sudafed Linctus is contra-indicated in patients with severe hypertension or severe coronary artery disease.

Sudafed Linctus should not be administered to patients where cough is associated with asthma or where cough is accompanied by excessive secretions.

Dextromethorphan, in common with other centrally acting antitussive agents, should not be given to patients in or at risk of developing respiratory failure.

Precautions: Although pseudoephedrine has virtually no pressor effect in patients with normal blood pressure, Sudafed Linctus should be used with caution in patients taking antihypertensive agents, tricyclic antidepressants, other sympathomimetic agents, such as decongestants, appetite suppressants and amphetamine-like psychostimulants. The effects of a single dose of Sudafed Linctus on the blood pressure of these patients should be observed before recommending repeated or unsupervised treatment.

As with other sympathomimetic agents, caution should be exercised in patients with uncontrolled diabetes, hyperthyroidism, elevated intraocular pressure and prostatic enlargement.

This product may potentiate the effects of alcohol and other CNS depressants.

Drug interactions: Concomitant use of Sudafed Linctus with sympathomimetic agents such as decongestants, tricyclic antidepressants, appetite suppressants and amphetamine-like psychostimulants, or with monoamine oxidase inhibitors which interfere with the catabolism of sympathomimetic amines, may occasionally cause a rise in blood pressure.

Because of its pseudoephedrine content, the effect of antihypertensive agents which modify sympathetic activity may be partially reversed by Sudafed Linctus.

The antibacterial agent furazolidone is known to cause a dose-related inhibition of monoamine oxidase and although there are no reports of a hypertensive crisis having occurred, it should not be administered concurrently with Sudafed Linctus.

Side- and adverse effects: In some patients, pseudoephedrine may occasionally cause insomnia. Rarely, sleep disturbance and hallucinations have been reported. Fixed drug eruption due to pseudoephedrine, taking the form of erythematous nummular patches, has been reported as a rare event.

Urinary retention may occasinally occur in male patients in whom prostatic enlargement could be an important predisposing factor.

Side-effects attributed to dextromethorphan are uncommon; occasionally dizziness, nausea, vomiting or gastro-intestinal disturbance may occur.

Use in pregnancy and lactation: Although pseudoephedrine and dextromethorphan have been in widespread use for many years without apparent ill consequence, there are no specific data on their use during pregnancy. Caution should therefore be exercised by balancing the potential benefit of treatment against any possible hazards.

Systemic administration of pseudoephedrine, up to 50 times the human dose in rats and up to 35 times the human dose in rabbits did not produce teratogenic effects.

It has been estimated that approximately 0.5–0.7% of a single dose of pseudoephedrine ingested by a mother will be excreted in the breast milk over 24 hours, but the effect of this on breast-fed infants is not known.

It is not known whether dextromethorphan or its metabolites are excreted in human milk.

Toxicity and treatment of overdosage: The effects of acute toxicity from Sudafed Linctus may include nystagmus, hypertension, irritability, restlessness, tremor, palpitations, visual and auditory hallucinations, convulsions, respiratory depression, difficulty with micturition, nausea and vomiting.

Gastric lavage and supportive measures for respiration and circulation should be performed if indicated. Convulsions should be controlled with an anticonvulsant. Catheterisation of the bladder may be necesary. If desired, the elimination of pseudoephedrine can be accelerated by acid diuresis or by dialysis.

Naloxone has been used successful as a specific antagonist to dextromethorphan toxicity in a child.

Pharmaceutical precautions Store below 25°C. Protect from light.

Legal category P.

Package quantities Bottle of 100 ml.

Further information Nil.

Product licence number 0003/0163.

SUDAFED* PLUS TABLETS AND SYRUP

Presentation Each tablet contains 2.5 mg Triprolidine Hydrochloride BP and 60 mg Pseudoephedrine Hydrochloride BP. Scored and coded 'WELLCOME M2A'. White in colour.

Each 5 ml of clear, golden-yellow syrup contains 1.25 mg Triprolidine Hydrochloride BP and 30 mg Pseudoephedrine Hydrochloride BP, and has a pleasant flavour.

Uses Symptomatic relief of allergic rhinitis.

Dosage and administration
Adults and children over 12 years: 1 tablet or 10 ml three times a day.

Children 6–12 years: 5 ml three times a day.

2–5 years: 2.5 ml three times a day.

Sudafed Plus may be diluted 1:1 (1 in 2) or 1:3 (1 in 4) with Syrup BP and these dilutions are stable for 4 weeks if stored at 25°C.

Use in the elderly: No specific studies have been carried out in the elderly, but triprolidine and pseudoephedrine have been widely used in older people. However, it may be advisable to monitor renal or hepatic function and if there is serious impairment then caution should be exercised.

Pharmacology: Pseudoephedrine has direct and indirect sympathomimetic activity and is an orally effective upper respiratory tract decongestant. Pseudoephedrine is substantially less potent than ephedrine in producing both tachycardia and elevation in systolic blood pressure and considerably less potent in causing stimulation of the central nervous system. Triprolidine provides antihistamine activity by antagonising H_1 receptors.

Contra-indications, warnings, etc
Contra-indications: Contra-indicated in patients with a known hypersensitivity to pseudoephedrine or triprolidine.

Contra-indicated in persons under treatment with monoamine oxidase inhibitors, and within two weeks of stopping such treatment.

It is also contra-indicated in patients with severe hypertension or severe coronary artery disease.

Precautions: Although pseudoephedrine has virtually no pressor effect in patients with normal blood pressure, Sudefed Plus should be used with caution in patients taking antihypertensive agents, tricyclic antidepressants, other sympathomimetic agents, such as decongestants, appetite suppressants and amphetamine-like psychostimulants. The effects of a single dose on the blood pressure of these patients should be observed before recommending repeated or unsupervised treatment.

As with other sympathomimetic agents, caution should be exercised in patients with uncontrolled diabetes, hyperthyroidism, elevated intraocular pressure and prostatic enlargement.

Drug interactions: Concomitant use of Sudafed Plus with sympathomimetic agents such as decongestants, tricyclic antidepressants, appetite suppressants and amphetamine-like psychostimulants, or with monoamine oxidase inhibitors which interfere with the catabolism of sympathomimetic amines, may occasionally cause a rise in blood pressure.

Because of its pseudoephedrine content, the effect of antihypertensive agents which modify sympathetic activity may be partially reversed by Sudafed Plus.

The antibacterial agent furazolidone is known to cause a dose-related inhibition of monoamine oxidase and although there are no reports of hypertensive crises having occurred, it should not be administered concurrently with Sudafed Plus.

Side- and adverse effects: In some patients, pseudoephedrine may occasionally cause insomnia. Rarely, sleep disturbance and hallucinations have been reported. Triprolidine may cause drowsiness. Patients should not drive a vehicle or operate machinery until they have determined their own response. In some patients, the drowsiness induced by antihistamines may be potentiated by alcohol or other central sedatives. Fixed drug eruption due to pseudoephedrine taking the form of erythematous nummular patches and lichenoid skin eruption due to triprolidine have been reported but these are rare events.

Urinary retention may occasionally occur in male patients in whom prostatic enlargement could be an important predisposing factor.

Use in pregnancy and lactation: Although pseudoephedrine and triprolidine have been in widespread use for many years without apparent ill-consequence, there are no specific data on their use during pregnancy. Caution should therefore be exercised by balancing the potential benefit of treatment against any possible hazards.

Systemic administration of triprolidine in rats and rabbits up to 75 times the human dose did not produce teratogenic effects.

Systemic administration of pseudoephedrine, up to 50 times the human dose in rats and up to 35 times the human dose in rabbits, did not produce teratogenic effects.

It has been estimated that approximately 0.5–0.7% of a single dose of pseudoephedrine and approximately 0.06–0.2% of a single dose of triprolidine ingested by a mother will be excreted in the breast milk over 24 hours, but the effect of this on breast-fed infants is not known.

Toxicity and treatment of overdosage: The effects of acute toxicity from Sudafed Plus may include drowsiness, lethargy, dizziness, ataxia, weakness, hypotonicity, respiratory depression, dryness of the skin and mucous membranes, tachycardia, hypertension, hyperpyrexia, hyperactivity, irritability, convulsions and difficulty with micturition. Gastric lavage and supportive measures for respiration and circulation should be performed if indicated. Convulsions should be controlled with an anticonvulsant. Catheterisation of the bladder may be necessary.

If desired, the elimination of pseudoephedrine can be accelerated by acid diuresis or by dialysis.

Pharmaceutical precautions
Tablets: Store below 25°C in a dry place. Protect from light.
Syrup: Store below 25°C. Protect from light.

Legal category P.

Package quantities
Tablets: Pack of 100 tablets.
Syrup: Bottle of 1 litre.

Further information Nil.

Product licence numbers
Tablets 0003/0248
Syrup 0003/0247

SYRAPRIM* TABLETS

Presentation White scored tablets coded 'WELLCOME Y3C' containing 300 mg Trimethoprim BP. White scored tablets coded 'WELLCOME 09A' containing 100 mg Trimethoprim BP.

Uses Syraprim is an antibacterial agent indicated for the treatment of infections due to trimethoprim-sensitive organisms, particularly those affecting the urinary and respiratory tracts. Also for the long-term prophylaxis of recurrent, or suppression of chronic, urinary tract infections caused by sensitive organisms.

Syraprim is active *in vitro* against a wide range of Gram-negative and Gram-positive organisms. It is not active against *Pseudomonas* spp., *Mycobacterium tuberculosis, Mycoplasma, Clostridium* spp., *Treponema pallidum* and anaerobes. It is relatively inactive against *Brucella* spp. and *Neisseria* spp.

Dosage and administration *Urinary Tract Infections: Treatment:*

Adults: 300 mg once daily.
Children over 12 years: as for adults.
6–12 years: 150 mg once daily.
Under 6 years: formulation inapplicable.

This dosage approximates to 6 mg/kg body weight/day.

Prophylaxis:

Adults: 100 mg once daily.
Children over 12 years: as for adults.
6–12 years: 50 mg once daily.
Under 6 years: formulation inapplicable.

This dosage approximates to 2 mg/kg body weight/day.

To ensure maximal urinary concentrations it may be advantageous to take the dose at bedtime.

Respiratory Infections:

Adults: 200 mg twice daily.
Children over 12 years: as for adults.
6–12 years: 100 mg twice daily.
6 months–6 years: 50 mg twice daily.

In acute infections, Syraprim should be given for at least five days or until the patient has been symptom-free for two days. Long-term administration may be continued for 3 to 12 months or more as appropriate.

Dosage recommendations in renal impairment: When creatinine clearance is below 15–20 ml/minute, trimethoprim levels should be monitored after approximately 3 days' treatment to provide guidance on the appropriate dosage reduction. When the clearance is below 10 ml/minute Syraprim should not be administered unless plasma concentrations can be estimated regularly and haemodialysis facilities are available.

Use in the elderly: No specific studies have been carried out in the elderly, although Syraprim has been widely used in older people. However, care is advised when treating the elderly because, as a group, they are more susceptible to adverse reactions. See also 'Precautions'.

Contra-indications, warnings, etc

Contra-indications: Syraprim should not be given to patients with a history of hypersensitivity to trimethoprim.

Contra-indicated in patients with severe impairment of renal function where repeated estimations of the plasma concentration, or haemodialysis, cannot be carried out.

Except in rare circumstances Syraprim should not be given to patients with serious haematological disorders.

Precautions: Syraprim should be discontinued if a skin rash appears.

Exercise caution when treating patients with severe hepatic parenchymal damage as changes may occur in the absorption and metabolism of trimethoprim.

Trimethoprim has been noted to impair phenylalanine metabolism but this is of no significance in phenylketonuric patients on appropriate dietary restriction.

Care should be taken when giving the drug to patients with blood dyscrasias.

Caution should be exercised in the administration of Syraprim to patients with actual or potential folate deficiency and administration of a folate supplement (e.g. 5–10 mg/day folinic acid) should be considered, especially in the elderly.

If Syraprim treatment is prolonged, especially in patients with suspected impairment of folate metabolism, it is suggested that complete blood counts including thrombocytes be performed at monthly intervals.

Drug interactions: Occasional reports suggest that patients receiving pyrimethamine as malarial prophylaxis at doses in excess of 25 mg weekly may develop megaloblastic anaemia should co-trimoxazole be prescribed concurrently. The same interaction is likely if trimethoprim be prescribed concurrently.

Trimethoprim may potentiate the anticoagulant activity of warfarin via stereo-selective inhibition of its metabolism. Careful control of the anticoagulant therapy during treatment with Syraprim is advisable.

Trimethoprim prolongs the half life of phenytoin and if co-administered the prescriber should be alert for excessive phenytoin effect. Close monitoring of the patient's condition and serum phenytoin levels is advisable.

Concurrent use of rifampicin and trimethoprim results in a shortening of the plasma half life of trimethoprim after a period of about one week. This is not thought to be of clinical significance.

Reversible deterioration in renal function has been observed in patients treated with trimethoprim and cyclosporin following renal transplantation.

Side- and adverse effects: Minor gastro-intestinal disturbances including nausea and vomiting, sore mouth/tongue, pruritus and skin rashes may occasionally occur. Although an effect on folate metabolism is possible, interference with haematopoiesis rarely occurs at the recommended dose. If any such change is seen, folinic acid should reverse the effect. Elderly patients may be more susceptible and a lower dosage may be advisable.

Use in pregnancy and lactation: The safety of trimethoprim in human pregnancy has not been established. Animal studies have shown, at high doses, teratogenic effects typical of a folate antagonist in rats but not rabbits; these were prevented by administration of dietary folates. The benefit of using Syraprim in pregnancy should be weighed against the possible hazard.

Despite its excretion in breast milk the administration of Syraprim to a lactating woman represents a negligible risk to the suckling infant.

Toxicity and treatment of overdosage: Nausea, vomiting, abdominal pain, dizziness and confusion are likely symptoms of overdosage. Stop therapy. Gastric lavage may be useful although absorption of trimethoprim from the gastro-intestinal tract is normally complete in approximately 2 hours. This may not be the case in gross overdosage. Calcium folinate (5–10 mg/day) given orally for five to seven days should counteract any folate deficiency effect on the bone marrow. Acidification of the urine will increase the elimination of trimethoprim. General supportive measures are recommended.

Trimethoprim is dialysable by renal dialysis.

Pharmaceutical precautions Store below 25°C and protect from light.

Legal category POM.

Package quantities
Bottle of 100 × 300 mg tablets.
Bottle of 100 × 100 mg tablets.

Further information Absorption by the oral route is rapid; significant plasma levels are obtained within half an hour; peak levels may be reached as early as one hour.

Excretion is predominantly in the urine in the form of unchanged drug. Urinary concentrations are generally well above the MIC of common pathogens for more than 24 hours after the last dose.

Trimethoprim may cause an apparent rise in serum creatinine levels due to (a) competition for the tubular secretory mechanisms; (b) chemical interference with the visual auto-analyser method of estimating creatinine.

Trimethoprim does not induce its own metabolism and therefore no dose modification is required on this account during long-term treatment.

Plasma or serum levels of trimethoprim may be determined by gas liquid chromatography and high performance liquid chromatography.

Product licence numbers
300 mg tablets 0003/0148
100 mg tablets 0003/0147

SYRAPRIM* INJECTION

Presentation Syraprim Injection is a sterile aqueous solution of trimethoprim lactate equivalent to 20 mg trimethoprim base in 1 ml of water. Each ampoule contains 5 ml. The pH is 4.0.

Uses Syraprim is an antibacterial agent indicated for the treatment of infections due to sensitive organisms, in particular Gram-negative infections. Syraprim injection may also be useful in acute urinary tract infections where oral therapy is inappropriate. Trimethoprim is effective *in vitro* against a wide range of Gram-negative and Gram-positive organisms. It is not active against *Pseudomonas* spp., *Mycobacterium tuberculosis, Mycoplasma, Clostridium* spp., *Treponema pallidum*, and anaerobes. It is relatively inactive against *Brucella* spp. and *Neisseria* spp.

Dosage and administration *Dosage: Adults and children over 12 years:* 150–250 mg every 12 hours. *Children under 12 years:* The total daily dose should approximate to 6–9 mg/kg of body weight divided into two or three equal doses and administered either 12-hourly or 8-hourly.

The severely ill patient may require initially higher, or more frequent, doses as may a person considerably in excess of the average weight for his/her height. Total doses up to 20 mg/kg of body weight per day in divided doses have been well tolerated.

Dosage recommendations in renal impairment: When creatinine clearance is below 15–20 ml/minute, trimethoprim levels should be monitored after approximately 3 days' treatment to provide guidance on the appropriate dosage reduction. When the clearance is below 10 ml/minute Syraprim should not be administered unless plasma concentrations can be estimated regularly and haemodialysis facilities are available.

Use in the elderly: No specific studies have been carried out in the elderly, although Syraprim has been widely used in older people. However, care is advised when treating the elderly because, as a group, they are more susceptible to adverse reactions. See also 'Precautions'.

Administration: Syraprim Injection should be administered slowly.

1. By direct intravenous injection, or
2. via the tubing (close to the vein) of an established intravenous infusion.

If it is necessary to add Syraprim Injection to the infusion fluid it is compatible with the following:

Glucose Intravenous Infusion BP 5% w/v.
Fructose Intravenous Infusion BP 5% w/v.
Sodium Lactate Intravenous Infusion BP.

Any chloride-containing solution is likely to cause precipitation of trimethoprim hydrochloride when used with Syraprim Injection.

Contra-indications, warnings, etc

Contra-indications: Syraprim should not be given to patients with a history of hypersensitivity to trimethoprim.

Contra-indicated in patients with severe impairment of renal function where repeated estimations of the plasma concentration, or haemodialysis cannot be carried out.

Except in rare circumstances Syraprim should not be given to patients with serious haematological disorders.

Precautions: Syraprim should be discontinued if a skin rash appears.

Exercise caution when treating patients with severe hepatic parenchymal damage as changes may occur in the absorption and metabolism of trimethoprim.

Trimethoprim has been noted to impair phenylalanine metabolism but this is of no significance in phenylketonuric patients on appropriate dietary restriction.

Care should be taken when giving the drug to patients with blood dyscrasias.

A folate supplement should be given when high doses of Syraprim are administered intravenously.

Caution should be exercised in the administration of Syraprim to patients with actual or potential folate deficiency, and administration of a folate supplement (e.g. 5–10 mg/day folinic acid) should be considered, especially in the elderly.

If Syraprim treatment is prolonged, especially in patients with suspected impairment of folate metabolism, it is suggested that complete blood counts including thrombocytes be performed at monthly intervals.

Drug interactions: Occasional reports suggest that patients receiving pyrimethamine as malarial prophylaxis at doses in excess of 25 mg weekly may develop megaloblastic anaemia should co-trimoxazole be prescribed concurrently. The same interaction is likely if trimethoprim be prescribed concurrently.

Trimethoprim may potentiate the anticoagulant activity of warfarin via stereo-selective inhibition of its metabolism. Careful control of the anticoagulant therapy during treatment with Syraprim is advisable.

Trimethoprim prolongs the half life of phenytoin and if co-administered the prescriber should be alert for excessive phenytoin effect. Close monitoring of the patient's condition and serum phenytoin levels is advisable.

Concurrent use of rifampicin and trimethoprim results in a shortening of the plasma half life of trimethoprim after a period of about one week. This is not thought to be of clinical significance.

Reversible deterioration in renal function has been observed in patients treated with trimethoprim and cyclosporin following renal transplantation.

Side- and adverse effects: Minor gastro-intestinal disturbances including nausea and vomiting, sore mouth/tongue, pruritus and skin rashes may occasionally occur. Although an effect on folate metabolism is possible, interference with haematopoiesis rarely occurs at the recommended dose. If any such change is seen, folinic acid should reverse the effect. Elderly patients may be more susceptible and a lower dosage may be advisable.

Nausea due to too rapid injection may occur and if so the time over which the injection is given should be prolonged.

Use in pregnancy and lactation: The safety of trimethoprim in human pregnancy has not been established. Animal studies have shown, at high doses, teratogenic effects typical of a folate antagonist in rats but not rabbits; these were prevented by administration of dietary folates. The benefit of using Syraprim in pregnancy should be weighed against its possible hazard.

Despite its excretion in breast milk the administration of Syraprim to a lactating woman represents a negligible risk to the suckling infant.

Toxicity and treatment of overdosage: Nausea, vomiting, abdominal pain, dizziness and confusion are likely symptoms of overdosage. Stop therapy. Calcium folinate (5–10 mg/day) given orally for five to seven days should counteract any folate deficiency effect on the bone marrow. Acidification of the urine will increase the elimination of trimethoprim. General supportive measures are recommended.

Trimethoprim is dialysable by renal dialysis.

Pharmaceutical precautions Store below 25°C and protect from light.

Syraprim Injection should not be added to any chloride-containing infusion fluid.

Syraprim Injection is incompatible with solutions of sulphonamides and the two should not be mixed.

Legal category POM.

Package quantities Box of 10 ampoules.

Further information Excretion is predominantly in the urine in the form of unchanged drug.

Trimethoprim may cause an apparent rise in serum creatinine levels due to (a) competition for the renal tubular secretory mechanism, (b) chemical interference with the usual auto-analyser method of estimating creatinine.

Trimethoprim does not induce its own metabolism and therefore no dose modification is required on this account during long-term treatment.

Syraprim Injection may be given in conjunction with, but separately from, parenteral aminoglycosides, metronidazole, or sulphonamides depending on the organism responsible for the infection.

Plasma or serum levels of trimethoprim may be determined by gas liquid chromatography and high performance liquid chromatography.

Product licence number 0003/0149.

TETANUS VACCINE BP (IN SIMPLE SOLUTION) WELLCOME* (Tet/Vac/FT)

Presentation Tetanus vaccine is prepared by formalin detoxification of *Clostridium tetani* exotoxin. Thiomersal BP is added as a preservative to a concentration of 0.01%. Each 0.5 ml dose contains not less than 14Lf toxoid.

The antigenic content and formulation of this vaccine has not been changed, although the labelled content has been altered to conform with the flocculation equivalence of the new British reference antitoxin preparation.

Uses For active immunisation against tetanus.

Administration of the antigenically more potent adsorbed vaccine is usually preferred for all injections. Tetanus vaccine in simple solution is insufficiently antigenic to be used as the first immunising dose but may be used instead of adsorbed tetanus vaccine if necessary for the second, third or later reinforcing injections. Tetanus vaccine in simple solution is now often reserved for administration to patients who have had some reaction to a previous dose of adsorbed vaccine and who are not thought to be adequately protected against infection.

Dosage and administration The dose of tetanus vaccine in simple solution is 0.5 ml given by deep subcutaneous or intramuscular injection. When Tetanus vaccine in simple solution is used for second or third doses in an immunising course, intervals of 6 to 12 weeks and 6 to 12 months respectively are recommended between the first and second and the second and third doses.

The United Kingdom Department of Health recommends the administration of reinforcing doses after five years and after a further 5 to 15 years with the administration of additional doses in the event of injuries which may give rise to tetanus. Tetanus vaccine should not be given to any patient who has received a booster dose in the preceding year.

A single dose of vaccine given several years after the completion of a primary course will rapidly stimulate the production of tetanus antitoxin in the circulation.

In subjects who have suffered a reaction to a previous dose of adsorbed vaccine it may be preferred to administer 0.1 ml of tetanus vaccine in simple solution intradermally.

Oral Poliomyelitis Vaccine BP may be given at the same time as tetanus vaccine.

Shake well before each dose is withdrawn. It is good practice to record the title, dose and lot numbers of all vaccines and dates of administration. Any untoward reactions should be reported to the regulatory authorities and to the manufacturer.

Use in the elderly: No special comment.

Contra-indications, warnings, etc
Contra-indications: The vaccine should not be administered to a subject who has experienced a serious reaction (e.g. anaphylaxis) to a previous dose of this vaccine or who is known to be hypersensitive to any component thereof. It is advisable to avoid vaccination during an acute infection. Tetanus vaccine in simple solution should not be given simultaneously with human tetanus immunoglobulin or tetanus antitoxin which may markedly depress its antigenicity.

Precautions: Although anaphylaxis is rare, facilities for its management should always be available during vaccination.

Side- and adverse effects: Local reactions consisting of swelling, redness and pain may develop at the injection site and persist for several days. Delays of up to 10 days before symptoms develop are reported. Occasionally these local reactions may be quite marked, with tenderness and swelling of a large area. Local reactions are rare in children and the incidence increases with age and according to the number of previously administered doses, but reactions may occur after the first dose. Subjects who develop reactions frequently have high titres of circulating antitoxin. Women develop reactions more frequently than men. General reactions are uncommon but may include headache, lethargy, malaise, myalgia and pyrexia. Acute anaphylactic reactions, urticaria, angioneurotic oedema, serum sickness and peripheral neuropathy occasionally occur.

Use in pregnancy and lactation: In developing countries tetanus vaccines are widely administered during pregnancy to prevent neonatal tetanus without significant apparent adverse effects on pregnancy or foetal development.

Toxicity and treatment of overdosage: Not applicable.

Pharmaceutical precautions Store at 2–8°C. Protect from light. *Do not freeze.* When multidose containers are employed it is good practice to discard any partly used vaccine vials at the end of the vaccinating session.

Legal category POM.

Package quantities Pack of 5 × 0.5 ml ampoules. Vial of 5 ml.

Further information Persons of all ages are susceptible to tetanus unless they have been immunised with tetanus vaccine. Rarely, if ever, does natural immunity develop even in persons who have recovered from severe tetanus. Since most tetanus cases follow trivial wounds all persons should be actively immunised against the disease.

Product licence number 0003/5190.

ADSORBED TETANUS VACCINE BP WELLCOME* (Tet/Vac/Ads)

Presentation Adsorbed tetanus vaccine is a suspension of highly purified toxoid prepared by formalin detoxification of *Clostridium tetani* exotoxin. The toxoid is adsorbed onto aluminium hydroxide. Thiomersal BP is added as a preservative to a concentration of 0.01%. Each 0.5 ml dose has an immunising potency of not less than 40 International Units (IU).

The immunising potency of this vaccine is now expressed in International Units in accordance with the requirements of the European and British Pharmacopoeias. These units measure the immunising activity of the vaccine whereas the previously used Lf units expressed the quantity of toxoid present. There is no simple numerical relationship between IU and Lf. No change has been made to the potency although it is now expressed in IU.

Uses For active immunisation against tetanus.

Dosage and administration Primary immunisation consists of three deep subcutaneous or intramuscular doses of adsorbed vaccine each of 0.5 ml administered at intervals of 6 to 12 weeks and 6 to 12 months respectively. Adsorbed tetanus vaccine may be used for the routine anti-tetanus immunisation of persons of all ages although it is usual to employ plain or adsorbed combined diphtheria/tetanus/pertussis vaccine (DTPer/Vac or DTPer/Vac/Ads) or adsorbed diphtheria and tetanus vaccine (DT/Vac/Ads) for immunisation of infants.

The United Kingdom Department of Health recommends the administration of reinforcing doses after five years and after a further 5 to 15 years with the administration of additional doses in the event of injuries which may give rise to tetanus. Tetanus vaccine should not be given to any patient who has received a booster dose in the preceding year.

A single dose of vaccine given several years after the completion of a primary course will rapidly stimulate the production of tetanus antitoxin in the circulation.

Adsorbed tetanus vaccine may be administered simultaneously with human tetanus immunoglobulin or tetanus antitoxin but must be given at separate sites. The antibody response of subjects to subsequent doses of vaccine is not significantly impaired by this procedure.

Oral Poliomyelitis Vaccine BP may be given at the same time as Tetanus Vaccine.

Shake well before each dose is withdrawn. It is good practice to record the title, dose and lot numbers of all vaccines and dates of administration. Any untoward reactions should be reported to the regulatory authorities and to the manufacturer.

Use in the elderly: No special comment.

Contra-indications, warnings, etc
Contra-indications: Adsorbed tetanus vaccine should not be administered intradermally.

The vaccine should not be administered to a subject who has experienced a serious reaction (e.g. anaphylaxis) to a previous dose of this vaccine or who is known to be hypersensitive to any component thereof. It is advisable to avoid vaccination during an acute infection.

Precautions: Although anaphylaxis is rare, facilities for its management should always be available during vaccination.

Side- and adverse effects: Local reactions consisting of swelling, redness and pain may develop at the injection site and persist for several days. Delays of up to 10 days before symptoms develop are reported. Occasionally these local reactions may be quite marked, with tenderness and swelling of a large area. Local reactions are rare in children and the incidence increases with age and according to the number of previously administered doses, but reactions may occur after the first dose. Subjects who develop reactions frequently have high titres of circulating antitoxin. Women develop reactions more frequently than men. General reactions are uncommon but may include headache, lethargy, malaise, myalgia and pyrexia. Acute anaphylactic reactions, urticaria, angioneurotic oedema, serum sickness and peripheral neuropathy occasionally occur.

Persistent nodules at the site of injection may occasionally follow administration of adsorbed vaccines especially if the inoculation is into the superficial layers of subcutaneous tissue.

Use in pregnancy and lactation: In developing countries tetanus vaccines are widely administered during pregnancy to prevent neonatal tetanus without significant apparent adverse effects on pregnancy or foetal development.

Toxicity and treatment of overdosage: Not applicable.

Pharmaceutical precautions Store at 2–8°C. Protect from light. *Do not freeze.* When multidose containers are employed it is good practice to discard any partly used vaccine vials at the end of the vaccinating session.

Legal category POM.

Package quantities Pack of 5 × 0.5 ml ampoules. Vial of 5 ml.

Further information Persons of all ages are susceptible to tetanus unless they have been immunised with tetanus vaccine. Rarely, if ever, is natural immunity developed even in persons who have recovered from severe tetanus. Since most tetanus cases follow trivial wounds all persons should be actively immunised against the disease.

Product licence number 0003/5191.

TINEAFAX* CREAM
TINEAFAX* POWDER

Presentation
Tineafax Cream contains 1.0% w/w tolnaftate in a white cream base.
Tineafax Powder is white and contains 1.0% w/w tolnaftate.

Uses Tineafax Cream is indicated for the treatment of tinea pedis ('athlete's foot') and other ringworm (dermatophytic) infections of the skin.

Tineafax Poweder is indicated for the prophylaxis of tinea pedis infections.

In vitro activity: Tolnaftate is active against a range of dermatophytic organisms including *Epidermophyton floccosum, Trichophyton rubrum, Trichophyton mentagrophytes* and *Microsporum canis*. It is not active against *Candida albicans* or *Aspergillus niger*.

Dosage and administration
Treatment: Adults and children: Tineafax Cream should be applied to the affected skin twice daily. Prior to applications, the skin should be washed and dried thoroughly.

Any dead or loose skin should be removed.

Treatment should be continued for 2–3 days after apparent clearance of lesions.

The feet should be kept clean and dry; walking barefooted in public dressing rooms should be avoided.

Prophylaxis: Adults and children: Tineafax Powder should be dusted onto the feet, and between the toes, twice daily. Prior to application, the feet should be washed and dried thoroughly.

Use in the elderly: No special comment.

Contra-indications, warnings, etc
Contra-indications: Tineafax is contra-indicated in patients with a known hypersensitivity to tolnaftate.

Precautions: For external use only.

Avoid contact of Tineafax with the eyes.

If a hypersensitivity reaction develops, or is suspected during therapy, the use of Tineafax should be stopped.

Side- and adverse effects: Allergic contact dermatitis following the use of topical tolnaftate has been reported rarely.

Use in pregnancy and lactation: There are no specific data on the use of tolnaftate formulations in pregnancy and lactation. Tineafax should be used only if the potential benefit of treatment to the patient outweighs any possible but unknown risk to the foetus.

Toxicity and treatment of overdosage: There are no reports of overdosage with tolnaftate.

Should untoward effects develop following excessive ingestion of tolnaftate, symptomatic and supportive therapy should be instigated.

Pharmaceutical precautions Store below 25°C.

Legal category GSL.

Package quantities *Tineafax Cream:* Tube of 25 g. *Tineafax Powder:* Puffer pack of 50 g.

Further information In clinical studies, tolnaftate has generally been found to be well tolerated and lacking in irritancy potential.

Product licence numbers

Tineafax Cream	0003/0250
Tineafax Powder	0003/0251

TRACRIUM* INJECTION

Presentation Tracrium injection contains atracurium besylate, 10 mg per ml, as a clear, faint-yellow solution for intravenous administration. Each 2.5 ml ampoule contains 25 mg atracurium besylate, each 5 ml ampoule contains 50 mg atracurium besylate and each 25 ml ampoule contains 250 mg atracurium besylate.

Uses Tracrium is a highly selective, competitive (non-depolarising) neuromuscular blocking agent.

It is used in anaesthesia to relax skeletal muscles during a wide range of surgical procedures and to facilitate controlled ventilation. Tracrium is highly suitable for endotracheal intubation especially where subsequent muscle relaxation is required. Tracrium is suitable for maintenance of muscle relaxation in Caesarean Section.

Tracrium is suitable for administration by continuous infusion to maintain neuromuscular block during long surgical procedures.

Metabolism: Tracrium is degraded spontaneously mainly by a non-enzymatic decomposition process (Hofmann elimination) which occurs at plasma pH and at body temperature and produces breakdown products which are inactive.

Tests with plasma from patients with pseudo-cholinesterase deficiency show that the inactivation of Tracrium proceeds unaffected. It is possible that some decomposition may occur by non-specific plasma esterases.

The termination of the neuromuscular blocking action of Tracrium is not dependent on metabolism and excretion by the liver or kidneys. The duration of action is therefore unlikely to be affected by impaired renal, hepatic or circulatory function.

Dosage and administration Tracrium is administered by intravenous injection.

The dosage range recommended for adults is 0.3–0.6 mg/kg depending on the duration of full block required and will provide relaxation for about 15–35 minutes.

Endotracheal intubation can usually be accomplished within 90 seconds of intravenous injection of 0.5–0.6 mg/kg.

Full block can be prolonged with supplementary doses of 0.1–0.2 mg/kg as required. Successive supplementary dosing does not give rise to accumulation.

The neuromuscular block produced by Tracrium can be rapidly and permanently reversed by standard doses of neostigmine, which should be preceded by the administration of atropine.

Recovery from the end of full block without the use of neostigmine occurs in about 35 minutes as measured by the restoration of the tetanic response to 95% of normal neuromuscular function.

Children: The dosage in children over the age of 1 month is similar to that in adults on a mg/kg basis.

Elderly and high-risk patients: Tracrium may be used at standard dosage in elderly patients and in those with respiratory, renal or hepatic failure.

Continuous infusion: Tracrium is suitable for administration by continuous infusion at rates of 0.005–0.01 mg/kg/minute (0.3–0.6 mg/kg/hour) to maintain neuromuscular block during long surgical procedures. Tracrium maintains acceptable physical and chemical stability in daylight at concentrations of 0.5 mg/ml and above at temperatures of up to 30°C for:

4 hours in Compound Sodium Lactate Intravenous Infusion BP.
8 hours in Ringer's Injection USP; Glucose Intravenous Infusion BP 5% w/v; or 0.18% w/v Sodium Chloride and 4% w/v Glucose Intravenous Infusion BP.
And for up to 24 hours in Sodium Chloride Intravenous Infusion BP.

Tracrium can be administered by infusion during cardiopulmonary bypass surgery, at the recommended infusion rates. Induced hypothermia to a body temperature of 25°C to 26°C reduces the rate of inactivation of atracurium, therefore full neuromuscular block may be maintained by approximately half the original infusion rates at these temperatures.

Contra-indications, warnings, etc

Contra-indications: There are no contra-indications to the use of Tracrium except known hypersensitivity to the drug.

Precautions: In common with all the other neuromuscular blocking agents, Tracrium paralyses the respiratory muscles as well as other skeletal muscles. Therefore it should be administered only by or under the close supervision of an anaesthetist and adequate facilities must be available for endotracheal intubation and artificial ventilation.

Tracrium should be used with caution in patients with myasthenia gravis, other neuromuscular disease and severe electrolyte disorders in which potentiation of other non-depolarising agents has been noted.

Patients with severe cardiovascular disease may be more susceptible to the effects of transient hypotension. In these patients slow intravenous injection in divided doses is recommended.

Drug interactions: The neuromuscular block produced by Tracrium may be increased by the concomitant use of inhalation anaesthetics such as halothane.

Neuromuscular block produced by Tracrium may be increased by the concomitant use of aminoglycosides (such as neomycin) and polypeptide antibiotics (such as polymyxin).

A depolarising muscle relaxant such as suxamethonium chloride should not be administered to prolong the neuromuscular blocking effects of non-depolarising blocking agents such as atracurium, as this may result in a 'mixed block' which is difficult to reverse with anticholinesterase drugs.

Side- and adverse effects: Tracrium does not have significant vagal or ganglionic blocking properties in the recommended dosage range. Consequently, Tracrium will not counteract the bradycardia produced by many anaesthetic agents, or by vagal stimulation during surgery.

In common with most neuromuscular blocking agents the potential exists for histamine release in susceptible patients. Associated with the use of Tracrium there have been reports of skin flushing, and transient hypotension which have been attributed to histamine release. Rarely, bronchospasm and, very rarely, anaphylactoid reactions have also been reported.

Use in pregnancy and obstetrics: Although animal studies have indicated that Tracrium has no adverse effects on foetal development, nevertheless, as with all neuromuscular blocking agents it should be used with caution in pregnant women.

Tracrium may be used to maintain neuromuscular relaxation in Caesarean Section as atracurium does not cross the placenta in clinically significant amounts.

Toxicity and treatment of overdosage: In the event of overdosage or delayed recovery, the patient should be given atropine and neostigmine and maintained on artificial ventilation until spontaneous respiration returns.

Pharmaceutical precautions Tracrium must not be mixed in the same syringe with thiopentone or any alkaline agent, as the high pH will inactivate Tracrium.

Where a small vein is selected as the injection site, Tracrium should be flushed through the vein after injection. Where other anaesthetic drugs are administered through the same in-dwelling needle or cannula as Tracrium, it is important that each drug is flushed through with Water for Injections BP or physiological saline.

Store at 2–8°C. Protect from light. Do not freeze. Opened ampoules of Tracrium should be discarded immediately after use.

Legal category POM.

Package quantities Box of 5 × 2.5 ml ampoules (each ampoule containing 25 mg atracurium besylate).

Box of 5 × 5 ml ampoules (each ampoule containing 50 mg atracurium besylate).

Box of 2 × 25 ml ampoules (each ampoule containing 250 mg atracurium besylate).

Further information Tracrium has no effect on the intra-ocular pressure, which makes it suitable for use in ophthalmic surgery.

Variations in the blood pH and body temperature of the patient within the physiological range will not significantly alter the duration of action of Tracrium.

Product licence number 0003/0166.

TRI-CICATRIN* OINTMENT

Presentation mTri-Cicatrin Ointment contains Neomycin Sulphate BP 3,400 units, Bacitracin Zinc BP 250 units, Nystatin (Dermatological) BP 100,000 units and Hydrocortisone BP 1% w/w per gram in a hydrocarbon ointment base.

Uses Tri-Cicatrin Ointment is indicated for the topical treatment of the following conditions: eczema/dermatitis including atopic eczema, primary irritant dermatitis, contact allergic dermatitis, seborrhoeic dermatitis, and intertriginous conditions in which bacterial or candidal infection is present or likely to occur, and secondarily infected insect bite reactions.

The use of Tri-Cicatrin Ointment does not exclude concomitant systemic therapy with other agents (for example antibiotics) where appropriate.

Dosage and administration The use of Tri-Cicatrin Ointment should not be continued for more than 7 days in the absence of any clinical improvement.

Adults: Prior to treatment, remove any debris such as pus, crusts, etc. from the affected area and then apply a thin film of ointment to the affected area one to three times per day, depending on the clinical condition.

Children: Tri-Cicatrin Ointment may be used in children with dosage and administration regimens as for adults. The maximum recommended dosages, however, should be reduced in proportion to bodyweight (see Precautions).

Use in the elderly: No specific studies have been carried out in the elderly. The maximum daily dosage should be reduced in cases where a decrease in renal function exists.

Contra-indications, warnings, etc The use of Tri-Cicatrin Ointment is contra-indicated in patients who are hypersensitive to neomycin sulphate, bacitracin zinc, nystatin, hydrocortisone, mineral oils or to cross-sensitising substances.

The presence of pre-existing nerve deafness is a contra-indication to the use of Tri-Cicatrin Ointment in circumstances in which significant systemic absorption could occur.

Viral, tuberculous, dermatophytic and primary bacterial and candidal infections of the skin are contra-indications to the use of Tri-Cicatrin Ointment.

Precautions: Avoid introduction of Tri-Cicatrin Ointment into the eyes.

Following the application of Tri-Cicatrin Ointment to large areas of raw or damaged skin, significant systemic absorption of the active ingredients may occur. Neomycin sulphate is the dose-limiting ingredient of Tri-Cicatrin Ointment because it can cause irreversible nerve deafness following significant systemic absorption. Both neomycin sulphate and bacitracin zinc have nephrotoxic potential following significant systemic absorption. The application of 60 g of ointment daily for 3 weeks should not be exceeded in adults. After such a course, treatment should not be repeated for at least three months.

In infancy, treatment with Tri-Cicatrin Ointment should not normally exceed 7 days.

The maximum recommended dosages should be reduced in patients with compromised renal function in accordance with the degree of impairment present.

In cases where there is established partial nerve deafness and where a significant degree of neomycin absorption could occur it might be inappropriate to use any neomycin-containing product and treatment with an antibacterial without an aminoglycoside constituent should be used if possible.

Concurrent administration of other aminoglycoside antibiotics is not recommended.

Cross-sensitisation to framycetin, kanamycin, gentamicin and other related antibiotics does occur.

The systemic absorption of hydrocortisone may lead to suppression of the function of the adrenal gland.

Patients with hypostatic leg ulcers or hypostatic leg eczemas may have an increased sensitivity to a large number of topically applied drugs, including neomycin.

Side- and adverse effects: Allergic hypersensitivity to neomycin is generally uncommon following topical use but may manifest itself as a reddening and scaling of the affected skin, as an eczematous exacerbation of the lesion or as a failure of the lesion to heal. Allergic hypersensitivity reactions following the topical administration of bacitracin zinc, hydrocortisone and nystatin are rare events but have been reported.

Topically applied hydrocortisone may produce skin atrophy as manifested by telangiectasiae, striae, etc. However, this effect only occurs following prolonged use, high dosage, occlusion of the topical site (for example by plastic or by natural occlusion as in the groin), and particularly applies to infants and young children.

Anaphylaxis following the topical application of bacitracin has been reported rarely.

As with other steroid/antimicrobial preparations, prolonged use may result in the overgrowth of non-susceptible organisms including fungi.

Drug interactions: The neuromuscular blocking activity of neomycin sulphate is unlikely to present any hazard in the topical use of this preparation.

Use in pregnancy and lactation: There is no evidence of safety of Tri-Cicatrin in human pregnancy. However, the active ingredients have been in use for many years without apparent ill-consequence, but there are no specific data on the use of the product as formulated.

Topical administration of corticosteroids to pregnant animals can cause abnormalities of foetal development. The relevance of this finding to human beings has not been established.

The use of Tri-Cicatrin cannot be recommended in circumstances where significant systemic absorption of the active ingredients may occur. Although topical administration is otherwise unlikely to be associated with risk, caution should be exercised by balancing the potential benefit of treatment against any possible hazards.

No information is available regarding the excretion of the active ingredients or their metabolites in human breast milk.

Toxicity and treatment of overdosage: In the event of toxic symptoms developing following significant systemic absorption of the active ingredients of Tri-Cicatrin Ointment, treatment with the product should be stopped and the patient's general status, hearing acuity and renal and neuromuscular functions monitored. Blood levels of neomycin sulphate and bacitracin zinc should be determined. A degree of adrenal suppression may occur following prolonged high dosage or application under occlusive dressing.

Serum levels of neomycin may be reduced by haemodialysis.

Pharmaceutical precautions Store below 25°C. Keep dry.

Legal category POM.

Package quantities Tubes of 15 g (OP) and 30 g (OP).

Further information Nil.

Product licence number 0003/0164.

TRIVAX* DIPHTHERIA, TETANUS AND PERTUSSIS VACCINE BP (DTPer/Vac)

Presentation Trivax is a sterile preparation consisting of a mixture of diphtheria and tetanus toxoids and killed whole *Bordetella pertussis*.

Each 0.5 ml of vaccine contains 25 Lf of purified diphtheria toxoid, 3.5 Lf of purified tetanus toxoid and not more than 20,000 million chemically killed Bordetella pertussis organisms with a potency of not less than 4 i.u., in an isotonic buffer solution. Organisms bearing all three pertussis agglutinogens are included. Vaccine of this composition has been shown to provide adequate immunising potency against each of the three diseases. Thiomersal is added as a preservative to a final concentration of 0.01%.

The antigenic content and formulation of this vaccine has not been changed, although the labelled content of the tetanus component has been altered to conform with the flocculation equivalence of the new British reference antitoxin preparation.

Uses For active immunisation against diphtheria, tetanus and whooping cough in infants and pre-school children. It is not recommended that pertussis-containing vaccines be used in older children except in areas where whooping cough is a serious problem.

Dosage and administration *Dosage: Adults:* Not recommended.

Children up to 5 years: Each dose is 0.5 ml, given by deep subcutaneous or intramuscular injection. The primary course consists of 3 doses of vaccine at intervals of not less than four weeks.

Use in the elderly: No special comment.

Administration: Since whooping cough can often be a serious disease in the early months of life the primary course should preferably be started between the third and sixth month of life. It is believed that immune responses are better if the interval between the first and second dose is extended to six to eight weeks and the interval between the second and third dose is four to six months. It is not considered necessary to repeat the full course of immunisation if these intervals are exceeded.

Reinforcing doses: Where primary immunisation was completed during the first six to eight months of life one reinforcing dose of 0.5 ml Diphtheria and Tetanus Vaccine (DT/Vac/FT or DT/Vac/Ads) should be given about 12 months later in order to boost immunity. Children over the age of five years do not normally require further immunisation with pertussis vaccine since whooping cough is rarely a problem in older children. However, reinforcement of immunity against diphtheria and tetanus is necessary. This can be achieved by giving 1 dose (0.5 ml) of Diphtheria and Tetanus Vaccine (DT/Vac/FT or DT/Vac/Ads) to five-year-old children and 1 dose (0.5 ml) of Tetanus Vaccine (Tet/Vac/Ads) at 15/19 years of age or on leaving school.

Shake well before withdrawing a dose. It is good practice to record the title, dose and lot numbers of all vaccines and dates of administration. Any untoward reactions should be reported to the regulatory authorities and to the manufacturer.

Contra-indications, warnings, etc
Contra-indications: Not for intradermal use. The administration of pertussis-containing vaccine is contra-indicated in children with a personal or family history in parents or siblings of idiopathic epilepsy or other familial or hereditary diseases of the central nervous system. Administration of pertussis vaccine is also contra-indicated in children with a history of seizures, convulsions, cerebral irritation in the neonatal period, developmental neurological defect or other disorder of the central nervous system. Children with acute infection or illness, particularly those with respiratory symptoms should not be immunised until they are fully recovered. Any child exhibiting a severe local or significant general reaction to a previous dose of a pertussis-containing vaccine should not be given a further dose. However, protection against diphtheria and tetanus is advisable and can be accomplished by giving Adsorbed Diphtheria and Tetanus Vaccine.

Precautions: Since combined diphtheria, tetanus and pertussis vaccines are widely used in a population in which sudden illnesses of undefined origin are not uncommon, intercurrent illness bearing a temporal but not a causal relationship to vaccination may be expected.

Although anaphylaxis is rare, facilities for its management should always be available during vaccination.

Side- and adverse effects: Local reactions, particularly erythema at the site of injection, are commonly seen during the 24 hours following vaccination. They normally subside without treatment. A nodule may be found at the site of injection; this occurs less frequently and is less persistent following the administration of plain vaccine.

A transient rise in temperature, restlessness, irritability, crying or loss of appetite may sometimes occur a few hours after vaccination, but does not generally call for treatment. Systemic reactions such as headache, malaise and somnolence have been reported. The incidence of these systemic reactions is lower following the administration of adsorbed vaccine. Allergic manifestations including pallor, dyspnoea and collapse have been observed rarely. Convulsions, infantile spasms and encephalopathy have been reported as rare complications after pertussis vaccination.

Convulsions may be precipitated by a febrile response to the pertussis component. In an individual case it may be difficult to distinguish between spontaneously occurring convulsions and those associated with vaccination.

Abnormal crying and persistent screaming have also been described as reactions which may be encountered after vaccination.

An increased incidence of reactions may occur due to failure to shake the container and re-suspend the vaccine before withdrawing a dose, to inadvertent intravenous administration or to an over-rapid injection.

Use in pregnancy and lactation: Since simultaneous vaccination against diphtheria, tetanus and pertussis in adults is uncommon there is no accurate information on the safety of this vaccine in pregnancy.

Toxicity and treatment of overdosage: Not applicable.

Pharmaceutical precautions Store between 2°C and 8°C, protected from light. *Do not freeze.*

When multi-dose containers are employed, it is good practice to discard any partly used vaccine vials at the end of the vaccinating session.

Legal category POM.

Package quantities Pack of 5 × 0.5 ml ampoules. Vial of 5 ml.

Further information Oral Poliomyelitis Vaccine BP may be given at the same time as Trivax.

Product licence number 0003/5192.

TRIVAX-AD* ADSORBED DIPHTHERIA, TETANUS AND PERTUSSIS VACCINE BP (DTPer/Vac/Ads)

Presentation Trivax-AD is a sterile preparation consisting of a mixture of diphtheria and tetanus toxoids and killed whole *Bordetella pertussis.*

Each 0.5 ml of vaccine has an immunizing potency of not less than 30 International units (IU) purified diphtheria toxoid and not less than 60 IU (mouse assay) purified tetanus toxoid, with not more than 20,000 million chemically killed *Bordetella pertussis* organisms with a potency of not less than 4 IU adsorbed onto aluminium hydroxide in an isotonic buffer solution. The aluminium content does not exceed 1.25 mg per dose. Organisms bearing all three pertussis agglutinogens are included. Vaccine of this composition has been shown to provide adequate immunizing potency against each of the three diseases. Thiomersal is added as a preservative to a final concentration of 0.01%

The potency of this vaccine is now expressed in International Units in accordance with the requirements of the European and British Pharmacopoeias. These units measure the immunizing activity of the vaccine, whereas the previously used Lf units expressed the quantity of toxoid present. There is no simple numerical relationship between IU and Lf. No change has been made to the potency although it is now expressed in IU.

Uses For active immunisation against diphtheria, tetanus and whooping cough in infants and pre-school children. It is not recommended that pertussis-containing vaccines be used in older children except in areas where whooping cough is a serious problem.

Dosage and administration *Dosage: Adults:* Not recommended.

Children up to 5 years: Each dose is 0.5 ml, given by deep subcutaneous or intramuscular injection. The primary course consists of 3 doses of vaccine at intervals of not less than four weeks.

Use in the elderly: No special comment.

Administration: Since whooping cough can often be a

serious disease in the early months of life the primary course should preferably be started between the third and sixth month of life. It is believed that immune responses are better if the interval between the first and second dose is extended to six to eight weeks and the interval between the second and third dose is four to six months. It is not considered necessary to repeat the full course of immunisation if these intervals are exceeded.

Reinforcing doses: Where primary immunisation was completed during the first six to eight months of life one reinforcing dose of 0.5 ml Diphtheria and Tetanus Vaccine (DT/Vac/FT or DT/Vac/Ads) should be given about 12 months later in order to boost immunity. Children over the age of five years do not normally require further immunisation with pertussis vaccine since whooping cough is rarely a problem in older children. However, reinforcement of immunity against diphtheria and tetanus is necessary. This can be achieved by giving 1 dose (0.5 ml) of Diphtheria and Tetanus Vaccine (DT/Vac/FT or DT/Vac/Ads) to five-year-old children and 1 dose (0.5 ml) of Tetanus Vaccine (Tet/Vac/Ads) at 15–19 years of age or on leaving school.

Shake well before withdrawing a dose. It is good practice to record the title, dose and lot numbers of all vaccines and dates of administration. Any untoward reactions should be reported to the regulatory authorities and to the manufacturer.

Contra-indications, warnings, etc
Contra-indications: Not for intradermal use. The administration of pertussis-containing vaccine is contraindicated in children with a personal or family history in parents or siblings of idiopathic epilepsy or other familial or hereditary diseases of the central nervous system. Administration of pertussis vaccine is also contraindicated in children with a history of seizures, convulsions, cerebral irritation in the neonatal period, developmental neurological defect or other disorder of the central nervous system. Children with acute infection or illness, particularly those with respiratory symptoms should not be immunised until they are fully recovered. Any child exhibiting a severe local or significant general reaction to a previous dose of a pertussis-containing vaccine should not be given a further dose. However, protection against diphtheria and tetanus is advisable and can be accomplished by giving Adsorbed Diphtheria and Tetanus Vaccine.

Precautions: Since combined diphtheria, tetanus and pertussis vaccines are widely used in a population in which sudden illnesses of undefined origin are not uncommon, intercurrent illness bearing a temporal but not a causal relationship to vaccination may be expected.

Although anaphylaxis is rare, facilities for its management should always be available during vaccination.

Side- and adverse effects: Local reactions, particularly erythema at the site of injection, are commonly seen during the 24 hours following vaccination. They normally subside without treatment. A nodule may be found at the site of injection, especially if the inoculation is introduced into the superficial levels of subcutaneous tissue; this occurs less frequently and is less persistent following the administration of plain vaccine.

A transient rise in temperature, restlessness, irritability, crying or loss of appetite may sometimes occur a few hours after vaccination, but does not generally call for treatment. Systemic reactions such as headache, malaise and somnolence have been reported. The incidence of these systemic reactions is lower following the administration of adsorbed vaccine. Allergic manifestations including pallor, dyspnoea and collapse have been observed rarely. Convulsions, infantile spasms and encephalopathy have been reported as rare complications after pertussis vaccination.

Convulsions may be precipitated by a febrile response to the pertussis component. In an individual case it may be difficult to distinguish between spontaneously occurring convulsions and those associated with vaccination.

Abnormal crying and persistent screaming have also been described as reactions which may be encountered after vaccination.

An increased incidence of reactions may occur due to failure to shake the container and re-suspend the vaccine before withdrawing a dose, to inadvertent intravenous administration, or to an over-rapid injection.

Use in pregnancy and lactation: Since simultaneous vaccination against diphtheria, tetanus and pertussis in adults is uncommon there is no accurate information on the safety of this vaccine in pregnancy.

Toxicity and treatment of overdosage: Not applicable.

Pharmaceutical precautions Store between 2°C and 8°C, protected from light. *Do not freeze.*

When multi-dose containers are employed, it is good practice to discard any partly used vaccine vials at the end of the vaccinating session.

Legal category POM.

Package quantities Pack of 5 × 0.5 ml ampoules. Vial of 5 ml.

Further information Oral Poliomyelitis Vaccine BP may be given at the same time as Trivax-AD.

Product licence number 0003/5193.

TUBARINE* INJECTION

Presentation Each ampoule of Tubarine Injection (miscible) contains 15 mg of Tubocurarine Chloride BP in 1.5 ml isotonic solution.

Uses Tubarine is used to relax skeletal muscles to facilitate a wide range of surgical, obstetric, and orthopaedic procedures under general anaesthesia. It is similarly used for investigatory procedures and in the intensive care of patients undergoing mechanical ventilation.

Dosage and administration Tubarine should be administered by intravenous injection over a period of about one minute.

Flaccid paralysis of skeletal muscle develops to reach a maximum within three to five minutes which persists for between twenty and forty minutes. This is followed by a recovery period during which full neuromuscular function progressively returns. The restoration of full neuromuscular function is usually accelerated by the injection of an anticholinesterase agent such as neostigmine (neostigmine is usually preceded by an injection of atropine). Tubarine does not affect the level of consciousness.

Since the dose response to Tubarine varies considerably from one patient to another the physician has to adjust the dose to meet each individual patient's needs.

The average dose for a 70 kg man is between 15 and 25 mg, but in individual patients the effective dose level may be as low as 10 mg or as high as 40 mg. Supplementary doses of 5 mg may be administered for the maintenance of muscle relaxation at intervals of between 25 and 60 minutes as necessary.

The average initial dose of Tubarine in children is between 0.3 and 0.5 mg/kg bodyweight and in neonates 0.25 mg/kg bodyweight. Supplementary doses of 20% of the initial dose may be administered at intervals to maintain muscle relaxation.

Use in the elderly: The hypotension produced by Tubarine is more common in the aged and is potentiated by dose and alveolar concentration of halothane and nitrous oxide. Use with caution in renal impairment.

Contra-indications, warnings, etc Tubarine is contra-indicated in persons who are known to be hypersensitive to d-tubocurarine.

Malignant hyperthermia.

Precautions: Tubarine should be administered only by or under close supervision of an anaesthetist familiar with its action, characteristics and hazards, who is skilled in the management of artificial respiration and only where there are adequate facilities for immediate endotracheal intubation with administration of oxygen by intermittent positive pressure ventilation.

Patients with myasthenia gravis have been shown to

be, on average, 5.5 times as sensitive to d-tubocurarine as non-myasthenic subjects. Marked sensitivity to d-tubocurarine has also been shown in patients with myasthenic syndrome complicating bronchial carcinoma, carcinomatous neuropathy, amyotrophic lateral sclerosis and von Recklinghausen's disease. The effect of d-tubocurarine is also prolonged in Duchenne muscular dystrophy.

Use in pregnancy and lactation: Tubarine in normal therapeutic doses does not cross the placental barrier in sufficient amounts to affect the respiration of the infant. It has not been established, however, that Tubarine is free from possible adverse effects on a pregnancy or the foetus. It should not be administered to pregnant women unless the potential benefit outweighs possible hazards.

A case has been reported in which arthrogryposis multiplex congenita followed the use of d-tubocurarine for a 10 day period at the 10th–12th week of pregnancy.

Side- and adverse effects: The most frequent side-effect of Tubarine is hypotension which is usually transient. A rapid intravenous injection of a large dose may cause a precipitous fall in blood pressure. Flushing of the skin of the neck and upper chest is not uncommon. This was unrelated to the degree of hypotension in individual patients. Hypotension is probably due to a combination of factors including peripheral vasodilation resulting from curare-induced release of histamine and diminished venous return from skeletal muscle.

Curare has the capacity to release histamine but signs of histamine release other than hypotension are rarely evoked by the therapeutic doses. Nevertheless Tubarine can provoke bronchospasm and circulatory collapse particularly in patients with a history of allergic disposition; asthma or urticaria have been reported as a rare complication.

The magnitude and/or duration of neuromuscular blockade due to Tubarine may be increased by the following:

1. Inhalation anaesthetics, for example isoflurane and halothane.
2. Various antibiotics including neomycin, streptomycin, dihydrostreptomycin, kanamycin, gentamicin, colistin, polymyxin B, certain tetracyclines and possibly bacitracin, clindamycin and lincomycin.
3. Other neuromuscular blocking agents.
4. Administration of Tubarine during the previous 24 hours.
5. Propranolol and other beta-blockers.
6. Frusemide, and possibly mannitol.
7. Myasthenic conditions such as myasthenia gravis (see Precautions) myasthenic syndrome complicating bronchial carcinoma, carcinomatous neuropathy, amyotrophic lateral sclerosis and multiple neurofibromatosis.
8. Respiratory acidoses.

Cooling decreases the magnitude of the neuromuscular blockade produced by Tubarine. Thus, in patients after operations under hypothermia, prolonged curarisation could occur on rewarming.

Decreased response to Tubarine may occur in patients with hepatic impairment or respiratory alkalosis.

Two cases have been reported in which malignant hyperpyrexia may have been triggered by d-tubocurarine.

Toxicity and treatment of overdosage: The important responses to overdosage are prolonged apnoea, cardiovascular collapse, and the effects of histamine release. The respiratory paralysis should be treated by the continuation of positive pressure artificial respiration with oxygen and maintenance of a patent airway until complete recovery of normal respiration is assured. Recovery may be hastened by the administration of neostigmine methyl sulphate, 2.5 mg to 5 mg. Atropine sulphate, 0.6–1.2 mg should be injected simultaneously or immediately before the neostigmine. Neostigmine antagonises the skeletal muscle blocking action but it may aggravate other side-effects of Tubarine such as hypotension and/or bronchospasm. Sympathomimetic amines may be given to support the blood pressure.

In neonates, one hour after the recommended initial dose, reversal may be obtained with atropine 0.018 mg/kg and neostigmine 0.08 mg/kg.

If neuromuscular blockade cannot be adequately reversed by the use of an anticholinesterase, then measures should be taken to maintain respiration and, if necessary, the circulation until neuromuscular function returns. Sedation may also be required since consciousness is retained.

Pharmaceutical precautions Although not recommended, up to 1 ml of Tubarine (Miscible) Injection may be mixed with not less than 20 ml of 2.5% thiopentone; the solution should be prepared immediately prior to injection and used only if it remains clear. Tubarine (Miscible) Injection should not be mixed with any other anaesthetic agents because differences in pH could cause precipitation or there may be chemical incompatibility.

Store below 25°C.

Legal category POM.

Package quantities Box of 5 × 1.5 ml ampoules.

Further information Nil.

Product licence number 0003/5065R.

TYPHOID VACCINE BP (MONOVALENT) WELLCOME* (Typhoid/Vac)

Presentation Typhoid (Monovalent) Vaccine contains heat-killed, phenol-preserved, *Salmonella typhi* organisms at a concentration of not less than 1,000 million organisms per ml.

Uses For active immunisation against typhoid fever.

Typhoid vaccine protects 70–90% of recipients against typhoid.

Dosage and administration

Wellcome Typhoid Vaccine (Monovalent) may be administered subcutaneously, intramuscularly or intradermally. Subcutaneous or intramuscular injection should be used for the first dose but intradermal injection reduces systemic reactions and may therefore be preferred for the second dose, particularly for persons who have experienced reactions in the past.

Shake well before withdrawing dose.

The interval between the first and second doses should be four to six weeks.

Initial dose to be administered by deep subcutaneous or intramuscular injection	*Time interval between administration of initial dose and second dose*	*Second dose*
Children 1–10 years		
0.25 ml	4–6 weeks	0.25 ml by i.m. or s.c. injection or 0.1 ml by intradermal injection
Children over 10 years and adults		
0.5 ml	4–6 weeks	0.5 ml by i.m. or s.c. injection or 0.1 ml by intradermal injection

Although two doses of vaccine are recommended for primary immunisation, the results of field trials indicate that one dose of typhoid vaccine is almost as effective, for a short period, as two doses.

Use in the elderly: No special comment.

Reinforcing doses: Under conditions of continued or repeated exposure to infection a reinforcing dose of vaccine should be given at least every three years. When more than three years have elapsed since the last dose, a single dose is sufficient to boost immunity.

It is good practice to record the title, dose and lot numbers of all vaccines and dates of administration. Any untoward reactions should be reported to the regulatory authorities and to the manufacturer.

Contra-indications, warnings, etc
Contra-indications: The vaccine should not be administered to a subject who has experienced a serious reaction (e.g. anaphylaxis) to a previous dose of this vaccine or who is known to be hypersensitive to any component thereof. It is advisable to avoid vaccination during an acute infection.

Precautions: Typhoid vaccine produces in some people constitutional or local reactions. These are often more marked in adults over the age of 35 years, especially where there is a history of previous vaccination against typhoid.

It is prudent to avoid administering vaccine to subjects with acute infections or chronic illness.

Vaccination of children under 12 months of age is not advised because of the risk of adverse reactions, the relatively low incidence of typhoid in this age group and the relatively mild course of the disease in infants.

Although anaphylaxis is rare, facilities for its management should always be available during vaccination.

Side- and adverse effects: Local redness, swelling, pain and tenderness may appear in two or three hours.

Systemic reactions, such as malaise, nausea, headache, or pyrexia may occur, but usually disappear in 36 hours, when they are severe the patient is best kept in bed. The incidence of systemic reactions is considerably reduced by giving the vaccine intradermally, but local reactions may still occur.

Neurological complications including polyneuritis, neuritis, myelitis or various manifestations of cerebral and meningeal disease have been described following the administration of typhoid-containing vaccines.

Use in pregnancy and lactation: While no specific effects on the foetus have followed the administration of Typhoid Vaccine, it is not considered advisable to administer vaccines which may cause pyrexia during pregnancy.

Toxicity and treatment of overdosage: Not applicable.

Pharmaceutical precautions Store at 2–8°C. Protect from light. *Do not freeze.* When multi-dose containers are employed it is good practice to discard any partly used vaccine vials at the end of the vaccinating session.

Legal category POM.

Package quantities Vial of 1.5 ml.

Further information Nil.

Product licence number 0003/5195.

VALOID* TABLETS
VALOID* INJECTION

Presentation Valoid Tablets each contain 50 mg Cyclizine Hydrochloride BP, scored, coded 'WELLCOME T4A', white in colour.

Valoid Injection contains 50 mg cyclizine lactate in each 1 ml ampoule.

Uses Anti-emetic. In the prevention and treatment of nausea and vomiting and drug-induced vomiting, especially that associated with the administration of narcotic drugs. It has been widely and effectively used in the prophylaxis and treatment of motion sickness, in the symptomatic management of vertigo and labyrinthine disorders (Meniere's syndrome), in postoperative vomiting and in radiation sickness, particularly when this is associated with the treatment of breast cancer.

Valoid Injection, by the intravenous route, is also indicated pre-operatively in patients undergoing emergency surgery in order to reduce the hazard of regurgitation and aspiration of gastric contents during induction of general anaesthesia.

Dosage and administration *Valoid Tablets: Adults and children over 12 years:* 1 tablet up to three times daily.
Children 6–12 years: ½ tablet up to three times daily.
Under 6 years: Formulation not applicable.
Valoid Injection: Adults: 50 mg intramuscularly or intravenously three times daily. When used intravenously, Valoid should be injected slowly into the bloodstream, with only minimal withdrawal of blood into the syringe.

25 mg Cyclizine, given intravenously (before induction of anaesthesia) to patients undergoing emergency surgery, increases tone in the lower oesophageal sphincter, thereby reducing the hazard of regurgitation and aspiration of gastric contents.

Use in the elderly: No specific information is available. Experience has indicated that normal adult dosage is appropriate.

For the prevention of postoperative nausea and vomiting, administer the first dose by slow intravenous injection 20 minutes before the anticipated end of surgery.

Contra-indications, warnings, etc
Contra-indications: Valoid should not be given to individuals with known hypersensitivity to cyclizine.

Precautions: Drowsiness, dryness of the mouth and blurred vision may occur in a small number of patients. It is, therefore, advisable that patients should determine their responses before driving or operating machinery. In some patients the action of Valoid may be potentiated by alcohol and other central sedatives.

Valoid may increase the side-effects of anticholinergic drugs and enhance the soporific effects of pethidine.

As with other anticholinergic agents, Valoid should be used with caution and appropriate monitoring in patients with glaucoma, obstructive disease of the gastrointestinal tract and in males with possible prostatic hypertrophy. Valoid Injection may have a hypotensive effect.

There have been no specific studies in hepatic and/or renal dysfunction.

Side- and adverse effects: Urticaria, drug rash, drowsiness, dryness of the mouth, nose and throat, blurred vision, tachycardia, urinary retention, constipation, restlessness, nervousness, insomnia and auditory and visual hallucinations have been reported, particularly when dosage recommendations have been exceeded. Cholestatic jaundice has occurred in association with cyclizine. Single case reports have been documented of fixed drug eruption, generalised chorea, hypersensitivity hepatitis and agranulocytosis.

Intravenous cyclizine may increase the incidence of tremors and muscle movements if given before propanidid and methohexitone anaesthesia.

Although very rare, anaphylaxis of a severe degree has been reported with the co-administration of intravenous cyclizine and propanidid.

Use in pregnancy and lactation: Some animal studies are interpreted as indicating that cyclizine may be teratogenic. The relevance of these studies to the human situation is not known, but in the absence of any certain human data the use of Valoid in pregnancy is not advised. No information is available on the use of cyclizine in lactating mothers.

In a study involving prolonged administration of cyclizine to male and female rats, there was no evidence of impaired fertility after continuous treatment for 90–100 days. There is no experience of the effect of cyclizine on human fertility.

Toxicity and treatment of overdosage: Symptoms: Symptoms of acute toxicity from cyclizine arise from peripheral anticholinergic effects and effects on the central nervous system.

Peripheral anticholinergic symptoms include, dry mouth, nose and throat, blurred vision, tachycardia and urinary retention. Central nervous system effects include drowsiness, dizziness, incoordination, ataxia, weakness, hyperexcitability, disorientation, impaired judgement, hallucinations, hyperkinesia, extrapyramidal motor disturbances, convulsions, hyperpyrexia and respiratory depression.

An oral dose of 5 mg/kg is likely to be associated with at least one of the clinical symptoms stated above. Younger children are more susceptible to convulsions. The incidence of convulsions, in children less than 5 years, is about 60% when the oral dose ingested exceeds 40 mg/kg.

Treatment: In the management of acute overdosage with Valoid, gastric lavage and supportive measures for respiration and circulation should be performed if necessary. Convulsions should be controlled in the usual way with parenteral anticonvulsant therapy.

Pharmaceutical precautions *Injection:* Store below 25°C. Protect from light.
Tablets: Store below 25°C.

Legal category Tablets P.
Injection POM.

Package quantities *Valoid Tablets:* Bottle of 100.
Valoid Injection: Box of 5 ampoules.

Further information Nil.

Product licence numbers
Tablets 0003/5213R
Injection 0003/5212R

VASOXINE* INJECTION

Presentation Each 1 ml ampoule contains 20 mg Methoxamine Hydrochloride BP (Methoxamine Injection BP).

Uses Methoxamine is indicated for counteraction of hypotension. The most common clinical application for methoxamine is the correction or prevention of hypotension associated with the use of antihypertensive drugs and spinal anaesthetics.

Methoxamine is indicated when pressor therapy is deemed appropriate during, and as a result of, the administration of cyclopropane or halogenated anaesthetics.

Dosage and administration
Adults: 5–10 mg (0.25–0.5 ml) Vasoxine intravenously at a rate of 1 mg/min. 5–20 mg (0.25–1.0 ml) Vasoxine by intramuscular injection.

Children: 80 micrograms Vasoxine per kg bodyweight intravenously. 250 micrograms Vasoxine per kg bodyweight by intramuscular injection.

A second dose should not be injected until the first dose has ceased to act.

Use in the elderly: Vasoxine may be used in the elderly provided there is no history of vascular disease or hypotension.

Contra-indications, warnings, etc
Contra-indications: Vasoxine is contra-indicated in cases of pre-existent severe hypertension.

Precautions: The effect of increased arterial pressure on a patient with pre-existing vascular disease or myocardial impairment should be considered before administering Vasoxine.

An exaggerated response to methoxamine may be expected in patients with hyperthyroidism, in patients who have received treatment with monoamine oxidase inhibitors within the previous two weeks, and in hypertensive patients with temporarily lowered arterial pressure due to spinal anaesthesia. The initial dosages should be decided accordingly.

Methoxamine should not be administered unless facilities are available to make repeated arterial pressure measurements.

The use of Vasoxine in combination with local anaesthetics to prolong their action at local sites is not recommended.

Concomitant use of Vasoxine with sympathomimetic agents, such as decongestants, some appetite suppressants and amphetamine-like psychostimulants or with monoamine oxidase inhibitors, which interfere with the catabolism of sympathomimetic amines, may cause an exaggerated response to methoxamine. Appropriate care should be taken therefore when administering methoxamine to patients who have received such drugs.

Side- and adverse effects: Subjective effects reported by patients receiving methoxamine include dull headaches, feelings of cold and other skin sensations resulting from piloerection, sensation of fullness in neck and chest and a desire to micturate.

Adrenergic receptor stimulation is inevitable but the unsought objective effects have little clinical importance.

Bradycardia may be excessive during the use of methoxamine. This can be abolished by 0.8 mg atropine given intravenously. This dosage may be reduced as appropriate for children.

Projectile vomiting may occur particularly after high dosage.

Topical methoxamine decongests mucous membranes but the effect is not usually apparent with the doses given systemically.

Use in pregnancy and lactation: When considering administering Vasoxine during pregnancy, any potential risk to which the foetus may be exposed must be weighed against the risk of the maternal disease process. (No record of use in human pregnancy is available). Vasoxine is poorly absorbed orally and is unlikely to present a problem to the breast-fed infant.

Toxicity and treatment of overdosage: Overdosage: If blood pressure does not return to normal, after waiting an appropriate time, management of associated hypertension can be achieved by phentolamine (5 mg) being administered intravenously and repeated as necessary.

Pharmaceutical precautions Store below 25°C. Do not freeze.

Legal category POM.

Package quantities Box of 5 ampoules.

Further information Because methoxamine is active only on alpha-adrenergic receptors it has little direct effect on cardiac adrenoreceptors which are predominantly beta. Hence it is appropriate for use with halogenated anaesthetics which cause beta receptor sensitisation.

Methoxamine has no central nervous system activity.

Product licence number 0003/5066R.

WELLFERON*
Interferon alfa-n1 (Ins)

Presentation Wellferon is a clear, colourless solution. Each vial contains either 3 or 10 mega units of purified Wellcome human lymphoblastoid interferon formulated in 1 ml of tris glycine buffered saline with Albumin Solution EP at a concentration of 1.5 mg/ml as a stabiliser.

(1 mega unit (MU) = 10^6 international units (IU) of lymphoblastoid interferon WHO Reference preparation Ga 23-901-532.)

Properties: Wellferon is a highly purified blend of natural human alfa-interferons, which is obtained from human lymphoblastoid cells following induction with Sendai virus. The final product has a purity of at least 95% and contains no detectable DNA (less than 10 picograms of Namalwa cell DNA per millilitre).

Wellferon resembles human leucocyte interferon in that it is a mixture of natural alfa subtypes; at least 22 have been detected. It also differs from recombinant alfa-interferon preparations made from bacteria or other genetically-engineered cells which contain only a single subtype.

Uses Wellferon is indicated for the treatment of patients with hairy cell leukaemia.

Wellferon is indicated for the treatment of adult patients with chronic active hepatitis B, who have markers for viral replication, e.g. those who are positive for HBV-DNA, DNA polymerase or HBeAg.

Mode of action: The mode of action of alfa-interferon in hairy cell leukaemia is not understood. The rapid rate of clearance of hairy cells from the blood on commencing treatment suggests a direct effect of interferon following cellular binding, particularly since malignant hairy cells are known to bear prolific interferon receptors on their surface membranes.

The mode of action of alfa-interferon in the treatment of chronic active hepatitis B is poorly understood, but seems to consist of both a direct antiviral effect and immune-modulatory actions.

Pharmacokinetics: There is considerable inter-patient variability in the handling of interferons; furthermore, absolute serum levels may be less meaningfull as a measure of interferon's biological activity than the induction of certain cellular enzymes such as 2', 5'-oligoadenylate synthetase (2-5A synthetase). Following intramuscular administration, maximum serum levels are usually reached within 4 to 8 hours after dosing, but may merge into a plateau phase as a result of rate-limited absorption from muscle. The measured serum half life also varies considerably as a result of this, being in the approximate range of 4 to 12 hours, although the true elimination half life can be estimated to be about 3 to 4 hours. When Wellferon is administered at the recommended daily dose for the treatment of hairy cell leukaemia, steady state accumulation results in maximum serum values lying in the approximate range of 30 to 90 IU per ml.

The range of doses suggested for the treatment of chronic active hepatitis B infection can be expected to result in maximum serum concentrations of 200 to 300 IU per ml. The main route of excretion and catabolism of alfa-interferons is known to be via the kidney following glomerular filtration. In one study, overall body clearance was found to be 57 ml/min/m^2.

Dosage and administration

Dosage in adults

Hairy cell leukaemia: For remission induction, the dose recommended is 3 MU given daily by intramuscular or subcutaneous injection, the latter being more convenient for patient self-administration.

After initial improvement in peripheral haematological indices (commonly 12–16 weeks), the dose may be administered thrice weekly, during which time further improvement in the bone marrow is to be anticipated.

Haematological recovery is to be expected in patients who have failed splenectomy as well as in those with palpable splenomegaly in whom a rapid reduction in spleen size is to be anticipated.

Alternative dosage regimens have also been used with effect. A randomised study comparing dosing at 2.0 MU/m^2 daily from one month and then thrice weekly, and 0.2 MU/m^2 according to the same schedule, has shown a greater anti-leukaemic effect at one year using the higher dosage regimen, although side effects were less using the lower dose.

Prolonged treatment for 6 months or more may be required to clear hairy cells from the bone marrow.

Chronic active hepatitis B infection: A twelve week course of thrice-weekly intramuscular or subcutaneous injections of 10 to 15 MU (up to 7.5 MU/m^2 body surface area) is generally recommended.

Longer periods of treatment for up to six months at lower doses (5 to 10 MU thrice weekly or up to 5 MU/m^2) have been employed and may be preferred for patients who do not tolerate higher doses.

An initial period, employing escalating daily doses, usually over five days (but up to 28 days with the longer treatment), may be a convenient way of introducing treatment.

Some patients appear to be less troubled by interferon-related side-effects if the dose is administered in the evening.

Dosage in Children: No information is available on the treatment of hairy cell leukaemia in children although preliminary clinical evidence shows that Wellferon is tolerated in other childhood conditions.

In the rare event of hairy cell leukaemia occurring in children, proportions of the adult dose based on body surface area would be appropriate.

Chronic active hepatitis B infection: Up to 10 MU/m^2 has been administered to children with chronic hepatitis B. However efficacy of therapy has not yet been demonstrated.

Use in the elderly: Elderly patients may be less tolerant of the side-effects of interferon and particularly those that are cumulative. These patients should be seen frequently whilst receiving treatment; Wellferon dosage should be reduced or even stopped if patients are unduly sensitive to side-effects.

Contra-indications, warnings, etc

Contra-indications: There are no absolute contra-indications to the use of Wellferon in hairy cell leukaemia. However, extreme caution is advised in treating patients with concurrent hepatic, renal, cardiovascular or central nervous system disease or with a history of pre-existing mental disturbance.

Chronic active hepatitis B infection: Wellferon is contra-indicated for patients with a history of hypersensitivity to interferon alfa-n1 (Ins), or any component of the preparation. It is also contra-indicated in patients with severe pre-existing cardiac disease; severe renal or hepatic dysfunction; epilepsy and/or compromised central nervous system function; chronic hepatitis with advanced decompensated cirrhosis of the liver; and chronic hepatitis in patients who are being or have recently been treated with immunosuppressive agents excluding short term 'steroid withdrawal'.

Precautions: It is important to monitor the blood count closely in patients during the first 6 weeks of treatment for hairy cell leukaemia, following which the suppressive effects of alfa-interferons on the bone marrow will be overtaken by the improving leukaemic state, leading towards a normalisation of haematological parameters. In patients with profound or potentially life-threatening neutropenia or thrombocytopenia at the outset, it may be preferable to initiate treatment using a lower dose of Wellferon, particularly for out-patients who are remote from immediate medical care.

During Wellferon treatment of chronic active hepatitis B infection, it is similarly important to monitor blood count and liver function throughout treatment.

Care should be exercised in patients with asthma, as exacerbation of the disease has been reported on isolated occasions following alpha-interferon administration.

As alfa interferons may affect central nervous system functions patients should be warned not to drive a vehicle or operate machinery until their tolerance of treatment has been assessed.

Efficacy in patients with chronic active hepatitis B co-infected with the human immunodeficiency virus (HIV) has not been demonstrated.

Side- and adverse effects: Wellferon is a highly active mediator of biological events, and its use may be associated with severe side-effects, particularly when larger doses are administered.

The most frequently reported side-effects of Wellferon and other alfa-interferon preparations consist of fever, chills (occasionally rigors), headache, malaise and myalgia, all reminiscent of an attack of influenza. These acute side-effects can usually be reduced or eliminated by concurrent administration of paracetamol and tend to diminish with continuing therapy. In contrast however, continuing therapy can lead to lethargy, weakness and fatigue accompanied by anorexia and weight loss.

Alfa-interferons have a suppressive effect on the bone marrow, leading to a fall in the white blood count, particularly the granulocytes, the platelet count and less commonly the haemoglobin concentration. Additionally, abnormalities in the blood clotting mechanism have occurred. This can lead to an increased risk of infection and haemorrhage.

Marked effects on the central nervous system may occur; these include abnormal EEGs with excess slow wave activity, severe depression, confusion, apathy and coma. Occasionally, seizures occur which may be precipitated by fever in children. A few reports of movement disorders (including extrapyramidal and cerebellar dysfunction) have been reported in cancer patients receiving Wellferon.

The administration of alfa interferons may give rise to hypotension, hypertension or arrhythmias in certain individuals. Severe cardiovascular events reported in patients receiving alfa-interferons include myocardial infarction, cerebrovascular accident and peripheral ischaemia.

Nausea, vomiting and diarrhoea occur sporadically. Alopecia occurs occasionally as a late side-effect.

Alfa-interferons can lead to an elevation in liver related enzymes; this is usually transient but occasionally is marked and persistent. Hepatic necrosis has been reported on very rare occasions.

Rare occurrences of renal failure and/or nephrotic syndrome have been seen in patients treated with Wellferon. These patients had all been suffering from myelomatosis and had varying degrees of prior renal dysfunction.

After repeated very high doses (100–200 MU) intravenously by infusion, hypocalcaemia and hyperkalaemia have occurred.

Reactions at injection sites have been reported in some patients.

Other events which have been reported in patients receiving alfa-interferons include arthralgia, Raynaud's phenomenon, urticaria, erythema nodosum, skin rashes, immune thrombocytopenia, haemolytic anaemia, hypothyroidism, mucositis and isolated peripheral nerve defects, and disturbances of antidiuretic hormone levels.

Use in pregnancy and lactation: Offspring from pregnant rhesus monkeys given daily Wellferon dosages of up to 2.5 MU/kg bodyweight (from Day 21 through to Day 50 in one group and from Day 51 through to Day 130 in the second group) did not reveal teratogenic or other adverse effects, although there was an increased incidence of abortion and stillbirth in those animals who received the highest dose (2.5 MU/kg bodyweight daily).

No information is available on the use of Wellferon in human pregnancy. In view of the profound effects of the drug on human metabolism and physiology however, Wellferon should be considered as a drug which might result in damage to the foetus and patients should therefore be advised accordingly. The expected clinical benefit of treatment to the patient must be balanced against any possible hazard to the developing foetus.

In view of the long clinical course of chronic hepatitis B infection and the availability of hepatitis B immunisation for the neonate, use of Wellferon to treat chronic active hepatitis B infection during human pregnancy is not recommended.

There is no information available on the effect of Wellferon on human lactation.

Drug interactions: Alfa-interferons may alter the activity of certain enzymes. In particular they reduce the activity of P-450 cytochromes. The metabolism of drugs such as cimetidine, phenytoin, warfarin, theophylline, diazepam and propranolol by these enzyme systems may therefore be impaired in patients receiving alfa-interferons. Several cytotoxic drugs are also metabolised by these systems.

In the treatment of chronic active hepatitis B infection, the occurrence of an acute, hepatitis-like illness presents the theoretical risk of additive interaction with hepatotoxic drugs and of further impairment of hepatic drug metabolism.

Concurrent administration of interferon with drugs which act on the central nervous system has occasionally resulted in unexpectedly severe changes in mental state.

Concurrent administration of immunosuppressive drugs (including corticosteroids), which may enhance viral replication, should be avoided during treatment of chronic active hepatitis B infection with Wellferon.

Toxicity and treatment of overdosage: There are no reports of overdosage but repeated large doses of alfa-interferons are associated with profound lethargy, fatigue, prostration, and coma. Such patients should be hospitalised for observation and appropriate supportive treatment given.

Pharmaceutical precautions Store at 2–8°C. Protect from light. The injection contains no preservative. Discard any partly used vials immediately after withdrawal of the dose.

Legal category POM.

Package quantities Individual vial containing 3 MU per ml or 10 MU per ml, packed singly.

Further information

Serum neutralising antibodies occur infrequently in patients receiving Wellferon, which would therefore appear to have low immunogenicity.

An overall antibody incidence of 1.8% was found in follow-up sera from approximately 900 patients who had received Wellferon for benign and malignant diseases. In the case of hairy cell leukaemia, no neutralising activity was present in follow-up sera received from over 70 patients despite high, cumulative Wellferon doses while for chronic hepatitis B infection, two of 97 patients (2.1%) developed neutralising antibodies.

Product licence number

3 mega units 0003/0221
10 mega units 0003/0220.

ZOVIRAX* CREAM

Presentation Zovirax cream is white and contains 5% w/w acyclovir in an aqueous cream base. It is supplied in tubes containing 2 g or 10 g.

Uses Zovirax cream is indicated for the treatment of herpes simplex virus infections of the skin including initial and recurrent genital herpes and herpes labialis.

Do not use in eyes.

Dosage and administration Zovirax cream should be applied five times daily at approximately four hourly intervals omitting the night-time dose. Treatment should be continued for 5 days. If, after 5 days, healing is not complete then treatment may be continued for a further 5 days. Therapy should begin as early as possible after the start of an infection, and for recurrent episodes this should preferably be during the prodromal period or when the lesions first appear.

Use in the elderly: No special comment.

Pharmacology: Acyclovir is an antiviral agent which is highly active *in vitro* against herpes simplex virus (HSV) types I and II and varicella zoster virus. Toxicity to mammalian host cells is low.

Acyclovir is phosphorylated after entry into herpes infected cells to the active compound acyclovir triphosphate. The first step in this process is dependent on the presence of the HSV-coded thymidine kinase. Acyclovir triphosphate acts as an inhibitor of, and substrate for, the herpes-specified DNA polymerase, preventing further viral DNA synthesis without affecting normal cellular processes.

Contra-indications, warnings, etc

Contra-indications: Zovirax Cream is contra-indicated in patients known to be hypersensitive to acyclovir or propylene glycol.

Precautions: Zovirax Cream is not recommended for application to mucous membranes such as in the mouth, eye or vagina, as it may be irritant.

Particular care should be taken to avoid accidental introduction into the eye.

Side- and adverse effects: Transient burning or stinging following application of Zovirax cream may occur. Erythema or mild drying and flaking of the skin have been reported in a small proportion of patients.

The results of a wide range of mutagenicity tests *in vitro* and *in vivo* indicate that acyclovir does not pose a genetic risk to man. Acyclovir was not found to be carcinogenic in long-term studies in the rat and the mouse. Largely reversible adverse effects on spermatogenesis in association with overall toxicity in rats and dogs have been reported only at doses of acyclovir greatly in excess of those employed therapeutically. Zovirax Tablets have been shown to have no definite effect upon sperm count, morphology or motility in man.

Use in pregnancy and lactation: Experience in humans is limited, so the clinical benefit to the patient must be balanced against any possible but unknown hazards to the developing foetus. Systemic administration of acyclovir in internationally accepted standard tests did not produce embryotoxic or teratogenic effects in rats, rabbits or mice.

In a non-standard test in rats, foetal abnormalities were observed, but only following such high subcutaneous doses that maternal toxicity was produced. The clinical relevance of these findings is uncertain.

There has been no experience of the effect of Zovirax Cream on human female fertility. Two-generation studies in mice did not reveal any effect of (orally administered) acyclovir on fertility.

No information is available on levels of acyclovir which may appear in breast milk after administration of Zovirax Cream. Limited human data show that the drug does pass into breast milk following systemic administration.

Drug interactions: Probenecid increases the mean half-life and area under the plasma concentration curve of systemically administered acyclovir. Other drugs affecting renal physiology could potentially influence the pharmacokinetics of acyclovir. However, clinical experience has not identified other drug interactions with acyclovir.

Toxicity and treatment of overdosage: No untoward effects would be expected if the entire contents of a Zovirax cream 10 g tube containing 500 mg of acyclovir were ingested orally. Doses of 800 mg five times daily (4 g per day), have been administered for seven days without adverse effects. Single intravenous doses of up to 80 mg/kg have been inadvertently administered without adverse effects. Acyclovir is dialysable.

Pharmaceutical precautions Store below 25°C. Zovirax Cream contains a specially formulated base and should not be diluted or used as a base for the incorporation of other medicaments.

Legal category POM.

Package quantities Tubes of 2 g (OP) and 10 g (OP).

Further information Nil.

Product licence number 0003/0180.

ZOVIRAX* I.V. for Intravenous Infusion

Presentation Vials containing the equivalent of 250 mg and 500 mg sterile acyclovir as the freeze-dried sodium salt, a white to off-white powder. When reconstituted as directed, Zovirax I.V. has a pH of about 11. The sodium ion content is approximately 26 mg and 52 mg per vial, respectively.

Uses

Non immunocompromised patients	*Immunocompromised patients*
Severe initial genital herpes	Herpes simplex infection
Recurrent varicella zoster virus infection	Primary and recurrent varicella zoster infection
	Prophylaxis of herpes simplex infection
Herpes simplex encephalitis	Herpes simplex encephalitis

Dosage and administration

Indication	*Immune status*	*Dosage*
Herpes simplex infection	Normal or immunocompromised	5 mg/kg every 8 hours
Recurrent varicella zoster infection	Normal	5 mg/kg every 8 hours
Primary and recurrent varicella zoster infection	Immunocompromised	10 mg/kg every 8 hours
Herpes simplex encephalitis	Normal or immunocompromised	10 mg/kg every 8 hours

The required dose of Zovirax I.V. should be administered by slow intravenous infusion *over a one hour period.*

A course of treatment with Zovirax I.V. usually lasts 5 days, but this may be adjusted according to the patient's condition and response to therapy. Treatment for herpes simplex encephalitis usually lasts 10 days.

The duration of prophylactic administration of Zovirax I.V. is determined by the duration of the period at risk.

In patients with renal impairment Zovirax I.V. should be administered with caution. The following modifications in dosage are recommended:

Creatinine clearance	*Dosage*
25–50 ml/min	The dose recommended above (5 or 10 mg/kg) should be given every 12 hours.
10–25 ml/min	The dose recommended above (5 or 10 mg/kg) should be given every 24 hours
0(anuric)–10 ml/min	In patients receiving continuous ambulatory peritoneal dialysis (CAPD) the dose recommended above (5 or 10 mg/kg) should be halved and administered every 24 hours. In patients receiving haemodialysis the dose recommended above (5 or 10 mg/kg) should be halved and administered every 24 hours and after dialysis.

Dosage in children: The dosage of Zovirax I.V. in neonates is calculated on the basis of bodyweight. Although its use in neonatal herpes is still experimental, doses of 10 mg/kg have been employed.

The dose of Zovirax I.V. for children aged between 3 months and 12 years is calculated on the basis of body surface area.

Children with herpes simplex (except herpes simplex encephalitis) or varicella zoster infections should be given Zovirax I.V. in doses of 250 mg per square metre of body surface area every 8 hours.

In immunocompromised children with varicella zoster infections or children with herpes simplex encephalitis, Zovirax I.V. should be given in doses of 500 mg per square metre of body surface area every 8 hours if renal function is not impaired.

Children with impaired renal function require an appropriately modified dose, according to the degree of impairment.

Dosage in the elderly: In the elderly, total acyclovir body clearance declines in parallel with creatinine clearance. Special attention should be given to dosage reduction in elderly patients with impaired renal function.

Reconstitution: Each vial should be reconstituted by the addition of either Water for Injections BP or Sodium Chloride Intravenous Infusion BP (0.9% w/v). 10 ml should be added to each 250 mg vial and 20 ml should be added to each 500 mg vial. This provides a solution containing 25 mg acyclovir per ml.

Administration: Zovirax I.V. after reconstitution, may be injected directly into a vein over 1 hour by a controlled rate infusion pump, or be further diluted for administration by infusion.

For intravenous injection by controlled rate infusion pump, a solution containing 25 mg acyclovir/ml is used.

For intravenous infusion, each vial of Zovirax I.V. should be reconstituted and then, wholly or in part (according to dosage required) added to and mixed with an appropriate volume of infusion fluid to give a concentration not greater than 0.5% w/v of acyclovir. Thus each vial containing 250 mg reconstituted acyclovir should be added to at least 50 ml of infusion fluid, and each vial containing 500 mg reconstituted acyclovir should be added to at least 100 ml of infusion fluid.

For practical purposes, however, most users will find an infusion bag containing 100 ml to be useful for any dose up to 500 mg acyclovir.

When diluted as above, Zovirax I.V. is known to be

compatible with the following infusion fluids and stable for up to 12 hours at room temperature (20°C).

Sodium Chloride Intravenous Infusion BP (0.45% and 0.9% w/v).
Sodium Chloride (0.18% w/v) and Glucose (4% w/v) Intravenous Infusion BP.
Sodium Chloride (0.45% w/v) and Glucose (2.5% w/v) Intravenous Infusion BP.
Compound Sodium Lactate Intravenous Infusion BP (Hartmann's solution).

After addition of Zovirax I.V. to an infusion solution, the mixture should be shaken to ensure thorough mixing.

Reconstitution or dilution should be carried out immediately before use and, as no preservative is included, any unused solution should be discarded. Should visible turbidity or crystallisation appear in the solution, before or during the infusion, the mixture should be discarded. The solution should not be refrigerated.

Pharmacology: Zovirax is an antiviral agent which is highly active *in vitro* against herpes simplex types I and II, and varicella zoster viruses. Toxicity to mammalian host cells is low.

Zovirax is phosphorylated to the active triphosphate after entry into a herpes-infected cell. The first step in this process requires the presence of the HSV-coded thymidine kinase. Acyclovir triphosphate acts as an inhibitor of, and substrate for, the herpes-specified DNA polymerase, preventing further viral DNA synthesis without affecting normal cellular processes.

In adults, the terminal plasma half-life of acyclovir after administration of Zovirax I.V., is about 2.9 hours. Most of the drug is excreted unchanged by the kidney. Renal clearance of acyclovir is substantially greater than creatinine clearance, indicating that tubular secretion, in addition to glomerular filtration, contributes to the renal elimination of the drug. 9-carboxymethoxymethylguanine is the only significant metabolite of acyclovir and accounts for 10–15% of the dose excreted in the urine. When acyclovir is given one hour after 1 gram of probenecid the terminal half-life, and the area under plasma concentration time curve, are extended by 18% and 40% respectively.

Mean steady state peak plasma concentrations (C^{ss} max) following a one hour infusion of 5 mg/kg or 10 mg/kg were 9.8 and 20.7 micrograms/ml respectively. The equivalent trough levels 7 hours later were 0.7 and 2.3 micrograms/ml respectively. In children over 1 year of age similar mean peak (C^{ss} max) and trough (C^{ss} min) levels were observed when a dose of 250 mg/m^2 was substituted for 5 mg/kg and a dose of 500 mg/m^2 was substituted for 10 mg/kg. In neonates (0–3 months of age) treated with doses of 10 mg/kg administered over a one hour infusion every 8 hours, the C^{ss} max was found to be 13.8 micrograms/ml and the C^{ss} min to be 2.3 micrograms/ml. The terminal plasma half-life in these patients was 3.8 hours. In the elderly, total body clearance falls with increasing age and is associated with decreases in creatinine clearance although there is little change in the terminal plasma half-life.

In patients with chronic renal failure the mean terminal half-life was found to be 19.5 hours. The mean acyclovir half-life during haemodialysis was 5.7 hours. Plasma acyclovir levels dropped approximately 60% during dialysis.

Cerebrospinal fluid levels are approximately 50 per cent of corresponding plasma levels. Plasma protein binding is relatively low (9 to 33%) and drug interactions involving binding site displacement are not anticipated.

Contra-indications, warnings, etc
Contra-indications: Zovirax I.V. is contra-indicated in patients known to be previously hypersensitive to acyclovir.

Precautions: Care should be observed when administering Zovirax to patients with abnormal renal function (see above), in order to avoid accumulation. In patients receiving Zovirax I.V. at higher doses (e.g. for herpes encephalitis), specific care regarding renal function should be taken, particularly when patients are dehydrated or have any renal impairment.

Reconstituted Zovirax I.V. has a pH of approximately 11 and should not be administered by mouth.

Side- and adverse effects: Rapid increases in blood urea and creatinine levels may occasionally occur in patients given Zovirax I.V. This is believed to be related to peak plasma levels and the state of hydration of the patient. To avoid this effect the drug should not be given as an intravenous bolus injection but by slow infusion over a one hour period. Adequate hydration of the patient should be maintained.

Renal impairment developing during treatment with Zovirax I.V. usually responds rapidly to rehydration of the patient and/or dosage reduction or withdrawal of the drug. Progression to acute renal failure, however, can occur in exceptional cases.

Severe inflammation, sometimes leading to ulceration, has occurred when Zovirax I.V. has been accidentally infused into extravascular tissues. Mechanical infusion pumps pose a greater risk than infusion by gravity feed.

Reversible neurological reactions such as confusion, hallucinations, agitation, tremors, somnolence, psychosis, convulsions and coma have been associated with I.V. therapy, usually in medically complicated cases.

Nausea and vomiting have been reported in patients receiving therapy with Zovirax I.V.

Other events reported in patients receiving Zovirax I.V. include increases in liver-related enzymes, decreases in haematological indices, rashes and fevers.

The results of a wide range of mutagenicity tests *in vitro* and *in vivo* indicate that acyclovir does not pose a genetic risk to man. Acyclovir was not found to be carcinogenic in long-term studies in the rat and mouse. Largely reversible adverse effects on spermatogenesis in association with overall toxicity in rats and dogs have been reported only at doses of acyclovir greatly in excess of those employed therapeutically. Zovirax Tablets have been shown to have no definite effect upon sperm count, morphology or motility in man.

Use in pregnancy and lactation: Experience in humans is limited so the use of Zovirax I.V. should be considered only when the potential benefits outweigh the possibility of unknown risks. Systemic administration of acyclovir in internationally accepted standard tests did not produce embryotoxic or teratogenic effects in rabbits, rats or mice.

In a non-standard test in rats, foetal abnormalities were observed but only following such high subcutaneous doses that maternal toxicity was produced. The clinical relevance of these findings is uncertain.

There is no experience of the effect of Zovirax I.V. on human female fertility. Two-generation studies in mice did not reveal any effect of (orally administered) acyclovir on fertility.

No information is available on levels of acyclovir which may appear in breast milk after administration of Zovirax I.V. Limited data on other formulations show that the drug does pass into the milk.

Drug interactions: Probenecid increases the acyclovir mean half-life and area under the plasma concentration curve. Other drugs affecting renal physiology could potentially influence the pharmacokinetics of acyclovir. However, clinical experience has not identified other drug interactions with acyclovir.

Toxicity and treatment of overdosage: Single doses of up to 80 mg/kg have been accidentally administered with no adverse consequences. Zovirax I.V. is dialysable.

Pharmaceutical precautions Store below 25°C.

Zovirax I.V. contains no antimicrobial preservative. Reconstitution and dilution should therefore be carried out under full aseptic conditions immediately before use and any unused solution discarded. The reconstituted or diluted solution should not be refrigerated. When reconstituted and diluted in accordance with the recommended procedure the infusion solution is stable for up to 12 hours at 20°C.

Legal category POM.

Package quantities
Zovirax I.V. 250 mg: pack of 5 vials.

Zovirax I.V. 500 mg: pack of 5 vials.

Further information Nil.

Product licence number 0003/0159.

ZOVIRAX* OPHTHALMIC OINTMENT

Presentation White to off-white sterile ointment containing 3 per cent w/w acyclovir in a white soft paraffin base.

Uses Treatment of herpes simplex keratitis.

Mode of action: Acyclovir is an antiviral agent which is highly active *in vitro* against herpes simplex (HSV) types I and II.

Dosage and administration *Adults:* 1 cm ribbon of ointment should be placed inside the lower conjunctival sac five times a day at approximately four hourly intervals, omitting the night-time application. Treatment should continue for at least 3 days after healing is complete.

Children: As for adults.

Use in the elderly: As for adults.

Pharmacology: Acyclovir is phosphorylated to the active compound acyclovir triphosphate after entry into a herpes infected cell. The first step in this process requires the presence of the HSV coded thymidine kinase. Acyclovir triphosphate acts as an inhibitor of, and substrate for, the herpes specified DNA polymerase, preventing further viral DNA synthesis without affecting normal cellular processes.

Pharmacokinetics: Acyclovir is rapidly absorbed from the ophthalmic ointment through the corneal epithelium and superficial ocular tissues, achieving antiviral concentrations in aqueous humor. It has not been possible by existing methods to detect acyclovir in the blood after topical application to the eye. However, trace quantities may be measured in the urine. These levels are not clinically significant.

Contra-indications, warnings, etc *Contra-indications:* Patients with a known hypersensitivity to acyclovir.

Side- and adverse effects: **For ophthalmic use only.** Transient mild stinging immediately following application may occur in a small proportion of patients. Superficial punctate keratopathy has been reported but has not resulted in patients being withdrawn from therapy, and healing has occurred without apparent sequelae. Local irritation and inflammation such as blepharitis and conjunctivitis have also been reported.

The results of a wide range of mutagenicity tests *in vitro* and *in vivo* indicate that acyclovir does not pose a genetic risk to man. Acyclovir was not found to be carcinogenic in long-term studies in the rat and the mouse. Largely reversible adverse effects on spermatogenesis in association with overall toxicity in rats and dogs have been reported only at doses of acyclovir greatly in excess of those employed therapeutically. Zovirax Tablets have been shown to have no definite effect upon sperm count, morphology or motility in man.

Drug interactions: Probenecid increases the acyclovir mean half-life and area under the plasma concentration curve of systemically administered acyclovir. Other drugs affecting renal physiology could potentially influence the pharmacokinetics of acyclovir. However, clinical experience has not identified other drug interactions with acyclovir.

Use in pregnancy and lactation: Experience in humans is limited, so the use of Zovirax Ophthalmic Ointment should be considered only when the potential benefits outweigh the possibility of unknown risks. Systemic administration of acyclovir in internationally accepted standard tests did not produce embryotoxic or teratogenic effects in rats, rabbits or mice.

In a non-standard test in rats, foetal abnormalities were observed, but only following such high subcutaneous doses that maternal toxicity was produced. The clinical relevance of these findings is uncertain.

There is no experience of the effect of Zovirax Ophthalmic Ointment on human female fertility. Two-generation studies in mice did not reveal any effect of (orally administered) acyclovir on fertility.

Limited human data show that the drug does pass into breast milk.

Toxicity and treatment of overdosage: No untoward effects would be expected if the entire contents of the tube containing 135 mg of acyclovir were ingested orally. Doses of 800 mg five times daily (4 g per day), have been administered for seven days without adverse effects. Single intravenous doses of up to 80 mg/kg have been inadvertently administered without adverse effects. Acyclovir is dialysable.

Pharmaceutical precautions Store below 25°C. Discard one month after opening.

Legal category POM.

Package quantities 4.5 g tube (OP).

Further information Nil.

Product licence number 0003/0150.

ZOVIRAX* TABLETS (Shingles Treatment Pack)

Presentation Each pale blue, biconvex, elongated tablet is impressed with the words 'ZOVIRAX 800' on one side, is scored on the other side, and contains 800 mg acyclovir.

Uses Zovirax Tablets (Shingles Treatment Pack) are indicated for the treatment of herpes zoster infections.

Pharmacokinetics: Acyclovir is only partially absorbed from the gut. Mean steady state peak plasma concentrations following doses of 800 mg acyclovir administered four-hourly were 8 microMolar (1.8 micrograms/ml), and equivalent trough plasma levels were 4 microMolar (0.9 micrograms/ml).

From studies with intravenous acyclovir, the terminal plasma half life has been determined as about 2.9 hours. Most of the drug is excreted unchanged by the kidney. Renal clearance of acyclovir is substantially greater than creatinine clearance, indicating that tubular secretion, in addition to glomerular filtration, contributes to the renal elimination of the drug.

9-carboxymethoxymethylguanine is the only significant metabolite of acyclovir, and accounts for 10–15% of the dose excreted in the urine. In patients with chronic renal failure, the mean terminal half-life was found to be 19.5 hours. The mean acyclovir half-life during haemodialysis was 5.7 hours. Plasma acyclovir levels dropped approximately 60% during dialysis. In the elderly, total body clearance falls with increasing age and is associated with decreases in creatinine clearance although there is little change in the terminal plasma half-life.

Pharmacology: Acyclovir is an antiviral agent that is highly active *in vitro* against varicella zoster virus. Toxicity to mammalian host cells is low.

Acyclovir is phosphorylated after entry into herpes-infected cells to the active compound acyclovir triphosphate. The first step in this process is dependent on the presence of the viral-coded thymidine kinase. Acyclovir triphosphate acts as an inhibitor of, and substrate for, the herpes-specified DNA polymerase, preventing further viral DNA synthesis without affecting normal cellular processes.

Dosage and administration For *treatment of herpes zoster* infections, 800 mg Zovirax should be taken five times daily at approximately four-hourly intervals, omitting the night-time dose. Treatment should continue for seven days.

In severely immunocompromised patients (e.g. after marrow transplant) or in patients with impaired absorption from the gut, consideration should be given to intravenous dosing.

Dosing should begin as early as possible after the start

of an infection: treatment yields better results if initiated as soon as possible after rash onset.

Dosage in children: No specific data are available on the *treatment of herpes zoster* infections in immunocompetent children. When treatment of herpes zoster infections is required in immunocompromised children, intravenous dosing should be considered.

Dosage in renal impairment: In the treatment of herpes zoster infections it is recommended that the dosage be adjusted to 800 mg Zovirax twice daily at approximately twelve-hourly intervals for patients with severe renal impairment (creatinine clearance less than 10 ml/minute), and to 800 mg Zovirax three or four times daily at intervals of approximately six to eight hours for patients with moderate renal impairment (creatinine clearance in the range 10–25 ml/minute).

Dosage in the elderly: In the elderly, total acyclovir body clearance declines along with creatinine clearance. Adequate hydration of elderly patients taking high oral doses of Zovirax should be maintained. Special attention should be given to dosage reduction in elderly patients with impaired renal function.

Contra-indications, warnings, etc
Contra-indications: Zovirax Tablets are contra-indicated in patients known to be hypersensitive to acyclovir.

Side- and adverse effects: Skin rashes have been reported in a few patients receiving Zovirax Tablets; the rashes have resolved on withdrawal of the drug.

Gastrointestinal effects including nausea, vomiting, diarrhoea and abdominal pains have been reported in some patients receiving Zovirax Tablets. In double-blind, placebo-controlled trials the incidence of gastrointestinal events has not been found to differ between placebo and acyclovir recipients.

Other events reported rarely in patients receiving oral formulations of Zovirax include mild, transient rises in bilirubin and liver related enzymes, small increases in blood urea and creatinine, small decreases in haematological indices, headaches, mild reversible neurological reactions and fatigue.

The results of a wide range of mutagenicity tests *in vitro* and *in vivo* indicate that acyclovir does not pose a genetic risk to man. Acyclovir was not found to be carcinogenic in long term studies in the rat and the mouse. Largely reversible adverse effects on spermatogenesis in association with overall toxicity in rats and dogs have been reported only at doses of acyclovir greatly in excess of those employed therapeutically. Zovirax Tablets have been shown to have no definite effect upon sperm count, morphology or motility in man.

Use in pregnancy and lactation: Experience in humans is limited so the use of Zovirax Tablets should be considered only when the potential benefits outweigh the possibility of unknown risks. Systemic administration of acyclovir in internationally accepted standard tests did not produce embryotoxic or teratogenic effects in rats, rabbits or mice.

In a non-standard test in rats, foetal abnormalities were observed, but only following such high subcutaneous doses that maternal toxicity was produced. The clinical relevance of these findings is uncertain.

There is no experience of the effect of Zovirax Tablets on human female fertility. Two-generation studies in mice did not reveal any effect of acyclovir or fertility.

There is some evidence that the drug does pass into breast milk.

Drug interactions: Probenecid increases the acyclovir mean half-life and area under the plasma concentration curve. Other drugs affecting renal physiology could potentially influence the pharmacokinetics of acyclovir. However, clinical experience has not identified other drug interactions with acyclovir.

Toxicity and treatment of overdosage: Acyclovir is only partly absorbed in the gastrointestinal tract. It is unlikely that serious toxic effects would occur if a dose of up to 5 g were taken on a single occasion. No data are available on the consequences of the ingestion of higher doses; such an occurrence warrants close observation of the patient.

Single intravenous doses of up to 80 mg/kg have been inadvertently administered without adverse effects. Intravenous overdosage could result in crystalluria. Acyclovir is dialysable.

Pharmaceutical precautions Zovirax Tablets (Shingles Treatment Pack): Store below 25°C. Keep dry.

Legal category POM.

Package quantities Zovirax Tablets (Shingles Treatment Pack): Pack of 35 tablets (OP) as 7 blister strips of 5 tablets.

Further information Nil.

Product licence number
Zovirax Tablets (Shingles Treatment Pack) 0003/0243.

ZOVIRAX* TABLETS (200 mg)
ZOVIRAX* TABLETS (400 mg)
ZOVIRAX* SUSPENSION

Presentation Each pale blue shield-shaped tablet is impressed with the word 'ZOVIRAX' on one side and a triangle on the obverse and contains 200 mg acyclovir.

Each pink shield-shaped tablet is impressed with the words 'ZOVIRAX 400' on one side and a triangle on the obverse and contains 400 mg acyclovir.

Zovirax Suspension is an off-white suspension with a banana odour and taste and contains 200 mg acyclovir for 5 ml.

Uses Zovirax Tablets and Zovirax Suspension are indicated for the treatment of herpes simplex virus infections of the skin and mucous membranes including initial and recurrent genital herpes.

Zovirax Tablets and Zovirax Suspension are indicated for the suppression (prevention of recurrences) of frequent and/or severe episodes of recurrent genital herpes or recurrent herpes simplex infections at other sites, in immunocompetent patients, who cannot be satisfactorily managed by intermittent treatment.

Zovirax Tablets and Zovirax Suspension are indicated for the prophylaxis of herpes simplex infections in immunocompromised patients.

Pharmacokinetics: Acyclovir is only partially absorbed from the gut. Mean steady state peak plasma concentrations (C^{ss} max) following doses of 200 mg acyclovir administered four hourly were 0.68 micrograms/ml and the equivalent trough plasma levels (C^{ss} min) were 0.36 micrograms/ml.

From studies with intravenous acyclovir, the terminal plasma half life has been determined as about 2.9 hours. Most of the drug is excreted unchanged by the kidney. Renal clearance of acyclovir is substantially greater than creatinine clearance, indicating that tubular secretion, in addition to glomerular filtration, contributes to the renal elimination of the drug.

9-carboxymethoxymethylguanine is the only significant metabolite of acyclovir, and accounts for 10–15% of the dose excreted in the urine. In patients with chronic renal failure, the mean terminal half-life was found to be 19.5 hours. The mean acyclovir half-life during haemodialysis was 5.7 hours. Plasma acyclovir levels dropped approximately 60% during dialysis. In the elderly, total body clearance falls with increasing age and is associated with decreases in creatinine clearance although there is little change in the terminal plasma half-life.

Pharmacology: Acyclovir is an antiviral agent that is highly active *in vitro* against herpes simplex virus (HSV) types I and II. Toxicity to mammalian host cells is low.

Acyclovir is phosphorylated after entry into herpes-infected cells to the active compound acyclovir triphosphate. The first step in this process is dependent on the presence of the viral-coded thymidine kinase. Acyclovir triphosphate acts as an inhibitor of, and substrate for, the herpes-specified DNA polymerase, preventing further viral DNA synthesis without affecting normal cellular processes.

Dosage and administration

Dosage in adults: For *treatment of herpes simplex* infections, 200 mg Zovirax should be taken five times daily at approximately four hourly intervals omitting the night time dose. Treatment should continue for 5 days, but in severe initial infections may have to be extended.

In severely immunocompromised patients (e.g. after marrow transplant) or in patients with impaired absorption from the gut the dose can be doubled to 400 mg Zovirax or alternatively intravenous dosing could be considered.

Dosing should begin as early as possible after the start of an infection; for recurrent episodes this should preferably be during the prodromal period or when lesions first appear.

For *suppression of herpes simplex* infections in immunocompetent patients, a starting dose of 200 mg Zovirax should be taken FOUR times daily at approximately six-hourly intervals.

Many patients may be conveniently managed on a regimen of 400 mg Zovirax twice daily at approximately twelve-hourly intervals.

Dosage titration down to 200 mg Zovirax two or three times daily may prove effective.

Some patients may experience break-through infections on total daily doses of 800 mg Zovirax.

Therapy should be interrupted periodically at intervals of six to twelve months, in order to reassess suitability for continued suppression.

For *prophylaxis of herpes simplex* infections in the immunocompromised 200 mg Zovirax should be taken FOUR times daily at approximately six hourly intervals.

In severely immunocompromised patients (e.g. after marrow transplant) or in patients with impaired absorption from the gut, the dose can be doubled to 400 mg Zovirax or, alternatively, intravenous dosing could be considered. The duration of prophylactic administration is determined by the duration of the period at risk.

Dosage in children: For *treatment of herpes simplex* infections, and for *prophylaxis of herpes simplex* infections in the immunocompromised, children over the age of two years should be given adult dosages and children below the age of two years should be given *half* the adult dose of Zovirax Suspension. No specific data are available on the *suppression of herpes simplex* infections in immunocompetent children.

Zovirax Suspension may be diluted with an equal volume of either Syrup BP or Sorbitol Solution BPC, non-crystallising grade. The diluted product is stable for 4 weeks at 25°C but it is recommended that all dilutions are freshly prepared.

Dosage in renal impairment: In the management of herpes simplex infections in patients with impaired renal function, the recommended oral doses will not lead to accumulation of acyclovir above levels that have been established by intravenous infusion. However, for patients with severe renal impairment (creatinine clearance less than 10 ml/minute) an adjustment of dosage to 200 mg Zovirax twice daily at approximately twelve-hourly intervals is recommended.

Dosage in the elderly: In the elderly, total acyclovir body clearance declines along with creatinine clearance. Adequate hydration of elderly patients taking high oral doses of Zovirax should be maintained. Special attention should be given to dosage reduction in elderly patients with impaired renal function.

Contra-indications, warnings, etc

Contra-indications: Zovirax Tablets and Zovirax Suspension are contra-indicated in patients known to be hypersensitive to acyclovir.

Side- and adverse effects: Skin rashes have been reported in a few patients receiving Zovirax Tablets; the rashes have resolved on withdrawal of the drug.

Gastrointestinal effects including nausea, vomiting, diarrhoea and abdominal pains have been reported in some patients receiving Zovirax Tablets. In double-blind, placebo-controlled trials the incidence of gastrointestinal events has not been found to differ between placebo and acyclovir recipients.

Other events reported rarely in patients receiving oral formulations of Zovirax include mild, transient rises in bilirubin and liver related enzymes, small increases in blood urea and creatinine, small decreases in haematological indices, headaches, mild reversible neurological reactions and fatigue.

The results of a wide range of mutagenicity tests *in vitro* and *in vivo* indicate that acyclovir does not pose a genetic risk to man. Acyclovir was not found to be carcinogenic in long term studies in the rat and the mouse. Largely reversible adverse effects on spermatogenesis in association with overall toxicity in rats and dogs have been reported only at doses of acyclovir greatly in excess of those employed therapeutically. Zovirax Tablets have been shown to have no definite effect upon sperm count, morphology or motility in man.

Use in pregnancy and lactation: Experience in humans is limited so the use of Zovirax Tablets or Zovirax Suspension should be considered only when the potential benefits outweigh the possibility of unknown risks. Systemic administration of acyclovir in internationally accepted standard tests did not produce embryotoxic or teratogenic effects in rats, rabbits or mice.

In a non-standard test in rats, foetal abnormalities were observed, but only following such high subcutaneous doses that maternal toxicity was produced. The clinical relevance of these findings is uncertain.

There is no experience of the effect of Zovirax Tablets or Zovirax Suspension on human female fertility. Two-generation studies in mice did not reveal any effect of acyclovir or fertility.

There is some evidence that the drug does pass into breast milk.

Drug interactions: Probenecid increases the acyclovir mean half-life and area under the plasma concentration curve. Other drugs affecting renal physiology could potentially influence the pharmacokinetics of acyclovir. However, clinical experience has not identified other drug interactions with acyclovir.

Toxicity and treatment of overdosage: Acyclovir is only partly absorbed in the gastrointestinal tract. It is unlikely that serious toxic effects would occur if a dose of up to 5 g were taken on a single occasion. No data are available on the consequences of the ingestion of higher doses; such an occurrence warrants close observation of the patient.

Single intravenous doses of up to 80 mg/kg have been inadvertently administered without adverse effects. Intravenous overdosage could result in crystalluria. Acyclovir is dialysable.

Pharmaceutical precautions

Zovirax Tablets (200 mg): Store below 25°C. Keep dry.
Zovirax Tablets (400 mg) and Zovirax Suspension: Store below 25°C.

Legal category POM.

Package quantities

Zovirax Tablets (200 mg): Pack of 25 tablets (OP).
Zovirax Tablets (400 mg): Pack of 56 tablets (OP) as 4 blister strips of 14 tablets.
Zovirax Suspension: Bottle of 125 ml (OP).

Further information Nil.

Product licence numbers

Zovirax Tablets (200 mg)	0003/0173
Zovirax Tablets (400 mg)	0003/0227
Zovirax Suspension	0003/0202

ZYLORIC* TABLETS
ZYLORIC-300* TABLETS

Presentation Zyloric Tablets each containing 100 mg Allopurinol BP imprinted 'WELLCOME' and coded 'U4A'. Creamy-white in colour. Zyloric-300 Tablets each containing 300 mg Allopurinol BP, imprinted 'ZYLORIC 300' and coded 'C9B'. Creamy-white in colour.

Uses Zyloric is indicated for the main clinical manifestations of urate/uric acid deposition. These are gouty arthritis, skin tophi and/or renal involvement through crystal deposition or stone formation. Such clinical manifestations occur in: idiopathic gout, uric acid lithiasis, acute uric acid nephropathy, neoplastic disease and myeloproliferative disease with high cell turnover rates, in which high urate levels occur either spontaneously or after cytotoxic therapy; certain enzyme disorders which lead to overproduction of urate and involve: hypoxanthine guanine phosphoribosyltransferase (including Lesch-Nyhan syndrome), glucose-6-phosphatase (including glycogen storage disease), phosphoribosylpyrophosphate synthetase, adenine phosphoribosyltransferase, glutathione reductase.

Zyloric is indicated for the management of 2,8-dihydroxyadenine (2,8-DHA) renal stones related to deficient activity of adenine phosphoribosyltransferase.

Zyloric is indicated for the management of recurrent calcium oxalate renal stones in the presence of hyperuricosuria, when fluid, dietary and similar measures have failed.

Allopurinol and its major metabolite, oxipurinol, act by inhibiting the enzyme xanthine oxidase which catalyses the end stage of the metabolism of purines to uric acid. Allopurinol and its metabolites are excreted by the kidney but the renal handling is such that allopurinol has a plasma half-life of about one hour whereas that of oxipurinol exceeds 18 hours. Thus therapeutic effect may be achieved by once-a-day dosage.

Dosage and administration *Adults:* 2 to 10 mg/kg bodyweight/day, or: 100 to 200 mg daily in mild conditions; 300 to 600 mg daily in moderately severe conditions; 700 to 900 mg daily in severe conditions.

The initial dosage should be in the range 100–300 mg per day which may be taken as a single dose preferably after food. Doses in excess of 300 mg should be administered in divided doses. It has rarely been found necessary to exceed 900 mg per day. The dose should be adjusted by monitoring serum uric acid and/or urinary uric acid levels at appropriate intervals until the desired effect is attained, which may take one to three weeks. The maintenance dose is normally 200–600 mg per day.

Children: 10–20 mg/kg bodyweight/day, or 100–400 mg daily.

Use in children is mainly indicated in malignant conditions especially leukaemia, and certain enzyme disorders (e.g. Lesch-Nyhan syndrome).

Initiation of therapy: In the early stages of treatment with Zyloric, as with the uricosuric agents, an acute attack of gouty arthritis may be precipitated. Therefore it is advisable to give a prophylactic dose of a suitable anti-inflammatory agent or colchicine for at least one month.

Use in the elderly: The dose should be maintained at the minimum necessary to maintain normal serum and urinary urate levels. (See *renal impairment* and *Precautions* sections.)

To prevent acute uric acid nephropathy in neoplastic conditions, treatment with Zyloric should precede treatment with cytotoxic drugs (see also sections under *Contra-indications, warnings, etc*).

Dose recommendations in impaired renal function: Since allopurinol and its metabolites are excreted via the kidney, impairment of renal function may lead to retention of the drug and its metabolites with consequent prolongation of action. In the presence of impaired renal function, serious consideration should be given to initiating treatment with a maximum dose of 100 mg/day and increasing it only if the serum and/or urinary urate response is unsatisfactory. In severe renal insufficiency, it may be advisable to use less than 100 mg per day or to use single doses of 100 mg at longer intervals than one day.

Alternative schedules based on creatinine clearances are unsatisfactory because of the imprecision of low clearance values.

If facilities are available to monitor plasma oxipurinol concentrations, the dose should be adjusted to maintain plasma oxipurinol levels below 100 micromol/litre (15.2 micrograms/ml).

Dose recommendations in renal dialysis: Allopurinol and its metabolites are removed by renal dialysis. If frequent dialysis is required, an alternative schedule of 300–400 mg Zyloric after each dialysis, with none in the interim, should be considered.

Contra-indications, warnings, etc

Contra-indications: Known intolerance of allopurinol. Zyloric is contra-indicated as a treatment for the acute attack of gout. Prophylactic therapy may be started when the acute attack has completely subsided, provided anti-inflammatory agents are also taken.

Precautions: Zyloric should be withdrawn IMMEDIATELY when a skin rash or other evidence of sensitivity occurs.

Dosage reduction should be considered in the presence of severe hepatic or renal disorder.

Asymptomatic hyperuricaemia *per se* is NOT an indication for use of Zyloric. Fluid and dietary modification with management of the underlying cause may correct the condition. If other clinical conditions suggest a need for Zyloric it must be introduced at low dosage (50 to 100 mg/day) to reduce the risk of adverse reactions and the dosage increased only if the serum urate response is unsatisfactory. Extra caution should be exercised if renal function is poor (see also *Dose recommendations in impaired renal function*). Zyloric must be withdrawn IMMEDIATELY and PERMANENTLY at the first signs of intolerance.

In conditions where the rate of urate formation is greatly increased (e.g. malignant disease and its treatment; the Lesch-Nyhan syndrome), xanthine deposition may occur in the urinary tract. This risk may be minimised by adequate hydration to achieve optimal urine dilution.

Adequate therapy with Zyloric will lead to dissolution of large renal pelvic uric acid stones with the remote possibility of impaction in the ureter.

Drug interactions: 6-mercaptopurine and azathioprine: When 6-mercaptopurine or azathioprine is given by mouth concurrently with Zyloric, only one-quarter of the usual dose of 6-mercaptopurine or azathioprine should be given because inhibition of xanthine oxidase will prolong their activity.

Adenine arabinoside: Evidence suggests that the plasma half-life of adenine arabinoside is increased in the presence of allopurinol. When the two products are used concomitantly extra vigilance is necessary, to recognise enhanced toxic effects.

Salicylates and uricosuric agents: Oxipurinol, the major metabolite of allopurinol and itself therapeutically active, is excreted by the kidney and in a similar way to urate. Hence drugs with uricosuric activity such as probenecid or large doses of salicylate may accelerate the excretion of oxipurinol. This may decrease Zyloric's therapeutic effect, but the significance needs to be assessed in each case.

Chlorpropamide: If Zyloric is given concomitantly with chlorpropamide when renal function is poor, there may be an increased risk of prolonged hypoglycamic activity.

Coumarin anticoagulants: There is no evidence that interaction between allopurinol and the coumarins seen under experimental conditions has any clinical significance. However, all patients receiving anticoagulants must be carefully monitored.

Phenytoin: Allopurinol may inhibit hepatic oxidation of phenytoin but the clinical significance has not been demonstrated.

Theophylline: Experimental studies of the effect of allopurinol on theophylline metabolism have produced contradictory findings. There have been no clinical reports of interactions.

Side- and adverse effects: Adverse reactions in association with Zyloric are usually rare and mostly of a minor nature. The incidence is higher in the presence of renal and/or hepatic disorders.

In the early stages of treatment with Zyloric, as with

the uricosuric agents, an acute attack of gouty arthritis may be precipitated. Therefore it is advisable to give a prophylactic dose of a suitable anti-inflammatory agent or colchicine for at least one month.

Skin reactions: These are the most common reactions and may occur at any time during treatment. They may be pruritic, maculopapular, sometimes scaly or purpuric and rarely exfoliative. Zyloric should be withdrawn immediately should such reactions occur. After recovery from mild reactions Zyloric may, if desired, be reintroduced at a low dose (e.g. 50 mg/day) which may be gradually increased. If the rash recurs, Zyloric should be permanently withdrawn.

Generalised hypersensitivity: Skin reactions associated with exfoliation, fever, lymphadenopathy, arthralgia and/or eosinophilia resembling Stevens–Johnson and/or Lyell syndrome occur rarely. Associated vasculitis and tissue response may be manifested in various ways including hepatitis, interstitial nephritis and, very rarely, epilepsy. If such reactions do occur, it may be at any time during treatment. Zyloric should be withdrawn *immediately and permanently*. Corticosteroids may be beneficial in overcoming them. When generalised hypersensitivity reactions have occurred, renal and/or hepatic disorder has usually been present particularly when the outcome has been fatal.

Angioimmunoblastic lymphadenopathy: Angioimmunoblastic lymphadenopathy has been described rarely following biopsy of a generalised lymphadenopathy. It appears to be reversible on withdrawal of Zyloric.

Granulomatous hepatitis: Very rarely granulomatous hepatitis, without overt evidence of more generalised hypersensitivity, has been described. It appears to be reversible on withdrawal of Zyloric.

Gastrointestinal disorder: In early clinical studies, nausea and vomiting were reported. Further reports suggest that this reaction is not a significant problem and can be avoided by taking Zyloric after meals.

Recurrent haematemesis has been reported as an extremely rare event, as has steatorrhoea.

Blood and lymphatic system: There have been occasional reports of transient reduction in the numbers of circulating formed elements of the blood, usually in association with renal and/or hepatic disorder. The clinical significance has yet to be demonstrated.

Miscellaneous: Exacerbation of acute gouty attacks may occur in the early stages of hypouricaemic therapy (see section under *Dosage and administration*). In those conditions where the body's miscible urate pool is greatly increased (e.g. malignant disease and its treatment; Lesch-Nyhan syndrome), the rise in the xanthine concentration resulting from the action of Zyloric may lead to tissue deposition of xanthine. Fluid intake should ensure adequate urinary output. Xanthine crystals have been seen in muscle tissue of patients receiving allopurinol, but this appears to have no clinical significance. The following complaints have been reported occasionally, but do not appear to have clear cause and effect relationship with allopurinol; fever, general malaise, asthenia, headache, vertigo, ataxia, somnolence, coma, depression, paralysis, paraesthesiae, neuropathy, visual disorder, cataract, macular changes, taste perversion, stomatitis, changed bowel habit, infertility, impotence, nocturnal emission, diabetes mellitus, hyperlipaemia, furunculosis, alopecia, discoloured hair, angina, hypertension, bradycardia, oedema, uraemia, haematuria.

Use in pregnancy and lactation: High dose intraperitoneal allopurinol in mice has been associated with foetal abnormalities but extensive animal studies with oral allopurinol have shown none. In human pregnancy there is no evidence that Zyloric taken orally causes foetal abnormalities; however, use in pregnancy only when there is no safer alternative and when the disease itself carries risks for the mother or child.

Based on data from a single individual, oxipurinol (126 micromol/l, 19.2 micrograms/ml), allopurinol (4.4 micromol/l, 0.6 micrograms/ml) and allopurinol riboside (5.6 micromol/l, 1.5 micrograms/ml) have been demonstrated in human breast millk four hours after a single dose of allopurinol 300 mg. There are no data concerning the effects of these metabolites on the breast-fed baby.

Toxicity and treatment of overdosage: Accidental or deliberate ingestion of up to 5 g allopurinol, or very rarely 20 g, has been reported. Symptoms and signs included nausea, vomiting, diarrhoea and dizziness. Recovery followed general supportive measures. The most likely reaction would be gastro-intestinal intolerance. Massive absorption of Zyloric may lead to considerable inhibition of xanthine oxidase activity, which should have no untoward effects unless Puri-Nethol* (6-mercaptopurine), adenine arabinoside, and/or Imuran* (azathioprine) is being taken concomitantly. In this case, the risk of increased activity of these drugs must be recognised. Adequate hydration to maintain optimum diuresis facilitates excretion of allopurinol and its metabolites. Dialysis may be resorted to if considered necessary.

Pharmaceutical precautions Store below 25°C. Keep dry.

Legal category POM.

Package quantities *Zyloric Tablets:* bottle of 100 tablets.

Zyloric-300 Tablets: Calendar pack of 28 tablets as 2 blister strips of 14 tablets (OP).

Further information Zyloric presents definite advantages over uricosuric agents or simple anti-inflammatory drugs, especially in patients with gouty nephropathy, in those who form renal urate stones and those with unusually severe disease. In most patients with extensive tophaceous deposits, progressive formation of tophi has been halted and draining urate sinuses have healed.

Product licence numbers

Zyloric Tablets	0003/5207R.
Zyloric-300 Tablets	0003/0092R.

**Trade Mark*

Wyeth Laboratories
Huntercombe Lane South
Taplow
Maidenhead, Berks SL6 0PH

Wyeth

APISATE*

Presentation Apisate tablets are two-layer tablets of 11.0 mm diameter. Both layers are yellow, with one face marked WYETH, and the other face marked 'WY 033'. Each tablet contains:

Diethylpropion hydrochloride (in a sustained action formulation)	75 mg
Thiamine Hydrochloride BP	5 mg
Riboflavine BP	4 mg
Pyridoxine Hydrochloride BP	2 mg
Nicotinamide BP	30 mg

Uses Apisate, containing diethylpropion hydrochloride, in a sustained action formulation, with a supplement of B-complex vitamins, is designed to give anorectic activity throughout the waking hours.

Apisate is suitable for short term use as an adjunct to the treatment of patients with moderate to severe obesity for whom close support and dietary supervision are also provided.

Dosage and administration *Route of administration:* Oral.

Dosage – Adults: One tablet swallowed whole mid-morning.

Elderly: Not recommended for the elderly.

Children: Not recommended for children.

Current medical opinion supports intermittent use of appetite suppressants. Apisate may be given for 4–8 weeks followed by a similar period without medication. This may reduce the risk of dependence. The stated dose should not be exceeded. Efficacy if used for more than 3–6 months, and safety in long-term use have not been established. Apisate should be discontinued if weight loss does not occur, or when patients stop losing weight.

Contra-indications, warnings, etc
Contra-indications:

1. Use in emotionally unstable individuals, including psychotics, who are known to be susceptible to alcohol or drug abuse.

2. Use in patients concomitantly treated with MAOIs or within two weeks of such treatment.

3. Use of diethylpropion is also contra-indicated in patients with advanced arteriosclerosis, hyperthyroidism, severe hypertension, glaucoma or idiosyncrasy to sympathomimetic amines.

4. Concurrent use with other appetite suppressant drugs.

5. There is inadequate evidence of safety in human pregnancy. The use of diethylpropion during any stage of pregnancy or lactation is not recommended. There is evidence from animal studies that the drug may be harmful to the foetus.

Isolated spontaneous reports of congenital malformations have been recorded in humans but no causal relationship to diethylpropion has been established.

Precautions: 1. Prolonged use of diethylpropion may induce dependence with a withdrawal syndrome on cessation of therapy. Several cases of toxic psychoses have been reported after excessive use of diethylpropion and a very small number have been reported in which the recommended dosage appears not to have been exceeded. The psychosis was temporary and cleared up when the drug was discontinued.

Since its introduction in 1958, diethylpropion has been used by at least 33,000,000 patients. Against this background of extensive clinical use, reports of abuse have been very rare. Most of the subjects who abused diethylpropion had previously misused other drugs, e.g. amphetamine or phenmetrazine, and many were described as having unstable personalities.

2. Diethylpropion should be used with caution in patients with hypertension, angina pectoris, cardiac arrhythmias and peptic ulceration. Caution should also be observed in patients with epilepsy, anxiety or tension states or severe depression.

3. Diethylpropion may interact with sympathomimetic agents. Care should be taken when treating hypertensive patients receiving anti-hypertensive drugs. Animal experiments suggest that anti-obesity agents can block or reverse the actions of such agents when taken together. Diethylpropion should not be given concurrently with psychotropic drugs, including sedatives.

Interactions between diethylpropion and hypoglycaemic agents are theoretically possible but no adverse interaction has so far been reported. A theoretical interaction between diethylpropion and alcohol may occur leading to an accentuation of uninhibited behaviour.

4. Patients should be warned against driving or operating machinery until it is established that they are not over-stimulated while taking Apisate or suffer from rebound tiredness after discontinuing treatment.

Side-effects: Diethylpropion has negligible effect on blood pressure, pulse rate or cardiac activity. Side-effects are infrequent and rarely severe enough to require discontinuation of treatment. Of those reported the more common effects include headache, allergic and other rashes and dependence. Less commonly reported effects include sleeplessness, increased nervousness, psychosis, hallucinations, tachycardia and constipation. Gynaecomastia has been reported rarely.

Overdosage: A few unsuccessful suicide attempts by deliberate overdosage of diethylpropion hydrochloride have been reported in adults. Dosage ranged from 450 to 2,250 mg. Transient sequelae included semi-coma or coma, lethargy, increased irritability and nausea.

A number of cases of accidental overdosage have been reported in children aged 6 months to $3\frac{1}{2}$ years. Known doses taken were from 50 to 1,100 mg. The most frequent effects were motor hyperactivity, excitability, tachycardia, rapid respiration, pupillary dilatation, and flushing.

Treatment of overdosage is initially by gastric lavage and close observation. The foregoing reports show that individual reactions may differ and further treatment will be symptomatic.

Recovery occurred in all patients with overdosage except one, in whom treatment with a large intravenous dose of sodium amobarbital was implicated.

Pharmaceutical precautions Store in a cool dry place, keep tightly closed.

Legal category CD (Sch 3), POM.

Package quantities Bottles of 30 and 100.

Further information Diethylpropion, including illegally manufactured tablets have been the subject of social abuse for euphoriant effect.

Product licence number 0011/5004R.

ATIVAN* TABLETS

Presentation Ativan tablets are capsule shaped containing 1 mg or 2.5 mg lorazepam BP, and are approximately 4 × 8 mm. The 1 mg tablets are blue with A1 on one side and a breakbar on the other. The 2.5 mg tablets are yellow with A2.5 on one side and a breakbar on the other.

Uses Ativan Tablets are recommended for short term use of approximately 2–4 weeks. As with all benzodiazepines doctors should be aware that long term use may lead to dependence and withdrawal symptoms in certain patients.

Ativan is indicated for the short-term treatment of moderate and severe anxiety, i.e. anxiety that is disabling or subjecting the individual to unacceptable distress. Ativan is also indicated for the short-term treatment of anxiety in psychosomatic, organic and psychotic illness and the short-term treatment of insomnia associated with anxiety. Ativan may also be used as premedication before operative dentistry and as a sedative for the anxious dental patient, and as premedication before general surgery.

All patients taking Ativan should be carefully monitored and routine repeat prescriptions should be avoided. Treatment in all patients should be withdrawn gradually with careful monitoring and reassessment to minimise possible withdrawal symptoms. Patients who have taken benzodiazepines for a long time may require a longer period during which doses are reduced. Should longer term therapy be necessary then intermittent treatment may be considered to minimise the risk of dependence.

Dosage and administration Route of administration: Oral.

In all cases the dosage of Ativan should be titrated according to the needs of the individual patient and the lowest effective dose necessary to control symptoms should be used.

Ativan should not be used for long-term chronic treatment.

Dosage: Adults: Moderate and severe anxiety – 1–4 mg daily in divided doses.

Insomnia – 1–2 mg before retiring.

Premedication – 2–3 mg the night before operation, 2–4 mg one to two hours before operation.

Elderly: The elderly may respond to lower doses and half the normal adult dose or less may be sufficient.

Children: Premedication – aged 5–13 years, 0.5–2.5 mg at 0.05 mg/kg to the nearest 0.5 mg according to weight, not less than one hour before operation.

Dentistry: 1–2.5 mg, 1½–2 hours before dental treatment. For operative dentistry dosage as for premedication.

Contra-indications, warnings, etc

Contra-indications: Ativan should not be given to patients with a previous history of sensitivity to benzodiazepines or patients with acute pulmonary insufficiency.

Use in pregnancy: Safety for use in pregnancy has not been established. Ativan tablets should not be administered during pregnancy or lactation unless in the judgement of the physician such administration is clinically justifiable. Ativan tablets are not recommended for use in the first three months of pregnancy. Use during the late phase of pregnancy or at delivery may require ventilation of the infant at birth.

Precautions and warnings: 1. Concomitant administration with central nervous system depressants, including alcohol, general anaesthetics, narcotic analgesics, monoamine oxidase inhibitors and antidepressants will result in an accentuation of their effects.

2. When used at the appropriate recommended dose for short term treatment of anxiety the dependence potential of Ativan is low. However, the risk of dependence increases with higher doses and longer-term use and is further increased in patients with a history of alcoholism, drug abuse or in patients with marked personality disorders.

Symptoms such as anxiety, depression, headache, insomnia, tension and sweating have been reported following abrupt discontinuation of benzodiazepines and these symptoms may be difficult to distinguish from the original symptoms of anxiety. Other symptoms such as persistent tinnitus, involuntary movements, paraesthesia, perceptual changes, confusion, convulsions, abdominal and muscle cramps and vomiting may be characteristic of benzodiazepine withdrawal syndrome.

3. As with other drugs acting on the central nervous system, patients should be cautioned against driving or operating machinery until it is established that they do not become dizzy or drowsy while taking Ativan tablets.

4. This product should be used with caution in patients with impairment of renal or hepatic function.

5. Elderly patients or those suffering from cerebral vascular changes such as arteriosclerosis are likely to respond to smaller doses.

6. Ativan tablets should be used with caution during labour. Respiratory depression, poor sucking and hypothermia in the neonate after delivery have occasionally been reported especially in infants who are at high risk.

7. Ativan does not depress respiration in most patients but the drug should be used with caution in patients with chronic pulmonary insufficiency.

8. The use of benzodiazepines may release suicidal tendencies in depressed patients. Lorazepam should not be used alone to treat depression, anxiety associated with depression or psychotic illness. Other rarely reported behavioural effects of the benzodiazepines include paradoxical aggressive outbursts, excitement, hallucinations and confusion. Amnesia may occur and in cases of loss or bereavement psychological adjustment may be inhibited by benzodiazepines.

Overdosage: As with other benzodiazepines, overdosage should not present a threat to life unless combined with other CNS depressants (including alcohol). General supportive measures should be used. Treatment is symptomatic and gastric lavage may be of use if performed shortly after ingestion. The patient is likely to sleep and a clear airway should be maintained.

Side-effects: Ativan is well tolerated and imbalance or ataxia is an indication of excessive dosage. Daytime drowsiness may be seen initially and is to be anticipated in the effective treatment of anxiety. It will normally diminish rapidly and may be minimised in the early days of treatment by giving the larger proportion of the day's dose before retiring.

Occasional confusion, hangover, headache on waking, dizziness, blurred vision, nausea, depression, change in appetite and sleep disturbance have been reported. In addition blood dyscrasias and increased liver enzymes have occasionally been reported.

On rare occasions visual disturbances, hypotension, gastrointestinal disturbances and mild, transient skin rashes have also been reported.

Pharmaceutical precautions Store in a cool dry place.

Legal category CD (Sch 4), POM.

Package quantities 1 mg and 2.5 mg tablets: boxes of 100 (5 × 20 blister strips) and containers of 1000.

Further information Ativan is a shorter acting benzodiazepine. It is rapidly absorbed from the gastro-intestinal tract and is metabolised by a simple one-step process to a pharmacologically inactive glucuronide. The elimination half-life of lorazepam is about 12 hours so that steady state plasma levels are quickly reached and there is minimal risk of excessive accumulation, giving a wide margin of safety.

The risk of benzodiazepine related dependence may be minimised by adopting the following guidelines for treatment:

1. Select patients carefully taking into account the precautions and warnings stated in this data sheet.
2. Adopt short-term or intermittent therapy.
3. Use lowest dose possible to achieve effective treatment.
4. Review treatment regularly; and especially before repeating prescriptions.

5. Discontinue treatment gradually taking into account patient reaction at each stage; i.e., "titrate downwards".

Product licence numbers
Tablets 1 mg 0011/0034R
Tablets 2.5 mg 0011/0036R

ATIVAN* INJECTION

Presentation Ativan injection is a clear, colourless solution containing Lorazepam BP at a concentration of 4 mg/ml supplied in 1 ml quantities in clear glass ampoules.

Uses Ativan injection is indicated for:

Pre-operative medication or premedication for uncomfortable or prolonged investigations, e.g. bronchoscopy, arteriography, endoscopy.

The treatment of acute anxiety states, acute excitement or acute mania. The control of status epilepticus.

Dosage and administration *Route of administration:* Ativan injection can be given intravenously or intramuscularly. However, the intravenous route is to be preferred. Care should be taken to avoid injection into small veins and intra-arterial injection.

Absorption from the injection site is considerably slower if the intramuscular route is used and as rapid an effect may be obtained by oral administration of Ativan tablets.

Ativan should not be used for long term chronic treatment.

Preparation of the injection: Ativan injection is slightly viscid when cool. To facilitate injection it may be diluted 1:1 with normal Saline or Water for Injections BP immediately before administration. If given intramuscularly it should always be diluted.

Ativan injection is presented as a 1 ml solution in a 2 ml ampoule to facilitate dilution.

Ativan injection should not be mixed with other drugs in the same syringe.

Dosage:
1. *Premedication: Adults:* 0.05 mg/kg (3.5 mg for an average 70 kg man). By the intravenous route the injection should be given 30–45 minutes before surgery when sedation will be evident after 5–10 minutes and maximal loss of recall will occur after 30–45 minutes. By the intramuscular route the injection should be given 1–1½ hours before surgery when sedation will be evident after 30–45 minutes and maximal loss of recall will occur after 60–90 minutes.
Children: Ativan injection is not recommended in children under 12.
2. *Acute anxiety: Adults:* 0.025–0.03 mg/kg (1.75–2.1 mg for an average 70 kg man). Repeat 6 hourly.
Children: Ativan injection is not recommended in children under 12.
3. *Status epilepticus: Adults:* 4 mg intravenously. *Children:* 2 mg intravenously.
Elderly: The elderly may respond to lower doses and half the normal adult dose may be sufficient.

Contra-indications, warnings, etc
Contra-indications:

1. Ativan injection should not be given to patients with a previous history of sensitivity to benzodiazepines or any of the vehicle constituents (polyethylene glycol, propylene glycol, benzyl alcohol), or to patients with acute pulmonary insufficiency.

2. Ativan injection is not recommended for out-patient use unless the patient is accompanied.

Use in pregnancy: Safety for use in pregnancy has not been established. Ativan injection should not be administered during pregnancy or lactation unless in the judgement of the physician such administration is clinically justifiable. Ativan injection is not recommended for use in the first three months of pregnancy. Use during the late phase of pregnancy or at delivery may require ventilation of the infant at birth.

Precautions and warnings:

1. Patients should remain under observation for at least eight hours and preferably overnight.

2. Patients should not drive or operate machinery within 24–48 hours of administration of Ativan injection and should be advised not to take alcohol.

3. The addition of scopolamine to Ativan injection is not recommended, since their combination has been observed to cause an increased incidence of sedation, hallucination and irrational behaviour.

4. The effects of centrally acting cerebral depressant drugs may be potentiated.

5. This product should be used with caution in patients with impairment of renal or hepatic function.

6. The injection should be given slowly except in the control of status epilepticus where rapid injection is required.

7. Airway obstruction may occur in heavily sedated patients and therefore equipment necessary to maintain a patent airway and to support respiration/ventilation should be available.

8. Extreme care must be taken in administering Ativan injection to elderly or very ill patients and to those with limited pulmonary reserve, because of the possibility that apnoea and/or cardiac arrest may occur. Care should also be exercised when administering Ativan injection to a patient with status epilepticus, especially when the patient has received other central nervous system depressants.

9. Elderly patients may require a lower dosage.

10. There is no evidence to support the use of Ativan injection in coma or shock.

11. There is insufficient data regarding obstetrical safety of parenteral Ativan, including use in cesarean section. Respiratory depression, poor sucking and hypothermia in the neonate after delivery have occasionally been reported, especially in infants who are at risk. Such use, therefore, is not recommended.

12. As with all benzodiazepines doctors should be aware of the possibility of dependence and withdrawal symptoms in certain patients. In normal acute usage dependence is unlikely to occur but the risk increases with higher doses and longer-term use and is further increased in patients with a history of alcoholism, drug abuse or in patients with marked personality disorders.

Symptoms such as anxiety, depression, headache, insomnia, tension and sweating have been reported following abrupt discontinuation of benzodiazepines. Other symptoms such as persistent tinnitus, involuntary movements, paraesthesia, perceptual changes, confusion, convulsions, abdominal and muscle cramps and vomiting may be characteristic of benzodiazepine withdrawal syndrome.

13. The use of benzodiazepines may release suicidal tendencies in depressed patients. Lorazepam should not be used alone to treat depression or anxiety associated with depression. Other rarely reported behavioural effects of the benzodiazepines include paradoxical aggressive outbursts, excitement and confusion.

Overdosage: As with other benzodiazepines, overdosage should not present a threat to life unless combined with other CNS depressants (including alcohol). General supportive measures should be used and the treatment of overdosage is symptomatic. The patient is likely to sleep and a clear airway should be maintained.

Side-effects: Lorazepam is well tolerated and imbalance or ataxia are signs of excessive dosage. Drowsiness may occur. Occasional confusion, hangover, headache on waking, dizziness, blurred vision, nausea, vomiting, restlessness, depression, crying, sobbing, hallucinations and diplopia have been reported. In addition blood dyscrasias and increased liver enzymes have occasionally been reported. On rare occasions visual disturbances, hypotension, hypertension, gastro-intestinal disturbances and mild transient skin rashes have also been reported.

Pharmaceutical precautions Store in a refrigerator between 0°C and 4°C. Protect from light.

Legal category CD (Sch 4), POM.

Package quantities 10 × 1 ml solution (in 2 ml ampoules) per pack (OP).

Further information Ativan is metabolised by a simple one-step process to a pharmacologically inactive glucuronide. There is minimal risk of accumulation after repeated doses, giving a wide margin of safety. Ativan injection can be administered concurrently with a wide range of other drugs and has minimal effect on blood pressure. Tolerance at the injection site is generally good although, rarely, pain and redness have been reported.

Product licence number 0011/0051R.

BARATOL*

Presentation Baratol tablets are round, convex, film coated tablets containing indoramin hydrochloride equivalent to 25 or 50 mg indoramin base. The 25 mg tablets are blue, 8.00 mm in diameter and marked WYETH on one face and '25' on the other. The 50 mg tablets are green, 9.5 mm in diameter, marked WYETH on one face and '50' on the other face which is also scored.

Uses *Actions:* Baratol is an alpha adrenoceptor blocking agent which acts selectively and competitively on post-synaptic alpha-1 receptors, causing a decrease in peripheral resistance.

Indications: Baratol tablets are indicated for the treatment of all grades of essential hypertension.

Dosage and administration
Adults: Initial dose: 25 mg twice daily for all patients.

Dose titration: The dosage of Baratol should be titrated as necessary to control blood pressure to a maximum of 200 mg daily in two or three divided doses. The daily dosage may be increased by the progressive addition of 25 mg or 50 mg, made at intervals of two weeks. When unequal doses are used, the largest dose should be given at night in order to avoid daytime sedation.

Elderly: Clearance of indoramin may be affected in the elderly. A reduced dose and/or reduced frequency of dosing may be sufficient for effective control of blood pressure in some elderly patients.

Children: Not recommended for children.

Combination with other anti-hypertensive agents: Baratol is effective in lowering blood pressure in all grades of hypertension, either used alone or when combined with other anti-hypertensive agents. The anti-hypertensive effect of Baratol is enhanced by concomitant administration of a thiazide diuretic or a beta-adrenoceptor blocking drug. Control of most cases of mild and moderate hypertension should be achieved by using Baratol alone or by adding Baratol to the regimen of a patient already under treatment with a thiazide diuretic. In severe hypertension, a combination of Baratol, a thiazide diuretic and a beta-adrenoceptor blocking drug is effective in many such patients.

When Baratol is used in combination with other anti-hypertensive agents, the dose of Baratol should be titrated in the same way as when it is used alone.

Contra-indications, warnings, etc
Contra-indications: Baratol tablets should not be prescribed for:

1. Patients with established heart failure.
2. Patients already under treatment with MAOIs.

Precautions and warnings:

1. Drowsiness is sometimes seen in the initial stages of treatment with Baratol or when dosage is increased too rapidly. Patients should be warned not to drive or operate machinery until it is established that they do not become drowsy while taking Baratol, and further cautioned to avoid the ingestion of alcohol or other central nervous system depressants.
2. The ingestion of ethanol has been shown to increase both the rate and extent of absorption of Baratol, and patients should be cautioned to avoid ingestion of alcohol.
3. Incipient cardiac failure should be controlled with diuretics and digitalis before treatment with Baratol.
4. Caution should be observed in prescribing Baratol for patients with hepatic or renal insufficiency.
5. A few cases of extrapyramidal disorders have been reported in patients treated with Baratol. Caution should be observed in prescribing Baratol in patients with Parkinson's disease.
6. In animals and in the one reported case of overdose in humans, convulsions have occurred. Due consideration should be given and great caution exercised in the use of Baratol in patients with epilepsy.
7. Caution should be observed in prescribing Baratol for patients with a history of depression.
8. Animal experiments indicate no teratogenic effects but Baratol tablets should not be prescribed for pregnant women unless considered essential by the physician.
9. There are no data available on the excretion of Baratol in human milk but the drug should not be administered during lactation unless in the judgement of the physician such administration is clinically justifiable.
10. Clearance of indoramin may be affected in the elderly. A reduced dose, and/or reduced frequency of dosing may be sufficient for effective control of blood pressure in some elderly patients.

Side-effects: Sedation occurs in some patients but is rarely intolerable and is usually overcome by a modest reduction in dosage. Less commonly, dry mouth, nasal congestion, weight gain, dizziness, failure of ejaculation and depression have also been noted.

Treatment of overdosage: The information available at present of the effects of acute overdosage in humans with Baratol is limited to one case. Effects seen in this case included deep sedation leading to coma, hypotension and fits. Results of animal work suggest that hypothermia may also occur.

Suggested therapy is along the following lines:

1. Recent ingestion of large numbers of tablets would require gastric lavage or a dose of ipecacuanha to remove any of the product still in the stomach of the conscious patient.
2. Ventilation should be monitored and assisted if necessary.
3. Circulatory support and control of hypotension should be maintained.
4. If convulsions occur diazepam may be tried.
5. Temperature should be closely monitored. If hypothermia occurs, rewarming should be carried out very slowly to avoid possible convulsions.

Legal category POM.

Pharmaceutical precautions Store below 25°C and protect from light.

Package quantities Bottles of 100.

Further information Baratol may be especially suitable for patients for whom beta-adrenoceptor blockade is contra-indicated, for example, in patients with a history of obstructive airways disease.

Reflex tachycardia is not associated with treatment with Baratol.

Postural hypotension is not a problem.

In one study, patients on Baratol who were treated with a tricyclic antidepressant showed no adverse effect on their blood pressure control.

Baratol has been used concomitantly with cardiac glycosides and other anti-hypertensive drugs with no interaction.

Rebound hypertension has not been observed after withdrawal of Baratol.

Selective alpha-1-blockade has been shown to be useful in the treatment of congestive heart failure. As yet, there is insufficient data to determine whether Baratol can also be indicated in this disorder.

Product licence numbers
25 mg tablets 0011/0071
50 mg tablets 0011/0058

EQUAGESIC*

Presentation Equagesic Tablets are three layer, flat bevel-edged tablets, 12.0 mm in diameter. A white layer is sandwiched between a yellow layer and a pink layer. The yellow face is marked WYETH and the pink face is plain. Each tablet contains:

Ethoheptazine citrate	75 mg
Meprobamate BP	150 mg
Aspirin BP	250 mg

Uses Equagesic is an analgesic with muscle-relaxant properties indicated for short-term symptomatic treatment of pain occurring in musculo-skeletal disorders.

Dosage and administration Route of administration: Oral.

Dosage – Adults: 2 tablets three or four times daily as needed for the relief of pain.

Elderly: The elderly may respond to lower doses and half the normal adult dose or less may be sufficient.

Children: Not recommended for children.

Contra-indications, warnings, etc
Contra-indications:

1. Equagesic should not be used in patients known to be hypersensitive to the active ingredients or to compounds related to meprobamate such as carisoprodol or carbromal.
2. Meprobamate should not be used in patients with a known propensity for dependence on drugs including alcohol and in patients susceptible to attacks of acute intermittent porphyria.
3. Aspirin should not be used in patients with active peptic ulceration, haemophilia or in renal disease.
4. Equagesic should not be used during lactation.
5. Equagesic should not be used concurrently with coumarin-type anticoagulants.
6. *Pregnancy:* There is no evidence as to drug safety in human pregnancy nor is there evidence that it is free from hazard. Do not use during pregnancy, especially during the first three months, unless there are compelling reasons.
7. Do not give to children under 12 unless your doctor tells you to, because of a possible association of aspirin with Reye's Syndrome.

Precautions and warnings:

1. This product may cause drowsiness. Patients receiving this medication should not drive or operate machinery unless the drug has been shown not to interfere with physical or mental ability.
2. Meprobamate may increase the effects of concurrently administered central nervous system depressants including alcohol.
3. The concurrent use of CNS depressant drugs should be avoided in hepatic or renal insufficiency.
4. Meprobamate may induce seizures in epileptic patients and meprobamate withdrawal may precipitate convulsions.
5. Like barbiturates, meprobamate causes induction of liver enzymes, so that the availability and blood levels of drugs given concurrently that are metabolised in the liver may be affected. These include the following: systemic steroids (including oral contraceptives), phenytoin, griseofulvin, rifampicin, phenothiazines (such as chlorpromazine) and tricyclic antidepressants. The clinical importance of the effect of enzyme induction by meprobamate on concurrently administered agents has not been established.
6. Individual response in overdosage with meprobamate is variable but in some cases the symptoms may be severe. It is therefore advisable that caution should be observed in prescribing drugs which contain meprobamate to patients with depression or to others who may be liable to suicidal ideation or intent.
7. Some degree of dependence may occasionally occur with meprobamate in certain cases if dosage recommendations are exceeded with withdrawal symptoms on sudden discontinuation. This is more likely in individuals with emotionally unstable personalities if the drug is taken over long periods, or in others liable to alcohol or other drug dependence. Treatment in these cases should be withdrawn gradually.

Equagesic is recommended for use for short periods only and therefore the risk of dependence occurring with this product is very small.

Aspirin: 8. (a) Aspirin may prolong labour and contribute to maternal and neonatal bleeding and is best avoided at term. It may precipitate bronchospasm and may induce attacks of asthma in susceptible subjects. Aspirin should only be used with great caution in patients with a history of peptic ulceration.

(b) Concomitant administration with certain other medications such as corticosteroids or oral hypoglycaemics may require adjustment of dosage of the various drugs. The action of uricosuric agents may be inhibited.

Overdosage: Meprobamate: Acute poisoning with meprobamate produces coma, shock, vasomotor and respiratory collapse. Very few suicide attempts have proved successful and documented fatal doses have ranged from 12 gm to 47.6 gm. Recovery has occurred after ingestion of similar large amounts (20–40 gm). Gastric lavage is only effective within a short period of drug ingestion as meprobamate is rapidly absorbed from the gastrointestinal tract. Blood concentrations may be reduced by a regime of forced alkaline diuresis or haemodialysis. Respiration may require assistance.

Aspirin: Overdosage with aspirin will result in the appearance of the signs and symptoms of salicylism. Treatment of aspirin poisoning is largely symptomatic and directed towards correction of the acid-base balance and electrolyte balance of the plasma.

Side-effects: Drowsiness, dizziness and nausea may be experienced with Equagesic but these symptoms usually disappear as treatment continues. Ataxia, vomiting, hypotension, paraesthesia and paradoxical excitement may also occur.

Hypersensitivity reactions have been reported in about 2% of patients being treated with meprobamate. These reactions include skin rashes, and may arise after one to four doses of the drug. They may be generalised or local, and include urticaria, itchy maculopapular rashes or erythema. Severe systemic reactions with shaking, chills and fever, nausea and vomiting, hypotension and collapse have occasionally occurred.

Blood disorders, including non-thrombocytopenic purpura, and rarely, thrombocytopenia, agranulocytosis, aplastic anaemia and pancytopenia have occurred. Rarely reported reactions, usually occurring as part of a generalised hypersensitivity reaction, include hyperpyrexia, angioneurotic oedema, bronchospasm, oliguria and anuria. Anaphylaxis, erythema multiforme, exfoliative dermatitis, stomatitis, proctitis, Stevens Johnson syndrome and bullous dermatitis have also been reported.

Hypersensitivity reactions to aspirin may manifest themselves as asthma, skin reactions and shock. Aspirin may induce gastro-intestinal haemorrhage, which is occasionally severe but in most cases blood loss is not significant.

Pharmaceutical precautions Store in a cool dry place. Keep tightly closed. Where necessary dispense Equagesic Tablets into suitable well-closed glass bottles.

Legal category CD (Sch 3), POM.

Package quantities Bottles of 100.

Further information Safety and efficacy have not been established beyond short-term use.

Product licence number 0011/5009R.

HRF*

Presentation HRF (gonadorelin hydrochloride) is a synthetic decapeptide that has a chemical composition and structure identical to the naturally-occurring luteinizing hormone-releasing hormone (LH-RH) isolated from porcine or ovine hypothalami, in a freeze-dried form. HRF is available in 2 strengths, 100 micrograms and 500 micrograms with 100 mg lactose. An ampoule

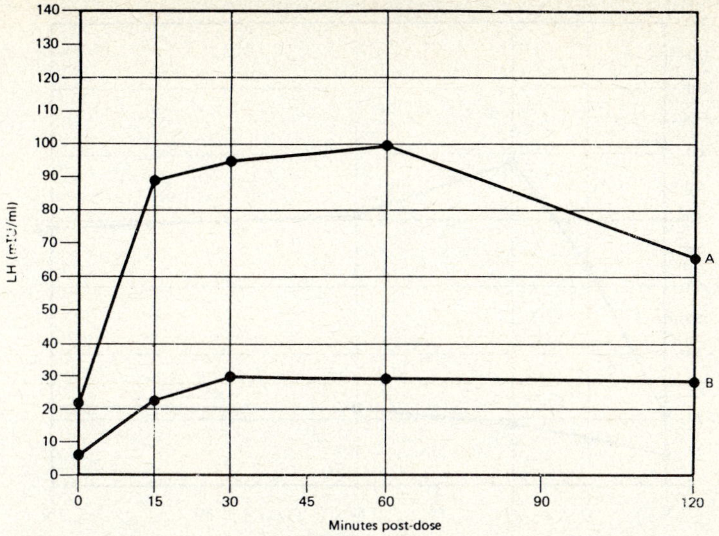

Figure 1. Normal male LH response after HRF 100 micrograms subcutaneous administration 10th and 90th percentiles.

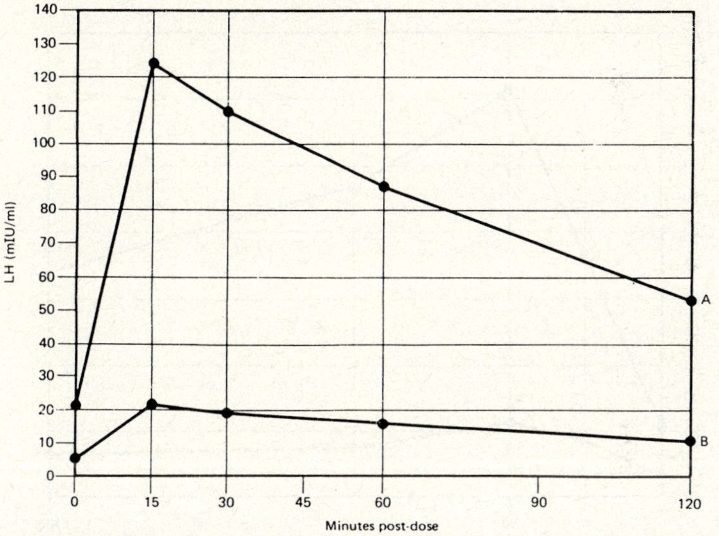

Figure 2. Normal male LH response after HRF 100 micrograms intravenous administration 10th and 90th percentiles.

of sterile diluent is supplied which contains 2% benzyl alcohol and water for injection.

Uses HRF as a single injection is indicated for evaluating the functional capacity and response of the gonadotropes of the anterior pituitary. The LH response is used in testing patients with suspected gonadotropin deficiency, whether due to the hypothalamus alone or in combination with anterior pituitary failure. HRF is also indicated for evaluating residual gonadotropic function of the pituitary following removal of a pituitary tumour or surgery and/ or irradiation.

Dosage and administration *Adults:* 100 micrograms dose, subcutaneously or intravenously. In females for whom the phase of the menstrual cycle can be established, the test should be performed in early follicular phase (days 1–7).

Test methodology: To determine the status of the gonadotropin secretory capacity of the anterior pituitary, a test procedure requiring seven venous blood samples for LH is recommended.

Procedure

1. Venous blood samples should be drawn at −15 minutes and immediately prior to HRF administration. The LH baseline is obtained by averaging the LH values of the two samples.
2. Administer a bolus of HRF subcutaneously or intravenously.
3. Draw venous blood samples at 15, 30, 45, 60 and 120 minutes after administration.
4. Blood samples should be handled as recommended by the laboratory that will determine the LH content. It must be emphasised that the reliability of the test is directly related to the inter-assay and intra-assay reliability of the laboratory performing the assay.

Interpretation of test results: Interpretation of the LH response to HRF requires an understanding of the hypothalamic-pituitary physiology, knowledge of the clinical status of the individual patient, and familiarity with the normal ranges and the standards used in the laboratory performing the LH assays.

Figures 1–4 represent the LH response curves after

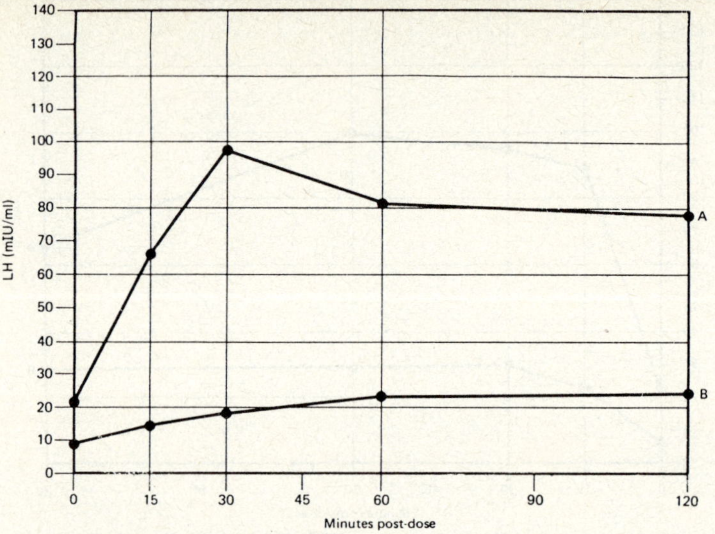

Figure 3. Normal female LH response after HRF 100 micrograms subcutaneous administration 10th and 90th percentiles.

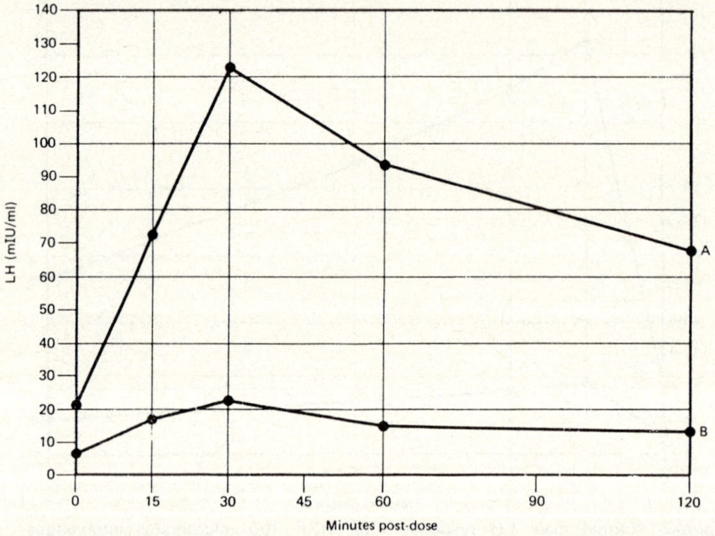

Figure 4. Normal female LH response after HRF 100 micrograms intravenous administration 10th and 90th percentiles.

HRF administration in normal subjects. The normal LH response curves were established between the 10th percentile (B line) and 90th percentile (A line) of all LH responses in normal subjects analysed from the results of clinical studies. Individual patient responses should be plotted on the appropriate curve. A subnormal response in patients is defined as three or more LH values which fall below the B line of the normal LH response curve.

In cases where there is a blunted or borderline response, the HRF test should be repeated.

The HRF test complements the clinical assessment of patients with a variety of endocrine disorders involving the hypothalamic-pituitary axis. In cases where there is a normal response, it indicates the presence of functional pituitary gonadotropes. The single injection test does not determine the pathophysiological cause for the subnormal response and does not measure pituitary gonadotropic reserve.

Contra-indications, warnings, etc *Contra-indications:* Hypersensitivity to HRF or any of the components. Known or suspected pregnancy. Do not use in children under one year of age as diluent contains 2% benzyl alcohol.

Precautions: Although allergic and hypersensitivity reactions have been observed with other polypeptide hormones, to date no such reactions have been encountered following the administration of a single 100 micrograms dose of HRF used for diagnostic purposes. Rare instances of hypersensitivity reactions have been reported (see Side Effects). Therefore, patients treated by intermittent pulsatile therapy in whom re-administration is considered, particularly by the intravenous route, should be carefully observed. Administration during the follicular phase of a normal cycle may result in premature ovulation and appropriate measures are advised to prevent an unwanted pregnancy in these circumstances.

Drug interactions: The HRF test should be conducted in

the absence of other drugs which directly affect the pituitary secretion of the gonadotropins. These would include a variety of preparations which contain androgens, oestrogens, progestins, or glucocorticoids. The gonadotropin levels may be transiently elevated by spironolactone, minimally elevated by laevodopa, and suppressed by oral contraceptives and digoxin. The response to HRF may be blunted by phenothiazines and dopamine antagonists which cause a rise in prolactin.

Side-effects: Systemic complaints such as headaches, nausea, lightheadedness, abdominal discomfort and flushing have been reported rarely following administration of HRF. Local swelling, occasionally with pain and pruritus at the injection site may occur if HRF is administered subcutaneously. Local and generalised skin rash have been noted after chronic subcutaneous administration.

Thrombophlebitis with septicaemia, mild and severe, has been reported in isolated cases at the site of intravenous injection. Rare instances of hypersensitivity reaction (bronchospasm, tachycardia, flushing, urticaria, swelling, itching and redness of face, eyelids and lips, induration at injection site) have been reported following multiple-dose administration of large doses. Antibody formation has also been reported rarely after chronic administration of large doses.

Overdosage: HRF has been administered parenterally in doses up to 3 mg bd for 28 days without any signs or symptoms of overdosage. In case of overdosage or idiosyncrasy, symptomatic treatment should be administered as required.

Pharmaceutical precautions Both the lyophilised powder vials and diluent ampoules have a shelf life of 3 years. Store at room temperature (approximately 25°C). Preparation for single injection administration: Reconstitute 100 micrograms vial with 1.0 ml of the accompanying sterile diluent of 2% benzyl alcohol. Reconstitute 500 micrograms vial with 2.0 ml of the accompanying sterile diluent of 2% benzyl alcohol. Prepare solution immediately before use. After reconstitution, refrigerate and use within 1 day. Discard unused reconstituted solution and diluent.

Legal category POM.

Package quantities Packs comprise a vial containing 100 micrograms or 500 micrograms freeze-dried material and a 2 ml ampoule of sterile diluent (OP).

Further information Nil.

Product licence numbers
HRF Ayerst 100 micrograms 0607/0016
HRF Ayerst 500 micrograms 0607/0017

Product licence holder: Ayerst Laboratories Limited.

ISORDIL*

Presentation Isordil Sublingual Tablets, containing isosorbide dinitrate 5 mg, are small, round, flat, bevel-edged pink tablets specially formulated for sublingual administration.

Isordil Tablets, containing isosorbide dinitrate 10 mg, are white, round, bi-convex tablets, scored on one side and engraved 'Isordil 10' on the other.

Isordil Tablets, containing isosorbide dinitrate 30 mg, are white, round, bi-convex tablets, scored on one side and engraved 'Isordil 30' on the other.

Isordil 10 mg tablet is 8 mm in diameter and the 30 mg tablet is 9.7 mm in diameter.

Uses Angina pectoris (classic effort associated angina, chronic stable angina, vaso-spastic angina, variant angina, unstable angina and angina decubitus).

Sublingual Isordil – for treatment of an attack and for prophylaxis in situations likely to provoke attacks.

Oral Isordil – for prophylactic treatment (not intended to abort the acute anginal episode).

Acute and chronic congestive heart failure including that associated with myocardial infarction as adjunctive therapy.

Dosage and administration
Angina Pectoris: Acute attack or prophylactically in situations likely to provoke attacks: One or two 5 mg Isordil tablets sublingually every 2 hours or as required.

Prophylaxis: 40 to 120 mg daily in divided doses or as required. In selected cases daily doses of up to 240 mg Isordil have been administered without undue adverse effects.

In order to obtain maximal therapeutic effect it is important that the dosages of sublingual and oral forms of Isordil be individualised in accordance with patients' needs, response and tolerance.

Congestive heart failure: Acute and chronic, including after myocardial infarction: Sublingual Isordil 5 to 15 mg every 2–3 hours or as needed. The oral form of Isordil may be administered in doses of 10 to 60 mg four times daily or as needed.

The therapeutic uses of Isordil in selected cases of acute and chronic congestive heart failure should be considered as an adjunct to the more conventional modes of therapy such as cardiac glycosides, diuretics and other vasodilators. In refractory cases Isordil may be used alone or concomitantly with other vasodilators. Haemodynamic monitoring of the patient under treatment is desirable and optimal dose regimens should be determined for individual cases depending on these results. Isordil therapy should begin with the lowest effective dose, based on assessment of the severity of heart failure and then adjusted as necessary. In both acute and chronic failure Isordil should be administered initially in the sublingual form to stabilise the patients' symptoms and determine the magnitude of haemodynamic response and then in the oral form for maintenance therapy.

Elderly: There are no special dosage requirements for elderly patients but as with all medicines the lowest effective dose should be used.

Children: Not recommended.

Contra-indications, warnings, etc
Contra-indications: Hypersensitivity to this drug.

Use in pregnancy and lactation: The product has not been studied in human pregnancy. The use of Isordil requires that the anticipated benefit be weighed against possible hazard. It is not known whether isosorbide dinitrate is excreted in human milk. It is unlikely that a nursing woman would require Isordil but the decision depends on the condition of the patient and caution should be exercised.

Precautions:

1. Tolerance to this drug and cross tolerance to other nitrates and nitrites, may occur; withdrawal restores the original sensitivity.
2. In congestive heart failure, as a rule, pulmonary capillary pressure should not be allowed to fall below 15 mmHg or systolic blood pressure below physiological range in normal or hypertensive patients. In patients with hypotension in the range of 90–100 mmHg of systolic pressure there should be no fall at all. As with other vasodilators in sensitive patients Isordil may cause paradoxical side-effects which may increase ischaemia and may even lead to extension of myocardial damage and advanced congestive heart failure. Treatment should therefore be discontinued.

Side effects: Side effects due to Isordil are common to all nitrates used for the treatment of angina pectoris.

1. Cutaneous vasodilation with flushing.
2. Headache is common and in some patients may be severe and persistent. Analgesics have been useful in some cases.
3. Transient episodes of dizziness and weakness and other signs of cerebral ischaemia associated with postural hypotension may occur.
4. This drug can act as a physiological antagonist to noradrenaline, acetylcholine, histamine and many other agents.
5. An occasional individual exhibits a marked sensitivity to the hypotensive effects of nitrate and severe responses (nausea, vomiting, weakness, restlessness,

pallor, perspiration and collapse) can occur even with the usual therapeutic dose. Appropriate treatment should be given. Alcohol may enhance this effect.

6. Drug rash and/or exfoliative dermatitis may occasionally occur.

Treatment of overdosage: The main manifestation is hypotension. In such an event treatment should be stopped and the patient carefully monitored. Passive exercise and elevation of legs of the recumbent patient will promote venous return. In life threatening situations administration of vasopressors should be considered. The LD_{50} of isosorbide dinitrate in rodents is of the order of 1000 mg/kg.

Pharmaceutical precautions *Storage:* Unlike glyceryl trinitrate, Isordil Tablets are stable and no special storage conditions are necessary.

Legal category P.

Package quantities Isordil Sublingual Tablets 5 mg in Securitainers of 100. Isordil Tablets 10 mg in Securitainers of 100 and 500. Isordil Tablets 30 mg in Securitainers of 100.

Further information Isordil has a very high solubility compared with other nitrates and therefore acts sublingually to abort the acute attack of angina pectoris quickly. In addition, Isordil can be administered orally to give a prolonged effect. Because Isordil is physically and chemically stable it is reliable in use.

Product licence numbers

Isordil Tablets 5 mg	0011/0172
Isordil Tablets 10 mg	0011/0173
Isordil Tablets 30 mg	0011/0174

ISORDIL* TEMBIDS* CAPSULES

Presentation Isordil Tembids capsules containing isosorbide dinitrate 40 mg in a sustained release formulation are gelatin capsules with a colourless, transparent body containing white irregular pellets and opaque blue cap for oral administration.

Uses Prophylaxis of angina pectoris (classic effort associated angina, chronic stable angina, vasospastic angina, variant angina, unstable angina, nocturnal angina and angina decubitus).

Dosage and administration *Adults:* For oral administration – One capsule 2 or 3 times a day. In selected cases daily doses of up to 240 mg oral isosorbide dinitrate have been administered. Capsules should be swallowed without chewing.

Elderly: There are no special dosage requirements for elderly patients but as with all medicines the lowest effective dose should be used.

Children: Not recommended.

Contra-indications, warnings, etc
Contra-indications: Hypersensitivity to this drug.

Precaution: Tolerance to this drug, and cross-tolerance to other nitrates and nitrites may occur; withdrawal restores the original sensitivity.

Use in pregnancy: The product has not been studied in human pregnancy. The use of Isordil Tembids requires that the anticipated benefit be weighed against possible hazard.

Side effects: Side effects due to Isordil are common to all nitrates used for the treatment of angina pectoris.

1. Cutaneous vasodilation with flushing.
2. Headache is common and in some patients may be severe and persistent. Analgesics have been useful in some cases.
3. Transient episodes of dizziness and weakness and other signs of cerebral ischaemia associated with postural hypotension may occur.
4. This drug can act as a physiological antagonist to noradrenaline, acetylcholine, histamine and many other agents.
5. An occasional individual exhibits a marked sensitivity to the hypotensive effects of nitrate and severe responses (nausea, vomiting, weakness, restlessness, pallor, perspiration and collapse) can occur even with the usual therapeutic dose. Alcohol may enhance this effect.
6. Drug rash and/or exfoliative dermatitis may occasionally occur.

Treatment of overdosage: The main manifestation is hypotension. In such event the drug should be withheld and the patient carefully monitored. Passive exercise and elevation of legs of the recumbent patient will promote venous return. In life threatening situations administration of vasopressors should be considered. The LD_{50} of isosorbide dinitrate in rodents is of the order of 1000 mg/kg.

Pharmaceutical precautions *Storage:* Unlike glyceryl trinitrate, Isordil Tembids are stable and no special storage conditions are necessary.

Legal category P.

Package quantities Securitainers of 100.

Further information Isosorbide dinitrate is released from the slow release formulation over a 6 hour period to provide up to 12 hours of sustained effect.

Product licence number 0607/0041.

Product licence holder: Ayerst Laboratories Limited.

LODINE*

Presentation Lodine capsules containing etodolac 200 mg are hard gelatin capsules with an opaque dark grey body and light grey cap, printed with two red bands and 'Lodine 200'.

Lodine capsules containing etodolac 300 mg are hard gelatin capsules with an Opaque light grey body and cap, printed with two red bands and 'Lodine 300'.

Lodine tablets contain etodolac 200 mg and are brown, oval biconvex film coated tablets, printed 'WYETH' or 'LODINE' and '200'.

Uses Lodine (etodolac) is indicated for acute or long-term use in rheumatoid arthritis and osteoarthritis.

Dosage and administration The recommended oral daily dosage of Lodine is 200 mg or 300 mg twice daily. Patients may also respond to 400 mg or 600 mg administered as a single daily dose.

The safety of doses in excess of 600 mg per day has not been established. No occurrence of tolerance or tachyphylaxis has been reported.

Elderly: No change in initial dosage required in the elderly (*see 'Precautions'*).

Children: A paediatric dosage has not been established.

Contra-indications, warnings, etc
Contra-indications: Lodine should not be used in patients who have previously shown hypersensitivity to it. Lodine should not be used in patients with active peptic ulceration or a history of peptic ulcer disease (including gastrointestinal haemorrhage due to another non-steroidal anti-inflammatory drug). Due to possible cross-reactivity, Lodine should not be administered to patients who experience asthma, rhinitis or urticaria during therapy with aspirin or other non-steroidal anti-inflammatory drugs.

Pregnancy: Drugs which inhibit prostaglandin biosynthesis may cause dystocia and delayed parturition as evidenced by studies in pregnant animals. Some inhibitors of prostaglandin biosynthesis have been shown to interfere with the closure of the ductus arteriosus. Safety in human pregnancy has not been established and Lodine should not be used during pregnancy. Safety of Lodine use during lactation has not been established and as such its use in nursing mothers should be avoided.

Precautions: Although non-steroidal anti-inflammatory drugs do not have the same direct effects on platelets as does aspirin, all drugs which inhibit the biosynthesis of prostaglandins may interfere, to some extent, with platelet function. Patients receiving Lodine who may be adversely affected by such actions should be carefully observed.

There has been no evidence of significant changes in renal or hepatic function with the use of Lodine in man. However, impairment of renal or hepatic functions due to other causes may alter drug metabolism; patients receiving long-term therapy, especially the elderly, should be observed for potential side-effects and their drug doses adjusted as needed, or the drug discontinued.

Drug interactions: Since Lodine is extensively protein-bound, it may be necessary to modify the dosage of other highly protein-bound drugs, *e.g.* anticoagulants when these are administered concurrently.

Bilirubin tests can give a false positive result due to the presence of phenolic metabolites of Lodine in the urine.

Side-effects: Lodine is well tolerated. Most side-effects are mild and transient and have only occasionally resulted in the discontinuation of therapy. Reported side-effects include nausea, epigastric pain, diarrhoea, indigestion, heartburn, flatulence, abdominal pain, constipation, vomiting, headaches, dizziness, drowsiness, tinnitus, rash, pruritis, fatigue, depression, insomnia, nervousness/anxiety, weakness/malaise, urinary frequency, angioedema, photosensitivity, urticaria, dyspepsia, malaena and rectal bleeding. More serious adverse reactions which may occur occasionally are gastro-intestinal bleeding and peptic ulceration.

Overdosage: The standard practices of gastric evacuation, activated charcoal administration and general supportive therapy should be undertaken.

Pharmaceutical precautions Store at room temperature (approximately 25°C).

Legal category POM.

Package quantities Lodine 200 mg capsules are available in Securitainers of 60 and 250. Lodine 300 mg capsules are available in blister packs containing 6 strips of 10 capsules. Lodine 200 mg tablets are available in white HDPE bottles of 60 and securitainers of 250 tablets.

Further information Nil.

Product licence numbers

Lodine 200 mg capsules	0011/0144
Lodine 300 mg capsules	0011/0145
Lodine 200 mg tablets	0011/0148

LORAZEPAM TABLETS

Presentation Lorazepam tablets are capsule shaped containing 1 mg or 2.5 mg Lorazepam BP, and are approximately 4 × 8 mm. The 1 mg tablets are blue with WYETH on one side and WY breakbar 19 on the other. The 2.5 mg tablets are yellow with WYETH on one side and WY breakbar 20 on the other.

Uses Lorazepam Tablets are recommended for short term use of approximately 2–4 weeks. As with all benzodiazepines doctors should be aware that long term use may lead to dependence and withdrawal symptoms in certain patients.

Lorazepam is indicated for the short-term treatment of moderate and severe anxiety, i.e. anxiety that is disabling or subjecting the individual to unacceptable distress. Lorazepam is also indicated for the short-term treatment of anxiety in psychosomatic, organic and psychotic illness and the short-term treatment of insomnia associated with anxiety. Lorazepam may also be used as premedication before operative dentistry and as a sedative for the anxious dental patient, and as premedication before general surgery.

All patients taking Lorazepam should be carefully monitored and routine repeat prescriptions should be avoided. Treatment in all patients should be withdrawn gradually with careful monitoring and reassessment to minimise possible withdrawal symptoms. Patients who have taken benzodiazepines for a long time may require a longer period during which doses are reduced. Should longer term therapy be necessary then intermittent treatment may be considered to minimise the risk of dependence.

Dosage and administration
Route of administration: Oral.

In all cases the dosage of Lorazepam should be titrated according to the needs of the individual patient and the lowest effective dose necessary to control symptoms should be used.

Lorazepam should not be used for long-term chronic treatment.

Dosage: Adults: Moderate and severe anxiety – 1–4 mg daily in divided doses.

Insomnia – 1–2 mg before retiring.

Premedication – 2–3 mg the night before operation; 2–4 mg one to two hours before operation.

Elderly: The elderly may respond to lower doses and half the normal adult dose or less may be sufficient.

Children: Premedication – aged 5–13 years, 0.5–2.5 mg at 0.05 mg/kg to the nearest 0.5 mg according to weight, not less than one hour before operation.

Dentistry: 1–2.5 mg, 1½–2 hours before dental treatment. For operative dentistry dosage as for premedication.

Contra-indications, warnings, etc
Contra-indications: Lorazepam should not be given to patients with a previous history of sensitivity to benzodiazepines or patients with acute pulmonary insufficiency.

Use in pregnancy: Safety for use in pregnancy has not been established. Lorazepam tablets should not be administered during pregnancy or lactation unless in the judgment of the physician such administration is clinically justifiable. Lorazepam tablets are not recommended for use in the first three months of pregnancy. Use during the late phase of pregnancy or at delivery may require ventilation of the infant at birth.

Precautions and warnings:

1. Concomitant administration with central nervous system depressants, including alcohol, general anaesthetics, narcotic analgesics, monoamine oxidase inhibitors and antidepressants will result in an accentuation of their effects.

2. When used at the appropriate recommended dose for short term treatment of anxiety the dependence potential of Lorazepam is low. However, the risk of dependence increases with higher doses and longer-term use and is further increased in patients with a history of alcoholism, drug abuse or in patients with marked personality disorders.

Symptoms such as anxiety, depression, headache, insomnia, tension and sweating have been reported following abrupt discontinuation of benzodiazepines and these symptoms may be difficult to distinguish from the original symptoms of anxiety. Other symptoms such as persistent tinnitus, involuntary movements, paraesthesia, perceptual changes, confusion, convulsions, abdominal and muscle cramps, and vomiting may be characteristic of benzodiazepine withdrawal syndrome.

3. As with other drugs acting on the central nervous system, patients should be cautioned against driving or operating machinery until it is established that they do not become dizzy or drowsy while taking Lorazepam tablets.

4. This product should be used with caution in patients with impairment of renal or hepatic function.

5. Elderly patients or those suffering from cerebral vascular changes such as arteriosclerosis are likely to respond to smaller doses.

6. Lorazepam tablets should be used with caution during labour. Respiratory depression, poor sucking and hypothermia in the neonate after delivery have occasionally been reported especially in infants who are at high risk.

7. Lorazepam does not depress respiration in most patients but the drug should be used with caution in patients with chronic pulmonary insufficiency.

8. The use of benzodiazepines may release suicidal tendencies in depressed patients. Lorazepam should not be used alone to treat depression, anxiety associated with depression, or psychotic illness. Other rarely reported behavioural effects of the benzodiazepines include paradoxical aggressive outbursts, excitement and confusion. Amnesia may occur and in cases of loss or bereavement psychological adjustment may be inhibited by benzodiazepines.

Overdosage: As with other benzodiazepines, overdosage should not present a threat to life unless combined with other CNS depressants (including alcohol). General supportive measures should be used. Treatment is symptomatic and gastric lavage may be of use if performed shortly after ingestion. The patient is likely to sleep and a clear airway should be maintained.

Side-effects: Lorazepam is well tolerated and imbalance or ataxia is an indication of excessive dosage. Daytime drowsiness may be seen initially and is to be anticipated in the effective treatment of anxiety. It will normally diminish rapidly and may be minimised in the early days of treatment by giving the larger proportion of the day's dose before retiring.

Occasional confusion, hangover, headache on waking, dizziness, blurred vision, nausea, depression, change in appetite and sleep disturbance have been reported. In addition blood dyscrasias and increased liver enzymes have occasionally been reported. On rare occasions visual disturbances, hypotension, gastrointestinal disturbances and mild transient skin rashes have also been reported.

Pharmaceutical precautions Store in a cool dry place.

Legal category CD (Sch 4), POM.

Package quantities 1 mg and 2.5 mg tablets: boxes of 100 (5 × 20 blister strips) and containers of 1000.

Further information Lorazepam is a shorter-acting benzodiazepine. It is rapidly absorbed from the gastrointestinal tract and is metabolised by a simple one-step process to a pharmacologically inactive glucuronide. The elimination half-life of lorazepam is about 12 hours so that steady state plasma levels are quickly reached and there is minimal risk of excessive accumulation, giving a wide margin of safety.

The risk of benzodiazepine related dependence may be minimised by adopting the following guidelines for treatment:

1. Select patients carefully taking into account the precautions and warnings stated in this data sheet.
2. Adopt short-term or intermittent therapy.
3. Use lowest dose possible to achieve effective treatment.
4. Review treatment regularly; and especially before repeating prescriptions.
5. Discontinue treatment gradually taking into account patient reaction at each stage; i.e., "titrate downwards".

Product licence numbers
Tablets 1 mg 0011/0108
Tablets 2.5 mg 0011/0109

LORMETAZEPAM TABLETS 0.5 mg and 1 mg

Presentation Lormetazepam tablets are white tablets containing 0.5 mg or 1 mg lormetazepam. The 0.5 mg tablets are round, white, 6.5 mm in diameter with "WYETH" embossed on one face, the other face plain. The 1 mg tablets are oval, white, 9.0 mm in length, 5.5. mm in width with "WYETH" embossed on one face and the other face plain.

Uses Lormetazepam tablets are indicated for the short-term (up to 4 weeks) treatment of insomnia, when it is disabling or subjecting the individual to extreme distress.

As with all benzodiazepines doctors should be aware that long-term use may lead to dependency and withdrawal symptoms in certain patients.

Dosage and administration Route of administration: Oral.

In all cases the lowest effective dose necessary to control symptoms should be used. Treatment should if possible be intermittent. Lormetazepam should not be used for long term chronic treatment.

Adults: Normally 0.5–1.5 mg before retiring. Subsequently the initial dosage may be increased in individual cases if this proves necessary.

Elderly: The lower adult dose is preferable for elderly patients.

Children: Lormetazepam has not been evaluated for the treatment of children.

All patients taking lormetazepam should be carefully monitored and routine repeat prescriptions avoided. Treatment in all patients should be withdrawn gradually with careful monitoring and reassessment to minimise possible withdrawal symptoms. Patients who have taken benzodiazepines for a long time may require a longer period during which doses are reduced.

Contra-indications, warnings, etc
Contra-indications:

1. Sensitivity to benzodiazepines.
2. Myasthenia gravis.
3. Acute pulmonary insufficiency.

Use in pregnancy: Safety for use in pregnancy has not been established. Lormetazepam tablets should not be administered during pregnancy unless in the judgement of the physician such administration is clinically justifiable. Lormetazepam tablets are not recommended for use in the first three months of pregnancy. Use during the late phase of pregnancy or at delivery may require ventilation of the infant at birth.

Precautions and warnings:

1. An underlying cause for insomnia should be sought before deciding on the use of benzodiazepines for symptomatic relief.

2. Concomitant administration with central nervous system depressants, including alcohol, general anaesthetics, narcotic analgesics, monoamine oxidase inhibitors and antidepressants may result in an accentuation of their effects.

3. When used at the appropriate recommended dose for short-term treatment of insomnia the dependence potential of lormetazepam is low. However, the risk of dependence increases with higher doses and longer-term use and is further increased in patients with a history of alcoholism, drug abuse or in patients with marked personality disorders.

Symptoms such as anxiety, depression, headache, insomnia, tension and sweating have been reported following abrupt discontinuation of benzodiazepines and these symptoms may be difficult to distinguish from the original ones. Other symptoms such as persistent tinnitus, involuntary movements, paraesthesia, perceptual changes, confusion, convulsions, abdominal and muscle cramps and vomiting may be characteristic of benzodiazepine withdrawal syndrome.

4. As with other drugs acting on the central nervous system, patients should be cautioned against driving or operating machinery until it is established that they do not become dizzy or drowsy while taking lormetazepam.

5. Elderly patients or those suffering from cerebral vascular changes such as arteriosclerosis are likely to respond to smaller doses.

6. The use of benzodiazepines may release suicidal tendencies in depressed patients. Lormetazepam should not be used alone to treat depression or anxiety associated with depression. Other rarely reported behavioural effects of the benzodiazepines include paradoxical aggressive outbursts, excitement, hallucinations and confusion. Amnesia may occur and in cases of loss or bereavement psychological adjustment may be inhibited by benzodiazepines.

Side-effects: Lormetazepam is generally well tolerated. However, in occasional sensitive patients, or because of overdosage, headache, drowsiness, dizziness and nausea may occur on the following morning.

On rare occasions hypotension, gastro-intestinal and visual disturbances, skin rashes, urinary retention, changes in libido, blood dyscrasias, jaundice and increased liver enzymes have been reported with some benzodiazepines.

Overdosage: As with other benzodiazepines, overdosage should not present a threat to life unless combined with other CNS depressants (including alcohol). General supportive measures should be used. Treatment is symptomatic and gastric lavage may be of use if performed shortly after ingestion. The patient is likely to sleep and a clear airway should be maintained.

Pharmaceutical precautions Store in a cool dry place.

Legal category CD (Sch 4), POM.

Package quantities 0.5 mg and 1 mg tablets are supplied in packs of 30 (OP) and 100.

Further information Lormetazepam is rapidly absorbed from the gastrointestinal tract and is metabolised by a simple one step process to a pharmacologically inactive glucuronide. There are no major metabolites and little risk of accumulation. Lormetazepam has a terminal phase half-life of about 11 hours. Clinical studies have shown minimal effects on REM sleep and on psychomotor performance on the day after treatment with lormetazepam.

The risk of benzodiazepine related dependence may be minimised by adopting the following guidelines for treatment:

1. Select patients carefully taking into account the precautions and warnings stated in this data sheet.
2. Adopt short-term or intermittent therapy.
3. Use lowest dose possible to achieve effective treatment.
4. Review treatment regularly; and especially before repeating prescriptions.
5. Discontinue treatment gradually taking into account patient reaction at each stage, i.e. 'titrate downwards'.

Product licence numbers
0.5 mg tablets 0011/0068.
1.0 mg tablets 0011/0069.

MEPTID* INJECTION

Presentation Meptid injection is a clear solution, containing meptazinol hydrochloride at a concentration equivalent to 100 mg meptazinol base per ml, supplied in 1 ml quantities in clear glass ampoules.

Uses Meptid injection is indicated for the treatment of moderate to severe pain, including post-operative pain, obstetric pain and the pain of renal colic.

Dosage and administration *Adults: Intramuscular dosage:* 75–100 mg Meptid. The injection may be repeated 2–4 hourly as required. For obstetric pain a dose of 100–150 mg should be used according to weight. This dose should approximate 2 mg/kg.

Intravenous dosage: 50–100 mg Meptid by slow intravenous injection. The injection may be repeated 2–4 hourly as required. If vomiting occurs, a suitable antiemetic should be given.

Epidural/Intrathecal use: This formulation is *not* suitable for these routes.

Elderly: The adult dosage schedule may be used in the elderly.

Children: Meptid Injection has not been evaluated for use in children.

Contra-indications, warnings, etc
Contra-indications: None known, except for individuals with known sensitivity to the product.

Precautions:
1. Caution should be observed in treating patients with hepatic or renal insufficiency.
2. Clinical studies have indicated absence of clinically significant respiratory depression but caution should be exercised in patients already severely compromised.
3. Safety for use in myocardial infarction has not been established.
4. Meptid injection is a useful analgesic in labour but in accordance with general medical principles it should not be given in other stages of pregnancy unless considered essential by the physician. There is no evidence from animal reproductive studies to anticipate a teratogenic risk.
5. Meptid should be used cautiously in patients with head injuries, as other drugs of this class have the potential to elevate cerebrospinal fluid pressure and to obscure the clinical course of such patients.

Warnings: Since dizziness and occasionally drowsiness have been reported, patients should be cautioned against driving or operating machinery until it is established that they do not become dizzy or drowsy while taking meptazinol. Other central nervous system depressants should be used with caution in patients receiving Meptid.

Treatment of overdosage: Overdosage with Meptid injection has not been reported. Large doses, including seven times the recommended therapeutic dose, have been given in balanced and total intravenous anaesthesia, without significant respiratory depressant effects.

In the event of cardiovascular and respiratory collapse, normal resuscitative procedures should be employed. Respiratory depression caused by overdosage with meptazinol may be reversed in part with therapeutic doses of Naloxone.

Side-effects: The most commonly reported adverse reactions after treatment with meptazinol are nausea, vomiting, dizziness, diarrhoea, increased sweating, abdominal pain, rash, vertigo, headache, somnolence and dyspepsia.

Pharmaceutical precautions Store below 25°C.

Meptid injection should *not* be mixed with other drugs in the same infusion solution or in the same syringe. Meptid injection is an acidic solution of the hydrochloride salt of meptazinol and is therefore pharmaceutically incompatible with injection solutions known to be strongly basic (for example thiopentone) as precipitation of the meptazinol base may occur.

Meptid at concentrations of 200 mg in 500 ml and 500 mg in 500 ml has been shown to be compatible with the following intravenous infusion fluids when added immediately prior to use:

Dextrose 5% w/v
Dextrose 10% w/v
Sodium chloride 0.9% w/v
Ringers solution
Hartmanns solution
Sodium chloride 0.9% w/v and dextrose 5% w/v

If Meptid is administered through an intravenous cannula, it is essential to flush the system with saline before and after administration.

Legal category POM.

Package quantities Cartons of 10 ampoules (OP).

Further information Nil.

Product licence number 0011/0046.

MEPTID* TABLETS

Presentation Meptid tablets are oval orange film coated tablets marked WYETH on one side, 14.5 mm in length and containing 200 mg meptazinol.

Uses Meptid tablets are indicated for the short term treatment of moderate pain.

Dosage and administration *Route of administration:* oral.

Dosage – Adults: 200 mg 3–6 hourly as required. Usually one tablet four hourly.

Elderly: The adult dosage schedule may be used in the elderly.

Children: Meptid tablets have not been evaluated for use in children.

Contra-indications, warnings, etc

Contra-indications: None known, except for individuals with known sensitivity to the product.

Precautions:

1. Caution should be observed in treating patients with hepatic or renal insufficiency.
2. Clinical studies have indicated absence of clinically significant respiratory depression but caution should be exercised in patients already severely compromised.
3. In accordance with general medical principles Meptid tablets should not be given to pregnant or lactating women unless considered essential by the physician. There is no evidence from animal reproductive studies to anticipate a teratogenic risk.
4. Meptid should be used cautiously in patients with head injuries, as other drugs of this class have the potential to elevate cerebrospinal fluid pressure and to obscure the clinical course of such patients.
5. Safety for use in myocardial infarction has not yet been established.

Warnings: Since dizziness and occasionally drowsiness have been reported, patients should be cautioned against driving or operating machinery until it is established that they do not become dizzy or drowsy while taking meptazinol. Other central nervous system depressants should be used with caution in patients receiving Meptid.

Treatment of overdosage: Meptid tablets are subject to a hepatic first pass metabolism which prevents systemic concentrations of the drug reaching levels achieved by parenteral administration. In the unlikely event of overdose producing respiratory depression naloxone is the treatment of choice.

Recommended treatment includes gastric lavage, supportive therapy and naloxone if required.

Side-effects: The most commonly reported adverse reactions after treatment with meptazinol are nausea, vomiting, dizziness, diarrhoea, increased sweating, abdominal pain, rash, vertigo, headache, somnolence and dyspepsia.

Pharmaceutical precautions None.

Legal category POM.

Package quantities Cartons of 100 tablets (5 blister packs of 20 tablets).

Further information Meptazinol is eliminated rapidly via the kidney. The main metabolite is a glucuronide conjugate and there is no accumulation of the drug or of active metabolites.

Product licence number 0011/0079.

MICROVAL*

Presentation Microval tablets are round white lustrous coated, convex tablets 5.0 mm in diameter. Each tablet contains 30 micrograms levonorgestrel.

Uses Oral contraception. Microval is particularly indicated for the older woman changing from combined oral contraceptives and for women for whom oestrogen treatment is considered unsuitable.

Dosage and administration The tablets are started on the first day of menstruation and taken daily without interruption for as long as contraception is desired. They should be taken at the same time each day, preferably after the evening meal or at bedtime so that the interval between tablets is always about 24 hours. Protection may be reduced when the interval increases beyond 27 hours.

During the first cycle additional contraceptive precautions should be taken for the first 14 days.

If a tablet is not taken at the usual time it should be taken as soon as possible and the next tablet taken at the usual time. If the interval between tablets is more than 27 hours protection may be impaired. The patient should take one tablet as soon as she remembers and thereafter one tablet daily as before but should use additional contraceptive measures until the tablets have been taken regularly for 14 days. If a tablet is missed, the patient should take 1 tablet daily as before but should use additional contraceptive measures until the tablets have been taken regularly for 14 days.

If vomiting occurs shortly after a tablet has been taken contraceptive protection can be maintained by taking another tablet, provided that it is taken within three hours of the normal time. The last tablet in the pack may be used for this purpose. If repeated vomiting or diarrhoea endanger absorption additional contraceptive precautions should be used for 14 days after the symptoms have disappeared.

Irregular spotting or bleeding may occur with a proportion of women initially but menstrual regularity is usually re-established after the first few cycles. Those patients whose menstrual patterns do not become reasonably regular after three to four cycles or who have prolonged bleeding or amenorrhoea lasting for two months should be instructed to return for advice.

Women who change from a combined oral contraceptive to Microval should stop taking the previous product, leave seven clear days and take the first Microval tablet on the eighth day, then continue to take 1 tablet daily. Additional contraceptive precautions should be taken until the fourteenth tablet has been taken.

Microval does not diminish the yield of breast milk and can be used from the seventh post-partum day.

Contra-indications, warnings, etc

Contra-indications: Microval should not be given –

1. To patients with established hepatic disease or to those in whom there is evidence of persistently abnormal liver function such as the Dubin–Johnson and Rotor syndromes, or to those who have a history during pregnancy of idiopathic jaundice or severe pruritis.
2. To patients with a history of infectious hepatitis until the liver function tests have returned to normal values.
3. To patients with abnormal vaginal bleeding of unknown aetiology.
4. To patients with suspected pregnancy.
5. Although the risk of thromboembolism has not been associated with progestogen-only contraceptives, it is at present required that a history of thromboembolic disorders should be regarded as a contra-indication.

Precautions:

1. Oral contraceptive medication should be discontinued if there is a gradual or sudden, partial or complete loss of vision, proptosis or diplopia, papilloedema or any evidence of retinal or vascular lesions.
2. Caution should be observed in prescribing oral contraceptives for any patients with a history of migraine, or if migraine is being treated with vasoconstrictor drugs. If migraine worsens or migraine or severe headache develops for the first time during treatment, medication should be discontinued immediately.
3. A small fraction of the progestogen has been identified in the milk of mothers receiving the drug. The long-range effect to the nursing infant is currently unknown.
4. Examination of the pelvic organs, breasts and blood pressure should precede prescription of Microval and should be repeated regularly.
5. Ectopic pregnancies appear to occur more frequently on progestogen-only oral contraceptives.

Side-effects: Microval is well tolerated but certain endocrine effects which are also characteristic of ovulatory cycles may occur. Those noted are headache, slight weight gain, nausea, breast tenderness and spotting between periods. The incidence of such effects with Microval is low and tends to decrease as treatment continues.

Drug interactions: Caution should be observed in prescribing oral contraceptives for patients taking other drugs since various interactions have been reported.

Pregnancies have been reported in women taking oral contraceptives concurrently with rifampicin and other antibiotics, anti-epileptic drugs, barbiturates and other sedative drugs.

Steroids affect drug metabolism and the therapeutic or toxic effects of other drugs may be modified. Interactions have been reported between oral contraceptives and tricyclic antidepressants, anticoagulants and corticosteroids.

Overdosage: No reports of serious ill-effects from overdosage with oral contraceptives have been reported. In general, therefore, treatment of overdosage is not necessary. If overdosage is, however, discovered within one hour and is so large that treatment seems desirable, gastric lavage or a suitable dose of ipecacuanha can be used. There are no specific antidotes and further treatment should be symptomatic.

Pharmaceutical precautions Store at or below room temperature.

Legal category POM.

Package quantities Microval tablets are supplied in memo packs of 35 tablets (OP).

Further information Estimates from clinical trials show that, if the tablets are taken correctly, out of 100 women taking them for one year, on average one woman may become pregnant during that year. Microval although not quite as effective as combined oral contraceptives, provides an extremely high degree of protection and is very much more effective than withdrawal, condom, rhythm method or chemicals and comparable to the I.U.C.D. and diaphragm.

Levonorgestrel is a totally synthetic progestogen which possesses no inherent oestrogenicity. It has anti-oestrogenic properties and has minimal effects on metabolic functions.

Product licence number 0011/0040.

MINULET*

Presentation Each white sugar coated tablet contains 30 micrograms ethinyloestradiol and 75 micrograms gestodene.

Uses Oral contraception and the recognised gynaecological indications for such oestrogen-progestogen combinations. The mode of action includes the inhibition of ovulation by suppression of the mid-cycle surge of luteinising hormone, the inspissation of cervical mucus so as to constitute a barrier to sperm, and the rendering of the endometrium unreceptive to implantation.

Dosage and administration
First treatment cycle: 1 tablet daily for 21 days, starting with the tablet marked number 1, on the first day of the menstrual cycle.

Subsequent cycles: Each subsequent course is started when seven tablet-free days have followed the preceding course.

Changing from another combined oral contraceptive: The first tablet of Minulet should be taken on the first day of the withdrawal bleed which follows the previous oral contraceptive course. Alternatively where it is desirable to retain the previous routine of tablet-taking, Minulet may be started on the same day that the previous combined oral contraceptive would have been resumed, provided the patient has had a withdrawal bleed. In this case, however, additional (non-hormonal) contraceptive precautions, other than the rhythm, temperature or cervical-mucus methods, should also be used for the first 14 days.

Post-partum use: After pregnancy oral contraception is usually started as soon as spontaneous menstruation has been resumed. Since the first post-partum ovulation may precede the first bleeding, another method of contraception should therefore be used in the interval between childbirth and the first course of pills, unless it is started within seven days of delivery.

Special circumstances requiring additional contraception:
Incorrect administration: If a tablet is delayed, it should be taken as soon as possible, and if it is taken within 12 hours of the correct time, additional contraception is not needed. Further tablets should then be taken at the usual time. However, if the delay exceeds 12 hours, ovulation may occur. In those circumstances, any tablet or tablets delayed more than 12 hours should be omitted, the remaining tablets should be taken on the correct days at the usual time, and extra precautions (except the rhythm, temperature or cervical-mucus methods) should be used until the next withdrawal bleed.

Gastro-intestinal upset: Vomiting or diarrhoea may reduce the effectiveness of the tablets by preventing them from being fully absorbed. Therefore, it is advisable that an additional method of contraception be used throughout the remainder of the course concerned. Mild laxatives do not impair contraceptive action.

Interaction with other drugs: Some drugs accelerate the metabolism of oral contraceptives taken concurrently. Drugs suspected of having the capacity to reduce the efficacy of oral contraceptives include barbiturates, phenytoin, phenylbutazone, rifampicin, ampicillin and other antibiotics. It is, therefore, advisable to use non-hormonal methods of contraception (except the rhythm, temperature or cervical-mucus methods) in addition to the oral contraceptive as long as an extremely high degree of protection is required during treatment with such drugs.

Contra-indications, warnings, etc
Contra-indications: Pregnancy. Thrombotic disorders and a history of these conditions, sickle-cell anaemia, disorders of lipid metabolism and other conditions in which, in individual cases, there is known or suspected to be a much increased risk of thrombosis. Acute or severe chronic liver diseases. Dubin-Johnson syndrome. Rotor syndrome. History, during pregnancy, of idiopathic jaundice or severe pruritus. History of herpes gestationis. Mammary or endometrial carcinoma, or a history of these conditions. Abnormal vaginal bleeding of unknown cause. Deterioration of otosclerosis during pregnancy.

Warnings: There is a general opinion, based on statistical evidence, that users of combined oral contraceptives experience, more often than non-users, venous thromboembolism, arterial thrombosis, including cerebral and myocardial infarction, and subarachnoid haemorrhage. Full recovery from such disorders does not always occur, and it should be realised that in a few cases they are fatal. How often these disorders occur in users of the modern low-dose pills is not known, but there are reasons for suggesting that they may occur less often than with older pills containing more oestrogen. Certain factors may entail some risk of thrombosis, e.g. smoking, obesity, varicose veins, cardiovascular diseases, diabetes and migraine. The suitability of a combined oral contraceptive should be judged according to the severity of such conditions in the individual case, and should be discussed with the patient before she decides to take it. The risk of arterial thrombosis associated with combined oral contraceptives increases with age, and this risk is aggravated by cigarette smoking. The use of combined oral contraceptives by women in the older age group, especially those who are cigarette smokers, should therefore be discouraged and alternative methods used. The possibility cannot be ruled out that certain chronic diseases may occasionally deteriorate during the use of combined oral contraceptives. (See 'Precautions'.)

The combination of ethinyloestradiol and gestodene, like other contraceptive steroids, is associated with an increased incidence of neoplastic nodules in the rat liver, the relevance of which to man is unknown.

Malignant liver tumours have been reported on rare occasions in long-term users of oral contraceptives. Benign hepatic tumours have also been associated with oral contraceptive usage. A hepatic tumour should be considered in the differential diagnosis when upper abdominal pain, enlarged liver or signs of intra-abdominal haemorrhage occur.

Numerous epidemiological studies have been reported on the risks of ovarian, endometrial, cervical and breast cancer in women using combined oral contraceptives. The evidence is clear that combined oral contraceptives offer substantial protection against both ovarian and endometrial cancer.

An increased risk of cervical cancer in long term users of combined oral contraceptives has been reported in some studies, but there continues to be controversy about the extent to which this is attributable to the confounding effects of sexual behaviour and other factors.

The evidence linking combined oral contraceptive use and breast cancer remains inconclusive. The results of some studies suggest an increased risk of breast cancer presenting below the age of about 35, the risk rising with duration of use. Any possible increased risk of breast cancer with combined oral contraceptives is however likely to be small and may be expected to be less with low dosage pills. This possible risk should be weighed against the many benefits of combined oral contraceptives, including their protective effects against ovarian and endometrial cancers.

Reasons for stopping oral contraception immediately: Occurrence of migraine in patients who have never previously suffered from it. Exacerbation of pre-existing migraine. Any unusually frequent or unusually severe headaches. Any kind of acute disturbance of vision. Suspicion of thrombosis or infarction. Six weeks before elective operations and during immobilisation, e.g. after accidents, etc. Significant rise in blood-pressure. Jaundice. Clear exacerbation of conditions known to be capable of deteriorating during oral contraception or pregnancy. Pregnancy is a reason for stopping immediately because it has been suggested by some investigations that oral contraceptives taken in early pregnancy may slightly increase the risk of foetal malformations. Other investigations have failed to support these findings. The possibility therefore cannot be excluded, but it is certain that if a risk exists at all, it is very small.

Precautions: Examination of the pelvic organs, breasts and blood-pressure should precede the prescribing of any combined oral contraceptive and should be repeated regularly. Before starting treatment, pregnancy must be excluded. The following conditions require careful observation during medication: a history of severe depressive states, varicose veins, diabetes, hypertension, epilepsy, otosclerosis, multiple sclerosis, porphyria, tetany, disturbed liver function, gall-stones, cardiovascular diseases, renal diseases, chloasma, uterine fibroids, asthma, the wearing of contact lenses, or any disease that is prone to worsen during pregnancy. The first appearance or deterioration of any of these conditions may indicate that the oral contraceptive should be stopped. The risk of the deterioration of chloasma, which is often not fully reversible, is reduced by the avoidance of excessive exposure to sunlight.

Side-effects: Occasional side-effects may include nausea, vomiting, headaches, breast tenderness, changed body weight or libido, depressive moods and chloasma.

Menstrual changes:

1. *Reduction of menstrual flow:* This is not abnormal and it is to be expected in some patients. Indeed, it may be beneficial where heavy periods were previously experienced.

2. *Missed menstruation:* Occasionally, withdrawal bleeding may not occur at all. If the tablets have been taken correctly, pregnancy is very unlikely, but should be ruled out before a new course of tablets is started.

Intermenstrual bleeding: Very light 'spotting' or heavier 'breakthrough bleeding' may occur during tablet-taking, especially in the first few cycles. It appears to be generally of no significance, except where it indicates errors of tablet-taking, or where the possibility of interaction with other drugs exists (q.v.). However, if irregular bleeding is persistent, an organic cause should be considered.

Effect on adrenal and thyroid glands: Oral contraceptives have no significant influence on adrenocortical function. The ACTH function test for the adrenal cortex remains unchanged. The reduction in corticosteroid excretion and the elevation of plasma corticosteroids are due to an increased cortisol-binding capacity of the plasma proteins.

The response to metyrapone is less pronounced than in untreated women and is thus similar to that during pregnancy.

The radio-iodine uptake shows that thyroid function is unchanged. There is a rise in serum protein-bound iodine, similar to that in pregnancy and during the administration of oestrogens. This is due to the increased capacity of the plasma proteins for binding thyroid hormones, rather than to any change in glandular function. In women taking oral contraceptives, the content of protein-bound iodine in blood serum should therefore, not be used for evaluation of thyroid function.

Effect on blood chemistry: Oral contraceptives may accelerate erythrocyte sedimentation in the absence of any disease. This effect is due to a change in the proportion of the plasma protein fractions. Increases in plasma copper, iron and alkaline phosphatase have also been recorded.

Overdosage: There have been no reports of serious ill-effects from overdosage, even when a considerable number of tablets have been taken by a small child. In general, it is, therefore, unnecessary to treat overdosage. However, if overdosage is discovered within two or three hours and is so large that treatment seems desirable, gastric lavage can be safely used. There are no specific antidotes and further treatment should be symptomatic.

Pharmaceutical precautions Store in cool, dry conditions.

Legal category POM.

Package quantities Individual packs containing 3 months' supply (OP).

Further information Nil.

Product licence number 0011/0135

MUCAINE*

Presentation Mucaine Suspension is a white suspension with the odour and flavour of peppermint. Each 5 ml contains:

Oxethazaine	10 mg
Magnesium Hydroxide BP	100 mg
Aluminium Hydroxide Mixture BP	4.75 ml

Uses Mucaine is an antacid mixture containing a topical anaesthetic and is indicated for oesophagitis whatever its cause, including peptic oesophagitis with or without hiatus hernia, radiation oesophagitis and the heartburn of late pregnancy.

The relief obtained in the symptomatic treatment of oesophagitis is due to the surface anaesthetic, oxethazaine, aided by the physical and antacid properties of the vehicle. Oxethazaine is stable at the levels of acidity or alkalinity found in the upper gastrointestinal tract and has relatively prolonged action.

Dosage and administration *Route of administration:* Oral.

Dosage – Adults: One to two 5 ml doses should be taken three or four times daily, 15 minutes before meals, and at bedtime, or as required. The dose should not be washed down with a drink.

Elderly: The adult dosage schedule may be used in the elderly.

Children: Not recommended for children.

Contra-indications, warnings, etc
Contra-indications: The aluminium ion combines with phosphate to form an insoluble complex which is not absorbed. When high doses are given together with a low phosphorus diet, phosphate depletion occurs. Phosphate depletion does not occur in patients on a normal diet. Mucaine is contra-indicated in patients with hypophosphataemia.

The use of magnesium containing antacids is contra-indicated in patients with severe renal impairment because hypermagnesaemia is more likely to occur.

Use in pregnancy and lactation: A rabbit study has shown a dose related reduction in litter size although the relevance of these findings to man is unknown. There is no evidence of safety of oxethazine in human pregnancy, therefore the product should not be used during the first trimester of pregnancy or during lactation.

Precautions:

1. The use of magnesium containing antacids in patients with mild to moderate renal impairment should be carefully observed due to the increased risk of hypermagnesaemia.
2. In patients with chronic renal failure, hyperaluminaemia may occur.

Interactions: The rate and/or extent of absorption of many drugs may be increased or decreased when they are used concurrently with aluminium-magnesium hydroxide containing antacids. Therefore, as a general rule, medication should not be taken within one to two hours of an antacid, if possible. This includes tetracycline, iron salts, chlorpromazine, levodopa, isoniazid, digoxin, H_2-antagonists, indomethacin, nitrofurantoin, and dicoumarol.

Side-effects: Mucaine is well tolerated and the side-effects which have been reported are almost invariably mild and transient in nature, consisting principally of constipation, dryness of the mouth and nausea. Hypersensitivity reactions including skin eruptions (dermatitis, urticaria), pruritis, glossitis and angioedema have been reported on rare occasions.

Action in case of overdosage: Not reported. Treatment should be symptomatic.

Pharmaceutical precautions Store in a cool place and discard contents of opened bottle after 14 days.

Legal category POM.

Package quantities Polypropylene bottles of 200 ml (OP).

Further information It is important to stress that Mucaine should not be washed down with a drink because maximal relief depends on good contact between the affected mucosal surface and the suspension as it passes down the oesophagus.

Product licence number 0011/5014.

NORMISON*

Presentation Normison capsules are yellow, opaque soft gelatin capsules containing 10 mg or 20 mg temazepam. The 10 mg capsules are No. 4 capsules printed with N10 in black lettering. The 20 mg capsules are No. 10 capsules printed N20 in red lettering.

Uses Normison is indicated for the short term (up to 4 weeks) treatment of insomnia when it is disabling or subjecting the individual to extreme distress, and for premedication before minor surgery or other procedures especially when hospital admission is not essential.

As with all benzodiazepines doctors should be aware that long term use may lead to dependence and withdrawal symptoms in certain patients.

Dosage and administration *Route of administration:* Oral.

Insomnia: In all cases the lowest effective dose necessary to control symptoms should be used. Treatment should if possible be intermittent. Normison should not be used for long term chronic treatment.

Adults: 10–30 mg half an hour before retiring. The dose may be increased to 40 or 60 mg in patients who do not respond to the lower dose because of severe or persistent insomnia.

Elderly: Elderly patients or those suffering from cerebral vascular changes such as arteriosclerosis are likely to respond to smaller doses, possibly half the normal adult dose.

Children: Not recommended.

All patients taking Normison should be carefully monitored and routine repeat prescriptions should be avoided.

Treatment in all patients should be withdrawn gradually with careful monitoring and reassessment to minimise possible withdrawal symptoms. Patients who have taken benzodiazepines for a long time may require a longer period during which doses are reduced.

Premedication:

Adults: 20–40 mg, 30–60 minutes before surgical or other procedures.

Elderly: Elderly patients are likely to respond to smaller doses, possibly half the normal adult dose.

Children: Not evaluated.

Contra-indications, warnings, etc

Contra-indications: Normison should not be given to patients with a previous history of sensitivity to benzodiazepines or patients with acute pulmonary insufficiency.

Use in pregnancy: Safety for use in pregnancy has not been established. Normison should not be administered during pregnancy or lactation unless in the judgement of the physician such administration is clinically justifiable. Normison is not recommended for use in the first three months of pregnancy. Use during the late phase of pregnancy or at delivery may require ventilation of the infant at birth.

Precautions:

1. An underlying cause for insomnia should be sought before deciding on the use of benzodiazepines for symptomatic relief.
2. Concomitant administration with central nervous system depressants, including alcohol, general anaesthetics, narcotic analgesics, monoamine oxidase inhibitors and antidepressants will result in an accentuation of their effects.
3. When used at the appropriate recommended dose for short term treatment of insomnia the dependence potential of Normison is low. However, the risk of dependence increases with higher doses and longer-term use and is further increased in patients with a history of alcoholism, drug abuse or in patients with marked personality disorders.

Symptoms such as anxiety, depression, headache, insomnia, tension and sweating have been reported following abrupt discontinuation of benzodiazepines and these symptoms may be difficult to distinguish from the original ones.

Other symptoms such as persistent tinnitus, involuntary movements, paraesthesia, perceptual changes, confusion, convulsions, abdominal and muscle cramps and vomiting may be characteristic of benzodiazepine withdrawal syndrome.

4. When used as a hypnotic, daytime drowsiness is unlikely to be a problem with Normison since the short half-life usually ensures that the effects disappear by the morning. As with other drugs acting on the central nervous system, however, patients should be cautioned against driving or operating machinery until it is established that they do not become dizzy or drowsy while taking Normison.
5. Elderly patients or those suffering from cerebral vascular changes such as arteriosclerosis are likely to respond to smaller doses.
6. After medication with Normison before surgical or other procedures, patients should be accompanied home.
7. The use of benzodiazepines may release suicidal tendencies in depressed patients. Benzodiazepines should not be used alone to treat depression or anxiety associated with depression. Other rarely reported behavioural effects of the benzodiazepines include paradoxical aggressive outbursts, excitement, hallucinations and confusion. Amnesia may occur and in cases of loss or bereavement psychological adjustment may be inhibited by benzodiazepines.

Side-effects: Because of its short half-life, the effects of temazepam are usually restricted to the night of ingestion. Drowsiness or dizziness on waking is rare. Morning headaches, transient rashes, mild gastro-intestinal disturbances, vivid dreams/nightmares, dry mouth or throat, depression, restless sleep and palpitations have occasionally been reported.

On rare occasions hypotension, gastro-intestinal and visual disturbances, skin rashes, urinary retention, changes in libido, blood dyscrasias, increased liver enzymes and jaundice have been reported with some benzodiazepines.

Overdosage: As with other benzodiazepines, overdosage should not present a threat to life unless combined with other CNS depressants (including alcohol). General supportive measures should be used. Treatment is symptomatic and gastric lavage may be of use if performed shortly after ingestion. The patient is likely to sleep and a clear airway should be maintained.

Pharmaceutical precautions Store in a dry place between 15°C and 25°C. Protect from light. Dispense Normison capsules into well-closed amber glass or amber/opaque plastic containers.

Legal category CD (Sch 4), POM.

Package quantities 10 mg: bottles of 50 (OP) and 100, securitainers of 500 and 1000. 20 mg: bottles of 100, securitainers of 500.

Further information Normison is a short acting benzodiazepine. It is rapidly absorbed from the liquid-filled soft gelatin capsules and peak plasma levels are usually reached in 20 to 40 minutes. Normison has a plasma half life of about eight hours. Normison is metabolised by a simple one-step process to a pharmacologically inert glucuronide. There are no major active metabolites and virtually no risk of accumulation. Clinical studies have shown minimal effects on REM sleep patterns and on psychomotor performance on the day after treatment with Normison.

The risk of benzodiazepine related dependence may be minimised by adopting the following guidelines for treatment:

1. Select patients carefully taking into account the precautions and warnings stated in this data sheet.
2. Adopt short-term or intermittent therapy.
3. Use lowest dose possible to achieve effective treatment.
4. Review treatment regularly; and especially before repeating prescriptions.
5. Discontinue treatment gradually taking into account patient reaction at each stage, ie 'titrate downwards'.

Product licence numbers
10 mg capsules 0011/0060
20 mg capsules 0011/0063

OVRAN*
OVRAN 30*
OVRANETTE*

Presentation Ovran tablets are round, white, convex tablets, 6.5 mm in diameter, both faces marked WYETH. Each tablet contains 250 micrograms levonorgestrel (d-norgestrel) and 50 micrograms Ethinyloestradiol BP.

Ovran 30 tablets are round, white, convex tablets, 6.5 mm in diameter, one face marked WYETH and the other plain. Each tablet contains 250 micrograms levonorgestrel (d-norgestrel) and 30 micrograms Ethinyloestradiol BP.

Ovranette tablets are round, white, convex tablets, 6.5 mm in diameter, one face marked WYETH and the other face marked '30'. Each tablet contains 150 micrograms levonorgestrel (d-norgestrel) and 30 micrograms Ethinyloestradiol BP.

Uses Oral contraception. Treatment of endometriosis, spasmodic dysmenorrhoea, pre-menstrual tension, oligomenorrhoea. Treatment of abnormal uterine bleeding such as menorrhagia, metropathia haemorrhagica. Emergency treatment of acute uterine bleeding.

Dosage and administration *Contraception:* For the first course of medication the tablets are started on the fifth day of the cycle, counting the first day of menstruation as day one. One tablet is taken at the same time each day for 21 days followed by seven days without medication. On the eighth day the tablets are started again. Additional contraceptive precautions should be taken until the fourteenth tablet of the first cycle has been taken. In subsequent cycles the protection covers every day of the cycle, provided that the tablets are taken correctly. During the seven clear days, withdrawal bleeding should occur. If a cycle with amenorrhoea occurs the patient should seek medical advice.

Women who change from another oral contraceptive to Ovran, Ovran 30 or Ovranette should stop taking the previous product, at the end of the pack leave seven clear days and take the first Ovran, Ovran 30 or Ovranette tablet on the eighth day, then continue to take 1 tablet daily for 21 days. Additional contraceptive precautions should be taken until the fourteenth tablet of the first cycle has been taken.

Occasionally spotting or bleeding may occur in some women initially, but menstrual regularity is usually re-established after the first few cycles. If medication is discontinued because of severe breakthrough bleeding a new course should be started on the fifth day from the start of bleeding. Additional contraceptive precautions should be taken until the fourteenth tablet of the new course has been taken.

If a tablet is forgotten the woman should take two on the following day at the usual time. If more than one tablet is missed, tablet taking should be resumed when remembered with the tablet appropriate for that day and additional precautions should be taken until the next withdrawal bleed. Withdrawal bleeding may occur as a result of missed tablets, but the patient should continue to take the tablets as directed.

Treatment with Ovran, Ovran 30 or Ovranette should be withdrawn six weeks before elective surgery or treatment of varicose veins by injection of sclerosant.

After childbirth oral contraception is usually started as soon as spontaneous menstruation has been resumed. Another method of contraception should be used in the interval between delivery and the first course, unless it is started within seven days of delivery.

Oral contraception may be started on the fifth day after an abortion or miscarriage.

If vomiting or diarrhoea impair absorption additional contraceptive precautions should be taken until the next withdrawal bleed.

Other indications: Ovran and Ovranette can be used for the indications listed below, but Ovran usually provides the more convenient dosage unit.

Endometriosis: Treatment should be continuous with 1 Ovran tablet daily. If spotting or breakthrough bleeding occurs it may be necessary to give 2 tablets daily or rarely 3 tablets daily in divided doses.

Spasmodic dysmenorrhoea, premenstrual tension, oligomenorrhoea: Dosage as for oral contraception.

Postponement of menstruation: If postponement of a withdrawal bleed is considered desirable, the woman should continue taking the tablets for the period during which delay is required. A seven-day gap should then be left before starting a new pack. If spotting or breakthrough bleeding occurs dosage should be increased to 2 tablets daily.

Functional uterine bleeding: When the diagnosis has been established dosage is similar to the dosage for oral contraception, but in the first one or two cycles it may be necessary to give 2 Ovran tablets (or in exceptional cases), 3 tablets daily in order to control the regularity of the cycle.

Emergency treatment of the acute uterine bleeding: 2 Ovran tablets are given immediately. If bleeding continues medication is continued at a dose of 4 tablets daily in divided doses. This can usually be reduced to 2 tablets within two to four days. Treatment should continue for 10 days and after this time it can either be discontinued to be followed after seven days by a complete course of 1 tablet daily for 21 days (see 'Functional uterine bleeding') or it can be continued for one to three months to inhibit the menses (see 'Postponement of menstruation'). In the latter case it should be possible to reduce the dosage to 1 tablet daily.

Contra-indications, warnings, etc
Contra-indications: Ovran, Ovran 30 and Ovranette, like other progestogen-oestrogen combinations, should not be given:

1. To patients with established hepatic disease or to those in whom there is evidence of persistently abnormal liver function such as the Dubin–Johnson and Rotor syndromes, or to those who have idiopathic recurrent jaundice of pregnancy.
2. To patients with a history or suspicion of carcinoma of the reproductive organs or breasts.
3. To patients with a history or evidence suggestive of thromboembolic or cerebrovascular disease or phlebitis.
4. To patients with cardiovascular disease.
5. To patients with a history of infectious hepatitis until the liver function tests have returned to normal values.
6. To patients with abnormal, vaginal bleeding of unknown aetiology.
7. To patients with known or suspected oestrogen-dependent neoplasia.
8. To patients with suspected pregnancy.
9. To patients with sickle cell anaemia.
10. To patients with deterioration of otosclerosis during pregnancy.
11. To patients with a history of herpes gestationis.

Precautions:

1. Under the influence of oestrogen-progestogen preparations, pre-existing uterine fibromyomata may increase in size.
2. Oestrogen-progestogen preparations may cause some degree of fluid retention. Conditions which might be influenced by this factor, such as epilepsy, migraine, asthma, cardiac or renal dysfunction, require careful observation.
3. Patients with a history of psychic depression should be carefully observed and the drug discontinued if the depression recurs to a serious degree.
4. A decrease in glucose tolerance has been observed in a significant percentage of patients on oral contraceptives. Diabetic patients should be carefully observed while receiving therapy.
5. Susceptible women may experience an increase in blood pressure following administration of contraceptive steroids. Caution should therefore be exercised in prescribing oral contraceptives for women with a history of hypertension.
6. Oral contraceptive medication should be discontinued if there is a gradual or sudden, partial or complete loss of vision, proptosis or diplopia, papilloedema or any evidence of retinal or vascular lesions.
7. Caution should be observed in prescribing oral contraceptives for any patient with a history of migraine, or if migraine is being treated with vasoconstrictor drugs. If migraine worsens or migraine or severe headache develops for the first time during treatment, medication should be discontinued immediately.
8. A small fraction of the hormonal agents in oral contraceptives has been identified in the milk of mothers receiving these drugs. The long-range effect to the nursing infant is currently unknown.
9. Malignant hepatic tumours have been reported on rare occasions in long-term users of oral contraceptives. Benign hepatic tumours have also been associated with oral contraceptive usage. A hepatic tumour should be considered in the differential diagnosis when upper abdominal pain, enlarged liver or signs of intra-abdominal haemorrhage occur.
10. Numerous epidemiological studies have been reported on the risks of ovarian, endometrial, cervical and breast cancer in women using combined oral contraceptives. The evidence is clear that combined oral contraceptives offer substantial protection against both ovarian and endometrial cancer.

    An increased risk of cervical cancer in long term users of combined oral contraceptives has been reported in some studies, but there continues to be controversy about the extent to which this is attributable to the confounding effects of sexual behaviour and other factors.

    The evidence linking combined oral contraceptive use and breast cancer remains inconclusive. The results of some studies suggest an increased risk of breast cancer presenting below the age of about 35, the risk rising with duration of use. Any possible increased risk of breast cancer with combined oral contraceptives is however likely to be small and may be expected to be less with low dosage pills. This possible risk should be weighed against the many benefits of combined oral contraceptives, including their protective effects against ovarian and endometrial cancers.
11. In breakthrough bleeding or irregular vaginal bleeding, non-functional causes should be borne in mind.
12. The risk of arterial thrombosis associated with combined oral contraceptives increases with age, and this risk is aggravated by cigarette smoking. The use of combined oral contraceptives by women in the older age group, especially those who are cigarette smokers, should therefore be discouraged and alternative methods advised.
13. Examination of the pelvic organs, breasts and blood pressure should precede prescription of an oral contraceptive and should be repeated regularly.
14. Certain conditions require careful observation during treatment with oral contraceptives. These are: a history of depression, varicose veins, diabetes, hypertension, epilepsy, otosclerosis, multiple sclerosis, porphyria, tetany, disturbed liver function, gall-stones, renal diseases, chloasma, uterine fibroids, asthma, the wearing of contact lenses or any condition prone to worsen during pregnancy.

Side-effects: Oral contraceptives produce certain endocrine effects characteristic of ovarian oestrogens and progesterone. The hormones secreted during an ovulatory cycle may produce similar effects including headache, slight weight gain, nausea, breast tenderness, changed libido, depressive moods, and spotting between periods. The overall incidence of such effects with Ovran, Ovran 30 and Ovranette is low and tends to decrease as treatment cycles continue. Cycle control is good and spotting and breakthrough bleeding occur only rarely. Extensive studies on considerable numbers of women taking oral contraceptives indicate some increased risks over non-pregnant women who are not taking oral contraceptives. These include thromboembolism, impaired glucose tolerance and even more rarely, liver dysfunction, hypertension and raised serum lipids.

Drug interactions: Caution should be observed in prescribing oral contraceptives for patients taking other drugs since various interactions have been reported. Pregnancies have been reported in women taking oral contraceptives concurrently with rifampicin and other antibiotics, anti-epileptic drugs, barbiturates and other sedative drugs.

Steroids affect drug metabolism and the therapeutic or toxic effects of other drugs may be modified. Interactions have been reported between oral contraceptives and tricyclic anti-depressants, anticoagulants and corticosteroids.

Overdosage: No reports of serious ill-effects from overdosage with combined oral contraceptives have been reported. In general, therefore, treatment of overdosage is not necessary. If overdosage is, however, discovered within one hour and is so large that treatment seems desirable, gastric lavage or a suitable dose of ipecacuanha can be used. There are no specific antidotes and further treatment should be symptomatic.

Pharmaceutical precautions Store at, or below, room temperature.

Legal category POM.

Package quantities Ovran, Ovran 30, and Ovranette are supplied in memo packs of 21 tablets (OP).

Further information Levonorgestrel is a totally synthetic progestogen which possesses no inherent oestrogenicity. It has anti-oestrogenic properties and has minimal effects on metabolic functions.

Pearl Index: Ovran, 0.19. Ovran 30, 0.13. Ovranette, 0.35.

Product licence numbers

Ovran	0011/0015
Ovran 30	0011/0050
Ovranette	0011/0041

OXAZEPAM TABLETS 10 and 15 mg

Presentation Oxazepam Tablets BP containing 10 or 15 mg oxazepam.

Oxazepam 10 mg tablets are white flat bevel edged tablets 6.5 mm in diameter, marked WYETH on one face and 'WY 012' on the other.

Oxazepam 15 mg tablets are white, flat, bevel edged tablets, 8.0 mm in diameter, marked 'WY 013' on one face and WYETH on the other.

Uses Oxazepam Tablets are recommended for short term use of approximately 2–4 weeks. As with all benzodiazepines doctors should be aware that long-term use may lead to dependence and withdrawal symptoms in certain patients.

Oxazepam is indicated for the short-term treatment of moderate anxiety i.e. anxiety that is disabling or subjecting the individual to unacceptable distress. Oxazepam is also indicated for the short term treatment of anxiety in psychosomatic, organic and psychotic illness and the short term treatment of insomnia associated with anxiety.

Dosage and administration Route of administration: Oral.

In all cases the dosage of Oxazepam should be titrated according to the needs of the individual patient and the lowest effective dose necessary to control symptoms should be used.

Oxazepam should not be used for long term chronic treatment.

Dosage: Adults: Moderate anxiety – one to two 15 mg tablets three (or four) times daily.

Elderly: Elderly patients or those who are particularly sensitive to the effects of benzodiazepines – 10–20 mg three or four times daily.

Insomnia: Most patients need a dose of 15–25 mg but some patients may need up to 50 mg. The dose should be taken 1 hour before retiring.

Children: Oxazepam is not recommended for the treatment of children.

All patients taking Oxazepam should be carefully monitored and routine repeat prescriptions should be avoided. Treatment in all patients should be withdrawn gradually with careful monitoring and reassessment to minimise possible withdrawal symptoms. Patients who have taken benzodiazepines for a long time may require a longer period during which doses are reduced. Should longer term therapy be necessary then intermittent treatment may be considered to minimise the risk of dependence.

Contra-indications, warnings, etc

Contra-indications:

1. Oxazepam should not be given to patients with a previous history of sensitivity to benzodiazepines.
2. Acute pulmonary insufficiency.

Use in pregnancy: Safety for use in pregnancy has not been established. Oxazepam should not be administered during pregnancy or lactation unless in the judgment of the physician such administration is clinically justifiable. Oxazepam is not recommended for use in the first three months of pregnancy. Use during the late phase of pregnancy or at delivery may require ventilation of the infant at birth.

Precautions and warnings:

1. Concomitant administration with central nervous system depressants, including alcohol, general anaesthetics, narcotic analgesics, monoamine oxidase inhibitors and antidepressants will result in an accentuation of their effects.

2. When used at the appropriate recommended dose for short term treatment of anxiety the dependence potential of oxazepam is low. However, the risk of dependence increases with higher doses and longer-term use and is further increased in patients with a history of alcoholism, drug abuse or in patients with marked personality disorders.

Symptoms such as anxiety, depression, headache, insomnia, tension and sweating have been reported following abrupt discontinuation of benzodiazepines and these symptoms may be difficult to distinguish from the original symptoms of anxiety. Other symptoms such as persistent tinnitus, involuntary movements, paraesthesia, perceptual changes, confusion, convulsions, abdominal and muscle cramps and vomiting may be characteristic of benzodiazepine withdrawal syndrome.

3. As with other drugs acting on the central nervous system, patients should be cautioned against driving or operating machinery until it is established that they do not become dizzy or drowsy while taking oxazepam.

4. The use of benzodiazepines may release suicidal tendencies in depressed patients. Oxazepam should not be used alone to treat depression, anxiety associated with depression, or psychotic illness. Other rarely reported behavioural effects of the benzodiazepines include paradoxical aggressive outbursts, excitement, hallucinations and confusion. Amnesia may occur and in cases of loss or bereavement psychological adjustment may be inhibited by benzodiazepines.

5. Oxazepam should not be used in labour unless considered essential. High single doses or repeated low doses of other benzodiazepines have been reported to produce hypotonia, poor sucking and hypotension in the neonate and irregularities in the foetal heart.

6. Caution should be observed in using oxazepam in chronic pulmonary insufficiency.

7. The pharmacokinetics of oxazepam in patients with liver disease differs little from that in normal subjects but caution should be observed in patients with liver damage. Oxazepam is conjugated in the liver.

Side-effects: Transient mild drowsiness is commonly seen in the first few days of therapy. If it becomes troublesome dosage should be reduced. In a few cases dizziness, ataxia, vertigo, headache and syncope have occurred either alone or with drowsiness; occasionally hypotension has occurred. Blurred vision, disorientation and fever have also been observed on occasion. Mild excitatory effects with stimulation of affect have sometimes been reported in psychiatric patients; these reactions usually appear in the first two weeks of therapy.

Other side effects include rare cases of minor diffuse skin rashes (morbilliform, urticarial and maculopapular), altered libido, nausea, lethargy, oedema, slurred speech and tremor. Blood dyscrasias, increased liver enzymes, jaundice and leukopenia have been rarely reported.

Overdosage: As with other benzodiazepines, overdosage should not present a threat to life unless combined with other CNS depressants (including alcohol). General supportive measures should be used.

Treatment is symptomatic and gastric lavage may be of use if performed shortly after ingestion. The patient is likely to sleep and a clear airway should be maintained.

Pharmaceutical precautions Store in a cool, dry place.

Legal category CD (Sch 4), POM.

Package quantities Oxazepam Tablets 10 mg and 15 mg – Packs of 100.

Further information Oxazepam may offer advantages in the treatment of the elderly because of its short half-life and lack of accumulation.

Oxazepam is a short-acting benzodiazepine. It is metabolised by a simple one-step process to a pharmacologically inert glucuronide. There are no major active metabolites. The elimination half-life is 6–8 hours and there is minimal risk of excessive accumulation.

The risk of benzodiazepine related dependence may be minimised by adopting the following guidelines for treatment:

1. Select patients carefully taking into account the precautions and warnings stated in this data sheet.
2. Adopt short-term or intermittent therapy.
3. Use lowest dose possible to achieve effective treatment.
4. Review treatment regularly; and especially before repeating prescriptions.
5. Discontinue treatment gradually taking into account patient reaction at each stage, i.e. 'titrate downwards'.

Product licence numbers
Oxazepam Tablets 10 mg 0011/0110
Oxazepam Tablets 15 mg 0011/0111

PENIDURAL* (ORAL)

Presentation Penidural Oral Suspension is a smooth, pink suspension with a sweet cherry flavour. Each 5 ml dose contains: 229 mg Benzathine Penicillin BP (equivalent to 300,000 units Penicillin G).

Penidural Oral Drops is a smooth pink suspension with a sweet cherry flavour. Each 1 ml contains 115 mg Benzathine Penicillin BP (equivalent to 150,000 units Penicillin G).

Uses Penidural Oral presentations are indicated for the treatment of mild to moderately severe penicillin-sensitive infections and prophylaxis of penicillin-sensitive secondary infections especially in children.

Dosage and administration *Route of administration:* Oral.

Dosage: Benzathine penicillin is a repository penicillin which gives effective blood levels for a long period, six- to eight-hourly dosage being adequate in most patients.

Penidural oral suspension: Adults: Two 5 ml doses three to four times daily.

Elderly: The adult dosage schedule may be used in the elderly.

Children: One 5 ml dose three to four times daily.

Penidural oral drops: Adults: Not recommended.

Children: up to 5 years of age: 1 or 2 dropperfuls three or four times daily. Each dropperful contains the equivalent of 100,000 units of Penicillin G.

Contra-indications, warnings, etc
Contra-indications: Benzathine penicillin is contra-indicated in patients with a previous history of penicillin hypersensitivity and in small babies whose mothers have such a history.

Precautions and warnings: 1. Prolonged use of an antibiotic may result in the development of super infection due to organisms resistant to that antibiotic.

2. Penidural oral suspension should not be administered during pregnancy or lactation unless in the judgement of the physician such administration is clinically justifiable. Special care should be taken in the first three months of pregnancy.

3. High doses of Penidural should be used with caution in patients with renal failure.

Interactions with other medicaments: Concurrent administration of penicillin and probenecid results in higher and more sustained serum antibiotic levels.

Side-effects: Pencillin may cause an acute anaphylactic reaction which can be fatal. This reaction appears to occur more frequently in patients with bronchial asthma or other allergic disorders. Reactions have been reported after the use of all forms of penicillin by all routes of administration but are less likely after oral penicillin because of slower absorption.

Penidural is otherwise virtually free from side-effects apart from occasional loose stools or borborygmi.

Pharmaceutical precautions *Penidural Oral Suspension:* Store in a cool place. Where necessary dispense Penidural Oral Suspension into suitable well-closed glass bottles. When required Penidural Oral Suspension may be diluted with Syrup BP (unpreserved or preserved with parahydroxybenzoates).

Penidural Oral Drops: Store in a cool place.

Legal category POM.

Package quantities Penidural Oral Suspension: Bottles of 100 ml (OP).

Penidural Oral Drops: Bottles of 10 ml (OP).

Further information Nil.

Product licence numbers
Suspension 0011/5019R
Drops 0011/5018R

PREMARIN* TABLETS

Presentation Premarin Tablets contain natural conjugated oestrogens.

Premarin Tablets 0.625 mg are maroon, oval, sugar-coated tablets.

Premarin Tablets 1.25 mg are yellow, oval, sugar-coated tablets.

Premarin Tablets 2.5 mg are purple, oval, sugar-coated tablets.

Uses Menopausal and post-menopausal oestrogen replacement therapy for vasomotor symptoms (sweating, flushes) and allied disorders such as post-menopausal osteoporosis, atrophic vaginitis, kraurosis vulvae, atrophic urethritis. Palliation of selected cases of breast cancer in women.

Dosage and administration *Menopausal and post-menopausal oestrogen deficiency:* Premarin 0.625–1.25 mg daily is the usual starting dose. Cyclic administration is recommended (three weeks' on followed by one week off). For maintenance the lowest effective dose should be used. If the patient has not menstruated within the last two months or more, cyclic administration is started arbitrarily. If the patient is menstruating, cyclic administration is started on day five of bleeding.

In women with an intact uterus and in particular in women with obesity, diabetes, low parity or a familial history of endometrial carcinoma, for whom hormone replacement therapy is required, the addition of a progestogen for 10–12 days per cycle is essential.

Before therapy commences it is recommended that the patient is fully informed of all the relative risks and benefits, and the question of continued need of treatment should be reviewed periodically. She should have a complete physical and gynaecological examination, including customary biochemical tests and special emphasis on blood pressure, breasts, abdomen and pelvic organs, including endometrial assessment, whenever possible. Regular follow-up examinations, including endometrial assessments, where possible, are recommended every 6–12 months. Any breakthrough bleeding is an indication for endometrial evaluation. Endometrial hyperplasia may persist following oestrogen therapy. Therefore, surveillance for bleeding is necessary.

Atrophic vaginitis, kraurosis vulvae and atrophic urethritis: Cyclically 0.625–1.25 mg daily depending on the response of the individual patient.

Post-menopausal osteoporosis: Cyclically 0.625–1.25 mg daily.

Breast cancer: In selected cases of mammary cancer oestrogens may be used for palliation in women who are at least five years post-menopausal. The suggested dose of Premarin is up to 10 mg three times a day for a period of at least three months.

Elderly: There are no special dosage requirements for elderly patients but as with all medicines the lowest effective dose should be used.

Children: Not recommended.

Contra-indications, warnings, etc

Contra-indications:

1. A history of, known or suspected cancer of the breast except in appropriately selected patients being treated for metastatic disease.
2. A history of, known or suspected oestrogen-dependent neoplasia.
3. Undiagnosed abnormal genital bleeding.
4. A history of, or active, thrombophlebitis, thrombosis or thromboembolic disorders especially when associated with previous oestrogen use (except when used in treatment of breast malignancy).
5. Acute or chronic liver disease or history of liver disease where the liver function tests have failed to return to normal. Rotor syndrome or Dubin-Johnson syndrome.
6. Severe cardiac or renal disease.

Use in pregnancy and lactation: Premarin Tablets should not be used in the event of known or suspected pregnancy. It is not known whether this drug is excreted in human milk. Many drugs are excreted in human milk, and therefore caution should be exercised when Premarin Tablets are administered to a nursing mother.

Warnings

1. In the female there is an increased risk of endometrial carcinoma associated with oestrogen administered long-term (for more than one year); the greatest risk appears to be associated with use over five years or more. However, the addition of a progestogen to an oestrogen regimen lowers the incidence of endometrial hyperplasia and cancer.

Animal data appear to indicate that there is a need for caution in prescribing oestrogens for women with a strong family history of breast cancer or who have breast nodules, fibrocystic disease or abnormal mammograms.

2. It has been reported that there is an increase in the risk of surgically confirmed gallbladder disease in women receiving postmenopausal oestrogens.
3. The increased risk of hypertension with oestrogen use is minimal in menopausal women. When oestrogens are administered, however, to patients with hypertension supervision is necessary and blood pressure should be monitored at regular intervals. As with oral contraceptives, blood pressure returns to normal on discontinuing the drug.
4. A worsening of glucose tolerance has been observed in patients on oestrogen containing oral contraceptives. For this reason, diabetic patients should be carefully observed while receiving oestrogen.
5. Administration of oestrogens may lead to hypercalcaemia in patients with breast cancer and bone metastases. If this occurs, the drug should be stopped and appropriate measures taken to reduce the calcium level.
6. Users of oral contraceptives have an increased risk of thrombophlebitis, pulmonary embolism, stroke, myocardial infarction and other thombotic vascular diseases, hepatic tumours, glucose intolerance and mental depression. These are questionable in the postmenopausal woman on oestrogen replacement therapy at the currently recommended low dosages but this does not rule out such possibility, particularly in sub-groups of women who have underlying risk factors or when large doses are used to treat cancer of the breast. They should be used with caution in patients with cerebral vascular or coronary artery disease and only for those in whom oestrogens are clearly needed.

Consideration should be given also to discontinue treatment at least four weeks prior to surgery if this entails a risk of thrombosis, or during periods of prolonged immobilisation.

Precautions

1. Oestrogens may cause fluid retention, therefore patients with epilepsy, migraine, asthma, and renal or cardiac dysfunction should be carefully observed.
2. Diseases that are known to be subject to deterioration during pregnancy (e.g. multiple sclerosis, epilepsy, porphyria, tetany and otosclerosis) should be carefully observed during treatment.
3. If jaundice or thrombosis develops in any patient receiving oestrogen, the medication should be discontinued while the cause is investigated.
4. Women of child-bearing potential should be advised to ahere to non-hormonal contraceptive methods.
5. Pre-existing uterine leiomyomata may increase in size during oestrogen therapy and symptoms associated with endometriosis may be exacerbated.
6. Since oestrogens influence the metabolism of calcium and phosphorus, they should be used with caution in patients with metabolic bone diseases that are associated with hypercalcaemia or in patients with renal insufficiency.
7. As larger doses of oestrogen may increase thyroid binding globulin leading to increased circulating total thyroid hormone, care should be taken in providing oestrogens for patients with thyrotoxicosis.
8. Larger doses of oestrogen may affect certain endocrine, liver function and coagulation tests.
9. Because of the effects of oestrogens on epiphyseal closure, they should be used judiciously in young patients in whom bone growth is not complete.
10. There is limited experience in the use of Premarin Tablets in children (e.g. Turner's Syndrome). If used in such cases the risk to benefit ratio must be considered. Doses lower than those recommended for adults should be used.

Side-effects: The following additional side-effects have been reported with oestrogenic therapy, including oral contraceptives:

1. Genitourinary system – breakthrough bleeding, spotting, change in menstrual flow, dysmenorrhoea, premenstrual-like syndrome, amenorrhoea during and after treatment, increase in size of uterine fibromyomata, vaginal candidiasis, change in cervical erosion and in degree of cervical secretion, cystitis-like syndrome.
2. Breasts – tenderness, enlargement, secretion.
3. Gastrointestinal – nausea, vomiting, abdominal cramps, bloating, cholestatic jaundice.
4. Skin – chloasma or melasma which may persist when drug is discontinued, erythema multiforme, erythema nodosum, haemorrhagic eruption, loss of scalp hair, hirsuitism.
5. Eyes – steepening of corneal curvature, intolerance to contact lenses.
6. CNS – headaches, migraine, dizziness, mental depression, chorea.
7. Miscellaneous – increase or decrease in weight, reduced carbohydrate tolerance, aggravation of porphyria, oedema, changes in libido.

Acute overdosage: Numerous reports of ingestion of large doses of oestrogen-containing oral contraceptives by young children indicate that acute serious ill effects do not occur. Overdosages of oestrogen may cause nausea, and withdrawal bleeding may occur in females.

Pharmaceutical precautions No special requirements for storage are necessary.

Legal category POM.

Package quantities

Premarin 0.625 mg: Blister packs of 21 (OP) and Securitainers of 100.

Premarin 1.25 mg: Blister packs of 21 (OP) and Securitainers of 100.

Premarin 2.5 mg: Securitainers of 100.

Further information Nil.

Product licence numbers

Premarin Tablets 2.5 mg	0607/0002
Premarin Tablets 1.25 mg	0607/5001
Premarin Tablets 0.625 mg	0607/5000

Product licence holder: Ayerst Laboratories Ltd.

PREMARIN* VAGINAL CREAM

Presentation Premarin Vaginal Cream contains 0.625 mg per gram of conjugated oestrogens in a non-liquefying base.

Uses For the short-term treatment of atrophic vaginitis, postmenopausal atrophic urethritis and kraurosis vulvae.

Dosage and administration The usual recommended dose is 1 to 2 g daily administered intravaginally or topically, depending on the severity of the condition. Administration should be cyclic (e.g. three weeks on and one week off). It should start on the fifth day of bleeding in the patient who is menstruating and arbitrarily if not.

The lowest effective dose which will control symptoms should be used and the need for continuing treatment should be reviewed periodically. Should long-term therapy be considered, an oral progestogen for 10–12 days at the end of each cycle is essential.

Before therapy commences it is recommended that the patient is fully informed of all the relative risks and benefits. She should have a complete physical and gynaecological examination, including customary biochemical tests with special emphasis on blood pressure, breasts, abdomen and pelvic organs, including endometrial assessment, whenever possible. Regular follow-up examinations where possible, are recommended. Any break-through bleeding is an indication for endometrial evaluation.

Elderly: There are no special dosage requirements for elderly patients, but as with all medicines, the lowest effective dose should be used.

Children: Not recommended.

Contra-indications, warnings, etc
Contra-indications:

1. A history of, known or suspected cancer of the breast except in appropriately selected patients being treated for metastatic disease.
2. A history of, known or suspected oestrogen-dependent neoplasia.
3. Undiagnosed abnormal genital bleeding.
4. A history of, or active, thrombophlebitis, thrombosis or thromboembolic disorders, especially when associated with previous oestrogen use (except when used in treatment of breast malignancy).
5. Acute or chronic liver disease or history of liver disease where the liver function tests have failed to return to normal. Rotor syndrome or Dubin-Johnson syndrome.
6. Severe cardiac or renal disease.

Use in pregnancy and lactation: Premarin Vaginal Cream should not be used in the event of known or suspected pregnancy. It is not known whether this drug is excreted in human milk. Many drugs are excreted in human milk, and therefore caution should be exercised when Premarin Vaginal Cream is administered to a nursing mother.

Due to oestrogen absorption following the application of Premarin Vaginal Cream, prolonged administration might result in systemic effects. Therefore, the following warnings and precautions should be considered.

Warnings

1. There is an increased risk of endometrial carcinoma associated with oestrogen administered long-term (for more than one year); the greatest risk appears to be associated with use over five years or more. However, the addition of a progestogen to an oestrogen regimen lowers the incidence of endometrial hyperplasia and cancer.

Animal data appear to indicate that there is need for caution in prescribing oestrogens for women with a strong family history of breast cancer or who have breast nodules, fibrocystic disease or abnormal mammograms.

2. It has been reported that there is an increase in the risk of surgically confirmed gallbladder disease in women receiving postmenopausal oestrogens.
3. The increased risk of hypertension with oestrogen use is minimal in menopausal women. When oestrogens are administered, however, to patients with hypertension supervision is necessary and blood pressure should be monitored at regular intervals. As with oral contraceptives, blood pressure returns to normal on discontinuing the drug.
4. A worsening of glucose tolerance has been observed in patients on oestrogen containing oral contraceptives. For this reason, diabetic patients should be carefully observed while receiving oestrogen therapy.
5. Administration of oestrogens may lead to hypercalcaemia in patients with breast cancer and bone metastases. If this occurs, the drug should be stopped and appropriate measures taken to reduce the calcium level.
6. Users of oral contraceptives have an increased risk of thrombophlebitis, pulmonary embolism, stroke, myocardial infarction and other thrombotic vascular diseases, hepatic tumours, glucose intolerance and mental depression. These are questionable in the postmenopausal woman on oestrogen replacement therapy at the currently recommended low dosages but this does not rule out such possibility, particularly in sub-groups of women who have underlying risk factors or when large doses are used to treat cancer of the breast. They should be used with caution in patients with cerebral vascular or coronary artery disease and only in those in whom oestrogen therapy is clearly needed.

Consideration should be given also to discontinue treatment at least four weeks prior to surgery if this entails a risk of thrombosis, or during periods of prolonged immobilisation.

Precautions

1. Oestrogen therapy may cause fluid retention, therefore patients with epilepsy, migraine, asthma, and renal or cardiac dysfunction should be carefully observed.
2. Diseases that are known to be subject to deterioration during pregnancy (e.g. multiple sclerosis, epilepsy, porphyria, tetany and otosclerosis) should be carefully observed during treatment.
3. If jaundice or thrombosis develops in a patient receiving oestrogen, the medication should be discontinued while the cause is investigated.
4. Women of child-bearing potential should be advised to adhere to non-hormonal contraceptive methods.
5. Pre-existing uterine leiomyomata may increase in size during oestrogen therapy and symptoms associated with endometriosis may be exacerbated.
6. Since oestrogens influence the metabolism of calcium and phosphorous, they should be used with caution in patients with metabolic bone diseases that are associated with hypercalcaemia or in patients with renal insufficiency.
7. As larger doses of oestrogen may increase thyroid binding globulin leading to increased circulating total thyroid hormone, care should be taken in providing oestrogens for patients with thyrotoxicosis.
8. Larger doses of oestrogen may affect certain endocrine, liver function and coagulation tests.
9. Because of the effects of oestrogens on epiphyseal closure, they should be used judiciously in young patients in whom bone growth is not complete.

Side-effects: The following additional side-effects have been reported with oestrogenic therapy including oral contraceptives:

1. Genitourinary system – breakthrough bleeding, spotting, change in menstrual flow, dysmenorrhoea, premenstrual-like syndrome, amenorrhoea during and after treatment, increase in size of uterine fibromyomata, vaginal candidiasis, change in cervical erosion and in degree of cervical secretion, cystitis-like syndrome.
2. Breasts – tenderness, enlargement, secretion.
3. Gastrointestinal – nausea, vomiting, abdominal cramps, bloating, cholestatic jaundice.
4. Skin – chloasma or melasma which may persist when drug is discontinued, erythema multiforme, erythema nodosum, haemorrhagic eruption, loss of scalp hair, hirsutism.
5. Eyes – steepening of corneal curvature, intolerance to contact lenses.
6. CNS – headaches, migraine, dizziness, mental depression, chorea.
7. Miscellaneous – Increase or decrease in weight, reduced carbohydrate tolerance, aggravation of porphyria, oedema, changes in libido.

Acute overdosage: Numerous reports of ingestion of large doses of oestrogen-containing oral contraceptives by young children indicate that acute serious ill effects do not occur. Overdosage of oestrogen may cause nausea, and withdrawal bleeding may occur in females.

Pharmaceutical precautions Store at room temperature (approximately 25°C).

Legal category POM.

Package quantities Each pack contains 42.5 g of the non-liquefying cream with one calibrated applicator (OP).

Further information Nil.

Product licence number 0011/0163.

PREMPAK*-C

Presentation Prempak-C 0.625 consists of 28 maroon tablets containing natural conjugated oestrogens 0.625 mg plus 12 light brown tablets containing norgestrel 0.15 mg.

Prempak-C 1.25 consists of 28 yellow tablets containing natural conjugated oestrogens 1.25 mg plus 12 light brown tablets containing norgestrel 0.15 mg.

Uses Menopausal and postmenopausal oestrogen replacement therapy for vasomotor symptoms (sweating, flushes) and allied disorders such as postmenopausal osteoporosis, atrophic vaginitis, kraurosis vulvae, atrophic urethritis.

Dosage and administration
Menopausal and postmenopausal oestrogen deficiency: Oestrogen 0.625 mg or 1.25 mg daily. One norgestrel tablet should be taken daily from day 17 to day 28 of oestrogen therapy. Oestrogen administration is continued without a break in therapy. Therapy may be initiated with either dose depending upon severity of symptoms: for maintenance, the lowest effective dose is recommended. Therapy may be commenced arbitrarily although, if the patient is menstruating regularly, commencement on first day of bleeding may be preferred.

In women with an intact uterus, and in particular in women with obesity, diabetes, low parity or a familial history of endometrial carcinoma, for whom hormone replacement therapy is required, Prempak-C should be considered in preference to unopposed oestrogen therapy. Prempak-C provides both oestrogens and a progestogen to avoid endometrial hyperstimulation. This also provides a form of cycle regulation in women who are still menstruating but irregularly.

Before therapy commences it is recommended that the patient is fully informed of all the relative risks and benefits, and the question of continued need of treatment should be reviewed periodically. She should have a complete physical and gynaecological examination, including customary biochemical tests and special emphasis on blood pressure, breasts, abdomen and pelvic organs, including endometrial assessment, where necessary. Regular follow-up examinations are recommended every 6–12 months. Any breakthrough bleeding is an indication for endometrial evaluation.

Elderly: There are no special dosage requirements for elderly patients, but as with all medicines, the lowest effective dose should be used.

Children: Not recommended.

Contra-indications, warnings, etc
Contra-indications:

1. Known or suspected pregnancy.
2. A history of, known or suspected cancer of the breast except in appropriately selected patients being treated for metastatic disease.
3. A history of, known or suspected oestrogen-dependent neoplasia.
4. Undiagnosed abnormal genital bleeding.
5. A history of, or active, thrombophlebitis, thrombosis or thromboembolic disorders (including coronary thrombosis, cerebrovascular accident, etc.), especially when associated with previous oestrogen use (except when used in treatment of breast or prostatic malignancy).
6. Acute or chronic liver disease or history of liver disease where the liver function tests have failed to return to normal. Rotor syndrome or Dubin-Johnson syndrome.
7. Severe cardiac or renal disease.

Precautions: Animal data appear to indicate that there is a need for caution in prescribing oestrogens for women with a strong family history of breast cancer or who have breast nodules, fibrocystic disease or abnormal mammograms.

Women who in the past received large doses of diethystilboestrol (DES) during pregnancy may be at increased risk for development of breast cancer. It is recommended that post-menopausal oestrogen replacement be used in these patients only for severe menopausal symptoms uncontrolled by other means and exposure to oestrogens be as short as possible. For women exposed to DES *in utero*, it is also recommended that oestrogen use be kept to a minimum.

It has been reported that there is an increase in the risk of surgically confirmed gallbladder disease in women receiving postmenopausal oestrogens.

When oestrogens are administered to patients with hypertension, supervision is necessary and blood pressure should be monitored at regular intervals. The increased risk of hypertension with oestrogen use is minimal in menopausal women. As with oral contraceptives, blood pressure returns to normal on discontinuing the drug.

Oestrogens may cause fluid retention, therefore patients with epilepsy, migraine, asthma, renal or cardiac dysfunction should be carefully observed.

Diseases that are known to be subject to deterioration during pregnancy (e.g. multiple sclerosis, epilepsy, porphyria, tetany and otosclerosis) should be carefully observed during treatment.

In a diabetic patient insulin requirement may be altered.

Consideration should be given to discontinue treatment at least four weeks prior to surgery if this entails a risk of thrombosis, or during periods of prolonged immobilisation.

If jaundice or thrombosis develops in any patients receiving oestrogen, the medication should be discontinued while the cause is investigated.

Oestrogen should be used with caution in patients with cerebral vascular or coronary artery disease.

Prempak-C is not an oral contraceptive, neither will it restore fertility. Women of child-bearing potential should be advised to adhere to non-hormonal contraceptive methods.

Endometriosis.

Since oestrogens influence the metabolism of calcium and phosphorus, they should be used with caution in patients with metabolic bone diseases that are associated with hypercalcaemia or in patients with renal insufficiency.

As larger doses of oestrogen may increase thyroid binding globulin leading to increased circulating total thyroid hormone, care should be taken in providing oestrogens for patients with thyrotoxicosis.

Changed oestrogen levels may theoretically affect certain endocrine and liver function tests.

There is the possibility that oestrogen and progestogen oral contraceptives may be associated with thromboembolic disease, benign and malignant hepatic neoplasms, glucose intolerance and mental depression, and that they may also occur following administration of natural oestrogens, particularly at high doses. This is questionable in the postmenopausal woman on oestrogen replacement therapy at the currently recommended low dosages. Similarly oral contraceptive use has been associated with an increased risk for non-fatal myocardial infarction in otherwise healthy women between the ages of 39 and 45 who smoke.

Side-effects: The following additional side-effects have been reported with oestrogen/progestogen therapy, including oral contraceptives but not necessarily with Prempak-C.

1. Genitourinary system – breakthrough bleeding,

spotting, change in menstrual flow, dysmenorrhoea, premenstrual-like syndrome, amenorrhoea during and after treatment, increase in size of uterine fibromyomata, vaginal candidiasis, change in cervical erosion and in degree of cervical secretion, cystitis-like syndrome.

2. Breasts – tenderness, enlargement, secretion.

3. Gastrointestinal – nausea, vomiting, abdominal cramps, bloating, cholestatic jaundice.

4. Skin – chloasma or melasma which may persist when drug is discontinued, erythema multiforme, erythema nodosum, haemorrhagic eruption, loss of scalp hair, hirsutism.

5. Eyes – steepening of corneal curvature, intolerance to contact lenses.

6. CNS – headaches, migraine, dizziness, mental depression, chorea.

7. Miscellaneous – increase or decrease in weight, reduced carbohydrate tolerance, aggravation of porphyria, oedema, changes in libido.

Acute overdosage: Numerous reports of ingestion of large doses of oestrogen-containing oral contraceptives by young children indicate that acute serious ill effects do not occur. Overdosage of oestrogen may cause nausea, and withdrawal bleeding may occur in females.

Pharmaceutical precautions No special requirements for storage are necessary.

Legal category POM.

Package quantities Blister strip of 28 oestrogen tablets 0.625 mg or 1.25 mg plus 12 norgestrel tablets 0.15 mg. There is also a triple pack of each strength containing 3 strips as above (OP).

Further information Prempak-C provides oestrogen/progestogen therapy for the menopausal syndrome and associated disorders. The blister strip contains 28 oestrogen tablets. From day 17 to day 28 inclusive each bubble contains in addition one norgestrel 0.15 mg tablet. The two tablets should be taken together for these twelve days. The specially designed pack avoids the use of tablets containing more than one active compound.

Product licence numbers
Prempak-C 0.625 0607/0053
Prempak-C 1.25 0607/0054

Product licence holder: Ayerst Laboratories Ltd.

SPARINE* SUSPENSION

Presentation Each 5 ml suspension contains promazine embonate equivalent to 50 mg Promazine Hydrochloride BP presented as a yellow suspension with an odour of pineapple.

Uses 1. As an adjunct to the short term management of moderate to severe psychomotor agitation.

2. Agitation and restlessness in the elderly.

Dosage and administration *Route of administration:* Oral.

Dosage: Psychomotor agitation: Adults: 100–200 mg four times daily.

Elderly: Half the normal dose may be sufficient for a therapeutic response in elderly patients.

Agitation and restlessness: Elderly: 25 mg initially. Increase if necessary up to 50 mg four times daily.

Children: Sparine Suspension is not recommended for children.

Contra-indications, warnings, etc
Contra-indications: 1. Use in patients hypersensitive to the active ingredient or other phenothiazines.

2. Sparine should not be used during lactation.

3. *Use in pregnancy:* Do not use during pregnancy, especially during the first three months, unless there are compelling reasons. There is insufficient evidence of the safety of promazine in human pregnancy nor is there evidence from animal studies that it is free from hazard.

Precautions and warnings:

1. Phenothiazines should only be used with great caution in patients with a history of jaundice or with existent liver dysfunction, or blood dyscrasias, coronary insufficiency or cardiac disease.

2. Respiratory depression may occur in patients with severe respiratory disease.

3. Promazine should be used with caution in patients with renal failure.

4. Patients receiving phenothiazines over a prolonged period require regular and careful surveillance with particular attention to potential for inducing eye changes, effects on haemopoiesis, liver dysfunction, myocardial conduction effects, particularly if other concurrently administered drugs also have potential effects on these systems.

5. Phenothiazines may impair alertness and induce drowsiness especially at the start of treatment. Persons taking these drugs should not drive or operate machinery unless the drug has been shown not to interfere with physical or mental ability.

6. Use of phenothiazines at high (relative or absolute) doses may induce extrapyramidal side-effects, dyskinesia, akathisia, dystonia. These are likely to be particularly severe in children. Caution should be exercised in patients with Parkinson's disease. Anti-Parkinson agents should not be prescribed routinely because of the risk of aggravating anticholinergic side-effects of promazine, of precipitating toxic-confusional states or of impairing its therapeutic efficacy. They should be given only as required.

7. Prolonged administration of phenothiazines may result in persistent or tardive dyskinesias particularly in the elderly.

8. Care should be exercised if Sparine is used for the treatment of patients with cerebral arteriosclerosis, coronary heart disease or other conditions in which a fall in blood pressure might be undesirable.

9. Caution should be observed with patients suffering from epilepsy or conditions predisposing to epilepsy.

10. Personal or family history of narrow angle glaucoma.

11. Phenothiazines may impair body temperature regulation. Caution should be observed in very hot weather.

12. Hypothyroidism.

13. Myasthenia gravis.

14. Phaeochromocytoma.

15. Prostatic hypertrophy.

16. Antipsychotic drugs may increase prolactin secretion.

17. Sparine suspension is formulated with aluminium hydroxide which may complex tetracyclines if given concomitantly.

18. *Drug interactions:* The concomitant administration of this product with other medication such as central nervous system depressants (including alcohol and anaesthetics) or antihypertensives, anticholinergic or dopaminergic drugs will result in accentuation of their effects, while potentiation of action will also occur with monoamine oxidase inhibitors, antidepressants and analgesics. Promazine may impair the effects of anticonvulsants.

Promazine may affect the control of diabetes. Undesirable anti-cholinergic effects can be enhanced by anti-Parkinson or other anticholinergic drugs.

Side-effects: Sparine is a member of the phenothiazine group of drugs and the side-effects associated with that group have been noted. These include drowsiness, sedation, dry mouth, nasal stuffiness. Other possible anticholinergic side-effects are blurred vision, tachycardia, constipation and urinary hesitancy or retention when due to enlarged prostate.

Confusional states, or epileptic fits can occur. Sexual function may be impaired. Agranulocytosis and transient leucopenia have rarely been reported. Allergic skin reactions have also been reported.

Promazine rarely causes obstructive jaundice associated with stasis in biliary canaliculi. Promazine treatment should be withdrawn and not given again. Transient abnormalities of liver function tests may occur without jaundice.

Some individuals may be susceptible to the drug in low dosage and show paradoxical effects of excitement, agitation, or insomnia and other minor side effects.

The elderly are particularly susceptible to side-effects of promazine, especially to the sedative, hypotensive and temperature regulation effects. These effects may be dose related.

Treatment of overdosages: Ingestion of large amounts of promazine is followed by deep sleep, with or without a pronounced fall in blood pressure and without particular change in respiration rate, other than the slowing attendant upon sedation. Occasionally an initial period of excitement may precede coma, followed by grand mal seizures.

In the absence of any specific antidote, treatment should be based on ordinary therapeutic principles with special emphasis on the following measures: (1) gastric lavage; (2) treat convulsions if present; (3) correction of acute hypotension if necessary; (4) counteraction of the effects of an excess of promazine hydrochloride on the central nervous system; (5) control and natural recovery of hypothermia.

Pharmaceutical precautions Store Sparine Suspension in a cool place and protect from light. When required Sparine Suspension may be diluted with Syrup BP (unpreserved or preserved with p-hydroxybenzoates).

Legal category POM.

Package quantities Bottles of 150 ml (OP) and 1 litre.

Further information Nil.

Product licence number 0011/5045R.

SPARINE* (PARENTERAL)

Presentation Sparine injection is a clear, colourless aqueous solution containing 50 mg Promazine Hydrochloride BP per millilitre.

Uses 1. As an adjunct to the short term management of moderate to severe psychomotor agitation.

2. Agitation and restlessness in the elderly.
3. Intractable hiccup.
4. Alleviation of nausea and vomiting, including that in labour.
5. Investigations in children, including cardiac and EEG examinations.

Dosage and administration *Route of administration:* Parenteral.

Dosage: Adults: Psychomotor agitation, 50 mg Sparine intramuscularly. Repeat if necessary after six to eight hours.

Intractable hiccup, 50 mg intramuscularly. Repeat if necessary with doses up to 100 mg 4 hourly. The daily dose should not exceed 1 g.

Labour, 50 mg Sparine intramuscularly. For convenience 50 mg Sparine may be mixed with 50 mg pethidine in the same syringe.

Elderly: Half the normal dose may be sufficient for a therapeutic response in elderly subjects.

Children: 0.7 mg/kg intramuscularly.

If Sparine is injected intravenously it should be diluted with an equal volume of saline.

Contra-indications, warnings, etc
Contra-indications: 1. Use in patients in coma.

2. Use in patients hypersensitive to the active ingredient or other phenothiazines.
3. Sparine should not be used during lactation.
4. *Use in pregnancy.* Do not use during pregnancy, especially during the first three months, unless there are compelling reasons. There is insufficient evidence of the safety of promazine in human pregnancy nor is there evidence from animal studies that it is free from hazard.

Precautions and warnings:

1. Phenothiazines should only be used with great caution in patients with a history of jaundice or with existent liver dysfunction, or blood dyscrasias, coronary insufficiency or cardiac disease.
2. Respiratory depression may occur in patients with severe respiratory disease.
3. Promazine should be used with caution in patients with renal failure.
4. Patients receiving phenothiazines over a prolonged period require regular and careful surveillance with particular attention to potential for inducing eye changes, effects on haemopoiesis, liver dysfunction, myocardial conduction effects, particularly if other concurrently administered drugs also have potential effects on these systems.
5. Phenothiazines may impair alertness and induce drowsiness, especially at the start of treatment. Persons taking these drugs should not drive or operate machinery unless the drug has been shown not to interfere with physical or mental ability.
6. Use of phenothiazines at high (relative or absolute) doses may induce extrapyramidal side-effects, dyskinesia, akathisia, dystonia. These are likely to be particularly severe in children. Caution should be exercised in patients with Parkinson's disease. Anti-Parkinson agents should not be prescribed routinely because of the risk of aggravating anticholinergic side-effects of promazine, of precipitating toxic-confusional states or of impairing its therapeutic efficacy. They should be given only as required.
7. Prolonged administration of phenothiazines may result in persistent or tardive dyskinesias particularly in the elderly.
8. Administration by the intravenous route may induce local vascular spasm or thrombophlebitis. The preparation must be diluted before use. Arteriolar spasm and gangrene have been reported following accidental intra-arterial injection of high concentrations.
9. Care should be exercised if Sparine is used for the treatment of patients with cerebral arteriosclerosis, coronary heart disease or other conditions in which a fall in blood pressure might be undesirable.
10. Caution should be observed with patients suffering from epilepsy or conditions predisposing to epilepsy.
11. Personal or family history of narrow angle glaucoma.
12. Phenothiazines may impair body temperature regulation. Caution should be observed in very hot weather.
13. Hypothyroidism.
14. Myasthenia gravis.
15. Phaeochromocytoma.
16. Prostatic hypertrophy.
17. Antipsychotic drugs may increase prolactin secretion.
18. *Drug interactions:* The concomitant administration of this product with other medication such as central nervous system depressants (including alcohol and anaesthetics) or antihypertensives, anticholinergic or dopaminergic drugs will result in accentuation of their effects, while potentiation of action will also occur with monoamine oxidase inhibitors, antidepressants and analgesics. Promazine may impair the effects of anticonvulsants.

Promazine may affect the control of diabetes. Undesirable anti-cholinergic effects can be enhanced by anti-Parkinson or other anticholinergic drugs.

Side-effects: Sparine is a member of the phenothiazine group of drugs and the side effects associated with that group have been noted. These include drowsiness, sedation, dry mouth, nasal stuffiness. Other possible anticholinergic side-effects are blurred vision, tachycardia, constipation and urinary hesitancy or retention when due to enlarged prostate.

Confusional states, or epileptic fits can occur. Sexual function may be impaired. Agranulocytosis and transient leucopenia have rarely been reported. Allergic skin reactions have also been reported.

Promazine rarely causes obstructive jaundice associated with stasis in biliary canaliculi. Promazine treatment should be withdrawn and not given again. Transient abnormalities of liver function tests may occur without jaundice.

Some individuals may be susceptible to the drug in low dosage and show paradoxical effects of excitement, agitation or insomnia and other minor side effects.

The elderly are particularly susceptible to side-effects of promazine, especially to the sedative, hypotensive and temperature regulation effects. These effects may be dose related.

Treatment of overdosages: Ingestion of large amounts of promazine is followed by deep sleep, with or without a pronounced fall in blood pressure and without particular change in respiration rate, other than the slowing attendant upon sedation. Occasionally an initial period of excitement may precede coma, followed by grand mal seizures.

In the absence of any specific antidote, treatment should be based on ordinary therapeutic principles with special emphasis on the following measures: (1) treat convulsions if present; (2) correction of acute hypotension if necessary; (3) counteraction of the effects of an excess of promazine hydrochloride on the central nervous system; (4) control and natural recovery of hypothermia.

Pharmaceutical precautions Sparine Injection should not be mixed with other injections with the exception of Pethidine Injection BP.

Legal category POM.

Package quantities Boxes of 10 by 1 ml or 2 ml ampoules (OP).

Further information Nil.

Product licence number 0011/5043R.

TEMAZEPAM CAPSULES

Presentation Temazepam capsules are opaque yellow, oval, soft gelatin capsules containing 10 mg or 20 mg temazepam. The 10 mg capsules are No. 4 capsules imprinted WYETH on one side and W10 on the reverse in black lettering. The 20 mg capsules are No. 10 oval capsules imprinted WYETH on one side and W20 on the reverse side in red lettering.

Uses Temazepam is indicated for the short term (up to 4 weeks) treatment of insomnia when it is disabling or subjecting the individual to extreme distress, and for premedication before minor surgery or other procedures especially when hospital admission is not essential.

As with all benzodiazepines doctors should be aware that long term use may lead to dependence and withdrawal symptoms in certain patients.

Dosage and administration Route of administration: Oral.

Insomnia

In all cases the lowest effective dose necessary to control symptoms should be used. Treatment should if possible be intermittent. Temazepam should not be used for long-term chronic treatment.

Adults: 10–30 mg half an hour before retiring. The dose may be increased to 40 or 60 mg in patients who do not respond to the lower dose because of severe or persistent insomnia.

Elderly: Elderly patients or those suffering from cerebral vascular changes such as arteriosclerosis are likely to respond to smaller doses, possibly half the normal adult dose.

Children: Not recommended.

All patients taking Temazepam should be carefully monitored and routine repeat prescriptions should be avoided.

Treatment in all patients should be withdrawn gradually with careful monitoring and reassessment to minimise possible withdrawal symptoms. Patients who have taken benzodiazepines for a long time may require a longer period during which doses are reduced.

Premedication

Adults: 20–40 mg, 30–60 minutes before surgical or other procedures.

Elderly: Elderly patients are likely to respond to smaller doses, possibly half the normal adult dose.

Children: Not evaluated.

Contra-indications, warnings, etc

Contra-indications: Temazepam should not be given to patients with a previous history of sensitivity to benzodiazepines, or to patients with acute pulmonary insufficiency.

Use in pregnancy: Safety for use in pregnancy has not been established. Temazepam should not be administered during pregnancy or lactation unless in the judgement of the physician such administration is clinically justifiable. Temazepam is not recommended for use in the first three months of pregnancy. Use during the late phase of pregnancy or at delivery may require ventilation of the infant at birth.

Precautions:

1. An underlying cause for insomnia should be sought before deciding on the use of benzodiazepines for symptomatic relief.
2. Concomitant administration with central nervous system depressants, including alcohol, general anaesthetics, narcotic analgesics, monoamine oxidase inhibitors and antidepressants may result in an accentuation of their effects.
3. When used at the appropriate recommended dose for short term treatment of insomnia the dependence potential of Temazepam is low. However, the risk of dependence increases with higher doses and longer-term use and is further increased in patients with a history of alcoholism, drug abuse or in patients with marked personality disorders.

Symptoms such as anxiety, depression, headache, insomnia, tension and sweating have been reported following abrupt discontinuation of benzodiazepines and these symptoms may be difficult to distinguish from the original ones.

Other symptoms such as persistent tinnitus, involuntary movements, paraesthesia, perceptual changes, confusion, convulsions, abdominal and muscle cramps and vomiting may be characteristic of benzodiazepine withdrawal syndrome.

4. When used as a hypnotic, daytime drowsiness is unlikely to be a problem with temazepam since the short half-life usually ensures that the effects disappear by the morning. As with other drugs acting on the central nervous system, however, patients should be cautioned against driving or operating machinery until it is established that they do not become dizzy or drowsy while taking temazepam.
5. Elderly patients or those suffering from cerebral vascular changes such as arteriosclerosis are likely to respond to smaller doses.
6. After medication with temazepam before surgical or other procedures, patients should be accompanied home.
7. The use of benzodiazepines may release suicidal tendencies in depressed patients. Benzodiazepines should not be used alone to treat depression or anxiety associated with depression. Other rarely reported behavioural effects of the benzodiazepines include paradoxical aggressive outbursts, excitement, hallucinations and confusion. Amnesia may occur and in cases of loss or bereavement psychological adjustment may be inhibited by benzodiazepines.

Side-effects: Because of its short half-life, the effects of temazepam are usually restricted to the night of ingestion. Drowsiness or dizziness on waking is rare. Morning headaches, transient rashes, mild gastro-intestinal disturbances, vivid dreams/nightmares, dry mouth or throat, depression, restless sleep and palpitations have occasionally been reported.

On rare occasions hypotension, gastro-intestinal and visual disturbances, skin rashes, urinary retention, changes in libido, blood dyscrasias, increased liver enzymes and jaundice have been reported with some benzodiazepines.

Overdosage: As with other benzodiazepines, overdosages should not present a threat to life unless combined with other CNS depressants (including alcohol). General supportive measures should be used. Treatment is symptomatic and gastric lavage may be of use if performed shortly after ingestion. The patient is likely to sleep and a clear airway should be maintained.

Pharmaceutical precautions Store in a dry place between 15°C and 25°C. Protect from light. Dispense Temazepam capsules into well closed amber glass or amber/opaque plastic containers.

Legal category CD (Sch 4), POM.

Package quantities 10 mg: securitainers of 250, 500 and 1000, bottles of 50 (OP).
20 mg: securitainers of 250 and 500.

Further information Temazepam is a short acting benzodiazepine. It is rapidly absorbed from the liquid-filled soft gelatin capsules and peak plasma levels are usually reached in 20 to 40 minutes. Temazepam has a plasma half life of about eight hours. Temazepam is metabolised by a simple one-step process to a pharmacologically inert glucuronide. There are no major active metabolites and virtually no risk of accumulation. Clinical studies have shown minimal effects on REM sleep patterns and on psychomotor performance on the day after treatment with temazepam.

The risk of benzodiazepine related dependence may be minimised by adopting the following guidelines for treatment:

1. Select patients carefully taking into account the precautions and warnings stated in this data sheet.
2. Adopt short-term or intermittent therapy.
3. Use lowest dose possible to achieve effective treatment.
4. Review treatment regularly; and especially before repeating prescriptions.
5. Discontinue treatment gradually taking into account patient reaction at each stage, i.e. 'titrate downwards'.

Product licence numbers
10 mg capsules 0011/0106
20 mg capsules 0011/0107

TEMAZEPAM* TABLETS

Presentation Temazepam tablets are white flat and bevel edged containing 10 mg or 20 mg temazepam. The 10 mg tablets are imprinted WYETH on one side, WY breakbar and 040 on the other. The 20 mg tablets are imprinted WYETH on one side and WY, breakbar and 041 on the other.

Uses Temazepam tablets are recommended for the short term treatment of insomnia only when it is severe, disabling or subjecting the individual to extreme distress.

For pre-medication prior to minor surgery and investigative procedures.

As with all benzodiazepines doctors should be aware that long term use may lead to dependence and withdrawal symptoms in certain patients.

Dosage and administration Route of administration: Oral.

Insomnia
Adults: 10–30 mg on or half an hour prior to retiring. The dose can be increased to 40–60 mg in unresponsive patients.

Elderly: Elderly patients may require lower doses, up to half the normal adult dose may be sufficient.

Children: The use of temazepam is not recommended in children.

Pre-medication
Adults: 20–40 mg between 30 and 60 minutes prior to surgery.

Elderly: Elderly patients may require lower doses, up to half the normal adult dose may be sufficient.

Children: The use of Temazepam tablets is not recommended in children.

Treatment should, if possible, be intermittent.

The lowest dose which can control symptoms should be used. It should not be continued beyond four weeks.

Long-term chronic use is not recommended.

Treatment should always be tapered off gradually.

Patients who have taken benzodiazepines for a long time may require a longer period during which doses are reduced.

Contra-indications, warnings, etc
Contra-indications: Benzodiazepines should not be used:

(a) To treat short-term 'mild' anxiety: their use here is inappropriate and unsuitable.

(b) Alone, to treat depression or anxiety associated with depression. Suicide may be precipitated in such patients.

(c) For phobic or obsessional states.

(d) For the treatment of chronic psychosis.

(e) In patients with known sensitivity to benzodiazepines.

(f) In acute pulmonary insufficiency and where there is respiratory depression.

Use in preganancy: There is no evidence as to drug safety in human pregnancy nor is there evidence from animal work that it is free from hazard. Do not use during pregnancy, especially during the first and last trimesters, unless there are compelling reasons.

The administration of high doses or prolonged administration of low doses of benzodiazepines in the last trimester of pregnancy or during labour has been reported to produce irregularities in the foetal heart rate, and hypotonia, poor sucking and hypothermia in the neonate.

If possible the use of benzodiazepines should be avoided during lactation.

Precautions and warnings
1. Temazepam will potentiate the effect of alcohol, general anaesthetics, narcotic analgesics, monoamine oxidase inhibitors, antidepressants and all other CNS depressants.

2. Temazepam can cause drowsiness and patients should be warned against driving or operating machinery until the absence of such drowsiness is established.

3. Dependence (and therefore withdrawal symptoms) can occur with therapeutic doses given for short periods of time, as well as with high doses or prolonged administration. Thus the lowest dose which can control symptoms should be used and long term chronic use is not recommended. When used as

(a) anxiolytics, benzodiazepines should not be continued beyond four weeks,

(b) as hypnotics, treatment should, if possible, be intermittent and the underlying cause for insomnia should be sought before resorting to benzodiazepines for symptomatic relief.

Whatever the indication treatment should always be tapered off gradually to negate withdrawal symptoms. Patients who have taken benzodiazepines for a long time may require a longer period during which the doses are reduced. Possible withdrawal symptoms include, anxiety, tremor, confusion, insomnia, perceptual disorders, fits, depression, gastro-intestinal and other somatic symptoms. These sometimes may be difficult to distinguish from the symptoms of the original illness.

Withdrawal effects usually appear shortly after stopping a benzodiazepine with a short half life, or up to several days after stopping one with a long life. Symptoms may continue for weeks or months.

4. Disinhibiting effects can occur with all benzodiazepines. These may be manifested in a number of ways. Suicide may be precipitated in patients who are depressed, and aggressive behaviour towards self and

others may be precipitated. Extreme caution should be used therefore in prescribing benzodiazepines in patients with personality disorders.

5. Amnesia also may occur. In cases of loss or bereavement psychological adjustment may be inhibited by benzodiazepines.

6. Benzodiazepines should be prescribed with caution in patients with chronic pulmonary insufficiency and chronic renal or hepatic disease.

7. The use of benzodiazepines with other centrally acting drugs is likely to increase the sedative effects. The elderly require special supervision.

8. It is advisable that patients receiving temazepam for pre-medication should be accompanied home.

Side-effects: Common adverse effects include drowsiness, sedation, blurring of vision, unsteadiness and ataxia. These effects can occur with single as well as repeated dosage and may persist well into the following day.

Rare adverse reactions have been reported, namely gastro-intestinal disturbances, visual disturbances, headache, vertigo, libido changes, hypotension, skin rashes, urinary retention, blood dyscrasias and jaundice.

Behavioural effects include paradoxical aggressive outbursts, excitement, hallucinations, confusion and the uncovering of depression with suicidal tendencies (see above).

Overdose: In the case of overdosage, treatment should be symptomatic with supportive measures. Gastric lavage can be performed shortly after ingestion, if it is felt necessary.

Pharmaceutical precautions Store in a cool, dry place.

Legal category CD (Sch 4), POM.

Package quantities 10 mg: Securitainers of 500.
20 mg: Securitainers of 250.

Further information The risk of benzodiazepine related dependence may be minimised by adopting the following guidelines for treatment:

1. Select patients carefully taking into account the precautions and warnings stated in this data sheet.
2. Adopt short-term or intermittent therapy.
3. Use lowest dose possible to achieve effective treatment.
4. Review treatment regularly; and especially before repeating prescriptions.
5. Discontinue treatment gradually taking into account patient reaction at each stage, i.e. 'titrate downwards'.

Product licence numbers
10 mg tablets 0011/0179
20 mg tablets 0011/0180

TRINORDIOL*

Presentation The memo pack holds six light brown tablets, containing 50 micrograms levonorgestrel and 30 micrograms Ethinyloestradiol BP, five white tablets containing 75 micrograms levonorgestrel and 40 micrograms Ethinyloestradiol BP and ten ochre tablets containing 125 micrograms levonorgestrel and 30 micrograms Ethinyloestradiol BP.

All tablets are round 5.6 mm in diameter with a lustrous sugar coating.

Uses Oral contraception.

Dosage and administration *Contraception:* For the first course of medication the tablets are started on the first day of the cycle, counting the first day of menstruation as day one. One tablet is taken at the same time each day for 21 days followed by seven days without medication. On the eighth day the tablets are started again. The protection covers every day of the cycle, provided that the tablets are taken correctly. During the seven clear days withdrawal bleeding should occur. If a cycle with amenorrhoea occurs the patient should seek medical advice.

Women who change from another oral contraceptive to Trinordiol should stop taking the previous product at the end of the pack and take the first tablet of Trinordiol on the day after taking the last tablet of their old pack, then continue to take 1 tablet daily for 21 days. If it is preferred to leave a seven-day gap before starting Trinordiol, then additional contraceptive precautions should be taken for the first 14 days of the first cycle.

Occasionally spotting or bleeding may occur in some women initially, but menstrual regularity is usually re-established after the first few cycles. If medication is discontinued because of severe breakthrough bleeding a new course should be started on the fifth day from the start of bleeding. Additional contraceptive precautions should be taken until the fourteenth tablet of the new course has been taken.

If a tablet is forgotten the woman should take it as soon as possible. If the delay is more than 12 hours additional precautions should be taken until the next withdrawal bleed. If more than one tablet is missed, tablet taking should be resumed when remembered with the tablet appropriate for that day and additional precautions should be taken until the next withdrawal bleed. Withdrawal bleeding may occur as a result of missed tablets, but the patient should continue to take the tablets as directed.

Treatment with Trinordiol should be withdrawn six weeks before elective surgery or treatment of varicose veins by injection of sclerosant.

After childbirth oral contraception is usually started as soon as spontaneous menstruation has been resumed. Another method of contraception should be used in the interval between delivery and the first course, unless it is started within seven days of delivery.

Oral contraception may be started on the fifth day after an abortion or miscarriage.

If vomiting or diarrhoea impair absorption, additional contraceptive precautions should be taken until the next withdrawal bleed.

Contra-indications, warnings, etc
Contra-indications: Trinordiol like other progestogen-oestrogen combinations, should not be given:

1. To patients with established hepatic disease or to those in whom there is evidence of persistently abnormal liver functions such as Dubin–Johnson and Rotor syndromes, or to those who have idiopathic recurrent jaundice of pregnancy.
2. To patients with a history or suspicion of carcinoma of the reproductive organs or breasts.
3. To patients with a history or evidence suggestive of thromboembolic or cerebrovascular disease or phlebitis.
4. To patients with cardiovascular disease.
5. To patients with a history of infectious hepatitis until the liver function tests have returned to normal values.
6. To patients with abnormal vaginal bleeding of unknown aetiology.
7. To patients with known or suspected oestrogen-dependent neoplasia.
8. To patients with suspected pregnancy.
9. To patients with sickle cell anaemia.
10. To patients with deterioration of otosclerosis during pregnancy.
11. To patients with a history of herpes gestationis.

Precautions:

1. Under the influence of oestrogen-progestogen preparations, pre-existing uterine fibromyomata may increase in size.
2. Oestrogen-progestogen preparations may cause some degree of fluid retention. Conditions which might be influenced by this factor, such as epilepsy, migraine, asthma, cardiac or renal dysfunction, require careful observation.
3. Patients with a history of psychic depression should be carefully observed and the drug discontinued if the depression recurs to a serious degree.
4. A decrease in glucose tolerance has been observed in a significant percentage of patients on oral contracep-

tives. Diabetic patients should be carefully observed while receiving therapy.

5. Susceptible women may experience an increase in blood pressure following administration of contraceptive steroids. Caution should therefore be exercised in prescribing oral contraceptives for women with a history of hypertension.

6. Oral contraceptive medication should be discontinued if there is a gradual or sudden, partial or complete loss of vision, proptosis or diplopia, papilloedema or any evidence of retinal or vascular lesions.

7. Caution should be observed in prescribing oral contraceptives for any patient with a history of migraine, or if migraine is being treated with vasoconstrictor drugs. If migraine worsens or migraine or severe headache develops for the first time during treatment, medication should be discontinued immediately.

8. A small fraction of the hormonal agents in oral contraceptives has been identified in the milk of mothers receiving these drugs. The long-range effect to the nursing infant is currently unknown.

9. Malignant hepatic tumours have been reported on rare occasions in long-term users of oral contraceptives. Benign hepatic tumours have also been associated with oral contraceptive usage. A hepatic tumour should be considered in the differential diagnosis when upper abdominal pain, enlarged liver or signs of intra-abdominal haemorrhage occur.

10. Numerous epidemiological studies have been reported on the risks of ovarian, endometrial, cervical and breast cancer in women using combined oral contraceptives. The evidence is clear that combined oral contraceptives offer substantial protection against both ovarian and endometrial cancer.

An increased risk of cervical cancer in long term users of combined oral contraceptives has been reported in some studies, but there continues to be controversy about the extent to which this is attributable to the confounding effects of sexual behaviour and other factors.

The evidence linking combined oral contraceptive use and breast cancer remains inconclusive. The results of some studies suggest an increased risk of breast cancer presenting below the age of about 35, the risk rising with duration of use. Any possible increased risk of breast cancer with combined oral contraceptives is however likely to be small and may be expected to be less with low dosage pills. This possible risk should be weighed against the many benefits of combined oral contraceptives, including their protective effects against ovarian and endometrial cancers.

11. In breakthrough bleeding or irregular vaginal bleeding, non-functional causes should be borne in mind.

12. The risk of arterial thrombosis associated with combined oral contraceptives increases with age, and this risk is aggravated by cigarette smoking. The use of combined oral contraceptives by women in the older age group, especially those who are cigarette smokers, should therefore be discouraged and alternative methods advised.

13. Examination of the pelvic organs, breasts and blood pressure should precede prescription of an oral contraceptive and should be repeated regularly.

14. Certain conditions require careful observation during treatment with oral contraceptives. These are: history of depression, varicose veins, diabetes, hypertension, epilepsy, otosclerosis, multiple sclerosis, porphyria, tetany, disturbed liver function, gall-stones, renal disease, chloasma, uterine fibroids, asthma, the wearing of contact lenses or any condition prone to worsen during pregnancy.

Side-effects: Oral contraceptives produce certain endocrine effects characteristic of ovarian oestrogens and progesterone. The hormones secreted during an ovulatory cycle may produce similar effects including headache, slight weight gain, nausea, breast tenderness, changed libido, depressive moods and spotting between periods. The overall incidence of such effects with Trinordiol is low and tends to decrease as treatment cycles continue. Cycle control is good and spotting and breakthrough bleeding occur only rarely. Extensive studies on considerable numbers of women taking oral contraceptives indicate some increased risks over non-pregnant women who are not taking oral contraceptives. These include thromboembolism, impaired glucose tolerance and even more rarely, liver dysfunction, hypertension and raised serum lipids.

Drug interactions: Caution should be observed in prescribing oral contraceptives for patients taking other drugs since various interactions have been reported. Pregnancies have been reported in women taking oral contraceptives concurrently with rifampicin and other antibiotics, anti-epileptic drugs, barbiturates and other sedative drugs.

Steroids affect drug metabolism and the therapeutic or toxic effects of other drugs may be modified. Interactions have been reported between oral contraceptives and tricyclic antidepressants, anticoagulants and corticosteroids.

Overdosage: No reports of serious ill-effects from overdosage with combined oral contraceptives have been reported. In general, therefore, treatment of overdosage is not necessary. If overdosage is, however, discovered within one hour and is so large that treatment seems desirable, gastric lavage or a suitable dose of ipecacuanha can be used. There are no specific antidotes and further treatment should be symptomatic.

Pharmaceutical precautions Store at, or below, room temperature.

Legal category POM.

Package quantities Trinordiol is supplied in packs of 3 blisters of 21 tablets (OP).

Further information Levonorgestrel is a totally synthetic progestogen which possesses no inherent oestrogenicity. It has anti-oestrogenic properties and has minimal effects on metabolic functions.

Research has shown that it is unnecessary to give the same doses of hormones throughout the cycle. The three-phase dosage mimics the secretion of hormones in a natural cycle and allows the total intake of steroids to be reduced while maintaining contraceptive efficacy and good cycle control.

Product licence number 0011/0066.

**Trade Mark*

Zyma (United Kingdom) Limited
Westhead
10 West Street
Alderley Edge
Cheshire SK9 7XP

EURAX*-HYDROCORTISONE

Presentation White to cream coloured soft cream with a faint odour of perfume, containing Crotamiton BP 10% and Hydrocortisone BP 0.25%.

Also contains: methyl hydroxybenzoate, propyl hydroxybenzoate, polyoxyl 40 stearate, propylene glycol, stearyl alcohol, white soft paraffin, water and fragrance (Givaudan No 45).

Uses
Mode of action: Eurax-Hydrocortisone combines the antipruritic action of crotamiton with the anti-inflammatory and anti-allergic properties of hydrocortisone.

Indications: Eczema and dermatitis of all types including atopic eczema, photodermatitis, otitis externa, primary irritant and allergic dermatitis, intertrigo, prurigo nodularis, seborrhoeic dermatitis and insect bite reactions.

Dosage and administration Eurax-Hydrocortisone is indicated for external application only.

Method of application: A thin layer of Eurax-Hydrocortisone cream should be applied to the affected area 2–3 times a day. Occlusive dressings should not be used. Treatment should be limited to 10–14 days or up to 7 days if applied to the face.

Use in the elderly: clinical evidence would indicate that no special dosage regime is necessary.

Use in children: Eurax-Hydrocortisone should be used with caution in infants and for not more than 7 days. Eurax-Hydrocortisone should not be applied more than once a day to large areas of the body surface in young children.

Contra-indications, warnings, etc
Contra-indications: Hypersensitivity to any component of the formulation. Bacterial, viral or fungal infections of the skin. Acute exudative dermatoses. Application to ulcerated areas.

Precautions: Eurax-Hydrocortisone should be used with caution in infants and for not more than 7 days; long-term continuous topical therapy should be avoided since this can lead to adrenal suppression even without occlusion.

Eurax-Hydrocortisone should not be allowed to come into contact with the conjunctiva and mucous membranes.

Side-effects: Occasionally at the site of application signs of irritation such as a burning sensation, itching, contact dermatitis/contact allergy may occur. Treatment should be discontinued if patients experience severe irritation or sensitisation.

Use in pregnancy and lactation: There is inadequate evidence of safety in human pregnancy. Topical administration of corticosteroids to pregnant animals can cause abnormalities of foetal development, including cleft palate and intra-uterine growth retardation. There may therefore be a very small risk of such effects in the human foetus.

It is not known whether the active substances of Eurax-Hydrocortisone and/or their metabolite(s) pass into the breast milk after topical administration. Use in lactating mothers should only be at the doctor's discretion.

Overdosage: Eurax-Hydrocortisone cream is for application to the skin only. If accidental ingestion of large quantities occurs, there is no specific antidote and general measures to eliminate the drug and reduce its absorption should be undertaken. Symptomatic treatment should be administered as appropriate.

Pharmaceutical precautions Protect from heat. Dilution of or addition to this formulation is not recommended.

Legal category POM.

Package quantities Tubes of 30 g (OP).

Further information Nil.

Product licence number 0001/0158.

FABROL*

Presentation Pale yellow, orange-flavoured granules in sachets containing 200 mg acetylcysteine.

Uses
Mode of action: Fabrol has an intense mucolytic action on mucoid and mucopurulent secretions due to its ability to split disulphide bonds in mucus glycoprotein. This property allows it to be used as adjuvant therapy in many clinical conditions characterised by the presence of viscous mucoid or mucopurulent secretions, particularly in the respiratory tract.

Indications: Fabrol is indicated in acute and chronic bronchitis and other respiratory conditions associated with the production of viscous mucus. Given on a long term basis in chronic bronchitis, it progressively improves symptoms due to mucus hypersecretion and substantially reduces the rate of infectious exacerbations.

Fabrol is also indicated for use in patients with abdominal complications associated with cystic fibrosis.

Dosage and administration The following dosage is recommended for the treatment of respiratory conditions:

Children up to 2 years: 1 sachet (200 mg) daily.

Children aged 2–6 years: 1 sachet (200 mg) twice daily.

Adults: 1 sachet (200 mg) three times daily.

Use in the elderly: There is no evidence to suggest that the dosage should be different in elderly patients.

In acute cases, a treatment period of 5–10 days is usually adequate but may be extended if necessary.

In chronic bronchitis, relief of symptoms may be noticeable after treatment for 1–2 months but treatment may be continued for up to six months, e.g. during the winter season.

For maintenance therapy in cystic fibrosis, the following dosage ranges are recommended:

Children up to 2 years: $\frac{1}{2}$ to 1 sachet (100 to 200 mg) three times daily.

Children aged 2–6 years: 1 sachet (200 mg) three times daily.

Adults: 1 or 2 sachets (200 or 400 mg) three times daily. In adults, a higher starting dose of 4 sachets (800 mg) three times daily is recommended for the acute treatment of abdominal complications associated with cystic fibrosis and, in severe cases, doses of up to 18 g acetylcysteine daily have been used and were well tolerated.

The granules should be dissolved before administration in a glass of water.

Fabrol can be administered concurrently with amoxycillin, doxycillin and erythromycin. When other oral antibiotics or drugs are required, they should be administered 1–2 hours apart from Fabrol.

Contra-indications, warnings, etc
Contra-indications: Hypersensitivity to acetylcysteine.

Precautions: Each Fabrol sachet contains the equivalent of 2.70 g sucrose. This should be taken into account when treating diabetic patients.

Side-effects: Nausea, heart-burn, vomiting, urticaria, headache and tinnitus have infrequently been reported but these rarely necessitate withdrawal of treatment.

Allergic skin reactions and bronchospasm, especially in asthmatic patients, have been reported rarely in patients taking oral acetylcysteine. High doses of acetylcysteine given intravenously have caused anaphylactoid reactions.

Pregnancy: The administration of acetylcysteine during pregnancy is advised only if there are compelling reasons.

Overdosage: There is no specific antidote for acetylcysteine and treatment is symptomatic. It consists of postural drainage, bronchial suction and supportive therapy as indicated.

Pharmaceutical precautions The addition of other drugs to the Fabrol solution should be avoided.

Legal category POM.

Package quantities Pack of 30 sachets.

Further information May be prescribed under the NHS Pharmaceutical Services as Acetylcysteine Granules for patients with abdominal complications associated with cystic fibrosis. Prescription must be endorsed 'S3B'.

Product licence number 0030/0038.

FENOSTIL* RETARD

Presentation *Fenostil-Retard Tablets:* Round, biconvex, greyish-white in colour, stamped on one face with the Zyma logo and on the reverse with the initials KA; diameter 9 mm, thickness 4.4 mm. Each tablet contains 2.5 mg dimethindene maleate in an inert slow release matrix.

Uses Antihistamine. Indicated for the relief of allergic conditions including pruritus of various aetiologies (e.g. eczema), urticaria, allergic dermatoses, allergic rhinitis and hay fever.

Dosage and administration For oral administration. The tablets should be swallowed whole and not chewed or crushed.

Adults: 1 tablet, morning and evening.

Children: No formulation of a dose suitable for children is available.

Use in the elderly: Since dimethindene maleate has a wide therapeutic index there are no specific precautions required when Fenostil Retard tablets are administered to elderly patients. The usual recommended adult dose is therefore considered suitable.

Contra-indications, warnings, etc
Contra-indications: Known hypersensitivity to dimethindene maleate.

Warnings: may cause drowsiness in susceptible individuals. Patients should be warned not to drive a vehicle or operate machinery during the early days of treatment until their own response has been determined. Avoid alcoholic drinks.

Precautions: Caution is recommended, as with other antihistamines, when Fenostil is administered to patients with glaucoma, bladder neck obstruction, e.g. prostatic hypertrophy, chronic obstructive pulmonary disease.

Care should be exercised during use in epileptic patients since Fenostil, like other antihistamines may act as a cerebral stimulant.

Interactions: As with other antihistamines, the sedative effect of CNS depressants including alcohol, hypnotics etc. may be enhanced.

The simultaneous administration of monoamine oxidase inhibitors may enhance the antimuscarinic and CNS depressant effects of antihistamines; concurrent use is not recommended.

Tricyclic antidepressants and anticholinergics may have an additive antimuscarinic effect with antihistamines, increasing the risk of aggravating glaucoma or urinary retention.

Use in pregnancy and lactation: as with other antihistamines, Fenostil Retard should not be used during pregnancy or in nursing mothers.

Side-effects: Fenostil is generally well tolerated.

Occasional: Drowsiness.

Rare: Dryness of the mouth or throat, dizziness, excitement, gastro-intestinal discomfort (including nausea), headache.

In isolated cases: Oedema, skin rashes, muscle spasm respiratory impairment.

Overdosage: In overdosage, as with other H_1-antihistamines, the following symptoms may occur: CNS depression with drowsiness (mainly in adults). CNS stimulation and antimuscarinic effects (especially in children), including excitement, ataxia, hallucinations, tonic–clonic spasms, mydriasis, dry mouth, flushed face, urinary retention and fever. Hypotension may also occur. Terminally, there may be deepening coma with cardiorespiratory collapse and death. No fatal outcome of overdosage has ever been reported with Fenostil.

There is no specific antidote to Fenostil.

Immediate treatment consists of forced emesis followed by gastric lavage with lukewarm water and instillation of approximately 10 g activated charcoal and 20–30 g sodium sulphate dissolved in water. Should convulsions or hypertonicity occur these may be treated with diazepam or phenobarbitone injection. Severe respiratory depression may necessitate mechanical respiration.

Pharmaceutical precautions Protect from light.

Legal category P.

Package quantities Containers of 100 tablets.

Further information Nil.

Product licence number 0030/5000R.

ISMELIN* EYE DROPS

Presentation A clear colourless odourless solution containing guanethidine sulphate 5% w/v, with Benzalkonium Chloride BP as a preservative.

Also contains: methocel, sodium chloride, dibasic sodium phosphate and water.

Uses *Mode of Action:* The precise mechanism of action of Ismelin in reducing intra-ocular tension has not yet been fully determined but a working hypothesis could be envisaged in which the therapeutic benefits are mediated by a local effect on the release of catecholamines, particularly those involved in the transmission of sympathetic impulses from terminal nerve fibres to target organs. This would be in line with the generally accepted concept of Ismelin activity in anti-hypertensive therapy. In relation to the eye one would have to postulate that to a greater or lesser extent the following ocular conditions are related to sympathetic overactivity: lid retraction following endocrine induced exophthalmos, lid retraction and lid lag in thyrotoxicosis and secretion of aqueous humor in glaucoma.

Indications: The reduction of intra-ocular pressure in glaucoma of the open angle type.

The treatment of lid retraction following exophthalmos and endocrine imbalance.

Dosage and administration Ismelin Eye Drops are intended for local administration to the eye.

The recommended adult dosages are as follows:

Open angle glaucoma: Initially one drop twice daily for at least a week. Dosage should then be adjusted according to the patient's needs, which may be one drop once or twice daily, or if necessary two drops once or twice daily, but rarely in excess of this.

Lid retraction: Initially one drop twice daily for at least one week, reducing thereafter to one drop daily. The dosage should be reduced as soon as possible to the minimum required to maintain the initial response – one drop on alternate days may be adequate.

Use in children: Ismelin Eye Drops are not recommended for use in children.

Use in the elderly: No specific studies have been performed in the elderly. Dosage in these patients is therefore at the discretion of the physician.

Contra-indications, warnings, etc *Contra-indications:* Use in narrow angle glaucoma or in patients with a shallow anterior chamber. Hypersensitivity to any of the components of the formulation. Ismelin Eye Drops should not be used during or within 14 days of treatment with a monoamine oxidase inhibitor. Use in combination with adrenaline.

Precautions: Soft contact lenses (hydrophilic lenses) should not be worn during treatment with Ismelin Eye Drops. It has been reported that patients receiving long-term guanethidine in combination with adrenaline may develop cicatrising conjunctivitis. Although the causative agent has not been identified, patients being treated with Ismelin Eye Drops should have regular (at least 6-monthly) examinations of the conjunctiva and cornea and treatment should be stopped if early signs of damage are seen to be developing.

Side-effects: Conjunctival vasodilation is regarded as a pharmacological side effect of Ismelin, but does not generally prove troublesome at the recommended dosage. Hyperaemia with discomfort is usually a sign of overdosage. Some degree of ptosis, valuable in the management of lid retraction, may represent an adverse effect in glaucoma but will usually respond to a reduction in dosage or frequency of administration. The slight miosis which occurs in most cases during Ismelin treatment causes little or no inconvenience and accommodation is not usually affected. At prolonged high dosage a tendency to superficial punctate keratitis has been reported, responding either to a reduction in dosage or interruption of treatment.

No systemic effects have been reported with Ismelin Eye Drops, even at maximum dosage.

Pharmaceutical precautions Protect from heat.

Do not exceed the stated dose.

The drops should not be used later than one month after first breaking the seal.

Legal category POM.

Package quantities Ismelin Eye Drops 5 ml (OP).

Further information The results of therapy with Ismelin Eye Drops have been in many cases dramatic, particularly in terms of cosmetic improvement of the unsightly eye manifestations such as lid retraction which occur in a high proportion of patients with exophthalmos and thyrotoxicosis.

There is minimal local irritation when the eye drops are used carefully according to the recommended dosage. Also considerable subjective relief of symptoms has been afforded even when the reduction in physical signs has been minimal.

Product licence number 0030/5901R.

LOCORTEN*-VIOFORM* EAR DROPS

Presentation A clear, yellowish solution containing 1% w/v clioquinol and 0.02% w/v flumethasone pivalate in polyethylene glycol.

Uses
Mode of action: Locorten-Vioform ear drops combine the anti-bacterial and anti-fungal properties of clioquinol with the anti-inflammatory activity of flumethasone pivalate.

Indications: Inflammatory conditions of the external ear where a secondary infection is suspected. Otorrhoea.

Dosage and administration
Method of application: instil 2 or 3 drops twice daily directly into the auditory canal of the affected ear. Treatment should be limited to 7–10 days.

If there is little improvement after 7 days treatment with Locorten-Vioform, appropriate microbiological investigations should be carried out and local or systemic antibiotic treatment given.

Use in the elderly: there is no evidence to suggest that dosage should be different in the elderly.

Use in children: Locorten-Vioform ear drops are contraindicated in children below the age of two years.

Contra-indications, warnings, etc
Contra-indications: Hypersensitivity to any component of the formulation, or iodine. Primary bacterial, viral or fungal infections of the outer ear. Perforation of the tympanic membrane. Use in children below the age of two years.

Precautions: Long-term continuous topical therapy should be avoided since this can lead to adrenal suppression.

Topical application of clioquinol-containing preparations may lead to a marked increase in protein-bound iodine (PBI). The results of thyroid function tests, such as PBI, radioactive iodine and butanol extractable iodine may be affected. However, other thyroid function tests, such as the T_3 resin sponge test or T_4 determination, are unaffected.

The ferric chloride test for phenylketonuria may yield a false-positive result when cliquinol is present in the urine.

Locorten-Vioform should not be allowed to come into contact with the conjunctiva.

Side-effects: Locorten-Vioform is generally well tolerated, but occasionally, at the site of application, there may be signs of irritation such as a burning sensation, itching, or skin rash. Hypersensitivity reactions may also occasionally occur. Treatment should be discontinued if patients experience severe irritation or sensitisation.

Locorten-Vioform may cause hair discolouration.

Use in pregancy and lactation: There is inadequate evidence of safety in human pregnancy. Topical administration of corticosteroids to pregnant animals can cause abnormalities of foetal development, including cleft palate and intra-uterine growth retardation. There may therefore be a very small risk of such effects in the human foetus.

It is not known whether the active substances of Locorten-Vioform and/or their metabolite(s) pass into breast milk after topical administration. Use in lactating mothers should only be at the doctor's discretion.

Overdosage: Locorten-Vioform is for topical (external) use only. If accidental ingestion of large quantities occurs, there is no specific antidote and general measures to eliminate the drug and reduce its absorption should be undertaken. Symptomatic treatment should be administered as appropriate.

Pharmaceutical precautions No special precautions.

Legal category POM.

Package quantities 7.5 ml dropper bottles (OP).

Further information Clothing stained with Locorten-Vioform should be washed immediately or soaked overnight.

Product licence number 0030/0049.

OTRIVINE-ANTISTIN* STERILE EYE DROPS

Presentation A clear colourless odourless solution containing xylometazoline hydrochloride 0.05% w/v and antazoline sulphate 0·5% w/v, with Benzalkonium Chloride BP as a preservative. Also contains: boric acid, disodium edetate, sodium tetraborate and water.

Uses Otrivine-Antistin is a combination of a long acting vasoconstrictor and antihistamine. The eye drops are for temporary relief of redness and itching of the eye due to seasonal and perennial allergies such as hay fever, or allergy due to house dust.

Dosage and administration Otrivine-Antistin Eye Drops are intended for local administration to the eye.

Adults: 1 or 2 drops instilled 2-3 times per day into the conjunctival sac.

Children 5–12 years and the elderly: no specific studies have been performed in these patients. Due to possible systemic effects caution must be exercised and the dosage reduced to 1 drop instilled 2–3 times per day.

The eye drops should not be used in children under the age of 5 years.

When necessary, mydriatics or miotics may be administered simultaneously with Otrivine-Antistin Eye Drops.

Contra-indications, warnings, etc
Contra-indications: Hypersensitivity to any of the components of the formulation. Presence of narrow angle glaucoma. The use of monoamine oxidase inhibitors within the last 14 days. Otrivine-Antistin is not recommended in patients who wear contact lenses of any type.

Precautions: in patients who are receiving medication for hypertension, cardiac irregularities, hyperthyroidism or diabetes mellitus particular caution should be exercised. Otrivine-Antistin is not suitable for patients suffering from dry eyes without first seeking medical advice. Rebound congestion may follow continued use. Inflammation arising from infection should receive appropriate antibacterial therapy.

No interactions with other drugs have been reported. There is a theoretical potential for interaction with clonidine.

Side effects: Otrivine-Antistin Eye Drops are well tolerated in the eye and for the majority of the patients will be non irritant, but in a few cases, slight transient local stinging may occur. Other side effects which have been reported very occasionally are blurred vision, headache and drowsiness.

Pharmaceutical precautions Protect from heat.

The drops should not be used later than one month after first breaking the seal.

Legal category P.

Package quantities Otrivine-Antistin Sterile Eye Drops 10 ml (OP).

Further information Nil.

Product licence number 0030/5900R.

PAROVEN*

Presentation Greyish-yellow, opaque, hard gelatin capsule (size No. 2) printed 'Paroven Zyma'. Each capsule contains 250 mg oxerutins.

Uses
Indications: Relief of symptoms of oedema associated with chronic venous insufficiency.

Dosage and administration For oral administration. The recommended dosages for adults and the elderly are as follows:

Chronic venous insufficiency (including adjuvant to support therapy): two capsules (500 mg) twice daily.

Use in children: As no specific indication exists, Paroven is not recommended for use in children below the age of 12 years.

If leg pain and swelling do not improve, or get worse, the patient should consult their doctor.

Contra-indications, warnings, etc
Contra-indications: hypersensitivity to oxerutins. Paroven should not be used for the treatment of leg oedema due to renal, hepatic or cardiac disease.

Side-effects: occasional mild adverse reactions (skin allergies, minor gastrointestinal disturbances, headaches and flushes) have been reported. These disappear rapidly on stopping treatment.

Use in pregnancy and lactation: clinical trials and animal studies have shown no increse in teratogenic (or other) hazard to the foetus if used in the recommended dosage during pregnancy. However, in keeping with current medical opinion, Paroven should not be used during the first trimester of pregnancy.

No information is available on excretion in breast milk. The use of Paroven in lactating women is therefore at the physician's discretion.

Overdosage: no cases of overdosage with symptoms have been reported. No specific antidotes are known.

Pharmaceutical precautions Protect from moisture.

Legal category P.

Package quantities Packs of 120 capsules.

Further information Nil.

Product licence number 0030/5002.

PECRAM*

Presentation Round, biconvex, pale yellow tablets imprinted on one face with the Zyma logo and on the other with the symbol SRA/225.

Each tablet contains 225 mg Aminophylline Hydrate BP in a slow release formulation.

Uses For the treatment and prophylaxis of asthmatic bronchospasm and that associated with emphysema and chronic bronchitis. For the treatment of cardiac asthma and left ventricular or congestive heart failure.

Dosage and administration For oral administration. The tablets should be swallowed whole and not chewed.

Standard dosing
Adults: The recommended initial dose is one tablet twice daily (one tablet to be taken in the morning and one in the evening).

The elderly: Reduced dosages may be required in elderly patients. The dosage should be titrated to attain optimum clinical response.

Children: Pecram tablets have not been fully evaluated in children.

Dose titration: The response to xanthines may vary between patients so that dosage must be individually titrated by clinical assessment and serum theophylline monitoring to a suitable dosage regimen, and when necessary the dose can be increased up to two tablets twice daily.

Steady state theophylline levels are generally reached with Pecram after 3–4 days. If satisfactory clinical response is not achieved, serum theophylline should be measured 4–6 hours after the last dose. Based on serum theophylline assay results, the dosage should be titrated using the following as a guide for twice daily administration.

Peak serum theophylline level	Dosage adjustment
< 10 micrograms/ml	Increase total daily dose by one tablet.
10–15 micrograms/ml	If the patient's symptoms persist, increase the total daily dose to a maximum of 2 tablets twice daily.
16–20 micrograms/ml	Do not adjust the dose unless side effects occur, in which case reduce the total daily dose by 1 tablet per day.
21–25 micrograms/ml	Decrease the total daily dose by 1 tablet per day
26–30 micrograms/ml	Miss the next dose and decrease the maintenance dose by one half.

It is advisable to re-check serum theophylline concentration after dose adjustment, when steady state is attained.

Pharmacokinetics: It has been demonstrated that twice-daily dosing produces minimal peak to trough variations. A dose regimen of 1 tablet twice daily for 6 days resulted in a peak plasma theophylline concentration of 9.5 mcg/ml (C_{Max}) at 4.0 hours (T_{Max}) and a minimum plasma concentration of 4.5 mcg/ml (C_{Min}) at 12 hours.

With appropriate dosage titration, plasma theophylline levels can be maintained in the range of 10–20 mcg/ml for 12 hours.

Smoking and alcohol consumption may increase theophylline clearance thus necessitating an increased dosage.

Other factors such as viral infections, liver disease and heart failure may reduce theophylline clearance requiring a reduction in dosage.

Transferability: It is not possible to ensure bioequivalence between different sustained release xanthine products. Once an effective dose has been established, patients should not be changed from Pecram to another preparation without re-titration and clinical assessment.

Contra-indications, warnings, etc
Contra-indications: Patients with a known hypersensitivity to the xanthine group of drugs.

Side-effects: Those associated with theophylline and xanthine derivatives such as nausea, gastric irritation, headache and CNS stimulation, are reduced when controlled release formulations such as Pecram are administered because the peak/trough variation is reduced.

Precautions: Suspected interactions have been documented between theophylline and the following drugs: Allopurinol, thiabendazole, halothane, lithium, oral contraceptives, erythromycin, triacetyloleandomycin, lomustine, phenobarbitone, propranolol, cimetidine, ciprofloxin and hydrocortisone. Care should be taken on its concomitant use with β-adrenergic agonists, glucagon and other xanthine drugs, as these will potentiate the effects of theophylline. The incidence of toxic effects may be enhanced by the concomitant use of ephedrine. Physicians should be aware that interaction may occur with influenza vaccine. Some reports have suggested that this may potentiate theophylline. The following drugs increase theophylline clearance and it may therefore be necessary to increase dosage to ensure a therapeutic effect: phenytoin, carbamazepine, rifampicin, sulphinpyrazone and barbiturates.

The prolonged release characteristic of this product should be kept in mind if intravenous aminophylline is to be administered, lest unintended high serum levels lead to toxicity.

Xanthines can potentiate hypokalaemia resulting from beta 2 agonist therapy, steroids, diuretics and hypoxia. Particular caution is advised in severe asthma. It is recommended that serum potassium levels are monitored in such situations.

Use in pregnancy and lactation: Theophylline crosses the placental barrier and is secreted in breast milk. It has been used during pregnancy without attributable adverse foetal effects. However, as with all drugs theophylline should only be used during pregnancy if considered essential by the physician.

Overdosage: In the event of overdosage, empty the stomach contents, monitor the patient's electrocardiogram and maintain fluid balance. Orally administer activated charcoal to reduce high theophylline plasma levels. With severe poisoning, charcoal column haemoperfusion should be used. Other treatment is symptomatic. Oxygen should be given as necessary.

Convulsions may be controlled by intravenous administration of diazepam 5 or 10 mg, or if necessary thiopentone sodium. The physician should be aware that tablets in the intestine will continue to release the drug over several hours.

In the event of blood monitoring showing low serum potassium levels it is recommended that potassium replacement therapy be instituted by mouth. Cases of acute hypokalaemia should be admitted to hospital.

Pharmaceutical precautions Protect from light. Store in a cool dry place.

Legal category P.

Package quantities Containers of 100 and 1000 tablets.

Further information Nil.

Product licence number 10013/0002.

PROFLEX* CREAM

Presentation Proflex cream contains Ibuprofen BP 5.0% w/w, a creamy white colouration, and of a soft consistency. Proflex cream also contains fractionated coconut oil, glyceryl stearate and PEG 100 stearate, PEG5 glyceryl stearate, propylene glycol, xanthan gum, sodium methyl hydroxybenzoate (E219), and water.

Uses
Indications: Proflex cream is a topical analgesic and anti-inflammatory treatment for the fast relief of the symptoms of rheumatic and muscular pain, backache, sprains, strains, lumbago and fibrositis.

Mode of action: Ibuprofen is a phenylpropionic acid derivative which has analgesic, anti-inflammatory and antipyretic actions. It is an inhibitor of prostaglandin synthetase (cyclo-oxygenase).

Pharmacokinetics: Percutaneous absorption of ibuprofen from Proflex cream amounts to approximately 5% that of oral ibuprofen. Maximum systemic concentrations, after about 2 hours, reach approximately 0.64 micrograms/ml, but with higher concentrations achieved locally.

Dosage and administration
Adults and elderly: Apply 4–10 cm (1½–4 inches) of cream (50–125 mg ibuprofen) 3 to 4 times daily, massaged into the skin over a large area of the affected site.

Children: Not recommended under 14 years.

Contra-indications, warnings, etc
Pregnancy and lactation: Use during pregnancy and in lactating mothers should if possible be avoided. No teratogenic effects have been demonstrated in animals with orally administered ibuprofen. Use of prostaglandin synthetase inhibitors may result in premature closure of the ductus arteriosus if given in the last trimester of pregnancy.

Contra-indications: Hypersensitivy to ibuprofen. Asthmatic patients in whom attacks of asthma, urticaria or acute rhinitis are precipitated by aspirin or other non-steroidal anti-inflammatory agents.

Precautions: Proflex cream should not be applied to broken skin, lips or near the eyes. Hands should be washed after use.

Drug interactions: None known via the topical route.

Side-effects: Slight erythema and occasional tingling at

the site of application has been reported, but rarely of sufficient seriousness to discontinue medication.

Overdosage: There is no specific antidote to ibuprofen. However, any overdose with a topical presentation of ibuprofen cream is extremely unlikely.

Pharmaceutical precautions Store in a cool place (store below 30°C).

Legal category P.

Package quantities Aluminium tubes, with a tamper-evident nozzle diaphragm, containing Proflex Cream 100 g.

Further information Nil.

Product licence number 0030/0052.

SABIDAL* SR

Presentation *Sabidal SR 270 tablets:* Round, convex, light yellow tablets, diameter 12 mm, thickness 6 mm. Each tablet contains 424 mg Choline Theophyllinate BP, equivalent to 270 mg anhydrous theophylline, in a sustained release formulation.

Uses For the relief and prevention of bronchospasm in asthma, chronic bronchitis and emphysema.

Dosage and administration For oral administration. The tablets should be swallowed whole and not chewed. The dosage should be adjusted to suit the individual patient, preferably on the basis of plasma theophylline levels (plasma concentrations of 10–20 mg/l are required for maximum therapeutic effect). The following initial dosage scheme is recommended:

Adults: The recommended adult dose is one tablet in the morning and two tablets at night. As with all theophylline preparations, it may be advisable in certain patients to commence treatment with one tablet twice daily for three days and then add the additional tablet at night.

Initially, treatment should be started at the above dose, which may be increased gradually if optimal bronchodilator effects are not achieved. If a higher dose is required, it is recommended that plasma theophylline levels should be monitored, since there is considerable individual variation in the rate of drug elimination. A plasma concentration of 20 mg/l should not be exceeded.

Use in the elderly: As with all theophylline-containing products, elimination of theophylline may be slightly retarded in elderly patients. However, the observed inter-individual variations at any age are far more important and, as with all patients, the dosage should be individually adjusted.

Use in children: Sabidal SR 270 tablets are not recommended for children.

Contra-indications, warnings, etc Known hypersensitivity to xanthines. Nursing mothers of premature infants.

Warnings: Theophylline should be given with caution in patients with active or previous peptic ulcer, tachycardia and/or arrhythmia, hypertension or other cardiovascular diseases, hyperthyroidism or epilepsy as these conditions may be exacerbated.

Several conditions may decrease theophylline clearance resulting in increased plasma concentrations. Therefore, careful monitoring of serum theophylline levels is recommended in the following conditions: congestive heart failure, hepatic dysfunction or chronic alcoholism, acute pulmonary oedema, acute febrile illness, severe hypoxia.

Theophylline clearance may be decreased by a low-protein, high-carbohydrate diet, and may be increased by a high-protein, low carbohydrate diet. Large amounts of caffeine containing food or beverages (coffee, tea, coca-cola or chocolate) should be avoided.

Precautions: Great caution must be exercised if intravenous aminophylline is administered and plasma theophylline concentrations should be monitored.

As with all sustained release methylxanthine preparations, tablets in the intestine will continue to release the drug over a period of hours.

Transferability: each patient should be individually titrated by clinical assessment and therapeutic monitoring to a suitable dosage regime for Sabidal SR tablets. After an effective therapeutic regime is obtained there is a danger of inefficacy or toxicity if an alternative sustained release methylxanthine preparation is substituted. It is not possible to ensure bioequivalence between different sustained release methylxanthine products for different patients. Inter-product substitution should not therefore be carried out after an effective stable regime of Sabidal SR tablets has been attained.

Interactions: Suspected interactions have been documented between theophylline and the following drugs: allopurinol, thiabendazole, halothane, lithium, oral contraceptives, erythromycin, triacetyloleandomycin, quinolones, lomustine, beta-adrenergic blocking agents, cimetidine, ranitidine and hydrocortisone. A reduced dosage may be necessary as these drugs reduce theophylline clearance, and plasma levels should be monitored.

The actions of theophylline and beta-2-adrenergic agents are additive and dosage should therefore be individually adjusted when these agents are co-administered. Association of theophylline with ephedrine or other sympathomimetics should be avoided because of a possible potentiation of cardiovascular toxicity. Potentiation of theophylline may occur with influenza vaccine.

Smoking and alcohol consumption may increase theophylline clearance thus necessitating an increased dosage. The following drugs increase theophylline clearance and it may be necessary to increase dosage to ensure therapeutic effect: phenytoin, carbamazapine, rifampicin, sulphinpyrazone and barbiturates.

Xanthines can potentiate hypokalaemia resulting from beta-2-agonist therapy, steroids, diuretics and hypoxia. Particular caution is advised in severe asthma. It is recommended that serum potassium levels are monitored in such situations.

Side-effects: If serious side-effects occur, Sabidal should be withdrawn. The incidence of serious theophylline toxicity increases at serum concentrations greater than 20 mg/l.

Gastro-intestinal tract: nausea, vomiting, diarrhoea, gastro-intestinal bleeding. These side-effects usually occur when serum theophylline concentrations are greater than 15–20 mg/l.

Central nervous system: restlessness, irritability, headache, insomnia.

Cardiovascular system: tachycardia, extrasystoles or palpitations.

Use in pregnancy and lactation: At high doses (over 100 mg/kg administered intraperitoneally) theophylline has been shown in mice to be embryotoxic and teratogenic (cleft palate, ectodactyly, syndactyly, micromelia and subcutaneous haematoma were the predominant malformations). A comparable teratogenic response has not been found in rats and the relevance of animal findings to human use is not clear. Theophylline does cross the placental barrier and in some neonates, tachycardia, irritability and nausea have been reported. Sabidal should not be administered during the first three months of pregnancy. Sabidal should be used after the first trimester only if clearly needed and if there is no safer alternative.

Methylxanthines are excreted in breast milk and irritability has been reported in breast-fed infants. Sabidal should therefore be used with caution in nursing mothers, and mothers taking Sabidal should not breast-feed premature infants.

Overdosage: This is characterised by nausea, vomiting, gastro-intestinal irritation, unusual thirst, tachycardia, fall in blood pressure and collapse. Severe overdosage may also lead to maniacal behaviour, diuresis and repeated vomiting with extreme thirst, tremor, delirium, hyperthermia, tachycardia, tachypnoea, electrolyte disturbances, convulsions and death.

Treatment should be by induced emesis or gastric

lavage, activated charcoal, saline laxative, or in severe cases (usually serum theophylline concentrations of 40 mg/l or more) by charcoal haemoperfusion. For fall in blood pressure, nurse in head-down position and give pressor drugs intravenously with general supportive measures. Convulsions should be treated with intravenous diazepam. Serum theophylline and potassium levels should be monitored and hypokalaemia corrected. The physician should be aware that tablets in the intestine will continue to release the drug over a period of hours.

Pharmaceutical precautions Protect from moisture.

Legal category P.

Package quantities Containers of 100 tablets.

Further information The sustained release properties of Sabidal SR tablets are due to pores in the membrane surrounding the tablet. Choline theophyllinate is released through these pores at a controlled rate as the tablet passes through the alimentary canal, where the active substance is completely absorbed. As a result of these features, effective plasma theophylline concentrations are obtained throughout the 12 hour dosage interval whilst the risk of side-effects associated with high-peaking formulations is reduced to a minimum.

Product licence number 0030/0023.

TANDERIL* EYE OINTMENT

Presentation A white to yellowish-white soft ointment, containing 10% Oxyphenbutazone BP as active ingredient and phenyl ethyl alcohol 0.5% as a preservative in a special paraffin base.

Also contains: anhydrous lanolin, liquid paraffin, white petroleum ophthalmic.

Uses Anti-inflammatory.

Disease of the anterior segment of the eye and conjunctival sac: blepharitis, conjunctivitis, kerato-conjunctivitis, episcleritis, keratitis and disease of the anterior uveal tract.

Inflammation following trauma: Traumatic injury, penetrating and non-penetrating.

Post Operative: Following cataract, squint or other surgical procedures.

Note: Herpes Simplex:

While Tanderil eye ointment is not recommended for the treatment of a simple dendritic ulcer it may prove particularly valuable in treating other stages of the disease which may develop, e.g. metaherpetic ulcer, disciform keratitis or anterior uveitis. In view of the serious nature of this disease, it is recommended that these patients be under close medical supervision and if necessary additional therapy be instituted.

Dosage and administration Apply to the inner surface of the lower lid of the affected eye two to five times a day.

Use in children and in the elderly: No specific studies have been performed in these patients. Dosage is therefore at the discretion of the physician. Tanderil eye ointment should not be administered to infants under 6 months of age. A treatment period of 2 weeks should not be exceeded.

Contra-indications, warnings, etc *Contra-indications:* Previous local or systemic sensitivity to pyrazole compounds such as phenylbutazone and oxyphenbutazone.

Precautions: Improvement can be expected within 8 days of starting treatment. If none is seen in this period, appropriate alternative therapy should be instituted.

In the treatment of purulent inflammatory eye conditions, appropriate anti-infective therapy should be given concurrently with Tanderil eye ointment. Although there is no evidence that Tanderil eye ointment increases intraocular pressure, it should be used with caution in cases of glaucoma secondary to injury or infection. To ensure maximum therapeutic benefit in the treatment of conditions involving the posterior uveal tract, retina or choroid, Tanderil eye ointment may be used in conjunction with a suitable systemic non-steroidal anti-inflammatory agent.

Tanderil eye ointment may be used in combination with antibiotics or anti-viral substances to treat eye inflammation caused by bacterial or viral infection.

If the patient is also receiving eye-drops, they should be administered at least 10 minutes before Tanderil eye ointment.

Side-effects: Intolerance to the eye ointment may develop after continued use, the signs being: oedema of the eyelid, epiphora (minimal), redness of the conjunctiva.

Use in pregnancy and lactation: Tanderil eye ointment should not be administered to pregnant and lactating women.

Overdosage: There is no experience of overdosage with Tanderil eye ointment. Should such an event occur, treatment should be symptomatic with general supportive measures.

Pharmaceutical precautions Store in a cool place. This is a sterile product and should be used within one month of opening the tube. Not to be diluted.

Legal category POM.

Package quantities Ophthalmic tubes of 5 g (OP).

Further information Experimental studies confirm that following local application of the ointment to the eye, Tanderil penetrates the corneoscleral barrier and is present in therapeutic concentrations in the aqueous humor, iris and ciliary body.

Animal studies have shown that in therapeutic concentrations, Tanderil does not affect lens metabolism, impede tissue healing, promote cataract formation or, in contrast to the anti-inflammatory corticosteroids, enhance viral replication or the invasiveness of bacterial pathogens. Furthermore, studies in man have shown that in therapeutic concentrations, Tanderil does not affect intra ocular pressure in the normal eye or in latent glaucoma.

Product licence number 0030/0017.

TANDERIL* CHLORAMPHENICOL EYE OINTMENT

Presentation A white to yellowish white soft ointment containing 10% Oxyphenbutazone BP and 1% Chloramphenicol BP as active ingredients and phenyl ethyl alcohol 0·5% as a preservative.

Also contains: anhydrous lanolin, liquid paraffin, white petroleum ophthalmic.

Uses Anti-inflammatory and antibacterial.

Disease of the anterior segment of the eye and conjunctival sac: blepharitis, conjunctivitis, episcleritis, keratitis and disease of the anterior uveal tract.

Inflammation of the eye following trauma and prophylaxis of secondary bacterial infection.

Post Operative: Following squint, cataract or other surgical procedures.

Note: Herpes Simplex:

The ointment is not contraindicated in the treatment of simple dendritic ulcer, but in view of the serious nature of this disease it is recommended that these patients be under close medical supervision and the necessary additional therapy be instituted.

Dosage and administration Apply to the inner surface of the lower lid of the affected eye two to five times daily.

Use in children and the elderly: No specific studies have been performed in these patients. Dosage is therefore at the discretion of the physician. Tanderil-Chloramphenicol eye ointment should not be administered to infants under 6 months of age. A treatment period of 2 weeks should not be exceeded.

Contra-indications, warnings, etc *Contra-indications:* Previous local or systemic sensitivity to pyrazole compounds such as phenylbutazone and oxyphenbutazone. Sensitivity to chloramphenicol. Severe blood dyscrasias and liver disease.

Precautions: Improvement can be expected within 8 days of starting treatment. If none is seen in this period, appropriate alternative therapy should be instituted.

Normal swabs should be taken before starting treatment and appropriate antibiotic therapy instituted when the results are known. Tanderil-Chloramphenicol eye ointment should not be used in conjunction with other local antibiotic therapy and only with caution if systemic antibiotics are required.

After topical use of chloramphenicol, isolated cases of aplastic anaemia have been observed. Because of this, Tanderil-Chloramphenicol eye ointment should not be given simultaneously with other drugs known to be associated with blood dyscrasias.

If the patient is also receiving eye-drops, they should be administered at least 10 minutes before Tanderil-Chloramphenicol eye ointment.

Side-effects: Intolerance to the eye ointment may develop after continued use, the signs being: oedema of the eyelid, epiphora (minimal), redness of the conjunctiva.

Use in pregnancy and lactation: Tanderil-Chloramphenicol eye ointment should not be administered to pregnant and lactating women.

Overdosage: There is no experience of overdosage with Tanderil-Chloramphenicol eye ointment. Should such an event occur, treatment should be symptomatic with general supportive measures.

Pharmaceutical precautions Store in a cool place. This is a sterile product and should be used within one month of opening the tube. Not to be diluted.

Legal category POM.

Package quantities Ophthalmic tubes of 5 g (OP).

Further information Nil.

Product licence number 0030/0018.

VIBROCIL*

Presentation *Nasal Spray and Nasal Drops:* a clear colourless solution with slight odour of lavender.

Nasal Gel: a colourless gel with a slight odour of lavender.

Each 100 ml of solution or 100 g of gel contains:

Dimethindene maleate	0.025 g
Phenylephrine base	0.250 g
Neomycin sulphate	0.350 g

with Benzalkonium Chloride BP as a preservative.

Uses Vibrocil has decongestant, antihistaminic and antibiotic properties. It is indicated for use in common colds, acute sinusitis, acute rhinitis, allergic rhinitis and vasomotor rhinitis, where these conditions are complicated by Staphylococcal infections.

Dosage and administration For topical application to the nasal mucosa. The duration of treatment should not exceed two weeks.

Spray: Adults and children over 6 years: 2 sprays in each nostril four times a day.

Children aged 2 to 6 years: the use of Drops or Gel is recommended.

Drops: Adults and children over 6 years: 3–4 drops in each nostril three to four times a day.

Children aged 2 to 6 years: 1–2 drops in each nostril three to four times a day.

Gel: Apply a small quantity as high up the nostrils as possible.

Adults and children over 6 years: three to four times a day.

Children aged 2 to 6 years: two to three times a day.

Use in infants: As with other sympathomimetic-containing preparations, Vibrocil is contra-indicated in infants below the age of two years.

Use in the elderly: No specific studies have been performed in the elderly population. However, the amount of active substance entering the systemic circulation following topical administration to the nasal mucosa is very low. The usual recommended adult dose is therefore considered suitable for the elderly patient.

Contra-indications, warnings, etc
Contra-indications: Use in patients with cardiovascular disease, thyrotoxicosis or closed angle glaucoma. Use in infants below the age of two years and in pregnant and breast-feeding women. Concurrent use in patients who are receiving monoamine oxidase inhibitors or who have received them in the previous 14 days. Hypersensitivity to any of the components.

Precautions: The physician or pharmacist should reassure himself that sympathomimetic-containing preparations are not simultaneously administered by several routes, i.e. orally and topically.

Topical administration of Vibrocil leads to only very low active constituent levels in the plasma. However, the following precautions concerning the constituents should be noted:

Neomycin, when used in large or prolonged doses, has been associated with ototoxicity and nephrotoxicity and can lead to the emergence of resistant strains of micro-organisms. Neomycin should not be used in patients receiving other aminoglycosides since immediate skin sensitivity reactions may occur in previously sensitised patients. Neomycin should be used with caution in patients receiving other drugs with neuromuscular blocking activity, anticoagulants, anti-emetics and other ototoxic drugs.

Phenylephrine is not recommended for use in patients with hypertension, cardiovascular disease or thyrotoxicosis. It should not be used by patients currently or recently taking monoamine oxidase inhibitors or tricyclic antidepressants and should be used with caution in patients taking β-adrenoceptor blocking agents.

Dimethindene maleate has potent antihistaminic activity with low toxicity and a high therapeutic ratio but the possibility of drowsiness, as with other antihistamines in hypersensitive patients, should be observed. If affected, the patient should not drive or operate machinery. As with all antihistamines, the sedative effect of central nervous system depressants, including alcohol, barbiturates, hypnotics, narcotic analgesics, sedatives and tranquillisers may be enhanced.

Side-effects: Rare cases of transient local reactions (e.g. stinging, dryness of the nose) have been reported. Rebound congestion may occur if the maximum recommended treatment period of two weeks is exceeded.

Use in pregnancy and nursing mothers: Vibrocil has not been studied in these patients and its use in these conditions is therefore contra-indicated.

Overdosage: Occasional cases of accidental oral ingestion have been reported. The majority of cases were symptom-free, but rarely tiredness, stomach ache, mild tachycardia, increased blood pressure, excitation, sleeplessness and pallor have been reported. Gastric lavage is not usually required and the administration of large quantities of fluid is usually sufficient.

Pharmaceutical precautions Protect from heat and light.

Legal category POM.

Package quantities

Spray:	10 ml plastic nebuliser (OP).
Drops:	15 ml amber glass dropper-bottle (OP).
Gel:	12 g in aluminium tube with lacquered interior (OP).

Further information Vibrocil is very well tolerated and does not interfere with the activity of the nasal cilia.

Product licence numbers
Gel 0030/5008
Spray 0030/5009
Drops 0030/5010

VIOFORM*-HYDROCORTISONE

Presentation The active ingredients Clioquinol BP 3% w/w and Hydrocortisone BP 1% w/w are presented as a white, water miscible cream and a smooth, off-white ointment.

Ointment also contains: light liquid paraffin and white soft paraffin.

Cream also contains: cetostearyl alcohol, cetyl palmitate, glycerol, sodium lauryl sulphate, 2-phenoxyethanol, white soft paraffin and water.

Uses
Mode of action: Vioform-Hydrocortisone combines the anti-fungal and anti-bacterial properties of clioquinol with the anti-inflammatory, anti-allergic and antipruritic effects of hydrocortisone.

Indications: Exudative and secondarily infected eczema and dermatitis, including atopic eczema, primary irritant dermatitis, allergic and seborrhoeic dermatitis. Infected insect bite reactions. Genital or perianal intertrigo.

Dosage and administration Vioform-Hydrocortisone is indicated for external application only.

Method of application: The preparation should be applied sparingly to the affected area, 1–3 times daily. Treatment should be limited to 7 days. Occlusive dressings should not be used.

If there is little improvement after 7 days treatment with Vioform-Hydrocortisone cream or ointment, the appropriate microbiological investigations should be carried out and local or systemic antibiotic treatment given.

Use in the elderly: there is no evidence to suggest that dosage should be different in the elderly.

Use in children: Vioform-Hydrocortisone is contraindicated in children below the age of two years.

Contra-indications, warnings, etc
Contra-indications: Hypersensitivity to any component of the formulation, or iodine. Primary bacterial, viral or fungal infections of the skin. Secondary infections due to yeasts. Application to ulcerated areas. Use in children below the age of two years.

Precautions: Long-term continuous topical therapy should be avoided since this can lead to adrenal suppression even without occlusion.

Application to relatively large and/or eroded areas of skin, use of occlusive dressings, and treatment for longer than one week, should be avoided, because this may lead to a marked increase in protein-bound iodine (PBI). Thyroid function tests such as PBI, radioactive iodine and butanol extractable iodine, may be affected, consequently it is advisable that such tests are not performed within one month of discontinuing treatment. However, other thyroid function tests, such as the T_3 resin sponge test or T_4 determination are unaffected.

The ferric chloride test for phenylketonuria may yield a false-positive result when clioquinol is present in the urine.

Vioform-Hydrocortisone should be used with caution in patients suffering from hepatic and/or renal failure.

Vioform-Hydrocortisone should not be allowed to come into contact with the conjunctiva.

Side-effects: Vioform-Hydrocortisone is usually well tolerated but occasionally, at the site of application, there may be signs of irritation such as a burning sensation, itching or skin rash. Hypersensitivity reactions may also occassionally occur. Treatment should be discontinued if patients experience severe irritation or sensitisation.

Vioform-Hydrocortisone may cause hair discolouration.

Use in pregnancy: There is inadequate evidence of safety in human pregnancy. Topical administration of corticosteroids to pregnant animals can cause abnormalities of foetal development, including cleft palate and intrauterine growth retardation. There may, therefore, be a very small risk of such effects in the human foetus.

It is not known whether the active substances of Vioform-Hydrocortisone and/or their metabolite(s) pass into the breast milk after topical administration. Use in lactating mothers should only be at the doctor's discretion.

Overdosage: Vioform-Hydrocortisone cream and ointment are for topical (external) use only. If accidental ingestion of large quantities occurs, there is no specific antidote and general measures to eliminate the drug and reduce its absorption should be undertaken. Symptomatic treatment should be administered as appropriate.

Pharmaceutical precautions Protect from heat. Dilution of or addition to these formulations is not recommended.

Legal category POM.

Package quantities Cream: Tubes of 30 g (OP). Ointment: Tubes of 30 g (OP).

Further information Clothing stained with Vioform-Hydrocortisone cream or ointment should be washed immediately or soaked overnight.

Product licence numbers
Vioform-Hydrocortisone cream 0030/0050
Vioform-Hydrocortisone ointment 0030/0051

ZYMAFLUOR*

Presentation *Zymafluor 1.00 mg:* Round, bi-convex tablets with bevelled edge and the Zyma logo imprinted on one face, slightly marbled yellow-beige in colour, diameter 5.0 mm, thickness 2.1 mm. Each tablet contains 2.21 mg sodium fluoride equivalent to 1.00 mg available fluoride.

Zymafluor 250 micrograms (0.25 mg): Round, bi-convex, white tablets, slightly sweet to the taste with odour of peppermint, diameter 4.0 mm, thickness 2.6 mm. Each tablet contains 550 micrograms sodium fluoride equivalent to 250 micrograms available fluoride.

Uses Prophylaxis of dental caries. Fluoride enhances the resistance of teeth to carious decay. The protective action of fluoride is due especially to its accumulation in the outer layers of the dental enamel. This process should begin before eruption of the teeth and continue for a long time afterwards.

Before eruption, Zymafluor when swallowed is carried to the developing teeth by the blood stream and thus permits effective pre-eruptive fluoridation. After their eruption the teeth take up fluoride both by internal channels and especially by way of direct contact with the fluoride contained in the saliva. Zymafluor tablets should thus not be swallowed whole: it is extremely important that they be allowed to dissolve slowly in the mouth.

Dosage and administration For oral administration. Not to be taken except on the advice of a dentist, doctor or pharmacist. Zymafluor should be given regularly, without interruption, from birth until about 16 years.

Intake of Zymafluor during pregnancy and feeding will protect the mother's teeth and lay down optimum conditions for a resistant set of milk teeth in her infant.

As soon as the age of the child permits, Zymafluor tablets should no longer be swallowed, but sucked slowly in the mouth, between the cheek and gum, sometimes on the left and sometimes on the right side. They are best taken in the evening before bedtime. For smaller infants 1 tablet should be crushed and dissolved in a little boiled and cooled water and added to one bottle or solid meal a day, or administered alone.

Zymafluor 250 micrograms: If not otherwise prescribed by the doctor or dentist.

From birth to two years of age: 1 tablet daily.

From two to four years: 2 tablets daily.

After the age of 4 years Zymafluor is best administered in the form of 1.00 mg tablets.

Zymafluor 1.00 mg: From the age of 4 years, adults and pregnant women: 1 tablet daily or as prescribed by the doctor or dentist.

In areas where there is fluoridation of the drinking water, the following doses are recommended:

Recommended Dose (fluoride ion/day)

Concentration of fluoride ion in drinking water (ppm)	*<0.3*	*0.3–0.7*	*>0.7*
Age			
2 weeks to 2 years	250 micrograms	0	0
2 to 4 years	500 micrograms	250 micrograms	0
4 to 16 years	1.0 mg	500 micrograms	0

Use in the elderly: The indication for Zymafluor is not applicable to elderly patients.

Contra-indications, warnings, etc There are no known contra-indications.

Precautions: The reduced doses recommended above should be given in areas where there is fluoridation of the drinking water.

Pharmaceutical precautions Store in a cool dry place.

Legal category P.

Package quantities *250 micrograms strength:* Containers of 400 tablets.
1.00 mg strength: Containers of 100 tablets.

Further information Nil.

Product licence numbers
250 micrograms strength 0030/5011
1.00 mg strength 0030/5012

***Trade Mark*

Physiological Values for some Body Fluids

This information concerning physiological values for certain body fluids is reproduced, by permission, from the Pharmaceutical Handbook, Nineteenth Edition, The Pharmaceutical Press, London, 1980.

The values given in the following pages have been taken from many sources and represent approximate normal ranges or typical normal values. In practice 'normal' values can vary considerably from laboratory to laboratory depending on the reagents and analytical methods used. Therefore when evaluating the results of laboratory tests the normal values from the laboratory which performed the test should be consulted.

Many factors affect the reliability of laboratory tests. The specimen must be withdrawn and stored in the correct manner, an appropriate preservative being used if necessary. Certain values fluctuate in every person according to diurnal, nocturnal, or seasonal influences. Other factors, such as exercise, posture, stress, or emotional disturbances, and the age and sex of the patient may also influence the results of laboratory tests.

Many drugs and foods can interfere with laboratory tests. This interference may be physical, chemical, or pharmacological. Dyes may interfere with colorimetric or spectrometric determinations. For example, ingestion of carrots, riboflavine, or foods containing yellow pigment prior to withdrawal of a sample will elevate estimates of total bilirubin in plasma. Many chemicals can cause test results to appear abnormally high or low. High values for catecholamines in urine may be obtained if the patient is taking drugs such as methyldopa. The pharmacological effects of drugs may interfere with laboratory test results. Antihistamines interfere with tests for allergies and mask hypersensitivities.

In the following tables these abbreviations are used: B = Blood; P = Plasma; S = Serum.

BLOOD

Physical Values

Circulation time	3 to 8 seconds (arm to lung)
Freezing-point	−0.52°
Osmolality, plasma	280 to 295 mmol per kg
pH, arterial	7.35 to 7.45
Pressure, arterial	
Systolic	< 140 mmHg
Diastolic	<90 mm Hg
Specific gravity	1.05 to 1.06
Volume, blood	50 to 80 ml per kg body-weight
Volume, plasma	31 to 55 ml per kg body-weight

Haematological Values

Blood count, complete	
Haematocrit (Packed cell volume)	Male: 40 to 54% Female: 35 to 47%
Haemoglobin	Male: 13 to 18 g per 100 ml Female: 12 to 16 g per 100 ml
Red cell count	Male: 4.5 to 6.5 million per mm^3 or 4.5 to 6.5 × 10^{12} per litre Female: 3.9 to 5.6 million per mm^3 or 3.9 to 5.6 × 10^{12} per litre
White cell count	4000 to 11 000 per mm^3
Coagulation tests	
Bleeding time	
Duke's method	<7 minutes
Ivy method	<7 minutes
Clotting time, Lee White method	5 to 11 minutes
Partial thromboplastin time, activated	35 to 60 seconds
Prothrombin time, Quick one stage	12 to 20 seconds
Erythrocyte sedimentation rate (ESR), Westergren method	Male: 3 to 5 mm in 1 hour Female: 4 to 7 mm in 1 hour
Haemoglobin A_2	1.5 to 3.5%
Haemoglobin F	<2%
Haptoglobin	0.3 to 2.0 g per litre
Platelet count	150 000 to 400 000 per mm^3 or per µl
Red cell diameter	6.7 to 7.7 µm average 7.2 µm
Red cell thickness	1.7 to 2.5 µm
Red cell volume	23 to 35 ml per kg body-weight
Reticulocyte count	0.5 to 2.0% of red cells
White cell count, differential	
Neutrophils, segmented	2500 to 7500 per mm^3 or per µl
Lymphocytes	1500 to 3500 per mm^3 or per µl
Monocytes	200 to 800 per mm^3 or per µl
Eosinophils	40 to 440 per mm^3 or per µl
Basophils	15 to 100 per mm^3 or per µl

BLOOD—*continued*

Blood Gases and Acid–Base Values

Base excess	±2.3 mmol per litre
Bicarbonate	
Plasma	21 to 30 mmol per litre
Standard	22 to 28 mmol per litre
Buffer base	45 to 50 mmol per litre
Carbon dioxide	
Arterial pCO_2	36 to 44 mmHg
Total CO_2	23 to 33 mmol per litre
Oxygen	
Arterial pO_2	90 to 110 mmHg

Chemical Values

		Metric	SI
Alpha-amino acid nitrogen	P	30 to 55 mg per litre	2.1 to 4 mmol per litre
Ammonium nitrogen (enzymatic method)	B	400 to 800 μg per litre	29 to 57 μmol per litre
Amylase	S	0.8 to 1.8 Somogyi units per ml	—
		3 to 10 Wohlgemuth units per ml	—
		86 to 268 iu per litre	—
Angiotensin II	B	12 to 36 ng per litre	11.6 to 34.9 pmol per litre
Ascorbic acid	B	5 to 20 mg per litre	28 to 114 μmol per litre
Bicarbonate	P	—	21 to 28 mmol per litre
Bilirubin,			
total	S	1 to 15 mg per litre	1.7 to 25 μmol per litre
total newborn	S	10 to 120 mg per litre	17 to 205 μmol per litre
Caeruloplasmin,			
adult	S	300 to 600 mg per litre	—
child	S	130 to 300 mg per litre	—
Calcium,			
total	S	85 to 105 mg per litre	2.1 to 2.6 mmol per litre
ionised	S	40 to 50 mg per litre	1 to 1.25 mmol per litre
Catecholamines, at rest			
Adrenaline	P	55 ng per litre	0.3 nmol per litre
Nor-adrenaline	P	254 ng per litre	1.5 nmol per litre
Chloride	S or P	3.368 to 3.723 g per litre (as chloride)	95 to 105 mmol per litre
Copper	S or P	0.7 to 1.5 mg per litre	11 to 24 μmol per litre
Cortisol 9 am	P	50 to 260 μg per litre	138 to 717 nmol per litre
5 pm	P	20 to 180 μg per litre	55 to 497 nmol per litre
Creatinine	S or P	6 to 15 mg per litre	53 to 133 μmol per litre
Cyanocobalamin	S	100 to 800 ng per litre	74 to 590 pmol per litre
Fibrinogen	P	2 to 4 g per litre	—
Folate	S	3 to 25 μg per litre	—
Gastrin	S, or P	5 to 290 ng per litre	—
Glucagon	P	0.4 to 1.4 μg per litre	115 to 402 pmol per litre
Glucose, fasting	S or P	0.7 to 1.1 g per litre	3.9 to 6.1 mmol per litre
Growth hormone	S	< 10 μg per litre	—
Immunoglobulins	S		
IgA		0.5 to 4 g per litre	—
IgD		5 to 50 mg per litre	—
IgE		0.1 to 1.3 mg per litre	—
IgG		8 to 16 g per litre	—
IgM		0.4 to 2.9 g per litre	—
Insulin	S	4 to 30 milliunits per litre	—
Iodine, protein-bound (PBI)	S	35 to 80 μg per litre	276 to 630 nmol per litre
Iron, total	S	0.5 to 1.8 mg per litre	9 to 32 μmol per litre
Iron-binding capacity	S	2.5 to 4.5 mg per litre	45 to 81 μmol per litre
Ketones (acetoacetate and acetone)	B	<30 mg per litre	—
Lactic acid,			
arterial	B	30 to 70 mg per litre	0.3 to 0.8 mmol per litre
venous	B	50 to 200 mg per litre	0.56 to 2.2 mmol per litre
Lead	B	<800 μg per litre	<3.9 μmol per litre
Lipids,			
total	S	4 to 10 g per litre	—
cholesterol	S	1.1 to 3.0 g per litre	2.8 to 7.8 mmol per litre
triglycerides	S	0.4 to 1.5 g per litre	—

BLOOD—*continued*

		Metric	SI
Magnesium	S	18 to 30 mg per litre	0.7 to 1.2 mmol per litre
Phenylalanine	S	<40 mg per litre	<242 μmol per litre
Phosphatase,			
acid, total	S	0.5 to 4 King-Armstrong units per 100 ml	—
alkaline, total	S	4 to 13 King-Armstrong units per 100 ml	—
Phosphorus, inorganic adults	S or P	25 to 45 mg per litre	0.8 to 1.5 mmol per litre
Potassium	P	137 to 196 mg per litre	3.5 to 5 mmol per litre
Prolactin	S	2 to 15 μg per litre	—
Proteins,			
total serum	S	60 to 84 g per litre	—
albumin	S	30 to 52 g per litre	—
globulin	S	23 to 37 g per litre	—
Pyruvic acid	B	3 to 10 mg per litre	34 to 114 μmol per litre
Sodium	P	3.1 to 3.4 g per litre	135 to 148 mmol per litre
Sulphate, inorganic	S	9 to 60 mg per litre	94 to 625 μmol per litre
Transaminases			
SGOT	S	0 to 30 iu per litre	—
SGPT	S	0 to 24 iu per litre	—
Thyroid hormone tests			
Thyroid stimulating hormones (TSH)	S	0.5 to 3.5 milliunits per litre	—
T_3 (Radio-immuno-assay)	S	0.7 to 1.9 μg per litre	—
T_4 (radio-immuno-assay)	S	40 to 120 μg per litre	—
T_4 Free	S	10 to 40 ng per litre	—
Urea nitrogen (BUN)	B or S	80 to 250 mg per litre	5.7 to 17.9 mmol per litre
Urea	B	171 to 535 mg per litre	2.9 to 8.9 mmol per litre
Uric acid	S	15 to 70 mg per litre	89 to 417 μmol per litre
Vitamin A	S	150 to 900 μg per litre	0.5 to 3.1 μmol per litre
Zinc	S	0.5 to 1.5 mg per litre	8 to 23 μmol per litre

CEREBROSPINAL FLUID

Physical Values	
Freezing-point	−0.540° to −0.603°
Osmolality	306 mmol per kg
pH	7.33 to 7.37
Pressure	60 to 180 mm of water
Specific gravity	1.0062 to 1.0082
Volume, adults	100 to 160 ml
Chemical Values	
Calcium	1 to 1.5 mmol per litre
Chloride	120 to 130 mmol per litre
Glucose	2.5 to 4.5 mmol per litre
Lactate dehydrogenase	0.2 to 4 iu per ml
Protein	
Lumbar	150 to 500 mg per litre
Cisternal	100 to 300 mg per litre
Ventricular	0 to 150 mg per litre
Albumin/Globulin ratio	2:1
Infants < 1 year	1:1
Albumin	100 to 300 mg per litre
Globulin	60 to 160 mg per litre
Urea	2 to 7 mmol per litre

URINE

Physical Values	
Glomerular filtration rate	100 to 150 ml per minute
Osmolality	100 to 1000 mmol per kg
pH	4.5 to 8.0
Specific gravity	1.010 to 1.025
Volume, normal adult	800 to 2000 ml per 24 hours

URINE—*continued*

Chemical Values

	Metric	*SI*
α Amino acid nitrogen	50 to 300 mg per 24 h	3.6 to 21.4 mmol per 24 h
δ Aminolaevulinic acid	0.1 to 7.5 mg per 24 h	0.8 to 57 μmol per 24 h
Calcium	100 to 300 mg per 24 h	2.5 to 7.5 mmol per 24 h
Catecholamines		
Adrenaline	< 20 μg per 24 h	< 109 nmol per 24 h
Nor-adrenaline	< 100 μg per 24 h	< 591 nmol per 24 h
Chloride	3.545 to 8.863 g per 24 h	100 to 250 mmol per 24 h
Creatine, adults	0 to 100 mg per 24 h	0 to 763 μmol per 24 h
Creatinine	1 to 2 g per 24 h	8 to 18 mmol per 24 h
Formiminoglutamic acid (FIGLU)	0 to 3 mg per 24 h	0 to 17 μmol per 24 h
After 15 g of L-Histidine	4 mg per 8 h	23 μmol per 8 h
Homovanillic acid (HVA)	0 to 15 mg per 24 h	0 to 82 μmol per 24 h
Hydroxyindole acetic acid (HIAA)	3 to 14 mg per 24 h	16 to 73 μmol per 24 h
Lead	< 100 μg per 24 h	< 483 nmol per 24 h
Magnesium	49 to 243 mg per 24 h	2 to 10 mmol per 24 h
Oxalate	15 to 40 mg per 24 h	167 to 444 μmol per 24 h
Phosphate, inorganic	0.5 to 1.5 g per 24 h	16 to 48 μmol per 24 h
Potassium	1.4 to 3.5 g per 24 h	35 to 90 mmol per 24 h
Protein	< 100 mg per 24 h	—
Urea	10 to 30 g per 24 h	167 to 500 mmol per 24 h
Uric acid,		
normal diet	0.2 to 0.5 g per 24 h	1.2 to 3 mmol per 24 h
high purine diet	up to 2 g per 24 h	up to 12 mmol per 24 h
Vanillylmandelic acid (VMA)	up to 9 mg per 24 h	up to 45 μmol per 24 h

Clearance Values

Serum and Urine

Aminohippuric acid (PAH) clearance	600 to 750 ml per min
Creatinine clearance (endogenous)	95 to 135 ml per min
Inulin clearance	100 to 150 ml per min
Urea clearance	
average standard	41 to 65 ml per min
average maximum	64 to 99 ml per min

Physiological Values During Pregnancy

The following table giving physiological values during pregnancy has been provided by Professor Geoffrey Chamberlain of the Department of Obstetrics and Gynaecology, St George's Hospital Medical School, London.

Haematological Functions	*Prepregnancy*	*Weeks of pregnancy*		
		20	*30*	*40*
Total Blood Volume (ml)	4000	4600	5500	5700
Erythrocyte Volume (ml)	1400	1500	1650	1800
Red Blood Cells (10^{12}/l)	4.5	4.0	3.7	4.0
White Blood Cells (10^{9}/l)	7.2	9.4	10.7	10.4
Haemoglobin (g/dl)	13.5	12.0	11.5	12.0
Serum Iron (mg/l)	1.2	1.0	0.9	0.9
Serum Folate (μg/l)	10	7	6	6
Total Iron Binding capacity (μmol/l)	50	40	60	70

Biochemical Functions	*Prepregnancy*	*Weeks of pregnancy*		
		20	*30*	*40*
Sodium (mmol/l)	138	136	137	136
Potassium (mmol/l)	4.26	4.00	4.10	4.21
Calcium (meq/l)	5.00	4.90	4.55	4.60
Colloid osmotic pressure (cm H_2O)	37	32	31	31
Albumen (g/l)	35	28	26	25
Total protein (g/l)	70	60	61	62
Plasma Osmolality (mmol/Kg)	281	283	280	280

Liver Function Tests	*Prepregnancy*	*Weeks of pregnancy*		
		20	*30*	*40*
Total Bilirubin (μmol/l)	4–16	0.5–16	0.5–16	0.5–16
Cholesterol (mmol/l)	4–8	6–8	7–9	8–10
Alkaline phosphatase (I.U./l)	16–24	16–44	16–60	20–100

Note: Pregnancy is associated with a large physiological change and many normal ranges of laboratory tests are expanded, some greatly. In these simplified charts, means are used from large series of normal pregnant women. This shows the trend of changes in later pregnancy; to include all ranges would have clouded the tables. For fuller and further details, the reader is referred to:

Hytten, F. & Lind, T. (1973) *Diagnostic Indices in Pregnancy*, Documenta Geigy, Basle.

Hytten, F. & Chamberlain, G. (1990) *Clinical Physiology in Pregnancy*, 2nd edition, Blackwells, Medical Publishers, Oxford.

1983 Metropolitan Height and Weight Tables for Men and Women

Weights at ages 25–59 based on lowest mortality. Weight in pounds according to frame (in indoor clothing weighing 5 lbs for men and 3 lbs for women; shoes with 1″ heels). Source of basic data: 1979 Build Study, Society of Actuaries and Association of Life Insurance Medical Directors of America, 1980.

MEN. Weight in pounds (in indoor clothing).

Height (in shoes)	*Small frame*	*Medium frame*	*Large frame*
5 ft. 2 in.	128 – 134	131 – 141	138 – 150
5 ft. 3 in.	130 – 136	133 – 143	140 – 153
5 ft. 4 in.	132 – 138	135 – 145	142 – 156
5 ft. 5 in.	134 – 140	137 – 148	144 – 160
5 ft. 6 in.	136 – 142	139 – 151	146 – 164
5 ft. 7 in.	138 – 145	142 – 154	149 – 168
5 ft. 8 in.	140 – 148	145 – 157	152 – 172
5 ft. 9 in.	142 – 151	148 – 160	155 – 176
5 ft. 10 in.	144 – 154	151 – 163	158 – 180
5 ft. 11 in.	146 – 157	154 – 166	161 – 184
6 ft. 0 in.	149 – 160	157 – 170	164 – 188
6 ft. 1 in.	152 – 164	160 – 174	168 – 192
6 ft. 2 in.	155 – 168	164 – 178	172 – 197
6 ft. 3 in.	158 – 172	167 – 182	176 – 202
6 ft. 4 in.	162 – 176	171 – 187	181 – 207

WOMEN. Weight in pounds (in indoor clothing).

Height (in shoes)	*Small frame*	*Medium frame*	*Large frame*
4 ft. 10 in.	102 – 111	109 – 121	118 – 131
4 ft. 11 in.	103 – 113	111 – 123	120 – 134
5 ft. 0 in.	104 – 115	113 – 126	122 – 137
5 ft. 1 in.	106 – 118	115 – 129	125 – 140
5 ft. 2 in.	108 – 121	118 – 132	128 – 143
5 ft. 3 in.	111 – 124	121 – 135	131 – 147
5 ft. 4 in.	114 – 127	124 – 138	134 – 151
5 ft. 5 in.	117 – 130	127 – 141	137 – 155
5 ft. 6 in.	120 – 133	130 – 144	140 – 159
5 ft. 7 in.	123 – 136	133 – 147	143 – 163
5 ft. 8 in.	126 – 139	136 – 150	146 – 167
5 ft. 9 in.	129 – 142	139 – 153	149 – 170
5 ft. 10 in.	132 – 145	142 – 156	152 – 173
5 ft. 11 in.	135 – 148	145 – 159	155 – 176
6 ft. 0 in.	138 – 151	148 – 162	158 – 179

Obstetric Table

Calculated from the first day of the last menstrual period.

January	1	2	3	4	5	6	7	8	9	10	11	12	13	14	15	16	17	18	19	20	21	22	23	24	25	26	27	28	29	30	31	*January*
October	8	9	10	11	12	13	14	15	16	17	18	19	20	21	22	23	24	25	26	27	28	29	30	31	1	2	3	4	5	6	7	*November*
February	1	2	3	4	5	6	7	8	9	10	11	12	13	14	15	16	17	18	19	20	21	22	23	24	25	26	27	28				*February*
November	8	9	10	11	12	13	14	15	16	17	18	19	20	21	22	23	24	25	26	27	28	29	30	1	2	3	4	5				*December*
March	1	2	3	4	5	6	7	8	9	10	11	12	13	14	15	16	17	18	19	20	21	22	23	24	25	26	27	28	29	30	31	*March*
December	6	7	8	9	10	11	12	13	14	15	16	17	18	19	20	21	22	23	24	25	26	27	28	29	30	31	1	2	3	4	5	*January*
April	1	2	3	4	5	6	7	8	9	10	11	12	13	14	15	16	17	18	19	20	21	22	23	24	25	26	27	28	29	30		*April*
January	6	7	8	9	10	11	12	13	14	15	16	17	18	19	20	21	22	23	24	25	26	27	28	29	30	31	1	2	3	4		*February*
May	1	2	3	4	5	6	7	8	9	10	11	12	13	14	15	16	17	18	19	20	21	22	23	24	25	26	27	28	29	30	31	*May*
February	5	6	7	8	9	10	11	12	13	14	15	16	17	18	19	20	21	22	23	24	25	26	27	28	1	2	3	4	5	6	7	*March*
June	1	2	3	4	5	6	7	8	9	10	11	12	13	14	15	16	17	18	19	20	21	22	23	24	25	26	27	28	29	30		*June*
March	8	9	10	11	12	13	14	15	16	17	18	19	20	21	22	23	24	25	26	27	28	29	30	31	1	2	3	4	5	6		*April*
July	1	2	3	4	5	6	7	8	9	10	11	12	13	14	15	16	17	18	19	20	21	22	23	24	25	26	27	28	29	30	31	*July*
April	7	8	9	10	11	12	13	14	15	16	17	18	19	20	21	22	23	24	25	26	27	28	29	30	1	2	3	4	5	6	7	*May*
August	1	2	3	4	5	6	7	8	9	10	11	12	13	14	15	16	17	18	19	20	21	22	23	24	25	26	27	28	29	30	31	*August*
May	8	9	10	11	12	13	14	15	16	17	18	19	20	21	22	23	24	25	26	27	28	29	30	31	1	2	3	4	5	6	7	*June*
September	1	2	3	4	5	6	7	8	9	10	11	12	13	14	15	16	17	18	19	20	21	22	23	24	25	26	27	28	29	30		*September*
June	8	9	10	11	12	13	14	15	16	17	18	19	20	21	22	23	24	25	26	27	28	29	30	1	2	3	4	5	6	7		*July*
October	1	2	3	4	5	6	7	8	9	10	11	12	13	14	15	16	17	18	19	20	21	22	23	24	25	26	27	28	29	30	31	*October*
July	8	9	10	11	12	13	14	15	16	17	18	19	20	21	22	23	24	25	26	27	28	29	30	31	1	2	3	4	5	6	7	*August*
November	1	2	3	4	5	6	7	8	9	10	11	12	13	14	15	16	17	18	19	20	21	22	23	24	25	26	27	28	29	30		*November*
August	8	9	10	11	12	13	14	15	16	17	18	19	20	21	22	23	24	25	26	27	28	29	30	31	1	2	3	4	5	6		*September*
December	1	2	3	4	5	6	7	8	9	10	11	12	13	14	15	16	17	18	19	20	21	22	23	24	25	26	27	28	29	30	31	*December*
September	7	8	9	10	11	12	13	14	15	16	17	18	19	20	21	22	23	24	25	26	27	28	29	30	1	2	3	4	5	6	7	*October*

Poisons Information Services

National Service

LONDON

Director:	Dr G N Volans
Address:	National Poisons Information Service National Poisons Unit Avonley Road London SE14 5ER
Telephone:	071 635 9191 (24-hour emergency service number) 071 955 5095 (laboratory enquiries and Unit Staff)
Fax:	071 639 2101

EDINBURGH

Director:	Dr A T Proudfoot
Address:	Scottish Poisons Information Bureau The Royal Infirmary Lauriston Place Edinburgh EH3 9YW
Telephone:	031 229 2477 (24-hour service)
Fax:	031 228 3332
Viewdata:	031 228 2441 (subscribers only)

CARDIFF:

Director:	Dr P Routledge
Address:	Welsh National Poisons Unit Ward West 5 Llandough Hospital Penarth South Glamorgan CF6 1XX.
Telephone:	0222 709901 (24-hour service)
Fax:	0222 708973

BELFAST

Director:	Dr D G Johnson
Address:	Poisons Information Centre Royal Victoria Infirmary Grosvenor Road Belfast BT12 6BB
Telephone:	0232 240503 (24-hour service) 0232 248095 (Regional Drug Information Service)
Fax:	0232 240899 (Hospital Fax number)

DUBLIN

Director:	Dr J A Tracy
Address:	Poisons Information Centre Beaumont Hospital PO Box 1297 Beaumont Road Dublin 9 Eire
Telephone:	0001 379966 0001 379964
Fax:	0001 376982

Regional Service

LEEDS

Director:	Dr A Judd
Address:	Leeds Poisons Bureau Pharmacy Department The General Infirmary Great George Street Leeds LS1 3EX
Telephone:	0532 430715 (Direct Line) 0532 432799 ext 3547
Fax:	0532 460517

BIRMINGHAM

Director:	Dr J A Vale
Address:	West Midland Poisons Unit Dudley Road Hospital Dudley Road Birmingham B18 7QH
Telephone:	021 554 3801 (24-hour service)
Fax:	021 551 5562

NEWCASTLE

Director:	Dr N Bateman
Address:	Poisons Information Service Royal Victoria Hospital Queen Victoria Road Newcastle upon Tyne NE1 4LP
Telephone:	091 232 1525 (Direct line, normal office hours) 091 232 5131 (24-hour service)
Fax:	091 232 3613

Monitoring of drug overdoses

The National Poisons Information Service at London monitors reports of drug overdosage in a similar manner to the monitoring of adverse reactions by the Committee on Safety of Medicines. Doctors are encouraged to report unusual or severe cases to this service (whether or not they need to use the service for information or advice). In particular, the service would be keen to hear reports of overdose of those drugs also highlighted by the CSM, using the black triangle, since experience of overdose with these drugs is bound to be limited.

Data sheets new to this edition

The following list comprises products which are the subject of data sheets in this edition of the Compendium but which were not included in the 1990–91 edition. It does not necessarily follow that they are recently introduced products.

Index of Products

*The brand name and non-proprietary name indices have been merged for this edition. Brand names are in ordinary type, generic names in italics. *Products with an asterisk contain a number of active ingredients and may be available in more than one formulation.*

Products without an asterisk contain a single active ingredient; in certain instances such products may also be available with added constituents and these formulations are often designated by the principal brand name with the addition of a suffix or other mark of distinction. Where several presentations of a product bear the same proprietary name, the page number given below is that of the first of the respective entries. It should be noted that although different products may contain the same active ingredient this does not imply that they are equivalent in regard to bio-availability or therapeutic activity.

Directory of participants

This directory is included in the Compendium so that doctors and other professional people may obtain additional information about products from participating companies.

page

Medical Information
Abbott Laboratories Ltd
Abbott House
Moorbridge Road
Maidenhead
Berkshire SL6 8JG

Telephone:
Maidenhead (0628) 773355

Telex: 96347 ABBOTT G

Facsimile: (0628) 773803 **1**

Alcon Laboratories (UK) Ltd
Imperial Way
Watford
Hertfordshire WD2 4YR

Telephone:
Watford (0923) 246133

Telex: 923709 ALCON G

Facsimile: (0923) 243331 **19**

Medical Information
Allen & Hanburys Ltd
Stockley Park West
Uxbridge
Middlesex UB11 1BT

Telephone: 081 990 9888 (including 24-hour emergency service)

Telex: 22134 GLXGFD G **26**

Technical Department
Allergan Limited
Crown Centre
Coronation Road
Cressex Industrial Estate
High Wycombe
Buckinghamshire HP12 3SH

Telephone:
High Wycombe (0494) 444722

Telex: 837621 ALLGAN G

Facsimile: (0494) 473593 **52**

Alpha Therapeutic UK Ltd
Howlett Way
Fison Way Industrial Estate
Thetford
Norfolk IP24 1HZ

Telephone:
Thetford (0842) 761942

Telex: 817321 ALPHA G

Facsimile: (0842) 766661 **57**

Regulatory Affairs Department
Approved Prescription Services Ltd
Water Street
Towngate
Wyke BD12 9AF

Telephone:
Wyke (0274) 606974

Telex: 518197 APSWYK G

Facsimile: (0274) 862237 **67**

page

Information Services Department
Armour Pharmaceutical Co Ltd
St Leonards House
St Leonards Road
Eastbourne
East Sussex BN21 3YG

Telephone:
Eastbourne (0323) 410200

Telex: 878536

Facsimile: (0323) 410306 **75**

Medical Information Department
Astra Pharmaceuticals Ltd
Home Park Estate
Kings Langley
Hertfordshire WD4 8DH

Telephone:
Kings Langley (0923) 266191 (including 24-hour emergency service)

Telex: 923442 ASTRA G

Facsimile: (0923) 270529 **81**

Bayer UK Limited
Pharmaceutical Business Group
Bayer House
Strawberry Hill
Newbury
Berkshire RG13 1JA

Telephone:
Newbury (0635) 39000

Telex: 847205 BAYNEW G
Facsimile: (0635) 39616 **124**

Medical Information Department
Beecham Research
Welwyn Garden City
Hertfordshire AL7 1EY

Telephone
Welwyn Garden (0707) 325111 (including 24-hour emergency service)

Telex: 261347

Facsimile: (0707) 325600/324935 **139**

Medical Information Department
Bencard
Welwyn Garden City
Hertfordshire AL7 1EY

Telephone
Welwyn Garden (0707) 325111 (including 24-hour emergency service)

Telex: 261347

Facsimile: (0707) 325600/324935 **158**

Regulatory Affairs Department
Berk Pharmaceuticals Ltd
Water Street
Towngate
Wyke BD12 9AF

page

Telephone:
Wyke (0274) 690696

Telex: 518351 BERWYK G

Facsimile: (0274) 690632 **170**

Medical Information
Bioglan Laboratories Ltd
1 The Cam Centre
Wilbury Way
Hitchin
Hertfordshire SG4 0TW

Telephone:
Hitchin (0462) 442242 (including 24-hour emergency service)

Telex: 826329 BIOGLN G

Facsimile: (0462) 442240 **195**

Information Services
Boehringer Ingelheim Ltd
Ellesfield Avenue
Bracknell
Berkshire RG12 4YS

Telephone:
Bracknell (0344) 424600 (including 24-hour emergency service)

Telex: 847634 BILWBP G

Facsimile: (0344) 481024 **200**

Information Services
Boehringer Ingelheim Hospital Division
Ellesfield Avenue
Bracknell
Berkshire RG12 4YS

Telephone:
Bracknell (0344) 424600

Telex: 847634 BILWBP G

Facsimile: (0344) 481024 **213**

Medical Information Department
Boehringer Mannheim UK (Pharmaceuticals) Ltd
Simpson Parkway
Kirkton Campus
Livingston
West Lothian EH54 7BH

Telephone:
Livingston (0506) 412512

Telex: 727306 BMPH G
Facsimile: (0506) 411395 **220**

Medical Services
Boots Pharmaceuticals
Research Department
Nottingham NG2 3AA

Telephone:
Nottingham (0602) 492900

Telex: 378431 BOOTS G

Facsimile: (0602) 492302 **231**

page

B Braun Medical Ltd
13/14 Farmbrough Close
Aylesbury Vale Industrial Park
Stocklake
Aylesbury
Buckinghamshire HP20 1DQ
Telephone:
Aylesbury (0296) 393900
Telex: 837086 BBMUK G
Facsimile: (0296) 435714 **247**

Medical Information Department
Bridge Pharmaceuticals
Welwyn Garden City
Hertfordshire AL7 1EY
Telephone:
Welwyn Garden (0707) 325111 (including 24-hour emergency service)
Telex: 261347
Facsimile: (0707) 325 600/ 324935 **253**

Medical Information Department
Bristol-Myers Pharmaceuticals
Bristol-Myers Squibb Pharmaceuticals Ltd
Bristol-Myers Squibb House
141-149 Staines Road
Hounslow
Middlesex TW3 3JA
Telephone:
Direct line: (081) 754 3740
BMS House and emergencies: (081) 572 7422
Telex: 261537 BMSHO G
Facsimile: 081-577 1756 **256**

Britannia Pharmaceuticals Ltd
Forum House
Brighton Road
Redhill
Surrey RH1 6YS
Telephone:
Redhill (0737) 773741
Telex: 939065 FORUM G
Facsimile: (0737) 762672 **271**

Medical Information Officer
Brocades (Great Britain) Ltd
Brocades House
Pyrford Road
West Byfleet
Surrey KT14 6RA
Telephone:
Byfleet (0932) 345535/342291
Telex: 917301 BROCAD G
Facsimile: (0932) 353458 **273**

Charwell Pharmaceuticals Ltd
Charwell House
Wilsom Road
Alton
Hampshire
Telephone:
Alton (0420) 84801
Facsimile: (0420) 89376 **281**

page

Ciba Consumer Pharmaceuticals
Wimblehurst Road
Horsham
West Sussex RH12 4AB
Telephone:
Horsham (0403) 50101 (including 24-hour emergency service)
Telex: 87430 CIGYPH G **283**

Information Services
CIBA Laboratories
Wimblehurst Road
Horsham
West Sussex RH12 4AB
Telephone:
Horsham (0403) 50101 (including 24-hour emergency service)
Telex: 87430 CIGYPH G **285**

Medical Information Department
Cilag Ltd
PO Box 79
Saunderton
High Wycombe
Buckinghamshire HP14 4HJ
Telephone:
Naphill (024024) 3541/9 (including 24-hour emergency service)
Telex: 83299 CILAG G
Facsimile: (024024) 5372 **325**

Medical Information Department
Cilag Biotech
PO Box 79
Saunderton
High Wycombe
Buckinghamshire HP14 4HJ
Telephone:
Naphill (024024) 3541/9 (including 24-hour emergency service)
Telex: 83299 CILAG G
Facsimile: (024024) 5372 **334**

Consolidated Chemicals Ltd
The Industrial Estate
Wrexham
Clwyd LL13 9PW
Telephone:
Wrexham (0978) 661351
Telex: 61497 CONCHEM G
Facsimile: (0978) 661673 **336**

Technical Department
Cox Pharmaceuticals
A. H. Cox & Co Limited
Whiddon Valley
Barnstaple
North Devon EX32 8NS
Telephone:
Barnstaple (0271) 75001 (including 24-hour emergency service)
Telex: 46531 COXPHM G
Facsimile: (0271) 46106 **339**

page

CP Pharmaceuticals Limited
Incorporating Weddel Pharmaceuticals
Ash Road North
Wrexham
Clwyd LL13 9UF
Telephone:
Wrexham (0978) 661261
Telex: 61507 CPWREX G
Facsimile: (0978) 660130

Medical Information
12 Derby Road
Loughborough
Leicestershire LE11 0BB
Telephone:
Loughborough (0509) 611001
Facsimile: (0509) 611116 **342**

Cutter Biological
Bayer House
Strawberry Hill
Newbury
Berkshire RG13 1JA
Telephone:
Newbury (0635) 39000
Facsimile: (0635) 39404 **356**

Medical Information
Davis & Geck
(A Division of Cyanamid of Great Britain Ltd)
Fareham Road
Gosport
Hampshire PO13 0AS
Telephone:
Fareham (0329) 224000
Telex: 86173 CYAMID G **357**

Degussa Pharmaceuticals Limited
ASTA Medical Ltd
ASTA House
168 Cowley Road
Cambridge CB4 4DL
Telephone:
Cambridge (0223) 423434
Telex: 818300 DGPL G
Facsimile: (0223) 420943 **361**

Technical Department
Delandale Laboratories Ltd
Delandale House
37 Old Dover Road
Canterbury
Kent CT1 3JF
Telephone:
Canterbury (0227) 766353/4
Facsimile: (0227) 470626 **370**

page

Medical Information
Dermal Laboratories Ltd
Tatmore Place
Gosmore
Hitchin
Hertfordshire SG4 7QR
Telephone:
Hitchin (0462) 458866
Emergency Medical Information Telephone: Dr M. Whitefield 081-455 4998
Telex: 826802 DERMAL G **376**

Dispersa (United Kingdom) Limited
Park West
Flanders Road
Hedge End
Southampton SO3 3LG
Telephone: (0489) 785399
Facsimile: (0489) 785245 **382**

Medical Information and Drug Surveillance Department
Dista Products Ltd
Dextra Court
Chapel Hill
Basingstoke
Hampshire RG21 2SY
Telephone:
Basingstoke (0256) 52011 (including 24-hour emergency service)
Telex: 858931 ELI EA G
Facsimile: (0256) 485858 **383**

Dumex Ltd
Longwick Road
Princes Risborough
Aylesbury
Buckinghamshire HP17 9UZ
Telephone: (0844) 274414
Facsimile: (0844) 274420 **399**

Duncan, Flockhart Division
A division of Glaxo Laboratories Ltd
Stockley Park West
Uxbridge
Middlesex UB11 1BT
Telephone: (081) 990 9333 (including 24-hour emergency service)
Telex: 22134 GLXGFD G **401**

The Medical Information Executive
Duphar Laboratories Ltd
Gaters Hill
West End
Southampton SO3 3JD
Telephone:
Southampton (0703) 472281
Telex: 47582 DUPHAR G
Facsimile: (0703) 465350 **418**

page

Medical Information Department
Du Pont Pharmaceuticals Ltd
Avenue One
Letchworth Garden City
Herts SG6 2HU
Telephone: (0462) 488200 **425**

Regulatory Affairs Department
Ethicon Limited
PO Box 408
Bankhead Avenue
Edinburgh EH11 4HE
Telephone: 031-453 5555
Telex: 727222/727993 ETHEDN G
Facsimile: 031-453 6011 **441**

Evans Medical Ltd
Langhurst
Horsham
West Sussex RH12 4QD
Telephone:
Horsham (0403) 41400
Telex: 877933 EMLHOR
Facsimile: (0403) 61101 **446**

Medical Information
Farmitalia Carlo Erba Ltd
Italia House
23 Grosvenor Road
St Albans
Hertfordshire AL1 3AW
Telephone:
St Albans (0727) 40041 (including 24-hour emergency service)
Telex: 22132 FICE UK G
Facsimile: (0727) 40290 **453**

Ferring Pharmaceuticals Ltd
11 Mount Road
Feltham
Middlesex TW13 6JG
Telephone (081) 898 8396
Telex: 935729
Facsimile: (081) 755 2254 **472**

UK Medical Department
Fisons plc
Pharmaceutical Division
12 Derby Road
Loughborough
Leicestershire LE11 0BB
Telephone:
Loughborough (0509) 611001 (including 24-hour emergency service)
Telex: 341055 FISONS G
Facsimile: (0509) 611116 **474**

Fournier Pharmaceuticals Ltd
116-120 London Road
Oxford OX3 9AT
Telephone: (0865) 741641
Facsimile: (0865) 741639 **487**

page

Galderma UK Ltd
Imperial Way
Watford
Hertfordshire WD2 4YR
Telephone:
Watford (0923) 210180
Telex: 923709
Facsimile: (0923) 210465 **488**

Information Services
Geigy Pharmaceuticals
Wimblehurst Road
Horsham
West Sussex RH12 4AB
Telephone:
Horsham (0403) 50101 (including 24-hour emergency service)
Telex: 87430 CIGYPH G **490**

Medical Information Department
Geistlich Sons Ltd
Newton Bank
Long Lane
Chester CH2 3QZ
Telephone:
Chester (0244) 347534
Facsimile: (0244) 319327 **513**

Medical Information
Glaxo Laboratories Ltd
Stockley Park West
Uxbridge
Middlesex UB11 1BT
Telephone: 081-990 9444 (including 24-hour emergency service)
Telex: 22134 GLXGFD G **522**

Glenwood Laboratories Ltd
Unit D
Jenkins Dale
Chatham
Kent ME4 5RD
Telephone: (0634) 830535
Telex: 966272 MEDCOM G
Facsimile: (0634) 831345 **557**

Medical Information Department
Gold Cross Pharmaceuticals
Division of G. D. Searle & Co Ltd
PO Box 53
Lane End Road
High Wycombe
Buckinghamshire HP12 4HL
Telephone:
High Wycombe (0494) 521124 (including 24-hour emergency service)
Telex: 837771 SEARLE G
Facsimile: (0494) 447872 **559**

page

Medical Information Department
Hoechst UK Ltd
Pharmaceutical Division
Hoechst House
Salisbury Road
Hounslow
Middlesex TW4 6JH
Telephone: 081-570 7712
Telex: 23284 HUKHLW G **566**

Medical Information Department
Hough, Hoseason & Co Ltd
20–22 Chapel Street
Levenshulme
Manchester M19 3PT
Telephone: 061- 224 3271
Telex: 666976 **591**

Medical Information
ICI Pharmaceuticals
King's Court
Water Lane
Wilmslow
Cheshire SK9 5AZ
Telephone: 0625 535999 or Freephone 0800 200 123 (both include 24-hour emergency service)
Telex: 668585
Facsimile: 0625 712450 **593**

Medical Information
Immuno Ltd
Arctic House
Rye Lane
Dunton Green
Nr. Sevenoaks
Kent TN14 5HB
Telephone:
Sevenoaks (0732) 458101
Telex: 95413 IMMUNO G
Facsimile: (0732) 455175 **624**

Innovex Medical Products Ltd
Innovex House
Reading Road
Henley-on-Thames
Oxon RG9 1EL
Telephone: (0491) 578171
Facsimile: (0491) 575057 **630**

Medical Information Department
International Laboratories Ltd
Floats Road
Wythenshawe
Manchester M23 9NF
Telephone:
061-945 4161
Telex: 665140 COLLAB G
Facsimile: 061-945 1830 **631**

Medical Information
Invicta Pharmaceuticals
A Division of Pfizer Ltd
Sandwich
Kent CT13 9NJ

page

Telephone:
Sandwich (0304) 616161 (including 24-hour emergency service)
Sandwich (0304) 616508 (medical information only)
Telex: 966555 PFIZER G **634**

The Medical Information Department
Janssen Pharmaceutical Ltd
Grove
Wantage
Oxon OX12 0DQ
Telephone:
Wantage (0235) 772966 (including 24-hour emergency service)
Telex: 837301 JANUK G **642**

Medical Information Department
Kabi Pharmacia Ltd
Davy Avenue
Knowlhill
Milton Keynes MK5 8PH
Telephone: (0908) 661101
Telex: 826778 PHGB G
Facsimile: (0908) 690091 **665**

Medical Information Department
Knoll Ltd
Fleming House
71 King Street
Maidenhead
Berkshire SL6 1DU
Telephone: (0628) 776360
Telex: 849451
Facsimile: (0628) 776579 **702**

Medical Department
Laboratories for Applied Biology Ltd
91 Amhurst Park
London N16 5DR
Telephone: 081-800 2252
Telex: 8812658 LABLON G
Facsimile: 081-809 6884 **708**

Medical Information Department
Lagap Pharmaceuticals Ltd
Woolmer Way
Bordon
Hampshire GU35 9QE
Telephone:
Bordon (0420) 478301
Telex: 859834 LAGAP G
Facsimile: (0420) 474427 **712**

Medical Information
Lederle Laboratories
Cyanamid of Great Britain Ltd
Fareham Road
Gosport
Hampshire PO13 0AS
Telephone:
Fareham (0329) 224000
Telex: 86173 CYAMID G **718**

page

Medical Department
Leo Laboratories Ltd
Longwick Road
Princes Risborough
Aylesbury
Buckinghamshire HP17 9RR
Telephone:
Princes Risborough (08444) 7333
Telex: 837017 LEOLAB G
Facsimile: (08444) 2278 **761**

Medical Information and Drug Surveillance Department
Eli Lilly & Co Ltd
Dextra Court
Chapel Hill
Basingstoke
Hampshire RG21 2SY
Telephone:
Basingstoke (0256) 473241 (including 24-hour emergency service)
Telex: 858931 ELI EA G
Facsimile: (0256) 485858 **784**

The Technical Department
Lipha Pharmaceuticals Ltd
Harrier House
High Street, Yiewsley
West Drayton
Middlesex UB7 7QG
Telephone:
West Drayton (0895) 449331 (including 24-hour emergency service)
Telex: 8952255 LIPHA G
Facsimile: (0895) 420605 **832**

Medical Information Department
Lorex Pharmaceuticals Ltd
PO Box 293
Lane End Road
High Wycombe
Buckinghamshire HP12 4HL
Telephone:
High Wycombe (0494) 526188 (including 24-hour emergency service)
Telex: 838724 LOREX G
Facsimile: (0494) 534156 **838**

LRC Products Ltd
North Circular Road
London E4 8QA
Telephone: 081-527 2377
Telex: 21644 LRILDN
Facsimile: 081-503 3100 **842**

Medical Department
Lundbeck Ltd
Lundbeck House
Hastings Street
Luton
Bedfordshire LU1 5BE
Telephone:
Luton (0582) 416565
Facsimile: (0582) 410392 **843**

page

Professional Services Department
3M Health Care Limited
Morley Street
Loughborough
Leicestershire LE11 1EP
Telephone:
Loughborough (0509) 611611 (including 24-hour emergency service)
Telex: 34587 HEALTH G **856**

Macfarlan Smith Ltd
Wheatfield Road
Edinburgh EH11 2QA
Telephone: 031-337 2434
Facsimile: 031-337 9813 **874**

Medical Department
Martindale Pharmaceuticals
Bampton Road
Harold Hill
Romford
Essex RM3 8UG
Telephone:
Romford (0708) 46033
Telex: 8953573 **876**

May & Baker Pharmaceuticals
See Rhône-Poulenc Rorer Ltd

Medical Information Department
Medo Pharmaceuticals Ltd
Schwarz House
East Street
Chesham
Buckinghamshire HP5 1DG
Telephone:
Chesham (0494) 772071
Telex: 837252 SANMED G
Facsimile: (0494) 773934 **880**

Medical Department
E. Merck Pharmaceuticals
(A Division of Merck Ltd)
Winchester Road
Four Marks
Alton
Hampshire GU34 5HB
Telephone:
Alton (0420) 87909 (including 24-hour answering service)
Telex: 858435 EMERCK G **882**

Medical Department
Merck Sharp & Dohme Ltd
Hertford Road
Hoddesdon
Hertfordshire EN11 9BU
Telephone:
Hoddesdon (0992) 467272 (including 24-hour emergency service)
Telex: 261915 MSDHOD G
Facsimile: (0992) 451066 **894**

page

Merieux UK Ltd
Clivemont House
Clivemont Road
Maidenhead
Berkshire SL6 7BU
Telephone:
Maidenhead (0628) 785291
Telex: 846583
Facsimile: (0628) 71722 **941**

Medical Information
Merrell Dow Pharmaceuticals Ltd
Lakeside House
Stockley Park
Uxbridge
Middlesex UB11 1BE
Telephone: 081-848 3456
Telex: 913338 MERRHQ G
Facsimile: (081) 848 5404 **946**

Medical Department
Thomas Morson Pharmaceuticals
Division of Merck Sharp & Dohme Ltd
Hertford Road
Hoddesdon
Hertfordshire EN11 9BU
Telephone:
Hoddesdon (0992) 467272 (including 24-hour emergency service)
Telex: 261915
Facsimile: (0992) 451066 **962**

Napp Laboratories Ltd
(A member of Napp Pharmaceutical Group)
Cambridge Science Park
Milton Road
Cambridge CB4 4GW
Telephone:
Cambridge (0223) 424444 (including 24-hour emergency service)
Telex: 817805 **980**

Regulatory Affairs Division
Nicholas Laboratories Ltd
225 Bath Road
Slough
Berkshire SL1 4AU
Telephone:
Slough (0753) 523971
Telex: 848388 NICLAB G
Facsimile: (0753) 570340 **999**

The Medical Department
Norgine Ltd
116–120 London Road
Headington
Oxford OX3 9BA
Telephone:
Oxford (0865) 750717
Telex: 837547 NOROXF G
Facsimile: (0865) 68826 **1010**

page

M...cal Information
Norwich Eaton Limited
New Sandgate House
PO Box IYD
City Road
Newcastle upon Tyne NE99 1YD
Telephone: (091) 222 1882
Facsimile: (091) 222 1593 **1016**

Novex Pharma
(A division of Innovex Medical Products Ltd)
Innovex House
Reading Road
Henley-on-Thames
Oxon RG9 1EL
Telephone: (0491) 578171
Facsimile: (0491) 575057 **1027**

Medical Information
Novo Nordisk Pharmaceuticals Ltd
Novo Nordisk House
Broadfield Park
Brighton Road
Pease Pottage
Crawley
West Sussex RH11 9RT
Telephone: (0293) 613555
Facsimile: (0293) 613535 **1028**

The Medical Information Officer
Organon Laboratories Limited
Cambridge Science Park
Milton Road
Cambridge CB4 4FL
Telephone: Daytime and Emergency Cambridge (0223) 423445
Telex: 818866 ORGCAM G **1038**

Ms C. Beaumont
Pharmaceutical Product Manager
Organon Teknika Ltd
Science Park
Milton Road
Cambridge CB4 4 FL
Telephone: Daytime and Emergency Cambridge (0223) 423650
Telex: 818866 ORGCAM G
Facsimile: (0223) 420264 **1064**

Medical Information Department
Ortho Division of Cilag Ltd
PO Box 79
Saunderton
High Wycombe
Buckinghamshire HP14 4HJ
Telephone:
Naphill (024 024) 3541/9 (including 24-hour emergency service)
Telex: 83299 CILAG G
Facsimile: (024024) 5372 **1068**

page

The Information Department
Paines & Byrne Ltd
Bilton Road
Perivale
Greenford
Middlesex UB6 7HG
Telephone: 081-997 1143/5
Telex: 267763
Facsimile: (081) 9970327 **1089**

Panpharma Limited
Hayes Gate House
27 Uxbridge Road
Hayes
Middlesex UB4 0JN
Telephone: 081-561 8774
Facsimile: 081-848 0738 **1095**

Medical Information Department
Parke-Davis Research Laboratories
Lambert Court
Chestnut Avenue
Eastleigh
Hampshire SO5 3ZG
Telephone:
Eastleigh (0703) 620500
Telex: 47226 WLUKCA G
Facsimile: (0703) 629819 **1098**

Perstorp Pharma Ltd
Intec 2
Wade Road
Basingstoke
Hampshire RG24 0NE
Telephone:
Basingstoke (0256) 477868
Facsimile: (0256) 21508 **1126**

Medical Information
Pfizer Ltd
Sandwich
Kent CT13 9NJ
Telephone:
Sandwich (0304) 616161 (including 24-hour emergency service)
Sandwich (0304) 616508 (medical information only)
Telex: 966555 PFIZER G **1128**

Information
Pharbita Ltd
Cavalry Hill Industrial Estate
Weedon
Northamptonshire NN7 4HP
Telephone: (0327) 349076
Facsimile: (0327) 41513 **1155**

Medical Department
Pharmax Limited
Bourne Road
Bexley
Kent DA5 1NX
Telephone: (0322) 550550
Telex: 896314 PHARMSA G
Facsimile: (0322) 558776 **1156**

page

Porton Products Ltd
Porton House
Vanwall Road
Maidenhead
Berkshire SL6 4UB
Telephone: (0628) 771417
Telex: 848296 LH FERM G
Facsimile: (0628) 770211 **1164**

Medical Information Department
Quinoderm Ltd
Manchester Road
Oldham
Lancashire OL8 4PB
Telephone: 061-624 9307
Facsimile: 061-627 0928 **1167**

Medical Information Unit
Reckitt & Colman Products
Dansom Lane
Hull HU8 7DS
Telephone:
Hull (0482) 26151 (including 24-hour emergency service)
Telex: 52166 RECCOL HULL
Facsimile: (0482) 25322 **1173**

Rhône-Poulenc Rorer Ltd
Rainham Road South
Dagenham
Essex RM10 7XS
Telephone: 081-592 3060
Telex: 28691 RPDAGN G
Facsimile: (081) 984 0575 **1181**

A. H. Robins Company Ltd
A Division of Wyeth Laboratories
Huntercombe Lane South
Taplow
Maidenhead
Berkshire SL6 0PH
Telephone: Burnham (Bucks) (0628) 604377 (including 24-hour emergency service)
Telex: 847640 WYLABS G
Facsimile:
(0628) 666368 **1224**

Medical Information Department
Roche Products Ltd
PO Box 8
Welwyn Garden City
Hertfordshire AL7 3AY
Telephone:
Welwyn Garden (0707) 328128
Telex: 262098 ROCHEW G **1233**

Information Services Department
Rorer Pharmaceuticals
St Leonards House
St Leonards Road
Eastbourne
East Sussex BN21 3YG
Telephone:
Eastbourne (0323) 21422
Telex: 878205 RORER G
Facsimile: (0323) 20666 **1296**

page

Medical Information Department
Roussel Laboratories Ltd
Broadwater Park
North Orbital Road
Uxbridge
Middlesex UB9 5HP
Telephone:
Uxbridge (0895) 834343 or dial 100 Freephone ROUSSEL MED-INFO
24-hour emergency service:
Uxbridge (0895) 834491
Telex: 23126 ROUSEL G
Facsimile: (0895) 834479 **1302**

Rybar Laboratories Ltd
30 Sycamore Road
Amersham
Buckinghamshire HP6 5DR
Telephone:
Amersham (0494) 722741
Telex: 837495 MEDBEC G
Facsimile: (0494) 728578 **1317**

Medical Information Services Department
Sandoz Pharmaceuticals
A division of Sandoz Products Ltd
Frimley Business Park
Frimley
Camberley
Surrey GU16 5SG
Telephone:
Camberley (0276) 692255 (including 24-hour answering service)
Camberley (0276) 698370 (medical information only)
Telex: 858685 SDZLON G
Facsimile: (0276) 692508 **1319**

Medical Information Department
Sanofi Pharma
Floats Road
Wythenshawe
Manchester M23 9NF
Telephone: 061-945 4161
Telex: 665140 COLLAB G
Facsimile: 061-945 1830 **1346**

Medical Information Department
Schering Health Care Limited
The Brow
Burgess Hill
West Sussex RH15 9NE
Telephone:
Burgess Hill (0444) 232323
Telex: 87577 SCHBH G
Facsimile: (0444) 246613 **1355**

The Medical Information Officer
Schering-Plough Ltd
Mildenhall
Bury St Edmunds
Suffolk IP28 7AX

page

Telephone:
Mildenhall (0638) 716321 (normal office hours)
(0638) 515096 (24-hour answering service)
Telex: 81471
Facsimile: (0638) 510832 **1387**

Medical Information Department
Schwarz Pharma Limited
Schwarz House
East Street
Chesham
Buckinghamshire HP5 1DG
Telephone:
Chesham (0494) 772071
Telex: 837252 SANMED G **1400**
Facsimile: (0494) 773934

Medical Information
Scotia Pharmaceuticals Ltd
Woodbridge Meadows
Guildford
Surrey GU1 1BA
Telephone: (0483) 574949
Telex: 859289
Facsimile: (0483) 506682 **1406**

Medical Information Department
Searle Pharmaceuticals
Division of G. D. Searle & Co Ltd
PO Box 53
Lane End Road
High Wycombe
Buckinghamshire HP12 4HL
Telephone:
High Wycombe (0494) 521124 (including 24-hour emergency service)
Telex: 837771 SEARLE G
Facsimile: (0494) 447872 **1408**

Serono Laboratories (U.K.) Ltd
99 Bridge Road East
Welwyn Garden City
Hertfordshire AL7 1BG
Telephone:
Welwyn Garden (0707) 331972
Telex: 8812831 SERONO G
Facsimile: (0707) 371873 **1417**

Medical Department
Servier Laboratories Ltd
Fulmer Hall
Windmill Road
Fulmer
Slough
Buckinghamshire SL3 6HH
Telephone:
Slough (0753) 662744
Telex: 849030 SERLAB G
Facsimile: (0753) 663456 **1427**

page

Shire Pharmaceuticals Ltd
1 Viscount Court
South Way
Andover
Hampshire SP10 5NW
Telephone:
Andover (0264) 333455
Facsimile: (0264) 333460 **1434**

Medical Department
Smith & Nephew Pharmaceuticals Ltd
Bampton Road
Harold Hill
Romford
Essex RM3 8SL
Telephone:
Ingrebourne (04023) 49333
Telex: 898058 SMINEP G
Facsimile: (04023) 71316 **1437**

Medical Information Department
Smith Kline & French Laboratories
Welwyn Garden City
Hertfordshire AL7 1EY
Telephone:
Welwyn Garden (0707) 325111 (including 24-hour emergency service)
Telex: 261347
Facsimile: (0707) 325600/ 324935 **1452**

Medical Information Department
SmithKline Beecham Pharmaceuticals
Welwyn Garden City
Hertfordshire AL7 1EY
Telephone:
Welwyn Garden (0707) 325111 (including 24-hour emergency service)
Telex: 261347
Facsimile: (0707) 325 600/ 324 935 **1473**

Solco Basle (UK) Ltd
3 Cliveden Office Village
Lancaster Road
High Wycombe
Buckinghamshire HP12 3Y2
Telephone:
High Wycombe (0494) 534991
Facsimile: (0494) 461205 **1475**

Medical Information
E. R. Squibb & Sons Ltd
Bristol-Myers Squibb House
141/149 Staines Road
Hounslow
Middlesex TW3 3JA
Telephone:
Direct line (081) 754 3740
BMS House and emergencies (081) 572 7422
Telex: 261537 ERSTW G
Facsimile: 081-577 1756 **1478**

page

Medical Products Manager
Stafford-Miller Ltd
45 Broadwater Road
Welwyn Garden City
Hertfordshire AL7 3SP
Telephone: (0707) 331001
Telex: 24470
Facsimile: (0707) 373370 **1523**

STD Pharmaceutical Products Ltd
Fields Yard
Plough Lane
Hereford HR4 0EL
Telephone:
Hereford (0432) 353684 and 272152
Telex: 35421
Facsimile: (0432) 342383 **1527**

Medical Information Services
Sterling-Winthrop Group Ltd
Sterling Winthrop House
Onslow Street
Guildford
Surrey GU1 4YS
Telephone:
Guildford (0483) 505515 (including 24-hour emergency service)
Telex: 859395 SWGUIL G
Facsimile: (0483) 35432 **1529**

Stiefel Laboratories (UK) Ltd
Holtspur Lane
Wooburn Green
High Wycombe
Buckinghamshire HP10 0AU
Telephone:
Bourne End (06285) 24966
Telex: 849312
Facsimile: (0628) 810021 **1563**

Medical Information
Stuart Pharmaceuticals
King's Court
Water Lane
Wilmslow
Cheshire SK9 5AZ
Telephone:
0625 535999 or Freephone 0800 200 123 (both include 24-hour emergency service)
Telex: 668585
Facsimile: 0625 712450 **1572**

Information Services Department
Syntex Pharmaceuticals Ltd
Syntex House
St Ives Road
Maidenhead
Berkshire SL6 1RD
Telephone:
Maidenhead (0628) 33191
Telex: 848387 SYNTEX G
Facsimile: (0628) 30198 **1588**

page

Thames Laboratories Ltd
Abbey Road
Wrexham Industrial Estate
Wrexham
Clwyd LL13 9PW

Telephone:
Wrexham (0978) 661351

Telex: 61497

Facsimile: (0978) 661673 **1608**

Medical Information
Tillotts Laboratories
23 Grosvenor Road
St Albans
Hertfordshire AL1 3AW

Telephone: (0727) 40041

Telex: 22132 FICE UK G

Facsimile: (0727) 40290 **1612**

Typharm Ltd
14 Parkstone Road
Poole
Dorset BH15 2PG

Telephone:
Poole (0202) 666626 **1624**

page

Medical Information
Upjohn Ltd
Fleming Way
Crawley
West Sussex RH10 2NJ

Telephone:
Crawley (0293) 531133 (switchboard and emergency)
Crawley (0293) 582368 (medical information only)

Telex: 87367 UPJOHN G
Facsimile: (0293) 548850 **1625**

Vifor (UK) Ltd
Bridgegate Pavilion
Chester Business Park
Chester CH4 9QH

Telephone:
(0244) 680982

Facsimile: (0244) 680985 **1661**

Scientific Services Division
Wellcome Medical Division
The Wellcome Foundation Ltd
Crewe Hall
Crewe
Cheshire CW1 1UB

page

Telephone:
Crewe (0270) 583151 (including 24-hour emergency service)

Telex: 36348 WELLCO G

Facsimile: (0270) 215387 **1666**

Medical Information Department
Wyeth Laboratories
Huntercombe Lane South
Taplow
Maidenhead
Berkshire SL6 0PH

Telephone:
Burnham (Bucks) (0628) 604377 (including 24-hour emergency service)

Telex: 847640 WYLABS G

Facsimile: (0628) 666368 **1756**

Zyma (UK) Ltd
Westhead
10 West Street
Alderley Edge
Cheshire SK9 7XP

Telephone:
Alderley Edge (0625) 584788

Facsimile: (0625) 583384 **1785**

IN CONFIDENCE – COMMITTEE ON SAFETY OF MEDICINES
REPORT ON SUSPECTED ADVERSE DRUG REACTION
(For advice on reporting reactions see The Reporting of Adverse Reactions section in this book)

NAME OF PATIENT (To allow for linkage with other reports for same patient. Please give record number for hospital patients)	Family name / Forename	Sex	AGE or DATE OF BIRTH	WEIGHT (Kg.)

SUSPECT DRUG (Please give brand name if known)	ROUTE	DAILY DOSE	DATE STARTED	DATE STOPPED	INDICATION

SUSPECTED REACTION

DATE OF ONSET ______ DATE STOPPED ______

OUTCOME (eg fatal, recovered) ______

REPORTING DOCTOR (BLOCK LETTERS)

Name: ______

Address: ______

Tel. No: ______ Specialty ______

Signature: Date:

If you would like information about other reports associated with the suspected drug, please tick box

SEND TO CSM, FREEPOST, London SW8 5BR
OR if you are in one of the following NHS regions:
TO CSM WestMidlands, FREEPOST, Birmingham B15 1BR
OR CSM Northern, FREEPOST 1085, Newcastle upon Tyne NE1 1BR
OR CSM Wales, FREEPOST, Cardiff CF4 1ZZ
OR CSM Mersey, FREEPOST, Liverpool L3 3AB

OTHER DRUGS
(Please record all other drugs, including self-medication, taken during the last 3 months, and give brand name if known)

DRUG	ROUTE	DAILY DOSE	DATE STARTED	DATE STOPPED	INDICATION

ADDITIONAL NOTES

IN CONFIDENCE – COMMITTEE ON SAFETY OF MEDICINES
REPORT ON SUSPECTED ADVERSE DRUG REACTION
(For advice on reporting reactions see The Reporting of Adverse Reactions section in this book)

NAME OF PATIENT (To allow for linkage with other reports for same patient. Please give record number for hospital patients)	Family name Forename				Sex	AGE or DATE OF BIRTH	WEIGHT (Kg.)
SUSPECT DRUG (Please give brand name if known)	ROUTE	DAILY DOSE	DATE STARTED	DATE STOPPED	INDICATION		

SUSPECTED REACTION

DATE OF ONSET ______ DATE STOPPED ______

OUTCOME (eg fatal, recovered) ______

REPORTING DOCTOR (BLOCK LETTERS)

Name: ______

Address: ______

Tel. No: ______ Specialty ______

Signature: Date:

If you would like information about other reports associated with the suspected drug, please tick box

SEND TO CSM, FREEPOST, London SW8 5BR
OR if you are in one of the following NHS regions:
TO CSM WestMidlands, FREEPOST, Birmingham B15 1BR
OR CSM Northern, FREEPOST 1085, Newcastle upon Tyne NE1 1BR
OR CSM Wales, FREEPOST, Cardiff CF4 1ZZ
OR CSM Mersey, FREEPOST, Liverpool L3 3AB

OTHER DRUGS
(Please record all other drugs, including self-medication, taken during the last 3 months, and give brand name if known)

DRUG	ROUTE	DAILY DOSE	DATE STARTED	DATE STOPPED	INDICATION

ADDITIONAL NOTES

IN CONFIDENCE – COMMITTEE ON SAFETY OF MEDICINES
REPORT ON SUSPECTED ADVERSE DRUG REACTION
(For advice on reporting reactions see The Reporting of Adverse Reactions section in this book)

NAME OF PATIENT (To allow for linkage with other reports for same patient. Please give record number for hospital patients)	Family name Forename	Sex	AGE or DATE OF BIRTH	WEIGHT (Kg.)

SUSPECT DRUG (Please give brand name if known)	ROUTE	DAILY DOSE	DATE STARTED	DATE STOPPED	INDICATION

SUSPECTED REACTION

DATE OF ONSET ______ DATE STOPPED ______

OUTCOME (eg fatal, recovered) ______

REPORTING DOCTOR (BLOCK LETTERS)

Name: ______

Address: ______

Tel. No: ______ Specialty ______

Signature: Date:

If you would like information about other reports associated with the suspected drug, please tick box

SEND TO CSM, FREEPOST, London SW8 5BR
OR if you are in one of the following NHS regions:
TO CSM WestMidlands, FREEPOST, Birmingham B15 1BR
OR CSM Northern, FREEPOST 1085, Newcastle upon Tyne NE1 1BR
OR CSM Wales, FREEPOST, Cardiff CF4 1ZZ
OR CSM Mersey, FREEPOST, Liverpool L3 3AB

OTHER DRUGS
(Please record all other drugs, including self-medication, taken during the last 3 months, and give brand name if known)

DRUG	ROUTE	DAILY DOSE	DATE STARTED	DATE STOPPED	INDICATION

ADDITIONAL NOTES

IN CONFIDENCE – COMMITTEE ON SAFETY OF MEDICINES
REPORT ON SUSPECTED ADVERSE DRUG REACTION
(For advice on reporting reactions see The Reporting of Adverse Reactions section in this book)

NAME OF PATIENT (To allow for linkage with other reports for same patient. Please give record number for hospital patients)	Family name ______ Forename	Sex	AGE or DATE OF BIRTH	WEIGHT (Kg.)

SUSPECT DRUG (Please give brand name if known)	ROUTE	DAILY DOSE	DATE STARTED	DATE STOPPED	INDICATION

SUSPECTED REACTION

DATE OF ONSET ______ DATE STOPPED ______

OUTCOME (eg fatal, recovered) ______

REPORTING DOCTOR (BLOCK LETTERS)

Name: ______

Address: ______

Tel. No: ______ Specialty ______

Signature: Date:

If you would like information about other reports associated with the suspected drug, please tick box

SEND TO CSM, FREEPOST, London SW8 5BR
OR if you are in one of the following NHS regions:
TO CSM WestMidlands, FREEPOST, Birmingham B15 1BR
OR CSM Northern, FREEPOST 1085, Newcastle upon Tyne NE1 1BR
OR CSM Wales, FREEPOST, Cardiff CF4 1ZZ
OR CSM Mersey, FREEPOST, Liverpool L3 3AB

OTHER DRUGS
(Please record all other drugs, including self-medication, taken during the last 3 months, and give brand name if known)

DRUG	ROUTE	DAILY DOSE	DATE STARTED	DATE STOPPED	INDICATION

ADDITIONAL NOTES

IN CONFIDENCE – COMMITTEE ON SAFETY OF MEDICINES
REPORT ON SUSPECTED ADVERSE DRUG REACTION
(For advice on reporting reactions see The Reporting of Adverse Reactions section in this book)

NAME OF PATIENT (To allow for linkage with other reports for same patient. Please give record number for hospital patients)	Family name Forename				Sex	AGE or DATE OF BIRTH	WEIGHT (Kg.)
SUSPECT DRUG (Please give brand name if known)	ROUTE	DAILY DOSE	DATE STARTED	DATE STOPPED	INDICATION		

SUSPECTED REACTION

DATE OF ONSET ______ DATE STOPPED ______

OUTCOME (eg fatal, recovered) ______

REPORTING DOCTOR (BLOCK LETTERS)

Name: ______

Address: ______

Tel. No: ______ Specialty ______

Signature: Date:

If you would like information about other reports associated with the suspected drug, please tick box

SEND TO CSM, FREEPOST, London SW8 5BR
OR if you are in one of the following NHS regions:
TO CSM WestMidlands, FREEPOST, Birmingham B15 1BR
OR CSM Northern, FREEPOST 1085, Newcastle upon Tyne NE1 1BR
OR CSM Wales, FREEPOST, Cardiff CF4 1ZZ
OR CSM Mersey, FREEPOST, Liverpool L3 3AB

OTHER DRUGS
(Please record all other drugs, including self-medication, taken during the last 3 months, and give brand name if known)

DRUG	ROUTE	DAILY DOSE	DATE STARTED	DATE STOPPED	INDICATION

ADDITIONAL NOTES

IN CONFIDENCE – COMMITTEE ON SAFETY OF MEDICINES
REPORT ON SUSPECTED ADVERSE DRUG REACTION
(For advice on reporting reactions see The Reporting of Adverse Reactions section in this book)

NAME OF PATIENT (To allow for linkage with other reports for same patient. Please give record number for hospital patients)	Family name / Forename			Sex	AGE or DATE OF BIRTH	WEIGHT (Kg.)
SUSPECT DRUG (Please give brand name if known)	ROUTE	DAILY DOSE	DATE STARTED	DATE STOPPED	INDICATION	

SUSPECTED REACTION

DATE OF ONSET ____ DATE STOPPED ____

OUTCOME (eg fatal, recovered) ____

REPORTING DOCTOR (BLOCK LETTERS)

Name: ____

Address: ____

Tel. No: ____ Specialty ____

Signature: Date:

If you would like information about other reports associated with the suspected drug, please tick box

SEND TO CSM, FREEPOST, London SW8 5BR
OR if you are in one of the following NHS regions:
TO CSM WestMidlands, FREEPOST, Birmingham B15 1BR
OR CSM Northern, FREEPOST 1085, Newcastle upon Tyne NE1 1BR
OR CSM Wales, FREEPOST, Cardiff CF4 1ZZ
OR CSM Mersey, FREEPOST, Liverpool L3 3AB

OTHER DRUGS
(Please record all other drugs, including self-medication, taken during the last 3 months, and give brand name if known)

DRUG	ROUTE	DAILY DOSE	DATE STARTED	DATE STOPPED	INDICATION

ADDITIONAL NOTES